WO 100

WEST ⬚ ⬚ HOSPITAL

Withdrawn

TEXTBOOK OF SURGERY

FOURTEENTH EDITION

TEXTBOOK OF SURGERY

The Biological Basis of Modern Surgical Practice

Edited by

DAVID C. SABISTON, Jr., M.D.

James B. Duke Professor and Chairman
Department of Surgery
Duke University Medical Center
Durham, North Carolina

W.B. SAUNDERS COMPANY
Harcourt Brace Jovanovich, Inc.
Philadelphia   London   Toronto   Montreal   Sydney   Tokyo

W. B. SAUNDERS COMPANY
Harcourt Brace Jovanovich, Inc.

The Curtis Center
Independence Square West
Philadelphia, PA 19106

Library of Congress Cataloging-in-Publication Data

Textbook of surgery: the biological basis of modern surgical
practice/[edited by] David C. Sabiston, Jr.—14th ed.

p.   cm.
Includes bibliographical references.
Includes index.
ISBN 0-7216-3492-3
1. Surgery.   [1. Surgery.]   I. Sabiston, David C., Jr.
   [DNLM: WO 100 T3552]
RD31.T473   1991
617—dc20
DNLM/DLC   90-8907

Listed here are the latest translated editions of this book together with the language of the translation
and the publisher.

Italian (*12th Edition*)—Piccin Nuova Libraria, Padova, Italy
Japanese (*11th Edition*)—Igaku Shoin Ltd., Tokyo, Japan
Portuguese (*11th Edition*)—Editora Guanabara-Koogan, Rio de Janeiro, Brazil
Spanish (*13th Edition*)—McGraw-Hill/Interamericana de España, Madrid, Spain

Editor: W. B. Saunders Staff

Developmental Editor: Kathleen McCullough

Designer: Ellen M. Bodner

Production Manager: Carolyn Naylor

Manuscript Editors: Jessie Raymond, Rose Marie Klimowicz, and Wynette Kommer

Illustration Coordinator: Margaret Shaw

Indexer: Julie Figures

Textbook of Surgery:
The Biological Basis of Modern Surgical Practice   ISBN   0-7216-3492-3

Last digit is the print number: 9   8   7   6   5   4   3   2   1

CONTRIBUTORS

Onye E. Akwari, M.D.
Associate Professor of Surgery and Associate Professor of Physiology in Cell Biology, Duke University Medical Center. Senior Attending Surgeon, Duke University Medical Center, Durham, North Carolina; Assistant Chief of Surgical Service, Durham Veterans Administration Medical Center, Durham, North Carolina; Consulting Surgeon, Durham County Hospital, Durham, North Carolina.
BENIGN TUMORS OF THE STOMACH; DISORDERS OF THE ANAL CANAL; PILONIDAL CYSTS AND SINUSES

Eben Alexander III, M.D.
Assistant Professor of Neurosurgery, Harvard Medical School, Boston, Massachusetts.
NEUROSURGICAL RELIEF OF PAIN

J. Wesley Alexander, M.D., Sc.D.
Professor of Surgery and Director, Transplantation Division, University of Cincinnati College of Medicine, Cincinnati, Ohio.
SURGICAL INFECTIONS AND CHOICE OF ANTIBIOTICS

James A. Alexander, M.D.
Director, Thoracic and Cardiovascular Residency Program, University of Florida College of Medicine; Professor and Chief, Division of Thoracic and Cardiovascular Surgery, University of Florida, Shands Teaching Hospital, Gainesville, Florida.
EBSTEIN'S ANOMALY

D. Bernard Amos, M.D.
James B. Duke Professor of Immunology and Experimental Surgery, Duke University Medical Center, Durham, North Carolina.
THE IMMUNOLOGY OF TRANSPLANT ANTIGENS; MECHANISMS AND CHARACTERISTICS OF ALLOGRAFT REJECTION

Robert W. Anderson, M.D.
Professor of Surgery and Biomedical Engineering, Northwestern University Medical School. Chief of Cardiothoracic Surgery, Northwestern Memorial Hospital, Chicago, Illinois; Chairman, Department of Surgery, Evanston Hospital, Evanston, Illinois.
THE USE OF CARDIOVASCULAR PHARMACOLOGIC AGENTS IN SURGICAL PATIENTS

Michael F. Angel, M.D.
Clinical Instructor, Department of Plastic Surgery, University of Virginia, Charlottesville, Virginia.
THE MOUTH, TONGUE, JAWS, AND SALIVARY GLANDS

Arnold J. Arem, M.D.
Clinical Assistant, University of Arizona College of Medicine; Clinical Associate, University of New Mexico. Active Staff, St. Josephs Hospital, Tucson, Arizona.
WOUND HEALING: BIOLOGIC AND CLINICAL FEATURES

Stanley W. Ashley, M.D.
Assistant Professor in Surgery, Washington University School of Medicine. Attending Surgeon, Barnes Hospital (St. Louis), St. Louis Children's Hospital, St. Louis, Missouri.
THE PARATHYROID GLANDS

Robert W. Bailey, M.D.
Assistant Professor, Department of Surgery, University of Maryland School of Medicine, Baltimore, Maryland.
DIVERTICULAR DISEASE OF THE COLON

William H. Baker, M.D.
Professor of Surgery, Stritch School of Medicine, Loyola University. Chief, Section of Peripheral Vascular Surgery, and Director, Peripheral Vascular Laboratory, Foster G. McGaw Hospital; Attending Physician, Hines Veterans Administration Hospital, Chicago, Illinois.
ARTERIAL INJURIES

Clyde F. Barker, M.D.
John Rhea Barton Professor and Chairman, Department of Surgery, University of Pennsylvania, School of Medicine. Chief of Surgery, Hospital of the University of Pennsylvania, Philadelphia, Pennsylvania.
RENAL TRANSPLANTATION

Robert H. Bartlett, M.D.
Professor of Surgery, University of Michigan. Director, Surgical Intensive Care Unit, and Chief of Trauma/Critical Care Division, University of Michigan Medical Center, Ann Arbor, Michigan.
EXTRACORPOREAL MEMBRANE OXYGENATION

James M. Becker, M.D.
Associate Professor of Surgery, Harvard Medical School. Chief, Division of General and Gastrointestinal Surgery, Brigham and Women's Hospital, Boston, Massachusetts.
ULCERATIVE COLITIS

Folkert O. Belzer, M.D.
Professor of Surgery, University of Wisconsin Medical School. Chairman, Department of Surgery, University of Wisconsin Hospital and Clinics, Madison, Wisconsin.
TRANSPLANTATION: ORGAN PRESERVATION

Harvey W. Bender, Jr., M.D.
Chairman, Department of Cardiac and Thoracic Surgery, Vanderbilt University School of Medicine. Professor of Surgery, Department of Cardiac and Thoracic Surgery, Vanderbilt University Medical Center, Nashville, Tennessee.
TRICUSPID ATRESIA

John J. Bergan, M.D.
Clinical Professor of Surgery, University of California, San Diego; Clinical Professor of Surgery, Uniformed Services University of Health Sciences, Bethesda, Maryland; Professor of Surgery Emeritus, Northwestern University Medical School, Chicago, Illinois. Attending Surgeon, Scripps Memorial Hospital, La Jolla, California.
VISCERAL ISCHEMIC SYNDROMES: OBSTRUCTION OF THE SUPERIOR MESENTERIC ARTERY, CELIAC AXIS, AND INFERIOR MESENTERIC ARTERY

F. William Blaisdell, M.D.
Professor of Surgery, University of California, Davis, School of Medicine. Chairman, Department of Surgery, University of California, Davis, Medical Center, Davis, California.
SHOCK: CAUSES AND MANAGEMENT OF CIRCULATORY COLLAPSE

R. Randal Bollinger, M.D., Ph.D.
Associate Professor of Surgery and Associate Professor of Immunology, Duke University Medical Center. Chief of Surgical Transplantation, Duke University Medical Center; Attending Surgeon and Consultant in Transplantation, Durham Veterans Administration Medical Center, Durham, North Carolina.
ACUTE RENAL FAILURE IN SURGICAL PATIENTS: PREVENTION AND TREATMENT; TRANSPLANTATION: HISTORICAL ASPECTS; AUTOTRANSPLANTATION

R. Morton Bolman III, M.D.
C. Walton and Richard C. Lillehei Professor and Chief, Division of Cardiovascular and Thoracic Surgery, University of Minnesota. Chief, Division of Cardiovascular and Thoracic Surgery, University of Minnesota Hospitals and Clinics, Minneapolis, Minnesota.
CARDIAC AND CARDIOPULMONARY HOMOTRANSPLANTS

C. Thomas Bombeck, M.D.
Late Professor of Surgery, University of Illinois College of Medicine. Late Chief of Surgery, West Side Veterans Administration Hospital, Chicago, Illinois.
HERNIAS

Gene D. Branum, M.D.
Senior Assistant Resident, General and Thoracic Surgery, Duke University Medical Center, Durham, North Carolina.
PYOGENIC AND AMEBIC LIVER ABSCESS; HEMOBILIA

Gert H. Brieger, M.D., Ph.D.
William H. Welch Professor and Director, Institute of the History of Medicine, The Johns Hopkins University School of Medicine, Baltimore, Maryland.
THE DEVELOPMENT OF SURGERY: HISTORICAL ASPECTS IMPORTANT IN THE ORIGIN AND DEVELOPMENT OF MODERN SURGICAL SCIENCE

Christopher Buller, M.D.
Clinical Fellow, Interventional Cardiology Program, Duke University Medical Center, Durham, North Carolina.
THE HEART: CARDIAC CATHETERIZATION AND PERCUTANEOUS CORONARY ANGIOPLASTY

John H. Calhoon, M.D.
Assistant Professor of Surgery and Chief of Pediatric Cardiac Surgery, University of Texas Health Science Center. Staff Surgeon, Medical Center Hospital; Staff Surgeon, Audie L. Murphy Memorial Veterans Hospital, San Antonio, Texas.
ANEURYSMS OF THE SINUS OF VALSALVA

John J. Callaghan, M.D.
Associate Professor, Department of Orthopaedics, University of Iowa Hospitals and Clinics, Iowa City, Iowa.
INFECTIONS AND NEOPLASMS OF BONE

John L. Cameron, M.D.
Professor and Chairman, Department of Surgery, The Johns Hopkins University School of Medicine. Chief of Surgery, The Johns Hopkins Hospital, Baltimore, Maryland.
THE PANCREAS

E. M. Camporesi, M.D.
Professor and Chairman, Department of Anesthesiology, and Professor of Physiology, SUNY Health Science Center of Syracuse. Anesthetist in Charge, SUNY Health Science Center, Syracuse, New York.
ANESTHESIA

Peter C. Canizaro, M.D.
Late Professor and Chairman, Texas Tech University Health Sciences Center. Late Chief of Surgical Services, Lubbock General Hospital, Lubbock, Texas.
FLUID AND ELECTROLYTE MANAGEMENT OF THE SURGICAL PATIENT

C. James Carrico, M.D.
Professor and Chairman, Department of Surgery, University of Texas Southwestern Medical School. Chief of Surgery, Parkland Memorial Hospital at Dallas, Dallas, Texas.
TRAUMA: MANAGEMENT OF ACUTE INJURIES

Aldo R. Castaneda, M.D.
William E. Ladd Professor of Surgery, Harvard Medical School. Surgeon-in-Chief, Children's Hospital, Boston, Massachusetts.
DISORDERS OF PULMONARY VENOUS RETURN

James Cerilli, M.D.
Professor of Surgery, University of Rochester Medical Center. Director of Transplantation, Strong Memorial Hospital, Rochester, New York.
VASCULAR ACCESS PROCEDURES FOR RENAL DIALYSIS

Ravi S. Chari, M.D.
Resident in Surgery, Duke University Medical Center, Durham, North Carolina.
CONGENITAL LESIONS OF THE CORONARY CIRCULATION

Laurence Y. Cheung, M.D.
Professor and Chairman, Department of Surgery, University of Kansas School of Medicine. Attending Surgeon, University of Kansas Hospital, Kansas City, Kansas.
THE PATHOGENESIS, PROPHYLAXIS, AND TREATMENT OF STRESS GASTRITIS

W. Randolph Chitwood, Jr., M.D.
Professor and Chief, Division of Cardiac Surgery, and Vice Chairman, Department of Surgery, East Carolina University School of Medicine. Chief of Cardiac Surgery and Director, Eastern Carolina Cardiovascular Heart Center, Pitt County Memorial Hospital, Greenville, North Carolina.
INTRA-AORTIC BALLOON COUNTERPULSATION: PHYSIOLOGY, INDICATIONS, AND TECHNIQUES

Frank W. Clippinger, M.D.
Professor of Surgery, Division of Orthopaedic Surgery, Duke University Medical Center. Staff Physician, Duke University Medical Center; Director, Duke Rehabilitation Center, Duke University Medical Center, Durham, North Carolina.
AMPUTATIONS AND LIMB SUBSTITUTIONS

John A. Collins, M.D.
Chidester Professor of Surgery, Stanford University School of Medicine. Attending Surgeon, Stanford University Hospital, Stanford, California.
BLOOD TRANSFUSIONS AND DISORDERS OF SURGICAL BLEEDING

Robert E. Condon, M.D.
Ausman Foundation Professor and Chairman, Department of Surgery, The Medical College of Wisconsin. Chief of Surgery, Froedtert Memorial Lutheran and Milwaukee County General Hospitals; Attending Surgeon, Zablocki Veterans Administration Medical Center, Milwaukee, Wisconsin.
APPENDICITIS

Rex B. Conn, M.D.
Professor and Vice Chairman, Department of Pathology and Cell Biology, Jefferson Medical College of Thomas Jefferson University. Active Staff, Director of Clinical Laboratories,

Thomas Jefferson University Hospital, Philadelphia, Pennsylvania.
APPENDIX: LABORATORY REFERENCE VALUES OF CLINICAL
    IMPORTANCE

Joel D. Cooper, M.D.
Professor of Surgery, Washington University School of Medicine, Seattle, Washington.
LUNG TRANSPLANTATION

James L. Cox, M.D.
Evarts A. Graham Professor of Surgery, Washington University School of Medicine at Barnes Hospital. Cardiothoracic Surgeon-in-Charge, Barnes Hospital, St. Louis, Missouri.
SURGICAL TREATMENT OF CARDIAC ARRHYTHMIAS

Fred A. Crawford, Jr., M.D.
Professor and Chairman, Department of Surgery, and Head, Division of Cardiothoracic Surgery, Medical University of South Carolina, Charleston, South Carolina.
PENETRATING CARDIAC INJURIES

Robert D. Croom III, M.D.
Professor of Surgery, University of North Carolina School of Medicine. Surgeon, University of North Carolina Hospitals, Chapel Hill, North Carolina.
THE SPLEEN

Haile T. Debas, M.D.
Professor, University of California, San Francisco. Chairman, Department of Surgery, Moffitt/Long Hospital, University of California, San Francisco, San Francisco, California.
THE SMALL INTESTINE: CARCINOID TUMORS AND THE CARCINOID
    SYNDROME

Jerome J. DeCosse, M.D., Ph.D.
Professor and Associate Chairman, Department of Surgery, Cornell University Medical College. Attending Surgeon, The New York Hospital–Cornell Medical Center, New York, New York.
RADIATION INJURY TO THE INTESTINE

Donald C. Dafoe, M.D
Associate Professor of Surgery, University of Pennsylvania School of Medicine. Associate Professor of Surgery and Chief, Transplantation Division, Hospital of the University of Pennsylvania, Philadelphia, Pennsylvania.
RENAL TRANSPLANTATION

Thomas A. D'Amico, M.D.
Research Fellow in Surgery, Duke University Medical Center, Durham, North Carolina.
KAWASAKI'S DISEASE

R. Duane Davis, Jr., M.D.
Senior Assistant Resident, Duke University Medical Center, Durham, North Carolina.
THE MEDIASTINUM; PERCUTANEOUS TRANSLUMINAL ANGIOPLASTY

Richard H. Dean, M.D.
Richard T. Myers Professor and Chairman, Department of General Surgery; Director, Division of Surgical Sciences, Bowman Gray School of Medicine. Chief of Surgery, North Carolina Baptist Hospital.
ANEURYSMS OF THE CAROTID ARTERY; CAROTID BODY TUMORS;
    CAROTID ARTERY OCCLUSIVE DISEASE

E. Patchen Dellinger, M.D.
Professor of Surgery, University of Washington School of Medicine. Attending Surgeon, University Hospital and Haborview Medical Center, Consulting Physician, Veterans Administration Medical Center, Seattle, Washington.
SURGICAL INFECTIONS AND CHOICE OF ANTIBIOTICS

Ralph G. DePalma, M.D.
Professor and Chairman, Department of Surgery, George Washington University School of Medicine. Chief of Surgery, George Washington University Hospital; Consultant in Surgery; Washington Veterans Administration Medical Center, Washington, D.C.
DISORDERS OF THE LYMPHATIC SYSTEM

Arnold G. Diethelm, M.D.
Professor and Chairman, Department of Surgery, University of Alabama School of Medicine. Surgeon in Chief, The University of Alabama Hospital, Birmingham, Alabama.
THE ACUTE ABDOMEN

James M. Douglas, Jr., M.D.
Assistant Professor of Surgery, Duke University Medical Center. Attending Surgeon, Duke University Medical Center; Attending Surgeon, Veterans Administration Medical Center, Durham, North Carolina, Consultant, Asheville Veterans Administration Medical Center, Asheville, North Carolina.
BENIGN TUMORS OF THE TRACHEA AND BRONCHI; BRONCHIAL
    ADENOMAS

Milton T. Edgerton, M.D.
Professor of Plastic and Maxillofacial Surgery, The University of Virginia Health Sciences Center. Professor of Plastic Surgery at University of Virginia Medical Center, Charlottesville, Virginia; Consultant in Plastic and Head and Neck Surgery, National Clinical Center, National Institutes of Health, Bethesda, Maryland.
THE MOUTH, TONGUE, JAWS, AND SALIVARY GLANDS

James M. Edwards, M.D.
Fellow, Vascular Surgery, University of Washington School of Medicine, Seattle, Washington.
RAYNAUD'S SYNDROME

John A. Feagin, M.D.
Associate Professor of Surgery, Division of Orthopaedic Surgery, Duke University Medical Center, Clinical Professor of Surgery, Uniformed Services University of Health Sciences, Bethesda, Maryland.
FRACTURES AND DISLOCATIONS: GENERAL PRINCIPLES

Aaron S. Fink, M.D.
Associate Professor of Surgery, University of Cincinnati Medical Center. Director, Surgical Endoscopy, and Co-Director, Gallstone Treatment Center; Attending Surgeon, University of Cincinnati Hospital; Staff Surgeon, Cincinnati Veterans Affairs Medical Center, Cincinnati, Ohio.
CARCINOMA OF THE STOMACH

Josef E. Fischer, M.D.
Christian R. Holmes Professor and Chairman, Department of Surgery, University of Cincinnati College of Medicine. Surgeon-in-Chief, University of Cincinnati Hospital, Consultant Staff, Veterans Administration Medical Center; Active Staff, Children's Hospital, Good Samaritan Hospital, and The Christ Hospital, Cincinnati, Ohio.
METABOLISM IN SURGICAL PATIENTS: PROTEIN, CARBOHYDRATE,
    AND FAT UTILIZATION BY ORAL AND PARENTERAL ROUTES

Robert D. Fitch, M.D.
Assistant Professor of Surgery, Division of Orthopaedic Surgery, Duke University Medical Center; Associate Professor, Department of Pediatrics, Duke University Medical Center. Consultant, Durham Veterans Administration Hospital, Durham, North Carolina; Consultant, Womack Army Hospital, Ft. Bragg, North Carolina.
FRACTURES AND DISLOCATIONS OF THE SHOULDER, ARM, AND FOREARM

J. Lawrence Fitzpatrick, M.D.
Assistant Professor, Department of Surgery, University of Maryland School of Medicine. Surgeon, University of Maryland Hospital; Surgeon, Mercy Medical Center, Baltimore, Maryland.
BENIGN NEOPLASMS OF THE COLON INCLUDING VASCULAR MALFORMATIONS

M. Wayne Flye, M.D., Ph.D.
Professor of Surgery, Molecular Microbiology, and Immunology, Washington University School of Medicine. Attending Staff, Barnes Hospital, St. Louis Children's Hospital, and Jewish Hospital of St. Louis, St. Louis, Missouri.
VENOUS DISORDERS

Thomas J. Fogarty, M.D.
Director, Cardiovascular Surgery, Sequoia Hospital, Redwood City, California.
ACUTE ARTERIAL OCCLUSION

Douglas L. Fraker, M.D.
Chief Resident in Surgery, University of California, San Francisco, San Francisco, California.
TUMOR MARKERS

Robert J. Freeark, M.D.
Professor and Chairman, Department of Surgery, Stritch School of Medicine of Loyola University. Chairman, Department of Surgery, Foster G. McGaw Hospital, Loyola University Medical Center, Maywood, Illinois.
ARTERIAL INJURIES

Allan H. Friedman, M.D.
Associate Professor of Surgery, Division of Neurosurgery, Duke University Medical Center, Durham, North Carolina.
NEUROSURGERY: SPONTANEOUS INTRACRANIAL AND INTRASPINAL HEMORRHAGE; CRANIOCEREBRAL INJURIES

David Fromm, M.D.
Penberthy Professor and Chairman, Department of Surgery, Wayne State University School of Medicine. Surgeon-in-Chief, Detroit Medical Center, Chief of Surgery, Harper Hospital, Detroit, Michigan.
CARCINOMA OF THE GALLBLADDER

William J. Fry, M.D.
Clinical Professor of Surgery, University of Michigan Medical School. Head, Department of General Surgery, Catherine McAuley Health System, Ann Arbor, Michigan.
FEMORAL ARTERY ANEURYSMS; POPLITEAL ARTERY ANEURYSMS

William E. Garrett, Jr., M.D., Ph.D.
Assistant Professor of Surgery, Division of Orthopaedic Surgery, Duke University Medical Center, Durham, North Carolina.
FRACTURES OF THE TIBIA, FIBULA, ANKLE, AND FOOT

William A. Gay, Jr., M.D.
Professor and Chairman, Department of Surgery, University of Utah School of Medicine. Chief of Surgical Services, University Hospital, Salt Lake City, Utah.
VENTRICULAR ANEURYSMS; THE ARTIFICIAL HEART

J. William Gaynor, M.D.
Chief Resident, General and Thoracic Surgery, Duke University Medical Center, Durham, North Carolina.
PATENT DUCTUS ARTERIOSUS, COARCTATION OF THE AORTA, AORTOPULMONARY WINDOW, AND ANOMALIES OF THE AORTIC ARCH

Gregory S. Georgiade, M.D.
Associate Professor of Surgery, General and Plastic Surgery, Duke University Medical Center; Associate Director, Trauma Service, Duke University Medical Center, Durham, North Carolina.
RECONSTRUCTIVE AND AESTHETIC BREAST SURGERY

Donald D. Glower, M.D.
Assistant Professor of Surgery, Duke University Medical Center, Durham, North Carolina.
BRONCHIECTASIS

J. Leonard Goldner, M.D.
James B. Duke Professor, Emeritus, Division of Orthopaedic Surgery, Duke University Medical Center. Consultant, Duke University Hospital, Durham Veterans Administration Hospital, Lenox Baker Childrens Hospital, Durham, North Carolina, and Womack Army Hospital, Ft. Bragg, North Carolina.
FRACTURE OF THE CARPAL SCAPHOID; FRACTURES AND DISLOCATION OF THE HAND; THE HAND: TENDON INJURY AND REPAIR; COMPRESSION NEUROPATHIES OF THE HAND AND FOREARM

Richard D. Goldner, M.D.
Assistant Professor of Surgery, Division of Orthopaedic Surgery, Duke University Medical Center, Durham, North Carolina.
FRACTURE OF THE CARPAL SCAPHOID; FRACTURES AND DISLOCATIONS OF THE HAND; THE HAND: COMPRESSION NEUROPATHIES OF THE HAND AND FOREARM

Cleon W. Goodwin, Jr., M.D.
Associate Professor of Surgery, Cornell University Medical College. Director, Burn Center, The New York Hospital–Cornell Medical Center, New York, New York.
BURNS: INCLUDING COLD, CHEMICAL AND ELECTRIC INJURIES

Robert D. Gordon, M.D.
Associate Professor of Surgery, University of Pittsburgh. Attending Surgeon, Children's Hospital of Pittsburgh, Presbyterian University Hospital, Veterans Administration Medical Center, Pittsburgh, Pennsylvania.
LIVER TRANSPLANTATION

John P. Grant, M.D.
Associate Professor of Surgery, Duke University Medical Center, Durham, North Carolina.
MALABSORPTION SYNDROMES

William J. Greeley, M.D.
Associate Professor of Anesthesiology and Pediatrics, Duke University Medical Center. Medical Director, Pediatric Intensive Care Unit, Duke University Medical Center, Durham, North Carolina.
ANESTHESIA

Paul D. Greig, M.D.
Assistant Professor, Department of Surgery, University of Toronto. Staff Surgeon, Toronto General Hospital, Toronto, Ontario, Canada.
PERITONEOVENOUS SHUNTS FOR INTRACTABLE ASCITES

Ward O. Griffen, Jr., M.D., Ph.D.
Professor of Surgery, Temple University School of Medicine. Attending Surgeon, Temple University Hospital, and Executive Director, American Board of Surgery, Philadelphia, Pennsylvania.
MECKEL'S DIVERTICULUM

Hermes C. Grillo, M.D.
Professor of Surgery, Harvard Medical School. Chief of General and Thoracic Surgery, Massachusetts General Hospital, Boston, Massachusetts.
TRACHEOSTOMY AND ITS COMPLICATIONS

Jay L. Grosfeld, M.D.
Lafayette Page Professor and Chairman, Department of Surgery, Indiana University School of Medicine. Surgeon-in-Chief, James Whitcomb Riley Hospital for Children, Indianapolis, Indiana.
PEDIATRIC SURGERY

Frederick L. Grover, M.D.
Professor of Surgery, Division of Cardiothoracic Surgery, University of Texas Health Science Center. Chief, Cardiothoracic Surgery Section, Audie L. Murphy Memorial Veterans' Hospital, Staff Surgeon, Medical Center Hospital, San Antonio, Texas.
ANEURYSMS OF THE SINUS OF VALSALVA

J. Caulie Gunnells, Jr., M.D.
Professor of Medicine, Nephrology Division, Duke University School of Medicine, Durham, North Carolina.
THE SURGICAL MANAGEMENT OF RENOVASCULAR HYPERTENSION

Carl E. Haisch, M.D.
Associate Professor of Surgery, University of Vermont College of Medicine. Director of Transplantation, Medical Center Hospital of Vermont, Burlington, Vermont.
VASCULAR ACCESS PROCEDURES FOR RENAL DIALYSIS

John D. Hamilton, M.D.
Professor of Medicine and Associate Professor of Microbiology and Immunology, Duke University Medical Center. Chief of Infectious Diseases and Assistant Chief of Medicine, Durham Veterans Administration Hospital, Durham, North Carolina.
VIRAL HEPATITIS AND THE SURGEON

Charles B. Hammond, M.D.
E.C. Hamblen Professor and Chairman, Department of Obstetrics and Gynecology, and Chief of Staff, Duke University Medical Center, Durham, North Carolina.
GYNECOLOGY: THE FEMALE REPRODUCTIVE ORGANS

William T. Hardaker, Jr., M.D.
Assistant Professor of Surgery, Division of Orthopaedic Surgery, Duke University Medical Center, Durham, North Carolina.
FRACTURES OF THE SPINE

Alfred Harding, M.D.
Vascular Resident, University of Missouri Hospital and Clinics, Columbia, Missouri.
THORACIC OUTLET SYNDROME

Alden H. Harken, M.D.
Professor of Surgery, University of Colorado School of Medicine. Chairman, Department of Surgery, University of Colorado Health Sciences Center, Denver, Colorado.
ACQUIRED DISORDERS OF THE AORTIC VALVE

John M. Harrelson, M.D.
Associate Professor of Surgery, Division of Orthopaedic Surgery, and Assistant Professor Pathology, Duke University Medical Center, Durham, North Carolina.
FRACTURES AND DISLOCATIONS: GENERAL PRINCIPLES; INFECTIONS AND NEOPLASMS OF BONE

Julio Hochberg, M.D.
Associate Professor, West Virginia University, School of Medicine. Section Chief for Plastic Surgery, West Virginia University Hospitals, Morgantown, West Virginia.
PRINCIPLES OF OPERATIVE SURGERY: ANTISEPSIS, TECHNIQUE, SUTURES, AND DRAINS

James W. Holcroft, M.D.
Professor of Surgery, University of California, Davis, School of Medicine. Director, Surgical Intensive Care Unit, University of California, Davis, Medical Center, Davis, California.
SHOCK: CAUSES AND MANAGEMENT OF CIRCULATORY COLLAPSE

William L. Holman, M.D.
Assistant Professor of Surgery, Division of Cardiothoracic Surgery, University of Alabama at Birmingham. University of Alabama Hospital, Veteran's Administration Medical Center, Birmingham, Alabama.
CARDIOPULMONARY BYPASS FOR CARDIAC SURGERY

Richard A. Hopkins, M.D.
Assistant Professor of Surgery, Georgetown University Medical School. Director, Pediatric Cardiac Surgery, Georgetown University Medical Center, Washington, D.C.
CLINICAL AND PHYSIOLOGIC EVALUATION OF PULMONARY FUNCTION; TRUNCUS ARTERIOSUS

Robert P. Iacono, M.D.
Assistant Professor of Neurosurgery, Section on Neurosurgery, University of Arizona Health Sciences Center, Tucson, Arizona.
STEREOTACTIC NEUROSURGERY

J. Dirk Iglehart, M.D.
Assistant Professor of Surgery, Duke University Medical Center, Durham, North Carolina.
THE BREAST

Suzanne T. Ildstad, M.D.
Assistant Professor, Department of Surgery, University of Pittsburgh, and Assistant Professor of Surgery, Children's Hospital of Pittsburgh, Pittsburgh, Pennsylvania.
PRINCIPLES OF IMMUNOSUPPRESSION

Anthony L. Imbembo, M.D.
Professor and Chairman, Department of Surgery, University of Maryland School of Medicine. Surgeon-in-Chief, University of Maryland Hospital, Baltimore, Maryland.
DIVERTICULAR DISEASE OF THE COLON; BENIGN NEOPLASMS OF THE COLON, INCLUDING VASCULAR MALFORMATIONS; VOLVULUS OF THE COLON; CARCINOMA OF THE COLON, RECTUM, AND ANUS

Bernard M. Jaffe, M.D.
Professor and Chairman, Department of Surgery, State University of New York Health Science Center at Brooklyn. Chief of Surgery, University Hospital of Brooklyn; Chief of Surgery,

Kings County Hospital Center, Attending Surgeon, Brooklyn Veterans Adminstration Medical Center, Brooklyn, New York.
THE ROLE OF PROSTAGLANDINS, THROMBOXANE, AND LEUKOTRIENES IN SURGERY

Richard A. Jonas, M.D.
Associate Professor of Surgery, Harvard Medical School. Senior Associate in Cardiac Surgery, Children's Hospital, Boston, Massachusetts.
DISORDERS OF PULMONARY VENOUS RETURN

Olga Jonasson, M.D.
Robert M. Zollinger Professor and Chair, Department of Surgery of The Ohio State University College of Medicine. Chief of Surgery, The Ohio State University Hospital; Consultant, Veterans Administration, Columbus, Veterans Adminstration Clinic, Columbus, Ohio.
SURGICAL ASPECTS OF DIABETES MELLITUS

R. Scott Jones, M.D.
Stephen H. Watts Professor and Chairman, Department of Surgery, University of Virginia Health Sciences Center. University of Virginia Hospital, Charlottesville, Virginia.
THE SMALL INTESTINE: ANATOMY; PHYSIOLOGY; INTESTINAL OBSTRUCTION

Robert H. Jones, M.D.
Mary and Deryl Hart Professor of Surgery and Associate Professor of Radiology, Duke University Medical Center. Attending surgeon, Duke University Medical Center, Durham, North Carolina.
RADIONUCLIDE EVALUATION OF CORONARY ARTERY DISEASE

Gregory J. Jurkovich, M.D.
Associate Professor, Department of Surgery, University of Washington. Director of Emergency Room Surgical Services, Harborview Medical Center, Seattle, Washington.
TRAUMA: MANAGMENT OF ACUTE INJURIES

Keith A. Kelly, M.D.
Chairman and Professor of Surgery, Department of Surgery, Mayo Medical School. Consultant in Surgery, St. Mary's Hospital and Rochester Methodist Hospital, Rochester, Minnesota.
CROHN'S DISEASE (REGIONAL ENTERITIS)

James K. Kirklin, M.D.
Professor, University of Alabama at Birmingham. Professor of Surgery, University of Alabama Hospital, Birmingham, Alabama.
VENTRICULAR SEPTAL DEFECTS; DOUBLE OUTLET RIGHT VENTRICLE; CARDIOPULMONARY BYPASS FOR CARDIAC SURGERY

John W. Kirklin, M.D.
Professor of Surgery, University of Alabama at Birmingham. Associate Chief of Staff, University of Alabama at Birmingham Hospitals, Birmingham, Alabama.
VENTRICULAR SEPTAL DEFECTS; DOUBLE OUTLET RIGHT VENTRICLE

Michael S. Klein, M.D.
Assistant in Surgery, University of Illinois. Staff Surgeon, University of Illinois Hospital, Chicago, Illinois.
HERNIAS

John J. Klosak, M.D.
Attending Vascular Surgeon, Franciscan Medical Center, Rock Island, Illinois.
ARTERIAL INJURIES

Thomas J. Krizek, M.D.
Professor and Chairman, Department of Surgery, University of Chicago. Surgeon-in-Chief, University of Chicago Hospital. Chicago, Illinois.
SURGICAL MANAGEMENT OF SUPPURATIVE MEDIASTINITIS

Terry C. Lairmore, M.D.
Research Fellow in Surgery, Washington University School of Medicine. Barnes Hospital, St. Louis, Missouri.
THE MULTIPLE ENDOCRINE NEOPLASIAS

Bernard Langer, M.D.
Professor and Chairman, Department of Surgery, University of Toronto. Attending Surgeon, Toronto General Hospital, Toronto, Ontario.
PERITONEOVENOUS SHUNTS FOR INTRACTABLE ASCITES

M. Lavelle-Jones, M.D.
Lecturer in Surgery, University of Dundee. Senior Registrar in Surgery, Ninewells Hospital, Dundee, Scotland.
SURGICAL COMPLICATIONS

John G. Lease, M.D.
Instructor of Plastic and Reconstructive Surgery, Department of Surgery, University of Chicago. Attending, University of Chicago Hospitals, Chicago, Illinois.
SURGICAL MANAGEMENT OF SUPPURATIVE MEDIASTINITIS

LaSalle D. Leffall, Jr., M.D.
Professor and Chairman, Department of Surgery, Howard University College of Medicine. Surgeon-in-Chief, Howard University Hospital, Washington, D.C.
SOFT TISSUE SARCOMAS

Alan T. Lefor, M.D.
Assistant Professor, Department of Surgery, University of Maryland School of Medicine. Surgeon, University of Maryland Hospital, Baltimore, Maryland.
CARCINOMA OF THE COLON, RECTUM, AND ANUS

George S. Leight, Jr., M.D.
Associate Professor of Surgery, Duke University Medical Center. Attending Surgeon, Duke University Medical Center; Consultant in Surgery, Durham Veterans Administration Hospital, Durham, North Carolina.
NODULAR GOITER AND BENIGN AND MALIGNANT NEOPLASMS OF THE THYROID

L. Scott Levin, M.D.
Chief Resident, Division of Plastic Surgery, Duke University Medical Center.
FRACTURES OF THE TIBIA, FIBULA, ANKLE, AND FOOT

Gary K. Lofland, M.D.
Associate Professor of Surgery and Associate Professor of Pediatrics, Medical College of Virginia, Virginia Commonwealth University. Director, Pediatric Cardiac Surgery, Medical College of Virginia Hospital, Richmond, Virginia.
TRANSPOSITION OF THE GREAT ARTERIES

William P. Longmire, Jr., M.D.
Professor of Surgery Emeritus, University of California, Los Angeles Medical Center. Attending Surgeon, University of California, Los Angeles Hospital, Los Angeles, California.
CARCINOMA OF THE STOMACH

Kim M. Loria, M.D.
Instructor in Medicine and Transplant Fellow, Evanston Hospi-

tal, Northwestern University Medical School, Chicago, Illinois.
THE USE OF CARDIOVASCULAR PHARMACOLOGIC AGENTS IN
SURGICAL PATIENTS

Donald E. Low, M.D.
Attending Surgeon, Department of Surgery, Section of General, Thoracic, and Vascular Surgery, Virginia Mason Medical Center, Seattle, Washington.
LUNG TRANSPLANTATION

James E. Lowe, M.D.
Associate Professor of Surgery and Pathology, Duke University Medical Center. Attending Surgeon and Director of Surgical Electrophysiology Service, Duke University Hospital.
CONGENITAL LESIONS OF THE CORONARY CIRCULATION; CARDIAC PACEMAKERS

Philip D. Lumb, M.B., B.S.
Professor of Anesthesiology and Professor of Surgery, Albany Medical College, Chairman, Department of Anesthesiology, Albany Medical College. Anesthesiologist in Chief, Co-Director, Surgical Intensive Care Unit, and Director, Pediatric Acute Care Unit, Albany Medical Center, Albany, New York.
ANESTHESIA

H. Kim Lyerly, M.D.
Assistant Professor of Surgery, Duke University Medical Center, Durham, North Carolina.
SURGICAL ASPECTS OF THE ACQUIRED IMMUNODEFICIENCY SYNDROME; THE THYROID GLAND: HISTORICAL ASPECTS AND ANATOMY; PHYSIOLOGY; HYPERTHYROIDISM; THYROIDITIS; CHRONIC PULMONARY EMBOLISM; ARTERIOVENOUS FISTULAS

Richard L. McCann, M.D.
Assistant Professor of Surgery, Duke University Medical Center. Attending Surgeon and Head, Section of Vascular Surgery, Duke University Medical Center, Durham, North Carolina.
PHYSIOLOGY OF THE ARTERIAL SYSTEM; FEMOROPOPLITEAL AND FEMOROINFRAPOPLITEAL BYPASS; SURGICAL MANAGEMENT OF RENOVASCULAR HYPERTENSION

Donald E. McCollum, M.D.
Professor of Surgery, Division of Orthopaedic Surgery, Duke University Medical Center. Professor of Orthopaedic Surgery, Duke Consultant, Durham County General Hospital, Durham, North Carolina.
FRACTURES OF THE PELVIS, FEMUR, AND KNEE

John C. McDonald, M.D.
Professor and Chairman, Louisiana State University Medical Center, Shreveport. Surgeon in Chief, Louisiana State University Medical Center, Shreveport, Louisiana.
ABDOMINAL WALL, UMBILICUS, PERITONEUM, MESENTERIES, OMENTUM, AND RETROPERITONEUM

James W. Mackenzie, M.D.
Professor and Chairman, Department of Surgery, University of Medicine and Dentistry of New Jersey–Robert Wood Johnson Medical School. Chief of Surgical Service, Robert Wood Johnson University Hospital, New Brunswick, New Jersey.
DIAGNOSTIC THORACOSCOPY

John W. Madden, M.D.
Clinical Professor of Orthopaedics, University of New Mexico, Albuquerque, New Mexico. Active Staff Privileges, El Dorado Hospital, St. Joseph's Hospital, and Tucson Medical Center, Tucson, Arizona.
WOUND HEALING: BIOLOGIC AND CLINICAL FEATURES

John A. Mannick, M.D.
Moseley Prof. of Surgery, Harvard Medical School. Surgeon-in-Chief, Brigham and Women's Hospital, Boston, Massachusetts.
SUBCLAVIAN STEAL SYNDROME

Daniel Mark, M.D., M.P.H.
Assistant Professor of Medicine, Duke University Medical Center. Co-Director, Cardiac Care Unit, Duke University Medical Center, Durham, North Carolina.
THE HEART: CARDIAC CATHETERIZATION AND PERCUTANEOUS CORONARY ANGIOPLASTY

G. Robert Mason, M.D., Ph.D.
Professor of Surgery, University of California, Irvine. Attending Surgeon, University of California Medical Center, Orange, California.
TUMORS OF THE DUODENUM AND SMALL INTESTINE

Douglas J. Mathisen, M.D.
Associate Professor of Surgery, Harvard Medical School. Associate Visiting Surgeon, Massachusetts General Hospital, Boston, Massachusetts.
TRACHEOSTOMY AND ITS COMPLICATIONS

A. David Mayer, M.S.
Tutor in Surgery, University of Birmingham. Senior Registrar in Surgery, Central Birmingham Health Authority, Birmingham, England.
SURGICAL COMPLICATIONS

William J. Meisler, M.D.
Assistant Professor of Radiology, University of Pittsburgh. Staff, Presbyterian University Hospital.
NEURORADIOLOGY

Anthony A. Meyer, Ph.D., M.D.
Professor of Surgery, University of North Carolina. Director, Surgical Intensive Care Unit, Assistant Director, Jaycee Burn Center, Medical Director of Critical Care, University of North Carolina Hospitals, Chapel Hill, North Carolina.
THE SPLEEN

William C. Meyers, M.D.
Chief, Gastrointestinal Surgery and Associate Professor of Surgery, Duke University Medical Center. Attending Surgeon, Duke University Medical Center, Durham, Veterans Administration Medical Center, Durham, North Carolina.
THE LIVER: ANATOMY AND PHYSIOLOGY; PYOGENIC AND AMEBIC LIVER ABSCESS; NEOPLASMS OF THE LIVER; HEMOBILIA

Gregory L. Moneta, M.D.
Assistant Professor of Surgery, Oregon Health Sciences University. Staff Vascular Surgeon, University Hospital and Veterans Affairs Medical Center, Portland, Oregon.
ARTERIAL SUBSTITUTES

Frank G. Moody, M.D.
Denton A. Cooley Professor and Chairman, Department of Surgery, The University of Texas Medical School at Houston. Surgeon-in-Chief, Hermann Hospital, Houston, Texas.
ULCERATIVE COLITIS

A. R. Moossa, M.D.
Professor and Chairman, Department of Surgery, University of California, San Diego. Surgeon-in-Chief, University of California, San Diego Medical Center, San Diego, California.
SURGICAL COMPLICATIONS

John J. Moossy, M.D.
Assistant Professor, University of Pittsburgh. Assistant Professor, Presbyterian University Hospital Veterans Administration Medical Center, Pittsburgh, Pennsylvania.
NEUROSURGICAL TREATMENT OF EPILEPSY

Jon F. Moran, M.D.
Associate Professor and Chairman, Department of Thoracic and Cardiovascular Surgery, University of Kansas Medical Center, Kansas City, Kansas.
SURGICAL TREATMENT OF PULMONARY TUBERCULOSIS

Raymond F. Morgan, M.D., D.M.D.
Distinguished Professor and Chairman, Department of Plastic Surgery, University of Virginia Health Sciences Center, Charlottesville, Virginia.
THE MOUTH, TONGUE, JAWS, AND SALIVARY GLANDS

Joseph A. Moylan, M.D.
Professor of Surgery, Duke University Medical Center. Director, Trauma Service, Duke University Medical Center; Chief of Surgery, Durham Veterans Administration Medical Center, Durham, North Carolina.
FAT EMBOLI SYNDROME

Gordon F. Murray, M.D.
Professor and Chairman, West Virginia University School of Medicine. Chief of Surgical Services, West Virginia University Hospitals; Cardiac Surgeon-in-Charge, Monongalia General Hospital, Morgantown, West Virginia.
PRINCIPLES OF OPERATIVE SURGERY: ANTISEPSIS, TECHNIQUE, SUTURES, AND DRAINS

David L. Nahrwold, M.D.
Loyal and Edith Davis Professor and Chairman, Department of Surgery, Northwestern University Medical School. Surgeon-in-Chief, Northwestern Memorial Hospital, Chicago, Illinois.
THE BILIARY SYSTEM: ACUTE CHOLECYSTITIS; CHRONIC CHOLECYSTITIS AND CHOLELITHIASIS; CHOLANGITIS

John S. Najarian, M.D
Regents' Professor and Jay Philips Chair in Surgery, University of Minnesota. Chairman, Department of Surgery, University of Minnesota Hospitals, Minneapolis, Minnesota.
PRINCIPLES OF IMMUNOSUPPRESSION

Ali Naji, M.D., Ph.D.
Professor of Surgery, Hospital of the University of Pennsylvania, Philadelphia, Pennsylvania.
RENAL TRANSPLANTATION

Blaine S. Nashold, Jr., M.D.
Professor of Surgery, Division of Neurosurgery, Duke University Medical Center, Durham, North Carolina.
NEUROSURGICAL RELIEF OF PAIN; NEUROSURGICAL TREATMENT OF EPILEPSY; STEREOTACTIC NEUROSURGERY

Jeffrey A. Norton, M.D.
Senior Investigator, Head, Surgical Metabolism Section, Surgery Branch, National Cancer Institute.
TUMOR MARKERS

William I. Norwood, M.D., Ph.D.
Professor of Surgery, University of Pennsylvania. Chief of Cardiac Surgery, Children's Hospital of Philadelphia, Philadelphia, Pennsylvania.
HYPOPLASTIC LEFT HEART SYNDROME

James A. Nunley, M.D.
Associate Professor of Surgery, Division of Orthopaedics, Duke University Medical Center, Durham, North Carolina.
THE HAND: TENDON INJURY AND REPAIR

Lloyd M. Nyhus, M.D.
Warren H. Cole Professor of Surgery, University of Illinois. Surgeon-in-Chief Emeritus, University of Illinois Hospital, Chicago, Illinois.
HERNIAS

Daniel J. O'Brien, Ph.D.
Assistant Professor, College of Nursing and the Division of Thoracic and Cardiovascular Surgery, University of Florida, Gainesville, Florida.
EBSTEIN'S ANOMALY

W. Jerry Oakes, M.D.
Assistant Professor of Surgery, Division of Neurosurgery, and Assistant Professor of Pediatrics, Department of Pediatrics, Duke University Medical Center. Attending Surgeon, Duke University Medical Center, Durham, North Carolina.
NEUROSURGERY: CONGENITAL ABNORMALITIES

C. Warren Olanow, M.D.
Professor of Neurology, University of South Florida. Section Chief, Neurology, Tampa General Hospital, Tampa, Florida.
SURGICAL MANAGEMENT OF MYASTHENIA GRAVIS

H. Newland Oldham, Jr., M.D.
Professor of Surgery, Duke University Medical Center, Durham, North Carolina.
SURGICAL TREATMENT OF HYPERTROPHIC CARDIOMYOPATHY

Don B. Olsen, D.V.M.
Professor of Surgery, Research Professor of Bioengineering, Research Professor of Pharmaceutics, and Director of the Institute for Biomedical Engineering, University of Utah, Salt Lake City, Utah.
THE ARTIFICIAL HEART

Susan L. Orloff, M.D.
Fifth Year, Surgical Resident, University of California, San Francisco, San Francisco, California.
THE SMALL INTESTINE: CARCINOID TUMORS AND THE CARCINOID SYNDROME

Mark B. Orringer, M.D.
Professor and Head, Section of Thoracic Surgery, University of Michigan Medical Center, Ann Arbor, Michigan.
THE ESOPHAGUS: HISTORICAL ASPECTS AND ANATOMY; PHYSIOLOGY; DISORDERS OF ESOPHAGEAL MOTILITY; DIVERTICULA AND MISCELLANEOUS CONDITIONS OF THE ESOPHAGUS; ESOPHAGOSCOPY; TUMORS OF THE ESOPHAGUS.

Albert D. Pacifico, M.D.
J. W. Kirklin Professor of Cardiovascular Surgery, University of Alabama at Birmingham. Director, Division of Cardiothoracic Surgery, University of Alabama at Birmingham, Birmingham, Alabama.
VENTRICULAR SEPTAL DEFECTS; DOUBLE OUTLET RIGHT VENTRICLE

Theodore N. Pappas, M.D.
Assistant Professor of Surgery, Duke University Medical Center. Staff Surgeon, Duke University Medical Center and Durham Veterans Administration Medical Center, Durham, North Carolina.
LYMPHOMA OF THE STOMACH

David F. Paulson, M.D.
Professor and Chief, Division of Urology, Department of Surgery, Duke University Medical Center, Durham, North Carolina.
THE URINARY SYSTEM

Leonard J. Perloff, M.D.
Professor of Surgery, Hospital of the University of Pennsylvania. Course Director, Department of Surgery, University of Pennsylvania Hospital; Staff, Children's Hospital of Philadelphia and Philadelphia Veterans Administration Medical Center, Philadelphia, Pennsylvania.
RENAL TRANSPLANTATION

Harry R. Phillips, M.D.
Associate Professor of Medicine, Duke University Medical Center. Director, Interventional Cardiac Catheterization Laboratory, Duke University Medical Center, Durham, North Carolina.
THE HEART: CARDIAC CATHETERIZATION AND PERCUTANEOUS CORONARY ANGIOPLASTY

Hiram C. Polk, Jr., M.D.
Ben A. Reid, Sr., Professor and Chairman, Department of Surgery, University of Louisville School of Medicine, Louisville, Kentucky.
PRINCIPLES OF PREOPERATIVE PREPARATION OF THE SURGICAL PATIENT

Walter J. Pories, M.D.
Professor and Chairman, Department of Surgery, East Carolina University School of Medicine. Chief of Surgeons, Pitt County Memorial Hospital, Greenville, North Carolina.
THE SURGICAL APPROACH TO MORBID OBESITY

John M. Porter, M.D.
Professor of Surgery and Chief, Division of Vascular Surgery, Oregon Health Sciences University. University Hospital, Portland, Oregon.
ARTERIAL SUBSTITUTES; RAYNAUD'S SYNDROME

Basil A. Pruitt, Jr., M.D.
Commander and Director, U.S. Army Institute of Surgical Research, Fort Sam Houston, Texas.
BURNS: INCLUDING COLD, CHEMICAL, AND ELECTRIC INJURIES

Scott K. Pruitt, M.D
Research Fellow, Department of Surgery, Duke University Medical Center, Durham, North Carolina.
BURNS: INCLUDING COLD, CHEMICAL, AND ELECTRIC INJURIES

Kenneth P. Ramming, M.D.
Professor of Surgery, University of California, Los Angeles Medical Center and John Wayne Cancer Clinic, Los Angeles, California.
BITES AND STINGS

J. Scott Rankin, M.D.
Professor of Surgery, Chief of Division of Cardiothoracic Surgery, University of California, San Francisco. Senior Associate, Cardiovascular Research Institute, University of California, San Francisco, San Francisco, California.
CARDIOPULMONARY RESUSCITATION; THE CORONARY CIRCULATION; MITRAL AND TRICUSPID VALVE DISEASE

Norman M. Rich, M.D.
Professor and Chairman, Department of Surgery, Uniformed Services University of the Health Sciences. Surgical Staff, Walter Reed Army Medical Center, Bethesda, Maryland.
VENOUS INJURIES

William J. Richardson, M.D.
Assistant Professor, Department of Surgery, Division of Orthopaedic Surgery, Duke University Medical Center, Durham, North Carolina.
FRACTURES OF THE SPINE

Wayne E. Richenbacher, M.D.
Assistant Professor, University of Utah. Staff Surgeon, University of Utah Health Sciences Center, Salt Lake City, Utah.
THE ARTIFICIAL HEART

Layton F. Rikkers, M.D.
Professor and Chairman, Department of Surgery, University of Nebraska Medical Center. Attending Physician, University of Nebraska Hospital and Clinic, Omaha, Nebraska.
SURGICAL COMPLICATIONS OF CIRRHOSIS AND PORTAL HYPERTENSION

William C. Roberts, M.D.
Clinical Professor of Pathology and Medicine (Cardiology), Georgetown University, Washington, D.C. Chief, Pathology Branch, National Heart, Lung, and Blood Institute, National Institutes of Health, Bethesda, Maryland.
CHANGES IN VENOUS AUTOGRAFTS USED AS AORTOCORONARY CONDUITS

Michael S. Rohr, M.D., Ph.D.
Professor of Surgery and Director of Transplantation Services, Bowman Gray School of Medicine. Staff, North Carolina Baptist Hospital, Winston-Salem, North Carolina.
ABDOMINAL WALL, UMBILICUS, PERITONEUM, MESENTERIES, OMENTUM, AND RETROPERITONEUM

Francis E. Rosato, M.D.
Professor and Chairman, Department of Surgery, Jefferson Medical College. Active Staff, Thomas Jefferson University Hospital, Philadelphia, Pennsylvania.
GALLSTONE ILEUS AND FISTULA

Joel J. Roslyn, M.D.
Associate Professor of Surgery, University of California, Los Angeles, School of Medicine. Attending Surgeon, Chief, General Surgery, Sepulveda Veterans Administration Hospital, Sepulveda, California.
THE COLON AND RECTUM: SURGICAL ANATOMY AND OPERATIVE PROCEDURES; PHYSIOLOGY; DIAGNOSTIC STUDIES; INTESTINAL ANTISEPSIS

Francis S. Rotolo, M.D.
Finney, Trimble and Associates, Baltimore, Maryland.
HEMOBILIA

David C. Sabiston, Jr., M.D.
James B. Duke Professor of Surgery and Chairman, Department of Surgery, Duke University Medical Center, Durham, North Carolina.
PULMONARY EMBOLISM: CHRONIC PULMONARY EMBOLISM; DISORDERS OF THE ARTERIAL SYSTEM: INTRODUCTION; ANATOMY; ANEURYSMS; SUBCLAVIAN ARTERY ANEURYSMS; VISCERAL ARTERIAL ANEURYSMS; AORTIC ABDOMINAL ANEURYSMS; THROMBO-OBLITERATIVE DISEASE OF THE AORTA AND ITS BRANCHES; TAKAYASU'S ARTERITIS; THROMBOTIC OBLITERATION OF THE ABDOMINAL AORTA AND ILIAC ARTERIES (LERICHE SYNDROME); ILIAC ARTERIAL OCCLUSION; ARTERIOVENOUS FISTULAS; CARCINOMA OF THE LUNG; CONGENITAL DEFORMITIES

OF THE CHEST WALL; THE MEDIASTINUM: PATENT DUCTUS ARTERIOSUS, COARCTATION OF THE AORTA, AORTOPULMONARY WINDOW, AND ANOMALIES OF THE AORTIC ARCH; THE TETRALOGY OF FALLOT; THE CORONARY CIRCULATION; CONGENITAL LESIONS OF THE CORONARY CIRCULATION; CARDIAC NEOPLASMS

Fred Sanfilippo, M.D., Ph.D.
Professor of Pathology, Immunology, and Experimental Surgery, Duke University Medical Center. Director, Immunopathology, Duke University Medical Center; Director, Transplantation Laboratory, Durham Veterans Administration Medical Center, Durham, North Carolina.
THE IMMUNOLOGY OF TRANSPLANT ANTIGENS; MECHANISMS AND CHARACTERISTICS OF ALLOGRAFT REJECTION

Bruce Schirmer, M.D.
Associate Professor of Surgery, University of Virginia. Attending Surgeon, University of Virginia Health Sciences Center, Charlottesville, Virginia.
VASCULAR COMPRESSION OF THE DUODENUM

Steve J. Schwab, M.D.
Associate Professor of Medicine, Duke University Medical Center. Director, Clinical Nephrology Service, Director of Dialysis Units, Duke University Medical Center, Durham, North Carolina.
ACUTE RENAL FAILURE IN SURGICAL PATIENTS: PREVENTION AND TREATMENT

Stewart M. Scott, M.D.
Consulting Professor of Surgery, Duke University Medical Center, Durham, North Carolina. Chief, Surgical Service, Veterans Administration Medical Center, Asheville, North Carolina.
PULMONARY INFECTIONS; THE PLEURA AND EMPYEMA

H. F. Seigler, M.D.
Professor of Surgery and Professor of Immunology, Duke University Medical Center. Co-Director, Transplantation Programs, Co-Program Director, Clinical Cancer Research Unit, and Staff Surgeon, Duke University Medical Center, Durham, North Carolina.
IMMUNOBIOLOGY AND IMMUNOTHERAPY OF NEOPLASTIC DISEASE; MELANOMA

Donald Serafin, M.D.
Professor and Chief, Division of Plastic Surgery, Department of Surgery, Duke University Medical Center, Durham, North Carolina.
THE SKIN: FUNCTIONAL, METABOLIC, AND SURGICAL CONSIDERATIONS

George F. Sheldon, M.D.
Professor of Surgery, University of North Carolina School of Medicine. Professor and Chairman, Department of Surgery, University of North Carolina Hospitals, University of North Carolina School of Medicine, Chapel Hill, North Carolina.
THE SPLEEN

G. Tom Shires, M.D.
Lewis Atterbury Stimson Professor and Chairman, Department of Surgery, Cornell University Medical College. Surgeon-in-Chief, The New York Hospital, New York, New York.
FLUID AND ELECTROLYTE MANAGEMENT OF THE SURGICAL PATIENT

Donald Silver, M.D.
Professor of Surgery and Chairman, Department of Surgery, University of Missouri Health Sciences Center. Attending Surgeon, Harry S. Truman Veterans Administration Hospital; Consulting Surgeon, Ellis Fischel State Cancer Hospital, Columbia, Missouri.
CIRCULATORY PROBLEMS OF THE UPPER EXTREMITY; THORACIC OUTLET SYNDROME

Norman A. Silverman, M.D.
Division Head, Cardiac and Thoracic Surgery, Henry Ford Hospital, Detroit, Michigan.
CARDIAC NEOPLASMS

Richard L. Simmons, M.D.
Professor and Chairman, University of Pittsburgh School of Medicine. Chief of Surgery, Presbyterian University Hospital; Active Staff, Children's Hospital of Pittsburgh, Active Staff, Monefiore University Hospital; Active Staff, Veterans Administration Hospital, Pittsburgh, Pennsylvania.
PRINCIPLES OF IMMUNOSUPPRESSION

James D. Sink, M.D.
Associate Clinical Professor of Surgery, University of Pennsylvania School of Medicine. Chief of Cardiothoracic Surgery, Philadelphia Heart Institute and Presbyterian Medical Center, Philadelphia, Pennsylvania.
CONGENITAL AORTIC STENOSIS

Kevin M. Sittig, M.D.
Assistant Professor of Surgery, Associate Director, Louisiana State University Burn Center, Louisiana State University Medical Center. Staff, Louisiana State University Medical Center, Shreveport, Louisiana.
ABDOMINAL WALL, UMBILICUS, PERITONEUM, MESENTERIES, OMENTUM AND RETROPERITONEUM

David B. Skinner, M.D.
Professor of Surgery, Cornell University College of Medicine. President, Chief Executive Officer and Surgeon, The New York Hospital, New York, New York.
PERFORATION OF THE ESOPHAGUS: SPONTANEOUS (BOERHAAVE'S SYNDROME), TRAUMATIC, AND FOLLOWING ESOPHAGOSCOPY; HIATAL HERNIA AND GASTROESOPHAGEAL REFLUX

Peter K. Smith, M.D.
Assistant Professor of Surgery and Assistant Professor of Biomedical Engineering, Duke University Medical Center, Durham, North Carolina.
THE ROLE OF COMPUTERS IN SURGICAL PRACTICE

James B. Snow, Jr., M.D.
Director, National Institute on Deafness and Other Communication Disorders, National Institutes of Health, Bethesda, Maryland.
SURGICAL DISORDERS OF THE EARS, NOSE, PARANASAL SINUSES, PHARYNX, AND LARYNX

Hans W. Sollinger, M.D., Ph.D.
Professor of Surgery and Pathology, University of Wisconsin School of Medicine. Attending Surgeon, University of Wisconsin Hospital, Madison, Wisconsin.
PANCREAS TRANSPLANTATION

James H. Southard, Ph.D.
Associate Professor, Department of Surgery, University of Wisconsin, Madison, Wisconsin.
TRANSPLANTATION: ORGAN PRESERVATION

David I. Soybel, M.D.
Assistant Professor of Surgery, Yale University School of Medicine. Staff Surgeon, Yale-New Haven Hospital and West Haven

Veterans Administration Medical Center, West Haven, Connecticut.
THE PITUITARY AND ADRENAL GLANDS

Thomas L. Spray, M.D.
Associate Professor of Surgery, Division of Cardiothoracic Surgery, Washington University School of Medicine. Attending Surgeon, Barnes Hospital, Washington University; Attending Surgeon, Children's Hospital; Staff Surgeon, Cochran Veterans Administration Hospital; Attending Surgeon, Jewish Hospital; Consulting Surgeon, St. Louis Regional Hospital, St. Louis, Missouri.
SURGICAL DISORDERS OF THE PERICARDIUM

Richard S. Stack, M.D.
Associate Professor, Department of Medicine, Division of Cardiology, Duke University Medical Center. Director, Interventional Cardiovascular Program, Duke University Medical Center, Durham, North Carolina.
THE HEART: CARDIAC CATHETERIZATION AND PERCUTANEOUS CORONARY ANGIOPLASTY

Robert J. Stanley, M.D.
Professor and Chairman, Department of Radiology, University of Alabama School of Medicine. Radiologist in Chief, University of Alabama Hospital, Birmingham, Alabama.
THE ACUTE ABDOMEN

Thomas E. Starzl, M.D., Ph.D.
Professor of Surgery, University of Pittsburgh School of Medicine. Staff Surgeon, Presbyterian University Hospital, Children's Hospital of Pittsburgh, and Veteran's Administration Medical Center, Pittsburgh, Pennsylvania.
LIVER TRANSPLANTATION

Mark Stegall, M.D.
Transplant Fellow, University of Wisconsin Hospital, Madison, Wisconsin.
PANCREAS TRANSPLANTATION

Delford L. Stickel, M.D.
Professor of Surgery, Duke University Medical Center. Attending Surgeon, Department of Surgery, Duke University Medical Center, Durham, North Carolina.
TRANSPLANTATION: HISTORICAL ASPECTS

James L. Talbert, M.D.
Professor of Surgery and Pediatrics and Chief of Children's Surgery, University of Florida College of Medicine. Staff, Shands Hospital at the University of Florida and Veterans Administration Medical Center, Gainesville, Florida.
CORROSIVE STRICTURES OF THE ESOPHAGUS

Gordon L. Telford, M.D.
Associate Professor of Surgery, Medical College of Wisconsin. Attending Surgeon, Milwaukee Veterans Administration Medical Center, Froedtert Memorial Lutheran Hospital and Milwaukee County Medical Center, Milwaukee, Wisconsin.
APPENDICITIS

James C. Thompson, M.D., M.A.
John Woods Harris Professor and Chairman, Department of Surgery, The University of Texas Medical Branch. Professor and Chairman, Department of Surgery, The University of Texas Medical Branch, Galveston, Texas.
THE STOMACH AND DUODENUM

James P. S. Thomson, M.S.
Dean of Postgraduate Studies, St. Mark's Hospital for Diseases of the Rectum and Colon; Honorary Lecturer in Surgery, The Medical College of St. Bartholomew's Hospital, University of London. Consultant Surgeon, St. Mark's and Hackney Hospitals; Honorary Consultant Surgeon, St. Mary's Hospital, London; Civil Consultant in Surgery (Rectal) to the Royal Air Force.
DISORDERS OF THE ANAL CANAL

Satoru Todo, M.D.
Associate Professor of Surgery, University of Pittsburgh School of Medicine. Surgeon, Children's Hospital of Pittsburgh, Presbyterian University Hospital, and Veterans Administration Medical Center, Pittsburgh, Pennsylvania.
LIVER TRANSPLANTATION

Douglas S. Tyler, M.D.
Chief Resident in Surgery, Duke University Medical Center, Durham, North Carolina.
SURGICAL ASPECTS OF THE ACQUIRED IMMUNODEFICIENCY SYNDROME

George S. Tyson, M.D.
Assistant Professor of Surgery, University of Pennsylvania School of Medicine. Surgeon, Hospital of the University of Pennsylvania, Philadelphia, Pennsylvania.
REOPERATION FOR CORONARY BYPASS

Andreas G. Tzakis, M.D.
Associate Professor of Surgery, University of Pittsburgh School of Medicine. Children's Hospital of Pittsburgh, Presbyterian University Hospital, and Veterans Administration Medical Center, Pittsburgh, Pennsylvania.
LIVER TRANSPLANTATION

James R. Urbaniak, M.D.
Professor and Chief, Division of Orthopaedic Surgery, Department of Surgery, Duke University Medical Center, Durham, North Carolina.
REPLANTATION OF AMPUTATED LIMBS AND DIGITS

Ross M. Ungerleider, M.D.
Assistant Professor of General and Thoracic Surgery and Assistant Professor of Pediatrics, Duke University Medical Center. Chief, Pediatric Cardiac Surgery, and Surgical Director, Pediatric Intensive Care Unit, Duke University Medical Center, Durham, North Carolina.
BRONCHOSCOPY; ATRIAL SEPTAL DEFECTS, OSTIUM PRIMUM DEFECTS, AND ATRIOVENTRICULAR CANALS; THE TETRALOGY OF FALLOT

Peter Van Trigt, M.D.
Assistant Professor of Surgery, Duke University Medical Center. Attending Surgeon, Duke University Medical Center, Durham, North Carolina.
SURGICAL MANAGEMENT OF FAILED ANGIOPLASTY

Robert B. Wallace, M.D.
Professor and Chairman, Department of Surgery, Georgetown University School of Medicine, Georgetown University Medical Center, Washington, D.C.
TRUNCUS ARTERIOSUS

W. David Watkins, M.D., Ph.D.
Professor of Anesthesiology, Duke University Medical Center. Chairman, Department of Anesthesiology, Duke University Medical Center, Durham, North Carolina.
ANESTHESIA

Andrew S. Wechsler, M.D.
Stuart McGuire Professor of Surgery and Chairman, Department of Surgery; Professor of Physiology, Medical College of Virginia, Virginia Commonwealth University. Chief of Surgery, Medical College of Virginia Hospitals; Attending Surgeon, Hunter Holmes McGuire Veterans Administration Medical Center; Attending Surgeon, Richmond Memorial Hospital, Richmond, Virginia.
SURGICAL MANAGEMENT OF MYASTHENIA GRAVIS

John L. Weinerth, M.D.
Associate Professor of Urology and Surgery, Duke University Medical Center. Attending Urologist, Duke University Medical Center, Durham, North Carolina.
THE MALE GENITAL SYSTEM

Samuel A. Wells, Jr., M.D.
Bixby Professor and Chairman, Department of Surgery, Washington University School of Medicine. Surgeon-in-Chief, Barnes Hospital (St. Louis); Surgeon, Children's Hospital and the Jewish Hospital of St. Louis, St. Louis, Missouri.
THE MULTIPLE ENDOCRINE NEOPLASIAS; THE PARATHYROID GLANDS; THE PITUITARY AND ADRENAL GLANDS

H. Brownell Wheeler, M.D.
Harry M. Haidak Distinguished Professor and Chairman, Department of Surgery, University of Massachusetts Medical School. Surgeon-in-Chief, University of Massachusetts Medical Center, Worcester, Massachusetts.
THROMBOANGIITIS OBLITERANS (BUERGER'S DISEASE)

Glenn J. R. Whitman, M.D.
Assistant Professor, Department of Cardiothoracic Surgery, University of Colorado, School of Medicine. Chief, Cardiothoracic Surgery, Denver Veterans Administration Hospital, Denver, Colorado.
ACQUIRED DISORDERS OF THE AORTIC VALVE

Robert H. Wilkins, M.D.
Professor and Chief, Division of Neurosurgery, Department of Surgery, Duke University Medical Center, Durham, North Carolina.
NEUROSURGERY: HISTORICAL ASPECTS; INTRACRANIAL TUMORS; SPONTANEOUS INTRACRANIAL AND INTRASPINAL HEMORRHAGE; INTRACRANIAL INFECTIONS; INTRASPINAL TUMORS; RUPTURED LUMBAR INTERVERTEBRAL DISC; CERVICAL DISC LESIONS; PERIPHERAL NERVE INJURIES

Douglas W. Wilmore, M.D.
Frank Sawyer Professor of Surgery, Harvard Medical School. Clinical Director, Nutrition Support Service, Brigham and Women's Hospital; Research Director, Laboratory for Surgical Metabolism and Nutrition, Boston, Massachusetts.
HOMEOSTASIS: BODILY CHANGES IN TRAUMA AND SURGERY

Walter G. Wolfe, M.D.
Professor of Surgery, Duke University Medical Center. Attending Surgeon, Duke University Medical Center, Durham, North Carolina.
TRAUMATIC ANEURYSMS OF THE AORTA; DISSECTING ANEURYSMS OF THE AORTA; ANEURYSMS OF THE THORACIC AORTA; DISORDERS OF THE LUNGS, PLEURA, AND CHEST WALL: ANATOMY; CLINICAL AND PHYSIOLOGIC EVALUATION OF PULMONARY FUNCTION

Bruce G. Wolff, M.D.
Associate Professor of Surgery, Mayo Medical School. Consultant, General Surgery and Colon and Rectal Surgery, Rochester Methodist Hospital and St. Marys Hospital, Rochester, Minnesota.
CROHN'S DISEASE (REGIONAL ENTERITIS)

Charles J. Yeo, M.D.
Associate Professor of Surgery, The Johns Hopkins University School of Medicine. Attending Surgeon, The Johns Hopkins Hospital, Baltimore, Maryland.
THE PANCREAS

Michael J. Zinner, M.D.
Professor and Chairman, Department of Surgery, University of California, Los Angeles, School of Medicine. Chairman, Department of Surgery, UCLA Medical Center; Attending Surgeon, Wadsworth Veterans Administration Hospital and Olive View Medical Center, Los Angeles, California.
THE COLON AND RECTUM: SURGICAL ANATOMY AND OPERATIVE PROCEDURES; PHYSIOLOGY; DIAGNOSTIC STUDIES; INTESTINAL ANTISEPSIS

Karl A. Zucker, M.D.
Associate Professor, Department of Surgery, University of Maryland School of Medicine. Surgeon, University of Maryland Hospital; Assistant Chief of Staff of Surgical Services, Loch Raven Veterans Administration Hospital, Baltimore, Maryland.
VOLVULUS OF THE COLON

PREFACE

The fourteenth edition of the *Textbook of Surgery* is a completely revised and updated version that provides a thorough description of the broad field of surgery. The first edition of this text was published in 1936, and it has since been regularly revised at appropriate intervals. The traditions of this text have been maintained in seeking internationally respected contributors for each chapter as well as the policy of presenting a complete update of each subject with new illustrations and bibliographic references. In this edition the basic scientific aspects of surgical disorders have been given prime attention in view of their increasing significance in the thorough understanding of clinical problems. The importance of this knowledge has been emphasized by the American Board of Surgery as well as in continuing education courses.

It is remarkable to reflect upon the many advances that have been made in surgery since the last edition was published in 1986. Remarkable achievements have been made in preoperative and postoperative care, nutrition, metabolism, cancer chemotherapy, antibiotics, tumor markers, open heart surgery, and the role of computers in the diagnosis and treatment of surgical disorders. To remain abreast of the field in the 1990s, twelve entirely new sections have been added to cover recent advances of special significance. These include

"Surgical Aspects of the Acquired Immunodeficiency Syndrome" by Drs. Douglas S. Tyler and H. Kim Lyerly

"Lung Transplantation" by Drs. Donald E. Low and Joel D. Cooper

"Tumor Markers" by Drs. Jeffrey A. Norton and Douglas L. Fraker

"Extracorporeal Membrane Oxygenation" by Dr. Robert H. Bartlett

"Surgical Management of Suppurative Mediastinitis" by Drs. Thomas J. Krizek and John G. Lease

"Penetrating Cardiac Injuries" by Dr. Fred A. Crawford, Jr.

"Hypoplastic Left Heart Syndrome" by Dr. William I. Norwood

"Surgical Management of Failed Angioplasty" by Dr. Peter Van Trigt

"Reoperation for Coronary Bypass" by Dr. George S. Tyson

"Kawasaki's Disease" by Dr. Thomas A. D'Amico

"Surgical Treatment of Hypertrophic Cardiomyopathy" by Dr. H. Newland Oldham, Jr.

"The Role of Computers in Surgical Practice" by Dr. Peter K. Smith

The sections have been arranged in a consistent format, beginning with a brief survey of the historic advances that have brought the subject to its present status, followed by the anatomic, pathologic, physiologic, biochemical, bacteriologic, immunologic, genetic, and pharmacologic features of each disorder. Following presentation of these basic scientific aspects of surgical problems, emphasis is then placed upon a review of the clinical manifestations, the findings on physical examination, and the diagnostic and therapeutic aspects of each condition.

The international impact of the *Textbook of Surgery* has been gratifying and continues to heighten each year. It has been translated into Spanish, Japanese, Portuguese, and Italian. For more than fifty years the fundamental goal of this text has been straightforward in its objective to serve the needs of all those involved in the science of surgery including medical students, surgical residents, practicing surgeons, and teachers of surgery throughout the world.

DAVID C. SABISTON, JR.

ACKNOWLEDGMENTS

The Editor is deeply indebted to the contributors to the fourteenth edition of the *Textbook of Surgery*. Each is well known for original contributions in the field represented, and all have been diligent in their insistence that both the basic scientific and clinical aspects of each disorder be thoroughly presented. Their inclusion of the most recent data in the literature is gratefully acknowledged.

Mr. Edward H. Wickland, Senior Medical Editor of the W. B. Saunders Company, is due much recognition for his steadfast commitment to achieving excellence in all aspects of this edition. He has been a much trusted advisor in the preparation of this text. It has been a particular privilege to work closely with Ms. Carolyn Naylor, Production Manager, and to thank her for skillful contributions based upon a very impressive knowledge of quality editing. Other members of the W. B. Saunders staff—including Ms. Ellen Bodner, Designer; Ms. Margaret Shaw, Illustration Specialist; Ms. Jessie Raymond, Senior Manuscript Editor; and Ms. Kathleen McCullough, Senior Developmental Editor—are due much recognition for their impressive contributions, which were essential for publication.

Ms. Kathryn Slaughter, Ms. Patricia Whitfield, and Ms. Beth Alley, of my personal editing staff, are deserving of enduring thanks for their contributions as well as painstaking reviews of each chapter in this edition. These efforts have been of monumental proportion, and their many hours of loyal dedication and enthusiasm for the entire work have made this edition a reality.

DAVID C. SABISTON, JR.

CONTENTS

THE DEVELOPMENT
OF SURGERY

Historical Aspects Important in the Origin and Development of Modern Surgical Science

Gert H. Brieger, M.D., Ph.D.

The history of surgery in the major surgical textbooks has a long and honorable tradition. Every field has its great contributors, and each its heroes. A history of surgery without Paré, Vesalius, Hunter, Lister, and Halsted would be a strange history indeed; the magnitude of the achievements of these men warrants discussion of their lives and work. Nevertheless, many justly famous names will be missing. Emphasis is placed on the *recent* past, *especially the last 100 years,* although the reader should bear in mind always that surgery's history is as old as that of human beings.

The history of disease is at least as old as the history of mankind. One can assume that surgical disease, or the surgical response to disease, is of similar antiquity. The basic forms of disease—tumors, infections, trauma, and congenital abnormalities—have existed unchanged.[55] Surgeons today obviously manage diseases differently from their colleagues of prehistoric time, yet some aspects of the surgeon's work are timeless. Ackerknecht, who has written extensively on primitive medicine, has emphasized that surgery was not defined as a special field by the primitives,[1] yet much of their medical treatment would be termed *surgical.* They treated wounds and tried to stop hemorrhage, and they trephined for injury to the head as well as for ritual reasons, such as the release of demons.

The single most important factor limiting the work of these early surgeons was their lack of knowledge of anatomy. It is true that evidence has been found of very successful bone setting for fractures in some tribes, but these good results may have been due to circumstances. The study of the anthropologist Adolph Schultz has shown that the efficacy of medical men cannot simply be assumed. Nature, too, as the ancients well knew, is a powerful healer in its own right. In 1939 Schultz reported finding healed fractures in wild apes; in one series of 118 wild adult gibbons, 42, or 36 per cent, had well-healed fractures.[81] Since these animals obviously did not have the benefit of surgical assistance, one must pause, then, before too quickly assigning credit for cures.

Ancient Egypt, long a fascinating subject for historians and archeologists, provides examples of some of the earliest known medical writings. The papyri that have been found consider medicine, surgery, obstetrics and gynecology, and veterinary problems. The Edwin Smith Papyrus, of greatest interest to surgeons, is one of the oldest. It was written in about 1600 B.C. but probably was copied from a still older version. It consists of 48 cases, mainly wounds, arranged in the order that later was to become the traditional one, *a capite ad calcem.*[82]

The strictures governing ancient surgery, from what is known of them, appear to have been stringent. In the code of Hammur-abi, for instance, the Babylonian law provided severe penalties for the surgeon whose operations were unsuccessful. If a free individual died as the result of an operation, the surgeon's right hand was cut off. It is doubtful whether surgeons could actually have practiced under such draconic conditions. Since social class may still today in some instances determine the amount and kind of medical care, it is of interest that the Babylonian laws provided that the surgeon who caused harm to or death of a slave was bound only to repay the owner an equal value. In ancient Persia, surgeons were not allowed to practice until they had performed three successful operations on infidels. If unsuccessful, the surgeon was declared forever unfit to practice the art.

Ancient India also has a rich medical legacy, all too often ignored by Western writers. Susruta described more than 100 surgical instruments, including scalpels, bistouries, lancets, scarifiers, saws, bone nippers, trocars, and needles. The Indian surgeons are best known for their great skill in plastic surgery, especially the restoration of noses and ears.

In Greek and Roman antiquity the surgeon existed as a specialist, but only when diet and drugs were of no avail did doctors resort to surgery. In cases of injury, of course, the surgeon might be called upon immediately. In the great Greek medical works that are ascribed to Hippocrates, but certainly not all written by him, there are books on fractures, dislocations, and other surgical disorders. One of the most interesting is simply entitled *On the Surgery.* Here the author described what the surgeon should know, how he should proceed with the treatment, and what general qualifications he should possess. Much of the work relates to bandaging of various types of injuries. "The things related to surgery are," the Hippocratic author wrote around 400 B.C., "the patient; the operator; the assistants; the instruments; the light; where and how; how many things, and how; where the body, and the instruments; the time; the manner; the place."

Besides the 70 books of the Hippocratic works, one of the best authorities on Greek medicine is the Roman encyclopedist of the early first century A.D., Aurelius Cornelius Celsus. His *De re medicina* reflects much learning, although its author was probably not a medical practitioner. This book was one of the earliest medical books to be printed (1478) after the invention of movable type. Of interest to surgeons is the classic description of inflammation Celsus left: "Now the characteristics of inflammation are four: redness and swelling, with heat and pain" (Book III). Of more direct interest, however, is what he had to say about surgery. He went into great detail regarding some surgical remedies, but his general comments found in the *Prooemium* of Book VII are timeless and bear repeating:

The third part of the Art of Medicine is that which cures by the hand. . . . It does not omit medicaments and regulated diets [the other two parts of medicine], but does most by hand. The effects of this treatment are more obvious than any other kind; in as much as in diseases since luck helps much, and the same things are often salutary, often of no use at all, it may be doubted whether recovery has been due to medicine or a sound body or good luck. . . . But in that part of medicine which cures by hand, it is obvious that all improvement comes chiefly from this, even if it be assisted somewhat in other ways. This branch, although very ancient, was more practiced by Hippocrates, the father of all medical art, than by his forerunners. . . .

Now a surgeon should be youthful or at any rate nearer youth than age; with a strong and steady hand which never trembles, and ready to use the left hand as well as the right; with vision sharp and clear, and spirit undaunted; filled with pity, so that he wishes to cure his patient, yet is not moved by his cries, to go too fast, or cut less than is necessary; but he does everything just as if the cries of pain cause him no emotion.

It is usually said that medicine in the Middle Ages slavishly followed the doctrines of Galen of the second century A.D. and that because of adherence to his humoral concept of disease, which he assumed and elaborated from the Hippocratic writers of five centuries earlier, no advances were made. The sins of the followers of Galen should not be attributed to Galen himself. Of importance, however, is that if one holds that disease is caused by the humors—yellow bile, black bile, blood, and phlegm—being either in excess or in the wrong location within the body, then surgery cannot be of much use. How can one operate on the humors? If the humoral excess should manifest itself as a pus-filled swelling, it might be incised and drained, but the likelihood of operative intervention was generally rare under this system of theory of pathology.

The surgery of the early Middle Ages has been described by Bishop as merely meddlesome.[11,12] Itinerant surgeons operated for stone, cataract, and hernia. Since these procedures were likely to be associated with complications, surgeons often operated and left town. Surgeons also cared for wounds and injuries, and later all skin diseases, especially syphilis, came within their province.

In the later Middle Ages, when medicine was in a stagnant state except for the contributions of the Arabs, surgery was the branch that began again to show progress. Surgery was separated from medicine during the time of Galen or before, and the two branches of medicine took quite different paths in the following 1500 years. There were probably many reasons why the surgeons were accorded less prestige and became a much less learned group than their medical colleagues, but the separation of surgery from medicine was not decreed by the church, as history books claimed for years. What misled historians of surgery was the phrase *Ecclesia abhorret a sanguine* (the Church abhors blood). This is not to be found in the text of the Council of Tours (1163), as was commonly claimed, or in any papal decree, although certainly the concept that the Church wished its monks to spend more time on matters of religion and less on secular things such as medicine and surgery appears reasonable. It was Quesnay, the eighteenth century French historian of surgery, who disseminated the mistaken idea that the Church actually forbade surgery, and the phrase and his interpretation were repeated over and over again.[86]

By the thirteenth and fourteenth centuries surgery was condemned and avoided by physicians who had received their education in the universities that were now arising all over Europe. Along with theology and law, medicine was usually one of the basic faculties. Surgeons, however, were often unlettered, lower-class men who were scorned in clerical circles. The surgeons were taught the ways of their craft by apprenticeship. However, as Sir Clifford Allbutt has written, "by the expulsion of surgery from the liberal arts medicine herself was eviscerated."[3]

That surgery had also declined there is no doubt. In the twelfth century, when a rebirth of medicine and surgery occurred, Salernitan surgeons believed that surgery's decadence could be ascribed to two causes: its division from medicine and the neglect of anatomy. It was not long thereafter, however, that two major developments greatly affected the future course of surgery. One was the invention of gunpowder and its use in human warfare beginning in the fourteenth century; the other was the beginning of a renewed interest in the study of anatomy. Thus, with greater call for their services and with the beginning of greater fundamental knowledge from which advances could be made, the surgeons can be credited with having carried medicine forward from the time of the fourteenth century. The texts of Guy de Chauliac, who unfortunately favored suppuration in healing, and the works of Theodoric and Henri de Mondeville, honored because they stressed clean wounds, reflected great credit upon the whole of medicine.

Guy de Chauliac, in his fourteenth century book on surgery, continued the custom begun by Celsus of including a history of surgery within his text. Moreover, he identified five different surgical schools existing at the time and differentiated one from the other on the basis of their treatment of wounds. The followers of Galen, who applied salves to promote pus formation, he called the orthodox school. A second group followed the teachings of Theodoric, who stressed clean wounds and healing by first intention. A third group deviated slightly by applying mild substances to the wound. A fourth group relied on charms and incantations to help them heal wounds, and the fifth were termed the "women and silly folk." They depended on nature or God.

There is little doubt that from the year 1200 on, surgeons existed as separate practitioners. They were especially to be found in the newly rising cities, where they joined guilds. Earlier, they had sometimes been admitted to the universities, where they could even lecture. As time passed, however, they were excluded and thus formed their own colleges, such as the Collège de St. Côme in Paris.[80] Along with these surgeons of the long robe, who were often clerics, the barbers existed, the even less learned surgeons. The physicians usually favored the barbers because, being simpler men, they were more likely to be willing to be at the beck and call of the learned doctors.

The barbers and surgeons of England had belonged to separate guilds since the fourteenth century. In 1540 a compromise as to the rights and duties of each was achieved, and a single company of Barbers and Surgeons was formed. Surgeons agreed to do no barbering, and the barbers restricted their surgery to dentistry. The union lasted 200 years. In 1745, it was dissolved and the surgeons' company again existed independently, jealously guarding its prerogatives and protecting its interests. In 1800, George III chartered the Royal College of Surgeons of London, which by charter from Queen Victoria in 1843 became the Royal College of Surgeons of England.

The works of many surgeons of the fourteenth to the seventeenth century were important, but space does not permit a review of them here. For greater detail the reader should see the references by Billings,[9] Bishop,[12] Graham,[45] Malgaigne,[63] and Zimmerman and Veith.[96] Suffice it to say that the surgeons of four centuries ago had the same aims as their counterparts today. Witness, for instance, what the British surgeon Peter Lowe (1550–1613) had to say in his *A Discourse of the Whole Art of Chirurgerie* (1597), the first genuine textbook of surgery written in English. Lowe asks: "What is chirurgerie?" The answer is as true today as four centuries ago: "It is a science or Arte that sheweth the manner howe to work on man's body, exercising all manuall operations necessary to heal man, or as much as is possible by using of most expedient medicines." Lowe's textbook, incidentally, is arranged under five headings, also used by Paré: (1) to take away; (2) to help and add; (3) to put in place that which is out; (4) to separate; and (5) to join what is separated.[30] These early surgeons also had a clear conception of what the surgeon should be. Who can improve upon the qualifications

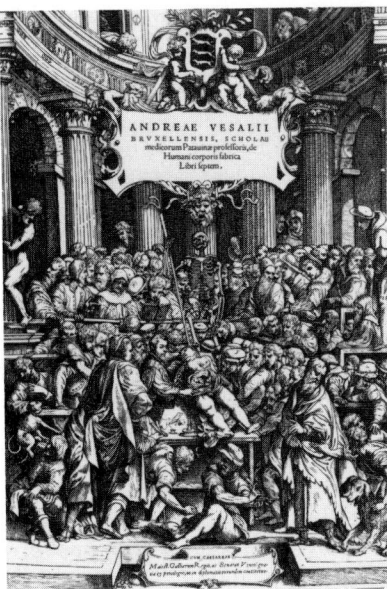

Figure 1. Frontispiece from Vesalius' *Fabrica*, published in 1543.

set forth by Thomas Vicary, mid–sixteenth century surgeon and author?

> Now then to know what properties and conditions this man must have before he be a perfect chirurgien. I doe note foure things most specially that every chirurgien ought so to have: the first, that he be learned; the second, that he be expert; the third, that he be ingenious; the fourth, that he be well mannered.[89]

Some physicians in the Renaissance saw clearly that medicine and surgery, united in ancient times, must be brought together again. During the Renaissance, surgery did slowly begin to regain a higher social position. No longer primarily in the hands of barbers, surgery was taught and practiced by some of the most illustrious physicians and anatomists. Vesalius and Fabricius of Aquapendente, the teacher of William Harvey, were but two of many.

Paracelsus, the sixteenth century rebel against the dead hand of the past, whom some have called the Luther of Medicine, called for a reunion of medicine and surgery:

> How can ye establish it as another faculty and profession? Ye wood doctor and fool! . . . In *judicando* ye are a physician, in *curando* a surgeon. The patient asks for cure—surgery—and not for theory—medicine—it is the doctor who needs the latter. That is: there can be no surgeon who is not also a physician; the latter begets the surgeon and the surgeon tests the physician by the result of his work. Where the physician is not also a surgeon, he is an idol that is nothing but a painted monkey.[73]

In this hurried survey, one must pause to recognize Ambroise Paré (1510–1590). Few men in the history of medicine have been more popular than this sixteenth century French surgeon. There are many reasons for his high standing. His superb work, his pleasing personality, his humility, and, not least, the loving study made of his life and work by the nineteenth century surgeon Joseph Malgaigne all are responsible for Paré's place in the history of surgery.

Born of humble parents in the province of Maine in 1510, Paré received his medical training as an apprentice barber-surgeon and then went to Paris where he was appointed a house surgeon at the Hôtel-Dieu, already a famous charity hospital. Here he learned anatomy and surgery and began to develop the superb manual dexterity and sound general knowledge of medicine of his time that led to his success. He served four successive kings of France as a military surgeon and wrote books in his own tongue instead of Latin, in which he and his fellow barber-surgeons were not schooled. Thus, in his writing as well as in his surgical treatment, Paré's achievement was a victory of experience over tradition.

The use of a digestive solution of egg yolk, rose oil, and turpentine to dress gunshot wounds was a discovery Paré made when the supply of hot oil usually used to cauterize wounds was exhausted during the war between Francis I and Charles V. Those men treated with Paré's improvised methods, he tells us, did much better, and he resolved to treat all gunshot wounds without boiling oil in the future.[74] Remarkable as were his results, of equal note is that Paré here knowingly challenged authority. The text of Giovanni da Vigo on wounds was widely followed by all the famous surgeons from whom Paré had learned and whom he was emulating in treating battle wounds. That he realized the meaning of his little chance experiment is no less wondrous then.

One can readily see in Paré's approach a great similarity to that of physicians today, doubtless still another reason he should be so revered today. For example, he stressed the importance of knowledge of anatomy, which in his time was beginning to emerge as a needed discipline.

ANATOMY

Anatomy, so avidly pursued in the school of Alexandria in Hellenistic times, was withdrawn from the medical curriculum. Its revival in the sixteenth century is closely related to several outside or nonmedical influences. One was the interest in the human form expressed by artists such as Leonardo da Vinci, Raphael, Donatello, and Michelangelo; another was the invention of printing and movable type, making books readily available. Even more important, illustrations so necessary to anatomic study could be faithfully reproduced and distributed. One need only look at the magnificent book by Vesalius to realize immediately the impact that illustrations could have made.

The origins of anatomy are obscure, but early surgeons who treated wounds and those who butchered animals must have had some concept of structure. The Greeks pursued the study of animal anatomy, and one must bear in mind that ancient anatomy, except for the school of Alexandria in the time of Herophilus and Erasistratus in the third century B.C., was largely animal anatomy. One of the great accomplishments of the Renaissance was the rediscovery of the fine structure of the body and the realization by the medical world that knowledge of anatomy was essential to all medical science.

Anatomic dissection began to be more frequent again at the end of the thirteenth century. With the first manual for dissection written by Mondino de Luzzi in 1316, students had some guide. The early dissections were still often confined to the bodies of animals; sometimes they were autopsies performed to ascertain the cause of death, especially if foul play was suspected. These dissections were usually the responsibility of the surgeon. Only by the middle of the fifteenth century had anatomic dissection become commonplace so that a special theater for it was built in Padua.

A basic requirement of any descriptive science is the ability to make illustrations that can be readily duplicated so that they can be used for instruction and for learning. Woodcuts began to be made in Europe probably late in the fourteenth century, mainly as a labor-saving device for producing sacred images. It was some time before biologists accepted the idea, but by the end of the fifteenth and early in the sixteenth century, occasional illustrated medical works began to appear. Johannes de Ketham's *Fasiculus medicinae*, Venice, 1491, and Berengario da Carpi's *Commentari . . . Super Anatomia Mundini · · ·* are two of the best known. Others appeared, but the best and most lasting proved to be Andreas Vesalius' *De humani corporis fabrica*. The publication of the *Fabrica* of 1543 coincided with the publication of another great book in the history of science, the *De revolutionibus orbium coelestium* of Nicolaus Copernicus. Thus, in a single year the modern understanding of both microcosm and macrocosm was under way.

The importance of Vesalius is that by his work and example he set forth a program. The famous frontispiece depicting him at the dissecting table, knife in hand, is itself programmatic. This young man, born in Louvain in 1514 and educated in Brussels and Paris, went to Padua to finish his medical studies. At the age of 23, upon receiving his degree, he was appointed professor of anatomy and surgery, an important academic combination for centuries to come. Vesalius was certainly not alone in his attack upon the ancients, particularly the anatomic-physiologic system of Galen. Yet his great achievements set a tone. One must also remember that in the same year as the *Fabrica* Vesalius also published the *Epitome*, a shorter book intended to serve as a guide for students. The great rarity of original editions of the *Epitome* probably attests to its heavy use.[72]

The relationship of Vesalius and his study of anatomy to the field of surgery was self-evident to him, yet he speaks of it in the preface of the *Fabrica*. "At Padua, in that most famous university of the whole world . . . I gave the lectures on surgical medicine, and because anatomy is related to this, I devoted myself to the investigation of man's structure."

The surgeon-anatomists, Vesalius being one of their number, had an increasingly important role as time and knowledge of anatomy advanced. Thomas Vicary in his anatomy text quoted Galen's statement that it is as possible for a surgeon not knowing anatomy to work in man's body without error as it is for a blind man to carve an image and make it perfect. The tradition of teaching both surgery and anatomy was continued by the professors of surgery in medical schools until the early twentieth century.

William Cheselden, the eighteenth century British surgeon, wrote a textbook of anatomy that was standard for nearly 100 years.[21,23] Henry Gray, a surgeon who in 1859, the year of Darwin's *Origin of Species*, introduced the first edition of his *Anatomy*, gave his book the title *Anatomy, Descriptive and Surgical.*[44]

PATHOLOGY AND EXPERIMENTAL SURGERY

The eighteenth century has often been termed the century of systems in the history of medicine. The work of William Cullen, John Brown, and Benjamin Rush affords proof for such an assertion, but in the history of surgery of the eighteenth century, the development of modern pathology and experimental surgery was associated with the name of John Hunter. To him, as much as to any single individual, must go the credit for introducing modern medicine of the nineteenth century. Again, because this essay is not a general history of medicine or a monograph on the history of surgery, a greatly simplified and somewhat distorted view of events is seen.

One of the great medical events of the eighteenth century was the publication of *On the Seats and Causes of Disease Investigated by Anatomy (De sedibus et causus morborum . . .)* in 1761 when the author was 79 years old—Giovanni Battista Morgagni, Padua's gifted professor of anatomy for nearly 60 years. It represented a lifetime of work and stands as one of the great classics of medicine. Morgagni insisted that clinical observations be correlated with postmortem findings. He intended his book to be a useful one and considered common diseases confronting physicians, not the rare and unusual ones usually written about by previous authors. Morgagni wrote his book as a series of 70 letters, composed in elegant Latin. Not until 1793 did Matthew Baillie, a nephew of the Hunters, write a book on morbid anatomy in English. In the tradition of Morgagni, John Hunter then brought pathologic study to surgery.

John Hunter, born in Scotland in 1728, was the youngest son in a large family.[31,59] He was a poor student and was little inter-

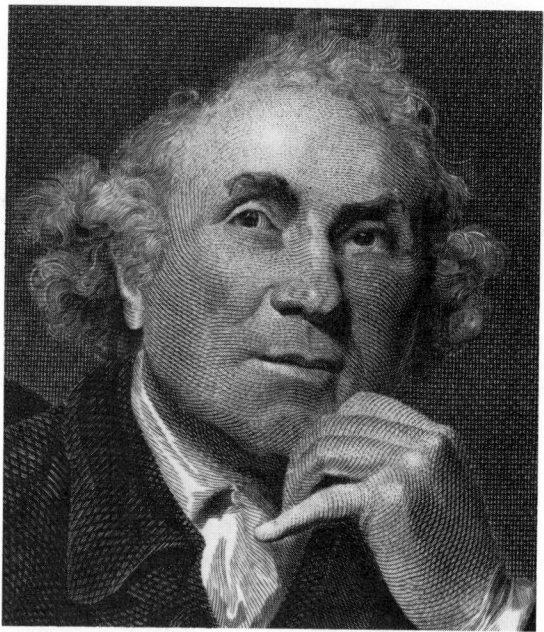

Figure 2. John Hunter (1728–1793), the father of experimental surgery and a superb anatomist and teacher.

ested in his studies except those having to do with natural history. At age 20 he was apprenticed to his brother William, 10 years his senior, who earlier that year had begun giving private anatomy lessons to surgeons in London. Such anatomy schools became legal in England in 1745 with the dissolution of the Barber-Surgeons' Company, and their founding introduced the great era of body snatching.[4]

John Hunter had been a poor student, but he became interested in dissection immediately, and his brother quickly recognized his talents. This was the beginning of a long illustrious career that found John Hunter to be a naturalist who collected a large museum of specimens, an anatomist and experimental surgeon, and a teacher of great influence. That he should have been the preceptor of so many pupils who later became famous in their own right is the more remarkable when one considers that he was a poor lecturer and an obtuse writer. Nevertheless, his precepts were stimulating and his writings widely read. His work on venereal disease confused syphilis and gonorrhea but was a major study of the subject. In 1794, a year after Hunter's death, his *Treatise on the Blood, Inflammation and Gun-Shot Wounds* appeared. Here one finds ample reason why Hunter's lectures on surgery, physiology, and pathology, often a combination of the three, were so successful. Hunter believed that "inflammation is not only occasionally the cause of disease, but it is often a mode of cure. . . . " Inflammation thus became "the first principle of surgery."

Equally well known was his study of ligation of arterial vessels in cases of aneurysm. By supposed experimental study on the antlers of deer, Hunter realized that collateral circulation would probably suffice if the vessel involved by aneurysm were ligated in its healthy part.[85] By this means, amputation, if the aneurysm was in the femoral or popliteal arteries, for example, could be avoided. This was a major advance in surgical therapy and was the beginning of what came to prominence in the nineteenth century as conservative surgery. Thus, Hunter amply earned the epitaph given him by the medical historian Fielding Garrison, who said, "With the advent of John Hunter, surgery ceased to be regarded as a mere technical mode of treatment, and began to take its place as a branch of scientific medicine, firmly grounded in physiology and pathology."[40]

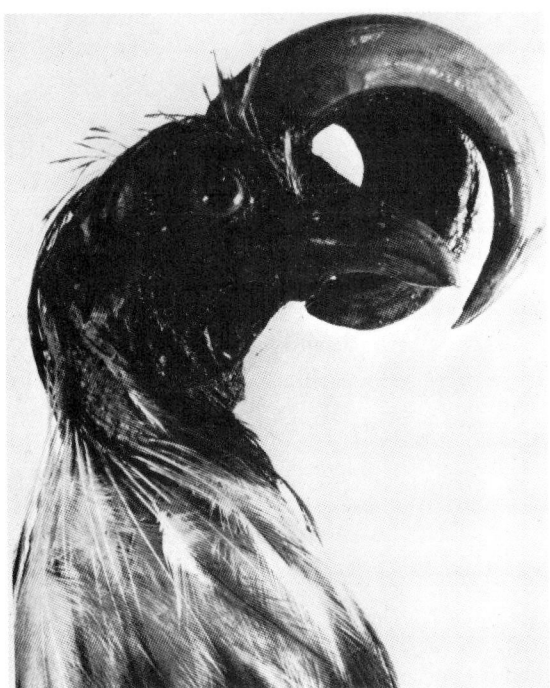

Figure 3. Photograph of a specimen from the Royal College of Surgeons of England of a spur that grew after being transplanted to the cock's comb by John Hunter (example of tissue transplantation).

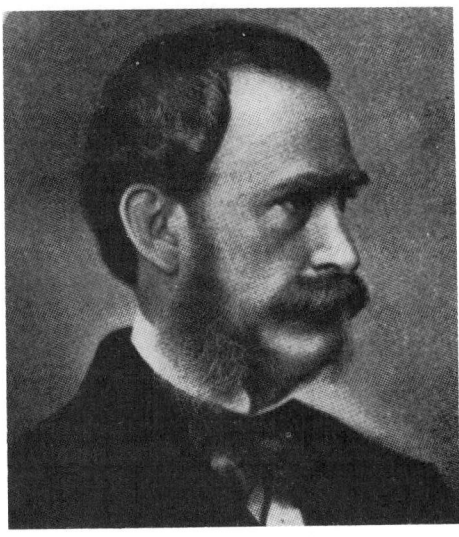

Figure 4. William T. G. Morton (1819–1868), a Boston dentist whose successful demonstration of ether anesthesia on October 16, 1846, at the Massachusetts General Hospital was a landmark in the history of surgery.

The influence of John Hunter was still keenly felt in the first half of the nineteenth century. Many of the leading surgeons of Britain and America had been his pupils. He made certain that all his students received thorough grounding in anatomy, physiology, and surgical pathology. And so medicine, surgery included, began gradually to assume a more scientific character.

Sir Astley Cooper, perhaps the most popular London surgeon of the first part of the nineteenth century, was a pupil of Hunter and a very fine operator. Part of his secret, no doubt, was his devotion to anatomic study, which he practiced and taught in his private dissecting room. "If I laid my head upon my pillow at night," Cooper said, "without having dissected something in the day, I should think that I had lost that day." [17]

ANESTHESIA AND ANTISEPSIS

Surgery of the twentieth century has been characterized by "a lifting of the eyes from the local lesion and the operation designed to deal with it to regard the more general aspects of surgical disorders," according to Churchill.[22] Whereas this approach is certainly a hallmark today, surgeons did not invent it. The institutes of surgery, as they were called in previous times, "are its settled principles," Henry J. Bigelow told his students in 1849.[8] Although the principles were still excessively general, discussion of constitution and disease was not entirely neglected by the surgeons. However, in the field of operative surgery, Bigelow confessed, "We occupy more directly what is popularly considered to be the province of the surgeon. The surgeon, with the public, is associated with surgical operations, and his notoriety is in measure with the belief which the world may entertain of the number of or magnitude of the operations he may perform."[8] The public may be impressed, warned Bigelow, and the surgeon should guard against much of the exaggerated sense of worth and of drama.

Both Bigelow and his Boston colleague, J. Mason Warren, wrote about the all too frequent sepsis that appeared after the drama in the amphitheater. "Primary healing," Warren wrote in 1864, "is seldom attained in city practice."[92] Union by first

intention had been rare for 20 years, he claimed. Part of the blame, Warren believed, could be attributed to the city fathers who were responsible for the unhygienic conditions then prevalent. Thus, some surgeons looked well beyond the local lesion, but they were usually powerless to make change.

The surgeons of the nineteenth century, incidentally, had an honorable part in the movement for sanitary reform. For example, Edmund Parke and John Simon in England and Stephen Smith and Willard Parker in New York were both surgeons and sanitarians. The French surgeon, E. Doyen, in his *Surgical Therapeutics and Operative Technique* of the early twentieth century, entitled one chapter "Parallelism of the Evolution of Surgical Asepsis and the Progress of Public Hygiene."

In the early nineteenth century surgical operations were still infrequent. Many hospitals in England and America had their weekly operating days, on which one or two procedures might be performed. In many major hospitals there were fewer operations in 1 year than are performed in 2 days in one of the modern busy surgical services. The surgical therapy of tuberculosis, especially its bony complications, represented a significant proportion of operations; accidents, strangulated hernias, abscesses, and aneurysms comprised most of the rest. Mortality varied from hospital to hospital and differed in different countries.[84] It was generally highest on the Continent, 40 to 60 per cent, depending on the operative procedure.

There were numerous obstacles to the advance of surgery. Pain, infection, hemorrhage, and shock were four of the most difficult to overcome. As each was considered, the bounds of surgery enlarged. As the limits of surgery were extended, the field of the individual surgeons appears to have become more and more restricted.

Since the fundamental aim of all medical art and science has always been to alleviate human pain and suffering, the development of anesthesia for use during surgical operations ranks as one of the most dramatic discoveries in the annals of medicine. The use of alcohol, mandrake root, opium, and even bleeding or reduction of blood flow to the brain to reduce sensibility was known to the ancients in a crude sense, but the effective use of general anesthesia can be precisely dated to the 1840s. In 1842 a rural Georgia practitioner, Crawford W. Long, used ether to remove small skin tumors, but he did not report his results until 3 years after William Morton successfully used ether in a patient for John Collins Warren on October 16, 1846, at the Massachusetts General Hospital. James Young Simpson of Edinburgh introduced chloroform in the next year, and a new age in surgery was born. Speed of operation would now no longer be the hallmark of the great surgeons.

The history of anesthesia, like that of most medical accomplishments, is quite long.[58] To disregard it in a simple paragraph does it an injustice, but the story, with its technical details and tragic priority conflicts, has been well told so often that it need not be repeated here. What should be emphasized is that the development of anesthesia and its very rapid acceptance after its introduction may be seen as part of a larger movement of humanitarianism. Reforms of prisons, public health, schools, almshouses, and mental hospitals; the crusades against the evils of drinking; and, in the United States especially, the abolitionist movement all had at root a genuine concern for human life and dignity. Also noteworthy in the story of anesthesia, especially in the twentieth century development of intratracheal and intravenous routes of administration as well as conduction or nerve block methods, is that physiology and surgery now became inseparably combined.

Although the mid–nineteenth century English physician John Snow, famous for his writing about cholera and the Broad Street pump, was one of the first to call himself an anesthesiologist, not until the years just before World War II did the specialty of anesthesiology begin to develop. No longer was it sufficient for a surgical house officer or even a medical student to be delegated the task of administering the anesthetic and monitoring the patient, who often was neglected as the student eagerly watched the surgeon operate.

Anesthesia found speedy acceptance. The same, unfortunately, cannot be said for the attempts to control infection. Wound healing in the days before Lister was a confused and depressing aspect of surgery. Wounding, either accidental or iatrogenic, was often followed by what was called irritative fever, usually lasting a few days followed by accumulation of pus in the wound. Sometimes the pus was creamy white; this thick exudate was often called "laudable pus." If the patient was fortunate, there was a slow healing process to recovery. This was the state of surgery seen from the patient's view, and it had existed for centuries.

The problem of surgical dressings was one of trial and error.[11] Surgeons in the early nineteenth century still used dressing materials that were as old as recorded surgical history. Some, of course, were very beneficial, but even with the most ingenious technique, the most agile and skilled operator all too often found that his work was ineffective because the patient succumbed to postoperative infection. The term *hospitalism* was used by surgeons to describe the postsurgical infections so commonly found in surgical wards: erysipelas, pyemia, septicemia, and hospital gangrene.[57,60] Whereas the cause of these infections may have been guessed by some shrewd surgeons of the prebacteriologic era, by and large most surgeons felt helpless in the wake of them. Sir James Simpson, the Scottish surgeon who introduced chloroform, strongly urged his colleagues to do their operating on kitchen tables or in small cottage hospitals, for here the patients were much less likely to become infected.

The history of the idea of so-called laudable pus is very difficult to trace. Some ancient writers mention pus formation as a normal part of healing, but the mere presence of pus does not make it laudable. What is certain, however, is that only with the last 100 or so years have surgeons been able to consider the problem effectively. The comments of Sir Clifford Allbutt about his experiences in the years just before antisepsis was introduced are typical of what may be found in the literature.

. . . in the third quarter of the nineteenth century, in my callow days as a physician, the apothecary of a large hospital showed me a row of amputations, with stumps pouring out pus in cataracts upon the cushions, and exclaimed — "That, Sir, is what I like to see; nothing so wholesome in a wound as a good discharge of laudable pus." As a university graduate, for as universities were then we knew nothing of surgery, — I assented in superior ignorance.[3]

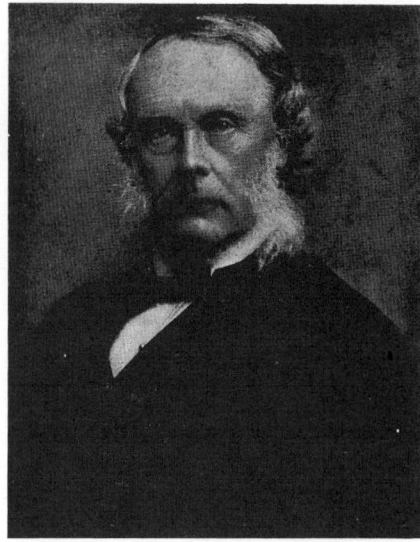

Figure 5. Joseph Lister (1827–1912), the originator of antiseptic surgery.

Joseph Lister was faced with these problems and watched the wretched patients in his surgical wards with increasing frustration and concern. Although he was not alone, he was the first to combat this major surgical obstacle successfully. The Hungarian obstetrician Ignaz Semmelweis and the American anatomist and writer Oliver Wendell Holmes had clearly shown in the 1840s that puerperal fever was carried to parturient women on the hands of their doctors. Simple washing in chlorinated lime solutions was extremely successful in Semmelweis' wards, but his Viennese colleagues and the world paid scant heed. Thus it was left to Lister determinedly to convince the world that wound infection was evil, not laudable, and that it could be effectively prevented.

Joseph Lister was born in Essex in 1827.[43] He was imbued with a love for science early in life by his father, Joseph Jackson Lister, a wine merchant who soon after his son's birth reported an important advance in microscopy to the Royal Society. An amateur scientist in the best tradition, the elder Lister perfected an achromatic lens that lessened the artifacts that had plagued the users of the earlier microscopes.

Young Lister attended University College, London, the common school for dissenters such as the Quaker Listers. He was graduated in 1847 and received his medical degree in 1852. In the following year he journeyed to Edinburgh to work and study with James Syme, one of the outstanding surgeons and surgical teachers of the midcentury. Syme was a leader in the movement toward conservative surgery, one that tried to conserve limbs by excision of parts of bone, with preservation of the limb as a whole. Lister remained in Edinburgh and became a member of the surgical staff of the Royal Infirmary, and he married Syme's eldest daughter, Agnes. In 1861 Lister moved to the chair of surgery at the Royal Infirmary in Glasgow, and it was during 8 fruitful years there that he began to develop his principles and practice of antisepsis. In 1869 he was recalled to Edinburgh to fill Syme's chair, and in 1877 he moved to King's College Hospital in London. In 1897 he became the first physician to be elevated to the peerage.

In his earlier Edinburgh and Glasgow years, Lister investigated a number of problems closely related to surgery, such as inflammation, wound healing, and the role of blood coagulation in both. His approach to the problems of surgery was distinctly modern, in the sense that it was scientific and physiologic. Despite Lister's attempts to sterilize his wards and to perform surgery as cleanly as possible, there was still an appalling rate of the common surgical complications of hospital gangrene, pyemia, and erysipelas among his patients.

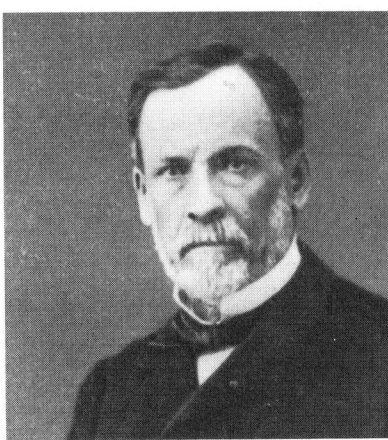

Figure 6. Louis Pasteur (1822–1895), the originator of the germ theory of disease.

In the years just prior to 1865, the French scientist Louis Pasteur slowly developed what came to be a germ theory of disease. He clearly showed that fermentation and putrefaction, observed since ancient days, were caused by living, multiplying matter. He reasoned that pus formation, wound infection, and some fevers must also be caused by minute organisms from the environment.[32]

It has never been entirely clear how Lister became aware of Pasteur's work. That he gave him specific credit there is no doubt. Rickman Godlee, Lister's surgical pupil, nephew, and biographer, claimed that it was a Glasgow colleague, a professor of chemistry, who suggested the practical implications of Pasteur's work to Lister and also suggested the use of carbolic acid. There is another possibility, however, although not provable without more information, that appears very plausible.

In the latter part of 1864, the year before Lister began to use carbolic acid on wounds, T. Spencer Wells, the eminent British surgeon, published a paper in the *British Medical Journal* entitled "Some Causes of Excessive Mortality After Surgical Operations." Wells described the work of Pasteur and said that it might well have an "important bearing upon the development of purulent infection and the whole class of diseases most fatal in hospitals and other overcrowded places."[94] Wells further suggested that germs might find their appropriate medium in wounds, causing pus and subsequent septicemia. Although clearly set forth, Wells' statement appears to have borne little fruit, unless, of course, Lister was indeed stimulated by it.

Lister's first papers describing his method and success appeared in 1867. In the following years, he changed the technical details of his method, added the steam-powered spray for the operating environment, and continued to fight for his concept in many publications. As years passed, he was able to perform operations safely that previously no capable surgeon would have dared attempt. The successful wiring of a fractured patella in 1877, which converted a closed fracture to an open one, brought much scorn upon him, but patience, determination, and scrupulous attention to detail led eventually to complete success. Lister admitted in the 1880s that the spray was not necessary and indeed may have been harmful to operators and patients alike. He gracefully accepted the development of aseptic surgery by the Germans and acknowledged that it was but a step beyond his own work and a logical extension of it.

The acceptance of listerism, as already indicated, was uneven and, with the advantage of retrospective view, was quite slow. There were many reasons for this, most of them not tied to simple conservatism or resistance to change. Lister's method was complicated; the carbolic acid was an unpleasant nuisance and could actually be harmful, and the method was time-consuming and expensive and required assistance. Some surgeons and physicians believed the germ theory to be mere speculation; therefore, the underlying theory or the rationale for Lister's technique was also slow to be accepted.[14] Also one must remember that many leading surgeons simply could not duplicate Lister's good results, hard as they might try. Theodor Billroth was one who tried the method, wanted to accept it, but found it somewhat frustrating. By the late 1870s he had adopted listerism fully, but not without much discouragement.[97]

Other surgeons reported that they used Lister's techniques but that their results were not much improved. In reading case reports in medical journals of the period, one must evaluate carefully such phrases as "listerism used" or "Lister's technique followed throughout." In the case of President James Garfield in 1881, for example, the extensive medical bulletins issued during his 2-month lingering battle with an abdominal gunshot wound inflicted through the back often reported "Lister's dressings used." Yet it is known, too, that fingers and instruments probed the wound from the first day on. Little real understanding of the germ theory can be ascribed to surgeons who carefully soaked their instruments in carbolic acid but then reused them without resoaking after they had dropped on the floor or, even more commonly, used them after they had been wiped on the operator's nonsterile apron or held between his teeth. Thus, the full realization by Lister of the meaning of Pasteur's work is perhaps his greatest achievement.

Rudolph Matas, one of the young American surgeons of the first generation of Lister disciples, emphasized that certain features of the typical Lister dressing routine were more readily adopted than parts of the doctrine itself. Carbolic acid was accepted as the preferred antiseptic; Chassaignac's rubber drainage tubes again came into wider use, and the ligatures, soaked in carbolic solution, were cut short. "But even this marvelous improvement in technique was slow in coming, for, in 1878 and 1879, I saw a number of amputation stumps from which long ligatures dangled, waiting to ripen in pus to drop off."[51,65]

In the 1880s, Matas recalled, the head, chest, and abdomen were still sanctuaries not to be opened, unless by accident.[65] It has frequently been stressed that the development of anesthesia and antisepsis greatly increased the numbers of operations performed, but a review of the statistics reveals that the increase was very slow. Halsted in 1904 showed that in the decade following the fairly wide acceptance of antisepsis in the United States (1878–1888), the numbers of operations performed increased only slightly.[47] This decade, it must be remembered, was the second after Lister's first enunciation of his principles in

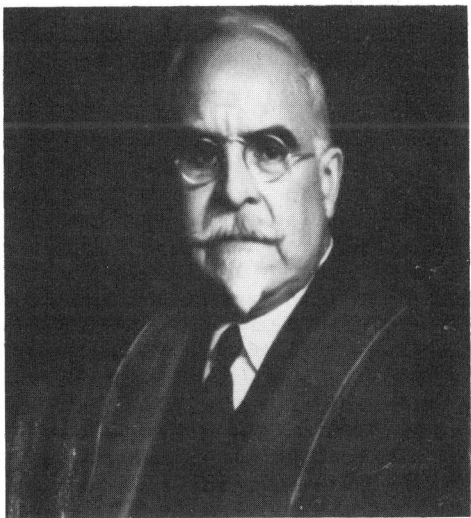

Figure 7. Rudolph Matas (1860–1957), Professor of Surgery at Tulane University in Louisiana and a pioneer in vascular surgery. He introduced the technique of endoaneurysmorrhaphy in the treatment of arterial aneurysm.

1867. Matas provided the figures for the Charity Hospital in New Orleans, where in 1881 only 172 operations were done among 5300 admissions, or about 3.2 per cent. In 1890, the Charity Hospital admitted 6083 patients, but only 291, or 4.7 per cent, had major surgical procedures. By 1939, about 40 per cent of admissions were surgical.[65] As Charles Rosenberg has so clearly shown in his history of hospitals, *The Care of Strangers*, it was the increasing use of hospitals by surgeons that helped to shift the locus of medical care in the early decades of this century increasingly to the hospital.[78]

In the decade after Lister's momentous papers on the efficacy of antisepsis, there was still much reticence, as has already been indicated, about accepting the method as well as its theoretical foundation, the germ theory of disease. There was also some reluctance to hope for much more improvement in the art of surgery. After the Napoleonic wars at the beginning of the century, the French surgeon and author of surgical texts, Alexis Boyer, supposedly said, "Surgery seems to have attained the highest degree of perfection of which it is capable."[75] Despite anesthesia and the development of many new techniques and despite the promise of antisepsis, John Eric Erichsen, one of the most perceptive and influential surgeons of latter nineteenth century Britain, came to similar conclusions in 1873:

> That there must be a final limit to development in this department of our profession there can be no doubt. . . . Like every other art, be it manipulative, plastic, or imitative, it can only be carried to a certain definite point of excellence. An art may be modified, it may be varied, but it cannot be perfected beyond certain attainable limits. . . . There cannot always be fresh fields for conquest by the knife; there must be portions of the human frame that will ever remain sacred from intrusion, at least in the surgeon's hands. That we have nearly, if not quite, reached these final limits there can be little question.[75]

The story of the last 100 or so years has proved Erichsen a poor prophet; yet most of those engaged in medicine have at one time or another shared his feelings. What Erichsen and his contemporaries could not foresee was that within 2 decades medicine (including surgery now) would join hands with biology as a whole and thereby be able to expand its horizon in ways previously unthought. Chemotherapy, cardiac surgery, and transplantation are but a few examples of significant teamwork between basic scientists and surgeons.

ABDOMINAL SURGERY

Among the many difficult technical problems confronted by nineteenth century surgeons was that of reconnecting the divided ends of hollow tubes, especially blood vessels and intestine. Just as cardiovascular surgery has captured both public and professional attention in the past 2 or 3 decades, 90 to 100 years ago it was abdominal surgery that had the same role. The successful removal of an inflamed appendix prior to rupture, the Billroth operations for esophageal and gastric cancer causing obstruction, the improved hernia operations of Bassini and Halsted, and abdominal operations for such other reasons as diseases of the ovary all caused great excitement in the medical world of the late nineteenth century.

The problem of intestinal obstruction confronted surgeons long before the 1880s. Strangulated hernia, for example, was not uncommon. Before the introduction of antisepsis, laparotomy was not usually performed. Ephraim McDowell, the Kentucky physician who successfully removed a huge ovarian tumor from Mrs. Jane Todd Crawford in 1809, was skilled, assuredly, but also very fortunate. An indication of what his townsmen thought is that they gathered in large numbers around his house on that Christmas Day in Danville, Kentucky, with a rope slung over a tree, ready for use if the doctor failed in the butchery they were convinced he was committing. They might well have hanged him had his patient died.[37]

The basic principle of intestinal suture, that the serous coats must be brought into contact, was not discovered until early in the nineteenth century and not put into use until some decades later. The British surgeon Benjamin Travers in 1812 published *An Inquiry Into the Process of Nature in Preparing Injuries of Intestines.* About the same time, Guillaume Dupuytren, one of the best trained and ablest surgeons of France, whose approach to surgery was much like John Hunter's in the use of experimental physiology and pathology, also concerned himself with intestinal suture. Although apparently quite a mean and unscrupulous man, he was a great teacher and surgical innovator. Unfortunately, his name is associated today mainly with an uncommon malady of the hand caused by contraction of the palmar fascia. Dupuytren's student, Antoine Lembert, is known for his suture, which followed the observation that careful approximation of the peritoneal coats of divided intestine would provide good healing. Not until the German and German-trained surgeons (including Swiss and Austrians) began putting antiseptic and aseptic principles to practice did the techniques of abdominal surgery become common.

In America, one of the important contributions to the advance of surgery stemmed from the work of a pathologist, Reginald Heber Fitz of Boston, and the surgeons Charles McBurney and Henry B. Sands of New York and John B. Murphy of Chicago. Fitz in 1886 published his classic paper on appendicitis, a term he coined.[35] Known for centuries under a variety of names such as *perityphlitis* and *iliac passion,* acute inflammation of the *vermiform* appendix was a surgical disease, according to Fitz.

Charles McBurney, professor of surgery at the College of Physicians and Surgeons, working mainly at Roosevelt Hospital in New York, in 1889 described the point of maximal tenderness, now bearing his name, and 5 years later proposed a new incision for appendectomy.[66,67] J. B. Murphy in the United States, Lord Moynihan of Leeds in England, and others at the turn of the century led the vigorous campaign for withholding purgatives and for resorting to prompt surgical therapy. It should be noted that the understanding of this common disease and the operative concept for it were accomplished by the cooperative efforts of physicians of several specialties.[83]

This use of surgery, self-evident to us today, required some years to become assimilated into standard medical practice. In 1900 abdominal surgery was not yet undertaken lightly by most doctors and patients. The successful drainage of an appendiceal abscess of King Edward VII of England, forcing the delay of his coronation in 1902, helped make appendicitis a fashionable disease and also helped break down further the resistance to surgery.

Another important contribution in the epoch of abdominal surgery of the last decades of the nineteenth century stemmed from work in pathologic physiology, especially in the various German medical centers. In these years the German physiologist Heidenhain devised his pouches for the study of gastric physiology and Nickolai Eck, a Russian, his anastomosis of the vena cava and portal vein. The latter experimental surgical procedure, devised in 1877, was then widely utilized by Mering, Minkowski, and other physiologists and internists in their study of digestion and liver function. During the decades after 1860 the German clinics made numerous advances in scientific medicine. Surgeons, with their new freedom to explore the abdomen, redirected the attention of the medical world to the importance of anatomic diagnosis.[34]

PHYSIOLOGY AND SURGERY

The alliance of surgery with physiology, although not as long-standing as that with anatomy, still has quite a history. The mid–eighteenth century Swiss, Albrecht von Haller, was professor of both surgery and physiology in Göttingen. Trained by the most famous medical teacher of his day, Hermann Boerhaave of Leyden, Haller wanted to teach medicine as a science in Göttingen as his master had done in Holland. To Haller must go the credit for animating anatomy and for stressing the importance of a systematic study of function. It must be admitted that although Haller taught the subject of surgery, he probably never took knife in hand except for anatomic dissection or physiologic experiment.

Many of the nineteenth century physiologists became superb experimental surgeons. François Magendie and Claude Bernard in France and Rudolph Heidenhain in Germany are good examples. Bernard joined Charles Huette in writing a manual of operative surgery. Similarly, some men who were primarily surgeons became well known for their contributions to physiology. Benjamin Collins Brodie, sergeant-surgeon to two kings of England, did important work on the effects of alcohol and curare as well as on the relationship of heat and respiration.

To William Beaumont's surgical skills and wound dressing is ascribed the fact that his patient, Alexis St. Martin, survived to become the most famous human experimental subject in the nineteenth century. St. Martin was wounded in the left lower chest by a musket shot at close range in 1822. Only after 3 years of constant and careful tending of the wounded area did Beaumont begin the famous investigations of gastric function.[5]

Not until the twentieth century, however, did surgeons begin to deal consistently with a variety of physiologic problems almost every time they operated. Early in this century, pain and infection were under control, but shock and the problem of maintaining respiration when the pleura was entered remained to be solved.

TRAINING OF THE SURGEON

Much has been written in the last 100 years about the training of the surgeon, the proper qualifications, and what it means to be a surgeon. Between the simple apprenticeship or even the transfer of knowledge from father to son that held sway until the nineteenth century and the thorough grounding in pathology, research, and operative and postoperative management required of today's surgeon, much surgical history has passed.[15,41,79]

The subject of surgical training in America invariably brings to mind the name of William S. Halsted, no doubt in part because of his famous address entitled "The Training of the Surgeon" delivered at Yale in 1904.[47] Halsted, who was born in New York City in 1852 and died in Baltimore 70 years later, made numerous important contributions to surgical technique and teaching.[53] After graduation from the College of Physicians and Surgeons and a trip to Europe, he quickly established himself as an energetic researcher, gifted operator, and popular young teacher in New York. While working with cocaine for nerve block anesthesia, he and some of his associates became addicted. Only after hospitalization and prolonged convalescence, and with the help of his faithful friend, William H. Welch, who invited him to Baltimore in 1886, did Halsted recover. Historians are still at work unraveling the circumstances of further addiction during his later and very productive years.

When the Johns Hopkins Hospital opened in 1889, Halsted was appointed acting surgeon and head of the outpatient clinic. He became professor of surgery in 1892, the year before admission of the first medical school class. Halsted developed improved methods for operating on hernias and cancer of the breast; he introduced the use of rubber gloves in surgery; and he constantly stressed the relationship of surgery to physiology. Careful handling of tissues and the minimization of blood loss were concepts he passed on to the many fine surgeons he trained during 30 years. Justifiable as has been his fame, Halsted was not solely responsible for establishing the surgical residency system as we know it. He would have been the first to note that the great German teachers of surgery, especially von

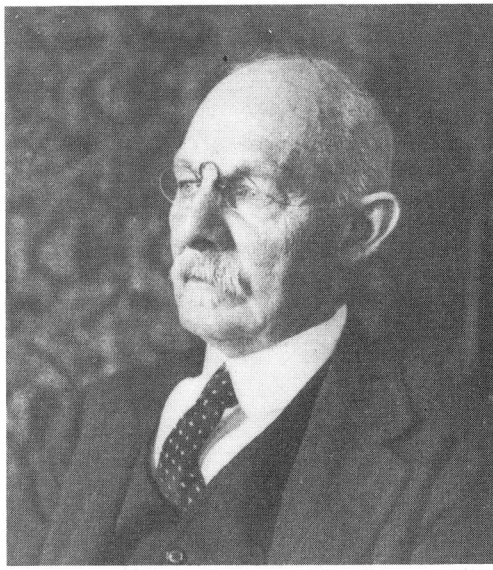

Figure 8. William S. Halsted (1852–1922), prominent American surgeon who introduced the German system of residency training to the United States. He also made fundamental contributions to the surgery of the thyroid, breast, and blood vessels and to the surgical treatment of hernia.

Langenbeck and his pupils, including Billroth, were his models. Moreover, Halsted's colleague William Osler deserves equal credit for instituting the system in medicine at Hopkins.

Why was it in Germany that the surgeons first adopted antisepsis? Halsted asked in his Yale lecture. The answer lay, he believed, "in the character of the scientific and practical training of surgeons in Germany." The assistants or "residents" in these programs enjoyed good research facilities, ample clinical material, and excellent instruction, and this is what Halsted successfully duplicated in Baltimore. "We need a system," he said at Yale in 1904, "and we shall surely have it, which will produce not only surgeons but surgeons of the highest type, men who will stimulate the first youths of our country to study surgery and to devote their energies and their lives to raising the standard of surgical science."[47] Reforms, Halsted stressed, had to come from both hospital and university, and the medical school should control a hospital of its own.

Halsted's German model was based mainly on the system founded by Bernhard Rudolf Konrad von Langenbeck (1810–1887), one of Germany's most distinguished nineteenth century surgeons. He received his degree in Göttingen in 1835, 7 years later became professor of surgery at Kiel, and in 1847 moved to Berlin. There he assumed what was probably the most prestigious chair in Germany, succeeding the illustrious Johann Friedrich Dieffenbach, who had done much to make orthopedic surgery and plastic surgery successful modes of treatment. Langenbeck thus followed in the footsteps of a superb operator, an imaginative innovator, and a highly popular teacher, but he was superbly equal to the task.

In 1861 Langenbeck, along with two of his pupils, Theodor Billroth, who became equally prominent, and Ernst Gurlt, the historian of surgery, founded the *Archive für klinische Chirurgie.* Langenbeck's editorial contributions and surgical improvements alone would assure him of a very high rank in the history of surgery, but perhaps his greatest contribution was his stress on a systematic way of training young surgeons. In general, this is what we now know as the surgical residency system.[10]

Halsted spent 2 years studying surgery, histology, and pathology in various German centers. He watched the work of Bergmann, Volkmann, Billroth, Esmarch, and Mikulicz in their surgical clinics. He was thus favorably inclined to the use of antisepsis, and the German thoroughness and insistence on

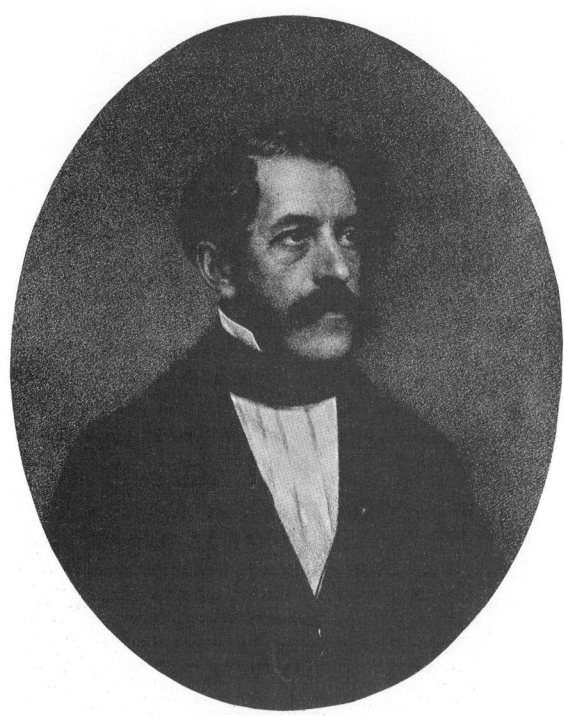

Figure 9. Bernhard von Langenbeck (1810–1887), master German surgeon who is acknowledged by many to be the father of the modern residency system in surgery. His students included Billroth and Kocher.

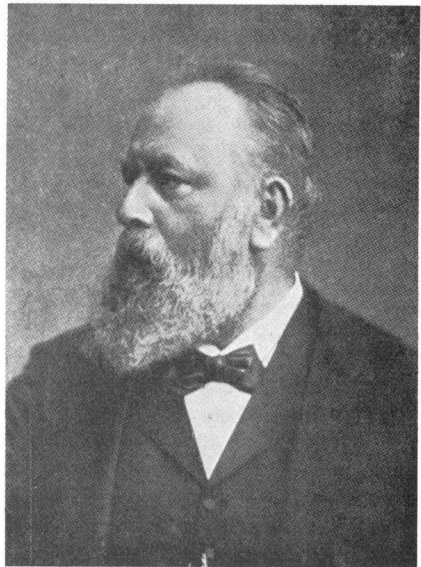

Figure 10. Theodor Billroth (1829–1894), Professor of Surgery at the University of Vienna and pioneer abdominal surgeon. Billroth was one of the most influential teachers of his time.

knowledge of the basic sciences as a foundation for surgery were to be the hallmarks of his own career as well. Halsted's 17 residents and more than 50 assistant residents carried this "German method" to many teaching centers in the United States. The second and third generations from this "Johns Hopkins School" are still to be seen in American academic centers.

William Halsted was a keen judge of surgical talent among both his peers and his students. That he considered Theodor Kocher of Berne perhaps the greatest surgeon of his time was one reason Kocher was very popular with American students. He was known for his work on the brain and spinal cord and especially for his careful techniques and study of the thyroid gland. His surgical treatment of goiter, a particularly severe disease in his native Switzerland, earned Kocher the Nobel Prize in 1909, the first time it was awarded to a surgeon.[61]

Kocher was born in Berne in 1841 and was trained in several European centers, although he considered himself a pupil of Theodor Billroth, the great surgical teacher of Vienna. Kocher was professor of surgery at the University of Berne and headed its surgical clinic for 45 years. Among his students were Harvey Cushing and many other Americans.

In his work on the surgical relief of goiter, Kocher not only developed the surgical technique necessary for removal of the thyroid but also added immeasurably to the understanding of its role in the body's metabolism. In his early patients, if removal of the thyroid was complete, myxedema, accompanied by all its unpleasant and stunting side effects, developed. When his colleagues pointed out this tragic aftereffect, Kocher took positive steps to learn from his mistake instead of engaging in scientific polemics, so common in his era.

NEUROSURGERY AND THORACIC SURGERY

It should be clear that the latter decades of the nineteenth century gave rise to numerous developments in surgery and that these developments clearly set the stage for advances in our own century. Changing concepts in pathology during the nineteenth century greatly influenced surgery. Especially important

was the idea that disease was localized and hence remediable by surgical attack. In addition to his many other talents, the pathologist Rudolf Virchow, who in 1858 published his *Cellular Pathology*, was also a superb historian. He wrote in his essays about the "anatomical idea," the progressive localization of life and disease in the body. The "anatomical idea" originated in the mid–eighteenth century with Morgagni, who believed disease had its seat within the organs of the body. At the beginning of the nineteenth century the French surgeon Xavier Bichat claimed that it was to the tissues that one must look.[2] He identified 21 types, such as muscle, bone, and nerve, and emphasized that when epithelium became inflamed, the reaction was similar no matter where in the body it might occur. Virchow took the last step and localized disease processes within the cell. This view has held sway since, although today disease is discussed also on the molecular or even the submolecular level.[87]

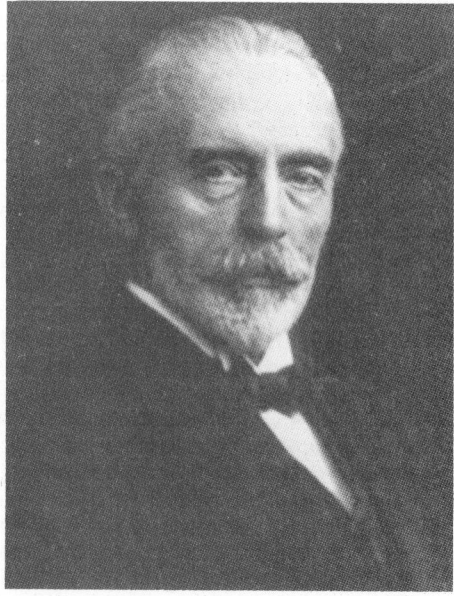

Figure 11. Theodor Kocher (1841–1917), Professor of Surgery at the University of Berne and pioneer in the development of surgery of the thyroid. He received the Nobel Prize in 1909.

Some aspects of the surgical approach to disease that the student of the 1990s may take for granted have actually a quite short history. The twentieth century is the century especially of neurosurgery, thoracic surgery, and the whole field of transplantation.

The field of neurosurgery, so much of it brought to its modern state by the work of Harvey Cushing, Walter Dandy, and others, is similar in its historical development to general surgery in a variety of ways. The operation of trephination of the skull is one of the oldest in the annals of surgery, but since it was done only to release evil spirits, to relieve pressure from injuries, or for the treatment of epilepsy, it hardly qualifies for pride of place as neurosurgery. Not until work on cerebral localization was done in the latter nineteenth century could the surgeon really begin to attack lesions within the cranium effectively. As in other branches of surgery, diagnostic means had to be developed along with safe and efficient operative measures.

Harvey Cushing, like all neurosurgeons until fairly recent times (after World War II), was trained in general surgery.[38] He was Halsted's resident, although emotionally and personally he felt much closer to the professor of medicine at Hopkins, William Osler. While still a medical student at Harvard, Cushing devised a chart for continuous recording of respiration and blood pressure by the anesthetist and some years later brought to American operating rooms the practice of sphygmomanometry. While at Hopkins, he helped found the "Hunterian" surgical laboratory, where the modern practice of experimental surgery in dogs began for medical students.[15,26]

In thoracic surgery, the story is much the same. Basic cardiac and pulmonary physiology had to be understood before surgical therapy could be contemplated. The problems of operating on a beating heart were as hard to overcome as the difficulty of maintaining pressure relationships within the chest. It was not until the 1890s that direct wounds of the heart were successfully sutured. Before this time chest surgery consisted primarily of evacuation of empyema or drainage of a pericardial sac filled with fluid or blood.

The story of the surgical treatment of cardiac lesions, traumatic, congenital, degenerative, or postinfective, has been told in some detail in books by Meade,[68] Richardson,[77] and Johnson.[56] There is no need to repeat the story here except to point out certain interesting aspects. It is almost entirely a twentieth century story. Historians, particularly thoracic surgeons, have taken some measure of pride from disproving the statement of Stephen Paget in *The Surgery of the Chest* in 1896:

Surgery of the heart has probably reached the limits set by Nature to all surgery: no new method, and no new discovery, can overcome the natural difficulties that attend a wound of the heart. It is true that "heart suture" has been vaguely proposed as a possible procedure, and has been done on animals; but I cannot find that it has ever been attempted in practice.

In the same year that Paget's book was published, Ludwig Rehn of Frankfurt became the first surgeon to suture a human heart laceration successfully.

The history of valvular surgery has been one of steady progress since the operations were reintroduced in the late 1940s. The progress relates not only to direct improvements in operative approach and technique, but also, as is the case in most thoracic surgery, to technical developments by which physiologic conditions can be made suitable for surgery. There is an interesting connection between surgeons and internists in the story of the surgical alleviation of valvular disease. As has been true throughout the history of medicine, the underlying theory regarding causation of disease has been closely intertwined with the therapy made available. In the case of mitral valve disease, for example, a great English clinician, the London cardiologist Sir Lauder Brunton, suggested in 1902 that animal experiments showed the feasibility of a surgical approach to the

disease. This suggestion was not well received, and no surgeon appears to have acted upon it until a London colleague, Henry Souttar, operated on a woman in 1925. Souttar, instead of inserting an instrument into the ventricle to reach the valve, used his finger to push through the valve from the atrium. The patient, a 19-year-old girl, lived in fair health for 5 years and died of a cerebral embolus.

New theories and innovations should not be accepted uncritically. The medical profession has been accused of being too conservative, but for the sake of patients this is a necessary trait. Other aspects of the resistance to change are not so defensible, as the story of listerism has shown. Once again, in the story of mitral valve surgery, a major theoretical hurdle had to be overcome before real progress could be made. James MacKenzie, who was Britain's leading cardiologist and a respected teacher, hastened to condemn Souttar's attempted treatment, basing his objections on the belief that the abnormality of mitral stenosis was in the myocardium, not in the valve. With this theory, as with that of a basically humoral pathology, surgical therapy made little sense. Theory must affect practice; one cannot be divorced from the other, as this example clearly illustrates.

By 1928 Elliot Cutler and Claude Beck could summarize only 12 known cases of valvular surgery, and the results were discouraging. Mortality was 83 per cent. The truly remarkable changes that have occurred in the years since 1955 are now known to all students of surgery.

Experimental cardiac surgery began approximately 100 years ago. M. H. Block, a German surgeon, published a report on wounds of the heart in 1882 in which he described successful suture of rabbit hearts, and he strongly urged that the procedure be used in humans. In the best surgical circles of the time, however, resistance to his innovation was strong. Billroth is reported to have said a year later, "A surgeon who would attempt such an operation should lose the respect of his colleagues." Here, too, the exact anatomic and functional relationships of various forms of heart disease had to be clearly understood before surgical intervention could be contemplated. In addition, the technical problems of pressure relationships in the chest, stilling the heart, and maintaining the circulation during surgery had to be mastered before practical application was possible. Claude Beck was perfectly correct in 1926 when he predicted, "These technical problems should be capable of solution, as were problems in the past, by methods, instruments, and gentleness."[6]

One of the very basic physiologic obstacles that had already been overcome was the problem of negative pressure within the pleural cavity. Ferdinand Sauerbruch, working in the clinic of his teacher, Mikulicz, in Breslau, devised an apparatus in which negative pressure for the open thorax could be maintained. These experiments in 1903 and 1904 led to the construction of a large chamber in the next years, and the technical difficulties involved were soon alleviated by the introduction of endotracheal or insufflation anesthesia around 1910. Not until the late 1930s was a reliable apparatus available that would provide good control of respiration.

Hypothermia and the heart-lung machine are even more recent developments. Hypothermia had been used in the treatment of cancer and other medical problems when it was adapted for surgery by groups in Philadelphia, Minneapolis, and Denver in the 1950s. Many of the same surgeons also did much to develop a safe and efficient means of extracorporeal circulation. John H. Gibbon began work on this problem before World War II.[42] He and others, especially C. Walton Lillehei and Clarence Dennis and their co-workers, made the possibility of extensive cardiac surgery an everyday reality in large hospital surgical services.

The problem of shock is important for all surgery, especially in times of war. Major surgical texts of the late nineteenth century rarely devoted more than a page to the subject. Loss of

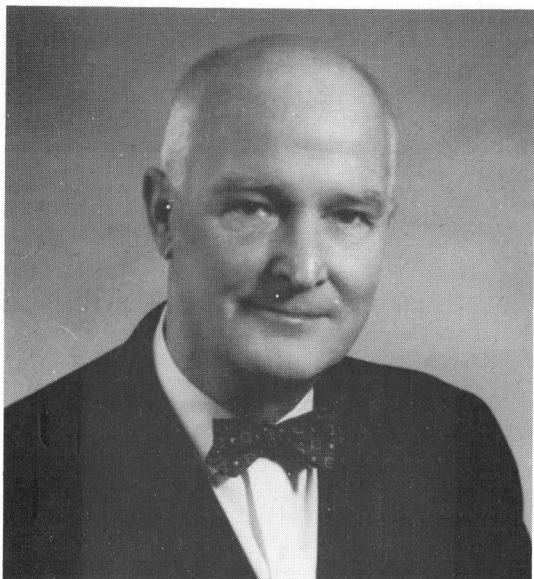

Figure 12. John H. Gibbon (1903–1973), pioneer cardiothoracic surgeon who developed extracorporeal circulation.

blood was known to be a cause, but beyond that not much more was known, nor could much have been done to counteract the effects. The list of credit for unraveling the story is a long one, but certainly two American surgeons, George Crile and Alfred Blalock, deserve special mention.[25]

Blalock, while he was at Vanderbilt University in the late 1920s and the 1930s, published significant papers on the cause and treatment of shock. The prevailing theory of the time was that the most likely cause of shock was release of a toxin, very

possibly histamine. In studies of shock produced by muscle injury, Blalock and his co-workers found a large accumulation of blood at the site of trauma, whether in an extremity or in the intestinal tract. In 1964, shortly before his death, Blalock summarized his work and added, "After thirty-four years have elapsed there still is much to be learned about shock."[13]

The contributions of surgical teachers and investigators such as Alfred Blalock, to single out just one among many, also illustrate the importance and influence of the scientific and academic environment. In Blalock's case, he was fortunate in having gone to Vanderbilt, a new medical center with many young men ambitious to do research. His former Hopkins roommate, Tinsley Harrison, was a resident in medicine at Vanderbilt when Blalock was a resident in surgery, and Harrison's influence, although hard to measure exactly, was doubtless important. After returning to Johns Hopkins in the early 1940s, Blalock worked in one of the finest medical research centers in any academic institution. His cooperation with the pediatrics department, particularly with Dr. Edwards A. Park and Dr. Helen Taussig, and with help from his gifted technician Vivien Thomas, culminated in the discovery of a successful method of surgical treatment of tetralogy of Fallot.[88] This in no way detracts from what Blalock or any other single individual may have contributed. It merely illustrates that an important change in scientific medicine has evolved since the time when Claude Bernard or Louis Pasteur worked in inadequate quarters with a handful of students and assistants. Science today is, more than ever before, a great cooperative venture. To conduct such a venture successfully, academic and scientific leadership of high quality is required. Perhaps it is for this kind of leadership, for the stimulus provided to a whole school of research rather than for individual surgical feats, that the recent great teachers such as Blalock and Owen Wangensteen will be best remembered. "My principal role," Dr. Wangensteen has said, "has been essentially that of trying to create an atmosphere friendly to learning."[62]

ELECTROLYTE AND FLUID BALANCE, NUTRITION, CHEMOTHERAPY, SURGICAL ENDOCRINOLOGY, AND RADIOLOGY

The concept of balance is an ancient one. The Greeks strove for a golden mean in life, and one of the pre-Socratic philosophers, Alcamaeon of Crotona, believed that the body's health depended on an equal combination of the four elements, earth, air, fire, and water. When this was achieved, there was *isonomia,* but when one element dominated a *monarchia* resulted.

Not until the 1850s and the work of Claude Bernard was a definition of the role of the blood and the body fluids clearly enunciated. In his *Liquids of the Organism,* a series of lectures published in 1859, Bernard first used the word *milieu* to express the internal environment. In the following years he elaborated his concept of the *milieu intérieur,* the physiologic state that allows the organism to exist independently.[71] In this century, these earlier ideas of Bernard were assumed by many, including Walter Cannon of Harvard, who coined the term "homeostasis,"[7,18] and Lawrence J. Henderson, also of Harvard, who wrote much on the mechanism of acid-base balance,[52] and whose name is familiar to all medical students who have mastered the Henderson-Hasselbalch equation at least for biochemistry examinations.

Neither Cannon nor Henderson was a surgeon, and although both were medically trained, neither practiced. Another Harvard physician, the Moseley Professor of Surgery, Francis D. Moore, early in his career became interested in the metabolic problems of surgical patients. The Coconut Grove fire in 1942 was a sad stimulus to learning for many. Moore continued to learn and to write and in 1952 published *Metabolic Response to*

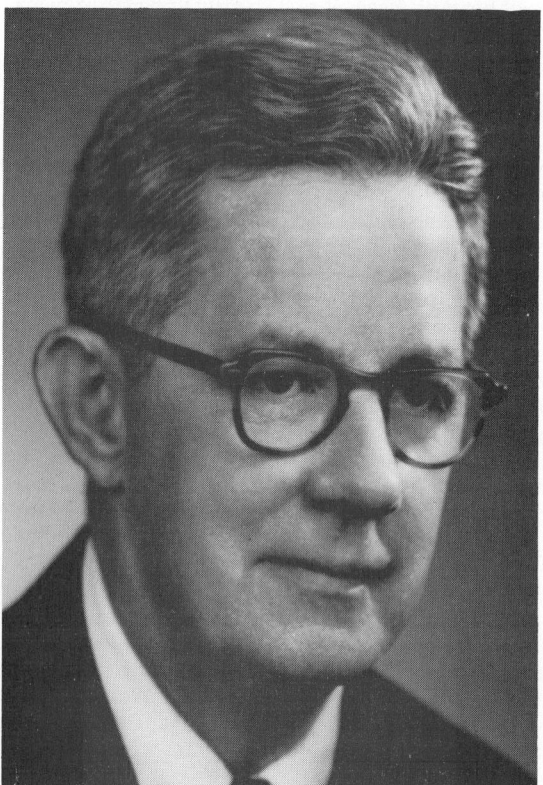

Figure 13. Alfred Blalock (1889–1964), noted investigator and clinical surgeon who made basic contributions to the understanding of the pathogenesis of shock. He also was a pioneer and innovator in the field of cardiac surgery.

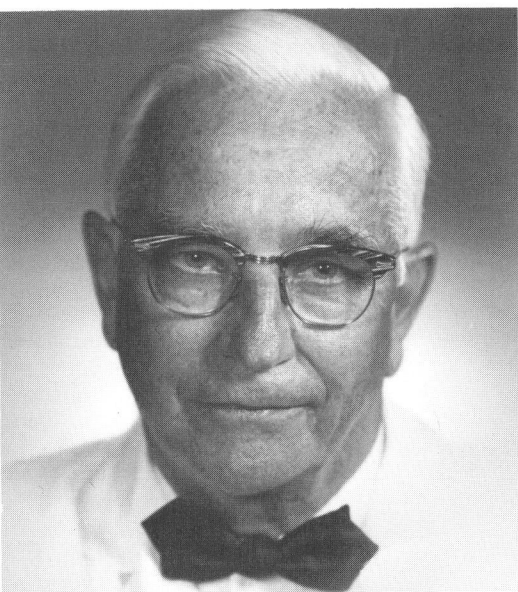

Figure 14. Owen H. Wangensteen, who for more than half a century was a leading teacher of surgeons at the University of Minnesota.

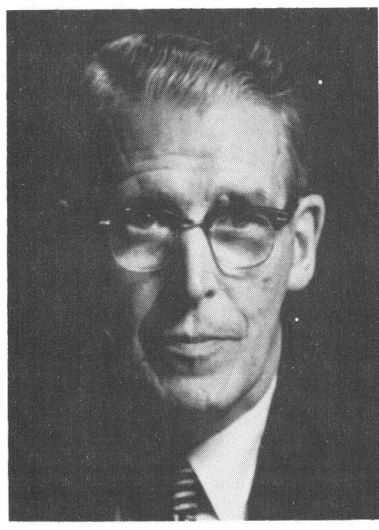

Figure 16. Jonathan Rhoads, distinguished Professor of Surgery at the University of Pennsylvania, editor, author, and investigative surgeon, who has made many contributions to surgery and teaching. His work in the field of surgical nutrition is outstanding, especially the introduction of total parenteral hyperalimentation. He is also known for his contributions to the field of surgical oncology.

Surgery,[70] a surgical landmark. He greatly expanded his ideas in *Metabolic Care of the Surgical Patient,*[69] which has been a standard work since it was published in 1959. Moore's definition of the boundaries of surgery is of interest to the historian as well, because it sets the task:

> The fundamental act of medical care is assumption of responsibility. Surgery has assumed responsibility for the cure of a large section of human illness: a segment of disease which is largely acute, focal, or traumatic. This is responsibility for the care of the entire range of injuries and wounds, local infections, benign and malignant tumors, as well as a large fraction of those various pathologic processes and anomalies which are localized in the organs of the body. The study of surgery is a study of these diseases, the conditions and details of their care.[69]

What should also be noted here is that the techniques and the outcome that patient and surgeon can reasonably expect have drastically changed over time, although the basic disease processes confronting the surgeon have changed very little.

The nutritive needs of surgical patients have been the subject of much attention and investigation. In this field, Jonathan Rhoads has been a pioneer and distinctive leader. Together with his colleague Stanley Dudrick, he introduced total parenteral hyperalimentation in the 1960s. This has become a very important aspect of preoperative and postoperative care, particularly in severely ill patients.[33]

The story of modern chemotherapy began with the successful use of the arsenical salvarsan or "606," introduced by Paul Ehrlich and his co-worker Sahachiro Hata in 1910. Actually, as Ehrlich described his approach to research, the concept began to evolve several decades earlier in his work on the development of tissue stains. The story continues with the work of the British pathologist Sir Alexander Fleming, who said in his Nobel Lec-

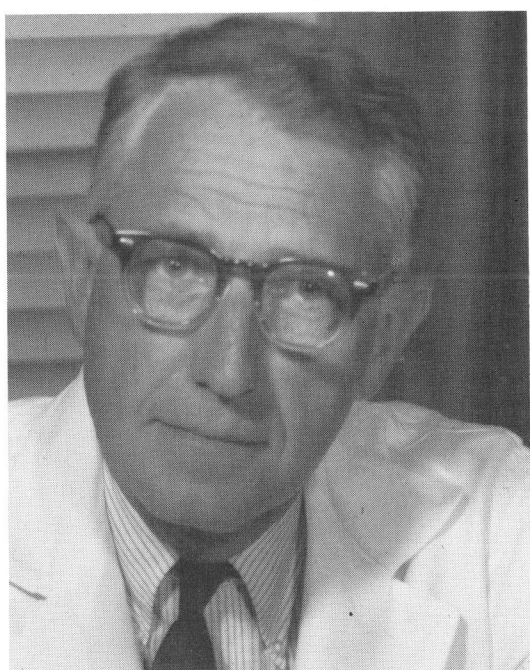

Figure 15. Francis D. Moore, leading investigative surgeon who defined objective aspects of metabolism in surgical patients.

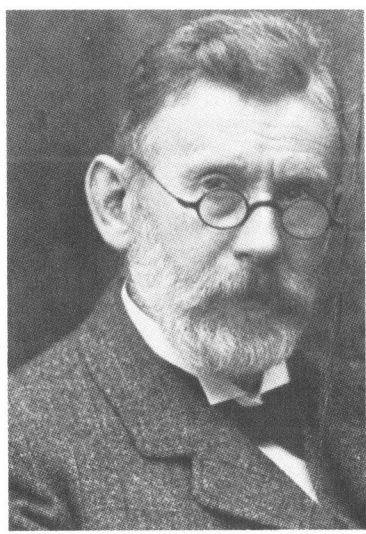

Figure 17. Paul Ehrlich (1854–1915), the father of modern chemotherapy, who introduced the use of the arsenicals (salvarsan) in 1910 for the treatment of syphilis.

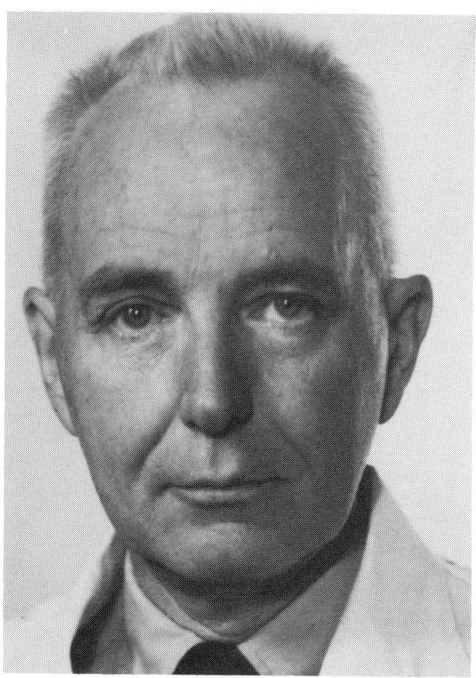

Figure 18. Charles B. Huggins, distinguished cancer researcher at the University of Chicago, who received the Nobel Prize in 1966 for his studies of the effects of hormones on tumor growth.

ture, "To my generation of bacteriologists the inhibition of one microbe by another was commonplace. We were all taught about these inhibitions and indeed it is seldom that an observant clinical bacteriologist can pass a week without seeing . . . very definite instances of antibacterial antagonism." [36]

The role of the endocrine glands in the pathogenesis and control of neoplastic disease has long been a subject of much interest. A major contribution in this area was made in 1940 when Charles Huggins showed that antiandrogenic treatment consisting of orchiectomy or the administration of estrogens could produce long-term regression in patients with advanced disseminated prostatic carcinoma.[54] His further studies of serum enzymes and protein chemistry, including the role of the renal glands in the control of metastatic neoplastic disease, have been monumental, and for these landmark observations he was awarded the Nobel Prize in 1966.

In 1921 Fleming described and isolated an inhibiting agent and called it lysozyme. Unfortunately, the bacteria inhibited by this natural enzyme are not those harmful to humans. However, the lysozyme work alerted him to search for other suitable antagonistic candidates. In the fall of 1928 Fleming noted that some of his plates of staphylococcal cultures contaminated by laboratory air grew a mold that inhibited growth of the bacteria.

Fleming's observation, so often ascribed to chance, was actually made in the course of careful laboratory investigation. Part of Fleming's goal was to find just such a substance. What did prove to be extremely fortuitous was that the product of the contaminating mold, penicillin, was a powerful antibacterial substance effective against some of the common human pathogens, yet remarkably free of toxicity for humans. Why Fleming's important discovery was not commercially produced until the war years is not entirely clear. Fleming claimed that physicians became interested in the possibility of antibiotics only after the demonstrated usefulness of the sulfonamide drugs introduced by Gerhard Domagk in 1935. Not until several American manufacturing plants became interested in the early 1940s was there enough penicillin for a clinical trial.

If Fleming fully recognized the momentous nature of his discovery, and every indication points to the fact that he did, the question still remains why he and others did not promote earlier penicillin synthesis or isolation.

Another development that deserves emphasis is the discovery of x-rays by Röntgen in 1895. Although part of a general physical investigation, this was a discovery that was accidental. Moreover, it was the first modern scientific discovery to receive banner headlines in the newspapers. The public was fascinated and frightened. "Old ladies," Derek Price relates, "went into their baths fully clothed, being convinced that the scientists now had mystery rays that could look through brick walls and round corners." [76] It was only a matter of months following the discovery that Frau Röntgen's hand and wrist bones could be clearly visualized when clinical application of the finding was made. Within a few years the use of rays was expanded to include physiologic studies, such as those of swallowing and intestinal motion. Walter B. Cannon used fluoroscopy for this purpose while he was still a medical student in 1901.[7]

ORGAN TRANSPLANTATION

Probably no recent development in surgery has so captured the public interest as has organ transplantation. Like some other contemporary aspects of medicine, transplantation has a long history.[95] An integral part of the story of transplantation is found in the annals of plastic surgery. The ancient Hindus were adept at transplanting skin from the buttocks area to refashion noses and ears. Even more common was the forehead flap method that was given wide publicity with a picture in *The Gentleman's Magazine* in 1794. This can be traced back to much earlier times.

In the sixteenth century the Italian surgeon Gasparo Tagliacozzi gained fame for his method of rhinoplasty. One sees in the history of plastic surgery a close connection between social customs and civilization as a whole and the surgeon's responses to the resultant needs. During the Renaissance and beyond, frequent street brawls, the cutting off of the nose or ears as punishment for thievery and adultery, and the devastating effects of leprosy, syphilis, and mercury treatment all made the need for a method to rebuild the face very evident. The history of plastic surgery can be seen in terms of an increasing facility in transplanting skin.

Another aspect of transplantation that has direct bearing on surgery is tissue and cell culture, more properly called explantation. Here medicine and biology met and joined forces in the early twentieth century. What happened in this one field is thus

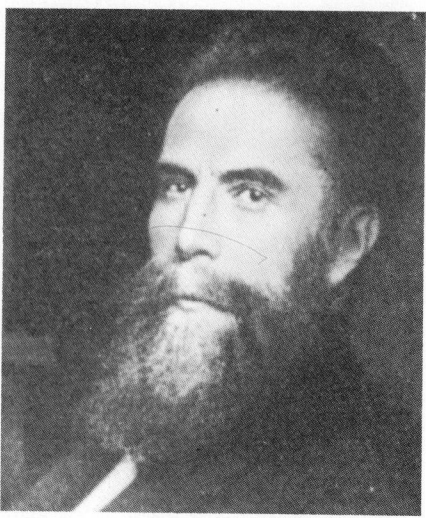

Figure 19. Wilhelm K. Röntgen (1845–1923), who discovered x-rays in 1895.

a typical case study for the development of twentieth century medicine and surgery generally. To understand the story of tissue culture and cell culture, one must go back into the history of botany, especially the history of plant grafting, and also into the history of experimental embryology, because it was the embryologists at the end of the last century who made extensive use of explantation of embryos to observe their subsequent growth and development. The history of tissue culture is really one of the more recent episodes in the history of medicine. It began with the work of Ross G. Harrison in the first decade of this century. Born in Germantown near Philadelphia in 1870, Harrison was among many illustrious students in the early years of the Johns Hopkins University, where he received his undergraduate degree in biology in 1889. After further study, including medical education, Harrison went to Yale in 1907 and in the same year published the paper that is generally considered to contain the rudiments of the method of modern tissue culture so widely used today.[49,50]

Harrison hoped to settle the controversy then being aired in the scientific journals over the growth of the nerve cell. Was its long process an outgrowth of the cell or was it an independent unit growing toward the cell body? By means of a hanging-drop preparation, Harrison was able to observe under direct vision the growth of frog embryo nervous tissue in clotted lymph. Soon after Harrison moved to New Haven, Montrose Burrows came from the newly established Rockefeller Institute in New York to learn about the method of independent cell growth.[24] Burrows suggested improvements in the medium and, incidentally, probably also deserves credit for suggesting the term "tissue culture." He returned to New York to report his findings to the man who had sent him to New Haven, the French-born surgeon, Alexis Carrel.

Carrel, born in Lyon in 1873, was one of the most colorful and most interesting figures in medicine in the first half of this century. He was trained in France and became a skilled and imaginative experimental surgeon who developed the finest of techniques. Carrel was much interested in Harrison's work because he saw its potential for his own work on wound healing and tissue proliferation. The problems could be much better studied if they were isolated from the body as a whole. Carrel and Burrows did indeed manage to grow tissues in flasks. The next step was to grow entire organs. Carrel had already been involved in extensive transplantation of organs in the decade from 1902 to 1912.

Here, in the work of this one man, there is a close connection between surgery and transplantation of organs and the growth of cells and tissues. What Carrel accomplished with the delicate instruments he devised was to suture blood vessels, end-to-end, without leaving tissue hanging into the lumen that could then act as a focus for clot formation. Previous attempts to transplant organs and to re-establish their blood supply had met with failure because of infection and thrombosis. Carrel first reported his technique in 1902, when he was not yet 30 and only 2 years after he had obtained his M.D. degree. His method was to use three retaining sutures, thereby converting a round hole to a triangular one, which could then be easily sutured — a simple but lasting technique for which he was awarded the Nobel Prize in 1912.[19]

Carrel came to the United States in 1905 and that summer worked with Charles Claude Guthrie at the Hull Physiological Laboratory at the University of Chicago. Guthrie, medically trained but a physiologist for most of his career, is the unsung hero in the story of vascular suture and hence organ transplantation. Guthrie suggested improvements in Carrel's technique, and the two men collaborated in numerous experiments and papers. Guthrie urged Carrel to include all layers of the vessel wall, even the endothelium, in the suture to prevent wrinkling.[48,93]

In 1906 Carrel presented the results of the work he and Guthrie had done on organ transplantation and discussed the clinical implications for cure of aneurysm and other conditions. Carrel said, in words that are very timely,

The question of the transplantation of organs in man is a very serious one and difficult, for will the transplanted organ remain and function normally after a long period of time? Another difficulty would be that of finding organs suitable for transplantation into man. A process of immunization would no doubt be necessary before the organs of animals would be suitable for transplantation into man. Organs from a person killed by accident would no doubt be suitable.[20]

One of the prime contributors to the field of cardiovascular surgery has been Michael E. DeBakey of Houston. In 1934 he

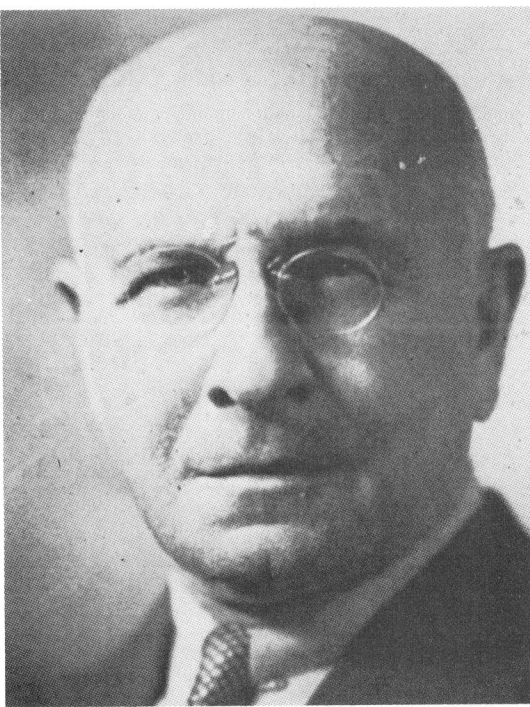

Figure 20. Alexis Carrel (1873–1944), an experimental surgeon interested in wound healing, tissue culture, organ transplantation, and blood vessel anastomosis. He was awarded the Nobel Prize in 1912.

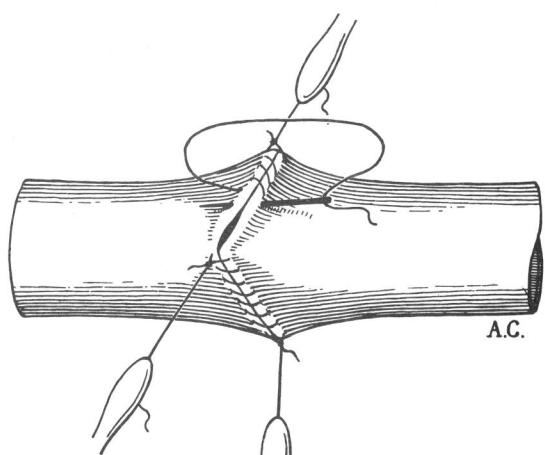

Figure 21. Joining blood vessels by suture anastomosis. Adapted from the line drawing by Alexis Carrel published in *Lyon Medical* in 1902. The walls of the two blood vessels (here drawn as about 5 mm. in diameter) are held together by three holding sutures. Another is then used to sew over and over, with very fine needles ("aiguilles extrêmement fines"). This method of suture anastomosis, demonstrated initially by Carrel, is still used throughout surgery, and particularly in the transplantation of organs.

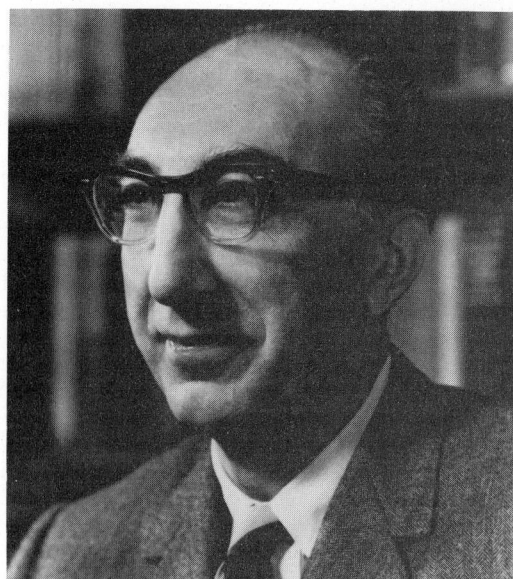

Figure 22. Michael E. DeBakey, American pioneer in cardiovascular surgery who has been a leading spokesman for medicine and medical research.

first described the occlusive roller pump, which has been widely used throughout the world in extracorporeal circulation.[28] After this basic contribution, he became a leader in the field of direct surgery for the treatment of thoracic and abdominal aneurysms, including complicated resections of lesions of the aortic arch. Moreover, he and his associates dedicated much time and effort to the development of plastic prosthetic arterial substitutes, which have been widely adopted and highly successful. He was the first to perform a successful carotid endarterectomy in 1953, and, in addition, he and his colleagues were also the first to report the successful use of a saphenous vein bypass graft for coronary arterial occlusion, a procedure they accomplished in 1964.[29]

In addition to his important surgical contributions, DeBakey has for more than 30 years been an influential member of an advisory group that has been important in shaping biomedical research. His influence on Mary and Albert Lasker and on members of Congress has been instrumental in the evolution of support for research and health care.

In reflecting on the history of surgery, one of the themes that stands out is progress. Although uneven over the years, and certainly not a straight line of advance after advance, the progress of human ability to contribute to the well-being of humanity by means of surgery appears impressive indeed.

Intimately related to this progress has been the increasing specialization in medicine as a whole and within the field of surgery itself. Surgery as a specialty began with the wound surgeons of early antiquity. From later antiquity to the early twentieth century, surgeons for the most part did not confine themselves to operative therapy; they were also charged with care for a variety of dermatologic disorders, especially syphilis. It is no accident that Sir Jonathan Hutchinson (1828–1913), a surgeon, described the triad of congenital syphilis: deformed incisor teeth, interstitial keratitis, and deafness. It was not until the great advances made by surgery in the nineteenth century that surgeons as a group began to regain prestige, which they did for themselves as well as for the medical profession as a whole.

In America, most historians have emphasized, no definite separation of medicine and surgery ever existed, despite the early attempts of John Morgan to have university-educated physicians desist from the work of the apothecary and the surgeon. The most widely known statement regarding the lack of

separation comes from a long review article by Samuel D. Gross on the achievements of surgery in the first 100 years of the country:

> Although this paper is designed to record the achievements of American surgeons, there are, strange to say, as a separate and distinct class, no such persons among us. It is safe to affirm that there is not a medical man on this continent who devotes himself exclusively to the practice of surgery. On the other hand, there are few physicians, even in our larger cities, who do not treat the more common surgical diseases and injuries. . . . In short, American medical men are general practitioners, ready for the most part, if well-educated, to meet any and every emergency, whether in medicine, surgery or midwifery.[46]

Interestingly, a few years later, Gross welcomed the newly founded American Surgical Association to its inaugural meeting in 1882. He justified the existence of the new society by pointing out that there were in the United States about 60,000 medical men, large numbers being surgeons.

In a general sense, surgeons doubtless practiced family medicine or the like, but there is evidence that they did exist as a distinct specialty even at the time of Gross and before. According to the *Seventh Census of the United States,* 1850, the State of New York, for example, is credited with 5060 physicians for a population of 3,097,394. In addition, listed separately among the occupations are 54 surgeons. Five years later, in a census of New York State, the City of New York claimed 1252 physicians and 19 surgeons. More and more, as the nineteenth century progressed, surgery was performed by those who called themselves surgeons. This became true especially in the urban areas and for the increasingly complex operations within the abdomen after the introduction of antisepsis. In rural areas there was less reluctance to do surgery among those not specifically trained. This is still true for some family practitioners today. The founding of the American Surgical Association in 1880, the American College of Surgeons in 1913, and the American Board of Surgery in 1937 has had an important part in setting and maintaining high professional standards and providing a forum for communication among men with similar scientific interests. Like their European predecessors, these surgical organizations have thus aided the process of professionalization by insisting on standards for both surgeons and hospitals.[16,27,64]

All of the people, events, and institutions discussed in this chapter have contributed to the science and the practice of surgery today. Perhaps nothing is more indicative of the great changes that have occurred, even in just the past 100 years, than to emphasize again that surgery has moved from the theatricality and the drama of the operating theater to the privacy and the relative sterility of the operating room. No longer is the drama of the operation nor the technical skill or the virtuosity of the surgeon on center stage. In the old surgery it was the art that predominated. In the new surgery it is science. The focus has thus shifted increasingly from the operation itself to the results that now provide the drama.[16]

SELECTED REFERENCES

Bennion, E.: Antique Medical Instruments. Berkeley, University of California Press, 1979.
A beautifully illustrated catalogue of instruments, especially surgical ones, from the eighteenth and nineteenth centuries with good explanatory text.

Bishop, W. J.: The Early History of Surgery. London, Robert Hale, 1960.
As suggested by the title, the history of surgery through the seventeenth century comprises two thirds of the book. It provides a general, not overly detailed, history of premodern surgery and its role in the history of medicine.

Cartwright, F. F.: The Development of Modern Surgery. New York, Thomas Y. Crowell Company, 1968.
This text stresses the last 100 years and is rich in detail and interpretation.

Comroe, J. H., Jr.: Exploring the Heart: Discoveries in Heart Disease and High Blood Pressure. New York, W. W. Norton, 1983.
Describes the work that has led to the understanding and treatment, both medical and surgical, of cardiovascular diseases.

Cope, Z.: A History of the Acute Abdomen. New York, Oxford University Press, 1965.
The author gives an excellent description of the evolution of surgical methods of treatment of abdominal emergencies.

Dale, W. A.: The beginnings of vascular surgery. Surgery, 76:849, 1974.
A fine review of an important aspect of twentieth century surgery with many references.

Earle, A. S.: Surgery in America: From the Colonial Era to the Twentieth Century. Philadelphia, W. B. Saunders Company, 1965.
Long excerpts from original papers in the American medical literature provide ready access to some of the best in surgical writing.

English, P. C.: Shock, Physiological Surgery, and George Washington Crile: Medical Innovation in the Progressive Era. Westport, Conn., Greenwood Press, 1980.
An excellent study describing the early growth of surgical research in the United States.

Forssmann, W.: Experiments on Myself, Memoirs of a Surgeon in Germany. Trans. H. Davies. New York, St. Martin's Press, 1974.
The autobiographic account of the Nobel Prize–winning surgeon, including the fascinating story of contrast radiography and catheterization of the heart.

Gelfand, T.: Professionalizing Modern Medicine: Paris Surgeons and Medical Science and Institutions in the Eighteenth Century. Westport, Conn., Greenwood Press, 1980.
A superior book that uses surgeons to illustrate the formation of modern medicine.

Gnudi, M. T., and Webster, J. P.: The Life and Times of Gasparo Tagliacozzi, Surgeon of Bologna 1545–1599. New York, Herbert Reichner, 1950.
The main emphasis of this book is on the accomplishments of Tagliacozzi in the field of plastic surgery. Other superb chapters consider the history of plastic surgery before and after Tagliacozzi and student life and the teaching of surgery in his time. There are many illustrations of sixteenth century medicine, particularly surgery.

Johnson, S. L.: The History of Cardiac Surgery 1896–1955. Baltimore, The Johns Hopkins Press, 1970.
This short but superior book describes the advances in physiology and technology that necessarily preceded or accompanied the development of cardiac surgery. The illustrations help make the story more readily understandable for those who are not specialists in thoracic surgery.

Majno, G.: The Healing Hand: Man and Wound in the Ancient World. Boston, Harvard University Press, 1975.
A superbly illustrated book describing wound care and the treatment of inflammation in the ancient cultures of Mesopotamia, Egypt, Arabia, China, India, and Greece.

Malgaigne, J. F.: Surgery and Ambroise Paré. Trans. W. B. Hamby. Norman, Okla., University of Oklahoma Press, 1965.
In 1840 Malgaigne brought out a large, three-volume Oeuvres de Paré. The first volume included a "History of Western Surgery from the Sixth to the Sixteenth Century," "Surgery During the First Half of the Sixteenth Century," and a long biographic sketch of Paré. These are here available in English for the first time. Although it is now over 140 years old, Malgaigne's is still a very useful history of early surgery.

Meade, R. H.: A History of Thoracic Surgery. Springfield, Ill., Charles C Thomas, 1960.
This large book considers the increasing complexity of thoracic surgery from antiquity to the 1950s, with an extensive bibliography.

Meade, R. H.: An Introduction to the History of General Surgery. Philadelphia, W. B. Saunders Company, 1968.
This is the most ambitious attempt in more recent years to cover the entire history of surgery. The 30 chapters are organized by individual organs or parts of the body, and each has an extensive list of references, with emphasis on the literature of the 25 years preceding publication.

Moore, F. D.: Give and Take, The Biology of Tissue Transplantation. Philadelphia, W. B. Saunders Company, 1964.
This is an excellent, concise description of the development of renal transplants and the surgical and biologic problems encountered by the pioneering group at Peter Bent Brigham Hospital.

Pernick, M. S.: A Calculus of Suffering, Pain, Professionalism and Anesthesia in Nineteenth Century America. New York, Columbia University Press, 1985.
As noted by the subtitle, this book explores how the use of anesthesia changed medicine in the nineteenth century.

Ravitch, M. M.: A Century of Surgery: The History of the American Surgical Association. 2 Vols. Philadelphia, J. B. Lippincott Company, 1981.
These magnificent volumes tell the story of the development of American surgery since 1880 through the work of its leading practitioners. An indispensable historical source.

Richardson, R. G.: Surgery: Old and New Frontiers. New York, Charles Scribner's Sons, 1969.
This revised edition of surgeon's tales is a very satisfactory book for a general understanding of the historical background of the more recent trends in surgery.

Richardson, R. G.: The Scalpel and the Heart. New York, Charles Scribner's Sons, 1970.
This book covers much the same ground as Johnson's, but has the added advantage of bringing the story to recent times, including many of the events since 1955.

Shryock, R. H.: The Development of Modern Medicine. New York, Alfred A. Knopf, 1947.
Despite its age, this is still the most satisfactory single volume on the history of medicine. The role of surgery in the development of medicine as a whole is well described.

Siraisi, N. G.: Taddea Alderotti and His Pupils: Two Generations of Italian Medical Learning. Princeton, Princeton University Press, 1981.
This book provides an excellent description of surgical practice and teaching in the period circa 1250.

Wangensteen, O. H., and Wangensteen, S. D.: The Rise of Surgery from Empiric Craft to Scientific Discipline. Minneapolis, University of Minnesota Press, 1978.
This is a major contribution to the history of surgery. Its 580 pages of text and 137 pages of notes and references make it the most extensive work in recent scholarship in the history of surgery.

Wertenbaker, L.: To Mend the Heart. New York, Viking Press, 1980.
A history of the developments of cardiac surgery in the last 40 years with a particular emphasis on the pioneering work of Dwight E. Harken.

Zimmerman, L. M., and Veith, I.: Great Ideas in the History of Surgery. Baltimore, Williams & Wilkins, 1961; 2nd ed., New York, Dover Publications, 1967.
Because of availability in a paperback edition, its judicious combination of readings from the great surgeons of antiquity to the early twentieth century with a well-written narrative by the authors, and the inclusion of many useful references, this book is highly recommended for further reading.

REFERENCES

1. Ackerknecht, E. H.: Primitive surgery. Am. Anthropol., 49:25, 1947.
2. Ackerknecht, E. H.: Medicine at the Paris Hospital 1794–1848. Baltimore, The Johns Hopkins Press, 1967.
3. Allbutt, T. C.: The Historical Relations of Medicine and Surgery to the End of the Sixteenth Century. London, Macmillan & Company, 1905.
4. Ball, J. M.:The Sack-em Up Men; an Account of the Rise and Fall of the Modern Resurrectionists. Edinburgh, Oliver & Boyd, 1928.
5. Beaumont, W.: Experiments and Observations on the Gastric Juice and the Physiology of Digestion, 1833. New York, Dover Publications, 1959.
6. Beck, C. S.: The operative story of the heart. Ann. Med. Hist., 8:224, 1926.
7. Benison, S., Barger, A. C., and Wolfe, E. L.: Walter B. Cannon, The Life and Times of a Young Scientist. Cambridge, Harvard University Press, 1987.
8. Bigelow, H. J.: Introductory Lecture. Boston, Mussey, 1850.
9. Billings, J. S.: The history and literature of surgery. In Dennis, F. (Ed.): System of Surgery. Vol. 1. Philadelphia, Lea, 1895, pp. 17–144.
10. Billroth, T.: The Medical Sciences in the German Universities. New York, The Macmillan Company, 1924.
11. Bishop, W. J.: A History of Surgical Dressings. Chesterfield, Robinson & Sons, 1959.
12. Bishop, W. J.: The Early History of Surgery. London, Robert Hale, 1960.
13. Blalock, A.: Reminiscence: Shock after thirty-four years. In Ravitch, M. (Ed.): The Papers of Alfred Blalock. Vol. 1. Baltimore, The Johns Hopkins Press, 1966, pp. 16–19.
14. Brieger, G. H.: American surgery and the germ theory of disease. Bull. Hist. Med., 40:135, 1966.
15. Brieger, G. H.: Surgery. In Numbers, R. L. (Ed.): The Education of American Physicians: Historical Essays. Berkeley, University of California Press, 1980, pp. 175–204.
16. Brieger, G. H.: A Portrait of surgery, surgery in America, 1875–1889. Surg. Clin. North Am., 67:1181, 1987.
17. Brock, R. C.: The Life and Work of Astley Cooper. Edinburgh, E. & S. Livingstone, 1952.
18. Cannon, W. B.: The Wisdom of the Body. New York, W. W. Norton, 1932.
19. Carrel, A.: La technique opératoire des anastomoses vasculaires et la transplantation des viscères. Lyon Med., 98:859, 1902.
20. Carrel, A.: Surgery of the blood vessels and its application to changes in circulation and transplantation of organs. Bull. Johns Hopkins Hosp., 17:236, 1906.
21. Cheselden, W.: The Anatomy of the Humane Body. London, 1713; 13th ed., 1792.
22. Churchill, E. D.: Surgery in the twentieth century. In Nardi, G. L., and Zuidema, G. D. (Eds.): Surgery, A Concise Guide to Clinical Practice, 2nd ed. Boston, Little, Brown & Company, 1965, pp. 1–8.
23. Cope, Z.: William Cheselden 1688–1752. Edinburgh, E. & S. Livingstone, 1953.
24. Corner, G. W.: A History of the Rockefeller Institute 1901–1953. New York, Rockefeller Institute Press, 1964.
25. Crile, G. W.: An Autobiography. 2 vols. Philadelphia, J. B. Lippincott Company, 1947.
26. Cushing, H.: Instruction in operative medicine with the description of a course given in the Hunterian Laboratory of experimental medicine. Bull. Johns Hopkins Hosp., 17:123, 1906.

27. Davis, L.: Fellowship of Surgeons, A History of the American College of Surgeons. Springfield, Ill., Charles C Thomas, 1960.
28. DeBakey, M. E.: A simple continuous-flow blood transfusion instrument. New Orleans Med. Surg. J., 87:383, 1934.
29. DeBakey, M. E.: Successful carotid endarterectomy for cerebrovascular insufficiency. Nineteen-year follow-up. J.A.M.A., 233:1083, 1975.
30. Dobson, J.: The training of a surgeon. Ann. R. Coll. Surg. Engl., 34:1, 1964.
31. Dobson, J.: John Hunter. Edinburgh, E. & S. Livingstone, 1969.
32. Dubos, R.: Louis Pasteur: Free Lance of Science. Boston, Little, Brown & Company, 1950; 2nd ed., 1976.
33. Dudrick, S. J., Wilmore, D. W., Vars, H. M., and Rhoads, J. E.: Long-term total parenteral nutrition with growth, development and positive nitrogen balance. Surgery, 64:134, 1968.
34. Faber, K.: Nosography in Modern Internal Medicine. New York, Paul B. Hoeber, 1923.
35. Fitz, R. H.: Perforating inflammation of the vermiform appendix; with special reference to its early diagnosis and treatment. Trans. Assoc. Am. Physicians, 1:107, 1886.
36. Fleming, A.: Penicillin. In Nobel Lectures, Physiology-Medicine. Vol. 3, 1942–1962. New York, American Elsevier Publishing Company, 1964, pp. 77–95.
37. Flexner, J. T.: Doctors on Horseback. New York, Dover Publications, 1969.
38. Fulton, J. F.: Harvey Cushing: A Biography. Springfield, Ill., Charles C Thomas, 1946.
39. Garrett, H. E., Dennis, E. W., and DeBakey, M. E.: Aortocoronary bypass with saphenous vein graft. Seven-year follow-up. J.A.M.A., 223:792, 1973.
40. Garrison, F. H.: History of Medicine, 4th ed. Philadelphia, W. B. Saunders Company, 1960.
41. Gelfand, T.: Empiricism and eighteenth century French surgery. Bull. Hist. Med., 44:40, 1970.
42. Gibbon, J. H.: Development of the artificial heart and lung extracorporeal blood circuit. J.A.M.A., 206:1983, 1968.
43. Godlee, R. J.: Lord Lister. London, Macmillan & Company, 1917.
44. Goss, C. M.: A Brief Account of Henry Gray, F.R.S., and his Anatomy, Descriptive and Surgical. Philadelphia, Lea & Febiger, 1959.
45. Graham, H.: The Story of Surgery. New York, Doubleday & Company, 1939.
46. Gross, S. D.: A Century of American medicine, 1776–1876. II. Surgery. Am. J. Med. Sci., 71:431, 1876.
47. Halsted, W. S.: The training of the surgeon. Bull. Johns Hopkins Hosp., 15:267, 1904.
48. Harbison, S. P.: Origins of vascular surgery: The Carrel-Guthrie letters. Surgery, 52:406, 1962.
49. Harrison, R. G.: Observations on the living developing nerve fiber. Anat. Rec., 1:116, 1907.
50. Harrison, R. G.: On the status and significance of tissue culture. Arch. Exp. Zellforsch., 6:4, 1928.
51. Harvey, S. C.: The history of hemostasis. Ann. Med. Hist., 1:127, 1929.
52. Henderson, L. J.: Blood; A Study in General Physiology. New Haven, Yale University Press, 1928.
53. Heuer, G. W.: Dr. Halsted. Bull. Johns Hopkins Hosp. (Suppl.), 90:1, 1952.
54. Huggins, C.: Endocrine-induced regression of cancers. In Nobel Lectures in Physiology-Medicine 1963–1970. Amsterdam, Elsevier Publishing Company, 1972.
55. Janssens, P. A.: Palaeopathology; Diseases and Injuries of Prehistoric Man. London, John Baker Publishers, 1970.
56. Johnson, S. L.: The History of Cardiac Surgery 1896–1955. Baltimore, The Johns Hopkins Press, 1970.
57. Jones, J.: Notes upon the history of hospital gangrene. South. Med. Surg. J., 1:55, 1866–67.
58. Keys, T. E.: The History of Surgical Anesthesia. New York, Dover Publications, 1963.
59. Kobler, J.: The Reluctant Surgeon. A Biography of John Hunter. New York, Doubleday & Company, 1960.
60. Koch, R.: Investigations into the Etiology of Traumatic Infective Diseases. Trans. W. W. Cheyne. London, New Sydenham Society, 1880.
61. Kocher, E. T.: Concerning pathological manifestations in lowgrade thyroid diseases. In Nobel Lectures, Physiology-Medicine. Vol. 1, 1901–1921. New York, American Elsevier Publishing Company, 1967, pp. 327–386.
62. Leonard, A. S.: Reflections of the Retiring Chief. Minneapolis, University of Minnesota Press, 1967.
63. Malgaigne, J. F.: Surgery and Ambroise Paré. Trans. W. B. Hamby. Norman, OK, University of Oklahoma Press, 1965.
64. Martin, F. H.: Fifty Years of Medicine and Surgery, An Autobiographical Sketch. Chicago, The Surgical Publishing Company, 1934.
65. Matas, R.: Surgical operations fifty years ago. Am. J. Surg., 82:111, 1951.
66. McBurney, C.: Experience with early operative interference in cases of disease of the vermiform appendix. N.Y. Med. J., 50:676, 1889.
67. McBurney, C.: The incision made in the abdominal wall in cases of appendicitis, with a description of a new method of operating. Ann. Surg., 20:38, 1894.
68. Meade, R. H.: A History of Thoracic Surgery. Springfield, Ill., Charles C Thomas, 1960.
69. Moore, F. D.: Metabolic Care of the Surgical Patient. Philadelphia, W. B. Saunders Company, 1959.
70. Moore, F. D., and Ball, M. R.: Metabolic Response to Surgery. Springfield, Ill., Charles C Thomas, 1952.
71. Olmsted, J. M. D., and Olmsted, E. H.: Claude Bernard and the Experimental Method. New York, Henry Schuman Publishers, 1952.
72. O'Malley, C. D.: Andreas Vesalius of Brussels 1514–1564. Berkeley, University of California Press, 1965.
73. Pagel, W., and Rattansi, P.: Vesalius and Paracelsus. Med. Hist., 8:309, 1964.
74. Paré, A.: The Apologie and Treatise of Ambroise Paré. G. Keynes (Ed.). New York, Dover Publications, 1968.
75. Poland, J.: A Retrospect of Surgery During the Past Century. London, Smith, Elder, 1901.
76. Price, D. J. D.: Science Since Babylon. New Haven, Yale University Press, 1961.
77. Richardson, R. G.: The Scalpel and the Heart. New York, Charles Scribner's Sons, 1970.
78. Rosenberg, C. E.: The Care of Strangers, The Rise of America's Hospital System. New York, Basic Books, 1987.
79. Sabiston, D. C., Jr.: A continuum in surgical education. Surgery, 66:1, 1969.
80. Schecter, D. C.: Role of the confraternity of St. Cosmas in the evolution of French surgery. Surgery, 64:1002, 1968.
81. Schultz, A. H.: Notes on diseases and healed fractures of wild apes and their bearing on the antiquity of pathological conditions in man. Bull. Hist. Med., 7:571, 1939.
82. Sigerist, H. E.: A History of Medicine. Vol. 1. Primitive and Archaic Medicine. New York, Oxford University Press, 1951.
83. Smith, D. C.: A Historical Overview of the Recognition of Appendicitis. Parts I and II. N.Y. J. Med., 86:571; 639, 1986.
84. Smith, S.: The comparative results of operations in Bellevue Hospital. Med. Rec., 28:427, 1885.
85. Stevenson, L. G.: The stag of Richmond Park: A Note on John Hunter's most famous animal experiment. Bull. Hist. Med., 22:467, 1948.
86. Talbot, C. H.: Medicine in Medieval England. New York, American Elsevier Publishing Company, 1967.
87. Temkin, O.: The role of surgery in the rise of modern medical thought. Bull. Hist. Med., 25:248, 1951.
88. Thomas, V.: Pioneering Research in Surgical Shock and Cardiovascular Surgery: Vivien Thomas and His Work with Alfred Blalock. Philadelphia, University of Pennsylvania Press, 1985.
89. Vicary, T.: The English-Man's Treasure. With the True Anatomie of Man's Body. London, 1633.
90. Wangensteen, O.: Reflections on the Blalock Papers. Bull. Hist. Med., 42:357, 1968.
91. Wangensteen, O. H., Smith, J., and Wangensteen, S. D.: Some highlights in the history of amputation reflecting lessons in wound healing. Bull. Hist. Med., 41:97, 1967.
92. Warren, J. M.: Recent Progress in Surgery. Boston, Clapp, 1864.
93. Watts, S. H.: The suture of blood vessels. Implantation and transplantation of vessels and organs. An historical and experimental study. Bull. Johns Hopkins Hosp., 18:153, 1907.
94. Wells, T. S.: Some causes of excessive mortality after surgical operations. Br. Med. J., 2:384, 1864.
95. Woodruff, M. F. A.: The Transplantation of Tissues and Organs. Springfield, Ill., Charles C Thomas, 1960.
96. Zimmerman, L. M., and Veith, I.: Great Ideas in the History of Surgery. Baltimore, Williams & Wilkins, 1961.
97. Zimmerman, L. M., and Veith, I.: Billroth's troubles with listerian antisepsis. Mod. Med., March 10:213, 1969.

2

HOMEOSTASIS
Bodily Changes in Trauma and Surgery

Douglas W. Wilmore, M.D.

Surgeons care for patients who experience sudden, rapid, and intense changes in normal physiologic function and metabolism. Such alterations occur following an elective operative procedure, an event that causes pain, interrupts normal food and fluid intake, and is usually associated with tissue removal and/or disruption, often involving a vital organ. A more dramatic perturbation occurs following major accidental injury, which is associated with rapid blood loss, tissue underperfusion, massive cellular damage, and disturbance of vital organ function.

The human body responds to these stresses with dramatic resilience. For example, following injury, clotting mechanisms are immediately activated to reduce blood loss; body fluids shift from the extravascular compartment to restore blood volume; blood flow is redistributed to ensure perfusion of vital organs; and respiratory and renal functions compensate to maintain acid-base neutrality and body fluid tonicity. Following these acute adaptations, other changes occur; these responses are more gradual and prolonged but are apparently necessary for recovery of the injured organism. A number of immunologic alterations are initiated; leukocytes are mobilized, macrophages and specialized T cells are produced, and "acute-phase" plasma proteins are synthesized by the liver. Inflammatory cells invade the injured area, set up a perimeter defense, and engulf the dead and dying cells and other wound contaminants. These initial steps are followed rapidly by ingrowth of blood vessels, appearance of fibroblasts that build collagen scaffolding, and a host of other local changes that aid wound repair.

Local changes that occur at the injury site are accompanied by systemic alterations in body physiologic processes and metabolism. Cardiac output is elevated, minute ventilation is increased, and the patient becomes febrile. Lipolysis and skeletal muscle proteolysis are accelerated, providing an ongoing fuel supply and an immediate source of amino acids that are utilized for wound healing and synthesis of "acute-phase" proteins and new glucose. The glucose provides essential energy for the brain and other vital organs and for healing of the wound.

These biologic functions following injury and other stresses are a reflection of a unique and indelible program that is encoded in higher species, particularly *Homo sapiens*. In strict Darwinian terms, these responses follow an evolutionary process that favors survival of the fittest in the struggle for existence. In teleologic terms, these responses have a purpose: to benefit the organism and aid recovery. Although a direct cause-and-effect relationship has not been established between many of these posttraumatic events and recovery, these adaptive responses occur during the same period when the wound heals and the patient returns to health. Elective operative procedures without complications, accompanied by appropriate anesthesia and adequate postoperative pain control, cause minimal changes in bodily functions in the low-risk patient. Thus, intervention on the part of the surgeon is rarely necessary and can even be meddlesome. However, critical illnesses secondary to major injury or infection necessitate significant therapy to aid eventual recovery. Knowledge of homeostatic adjustments that occur in critically ill patients is essential for optimal patient care and reflects the physician's insight into blood volume regulation, nutritional requirements, cardiovascular resuscitation, wound healing, and physical and psychological rehabilitation and recovery from a life-threatening illness.

Whereas constancy of biologic systems was appreciated as early as the time of Hippocrates, it was not until the 1800s, when Claude Bernard established physiology as a new discipline, that regulation of body systems to maintain internal constancy was actually proposed. Bernard suggested that all living processes were attributable to biochemical and physiologic reactions and that a detailed analysis of these functions would allow a more complete understanding of the process of life. In his *Introduction to the Study of Experimental Medicine*, Bernard detailed a number of studies that described the digestion of food, the maintenance of blood glucose, and the vasomotor control of circulation. He proposed that living organs did not exist "in the *milieu exterieur* (the atmosphere, or salt or fresh water), but in a liquid *milieu interieur* formed by circulating organic liquid that surrounds and bathes all of the tissue elements; this is the lymphoplasma, the liquid part of the blood, which in the higher animals is perfused through the tissue and is the basis of all local nutrition and the common factor of all elementary metabolic changes. The stability of the *milieu interieur* is the primary condition for freedom and independence of existence.[4] Thus, Claude Bernard's description of the constancy of the chemical composition of the body formed the basis for understanding the uniqueness of animal life.

The next major contributor to the field of body homeostasis was Walter B. Cannon, an American who served as a physiologist at the Harvard Medical School for most of his professional career. Much like Bernard, Cannon worked in a number of different areas, including digestion, metabolism, control of hunger and thirst, maintenance of blood glucose, tissue energetics, thermoregulation, and maintenance of oxygen supply. Cannon, however, is best known for his detailed studies of the autonomic nervous system; he described the sympathetic and parasympathetic nervous system and proved that autonomic nervous system control was responsible for the maintenance of constancy and autoregulatory adjustments following stress. Cannon coined the word "homeostasis" and defined it as "the coordinated physiological process which maintains most of the steady states in the organisms."[9] He noted that homeostatic responses were extremely complex, involving brain, nerves, heart, lungs, kidneys, and spleen; these organs worked cooperatively to maintain body constancy.

While these physiologic mechanisms were evolving, the description and categorization of responses that occurred in patients following injury and other critical illnesses were also being recorded. John Hunter, an English surgeon and biologist in the eighteenth century, commented on the biologic response that occurred following tissue injury and noted, "There is a circumstance attending accidental injury which does not belong to disease, namely that the injury done, has in all cases a tendency to produce, both the deposition and means of cure."[14] This was the first suggestion that the responses to injury were beneficial to the host.

In the latter part of the nineteenth century, an extremely imaginative and creative group of German scientists focused their energies on the study of protein metabolism and the thermogenesis of food. These individuals, led by Carl Voit, performed nitrogen balance studies and built large calorimeters for the study of food oxidation and heat production. Both energy and nitrogen balance studies were performed under a variety of experimental conditions in animals and humans. Using these techniques, the impact of infection on protein metabolism was studied and a view contrary to that suggested by Hunter was proposed.[29] The German scientists described the accelerated proteolysis that accompanies infection as the "toxic destruction of protein," implying that this process was maladaptive rather than an appropriate response to illness.

The "modern era" of understanding injury responses was initiated by the careful and thorough studies of David Patton Cuthbertson, a young Scottish clinical chemist working in Glasgow in the early 1930s. Cuthbertson studied the urinary excretion of calcium and phosphorus in patients who sustained long bone fractures. He hoped to relate abnormal mineral excretion to delayed fracture healing. Extensive balance studies were performed in normal individuals confined to bed and in patients with long bone fractures. He noted that the injured patients had increased urinary excretion of phosphorus and exaggerated urinary losses of nitrogen and potassium.[11] He also determined energy requirements, using indirect calorimetry in the injured patients, and found that increased oxygen consumption accom-

panied the protein catabolic response. Cuthbertson described a constant rise in body temperature in uninfected, injured patients and characterized this response as "posttraumatic fever." In subsequent studies he attempted to modify the injury response by altering food intake but noted that the increased nitrogen excretion could not be diminished by nutrient intake. Because of the large quantity of nitrogen lost, he suggested that the nitrogen excreted in the urine was due to a generalized proteolytic response throughout the skeletal muscle mass and did not follow protein breakdown at the site of injury.

Some years later, Francis D. Moore, Moseley Professor of Surgery at the Harvard Medical School, collected, tabulated, categorized, and applied much of the knowledge concerning homeostatic responses following trauma and surgery to patient care. Dr. Moore spent over 30 years of his professional life working in this area. He brought sophisticated scientific techniques to the bedside, used isotopic dilution methodology to measure body composition in patients, and developed an intensive care unit where careful balance studies could be performed in critically ill patients. He evaluated the impact of specific components of the injury response such as bed rest, anesthesia, volume loss, and starvation on metabolic responses and described various stages of convalescence following injury. His introduction of isotopic methodology to the practice of clinical medicine, coupled with meticulous balance techniques, is detailed in his classic volume *The Metabolic Care of the Surgical Patient*.[21] More important, however, this information was translated into knowledge that could be applied by the practicing surgeon to improve the care of the critically ill surgical patient.

Many others have contributed to the field of homeostatic alterations following injury. A few of these individuals and their contributions are listed in Table 1. Recent authorities have directed their attention to specific areas, and much of this knowledge serves as the basis for chapters in this textbook. In

TABLE 1. Other Important Contributors to Homeostatic Responses

Area of Research	Contributor	Area of Specific Contribution
Maintenance of blood volume and fluid and electrolyte balance	L. J. Henderson	Oxygen-carrying capacity of blood
	J. L. Gamble	Fluid and electrolyte homeostasis
	D. B. Dill	Water homeostasis
	C. A. Moyer	Salt replacement following shock
	G. T. Shires	
Hormonal and metabolic responses to injury	H. Selye	Adrenal cortical response to stress
	F. Albright	Balance and isotopic techniques to study patients with endocrine disorders
	D. Hume	Central nervous system control following stress
	M. Kleiber	Animal energetics, food, and environmental interaction
	H. Munro	Regulation of protein and amino acid metabolism
	J. M. Kinney	Energy balance, effect of nutrition on energetics, and substrate regulation
Nutrition	F. G. Benedict	Energy balance, caloric values of food
	E. F. Dubois	
	R. Elman	Parenteral nutrition
	A. R. Behnke	Body composition
	A. Wretlind	Fat emulsions
	J. E. Rhoads	Nutrition in surgical patients
	J. T. Randall	Defined formula diets
Environmental influences on injury	S.-O. Liljedahl	Optimal ambient temperature for burn patients
	H. B. Stoner	Thermal regulation following shock
Immunologic responses, inflammation, wound healing	P. B. Beeson	"Endogenous" pyrogen
	J. E. Dunphy	Wound healing
	W. A. Altemeier	Infection in surgical patients
	W. R. Beisel	Metabolic responses to systemic infection
	S. M. Levenson	Wound healing, nutrition, and infection

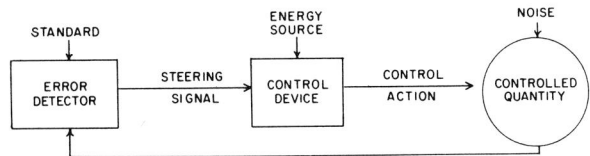

Figure 1. An early model of a biologic control system. The error detector serves as a monitor and elicits signals (usually hormonal or nervous), which affect the control device that imparts a change. This perturbation is generally larger than the background "noise" level, and the correction is perceived by the detector. A biologic example would be the response to hypoglycemia (glucose being the "controlled quantity"). This would be detected in the hypothalamus, which would "signal" via hormones and the sympathetic nervous system to the liver ("control device") to liberate more glucose. When the blood glucose level is corrected, the "error detector" diminishes its signal. (From Brookhaven Symposia in Biology, #10, Homeostatic Mechanisms. Office of Technical Services, Washington, D.C., 1958.)

addition to focusing on specific areas, a body of knowledge has evolved that is directed toward the understanding of responses to stress and the control of biologic systems.

Proposed models for the regulation of homeostasis define a signal detector, a processor, and an effector organ, all elements necessary for maintenance of the internal milieu. In classic physiologic terms, such systems are controlled by negative feedback servomechanisms (Fig. 1). In addition, open loop controllers may function in the trauma patient. One example is the constant demand for glucose by the healing wound; provision of dietary glucose fails to suppress the accelerated gluconeogenesis and marked insulin resistance that occur following injury, suggesting that the usual feedback signal is absent. Only wound closure and/or healing returns these alterations to normal, indicating that an open loop stimulus-response system may be operative. Much of the knowledge of biochemical control is incorporated in the field of endocrinology, but more specific areas of

study have evolved and include cybernetics and control therapy. These areas of knowledge have improved understanding of biologic processes and with computer application may lead to the development of artificial intelligence.

ANATOMY

BODY COMPOSITION AND ITS RESPONSE TO SURGICAL STRESS. The body is composed of two major components: a *nonaqueous* and an *aqueous* phase.[21] Body fat and extracellular solids such as bone matrix, tendon, fascia, and collagen comprise the nonhydrous portion. The aqueous phase is, in general, the sum of three compartments: extracellular water, blood volume, and intracellular fluid. Cells of the body are supported within the aqueous phase, and the heterogeneous mass of body cells and the supporting aqueous environment is called the *lean body mass*. The *body cell mass* is the metabolically active portion of the body and is composed of the lean body mass minus the extracellular fluid. Body cell mass was defined by Moore as that portion of the body that consists of all hydrated cells and represents the functioning, actively exchanging component of the body. The body cell mass consists of skeletal muscle, visceral organs, and a smaller portion of cells that lies on the periphery and includes connective tissue, skin, and areolar cells, and the red cell mass. The body cell mass is most easily quantitated by determining total exchangeable potassium. Since potassium is primarily maintained within this intracellular aqueous environment of the body cell mass, it is quantitatively related to the size of this compartment. The quantity of intracellular potassium is also related to nitrogen content, and the measure of total body nitrogen by neutron activation analysis also allows quantitation of the body cell mass. In contrast, extracellular fluid is relatively depleted of potassium but is rich in sodium. Extracellular fluid is determined by one of a variety of isotope dilutional techniques

TABLE 2. Normal Adult Body Composition

	Male, 70 kg.		Female, 60 kg.	
	Absolute	*Relative (% Body Weight)*	*Absolute*	*Relative (% Body Weight)*
Nonaqueous Phase				
Total body fat*	16.0 kg.	22.8	19.0 kg.	31.7
Bone mineral mass†	4.8 kg.	6.9	4.0 kg.	6.7
Aqueous Phase				
Total body water	39.4 L.	56.3	29.5 L.	49.2
Intracellular water	22.1 L.	31.6	15.5 L.	25.8
Extracellular water	17.3 L.	24.7	14.0 L.	23.3
Interstitial water	14.3 L.	20.4	11.4 L.	19.0
Blood volume	5.08 L.	7.3	4.03 L.	6.7
Plasma volume	3.15 L.	4.5	2.63 L.	4.4
Red cell volume	1.93 L.	2.8	1.40 L.	2.3
Lean body mass‡	54.0 kg.	77.1	41.0 kg.	68.3
Body cell mass†	30.9 kg.	44.1	21.7 kg.	36.2
Muscle mass	17.4 kg.	24.3	9.6 kg.	16.0
Nonmuscle mass	32.8 kg.	46.8	27.1 kg.	45.1
Other Measurements				
Total exchangeable potassium	3380 mEq.		2380 mEq.	
Total exchangeable sodium	2980 mEq.		2360 mEq.	
Total body nitrogen	1.7 kg.		1.3 kg.	
Total body calcium	1.0 kg.		0.8 kg.	

*Total body fat = body weight − lean body mass.
†Derived from primary measurement, unless noted.

‡Lean body mass = $\dfrac{\text{total body water}}{0.73}$.

Data from references 10 and 21.

or other body compositional measurements that quantitate the size of the extracellular fluid compartments. Body composition of normal individuals varies with age and sex.[10,21] Normal values are shown in Table 2.

ALTERATION IN BODY COMPOSITION WITH DISEASE. The components of the body change with disease. For example, obesity causes an increase in the absolute (or relative) quantity of adipose tissue, whereas starvation causes loss of both fat and lean body mass. Patients with disorders of fluid homeostasis have alterations in the size of the aqueous compartments. For example, an individual with congestive heart failure has an expanded extracellular fluid volume associated with an increase in total exchangeable body sodium. A common response also occurs following loss of body protoplasm. This is characterized by loss of body cell mass as measured by a decrease in total exchangeable potassium and an observable diminution of skeletal muscle mass associated with loss of body fat, expansion of the extracellular fluid compartment, and increase in total exchangeable sodium. Thus, the extracellular fluid compartment enlarges and salt is retained, while the body mass (functional tissue) is reduced (Table 3). These changes may be greatly exaggerated by specific organ dysfunction (such as heart or renal failure) and/or accelerated weight loss, which occurs in unfed patients following severe injury or infection. Because of the avidity of the body to retain water and sodium, critically ill patients become extremely sensitive to volume and sodium loads; sodium-containing solutions should be administered judiciously in such individuals.

BODY ENERGY STORAGE. The components of the body cell mass represent active, functioning tissue. These cells and the adipose tissue also represent a form of stored energy. The greatest energy component is fat, which is a nonhydrous portion of the body and yields approximately 9 calories per gm. (Table 4). Thus, this calorically dense storage form of energy provides a source of lightweight and transportable fuel to be utilized by highly mobile species. The protein component of the body is the next largest substrate mass but yields considerably fewer calories than body fat because of its caloric content of only 4 calories per gm. Moreover, because the body cell mass is hydrated, body protein, when expressed as caloric potential, is quite different from fat on a weight basis. This is because hydrated muscle tissue contains three parts water and one part protein, which yield only 1 calorie per gm. of hydrated protein. These differences between nonhydrous fat and hydrated protein highlight the relative inefficiency of body protein as a transportable caloric source. Body protein is thus not a primary storage fuel but rather serves as structural and functional components of the body; *loss of body protein is associated with loss of body function.* Reduction of body protein is not without consequence. During catabolic states, protein is broken down and utilized primarily for the synthesis of new glucose, which does not exist in storage form to a great extent and is rapidly oxidized following stress (Table 4). Because a number of vital organs, including the brain, peripheral nerves, renal medulla, red cells, white cells, and in-

TABLE 4. Estimated Fuel Consumption of Normal Individuals

	kg.	kcal.
Tissues		
Fat	15.0	141,000
Protein	6.0	24,000
Glycogen (muscle)	0.150	600
Glycogen (liver)	0.075	300
Total		165,900
Circulating		
Glucose (extracellular water)	0.020	80
Free fatty acids (plasma)	0.0003	3
Triglyceride (plasma)	0.003	30
Total		113

Adapted from Cahill, G. F., Jr.: Starvation in man. N. Engl. J. Med., *282:* 668, 1970.

flammatory tissue, all utilize glucose as a primary fuel, the need for an ongoing glucose supply is imperative if the organism is to survive. An ongoing glucose supply is provided via proteolysis (primarily skeletal muscle) and accelerated hepatic gluconeogenesis. The conversion of amino acids to glucose is a necessary step because the enzymatic machinery is not present in humans to convert long-chain fatty acids to glucose.

The alterations in body compartments following critical illness have been quantitated utilizing compositional studies and balance techniques. Whereas most normal individuals can lose up to 10 per cent of body weight with minimal changes in physiologic function, weight loss greater than this compromises normal responses and may limit survival. Approximately one half of the weight loss following a catabolic illness reflects a decrease in body fat; the remaining portion reflects loss of protein and its associated water (body cell mass).[21] Limitations in body function are reflected primarily by loss of body protein, excreted in the urine as nitrogen, and large losses may be extensive in a critically ill patient. If a normal individual undergoes 5 days of starvation, total protein loss may average approximately 1600 gm. of muscle tissue. If this same individual sustains an injury and cannot eat, total protein loss is accelerated to 550 to 600 gm. over the same period, representing loss of more than 2 kg. of muscle tissue. Whereas these quantities are relatively small in terms of overall body protein, it should be realized that associated complications that may occur in the traumatized patient, coupled with inadequate food intake, further accelerate proteolysis. Since death, secondary to starvation, is associated with losses of body protein of approximately 30 to 40 per cent, such a tremendous drain on body nitrogen stores exerts an additional stress on the patient and may be associated with the inability to survive major injury.

HOMEOSTATIC RESPONSES TO SPECIFIC COMPONENTS OF INJURY

Critical illness results in a variety of complex interacting homeostatic responses. The clinical features observed are the sum of changes known to occur following single perturbations. In the following section, events frequently observed in surgical patients are discussed as responses to one single change. These adjustments include volume loss, underperfusion, starvation, tissue damage, and invasive infection.

VOLUME LOSS. Acute volume reduction associated with accidental injury or an elective surgical procedure is a nonlethal stimulus for the mechanisms that maintain circulation and restore blood volume. Volume loss signifies the decrease of effec-

TABLE 3. Body Composition in Normal Individuals and Catabolic Surgical Patients

	Normal Individuals (% Total Body)	Catabolic Patients (% Total Body)
Body weight (kg.)	70.4	58.9
Extracellular fluid (L.)	25.6 (36)	31.9 (54)
Body cell mass (kg.)	24.7 (35)	14.7 (25)
Estimated fat mass (kg.)	20.1 (29)	12.3 (21)

Data from Shizgal, H. M.: Body composition. *In* Fischer, J. E. (Ed.): Surgical Nutrition. Boston, Little, Brown & Company, 1983, pp. 1–17.

tive circulating blood volume. The most frequent form of volume reduction in the surgical patient is simple hemorrhage. With blood loss there is no initial change in plasma osmolality or tonicity, and serum sodium and/or osmolality remains normal (this is referred to as *isotonic volume reduction*). A variety of responses are initiated following simple volume reduction.

First, pressor receptors in the carotid artery and aortic arch and volume (stretch) receptors in the wall of the left atrium initiate afferent nerve signals that eventually stimulate the release of both aldosterone and vasopressin (antidiuretic hormone [ADH]). ADH also responds to osmoregulation, and small alterations in plasma tonicity stimulate the release of ADH from the posterior pituitary gland. Other afferent neurogenic stimuli related to the trauma itself (such as pain) may also stimulate ADH output; alcohol blocks its release. ADH acts directly on the renal tubules, permitting passive diffusion of water along an osmotic gradient across the cell and into the peritubular vessel. Clinically, this is manifest as fluid retention. Administration of water under these circumstances may produce hypotonicity rather than diminishing ADH release via the normal servo-feedback loop. Such hypotonicity is frequently observed following an elective operation and is due in part to the afferent nervous stimulation from the procedure and the isotonic volume reduction that stimulates elaboration of ADH.

Aldosterone is released by one of several mechanisms. First, decreased pulse pressure stimulates the juxtaglomerular apparatus of the kidney, activating the renin-angiotensin system. This system is a major controller of extracellular fluid volume via the regulation of aldosterone production. Aldosterone has a direct effect on the renal tubule to reabsorb sodium and, hence, to conserve water. In addition, afferent nerve stimuli cause elaboration of adrenocorticotropic hormone (ACTH), which has a minor role in regulating aldosterone release. The augmented aldosterone response following volume loss is fundamental to maintenance and restoration of plasma volume.

In addition to the hormonal responses to a volume loss, there is a marked shift of fluid across capillary beds into the bloodstream.[21] This "refill" phenomenon decreases concentration of red cells (as measured by the hematocrit) and may cause a slight dilution in the serum protein concentration. Transcapillary refill is stimulated by as little as a 15 to 20 per cent loss in blood volume and, with other mechanisms, requires about 24 hours for restoration of blood volume.

In addition to hemorrhage, volume reduction occurs by other mechanisms. There may be acute *de-salting water loss* associated with vomiting, diarrhea, pancreatic fistula, uncontrolled ileostomy loss, or intestinal obstruction. In these cases, there is minimal loss of red cell mass but often a decrease in tonicity following mobilization of cell water, which is relatively free of sodium. If osmotic changes in the plasma are marked, the plasma electrolyte alterations become quite distinct from those of isotonic volume reduction, as seen with mild to moderate hemorrhage.

Fluid losses may also cause the *desiccation-dehydration syndrome*, in which there is excessive water loss from the skin or lungs without accompanying salt loss. Such marked dehydration is characteristic of exposure to heat but can also occur with acute renal dysfunction, diarrhea associated with tube feedings, diabetic ketoacidosis, and simple dehydration. A rise in serum sodium, and thus in plasma tonicity, is characteristic of these states.

UNDERPERFUSION. Volume reduction is characterized by a set of compensatory responses that attempt to maintain circulating volume and plasma tonicity. However, blood volume reduction of any type, if severe enough, causes a prolonged low-flow state. During a low-flow state, oxygen delivery is inadequate for oxygen demands of the tissues, despite compensatory mechanisms, and cell deterioration occurs. Inadequate perfusion causes accumulation of acid products, particularly lactic acid, within the body, and this is associated with a profound acidosis of both the intracellular and the extracellular fluid compartments. Compensatory adjustments are stimulated by the kidney and respiratory tract. However, with underperfusion minimal quantities of urine are excreted, and this, accompanied by the presence of abnormal pigments in the plasma such as hemoglobin or myoglobin, may cause acute renal failure. If a low-flow state persists, cellular damage increases, distributing membrane function. This effect is manifest by the requirement for large volumes of fluid to resuscitate the patient, referred to in animal shock models as the "reuptake phenomenon." In addition, reperfusion may be associated with the generation of free oxygen radicals, which cause tissue oxidative injury and cellular disruption. Thus, recovery from low-flow states depends on the extent and duration of the insult. Brief periods of underperfusion cause little sustained cellular damage, whereas more prolonged episodes cause marked acidosis, renal failure, central nervous system hypoxia, and generalized disruption of cell function. Often, the patient does not recover if these alterations are irreversible.

STARVATION. In many surgical patients, fluid and nutrient intake is interrupted and inadequate, or insufficient energy and protein are provided. When this occurs during simple starvation, fat mobilization proceeds and ketosis results. Plasma substrate concentration generally reflects the decrease in glucose as a primary oxidizable fuel and the increase in fatty acids as the body's major energy source.[8] Insulin appears to have a central role in adaptation to fasting. As glucose and insulin levels fall, fatty acid mobilization and utilization are favored at high rates of oxidation. Increased concentrations of fatty acid compete

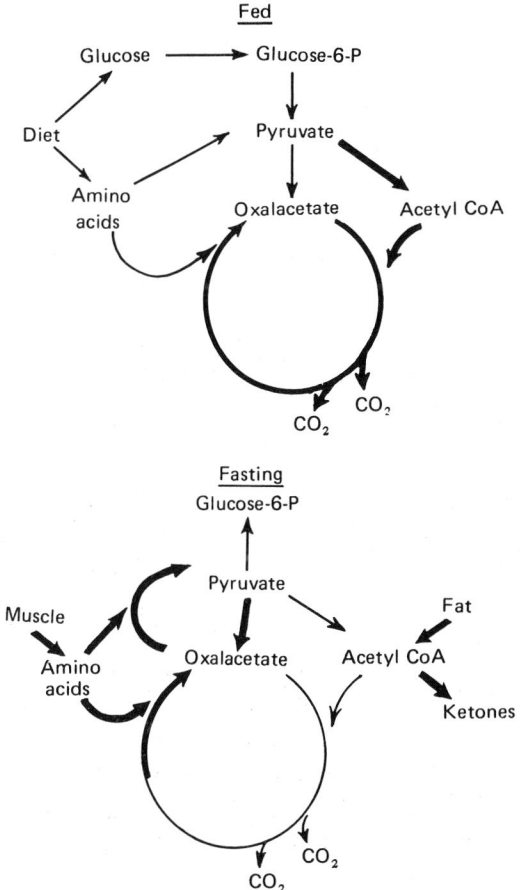

Figure 2. The flow of substrate during the fed and fasting states. The hormonal environment associated with critical illness attenuates the ketosis of starvation, and starvation adaptation does not occur following injury or sepsis. (From Wilmore, D. W.: The Metabolic Management of the Critically Ill. New York, Plenum Medical Book Company, 1977.)

with glucose for entry into muscle cells and therefore are potent peripheral glucose antagonists. After several days of starvation, fatty acids are primarily oxidized in the liver to form acetoacetate, acetone, or beta-hydroxybutyrate, all referred to as "ketone bodies." The parent molecule of ketones, acetoacetyl coenzyme A (CoA), is a normal intermediate of lipolysis and lipogenesis. Fatty acid oxidation is unimpaired to the level of the acetyl CoA. However, acetyl CoA cannot enter into the citric acid cycle because it must combine with oxalacetate. This endproduct of carbohydrate breakdown is preferentially incorporated into the gluconeogenic sequence and is thus relatively unavailable to combine with acetyl CoA to form citric acid. Thus, this step becomes rate-limiting and the fatty acid breakdown products are shunted via acetyl CoA into ketone body formation (Fig. 2). Blood ketone concentrations rise markedly and serve as signals to a variety of tissues to decrease glucose utilization or minimize protein breakdown. These compounds are essential substrates that diminish skeletal muscle proteolysis during prolonged starvation. In addition, ketone bodies serve as an oxidizable fuel, since these compounds are a water-soluble form of fat and can be utilized by the central nervous system during prolonged starvation.

Because carbohydrate stores are limited and because these glycogen stores are utilized rapidly following stress, an ongoing supply of glucose must be provided. Skeletal muscle proteolysis provides amino acids that serve as glucose precursors, although glycerol from triglyceride breakdown may also be used as a carbon source for new glucose.[8] Gluconeogenesis results and is generally proportional to the proteolysis and increased loss of urea in the urine. Ammonia is also excreted in the urine as a method of buffering the acid load that accompanies ketoacidosis. All of these mechanisms are reversed by providing small quantities of carbohydrate calories.

TISSUE DAMAGE. Unlike the responses to simple starvation, which are characterized by a generalized decrease in metabolism, injured patients demonstrate heightened metabolic responses. This is due to the increased elaboration of catabolic hormones that stimulate respiration, cardiac output, and fuel mobilization and utilization. All of the processes contribute to the accelerated loss of body tissue. This response is characterized by increased fat oxidation and marked proteolysis, causing increased loss of nitrogen in the urine. Volume loss, underperfusion, and simple starvation may be additional components of this response, but the specific presence of damaged tissue appears to be the initiator of this hypercatabolic response. Tissue injury causes afferent nerve signals that increase elaboration of ACTH and other pituitary hormones. However, other substances, such as cell breakdown products or mediators released during inflammation, may have additional metabolic effects. Many new inflammatory cells appear in the wound soon after injury. Initially leukocytes predominate but later macrophages and fibroblasts are the major cell types present. These cells release a variety of mediator substances including cytokines, soluble biochemical signals that influence the proliferation, development, and function of surrounding cells to aid host resistance and wound repair. Many of these substances have been identified and include the interleukins (IL-1 to IL-8), tumor necrosis factor-alpha (also referred to as cachectin), the interferons, and a variety of other growth factors (Table 5). These factors predominantly modify local cellular proliferation and regulate wound repair, through their paracrine action, but they may also reach the bloodstream to exert systemic effects, such as mediating fever, stimulating the elaboration of acute-phase proteins, and causing redistribution of trace elements. These responses to inflammation are collectively referred to as the acute-phase response. In addition, cytokines may stimulate the elaboration of pituitary hormones and activate the cyclo-oxygenase pathway, causing prostaglandin synthesis. Elaboration of prostaglandins, particularly PGE_2, may also contribute to some of the systemic responses observed following tissue injury.

TABLE 5. Sources and Targets of Some Cytokines and Other Peptide Regulatory Factors

Regulatory Factor*	Sources	Target Tissues/Cells
Interleukins (ILs)		
IL-1α, IL-1β (endogenous pyrogen, lymphocyte-activating factor, leukocyte endogenous mediator, hemopoietin-1)	Monocytes/macrophages; many endothelial, epithelial, and hematopoietic cells	Thymocytes, T and B cells, hematopoietic cells, fibroblasts, chondrocytes, receptors in brain and liver
Il-2 (T cell growth factor)	T cells	T and B cells, thymocytes, natural killer cells
IL-6 (B cell–stimulating factor 2, interferon-beta$_2$, hepatocyte-stimulating factor, hybridoma growth factor, B cell differentiation factor, 26-kd. protein)	Monocytes/macrophages, T cells, fibroblasts, epithelial cell types	T and B cells, fibroblasts, hepatocytes, hematopoietic stem cells
Tumor Necrosis Factors (TNFs)		
TNF (TNF-α, cachectin)	Monocytes/macrophages, lymphocytes, natural killer cells, glial cells, Kupffer cells	Endothelial cells, monocytes/macrophages, neutrophils, fibroblasts, receptors in liver, muscle, lung, gut, kidney
Interferons		
Gamma interferon (immune interferon, macrophage-activating factor)	Multiple cell types (antigen-antibody reaction)	T and B cells, phagocytic cells
Other Growth and Regulatory Factors		
Epidermal growth factor	Salivary gland, kidney, ? mammary tissue	Epidermal/epithelial cells, angiogenesis factor
Platelet-derived growth factor	Platelets, macrophages, vascular endothelium, astrocytes	Fibroblasts, skeletal muscle
Transforming growth factors (TGFs)		
TGF-α	Embryonic cells, placenta, keratinocytes	Epidermal/epithelial cells, angiogenesis factor
TGF-β	Macrophages, neural cells, platelets, bone, connective tissue	Many cell types (stimulates extracellular matrix components)

The terms in parentheses are terms that have been, and in some cases are, used for the same substance or group of substances.

INVASIVE INFECTION. The major complication observed in surgical patients is infection. The infective organisms are generally opportunistic bacteria that, under normal circumstances, are ubiquitous, noninvasive, and, therefore, benign. However, the multiple sites of entry via wounds and tubes that are present in the critically ill patient, coupled with alterations in host defense mechanisms, cause increased susceptibility of injured patients to infection. Infection alone initiates catabolic responses that are similar to (but not the same as) those described following injury in noninfected patients.[3] Both processes cause fever, hyperventilation, tachycardia, accelerated gluconeogenesis, increased proteolysis, and lipolysis, with fat utilized as the principal fuel. If the infection is sudden and severe (such as would occur with dehiscence of a colonic anastomosis), hypotension and *septic shock* may result. It has recently been found that the mediators for all of these events are cytokines, products of the host's own cells. In most cases, the signal that initiates these alterations is bacterial endotoxin, a lipopolysaccharide elaborated by gram-negative organisms. However, antigen-antibody reactions may also trigger these events, and this mechanism is thought to be responsible for the responses observed following gram-positive infections and antigenic stimulation, such as blood transfusion reactions and responses following organ rejection.

Following endotoxin, monocytes, macrophages, and lymphocytes are stimulated to produce tumor necrosis factor (TNF), which mediates many of the systemic responses associated with infection (Fig. 3). Many of the cellular events are mediated via the cyclo-oxygenase reaction and can be markedly attenuated by administration of nonsteroidal anti-inflammatory agents, which block the generation of prostaglandins. The systemic responses observed following infection are related to the amount of TNF elaborated; this has been demonstrated by studies that examined the response characteristics following infusion of increasing doses of TNF into patients (Table 6). In addition, other factors may affect the final responses observed, and these include the presence of other cytokines that may amplify the responses[22] and the time and duration of TNF in the bloodstream.

Other cytokines have also been identified as postinflammatory circulating signals, and these include IL-1, IL-2, and gamma-interferon. The relative elaboration of various cytokines probably depends on the specific disease process, the size of the initial inflammatory focus, and the extent of bacterial colonization or infection.

RESPONSES TO ELECTIVE OPERATIVE PROCEDURES

ENDOCRINE CHANGES AND THEIR METABOLIC CONSEQUENCES. Most patients requiring elective operative procedures are adequately nourished. They are fasted overnight and receive intravenous solution containing 5 per cent glucose. They then receive a general anesthetic; the patient's skin is prepared, and the operative site is draped. An incision is then made.

One of the earliest consequences of the surgical incision is the rise in levels of circulating cortisol that occurs in response to a sudden outpouring of ACTH from the anterior pituitary gland.[27] Activation of the pituitary gland occurs when afferent nervous signals from the operative site reach the hypothalamus to initiate the stress response, which then stimulates the elaboration of cortisol. This hormone remains at two to five times normal levels for approximately 24 hours after a major operation. Cortisol has generalized effects on tissue catabolism and mobilizes amino acids from skeletal muscle that provide substrates for wound healing and serve as precursors for the hepatic synthesis of acute-phase proteins or new glucose. Associated with the activation of the adrenal cortex is stimulation of

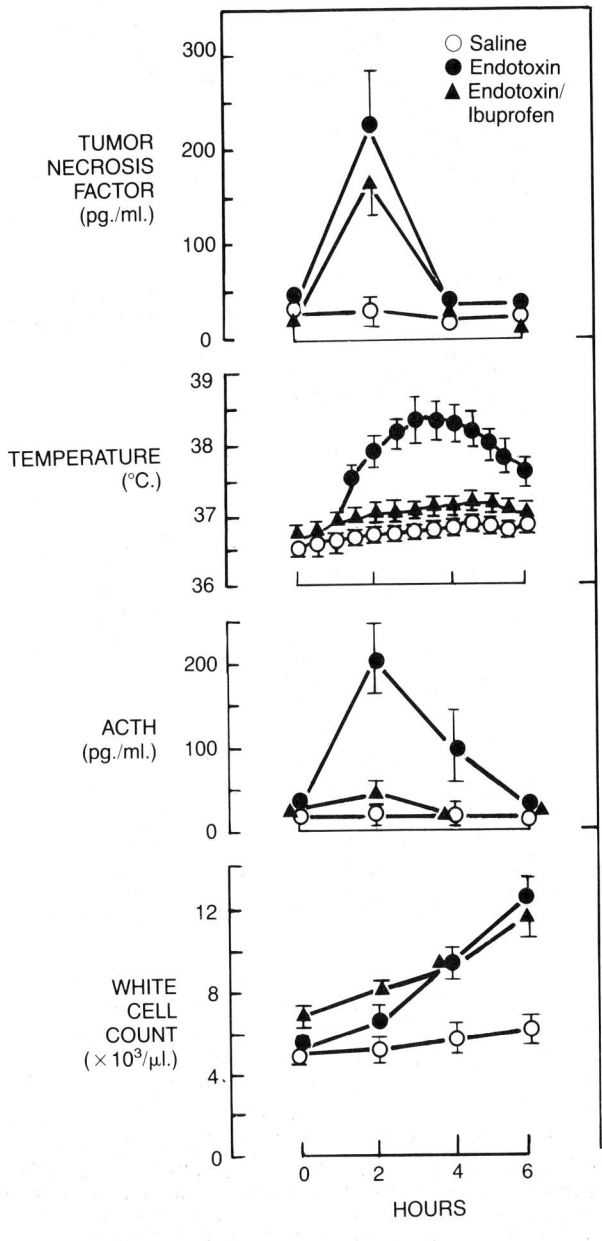

Figure 3. Changes in plasma concentrations of tumor necrosis factor and metabolic responses after endotoxin administration in 13 subjects without ibuprofen pretreatment and in 8 subjects with ibuprofen pretreatment. The data obtained in the group pretreated with ibuprofen were similar to those obtained during saline studies in the group that was not pretreated, and the data from both groups have been pooled. (Redrawn from Michie, H. R., Manogue, K. R., Spriggs, D. R., Revhaug, A., O'Dwyer, S. T., Dinarello, C. A., Cerami, A., Wolff, S. M., and Wilmore, D. W.: Detection of circulating tumor necrosis factor during endotoxemia in humans. N. Engl. J. Med., *318*:1481, 1988.)

the adrenal medulla through the sympathetic nervous system, with elaboration of epinephrine. Urinary catecholamines may be elevated for 24 to 48 hours after operation and may then return to normal. This circulating neurotransmitter has an important role in circulatory adjustment, but it may also stimulate hepatic glycogenolysis and gluconeogenesis in concert with glucagon and glucocorticoids.

The neuroendocrine responses to operation also modify the various mechanisms in salt and water excretion. Alterations in serum osmolarity and tonicity of body fluids secondary to anesthesia and the operative stress stimulate the secretion of aldos-

TABLE 6. Host Responses to Various Doses of Tumor Necrosis Factor

Dose of TNF Infused (μg./m.²/24 hr.)	Response	Clinical Correlate
1	Hypoferremia	Subclinical infection
20	Myalgia and headache, anorexia, fever, tachycardia, elevated acute-phase proteins	Influenza, acute appendicitis
>500	Rigors, elevated stress hormones, fluid retention, lymphopenia, hypotension	Intra-abdominal abscess, major thermal injury
>620	Decreased consciousness, profound hypotension, pulmonary edema, oliguria	Septicemia, severe acute pancreatitis, infected massive burns

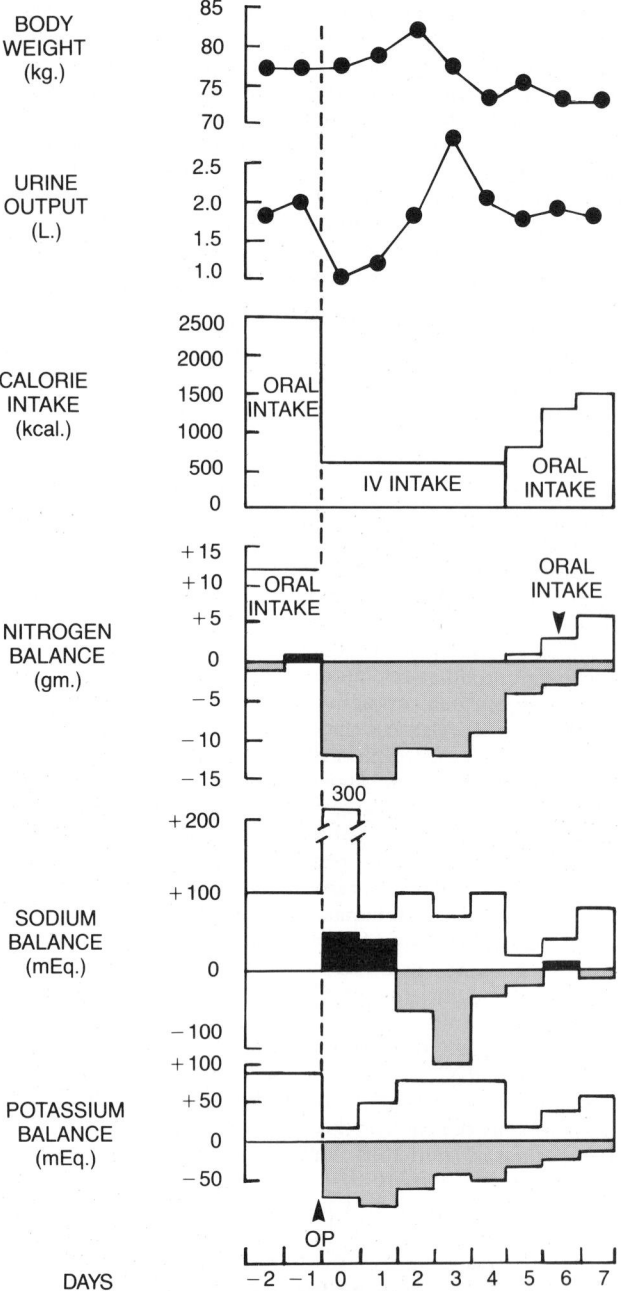

Figure 4. The metabolic response of a previously healthy subject to an elective operative procedure. Intake is plotted upward from zero, output downward from the top of the intake line. Negative balance is represented by the shaded, with positive balance solid black. (Redrawn from Wilmore, D. W., and Souba, W. W.: Diet and nutrition in the care of the patient with surgery, trauma and sepsis. *In* Shils, M. E., and Young, V. R. (Eds.): Modern Nutrition in Health and Disease. Philadelphia, Lea & Febiger, 1988, p. 1309.)

terone and ADH.[23,27] The ability to excrete a water load after elective surgical procedures is restricted. The usual postoperative patient concentrates urine to 1 to 2 ml. water per mOsm. solute excreted, corresponding to a urine osmolarity of 500 to 1000 mOsm. per liter, even in the presence of adequate hydration. Hence, weight gain secondary to salt and water retention is usual following operation (Fig. 4). Edema occurs to a varying extent in all surgical wounds, and this accumulation is proportional to the extent of tissue dissection and local trauma. Administration of sodium-containing solutions during operation replaces this functional volume loss as extracellular fluid redistributes in the body. This "third-spaced" fluid eventually returns to the circulation as the wound edema subsides and diuresis commences 2 to 4 days following the operation.

Alterations occur in the response of the endocrine pancreas following elective operation. In general, insulin elaboration is diminished, and glucagon concentrations rise.[27] This response may be related to increased sympathetic activity or to the rise in levels of circulating epinephrine, which is known to suppress insulin release. The increased elaboration of glucagon may be related to increased sympathetic nervous system stimulation or to alterations in circulating mediators. The rise in glucagon and the corresponding fall in insulin are a potent signal to accelerate hepatic glucose production, and, with other hormones (epinephrine and glucocorticoids), gluconeogenesis is maintained.

The postoperative hormonal responses are thought to orchestrate physiologic and biochemical changes that benefit the host. Salt and water conservation support the circulating blood volume. Augmented hepatic glucose production provides adequate essential fuel for the nervous system, the red and white blood cells, and the healing wound. Skeletal muscle proteolysis provides amino acid precursors for gluconeogenesis and hepatic protein synthesis although negative nitrogen balance occurs. Postoperative lipolysis provides abundant quantities of free fatty acid, as an additional energy source. Current techniques of postoperative care minimize, but do not reverse, these responses.

STAGE OF SURGICAL CONVALESCENCE. The period of catabolism initiated by operation, a combination of inadequate nutrition and alteration of the hormonal environment, has been termed the adrenergic-corticoid phase.[21] This period is followed by the onset of anabolism, which occurs at a variable time in the patient's convalescence. In general, in the absence of postoperative complications, this phase starts 3 to 6 days after an abdominal operation of the magnitude of a colectomy or gastrectomy, often concomitant with the commencement of oral feedings.

This "turning point" from catabolism to anabolism is referred to as the corticoid-withdrawal phase because it is characterized by a spontaneous sodium and free-water diuresis, a positive potassium balance, and a reduction in nitrogen excretion. This transitional phase usually lasts only 1 to 2 days.

The patient then enters a prolonged period of early anabolism characterized by positive nitrogen balance and weight gain. Protein synthesis is increased following sustained enteral feedings, and this change is related to the return of lean body mass and muscular strength.

The fourth and final phase of surgical convalescence is late anabolism, the hallmark of which is much slower weight gain.

During this period, the patient is in nitrogen equilibrium but in positive carbon balance, which follows deposition of body fat.

MODIFYING POSTOPERATIVE RESPONSES. Early investigators who studied the catabolic responses following operation concluded that these responses were "obligatory" and irreversible. However, Riegel and associates supplied adequate energy and nitrogen to postoperative patients by feeding tube and greatly diminished the catabolic response to operation.[24] Holden and associates supported gastrectomy patients with intravenous nutrients and noted that weight was maintained and near nitrogen balance was achieved.[12] Thus, the catabolic response to an elective operation is due in large part to inadequate food intake and is not an obligatory consequence of operative stress.

A variety of human studies have shown that many postoperative responses can be ablated following denervation of the wound. Kehlet and colleagues used epidural or spinal anesthesia in women undergoing elective abdominal hysterectomy.[17] With epidural anesthesia extending from S5 to T4, plasma concentrations of cortisol, aldosterone, glucose, and free fatty acids remained normal, in contrast to increased concentrations in patients receiving general anesthesia alone. Other workers have extended these observations and have reported that low spinal anesthesia blocks the elevation of catecholamines, hyperglycemia, and inhibition of insulin release observed in patients undergoing surgical procedures on the lower half of the body. These observations suggest that regional anesthetic techniques block afferent signals from the wound and interrupt sympathetic nervous efferent signals to the adrenal gland and possibly the liver. The effect of sympathetic blockade is a reduction in the apparent magnitude of the stress response.

Increased insulin administration in patients receiving parenteral nutrition may also be beneficial. Insulin attenuates cortisol-induced breakdown of skeletal muscle protein *in vitro*, and Finley and associates demonstrated improved nitrogen utilization in patients receiving total parenteral nutrition and insulin after operation.[15] Critically ill patients are much less sensitive to the hypoglycemic effects of insulin than are normal individuals; therefore, exogenous insulin administration at levels higher than those required to prevent excessive hyperglycemia may be of clinical benefit.

Growth hormone is another anabolic hormone that may improve the response to injury. Manson and co-workers administered a hypocaloric diet (with an adequate amount of nitrogen) to normal individuals.[18] Subjects who also received daily doses of recombinant human growth hormone achieved positive nitrogen balance. Small doses of growth hormone (approximately 3 to 4 mg. per day) and a hypocaloric diet were administered to patients after elective gastrectomy or colectomy.[16] The subjects received parenteral nutrition containing 20 calories per kg. per day and 1 gm. protein per kg. per day. Injections of drug or placebo were given daily during the first week after operation. The 9 control subjects lost 3.3 kg. (5.9 per cent of preoperative weight) and had a cumulative nitrogen loss of 32.6 ± 4.2 gm. per 8 days. The patients receiving growth hormone lost significantly less weight (1.3 kg.), and nitrogen loss was 7.1 ± 3.1 gm. per 8 days (p < 0.001) (Fig. 5). Kinetic studies showed that the anabolic effects of growth hormone were associated with increased protein synthesis, and amino acid flux studies across the forearm revealed increased uptake of amino acid nitrogen in the patients treated with growth hormone. Body compositional analysis revealed that the patients receiving growth hormone maintained their lean body mass despite the major surgical procedure.

RESPONSES TO ACCIDENTAL INJURY

GENERAL FEATURES AND TIME COURSE. Events that occur following injury are generally graded responses: the more

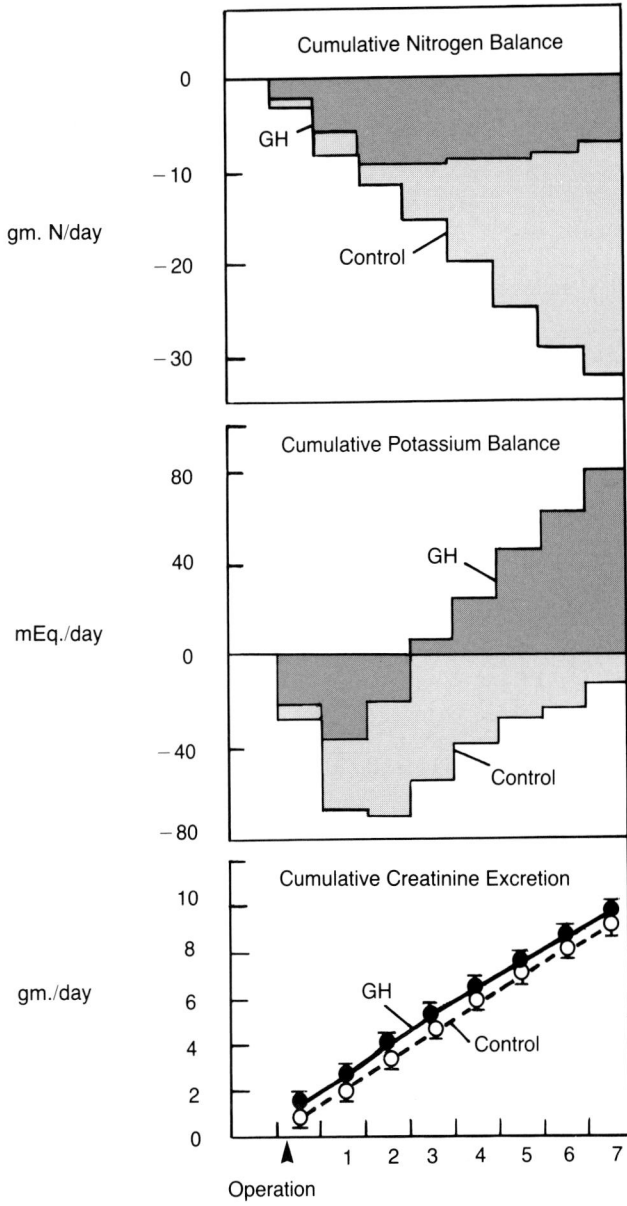

Figure 5. The cumulative nitrogen balance was significantly different between groups from postoperative days 3 to 7. Potassium balance tended to follow nitrogen balance. Creatinine excretion was similar in both groups of patients, confirming the adequacy of urinary collection. (Redrawn from Jiang, Z.M., He, G. Z., Zhang, S. Y., Wang, X. R., Yang, N. F., Zhu, Y., and Wilmore, D. W.: Low-dose growth hormone and hypocaloric nutrition attenuate the protein-catabolic response after major operation. Ann. Surg., *210*:514, 1989.)

severe the injury, the greater the response (Fig. 6). The response generally increases until a maximal level is reached; injury severity over and above this level simply causes a maximal response.

Responses to injury change with time, and events occurring at various points in time were initially described as periods of "ebb" and "flow." The early phase ("ebb" phase or low-flow phase) occurred immediately after injury and was characterized by a fall in metabolic functions and a decrease in core temperature but increased levels of stress hormones.[31] Blood glucose might fall to hypoglycemic levels if the patient could not be resuscitated and measurements were made in the terminal state. With restoration of blood flow and with time, the patient's responses changed (Table 7). The metabolic rate rose, body tem-

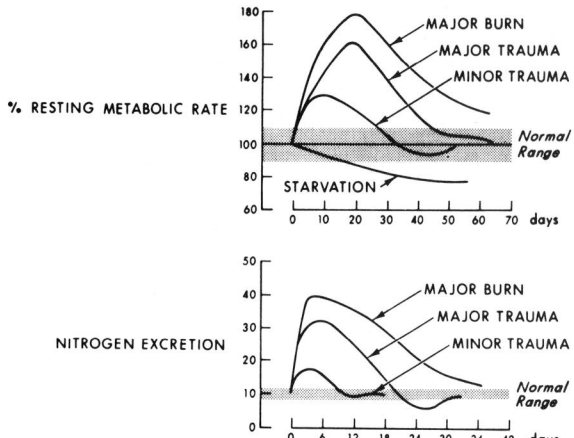

Figure 6. Hypermetabolism and increased nitrogen excretion are closely related following minor or major trauma or major burn injury. Patients received 12 gm. of nitrogen intake per day. (Adapted from Kinney, J. M.: Energy deficits in acute illness and injury. *In* Morgan, A. P. (Ed.): Proceedings of a Conference on Energy Metabolism and Body Fuel Utilization. Cambridge, Harvard University Press, 1966, p. 174.)

perature became elevated, and blood insulin levels were normal or even increased, as were catecholamines, glucose, and blood lactate. Free fatty acid levels were generally normal or decreased. These changes occurred during the "flow" phase, which is also referred to as the chronic or hyperdynamic phase of injury. It was later realized that many of the early changes were related to hypovolemia and organ perfusion; with resuscitation of the patient and restoration of circulating blood volume, flow phase responses occurred rapidly. Aside from research directed toward improved shock resuscitation, most investigative work has now been focused on the later or hyperdynamic phase of injury when wound closure, nutritional support, prevention of infection, and respiratory support are central to patient care.

Several other characteristics of the metabolic responses to injury may confound interpretation of the patient's response. *Complications* occur in injured patients, particularly the complication of infection, and these effects appear additive to injury responses. *Treatment variables* alter injury responses, and factors such as repeated operative procedures, use of steroids, patient paralysis during mechanical ventilation, use of positive end-expiratory pressure, and administration of pressor drugs are therapies that alter hemodynamics and metabolism and thus may influence usual responses.

A variety of factors unique to each individual patient influence the metabolic responses to injury. For example, *body com-*

positional status reflects the quantity of fat and protein available for metabolic pathways. A muscular male weight lifter loses more protein following a standard stress than does a nonexercising individual of comparable size. Because muscle mass is reduced with age, elderly patients lose less protein following operation than do younger individuals. Age also influences a variety of other homeostatic responses, since maximal function of most vital organ systems (heart, kidneys, lungs) is reduced in the elderly. These alterations limit the ability of the aged patient to adjust to stresses of critical illness to the extent comparable to that observed in a younger person. Diminished physiologic responses in the elderly may represent the high mortality that occurs in this age group when complications occur.

INITIATION OF INJURY RESPONSES: HOW DO WE KNOW WHEN WE ARE INJURED? Following injury, three general types of stimuli signal the central nervous system to initiate homeostatic adjustment.

1. *Afferent sensory nerve fibers* provide the most direct and the quickest route for signals to arrive at the central nervous system (CNS) following stress. It has frequently been suggested that pain may serve as the initial afferent signal following injury, and a variety of studies suggest that the afferent nerve signals from the injured area are essential for the stimulation of the pituitary-adrenal axis.[13] The adrenocortical response to injury was not observed in animals after section of the peripheral nerves to the area of injury, transection of the spinal cord above the injury, or section through the medulla oblongata (Fig. 7). A similar pattern of response to denervation before injury has been described in humans. Both growth hormone and ACTH levels in the serum rise within 1 hour following incision in patients receiving general anesthesia and undergoing cholecystectomy or inguinal herniorrhaphy. However, this hormonal response did not occur in patients undergoing herniorrhaphy who received spinal anesthesia, nor did the usual rise in serum cortisol levels occur in patients undergoing abdominal procedures when epidural blockade was utilized in conjunction with the general anesthetic.[17,27] Studies of the pituitary-adrenal axis following operation in paraplegic patients demonstrate a markedly diminished cortisol response when the operation is performed in a denervated area. Nerve afferents also appear to stimulate the elaboration of ADH following trauma. In addition, a number of factors that accompany the "stress" of critical illness — restraint, immobilization, environmental disturbances — most likely alter afferent nerve impulses and affect the response to injury.

2. *Fluid loss from the vascular compartment* causes stimulation of volume and pressure receptors, initiating a series of CNS-mediated cardiovascular adjustments. Cardiac output falls, pe-

TABLE 7. Alterations that Occur Following Injury

"Ebb" Phase	"Flow" Phase
Blood glucose elevated	Glucose normal or slightly elevated
Normal glucose production	Increased glucose production
Free fatty acids elevated	Free fatty acids normal or slightly elevated — flux increased
Insulin concentration low	Insulin concentration normal or elevated
Catecholamines and glucagon elevated	Catecholamines high-normal or elevated; glucagon elevated
Blood lactate elevated	Blood lactate normal
Oxygen consumption depressed	Oxygen consumption elevated
Cardiac output below normal	Cardiac output increased
Core temperature below normal	Core temperature elevated

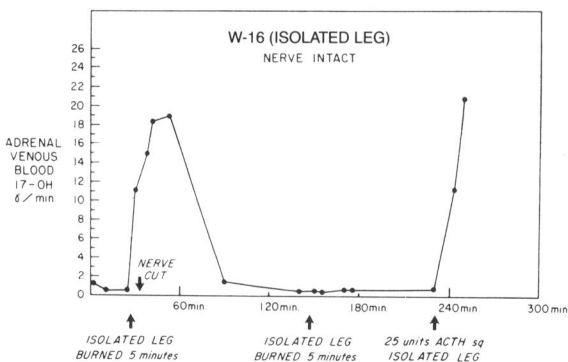

Figure 7. Glucocorticoids are stimulated following injury to the isolated leg, which is attached to the body by only one artery, one vein, and one nerve. The nerve is cut, and the leg is reinjured; a second burn causes no adrenocortical response, demonstrating the importance of sensory nerve stimulation in mediating glucocorticoid output. (From Hume, D. M., and Egdahl, R. H.: The importance of the brain in the endocrine response to injury. Ann. Surg., *150*:697, 1959.)

ripheral resistance increases, and blood is redistributed to vital organs to maintain function. With progressive volume loss into the area of injury, the resulting hypoperfusion reduces tissue oxygenation and causes disturbances in the acid-base equilibrium. Chemoreceptor stimulation thus serves as additional afferent input to both vasomotor and respiratory centers during hypovolemia. Because loss of fluid volume following injury is closely related to the extent of tissue damage, these specific mechanisms allow a quantitative response to occur following trauma (i.e., the response is directly proportional to the size of the injury).

3. *Circulating substances* may directly or indirectly stimulate the CNS and set in motion the injury response. Alterations in serum electrolytes, release of cell breakdown products, changes in the amino acid pattern, and elaboration of endotoxin and the release of cytokines, all originating from or a direct result of the wound, may initiate homeostatic adjustments that develop following injury.

SIGNAL INTEGRATION AND EFFECTOR MECHANISMS: ROLE OF THE CNS, HORMONES, AND TISSUE FACTORS. The brain receives a variety of signals that a "stress" has occurred and integrates this afferent input. Although the sympathetic nervous system is not essential to the adaptation to simple starvation, the CNS is essential to the hypermetabolic response to injury; patients with "brain death" and associated soft tissue injury failed to mount a "flow" phase response. Similarly, in severely burned patients, morphine anesthesia, which markedly reduced hypothalamic function, caused a prompt decrease in hypermetabolism, rectal temperature, and cardiac output.[31] In contrast, however, quadriplegic patients with high spinal cord transections that totally interrupted sympathetic efferent activity failed to generate a febrile response to infection but were able to increase the leukocyte count and blood glucose concentration during sepsis. Moreover, when low-molecular-weight extracts from granulation tissue were injected (both intravenously and subcutaneously) into normal animals, fibroblast proliferation and collagen biosynthesis were observed. These findings suggest that several circulating mediators with direct and specific cellular effects may exist and initiate catabolic responses. However, in all patients with an intact CNS, a variety of adjustments are observed within the hypothalamus and pituitary gland; these alterations in neurohumoral control appear to be specific compensatory adjustments to stress. These alterations in CNS control have an impact on thermoregulation, substrate mobilization, and intraorgan energy transfer.

The most prominent clinical expressions of the hypothalamic alterations are the marked adjustments in thermoregulation that occur following infection and severe injury. At any ambient temperature studied, core and mean skin temperatures of injured patients are above those observed in normal individuals.[2] When allowed to adjust ambient temperature, these febrile patients select a warmer environment than normal persons do to achieve comfort, despite the fact that the patients have elevated core and mean skin temperatures (Table 8). The ambient temperature selected is generally related to the extent of injury or

severity of infection. Administration of a variety of pharmacologic agents known to affect the temperature "set point" in humans has not generally reduced the hypermetabolism and hyperpyrexia that occur following injury, although the newer generation of prostaglandin inhibitors has not been studied.

Other alterations in normal hypothalamic neuroendocrine regulation, such as altered growth hormone release, are observed in starved individuals and in critically ill surgical patients, and these adjustments undoubtedly affect the metabolic responses that are observed.

THE HORMONAL ENVIRONMENT. A variety of hormonal alterations occur in patients following injury; however, cause-and-effect relationships between the hormonal environment and the posttraumatic metabolic alterations have only recently been established. In all phases of injury there is a marked rise in the counterregulatory hormones glucagon, glucocorticoids, and catecholamines. In contrast, plasma concentrations of the patient's anabolic hormone insulin may be low, normal, or elevated (Fig. 8). During the "ebb" phase of injury, the sympatheticoadrenal axis primarily serves to maintain the pressure-flow relationships necessary for maintenance of organ perfusion. With the onset of hypermetabolism, characteristic of the "flow" phase of injury, these and other hormones exert a variety of metabolic effects, detailed in the following.

INSULIN. During the "ebb" (shock) phase of injury, insulin concentrations are low, even in the presence of hyperglycemia. This effect is due to the regulation of the endocrine pancreas by the sympathetic nervous system; in this case, insulin release is inhibited by alpha-adrenergic stimulation, whereas beta-receptor stimulation augments insulin elaboration. Insulin inhibition accounts in part for the posttraumatic hyperglycemia and thus allows glucose to be utilized primarily by non-insulin-mediated tissues, i.e., the brain and the peripheral nervous system.

During the "flow" or hypermetabolic phase of injury, insulin concentrations are normal or increased. However, the effects of these elevated insulin concentrations on peripheral tissues (skeletal muscle and fat) are blunted.[7] The cause of the marked insulin resistance is related to diminished food intake and an altered hormonal environment that exerts anti-insulin activity.[5] The "counterregulatory" hormones *glucagon, cortisol,* and *catecholamines* oppose the storage or anabolic functions of insulin. In the short term, they maintain blood glucose levels and prevent hypoglycemia. More chronic hormonal elaboration accelerates body catabolism.

GLUCAGON. Glucagon elaboration is regulated by blood glucose concentration (hypoglycemia stimulates glucagon release) and the sympathetic nervous system (beta-agonists stimulate glucagon release), signals that also influence insulin elaboration. However, these pancreatic hormones are generally released in a reciprocal manner: when insulin is stimulated, glucagon is suppressed, favoring anabolism and protein conservation, and when glucagon is elaborated relative to insulin, there is increased glycogenolysis, gluconeogenesis, and ureagenesis at the expense of protein biosynthesis.

GLUCOCORTICOIDS. Glucocorticoids are also released following

TABLE 8. Ambient Comfort Temperature Selected by Normal Subjects and Injured Patients (mean ± S.E.M.)

	Number	Burn Size*	Room Comfort Temperature (°C)	Mean Skin Temperature (°C)	Core Temperature (°C)
Normal subjects	5	0	27.8 ± 0.6	33.4 ± 0.6	36.9 ± 0.1
Burn patients	9	39	30.4 ± 0.7	35.2 ± 0.4	38.4 ± 0.3
			p < 0.05	p < 0.05	p < 0.01

*Burn size expressed in percentage of total body surface.
Adapted from Wilmore, D. W., Orcutt, T. W., Mason, A. D., Jr., and Pruitt, B. A., Jr.: Alterations in hypothalamic function following thermal injury. J. Trauma, 15:697, 1975.

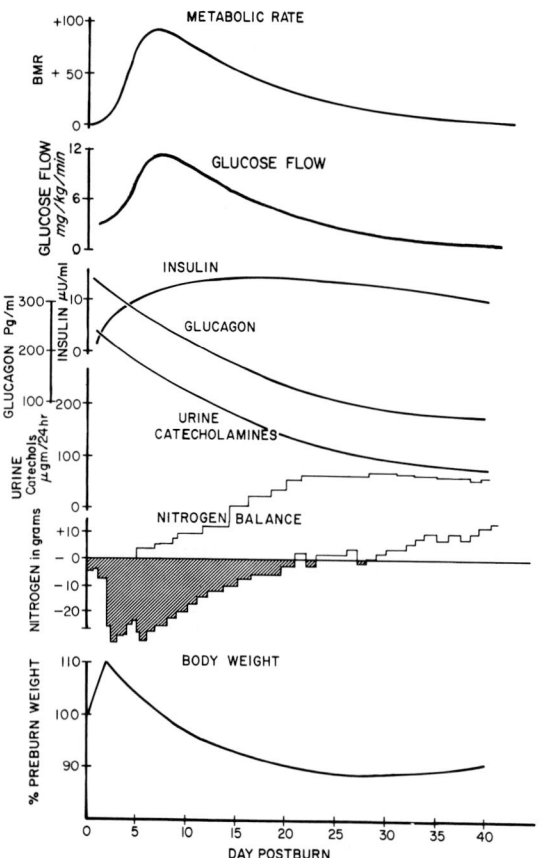

Figure 8. The increased rate of hepatic glucose production (glucose flow) parallels the hypermetabolic response following thermal injury. Increased gluconeogenesis is associated in time with negative nitrogen balance and high levels of glucagon and catecholamines relative to insulin. Cortisol concentrations (not shown) parallel glucagon and catecholamine alterations. As these hormonal mediators return to normal, oxygen consumption and hepatic glucose production fall and nitrogen balance becomes positive.

stress, and steroids have potent effects on substrate and mineral metabolism. Cortisol is elaborated in response to increasing concentrations of ACTH released from the anterior pituitary gland. Cortisol mobilizes amino acids from skeletal muscle and increases hepatic gluconeogenesis. Cortisol also causes marked insulin resistance, and these effects cause the marked hyperglycemia associated with acute illness.[5]

CATECHOLAMINES. Elaboration of catecholamines—epinephrine and norepinephrine—may be the most basic of the hormonal responses to stress.[31] Epinephrine is stored in the adrenal medulla and liberated into the bloodstream in response to nerve stimulation. This circulating hormone is a potent beta-receptor stimulant, particularly at lower concentrations, and exerts a variety of regulatory effects on cardiac output, regional circulation, blood glucose, and oxidative metabolism. Epinephrine stimulates glycogenolysis, which, in skeletal muscle, promotes lactate production. In addition, epinephrine at higher concentrations markedly inhibits insulin elaboration, thus facilitating amino acid and fat mobilization.

Norepinephrine is elaborated from nerve endings, and this neuromediator exerts direct effects on innervated tissue, such as blood vessels and visceral organs. Sympathetic nerve stimulation causes a discrete effect, depending on the localization of the nerve ending. With sustained stimulation, some norepinephrine diffuses from the synaptic cleft into the bloodstream and thus may exert regulatory effects on distant organs.

The infusion of any one of these "catabolic" hormones alone in normal individuals caused only minimal alterations in metabolism and circulation. However, when the three hormones were infused together, the effects were synergistic, and sustained hepatic glucose production was observed. Bessey and associates utilized similar infusions in fed normal subjects infused over 74 hours.[5] Negative nitrogen balance, gluconeogenesis, and hypermetabolism were observed, associated with salt and water retention, all major components of the injury response (Table 9). Watters and associates administered a similar hormonal mix to fasting volunteers. In addition to the catabolic responses just noted, hyperglycemia occurred and ketosis of fasting was attenuated.[30] Thus, it appears that the simultaneous elaboration of the counterregulatory hormones glucagon, cortisol, and epinephrine is responsible in part for the posttraumatic changes.

THE ROLE OF CYTOKINES. Another regulatory component appears to mediate other changes that occur following injury. Inflammation associated with wound repair generates a variety of signals such as substance P, bradykinin, and prostaglandins. Whereas most of these signals serve to direct local inflammatory events, some may reach the bloodstream and alter systemic metabolism. Such a molecule is the lymphokine interleukin-1 (IL-1), a substance generated by stimulated macrophages, both in the wound and in those cells fixed in the reticuloendothelial system. IL-1 stimulates a variety of responses commonly observed in the critically ill host, including the mobilization of leukocytes, the stimulation of fever, the redistribution of circulating iron and other trace minerals, and the hepatic stimulation of acute-phase protein synthesis.

Tumor necrosis factor, also known as cachectin, is another substance elaborated by activated macrophages that mediates many of the responses following endotoxin and severe infection.[19] This factor may serve primarily as an autocrine and paracrine mediator, aiding local host defense and wound repair. However, when this substance overflows into the bloodstream, severe systemic responses may be observed, including hyperpyrexia, rigors, and septic shock (Fig. 9). Other substances that participate in the stress response and may be viewed as systemic mediators include IL-2,[20] IL-6, and interferon-gamma. The cytokines may amplify a variety of immunologic and hormonal signals, and thus act synergistically to mediate inflammatory responses. Thus, in addition to hormonal regulation, the presence of a wound elicits additional signals that stimulate additional responses or augment hormone-directed changes in metabolism.

CHARACTERISTICS OF THE FLOW PHASE OF THE INJURY RESPONSE

HYPERMETABOLISM. Following injury, oxygen consumption rises above basal levels predicted on the basis of age, sex, and body size. The metabolic rate is usually determined by measuring the exchange of respiratory gases and calculating heat production from oxygen consumption and carbon dioxide produc-

TABLE 9. Effect of Infusion of Cortisol, Glucagon, and Epinephrine on Metabolism

	Saline	Hormones*
Metabolic rate (kcal./m.²/hr.)	32.24 ± 1.05	38.42 ± 1.31
Nitrogen balance (gm./day)	-0.2 ± 0.4	-3.2 ± 0.4
Protein catabolic rate (gm. N/day)	38.4 ± 1.9	46.5 ± 2.5
Plasma glucose (mg./100 ml.)	94 ± 2	133 ± 4
Serum insulin (μunit/ml.)	8 ± 1	22 ± 3
Glucose production rate (mg./kg./min.)	2.08 ± 0.06	2.55 ± 0.06
Insulin-mediated glucose disposal (mg./kg./min.)	8.62 ± 0.51	3.22 ± 0.51
Insulin-mediated forearm glucose uptake (mg./100 ml. forearm/min.)	1.03 ± 0.09	0.48 ± 0.12

*All significantly different from control values.

Adapted from Bessey, P. Q., Watters, J. M., Aoki, T. T., and Wilmore, D. W.: Combined hormone infusion simulates the metabolic response to injury. Ann. Surg., *200*:264, 1984.

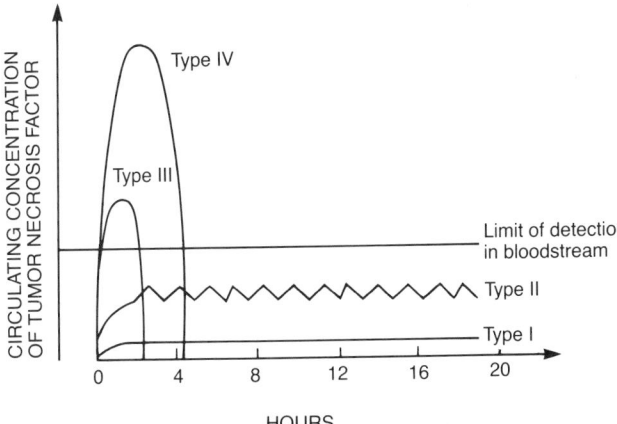

Figure 9. Different states of inflammation/infection are likely to be associated with different patterns of cytokine release into the bloodstream. For example, Type I demonstrates responses that occur with a small wound or localized cellulitis; local responses predominate and systemic levels are absent. Type II is representative of a larger wound (femoral fracture) or infection (appendiceal abscess) that persists for some time to stimulate systemic manifestations of the inflammatory state. The cytokine signal is weak, undetectable in the bloodstream by current techniques, but sufficient to stimulate other tissues. Type III response might follow an infection of the biliary tree or bladder. With operation to resolve the obstruction, endotoxin occurs producing a short-lived but high-amplitude signal. Hyperpyrexia, rigors, and other symptoms occur. Type IV is the manifestation of severe sepsis, such as following peritoneal decontamination. A very high amplitude signal occurs, causing vasodilation, increased vascular permeability, and irreversible septic shock. (From Michie, H. R., and Wilmore, D. W.: Sepsis: Signals and surgical sequelae. Arch. Surg. 125:531, 1990.)

tion. The degree of hypermetabolism (i.e., increased oxygen production) is generally related to the severity of the injury. Patients with long bone fractures exhibit a 15 to 25 per cent increase in metabolic rate, whereas those with multiple injuries increase metabolic needs by 50 per cent. Patients with severe burn injuries (greater than 50 per cent of the body surface area) demonstrate resting metabolic rates that may reach twice basal levels. These rates of heat production in trauma patients are contrasted with those that occur in postoperative patients, who rarely increase their basal metabolic rate by more than 10 to 15 per cent following operation.

Concomitant with the development of hypermetabolism, the trauma patient usually develops a 1 to 2° C. elevation in body temperature. This posttraumatic fever is a well-recognized component of the injury response, represents an upward shift in the thermoregulatory set point of the brain,[2] and is probably the consequence of increased levels of circulating IL-1. In general, if this febrile response is not marked (less than 38.5° C.) and the patient is asymptomatic, the fever is rarely treated.

ALTERATIONS IN PROTEIN METABOLISM. Extensive urinary nitrogen loss occurs following major injury. Because of the magnitude of these losses and the progressive wasting of skeletal muscle mass and associated muscle weakness, it was originally hypothesized that the nitrogen loss was a generalized and accelerated breakdown of muscle protein.[11] Like other responses, the loss of nitrogen following injury is related to the extent of the trauma but also depends on the age, sex, and previous nutritional status of the patient, since these factors determine, in part, the size of the muscle mass.

Whereas nitrogen balance studies demonstrate marked negative nitrogen balance following injury, these studies reflect only *net* nitrogen catabolism and not the absolute rate of nitrogen breakdown. In normal individuals, nitrogen equilibrium is maintained by a careful balance between rates of protein synthesis and degradation. Negative nitrogen balance occurs if the breakdown rate increases and protein synthesis remains the same or if the breakdown rate remains the same and the rate of synthesis decreases. The use of isotopically labeled, nonra-

dioactive amino acids allows quantification of the alterations in synthesis and breakdown rates associated with a wide variety of disease processes. Such studies have demonstrated that protein synthesis is *diminished in normal subjects* when food is restricted or prolonged bed rest is imposed. In contrast, protein breakdown is *accelerated* in *injured* or *septic patients*. Feeding these individuals *elevates* protein synthesis to match breakdown and therefore achieves nitrogen balance (Table 10).

That muscle is the origin of the nitrogen loss in the urine following extensive injury was initially suggested by Cuthbertson.[11] However, it has only recently been recognized that the composition of amino acid efflux from skeletal muscle does not reflect the composition of muscle protein. Alanine and glutamine constitute the majority of amino acids released, whereas each comprises only about 6 per cent of muscle protein. The branched chain amino acids (valine, leucine, and isoleucine), however, comprise approximately 6 per cent of the released amino acids but constitute nearly 15 per cent of muscle protein. Glutamate can serve as a precursor for glutamine synthesis or as an amino donor for alanine synthesis. These coupled reactions could explain the synthesis and increased release of alanine and glutamine, as well as the diminished release of branched chain amino acids. Oxidation of branched chain amino acids by skeletal muscle is accelerated following injury, and skeletal muscle release of glutamine and alanine is increased.[1,9] Glutamine is extracted by the kidneys, where it contributes ammonium groups for ammonia generation, a process that produces the net loss of acid, and this effect can be augmented by the administration of glucocorticoids.[26] Glutamine is also taken up by the gastrointestinal tract, where it serves as an oxidative fuel. The gut enterocytes convert glutamine primarily to ammonia and alanine, and these two substances are released into the portal venous blood. The ammonia is then removed by the liver and converted to urea, and the alanine may also be removed by the liver and serve as a gluconeogenic precursor. Following the stress of a standard laparotomy, glutamine consumption by the bowel and the kidneys is accelerated,[25] and the reaction appears to be regulated by the increased elaboration of the glucocorticoids.[26] While skeletal muscle releases alanine at an accelerated rate, the gastrointestinal tract and kidneys also accelerate the production of alanine. This amino acid is extracted by the liver and used in the synthesis of glucose and acute-phase proteins. Therefore, glutamine and alanine are important compounds that participate in the transfer of nitrogen from skeletal muscle to visceral organs. However, their metabolic pathways favor the production of urea and ammonia, which are lost from the body (Fig. 10).

ALTERATIONS IN GLUCOSE METABOLISM. Hyperglycemia commonly occurs following injury. Hepatic glucose production is increased, and the accelerated gluconeogenesis tends generally to be related to the extent of the injury.[33] Much of the new glucose generated by the liver in injured patients arises from 3-carbon precursors (lactate, pyruvate, amino acids, and glycerol) released from peripheral tissues.

TABLE 10. Alterations in Rates of Protein Synthesis and Catabolism that May Affect Hospitalized Patients

	Synthesis*	Catabolism*
Normal—starvation	↓	0
Normal—fed, bed rest	↓	0
Elective surgical procedure	↓↓	0
Injury/sepsis—IV dextrose	↑↑	↑↑↑
Injury/sepsis—fed	↑↑↑	↑↑↑

*Key: ↓ decrease; ↑ increase; 0, no change.
Adapted from Wilmore, D. W.: The Metabolic Management of the Critically Ill. New York, Plenum Medical Book Company, 1977.

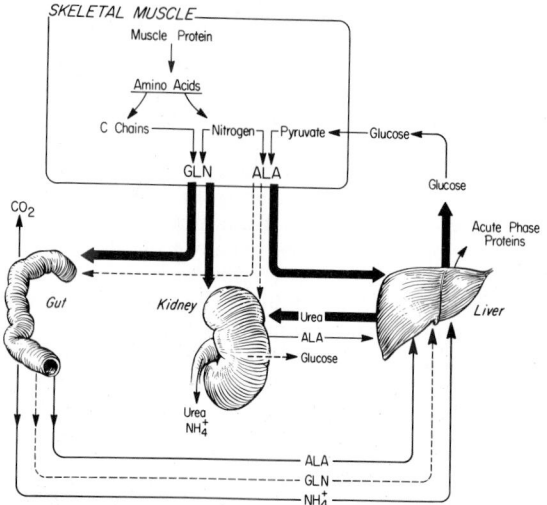

Figure 10. The pathways involved for the handling of amino acids following skeletal muscle proteolysis. Alanine and other amino acids are converted in the liver to glucose, with the nitrogen residue forming urea. Glutamine is oxidized by the bowel as a primary fuel; the ammonia liberated is transported via the portal system to the liver to form urea. The kidney utilizes the glutamine nitrogen to form ammonia and buffer organic acids. All these pathways represent the "obligatory" loss of nitrogen from the body during stress.

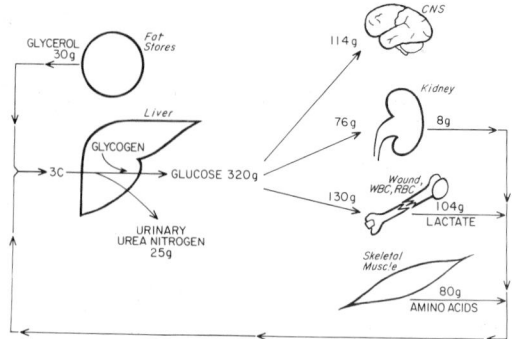

Figure 11. Accelerated hepatic glucose production following injury supplies the increased glucose requirements for the kidney and inflammatory cells of the wound. Normal glucose uptake occurs in the central nervous system. The wound converts most of the glucose to lactate, which is recycled to the liver (the Cori cycle) and reconverted to glucose. Glucose oxidized by the brain and kidney is replaced by amino acids arising from skeletal muscle, with a smaller portion coming from glycerol released during lipolysis.

Studies have been performed to determine the sites of utilization of the glucose produced by the liver. First, glucose uptake was measured across injured and uninjured extremities. Net glucose flux across uninjured extremities was low, suggesting that fat, not glucose, was the primary fuel for resting skeletal muscle in the postabsorptive state. Similar observations have been made in normal volunteers. However, increased glucose uptake occurred across the injured extremity.[32] In addition, the injured extremity released large quantities of lactate, which represented as much as 80 per cent of the glucose consumed. This is consistent with knowledge of the biochemistry of the highly specialized cells of the wound and inflammatory tissue (fibroblasts, macrophages, leukocytes), which undergo anaerobic metabolism and demonstrate a large capacity for lactate production. Additional measurements of blood flow and substrate concentration differences across the kidneys and brain further characterize the glucose disposal in resting patients after injury. The glucose consumed by the CNS in the injured patient is approximately normal (120 gm. per day), whereas the rate of glucose consumed by the kidneys is approximately twice normal (75 gm. per day). Only a small fraction of the glucose is taken up by the resting skeletal muscle, and the remainder is consumed by the wound (Fig. 11). The wound converts most of the glucose to lactate, which is recycled to the liver in the Cori cycle. For example, infusion of a small glucose load (2 mg. per kg. per minute) generally suppresses hepatic glucose production in normal individuals. Similar infusions in trauma patients fail to inhibit hepatic glucose production. In other studies, insulin was infused and blood glucose was maintained by a variable infusion of 20 per cent glucose. Hyperinsulinemia completely suppresses glucose production in normal subjects, whereas endogenous glucose production is only partially reduced in trauma patients despite high concentrations of insulin.[6]

To quantitate the extent of insulin resistance in peripheral tissues, Brooks and associates measured glucose uptake across the uninjured forearm in conjunction with insulin infusions and euglycemia.[7] Glucose uptake by uninjured forearm skeletal muscle of trauma patients was markedly diminished when compared with the uptake observed in controls.

Thus, profound insulin insensitivity occurs in injured patients. These effects do not occur because of inadequate quantities of insulin released from the endocrine pancreas, for in most cases hyperinsulinemia exists. However, similar effects are observed following alterations in the hormonal environment. For example, insulin-mediated forearm glucose uptake is markedly diminished in normal subjects following 2 hours of epinephrine infusion. Similarly, 3 days of glucocorticoid administration decreases insulin-stimulated forearm glucose uptake.[6]

ALTERATIONS IN FAT METABOLISM. To support hypermetabolism, increased gluconeogenesis, and interorgan substrate flux, stored triglyceride is mobilized and oxidized at an accelerated rate. This may be the result of continuous sympathetic nervous system stimulation. Although there is accelerated mobilization and utilization of free fatty acids in injured subjects, ketosis during brief starvation is blunted, and the accelerated protein catabolism remains uncontrolled. If severely injured patients are unfed, their fat and protein stores are rapidly depleted. Such malnutrition increases susceptibility to added stresses of hemorrhage, operation, and infection and may contribute to organ system failure, sepsis, and death.

CIRCULATORY ADJUSTMENTS. In the initial phase of injury, blood volume is reduced, peripheral resistance increases, and cardiac output falls. With resuscitation and restoration of blood volume, cardiac output returns to normal and then increases, a characteristic of the "flow" of hyperdynamic phase of injury. This augmented blood flow is necessary to maintain wound perfusion and increased demands of visceral organs. Marked vasodilation occurs in vessels that perfuse injured areas, and this is accompanied by the ingrowth of new capillaries.

The neurovasculature of a large wound appears to be released from central neurogenic regulation, although it is not known if this effect is the result of actual physical disruption of vasomotor efferent nerves or interference with neuromuscular transmission in innervated vessels due to the local inflammatory factors. This loss of neural control allows local environmental factors to exert a major influence on wound blood flow. Control of wound circulation is similar to other critical tissues (heart, brain, working skeletal muscle), in which blood flow varies as a function of local metabolic conditions rather than being part of integrated central vasoregulatory reflexes. This implies that as long as blood pressure is maintained, wound perfusion is ensured.

SUMMARY

Homeostatic adjustments constantly occur in surgical patients in an effort to maintain the *milieu interieur* and ensure wound healing. Multiple factors, including diminished blood volume, tissue underperfusion, reduced food intake, extensive tissue damage, and invasive infection, initiate these responses via the neuroendocrine system. As a result of these physiologic adjustments, tissue perfusion is maintained, which supports the increased metabolic demands accompanying critical illness. Increased skeletal muscle proteolysis and accelerated gluconeogenesis are coupled responses that also occur; these biochemical alterations provide essential nutrients to support vital organ function and wound repair.

An elective or semielective operative procedure in the previously healthy patient stimulates minor catabolic changes when present-day anesthetic and operative techniques are successfully employed. However, multiple injuries, large burns, invasive infections, and major operative procedures in patients with minimal "physiologic reserve," such as the elderly, require constant intervention on the part of the surgeon to help maintain the internal environment and aid recovery. As a result, patients with catabolic illnesses can sustain near-maximal stresses and yet heal their wounds and resolve their infections. With appropriate support of bodily changes, body composition and function are restored, and the patients return to a useful and normal life.

SELECTED REFERENCES

Cannon, W. B.: The Wisdom of the Body. New York, W. W. Norton and Company, 1939.
A condensation of many experiments by the author, describing how the body adjusts to "stresses." After spending a lifetime of work in the area of physiologic regulation, the author summarized his views on the importance of neuroendocrine regulation in body homeostasis.

Cuthbertson, D. P.: The disturbance of metabolism produced by bony and non-bony injury, with notes on certain abnormal conditions of bone. Biochem. J., 24:1244, 1930.

Cuthbertson, D. P.: Observations on the disturbance of metabolism produced by injury to the limbs. Q. J. Med., 1:233, 1932.
These papers present the first major quantitative evidence that altered metabolism occurs following accidental injury of the long bones. These works serve as the bases for all modern-day investigations of endocrine, biochemical, and metabolic responses to catabolic illness.

Hume, D. M., and Egdahl, R. H.: The importance of the brain in the endocrine response to injury. Ann. Surg., 150:697, 1959.
The authors describe for the first time the importance of neural pathways to activate responses following injury and other stress. Nerve transection and central nervous system ablation experiments demonstrated that specific injury responses could be attenuated when the central nervous system was removed from the reflex arc. This paper serves as the experimental basis for pharmacologic therapy that diminishes responses to stress.

Moore, F. D.: The Metabolic Care of the Surgical Patient. Philadelphia, W. B. Saunders Company, 1959.
An overwhelming accumulation of knowledge written in orderly, logical, and understandable manner, with implications for patient treatment clearly outlined. The author presents his own data and reviews other published studies to reach his conclusions. There are few surgical texts that represent "landmarks" in personal accomplishment. This is one!

REFERENCES

1. Aulick, L. H., and Wilmore, D. W.: Increased peripheral amino acid release following burn injury. Surgery, 85:560, 1979.
2. Aulick, L. H., and Wilmore, D. W.: Hypermetabolism in trauma. *In* Girardier, L., and Stock, M. J. (Eds.): Mammalian Thermogenesis. London, Chapman and Hall, 1983, p. 259.
3. Beisel, W. R.: Metabolic response to infection. Ann. Rev. Med., 26:9, 1975.
4. Bernard, C.: Introduction to the Study of Experimental Medicine. Green, H. C. (Trans). New York, The Macmillan Company, 1927.
5. Bessey, P. Q., Watters, J. M., Aoki, T. T., and Wilmore, D. W.: Combined hormonal infusion simulates the metabolic response to injury. Ann. Surg., 200:264, 1984.
6. Black, P. R., Brooks, D. C., Bessey, P. Q., Wolfe, R. R., and Wilmore, D. W.: Mechanisms of insulin resistance following injury. Ann. Surg., 196:420, 1982.
7. Brooks, D. C., Bessey, P. Q., Black, P. R., Aoki, T. T., and Wilmore, D. W.: Posttraumatic insulin resistance in uninjured skeletal muscle. J. Surg. Res., 37:100, 1984.
8. Cahill, G. F., Jr.: Starvation in man. N. Engl. J. Med., 282:668, 1970.
9. Cannon, W. B.: The Wisdom of the Body. New York, W. W. Norton and Company, 1939.
10. Cohn, S. H., Vartsky, D., Yasumura, S., Sawitsky, A., Zanai, I., Vaswani, A., and Ellis, K. J.: Compartmental body composition based on total body nitrogen, potassium, and calcium. Am. J. Physiol., 239:E524, 1980.
11. Cuthbertson, D. P.: The disturbance of metabolism produced by bone and non-bony injury, with notes on certain abnormal conditions of bone. Biochem. J., 24:1244, 1930.
12. Holden, W. D., Krieger, H., Levey, S., and Abbott, W. E.: The effects of nutrition on nitrogen metabolism in surgical patients. Ann. Surg., 146:563, 1957.
13. Hume, D. M., and Egdahl, R. H.: The importance of the brain in the endocrine response to injury. Ann. Surg., 150:697, 1959.
14. Hunter, J.: A Treatise on the Blood Inflammation and Gunshot Wounds. London, 1794.
15. Inculet, R. I., Finley, R. J., Duff, J. H., Pace, R., Clive, R., Groves, A. C., and Woolf, L. I.: Insulin decreases muscle protein loss after operative trauma in man. Surgery, 99:752, 1986.
16. Jiang, Z.-M., He, G.-Z., Zhang, S.-Y., Wang, X.-R., Yang, N.-F., Zhu, Y., and Wilmore, D. W.: Low-dose growth hormone and hypocaloric nutrition attenuate the protein-catabolic response after major operation. Ann. Surg., 210:514, 1989.
17. Kehlet, H.: Modification of responses to surgery and anesthesia by neural blockade. *In* Cousins, M. J., and Bridenbaugh, P. O. (Eds.): Neural Blockade in Clinical Anesthesia and Management of Pain. Philadelphia, J. B. Lippincott Company, 1987, p. 145.
18. Manson, J., and Wilmore, D. W.: Positive nitrogen balance with human growth hormone and hypocaloric intravenous feedings. Surgery, 100:188, 1986.
19. Michie, H. R., Manogue, K. R., Spriggs, D. R., Revhaug, A., O'Dwyer, S. T., Dinarello, C. A., Cerami, A., Wolff, S. M., and Wilmore, D. W.: Detection of circulating tumor necrosis factor during endotoxemia in humans. N. Engl. J. Med., 318:1481, 1988.
20. Michie, H. R., Eberline, T. J., Spriggs, D. R., Manogue, K. R., Cerami, A., and Wilmore, D. W.: Interleukin-2 initiates metabolic responses associated with critical illness in humans. Ann. Surg., 208:493, 1988.
21. Moore, F. D.: The Metabolic Care of the Surgical Patient. Philadelphia, W. B. Saunders Company, 1959.
22. Okusawa, S., Gelfand, J. A., Ikejima, T., Connoly, R. J., and Dinarello, C. A.: Interleukin 1 induces a shock-like state in rabbits: Synergism with tumor necrosis factor and the effect of cyclooxygenase inhibition. J. Clin. Invest., 81:1162, 1988.
23. Philbin, D. M., and Coggins, C. H.: Morphine suppresses effects of antidiuretic hormone following operation. Anesthesiology, 49:95, 1978.
24. Riegel, C., Koop, C. E., Drew, J., Stevens, L. W., and Rhoads, J. E.: The nitrogen requirements for nitrogen balance in surgical patients during the early postoperative period. J. Clin. Invest., 26:18, 1947.
25. Souba, W. W., and Wilmore, D. W.: Postoperative alterations of arteriovenous exchange of amino acids across the gastrointestinal tract. Surgery, 94:342, 1983.
26. Souba, W. W., Smith, R. J., and Wilmore, D. W.: Effects of glucocorticoids on glutamine metabolism in visceral organs. Metabolism, 34:450, 1985.
27. Traynor, C., and Hall, G. M.: Endocrine and metabolic changes during surgery: Anesthetic implications. Br. J. Anesth., 53:153, 1981.
28. Unger, R.: Glucagon and the insulin:glucagon ratio in diabetes and other catabolic illnesses. Diabetes, 20:834, 1971.
29. Voit, F.: Über den Eiweissumatz bei kunstlich erhohter Korpertemperature. Gesellsch. Morphol. Physiol. (München), 11:120, 1895.
30. Watters, J. M., Bessey, P. O., Aoki, T. T., and Wilmore, D. W.: Catabolic hormones suppress adaptation to starvation. Br. J. Surg. 73:108, 1986.
31. Wilmore, D. W.: The Metabolic Management of the Critically Ill. New York, Plenum Medical Book Company, 1977.
32. Wilmore, D. W., Aulick, L. H., Mason, A. D., Jr., and Pruitt, B. A., Jr.: The influence of the burn wound on local and systemic response to injury. Ann. Surg., 186:444, 1977.
33. Wilmore, D. W., Goodwin, C. W., Aulick, L. H., Powanda, M. C., Mason, A. D., Jr., and Pruitt, B. A., Jr.: Effect of injury and infection on visceral metabolism and circulation. Ann. Surg., 192:491, 1980.

3

SHOCK

Causes and Management of Circulatory Collapse

James W. Holcroft, M.D., and F. William Blaisdell, M.D.

HISTORICAL ASPECTS

Insofar as can be determined, the concept of shock was first recognized in the early 1700s. The term *shock* was used in 1743 by an unknown translator of the treatise of LeDran on the management of gunshot wounds.[65] Guthrie, in 1815, as credited by Morris, used the term shock in his book on gunshot wounds of the extremities.[50] In 1872, Samuel D. Gross referred to shock as a "rude unhinging of the machinery of life."[65] John Collins Warren applied the term to "a momentary pause in the act of death" and postulated that shock was a reaction to major injury.[68]

Most of the clinical observations that led to development of the concept of shock were made on the battlefield. When external hemorrhage was massive, the cause of death was easily recognized as hemorrhage. If the patient survived the initial bleeding episode, however, the concept that the patient could still die as a consequence of the initial blood volume loss was difficult to grasp. Indeed, many illnesses were treated by bleeding to remove "toxins in the blood." In 1534, Ambroise Paré, the surgeon who saved battlefield casualties by the judicious use of ligature rather than boiling oil or cautery, believed that phlebotomy was required to treat certain war wounds.[68] In the late 1700s, John Hunter, the founder of many modern surgical concepts, assumed that toxic factors caused death after injuries and advocated bleeding to treat gunshot wounds, provided there was no overt hemorrhage.[39] By the time of the American Civil War, phlebotomy was no longer used to treat shock, but the concept that toxic factors were the primary cause of shock still dominated. Soldiers with major wounds of the extremities died when managed nonoperatively, and extremities were amputated (amputation being the most common operation during the war) to prevent toxic and septic causes of death. Thus, based largely on battlefield observations, the concept of shock became "a term used to describe the morbidity following physical violence to the body."[65]

The laboratory investigations of shock by George W. Crile at the end of the nineteenth century demonstrated in experimental animals that the likelihood of shock increased with the magnitude of injury and that a small hemorrhage preceding injury impaired the animal's ability to survive.[23] Crile found that the central venous pressure fell in shock and that intravenous infusions of saline improved survival rates. He hypothesized that the fluid acted to increase the venous pressure, thereby restoring cardiac filling, cardiac output, blood pressure, and organ perfusion. He erroneously concluded, however, that the final common pathway of shock was failure of autonomic control of the cardiovascular system, as opposed to a deficiency of blood volume. In 1910, Yandel Henderson reiterated the importance of venous return to the heart.[33] He, too, noted the important

relationship between venous return, cardiac output, and arterial blood pressure, but he also failed to recognize that internal loss of plasma or blood could deplete the blood volume and impair filling of the heart.

Perhaps the first major clinical breakthrough in the treatment of shock, beyond control of hemorrhage and debridement of dead tissue, came in World War I. In the beginning of that war, simple fractures of the femur had a mortality of 70 per cent. Introduction of the Thomas splint lowered the mortality to 10 per cent, even in the absence of aggressive fluid resuscitation. The reduced mortality was attributed to reduction of tissue damage and curtailed production of toxic factors.

The battlefield observation that fracture immobilization lowered mortality rates prompted further physiologic investigation. Cannon, an American physiologist, and Bayliss, a British physiologist, studied battlefield casualties, collected clinical descriptions, and measured the physiologic and biochemical changes of patients in shock. In addition, Cannon conducted parallel studies in animals, his models consisting of animals with lacerations and crush injuries. He believed that the systemic effects of shock were caused by toxic products of tissue breakdown. He ascribed shock-induced hypotension to cardiac failure and attributed stagnation of blood in venous reservoirs to loss of vasomotor tone. Cannon noted that shock produced a metabolic acidemia and that the circulation improved with administration of sodium bicarbonate. He postulated that toxic factors, one of them being hydrogen ion, paralyzed vascular tone and hindered venous return.[20]

CURRENT CONCEPTS

At the same time, however, and during the next 20 years between the two great wars, investigators also turned more attention to occult blood volume loss as a primary cause of the hemodynamic abnormalities of shock. In 1917, Archibald and McLean reviewed their experience with blood pressure measurements from casualties of World War I and concluded that hypotension, although one of the signs of severe shock, was not the cause of shock.[3] They emphasized that too much attention had been placed on the significance of blood pressure. Keith, in 1919, documented that blood volume, determined by dye dilution, was decreased in shock.[40] Subsequently, in 1930, Blalock, in experiments on dogs with crush injuries to the thigh, convincingly refuted the toxic theory of Cannon and found that the thigh swelling that followed injury was caused by internal hemorrhage and plasma loss.[15] These internal losses of red blood cells and plasma were sufficient to explain the decrease in blood volume.

During World War II, a board headed by Beecher performed biochemical studies on the wounded at the front line in the

Mediterranean Theater.[8] The major cause of shock was found to be loss of blood volume, which, when severe and protracted, led to metabolic acidosis. The hypothesis that shock was caused by blood volume loss was supported by the advent of blood banks. Mortality rates for simple femoral fractures treated not only by immobilization but also by blood transfusion declined to negligible levels. The blood volume depletion hypothesis was also supported by cardiac catheterization studies by Cournand and colleagues, which showed that the fall in cardiac output paralleled shock-induced fluid loss.[22]

During and after the war, Wiggers developed a hemorrhagic shock model in dogs that consisted of arterial cannulation, with connection of the cannula to a reservoir that was maintained at a constant height above a dog's heart.[75] The animal was anticoagulated and bled into the reservoir so that a constant level of hypotension was maintained. Increments of arterial blood accumulated in the reservoir over a period of hours, and then the level of blood in the reservoir began to fall as the animal accumulated fluid, even though the systemic arterial pressure remained the same. Wiggers called this the decompensatory phase of shock. Subsequent reinfusion of the shed blood at this time was not sufficient to resuscitate the animal.

The failure of animals to recover from hemorrhagic shock after reaching the decompensatory phase in Wiggers' model determined the concept of irreversible shock. This concept was reinforced during the first several years of the Korean conflict. At that time, renal failure became a major cause of death after what was thought to have been successful resuscitation from injuries. The renal failure was considered inevitable in some patients, because it was believed that they had been initially subjected to an irreversible insult.

Later in the Korean conflict, it became evident that the renal failure was, in most instances, prerenal in origin and could be prevented by infusing large volumes of fluid during resuscitation. It was not clear, however, why so much fluid was needed. Shires and associates then demonstrated that as hypovolemic shock progressed, an advancing interstitial fluid deficit developed.[62] Sodium and water moved into the cell following changes in cell membrane function. Successful resuscitation followed administration of balanced salt solutions to animals in "irreversible shock."

Recognition of interstitial fluid depletion was well established by the time of the Vietnam conflict, leading to usually successful shock resuscitation. Aggressive resuscitation and rapid transport to base hospitals enabled victims of massive injuries to survive for at least a few days. This led to the recognition of a new shock lesion, the respiratory distress syndrome.[51] Because many of the patients had received large volumes of fluid during resuscitation and because the lungs at autopsy were noted to be edematous, it was initially believed that this lesion was caused by the excessive administration of fluid. Subsequently, through the development and use of the Swan-Ganz catheter, it was demonstrated that certain advanced forms of shock, particularly those associated with massive soft tissue injury, were followed by a diffuse increase in vascular permeability and an obligatory loss of fluid from the vascular space into the interstitium. The interstitial edema found in the lung was therefore caused by shock-generated increases in vascular permeability and not by overly vigorous resuscitation.[11]

The invention and use of the Swan-Ganz catheter finally resolved the controversy as to whether the respiratory distress syndrome was caused by too much or too little volume resuscitation. Previously, the central venous pressure had been regarded as an accurate reflection of left atrial pressure. With the development of the respiratory distress syndrome, however, it became evident that a discrepancy often occurred between right-sided and left-sided pressures, and that reliance on right-sided filling pressures sometimes curtailed adequate resuscitation. The pulmonary edema of the respiratory distress syndrome was found to be caused by increased capillary permeability, not by high pulmonary microvascular pressures.[11]

The etiology of the increased capillary permeability of the shock lung lesion still required explanation and prompted new efforts to find a shock toxic factor. Excluding one lung of an experimental animal from the circulation during the period of shock and resuscitation reduced pulmonary damage in the excluded lung.[11] This procedure suggested that some blood-borne particle or substance or both were responsible for the pulmonary damage. A search began again for toxic factors.[13] It now appears likely that toxic factors are produced in some forms of shock and that these factors arise from damaged, ischemic, or infected tissues. After soft tissue injury or infection, fragments of tissue entering the bloodstream are capable of initiating an intravascular inflammatory response through the mechanism of disseminated intravascular coagulation and through activation of platelets and white blood cells, with subsequent release of inflammatory mediators such as tumor necrosis factor, interleukin I, complement, prostaglandins, leukotrienes, histamine, kinins, and oxygen radicals. This inflammatory response causes a generalized increase in vascular permeability, manifested by generalized interstitial edema.[13]

Aggressive débridement of damaged, ischemic, or infected tissue, combined with aggressive support of the cardiovascular system, remains the best means of reducing the production of toxic factors and of preventing organ failure and death. As yet, there is no specific treatment for the intravascular coagulation and inflammatory response that accompany inadequately treated or untreatable shock. The search for such treatment continues today.

DEFINITION AND CLASSIFICATION

Shock can be concisely defined as a condition in which the metabolic needs of the body are not met because of an inadequate cardiac output. The definition, although concise, is not as helpful in the care of patients as it might appear initially. In most patients, inadequate cardiac output refers to a cardiac output (indexed to body surface area) that is much lower than the normal 3 liters per minute per sq. m., but occasionally, as in the hypermetabolic septic state, the output might be higher than normal and still inadequate to meet the metabolic needs of the body. Failure to meet the metabolic needs of the body is always associated with the accumulation of abnormal amounts of lactic acid in some tissues of the body, but detection of cellular acidosis is not usually practicable (noninvasive measurements of tissue acidosis require nuclear magnetic spectroscopy[49]) and measuring concentrations of lactic acid in circulating blood is not sensitive enough — perfusion to many organs during shock can be so poor that the accumulated lactic acid is not washed out into the systemic circulation until resuscitation is under way. Overall oxygen consumption, as an indicator of the body's metabolic needs, is usually less than the normal resting value of 150 ml. per minute per sq. m., but it can be elevated in shock — as in the agitated hypovolemic patient, the shivering septic patient, or the hyperventilating patient — because of oxygen use by contracting muscles. The oxygen *needs* in shock are not met by the cardiac output, by definition, but oxygen consumption is not always the same as oxygen needs, and oxygen needs cannot be determined by any simple clinical measurement.

Thus, the definition of shock does not easily lend itself to any single, straightforward, clinically usable criterion, and some of the challenge facing the physician who cares for patients in shock is to recognize the entity in the absence of such a criterion. Recognition can be simplified, however, by first considering shock in one of three categories, based on the three main causes of an inadequate cardiac output in such patients: (1) inadequate circulating blood volume, (2) loss of autonomic control of the vasculature, or (3) impaired cardiac function. Shock can then be placed in a category that links the shock with a clinical condition, to provide a working classification of shock as hypovolemic, traumatic, septic, neurogenic, cardiac compressive, cardiogenic, or cardiac obstructive (Table 1).

Inadequate blood volume, the first of the three main causes of shock, can develop from intravascular loss of salt and water, loss of plasma, or loss of blood. The losses deplete the venous capacitance bed (Table 2)[59] and decrease ventricular end-diastolic volumes, stroke volumes, and cardiac output. The losses can be primarily external, as in *hypovolemic shock;* partially external and partially internal, as in *traumatic shock;* or primarily internal, as in *septic shock.* Loss of autonomic control, the second of the three causes of shock, is referred to as *neurogenic* shock. Impaired cardiac function, the third cause, can follow impaired filling *(cardiac compressive shock),* impaired cardiac pump function *(cardiogenic shock),* or impaired emptying *(cardiac obstructive shock).*

Hypovolemic shock can be hemorrhagic or nonhemorrhagic and caused by hemorrhage, vomiting, diarrhea, loss of water and electrolytes into the gut lumen, or dehydration. *Traumatic shock* (including shock caused by burns) begins with external blood or fluid losses from a wound and is then complicated by internal fluid losses, which arise from wound-produced inflammatory mediators, disrupted microvascular endothelium, and plasma extravasation into the interstitium. *Septic shock* can be caused by any severe bacterial infection, such as cholangitis, pyelonephritis, peritonitis, meningitis, abscesses, or soft tissue infection. As in traumatic shock, inflammatory mediators disrupt the microvascular endothelium, leading to plasma extravasation and vascular volume depletion. The inflammatory mediators, which arise from the infected tissues, produce a hypermetabolic state and increased tissue oxygen needs. In the early stages of sepsis, the hypermetabolic component of the sepsis usually dominates, and the cardiac output can usually increase sufficiently to meet tissue oxygen needs. As such, the patient is not yet in shock. The hypermetabolic state is made evident, however, by fever and compensating cutaneous vasodilation (to rid the body of excess heat). As plasma extravasation depletes the vascular volume to the point that the cardiac output becomes inadequate to meet the body's increased metabolic needs, a true shock state develops. This shock state is characterized by cutaneous vasoconstriction and clinically has much the same appearance as hypovolemic or traumatic shock. The main cardiovascular abnormality at this point is vascular depletion.

In severe forms of shock caused by vascular volume depletion — hypovolemic, traumatic, or septic shock — the volume depletion is worsened by an intracellular shift of sodium, chloride, and water.[62,70] This shift probably serves to help buffer the intracellular acidosis of the severe shock state, but it has a price, in that it further depletes an already depleted vascular volume of needed water and electrolytes. Severe hypovolemia produces intracellular shifts that worsen the hypovolemia.

Neurogenic shock is caused by a loss of autonomic control of the vasculature. It can be due to injuries to the spinal cord,

TABLE 1. Shock

Primary Cause	Type	Mechanisms Underlying Primary Cause	Associated Clinical Conditions
Inadequate circulating blood volume	Hypovolemic shock	Hemorrhage (hemorrhagic shock) Loss of fluid into gut or dehydration (nonhemorrhagic hypovolemic shock)	Hemorrhage Vomiting Diarrhea Bowel obstruction
	Traumatic shock (including burn shock)	External blood or plasma loss combined with internal losses	Trauma Burns
	Septic shock	Loss of plasma into tissues and sequestration of blood in the cutaneous vasculature	Systemic sepsis
Loss of autonomic control of the vasculature	Neurogenic shock	Pooling of blood in denervated venous beds and excess perfusion of relatively unessential vascular beds	Spinal cord injury Regional anesthetic
Impaired cardiac function	Cardiac compressive shock	Compression of great veins or cardiac chambers or both	Pericardial tamponade Tension pneumothorax Ascites Hemoperitoneum Inflation of abdominal portion of pneumatic antishock garment Diaphragmatic rupture Mechanical ventilation
	Cardiogenic shock	Intrinsic abnormality of the heart	Congenital abnormalities Arrhythmias Myocardial ischemia Valvular or septal defects Cardiomyopathies Coronary air embolism
	Cardiac obstructive shock	Obstruction of either the pulmonary or systemic circulation	Pulmonary embolism Mechanical ventilation Pulmonary vascular disease Engorgement of pulmonary vasculature Mechanical obstruction of aorta Systemic arteriolar constriction Polycythemia

TABLE 2. Pressure-Volume Characteristics of the Cardiovascular System in a 70-Kg. Man*

Vessel	Intracavitary Pressure (mm. Hg)	Extracavitary Pressure (mm. Hg)	Volume (mm.)	Volume (% of total)
Systemic arteries	120/80	0	700	14
Systemic capillaries	20	0	300	6
Systemic small veins	14	0	2300	46
Systemic large veins	5	0	900	18
Right atrium	4	−3	70	1
Right ventricle	25/4	−4	110	2
Pulmonary arteries	25/10	−3	130	3
Pulmonary microvasculature	15/10	−3	110	2
Pulmonary veins	8	−3	200	4
Left atrium	7	−3	70	1
Left ventricle	120/7	−2	110	2
Total			5000	99

* All pressures measured with respect to atmosphere with transducer zeroed at the midaxillary line. Heart volumes measured at end-diastole.
Data extrapolated in part from Rothe, C. F.: Venous system: Physiology of the capacitance vessels. *In* Shepherd, J. T., Abboud, F. M., and Geiger, S. R. (Eds.): Handbook of Physiology, Section 2: The Cardiovascular System. Vol. 3, Peripheral Circulation and Organ Blood Flow, Part 1. Bethesda, Md., American Physiological Society, 1983, pp. 397–452.

regional anesthetics, or administration of autonomic blocking agents. The resultant expansion of the vasculature leads to inappropriate perfusion and pooling of blood in vascular beds that do not need it at the expense of those that do.

Cardiac compressive shock is caused by compression of the heart or great veins, which decreases ventricular end-diastolic volumes. Causes include pericardial tamponade; tension pneumothorax; positive-pressure ventilation; compression of the heart by bowel that has eviscerated through a ruptured diaphragm; and compression caused by any process associated with high abdominal pressures, such as tense ascites, abdominal bleeding, or inflation of the abdominal portion of a pneumatic antishock garment. These last conditions compress both the inferior vena cava, to limit venous return, and the heart, by pushing the diaphragm into the chest. *Cardiogenic shock*, or shock arising primarily from an intrinsic abnormality of the heart, can be caused by congenital abnormalities, arrhythmias, ischemia-induced myocardial failure, valvular and septal defects, cardiomyopathies, or coronary air embolism. Cardiac *obstructive* shock is caused by obstruction of either the pulmonary or the systemic vasculature. Pulmonary vascular obstruction can arise from a pulmonary embolus, mechanical ventilation, intrinsic pulmonary vascular disease, or the pulmonary vascular engorgement that originates from left-sided congestive heart failure. Systemic vascular obstruction can arise from a surgically placed aortic clamp or from systemic arteriolar constriction. Both sides of the heart can be functionally obstructed by excessively viscous blood, as in a patient with polycythemia.

HYPOVOLEMIC SHOCK

DIAGNOSIS

The symptoms and signs of hypovolemic shock depend upon the degree of blood volume depletion, the duration of shock, and the body's compensatory reactions to the shock itself. These compensatory reactions begin with cardiovascular adrenergic discharge. The systemic venules and small veins go into spasm. Residual blood is displaced to the heart, ventricular end-diastolic volumes are partially restored, and stroke volumes and cardiac output are partially re-established. The arterioles in the skin, fat, skeletal muscle, and, eventually, the splanchnic organs and kidneys, constrict to maintain blood flow to the heart and brain.[71] Angiotensin and vasopressin are generated to add to the constriction of the noncardiac and noncerebral arterioles.[35,54] Release of vasopressin and aldosterone augments reabsorption of water and sodium from the glomerular filtrate to preserve the remaining blood volume.

The symptoms and signs of hypovolemic shock are thus manifested progressively by (1) signs of adrenergic discharge to the skin, (2) oliguria, (3) hypotension and electrocardiographic signs of myocardial ischemia, and (4) neurologic signs and symptoms. The findings in shock correlate with the organs that are compromised—that is, the findings correlate with the severity of the shock. Flow to the skin is sacrificed first, then flow to the kidneys and viscera, and finally flow to the heart and brain (Table 3).

In *mild shock* (loss of less than 20 per cent of blood volume), the most sensitive clinical findings are caused by adrenergic constriction of blood vessels in the skin. The extremities, particularly the feet, become pale and cool. The subcutaneous veins collapse. Capillary filling decreases, and the feet may become damp with sweat. Blood pressure with the patient in the supine position remains normal, as does the urinary output (although the urine may be concentrated). The patient feels cold and may complain of thirst.

In addition to the symptoms and signs of mild hemorrhagic shock, the patient in *moderate shock* (loss of 20 to 40 per cent of blood volume) develops a low urinary output (defined as less than 0.5 ml. per kg. per hour in the adult or less than 2.0 ml. per kg. per hour in the infant). This oliguria reflects the effects of circulating aldosterone and vasopressin. The supine blood pressure usually remains normal, and the patient may be restless.

The patient in *severe shock* (loss of more than 40 per cent of blood volume) shows signs of adrenergic discharge to the skin, with decreased urinary output and low blood pressure. The electrocardiogram may show signs of myocardial ischemia, with Q waves and depressed ST-T segments. The patient may be agitated, restless, or obtunded solely on the basis of hypovolemia.

Moderately severe and severe shock are usually easy to recognize, but early or mild hypovolemic shock can pose a problem in diagnosis—the signs of adrenergic discharge to the skin can be subtle and difficult to detect. Yet recognition of early or mild shock can be critical, not because mild shock in itself threatens the patient but because the pathologic process causing the mild shock may lead to severe shock. To help detect mild or progressing hypovolemic shock, the urinary output should be monitored and serial hematocrit levels measured. In addition, in selected patients, postural changes in blood pressure should be elicited.

Assessment of urinary output is almost as sensitive as detection of the signs of cutaneous adrenergic discharge in diagnosing early and progressing hypovolemic shock, and it has the

TABLE 3. Characteristics of Shock States

| | Hypovolemic or Traumatic Shock | | | Early Septic Shock | Late Septic Shock | Neurogenic Shock | Cardiac Compressive Shock | Cardiogenic Shock | Cardiac Obstructive Shock |
	Mild	Moderate	Severe						
Skin perfusion	Pale	Pale	Pale	Pink	Pale	Pink*	Pale	Pale	Pale
Urinary output	Normal	Low	Low	Low	Low	Low	Low	Low	Low
Blood pressure	Normal	Normal	Low	Low	Low	Low	Low	Low	Normal
Mental status	Thirsty	Restless	Obtunded	Abnormal	Abnormal	Normal†	Normal†	Normal†	Normal†
ECG	Normal	Normal	Abnormal	Normal	Normal†	Normal†	Normal†	Abnormal	Abnormal
Neck veins	Flat	Flat	Flat	Flat	Flat	Flat	Distended	Distended	Distended
Cardiac output	Low	Low	Low	High	Low	Low	Low	Low	Low
Systemic vascular resistance	High	High	High	Low	High	Low	High	High	High
Mixed venous oxygen content	Low	Low	Low	High	Low	Low	Low	Low	Low
Oxygen consumption‡	Low	Low	Low	Low	Low	Low	Low	Low	Low

* In denervated areas.
† Will be abnormal if shock is severe.
‡ In relation to oxygen needs.

advantage that little clinical skill is needed to interpret the findings. A Foley catheter should be placed for monitoring purposes in any patient who manifests mild shock and whose future status is uncertain. Such a catheter can be placed safely in all patients, except in those with a torn urethra and those with pathologic lesions in the urethra or bladder.

A fall in the hematocrit with intravenous administration of asanguineous fluid is another interpretable sign of hypovolemia. The initial hematocrit obtained immediately after hemorrhage is normal, and the hematocrit in a patient with a bowel obstruction or major burn may be high. Asanguineous fluid resuscitation that restores peripheral perfusion, urinary output, and blood pressure, however, decreases the hematocrit. Generally in an adult patient, a fall in the hematocrit of three or four points with fluid resuscitation indicates that the patient's blood volume before resuscitation was depleted by 500 ml. Failure of the hematocrit to reach equilibration implies continuing volume loss. Overenthusiastic volume expansion with asanguineous fluid can make interpretation of a falling hematocrit somewhat problematic but should not often pose difficulties. Administration of excessive fluid decreases the hematocrit by several points; the kidneys rapidly excrete the excess water and salt.

Postural changes in blood pressure are a simple and sensitive indicator of early shock. Unfortunately, elicitation of such changes is impracticable in many surgical patients, in whom serious injuries or illness may preclude rapid assumption of the upright position. Postural changes in the blood pressure can be obtained, however, in many patients in whom hypovolemia is suspected on the basis of dehydration or occult gastrointestinal blood loss, and the blood pressure should be measured in such patients in both supine and upright positions. A fall in the systolic pressure of 10 mm Hg that persists for more than 30 seconds suggests hypovolemia.

Contrary to time-honored tradition and to experiments in anesthetized animals, the pulse rate does not consistently increase in response to graded volume loss.[41] Hypovolemic patients frequently have heart rates within the normal range, and in severely hypovolemic patients bradycardia can develop as a preterminal event. A rapid heart rate can indicate possible hypovolemia; a normal or slow heart rate is inconsequential or, on occasion, may reflect myocardial ischemia and impending cardiac arrest.

Signs of adrenergic discharge to the skin and oliguria are not reliable indicators of hypovolemia in the inebriated patient.

High blood alcohol levels induce a generalized vasodilation that can override the effects of discharge of the adrenergic nervous system. Alcohol also inhibits the secretion of vasopressin from the pituitary, so that the hypovolemic patient may still have adequate urinary output. Thus, the two most sensitive signs of hypovolemia — constriction of the cutaneous vasculature and oliguria — are masked by the presence of alcohol. The generalized vasodilation of alcohol intoxication, however, causes systemic arterial hypotension, even in mild-to-moderate shock. Hypotension in the noninebriated patient is a late sign of hypovolemia, whereas in the inebriated patient it can be an early sign.

Blood flow to both the heart and the brain is decreased in severe shock. In older patients, the heart is usually affected more than the brain. Hypotension is more likely to be present than cerebral signs. In young patients, however, the brain is more often affected. Hypovolemia should be excluded with absolute certainty in any patient who presents with cerebral symptoms after any injury, even if the patient has an obvious head injury. Correction of hypovolemia sometimes completely corrects all abnormalities in mental status. As a corollary, cardiovascular instability should never be ascribed to a head injury. Although normovolemic patients with preterminal head injuries pass through a stage of cardiovascular instability before they die, the most patients with head injuries and hypotension are hypotensive because they are hypovolemic. Normovolemic patients with severe head injuries usually have a *high* blood pressure and a *low* pulse rate (the Cushing reflex). The surgeon should search for conditions that can be treated, such as hypovolemia, in contrast to attributing the hypotension to an untreatable lesion, such as a fatal head injury.

Hypoglycemic shock may present with signs and symptoms similar to those of hypovolemic shock, the common signs and symptoms in both conditions being caused by discharge of the adrenergic nervous system and by cerebral hypoxia. A hypoglycemic patient typically is cool, vasoconstricted, pale, and sweaty and, with severe hypoglycemia, may be hypotensive, oliguric, irritable, obtunded, or unconscious. The urinalysis is normal. Any patient in shock in whom insulin-dependent diabetes is suspected should have the blood glucose measured by a Dextrostix and should be given an infusion of 25 gm. of glucose to treat possible hypoglycemia. Although the patient may have been in an accident, it may have been caused by the lethargy of hypoglycemia.

TREATMENT

Initial Resuscitation and Venous Access

The principles of treatment for hemorrhagic and nonhemorrhagic forms of hypovolemic shock are similar. This discussion concentrates on the treatment of hemorrhagic shock, the most common form of hypovolemic shock seen by the surgeon.

Resuscitation should begin with ensuring adequate ventilation and oxygenation. If the patient is unconscious, lowering the head with support of the jaw to prevent airway obstruction and administering supplemental oxygen may be all that are needed. In patients with obtundation or airway obstruction, the trachea should be intubated and mechanical ventilation initiated.

Hypovolemic shock caused by hemorrhage is best treated by prompt identification of the source, followed by immediate control of bleeding. External hemorrhage should be tamponaded by compression. The source of internal hemorrhage caused by trauma should be surgically exposed and the bleeding controlled. That from the gastrointestinal tract should have the source identified, and specific treatment should be initiated.

Intravenous fluid should be administered simultaneously or as preparations are being made to control bleeding. Administering fluid requires access to the venous system, the type of access depending on the clinician's assessment of the degree of hypovolemia. If the patient's only sign of hypovolemia is cutaneous vasoconstriction, percutaneously placed venous cannulas in the upper extremities are adequate, at least initially. If the hypovolemia is severe, to the point that urinary output is diminished, two or three large-bore intravenous catheters should be inserted.

The best large-bore catheter is a cut-off length of intravenous tubing or a large-bore (12-gauge or larger) catheter, ideally placed into a surgically exposed saphenous vein at the ankle. At that level, the saphenous vein has no important structures near it and accepts a large-bore catheter with ease. A cutdown on the saphenous vein should not be used in a severely injured extremity but can be used in patients with other more proximal injuries, including injuries to the iliac veins or to the abdominal vena cava. Collateral flow around these great veins is excellent, and fluid infused into a saphenous vein flows into the central circulation even in the presence of a major abdominal venous injury. The saphenous vein catheter should be removed the next day because it can produce thrombophlebitis if left in place longer than 24 hours.

A percutaneously placed central venous catheter is of value for measuring right atrial pressure but is best placed semi-electively once resuscitation has restored venous filling. The usual 16-gauge catheter passed through a 14-gauge needle into the subclavian or internal jugular vein is too long and too narrow to permit the rapid administration of fluid. Percutaneous central punctures are associated with several risks. Puncture of the parietal pleura can induce a pneumothorax, a complication that is well tolerated in an otherwise healthy patient but can be fatal in a patient with multiple injuries and shock. Puncture of an artery near the pleural cavity with bleeding into the pleural space can be catastrophic. Placement of such catheters under emergency circumstances can be difficult. This difficulty increases in proportion to the severity of shock. In advanced shock, the venous system is constricted and empty. Percutaneous central catheters should be placed only by surgeons who are positive that they can place such catheters with a very low incidence of complications. If such a catheter is to be used, it should be 12-gauge or larger so that it can be used for rapid administration of fluid.

Crystalloid Infusion

A nonsugar, nonprotein crystalloid solution with an electrolyte composition approximating that of plasma is preferable in the initial resuscitation of patients with all forms of shock, except cardiogenic shock, assuming that large-bore vascular access has been obtained and that large volumes of fluid can be given quickly. The authors prefer lactated Ringer's solution, but the solution can be acetated Ringer's or normal saline supplemented with administration of an ampule of sodium bicarbonate for each liter of fluid. The lactate, acetate, or bicarbonate buffers the hydrogen ion that is washed out of the ischemic tissues when reperfusion is first established. In the case of bicarbonate, combination with hydrogen ion produces carbonic acid, which breaks down to water and carbon dioxide, the carbon dioxide being eliminated by the lungs. In the case of lactate or acetate, combination with hydrogen ion produces lactic or acetic acid, which requires enough liver function to convert the acid to water and carbon dioxide, by the Krebs cycle. The required amount of hepatic function is usually no problem in surgical patients, even if the patient is in deep shock and has poor liver perfusion because of that shock. The initial volume expansion with the balanced salt solution is more than enough to re-establish liver blood flow and allow metabolism of the lactic or acetic acid.[19] Lactated and acetated Ringer's solution should not be used, however, in patients with severe pre-existing cirrhosis. In these patients, normal saline supplemented with sodium bicarbonate is safer.

Colloid solutions, such as albumin, hydroxyethyl starch, or dextran compounds, may prove to be useful in plasma volume expansion in those circumstances in which it is impossible to give large amounts of resuscitative fluids, such as in the prehospital treatment of trauma patients. Colloid administration provides more vascular volume expansion, on a temporary basis, than does administration of an equivalent amount of an isotonic crystalloid solution. The advantage of the colloid is transient, however, because severe shock is accompanied by a generalized disruption of the microvascular endothelium. The colloid leaks out of the vascular space into the interstitium within a matter of an hour or two.[42,72,74] Fresh frozen plasma should not be used for plasma volume expansion because, with time, it too leaks out of the vascular space and because it has the risk of transmitting AIDS or hepatitis to the patient.

Hypertonic saline solutions in combination with a synthetic colloid, in experimental animals and in preliminary patient trials, are much more effective than isotonic crystalloid solutions for the resuscitation of hypovolemic shock, on a volume-per-volume basis.[37] The hypertonic saline draws water out of the cells, and perhaps out of the gut lumen, and into the extracellular space; the colloid helps hold the recovered volume in the vascular space for an hour or so. Such solutions may be particularly effective in those situations, such as the prehospital setting, in which large-volume resuscitation is impossible. When large-volume resuscitation is possible, however, isotonic crystalloid resuscitation is probably just as effective.

The lactated Ringer's or other crystalloid solution should not be given in glucose solution unless the patient is thought to be in hypoglycemic shock from an insulin reaction. Rapid administration of glucose, even as a 5 per cent solution, can induce an osmotic diuresis. The diuresis further depletes the patient's vascular volume; it also confuses the clinical presentation by eliminating urinary output as an index of adequacy of resuscitation.

Administration of fluid not only helps resuscitate patients in hemorrhagic shock but also serves as a diagnostic test to detect continuing bleeding. Two to three liters of fluid given over 5 to 15 minutes resuscitates any patient with arrested hemorrhage. The need for administration of more fluid indicates continuing bleeding. Such hemorrhage usually needs surgical control.

Blood Administration

If the patient can be operated on promptly, it is best to withhold administration of blood until surgical control of the bleeding is obtained or at least until just before induction of anesthesia. A young patient with a normal heart can tolerate hematocrit values as low as 15 per cent even when the anemia is induced rapidly, as long as the blood volume is kept normal by administering adequate volumes of asanguineous solutions.[76] The restoration of circulation following the initial administration of fluid for the patient in hypovolemic shock leads to the release of products of anaerobic and catabolic metabolism into the central circulation. As these products are washed into the coronary arteries, transient myocardial dysfunction can result. If resuscitation is initiated with acidotic, cold bank blood with a high potassium concentration, the myocardium can be compromised even more. Too early administration of blood before surgical control of hemorrhage also means a waste of blood bank resources—at least some of the administered blood will end up in the suction canisters in the operating room or in the tissues. Rapid replacement of the freshest blood available after control of hemorrhage leads to the most efficient use of blood products and the least risk of transfusion complications.

At times, however, blood has to be given before surgical control of hemorrhage is obtained (see Chapter 6, Blood Transfusions and Disorders of Surgical Bleeding). Type-specific blood, which can be obtained within 10 minutes from most blood banks, should be given if cross matched units are not available. It has a negligible risk for transfusion reaction in massively injured patients. These patients have little of their own blood remaining in their vascular space after resuscitation, and clinically evident transfusion reactions are rare.

If type-specific blood is not available, O-negative blood can be given. In the confusion often associated with the treatment of mass casualties, its use minimizes the risk of transfusing the wrong blood type to a patient. Its administration depletes a valuable blood bank resource, however, and complicates typing of blood after the patient's initial resuscitation.

The amount of blood given depends on the presumed status of the patient's coronary arteries and on the circumstances that indicate the need for transfusion.[26,31] Initial crystalloid resuscitation from hemorrhagic shock produces a hemodiluted state. Hemodilution, to a certain degree, is beneficial: it reduces blood viscosity, which improves circulation to the microvasculature and decreases both systemic and pulmonary vascular resistances. Although anemia reduces the amount of oxygen transported by the blood, a decreased delivery of oxygen to most organs is usually of little consequence, because only a small amount of the oxygen delivered to them is ordinarily used as long as flow is maintained. Moreover, under conditions of shock, local accumulations of hydrogen ion and carbon dioxide facilitate off-loading of oxygen to ischemic tissues. Low hemoglobin concentrations are usually not a limiting factor.

The heart is the exception, however, because under resting circumstances in normal persons with normal hematocrits, it uses approximately one-half the oxygen delivered to it. If the hematocrit falls too far, its needs will exceed the supply. Hematocrit values of 20 per cent after resuscitation are usually adequate if control of hemorrhage is assured, but the generally accepted desired hematocrit is 25 per cent. Lower levels might be dangerous if the patient unexpectedly starts to bleed again. Patients with coronary artery disease should be transfused to hematocrits of approximately 30 to 35 per cent, because their hearts do not have the reserve to tolerate even transient episodes of ischemia.

Pneumatic Antishock Garment

Pneumatic antishock garments—inflatable overalls that are placed around the legs, thighs, and abdomen of trauma patients or patients with leaking abdominal aneurysms—have been adopted by many prehospital paramedical personnel to assist in the resuscitation of hemorrhagic shock. Inflating the garment can tamponade bleeding and theoretically could help the patient compensate for acute blood loss by compressing the veins in those parts of the body enclosed by the garment, to displace

residual venous blood to the heart and to increase ventricular end-diastolic volumes and stroke volumes.

Pneumatic antishock garments should be used only in selected patients, however, until more information about them becomes available.[36,45] Although inflation of the garment compresses the systemic venules and small veins and thus might translocate some blood to the heart, moderately severe or severe degrees of hypovolemia and adrenergic discharge will already have emptied the veins of most of their displaceable blood. Inflation around the abdomen compresses the inferior vena cava and impedes return of blood to the right heart. Inflation of the garment compresses the arterioles in the abdomen and lower extremities and hinders left ventricular emptying. Compression of the abdomen pushes the diaphragm into the chest, compresses the heart, and limits ventricular filling during diastole. Discharge of the adrenergic nervous system in hemorrhagic shock deprives infradiaphragmatic organs of all but a residual blood flow. Inflation of the garment to high pressures can deprive the organs encompassed within of any residual blood flow that they might be receiving. Such deprivation can cause production and then release of toxic products from the ischemic organs when the garment is deflated or when perfusion is re-established. High blood concentrations of these toxic factors can prove fatal. Probably no organs are totally expendable during shock. The organs beneath the diaphragm are just as essential to survival as those above.

In summary, pneumatic antishock garments may be useful in controlling hemorrhage and in immobilizing fractures, particularly pelvic fractures. Other indications for use of the garments are still controversial. For the time being, their use should be restricted to selected patients until prospective trials have demonstrated whether they have any role in shock resuscitation.

Occlusion of Descending Thoracic Aorta

Occlusion of the descending thoracic aorta through an anterolateral thoracotomy is occasionally useful in the resuscitation of patients who are close to cardiac arrest because of hemorrhage from abdominal or pelvic injuries. Cardiac compression can be used at the same time to maintain perfusion of the brain and myocardium. Aortic occlusion under these circumstances should be used primarily as a means of controlling hemorrhage, as opposed to primarily restoring cardiovascular function. The occlusion should be brief and limited to a maximum of 15 minutes. More prolonged occlusion risks irreversible ischemic damage to the abdominal viscera. The disadvantages of occluding the aorta are similar to those of inflating a pneumatic antishock garment to high pressures.

Trendelenburg's Position

Elevation of the lower extremities above the level of the heart is of no value in treating hypovolemic shock.[64] Although one might theorize that such elevation could provide some transient dislocation of blood from the elevated parts to the heart, in fact the peripheral venules and small veins in even moderately severe shock are already fully depleted from the volume loss and from venoconstriction. The elevated extremities place an added burden on the heart, by forcing it to pump some of its output upward.

Nonhemorrhagic Hypovolemic Shock

Nonhemorrhagic hypovolemic shock is treated with the same goals in mind as those used for hemorrhagic shock, except that blood is usually not necessary. In shock caused by loss of fluid into the gut lumen, asanguineous fluids should be given to establish a normal urinary output and to bring the hematocrit down into the mid-30s range. The fluid used for replenishment of the vascular volume should have an electrolyte composition similar to that which was lost.[43]

TRAUMATIC SHOCK

DIAGNOSIS

Traumatic shock, including shock caused by burns, is a more virulent form of hypovolemic shock. It is initially caused by both internal and external volume losses — from loss of blood or plasma externally, from the wound or burn surface, and from loss of blood or plasma into the damaged tissues. These volume losses are worsened by plasma extravasation into tissues distal to the injured areas.[16,66] This extravasation arises from a generalized systemic intravascular inflammatory response, which is generated by the release of inflammatory mediators from the damaged tissues when they are reperfused during resuscitation.[13]

Hypovolemia caused by the injury catalyzes this response, which appears to be mediated through activation of the coagulation system.[11] Activation of factor XII activates complement, kinins, and thromboxanes. Moreover, tissue injury mobilizes and activates white blood cells and platelets with release of tumor necrosis factor, interleukin I, oxygen radicals, leukotrienes, kinins, serotonin, and histamine. The consequence is the development of a generalized increase in systemic vascular permeability, with loss of plasma into the interstitial tissues and aggravation of any pre-existing hypovolemia.

The major consequences of traumatic shock do not manifest fully until 24 to 48 hours following the initial injury, since the inflammation-mediated vascular permeability develops gradually over many hours. Initially, right-sided venous pressure provides a guide to the adequacy of volume therapy. As the pulmonary microvasculature becomes occluded with particulate matter generated by intravascular coagulation, however, and as the vasculature constricts in response to vasoactive inflammatory mediators from white cells and platelets, the right ventricle can fail. Left-sided and right-sided filling pressures can diverge, and measurement of left-sided pressures with a Swan-Ganz catheter can become essential for guiding fluid administration.

TREATMENT

The primary initial treatment of traumatic shock is immediate correction of hypovolemia. Hypovolemia, in the presence of tissue fragments in the blood, escalates and perpetuates the intravascular inflammatory process, thus exacerbating the increased vascular permeability that characterizes this form of shock. Further treatment includes prompt debridement of ischemic or devitalized tissue and immobilization of fractures to prevent further tissue damage — to be accomplished within the first 24 hours following injury.

As fluid is given to maintain vascular volume, the increases in vascular permeability are most prominently manifest in the lung, and the status of pulmonary function should be monitored closely. There is a progressive loss of compliance and closure of alveoli, with a progressive fall in arterial P_{O_2} despite supplemental oxygen. When the respiratory rate exceeds 30 to 35 breaths per minute or when the P_{O_2} cannot be maintained above 70 mm. Hg, intubation and ventilatory support are indicated.

As is true with simple hypovolemic shock, the kidneys remain the best organs to monitor for adequacy of vital organ perfusion. A urinary output of between 0.5 and 1.0 ml. per kg. per hour provides assurance that resuscitation is adequate. Urine output below this level indicates circulatory inadequacy and the need for more volume. If fluid requirements appear excessive, a Swan-Ganz catheter should be placed to determine left-sided filling pressures. If low, the pulmonary artery wedge pressure should be raised gradually, by balanced salt crystalloid infusion, to 12 to 15 mm. Hg and the effect on cardiac output and urinary output determined. The lowest wedge pressure consistent with a hyperdynamic cardiac output and an adequate urine volume should be used. An additional 5 to 10 mm. Hg filling pressure on a rare occasion may be necessary if the patient requires high positive end-expiratory pressure (150 mm. H_2O or above). Under these circumstances, if cardiac output appears to be plateauing, the administration of cardiotonic agents, such as low-dose dopamine or dobutamine, may be indicated (see cardiogenic shock section). In the unstable resuscitation phase, the hematocrit should be kept above 30 per cent with whole blood or packed cells and lactated Ringer's solution. The presence of increased microvascular permeability is a relative contraindication for colloid utilization, because the colloid extravasates into the interstitium. When spontaneous diuresis starts, fluids should be reduced to maintenance levels.

SEPTIC SHOCK

DIAGNOSIS

As the systemic infection that leads to septic shock progresses, the initial manifestations are those that arise from the development of a hypermetabolic state (see Table 3).[14] Heat production increases, and heat loss is accomplished by the diversion of blood flow to the skin through the opening of cutaneous arteriovenous shunts. The capacitance of the cutaneous vascular bed expands so that unless fluid volume is provided simultaneously other areas of the body become deprived of blood flow.[60]

As systemic sepsis develops, an intravascular inflammatory process is activated similar to that seen in traumatic shock, but in this instance the initiating inflammatory mediator appears to be endotoxin, rather than tissue fragments.[48] Activation of the clotting cascade causes release of all the inflammatory factors previously described. These produce an intense reaction within the vascular system with damage to endothelial cells, the end result being a diffuse increase in microvascular permeability.[4] The circulatory system is unable to hold volume within the vascular space, and hypovolemia develops. Acidosis and catecholamine release following shock further activate the clotting cascade and the associated intravascular inflammatory reaction, and a vicious cycle is initiated. In the absence of effective treatment, fatal shock ensues.

The first manifestation of systemic sepsis is usually an increased fluid requirement to maintain urinary output and peripheral perfusion, as early in the septic process fluid starts to leak out of the vascular system. At this stage, two factors — hypovolemia and increased metabolism — work in opposition to one another. Sepsis-induced hypermetabolism causes a fever, which activates the hypothalamic temperature control center. Cutaneous arteriovenous shunts open, blood flow is diverted to the skin, and the heat produced by the hypermetabolism is dissipated externally. The cutaneous vasodilation, however, causes a fall in the blood pressure and a pooling of blood in the cutaneous venous capacitance bed. Perfusion of vital organs becomes compromised. Urinary output decreases. This stage constitutes early septic shock, or "red shock."

Eventually, hypoperfusion of vital organs activates cutaneous pressor mechanisms, diverting blood away from the less essential skin and subcutaneous tissue and transiently restoring vital organ perfusion. Decreased skin perfusion causes a fall in skin temperature and a cold sensation perceived by the patient, which progresses to shaking chills. This vasoconstriction, which is required to maintain blood pressure and splanchnic perfusion, compromises the body's ability to dissipate heat and leads to another rapid rise in body temperature. The increased temperature once again activates the hypothalamic temperature control center, which reinitiates a cycle of cutaneous vasodilation, hypotension, and splanchnic hypoperfusion (Figs. 1 and 2).

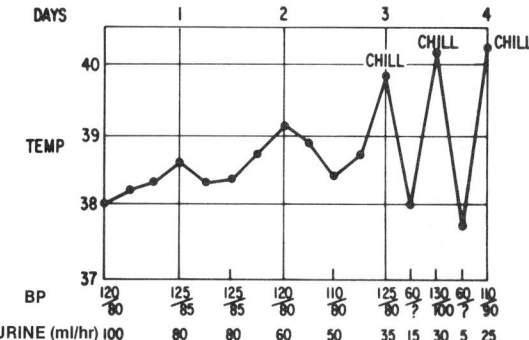

Figure 1. Vital signs of a patient who became septic and then went into warm septic shock over a 4-day period. Beginning on day 3, he developed shaking chills followed immediately by temperature spikes. His skin then became warm, and his blood pressure and urinary output fell. (From Blaisdell, F. W.: Controversy in shock research. Con: The role of steroids in septic shock. Circ. Shock, *68:*1, 1983.)

In the terminal phase of sepsis, inflammatory mediators disrupt the microvascular endothelium, leading to hypovolemia and a marked decrease in the cardiac output ("white septic shock") (see Table 3). Inadequate splanchnic perfusion causes gastrointestinal, pancreatic, hepatic, and renal ischemia and failure. Marked arterial oxygen desaturation occurs following progressive pulmonary dysfunction, further compromising function of all organs, including the brain. The final event is coronary insufficiency, manifested by arrhythmias, cardiac fibrillation, and arrest.

TREATMENT

Septic shock is best treated by prevention, with the early recognition of sepsis and definitive treatment of the infection. This prevention requires identification of the source of infection, administration of specific antibiotics, and institution of surgical drainage if possible.

Circulatory resuscitation must be prompt, and large volumes of fluid may be needed to correct the hypovolemia that is responsible for the shock. In almost all instances, a Swan-Ganz catheter should be passed to facilitate the prompt optimization of the circulation without overinfusion of fluids. Fluid administration should begin with 2 liters of a balanced salt solution, which can be administered over 10 to 15 minutes to most adult patients with safety, but as much as 10 to 15 liters of fluid may be required in the first 24 hours of resuscitation. If the circulation does not respond to the first few boluses of fluid, a Starling curve of cardiac function should be obtained by determining the optimal filling pressures that generate an adequate cardiac output, the end point being the restoration of vital organ perfusion as evidenced by a good urinary output. Because of the presence of wide-open skin shunts, adequate organ flow requires cardiac outputs far in excess of normal. The guidelines for fluid admin-

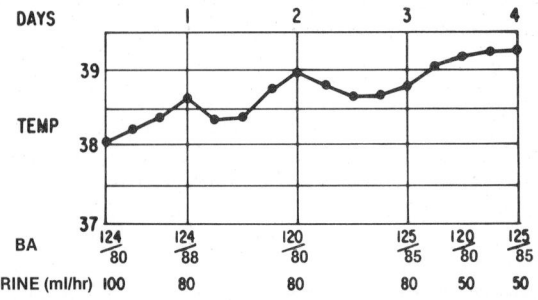

Figure 2. Compare the type of septic course now being seen in septic patients who have careful maintenance of vascular volume with the course of the patient shown in Figure 1. When the Swan-Ganz catheter is used and fluid administration is adequate, shock is not seen except as a terminal clinical event. (From Blaisdell, F. W.: Controversy in shock research. Con: The role of steroids in septic shock. Circ. Shock, *68:*1, 1983.)

istration are similar to those discussed under "Hypovolemic Shock." Filling pressures of the heart should be restored to 12 mm. Hg or more and may have to be brought to as much as 18 mm. Hg. If cardiac output still appears inadequate, cardiotonic agents such as dopamine or dobutamine should be administered.

Cultures of all suspicious sources should be obtained immediately. Unless the organism has been previously identified, broad-spectrum antibiotics should be administered. Most commonly the bacteria responsible for septic shock are gram-negative, and therapy should be directed so as to include the spectrum of enteric organisms. The antibiotics can be adjusted subsequently on the basis of identification of the offending organisms. All pathogenic organisms identified in the blood must be eradicated—with the most specific and least toxic antibiotic available.[29] Organisms recovered from other sites should be eradicated with antibiotics if the clinical circumstances indicate that an infection from the site is probably causing the systemic sepsis.[21] If no source is apparent, the cause probably lies in the abdomen. Direct assessment, with ultrasonography, computed tomography, or magnetic resonance imaging, may be of value, particularly if there is reason to believe that the infection is localized and might be susceptible to percutaneous catheter or operative drainage.

The monitoring catheters of all intensive-care patients should be viewed with suspicion. Such catheters are frequently a source of sepsis and should be removed unless another source has been unequivocally identified. When there is doubt as to source, intravenous lines should be changed and the tips Gram-stained and cultured; pulmonary arterial catheters also should be changed, but systemic arterial catheters are rarely the source of systemic sepsis and usually do not have to be replaced, unless the skin and tissues overlying the catheter are inflamed or unless peripheral embolism develops, as evidenced by petechiae in the skin supplied by the cannulated artery. Ultrasound examination of the kidneys may be indicated to exclude an obstructive uropathy and urinary tract sepsis. Ultrasound survey of the biliary tract and percutaneous aspiration of the gallbladder may be used to exclude acalculous cholecystitis.

The patient's pulmonary function should be carefully monitored, because the increases in permeability generated by severe sepsis cause pulmonary dysfunction.[25] Almost all patients in septic shock require endotracheal intubation and mechanical ventilation to ensure adequate arterial oxygenation.

Adequate volume resuscitation usually causes re-establishment of renal function. If the septic process continues for more than 24 hours, however, renal tubular necrosis may develop. Failure of the kidneys to respond to adequate circulatory resuscitation may require hemofiltration or dialysis.

In the past, steroids have been advocated for the treatment of septic shock and its consequences, but recent studies have shown no benefit.[9,17,73] Cardiovascular function may be improved temporarily but only at the price of immune suppression and increased vulnerability to overwhelming sepsis.

A number of other agents, including prostaglandins, opiate inhibitors, anticoagulants, oxygen radical scavengers, and blockers of tumor necrosis factor, have been used experimentally and clinically for the treatment of sepsis and may ultimately prove efficacious.[34,69] It is possible that vascular damage from sepsis may be modified by early use of these drugs, but it is unlikely that they are of benefit in fulminant septic shock unless infection can be controlled. In the last analysis, infection must be controlled. Unless control is possible, all therapeutic interventions are unsuccessful.

NEUROGENIC SHOCK

DIAGNOSIS

Diagnosis of neurogenic shock is usually based on the neurologic examination or on the knowledge that the patient has had a regional anesthetic agent or has received an autonomic blocker. The degree of shock directly relates to the level and duration of the denervation. Loss of vasomotor control can cause a severalfold expansion of the venous capacitance bed with peripheral pooling and inadequate ventricular filling. The shock state resembles that seen in patients with warm septic shock (see Table 3). The skin of the denervated portions of the body is warm, pink, and well perfused. The blood pressure is low. Urinary output may be normal or low. The heart rate is usually rapid but may be slow if the adrenergic nerves to the heart are blocked. Because vasomotor control is lost, heat loss can be a major problem, and many patients are hypothermic at the time of initial presentation, especially when the duration of denervation has been prolonged prior to treatment.

TREATMENT

Filling of the heart should be corrected by administering a balanced salt solution in a volume of several liters (in an adult). If the blood pressure does not respond promptly, a vasoconstrictor should be given to restore venous tone, ventricular end-diastolic volumes, and cardiac output. Vasoconstrictor-induced constriction of the systemic arterioles also increases arterial blood pressure, but this effect is less important than the effect on the venous capacitance bed and on cardiac filling. Neurogenic shock is the only form of shock that can be safely treated with a vasoconstrictor without having a Swan-Ganz catheter in place. Even in neurogenic shock, however, the patient is at some risk with vasoconstrictor use, because the vasculature to those parts of the body with an intact autonomic nervous system may constrict excessively. Vital organs, such as the kidneys or the gut, can be compromised; ischemic necrosis of the fingers can develop.

Elevation of the legs is effective in the initial treatment of patients in neurogenic shock while fluid therapy is being initiated. Assumption of Trendelenburg's position displaces blood from the systemic venules and small veins to the heart and thus serves to increase stroke volume and cardiac output. Left ventricular emptying is not impaired, even though the heart has to pump the blood upward into the extremities. In the case of neurogenic shock, the systemic vascular resistance is low. Left ventricular emptying is efficient despite the elevated legs.

Body temperature should be monitored and excessive heat loss prevented by appropriate cover. If the patient is hypothermic, heating blankets should be used to restore a reasonably normal temperature.

CARDIAC COMPRESSIVE SHOCK

DIAGNOSIS

The key to the diagnosis of cardiac compressive shock in acutely injured patients is observing distended neck veins or an elevated central venous pressure in a patient who presents with a history and findings that are otherwise consistent with hypovolemic or traumatic shock (see Table 3). To emphasize the point by repetition—distended neck veins in the injured patient suggest cardiac compression. The surgeon should search for a tension pneumothorax, pericardial tamponade, or rupture of the diaphragm. The absence of distended neck veins, however, does not exclude cardiac compressive shock in the hypovolemic injured patient. Distention of the neck veins may become evident only after the patient's blood volume is replenished.

The conditions that produce cardiac compressive shock have distinctive clinical characteristics. Patients with a tension pneumothorax have a shift of the trachea to the uninvolved side, a hyperresonant percussion note and decreased breath sounds on the involved side, and distended neck veins. Discharge of the adrenergic nervous system makes the skin pale, cool, and clammy, although the superficial veins may be distended because of high venous pressures. Oliguria and hypotension develop as the shock increases. Time usually does not permit a chest film, although if obtained, it usually makes the diagnosis obvious.

Patients with pericardial tamponade also present with pale, cool, clammy skin, oliguria, hypotension, and distended neck veins. Heart sounds may be muffled. A chest film may show enlargement of the cardiac shadow if the tamponade is chronic; a characteristic "water bottle" shape may be seen in which the base of the heart shadow is widened in a transverse direction on an upright film. Voltage on the electrocardiogram may be diminished. In many cases, the findings on physical examination may be subtle, but the diagnosis can be established by an echocardiogram. In patients with pericardial tamponade, and sometimes those with other forms of cardiac compressive shock, a pulsus paradoxus—a drop in the systolic systemic arterial blood pressure of more than 10 mm. Hg with a spontaneous breath—can also develop. Kussmaul's sign, a rise in the central venous pressure with a spontaneous inspiration, is highly suggestive of tamponade but infrequently present.

The specific clinical findings associated with diaphragmatic herniation may be demonstrated on the admission chest film. The left costophrenic angle may be blunted, and a double-air density may be seen in the left lower lung field or in the upper abdomen. A nasogastric tube may be curled in the left chest. In many patients, however, the chest film may appear normal. Stab wounds and gunshot wounds near the diaphragm need exploration to exclude this entity.

Positive-pressure ventilation with large tidal volumes can produce compressive shock in hypovolemic patients (1) by compressing the cavae, right atrium, and right ventricle, to limit right ventricular filling; (2) by compressing the pulmonary microvasculature between inflated alveoli, to hinder right ventricular emptying; and (3) by compressing the large pulmonary veins, left atrium, and left ventricle, to limit left ventricular filling.[57] Definitive diagnosis usually requires measurements from a Swan-Ganz catheter, which document a low cardiac output with modestly elevated right atrial and pulmonary artery wedge pressures. The right atrial and wedge pressures are usually within a few millimeters of mercury of each other. Cardiac compression can be assumed to be present in patients without a Swan-Ganz catheter if they are oliguric and if they are receiving tidal volumes in excess of 12 ml. per kg. or positive end-expiratory pressure greater than 100 mm. H_2O, provided that other causes of shock and oliguria have been excluded.

TREATMENT

Treatment of cardiac compressive shock consists of fluid administration to increase ventricular filling pressures and correction of the underlying mechanical cause of the shock. A tension pneumothorax should be decompressed either by the immediate insertion of a chest tube or by insertion of a 14-gauge needle in the second intercostal space in the midclavicular line. Treatment in the emergency setting should proceed on the basis of the physical examination and should not wait for radiographic confirmation; confirmation of the diagnosis comes after treatment, with a rush of air out of the site of thoracic decompression and with resolution of the shock.

Chest tubes should be inserted in the fourth intercostal space in the midaxillary line. The fourth intercostal space should be used because insertion through a lower intercostal space, without benefit of a chest radiograph, might perforate the diaphragm and damage intra-abdominal organs. The midaxillary line should be used because it is the least muscular part of the thorax. The skin, fat, and muscle over the fourth rib should be cut sharply and a large clamp inserted over the rib and into the pleural cavity. Entry into the cavity should be confirmed by inserting a finger and palpating the collapsed lung and by sweeping the finger around inside the chest to feel the smooth parietal pleura and break down any adhesions. The tube should be directed posteriorly and toward the apex of the pleural cavity. The part of the tube in the posterior thorax drains blood; the tip of the tube drains air. Care should be taken during insertion not to unintentionally slide the tube outside the ribs and underneath the scapula.

If insertion of a needle or tube on one side does not reverse the hemodynamic abnormalities and if suspicion remains that the shock is still caused by a tension pneumothorax, a needle should be inserted on the opposite side. Tension pneumothoraces can be difficult to lateralize in some patients, especially in those on mechanical ventilation. Breath sounds can be transmitted into a collapsed lung, and, in a noisy emergency setting, hyperresonance can be missed.

Acute pericardial tamponade in an unstable patient should be treated by a left anterolateral thoracotomy, with decompression of the tamponade and surgical control of the underlying abnormality. In a stable patient, a pericardiocentesis can be accomplished by inserting a needle to the left of the xiphoid process and directing it longitudinally upward and posteriorly, at a 45-degree angle, toward the vertebral column. The location of the needle tip can be monitored by connecting its hub to the V-lead of an electrocardiograph. If the needle touches the myocardium, the voltage indicator on the electrocardiograph easily exceeds the width of the paper (the giant complex of injury). Regardless of whether electrocardiographic monitoring is used, when blood is encountered, it should be aspirated. Withdrawal of 50 ml. of blood should return cardiovascular dynamics to normal. Failure of the patient to respond to the withdrawal of 50 ml. of blood suggests that the end of the needle has aspirated blood from the heart rather than from the pericardial sac.

Acute rupture or laceration of the diaphragm requires immediate surgical correction, usually through the abdomen. The abdominal approach allows inspection of the abdominal viscera and repair of other organs that may be damaged.

Treatment of cardiac compression caused by mechanical ventilation usually requires volume expansion combined with adjustment of the ventilator.[7] In the acute situation, when Swan-Ganz catheterization is not available, the tidal volumes should be kept small (10 ml. per kg.), the inspiratory to expiratory ratios short (I:E ratios of 1:3), and end-expiratory pressures zero. Inspiratory oxygen concentrations have to be kept high. In patients with a Swan-Ganz catheter in place, treatment should be titrated to produce the highest cardiac output with the lowest filling pressures and the least compromise of pulmonary support. This titration is accomplished by volume administration combined with ventilator adjustments. Measurements with the different combinations include urinary output; blood gases; cardiac output; and right atrial, wedge, and systemic arterial pressures.

CARDIOGENIC SHOCK

DIAGNOSIS

Patients with cardiogenic shock on the basis of either right or left ventricular dysfunction present with clinical findings associated with discharge of the adrenergic nervous system and with release of angiotensin and vasopressin (see Table 3). The skin is pale and cool, and urinary output is low. In severe cases, the systemic arterial blood pressure is low. In shock caused by right ventricular dysfunction, the neck veins are distended. In shock caused by left ventricular dysfunction, the patient has rales and a third heart sound or gallop rhythm. If the dysfunction is chronic or severe, the heart may be enlarged, and signs of right ventricular dysfunction, such as distended neck veins, may be present as well.

Cardiogenic shock can be produced by intrinsic cardiac disease, penetrating cardiac trauma, or, rarely, blunt trauma. Intrinsic cardiac disease can include congenital defects, valvular abnormalities, coronary artery disease, myocardiopathies, and arrhythmias. Penetrating injuries to the heart can damage the myocardium, cardiac valves, or coronary arteries.

Blunt trauma can also damage any part of the heart, but a note of caution is in order here. In the great majority of cases, blunt trauma to the heart either produces an arrhythmia or a cardiac rupture that is immediately fatal or produces no injury of any clinical consequence.[79] Hemodynamically stable patients with no conduction abnormalities on electrocardiograms in the emergency department will only rarely have cardiogenic shock on the basis of a blunt cardiac injury. The point to bear in mind is that shock in the patient with a blunt injury is almost always caused by hypovolemia, autonomic dysfunction, or cardiac compression and almost never by a myocardial contusion, even in patients with severe blunt injuries to the chest. Thus, patients in shock after blunt trauma (or penetrating trauma, for that matter) should be treated with blood volume expansion; fluids should not be withheld because of the possibility that the patient might have cardiogenic shock on the basis of a myocardial contusion. On a rare occasion a patient with a cardiac rupture might be hemodynamically stable on admission to the emergency department. Such patients deteriorate within the first 24 hours in the hospital, however; echocardiography makes the diagnosis at that time.

Myocardial infarction with cardiac failure can mimic a ruptured abdominal aortic aneurysm. If the infarcted left ventricle does not create an engorged pulmonary vasculature and a failing right ventricle, the neck veins may not be distended and the pain may be in the upper abdomen or back. Conversely, a ruptured aneurysm can mimic myocardial infarction. Hypovolemia can induce ischemic changes, which are observed on the electrocardiogram, especially in a patient with a pre-existing coronary artery disease. The physician may focus on the abnormal electrocardiogram and mistakenly ascribe the thoracic, abdominal, or back pain to an infarction.

If a patient presents with features consistent with a myocardial infarction and distended neck veins, it is safe to accept a diagnosis of infarction. If the neck veins are flat, however, a more thorough work-up is necessary before accepting this diagnosis. Palpation of the abdominal aorta and femoral and popliteal arteries may reveal aneurysmal disease. Peripheral aneurysms suggest the coexistence of an aortic aneurysm. Cross-table radiographs of the abdomen may reveal calcifications in the wall of the abdominal aortic aneurysm. Hematocrit values should be followed serially.

TREATMENT

Optimization of Heart Rate

The initial treatment of cardiogenic shock begins with administration of oxygen by nasal prongs or mask. Treatment beyond that depends on the cause of myocardial failure but can usually be approached sequentially by (1) correcting arrhythmias and optimizing the heart rate, (2) optimizing ventricular end-diastolic volumes, (3) providing adequate peripheral vasodilation, (4) maximizing myocardial contractility, (5) preserving marginal myocardium with the use of beta-blocking agents, (6) assuring adequate perfusion of the coronary vasculature with the use of vasoconstrictors, (7) providing mechanical assistance to the heart, and (8) surgical correction of cardiac lesions.[32,38,56,58]

Optimization of the heart rate is first in treatment of cardiogenic shock, because the cardiac output equals the heart rate times the stroke volume. In addition, a rapid rate increases velocity of the blood. Increasing velocity decreases blood viscosity and decreases resistance to blood flow. However, too rapid rates lead to inefficient cardiac function. Hindrance to ventricular contraction depends in part on the frequency of contraction. Rapid rates decrease the time available for diastolic ventricular filling. Rapid rates also allow less time for perfusion of the coronary vasculature, which depends on flow during diastole.

The optimal heart rate varies with age and with the status of the coronary arteries. As an individual grows older, the large arteries (aorta and its main bronchus) stiffen and pose an increasing hindrance to ventricular ejection, which increases the work load superimposed on the heart.[5,53] The myocardial oxygen needs for a constant stroke volume thus increase with increasing age. A rapid heart rate that is tolerated in a young patient with compliant large arteries and minimal myocardial oxygen demands may not be tolerated in an older patient, especially a patient with stenotic coronary arteries. The limited time for perfusion of the coronary vasculature with rapid heart rates is also a major problem for the patient with coronary artery disease. A patient with normal coronary arteries can mount a pulse rate equal to the difference of 220 and his age in years multiplied by three fourths. Thus, a 60-year-old patient with normal coronaries can maintain a pulse rate of 120 beats per minute indefinitely. In the presence of coronary disease, the rate should not exceed this number minus 30. Thus, the heart rate in a 60-year-old patient with coronary artery disease should not be allowed to exceed 90 beats per minute. The definitive test for determining whether a heart rate is excessively rapid is to observe the patient for signs of myocardial ischemia, as the heart is the first organ to show the ill effects of an inappropriately rapid rate. Anginal chest pain and electrocardiographic signs of ischemia are the most sensitive indicators.

Life-threatening bradycardias in unstable patients should undergo cardioversion (Fig. 3).[32] More stable patients with a bradyarrhythmia can be treated with a chronotropic agent. Atropine is the drug of first choice. External pacing, followed if necessary by transvenous pacing, is the second choice if atropine fails. On occasion, isoproterenol can be used to increase the heart rate, but it frequently causes arrhythmias, particularly in patients with coronary artery disease.[58]

With the exception of asystole, all tachyarrhythmias that create hemodynamic instability should be cardioverted.[32] In the case of asystole, the patient should be treated first with epinephrine and atropine, to produce ventricular fibrillation, which should then be cardioverted. If the patient with a tachyarrhythmia is relatively stable, a full 12-lead electrocardiogram should be obtained (Fig. 3). If the QRS complex is longer

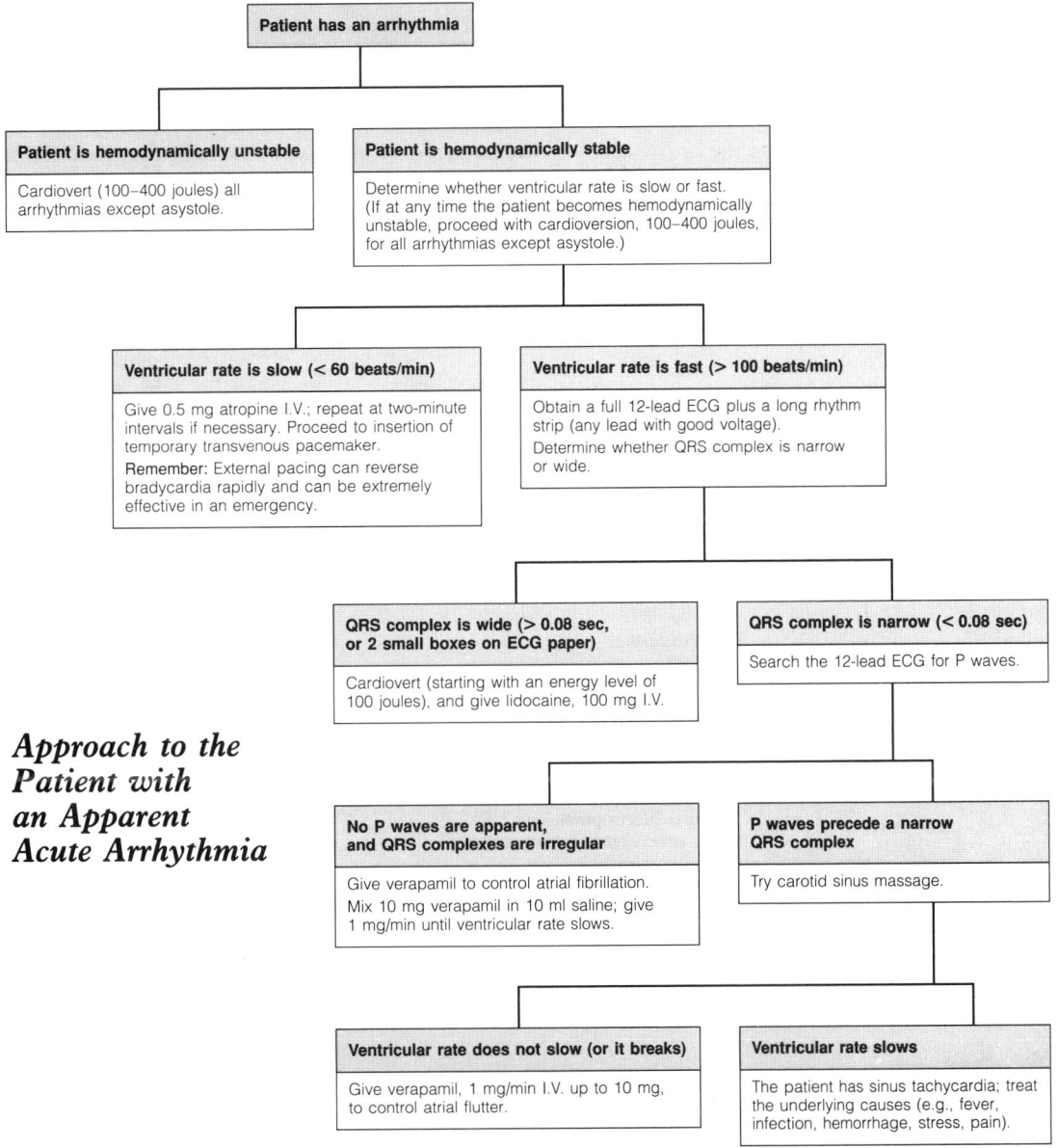

Approach to the Patient with an Apparent Acute Arrhythmia

Figure 3. Algorithm for treatment of arrhythmias. (From Harken, A. H.: Cardiac arrhythmias. *In* Wilmore, D. W., Brennan, M. F., Harken, A. H., Holcroft, J. W., and Meakins, J. L. (Eds.): Care of the Surgical Patient. Vol. 1. Critical Care, A Publication of the Committee on Pre- and Postoperative Care, American College of Surgeons. New York, Scientific American, Inc., 1989.)

than 0.08 second, the patient should undergo cardioversion. If the complex is shorter than 0.08 second, the electrocardiogram should be searched for P waves. If no P waves are apparent and the QRS complexes are irregular, verapamil should be given, to slow the ventricular rate. If P waves are present, the carotid bulb should be compressed. In response to the compression, the ventricular rate slows, reverts, or remains unchanged. If compression reverts or has no influence on the arrhythmia, verapamil should be given; if the rate slows, the patient has a sinus tachycardia, and treatment should be directed toward the underlying cause.

The uncommon arrhythmia with a ventricular response in the physiologic range may not cause any hemodynamic instability and may even produce a supranormal cardiac index. These arrhythmias do not need to be immediately treated, although their etiology should be determined.

Adjustment of Ventricular End-Diastolic Volumes

Optimization of ventricular end-diastolic volumes—by either augmentation or diminution—is next. Increasing the end-diastolic volumes, by the administration of fluids, should usually be tried initially. An increase in end-diastolic volumes increases the stroke volumes, as long as the patient is on the ascending limb of the Frank-Starling curve and as long as myocardial contractility and vascular resistances do not change to make cardiac function less effective. Increasing the blood volume, however, can engorge the pulmonary vasculature and hinder right ventricular emptying. Increasing the stroke volume can increase the stroke work and increase myocardial oxygen demands. Increasing ventricular end-systolic volume can lead to excess myocardial heat dissipation during isovolumetric ventricular relaxation and to increased myocardial oxygen needs.[67] Distention of the ventricular walls during diastole can compress the coronary vasculature and limit myocardial perfusion. Distention of the right atrium can impede flow of blood from the coronaries into the coronary sinus. Distention of the atria can also lead to pulmonary or peripheral edema.

Thus, expansion of the blood volume and increasing end-diastolic volumes do not always cause an increase in stroke volumes or an improvement in the patient's condition. If fluid administration does not produce beneficial effects or if the patient's clinical condition suggests that the vascular volume is already fully expanded, then the blood volume and end-diastolic volumes should be decreased, as a trial, with a diuretic. Reducing pulmonary vascular engorgement can ease right ventricular emptying[55]; a modest decrease in stroke volume can decrease stroke work and myocardial oxygen consumption (which might be critical in a patient with compromised myocardial perfusion); decreasing end-systolic volumes can decrease myocardial heat dissipation and oxygen needs; decreasing diastolic ventricular distention can decompress the coronary vas-

culature; decreasing right atrial distention can augment flow into the coronary sinus; and decreasing atrial distention can help mobilize pulmonary and peripheral edema.

If the patient is thought to be hypovolemic, a fluid bolus of 250 ml. should be given over a period of 10 minutes for determining whether the cardiac status improves with augmentation of end-diastolic volumes. If the patient's condition worsens with the bolus or if, at initial evaluation, the patient is thought to be hypervolemic, a single intravenous dose of furosemide, 40 mg., should be given. A prompt diuresis with resolution of shock supports the diagnosis of cardiac failure and volume overload. Minimal or no response should prompt reconsideration of the diagnosis.

The decision to use volume expansion or reduction is simplified if a Swan-Ganz catheter is in place. The goal is to produce the highest cardiac output with the lowest filling pressures; that is, the goal is to maximize delivery of oxygen to the tissues while minimizing formation of edema. The goal is not primarily to increase urine output. Oliguria develops in all types of shock, if the shock is severe enough. A diuretic-induced urinary output in a trauma or septic patient who is thought to have an element of cardiogenic shock may be seen as encouraging to the treating physician, but diuretics are almost never indicated under such conditions. They should be used only when the atrial filling pressures are high and it is thought that an engorged pulmonary vasculature is impeding efficient function of the right ventricle. The pitfalls of measuring atrial pressures with the Swan-Ganz catheter should also be borne in mind.[1] A misplaced transducer, placement of the catheter in a zone of the pulmonary vasculature that is occluded by inflated alveoli, and miscalibration can lead to the mistaken impression that filling pressures of the heart are high, when indeed they may be low. Moreover, measurements of the filling pressures are determinations of intracavitary pressures only. Many critically ill surgical patients have an associated element of cardiac compression. The pressures inside the chambers of the heart may be high, but the end-diastolic volumes may be low if the heart is compressed by an elevated diaphragm or by high airway pressures induced by positive-pressure ventilation.

Vasodilators

Vasodilators have several attractive features and very few disadvantages if used carefully.[58] They can decrease the systemic and pulmonary vascular resistances and ease ventricular contraction. Nitroglycerin and, to a lesser extent, nitroprusside dilate the systemic venules and small veins and thus decrease filling of the right heart, pulmonary vasculature, and left heart. Decreased filling of the cardiac chambers, induced by venodilation, combined with more efficient emptying of the ventricles, induced by low resistances, serves to decrease filling pressures and volumes in all chambers of the heart. Decreased right atrial

TABLE 4. Effects of Some Therapeutic Interventions
on Circulatory Derangements in Shock

Intervention	Cardiac Output	Atrial Pressures	Myocardial Oxygen Needs
Inflation of pneumatic antishock garment	↓↑	↑	↑
Trendelenburg's position	↓↑	↑	↑
Correction of bradycardia	↑	↓	↓
Correction of tachyarrhythmia	↑	↓	↓
Administration of fluid	↑	↑	↑
Administration of diuretic	↓↑	↓	↓
Administration of vasodilator	↑	↓	↓
Administration of inotrope	↑	↓	↑
Administration of beta-blocker	↓	↓↑	↓
Administration of vasoconstrictor	↓↑	↑	↑
Use of intra-aortic balloon pump	↑	↓	↓

and coronary sinus pressures and reduced tension in the ventricular wall increase coronary blood flow as well. The heart benefits from decreased myocardial work and myocardial oxygen demands and from increased oxygen supplies. Administration of nitroglycerin or nitroprusside to patients in cardiogenic shock with high systemic vascular resistances, high filling pressures of the heart, and large cardiac chambers can be a nearly ideal therapeutic maneuver (Table 4).

In some patients, however, administration of nitroglycerin or nitroprusside excessively dilates the systemic venules and small veins and excessively decreases end-diastolic volumes. Excessive arteriolar dilation can also lower aortic diastolic pressures to the point that coronary perfusion is compromised. These potential adverse effects should be sought by measuring filling pressures and cardiac outputs before and after establishment of the infusion and by noting the presence or absence of chest pain and electrocardiographic evidence of myocardial ischemia during the infusion.

Morphine can be extremely effective in treating patients in cardiogenic shock after an acute myocardial infarction. The drug dilates both the systemic arterioles and venules and relieves pain. There is little concern about the volume status in these patients, and the drug is usually safe to use even without Swan-Ganz monitoring. Opiates can be used in potentially hypovolemic patients, but only judiciously, as they can further impair filling of the heart and lead to catastrophic lowering of cardiac output. Most patients in shock do not require pain relief, as agitation and expressions of discomfort are usually caused by hypoxemia or by the shock itself rather than by pain. However, small intravenous doses of a narcotic can be used with care in selected patients in whom volume resuscitation is deemed adequate. A subsequent fall in blood pressure with administration of an opiate strongly suggests inadequate volume replenishment and should lead to administration of more fluid and to a search for the cause of the presumed hypovolemia.

Inotropic Agents

Inotropic agents are next to be considered, after control of arrhythmias, adjustment of end-diastolic volumes, and consideration of a vasodilator. Dopamine and dobutamine are the most useful.[58] In low doses, they increase myocardial contractility, and dopamine can dilate the renal vasculature, thus selectively increasing renal blood flow and urinary output. Dopamine can raise the heart rate excessively; dobutamine usually does not. Both drugs have to be used with caution. Low-dose dopamine (less than 5 μg. per kg. per minute, for example) is thought to have minimal alpha-adrenergic effects. This belief is based on studies in which the drug has been infused in normal subjects at different doses and the cardiovascular effects measured at these different doses. Normal subjects differ from patients in shock, however. In some patients in shock, even low doses of dopamine can augment underlying vasoconstriction to a dangerous degree, causing an increased systemic vascular resistance and even causing ischemic necrosis of the digits or extremities.

Patients who require dopamine or dobutamine should be monitored in an intensive care unit. Excessive cutaneous vasoconstriction should lead to reassessment of the need for the drug. If the drug is used for more than 1 hour, a Swan-Ganz catheter should be placed to ensure that the patient's shock is truly on the basis of myocardial dysfunction. Filling pressures and cardiac indices should be measured at different infusion rates. If any question remains about adequacy of volume resuscitation, the filling pressures and cardiac output should be measured before and after a fluid bolus.

In most surgical patients, the goal of any therapeutic intervention in the cardiovascular system is to increase the cardiac index to a slightly hyperdynamic state (5.0 liters per minute per sq. m. for young patients and 3.5 liters per minute per sq. m.

for old patients) while maintaining pulmonary artery wedge pressures at low levels (7 mm. Hg for patients breathing spontaneously and 12 mm. Hg for those on positive-pressure ventilation).[63] Effects on systemic arterial blood pressure and urinary output are usually secondary. Dopamine and dobutamine should be used to increase flow in the cardiovascular system. These drugs should not be used as vasoconstrictors or as diuretics.

Digitalis compounds should not be used in the shock setting because their inotropic actions offer nothing beyond that of dopamine and dobutamine. They also have the potential for toxicity, especially in circumstances of overall cardiovascular instability, when pH and electrolyte changes are unpredictable.

Beta-Blocking Agents

An occasional patient in cardiogenic shock, with an ischemic myocardium and a rapid heart rate, benefits from administration of a beta-blocker, such as propranolol, even though such agents usually decrease the cardiac output. Decreasing myocardial contractility and the heart rate and dilating the peripheral vasculature decrease myocardial oxygen requirements (Table 4). Smaller stroke volumes and diminished stroke work also decrease oxygen needs. This state of myocardial hibernation can be beneficial for a patient who has had a recent myocardial infarction and in whom the surrounding tissue is of marginal viability, and might be useful temporarily while one is preparing a patient for urgent revascularization. Beta-blockers should not be used in noncardiac patients with large wounds or septic foci. These patients need the highest possible output to heal their tissues and to fight off infection.

Vasoconstrictors

Vasoconstrictors, such as norepinephrine, phenylephrine, or metaraminol, are sometimes of value in treating patients with cardiogenic shock. Their main role in this condition is that they increase aortic diastolic blood pressure and increase perfusion of the coronary circulation. They may also increase myocardial contractility. Constrictors are most likely to be useful in patients with coronary disease who need high aortic pressures during diastole to perfuse the myocardium. Constrictors can also be useful in treating air embolism—to break up air bubbles trapped in the microvasculature of the heart and brain and force the bubbles into the venous side of the circulation. Other patients may need a vasoconstrictor to increase perfusion pressure of the coronary arteries during open or closed cardiac massage.

The beneficial effects of increased coronary artery pressure and increased contractility, however, are frequently offset by increased myocardial work. On balance, vasoconstrictors usually do more harm than good (Table 4). Most patients in shock have more than adequate discharge of the adrenergic nervous system and appropriate vasoconstriction of the vascular beds. Vascular beds have autoregulatory capabilities that accurately modulate blood flow to potentially compromised organs. If such beds are not maximally constricted, it is usually for good reason. Administration of a vasoconstrictor may shut off critical residual flow that is just maintaining metabolic integrity of the organ in question.

Intra-aortic Balloon Pump

Mechanical circulatory assistance with an intra-aortic balloon pump can be of substantial value in selected patients with severe left ventricular dysfunction.[56] By inflating the balloon in diastole and deflating it in systole, the intra-aortic balloon pump augments coronary filling and aids ventricular contraction. It can be highly effective in treating cardiogenic shock; it is usually preferable to long-term use of inotropic agents and is almost always preferable to use of vasoconstrictors. Its effects on the cardiovascular system are all positive. It decreases ventricular volumes, relieves compression on the coronary microvasculature, reduces myocardial oxygen needs, and reduces the tendencies to form pulmonary and peripheral edema (Table 4). Its main disadvantages are that it is cumbersome to use and that its use can damage the frequently atherosclerotic arteries of the patient who is likely to need it. Indications for such devices are currently being evaluated. They should be used only in patients with Swan-Ganz catheters in place.

Reconstructive Surgery

Although listed last in this discussion of shock treatment, reconstructive surgery should be an early option for some patients in cardiogenic shock. It can be particularly effective in selected cases of coronary insufficiency, ventricular septal rupture, papillary muscle rupture, and mitral valve dysfunction. (See Chapter 56, The Heart.)

CARDIAC OBSTRUCTIVE SHOCK

DIAGNOSIS

The conditions that produce cardiac obstructive shock usually affect one ventricle much more than the other, and the diagnosis frequently arises from the findings of single ventricle dysfunction combined with the clinical characteristics of the condition causing the dysfunction. The diagnosis (and treatment) of pulmonary embolism is discussed in Chapter 50. The diagnosis of right-sided cardiac dysfunction that arises from mechanical ventilation is discussed in this chapter in the section on cardiac compressive shock. It is necessary to point out here only that mechanical ventilation has several adverse effects on cardiac function, and that compression of the pulmonary vasculature is one of them.[57] Pulmonary microvascular constriction or obstruction can arise from congenital abnormalities, acute lung disease such as the adult respiratory distress syndrome, or long-standing left-sided congestive heart failure. When severe or

when exacerbated by acute pulmonary infection, the construction or obstruction can produce right-sided failure. The diagnosis is usually obvious and based on a previously established recognition of the underlying disease. Right-sided congestive failure can also arise from left-sided failure because of pulmonary vascular engorgement. In these circumstances, the microvasculature may be widely patent, but the larger vessels are so distended that their walls stiffen to the point that the right ventricle can no longer pump effectively.[38] The diagnosis is usually made by the findings of left-sided congestive failure with an engorged pulmonary vasculature on the chest film, combined with the findings of right-sided failure. The diagnosis of cross-clamp–induced left ventricular failure is best made in elective aortic surgery by using a previously placed Swan-Ganz catheter to measure cardiac output before and after application of the clamp; in emergency cases without a Swan-Ganz catheter in place, usually the diagnosis can be made only if the failure is severe enough to produce electrocardiographic abnormalities or hypotension. Failure caused by systemic arteriolar constriction is always associated with systemic hypertension; failure caused by the excessively viscous blood of polycythemia arises only with hematocrits of at least 50 per cent.

TREATMENT

Treatment of cardiac obstructive shock should be directed toward the cause of the shock; adjuvant treatment of the heart failure itself—with inotropes, fluid administration, or, conversely, diuretics—is sometimes helpful and sometimes not. Anticoagulation with large-dose heparin can sometimes dramatically reverse obstruction to right ventricular output. Adjustment of the ventilator, along with fluid administration, can usually overcome the ill effects of mechanical ventilation on a compromised right heart. Treatment of pulmonary vascular disease may require surgical correction of a congenital defect or medical treatment of a superimposed pulmonary infection. Engorgement of the pulmonary vasculature from left-sided failure

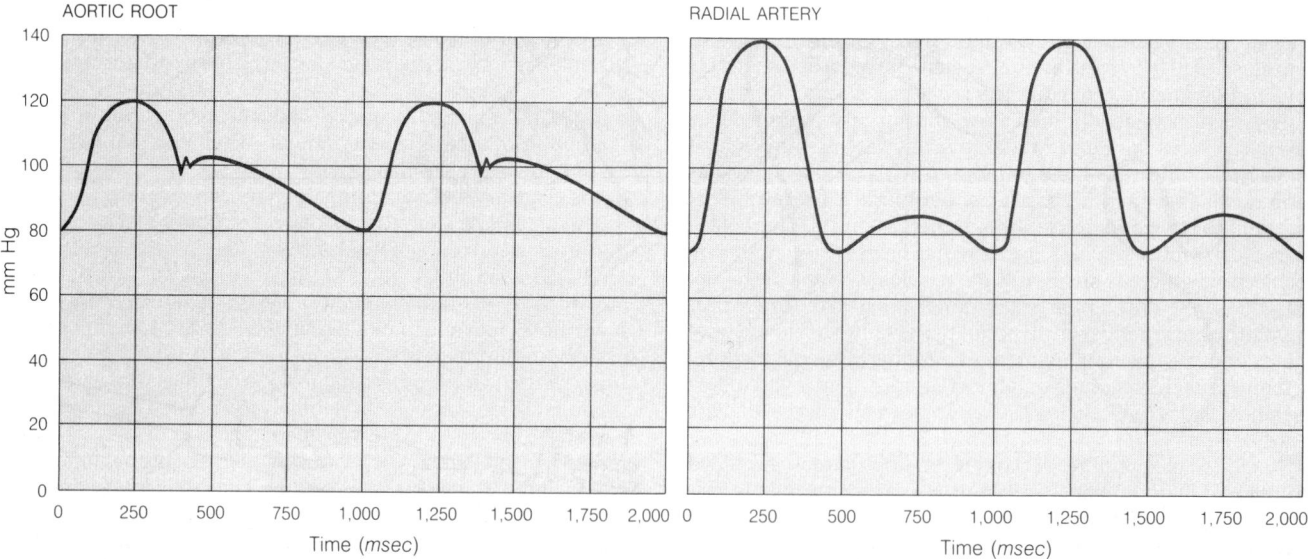

Figure 4. The mean pressure is defined as the area under a pressure tracing over an entire cycle, divided by the time needed to produce that cycle. A pressure wave in the ascending aorta with a blood pressure of 120/80 has the same mean pressure as a pressure wave in the radial artery of the same patient, even though the radial artery pressure might be 140/75, because the systolic pressure in the radial artery is usually inscribed more rapidly than the systolic pressure in the aorta. The areas underneath the aortic pressure and radial artery pressure curves are identical. A useful but not infallible approximation of the mean pressure is to take the diastolic pressure plus one third of the difference between the systolic and diastolic pressures. In these examples, this formula would not work. The mean aortic pressure would be approximated at 93 mm. Hg, whereas the mean radial artery pressure would be approximated as 97 mm. Hg. Such results would be impossible: if the mean pressure in the radial artery actually were greater than the mean pressure in the aorta, blood would flow backward. This confusion is avoided by actually measuring the area under the curve and calculating the mean pressure exactly. Computer circuits in most pressure-monitoring systems make exact calculations of the mean pressure. Thus, the mean pressure, taken from the digital readout of the pressure monitor, is the single most accurate indicator of the actual pressure being measured and should be used for measurements of systemic pressure. (From Abrams, H. J., Cerra, F., and Holcroft, J. W.: Cardiopulmonary monitoring. In Wilmore, D. W., Brennan, M. F., Harken, A. H., Holcroft, J. W., and Meakins, J. L. (Eds.): Care of the Surgical Patient. Vol. 1. Critical Care, A Publication of the Committee on Pre- and Postoperative Care, American College of Surgeons. New York, Scientific American, Inc., 1989.)

usually responds well to diuresis. Vasodilators can sometimes reverse the failure produced by an aortic cross-clamp. Vasodilators can almost always reverse the failure of extreme arteriolar constriction, unless the heart has become irretrievably damaged by long-standing hypertension. Polycythemia is effectively treated by phlebotomy.

MONITORING IN THE ICU

The discussion so far has approached the diagnosis and treatment of shock by placing the shock into specific categories and then describing treatment for that particular type of shock. This approach is useful in the initial management of shock and is all that is necessary in the majority of patients who present to the emergency department. Those who do not respond well have to be managed in conjunction with information obtained from arterial catheters and sometimes pulmonary arterial catheters, which usually leads to a more fundamental understanding of the shock state. Such an understanding of the pathophysiology can be particularly useful when a proposed treatment for one abnormality might produce a new abnormality. For example, fluid administration might be needed for resuscitating a patient in shock from musculoskeletal and cranial injuries, but too much fluid might unnecessarily increase intracranial pressure. Fluid might be needed to maintain renal perfusion and urinary output in the same patient, but too much might produce pulmonary edema. Use of a vasoconstrictor might be logical in some types of shock and dangerous in others. Use of other therapeutic modalities, such as vasodilators, inotropic agents, beta-blockers, diuretics, blood administration, and mechanical ventilation, can also be beneficial or dangerous, depending on the circumstances. Treatment of these more complicated pathophysiologic states requires an understanding of how to use systemic arterial and Swan-Ganz catheters.[1]

ARTERIAL CATHETERS

Intra-arterial catheters are frequently useful in managing patients in shock who do not respond quickly to therapy. Because these catheters can lead to thrombosis of the vessel in which they are inserted, they are most safely placed in arteries with abundant collateral circulation. The radial artery is safer to use than the brachial, and the dorsalis pedis is safer than the femoral. The catheters should be continuously flushed with a dilute heparin solution, but bolus flushing should be kept to a minimum, especially with radial and brachial artery catheters. Retrograde embolization of clot and other atherosclerotic debris to the vertebral artery and brain stem can occur with rapid infusion of volumes as small as 2 ml.

The most reliable pressure obtained from the arterial catheter is the mean pressure, which can be taken from the digital readout of an electronic pressure monitoring module (Fig. 4).[1] It is best not to place much reliance on the systolic and diastolic values, which can be misleading for three reasons. First, the systolic and diastolic pressures measured at the transducer are frequently different from the pressures in the artery itself. If the transducer-tubing-catheter system is very compliant compared with the arterial system, or if it has a high resistance, the pressures at the transducer are damped. Air bubbles are probably the most common cause of an excessively compliant system; partially occluding clots are the most common cause of a too high resistance. Conversely, a system that is too stiff or that has a resistance that is very low, compared with the patient's vascular system, produces exaggerated "ringing" pressure waves at the transducer. The mean pressure, however, is unaffected by mismatching of the compliances and resistances.

The second reason to be wary of systolic and diastolic pressure measurements has to do with amplification of the pulse pressure as the measuring site moves distally from the root of the aorta. As the distance increases, the systolic pressure increases and the diastolic pressure decreases, because pulse wave reflection from the arterioles comes back more in phase with the antegrade wave as distance from the root of the aorta increases. The mean pressure, however, is unaffected (Fig. 5).

Third, the diastolic pressure can be misinterpreted because of catheter whip or fling. Rapid movements of the catheter generate drops in pressure at the tip of the catheter. The artifactual drop can be misinterpreted as a diastolic pressure. Although use of the mean pressure does not completely solve this problem, it will be influenced less than the apparent diastolic pressure.

In brief, in the measurement of systemic arterial pressures, the mean pressure is the value to use.

SWAN-GANZ CATHETER

The Swan-Ganz catheter, in selected patients, can give valuable information about the diagnosis and treatment of the circulatory derangements of shock. The catheter allows measurement of (1) flow in the cardiovascular system, as measured by thermodilution, (2) blood gases in mixed venous blood, and (3) filling pressures of both the right and left sides of the heart. From these primary data, derived quantities can be calculated

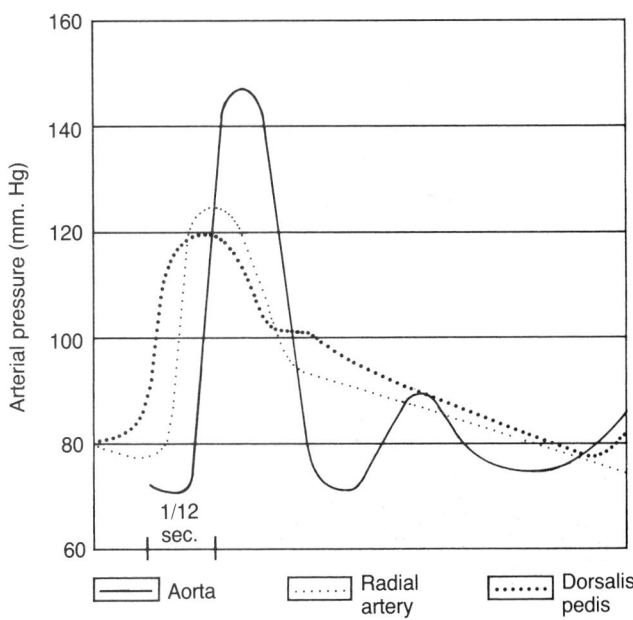

Figure 5. There are true differences in systolic and diastolic pressures in arteries at different distances from the heart. These differences result when pressure waves reflected from distal arteriolar sites are superimposed onto the forward-traveling pressure waves from the aorta. As the measuring point (i.e., the catheter) moves closer to the distal reflecting site, systolic pressures increase and diastolic pressures decrease, because the reflected pressure waves from the periphery return sooner to a catheter that is placed distally. The result of this in-phase superimposition of reflected waves onto antegrade waves is augmentation of systolic pressures and diminution of diastolic pressures. The systolic pressure in the radial artery, therefore, can be 10 to 20 mm. Hg higher than the systolic pressure in the ascending aorta, leading to confusion. Moreover, the pressure tracing at the root of the aorta is wider than the pressure tracing in the radial artery, because reflected waves are returning from the periphery at different times; their effect is thus distributed over a larger portion of the cardiac cycle, and the pressure wave in the aorta is broad. The pressure wave in the radial artery is narrow, because the reflected waves tend to be superimposed on the forward-traveling waves, in phase. The mean pressures, however, are almost the same in the two vessels, with the mean pressure in the radial artery being just slightly less than the mean pressure in the ascending aorta. Use of the mean pressure eliminates inaccuracies introduced by catheter-vascular mismatching and confusion introduced by pulse wave reflection; inspection of the tracing usually reveals aberrations introduced by catheter whip. (From Abrams, J. H., Cerra, F., and Holcroft, J. W.: Cardiopulmonary monitoring. *In* Wilmore, D. W., Brennan, M. F., Harken, A. H., Holcroft, J. W., and Meakins, J. L. (Eds.): Care of the Surgical Patient. Vol. 1. Critical Care, A Publication of the Committee on Pre- and Postoperative Care, American College of Surgeons. New York, Scientific American, Inc., 1989.)

TABLE 5. Normal Values Obtained from Commonly Used Monitors

Variable	Abbreviation or Derivation	Normal Value	Units
Partial pressure of oxygen in systemic arterial blood	Pao_2	Varies with age (e.g., 95 for young adults, 80 for elderly)	mm. Hg
Partial pressure of carbon dioxide in arterial blood	$Paco_2$	40 (does not vary with age)	mm. Hg
Oxygen saturation in arterial blood	Sao_2	97%	Dimensionless
Oxygen content in arterial blood	Cao_2* $4/3 \times [Hb] \times Sao_2$	20	ml. O_2/100 ml. blood, or vol. %
Partial pressure of oxygen in mixed venous blood	$Pmvo_2$	40	mm. Hg
Partial pressure of carbon dioxide in mixed venous blood	$Pmvco_2$	46	mm. Hg
Oxygen saturation in mixed venous blood	$Smvo_2$	75%	Dimensionless
Oxygen content in mixed venous blood	$Cmvo_2$* $4/3 \times [Hb] \times Smvo_2$	15	ml. O_2/100 ml. blood, or vol. %
pH	—	7.4	dimensionless
Hydrogen ion concentration	—	40	nmol./L.
Bicarbonate ion concentration	$24 \times Pco_2 \div [H^+]$	24	mmol./L.
Cardiac index	CI	3	L./min./sq. m.
Mean systemic arterial pressure	Pa	93	mm. Hg
Mean right atrial pressure	Pra	3†	mm. Hg
Mean pulmonary arterial pressure	Ppa	15†	mm. Hg
Mean wedge pressure	$Pwedge$	8†	mm. Hg
Systemic vascular resistance index	$(Pa - Pra) \div CI$	30	mm. Hg/min./sq. m./L.
Pulmonary vascular resistance index	$(Ppa - Pwedge) \div CI$	2	mm. Hg/min./sq. m./L.
Oxygen transport	$CI \times Cao_2$	600	ml. O_2/min./sq. m.
Oxygen return	$CI \times Cmvo_2$	450	ml. O_2/min./sq. m.
Oxygen consumption	$CI \times (Cao_2 - Cmvo_2)$	150	ml. O_2/min./sq. m.

* Oxygen contents calculated on the assumption that [Hb] equals 15 gm. per 100 ml. and that O_2 consumption and cardiac index are normal.

† Values given are for when the patient is breathing spontaneously. Pressures, on average, will be 5 mm. Hg higher if the patient is being mechanically ventilated.

From Abrams, J. H., Cerra, F., and Holcroft, J. W.: Cardiopulmonary monitoring. *In* Wilmore, D. W., Brennan, M. F. Harken, A. H., Holcroft, J. W., and Meakins, T. L. (Eds.): Care of the Surgical Patient. Vol. 1. Critical Care, A Publication of the Committee on Pre- and Postoperative Care, American College of Surgeons. New York, Scientific American, Inc., 1989.

(Table 5). The systemic vascular resistance is the difference between the mean systemic arterial and right atrial pressures divided by the cardiac output or index. The pulmonary vascular resistance is the difference between the mean pulmonary artery and pulmonary artery wedge pressures divided by the cardiac output or index. Oxygen consumption is the difference between systemic and pulmonary arterial oxygen contents multiplied by the cardiac output or index.

The findings expected in various states of shock are summarized in Table 3. Although the Swan-Ganz catheter is sometimes helpful in diagnosing these states, it is even more helpful in guiding therapy. It is useful in this regard, however, only if measurements are made with care. The next three sections describe some precautions to be taken to assure accurate measurements with the Swan-Ganz catheter.[1]

CARDIAC OUTPUT. Cardiac output, as measured by thermodilution, is obtained by injecting a known volume of a cold crystalloid solution into the right atrium and measuring the resulting temperature drop in the pulmonary artery as the cool blood flows past a thermistor located on the end of the catheter. The greater the temperature drop over a given period of time, the slower the flow through the right heart. Computers specifically designed to calculate cardiac output from thermodilution measurements are available. The computers can make accurate computations, however, only if certain precautions are taken when injecting the solution. Room temperature or ice-cold solutions can be used as injectates. The advantage of a room temperature injectate is that a solution of precisely known temperature is delivered to the right atrium with a minimum of apparatus.

The advantage of injecting an ice-cold solution is that the resulting temperature drop in the pulmonary artery is large, thus maximizing the signal-to-noise ratio. The amount injected should be precisely known. Injections should be made at the same time in the ventilatory cycle, as flow in the cardiovascular system depends on the phase of the ventilatory cycle. Injection at end-expiration is recommended, with the patient either breathing spontaneously or on positive-pressure ventilation.

MIXED VENOUS OXYGEN LEVELS. The catheter can be used for drawing blood for determination of mixed venous oxygen contents. The balloon should be deflated when blood is withdrawn, and the blood should be withdrawn slowly. If blood is withdrawn too quickly, the wall of the pulmonary artery surrounding the tip of the catheter can collapse around the end of the catheter (Fig. 6). Blood withdrawn through the catheter has a falsely high oxygen content because, under these circumstances, the blood is drawn back past ventilated alveoli, absorbing oxygen from these alveoli. This potential problem can, and should, be assessed by measuring the partial pressure of carbon dioxide in the specimen. Normally, the Pco_2 of mixed venous blood is approximately 6 mm. Hg higher than the Pco_2 of simultaneously drawn systemic arterial blood. If blood is drawn back past nonperfused but ventilated alveoli, the Pco_2 in that blood falls. Thus, if blood is drawn back too fast, the Pco_2 of the withdrawn blood approaches the Pco_2 of simultaneously drawn systemic arterial blood; it may even become less. This abnormal difference in Pco_2 alerts the physician that the partial pressure of oxygen in the specimen is falsely high.

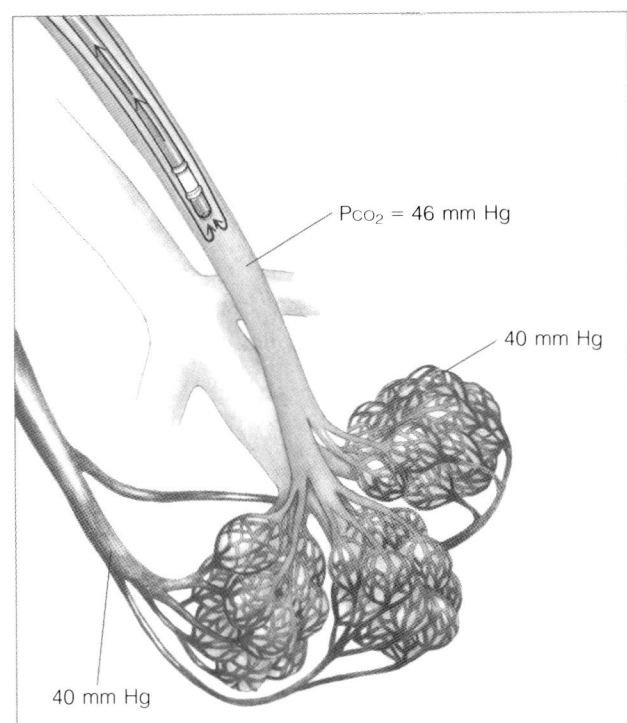
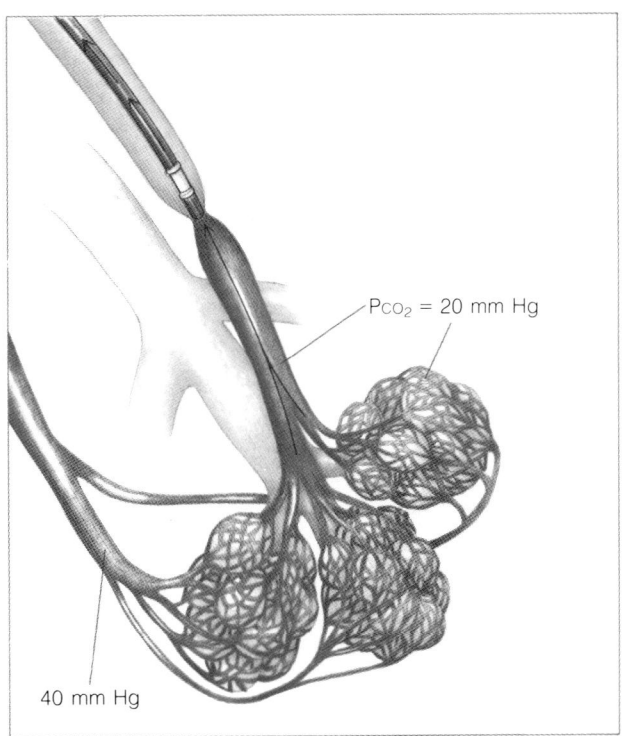

Figure 6. The Swan-Ganz catheter allows collection of mixed venous blood for measurement of mixed venous oxygen saturation and content *(A)*. If blood from the pulmonary artery is withdrawn through the catheter too forcefully, however, arterial walls can collapse around the tip of the catheter *(B)*. The blood that is withdrawn for sampling, in that case, consists of blood from the distal pulmonary vasculature that has been pulled back past ventilated alveoli. To determine whether pullback of blood through the catheter has led to retrograde flow *(B)*, the partial pressure of carbon dioxide in the sample can be assessed. PCO_2 in mixed venous blood is typically some 6 mm. Hg greater than PCO_2 in systemic arterial blood. If the artery walls have collapsed around the catheter, the sample consists of blood from which much of the CO_2 already has been excreted into the ventilated alveoli, and the recovered blood has a PCO_2 that might be as much as 20 mm. Hg lower than simultaneously obtained arterial blood. Specimens of this sort should be discarded and new ones obtained. (From Abrams, J. H., Cerra, F., and Holcroft, J. W.: Cardiopulmonary monitoring. *In* Wilmore, D. W., Brennan, M. F., Harken, A. H., Holcroft, J. W., and Meakins, J. L. (Eds.): Care of the Surgical Patient. Vol. 1. Critical Care, A Publication of the Committee on Pre- and Postoperative Care, American College of Surgeons. New York, Scientific American, Inc., 1989.)

CENTRAL PRESSURES. All pressures obtained with the Swan-Ganz catheter should be measured at end-expiration, without regard to the mode of ventilation. The right atrial pressure is measured through the proximal port of the Swan-Ganz catheter and is the most reliable of all the pressures obtained with the catheter. It, and all central pressures, should be measured at end-expiration (Fig. 7).

Measurements of the pulmonary artery systolic and diastolic pressures may be inaccurate. If the catheter system and its connecting tubing are stiff or noncompliant compared with the stiffness of the pulmonary vasculature, the systolic and diastolic pressures recorded at the level of the pressure transducer are exaggerated. If the catheter and the connecting tubing are compliant, compared with the pulmonary vasculature, the recorded pressures are dampened. The pulmonary artery systolic and diastolic pressures measured with a pulmonary artery catheter are accurate only if the compliance and resistance of the catheter-transducer system are similar to those of the pulmonary vasculature. Most intensive care units do not make a correction for this mismatch of impedances. Unless such a correction is made, it is best not to use the systolic or diastolic pressures obtained from the pulmonary artery catheter.

The mean pulmonary artery pressure, however, is accurate and does truly reflect the mean pressure in the pulmonary vasculature, no matter what the impedance of the catheter and the transducer system may be. The mean pulmonary artery pressure should be taken at one point in the ventilatory cycle because it varies with the changes induced by airway pressure on the cardiovascular system. Pressure measurements should be obtained at end-expiration in all patients, whether they are breathing spontaneously or on positive-pressure ventilation (Fig. 8). Generally, with a patient breathing spontaneously, the pressure that should be recorded is the highest of the pressures recorded on the oscilloscope. With the patient on positive-pressure ventilation, the pressure recorded should be the lowest of the recorded pressures.

The pulmonary artery wedge pressure accurately reflects left atrial pressure as long as the pulmonary artery catheter is in a portion of the vasculature that communicates directly with the left atrium and as long as inflation of the balloon occludes all flow going through that portion of the vasculature. For example, if the catheter is in a portion of the lung where inflation of the lung occludes the pulmonary capillaries, the end of the Swan-Ganz catheter "sees" the pressure in the alveoli rather than the pressure in the left atrium. Therefore, the end of the catheter has to be in a portion of the pulmonary vasculature that is not compressed by the lung. Most of the lung of patients in the supine position is adequately perfused, and occlusion of the vasculature by hyperinflated alveoli is not often a problem. The main point to bear in mind is that the wedge pressure does not always accurately reflect the left atrial pressure. Wedge pressures should be measured at end-expiration (see Fig. 8).

SYSTEMIC RESPONSES TO SHOCK

Shock elicits systemic responses that help compensate for the shock insult but that sometimes contribute to shock-induced organ failure. Adrenergic discharge and exposure to vasopressin and angiotensin, by constricting the venules and small veins, displaces blood to the heart, to increase ventricular end-diastolic volumes; constriction of the noncerebral and noncardiac arterioles maximizes blood flow to the brain and heart while sacrificing flow to the rest of the body. Vasopressin and aldosterone maximize renal conservation of vascular volume. Spon-

SPONTANEOUS VENTILATION

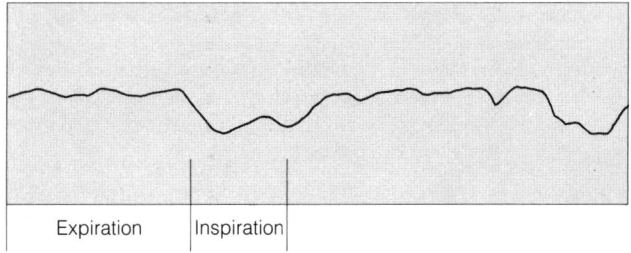

Expiration | Inspiration

MECHANICAL VENTILATION

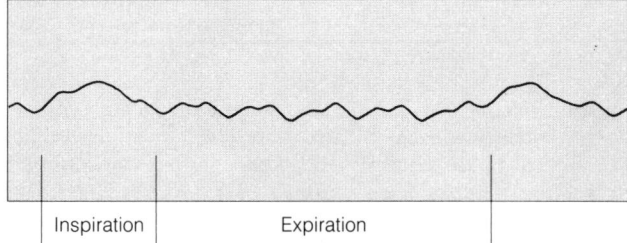

Inspiration | Expiration

INTERMITTENT MANDATORY VENTILATION

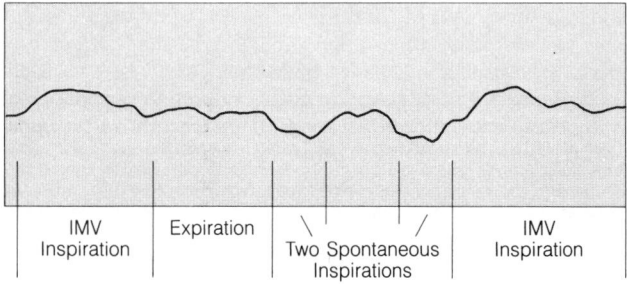

IMV Inspiration | Expiration | Two Spontaneous Inspirations | IMV Inspiration

Figure 7. End-expiratory pressure is relatively independent of the patient's ventilatory status and thus is most representative of the patient's vascular volume. For example, in a patient breathing spontaneously *(top)*, central venous pressure (or equivalently, right atrial pressure) falls as the lungs pull away from the intrathoracic great veins and right atrium. In these patients, the end-expiratory pressure is the highest pressure measured during the ventilatory cycle. During mechanical ventilation *(middle)*, the lungs are pushed against the outside of the heart and great veins; intracavitary and intravascular pressures are thereby increased during inspiration, and the end-expiratory pressure is the lowest pressure measured during the ventilatory cycle. During intermittent mandatory ventilation *(bottom)*, the machine-generated breaths produce increases in the central venous pressure and spontaneous breaths produce decreases; the end-expiratory pressure is the plateau pressure between the two extremes. (From Abrams, J. H., Cerra, F., and Holcroft, J. W.: Cardiopulmonary monitoring. *In* Wilmore, D. W., Brennan, M. F., Harken, A. H., Holcroft, J. W., and Meakins, J. L. (Eds.): Care of the Surgical Patient. Vol. 1. Critical Care, A Publication of the Committee on Pre- and Postoperative Care, American College of Surgeons. New York, Scientific American, Inc., 1989.)

taneous hyperventilation, in response to the metabolic acidemia of shock, augments cardiac output by placing traction upon the walls of the great veins and cardiac chambers to increase ventricular end-diastolic volumes.

Adrenergic discharge, vasopressin, and angiotensin lead to resorption of fluid from the interstitium into the vascular space. The arterioles, the postcapillary sphincters, and the venules and small veins in the skin, skeletal muscle, kidneys, and splanchnic organs all constrict. The main effect, however, is on the arterioles. Capillary hydrostatic pressure decreases because the arterioles constrict more than the venules and small veins and because of systemic arterial hypotension. Moreover, the low cardiac output of shock decreases the surface area of perfused capillaries. The decreases in intravascular capillary hydrostatic pressure and surface area of perfused capillaries lead to influx of water, sodium, and chloride from the interstitium into the vascular space.[46]

Vascular volume is also replenished by a hyperosmolar-induced shift of fluid from the cells into the extracellular space.[30] Release of epinephrine, cortisol, and glucagon and inhibition of release of insulin all lead to high extracellular glucose concentrations and to an increased extracellular hyperosmolality.[10] This hyperosmolality draws water out of the cells. Interstitial pressure increases, forcing water, sodium, and chloride across the capillary endothelium into the vascular space. The increased interstitial pressure also forces interstitial protein into the lymphatics (interstitial protein stores constitute at least one half, if not three fourths, of the total extracellular protein). The lymphatics then deliver the protein into the vascular space. Increased intravascular oncotic pressure associated with decreased interstitial oncotic pressure draws still more water, sodium, and chloride out of the interstitium and into the vascular space.

In late or severe shock, two mechanisms can worsen the shock state: relaxation of arteriolar spasm and cell swelling. The postcapillary sphincters maintain their spasm in late or severe shock, but the arterioles lose their capability to maintain spasm. With loss of vascular spasm proximal to the capillaries, hydrostatic pressure in the capillaries increases. Sodium, chloride, and water are forced from the vascular space into the interstitium, and the intravascular volume decreases even further.[46] In addition, the cells swell in late or severe hypovolemic shock. Sodium, chloride, and water shift from the interstitium into the cell to further deplete the extracellular space.[62]

A multitude of metabolic and inflammatory abnormalities also develop in response to severe shock, especially in septic shock and in shock associated with major injuries. The point emphasized is that these pathologic processes initiate inflammation throughout the body and lead to a generalized increase in microvascular permeability.[13] Protein extravasates into the interstitium, depleting the vascular volume further and worsening interstitial edema. The edema can compromise function of any organ in the body.

ORGAN FAILURE SYNDROMES OF SHOCK

Profound, prolonged, or poorly treated shock may result in permanent damage to any organ of the body.[44,80]

BRAIN

Four minutes of total circulatory arrest at normothermia usually causes permanent cerebral damage. However, many patients who appear to have had circulatory arrest for more than 10 minutes have been successfully resuscitated without irreversible brain damage. Children, particularly those rendered hypothermic during accidents such as near-drowning, have survived prolonged periods of hypoxemia. The primary problem may be injury to the microcirculation of the brain itself, because brain cells in tissue culture have been shown to withstand prolonged periods of hypoxia, whereas clinical experience has documented that 4 to 5 minutes of circulatory arrest may produce irreversible cerebral ischemia at normothermia.

Because all the physiologic responses of shock are designed to preserve blood flow to the brain, this organ may still be perfused even when there is little clinical evidence of circulatory activity. For this reason, if the period of apparent arrest is short, every effort should be made to resuscitate the shock victim. It is surprising that only a very small percentage of patients successfully resuscitated from profound shock with cardiac arrest have permanent brain damage.

HEART

In experimental animals, the isolated heart can be resuscitated after 30 minutes of circulatory arrest. Myocardial factors

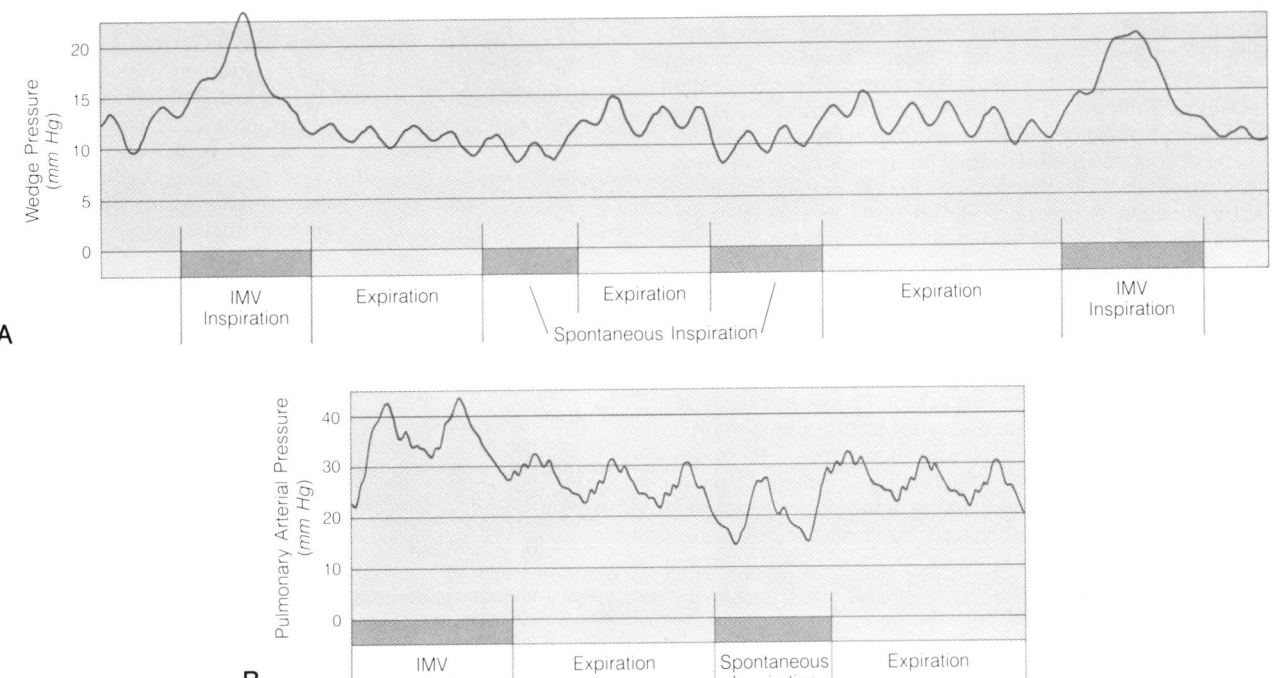

A

B

Figure 8. Mechanical ventilation can generate wide swings in pressure and make it difficult to assign a value to wedge or pulmonary arterial pressures. When the wedge tracing shown here *(a)* was obtained, the patient was on intermittent mandatory ventilation (IMV). The mechanical breaths generated pressure peaks of more than 20 mm. Hg; spontaneous inspiratory efforts by the patient developed trough pressure readings of 8 mm. Hg. The correct value, which should be taken at the plateau between the matching and spontaneous breaths, in this patient is 12 mm. Hg. Similar difficulties arise with interpretation of pulmonary arterial pressure *(b)*. Wide swings in pressure between systole and diastole in the pulmonary artery compound the problem even more. The mean pressure is somewhere between the two extremes; during the IMV inspiration shown here, the mean pressure is between 32 and 43 mm. Hg. Approximating the mean pressure as the diastolic pressure plus one third of the pulse pressure would give a value of 36 mm. Hg. During the spontaneous inspiration, the mean pressure is between 15 and 28 mm. Hg; approximating the mean pressure would give a value of 19 mm. Hg. The ideal is to read the mean pressure during expiration, toward the end of the expiratory cycle, but this can be a challenge for even the most experienced ICU nurse. Here, the mean pressure during expiration is between 23 and 31 mm. Hg; the approximated mean pressure is 26 mm. Hg. (From Abrams, J. H., Cerra, F., and Holcroft, J. W.: Cardiopulmonary monitoring. *In* Wilmore, D. W., Brennan, M. F., Harken, A. H., Holcroft, J. W., and Meakins, J. L. (Eds.): Care of the Surgical Patient. Vol. 1. Critical Care, A Publication of the Committee on Pre- and Postoperative Care, American College of Surgeons. New York, Scientific American, Inc., 1989.)

are rarely the cause of irreversible shock except in patients with primary cardiogenic shock. Part of the problem in achieving cardiac resuscitation in patients in noncardiogenic shock may be brain damage with secondary depression of cardiac function. Another factor that may interfere with successful resuscitation is microcirculatory damage, since platelet aggregation can occur in coronary arteries in shock and transiently obstruct the microcirculation.

LUNGS

Most of the late deaths after initial successful resuscitation from shock are caused by pulmonary damage and respiratory failure (Fig. 9).[12,24] In fact, the development of intensive care units for surgical patients resulted from the need for prolonged mechanical ventilatory support for victims of trauma and major surgical procedures in which shock has had a part. Many types of respiratory failure are seen following shock, including aspiration of gastric contents, airway obstruction, atelectasis from bronchial obstruction by mucus or blood, pulmonary edema from inappropriate fluid administration, chest wall injury, pulmonary contusion, pulmonary embolism, and infection. In addition, a specific syndrome, that is a shock lesion, may occur in pure form or in association with any of the conditions just mentioned. It is now referred to as the respiratory distress syndrome. This syndrome usually becomes evident within the first 24 hours after an episode of shock. The early clinical signs are tachypnea and increased respiratory effort. Evaluation reveals a progressive decrease in pulmonary compliance, increased ventilatory dead space, and evidence of increased pulmonary arteriovenous shunting manifested by a fall in the arterial Po_2. Rales are absent, and pulmonary secretions are minimal. The

findings on the chest film follow some 12 to 24 hours after the clinical symptoms. Initially the chest film is clear but later shows diffuse alveolar infiltrates that may progress to complete consolidation. As the pulmonary lesion progresses, increased ventilatory pressures are needed to maintain normal tidal volume, and greater inspiratory oxygen concentrations are required to provide adequate arterial oxygenation.

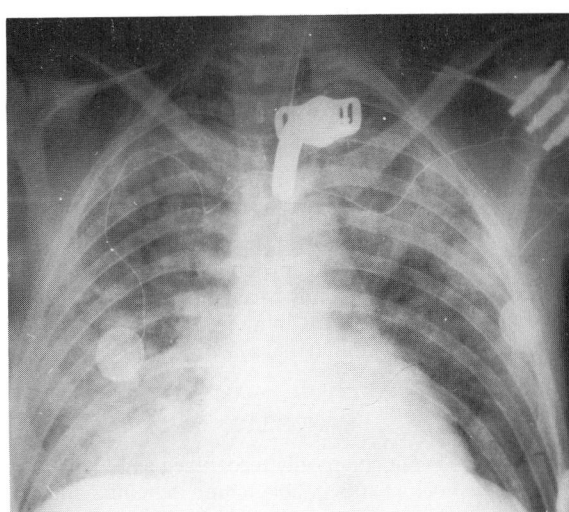

Figure 9. Chest film shows the diffuse reticular infiltrates associated with the respiratory distress syndrome. Cardiac size is not increased, and pulmonary vascular markings are not particularly prominent, both of which help differentiate the changes from those of classic pulmonary edema, with which the respiratory distress syndrome is often confused.

With intensive respiratory care—most often requiring endotracheal intubation, mechanical ventilation, and positive end-expiratory pressure—the patient usually recovers gradually over 3 to 5 days. Failure to respond or progressive exacerbation is usually attributed to the development of superimposed infection with septicemia or endotoxemia from sources remote from the lung or from diffuse infiltrating pulmonary infection. In the latter circumstances, unless the infection can be controlled, pulmonary function is progressively impaired so that the lungs become stiff and difficult to ventilate, and high inhalation pressures are required. Despite the administration of 100 per cent oxygen and high positive end-expiratory pressure, oxygen tension in the blood falls to critical levels, cardiac arrhythmias ensue, and the patient dies.

The pulmonary lesion develops from a combination of shock and conditions that activate coagulation or inflammation, including dead or devitalized tissue, infection, and hemolytic transfusion reactions. With profound shock, even if these conditions are minor, a virulent coagulopathy or inflammatory reaction can develop. This coagulopathy or intravascular reaction damages the microvasculature, causing a diffuse increase in vascular permeability. The increased permeability is reflected most prominently in the lung and is the mechanism by which pulmonary dysfunction is produced.

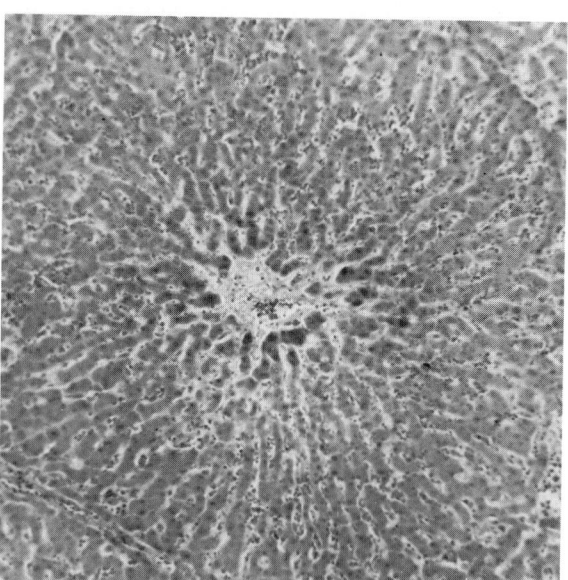

Figure 10. Microscopic section of a liver biopsy in a patient with jaundice following severe traumatic shock. Central lobular necrosis characterizes the changes seen in the lesion.

KIDNEYS

Patients in shock almost immediately manifest a fall in urinary output. As shock progresses, blood shunts to the medulla and bypasses the cortex. If the cortex is deprived of blood flow for more than 24 hours, cortical necrosis and renal failure result.[47] Resuscitation of the circulation within this critical period prevents permanent tubular damage, however. Hemodialysis can be used as necessary to support the patient until renal function returns; however, the mortality from renal failure in surgical patients varies between 50 and 100 per cent and has not changed appreciably in the last 2 decades. When renal failure develops in the postresuscitation period, it is usually caused by nephrotoxic drugs, the most common of which are the aminoglycoside antibiotics.[28] If the blood urea nitrogen and creatinine begin to rise, drug administration should be assessed and potential nephrotoxic agents discontinued.

LIVER

Shock-induced liver failure is rarely severe enough to cause death, but some degree of liver failure, as manifested by elevation of the serum bilirubin concentration and by changes in liver enzymes, frequently complicates severe shock (Fig. 10).[27,52] Central lobular necrosis of the liver develops in severe cases, and the jaundice presumably follows a high pigment load in the presence of a damaged liver. If the patient does not develop any other complications, the most common of which is infection, liver function improves. The liver is essential for protein synthesis, and compromise of liver function is associated with a high incidence of infections, possibly because of nutritional compromise, decreased synthesis of immune proteins, and perhaps damage to the reticuloendothelial system.

PANCREAS

The pancreas is not commonly recognized as a shock organ. Nonetheless, shock results in splanchnic ischemia, and when laparotomy is necessary in the shock patient, the pancreas frequently appears edematous, ischemic, or occasionally necrotic. Toxins released by the ischemic pancreas may well contribute to increases in vascular permeability and pulmonary damage.

GASTROINTESTINAL TRACT

Factors similar to those that compromise the liver and pancreas also affect the gastrointestinal tract.[78,81] If a patient dies a day or two after severe shock, ischemic damage of the mucosa may be evident when the stomach or bowel is inspected at autopsy. Intestinal mucosal damage is difficult to assess at laparotomy, because the mucosa is much more active metabolically than the remainder of the intestinal wall, and, externally, the intestine may appear normal to observation. When the distal colon is involved, sigmoidoscopy provides clues that an ischemic intestine exists.

Gastric mucosal ulceration, often referred to as "stress ulcer," very commonly complicates severe shock states and is clinically manifested by gastrointestinal hemorrhage. This complication has largely been prevented in the intensive care setting by the routine use of antacids and H_2-blockers.

Ulceration and damage to the mucosa of the gastrointestinal tract may be an important cause of secondary complications that arise from the shock state. Products of bacterial action entering the portal circulation may be responsible for systemic endotoxemia and the high incidence of systemic sepsis following shock.[6,77]

ADRENALS

On rare occasions following severe shock, hemorrhagic necrosis of one or both adrenal glands may develop. When both adrenal glands are involved, acute adrenal insufficiency occurs. The inability to retain sodium causes a refractory form of shock, which may be difficult to recognize. When this form of shock is suspected, a trial of physiologic doses of steroids is indicated.

HEMATOPOIETIC AND COAGULATION SYSTEMS

After resuscitation from severe shock, patients have a tendency to develop refractory anemias even when no further blood loss occurs.[61] This probably follows changes in the red cell membrane that affect deformability and cause red cell aggregation and trapping in the microcirculation. Low-grade intravascular coagulation may coat the red cells with fibrin, leading to the tendency for rouleaux formation, which obstructs the microcirculation.

Intravascular coagulation is a frequent but usually poorly documented phenomenon associated with shock, tissue injury, and sepsis.[2,18] It varies from simple hypercoagulability seen in the injured patient, which causes a tendency for thrombosis in areas of vascular stasis such as leg veins with attendant risk of pulmonary embolism, to fulminating disseminated intravascular coagulation and activation of fibrinolysis. This causes a massive bleeding syndrome, "consumption coagulopathy," that is often uncontrollable. It is the most common cause of immediate fatality following shock resuscitation.

IMMUNE SYSTEM

Sepsis is the most common cause of late death in shock patients. The likelihood of secondary infection increases with the severity of initial shock and tissue injury. The immune mechanism is activated by contact of macrophages with bacteria, which initiates the immune response. Immune blockade may result when a large number of tissue fragments or the products of intravascular coagulation are engulfed by and block the reticuloendothelial system. At present, the factors that are responsible for the immune depression following severe shock and injury are not well understood. Antibiotics may be helpful but in themselves are not the answer, since immune function in the host is essential for maximizing antibiotic effect. Many new techniques for support of the immune system are being evaluated currently, but none have yet proved effective.[34,69]

SELECTED REFERENCES

Simeone, F. A.: Shock, trauma, and the surgeon. Ann. Surg., 158:759, 1963.
This classic paper reviews the development of the "shock concept," including the nomenclature and classification of shock. It defines "wound shock" and "septic shock." The author considers the heart to be the weak link in shock and discusses at length the cardiac degenerative changes associated with shock.

Wiggers, C. J.: Physiology of Shock. New York, The Commonwealth Fund Publications, 1950.
This monograph on shock by a noted physiologist presents a classic historical review. It presents the various models that have been used to study shock as well as the "state of the art" as of 1950.

Wilmore, D. W., Brennan, M. F., Harken, A. H., Holcroft, J. W., and Meakins, J. L. (Eds.): Care of the Surgical Patient. Vol. 1. Critical Care, A Publication of the Committee on Pre- and Postoperative Care, American College of Surgeons. New York, Scientific American, Inc., 1989.
This publication from the Pre- and Postoperative Care Committee of the American College of Surgeons has several up-to-date monographs on various aspects of shock. The manual is kept current with frequent revisions of the individual monographs as new information becomes available.

REFERENCES

1. Abrams, J. H., Cerra, F., and Holcroft, J. W.: Cardiopulmonary monitoring. In Wilmore, D. W., Brennan, M. F., Harken, A. H., Holcroft, J. W., and Meakins, J. L. (Eds.): Care of the Surgical Patient. Vol. 1. Critical Care, A Publication of the Committee on Pre- and Postoperative Care, American College of Surgeons. New York, Scientific American, Inc., 1989.
2. Addonizio, V. P.: Hematologic failure. In Wilmore, D. W., Brennan, M. F., Harken, A. H., Holcroft, J. W., and Meakins, J. L. (Eds.): Care of the Surgical Patient. Vol. 1, Critical Care, A Publication of the Committee on Pre- and Postoperative Care, American College of Surgeons. New York, Scientific American, Inc., 1989.
3. Archibald, E. W., and McLean, W. S.: Observations upon shock with particular relevance to the condition as seen in war surgery. Ann. Surg., 66:281, 1917.
4. Avila, A., Warshawski, F., Sibbald, W., Finley, R., Wells, G., and Holliday, R.: Peripheral lymph flow in sheep with bacterial peritonitis: Evidence for increased peripheral microvascular permeability accompanying systemic sepsis. Surgery, 97:685, 1985.
5. Avolio, A. P., Chen, S.-G., Wang, R.-P., Zhang, C.-L., Li, M.-F., and O'Rourke, M. F.: Effects of aging on changing arterial compliance and left ventricular load in a northern Chinese urban community. Circulation, 68:50, 1983.
6. Baker, J. W., Deitch, E. A., Li, M., Berg, R. D., and Specian R. D.: Hemorrhagic shock induces bacterial translocation from the gut. J. Trauma, 28:896, 1988.
7. Bartlett, R. H.: Use of the mechanical ventilator. In Wilmore, D. W., Brennan, M. F., Harken, A. H., Holcroft, J. W., and Meakins, J. L. (Eds.): Care of the Surgical Patient. Vol. 1, Critical Care, A Publication of the Committee on Pre- and Postoperative Care, American College of Surgeons. New York, Scientific American, Inc., 1989.
8. Beecher, H. K.: The Physiologic Effects of Wounds. Washington, D.C., Medical Department, U.S. Army, 1952.
9. Bernard, G. R., Luce, J. M., Sprung, C. L., Rinaldo, J. E., Tate, R. M., Sibbald, W. J., Kariman, K., Higgins, S., Bradley, R., Metz, C. A., Harris, T. R., and Brigham, K. L.: High-dose corticosteroids in patients with the adult respiratory distress syndrome. N. Engl. J. Med., 317:1565, 1987.
10. Bessey, P. Q.: Metabolic response to critical illness. In Wilmore, D. W., Brennan, M. F., Harken, A. H., Holcroft, J. W., and Meakins, J. L. (Eds.): Care of the Surgical Patient. Vol. 1, Critical Care, A Publication of the Committee on Pre- and Postoperative Care, American College of Surgeons. New York, Scientific American, Inc., 1989.
11. Blaisdell, F. W., and Lewis, F. R., Jr.: Respiratory Distress Syndrome of Shock and Trauma. Philadelphia, W. B. Saunders Company, 1977.
12. Blaisdell, F. W., Lim, R. C., Amberg, J. R., Choy, S. H., Hall, A. D., and Thomas, A. N.: Pulmonary microembolism. Arch. Surg., 93:776, 1966.
13. Blaisdell, F. W.: Traumatic shock: The search for a toxic factor. Bull. Am. Coll. Surg., 68:1, 1983.
14. Blaisdell, F. W.: Controversy in shock research. Con: The role of steroids in septic shock. Circ. Shock, 8:673, 1981.
15. Blalock, A.: Experimental shock: The cause of low blood pressure produced by muscle injury. Arch. Surg., 20:959, 1930.
16. Bock, J. C., Barker, B. C., Clinton, A. G., Wilson, M. B., and Lewis, F. R.: Post-traumatic changes in, and effect of colloid osmotic pressure on, the distribution of body water. Ann. Surg., 210:395, 1989.
17. Bone, R. C., Fisher, C. J., Jr., Clemmer, T. P., Slotman, G. J., Metz, C. A., Balk, R. A., and the Methylprednisolone Severe Sepsis Study Group: A controlled clinical trial of high-dose methylprednisolone in the treatment of severe sepsis and septic shock. N. Engl. J. Med., 317:653, 1987.
18. Cafferata, H. T., Aggeler, P. M., Robinson, A. J., and Blaisdell, F. W.: Intravascular coagulation in the surgical patient: Its significance and diagnosis. Am. J. Surg., 118:281, 1969.
19. Canizaro, P. C., Prager, M. D., and Shires, G. T.: The infusion of Ringer's lactate solution during shock. Am. J. Surg., 122:494, 1971.
20. Cannon, W. B.: Traumatic Shock. New York, Appleton and Company, 1923.
21. Christou, N. V., and Solomkin, J. S.: Antibiotics. In Wilmore, D. W., Brennan, M. F., Harken, A. H., Holcroft, J. W., and Meakins, J. L. (Eds.): Care of the Surgical Patient. Vol. 2, Critical Care, A Publication of the Committee on Pre- and Postoperative Care, American College of Surgeons. New York, Scientific American, Inc., 1989.
22. Cournand, A., Riley, R. L., Bradley, S. E., Breed, E. S., Noble, R. P., Lauson, H. D., Gregersen, M. I., and Richards, D. W.: Studies of the circulation in clinical shock. Surgery, 13:964, 1943.
23. Crile, G. W.: Experimental Research into Surgical Shock. Philadelphia, J. B. Lippincott Company, 1899.
24. Demling, R. H., and Goodwin, C. W.: Pulmonary dysfunction. In Wilmore, D. W., Brennan, M. F., Harken, A. H., Holcroft, J. W., and Meakins, J. L. (Eds.): Care of the Surgical Patient. Vol. 1, Critical Care, A Publication of the Committee on Pre- and Postoperative Care, American College of Surgeons. New York, Scientific American, Inc., 1989.
25. Demling, R. H.: Early postoperative pneumonia. In Wilmore, D. W., Brennan, M. F., Harken, A. H., Holcroft, J. W., and Meakins, J. L. (Eds.): Care of the Surgical Patient. Vol. 2, Critical Care, A publication of the Committee on Pre- and Postoperative Care, American College of Surgeons. New York, Scientific American, Inc., 1989.
26. Federal Drug Administration Drug Bulletin: Use of blood components. FDA Drug Bull. 19:14, 1989.
27. Fischer, J. E.: Hepatic failure. In Wilmore, D. W., Brennan, M. F., Harken, A. H., Holcroft, J. W., and Meakins, J. L. (Eds.): Care of the Surgical Patient. Vol. 1, Critical Care. A Publication of the Committee on Pre- and Postoperative Care, American College of Surgeons. New York, Scientific American, Inc., 1989.
28. Flint, L. M., Gott, J., Short, L., Richardson, D., and Polk, H. C., Jr.: Serum level monitoring of aminoglycoside antibiotics. Arch. Surg., 120:99, 1985.
29. Fry, D. E.: The positive blood culture. In Wilmore, D. W., Brennan, M. F., Harken, A. H., Holcroft, J. W., and Meakins, J. L. (Eds.): Care of the Surgical Patient. Vol. 2: Critical Care, A Publication of the Committee on Pre- and Postoperative Care, American College of Surgeons. New York, Scientific American, Inc., 1989.
30. Gann, D. S., Carlson, D. E., Byrnes, G. J., Pirkle, J. C., Jr., and Allen-Rowlands, C. F.: Role of solute in the early restitution of blood volume after hemorrhage. Surgery, 94:439, 1983.
31. Greenburg, A. G.: Indications for transfusion. In Wilmore, D. W., Brennan, M. F., Harken, A. H., Holcroft, J. W., and Meakins, J. L. (Eds.): Care of the Surgical Patient. Vol. 1, Critical Care, A Publication of the Committee on Pre- and Postoperative Care, American College of Surgeons. New York, Scientific American, Inc., 1989.
32. Harken, A. H.: Cardiac arrhythmias. In Wilmore, D. W., Brennan, M. F., Harken, A. H., Holcroft, J. W., and Meakins, J. L. (Eds.): Care of the Surgical Patient. Vol. 1, Critical Care, A Publication of the Committee on Pre- and

Postoperative Care, American College of Surgeons. New York, Scientific American, Inc., 1989.

33. Henderson, Y.: Acapnea in shock, the failure of the circulation. Am. J. Physiol., 27:152, 1910.

34. Hinshaw, L. B., Archer, L. T., Beller, B. K., Change, A. C. K., Flournoy, D. J., Passey, R. B., Long, J. B., and Holaday, J. W.: Evaluation of naloxone therapy for *Escherichia coli* sepsis in the baboon. Arch. Surg., 123:700, 1988.

35. Hock, C. E., Su, J.-Y., and Lefer, A. M.: Role of AVP in maintenance of circulatory homeostasis during hemorrhagic shock. Am. J. Physiol., 246:H174, 1984.

36. Holcroft, J. W., Link, D. P., Lantz, B. M. T., and Green, J. F.: Venous return and the pneumatic antishock garment in hypovolemic baboons. J. Trauma, 24:928, 1984.

37. Holcroft, J. W., Vassar, M. J., Turner, J. E., Derlet, R. W., and Kramer, G. C.: 3% NaCl and 7.5% NaCl/Dextran 70 in the resuscitation of severely injured patients. Ann. Surg., 206:279, 1987.

38. Holcroft, J. W.: Shock. In Wilmore, D. W., Brennan, M. F., Harken, A. H., Holcroft, J. W., and Meakins, J. L. (Eds.): Care of the Surgical Patient. Vol. 1. Critical Care, A Publication of the Committee on Pre- and Postoperative Care, American College of Surgeons. New York, Scientific American, Inc., 1989.

39. Hunter, J.: Observations on Certain Parts of the Animal Oeconomy. London, Nicol and Johnson, 1792.

40. Keith, N. M.: Blood Volume in Wound Shock. London, Medical Research Committee Special Report, Series 26, 1919.

41. Little, R. A.: 1988 Fitts Lecture: Heart rate changes after haemorrhage and injury: A reappraisal. J. Trauma, 29:903, 1989.

42. Lowe, R. J., Moss, G. S., Jilek, J., and Levine, H. D.: Crystalloid vs. colloid in the etiology of pulmonary failure after trauma: A randomized trial in man. Surgery, 81:676, 1977.

43. Lowry, S. F., and Brennan, M. F.: Life-threatening electrolyte abnormalities. In Wilmore, D. W., Brennan, M. F., Harken, A. H., Holcroft, J. W., and Meakins, J. L. (Eds.): Care of the Surgical Patient. Vol. 1, Critical Care, A Publication of the Committee on Pre- and Postoperative Care, American College of Surgeons. New York, Scientific American, Inc., 1989.

44. Marshall, J. C., and Meakins, J. L.: Multiorgan failure. In Wilmore, D. W., Brennan, M. F., Harken, A. H., Holcroft, J. W., and Meakins, J. L. (Eds.): Care of the Surgical Patient. Vol. 1: Critical Care, A Publication of the Committee on Pre- and Postoperative Care, American College of Surgeons. New York, Scientific American, Inc., 1989.

45. Mattox, K. L., Bickell, W. H., Pepe, P. E., and Mangelsdorff, A. D.: Prospective randomized evaluation of antishock MAST in post-traumatic hypotension. J. Trauma, 26:779, 1986.

46. Mellander, S., and Johansson, B.: Control of resistance, exchange, and capacitance functions in the peripheral circulation. Pharmacol. Rev., 20:117, 1968.

47. Meyer, A.: Acute renal failure. In Wilmore, D. W., Brennan, M. F., Harken, A. H., Holcroft, J. W., and Meakins, J. L. (Eds.): Care of the Surgical Patient. Vol. 1: Critical Care, A Publication of the Committee on Pre- and Postoperative Care, American College of Surgeons. New York, Scientific American, Inc., 1989.

48. Michie, H. R., Guillou, P. J., and Wilmore, D. W.: Tumour necrosis factor and bacterial sepsis. Br. J. Surg., 76:670, 1989.

49. Moore, J. S., Bogusky, R. T., Kramer, G. C., and Holcroft, J. W.: Nuclear magnetic resonance spectroscopy and tissue analysis of skeletal muscle during hemorrhagic shock. Surg. Forum 38:59, 1987.

50. Morris, E. A.: A Practical Treatise on Shock After Operations and Injuries. London, Hartwicke Publishers, 1867.

51. National Academy of Sciences—National Research Council: Pulmonary effects of non-thoracic trauma. Eiseman, B., and Ashbaugh, D. G. (Eds.). J. Trauma, 8:623, 1968.

52. Nunes, G., Blaisdell, F. W., and Margaretten, W.: Mechanism of hepatic dysfunction following shock and trauma. Arch. Surg., 100:546, 1970.

53. O'Rourke, M. F.: Vascular impedance in studies of arterial and cardiac function. Physiol. Rev., 62:570, 1982.

54. Pang, C. C. Y.: Effect of vasopressin antagonist and saralasin on regional blood flow following hemorrhage. Am. J. Physiol., 245:H749, 1983.

55. Piene, H.: Pulmonary arterial impedance and right ventricular function. Physiol. Rev., 66:606, 1986.

56. Rankin, J. S.: Hemodynamic management. In Wilmore, D. W., Brennan, M. F., Harken, A. H., Holcroft, J. W., and Meakins, J. L. (Eds.): Care of the Surgical Patient. Vol. 1, Critical Care, A Publication of the Committee on Pre- and Postoperative Care, American College of Surgeons. New York, Scientific American, Inc., 1989.

57. Rankin, J. S., Olsen, C. O., Arentzen, C. E., Tyson, G. S., Maier, G., Smith, P.

K., Hammon, J. W., Jr., Davis, J. W., McHale, P. A., Anderson, R. W., and Sabiston, D. C., Jr.: The effects of airway pressure on cardiac function in intact dogs and man. Circulation, 66:108, 1982.

58. Rice, C. L.: Pharmacologic support of the failing heart. In Wilmore, D. W., Brennan, M. F., Harken, A. H., Holcroft, J. W., and Meakins, J. L. (Eds.): Care of the Surgical Patient. Vol. 1, Critical Care, A Publication of the Committee on Pre- and Postoperative Care, American College of Surgeons. New York, Scientific American, Inc., 1989.

59. Rothe, C. F.: Venous system: Physiology of the capacitance vessels. In Shepherd, J. T., Abboud, F. M., and Geiger, S. R. (Eds.): Handbook of Physiology, Section 2: The Cardiovascular System. Vol. III: Peripheral Circulation and Organ Blood Flow, Part 1. Bethesda, Md., American Physiological Society, 1983, pp. 397–452.

60. Rowell, L. B.: Cardiovascular aspects of human thermoregulation. Circ. Res., 52:367, 1983.

61. Sheldon, G. F., Sanders, R., Fuchs, R., Garcia, J., and Schooley, J.: Metabolism, oxygen transport, and erythropoietin synthesis in the anemia of thermal injury. Am. J. Surg., 135:406, 1978.

62. Shires, G. T., Cunningham, J. N., Baker, C. R. F., Reeder, S. F., Illner, H., Wagner, I. Y., and Maher, J.: Alterations in cellular membrane function during hemorrhagic shock in primates. Ann. Surg., 176:288, 1972.

63. Shoemaker, W. C., Appel, P. L., Waxman, K., Schwartz, S., and Chang, P.: Clinical trial of survivor's cardiorespiratory patterns as therapeutic goals in critically ill postoperative patients. Crit. Care Med., 10:398, 1982.

64. Sibbald, W. J., Paterson, N. A. M., Holliday, R. L., and Baskerville, J.: The Trendelenburg position: Hemodynamic effects in hypotensive and normotensive patients. Crit. Care Med., 7:218, 1979.

65. Simeone, F. A.: Shock, trauma, and the surgeon. Ann. Surg., 158:759, 1963.

66. Sturm, J. A., Wisner, D. H., Oestern, H.-J., Kant, C. J., Tscherne, H., and Creutzig, H.: Increased lung capillary permeability after trauma: A prospective clinical study. J. Trauma, 26:409, 1986.

67. Suga, H.: Total mechanical energy of a ventricle model and cardiac oxygen consumption. Am. J. Physiol., 236:H498, 1979.

68. Thal, A. P.: Shock: A Physiologic Basis for Treatment. Chicago, Year Book Medical Publishers, 1971.

69. Tracy, K. J., Fong, Y., Hesse, D. G., Manoque, K. R., Lee, A. T., Kuo, G. C., Lowry, S. F., and Cerami, A.: Anti-cachectin/TNF monoclonal antibodies prevent septic shock during lethal bacteraemia. Nature, 330:662, 1987.

70. Trunkey, D. D., Illner, H., Wagner, I. Y., and Shires, G. T.: The effect of septic shock on skeletal muscle action potentials in the primate. Surgery, 85:638, 1979.

71. Vatner, S. F.: Effects of hemorrhage on regional blood flow distribution in dogs and primates. J. Clin. Invest., 54:225, 1974.

72. Velanovich, V.: Crystalloid versus colloid fluid resuscitation: A meta-analysis of mortality. Surgery, 105:65, 1989.

73. Veterans Administration Systemic Sepsis Cooperative Study Group: Effect of high-dose glucocorticoid therapy on mortality in patients with clinical signs of systemic sepsis. N. Engl. J. Med., 317:659, 1987.

74. Virgilio, R. W., Rice, C. L., Smith, D. E., James, D. R., Zarins, C. K., Hobelmann, C. F., and Peters, R. M.: Crystalloid vs. colloid resuscitation: Is one better? Surgery, 85:129, 1979.

75. Wiggers, C. J.: Physiology of Shock. New York, The Commonwealth Fund Publications, 1950.

76. Wilkerson, D. K. Rosen, A. L., Sehgal, L. R., Gould, S. A., Sehgal, H. L., and Moss, G. S.: Limits of cardiac compensation in anemic baboons. Surgery, 103:665, 1988.

77. Wilmore, D. W., Smith, R. J., O'Dwyer, S. T., Jacobs, D. O., Ziegler, T. R., and Wang, X.-D.: The gut: A central organ after surgical stress. Surgery, 104:917, 1988.

78. Wilson, S., and Blaisdell, F. W.: Superficial gastric erosion. Am. J. Surg., 126:136, 1973.

79. Wisner, D. H., Reed, W. H., and Riddick, R. S.: Suspected myocardial contusion: Triage and indications for monitoring. Ann. Surg., 212:82–86, 1990.

80. Wolfe, B. M., and Suda, S.: Preparation of the ICU patient for operation. In Wilmore, D. W., Brennan, M. F., Harken, A. H., Holcroft, J. W., and Meakins, J. L. (Eds.): Care of the Surgical Patient. Vol. 1, Critical Care, A Publication of the Committee on Pre- and Postoperative Care, American College of Surgeons. New York, Scientific American, Inc., 1989.

81. Yeo, C. J., and Zinner, M. J.: Gastrointestinal failure. In Wilmore, D. W., Brennan, M. F., Harken, A. H., Holcroft, J. W., and Meakins, J. L. (Eds.): Care of the Surgical Patient. Vol. 1, Critical Care, A Publication of the Committee on Pre- and Postoperative Care, American College of Surgeons. New York, Scientific American, Inc., 1989.

4

FLUID AND ELECTROLYTE MANAGEMENT OF THE SURGICAL PATIENT

G. Tom Shires, M.D., and Peter C. Canizaro, M.D.

Fluid and electrolyte management is an integral part of the care of surgical patients, and it may be a critical factor in certain patients. Many diseases, injuries, and operative trauma impose a great impact on the physiology of body fluids and electrolytes, far greater than the changes associated with a simple lack of alimentation. Therefore, a thorough understanding of the metabolism of salt, water, and other electrolytes and of certain metabolic responses is essential to the care of surgical patients.

This chapter addresses definition of the anatomy of body fluid compartments and the physiologic principles relating to fluids and electrolytes. In addition to normal functions, a classification of derangements is provided so that therapy may be described.

ANATOMY OF BODY FLUID COMPARTMENTS

A prerequisite to the understanding of fluid and electrolyte management is knowledge of the extent and composition of the various body fluid compartments. Early attempts to define these compartments were relatively accurate, but a more precise definition has been obtained by many investigators through the use of isotopic tracer techniques. The wide range of normal values is a function of body size, weight, and sex; but these compartments are relatively constant in size for the individual patient in the normal steady state. The figures used in this section are approximate and reported as percentages of body weight.

Total Body Water

Water constitutes between 50 and 70 per cent of total body weight. With deuterium oxide or tritiated water for measurement of total body water (TBW), the average normal value is 60 per cent of body weight for young adult males and 50 per cent for young adult females. A normal variation of ±15 per cent applies to both groups. The actual figure for a healthy individual is remarkably constant and is a function of several variables, including lean body mass and age. Since fat contains little water, the lean individual has a greater proportion of water to total body weight than the obese person. Thus, an extremely obese individual may have 25 to 30 per cent less body water than a lean individual of the same weight. The lower percentage of total body water in females correlates with a larger amount of subcutaneous adipose tissue and smaller muscle mass. Moore and associates have shown that total body water, as a percentage of total body weight, decreases steadily and significantly with age to a low of 52 and 47 per cent in males and females, respectively.[29] Conversely, the highest proportion of total body water is found in newborn infants, with a maximum of 75 to 80 per cent. During the first several months following birth, there is a gradual "physiologic" loss of body water as the infant adjusts

to his environment. At 1 year, the total body water averages approximately 65 per cent of the body weight and remains relatively constant throughout the remainder of infancy and childhood.

The water of the body is divided into three functional compartments (Fig. 1). The fluid within the body's diverse cell population, intracellular water, represents between 30 and 40 per cent of the body weight. The extracellular water represents approximately 20 per cent of the body weight and is divided between the intravascular fluid or plasma (5 per cent of body weight), and the interstitial, or extravascular, extracellular fluid (15 per cent of body weight).

INTRACELLULAR FLUID. Measurement of intracellular fluid is determined indirectly by subtraction of the measured extracellular fluid from the measured total body water. The intracellular water is between 30 and 40 per cent of the body weight, with the largest proportion in the skeletal muscle mass. Because of the smaller muscle mass in the female, the percentage of intracellular water is lower than in the male.

The chemical composition of the intracellular fluid is shown in Figure 2, with potassium and magnesium the principal cations and phosphates and proteins the principal anions. This is an approximation, since so few data concerning the intracellular fluid are available.

EXTRACELLULAR FLUID. The total extracellular fluid volume represents approximately 20 per cent of the body weight. The extracellular fluid compartment has two major subdivisions. The plasma volume is approximately 5 per cent of the body weight in the normal adult. The interstitial, or extravascular, extracellular fluid volume, obtained by subtracting the plasma volume from the measured total extracellular fluid volume, represents approximately 15 per cent of the body weight.

The interstitial fluid is further complicated by having a rapidly equilibrating or functional component as well as several more slowly equilibrating, or relatively nonfunctioning, components. The nonfunctioning components include connective tissue water as well as water that has been termed *transcellular*, including cerebrospinal and joint fluids. This nonfunctional component normally represents only 10 per cent of the interstitial fluid volume (1 to 2 per cent of body weight) and is not to be confused with the relatively nonfunctional extracellular fluid, often termed a third space, found in burns and soft tissue injuries.

The normal constituents of the extracellular fluid are shown in Figure 2, with sodium the principal cation and chloride and bicarbonate the principal anions. There are minor differences in ionic composition between the plasma and the interstitial fluid occasioned by the difference in protein concentration. Because of the higher protein content (organic anions) of the plasma, the total concentration of cations is higher and the concentration of

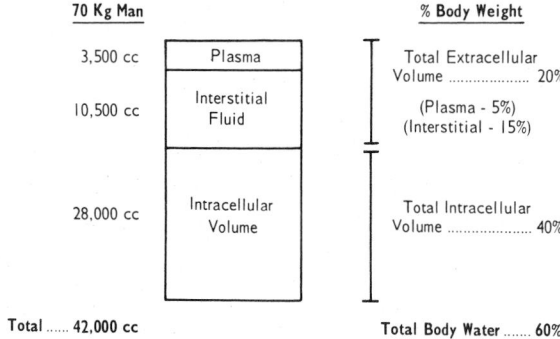

Figure 1. Functional compartments of body fluids.

inorganic anions somewhat lower than in the interstitial fluid, as explained by the Gibbs-Donnan equilibrium equation.* For practical consideration, however, they may be considered equal. The total concentration of intracellular ions exceeds that of the extracellular compartment and would appear to violate the concept of osmolar equilibrium between the two compartments. This apparent discrepancy is due to the fact that the concentration of ions is expressed in milliequivalents without regard to osmotic activity. In addition, some of the intracellular cations probably exist in undissociated form.

OSMOTIC PRESSURE. Relevant to a discussion of the complicated interactions between the various body fluid compartments is the definition of commonly used terms: The physiologic and chemical activity of electrolytes depends on (1) the *number of particles* present per unit volume (moles or millimoles per liter), (2) the *number of electrical charges* per unit volume (equivalents or milliequivalents per liter), and (3) the *number of osmotically active particles*, or ions per unit volume (osmoles or milliosmoles per liter). The use of the term *grams* or *milligrams per 100 milliliters* expresses the weight of the electrolytes per unit volume but does not allow a physiologic comparison of the solutes in a solution.

A mole of a substance is the molecular weight of that substance in grams, and a millimole is that figure expressed in milligrams. For example, a mole of sodium chloride is 58 grams (Na, 23; Cl, 35), and a millimole is 58 milligrams. This expression, however, provides no direct information as to the number of osmotically active ions in solution or the electrical charges that they carry.

The electrolytes of the body fluids then may be expressed in terms of chemical combining activity, or equivalents. An equivalent of an ion is its atomic weight expressed in grams divided by the valence, whereas a milliequivalent of an ion is that figure expressed in milligrams. In the case of univalent ions, a milliequivalent is the same as a millimole. However, in the case of divalent ions, such as calcium or magnesium, 1 mmol. equals 2 mEq. The importance of this expression is that a milliequivalent of any substance combines chemically with a milliequivalent of any other substance; in any solution, the number of milliequivalents of cations present is balanced precisely by the same number of milliequivalents of anions.

When the osmotic pressure of a solution is considered, it is more descriptive to employ the terms *osmole* and *milliosmole*. These terms refer to the actual number of osmotically active particles present in solution but are not dependent on the chemical combining capacities of the substances. Thus, 1 mmol. of sodium chloride, which dissociates nearly completely into sodium and chloride, contributes 2 mOsm., and 1 mmol. of so-

dium sulfate (Na_2SO_4), which dissociates into three particles, contributes 3 mOsm. One millimole of an un-ionized substance such as glucose is equal to 1 mOsm. of the substance.

The differences in ionic composition between intracellular and extracellular fluid are maintained by the cell wall, which functions as a semipermeable membrane. The total number of osmotically active particles is 290 to 310 mOsm. in each compartment. Although the osmotic pressure of a fluid is the sum of the partial pressures contributed by each of the solutes in that fluid, the *effective* osmotic pressure is dependent on those substances that fail to pass through the pores of the semipermeable membrane. The dissolved proteins in the plasma, therefore, are primarily responsible for effective osmotic pressure between the plasma and the interstitial fluid compartments. This is frequently referred to as the *colloid osmotic pressure*. The effective osmotic pressure between the extracellular and intracellular fluid compartments would be contributed to by any substance that does not traverse the cell membranes freely. Thus, sodium, which is the principal cation of the extracellular fluid, contributes a major portion of the osmotic pressure; but any substance that fails to penetrate the cell membrane freely, such as glucose, also increases the effective osmotic pressure.

Since the cell membranes are completely permeable to water, the effective osmotic pressures in the two compartments are considered equal. Any condition that alters the effective osmotic pressure in either compartment results in redistribution of water between the compartments. Thus, an increase in effective osmotic pressure in the extracellular fluid, which would occur most frequently as a result of increased sodium concentration, causes a net transfer of water from the intracellular to the extracellular fluid compartment. This transfer of water continues until the effective osmotic pressures in the two compartments are equal. Conversely, a decrease in the sodium concentration in the extracellular fluid causes a transfer of water from the extracellular to the intracellular fluid compartment. Depletion of the extracellular fluid volume *without a change in the concentration* of ions, however, does not cause transfer of free water from the intracellular space.

Thus, the intracellular fluid shares in losses that involve a change in concentration or composition of the extracellular fluid but shares slowly in changes involving loss of isotonic volume alone. For practical consideration, most losses and gains of body fluid are directly from the extracellular compartment.

---

* The product of the concentrations of any pair of diffusible cations and anions on one side of a semipermeable membrane equals the product of the same pair of ions on the other side.

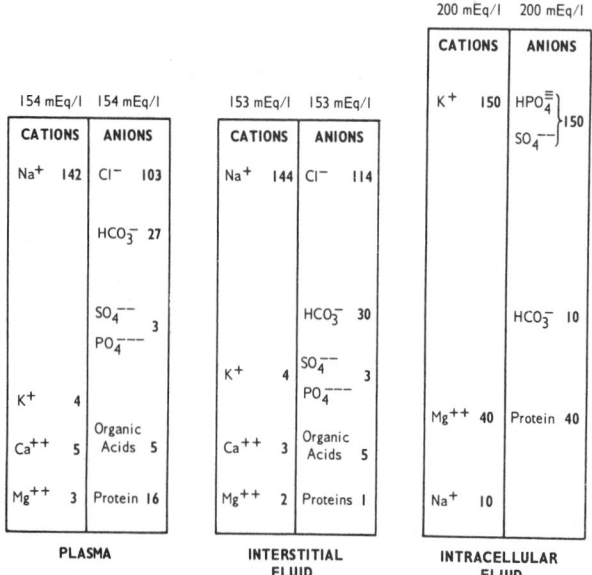

Figure 2. Chemical composition of body fluid compartments.

CLASSIFICATION OF BODY FLUID CHANGES

The disorders in fluid balance may be classified in three general categories: disturbances of (1) volume, (2) concentration, and (3) composition. Of primary importance is the concept that although these disturbances are interrelated, each is a separate entity.

If an isotonic salt solution is added to or lost from the body fluids, only the *volume* of the extracellular fluid is changed. The acute loss of an isotonic extracellular solution, such as intestinal juice, is followed by a significant decrease in the extracellular fluid volume and little if any change in the intracellular fluid volume. Fluid will not be transferred from the intracellular space to refill the depleted extracellular space as long as the osmolality remains the same in the two compartments.

If water alone is added to or lost from the extracellular fluid, the *concentration* of osmotically active particles changes. Sodium ions represent a majority of the osmotically active particles in the extracellular fluid and generally reflect the tonicity of other body fluid compartments. If the extracellular fluid is depleted of sodium, water passes into the intracellular space until osmolality is again equal in the two compartments.

The concentration of most other ions within the extracellular fluid compartment can be altered without significant change in the total number of osmotically active particles, thus producing only a *compositional* change. For example, a rise of the serum potassium concentration from 4 to 8 mEq. per liter would have a significant effect on the myocardium, but it would not significantly change the effective osmotic pressure of the extracellular fluid compartment. Normally functioning kidneys minimize these changes considerably, particularly if the addition or loss of solute or water is gradual.

An internal loss of extracellular fluid into a nonfunctional space, such as the sequestration of isotonic fluid in a burn, peritonitis, ascites, or muscle trauma, is termed a *distributional* change. This transfer or functional loss of extracellular fluid internally may be extracellular (e.g., as in peritonitis) or intracellular (e.g., as in hemorrhagic shock).[33,35] In any event, all distributional shifts or losses cause a contraction of the *functional* extracellular fluid space.

Volume Changes

An excess or deficit of extracellular fluid (ECF) volume must be diagnosed by clinical examination of the patient. Direct measurement of the ECF volume using sodium bromide or radioactive sodium sulfate is feasible in a research setting but is of limited use clinically because of the complexity of the tests. There are several laboratory tests, however, that indirectly reflect changes in ECF volume. The blood urea nitrogen rises with an ECF deficit of sufficient magnitude to reduce glomerular filtration. The serum creatinine may not increase proportionally in young people with healthy kidneys, and this discrepancy is often used as one test to differentiate prerenal and renal azotemia. (Importantly, the rise in serum creatinine often parallels the increase of blood urea nitrogen in elderly patients and those with chronic renal disease.)

The concentration of formed elements in the blood (erythrocytes (RBC), leukocytes (WBC), platelets, plasma proteins) increases with an ECF deficit and decreases with an ECF excess. The concentration of serum sodium, however, is not related to the volume status of extracellular fluid: a severe ECF volume deficit may exist with a normal, low, or high serum sodium level.

VOLUME DEFICIT. Extracellular fluid volume deficit is by far the most common fluid disorder in the surgical patient. The fluid lost is not water alone, but water and electrolytes in approximately the same proportion as that in which they exist in normal extracellular fluid. The most common disorders leading to an extracellular fluid volume deficit include losses of gastrointestinal fluids due to vomiting, nasogastric suction, diarrhea, and fistula drainage. Other common causes include sequestration of fluid in soft tissue injuries and infections, intra-abdominal and retroperitoneal inflammatory processes, peritonitis, intestinal obstruction, and burns. The signs and symptoms of this state are easily recognized and are listed in Table 1. The central nervous system and cardiovascular signs occur early with acute rapid losses, whereas tissue signs may be absent until the deficit has existed for at least 24 hours. The central nervous system (CNS) signs are similar to barbiturate intoxication and may be overlooked by the casual observer if the volume deficit is mild. The cardiovascular signs are secondary to a decrease in plasma volume and may be associated with varying degrees of hypotension in a patient with severe ECF volume deficit. Skin turgor may be difficult to assess in an elderly patient or in a patient with recent weight loss and is not diagnostic in the absence of other confirmatory signs. The body temperature tends to vary with the environmental temperature. In a cool room, a patient may be slightly hypothermic, and the febrile response and increased WBC count expected with infection may be suppressed. This occurs frequently and can be misleading during clinical evaluation of a septic patient. After partial correction of the volume deficit, the temperature and WBC count usually rise to appropriate levels.

Severe volume depletion depresses all body systems (including the CNS) and interferes with the clinical evaluation of a patient. For example, a volume-depleted patient with severe sepsis from peritonitis may have a normal temperature and WBC count, complain of little pain, and have unimpressive findings on abdominal examination. The clinical presentation changes dramatically, however, as the ECF volume is restored.

The oliguria is secondary to renal hypoperfusion (prerenal azotemia) and occasionally may be difficult to distinguish from oliguria caused by intrinsic renal disease (renal azotemia). In addition to the clinical setting and examination of urinary sediment, the tests of urinary function listed in Table 2 may be beneficial.[27] Some of these tests are of limited value in the differential diagnosis of oliguria in elderly patients because of the diminished ability to concentrate urine generally associated with aging.[40] Many, however, retain the ability to conserve sodium. Of the listed tests, the *renal failure index* and the *fractional excretion of filtered sodium* are the most accurate.

VOLUME EXCESS. Extracellular fluid volume excess is generally iatrogenic or secondary to renal insufficiency. Both the plasma and the interstitial fluid volumes are increased. In a healthy young adult, the signs are generally those of circulatory overload, manifested primarily in the pulmonary circulation, and of excessive fluid in other tissues (see Table 1). In an elderly patient, for example, congestive heart failure with pulmonary edema may develop rather quickly with a moderate volume excess.

Concentration Changes

The serum sodium level is used in estimating total body fluid osmolality. Since the extracellular and intracellular fluid compartments are separated by a membrane that is freely permeable only to water, osmolality is approximately the same in the two spaces. Any change in the number of particles (osmolality) in one compartment will initiate an appropriate transfer of water between the two spaces. Therefore, even though the sodium ion is largely confined to the extracellular compartment, its level reflects total body fluid osmolality. Hyponatremia and hypernatremia can be diagnosed by clinical manifestations (Table 3), but discernible signs and symptoms are not generally present until the changes are severe. Changes in concentration should be noted early by appropriate laboratory tests and corrected promptly. Clinical signs of hyponatremia or hypernatremia tend to occur early and with greater severity if the rate of change is rapid.

TABLE 1. Extracellular Fluid Volume

| | Deficit | | Excess | |
	Moderate	Severe	Moderate	Severe
CNS	Sleepiness Apathy Slow responses Anorexia Cessation of usual activity	Decreased tendon reflexes Anesthesia of distal extremities Stupor Coma	None	None
Gastrointestinal	Progressive decrease in food consumption	Nausea, vomiting Refusal to eat Silent ileus and distention	*At Operation:* Edema of stomach, colon, lesser and greater omenta, and small bowel mesentery	
Cardiovascular	Orthostatic hypotension Tachycardia Collapsed veins Collapsing pulse	Cutaneous lividity Hypotension Distant heart sounds Cold extremities Absent peripheral pulses	Elevated venous pressure Distention of peripheral veins Increased cardiac output Loud heart sounds Functional murmurs Bounding pulse High pulse pressure Increased pulmonary second sound Gallop	Pulmonary edema
Tissue signs	Soft, small tongue with longitudinal wrinkling Decreased skin turgor	Atonic muscles Sunken eyes	Subcutaneous pitting edema Basilar rales	Anasarca Moist rales Vomiting Diarrhea
Metabolism	Mild decrease of temperature, 97–99°F.	Marked decrease of temperature, 95–98°F.	None	None

HYPONATREMIA. Acute *symptomatic* hyponatremia clinically is characterized by central nervous system signs of increased intracranial pressure and tissue signs of excessive intracellular water. There are no cardiovascular signs *per se*. The hypertension is induced by the rise in intracranial pressure, since the blood pressure generally returns to normal after correction of the sodium level. Of importance with severe hyponatremia is the relatively rapid development of oliguric renal failure, which may not be reversible if therapy is delayed.

TABLE 2. Oliguria

	Prerenal	Renal
Urine osmolality (mOsm./ kg. H$_2$O)	>500	<350
Urine sodium (mEq./L.)	<20	>40
BUN/serum creatinine	>15	<10
Urine/plasma urea	>8	<3
Urine/plasma creatinine	>40	<20
Renal Failure Index RFI = $\dfrac{\text{Urine Na}}{\text{U/P creatinine}}$	<1	>1.5
Fractional excretion sodium FE$_{Na}$ = $\dfrac{\text{U/P Na}}{\text{U/P Cr}} \times 100$	<1	>1.5

Patients with early acute glomerulonephritis may have indices similar to prerenal patients. Indices are not reliable in patients with obstructive uropathy.

Adapted from Miller, T. R., et al.: Urinary diagnostic indices in acute renal failure. Ann. Int. Med., *89:*47, 1978.

Many *hyponatremic* states are asymptomatic until the serum sodium level falls well below 120 mEq. per liter. One important exception is the patient with increased cerebrospinal fluid pressure, such as following closed head injury, in which mild hyponatremia may be extremely deleterious, even fatal. This is due to the progressive increase in intracellular water (further increasing intracranial pressure) as the extracellular fluid osmolality falls.

HYPERNATREMIA. Central nervous system and tissue signs (listed in Table 3) characterize acute symptomatic hypernatremia. This is the only state in which dry, sticky mucous membranes are characteristic. This sign does not occur with extracellular fluid volume deficit alone and usually is only an indication that the patient is breathing through the mouth. Body temperature is generally elevated and may approach a lethal level, as in the patient with heat stroke, while volume changes occur frequently without a change in serum sodium concentration (osmolality), the reverse is not true. Disease states that cause acute alterations in serum sodium levels frequently produce concomitant changes in the extracellular fluid volume.

Mixed Volume and Concentration Abnormalities

Mixed volume and concentration abnormalities may develop as a consequence of the disease state or occasionally from inappropriate parenteral fluid therapy. Moyer noted that the clinical presentation associated with a combination of fluid abnormalities tends to be an algebraic composite of the signs and symptoms of each state.[44] Equal signs produced by both abnormalities are additive, and opposing signs tend to nullify one another.

One of the more common mixed abnormalities is an extracellular fluid deficit and hyponatremia. This state is readily produced in a patient who continues to drink water while losing

TABLE 3. Acute Changes in Osmolar Concentration

	Hyponatremia (Water Intoxication)		Hypernatremia (Water Deficit)	
CNS	*Moderate* Muscle twitching Hyperactive tendon reflexes Increased intracranial pressure (compensated phase)	*Severe* Convulsions Loss of reflexes Increased intracranial pressure (decompensated phase)	*Moderate* Restlessness Weakness	*Severe* Delirium Maniacal behavior
Cardiovascular	Changes in blood pressure and pulse secondary to increased intracranial pressure		Tachycardia Hypotension (if severe)	
Tissue signs	Increased salivation, lacrimation Watery diarrhea "Fingerprinting" of skin (sign of intracellular volume excess)		Decreased saliva and tears Dry and sticky mucous membranes Red, swollen tongue Flushed skin	
Renal	Oliguria progressing to anuria		Oliguria	
Metabolic	None		Fever	

large volumes of gastrointestinal fluids. It may also occur in the postoperative period when gastrointestinal losses are replaced with only 5 per cent dextrose in water or a hypotonic sodium solution. An extracellular volume deficit accompanied by hypernatremia may be produced by the loss of a large amount of hypotonic salt solution, such as an osmotic diuresis due to glucosuria in a hyperglycemic patient.

The prolonged administration of excessive quantities of sodium salts may eventually cause an extracellular volume excess and hypernatremia. This may also occur when pure water losses (such as insensible loss of water from the skin and lungs) are replaced with only sodium-containing solutions. Similarly, the excessive administration of water or hypotonic salt solutions to a patient with oliguric renal failure may rapidly produce an extracellular volume excess and hyponatremia.

Normally functioning kidneys minimize these changes to some extent and compensate for many of the errors associated with parenteral fluid administration. In contrast, the patient in anuric or oliguric renal failure is particularly prone to development of these mixed volume and osmolar concentration abnormalities. Fluid and electrolyte management in these patients, therefore, must be precise. Unfortunately, the fact that a patient with normal kidneys in whom a significant volume deficit develops may be in a state of "functional" renal failure is often not recognized. As the volume deficit progresses, the glomerular filtration rate falls precipitously, and the kidneys' unique mechanisms for maintaining fluid and electrolyte homeostasis are compromised. Such changes may occur with only mild volume deficits in elderly patients with borderline renal function. In these patients, the blood urea nitrogen level may rise higher than 100 mg. per 100 ml. in response to the fluid deficit, with a concomitant rise in the serum creatinine level. Fortunately, the changes are usually reversible with early and adequate correction of the extracellular fluid volume deficit.

Composition Changes

Compositional abnormalities of importance include changes in acid-base balance and concentration changes in potassium, calcium, and magnesium.

ACID-BASE BALANCE. The pH (the negative logarithm of the hydrogen ion concentration) of the body fluids is normally maintained within narrow limits despite the rather large load of acid produced endogenously as a by-product of body metabolism. The acids are neutralized efficiently by several buffer systems and subsequently excreted by the lungs and kidneys. The important buffers include proteins and phosphates, which have

a primary role in maintaining intracellular pH, and the bicarbonate-carbonic acid system, which operates principally in the extracellular fluid space. Proteins have only minor influence in the extracellular fluid space, but hemoglobin is of prime significance as a buffer in the red cell.

A buffer system consists of a weak acid or base and the salt of that acid or base. The buffering effect is the result of the formation of an amount of weak acid or base equivalent to the amount of strong acid or base added to the system. The resultant change in pH is considerably less than it would be if the substance were added to water alone. Thus, inorganic acids (e.g., hydrochloric, sulfuric, phosphoric) and organic acids (e.g., lactic, pyruvic, keto) combine with base bicarbonate, producing the sodium salt of the acid and carbonic acid:

$$(HCl + NaHCO_3 \longrightarrow NaCl + H_2CO_3)$$

The carbonic acid formed is then excreted via the lungs as CO_2. The inorganic acid anions are excreted by the kidneys with hydrogen or as ammonium salts. The organic acid anions generally are metabolized as the underlying disorder is corrected, although some renal excretion may occur with high levels.

The functions of the buffer systems are expressed in the Henderson-Hasselbalch equation, which defines the pH in terms of the ratio of the salt and acid. The pH of the extracellular fluid is defined primarily by the ratio of the amount of base bicarbonate (majority as sodium bicarbonate) to the amount of carbonic acid (related to the CO_2 content of alveolar air) present in the blood:

$$pH = pK + \log \frac{BHCO_3}{H_2CO_3} = [6.1] +$$

$$[\log \frac{27 \text{ mEq./L.}}{1.35 \text{ mEq./L.}} = \frac{20}{1} = 1.3] = 7.4$$

pK represents the dissociation constant of carbonic acid in the presence of base bicarbonate and by measurement is 6.1. At a body pH of 7.4, the ratio must be 20:1, as depicted. From a chemical standpoint this is an inefficient buffer system, but the unusual property of CO_2 to behave as an acid or to change to a neutral gas subsequently excreted by the lungs makes it quite efficient biologically.

As long as the 20:1 ratio is maintained, regardless of the absolute values, the pH remains at 7.4. When an acid is added to the system, the concentration of bicarbonate (the numerator in the Henderson-Hasselbalch equation) decreases. Ventilation immediately increases to eliminate larger quantities of CO_2 with

TABLE 4. Acidosis-Alkalosis

	Defect	Common Causes	$\dfrac{BHCO_3}{H_2CO_3} = \dfrac{20}{1}$	Compensation
Respiratory acidosis	Retention of CO_2 (decreased alveolar ventilation)	Depression of respiratory center by morphine CNS injury Pulmonary disease — emphysema, pneumonia	↑Denominator Ratio less than 20:1	Renal Retention of bicarbonate, excretion of acid salts, increased ammonia formation Chloride shift into red cells
Respiratory alkalosis	Excessive loss of CO_2 (increased alveolar ventilation)	Hyperventilation: emotional disturbances, severe pain, assisted ventilation, encephalitis	↓Denominator Ratio greater than 20:1	Renal Excretion of bicarbonate, retention of acid salts, decreased ammonia formation
Metabolic acidosis	Retention of fixed acids or loss of base bicarbonate	Diabetes, azotemia, lactic acid accumulation, starvation Diarrhea, small bowel fistulas	↓Numerator Ratio less than 20:1	Pulmonary (rapid): increased rate and depth of breathing Renal (slow): as in respiratory acidosis
Metabolic alkalosis	Loss of fixed acids Gain of base bicarbonate Potassium depletion	Vomiting or gastric suction with pyloric obstruction Excessive intake of bicarbonate Diuretics	↑Numerator Ratio greater than 20:1	Pulmonary (rapid): decreased rate and depth of breathing Renal (slow): as in respiratory alkalosis

a subsequent decrease in the carbonic acid (the denominator in the Henderson-Hasselbalch equation) until the 20:1 ratio is re-established. Slower, more complete compensation is effected by the kidneys with increased excretion of acid salts and retention of bicarbonate. The reverse occurs if an alkali is added to the system. Respiratory acidosis and alkalosis are produced by disturbances of ventilation, with an increase or decrease in the denominator and a resultant change of the 20:1 ratio. Compensation is primarily renal, with a retention of bicarbonate and increased excretion of acid salts in respiratory acidosis and the reverse process in respiratory alkalosis.

The four types of acid-base disturbances are listed in Table 4. Use of the CO_2 combining power (approximates the plasma bicarbonate) or CO_2 content (includes bicarbonate, carbonic acid, and dissolved CO_2) and knowledge of the patient's disease may allow an accurate diagnosis in the uncomplicated case. However, use of the CO_2 content or CO_2 combining power alone is generally inadequate as an index of acid-base balance. Both these tests principally reflect the level of plasma bicarbonate, since dissolved CO_2 and carbonic acid contribute no more than a few millimoles under most circumstances. In the acute phase, therefore, respiratory acidosis or alkalosis may exist without any change in the CO_2 content; determinations of the pH and P_{CO_2} from a freshly drawn arterial blood sample are necessary for diagnosis. Thus, measurements of pH, bicarbonate concentration, and P_{CO_2} are required for a more complete understanding of the acid-base status in most patients (Table 5).

Unfortunately, more complex acid-base disturbances are frequently encountered. Combinations of respiratory and metabolic changes occur and may represent compensation for the initial acid-base disturbance or may indicate two or more coexisting primary disorders (e.g., a *primary* respiratory acidosis complicated by a *primary* metabolic acidosis or alkalosis).

Usually, primary acid-base disturbances are compensated to some extent. A primary metabolic disturbance is initially compensated by changes in pulmonary ventilation, while respiratory disturbances are compensated by renal mechanisms. For example, the initial compensation for an acute metabolic acidosis is an increase in the rate and depth of breathing to lower the arterial P_{CO_2}. As emphasized by Astrup and associates, the actual state of the acid-base disorder may be characterized by the degree of compensation — *not compensated* (early or compensatory mechanisms not functioning), *partially compensated* (pH has not returned to a normal value), *compensated, or overcompensated*.[3] Physiologically, *complete compensation or overcompensation* cannot occur; when tempted to draw this conclusion, one should consider the presence of a mixed acid-base disturbance as the explanation.[30]

As previously noted, a knowledge of the pH, bicarbonate concentration, and P_{CO_2} allows an accurate diagnosis of most acid-base disturbances. However, the clinical interpretation of these measurements is associated with some inherent problems. Although the arterial P_{CO_2} is considered an accurate index of primary respiratory disturbances, changes in the level may rep-

TABLE 5. Respiratory and Metabolic Components of Acid-Base Disorders

	Acute (Uncompensated)			Chronic (Partially Compensated)		
	pH	P_{CO_2} (respiratory component)	Plasma HCO_3^-* (metabolic component)	pH	P_{CO_2} (respiratory component)	Plasma HCO_3^-* (metabolic component)
Respiratory acidosis	↓↓	↑↑	N	↓	↑↑	↑
Respiratory alkalosis	↑↑	↓↓	N	↓	↓↓	↑
Metabolic acidosis	↓↓	N	↓↓	↑		↓
Metabolic alkalosis	↑↑	N	↑↑	↑	↑?	↑

* Measured as standard bicarbonate, whole-blood buffer base, CO_2 content or CO_2-combining power. The *base excess value* is positive when the standard bicarbonate is above normal and negative when the standard bicarbonate is below normal.

resent compensation for a primary metabolic alteration. Thus, a depressed P_{CO_2} (below 40 mm. Hg) is characteristic of respiratory alkalosis but also represents the normal compensatory response to a metabolic acidosis. Similarly, the level of plasma bicarbonate cannot be regarded exclusively as an index of metabolic disturbances. An elevated plasma bicarbonate level may indicate a primary metabolic alkalosis or a compensatory response to chronic respiratory acidosis.

In an effort to separate the respiratory and metabolic components of acid-base disorders, two other approaches have been introduced: In 1948 Singer and Hastings[39] introduced the concept of *whole blood buffer base,* and later Astrup and colleagues proposed the use of the *standard bicarbonate* and *base excess* values.[2,3,25] The approach advocated by Astrup has been the more popular of the two, although both are attempts to quantify the metabolic, or nonrespiratory, component in an acid-base disturbance and separate it from the respiratory component.

The standard bicarbonate is defined as the concentration of bicarbonate in plasma, when whole blood with fully oxygenated hemoglobin has been equilibrated with CO_2 at a P_{CO_2} of 40 mm. Hg at a temperature of 38°C. This value may be rapidly determined by means of the Astrup technique by measuring pH values at two known levels of P_{CO_2} and reading the standard bicarbonate directly from a nomogram. The normal mean value for standard bicarbonate is 24.5 mEq. per liter of plasma. Base excess (or deficit) directly expresses the amount, in milliequivalents, of fixed base (or fixed acid) added to each liter of blood. This value is obtained by multiplying the deviation of standard bicarbonate from the normal mean by a factor of 1.2. This factor corrects for the buffering capacity of the red cells and varies slightly with changes in hemoglobin concentration.[3] To avoid calculations, the base excess may be read directly from a nomogram. When the term *base excess* is used exclusively, the *positive* values represent the excess of base, and the *negative* values reflect the deficit of base (or excess of acid).*

In an excellent review of the Singer-Hastings and the Astrup systems, Schwartz and Relman state that neither system offers any advantage over the classic approach for the diagnosis of acid-base disorders.[34] They question the validity of using an *in vitro* CO_2 titration curve as a measure of *in vivo* acid-base changes. Additionally, they note that the use of either of the two systems may be misleading in the analysis of chronic disorders. For example, a low pH with an elevated P_{CO_2}, a normal standard bicarbonate value, and a base excess value of zero are compatible with a diagnosis of primary uncompensated respiratory acidosis. After several hours or days, compensatory renal mechanisms would cause elevation of the standard bicarbonate level above normal, causing a positive base excess value. This partially compensated respiratory acidosis, then, could be erroneously interpreted as a respiratory acidosis *plus* a metabolic alkalosis as indicated by a significant base excess.

Despite these shortcomings, either approach may be useful when properly interpreted as a single laboratory test. Other systems have been recommended, some with ingeniously devised nomograms, but all are subject to misinterpretation. Unfortunately, there are no shortcuts. Regardless of the methods used, the proper analysis of complex acid-base disorders requires a thorough knowledge of the clinical situation, good judgment, and a sound understanding of acid-base physiology.

RESPIRATORY ACIDOSIS. In most instances the underlying cause of a respiratory disorder is readily apparent by history and physical examination (Table 6), and special tests are generally not required. Respiratory acidosis is caused by retention of CO_2

---

* The deficit or excess of base in the extracellular compartment can be estimated in milliequivalents by multiplying the negative or positive value for base excess, in milliequivalents per liter of blood, by 0.3 times the body weight in kilograms.[25]

TABLE 6. Causes of Respiratory Disturbances

Acidosis (Hypoventilation)	Alkalosis (Hyperventilation)
Airway obstruction Foreign body, pneumonia, emphysema, laryngospasm	Central nervous system disorders Injury, tumor, stroke, anxiety
Central nervous system depression Narcotics, anesthetics, injury, tumor	Hypoxia Adult respiratory distress syndrome, pulmonary embolus, atelectasis, anemia
Thoracic injury Pneumothorax, flail chest, tracheal tear	Mechanical ventilation Excess tidal volume and/or rate
Mechanical ventilation Inadequate rate and/or tidal volume, increased dead space	Hypermetabolism Fever, injury, sepsis
Miscellaneous Congestive heart failure, myopathy, severe obesity	Miscellaneous Congestive heart failure, salicylate intoxication, cirrhosis

secondary to decreased alveolar ventilation. Initially P_{CO_2} is elevated and plasma bicarbonate concentration is normal. In the chronic form, P_{CO_2} remains elevated and bicarbonate concentration rises as renal compensation occurs.

A number of conditions causing inadequate ventilation (airway obstruction, pneumonia, atelectasis, pleural effusion, and hypoventilation due to the pain of abdominal incisions or to abdominal distention limiting diaphragmatic excursion) may exist singly or in combination to produce respiratory acidosis. The problem is particularly serious in patients with chronic pulmonary disease, in whom pre-existing respiratory acidosis may be accentuated by another illness or injury. With surgical patients a not infrequent problem in the postoperative period is restlessness, hypertension, and tachycadia. These findings may be due to pain, although similar signs are associated with inadequate ventilation and hypercapnia compounded by the use of narcotics.

Management of respiratory acidosis involves prompt correction of the pulmonary defect, when feasible, and measures to ensure adequate ventilation. This is particularly important in trauma patients with closed head injury or hypoxic brain damage. Acute hypercarbia aggravates existing cerebral edema because it causes cerebral vasodilatation and increased cerebral blood flow. Maintenance of mild hypocarbia to temporarily reduce cerebral edema in such patients has been suggested.[47] In contrast, correction of a chronic well-compensated respiratory acidosis should be accomplished slowly.[10] Sudden lowering of P_{CO_2} in such patients may produce a severe alkalosis since bicarbonate concentration is already greatly elevated (as compensation for the original disorder) and will not return to normal for many hours. Additionally, administration of oxygen may depress or arrest ventilation if the P_{CO_2} is above 65 mm Hg. Normally, increased P_{CO_2} stimulates the respiratory center; above 65 mm Hg, however, the respiratory center is depressed and hypoxia is the principal stimulus for respiration.

RESPIRATORY ALKALOSIS. Hyperventilation due to apprehension, pain, hypoxia, CNS injury, and assisted ventilation are common causes of respiratory alkalosis. Any of these conditions may cause rapid depression of arterial P_{CO_2} and elevation of pH. Plasma bicarbonate concentration is normal in the acute phase but falls with renal compensation if the condition persists.

The majority of patients who require ventilatory support develop varying degrees of respiratory alkalosis. This may be inadvertent, due to improper use of a mechanical ventilator, or it may occur during attempts to raise the PO_2 in a hypoxic patient.

Proper management requires frequent measurements of blood gases and appropriate corrections of the ventilatory pattern when indicated. Generally, the P_{CO_2} can be maintained at an acceptable level by adjustments of the ventilatory rate and volume. Increasing the pulmonary dead space to raise P_{CO_2} is of doubtful benefit, and adding 5 per cent CO_2 to inspired air is potentially dangerous and poorly tolerated by many patients.

Severe respiratory alkalosis may cause serious impairment of both cardiovascular and cerebral functions. The predisposition for development of cardiac arrythmias and cardiac arrest is particularly acute in patients who are receiving digitalis or have pre-existing hypokalemia. Hypokalemia may develop suddenly and is related to entry of potassium ions into cells in exchange for hydrogen and excessive urinary potassium loss in exchange for sodium. Additionally, an abrupt fall in the level of ionized calcium (caused by acute alkalosis) alone may produce serious arrythmias. Cerebral ischemia and acidosis due to cerebral vasoconstriction may also occur with the sudden onset of severe respiratory alkalosis.[21] This is of little consequence in some patients but may cause irreparable damage in patients with impaired cerebral blood flow from obstructive arterial disease or during performance of a carotid endarterectomy. Another effect of alkalosis that is often not appreciated is a shift of the oxygen dissociation curve to the left, which may limit the ability of hemoglobin to unload oxygen to tissues.[8]

Severe and persistent respiratory alkalosis is often difficult to correct and may be associated with a poor prognosis because of the underlying cause of hyperventilation (e.g., intracranial injury). Treatment is directed primarily toward the cause of the disorder. Additionally, preventing the condition by proper use of mechanical ventilators and correction of any existing potassium deficit are important.

METABOLIC ACIDOSIS. Metabolic acidosis follows retention or production of acids (diabetic ketoacidosis, lactic acidosis, azotemia) or loss of bicarbonate (diarrhea, pancreatic or small bowel fistula). The excess hydrogen ion causes lowering of pH and plasma bicarbonate concentration. Initial compensation is pulmonary, with an increase in the rate and depth of breathing and depression of arterial P_{CO_2}; more definitive control is effected by the kidneys. Coexisting renal insufficiency, however, compounds the problem. Decreased glomerular filtration causes retention of acid metabolites, and renal tubular dysfunction interferes with the excretion of hydrogen in exchange for sodium and the production of ammonia. The acidosis may be greatly accentuated and difficult to control.

The causes of metabolic acidosis can be divided into two manageable groups by determining the anion gap.[6] This value should be determined routinely when evaluating a set of serum electrolytes; one simply subtracts the sum of serum chloride and bicarbonate from the serum sodium concentration. The normal value is 10 to 15 mEq. per liter. The anion gap is a laboratory anomaly, since routine clinical laboratory tests measure the cations sodium and potassium and the anions chloride and bicarbonate. The unmeasured anions that represent the gap are sulfate and phosphate plus lactate and other organic anions (Fig. 3). If the acidosis is due to loss of bicarbonate (e.g., diarrhea) or gain of a chloride acid (e.g., administration of ammonium chloride), the anion gap is normal. Conversely, if the acidosis is due to increased production of an organic acid (e.g., lactic acid in circulatory shock) or the retention of sulfuric or phosphoric acid (e.g., renal failure), the concentration of unmeasured anions (anion gap) is increased.

Conditions associated with an elevated anion gap are listed in Table 7. By far the most common is shock or inadequate tissue perfusion from any number of causes, causing accumulation of large quantities of lactic acid. Diabetic ketoacidosis, starvation, and ethanol intoxication cause elevation of the anion gap by the formation of ketoacids; renal failure and uremia cause such elevation by the retention of sulfuric and phosphoric acids. Poi-

Figure 3. The anion gap.

soning by methanol, ethylene glycol, and aspirin produces increased anion gaps by elevation of their organic acid counterparts (formic, oxalic, and salicylic acids). In a patient with an elevated anion gap, therefore, one or more of these causes should be considered.

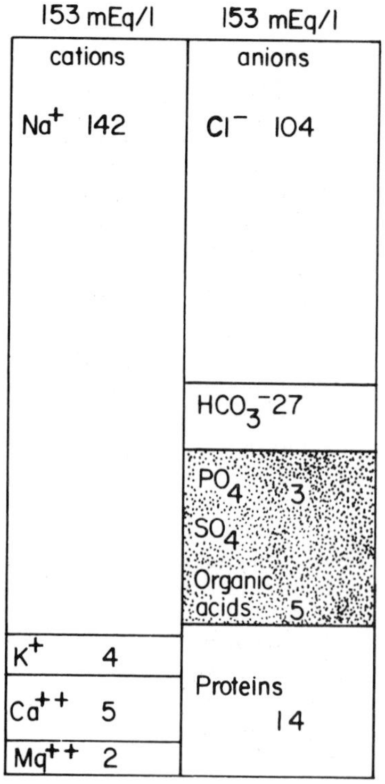

Metabolic acidosis associated with a loss of bicarbonate or retention of chloride acids is characterized by a normal anion gap. Diarrhea, small bowel fistula, and ureterosigmoidostomy cause significant losses of bicarbonate; whereas the resorption of bicarbonate is decreased in patients with proximal renal tubular acidosis. The anion gap is also normal in patients with distal renal tubular acidosis, in whom the excretion of fixed acids (containing chloride) is decreased. Metabolic acidosis may also develop in patients who have large losses of gastrointestinal fluids containing bicarbonate (biliary, pancreatic, and small bowel secretions) replaced with normal saline. Use of a bal-

TABLE 7. Causes of Metabolic Acidosis

Causes	Mechanisms
Normal Anion Gap	
Diarrhea, small bowel fistula, uterosigmoidostomy	Loss of HCO_3
Proximal renal tubular acidosis	Decreased tubular reabsorption of HCO_3
Distal renal tubular acidosis	Decreased acid excretion
Acid administration (NH_4Cl, HCl)	Increased acid load
"Dilutional" acidosis	Volume expansion with HCO_3^- free fluids
Elevated Anion Gap	
Shock (inadequate perfusion)	Increased lactic acid
Diabetes, starvation, alcohol intoxication	Increased ketoacids
Uremia	Retention of sulfuric and phosphoric acids
Ingestion of methanol, ethylene glycol, aspirin	Conversion to formic, oxalic, and salicylic acids

anced salt solution containing sodium lactate or bicarbonate is more appropriate. Additionally, massive replacement of extracellular fluid volume with bicarbonate-free solutions may cause dilutional acidosis associated with a normal anion gap.[36]

The most common cause of severe metabolic acidosis in surgical patients is acute circulatory failure with accumulation of lactic acid. Acute hemorrhagic shock causes a rapid and profound drop in pH, and attempts to raise the blood pressure with vasopressors simply compound the problem. Attempts to correct the acidosis by infusion of large quantities of sodium bicarbonate without restoration of flow are futile. Following restoration of adequate tissue perfusion by volume replacement, lactic acid is cleared rapidly and the pH returns toward normal. Concomitant with administration of blood, use of lactated Ringer's solution to replace the extracellular fluid deficit caused by severe, prolonged hemorrhagic shock and associated injuries does not accentuate the lactic acidosis. Instead, there is a rapid decrease in the lactic acid level and return of pH toward normal, as opposed to the results of using blood alone.[9,24]

Routine use of sodium bicarbonate during resuscitation of patients in hypovolemic shock is discouraged. A mild metabolic alkalosis is a common finding following resuscitation, which is in part due to the alkalinizing effects of blood transfusions and administration of lactated Ringer's solution. After infusion (and partial restoration of hepatic blood flow), the citrate contained in the transfused blood and the lactate in lactated Ringer's solution are metabolized, producing bicarbonate. Lactic acid production ceases, excess hydrogen ion is buffered and excreted, and the organic anion lactate is metabolized by the liver. If excessive quantities of sodium bicarbonate are administered during resuscitation, severe metabolic alkalosis can follow. A highly alkaline pH is undesirable, particularly in patients with hypoxia or low fixed cardiac outputs, since the oxygen dissociation curve is shifted to the left. Other factors tending to shift the curve to the left that may be operative in such patients include hypothermia and depressed levels of erythroctye 2,3-diphosphoglycerate in stored transfused blood. If the curve shifts sufficiently far to the left, interference with oxygen unloading at the cellular level may occur.

The treatment of metabolic acidosis is directed toward correction of the underlying disorder when possible. Bicarbonate therapy is appropriately reserved for the treatment of severe metabolic acidosis, particularly following cardiac arrest, when partial correction of pH may be essential to restore myocardial function. Previous studies[7,23] have indicated that the acidosis accompanying cardiac arrest is compensated for a period of time if the patient is well ventilated and not previously acidotic (although cardiac arrest following prolonged hypovolemic shock is invariably associated with severe metabolic acidosis). Additionally, administration of bicarbonate in the usually recommended doses may induce an acute, severe hypernatremia and hyperosmolar state. Thus, bicarbonate should be used judiciously during cardiac arrest; Mattar and associates[23] recommended that the initial dose of bicarbonate not exceed 50 ml of 7.5 per cent solution (45 mEq. $NaHCO_3$ containing 90 mOsm.) and that the decision for additional doses be based on measurements of pH when possible.

Correction of pH in more protracted states of metabolic acidosis may be indicated and should be accomplished slowly. Frequent measurements of bicarbonate and blood pH are the best guides to therapy, since a satisfactory formula for estimating the amount of alkali needed has not been devised.

METABOLIC ALKALOSIS. Metabolic alkalosis follows loss of fixed acids or gain of bicarbonate and is aggravated by any existing potassium deficit. Both the pH and the plasma bicarbonate concentration are elevated. Compensation is primarily by renal mechanisms, since respiratory compensation is generally small and cannot be detected in many patients. The expected respiratory response is a decrease in ventilation to retain CO_2. Po_2

would also fall, however, so that hypoxia imposes a limit on the amount of respiratory compensation that can occur.[43] In the rare situation in which hypercapnia is thought to represent a compensatory response to metabolic alkalosis, rapid reduction of Pco_2 by mechanical ventilation should be avoided. Rather, the Pco_2 falls as the metabolic alkalosis is corrected.

The causes of metabolic alkalosis can be divided into two major groups, *chloride-responsive* (urine chloride less than 10 to 20 mEq. per liter) and *chloride-resistant* (urine chloride more than 10 to 20 mEq. per liter), depending on the amounts of chloride in the urine of untreated patients (Table 8).[6] States of chloride-resistant metabolic alkalosis are usually associated with a normal or slightly increased extracellular fluid volume. Most are secondary to adrenal disorders, in which the high levels of steroid secretion cause maximal tubular resorption of sodium and bicarbonate and an excessive loss of chloride in the urine. The result is metabolic alkalosis and (because of increased sodium reabsorption) expansion of the extracellular fluid compartment. Therapy is directed toward the underlying cause.

Chloride-responsive types of metabolic alkalosis are considerably more common and are often associated with extracellular fluid volume deficits. In addition to volume replacement, the provision of an adequate quantity of chloride is a prerequisite to restoration of normal acid-base and potassium equilibrium, for the following reasons: (1) Sodium reabsorption occurs along the entire renal tubule, although the responsible mechanisms vary in the proximal and distal portions of the tubule. The majority of sodium filtered by the glomerulus is removed in the proximal tubule; electroneutrality is maintained by the simultaneous reabsorption of an anion, principally chloride. If there is a deficit of chloride ion, more sodium must be reabsorbed in the *distal* tubule in exchange for hydrogen or potassium. (2) In the distal tubule, sodium is reabsorbed in exchange for hydrogen or potassium, depending on their relative availability. This process also involves the generation of one bicarbonate ion for each sodium ion that is reabsorbed, which perpetuates the alkalosis. Administering the patient an adequate quantity of chloride is critical to reverse this imbalance and allow more sodium to be reabsorbed with chloride in the proximal tubule.[18]

The prototype for a chloride-responsive, hypochloremic, hypokalemic metabolic alkalosis is that which occurs from persistent vomiting or prolonged nasogastric suction in the presence of an obstructed pylorus. Unlike vomiting with an open pylorus (involving a loss of gastric, pancreatic, biliary, and intestinal secretions), this entity causes loss of fluid with high chloride and hydrogen ion concentrations in relation to sodium. In addition to a chloride deficit, the accompanying depletion of extracellular fluid volume (often marked) stimulates maximal reabsorption of sodium in the distal renal tubule to maintain volume. Since there is less chloride in the glomerular filtrate for reabsorption of sodium in the proximal tubule, more sodium by necessity must be reabsorbed in the distal tubule in exchange for

---

TABLE 8. Metabolic Alkalosis

Chloride-Responsive
(Urine Chloride < 10 – 20 mEq./L.)
    Vomiting, gastric suction with obstructed pylorus
    Diuretics
    Villous adenoma of colon

Chloride-Resistant
(Urine Chloride > 10 – 20 mEq./L.)
    Primary hyperaldosteronism
    Cushing's disease
    Exogenous corticosteroids
    Chronic hypokalemia

Unclassified
    Alkali ingestion or infusion

hydrogen and potassium. The developing hypokalemia from continued vomiting causes even greater excretion of hydrogen, since less potassium is available for exchange. If severe enough, the initially alkaline urine becomes acid (paradoxic aciduria). Treatment involves replacing the extracellular fluid volume deficit with isotonic sodium chloride solution and potassium. The provision of chloride allows increased sodium reabsorption in the proximal tubule, and less sodium is presented to the distal tubule. As the amount of sodium reabsorbed in the distal tubule decreases, the alkalosis begins to resolve as less hydrogen ion is secreted and less bicarbonate is generated. Additionally, hydrogen secretion is decreased further as hypokalemia is corrected, since more potassium is now available for exchange with sodium. Although severe potassium depletion is invariably present, volume repletion should be started and good urinary output obtained before potassium is administered.

Rarely, severe metabolic alkalosis in a patient with pyloric outlet obstruction may be refractory to standard therapy. This occurs most often in patients who also have severe hypochloremia and several liters of nasogastric drainage daily. The infusion of ammonium chloride or arginine hydrochloride has been the usual method of increasing the level of nonvolatile acids in this situation. However, use of the first may produce ammonia toxicity, and the latter solution is no longer available commercially. The use of 0.1 N to 0.2 N hydrochloric acid has been shown to be safe and effective therapy for the correction of severe, resistant metabolic alkalosis.[1,15,20,46] A 0.15 N hydrochloric acid solution is prepared by addition of 150 ml. of 1 N hydrochloric acid to 1 liter of isotonic saline or 5 per cent dextrose solution. This is infused into a large vein at a rate of 25 to 50 ml. per hour, and measurements of pH, P_{CO_2}, and serum electrolytes are obtained every 4 to 6 hours. Generally, 1 or 2 liters of solution over a period of 24 hours is sufficient, although one should not hesitate to give additional hydrochloric acid when the need is based on appropriate clinical and laboratory evidence. Temporary control of alkalosis is usually successful, but the pyloric outlet obstruction should be corrected as soon as possible.

It should be emphasized that alkalotic patients are invariably hypokalemic, and potassium depletion itself may induce metabolic alkalosis. In the latter instance, potassium lost from body cells is replaced in part by hydrogen, which causes extracellular fluid alkalosis. The same process occurs in the distal renal tubular cells, so there is less potassium to exchange for sodium; therefore, more hydrogen must be excreted in the urine in exchange for sodium. Conversely, an alkalosis (affecting both the intracellular and extracellular fluid compartments) increases the urinary loss of potassium. As hydrogen leaves the cell, it is replaced in part by potassium. In the renal tubular cell, more potassium than hydrogen is available for exchange with sodium, causing a rise in urinary potassium. As a matter of fact, the secretion of potassium is so closely related to alkalosis that simple hyperventilation (producing respiratory alkalosis) immediately increases renal excretion of potassium approximately threefold.[31]

POTASSIUM ABNORMALITIES. The normal dietary intake of potassium is approximately 50 to 100 mEq. daily, and in the absence of hypokalemia most is excreted in the urine. Ninety-eight per cent of the potassium in the body is located in the intracellular compartment at a concentration of approximately 150 mEq. per liter, and it is the major cation of intracellular water. Although the total extracellular potassium in a 70-kg. male would approximate only 63 mEq. (4.5 mEq. per liter × 14 liters), this small amount is critical to cardiac and neuromuscular function. In addition, the turnover rate in the extracellular fluid compartment may be extremely rapid.

The intracellular and extracellular distribution of potassium is influenced by many factors. Significant quantities of intracellular potassium are released into the extracellular space in response to severe injury or surgical stress, acidosis, and the cata-

bolic state. A significant rise in serum potassium may occur in these states in the presence of oliguric or anuric renal failure, but dangerous hyperkalemia (greater than 6 mEq. per liter) is rarely encountered if renal function is normal. After severe trauma, however, normal or excessive urinary volumes may not reflect the ability of the kidneys to clear solutes or to excrete potassium. (See the later section High-Output Renal Failure.)

HYPERKALEMIA. The signs of significant hyperkalemia are limited to the cardiovascular and gastrointestinal systems. The gastrointestinal symptoms include nausea, vomiting, intermittent intestinal colic, and diarrhea. The cardiovascular signs are apparent on the electrocardiogram initially, with high peaked T waves, widened QRS complex, and depressed S-T segments. Disappearance of T waves, heart block, and diastolic cardiac arrest may develop with increasing levels of potassium.

Treatment of hyperkalemia consists of immediate measures to reduce the serum potassium level, withholding of exogenously administered potassium, and correction of the underlying cause when possible. Temporary suppression of the myocardial effects of a sudden rapid rise of potassium can be accomplished by the intravenous administration of 1 gm. of 10 per cent calcium gluconate under electrocardiographic (ECG) monitoring. Infusion of calcium ions does not affect serum potassium concentration but does counteract the effects of hyperkalemia on cardiac cells by restoring a more normal differential between threshold and resting cellular transmembrane potential. Serum potassium levels may be transiently decreased by administration of bicarbonate and glucose with insulin (45 mEq. $NaHCO_3$ in 1000 ml. of $D_{10}W$ with 20 units regular insulin). The administration of dextrose stimulates insulin release, which augments cellular potassium uptake. Rapid alkalinization of the extracellular fluid with either sodium lactate or bicarbonate promotes transfer of potassium into cells; it is particularly valuable when hyperkalemia is partially due to a metabolic acidosis. These maneuvers are temporary and allow time for definitive removal of excess potassium by cation-exchange resins, peritoneal dialysis, or hemodialysis.

HYPOKALEMIA. A more common problem in the surgical patient is hypokalemia, which may occur as a result of (1) excessive renal excretion, (2) movement of potassium into cells, (3) prolonged administration of potassium-free parenteral fluids with continued obligatory renal loss of potassium (more than 20 mEq. per day), (4) parenteral nutrition with inadequate potassium replacement, and (5) loss of gastrointestinal secretions.

Potassium has an important role in the regulation of acid-base balance. Increased renal excretion occurs with both respiratory and metabolic alkalosis. Potassium is in competition with hydrogen ion for renal tubular excretion in exchange for sodium ion. Thus, in alkalosis, the increased potassium ion excretion in exchange for sodium ion permits hydrogen ion conservation. Hypokalemia itself may produce a metabolic alkalosis, since an increase in excretion of hydrogen ions occurs when the concentration of potassium in the tubular cells is low. In addition, movement of hydrogen ions into the cells as a consequence of potassium loss is partly responsible for the alkalosis. In metabolic acidosis the reverse process occurs, and the excess hydrogen ion exchanges for sodium with retention of greater amounts of potassium.

Renal tubular excretion of potassium ion is increased when large quantities of sodium are available for excretion. The more sodium ion available for resorption, the more potassium is exchanged for it in the lumen. Potassium requirements for prolonged or massive isotonic fluid volume replacement are increased, probably on this basis. The same mechanism may also explain the increased potassium ion excretion with steroid administration.

The renal excretion of potassium may be small when compared with the amount of potassium that can be lost in gastrointestinal secretions. The amount per liter in various types of gas-

TABLE 9. Composition of Gastrointestinal Secretions

	Volume (ml./24 hr.)	Na (mEq./L.)	K (mEq./L.)	Cl (mEq./L.)	HCO$_3$ (mEq./L.)
Salivary	1500 (500–2000)	10 (2–10)	26 (20–30)	10 (8–18)	30
Stomach	1500 (100–4000)	60 (9–116)	10 (0–32)	130 (8–154)	—
Duodenum	(100–2000)	140	5	80	—
Ileum	3000 (100–9000)	140 (80–150)	5 (2–8)	104 (43–137)	30
Colon	—	60	30	40	—
Pancreas	(100–800)	140 (113–185)	5 (3–7)	75 (54–95)	115
Bile	(50–800)	145 (131–164)	5 (3–12)	100 (89–180)	35

trointestinal fluids is shown in Table 9. Although the average potassium concentration of some of these fluids is relatively low, significant hypokalemia results if potassium-free fluids are used for replacement.

Hypokalemia may also be a problem in the patient maintained on intravenous nutrition. Large quantities of supplemental potassium generally are necessary to restore depleted intracellular stores and to meet the requirements for tissue synthesis during the anabolic phase.

In summary, most of the factors that tend to influence potassium metabolism cause excess excretion, and a tendency toward hypokalemia occurs frequently in the surgical patient except when shock or acidosis interferes with the normal renal management of potassium.

The signs of potassium deficit are related to failure of normal contractility of skeletal, smooth, and cardiac muscle and include weakness that may progress to flaccid paralysis, diminished to absent tendon reflexes, and paralytic ileus. Sensitivity to digitalis with cardiac arrhythmias and electrocardiographic signs of low voltage, flattening of T waves, and depression of S-T segments are characteristic. However, signs of potassium deficit may be masked by those of a severe extracellular fluid volume deficit. Repletion of the volume deficit may further aggravate the situation by lowering the serum potassium level secondary to dilution.

The treatment of hypokalemia involves, first, prevention of this state. In the replacement of gastrointestinal fluids, it is safe to replace the upper limits of loss, since an excess is readily managed by the patient with normal renal function. No more than 40 mEq. should be added to 1 liter of intravenous fluid, and the rate of administration should not exceed 40 mEq. per hour unless the electrocardiogram is being monitored. In the absence of specific indications, potassium should not be given to an oliguric patient or during the first 24 hours following severe surgical stress or trauma.

CALCIUM ABNORMALITIES. The majority of the 1000 to 1200 gm. of body calcium in the average-sized adult is found in the bone in the form of phosphate and carbonate. Normal daily intake of calcium is between 1 and 3 gm. Most of this is excreted via the gastrointestinal tract, and 200 mg. or less is excreted in the urine daily. The normal serum level is between 8.5 and 10.5 mg. per 100 ml. (depending on the individual laboratory's normal range), and approximately half of this is not ionized and is bound to plasma protein. An additional nonionized fraction (5 per cent) is bound to other substances in the plasma and interstitial fluid, whereas the remaining 45 per cent is the ionized portion that is responsible for neuromuscular stability. Determination of the plasma protein level, therefore, is essential for proper analysis of the serum calcium level. The ratio of ionized to nonionized calcium is also related to the pH; acidosis causes an increase in the ionized fraction, whereas alkalosis causes a decrease.

Disturbances of calcium metabolism generally are not a problem in the postoperative patient without complications, with the exception of skeletal loss during prolonged immobilization. Routine administration of calcium to the surgical patient, therefore, is not needed in the absence of specific indications.

HYPOCALCEMIA. The symptoms of hypocalcemia (serum level less than 8 mg. per 100 ml.) are numbness and tingling of the circumoral region and the tips of the fingers and toes. The signs are of neuromuscular origin and include hyperactive tendon reflexes, a positive Chvostek sign, muscle and abdominal cramps, tetany with carpopedal spasm, convulsions (with severe deficit), and prolongation of the Q-T interval on the ECG.

The common causes include acute pancreatitis, massive soft tissue infections (necrotizing fasciitis), acute and chronic renal failure, pancreatic and small intestinal fistulas, and hypoparathyroidism. Transient hypocalcemia is a frequent occurrence in the hyperparathyroid patient after removal of a parathyroid adenoma until the remaining parathyroid tissue resumes normal hormone secretion. Severe postoperative hypocalcemia is likely if marked bone resorption was present preoperatively or if the normal parathyroid glands were injured during surgical therapy. Asymptomatic hypocalcemia may occur with hypoproteinemia (normal ionized fraction), whereas symptoms may appear with a normal serum calcium level in a patient with severe alkalosis. The latter is due to a decrease in the physiologically active or ionized fraction of total serum calcium. Calcium levels also may fall with a severe depletion of magnesium.

Treatment is directed toward correction of the underlying cause with concomitant repletion of the deficit. Acute symptoms may be relieved by the intravenous administration of calcium gluconate or calcium chloride. Calcium lactate may be given orally, with or without supplemental vitamin D, in the patient requiring prolonged replacement.

The routine administration of calcium during massive transfusions of blood remains controversial. At present, available data indicate that the majority of patients receiving blood transfusions do not require calcium supplementation.[11,12] The binding of ionized calcium by citrate is generally compensated for by the mobilization of calcium from body stores. For patients receiving blood as rapidly as 100 ml. per minute, however, calcium administration may be indicated. An appropriate dose, obtained from the data of Moore and associates, is 0.2 gm. of calcium chloride (2 ml. of 10 per cent calcium chloride solution), administered intravenously in a separate line, for every 500 ml. of blood transfused.[29] To avoid dangerous levels of hypercalcemia, this dose of calcium is recommended only while blood is being transfused at the rate just noted. Additionally, the total dose of calcium generally should not exceed 3 gm. unless there is objective evidence of hypocalcemia. Larger doses are rarely indicated, since there is some mobilization of calcium and citrate breakdown with release of calcium ion, even with shock and inadequate peripheral perfusion. During massive transfusions, some attempt should be made to monitor the calcium level. An approximation of calcium ion concentration can be obtained by monitoring the Q-T interval on the electrocardiogram, although techniques for the rapid measurement of calcium ion concentration are now available.

HYPERCALCEMIA. The symptoms of hypercalcemia are rather vague and of gastrointestinal, renal, musculoskeletal, and central nervous system origin. The early manifestations of hypercalcemia include easy fatigue, lassitude, weakness of varying degree, anorexia, nausea, vomiting, and weight loss. With higher serum calcium levels, lassitude gives way to somnolence, stupor, and finally coma. Other symptoms include severe headaches, pains in the back and extremities, thirst, polydipsia, and polyuria. The critical level for serum calcium is between 16 and 20 mg. per 100 ml.; and unless treatment is instituted promptly, the symptoms may rapidly progress to death. The two major causes of hypercalcemia are hyperparathyroidism and cancer with bony metastasis. The latter is most frequently seen in a patient with metastatic breast cancer.

A serum calcium concentration of 15 mg. per 100 ml. or higher requires emergency treatment. Most of the patients have an extracellular fluid volume deficit due to the effects of hypercalcemia (vomiting, polyuria), and vigorous volume repletion with salt solutions lowers the calcium level by dilution and increased urinary calcium excretion. Concomitant use of large doses of intravenous furosemide has been recommended to increase urinary calcium excretion, but careful monitoring and replacement of resulting fluid and electrolyte losses are necessary.

Oral or intravenous inorganic phosphates effectively lower serum calcium by inhibiting bone resorption and forming calcium-phosphate complexes that are deposited in soft tissues and bone. Intravenous use may cause an abrupt fall in calcium, however, and tetany, hypotension, and acute renal failure have been reported with this form of therapy. If used, intravenous phosphorus should be given slowly over a period of approximately 12 hours once daily for no more than 2 or 3 days. Inorganic phosphates are contraindicated in patients with hyperphosphatemia or renal failure. Intravenous sodium sulfate also lowers serum calcium by increasing urinary excretion of this ion. It is less effective than phosphate salts, however, and is probably no more effective than normal saline.

Corticosteroids decrease resorption of calcium from bone and reduce the intestinal absorption of vitamin D. They have been found useful in treating hypercalcemic patients with sarcoidosis, myelomas, lymphomas, and leukemias, although the reduction in serum calcium may not be apparent for 1 or 2 weeks. Mithramycin, a cytotoxic drug, effectively lowers serum calcium in 24 to 48 hours by direct action on the bones. The drug is relatively safe in the small doses used, and the calcium level may remain normal for several days to weeks following a single dose.[14,41] Calcitonin induces a moderate decrease in serum calcium, but the effect is diminished with repeated administration. The definitive treatment of acute hypercalcemic crisis in patients with hyperparathyroidism is immediate surgical therapy.[4]

Treatment of hypercalcemia in a patient with metastatic cancer is primarily that of prevention. The serum calcium level is assessed frequently; if it is elevated, the patient is placed on a low-calcium diet, and measures to ensure adequate hydration are instituted.

MAGNESIUM ABNORMALITIES. The total body content of magnesium in the average adult is approximately 2000 mEq., about half of which is incorporated in bone and only slowly exchangeable. The distribution of magnesium is similar to that of potassium, the major portion being intracellular. Serum magnesium concentration normally ranges between 1.5 and 2.5 mEq. per liter. The normal dietary intake of magnesium is approximately 20 mEq. (240 mg.) daily. The larger part is excreted in the feces, and the remainder in the urine. The kidneys have a remarkable ability to conserve magnesium; on a magnesium-free diet, renal excretion of this ion may be less than 1 mEq. per day.

MAGNESIUM DEFICIENCY. Magnesium deficiency is known to occur with starvation, malabsorption syndromes, protracted losses of gastrointestinal fluid, prolonged parenteral fluid therapy with magnesium-free solutions, and parenteral nutrition when inadequate quantities of magnesium have been added to the solution. Other causes include acute pancreatitis, diabetic acidosis during treatment, primary aldosteronism, and chronic alcoholism.

The magnesium ion is essential for proper function of most enzyme systems, and depletion is characterized by neuromuscular and central nervous system hyperactivity. The signs and symptoms are quite similar to those of calcium deficiency, including hyperactive tendon reflexes, muscle tremors, and tetany with a positive Chvostek sign. Progression to delirium and convulsions may occur with a severe deficit. A concomitant calcium deficiency occasionally is noted and is refractory to treatment in the absence of magnesium repletion.

The diagnosis of magnesium deficiency depends on an awareness of the syndrome and clinical recognition of the symptoms. Laboratory confirmation is available but not reliable, because the syndrome may exist in the presence of a normal serum magnesium level. The possibility of magnesium deficiency should always be considered in a surgical patient who exhibits disturbed neuromuscular or cerebral activity in the postoperative period. This is particularly important in patients who have had protracted dysfunction of the gastrointestinal tract with long-term maintenance on parenteral fluids and in patients on total parenteral nutrition. Routine administration of magnesium is always indicated in the management of these patients.

Treatment of magnesium deficiency is by the parenteral administration of magnesium sulfate or magnesium chloride solution. If renal function is normal, as much as 2 mEq. of magnesium per kilogram of body weight can be administered in a day in the presence of severe depletion. Magnesium sulfate (50 per cent solution contains approximately 4 mEq. of magnesium ion per milliliter) may be given intravenously or intramuscularly. The intravenous route is preferable for the initial treatment of a severe symptomatic deficit. This can be accomplished by the addition of 80 mEq. of magnesium sulfate (20 ml. of 50 per cent solution) to 1 liter of intravenous fluid administered over a 4-hour period.[16] If the patient is not symptomatic, the infusion should be given over a longer period of time. The possibility of acute magnesium toxicity should be borne in mind when one is administering this ion intravenously. When large doses are administered, the heart rate, blood pressure, respiration, and ECG should be monitored closely for signs of magnesium toxicity, which could lead to cardiac arrest. It is advisable to have calcium chloride or calcium gluconate available to counteract any adverse effects of a rapidly rising serum magnesium level.

Partial or complete relief of symptoms may follow this infusion as a result of increased concentration of magnesium ion in the extracellular fluid compartment, although continued replacement over a 1- to 3-week period is necessary to replenish the intracellular compartment. For this purpose and for an asymptomatic patient who is likely to have significant magnesium depletion, 10 to 20 mEq. of 50 per cent magnesium sulfate solution is given daily by the intramuscular route or in infusion fluids. When magnesium sulfate is used, it should be given in divided doses or at multiple sites, since the intramuscular injection of this salt is painful. Following complete repletion of intracellular magnesium and in the absence of abnormal loss, balance may be maintained by the administration of as little as 4 mEq. of magnesium ion daily. The amount of magnesium supplementation required for patients on total parenteral nutrition varies, but is approximately 12 to 24 mEq. daily for the average patient.[13]

Magnesium should not be given to an oliguric patient or in the presence of severe volume deficit unless actual magnesium depletion is present. If given to a patient with renal insufficiency, considerably smaller doses are used, and the patient is carefully observed for signs or symptoms of toxicity.

MAGNESIUM EXCESS. Symptomatic hypermagnesemia, although rare, is most commonly seen with severe renal insufficiency. Retention and accumulation of magnesium may occur in any patient with impaired glomerular or renal tubular function, and the presence of acidosis may rapidly compound the situation. Serum magnesium levels tend to parallel changes in potassium concentration in these cases. Therefore, magnesium levels should be carefully monitored in patients with acute and chronic renal failure and in selected patients with borderline renal function. Randall and associates have shown in patients on ordinary dietary intakes of magnesium that increased serum concentrations of the ion do not occur until the glomerular filtration rate falls below 30 ml. per minute.[32] As noted by Henzel and colleagues, however, magnesium-containing antacids and laxatives (Milk of Magnesia, Epsom Salts, Gelusil, Maalox) are commonly administered in quantities sufficient to produce toxic serum levels of magnesium when impaired renal function is present.[16] Other conditions that may be associated with symptomatic hypermagnesemia include early-stage burns, massive trauma or surgical stress, severe extracellular volume deficit, and severe acidosis.

The early signs and symptoms include lethargy and weakness, with progressive loss of deep tendon reflexes. Interference with cardiac conduction occurs with increasing levels of magnesium, and ECG changes (increased P-R interval, widened QRS complex, and elevated T waves) resemble those seen with hyperkalemia. Somnolence leading to coma and muscular paralysis occur in the later stages, and death is usually caused by respiratory or cardiac arrest.

Treatment consists of immediate measures to lower the serum magnesium level by correcting any acidosis, replenishing any pre-existing extracellular volume deficit, and withholding exogenously administered magnesium. Acute symptoms may be temporarily controlled by the slow intravenous administration of 5 to 10 mEq. of calcium chloride or calcium gluconate. If elevated levels or symptoms persist, peritoneal dialysis or hemodialysis is indicated.

NORMAL EXCHANGE OF FLUID AND ELECTROLYTES

Knowledge of the basic principles governing both the internal and the external exchanges of water and salt is mandatory for care of the patient undergoing major operative procedures. The stable internal fluid environment, which is maintained by the kidneys, brain, lungs, skin, and gastrointestinal tract, may be compromised by severe surgical stress or direct damage to any of these organs.

WATER EXCHANGE. The normal individual consumes an average of 2000 to 2500 ml. of water per day; approximately 1500 ml. of water is taken by mouth, and the rest is extracted from solid food, either from the contents of food or as the product of oxidation (Table 10). The daily water losses include 250 ml. in stools, 800 to 1500 ml. as urine, and approximately 600 to 900 ml. as insensible loss. A patient deprived of all external access to water must still excrete a minimum of 500 to 800 ml. of urine per day in order to excrete the products of catabolism, in addition to the mandatory insensible loss through the skin and lungs.

Insensible loss of water occurs through the skin (75 per cent) and the lungs (25 per cent) and is increased by hypermetabolism, hyperventilation, and fever. The insensible water loss through the skin is not from evaporation of water from sweat glands but from water vapor formed within the body and lost through the skin. With excessive heat production (or excessive environmental heat), the capacity for insensible loss through the skin is exceeded, and sweating occurs. These losses may, but seldom do, exceed 250 ml. per day per degree of fever. An unhumidified tracheostomy with hyperventilation increases the loss through the lungs and causes a total insensible loss up to 1.5 liters per day.

A frequently overlooked source of gain is the "water of solution," which is another term for cell water. Normally, gain of water from this source is zero, but after 4 to 5 days without food intake, a patient may begin to gain significant quantities of water (maximum 500 ml. daily) from excessive cell catabolism and release of its water. The amount depends on the degree of trauma and the complications occurring postoperatively.

SALT GAIN AND LOSSES. In a normal individual, the daily salt intake varies between 50 and 90 mEq. (3 to 5 gm.) as sodium chloride (Table 11). Balance is maintained primarily by the kidneys, which excrete the excess salt. Under conditions of reduced intake or extrarenal losses, normal kidneys can reduce sodium excretion to less than 1 mEq. per day within 24 hours after restriction. In a patient with salt-wasting kidneys, however, the loss may exceed 100 mEq. per liter of urine. Sweat represents a

TABLE 10. Water Exchange (60- to 80-kg. Man)

	Average Daily Volume (ml.)	Minimal (ml.)	Maximal (ml.)
H₂O Gain – Routes			
Sensible			
Oral fluids	800–1500	0	1500/hr.
Solid foods	500–700	0	1500
Insensible			
Water of oxidation	250	125	800
Water of solution	0	0	500
H₂O Loss – Routes			
Sensible			
Urine	800–1500	300	1400/hr. (diabetes insipidus)
Intestinal	0–250	0	2500/hr.
Sweat	0	0	4000/hr.
Insensible			
Lungs and skin	600–900	600–900	1500

TABLE 11. Sodium (Salt) Exchange (60- to 80-kg. Man)

Sodium Exchange	Average	Minimal	Maximal
Sodium gain			
Diet	50–90 mEq./day	0	75–100 mEq./hour (oral)
Sodium loss			
Skin (sweat)	10–60 mEq./day*	0	300 mEq./hour
Urine	10–80 mEq./day	<1 mEq./day†	110–200 mEq./L.‡
Intestine	0–20 mEq./day	0	300 mEq./hour

* Depending on the degree of acclimatization of the individual.
† With normal renal function.
‡ With renal salt wasting.

hypotonic loss of fluids with an average sodium concentration of 15 mEq. per liter in an acclimatized patient. In an unacclimatized individual, the sodium concentration in sweat may be 60 mEq. per liter or more. Insensible fluid lost from the skin and lungs, by definition, is pure water. For practical considerations, then, normal losses may be relatively free of salt in the healthy individual with normal renal function.

The volume and composition of various types of gastrointestinal secretions are shown in Table 9. Gastrointestinal losses are usually isotonic, although there is considerable variation in their compositions. These should be replaced by isotonic salt solutions. It is also important to reiterate that distributional or sequestration losses of extracellular fluid at any point in the operative or postoperative course also represent isotonic losses of salt and water.

FLUID AND ELECTROLYTE THERAPY

Parenteral Solutions

The composition of various parenteral fluids is shown in Table 12. There is sufficient variety to satisfy the majority of fluid requirements in the surgical patient. The proper choice of parenteral fluid in a specific situation corrects the abnormalities but imposes minimal demands on the kidneys.

A good available isotonic salt solution for replacing gastrointestinal losses and extracellular fluid volume deficits, in the absence of gross abnormalities of concentration and composition, is lactated Ringer's solution. This solution is "physiologic" and contains 130 mEq. of sodium balanced by 109 mEq. of chloride and 28 mEq. of lactate. Lactate is used instead of bicarbonate, since the former is more stable in intravenous fluids during storage. The lactate is readily converted to bicarbonate by the liver after infusion. Concern about the ability of the liver to metabolize lactate is unwarranted even when one is infusing large quantities of lactated Ringer's solution to patients in hemorrhagic shock.[9] This fluid has minimal effects on normal body fluid composition and pH even when infused in large quantities. There are other balanced salt solutions available, some with sodium acetate or bicarbonate instead of lactate; all are considered interchangeable.

The remainder of the solutions listed in Table 12 are used to correct specific deficits. Choice of a particular fluid depends on the volume status of the patient and the type of concentration or compositional abnormality present.

Isotonic sodium chloride contains 154 mEq. of sodium and 154 mEq. of chloride per liter. The high concentration of chloride above the normal serum concentration of 103 mEq. per liter imposes on the kidneys an appreciable load of excess chloride that cannot be rapidly excreted. Thus, a dilutional acidosis may develop.* This solution is ideal, however, for the initial correction of an extracellular fluid volume deficit in the presence of hyponatremia, hypochloremia, and metabolic alkalosis. In a similar situation with moderate metabolic acidosis, M/6 sodium lactate (167 mEq. per liter each of sodium and lactate) may be given.

A frequent choice for maintenance fluid in the postoperative period, 0.45 per cent sodium chloride in 5 per cent dextrose solution provides free water for insensible losses and some sodium for renal adjustment of serum concentration. With added potassium, this is a reasonable solution to use for maintenance requirements in a patient without complications who requires only a short period of parenteral fluids.

A 5 per cent sodium chloride solution may be used to correct symptomatic hyponatremic states. After the correction of concentration and compositional abnormalities by means of specific electrolyte solutions, a balanced salt solution is used to replenish the remaining volume deficit.

Preoperative Fluid Therapy

Preoperative evaluation and correction of existing fluid disorders are integral parts of surgical care. An orderly approach to these problems requires both an understanding of the common fluid disturbances associated with surgical illness and adherence to a few simple guidelines. There are no quick methods; close observation of the patient and frequent re-evaluation of the clinical situation are the most rewarding approaches.

The analysis of a fluid disorder may be facilitated by categorizing the abnormalities into *volume, concentration,* and *compositional changes.* Although some disease states produce characteristic changes in fluid balance, much confusion may be avoided by regarding each disturbance as a separate entity. For example, volume changes cannot be accurately predicted from a knowledge of the level of serum sodium, since an extracellular fluid volume deficit or excess may exist with a normal, low, or high sodium concentration. Similarly, any of the four primary acid-base disturbances may be associated with any combination of volume and concentration abnormalities.

CORRECTION OF VOLUME CHANGES. Changes in the volume of extracellular fluid are the most frequent and important abnormalities encountered in the surgical patient. Depletion of the extracellular fluid compartment without changes in concentration or composition is a common problem. The diagnosis of volume changes is made almost entirely on clinical grounds. The signs that are present in an individual patient depend not only on the relative or absolute quantity of extracellular fluid loss but also on the rapidity with which it is lost and the presence or absence of signs of associated disease.

Volume deficit in the surgical patient may follow external loss of fluids or an internal redistribution of extracellular fluid into nonfunctional compartments. Often, it involves a combination of the two, but the internal redistribution is frequently overlooked.

The phenomenon of internal redistribution or translocation of extracellular fluid is peculiar to many surgical diseases; in the

---

* Infusion of a large volume of isotonic sodium chloride solution may induce or aggravate an existing acidosis by reducing the amount of base bicarbonate in the body relative to the carbonic acid content.[36]

TABLE 12. Composition of Parenteral Fluids:
Electrolyte Content (mEq./L.)

Solution	Cations				Anions	
	Na	K	Ca	Mg	Cl	HCO$_3^-$
Extracellular fluid	142	4	5	3	103	27
Lactated Ringer's	130	4	2.7		109	28*
0.9% sodium chloride (saline)	154				154	
D$_5$/0.45% sodium chloride	77				77	
M/6 sodium lactate	167					167*

* Present in solution as lactate, which is converted to bicarbonate.

individual patient, the loss may be quite large. Although the concept of a "third space" is not new, it is generally considered only in relation to patients with massive ascites, burns, or crush injuries. Of more importance, however, is the "third space" loss into the peritoneum, the bowel wall, and other tissues associated with inflammatory lesions of the intra-abdominal organs. The magnitude of these losses may not be fully appreciated without realization of the fact that the peritoneum alone has approximately 1 sq. meter of surface area. A slight increase in thickness from sequestration of fluid, which would not be appreciated on casual observation, may cause a functional loss of several liters of fluid. Swelling of the bowel wall and mesentery and secretion of fluid into the lumen of the bowel causes even larger losses. Similar deficits may occur with massive infection of the subcutaneous tissues (necrotizing fascitis) or with severe crush injury.

These "parasitic" losses remain a part of the extracellular fluid space and may be measured as a slowly equilibrating volume. The term *nonfunctional* is used because the fluid is no longer able to participate in the normal functions of the extracellular fluid compartment. Any transfer of intracellular fluid to the extracellular compartment for replenishment of the loss is insignificant. The patient with ascites may have an enormous total extracellular fluid volume even though the functional component is severely depleted. The same is true of extensive inflammatory or obstructive lesions of the gastrointestinal tract, although the loss is not as obvious. These losses evoke the signs and symptoms of an extracellular fluid volume deficit with or without the concomitant external loss of fluids.

Exact quantification of these deficits is impossible. The defect can be estimated on the basis of the severity of the clinical signs. A mild deficit represents a loss of approximately 4 per cent of body weight (e.g., 70 kg. × 0.04 = 2.8-liter deficit); a moderate deficit, a loss of 6 to 8 per cent of body weight; and a severe deficit, a loss of approximately 10 per cent of body weight. It is important to emphasize the fact that cardiovascular signs predominate when there is acute rapid loss of fluid from the extracellular compartment with few or no tissue signs. In addition to the estimated deficit, fluids lost during the period of treatment must be replaced.

Fluid replacement should be started and changed according to the response of the patient noted on frequent clinical observation. Reliance on a formula or single clinical sign for determining the adequacy of resuscitation is unwise. Rather, reversal of the signs of the volume deficit, combined with stabilization of the blood pressure and pulse, and an hourly urine volume of 30 to 50 ml. are used as general guidelines. An adequate hourly urinary output, although usually a reliable monitor for volume replacement, may be totally misleading, however. For example, the excessive administration of glucose (over 50 gm. in a 2- to 3-hour period) may cause osmotic diuresis, whereas an osmotic agent such as mannitol produces urine at the expense of the vascular volume. Patients with chronic renal disease or incipient acute renal damage from shock and injury also may have inappropriately high urinary volumes. Additionally, the rapid administration of salt solutions may transiently expand the intravascular volume, increase the glomerular filtration rate, and cause an immediate outpouring of urine, although the total extracellular fluid space remains quite depleted.

The choice of a proper fluid for replacement depends on the existence of concomitant concentration or compositional abnormalities. With pure extracellular fluid volume loss or when only minimal concentration or compositional abnormalities are present, the use of a balanced salt solution is desirable.

RATE OF FLUID ADMINISTRATION. This varies considerably, depending on the severity and type of fluid disturbance, the presence of continuing losses, and the cardiac status. In general, the most severe volume deficits may be safely replaced initially with isotonic solutions at a rate of 1000 ml. per hour, reducing the rate as the fluid status improves. Constant observation by a physician is mandatory when administration exceeds 1000 ml. per hour. At these rates, however, a significant portion may be lost as urinary output owing to a transient overexpansion of the plasma volume.

In elderly patients, associated cardiovascular disorders do not preclude correction of existing volume deficits; but they do require slower, more careful correction with appropriate monitoring, including the central venous, pulmonary arterial, and pulmonary capillary wedge pressures.

CORRECTION OF CONCENTRATION CHANGES. If severe *symptomatic* hyponatremia or hypernatremia complicates the volume loss, prompt correction of the concentration abnormality to the extent that symptoms are relieved is the first step. Volume replenishment then should be accomplished, with slower correction of the remaining concentration abnormality. For immediate correction of severe symptomatic hyponatremia, a 5 per cent sodium chloride solution is used. The sodium deficit can be estimated by multiplying the decrease in serum sodium concentration below normal (in milliequivalents per liter) *times* the liters of total body water. Total body water averages 60 per cent of the body weight in young adult males and 50 per cent in young adult females.

Example: A 24-year-old female with symptomatic hyponatremia; weight = 60 kg.; serum sodium = 120 mEq. per liter:
Total body water = 60 kg. × 0.50 = 30 liters
Sodium deficit = (140 − 120 mEq. per liter) × 30 liters = 600 mEq.

Note that this estimate is based on total body water, since the effective osmotic pressure in the extracellular compartment cannot be increased without increasing this fraction proportionally in the intracellular compartment. Although absolute reliance on any formula is undesirable, proper use of this estimate allows a safe quantitative approximation of the sodium deficit. Generally, only a portion of the total deficit is replaced initially to relieve acute symptoms. Further correction is facilitated when renal function is restored by correction of the volume deficit. If the total calculated deficit is given rapidly, symptomatic hypervolemia may occur, particularly in patients with limited cardiac reserve. Of more importance, central pontine and extrapontine myelinolysis may occur during *rapid* correction of hyponatremia and cause irreversible CNS damage or death.[22] It is recommended, therefore, that the serum sodium level not be increased more than 12 mEq. per liter during the first 24 hours and even less during each subsequent 24-hour period. In practice, the infusion of small, successive increments of hypertonic saline solution with frequent evaluation of the clinical response and serum sodium concentration is recommended.

In the treatment of moderate hyponatremia with an associated volume deficit, volume replacement can be initiated immediately with concomitant correction of the serum sodium deficit. Isotonic sodium chloride solution (normal saline) is used initially in the presence of metabolic alkalosis, whereas M/6 sodium lactate is used to correct an associated acidosis. Only a few liters of these solutions may be necessary to correct the serum sodium concentration; the remainder of the volume deficit can be repaired with a balanced salt solution.

Treatment of hyponatremia associated with *volume excess* is by restriction of water. In the presence of severe symptomatic hyponatremia, a small amount of hypertonic salt solution may be infused cautiously to alleviate symptoms. Since this causes additional volume expansion, it is contraindicated in patients with limited cardiac reserve; peritoneal dialysis or hemodialysis is preferred in this situation.

For the correction of severe, symptomatic hypernatremia with an associated volume deficit, 5 per cent dextrose in water may be infused slowly until symptoms are relieved. If the extracellular osmolarity is reduced too rapidly, however, convulsions and coma may result. For this reason, correction of hypernatremia concomitant with repletion of the volume deficit by half-strength sodium chloride or half-strength balanced salt solution is safer in most cases. In the absence of a significant volume deficit, water should be administered cautiously, since hypervolemia may result; constant observation and frequent determinations of the serum sodium concentration are indicated. The problem is somewhat simplified when a sufficient quantity of fluid has been given to permit renal excretion of the solute load.

COMPOSITION AND MISCELLANEOUS CONSIDERATIONS. Correction of potassium deficits should be started *after* an adequate urinary output is obtained. The concentration of potassium chloride should not exceed 40 mEq. per liter of intravenous fluids, with rare exceptions, such as the treatment of digitalis intoxication, during which the ECG must be monitored. Calcium and magnesium rarely are needed during preoperative resuscitation but should be given if indicated, particularly to patients with massive subcutaneous infections, those with acute pancreatitis, and those who have been chronically starved.

Fluid abnormalities also must be suspected in the patient for whom an elective procedure is planned. Chronic illnesses frequently are associated with extracellular fluid volume deficits, and concentration and compositional changes are not uncommon. Correction of anemia and recognition of the fact that a contracted blood volume may exist in the chronically debilitated patient are of obvious importance.

Of equal importance is the prevention of volume depletion during the preoperative period. Prolonged periods of fluid restriction in preparation for various diagnostic procedures, the use of cathartics and enemas for preparation of the bowel, and osmotic diuresis from contrast agents may cause a significant acute loss of extracellular fluid. Prompt recognition and treatment of these losses are necessary to prevent complications during the operative procedure.

Intraoperative Management of Fluids

If preoperative replacement of extracellular fluid volume has been incomplete, hypotension may develop promptly with the induction of anesthesia. This can be quite insidious, because the ability of the awake patient to compensate for a mild volume deficit is revealed only when compensatory mechanisms are abolished with anesthesia. This problem is prevented by maintaining baseline requirements and replacing abnormal losses of fluids and electrolytes by intravenous infusions in the preoperative period.

Blood loss during the operative procedure should be replaced steadily. It is usually unnecessary to replace blood loss of less than 500 ml. (even more in young, healthy patients), but after the loss has exceeded this, replacement should begin. The warnings against the use of a single transfusion during operation have been somewhat confusing. There may be a definite need for a single-unit transfusion in the patient who loses between 500 and 1000 ml. of blood during operation.

In addition to blood losses during operation, there are extracellular fluid losses during major operative procedures. Some of these, including edema from extensive dissection, fluid collections within the lumen and the wall of the small bowel, and accumulations of fluid in the peritoneal cavity, are clinically discernible and well recognized. They are generally thought to represent distributional shifts, in that the functional volume of extracellular fluid is reduced but not externally lost from the body. These functional losses are often referred to as "a parasitic loss of extracellular fluid," "third-space edema," or "sequestration" of extracellular fluid. Another source of extracellular fluid loss during major operative trauma is the wound itself. This is a relatively small loss that is difficult to quantify except in extensive operative procedures.

At the beginning of this century, surgeons became aware that many changes occurred in urinary output, blood volume, and fluid and electrolyte composition during and after surgical therapy. Assessment of these changes, however, awaited the development of analytic techniques and their application to patient studies. In the following 25 years, saline solutions in varying combinations were given to patients undergoing operation, often in excessive amounts. Work in the late 1930s and early 1940s by Moyer and others indicated that during and after operative procedures saline and water solutions should be withheld entirely because most of the fluid administered is retained.[26]

The possibility existed, however, that the operative and postoperative retention of salt and water might simply be physiologic retention to replace a deficit of salt and water incurred by the operative procedure.[49] Subsequent studies revealed that functional extracellular fluid decreases with major abdominal operations, largely as a sequestered loss into the operative site.[33,37,38] Intraoperative correction of this volume deficit with a balanced salt solution eliminates "postoperative salt intolerance." The use of salt solution is not intended to be a substitute for blood replacement; rather, it is to replace the extracellular fluid volume deficit.

Thus, the indiscriminate use of salt solutions in the first quarter of this century changed to almost total withholding of fluids and electrolytes from surgical patients in the second quarter of the century; indications at present are that proper management lies somewhere between these two extremes. Some guidelines are necessary, since exact quantification of the deficit is not possible. The amount of lost or sequestered extracellular fluid directly correlates with the amount of operative trauma, for example, only a few hundred milliliters during a 1-hour cholecystectomy in a thin patient, compared with several liters during a prolonged and difficult low anterior colon resection in an obese one. The loss also is directly related to the amount of surface area of the traumatized tissues. Characteristically, the largest losses occur during intra-abdominal surgical procedures because of the extensive surface area of the peritoneum, bowel, and mesentery. Smaller losses are incurred during thoracic and orthopedic procedures, since fluid is sequestered primarily into retracted muscle and subcutaneous tissues. Losses during head and neck surgery are negligible.

Some arbitrary but clinically useful guidelines are the following: (1) Blood should be replaced as lost, irrespective of any additional fluid and electrolyte therapy. (2) The replacement of extracellular fluid should begin during the operative procedure. (3) Balanced salt solution needed during operation is approximately 0.5 to 1 liter per hour, but only to a maximum of 2 to 3 liters during a 4-hour major abdominal procedure, unless there are other measurable losses. Using a similar fluid regimen, Thompson and associates reported their experiences in a series of 670 patients undergoing major aortoiliac reconstructive procedures.[42] In this group, the average amount of lactated Ringer's solution administered was 3555 ml., giving an average intraoperative replacement of salt solution of 677 ml. per hour of operative procedure. In the last 6 years of this study, there were only 2 deaths in 298 operations, an operative mortality of 0.67 per cent. Among the entire 670 patients, only 2 patients died of renal failure, an incidence of 0.3 per cent. No patient died of pulmonary insufficiency. This extremely low incidence of renal failure, even in the presence of extensive operative trauma, is similar to the authors' data for major abdominal operative procedures.

The use of albumin solutions, in addition to balanced salt solutions, to replace extracellular fluid deficits incurred during operative procedures is not only unnecessary but potentially harmful. Measurements of cardiac function and extravascular lung water indicate optimal function following replacement of blood loss and the administration of balanced salt solution without the addition of albumin.[45]

In summary, the replacement of ECF deficits during operation with an appropriate volume of balanced salt solution, in addition to blood replacement, has markedly improved the ability to maintain intraoperative homeostasis and avoid organ injury associated with inadequate volume replacement.

Postoperative Management of Fluids

IMMEDIATE POSTOPERATIVE PERIOD. Orders for postoperative fluids are not written until the patient is in the recovery room and the fluid status has been assessed. Evaluation at this point should include a review of preoperative fluid status, the amount of fluid loss and gain during operation, and clinical examination of the patient with assessment of vital signs and urinary output. Initial fluid orders are written to correct any existing deficit, followed by maintenance fluids for the remainder of the day. For a patient with complications who has received or lost large amounts of fluid, it is frequently difficult to estimate the fluid requirements for the ensuing 24 hours. In this situation, intravenous fluids are ordered 1 liter at a time, and the patient is examined frequently until the situation is clarified. Proper replacement of fluids during this relatively short period facilitates subsequent fluid management.

After operation, sequestration of extracellular fluid into the sites of injury or operative trauma may continue for 12 hours or more. Unrecognized deficits of extracellular fluid volume during the early postoperative period are not uncommon and are manifest primarily as circulatory instability. Evaluation of the level of consciousness, pupillary size, airway patency, breathing patterns, pulse rate and volume, skin warmth, color, body temperature, and a 30- to 50-ml. hourly urinary output, combined with critical review of the operative procedure and the operative fluid management, is usually rewarding. Operative blood loss is usually estimated by the surgeon to be 15 to 40 per cent less than the isotopically measured blood loss from the patient.[17] In addition, several liters of extravascular, extracellular fluid can be sequestered in areas of injury and manifested only by oliguria and mild depression of the blood pressure with a rapid pulse. For a patient with circulatory instability, further volume replacement of an additional 1000 ml. of balanced salt solution, while determining whether continuing losses or other causes are present, often resolves the problem.

It is unnecessary and probably unwise to administer potassium during the first 24 hours postoperatively unless a definite potassium deficit exists. This is particularly important for a patient subjected to prolonged operative trauma involving one or more episodes of hypotension and for a posttraumatic patient with hemorrhagic hypotension. Oliguric renal failure or the more insidious high-output renal failure may develop, and the administration of even a small quantity of potassium may be detrimental.

LATE POSTOPERATIVE PERIOD. The problem of volume management during the postoperative convalescent phase is one of accurate measurement and replacement of all losses. In the otherwise healthy individual, this involves the replacement of measured sensible losses, which are generally of gastrointestinal origin, and the estimation and replacement of insensible losses.

The insensible loss is usually relatively constant and averages 600 to 900 ml. daily. This may be increased by hypermetabolism, hyperventilation, and fever to a maximum of approximately 1500 ml. daily. The estimated insensible loss is replaced with 5 per cent dextrose in water. This loss may be partially offset by an insensible water gain from excessive tissue catabolism in the postoperative patient with complications, particularly if associated with oliguric renal failure.

Approximately 1 liter of fluid should be given to replace that volume of urine required to excrete the catabolic end products of metabolism (800 to 1000 ml. per day). In the individual with normal renal function, this may be given as 5 per cent dextrose in water, since the kidneys are able to conserve sodium, with excretion of less than 1 mEq. daily. It is probably unnecessary to stress the kidneys to this degree, however, and a small amount of salt solution may be given in addition to water to cover urinary loss. In an elderly patient with salt-losing kidneys or in patients with head injuries, an insidious hyponatremia may develop if urinary losses are replaced with water. Urinary sodium in these circumstances may exceed 100 mEq. per liter and cause daily loss of significant amounts of sodium. Measurement of urinary sodium facilitates accurate replacement. Urine volume is not replaced on a milliliter-for-milliliter basis. A urinary output of 2000 to 3000 ml. on a specific day may simply represent diuresis of fluids given during operation or may represent excessive fluid administration. If these large losses are completely replaced, the urinary output progressively increases.

Sensible losses, by definition, can be measured or, as in the case of sweating, the amount can be estimated. Gastrointestinal losses are usually isotonic or slightly hypotonic, and they are replaced with an essentially isotonic salt solution. When the estimated loss is slightly above or below isotonicity, appropriate corrections can be made in the daily water administration, while isotonic salt solutions are used to replace these losses volume for volume. Sweating is not usually a problem except with the febrile patient, in whom losses may, but seldom do, exceed 250 ml. per day per degree of fever. Excessive sweating may, in addition, represent a considerable loss of sodium in the unacclimatized individual.

Determination of serum electrolyte levels is generally unnecessary in a patient with an uncomplicated postoperative course maintained on parenteral fluids for 2 to 3 days. A more prolonged period of parenteral replacement or one complicated by excessive fluid losses requires frequent determinations of the serum sodium, potassium, and chloride levels and carbon dioxide combining power. Adjustments then can be made with intravenous fluid of appropriate composition. For example, gastrointestinal losses should be replaced with isotonic sodium chloride solution in a patient with hyponatremia, hypochloremia, and mild metabolic alkalosis, and this should be continued until these abnormalities are corrected. In a hyponatremic patient with obvious volume overload, the amount of free water given is restricted. In the presence of hyponatremia and mild metabolic acidosis, lactated Ringer's solution with added sodium bicarbonate may be used. In this way, severe concentration and compositional changes can be avoided while an adequate extracellular fluid volume is maintained by appropriate maintenance fluids.

Maintenance fluids are administered at a steady rate over an 18- to 24-hour period as the losses are incurred. If given over a shorter period of time, renal excretion of the excess salt and water may occur while the normal losses continue over the full 24-hour period. For the same reason, fluids of different composition are alternated, and additives to intravenous fluids are evenly distributed in the total volume of fluid given.

In summary, daily fluid orders should begin with an assessment of the patient's volume status and for possible concentration or compositional disorders as reflected by proper laboratory determinations. All measured and insensible losses are replaced with fluids of appropriate composition, allowing for any pre-existing deficit or excess. The amount of potassium replacement is 40 mEq. daily for baseline renal excretion of potassium, in addition to approximately 20 mEq. per liter for replacement of gastrointestinal losses. Inadequate replacement may prolong the usual postoperative ileus and contribute to the insidious development of a resistant metabolic alkalosis. Calcium and magnesium are replaced when needed, as previously discussed.

SPECIAL CONSIDERATIONS IN THE POSTOPERATIVE PATIENT. VOLUME EXCESS. The administration of isotonic salt solutions in excess of volume losses (external or internal) may cause overexpansion of the extracellular fluid space. The otherwise normal person in a postoperative state tolerates an acute overexpansion extremely well. Excesses administered over a period of several days, however, soon exceed the kidneys' ability to excrete sodium; since water losses continue, hypernatremia may ensue. Therefore, it is important to determine as accurately as possible from intake and output records and serum sodium concentrations the actual needs of the patient managed over several postoperative days. Attention to the signs and symptoms of overload usually prevents this fluid abnormality. It arises most frequently with attempts to meet excessive volume losses that are not measurable, such as those occurring from incompletely controlled fistula drainage.

The earliest sign is a weight gain (when measurable) during the catabolic period, when the patient should be losing $\frac{1}{4}$ to $\frac{1}{2}$ pound per day. Heavy eyelids, hoarseness, or dyspnea on exertion may rapidly appear. Circulatory and pulmonary signs of overload appear late and represent a rather massive overload. Peripheral edema may be a sign, but it does not necessarily indicate an excess of *functional* extracellular volume. In the absence of additional evidence for volume overload, other causes for peripheral edema should be considered. Of particular importance is the fact that overexpansion of the *total* extracellular fluid may coexist with *depletion* of the functional extracellular fluid compartment (e.g., patient with ascites). Central venous pressure measurements may be helpful during volume replacement but may be misleading, because a rapid rise may indicate an excessive rate of fluid administration or primary pump failure, but it may not accurately establish volume status. Measurement of pulmonary wedge pressure is a more sensitive indicator of volume status.

HYPONATREMIA. Significant postoperative alterations in serum sodium concentration are not frequently observed if the fluid resuscitation during operation has included adequate volumes of isotonic salt solutions. The kidneys retain the ability to excrete moderate excesses of salt water administered in the early postoperative period if functional extracellular fluid has been adequately replaced during the operative or immediate postoperative period. Previous studies of sodium balance have revealed that patients do excrete sodium after the functional deficit incurred by the shift of extracellular fluid has been replaced. Wright and Gann demonstrated normal capacity to excrete

water postoperatively when isotonic salt solutions are administered prior to a challenge with a water load.[49] Thus, the commonly described hyponatremia associated with surgical procedures and traumatic injury is prevented by the replacement of extracellular fluid deficits. Thereafter, the daily maintenance of normal osmolarity is simplified by the replacement of observable losses of known sodium content.

Hyponatremia may easily occur when water is given to replace losses of sodium-containing fluids or when water administration consistently exceeds water losses. The latter may occur with oliguria or in association with decreased water loss through the skin and lungs, intracellular shifts of sodium, or the cellular release of excessive amounts of endogenous water. Severe or refractory hyponatremia, however, is difficult to produce if renal function remains normal.

In the presence of hyperglycemia, knowledge of the glucose concentration is necessary to evaluate the significance of a depressed serum sodium level. Since glucose does not enter cells by passive diffusion, it exerts an osmotic force in the extracellular compartment. This contribution to osmotic pressure is normally small; but with an elevated glucose concentration, the increased osmotic pressure causes the transfer of cellular water into the extracellular compartment, causing a dilutional hyponatremia. Hyponatremia, therefore, may be observed when the total effective osmotic pressure in the extracellular compartment is normal or even above normal. In terms of tonicity, each 100-mg. per 100 ml. rise in blood glucose above normal causes a fall in serum sodium concentration variously estimated to be between 1.6 and 2.8 mEq. per liter. The figure 2.8 is based on the assumption that the shift of water from the cells continues until osmolality is restored to normal in the extracellular compartment. This does not occur because the flow of water will cease before normal osmolality is obtained (i.e., the addition of solute to the extracellular compartment increases osmolality in both compartments after equilibration). Katz, therefore, has suggested use of the lower figure 1.6.[19] This may also be inaccurate, since renal and thirst mechanisms usually have already been activated in attempts to normalize extracellular fluid osmolality. To resolve the dilemma, the authors have arbitrarily chosen a whole number between the two extremes for use in clinical practice; that is, serum sodium falls approximately 2 mEq. per liter for each 100-mg. per 100 ml. rise of serum glucose above normal. Consider a patient with a serum sodium concentration of 128 mEq. per liter and a blood glucose levels of 500 mg. per 100 ml. The glucose is approximately 400 mg. per 100 ml. above normal, which should cause an 8-mEq. per liter fall in serum sodium; the low sodium level is, therefore, primarily due to a high glucose concentration. In this instance, therapy is directed toward lowering the glucose concentration; once accomplished, the serum sodium rises (to approximately 136 mEq. per liter in the example above) as the excess water leaves the extracellular compartment. In a similar manner, urea elevation causes a fall in extracellular sodium concentration. For clinical purposes, each 30-mg. per 100 ml. rise in blood urea nitrogen concentration *above normal* is expected to reduce the serum sodium concentration 2 mEq. per liter.

Replacement of Sodium Losses with Water. A common error is replacement of gastrointestinal and other isotonic salt losses with D_5W or a hypotonic salt solution. Additionally, patients with head injury or renal disease (loss of concentrating ability) may elaborate urine with a high salt concentration (50 to 200 mEq. per liter) that must be replaced. The former is usually secondary to excessive secretion of antidiuretic hormone, with consequent water retention, and the latter ("salt-wasting kidneys") is a common problem in elderly patients. This source of sodium loss is frequently not anticipated, since the blood urea nitrogen and creatinine levels may be normal. Continued replacement of these urinary losses with D_5W may eventually cause marked hyponatremia. The urine sodium concentration should be determined if the diagnosis is in doubt; with hyponatremia and normal renal function, the urine should be nearly free of sodium.

Decreased Urinary Volume. Oliguria, of whatever cause (prerenal or renal), reduces the daily water requirements if not corrected. Cellular catabolism and the metabolic acidosis produced by the retention of nitrogenous waste products increase the cellular release of water. Therefore, the gain of endogenous water decreases the total water requirement beyond that expected when the urinary volume is low.

Endogenous Water Release. The patient maintained on intravenous fluids without adequate caloric intake, between the fifth and tenth postoperative days, gains significant quantities of water (maximum, 500 ml. daily) from excessive cellular catabolism, thus decreasing the quantity of exogenous water required per day.

Intracellular Shifts. Systemic bacterial sepsis is often accompanied by a precipitous drop in serum sodium concentration. This sudden change is poorly understood but usually accompanies loss of extracellular fluid as either interstitial or intracellular sequestrations. This can be treated by withholding free water, restoring extracellular fluid volume, and initiating treatment of the sepsis.

HYPERNATREMIA. Hypernatremia (serum sodium concentration above 150 mEq. per liter), although uncommon, is a dangerous abnormality. In contradistinction to decreased serum sodium concentration, hypernatremia is easily produced when renal function is normal. The extracellular fluid hyperosmolarity causes a shift of intracellular water to the extracellular fluid compartment; in this situation, a high serum sodium level may indicate a significant deficit of total body water. In surgical patients hypernatremia arises most often from excessive or unexpected water losses, although it may follow use of salt-containing solutions to replace water losses. The following classification of water losses may be helpful in preventing and treating this abnormality.

Excessive Extrarenal Water Losses. With increased metabolism from any cause, but particularly associated with fever, the water loss through evaporation of sweat may reach several liters daily. Patients with tracheostomies in dry environments can (with excessive minute volume air exchange) lose as much as 1 to 1.5 liters of water per day by this route. Increased water evaporation from a burn wound is often of significance in the thermally injured patient; losses may be as great as 3 to 5 liters per day.[28]

Increased Renal Water Losses. Extremely large volumes of solute-poor urine may follow hypoxic damage to the distal tubules and collecting ducts or loss of antidiuretic hormone stimulation from damage to the central nervous system. In both instances, facultative water resorption is impaired. The former occurs in high-output renal failure; in the authors' experience, this is the most common type of renal failure following severe injury or operative trauma. The latter occurs with extensive head injuries accompanied by temporary diabetes insipidus.

Solute Loading. High protein intake may produce an increased osmotic load of urea, which necessitates the excretion of large volumes of water. Hypernatremia, azotemia, and extracellular fluid volume deficits follow. In general, these can be prevented by an intake of 7 ml. of water per gram of dietary protein.

Osmotic diuretics such as mannitol, urea, and glucose cause the obligatory excretion of large volumes of urine, with free water losses greatly exceeding those of sodium. Uncontrolled hyperglycemia during intravenous nutrition is a most common cause of serious hypernatremia. The associated glucosuria causes an osmotic diuresis of large volumes of salt-poor urine, causing hypernatremia and an extracellular fluid volume deficit. If not corrected for several days, nonketotic, hyperosmolar coma may ensue. Treatment involves measures to lower serum glucose and replacement of the severe volume deficit with 0.45 per cent sodium chloride solution.

HIGH-OUTPUT RENAL FAILURE. Acute renal insufficiency following trauma or surgical stress may be a lethal complication. The diagnosis is classically based on persistent oliguria and chemical evidence of uremia after stabilization of the circulation. The clinical course is characterized by oliguria lasting from several days to several weeks, followed by a progressive rise in daily urinary volume until both the excretory and the concentrating functions of the kidneys are gradually restored.

Uremia, occurring without a period of oliguria and accompanied by a daily urinary volume greater than 1000 to 1500 ml. per day, is a more frequent but less well recognized entity.[5] Clinical experience and laboratory experiments suggest that high-output renal failure represents the renal response to a less severe or modified episode of renal injury than that required to produce classic oliguric renal failure. Its importance lies in the fact that it is a milder form of renal insufficiency, and realization of its presence by serial measurements of blood urea nitrogen and serum electrolytes permits intelligent chemical and fluid volume management with a much greater latitude because of the daily urinary volume excretion. Normal extracellular fluid volume and serum sodium concentration, therefore, are quite easily maintained when accurate daily outputs of each are obtained and replaced accordingly. The sodium-containing fluids may be administered as lactate to control the mild metabolic acidosis that occurs. More severe acidosis may develop if isotonic losses from the gastrointestinal tract or from renal excretion of sodium are replaced with sodium chloride.

Two common errors made in patients with high-output renal failure are (1) failure to recognize its existence because of normal urinary output and (2) the intravenous administration of potassium salts. Initially, the patient may be very sensitive to exogenously administered potassium, not unlike an individual in oliguric renal failure. Later in the course of the disease, normal amounts of maintenance potassium are usually required.

The typical course of high-output renal failure begins without a period of oliguria. The daily urinary volumes are normal or greater than normal, often reaching levels of 3 to 5 liters per day, while blood urea nitrogen is increasing. An attempt to decrease urinary output by water restriction rapidly causes hypernatremia without a change in urinary volume. On average, blood urea nitrogen continues to increase for 8 to 12 days before a downward trend occurs. The blood/urine urea ratio is about 1 : 10 until a decrease occurs in the blood urea nitrogen concentration.

Functionally, the lesion is characterized by a glomerular filtration rate of less than 20 per cent of normal and complete resistance to vasopressin for 1 to 3 weeks after the blood urea nitrogen has declined. During the next 6 to 8 weeks, the glomerular filtration rate gradually rises, and the response to vasopressin becomes normal. The early recognition of high-output renal failure by serial blood determinations of blood urea nitrogen is important. Failure to recognize its presence may have as its result death caused by hyperkalemia, hypernatremia, or acidosis.

SELECTED REFERENCES

1. Bear, R. A., and Dyck, R. F.: Clinical approach to the diagnosis of acid-base disorders. Can. Med. Assoc. J., 120:173, 1979.
   A unique and instructive approach to this topic.
2. Brenner, B. M., and Rector, F. C., (Eds): The Kidney, 3rd ed. Philadelphia, W. B. Saunders Company, 1987.
   Extensive coverage of renal physiology and renal diseases.
3. Collins, J. A., Murawski, K., and Shafer, W. A. (Eds.): Massive Transfusion in Surgery and Trauma. New York, Alan R. Liss, Inc., 1982.
   A collaborative effort detailing the pathophysiology and treatment of hemorrhagic shock, including complications associated with massive blood transfusions.
4. Guyton, A. C., Taylor, A. E. and Granger, H. J.: Circulatory Physiology II. Dynamics and Control of the Body Fluids. Philadelphia, W. B. Saunders Company, 1975.
   An in-depth review of this subject for the serious student of fluid and electrolyte metabolism.
5. Maxwell, M. H., Kleeman, C. R., and Narins, R. G. (Eds.): Clinical Disorders of Fluid and Electrolyte Metabolism, 4th ed. New York, McGraw-Hill, 1987.
   Encyclopedic coverage of fluid and electrolyte metabolism.

6. Mengoli, L. R.: Excerpts from the history of postoperative fluid therapy. Am. J. Surg., 121:311, 1971.

An interesting historical review, beginning in 1831 with W. B. O'Shaughnessy's suggestion that saline solution be given intravenously for the treatment of cholera and ending with a discussion of the work of Shires and associates advocating the replacement of extracellular fluid volume deficits incurred during surgery. The seesaw pattern of recommendations made between 1913 and 1967 for the administration or withholding of salt solutions during operative procedures is particularly illuminating.

7. Pitts, R. F.: Acid-base regulation by the kidneys. Am. J. Med., 9:356, 1950.

A clear and concise treatise on the renal mechanisms involved in regulation of acid-base balance.

8. Roberts, J. P., Roberts, J. B., Skinner, C., Shires, G. T., III, Illner, H., Canizaro, P. C., and Shires, G. T.: Extracellular fluid deficit following operation and its correction with Ringers Lactate: A reassessment. Ann. Surg., 202:1, 1985.

An update of the original report by the senior author of this chapter quantitating the loss of functional extracellular fluid during abdominal surgical procedures.

9. Schwartz, W. B., and Relman, A. S.: A critique of the parameters used in the evaluation of acid-base disorders. N. Engl. J. Med., 268:1382, 1963.

This is an excellent critique of the systems for analysis of acid-base problems advocated by Singer and Hastings (buffer base) and Astrup (standard bicarbonate and base excess). Specifically, the authors discuss the limitations of these techniques and conclude that traditional measurements of pH, PCO_2, and plasma bicarbonate, combined with appropriate clinical information, allow proper evaluation of even the most complicated acid-base disorders.

10. Thompson, J. E., Vollman, R. W., Austin, D. J., and Kartchner, M. M.: Prevention of hypotensive and renal complications of aortic surgery using balanced salt solution: Thirteen-year experience with 670 cases. Ann. Surg., 167:767, 1968.

An excellent clinical report emphasizing the need for replacement of both extracellular fluids and blood during major operative procedures. In this large series of aortoiliac reconstructive procedures, only two patients died of renal failure, an incidence of 0.3 per cent.

11. Vanatta, J. D., and Fogelman, M. J.: Moyer's Fluid Balance, 3rd ed. Chicago, Year Book Medical Publishers, 1982.

The authors have successfully updated this classic manual, retaining the basics of Moyer's method for the diagnosis and treatment of fluid and electrolyte disorders.

12. Welt, L. G.: Clinical Disorders of Hydration and Acid-Base Equilibrium, 2nd ed. Boston, Little, Brown and Company, 1959.

Although somewhat dated, this book is a valuable reference for many of the basics of fluid and electrolyte metabolism.

REFERENCES

1. Abouna, G. M., Veazey, P. R., and Terry, D. B.: Intravenous infusion of hydrochloric acid for treatment of severe metabolic alkalosis. Surgery, 75:194, 1974.
2. Andersen, O. S., and Engel, K.: A new acid-based nomogram: An improved method for the calculation of the relevant blood acid-base data. Scand. J. Clin. Lab. Invest., 12:177, 1960.
3. Astrup, P., Jorgensen, K., Anderson, O. S., and Engel, K.: The acid-base metabolism: A new approach. Lancet 1:1035, 1960.
4. Bartlett, W. C.: Acute hyperparathyroid crisis. Am. J. Surg., 114:796, 1967.
5. Baxter, C. R., Zedlitz, W. H., and Shires, G. T.: High output acute renal failure complicating traumatic injury. J. Trauma, 4:467, 1964.
6. Bear, R. A., Dyck, R. F.: Clinical approach to the diagnosis of acid-base disorders. Can. Med. Assoc. J., 120:172, 1979.
7. Bishop, R. L., and Weisfeldt, M. L.: Sodium bicarbonate administration during cardiac arrest: Effect of arterial pH, PCO_2, and osmolality, J.A.M.A., 235:506, 1976.
8. Canizaro, P. C.: Oxygen transport in shock. *In* Shires, G. T. (Ed.): Shock and Related Problems. Edinburgh, Churchill Livingston, 1984, p. 95.
9. Canizaro, P. C., Prager, M. D., and Shires, G. T.: The infusion of Ringer's lactate solution during shock. Am. J. Surg., 122:494, 1971.
10. Christensen, M. S., Brodersen, P., Olesen, J., et al: Cerebral apoplexy (stroke) treated with or without prolonged artificial hyperventilation. II. Cerebrospinal fluid acid-base balance and intracranial pressure. Stroke, 4:620, 1973.
11. Collins, J. A.: Problems associated with the massive transfusion of stored blood. Surgery, 75:274, 1974.
12. Cooper, N., Brazier, J. R., Hottenrott, C., Mulder, D. G., Maloney, J. V., and Buckberg, C. D.: Myocardial depression following citrated blood transfusion. Arch. Surg., 107:756, 1973.
13. Dudrick, S. J., et al.: General principles and techniques of intravenous hyperalimentation, *In* Cowan, G. S. M., and Schutz, W. L. (Eds.): Intravenous Hyperalimentation. Philadelphia, Lea & Febiger, 1972.
14. Elias, E. G., and Evans, J. T.: Hypercalcemic crisis in neoplastic disease: Management with mithramycin. Surgery, 71:631, 1972.
15. Harken, A. H., Gabel, R. A., Fencl, V., and Moore, F. D.: Hydrochloric acid in the correction of metabolic acidosis. Arch. Surg., 110:819, 1975.
16. Henzel, J. H., DeWeese, M. S., and Ridenhour, C.: Significance of magnesium

and zinc metabolism in the surgical patient. I. Magnesium. Arch. Surg., 95:974, 1967.
17. Jenkins, M. T., and Beck, G. P.: Differential diagnosis of hypotension occurring during anesthesia and surgery. Clin. Anesth., 3:106, 1963.
18. Kassirer, J., Berkman, P., Lawrenz, D., et al.: The critical role of chloride in the correction of hypokalemic alkalosis in man. Am. J. Med., 38: 172, 1965.
19. Katz., M. A.: Hyperglycemia-induced hyponatremia: Calculations of expected serum sodium depression. N. Engl. J. Med., 289:843, 1973.
20. Kwun, B. K., Boucherit, T., Wong, J., et al.: Treatment of metabolic alkalosis with intravenous infusion of concentrated hydrochloric acid. Am. J. Surg., 146:328, 1983.
21. Lassen, N. A.: Control of cerebral circulation in health and disease. Circ. Res., 34:749, 1974.
22. Laurens, R., and Karp, B. I.: Pontine and extrapontine myelinolysis following rapid correction of hyponatremia. Lancet, 1:1439, 1988.
23. Mattar, J. A., Weil, M. H., Shubin, H., and Stein, L.: Cardiac arrest in the critically ill: II Hyperosmolal states following cardiac arrest. Am. J. Med., 56:162, 1974.
24. McClelland, R. N., Shires, G. T., Baxter, C. R., Coln, C. D., and Carrico, C. J.: Balanced salt solution in the treatment of hemorrhagic shock studies in dogs. J.A.M.A., 199:830, 1967.
25. Mellemgaard, K., and Astrup, P.: The quantitative determination of surplus amounts of acid or base in the human body. Scand. J. Clin. Lab. Invest., 12:187, 1960.
26. Mengoli, L. R.: Excerpts from the history of postoperative fluid therapy. Am. J. Surg., 121:311, 1971.
27. Miller, T. R., Anderson, R. J., Linas, S. L., Henrich, W. L., Berns, A. S., Gabow, P. A., and Schrier, R. W.: Urinary diagnostic indices in acute renal failure. Ann. Int. Med., 89:47, 1978.
28. Moncrief, J. A., and Mason, A. D.: Water vapor loss in the burned patient. Surg. Forum, 13:38, 1962.
29. Moore, F. D., Olesen, K. H., McMurrey, J. D., Parker, H. V., Ball, M. R., and Boyden, C. M.: The Body Cell Mass and Its Supporting Environment. Philadelphia, W. B. Saunders Company, 1963.
30. Narins, R. G., and Emmett, M.: Simple and mixed acid-base disorders: A practical approach. Medicine, 59:161, 1980.
31. Pitts, R. F.: Acid-base regulation by the kidneys. Am. J. Med., 9:356, 1950.
32. Randall, R. E., Jr., Cohen, M. D., Spray, C. C., Jr., and Rossmeisl, E. C.: Hypermagnesemia in renal failure: Etiology and toxic manifestations. Ann. Intern. Med., 61:73, 1964.
33. Roberts, J. P., Roberts, J. B., Skinner, C., Shires, G. T., III, Illner, H., Canizaro, P. C., and Shires, G. T.: Extracellular fluid deficit following operation and its correction with Ringers Lactate: A reassessment. Ann. Surg., 202:1, 1985.
34. Schwartz, W. B., and Relman, A. S.: A critique of the parameters used in the evaluation of acid-base disorders. N. Engl. J. Med., 268:1382, 1963.
35. Shires, G. T., Cunningham, J. N., Baker, C. R. F., Reeder, S. F., Illner, H., Wagner, I. Y., and Maher, J.: Alterations in cellular membrane function during hemorrhagic shock in primates. Ann. Surg., 176:288, 1972.
36. Shires, G. T., and Holman, V.: Dilutional acidosis. Ann. Intern. Med., 28:551, 1948.
37. Shires, G. T., and Jackson, D. E.: Postoperative salt tolerance. Arch. Surg., 84:703, 1962.
38. Shires, G. T., Williams, J., and Brown, F.: Acute changes in extracellular fluids associated with major surgical procedures. Ann. Surg., 154:803, 1961.
39. Singer, R. B., and Hastings, A. B.: An improved clinical method for the estimation of disturbances of the acid-base balance of human blood. Medicine, 27:223, 1948.
40. Sporn, N., Lancestremere, R. G. and Papper, S.: Differential diagnosis of oliguria in aged patients. N. Engl. J. Med., 267:130, 1962.
41. Stewart, A. F.: Therapy of malignancy-associated hypercalcemia. Am. J. Med., 74:475, 1983.
42. Thompson, J. E., Vollman, R. W., Austin, D. G., and Kartchner, M. M.: Prevention of hypotensive and renal complications of aortic surgery using balanced salt solution. Ann. Surg., 167:767, 1968.
43. Tuller, M. A., and Mehdi, F.: Compensatory hypoventilation and hypercapnia in primary metabolic alkalosis. Am. J. Med., 50:281, 1971.
44. Vanatta, J. D., and Fogelman, M. J.: Moyer's Fluid Balance. 3rd ed. Chicago, Year Book Medical Publishers, Inc., 1982.
45. Virgilio, R. W., Rice, C. L., Smith, D. E., et al.: Crystalloid vs colloid resuscitation: Is one better? Surgery, 85:129, 1979.
46. Williams, D. B., and Lyons, J. H.: Treatment of severe metabolic alkalosis with intravenous infusion of hydrochloric acid. Surg. Gynecol. Obstet., 150:315, 1980.
47. Wilson, R. F., and Sibbold, W. J.: Approach to acid-base problems in the critically ill and injured. J. Am. Coll. Emerg. Physicians, 5:515, 1976.
48. Wong, E. T., Rude, R. K., Singer, F. R., et al.: A high prevalence of hypomagnesemia and hypermagnesemia in hospitalized patients. Am. J. Clin. Path., 79:348, 1983.
49. Wright, H. K., and Gann, D. S.: Correction of defect in free water excretion in postoperative patients by extracellular fluid volume expansion. Ann. Surg., 158:70, 1963.

5

PRINCIPLES OF PREOPERATIVE PREPARATION OF THE SURGICAL PATIENT

Hiram C. Polk, Jr., M.D.

The modern preparation of the patient for operation characterizes the emergence of the surgical disciplines from an art to science. The development of *anesthesia*, followed by the introduction of the *antiseptic concepts* of Semmelweis and Lister, was a monumental achievement, but it can be viewed best as providing the basis for the healthy growth and development of modern surgery.

ASSESSMENT OF OPERATIVE RISK

Inherent in a discussion of operative risk is the determination each physician must make regarding the relative rewards and risks of treatment of a specific illness. Surgeons are perhaps fortunate that the dramatic nature of their methods magnifies the significance of adverse results and permits clear understanding of this expression in the therapeutic ratio. In its simplest terms, such a ratio defines the relative harm (risk) and the relative good (benefit) that are likely to follow a specific operation for a specific illness in a specific patient. There are few more valuable parameters than the *natural history* of the disease process — that is, the course of the disease and its ultimate outcome if untreated. Especially good examples concern the natural history of abdominal aortic aneurysms,[7] the course of untreated mammary carcinoma,[13] and the description of iliofemoral atherosclerosis.[35] Such data are of particular significance in an era of therapeutic chauvinism.

One must further ascertain that the *stages* of disease being considered are *clinically* comparable. Errors in clinical staging produce the greatest number of controversies regarding medical or surgical therapy, or both. More often than not, alleged differences between treatments are attributable to differences in clinical staging of the patient populations under comparison[26] and not due to different results of the putative therapies.

Special problems that influence operative risk are of major concern in the preoperative preparation of the patient. The therapeutic ratio of appendectomy for *suspected* appendicitis is quite clearly in favor of intervention. Treating appendicitis by excision, even with a 20 per cent incidence of normal appendices, is much better than allowing a single appendix to perforate, in view of the exaggerated morbidity and geometric effect upon mortality if the latter occurs. This potential for an adverse effect has been recently redefined in a current analysis of the gatekeeper and managed care trends in American practice today.[2] Similarly, the urgency of a specific procedure is in part a function of the relative risks and rewards. In suspected appendicitis, the rewards of treatment entail prompt control of an inflamed focus or management of a systemic complication that is very likely to be fatal if untreated. The benefits compared with nonoperative treatment or diagnostic delay point strongly toward prompt operation.

Those benefits depend upon the promptness with which contamination is terminated or otherwise treated. Whereas urgency of an operation may determine the period of time for and indirectly limit the measure taken to prepare the patient, it is all the more important that these preparations be accomplished promptly. Although one cannot correct chronic malnutrition in 2 to 3 hours, it is possible to initiate significant correction of certain concentration and volume deficiencies.

The nature of the illness being treated sharply influences outcome. For example, a patient with advanced neoplastic disease often presents with anemia, profound weight loss, and evidence of metastases that alter hepatic, pulmonary, or cerebral function. When a decision is made for operation, each consideration becomes important in preparing the individual for definitive treatment. However, the nature of the illness is such that definitive correction of all its manifestations cannot be achieved, preoperatively or even postoperatively. By contrast, the systemic effects of an inflammatory process that has caused contamination of the entire peritoneal cavity may be treated vigorously with parenteral fluids, antibiotics, and intestinal decompression, with full knowledge that operative correction of the offending focus, regardless of cause, is definitive in eliminating the source of continuing contamination.

Similarly, elderly patients often require concurrent management of multiple organ degenerative disease. When one disease produces a complication that can be controlled only by operation, particular attention should be given to the often subtle but physiologically important alterations of the other organs essential for life support. The influence of age upon operative risk is very important. Some elderly individuals may appear physiologically young, but it is often said that an operation or an injury quickly brings them up to chronologic age.

Among the specific considerations that markedly influence operative risk are cardiovascular, respiratory, renal, and gastrointestinal disease. Significant impairment of more than one organ system profoundly influences operative risk. For example, an individual with severe respiratory disease plus major renal insufficiency bears only 1 chance in 50 of surviving definitive surgical treatment of a duodenal ulcer.[16]

The capacity for sound clinical *judgment* is the ultimate characteristic of the mature physician. The parameters involved in clinical decisions are difficult to define, but quantification of these factors is desirable, both to affirm the physician's initial professional judgment and to provide the younger physician with a means of more promptly learning this attribute of professional excellence. Some have criticized a quantitative approach as unnecessary, because all good physicians are assumed to be capable of sound clinical judgment, but there is continuing evidence that more is required in this area. Linn and associates[18] found that the presence of systemic and local disease is generally additive in determining the probability of death during hospitalization, profoundly influencing some decisions for operation. In prospective and retrospective studies of peptic ulcer disease, the effects of multiple organ system disease were shown to be so profound as to *eliminate* from surgical consideration some patients previously recognized as having an increased but tolerable risk. Despite general agreement about principles of *intra*operative decisions in a common major operation, practicing Board-certified surgeons often deviated from accepted standards; those deviations were associated with significant increases in death after operation and in decreased cure of some colorectal cancers.[17] Algorithms may be helpful in delineating more of these crucial but often overlooked concepts (Table 1) and a logarithmic growth of such literature has been noted.

For the determination of operative risk and factors requiring specific preoperative correction, a simple list should be made part of each physical examination, including (1) personal and familial history of any past bleeding tendency, with laboratory definition of its significance; (2) allergic responses to medication or prior treatment; and (3) current medications, with awareness that patients often forget to list some drugs or to recognize that nonprescription products may contain active medicinal agents. Examples are the intermittent use of corticosteroids, with the real possibility of adrenal insufficiency at the time of stress, and the use of diuretics associated with induced hypokalemia and its obvious systemic effects at the time of anesthesia and operation.

PERSONAL RELATIONSHIPS

When a surgical procedure is being considered, a genuine bond of communication and personal responsibility must be established between the surgeon and the patient. The patient's confidence is based upon true understanding, allowing him to participate, when appropriate, in judgments affecting risks, future lifestyle, and the process of postoperative recovery. The rarity of legal action taken by a patient when a careful effort has been made by the physician to achieve such understanding prior to operation is noteworthy and depends upon a carefully informed and accurate statement of the relative risks and rewards of the operation. Many patients today have growing insight regarding such matters and should be allowed to participate actively in the decisions. In achieving this goal, the physician must not convey a sense of hurry or inadequate time for explanations, no matter how small or seemingly minor the operation might be. Finally, there are occasions when a direct answer may not be possible, and it has been said that a measure of a physician is a capacity to say "I don't know."

Another attribute of the mature and capable physician is the desire to involve consultants who may have additional or parallel skills to contribute to diagnosis and treatment. From largely unfounded recriminations about so-called unnecessary operations, there has evolved a desire for and understanding of the occasional value of a *second opinion* concerning the need for some operative procedures.[32] If there is reasonable question on the part of a patient that an operation is indicated, the surgeon should seek confirmation by obtaining the independent view of another surgeon.

The patient in a teaching institution finds illness and operation a focal point for the education of students at several levels.

TABLE 1. Basic Factors Affecting Operative Risk

Age over 70 years
Overall physical status
Elective versus emergency operation
Physiologic extent of procedure
Number of associated illnesses

Properly conducted, this can be a positive influence for the patient psychologically, as many enjoy such attention, so long as it involves the patient personally and considers the medical problems in a tactful manner. Most discussions can be done at the bedside and do much to reassure the patient as to the total understanding of the illness and of the projected treatment.

For the young surgeon, few concepts are less well understood than effective relationships with referring physicians. In most situations, patients are referred to surgeons by physicians in other disciplines; it is important to have an understanding of the wishes and views of the referring physician at the outset. On some occasions the referring physician will have made certain judgments that are at variance with those of the surgeon— differences that must be discussed with the surgeon and, occasionally, with the patient. Further, it is very helpful to have a clear understanding of the projected course of treatment and the relative participation of the referring physician in the postoperative care, so that duplicative or, more important, contradictory efforts and orders are avoided.

The *specific permission* for conduct of an operative procedure is a focal point of medical, legal, and sociologic discussion. Local custom and recent legal practice often determine which of these is most appropriate. The surest perception of true *informed consent* can be attained in a setting in which there is a full and frank discussion with the patient as well as a close relative and an appropriate professional witness. One should concisely record a summary of this encounter in the hospital chart. Moreover, when writing such a note, the surgeon will often wish to enumerate those patient characteristics that determine the need for operation; the special risk factors recognized, with further notation as to their amelioration; and the special intra- and postoperative problems anticipated. This also serves as a checklist for possible errors of omission.

Some procedures have such major measurable risk that the real possibility of death or disability must be discussed as part of the mutual decision-making process. It is usually sufficient to inform the patient that there are risks of both complication and death, no matter how well or carefully the operation is conducted. One must truly respect the patient's options, but it is also important to avoid undue arousal of fear.

GENERAL PREPARATION OF THE PATIENT

The basic principles of preparation of the patient for a major operative procedure can be readily enumerated, but it is much more difficult to determine the rapidity with which such preparation must be accomplished. For example, time may be of minor importance when an operation is being planned for a patient with a chronic intractable duodenal ulcer; this is more often a matter of personal convenience for the patient, the family, and the surgeon. In contrast is the patient with a radiographically demonstrated carcinoma of the colon, who should undergo definitive operation within a reasonable time in order to prevent development of obstruction and/or metastases from the lesion. In the patient suspected of having acute appendicitis, operation should be performed within a few hours. Moreover, in a patient with rupture of an abdominal aortic aneurysm or with mesenteric vascular occlusion, the lethality of uncontrolled hemorrhage in the first and the rapid progression of intestinal gangrene in the second require surgical treatment within a few minutes at most. Thus, there is a measurable *spectrum of urgency* that substantively determines the rapidity and completeness of preoperative preparation.

Psychologic Preparation

A frank, but optimistic, discussion of the possibilities ahead is of great value for the patient who is to undergo a major surgical procedure. The preoperative steps should be enumerated, justified, and explained in detail. The use of drainage devices and various forms of intubation is better tolerated, both physiologically and psychologically, if their need has been previously explained. The patient then anticipates and understands the benefits and realizes that the discomfort serves an identifiable purpose.

The surgeon must not equivocate in discussing possible disfiguring operations, such as upon the head and neck, the breasts, or genital organs, and most especially with respect to methods of urinary or fecal elimination.

PLANS FOR FURTHER CARE IN CERTAIN CHRONIC ILLNESSES. When an illness is apt to have a clinically significant course beyond the duration of the early posthospital follow-up, it is usually very reassuring for the surgeon to explain the continuing commitment to the patient. This is particularly helpful for the patient with neoplastic disease, who may correctly or incorrectly perceive life expectancy to be 6 months or less. The surgeon should make realistic projections about continuing office visits at progressively longer intervals as the patient continues to do well after treatment. Both the reassurance of anticipated longevity on the part of the patient and the assurance that the surgeon will be a partner in the long-term management of the disease or any complication that may arise from the treatment are most reassuring. In neoplastic disease, the issue of honesty as to preoperative and postoperative diagnosis always arises.

Well-intentioned friends or family members often wish to shield the patient from unpleasant facts. This is generally unwise, and the surgeon's contract ordinarily is with the patient. When the medical facts are unpleasant, it is wise to allow the patient an opportunity to recover from the immediate effects of the operation and to ascertain that he is alert before such information is provided. Often it is useful to allow the patient to ask about the status of the disease spontaneously. However, if this has not occurred within a period of several days, the surgeon should take the initiative and review with the patient the operative finding and the probable prognosis. Such gentle frankness guarantees that the patient who may reach even more difficult stages of illness will once again turn to the surgeon as a person who has been honest about the prospects. The patient likewise will once more expect the surgeon to be thoroughly honest about the treatments available in difficult circumstances. At the point of first information, the prognosis, if poor, should *not* be presented as hopeless. This is unjustified biologically and also denies the patient that small degree of justifiable optimism that supports an individual with a grim prognosis surprisingly well.

Physiologic Preparation

BLOOD VOLUME CONSIDERATIONS. A variety of chronic disease processes are associated with anemia. In some instances, these represent visible external losses, as in carcinoma of the cecum. Other instances are far less clear and are associated with chronic infection or with chronic inflammatory processes of the bowel. These patients all fit a pattern in which there is substantial blood loss producing reduction of red cell mass. Indeed, such patients have a normal *total blood volume*. They have compensated for a significantly decreased red blood cell volume by expansion of the plasma volume to supernormal levels.[25] While *acute* intravascular volume deficiencies are manifested by an increased pulse rate or decreased blood pressure, on a chronic basis volume is restored by expanding the plasma volume, often at the expense of the extracellular fluid, to compensate for the loss of or nonproduction of red cell mass.

Correction of these concentration deficits prior to an elective operation requires recognition that even large deficits in red cell mass occurring over a long period are well tolerated. A patient may enter the hospital with a hemoglobin concentration of 5 gm. per 100 ml. with no evidence of tachycardia or hypovolemia, the anemia having been sustained over an extended period. Although 10 gm. per 100 ml. of hemoglobin is regarded by

many as minimal for general anesthesia, what must be determined are the physiologic limits safe for tissue oxygen delivery. Enhanced oxygen delivery can be achieved in the following ways: (1) increase in heart rate, (2) increase in stroke volume, and (3) increase in oxygen extraction. The last may be least amenable to improvement, and to increase stroke volume or pulse rate places a definite physiologic stress upon the heart, which often is diseased itself in the elderly patients who acquire such chronic illnesses. Therefore, there is a reasonable limit to the hemoglobin concentrations that are safe for a major operation. Indeed, if one could ascertain that no unforeseen blood losses or inadvertent hypoxia would occur, a patient could expect to safely undergo an elective operation with a very low hemoglobin concentration. However, the risk of one of these untoward events is greater than the hazard of transfusion. Thus, patients being prepared for operation who have an anemia commonly associated with chronic disease should have replacement of the red cell mass up to 10 gm. per 100 ml., or even to more nearly normal values when there is evidence of associated heart disease.

A useful rule when attempting physiologic correction of chronic anemia is seldom to administer more than 1 unit of blood per day, thereby allowing time for excretion of excess plasma. An anemia that has been acquired over months is not ordinarily corrected in a matter of hours.

OTHER FLUID DEFICITS. Whereas blood deficits are primarily concentrational, plasma and extracellular fluid deficits are significant in both volume and concentration in terms of the preparation of most patients preoperatively. Special problems are presented when the volume deficiencies are *pre-existing* or *concealed*. For example, *pre-existing* losses may represent vomitus and/or diarrhea occurring for 3 to 4 days before hospitalization. It is very difficult for the patient to estimate the volume of such losses. Although some losses occur visibly, as in a fracture of the femur or in a major third-degree burn of an extremity, and are manifested by visible swelling, more often such fluid losses are concealed and thus inadequately estimated. A patient with intestinal obstruction may present with vomiting of 3 days' duration with signs of dry mucous membranes and tongue and complaining of thirst. Although he has taken reasonable amounts of liquid orally over each of the 3 days, the patient has continued to vomit. His hemoglobin concentration might well be an index of dehydration, but this requires a recent known normal value for that patient. For example, if the hemoglobin is normal, one could postulate either that there had been very little volume loss or that there had been a major plasma volume loss superimposed upon pre-existing anemia. This occurs with a colonic carcinoma, which may produce significant red blood cell deficiency and then causes intestinal obstruction, which produces an extracellular fluid volume deficit. These offsetting losses produce a misleading hemoglobin concentration that is in the normal range.

The problem of *concealed* loss is particularly difficult. These "third-space losses" in which blood, plasma, and/or extracellular fluid are extravasated, are often associated with fractures, and it is only upon careful comparison of the fractured and unfractured limb for circumference that one can appreciate the magnitude of such losses. Objective estimation of pre-existing and continuing fluid deficits should be obtained, and one of the most ubiquitously useful is hourly urinary output through a urinary catheter as a measure of efficacy of replenishment. As difficult as estimation of pre-existing or concealed losses may be, this first step to assess continuing losses is essential for correction of that deficit. Hemoglobin concentration, appearance of the mucous membranes, and skin turgor assist in such a judgment. It is emphasized that standard losses in these circumstances total approximately 3 liters a day, or 125 ml. an hour in adults. Therefore, the rate of fluid resuscitation in a *deficit* situation should begin at twice that rate. The hourly urinary output should be assessed over a period of 3 to 4 hours for determination of volume deficiency and the rate at which replenishment should continue.

A common error in quantitating concentrational deficits is to assume that the normal serum concentration of a specific electrolyte assures that there has been no loss. Isotonic losses of water, salt, chloride, and potassium may produce profound volume deficiencies with maintenance of normal concentrations of the commonly measured serum electrolytes. When concentrational abnormalities exist, they imply only that the loss of electrolyte concentration has been relatively greater than the loss of water, or vice versa. Although administration of any fluid containing the deficient electrolytes ultimately is of value, it may be very inefficient, as, for example, replenishing sodium chloride and potassium deficits by administration of 5 per cent dextrose in half-normal (0.45 per cent) saline. Reasonably normal kidneys conserve all sodium and chloride administered. However, to do so is metabolically expensive, because the kidneys must excrete large amounts of free water. Ultimately, correction is accomplished, but infusion of solutions proportionate to losses is much more precise and definitive.

Under what circumstances should hypertonic resuscitative solutions be used? Seldom. In the presence of severe cerebral dysfunction attributed to hyponatremia (e.g., coma), the limited administration of a hypertonic solution is therapeutically acceptable. Unless there is clear evidence of renal disease, potassium replenishment should proceed along with sodium infusion.

TIMING AND PARAMETERS. Again, urgency of the operation is the major determinant in the time available for correction of fluid and electrolyte balance. All volume and concentrational deficits need not be corrected before operation is undertaken, but a significant fraction of the total deficit should be replaced in order to enhance the safety of anesthesia and operation. For example, in a patient with nonstrangulating intestinal obstruction of 3 days' duration and normal electrolyte concentrations without signs of urinary or hemoconcentration, one should assume that there has been a significant isotonic loss of electrolytes and water. Resuscitation may be initiated with lactated Ringer's solution with added potassium at a rate of 500 ml. in the first hour. If the urinary response to such administration is only 10 ml., another 500 ml. should be infused during the next hour. Should urinary output increase to 20 ml. per hour, one might reasonably anticipate operation. In general, the longer a patient has been ill, the more time one can take to correct the deficiencies. In other words, the patient has adjusted physiologically to the deficiency induced by the illness. One must be certain that the rapid replenishment of those deficits does not impose a risk greater than the illness itself. The overly rapid correction of fluid deficits and induction of pulmonary edema, particularly in elderly patients with marginal cardiovascular compensation, is a risk that could be tolerated in the young patient with a normal cardiovascular system and an acutely encountered disease.

Nutrition

Nutrition has been a major component in previous editions of this chapter. It is now substantively covered in detail elsewhere (Chapter 7). Although nutritional replenishment and supplementation have become a common (and expensive) worldwide surgical practice, their specific role in improved survival from certain illnesses or after certain operations continues to defy documentation and certainly defies cost-benefit analysis. As a skeptic, the author recommends accepting the tide of surgical opinion about the value of aggressive nutrition in certain situations, perhaps assuming that such supportive measures are providing the basis for prolonged in-hospital survival and that some future advance is required to convert longer in-hospital courses to ultimate improvement in hospital discharge data.

Such a sequence occurred in burn care earlier in this century; better resuscitation produced longer survival but no improvement in overall burn survival as measured by hospital discharges. When burn care was combined with topical antimicrobial therapy 25 years later, a sudden and precipitous improvement in burn survival evolved. So it may be for nutrition.

Prevention of Infection

Infection continues to be a major source of morbidity and a disconcerting source of mortality in the surgical patient. The patient who is badly injured or who undergoes a major operation and survives despite the development of secondary shock and electrolyte disturbances is at very high risk for serious infection. Therefore, control of infection is a major consideration before, during, and after every operation. Only certain aspects of the problem of infection as it particularly pertains to the preoperative assessment of the patient are here reviewed.

The first consideration is identification of the *genuine* high-risk factors for infection (Table 2). For example, diabetics have long been considered particularly prone to infection. As a matter of fact, this is correct, as long as one considers their well-known propensity to develop infection in the lower extremities related to small vessel arteriosclerosis and peripheral neuropathy. If these possibilities are eliminated, the well-controlled diabetic is probably no more prone to infection than any other individual of similar age and illness.[24] Nevertheless, clinical compromises are often inescapable. Termination of steroid medication must be considered carefully in view of the obvious risk of acute adrenal insufficiency in the intra- or postoperative patient who has been receiving exogenous steroids for a long period.

During preoperative evaluation, the patient should be protected from any patient with extramural or hospital-acquired infections. The proposed operative site should be washed with an appropriate antiseptic agent on several occasions before operation, and shaving should be done either as close to the time of operation as feasible or not at all, substituting either clipping or depilatory agents when removal of hair is desired.[28]

A primary factor that should be considered in preparation of the patient is antibiotic prophylaxis. Proper evidence finally demonstrated the commonly accepted efficacy of preoperative intestinal preparation with poorly absorbed oral antimicrobial agents for colon operations.[36] Explicit laboratory studies[22] were confirmed by a now seemingly endless flow of randomized clinical trials that showed *systemic* antibiotics highly effective

TABLE 2. Factors Influencing Likelihood of Infection After Operation

Definite Decreased Host Resistance
Increasing age
Obesity/malnutrition
Diabetic ketoacidosis
Acute/chronic steroid therapy
Immunosuppressive drugs
Remote, synchronous infection

Possible Decreased Host Resistance
Cancer (some forms)
Radiation therapy
Adrenocortical deficiency
Percutaneous foreign bodies
Early shaving of operative site

No Effect on Host Resistance
Patient's gender
Patient's race
Controlled diabetes mellitus
Acute nutritional deprivation

TABLE 3. Operations Benefiting from Systemic Antibiotic Prophylaxis

Head and neck, which open upper aerodigestive tract
Esophageal, excluding hiatal hernia repair
Gastroduodenal, except for complications of uncorrected hyperacidity
Biliary tract for patients
    Over 70 years old
    With acute cholecystitis, and/or
    Requiring choledochostomy
Small and large bowel resections
Gangrenous or perforated appendicitis
Hysterectomy
Abdominal and lower extremity revascularizations, including a prosthetic graft
Other clean operations implanting a high-risk prosthesis, e.g., hip, knee, aortic valve

when used just before, during, and immediately after an operation.[1, 27] However, one must always balance the risk of an adverse effect of an antibiotic with its potential benefit. To date, most studies showing clear-cut benefit from such antibiotic use have been in operations that bore an appreciable risk of infection; the other characteristics varied considerably (Table 3).

The agent selected should manifest sustained antibiotic activity in the surgical wound.[29] Declining wound antibiotic activity is an indication to readminister the agent or to seek a drug producing more sustained activity levels. Another major factor is unanticipated delays in elective operations.[9] Agents selected must also have been subjected to stringent randomized clinical trials.

Urgency of operation, reflecting limited time for preparation; the nature of the illnesses requiring immediate intervention; and the degree of likely operative contamination determine the probability of postoperative infection. If preoperative preparation has been ideal, operative maneuvers likely to control infection are obviously important (Table 4). The elimination of unnecessary conversation and traffic in the operating room, strict adherence to sterile technique, and the precise use of noninjurious methods of handling tissue are also important.

With regard to delivery of antimicrobial protection to the wound itself, one may administer systemic antibiotics or choose topical antibiotics in the wound.[30] A method of wound management that has stood the test of time in badly contaminated cases is *delayed* primary closure of the wound.[5] The peritoneum and muscle layers are closed securely, and the subcutaneous fat and skin are left open and covered with gauze treated with either saline or an antimicrobial agent. At a suitable time postoperatively, when the wounds are shown to be free of infection by inspection or culture, the subcutaneous fat and skin are closed with tape or previously placed sutures. Although cumbersome, this method has been the standard for many years and should continue to be so.

No single technical complication is as frequently associated with infection as is the presence of a *hematoma,* implying incomplete hemostasis. It is often thought to provide a medium for bacterial growth, and iron-binding proteins contribute di-

TABLE 4. Operative Techniques to Minimize Infection

Eliminate hair, if indicated, just prior to incision time
Effective skin preparation, i.e., iodophor chlorhexidine
Gentle tissue handling
Effective hemostasis
Eradicate dead spaces
Operation lasting less than 2 hours
Closed suction drainage, if indicated, at a distance from the incision

rectly to the nonspecific host defense response to a number of microorganisms, probably competing with the potential pathogen for ferric iron, a known requirement for pathogenicity of numerous microbes. A hematoma of the wound has the theoretical and probably the practical capacity to impair this important defense mechanism. Therefore, hematoma must be avoided by meticulous technique and by closed suction drainage at a distance from the wound when avoidance appears otherwise impossible.

Numerous workers have assessed the impact of overt and occult malnutrition on the frequency of postoperative infectious complications, including death associated with infection. MacLean and associates have related skin test anergy to subsequent infection and appear to have shown that nonspecific nutritional repletion reverses both anergy and the tendency to infection.[21,34] More probing analysis in other systems appears to indicate that there is a measurable opsonic deficiency in diluted serum of malnourished individuals. Further pursuit and verification are warranted, but most clinicians accept preoperative initiation of nutritional repletion as an effective anti-infective maneuver.

SPECIFIC ORGANS AND SYSTEMS

CARDIOVASCULAR. Every patient scheduled for any operation should have specific, careful cardiovascular evaluation. In young people, previously overlooked congenital lesions may be discovered; in elderly patients, prevalent atherosclerosis must be sought. Initial efforts to quantify what appeared to be subjective impressions were enhanced by the work of Mauney and co-workers.[19] The efforts of Goldman and associates did much to advance this whole line of inquiry toward precise determination of operative risk[12] and has recently been updated.[31] The capacity of the patient to increase cardiac output in response to intra- and postoperative challenges is perhaps the most fundamental determinant of survival following complex operations.[4]

The risk factors found to be useful predictions of both fatal and nonfatal but life-threatening complications of cardiac origin after *noncardiac* operations are listed in Table 5. These variables of cardiac status are also associated with unfavorable characteristics of the operation itself, and the need for emergency operation. Such factors allowed Goldman and associates to develop a weighting scheme for these factors, which then correlated accurately with the likelihood of significant cardiac risk (Table 6), as has been discussed elsewhere in this chapter. This work is a useful advance compared with prior methods to

TABLE 5. Preoperative Factors Associated with Postoperative Cardiac Complications in Order of Discovery Significance

Jugular vein distention or S_3 gallop
Myocardial infarct in previous 6 months
Premature atrial contractions or rhythm other than sinus on ECG
Three to five premature ventricular contractions per minute
Age over 70 years
Significant aortic valvular stenosis
Poor general medical condition
    $Pao_2 < 60$ mm. Hg; $Paco_2 > 50$ mm. Hg
    $K^+ < 3.0$ mEq./L.; $HCO_3 < 20$ mEq./L.
    BUN > 50 mg./100 ml.; creatinine > 3.0 mg./100 ml.
    Elevated transaminase
    Signs of chronic liver disease
    Patient bedridden from noncardiac causes

Modified from Goldman, L., Caldera, O. L., Nussbaum, S. R., et al.: Multifactorial index of cardiac risk in noncardiac surgical procedures. N. Engl. J. Med., 297:845, 1977.

TABLE 6. Weighting of Cardiac Risk Factors

Criteria	Points
Historical	
Age over 70 years	5
Myocardial infarction previous 6 months	10
Examination	
S_3 gallop/jugular venous distention	11
Significant aortic valvular stenosis	3
ECG	
Premature atrial contractions or rhythm other than sinus	7
More than 5 premature ventricular contractions/min.	7
General Status	3
Abnormal blood gases	
K^+/HCO_3 abnormalities	
Abnormal renal function	
Liver disease/bedridden	
Operation	
Emergency	4
Intraperitoneal/intrathoracic/aortic	3
Total possible	53

Modified from Goldman, L., Caldera, D. L., Nussbaum, S. R., et al.: Multifactorial index of cardiac risk in noncardiac surgical procedures. N. Engl. J. Med., *297*:845, 1977.

the same end and is as important for what it did not find as for its positive observations. Although the statistical soundness of a negative observation is dependent upon limited numbers' fulfilling such "negative criteria," Goldman and associates did *not* confirm the significance of diabetes mellitus, smoking, hypertension, hyperlipidemia, stable angina pectoris, remote myocardial infarcts, ST-segment or T-wave changes on the electrocardiogram (ECG), bundle branch blocks, mitral valvular disease, or cardiomegaly. These must not be ignored but are apparently less pertinent determinants of *cardiac* risk than had been thought.

Note further that 28 of the 53 points in the cardiac risk weighting scheme are potentially treatable. Improvement in the overall cardiac status could defer operation until a time when prognosis is more favorable. One of the risk factors reflective of congestive failure and susceptible to preoperative cure is that associated with profound anemia, as from chronic gastrointestinal blood loss, which produces a secondary demand for increased cardiac output. When the hemoglobin concentration is returned to normal, these patients are readily converted to a much lower risk category.

There is a steady increase in life-threatening complications as the point total rises but a precipitous one in cardiac deaths in patients with more than 25 points.

Also significant in detecting the unsuspected high-risk patient is the work of DelGuercio and Cohn on preoperative pulmonary wedge pressure monitoring with and without challenge. More important, their method has unmasked some patients with prohibitive cardiac risk and allowed others to be improved prior to operation.[6] Successful myocardial revascularization, not surprisingly, ameliorates much of the excess risk of coronary ischemia.[8]

Thromboembolism is a generally infrequent clinical event; the value of brief or mini-anticoagulation for some patients is widely debated and is discussed in detail elsewhere in this text. Patients at increased risk include (1) those with a clear history of clinical signs of prior thrombosis or embolism; (2) those likely to have prolonged operations, with special emphasis upon procedures that temporarily interfere with lower extremity blood

TABLE 7. Risk Factors for Postoperative Pulmonary Complications

Thoracic and upper abdominal surgery
Preoperative history of chronic obstructive pulmonary disease
Preoperative purulent productive cough
Anesthesia time greater than 3 hours
History of cigarette smoking
Age greater than 60 years
Obesity
Poor preoperative state of nutrition
Symptoms of respiratory disease
Abnormal findings on physical examination
Abnormal chest film findings

Modified from Houston, M. C., Ratcliff, D. G., Hays, J. T., and Gluck, F. W.: Preoperative medical consultation and evaluation of surgical risk. South. Med. J., *80*:1385, 1987.

flow, such as some aortic reconstructions or perineal operations requiring the use of stirrups; and (3) those with certain reconstructive operations upon the hip. Based upon these and other parameters, the clinician may then employ a variety of methods to reduce the risk of thromboembolism, including elastic stockings, exercises, early ambulation, and variable degrees of anticoagulation.

RESPIRATORY. Respiratory complications of operations constitute two major groups: (1) the development of respiratory abnormalities secondary to anesthetic agents and operation in patients with grossly normal lungs; (2) the increasing number of patients with overt chronic lung disease who require operation, thus superimposing the problems of anesthesia and operation upon intrinsically diseased pulmonary tissue. Some risk factors are outlined in Table 7.

Preoperative pulmonary insufficiency requires the surgeon to determine whether operation can be tolerated at all and the optimal preparation if operation is to be undertaken. The distinction between nonobstructive and obstructive pulmonary emphysema can be made with the standard tests of pulmonary function. In general, patients below the age of 40 years who have no pulmonary signs or symptoms do not require special tests. In older patients and those with pre-existing disease, especially lesions requiring upper abdominal operations, tests of pulmonary function may provide useful information. Abnormalities of the lungs and tracheobronchial tree are detected in some patients despite a history negative for pulmonary disease. Pulmonary function that permits toleration of a major operation comes into special focus with respect to patients who require excision of functioning or nonfunctioning lung tissue and those who undergo nonpulmonary operation. Although a number of specific tests delineate minimal function, careful evaluation by the surgeon, in consultation with pulmonary medicine specialists, is often indicated.[33] A simple, useful test is a brisk walk of the patient up a flight of stairs with observation of tolerance.

TABLE 8. Perioperative Prophylactic Pulmonary Maneuvers

Cessation of smoking
Bronchodilators
Chest physiotherapy and postural drainage
Preoperative education and postoperative use of incentive spirometer and deep breathing exercises
Preoperative antibiotics if sputum is purulent
Early postoperative ambulation

Modified from Houston, M. C., Ratcliff, D. G., Hays, J. T., and Gluck, F. W.: Preoperative medical consultation and evaluation of surgical risk. South. Med. J., *80*:1385, 1987.

TABLE 9. Preoperative Variables Differ Between Survivors
and Nonsurvivors

Variable	Mortality If Variable Present (%)	Mortality If Variable Present (%)
Child's classification		
A	10	50
B	31	30
C	76	18
Ascites	58	11
Infection/contamination	64	21
Emergency procedure	57	10
Poor nutrition	62	22
Bilirubin $\geq$ 3 mg./100 ml.	62	17
Albumin < 3 mg./100 ml.	58	12
PT > control	47	7
PT > 1.5 sec./control	63	18
PTT > control	54	18
WBC > 10,000	54	19

$p < 0.01$ for all variables listed.
Listed in order of decreasing importance in predicting survival.
Modified from Garrison, R. N., Cryer, H. M., Howard, D. A., and Polk, H. C., Jr.: Clarification of risk factors for abdominal operations in patients with hepatic cirrhosis. Ann. Surg., 199:648, 1984.

One test of proven value is preoperative documentation of the normal resting *arterial blood gases.* There is no "normal" blood gas profile for all patients. Whereas consideration of standard age-related changes in $P(A-a)o_2$ may be the only resource in an emergency, there is no excuse for failure to determine a patient's normal range of blood gases prior to an elective operation when the procedure is of great magnitude or when other clear factors, including age, suggest the possibility of respiratory complications.

Maneuvers of variable benefit to the patient with documented chronic pulmonary disease undergoing elective operation are noted in Table 8. How much the carefully regulated use of assisted respiration such as "incentive spirometry"[14] adds is conjectural. What is well documented is the lack of value of routine postoperative respiratory treatments in lieu of interested and specific attention by the nursing staff and physician.[20]

RENAL. With appropriate perioperative hydration, renal complications of major surgical endeavors have become relatively uncommon. A normal blood urea nitrogen (BUN), however, may be misleading. Surely, when there is the slightest suspicion of intrinsic renal disease, appropriate creatinine stud-ies should be undertaken. Conversely, the most common erroneous consideration in the surgical patient is the fear that renal disease exists. Renal disease is not nearly as frequent in the apparently asymptomatic population as are cardiovascular and respiratory diseases. With the screening procedures of BUN, creatinine determination, and urinalysis, one may proceed to an operation and subsequent fluid therapy reasonably confident that the patient will tolerate judiciously managed fluid loads with ease. The most common cause of oliguria on surgical services continues to be *hypo*volemia rather than incipient renal failure.

A special type of renal disease is associated with obstruction in the lower urinary tract, exemplified by prostatic hypertrophy in elderly men. If time permits, catheter drainage of the obstructed urinary tract and elimination of infection should be done before an elective procedure, allowing return of adequate function.

HEPATIC. The signs and symptoms of significant liver impairment are detectable on a number of standard examinations. The typical patient has obvious signs of advanced nutritional cirrhosis or widespread metastatic liver disease. In many instances, these abnormalities can be corrected only marginally before operation. With cirrhotic patients, a substantial preoperative period must be allowed if any recovery of function is to be achieved, again concentrating on nutrition and avoidance of hepatotoxins in any form. The overwhelming risk of cirrhosis in nonshunting operations has been a subject of great importance and wide discussion.[10] Some factors are especially important and often preclude all but absolute immediate life-saving operations (Table 9).

NEUROLOGIC. Maintenance of cerebral function via appropriate oxygenation and circulation is of vital concern to the anesthesiologist and the surgeon. Of special concern is the prevalence of occult cerebrovascular disease in elderly people, who constitute a major proportion of patients requiring surgical attention. Earlier editions of this textbook emphasized the detection and correction of minimal carotid disease prior to another warranted procedure—for example, carotid correction before abdominoperineal resection with its usual hypotension.[23] Several lines of evidence now suggest that the significant occult asymptomatic carotid lesion is rare and that corrective procedures undertaken prior to the primary operation are seldom justified.[3]

Just as was the case with the more specific and probing study of cardiac risk factors, it is now clear that asymptomatic carotid stenoses rarely produce problems without prior development of symptoms,[15] ulcerated plaques may be reliably segregated into groups that bear little or no significant risks, and patients with

TABLE 10. A Sample Preoperative Checklist

Operative permit—appropriately signed and witnessed
Dietary considerations
    For abdominal operation, liquid diet and laxatives to ensure clean, collapsed bowel
    Nothing by mouth at least 6 hours before operation
Review of life-support systems
    Vital signs recorded often enough to establish "normal"
    Pulmonary system—chest films; other studies as indicated
    Cardiac function—ECG; other studies as indicated
    Renal function—urinalysis; BUN and possibly creatinine determinations
Adequate hydration up to time of operation—especially to compensate for laxatives and fasting
Area of operation washed with appropriate germicidal detergent and shaved, clipped, or cleansed with
    depilatory agent
Blood transfusions prepared as anticipated
Order that patient should void on call to operating room
Preoperative medications—vagolytic and sedative drugs
Special medications—digitalis, insulin, and so on

Modified from Houston, M. C., Ratcliff, D. G., Hays, J. T., and Gluck, F. W.: Preoperative medical consultation and evaluation of surgical risk. South. Med. J., 80:1385, 1987.

asymptomatic carotid bruits are not as susceptible to stroke as are patients with transient ischemic attacks.[23] All in all, a careful history remains the best determinant of whether cerebrovascular disease poses a real or imagined risk to the patient requiring another operation.

SPECIAL PROBLEMS

A number of special problems demand preoperative correction. Foremost among these is incomplete cleansing of the alimentary tract. Pulmonary aspiration is a dreaded surgical complication, the treatment of which remains inadequate, whereas prevention is simple. There are almost no circumstances when general anesthesia should be induced without specific attention to evacuation of the patient's stomach, ascertained in any questionable case by the surgeon. Although so simple to prevent, aspiration remains one of the more common causes of surgical mortality. A useful checklist of preoperative considerations that should be reviewed at the time of writing preoperative hospital orders is provided in Table 10.

SELECTED REFERENCES

Bolt, R. J.: Medical Evaluation of the Surgical Patient. Mount Kisco, N.Y., Futura Publishing Company, 1987.
Although organized as a medical consultant's handbook, this monograph brings the current, largely medical, literature to bear on risk factors, correction thereof, and the "tuning up" of the surgical patient.

Moore, E. E., Eiseman, B., van Way, C. W., III.: Critical Decisions in Trauma. St. Louis, C. V. Mosby Company, 1984, and Norton, L. W., and Eiseman, B.: Surgical Decision Making, Two. Philadelphia, W. B. Saunders Company, 1986.
The use of algorithms is especially helpful in determining options in the surgical patient with multiple associated or underlying illnesses.

Feinstein, A. R.: Clinical Judgment. Baltimore, Williams & Wilkins Company, 1967.
The process of assessing operative risk is discussed in detail in this rambling but incisive monograph. Clinical examples are drawn to provide objectivity and specificity, and most apply directly or indirectly to the surgical setting even today.

Moyer, C. A.: The assessment of operative risk. In Rhoads, J. E., Allen, J. G., Harkins, H. N., and Moyer, C. A. (Eds.): Surgery. Principles and Practice, 4th ed. Philadelphia, J. B. Lippincott Company, 1970, pp. 232–243.
The requisite process for evaluating factors that genuinely influence operative risk is explicitly reviewed and documented. Mechanisms by which future risk factors can be evaluated are also presented in detail in the first systematic analysis of operative risk.

Polk, H. C., Jr. (Ed.): Infection and the Surgical Patient. Edinburgh, Churchill Livingstone, 1982.
A complete and current overview of factors influencing infection in the surgical setting is provided by an international assembly of major contributors to the field.

REFERENCES

1. Bernard, H. R., and Cole, W. R.: The prophylaxis of surgical infection: The effect of prophylactic antimicrobial drugs on the incidence of infection following potentially contaminated operations. Surgery, 56:151, 1964.
2. Cacioppo, J. C., Diettrich, N. A., Kaplan, G., Nora, P. F.: The consequences of current constraints on surgical treatment of appendicitis. Am. J. Surg., 157:276, 1989.
3. Carney, W. I., Jr., Stewart, W. B., DePinto, D. J., et al.: Carotid bruit as a risk factor in aortoiliac reconstruction. Surgery, 81:567, 1977.
4. Clowes, G. H. A., Jr., DelGuercio, L. R., and Barwinsky, J.: The cardiac output in response to surgical trauma. A comparison between patients who survived and those who died. Arch. Surg., 81:212, 1960.
5. Coller, F. A., and Valk, W. L.: The delayed closure of contaminated wounds: a preliminary report. Ann. Surg., 112:256, 1940.
6. DelGuercio, L. R., and Cohn, J. D.: Monitoring operative risk in the elderly. J.A.M.A., 243:1350, 1980.
7. Estes, J. E., Jr.: Abdominal aortic aneurysms: A study of 102 cases. Circulation, 2:258, 1950.
8. Fudge, T. L., McKinnon, W. M. P., Schoette, G. P., et al.: Improved operative risk after myocardial revascularization. South. Med. J., 74:799, 1981.
9. Galandiuk, S., Polk, H. C., Jr., Jagelman, D. G., Fazio, V. W.: Re-emphasis of priorities in surgical antibiotic prophylaxis. Surg. Gynecol. Obstet., 169:219, 1989.
10. Garrison, R. N., Cryer, H. M., Howard, D. A., and Polk, H. C., Jr.: Clarification of risk factors for abdominal operations in patients with hepatic cirrhosis. Ann. Surg., 199:648, 1984.
11. Goldman, L., Caldera, D. L., Nussbaum, S. R., et al.: Multifactorial index of cardiac risk in noncardiac surgical procedures. N. Engl. J. Med., 297:845, 1977.
12. Goldman, L.: Cardiac risks and complications of noncardiac surgery. Ann. Surg., 198:780, 1983.
13. Greenwood, M.: A Report on the Natural Duration of Cancer. Ministry of Health Reports on Public Health and Medical Subjects. No. 33. London, Her Majesty's Stationery Office, 1926.
14. Houston, M. C., Ratcliff, D. G., Hays, J. T., and Gluck, F. W.: Preoperative medical consultation and evaluation of surgical risk. South. Med. J., 80:1385, 1987.
15. Humphries, A. W., Young, J. R., Santilli, P. H., Beven, E. G., and deWolfe, V. G.: Unoperated, asymptomatic significant internal carotid artery stenosis: A review of 182 instances. Surgery, 80:695, 1976.
16. Irvin, G. L., III, and Zeppa, R.: Predicted survival in peptic ulcer patients based on computer analysis of preoperative variables. Ann. Surg., 183:594, 1976.
17. Knutson, C. O., Fry, D. E., Barbie, R. D., et al.: Reassessment of intraoperative decisions. Why operations for cancer of the large bowel fail. Ann. Surg., 187:549, 1978.
18. Linn, B. S., Linn, M. W., and Wallen, N.: Evaluation of results from studies of surgery in the elderly. Ann. Surg., 195:90, 1982.
19. Mauney, F. M., Ebert, P. A., and Sabiston, D. C.: Postoperative myocardial infarction: A study of predisposing factors, diagnosis and mortality in a high risk group of surgical patients. Ann. Surg., 172:497, 1970.
20. McConnell, D. H., Maloney, J. V., Jr., and Buckberg, G. D.: Postoperative intermittent positive-pressure breathing treatments. Physiological considerations. J. Thorac. Cardiovasc. Surg., 68:944, 1974.
21. Meakins, J. L., Pietsch, J. B., Christou, N. V., MacLean, L. D.: Predicting surgical infection before the operation. World J. Surg. 4:439, 1980.
22. Miles, A. A., Miles, E. M., and Burke, J.: The value and duration of defense reactions of the skin to primary lodgement of bacteria. Br. J. Exp. Pathol. 38:79, 1957.
23. Moore, W. S., Boren, C., Malone, J. M., et al.: Natural history of nonstenotic, asymptomatic ulcerative lesions of the carotid artery. Arch. Surg., 113:1352, 1978.
24. National Academy of Sciences–National Research Council: Post-operative wound infections: The influence of ultraviolet irradiation of the operating room and of various other factors. Ann. Surg., 160(Suppl):1, 1964.
25. Peden, J. E., Jr., Maxwell, M., Ohin, A., et al.: A consideration of indications for preoperative transfusion based on analysis of blood volumes and circulating proteins in normal and malnourished patients with or without cancer. Ann. Surg., 151:303, 1960.
26. Polk, H. C., Jr.: The mathematics of clinical judgment, including an evaluation of operative risk. In Polk, H. C., Jr. (Ed.): Basic Surgery, 3rd ed. Norwalk, Appleton-Century-Crofts, 1987, pp. 9–21.
27. Polk, H. C., Jr., and Lopez-Mayor, J. F.: Postoperative wound infection: A prospective study of determinant factors and prevention. Surgery, 66:97, 1969.
28. Polk, H. C., Jr., Simpson, C. J., Simmons, B. P., and Alexander, J. W.: Guidelines for prevention of surgical wound infection. Arch. Surg., 118:1213, 1983.
29. Polk, H. C., Jr., Trachtenberg, L., and Finn, M. P.: Human incisional antibiotic activity. J.A.M.A., 244:1353, 1980.
30. Pollock, A. V.: Topical antibiotics. In Polk, H. C., Jr. (Ed.): Infection and the Surgical Patient. Edinburgh, Churchill Livingstone, 1982, pp. 91–100.
31. Rose, S. D.: Cardiac risk factors in patients undergoing non-cardiac surgery. In Bolt, R. J. (Ed.): Medical Evaluation of the Surgical Patient. Mount Kisco, N.Y., Futura Publishing Company, 1987, pp. 253–280.
32. Rutkow, I., Gittlesohn, A., and Zuidema, G.: Surgical decision making: The reliability of clinical judgment. Ann. Surg., 190:145, 1979.
33. Siefkin, A. D., Lillington, G. A.: Pulmonary complications of surgery. In Bolt, R. J. (Ed.): Medical Evaluation of the Surgical Patient. Mount Kisco, N.Y., Futura Publishing Company, 1987, pp. 307–326.
34. Tchervenkov, J. I., Diano, E., Meakins, J. L., Christou, N. V.: Susceptibility to bacterial sepsis. Accurate measurement by the delayed-type hypersensitivity skin test score. Arch. Surg. 121:37, 1986.
35. Warren, R., and Kihn, R. B.: A survey of lower extremity amputations for ischemia. Surgery, 63:107, 1968.
36. Washington, J. A., II, Dearing, W. H., Judd, E. S., et al.: Effect of preoperative antibiotic regimen on development of infection after intestinal surgery: Prospective, randomized, double-blind study. Ann. Surg., 180:567, 1974.

6

BLOOD TRANSFUSIONS AND DISORDERS OF SURGICAL BLEEDING

John A. Collins, M.D.

Adequate hemostasis is fundamental in operative procedures. If the patient has a faulty hemostatic mechanism, the surgeon must have sufficient understanding of hemostasis, the nature of the injuries produced, and the remedies available in order to estimate the risks and proper timing of anticipated procedures, to modify surgical technique as necessary, and to help direct correction of the hemostatic defects. The advice of experts in coagulation is often necessary, but a surgeon cannot be ignorant in matters so necessary for the practice of his craft and the health of his patients.

The decision to transfuse is a serious one because of the risks involved. Modern blood banking has made great advances in what can be offered for treatment. Unfortunately, the sophistication of many practitioners has not kept pace. Many harmful practices and attitudes persist. One frequently hears the following statements and sees patients treated accordingly: "If the hematocrit is below 30, transfuse"; "If you need one unit, you need two"; "If the platelet count is below 100,000, give some"; "For every five units of blood transfused, give some fresh frozen plasma and platelets." Every one of these statements is wrong; every one of them is harmful. What comes out of the blood bank is potent but dangerous material. Knowledge of its proper use is mandatory in order to properly care for surgical patients.

This chapter addresses hemostatic mechanisms and focuses on the conditions likely to cause excessive bleeding. Blood and the products that relate to hemostasis in the modern blood bank are discussed in this context. Arterial thrombosis and embolism, venous thrombosis and pulmonary embolism, and the treatment of hypovolemia and shock are discussed elsewhere in this text. (Abbreviations used are listed in Table 1.)

NORMAL HEMOSTASIS

The surgeon's concern with hemostasis begins with injury to a blood vessel. Contraction of injured vessels, including capillaries, is a very early protective response. Thromboxane (TxA_2) is produced locally very soon after injury and is the most powerful constrictor of smooth muscle yet identified. Vasoconstriction in larger vessels is reinforced by direct innervation and by circulating vasoconstrictors such as norepinephrine. Medium-sized arteries can be surprisingly effective in sealing off by constriction when they have been transected—if hemostatic mechanisms are normal. Diseased arteries, especially those stiffened by atherosclerosis, cannot contract and will remain open and hemorrhaging until there is tamponade by the bleeding, control by the surgeon, or death of the patient. Large veins are less efficient at constricting when injured because of their much less muscular walls, but they are easier to seal by tamponade because of the lower intraluminal pressures. The most dangerous injury occurs in areas where tamponade occurs late or not at all (thoracic cavity, external bleeding, free intraperitoneal bleeding). Incomplete transection, paradoxically, is less likely to be controlled by vascular constriction than is complete transection. Major arteries and veins tend to lie next to each other, and partially transected vessels tend to remain open. Thus, post-traumatic arteriovenous fistulas are found with appreciable incidence in long-term follow-up of patients with penetrating wounds to appropriate areas.

Current views of normal hemostasis correctly focus on four major components: the vascular endothelium, platelets, coagulation, and inhibition and lysis of coagulation. There has been a great increase in knowledge of each of these subsystems in recent years, especially in the molecular biology of previously obscure processes. As a result, scientific knowledge is rapidly accumulating. The following description is an overview only; the details are certain to change.

Not long ago vascular endothelium was viewed as little more than a nonclotting surface through which blood flowed. Illustrating the recent activity in this field, vascular endothelium is now known to be a specialized biochemical powerhouse that begins and fine-tunes many of the essential processes of hemostasis and that produces some of the key components of other subsystems.[43] In addition, it has an active role in lipid metabolism and in the lung forms an important barrier to protect the systemic circulation from spillover effects of inflammatory mediators released at sites of injury. Vascular endothelium is nonthrombogenic because of several properties. The luminal surface is strongly negatively charged; this may serve to repel similarly charged platelets. Vascular endothelium synthesizes and releases prostacyclin (PGI_2), a powerful local vasodilator and inhibitor of platelet aggregation; thrombomodulin, which binds circulating thrombin to the cell surface, blocking its ability to activate coagulation factors and promoting activation of protein C; heparan sulfate, very similar to heparin, which combines with circulating antithrombin III (AT-III) to block the action of local thrombin and inactivate certain other activated coagulation components; and tissue plasminogen activator (tPA), which produces local fibrinolysis. In addition, the release of PGI_2 is stimulated by thrombin itself, epinephrine, injury, and vigorous exercise. When the integrity of the vessel is destroyed, blood comes in contact with the subendothelial environment, or even deeper. This allows platelets to adhere to collagen and become activated, and hemostasis begins. On the thrombogenic side of the scales, endothelial cells produce factor V, factor VIII, and von Willebrand factor (vWF), all necessary components of coagulation; fibronectin, which helps bond fibrin to the surrounding tissue; collagen; and extracellular matrix. Endothelium contains abundant contractile proteins, so even muscleless capillaries can constrict.

TABLE 1. Abbreviations and Codes Used

Code	Full Name
TxA_2	Thromboxane, thromboxane A_2
PGI_2	Prostacyclin, prostaglandin I_2
AT-III	Antithrombin III, heparin cofactor
tPA	Tissue plasminogen activator
vWF	von Willebrand factor
ADP	Adenosine diphosphate
ATP	Adenosine triphosphate
HMWK	High-molecular-weight kininogen, Williams-Fitzgerald-Flaujeac factor
cAMP	cyclic AMP, 3′,5′-adenosine monophosphate
PGD_2	Prostaglandin D_2
DIC	Disseminated intravascular coagulation
C1	First component of complement
DDAVP	Desmopressin, 1-diamino-8-D-arginine vasopressin
PT	One-stage prothrombin time
PTT	Partial thromboplastin time
FFP	Fresh frozen plasma
CPD-A	Citrate-phosphate-dextrose-adenine anticoagulant
NANB	Non-A, non-B hepatitis
HIV	Human immunodeficiency virus
2,3-DPG	2,3-diphosphoglyceric acid
DNA	Deoxyribonucleic acid

Platelets adhere to exposed collagen. At high rates of flow, this requires vWF, which bonds to a specific cell surface receptor. Even when the exposed collagen is covered by a layer of platelets, more platelets "pile on," forming a substantial mass. This aggregation reaction can be caused by a wide variety of substances, the most physiologically relevant of which are epinephrine, collagen, thrombin, and adenosine diphosphate (ADP), which bind to specific membrane receptors on the platelets. These agonists can also cause synthesis and/or release of certain important substances: TxA_2, a potent platelet aggregator and vasoconstrictor; serotonin, ADP, and calcium; fibrinogen, vWF, and factor V; fibronectin, high-molecular-weight kininogen (HMWK), alpha$_1$-antitrypsin, beta-thromboglobulin, and platelet factor 4. Activation by agonists also results in exposure of certain membrane receptors; binding of fibrinogen to the glycoprotein IIb and IIIa surface complex is necessary for platelet aggregation *in vivo*. Activation of platelets also uncovers receptors on their surfaces for activated factor V (Va). The bound Va acts in turn as a binding site for activated factor X (Xa), almost certainly contributing substantially to local coagulation. Platelet aggregation and activation may be largely modulated by 3′, 5′-adenosine monophosphate (cAMP), which counteracts the effects of platelet agonists. Production of cAMP in platelets is powerfully stimulated by prostaglandin D_2 (PGD_2), produced in activated platelets, and PGI_2, produced in endothelial cells. Vascular endothelium also can rapidly destroy ADP, probably the most important platelet agonist.

Some of the products produced or released by platelets have not been studied well enough for us to be sure of their physiologic roles (e.g., thrombospondin and platelet factor 4). Platelet-activating factor is an interesting substance produced by leukocytes, platelets, and vascular endothelium that activates platelets in most mammalian species, including human, and whose action is not blocked by aspirin.[4] The exact physiologic role of this substance in hemostasis is still uncertain and debated. Other actions include hypotension and a generalized increase in vascular permeability. Platelets may also be linked to inflammatory processes through additional effects of TxA_2, which appears to be involved in the entrapment and oxidative burst of neutrophils that have traversed areas of ischemic injury.[32]

The formation of a fibrin clot is the next important step in hemostasis. The mechanisms by which this occurs, called coagulation, are a series of linked reactions involving circulating proteins (Fig. 1, Table 2). Most steps involve enzymatic conversion of inactive precursors to active forms, which in turn cause the activation of the next step in the sequence. Most steps require one to four cofactors, of which ionized calcium is a near constant requirement. There is a general increase in effect from step to step, so that the overall sequence forms a biologic amplification device. Various control mechanisms are active at most steps and there are substantial feedback loops and crossover effects of both amplification and inhibition. The coagulation sequence leads to the formation of thrombin, which splits fibrinogen to form soluble fibrin monomers. The monomers polymerize to form insoluble fibrin, which is acted upon by factor XIII to increase cross-linking, forming a firmer clot more resistant to lysis.

Two initiating pathways are described: the intrinsic, which involves substances already in the blood and begins with factor XII; and the extrinsic, which begins with an extravascular lipoprotein that is strongly thromboplastic, currently called *tissue factor*, interacting with factor VII. The intrinsic pathway has been investigated in considerable detail although its clinical significance is not clear. In some manner, factor XII binds to negatively charged surfaces (but not normal endothelium) and initiates its own activation. The materials that are known to initiate the intrinsic cascade are not those encountered in the ordinary course of injury and repair; endotoxin might be an exception, but even that hardly constitutes a clinically useful trigger for initiating coagulation. Even more to the point, congenital or acquired absence of any of the proteins involved in initiating the intrinsic pathway is associated with prolonged whole blood clotting times and partial thromboplastic times, but no major defect in clinical hemostasis! This may be evidence that factor XI or factor IX can be activated more directly when tissues are injured. There is some evidence that tissue factor can activate

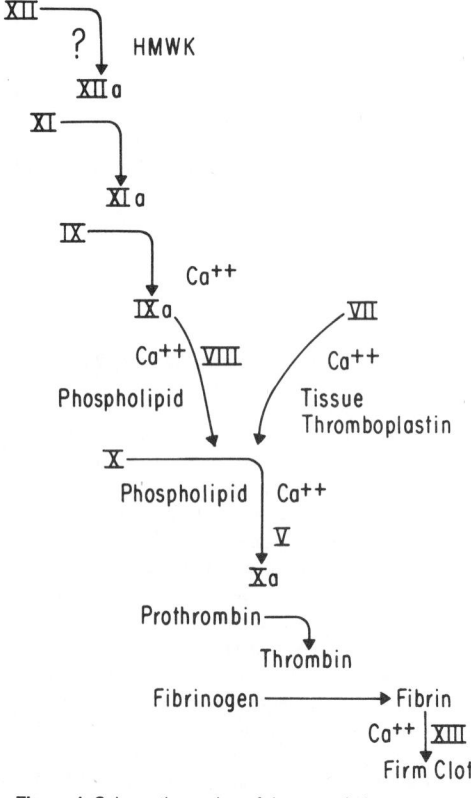

Figure 1. Schematic version of the coagulation system.

TABLE 2. Clinically Important Characteristics of Coagulation Factors

Coagulation Factor	Name	Site of Production	Level Needed for Hemostasis (% Normal)	Immediate Recovery in Circulation (% Infused)	Half-Life (hr.)	Stable in Plasma at 4° C.
I	Fibrinogen	Liver	10–25	50	100	Yes
II	Prothrombin	Liver (K)*	40	50	72	Yes
V	Proaccelerin	Liver, endothelium	15	50	15	No
VII	Proconvertin	Liver (K)*	10	100	4	Yes
VIII	Antihemophiliac factor	Endothelium	>30	70	8–12	No
vWF	von Willebrand factor	Endothelium	25–50	?	<10	No
IX	Christmas factor	Liver (K)*	>30	40	12–24	Yes
X	Stuart factor	Liver (K)*	10	50	50	Yes
XI	Plasma thromboplastin antecedent	Liver	25	90	60	Yes
XII	Hageman factor	?	—	?	60	Yes
XIII	Fibrin-stabilizing factor	?Liver	2	50–100	>100	Yes

Adapted from Smith, J. K., and Bidwell, E.: Therapeutic materials used in the treatment of coagulation defects. Clin. Haematol., *8*:183, 1979; and Technical Manual, 9th ed. Arlington, VA, Am. Assoc. Blood Banks, 1985.

* Signifies dependency upon vitamin K for synthesis.

factor IX. Activation of factor XII has other pertinent effects: prekallikrein is converted to kallikrein, which in turn activates many kinins, and the first component of complement may be activated. The link between coagulation and inflammation is becoming progressively more clear.[25]

Disruption of tissue exposes blood to tissue factor, which leads to the activation of factor VII.[31] Activated factor VII (VIIa) and activated factor IX (IXa) both lead to the activation of factor X (Xa), which is the beginning of the final common pathway of coagulation. There are other interactions between the intrinsic and extrinsic pathways, however. The effects of factor VII are increased by XIIa or IXa and are affected both ways by Xa. Tissue factor may activate factor IX. The steps in the final pathway are more complex than those preceding. Conversion of factor X to Xa is too slow to be effective without the participation of cofactors. When activated via the intrinsic pathway, phospholipid and factor VIII, a large protein, serve that role; when activated via VIIa, tissue factor serves as the cofactor. With either pathway, the conversion of X to Xa appears to be identical. Xa converts prothrombin to thrombin, but this also requires phospholipid and a large protein, factor V, to be effective. These reactions requiring phospholipid occur largely on the membranes of activated platelets, further linking platelets and coagulation and positioning the ensuing clot where it is needed. The main role of thrombin is to convert fibrinogen to fibrin, but it has many other effects: to "activate" factors V, VIII, and XIII; to activate protein C; to cleave prothrombin to prethrombin; and to interact with endothelium and platelets as already described. The conversion of fibrinogen to fibrin, which then polymerizes and cross-links under the influence of factor XIII, is the immediate "goal" of the coagulation cascade. The fibrin mesh helps seal the breaks in blood vessels and stop the loss of blood through its immediate physical effect, through its strengthening of the platelet plug and aiding the recruitment of more platelets, and through the improved binding of the entire hemostatic plug via its interaction with platelets, vessel wall and collagen, and other adhesive proteins such as vWF, fibronectin, and thrombospondin.

The coagulation system appears less intimidating in its complexity if one considers various similarities and functional groupings. The factors directly involved in the intermediate steps of the final common pathway, II, X, VII, and IX, are all dependent on vitamin K; all share the unusual amino acid gamma-carboxyglutamic acid, which helps form the calcium binding site; and the two main reactions in which they partici-

pate, generation of Xa and thrombin, require phospholipid and large molecular cofactors. Those large molecular cofactors, V and VIII, are produced in endothelial cells and, like fibrinogen and prothrombin, are used up in the course of coagulation and are digested by plasmin and converted by thrombin.

Producing clots is necessary in order to stop bleeding; controlling clots is necessary in order to preserve circulation and control healing. This fourth component system of hemostasis is probably the least understood, but enough is known to describe the outlines of the controlling processes. The balanced opposing control mechanisms in vascular endothelium and platelets have been mentioned: TxA_2 versus PGI_2, ADP versus endothelial ADPase, surface receptors on platelets for agonists and certain coagulation proteins that are hidden or exposed according to other signals, thrombin versus thrombomodulin (endothelial), heparan (endothelial) versus coagulation, tPA (endothelial) versus fibrin, and others (Table 3). When a fibrin clot is formed it contains within itself the seeds of its own destruction in the form of adsorbed plasminogen, which has its greatest efficacy against fresh clots. In addition to these controlling mechanisms that act locally at the site of injury, it is essential to prevent systemic activation of the coagulation cascade. This is accomplished by two approaches, inhibiting various activated components of the coagulation cascade and activating fibrinolytic enzymes (Table 4). AT-III is the most important of the circulating inhibitors of coagulation. It is the major circulating inhibitor of IXa, Xa, and thrombin. Heparin binds to AT-III and increases its activity; this is how the pharmacologic effects of heparin are produced. Recently, a second heparin cofactor has been identified, but it appears much less important than AT-III. There is enough AT-III circulating to neutralize several times the amount of thrombin that could be produced, yet levels below 50 per cent of normal are associated with increased thrombosis. Congenital deficiencies of AT-III are associated with a marked increase in venous thromboembolism. C1 inhibitor neutralizes XIIa and kallikrein, but deficiencies result in angioedema rather than excess coagulation, reinforcing the doubts about the importance of the classic intrinsic activation pathway in hemostasis and reinforcing the connection between coagulation and inflammation via this pathway. Alpha$_1$-antitrypsin inhibits XIa but also inhibits neutrophil elastase. Deficiencies result in emphysema owing to the effects of elastase from circulating stimulated neutrophils on the pulmonary alveoli. Again, there is little excess thrombosis because of lack of an inhibitor of an activated component of the intrinsic pathway. Alpha$_2$-macroglobulin in-

TABLE 3. Some of the Counteracting Effects Produced or Released at Various Levels in the Hemostatic Process

	Effect	
Level	Hemostatic	Antithrombotic
Vascular endothelium	Contractile proteins Factors V, VIII, vWF tPA inhibitor Collagen and matrix (fibronectin)	PGI_2 Thrombomodulin, heparan tPA ADPase, PGI_2
Platelets	*Synthesis/Release* TxA_2, Serotonin, ADP, calcium, factors I, V, vWF, proco- agulants ("factor 3"), ?thrombospondin, ?platelet factor 4, ?tPA inhibitor	*Synthesis/Release* C1-inhibitor, alpha$_1$-antitrypsin, alpha$_2$-macroglobulin Antirelease: cAMP (PGD_2)
	Surface receptors Adherence (collagen)? Aggregation (ADP, collagen, thrombin, epinephrine) Coagulation (Va, Xa, I, fibronectin, HMWK)	Anti-adherence: cAMP Anti-aggregation: cAMP, (PGI_2)
Coagulation	Thrombin Tissue factor Factor XII activators Other activated coagulation components	Thrombomodlin, AT-III, second heparin cofactor Alpha$_1$-antitrypsin, C1-inhibitor AT-III, protein C (and S)
Fibrinolysis	Alpha$_2$-plasmin inhibitor, alpha$_2$-macroglobulin, tPA in- hibitor (plasmin activates XII)	Plasmin (tPA, urokinase)

hibits most of the activated factors mentioned for the other inhibitors and developmentally appears to be the oldest and perhaps the direct descendant of the ancient original of this family of proteins. Its actions are slower, however, and some enzymes retain some reduced activity even after they are bound. No disorder resulting from deficiency has been identified. The most recently discovered coagulation inhibitor is protein C, a vitamin K–dependent protein that works with a cofactor called protein S. Protein C is bound by the thrombin-thrombomodulin complex on the endothelial cell surface when this is formed, which activates and releases it. Activated protein C destroys the coagulant properties of factors V and VIII. Deficiencies of protein C or protein S are associated with thromboembolic disease.

The primary mechanism for removing fibrin is lysis by plasmin. Plasmin is a serine protease, like many of the active components of the coagulation cascade. It circulates in the inactive form of plasminogen, which can be activated by a variety of stimuli. Plasminogen is adsorbed to the surfaces of a forming fibrin plug. During the process of adsorption, the plasminogen becomes much more susceptible to cleavage to plasmin. This process appears greatest with fresh fibrin clots. Adsorbed plasminogen and locally released plasmin are much less susceptible to the action of circulating inhibitors, allowing local fibrinolysis while maintaining protection against the development of a generalized activation. Alpha$_2$-plasmin inhibitor is also bound to fresh fibrin by factor XIII, presumably to provide a potential rein on unwanted local fibrinolysis. The agents that convert plasminogen to plasmin that have received the most attention are tPA, produced by endothelium and a variety of other cell types; urokinase, produced by renal tubular cells and normally found in urine; and various pharmacologic activators such as streptokinase. The most important action of plasmin is the dissolution of fibrin clots, but it is far from a specific enzyme. In addition to fibrin, plasmin attacks fibrinogen and factors II, V, VIII, and possibly IX and XI and can digest adrenocorticotropic hormone, growth hormone, insulin, and complement. Plasmin activates factor XII and via XIIa amplifies coagulation and activates the kinin and complement systems. Plasmin even acts on plasminogen, making it more susceptible to activation. Clearly, something with this power must be carefully controlled. The primary circulating inhibitor is alpha$_2$-plasmin inhibitor, which is rapid

TABLE 4. Major Circulating Protease Inhibitors

Substance	Mol. Wt.	Concentration (μM.)	Inhibitory Activity*	Congenital Absence
Antithrombin III†	58,000	2.5–5	**Thrombin, Xa, IXa**	Arterial and venous thromboses
Alpha$_2$-plasmin inhibitor	67,000	1	**Plasmin**	Excessive bleeding
Alpha$_1$-antitrypsin	54,000	25–45	**XIa, elastase**	Pulmonary emphysema, cirrhosis
C1-inactivator	105,000	2	**XIIa, kallikrein, activated C1**	Angioneurotic edema
Alpha$_2$-macroglobulin	725,000	3	Thrombin, plasmin, kallikrein	?
Heparin cofactor II†	66,000	0.14	Thrombin	?Thromboses
tPA inhibitor	67,000	0.1–1 nM	**tPA**	Excessive bleeding
Protein C	62,000	?	**Va, VIIIa**	Fatal thromboses
Activated protein C inhibitor†	57,000	0.1	**Protein C**	?

* Bold type indicates the main physiologic role.
† Activity greatly augmented by heparin.
Adapted from Aoki, N.: Natural inhibitors of fibrinolysis. Prog. Cardiovasc. Dis., 21:267, 1979; and Harpel P. C.: Blood proteolytic enzyme inhibitors: Their role in modulating blood coagulation and fibrinolytic enzyme pathways. *In* Colman, R. W., Hirsh, J., Marder, V. J., and Salzman, E. W. (Eds.): Hemostasis and Thrombosis: Basic Principles and Clinical Practice, 2nd ed. Philadelphia, J. B. Lippincott, 1987, p. 219.

and effective. It is becoming apparent that there are inhibitors of activators and activators of inhibitors. It remains to be seen through how many layers this complex control mechanism extends. Congenital defects of plasminogen result in a thrombotic tendency, whereas defects in alpha$_2$-plasmin inhibitor result in a hemorrhagic disorder. One of the most important and fundamental questions in hemostasis remains unanswered: how are beneficial clots maintained while harmful or rogue clots are usually lysed? Potential antagonistic controlling mechanisms have been identified, but it is not clear how they are so precisely orchestrated.

CONGENITAL ABNORMALITIES OF HEMOSTASIS

The best known congenital disorders of hemostasis are in the realm of coagulation.[28] Of these the most frequent and important to surgeons are the hemophilias and von Willebrand's disease. Congenital abnormalities of platelet function are much less common. Inherited disorders of the fibrinolytic system and its inhibitors are being described with increasing frequency and are variably associated with either increased bleeding or increased thromboembolic events.

The most common congenital abnormality of hemostasis is classic hemophilia (hemophilia A), a sex-linked inherited disorder that also occurs spontaneously in about 1 in every 25,000 births. The disorder results in an almost total lack of factor VIII activity. It is now apparent that the clinical manifestations, although always present and always serious, do vary in severity. Bleeding, spontaneous and after even slight trauma, is the main problem. The surgical problems are most often orthopedic, with severe disabilities resulting from repeated bleeding into joints. There is a pattern of which general surgeons should be aware. Spontaneous retroperitoneal bleeding is often manifested by severe abdominal pain, tenderness, and ileus. A falling hematocrit, laboratory evidence of poor control of the hemostatic disorder, and other evidence of spontaneous bleeding (often hematuria) are the clues. It is advisable not to operate, but careful observation is necessary because other conditions that require operation may present in the same way. Death in hemophiliacs often results from bleeding into the central nervous system. Suicide is common in young adults, as is serious trauma, some of which may be unrecognized attempted suicide. Treatment consists of maintenance of factor VIII levels by periodic infusion of an appropriate material to prevent spontaneous bleeding. Higher levels of infused factor VIII are needed for surgical procedures or if the patient is bleeding. Antibodies to infused material develop in some patients and create significant problems in management. As hemophiliacs live longer, more problems with chronic liver disease are occurring and increasing numbers of patients (up to one third in some series) have the acquired immune deficiency syndrome (AIDS). Both of these relate to the necessary prolonged use of plasma products pooled from large numbers of donors. It is hoped that recent improvements in the production of products containing factor VIII will improve this dismal record of iatrogenic transmitted viral disease.

Hemophilia B (Christmas disease) is a congenital deficiency of factor IX and is the second most common congenital disorder of coagulation. The clinical manifestations may be milder than in hemophilia A but can be severe, especially with operative or accidental injury. Some patients require maintenance therapy to prevent spontaneous bleeding. Although hemophilia B is easily confused with hemophilia A on screening tests and may resemble it clinically, it will not respond to the administration of factor VIII. Accurate diagnosis is therefore essential.

Von Willebrand's disease, which is lack of the factor of the same name, is the third most common inherited disorder of coagulation. It is easily mistaken for one of the hemophilias. Clinically it has the added problem of platelet dysfunction. It varies in severity, but the bleeding tends to be more from mucous membranes than from the musculoskeletal system. The platelet disorder responds to the infusion of material containing factor VIII and von Willebrand factor, which raises interesting questions about the details of platelet function.

There are many other congenital disorders of coagulation, most of them rare.

ACQUIRED DISORDERS OF HEMOSTASIS

Among the acquired disorders of coagulation, probably the most common in the United States today are those related to drugs. Vitamin K antagonists (warfarin-like drugs) inhibit the production by the liver of factors II, VII, IX, and X and proteins C and S. All these factors contain an unusual amino acid, gamma-carboxyglutamic acid, that helps form the calcium-binding site. Levels of coagulation factors above 30 per cent of normal are usually not associated with prolonged bleeding, whereas levels below 10 per cent are dangerous and spontaneous bleeding is likely. The one-stage prothrombin time is the most frequently used test for managing therapeutic use of these drugs but the correlation between the results of the laboratory test and clinical bleeding and thrombosis is poor. Most of the vitamin K that we normally use is produced by the microbial flora of the gut and is absorbed as fat in the ileum. Deficiency of vitamin K can result from obstructive jaundice, use of antibiotics that suppress gut flora, prolonged inanition, short gut syndromes, malabsorption of fat, and other causes. Some antibiotics (e.g., moxalactam and cefamandole) contain a moiety, N-methylthiotetrazole, that may interfere with the utilization of vitamin K by the liver, thereby greatly augmenting and accelerating the effect of antibiotics on production of vitamin K–dependent factors.[3] Newborns are unable to synthesize normal amounts of these vitamin K–dependent factors, and they lack the gut flora needed for synthesis of vitamin K. Supplementation with vitamin K is now commonly practiced. In these days of ill-informed nutritional self-manipulation, it may be worth remembering that excess intake of vitamins A or E can interfere with the utilization of vitamin K.

Heparin exerts its effects by combining with AT-III to inhibit thrombin, plasmin, kallikrein, and the activated forms of factors IX, X, XI, and XII. The effects against plasmin, kallikrein, and XIIa account for the anti-inflammatory activity of heparin. The effects of heparin are therefore dependent on the circulating level of AT-III, an important discovery that explains some of the previous difficulties in establishing dose-response relationships in clinical settings. Levels of AT-III are decreased after trauma or operation, with active clotting, during prolonged treatment with heparin, and during episodes of DIC. The effective dose of heparin is uncertain and may vary with time in the same patient as the level of AT-III changes. More important, no laboratory test appears to predict effectiveness or risk of hemorrhage. An important obsevation is that bleeding complications are very unusual during the first 24 hours of treatment. AT-III can now be measured in most centers, and plasma fractions rich in AT-III for therapeutic use are being evaluated clinically. Thrombocytopenia occurs in about 1 to 2 per cent of patients receiving heparin, sometimes associated with arterial thromboses.[8] There may be several mechanisms involved including an immune mechanism and a platelet aggregating effect in susceptible patients. The thrombocytopenia usually appears after about a week of treatment and may be more common in older women. Heparin is not a single substance. Recently there has been considerable interest in the lower molecular weight fractions, which theoretically may have a better ratio of therapeutic effects to unwanted bleeding.[5] These fractions have a longer duration of action than does native heparin. Therapeutic superiority has not yet been demonstrated, and they are more expensive.

Dextran and, to a lesser extent, hydroxyethyl starch interfere with formation of firm fibrin clots and probably have some inhibitory effects on platelet function.[48] Both are used for expansion of plasma volume when a colloid effect is sought. They are cheaper than albumin; but the side effects on hemostasis are often forgotten, even though dextran is now specifically used to help prevent postoperative deep venous thrombosis, especially following operations on the hip. It is because of the effects on hemostasis that a maximal recommended dose has been set at 1 liter in 24 hours. In the extensively bleeding patient, more may be used inadvertently. This might very well worsen the situation significantly.

Hepatic insufficiency can be devastating in its impact on hemostasis. The liver is the sole site of production of fibrinogen and of the vitamin K–dependent coagulation factors II, VII, IX, X, and proteins C and S; it is the main site of production of circulating factor V and probably of prekallikrein and HMWK, plasminogen, AT-III, antiplasmin, alpha$_1$-antitrypsin, and perhaps alpha$_2$-macroglobulin. Although synthesis of fibrinogen is usually preserved until end-stage disease is reached, the fibrinogen produced may be functionally defective. In addition, the liver is normally the primary site for clearance from the circulation of activated coagulation components, plasminogen activators, and fibrin degradation products. Furthermore, many forms of chronic liver disease result in portal hypertension, esophageal varices, and secondary hypersplenism with its thrombocytopenia. The impact of hepatic insufficiency is thus usually multifactorial and can be extensive, involving platelets, coagulation components, the regulation of fibrinolysis, and the clearance of potentially destructive circulating by-products of hemostasis. When the patient is bleeding actively, it is usually necessary to liberally administer both platelets and coagulation factors in the form of fresh frozen plasma (to include factor V), but this is often relatively futile. Lack of synthesis is often compounded by accelerated consumption in the form of disseminated intravascular coagulation (DIC) in patients with severe hepatic insufficiency. The management of bleeding in such patients can be extremely difficult.

Uremia is often accompanied by a prominent bleeding tendency. Coagulation factors may be deficient because of inanition or malabsorption, and in a few patients because of accelerated losses through the urine. Many patients have evidence of a chronic, low-grade DIC. The main hemostatic defect in uremia relates to platelets. Almost all tests of platelet function are markedly abnormal in some patients, and the prolonged bleeding times do not correlate with platelet counts, which are usually normal. Infused platelets quickly become as dysfunctional as the patient's own. Many of these platelet defects improve with dialysis, and several dialyzable substances have been proposed as the agents responsible for the dysfunction, but the clinical bleeding tendency does not always respond. The bleeding of uremic patients can also be shortened by administration of conjugated estrogens or 1-diamino-8-D-arginine vasopressin (DDAVP, see later), reinforcing speculation that the interaction between platelets and factor VIII and vWF is the primary hemostatic defect in uremia. In some uremic patients, prolonged bleeding times can be markedly shortened simply by raising the hematocrit.[40] On the other side of the hemostatic scales, fibrinolytic activity of the blood is often decreased in uremic patients, apparently because of increased concentrations of fibrinolytic inhibitors. Some patients with the nephrotic syndrome develop thromboembolic complications, perhaps related to loss of AT-III in the urine.

A significant number of patients exhibit prolonged abnormal bleeding after cardiopulmonary bypass. The incidence was higher with older equipment and when the equipment was primed primarily with whole blood. Currently, the incidence appears to be related to the duration of bypass and the complexity of the procedure, especially a repeat procedure. The causes are many, but platelet dysfunction is probably the most common.[22]

Some systemic diseases are accompanied by the formation of paraproteins or immunoglobulins that interfere with various aspects of hemostasis. Probably the best studied is the "lupus anticoagulant," an immunoglobulin produced by some patients with systemic lupus erythematosus that is a model for this effect in patients with autoimmune diseases. These patients have prolonged coagulation screening tests and may have excessive bleeding. This effect is now thought to be due to action against the prothrombin activation mechanism, in particular against the phospholipid component. Interestingly, such patients may be more likely to experience serious thrombotic complications also, perhaps because of inhibition of release of PGI$_2$.

Acquired disorders of platelet function are most commonly related to drugs, many of which interfere with the synthesis of arachidonic acid metabolites. Aspirin is the prototype, but there are many others. Ingestion of these agents is so common that many patients do not even consider them drugs and may give inadvertently false answers unless questioned carefully and explicitly. With many of these drugs, all platelets circulating at the time of effective blood levels are permanently impaired. Platelet function recovers with the production and release of new platelets not exposed to the drug(s) in question.[39] In view of the nature of the lesion and the ease with which such drug effects can be detected with platelet function tests and the bleeding time, it is surprising that the clinical bleeding disorder that results is not more impressive than it is. There may be differential effects that help offset the platelet defect; the production of TXA$_2$ and PGI$_2$, for example, may be unequally altered by aspirin. It is also possible that relatively few normally functioning platelets can recruit at least some drug-impaired platelets that could not initiate the platelet response on their own. Some classes of drugs are rarely thought of as platelet-inhibiting agents, yet occasionally can cause severe disorders. The penicillins and chemically related antibiotics (carbenicillin, cephalosporins) are examples. The mechanisms involved are unknown. Entirely different classes of drugs suppress the production of platelets without altering function. Production of platelets can also be impaired by replacement of marrow with tumor, radiation effects on marrow, and many forms of failure of synthesis of one or more cell lines that are not yet understood. At the other end of the cell-production spectrum, patients with a wide variety of myeloproliferative disorders often have markedly disordered platelet function, again with mechanisms not understood. Erythrocythemia, even of the secondary type, is associated with increased bleeding during injury or operation, and later with thromboembolism.

Accelerated destruction of platelets occurs in many disorders that cause enlargement of the spleen (secondary hypersplenism) and in idiopathic thrombocytopenic purpura. In the latter, the spleen is the site not only of destruction of platelets but also often of production of the antibodies that lead to accelerated destruction. Thrombotic thrombocytopenic purpura and its variants are even more complex diseases characterized by small vessel thromboses and thrombocytopenia. The distinction between thrombocytopenia due to accelerated destruction and that due to impaired production is functionally significant. With accelerated destruction and normal production, the circulating population of platelets is younger, larger, and functionally superior. With impaired production, the circulating population of platelets tends to be older and functionally poorer. Thus, the same platelet count may be associated with no spontaneous bleeding and reasonable hemostasis during operation in a patient with a platelet-destructive disorder, but with significantly worsened bleeding in a patient with impaired production of platelets (Fig. 2).

DIC (consumption coagulopathy, defibrination syndromes) is perhaps the most troublesome of the acquired disorders of

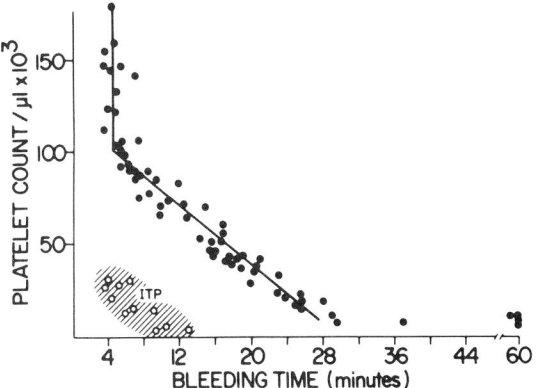

Figure 2. Intraoperative platelet counts and hemostasis (see text). (From Slichter, S. J.: Controversies in platelet transfusion therapy. Ann. Rev. Med., 31:514, 1980.)

hemostasis. The mechanisms, causes, incidence, and even definition are still subject to disagreement, but a considerable amount is known. There are at least two forms. In one, coagulation and its sequel, fibrinolysis, are triggered diffusely throughout the circulation by the introduction of potent thrombogenic materials into the circulation, usually in a continuing or repeated pattern. Inciting causes include a variety of malignant tumors, most commonly those arising from sites normally rich in thromboplastin (pancreas, prostate, lung); intravascular hemolysis (red cell stroma contains a very thromboplastic phospholipid); various kinds of tissue embolism (amniotic fluid, brain, perhaps fat and bone marrow); crushing injuries and retained dead tissue (which may be varieties of tissue embolism); and others.

The mechanism appears straightforward. Once intravascular coagulation and fibrinolysis occur and are sustained, the production of fibrin and fibrinogen degradation products and the depletion of various clotting factors result in a hypocoagulable state that can cause spontaneous bleeding. Active fibrinolysis makes hemostasis very difficult to achieve. These vicious circles can sometimes be broken by the seemingly paradoxical use of heparin, usually in less than full anticoagulating doses. This slows the consumption of various coagulation factors, allowing their replenishment, and stops the active fibrinolysis and production of fibrin/fibrinogen degradation products. The stimuli produced by severed vessels are still sufficient to allow coagulation to occur where needed. This sounds appealing in concept, but the proper balance between harmful and helpful coagulation is unlikely to be easily found. Removal of the cause is more effective and eventually necessary.

The other type of DIC is less well understood and much more resistant to treatment. It carries a very poor outlook for recovery. It is also characterized by ongoing intravascular consumption and fibrinolysis with a breakdown in hemostasis. Spontaneous bleeding and bleeding from recent wounds, even trivial ones, are very common. Characteristically, even venipuncture sites become loci of hemorrhage. Bleeding from the skin is very common, but bleeding into body cavities is the most difficult to control. Reoperation for hemostasis at this stage usually is futile and may initiate bleeding from new sites. Often the antecedent events are (1) severe infection, especially with gram-negative organisms, usually persisting for at least several days with poor control and often with hypotension; (2) severe and sustained hypoperfusion, often in conjunction with serious tissue damage; and (3) severe liver disease, especially acute ischemic injury to the liver (some of the most spectacular examples are seen following transplantation of the liver).

These conditions carry the possibility of the release of thromboplastic material. Endotoxin has such properties: it activates factor XII and it causes the aggregation and release reaction in platelets. Ischemia may cause the release of thromboplastic materials from damaged cells and may even trigger the release of plasminogen activators as a response to impaired flow of blood. The central role of the liver in coagulation and fibrinolysis has been described. Hypoperfusion of the liver may be an important factor in the DIC that occurs during severe hemorrhage. Whatever the cause, the use of heparin in this setting has not been successful, and some think it contraindicated. Use of heparin in combination with fibrinolytic inhibitors has more appeal in theory, but the complexity of the disorder is so great that little success has followed this approach. Use of fibrinolytic inhibitors without heparin is unwise because the fibrinolytic response is protecting the circulation from unnecessary coagulation. The few survivors of florid posttraumatic or postseptic DIC have been mainly relatively young patients in otherwise good health whose perfusion could be sustained by infusion of the appropriate materials and in whom the inciting factors could be removed or controlled. Under those circumstances, reversal of the severe disorders of coagulation usually occurred after several hours of adequate perfusion.

There are a number of unfortunate coincidences that make DIC difficult to reverse, once established. Factors I, II, V, and VIII are consumed during coagulation and are also attacked by plasmin; factors V and VIII deteriorate during storage of blood in the liquid state; factors I, II, and V are produced in the liver, making synthesis vulnerable to changes in hepatic perfusion. Some of the products of fibrin/fibrinogenolysis interfere with platelet function and with polymerization of fibrin; these products are cleared from the circulation primarily by the liver.

It is highly likely that the term DIC as now used covers a disparate group of acute and chronic disorders with different mechanisms, courses, and optimal treatments, including the acute disorder in surgical patients now thought to be a single entity. Better classification, characterization, understanding, and treatment will probably follow the development of reliable tests specific for various events in the hemostatic sequences.

Therapeutic use of fibrinolytic drugs is becoming more common.[46] Such drugs induce activation of plasmin with the aim of lysing recently formed clots. Such agents are particularly hazardous in patients who have had operations within a week to 10 days, especially in deep body cavities where bleeding cannot be easily detected or controlled by direct pressure. One must be particularly well informed in this area to safely use these drugs in postoperative or posttraumatic patients. It was hoped that one of the forms of tPA used therapeutically would produce lysis of recent clots with fewer hemorrhagic side effects, but there is some doubt now that this expensive agent is significantly superior to streptokinase, which is less expensive but very antigenic.

LABORATORY TESTS AND EVALUATION OF THE PATIENT'S CONDITION

Although there is a seemingly bewildering array of tests of hemostatic function, relatively few are in general use and of interest to those who are not expert in this area.

The tests relating to coagulation are the most familiar. Whole blood clotting time theoretically measures the intrinsic and common pathways, but the test is too variable, too insensitive to important changes, and too sensitive to unimportant changes. The recalcification time using citrated whole blood or separated platelet-rich plasma is more reproducible but shares the same problems of sensitivity. The one-stage prothrombin time (PT) measures the time required to form clot in citrated plasma at 37° C. after calcium and a standardized tissue thromboplastin are added. This reflects the extrinsic and common pathways, factors I, II, V, VII, and X, but is most sensitive to deficiencies in VII. This makes it suitable for following therapy with vitamin K antagonists but allows only an approximate correlation with clinical thrombosis or bleeding. A variant usually called the "P and P" test or Thrombotest measures the vitamin K–dependent factors more exclusively by adding factor V from adsorbed bovine plasma. If Russell's viper venom (Stypven) is used as the thromboplastin in the PT, factor VII is bypassed and the common pathway is measured. The partial thromboplastin time (PTT) is similar to the PT but uses a phospholipid similar to platelet factor III instead of a tissue thromboplastin. The activated PTT is used in most centers; this includes use of kaolin to ensure complete activation of factor XII. The intrinsic and common pathways are measured. The results are very reproducible, but the greatest sensitivity is to the intrinsic pathway factors, which correlate poorly with clinical events. The test is quite useful, however, for screening for the hemophilias and following treatment in such patients, for detecting coagulopathies in patients with hepatic insufficiency and following treatment, and for following serial changes in patients with DIC. Recently the test has been popular for regulating the dose of heparin. The theoretical basis for this is questionable, but some evidence of efficacy has been reported.[23] The thrombin time measures the time required for plasma to form a gross clot after addition of a standard solution of thrombin. This is primarily sensitive to the conversion of fibrinogen to fibrin and the polymerization of fibrin, but the test is sensitive to the concentration of fibrinogen only when it is very low (below 90 mg. per 100 ml.). The test is very sensitive to the presence of circulating anticoagulants or abnormalities in fibrinogen, which includes the presence of fibrin(ogen) breakdown products. Reptilase-R can be used instead of thrombin in the test, making it less sensitive to heparin.

Fibrinogen is the easiest of the individual coagulation factors to measure, but the results can be misleading. Chemical assays may measure nonclottable fibrinogen, whereas methods that rely on conversion to fibrin by the action of thrombin are subject to the same influences as is the thrombin time. Factor VIII can now be measured readily in most centers. The other coagulation components can be measured individually with varying degrees of difficulty; prothrombin is still very difficult to measure directly.

In assessing platelets one usually begins with the platelet count.[16] As noted previously, the relationship of the platelet count to the bleeding time, much less to clinical bleeding, is complex and is very sensitive to the functional status of the platelets. The template bleeding time may be the most useful screening test for platelet function, but it is very sensitive to variations in technique. More sophisticated and specific tests involve measurement of aggregation in response to various stimuli and agonists; collagen, ADP, and epinephrine are the most frequently used. Assays of the release reactions are more expensive and laborious; serotonin and platelet factor III are often measured. Recently, an assay for a component of platelet cell walls that circulates during platelet destruction has been reported. This may help distinguish platelet-destructive disorders from those due to failure of production.[42]

The most rapidly developing area is that dealing with the fibrinolytic and inhibitor side of coagulation. Most of the major circulating inhibitors can now be measured independently, including protein C. Measurements of fibrinolytic components are still largely indirect.[46] The euglobulin lysis time is an older test that reflects the concentration of plasminogen and was the most frequently used test for detecting fibrinolytic effects in the various controlled trials of fibrinolytic agents. Fibrin plate lysis measures the fibrinolytic activity of plasma and with modifications can measure plasminogen, plasmin, or plasmin inhibitors. The test requires nearly 24 hours for completion, but use of a radiolabeled substrate can hasten the production of reproducible results in exchange for an increased cost. Casein is substituted for fibrin in some versions.

Tests for measurement of specific products of the activity of plasmin and of thrombin are being developed. These are largely research tools, but in theory they would allow a much more detailed analysis of hemostatic events in vivo. At the moment, clinical use of tests such as these is largely limited to the measurement of products of fibrinolysis by indirect methods. These rely on reactions whose mechanisms are not fully understood, such as clumping of certain strains of staphylococci or formation of clots in ethanol gel or protamine gel when fibrin monomers or complexes or split products of fibrin(ogen) are added. These tests are difficult to evaluate but usually appear helpful despite an occasional false-positive or false-negative reaction. More specific, quantitative, and reproducible assays would be welcome, and some are under development.

Screening tests for circulating anticoagulants are based on various schemes combining the patient's plasma with normal pooled plasma. In general, prolongation of various screening tests due to deficiencies in the patient's plasma will be corrected by addition of relatively small amounts of pooled normal plasma. Prolongations due to circulating anticoagulants may not be corrected by addition of even large amounts of normal plasma.

Surgical patients undergoing evaluation of their hemostatic status form two distinct groups: patients who are bleeding and those who are not. Surgical patients who are not bleeding vastly outnumber those who are, and the most common hemostatic evaluation occurs in the setting of a patient about to undergo an operation. There has perhaps been more money wasted and blood unnecessarily shed in this setting than in any other in medicine. It has been known for a long time that the best screening test for hemostasis in surgical patients is a carefully obtained history soliciting evidence of hemostatic defects in the patient and in close relatives. Past responses to planned or accidental injuries should be known; if none can be recalled, family members should be questioned. Brushing the teeth can constitute a significant test of hemostasis in some settings. Almost as important today is a history of drugs taken regularly and irregularly; platelet-impairing drugs are quite numerous. Most of these do not substantially increase surgical bleeding, but some can lead to unnecessary confusion and consternation if certain laboratory tests of hemostasis are performed. The history is so valuable a screen that it makes laboratory screening of hemostasis unnecessary in most patients who can give an adequate history. Despite this fact, such patients are routinely submitted to a "preoperative screen" of hemostatic function in many practices. To this author's knowledge, the balance of evidence is that such a practice can be very wasteful.[35] Even attempts to rationalize the approach are suspect. Rapaport proposed a scheme for evaluating hemostatic function in preoperative patients that has received considerable favorable comment.[33] The scheme categorizes patients into one of four groups and determines the need for evaluation by the grouping. Group 1 is patients with a reassuring history who are facing relatively bloodless operations. No screening is indicated; no argument there. Group 2 is patients with a reassuring history who are to undergo major operative procedures. A battery of hemostatic screening tests is proposed for such patients. This is a relatively large number of patients each year in the United States and there is almost no evidence that they need or benefit from such screening. Groups 3 and 4 have reasons to suspect hemostatic disorders or are to undergo procedures at high risk for abnormal bleeding (e.g., cardiopulmonary bypass) or in which even small increases in bleeding could be disastrous (e.g., central venous system). The recommendations for laboratory evaluation are reasonable. The problems with unnecessary screening tests go beyond economics. A large number of tests in a normal population involve some abnormalities in laboratory results where no disease or disorder exists. Having obtained nonindicated screening tests, relatively minor abnormalities are too often pursued with vigor, greatly increasing the waste of money and unnecessary apprehension in a patient who has successfully withstood a lifetime of the slings and arrows of outrageous fortune only to be told that there is something wrong with his clotting ability that must be pursued. Tragically, some patients eventually receive potentially dangerous material to correct an abnormality that never existed and should never have been sought.

For the bleeding patient, the history is at least as important. In addition, the setting in the patient must be carefully and fully elucidated: hepatic, renal, immunologic, circulatory function, the presence of conditions associated with acquired disorders of hemostasis (dead tissue, malignancies, uncontrolled infection, marrow-suppressing drugs, drugs that can impair platelet function or suppress vitamin K–dependent proteins), local factors such as reoperation through dense scar or previously irradiated tissues. In the setting of the bleeding patient, laboratory testing is mandatory, even if a plausible hypothesis has already been formed. Treatment should be chosen in conjunction with the results of appropriate tests and guided by serial changes in those tests. The significantly bleeding patient should be treated empirically only when appropriate tests are not available in a timely manner or no clear pattern to guide treatment can be discerned. Most often the latter situation arises when the cause of the bleeding is mechanical. Poor mechanical hemostasis is the most common cause of significant bleeding in a postoperative patient. Stated another way, the most common postoperative coagulation defect is silk. There is always a temptation to shift the blame for a poor result to the patient. The good surgeon knows when to stop seeking unusual conditions and to face the need for re-exploration and better surgical hemostasis. In the unusual situation, knowledge of the various hemostatic disorders and the methods of diagnosis and management is invaluable, but more often the craft of surgery is the critical variable.

PRODUCTS THAT AID HEMOSTASIS

Products that augment or replace components of the coagulation system are available from the blood bank in most hospitals (Table 5). Usually, expert advice on many aspects of their use is available from the same source. Some of the clinically important features of various members of the coagulation system are depicted in Table 2.

Fresh frozen plasma (FFP) is the plasma component of whole blood separated soon after collection and immediately frozen and stored in the frozen state. Most of the coagulation factors approach the concentration in normal plasma when the product is thawed and infused. The longer the interval between thawing and infusion, the greater the loss of labile factors (such as V and VIII). None of the factors is in a concentration greater than normal. Therefore, FFP (and very fresh whole blood) provides an excellent spectrum of coagulation components, but rather large volumes are required to raise levels appreciably in recipients. As indicated in Table 5, FFP is the most usable source of factor V; there is no concentrated form of factor V currently

available. FFP thus has an important role in the management of patients with multiple coagulation defects resulting from hepatic insufficiency, patients with DIC who need replacement of consumed and lysed factors, and rarely (and doubtfully) the patient in whom the labile coagulation components have been depleted by the transfusion of very large amounts of old stored blood. In practice, liquid stored plasma is now available only in the form of FFP, so it is used in other situations, for example, to rapidly reverse the deficits in patients who have been taking vitamin K antagonists. The use of FFP in the United States has risen dramatically in the past decade, seemingly far out of proportion to reasonable estimates of need. The recent consensus conferences of the National Institutes of Health confirmed the preceding group of indications for use and questioned the safety of its use in other circumstances. FFP is a single-donor product with the same risk of transmitting viral diseases as that of whole blood. It contains the major anti-A, B, and Rh antibodies, so type- and Rh-specific plasma should be used.

Cryoprecipitate is probably the next most used aid to coagulation in the blood bank. It is a source of factor VIII and vWF in concentrated form. It also contains about one third the amount of fibrinogen found in a unit of whole blood, which is potentially important because fibrinogen is no longer available in concentrated form. Cryoprecipitate is also a source of factor XIII and fibronectin. The major advantages of cryoprecipitate are its small volume and its single-donor status. Cryoprecipitate contains small amounts of anti-A, B, and Rh antibodies. These usually cause no problems unless large amounts of cryoprecipitate are used. Hemolytic anemia can then occur and be confused with hidden hemorrhage.

There are various commercially prepared factor VIII concentrates, which contain factor VIII and variable amounts of vWF. Their advantages are ease of handling and storage and their high concentrations of factor VIII without fibrinogen. The disadvantage is their rate of transmitting disease—these are plasma products pooled from large populations. Recent methods of controlled heating appear to have eliminated the risk of transmitting human immunodeficiency virus (HIV), a major problem for hemophiliacs in the last decade. The impact of these controlled heating methods on the transmission of hepatitis may also be beneficial.[37] Over a lifetime of use, the risk of hepatitis may well be the same for the pooled products as for single-donor cryoprecipitate because the cumulative exposure to donors will be great in either case.

The other category of commercially prepared coagulation factor concentrate involves the prothrombin complex factors: II, VII, IX, and X. Factor VII is usually present in somewhat lower concentrations than the others. This product was designed for use in patients with factor IX deficiency (hemophilia B), for whom there is no other product that has factor IX in concentrated form. It is obviously also suited to patients who need

TABLE 5. Hemostatic Factors in Commonly Available Blood Component Products (units/ml.)

Hemostatic Factor	Fresh Frozen Plasma (250 ml.)	Cryoprecipitate (10 ml.)	Factor VIII Concentrate (10–30 ml.)	Prothrombin Complex Concentrate (20–30 ml.)	Platelet-Rich Plasma (250 ml.)	Platelet Concentrate (25 ml.)
I	(3 mg./ml.)	(150 mg./bag)	Small	0	3 mg./ml.	3 mg./ml.
II	0.9	0	0	<10	0.9	0.9
V	0.6	0	0	0	<0.3	<0.3
VII	0.9	0	0	<25	0.9	0.9
VIII	0.8	80 Units/bag	High; labeled	0	?0.5	?0.5
von Willebrand	?Normal	High	Variable	0	?Normal	?Normal
IX	0.9	0	0	25	0.9	0.9
X	0.9	0	0	<25	0.9	0.9
XI	0.9	0	0	0	<0.9	<0.9
XII	0.9	0	0	0	0.5	0.5
Platelets	0	0	0	0	Labeled	Labeled

rapid reversal of the effects of vitamin K antagonists. Its detrimental effects were the high risk of transmitting hepatitis and HIV, but the latter has probably also been eliminated by production methods using controlled heating. This product had an unusual additional problem: some lots caused a high incidence of serious thromboembolic events, especially with rapid infusion after injury. Various *in vitro* and experimental *in vivo* assays for hypercoagulability correlated approximately with the reported incidence of thromboembolic complications. Lots are now screened for this effect and suspicious lots are eliminated. Some of the most active were reserved for use in patients with hemophilia A who had high levels of inhibitors to infused factor VIII, an interesting example of turning a disadvantage to good use. This use is not proven in rigidly controlled trials, but enjoys some popularity. These "hypercoagulable" products have also been used by some in patients with severe diffuse oozing after cardiopulmonary bypass. Unusual thrombotic complications have not been reported in this setting; it may be that the several hemostatic defects after bypass are protective.[22] This use is unproven by anything approaching a controlled trial, however, and such patients, unlike hemophiliacs, are at considerable risk of contracting hepatitis from such exposures.

Fibrinogen is no longer a licensed product in the United States. The indications for use have always been uncertain, the incidence of hepatitis following use has been very high, and a safer alternative is now available in cryoprecipitate.

Platelets are prepared in each blood bank or regional blood center as needed because platelets cannot be stored for more than a few days.[39] Methods allowing longer periods of storage are being investigated and may be available soon. Most of the time platelets are used in "packs" containing the platelets from a single donor in 30 to 50 ml. plasma. The number of platelets recovered varies with the techniques used, and it is well to inquire periodically with local sources as to the average concentration of platelets in their products. It is highly advisable to measure the platelet concentration in the recipient's blood several times after infusion (1 and 24 hours are useful) to determine the immediate response to the infused platelets and their persistence after infusion. The effect of infusing platelets varies with the hemostatic status of the patient. Large oozing areas can consume administered platelets very rapidly, and the amount required for clinical effect may be impossible to predict before infusion. Infection, fever, previous infusion of platelets, enlarged spleen, and active bleeding are all associated with a less-than-expected response to infused platelets.

The prophylactic use of platelets, that is, giving platelets to prevent possible bleeding, is a very uncertain area. The concentration of platelets in the patient's blood is certainly important, but a significant increase in the amount of blood lost spontaneously into the gastrointestinal tracts of patients with suppressed production of platelets was found only at platelet concentrations below 10,000 per μl. Prospective studies in patients with leukemia showed beneficial effects of administering platelets when the patient's platelet count fell below 20,000 per μl., but lower concentrations were not tested and many think this "trigger" can be safely set at a lower level. Patients with idiopathic thrombocytopenic purpura usually have their platelet disorder corrected or at least improved by splenectomy. If such patients are not bleeding spontaneously before operation, they can usually safely undergo splenectomy even with extremely low concentrations of platelets, down to 5000 per μl. Some compound the error of giving platelets unnecessarily to these patients by giving the platelets when the spleen is still in the circulation, which is less beneficial than throwing the platelets away — at least then the patient would not be risking serious disease unnecessarily. Two prospective controlled studies in patients undergoing cardiopulmonary bypass showed no benefit from prophylactic use of platelets, and an important prospective controlled study in heavily transfused trauma patients yielded the same negative results.[34] Thus, prophylactic use of platelets

in surgical patients appears rarely if ever indicated, a conclusion shared by the recent NIH consensus conference on the use of platelets. Platelets are usually given as the recovered platelets from several donors. The risk of transmitted disease is directly proportional to the number of donors. An additional disadvantage to unnecessary use is the considerable immunizing potential of platelets; if subsequently truly needed, they may be much less effective because of the production of platelet-specific antibodies. Because of the donor plasma present, platelets must be ABO-compatible with the recipient's blood. In addition, there are a few red cells present in the platelet preparations, so they should be Rh-compatible, especially in recipients with the potential for pregnancy.

Topical hemostatic aids are supposed to promote clotting at the level of the bleeding vessel. Actually, most promote the coagulation of shed blood. Topical thrombin is prepared from bovine blood and is probably most extensively used in dentistry. Gelatins come in various forms, including sponges and sheets. They promote the coagulation of blood on contact and provide some biodegradable bulk that can be pressed against a bleeding surface. In practice, topical thrombin is often used with a gelatin sponge rather than alone. A more recent product, microfibrillar collagen, is a powder derived from bovine collagen that promotes platelet aggregation and the release reaction on contact. This has certain theoretical advantages over products that act on coagulation alone, but it should be remembered that application on the surface of a bleeding wound does not necessarily mean contact with the cut ends of bleeding vessels. The main disadvantage of many of these materials is the addition of foreign material to an area of uncertain hemostasis, which creates an added hazard of infection. A more subtle disadvantage is the belief that hemostasis is being produced in some situations when it is not. The cost of these products can be significant. Recently, various mixtures of fibrinogen and thrombin, freshly mixed, have been developed for local injection into oozing surfaces. This is a somewhat strange approach to hemostasis, and the potential for transmitting disease by these components must be very carefully monitored. Finally, advances continue to be made in an old but proven hemostatic aid, electrocautery. Variations now include laser coagulation at various wavelengths and, recently, a controllable jet of "activated" argon. The more exotic these approaches become, the more one is compelled to emphasize that gentle handling, precise dissection, and accurately applied hemostasis involving minimal destruction of tissue and the least possible addition of foreign material constitute much of the art of surgery. Injecting, burning, stuffing, and scorching wounds is not likely to lead to a higher plateau of accomplishment.

RED BLOOD CELL PRODUCTS

Eventually, continuing hemorrhage requires the transfusion of red cells. The red blood cell products are the most commonly used products of the blood bank. Like the coagulation products, their use is steadily increasing but not as rapidly.

The most common indication for transfusing red cells is to increase the recipient's mass of red cells. Transfused red cells are removed from the circulation in two ways: rapid (within 24 hours) removal of dead or damaged red cells, and removal of the remainder at the normal rate as they reach senescence. The amount that is rapidly removed is a function of the age of storage and varies with individual units, but should rarely be as much as 25 per cent of the transfused cells. With relatively fresh blood it will be less than 10 per cent. Transfused red cells are thus only a temporary supplement to the recipient's supply. As this temporary increment is achieved at some risk, the indications for this temporary increase should be clear-cut and imperative.

The indications for transfusion for the correction of anemia are not simple. The problem is one of deciding when and to what degree oxygen delivery needs improvement. Oxygen delivery involves pulmonary, circulatory, and cellular metabolic components. The oxygen-carrying capacity of the blood is an important, but not the only, component, and it is not the only one altered by transfusion. If the recipient is also hypovolemic, the expansion of the blood volume achieved by transfusion may be more beneficial to oxygen delivery than the increase in the red cell mass. If the patient is hypervolemic, transfusion may precipitate pulmonary edema and thereby worsen oxygen delivery. Nevertheless, the change in hematocrit is usually the most decisive impact that transfusion of red cells has on oxygen delivery.

The relationship between hematocrit and oxygen delivery is complex. The oxygen content of blood varies directly and linearly with changes in the hematocrit, but the resistance of blood to flow varies inversely with changes in hematocrit. This latter relationship is very complex and still not completely understood. Some fairly simple extrapolations to clinical situations have been proposed based on experiments *in vitro*, but it is clear that important variables, such as the geometry of the system, the surfaces in contact with the blood, and the velocity of flow, all differed significantly from the conditions that apply *in vivo*. Such analyses and predictions may be possible when more sophisticated techniques of studying the flow properties of blood become available.

Studies in intact animals are also somewhat contradictory. Anemia is always accompanied by an increase in cardiac output if blood volume is kept constant. Some believe that this occurs not in response to peripheral hypoxic signals but instead represents increased flow because of decreased resistance of the anemic blood to flow. In this scheme there is no new work by the heart, which means that anemia is self-correcting, at least within limits, because the cost-free increase in flow compensates for the decrease in oxygen content per unit of blood. Although an element of such self-correction may be operative in anemic states, most chronically anemic patients and animals develop left ventricular hypertrophy. This is very strong evidence of increased work by the heart during anemia and is clearly incompatible with the completely self-correcting hypothesis.

Numerous experiments in animals have dealt with a variety of challenges (hemorrhage, stopping the heart, acute hypoxia), a variety of end points (survival, neurologic function, cardiac function, tissue oxygen tension), and a variety of mammalian species, all testing the effects of different hematocrits. Most, but not all, of these experiments indicated the most favorable results at hematocrits that were near normal at the time of the challenge. Stress testing of anemic human volunteers, however, in sophisticated crossover studies with patients serving as their own controls, indicated little impairment of work performance or intellectual functioning at hematocrits down to about 60 per cent of normal. The remarkable discrepancy between the results of these two groups of experiments was explained when the autoregulatory functions of the red cell became known. By increasing the production of 2,3-diphosphoglyceric acid (2,3-DPG), most mammalian red cells (including human) lower the affinity of their hemoglobin for oxygen. Because of the shape of the oxyhemoglobin dissociation curve, this results in slightly less oxygen being picked up in the lungs, but much more oxygen being released in the capillary bed. Thus, oxygen delivery is increased with no change in the amount of hemoglobin or in the oxygen tensions in the pulmonary alveoli or the peripheral tissues and no increased work by the heart. It is a marvelously efficient response. At maximal production of 2,3-DPG, human red cells can nearly double their efficiency as oxygen-delivering agents under physiologic conditions at the cost of consumption of a bit more glucose. This explains the findings in the human volunteers, most of whom were chronically anemic. The studies in animals were almost all done with acutely induced anemia. This compensatory mecha-

nism also explains the well-known benignity of chronic anemia, and it suggests caution in the zealous approach to correcting anemia in patients. The response is not immediate, but it is usually well developed by several days after hemorrhage. The rate of response is affected by blood pH (increased by alkalosis) and serum phosphate (impaired by hypophosphatemia). Even under the best circumstances, it cannot compensate for the loss of more than half the normal amount of hemoglobin.

In recent years, several studies on agricultural field workers in economically poor countries have produced results that appear to contradict those just described.[2,18] In these studies, the ability to produce by manual labor appeared to be directly related to the concentration of hemoglobin in the laborer's blood. It appears clear in several of these studies, however, that the laborers were suffering from multiple nutritional deficiencies, parasitic infections, and perhaps other significant illnesses. In one study, productivity increased almost as much in the control group given a placebo containing several hundred calories per day as in the study group given iron to correct the anemia. The studies done in industrialized countries, which found little effect of moderate degrees of anemia, were performed in well-nourished, otherwise healthy subjects. The results of the studies in economically poor countries suggest that the ability to compensate for anemia may not be as great in patients with multiple deficiencies.

The vulnerability of the heart in some anemic patients deserves emphasis. The mixed venous oxygen tension of the human heart is always near its minimal functioning value. This peculiar situation means the heart cannot extract more oxygen from the available blood in times of stress by working at a lower oxygen tension, but must instead rely on increased flow of blood. This points to the great importance of coronary artery dilation in times of stress. Experiments nearly 40 years ago on isolated perfused hearts showed that these hearts could function quite well when the hematocrit of the blood perfusing them was lowered significantly.[7] If the coronary arteries were banded so that they could not expand, however, every decrease in hematocrit was accompanied by a decrease in left ventricular function. The clinical equivalent of these experiments is the patient with anemia and coronary arterial insufficiency. Such patients can often detect when their anemia reaches a certain level because at that point they develop ischemic pain or congestive failure, which can be relieved by judicious transfusion of red cells. Studies in patients with arterial insufficiency in other areas have been somewhat contradictory, but at least some found that lowering the hematocrit even moderately in patients with intermittent claudication impaired rather than improved performance.[50]

In trying to devise a rational set of guidelines for the treatment of anemia by transfusion, one finds several circumstances that favor transfusion and several that weigh against it. Militating against transfusion are the facts that transfusion involves significant risk to the recipient, the benefit gained is temporary, and the supply of red cells for transfusion is tenuous at certain times of the year. Under the proper circumstances, anemia down to half the normal level of hemoglobin can be very well tolerated. Even lower levels may be acceptable if no undue demands are made on the oxygen-delivering system and endogenous replacement is likely. Patients who are stable and doing well should be allowed to replace their own red cell mass. Favoring transfusion for anemia are conditions in which the patient might soon face increased demands or further significant blood loss or in which there are pre-existing disorders, especially coronary arteriosclerosis, that make anemia less well tolerated. Thus, a 20-year-old man doing well on the day after a splenectomy for trauma should not be transfused for a hematocrit in the low 20s, whereas an elderly woman with known heart disease may well require transfusion for a hematocrit 10 points higher on the day following exploration for a perforated colonic diverticulum with extensive peritonitis. The key should be individualization, with emphasis on how the patient is tolerating the anemia and what challenges are faced before endogenous correction can occur. The too common practice of using a single trigger for transfusing all patients, commonly a hematocrit of 30 per cent, is to be firmly condemned. There is no good evidence supporting such a practice, and by its very nature it is unscientific and clinically harmful.[6]

Massive hemorrhage (hemorrhage that threatens to result in exsanguination) is best treated by transfusion with whole blood, which simultaneously provides oxygen-delivering capacity and volume. Most transfusions are not for imminent exsanguination, however. These are better performed with red cell concentrates or the equivalent. This reduces the volume required for administration, reduces the recipient's exposure to some of the potentially harmful substances in the plasma phase, and allows separation, salvage, and specific use of components that would be lost during liquid storage as whole blood (platelets, cryoprecipitate, fresh frozen plasma). Thus, one donation of blood can serve several purposes, and the flexibility and range of products offered by the modern blood bank becomes possible. Most surgeons understand the added tragedy of not harvesting potentially transplantable organs when a young patient dies. Storing blood as whole blood is exactly analogous: potentially useful components are lost to everyone.

Most red cell products are currently stored in the liquid state in a citrate-based anticoagulant. Citrate binds calcium sufficiently to prevent clotting, is not metabolized during storage, and is a normal intermediary metabolite that is rapidly consumed after transfusion. It has been the basis of storage solutions since the inception of modern blood banking, and it would be difficult to find a more ideal substance. As now used, the preservative solution contains added adenine and glucose, which allows the storage of red cells for up to 5 weeks in the liquid state. Recently, a new method of storage has gained some popularity. The blood is collected in a citrate-based anticoagulant, but most of this is separated for storage of the various hemostatic components. The red cell fraction is then stored in a simpler electrolyte solution that may contain some citrate (much less than previously) and a small amount of mannitol for its osmotic effect. In this form, the amount of citrate is much less, as is the amount of plasma. The resulting solution, largely red cells suspended in a simple electrolyte solution, is much easier to infuse rapidly because of the lower viscosity.

Except in this newer form, red cell concentrates are whole blood with 70 to 80 per cent of the plasma removed. There is otherwise little difference from stored whole blood. A unit of whole blood consists of 450 ml. of donor blood in 63 ml. of citrate-phosphate-dextrose-adenine (CPDA) anticoagulant. Potentially significant changes occur in blood during storage, some of which are listed in Table 6. A less commonly used preparation is "whole blood, modified," which means that platelets and cryoprecipitate were removed soon after collection and the remaining plasma was rejoined with the red cells. As both platelets and factor VIII lose their activity during storage, this makes the product little different from stored whole blood. Whole blood is sometimes collected in heparin for special purposes, e.g., for neonatal exchange transfusion. Heparin is useful for no more than 48 hours of storage.

Frozen red cells are red cells separated from plasma and maintained frozen in a cryopreservative (glycerol). To be used they must be thawed and repeatedly washed to remove the cryopreservative. They are transfused in a simple electrolyte solution within 24 hours of thawing. The cells maintain the functional characteristics in effect when they were frozen while they remain frozen. Thus, if frozen directly after collection, they are the functional equivalent of freshly drawn red cells, even if thawed several years later. This functional preservation and the very long allowable period of storage in the frozen state are the main advantages of this method of preservation. The main dis-

TABLE 6. Metabolic and Related Changes During Storage; Value for Third Week of Storage of Whole Blood in CPD

Metabolic acid load	25–40 mEq./L.
Citrate	5 mEq./L.
Phosphate	6–10 mg./L. plasma
Ammonia	Up to 1 mg./100 ml.
Plasma hemoglobin	20 mg./100 ml.
Particulate matter	Up to 2–4 gm./unit
Negative thermal load	14.4 kcal./unit at 4° C.
Plasticizer	20–25 mg./unit
Red cells	
Posttransfusion early loss	20–25%
2,3-DPG	0
ATP	Very low
Membrane lipids	Depleted
Osmotic fragility	Increased
Coagulation	
Factor V	Probably 10% or less
Factor VIII	Probably 30% or less
Platelets	0
Antigenic debris	Considerable (HL-A, platelet, red cell, leukocyte, plasma protein antigens)
Transmissible diseases	See text
Denatured proteins	Likely but undefined
Vasoactive substances	Serotonin, bradykinin, histamine, ?others

advantages are cost (probably at least double that of liquid storage) and the loss of at least 10 per cent of the red cells in processing.

Washing red cells, either as part of deglycerolization or as applied to liquid-stored red cells, removes most of the plasma, in excess of 99 per cent by some methods. This means removal of most of the potentially harmful elements of the plasma fraction. Unfortunately, this appears not to eliminate the transmission of hepatitis; data on the transmission of HIV are not available. Red cell concentrates do not have a lesser risk of transmitting viral diseases than does whole blood; the amount of plasma remaining is much too large. Red cells treated in a number of ways to reduce the amount of leukocyte and platelet debris are useful for patients requiring transfusion who react to such antigens (the most common cause of febrile transfusion reactions in the United States) and for patients who are likely to require red cell transfusions repeatedly over long periods in order to minimize immunization against such antigens.

RISKS OF TRANSFUSION

The human blood group antigens A and B are widely distributed in plants and in microbial products. Therefore, almost all humans form antibodies to these antigens at an early age if they lack the antigen as part of their normal body composition.[30] The antibodies formed are usually hemolytic. Thus, infusing red cells of blood group A or B into a recipient lacking that blood group antigen is likely to produce acute intravascular hemolysis, which, in turn, often results in DIC and acute renal failure. The chance of dying from such an event is not clearly known, but under the best of circumstances it is estimated to be greater than 10 per cent and in the absence of prompt recognition and treatment will be much greater. The reverse problem also exists: if enough plasma products containing anti-A or anti-B are infused into a recipient whose red cells contain A or B, hemolysis will also occur. Because the number of targets in such a situation greatly exceeds the amount of antibody, hemolysis is usually less explosive and less likely to produce serious complications, but this reaction should not be assumed to be safe. In the United States, most hemolytic reactions caused by transfusion result from misidentification that occurs outside the blood bank: either the blood product or the patient is misidentified, or the blood sample sent for typing and crossmatching is mislabelled. It is because of the gravity of such an error that most hospitals have somewhat elaborate and rigid requirements for identification of the recipient and confirmation of the product before infusion, usually by at least two people. These safeguards should not be bypassed.

The other blood group antigens, including those of the Rh system, are usually clinically important only in patients who have been transfused previously or who have had multiple pregnancies. These observations led to the concept of safe donor blood for dire emergencies when crossmatching or even typing would require too much time. One can use type- and Rh-specific blood, which requires about 10 minutes after a clotted sample arrives in the blood bank to determine the recipient's type, or one can use type O blood, which can be given immediately. The use of type O is preferable when there are multiple casualties and the risk of mix-up is therefore greater; this was the approach used by the United States military in Korea and in Vietnam. Waiting longer and accepting a slightly higher risk of misidentification with the use of type- and Rh-specific blood avoids overuse of type O and the immunization of the 15 per cent of recipients who are Rh-negative.

A list of transfusion reactions is given in Table 7. The important points are that most hemolytic transfusion reactions are serious, carrying significant morbidity and mortality, and most are due to human error. Giving blood at random from one human to another has about one chance in three of resulting in major intravascular hemolysis. Most such patients can die of that event. Few things in clinical medicine are as dangerous as giving one person's blood to someone else: *great care must be taken.*

The most frequent serious complication directly attributable to transfusion is the transmission of disease. Whereas many diseases have been transmitted by transfusion, the most important is hepatitis. At least 80 per cent of the hepatitis transmitted by transfusion in the United States is not among the recognized types.[1] It is called non-A, non-B hepatitis (NANB) because it appears to be several viral diseases. It is less deadly than hepatitis B initially and is more often subclinical, but it is prominently associated with chronic active hepatitis and posthepatitis cirrhosis.[38] With an all-volunteer donor population, about 7 per cent of transfused patients develop laboratory evidence of hepatitis within 6 months after transfusion. The incidence after exposure to a single donor is not clear because so few transfused patients are now exposed to only one donor (an interesting observation in itself), but evidence from some prospective studies indicates an incidence of about 1.5 to 4 per cent. Evidence from several sources suggests the incidence of hepatitis is proportional to the exposure to donors, at least up to about 6 to 10 units transfused, but data from other studies found no such relationship. The difficulty again is the skewed distribution of exposure in transfused patients; the great majority are exposed to 3 or 4 donors and there are relatively few survivors at other levels of exposure. The level of alanine aminotransferase in the

TABLE 7. Characteristics of Various Types of Transfusion Reactions

Type	Incidence	Inciting Component	Manifestations	Course, Treatment, or Prevention
Non–Red Cell				
Allergic	About 1%	Plasma proteins	Hives, pruritus	Usually mild; antihistamines; use washed red cells
Febrile	Not rare with repeated transfusions	Leukocyte antigens	Fever, chills, flushing, occasionally fatal	Stop transfusion if severe; use buffy coat–poor red cells
Anaphylactoid	Rare	IgA	Vascular collapse, abdominal pain, diarrhea, bronchospasm, chills, fever	Stop transfusion, support circulation
Pulmonary "hyper-sensitivity"	Rare	Usually leukocyte antigen	Normovolemic pulmonary edema	Stop transfusion, support ventilation
Graft vs. host	Very rare	Donor lymphocytes vs. immunosuppressed recipient	Late: bone marrow, gastrointestinal, liver, skin manifestations	Irradiate blood for transfusion
Purpura	Very rare	Platelet antigen and antibody (usually $P1^{A1}$)	Purpura 1 week after transfusion	Exchange transfusion or plasmapheresis
Red Cell				
Immediate hemolysis	Infrequent	A, B, occasionally Rh incompatibility	Hemoglobinemia, hemoglobulinuria, DIC, acute renal failure	Care in using blood—almost always due to human error; stop transfusion, back-check; expand blood volume
Delayed hemolysis	Infrequent	Red cell antigen other than A, B	Anemia, perhaps icterus, occasionally renal failure	General support; back-check to find offending antigen
Iatrogenic hemolysis	?	Administering blood through 5% dextrose/water	Same as immediate hemolysis	Same as immediate hemolysis
Iatrogenic clotting	?	Administering blood through calcium-containing solution (usually lactated Ringer's)	Clotting of line; pulmonary emboli if pushed	Common sense
OtherTypes of Reactions				
Contaminated blood	Very rare	Bacteria, endotoxin in stored blood	Septic shock	Stop transfusion; support circulation; culture recipient's blood (include cold-growing organisms); Gram stain bank blood
Circulatory overload	Medium	Overloading the recipient's circulation	Pulmonary edema	Monitor patient; choose proper component; diuresis; ? phlebotomy

donor's blood also relates to the incidence of hepatitis in the recipients. This and antibody to hepatitis B core antigen are now tested for in essentially all donors in the U.S. This is a form of surrogate testing, hoping to thereby reduce the transmission of NANB and human immunodeficiency virus (HIV) by transfusion. The impact of such surrogate testing has not yet been well documented. It will probably lower the incidence of transmitted disease but cannot eliminate it. All potential blood donors are now tested for the hepatitis B antigen. This has eliminated most but not quite all of the posttransfusion hepatitis B because the sensitivity of the method is less than the minimal infective dose of the virus. Hepatitis B is found in less than 1 per cent of the transfused patients in the U.S.

Of the transmitted diseases, HIV infection has received by far the most attention from the public and even from the profession. Whereas significant numbers of patients were and will be killed by HIV transmitted by transfusion, their number probably does not even approach the number who have been and will be killed by NANB. There is now a test for anti-HIV antibody that is applied to all blood donors at each donation. This has certainly lowered the incidence of transmission by transfusion, but has not eliminated it. The problem here is that infectivity precedes the appearance of circulating antibodies. Voluntary exclusion of donors in groups at high risk of contracting (and transmitting) HIV appears to have been effective in some parts of the country but not in others.

Recently, a new concern about transfusion has arisen. Prompted by the evidence that prior transfusion appeared to make uremic patients less likely to reject a renal homograft, several centers have reviewed the relationship between transfusion at the time of surgical treatment and the subsequent clinical course of solid cancers.[9] The results have been mixed, with some finding that transfusion appeared to impair the chance of being cured of cancer, whereas others found no such relationship, even with the same types of cancer. The problems with such reviews are that they are all necessarily retrospective and uncontrolled. Even more important, transfusion does not occur randomly. In the treatment of many cancers, transfusion is linked to unfavorable factors such as the need for larger operations, ulcerated tumors, and others. Thus, great caution is needed before accepting a direct causal relationship when association is found, and skepticism is warranted by the failure to find even association in many series. Nevertheless, the question is an important one, and an attempt at a prospective trial will be made in the United Kingdom, contrasting whole blood with washed red cell transfusions (the causative mechanism, if any, is thought to reside in the leukocyte components).[44]

Massive transfusion means the continuous, rapid infusion of large amounts of blood.[11] The term generally implies a total at least equal to the recipient's normal blood volume continuously infused over no more than 6 to 8 hours. In fact, infusion of stored blood at the rate of 1 to 2 units per hour will produce little in the way of metabolic abnormalities, even if continued for long periods of time. The metabolic problems discussed for massive transfusion should be considered only in situations of very rapid sustained rates of transfusion.

Massive transfusion occurs as simultaneous rapid hemorrhage and transfusion. It is thus a situation of exchange transfusion, with roughly equal volumes in and out of a relatively closed system. As such, it can be analyzed by several different mathematical approaches, using a variety of "boundary" conditions that must apply if the recipient is still alive, and other conditions that have been observed to apply in most clinical circumstances. The results of such analyses are in close agreement with each other and have had some degree of experimental verification. They indicate a degree of exchange that is less than most clinicians assume. The percentage of the recipient's original blood volume that will remain after hemorrhage and the transfusion of one, two, and three blood volumes in three

TABLE 8. Percentage of Recipient's Blood Volume Remaining after Hemorrhage and Transfusion as Indicated

Situation	1 Blood Volume	2 Blood Volumes	3 Blood Volumes
Perfect exchange	35%	14%	5%
Clinically likely	30%	10%	3–4%
Fatal delay	18%	3%	0.4%

From Collins, J. A.: Massive blood transfusion. Clin. Haematol., 5:201, 1976.

different situations is shown in Table 8. "Perfect exchange" means blood is infused at the same rate and at the same time that it is lost. "Fatal delay" means that the subject loses half a blood volume, then bleeds and is transfused at the same rates, with blood volume restored to normal only after the hemorrhage stops; such a situation is probably always fatal. "Clinically likely" is a combination of circumstances between these two extremes and probably approximates the majority of clinical situations. In this case, transfusion and hemorrhage equal to one blood volume means that the recipient still has about 30 per cent of the original blood elements remaining, and even at two blood volumes 10 per cent still remains. Any endogenous replacement during transfusion and the presence of any of the pertinent elements in the transfused blood will of course result in higher levels in the recipient.

These considerations of the degree of exchange that actually occurs are pertinent to many of the potential metabolic and related problems that can arise after transfusion (Table 9), but they are most relevant to the problem of hemostatic breakdown. This is a distressing, often disastrous abnormal diffuse bleeding that occurs in some heavily transfused patients.[10] The traditional wisdom is that the breakdown is due to replacement of the patient's blood with hemostatically defective blood bank products. There have not been many objective studies of this phenomenon, and many of those that have been reported were done in combat casualties.

The results of these studies are not completely consistent and they are not easy to summarize, but several patterns are discernible. First, in patients clearly bleeding abnormally, the quantitative studies on various hemostatic components (platelets, occasionally factors V and VIII) indicate greater degrees of depletion than can be accounted for by exchange transfusion. For example, a platelet count of 15,000 per μl. is less than 10 per cent of normal and therefore cannot be explained by transfusion of 10 units of blood in a normal-sized adult. Further, studies of certain elements give qualitative evidence against a simple replacement lesion. Fibrinogen levels are often severely low in these patients, but the fibrinogen levels in stored blood are normal, and even red cell concentrates contain about one third the normal amount

TABLE 9. Potential Metabolic and Related Problems of Massive Transfusion

Hemostatic failure
Impaired oxygen delivery
Acidosis
Hyperkalemia
Citrate toxicity
Pulmonary insufficiency
Uncertain
    Plasticizer toxicity
    Impaired antibacterial defenses
    Denatured proteins
    Impaired red cell deformability
    Elevated phosphate, ammonia

of fibrinogen. Fibrin(ogen) degradation products and complexes are often elevated in the blood of these patients to levels greater than are found in stored blood. Finally, rapid air evacuation of the massively injured in Vietnam allowed the acquisition of some interesting temporal data. Most patients who developed serious coagulation abnormalities had evidence of these abnormalities before they were transfused, improved while receiving blood, and worsened when the transfusions stopped.

All these lines of evidence point toward something other than the transfused blood as the cause of the hemostatic breakdown. Most evidence suggests that patients who bleed diffusely during hemorrhage and resuscitation have developed DIC. The distinction as to cause is important because DIC in this setting is at least in part a disease of hypoperfusion. In the acutely injured patient it is a consequence of not receiving enough blood soon enough, quite the opposite of the popular assumption that transfusion is the cause. Confirmation of this hypothesis came from studies on injured patients in West Germany.[21] There was no particular correlation between measured coagulation abnormalities and the amount of blood transfused, but when heavily transfused patients were grouped according to the duration of hypotension, a strong correlation was evident. Large amounts of transfused blood were associated with coagulation abnormalities only in proportion to the duration of hypotension, not the amount of blood transfused. Several fine studies from Seattle on changes in coagulation during extensive transfusion further indicated the difficulty in producing "washout" by transfusion. Factor V rarely fell below half normal, and factor VIII tended to increase above normal concentrations even during massive transfusion.[15] The interpretation of changes in platelet count in the first of these studies was unfortunate because it assumed a straight linear relationship between transfusion and platelet count when theory predicted and the data clearly showed the expected semilogarithmic relationship. Correctly interpreted, the data confirm almost every other such study: the platelet count rarely drops below 50,000 per μl. as a result of transfusion alone. A subsequent study addressed the platelet issue definitively.[34] It is the only prospective controlled study testing the administration of platelets prophylactically to massively transfused patients. There were very small differences in the platelet counts of those supplemented and those not. In both groups, the platelet counts were much higher than would have occurred with uncompensated washout and tended to level off at 50,000 per μl. even with enormous volumes of transfusion. Most important, there was no difference in clinical bleeding pattern between those supplemented and those not. In other words, the exposure of the supplemented patients to many more donors was done with no evident benefit to the recipient.

In summary, the relationship between transfusion and hemostatic breakdown appears primarily to be one of shared causes, not direct cause and effect. Rapid and effective restoration of blood volume is probably the most effective way of preventing this hemostatic breakdown. There is no evidence that supplementing transfusion of red cells with fresh frozen plasma and/or platelets prevents this complication; the controlled trials that have been done do not show any benefit. Since there is risk, the practice should be abandoned and patients should be treated on the basis of specific findings and demonstrated needs, not by formulas based on presumptions that lack validity.

The function of hemoglobin in stored blood presents an interesting problem. As duration of storage in most liquid media increases, the amount of 2,3-diphosphaglycerate (2,3-DPG) decreases and red cells become less efficient as oxygen-delivering agents. Restoration of 2,3-DPG begins immediately after infusion but is not complete for at least 12 hours. Thus, with massive transfusion, a less efficient oxygen-delivering carrier is placed in the circulation at a time when life is threatened by a breakdown in oxygen delivery. Despite these theoretical considerations, it has been difficult to show that transfusion of red cells depleted

of 2,3-DPG is harmful. Much of the blood transfused in the U.S. is transfused during the fist week of storage when levels of 2,3-DPG have not disappeared completely. Even blood totally depleted of 2,3-DPG delivers oxygen and supports life. Studies in experimental animals indicated that recovery from hemorrhage was not impaired by the use of red cells depleted of 2,3-DPG provided that hematocrit was kept near normal.[14] Combinations of anemia and depletion of 2,3-DPG did impair survival after hemorrhage, implying a critical level of oxygen-delivering capacity of the blood, above which survival after hemorrhage is not altered but below which oxygen delivery by blood becomes a limiting factor in survival. As noted in the discussion of anemia, there are grounds for concern about the oxygen-delivering capacity of blood in patients with coronary arterial insufficiency. Several studies have addressed this point, none convincingly. Once proved, it may be that red cell function will have to be a consideration in choosing blood for transfusion in some patients.

Acid-base imbalance might reasonably be expected during massive transfusion. Blood is increasingly acidotic during storage and many exsanguinating patients have a marked lactic acidosis. Paradoxically, transfusion of even old stored red cells usually results in correction of the acidosis. The reason is that the acids of the patient and the blood are normal intermediary metabolites that are rapidly "burned off" when perfusion is restored, which is one of the effects of transfusion. Extensive transfusion, in fact, usually results in significant metabolic alkalosis because most of the citrate anticoagulant is present as sodium citrate, which becomes sodium bicarbonate as the citrate is metabolized. This effect will be less in products with less citrate. There is no need to alkalinize heavily transfused patients unless blood gas analysis clearly shows it to be necessary; even then caution is warranted because the most likely cause by far of severe metabolic acidosis would be hypoperfusion, which is not treated by alkalinization. The acid-base changes during massive transfusion nicely illustrate several important principles: the system is a very complex one and changes must be measured, not assumed, and a well-perfused patient is very well able to defend against the metabolic challenges of massive transfusion.[13]

Hyperkalemia is also theoretically possible because the concentration of potassium in the plasma in stored red cell products can be very high. Most of this potassium has shifted out of the red cells because of the low temperature of storage. This shift is corrected after transfusion, when the transfused red cells take back as much potassium as they released during storage, so that the truly additional potassium load is only that released from hemolyzed cells, which is rather small. Almost all studies show that most patients at the end of massive transfusion are mildly hypokalemic, probably because of the alkalosis induced by transfusion. Those patients who are hyperkalemic are probably so because of acidosis and poor perfusion; this represents a need for more blood, not a lesion produced by transfused blood.

Citrate toxicity is possible during massive transfusion because much of the citrate is in excess of the molar amount necessary to bind all the calcium in blood in order to ensure nearly complete binding of the ionized calcium.[17] Thus, transfusion represents the infusion of free citrate. Experimentally it is almost impossible to cause difficulty by exchange transfusion with blood that is totally free of calcium, but it is possible to kill experimental animals with infusions of citrated blood. The lethal effects are entirely rate-dependent and usually require very rapid and sustained rates of infusion, probably in excess of 1 unit of whole blood every 5 minutes for an hour or more in a warm, normal-sized, well-perfused adult. Such rates are rarely sustained clinically. There is disagreement about the use of supplemental calcium during transfusion. Calcium infusions can be lethal in themselves. The citrate infused with transfusion is usually rapidly metabolized, and the body mobilizes calcium rapidly from skeletal stores. Clinical experience without the use of supplemental calcium has been very reassuring. Studies with the calcium ion–sensitive electrode, however, clearly show that most transfused patients have decreased ionized calcium levels during rapid transfusion. It is not clear at what level intervention is needed and under what circumstances it is safe. Generally, calcium is not needed if the patient appears to be responding to transfusion satisfactorily. Persistent circulatory collapse in massively transfused patients is almost always due to persistent hypovolemia and thus is another example of too little transfusion rather than too much. If there is objective evidence of failing cardiac function despite correction of hypovolemia, a cautious trial of intravenous calcium may be warranted along with a search for other possible causes, e.g., pericardial tamponade. One should use only enough to achieve the desired effect, remembering that in large doses calcium is a potentially dangerous drug.

Hypothermia frequently accompanies massive transfusion, often with serious consequences. The specific heat of blood is such that it requires 145 kcal. to raise 10 units of whole blood from 4 °C. (the temperature of storage) to 37° C. This represents a metabolic requirement for 30 liters of oxygen plus the fuel substrates. For these reasons, considerable attention has been given to the problem of rapidly heating blood from the blood bank. Red blood cells hemolyze at temperatures above 45° C., so heating by exposure to a hot surface is not permissible. This means that there must be either slow flow, which is not acceptable clinically, or a large surface of contact, which means a large "dead space" and some delay. Recently, there has been a revival of interest in mixing the red cells for transfusion with preheated saline, which would not only heat the red cells but also lower the viscosity of the product and facilitate rapid infusion.[49] In fact, the efforts spent on heating red cells may be misplaced. In modern practice, far more fluid is given as non–red cell solutions, which usually can be easily prewarmed to some suitable temperature. Perhaps even more important is the environment, both the accident room and the operating room. Unconscious or paralyzed patients can lose heat very quickly, as can some patients with serious head injuries. Maintaining the temperatures of these often cold, air conditioned rooms closer to body temperature is uncomfortable for the staff but far more effective at preserving body heat in the patients. Hypothermia is almost unique among the metabolic complications of transfusion because of its great potential for making so many other complications worse. It shifts the affinity of hemoglobin for oxygen in the wrong direction, further impairing the delivery of oxygen. It impairs the metabolism of citrate and lactate. It stimulates the release of potassium from cells into the extracellular space, which is further promoted by acidosis and poor perfusion, which in turn can be worsened by the effects on citrate and lactate. It impairs coagulation in ways that are incompletely understood and it impairs the function of platelets to the extent of prolonging the bleeding time. Although surprisingly sparingly examined by experimental efforts or clinical reviews, hypothermia seems well worth the efforts required to prevent it.

Considerable interest has been shown in the possible relationship between massive transfusion and pulmonary insufficiency. In many clinical series, those two events tend to occur together. There are a number of ways by which transfusion might impair pulmonary function: overloading the circulation, DIC, activated inflammatory mediators, plasticizers, and metabolic abnormalities. All of these mechanisms have varying degrees of experimental support. The factor that has received the greatest attention is microembolization. Stored blood contains considerable particulate debris that slips through the relatively coarse (170-μ mesh) standard filters. No one thinks this material does any good, but it is not clear that it does any harm or that use of special filters, which are more expensive and which slow the rate of transfusion, is warranted.[41] Experiments in dogs support the use of fine filters, but those in primates are inconclusive at best. The best controlled clinical study did not reveal any benefit from the use of fine filters. Combat casualties in Vietnam were treated with large amounts of whole blood without the use of fine filters, and there was little evidence of pulmonary insufficiency associated with transfusion.[12] This observation is pertinent to the question of microembolization and also to the broader relationships between transfusion and pulmonary function.

Other potentially harmful effects of massive transfusion are either still poorly documented or unlikely to be important.

Autologous transfusion, the return of the patient's own blood, occurs in two ways. Electively, the patient can be bled several days to weeks before operation, and the blood can be stored for use then if needed. The hypovolemia after donation is rapidly repaired, most proteins are replaced fairly rapidly, and red cell production is increased by the time of operation. Blood shed at operation or recovered from a variety of closed, sterile drainage systems can be processed by a variety of devices and reinfused as needed. The safest method involves washing the shed red cells and reinfusing them in a simple electrolyte solution, avoiding the potential problems from tissue thromboplastins, hemolyzed red cells, and altered plasma proteins. All forms of autologous transfusion have received considerable increases in interest and use because of the public's fear of HIV. The effect is desirable, but the profession should have been more a leader than a follower.[45]

FUTURE DEVELOPMENTS IN BLOOD BANKING

Potentially the most important development in blood banking in the United States in recent years is the reported development of an effective test for the antibody against the most common form of NANB.[26] If this is confirmed, it could improve very substantially the safety of transfused blood products. The most impressive scientific development recently confirmed is the identification, isolation, and use of the genetic mechanism responsible for producing factor VIII to produce this material on a low-volume commercial basis.[47] This is such a complex mechanism that it was widely assumed that a much longer period of time would be necessary before a "manufactured" effective and safe product could be produced. Similar approaches are now anticipated for other important noncellular blood components. Such methods of production ensure supply and vastly increase safety. Monoclonal antibodies continue to replace many of the older style reagents used in blood banking, thereby improving quality control. In the more mundane realm, more of the components of blood are being separated and developed as specific transfusion products. AT-III and fibronectin will soon be available.

On the cellular side, non–red cell oxygen-delivering agents are being developed and evaluated.[24] The fluorocarbons as a group hold promise in this area, but the agents developed to date have been ineffective. Stroma-free hemoglobin, modified to delay excretion and improve oxygen-delivering characteristics, holds great promise for use as a resuscitative fluid at the scene of accidents and as a limited substitute for red cells. The product continues to be plagued by problems in manufacture, however.[20] More exotic strategies involve microencapsulating oxygen-delivering material in lipid-based particles ("artificial red cells"); these are still in early stages of development. Although artificial platelets are less likely at the moment, several drugs have proved surprisingly effective in reducing bleeding when platelet function was impaired. DDAVP (1-diamino-8-D-arginine vasopressin) promotes the release of factor VIII and vWF.[36] It has been found to shorten the bleeding time and lessen clinical bleeding in uremic patients and in patients with von Willebrand's disease,[29] and to lessen blood loss in patients undergoing cardiopulmonary bypass for complex operations.[36]

Conjugated estrogens shorten the bleeding time in uremic patients with a longer duration of effect than DDAVP.[27] Estrogens do not appear to affect vWF, but may inhibit release of PGI_2.[51] PGI_2 has been used during cardiopulmonary bypass and hemodialysis to inhibit platelet aggregation during contact of the blood with foreign surfaces. After contact ceases, platelet function is better than if aggregation had been allowed to occur, but the other effects of PGI_2 can be troublesome. Intravenous immune globulin temporarily improves platelet count in many patients with immune thrombocytopenia, often allowing splenectomy to be performed without platelet transfusions in patients with severe disease bleeding spontaneously and resistant to steroids.

These examples illustrate a trend toward development of drugs to improve disordered hemostasis and eliminate or lessen the need for replacement with dangerous and/or scarce blood components. On a slightly different front, human erythropoietin manufactured by recombinant DNA techniques promises to greatly reduce the need for red cell transfusions in uremic patients; what role it might have in the treatment of other anemias is not known.[19]

SELECTED REFERENCES

Collins, J. A. Murawski, A., and Shafer, W. (Eds.): Massive transfusion in surgery and trauma. Progr. Clin. Biol. Res., 108, 1982.
An Annual Red Cross Scientific Symposium, this time on a subject of great interest to surgeons.

Colman, R. W., Hirsh, J., Marder, V. J., and Salzman, E. W. (Eds.): Hemostasis and Thrombosis: Basic Principles and Clinical Practice, 2nd ed. Philadelphia, J. B. Lippincott, 1987.
The definitive comprehensive text in the area; most chapters are very good, some are superb; the "overlook" chapters are especially valuable for the non-expert. Much of the material in this chapter is based on material from this excellent reference.

Mollison, P. L., Engelfriet, C. P., and Contreras, M.: Blood Transfusion in Clinical Medicine, 8th ed. Oxford, Blackwell, 1987.
The classic text on transfusion medicine, now multi-authored but with no loss of readability.

National Institutes of Health Consensus Development Conference Statement: Fresh frozen plasma: indications and risks, vol. 5, no. 5, 1985; Platelet transfusion therapy, vol. 6, no. 7, 1986; Perioperative red cell transfusion, vol. 7, 1987.
The consensus conference statements of the NIH are intended to reflect a reasonable consensus of opinion among experts in areas of clinical practice where scientific data may not be complete or conclusive; those dealing with transfusion are worthwhile for putting the scientific context around what are sometimes difficult clinical decisions.

Technical Manual of the American Association of Blood Banks, 9th ed. Arlington, VA, Am. Assoc. Blood Banks, 1985.
A wealth of practical information about what the blood bank has to offer, in a very understandable form.

Thurer, R. L., and Hauer, J. M. Autotransfusion and blood conservation. Curr. Probl. Surg., 19:97, 1982.
Fine review of methods and techniques of giving patients the safest blood—their own.

REFERENCES

1. Aach, R. D., and Kahn, R. A.: Post-transfusion hepatitis: Current perspectives. Ann. Intern. Med., 92:539, 1980.
2. Basta, S. S., Soekirman, M. S., Karyadi, D., and Scrimshaw, N. S.: Iron deficiency anemia and the productivity of adult males in Indonesia. Am. J. Clin. Nutr., 32:916, 1979.
3. Baxter, J. G., Marble, D. A., Whitfield, L. R., Wels, P. B., Walczak, P., and Schentag, J. J.: Clinical risk for prolonged PT/PTT in abdominal sepsis patients treated with Moxalactam or Tobramycin plus Clindamycin. Ann. Surg., 201:96, 1985.
4. Braquet, P., Touqui, L., Shen, T. Y., and Vargaftig, B. B.: Perspectives in platelet-activating factor research. Pharmacol. Rev., 39:97, 1987.
5. Breddin, H. K., Fareed, J., and Bender N. (Eds.): Low-Molecular-Weight Heparins. Basel, Karger, 1987.
6. Carson, J. L., Poses, R. M., Spence, R. K., and Bonavita, G.: Severity of anemia and operative mortality and morbidity. Lancet, 1:727, 1988.
7. Case, R. B., Berglund, E., and Sarnoff, S. J.: Ventricular function. VII. Changes in acute coronary resistance and ventricular function resulting from acutely

8. induced anemia and the effect thereon of coronary stenosis. Am. J. Med., 18:397, 1955.
8. Cines, D. B., Tomaski, A., and Tannenbaum, S. T.: Immune endothelial-cell injury in heparin-associated thrombocytopenia. N. Engl. J. Med., 316:581, 1987.
9. Collins, J. A.: Current status of blood therapy in surgery. Adv. Surg., 22:75, 1989.
10. Collins, J. A.: Recent developments in the area of massive transfusion. World J. Surg., 11:75, 1987.
11. Collins, J. A.: Massive blood transfusion. Clin. Haematol., 5:201, 1976.
12. Collins, J. A., James, P. M., Bredenberg, C. E., Anderson, R. W., Heisterkamp, C. A., and Simmons, R. L.: The relationship between transfusion and hypoxemia in combat casualties. Ann. Surg., 188:513, 1978.
13. Collins, J. A., Simmons, R. L., James, P. M., Bredenberg, C. E., Anderson, R. W., and Heisterkamp, C. A.: Acid-base status of seriously wounded combat casualties. II. Resuscitation with stored blood. Ann. Surg., 173:6, 1971.
14. Collins, J. A., and Stechenberg, L.: The effects of the concentration and function of hemoglobin on the survival of rats after hemorrhage. Surgery, 85:412, 1979.
15. Counts, R. B., Haisch, C., Simon, T. L., Maxwell, N. G., Heimbach, D. M., and Carrico, C. J.: Hemostasis in massively injured trauma patients. Ann. Surg., 198:91, 1979.
16. Day, H. J., and Rao, A. K.: Platelets and megakaryocytes. V. Evaluation of platelet function. Semin. Hematol., 23:89, 1986.
17. Dzik, W H., and Kirkley, S A.: Citrate toxicity during massive transfusion. Transfusion Med. Rev., 2:76, 1988.
18. Edgerton, V. R., Gardner, G. W., Ohira, Y, Gunawardena, K. A., and Senewiratne, B.: Iron-deficiency anemia and its effect on worker productivity and activity patterns. Br. Med. J., 2:1546, 1979.
19. Eschbach, J. W., Egrie, J. C., Downing, M. R., Browne, J. K., and Adamson, J. W.: Correction of the anemia of end-stage renal disease with recombinant human erythropoietin: Results of a combined phase I and phase II clinical trial. N. Engl. J. Med., 316:1109, 1986.
20. Gilroy, D., Shaw, C., Parry, E., and Odling-Smee, W.: Detection of a vasoconstrictor factor in stroma-free haemoglobin solutions. J. Trauma, 28:1312, 1988.
21. Harke, H., and Rahman, S.: Coagulation disorders in massively injured patients. Progr. Clin. Biol. Res., 108:213, 1982.
22. Harker, L. A.: Bleeding after cardiopulmonary bypass. N. Engl. J. Med., 314:1446, 1986.
23. Hull, R. D., Raskob, G. E., Hirsh, J., et al.: Continuous intravenous heparin compared with intermittent subcutaneous heparin in the initial treatment of proximal-vein thrombosis. N. Engl. J. Med., 315:1109, 1986.
24. Kahn, R. A., Allen, R. W., and Baldassare, J.: Alternate sources and substitutes for therapeutic blood components. Blood, 66:1, 1985.
25. Kaplan, A. P., and Silverberg, M.: The coagulation-kinin pathway of human plasma. Blood, 70:1, 1987.
26. Kuo, G., Choo, Q.-L., Alter, H. J., et al.: An assay for circulating antibodies to a major etiologic virus of human non-A, non-B hepatitis. Science, 244:362, 1989.
27. Livio, M., Mannucci, P. M., Vigano, G., Mingardi, G., Lombardi, R., Mecca, R., and Remuzzi, G.: Conjugated estrogens for the management of bleeding associated with renal failure. N. Engl. J. Med., 315:731, 1986.
28. Mammen, E. F. (Ed.): Congenital coagulation disorders. Semin. Thromb. Hemost., 9:1, 1983.
29. Mannucci, P. M.: Desmopressin: A nontransfusional form of treatment for congenital and acquired bleeding disorders. Blood, 72:1449, 1988.
30. Mourant, A. E., Kopec, A. C., and Domaniewska-Sobczak, K.: The Distribution of Human Blood Groups and Other Biochemical Polymorphisms, 2nd ed. New York: Oxford University Press, 1976.
31. Nemerson, Y.: Tissue factor and hemostasis. Blood, 71:1, 1988.
32. Paterson, I. S., Klausner, J. M., Goldman, G., Kobzik, L., Welbourn, R., Valeri, C. R., Shepro, D., and Hechtman, H. H.: Thromboxane mediates the ischemia-induced neutrophil oxidative burst. Surgery, 106:224, 1989.
33. Rapaport, S. I.: Preoperative hemostatic evaluation: Which tests, if any? Blood, 61:229, 1983.
34. Reed, R. L., Heimbach, D. M., Counts, R. B., Ciavarella, D., Baron, L., Carrico, C. J., and Pablin, E.: Prophylactic platelet administration during massive transfusion. Ann. Surg., 203:40, 1986.
35. Rohrer, M. J., Michelotti, M. C., and Nahrwold, D. L.: A prospective evaluation of the efficacy of preoperative coagulation testing. Ann. Surg., 208:554, 1988.
36. Salzman, E. W., Weinstein, M. J., Weintraub, R. M., et al.: Treatment with desmopressin acetate to reduce blood loss after cardiac surgery: A double randomized trial. N. Engl. J. Med., 314:1402, 1986.
37. Schimpf, K., Mannucci, P. M., Kreutz, W., et al.: Absence of hepatitis after treatment with a pasteurized factor VIII concentrate in patients with hemophilia and no previous transfusions. N. Engl. J. Med., 316:918, 1987.
38. Seef, L. B., and Dienstag, J. L.: Transfusion-associated non-A, non-B hepatitis: Where do we go from here? Gastroenterology, 95:530, 1989.
39. Slichter, S.: Controversies in platelet transfusion therapy. Ann. Rev. Med., 31:509, 1980.
40. Small, M., Lowe, G. D. O., Cameron, E., and Forbes, C. D.: Contribution of the haematocrit to the bleeding time. Haemostasis, 13:379, 1983.
41. Snyder, E. L., and Bookbinder, M.: Role of microaggregate blood filtration in clinical medicine. Transfusion, 23:460, 1983.
42. Steinberg, M. H., Kelton, J. G., and Coller, B. S.: Plasma glycocalicin: An aid in

the classification of thrombocytopenic disorders. N. Engl. J. Med., *317*:1037, 1987.

43. Stern, D. M., Kaiser, E., and Nawroth, P. P.: Regulation of the coagulation system by vascular endothelial cells. Haemostasis, *18*:202, 1988.

44. Taylor, R. M. R., and Parrott, N. R.: Red alert. Br. J. Surg., *75*:1049, 1988.

45. Toy, P. T. C. Y., Strauss, R. G., Stehling, L. C., et al.: Predeposited autologous blood for elective surgery: A national multicenter study. N. Engl. J. Med., *316*:517, 1987.

46. Verstraete, M., and Collen, D.: Thrombolytic therapy in the eighties. Blood, *67*:1529, 1986.

47. White, G. C., McMillan, C. W., Kingdom, H. S., and Shoemaker, C. B.: Use of recombinant antihemophilic factor in the treatment of two patients with classic hemophilia. N. Engl. J. Med., *320*:166, 1989.

48. Wieslander, J. B., Dougan, P., Stjernquist, U., Aberg, M., and Bergentz, S. E.: The influence of dextran and saline solution upon platelet behavior after microarterial anastomosis. Surg. Gynecol. Obstet., *163*:256, 1986.

49. Wilson, E. B., Knauf, M. A., Donohoe, K., and Iverson, K. V.: Red blood cell survival following admixture with heated saline: Evaluation of a new blood warming method for rapid transfusion. J. Trauma, *28*:1274, 1988.

50. Wolfe, J. H. N., Waller, D. G., Chapman, M. B., Blackford, H. N., and Prout, W. G.: The effects of hemodilution upon patients with intermittent claudication. Surg. Gynecol. Obstet., *160*:347, 1985.

51. Ylikorkala, O., Puolakka, J., and Vienikka, L.: The effect of oral contraceptives on antiaggregatory prostacyclin and proaggregatory thromboxane A_2 in humans. Am. J. Obstet. Gynecol., *142*:573, 1982.

7

METABOLISM IN SURGICAL PATIENTS

Protein, Carbohydrate, and Fat Utilization by Oral and Parenteral Routes

Josef E. Fischer, M.D.

The inclusion of this chapter is testimony to the contribution that nutritional supplementation makes to the care of sick patients. This current view represents a remarkable turnabout. In previous centuries, therapy included catabolic stimuli such as purging and blood-letting, which undoubtedly contributed to the demise of the patient. "Starving a fever" was so entrenched that Graves, of nineteenth century fame, preferred to be remembered as a physician "who would feed a fever." However, despite extensive progress by Dubois and others in the early twentieth century, principles of metabolic and nutritional support have only recently attained full acceptance. Indeed, even at present, nutritional support, even in those patients with the most dire need, is universally practiced neither geographically nor across disciplinary lines. Surgeons remain most concerned and aggressive about nutritional support of critically ill patients.

The history of parenteral nutrition is largely the history of infusion of substances that may be loosely regarded as nutritionally beneficial. Discounting the disastrous attempt of an elderly fourteenth-century Pope to regain his youth by the transfusion of blood from three young boys (all four died), the history of parenteral infusion begins shortly after William Harvey described circulation, with Christopher Wren infusing morphine to a dog and oleic acid to a horse, using hollowed goose quills as needles. Thereafter, sporadic experiments using infusions of alcohol or milk persisted until the twentieth century when Henriques and Anderson hydrolyzed casein to avoid an allergic reaction to foreign protein and infused it in a goat, claiming nitrogen equilibrium. In 1936, Robert Ellman reported the first successful administration of protein hydrolysate in humans, and parenteral nutrition in an infant was reported in 1944 with Helfrick and Abelson's support of an infant with intractable diarrhea by the intravenous administration of fat and protein.

When the history of medicine in the twentieth century is written, it is likely that nutritional support, along with antibiotics, blood transfusions, critical care monitoring and support, advances in anesthesia, and cardiopulmonary bypass, will rank high among surgical advances. It is rare for priorities to be so clearly established, but, in this case, they are. Although in Europe safe parenteral fat emulsions made it possible to support patients with protein hydrolysates, small amounts of glucose, and intravenous fat emulsions, it remained for Dudrick, working in Rhoads' laboratory at the University of Pennsylvania, to realize total nutritional support, first in animals and then in man. This fundamental contribution to medicine was first demonstrated in simple, yet elegant, experimental studies. This is superbly illustrated in Figure 1 showing two puppies that were littermates, one of which was fed by total parenteral alimentation and the other by the normal oral route. At 5 months their appearance is astonishingly similar (Fig. 1). Characteristically, military conflict contributed significantly to the development of this technique, as it so often has in surgical history. The practicality of infusing hypertonic dextrose with a calorie:nitrogen ratio that would support nitrogen equilibrium and protein synthesis was aided by application of Aubiniac's subclavian venipuncture, originally proposed during the French-Vietnam conflict in 1952 as a method of achieving rapid blood transfusion. The widespread application of nutritional support began.

Although the field of parenteral nutrition is but 20 years old, it has evolved from an initial period of enthusiastic, uncritical acceptance to a more critical review, with demands for demonstrable efficacy. The definition of nutritional needs in specific disease states has begun in earnest. A more recent phase, nutritional pharmacology, is the use of specific nutrient components as drugs. The targeted use of such specific components and/or modifications of the physiologic milieu is possible only when pathophysiologic mechanisms are defined.

The author believes the significance of nutritional support to operative procedures is of the same magnitude as antibiotics, fluid and blood transfusion, and critical care monitoring. These parasurgical techniques extend the frontiers of surgery, enabling the performance of more extensive procedures on sicker patients, and expectations of a better outcome.

SURGICAL ANATOMY: INTERORGAN RELATIONSHIPS

Interorgan relationships, the anatomic arrangements of the various metabolic organs, have not been stressed but must be extremely important. The liver, the central metabolic powerhouse, occupies a position astride the portal vein, receiving, processing, and storing ingested nutrients for later release in response to appropriate hormonal signals. It is not clear that the liver, which may process between 75 and 100 per cent of all portal vein nutrients in one pass, requires this massive input to maintain its functional integrity or requires considerably less. Certainly, many processes appear wasteful, such as the enormous postprandial urea production (56 per cent) from absorbed amino acids, with the result that only one fourth of ingested protein ever becomes available to the periphery as amino acids. If, however, this massive nutrient supply is required for hepatic functional integrity, this would have implications for routes of nutrient administration that do not primarily flow to the liver.

The anatomic relationship between the gut and the liver is important with respect to the recent proposal of glutamine as the major fuel source of the gut,[106] and the ability of the gut to

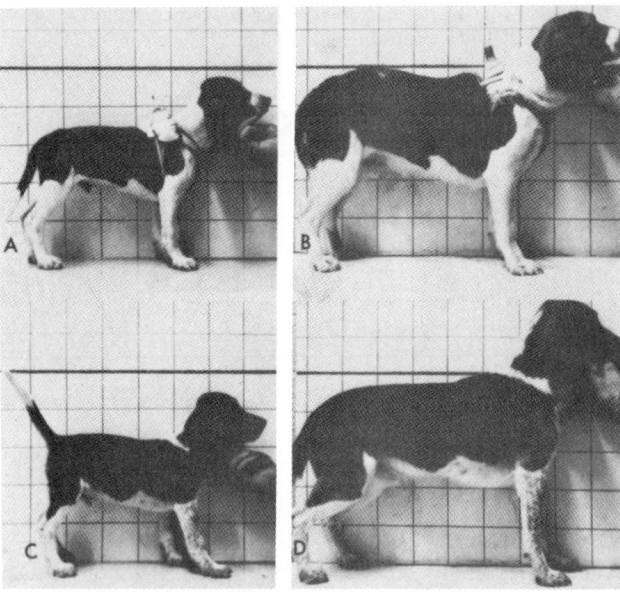

Figure 1. The growth and development of a puppy fed entirely by vein (*A* and *B*) was normal, comparable to that of a littermate (*C* and *D*) fed an optimal oral diet during the study period, which began at 12 weeks of age (*A* and *C*) and was completed 235 days later (*B* and *D*). (From Dudrick, S. J., and Rhoads, J. E.: Metabolism in surgical patients: Protein, carbohydrate, and fat utilization by oral and parenteral routes. *In* Sabiston, D. C., Jr. (Ed.): Davis-Christopher Textbook of Surgery, 12th ed. Philadelphia, W. B. Saunders Company, 1981.)

transpose glutamine to alanine with the release of ammonia "under cover" of the liver's detoxifying ability for ammonia. Moreover, the interposition of liver between gut and lung protects the lung. When the liver fails to perform its detoxifying role, as in liver disease and/or portosystemic shunting, the lung may acquire a detoxifying role as well. This may be deleterious to pulmonary function, as in the carcinoid syndrome, in which kinins, serotonin, and substance P, among others, which normally are cleared by the liver, adversely affect the heart and lung.

Other functions are enhanced by the anatomic arrangement. The trophic role of insulin and glucagon in maintenance of hepatic function is well known, but other gut-produced hepatotrophic substances may exist as well. The recently described relationships between Kupffer cells and hepatocytes,[10] and possible deleterious effects of gut products on Kupffer cell and hepatocyte function, make this a fruitful research area.

Both liver and kidney have a role in the disposition of nitrogen excess to urea for subsequent excretion in the urine. Less fully appreciated is the metabolic cycle between skeletal and visceral muscle (such as the heart) in which the liver metabolizes amino acids released during proteolysis, with the subsequent formation of glucose. Other anatomic and functional cycles are probably equally important, such as the relationship between brown fat pads and the liver, for example. Such cycles will undoubtedly be investigated more in the future.

PROTEIN

Of the three major foods — protein, carbohydrate, and fat — protein is most important, because it is the effector of all organic functions, whether enzymatic, contractile, or immunologic. Protein is unique, because, of all the food materials, it alone is specific for genus and perhaps species.

The balance between protein synthesis and degradation is critical. Synthesis is energy-requiring, whereas breakdown, particularly for gluconeogenesis, yields only one fourth of the

energy in energy-rich phosphate as synthesis requires; the remainder is expended as heat. Thus, utilization of protein for energy is clearly wasteful. The demonstration by Sir David Cuthbertson that nitrogen excretion and presumably proteolysis were increased after injury[28] was possibly the beginning of contemporary metabolic history.

AMINO ACIDS

BASIC STRUCTURE. The basic units of protein, the amino acids, have a core configuration of an amino and a carboxyl group adjacent to a single carbon atom from which a side chain extends. In glycine, this side chain is a hydrogen atom, but in all other amino acids, one or more carbon atoms are present. Amino acids also exist as optically active isomers that rotate a plane of polarized light to the left (levorotatory, or L-form) or to the right (dextrorotatory, or D-form). The L-forms are more important in mammalian life, as they are used preferentially to the D-forms. Amino acids are grouped based on the nature and electrical charge of the side chain.

The neutral amino acid group comprises 12 amino acids, including glycine and alanine; the hydroxy amino acids serine and threonine; the branched chain amino acids valine, leucine, and isoleucine; and the aromatic amino acids phenylalanine, tyrosine, and tryptophan (more properly, a heterocyclic amino acid); as well as the sulfur-containing amino acids methionine and cysteine. Two amino acids — aspartic and glutamic acid — are diacidic, whereas three amino acids — arginine, lysine, and histidine — are dibasic. These structural and charge features determine the characteristics of transport across membranes and into cells.

ESSENTIAL VERSUS NONESSENTIAL AMINO ACIDS. The essential or indispensable amino acids are those whose carbon skeleton cannot be synthesized. These include the classic eight (as determined by Rose and colleagues): the three branched chain amino acids valine, leucine, and isoleucine; lysine; methionine; phenylalanine; threonine; and tryptophan. In addition, cysteine and tyrosine are synthesized from the essential amino acids methionine and phenylalanine, respectively. Histidine and arginine are probably essential, certainly in infants and when needs are increased, as synthetic rates fall short of requirements.

The remaining eight amino acids — alanine, aspartic acid, asparagine, glutamic acid, glutamine, glycine, proline, and serine — are not essential.

BASIC PRINCIPLES. Three major fates of amino acids are (1) protein synthesis or turnover; (2) catabolic reactions leading to the production of CO_2 and energy or storage of the carbon as carbohydrate and/or fat while the nitrogen is eliminated as urea; and (3) utilization of the nitrogen to synthesize nonessential amino acids and other small molecules, such as purines and pyrimidines.

TRANSPORT. Transport of free amino acids across the cell membranes has been studied in only a few types of cells, although it is probably universal. Christensen has proposed several transport systems:

1. The A-system is an energy- and sodium-dependent system with a high affinity for alanine and other neutral amino acids, including the synthetic amino acids alpha-amino-isobutyric (AIB) acid and, more specifically, alpha-methyl-amino-isobutyric acid (MeAIB). It is concentrative against a gradient and is stimulated by insulin.

2. The L-system transports the branched chain amino acids — leucine, isoleucine, and valine, and the aromatic amino acids — phenylalanine, tyrosine, and tryptophan — and probably methionine and histidine. It is neither energy- nor sodium-requiring, but operates by exchange for intracellular amino acids, such as methionine. It is competitive.

3. Two transport systems are available for the basic amino acids. The carriers for transport of dibasic amino acids and the L-system may be linked in some as yet unknown way.[61]

4. Dicarboxylic amino acids have their own transport system.

Although brain amino acid transport has been studied to a considerably greater extent than muscle transport, changes in muscle amino acid transport in conditions such as sepsis[52,53] may prove important in fully understanding some of the metabolic changes.

TURNOVER: SYNTHESIS AND DEGRADATION. Synthesis of protein is energy-requiring. It is highly complex, beginning with the genetic-coded material contained in DNA, through a series of mostly energy-requiring transfers transmitting the message through messenger RNA to charge tRNA, and finally to the polysomes where amino acids are aligned on a template and then split off as the protein is synthesized.

Degradation of protein under normal equilibrium conditions is a mechanism by which worn-out, three-dimensionally damaged protein is recycled back to free amino acids so that they may be reutilized. Amino acids are catabolized to small nitrogen molecules, ammonia and urea, CO_2, energy, and glucose. Of the essential, or indispensable, amino acids, 7 of the 10 are degraded by the liver, the exceptions (in the conventional wisdom) being the three branched chain amino acids valine, leucine, and isoleucine.[99] This view, however, has been challenged.[91] Skeletal muscle has a major role in the catabolism of the branched chain amino acids.[79]

There are several processes by which amino acids are degraded. Twelve of the 20 amino acids are transaminated initially to an alpha-ketoacid, which then has two fates: (1) conversion to glucose and (2) oxidation to CO_2 (and high-energy phosphate) via the tricarboxylic acid cycle.

In addition, two amino acids—alanine and glutamine—are the nitrogen carriers for a complex series of organ exchanges of nitrogen. Thus, the branched chain amino acids undergo their first step in catabolism in muscle by transamination with pyruvate to alanine and, with glutamate, to glutamine (Fig. 2). A less important pathway involves oxidative deamination. A third protein degradative pathway involves urea synthesis, in which both the liver and the kidney participate.

REGULATION OF AMINO ACID LEVELS. The liver is most important in regulation of plasma amino acid levels. Sitting astride the portal vein, it filters the blood and extracts nutrients for processing or storage and controlled release to the periphery following neurogenic or hormonal stimuli. Most hepatic regulation appears designed to prevent excessive accumulation of plasma amino acids. This is understandable in view of the sudden postprandial peaks of amino acids, which conceivably could result in dramatic increases in amino acid brain neurotransmitter precursors that may damage the brain. Thus, the liver's ability to quickly increase the degradative ability for, in particular, the aromatic amino acids is understandable. Only 25 per cent of ingested protein reaches the general (nonportal) circulation as free amino acids. Most (almost 60 per cent) is converted to urea,[34] a small amount (6 per cent) is synthesized to plasma protein, and 14 per cent is synthesized to liver protein. With such a small percentage of the plasma amino acid pool derived from exogenous oral intake, most of the free amino acid pool is derived from breakdown of endogenous protein.

In parenteral nutrition, nutrients are first supplied to the systemic rather than the portal circulation, thus overriding the liver, normally the principal controlling factor. This is because only 20 per cent of cardiac output goes to the liver, and of that, one third is supplied by the hepatic artery, the remainder via portal flow that has already gone through another organ, the gut. Thus, a critical aspect of at least amino acid and probably most nutrient regulation is bypassed by parenteral nutrition.

OTHER REGULATION. In addition to hepatic regulation, the

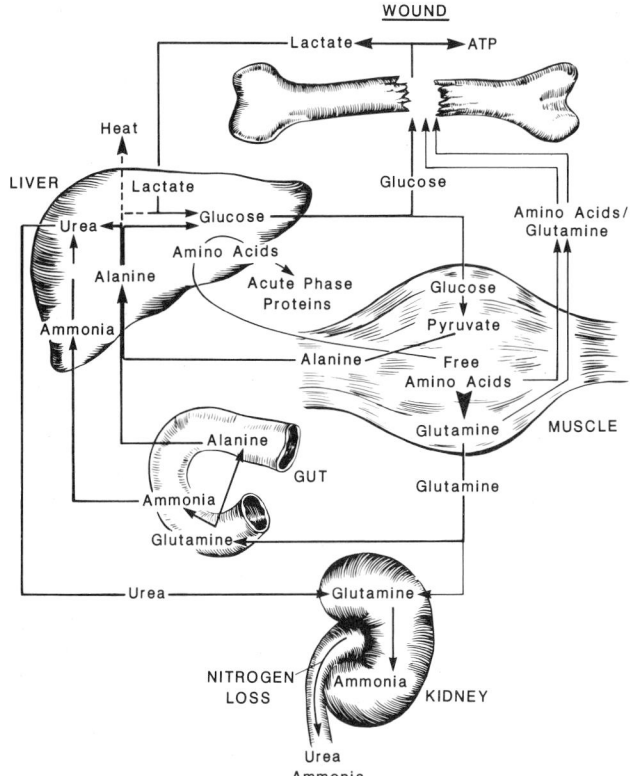

Figure 2. An overall scheme of the metabolic response to illness. This scheme includes one feature that heretofore has not been very prominently addressed, that is, the metabolic relationship between organs, now receiving increased attention. One of the articles of faith is that teleologically such responses occur in response to injury and are teleologically correct and beneficial. Thus, the wound requires glucose, probably glutamine, and certainly arginine with respect to certain cellular elements. The movement of amino acids from the periphery (muscle) to the liver presumably results in the secretion of acute-phase protein, the purpose of which in turn is to fight infection. The muscle-gut-liver-alanine-glutamine-glucose cycle is prominently displayed. (Adapted from Bessey, P. Q.: Metabolic response to critical illness. *In* Wilmore, D. W., Brennan, M. F., Harken, A. H., Holcroft, J. W., and Meakins, J. L. (Eds.): Care of the Surgical Patient. Section II, Chapter 11, © 1990 Scientific American, Inc. All rights reserved.)

plasma amino acid pool is also influenced by exchange of nitrogen and amino acids between skeletal muscle and gut. In muscle, the branched chain amino acids are transaminated to alanine and glutamine. Alanine is processed by the liver to glucose (among other things) and glutamine to alanine by the gut, alanine going to the liver.

REGULATION OF AMINO ACID LEVELS WITHIN ORGANS. Although transport of amino acids across cell membranes of brain, kidney, and gut has received some attention, the study of transport systems into other organs such as skeletal muscle, which contains the bulk of amino acids, has been comparatively neglected.

REGULATION OF AMINO ACIDS IN MUSCLE. Skeletal muscle contains the bulk of the body's amino acids, with glutamine comprising between 50 and 60 per cent of muscle free amino acids. Within 24 hours of operation or trauma, much of this glutamine store has disappeared from muscle, and is not fully replaced until as long as 8 weeks later. Stoichiometrically, the glutamine that has disappeared is equivalent to the urinary excretion of urea within the first postoperative 36 hours. The significance of the glutamine export is not clear, nor is it clear why refilling this store takes so long.

Recent attempts to prevent depletion of muscle free glutamine by glutamine supplementation in parenteral nutrition solutions have shown some glutamine sparing.[94] However, the marginal improvements in nitrogen balance are of such small magnitude that they are unlikely to improve outcome.[50,94]

Control of protein synthesis and degradation in muscle is being increasingly explored because of its importance in starvation and sepsis. Muscle protein synthesis is presumably not identical in the white fast-twitch muscle as opposed to the red slow-twitch muscle in its response to various stimuli; however, they are likely qualitatively similar. Protein synthesis is stimulated by insulin, administration of amino acid nitrogen with adequate calories, increased concentration of branched chain amino acids, and possibly human growth hormone and its release of somatomedin, a product closely related to the secretion of insulin. Release of insulin and human growth hormone is stimulated by individual amino acids, such as arginine, also a preferred fuel for macrophages, especially within the healing wound. The branched chain amino acids have a special role since, in a healthy individual in nitrogen equilibrium, the postprandial uptake of branched chain amino acids into skeletal muscle represents between 60 and 100 per cent of daily nitrogen retention. Plasma levels of the branched chain amino acids are a tertiary but real controlling factor in the efflux of amino acids from muscle.[15,79]

In sepsis, the response to normal stimuli is altered. Protein synthesis is increased by the branched chain amino acids, but only at twice-normal concentrations.[54] The slope of the response to insulin is normal, but the baseline is depressed, so that the actual response to insulin is about half that of the normal muscle.[56]

The ability to study breakdown of muscle has until recently been inhibited by the absence of sensitive methods to measure small concentrations of 3-methylhistidine, and the reliance on tyrosine, which reflects total muscle breakdown, may have given an inaccurate view of what is actually transpiring. All agree that in sepsis and trauma, proteolysis is increased. Substances that encourage proteolysis include the classic counterregulatory hormones—glucagon, steroids, and epinephrine (Fig. 3). In addition, a newly discovered class of compounds—cytokines, such as interleukin 1, tumor necrosis factor (TNF)/cachectin, and perhaps proteolysis-inducing factor, a protein of molecular weight 4200 described by Clowes and co-workers[26]—possibly also contribute to proteolysis, although most data suggest that alone, they do not. The Cincinnati studies suggest that, at least in rats, perhaps 50 per cent of muscle breakdown is due to corticosterone, the normal rat

steroid that is increased in trauma and sepsis, and other studies suggest that at least some of the actions previously attributed to TNF/cachectin require the presence of and perhaps are mediated by steroids.[72] Another issue complicating the process is a new apparent cytokine of approximate molecular weight 1500 that prevents the muscle transport of amino acids by system A in septic or endotoxemic animals and perhaps man.[52,53,102] Since amino acids cannot enter the muscle, they cannot be incorporated into muscle protein synthesis. This cytokine, which is produced by macrophages and also by injection of endotoxin, thus diverts plasma amino acids derived from muscle breakdown or other sources to the liver for hepatic protein synthesis.

An elegant series of studies by Abumrad has shed new light on some of the controlling mechanisms that normally affect muscle protein breakdown. The provision of exogenous glucose can decrease muscle amino acid appearance (breakdown) maximally 50 per cent, but it has not been clear that one can shut off muscle amino acid efflux entirely. Using both glucose and amino acid clamps, Abumrad has demonstrated that the non–glucose-responsive portion of muscle protein breakdown is responsive to leucine. However, in sepsis, muscle protein breakdown is not responsive to glucose, and the Cincinnati studies indicate that the muscle proteolysis is not responsive to even pharmacologic doses of leucine.[54] Thus, these studies emphasize the altered control systems in sepsis. Additionally, recent findings from this laboratory suggest that nonconventional fuels, such as short-chain fatty acids, may be effective in decreasing muscle proteolysis in sepsis when conventional fuels fail (unpublished observations). Whether these are clinically applicable is not yet clear.

When hypocaloric feeding and "safe amounts" of amino acids are given in association with recombinant growth hormone to patients with ample fat stores, the remainder of the calories are to be provided by the utilization of fat. In one study, there was significant retention of nitrogen, phosphorus, and potassium, suggesting the accretion of small amounts of lean body mass.[70] Unfortunately, such studies must be very carefully controlled for dietary components, because paradoxical results have been reported. For example, in one recent study, loss of lean body mass was decreased in patients subjected to severe dietary restriction and given growth hormone, but fat loss remained unchanged, in contrast to what had been predicted. In another study, no effect of growth hormone was seen on fatty acid flux across the forearm in patients receiving total parenteral nutrition. Thus, the use of growth hormone remains open. Moreover, the beneficial effects on nitrogen balance are so small that differences in clinical outcome are unlikely.

Appreciation of metabolic processes in muscle is achieved by measuring arteriovenous differences of amino acids and 3-methylhistidine and urinary 3-methylhistidine (3-MH) excretion. 3-MH, a breakdown product of actin and myosin, is not reutilized for protein synthesis after it is released, and it is excreted in the urine provided renal function is normal. Although it has been proposed as a measure of muscle turnover or synthesis, it is now clear that 3-MH also comes from the gut, whose rapid turnover invalidates the use of 3-MH for measuring muscle turnover alone although use of urinary 3-MH as a reflection of lean body mass turnover may still be valid.[109] Arteriovenous differences do not reflect the recycling of various amino acids within muscle.

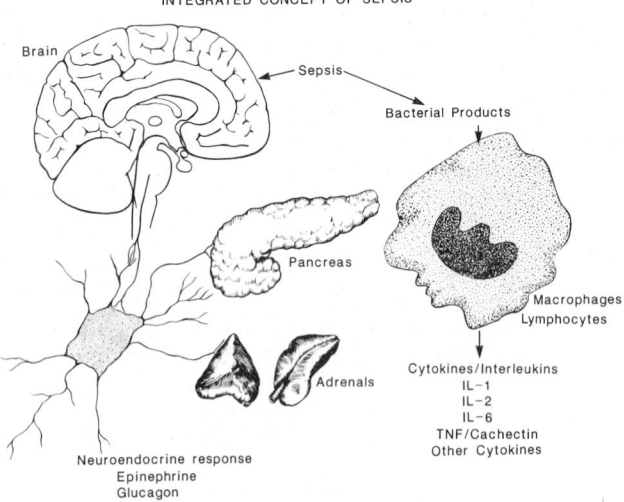

INTEGRATED CONCEPT OF SEPSIS

Brain

Sepsis

Bacterial Products

Pancreas

Macrophages
Lymphocytes

Cytokines/Interleukins
IL-1
IL-2
IL-6
TNF/Cachectin
Other Cytokines

Adrenals

Neuroendocrine response
Epinephrine
Glucagon
Steroids

Figure 3. An emerging concept of the response to stress and sepsis. In previous years, the neurosympathetic response to sepsis was emphasized, with the secretion of epinephrine, glucagon, and steroids—the so-called counterregulatory hormones. It is now clear that this is but one half of the efferent limb, and that cytokines, including those listed here and in Table 2, are extremely important.

ROLES OF THE KIDNEY

The roles of the kidney in protein metabolism include (1) the production of urea (with the liver) from ammonia via the argininosuccinate cycle; (2) the production of ammonia (largely from glutamine) in response to acidification of the urine; and (3) to a

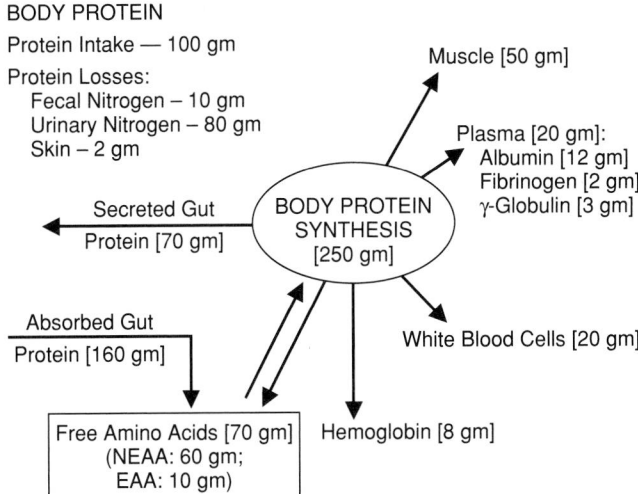

BODY PROTEIN

Protein Intake — 100 gm

Protein Losses:
Fecal Nitrogen – 10 gm
Urinary Nitrogen – 80 gm
Skin – 2 gm

Secreted Gut
Protein [70 gm]

Absorbed Gut
Protein [160 gm]

BODY PROTEIN
SYNTHESIS
[250 gm]

Muscle [50 gm]

Plasma [20 gm]:
Albumin [12 gm]
Fibrinogen [2 gm]
γ-Globulin [3 gm]

White Blood Cells [20 gm]

Hemoglobin [8 gm]

Free Amino Acids [70 gm]
(NEAA: 60 gm;
EAA: 10 gm)

Figure 4. Diagram to show the daily flux of amino acids on the body of a 70-kg. man. Note that total body protein synthesis is 250 gm. per 24 hours, of which 50 gm. is muscle; proteolysis contributes approximately the same. Thus, with adequate amounts of energy, nitrogen equilibrium is the result. (Data from Munro, H. N.: Parenteral nutrition: Metabolic consequences of bypassing the gut and liver. *In* Clinical Nutrition Update: Amino Acids. Chicago, American Medical Association, 1977, p. 141.)

lesser degree, metabolism of other amino acids, such as the branched chain amino acids, principally in acid-base regulation.

TOTAL INTEGRATION OF BODY PROTEIN

In a 70-kg. man, there are between 10 and 11 kg. of protein, largely as muscle but also as viscera. Daily protein turnover is 250 to 300 gm., or 3 per cent; the gut is the largest component, mainly shed enterocytes and secreted digestive enzymes. After digestion, all amino acids are absorbed, except for 1 gm. of nitrogen excreted in the stool. Proteolysis represents another 50 to 70 gm. of amino acids, most of which are resynthesized if adequate energy is present. Twenty gm. of plasma protein, 8 gm. of hemoglobin, 20 gm. of white cells, and a few grams of skin constitute the remainder of total body synthesis (Fig. 4). Ingested amino acids contribute only 25 gm. to the free amino acid pool (Fig. 5), whereas 250 gm. of amino acids are provided by endogenous breakdown. Whether protein synthesis is ade-

quate if only a source of energy and a small amount of essential amino acids are supplied is still controversial. Under such circumstances it is proposed that the other nonessential amino acids are synthesized from carbon skeletons and readily available sources of nitrogen such as glutamine.

Protein turnover decreases with age. Thus, turnover in a neonate approximates 25 gm. of protein per kg. per day, which decreases to 7 gm. per kg. per day at the age of 1 year. The rate in adults falls to approximately 3 gm. per kg. per day, slightly greater in males. Thus, as people age, the rate of turnover decreases, but as lean body mass increases, total body turnover remains approximately the same.

Caloric supply is important. Carbohydrate increases muscle protein synthesis, probably under the influence of insulin, whereas fat increases hepatic protein synthesis. Carbohydrate depresses albumin synthesis compared with an optimal amount of calories as fat.

PROTEIN REQUIREMENTS

One can approach protein requirements by assuming that after some days on a protein-free diet, nitrogen excretion is minimal and represents true requirements. Thus, on a calorically adequate protein-free diet, 37 mg. of nitrogen per kg. are excreted into the urine, whereas 12 mg. of nitrogen per kg. are lost in the feces. Integumentary losses constitute another 5 mg. per kg., and skin contributes another 2 to 3 mg. per kg. by evaporation, making a total of 56 to 57 mg. per kg. of nitrogen or, in terms of whole protein, 0.34 gm. per kg. per day. With various corrections and allowances for low-biologic-value protein, the average normal requirement is 0.8 gm. of protein per kg. or between 56 and 60 gm. of protein per day. Trauma increases the requirement. Normal intake is twice that amount in affluent American society.

Parenteral nutrition overrides the principal controlling mechanism, the liver. Also, the effects of recycling have not been comprehensively studied, but most of the amino acids can be recycled provided there is an adequate source of energy. Thus, small amounts of essential amino acids with adequate energy are sufficient for nitrogen equilibrium. In infants, between 40 and 50 per cent of the protein intake should be essential amino acids, whereas in an adult in nitrogen equilibrium without stress, sepsis, or trauma, 19 to 20 per cent is sufficient. The percentage of essential amino acids should increase with injury or depletion. A "safe" intake figure for patients on parenteral nutrition is 250 mg. of nitrogen per kg. or 1.7 gm. of protein equivalent per kg. per day.

CALORIES

CALORIC SOURCES. The body can utilize three sources of energy—protein, carbohydrate, and fat. Amino acids contribute 15 per cent of normal energy expenditure. The branched chain amino acids, which can be oxidized directly to high-energy phosphate without going through glucose, contribute 6 to 7 per cent of the normal energy requirements, the remaining 8 to 9 percent derived from gluconeogenesis. The remaining 85 per cent of normal energy expenditure is derived from carbohydrate or fat. Normally, 70 to 75 per cent of the resting metabolic expenditure is derived from fat utilization, either oxidized directly or metabolized via the liver to ketone bodies and, in turn, energy. Most of the body's energy stores exist as fat, there being very little carbohydrate (glycogen) after a 24-hour fast.

Most calories in total parenteral nutrition (TPN) are administered as glucose; it is not clear to what extent fat is used in all states, particularly in sepsis. Utilization of various caloric sources is estimated from the respiratory quotient (R.Q.), which

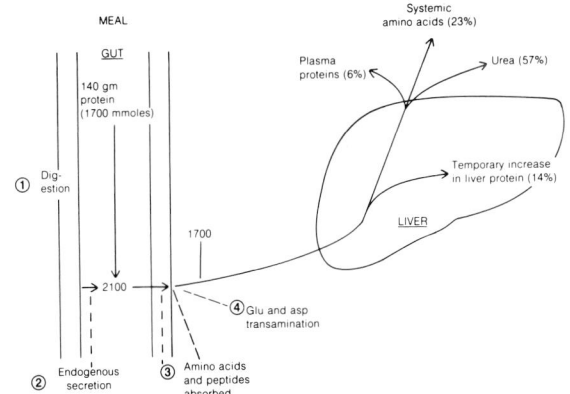

MEAL

GUT

140 gm
protein
(1700 mmoles)

① Digestion

1700

2100

② Endogenous
secretion

③ Amino acids
and peptides
absorbed

④ Glu and asp
transamination

LIVER

Plasma
proteins (6%)

Systemic
amino acids (23%)

Urea (57%)

Temporary increase
in liver protein (14%)

Figure 5. Absorption and metabolism of amino acids after a meal of meat eaten by a dog, based on data of Elwyn. Note that of ingested protein only 23 per cent appears in the plasma as free amino acids. (From Munro, H. N., and Crim, M. C.: The proteins and amino acids. *In* Goodhart, R. S., and Shils, M. E. (Eds.): Modern Nutrition in Health and Disease, 6th ed. Philadelphia, Lea & Febiger, 1980.)

TABLE 1. R.Q.s Commonly Seen in Clinical Practice and Their Implications

R.Q. Observed	Interpretation
>1.0	Lipogenesis
1.0	Reliance on carbohydrate calories
0.75–0.85	Mixed fuel utilization
0.70	"Pure" fat utilization
0.62–0.65	Ketogenesis

is the relationship between CO_2 produced and O_2 consumed, given by the following equation.*

$$R.Q. = \frac{V_{CO_2}}{V_{O_2}}$$

Metabolic carts make it possible to determine in a clinical setting which fuel is being consumed. An R.Q. of 1 or greater indicates pure carbohydrate utilization, and although theoretically the R.Q. with lipogenesis can be as high as 9, an R.Q. of greater than 1 is rarely seen clinically. Alternatively, an R.Q. of 0.7 indicates fat utilization. An R.Q. of less than 0.7 generally indicates ketogenesis (Table 1).

Without such measurements, when fat is administered intravenously, it is necessary to use indirect measures of fat utilization, such as absence of plasma lipemia and the presence of ketone bodies, to make certain the administered fat is being utilized.

CALORIE/NITROGEN RATIO. The energy required for protein synthesis has been estimated as a calorie/nitrogen ratio of 100 to 150/1 (i.e., 100 to 150 nonprotein calories per gm. of nitrogen) in normal patients. The calorie/nitrogen ratio probably changes in different disease states; in sepsis, a higher amount of nitrogen and decreased nonprotein calories are appropriate, whereas in uremia, a calorie/nitrogen ratio of between 300 and 400/1 (calorie per gm. of nitrogen) has been advocated. However, the manner of investigation is critical, that is, keeping nitrogen adequate and varying the calorie/nitrogen ratio is the preferred method of investigation. When inadequate amounts of protein have been given while caloric intake has varied, erroneous data have resulted.

ENERGY REQUIREMENTS. Metabolic carts help determine caloric requirements at the bedside. With such measurements, it is clear that in the past oversupplementation was the rule, resulting in excessive lipid deposition. Whereas 15 years ago it was common for patients to receive 3500 to 4000 calories per day, at present, mean caloric supplementation is closer to 1800 to 2000 calories per day, with an increase to 2500 calories per day if required in stress states. The Harris-Benedict equation may also be used:

$$BEE = \frac{66.5 + 13.7\ W + 5.0\ H - 6.8\ A\ [male]}{65.5 + 9.6\ W + 1.7\ H - 4.7\ A\ [female]}$$

where W = weight in kg.; H = height in cm.; and A = age in years.

The estimate shown in Figure 6 may be used, although it may overestimate caloric requirements, because when measurements have been applied to patients, requirements have been

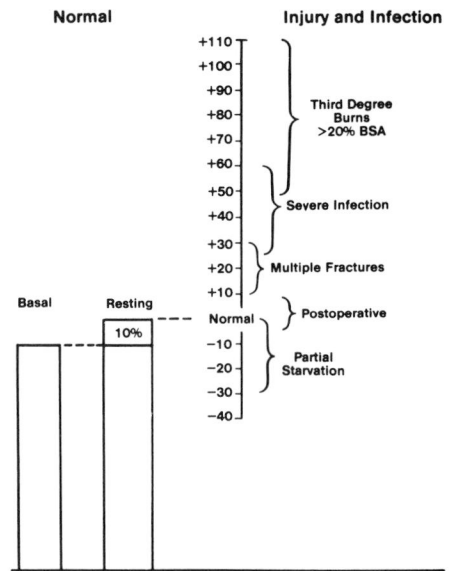

Figure 6. The increases in resting energy expenditure that have been shown to occur during the acute catabolic phase of injury or infection, when compared with the decreases that develop during partial starvation. (From Kinney, J. M.: The application of indirect calorimetry to clinical studies. *In* Kinney, J. M. (Ed.): Assessment of Energy Metabolism in Health and Disease. Columbus, Ohio, Ross Laboratories, 1980.)

lower than calculated. When metabolic cart measurements have been used, patients are in a basal state; thus, it is customary to increase the metabolic cart estimation of caloric requirements by 15 per cent to compensate for activity. Studies in the Cincinnati unit suggest that reasonable accuracy can be achieved by either method.[13]

CARBOHYDRATES. Glucose is the preferred carbohydrate source in traditional TPN. Other carbohydrates include fructose, sorbitol, xylitol, and glycerol. Several facts are important: First, there are no carbohydrate stores beyond a 24-hour fast. Liver glycogen is exhausted, although small amounts of muscle glycogen may remain; it soon disappears. Second, oxidizing glucose completely through the Krebs tricarboxylic acid cycle results in a much higher production of high-energy phosphate (aerobic glycolysis) than incomplete oxidation to lactate (anaerobic glycolysis). The exact circumstances of aerobic and anaerobic glycolysis are vague; in sepsis, low-flow states, and neoplasia, gluconeogenesis is increased, and yet the maximal energy value from the produced glucose is not obtained because of anaerobic (incomplete) glycolysis.

Glucose is the "gold standard" for protein sparing. A minimum of 400 calories per 24 hours (based on Gamble's classic work) and up to 1800 calories in the resting fasting state minimizes protein breakdown, particularly after adaptation to starvation. Glucose will not decrease proteolysis beyond 50 per cent; the remainder is apparently amino acid–sensitive. In addition, red cells, white cells, and the central nervous system "prefer" glucose—the red and white cells because of limited metabolic apparatus; the central nervous system ultimately "prefers" glucose, although it can adapt to other energy sources. Wound repair requires glucose, although some cellular elements utilize amino acids such as arginine extensively.

Deleterious effects of excessive glucose include hepatic steatosis (see later, under Metabolic Complications). Blood sugars in excess of 300 to 350 adversely affect neutrophil function.

Other carbohydrate sources have not achieved popularity in the United States. Fructose, which some have proposed as a preferred carbohydrate source under circumstances of glucose resistance, may cause fatal lactic acidosis. Moreover, fructose requires expenditure of high-energy phosphate through the

---

*Metabolic rate = 4.83 × V_{O_2} (resting subject, average American diet—4.83 kcal. generated for every liter of oxygen consumed). Heat per unit time (energy equivalent—kcal. per min.) = 3.941 V_{O_2} + 1.106 V_{CO_2}. Heat per unit time (energy equivalent—kcal. per min.) = V_{O_2} (3.941 + 1.106 respiratory quotient). If urinary nitrogen measurements are included, the formula described by Weir[104] can be used: heat production per unit time (energy equivalent—kcal. per min.) = 3.94 V_{O_2} + 1.11 V_{CO_2} − 2.17 urinary nitrogen.

pentose-monophosphate shunt for conversion to glucose; 80 per cent of the administered fructose is finally metabolized as glucose. Thus, use of fructose in the presence of glucose resistance appears illogical.

The polyalcohols xylitol and sorbitol also undergo transformation to glucose. Xylitol is hepatotoxic and has caused several deaths in the Australian experience. Despite this, xylitol and sorbitol are again being examined as substrates for specialized circumstances.

Glycerol is another potential source of glucose. It has the advantage that it may be sterilized in solution with amino acids, without the amino acids undergoing the caramelization reaction. In addition, its osmolality is low. These properties of glycerol have been recently utilized in a new solution, Procalamine,* which does not require mixing and thus saves pharmacy costs. This solution, administered peripherally, is intended as an intermediate solution for temporary nutritional support in patients who are not terribly ill and in whom it is not clear TPN will be needed, and at relatively low cost. Its place in the armamentarium remains to be determined. Glycerol in large doses may cause renal failure in experimental animals. Although the doses of glycerol administered clinically do not approach those in experimental renal failure, deleterious effects may result in patients with already compromised organ function; caution is appropriate.

CONTROLLING MECHANISMS. Under normal circumstances, administration of glucose inhibits lipolysis; this is presumbly mediated by insulin. In sepsis, and possibly stress, these "shut-off" valves do not function adequately, and gluconeogenesis continues, despite the administration of either fat or perhaps even carbohydrate.

FAT AS A CALORIC SOURCE. In normal resting starvation, fat provides the bulk of caloric expenditure, mostly as ketone bodies manufactured by the liver from long-chain fatty acids. Lipolysis is encouraged by steroids, catechols, and glucagon and is extremely sensitive to inhibition by insulin. Following stress, generous lipolysis occurs, presumably to provide energy. Between 25 and 45 per cent of the calories in the American diet are normally supplied by fat. The omission of fat in the early history of parenteral nutrition was largely due to the lack of availability of a safe fat emulsion. When it was realized that the practice of administering plasma was an insufficient source of trace metals and essential fatty acids, administration of fat was directed toward supplying 4 per cent of the calories as fat emulsion to prevent essential fatty acid deficiency. Currently, fat is administered both as a caloric source and as a source of essential fatty acids. Since fatty acids are the precursors of the prostaglandins, alternative types of fat are currently being investigated in an attempt to modify the inflammatory and immunologic response (see later).[96]

One remaining area of controversy is the use of fat in severe stress and sepsis. It is agreed that under normal circumstances or in patients with only moderate stress, fat and carbohydrate are indistinguishable with respect to nitrogen accumulation and balance, with 25 per cent of nonprotein calories as fat apparently optimal for hepatic protein synthesis. If all nonprotein calories are given as carbohydrate, amino acids are preferentially diverted to muscle protein synthesis under the influence of insulin. It is not clear, however, at which point in stress and/or sepsis that fat oxidation and/or utilization becomes impaired. Most investigators agree that fat clearance remains relatively normal until comparatively late in sepsis, but fat oxidation is impaired somewhat earlier. Unfortunately, when fat oxidation is impaired, multiple defects in metabolism usually have impaired utilization of most other substrates as well.

The specific dynamic action of carbohydrate when given with amino acids appears trivial at physiologic concentrations. The author's practice, other than in patients with severe sepsis, is to administer 25 per cent of the nonprotein calories as fat emulsion. In patients with severe sepsis, it is necessary either to measure R.Q. and/or to continually monitor the lipemia to ensure that fat is being both cleared and oxidized. The accumulation of fat within the plasma indicates lack of utilization. A limitation of 2 gm. of fat emulsion per kg. per day in adults prevents fat overload syndrome, manifested by fever, back pain, chills, pulmonary insufficiency secondary to fat accumulation and fat embolism, and blocking of the reticuloendothelial system. In babies, who are anatomically mainly viscera with little skeletal muscle, up to 4 gm. per kg. per day is tolerated, because the principal metabolic fuel of viscera is fat. At present, it is not clear whether in severe sepsis normal amounts of fat block the reticuloendothelial system.

ALTERNATIVE OR NONCONVENTIONAL FUELS. Dissatisfaction with the current standard caloric sources as well as their inability to sustain certain organ systems, such as the gut, in fully functional state has led to consideration of nonconventional substrates. Glutamine (which will be discussed subsequently) as a fuel for enterocytes has received much attention, with several clinical trials. Small changes in nitrogen balance result from the administration of a dipeptide glutamine ester.[50,94] The advantages appear so small that differences in outcome are unlikely. The ketone bodies—acetoacetate, proprionate, and butyrate—are the subjects of considerable investigation, again with respect to their beneficial effect on the gut and especially the effect of butyrate on the ileum and colon.

No clinical studies are as yet available using ketone bodies, but several experimental studies have been reported. Monoacetoacetin, a water-soluble neutral monoacylglycerol ester of acetoacetate, is nontoxic when given intravenously. It is hydrolyzed to glycerol, which in turn may be used as a fuel, and to acetoacetate. Acetoacetate has a minimal effect on the colonic mucosa, with only 10 per cent being consumed locally and 90 per cent being distributed to the portal system. Yet is it interesting that animals receiving monoacetin showed greater preservation of jejunal mucosal weight, protein, RNA, and DNA. An effect on colonic DNA was lacking. No differences in nitrogen balance or weight gain were noted, despite a predominance of calories furnished by monoacetin.[65] In burned rats, the administration of monoacetin appeared as efficacious as a dextrose-based TPN solution. From the literature, it would appear that judiciously supplied butyrate might be more efficacious, since the beneficial effect appears to extend to both colonocytes and ileal enterocytes. In addition, when produced from soluble pectin by gut bacteria, 80 per cent of the butyrate is utilized locally by colonocytes and only 20 per cent is released into the portal vein, suggesting that on a trophic basis, butyrate may be more effective. The author is not aware of any completed studies testing butyrate in patients.

CATABOLISM

CAUSES OF INADEQUATE NUTRITION. Lack of food is a cause of malnutrition in poor urban populations, especially in alcoholics. In lesser developed countries, lack of food is commonly a cause of malnutrition. In the United States hospital setting, however, starvation is the result of either anorexia, such as occurs with cancer, sepsis, or liver disease, or a lack of intake due to obstruction. Obstruction may, in turn, be due to neoplasia or stricture of the esophagus secondary to reflux or lye or may be distal in the gastrointestinal tract, such as carcinoma of the colon. Less common intra-abdominal illness, such as scleroderma, motility disorders, pseudo-obstruction, major gastric resection, or a short bowel syndrome also result in inadequate absorption. Inadequate nutrition may also be caused by exces-

---

*Kendall-McGaw, Irvine, California.

sive losses, as with gastrointestinal fistulas, or from malabsorption, as with inflammatory bowel disease or protein-losing enteropathies. However, the most common causes of in-hospital malnutrition are unfortunately those that are easily correctable with some thought. Food served in hospitals is unappetizing, timed poorly, and apparently served for the benefit of personnel rather than patients. (How else can one explain meals offered at 8:30 A.M., 11:30 A.M., and 5 P.M.?) Patients are kept *nil per os* for the most trivial reasons (chest or abdominal films). Diets are not advanced rapidly following the most trivial operations (why "clear liquids" for 2 days?). Food is served cold. The hospital administration looks upon food as an area in which to save money. Given the importance of nutrition, changes are needed.

REASONS FOR PROTEIN LOSS. There are probably different controls for protein metabolism in "red" and "white" muscle, but most understanding of muscle metabolism has been derived from *in vitro* preparations, such as rat hemidiaphragm. This is an atypical muscle that is highly catabolic and probably partially dying in this *in vitro* preparation. Subsequent work in other preparations such as epitrochlearis and soleus has revealed somewhat different results. In general, however, the major controls of nitrogen accrual in muscle include (1) tension-exercise, probably the most potent controlling mechanism[79]; (2) presence of insulin, the principal storage hormone; (3) presence of glucose; and (4) presence of branched chain amino acids.[47]

Branched chain amino acids will subsequently be discussed more completely. However, both the *in vitro* and *in vivo* effects of the branched chain amino acids on positive nitrogen accrual and decreasing amino acid efflux have been performed in hypercatabolic and/or metabolically rapid turnover situations. The effects of the branched chain amino acids have been much more difficult to establish in normal patients and in less catabolic experimental preparations.

HORMONAL CHANGES. The hormonal milieu provides either a storage or a breakdown state (Fig. 7). Insulin is the single most potent metabolic storage factor, decreasing lipolysis and increasing nitrogen accrual in peripheral muscle. The effect of insulin on the liver is less well studied but probably also increases protein synthesis and fat storage, especially portal insulin.[69] Increased secretion of glucagon, catecholamines, and steroids results in gluconeogenesis and breakdown of muscle. These hormones also increase hepatic protein synthesis.

CYTOKINES. A traditional concept of the metabolic response to trauma or sepsis includes the so-called counterregulatory hormones—glucagon, steroids, and catecholamines. In the past 5 years, there has been much research activity in the area of substances known as cytokines, materials produced by macrophages and at least T lymphocytes (Table 2; Fig. 3). Although there are probably more than 100 products of macrophages, attention has focused largely on only a few—interleukin-1, interleukin-2, interleukin-6, TNF/cachectin, and gamma-interferon. Investigators have studied etiocholanolone (as a cause of fever)[103] with interleukin-1 and TNF/cachectin in an attempt to elucidate some of the metabolic responses to sepsis.[41] Summarizing both *in vivo* and *in vitro* studies, it is possible to state: First, prostaglandins probably have little role in the control of skeletal muscle proteolysis, although this is controversial.[57,84] Second, TNF has little role *in vitro* in muscle proteolysis. The role of TNF *in vivo* probably requires steroids, either as a permissive or cofactor in promoting muscle breakdown.[72] The Cincinnati studies using *in vitro* preparations suggest that at least 50 per cent of the proteolytic activity in sepsis is due to steroids.

The effects of cytokines on the liver are complex, with different cytokines having different effects. Interleukin-1 is associated with increased hepatic protein synthesis of some of the complement intermediates,[80] whereas synthesis of transferrin is steroid-dependent. Interleukin-6 (hepatocyte-stimulating factor) increases synthesis of some of the alpha-glycoproteins.[8] Probably as yet unknown cytokines are involved as well.

Many if not all of these effects can be induced by the *in vivo* injection of endotoxin. The incubation of pharmacologic quantities of endotoxin *in vitro* is without effect, suggesting that a synergism with other substances is necessary. Most reagents are not endotoxin-free, that is, almost all chemical reagents and much of the water used in various experiments has picogram quantities of endotoxin present. Their role is not clear, but many experiments are currently being repeated with endotoxin-free materials. It is of interest that Jacob Fine's endotoxin hypothesis is now being revisited 50 years after it was discredited.

The proposal by Clowes[26] that proteolysis-inducing factor (PIF), a substance of molecular weight 4200 and thought to be a split product of interleukin-1, was responsible for both proteolysis and increased hepatic protein synthesis probably did more than any recent paper to stimulate interest (at least in surgery) in the cytokines. Consequently, it is ironic that subsequent studies, including experiments in the Cincinnati laboratory, attempting to confirm PIF have proved very difficult.[55] It appears that the very peculiar experimental conditions used by Clowes may produce the effects attributed to PIF.[55] Unfortunately controls were not done in the initial study. Nonetheless, the contribution of Clowes is enormous. The amount of other work stimulated, rather than whether it is correct or incorrect, is often the major factor in assessing the significance of research work.

CAUSES OF INCREASED PROTEIN LOSS. The normal turnover of protein is 2.5 to 3 per cent of lean body mass per day (see Fig. 4). Nitrogen equilibrium exists with normal protein and calorie intake, and without strenuous exercise to build up muscle, only a minuscule accrual of nitrogen occurs. Proteolysis is far more frequent and occurs in response to starvation, stress, and sepsis and is mediated by hormonal changes; increased secretion of glucagon, catechols, and steroids, with a considerably smaller increase in insulin; and (in trauma or sepsis) the presence of various cytokines. Proteolysis supplies the liver with the necessary amino acids to increase protein synthesis for host defense and for glucose production by gluconeogenesis, the so-called alanine-glucose cycle. The alanine-glucose cycle is not a true cycle, because nitrogen is lost from the amino acids during each turn of the cycle, with ammonia going to urea. Thus, although glucose, which originates from pyruvate, is returned to the periphery, there is net destruction of muscle.

The importance of the endogenous amino acid recirculation in supplying 250 gm. of amino acids available for protein synthesis is again emphasized, because under normal circum-

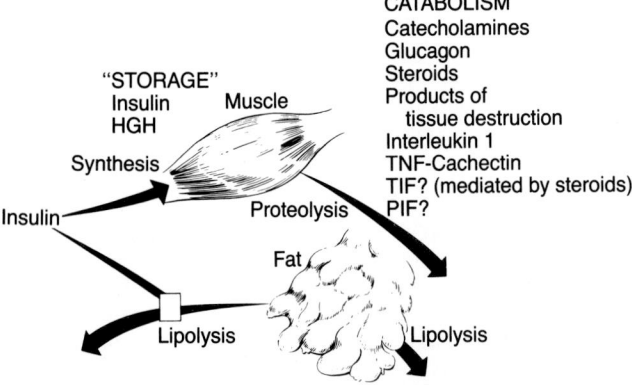

Figure 7. A graphic presentation of the balance between storage and catabolism. Insulin, the single storage hormone, blocks lipolysis and encourages muscle protein synthesis. Catabolism including lipolysis and proteolysis is favored by many factors, of which the most prominent are glucagon, catecholamines, and steroids, especially when present in combination, as well as interleukin 1 and, undoubtedly, various other products of tissue destruction and infection. (HGH, human growth hormone; TNF, tumor necrosis factor; TIF, amino acid transport–inhibiting factor; PIF, proteolysis-inducing factor.)

TABLE 2. Sources and Targets of Cytokines and Other Peptide Regulatory Factors

Regulatory Factor*	Sources	Target Tissues/Cells
Interleukins (ILs)		
IL-1α, IL-1β (endogenous pyrogen, lymphocyte-activating factor, leukocyte endogenous mediator, hemopoietin-1)	Monocytes/macrophages; many endothelial, epithelial, and hematopoietic cells	Thymocytes, T and B cells, hematopoietic cells, fibroblasts, chondrocytes, receptors in brain and liver, hepatocytes
IL-2 (T cell growth factor)	T cells	T and B cells, thymocytes, natural killer cells
IL-3 (multipotential colony-stimulating factor, hematopoietic growth factor)	T cells, myelomonocytic cells	Hematopoietic cells, pre-B cells
IL-4 (B cell-stimulating factor 1, B cell growth factor I)	T cells, mast cells	T and B cells, mast cells, other hematopoietic cells
IL-5 (T cell-replacing factor, eosinophil differentiation factor, B cell growth factor II, eosinophil colony-stimulating factor, IgA-enhancing factor)	T cells	B cells, eosinophils, thymocytes
IL-6 (B cell-stimulating factor 2, beta₂ interferon, hepatocyte-stimulating factor, hybridoma growth factor, B cell differentiation factor, 26 kd. protein)	Monocytes/macrophages, T cells, fibroblasts, epithelial cell types	T and B cells, fibroblasts, hepatocytes, hematopoietic stem cells
IL-7 (lymphoprotein-1, pre-B cell growth factor)	Stomal cells, thymus	Pre-B cells, thymocytes
Tumor Necrosis Factors (TNFs)		
TNF (TNF-α, cachectin)	Monocytes/macrophages, lymphocytes, natural killer cells, glial cells, Kupffer's cells	Endothelial cells, monocytes/macrophages, neutrophils, fibroblasts, receptors in liver, muscle, lung, gut, kidney
Lymphotoxin (TNF-β)	Monocytes/macrophages	? Same receptors as TNF
Interferons		
Interferon-α (leukocyte interferon)	Monocytes/macrophages	Multiple immune cells
Interferon-β (fibroblast interferon)	Fibroblasts, epithelial cells	Multiple immune cells
Interferon-β [see IL-6]		
Interferon-γ (immune interferon, macrophage-activating factor)	Multiple cell types (antigen/antibody reaction)	T and B cells, phagocytic cells
Other Growth and Regulatory Factors		
Insulin-like growth factors (IGFs)		
IGF-1 (somatomedin C)	Fibroblasts, astrocytes, other neuronal and non-neuronal cells	Most cell types (necessary for cell survival), muscle and cartilage, precursor cells
IGF-2 (somatomedin A)	Astrocytes	Most cell types

* The terms in parentheses are alternative terms that have been, and in some cases still are, used for the same substance or group of substances. Adapted from Bessey, P. Q.: Metabolic response to critical illness. *In* Wilmore, D. W., Brennan, M. F., Harken, A. H., Holcroft, J. W., and Meakins, J. L. (Eds.): Care of the Surgical Patient. Section II, Chapter 11. © 1990, Scientific American, Inc. Data drawn from Old, L. J.: Tumor necrosis factor. Scientific American, *258*(5):59, and from Peptide regulatory factors. *Lancet, 1:* 705, 765, 825, 885, 943, 1003, 1060, 1122, 1179, 1243, 1312, 1373, and 1432 and 2:30, 1989.

stances, only 25 per cent (or 20 gm.) of the normal exogenous intake of 100 gm. of protein per day enters the free amino acid pool for protein synthesis (Fig. 5).

In starvation, the loss of protein may be as much as 300 gm. of protein per day for an average man. However, the body rapidly adapts to resting starvation, so that proteolysis becomes minimal after as little as 4 days. The metabolic tragedy of sepsis is that this adaptation to starvation does not occur, and breakdown of protein, to supply amino acids either for hepatic protein synthesis for host defense or for gluconeogenesis for the energy needs of the organism, continues.

The bodily calorie stores are given in Table 3, with fat constituting the bulk of calories available. The additional metabolic tragedy of stress and sepsis is that fat is not utilized to its maximal potential and protein is continually broken down for glucose. Because the control mechanisms appear inoperative, the administration of either fat or glucose, although slightly decreasing the breakdown of protein, does not abolish proteolysis.

Recent data from this laboratory suggest that, in the muscle from a septic animal or patient, the branched chain amino acids, which normally decrease the efflux of amino acids from muscle, do not decrease muscle breakdown even in pharmacologic

TABLE 3. Normal Stores of Available Energy and Rates of Utilization in a Man Weighing 65 Kg.

	Total Body Content (gm.)	Available Store			Daily Utilization* (gm.)	Exhaustion Time (days)
		Grams	Millijoules	Kilocalories		
Carbohydrate	500	150	2.5	600	All used in first 24 hours	<1
Protein	11,000	2400	40	9600	60	About 40†
Fat	9000	6500	235	58,500	150	About 40†

* Assuming an energy expenditure of about 6.7 mj. (1600 kcal.) per day.

† Recent experience in voluntary starvation suggests that the limit of resting starvation in young men in excellent physical condition may be as much as 60 to 70 days (Maize Prison).

From Passmore, R., and Robson, J. S.: A Companion to Medical Studies. Vol. 3. Oxford, Blackwell Scientific Publications, 1974.

quantities (5 mM.).[54] Leupeptin, an inhibitor of lysosomal breakdown, diminishes protein breakdown.[59]

NUTRITIONAL ASSESSMENT
METHODS OF ASSESMENT

LEAN BODY MASS. Accumulation of lean body mass is the principal objective of nutritional support; thus, determination of lean body mass would be the most appropriate means of nutritional assessment. Such determinations are complicated and usually available only on a research basis.

DISPLACEMENT. This is probably the most sensitive determination of lean body mass. In this procedure, the various body components are estimated by immersion in a tank with displacement of water volume. This is beyond the capacity of most institutions.

EXCHANGE OF LABELED IONS. Although more common, this procedure is available only in research centers. Total body water may be determined by administration of tritiated water. Lean body mass may be estimated by the determination of exchangeable potassium (^{42}K) and extracellular water by total exchangeable sodium (^{22}Na). Shizgal has suggested that a ratio of exchangeable sodium to exchangeable potassium of greater than 1.22 indicates the increased extracellular water and decreased body mass accompanying malnutrition. Shizgal also suggested derivative ratios to estimate total body fat, but because of compounded error in the ratios, these are probably inaccurate.[92]

NEUTRON ACTIVATION ANALYSIS. This technique is accurate but requires sophisticated apparatus in which the body is bombarded with activated neutrons. Nitrogen, especially that of lean body mass, is then measured. Other ions may also be determined.[51]

TOTAL BODY COUNTERS. There are approximately 13 body counters in the United States. These large installations measure spontaneous decay of naturally occurring isotopes, such as ^{40}K, which reflect lean body mass. However, these measurements are not suitable for patients who are ill, because one must remain stationary within the counter for prolonged periods of time, and the locations, such as the counter in the institution in Cincinnati, are remote.

NUCLEAR MAGNETIC RESONANCE. The advent of nuclear magnetic resonance may enable accurate measurement of lean body mass. Most of the current work has not focused on lean body mass, but on energy stores and the relationships between phosphocreatinine, ATP, ADP, creatine, and AMP, especially in starvation and refeeding. In rats, changes are detected following 6 to 8 days of starvation, with a decrease in phosphocreatinine that has been teleologically interpreted as being utilized to maintain ATP. Other studies suggest that there may be some decrease in efficiency in the starved muscle, but this has not been confirmed.

HISTORY AND PHYSICAL EXAMINATION. A history of weight loss, anorexia, or a disease process that interferes with intake such as esophageal carcinoma should alert the examiner to the possibility of malnutrition. This can be verified on physical examination by muscle wasting, loss of thenar muscles, loose flabby skin, and the edema of hypoproteinemia. More detailed physical examination will reveal weakness, loss of body fat, and pallor, to name a few confirming features. Several studies have revealed that a careful history and observation from a seasoned clinician are as accurate as multiple complex tests.[6,107]

CLINICAL METHODOLOGIES. Most attempts at nutritional assessment have utilized simple tests available in most hospitals. These include, first and foremost, nitrogen balance.

Nitrogen Balance. Nitrogen balance for research purposes is a tedious technique that requires the measurement of expired nitrogen in the breath as well as the collection of all integumentary, wound, and excretory losses. In the clinical setting, nitrogen balance is generally determined by measuring urinary and gastrointestinal losses. However, because most patients on parenteral nutrition are not eating, stool nitrogen, which is more difficult to determine, can be disregarded. One can measure nitrogen balance in two ways, depending upon the instrumentation available. Urinary urea nitrogen excretion is within the capacity of any hospital laboratory, but urinary collection must be accurate; this can be monitored by the simultaneous measurement of urinary creatinine. If one measures total urinary urea nitrogen excretion, 2 to 3 gm. of nitrogen should be added for insensible and non-urea losses. An alternative is to measure total urinary nitrogen excretion by the increasingly available technique of chemiluminescence, in which case a small amount of nitrogen, less than 1 gm., should be added for insensible losses. This is compared with nitrogen intake, and nitrogen balance is obtained.

Nitrogen Breakdown. Nitrogen breakdown and turnover, particularly that of lean body mass, had been initially estimated by urinary excretion of 3-methylhistidine (3-MH), a methylated derivative of histidine. Whereas 3-MH, a product of actin and myosin, which once methylated is not reutilized for nitrogen synthesis,[109] does not merely measure breakdown but probably turnover as well, it is likely that 3-MH measures not only muscle lean body mass but also a relatively small, rapidly turning-over protein pool derived from the gut. This does not invalidate 3-MH as a measurement of breakdown or turnover of lean body mass; it does invalidate it as a measurement of turnover of skeletal muscle. Most authorities now believe that 3-MH reflects lean body mass, but not skeletal muscle alone.

Indirect Calorimetry. Indirect calorimetry, now available as bedside metabolic carts, is used increasingly to measure energy balance, which, according to most recent data from Elwyn and Kinney, may be as important as nitrogen balance in determining equilibrium. Metabolic carts are also used to estimate caloric requirements. The measurement is usually obtained in the resting state and must be increased by approximately 15 per cent for activity. In a recent study from the author's institution, use of the Harris-Benedict equation, with some correction for the clinical state, compared favorably with metabolic cart measurements as an estimation of patient requirements.[13] The caloric requirement is considerably lower than it was originally thought to be 10 or 15 years ago, more in the range of between 1800 and 2200 kcal. per 24 hours than the 3500 or 4000 kcal. per 24 hours as was common practice at that time.

Delayed Cutaneous Hypersensitivity or Anergy. During the initial years when nutritional assessment was attempted on a large scale, delayed cutaneous hypersensitivity was widely used. Although there was a statistical relationship in most studies between anergy and mortality,[24] recent reviews[74,97] concluded that delayed cutaneous hypersensitivity was without value for measuring operative risk. More recent data by Christou and co-workers, using different antigens and technique, suggest that this view is too simplistic. When carefully performed and observed by trained personnel, and done at defined times— upon entry into the hospital rather than at random times throughout the hospital course—this test has proved valuable.[25] In patients entering the hospital after trauma or with infection, anergy to cutaneous recall antigens is associated with a high mortality and morbidity. This is associated with, but certainly not coincident with, patients with severe malnutrition. Moreover, as Christou has painstakingly emphasized, not all patients who are malnourished are at risk; the defect is not nutritional but immunologic. In subsequent, as yet unpublished studies, Christou and co-workers have related anergy to malnutrition and obtained yet another logit function, using albumin (ALB) and reactivity to recall antigens as a specific function:

$$P|death| = 1/\{1 + e^{(-3.45 + 1.75*(ALB) + 0.3*(ln[DTH\ score])}\}$$

Thus, it now appears that the group of patients with severe malnutrition at risk can be identified by the use of injected recall antigens under carefully controlled conditions.[25]

Delayed cutaneous hypersensitivity is complicated by extraneous factors that have no relationship to nutrition. Operation is followed by immediate anergy in many patients. Cancer is associated with anergy that is reversed upon successful resection. Thus, delayed cutaneous hypersensitivity is not a pure model but needs to be assessed in concert with other tests.

Functional Studies of Muscle Function. Since many of the tests described are not readily available, several investigators have been accumulating experience with muscle strength either as evaluated by hand-grip dynamometry or as force frequency characteristics and rate of recovery from fatigue following electrical stimulation of the ulnar nerve.[86] Although not perfect, both of these studies, if properly conducted, may provide an approximate guide to a functional counterpart of severe protein-calorie malnutrition. In most studies, however, patients with deficits in hand dynamometry are easily identifiable by other means such as a simple functional history, physical examination, or "global nutritional assessment."[6,107]

NUTRITIONAL ASSESSMENT

Nutritional assessment, a clinical term, is a method of estimating changes in body nutritional composition in order to predict risk for a given treatment, usually surgical therapy but at times chemotherapy and/or radiation. Nutritional assessment at present is disappointing but shows some hope of improvement. Although the ability to predict risk in a large population, such as severely malnourished populations in Third World Countries, has been well established in the nonsurgical nutritional literature, risk for an individual patient cannot be predicted accurately in a United States hospital setting. In other words, outcome has not been predictable except in a statistical sense.

It is thought that confusion in this area is due to inaccuracies of concept, such as confusion between measuring structure and function. Theoretically, one should measure lean body mass functionally. For example, how does loss of lean body mass affect muscular, respiratory, cardiac, hepatic, and renal functions? More important, how have immunologic and host defense functions, including neutrophil function,[4] been affected?

If one views current practices in the light of the aforementioned goals, the parameters commonly used are disappointing. Structural measurements including midarm muscle circumference and height/weight ratio, indicate stores but do not reflect function, and triceps skinfold thickness measures fat stores, which has little to do with function. Neutrophil function is at least one order of magnitude removed from cell-mediated immunity, most commonly tested by delayed hypersensitivity to skin recall antigens. Although recent reviews discounted the value of skin recall antigen testing,[74,97] better-directed studies may identify the individual patient at risk.[25]

Acceptable studies, in the author's opinion, should be randomized and prospective, include a large number of *consecutive* nonselected patients, and have blinded observers. When these criteria are applied, few studies qualify. Most published studies are retrospective for selected patients, usually specifically those patients judged severely at risk. More recent studies that emphasize hepatic synthesis of short-turnover proteins, immunologically related proteins, and neutrophil function may be more successful in identifying patients at risk for infection.[4] Buzby, Mullen, and co-workers have suggested a "prognostic nutritional index," but the patients were selected nonconsecutively and studied retrospectively.[17,76] Consecutive patients studied prospectively in equally large numbers failed to reveal a group at risk.[88] Other investigators have convincingly shown that accurate observation by experienced observers not particularly skilled in "nutritional assessment" provides the same accuracy as extensive tests.[6]

Recent studies have stressed the importance of a careful functional history.[107] Christou and co-workers have emphasized

that it is not the malnutrition, *per se*, but apparently an immunologic defect associated with severe malnutrition that places patients at risk.[25] Once this subset of patients can be identified, one can then concentrate on repairing the defect. Buzby and co-workers, in the recent Veterans Administration Hospital cooperative study, have identified a group of severely malnourished patients at risk, and decreased operative morbidity with perioperative parenteral nutrition.[16] If all of these studies are collated, the potential for identification of the patient at risk is quite close. Clearly, while many of the large demographic studies using commercially available skin-testing apparatus are nonspecific, carefully done studies may soon identify the individual patient at risk, which is the goal of nutritional assessment.

When all studies are evaluated, the patient at risk can be recognized, in the author's opinion, in the following manner:

1. Recent weight loss of greater than 15 per cent body weight and/or body weight of 80 to 85 per cent ideal body weight.
2. Serum albumin in a stable, hydrated patient of less than 3.0 gm. per 100 ml.

These two simple parameters will probably define the population at risk. Additional corroborative information includes:

3. Anergy to *injected* skin recall antigen by the technique of Christou.[25]
4. True transferrin of less than 200 mg. per 100 ml.
5. A history of functional impairment.
6. Significant deficits in hand dynamometry.

The importance of albumin is shown by juxtaposing two logit functions that attempt to identify the patient at risk:

From Mullen and co-workers:

$$PNI = 158 - 16.6 \, ALB - 0.78 \text{ triceps skinfold} - 0.20 \, TFN - 5.8 \, DTH$$

PNI is prognostic nutritional index, DTH is delayed-type hypersensitivity, and TFN is transferrin.

From Christou's work:

$$P|death| = 1/\{1 + e^{(-3.45 + 1.75 \cdot (ALB) + 0.3 \cdot (\ln[DTH \, score])\}}$$

INDICATIONS FOR NUTRITIONAL SUPPORT

In the absence of ability to accurately predict the risk in a given patient, indications for parenteral nutrition should include the following considerations: (1) the premorbid state (healthy or otherwise), especially the nutritional status; (2) age of the patient; (3) duration of starvation; (4) degree of the anticipated insult; (5) the likelihood of resuming normal intake soon; (6) weight loss of 15 per cent; and (7) a serum albumin less than 3.0 gm. per 100 ml. Confirmatory values indicating a possible problem with sepsis include a true transferrin of less than 200 mg. per 100 ml. and anergy to injected antigens. These criteria indicate a type of patient, 60 per cent of whom may develop septic complications. However, the ability to predict the individual patient at risk is still lacking.

Each practitioner must choose the criteria in a given patient. However, patients in the seventh and eighth decades lose lean body mass, although their percentage of lean body mass as a percentage of total body composition is greater with fewer fat reserves. Patients up to 60 years of age can tolerate a 12- to 14-day period of fast, beyond which continued starvation is deleterious. It is not suggested that such patients should be allowed to starve for 12 to 14 days, merely that this can perhaps be tolerated. In septuagenarians, 7 to 8 days is the limit, and probably 5 to 6 days is the limit in patients of 80 years or more. Obviously, in critically ill patients, nutritional supplementation should be undertaken more readily than in those less severely stressed.

ROUTES OF ADMINISTRATION

Two routes are possible: the enteral route, using either the stomach or small intestine, and the parenteral route. The enteral route is more physiologic in that the liver is not bypassed and hepatic ability to take up, process, and store the various nutrients for later release upon nervous or hormonal command is maintained. Furthermore, there is some evidence that additional work, such as increased cardiac output, is required when the gut is bypassed. With parenteral nutrition, gut blood flow increases about 15 to 20 per cent, presumably to allow the gut to perform its usual metabolic functions, such as transamination.

It is often said that enteral nutrition is safer and more efficacious than the parenteral route. However, not a single study, in either experimental animals or man,[75] has demonstrated an improved outcome using enteral nutrition. Enteral nutrition is not more efficacious than parenteral nutrition when the unavoidable catheter sepsis in experimental animals is taken into account, that is, when animals in which the catheters are septic (as judged either by mediastinal culture or section) are eliminated. Similar results are obtained in patients in whom enteral and parenteral feeding are compared.[19,20,75] Nor is it true that enteral nutrition is safer. Deaths with enteral nutrition are generally due to aspiration; gastric motility suddenly changes with the onset of sepsis. One death from aspiration is equivalent to the mortality over 2 to 3 years of a well-operated parenteral nutrition program, despite the danger of catheter sepsis (which in well-operated units is now less than 1 per cent).

Despite this, there is greater emphasis on the use of the gut, if available. There are several reasons for this, including that enteral nutrition is "cheaper," it is a more physiologic route of administration, it likely protects and improves hepatic function, and it mimics the normal ingress of nutrients so that the liver can store, process, and release nutrients as it normally does. There is also increased appreciation for maintenance of gut mucosal integrity, particularly in burns and hemorrhagic shock. When mucosal integrity is not protected, increased translocation of bacteria or their products may occur.

THE TRANSLOCATION HYPOTHESIS. A possible deleterious role of the gut and/or its contents in the pathophysiology of severe injury, particularly burns, was first proposed by Alexander and co-workers, who prevented hypercatabolism by immediate enteral feeding in burned guinea pigs.[33] When feedings were delayed by 24 hours, even increases in the caloric intake from 175 calories per kg. to 200 calories per kg. did not prevent hypercatabolism and weight loss as well as early feeding. Similar results have been obtained in patients.[64]

Translocation is a normal process, which teleologically may be important in releasing small amounts of endotoxin to prime the immune systems. It is increased in burns and by hemorrhagic shock,[85] but not by pure starvation.[31] Whereas the bacteria may normally be cleared by the lymph nodes, it is the bacterial products in the portal circulation, presumably interacting with the Kupffer cells and hepatocytes, that *may* contribute to the hepatic dysfunction and multiple organ system failure.[9] The one study comparing enteral with parenteral nutrition in critically ill patients showed no improvement in outcome or decrease in frequency of multiple organ system failure.[19] Thus, caution is appropriate. It may well be that translocation is important in severe illness, as its enthusiasts propose, but for the present, confirmatory data exist only for burns and perhaps hemorrhagic shock; it remains a field of active investigation.

ENTEROCYTE-SPECIFIC NUTRITIONAL SUBSTRATES. Enterocyte-specific nutrients, such as glutamine and the short-chain fatty acid products of bacterial action on soluble pectin, have received much recent attention. The inclusion of such substrates in routine parenteral nutrition will, it is hoped, prevent gut atrophy and maintain the gut barrier.

GLUTAMINE. It has recently been proposed that the addition of glutamine to parenteral nutrition solutions may prevent the gut atrophy that normally accompanies parenteral nutrition. In some studies, addition of 2 per cent glutamine to parenteral nutrition solution has shown maintenance of jejunal or ileal mucosal thickness, protein content, and DNA.[60,101,105] Not all agree, however. It is difficult to obtain reproducible sections through the gut mucosa to measure thicknesses, and similar inconsistencies plague the scraping techniques by which gut mucosal protein, DNA, and RNA are measured. The beneficial results occur after 2 weeks, a biologically long time for a rat, and likely longer in humans. In the Cincinnati studies, in which such measurements were done incidentally, gut DNA was slightly increased at 1 week, but gut protein, RNA, and wall thickness were unchanged.[68] Additionally, epidermal growth factor is much more efficacious in preventing gut wall atrophy than is glutamine.[60] Glutamine's effects in either preventing or healing chemotherapeutic or radiation toxicity,[42] and the regrowth following massive small bowel resection, are more impressive. However, in neoplastic disease, one should remember that glutamine is a principal nitrogen source for many tumors, thus raising a cautionary flag. Glutamine constitutes between 50 and 60 per cent of the muscle free amino acids. Within 24 hours after stress or injury, much of this disappears, the nitrogen component of which can represent the increased urea excretion in the first 36 hours following stress and trauma. Kinney has suggested that replacement of intramuscular glutamine takes approximately 2 months and is the last value to return to normal following trauma. Early studies in postoperative patients whose TPN was supplemented with a glutamine dipeptide show a small positive difference in nitrogen balance in the group supplemented with glutamine, but these small differences are unlikely to be clinically significant.[50,94] Further studies are indicated.

SHORT-CHAIN FATTY ACIDS. Acetoacetate, proprionate, and butyrate are produced by the fermentation of soluble pectin by colonic bacteria. Only 10 per cent of acetoacetate is utilized locally, with 90 per cent exported into the portal vein. With proprionate, 50 per cent is exported, and of beta-hydroxybutyrate 80 per cent is consumed locally by the colonocytes and only 20 per cent enters the portal vein. The administration of intravenous beta-hydroxybutyrate results in wall thickening and increased protein content of both the colon and ileum.[66] Preliminary uses of ketone bodies in preventing diversion colitis have been promising. More studies undoubtedly will be forthcoming, particularly in areas of gut dysfunction.

GENERAL PRINCIPLES OF ENTERAL FEEDING

The stomach is the principal defense against an enteral osmotic load. Following bolus administration of hyperosmotic fluid, gastric motility decreases and gastric secretion proceeds until gastric contents are iso-osmotic, at which point transfer across the pylorus begins. The small bowel is less able to dilute osmotic loads when administered directly. Moreover, gastric acid secretion, which normally prevents bacterial contamination of the gastrointestinal tract, may be neutralized by constant infusion into the stomach; thus, bacterial overgrowth in the gastrointestinal tract may occur. If nutritional solutions are not properly refrigerated or are suspended unprotected for prolonged periods of time, bacterial overgrowth may occur in the container.

The small bowel is the principal area for nutrient absorption. Dipeptides are the preferred configuration for protein absorption, not, as commonly thought, single amino acids. With normal gut function, this is unimportant, because protein is completely absorbed in the first 120 cm. of jejunum. With short or diseased bowel, there may be a decided advantage of diets in the dipeptide form. Carbohydrate is also absorbed high in the jejunum, with simple sugars preferred. Complex sugars, such as disaccharides, require enzymatic cleavage. A common difficulty with patients who are seriously ill is acquired lactase deficiency, which often corrects itself in time, but in the early post-injury recovery phase, lactose-containing products may cause diarrhea. Fat is the most difficult nutrient to absorb, being dependent upon proper release and mixing of bile and pancreatic enzymes. Following gastrectomy, pancreatic resection, or upper abdominal complex operative procedures, such relationships are disturbed. Calcium, iron, and other metals are absorbed in the duodenum. Consequently, duodenal bypass (as following Billroth II gastrectomy) may result in long-term deficiencies.

OTHER FUNCTIONS OF THE GUT. At least 22 putative gut hormones have been described and immunohistochemical examinations have revealed an equally complex series of endocrine-like cells. The gut also performs important immunologic functions, producing large amounts of globulins.

PRACTICALITIES OF ENTERAL FEEDING

Because hyperosmolar solutions are better tolerated by the stomach than by the intestine, enteral feeding is best given by the smallest possible nasogastric tube, although to prevent aspiration many prefer nasoduodenal tubes. A No. 10 French Silastic catheter is adequate for most enteral diets, whereas a No. 8 French tube can be used for some diets but not for some of the thicker hydrolysates because it obstructs easily. Long-term indwelling tubes probably render the cardia incompetent, and the resultant prolonged reflux may (rarely) yield an esophageal stricture. Patients should be infused constantly, with the bolus technique reserved for special situations. To prevent reflux and aspiration, patients should be maintained at a 30-degree angle, and, in general, gastric tube feedings should cease at approximately 11 P.M., when only skeletal nursing shifts are present. Gastric and/or intestinal motility may change rapidly with the onset of sepsis; with continued feeding, aspiration may result. From the standpoint of safety but not physiology, it is safer to give diets into the small intestine, either by passing a tube via mouth or nostril, through a gastrostomy into the duodenum, or by needle catheter jejunostomy (Fig. 8), or, as the author now prefers, a small (No. 12 French) catheter jejunostomy, which has greater flexibility with a variety of diets.

ADMINISTRATION. For gastric feeding, first osmolality and then volume is increased. One third or one fourth strength, especially with the extremely hyperosmolar solutions, is generally initiated. With formulations that are almost iso-osmolar, additional water is essential. If administration is into the small bowel, volume should be increased first and then osmolality should be increased. Most patients do not tolerate small bowel administration of osmolar concentrations greater than 500 to 600 mOsm.

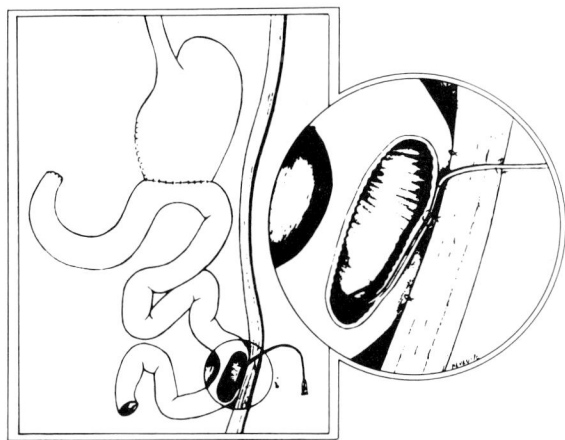

Figure 8. Diagrammatic representation of a needle catheter jejunostomy placed just distal to the gastrojejunostomy. (From Page, C. P., Ryan, J. A., Jr., and Haff, R. C.: Continual catheter administration of an elemental diet. Surg. Gynecol. Obstet., 142:184, 1976.)

DIETS AVAILABLE. There are a wide variety of enteral products available. For patients with normal gut function, a sterilized and less expensive commercial version of the familiar blenderized meal, a "hydrolysate," is usually well tolerated and all that is required. Patients in this category include those who simply cannot eat, such as the elderly, those with carcinoma of the head and neck, and those with neurologic disease. Additionally, there are products with various degrees of complexity and predigestion, ranging from oligopeptides to individual amino acids. The caloric supply varies from dextrose to complex starches (Table 4). Modular diets are those in which the protein, fat, and carbohydrate components can be individually supplied. A listing of the common products available is given in Table 4.

There has been much discussion of the advantages and disadvantages of elemental diets over hydrolysates. With reasonably normal gut function, there appears to be no advantage. Elemental diets, however, are more easily administered through needle catheter jejunostomies or No. 8 French catheters.

COMPLICATIONS OF ENTERAL ADMINISTRATION. In addition to the technical problems of administration, such as malposition of the catheter (i.e., within the pharynx or trachea) and/or aspiration due to changes in gastric motility or overloading, the most common complications of enteral feedings result from solute overload. Inappropriately rapid administration of hyperosmolar solutions results in diarrhea, dehydration, electrolyte imbalance, and hyperglycemia (with glucose-containing solutions) as well as loss of potassium, magnesium, and other ions lost in diarrhea. Hyperosmolar nonketotic coma can occur with enteral feedings as well as with parenteral nutrition. Perforation, although rare, may occur, particularly with the new catheters with rigid styluses to aid in their passage. Malposition, such as in the bronchus with perforation into the pleural cavity, appears associated with the more rigid Enteriflex tube.[108]

All these complications are avoidable. As stated previously, aspiration can be prevented by the head-up position of 30 degrees, placing the catheter into the duodenum, the judicious advancing of enteral diets, and monitoring of gastric residual, particularly in the presence of fever. Dehydration can be prevented by carefully increasing osmolality and using Kaopectate and opiate-like medications to prevent excessive diarrhea. Dehydration and hyperosmolality can be prevented by the addition of free water.

Enteral feeding is much less expensive than parenteral nutrition. In some institutions in the United States, the hydrolysates cost as little as $25 to $50 per day, compared with up to $200 per day for total parenteral nutrition. In the Cincinnati studies, comparable nitrogen retention could be achieved at 30 to 50 per cent of the cost. However, enteral nutrition is often not possible in patients who are very ill and whose situation is complicated by intra-abdominal sepsis; it is then necessary to use a parenteral approach.

THE PARENTERAL ROUTE

In discussing the parenteral route, several assumptions will be made:

1. The protein component is a mixture of single amino acids of synthetic origin, largely produced from "intelligent bacteria" cultures. At present, Japan is the sole source. Although hydrolysates are available, there is much protein wastage in the hydrolysates, because hydrolysis is incomplete. Legally, 55 per cent of the protein should be hydrolyzed to amino acids to qualify as a hydrolysate, and few firms continue hydrolysis beyond this point. The residual di- and tripeptides are not efficiently utilized. A further advantage of synthetic amino acid solutions is the ability to tailor solutions for different disease states (such as hepatic and renal disease).

Text continued on page 125

TABLE 4. Enteral Nutritional Products

Blenderized Formulas

	Compleat-Regular (Sandoz)		Compleat-Modified (Sandoz)		Vitaneed (Sherwood)	
kcal./ml.	1		1		1	
Protein, gm./L. (source)	43	(beef, nonfat milk)	43	(beef, Ca caseinate)	40	(beef, Na + Ca caseinates)
Fat, gm./L. (source)	43	(corn oil, beef fat)	37	(corn oil, beef fat)	40	(soy oil, beef fat)
Carbohydrate, gm./L. (source)	128	(hydrolyzed cereal, fruit, vegetables, maltodextrin, lactose)	141	(hydrolyzed cereal, fruit, vegetables)	128	(pureed fruit + vegetables, maltodextrin)
Lactose, gm./L.	24		0		0	
Minerals/L.						
Calcium, mg.	670		670		667	
Phosphorus, mg.	1300		930		667	
Magnesium, mg.	267		267		200	
Iron, mg.	12		12		12	
Sodium, mEq.	57		29		30	
Potassium, mEq.	36		36		32	
Chloride, mEq.	25		13		28	
Iodine, μg.	100		100		100	
Zinc, mg.	10		10		20	
Copper, mg.	1		1		1.5	
Manganese, mg.	3		3		3	
Volume required to meet 100% RDA, ml.	1500		1500		1500	
kcal./gm. N_2	131/1		131/1		154/1	
mOsm./kg. H_2O	405		300		300	
Preparation	Ready to use		Ready to use		Ready to use	
Comments	Commercially prepared blenderized tube feeding		Commercially prepared blenderized tube feeding, lactose free		Commercially prepared blenderized tube feeding, lactose free	

Milk-Based Formulas

	C.I.B. (Carnation)		Meritene Liquid (Sandoz)		Sustagen (Mead Johnson)	
kcal./ml.	1		1		1.8	
Protein, gm./L. (source)	58	(nonfat dry milk, Ca caseinate, sweet dairy whey)	58	(nonfat milk)	111	(nonfat milk, powdered whole milk, Ca caseinate)
Fat, gm./L. (source)	31	(milk fat)	32	(corn oil)	17	(milk fat)
Carbohydrate, gm./L. (source)	135	(lactose, sucrose, maltodextrin)	110	(lactose, corn syrup solids, sucrose)	312	(corn syrup solids, lactose, dextrose)
Lactose, gm./L.	100		57		105	
Minerals/L.						
Calcium, mg.	1371		1200		3328	
Phosphorus, mg.	1105		1200		2500	
Magnesium, mg.	459		320		416	
Iron, mg.	18		14		19	
Sodium, mEq.	42		38		45	
Potassium, mEq.	72		41		85	
Chloride, mEq.	51		45		79	
Iodine, μg.	147		120		156	
Zinc, mg.	16		12		21	
Copper, mg.	2		2		2	
Manganese, mg.	3		3		5	
Volume required to meet 100% RDA, ml.	1373		1250		1030	
kcal./gm. N_2	108/1		79/1		102/1	
mOsm./kg. H_2O	671– 758		505		1100	
Preparation	Powder		Ready to use		Powder	
Comments	Palatable, easily available, inexpensive		Supplemental, high-protein		Supplemental, high-calorie, high-protein	

TABLE 4. Enteral Nutritional Products *Continued*

	Supplements				**Defined Formula Diet**	
	Ensure Pudding (Ross)		**Sustacal Pudding (Mead Johnson)**		**Reabilan (O'Brien)**	
kcal./ml.	1.7		1.6		1	
Protein, gm./L. (source)	45	(nonfat milk)	45	(nonfat milk)	32	(casein + whey peptides)
Fat, gm./L. (source)	65	(soy oil)	63	(partially hydrogenated soy oil)	39	(MCT, primrose oil, soy lecithin, mono- and distearate glycerin)
Carbohydrate, gm./L.	227	(modified starch, sucrose)	213	(sucrose, modified starch, lactose)	132	(dextrin, maltose, tapioca)
Lactose, gm./L.	60		646		0	
Minerals/L.						
Calcium, mg.	1333		1467		499	
Phosphorus, mg.	1333		1467		499	
Magnesium, mg.	454		400		251	
Iron, mg.	20		18		10	
Sodium, mEq.	70		35		30	
Potassium, mEq.	56		55		32	
Chloride, mEq.	43		38		56	
Iodine, μg.	400		147		75	
Zinc, mg.	26		15		10	
Copper, mg.	2		2		2	
Manganese, mg.	6		4.5		2	
Volume required to meet 100% RDA, ml.	880		1000		2000	
kcal./gm. N_2	230/1		226/1		175/1	
mOsm./kg. H_2O						
Preparation	Ready to use		Ready to use		Ready to use	
Comments	Supplemental		Supplemental		Tube feeding, high peptide content, absorbed in upper gut	

Lactose-Free Formulas

	Citrotein (Sandoz)		**Isocal HN (Mead Johnson)**		**Ensure (Ross)**	
kcal./ml.	0.7		1.06		1	
Protein, gm./L. (source)	41	(egg albumin)	44	(Na + Ca caseinates, soy protein isolates)	37	(Na + Ca caseinates, soy protein isolates)
Fat, gm./L. (source)	2	(partially hydrogenated soy oil)	45	(soy oil, MCT)	37	(corn oil)
Carbohydrate, gm./L.	122	(maltodextrin, sucrose)	124	(maltodextrin)	145	(corn syrup, sucrose)
Lactose, gm./L.	0		0		0	
Minerals/L.						
Calcium, mg.	1060		850		500	
Phosphorus, mg.	1060		850		500	
Magnesium, mg.	420		340		200	
Iron, mg.	38		15.2		9	
Sodium, mEq.	31		40		35	
Potassium, mEq.	18		41		38	
Chloride, mEq.	27		41		38	
Iodine, μg.	158		127		35	
Zinc, mg.	16		12.7		11	
Copper, mg.	2		1.7		1	
Manganese, mg.	5.1				3	
Volume required to meet 100% RDA, ml.	1180		1250		1887	
kcal./gm. N_2	76/1		151/1		178/1	
mOsm./kg. H_2O	480		300		470	
Preparation	Powder		Ready to use		Ready to use	
Comments	Protein, vitamin, mineral supplement		High-protein, ultra–trace elements		Supplemental, tube feeding	

Table continued on following page

TABLE 4. Enteral Nutritional Products *Continued*

Lactose-Free Formulas

	Ensure HN (Ross)		Ensure Plus (Ross)		Ensure Plus HN (Ross)	
kcal./ml.	1		1.5		1.5	
Protein, gm./L. (source)	44	(Na + Ca caseinates, soy protein isolates)	55	(Na + Ca caseinates, soy protein isolates)	63	(Na + Ca caseinates, soy protein isolates)
Fat, gm./L. (source)	35	(corn oil)	53	(corn oil)	50	(corn oil)
Carbohydrate, gm./L.	141	(corn syrup, sucrose)	200	(corn syrup, sucrose)	200	(hydrolyzed corn starch, sucrose)
Lactose, gm./L.	0		0		0	
Minerals/L.						
Calcium, mg.	756		706		1057	
Phosphorus, mg.	756		706		1057	
Magnesium, mg.	302		283		423	
Iron, mg.	14		13		19	
Sodium, mEq.	41		50		52	
Potassium, mEq.	40		54		47	
Chloride, mEq.	41		56		45	
Iodine, μg.	113		106		159	
Zinc, mg.	17		16		24	
Copper, mg.	2		1		2	
Manganese, mg.	4		1		5	
Volume required to meet 100% RDA, ml.	1400		1420		947	
kcal./gm. N_2	150/1		171/1		150/1	
mOsm./kg. H_2O	470		690		650	
Preparation	Ready to use		Ready to use		Ready to use	
Comments	Supplemental, tube feeding		Supplemental, tube feeding, high-calorie		Supplemental, tube feeding, high-calorie	

	Sustacal Liquid (Mead Johnson)		Sustacal HC (Mead Johnson)		Isocal (Mead Johnson)	
kcal./ml.	1		1.5		1	
Protein, gm./L. (source)	61	(Na + Ca caseinates, soy protein isolates)	61	(Na + Ca caseinates)	34	(Na + Ca caseinates, soy protein isolates)
Fat, gm./L. (source)	23	(partially hydrogenated soy oil)	58	(corn oil)	44	(soy oil, MCT)
Carbohydrate, gm./L.	140	(sucrose, corn syrup)	190	(corn syrup solids, sucrose)	133	(maltodextrin)
Lactose, gm./L.	0		0		0	
Minerals/L.						
Calcium, mg.	1010		850		630	
Phosphorus, mg.	930		850		530	
Magnesium, mg.	380		340		210	
Iron, mg.	17		15		9	
Sodium, mEq.	41		36		23	
Potassium, mEq.	54		38		34	
Chloride, mEq.	42		36		30	
Iodine, μg.	140		130		79	
Zinc, mg.	14		13		11	
Copper, mg.	2		2		1	
Manganese, mg.	3		3		3	
Volume required to meet 100% RDA, ml.	1080		1200		1887	
kcal./gm. N_2	104/1		160/1		190/1	
mOsm./kg. H_2O	620		650		300	
Preparation	Ready to use		Ready to use		Ready to use	
Comments	Supplemental, high-protein		Supplemental, high-calorie		Supplemental, tube feeding	

TABLE 4. Enteral Nutritional Products *Continued*

Lactose-Free Formulas

	Isocal HCN (Mead Johnson)		Isotein HN (Sandoz)		Osmolite (Ross)	
kcal./ml.	2		1		1	
Protein, gm./L. (source)	75	(Na + Ca caseinates)	68	(delactosed lactalbumin)	37	(Na + Ca caseinates, soy protein isolates)
Fat, gm./L. (source)	102	(soybean oil, MCT)	34	(soy oil, MCT)	38	(corn oil, soy oil, MCT)
Carbohydrate, gm./L.	200	(corn syrup)	156	(maltodextrins, monosaccharides)	145	(glucose polymers)
Lactose, gm./L.	0		0		0	
Minerals/L.						
Calcium, mg.	1000		560		528	
Phosphorus, mg.	1000		560		528	
Magnesium, mg.	400		226		211	
Iron, mg.	18		10		9	
Sodium, mEq.	35		27		28	
Potassium, mEq.	43		27		26	
Chloride, mEq.	34		27		24	
Iodine, μg.	150		85		80	
Zinc, mg.	30		9		12	
Copper, mg.	3		1		1	
Manganese, mg.	3		2		3	
Volume required to meet 100% RDA, ml.	1000		1770		1887	
kcal./gm. N_2	170/1		86/1		178/1	
mOsm./kg. H_2O	690		300		300	
Preparation	Ready to use		Powder		Ready to use	
Comments	Supplemental, tube feeding, high-calorie, high-protein		Supplemental, tube feeding, high-protein, isotonic		Tube feeding	

	Osmolite HN (Ross)		Magnacal (Sherwood)		Portagen (Mead Johnson)	
kcal./ml.	1		2		1	
Protein, gm./L. (source)	37	(Na + Ca caseinates, soy protein isolates)	70	(Na + Ca caseinates)	35	(Na caseinate)
Fat, gm./L. (source)	39	(MCT, corn oil, soy oil)	80	(partially hydrogenated soy oil)	48	(86% MCT, corn oil, soy lecithin)
Carbohydrate, gm./L.	145	(glucose polymers)	250	(maltodextrin, sucrose)	115	(corn syrup solids, sucrose)
Lactose, gm./L.	0		0		0	
Minerals/L.						
Calcium, mg.	758		1000		936	
Phosphorus, mg.	758		1000		707	
Magnesium, mg.	304		400		208	
Iron, mg.	14		18		19	
Sodium, mEq.	40		43		24	
Potassium, mEq.	40		32		32	
Chloride, mEq.	41		27		24	
Iodine, μg.	114		150		73	
Zinc, mg.	17		30		9	
Copper, mg.	2		2		2	
Manganese, mg.	4		5		1	
Volume required to meet 100% RDA, ml.	1321		1000		2000	
kcal./gm. N_2	150/1		154/1		178/1	
mOsm./kg. H_2O	300		590		320	
Preparation	Ready to use		Ready to use		Powder	
Comments	Supplemental, tube feeding, high-protein		Supplemental, tube feeding, high-calorie, high-protein		Supplemental, tube feeding, indicated in fat malabsorption	

Table continued on following page

TABLE 4. Enteral Nutritional Products *Continued*

Lactose-Free Formulas

	Precision Isotonic (Sandoz)		*Attain (Sherwood)*		*TraumaCal (Mead Johnson)*	
kcal./ml.	1		1		1.5	
Protein, gm./L. (source)	30	(egg albumin)	40	(Na + Ca caseinates)	83	(Na + Ca caseinates)
Fat, gm./L. (source)	31	(soybean oil)	40	(corn oil)	68	(soy oil, MCT)
Carbohydrate, gm./L.	150	(glucose oligosaccharides, sucrose)	120	(maltodextrin)	143	(corn syrup, sucrose)
Lactose, gm./L.	0		0		0	
Minerals/L.						
Calcium, mg.	667		500		750	
Phosphorus, mg.	667		500		750	
Magnesium, mg.	267		200		200	
Iron, mg.	12		9		9	
Sodium, mEq.	35		22		52	
Potassium, mEq.	27		32		36	
Chloride, mEq.	30		24		45	
Iodine, μg.	100		75		75	
Zinc, mg.	10		15		15	
Copper, mg.	1		1		2	
Manganese, mg.	3		2		3	
Volume required to meet 100% RDA, ml.	1560		1600		3000	
kcal./gm. N_2	200/1		131/1		116/1	
mOsm./kg. H_2O	300		300		490	
Preparation	Powder		Ready to use		Ready to use	
Comments	Supplemental, tube feeding, high–biologic value protein, isotonic, absorbed in upper gut		Supplemental, tube feeding		Supplemental, tube feeding	

	Isosource (Sandoz)		*Isosource HN (Sandoz)*		*Jevity (Ross)*	
kcal./ml.	1.2		1.2		1	
Protein, gm./L. (source)	43	(Na + K caseinates)	53	(Na + K caseinates)	44	(Na + Ca caseinates)
Fat, gm./L. (source)	41.6	(MCT, carrola oil)	41.6	(MCT)	37	(MCT 50%, corn oil, soy oil)
Carbohydrate, gm./L.	167	(maltodextrin	145	(maltodextrin)	152	(hydrolyzed corn starch, soy polysaccharide)
Lactose, gm./L.	0		0		0	(14 gm. fiber/1000 cal.)
Minerals/L.						
Calcium, mg.	667		667		917	
Phosphorus, mg.	667		667		763	
Magnesium, mg.	266		266		305	
Iron, mg.	12		12		14	
Sodium, mEq.	32		32		40	
Potassium, mEq.	43		43		40	
Chloride, mEq.	32		32		40	
Iodine, μg.	100		100		114	
Zinc, mg.	17		17		17	
Copper, mg.	1.3		1.3		2	
Manganese, mg.	3		3		4	
Volume required to meet 100% RDA, ml.	1500		1500		1321	
kcal./gm. N_2	173/1		140/1		150/1	
mOsm./kg. H_2O	390		390		310	
Preparation	Ready to use		Ready to use		Ready to use	
Comments	Supplemental, tube feeding		Supplemental, tube feeding		Tube feeding, increased fiber	

TABLE 4. Enteral Nutritional Products *Continued*

Lactose-Free Formulas

	Enrich (Ross)		Nutren (Clintec)		Replete (Clintec)	
kcal./ml.	1		1		1	
Protein, gm./L. (source)	40	(Na + K caseinates, soy protein)	40	(Ca + K caseinates)	62	(K + Ca caseinates)
Fat, gm./L. (source)	37	(corn oil)	38	(MCT, corn oil)	33	(corn oil)
Carbohydrate, gm./L.	162	(hydrolyzed corn starch, sucrose, soy polysaccharides)	127	(maltodextrin, corn syrup)	113	(maltodextrin, sucrose)
Lactose, gm./L.	0	(23 gm. fiber/1000 cal.)	0		0	(14 gm. fiber/1000 cal.)
Minerals/L.						
Calcium, mg.	718		500		600	
Phosphorus, mg.	718		500		540	
Magnesium, mg.	288		250		300	
Iron, mg.	13		9		9	
Sodium, mEq.	38		22		22	
Potassium, mEq.	43		32		40	
Chloride, mEq.	41		28		17	
Iodine, μg.	108		76		76	
Zinc, mg.	16		10		10	
Copper, mg.	1		1		1	
Manganese, mg.	3		2		2	
Volume required to meet 100% RDA, ml.	1416		2000		2000	
kcal./gm. N_2	148/1		131/1		100.1	
mOsm./kg. H_2O	480		300		350	
Preparation	Ready to use		Ready to use		Ready to use	
Comments	Supplemental, tube feeding, increased fiber		Supplemental, tube feeding, increased fiber		Supplemental, tube feeding, high-protein	

	Travasorb MCT (Clintec)		Criticare HN (Mead Johnson)	
kcal./ml.	1		1	
Protein, gm./L. (source)	49	(lactalbumin, K + Na caseinates)	38	(hydrolyzed casein, 60% free amino acids, 40% peptides)
Fat, gm./L. (source)	33	(MCT, sunflower oil)	5	(safflower oil, soy oil)
Carbohydrate, gm./L.	123	(corn syrup solids)	220	(maltodextrin, modified corn starch)
Lactose, gm./L.	0		0	
Minerals/L.				
Calcium, mg.	500		530	
Phosphorus, mg.	500		530	
Magnesium, mg.	200		210	
Iron, mg.	9		10	
Sodium, mEq.	15		27	
Potassium, mEq.	26		34	
Chloride, mEq.	34		30	
Iodine, μg.	75		79	
Zinc, mg.	15		11	
Copper, mg.	1		10	
Manganese, mg.	2		3	
Volume required to meet 100% RDA, ml.	2000		1890	
kcal./gm. N_2	127/1		173/1	
mOsm./kg. H_2O	312		650	
Preparation	Powder		Ready to use	
Comments	Supplement, tube feeding, for patients with fat intolerance		Tube feeding, uses peptide carrier system + free amino acids, absorbed in upper gut	

Table continued on following page

TABLE 4. Enteral Nutritional Products *Continued*

	Lactose-Free Formulas				Defined Formula Diet	
	Travasorb HN *(Clintec)*		**Travasorb STD** *(Clintec)*		**Vital HN** *(Ross)*	
kcal./ml.	1		1		1	
Protein, gm./L. (source)	45	(hydrolyzed lactalbumin, 25% 5–10 peptide links, 25% 2–3 peptide links, 50% free amino acids)	30	(hydrolyzed lactalbumin, 25% 5–10 peptide links, 25% 2–3 peptide links, 50% free amino acids)	42	(whey, soy + meat protein hydrolysate; free essential amino acids)
Fat, gm./L. (source)	13	(MCT, sunflower oil)	13	(MCT, sunflower oil)	11	(MCT, safflower oil)
Carbohydrate, gm./L.	175	(glucose oligosaccharides)	190	(glucose oligosaccharides)	185	(hydrolyzed corn starch, sucrose)
Lactose, gm./L.	0		0		1	
Minerals/L.						
Calcium, mg.	500		500		667	
Phosphorus, mg.	500		500		667	
Magnesium, mg.	200		200		267	
Iron, mg.	9		9		12	
Sodium, mEq.	40		40		20	
Potassium, mEq.	30		30		34	
Chloride, mEq.	38		42		25	
Iodine, μg.	75		75		100	
Zinc, mg.	8		8		15	
Copper, mg.	1		1		1	
Manganese, mg.	1		1		3	
Volume required to meet 100% RDA, ml.	2000		2000		1500	
kcal./gm. N_2	126/1		202/1		150/1	
mOsm./kg. H_2O	560		560		500	
Preparation	Powder		Powder		Powder	
Comments	Supplemental, tube feeding, uses peptide carrier system + free amino acids, absorbed in upper gut		Supplemental, tube feeding, uses peptide carrier system + free amino acids, absorbed in upper gut		Supplemental, tube feeding, uses peptide carrier system + free amino acids, absorbed in upper gut	

	Defined Formula Diets					
	Tolerex *(Norwich Eaton)*		**Vivonex HN** *(Norwich Eaton)*		**Peptamen** *(Clintec)*	
kcal./ml.	1		1		1	
Protein, gm./L. (source)	21	(L-amino acids)	42	(L-amino acids)	40	(whey protein hydrolysate)
Fat, gm./L. (source)	1.5	(safflower oil)	0.9	(safflower oil)	39	(MCT, sunflower oil)
Carbohydrate, gm./L.	226	(glucose oligosaccharides)	210	(glucose oligosaccharides)	127	(maltodextrin, starch)
Lactose, gm./L.	0		0		0	
Minerals/L.						
Calcium, mg.	555		333		600	
Phosphorus, mg.	555		333		500	
Magnesium, mg.	222		133		300	
Iron, mg.	10		6		9	
Sodium, mEq.	20		23		22	
Potassium, mEq.	30		30		32	
Chloride, mEq.	27		23		28	
Iodine, μg.	83		50		75	
Zinc, mg.	8		5		10	
Copper, mg.	1		1		1	
Manganese, mg.	2		1		2	
Volume required to meet 100% RDA, ml.	1800		3000		2000	
kcal./gm. N_2	231/1		150/1		156.1	
mOsm./kg. H_2O	550		810		260	
Preparation	Powder		Powder		Ready to use	
Comments	Supplemental, tube feeding, absorbed in upper gut		Supplemental, tube feeding, high-protein, absorbed in upper gut		Tube feeding, elemental	

TABLE 4. Enteral Nutritional Products *Continued*

Branched Chain–Enriched Solutions

	Trauma-Aid HBC (Kendall-McGaw)		Vivonex TEN (Norwich Eaton)		Stresstein (Sandoz)	
kcal./ml.	1		1		1.2	
Protein, gm./L. (source)	56	(amino acids, 50% of total as branched chain amino acids)	38	(amino acids, 30% of total as branched chain amino acids)	70	(amino acids, 44% of total as branched chain amino acids)
Fat, gm./L. (source)	6	(soy oil, MCT)	3	(safflower oil)	28	(MCT, soy oil)
Carbohydrate, gm./L.	186	(maltodextrins)	206	(maltodextrins and modified food starch)	170	(maltodextrin
Lactose, gm./L.	0		0		0	
Minerals/L.						
Calcium, mg.	400		500		500	
Phosphorus, mg.	400		500		500	
Magnesium, mg.	133		200		200	
Iron, mg.	6		9		9	
Sodium, mEq.	23		20		28	
Potassium, mEq.	30		20		31	
Chloride, mEq.	23		23		26	
Iodine, μg.	50		75		75	
Zinc, mg.	7		10		8	
Copper, mg.	1		1		1	
Manganese, mg.	1		1		2	
Volume required to meet 100% RDA, ml.	3000		2000		2000	
kcal./gm. N_2	100/1		175/1		100/1	
mOsm./kg. H_2O	675		630		910	
Preparation	Powder		Powder		Powder	
Comments	Supplement, tube feeding, enriched with branched chain amino acids		Supplement, tube feeding, enriched with branched chain amino acids, absorbed in upper gut		Tube feeding, enriched with branched chain amino acids	

Special Formulations

	Hepatic-Aid II (Kendall-McGaw)		Travasorb Renal (Clintec)		Travasorb Hepatic (Clintec)	
kcal./ml.	1		1.35		1.1	
Protein, gm./L. (source)	44	(amino acids, 40% of total as branched chain amino acids, low in aromatic amino acids)	23	(crystalline amino acids)	28	(amino acids, 50% of total as branched chain amino acids, low in aromatic amino acids)
Fat, gm./L. (source)	36	(soy oil, mono- and diglycerides)	18	(MCT, sunflower oil)	14	(MCT, sunflower oil)
Carbohydrate, gm./L.	169	(maltodextrins, sucrose)	271	(glucose oligosaccharides, sucrose)	209	(glucose oligosaccharides, sucrose)
Lactose, gm./L.	0		0		0	
Minerals/L.						
Calcium, mg.	negligible				440	
Phosphorus, mg.	negligible				440	
Magnesium, mg.	negligible				176	
Iron, mg.	negligible				9	
Sodium, mEq.	negligible				19	
Potassium, mEq.	negligible				29	
Chloride, mEq.	negligible				19	
Iodine, μg.	negligible				71	
Zinc, mg.	negligible				7	
Copper, mg.	negligible				1	
Manganese, mg.	negligible				1	
Volume required to meet 100% RDA, ml.	NA		2100		2100	
kcal./gm. N_2	174/1		363/1		218/1	
mOsm./kg. H_2O	560		590		600	
Preparation	Powder		Powder		Powder	
Comments	Supplement, tube feeding, low electrolytes, indicated for liver disease, contains aspartame		Supplement, tube feeding, low electrolytes, indicated for renal disease		Supplement, tube feeding, indicated for liver disease	

Table continued on following page

TABLE 4. Enteral Nutritional Products *Continued*

Special Formulations

	Impact (Sandoz)		Pulmocare (Ross)		Amin-Aid (Kendall-McGaw)	
kcal./ml.	1		1.5		1.9	
Protein, gm./L. (source)	56	(Na + Ca caseinates, arginine)	62	(Na + Ca caseinates)	19	(crystalline essential amino acids)
Fat, gm./L. (source)	28	(vegetable oil, MCT, fish oil)	91	(corn oil)	66	(partially hydrogenated soybean oil)
Carbohydrate, gm./L.	132	(maltodextrin)	104	(sucrose, corn starch)	330	(maltodextrin, sucrose)
Lactose, gm./L.	0		0		0	
Minerals/L.						
Calcium, mg.	800		1074			
Phosphorus, mg.	800		1074			
Magnesium, mg.	267		423			
Iron, mg.	12		19			
Sodium, mEq.	46		57		<15	
Potassium, mEq.	32		49			
Chloride, mEq.	38		48			
Iodine, μg.	100		159			
Zinc, mg.	15		24			
Copper, mg.	1.6		2			
Manganese, mg.	2		5			
Volume required to meet 100% RDA, ml.	1500		947		NA	
kcal./gm. N_2	91/1		150/1		625/1	
mOsm./kg. H_2O	375		490		900	
Preparation	Ready to use		Ready to use		Powder	
Comments	Contains RNA, ultra–trace elements		Supplement, tube feeding, high-fat, low-carbohydrate formula		Supplement, tube feeding, low electrolytes, indicated for renal disease	

Special Formula

	Glucerna (Ross)	
kcal./ml.	1	
Protein, gm./L. (source)	42	(Na + Ca caseinates)
Fat, gm./L. (source)	56	(high oleic safflower oil, soybean oil)
Carbohydrate, gm./L.	94	(glucose polymers, fructose, soy polysaccharides)
Lactose, gm./L.	0	
Minerals/L.		
Calcium, mg.	704	
Phosphorus, mg.	704	
Magnesium, mg.	282	
Iron, mg.	13	
Sodium, mEq.	40	
Potassium, mEq.	40	
Chloride, mEq.	41	
Iodine, μg.	106	
Zinc, mg.	16	
Copper, mg.	2	
Manganese, mg.	4	
Volume required to meet 100% RDA, ml.	1422	
kcal./gm. N_2	150/1	
mOsm./kg. H_2O	375	
Preparation	Ready to use	
Comments	Supplement, tube feeding, increased fiber, for patients with abnormal glucose tolerance	

MCT, medium-chain triglycerides; NA, not available.

This table was originally prepared by Carol Lang, R. D., and revised 11/17/89, by Joseph Lacy, M.S., R.D., University of Cincinnati Medical Center Nutritional Support Team.

2. In the United States, the caloric supply is predominantly carbohydrate, usually hypertonic dextrose. A few solutions, especially those intended for peripheral use, use fructose and/or glycerol.

3. Fat emulsions consist of 10 or 20 per cent emulsions of soy or safflower oil emulsions, usually emulsified and stabilized with egg phosphatide and lecithin. Newer fat sources using omega-3 sources are not yet available for intravenous use.

THE PERIPHERAL ROUTE

PARENTERAL ADMINISTRATION. The central venous approach is most common, particularly in patients who require parenteral nutrition for 2 to 3 weeks. The peripheral route is used largely in situations without formal nutritional support programs. The peripheral route is useful only under very limited circumstances, such as when the duration of parenteral nutrition will be limited or one is not certain that full parenteral nutrition will be required. When the risk of catheter sepsis is significant because of the lack of a protocol and a nutritional support team to enforce that protocol, "peripheral hyperalimentation" may be safer, but the needs of sick patients are rarely satisfied by this approach.

The peripheral approach may involve the use of the "lipid system," in which caloric need is largely satisfied by the use of fat emulsions given in conjunction with amino acids and 5 per cent dextrose. There is nothing magical about amino acids given in water without dextrose. The hypothesis of Flatt and Blackburn,[40] which proposed the administration of dextrose-free amino acids to be of greater advantage by allowing the utilization of endogenous fat secondary to lower plasma levels of insulin, has been thoroughly discredited by at least 12 laboratories that have found that amino acids and 5 per cent dextrose is at least as effective as amino acids in water. The rationale for (hypocaloric) amino acids and 5 per cent dextrose, or glycerol, is an attempt to minimize nitrogen breakdown for limited periods of time. In using the lipid system, which is not synonymous, full caloric supplementation is intended. Most institutions use a Y tube with 10 or 20 per cent lipid emulsion to meet the caloric requirements in patients who are not severely ill or septic. In the author's experience, the lipid system exhausts peripheral arm veins very quickly, and fat emulsions have not protected against phlebitis. Thus, after 1 or 2 weeks, the necessity for a central line becomes obvious.

This technique cannot be used to meet high caloric demands or in severe sepsis, because of limited caloric supply by this technique; nor is it clear that fat is completely utilized in sepsis. The advantages are the avoidance of the central line and the attendant complications of placement (about 4 to 6 per cent in most institutions), and the ever-present possibility of sepsis, especially *Candida* sepsis.

It is not clear what the new mixture of amino acids and glycerol (Procalamine)* will mean to the peripheral technique, because insufficient data are available to document its efficacy. On a theoretic basis, glycerol is an acceptable carbohydrate, and the avoidance of expense of pharmacy mixing is an advantage.

CENTRAL APPROACH. In central hyperalimentation (total parenteral nutrition, or TPN), the central venous catheter usually terminates in the superior vena cava, although with care the inferior vena cava may be used. For short-term parenteral nutrition, Silastic or Teflon-coated catheters have largely replaced polyvinyl chloride–coated catheters, because they are less reactive and probably associated with a lower incidence of thrombosis. With percutaneous (or open via the axilla, which is preferred) placement of indwelling "permanent" (Broviac or Hickman) catheters, catheters are being placed early in patients in whom the need of a central indwelling line for weeks is

---

* Kendall-McGaw, Irvine, California.

obvious. It is likely that the incidence of thrombosis and/or sepsis is lower when these catheters are used.

Safe TPN requires an organization composed of nurses, physicians, and pharmacists and an enforced protocol. In this institution, the advent of such an organization decreased the catheter sepsis rate from 27 to 0.64 per cent.

REQUIREMENTS FOR NUTRITION. "Safe" protein requirements are in the range of 250 mg. of nitrogen per kg. per day or 1.7 gm. of protein equivalent per kg. per day. In the absence of severe sepsis or major burn, 35 kcal. per kg. per day is probably adequate. Twenty per cent of nonprotein calories as fat is probably optimal for hepatic protein synthesis. Vitamins and trace minerals should be given in adequate amounts, but knowledge is incomplete as to what amounts. Most authorities advocate two to five times the requirement for water-soluble vitamins and minimal daily requirements for the fat-soluble vitamins that may be toxic when given in excess. Thiamine deficiency in patients receiving normal amounts of thiamine has occasionally been seen. The setting is usually a very depleted patient given a sudden carbohydrate load. The clinical syndrome consists of disturbed mentation, diabetes insipidus, hyperbilirubinemia, thrombocytopenia, and lacticacidosis. The plasma amino acid pattern is very distorted, with high levels of proline and the appearance of hydroxyproline. Once recognized, thiamine deficiency is easily treated with 100 mg. of thiamine per day. Trace metals are given in sufficient quantities to prevent deficiency states and meet increased needs (Table 5).

INDICATIONS FOR PARENTERAL NUTRITION

Indications for parenteral nutrition may be organized into three categories, depending upon the desired outcome: (1) primary therapy, in which parenteral nutrition is thought to influ-

TABLE 5. Suggested Dosage of
Vitamins and Trace Metals
During Severe Illness

Vitamin	mg./day
Water-Soluble	
Thiamine	25
Riboflavin	25
Niacin	200
Pantothenic acid	50
Pyridoxine	50
Folic acid*	2.5
B$_{12}$†	5
Fat-Soluble	
A†	5000 μg.
D†	400 μg.
E†	100 μg.
K*	10

Trace Metal	mg./day
Zinc	10–20
Copper	0.5–2.0
Chromium	20 μg.
Selenium	70–150 μg.
Manganese	2–2.5
Iron	25

* Inactivated (oxidized) by addition to hypertonic glucose amino acid solutions.

† Sufficient stores of these vitamins exist so that deficiency states are unlikely during short-term (2 to 4 weeks) parenteral nutrition. In practice, however, it is wise to provide them.

TABLE 6. Indications for Parenteral Nutrition

Primary Therapy
Efficacy shown*
  Gastrointestinal cutaneous fistulas
  Renal failure (acute tubular necrosis)
  Short bowel syndrome
  Acute burns
  Hepatic failure (acute decompensation superimposed on cirrhosis)
Efficacy not shown
  Crohn's disease
  Anorexia nervosa

Supportive Therapy
Efficacy shown*
  Acute radiation enteritis
  Acute chemotherapy toxicity
  Prolonged ileus
  Weight loss preliminary to major operation
Efficacy not shown
  Prior to cardiac surgery
  Prolonged respiratory support
  Large wound losses

Areas Under Intensive Study
Patients with cancer
Patients with sepsis

* This indicates that randomized prospective trials or similar investigations have suggested that such nutritional intervention results in changed (improved) outcome.

ence disease process; (2) supportive therapy, in which nutritional support is achieved, but alterations in disease processes have not been established; and (3) controversial or under intensive study. These indications are listed in Table 6.

PRIMARY THERAPY: EFFICACY SHOWN

GASTROINTESTINAL-CUTANEOUS FISTULAS. Patients with gastrointestinal-cutaneous fistulas represent the classic indication for TPN. Gut failure is obvious, and increased oral intake increases fistula output. Two longitudinal reviews[82,93] of fistulas concluded the following:

1. TPN increases spontaneous closure of fistulas.
2. TPN has not resulted in a *dramatic* decrease in mortality in most centers experienced in the treatment of fistulas. The major decrease in mortality in the series at Massachusetts General Hospital[93] and the University of California at San Francisco[82] occurred in the 1960s, probably the result of improved parasurgical intensive care, including monitoring, respiratory care, and better understanding of fluid and electrolyte balance.
3. TPN probably has contributed to decreased mortality in patients with fistulas in most other institutions.
4. The treatment of patients with fistulas has been altered by nutritional support. If spontaneous closure does not occur because of the anatomic circumstances of the fistula, patients are much better prepared for operation.

RENAL FAILURE. TPN has resulted in decreased mortality in patients with acute renal failure, but controversy persists concerning the amino acid solution used. Abel and co-workers,[1] using a mixture of essential amino acids with hypertonic dextrose largely in patients with surgically related renal failure, described decreased urea appearance, earlier diuresis, and a statistically significant improvement in survival in treated patients as opposed to dextrose alone. Others have argued for a more complete amino acid formula, dealing with the rise in blood urea nitrogen by dialysis. The author's practice is as follows.

In patients in whom it is not clear whether dialysis will be necessary or particularly those in non-oliguric renal failure in whom dialysis may be averted or delayed, a solution of essential amino acids and hypertonic dextrose is used. An additional advantage is that soon after operations, such as for ruptured abdominal aortic aneurysm, patients may not tolerate the cardiovascular stress of hemodialysis, and the retroperitoneum may not be sufficiently sealed to tolerate peritoneal dialysis. Dialysis may be delayed until better tolerated, as accumulation of blood urea nitrogen and hyperkalemia is decreased by the use of the essential amino acid solution. After the need for regular dialysis has been established, a conventional mixture of essential and nonessential amino acids is used. Essential amino acid solutions and mixtures of essential and nonessential amino acid solutions have been compared, but the number of patients is small, thus preventing conclusions from being drawn.[35,73]

Recently, it has been proposed that protein excesses may be injurious to patients with renal failure. Patients with chronic renal failure on a low-protein diet deteriorated more slowly, while the use of alpha-ketoanalogs maintained renal function over a period of several years without deterioration. Although the use of ketoanalogs in renal failure was proposed more than a decade ago, their use in hepatic or renal failure is not widely practiced.[100] This does, however, suggest that the use of essential amino acids may have other advantages.

THE SHORT BOWEL SYNDROME. Repeated small bowel resections for Crohn's disease or major enterectomy following mesenteric thrombosis or volvulus are the three major causes of short bowel syndrome. There is little alternative to long-term (generally home) TPN. No randomized prospective trials have been undertaken, but patients with short bowel syndrome have no alternative. It is now common for patients on home TPN who would otherwise almost certainly have died to survive for 10 years.[48] Some of these patients have exhibited sufficient hypertrophy of remaining small bowel to decrease or obviate the need for home TPN after a period of time. If a patient is left with 1½ feet of small bowel anastomosed to the left colon, hypertrophy of 1 or 2 years will in most cases enable survival without daily parenteral nutritional support, although twice-weekly supplementation may be necessary.

BURNS. The sharp decrease in mortality in patients with burns from 1965 to 1970 is likely the result of aggressive nutritional support. A prospective trial by Alexander and colleagues[4] randomized children with major burns for normal protein (15 per cent of calories as protein) versus a high-protein (25 per cent of calories as protein) diet, with all other treatment identical. The group receiving the high-protein diet showed improved survival as well as improved immunologic protein synthesis parameters and improved neutrophil function. The group receiving the high-protein diet received more of their nutrition enterally. Early aggressive nutritional support (particularly an increased amount of protein) in patients with major burns is associated with improved survival.[64]

With the striking finding by Alexander and co-workers that early enteral feeding in a guinea pig burn model prevented hypercatabolism,[33] and with the verification of this work by Warden, Alexander, and co-workers in burned patients,[64] aggressive enteral feeding beginning within 3 hours of burn injury is being increasingly adopted. Parenteral nutritional support is reserved for those few patients in whom enteral nutrition cannot meet the patient's caloric needs. Moreover, "nutritional pharmacology" (see later) is increasingly utilized in enteral diets specifically designed for burned patients. Thus, increasing the concentration of arginine as well as changing the composition of the fatty acid source to omega-3 fats in fish oil, with the resultant production of the PGE$_3$ series of prostaglandins and thromboxanes, and thus using eicosapentaenoic acid rather than the arachidonic acid metabolites, have drastically altered nutritional support of burned patients. A new product pioneered by Alexander and co-workers, known as Impact,* is currently being tested in a multicenter trial. Early results have suggested that patients receiving this enteral diet have a lower sepsis rate, fewer days of bacteremia, perhaps earlier wound healing, a lower mortality, and shorter hospital stay.

HEPATIC FAILURE. Improved survival is also seen in patients with hepatic failure given aggressive parenteral nutritional support.[18,36] Patients with liver disease are often malnourished secondary to excessive alcohol and decreased food intake and have decreased tolerance to stress. Protein is the important nutritional component that they require, and yet they are specifically intolerant to protein because of hepatic encephalopathy. The amino acid–neurotransmitter hypothesis proposed by Fischer and Baldessarini[39,62] proposes that under circumstances of decreased hepatic function and functional or anatomic shunting of portal blood around the liver, amino acid imbalance in the plasma, specifically of the amino acid precursors of central monoamine neurotransmitters, leads to deranged neurotransmitters within the central nervous system. Correcting the plasma amino acid imbalance by the administration of solutions enriched with branched chain amino acids and deficient in aromatic amino acids results in increased tolerance to administered protein and arousal from hepatic encephalopathy.[43] (A complete discussion of this hypothesis is beyond the scope of this chapter; the interested reader is referred to the references.) Of the seven randomized prospective trials performed thus far, in the five in which hypertonic dextrose was used as the caloric source, branched chain–enriched amino acid solutions were at least as effective as lactulose or neomycin in the treatment of hepatic encephalopathy. In two of those studies improved survival against lactulose and/or neomycin was seen. In the studies in which the major caloric source was fat, efficacy for the branched chain–enriched amino acid solutions was not seen.[38] A similar conclusion was reached by Naylor and colleagues using the technique of metanalysis of all the published studies.[78]

The mechanism of this apparently improved survival may be improved healing and possibly regeneration of the liver,[83] better cooperation of the patient with therapy, and decreased infection as a result of improved nutritional support.

PARENTERAL NUTRITION AS PRIMARY THERAPY: EFFICACY NOT SHOWN

INFLAMMATORY BOWEL DISEASE. In patients with inflammatory bowel disease, oral intake often provokes diarrhea, protein-losing enteropathy, bleeding, and so on. Although TPN and bowel rest are useful in the treatment of Crohn's disease (particularly limited to the small bowel, in which a remission rate of 75 per cent can be expected), such therapy has never been subjected to a randomized prospective trial. The mean duration of remission in the Cincinnati experience is approximately 11 months. Patients with colonic involvement do less well; their rate of initial remission is considerably less and the duration of remission is shorter than that of patients with small bowel disease alone. In the author's experience, such recurrences can be prevented by maintaining patients who go into remission on small doses of prednisone, about 5 or 10 mg. per day, a point of view that has not been generally accepted. A recent long-term study analyzing the results of parenteral nutrition for acute exacerbations of Crohn's disease has revealed that after 15 months only 26 per cent of these patients had avoided operation.[90]

Some patients with extensive, severe, and chronically recurrent Crohn's disease are suitable subjects for home hyperalimentation, particularly when surgical therapy would entail massive small bowel resection, leaving the patient almost anenteric.

Ulcerative colitis does not generally respond to short-term parenteral nutrition, nor is long-term TPN indicated to induce remission, as sphincter-saving operation produces long-term cure. However, the author has found TPN useful in preparation for the Soave procedure.[71] In-hospital TPN for usually less than 2 weeks, but occasionally longer, in conjunction with intravenous antibiotics (chloromycetin or metronidazole) allows rectal mucosa to heal, thereby facilitating rectal mucosal stripping. Home parenteral nutrition in ulcerative colitis is a misuse of an expensive technique.

ANOREXIA NERVOSA. Patients with anorexia nervosa often starve themselves to a moribund state, with enormous losses of lean body mass. Similar protein depletion likely occurs in the brain, and, for psychotherapy to be successful, some repletion of brain protein is essential. However, anorectic patients are difficult to treat; they are destructive and often attempt suicide by disconnecting their intravenous lines, inviting air embolism. To the author's knowledge, a prospective trial has never been performed with anorexia nervosa, but TPN appears efficacious as an adjunct without affecting the primary disease state.

SUPPORTIVE THERAPY

SUPPORTIVE THERAPY: EFFICACY SHOWN

ACUTE RADIATION ENTERITIS OR CHEMOTHERAPY TOXICITY. Acute radiation enteritis and/or gastrointestinal complications of chemotherapy may prevent oral intake. Elemental diets have not been found of much value. A period of TPN until the gut mucosa heals enables the patient to survive this difficult period. Chronic radiation enteritis with multiple strictures may render the patient unsuitable for operative intervention, a candidate for home parenteral nutrition or, rarely, enteral feeding with minimal residue diets, provided the original neoplasm has been cured.

PROLONGED ILEUS. Prolonged ileus following an abdominal procedure may necessitate a course of TPN until the ileus subsides. Obviously, this is but supportive.

SUPPORTIVE THERAPY: EFFICACY PROBABLY PRESENT BUT NOT CLEARLY ESTABLISHED

WEIGHT LOSS PRELIMINARY TO MAJOR OPERATIONS (PERIOPERATIVE PARENTERAL NUTRITION). There are four major questions concerning the use of parenteral nutrition in patients who have lost weight prior to major operations: (1) Are operative complications of major surgical procedures increased in patients who have lost weight? (2) If so, can this group be identified? (3) If this group can be identified, does short-term parenteral nutrition change the outcome? (4) If all of these conditions are met, what mode of nutritional repletion should be used and/or for how long?

1. *Are surgical complications of major operative procedures increased in patients who have lost weight?* A large number of studies have been done. In a nice review analyzing 18 randomized and pseudorandomized studies, Detsky and colleagues concluded that the case had not yet been made for the use of total parenteral nutrition prior to major operation.[32] Yet the Veterans Administration study appears to identify a group at risk.[16] This group of patients has lost greater than 15 per cent of body weight. The operant defect is not malnutrition, *per se*, but immunologic dysfunction.[25] The two are different; there are pa-

---

* Sandoz Pharmaceuticals, Minneapolis, Minnesota.

tients who are malnourished and have lost 15 per cent of their body weight, who remain immunologically capable; other patients with similar weight loss are immunologically dysfunctional. Similar support has come from Graham Hill's work, in which the group who lost greater than 15 per cent of their body weight and functional impairment was most likely at risk.

2. *Can this group be identified?* Studley suggested that patients with profound (20 per cent) weight loss and low serum albumin experienced increased complications and mortality following gastrectomy.[95] As detailed in the discussion of nutritional assessment, the group at risk statistically can probably be identified, but the individual patient cannot yet be identified.

Thus, identifying the group at risk would include careful history and a global assessment. A history of greater than 15 per cent weight loss and albumin of less than 3 gm. per 100 ml. would place these patients into a high-risk group (see earlier). Delayed cutaneous hypersensitivity testing (as proposed by Christou),[25] hand dynamometry, and serum transferrin are optional.

3. *Does short-term nutritional intervention change the outcome?* The answer to this question appears increasingly *yes*, provided nutritional intervention is limited to the group with severe malnutrition and immunologic dysfunction. In the Veterans Administration multicenter trial, in patients judged severely malnourished, who had lost greater than 15 per cent of their body weight, preoperative nutritional intervention for 7 to 10 days decreased septic complications. In the group stratified as having mild to moderate malnutrition, the decrease in surgical complications was more than offset by the increase in non–catheter-related infectious complications. Thus, TPN, even in the absence of hyperglycemia of greater than 300 mg. per 100 ml. (which interferes with neutrophil function, and which it is presumed was not the case in these studies), increased the risk of non–catheter-related infection.

4. *How long should these patients be treated preoperatively?* The proper duration of preoperative parenteral nutrition is likely 5 to 7 days. In previous studies, with 3 days of parenteral nutritional support prior to operation, there was a trend toward decreased sepsis, but it did not reach statistical significance, possibly owing to a small number of patients.[58] If one carefully observes such depleted patients preoperatively, they begin to feel better at approximately 5 days. This generally coincides with an increase in the shortest turnover proteins, retinol-binding protein and thyroxin-binding prealbumin. In the Veterans Administration cooperative study,[16] the duration of preoperative parenteral nutrition was between 7 and 10 days. Thus, 5 to 7 days should be used for preoperative nutritional preparation.

THE PATIENT WITH MALIGNANT DISEASE. Special considerations are appropriate, as it is likely that the current form of total parenteral nutrition, especially with overfeeding, may increase growth of the tumors (see later). The author's current practice is to limit preoperative TPN for 5 days.

CARDIAC SURGERY. Patients with cardiac cachexia are at increased risk for complications and mortality following cardiac surgery. The conventional wisdom is based on Starling's pronouncement in 1912 that the heart is spared the ravages of starvation. This is not true. Protein depletion in experimental animals results in decreased myocardial contractility, which has its anatomic counterpart in distortion of cardiac histology, edema, disruption, and necrosis of myofibrils, findings that are not totally reversed, even after prolonged nutritional repletion.[3] In the single available prospective randomized trial in which nutritional supplementation was begun on the day of operation, and thus in the current state of knowledge was unlikely to show efficacy, there was no improvement in outcome.[2] A study in which patients with cardiac cachexia about to undergo operation are subjected to prolonged nutritional repletion with appropriate solutions has yet to be done. Anecdotal clinical evidence suggests that patients with cardiac cachexia require prolonged nutritional supplementation (about 2 to 3 weeks) prior to operation, a finding supported by experimental evidence. Fluid limitations in such patients require more concentrated solutions.

RESPIRATORY FAILURE AND REQUIREMENTS FOR PROLONGED RESPIRATORY SUPPORT. It is barely conceivable that while severely ill patients are receiving the best in intensive care support, nutritional support is neglected, but it commonly occurs. The author is not aware of evidence that pulmonary function itself, rather than muscles of respiration, is improved by nutritional support. Furthermore, there is little information concerning the metabolic needs of the alveolar cells responsible for surfactant production, gas exchange, and so on. Because these cells represent such a small proportion of the actual structure of the lung, any attempt to derive the metabolic needs of alveolar cells will more likely identify the metabolic needs of the supportive elements but not of the pneumocytes.

Weaning from ventilators may improve with nutritional support. However, a potential deleterious effect of hypertonic dextrose on weaning from the ventilators is CO_2 overproduction, especially in patients who are septic, very depleted, and given a sudden glucose load.[5] Although this has been given extensive publicity, occasionally in patients with marginal pulmonary function, CO_2 overproduction may require replacing glucose calories with fat calories in order to promote weaning. Simple awareness of this potential problem is all that is necessary, because CO_2 production can be measured in most intensive care units.

LARGE WOUNDS AND OTHER SOURCES OF NITROGEN LOSS. Many hospitalized patients with large wounds such as decubiti are unable to eat. Provision of nutritional support to improve wound healing is logical, but few studies exist.

AREAS UNDER INTENSE STUDY

PATIENTS WITH CANCER. Patients with neoplastic disease may suffer profound weight loss. Anorexia is common, even when the tumor is small, suggesting deranged central nervous system satiety mechanisms.[23] In addition, obstruction of the gastrointestinal tract and mechanical interference with digestion and absorption also contribute to cachexia. During the past decade, the initial enthusiasm for adjunctive nutritional support in patients with cancer has waned.[27] Experimental evidence suggests that tumor growth is stimulated at least in direct proportion to supply of protein and calories.[81] Indeed, some clinical evidence suggests that nutritional supplementation of patients undergoing chemotherapy and/or radiation may decrease survival and/or remission-free interval,[37] and alter cell kinetics.[7]

This important area is plagued by a lack of uniformity in experimental studies, in differences that may exist between patient populations, that both malnourished and normally nourished patients have been included in these studies, and that respone to adjunctive nutritional support may differ depending upon whether the treatment modality is to be radiation or chemotherapy and/or resection (see Table 7).[37] Moreover, the types of calories currently supplied to most patients may be inappropriate in the patient with cancer. Although different tumors require different growth factors, glucose may be utilized preferentially by tumors as opposed to fat. Recent studies from this laboratory in specific tumor models indicate that by identifying the substrates that are useful to the tumors and by employing specific blocking agents, it may be possible to treat animals with TPN, adding nitrogen to the carcass without increasing the growth of such tumors.[22] For example, TPN in the presence of acivicin, a glutamine blocker (glutamine is a preferred fuel for such tumors), and insulin, which diverts glucose from the tumor to the normal body mass, added lean body mass of the host rat, while averting tumor growth. Unfortu-

TABLE 7. Studies of the Effects of Parenteral Nutrition on Patients with Cancer Undergoing Surgery, Radiation, or Chemotherapy

	No. of Patients	Type of Tumor	Type of Therapy	Nutritional Effects*		Response to Therapy (%)		Complications of Therapy (%)		Survival (%)		Comments
				PN	Control	PN	Control	PN	Control	PN	Control	
Holter and Fischer (1977)	56	GI cancer	Surgery	Decreased wt. loss and increased albumin level with PN		same		13	19	93.4	92.4	Lower major complication rate with PN
Moghissi et al. (1977)	15	Esophageal cancer	Surgery	Better N balance with PN		same		0	20	NA	NA	Lower rate of wound infection with PN
Issell et al. (1978)	26	Squamous cell lung cancer	Chemotherapy	Improved wt. gain and arm circumference with PN		31	7	15	77	NA	NA	Less myelosuppression, less toxic effects of chemotherapy with PN
Heatley et al. (1979)	74	Esophageal/gastric cancer	Surgery	same		same		35	83	15	22	Significant reduction in postoperative wound infection
Simms et al. (1980)	30	Esophageal/gastric cancer	Surgery	Improved N balance and albumin level with PN		same		NA	NA	10	10	
Lanzotti et al. (1980)	56	Non–oat cell lung cancer	Chemotherapy	NA	NA	10	23	NA	NA	11 wk median	12 wk NA	
Sako et al. (1981)	69	Head and neck cancer	Surgery	Wt. gain and better N balance with PN		same		50	56	NA	NA	Significantly better long-term survival curve for PN
Valdivieso et al. (1981)	49	Small cell bronchogenic cancer	Chemotherapy	Wt. gain with PN		85	59	NA	NA	Survival advantage for PN		PN did not ameliorate hematologic, GI, or infectious morbidity
Thompson et al. (1981)	41	GI cancer	Surgery	Improved wt. gain with PN		same		17	11	100	100	
Popp et al. (1981)	36 42	Diffuse lymphoma	Chemotherapy	Marked wt. gain with PN; lean body mass, anthropometry, albumin, transferrin, and total lymphocytes similar for both groups				11% subclavian vein thrombosis		69	66	No difference in drug tolerance or total drug dose between control and TPN
Nixon et al. (1981)	45	Metastatic colon cancer	Chemotherapy	Wt. gain with PN; no other differences		15	12			79 days	308 days	
Serrou et al. (1981)	19	Anaplastic lung cancer	Chemotherapy	same		83	80	same		84	80	
Samuels et al. (1981)	30	Metastatic testicular cancer	Chemotherapy	Less wt. loss with PN		63	79	Increased incidence of noncatheter infections with PN		75	79	
Linn et al. (1981)	24	Esophageal cancer	Surgery	Better wt. gain and N balance with PN				6 complications 17	12 complications 32	90	80	Preoperative TPN and gastrostomy feeding compared
Muller et al. (1982)	125	GI cancer	Surgery	Improved wt. gain, visceral proteins, and immunologic status with PN				17	32	96	81	
Shamberger et al. (1983)	27	Sarcomas	Chemotherapy	Improved N balance with PN, but similar visceral proteins				42	33			Similar granulocyte and platelet recovery following chemotherapy-induced myelosuppression
Shamberger et al. (1984)	32	Sarcomas	Chemotherapy	Improved N balance with PN		71	86			Long-term survival rate similar		Shorter remissions for PN
Clamon et al. (1985)	119	Small cell lung cancer	Chemotherapy	Higher colonic and protein intake with PN		48	43	NA	NA	same		Significantly more febrile episodes with TPN
Muller et al. (1986)	110	Gastroesophageal	Surgery	Improved visceral proteins and immunocompetence with PN		NA	NA	8	17	4	11	Improvement in surgical technique limited value of TPN

* PN, parenteral nutrition; NA, not available.

nately, this particular combination is too toxic to be utilized in patients, but others will be effective. Thus, in the future, it is likely that patients will be receiving TPN and a combination of medications that prevent the growth of tumors. Whatever the ultimate combination, these studies suggest that the primacy of the tumor as a magical entity is not correct, and that metabolic analysis of tumor needs may become an important therapeutic maneuver.

In only one randomized prospective trial in patients with carcinoma of the esophagus or gastric cardia was there benefit from the preoperative and perioperative application of nutritional support, with decreased mortality and morbidity without apparent stimulation of the tumor.[77] Caution is justified; adjunctive nutritional therapy is indicated only for patients who are severely malnourished and unable to survive a contemplated course of therapy or operative procedure.[16] In the pediatric age group, however, in whom the needs of growth are additive to the requirements of stress of operative or other therapy, adjunctive nutritional support results in decreased concurrent infection.[98]

SEPSIS. Sepsis is the major current cause of mortality. The metabolic response to sepsis includes proteolysis, with a flow of amino acids from muscle to the liver. Hepatic protein synthesis is increased. The metabolic stimuli for accelerated breakdown of lean body mass include hyperglucagonemia greater than the corresponding hyperinsulinemia, increased steroids and catecholamines, and cytokines such as interleukin 1 and 6, TNF/cachectin, gamma interferon, and additional cytokines such as that which blocks amino acid transport into the muscle (see Table 2).[53] There appears to be tremendous wastage of amino acids supplied to the liver, because much of the amino acids supplied is metabolized to urea. Is this excess required for a specific purpose? Are the excessive amounts of glucose generated by muscle breakdown via gluconeogenesis completely appropriate in view of the accompanying glucose resistance? Several years ago, the author and associates (among others) suggested that modified nutritional substrate might be more appropriate for patients with sepsis.[46] In overwhelming sepsis, glucose resistance, the failure of ketone body manufacture, and inefficiencies in the utilization of lipid fuels suggested that an alternative fuel that did not require metabolism through glucose might be more efficient. In addition, with the aforementioned evidence that the amount of amino acids supplied to the liver may be excessive, provision of substrates, such as the branched chain amino acids, that supply energy and decrease the breakdown of lean body mass might be more appropriate.

The branched chain amino acids, valine, leucine, and isoleucine, have the ability to be utilized as energy without going through glucose, stimulate protein synthesis, and decrease proteolysis in skeletal muscle. In a series of studies in experimental animals and subsequently in man, high–branched chain amino acid solutions were administered to experimental animals with sepsis and finally in patients with severe sepsis. The results of prospective randomized trials indicate that a high–branched chain solution that is either balanced with respect to all three—leucine, isoleucine, and valine—or containing more leucine is only marginally more efficacious in preventing breakdown of lean body mass and perhaps increasing hepatic protein synthesis in patients with overwhelming sepsis.[12,14] No difference in outcome was seen, although the number of patients studied was small. Similar results were reported by Cerra and co-workers[21] and by Brennan and his group.[29] The sicker the patient, the more likely one is to see marginal improvement in amino acid flux, nitrogen balance, short-turnover proteins, and decreased requirement for insulin following administration of high (45 per cent) branched chain amino acid solutions; however, the differences are too small to result in improved outcome.

Such solutions represent only an initial attempt; future attempts to provide nutritional support in septic patients should

stimulate hepatic protein synthesis and improve neutrophil function and other forms of host defense. Given the apparently specific cytokine blocking amino acid transport into muscle, it may be difficult to maintain lean body mass. Investigations toward these goals are currently under way in several laboratories.

COMPLICATIONS OF PARENTERAL NUTRITION

Complications of parenteral nutrition may be grouped into three categories: technical, metabolic, and septic.

TECHNICAL COMPLICATIONS

EARLY TECHNICAL COMPLICATIONS. The most common complications of TPN are related to catheter placement through a crowded thoracic inlet. These complications decrease with experience, but even the most experienced physician may occasionally elicit one of the following complications:

1. Pneumothorax, more common in elderly and/or cachectic patients.
2. Arterial lacerations, rare, can be avoided by keeping the needle no deeper than 10 degrees to the horizontal.
3. Hemothorax, the result of leakage of blood from the subclavian vein.
4. Mediastinal hematoma, especially in patients with deficient clotting factors.
5. Nerve injury to the brachial plexus.
6. Hydrothorax, the result of catheter malposition and fluid administration into the thoracic cavity.
7. Sympathetic effusions (usually bilateral transudates in response to mediastinal hematoma), substernal pain, and fever.
8. Injury to the thoracic duct following left-sided cannulation.
9. Air embolism, usually the result of improper technique, with the patient not being sufficiently dependent or adequately hydrated prior to catheter placement.
10. Catheter embolism, due to shearing of the catheter by the needle when a catheter thought to be improperly placed is removed without removing the needle.

LATE TECHNICAL COMPLICATIONS

1. Erosion of the catheter into bronchus, right atrium, or other structures.
2. Subclavian thrombosis occurs in about 5 to 10 per cent of patients; signs may be subtle, such as upper arm swelling and/or pain at the base of the neck. When thromobosis is suspected, the catheter should be removed, and after confirmation, thrombolytic therapy begun. After completion of streptokinase therapy, heparin should be continued for 1 or 2 weeks, followed by coumadin therapy for 6 months.
3. Septic thrombosis is a life-threatening complication. Excision of the subclavian vein is a technical *tour de force* that is sometimes successful. Massive antibiotic therapy and Fogarty catheter embolectomy of septic thromboses may occasionally be successful.

METABOLIC COMPLICATIONS

Metabolic complications may be categorized as (1) prevention of deficiency states, generally due to inadequate administration of needed nutrients; (2) disorders of glucose metabolism; and (3) those metabolic complications that are specific for parenteral nutrition.

ABNORMAL PLASMA ELECTROLYTE CONCENTRATIONS. Abnormalities in plasma concentrations of electrolytes are relatively common and may be minimized by careful monitoring and the administration of at least 50 mEq. of sodium, 40 mEq. of potassium per liter of 25 per cent dextrose, 90 to 100 mEq. of phosphorus, and 28 to 32 mEq. of magnesium and calcium per day to all patients receiving parenteral nutrition. Patients who are rapidly anabolic may require additional potassium. Acid-base imbalance may be prevented by giving acetate to patients with acidosis and by administration of potassium chloride to patients with large volumes of gastric drainage. If potassium chloride is insufficient to prevent metabolic alkalosis, administration of hydrochloric acid or arginine hydrochloride may be necessary.

TRACE METAL DEFICIENCIES

ZINC DEFICIENCY. Patients who are very catabolic or have excessive diarrhea may develop zinc deficiency. Neither plasma nor hair zinc is an accurate reflection of total body stores. Three to 6 mg. of elemental zinc per day is required in patients with normal stool losses, and between 12 and 20 mg. in patients with short bowel syndrome or excessive diarrhea. A characteristic perioral pustular rash, darkening of the skin creases, and neuritis are the principal clinical manifestations of zinc deficiency.

COPPER DEFICIENCY. Copper deficiency has been observed in a few patients receiving home parenteral nutrition as a microcytic anemia, which may be mistaken for pyridoxine deficiency. Copper supplementation may require up to 2 mg. per day of the sulfate.

CHROMIUM DEFICIENCY. This has been reported in two patients on long-term parenteral nutrition, and the author is aware of a third. It is likely to occur only in patients on long-term TPN with minimal or no oral intake. Chromium is necessary for the adequate utilization of glucose. Deficiency may be associated with a sudden diabetic state in which blood sugar is difficult to control, with peripheral neuropathy and encephalopathy. Fifteen to 20 μg. per day of chromium is adequate to meet daily requirements. To treat chromium deficiency, 150 μg. of chromium per day should be supplemented for several days.

SELENIUM DEFICIENCY. Selenium deficiency has not been clearly established. Abnormalities in basement and plasma membranes have been seen in skeletal muscle biopsies. It is rare.

BIOTIN DEFICIENCY. This has been reported by Dudrick (personal communication). Since biotin is ubiquitous, deficiency almost never occurs in patients taking anything by mouth.

ESSENTIAL FATTY ACID DEFICIENCY. Essential fatty acid deficiency may be prevented by administration of between 4 and 6 per cent of the daily calories as either soybean or safflower oil fat emulsion. The biochemical manifestations occur within 1 week of fat-free parenteral nutrition and are generally associated with lower levels of linoleic and arachidonic acid, high levels of 5,8,11-eicosatrienoic acid, and an increase in the triene/tetraine ratio; the latter is not uniform. The principal lesion is dry, flaky skin with small reddish papules and alopecia. Biochemical evidence of prostaglandin deficiency results in decreased intraocular pressure (a convenient noninvasive clinical method of testing for essential fatty acid deficiency).[44] Essential fatty acid deficiency can also be prevented by the ingestion of approximately 25 to 50 ml. of corn, sunflower, or safflower oil or margarine per day, made palatable with toast, orally. Patients with essential fatty acid deficiency will absorb essential fatty acids through the skin, but this is not practical except in babies.

DISORDERS OF GLUCOSE METABOLISM

HYPOGLYCEMIA. The most common cause of hypoglycemia, other than excessive insulin administration, is a sudden slowing of the glucose infusion. A curious form of hypoglycemia may be caused by the oversecretion of endogenous insulin at high infusion rates. Slowing of the infusion will decrease the hyperinsulinism.

HYPERGLYCEMIA. This is the most dangerous metabolic complication, most commonly caused by too rapid initiation of the infusion. This may be prevented by the initiation of the infusion at 60 ml. per hour (25 per cent glucose base) and an increase of 20 ml. per hour every 24 or 48 hours, depending upon the age of the patient, the degree of sepsis, and tolerance to infused glucose. Patients with normal glucose tolerance may manifest glycosuria for the first 24 to 48 hours of parenteral nutrition, but prior to initiating insulin, one must be certain that the blood sugar is high and that the glycosuria is not secondary to a reduced renal threshold for glucose; blood sugar is often normal, and the glycosuria disappears with continued parenteral nutrition. The most common cause of sudden hyperglycemia is sepsis, and hyperglycemia may antedate sepsis by up to 24 hours. Sudden appearance of hyperglycemia in a previously stable patient should initiate a thorough search for the source of infection.

THE DIABETIC PATIENT. Patients with diabetes, especially adult-onset diabetes, have not been difficult to control. Although secretion of insulin in response to glucose is deranged in these patients, adequate insulin release is elicited by amino acid administration. However, in both spontaneous hyperglycemia and diabetes, hyperosmolar nonketotic coma may suddenly occur. Blood sugars well in excess of 700 mg. per 100 ml. result in osmotic diuresis followed by dehydration, fever, obtundation, and coma. Death may follow unless the situation is corrected by the administration of heroic amounts of insulin, up to 200 units per day, and the administration of large amounts of dextrose-free hypo-osmotic solution, generally 0.45 per cent saline with added potassium.

LIVER FUNCTION DERANGEMENTS. Patients receiving any hyperalimentation solution, regardless of composition, may manifest abnormalities in aspartate aminotransferase, alanine aminotransferase, gamma-glutamyl transferase, and alkaline phosphatase. Hyperbilirubinemia, however, is rare, and, when it occurs in a patient on TPN, the cause is generally sepsis rather than hyperalimentation. All components of parenteral nutrition have at one time or another been accused of being responsible for the hepatic steatosis that occurs with parenteral nutrition. Metabolic products of tryptophan and preservatives have each been blamed in turn. Several facts, however, should be borne in mind. Hepatic steatosis occurs most commonly secondary to excessive glucose administration. Whereas other investigators have proposed that either translocation of gut bacteria or, more important, their products such as endotoxin are responsible for increased hepatic fat, using a very specific chromogenic assay, the group at Cincinnati has been unable to identify endotoxin in the portal circulation.[89]

The relationship between insulin and glucagon is an attractive hypothesis, but correlations between peripheral venous concentrations of insulin and glucagon and hepatic steatosis have not been identified. However, there is an excellent correlation between the portal vein insulin and glucagon molar ratio and hepatic fat content. This appears logical, because the portal concentrations of insulin and glucagon are what the liver "sees." Insulin results in hepatic lipogenesis, and glucagon in fat mobilization. Incubation of mice hepatoma cells with insulin and glucagon decreases the number of insulin receptors, thus decreasing the fat storage function of insulin by the presence of glucagon. Subsequent work in this laboratory has also confirmed that even once established, hepatic steatosis is cleared by the addition of small amounts (15 μg.) of glucagon to TPN in experimental animals despite continuing glucose overload.[67] Similarly, when fat is added to parenteral nutrition or enteral feedings, or, as recently suggested, glutamine, the decrease in the portal vein insulin/glucagon molar ratio to normal is associated with clearance of hepatic steatosis.

In infants, hepatic dysfunction is more serious and is frequently associated with cholestasis. Even when TPN is discontinued, hepatic dysfunction may persist and progress to cirrhosis and even death. Whether translocation of gut bacteria or their products across the immature gut, immaturity of other enzyme systems, or other factors have a role is not clear, but the disease in infants clearly is different from that seen in adults.

SEPTIC COMPLICATIONS

CATHETER INFECTION. Catheter sepsis is potentially the most lethal complication in patients receiving TPN. Bacterial catheter sepsis is directly related to catheter care and can be reduced to the current minimum of less than 1 per cent by careful attention to detail and the avoidance of multi-use catheters.[87] Fungemia, a far more serious complication, represented more than 50 per cent of the septicemias in a recent study, but the rate of disseminated candidiasis was low.[11] The entry site of *Candida*, the most common fungal pathogen, is probably the gastrointestinal tract. Large doses of oral nystatin may prevent *Candida* colonization and suprainfection.

Most hyperalimentation patients are malnourished and debilitated, which makes them more prone to infection. Steroid administration apparently also predisposes patients to infection, as do multiple antibiotics and chemotherapy. The following factors are important in the development of catheter sepsis:

1. The absence of a protocol. At the University of Cincinnati Medical Center, the sepsis rate decreased from 27 per cent, prior to the establishment of a hyperalimentation team and a rigid protocol, to 0.6 per cent at present.

2. Catheter sepsis is correlated with the degree of colonization of the pericatheter skin. When the skin around catheters was serially and quantitatively cultured, those catheters with surrounding skin which showed colonization of 10^3 organisms or greater had associated sepsis. There was a gradient of colonization from the skin to the intravascular portion of the catheter, especially along the fibrin sleeve.[11]

3. Gram-positive organisms originating from other sites may seed the fibrin sleeve along the catheter. Consequently, in a patient with established gram-positive bacteremia, the catheter should be removed. Gram-negative organisms do not seem to implant as readily, and antibiotic treatment may be sufficient to sterilize the catheter.

4. *Candida* seeds the bloodstream through the gut. Once *Candida* infection is well established, all intravenous nutritional regimens must be stopped, as they all support *Candida* sepsis. Nutrition must be given enterally.

MANAGEMENT OF THE PATIENT WITH SUSPECTED CATHETER SEPSIS. In the Cincinnati unit, a catheter in a patient whose skin shows colonization of greater than 10^3 organisms per sq. cm. is removed. In patients who have suspected catheter sepsis but whose quantitative cultures are less than 10^3, removal of a catheter has rarely (less than 5 per cent of the time) confirmed catheter sepsis. However, in situations in which rigid protocols are not followed and quantitative cultures are not obtained, the following protocol is proposed: If a patient who was previously afebrile suddenly spikes a fever when receiving hyperalimentation, the bottle should be taken down, the tubing and filter changed, and a new bottle suspended; the bottle and tubing should then be cultured. Blood cultures should be drawn and a thorough search made of other possible sources of fever, such as pneumonia, intra-abdominal abscess, urinary tract infection, and wound infection. If the fever persists after an 8-hour period, the catheter should be removed and the tip cultured. Four out of the 5 catheters removed under these circumstances will be innocent, and sources of sepsis ultimately found elsewhere. When a septic catheter is removed, it is not necessary to treat the patient with antibiotics unless the fever persists for longer than 24 hours. At the Cincinnati Medical Center, catheters are not changed over guidewires when catheter infection is suspected, because the causative infected skin tract is still present. However, when another source is suspected, it is reasonable to change catheters over guidewires.

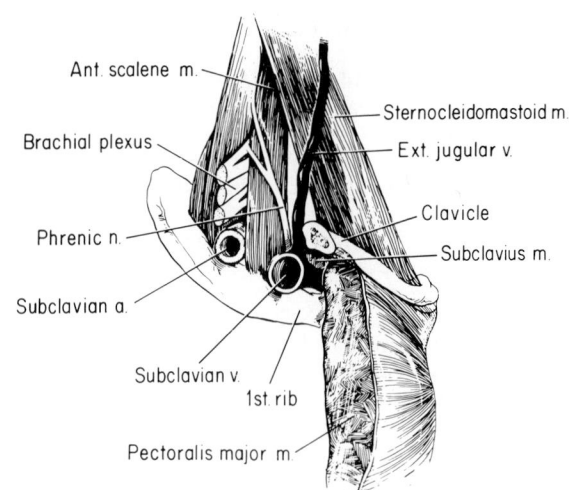

Figure 9. A section of the thoracic inlet through the area of the subclavian vein. Note that the subclavian vein is the most anterior structure in a thoracic inlet. (From Fischer, J. E., and Freund, H. R.: Central hyperalimentation. *In* Fischer, J. E. (Ed.): Surgical Nutrition. Boston, Little, Brown & Company, 1983, p. 695.)

When triple-lumen catheters are used, they should be changed every 72 hours over a guidewire to reduce infection.

PREVENTION OF CATHETER COMPLICATIONS IN PATIENTS

PLACEMENT OF THE CATHETER. Hyperalimentation catheter placement is never an emergency procedure and should be done only under proper conditions, with the patient well hydrated and lightly sedated and with adequate assistance. The author prefers a subclavian approach: The patient should be positioned with a roll between the shoulder blades, arms at the sides, head relaxed, and the bed tilted at 15 degrees in the Trendelenburg position. The subclavian vein is the most anterior structure in the thorax (Fig. 9). On the left side, the subclavian catheter takes a more transverse arch through the apex of the chest compared with the right side (Fig. 10). Right-handed people will find it easier to pass a left subclavian catheter. After carefully preparing and draping the patient, the vein is found with a No. 22 needle through which lidocaine (Xylocaine) is infiltrated along the anticipated track, infiltrating the periosteum as well. The point of insertion is 1 cm. medial and 1 cm. caudad to the midpoint of the clavicle (Fig. 11). The needle is aimed no more than 10 to 15 degrees to the horizontal immediately beyond the clavicle and to a point one fingerbreadth above the suprasternal

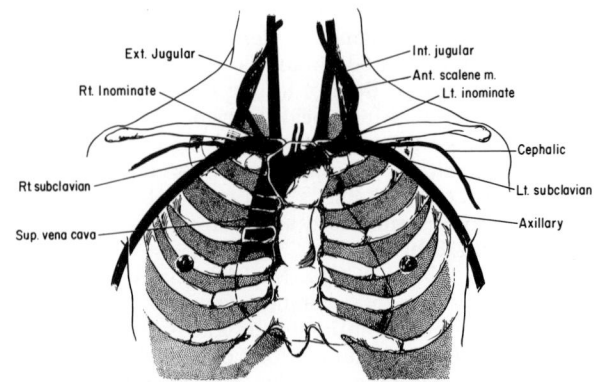

Figure 10. The venous anatomy of the thoracic inlet. Note the transverse position of the subclavian veins. The horizontal course of the subclavian vein is longer on the left than on the right. It is also easier for a right-handed person to cannulate the left subclavian vein. (From Fischer, J. E., and Freund, H. R.: Central hyperalimentation. *In* Fischer, J. E. (Ed.): Surgical Nutrition. Boston, Little, Brown & Company, 1983, p. 696.)

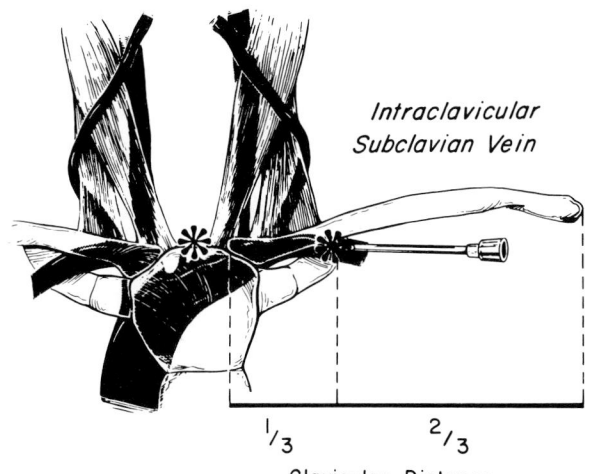

Intraclavicular Subclavian Vein

$1/3$ $2/3$

Clavicular Distance

Figure 11. The position of the needle in cannulating the subclavian vein. Note that one approaches the subclavian vein through the medial third of the thoracic inlet, aiming for that portion of the subclavian vein behind the clavicle. (From Fischer, J. E., and Freund, H. R.: Central hyperalimentation. *In* Fischer, J. E. (Ed.): Surgical Nutrition. Boston, Little, Brown & Company, 1983, p. 697.)

notch. After the vein is located with the small needle, the larger needle is inserted; a pop will be felt. After blood is aspirated freely with a syringe, the patient is asked to do a Valsalva maneuver, the hub of the needle is tipped cephalad, and the catheter is inserted with the patient still holding his breath. If the catheter does not thread and is not easily withdrawn, both the needle and the catheter should be withdrawn together to prevent the catheter from shearing off. If the Seldinger technique is used, the wire is placed though the needle, and the catheter is inserted over the wire after the needle has been withdrawn. When the catheter is in place, it is secured with a single 3–0 or 4–0 suture. After the dressing, tubing, and intravenous line have been hung, the bottle should be depressed to confirm backflow of blood through the catheter, and a confirmatory chest film is taken. In placing an internal jugular catheter, the operator uses a point 2 cm. above the clavicle at the posterior edge of the posterior belly of the sternocleidomastoid. The internal jugular vein may be approached by aiming the needle toward the supersternal notch with a lifting motion immediately under and in the plane of the fissure of the the the sternocleidomastoid (Fig. 12). In the anterior approach, the internal jugular vein may be entered at a point directly posterior where the external jugular vein crosses the sternoclavicular head. The in-

ternal jugular approach is not preferred, because it is less comfortable for patients and dressings are more difficult.

NUTRITIONAL SUPPORT TEAMS AND PROTOCOLS. Because of current cost constrictions, many hospital administrators are resistant to the concept of a nutritional support team, which should include physicians, pharmacists, one or two dieticians, and nurse clinicians for the supervision of safe parenteral nutritional support throughout the hospital. Rigid protocols must be established in the care of the catheters, because once established, clinical catheter sepsis may require at least 2 and possibly 6 weeks in the hospital and expensive intravenous antibiotics. Endophlebitis or endocarditis must be treated in a vigorous, long-term manner. If the infection rate could be decreased from an average of approximately 10 to 2 per cent by a nutritional support team and a protocol, the nutritional support team becomes cost effective.

The pharmacy is responsible for the manufacture and quality control of solutions supplied for nutritional support. This process is generally performed in a clean room, using a laminar-flow hood to minimize contamination. A variety of mechanisms may be utilized to obtain safe ordering techniques for parenteral nutrition. At the University of Cincinnati Medical Center, a multiple-copy order form (Fig. 13) is used on which orders before 9:30 A.M. are taken down to the pharmacy so that they may be promptly hung at 2 P.M. when staffing is most plentiful. A list of maximal allowable additives is given in Table 8. The protocol is placed in the patient's orders (Fig. 14).

OTHER CONSIDERATIONS

THE PEDIATRIC PATIENT POPULATION

The requirements for pediatric patients differ considerably from those for adults. Growth is more rapid. The distribution of viscera versus lean body mass is considerably different in an infant—an infant is all viscera in a skin envelope, with very little fat or skeletal muscle. In the very young, enzyme systems are incompletely developed and excessive administration of certain amino acids may result in abnormally high concentrations of potentially toxic amino acids in the brain and perhaps other viscera. In addition, the surface area of the infant is proportionally greater compared with adults, with little fat insulation, and heat loss is thus more of a problem.

Requirements for nutritional support in infants are given in Table 9. Note that the requirement for protein is far in excess of that for adults and that it decreases progressively with age. Energy requirements are also far greater than for adults. This requirement may be decreased by careful attention to heat loss and by providing a thermoneutral environment. The amount of lipid that can safely be administered is approximately 4 gm. per kg. in the infant, whereas the upper normal limit in the adult is thought to be 2 gm. per kg. Whether this is due to the presence of proportionally larger amounts of viscera, the caloric requirements of which are largely met by fat, is unclear.

Vitamins and trace metals must be carefully administered because stores are limited; yet the opportunity for toxicity is greater. Access is a problem; the use of the umbilical artery or vein is mentioned only to be condemned, because catheter sepsis here is a disaster in small infants.

In certain catastrophes, such as meconium ileus, gastroschisis, and neonatal enterocolitis, the increased survival now seen is almost certainly the result of aggressive nutritional support as well as contributions in the areas of monitoring and perioperative care. The contribution of nutritional support to the survival of low-birth-weight babies is suggestive but yet to be proved.

HOME HYPERALIMENTATION. Patients have been maintained in a functional state on parenteral nutrition for more than a decade with minimal intake by mouth. Home hyperalimenta-

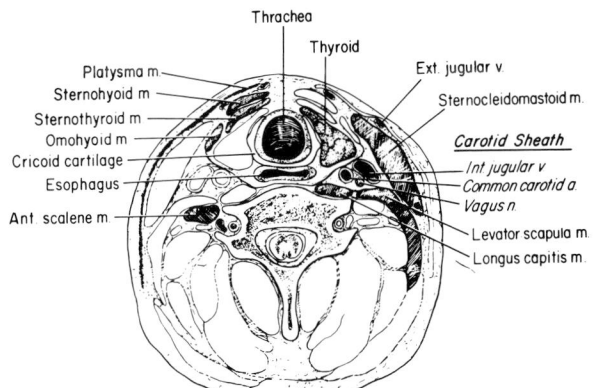

Thrachea

Thyroid

Platysma m.
Sternohyoid m
Sternothyroid m
Omohyoid m
Cricoid cartilage
Esophagus

Ant. scalene m.

Ext. jugular v.

Sternocleidomastoid m.

Carotid Sheath

Int jugular v
Common carotid a
Vagus n.

Levator scapula m.
Longus capitis m.

Figure 12. A cross section of the neck at the level of insertion of an internal jugular catheter. Note that the internal jugular vein lies in relationship to the sternocleidomastoid muscles and is lateral to the common carotid artery. (From Fischer, J. E.: Nutritional support in the seriously ill patient. *In* Ravitch, M. M., and Steichen, F. M. (Eds.): Current Problems in Surgery, Vol. XVII, No. 9, Sept. 1980, p. 515. Copyright © 1980 by Year Book Medical Publishers, Inc., Chicago.)

UMC-375
11/85

UNIVERSITY OF CINCINNATI HOSPITAL

☐ University Hospital

☐ Christian R. Holmes Division

PHYSICIAN'S ORDER FORM
Parenteral Nutrition

CENTRAL FORMULATION

2

Each 1000ml contains:

Amino Acids (4.25%)	42.5 GM
Dextrose (25%)	250 GM
Non-Protein Calories	850 KCAL
Total Calories	1020 KCAL

TRACE ELEMENTS (3ml)
added to bottle #1 ONLY

Zn - 3.0mg
Cu - 1.2mg
Cr - 12mcg
Mn - 0.3mg
Se - 60mcg

In addition
on Monday in
Bottle #2 ONLY
(for patients not receiving
anticoagulants)

Vit K - 5mg

VITAMINS (10 ml) ———— MVI-12
added to bottle #1 ONLY

	K	Na	Mg	Ca	P(mM)	Cl	Acetate	**Human Regular Insulin
STANDARD	13	20	8	4.7	14	10	45	0
WITH ADDED Na	13	52	8	4.7	14	27	59	0
WITH ADDED INSULIN	13	20	8	4.7	14	10	45	15
WITH ADDED Na + INSULIN	13	52	8	4.7	14	27	59	15
WITH ADDED K	40	20	8	4.7	17	17	59	0
WITH ADDED K + Na	40	52	8	4.7	17	27	81	0
WITH ADDED K + INSULIN	40	20	8	4.7	17	17	59	15
WITH ADDED K + Na + INSULIN	40	52	8	4.7	17	27	81	15

*Values expressed in mEq/liter unless otherwise noted.

**Expressed as units. (Other Insulin Species must be specified if desired.)

DATE _____ TIME _____

SOLUTIONS FROM PHARMACY
CHECK **ONE** FORMULA FOR EACH BOTTLE

ORDERS MUST BE IN THE PHARMACY BEFORE 9:30 A.M.

ADDITIONAL ADDITIVES:

INDICATE **TOTAL** AMOUNT OF EACH **ADDITIONAL**
ADDITIVE DESIRED PER BOTTLE.

SEQ.#	BOTTLE	STANDARD	ADDED Na	ADDED INSULIN	ADDED Na & INSULIN	ADDED K	ADDED K & Na	ADDED K & INSULIN	ADDED K, Na & INSULIN	
	#1									
	#2									
	#3									
	#4									
	#5									

RATE _____ ML/HR

INTRAVENOUS FAT EMULSION

check appropriate box

		250 ML	500 ML	1000 ML
Each ml contains 1.1 KCAL	10%			
Each ml contains 2.0 KCAL	20%			

infuse over _____ hours.

_____ M.D.

WHITE–CHART   YELLOW–PHARMACY

Figure 13. Physician's order form for central formulation used at the University of Cincinnati Medical Center. Carbon copies are collected by the pharmacy each morning and are manufactured and delivered by 2 P.M. The variety of solutions minimizes the chance of error and enables one to handle almost any metabolic situation. Note that the various possible contents of each solution are given.

TABLE 8. Allowable Additive Supplementation
(at University of Cincinnati Hospital)

Additives	Available Products (Injection)	Maximal Allowable Total per Liter
Calcium	Calcium gluconate	9 mEq.
	Calcium chloride	
Magnesium	Magnesium sulfate	12 mEq.
Phosphate	Sodium phosphate	21 mmol.
	Potassium phosphate	
Potassium	Potassium chloride	80 mEq.
	Potassium acetate	
Sodium	Sodium chloride	Patient tolerance and/or need
	Sodium acetate	
Chloride	Sodium chloride	Limited by amount of cation
	Calcium chloride	
	Potassium chloride	
Acetate	Sodium acetate	Limited by amount of cation
	Potassium acetate	
Insulin	Regular insulin	50 units

Some points to remember:

1. Bicarbonate salts *must not* be added to parenteral nutrition formulations since they create a number of incompatibilities and are ineffective given in this manner.

2. Medicinal agents not mentioned *must not* be admixed or administered with parenteral nutrition formulations unless compatibility data are available.

3. Phosphate supplementation *must* be ordered in terms of millimoles of phosphate. Note that phosphate is available only as the sodium or potassium salts and that when the potassium salt is used for "added" phosphate it must not exceed the maximal allowable concentration of potassium (i.e., 80 mEq.).

tion has now been standardized, using Silastic catheters with long subcutaneous tunnels and caps; these catheters may be used only intermittently, provided they are regularly filled with heparin. Mean catheter life of a properly cared for catheter is now approaching 7 years in well-operated programs. The Cincinnati experience with the various subcutaneous ports has not been as happy, with sepsis more frequent, which is unfortunate because patients can swim with the ports. Although 24-hour parenteral nutrition is the choice of one or two units, the overwhelming majority of home hyperalimentation is performed overnight, using sophisticated pumps with an impressive array of protective alarms.

Most patients requiring home parenteral nutrition have lost a large portion of the gastrointestinal tract, either by repeated resections for Crohn's disease, by the presence of fistulas in Crohn's disease that do not respond to conservative or surgical therapy, or by massive small bowel resection following midgut volvulus and/or mesenteric thrombosis. Rare indications for home parenteral nutrition include peculiar malabsorption diseases such as sprue, pseudo-obstruction, and scleroderma. In the author's opinion, home hyperalimentation for patients with cancer is rarely indicated except for patients in whom leukemia has been successfully treated and who are on continued suppressive therapy, or in patients on aggressive therapy in whom there is a reasonable chance for survival.

A Silastic catheter is placed either in open manner or percutaneously through an introducer. Whereas most institutions are now doing percutaneous placement directly into the subclavian vein, the author still favors an axillary approach using a small branch of the axillary vein and a long tunnel into the abdominal wall (Fig. 15). In this unit, the average life of a catheter is greater than 7 years, and catheters are most often changed for material fatigue and breakage. Although many patients no longer require parenteral nutrition after gut hypertrophy in the first 1 or 2 years, there will be a number of patients in whom several cath-

eter sites will be required. It is logical to sacrifice as few of the large veins as necessary, because one may have to rotate catheters using the axilla and branches of the internal jugular vein over the years.

Patients with home hyperalimentation manifest a special series of complications. Deficiency states that are almost never seen in human nutrition, such as biotin deficiency (because of biotin's ubiquitous nature), may be seen in patients in whom the only nutrient supply is from the intravenous fluid administered. Catheter complications are largely those of sepsis. Thrombosis of the superior vena cava and subclavian vein is rarely seen because of the inert nature of the Silastic catheter inserted. Infection of the external site of the catheter can be treated with appropriate antibiotics, and if the tunnel of the catheter is not severely infected, these infections may be successfully treated without the loss of the catheter.

The cost of home hyperalimentation is a source of consternation to most working in that field. Depending upon the area of the country and the technique used, such costs may run anywhere from $30,000 to $60,000 per year. Clearly, patient function, rehabilitation, quality of life, and other considerations enter the cost/benefit ratio. In the Cincinnati experience, such patients are extremely well motivated and almost all of them work and/or have returned to their premorbid situation.

ACQUIRED IMMUNE DEFICIENCY SYNDROME (AIDS). The place of home TPN in the treatment of patients with AIDS is controversial. It is probably dependent on the outcome of the current debate on the proper locale for treatment. Although this is not an area of the author's expertise, it is understood from infectious disease authorities that it may be appropriate to treat AIDS patients in an acute hospital setting for the first infection; thereafter, the issue becomes uncertain.

ADVANCES IN NUTRITIONAL PHARMACOLOGY. Nutritional pharmacology is a relatively new term that emphasizes the use of nutritional support to change either the milieu or the pathophysiology of a disease process in an effort to affect outcome. Early examples of what are now recognized as nutritional pharmacology include the application of the Giordano-Giovanetti diet as essential amino acids to patients in acute renal failure, and the modified amino acid mixtures for the treatment of patients with acute hepatic failure superimposed on cirrhosis. The areas of nutritional pharmacology currently under investigation involve the use of specific nutrients to alter certain conditions or enhance host defenses in certain situations.

GLUTAMINE AND KETONE BODIES. These have been discussed previously.

ARGININE. A deficiency of arginine and the dibasic amino acids in the plasma of patients with overwhelming sepsis was observed as early as 1978.[48] Although arginine was thought to be a nonessential amino acid, it is now recognized that the ability to synthesize arginine in the presence of increased requirements may be exceeded, and it probably is semiessential. Arginine is used not only by the host but apparently by macrophages, lymphocytes, and perhaps other cells in healing wounds. Arginine-supplemented diets are utilized in patients with burns as a new enteral formula and may also be useful in trauma. Arginine enhances the responsiveness of T lymphocytes to mitogenic stimulation. There has also been recent interest in the use of the response of the T lymphocytes to arginine in patients with cancer. Daly and co-workers,[30] in a controlled study, administered arginine in an enteral diet to 30 cancer patients; the controls received an L-glycine–supplemented, isonitrogenous enteral diet. Whereas nitrogen accumulation was no different between the two groups, the beneficial effect of arginine on T lymphocyte response to concanavalin A was verified, but it was also associated with increased T helper cell activity. There was an increased T cell proliferation to both concanavalin A and phytohemagglutinin in the arginine-supplemented patients.

UMC-374
Revised 5/88
                University of Cincinnati Hospital
                Physician's Checklist/Order Sheet

All applicable orders have been checked. A line has been placed
through orders that have been voided. ORDERS NOT CHECKED
ARE NOT TO BE FOLLOWED. Orders have been modified
according to the medical condition of the patient. These orders
have been dated, timed and signed by a physician. As an order is
filled, the individual doing so must date/time and initial in the
space provided. Further orders will be added as needed.

PAGE __1__ OF __1__

ORDER NUMBER	✓	PHYSICIAN'S STANDING ORDERS PARENTERAL NUTRITION	ORDER NOTED (DATE/TIME)	(INITIAL)
1.	✓	Infuse only through a new subclavian or internal jugular		
		or existing implanted catheter which terminates in		
		superior vena cava or brachiocephalic vein.		
2.	✓	STAT portable chest x-ray.		
3.	✓	Initial and subsequent dressing by nurse (per Nursing		
		Procedure).		
4.	✓	Infuse D_5W at 40 ml/hr until TPN is available.		
5.	✓	Administration via infusion device.		
6.	✓	Catheter may be used only for TPN except by order of		
		Nutritional Support physician.		
7.	✓	Vital signs Q 6 hours.		
8.	✓	Urine sugars Q 6 hours with Diastix.		
9.	✓	Intake and Output Q 24 hours.		
10.	✓	Weights Monday, Wednesday, and Friday.		
11.	✓	Blood Work:		
		MONDAY: Renal (4203), Bone (4041) & Hepatic (4162)		
		Profiles.		
		THURSDAY AND PRIOR TO STARTING PARENTERAL NUTRITION:		
		Renal (4203), Bone (4041) & Hepatic (4162) Profiles,		
		CBC (4032), Prothrombin Time (4204), Transferrin (4706),		
		Prealbumin (4705), Retinol Binding Protein (4707),		
		Magnesium (4229), Cholesterol & Triglyceride (4726),		
		Amino Acid Profile (4265).		
12.	✓	STAT blood glucose for 1/4% or greater glycosuria.		
13.	✓	If parenteral nutrition solution is interrupted, infuse		
		D_5W at the same rate until it is restarted.		
14.	✓	Notify Nutritional Support for catheter removal and		
		culture Mon.-Fri. 9:00 a.m.-4:00 p.m.		

Physician's signature _____

White-Chart   Yellow-Kardex
                                Date _____ Time _____

Developed by ___Robert H. Bower, M.D.___   Date ___4/88___

Figure 14. Standard hyperalimentation orders at the University of Cincinnati Medical Center.

TABLE 9. Nutritional Requirements in Infants

Protein (gm./kg./day)	Newborn to 6 months 2.5	6–12 months 2.0	School age 1.75	Adolescent 1.2	Kcal./Nitrogen 150:1
Calories (kcal./kg./day)	Newborn or premature 120	Infant (to 10 kg.) 100	10–20 kg. 100 + 50	Over 20 kg. 100 + 50 + 20	
Fat	? 35% of calories (up to 3.5 gm./kg./day)				

Electrolytes (mEq./M²/day)	Trace Elements (per day)		Vitamins (per day) (MVI/L.)	
Na^+ 50	Ca^{++}	9.4 mEq./L.	A	2000 IU
K^+ 30	Mg^{++}	8.1 mEq./L.	C	100 mg.
Urine Na^+:K^+ > 1.0 adequate	P	6.0 mM./L.	D	200 IU
	Zn	800 g./L.	B_1	10 mg.
	Cu	100 g./L.	B_2	2 mg.
			B_6	3 mg.
			E	1 IU
			Niacin	20 mg.
			Dexpanthenol	5 mg.
			Folic acid	3 mg.
			B_{12}	50 μg.
			K	2 mg.

MVI, multivitamins.

ALTERATIONS IN LIPID PROFILE AND THEIR POSSIBLE EFFECTS ON THE INFLAMMATORY RESPONSE. The synthesis of prostaglandins, thromboxanes, and leukotrienes through lipoxygenase-mediated pathways has arachidonic acid as the source material. Although the evidence that prostaglandins themselves are involved in the proteolysis and catabolism that follow sepsis has been extensively challenged recently, there is good evidence that the prostaglandins may have a role in the immunologic response to transplantation rejection, for example. The use of fish oil as a lipid source in patients with burns, in trauma, and particularly in experimental animals in investigating the rejection phenomenon has been investigated. Recent preliminary studies in patients with burns using a fish oil derivative as a lipid source, instead of the traditional arachidonic acid–based deriv-

atives, suggest that the inflammatory response is modified. In the area of transplantation immunology, at least in experimental animals, the substitution of a fish oil lipid source together with cyclosporine and pretransplantation transfusion has resulted in indefinite survival of transplanted rat hearts. This very exciting development suggests that in patients with inflammatory disease and in patients about to undergo transplantation, dietary manipulation by substitution of the lipid source may result in a dramatic improvement in outcome. One word of caution: When one modifies essential responses, timing may be very important; it is conceivable that with improper timing, as with all immunomodulation, harm may result as well.

It is clear that as surgeons become more facile biochemically and continue to investigate the basis for some of the pathophys-

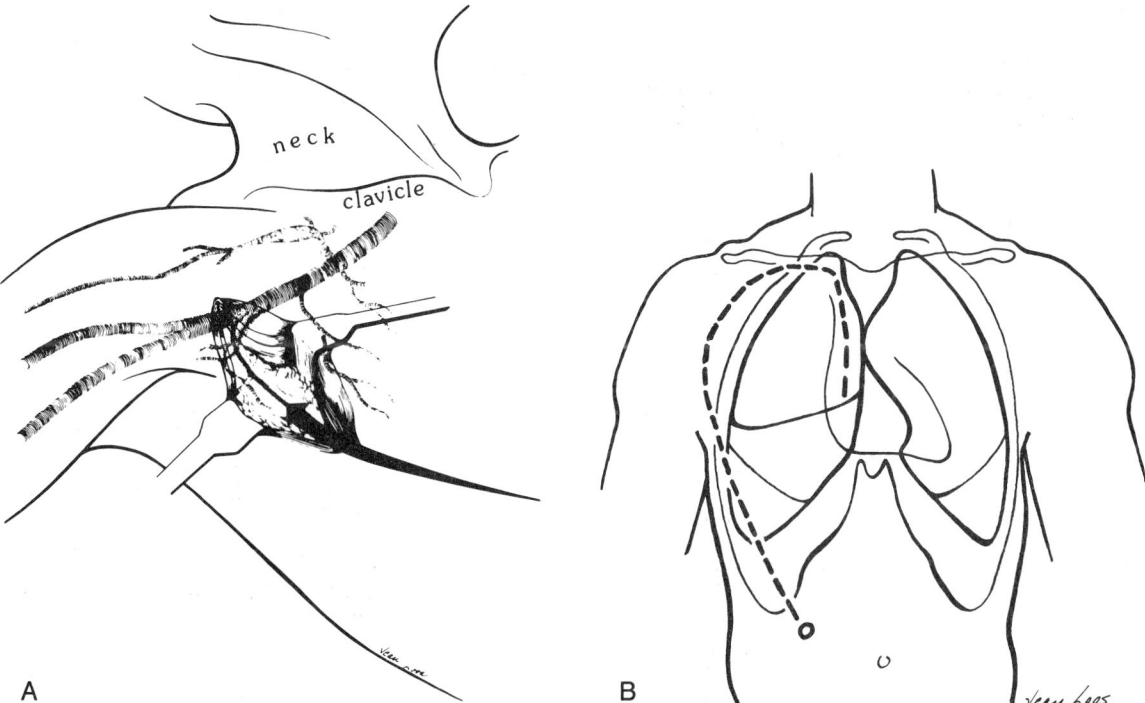

A   B

Figure 15. *A,* Open axillary approach to placement of long-term indwelling catheter. The incision is posterior and parallel to the pectoralis major, and is hidden (an important consideration in females). A branch of the axillary vein is cannulated under direct vision. This approach is especially useful in patients with bleeding tendencies. *B,* Hickman catheter in place, with tip in right atrium and exit site over right upper quadrant of the abdomen. (From Freund, H. R., Benson, D. W., Bower, R. H., and Fischer, J. E.: Enteral and parenteral nutrition. *In* Moody, F. G., Carey, L. C., Jones, R. S., Kelly, K. A., Nahrwold, D. L., and Skinner, D. B. (Eds.): Surgical Treatment of Digestive Disease, 2nd ed. Chicago, Year Book Medical Publishers, 1990, p. 864.)

iologic responses in sepsis and injury, the ability to modify the milieu will yield enormous dividends to patients in various disease states.

SUMMARY

Total nutritional support has been available on a prolonged basis for approximately 2 decades. It has already proved its value as one of the most important therapeutic modalities in this century and perhaps in the history of medicine. While still in its infancy, a new phase of nutritional support is emerging. As investigators have been trained who are equally familiar with the operating room and biochemistry, physiology, and immunology laboratories, the basic mechanisms and pathophysiology of disease at a biochemical and even molecular level are being elucidated. Advances in nutritional pharmacology are due to the attempt on the part of various investigators, but largely surgeons, to elucidate some of the mechanisms responsible for the responses in disease states. It is clear that only the surface of the ability to modify the internal milieu of patients, the response to certain cytokines, or some of the pathophysiologic and biochemical mechanisms that occur in patients and in diseases has been achieved. The next several decades should prove very exciting, and nutritional support and especially advances in nutritional pharmacology will almost certainly contribute to an improvement in outcome in various disease states that are today the cause of significant mortality in patients.

Acknowledgments. The author wishes to thank Steve Wiesner, B.A., for his excellent editorial work and Joseph A. Lacy, M.S., R.D., for his assistance in collating the enteral preparations.

SELECTED REFERENCES

Abel, R. M., Beck C. H., Jr., Abbott, W. M., Ryan, J. A., Barnett, G. O., and Fischer, J. E.: Improved survival from acute renal failure after treatment with intravenous essential L-amino acids and glucose: Results of a prospective, double-blind study. N. Engl. J. Med., 288:695, 1973.
An early, randomized, double-blind trial showing improved survival following the application of techniques of parenteral nutrition and a specialized solution to patients with renal failure. The eight essential L-amino acids in hypertonic dextrose were administered to patients with renal failure and compared with a group receiving isocaloric hypertonic dextrose alone. Improved survival and perhaps early healing of the renal lesion were seen. At present, because dialysis techniques are more widely used, there is controversy as to what solution should be used in patients with renal failure: essential amino acids alone or a low dose of a standard solution. This article, however, represents an excellent early effort in defining needs of patients wth specialized disease states.

Askanazi, J., Rosenbaum, S. H., Hyman, A. I., Silverberg, P. A., Milic-Emili, J., and Kinney, J. M.: Respiratory changes induced by the large glucose loads of total parenteral nutrition. J.A.M.A., 243:1444, 1980.
In this paper, the effect of glucose in generating excess CO_2, particularly in patients with sepsis, is described. Although one should be aware of this phenomenon, which has been given wide publicity, it occurs largely in patients who are septic and whose glucose loads are increased rather suddenly and dramatically as in this study. Nonetheless, in patients with marginal pulmonary reserve who have difficulty weaning from the ventilator because of carbon dioxide retention, decreasing the glucose load and substitution of fat calories sometimes enables successful weaning. If possible, CO_2 production should be measured.

Clowes, G. H. A., George, B. C., Villee, C. A., and Saravis, C. A.: Muscle proteolysis induced by a circulating peptide in patients with sepsis or trauma. N. Engl. J. Med., 308:545, 1983.
Few papers have inspired as much interest and excitement as this description of a molecular weight 4200 protein isolated in the plasma of patients with sepsis. This hypothetical cytokine, PIF, increased hepatic protein synthesis and muscle breakdown. Subsequent experiments have revealed that the particular conditions used in these experiments may have contributed to these findings. Nonetheless, this paper probably contributed more to the research in surgical investigation of cytokines than any other paper, exciting a great deal of work over the subsequent 6 years.

Cuthbertson, D. P.: Observations on the disturbance of metabolism produced by injury to the limbs. Q. J. Med., 1:233, 1932.
This study may well have begun contemporary nutritional support. A classic description of loss of nitrogen and breakdown of lean body mass following injury. A careful study in a classic tradition.

Dominioni, L., Trocki, O., Mochizuki, H., Fang, C. H., and Alexander, J. W.: Prevention of severe postburn hypermetabolism and catabolism by immediate intragastric feeding. J. Burn Care Rehab., 5:106, 1984.
The first demonstration that changes in gut flora and the translocation of bacteria or absorption of bacterial products following thinning of mucosa in burns contribute to hypermetabolism. With the confirmation of similar results in patients with burns, it is clear that this hypothesis with respect to gut products is operant in patients as well.

Dudrick, S. J., Wilmore, D. W., Vars, H. M., and Rhoads, J. E.: Long-term total parenteral nutrition with growth, development, and positive nitrogen balance. Surgery, 64:134, 1968.
One of the classic papers originally describing high-glucose central total parenteral nutrition from which the current popularity of parenteral nutrition in the United States stems. In this ambitious project, the biochemical requirements for growth in puppies were investigated with astounding results: normal growth comparable to puppies eating ad lib could be achieved without any oral intake provided that one infused the necessary nutrients by vein.

Fischer, J. E., Rosen, H. M., Ebeid, A. M., James, J. H., Keane, J. M., and Soeters, P. B.: The effect of normalization of plasma amino acids on hepatic encephalopathy in man. Surgery, 80:77, 1976.
In this study, an approach to liver disease and the intolerance to protein in patients with hepatic encephalopathy are described. This study represents the culmination of a hypothesis of hepatic encephalopathy, depending upon altered plasma amino acid patterns, changes subsequently discovered to be amplified by changes in the blood-brain barrier secondary to disturbed metabolism in liver disease. It represents an early anecdotal attempt to enable patients with severe hepatic deficiency to receive adequate nutrition at the same time as awakening from hepatic encephalopathy while receiving increased protein equivalent in the form of a branched chain-enriched (to 36 per cent) amino acid solution now commercially available as hepatamine.

Ryan, J. A., Jr., Abel, R. M., Abbott, W. M., Hopkins, C. C., Chesney, T., Colley, R., Phillips, K., and Fischer, J. E: Catheter complications in total parenteral nutrition: A prospective study of 200 consecutive patients. N. Engl. J. Med., 290:757, 1974.
A study of the complications of parenteral nutrition in a large hospital with one of the first centralized nutritional support teams. This study confirmed that rigid asepsis in the care of catheters and minimizing catheter manipulation were the most important factors in preventing line catheter sepsis.

Wilmore, D. W., and Dudrick, S. J.: Treatment of acute renal failure with intravenous essential L-amino acids. Arch. Surg., 99:669, 1969.
This study represents the earliest approach to disease-specific parenteral nutrition. The principle of attempting to define the metabolic abnormalities in a given patient and infusing an appropriate nutritional substrate was first proposed in this study. The intravenous equivalent of a Giordano-Giovanetti diet, containing only the eight L-essential amino acids—a "high biologic value" oral diet—was used.

BOOKS

Fischer, J. E. (Ed.): Total Parenteral Nutrition. Boston, Little, Brown & Company, 1976.
This book represents an early attempt to standardize the practical approach to total parenteral nutrition. It is still current. A second edition is being prepared.

Fischer, J. E. (Ed.): Surgical Nutrition. Boston, Little, Brown & Company, 1983.
An attempt to collate basic science knowledge and practical knowledge in one volume. The various chapters also address efficacy of parenteral nutrition.

Grant, J. P. (Ed.): Handbook of Total Parenteral Nutrition. Phildelphia, W. B. Saunders Company, 1980.
A somewhat shorter version in an attempt to detail knowledge in the area of parenteral nutrition. The bibliography is particularly exhaustive and quite useful. A second edition is being prepared.

Greep, J. M., Soeters, P. B., Wesdorp, R. I. C., Phaf, C. W. R., and Fischer, J. E. (Eds.): Current Concepts in Parenteral Nutrition. The Hague, Martinus Nijhoff Medical Division, 1977.
A record of historic interest. The meeting was held at a time when there were many controversies in parenteral nutrition, and many authorities were present at this meeting. The discussion, which is published in its entirety, is of particular interest.

Rombeau, J. L., and Caldwell, M. D. (Eds.): Enteral Nutrition (Vol. 1) and Parenteral Nutrition (Vol. 2). Philadelphia, W. B. Saunders Company, 1986.
This is the most recent large textbook on enteral and parenteral nutrition. It is well done and reasonably current. There are a large number of specialized chapters.

Wilmore, D. W. (Ed.): The Metabolic Management of the Critically Ill. New York, Plenum Press, 1977.
An excellent summary that goes into great detail in certain metabolic areas, particularly in critically ill patients. It is still current and, although much of the "basic" science components have subsequently been enlarged upon, can still be read with profit.

REFERENCES

1. Abel, R. M., Beck, C. H., Jr., Abbott, W. M., Ryan, J. A., Barnett, G. O., and Fischer, J. E.: Improved survival from acute renal failure following treatment

with intravenous essential L-amino acids and glucose: Results of a prospective, double-blind study. N. Engl. J. Med., 288:695, 1973.

2. Abel, R. M., Fischer, J. E., Buckley, M. J., Barnett, G. O., and Austen, W. G.: Malnutrition in cardiac surgical patients: Results of a prospective, randomized evaluation of early postoperative parenteral nutrition. Arch. Surg., 111:45, 1977.

3. Abel, R. M., Grimes, J. B., Alonso, D., Alonso, M. L., and Gay, W. A., Jr.: Adverse hemodynamic and ultrastructural changes in dog hearts subjected to protein-calorie malnutrition. Am. Heart J., 97:733, 1979.

4. Alexander, J. W., MacMillan, B. G., Stinnett, J. D., Ogle, C. K., Bozian, R. C., Fischer, J. E., Oakes, J. B., Morris, M. J., and Krummel, R.: Beneficial effects of aggressive protein feeding in severely burned children. Ann. Surg., 192:505, 1980.

5. Askanazi, J., Rosenbaum, S. H., Hyman, A. I., Silverberg, P. A., Milic-Emili, J., and Kinney, J. M.: Respiratory changes induced by the large glucose loads of total parenteral nutrition. J.A.M.A., 243:1444, 1980.

6. Baker, J. P., Detsky, A. S., Wesson, D. E., Wolman, S. L., Stewart, S., Whitewell, J., Langer, B., and Jeejeebhoy, K. N.: Nutritional assessment: A comparison of clinical judgment and objective measurements. N. Engl. J. Med., 306:969, 1982.

7. Baron, P. L., Lawrence, W., Jr., Chan, W. M. Y., White, F. K. H., and Banks, W. L., Jr.: Effects of parenteral nutrition on cell cycle kinetics of head and neck cancer. Arch. Surg., 121:1282, 1986.

8. Baumann, H., Onorato, V., Gauldie, J., and Jahreis, G.: Distinct sets of acute-phase plasma proteins are stimulated by separate human hepatocyte stimulating factors and monokines in rat hepatoma cells. J. Biol. Chem., 262:9756, 1987.

9. Billiar, T. R., Curran, R. D., Stuehr, D. J., Ferrari, F. K., and Simmons, R. L.: Evidence that activation of Kupffer cells results in production of L-arginine metabolites that release cell-associated iron and inhibit hepatocyte protein synthesis. Surgery, 106:364, 1989.

10. Billiar, T. R., Maddaus, M. A., West, M. A., Curran, R. D., Wells, C. A., and Simmons, R. L.: Intestinal gram-negative bacterial overgrowth in vivo augments the in vitro response of Kupffer cells to endotoxin. Ann. Surg., 208:532, 1988.

11. Bjornson, H. S., Colley, R., Bower, R. H., Duty, V. P., Schwartz-Fulton, J. T., and Fischer, J. E.: Association between microorganism growth at the catheter insertion site and colonization of the catheter in patients receiving total parenteral nutrition. Surgery, 92:720, 1982.

12. Bower, R. H., Muggia-Sullam, M., Vallgren, S., Hurst, J. M., Kern, K. A., LaFrance, R., and Fischer, J. E.: Branched chain amino acid–enriched solutions in the septic patient: A randomized, prospective trial. Ann. Surg., 203:13, 1986.

13. Branson, R. D., Hurst, J. M., Warner, B. W., Bower, R. H., and Arita, A.: Measured versus predicted energy expenditure in mechanically ventilated patients with chronic obstructive pulmonary disease. Respiratory Care, 32:748, 1987.

14. Brennan, M. F., Cerra, F., Daly, J. M., Fischer, J. E., Moldawer, L. L., Smith, R. J., Vinnars, E., Wannemacher, R., and Young, V. R.: Report of a research workshop: Branched chain amino acids in stress and injury. J. Parent. Enteral Nutr., 10:446, 1986.

15. Buse, M. G., and Reid, S. S.: Leucine: A possible regulator of protein turnover in muscle. J. Clin. Invest., 56:1250, 1975.

16. Buzby, G. P.: Case for preoperative nutritional support. Presented at the American College of Surgeons 1988 Clinical Congress Postgraduate Course on "Pre- and Postoperative Care: Metabolism and Nutrition," Chicago, IL, October 25–28, 1988.

17. Buzby, G. P., Mullen, J. L., Matthews, D. C., Hobbs, C. L., and Rosato, E. F.: Prognostic nutritional index in gastrointestinal surgery. Am. J. Surg., 139:160, 1980.

18. Cerra, F. B., Cheung, N. K., Fischer, J. E., Kaplowitz, N., Schiff, E. R., Dienstag, J. L., Bower, R. H., Mabry, C. D., Leevy, C. M., and Kiernan, T.: Disease-specific amino acid infusion (F080) in hepatic encephalopathy: A prospective, randomized, double-blind, controlled trial. J. Parent. Enteral Nutr., 9:288, 1985.

19. Cerra, F. B., McPherson, J. P., Konstantinides, F. N., Konstantinides, N. N., and Teasley, K. M.: Enteral nutrition does not prevent multiple organ failure syndrome (MOFS) after sepsis. Surgery, 104:727, 1988.

20. Cerra, F. B., Shronts, E., Konstantinides, N., Konstantinides, F., and Teasley, K. M.: Enteral feeding in sepsis: A prospective, randomized, double-blind trial. Surgery, 98:632, 1985.

21. Cerra, F. B., Upson, D., Angelico, R., Wiles, C., Lyons, J., and Paysinger, J.: Branched chains support postoperative synthesis. Surgery, 92:192, 1982.

22. Chance, W. T., Cao, L., and Fischer, J. E.: Insulin and acivicin improve host nutrition and prevent tumor growth during total parenteral nutrition. Ann. Surg., 208:524, 1988.

23. Chance, W. T., Cao, L., Nelson, J. L., Foley-Nelson, T., and Fischer, J. E.: Reversal of neurochemical aberrations after tumor resection in rats. Am. J. Surg., 155:124, 1988.

24. Christou, N. V., Meakins, J. L., and MacLean, L. D.: The predictive role of delayed hypersensitivity in preoperative patients. Surg. Gynecol. Obstet., 152:297, 1981.

25. Christou, N. V., and Tellado, J. M.: In vitro polymorphonuclear neutrophil function in surgical patients does not correlate with anergy but with "activating" processes such as sepsis or trauma. Surgery, 106:718, 1989.

26. Clowes, G. H. A., Jr., George, B. C., Villee, C. A., Jr., and Saravis, C. A.: Muscle proteolysis induced by a circulating peptide in patients with sepsis or trauma. N. Engl. J. Med., 308:545, 1983.

27. Copeland, E. M., MacFayden, B. V., and Dudrick, S. J.: Effect of intravenous hyperalimentation on established delayed hypersensitivity in the cancer patient. Ann. Surg., 184:60, 1976.

28. Cuthbertson, D. P.: Observations on the disturbance of metabolism produced by injury to the limbs. Q. J. Med., 1:233, 1932.

29. Daly, J. M., Mihranian, M. H., Kehoe, J. E., and Brennan, M. F.: Effects of post-operative infusion of branched chain amino acids on nitrogen balance and forearm muscle substrate flux. Surgery, 94:151, 1983.

30. Daly, J. M., Reynolds, J., Thom, A., Kinsley, L., Dietrick-Gallagher, M., Shou, J., and Ruggieri, B.: Immune and metabolic effects of arginine in the surgical patient. Ann. Surg., 208:512, 1988.

31. Deitch, E. A., Berg, R., and Specian, R.: Endotoxin promotes translocation of bacteria from the gut. Arch. Surg., 122:185, 1987.

32. Detsky, A. S., Baker, J. P., O'Rourke, K., and Goel, V.: Perioperative parenteral nutrition: A meta-analysis. Ann. Intern. Med., 107:195, 1988.

33. Dominioni, L., Trocki, O., Mochizuki, H., Fang, C. H., and Alexander, J. W.: Prevention of severe postburn hypermetabolism and catabolism by immediate intragastric feeding. J. Burn Care Rehab., 5:106, 1984.

34. Elwyn, D. H.: The role of the liver in regulation of amino acid and protein metabolism. In Munro, H. N. (Ed.): Mammalian Protein Metabolism. Vol. 4. New York, Academic Press, 1970, pp. 523–557.

35. Feinstein, E. I., Blumenkrantz, M. J., Healy, H., Koffler, A., Silberman, H., Massry, S. G., and Kopple, J. D.: Clinical and metabolic responses to parenteral nutrition in acute renal failure: A controlled double blind study. Medicine (Baltimore), 60:124, 1981.

36. Fiaccadori, F., Ghinelli, F., Pedretti, G., Pelosi, G., Sacchini, D., Zeneroli, M. L., Rocchi, E., Gibertini, P., and Ventura, E.: Branched chain amino acid enriched solutions in the treatment of hepatic encephalopathy: A controlled trial. In Capocaccia, L., Fischer, J. E., and Rossi-Fanelli, F. (Eds.): Hepatic Encephalopathy in Chronic Liver Failure. New York, Plenum Press, 1984, pp. 323–334.

37. Fischer, J. E.: Adjuvant parenteral nutrition in the patient with cancer. Editorial. Surgery, 96:578, 1984.

38. Fischer, J. E.: Branched chain amino acids in hepatic encephalopathy: Results of parenteral trials. In Holm, E., and Kaspar, H. (Eds.): Metabolism and Nutrition in Liver Disease. Lancaster, MTP Press, 1985, pp. 259–273.

39. Fischer, J. E., and Baldessarini, R. J.: False neurotransmitters and hepatic failure. Lancet, 2:75, 1971.

40. Flatt, J. P., and Blackburn, G. L.: The metabolic fuel regulatory system: Implications for the design of protein-sparing therapies during periods of caloric deprivation and disease. Am. J. Clin. Nutr., 27:175, 1974.

41. Flores, E. A., Bistrian, B. R., Pomposelli, J. J., Dinarello, C. A., Blackburn, G. L., and Istfan, N. W.: Infusion of tumor necrosis factor/cachectin promotes muscle catabolism in the rat: A synergistic effect with interleukin-1. J. Clin. Invest., 83:1614, 1989.

42. Fox, A. D., Kripke, S. A., De Paula, J. A., Berman, J. M., Settle, R. G., and Rombeau, J. L.: Effect of a glutamine-supplemented enteral diet on methotrexate induced enterocolitis. J. Parent. Enteral Nutr., 12:325, 1988.

43. Freund, H. R., Dienstag, J., Lehrich, F., Yoshimura, N., Bradford, R. R., Rosen, H., Atamian, S., Slemmer, E., Holroyde, J., and Fischer, J. E.: Infusion of BCAA solution in patients with hepatic encephalopathy. Ann. Surg., 196:209, 1982.

44. Freund, H. R., Floman, N., Schwartz, B., and Fischer, J. E.: Essential fatty acid deficiency in total parenteral nutrition. Ann. Surg., 190:139, 1979.

45. Freund, H. R., James, J. H., and Fischer, J. E.: Nitrogen-sparing mechanisms of singly administered branched chain amino acids in the injured rat. Surgery, 90:237, 1981.

46. Freund, H. R., Ryan, J. A., and Fischer, J. E.: Amino acid derangements in sepsis: Treatment with branched chain amino acid rich infusions. Ann. Surg., 188:423, 1978.

47. Fulks, R. M., Li, J. B., and Goldberg, A. L.: Effects of insulin, glucose, and amino acids on protein turnover in rat diaphragm. J. Biol. Chem., 250:280, 1975.

48. Galandiuk, S., O'Neill, M., McDonald, P., Fazio, V., and Steiger, E.: A century of home parenteral nutrition for Crohn's disease. Am. J. Surg., 159:540, 1990.

49. Gimmon, Z., Murphy, R. F., Chen, M. H., Nachbauer, C. A., Fischer, J. E., and Joffe, S. N.: The effect of parenteral and enteral nutrition on portal and systemic immunoreactivities of gastrin, glucagon, and vasoactive intestinal polypeptide (VIP). Ann. Surg., 196:571, 1982.

50. Hammarqvist, F., Wernerman, J., Ali, R., von der Decken, A., and Vinnars, E.: Addition of glutamine to total parenteral nutrition after elective surgery spares free glutamine in muscle, counteracts the fall in muscle protein synthesis, and improves nitrogen balance. Ann. Surg., 209:455, 1989.

51. Harvey, T. C., Jain, S., Dykes, P. W., James, H., Chen, N. S., Chettle, D. R., Ettinger, K. V., Fremlin, J. H., and Thomas, B. J.: Measurement of whole body nitrogen by neutron activation analysis. Lancet, 2:395, 1973.

52. Hasselgren, P. O., James, J. H., and Fischer, J. E.: Inhibited muscle amino acid uptake in sepsis. Ann. Surg., 203:360, 1986.

53. Hasselgren, P. O., James, J. H., Warner, B. W., Ogle, C. K., Takehara, H., and Fischer, J. E.: Reduced muscle amino acid uptake in sepsis and the effects in vitro of septic plasma and interleukin-1. Surgery, 100:222, 1986.

54. Hasselgren, P. O., James, J. H., Warner, B. W., Hummel, R. P., III, and Fischer, J. E.: Protein synthesis and degradation in skeletal muscle from

septic rats: Response to leucine and alpha-ketoisocaproic acid. Arch. Surg., 123:640, 1988.

55. Hasselgren, P. O., James, J. H., Benson, D. W., Li, S., and Fischer, J. E.: Is there a circulating proteolysis inducing factor (PIF) during sepsis? Arch. Surg., 125:510, 1990.

56. Hasselgren, P. O., Warner, B. W., James, J. H., Takehara, H., and Fischer, J. E.: Effect of insulin on amino acid uptake and protein turnover in skeletal muscle from septic rats: Evidence for insulin resistance of protein breakdown. Arch. Surg., 122:228, 1987.

57. Hasselgren, P. O., Warner, B. W., Hummel, R. P., III, James, J. H., Ogle, C. K., and Fischer, J. E.: Further evidence that accelerated muscle protein breakdown during sepsis is not mediated by prostaglandin E$_2$. Ann. Surg., 207:399, 1988.

58. Holter, A., and Fischer, J. E.: Effects of perioperative hyperalimentation on complications in patients with carcinoma and weight loss. J. Surg. Res., 23:31, 1977.

59. Hummel, R. P., III, James, J. H., Warner, B. W., Hasselgren, P. O., and Fischer, J. E.: Evidence that cathepsin B contributes to skeletal muscle protein breakdown during sepsis. Arch. Surg., 123:221, 1988.

60. Hwang, T. L., O'Dwyer, S. T., Smith, R. J., and Wilmore, D. W.: Preservation of the small bowel mucosa using glutamine-enriched parenteral nutrition. Surg. Forum, 37:56, 1986.

61. James, J. H., Escourrou, J., and Fischer, J. E.: Blood-brain neutral amino acid transport activity is increased after portacaval anastomosis. Science, 200:1395, 1978.

62. James, J. H., Jeppsson, B., Ziparo, V., and Fischer, J. E.: Hyperammonemia, plasma amino acid imbalance and blood-brain amino acid transport: A unified theory of portal-systemic encephalopathy. Lancet, 2:772, 1979.

63. Jeejeebhoy, K. N., Baker, J. P., Wolman, S. L., et al.: Critical evaluation of the role of clinical assessment and body composition studies in patients with malnutrition and after total parenteral nutrition. Am. J. Clin. Nutr., 35:1117, 1982.

64. Jenkins, M., Gottschlich, M., Alexander, J. W., and Warden, G. D. Effect of immediate enteral feeding on the hypermetabolic response following severe burn injury. J. Parent. Enteral Nutr., 13(Suppl. 1):12s, 1989.

65. Kripke, S. A., Fox, A. D., Berman, J. M., De Paula, J., Birkhahn, R. H., Rombeau, J. L., and Settle, R. G.: Inhibition of TPN-associated intestinal mucosal atrophy with monoacetoacetin. J. Surg. Res., 44:436, 1988.

66. Kripke, S. A., Fox, A. D., Berman, J. M., De Paula, J. A., Rombeau, J. L., and Settle, R. G.: Inhibition of TPN-associated colonic atrophy with beta hydroxybutyrate. Surg. Forum, 39:48, 1988.

67. Li, S., Nussbaum, M. S., McFadden, D. W., Dayal, R., and Fischer, J. E.: Reversal of hepatic steatosis in rats by addition of glucagon to total parenteral nutrition (TPN). J. Surg. Res., 46:557, 1989.

68. Li, S., Nussbaum, M. S., McFadden, D. W., Zhang, F. S., LaFrance, R. J., Dayal, R., and Fischer, J. E.: Addition of L-glutamine to total parenteral nutrition (TPN) and its effects on portal insulin and glucagon and the development of hepatic steatosis in rats. J. Surg. Res., 48:421, 1990.

69. Li, S., Nussbaum, M. S., Teague, D., Gapen, C. L., Dayal, R., and Fischer, J. E.: Increasing dextrose concentrations in total parenteral nutrition (TPN) causes alterations in hepatic morphology and plasma levels of insulin and glucagon in rats. J. Surg. Res., 44:639, 1988.

70. Manson, J., and Wilmore, D. W.: Positive nitrogen balance with human growth hormone and hypocaloric intravenous feeding. Surgery, 100:188, 1986.

71. Martin, L. W., Fischer, J. E., Sayers, H. J., Alexander, F., and Torres, M. A.: Anal continence following Soave procedure: Analysis of results in 100 patients. Ann. Surg., 203:525, 1986.

72. Mealy, K., van Lanschot, J. J. B., Robinson, B., Rounds, J., and Wilmore, D. W.: Are the catabolic effects of tumor necrosis factor mediated by glucocorticoids? Arch. Surg., 125:42, 1990.

73. Mirtallo, J. M., Schneider, P. J., Mavko, K., Ruberg, R. L., and Fabri, P. J.: A comparison of essential and general amino acid infusions on the nutritional support of patients with compromised renal function. J. Parent. Enteral Nutr., 6:109, 1982.

74. Moore, F. D.: Delayed scientific hypersensitivity. Editorial. J. Parent. Enteral Nutr., 6:1, 1982.

75. Muggia-Sullam, M., Bower, R. H., Murphy, R. F., Joffe, S. N., and Fischer, J. E.: Postoperative enteral versus parenteral nutritional support in gastrointestinal surgery: A matched prospective study. Am. J. Surg., 149:106, 1985.

76. Mullen, J. L., Buzby, G. P., Matthews, D. C., Small, B. F., and Rosato, E. F.: Reduction of operative morbidity and mortality by combined preoperative and postoperative nutritional support. Ann. Surg., 192:604, 1980.

77. Muller, J. M., Dienst, C., Brenner, V., and Pichlmaier, H.: Preoperative parenteral feeding in patients with gastrointestinal carcinoma. Lancet, 1:68, 1982.

78. Naylor, C. D., O'Rourke, K., Detsky, A. S., and Baker, J. P.: Parenteral nutrition with branched-chain amino acids in hepatic encephalopathy: A meta-analysis. Gastroenterology, 97:1033, 1989.

79. Odessey, R., and Goldberg, A. L.: Oxidation of leucine by rat skeletal muscle. Am. J. Physiol., 223:1376, 1972.

80. Pedersen, P., Hasselgren, P. O., Li, S., Hiyama, D. T., and Fischer, J. E.:

Synthesis of acute-phase proteins in perfused liver following the administration of recombinant interleukin-1 to normal or adrenalectomized rats. J. Surg. Res., 45:333, 1988.

81. Popp, M. B., Wagner, S. C., and Brito, O. J.: Host and tumor responses to increasing levels of intravenous nutritional support. Surgery, 94:300, 1983.

82. Reber, H. A., Roberts, C., Way, L. W., and Dunphy, J. E.: Management of external gastrointestinal fistulas. Ann. Surg., 188:460, 1978.

83. Rigotti, P., Peters, J. C., Tranberg, K. G., and Fischer, J. E.: Effects of amino acid infusions on liver regeneration after partial hepatectomy in the rat. J. Parent. Enteral Nutr., 10:17, 1986.

84. Rodemann, H. P., and Goldberg, A. L.: Arachidonic acid, prostaglandin E$_2$ and F$_{2\alpha}$ influence rates of protein turnover in skeletal and cardiac muscle. J. Biol. Chem., 257:1632, 1982.

85. Rush, B. F., Jr., Redan, J. A., Flanagan, J. J., Jr., Heneghan, J. B., Hsieh, J., Murphy, T. F., Smith, S., and Machiedo, G. W.: Does the bacteremia observed in hemorrhagic shock have clinical significance? A study in germ-free animals. Ann. Surg., 210:342, 1989.

86. Russell, D. M., Leiter, L. A., Whitwell, J., Marliss, E. B., and Jeejeebhoy, K. N.: Skeletal muscle function during hypocaloric diets and fasting: A comparison with standard nutritional assessment parameters. Am. J. Clin. Nutr., 37:133, 1983.

87. Ryan, J. A., Jr., Abel, R. M., Abbott, W. M., Hopkins, C. C., Chesney, T., Colley, R., Phillips, K., and Fischer, J. E.: Catheter complications in total parenteral nutrition: A prospective study of 200 consecutive patients. N. Engl. J. Med., 290:757, 1974.

88. Ryan, J. A., Jr., and Taft, D.: A preoperative nutritional assessment does not predict morbidity and mortality in abdominal operations. Surg. Forum, 31:96, 1980.

89. Sax, H. C., Talamini, M. A., Brackett, K., and Fischer, J. E.: Hepatic steatosis in total parenteral nutrition: Failure of fatty infiltration to correlate with abnormal serum hepatic enzyme levels. Surgery, 100:697, 1986.

90. Shiloni, E., Coronado, E., and Freund, H. R.: The role of total parenteral nutrition in the treatment of Crohn's disease. Am. J. Surg., 157:180, 1989.

91. Shinnick, F. L., and Harper, A. E.: Branched chain amino acid oxidation by isolated rat tissue preparation. Biochim. Biophys. Acta, 437:477, 1976.

92. Shizgal, H. M.: Body composition. In Fischer, J. E. (Ed.): Surgical Nutrition. Boston, Little, Brown & Company, 1983, pp. 3–19.

93. Soeters, P. B., Ebeid, A. M., and Fischer, J. E.: Review of 404 patients with gastrointestinal fistulas: Impact of parenteral nutrition. Ann. Surg., 190:189, 1979.

94. Stehle, P., Zander, J., Mertes, N., Albers, S., Puchstein, C., Lawin, P., and Fürst, P.: Effect of parenteral glutamine peptide supplements on muscle glutamine loss and nitrogen balance after major surgery. Lancet 1:231, 1989.

95. Studley, H. O.: Percentage of weight loss: A basic indicator of surgical risk in patients with chronic peptic ulcer. J.A.M.A., 106:458, 1936.

96. Trocki, O., Heyd, T. J., Waymack, J. P., and Alexander, J. W.: Effects of fish oil on postburn metabolism and immunity. J. Parent. Enteral Nutr., 11:521, 1987.

97. Twomey, P., Ziegler, D., and Rombeau, J.: Utility of skin testing in nutritional assessment: A critical review. J. Parent. Enteral Nutr., 6:50, 1982.

98. Van Eys, J., Copeland, E. M., Cangir, A., Taylor, G., Teitell-Cohen, B., Carter, P., and Ortiz, C.: A randomized controlled clinical trial of hyperalimentation in children with metabolic malignancies. Med. Pediatr. Oncol., 8:63, 1980.

99. Wahren, J., Felig, P., and Hagenfeldt, L.: Effect of protein ingestion on splanchnic and leg metabolism in normal men and in patients with diabetes mellitus. J. Clin. Invest., 57:987, 1976.

100. Walser, M., Coulter, A. W., Dighe, S., and Crantz, F. R.: The effect of ketoanalogues of essential amino acids in severe chronic uremia. J. Clin. Invest., 52:678, 1973.

101. Wang, X., Jacobs, D. O., O'Dwyer, S. T., Smith, R. J., and Wilmore, D. W.: Glutamine-enriched parenteral nutrition prevents mucosal atrophy following massive small bowel resection. Surg. Forum, 39:44, 1988.

102. Warner, B. W., Hasselgren, P. O., James, J. H., Hummel, R. P., III, Rigel, D. F., and Fischer, J. E.: Reduced amino acid transport in skeletal muscle caused by a circulating factor during endotoxemia. Ann. Surg., 211:323, 1990.

103. Watters, J. M., Bessey, P. Q., Dinarello, C. A., Wolff, S. M., and Wilmore, D. W.: The induction of interleukin-1 in humans and its metabolic effects. Surgery, 98:298, 1985.

104. Weir, J. B. de V.: New methods for calculating metabolic rate with special reference to protein metabolism. J. Physiol., 109:1, 1949.

105. Windmueller, H. G.: Glutamine utilization by the small intestine. Adv. Enzymol., 53:201, 1982.

106. Windmueller, H. G., and Spaeth, A. E.: Uptake and metabolism of plasma glutamine by the small intestine. J. Biol. Chem., 249:5070, 1974.

107. Windsor, J. A., and Hill, G. L.: Weight loss with physiologic impairment: A basic indicator of surgical risk. Ann. Surg., 207:290, 1988.

108. Woodall, B. H., Winfield, D. F., and Bisset, G. S., III: Inadvertent tracheobronchial placement of feeding tubes. Radiology, 165:727, 1987.

109. Young, V. R., and Munro, H. N.: N$^+$-methylhistidine (3-methylhistidine) and muscle protein turnover: An overview. Fed. Proc., 37:2291, 1978.

8

SURGICAL ASPECTS OF DIABETES MELLITUS

Olga Jonasson, M.D.

Diabetes mellitus is a disorder of carbohydrate metabolism that causes hyperglycemia. It is the result of a deficiency of insulin or resistance to the action of insulin. The consequences of diabetes are due to elevated levels of blood glucose, frequently complicated by other factors. The major aim of long-term therapy for the diabetic patient is consistent control of blood glucose levels within the normal range through diet, oral hypoglycemic agents, and, when necessary, exogenous insulin administration. Strict control of the blood glucose level is a basic requirement for successful management of the ill or injured diabetic patient requiring surgical treatment; exogenous insulin is required in the majority of patients.

PATHOPHYSIOLOGY

Insulin is normally produced in the beta cells of islets of Langerhans by a process involving cleavage of a proinsulin molecule into equimolar amounts of insulin and a connecting peptide (C peptide). Whenever it is necessary to measure insulin production in patients receiving exogenous insulin, it is advisable to measure the C peptide molecule, since both endogenous and exogenous insulin are measured in an insulin assay. Glucose is the main stimulus for insulin release, although neuroendocrine actions and other factors also regulate insulin secretion. Insulin acts on peripheral tissues through binding to specific insulin receptors on target tissue cells, followed by internalization and intracellular processes causing peripheral glucose utilization. Glucagon, produced by the pancreatic alpha islet cells, is a counterregulatory hormone, acting to promote glycogenolysis and hepatic gluconeogenesis. Diabetes can be the result of failure of insulin production, deficiencies in binding of insulin to its receptor, or intracellular defects in insulin action. The net effect is hyperglycemia.

Diabetes mellitus is diagnosed by measurement of the blood glucose. Fasting levels of greater than 140 mg. per dl. on at least two occasions indicate the presence of diabetes. Some individuals have fasting blood glucose levels of less than 140 mg. per dl. but have abnormal glucose tolerance tests; these patients do not maintain consistent blood glucose control and should be treated as diabetics, especially during an acute illness or a perioperative period. Many factors, such as starvation, infection, pregnancy, medical illnesses, inactivity, medications such as steroids, thiazide diuretics, and oral contraceptives, and age, influence the glucose tolerance test and make the results difficult to interpret. Nonetheless, hyperglycemic patients must be appropriately treated to normalize their blood glucose levels during any acute illness, stress, or operation.

CLASSIFICATION

Diabetes mellitus is classified into several categories (Table 1). Type I diabetes mellitus or insulin-dependent diabetes mellitus (IDDM) usually develops in childhood or adolescence and was formerly known as juvenile onset diabetes. It represents about 20 per cent of all types of diabetes. These patients are entirely dependent on daily insulin administration and are prone to develop severe hyperglycemia, ketosis, and dehydration. Generally, they are not obese. Hypoglycemia is a frequent complication of insulin administration, especially in patients who do not eat properly. Hypoglycemic episodes are life-threatening due to permanent central nervous system damage, and they must be suspected in all obtunded or neurologically impaired diabetic patients receiving insulin.

Patients with Type II diabetes mellitus, or non–insulin-dependent diabetes (NIDDM), have retained some degree of endogenous insulin production and, therefore, are not dependent on exogenous insulin administration. Insulin levels may be normal or supernormal. In some patients much of the capacity for endogenous insulin production is lost as the disease progresses, and many Type II diabetics eventually require insulin. Most patients with Type II diabetes who are septic or who are undergoing stress or surgical treatment also require insulin during their illness and perioperative period.

The onset of Type II diabetes is in adulthood. Many patients are essentially asymptomatic, and most are overweight. Ketosis and ketoacidosis are rare. Patients fail to respond to an oral glucose load with appropriate insulin secretion, and also demonstrate resistance of peripheral tissue cells to the action of insulin, apparently in the intracellular events to be triggered by insulin receptor binding or in defects of the binding action itself of insulin to its receptor.

A third category of diabetes is secondary diabetes. Pancreatic diabetes is found in patients with pancreatic disease, such as chronic pancreatitis or hemachromatosis, or following total pancreatectomy. These patients have lost all islet cell function and are "brittle," in that counterregulatory hormones such as glucagon are also absent. Patients with pancreatic diabetes are entirely dependent on insulin but, because of the absence of glucagon and the presence of pancreatic exocrine insufficiency and poor food absorption, are especially prone to the development of hypoglycemia. Diabetes also occurs as the result of hormonal excess, as in Cushing's disease or funtional adrenal cortical neoplasms, or following administration of corticosteroids or thiazide diuretics. Other causes of diabetes are less common.

COMPLICATIONS

Regardless of the cause, the net result of the diabetic state is hyperglycemia. Diabetic patients are at risk for the development of complications related to hyperglycemia, and all are treated similarly during periods of stress and the perioperative period.

Acute

METABOLIC. Hyperglycemia causes a number of pathophysiologic conditions causing both acute and chronic disease

TABLE 1. Classification of Diabetes Mellitus

Type I   Insulin-dependent diabetes mellitus
(also termed IDDM, previously termed juvenile-onset diabetes)

    20% of all diabetes mellitus
Onset in childhood or adolescence; patients not obese
Entirely dependent on exogenous insulin
Prone to develop ketosis and acidosis

Type II   Non–insulin-dependent diabetes
(also termed NIDDM, previously termed adult-onset diabetes)

    Onset after age 30 years; patients usually obese
Not dependent on insulin; insulin levels may be normal or high. Insulin resistance common
Not prone to ketosis or acidosis

Secondary diabetes

    Pancreatic diabetes
      Occurs with pancreatic insufficiency, such as chronic pancreatitis, hemochromatosis, pancreatectomy
      Entirely insulin-dependent
      "Brittle"—no glucagon, exocrine insufficiency, poor food absorption

    Hormonal excess diabetes
    Drug-induced diabetes
      Increased insulin resistance due to excess corticosteroids or drugs such as thiazide diuretics

(Table 2). Many of these conditions require surgical intervention, and many seriously complicate the medical condition of the patient who undergoes operative therapy. The immediate effect of hyperglycemia is glucosuria and osmotic diuresis. Patients note polyuria and polydipsia and may become dehydrated to the point of shock because of depletion of extracellular volume. Absence of insulin promotes release of free fatty acids, which are metabolized in the liver to ketone bodies and appear in the plasma and urine. Severe electrolyte losses occur in the urine to buffer the ketone body acids. If uncorrected, the condition of diabetic ketoacidosis occurs: extreme hyperglycemia, ketosis, and acidosis. Patients become obtunded and display deep and prolonged Kussmaul respirations. Leukocytosis and abdominal pain due to delayed gastric emptying are often present. The basic cause, such as sepsis or stress, is usually found, and this must be corrected to treat the patient successfully. During the course of their lives, the majority of patients with Type I diabetes experience diabetic ketoacidosis.

INFECTIONS. Hyperglycemia appears to be directly related to the well-known heightened susceptibility of diabetics to infections. Although the precise reasons for this effect are not known, there is evidence that polymorphonuclear leukocyte

TABLE 2. Complications of Diabetes Mellitus

Acute	Chronic
Susceptility to infections	Retinopathy
Metabolic derangements	Nephropathy
Hyperglycemia	Proteinuria
Acidosis	Renal failure
Hyperlipidemia	Neuropathy
	Peripheral
	Autonomic
	Macrovascular disease
	Peripheral arterial insufficiency
	Coronary artery disease
	Mesenteric vascular insufficiency
	Cerebral artery insufficiency

function is abnormal when the blood glucose level is elevated. Chemotaxis of leukocytes to the site of inflammation is less than in nondiabetics, phagocytic activity is depressed, and intracellular bactericidal activity is reduced. There is no measurable effect of diabetes on the immune system.

The most common site of infection in diabetic patients is the urinary tract. Pyelonephritis, papillary necrosis, emphysematous pyelonephritis, and perinephric abcesses are more common in diabetic than in nondiabetic patients. Pulmonary infections with common organisms such as *Streptococcus pneumoniae, Escherichia coli,* and *Staphylococcus aureus* also occur frequently and are associated with high mortality in diabetics. Unusual infections may occur predominantly in diabetics. These include rhinocerebral mucormycosis, which is an invasive fungal infection of the nose and sinuses, and malignant external otitis, which is an invasive bacterial infection of the auditory canal, usually due to *Pseudomonas aeruginosa.* Necrotizing cellulitis and fasciitis can occur, especially in the perineal region of elderly male diabetics who have recently had urethral catheterization. Known as Fournier's gangrene, this polymicrobial infection with aerobic and anaerobic organisms must be treated with aggressive surgical debridement, colostomy, and systemic antibiotics.[9]

A troublesome complication of hyperglycemia is gingivitis and pyorrhea, with periodontal infections, abscesses, and loss of teeth. Dental sepsis often may cause systemic symptoms and precipitate hyperglycemia and even diabetic ketoacidosis. Great care must be taken with oral hygiene, including professional control of plaque and hypertrophic gingivitis.

POLYOL PATHWAY. Hyperglycemia may be responsible for the development of lesions of the lens of the eye, peripheral nerves, and possibly the vascular endothelium. According to this hypothesis, when blood glucose is elevated, it enters the cells of the lens, the Schwann cells, or the endothelium, where, in the presence of aldose reductase, it is converted to sorbitol and then to fructose, creating intracellular hyperosmolarity. Water influx into these cells, with cell swelling and injury, causes cataract formation in the lens and may be responsible for the peripheral neuropathy so prevalent in diabetics. The initiating lesion for the development of accelerated atherosclerosis of diabetes has also been attributed to the sorbitol (or polyol) pathway and endothelial cell injury.

Chronic

The major effects of chronic hyperglycemia are the long-term complications of diabetes, including blindness, neuropathy, renal failure, and accelerated advanced atherosclerosis.[1,6] These long-term complications shorten life expectancy for diabetics and severely compromise their quality of life. Surgical intervention is needed in many diabetics, and the presence of diabetes adds considerably to the patient's operative risk. The economic costs of Type II diabetes in the United States have been estimated recently at nearly $20 billion annually, including health care expenditures and premature disability and mortality.[5] Type I diabetes is associated with an even higher frequency of blindness and renal failure; although only 20 per cent as frequent as Type II, it could be assumed to have economic costs nearly as high.

VISION IMPAIRMENT AND BLINDNESS. After 15 years, essentially all patients with Type I diabetes have some visual impairment because of diabetic retinopathy, cataracts, or both.[7] Blindness occurs in nearly one half of these patients; diabetes is the leading cause of new blindness in adults. The precise etiology of the retinopathy has not been determined, but loss of the supportive structure of pericytes about the retinal arterioles, capillary dropout and ischemia, and macular edema are frequently identified. Proliferative retinopathy is a more advanced stage and often causes vitreous hemorrhage and retinal detachment. The development of retinopathy has been strongly linked to the presence of systemic hypertension. Anticoagulation of the diabetic patient with proliferative retinopathy is considered to be hazardous, especially in the presence of hypertension.

NEUROPATHY AND THE DIABETIC FOOT. Peripheral neuropathy is a devastating complication of chronic hyperglycemia and causes considerable disability. Neuropathy develops in both Type I and Type II patients with long-standing diabetes and can affect autonomic as well as peripheral nerves. The most common manifestation is peripheral neuropathy of the feet and distal lower extremity, with loss of sensation in the foot. Normal adjustments of the foot in weight bearing then do not occur, and heavy calluses form over pressure points, which add to the pressure and cause necrosis under the callus. Ulcers of the weight-bearing surface then appear. Even minor trauma may develop into a serious necrotizing infection with tissue loss. Patients with diabetes must be enthusiastically and continuously encouraged to take care of their feet to avoid trauma or irritation from any source (Table 3). Because the foot is anesthetic, they must avoid hot soaks or baths. Their toenails, corns, and calluses should be expertly trimmed. Many clinics caring for diabetic patients employ a podiatrist to collaborate in management of these problems. Shoes must be roomy and well padded. Diabetic patients should never walk barefoot. They must thoroughly inspect their feet daily; if their vision is poor, someone else must do the inspection. The feet and web spaces between the toes must be kept dry and clean.

Diabetic foot ulcers and infection are usually initiated by minor trauma but can become extensive, deep, and spreading. These infections require surgical drainage and débridement, which frequently involves amputation at the level of the toes, the transmetatarsal level, or even the foot or leg. The most common organisms involved in diabetic foot ulcers and infections are gram-positive cocci, but as the ulcer becomes more extensive and necrotic, gram-negative organisms and anaerobes become more numerous. In patients with major foot infections and signs of spreading sepsis, antibiotics active over a wide spectrum of organisms, including anaerobes, are indicated. Patients with a large amount of necrotic tissue must also be given tetanus prophylaxis. It is common to find gas in the tissues of the foot and even the lower leg in patients with an extensive infection, usually due to anaerobic organisms. These infections are especially virulent and must be treated with aggressive surgical debridement and drainage. Clostridial species may be present and must be sought with Gram's stains and cultures; if identified, appropriate treatment must include wide débridement or amputation and penicillin.

Necrobiosis lipoidica diabeticorum is an unusual lesion occurring in the lower leg in association with severe peripheral neuropathy and local areas of anesthesia. This ulcerating lesion is resistant to local treatment and may require radical excision and skin grafting.

GASTROINTESTINAL AND CARDIAC NEUROPATHY. Autonomic neuropathy is very troublesome and may occur in nearly one third of diabetic patients. Gastroparesis occurs in patients with peripheral neuropathy and other complications of chronic diabetes, such as visual impairment and diabetic renal disease. Ineffectual peristalsis and depressed antral motor function cause gastric retention and dilatation. Hypoglycemic episodes and poor diabetic control are common. Bethanechol and metoclopramide have been used with some effect to increase gastric motility, but surgical procedures such as gastric resection or pyloroplasty have been ineffective. Similar hypotonicity and failure to empty occur in the urinary bladder. A neurogenic bladder is often present in diabetic patients undergoing kidney transplantation.

Intractable diarrhea and steatorrhea are advanced manifestations of gastrointestinal autonomic neuropathy. Diarrhea is often nocturnal, profuse, and watery and is related not only to disordered neurologic control of intestinal motility but also to bacterial overgrowth occurring in poorly draining segments, including the stomach. Oral antibiotics and cholestyramine to bind bile acids may be of some benefit, but there is no effective surgical treatment.

Dysmotility may also occur in the esophagus and is usually found in patients who have advanced peripheral neuropathy and other complications of diabetes. Moreover, *Candida* infection of the esophagus is commonly found in poorly controlled diabetic patients who have oral candidiasis (thrush). Esophageal candidiasis may be invasive and cause deep mucosal ulcerations in the distal esophagus, which may bleed extensively. In diabetic patients with dysphagia, fiberoptic esophagoscopy is indicated to determine whether candidiasis is present. Mucosal brushings and biopsies establish the diagnosis. Treatment with oral ketoconazole is indicated; and if the infection is invasive, low-dose amphotericin B should be given. Patients with oral candidiasis should be given nystatin as a mouthwash to "swish and swallow" as prophylaxis against esophageal infection. Nystatin mouthwashes and swallows are often used routinely in diabetic surgical patients throughout the period of perioperative stress.

Cardiac autonomic neuropathy may also occur and is usually associated with other manifestations of peripheral and autonomic neuropathy. Cardiac symptoms are principally those of postural hypotension or hemodynamic instability during hemodialysis and mild tachycardia.

DIABETIC NEPHROPATHY. Most insulin-dependent diabetics and Type II diabetics with constant hyperglycemia display glomerular hyperfiltration and microproteinuria. Their kidneys and the glomeruli are visibly enlarged, and measurements of renal plasma flow and glomerular filtration rates are elevated. Albumin, a small molecule, is present in the urine in amounts detectable only with sensitive assays and in insufficient amounts (less than 0.5 gm. per 24 hours) to give a positive "dipstick" test. The amount of albumin excreted in the urine is related to the degree of hyperfiltration and increases with exercise and with hypertension. Especially in hyperglycemic patients who consume large amounts of dietary protein, mesangial matrix expansion within the glomeruli occurs and gradually the filtration surfaces of the capillary loops become compromised. Diabetic nephrosclerosis then ensues. At this point, usually more than 15 years after the onset of diabetes, overt proteinuria appears (greater than 0.5 gm. per 24 hours, positive dipstick test), and the composition of the proteinuria changes to include many larger plasma proteins (global proteinuria). Renal function then fails at a rapid and accelerating rate as additional nephrons are lost and the remaining glomeruli are exposed to even more severe hyperfiltration. When overt proteinuria appears, median survival is reduced to 7 to 8 years.[2] Because of the pre-existing hyperfiltration in poorly controlled diabetic patients and their chronic osmotic diuresis, they are highly susceptible to the nephrotoxic effects of iodinated radiologic contrast agents, especially (but not exclusively) when these are given intravenously. Diabetic patients who are scheduled for angiography, computed tomographic scanning, or even oral cholecystography must be prepared by correction of pre-existing dehydration and normalization of blood glucose levels.

TABLE 3. Rules for Care of Diabetic Patients' Feet

1. Always wear roomy and comfortable shoes, well padded.
2. Keep feet warm, dry, and clean.
3. Inspect feet daily, cotton between toes. (If vision is poor, have someone else do this.)
4. Avoid hot soaks or baths.
5. Trim toenails and calluses expertly.
6. Never walk barefoot.
7. Get prompt medical attention for any injury or blister.

Chronic renal failure as the result of diabetic nephrosclerosis occurs in up to 40 per cent of patients with Type I diabetes. Although less common in patients with Type II diabetes, renal failure also develops in patients with long-standing poorly controlled disease. Currently, at least 25 per cent of new patients enrolled in hemodialysis and renal transplant programs are diabetic. Predisposing causes for progression into renal failure appear to be poor control of blood glucose levels (with resultant hyperfiltration) and systemic hypertension. Patients who are genetically predisposed to the development of hypertension may be especially at risk.[8] There is evidence that the progression of diabetic renal disease can be slowed by strict reduction in dietary protein and control of hypertension with an angiotensin-converting enzyme inhibitor.

ATHEROSCLEROSIS

The greatest risk to survival and to quality of life of diabetic patients is the development of macrovascular atherosclerotic disease.[8] Atherosclerosis and coronary artery disease have a considerably higher prevalence in diabetic than in nondiabetic patients of a similar age. Vascular insufficiency of the lower extremities, together with the propensity of diabetic patients for foot infections and ulcers (discussed earlier) is responsible for the observation that nearly two thirds of patients requiring amputation of the lower extremity are diabetic. Large-vessel atherosclerotic lesions occur at an earlier age than in a normal population, and tibial artery occlusion is often the first lesion to appear. In addition to large-vessel occlusion, small arteries are diseased, perhaps because of abnormalities in formation of capillary basement membranes during conditions of hyperglycemia. Abnormalities in plasma lipoproteins and endothelial cell transport have been suggested as contributing factors, as has increased platelet aggregation and hyperviscosity of the blood.

The principal threat to life of the diabetic patient is coronary artery disease. The incidence is high, and mortality from an acute myocardial infarction is twice that in nondiabetics; the combination of increased frequency of occurrence and increased mortality from a myocardial infarction makes coronary artery disease the major cause of premature death in diabetic patients. Patients with Type II diabetes are as likely to die of coronary artery disease as Type I patients. Women are also at high risk; compared with a nondiabetic group of a similar age range, diabetic women who were aged 40 to 54 years at the time of diagnosis had a 39 per cent mortality from heart disease by age 70 years, whereas nondiabetic women had 10 percent mortality in the same period. An angiographic study of diabetic patients awaiting kidney transplantation revealed a 40 per cent incidence of significant coronary artery occlusive disease or left ventricular dysfunction.[3]

The strong likelihood of significant coronary artery occlusive disease must be considered when undertaking surgical treatment of any diabetic patient (Table 4). A thorough history must be obtained for one to detect angina or previous myocardial infarction, treatment with antihypertensive drugs, beta blockade, coronary vasodilators, calcium channel blocking agents, and diuretics, because all these factors influence perioperative management. Electrocardiography, echocardiography, stress myocardial function tests, and coronary angiography are indicated should any evidence of heart disease be determined, or when the diabetic patient is over 30 years of age. Perioperative management in a facility in which heart rate, rhythm, and blood pressure can be continuously monitored is required. Invasive monitoring of hemodynamic status with a pulmonary artery catheter may be indicated in a patient with existing heart damage who has undergone a major surgical procedure.

TABLE 4. Preoperative Workup of the Diabetic Patient

History
  Duration of diabetes; insulin, diet, or oral hypoglycemic therapy; episodes of diabetic ketoacidosis or hypoglycemia
  Complications: visual impairment, neuropathy, symptoms of renal or peripheral vascular disease
  History of heart disease: angina, congestive failure, myocardial infarction
  Drug history: antihypertensive drugs, calcium channel blockers, beta blockade, coronary vasodilators, diuretics
  Symptoms of infection at any site: urinary tract, lungs, skin and subcutaneous tissues, gums, feet, intra-abdominal
Physical Examination
  Ophthalmoscopy: the eye is the window to the kidney
  Blood pressure: often elevated
  Circulation: evidence of congestive failure or peripheral vascular insufficiency
  Neurologic examination: evidence of peripheral neuropathy, mental status evaluation
  Status of feet: ulcers, infection, sensation
Laboratory Evaluation
  Blood glucose, serum Na, K, and $NaHCO_3$ levels
  Renal function: proteinuria, BUN, and creatinine levels
  Cardiac evaluation: electrocardiogram, radioisotope myocardial stress studies, possible coronary angiogram

MANAGEMENT OF THE DIABETIC PATIENT

The basic goal of management of diabetes is the consistent maintenance of a normal blood glucose level. The cornerstone of long-term therapy is diet. Type II (NIDDM) patients are obese and hyperlipidemic; the objective of dietary management in these patients is weight reduction to ideal body weight. At least half the daily caloric requirement of 20 to 30 kcal. per kg. ideal body weight per day should be provided as carbohydrates. Saturated fats should be minimal because hyperlipidemia probably contributes to the excessively high incidence of vascular disease in these patients. Most Type II diabetic patients respond well to dietary management alone if they are cooperative. If hyperglycemia persists (fasting blood glucose levels greater than 160 mg. per dl.), Type II patients benefit from sulfonylurea drugs (oral hypoglycemic agents). In time, some Type II patients become insulin-dependent, although still retaining some insulin-secreting capacity.

Type I (IDDM) and other insulin-dependent patients require daily insulin. Their meals must be carefully balanced throughout the day so that insulin administration can mimic a normal physiologic beta cell response. Insulin is available in human recombinant, beef, pork, or semisynthetic preparations. Only the rapid-acting regular insulin can be administered intravenously; intermediate and long-acting insulins are given subcutaneously or intramuscularly. Various preparations have different times of peak activity and duration, so an individualized regimen can be chosen for each patient, related to diet and activity habits (Table 5).

The efficacy of the long-term treatment program with diet, oral hypoglycemics, and insulin can be assessed by periodic measurement of the level of glycosylated hemoglobin (HgA_{1c}) in erythrocytes. Hemoglobin becomes irreversibly glycosylated during periods of hypoglycemia. This measurement better reflects total exposure to hyperglycemia than do random blood glucose values.

HYPOGLYCEMIA. Severe hypoglycemia associated with coma or requiring assistance to reverse is now the most common metabolic emergency encountered in insulin-dependent diabetics. This has been the consequence of emphasis on maintaining constant euglycemia by use of multiple insulin injection regimens or insulin infusion pumps (constant subcutaneous in-

TABLE 5. Insulin Preparations* and Regimens

	Peak (Hr.)	Duration (Hr.)
Rapid-acting—regular†	0.5–4	5–7
Semilente	4–6	12–16
Intermediate—NPH, Lente	4–12	18–24
Long-acting—PZI, Ultralente	18–24	>36

Regimens
1. Intermediate + regular (⅔ + ⅓) in A.M., 0.5 unit/kg. ideal body weight. Check blood glucose at 4–5 P.M. to regulate next day's dose.
2. Intermediate ⅔ in A.M. and ⅓ in P.M. plus supplemental regular for late A.M. or bedtime hyperglycemia. REGULAR IS NEVER GIVEN AT BEDTIME.
3. Single small dose of intermediate in A.M. and 5–10 units subcutaneously before each meal.
4. CSII‡ with an open loop pump set at a basal infusion of 1 unit/hr. with 5- to 10-unit bolus 15 minutes before each meal.

*Available as pork or beef extracts, semisynthetic, or human recombinant.
†Only regular insulin can be administered intravenously.
‡Continuous subcutaneous insulin infusion.

sulin infusion, CSII). According to diabetologists who manage many such patients with close control, 10 per cent of insulin-dependent patients have one or more episodes of severe hypoglycemia each year, and hypoglycemia contributes to 3 to 6 per cent of premature deaths. Patients with gastroparesis or those with pancreatic exocrine insufficiency who absorb food poorly are especially at risk. Severe hypoglycemia should be treated by oral carbohydrates, but an unconscious patient requires an intravenous bolus of 20 ml. of 50 per cent glucose, repeated as necessary, and an intravenous infusion of 5 or 10 per cent dextrose until the blood sugar is above 100 mg. per dl. and the patient is conscious.

Perioperative Management

Approximately half of the 6 to 10 million diabetic patients in the United States undergo at least one operation during their lifetime. Most operations are for infections, and a substantial number are for emergency conditions. Many patients presenting for elective or emergency operations have previously undiagnosed Type II diabetes. The acute management of diabetic patients in the perioperative period has the same basic goal as for long-term care, that is, maintenance of a normal blood glucose level. Except for the Type II patient who is easily managed by diet alone, diabetic patients require insulin infusions to achieve and maintain euglycemia during illness and operative stress (Table 6). Any patient with preoperative hyperglycemia

TABLE 6. Perioperative Management of Diabetic Patients

Discontinue oral hypoglycemic agents 24 hours before operation.
  Give no intermediate or long-acting insulin on the day of operation.
Give nothing by mouth after midnight.
Start IV infusion of D_5W or D_5NS with 20 mEq. KCl/L. at 6 A.M. Administer at 100–200 ml./hr.
Start second IV infusion of insulin, 25 units/250 ml. NS. Run 75 ml. through the IV tubing (to occupy protein binding sites on tubing), then discard. Administer at 1–2 units/hr. via infusion pump.
Monitor blood glucose at 30-min. intervals until stable at 150–200 mg./dl., then monitor hourly until patient is awake, every 4 hours until diet is resumed.
Convert to maintenance regimen when diet has resumed by giving 80% of previous day's total insulin, ⅔ as intermediate and ⅓ as regular. Adjust daily, using blood glucose values (see Table 5).

should be treated before operation for normalization of the blood glucose level and must be constantly monitored during and after operation.

For elective procedures, patients who have had nothing by mouth for more than one meal should have oral hypoglycemic agents discontinued at least 24 hours prior to operation. Insulin-dependent patients should not receive their full dose of either intermediate or long-acting insulin on the day of operation. Glucose is given intravenously at a rate of 5 to 10 gm. per hour (D_5W at 100 to 200 ml. per hour; potassium chloride, 20 mEq. per liter, is added), and another infusion of insulin is begun (25 units per 250 ml. of normal saline: the first 75 ml. is flushed through the tubing and discarded) at a rate of 1 to 2 units per hour. The blood glucose level is measured by venous or capillary blood samples 1 hour after beginning this infusion and at intervals thereafter, and the rate of insulin is adjusted to maintain the blood glucose level between 150 and 200 mg. per dl.

Postoperatively, the patient is maintained with glucose, potassium, and insulin until a normal diet is resumed and then returned to an intermediate or long-acting subcutaneous insulin regimen. One does this by measuring 80 per cent of the previous day's total insulin and administering two thirds as long-acting and one third as regular, then measuring fasting and late afternoon blood glucose values in order to adjust and regulate the regimen. It is incorrect to use urine glucose levels to determine insulin doses, because a number of factors relating to renal threshold for glucose, urinary flow rates, and concentration of the urine influence the results. Urinary glucose values provide only an approximation of the blood glucose.

HYPERGLYCEMIC CRISES

In diabetic patients who have infections or other acute illnesses and stress, and in some who have simply been noncompliant with medical management, severe hyperglycemia may develop (Table 7). Insulin-dependent diabetics who have not had sufficient insulin may present with diabetic ketoacidosis (DKA). In these patients, insulin deficiency leads to accelerated gluconeogenesis with hyperglycemia and the production of ketone bodies with acidosis. Vomiting, abdominal pain and cramps, and abdominal rigidity on physical examination are often present. The characteristic physical findings of DKA are severe dehydration, mental status changes, Kussmaul respirations, a "fruity" (acetone) odor to the breath, and hypotension. Laboratory findings include severe acidosis with a markedly

TABLE 7. Hyperglycemic Crises in the Surgical Patient

Symptoms	Signs	Laboratory Values
Diabetic Ketoacidosis		
Type I diabetic	Hypotension	Blood glucose >350 mg./dl.
Missed insulin doses	Hypothermia	Arterial pH <7.3
Vomiting	Kussmaul breathing	Elevated plasma ketones
Polyuria, polydipsia	Fruity odor	$NaHCO_3$ <15 mEq./L.
Weakness	Mental status changes	Leukocytosis
Blurred vision	Abdominal rigidity	Osmoles >300
Abdominal pain		
Nonketotic Hyperosmolar Syndrome		
Type II diabetic	Obtundation or coma	Blood glucose >600 mg./dl.
Complicating medical illness	Severe dehydration	Osmoles >330
Mental status changes	Oliguria	Arterial pH >7.3
	Urosepsis, pneumonia, CHF, or MI	Elevated BUN, creatinine levels

low bicarbonate value, hyperglycemia, hyperosmolarity of the serum, initial hyperkalemia followed by hypokalemia, elevated plasma ketones, and a leukocytosis. Certain tests, such as the serum creatinine and liver enzymes, may be falsely elevated because of chemical interference in the automated blood chemistry methods, although renal failure is common, based on prerenal causes and underlying diabetic nephropathy. It is important to establish the diagnosis of DKA and treat this condition before concluding that an emergency surgical procedure is required, although it must be borne in mind that the precipitating cause for the development of DKA might be an acute abdominal condition.

Non–insulin-dependent diabetics (Type II) may develop even more serious hyperglycemia associated with coma. Because these patients produce enough endogenous insulin to prevent lipolysis and ketogenesis but insufficient insulin to utilize glucose, the syndrome is that of nonketotic hyperosmolar hyperglycemia. It is associated with serious medical complications, such as bacterial or viral sepsis or myocardial infarction, and usually occurs in elderly patients. The syndrome is characterized by extreme hyperglycemia (blood glucose levels may exceed 1000 mg. per dl.). Osmolarity may exceed 350 mOsm. per liter. There is only mild acidosis, and ketonemia is absent. Dehydration is severe, and prerenal azotemia is common. Mental status changes, obtundation, or coma is present. Since these patients are elderly and there is usually a serious underlying condition, the mortality for the nonketotic hyperosmolar syndrome is at least 50 per cent.

The treatment of severe hyperglycemia must precede any operative intervention in patients with DKA or the nonketotic hyperosmolar syndrome and should be accomplished as expeditiously as possible, since an infectious process requiring surgical treatment is frequently the cause of this serious complication. The basic principles of treatment include intravenous administration of insulin, resuscitation with intravenous fluids and electrolytes, treatment of the underlying medical conditions, and avoidance of complications. It is most important to treat the acidosis and dehydration; correction of the blood glucose levels follows. Resuscitation should take place in a monitored setting, such as the intensive care unit. Invasive monitoring with a pulmonary artery catheter is advisable; many of the patients with DKA have coronary artery disease, and all the patients with nonketotic hyperosmolar syndrome can be assumed to have established organic heart disease. Patients with mental status changes probably require endotracheal intubation, and a nasogastric tube must be placed, because all severely hyperglycemic patients have gastric stasis.

Fluid resuscitation is begun with normal saline supplemented with potassium chloride (lactated solutions are avoided) (Table 8). As much as 10 to 12 liters of electrolyte solution may eventually be required. Replacement is based on hemodynamic parameters, not on urinary flow rate, because renal dysfunction and osmotic diuresis are usually present. When the serum sodium approaches 150 mEq.per liter, the solution is changed to 0.45 per cent NaCl. A separate intravenous infusion of regular insulin in normal saline is begun, with an intravenous loading dose of 0.1 to 0.2 unit per kg. (10 to 15 units). The insulin is then infused at a rate of 5 to 10 units per hour until the blood glucose level is about 300 mg. per dl.; the rate is then reduced to 1 to 2 units per hour, and the intravenous fluids are changed to 5 per cent dextrose in 0.45 per cent NaCl with KCl, 20 mEq. per liter. Blood glucose may respond sooner than the ketonemia, but intravenous fluid resuscitation must continue until plasma ketones become undetectable. A simple bedside method for monitoring ketonemia is to dilute serially the patient's serum from 1:1 to 1:32 and place a drop onto an Acetest tablet. This test should be negative; that is, there should be no purple color. Sodium bicarbonate, 44 to 88 mEq., is given for acidosis (pH <7.1). Potassium should always be given cautiously in patients

TABLE 8. Treatment of Hyperglycemic Crises in the Surgical Patient

1. Admit to intensive care unit.
   Insert nasogastric tube.
   Consider endotracheal intubation.
   Institute cardiac monitoring, including central venous pressure measurement or placement of a Swan-Ganz pulmonary artery catheter for hemodynamic monitoring.

2. Begin IV infusion of NS solution through large-bore catheter. Base fluid requirements on hemodynamic and biochemical parameters. Plan on 5–10 L. of fluid for resuscitation.

3. Through a separate IV, begin insulin infusion, using solution of 1 unit insulin/10 ml. NS. Discard first 75 ml. after running through the tubing. Give loading dose of 1–2 units/kg. and then infuse at 0.1 unit/kg./hr. Rate can be doubled if necessary.

4. Monitor blood glucose hourly. Goal is to reduce hyperglycemia by 100 mg./dl./hr. More rapid reduction is likely to cause cerebral edema.
   When serum Na >150 mEq./L., change IV fluids to 0.45% saline with 20 mEq. KCl/L. Monitor serum K closely.

5. When blood glucose is ≤250 mg./dl., reduce insulin infusion to 1–2 units/hr. and change IV fluids to D_5W with 20 mEq. KCl, at 50–100 ml./hr.

Monitor serial 1:2 dilutions of patient's plasma for ketones and continue to resuscitate with glucose-potassium-insulin solutions until reaction is negative (Acetest tablets).

with renal failure. Magnesium may also be necessary, although replacement of phosphorus is not advised.

Throughout resuscitation, the capillary or venous blood glucose is monitored every 30 to 60 minutes until it is near normal and the insulin infusion rate adjusted accordingly. The goal is to reduce the blood glucose by approximately 100 mg. per dl. per hour. A more rapid decrease in the blood glucose is ill-advised, since cerebral edema may ensue. The response of ketoacidosis and hyperglycemia to insulin is usually prompt and reliable.

The nonketotic hyperosmolar syndrome is treated similarly, although the factor of acidosis is not a concern. These patients are usually much more severely hyperglycemic and dehydrated. They are treated with fluid and electrolyte resuscitation and an intravenous insulin infusion, as just described. Urosepsis, pneumonia, myocardial infarction, or other serious medical illness is usually present, and it is essential to correct the problem.

TRANSPLANTATION OF THE PANCREAS

Replacement of the pancreatic beta cells by transplantation of the vascularized pancreas or isolated islets of Langerhans in Type I (IDDM) patients would be highly desirable. The disadvantages of exogenous insulin administration, such as hypoglycemia, inconvenience, and the need for frequent blood glucose measurements, could be avoided if beta cells were present to respond normally to a glucose stimulus. In recent years, technical improvements in methods of anastomosis and drainage of exocrine secretions have achieved a reasonable rate of patient and graft survival. The Pancreas Transplant Registry now reports patient survival of 95 per cent or greater in several centers, with 1-year graft survival in some programs of 70 to 80 per cent.[11] With further improvements in immunosuppression and technique, it will become feasible to offer pancreatic transplantation to Type I diabetic patients at a sufficiently early stage in their diabetes to prevent the development of devastating microvascular and macrovascular lesions. Transplantation of isolated islets of Langerhans is less hazardous but awaits technical successes in purification and implantation techniques. The nature of the autoimmune islet lesions of Type I patients also awaits clarification.

SUMMARY

Diabetes mellitus is a serious disease affecting millions of individuals. Approximately one half of the diabetics in the United States undergo at least one operation in their lifetime, largely for infections; and nearly one quarter of adults coming to elective or emergency operations have undiagnosed diabetes (Type II, NIDDM). One half of the operative mortality of diabetic patients is attributed to myocardial infarction, heart failure, or stroke. Acute complications, such as infection and metabolic disorders of glucose and acid-base homeostasis, pose major problems in medical management and surgical therapy. Long-term complications of the microcirculation and large vessel atherosclerotic disease cause blindness, renal failure, and vascular insufficiency, particularly in the coronary artery circulation and the legs. Peripheral and autonomic neuropathy adversely affect the quality of life.

The goal of management of the diabetic patient at any stage is maintenance of blood glucose within the normal range. Exogenous insulin administration is required in all patients with insufficient endogenous production and in many patients with insulin resistance, especially in the perioperative period. Infections must be treated with systemic antibiotics and aggressive surgical debridement and drainage. Frequent monitoring of the blood glucose is required for proper management of the patient, and insulin administration is based on these values.

SELECTED REFERENCES

Kitabchi, A. E., and Murphy, M. B.: Diabetic ketoacidosis and hyperosmolar hyperglycemic nonketotic coma. Med. Clin. North. Am., 72:1543, 1988.
  This is a review of the pathophysiology and management of hyperglycemic crises. The paper is well illustrated and clear. Safe and expeditious algorithms for treatment are outlined.

Levin, M. E., and O'Neal, L. W.: The Diabetic Foot, 4th ed. St. Louis, C. V. Mosby Company, 1988.
  A complete and most useful text considering all aspects of diabetic foot problems, including vascular assessment and treatment and general management with orthotics, podiatry, and operation. Well illustrated and well written.

Olefsky, J. M.: Diabetes Mellitus. *In* Wyngaarden, J. B., and Smith, L. H., Jr. (Eds.): Cecil Textbook of Medicine, 18th ed. Philadelphia, W. B. Saunders Company, 1988, pp. 1360-1381.
  An up-to-date review of diabetes from an expert in Type II disease and insulin resistance. The pathophysiology, genetics, biochemistry, and etiology of the disease and its complications are clearly presented and well illustrated.

Wheelock, F. C., Jr., Gibbons, G. W., and Marble, A.: Surgery in diabetes. *In* Marble, A., Krall, L. P., Bradley, R. F., Christlieb, A. R., and Soeldner, J. S. (Eds.): Joslin's Diabetes Mellitus, 12th ed. Philadelphia, Lea & Febiger, 1985, pp. 712-731.
  From the classic text of diabetes, this chapter is written by a most experienced group of surgeons and internists. The diabetic foot and its complications are well described. Other aspects of diabetic vascular disease are thoroughly discussed, and practical suggestions for surgical treatment are given.

REFERENCES

1. Bilous, R. W., Mauer, S. M., Sutherland, D. E. R., Najarian, J. S., Goetz, F. C., and Steffes, M. W.: The effects of pancreas transplantation on the glomerular structure of renal allografts in patients with insulin-dependent diabetes. N. Engl. J. Med. 321:80, 1989.
2. Borch-Johnsen, K., Andersen, P. K., and Deckert, T.: The effect of proteinuria on relative mortality in Type I (insulin-dependent) diabetes mellitus. Diabetologia 28:590, 1985.
3. Braun, W. E., Phillips, D., Vidt, D. G., Novick, A. C., Nakamoto, S., Popowniak, K., Magnusson, M., Pohl, M., Paganini, E., Steinmuller, D., Protiva, D., and Buszta, C.: The course of coronary artery disease in diabetics with and without renal allografts. Transplant Proc. 15:1114, 1983.
4. Hostetter, T. H., Rennke, H. G., and Brenner, B. M.: The case for intrarenal hypertension in the initiation and progression of diabetic and other glomerulopathies. Am. J. Med. 72:375, 1982.
5. Huse, D. M., Oster, G., Killen, A. R., Lacey, M. J., and Colditz, G. A.: The economic costs of non-insulin-dependent diabetes mellitus. JAMA 262:2708, 1989.
6. Klein, R., Klein, B. E. K., Moss, S. E., Davis, M. D., and DeMets, D. L.: Glycosylated hemoglobin predicts the incidence and progression of diabetic retinopathy. JAMA 260:2864, 1988.
7. Krolewski, A. S., Warram, J. H., Rand, L. I., and Kahn, C. R.: Epidemiologic approach to the etiology of type I diabetes mellitus and its complications. N. Engl. J. Med. 317:1390, 1987.
8. Krolewski, A. S., Canessa, M., Warram, J. H., Laffel, L. M. B., Christlieb, A. R., Knowler, W. C., and Rand, L. I.: Predisposition of hypertension and susceptibility to renal disease in insulin-dependent diabetes mellitus. N. Engl. J. Med. 318:140, 1988.
9. Simmons, R. L., and Ahrenholz, D. H.: Infections of the skin and soft tissues. *In* Howard, R. J., and Simmons, R. L. (Eds.): Surgical Infectious Diseases, 2nd ed. Norwalk, Conn., Appleton & Lange, 1988, pp. 400–408.
10. Stern, M. P., and Haffner, S. M.: Prospective assessment of metabolic control in diabetes mellitus: The complications question. JAMA 260:2896, 1988.
11. Sutherland, D. E. R., and Moudry, K. C.: Pancreas transplantation registry report. Transplant Proc. 21:2759, 1989.

9

ANESTHESIA

*E. M. Camporesi, M.D., William J. Greeley, M.D.,
Philip D. Lumb, M.B., B.S., and W. David Watkins, M.D., Ph.D.*

HISTORICAL ASPECTS

General anesthesia was first recognized during a public surgical demonstration on October 16, 1846, by William Morton, a medical student and a practicing dentist who administered vapors of sulfuric ether to a young man, Gilbert Abbott, for the removal of a tumor of the jaw. The surgeon, John C. Warren, and his colleagues at Massachusetts General Hospital successfully validated the use of diethyl ether in several subsequent days. The first printed scientific report of alleviation of pain in the surgical theater was published on November 18 of that year. News spread rapidly, and the use of general anesthesia developed in Europe: ether was administered in Paris on December 15 and in London on December 19. The famous English surgeon Robert Liston ensured the acceptance of general anesthesia following his first successful operation using ether anesthesia on December 21, 1846.

These events initiated an intense and uncoordinated period of discovery, which offers valuable lessons in the principles of medical research and development. Crawford Long used ether for surgical practice in 1842, in Athens, Georgia, but failed to report it; and Morton, Wells, and Jackson, all variously involved in its first public demonstration, became consumed by a battle of priority and patents. In England, John Snow became the first physician to devote his clinical practice to the administration of anesthetics and most clearly first described the clinical signs of anesthetic depth. Simpson introduced the use of chloroform's analgesia during Queen Victoria's fifth labor and delivery, thereby leading to wide acceptance of general anesthesia in both surgery and obstetrics.

During the first half of this century, anesthetic advances were marked by a quest for the "ideal" anesthetic agent. Such a compound was considered to exhibit pharmacologic potency, inertness, and therapeutic safety. No product met these criteria. In parallel, it was appreciated that other adjunctive therapeutic drugs would be valuable in general anesthesia. The effectiveness of narcotics for premedication and the clinical usefulness of intravenous barbiturates and tranquilizers were recognized.

Rather than a single ideal anesthetic agent, practitioners from every country confirmed the efficacy of the use of multiple agents for achieving selected effects, each suited to unique surgical requirements. Attention was focused on recovery from anesthesia and on intra- and perioperative maintenance of physiologic functions. At the same time that a wider array of drugs was incorporated into the armamentarium for use in general anesthesia, advances in regional anesthetic techniques were realized after the introduction of safer and more potent local anesthetic drugs.

PHARMACOLOGIC PRINCIPLES

The current practice of anesthesiology incorporates recent developments in quantitative pharmacology. Some important definitions follow.

PHARMACOKINETICS. Pharmacokinetics is that scientific knowledge involved with the mathematic description of drug movement from the site of administration into the blood, distribution into the tissues, and elimination by metabolism or excretion. *Pharmacodynamics* relates drug concentration in the various body compartments to the pharmacologic effects.

Rapid advances in analytical chemistry have broadened the scope of both of these disciplines, permitting sophisticated compartmental analysis with computer simulation. Among the newer concepts introduced in clinical sciences are the principles of drug distribution and biotransformation with which clinicians are attempting to rationalize drug dosage and administration profiles.

VOLUME OF DISTRIBUTION. The apparent volume of distribution is a pharmacokinetic parameter relating the plasma concentration of a drug to the total amount of the drug in the body. It measures the extent of drug distribution. An apparent volume of distribution exceeding anatomic size occurs when drug tissue concentrations are greater than plasma concentrations; this suggests extensive tissue affinity. Several pathophysiologic states can significantly alter the volume of distribution of a drug. For example, a decrease in the volume of distribution of lidocaine has been demonstrated to exist in patients with congestive heart failure, possibly because of alterations in tissue perfusion that follow the low cardiac output state. Also, alterations in body composition at the extremes of age can alter the volume of distribution.

Removal of a drug from the body can be characterized by a pharmacokinetic parameter termed *drug clearance*, that is, the volume of blood or plasma from which a drug is completely removed per unit of time. Morphine and meperidine have a high hepatic extraction ratio, indicating that a substantial fraction of an oral dose undergoes hepatic biotransformation during the first passage through the liver, thus failing to reach the systemic circulation. Conversely, general anesthesia, with the attendant depression of cardiac output and redistribution of regional blood flow, may alter hepatic clearance. Splanchnic vascular resistance tends to increase in anesthetized human beings, possibly related to artificial ventilation, which causes a reduction in hepatic blood flow. The potent inhalation anesthetics, such as halothane and enflurane, cause a decrease in hepatic blood flow secondary to depression of cardiac output; and spinal anesthesia may reduce hepatic blood flow from hypotension. The effects of anesthesia and surgical therapy on the disposition of certain drugs in humans are definitely important clinically but have not been fully studied.

DRUG-PROTEIN INTERACTION. Drugs bind to serum and tissue proteins in a manner that has important implications for drug distribution and elimination. For example, although only 5 per cent of plasma diazepam is bound to proteins, more than 40 per cent of lidocaine and 80 per cent of digoxin are protein-bound.

The role of plasma protein binding in drug distribution and elimination has been defined, but the exact role of drug binding to tissue remains uncertain. Nevertheless, it is well known that clinically significant drug interactions involving protein binding tend to occur with drugs that are highly bound, that have a small apparent volume of distribution, and that display a relatively narrow therapeutic index. Moreover, some diseases can alter drug binding to plasma proteins by numerous mechanisms. For example, hypoalbuminemia can follow reduced synthesis or excessive loss or catabolism in various diseases. This is clinically important after bolus injection of powerful agents, which unexpectedly have a greater pharmacologic effect and may demonstrate toxic effects.

MONITORING

The essential goal of physiologic monitoring is careful observation of vital functions by periodic or continuous assessment. Historically, the measurement of depth of surgical anesthesia was the primary intent. More recently, the control of vital systems such as respiration and circulation has diverted the emphasis to new methods of quantitating anesthetic action and the patient's condition. The anesthesiologist's responsibility and training include monitoring drug effects during pre-, intra-, and postoperative care of patients. This evaluation of patient status is achieved qualitatively (e.g., monitoring by means of the senses of touch, hearing, and sight) and quantitatively (by means of specialized equipment). Repetitive assessment defines important physiologic trends necessary for possible therapeutic intervention.

Physiologic monitoring during anesthesia can be divided into the essential and the specialized. Various monitoring techniques have become standard medical practice and are selected in a manner appropriate to each patient, based on the severity of disease and the nature of the surgical procedure. Conventional monitoring includes continuous assessment by the anesthesiologist with regard to inspection, palpation, and auscultation. Additionally, essential monitoring includes a continuous electrocardiogram (ECG), a blood pressure measurement device, a temperature probe, a precordial or esophageal stethoscope, and an oxygen analyzer in the inspiratory branch of the anesthesia machine. In addition, specialized monitoring is incorporated for the patient with a particular disease, for the use of a specialized anesthetic technique, or for certain surgical procedures. This is demonstrated best with the comprehensive monitoring of the critically ill surgical patient, in which case the intensive care environment is duplicated in the operating room.

VENTILATION. Ventilation is a vital function that is altered by most anesthetic techniques and by many surgical procedures. Continuous auscultation of the chest with a precordial or esophageal stethoscope is essential during anesthesia. Changes in breath sounds may reveal the development of airway obstruction, bronchospasm, or anesthesia circuit disconnection. In patients with significant pulmonary disease or during certain operations such as thoracotomy, better quantification of respiratory adequacy may be necessary. This specialized monitoring may include serial arterial blood gas measurements, end-tidal CO_2 monitoring, transcutaneous oximetry, respirometry, or mass spectrometry of inspired and exhaled gases.

CARDIOVASCULAR SYSTEM. Basic monitoring for all patients should include noninvasive blood pressure measurement, which can be accomplished by use of a sphygmomanometer, oscillotonometry, or a flow detection device such as a Doppler device. Automated devices are available for serial, noninvasive blood pressure determinations. Additionally, the ECG should be monitored during the administration of any anesthetic. The ECG is useful for diagnosing various dysrhythmias as well as providing an audible indicator of the electrical activity of the heart when the QRS complex is acoustically coupled. In certain circumstances, such as when a patient is critically ill or has significant cardiac or pulmonary disease, or for specialized techniques such as deliberate hypotension or cardiopulmonary bypass, an intra-arterial pressure monitoring system is mandatory. When appropriate, central venous pressure measurement or pulmonary artery pressure measurements provide useful indices of the adequacy of circulating blood volume. An overall quantitative estimate of cardiovascular performance may be obtained by measuring cardiac output with a thermodilution pulmonary artery catheter or by the serial measurement of central venous oxygen saturation.

CENTRAL NERVOUS SYSTEM. The central nervous system is monitored by the anesthesiologist, who carefully observes the clinical signs of anesthetic depth and adjusts the anesthetic agents accordingly. Specialized monitoring such as an electroencephalogram (EEG) can be utilized during anesthesia for those patients at risk for regional brain ischemia. Cerebral blood flow determination and intracranial pressure monitoring are available but are limited in their application.

RENAL FUNCTION. A bladder catheter should be used in all major operations for observation and quantitation of urinary flow. Qualitative urinalysis should also be evaluated, especially during periods of oliguria.

BODY TEMPERATURE. It is essential to monitor body temperature during anesthesia. The temperature is usually monitored in the esophagus or rectum, although occasionally, the axilla, nasopharynx, or tympanic membrane is employed as an alternative site. Because of the morbidity and mortality associated with hypothermia and hyperthermia, it has become standard practice to monitor body temperature in all patients during anesthesia.

GENERAL. In addition to monitoring the various vital organ systems just mentioned, the anesthesiologist must observe and assess the general condition of the patient. This includes an assessment of various body sites vulnerable to injury because of positioning of the anesthetized patient and the application of protective padding to those sites at risk. The eyes and ears must be protected from pressure, and the various nervous and vascular plexuses must be protected from overextension. Extraneous, dangerous objects such as needles should be removed around the patient, and precautions against electrical burns should be taken.

Vigilance by the anesthesiologist, together with the appropriate and precise application of monitoring devices, provides safe anesthesia for the patient and minimizes perioperative complications.

GENERAL ANESTHESIA

The anesthesiologist's attention is directed toward both the patient he is attending and the surgeon performing the operation. The anesthesiologist's goals are to render the patient pain-free and amnesic, to preserve vital functions during the operation, and to offer to the surgeon a quiet, relaxed field. Modern anesthesia achieves this with the use of potent inhalation agents or intravenous drugs. In this section, specific agents that are currently in use and the principles of their application are discussed.

Nitrous oxide (N_2O) is an odorless gas with weak anesthetic potency. Although 80 per cent N_2O induces unconsciousness, only higher concentrations can produce a real anesthetic state. These can be administered only at increased environmental pressure in order to supplement the gas mixture with sufficient concentrations of oxygen. Despite limited potency, N_2O is still a component of many anesthetic regimens, supplementing intravenous analgesics and muscle relaxants. It is the most widely used inhalation anesthetic.

In healthy individuals and in various animal populations, it has been demonstrated that 50 per cent N_2O has limited but significant cardiodepressant properties. Peripheral resistances are usually elevated, as are the levels of circulating catecholamines, suggesting an activation of the sympathetic nervous system. In patients with a compromised cardiac reserve, all these effects are undesirable. The reason for the widespread use of N_2O is that the dosage of other drugs (usually more cardiodepressant) can be reduced when combined with N_2O. This is also observed when volatile anesthetics are used additively. The limited solubility of N_2O in body fluids may induce expansion of air-filled spaces in body cavities, such as in an occluded middle ear or in a pneumothorax cavity, and it may increase the size of gas emboli in the circulation. This may be a clinically important phenomenon in patients after cardiopulmonary bypass surgery, where small emboli may enlarge to produce circulatory obstruction after N_2O administration. Another disadvantage of N_2O is its potential for "diffusion hypoxia" when room air, rather than oxygen, is suddenly substituted for elevated N_2O mixtures. Moreover, although for a long time N_2O was thought to be completely inert, more recent evidence indicates that it interferes with the synthesis of methionine and thymidine, a DNA component. Megaloblastic erythropoiesis was found in patients exposed to N_2O for several days for alleviation of tetanus symptoms, and chronic abusers of N_2O develop a neuropathy similar to that associated with vitamin B_{12} deficiency. Also, chronic exposure to N_2O has been implicated in the increased incidence of congenital anomalies and fetal deaths among the offspring of exposed personnel. Because of these problems, it appears that the use of N_2O will be reduced in the future, although scavenging devices are usually applied during its utilization to prevent environmental contamination.

INHALATION AGENTS

Halogenated Anesthetic Drugs

Halogenated compounds (almost exclusively halothane, enflurane, and isoflurane) represent the bulk of contemporary inhalational general anesthetics. Fluorination of aliphatic compounds lowers flammability and increases anesthetic potency. At room temperature and atmospheric pressure, all the fluorinated agents are colorless, volatile liquids with odors qualified as sweet, fruity, or ethereal. These agents are altered by sun and ultraviolet light and are stored in amber-colored bottles.

All three agents are administered as vapors. The ease of vaporization of the liquid anesthetic is associated with a high vapor pressure, a low boiling point, and a low heat of vaporization.

Clinically, the solubility of an anesthetic agent in different body constituents is an important physical characteristic. For example, the blood gas partition coefficient for halothane is 2.3, signifying that for an alveolar concentration of 1 volume/per cent, the blood concentration at equilibrium is 2.3 volumes of gaseous halothane per 100 ml. of blood.

The blood solubility of the volatile anesthetic drugs is a major determinant of their uptake and elimination (assuming a constant cardiac output). For example, a low blood solubility permits the alveolar concentration to track closely the inspired concentration. Because the concentration of the vapor in the alveoli is representative of the cerebral concentration at equilibrium, rapid increase or decrease of alveolar concentration produces a short induction time and rapid recovery.

Vaporizers

Because of their potency, halogenated anesthetic vapors must be diluted precisely to be administered reliably. Most popular vaporizers incorporate a constant temperature chamber in which a fully saturated vapor is produced, which is then diluted into a carrier gas flow. Vaporizers maintain the stored anesthetic at constant (ambient) temperature. They are usually constructed with a large heat sink and with chambers automatically compensating for gas flow.

The gas exposed to the anesthetic vapor is always completely saturated at the temperature of the vaporizer and is therefore variously diluted by the total flow of gas. Modern anesthesia machines monitor the oxygen content of the final gas mixture flowing into the patient's breathing circuit. Other fail-safe devices are incorporated into current equipment to minimize the possibly disastrous consequences of malfunction.

Principles of Anesthetic Uptake and Distribution

Diffusion of anesthetics across alveolar-capillary and blood-brain membranes is rapid, and the cerebral blood flow represents a substantial elevated proportion of the total flow to the tissues. For these reasons, the alveolar concentration of an anesthetic may be used to define the potency of volatile agents: the minimal alveolar concentration (MAC) of an anesthetic is that concentration which produces immobility in 50 per cent of patients subjected to a painful surgical stimulus. This clinically useful term is in common use. The various factors influencing the alveolar concentration of the inhalation anesthetic include (1) alveolar ventilation (the greater the alveolar ventilation, the more rapidly alveolar concentration increases to match inspired concentration; in this respect, the larger the functional residual capacity, the larger dilution it imposes on inspired gas, delaying the attainment of elevated alveolar levels) and (2) the rate of transfer of alveolar anesthetic to blood and tissues. Only a small fraction of the inhaled dose is absorbed by lung tissue, because pulmonary tissue volumes are small. The remainder enters the systemic circulation, where individual tissue uptake depends upon blood solubility, alveolar-venous difference in anesthetic concentration, and cardiac output. An increase in cardiac output accelerates the loss of anesthetic from the alveoli and slows the rate of increase of alveolar concentration. The volume of the various storage compartments varies according to the solubility of the agents. The vessel-rich group of tissues receives 75 per cent of the cardiac output, but it has a limited storage capacity. It comprises the brain, heart, kidneys, digestive tract, and the endocrine glands.

Elimination of gas during emergence from anesthesia follows a sequence of events that is the reverse of that during induction. In this phase, the alveolar concentration diminishes more rapidly with higher cardiac output and alveolar ventilation. Emergence after inhalation of very poorly soluble gases such as N_2O is very rapid. In contrast, emergence is delayed when soluble agents are used, especially following prolonged exposures that saturate body stores. The ventilatory depression produced by narcotic analgesics delays emergence due to the predicted decrease in ventilatory drive and alveolar ventilation.

Thus far, uptake and distribution of anesthetic vapors have been discussed with the assumption that anesthetic agents act as inert gases. However, studies on anesthetic metabolism during the past decade have demonstrated that all clinically used inhalation anesthetics are biodegraded. This is unimportant during administration because it is common to provide fresh inhalation anesthetic in amounts far in excess of biodegradation. However, a possible association between anesthetic metabolism and biotoxicity of anesthetic agents is suggested. In fact, most drugs undergo detoxification during their metabolism. Unfortunately, there are examples of drug metabolism in which the end result is not drug detoxification, but rather formation of metabolites of greater toxicity than the parent compound.

It is of interest that of the anesthetic agents, only chloroform is capable of producing direct cellular damage. A long-standing concern regards the possible association of halothane administration and hepatotoxicity. Evidence from animal studies and from the analysis of several million cases remains inconclusive regarding the pathophysiologic basis of this phenomenon. There is laboratory evidence that anesthetic metabolism is increased by enzyme induction and in the presence of hypoxia a more toxic reductive pathway is encouraged.

The administration of inhalation anesthetics is a versatile and controllable technique, because it is centered on the lungs, which act as entry and elimination pathways of the anesthetic. As such, the anesthetic level can be altered rapidly, provided the patient sustains voluntary ventilatory efforts or that ventilation is controlled. Respiratory obstruction due to pharyngeal soft tissue relaxation, excessive secretions, or laryngospasm must be avoided. Additionally, abnormalities of pulmonary ventilation-perfusion matching must be assessed, and the extent of circulatory depression and production of adequate brain concentration of the agent depend upon a balance of these factors. The development of inhalation anesthetics historically contributed to many technical developments related to airway maintenance and breathing circuits. These developments range from apparently simple concepts to sophisticated physiologic principles, all of which find application in anesthetic practice. Some of the important concepts are mask fitting, prevention of respiratory obstruction, the use of oral and nasal airways, prevention of bronchospasm, disposition of mucous secretions and vomitus, and intubation of the trachea and the mainstem bronchi. A host of principles of applied respiratory physiology, from the clinical use of blood gases to the use of breathing gas analysis, have contributed to the expertise of anesthesiologists in providing prolonged ventilatory support both inside and outside the operating room.

INTRAVENOUS ANESTHESIA

Administration of potent intravenous anesthetic agents has several advantages in clinical practice and offers the alternatives of single-bolus injections or continuous infusion. This method is generally well accepted by patients and is relatively easy for the practitioner. However, in contrast to the inhalation agents, whose concentration in brain and cardiac tissues may be reduced by altering the inspired concentration, usually there is no practical way to antagonize or remove intravenous agents. Termination of pharmacologic effect depends upon redistribution, metabolism, and excretion of the agent.

Intravenous drugs may be used as induction agents, as in the case of barbiturates; as supplementary or main anesthetic agents, as in the case of ketamine; and, in special situations, as sole anesthetic agents, as recently demonstrated with high-dose narcotics.

Barbiturates

Barbiturates represent the main class of compounds which have gained widespread acceptance as anesthetics during the last 40 years. By far, thiopental and methohexital, two ultra-short-acting compounds, are the most used agents, and thiopental sodium has long been the standard against which all other intravenous agents have been compared. Control of individual responses to injection can be improved by using dilute solutions (2.5 per cent usually), by injection of small test doses to assess the effect, and by waiting a sufficient time to allow differences in circulation time from the venous site of injection in order to observe cerebral and myocardial effects. Requirements are approximated to body weight and are reduced with advancing age.

Thiopental, as well as other barbiturates, exerts a depressant effect on the myocardium and produces peripheral vasodilation. These factors may adversely affect coronary blood flow, especially in patients with pre-existing cardiac disease and in situations in which the intravascular circulating blood volume is restricted, as in shock. In obstetrics, it is wise to reduce to a minimum the dosage of barbiturate administered to the mother, because these agents cross the placental barrier and may cause depression of the newborn.

The thiobarbiturates undergo metabolic degradation by desulfuration and oxidation, principally in the liver, but some biotransformation also occurs in other organs. The principal pathway of excretion is the urine. However, redistribution in the body, rather than biotransformation, is the main mechanism terminating thiobarbiturate effects. Thus, after a rapid equilibration period in all organs (e.g., peak concentrations following single-bolus injection are measured in the brain in 50 seconds and associated with unconsciousness), recirculation removes thiopental from the blood and redistributes the drug in other tissues. Muscle equilibrates in several minutes, whereas the final pool of fat does not reach equilibrium with plasma for several hours. Through redistribution, the cerebral concentration decreases sufficiently such that awakening may begin 5 to 10 minutes after injection, despite the fact that only a small amount of the drug has undergone biotransformation.

The fraction of thiopental that is not protein-bound or not ionized can pass freely through membranes. Therefore, physical properties affect the onset and extent of thiopental's effects. In healthy surgical patients, thiopental is moderately bound to albumin (15 to 25 per cent). An elevated thiopental-free fraction can occur if a second drug has increased affinity for the thiopental binding sites on albumin, such as aspirin, although the blood concentrations of these competing drugs must be elevated to demonstrate clinically important differences.

Ketamine

Ketamine is a powerful intravenous dissociative agent related chemically to phencyclidine. In sufficient dosage, ketamine produces good analgesia. The characteristic "cataleptic" properties of this compound can be defined as a combination of little hypnotic potency and good analgesia. Hypertonus may often be present. Its original use for neuroradiologic and cardiovascular investigations in children was limited to short procedures. However, higher doses associated with neuromuscular blocking drugs and the alleviation of psychic disturbances during the recovery phase by pretreatment with benzodiazepines have substantially widened its spectrum of useful applications.

Ketamine is unique among the intravenous agents in its cardiovascular stimulation, which mimics increased activity of the sympathetic nervous system. In unpremedicated healthy volunteers, 2 mg. per kg. intravenously increases heart rate, systemic pressure, and cardiac output without changes in cardiac filling pressures. Such an increase in myocardial oxygen requirement can be compensated easily in healthy subjects but limits ketamine use in patients with reduced coronary reserve. The usual pattern of response follows a combination of vagal inhibition and adrenergic stimulation. A useful property of ketamine is its apparent ability to maintain hypoxic pulmonary vasoconstriction reflexes. This makes it a useful agent during performance of endobronchial anesthesia in thoracic surgery.

Benzodiazepines

Diazepam and, more recently, lorazepam have been used variously as intravenous induction or adjuvant agents. Various dosages and administration regimens may cause a variety of conscious levels, from heavy sedation to complete unconsciousness associated with profound amnesia.

The cardiovascular responses to intravenous administration of these compounds are usually small, with a moderate reduction in stroke volume and usually an unchanged cardiac output with 100 per cent oxygen. In fact, myocardial oxygen balance may be favorably altered, even in patients with coronary occlusive disease. Diazepam lacks significant analgesic properties, and it is often used in association with a narcotic to produce a pain-free, amnesic period that would not be possible with a lower dose of either compound alone. In most patients, the hemodynamic alterations observed with such combinations are small. The major limitations for anesthetic use are due to prolonged duration of action, disorientation, and often apnea, even in minimal doses when administered to the elderly or cachectic patient.

Narcotics

Although the use of oral and parenteral opiates is recorded historically, narcotics were considered adjuvant agents in anesthesia. Only recently have narcotics been used in sufficiently high doses to manifest their complete anesthetic properties. These doses are significantly larger than the amounts used to produce reliable analgesia and sedation. For example, 10 to 20 mg. of morphine produces analgesia in the average man but rarely complete anesthesia without supplementation with other agents. In contrast, a 10 to 30 times larger dose must be administered to produce anesthesia. The use of larger doses of narcotics is not without side effects. Rapid injection may induce prolonged hypotension, anaphylactoid reactions (histamine degranulation is common upon rapid injection of morphine), and, usually, prolonged respiratory depression. In the early 1970s, it was demonstrated that slow administration of large (up to 3 mg. per kg.) doses of morphine did not alter cardiovascular dynamics in patients with normal ventricles, provided adequate ventilation sustained proper gas exchange. This technique gained popularity, especially for cardiac valvular surgery, because of the cardiovascular stability offered, despite the frequently incomplete amnesia. Similar side effects are less frequent with more potent narcotics. Therefore, it is understandable that widespread use of large-dose narcotic anesthesia depended upon confirmed respiratory support measures easily available in the postoperative period, and the technique gained in popularity with the clinical availability of shorter-acting narcotics such as fentanyl.

Fentanyl, a synthetic narcotic, has been found to exert very little effect on ventricular performance. Addition of diazepam or of N_2O to the inspired gas produces significant cardiovascular depression. Single, large-dose injections of fentanyl in patients undergoing coronary artery surgery do not produce cardiovascular depression. Cardiovascular stability is maintained even in patients in whom fentanyl is used as the sole anesthetic.

All opiates induce a dose-related respiratory depression of responsiveness to increasing carbon dioxide levels and to hypoxia. Also, narcotics affect respiratory rhythmicity and respiratory reflexes. Respiratory depression can continue by several hours the shorter duration of analgesia, even with fentanyl, and patients may have to be ventilated for 12 to 18 hours postoperatively. Opioid antagonists such as naloxone can reverse opioid-induced respiratory depression. However, the half-life of naloxone is shorter than that of all agonists. Analgesic effects can be reversed by an antagonist; therefore, extreme caution must be taken when administering naloxone to reverse the depressant effects of opioids, particularly when these have been administered in large doses to prevent sudden awareness and return of surgical pain.

It is difficult to define the neurologic state obtained by use of large doses of opioid analgesics. Whereas inhalation of volatile anesthetic agents induces a state of general anesthesia through a dose-related generalized depression of the central nervous system, high-dose fentanyl anesthesia is more selective in action and induces a very specific EEG response (high voltage, slow delta waves). This typical EEG appearance is consistent with deep surgical anesthesia. Additionally, narcotic analgesics do not produce muscle relaxation but increase muscle tone, sometimes resulting in truncal rigidity. Neuromuscular blocking agents can be used to abolish the rigidity, which is highest in patients who are in the younger decades of life; it decreases in frequency as patients advance in age. However, one of the most troublesome problems of narcotic anesthesia is the subtlety of responses in different patients. Only careful monitoring of all clinical signs such as blood pressure, heart rate, cardiac output, and peripheral vascular resistance allows maintenance of acceptable anesthesia. Several new fentanyl derivatives, which are now undergoing clinical investigation, have been synthesized. Alfentanyl is a less potent but shorter-acting drug than fentanyl. The pharmacokinetics of alfentanyl indicate a shorter elimination half-life than that of related compounds. The rapid elimination and shorter duration of clinical action suggest that it might be well suited for repeated administration or continuous infusion.

MUSCLE RELAXANTS

The introduction of curare into the field of anesthesia by Griffith and Johnson in 1942 revolutionized patient management. Suddenly it was possible to obtain abdominal wall relaxation without resorting to dangerously toxic levels of general inhalation agents. Administration of muscle relaxants to a large section of the surgical population contributed significantly to a refinement of the studies on pharmacologic principles and advanced the quest for the ideal muscle relaxant.

The effect of drug action on neuromuscular transmission is best understood as an alteration of the normal chemistry of the myoneural junction. It is well established that the acetylcholine-acetylcholinesterase system is centrally involved in cholinergic transmission. The general mechanism can be summarized as the chemistry of synthesis, dissociation, and metabolism of the transmitter, acetylcholine. The presynaptic area is the site of synthesis and storage of acetylcholine. When the nerve impulse arrives, a wave of depolarization reaches the nerve terminal, and specific calcium gates open on the axon membrane, which leads to an influx of calcium ions. Calcium causes the attachment and local fusion between the vesicular and axon membranes, producing the discharge of the vesicular content (acetylcholine) into the synaptic cleft. The liberated acetylcholine diffuses to react with the cholinergic receptor on the postsynaptic membrane. The alterations induced on the receptor by the acetylcholine affect the change in conductance of sodium and potassium ions at the postsynaptic membrane, which is sufficient to generate a self-propagating action potential.

The activity of acetylcholine can be terminated by reducing its concentration in the receptor area. Principally, the enzyme acetylcholinesterase is responsible for this by rapidly hydrolyzing the free acetylcholine ester. With the concentration of acetylcholine falling, the ester-receptor complex dissociates in accordance with mass action laws.

Succinylcholine mimics the action of the physiologic depolarizer acetylcholine and keeps the postsynaptic membrane depolarized. For this reason, it is described as a "depolarizing" muscle relaxant. Nondepolarizing relaxants such as curare compete with acetylcholine for the receptor and reduce the number of available calcium channel openings, thereby preventing depolarization. Neostigmine and edrophonium, potent anticholinesterase agents, inhibit the essential enzyme acetylcholinesterase, thereby increasing the local, active concentration of acetylcholine and reversing the block induced by this class of muscle relaxants.

The criteria for choice of a muscle relaxant are primarily dependent upon the duration of action and the pharmacokinetic profile of the various available agents and on the cardiovascular side effects they might produce. The main depolarizing agent in use, succinylcholine, may cause significant hyperkalemia in certain conditions (e.g., burns, massive trauma, and some neurologic diseases) because of membrane depolarization. The nondepolarizing agents in clinical use abound and differ significantly in the amount of stimulation of autonomic ganglia and cardiac muscarinic receptors and in the potential for histamine release. Briefly, curare and, to a lesser extent, metocurine may produce hypotension, primarily by liberation of histamine and, in larger doses, by ganglionic blockade. Pancuronium causes an increase in heart rate due to a vagolytic effect. This might be desirable, such as in the setting of large doses of fentanyl, which may produce bradycardia. Newer muscle relaxants, such as vecuronium and atracurium, have no effect on autonomic ganglia and cardiac muscarinic receptors, do not induce significant release of histamine, and appear to lack any cumulative effect.

The degree of muscular relaxation depends upon the number of muscle units blocked compared with the total number of available units. By the response of a partially blocked muscle to electrical stimulation of its motor nerve, one can differentiate a depolarizing block from a competitive block (nondepolarizing, curare-like) and quantitate the intensity of the block. In the nondepolarizing block, if tetanic stimulation is applied via a nerve stimulator, the resulting contraction is a fused tetanus, reduced from a control or pre-drug stimulus in a manner proportional to the intensity of the block. The early tetanic twitches are reduced, and the subsequent tetanic twitches decline in amplitude. This is the phenomenon of "fade." Another typical feature is "posttetanic facilitation" or augmentation of the early posttetanic stimulated single twitches. Therefore, electrical stimulation of a muscle partially blocked by a nondepolarizing competitive drug demonstrates fade on tetanus and posttetanic facilitation. Clearly, complete paralysis produces no twitch and the absence of tetanus. In the case of a depolarizing block, the tetanus is sustained, there is no fade, and there is no posttetanic facilitation, but the amplitude of the response is reduced. Similar tests are used to monitor the degree of neuromuscular blockade and to monitor the return to normal after administration of relaxant and reversal drugs.

REVERSAL OF NEUROMUSCULAR BLOCK. Nondepolarizing muscle relaxants can be antagonized by agents such as edrophonium, neostigmine, or pyridostigmine. These drugs act by interfering with cholinesterase action, thus preventing acetylcholine metabolism. The effect of acetylcholine is not limited to the end-plate of striated muscle but also extends to structures innervated by the parasympathetic nervous system. Therefore, in order to prevent muscarinic responses such as bradycardia, bronchospasm, and excessive salivation, atropine is usually administered before or in combination with the selected anticholinesterase drugs.

No reliable antagonist of depolarizing muscle relaxants exists. For safety measures, ventilation should be maintained until spontaneous recovery occurs.

REGIONAL ANESTHESIA

In contrast to general anesthetics, which are directly or indirectly deposited in the circulation with the primary goal of reaching receptors located in the central nervous system, local anesthetics are delivered directly to peripheral neural targets with the primary goal of interrupting conduction of afferent nerve impulses.

Pharmacology of Local Anesthetic Agents

Local anesthetics are drugs that produce reversible neural blockade by impeding impulse transmission in peripheral nerves, spinal roots, or nerve endings. These drugs obtund sensation and reduce motor tone in the innervated areas distal to the site of application without depressing consciousness or sensation in other parts of the body. Although excellent local analgesic drugs are used worldwide, the search for the ideal drug continues. Its properties should include short latency, adequate potency, superior penetration, controllable duration of action with complete reversibility, low toxicity, topical activity, solubility in water, and stability in solution to permit heat sterilization. It should have no side effects and should be nonaddictive, nonirritating, and nonantigenic and should not interfere with the process of wound healing.

A local anesthetic produces a nondepolarizing block that takes effect at the surface membrane of excitable tissue cells. Smooth and striated muscle (blood vessels and myocardium) as well as nerve fibers are affected. The site of action of a local anesthetic in a myelinated nerve is at the node of Ranvier, and 2 to 3 adjacent nodes must be exposed to the local anesthetic to prevent saltatory conduction. At least 6 mm. and preferably 1 cm. of a nerve length must be exposed to the anesthetic solution to deter impulses from bypassing the blocked segments. Nerve conduction is interrupted because generation of an action potential is prevented by obstruction of the inward flow of sodium ions through the nerve membranes. A low concentration of local anesthetic may simply delay the migration of ions, without completely preventing it. The electrical excitability of myocardial tissue is reduced by agents such as lidocaine or procainamide, which hinder the transmission of stimuli and inhibit the appearance of ectopic foci. In the central nervous system, it has been demonstrated that a subconvulsive dose of lidocaine can have an anticonvulsant effect due to its stabilizing properties on excitable membranes.

There are three main types of nerve fibers: A, B, and C. Myelinated somatic nerve fibers are classified as A fibers and subdivided into alpha, beta, gamma, and delta, according to decreasing diameter and conduction velocity. Alpha fibers are the largest and most rapidly conducting; delta fibers are the smallest and slowest conducting. B fibers are myelinated autonomic preganglionic fibers. C fibers are nonmyelinated, easily blocked small fibers, both somatic and autonomic. Local anesthetic agents block the fibers in the following order: B, C, delta, gamma, beta, and alpha fibers. Recovery occurs in the reverse order. Compression of a nerve, on the contrary, blocks A fibers before C fibers. Large A fibers, alpha and beta groups, subserve motor function, proprioception, and touch; small A fibers, the delta group, and C fibers subserve pain and temperature sensations.

Local analgesic solution must diffuse from the site of injection to the nerve and penetrate fibers and connective tissues before reaching the individual axons within the nerve. Intraneural diffusion then proceeds from the nerve mantle to the core, as manifested clinically by nerve blocks spreading from proximal to distal parts of the body. Recovery of function occurs in the same order when the analgesic solution is effectively exhausted by dilution with tissue fluids, dispersion away from the nerve, uptake by the bloodstream, and metabolic inactivation. The latency depends upon nerve diameter, pH, diffusion rate, and analgesic concentration. The higher the concentration of the analgesic solution, the more rapid is the onset of the block.

Chemical Considerations

Most injectable local anesthetics are tertiary amines; a few are secondary amines. The general configuration of a local anesthetic is composed of two key structural components: one imparting lipid solubility (lipophilic) and the other imparting water solubility (hydrophilic). These two components are joined by an intermediate hydrocarbon chain, which is usually either an *ester* or an *amide* linkage. Compounds that lack the hydrophilic portion of the molecule are almost insoluble in water and therefore not suitable for injection, but they are frequently used in topical analgesia of mucous membranes (e.g., benzocaine).

Local analgesics are weak bases with a dissociation constant (pK) between 7 and 10. Because they are poorly soluble and unstable in water, they are usually clinically available as the water-soluble acid salt. The degree of ionization of the molecule is determined by the pK and the pH of the tissues. When the pH of a solution has the same value as the pK of the analgesic agent, half the drug exists as the cation and the other half as the base. Apparently only the base form can penetrate the nerve membrane. Alkalinization of local anesthetic solutions speeds the onset and effectiveness of a block, albeit rendering the solution too unstable for clinical practice.

The buffer reserve in normal tissues tends to maintain a constant pH, delaying neutralization and therefore full effect of the local anesthetic. Anesthesia might be inadequate in inflamed tissues because of the low pH of the interstitial fluid, causing reduced liberation of free anesthetic base.

Toxic Effects

The major target organs for the toxicity of local anesthetics are the central nervous system and the cardiovascular system. Plasma concentration of a drug is mainly dependent upon absorption of the drug from the injection site, clearance of the drug from the bloodstream to the tissue (tissue distribution), and elimination of the drug through metabolism and urinary excretion. Tissue areas with a good blood supply cause rapid absorption of the drug and a rapid increase in plasma concentration, similar to intravascular injections. Rapid absorption also occurs after application to the mucous membrane of the respiratory tract, and intrabronchial spray of local anesthetic produces serum levels comparable to those produced by an intravenous injection. Local anesthetics of the amide type are largely bound to plasma proteins. Nevertheless, the concentration of the unbound drug determines the rate of disappearance of the drug from the bloodstream and is also responsible for the biologic action of the drug and its passage across the placenta.

Local analgesics are removed from the bloodstream by redistribution, metabolism, and excretion. Highly perfused organs such as the brain, heart, lungs, and liver receive the initial bulk. Procaine and the related ester-linked analgesics are hydrolyzed by esterases. Any interference with their metabolism by pathologic processes or drugs increases their systemic toxicity (e.g., hereditary changes of plasma cholinesterase or decreased cholinesterase activity caused by pregnancy, liver disease, or anticholinesterase drugs).

The amide-linked drugs are the most widely used local anesthetics and have been subjected to extensive study. They are almost completely metabolized by the liver before excretion. Their metabolism is slower than that of the ester-linked agents. Hepatic blood flow is most important, and, if liver perfusion is decreased as in congestive cardiac failure or if the liver is diseased, plasma clearance is decreased.

The central nervous system effects of toxicity are anxiety, tinnitus, restlessness, tremors proceeding to convulsions, and respiratory failure. Toxicity usually follows overdosage, accidental intravenous injection, a prematurely released tourniquet, or rapid absorption from vascular sites. Treatment should be prompt, ensuring ventilation with oxygen, and should include the use of intravenous diazepam and/or barbiturates to control seizures.

Clinically Relevant Local Anesthetics

ESTER-LINKED. PROCAINE. Synthesized by Einhorn in 1904, procaine is a marked vasodilator and is rapidly hydrolyzed in plasma and in the liver. Procaine lacks the central and sympathomimetic effects of cocaine; it has a quinidine-like influence on the heart but, in large doses, depresses the myocardium and causes peripheral vasodilation. It is an inexpensive, relatively safe local anesthetic, used often for perivascular infiltration prior to cannulation procedures. The maximal safe dose for an adult may be up to 1000 mg., provided absorption is reasonably slow.

TETRACAINE. First synthesized in 1928, tetracaine, like procaine, is an ester of p-aminobenzoic acid, and it is hydrolyzed into procaine by plasma cholinesterase. It is approximately 10 times more toxic than procaine. Because of its longer duration of action, it is still one of the preferred agents for subarachnoid block. It is also an optimal topical anesthetic of the tracheobronchial tree. The maximal safe dosage is 1 mg. per kg.

AMIDE-LINKED. LIDOCAINE. Synthesized in 1943, lidocaine is very stable and probably the most widely used agent by all routes of administration. It has great penetrating powers, excellent topical action (4 per cent solution), and is very useful for peridural and plexus blocks (0.5 to 2 per cent solutions). It

has marked central effects, inducing drowsiness, amnesia, and sedation. Nerve blocks are optimally performed with 1.5 to 2 per cent solutions with the addition of epinephrine (1 part per 200,000). Maximal safe dose is 200 mg. without and 500 mg. with the addition of epinephrine.

BUPIVACAINE. Synthesized in 1957, bupivacaine is a very stable compound, 80 to 95 per cent protein-bound. It is a highly lipid-soluble substance, approximately four times more potent than lidocaine; it has longer latency but is considerably longer lasting. It is one of the agents of choice for continuous epidural anesthesia and for intercostal block. The comparatively long duration of action is a valuable characteristic for obstetrics and postoperative analgesia. The maximal safe dose is 2 mg. per kg.

Complications and Risks of Regional Anesthesia

The choice of regional anesthesia for several operative procedures is steadily increasing. Patient acceptance and popularity in the belief of reduced recovery times often free from postoperative malaise is one of the reasons for this choice. This trend must be carefully assessed, because regional anesthesia may expose patients to additional risks and complications, especially if proper precautionary measures are not taken. Undesirable adverse reactions observed as consequences of different types of block may be ascribed to the specific agent used (toxic reactions), to the anatomy of the puncture site (e.g., a subarachnoid massive infusion of local anesthetic during attempted epidural anesthesia or pneumothorax following supraclavicular brachial plexus block), and to positioning-related complications. Prevention and treatment of regional anesthetic mishaps require scrupulous observance of antisepsis procedure, a sound anatomic knowledge and common prudence, the presence of an intravenous access, and availability of general resuscitative measures to control ventilation and to sustain circulation. Generally, it must be remembered that the same resuscitative equipment and standard materials should be readily available for regional anesthesia as for general anesthesia.

Spinal Anesthesia

During the late 1890s, lumbar puncture became a commonly used clinical procedure, following Quincke's studies at the University Hospital in Kiel, Germany. Cocaine was first injected intradurally in 1899 by August Bier, a colleague of Quincke and an adventurous young surgeon.

Some essential points in the practice of this useful technique follow. Because the spinal cord usually ends at the upper border of the body of the second lumbar vertebra, at the same level as the second lumbar spine, a needle inserted any higher than the L2–L3 interspace may transfix the spinal cord. Therefore, the safest approach to lumbar puncture should be considered to be below this level. The specific gravity of the cerebrospinal fluid (CSF) is low, very near to that of water. The opening pressure of the CSF at the lumbar puncture level depends upon the position of the vertebral column. It is usually 50 mm. H_2O in the lateral and up to 500 mm. H_2O in the sitting position, because of the hydrostatic pressure in the vertical column of CSF. Pressure is also increased as cerebral venous pressure increases, and it is crucially important not to withdraw CSF from patients who could have a tumor or other space-occupying lesions in the brain or from those who exhibit signs of raised intracranial pressure. If CSF is removed in these patients, a sudden decrease in intracranial pressure may cause herniation of brain contents through the tentorium, producing respiratory arrest and death.

When local anesthetic solutions are injected into the intradural space, the spread of anesthesia is determined by the specific gravity of the solution, the force of injection, and its volume. Gravity might be used to spread the drug in either direction by changing the position of the patient. Moreover, the actual mass of local anesthetic injected, irrespective of both the concentration and specific gravity of the solution, directly relates to the extent of the block produced.

Hypobaric solutions can be used in a fairly large injection volume if the patient is lying supine with the head of the table tilted downward.

Paralysis of the preganglionic sympathetic fibers leaving the cord with anterior roots of the spinal nerves from T1–L2 is the cause of the vasodilation and potential hypotension observed in the presence of spinal block. Traditionally, patients are positioned in the Trendelenburg position so that the return flow of blood to the right atrium is increased. If the hypotension is severe, the legs should be elevated without lowering the patient's head. In the presence of hypotension, any movement of the patient must be gentle in order to avoid blood pooling in dependent areas. Vasoactive drugs, oxygen, and always the necessary equipment for resuscitation and intubation should be available immediately.

Even with meticulous care and faultless technique, experienced workers may obtain too high or too low a block. Unilateral analgesia can be produced by very slow injection of small amounts of a hyperbaric solution. This is a useful block for lower extremity amputation, and, if sufficient time is allowed for the anesthesia to be localized, cardiovascular alterations can be kept to a minimum, even in very debilitated patients.

This relatively simple procedure provides excellent anesthesia for surgical procedures involving the lower abdomen, pelvis, and lower extremities; for urologic procedures; and for vaginal delivery.

Lumbar Epidural Anesthesia

The extradural space occupies the vertebral canal between the periosteum lining the canal and the dura. Superiorly, it is limited by the fusion of the periosteum and the dura in the upper cervical region. Fluid injected in the epidural space in the cervical region cannot pass above the foramen magnum. Inferiorly, the space ends at the sacrococcygeal membrane. The space is widest in the midline posteriorly in the lumbar region. The anterior and posterior nerve roots, with their dural coverings, pass across this space.

Most frequently, the epidural space is approached through the lumbar area. When inserted in the midline, the needle must pass through skin, fascia, supraspinous and interspinous ligaments, and the ligamentum flavum prior to reaching the extradural space. The thoracic approach is more complex because of the need to insert the needle at an acute angle to the skin. A potential danger is the presence of the spinal cord at this level of the spine.

Solutions of anesthetic drugs injected in the extradural space, either directly through a needle or through a catheter positioned through the needle, block a variable number of spinal segments, depending upon the volume of the solution injected and the concentration of the anesthetic. Dose requirements are greatest in the adolescent and young adult, and they decrease with age. Smaller doses are required in the presence of occlusive arterial disease, in pregnancy, and in the very young.

The mass of local anesthetic drug in the epidural space far exceeds that required for comparable effect with an intradural injection. The site of action of the local anesthetics injected in the epidural space is multifocal, both at the nerve root level and at the spinal cord level.

A high epidural block is usually accompanied by a fall in mean pressure, a fall in stroke volume, reduction of cardiac output, and a reduction in peripheral resistance. Because the mass of local anesthetic injected in the epidural space is usually large, systemic effects due to reabsorption of considerable amounts of anesthetic are usually superimposed on the direct neuroplegic effects. It is usual to combine large doses of epidural local anesthetics with epinephrine, 1:200,000, to reduce the speed of anesthetic reabsorption into the circulation.

If sufficient time is available to observe the onset of anesthesia, epidural anesthesia is usually more controllable in extension than is intrathecal anesthesia. The complications are usually more limited and less severe. Nevertheless, the same precautionary measures should be adopted as for intradural injection. The use of the epidural technique has one further advantage in the complete absence of post–lumbar puncture headache following extradural block. The technique is an extremely useful one for operations involving the lower abdomen, pelvis, or lower extremities; for obstetric procedures, including cesarean section as well as vaginal delivery; and for radiologic studies of the large vessels branching from the abdominal aorta into the lower limbs. Extreme caution should be observed when epidural (and spinal) anesthesia is contemplated in patients with existing neurologic disease, spinal deformities, or septicemia or those receiving anticoagulant therapy, and a detailed risk-benefit analysis should be made before proceeding.

Caudal anesthesia, a form of epidural anesthesia infrequently employed, is practiced when the epidural space is entered by way of the sacral hiatus. This technique is useful for perineal, urologic, and gynecologic procedures as well as for vaginal delivery; however, usually larger volumes of solutions are necessary in order to extend the anesthetic level up to T10–T12.

EPIDURAL NARCOTICS. The discovery of specific opiate receptors within the central nervous system in the early 1970s led to a better appreciation of the selective actions of the opiates. It is now known that there are several types of opiate receptors, and their anatomic locations within the central nervous system have been described. The analgesic actions of opiates appear to be due, at least in part, to the close association of the receptors with major regions in the spinal cord and brain involved in pain sensation. The two most studied locations in recent years have been (1) a local system within the dorsal horn of the spinal cord, modulating on the substantia gelatinosa, and (2) descending systems from the brain stem to the dorsal horn, such as the periaqueductal gray.

Narcotics, like local anesthetics, when injected into the epidural space reach their site of action by diffusion across the dura. As with all bases, the lower the pKa, the greater the percentage of a specific dose that is in the diffusable, undissociated form. The narcotic, once in the CSF and bathing the spinal cord, spreads into the cord to the opiate receptors. The more lipid-soluble the compound, the greater the spread into the nervous tissue and the more rapid the clearance from the CSF. Thus, drugs such as fentanyl and meperidine, drugs with low pKa and high lipid solubility, penetrate the dura rapidly and have a rapid onset, shorter duration of action, and rapid clearance from the CSF. In contrast, morphine, a polar hydrophilic agent, penetrates the dura slowly and has a slow onset, a long duration of action, and a slow clearance from the CSF. This explains the potential danger of delayed respiratory depression with epidural morphine.

At present, use of epidural and spinal narcotics is an active area of research with collaboration among pharmacologists, neuroscientists, and clinicians. Currently, postoperative analgesia without sympathetic blockade appears the most fruitful application of epidural narcotics.

PREOPERATIVE ASSESSMENT

Current anesthetic practice requires that anesthetic management extend into the pre- and postoperative periods in addition to its use in the time between induction and emergence from anesthesia. The multiplicity of preoperative medications and the possibility of pharmacologic interactions among the wide variety of anesthetic, hypnotic, and analgesic medications used in the operating room demand close preoperative scrutiny. Additionally, plans must be made to discontinue, substitute, or reinstitute various medications during the operation itself and in the immediate postoperative period. Therefore, a preanesthetic assessment must include an appropriate history, with special emphasis on previous anesthetic mishaps and anesthetic complications involving direct relatives, a full drug history, and attention to details that could complicate induction of anesthesia (e.g., recessed chin, poor dentition, cervical spine disease, obesity with lack of peripheral venous access). In addition, plans must be made at this stage that ensure the rapid progression of the patient through the perioperative period.

The changing practice of anesthesia reflects several new constraints posed on surgical practice by limitations in reimbursement and reduction or absence of preoperative hospital admission days. The older patient population, with the attendant increased frequency of concurrent diseases, also provides a more challenging task for the anesthesiologist.

Preoperative evaluation provides an important opportunity for physicians to gain the patient's confidence and to reduce perioperative morbidity. This is accomplished by optimizing preoperative status and planning the anesthetic and recovery management. The attempt to maximize preoperative diagnostic screening of the patient by ordering a battery of laboratory tests, however, has proved inefficient and of limited values, when a proper history and rational assessment are not elicited.

Most studies agree that approximately 60 per cent of current preoperative testing could be eliminated without compromising patient care. It has been demonstrated also that unnecessary testing causes additional risk to the patient, inefficiency in operating room scheduling, and unnecessary costs to society. Several studies on thousands of patients, performed with appropriate controls, demonstrate that preconceived batteries of screening tests frequently fail to reveal pathologic conditions; if an abnormality is detected, it often remains unrecorded, or it is not appropriately pursued. Even in a subset of intact elderly patients screened by routine batteries of preoperative tests, it has been demonstrated that much less than 1 per cent of all tests ordered change patient management.

History and physical examination remain the best measures for screening for disease, and they usually indicate the probability of abnormality in all patients subsequently found to have abnormalities detected through laboratory testing.

Patient Assessment

The American Society of Anesthesiologists (ASA) has provided a graded scale into which all patients are placed prior to anesthesia. This scale represents the significance of a patient's illness prior to anesthesia, and, as would be expected, emergency procedures require special weighting to reflect the increased risk inherent in an imperfectly controlled situation. The following is a description of the ASA scale:

ASA I — Healthy individual *with no systemic disease,* undergoing elective surgery. Patient not at extremes of age. (*Note: Age is often ignored as affecting operative risk; however, in practice, patients at either extreme of age are thought to have increased risk.*)

ASA II — Individual with *one-system, well-controlled disease.* Disease does not affect daily activities. Other anesthetic risk factors, including mild obesity, alcoholism, and smoking, can be incorporated at this level.

ASA III — Individual with *multiple-system disease* or *well-controlled major system disease.* The disease status limits daily activity. However, there is no immediate danger of death due to any individual disease.

ASA IV — Individual with *severe, incapacitating disease.* Normally, the disease state is poorly controlled or end-stage. Danger of death due to organ failure is always present.

ASA V — Patient in *imminent danger of death.* Operation deemed to be a last-resort attempt at preserving life. The patient is not expected to live through the next 24 hours. In some cases, the patient may be relatively healthy prior to a catastrophic event that led to the current medical condition.

All these classifications can be modified if the case is treated as an emergency, although it can be argued that surgery in ASA V patients can never be elective. Specific considerations in emergency and trauma surgery are discussed later in this chapter.

When an appreciation of anesthetic risk is reached, completion of the preoperative assessment requires a brief general physical examination, which includes assessment of the following:

1. *Neurologic function* — Cranial nerves, peripheral reflexes, any neurologic symptoms. Abnormalities should be carefully noted. In patients in whom regional epidural or subarachnoid block is contemplated, a complete examination of the neurologic function of the areas to be affected is performed.

2. *Airways* — Potential for difficult management should be sought (e.g., poor dentition with loose teeth, short neck, cervical spine abnormalities, deviated trachea, neck masses, dysfunction of jaw motion, macroglossia).

3. *Lungs* — Preoperative smoking history, presence of longstanding or acute disease; asthma; presence of productive cough and hemoptysis; chest wall abnormalities, restrictive components; dyspnea; preoperative blood gases and pulmonary function tests.

4. *Cardiovascular* — Presence of organic or symptomatic cardiac or peripheral vascular disease, hypertension, recent myocardial infarction, or uncontrollable angina.

5. *Renal function* — Presence of chronic renal disease or acute insults. Radiocontrast studies should be noted. Preoperative diuretic anesthetic management and early postoperative diuretic use may be indicated.

6. *Nutrition/metabolism* — The patient's general physical status must be carefully assessed. Nutritional deficiency may be reason for surgical delay; increased risks and decreased wound healing are observed in malnourished patients. Endocrine diseases should be carefully noted prior to anesthesia induction, because no anesthetic procedure is stress-free and a patient's response to stress must be accurately predicted. Diabetic patients require careful assessment and special management.

7. *Pharmacologic history* — A full list of current medications and all known allergies is mandatory. Plans for medication continuance during the perioperative period should be made.

POSTOPERATIVE CARE

The Recovery Unit

The postoperative period is one of multiple physiologic and pharmacologic changes. Too often, reversal of the anesthetic is regarded as a prime determinant of success, and most traditional assessments of patient progress ignore features that may have significant impact on the quality of the postoperative course. Anesthetic management affects not only the patient's conscious state but also fluid and electrolyte balance, renal and hepatic function, neurologic function, and immune characteristics. Postanesthetic management traditionally began as an unsupervised period through which a patient survived while spontaneous reversal of poorly understood agents occurred. With increasing sophistication, a more responsible attitude toward patient care emerged, which paralleled the increased sophistication of surgical and anesthetic techniques and formed the development of new areas of expertise. The first movement was a nursing realization that patients could not be left unsupervised following any surgical procedure (even the most simple), because, during the time of depressed protective reflexes and large fluid and electrolyte changes, the patient was at extreme risk from relatively simple and, in large part, preventable occurrences (e.g., vomiting with aspiration and suffocation; unrecognized dysrhythmias with sudden cardiac death). Therefore, postanesthetic observation units were developed, into which all postoperative patients were placed for several hours until they were capable of self-protection in general ward situations. Gradually, the postanesthetic recovery area became viewed as a haven in which great expertise had developed in postoperative care and prolonged patient management. The immediate postoperative period is one of major physiologic changes for the patient, because of both the pharmacology surrounding reversal of anesthetic agents and the ongoing physiologic changes secondary to surgical trauma.

ANESTHESIA-RELATED COMPLICATIONS. The postanesthetic report must include complete details of the patient's preoperative condition and intraoperative management. Anesthetic agents, premedicants, previous drug therapy, and patient allergies are of prime importance. Additionally, significant medical history, especially as it affects postoperative outcome, must be included (e.g., significant cardiac or pulmonary disease obviously affects the postoperative monitoring requirements and fluid management).

The immediate postsurgical period is a period of time that is beginning to attract the attention and research interest it deserves. It is now considered to be a time requiring close physiologic monitoring, active pharmacologic intervention, and vigorous attempts to minimize adverse effects. A major difficulty in assessing a patient's postoperative recovery resides in attempting to define an adequate scale against which recovery progress can be measured. At all times, the distinction between appropriate responses to the withdrawal of residual anesthetic effects versus inappropriate behavior or hemodynamic instability secondary to a new physiologic process or complications related to the operation itself must be made. No absolute recovery scales exist, but a postanesthesia recovery score (PARS), introduced by Aldrete, has provided an impetus to analyze the recovery period. Based on motor performance, respiratory and hemodynamic stability, and level of consciousness in a manner similar to that used in the Apgar score of the neonate, the PARS system enables recovery room staff nurses to qualify recovery for an individual patient, and, in some instances, the system enables comparison of anesthetic techniques on recovery, in both the quality and duration of the process. A major variable left unexamined on this score is patient temperature, which may have a marked effect on recovery time and the hemodynamic stability of the period. An example of the importance of temperature is seen following aortic aneurysm surgery, during which time the perfusion of the lower extremities distal to the grafted area is of major concern. Although a patient with low core temperature and peripheral vasoconstriction may appear to have a stable pulse rate and stable blood pressure, the blood flow to the extremities is compromised. Not only must rewarming be accomplished expeditiously, but the need for vigorous volume resuscitation must be supported as the core temperature increases with concomitant peripheral vasodilatation. If the blood volume is not supported, relative hypovolemia may progress to hypotension, decreased peripheral perfusion and blood flow throughout the new graft, possible renal compromise, and increased strain on myocardial oxygen delivery. Singly or in concert, these changes can severely compromise the surgical result and cause significant postoperative morbidity.

SURGICAL COMPLICATIONS. These must be rapidly diagnosed, accurately assessed, and expeditiously treated for prevention of morbidity or mortality. In some instances, such as postthyroidectomy hemorrhage with resultant airway compromise, the residual anesthetic effects have a minor role in obscuring the problem. However, in other situations, such as postsurgical intra-abdominal hemorrhage, postoperative hemodynamic instability may be confused with a period of rewarming and increased blood volume supplementation. Also, pain, which may be an important symptom, is also an expected accompaniment of surgical therapy. Therefore, prior to the administration of analgesics, it is just as important to obtain a brief pain history in the recovery room as it is elsewhere. In most instances, the patient, with appropriate coaching, is able to distinguish incisional pain from other and perhaps more significant complaints (e.g., acute onset of angina in a patient following thoracotomy or abdominal surgery).

PRE-EXISTING MEDICAL DISEASE. As the patient population ages and surgical and anesthetic techniques improve, longer and more complex procedures are being performed on a less stable, sicker patient population with complex preoperative pharmacology. The preanesthetic visit identifies areas of special concern, and it is of vital importance that an adequate preparation be given to the recovery room team to ensure their full anticipation of the complexities of the case. Requirements for adequate postoperative monitoring and plans for active pharmacologic intervention must be met.

Surgical Intensive Care Unit

Although initially modeled on the postanesthesia recovery room, surgical intensive care units (ICUs) have acquired a place, character, and responsibility distinct from and yet complementary to that of the recovery room. Although the operating room provides most admissions to this area, the unit also functions as a preoperative stabilization and diagnostic area and as a resuscitative area following trauma and sepsis (conditions that may or may not lead to the operating room). The usual candidate for admission is a patient unlikely to recover completely in the usual 2- to 4-hour recovery time because of pre-existing medical problems, complexity of operation and anesthesia, or duration of operation alone. Postcardiac surgical ICUs provide an example of the further development of specialized surgical ICUs for specific surgical candidates. The common denominator that should characterize all intensive care areas includes specialized nursing services with highly motivated and continually updated nursing staff; continuous in-unit physician surveillance; ready access to all hospital support services, including respiratory therapy, diagnostic radiology, and a designated unit medical director who provides continuity of care and coordination of resident instruction and consultation services. In many respects, the modern surgical ICU parallels the operating room in that multiple illnesses and procedures must be performed in a highly specialized environment. Specialized units such as those for neurosurgery or cardiothoracic surgery, by the nature of the relatively uniform and predictable patient population, are, in general, easier to staff and equip than a multidisciplinary or general surgical ICU.

Training in intensive care medicine is now recognized as a multidisciplinary responsibility because of the necessity of specialty boundary crossing and elimination of the territorial attitudes of traditional medical practice. Current controversies surrounding patient management underscore the point that there can be no absolutes and that good care must explore all possible avenues of treatment. Ultimately, a management decision will be reached and the role of the intensive care team will be to provide adequate surveillance and direction to incorporate the goals of the management protocol.

Preoperative physiologic and hemodynamic assessment is assuming an increasingly important place in the complete management of the high-risk operative candidate. In a manner similar to diagnostic cardiac catheterization, the preoperative patient may be admitted to the surgical ICU for hemodynamic assessment. This may include placement of pulmonary artery and radial arterial catheters and subsequent manipulation of physiologic variables that stress the patient and provide valuable insight into the ability to withstand subsequent anesthetic and surgical manipulation. Data collected may include information on preloading and cardiac performance, intrapulmonary shunt, renal failure, and, in some cases, patient motivation. There is great practical importance to these manipulations in terms of the subsequent anesthetic management and postsurgical ICU course of monitored patients. There is also evidence suggesting that some patients can be identified who, despite aggressive preoperative preparation and physiologic manipulation, are at such great risk that operative mortality in elective surgery is unacceptable. In this group, surgical therapy should not be performed unless it is designed to correct the limiting physiologic variable. In this sense, the ICU is developing a role as a diagnostic, physiologic preparation unit.

In the postoperative period, ICU staff must cope with problems inherent in acute patient management and also with the complex challenges of chronic, recuperative care, including innovative home care and in-hospital activities for chronically ill but stable patients.

CARDIOPULMONARY ANESTHESIA

Cardiac Surgery

The principles of anesthetic management of patients for cardiac surgery differ little from those required for other types of surgical procedures. However, specific procedure-related knowledge is essential for optimal management. Understanding of the underlying hemodynamic abnormalities and their functional effects on the patient dictates the choice of anesthetic drugs.

The general approach to anesthetizing the patient who has heart disease should focus upon the individual patient and the functional hemodynamic state. A pre-anesthetic evaluation should include a thorough history, reviewing current and past medical illnesses, and previous anesthetic and surgical procedures. Current drug therapy should be carefully detailed. The potential benefits and risks of continuing or discontinuing the medication before operation should be evaluated. For example, the abrupt discontinuation of propranolol prior to operation is known to cause rebound hypertension and exacerbate cardiac symptoms. Of paramount importance is ascertaining the presence or absence of cardiac failure and assessing functional performance with stress such as exercise.

Routine laboratory data should be reviewed, minimal requirements being a complete blood count, serum electrolytes, a renal function screen, and a coagulation survey. More important, special laboratory investigations should be reviewed, because they are informative and prognostic in the assessment of dysfunction, infarction, and dysrhythmias. The presence of cardiomegaly on chest films is predictive of poor ventricular function in most patients. Rest and exercise ECGs are predictive for detection of both dysrhythmia and ischemia. With M-mode and two-dimensional echocardiography, an assessment of wall motion abnormalities and left ventricular dysfunction can be made. The use of radioisotope imaging is useful for the detection of ventricular dysfunction, but the prognostic value is yet to be determined. Finally, cardiac catheterization and angiography data should be reviewed, because they are the most accurate and informative techniques for definition of structural abnormalities and quantification of ventricular function. Data yielded by these models are both informative and prognostic in terms of ventricular function such as ejection fraction, cardiac output, and the presence or absence of wall motion abnormalities, as well as angiographic information regarding structural defects, whether acquired or congenital.

Anesthetic Management

A safe and effective anesthetic plan should be developed based on the individual patient and the disease state, the surgical procedure, the available anesthetic drugs and techniques, and the anticipated requirements for postoperative care.

The goal of a preanesthetic medication is a calm, cooperative patient during the preinduction period. The preoperative medication should suppress anxiety and pain associated with the placement of invasive monitoring devices and provide some amnesia of the preoperative period. Most premedication schedules are designed to provide sufficient sedation to allow an atraumatic, smooth induction of anesthesia. A typical regimen might be a combination of diazepam and a narcotic such as morphine.

Monitoring

Although the entire spectrum of monitoring capability is available, application should be individualized to each patient and to the surgical procedure after evaluating the benefits and the risks. Both invasive and noninvasive techniques are used, depending upon which is appropriate. Minimal requirements for monitoring include a precordial stethoscope, blood pressure cuff, temperature probe, urinary bladder catheter, a continuous ECG with a recorder and a precordial (V5) lead, a continuous arterial blood pressure monitor, blood gas analysis, and a method for determining anticoagulant activity. Specialized monitoring is indicated in certain circumstances for some patients. This monitoring may include use of a pulmonary artery catheter for assessment of ventricular filling pressures, cardiac output determinations, and mixed venous oxygen saturations. Newer techniques such as intraesophageal echocardiography are still in the evaluation phase.

Anesthetic Technique

As stated previously, the choice of a specific anesthetic technique is governed by the patient's medical condition and the surgical procedure, as well as by the anesthesiologist's ability to control hemodynamic variables at the time of operation. There are no absolute indications for or against any type of anesthetic agent currently used in cardiac anesthesia. The halogenated agents (halothane, enflurane, isoflurane) offer rapidity of induction and recovery, minimal side effects, and good muscle relaxation, and they suppress the sympathoadrenal stress response to surgical intervention. Levels required for anesthesia during operations are well tolerated hemodynamically in the patient with good left ventricular function. Because these agents are direct myocardial depressants, their use in patients with poor ventricular function should be avoided. In such patients, hemodynamic deterioration may occur before the anesthetic state is achieved.

Intravenous agents, specifically the narcotics, are chosen when minimal cardiovascular depression is particularly important. The narcotic analgesics have become the primary anesthetic for patients with impaired ventricular function. Included in this group of agents are morphine and fentanyl, and the fentanyl derivatives, alfentanil and sufentanil. The major advantage of the narcotic agents is the hemodynamic stability provided, especially in patients at risk of cardiac decompensation. The major disadvantage of the narcotic analgesics as anesthetics is the requirement for high doses to reliably achieve amnesia and a stress-free state, often necessitating the need for postoperative ventilation. Muscle relaxants are an integral part of anesthetic management for operations in these patients, because they permit the use of smaller amounts of potent, depressant anesthetics.

Cardiopulmonary Bypass

A knowledge of the fundamentals of cardiopulmonary bypass (CPB) is essential for the safe and effective management of extracorporeal circulation. The anesthesiologist must understand the CPB circuit, the various oxygenators, and the requirements for pump priming solutions. Prior to the cannulation of the great vessels, intravenous heparin (3 mg. per kg.) is administered to ensure proper anticoagulation prior to CPB. Serial measurements of activated clotting time (ACT) are performed before and during CPB, maintaining the ACT level above 400 seconds.

Several important problems that should be familiar to the anesthesiologist may develop during the initiation of CPB. Initiation of CPB is a physiologic stress for the patient, and the hemodynamic alterations may require pharmacologic intervention. Another problem that may be encountered is obstruction of venous return due to venous cannulas. Malpositioning of the aortic cannula may also cause significant reduction of perfusion. Pump flow should be set at or above the calculated normal resting cardiac output for the individual patient, with adjustments made depending upon the degree of body temperature and the perfusion hematocrit. Mean blood pressure during CPB can then be adjusted into a range of 40 to 90 mm. Hg by using vasopressors and vasodilators. A working knowledge of CPB should also include an understanding of myocardial preservation and the role of cardioplegia.

During the rewarming phase of CPB, the anesthesiologist must address the need to administer additional anesthetic drugs, evaluate the adequacy of anticoagulation, and make an assessment of hematocrit, serum potassium, and arterial blood gas data. Just before discontinuing CPB, the core temperature should be greater than 36° C., spontaneous or pacemaker-produced cardiac rhythm must be capable of generating cardiac output, ventilation of the lungs should be initiated, and venting of arterial air should be accomplished prior to ventricular ejection. With the gradual discontinuation of CPB, preload, ventricular ejection, and afterload conditions should be optimized. If indicated, inotropic or vasodilator therapy may be initiated and titrated to optimal cardiac performance. After the discontinuation of CPB and decannulation of the vena cava and aorta, protamine reversal of heparin is accomplished. Maintenance of circulating blood volume is achieved by blood transfusion, administration of fresh frozen plasma, and platelet infusion as indicated. Hemodynamic adjustments are made on the basis of cardiac output determinations, systemic and pulmonary artery pressure measurements, and cardiac rhythm. Also, attention should focus on adequate ventilation, urinary output, and body temperature after CPB. The anesthetic requirements after CPB are guided by the same principles as those before CPB.

Postoperative Care

The major requirements for safe transportation of the postoperative cardiac patient include adequate airway maintenance, monitoring of a continuous ECG and arterial pressure, and pharmacologic or electrical therapy. The immediate postoperative care of these patients necessitates an intensive care unit with experienced personnel to provide circulatory and ventilatory support. From observations made in the operating room, the anesthesiologist possesses valuable information concerning the patient's condition in the early postoperative period. This information should be carefully relayed to surgical colleagues and others caring for the patient in the ICU. Full ventilatory support should be maintained until the patient achieves hemodynamic stability and the absence of significant postoperative bleeding. When these conditions are met and the patient is awake, with protective airway reflexes intact, ventilatory support can be withdrawn and the patient can be extubated.

Pulmonary Surgery

Careful assessment and management of patients with pulmonary disease are essential parts of anesthesia for thoracic operations. Preoperative assessment focuses on the nature and degree of cardiopulmonary function. Inquiries regarding exercise tolerance, cyanosis, and symptoms of respiratory distress delineate those patients at risk during anesthesia. A number of common laboratory tests are helpful in the preoperative evaluation of these patients and should include chest films, a complete blood count, sputum analysis, ECG, and pulmonary function testing.

Thoracic surgical patients are at high risk of postoperative complications. The incidence of postoperative pulmonary complications is correlated with the degree of preoperative respiratory dysfunction. Vigorous preoperative pulmonary preparation can significantly reduce these complications. These preoperative measures should include discontinuation of smoking, antibiotic treatment of acute infection, the use of bronchodilators, chest physiotherapy, deep breathing and coughing exercises, and incentive spirometry.

Close communication between the anesthesiologist and the surgeon preoperatively and intraoperatively is essential, because the surgical procedure often requires a shared airway and respiratory tract. Constant observation of the surgical field by the anesthesiologist is very important. An ECG should be done; and blood pressure, body temperature, inspired oxygen tension, and breath sounds must be monitored. Additionally, radial artery catheterization allows frequent assessment of blood gases and continuous observation of blood pressure. The use of a pulmonary artery catheter is reserved for patients with left ventricular dysfunction.

General anesthesia with controlled ventilation is the safest method of anesthetizing these patients. Although a variety of general anesthetic techniques can be used, the preferred method of most anesthesiologists is one using halogenated anesthetics, because they permit high inspired oxygen concentrations, relaxation of bronchomotor tone, and rapid elimination at the termination of the procedure. Special anesthetic techniques may be used in pulmonary surgery, especially one-lung anesthesia. The absolute indications for one-lung anesthesia with an endobronchial tube include massive hemorrhage, bronchopleural fistula, unilateral infection, pulmonary air cysts, and unilateral bronchopulmonary lavage. Relative indications for one-lung anesthesia include the need for surgical exposure, especially for pneumonectomy and thoracic aortic aneurysm. Patients with poor respiratory function or cardiac disease may be poorly suited for one-lung anesthesia.

The timing of extubation is based on the degree of preoperative pulmonary disease, the nature of the operation, and the postoperative status of the patient. The major abnormality in the postoperative period is that of gradual and progressive alveolar collapse. For minimizing this effect, pain should be treated so that deep breathing can take place. Additional postoperative maneuvers may include voluntary expiratory maneuvers, chest physiotherapy, deep-breathing exercises, and incentive spirometry.

ANESTHESIA FOR NEUROSURGERY

Optimal anesthetic management of the neurosurgical patient requires a knowledge of cerebral blood flow, intracranial pressure control, and the dynamics of brain injury. A detailed knowledge of the physiologic and pharmacologic control of the cerebral circulation is essential in order to preserve the patient's neurologic function. Of paramount importance is the alteration of the cerebral circulation and intracranial pressure by drugs and disease states.

Physiologic Considerations

The intracranial contents consist of brain matter, cerebral blood volume, and CSF. The contents are essentially incompressible. The translocation of the CSF to extracranial areas serves as a major mechanism for volume equilibration during brain expansion. When this volume-buffering capacity is exhausted, no further room exists to accommodate any expanding intracranial mass. Thereafter, the intracranial pressure rises rapidly. At this point, small changes in volume are associated with large changes in intracranial pressure. Therefore, it is necessary to reduce cerebral blood flow and consequently cerebral blood volume to limit the rise in intracranial pressure.

The major determinants of cerebral blood flow are arterial CO_2 and O_2, systemic arterial pressure, and temperature. $Paco_2$ is linearly related to cerebral blood flow. High $Paco_2$ leads to increased cerebral blood flow, whereas hypocarbia decreases cerebral blood flow. Arterial oxygen tension has little effect on cerebral blood flow except when the Pao_2 is below 50 mm. Hg, at which level cerebral blood flow increases. The arterial pressure has minimal effect on cerebral blood flow between 60 and 160 mm. Hg due to autoregulatory reflexes which preserve uniform blood flow. Elevation of arterial pressure above 160 mm. Hg leads to increased cerebral blood flow, and arterial pressure below 60 mm. Hg leads to decreased cerebral blood flow. Factors that increase intracranial pressure by increasing cerebral blood volume include hypercapnia, hypoxia, head-down position, jugular venous obstruction, positive end-expiratory pressure (PEEP), hyperthermia, volatile anesthetics, muscle activity, pain, and arterial hypertension. Factors that decrease intracranial pressure by reducing cerebral blood volume include hypocapnia, head-up position, neutral position of the head, hypothermia, barbiturates, neuromuscular blockade, hyperventilation, analgesia, and arterial hypotension.

Neurosurgical Anesthesia Management

The purpose of the preoperative visit is for the anesthesiologist to become familiar with the patient's neurologic condition and to institute corrective measures so that the patient is in an optimal physiologic state prior to operation. Preoperative evaluation should include a thorough medical history and physical examination that focus on a detailed neurologic assessment, an assessment of intracranial pressure, and current drug therapy. The computed tomography (CT) scan should be reviewed for evidence of brain displacement and of previous intraventricular catheter insertion, and intracranial compliance should be assessed. Preoperative medication may be limited to a barbiturate. Narcotics should be avoided in patients with increased intracranial pressure. The safest course is to omit premedication altogether when feasible.

Monitoring

Essential monitoring of the neurosurgical patient includes blood pressure measurement, a continuous ECG, a precordial stethoscope, a temperature probe, and an O_2 analyzer on the inspiratory limb of the anesthesia machine. Operations involving intracranial trauma, vascular tumors, mass lesions, patients in the sitting position, and induced hypotension are all indications for more specialized monitoring, including continuous measurement of intra-arterial pressure, central venous pressure, an end-tidal CO_2 monitor, a urinary bladder catheter, and an intracranial pressure monitor. During operations in which air embolism is a risk, that is, where the site of operation is higher than the heart (e.g., sitting position), a precordial Doppler ultrasound transducer and a pulmonary artery pressure monitor may be helpful for the detection of air embolism.

Anesthetic Management

The essential elements of a smooth and safe anesthetic procedure are maintenance of an adequate airway and ventilation, the absence of coughing or straining, appropriate anesthetics that reduce or do not alter cerebral blood flow, and a rapid return to consciousness at the end of the surgical procedure. In patients with elevated intracranial pressure, measures to improve intracranial compliance prior to induction include elevation of the head, administration of osmotic diuretics (e.g., mannitol), and avoidance of drugs that reduce compliance. In patients with closed head trauma or with altered states of consciousness, it is best to assume a noncompliant response and to take precautions against any further increases in intracranial volume.

Induction of anesthesia should be rapid and smooth after voluntary hyperventilation and accomplished with agents that reduce intracranial pressure. Thiopental is the usual induction agent used, followed by passive hyperventilation, combined with intravenous doses of a narcotic such as fentanyl and a muscle relaxant. Thereafter, anesthetic depth is adjusted to

known stimulation patterns such as endotracheal intubation, head clamping, incision, dural opening and closing, and skin closure. The stimuli during these events may cause blood pressure elevation, coughing, or straining, and these responses should be blunted by maintenance anesthetics such as fentanyl and continual neuromuscular blockade. All volatile anesthetics may increase cerebral blood flow and intracranial pressure, although the effect is dose-related and, in the case of isoflurane, may be prevented by hyperventilation before its use. Hyperventilation is continued when N_2O is used. Osmotherapy is used when a negative fluid balance is desirable. Isotonic solutions are preferred so that rebound cerebral edema is avoided.

It is essential that "bucking" on the endotracheal tube during emergence from anesthesia be avoided. Neuromuscular blockade is not reversed until the application of the head bandage in order to ensure a smooth emergence and extubation. Small, intermittent doses of thiopental or lidocaine may also further control emergence from anesthesia. Having an alert, cooperative patient with an adequate airway at termination of the operation is the goal of safe anesthetic management.

In the recovery room, careful observation of vital signs as well as repeated neurologic examinations and assessment of consciousness are mandatory. Additionally, continuous monitoring of arterial blood pressure, ECG, and urinary output provides valuable guides to postoperative management. When appropriate, intracranial pressure monitoring is of valuable assistance in monitoring selected neurosurgical patients. Patients are generally permitted to recover in a semisitting position, and sedatives and analgesics are generally avoided because of the minimal postoperative pain associated with neurosurgical operations. Also, these drugs may cause decreased ventilation and may interfere with the evaluation of neurologic function. Initial postoperative problems include cerebral edema, intracranial hemorrhage, seizures, fluid and electrolyte disturbances, inadequate ventilation, hypertension, and fever. Rapid recognition of these problems and appropriate therapy are the cornerstones of management of the postoperative neurosurgical patient.

PEDIATRIC ANESTHESIA

Mortality in infants and children has decreased dramatically over the past 50 years, largely because of advances in pediatric medicine, including antibiotic therapy, a better understanding of pathophysiologic states in children, and advances in surgical therapy and intensive care. The increased survival of small infants has been accompanied by an increased number of problems requiring anesthesia and surgical therapy, for example, patent ductus arteriosus, necrotizing enterocolitis, and inguinal hernia. With further advances, it is expected that many more infants and children with congenital anomalies will survive and that increasing numbers of infants and young children will be anesthetized for operation.

The risks of a specific anesthetic for a surgical procedure are greater in patients who are younger than 1 year of age, compared with the risks in older patients and adults. During the past decade, there has been a significant reduction in the combined anesthetic and surgical mortality among children, even patients who are seriously ill. The reduction in anesthetic mortality is largely due to major medical advances affecting pediatric anesthesia, including improved understanding of the physiology and adaptation of the neonate to extrauterine life, advances in clinical pharmacology of various inhalation and intravenous anesthetic agents and muscle relaxants, improved technology of monitoring equipment, and extensive improvement in postoperative intensive care, including respiratory therapy.

Equipment

Maintenance of an airway in children requires an appreciation of both quantitative and qualitative differences in anatomy and physiology. Special anesthesia circuits for the pediatric patient are designed to minimize apparatus dead space and flow resistance as well as to provide adequate humidification. Appropriately sized endotracheal tubes should be uncuffed in children younger than 8 years of age and should allow a small leak during positive pressure ventilation to avoid mechanical trauma to the trachea and possible later subglottic edema. Older children usually require a cuffed endotracheal tube, because the narrowest portion of their larynx is at the level of the vocal cords and not in the subglottic region, as in young infants.

Monitoring

The principles of monitoring are the same in both the pediatric and adult populations, but the differences in physiology and anatomy require modification of method. Basic monitoring of any anesthetized child should include a continuous ECG monitor, a method for blood pressure measurements, a rectal or esophageal temperature probe, an inspiratory O_2 analyzer, and a precordial stethoscope that allows continuous monitoring of heart rate and breath sounds. For certain operations, such as thoracotomies or open heart surgery, or specialized techniques, such as deliberate hypotensive anesthesia for operations with a large expected blood loss, one should consider continuous arterial pressure monitoring, central venous pressure measurements, or pulmonary artery catheterization.

Preoperative Evaluation and Preparation

The preoperative visit allows the physician not only to evaluate the child but also to prepare the child and the parent psychologically for anesthesia and operation. A preoperative review of systems should focus on the child's present illness and his functional capabilities; an assessment of underlying medical diseases and therapy; prior anesthetic history; the presence of any associated congenital anomalies; an assessment of any recent intercurrent illnesses, such as an upper respiratory infection; and a review of anesthetic complications in parents, siblings, or relatives. The physical examination should include an assessment of the patient's general health and exercise tolerance, the cardiopulmonary system, and the state of hydration. Minimal laboratory work-up on pediatric patients consists of a hemoglobin measurement and a hematocrit.

Preoperative feeding should be individualized for each patient, with the following factors taken into consideration: the timing of the surgical procedure and seeking a balance between the need for an empty stomach and the fluid and glucose requirements of the child.

Preoperative medication for the pediatric patient should be individualized according to the patient's needs and institutional practices. Preoperative sedation may be provided by intramuscular narcotics or by an oral regimen of a narcotic, a sedative, and a minor tranquilizer such as meperidine, pentobarbital, and diazepam. These premedications should be individualized and should be given approximately 1 hour prior to the induction of anesthesia. In some circumstances, a skillful preoperative visit with a cooperative patient may obviate the need for a preoperative medication altogether.

Anesthetic Management

All the common inhalation and intravenous agents and techniques have been used in children. However, one of two general anesthetic techniques is usually chosen for children, and ventilation is usually controlled: (1) oxygen, N_2O, a narcotic, and an intravenous nondepolarizing muscle relaxant or (2) oxygen, N_2O, and a halogenated agent, with or without a nondepolarizing muscle relaxant. The technique for induction of anesthesia depends upon the age, size, hazard of regurgitation, and physical status of the patient. For young children and those who are apprehensive of needles, a mask induction of anesthesia is preferred by most anesthesiologists. When the child loses consciousness, an intravenous cannula may be placed. For older children, a routine intravenous induction is normally used. Tracheal intubation and controlled ventilation are indicated in (1) operations of the head and neck, (2) intrathoracic and intraperitoneal procedures, (3) operations in the prone position, (4) most procedures in infants younger than 1 year of age, and (5) all emergency procedures.

The goal of intravenous therapy in this group of patients is to meticulously avoid either deficits or excesses of fluids and electrolytes throughout the perioperative period. The fluid therapy calculations should include estimates of preoperative deficits, intraoperative maintenance fluid requirements, intraoperative third space losses, and estimated blood loss. Careful administration and monitoring of fluid therapy are very important and are instituted with the use of a calibrated infusion pump or a calibrated gravity-dependent infusion system. Intraoperative fluid therapy demands attention to detail, with consideration given to the preoperative state of the patient, the extent of surgical procedure, and the choice of anesthetic agents and techniques.

At the conclusion of the surgical procedure, neuromuscular blockade should be reversed in most circumstances. Extubation should be accomplished, usually when the patient is fully awake and exhibits complete return of muscle strength, thus ensuring a patent, functional airway upon withdrawal of the endotracheal tube. Children should be transported to the recovery room with a precordial stethoscope in place to monitor heart rate and breath sounds. Oxygen is administered in the recovery room until consciousness is regained. Common recovery room problems include emergence delirium, pain, anxiety, nausea and vomiting, airway obstruction, and intravenous disruption. Each of the problems, when present, should be treated in an emergent and appropriate manner.

GERIATRIC ANESTHESIA

The risks of a specific anesthetic and surgical procedure are greater in the geriatric population, defined as age 70 or older, when compared with all other age groups except the very young. In large part, this is due to the deterioration of various physiologic functions that have a significant impact upon the perioperative management of these patients. Additionally, most operations performed in this population are major or emergent or involve major organ systems. As with the very young patient, it is better to assess the anesthetic and surgical risks on the basis of the patient's physiologic state, rather than chronologic age. Functional differences in the cardiovascular system of the elderly patient include physiologic changes in characteristics of the myocardium, the vascular tone, the autonomic nervous system, and the stress response. In general, the autonomic nervous system demonstrates attenuated response to significant circulatory changes in blood pressure. This is especially true of the baroreceptor responses that are diminished in the aged. There is a decreased end-organ response to the circulating catecholamines secreted during stress. Both cardiac output and cardiac index slowly decline with age, achieving their lowest levels in the elderly. This decline is largely due to the progressive process of atherosclerosis, which causes the increased afterload observed in the elderly. Functional abnormalities of wall motion and ejection fraction are observed in this group of patients during exercise. The gradual change in the systemic arterial circulation toward the development of noncompliant and inelastic vessels causes hypertension. The net result of these changes is the limited response to cardiac compromise, which decreases the margin of safety for anesthetic agents and surgical stress.

The respiratory system of the elderly patient demonstrates important physiologic changes due to the aging process. There are functional differences in respiratory control. These changes are manifested by an altered CO_2 response curve, which is markedly depressed in the presence of narcotics. Abnormal breathing patterns during natural sleep are characterized by periods of apnea and by periodic breathing. Elderly patients possess diminished protective reflexes, especially gag and cough, and may aspirate fluids. When compared with the normal adult, the geriatric patient exhibits an increase in functional residual capacity and residual volume, as well as closing volume. These changes are secondary to decreased lung elastic recoil and decreased chest compliance. The net result is a closing capacity that operates in the tidal breathing range, which causes an increase in ventilation-perfusion mismatching. The clinical effect of these changes is a reduction of arterial Po_2. These specific changes in respiration are potential sources of perioperative problems and, therefore, place the geriatric patient at risk.

Pharmacology

The changes in pharmacology observed in the elderly patient may be attributed to both different pharmacokinetic parameters and an altered physiologic state associated with age. The pharmacokinetic changes are due, in part, to alterations in renal function and to diminished hepatic metabolic functions. Basically, the changes alter drug redistribution, clearance, and excretion, usually prolonging drug action. Moreover, the increased pain threshold of the elderly patient reduces the dose response for various agents, including analgesics. It is now well accepted that there is a reduced requirement for inhalation and intravenous anesthetics in older patients. The reduction in cardiac output and respiratory reserve requires a prolonged recovery from various intravenous drugs. The clinical consequence is that the elderly patient is more susceptible to the action of all drugs when compared with patients in other age groups.

Anesthetic Management

The preanesthetic evaluation in this group of patients is no different from that of any other age group. Review of the patient's past medical history as well as the physical examination should focus on the physiologic changes in the patient's condition, which were previously discussed. A working knowledge of the patient's physiologic abnormalities helps assess the patient's capability of tolerating the effects of anesthesia and operation and assists in devising a safe anesthetic plan. There is a potential for excessive sedation; thus, premedication in this group of patients should be eliminated or used sparingly.

The monitoring requirements should be individualized, and the patient's medical condition and attendant risk, as well as the particular surgical procedure, should be considered. Essential monitoring in all patients should include measurement of blood pressure, ECG, and the use of a precordial stethoscope, an oxygen analyzer, and a temperature probe. Special monitoring of continuous arterial pressure or the use of a pulmonary artery catheter may be warranted during certain surgical procedures or in a patient who is at high risk for major complications.

There is no proven benefit to one anesthetic technique over another in managing these patients. Morbidity and mortality appear to be the same whether a general or a regional anesthetic is chosen.

Other considerations during anesthetic management should include avoidance of hypothermia during the surgical procedure, which increases oxygen consumption during rewarming and raises systemic vascular resistance at the same time as prolonging drug effects. Additionally, careful fluid and electrolyte management in the perioperative period is essential because of the limited renal reserve in these patients.

Finally, optimal cerebral blood flow must be maintained. This is accomplished by maintenance of normal arterial pressure, keeping the head in the neutral position, and maintaining normocarbia.

Upon emergence from general anesthesia, the usual concerns regarding laryngospasm, vomiting, and excitement should be observed. Additionally, these patients may hypoventilate for long periods of time because of delayed metabolism and excretion of chosen anesthetic agents.

OUTPATIENT ANESTHESIA

Outpatient surgery is defined as provision of surgical services that require anesthesia and a period of postoperative observation to patients who are not expected to require overnight hospitalization. In recent years, the concept of outpatient surgery has enjoyed renewed interest for providing an alternative means of performing procedures that are too demanding for the surgeon's office, yet not sufficiently complex to require inpatient hospitalization. Historically, many of the earliest general anesthetics were administered to outpatients, with excellent clinical outcome. Nicolo reported a series of almost 9000 outpatient operations in 1909 with 50 per cent of the patients less than 3 years of age. Procedures in this series included repair of cleft lip and palate, myelomeningocele, depressed skull fracture, pyloromyotomy, and herniorrhaphy. Although contemporary outpatient selection is more restricted, these programs may provide enhanced utilization of hospital facilities, thus serving as a safe cost-effective alternative to traditional hospitalization.

The advantages of outpatient surgery include reducing the cost of medical care; bed availability for those patients requiring hospitalization; decreased hospital-acquired infections; a timely surgical schedule with no undue delays due to complex cases; and, most important, an abbreviated hospital stay, obviating the need for extended separation from one's family or job. The disadvantages of such a surgical unit include the potential for problems in the patient with undiagnosed acute or chronic illness.

The selection of patients for outpatient surgery varies from institution to institution. Factors that influence the selection of these patients include the patient's condition, the type of surgical procedure, the incidence of postoperative complications, the reliability of the patient, the patient's psychologic acceptance of the situation, and the cooperation of the surgeon. The patient should be healthy, with stable control of any chronic illness such as seizures, asthma, or diabetes mellitus. The planned surgical procedure should be short and should not require major intervention in the abdomen, thorax, or cranium. The patient who needs prolonged postoperative observation either because of pre-existing illness or because of the surgical procedure is not considered a candidate for outpatient surgery.

A preoperative screening visit is an essential requirement for all patients. During this visit, a complete history and physical examination are obtained, as well as appropriate laboratory studies and consultations when indicated. This preanesthetic evaluation can occur from a few days up to 1 month prior to operation. It is best to accomplish this evaluation before the patient arrives in the hospital so as to minimize delays. Also, during this visit, anesthetic management is explained and specific preoperative instructions are given. An interval history is obtained on the day of operation for ascertaining changes from the original work-up, as well as diagnosing any potential intercurrent illness.

The essence of anesthetic management is rapid recovery. A variety of anesthetic agents and techniques have been chosen for outpatient anesthesia, attesting to the fact that there is no uniform anesthetic for outpatient surgery. Although requirements for these patients may be different, the approach and techniques should be the same as for any anesthetic in which the particular agent or technique is individualized to the needs of the patient in order to ensure a smooth induction, safe maintenance, and a rapid and comfortable recovery without compromising safety. Each patient should be carefully evaluated for need of postoperative pain relief. No patient should be denied an appropriate dose of narcotic because of fear of slightly delaying discharge. The surgical procedures that require frequent use of potent intravenous narcotics or major intravenous fluid administration for a translocation of body fluids are, by definition, not appropriate for outpatient surgery.

Recovery and early ambulation are major objectives in outpatient surgery. In managing outpatients, a safe discharge from the recovery room must be viewed as a safe discharge to home. Discharge criteria should include the following:

A physician available to personally discharge all patients.
Stable vital signs.
Return of protective reflexes, including cough, gag, and swallow.
Ability to ambulate.
Absence of airway or respiratory problems.
The patient's being fully awake and oriented to time and place.
Minimal nausea and vomiting.
An extended period of observation for those patients requiring endotracheal intubation or those receiving depressant medication for pain relief or vomiting.

The most frequent complications following outpatient anesthesia and surgical therapy are sore throat, croup, headache, nausea and vomiting, pain, bleeding, and slow emergence. Although life-threatening complications are rare, hospital admission criteria should be formulated to treat objectively these infrequent complications. It is clear that outpatient anesthesia and surgical procedures result in rare morbidity and mortality when the criteria for this form of practice are strictly formulated and followed. Anesthetic management of the surgical outpatient can be conducted safely and may offer cost-saving alternatives to traditional hospital practice. Maintenance of high standards of safety in the ambulatory setting is the mainstay for its continued success.

SUMMARY

The art and science of anesthetic practice has existed as a unique medical discipline for less than 150 years. During that time, the focus has changed from helping the patient tolerate surgical stress by rendering him insensible to pain to controlling stress and the patient's physiologic responses in the perioperative period by careful titration of powerful pharmacologic means and the appreciation of sound medical judgment. The anesthesiologist is an integral member of the patient's physician group and provides expertise in preoperative evaluation, preparation, resuscitation, intraoperative management, and postoperative outcome. Peripheral activities associated with this discipline include pain diagnosis and management, neonatology, critical care medicine, medical evacuation and transport programs, and others. New advances in pharmacology and microbiology will broaden future avenues of drug synthesis and mechanisms of anesthetic action. The search for the ideal agent or agents continues, and, as more powerful chemicals are synthesized, the requirement for increasingly sophisticated physician practitioners will increase.

SELECTED REFERENCES

Bromage, P. R.: Epidural Anesthesia. Philadelphia. W. B. Saunders Company, 1978.

This text gives a detailed account of epidural analgesia and anesthesia, bringing together clinical and laboratory information. Included is a section on the pharmacology of local anesthetics, which serves as a basis for logical use of these drugs in practice. Several clinical illustrations and actual case descriptions make this a complete resource.

Cottrell, J. E., and Turndof, H.: Anesthesia and Neurosurgery. St. Louis, C. V. Mosby Company, 1980.
This multiauthored text presents the application of basic information concerning central nervous system disease in a context of understanding the intracranial effects of anesthetic drugs and techniques. The text presents neuroanesthesia practice as an amalgam of neurology, neurosurgery, and anesthesia.

Dripps, R. D., Eckenhoff, J. E., and Vandam, L. K.: Introduction to Anesthesia, 6th ed. Philadelphia, W. B. Saunders Company, 1982.
This is the best introductory text in the field of anesthesiology. An overall view of the important aspects of anesthesia is presented in a uniform and concise style.

Gregory, G. A. (Ed.): Pediatric Anesthesia. New York, Churchill Livingstone, 1981.
This is the most comprehensive text for anesthetic care of the infant and child. It provides a physiologic and pharmacologic approach to anesthesia for the pediatric patient.

Miller, R. D. (Ed.): Anesthesia. New York, Churchill Livingstone, 1981.
The most current, comprehensive textbook of anesthesia that is available. Its two volumes were written by 31 contributors, all recognized experts in their particular subspecialty of anesthesia. This book is invaluable as a resource for both theoretical and practical knowledge.

Ream, A. K., and Fogdall, R. P.: Acute Cardiovascular Management. Anesthesia and Intensive Care. Philadelphia, J. B. Lippincott Company, 1982.
An excellent text that collates known principles of the care of the acutely unstable cardiovascular patient and presents a scientific basis for their medical management. Considerable effort has been expended to ensure that each major topic is covered thoroughly by experienced investigative anesthesiologists, cardiologists, and surgeons.

Scurr, C., and Feldman, S. (Eds.): Scientific Foundations in Anaesthesia, 2nd ed. London, Heinemanor Medical Books Ltd, 1974.
An excellent review of the scientific principles upon which are based the clinical practice of anesthesia, resuscitation, and intensive care. It details the physics, mathematics, and measurement techniques of practice with emphasis on practical knowledge.

Shoemaker, W. C., Thompson, W. L., and Holbrook, P. R. (Eds.): Textbook of Critical Care. Philadelphia, W. B. Saunders Company, 1984.
This text serves as the data base for a unique and comprehensive approach to the care of the critically ill, especially the patient with multiple organ system failure. The knowledge, skills, and attitudes necessary to the practice of critical care medicine are reviewed in this benchmark book.

Stanski, D. R., and Watkins, W. D.: Drug Disposition in Anesthesia. New York, Grune & Stratton, 1982.
This text describes both the mechanisms and the kinetics of drug disposition for intravenous drugs used in the practice of anesthesia and facilitates the application of pharmacokinetics reasoning to the practice of anesthesiology.

Critical Care Medicine

Blitt, C. D. (Ed.): Monitoring in Anesthesia and Critical Care Medicine. New York, Churchill Livingstone, 1985.
Chernow, B. (Ed.): The Pharmacologic Approach to the Critically Ill Patient, 2nd ed. Baltimore, Williams & Wilkins, 1988.
Civetta, J. M., Taylor, R. W., and Kirby, R. R. (Eds.): Critical Care. Philadelphia, J. B. Lippincott Company, 1988.
Lyerly, H. K. (Ed.): The Handbook of Surgical Intensive Care, 2nd ed. Chicago, Year Book Medical Publishers, 1989.
Shoemaker, W. C., Thompson, W. L., and Holbrook, P. D. (Eds.): Textbook of Critical Care, 2nd ed. Philadelphia, W. B. Saunders Company, 1988.
Snyder, J. V., and Pinsky, M. P. (Eds.): Oxygen Transport in the Critically Ill. Chicago, Year Book Medical Publishers, 1987.
It is hoped that these references provide a stimulating insight into the variegated field of Critical Care Medicine, and that interested students will continue their studies by adding to the current knowledge base.

10

WOUND HEALING
Biologic and Clinical Features

John W. Madden, M.D., and Arnold J. Arem, M.D.

The response of living tissues to injury forms the foundation of all surgical practice. Indeed, from a biologic viewpoint, tissue injury and its sequelae participate in a majority of general medical problems. Although the cardiologist discusses complications of myocardial infarction in physiologic terms (congestive heart failure, chronic arrhythmia, embolism, and so forth), the ultimate outcome may depend entirely on the healing reactions of the heart. The gastrointestinal surgeon attacks abnormal physiology by removing or rerouting segments of gut; the vascular surgeon restores peripheral blood flow with clever reconstructions or replacement of peripheral blood vessels. Although directed toward correcting physiologic abnormalities, these therapeutic manipulations depend entirely on the body's ability to repair tissue damage. Unfortunately, because wound healing represents such a basic response of living organisms to life and, generally, produces successful restoration of tissue integrity, the biology of repair is taken for granted or ignored by some physicians.

HISTORICAL ASPECTS

The passive attitude toward the biology of repair has historical roots. The earliest medical writings extensively consider wound care. Seven of the 48 case reports included in the Smith Papyrus (1700 B.C.) describe wounds and their management. Empirically, the ancient physicians of Egypt, Greece, India, and Europe developed gentle methods of treating wounds. They appreciated the necessity of removing foreign bodies, suturing, covering wounds with clean materials, and protecting injured tissues from corrosive agents.

During the fourteenth century, with the widespread use of gunpowder and the increasing frequency of bullet wounds, a new era of wound treatment emerged. Instead of maintaining a caretaker's attitude in wound management and relying on natural processes for repair, surgeons assumed an aggressive posture. Active and dramatic action was taken to "help wounds heal." Applications of boiling oil, burning oil, hot cautery, and scalding water replaced gentle washing with warmed, boiled water and the application of mild salves. Cleanliness was forgotten. Needless to say, this "lets-do-something-about-it" attitude toward wound healing produced disastrous results.

In the mid sixteenth century, Ambroise Paré, the great French army surgeon, rediscovered gentle methods. As in so many great biologic contributions, chance had a key role. During the Battle of Villaine, the supply of oil was exhausted, and Paré was forced to apply milder treatments to amputation wounds. To his surprise these wounds healed rapidly without the expected complications. From this beginning, the modern era of gentle wound care evolved. John Hunter, William Stewart Halsted, Alexis Carrel, and many other great clinical biologists demonstrated that minimizing tissue injury produces rapid and effective healing. The majority of technical advances in wound care over the past century have been based on a "minimal interference" concept: If the surgeon can remove all impediments, normal wound healing processes produce the best possible result

In most clinical situations this elegant, simple concept is sound. The greatest portion of this chapter is devoted to exploring the normal phenomenon of wound healing and demonstrating ways to allow the normal course of events to occur. Unfortunately, however, the normal response of tissues to injury does not always produce a perfectly functional result. The same processes that establish strength and integrity in incisions of the bowel or abdominal wall also produce fibrous stricture of the esophagus, rheumatic valvular disease, cirrhosis of the liver, incarcerated tendons, keloids, intestinal adhesions, and a host of other abnormalities. If effective methods of controlling shape, size, and physical properties of scars existed, a new phase of wound management could evolve. The pathophysiologic phenomena created by scar formation would no longer be considered inevitable. Effective control would replace minimal interference as a guiding principle. To some observers, this new era in wound management appears imminent. Experimentally, the wound healing process can be altered effectively, eliminating or reducing the pathophysiologic consequences of scar formation. Current methods of controlling scar formation are discussed briefly at the close of this chapter.

BIOLOGIC CONSIDERATIONS

Wound healing represents a highly dynamic, integrated series of cellular, physiologic, and biochemical events that occur exclusively in whole organisms. Although individual components of the wound healing reaction (cell multiplication, cell migration, collagen synthesis, collagen cross-linking, and so forth) occur in tissue culture or even in cell-free systems, wounds do not heal in a bottle, nor do single events occur in isolation. Examining all processes simultaneously, however, can be confusing. For the purposes of this discussion, wound healing is separated into several natural components and later discussed as an integrated whole. Again, although all wounds heal by the same basic processes, clinical wounds are of two distinct types – simple closed wounds and open wounds with or without tissue loss. For organizational purposes, each of these clinical situations is discussed separately.

CLOSED WOUNDS

Morphologic Events

INFLAMMATION. Disrupting tissue integrity by accidental trauma or the surgeon's knife initiates a series of striking morphologic changes. After a transient vasoconstriction, all local small vessels dilate. As dilatation occurs, capillaries become abnormally permeable to proteins and plasma leaks into the site of injury. Coincident with vasomotor changes, alterations occur at the interface between white blood cells and endothelium. White cells adhere to endothelial surfaces, particularly small venules, and actively migrate through the vessel walls. Within hours after injury, the wound space fills with a highly cellular, inflammatory exudate composed of white cells, red cells, soluble plasma proteins, and fibrin strands. The duration and intensity of this inflammatory response depend on the amount of local tissue damage. Extensive tissue injury or the presence of foreign materials or bacteria can prolong the inflammatory phase for months. In the usual clean incision, however, acute inflammation subsides within a few days.

In the early stages of inflammation, actively motile white cells migrate into the wound and begin engulfing and removing cellular debris and injured tissue fragments. At first, polymorphonuclear leukocytes appear to predominate, even though the ratio of granulocytes to monocytes in blood and extracellular exudate is identical. As the transient phase of white cell migration ends and the shorter-lived granulocytes die, lyse, and release acid hydrolases into the local environment, the proportion of monocytes increases significantly, differential survival rates representing the shift in cell population.[92] Monocytes can continue their scavenging activity for weeks.

The precise role that each inflammatory cell type has in the wound healing process remains obscure, but studies using specific anticellular antisera suggest that wound healing proceeds normally in the absence of both polymorphonuclear granulocytes and lymphocytes. In contrast, monocytes must be present to create normal fibroblast production and invasion of the wound space.[33,51]

EPITHELIALIZATION. While dead material is being removed from deeper areas, important events occur at the edges of epithelial wounds. In skin wounds, the epidermis immediately adjacent to the wound edge begins thickening within 24 hours after injury. Marginal basal cells lose their firm attachment to underlying dermis, enlarge, and begin to migrate down and across the defect. Fixed basal cells in a zone near the cut edge undergo a series of rapid mitotic divisions, and daughter cells emigrate, presumably directed in their migrations by contact guidance along fibrin strands and by contact inhibition.[67] Within 48 hours, the entire wound surface is re-epithelialized. Deeper recesses of the wound contain only fibrin strands and inflammatory cells at this point. After bridging the wound defect, migrating epithelial cells lose their flattened appearance, become more columnar in shape, and increase mitotic activity. Layering of epithelium is re-established, and surface cells keratinize. The epithelial-mesenchymal interface, however, never regains a normal architecture.[43]

This remarkable response of epithelial cells to injury is not confined to surface areas. Injury to any epithelial element can initiate epithelial cell migration. For example, if sutures remain in skin wounds for more than a few days, epithelial cells migrate down the suture tracts. Subsequent epithelial thickening and keratinization may produce marked foreign body reactions and sterile abscesses. Even subcuticular sutures that incise hair follicles or sweat glands can become surrounded by epithelial tracts and produce epithelial cysts.[68]

CELLULAR PHASE. As the inflammatory reaction subsides and the epithelial surface thickens, a new cell type appears in the wound depths. Beginning on the second or third day, spindle-shaped cells with oval nuclei become increasingly abundant and by 10 days dominate the cell population. Shortly after this cellular invasion, collagen fibers appear in the wound. Conclusive data indicate that this new cell type, the fibroblast, synthesizes and secretes collagen molecules. Although usually the active fibroblast is described as a stellate or spindle-shaped cell, direct observations of living material demonstrate that fibroblasts can assume almost any configuration. The electron microscopic appearance, however, is characteristic (Fig. 1). In addition to a diffuse Golgi apparatus and large mitochondria with irregular cristae, fibroblasts contain an extensively developed and dilated rough endoplasmic reticulum. The long intercommunicating cisternae are bound by curved double rows of polysomes attached to ergastoplasmic membranes.

Although the origin of wound fibroblasts is controversial, data indicate that almost all fibroblasts observed in healing wounds are derived from local mesenchymal cells, particularly those associated with blood vessel adventitia. If circulating cells are capable of becoming fixed fibroblasts, as some authors suggest, they have a negligible role in wound healing. The most convincing evidence for the local origin of fibroblasts originates from Ross's experiments with parabiotic rats.[77]

At the time local fibroblasts begin moving into the wound, the wound space is filled with fibrin strands. Although migratory fibroblasts appear to use the fibrin network as a scaffolding, whether or not the fibrin strands provide orientation or contact guidance is still debated. Unlike ameboid cells, however, epithelial cells and fibroblasts require a solid or semisolid substrate for their gliding movements. Fibroblasts and epithelial cells move by forming adhesive contacts with the substratum, not by cytoplasmic flow. The leading edge of a moving fibroblast demonstrates the largest number of attachments and consists of a thin, fanlike membrane, 5 to 10 μ wide. This ruffled membrane undergoes continual folding movements that beat inward from the edge. Moving cells require a normal endoplasmic, microtubular architecture, and power is generated by contracting microfilaments within the cell.[7]

In isolated cells, ruffled membranes form intermittently on all areas of the cell surface, and the cell moves randomly within a small area. When the ruffled membranes of two cells meet, each cell contracts slightly, the ruffled membranes disappear at the area of contact, and cell migration in that direction ceases. Cell edges free of cellular contact, however, continue to form ruffled membranes, and cells move in the direction of ruffling. Although ruffled membrane formation and contact inhibition force populations of cells to migrate into cell-free spaces, neither phenomenon provides orientation or directional movement to single cells. In tissue culture, cell orientation and movement are influenced significantly by substrate orientation. Fibrin strands, glass fibers, and even grooves cut in glass or plastic surfaces orient cells. This peculiar behavior, termed contact guidance, may operate on many levels of substrate organization. Thus, the phenomena of contact inhibition and contact guidance may direct the fibroblast invasion of the wound space by means of either the fibrin network or an undetected substrate orientation.

Because the first recognizable collagen fibers are associated with fibrin strands, some observers have suggested that fibrin is somehow converted to collagen. Quite the opposite is true. Fibroblasts do not contain fibrinolytic enzymes. Large amounts of fibrin, blood clots, or dead tissue actually produce a physical barrier, preventing fibroblast penetration and delaying collagen fiber production. Fortunately, the fibroblast has help.

Rapid capillary proliferation is a prominent feature of all early wound healing. In closed or open wounds, new capillaries form by the budding of existing venules. Endothelial cells proximal to the injury undergo rapid mitosis. The distal cells lose their attachments to the basement membrane and move out into the injured area. Unlike fibroblasts, endothelium moves as a contiguous sheet. Only the leading cells develop ruffled membranes; cell membranes of the followers remain in intimate contact. Because endothelial cells proliferate from many points, a rich network of small vessels is established rapidly. Endothelial cells contain a potent plasminogen activator. Thus, as fibroblasts advance into the injured area, followed closely by proliferating capillaries, fibrinolysis occurs, destroying the fibrin network.

FIBROPLASIA. The fixed cellular phase of wound healing lasts several weeks. By the fourth or fifth week, however, the absolute number of wound fibroblasts has decreased markedly. In addition, the rich capillary network has dwindled to a few well-defined capillary systems. Throughout the life of the scar, a modest number of cells remain associated with scar material, but these fibrocytes no longer possess the active endoplasmic reticulum characteristic of fibroblasts.

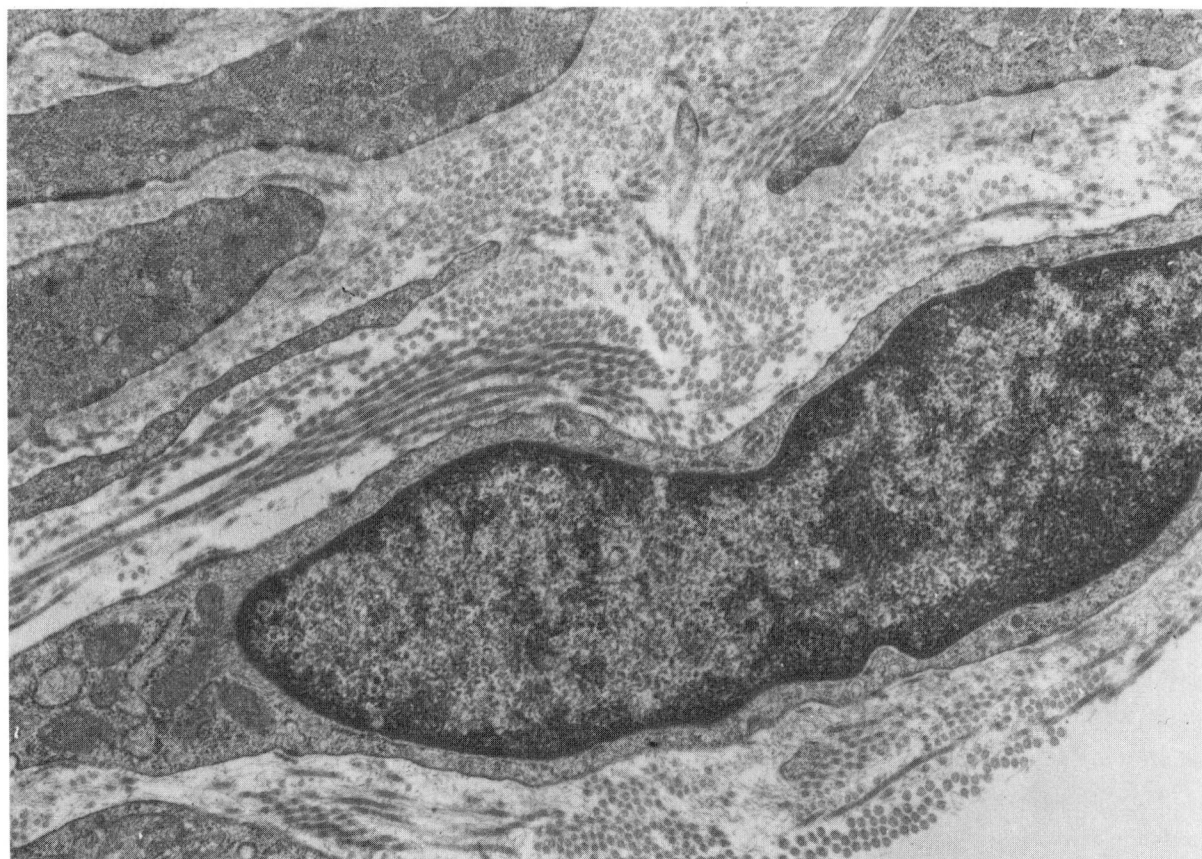

Figure 1. Normal resting fibroblast from human connective tissue. Note the large, smooth, oval nucleus; normal mitochondria; and a small amount of rough endoplasmic reticulum. The cell is surrounded by collagen fibrils cut in longitudinal and cross section. The cell fragments seen in the upper left are typical smooth muscle cells. Electron micrograph, ×22,000. (Courtesy of Edward C. Carlson, Ph.D.)

As the fibroblast population decreases, collagen fibers become the dominant anatomic feature of wounds (Fig. 2). The first collagen fibers appear at 4 or 5 days after injury. Rapidly, the wound space fills with small, randomly oriented fiber bundles. Fiber bundles enlarge gradually and produce a massive, dense collagenous structure (the scar) binding the severed tissues together firmly.

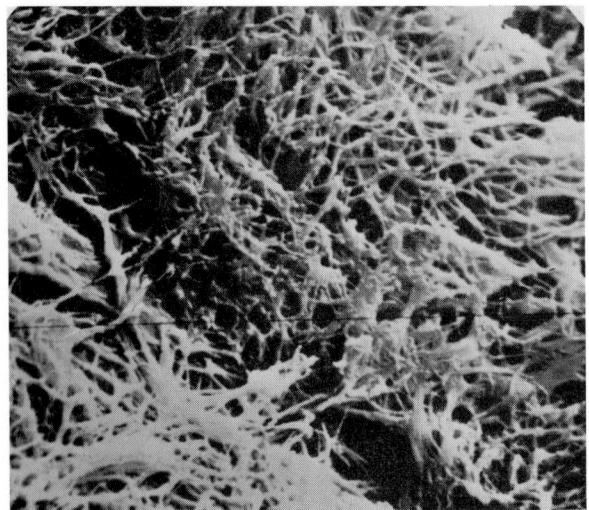

Figure 2. Collagen fibers in a 10-day-old sutured rat skin wound. Note the small size and random arrangement of fibers. Scanning electron micrograph, ×4500. (From Forrester, J. C., Zederfeldt, B. H., Hayes, T. L., and Hunt, T. K.: Wolff's law in relation to the healing skin wound. J. Trauma, *10*:770, 1970. © Williams & Wilkins, 1970.)

In the past, the morphologic discussion of wound healing might have ended here. For years, many biologists suggested that the important events in wound healing occurred quickly and stopped abruptly. Every careful observer with a personal wound knows this statement is false. All scars, deep or superficial, slowly and progressively change in bulk and form over many years. In certain unfortunate individuals, skin wounds enlarge, producing massive keloids or hypertrophic scars; in others, color fades, bulk decreases, normal pigmentation returns, and the scar all but disappears. Scar tissue in most abdominal incisions remains firm and strong forever; occasionally, however, abdominal scars thin, spread, and lose strength, and incisional hernias develop.

The phenomenon of scar remodeling is basic to the function of injured tissues. The gross appearance of remodeling scars suggests that collagen fibers are, in some manner, altered or rewoven into different architectural patterns with time. Unfortunately, classic light and electron microscopic techniques are not adequate for investigating remodeling except in unusual situations. Development of the scanning electron microscope, however, has provided a powerful method suitable for investigating fiber architectural changes. Scanning electron micrographs demonstrate that scar fiber patterns do change slowly for many months.[26] Because remodeling represents such an important clinical property of scars, the phenomenon is discussed in greater depth in connection with wound chemistry.

Chemical Events

INFLAMMATION. Although investigated extensively, the chemistry of local inflammation remains controversial. Since the early 1900s, a series of experimental studies have demonstrated conclusively that local substances released by injury produce vasodilatation and increased small vessel permeability. Initially, histamine was considered the primary mediator of inflammatory vascular responses. Histamine, liberated from mast cells, granulocytes, and platelets, produces local vasodilatation and increases small vessel permeability. Although present in early inflammatory exudates, histamine acts for short periods (less than 30 minutes) and local sources are depleted rapidly. In the rat, serotonin (5-hydroxytryptamine), also found in mast cells, has a local action similar to that of histamine. In man, however, the local effects of serotonin are negligible. Because of their short duration of action, it appears unlikely that these amines are responsible for prolonged inflammatory reactions.[92]

More recently, the kinins, a series of biologically active peptides, and the prostaglandins, principally PGE_1 and PGE_2, have been implicated in local inflammatory vascular responses. Kallikrein, an enzyme found in plasma and in granulocytes, releases bradykinin and kallidin from the α_2-globulin of plasma. In the presence of kinins and the complement system, local cells produce a variety of prostaglandins. Prostaglandins probably act by regulating cell cyclic nucleotide levels.[30] The prostaglandins appear to be the final mediators of acute inflammation, including the reversible small vessel permeability, and may have a chemotactic role for fibroblasts and white cells as well.[88] Aspirin and indomethacin are potent inhibitors of prostaglandin biosynthesis, and the anti-inflammatory action of these drugs may follow their effects on prostaglandin metabolism.

The second phase of inflammatory response, local invasion by white blood cells, may also have chemical mediators. The evidence, however, is even more controversial. Leukotaxine, claimed to be a peptide formed in damaged tissue by the enzymatic destruction of albumin, was thought to be a chemotactic agent, attracting leukocytes into the damaged area. Although large concentrations of certain isolated peptides can cause leukocyte attraction in tissue culture and other experimental preparations, they do not demonstrate chemotactic activity in concentrations found in damaged tissue. Extracts of white blood cells and even certain forms of collagen cause leukocyte chemotaxis in experimental situations. Their role in wound healing, however, is unclear.

GROUND SUBSTANCE. Mature and developing scars contain the same basic extracellular components as all mesenchymal tissue: fibrous proteins, principally collagen; and glycosaminoglycans–mucopolysaccharides, mucoproteins, and glycoproteins. Although the metabolism of both classes may be highly interrelated, their chemistry and kinetics are discussed separately.

All connective tissues contain variable amounts of glycosaminoglycans (Table 1). These huge macromolecules, composed primarily of carbohydrate and a variable amount of protein, are of seven major types. Heparin may be included in this classification, but it is not a structural component of connective tissue. All glycosaminoglycans occur in the form of protein polysaccharide complexes with molecular weights between 7.5×10^5 and $10 \times$

10^5. The polysaccharide components are attached to a central protein core, and the whole molecule has the configuration of a test tube or bottle brush. The highly charged, sulfated compounds influence local cellular environment significantly. For example, the water or hydration shell around these molecules is huge and must produce significant effects on extracellular fluid composition.[48]

Early histochemical studies and hexosamine determinations suggested that during the first 3 or 4 days of healing wounds synthesized large amounts of glycoaminoglycans. During the next few days, as collagen appeared in the wound, hexosamine content decreased sharply. Investigators concluded that the production and deposition of mucopolysaccharides prepared and directed the fibroblasts to produce collagen. Unfortunately, hexosamine values alone do not reflect accurately the glycosaminoglycan content of wounds. Detailed analysis of the types of hexosamine-containing compounds present demonstrates conclusively that the early increase reflects the appearance of serum glycoproteins carried into the wound with the initial inflammatory exudate rather than the appearance of locally synthesized compounds.[19]

Although human wounds have not been analyzed rigorously, careful studies of animal wounds provide an entirely different pattern of glycosaminoglycan metabolism. Minor differences occur in various animal models, but, generally, the hyaluronic acid content of wound tissue remains relatively constant or decreases during the first 3 weeks of healing. In contrast, chondroitin-4-sulfate and dermatan sulfate concentrations increase progressively from the fourth through the twenty-first day.[6] No sharp drop in concentration occurs with the appearance of collagen fibers. As yet, no clear-cut role has been established for glycosaminoglycans in wound healing. Several important possibilities exist, however, and are discussed in a subsequent section.

Physical Events

From the surgeon's point of view, all of the morphologic and chemical events of wound healing lead to a single important conclusion: *wounds become stronger with time.* The re-establishment of tissue integrity and strength produced by normal healing reactions allows the surgeon to perform modern manipulative therapy. The rate of strength gain and the ultimate strength of wounds determine what suture material should be used, when sutures should be removed, how patient activity should be resumed, and why certain incisions may be more appropriate than others.

Like so much of the data presented here, most of the information on strength relationships in healing wounds is derived from animal experimentation (Fig. 3). Although major clinical differences exist between all species, most biologic events in healing appear comparable. The magnitude and timing of specific features, however, may differ significantly.

All measurable mechanical properties of physical objects depend on the direction and rate of application of force. Although

TABLE 1. Mucopolysaccharides of Connective Tissue

	Synonyms	Disaccharide Repeating Unit
Chondroitin	—	Glucuronic acid + galactosamine
Chondroitin 4-sulfate	Chondroitin sulfate A	Glucuronic acid + 4 sulfo-galactosamine
Chondroitin 6-sulfate	Chondroitin sulfate C	Glucuronic acid + 6 sulfo-galactosamine
Dermatan sulfate	Chondroitin sulfate B, heparin	Iduoronic acid + 4 sulfo-galactosamine
Heparan sulfate	Heparitin sulfate Heparan monosulfate	Glucuronic acid + glucosamine (contains N and O sulfate groups)*
Hyaluronic acid	—	Glucuronic acid + glucosamine
Keratan sulfate	Kerato sulfate	Galactose + 6 sulfo-glucosamine

* The structure of this compound is not completely clear.

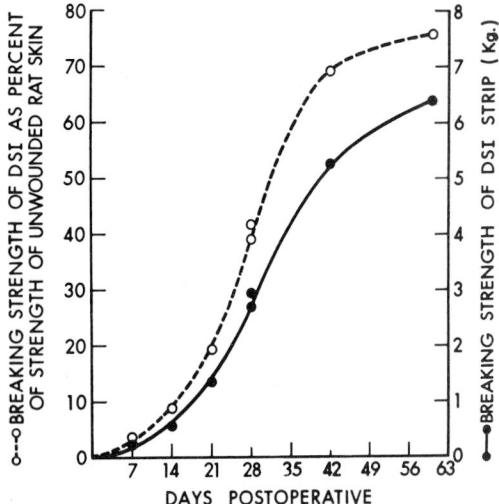

Figure 3. Increase in breaking strength of a healing rat skin wound shown in absolute terms and as a percentage of comparable unwounded skin. Note the prolonged gain in strength. The strength of the wound reached only 80 per cent of the strength of unwounded skin. DSI, dermal skin incision. (From Levenson, S. M., et al.: The healing of rat skin wounds. Ann. Surg., *161*:293, 1965.)

many mechanical parameters, including stress-strain curves, elastic versus inelastic or plastic stretch, and energy absorption curves, have been utilized to measure physical properties of scars, the two most commonly used parameters are burst strength and tensile strength (Fig. 4). These measurements are not interchangeable. Tensile strength measures load per cross-sectioned area at rupture; burst strength measures load required to break the wound regardless of dimension. Failure to appreciate this simple difference produces erroneous interpretation of available data. For example, because of thickness, the burst strength of back skin and eyelid skin differs significantly; the tensile strength, however, is comparable. Burst strength can provide valid comparisons between tissues and wounds only if the physical dimensions are comparable.

Strength gain in incised wounds begins immediately after

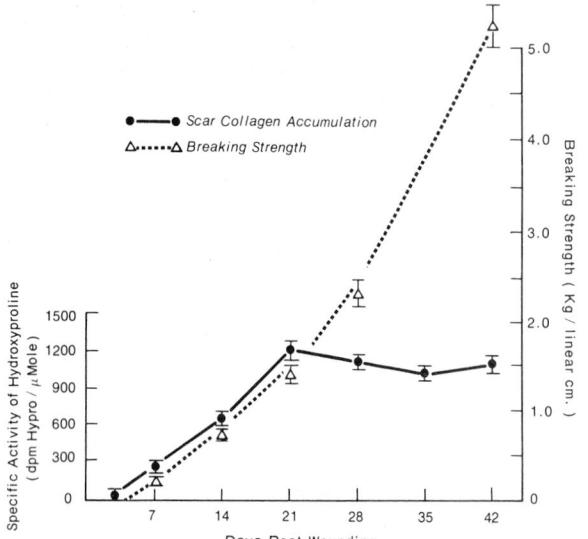

Figure 4. The breaking strength of rat skin wounds compared with net scar collagen accumulation. Note that over the first 3 weeks, strength and collagen content correlate. After 3 weeks, however, the wound continues to gain strength rapidly, but net scar collagen accumulation stops. There is no correlation between content and strength after 3 weeks. (From Madden, J. W., and Peacock, E. E., Jr.: Studies on the biology of collagen during wound healing. III. Dynamic metabolism of scar collagen and remodeling of dermal wounds. Ann. Surg., *174*:511, 1971.)

suture. By 2 days, burst strength in incised rat skin wounds reaches 50 to 100 gm. per linear centimeter. Note that the wound space contains only fibrin strands, a few capillary loops, white cells, and a few fibroblasts at this point. The epithelial surface, however, does consist of a confluent sheet of cells. Experimental studies indicate that intercellular forces, adhesion of globular proteins, and fibrin polymerization can produce forces of this magnitude.[78]

With the appearance of collagen fibers on the third day, rate of gain in strength increases rapidly (Figs. 5 & 6). By 21 days, burst strength has reached over 1 kg. per linear centimeter.[36] Despite a generally held misconception, gain in strength does not cease here. Carefully performed studies even fail to reveal a plateau in strength at this point.[52] Instead, skin wounds continue to gain strength at a relatively rapid and constant rate for over 4 months and at a slower rate for over 1 year. Despite its rediscovery every 10 or 15 years, this significant behavior, first measured experimentally by Howes and co-workers in 1939, is still omitted from many discussions of wound healing.[35] Prolonged gain in strength is not limited to skin wounds. Muscle and fascial wounds gain strength slowly,[18] and rate or gain in strength for tendon injuries is even slower.[63] Despite prolonged strength gain, wounds rarely, if ever, regain the strength of normal tissues. In addition, strength is not the only important physical parameter of scars. Normal elasticity, so important in tissue function, is lost in scars. The products of wound healing, although strong, often convert an elastic, pliable tissue to an inelastic, brittle mass.

OPEN WOUNDS

Open wounds with or without tissue loss present clinical problems entirely different from those of incised and sutured wounds. Although the basic morphologic and chemical processes operating in the closed wound participate in healing open wounds, contraction becomes an important feature in open wounds, and epithelialization assumes a more prominent role. Interestingly, these two processes appear independent.[85]

Incised wounds allowed to remain open begin the healing process normally. An inflammatory exudate collects on the surface; marginal epithelial cells mobilize, divide, and migrate down the edges; injured venules bud, forming capillary networks; and fibroblasts invade the injured area. Early physicians, impressed with the finely granular nature of the new surface, termed this material granulation tissue. After 3 or 4 days, the wound surfaces can be closed with sutures or other mechanical devices, and healing proceeds normally. Careful bacteriologic investigations demonstrate that heavily contaminated wounds left open can show a marked reduction in bacterial concentration during the first 3 to 6 days. In many instances, delayed closure of contaminated wounds can prevent clinical infection. This technique, developed during World War II, has become increasingly popular.

If delayed closure is not performed or if tissues have been lost, a remarkable change in the physical dimensions of the wound occurs with time. After a delay of 2 or 3 days, the wound margins move toward each other, making the surface defect smaller. The remarkable propensity of open wounds to contract has been recognized for centuries. Only recently, however, have the mechanisms responsible for wound contraction been investigated extensively.

Clinical observations in animals and man demonstrate that skin wounds contract by stretching the surrounding skin to close the defect, not by the production of new skin. In areas where skin is relatively loose and mobile structures are not nearby, wound contraction produces minimal deformity. For example, a 10 by 10-cm. defect high on one buttock contracting to 2 by 2 cm. causes little functional impairment. In contrast, where mobile skin is important, contraction produces serious

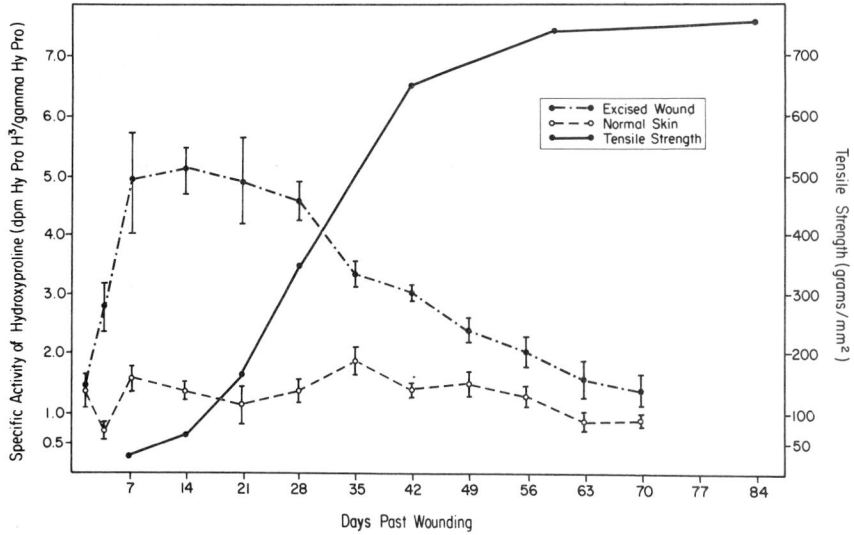

Figure 5. The relationship of rate of collagen synthesis to tensile strength of rat skin wounds. Note that the net rate of collagen synthesis and deposition remains elevated throughout the study period. Despite a stable collagen content, incised wounds continued to synthesize and deposit collagen rapidly for prolonged intervals. Unlike net scar collagen content, net rate of new collagen deposition correlates with strength gain throughout the study interval. (From Madden, J. W., and Peacock, E. E., Jr.: Studies on the biology of collagen during wound healing. I. Rate of collagen synthesis and deposition in cutaneous wounds of the rat. Surgery, *64*:288, 1968; tensile strength curve taken from Levenson, S. M., et al.: The healing of rat skin wounds. Ann. Surg., *161*:293, 1965.)

functional abnormalities. A 4 by 4-cm. defect on the dorsum of the hand contracting to 2 by 2 cm. can cause a permanent extension deformity of the fingers. Because contraction appears limited by the tension developed in skin surrounding the defect, simply pulling the wound edges together with skin hooks reproduces the ultimate deformity. Thus, contraction of a defect in the upper eyelid can produce ectropion; of the antecubital space, a flexion contracture of the elbow; of the axillary skin, an adduction contracture of the arm. Obviously, the contraction of open wounds produces serious deformity, and controlling this relentless process becomes an important part of the surgeon's task.

Because skin is normally under mild tension, excision of full-thickness skin produces a defect slightly larger than the sample removed.[8] After a delay of 2 or 3 days, the dermal edges begin moving toward each other. Between days 5 and 10, wound edges move rapidly but slow again by 2 weeks. In a rectangular or square defect, the midpoints of the sides move more rapidly than the corners, and the ultimate scar is stellate. Only three possible explanations for this event exist: the dermal wound edges are pulled together by a force originating in the open bed, the edges are pushed toward the center by forces at the periphery, or contraction occurs by a combination of both. Although initially a rather simple problem, distinguishing between the possibilities is difficult.

Even though large amounts of collagen are produced by the granulating surface, neither normal collagen synthesis nor strong covalent bonding between collagen fibers is required for normal wound contraction.[41] Open skin wounds in scorbutic animals and man produce small amounts of collagen but contract normally.[1] In addition, inhibiting covalent bonding with lathyrogenic agents has no effect on contraction.[40] Collagen fibers themselves are not composed of contractile proteins. Where, then, does the force originate?

Wherever the application occurs, the force of wound contraction is derived from living cells. Cytotoxic agents in nonlethal doses, particularly the cytochrome poisons, inhibit wound contraction significantly, and the effect is reversible. Any treatment that inhibits cell motility has significant effects on wound contraction. Moreover, single cells and cell sheets moving on solid substrates can generate forces capable of closing open wounds. Where the cells responsible for wound contraction reside, however, is debated.

Grillo and associates implicated a group of large cells immediately beneath the advancing dermal edge.[31] Excising the central granulating surface of open wounds in guinea pigs had no effect on contraction. Excising the dermal edge itself, however, re-established the initial size of the wound, leaving a smaller central area.[87] Repeated excisions of central mass had no effect; repeated excisions of the frame area always eliminated contraction. Irradiating the local area during the phase of active fibroblast division retarded contraction significantly. Although

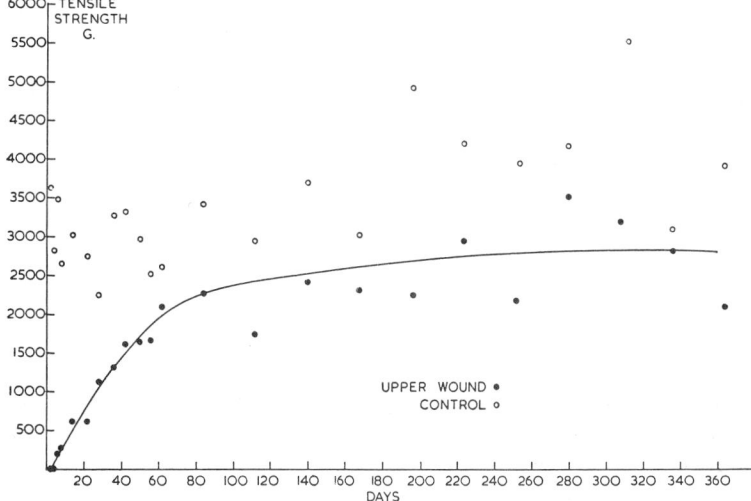

Figure 6. Breaking strength of a wound in the upper dorsal aponeurosis compared with the strength of unwounded fascia (open circles). Note that fascial wounds behave as skin wounds and gain strength steadily for months. (From Douglas, D. M.: The healing of aponeurotic incisions. Br. J. Surg., *40*:79, 1952.)

irradiation of wound margin and central granulation tissue separately was not possible, these studies support the involvement and local origin of living cells.

Unfortunately, repeating the excision experiments in other species produces different results. In rabbits, excising the central granulating mass or separating the dermal edge from the wound base enlarges the contracting wound to the original dimensions.[2] In addition, inhibiting contraction with external splints and releasing the wound edges after a few days produces contraction at a rate far too rapid to be explained by cell movements alone. Incising the wound base prior to releasing the splint eliminates the rapid marginal movement. Therefore, rapid contraction in the splinted wound appears to follow forces built up during splinting.

Gabbiani and co-workers have identified a specific cell type in granulation tissue that may represent the contractile element responsible for wound contraction.[29] This unique cell combines the ultrastructural features of the fibroblast and smooth muscle cell. Modified fibroblasts (myofibroblasts) have been identified in contracting tissues from several animal species and in a number of human fibrocontractive diseases (Fig. 7).[55-57] Although impossible to prove using morphologic criteria alone, data support the concept that atypical cells resembling smooth muscle supply the motive force for wound contraction. Biochemical measurements demonstrate that granulation tissue from contracting wounds contains as much actomyosin as does the uterus.[28] Human anti–smooth muscle sera label the cytoplasm of myofibroblasts.[34] Granulation tissue containing significant numbers of modified fibroblasts contracts actively *in vitro*, behaving as vascular smooth muscle tissue.[62] The life cycle of these cells in an open, granulating wound parallels the time span of wound contraction.[79,80] Finally, topically applied anti–smooth muscle agents inhibit wound contraction completely.[60]

The mechanism of wound contraction remains an exciting area for investigation. Over the next few years, the nature of the cells involved in wound contraction and their relationship to pathophysiologic conditions will be clarified.

Although the precise mechanism of wound contraction remains controversial, the factors responsible for initiating and inhibiting the contraction process are central to wound management. Forces of contraction act to close the wound until balanced by equal tension in the surrounding skin. Although tensions in surrounding tissue may lessen with time, for all practical purposes, the wound contracts until fixed tissues prevent further contraction. Certain biologic manipulations are known to influence the contraction process. Contrary to popular opinion, epithelialization *per se* does not inhibit wound contraction.[86] Contraction can be minimized by replacing missing skin immediately with thick skin grafts or pedicle flaps. The ultimate area of the defect following coverage depends upon several important factors. Full-thickness skin grafts inhibit the contraction mechanism most effectively.[83] Thin split-thickness grafts inhibit wound contraction, but only slightly. The thicker the graft, the larger the ultimate area. When contraction has begun, replacing missing skin is much less effective in inhibiting the contraction process.[85] A combination of immediate skin coverage plus mechanical splinting, by skeletal structures in the area or by external devices, is the most effective method of minimizing wound contraction.[86] Obviously, the control of wound contraction resides in the interphase between the injured area and the moving dermal margin or grafted dermal tissue. The precise mechanism of this interaction, however, has not been defined.

In areas of fixed tissues and little excess skin (the skin over the skull or lower leg), maximal contraction cannot close a significant defect. Sufficient skin simply cannot be pulled into the

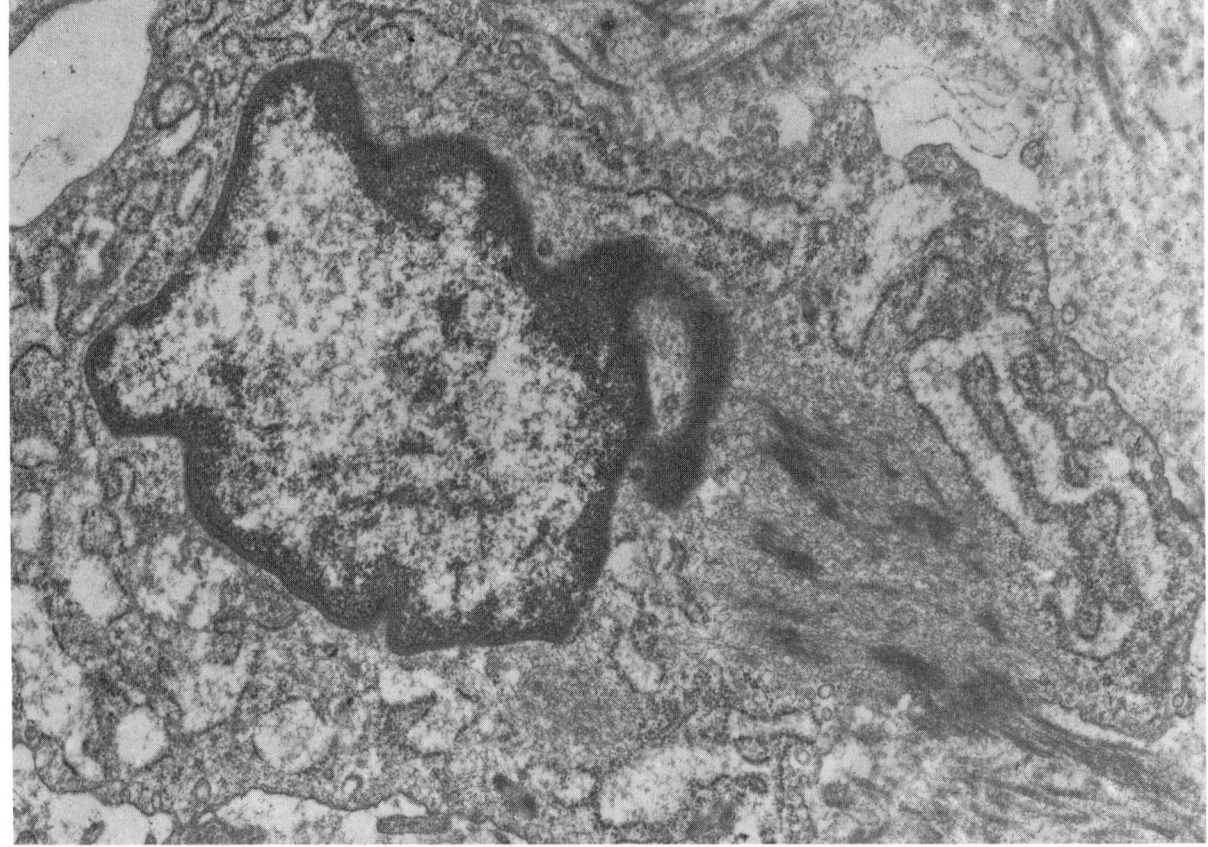

Figure 7. Atypical fibroblast (myofibroblast) from patient with plantar fasciitis. Compare this cell with the fibroblast illustrated in Figure 1. Note the highly irregular nucleus, the large amount of rough endoplasmic reticulum, and, most important, the dense collection of myofilaments. There are numerous dense bodies adjacent to and intermingled with the myofilaments. No basal lamina is seen, and the cell is surrounded by numerous collagen fibrils. This cell has ultrastructural features intermittent between a fibroblast and smooth muscle cell. Electron micrograph ×25,000. (Courtesy of Edward C. Carlson, Ph.D.)

wound. The wound surface either remains uncovered as a chronic open ulcer or closes by epithelialization. In full-thickness defects, epithelialization occurs by the same mechanisms discussed under the closed wound. The magnitude of the process and its consequences, however, are entirely different. Even in partial-thickness injuries, in which cells from the dermal appendages aid in epithelialization, the results are far from satisfactory.

Open wounds are covered by dried or denatured plasma proteins and dead cells, the scab. In thermal injuries, denatured dermal collagen may remain in place and constitute an eschar. In either case, epithelialization occurs beneath the surface covering. In thermal injuries with an intact eschar, migrating epithelial cells secrete collagenase, destroying the intact collagenous connections. Underneath a scab, the epithelial cells migrate on the collagenous tissue in the wound base.

Although epithelial sheets have remarkable migratory capacities, the extent of their migrations is not infinite. Cells can migrate 1, 2, and even 3 cm. from the wound edge under special circumstances, but they rarely cover larger defects. If the area is too large to be covered by epithelialization and contraction, the wound becomes a chronic open ulcer. Over long periods of time, open wounds of this type can develop a highly malignant form of squamous cell carcinoma. Adequate coverage can prevent this disastrous complication.

Like normal skin, epithelialized scar tissue represents a superficial epidermal layer and a deeper collagenous base. Epithelial cells on a base of scar tissue, however, have little resemblance to skin. Normally, epidermis is bound tightly to dermis through a strong undulating basement membrane. The rete pegs and epidermal appendages (hair follicles, sweat glands, sebaceous glands) provide a strong epidermal-dermal junction. Junction of epithelium with scar tissue, however, is poor, with little strength. Even minor shearing forces produce epithelial separation and loss. Under normal skin, epithelialized scar tissue responds to stress by deteriorating, not by a compensatory increase in strength. Although some animals can regenerate a few hair follicles and sebaceous glands with time, scar tissue in man lacks epidermal appendages. Epithelialized scar remains a poor substitute for skin.

Local and Systemic Factors

SECONDARY WOUND HEALING AND WOUND HORMONES. A number of imaginative biologists have suggested through the years that injured tissues produce specific wound hormones. These substances, allegedly circulating freely in blood, increase the rate of healing at distant sites. To date, there are no critical experimental data to support this contention. In most instances, observed differences in healing rates follow other factors. These experiments, however, did produce a significant observation on the behavior of dehisced and resutured wounds.

Botsford noted that incised wounds allowed to heal for short periods undisturbed, then dehisced and immediately resutured, developed strength at a significantly faster rate than primary wounds.[10] The experiments of Dunphy, his associates, and others established that this secondary wound healing phenomenon was related entirely to local factors at the wound site and was not associated with circulating wound hormones.[82] Interestingly, excising the skin wound as a strip 14 mm. wide with the wound at the center and reapproximating the fresh edges abolishes rapid gain in strength. Excising a narrower skin strip with the wound reduces but does not completely inhibit increased rate of gain in strength. Small increases in rate have been noted in wounds dehisced months after the original incision. Collagen content of excised secondary wounds appears to be the same as or even lower than that of primary wounds of the same age. Time-related features of scar collagen metabolism, however, appear to explain secondary healing. As discussed previously, primary wounds require several days to prepare for

collagen synthesis and continue to synthesize and deposit collagen at elevated rates for prolonged periods. Dehiscing and resuturing wounds appear to have no effect on rate of new collagen deposition.[61] Experiments in rats demonstrate that strength gain on wounds dehisced and resutured at different times correlates with the rate of collagen deposition at the time of dehiscence. Thus, in the dehisced and resutured wound, as well as the primary wound, gain in strength appears to depend less on collagen content than on rate of new collagen deposition.

GENERAL NUTRITIONAL FACTORS. Incised wounds in animals fed a protein-free diet for prolonged periods gain strength slowly. Although plasma restores normal wound kinetics, the plasma protein concentration fails to correlate with local wound abnormalities. Feeding DL-methionine or cystine alone prevents delayed healing.[91] This effect appears unrelated to collagen synthesis, and the mechanism of protein depletion effects on wound healing is obscure. Although discussed frequently, the magnitude of the effect of protein depletion on wound healing in man remains unknown.[39,54] Advanced age has also been thought to adversely affect wound healing. Although data suggest that wound healing mechanisms are more efficient in the young,[72] wound complications in the aged appear more related to pulmonary and cardiovascular problems than to factors inherent in the wound.[38]

VITAMIN AND TRACE ELEMENT DEFICIENCIES. Although most species synthesize adequate amounts of ascorbic acid, primates and the guinea pig lack this ability. Experimental studies indicate that collagen synthesis can proceed at low rates in ascorbic acid–deficient animals. When circumstances require rapid synthesis, however, ascorbic acid depletion has profound effects on collagen production. Providing relatively small amounts of vitamin C restores normal healing; saturation is unnecessary. Physiologic abnormalities in scurvy are not limited to collagen metabolism. Ascorbic acid, a strong reducing agent, appears to be involved in several other oxidation-reduction systems. Normal wound healing requires adequate amounts of ascorbic acid, but deficiency states are rare in the Western world except in alcoholics or severely malnourished individuals. Vitamin A and vitamin A deficiencies have been implicated in abnormal wound healing phenomena. Although the full implications of vitamin A deficiency have yet to be explored, vitamin A appears to be a specific antagonist to certain abnormalities created by cortisone and its derivatives.[21,37] The effect of supplemental vitamin A on the healing of colonic anastomoses was evaluated experimentally in animals that were irradiated preoperatively. The bursting strength and hydroxyproline determinations performed on both the anastomotic segment and a normal proximal segment of adjacent colon demonstrated a significant increase in the bursting strength at the colon anastomosis and in the collagen content after preoperative irradiation. This effect was mitigated by dietary supplementation of vitamin A.[93] In another experimental study, supplemental vitamin A was also shown to prevent acute radiation-induced defects in wound healing.[53]

The role of metals in wound healing is being studied intensively. Copper and ferrous iron are required for normal collagen metabolism, but deficiency states are rarely, if ever, observed. Zinc and other divalent cations are co-factors in many metabolic reactions, and deficiency states in animals retard epithelialization and strength gain. Relative zinc deficiency has been suggested as one cause of poor epithelialization in children with large burns. The data, however, are equivocal at present.[11,71]

The effects of elevated calcium were evaluated in cultured keratinocytes in vitro on two of the rate-limiting steps of wound healing, specifically chemotaxis and adhesion.[81] It was found that elevated calcium prohibited both chemotaxis and adhesions, whereas pretreatment with the calcium channel blocker verapamil partially reversed this phenomenon. The addition of verapamil to chronic wounds caused improved wound closure.

ANEMIA, BLOOD LOSS, AND OXYGEN TENSION. Many

clinicians believe strongly that significant anemia delays healing. Unfortunately, this hypothesis is difficult to verify experimentally. The literature contains data to support both sides of a debate. The importance of tissue oxygen tension in healing, however, is established. Prolonged low tissue oxygen tension impairs healing significantly.[84]

The effect of hemodialysis on subcutaneous tissue oxygen tension was studied in a clinical series.[42] The subcutaneous oxygen tension decreased from 52 to 28 mm. Hg, a decrease sufficient to make likely the fact that hemodialysis may contribute to wound morbidity frequently observed in dialyzed patients because of the low tissue oxygen. The effect of local hyperthermia on subcutaneous tissue oxygen tension was investigated in a series of patients with subcutaneously implanted oxygen tonometers.[75] The temperature increased, partial pressure of subcutaneous oxygen rose, and there was a threefold increase in local perfusion. The data reaffirmed the value of local hyperthermia in treating contaminated wounds and suggest a mechanism for its ability to ameliorate infections. Local heat may also have *prophylactic* value.

As noted earlier, data suggest that relative concentrations of lactic dehydrogenase (LDH) isoenzymes, varying with wound tissue Po_2, may be important in regulating collagen synthesis.[38] Perhaps the equivocal results with experimental anemias may be explained by differences in local oxygen tension. Adequate tissue perfusion appears to be more important than the oxygen-carrying capacity of the blood for normal healing. Hemorrhage or anemia alone may not alter tissue oxygen tension; hypovolemia, vasoconstriction, and elevated blood viscosity, however, can have profound effects on local oxygen tension. Environmental temperature also influences local oxygen tension in the skin and affects wound healing. Wounds gain strength significantly faster at higher than at lower room temperatures. Local blood flow appears critical because reducing local vasoconstriction by denervating the skin abolishes the effect of temperature on healing.

STRESS, STEROIDS, AND ANTI-INFLAMMATORY AGENTS. Although wide variations exist between species and between individuals, ACTH, cortisone, and other glucocorticoids can have profound effects on healing rate.[3] Cortisone and its derivatives decrease the rate of protein synthesis, stabilize lysosomal membranes, and inhibit the normal inflammatory reaction. In most species studied, including man, high doses of corticoids limit capillary budding, inhibit fibroblast proliferation, and decrease the rate of epithelialization. Experimentally, steroids given prior to or immediately after wounding have the greatest effect.[64] Generally, even with high doses of steroids, wound healing reactions go to completion; only the time scale is altered. All phases of healing proceed much more slowly, and most clinicians agree that patients receiving chronic steroid therapy who undergo surgical procedures have a greater risk of delayed healing. If careful adjustments are made for the altered time scale, however, wound complications can be minimized.

The effects of cyclosporine A, azathioprine, and prednisone on wound healing were assessed in an experimental study.[23] The data indicated that cyclosporine A in clinical dosages did not inhibit skin or fascial healing, whereas azathioprine and prednisone significantly retarded skin healing but did not affect musculofascial healing. Patients with leprosy and cutaneous ulcers associated with this disease were treated with porcine xenografts and achieved healing in ulcers that had been present for as long as three decades.[24]

The other commonly used anti-inflammatory agents (salicylate derivatives, phenylbutazone) have minimal effects on healing. Experimentally, huge doses of aspirin delay strength gain significantly, but pharmacologic doses have no effect.[50]

In a study of patients with brown recluse spider bites treated either by immediate surgical excision or with the leukocyte inhibitor dapsone followed by delayed surgical excision, it was shown that pretreatment with dapsone reduced the incidence of wound complications and scarring.[76]

GROWTH FACTOR. The potential influence of platelet-derived growth factor–BB hemodimers (PDGF-BB) on surgical incisions in radiated animals with depressed wound healing was evaluated in a recent study.[65] PDGF-BB–treated wounds were 50 per cent stronger than the controls. The results suggested that PDGF requires bone marrow–derived cells, like wound macrophages, for activity and that it may be useful as a topical agent in postradiation surgical incisions. In a clinical study, topical application of platelet-derived growth factors on the repair of chronic nonhealing ulcers indicated a highly statistically significant positive effect,[46] confirmed in another study.[45]

CYTOTOXIC DRUGS AND RADIATION. Chronic tissue changes induced by radiant energy of short wavelength have profound effects on healing and are discussed elsewhere in this volume. Acute radiation effects and effects of other cytotoxic agents, however, also influence healing rate. Most cytotoxic agents demonstrate their greatest effect on dividing cells. From previous discussion it is clear that any agent that inhibits the division of local fibroblasts or epithelial cells should prevent or delay healing. Fortunately, the systemic administration of nitrogen mustard, thioTEPA, 5-fluorouracil, and other antimetabolites rarely causes high enough tissue concentrations to influence cell division in wounds. However, the chronic, local application of these agents (particularly 5-fluorouracil) can completely prevent healing. Similarly, high doses of radiation, especially during the first 3 days, delay strength gain significantly.

In an experimental study, the administration of perioperative doxorubicin hydrochloride (Adriamycin) also had profound effects on wound healing for 5 of 7 patients with breast cancer and 5 of 5 patients with melanoma after intravenous and intra-arterial infusional chemotherapy.[9] To determine whether or not any interval between preoperative or postoperative administration of doxorubicin hydrochloride (Adriamycin) and wounding would limit the impairment in healing induced by Adriamycin, the results of a study demonstrated data that warned against the use of preoperative Adriamycin and supported the use of postoperative Adriamycin administered 28 days after a surgical procedure. A greater impairment was noted when postoperative Adriamycin was administered up to 21 days after wounding.[49]

WOUND CARE

Because almost all biologic phenomena associated with healing require the active participation of cells, local enviromental conditions must be optimal for cellular metabolism. Any local diminution of blood supply delays or prevents healing. Gross alterations in local tissue perfusion are easily recognized, but significant changes in tissue oxygen tension may be caused by subtle factors. Drying of exposed tissues not only kills surface cells but also destroys normal blood flow in small vessels some distance from the surface. Because local inflammation alters vessel permeability, a suture initially encircling tissue under slight tension may become a garrot, choking off all local blood flow, as injured tissues swell. In addition, external pressure from carelessly applied dressings can decrease local tissue perfusion significantly. In order for healing to proceed normally, care must be taken to ensure adequate tissue perfusion.

Preparing local tissues for operation requires a thoughtful surgical biologist. The thick cornified layer of epidermis protects intact skin and underlying tissues from many noxious substances. When the epidermal layer is injured, deeper tissues are exposed to the surgeon's mistakes. Ethyl alcohol, iodine, ether, and other commonly used preparation solutions placed on the intact skin have minor effects; the same materials poured into an open wound kill cells on contact. Open wounds must be protected from all substances harmful to living cells.

Rapid and complete invasion of the wound space by fibroblasts is a critical step in normal healing. As noted, dead tissue fragments, hematomas, foreign bodies, and fluid collections act as physical barriers, preventing normal fibroblast penetration. Space-occupying lesions prolong inflammation, encourage bacterial growth, and delay gain in strength significantly. Therefore, thorough removal of all dead materials and prevention of fluid collections are primary goals in good wound management. Tissue fragments and foreign objects loosely attached to the wound surface can be removed with careful saline irrigations. Usually, however, dirty, traumatic wounds must be débrided carefully by means of forceps, sharp tools, and, most important, adequate time. Primarily healed abdominal wounds, functional extremities, and cosmetically acceptable facial scars are the surgeon's reward for the hours spent meticulously debriding traumatic wounds; infection, fibrosis, hypertrophic scars, and foreign body granulomas await the careless operator.

Although not discussed specifically, the rational choice of suture materials was implicit in the discussion of the biologic behavior of wounds. Only two questions need be asked: How much strength is needed? How long must the suture supply mechanical strength? Because wounds gain strength and remodel slowly, tissue unions requiring initial and prolonged strength should be made with suture material that retains strength for the desired period. In addition, the tissues coapted should be of sufficient mechanical strength to produce the desired result. Although several absorbable synthetic materials are available, a commonly used absorbable suture is catgut, a collagenous preparation made from the submucosa of sheep intestines. Plain or untanned catgut retains strength for approximately 3 weeks, depending upon the local environment. As noted, most wounds develop less than 15 per cent of their ultimate tensile strength by 3 weeks. If this degree of physical integrity is sufficient, absorbable sutures are appropriate. If suture material must supply appreciable amounts of wound strength for longer periods, nonabsorbable materials are indicated.

Determining how much strength a suture must supply in each specific instance is difficult. Like most biologic systems, the human body is overengineered. Dense connective tissues are probably ten times stronger than needed to absorb the stresses of everyday living. Even when disease alters the physical properties of connective tissues significantly (e.g., the Ehlers-Danlos syndrome), affected individuals do not have gaping wounds constantly. In many clinical situations, including the majority of abdominal incisions, 15 per cent of the ultimate tensile strength may be sufficient to resist normal stress.

A comparison was made in laser-welded and sutured arteriotomies. The results showed that there were no significant differences in the rate of collagen synthesis and there was no evidence of abnormal healing in the laser-welded specimens, contrasted with those closed by sutures. It was concluded that argon laser welding may be an alternative to suture repair of arteriotomies on the basis of these experimental studies.[90] The histologic and biochemical effects of carbon dioxide and neodymium (Nd)-YAG laser welding on the healing of venotomies were studied. It was concluded that the CO_2 and Nd-YAG lasers can be used successfully to weld venotomies and provide an alternative to conventional suture techniques.[89]

One additional factor determines the magnitude of strength required. Significant pain inhibits the full activity of most voluntary muscles. Therefore, injured tissues are splinted internally if normal pain mechanisms are functioning. If pain is totally eliminated, generated stresses can be much higher. As an example, many have had the unfortunate experience of having an entire inguinal hernia repair disrupted at the close of a procedure. Characteristically, the patient strains maximally during extubation and a frightening series of pops is palpated or heard! On immediate re-exploration, it is found that the sutures have either broken or, more commonly, have actually pulled out of the dense connective tissue in which they were placed. Because the patient is without pain during this interval, he can make stresses sufficient to disrupt the repair. When the full pain mechanism is restored, however, the same mechanical repair is entirely sufficient to resist the stresses applied by the patient. Overengineering and protective behavior following injury enable surgeons to close abdominal incisions and other stressed wounds successfully using a number of materials.

Because a nonabsorbable suture, even monofilament steel or nylon, can act as a nidus for infection, absorbable materials have an advantage in contaminated or potentially contaminated wounds.[20] Absorbable materials, however, create a more intense tissue reaction. If minimal reaction is desired, nonabsorbable materials should be used.

A thorough understanding of wound healing biology provides a rational approach to suture removal. As noted, skin epithelial cells migrate down suture tracts, causing inflammation and sterile abscesses. In addition, skin sutures present for long periods tend to injure underlying skin, creating additional scarring. Therefore, when cosmesis is important, skin sutures should be removed early. Adequate strength to prevent wound spreading during remodeling can be obtained by placing permanent buried subcuticular sutures in the lowest portion of the dermis. Where cosmesis is not a problem, skin sutures should remain in place until strength sufficient to resist local tissue tension and minor trauma has been attained. Timing varies widely in different areas of the body and in different individuals. The surgeon who always removes skin sutures on the same day in all areas and in all individuals eventually has wound problems. For example, the tensions on a simple horizontal laceration of the upper eyelid are minimal. Strength attained by fibrin strands and epithelialization is usually sufficient to prevent dehiscence, and sutures can be removed in 24 to 48 hours. In contrast, a vertical wound on the dorsal thorax may require 21 days to acquire sufficient strength to resist local tissue tension and strain produced by body movements. When doubt exists, removing several sutures and testing wound strength gently is helpful.

Epithelial cells will not spread on surfaces composed of dead material or tissue burdened with an excessive number of bacteria. Granulating wounds awaiting epithelialization must be kept free of dead material. Careful débridement with forceps and sharp instruments can be invaluable. If small areas of dead tissue are too numerous or too small for gross mechanical removal, frequent wet-to-dry dressings can produce effective débridement. Dressings on epithelializing wounds must be applied carefully, however. As noted, the interface between epithelial cells and deeper scar is fragile and never regains normal epidermal-dermal strength. Migrating cells and recently epithelialized surfaces must be protected from mechanical trauma. Moreover, epithelialized scar tissue and fresh skin grafts are quite susceptible to bacterial invasion. As crusts develop and small suture abscesses occur, they must be removed mechanically. The care of skin grafts and consideration of dressings are covered in greater depth in other chapters.

Wound contraction can produce serious functional impairment. The most effective method of preventing contraction is early coverage of open surfaces. The techniques used are discussed in detail elsewhere. The timing, however, is equally important. Although fresh wounds covered with thick split-thickness or full-thickness grafts do remodel and contract with time, the magnitude of contraction is small. Wounds allowed to remain open for long periods contract to a maximum. The only effective method of preventing contraction at present is early coverage. Treating a fully contracted and epithelialized wound requires the excision of all the products of wound healing, recreation of the original defect, and resurfacing of the newly created wound as soon as possible.

For the past 20 years military practices included the principle of excision of all injured tissues around the path of a penetrating projectile. In an experimental study, healing of bullet paths in experimental animals was evaluated. The study demonstrated that the simple extremity wound caused by the modern generation assault rifle, provided with adequate open drainage and systemic penicillin, healed as rapidly when the body defense mechanisms handled the disrupted tissue as when an attempt was made to excise it surgically.[25]

Finally, the prolonged metabolic activity of wounds can be used to the surgeon's advantage. As discussed, wounds reopened months after the initial incision gain strength at a more rapid rate than primary wounds. Even though strength increases may be minimal, the secondary wound healing phenomenon can be used profitably. When rapid gain in strength is desirable, old incisions should not be excised. Rather, the new incision should remain with the old scar. In addition, because wounds change slowly in color, bulk, and strength, scar revision or reconstructive procedures should be delayed until scar reactivity is minimal. Bulky, prominent scars present 3 months after injury may become smooth, flat, and inconspicuous by 1 year. When reconstructive or cosmetic procedures are contemplated, patience is a virtue.

CONTROLLING THE HEALING PROCESS

In most cases, normal healing re-establishes tissue integrity quickly and effectively. Organ function is preserved, satisfying both the patient and the surgeon. There are situations, however, in which the surgeon wishes he had some control over the healing process. For example, an effective method of increasing rate of gain in strength could prevent dehiscence and evisceration, disastrous complications of abdominal surgery. Increasing the rate of epithelialization in open wounds could reduce mortality in burned patients. Effective control of the remodeling process could ensure normal function after tendon injury, prevent fibrous stricture of the esophagus following lye burns, and eliminate stenosis of hollow organs. More important, the same scarring process observed in healing wounds appears to be involved in a variety of human diseases. Cirrhosis of the liver, retroperitoneal fibrosis, Dupuytren's contracture, interstitial pulmonary fibrosis, posttraumatic epilepsy, rheumatic valvular disease, and a host of other pathologic conditions follow inappropriate fibrous tissue production. Effective methods of controlling scar formation would be extremely valuable.

Because of the obvious practical implications, many surgeons have searched for methods of accelerating healing through the years. In the early 1900s, Alexis Carrel noted that extracts of embryonic tissues increased mitotic activity of cultured fibroblasts. This simple observation stimulated surgeons to homogenize tissues of all varieties, both embryonic and adult, and to inject or apply extracts to wounds. After decades of experimentation, only one of these substances, cartilage powder, has been shown to affect healing unequivocally. Dried powdered cartilage from many species produces significant increases in breaking strength of animal and human wounds.[74] The effect, dose-related and demonstrable within 4 days, can be produced with local applications or by injecting saline extracts at a distance from the wound. Data suggest that polymers of N-acetyl-glucosamine may be the effective agent.[73] By 7 days, cartilage-treated wounds are 20 per cent stronger than controls. Although the absolute strength gain remains constant for several weeks, the percentage change drops to a small value as the absolute strength of the wound increases. The mechanism of cartilage action is unknown. However, histologic studies suggest that fibroblast density and collagen formation are increased during the early phases of repair. Cartilage powder, implanted within polyvinyl sponges, stimulates rapid production of collagen. No direct measurements of rate of scar collagen synthesis or of scar collagen turnover have been performed, however.

Although supplying supernormal amounts of ascorbic acid, protein, or methionine fails to accelerate gain in strength, increasing local oxygen tension stimulates healing significantly. Animals in a 40 per cent oxygen environment have stronger wounds at 7 days than animals breathing air.[84] The oxygen effect appears unrelated to carbon dioxide concentrations. Again, however, the magnitude of acceleration is slight, amounting to less than 15 per cent at 7 days.

Unfortunately, neither cartilage powder nor increased oxygen tension increases strength gain sufficiently to satisfy most clinicians. As discussed, incised wounds gain less than 5 per cent of their ultimate strength by 7 days and less than 15 per cent by 3 weeks. A 20 per cent increase or even a 100 per cent increase at 2 or 3 weeks may be of little clinical significance. Even with the increase, suture material would provide significant strength to the wounds. Gains of 300 per cent or 500 per cent by 3 weeks, however, could be of tremendous value.

Although of limited clinical usefulness, these experiments demonstrate that wounds can be induced to gain strength more rapidly. Because the ultimate strength of scars depends on collagen molecules, cross-linking density, and fiber weave, agents influencing collagen metabolism should have significant effects on healing. Currently, agents known to affect cross-linking are much too nonspecific and toxic for clinical application. However, biologic agents may exist that influence cross-linking even under normal conditions. For instance, the rate of conversion of non-cross-linked collagen to insoluble collagen differs significantly between tissues, between individuals, and even in the same individual at different ages. Data suggest that these differences may be due entirely to altered environmental conditions. However, if rate of cross-linking is determined, even in part, by enzymatic reactions, pharmacologic agents might be found that alter cross-linking rates and influence wound strength significantly. Influencing fiber weave in soft tissue healing remains an unexplored area. In bone remodeling, local electrical field changes appear to influence the architecture of bone matrix significantly.[5] Electrical fields, of course, can direct molecular orientation in vitro. Their influence on collagen fiber architecture in scars, however, is unknown. Tension and stress appear to produce significant alterations in scar metabolism, but as yet too little is known to use these modalities rationally.[4]

Although methods of effectively accelerating wound healing are desirable, techniques of inhibiting the fibrotic process might be more beneficial to man. Pathologic fibrosis produces significant pathophysiologic change by altering the form or physical properties of tissue. Normally pliant heart valves stiffened with scar become incompetent. Distensible gut replaced by firm, unyielding scar becomes an inefficient conduit. Therefore, methods of preventing collagen synthesis or altering the physical properties of collagen fibers might reverse or prevent pathophysiologic changes.

The techniques used must be specific in their effects on collagen and selective in their effects on scar tissue. All metabolic inhibitors of protein synthesis (puromycin, actinomycin D) decrease collagen synthesis. Unfortunately, they also inhibit the synthesis of other proteins; the effect is nonspecific and quite toxic to living cells. Selectivity can occur only by interference with metabolic processes unique to collagen. As discussed, the hydroxylation of proline is unique. Peptidyl proline hydroxylase activity requires molecular oxygen, α-ketoglutarate, ascorbic acid, and ferrous iron. No method of producing instant scurvy exists, but altering ferrous iron metabolism has profound effects on collagen synthesis. In tissue culture preparations, ferrous iron chelators specifically inhibit the synthesis of collagen without affecting noncollagenous protein metabolism.[14] More important, systemic administration of ferrous iron chelators in animals prevents silica-induced hepatic fibrosis, alters collagen intent in implanted polyvinyl sponges, and reduces wound strength significantly.[12] Because most of the iron chelators tested so far have disturbing side effects, no human data are available; the effects of ferrous iron chelation on collagen metabolism in man are unknown.

Several other techniques can specifically inhibit collagen synthesis. Because the oxygen utilized in proline hydroxylation is derived from molecular oxygen, cells grown in a nitrogen atmosphere fail to hydroxylate protocollagen, and secretion of collagen ceases. This technique has no future in clinical medicine. More recent observations, however, suggest use of another technique with wider application. Several analogs of proline (3,4-dehydroproline, cis-hydroxyproline) are incorporated into proteins but not hydroxylated.[12] In high enough concentrations, proline analogs prevent collagen formation and appear to have minimal effects on noncollagenous protein synthesis. Several authors have claimed that administering proline analogs to animals inhibits collagen synthesis and affects scar formation significantly.[16,47] The effects of proline analogs in vivo, however, are controversial and the effects in human beings remain unknown.[13,58]

The physical properties of scars can be altered without affecting the rate of collagen synthesis. As noted, collagen fibers achieve their tremendous tensile strength by forming intermolecular covalent cross-links. A class of compounds, the osteolathyrogens, specifically inhibits intermolecular covalent cross-linking in newly synthesized collagen. Beta-aminopropionitrile (BAPN), a compound found in the stems and seeds of plants of the genus Lathyrus, prevents the formation of lysine-derived aldehydes by inhibiting lysyl amine oxidase activity. Under the influence of lathyrogens, collagen molecules are synthesized and excreted at normal rates, but the aggregated fibers fail to form cross-links. Lathyrogenic collagen, therefore, has little tensile strength and is disrupted easily. Penicillamine, a powerful copper chelator liberated during the alkaline hydrolysis of penicillin, is lathyrogenic but produces its effects by a different mechanism.[66] Rather than inhibiting aldehyde formation, penicillamine chelates the resultant aldehydes, preventing aldol condensation reactions or Schiff base formation. In animals, systemic administration of BAPN or penicillamine inhibits gain in strength of incised wounds.[69] More important, BAPN prevents or reverses pathophysiologic changes in animal models of fibrotic diseases. Induced lathyrism prevents the stiff joint of immobility, improves gliding after tendon injury, prevents esophageal stenosis following lye burns, and restores esophageal diameter in fixed esophageal stenosis.[15,17,27,59] Experience with BAPN in man is limited, but systemic administration does inhibit intermolecular cross-linking in scar collagen.[70] In one clinical series, BAPN produced significant allergic reactions; in another, no toxicity was demonstrated.[44] Whether or not lathyrogenic agents can alter pathophysiology in man remains untested.

Each of the anticollagenous agents discussed affects collagen metabolism specifically. To be clinically effective, however, specificity alone is insufficient; agents must selectively affect the scar. The dynamic metabolism of scar collagen, however, can provide selectivity and establish a useful therapeutic ratio. Because the techniques described affect only newly synthesized collagen, a differential turnover rate between scar collagen and normal tissue produces selectivity. Scar tissue turning over five times as rapidly as normal tissue responds selectively to short periods of anticollagenous therapy.[69] Theoretically, any fibrotic condition meeting the following criteria could be treated with effective anticollagenous agents: (1) Pathophysiologic features should be related directly to alterations in form or physical properties of fibrotic tissues. (2) The rate of new collagen deposition or turnover should be significantly higher in diseased than in normal tissues. (3) Formation of pathologic fibrous tissue should be limited to a short period of time. Interestingly, many common surgical problems meet these criteria.

To date, effective control of the healing process in man has not been achieved. However, experimental data suggest that clinical control of the healing process is feasible. With time,

clinically useful methods of controlling scar formation and wound contraction will be developed. Until these are available, the skillful surgeon must utilize the biologic information covered in this chapter to regain maximal function in injured parts. At present there is no pharmacologic crutch to support poor wound management.

SELECTED REFERENCES

International Review of Connective Tissue Research. New York, Academic Press. 1963 to current.
A continuing series of volumes is published under this title. Each volume contains monographs by several authors devoted to current connective tissue research problems. Most of the articles will interest serious students.

McMinn, R. M. H.: Tissue Repair. New York, Academic Press, 1969.
This scholarly monograph reviews the morphologic aspects of injury and repair in detail. Although the book is not oriented toward the surgeon, McMinn provides a rich source of anatomic information invaluable for the serious student.

Nimni, M. E.: Collagen: Structure, Function, and Metabolism in Normal and Fibrotic Tissues. Semin. Arthritis Rheum., 13:1, 1983.
An extensive review of connective tissue chemistry with over 750 references. An excellent reference work.

Peacock, E. E., Jr., and Van Winkle, W., Jr.: Surgery and Biology of Wound Repair, 2nd ed. Philadelphia, W. B. Saunders Company, 1976.
This monograph is by far the most comprehensive work on wound healing available. Written by a surgeon and a biologist, this volume reviews current data on the biology of repair and extends basic biologic concepts to all phases of surgical therapy. The practical consideration given to difficult wound healing problems should be valuable to any practicing clinician. This volume is recommended to all physicians with more than a passing interest in repair.

Trinkaus, J. P.: Cells into Organs, 2nd ed. Englewood Cliffs, N.J., Prentice-Hall, Inc., 1984.
Although written for the student embryologist, this monograph contains a superb review of cell behavior. The author discusses mechanisms of cell locomotion, directional movements, chemotaxis, mechanisms of cell adhesion, and cell segregation in a clear, authoritative manner. This small volume makes fascinating reading for any physician, but is particularly useful for the student of wound healing.

REFERENCES

1. Abercrombie, M., Flint, M. H., and James, D. W.: Wound contraction in relation to collagen formation in scorbutic guinea pigs. J. Embryol. Exp. Morphol., 4:167, 1956.
2. Abercrombie, M., James, D. W., and Newcombe, J. F.: Wound contraction in rabbit skin studied by splinting the wound margins. J. Anat., 94:170, 1960.
3. Alrich, E. M., Carter, J. P., and Lehman, E. P.: The effect of ACTH and cortisone on wound healing. Ann. Surg., 133:783, 1951.
4. Arem, A., and Madden, J. W.: Effects of stress on healing wounds: I. Intermittent non-cyclical tension. Surg. Res., 20:93, 1976.
5. Becker, R. O., and Bassett, C. A. L.: Generation of electric potential by bone in response to mechanical stress. Science, 137:1063, 1962.
6. Bentley, J. P.: Rate of chondroitin sulfate formation in wound healing. Ann. Surg., 165:186, 1967.
7. Bhisey, A. N., and Freed, J. J.: Ameboid movement induced in cultured macrophages by colchicine or vinblastine. Exp. Cell Res., 64:419, 1971.
8. Billingham, R. E., and Russel, P. S.: Studies on wound healing with special reference to the phenomenon of contracture in experimental wounds in rabbits' skin. Ann. Surg., 144:961, 1956.
9. Bland, K. I., Palin, W. E., von Fraunhofer, J. A., Morris, R. R., et al.: Experimental and clinical observations of the effects of cytotoxic chemotherapeutic drugs on wound healing. Ann. Surg., 199:782, 1984.
10. Botsford, T. W.: The tensile strength of sutured skin wounds during healing. Surg. Gynecol. Obstet., 72:690, 1941.
11. Chvapil, M.: Zinc and wound healing. In Zederfeldt, B. (Ed.): Symposium on Zinc. Lunds, Sweden, A. B. Tika, 1974.
12. Chvapil, M.: Pharmacology of fibrosis: Definitions, limits, and perspectives. Life Sci. 16:1345, 1975.
13. Chvapil, M., Madden, J. W., Carlson, E. C., and Peacock, E. E., Jr.: Effect of cis-hydroxyproline on collagen and other proteins in skin wounds, granuloma tissue, and liver of mice and rats. Exp. Mol. Pathol., 20:363, 1974.
14. Chvapil, M., Ryan, J. N., Madden, J. W., and Peacock, E. E., Jr.: Effect of chelating agents, proline analogs, and oxygen tension in in vivo and in vitro experiments on hydroxylation, transport, degradation, and accumulation of collagen. In Vogel, H. G. (Ed.): Connective Tissue and Ageing, 1:195, 1973. International Congress Series, No. 264. Amsterdam, Excerpta Medica.
15. Craver, J. M., Madden, J. W., and Peacock, E. E., Jr.: Biological control of physical properties of tendon adhesions: Effect of β-aminopropionitrile in chickens. Ann. Surg., 157:697, 1968.
16. Daly, J. M., Steigher, E., Prockop, D. J., and Dudrick, S. J.: Inhibition of collagen synthesis by the proline analogue cis-4-hydroxyproline. J. Surg. Res., 14:551, 1973.

17. Davis, W. M., Madden, J. W., and Peacock, E. E., Jr.: A new approach to the control of esophageal stenosis. Ann. Surg., *176*:469, 1972.
18. Douglas, D. M.: The healing of aponeurotic incisions. Br. J. Surg., *40*:79, 1952.
19. Dunphy, J. E., and Jackson, D. S.: Practical applications of experimental studies in the care of primarily closed wounds. Am. J. Surg., *104*:273, 1962.
20. Edlich, R. F., Panek, P. H., Rodehaver, G. T., Turnbull, V. G., Kurtz, L. D., and Edgerton, M. T.: Physical and chemical configuration of sutures in the development of surgical infection. Ann. Surg., *177*:679, 1973.
21. Ehrlich, H. P., and Hunt, T. K.: Effects of cortisone and vitamin A on wound healing. Ann. Surg., *167*:324, 1968.
22. Eisen, A. Z., Bauer, E. A., and Jeffrey, J. J.: Animal and human collagenases. J. Invest. Dermatol., *55*:359, 1970.
23. Eisinger, D. R., and Sheil, A. G. R.: A comparison of the effects of cyclosporin A and standard agents on primary wound healing in the rat. Surg. Gynecol. Obstet., *160*:135, 1985.
24. Ersek, R. A., and Lorio, J.: The most indolent ulcers of the skin treated with porcine xenografts and silver ions. Surg. Gynecol. Obstet., *158*:431, 1984.
25. Fackler, M. L., Breteau, J. P., Courbil, L. J., et al.: Open wound drainage versus wound excision in treating the modern assault rifle wound. Surgery, *105*:576, 1989.
26. Forrester, J. C., Zederfeldt, B. T., Hayes, T. L., and Hunt, T. K.: Wolff's law in relation to the healing skin wound. J. Trauma, *10*:770, 1970.
27. Furlow, L. T., Jr., and Peacock, E. E., Jr.: Effect of β-aminopropionitrile on joint stiffness in rats. Ann. Surg., *165*:442, 1967.
28. Gabbiani, G., Hirschel, B. J., Ryan, G. B., Statkov, P. R., and Majno, G.: Granulation tissue as a contractile organ: A study of structure and function. J. Exp. Med., *135*:719, 1972.
29. Gabbiani, G., Ryan, G. B., and Majno, G.: Presence of modified fibroblasts in granulation tissue and their possible role in wound contraction. Experimentia, *27*:549, 1971.
30. Gorman, R. R.: Prostaglandins, thromboxanes and prostacyclin. Int. Rev. Biochem., *20*:81, 1978.
31. Grillo, H. C., Watts, G. T., and Gross, J.: Studies in wound healing: I. Contraction and wound contents. Ann. Surg., *148*:145, 1958.
32. Gross, J., and Lapiere, C. M.: Collagenolytic activity in amphibian tissues: A tissue culture assay. Proc. Nat. Acad. Sci., *48*:1014, 1962.
33. Heppelston, A. G., and Styles, J. A.: Activity of a macrophage factor in collagen formation by silica. Nature, *214*:521, 1967.
34. Hirschel, B. J., Gabbiani, G., Ryan, T. B., and Majno, G.: Fibroblasts of granulation tissue: Immunofluorescent staining with anti-smooth muscle serum. Proc. Soc. Exp. Biol. Med., *138*:466, 1971.
35. Howes, E. L., Harvey, S. C., and Hewitt, W. J.: Rate of fibroplasia and differentiation in the healing of cutaneous wounds in different species of animals. Arch. Surg., *38*:934, 1939.
36. Howes, E. L., Sooy, J. W., and Harvey, S. C.: The healing of wounds as determined by their tensile strength. J.A.M.A., *92*:242, 1929.
37. Hunt, T. K.: Control of wound healing with cortisone and vitamin A. *In* Longacre, J. J. (Ed.): The Ultrastructure of Collagen. Springfield, Ill., Charles C Thomas, Publisher, 1976, pp. 497–503.
38. Hunt, T. K., Connolly, W. B., Aronson, S. B., and Goldstein, P.: Anaerobic metabolism and wound healing. A hypothesis for the initiation and cessation of collagen synthesis in wounds. Am. J. Surg., *135*:328, 1978.
39. Irvin, T. T.: Effects of malnutrition and hyperalimentation on wound healing. Surg. Gynecol. Obstet., *146*:33, 1978.
40. Jacques, J.: Wound contraction in experimental lathyrism. Br. J. Exp. Pathol., *50*:486, 1969.
41. James, D. W., and Newcombe, J. F.: Granulation tissue resorption during free and limited contraction of skin wounds. J. Anat., *95*:247, 1961.
42. Jensen, J. A., Goodson, W. H., III, Omachi, R. S., et al.: Subcutaneous tissue oxygen tension falls during hemodialysis. Surgery, *101*:416, 1987.
43. Johnson, F. R., and McMinn, R. M. H.: The cytology of wound healing of body surfaces in mammals. Biol. Rev., *35*:364, 1960.
44. Keiser, H. R., and Sjoerdsma, A.: Studies on beta-aminopropionitrile in patients with scleroderma. Clin. Pharmacol. Ther., *8*:593, 1968.
45. Knighton, D. R., Ciresi, K. F., Fiegel, V. D., Austin, L. L., and Butler, E. L.: Classification and treatment of chronic nonhealing wounds: Successful treatment with autologous platelet-derived wound healing factors (PDWHF). Ann. Surg., *204*:322, 1986.
46. Knighton, D. R., Ciresi, K., Fiegel, V. D., et al.: Stimulation of repair in chronic, nonhealing, cutaneous ulcers using platelet-derived wound healing formula. Surg. Gynecol. Obstet., *170*:56, 1990.
47. Lane, J. M., Bora, F. W., Prockop, D. J., Heppenstall, R. B., and Black, J.: Inhibition of scar formation by the proline analog cis-hydroxyproline. J. Surg. Res., *13*:135, 1972.
48. Laurent, T. C.: The interaction between polysaccharides and other macromolecules. 9. The exclusion of molecules from hyaluronic acid gels and solutions. Biochem. J., *93*:106, 1964.
49. Lawrence, W. T., Talbot, T. L., and Norton, J. A.: Preoperative or postoperative doxorubicin hydrochloride (Adriamycin): Which is better for wound healing? Surgery, *100*:9, 1986.
50. Lee, K. H.: Studies on the mechanism of action of salicylate. II. Retardation of wound healing by aspirin. J. Pharm. Sci., *57*:1042, 1968.
51. Leibovich, S. J., and Ross, R.: The role of the macrophage in wound repair. Am. J. Pathol., *78*:71, 1975.
52. Levenson, S. M., Geever, E. F., Crowley, L. V., Oates, J. F., Berard, C. W., and Rosen, H.: The healing of rat skin wounds. Ann. Surg., *161*:293, 1965.
53. Levenson, S. M., Gruber, C. A., Rettura, G., et al.: Supplemental vitamin A prevents the acute radiation-induced defect in wound healing. Ann. Surg., *200*:494, 1984.
54. Levenson, S. M., and Seifter, E.: Dysnutrition, wound healing and resistance to infection. Clin. Plast. Surg., *4*:375, 1977.
55. Madden, J. W.: On the contractile fibroblast. Plast. Reconstr. Surg., *52*:291, 1973.
56. Madden, J. W., and Carlson, E. C.: Atypical fibroblasts, wound contraction and human fibrocontractive disease. Proceedings of the International Symposium on Wound Healing. Rotterdam, 1974.
57. Madden, J. W., Carlson, E. C., and Hines, J.: Presence of modified fibroblasts in ischemic contracture of intrinsic musculature of the hand. Surg. Gynecol. Obstet., *140*:509, 1975.
58. Madden, J. W., Chvapil, M., Carlson, E. C., and Ryan, J. N.: Toxicity and metabolic effect of 3,4-dehydroproline in mice. J. Toxicol. Appl. Pharmacol., *26*:426, 1973.
59. Madden, J. W., Davis, W. M., Butler, C., II and Peacock, E. E., Jr.: Experimental esophageal lye burns. 2. Correcting established strictures with β-aminopropionitrile and bougienage. Ann. Surg., *178*:277, 1973.
60. Madden, J. W., Morton, D., Jr., and Peacock, E. E., Jr.: Contraction of experimental wounds. I. Inhibiting wound contraction using a topical smooth muscle antagonist. Surgery, *76*:8, 1974.
61. Madden, J. W., and Smith, H. C.: Rate of collagen synthesis and deposition in dehisced and resutured wounds. Surg. Gynecol. Obstet., *130*:487, 1970.
62. Majno, G., Gabbiani, G., Hirschel, B. J., Ryan, G. B., and Statkov, P. R.: Contraction of granulation tissue *in vitro*: Similarity to smooth muscle. Science, *173*:548, 1971.
63. Mason, M. L., and Allen, H. S.: The rate of healing of tendons. An experimental study of tensile strength. Ann. Surg., *113*:424, 1941.
64. Meadows, E. C., and Prudden, J. F.: A study of the influence of adrenal steroids on the strength of healing wounds. Surgery, *33*:841, 1976.
65. Mustoe, T. A., Purdy, J., Gramates, P., et al.: Reversal of impaired wound healing in irradiated rats by platelet-derived growth factor-BB. Am. J. Surg., *158*:345, 1989.
66. Nimni, M. E.: A defect in the intramolecular and intermolecular cross-linking of collagen caused by penicillamine. J. Biol. Chem., *743*:1457, 1967.
67. Odland, G., and Ross, R.: Human wound repair. I. Epidermal regeneration. J. Cell. Biol., *39*:135, 1968.
68. Ordman, L. J., and Gillman, T.: Studies on the healing of cutaneous wounds. I. The healing of incisions through the skin of pigs. Arch. Surg., *93*:857, 1968.
69. Peacock, E. E., Jr., and Madden, J. W.: Some studies on the effect of β-aminopropionitrile on collagen in healing wounds. Surgery, *60*:7, 1966.
70. Peacock, E. E., Jr., and Madden, J. W.: Some studies on the effect of β-aminopropionitrile in patients with injured flexor tendons. Surgery, *66*:215, 1969.
71. Pories, W. J., Henzel, J. H., Rob, C. G., and Strain, W. H.: Acceleration of healing with zinc sulfate. Ann. Surg., *165*:432, 1967.
72. Prockop, D. J., et al.: The biosynthesis of collagen and its disorders. Part II. N. Engl. J. Med., *301*:77, 1979.
73. Prudden, J. F., Migel, P., Hanson, P., Friedrich, L., and Balarsa, L.: The discovery of a potent pure chemical wound-healing accelerator. Am. J. Surg., *119*:560, 1970.
74. Prudden, J. F., Wabarsky, E. P., and Balarsa, L.: The acceleration of healing. Surg. Gynecol. Obstet., *128*:1321, 1969.
75. Rabkin, J. M., and Hunt, T. K.: Local heat increases blood flow and oxygen tension in wounds. Arch. Surg., *122*:221, 1987.
76. Rees, R. S., Altenbern, D. P., Lynch, J. B., and King, L. E., Jr.: Brown recluse spider bites. A comparison of early surgical excision versus dapsone and delayed surgical excision. Ann. Surg., *202*:659, 1985.
77. Ross, R., Everett, N. B., and Tyler, R.: Wound healing and collagen formation. VI. The origin of the wound fibroblast studied in parabiosis. J. Cell Biol., *44*:645, 1970.
78. Rovee, D. T., and Miller, C. A.: Epidermal role in the breaking strength of wounds. Arch. Surg., *96*:43, 1968.
79. Rudolph, R.: Location of the force of wound contraction. Surg. Gynecol. Obstet., *148*:547, 1979.
80. Rudolph, R., Guber, S., Suzuki, M., and Woodward, M.: The life cycle of the myofibroblast. Surg. Gynecol. Obstet., *145*:389, 1977.
81. Sank, A., Chi, M., Shima, T., Reich, R., and Martin, G. R.: Increased calcium levels alter cellular and molecular events in wound healing. Surgery, *106*:1141, 1989.
82. Savlov, E. D., and Dunphy, J. E.: The healing of the disrupted and resutured wound. Surgery, *36*:362, 1954.
83. Sawhney, C. P., and Monga, H. L.: Wound contraction in rabbits and the effectiveness of skin grafts in preventing it. Br. J. Plast. Surg., *23*:318, 1970.
84. Stevens, F. O., and Hunt, T. K.: Effect of changes in inspired oxygen and carbon dioxide tensions on wound tensile strength: An experimental study. Ann. Surg., *173*:515, 1971.
85. Stone, P. A., and Madden, J. W.: Effect of primary and delayed split skin grafting on wound contraction. Surg. Forum, *25*:41, 1974.
86. Stone, P. A., and Madden, J. W.: Biological factors affecting wound contraction. Surg. Forum, *26*:547, 1975.
87. Watts, G. T., Grillo, H. C., and Gross, J.: Studies in wound healing: II. The role of granulation tissue in contraction. Ann. Surg., *148*:153, 1958.
88. Weeks, J. R.: Prostaglandins. Ann. Rev. Pharmacol., *12*:317, 1972.
89. White, R. A., Abergel, R. P., Klein, S. R., et al.: Laser welding of venotomies. Arch. Surg., *121*:905, 1986.

90. White, R. A., Kopchok, G., Donayre, C., et al.: Comparison of laser-welded and sutured arteriotomies. Arch. Surg., *121*:1133, 1986.

91. Williamson, M. B., and Fromm, H. J.: Effect of cystine and methionine on healing experimental wounds. Proc. Soc. Exp. Biol. Med., *80*:523, 1957.

92. Willoughby, D. A.: Some views on the pathogenesis of inflammation. *In* Montagna, W., Bentley, J. P., and Dobson, R. (Eds.): The Dermis, Advances in Biology of Skin, Vol. 10. New York, Appleton-Century-Crofts, 1970, pp. 221–230.

93. Winsey, K., Simon, R. J., Levenson, S. M., et al.: Effect of supplemental vitamin A on colon anastomotic healing in rats given preoperative irradiation. Am. J. Surg., *153*:153, 1987.

11

BURNS

Including Cold, Chemical, and Electric Injuries*

Basil A. Pruitt, Jr., M.D., Cleon W. Goodwin, Jr., M.D., and Scott K. Pruitt, M.D.

THERMAL INJURY

More than 2 million people are burned in the United States each year, and among those there are 6500 burn- and fire-related deaths.[78] The cause of injury and the risks of burn injury and burn death are influenced by age, economic circumstances, and occupation, with the risk of burn injury and fire death greatest in the economically disadvantaged. Seventy-five per cent of all burn-related deaths follow house fires, and the death rates are highest among young children and the elderly, who have difficulty escaping from the fire. Flame injury, most commonly that following a house fire or ignition of clothing, is the predominant type of burn injury in patients admitted to burn centers, but approximately 30 per cent of all burns requiring hospital treatment are caused by scalding with hot liquids.

The majority of burn injuries are of sufficiently limited extent and severity that patients can be cared for on an outpatient basis. The remainder, amounting to approximately 300 burn patients per million people per year, require hospital care because of the extent of the burn or a complicating factor such as associated injury or extreme age or youth. Even within this subset of burn patients, the majority, or 75 per cent, have burn injuries that involve less than 20 per cent of the total body surface, and most of those are adequately cared for in a general hospital by personnel experienced in burn care. Within the group of burn patients requiring in-hospital care is a smaller group (82 per million people per year) who are classified, on the basis of burn size and complicating co-morbid factors, as having major burn injuries. The American Burn Association has defined major burn injuries as (1) burns that involve more than 10 per cent of the total body surface area in patients younger than 10 years and older than 50 years; (2) burns that involve more than 20 per cent of the total body surface in patients of intervening age; (3) significant burns of the face, hands, feet, genitalia, perineum, or major joints; (4) full-thickness burns that involve more than 5 per cent of the total body surface area in patients of any age; (5) significant electric injury, including lightning injury; and (6) significant chemical injury. Inhalation injury, concomitant mechanical trauma, and significant pre-existing medical disorders mandate burn center care for patients with burns of lesser extent. All patients with major burn injuries are best cared for in a burn center where the specialized skills of a multidisciplinary staff and burn-specific equipment and facilities ensure optimal salvage.

Pre-Hospital and Emergency Room Care of Burn Patients

At the scene of the injury the first responder should remove the patient from the source of heat; extinguish burning clothing; remove the patient from electrical contact without making contact with the current; dilute with copious lavage any chemical agent causing tissue injury; and remove all clothing, including footwear and gloves, contaminated by a chemical agent. Cardiopulmonary function must be maintained in the burn patient as in any other trauma patient. Early postinjury cardiorespiratory arrest and the resulting need for cardiopulmonary resuscitation are uncommon in burn patients except for those who have sustained high-voltage electrical injury. If transport to a treatment facility requires less than 30 to 45 minutes, the first responder should not attempt to place an intravenous line unless the patient has evidence of cardiac irregularity or has sustained significant blood loss due to associated mechanical trauma.

The application of ice or cold water soaks is effective in decreasing pain in areas of second-degree burn and should be used for analgesic effect if the burns involve less than 25 per cent of the total body surface. Cold soaks or ice should be used only for the length of time necessary to relieve pain, and systemic hypothermia should be avoided. Cold applications may also be used to reduce tissue heat content, and thus thermal injury, in patients with severe burns if the patient is seen within 10 minutes of the time of burning but exert little effect beyond that time. Following cooling procedures, the burns should be covered with a clean sheet, over which a blanket can be placed to conserve body heat. If feasible, the burned parts should be elevated to minimize edema formation both before and during transport.

Carbon monoxide poisoning, most apt to be present in patients who were burned in a closed space, impairs tissue oxygenation by reducing the oxygen-carrying capacity of the blood, shifting the oxygen-hemoglobin dissociation curve to the left, binding to myoglobin, and binding to the terminal cytochrome oxidase. Since symptoms of carbon monoxide poisoning correlate poorly with measured carboxyhemoglobin levels, little purpose is served by attempting to estimate carboxyhemoglobin levels in the field. The first responder should begin the administration of 100 per cent oxygen by nonrebreathing mask to accelerate the dissociation of carboxyhemoglobin in any patient in whom inhalation of significant amounts of carbon monoxide is suspected. An endotracheal tube should be inserted to maintain airway patency in patients with severe inhalation injury and those in whom edema of the upper airway may develop rapidly.

Hyperbaric oxygen therapy has been advocated for those pa-

---

* The opinions or assertions contained herein are the private views of the authors and are not to be construed as official or as reflecting the views of the Department of the Army or the Department of Defense.

TABLE 1. Characteristics of First-, Second-, and Third-Degree Burns

	First-Degree	Second-Degree	Third-Degree
Cause	Exposure to sunlight	Limited exposure to hot liquid, flash, flame, or chemical agent	Prolonged exposure to flame, hot object, or chemical agent Contact with high-voltage electricity
Color	Red	Pink or mottled red	Pearly white, charred, translucent, or parchment-like Deeply tanned—strong acid burns Dark red—in young children
Surface	Dry or small to moderate-sized blisters	Bullae or moist weeping surface	Dry, with thrombosis of superficial vessels Focal tissue loss—high-voltage electric injury Soapy tissue necrosis—strong alkali
Sensation	Painful	Painful Deep second-degree burns may be anesthetic to pinprick with intact pressure sensation	Insensate surface
Healing	3–6 days	10–21 days—superficial second-degree > 21 days—deep second-degree	Requires grafting

tients with carbon monoxide poisoning who are comatose. Such treatment unquestionably accelerates the dissociation of carbon monoxide from hemoglobin, but improvement in neurologic outcome remains undocumented.

Hydrogen cyanide, present in the smoke generated by the combustion of natural or synthetic nitrogen-containing polymers, inhibits cellular respiration and impairs generation of adenosine triphosphate (ATP). Since cyanide poisoning is rare in patients without carbon monoxide poisoning, treatment for cyanide poisoning need be considered only for unconscious burn patients with signs of hypoxia. Chelating agents that form cyanide complexes that can be excreted by the kidneys are more effective than other antidotes. Hydroxycobalamine, the antidote of choice, has few toxic effects and is preferred over cobalt edetate, which commonly induces vomiting and occasionally induces anaphylactic reactions. Sodium thiosulfate, an agent that enhances enzymatic detoxification of cyanide to thiocyanate and has no significant side effects, can be administered

intravenously but acts slowly. The beneficial effects of both agents are realized if 80 ml. of a solution containing 4 gm. of hydroxycobalamine and 8 gm. of sodium thiosulfate are given intravenously over 3 to 5 minutes. Antidotes that cause the formation of methemoglobin—i.e., amyl nitrite aerosol, parenteral sodium nitrites, and 4-dimethylaminophenol—should be administered only in the hospital where methemoglobin levels can be monitored and the dosage adjusted to prevent critical reduction of the oxygen-carrying capacity of the blood.

In the emergency room, fluid resuscitation should be initiated by infusing a balanced salt solution through a large-caliber intravenous cannula placed in a peripheral vein underlying unburned skin, a peripheral vein underlying the burn wound, or a central vein in that order of preference. Patency of the airway should be assessed and adequate ventilation ensured by endotracheal intubation, if necessary. Insofar as possible, a history should be obtained with emphasis on determining the circumstances of the injury, the presence of pre-existing disease and allergies, and any medications taken prior to injury. A swift but thorough physical examination should be performed to identify any associated injuries. An arterial blood sample for determination of pH, blood gases, carboxyhemoglobin, electrolytes, urea nitrogen, glucose, and hematocrit should be obtained for any patient with a major burn injury.

The patient should be weighed, the depth of the burns assessed (Table 1 and Fig. 1), and the extent of burn estimated by the rule of nines* or any of several burn diagrams that relate skin surface area of various body parts to total body surface area (Fig. 2). Fluid needs are then estimated on the basis of the total extent of second- and third-degree burns and body weight, and the fluid infusion rate is adjusted accordingly. The volume and type of all fluids administered must be recorded on a flow sheet.

Ventilatory status should again be assessed to determine the need for endotracheal intubation, oxygen administration, and mechanical ventilatory support. A urethral catheter should be placed in all burn patients requiring intravenous fluid therapy, and the hourly urinary output should be measured and re-

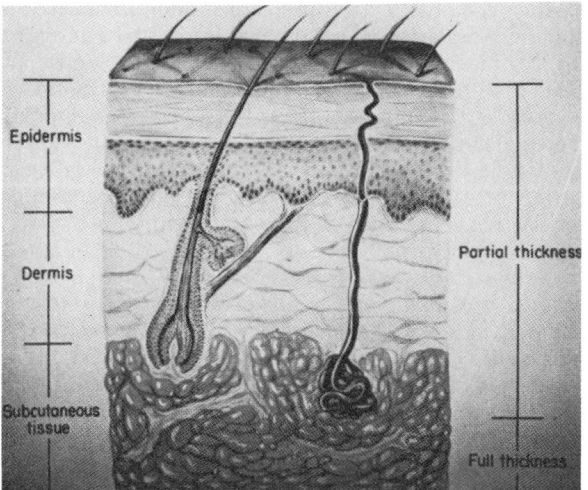

Figure 1. Diagram of skin and subcutaneous tissue showing the relationship of the depth of the burn to the location of adnexal structures. A partial-thickness or second-degree burn, if protected from infection, desiccation, and subsequent ischemia, will heal spontaneously as epithelial cells migrate from residual viable hair follicles and sweat glands. Because all adnexa are destroyed in full-thickness or third-degree burns, such wounds will not re-epithelialize and must be closed by skin grafting.

* The rule of nines describes that percentage of the body surface represented by various anatomic areas—i.e., each upper limb, 9 per cent; each lower limb, 18 per cent; anterior and posterior trunk, each 18 per cent; head and neck, 9 per cent; and perineum and genitalia, 1 per cent.

BURN ESTIMATE AND DIAGRAM
AGE vs. AREA

Area	Birth 1 yr	1–4 yr	5–9 yr	10–14 yr	15 yr	Adult	2°	3°	Total	Donor Areas
Head	19	17	13	11	9	7				
Neck	2	2	2	2	2	2				
Ant. Trunk	13	13	13	13	13	13				
Post. Trunk	13	13	13	13	13	13				
R. Buttock	2½	2½	2½	2½	2½	2½				
L. Buttock	2½	2½	2½	2½	2½	2½				
Genitalia	1	1	1	1	1	1				
R.U. Arm	4	4	4	4	4	4				
L.U. Arm	4	4	4	4	4	4				
R.L. Arm	3	3	3	3	3	3				
L.L. Arm	3	3	3	3	3	3				
R. Hand	2½	2½	2½	2½	2½	2½				
L. Hand	2½	2½	2½	2½	2½	2½				
R. Thigh	5½	6½	8	8½	9	9½				
L. Thigh	5½	6½	8	8½	9	9½				
R. Leg	5	5	5½	6	6½	7				
L. Leg	5	5	5½	6	6½	7				
R. Foot	3½	3½	3½	3½	3½	3½				
L. Foot	3½	3½	3½	3½	3½	3½				

TOTAL

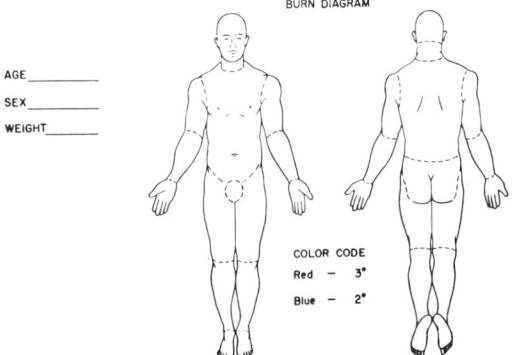

BURN DIAGRAM

AGE _____
SEX _____
WEIGHT _____

COLOR CODE
Red — 3°
Blue — 2°

Figure 2. Burn diagram and table used in estimating the extent of the burn. Note that the fractions of total body surface represented by the head and lower limbs change with age and assume constant proportions after age 15.

corded. Electrocardiographic (ECG) monitoring of patients who have sustained high-voltage electric injury should also be initiated in the emergency room.

Initial burn wound care should be accomplished in the emergency room for those patients whose burns are of such limited extent that they do not require in-hospital care. The burned areas should be gently cleansed with a surgical soap or detergent, and loose, nonviable skin should then be débrided. Bullae that are less than 2 cm. in diameter can be left intact, but larger bullae should be excised, because they frequently rupture and are thereafter easily infected. Burns of limited extent are not at significant risk of infection, and topical antimicrobial agents need not be used. Such small burns can be dressed with fine-mesh gauze thinly impregnated with petrolatum, over which a dry bulky dressing is applied and held in place with a semielastic gauze wrap. Alternatively, if the site of the burn permits rapid formation of a protective crust and the rapid drying of that crust after daily soap and water cleansings, the wound can be left exposed. The patient should be seen in follow-up at least every 3 days, at which time dressings, if utilized, are changed and the wound inspected. If healing is proceeding uneventfully and the wound is free of infection, a clean dressing is applied and that sequence repeated as many times as necessary until healing has occurred. If, at the time of follow-up examination, infection is evident, the dressing should be removed, the patient admitted to the hospital, and topical antimicrobial chemotherapy initiated.

In the case of patients requiring in-hospital care, transfer to the appropriate treatment facility is made after completion of emergency room procedures. The wounds should be covered by a clean dry sheet (and a blanket if necessary) during transfer. Débridement is performed and specific wound care is initiated at the definitive treatment center.

TABLE 2. Extent of Burn Associated with a 50 Per Cent Mortality, LA$_{50}$, as Related to Age: 1985–1989 (U.S. Army Institute of Surgical Research)

Age	Number of Patients	LA$_{50}$
0–14	222	53.4%
15–40	556	75.6%
41+	231	44.0%

Pathophysiology of Thermal Injury

Thermal energy causes cell injury of variable degree and coagulation necrosis of the skin and underlying tissues to variable depth, depending upon both the temperature to which the tissue is exposed and the duration of heat application. Burn injury also exerts deleterious effects on all other organ systems with the extent and duration of organ dysfunction proportional to the extent of burn.[75] The biphasic changes (early hypofunction and later hyperfunction) in organ function may be clinically inapparent in patients with burns of less than 25 per cent of the total body surface but are readily identified in patients with more extensive burns. Mortality is similarly related to the extent of the burn in a sigmoid dose-response manner and is further influenced by the patient's age (Table 2).

Immediately after thermal injury, the changes that occur in the cardiovascular system predominate and assume treatment priority in order to limit volume deficits, prevent the development of burn shock, and achieve maximal salvage (Fig. 3). The direct effect of heat as well as the liberation of vasoactive materials from the area of injury alter transvascular pressure relationships and capillary permeability, both of which promote loss of fluid and protein from the intravascular into the extravascular compartment. These volume shifts occur in direct proportion to the extent of the burn and are clinically apparent as edema, which develops in areas of thermal injury and may also occur in unburned tissues as resuscitation proceeds in patients with extensive burns, i.e., those of over 25 per cent of the total body surface.[7]

Within minutes after burning, cardiac output falls in proportion to burn size in association with an increase in peripheral vascular resistance.[79] Later (but still early after the burn) cardiac output remains depressed or is further reduced by the combined

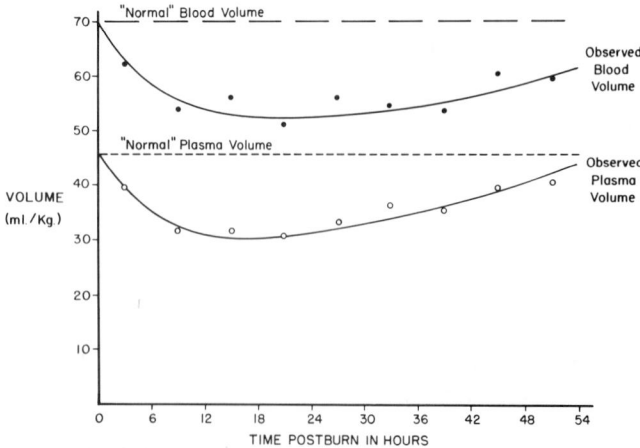

Figure 3. Mean blood and plasma volume changes during the first 54 hours after injury in 10 patients with burns involving an average of 65 per cent of the total body surface. Fluid resuscitation guided by the Brooke formula permitted an early modest volume loss (the velocity of which decreased with time), defended against further loss, and restored plasma volume to near predicted levels by 54 hours.

effect of a decreasing blood volume and increasing blood viscosity, as indexed by a rising hematocrit. Although a circulating myocardial depressant factor has been implicated as the cause of impaired myocardial function, animal studies have demonstrated that the depressed cardiac function is associated with a decrease in myocardial ATP that is prevented by resuscitation,[60] is most prominent in older animals with extensive burns and is ameliorated by increasing coronary blood flow,[42] is partially corrected by administration of oxygen radical scavengers or histamine H_2 receptor antagonists,[9,43] and is completely reversed by fluid resuscitation.[15] Clinical studies in burn patients without heart disease in whom cardiac output was depressed in the first 24 postburn hours have revealed no evidence of myocardial depression. In those patients, the heart was hyperdynamic, indicated by elevation of ejection fraction and velocity of myocardial fiber shortening. Hypovolemia, as manifested by a depressed left ventricular end-diastolic volume, was an obvious cause of the depressed cardiac output in those patients.

The loss of fluid from the vascular tree has been generally attributed to an increase in microvascular permeability due to the direct effects of heat and the effects of a variety of humoral factors liberated from damaged tissue and cytokines produced by activated leukocytes. The most frequently incriminated cell product is histamine, present in abundance in mast cells. The plasma histamine concentration rises in proportion to burn size within 1 minute of thermal injury. Preburn depletion of histamine by administration of polymyxin B has been reported to partially inhibit edema formation in the unburned ear of a mouse after a burn of the opposite ear. However, Yurt and associates using a murine model of a larger (30 per cent) burn found that preburn administration of polymyxin B degranulated mast cells and significantly reduced the number of mast cells per vessel in the burn wound but failed to reduce edema formation in the wound.[97] These studies suggest that histamine contributes to the systemic vascular changes consequent to burn injury but is of minor importance in the formation of edema in the burn wound.

Arachidonic acid metabolites (principally thromboxane A_2 and leukotrienes), substance P (apparently originating in sensory nerve endings), fibrin degradation product D, and activated proteases have been reported to increase vascular permeability. Antagonists of each of those agents (when administered prior to burn injury) have been reported to reduce but not eliminate the increase in transcapillary filtration that occurs after burn injury. Although pretreatment in animal models of burn injury with indomethacin suppresses lymph flow from the burn wound and transcapillary transport of macromolecules, and topical application of thromboxane synthetase inhibitors has been reported to reduce tissue damage, as evidenced by more rapid wound healing, such inhibitors appear to exert little effect on microvascular permeability. Animal studies have demonstrated that the leukotriene receptor antagonist FPL 55712 decreases edema in burned skin even when administered after injury.[1] However, that finding does not confirm a primary effect of leukotrienes on microvascular permeability, since they are strong vasoconstrictors.

Activation of the immune system also causes the production of factors that can increase microvascular permeability, i.e., products of complement activation, lysosomal enzymes,[87] increased xanthine oxidase activity, oxygen radicals,[87] and activated killer lymphocytes.[20] Administration of neutrophil cathepsin G produces an increase in weight of the isolated perfused lung and an increase in albumin movement across cultured endothelial cell monolayers, effects that could be attenuated by heparin, dextran sulfate, and human serum.[68] Similarly, interleukin-2 (IL-2)–activated human killer lymphocytes in contact with cultured endothelial cells increase albumin flux across monolayers of such cells.[20] Till and associates have reported that neutrophil depletion protects against postburn lung

injury but has no effect on burn wound edema formation.[88] Using a murine model of burn injury, they found that inhibitors of xanthine oxidase decreased edema formation in burned skin and that excision of the burn within 3 minutes of burning significantly attenuated the rise in plasma xanthine oxidase activity. The location-specific effects of neutrophil depletion, enzyme inhibitors, and oxygen radical scavengers are consistent with studies by Yurt and Pruitt showing that neutrophil accumulation in the burn decreases and indiscrete margination increases as burn size increases.[98]

A variety of materials that have cytotoxic, vasoactive, immunologic, and antifibrinolytic effects have been identified in burn blister fluid. The thromboxane A_2, complement activation products, proteases, IL-1, and inhibitor of fibrinolysis present in burn blister fluid may contribute to the progression of cell damage in the injured tissue underlying the blister, but the nonviable tissue that forms the base of the blister and the impaired blood supply of that tissue appear to limit the access of the blister fluid constituents to the general circulation. Oxygen-derived free radicals appear to be of little importance in local vascular changes. Melikian and associates found that oxygen radical scavengers administered parenterally or topically and parenteral administration of a xanthine oxidase inhibitor did not influence the rate or quality of healing of partial-thickness burns.[55]

Recent studies have focused attention on changes of capillary pressure and interstitial fluid hydrostatic pressure as etiologic factors in the formation of postburn edema. Pitt and associates have reported that following a scald burn 53 per cent of the increased capillary filtration observed during the first 3 hours was due to increased capillary pressure with a threefold increase in the fraction of filtrate that passed through large pores.[69] The proportion of the increased capillary filtration due to increased permeability increased with time. Lund and associates have measured, in an animal model of burn injury, a strongly negative interstitial fluid hydrostatic pressure within 15 to 30 minutes after burning.[49] The negativity of the pressure was proportional to burn size, as was its duration. That investigative group has also reported an early temporary reversal of transcapillary osmotic pressure gradient with an early increase in interstitial fluid colloid osmotic pressure following a burn of 10 per cent of the total body surface.[48] The reversed transcapillary osmotic pressure gradient persisted for up to 12 hours. After a larger (40 per cent) burn, the plasma leak increased in intact unburned tissues, as indicated by increased filtration coefficients measured in unburned skin and muscle.[7]

The rate of edema formation is greatest immediately after burning and has been reported to reach peak values 3 to 24 hours after burning. The subsequent time-related decrease in edema formation has been related to restoration of capillary integrity.[79] Studies by Lund and Reed, using a murine model of a 10 per cent burn, demonstrated that without resuscitation the major portion of fluid translocation occurred in the first 60 minutes after injury.[48] However, other studies, using a murine model of a 20 per cent full-thickness burn, have revealed a rapid progressive rise in burn wound edema for the first 6 hours and a subsequent slow rise over the next 18 hours to reach a peak of burn wound water and protein content at 24 hours after injury. At that time, capillary permeability, as measured by albumin flux rates, was still elevated, but edema formation ceased because a new equilibrium of fluid and protein flow through the wound had been established.

Diminished blood volume and cardiac output cause a postburn decrease in renal blood flow and glomerular filtration rate. The resulting oliguria, if untreated, may progress to acute renal failure. Postburn hypovolemia may also impair flow to other organs as well, and restlessness (a reflection of impaired cerebral blood flow) is a frequent early sign of blood volume depletion. After resuscitation, renal blood flow and glomerular filtration rate increase to supranormal levels in concert with the increase in cardiac output characteristic of postburn hypermetabolism. The hyperdynamic renal circulation often necessitates adjustment of the dose of antibiotics and other drugs that are primarily excreted by the kidney.

Studies in burn patients have demonstrated that the postresuscitation increase in cardiac output is wound-directed. The blood flow to a burned limb is significantly greater than that to an unburned limb in the same patient, and the increase is proportional to the extent of burn on the involved limb.[5] Consequently, pharmacologic reduction of cardiac output might well compromise burn wound healing by reducing the local delivery of oxygen and other nutrients necessary for tissue repair.

Alterations of pulmonary function following burn injury vary according to the extent and location of the burn and the presence or absence of inhalation injury. In those patients with circumferential burns of the thorax, the constricting eschar and underlying edema may produce a restrictive ventilatory defect requiring relief by placement of escharotomy incisions as described later. In patients without burns of the thorax or inhalation injury, the initial hypovolemia may cause rapid shallow respirations. After resuscitation, hyperventilation (two to two and one-half times normal minute ventilation) with modest, if any, evidence of parenchymal dysfunction is customarily observed. This response, considered to be a reflection of postinjury hypermetabolism, may be associated with modest hypoxemia, especially during the period of edema resorption. As a consequence of this hyperventilation, a mild respiratory alkalosis is the most frequent acid base disturbance in burn patients after resuscitation. If secondary pulmonary complications supervene, the hyperventilation may be accentuated. If pulmonary reserve is exceeded, the acid base status may quickly change from alkalosis to acidosis, hypoxemia (at times profound) may develop, and pulmonary insufficiency may be of such severity as to require mechanical ventilatory support. The hyperventilation recedes as the burn wound heals.

Pulmonary vascular resistance increases in the immediate postburn period, and the magnitude and duration of this pressure increase in the lesser circulation exceed those in the systemic circulation. The rarity of pulmonary edema during the resuscitation phase, even when large volumes of fluid are infused, is consistent with the site of increased resistance being in a precapillary location and being protective in nature.

Studies using an ovine model have identified differential changes in the lymph/plasma protein ratios in the lymph draining from burned tissue, unburned subcutaneous tissue, and the lung, indicating that burned injury has no apparent effect on pulmonary capillary permeability.[23] An increase in the lymph/plasma ratios for proteins with radii of 35 to 108 angstroms was noted in the lymph draining burn tissue, while the lymph/plasma ratio for proteins with a 58-angstrom radius was increased (for only 12 hours) in the lymph draining unburned subcutaneous tissue, and the lymph/plasma ratio for all protein fractions was decreased in the lung in which there was no apparent change in protein sieving.[38]

Burn injury itself as well as initial fluid therapy appear to evoke other immediate and delayed changes in the pulmonary vasculature and alter pulmonary function. Laboratory studies have shown that postburn generation of the chemotactic peptide C5a, as a result of progressive activation of complement, is temporally related to neutropenia, aggregation of leukocytes in pulmonary capillaries, and intra-alveolar hemorrhages.[87] The eicosanoids appear to be involved in the lung injury induced by complement activation but to have no role in the associated pulmonary hypertension, since both cyclooxygenase and lipoxygenase inhibitors attenuate the former and exert little if any effect on the latter.[25,57] During the period of lung dysfunction, thromboxane levels in the lymph from the burned areas and in venous plasma were increased and the preburn administration

of ibuprofen reduced postinjury lung dysfunction.[25] Protection was also afforded by preburn depletion of complement, neutrophils, or platelets and by systemic therapy with catalase and superoxide dismutase.[87] Those findings have implicated toxic oxygen products, produced by activated neutrophils, as agents contributing to postburn pulmonary pathophysiology.

Hypoproteinemia induced by the infusion of large volumes of colloid-free fluid in the course of resuscitation has been both implicated and exonerated as a cause of postburn pulmonary changes. In an ovine model of a 50 to 60 per cent full-thickness burn injury, resuscitation-induced hypoproteinemia did not appear to alter pulmonary transvascular filtration rate independent of changes in hydrostatic pressure. In other studies using that same model, a postburn increase in lymph flow in both lung and unburned tissue was observed that was eliminated by resuscitation with the use of plasma to restore plasma protein levels.[23] Lymph flow in burned tissue was unchanged by such treatment. Pulmonary hypertension and associated depression of arterial oxygen tension occurred in animals with burns of from 50 to 70 per cent of the total body surface, and lung lymph flow was increased in proportion to burn size. Resuscitation with dextran and protein prevented the postburn increase in lung lymph flow but exerted no effect on postburn hypoxia or hypertension. In other studies using that model of burn injury in which lactated Ringer's solution was infused to return cardiac filling pressures to baseline levels, dynamic lung compliance decreased by 40 per cent at 12 hours and was associated with an increase in protein-poor lung lymph flow and evidence of lipid peroxidation of lung tissue, but no increase in extravascular lung water was observed. Inasmuch as preburn administration of ibuprofen attenuated the decrease in dynamic compliance, that alteration was attributed to mediator-induced bronchoconstriction and not pulmonary edema.[45]

The burn wound may also serve as the source of cell metabolites that are produced by infection and exert deleterious effects on the lungs. In laboratory studies, the injection of endotoxin into the subcutaneous tissue beneath a burn increased the thromboxane B_2 content in lymph draining from the burned area and in venous plasma and was associated with a coincident increase in pulmonary artery pressure and a decrease in mean arterial oxygen tension. Topical application of ibuprofen prior to endotoxin challenge significantly reduced the increase of thromboxane in the lymph draining from the burned area and prevented the increase of thromboxane B_2 in venous plasma and subsequent pulmonary dysfunction.[47] These studies, indicating that lung dysfunction can be induced by thromboxane products generated locally after injection of endotoxin into the burned tissue, even in the absence of circulating endotoxin, provide insight into the pathogenesis of pulmonary dysfunction in patients with remote infections caused by endotoxin-producing organisms.

In addition to the loss of plasma from the circulation in the early postburn period, there is immediate red cell destruction in direct proportion to the extent of burn, particularly the extent of third-degree burn. In patients with extensive burns there is a continuing red cell loss of variable extent (8 to 12 per cent of red cell mass per day) due to the aggregate effect of lysis of cells damaged by heat, microvascular thrombosis in areas of damaged tissue that subsequently undergo necrosis, and blood sampling necessitated by care requirements.

A biphasic alteration of the coagulation system also characterizes the response to thermal injury. Animal studies have identified vascular occlusion by platelet microthrombi, not leukocyte adherence, as the major factor causing progressive postburn dermal ischemia. That process is reflected in the early marked depression of platelet and fibrinogen levels accompanied by a parallel increase in fibrin split product levels that is observed in patients with extensive burns. These changes are followed by a prompt postresuscitation return to normal and subsequent elevation of those coagulation factors in association with an increase in factors V and VIII. As early as 3 days after burning, marked depression of antithrombin III and protein C levels has been identified. Although thromboembolic disease is surprisingly rare in patients with extensive burns, when such occurs and anticoagulation is necessary, the antithrombin III deficit may markedly elevate the dose of heparin required for effective anticoagulation. Secondary alterations in clotting factor levels may occur later in the postburn course, commonly in association with infection. Fibrinogen appears relatively insensitive to sepsis *per se* unless the infection is accompanied by intravascular coagulation.

The gastrointestinal tract also responds in a stereotypic burn-size–related manner to thermal injury. Ileus is nearly universal in patients with burns of more than 25 per cent of the total body surface, presumably because of the combined effects of hypovolemia and neurohormonal changes. After resuscitation, gastrointestinal motility returns by the third to fifth postburn day. Animal studies have identified an early diminution of gastric mucosal blood flow after injury that is corrected by fluid resuscitation. Gastric and duodenal mucosal damage, secondary to focal ischemia, can be observed as early as 3 to 5 hours after burning. If the mucosa is unprotected, the early erosions may progress to frank ulceration. Later in the postburn period, sepsis and/or hypovolemia can produce similar ischemic mucosal and even transmural changes throughout the gastrointestinal tract.

In the early postburn period, a catabolic endocrine pattern develops, characterized by elevated glucagon, cortisol, and catecholamine levels and depressed insulin and triiodothyronine levels. These changes are associated with a burn size–related increase in metabolic rate, glucose flow, and negative nitrogen balance. Circulating hormone levels return toward normal in the patient with an uncomplicated burn as the wound is closed or grafted, after which anabolism and reconstitution of body mass begin. Endocrine function in injured patients can be further influenced by sepsis or other complications. The injury-induced changes may be either exaggerated or attenuated, depending upon the severity of the complicating disease.

Specific neurologic changes are most commonly observed in patients with high-voltage electric injury or in association with mechanical trauma. Nonspecific neurologic changes, such as disorientation, obtundation, or seizures, may reflect infection, electrolyte or fluid imbalance, or the toxic effects of medication and are similar to those that can occur after any other form of injury.

The global effects of burn injury on the immune system are reflected by the fact that infection remains the major cause of death in burn patients.[74] Destruction of the mechanical barrier of the skin contributes to susceptibility to infection, but postburn alterations in immune function may also be of critical importance. Depression of the cellular immune response, as demonstrated by prolonged skin allograft survival in both thermally injured experimental animals and patients, has long been recognized. Delayed hypersensitivity as well as peripheral blood lymphocyte proliferation in the mixed lymphocyte reaction in burn patients is also inhibited.[12,52,81] With burns of 20 per cent or more of the body surface area, impairment of cell-mediated immunity is proportional to burn size.

After thermal injury many alterations in lymphocyte number and function occur. During the first week after burning, while the total white blood cell count is increased, peripheral blood lymphocyte counts are reduced, as are the numbers of CD3-positive T cells, CD4-positive helper/inducer T cells (Th/i), and CD8-positive suppressor/cytotoxic T cells (Ts/c), with inversion of the normal Ts/c-to-Th/i ratio.[12,52,81] All of these indices normalize over the second postburn week in normally recovering patients. A late (more than 14 days after burning) increase in the Ts/c-to-Th/i ratio has been shown by McIrvine and associates to correspond to patient death from sepsis,[52] but experimental studies suggest that this alteration may be an effect, rather than a cause, of sepsis.[10]

Monocytosis, granulocytosis, and B-lymphocytosis also occur early in the postburn course (beginning on postburn day 1)[12]; but serum immunoglobulin G (IgG) levels are decreased after burn injury and gradually return to normal over the next 2 to 4 weeks. Exogenous administration of IgG to burned patients promptly restores IgG to normal levels but exerts no demonstrable effect on morbidity or mortality.

As an assay of lymphocyte responsiveness, blast transformation assays of lymphocytes from thermally injured patients have produced contradictory results. In 38 patients with a mean body surface area of burn of 38 per cent, Munster and associates performed serial determinations of peripheral blood lymphocyte blast transformation and found that decreased responsiveness to streptokinase-streptodornase, purified protein derivative (PPD), mumps, and allogeneic stimulator cells, but not the mitogen phytohemagglutinin (PHA), accurately predicted patient survival.[61] On the basis of studies of peripheral blood lymphocytes from thermally injured patients showing both increased spontaneous blast transformation and reduced responsiveness to mitogen stimulation, Deitch suggests that this immune defect in burn patients is due not to the functional inability of lymphocytes to become activated, but instead to the resistance of already activated cells to further immune stimulation.[22] Conversely, more recent investigations suggest that the diminished responsiveness in these assays may be due to the presence of nonlymphoid cells contaminating the lymphocyte preparations.[10,21] When these contaminated cells are removed, burn patient peripheral blood lymphocytes have been found to respond normally to mitogens and alloantigens.[21]

Alterations in IL-2 production and IL-2 receptor (IL-2R) expression by lymphocytes from burn patients have also been noted. In a murine model of thermal injury, Gadd and associates found marked defects in mitogen-induced IL-2R expression by cultured splenocytes, unresponsive to exogenously added IL-2.[29] Peripheral blood lymphocytes from burn patients show a similar defect in mitogen-induced IL-2R expression, but exogenously added IL-2 significantly increases the percentage of IL-2R–expressing cells. Because this increase in IL-2R expression with exogenous IL-2 is not paralleled by enhanced lymphocyte proliferation in response to added IL-2, Teodorczyk-Injeyan and associates suggest that thermal injury reduces the ability of lymphocytes to express functional high affinity IL-2R and that the IL-2R present on these cells is of low affinity and is nonfunctional.[85]

Gough and co-workers have noted impairment of IL-2 production by splenocytes from thermally injured animals. Mitogen responsiveness of these cells was also impaired but was normalized by the *in vitro* addition of IL-2 to the culture medium.[32] In thermally injured patients, Wood and associates found a direct correlation between burn size and the reduction of IL-2 production by peripheral blood lymphocytes. During septic episodes in these patients, IL-2 production was further reduced.[95]

Similarly Teodorczyk-Injeyan and associates found a significant reduction in mitogen-induced IL-2 production by peripheral blood lymphocytes in burn patients. Further investigations by that group and by Xiao and associates have shown markedly elevated levels of soluble IL-2R in serum from burn patients in proportion to burn size.[86,96] Soluble IL-2R in burn serum may bind IL-2 and competitively inhibit IL-2–dependent immune responses, representing some of the immune dysfunction in burn patients. *In vivo* administration of IL-2 to thermally injured mice prior to septic challenge produces significantly improved survival following cecal ligation and puncture, suggesting the potential for therapeutic applications of IL-2 administration to enhance host immune competence in the burned patient.[32] Conflicting results have been obtained in an animal model of burn wound sepsis in which the administration of IL-2 had no effect on mortality.

In addition to lymphocytes, other populations of immune cells are known to be adversely affected by burn injury. Natural killer cell activity of peripheral blood lymphocytes is reduced in thermally injured patients, possibly because of circulating endotoxin. Polymorphonuclear leukocytes from burn patients exhibit a reduction in chemotactic activity, which is proportional to burn size and can be restored by incubation with normal serum, and also demonstrate defects in phagocytosis.[2] Studies of neutrophil function using chemiluminigenic probes have demonstrated a variable immediate response to burn injury with a generally greater depression of granulocyte oxidative activity in patients with burns of over 40 per cent of the body surface.[4] After resuscitation, neutrophil oxidative activity is influenced by the patient's clinical condition. In burn patients with infection, granulocyte peroxidase activity is typically elevated in association with toxic granulation. Granulocyte membrane–associated oxidase is depressed and progressively decreases in patients who die. A preterminal decrease in peroxidase activity appears to reflect bone marrow exhaustion.

Moreover, numerous investigators, utilizing a number of experimental methods, have demonstrated immunosuppressive factors in serum from burn patients. Both Hakim and Constantian have described an immunosuppressive polypeptide of approximately 10,000 daltons molecular weight obtained from burn patient serum that inhibits mitogen-stimulated lymphocyte proliferation.[18,34] Similar but elevated immunosuppressive activity has also been detected in subeschar fluid and may be a contributing factor to burn wound invasion.[27] Burn serum has also been noted to inhibit neutrophil chemotaxis and to impair neutrophil chemiluminescence.[4]

In addition to a suppressive peptide, other proposed immunosuppressive factors in burn serum include complement degradation products which inhibit phagocyte function,[2] immunoglobulin fragments, breakdown products of the coagulation and fibrinolytic systems,[67] prostaglandins, and endotoxin.[91] Although serum suppressive activity appears to be present in all severely burned patients, levels of activity do not correlate with patient survival.

Although it is difficult to define the specific cause-and-effect relationship between changes in various components of the immune system and infection in human burn patients, Moss and associates, using an animal model of thermal injury, have convincingly demonstrated a correlation between defects in cellular immune function and susceptibility to sepsis.[58] Thus, to reduce the susceptibility to infection in the burn patient, methods to favorably enhance depressed immune function are being developed. Among the therapies investigated, early burn wound excision with grafting has been shown to restore defective neutrophil migration in an animal model.[84] Administration of polymyxin B to severely burned patients has been shown to enhance depressed natural killer cell activity; and, as previously mentioned, administration of recombinant IL-2 has been shown to improve resistance to a secondary septic challenge in a murine model of thermal injury.[32] The limited or total lack of effectiveness of various vaccines, immunomodulators, and serologic agents, such as IgG and IL-2, in preventing invasive burn wound infection and improving survival of burn patients may simply represent the inability of any single agent to correct the multiple immune deficits induced by an extensive burn. Newly developed immunomodulatory drugs and recombinant lymphokines, used in combination therapy, may have a future clinical role in reducing the burn patient's susceptibility to infection.

Fluid Resuscitation

Fluid resuscitation should be initiated as soon as possible after injury in all patients with burns of 15 per cent or more of the total body surface. Since ileus occurs in nearly all such patients, oral resuscitation is precluded and the fluids must be infused intravenously. A large-caliber cannula should be placed in a vein (preferably a vein beneath unburned skin) of sufficient size to permit unimpeded fluid flow. Several formulas, most of which are based on the weight of the patient and the extent of the burn, have been proposed for estimating a burn patient's fluid needs. The fluid estimates of each of the commonly used formulas are shown in Table 3.

Studies by several investigators have indicated that during the first 24 hours after burning colloid-containing fluids are not essential for resuscitation. During that period, colloid-containing fluids appear to be retained within the circulation to no greater extent than an equal volume of colloid-free electrolyte-containing fluid, such as lactated Ringer's solution.[79] In a randomized prospective clinical trial, resuscitation using only crystalloid fluids during the first 24 hours was compared with resuscitation using a combination of crystalloid- and colloid-containing fluid (2.5 per cent albumin in Ringer's lactate).[30] When resuscitation was guided by hourly urinary output, as an index of adequate organ perfusion, the colloid-containing regimen restored cardiac output more rapidly than did crystalloid solution alone. This earlier restoration of cardiac output in the patients receiving the colloid solution was associated with a more rapid replacement of plasma volume deficits, as evidenced by stroke index and end-diastolic volume index measurements (Table 4). However, by the end of the first 48 postburn hours the two resuscitation regimens were equally effective in restoring cardiac output and intravascular volume. The potential advantages of the colloid-containing resuscitation regimen appeared to be offset by deleterious effects of colloid-containing fluids on the lung. Extravascular lung water remained essentially unchanged during the first postburn week in those patients who initially received only crystalloid-containing fluids but increased significantly above normal in those patients who received colloid-containing fluids as a component of initial resuscitation. Late pulmonary complications and mortality were also higher in the colloid-treated patients.

Although the volume and composition of the resuscitation fluid estimated by the formulas in Table 3 vary considerably, each formula has been found to be clinically effective. It is evident that the physiologic tolerance of the majority of burn patients allows them to adapt to the variations in formula-based fluids. Conversely, none of the formulas uniquely satisfies the fluid needs of all burn patients, and there are subsets of patients who predictably require modification of the resuscitation regimen and individualized treatment. Patients who characteristically require volumes of fluid greater than those estimated by the formulas include those with high-voltage electrical injury, those with inhalation injury, those with delayed resuscitation, and those who are burned while inebriated. Conversely, "volume-sensitive" patients who require the least possible resuscitation volume consistent with maintenance of organ function include those above 50 years of age, those under 2 years of age, and those with pre-existing cardiopulmonary disease. Although there is no documented need for salt in excess of water in burn patients, the use of concentrated salt solution for burn patient resuscitation has been recommended by some.[8] Hypertonic salt solution may be of value in diminishing volume loading and promoting kaliuresis in "volume-sensitive" burn patients. There appear, however, to be limits to both serum sodium concentration elevation (160 mEq. per liter) and cellular dehydration (15 per cent) that, when reached, interfere with cell, tissue, or organ function and necessitate that resuscitation be continued with more dilute fluids. In some reports those limitations appear to have been fortuitously avoided by allowing the patient access to hypotonic oral fluids. The sodium content of the total fluid dose received by such patients approximated isotonicity.[72]

The goal of burn patient resuscitation is the maintenance of vital organ function at the least immediate or delayed physio-

TABLE 3. Commonly Used Burn Resuscitation Formulas for Adult Patients

Formula	First 24 Hours Postburn			Second 24 Hours Postburn		
	Electrolyte-Containing Solution	Colloid-Containing Fluid Equivalent to Plasma	Glucose in Water (D5W)	Electrolyte-Containing Solution	Colloid-Containing Fluid Equivalent to Plasma	Glucose in Water (D5W)
Burn budget of F.D. Moore	Lactated Ringer's, 1000–4000 ml. 0.5 normal saline, 1200 ml.	7.5% of body weight	1500–5000 ml.	Lactated Ringer's, 1000–4000 ml. 0.5 normal saline, 1200 ml.	2.5% of body weight	1500–5000 ml.
Evans	Normal saline, 1.0 ml./kg./% burn	1.0 ml./kg./% burn	2000 ml.	½ of first 24-hour requirement	½ of first-24hour requirement	2000 ml.
Brooke	Lactated Ringer's, 1.5 ml./kg./% burn	0.5 ml./kg./% burn	2000 ml.	½ to ¾ of first 24-hour requirement	½ to ¾ of first 24-hour requirement	2000 ml.
Parkland	Lactated Ringer's, 4.0 ml./kg./% burn	—	—	—	20% to 60% of calculated plasma volume	As necessary to maintain urinary output
Hypertonic sodium solution	Volume of hypertonic lactated saline (HLS) containing 250 mEq. sodium per liter to maintain hourly urinary output of 30 ml.	—	—	0.6 ml. HLS/kg./% burn plus oral Haldane's solution to replace insensible water loss or ⅓ isotonic salt solution orally up to 3500 ml. limit		
Modified Brooke	Lactated Ringer's, 2.0 ml./kg./% burn	—	—	—	0.3–0.5 ml./kg./% burn	As necessary to maintain urinary output

logic cost. The authors believe this can be achieved by using only a balanced salt solution for fluid replacement during the first 24 hours after burning. The quantity to be infused in the adult, estimated by the commonly used formulas, ranges from 2 to 4 ml. per kg. body weight per per cent burn but the authors recommend using 2 ml. for the initial estimate in order to minimize volume loading, increasing the infused volume only if necessary. For children under 15 years of age who have a larger surface area per unit of body mass, 3 ml. per kg. body weight per per cent burn is employed for calculating fluid needs for the

TABLE 4. Left Ventricular Indices During Postburn Resuscitation

Time Period (hours)	Treatment	Cardiac Index*	End-Diastolic Volume Index†	Stroke Index‡
0–12	Colloid	3.05	42	32
	Crystalloid	3.11	43	34
12–24	Colloid	4.67	56	40
	Crystalloid	2.75	36	27
24–48	Colloid	4.42	52	39
	Crystalloid	4.03	51	37

* Normal = 3.40 L./min./sq. m.
† Normal = 60 ml./sq. m.
‡ Normal = 44 ml./cycle/sq. m.

first 24 hours. As noted above, capillary permeability is maximally increased immediately postburn with gradual restoration of functional capillary integrity during the first 24 hours thereafter. These time-related changes in capillary permeability dictate administering, in the first 8 hours after injury, half of the volume calculated for infusion during the first 24 hours and the remaining half over the succeeding 16 hours. The volume actually infused is governed by the patient's response to his injury and resuscitation.

Moore and associates reported that in a porcine model of burn injury infusion in the first 2 hours after injury of one half of the first 24-hour resuscitation volume more rapidly returned the cardiac index to 88 per cent of baseline.[56] Infusion of such large volumes during the period when intravascular pressure is the predominant determinant of capillary filtration may serve only to accentuate edema formation. Consistent with that possibility was those authors' observation that when the infusion rate of resuscitation fluid was thereafter decreased so that the remaining half of the calculated volume would be administered over the next 22 hours, the salutary effect on cardiac index promptly dissipated and the hemodynamic indices became identical to those in animals that received resuscitation according to the standard clinical regimen. Laboratory studies have also demonstrated that the administration of cimetidine within a half hour of burn injury reduces the amount of resuscitation fluid required for cardiovascular support, but the clinical usefulness of that agent remains undefined.[9]

The administration of additional electrolyte-free water in the first 24 hours after burn injury appears to be unnecessary because evaporative water loss is, at most, modest during that period of hypovolemia and peripheral vasoconstriction and because the balanced salt solutions commonly employed for burn patient resuscitation are hypotonic with respect to sodium. In burned children it may be necessary to administer maintenance fluids in addition to those administered for burn resuscitation. The need for additional maintenance fluid is greatest in small children with small burns and decreases as the size of the child increases and the size of the burn increases. Since the endocrine response to burn injury commonly induces hyperglycemia, glucose-containing fluids should not be used for resuscitation in burned adults. The limited glycogen reserves and relatively small blood volume of the burned child mandate scheduled monitoring of blood glucose levels and the use of lactated Ringer's solution containing glucose to avoid hypoglycemia.

During the second 24 hours after injury any persistent plasma volume deficit should be replaced by infusion of colloid-containing fluids. The plasma volume deficit can be measured directly or estimated to be 0.3 to 0.5 ml. per kg. body weight per per cent burn (0.3 ml. in patients with 30 to 50 per cent burns, 0.4 ml. in patients with 50 to 70 per cent burns, and 0.5 ml. in patients with burns of over 70 per cent of the total body surface). The colloid-containing solution should be administered as a plasma equivalent with the use of salt-free albumin diluted to physiologic concentration in normal saline (5 gm. per 100 ml.). The administration of other colloid-free, salt-containing fluids can usually be discontinued. Even though a 10 per cent pentastarch form of hydroxyethyl starch, infused at the end of the first 24 hours after burn injury, has been reported to be as effective in expanding plasma volume as a 5 per cent albumin solution, the greater prolongation of prothrombin time and plasma thromboplastin following infusion of as little as 500 ml. of pentastarch speaks against use of larger volumes of that solution.[92] Electrolyte-free fluid, such as 5 per cent dextrose in water, is infused in a volume sufficient to maintain urinary output while covering evaporative water loss and meeting metabolic needs. In small children, hyponatremia and the associated risk of cerebral edema should be avoided by administering 5 per cent glucose in one-quarter normal saline to maintain urinary output.

MONITORING OF FLUID RESUSCITATION. Resuscitation fluids should be infused during the first and second postburn days in amounts sufficient to maintain vital signs, a satisfactory general condition, and an hourly urinary output of 30 to 50 ml. in the adult and 1 ml. per kg. per hour in children weighing less than 30 kg. The fluid infusion rate should be adjusted if the hourly urinary output falls below or exceeds the desired urinary output by more than 33 per cent. If a burn patient requires more than twice the estimated resuscitation volume during the first 12 hours after injury and that need extends into the latter half of the first postburn day, colloid-containing fluid should be administered. The remainder of the calculated first 24-hour electrolyte-containing fluid dose should be decreased by a volume of three times the amount of colloid infused in order to reduce the total volume of infusate.

Anxiety and restlessness may be early signs of hypovolemia and hypoxemia that require correction. Sphygmomanometric measurement of blood pressure in a burned limb can be misleading because the auditory blood pressure signal may be progressively attenuated as edema develops beneath the burn wound. Massive fluid overloading can occur if more fluid is administered, which produces yet more edema, which further dampens the auditory blood pressure signal in the burned limb. Even blood pressure measurements obtained by the use of an intra-arterial cannula may be inaccurate in patients with extensive burns in whom markedly elevated circulating levels of catecholamines and other vasoactive materials cause severe vasospasm. If repeated arterial blood sampling is required, as may be necessary in patients with inhalation injury, an artery in the forearm should be cannulated in an attempt to decrease the risk

of complications associated with repetitive arterial puncture. In elderly and very young burn patients in whom the risk of femoral artery thrombosis and limb ischemia as a consequence of repeated arterial sampling are greatest, an arterial cannula should be placed.

Invasive monitoring of cardiac function should be reserved for those patients who do not respond to resuscitation in the anticipated manner and in whom the value of hemodynamic monitoring outweighs the risks of intravascular contamination and pulmonary parenchymal injury. In these patients a Swan-Ganz catheter should be placed to measure pulmonary capillary wedge pressure in order to assess myocardial function and intravascular volume. If a burn patient continues to require significantly more than the estimated resuscitation volume, has no evidence of a significant blood volume deficit, and has a pulmonary capillary wedge pressure within or above the physiologic range, dopamine or another inotropic agent can be used to improve myocardial function.

Occasionally oliguria persists in association with persistent or recurrent elevation of systemic vascular resistance and diminution of cardiac output in patients who have received more than estimated fluid needs and appear to be adequately resuscitated. Administration of hydralazine in a dosage of 0.5 mg. per kg. decreases systemic vascular resistance and increases the hourly urinary output in such patients.[79] Hydralazine should be administered only to patients who have received adequate fluid loading lest the resulting vasodilatation unmask hypovolemia and further depress cardiac output. Although investigators, using animal models of 15 to 40 per cent full-thickness burn injury, have demonstrated that the intravenous administration of either sodium nitroprusside or verapamil, beginning 30 minutes after injury, reduces peripheral vascular resistance and increases cardiac output, the clinical role of those agents remains undefined.

Since oliguria during the resuscitation period (first 48 hours after injury) is commonly due to inadequate resuscitation and is rarely an indication of acute renal failure, it should be treated by increased fluid administration, not by fluid restriction or administration of a diuretic. However, there are four categories of burn patients in whom administration of a diuretic may be necessary: those with high-voltage electrical injury, those with associated mechanical soft tissue injury, those with particularly deep burns involving muscle, and those with extensive burns who remain oliguric despite receiving fluid volumes in excess of estimated needs. Patients in the first three categories characteristically have heavy loads of hemochromogens in their urine and are prone to develop acute renal failure unless a brisk urinary output is maintained until the pigment concentration is reduced to insignificant levels. Fluid should be infused in these patients at the rate needed to achieve an hourly urinary output of 75 to 100 ml.; but if the patient does not respond to increased fluid input with an increase in urine volume and clearing of the heme pigments, a diuretic should be administered. One ampule (12.5 gm.) of mannitol is added to each liter of intravenous fluid until the desired level of urinary output is achieved and the pigment clears. After administration of a diuretic, urinary output is no longer a reliable guide to the adequacy of resuscitation, and one must rely on other indices, such as vital signs and the general condition and appearance of the patient.

During the second postburn day, to minimize volume loading in those patients with a satisfactory urinary output, one should arbitrarily reduce the volume of fluids infused per hour by 25 to 50 per cent. If the urinary output remains satisfactory, that reduced rate of fluid infusion should be maintained over the next 3 hours, at which time the infusion volume should be further reduced in stepwise fashion.

A chest roentgenogram should be obtained at least daily during the resuscitation and edema resorption periods and later in the postburn course if pneumonia or other pulmonary complications develop. Serum chemistries, blood urea nitrogen, blood glucose, arterial blood gases, and other baseline blood studies should be obtained upon admission with the frequency of subsequent determinations dictated by the patient's response to injury and treatment. The patient should be weighed upon admission and daily thereafter as a means of monitoring fluid balance.

Escharotomy and Fasciotomy

Monitoring of the peripheral circulation and ventilatory exchange is required in those patients with circumferential full-thickness burns of the extremities or thoracic wall, respectively. The edema that forms beneath inelastic eschar may increase tissue pressure to a point at which it exceeds venous pressure (thereby increasing edema formation), approaches arteriolar pressure, and severely impairs blood flow to unburned tissue in the underlying muscle compartments. The clinical indications of compromised limb blood flow include cyanosis, impaired capillary refilling, and progressive neurologic signs, particularly paresthesias and deep tissue pain. Absence of flow or progressive diminution of the flow signal on serial ultrasonic flowmeter examination of the palmar arch vessel in the upper limb or the posterior tibial artery in the lower limb is a much more reliable indication of the need for escharotomy than are the previously noted clinical signs. A decrease in perception of a vibratory stimulus generated by a 256–cycles per second tuning fork has been reported to be another reliable diagnostic criterion of muscle compartment pressures exceeding 35 mm. Hg.

Invasive techniques that have been utilized to determine elevated muscle compartment pressure include intramuscular injection of xenon-133 for "washout" determination of muscle blood flow. A muscle blood flow of less than 1.5 ml. per minute per 100 gm. of muscle has correlated well with positive ultrasonic examination findings in burn patients requiring limb escharotomy. That correlation and the relative complexity of the muscle blood flow determination speak for use of the more easily performed ultrasonic assessment. Muscle compartment pressure can also be directly measured by insertion of either a slit or wick catheter. Both of the invasive techniques are associated with a risk of microbial seeding of the muscle compartment by passage of the catheters or isotope injection needle through the contaminated eschar. Edema formation in a burned limb and the need for escharotomy are reduced by continuous elevation of the burned part and active motion of the part for 5 minutes every hour.

Escharotomy is performed as a ward procedure; and neither general nor local anesthesia is required, because only the insensate eschar is incised. The eschar on a circumferentially burned limb is incised in either the mid-lateral or the mid-medial line, with the excision extending the entire length of the burned area and carried down through the eschar and the superficial fascia to a depth sufficient to allow the cut edges of the eschar to separate without incising other unburned subcutaneous tissue (Fig. 4). When the incision is performed in this manner, bleeding is minimal and can be controlled by electrocoagulation or a briefly applied compression dressing. If, after one incision, distal flow is not restored, a second, similar incision should be made in the contralateral midline of the limb. Mid-lateral escharotomies should also be performed on a circumferentially burned digit in which digital arterial flow is absent and the subeschar tissues are viable. If the digit is burned so severely as to be desiccated, such incisions are of no value.

Impairment of ventilatory exchange by restriction of chest wall motion due to edema is an indication of the need for a chest wall escharotomy. Chest wall escharotomies should be placed in the anterior axillary line bilaterally, extending from the clavicle to the costal margin. If the eschar involves the skin of the anterior abdominal wall, the anterior axillary line escharotomies should be connected by a similar costal margin incision (Fig. 5).

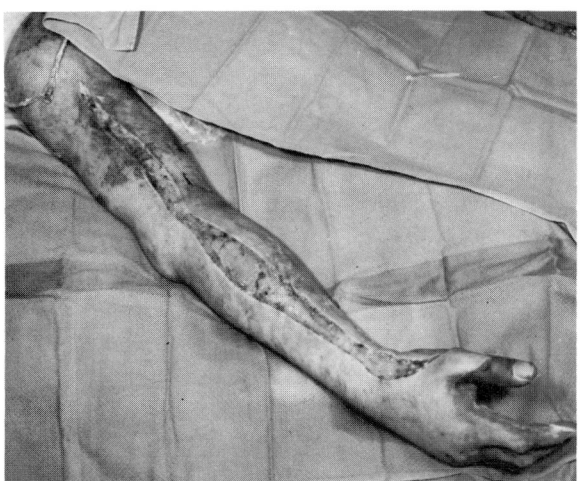

Figure 4. Escharotomy incision in the midlateral line of the circumferentially burned arm. Note the separation of the incised edges of the eschar, particularly at the level of the wrist. Desiccation of distal phalanges ruled out escharotomies of the severely burned digits.

Rarely, mid-lateral line escharotomies may be needed for circumferential burns of the neck and a mid-dorsal escharotomy for a circumferential penile burn. After escharotomy has been performed, it is important to maintain constant coverage of the escharotomy wound with the topical antimicrobial agent used on the adjacent burn wound to prevent invasion of the exposed subcutaneous tissue by the burn wound flora.

Infrequently, escharotomy does not restore blood flow to unburned tissue, and fasciotomy is required. A muscle compartment requiring fasciotomy is characteristically stony hard to palpation. The patients who most often require fasciotomy are those in whom edema occurs beneath the investing fascia, i.e., those with high-voltage electrical injury, those with associated soft tissue, long bone, or vascular injury, and those with burns involving muscle. Fasciotomy should be performed with the use of general anesthesia, and the fascia of all involved compartments must be adequately released. In the lower limb, fibulectomy effectively opens all four tissue compartments of the lower leg, but in the authors' experience the deep posterior

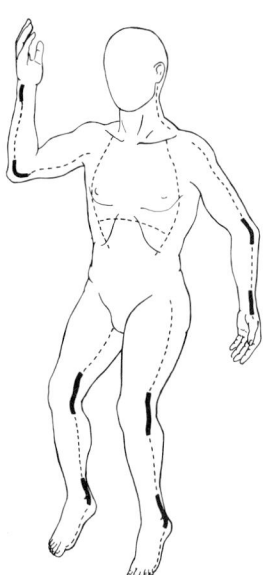

Figure 5. Diagram showing preferred sites of escharotomy incisions. Heavy portions of lines emphasize the necessity of extending escharotomy incisions across involved joints where the vessels and nerves are readily compressed by subeschar edema.

compartment has seldom been involved and the problem has been adequately managed by fascial incisions. The anterior tibial compartment is the muscle compartment most frequently requiring fasciotomy in burn patients, and a single fasciotomy incision suffices to relieve the increased tissue pressure in that compartment. Hypoesthesia of the skin of the first web space of the foot is an early sign of anterior tibial compartment compression. Autopsy studies of hands with full-thickness dorsal and palmar burns have revealed a high incidence of intrinsic muscle necrosis. On the basis of those findings, the authors perform dorsal interosseus fasciotomies in patients with such burns. Fasciotomy incisions, like escharotomy incisions, should be protected from microbial invasion by generous application of the topical agent being used on the adjacent burn wound.

Inhalation Injury

Direct thermal injury of the tracheobronchial tree, except in the case of steam burns (water has a heat-carrying capacity 4000 times that of air), is rarely encountered in clinical practice but is not infrequently observed by the forensic pathologist in patients who die in a fire. Inhalation injury, a chemical tracheobronchitis and acute pneumonitis due to the inhalation of smoke and other irritative products of incomplete combustion, is frequently present in patients admitted to burn centers (35 per cent of patients treated at the United States Army Institute of Surgical Research during a recent 5-year period[83]).

Studies of inhalation injury in animal models suggest that inhaled smoke exerts through multiple pathways deleterious effects on both the airways and the pulmonary vasculature. The inhalation of wood smoke has been reported to cause an increase in pulmonary microvascular permeability, and acrolein smoke appears to exert a toxic effect on peribronchial vessels as manifested by peribronchial edema that can be reduced and delayed in onset by occlusion of the bronchial arteries prior to exposure.[35,63] In a goat model of inhalation injury, arterial levels of thromboxane A_2 were found to increase within 5 minutes of inhalation injury and to peak at 2 hours in concert with an increase in both the flow and lymph/plasma protein ratio of lung lymph and extravascular lung water.[44] Pulmonary vascular changes appear to represent local effects of absorbed toxic material, since lung lesions are confined to the involved lung when only one lung is insufflated with smoke.[70]

The role of surfactant in the pathophysiology of inhalation injury is uncertain and may be smoke component–specific. Studies in a canine model have demonstrated significant surfactant reduction (minimal surface tension increased from 7 to 22 dynes per cm.) after smoke inhalation, whereas other studies in a sheep model have shown no decrease in phosphatidylcholine in alveolar lavage fluid 24 hours after inhalation injury.[64,71] Other studies have implicated leukocytes, since leukopenia induced by preinjury nitrogen mustard treatment has been reported to attenuate significantly the increases in pulmonary artery pressure, pulmonary vascular resistance, and pulmonary lymph flow following inhalation injury. Herndon and associates, on the basis of clinical experience, have recommended the administration of 50 per cent more than the calculated resuscitation fluid volume to maintain cardiac output at normal levels in patients with inhalation injury.[41] These authors reported that the additional resuscitation volume was not associated with the development of pulmonary edema and might even decrease lung edema by increasing shear rate in the pulmonary capillaries, thereby reducing neutrophil margination and the deleterious local effects of such cells.

This injury should be suspected in any patient burned in a closed space or burned during a period of impaired mentation due to inebriation, drug overdose, or head trauma. Although head and neck burns and singeing of the nasal vibrissae are commonly present in patients with inhalation injury, they are nonspecific, compared with frank inflammatory change of the oropharyngeal mucosa. Other signs of inhalation injury include

a brassy cough, hoarseness and wheezing, bronchorrhea, unexplained hypoxemia, and the production of carbonaceous sputum, the last being specific. Unfortunately, carbon-stained bronchial secretion may be cleared from the airway by the time of admission, and the other signs may not be evident for 2 to 3 days after injury. Consequently, the diagnosis of inhalation injury is commonly delayed and the second postburn day has been the mean time of diagnosis on the basis of clinical signs.

The chest roentgenogram is notoriously insensitive in detecting even severe lung injury. Even though changes may be evident on the chest roentgenographs obtained during the first 5 days following severe inhalation injury, it is difficult to differentiate changes due to inhalation injury from those due to aspiration, pneumonia, and pulmonary edema. In a recently reported study, chest radiographs obtained on the day of injury were considered to be falsely negative in 92 per cent of 106 patients with inhalation injury.[17] The use of three modalities has enhanced the timeliness and reliability of the diagnosis of inhalation injury: fiberoptic bronchoscopic examination, ^{133}Xe ventilation-perfusion pulmonary scintiphotography, and pulmonary function testing.

Fiberoptic bronchoscopy can be performed as a bedside procedure as soon as the burn patient with suspected inhalation injury is hemodynamically stable. An appropriately sized endotracheal tube should be placed over the bronchoscope before performing the examination so that the tube can be placed during the course of the examination if the inflammatory reaction threatens airway patency. A topical anesthetic should be applied to the upper airway to facilitate the examination. The supraglottic airway is examined for signs of inflammation and for the presence and severity of glottic edema. If edema of the cords and upper airway threatens airway occlusion, the endotracheal tube should be placed immediately and the examination continued by passage of the bronchoscope through the tube into the lower airway. Evidence of mucosal inflammation and ulceration of the infraglottic airway as well as deposition of carbon particles on the endobronchial mucosa indicate inhalation injury. Bronchoscopic examination of burn patients may be misleading, and both falsely negative and falsely positive results have been reported; the former are due to failure of inflammatory changes to develop in the hypovolemic patient with impaired mucosal perfusion, and the latter are due to pre-existing bronchitis.

Since the site of aerosol particle deposition within the airways is strongly influenced by particle size, it is possible for the large endoscopically visible airways to be relatively uninjured in the presence of significant terminal bronchiolar and alveolar inflammatory damage when the smoke particle mass median diameter is less than .05 μ. If a burn patient is suspected of having inhalation injury but has no or minimal inflammatory changes evident on bronchoscopic examination, a ^{133}Xe ventilation-perfusion lung scan should be performed after hemodynamic stability is achieved but before postburn hyperventilation reaches significantly elevated levels (usually beyond 72 hours after injury). Serial scintiphotographs are obtained after injection of 10 μC. of the insoluble gas into a peripheral vein. Unequal radiation density and retention of the gas in the lungs beyond 90 seconds after injection are considered positive indications of inhalation injury (Fig. 6). Both false-negative (5 per cent) and false-positive (8 per cent) lung scan results may be obtained, the former because the test was performed in the presence of pronounced hyperventilation and the latter because of pre-existing bronchitis (common in heavy smokers).

Pulmonary function tests of varying degrees of complexity, ranging from the determination of arterial blood oxygen tension to the measurement of maximum expiratory flow-volume curves are also helpful in making the diagnosis of inhalation injury. The pulmonary function tests listed in Table 5 have been found to be significantly altered in those patients with inhalation injury. The exclusion of compliance measurements from high-frequency positive pressure ventilation as a means of minimizing airway collapse, atelectatic change, and the development of pneumonia.[16] The incidence of pneumonia in the first 30 patients entered in that trial, all with bronchoscopic evidence of inhalation injury, has been 30 per cent, as contrasted with 46 per cent in historical controls. The prophylactic systemic administration of steroids has had no influence on the morbidity or mortality of patients with inhalation injury; in fact, such prophylaxis has been reported to increase the occurrence of infection.

Pulmonary infection, especially bronchopneumonia, is the most frequent cause of morbidity and mortality in patients with inhalation injury. At the first sign of pulmonary infiltrates on the chest roentgenogram, endobronchial cultures should be obtained and systemic antibiotic therapy initiated as described for bronchopneumonia (see below). Prophylactic administration of antibiotics by aerosol has been ineffective in altering the pulmonary complications or mortality in burn patients with inhalation injury. In fact, such prophylaxis was found to exert no detectable effect on the endobronchial flora, since *Pseudomonas* species were the predominant organisms in the sputum in both treatment and control groups.

Long-term morbidity of burn patients with inhalation injury who survive is related to both the severity of the airway injury and the treatment employed, particularly the use of invasive airway devices necessary to preserve respiratory function. In general, the sequelae of tracheotomy are more common and more severe than those associated with translaryngeal intubation. The duration of intubation, regardless of route, and the presence of a tracheal stoma are the most important etiologic factors in permanent airway damage. Granuloma formation and tracheal stenosis are the most frequently observed lesions. Spirometric determination of flow-volume loops, although somewhat insensitive, may be used as a noninvasive means of identifying patients with functionally significant narrowing of the airway. Xeroradiography may provide additional information about the degree of tracheal stenosis. Fiberoptic bronchoscopy is required to document airway lesions and should be performed in all patients in whom the duration of airway intubation has exceeded 10 days and evidence of airway compromise exists. Saccular bronchiectasis has been identified in patients who have survived severe inhalation injury and has been the cause of recurrent bronchitis in these patients. Bronchography confirms this sequela of severe inhalation injury and indicates the need for close follow-up and antibiotic treatment of recurrent bronchitic infection.

Mortality in burn patients with inhalation injury is greater overall than in patients with burns of similar size who have no inhalation injury. The mortality-enhancing effect of inhalation injury is both age- and burn size–related, rising to a maximal increase in expected mortality of 20 per cent in patients whose predicted mortality from burn injury alone would be 50 per cent.[83] Mortality appears to be less affected by the addition of inhalation injury to the relatively minor physiologic stress in patients with progressively smaller burns. In patients with burns associated with an anticipated mortality of more than 50 per cent, the increasing burn-related mortality progressively obscures the effect of inhalation injury. Maximal therapeutic effort therefore should be directed to the group in whom inhalation injury exerts its greatest effect, that is, those with significant burn injury in whom salvage is not only possible but is improved by treatment of both the burn and the inhalation injury.

Other Considerations in Early Care

The almost universal occurrence of ileus during the immediate postburn period in patients with burns of more than 25 per cent of the total body surface precludes oral resuscitation and necessitates insertion of a nasogastric tube to evacuate gastric contents and thereby prevent emesis and aspiration. Prophy-

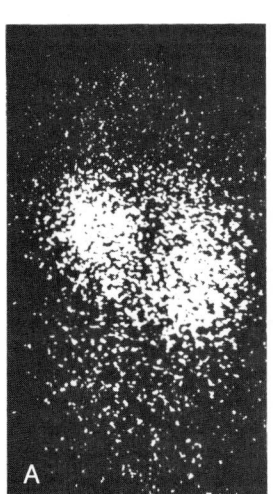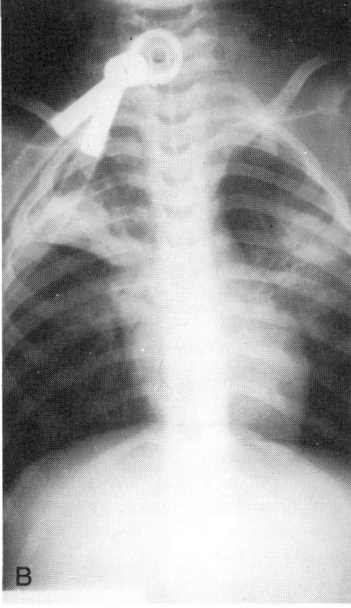

Figure 6. *A*, Scintiphotograph taken after injection of ^{133}Xe in a peripheral vein of a patient burned in a house fire. The initial standard chest roentgenogram was normal. Note the retention and focal increase in radiation density in both upper lung fields. *B*, Standard chest roentgenogram of the same patient showing subsequent development of pulmonary infiltrates in areas positive on the lung scan.

that list reflects the authors' experience demonstrating that compliance has been insensitive to inhalation injury. When performed serially, maximum expiratory flow-volume curves are of prognostic value and are useful in assessing the effects of treatment. The necessity for full patient cooperation and the complexity of the equipment required for some of the pulmonary function tests severely limit their clinical usefulness in critically ill patients. The use of all three diagnostic modalities permits the diagnosis of inhalation injury with 96 per cent accuracy, the residual error being that of overdiagnosis.

The treatment of inhalation injury is guided by the severity of pulmonary insufficiency in the individual patient. In patients with mild disease, the administration of warm, humidified, oxygen-enriched air and the use of incentive spirometry may be adequate. Repeated bronchoscopy (using the rigid bronchoscope) may be required for patients with extensive mucosal sloughing who are unable to clear their airways spontaneously. Progressive hypoxemia necessitates endotracheal intubation and the use of mechanical ventilatory assistance. Studies in an ovine model of inhalation injury have demonstrated the importance of small airway disease in the development of poorly aerated lung segments and have prompted a clinical trial of

TABLE 5. Pulmonary Function Tests Significantly Altered in Patients with Inhalation Injury*

Test	Burn Patients With Inhalation Injury (n = 7)	Burn Patients Without Inhalation Injury (n = 8)
Arterial Po$_2$ (torr)	69.4	85.5
Ventilation perfusion gradient (torr)	37.4	27.2
Resistance (cm. H$_2$O/L./sec.)	4.85	3.05
Nitrogen washout slope (% rise)	3.1	1.6
Peak flow (% of predicted)	61.9	99.1

* Patients treated at the U.S. Army Institute of Surgical Research.

laxis against stress ulcer complications should be initiated as described below. The nasogastric tube should be removed as soon as gastrointestinal motility returns, usually on the third or fourth postburn day, at which time oral fluids should be administered and the patient advanced to a diet as tolerated.

Tetanus prophylaxis is determined by the patient's immunization status. Burn patients who have undergone previous active immunization and have had a toxoid booster injection within 5 years of the time of injury require no further prophylaxis unless they have an associated tetanus-prone wound, in which case a toxoid booster injection should be administered. Patients who have received their most recent booster injection more than 5 years before injury should also be given a booster dose of toxoid. Those who have not undergone prior immunization (most commonly elderly patients and patients from developing countries) should be given 250 to 500 units of human antitetanus globulin at one site with an initial immunizing dose of toxoid administered at another site. Active immunization is thereafter completed with the use of the routine dosage schedule.

Beta hemolytic streptococcal infection prophylaxis is no longer employed by the authors, since such infections are now uncommon in burn patients and respond promptly to penicillin treatment if they do occur. Some physicians, those dealing principally with pediatric burn patients and those involved in the out-of-hospital treatment of patients with second-degree burns of 10 to 15 per cent of the body surface, still employ penicillin prophylaxis using 20,000 units per kg. body weight per day in the child and 3 to 5 million units per day in the adult.

The severity of pain in the immediate postburn period is related to the depth of the burn. Second-degree burns may be very painful, and patients with such burns complain of even a draft of air crossing the burn surface. Third-degree burns, however, because of coagulation necrosis of sensory nerve endings, are insensate. Analgesia in the immediate postburn resuscitation and edema-formation period must be effected by the intravenous administration of small doses of morphine. Subcutaneous or intramuscular administration of narcotics during the period of hypovolemia and impaired tissue flow is ineffective; and the resulting lack of pain relief can lead to the administration of multiple doses, which, when mobilized, may cause life-threatening or fatal respiratory depression. Pain associated with second-degree burns abates when a serous crust forms on the burn surface. In such patients and in those with third-degree burns, wound pain is subsequently associated with wound manipulations, such as cleansing, débridement, and dressing changes. Analgesics should be administered at an appropriate interval prior to wound manipulation to reduce pain and minimize pain-related stress.

Postresuscitation Fluid Management

Fluid management after resuscitation is completed should permit excretion of the salt load infused during resuscitation while permitting a daily loss of 10 to 12 per cent of the weight gained during resuscitation, so that the patient returns to pre-burn weight by the eighth to tenth postburn day. Any departure from that weight loss trajectory necessitates review of the patient's intake and output records and adjustment of fluid therapy. The development of secondary disturbances of fluid and electrolyte imbalance should also be prevented. The modest hyponatremia present at the end of resuscitation that is caused by infusion of large volumes of lactated Ringer's requires no treatment, since appropriate fluid management permits increased evaporative water loss to correct that imbalance.

Hyponatremia may occur in patients treated with 0.5 per cent silver nitrate soaks. The administration of supplemental sodium chloride and sodium lactate prevents or corrects this complication. Inappropriate secretion of antidiuretic hormone is a rare cause of generally asymptomatic hyponatremia in burn patients and usually responds to reduction in the amount of administered electrolyte-free fluid. Early in the course of infection, modest hyponatremia may follow reduction in free water clearance. In addition to adjustment of the fluid therapy of these patients, identification of the causative infection should be made and the infection controlled.

The most common postresuscitation fluid and electrolyte disturbance is hypernatremia associated with dehydration due to inadequate replacement of insensible water loss. Burn injury destroys the water vapor barrier of the skin, and evaporative water loss from the burned area is markedly elevated because the wound acts as a free water surface. Fluid needs can be estimated on the basis of total insensible water loss calculated as follows: insensible water loss (milliliters per hour) = (25 + per cent body surface burned) × total body surface area in square meters. The formula estimates water loss at the low end of the range of observed water losses; and the patient's body weight, serum sodium concentration, and serum osmolality should be monitored on a daily basis for assessment of the adequacy of hydration and the need to adjust fluid therapy. Other less frequent causes of dehydration and associated hypernatremia include: osmotic diuresis caused by glucosuria and increased urinary nitrogen, treated by dietary manipulation or therapy of underlying diabetes mellitus; diabetes insipidus, treated by the administration of vasopressin; and sepsis, treated by control of the infection.

The release of potassium from red cells and other tissues injured by the burn commonly produces a modest hyperkalemia during the resuscitation period that usually requires no specific therapy. If acidosis, due to inadequate resuscitation, supervenes, the serum potassium concentration may be elevated to symptomatic levels necessitating rapid fluid infusion and specific therapy to effect reduction of the potassium concentration.

After resuscitation, increased potassium loss may cause hypokalemia. In patients treated with Sulfamylon burn cream, the kaliuretic effect of that agent may accentuate those losses. Patients treated with 0.5 per cent silver nitrate soaks that exaggerate transeschar potassium losses and patients with profuse diarrhea induced by enteral feeding may also become hypokalemic. In all burn patients, the serum potassium concentration and urinary potassium losses should be monitored and potassium supplements administered to prevent or correct deficits.

BURN WOUND CARE

Initial Treatment and Topical Therapy

Attention should be directed to the burn wound itself only after resuscitation has effected hemodynamic and respiratory stability. The burn wound should be cleansed using a surgical detergent, all loose nonviable skin trimmed away, and all hair shaved from the burned areas and a generous margin of unburned skin. The initial débridement can best be performed in a shower-like area with a hand-held showerhead with the patient lying on a litter or, alternatively, on a slanted plinth suspended over (but not immersed in) a Hubbard or other physical therapy tank. Thereafter the burns are similarly cleansed each day in a tank or shower, depending upon the patient's general status and the location of the burns. Daily wound care of patients whose general condition is too critical to permit them to be moved can be performed at the patient's bed. Following cleansing and débridement, the topical agent of choice is applied. In the case of patients treated with topical creams by the exposure technique, the agent is reapplied 12 hours later to those areas from which it has been abraded. In the case of patients treated with 0.5 per cent silver nitrate soaks, the occlusive dressings are changed two or three times daily and kept moistened between dressing changes by application of additional 0.5 per cent silver nitrate solution every 2 hours.

Both burn wound and microbial factors influence the rate of microbial proliferation in and penetration of the eschar. The burned tissue, which is rich in protein and moist by virtue of the transeschar movement of fluid and serum, serves as an excellent microbial culture medium. The avascularity of the burned tissue following thermal thrombosis limits both the delivery of endogenous phagocytic cells and the effectiveness of systemically administered antibiotics. Wound maceration and pressure necrosis may also favor microbial proliferation and should be avoided by frequently changing the position of the patient. Later in the postburn course, exposure and desiccation of granulation tissue may cause formation of a neoeschar, which supports bacterial growth and proliferation. Systemic impairment of blood flow, as may occur with septic or hypovolemic shock, further predisposes the patient to invasive infection by reducing delivery of oxygen, energy substrates, and phagocytic cells to the viable tissue underlying the wound.

Microbial factors that influence the natural history of the burn wound and the likelihood of infection or systemic sepsis include density of organisms (invasion is uncommon unless the number of bacteria equals or exceeds 10^5 per gm. of tissue) and a variety of strain-specific factors. Relatively few organisms can be recovered from the burn surface immediately after injury, and those that are present are predominantly gram-positive. The type and density of organisms present in the untreated burn wound change with time, so that by the fifth postburn day gram-negative organisms can be recovered from 60 per cent of patients. By the middle of the second postburn week, the burn wound organisms are predominantly gram-negative and have increased to levels of 10^2 to 10^4 per sq. cm. of wound surface. Without topical therapy, the organisms penetrate the eschar by migration along hair follicles and sweat glands and extend down to the viable-nonviable tissue interface (termed by some the subeschar space). At this site, further microbial proliferation commonly occurs and promotes lysis of denatured collagen and spontaneous slough of the eschar. In those patients with inadequate host defense capacity or those in whom topical therapy is ineffective, the subeschar organisms invade the underlying unburned tissue and may spread systemically. Strain-specific factors that appear to be important in the pathogenesis of invasive burn wound infection include both endotoxins and exotoxins and a variety of enzymes such as collagenase, protease, elastase, esterase, lipase, hemolysin, and nucleases. Bacterial motility and antibiotic resistance also appear to be important in the development of invasive wound infections.[74]

The aforementioned factors as well as the depression of host defense mechanisms in the burn patient were responsible for the development of burn wound infection and invasion in 60 per cent of all patients who died after burn injury prior to 1964. The incidence of burn wound sepsis (defined as invasive burn wound infection associated with systemic sepsis) is related to burn depth, burn size, and patient age. Invasive infection is uncommon in second-degree burns. The incidence of burn wound sepsis is low in patients with burns of less than 30 per cent of the body surface and rises as burn size increases above that level. Burn wound sepsis has been most common in children, less common in the elderly, and least common in young adults.

The use of clinically effective topical antimicrobial agents developed in the mid 1960s has significantly decreased the occurrence of invasive burn wound infection and burn wound sepsis, an effect that has been associated with the improved survival of burn patients.[74] At the present time, even in patients with massive burns, the cause of death is seldom burn wound sepsis and is commonly infection at another site. Three topical agents are in wide clinical use, and each has specific advantages and limitations. The agents should be used selectively to meet the individual patient's wound care needs. Mafenide acetate (Sulfamylon) burn cream and 0.5 per cent silver nitrate soaks were developed

contemporaneously, and several years later silver sulfadiazine burn cream was formulated in an attempt to combine the favorable effects and reduce the side effects of the two agents developed earlier.

Sulfamylon burn cream is an 11.1 per cent suspension of mafenide acetate, which is bacteriostatic, is freely soluble, and readily diffuses through the eschar to establish an effective concentration at the nonviable-viable tissue interface. This agent also has the broadest spectrum of activity against *Pseudomonas* organisms in particular and gram-negative organisms in general. These characteristics make it the best agent for treating patients in whom a dense bacterial population has developed in the eschar or those whose prior wound care regimens have failed to control the bacterial proliferation in the wound. The principal limitations of Sulfamylon burn cream result from its inhibition of carbonic anhydrase, which promotes wasting of bicarbonate by the kidney and accentuates postburn hyperventilation. Both of these derangements predispose the patient to the development of acidosis—directly by the first mechanism and indirectly (if pulmonary complications intervene) by the second mechanism.

Silvadene burn cream, a 1 per cent suspension of silver sulfadiazine, is bacteriostatic but poorly diffusible and penetrates the eschar to a lesser extent than Sulfamylon burn cream. This agent, in contradistinction to Sulfamylon burn cream, produces no pain when applied to second-degree burns and causes no electrolyte or acid-base disturbances. The principal limitations of this agent include development of neutropenia (the granulocyte count commonly returns to "normal" levels after change of topical agents) and ineffectiveness against certain gram-negative organisms (some *Pseudomonas* strains and nearly all *Enterobacter cloacae* species). At present, most gram-negative organisms recovered from the burn wounds of patients treated with this agent are resistant to sulfadiazine but sensitive to silver ions. The sensitivity of the microorganisms to silver maintains effectiveness of the compound as a topical antimicrobial agent. However, the sulfadiazine resistance is plasmid-mediated and confers resistance to multiple antibiotics as well as to other antimicrobial agents, thus making the treatment of other complicating infections in the burn patient more difficult.

One-half per cent silver nitrate solution has, as do the other agents, a broad spectrum of antibacterial activity. This agent, which is applied in the form of many-layered soaks, causes no wound pain, but the soaks impede motion of involved joints, and their removal at the time of dressing changes can cause pain. This agent does not penetrate the eschar; in fact, the silver ions are immediately precipitated upon contact with any proteinaceous or other foreign material, a reaction responsible for the discoloration of the unburned skin of the patient, the skin of attending personnel, and nearly anything else in the environment. The principal limitations of this agent consist of the leeching of sodium, potassium, chloride, and calcium from the wound and the transeschar absorption of the aqueous vehicle, which may cause mineral deficits, alkalosis, and water loading. Supplements of sodium and the other minerals must be administered to prevent or correct these electrolyte deficits, and fluid administration must be adjusted to prevent overhydration.

All three agents have been found to be effective in the control of invasive burn wound infection and burn wound sepsis, although the silver nitrate soaks and Silvadene burn cream, because of minimal or no eschar penetration, are most effective when initiated immediately after burning, before significant microbial colonization has occurred. Several other topical agents have been advocated, but they have either been used in so few patients or have been evaluated in such an uncontrolled manner that their effectiveness remains unconfirmed.

The microbial ecology of the burn wounds of the patients cared for at any burn unit changes with time, and alterations in the flora assume the form of mini-epidemics with a succession of predominant organisms. In the 1960s *Pseudomonasa aeruginosa* was the most common cause of infection in severely burned patients; and since that time, mini-epidemics caused by *Providencia stuartii, Enterobacter cloacae, Klebsiella,* and recrudescent *Pseudomonas* spp. have occurred. Since 1977 recovery of *Pseudomonas* spp. from the wounds and blood of patients treated at the U.S. Army Institute of Surgical Research has decreased precipitously.[53] The near disappearance of invasive *Pseudomonas* burn wound infection has occurred during a period in which the wounds are cleansed daily with chlorhexidine and Sulfamylon burn cream and Silvadene burn cream applied alternately every 12 hours to minimize the side effects of each while advantage is taken of the superior gram-negative activity of the former and the superior anticandidal activity of the latter. In patients with sulfa drug allergy, 0.5 per cent silver nitrate soaks are the treatment of choice.

Topical antimicrobial chemotherapy is utilized to limit microbial proliferation in the burn wound until the burned tissue can be surgically removed, and burn wound excision of even extensive burn wounds should be initiated as soon after resuscitation as the patient's physiologic status permits. In patients whose wounds cannot be completely excised at a single procedure, topical chemotherapy is continued to the burn wounds that remain unexcised. In patients whose physiologic status does not permit early excision, topical chemotherapy is continued until excision can be accomplished or until daily débridement removes the eschar.

Burn Wound Excision

Excision of the burned tissue in full-thickness and most deep partial-thickness burns should be performed as soon as possible after resuscitation is complete. Although immediate excision within the first 24 postburn hours has been reported to be possible, anesthetic ablation of the early postburn physiologic compensations may complicate anesthetic and fluid management, and there is no documentation that such timing alters outcome in patients with extensive burns. The adverse effects of excision include the anesthetic risk and the operative stress associated with what can be prodigious blood loss (amounts equal to or exceeding the blood volume) when excisions of more than 20 per cent of the total body surface are done as a single procedure. These effects speak for undertaking excision only when the patient's physiologic reserve has been re-established and for limiting an excision procedure to 20 per cent of the total body surface or 2 hours operative time. Other adverse effects include the susceptibility of the excised wound to infection from adjacent unexcised burn; the sacrifice, when excision is at the level of the investing fascia, of viable skin in areas of partial-thickness burn that are intermixed with areas of full-thickness burn; and the uncertainty of graft take, particularly on fatty tissue that is exposed in the wound produced by tangential excision. Also limiting are the immunosuppressive effects of the transfusions needed to replace excision-related blood loss. The inability to effect immediate definitive closure following excision because of the paucity of available donor sites limits the usefulness of excision in patients with massive burns.

The advantages of burn wound excision that have led to its acceptance and current widespread use in the treatment of patients with burns of less than 20 per cent of the total body surface include decreased hospital stay and associated lesser costs, an earlier return to work, a greater likelihood that the patient will return to work, and fewer complications. In patients with burns of between 20 and 40 per cent of the total body surface, excision is associated with a shorter hospital stay and a reduction of the time during which the wound is at risk to invasive infection. In patients with burns of more than 40 per cent of the total body surface, burn wound excision has been credited with decreasing the duration and magnitude of injury-related physiologic stress by reducing the extent of the burn.

However, laboratory studies indicate that reduction of postburn hypermetabolism is achieved only when the entire burn wound can be excised and closed by grafting at a single procedure.[24] Immunologic benefits have also been attributed to excision in patients with extensive burns, but the earlier restoration of lymphocyte responsiveness appears to be related to the improved function of the lymphocytes contained in the transfusions the patients received perioperatively. Randomized prospective controlled trials have documented no effect of burn wound excision on mortality, and one study found no difference in postburn scarring or the need for reconstructive surgery within 3 years.[46]

Since at least the mid 1950s, scalpel excision at the level of the investing fascia has been used to remove full-thickness burn wounds. A tourniquet can be used to reduce the blood loss associated with excision of burns on a limb. The carbon dioxide laser and standard electrocautery instruments have also been used for burn wound excision at the level of the investing fascia to reduce the associated blood loss. The use of the laser is attended by lesser blood loss than is the use of an electrocautery device, but the former is a more expensive instrument, and the time required for excision has been reported to be longer. The take of immediately applied autograft skin is similar following use of the scalpel, laser, or electrocautery device.

In the mid 1960s a technique termed tangential excision was introduced for the treatment of partial-thickness burns of generally limited extent. In recent years, the technique has been applied to the treatment of patients with extensive partial-thickness and even full-thickness burns. Successive thin layers of burned tissue are removed by means of a guarded skin knife or dermatome until all nonviable tissue is excised, as indicated by uniformly dense capillary bleeding from the entire wound bed. The wound produced by any form of excision must be closed by autografting or, if donor sites are limited, by application of a biologic dressing or skin substitute as described below. The blood loss associated with this form of excision can also be formidable (as much as 9 per cent of the circulating blood volume per percentage of body surface excised), but the use of a tourniquet obliterates capillary bleeding from the wound bed, which is used as the end point for the operative procedure. The loss of blood can be reduced by topical application of gauze sponges moistened with a warm solution of thrombin with or without epinephrine or by intravenous infusion or subeschar infiltration of vasopressin.

A variant of tangential excision has been used to reduce the associated blood loss. The excision of successive layers of burned tissue is terminated at the first sign of capillary bleeding, following which the wound is covered with either a biologic dressing or gauze dressing soaked with an antimicrobial solution, depending upon the amount of nonviable tissue remaining. If little nonviable tissue remains after this form of excision, a biologic dressing is applied and the patient is returned to the operating room 5 to 7 days later, at which time the biologic membrane is removed and autografting accomplished after any necessary further excision. If the residual nonviable tissue precludes application of a biologic dressing at conclusion of the initial excision, a dressing is applied and the patient is returned to the operating room every 3 days until the sequential excisions produce a graftable wound bed.

The excision technique employed should be based on the depth and microbial status of the patient's burns. Scalpel or electrocautery excision at or below the level of the investing fascia should be employed in the treatment of full-thickness burns of limited extent, the débridement of high-voltage electrical injuries, and excision of areas of burn wound infection. Tangential excision is indicated in the treatment of deep partial-thickness burns of 20 per cent or less of the total body surface (particularly burns involving the dorsum of the hand), and for the staged excision of more extensive partial- and full-thickness burns. The lesser variant of tangential excision may be used to reduce blood loss and conserve tissue in the treatment of second- and third-degree burns in areas of cosmetic and functional importance and in the removal of persistent eschar.

A recent review of 381 patients with burns of more than 30 per cent of the total body surface treated at the U.S. Army Institute of Surgical Research during a 5½-year period has revealed that burn wound excision was performed in all but 17 (7 per cent) of the 235 surviving patients but was precluded by a complication in 75 (51 per cent) of the 146 patients who died. The physiologic instability that either prevented movement of the patient to the operating room or limited the patient's ability to withstand the operative stress was pulmonary insufficiency in 58, hemodynamic insufficiency in 14, and sepsis with disseminated intravascular coagulation in 3 of the 75 patients who died with their burn wounds unexcised. A temporary delay in excision may be necessitated by the need to control burn wound cellulitis or correct acid-base and electrolyte disturbances.

Nonexcisional Therapy

Burn wound care for those patients with superficial partial-thickness burns or deep partial-thickness and full-thickness burns that are not or cannot be excised consists of daily cleansing and repeated application of topical antimicrobial agents as described. As wound maturation proceeds, crusts separate from areas of second-degree burn as re-epithelialization occurs and the eschar loosens and sloughs from areas of third-degree burn as granulation tissue develops at the viable-nonviable tissue interface. These processes can be hastened by débridement to the point of bleeding or pain at the time of daily wound cleansing. Analgesia may be necessary for daily débridement, but anesthesia is not used for such procedures because of its adverse effects on gastrointestinal motility. Treatment of the wound following débridement depends upon the maturity of the granulation tissue, the amount of residual necrotic debris, and the extent of the débrided area. If there is significant residual necrotic debris, the wound is covered with a topical antimicrobial agent. If there is less residual debris, only a small fully débrided area, or inadequate granulation tissue, the wound can be covered with a dressing soaked in an antimicrobial solution (5 per cent mafenide acetate) that is changed 2 or 3 times a day and kept moist by application of additional antimicrobial solution between dressing changes. If there is little residual nonviable tissue and well-established granulation tissue covering an area of more than 1 to 2 per cent of the body surface, a biologic dressing can be applied.

Wound Closure

The goal of burn wound care is the timely definitive closure of the wound. Those wounds ready for split-thickness autograft closure are those that have been excised or those treated by the nonexcisional method that are characterized by absence of residual nonviable tissue and pooled secretions; firm, red, finely granular granulation tissue; a surface bacterial count of less than 10^5 organisms per sq. cm. of wound surface; and absence of beta hemolytic streptococci. Adherence of viable cutaneous allograft to the wound bed can be used as an index of the readiness for autografting of wounds treated by the daily débridement technique. General adherence and vascularization of allograft skin are customarily associated with universal adherence of subsequently applied autograft skin (Fig. 7). The biologic dressing is removed in the operating room; and after the establishment of hemostasis by the application of warm packs, autograft skin is applied directly to the areas from which the cutaneous allografts were removed.

Autografts of 0.012 to 0.015 inch in thickness (a compromise between "the thicker the skin, the better the cosmetic results" and "the thinner the skin, the better the take") are generally used for initial skin coverage in patients with extensive burns.

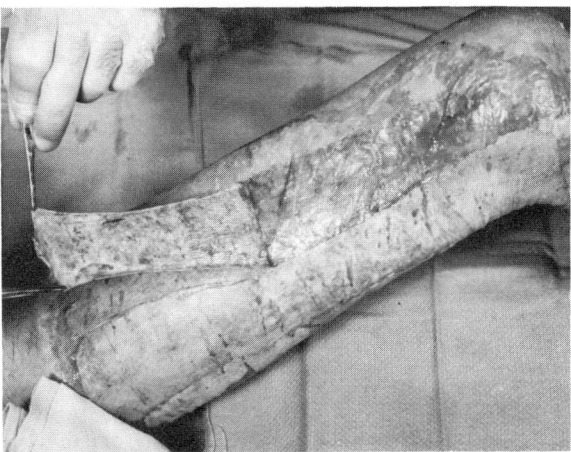

Figure 7. Removal, 5 days after application, of viable cutaneous allografts, which are generally adherent and free of subgraft suppuration. A mature, finely granular bed of fresh granulation tissue indicates that immediately applied autografts will invariably adhere.

Donor sites are dressed with a single layer of fine mesh gauze; and initial hemostasis of the donor site is obtained by application, in the operating room, of warm laparotomy packs over the fine mesh gauze. Alternatively, a variety of treated dressings that maintain better flexibility and elasticity can be applied to reduce donor site discomfort. Upon return of the patient to the recovery room or the ward, the laparotomy packs are removed and the donor site dressing is exposed to a heat lamp to hasten drying.

In patients with burns associated with an anticipated mortality of less than 50 per cent, priority of skin grafting is given to burn wounds involving the hands, feet, face, and joints. In patients with more extensive burns, priority is given to area coverage of flat planar surfaces, such as the anterior and posterior trunk and the thighs, to reduce as soon as possible the extent of the total burn and the associated physiologic derangements. In patients with extensive burns and limited donor sites, the quality of skin graft harvested from donor sites overlying bony areas can be improved by the subcutaneous infiltration of saline, but this salt load must be considered in planning postoperative fluid management. The scalp can be utilized as a donor site in patients with extensive burns and limited donor sites; scalp donor sites are characterized by rapid re-epithelialization and freedom from hypertrophic scar formation. Consequently, the scalp can be used for repeated harvest of autograft skin with greater frequency than other areas. When taking skin grafts from the scalp, it is important to leave a fringe of hair at the anterior hair line so the donor site is not extended onto the forehead. The quality of skin grafts obtained with each subsequent harvest of a previously used donor site progressively declines. Since the residual dermis is progressively thinner and the overlying epithelium is relatively immature, the grafts must be thinner with each successive harvest. Treated as described, a donor site heals in approximately 14 to 21 days, but the interharvest intervals should be as long as is consistent with skin graft coverage needs to permit maximal donor site maturation between harvests.

Mesh grafts can be utilized to increase the extent of wound covered by skin obtained from a donor site of a given size. By use of the appropriate "carrier board" or mesh dermatome, it is possible to prepare grafts that can be expanded at ratios of 1½:1, 2:1, 3:1, 4:1, 6:1, and even 9:1. Expansion ratios of 1½:1 up to 4:1 appear adequate for nearly all needs. In general, mesh grafts should not be applied to the face or over joints, although after excision of burns of the dorsum of the hand, unexpanded 1½:1 mesh grafts that allow egress of serum and blood have been used to good effect. Use of the larger expansion ratios is associated with an excessive time for closure of the interstices and excessive scar epithelium formation. Generally, mesh grafts are covered with occlusive dressings, kept wet with an antimicrobial solution such as 0.5 per cent silver nitrate or 5 per cent mafenide acetate solution to prevent desiccation of the interstices and microbial proliferation in the exposed tissue. Alternatively, sheets of cutaneous allograft or sheets of the synthetic biologic dressing Biobrane can be applied over mesh grafts to prevent desiccation and protect them from dislodgment by shearing.

Biologic Dressings

Viable cutaneous allograft is the biologic dressing of choice against which all other available materials must be evaluated (see Fig. 7). Allograft skin is typically harvested in the operating room with sterile technique from cadavers free of jaundice, cutaneous malignancy or infection, and viral disease. The harvested grafts are spread on fine-mesh gauze that is thinly impregnated with petrolatum, placed in sterile containers, and then refrigerated for up to 2 weeks. Alternatively, the tissue can be frozen with cryoprotective agents and techniques. If refrigerated, such tissue performs better as a biologic dressing the sooner after harvest it is used. Viable cutaneous allografts and any other biologic dressings or skin substitutes should be applied only to a burn wound from which most of the nonviable tissue has been débrided or spontaneously sloughed lest the membrane convert an open contaminated wound to a closed infected one.

Cutaneous allograft prevents wound desiccation; promotes maturation of granulation tissue; limits bacterial proliferation in the burn wound; prevents exudative protein and red cell loss; decreases wound pain, thereby facilitating movement in involved joints; diminishes evaporative water loss from the burn, thus decreasing heat loss; and serves to protect tendons, vessels, and nerves.[77] If small areas of necrotic debris are covered, subgraft suppuration in those areas appears to effect more rapid débridement. When applied to superficial second-degree burns, cutaneous allografts accelerate re-epithelialization and enhance the quality of healing. Because of the limitations of cutaneous allografts, i.e., a finite shelf life, refrigeration requirements, potential transmission of diseases such as hepatitis and the acquired immunodeficiency syndrome, and uncertain availability, other biologic dressings have been developed.

Lyophilized allograft skin has an indefinite shelf life and is easily reconstituted. However, it, too, is in limited supply; shows less adherence to the wound than viable allograft skin; and, if harvested at too great a thickness, undergoes dermal-epidermal separation after application to the wound, with subsequent desiccation of the exposed dermis. Cutaneous xenografts suffer no shortage of supply but are less effective as physiologic dressings and allow survival of greater numbers of subgraft bacteria, presumably because such tissue is not vascularized by the host. Studies of porcine cutaneous xenografts have shown that biologic union is formed by the growth of fibrovascular tissue from the host into the dermis of the graft without vessel-to-vessel attachment. Such tissues are not rejected, but slough after necrosis. Amnion is another physiologic dressing that is readily available and inexpensive. Since the amniotic tissue desiccates and spontaneously separates from the wound bed if left exposed, it must be covered with occlusive dressings that preclude continuous observation of the dressing and underlying wound bed. Amnion, like cutaneous xenografts, is not vascularized by the host, and biologic union occurs by ingrowth of granulation tissue.

A number of synthetic membranes have been proposed for use as skin substitutes, i.e., polymers of polyvinyl alcohol, polyurethane foam, collagen films, collagen sponges, Dacron velours, and amino acid films. All such unilamellar skin substitutes have either had draping characteristics that limited conformity of the membrane to the irregularities of the wound bed or permeability characteristics that promoted submembrane seroma formation and suppuration.

Studies in several laboratories have indicated that a bilaminate structure is required for a skin substitute to function effectively. The thin outer layer (epidermal analog) should have pores less than 5 μ in diameter to permit passage of water vapor but no liquid water or bacteria. The thicker inner layer (dermal analog) should have pores at least 80 μ in diameter that permit ingrowth of fibrovascular tissue from the wound surface to form a satisfactory biologic union.[66] Studies of a totally synthetic bilaminate membrane have demonstrated that when applied to clean wounds it functioned as well as cutaneous xenograft. When the membrane was applied to areas where nonviable tissue remained, purulent material generated by subgraft suppuration migrated through the skin substitute, indicating the need to remove or change the membrane.[77] Used in that manner, the skin substitute hastens débridement of limited areas of burn wound from which the bulk of the eschar has separated but upon which nonviable tenaciously adherent dermis remains.

Clinical effectiveness has also been demonstrated for two collagen-based bilaminate skin substitutes. Biobrane consists of a collagen gel dermal analog and a Silastic epidermal analog. This material is indistinguishable from porcine cutaneous xenograft when applied to a freshly excised burn wound in terms of submembrane formation of granulation tissue, submembrane suppuration, wound adherence, conformation to the wound surface, and membrane pliability. When applied to the clean superficial partial-thickness burns of a child immediately following injury, Biobrane strikingly reduces wound pain. If submembrane suppuration does not occur, the Biobrane need not be changed and separates as the wound re-epithelializes. Another bilaminate skin substitute that has been used to provide immediate coverage of excised burn wounds consists of a dermal analog of fibrils of collagen enriched with chondroitin-6-sulfate and a Silastic epidermal analog.[40] When the dermal analog of the skin substitute is adequately vascularized (3 to 4 weeks) by the ingrowth of granulation tissue, the Silastic membrane is removed and the wound closed by direct application of "ultra-thin" split-thickness skin grafts to the vascularized dermal analog. The residual exogenous tissue is apparently gradually resorbed and replaced by host tissue.

Signs of systemic sepsis following application of any biologic dressing or skin substitute dictate removal of such material and resumption of topical antimicrobial therapy. Particular care must be exercised when such membranes are placed on what are judged to be superficial second-degree burns, particularly in children in whom the initial appearance of the wound can be misleading. Application of these membranes to deep second- or third-degree burns may serve only to convert an open contaminated wound to a closed infected one and promote the development of invasive burn wound infection and systemic sepsis. After initial application of a biologic dressing to other than a freshly excised wound, subgraft suppuration may be quite extensive within as brief a period as 24 hours. If this occurs, in the absence of signs of systemic sepsis, the membrane should be removed, the wound gently cleansed, and fresh biologic dressings reapplied. As the wound matures with such treatment, subgraft suppuration decreases and graft adherence increases. The frequency with which the biologic dressing must be changed likewise decreases. With the exception of patients in whom prolonged biologic dressing adherence is desirable, as in those patients with massive burns following excision, cutaneous allografts should be changed at least every 5 to 7 days to avoid the hazards of rejection or the need at the time of autografting to excise the foreign tissue, a procedure often associated with considerable blood loss. In the absence of submembrane suppuration and infection, cutaneous xenografts and synthetic skin substitutes need not be changed.

Culture-Derived Epidermal Sheets

Cultured autologous keratinocytes have been used to close the wounds after excision in extensively burned patients with few available donor sites. Since it requires 3 to 4 weeks for a clinically useful amount of epidermal tissue to be produced by culture, the patient must survive that long for the epidermal sheets to be applied. Susceptibility to microbial lysis, low resistance to mechanical trauma, and the late occurrence of wound contraction and scar formation limit the clinical usefulness of the material. A recently developed bilaminate tissue composite consisting of cultured autologous keratinocytes attached to a collagen-glycosaminoglycan membrane seeded with cultured autologous fibroblasts appears to have overcome some of the limitations of sheets of cultured epidermal cells.[37] When applied to the wound bed immediately after excision of full-thickness burns, approximately two thirds of such grafts survived and demonstrated the development of a "basement membrane" within 9 days of grafting. Stimulation of angiogenesis and epithelial growth by the addition of basic fibroblast growth factor to the culture medium immediately before application of the grafts to the wound has been proposed as the mechanism by which the grafts accelerated wound closure.

ELECTRIC INJURY

Electricity exerts its tissue-damaging effects by conversion to thermal energy. Tissue damage following a high-voltage electrical injury not only occurs at the cutaneous contact site but may also involve underlying tissues and organs along the route taken by the current between the entrance and exit sites. This characteristic necessitates modification of the previously described treatment in patients who have sustained high-voltage (more than 1000 volts) electric injury. Although heat is the principal mediator of tissue damage in high-voltage injury and heat production is related to tissue resistance, the differences of tissue resistance are so small that the body acts as a volume conductor. The heat generated in this conducting tissue is a function of current density, i.e., voltage drop and current flow per unit of cross-sectional area. The relationship of heat generation to cross-sectional area is responsible for the frequency of severe injury to the extremities and the rarity of significant injury to the trunk in high-voltage electric injury. At the points of electric contact (the sites of greatest current density), the skin is severely injured and charred. When this occurs, resistance increases sharply with limitation of further passage of current and limitation of tissue heating if the voltage is 1000 or less. At higher voltages reduction of current flow does not occur and tissue injury continues. As the heated tissue cools, it acts as a volume radiator, i.e., the deeper portions cool more slowly than the superficial portions; therefore, the deeper tissues are more liable to severe injury. Although progressive tissue necrosis following electric injury has been attributed to an injury-specific vasculitis, recent laboratory studies of skeletal muscle energy metabolism identified no extension of the metabolic deficits to muscles deemed viable immediately after injury.

As a consequence of these characteristics of electric injury, misleadingly small cutaneous lesions may overlie extensive areas of devitalized muscle, which may liberate significant quantities of myoglobin and cause acute renal failure if an adequate urinary output is not maintained. Fluid estimates based on the limited cutaneous injury will cause underresuscitation and further predispose the patient to acute renal failure. To avoid this complication, fluid management may have to be modified as described previously in the section on resuscitation. Hyperkalemia may develop as a consequence of extensive tissue necrosis and require treatment based on its severity.

Both high-voltage electric injury and lightning injury can induce cardiopulmonary arrest. Cardiopulmonary resuscitation must be initiated immediately for the treatment of cardiac arrest, which may be due to asystole or fibrillation. Since cardiac arrhythmias may also occur following resuscitation, patients with high-voltage injuries who have lost consciousness or have an abnormal ECG should be monitored for at least 48 hours after injury even in the absence of arrhythmias and for 48 hours beyond the last electrocardiographic evidence of dysrhythmias if such are documented.

Patients who have sustained high-voltage electric injury may require operative treatment as soon as hemodynamic stability is achieved. Edema formation in injured tissue beneath the investing fascia may increase muscle compartment pressure to the point where it impairs the blood supply of distal unburned tissue, in which case fasciotomy should be performed to prevent ischemic necrosis of the unburned tissue. Physical examination and several diagnostic modalities have been used in determining the need for fasciotomy and surgical exploration of extremities involved in high-voltage electric injury. Stony hard edema of muscle compartments should prompt fasciotomy and exploration, as should absence of peripheral pulses distal to the site of electric contact. The other noninvasive and invasive techniques used to assess the need for escharotomy as described previously can also be used to determine the need for fasciotomy.

Even if fasciotomy is not required, it may be necessary to débride nonviable tissue or even amputate a severely burned limb. Several diagnostic modalities have been used to assess the viability of muscle in a limb with high-voltage electric injury. Scintiphotographic findings following intravenous injection of technetium-99m pyrophosphate have been difficult to interpret. The fact that both absence of tissue uptake and increased uptake with delayed washout have been correlated with tissue injury confounds diagnosis. Arteriography may be helpful in determining the need for exploration of a limb in which clinical findings are equivocal. Narrowing of the arteries of an involved limb is used as an indication for exploration, and pruning of the nutrient vessels of muscle may also assist in determining the need for and the required level of amputation. Histologic examination of muscle at the time of exploration has been reported to be useful in determining the necessary level of amputation, but the morphologic changes observed are not specific for electric injury. Since the described histologic changes in the nuclei of electrically injured cells are seldom evident within 24 hours of injury, this procedure may be of marginal value if amputation is to be performed in the immediate postinjury period. Tissue resistivity to 60 Hz. current has also been proposed as a means of assessing the severity of tissue damage following electric injury and identifying the necessary extent of débridement. Laboratory studies have shown that within 1 hour resistivity decreases in proportion to the severity of injury with the greatest decrease in grossly destroyed tissue.[14] The ability of such measurements to distinguish between reversible and irreversible change in tissue with lesser injury must be confirmed by longer-term studies prior to clinical use.

At the time of exploration of a limb that has been the site of high-voltage electric injury, all muscles, particularly those in the periosseous region, must be thoroughly explored, since even in the presence of viable superficial muscle the underlying periosseous muscles may be necrotic. If amputation is necessary, the amputation wound is left open and the patient is returned to the operating room in 24 to 48 hours for re-examination of the amputation site and any other débrided wounds. If no residual tissue necrosis is evident, the amputation wound may be closed. If further débridement is required, the wound should again be packed loosely open and dressed or covered with cutaneous allografts. The patient is scheduled for repeat operative examination of the wounds or amputation site 48 to 72 hours later.

A number of neurologic changes may occur in patients with

high-voltage electric injury ranging from immediate peripheral deficits due to the direct effects of the electric current, from which recovery is rare, to relatively late-appearing deficits that may be part of a polyneuritic syndrome involving remote nerves. In general, motor nerves appear to be more commonly affected than sensory nerves. Spinal cord function deficits can also be of immediate or delayed onset, with the delayed deficits assuming the form of quadriplegia, hemiplegia, localized nerve deficits, ascending paralysis, transverse myelitis, or a syndrome resembling amyotrophic lateral sclerosis. Thrombosis of the nutrient vessels of nerve trunks or the spinal cord may play a role in the late-occurring spinal cord deficits, whereas the early-onset deficits appear to be related to direct neuronal injury. Spinal cord deficits of late onset are more likely to be permanent, whereas those of immediate onset are more likely to be transient.

A complete neurologic examination must be performed on admission and at scheduled intervals thereafter to document the presence and time of occurrence of neurologic deficits in all patients with high-voltage electric injury. Physical therapy should be initiated upon admission and continued thereafter to prevent contractures, particularly for those patients with paralyzed limbs in whom some return of nerve function is anticipated.

Although visceral injury is rare, liver necrosis, intestinal perforation, focal pancreatic necrosis, and focal gallbladder necrosis have all been reported in patients with high-voltage electric injury. An increased incidence of cholelithiasis has also been reported to occur within 2 years of electric injury. Compression fractures of the vertebrae may also occur as a result of tetanic contractions at the time of electric contact, and fractures of the skull, spine, and long bones may result from falls subsequent to the electric injury.

Late complications include delayed hemorrhage from even moderate-sized blood vessels. Such hemorrhage has been attributed by some to "arteritis" produced by the electric current but appears more commonly to be the result of inadequate wound débridement or exposure of the involved vessel. Cataracts may form early after electric injury or up to 3 or more years thereafter and have been most frequent in patients in whom the electric contact has been on the head or the neck.

An electric burn peculiar to children typically involves the commissure of the mouth and usually results from the child's sucking on the end of a live extension cord or an electric outlet or biting an electric cord. The lesion typically has the pearly white appearance characteristic of a full-thickness burn, and bleeding from the labial artery is of sufficient frequency to justify at least initial in-hospital care. Although some authors favor early débridement and even excision, most prefer conservative treatment with delayed grafting if necessary. Even those injuries that initially appear to be of striking severity usually heal with minimal cosmetic defects, which can be repaired electively after spontaneous healing.

Cardiopulmonary arrest is common following lightning injury and must be treated by prompt cardiopulmonary resuscitation. Immediate postinjury coma and neurologic defects are also common but characteristically clear in a few hours or days. The lightning strike may rupture the tympanic membrane, with resultant hearing loss. Myoglobinuria may also be a prominent feature in patients who have sustained lightning injury and is treated as previously described. Lightning burns are characteristically superficial and present a spidery or arborescent pattern. Adequate fluid resuscitation has largely eliminated the cutaneous mottling and other signs of vasoconstriction that were formerly considered specific attributes of lightning injury. Lightning injury, contrary to popular belief, is lethal in only approximately one third of patients.

Electric energy in the form of microwave radiation damages tissue by a heating effect. Microwave burns have been caused by malfunction of appliances and by intentional child abuse. The sparing of subcutaneous fatty tissue between more severely damaged overlying and underlying tissue said by some to be characteristic of microwave burns may simply reflect the lower water content of fat. Such injuries are treated as are other burns.

CHEMICAL INJURIES

The reaction of a strong acid or base with tissue constituents liberates thermal injury that damages tissue. Other agent-specific mechanisms of local tissue damage include liquefaction necrosis caused by strong alkalis, delipidation caused by petroleum products, and vesicle formation caused by the vesicant gases. The severity of tissue damage secondary to contact with chemicals is related to the concentration of the chemical agent, the amount of agent in contact with the tissue, and the duration of contact. Thus, contrary to the case in all other burn patients, immediate wound care takes priority in patients with chemical injury, and initial treatment consists of removal of the offending material from further contact with tissue. This is best done by the removal of *all* clothing contaminated by the chemical agent and by immediate copious water lavage to dilute the agent and reduce the heat content of injured tissue. The application of neutralizing agents has no advantage over copious water lavage and may even be counterproductive, since time may be lost searching for the agent, and the heat of reaction between the chemical agent and the neutralizing solution may accentuate tissue damage.

Tissue injury may also occur after ingestion of chemical agents. Severe esophageal injury is unusual, but pyloric and antral stenosis are common after acid ingestion. Conversely, esophageal perforation and stricture are common after ingestion of strong alkali, but distal upper gastrointestinal tract injury is rare unless there are severe circumferential esophageal burns. Emetics are proscribed in the early treatment of patients following chemical ingestion lest additional injury of the esophagus, oropharynx, and upper airway occur as the chemical is regurgitated. Early endoscopic examination of the oropharynx, upper airway, and esophagus is essential for assessment of the severity of tissue injury. Although panendoscopy has been advocated by some, most authors recommend that the endoscopic examination be terminated as soon as circumferential injury of the esophagus is encountered. Treatment of patients with extensive esophageal injury without perforation includes systemic administration of broad-spectrum antibiotics and steroids and total parenteral nutrition. In patients who have injury that involves the entire wall of the esophagus or stomach, surgical intervention may be required for the prevention or treatment of perforation.

The inhalation of volatile chemical agents, such as anhydrous ammonia, the ignition products of white phosphorus, and the vapors of strong acids, mustard gas, and chlorine, can cause varying degrees of pulmonary insufficiency as a result of agent-specific airway edema formation, mucosal desquamation, and bronchospasm. The pulmonary status of patients with such inhalation injuries must be frequently monitored. If pulmonary insufficiency develops, treatment is severity-related, as described previously. A variety of chemical agents, such as petroleum distillates, phenol, mustard gas, and several of the strong acids also exert systemic effects that may necessitate pharmacologic intervention and organ system support of variable duration.

Common pitfalls in the treatment of patients with chemical injury, in addition to the failure to remove all contaminated clothing and a delay in water lavage, include inadequate lavage and inaccurate assessment of tissue injury. Skin damaged by contact with strong acids may have a tanned appearance and a silky smooth texture. If such areas are mistaken for a "suntan," rather than the full-thickness tissue loss they represent, fluid needs are underestimated, and hypovolemia and oliguria result. Wound irrigation should in general be carried out for at least 30 minutes; and in the case of strong alkali injury in which rapid tissue penetration occurs, irrigation of even longer duration may be necessary. Some authors have recommended treating such patients under a continuous shower for 24 to 48 hours, but in the authors' experience this has seldom been required. In patients in whom a strong alkali has been in prolonged contact with tissue, early excision may be necessary to limit extension of tissue damage.

There are several chemical agents for which more specific treatment is necessary. Hydrofluoric acid injury is an occupational hazard of petroleum refinery workers and those engaged in etching processes, the cleaning of air conditioning equipment, and certain chemical manufacturing processes. Contact with this agent is typically followed by a pain-free interval with subsequent focal pallor progressing to penetrating necrosis in association with severe tissue pain. Initial treatment consists of prolonged irrigation with benzalkonium chloride solution or application of calcium gluconate gel. If the pain does not relent or recurs, local injection of 10 per cent calcium gluconate into the tissue damaged by hydrofluoric acid may afford prompt pain relief, but care must be taken not to compromise the circulation.[33] Intra-arterial infusion of calcium gluconate has also been reported to limit tissue damage and relieve pain, but local excision with skin grafting may be necessary for definitive pain control and removal of damaged tissue. Hypocalcemia produced by extensive hydrofluoric acid injury is treated by intravenous infusion of calcium.

Burns caused by phenol should be treated as is any other chemical injury, by initial water lavage followed by washing of the entire area with a lipophilic solvent such as polyethylene glycol, propylene glycol, or glycerol to remove residual phenol, which is only slightly soluble in water. If phenol burns are of such extent as to permit absorption of sufficient phenol, central nervous system depression, hypothermia, hypotension, intravascular hemolysis, and even death may occur.[59] In patients injured by contact with dry alkali powders or the condensate of anhydrous ammonia, any residual powder should be quickly brushed off the skin surface before lavage is instituted.

The injury caused by contact with white phosphorus is in the majority of cases due to burning, because white phosphorus ignites at 34° C. Systemic phosphorus toxicity is rarely a problem unless significant amounts of particulate phosphorus are retained within tissue. Most white phosphorus injuries have resulted from ignition of military munitions, and particles of phosphorus may be embedded in tissue because of the explosive force of the device. Such wounds should be irrigated with saline and then covered with a dressing moistened with water or saline to prevent subsequent ignition of retained particles. More harm than good has probably been done by the inappropriate use of copper sulfate in the treatment of phosphorus injuries, i.e., the use of a solution of greater than 1 per cent concentration or the use of the solution as a soak. Use of a dilute 0.5 to 1 per cent solution of copper sulfate as a wash, followed by copious rinsing with water or saline, results in the formation of a blue-gray cupric phosphide coating on the retained phosphorus particles that facilitates identification and impedes ignition. Alternatively, retained particles of white phosphorus can be identified by their phosphorescence when exposed to ultraviolet light in a darkened operating room. Removed phosphorus particles must be placed under water lest they ignite and cause a fire.

Chemically injured eyes must be irrigated with water, saline, or phosphate buffer immediately (even before leaving the site of the accident) to minimize corneal damage. Prolonged irrigation, 12 to 72 hours, is recommended for eyes injured by strong alkalis because of the rapidity with which such agents penetrate ocular tissue. Blepharospasm secondary to the injury makes irrigation difficult unless small-caliber irrigating cannulas are placed in the conjunctival sulci or a modified scleral contact lens with an irrigating sidearm is used. After irrigation, a cycloplegic, such as 1 per cent atropine, should be instilled on a scheduled basis to counteract iritis, and some authors recommend simultaneous instillation of a miotic agent as well. Corneal damage can be severe despite such treatment, presumably as a consequence of collagenase activation, and various authors recommend instillation of cysteine or edetic acid sodium, subconjunctival injection of autologous serum, and even removal of necrotic tissue with mucosal grafts used for coverage of the resulting defect. Xerophthalmia and symblepharon formation are late complications of severe alkali injury of the eye. The former is treated with variable results by the use of artificial tear solutions and "bandage" lenses, and the latter is treated by surgical release and repair after the acute process resolves. The results of corneal transplantation to restore vision in eyes severely damaged by alkali have been discouraging.

Tar and Bitumen Burns

Tar and bitumen injuries are actually contact burns. Immediate treatment consists of cooling the hot adherent material with cold water. Petroleum-based solvents should not be used to remove adherent bitumen, because they may cause further tissue injury and even systemic toxic effects. After cooling, material adherent to blisters is removed when the blisters are débrided, but that adherent to unblistered tissue should be covered with a petrolatum-based ointment and dressed. Daily reapplication of the ointment and the dressing effects emulsification and atraumatic removal of the bitumen following which the burn is treated as is any other burn.

METABOLIC ALTERATIONS AND NUTRITIONAL SUPPORT

The metabolic response following burn injury is related to burn size, with the metabolic rate rising in a curvilinear fashion. In patients with burns of more than 50 per cent of the total body surface, metabolic rates rise to levels 2 to 3 times normal and far exceed those associated with any other injury or illness. Postburn hypermetabolism is manifested by increased oxygen consumption, elevated cardiac output and minute ventilation, increased core temperature, wasting of lean body mass, and increased urinary nitrogen excretion. Recent studies have shown that the burned patient is not externally cold because of increased evaporative heat loss but is internally warm, with an upward resetting of thermal regulatory mechanisms. This hypermetabolism is temperature-sensitive in patients with burns over 50 per cent of the total body surface but is not temperature-dependent. The core temperature, skin temperature, core-to-skin heat transfer, and metabolic rate remain elevated at and above thermal neutral temperature, but the metabolic rate in patients with burns over one half of the total body surface can be diminished by up to 10 per cent by ambient temperatures above 30° C. (Fig. 8). Regional blood flow to the viscera likewise increases, although its fraction of the total flow remains unchanged or slightly increased.[93] Similarly, visceral oxygen utilization, although increased, remains an unchanged slightly elevated fraction of total body oxygen consumption. By contrast, blood flow to the wound is markedly exaggerated in relation to total body blood flow. In studies of patients with leg burns, blood flow to the injured extremity increased as burn wound size increased.[5] However, blood flow to the underlying muscle was normal, indicating that the entire increment in extremity blood flow was directed to the overlying wound. These findings, in part, explain the direct influence of the burn wound on the postinjury hypermetabolic and cardiodynamic response.

The postburn elevation in metabolic rate is associated with, and appears to be mediated by, increases in catecholamine (pri-

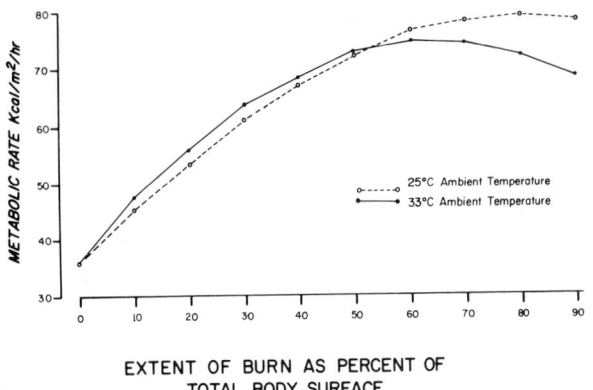

EXTENT OF BURN AS PERCENT OF
TOTAL BODY SURFACE

Figure 8. Graph illustrating the relationship between burn size and metabolic rate. Note the temperature sensitivity (divergence of curves above 50 per cent burn) and temperature independence (elevation of metabolic rate at both ambient temperatures) of postburn hypermetabolism.

marily norepinephrine) production and excretion.[94] These hormones influence the disposition and utilization of nutrients both directly and as a result of their secondary effect on other hormones. Studies have identified a reciprocal relationship between thyroid hormone and catecholamine levels, with an initial depression of thyroid hormone levels followed by a gradual return to normal as catecholamine levels recede. In the early postburn period, glucagon levels are elevated and insulin levels are absolutely or relatively decreased, causing a markedly lowered insulin-glucagon molar ratio that, in the absence of complications, gradually increases and returns to the normal value of 3 to 4 when the burn wound heals or is grafted and convalescence begins. Rather than being a secondary response to the early elevations of catecholamine concentrations, glucagon is probably one of the primary mediators of the increase in catabolic biochemical pathways, particularly those in muscle.[90] As a result of these hormonal changes, glucose flow rises, as does glucose distribution space. Urinary urea nitrogen excretion increases as muscle protein is broken down to provide amino acid gluconeogenic precursors (principally alanine and glutamine), which are transported to the liver and gut, where they are deaminated and converted to glucose to provide the energy substrate needed to satisfy the metabolic needs. Severe infection, particularly gram-negative infection, may exaggerate metabolic needs but may also impair hepatic gluconeogenesis, thereby decreasing blood glucose levels and glucose flow, altering glucose distribution space, and reducing the insulinogenic index. These effects of sepsis can, in part, be counteracted by administration of exogenous glucose and insulin to maintain the necessary supply of nutrients to peripheral tissues.

Although postburn hypermetabolism can be significantly reduced by beta adrenergic blockade and pharmacologic doses of morphine, the hypermetabolic response appears in large part to be driven by the needs of the wounds. Blood flow to the wound is significantly and disproportionately (with respect to visceral and other soft tissue blood flow) elevated.[93] Glucose consumption and lactate production are significantly increased in the area of burn without a significant change in oxygen consumption, as compared with unburned tissue, and this metabolic milieu is characteristic of granulation tissue.[5] Since pharmacologic attenuation of this response to injury would diminish delivery of the nutrients and energy needed for wound healing, it appears physiologically sound to meet the elevated calorie and protein needs of the burned patient, rather than to attempt suppression of the accelerated metabolic process.

The nutritional needs of the burned patient can be measured by indirect calorimetry, predicted by use of a variety of nomograms, or estimated (for adult patients with burns of over 40 per cent of the total body surface) as being 2000 to 2200 calories per

sq. m. of body surface daily and 12 to 18 gm. of nitrogen per sq. m. of body surface daily. Since spontaneous nutritional intake at the usual mealtimes appears to be fixed at preinjury levels, it is commonly necessary to provide severely burned patients with any of several liquid dietary supplements at scheduled intervals (usually every 2 hours) around the clock in order to meet their nutritional requirements. If the patient cannot or will not take adequate nutrients and has intact gastrointestinal function, tube feeding should be utilized, with care taken to avoid aspiration. If diarrhea or ileus precludes enteral feeding, or if the patient has lost more than 10 per cent of his preburn weight, and closure of the wounds is deemed unlikely within 7 to 10 days, parenteral nutrition should be initiated by means of an intravenous cannula placed in a large-caliber, high-flow central vein.

Nitrogen loss increases after major burns, and 80 to 90 per cent of the nitrogen appears in the urine as urea, which may exceed 40 gm. per day in patients with severe burns who are being fed. Although the extent of nitrogen loss is proportional to the postinjury increase in energy expenditure, the nitrogen-containing lean body mass is not the major source of metabolic fuel oxidized for energy. Over a wide range of metabolic response, body protein in burned patients contributes only 15 to 20 per cent of the energy required to meet metabolic needs. In the absence of exogenously administered calories, lipid stores are the major source of energy for meeting metabolic requirements. Visceral proteins are quite labile and rapidly exhausted. Skeletal muscle is the primary source of nitrogen lost in the urine, and muscle proteolysis is reflected by increased excretion of creatinine and 3-methyl histidine. The intake of nitrogen alone spares protein and improves nitrogen balance after burn. The addition of nonprotein calories to the source of nitrogen further improves nitrogen balance and enables more calories to be utilized for the restoration of nitrogen equilibrium. Calories and protein cooperatively contribute to this improvement in nitrogen economy. The addition of glucose to a previously carbohydrate-free protein diet causes enhanced amino acid incorporation into protein and improves nitrogen balance.

Total protein intake appears to be more important than the source from which the protein is derived or the form in which it is administered. Alexander and co-workers have demonstrated that protein intake in burned patients improves immunologic response and increases survival.[3] The optimal calorie to nitrogen ratio varies between 150:1 to 100:1. Branched chain amino acids have been found to improve nitrogen retention, restore immunologic function, and increase plasma transport proteins; no beneficial effect on morbidity or mortality was observed.[13] This failure of branched chain amino acids to improve outcome may be related, in part, to the inability of burned patients to completely oxidize branched chain amino acids in muscle.[6] Glutamine may have uniquely beneficial effects on total body nitrogen economy and organ function, particularly in the intestinal tract. After severe injury, gut mucosa utilizes glutamine, thereby sparing glucose and allowing it to be utilized for tissues with obligatory glucose requirement. Glutamine levels decrease in both tissue and plasma pools; and in the absence of glutamine administration, the gut mucosa becomes atrophic. Addition of glutamine to the nutritional support regimen increases mucosal cellularity and decreases extremity glutamine efflux. The significance of this major metabolic pathway and its implications on dietary support strategies are illustrated by the effect of enterectomy in critically ill patients.[28] Removal of large portions of the intestine decreases extremity glutamine efflux, indicating that the gut provides a feedback signal to peripheral tissues to maintain glutamine mobilization. The addition of glutamine to total parenteral nutrition after surgical stress spares glutamine in muscle, counteracts the fall in muscle protein synthesis, and improves nitrogen balance.[36] Such studies indicate that glutamine supplementation may be beneficial in the nutritional support of thermally injured patients.

The roles of carbohydrate and fat as sources of nonprotein calories depend on the extent of injury and the associated metabolic response. In general, carbohydrate and fat can be used interchangeably as effective nonprotein calorie sources for feeding patients with relatively small burns. However, as the hypermetabolic response becomes more pronounced in patients with larger burns, carbohydrate is more effective in maintaining body protein than fat when each food source is used alone.[31] If fat alone is administered parenterally as a long-chain triglyceride emulsion, the reduced nitrogen excretion is due to the glycerol in the emulsion. Studies have shown that emulsions of medium-chain triglycerides, in contrast to long-chain triglycerides, are much more effective in maintaining lean body mass. The medium-chain triglycerides demonstrate more rapid elimination kinetics and increased ketone production and are associated with less fat deposition in the tissues.[19]

In practice, enteral intake is instituted on postburn day 3 and increased to meet predicted calorie requirements by postburn day 5. Any of the commercially available enteral formulas with an appropriate nitrogen : calorie ratio can be used. In patients who are unable to utilize the gastrointestinal tract by postburn day 5, parenteral nutrition is instituted with standard glucose–amino acid solutions. Lipid emulsions are utilized only to prevent the development of essential fatty acid deficiencies. Five hundred to 1000 ml. of fat emulsions are given twice a week. At this dose, the fat overload syndrome rarely occurs. Blood sugar levels should be monitored frequently and kept below 200 ml. per 100 ml. Sudden intolerance of previously well-tolerated glucose loads is an early sign of sepsis and should prompt careful search for a source of infection. The high risk of cannula-related sepsis makes change of the intravenous cannula necessary every 48 to 72 hours. Total metabolic support of the burned patient also entails measures to minimize pain, to maintain muscle activity in order to prevent disuse atrophy, to promptly diagnose and treat infection, and to maintain a warm microenvironment in order to minimize cold stress.

INFECTIONS AND SEPTIC COMPLICATIONS OF BURN PATIENTS

Diagnosis and Treatment of Burn Wound Infections

The available topical agents maintain the bacterial density in the burn wounds of most patients below the level of 10^5 organisms per gm. of tissue but do not sterilize the wound. Consequently, the bacteria in the burn wounds of any patient may escape control and invade the underlying tissue. This complication occurs most commonly in patients with burns of more than 30 per cent of the body surface, part or all of which have not been excised, or those in whom skin graft failure has occurred after initial excision. To identify invasive burn wound infection at the earliest possible time, it is mandatory that the entire burn wound be examined each day, with any change in wound appearance noted. Conversion of an area of partial-thickness burn to full-thickness necrosis and the appearance of focal areas of black or dark hemorrhagic discoloration are the most common changes indicative of burn wound infection (Fig. 9). If those or any of the other clinical signs of burn wound infection listed in Table 6 are identified, it is necessary to assess the microbial status of the burn wound to confirm the diagnosis of invasive infection, since similar changes in wound appearance can be caused by hemorrhage due to local trauma or maceration.[74]

Surface cultures of the burn wound may provide useful epidemiologic information but are not helpful in making the diagnosis of invasive infection. Even quantitative cultures of wound tissue are of limited usefulness. Quantitative counts of less than 10^5 per gm. of biopsy tissue correlate well with the absence of invasive burn wound infection, but quantitative counts above that level correlate poorly with the presence of invasive burn wound infection—i.e., invasive infection cannot be confirmed

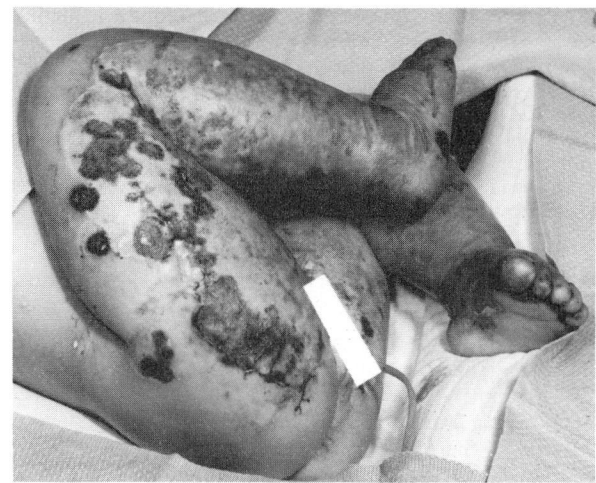

Figure 9. Focal hemorrhagic changes in burn wound characteristic of *Pseudomonas* burn wound sepsis. These lesions appeared on the tenth postburn day in this child aged 1 year and 4 months with burns over 25 per cent of the total body surface. Note the edema and hemorrhagic change in the wound margin of the right buttock and extension of hemorrhage into unburned skin at the periphery of this lesion on the midlateral thigh.

by histologic examination in more than half of biopsy specimens with such high counts.[54]

The histologic examination of a burn wound biopsy is the most rapid and only reliable means of making the critical differentiation between microbial colonization of nonviable tissue, which is present in all burn wounds, and the presence of microorganisms in unburned viable tissue that is characteristic of invasive burn wound infection. By scalpel dissection, a 500-mg. lenticular tissue sample, including both eschar and underlying unburned tissue, is obtained from that area of the wound showing the most pronounced changes. The biopsy is performed as a ward procedure, and hemostasis is seldom a problem. Blood loss is readily controlled by a brief application of direct pressure or by electrocoagulation. If local anesthesia is necessary, the anesthetic agent should be injected at the periphery of the intended biopsy site to minimize distortion of the morphologic characteristics of the tissue in the biopsy sample. One half of the biopsy sample is submitted to the microbiology laboratory for culture identification of the organisms present and their antibiotic sensitivities. The other half of the specimen is submitted to the pathology laboratory, where histologic sections are prepared by rapid section technique requiring 3 to 4 hours or a frozen section technique requiring 30 minutes. A specimen originally processed by the frozen section technique should be subsequently processed by regular section technique to correct the 4 per cent falsely negative diagnosis rate of frozen sections. The pathologist examines the histologic preparations for the presence of microorganisms in unburned viable tissue, which confirms the diagnosis of invasive burn wound infection. The other histologic findings listed in Table 7 are not diagnostic of inva-

TABLE 6. Clinical Signs of Burn Wound Infection

Conversion of second-degree burn to full-thickness necrosis
Focal dark brown or black discoloration of wound
Degeneration of wound with "neoeschar" formation
Unexpectedly rapid eschar separation
Hemorrhagic discoloration of subeschar fat
Erythematous or violaceous edematous wound margin
Crusted serrations of wound margin*
Metastatic septic lesions in unburned tissue†

* Characteristic of herpetic infections.
† Ecthyma gangrenosum characteristic of *Pseudomonas* burn wound sepsis.

TABLE 7. Histologic Criteria of Burn Wound Infection

Microorganisms in unburned tissue
Hemorrhage in unburned tissue
Heightened inflammatory reaction in adjacent viable tissue
Small vessel thrombosis or ischemic necrosis of unburned tissue
Perineural and intralymphatic migration of organisms*
Vasculitis with perivascular "cuffing" of organisms*
Intracellular viral inclusions

---

* Characteristic of invasive *Pseudomonas* infections.

---

sive burn wound infections, but should raise the pathologist's index of suspicion and prompt a careful search of the specimen for microorganisms in the unburned tissue.

The microbial status of a burn wound can be staged according to microscopic findings as noted in Table 8. If only colonization is evident in the first biopsy specimen obtained from a burn patient, no change in wound care is required. If examination of serially obtained biopsy specimens reveals evidence of microbial proliferation and penetration, i.e., progression from Stage IA to Stage IC, wound care should be altered. A histologic diagnosis of Stage II mandates prompt intervention as described below. Microscopically evident involvement of the microvasculature and lymphatics, i.e., Stage IIC, is associated with a high likelihood of hematogenous spread to remote tissues and organs and mandates close monitoring of the lungs and the heart (Fig. 10).

Burn wound biopsies can be misleading but are less commonly so than wound cultures. The limitations of burn wound biopsies are principally technical ones e.g., sampling of a noninfected area, failing to include unburned tissue by sampling only the eschar, and erroneous histologic interpretation. Consequently, burn wound biopsy results should be interpreted in terms of the patient's hospital course. Negative biopsy results in the presence of clinical deterioration should prompt re-examination of the burns and biopsy sampling of other areas showing changes indicative of infection.

Histologic confirmation of invasive infection requires an immediate therapeutic response with the treatment depending upon both the extent and the depth of the septic process. If the infection is bacterial and one of the nondiffusible topical agents is being used, it should be discontinued and topical therapy continued with mafenide acetate burn cream. Systemic antimicrobial therapy should be instituted based on the sensitivity

**TABLE 8. Histologic Staging of Microbial Status
of Burn Wounds**

Stage	Histologic Findings
I. Colonization	
A. Superficial	Microorganisms confined to surface of burn wound
B. Penetrating	Microorganisms extending into variable thickness of eschar
C. Proliferating	Variable density of microorganisms in subeschar space
II. Invasion	
A. Microinvasion	Microorganisms present in viable tissue
B. Deep invasion	Penetration of microorganisms deep into viable subcutaneous tissue
C. Microvascular invasion	Involvement of small blood vessels and/or lymphatics

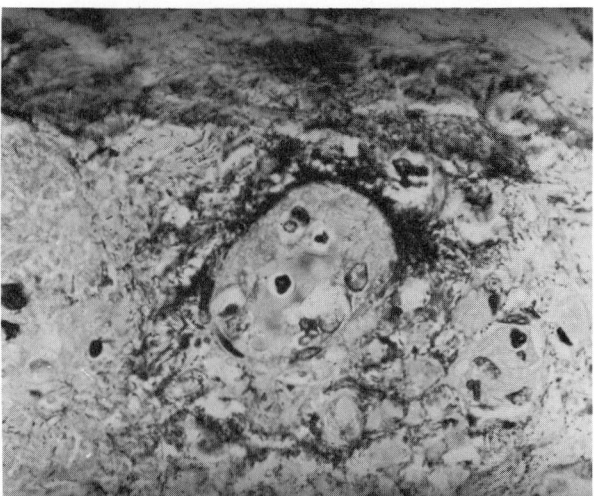

Figure 10. Photomicrograph of biopsy specimen obtained from a patient with invasive *Pseudomonas* burn wound sepsis. Note the perivascular cuffing of bacteria characteristic of *Pseudomonas* vasculitis. Even though the involved vessel is thrombosed in this area, such a finding makes hematogenous dissemination likely and mandates systemic antibiotic therapy.

patterns of the microbial flora resident on the burn unit at that time as determined by the microbial surveillance program. When the patient's culture and sensitivity results are available, systemic antimicrobial therapy should be adjusted accordingly.

Although the incidence of invasive burn wound infection has decreased markedly in recent years, *Pseudomonas aeruginosa* remains the most common causative organism. Since such organisms are typically sensitive to high concentrations of broadspectrum penicillins, one half of the daily dose of a broadspectrum penicillin, such as piperacillin, suspended in 1000 ml. of normal saline, should be immediately infused into the subeschar tissues beneath all infected areas of the wound by means of a number 20 spinal needle to minimize the number of injection sites. The patient should be scheduled for excision of the infected tissue within the next 12 hours and a second subeschar antibiotic infusion carried out immediately prior to the excision in order to protect the patient from hematogenous dissemination of viable bacteria that may occur during the excision. Wide local excision, superficial to the fascia, is carried out if the process is confined to the subcutaneous tissue, as is commonly the case with bacterial infections. Excision of involved fascia and muscle is required for the treatment of deeper invasion.

As the incidence of bacterial burn wound infections has decreased over the past 25 years, the incidence of nonbacterial burn wound infections has increased.[53] *Candida* species, the most common nonbacterial burn wound colonizers, seldom invade and typically remain confined to the burned tissue and consequently require no specific treatment. Candidal infection may occur in the interstices of a mesh graft or an excised burn wound exposed by skin graft loss and require treatment by twice-daily application of a topical antifungal agent, such as clotrimazole cream or ciclopirox olamine cream. If such treatment is ineffective in preventing extension of this usually superficial infection, excision should be carried out and amphotericin B administered systemically.

Filamentous fungi are much more aggressive burn wound invaders and may cause infections of grave consequence. *Aspergillus* species, the fungi that most often cause invasive burn wound infections (42 cases in a recent 6½-year period), seldom traverse fascial planes and commonly remain confined to the subcutaneous tissues. The Phycomycetes are the most aggressive true fungi, and these organisms spread rapidly along tissue planes, readily traverse fascia, and have a predilection for invading vessels. Infections caused by the Phycomycetes are characterized by rapidly expanding soft tissue ischemic necrosis with a peripheral rim of subcutaneous edema and frequent hematogenous dissemination to remote tissues.[73] The diagnosis of invasive fungal infection is best made by the histologic examination of a burn wound biopsy specimen. Treatment of such infections consists of twice-daily topical application of an antifungal agent, systemic administration of amphotericin B, and prompt wide excision of the infected tissue. When a phycomycotic infection on a limb has traversed the investing fascia and involves significant amounts of underlying muscle, amputation is necessary to control the infectious process.

Viral burn wound infections are relatively uncommon and are caused most often by herpes simplex virus I. Herpetic infections occur most frequently in healing or recently healed partial-thickness burns, particularly those in the nasolabial area. Herpetic burn wound infection is most reliably diagnosed by the histologic examination of a biopsy or scrapings from the cutaneous lesions. There is currently no effective topical therapy for such lesions. Systemic herpesvirus infections involving multiple organs, such as the liver, lungs, spleen, adrenals, and bone marrow, may also occur. Systemic signs of sepsis and unexplained hypotension in a burn patient with rapidly spreading cutaneous herpetic lesions should direct attention to the possibility of systemic herpes infection, which, if confirmed, is treated by systemic antiviral therapy using either adenine arabinoside or acyclovir.

Other Septic Complications

Although invasive burn wound infection has become uncommon, infection may occur in other organs and tissues as a reflection of the immunologic effects of both the injury and treatment. Infections in sites other than the burn wound have actually increased as principal causes of death because of the decrease in fatal burn wound sepsis. As *Pseudomonas* spp. have decreased in importance, *Staphylococcus aureus* has emerged as the most common organism recovered from infections in burn patients today[53] (Fig. 11).

PNEUMONIA. The most common site of infection in the burn patient is at present the lungs. During a recent 5-year period, pneumonia was present in 55 per cent of 166 fatal burns and was considered to be the primary cause of death in 83, or 50 per cent, of those patients. The reduction of invasive burn wound infection has been attended by a change in the predominant type of pneumonia from hematogenous to airborne (bronchopneumonia).[74] Bronchopneumonia in the burn patient, as in any other critically ill patient, is commonly caused by *Staphylococcus aureus* and gram-negative opportunistic bacteria and occurs relatively early in the postburn period (average onset,

tenth postburn day). Atelectasis often precedes this complication, and the pneumonic process may first be evident on the chest roentgenogram as an ill-defined infiltrate of irregular outline. When such an infiltrate appears and the patient has clinical signs of pneumonia, the endobronchial secretions must be cultured and antibiotic treatment initiated on the basis of the sensitivity of the treatment facility's resident flora as determined by the microbiologic surveillance program. Antimicrobial treatment is adjusted as necessary when the results of the patient's culture and sensitivity testing are obtained.

Hematogenous pneumonia commonly begins relatively late in the postburn course (average time of diagnosis, seventeenth postburn day) and is caused by microorganisms arising from a remote septic focus. The sudden appearance of a solitary rounded infiltrate on the chest roentgenogram (Fig. 12) may be the first manifestation of this pulmonary infection. While an occult visceral perforation or an inapparent soft tissue abscess is a rare source of the microorganisms causing this infection, an infected wound or a vein harboring a focus of intraluminal suppuration is the source of infection in the majority of cases (98 per cent). All possible sites must be examined if a characteristic pulmonary infiltrate appears. An identified source of infection must be removed or controlled and the pneumonic process treated by systemic administration of antibiotics active against the causative organisms. Hematogenous pneumonitis is more often associated with a fatal outcome than is airborne pneumonia but as a reflection of its secondary nature is less often the principal cause of death.

SUPPURATIVE THROMBOPHLEBITIS. Suppurative thrombophlebitis can occur in any previously cannulated peripheral or even central vein (Fig. 13). The likelihood of occurrence increases with the duration of cannulation. Strict limitation of cannula residence to 3 days or less in burn patients has been associated with a reduction of the incidence of this complication from 4.3 per cent to 2.5 per cent in recent years. Because of the presence of an overlying burn and the immunosuppressive effect of the burn injury itself, local signs of this disease are present in less than half the patients so afflicted. The appearance of a pulmonary infiltrate characteristic of hematogenous pneumonia or the occurrence of septicemia in the absence of any other obvious source of infection should prompt exploration of every previously cannulated vein. The most frequent site of intraluminal suppuration is the area of the vein where the cannula tip resided, and that region must be examined before suppurative thrombophlebitis can be excluded. Identification of purulent material within a vein mandates surgical removal of the entire length of vein involved in the suppurative process and the systemic administration of antibiotics to which the

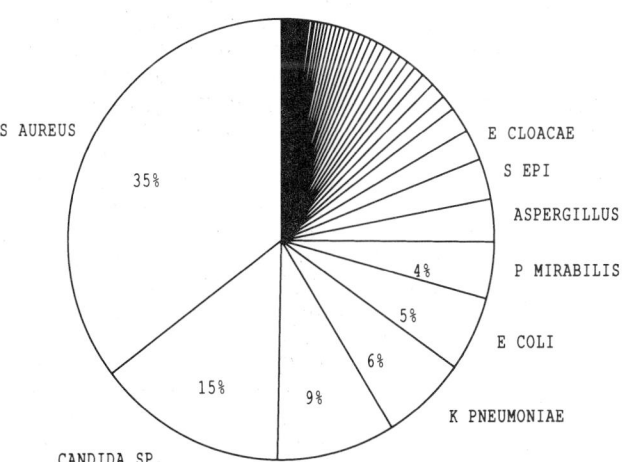

Figure 11. Frequency of recovery of microorganisms from infections in burn patients treated at the United States Army Burn Center 1984 to 1989.

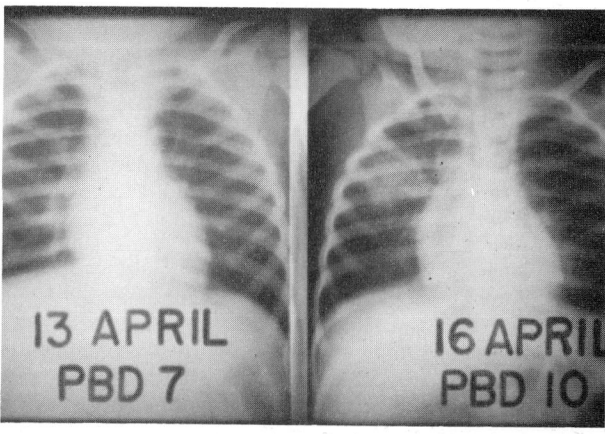

Figure 12. Chest roentgenograms documenting the sudden appearance, on the tenth postburn day, of nodular infiltrate characteristic of hematogenous pneumonia in the right lung. The patient died 2 days later, and the source of disseminated bacteria was found to be suppuration in a previously cannulated vein.

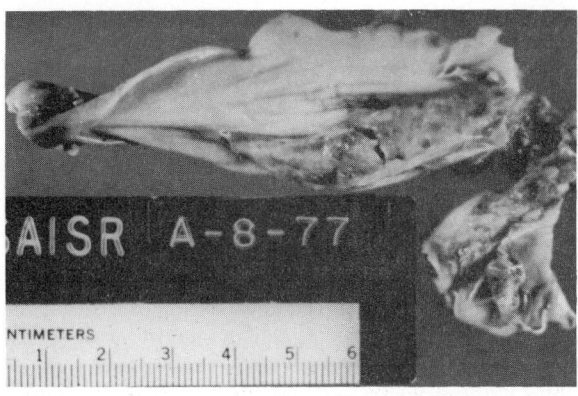

Figure 13. Autopsy specimen showing infected thrombi in both iliac veins at sites of previously resident cannula tips. The patient, aged 72 years, died with overwhelming sepsis on the eighty-fourth postburn day.

causative organism is sensitive. Failure of sepsis to clear after vein excision can be due to inadequate extent of the excision, suppuration within another vein, or hematogenous dissemination of the organism to other organs, such as the heart or lungs, prior to or during excision of the infected vein.

ACUTE ENDOCARDITIS. The incidence of acute endocarditis is relatively high in burn patients (1.3 per cent of 1699 patients treated from 1969 to 1974) because of the frequent need for prolonged intravenous infusions, the high incidence of suppurative thrombophlebitis, and the frequency of bacteremia associated with wound manipulation. Identification of characteristic murmurs is difficult in burn patients because of their hyperdynamic circulation. Two-dimensional echocardiographic examination may detect valvular lesions, but small vegetations may remain undetected. Although this infectious complication most frequently involves the right side of the heart, it may occur on either or both sides. *Staphylococcus aureus* is the most common causative agent, and the presence of that organism in two or more blood cultures from a burn patient with sepsis and no other apparent infection should suggest the diagnosis. When this complication is diagnosed, systemic maximal-dose antibiotic therapy should be initiated and continued for at least 3 weeks and longer as needed to clear blood cultures.

SUPPURATIVE SINUSITIS. Suppurative sinusitis is most likely to occur in patients who require long-term transnasal intubation, particularly those with tubes in both the airway and the gastrointestinal tract. This complication may be inapparent clinically, and radiologic studies are required for confirmation of the diagnosis. Therapy is initiated with broad-spectrum antibiotics, but surgical drainage of the involved sinuses may be necessary if the infection is unresponsive to antibiotic therapy. A tracheostomy and/or gastrostomy may be necessary if continued intubation of the airway and/or the gastrointestinal tract is required.

BACTEREMIA AND SEPTICEMIA. In order to minimize the development of antibiotic resistance in the bacteria present on the burn wound and elsewhere, systemic antibiotics should not be administered prophylactically, but should be administered only on the basis of a secure clinical or laboratory diagnosis of infection. Wound care procedures may cause hematogenous dissemination of microorganisms. Twenty-one per cent of blood cultures obtained during burn wound manipulations are positive, with the recovery rate related to both the extent of the burn and the magnitude of the procedure. To minimize the seeding of remote tissues and organs due to such bacteremias, antibiotics active against both gram-positive and gram-negative organisms should be administered perioperatively to patients undergoing surgical débridement or excision of the burn wound.

In burn patients with sepsis, initial antibiotic therapy should

be based on the results of the institution's microbial surveillance program and, if available, the histologic findings of burn wound biopsy specimens or Gram stain preparations of secretions and other infected material. Blood cultures should be obtained on a scheduled basis and the antibiotic regimen changed if necessary on the basis of that patient's culture and sensitivity test results. Blood cultures from critically ill extensively burned patients may show growth of multiple organisms or growth of different organisms in serial cultures. Those culture results reflecting the immunologic incompetence of such patients, should not be regarded as indicative of technical error; and even though the survival of such patients is low, they should be treated with antibiotics active against all the organisms recovered.

GASTROINTESTINAL COMPLICATIONS

The gastrointestinal complications of the burn patient are the same as those of other severely injured patients and include acalculous cholecystitis, pancreatitis (usually associated with a posterior penetrating ulcer, pre-existing alcoholism, sepsis, or disseminated intravascular coagulation), and ulceration of the gastrointestinal tract. Acute ulceration of the stomach and duodenum (Curling's ulcer), formerly the most frequent life-threatening gastrointestinal complication of burn patients, is now effectively controlled by prophylactic antacid or H_2 histamine receptor antagonist therapy. As a result of such prophylaxis, hemorrhage or perforation requiring surgical intervention is now exceedingly rare.[76] During the early postburn period, when ileus is present, the quantity of antacid necessary to maintain gastric aspirate pH above 5 is instilled hourly through the nasogastric tube in all patients with burns of more than 35 per cent of the body surface. After return of gastrointestinal motility, similar doses of antacid are given orally until the extent of burn is reduced by healing or by grafting to less than 35 per cent of the body surface. Alternatively, 400 mg. of cimetidine can be administered parenterally every 4 hours during the period of ileus, with oral dosage of 300 mg. every 6 hours continued after the ileus abates. Occasionally, both forms of prophylaxis are necessary to maintain gastric aspirate pH above 5 in patients with extensive burns or patients with septic complications. Although the gastric anacidity following such prophylaxis has been implicated as a factor contributing to the high incidence of bronchopneumonia in critically ill patients, the data supporting that hypothesis are tenuous.

Acute dilatation of the colon may occur in burn patients in whom sepsis develops. Additionally, focal necrosis with acute ulceration of the colon has been identified in burn patients with severe complications, particularly those with sepsis-related episodes of hypotension. Certain of these lesions have penetrated the full thickness of the colonic wall to the level of the serosa, but no free perforations have as yet been observed. Healing of the more superficial of the ulcers of the large bowel can apparently occur when the underlying condition has been corrected, since distortion of the colonic mural architecture indicating healing of lesions of varying age has been noted in some burn patients who have died. Endoscopic examination should be performed if the dilatation reaches significant proportions. If the dilatation does not relent with conservative therapy or if significant mucosal necrosis is endoscopically evident, operative intervention is indicated. Because of the increased risk of postoperative wound infection and dehiscence, retention sutures should be used in closing any abdominal incision in a burn patient.

BURN SCAR CARCINOMA

Burn scar carcinoma or Marjolin's ulcer is a rare neoplasm that occurs in the unstable scar of a full-thickness burn. Subsequently, this unstable scar is susceptible to trauma and continuously breaks down and heals. The latent period is 1 to 75 years, with a mean of approximately 35 years. Although basal cell carcinomas have occurred in old burn scars, they are exceedingly rare, and most Marjolin's ulcers are squamous cell carcinomas. These tumors are highly invasive, and regional node metastases were present in 35 per cent of 46 cases reported by Novick and associates.[65] Metastases are more frequent in patients with primary lesions located on the extremities than in patients with primary lesions on the trunk. All ulcerative lesions in burn scars should be biopsied. If no tumor is found, the ulcerated area, with a 2-cm. margin, is excised and the defect closed with a skin graft. If carcinoma is found, extirpation of the tumor must include all involved tissue as verified by histologic examination of the wound margins.

SUN AND HEAT OVEREXPOSURE

Overexposure to sunlight is a common cause of mild cutaneous burn injury but can also cause more severe injury. Erythema and pain from sunburn reaches a maximum at 10 to 24 hours after exposure and resolves within 72 to 96 hours.[82] Treatment is largely symptomatic, utilizing cooling showers, cold soaks, or topical analgesics to reduce pain, oral acetylsalicylic acid to reduce prostaglandin-mediated inflammation, and antihistamines or hydroxyzine to reduce histamine-mediated pruritus occurring on the second to fourth postburn days. The patient should also be warned of possible postural hypotension. A severe sunburn with pain, erythema, and bullae should be treated like any other partial-thickness injury, as outlined previously.

Heat stroke usually occurs in the elderly during heat waves or in younger, otherwise healthy, individuals performing strenuous exercise in a hot environment. It represents a total loss of the body's thermoregulatory control, occurring because the demands for maintenance of blood pressure dominate the requirements for body temperature maintenance. By definition, the core body temperature exceeds 40.6° C. (105° F.), with associated anhidrosis and central nervous system dysfunction.

Pathophysiologic changes commonly encountered include disorientation and bizarre behavior, hypovolemia, hemoconcentration, and hypotension. Variable disturbances of acid-base and electrolyte balance may occur, depending upon the duration of heat exposure and the patient's compensatory response. Compensatory hyperventilation may cause respiratory alkalosis; but if hypovolemia is so severe as to impair tissue blood flow and cause shock, lactic acidosis results. Hypernatremia may be present with severe dehydration; but in unacclimated patients, hyponatremia may occur due to salt loss in sweat and can be exaggerated by intake of electrolyte-free water. Hypokalemia may result from the combined effect of respiratory alkalosis and hypovolemia-induced activation of renin, angiotensin, and aldosterone. Conversely, hyperkalemia may occur in those patients in whom acidosis develops or in whom heat stroke causes skeletal muscle necrosis. Mortality rates as high as 18 per cent have been reported. The presence of coma, coagulopathy, hypotension, or renal failure, the need for intubation, and a high degree and long duration of hyperthermia are associated with a poor prognosis.

Vital to treatment is rapid cooling of the patient to a body temperature of 38.9° C. (102° F.) utilizing ice packs, cool water sprays, and intravenous administration of cold saline. Immersion in ice water can decrease body cooling because of cutaneous vasoconstriction and is therefore not recommended. During cooling, cardiac activity should be monitored continuously and any dysrhythmias treated accordingly. If hypotension does not resolve with cooling and intravenous saline, vasopressors may be necessary, but pure alpha-agonists should be avoided because of their peripheral vasoconstrictive effects. Metabolic acidosis should be corrected, as should any coagulopathy; but hypokalemia should be corrected only if acidosis is present.

Hyperkalemia is treated as in other patients. Hyponatremia responds to administration of salt-containing fluids. Hypernatremia also responds to the infusion of cool lactated Ringer's solution. Intubation may be required to maintain adequate oxygenation. Administration of dantrolene, effective in the treatment of malignant hyperthermia, is controversial, with no proven efficacy in patients with heat stroke. On an empiric basis, seizure prophylaxis with phenytoin is recommended.

COLD INJURY

Exposure to cold environments can produce a spectrum of physiologic derangements, varying from direct tissue damage to severe total body hypothermia. The injury produced by exposure to cold depends upon the degree of low temperature, the duration of exposure, and environmental conditions that can influence the effects of low temperature. Although resembling heat injury in many ways, cold injury induces unique pathophysiologic alterations and requires a therapeutic approach distinct from that of heat injury. Always a concern in military populations, such injuries are now observed with increasing frequency as the popularity of winter sports rises, the elderly population grows, and the number of homeless individuals expands.

Frostbite

Frostbite causes freezing of tissue and produces damage by tissue ice crystallization, cellular dehydration, and microvascular occlusion. The skin and subcutaneous tissue of exposed body parts, especially the hands, feet, nose, and ears, are most often affected and the severity of the injury is enhanced by wet clothing, air movement (chill factor), peripheral vascular disease, and decreased level of consciousness. When less insulated parts of the body are exposed to below freezing temperatures for prolonged periods of time, freezing begins distally at a relatively slow pace. Rarer and more devastating injuries follow contact with liquid petroleum products and metal surfaces at subfreezing temperature: subsequent tissue freezing is rapid, is often extensive, and can involve any part of the body.

PATHOGENESIS. Tissue necrosis following frostbite is related primarily to the mechanical effects of ice crystals, loss of cellular water, and microvascular thrombosis (Table 9). With loss of heat, water freezes and forms crystals which can appear both within the cells and the extracellular space in any tissue. Rapid lowering of tissue temperature causes supercooling, with tissue temperature reaching −10° to −15° C. before freezing occurs, and the formation of intracellular ice crystals, which irreversibly disrupt cellular architecture and cause cell death.[51] Because of circulatory reflexes in response to cold, freezing usually is much slower, and ice crystals form primarily in the extracellular space with comparatively less structural damage to the cell. As freezing progresses, intracellular water shifts to the extracellular space and causes intracellular dehydration, with an increase in the intracellular concentrations of electrolytes, proteins, sugars, and enzymes. The resulting hyperosmolarity causes intracellular protein denaturation. While skin is relatively resistant to these damaging effects, other tissues, including nerves and blood vessels, are quite sensitive.

TABLE 9. Pathogenesis of Frostbite

Freezing
    Intracellular ice crystallization
    Cellular dehydration
    Microvascular occlusion
Thawing
    Extracellular loss of high-protein fluid
    Vasospasm only in narrow border of frozen tissue
    Surrounding vasodilatation

At subzero environmental temperatures, exposed tissue temperature begins to decrease. Sensation in cooling skin is reduced and is finally abolished when tissue temperatures reach 10° C. During this phase, cutaneous vasculature exhibits vasoconstriction. If tissue temperatures stabilize at this level, the microcirculation displays alternating periods of vasoconstriction and vasodilation (hunting reaction, see below). However, with a further loss of heat, microvascular flow ceases and tissue temperature falls to below freezing.

The vascular system is particularly susceptible to freeze injury and appears to be the primary target organ of frostbite.[80] Although cooling increases viscosity and causes sludging of blood before tissue freezing, only after thawing do the detrimental vascular changes induced by freezing become evident. Endothelium is particularly vulnerable to cold injury, and microvascular permeability increases, with loss of plasma and hemoconcentration. Within minutes of thawing and restoration of blood flow, platelet aggregates form and begin to occlude venules.[99] Subsequently, red cells begin to aggregate and contribute to venular occlusion, which within 1 to 2 hours begins retrograde extension into capillary and arteriolar vascular beds of the damaged tissue. The net effect is decreased capillary flow in the thawed tissue. During this interval, arteriovenous shunts open; and while total blood flow to an injured body part characteristically rises above normal levels, flow in the damaged tissue remains compromised. If injury to the tissue is severe, arteriovenous shunt flow begins to fall after 24 to 48 hours and eventually ceases. This cessation of flow is followed by occlusion of major arteries and finally gangrene.

After thawing, high-protein, plasma-like fluid leaks from the injured capillary bed into the interstitial space in a manner similar to that in burn injury. Tissue pressure increases to some degree, promoting venular stasis and occlusion. Swelling is maximal in 2 to 6 hours and thereafter slowly subsides. Although the vessels in the thawed tissue retain the ability to constrict in response to adrenergic stimulation, the majority of vessels are dilated. Except in the narrow border zone surrounding the previously frozen tissue, persistent vasospasm of the nutritional vasculature is absent,[99] which explains in part the ineffectiveness of therapeutic modalities designed to alleviate vasoconstriction. Blood viscosity changes following thawing are short-lived and relatively unimportant, and the use of antiviscosity agents would be expected to provide little benefit to microcirculatory blood flow.

Because of circulatory alterations that sacrifice core heat to keep peripheral structures warm, tissue freezing usually is a slow process. Maximal vasoconstriction occurs with tissue temperatures of approximately 15° C. As cooling falls below 10° C., peripheral tissues alternately vasoconstrict and then vasodilate, often in a cyclic manner. This cold vasodilatation response, or "hunting reaction," prevents or retards tissue freezing at the expense of body heat loss. If the individual is warm and well insulated, cold vasodilatation is pronounced and exposed body parts are partially protected from the effects of low ambient temperatures. If the individual is cold and inadequately clothed or if he is rapidly cooled, cold vasodilatation does not occur, and tissues can freeze rapidly. Constricting clothing, peripheral vascular disease, and open wounds prevent these circulatory adaptations and increase the likelihood of tissue freezing.

Rapid freezing promotes supercooling and intracellular ice crystallization, both of which augment tissue destruction and blunt protective circulatory adjustments. Prolonged freezing increases both the depth and the extent of damage; by accentuating intracellular dehydration, very low temperatures are more injurious than higher subzero temperatures. Wet skin cools faster than dry skin and freezes at a higher ambient temperature. Air movement accelerates heat loss, and wind velocity determines what is termed the wind chill factor. Thus, the chilling effect of a temperature of −6° C. (20° F.) when the wind velocity is 45 miles per hour is equivalent to that of a temperature of −40° C. (−40° F.) when winds are calm. However, wind velocity does not determine the final tissue temperature, which cannot fall below the ambient temperature. In order for freezing to occur, the ambient temperature must fall below −2° to −3° C. Nevertheless, increasing wind chill promotes nonfreezing cold injury and is a major contributing factor to body heat loss.

EPIDEMIOLOGY OF FROSTBITE. In an excellent epidemiologic study, Urschel evaluated a large series of patients with severe frostbite.[89] Most patients were males who were poorly clothed during the winter months. Fewer than 20 per cent displayed a normal mental status, and acute alcoholism and psychiatric illness were major predisposing factors. The arms and legs were involved with equal frequency. A past history of frostbite predisposed the patients to reinjury of the previously frostbitten body parts, and such areas more frequently required surgical ablation. The local environment and social conditions influence the presentation of severe frostbite. Occupational or recreational exposure often causes injury in frigid climates, and the increasingly large homeless population of urban centers is subject to an escalating incidence of frostbite in more temperate environments.

CLINICAL PRESENTATION. The depth of frostbite is classified into four levels of severity based on appearance after thawing. *First-degree frostbite* causes hyperemia, edema, and often very superficial freezing of the epidermis (frost nip). Necrosis is minimal and vesicles do not form. *Second-degree frostbite* causes hyperemia, edema, and usually vesicle formation, resulting in a partial-thickness injury (Fig. 14). As in partial-thickness burns, cutaneous sensation remains intact. *Third-degree frostbite* causes necrosis of the entire skin thickness and extends to a variable depth into the underlying subcutaneous tissue. Vesicles formed with this severity of injury tend to be much smaller than those with second-degree injury. *Fourth-degree frostbite* causes full-thickness necrosis of the skin and extends into underlying muscle and bone. Such injuries commonly terminate with gangrene of the body part and require amputation.

Frozen tissue usually is cold to the touch and appears pale, gray, and bloodless. If frostbite is superficial, soft and pliable tissue can be palpated beneath the stiff frozen skin. The deeply frozen body part is stony hard. Although prediction of tissue loss is usually not possible for weeks following frostbite injury, the appearance of the tissue after thawing denotes the severity of tissue damage (Table 10). In *mild injuries*, capillary flow in the previously frozen tissue rapidly returns toward normal, and total flow to the body part increases to supranormal levels as arteriovenous shunts open. The involved part, usually a hand or foot, becomes bright red and warm, and capillary pulsations may be visibly associated with throbbing pain. Paresthesias appear, and sensation and motor function return. Although swelling and edema rapidly develop a few hours after thawing, the underlying tissue does not become as tense as it does in a circumferential full-thickness burn. Large vesicles appear within a few hours, are filled with straw-colored fluid, and extend to the tips of affected extremities. Most of these changes resolve in 1 to 2 weeks with little or no tissue loss. The blisters may form a black eschar, which eventually sloughs; the underlying regenerated skin is initially fragile and hypersensitive but later develops the characteristics of normal skin. After thawing of *severely frostbitten tissue*, blood flow remains depressed; although total flow to the injured part may transiently approach normal values, nutritional capillary flow is never restored. Because the majority of blood flow occurs through deep arteriovenous shunts, the injured area is cool to the touch and deep red to purple in appearance. Although sensation and distal muscle function are absent, the patient may still be able to move distal parts because the tendons and proximal muscles remain intact. Blisters are small, dark, and hemorrhagic and may require weeks to form, if they occur at all. Except for very deep injury

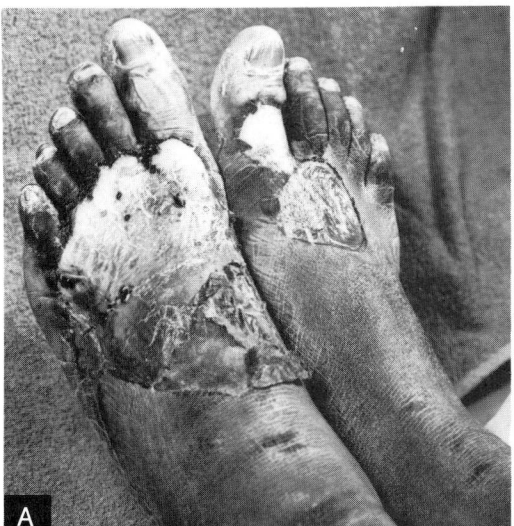 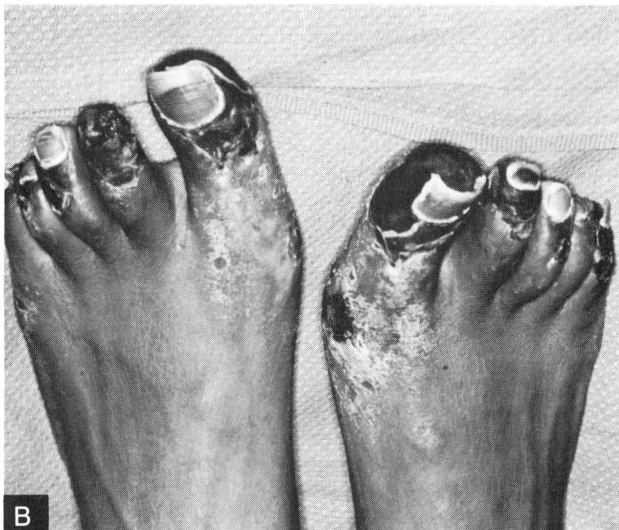

Figure 14. Frostbite of the feet. *A*, Thirteen days after injury. Bullae have desiccated and formed a crustlike eschar on each foot. *B*, Seventy days after injury. Clear demarcation of necrotic tissue is now established. The distal phalanges of the toes were eventually amputated. Note that the final extent of tissue loss is considerably less than would have been estimated during the first weeks after injury. Unnecessary débridement was avoided and tissue loss was minimized by meticulous wound care that prevented maceration and infection.

with primary arterial occlusion, edema formation is slow but extensive and may persist for months. Eventually, the nonviable skin and deep structures demarcate and mummify.

Most cases of frostbite are between the two extremes described, and an involved extremity may display all degrees of freezing injury. Determination of tissue viability is all but impossible during the first several weeks following injury and often can be made only after the gangrenous tissue has demarcated and sloughed. Superimposed infection can amplify tissue loss. Since clinical signs and symptoms provide inaccurate guidelines for the estimation of potential tissue loss following frostbite, a number of laboratory procedures have been used to define nonviable tissue. Radionuclide scanning with technetium 99m methylene diphosphonate accurately identifies nonviable bone, and Doppler ultrasonography and pulse-volume plethysmography appear to distinguish mild from severe frostbite soon after thawing. Angiographic techniques have been used primarily to evaluate chronic vascular abnormalities of freeze-injured tissue. These modalities may prove useful in evaluating the effectiveness of therapeutic interventions to increase tissue salvage following rewarming.

A rare form of cold injury may be encountered when liquid propane, butane, and other extremely low temperature liquids spill onto the skin. These cold injuries occur predominantly as an occupational accident in petroleum industry workers. Immediately after exposure, the cutaneous injury appears to be similar to a relatively benign second-degree burn, displaying a pink

color with no obvious evidence of deep tissue necrosis. However, as this form of cold injury matures over the next 48 to 72 hours, the wound assumes the appearance of an eschar typical of a deep full-thickness burn. The clinical course also resembles that of a deep thermal injury, with early large fluid resuscitation requirements. Wound care consists of topical antimicrobial agents and excision and grafting.

TREATMENT. Treatment of frostbite should begin as soon as feasible to decrease the duration of tissue freezing. All wet and constricting clothing, including socks, boots, and gloves, should be removed. Because frostbitten patients often are hypothermic to some degree, they should be wrapped in warm blankets and given hot fluids. Alcohol promotes further heat loss by causing vasodilatation and should not be used.

Rapid rewarming of the frozen part is the single most effective therapeutic maneuver for preserving potentially viable tissue. However, a frozen body part should not be thawed if refreezing of the injured extremity is possible. If it can be arranged expeditiously, transport to a medical facility is preferable before instituting rewarming procedures. The frozen part is placed in water at 40° C., which is circulated to prevent the formation of temperature gradients. When the tissue is completely thawed, as reflected by the return of pink color and obvious perfusion, it should be removed from the heated water. Rewarming usually requires 20 to 30 minutes, and prolonged heating and the use of water temperatures above 42° C. decrease tissue salvage. Warmed water provides a well-regulated constant level of heat by virtue of its high heat capacity and thermal conductivity. Rapid rewarming causes a rapid increase in the tissue temperature, prevents the long persistence of tissue temperature at a level just below freezing that occurs with euthermic conversion of ice to water, and promotes vasodilatation and a rapid return of tissue perfusion. Slow rewarming is not as effective in maintaining tissue viability and causes more extensive microvascular damage than that occurring with rapid rewarming. The use of dry heat, such as from a fire, is dangerous and not nearly as effective for rapidly thawing frozen tissue. The injured part lacks sufficient sensation for temperature to be judged, and a serious burn injury can occur. The frozen part should not be rewarmed in ice water, rubbed with ice, or massaged. Such procedures invariably extend tissue damage. Refreezing thawed tissue further augments tissue loss; and if permanent thawing and subsequent treatment are not feasible, the frozen limb is best left alone until proper facilities and treatment are

TABLE 10. Signs and Symptoms of Frostbite

Mild injury
  Bright red and warm
  Painful
  Paresthesias
  Rapid onset of edema
  Large vesicles (early)
  Superficial eschar (later)
Deep injuries
  Deep purple and cool
  Minimal pain
  Small hemorrhagic vesicles
  Slow onset of edema
  Deep structures demarcate and mummify

available. Prior to definitive treatment, less injury ensues from walking on a frozen foot than on one that has been thawed; local destruction of tissue and refreezing invariably occur. The pain during and after rewarming is relieved by narcotics.

Local care is directed toward preserving damaged tissue and preventing infection. Unless infected or leaking, vesicles should be left intact and allowed to dry into a black eschar. The patient is placed at bed rest and the wounds exposed to the air. Mechanical trauma by overlying bed sheets is prevented by a foot cradle, and lamb's wool is inserted between affected digits. Weight bearing on injured lower extremities is proscribed until complete healing has occurred. The wound is gently cleansed daily with an antibacterial solution in a whirlpool bath. The use of pressure dressings to decrease wound edema may cause extensive tissue destruction and is contraindicated. Smoking is not permitted.

Because assessment of tissue viability is difficult and often inaccurate, surgical intervention must be delayed until clear demarcation of dead tissue has occurred. Early débridement increases tissue damage and removes the protective covering of mummified tissue. Although "watchful waiting" for demarcation may require months, tissue loss is often much less than initial estimates (see Fig. 14). However, supervening infection with wet gangrene requires immediate surgical removal of the source of sepsis. The role of escharotomy and fasciotomy in the acute treatment of a previously frozen extremity is controversial, and these procedures probably should not be utilized in most situations. Since freezing directly damages blood vessels, the loss of circulation following thawing is more likely to be caused by primary vascular occlusion than by constriction of edematous tissues. Available studies document no benefit and suggest that such decompression procedures may increase tissue loss.

Tetanus prophylaxis is based on the patient's prior immunization status and the condition of the wound. Antibiotics are indicated when infection is evident or when an open wound was present before freezing.[11] In the rare situation in which a large volume of tissue has been frozen, massive fluid loss into the injured tissues after thawing may require intravenous fluid resuscitation.

A number of controversial treatments have been employed in an attempt to promote survival of marginally viable tissue following thawing. Sympathectomy by nerve trunk section and more recently by intra-arterial injection of vasodilators has enjoyed considerable popularity on the basis of the assumptions that resistant vasospasm in recently frozen tissue promotes ischemic tissue loss and that therapeutic sympathetic blockade induces vasodilatation and increased nutritional blood flow. However, histologic studies indicate that the vasculature in the freeze-injured wound is dilated, not constricted, and that inadequate perfusion is a consequence of endothelial injury and intravascular cellular platelet aggregation.[99] Vessels in the narrow border zone surrounding the injured tissue may initially be constricted but soon dilate as total blood flow increases. Sympathectomy may accentuate the damage of the freeze injury by diverting nutritional blood flow from the wound into arteriovenous channels. No rigorous studies to date have documented that the use of sympathetic blockade is better than rapid rewarming alone in promoting survival of recently thawed tissue. Although experimental studies have described beneficial tissue preservation effects from the use of heparin and low-molecular-weight dextran, especially if administered before the onset of freezing, no clinical studies have demonstrated clear evidence of increased tissue salvage. Although rarely practical, low-molecular-weight dextran may be beneficial if administered before thawing. The efficacy of dimethyl sulfoxide, anti-inflammatory agents, and hyperbaric oxygen is unproved. Perhaps the most promising pharmacologic agents for treating frostbite are the antiprostanoid and antithromboxane agents.[39]

These drugs block the arachidonic acid cascade and appear in human studies to inhibit vasospasm and platelet aggregation responsible for the progressive ischemia in frostbite. In animal studies, intravenous administration of streptokinase, by reversing early thrombosis of damaged vessels, significantly reduced tissue loss after rewarming.

In contrast to acute frostbite, the use of sympathetic blockade is quite effective for the treatment of chronic postfrostbite sequelae. The most frequent complaints are hyperhidrosis, paresthesias, cool extremities, cold sensitivity, and edema, which are exacerbated by exposure to cold. These vasospastic sequelae must be differentiated from neuropathic sequelae, especially the intense constant burning pain of postfrostbite neuritis, which is unresponsive to and may be aggravated by sympathetic blockade. Angiography is useful for demonstrating vasospasm, which, if present, can be treated by the intra-arterial injection of reserpine, 0.25 to 0.5 mg., into the brachial, femoral, or radial artery. A beneficial response is reflected by hyperemia and increased warmth in the distal extremity. Injection into the arterial inflow of an injured extremity allows the use of a small dose and minimizes systemic effects. Reserpine produces vasodilatation by causing vascular depletion of norepinephrine and provides prolonged relief from vasospastic symptoms. If these chronic symptoms recur after several injections of reserpine, surgical division of the regional sympathetic trunks provides long-term relief. Other postfrostbite sequelae, such as depigmentation and bone changes, are permanent. A rare long-term complication of deep frostbite injuries is squamous cell carcinoma in the frostbite scar. Clinical presentation, treatment, and prognosis are similar to those of Marjolin's ulcer in chronic burn scars. Wide local excision should be performed after biopsy and histologic confirmation of squamous cell carcinoma.

Nonfreezing Cold Injury

Exposure to low environmental temperatures more commonly causes nonfreezing tissue injury than frostbite in both civilian and military settings. Tissue loss is usually not extensive and is due to microvascular injury with endothelial damage, capillary stasis, and eventual vascular occlusion. Trench foot and immersion foot occur after prolonged exposure to a wet and cold environment with ambient temperatures above freezing, and both conditions affect lower extremities that have been continuously immobile and dependent. Trench foot develops after 1 to several days' exposure to dampness at or near freezing. Immersion foot develops more slowly, after a few days to several weeks of immersion in cool or cold water at temperatures usually higher than those causing trench foot. The entire foot may turn black from superficial gangrene, but deep tissue destruction is unusual. Following rewarming, the injured limb is initially anesthetic and anhidrotic, and massive edema rapidly develops. Blood flow increases to above normal levels, and this hyperemia may persist for weeks. Paresthesias are common, and in deeper injuries ulceration, vesiculation, and occasionally gangrene may develop. Long-term sequelae are similar to those following frostbite and include paresthesias, cold sensitivity, muscle weakness, and pain on weight bearing. If persistent vasospasm is demonstrated, sympathetic blockade usually provides effective relief.

Pernio, or chilblain, is a less severe injury and develops after prolonged exposure to dry cold above freezing. It is more commonly observed in women and participants in certain winter sports, such as mountain climbers. Small superficial ulcers develop on chronically exposed body surfaces, especially the legs, and may be accompanied by hemorrhages, bullae, and areas of localized cyanosis.

Treatment of all three variations of nonfreezing cold injury is supportive and consists of rapid rewarming and meticulous local care, as described previously for frostbite. Shoes and wet clothing should be removed from the injured extremity. The local injuries should be protected from further trauma by soft dressings, and injured extremities should be elevated. Some patients develop acrocyanosis and persistently painful nodules in exposed areas, and these symptoms may respond to the calcium channel blocker nifedipine.[26]

Other nonfreezing cold injuries occasionally may be encountered. Extensor tenosynovitis may follow prolonged exposure of the hands to cold. Erythema, edema, and crepitation are present under the undamaged skin of the dorsum of the hand, and movement of the fingers produces pain along the extensor tendons. Treatment consists of warming and splinting the hand. If the pain and swelling do not resolve within 48 hours, aspirin and, if required, intrasynovial injection of corticosteroid produce prompt relief of symptoms.

Hypothermia

Because of a variety of social phenomena, total body hypothermia following prolonged exposure to low environmental temperatures is being encountered with increasing frequency. When the onset of hypothermia is rapid, as by immersion in near-freezing water, the signs and symptoms are obvious and should elicit prompt treatment. When the fall in body temperature occurs more slowly in environmental conditions that are temperate or only moderately cool, the more obvious clinical manifestations of hypothermia are often absent and the diagnosis is often overlooked. Unsuspected hypothermia particularly affects the elderly, whose ability to increase heat production and to decrease heat loss by vasoconstriction in response to cold is impaired.

The diagnostic hallmark of generalized hypothermia is a core temperature (clinically approximated by rectal temperature) below 34° C. Because standard clinical thermometers do not register below that level, special thermometers are required. An altered level of consciousness is the most constant symptom of hypothermia and ranges from confusion, poor judgment, and mood changes to severe agitation and coma. More than 90 per cent of patients with rectal temperatures at or below 32° C. demonstrate these mental aberrations. Hypothermic patients often do not shiver, especially if heat loss has occurred slowly. In addition to having low body temperature, the patient appears gray and cyanotic and is cool to the touch. Blood pressure, pulse rate, and respiratory rate are frequently decreased; a Doppler ultrasonic flowmeter is most useful in assessing the adequacy of circulation. However, vital signs correlate poorly with body temperature and ultimate recovery, and the absence of respiratory or cardiac activity early after exposure does not preclude recovery.

Prompt initiation of rewarming is the most important therapeutic intervention, and the patient's temperature and vital signs should be monitored during this process. All wet clothing is removed; and the patient, if alert, is given warm fluids to drink. Alcohol causes peripheral vasodilatation, depresses shivering, promotes additional heat loss, and therefore is never used. The choice of rewarming technique depends on the patient's response to low body temperature and to the initial attempts at rewarming. Patients with mild hypothermia (32° to 35° C.) can be passively rewarmed by wrapping in warm clothes and blankets, drinking hot fluids, and allowing shivering to generate body heat. For moderately severe hypothermia (28° to 32° C.), passive rewarming is effective if shivering is present. Because the level of consciousness is usually depressed in such patients, warm fluids are administered intravenously. Active rewarming is necessary when passive rewarming fails to elevate body temperature faster than 1° to 2° C. per hour, when the initial body temperature is below 28° C., and when cardiac activity has ceased before or during rewarming treatment.

Active rewarming is most easily accomplished by placing the patient in a circulating water bath warmed to 40° C. This method of surface warming allows rapid gain of body heat, decreases shivering, with its obligatory metabolic demands, and improves venous return and cardiac output by hydrostatic pressure, which may be beneficial to the hypovolemic patient. A heating blanket, although less efficient in heat transfer, may be used if a water bath is not available. The theoretic objection to surface rewarming is that external heat relieves peripheral vasoconstriction, thus accentuating hypovolemia and allowing cold blood and tissue metabolites to flow to the heart, which may cause subsequent ventricular fibrillation. However, this vasodilatory response may be mitigated by heat-induced cutaneous vasoconstriction and reflex opening of proximal arteriovenous anastomoses.[62] This effect is mediated by postganglionic sympathetic fibers in the glabrous tissue. Core heating with cardiopulmonary bypass, peritoneal dialysis, or mediastinal lavage has been advocated for active rewarming because it directly warms the heart and avoids rewarming collapse; it may be indicated in the patient with cardiac arrest who does not respond to cardioversion. Cardiopulmonary bypass, if available, appears to be the most logical method, because it both supports the circulation and allows heating.[50] However, no available data indicate the superiority of core rewarming over surface rewarming, and the complications of such procedures may outweigh any potential advantages.

The patient's vital functions must be appropriately supported during treatment. The hypothermic patient who is asystolic and apneic when brought to the hospital or who suffers cardiac arrest during therapy should be treated with intubation, closed chest massage, and rewarming. These efforts should be continued if necessary until the core temperature is over 30° C. Hypovolemia and electrolyte imbalance, usually hypokalemia, may be particularly severe if hypothermia was slow in onset and usually become evident during rewarming. Warmed balanced electrolyte solutions with supplemental potassium as indicated by laboratory monitoring provide adequate replacement of the depleted plasma volume. Most electrocardiographic abnormalities are supraventricular in origin, require no treatment, and revert to normal as body temperature increases. Occasionally, rhabdomyolysis and pancreatitis develop after rewarming and accentuate fluid requirements.

After the body temperature has been raised above 35° C., clinical assessment of the patient should be completed. Precipitating causes of hypothermia, such as sepsis, uncontrolled diabetes mellitus, pronounced malnutrition, neurologic disease, myxedema, drug overdose, and associated injuries, including frostbite, must be identified and treated. Signs of drug withdrawal may develop during hospitalization. The outcome of severe hypothermia is related to associated medical conditions and not to the method of rewarming. Therefore, the mortality is over 80 per cent in the elderly and only 10 per cent in otherwise healthy young individuals, who typically have no sequelae.

SELECTED REFERENCES

Boswick, J. A., Jr.: The art and science of burn care. Rockville, Md., Aspen Publishers, 1987.
This text, by a group of authors selected on the basis of experience and expertise, provides a current and thorough overview of all aspects of burn care, from the organization of burn centers to rehabilitation and reconstruction.

Demling, R. H., and LaLonde, C.: Burn Trauma. New York, Thieme Medical Publishers, 1989.
This text relates burn care treatment priorities to time after injury. The pathophysiologic basis of the treatment recommendations is detailed.

Goodwin, C. W., and Wilmore, D. W.: Surgery and Burns. In Paige, D. M. (Ed.): Clinical Nutrition, 2nd ed. St. Louis, C. V. Mosby Company, 1988, pp. 372–391.
The metabolic response to injury is described in relation to time of onset and its integration into other aspects of patient treatment. The major role of carbohydrate and nitrogen for nutritional support of the severely hypercatabolic patient is related to the neuroendocrine response to major injury.

Pruitt, B. A., Jr.: The Burn Patient. I. Initial Care. II. Later Care and Complications of Thermal Injury. Curr. Prob. Surg. 16 (4 and 5), April and May 1979.
The first monograph provides a detailed discussion of burn resuscitation and early care, including treatment of electric and chemical injury, inhalation injury, and postresuscitation fluid and electrolyte disturbances (124 references). The second monograph describes burn wound care, including early studies of excisional therapy. Detailed descriptions of postburn metabolic and host resistance changes are provided. The diagnosis and treatment of common postburn complications are discussed (228 references).

Pruitt, B. A., and Mason, A. D.: Lightning and electric shock. *In* Weatherall, D. J., Ledingham, J. G. G., and Warrell, D. A. (Eds.): Oxford Textbook of Medicine, 2nd ed. Oxford, Oxford University Press, 1987, pp. 6.126–6.129.
The clinical effects of electric injury are related to the physical characteristics of electric current and its interaction with tissue. The diagnosis and treatment of local injury as well as anatomically and temporally remote injuries are described.

Pruitt, B. A., Jr., McManus, A. T., and Kim, S. H.: Burns. *In* Gorbach, S. L., Bartlett, J. G., and Blacklow H. R. (Eds.): Infectious Diseases in Medicine and Surgery. Philadelphia, W. B. Saunders Company, in press.
The changing epidemiology and incidence of infections in burn patients are presented. The pathogenesis, diagnosis, and treatment of infections in the burn wound and elsewhere are presented in detail.

Pruitt, B. A., Jr., McManus, W. F., and McDougal, W. S.: Surgical management of burns. *In* Nora, F. P. (Ed.): Operative Surgery: Principles and Techniques. Philadelphia, W. B. Saunders Company, 1990, pp. 1283–1308.
A detailed, well-illustrated presentation of the surgical principles and techniques used in burn care from the time of admission until wound closure.

Pruitt, S. K.: Burns. *In* Lyerly, H. K. (Ed.): The Handbook of Surgical Intensive Care: Practices of the Surgery Residents at the Duke University Medical Center. Chicago, Year Book Medical Publishers, 1989, pp. 487–502.
A concise outline that provides the house officer with complete information on the resuscitation and early care of burn patients.

Shirani, K. Z., Moylan, J. A., Jr., and Pruitt, B. A., Jr.: Diagnosis and treatment of inhalation injury. *In* Loke, J. (Ed.): Pathophysiology and Treatment of Inhalation Injuries. New York, Marcel Dekker, 1988, pp. 239–280.
This chapter thoroughly reviews the pathophysiology, diagnosis, and treatment of inhalation injury (including carbon monoxide poisoning) and its complications.

Waymack, J., and Pruitt, B. A., Jr.: Burn wound care. Adv. Surg., 23:261, 1990.
A detailed description of current techniques of burn wound care, including discussion of topical chemotherapy, the advantages and limitations of burn wound excision, the use of biologic dressings and skin substitutes, and the prevention and treatment of hypertrophic scars.

REFERENCES

1. Alexander, F., Mathieson, M., Teoh, K. H., et al.: Arachidonic acid metabolites mediate early burn edema. J. Trauma, 24:709, 1984.
2. Alexander, J. W.: Alteration of opsonic activity after burn injury. Proceedings of the 40th Anniversary Symposium, U.S. Army Institute of Surgical Research, Fort Sam Houston, Texas, 1989, p. 126.
3. Alexander, J. W., MacMillan, B. G., Stinnett, J. D., et al.: Beneficial effects of aggressive protein feeding in severely burned children. Ann. Surg., 192:505, 1980.
4. Allen, R. C., and Pruitt, B. A., Jr.: Humoral-phagocyte axis of immune defense in burn patients: Chemiluminigenic probing. Arch. Surg., 117:133, 1982.
5. Aulick, L. H., Wilmore, D. W., Mason, A. D., et al.: Influence of the burn wound on peripheral circulation in thermally injured patients. Am. J. Physiol., 233:H520, 1977.
6. Aussel, C., Cynober, L., Lioret, N., et al.: Plasma branched-chain keto acids in burn patients. Am. J. Clin. Nutr., 44:825, 1986.
7. Bowen, B. D., Bert, J. L., Gu, X., et al.: Microvascular exchange during burn injury: III. Implications of the model. Circ. Shock, 28:221, 1989.
8. Bowser-Wallace, B. H., Cone, J. B., and Caldwell, F. T., Jr.: Hypertonic lactated saline resuscitation of severely burned patients over 60 years of age. J. Trauma, 25:22, 1985.
9. Boykin, J. V., Jr., Crute, S. L., and Haynes, B. W., Jr.: Cimetidine therapy for burn shock: A quantitative assessment. J. Trauma, 25:864, 1985.
10. Burleson, D. G., Vaughan, G. M., Mason, A. D., Jr., et al.: Flow cytometric measurement of rat lymphocyte subpopulations after burn injury and burn injury with infection. Arch. Surg., 122:216, 1987.
11. Butson, A. R.: Effects and prevention of frostbite in wound healing. Can. J. Surg., 18:145, 1975.
12. Calvano, S. E., DeRiesthal, H. F., Marano, M. A., et al.: The decrease in peripheral blood CD4+ and T cells following thermal injury in humans can be accounted for by a concomitant decrease in suppressor-inducer CD4+ and T cells as assessed using anti-CD45R. Clin. Immunol. Immunopathol., 47:164, 1988.
13. Cerra, F. B., Mazuski, J. E., Chute, E., et al.: Branched chain metabolic support: A prospective, randomized, double-blind trial in surgical stress. Ann. Surg., 199:286, 1984.
14. Chilbert, M., Maiman, D., Sances, A., Jr., et al.: Measure of tissue resistivity in experimental electrical burns. J. Trauma, 25:209, 1985.
15. Cioffi, W. G., DeMeules, J. E., and Gamelli, R. L.: The effects of burn injury and fluid resuscitation on cardiac function in vitro. J. Trauma, 26:638, 1986.
16. Cioffi, W. G., Graves, T. A., McManus, W. F., et al.: High-frequency percussive ventilation in patients with inhalation injury. J. Trauma, 29:350, 1989.
17. Clark, W. R., Bonaventura, M., and Myers, W.: Smoke inhalation and airway management at a regional burn unit: 1974–1983. Part I. Diagnosis and consequences of smoke inhalation. J. Burn Care Rehabil., 10:52, 1989.
18. Constantian, M. B.: Association of sepsis with an immunosuppressive polypeptide in the serum of burn patients. Ann. Surg., 188:209, 1978.
19. Cotter, R., Taylor, C. A., Johnson, R., et al.: A metabolic comparison of a pure long-chain triglyceride lipid emulsion (LCT) and various medium-chain triglyceride (MCT)-LCT combination emulsions in dogs. Am. J. Clin. Nutr., 45:927, 1987.
20. Damle, N. K., and Doyle, L. V.: IL-2-activated human killer lymphocytes but not their secreted products mediate increase in albumin flux across cultured endothelial monolayers. J. Immunol., 142:2660, 1989.
21. Xu, D. Z., Deitch, E. A., Sittig, K., et al.: In vitro cell-mediated immunity after thermal injury is not impaired: Density gradient purification of mononuclear cells is associated with spurious (artifactual) immunosuppression. Ann. Surg., 208:768, 1988.
22. Deitch, E. A., Landry, K. N., and McDonald, J. C.: Postburn impaired cell-mediated immunity may not be due to lazy lymphocytes but to overwork. Ann. Surg., 201:793, 1985.
23. Demling, R. H., Kramer, G., and Harms, B.: Role of thermal injury-induced hypoproteinemia on fluid flux and protein permeability in burned and non-burned tissue. Surgery, 95:136, 1984.
24. Demling, R. H., and Lalonde, C.: Effect of partial burn excision and closure on postburn oxygen consumption. Surgery, 104:846, 1988.
25. Demling, R. H., Wong, C., Jin, L. J., et al.: Early lung dysfunction after major burns: Role of edema and vasoactive mediators. J. Trauma, 25:959, 1985.
26. Dowd, P. M., Rustin, M. H., and Lanigan, S.: Nifedipine in the treatment of chilblains. Br. Med. J., 293:923, 1986.
27. Ferrara, J. J., Dyess, D. L., Luterman, A., et al.: The suppressive effect of subeschar tissue fluid upon in vitro cell-mediated immunologic function. J. Burn Care Rehabil., 9:584, 1988.
28. Fong, Y., Tracey, K. J., Hesse, D. G., et al.: Influence of enterectomy on peripheral tissue glutamine efflux in critically ill patients. Surgery, 107:321, 1990.
29. Gadd, M. A., Hansbrough, J. F., Hoyt, D. B., et al.: Defective T-cell surface antigen expression after mitogen stimulation: An index of lymphocyte dysfunction after controlled murine injury. Ann. Surg., 209:112, 1989.
30. Goodwin, C. W., Dorethy, J., Lam, V., et al.: Randomized trial of efficacy of crystalloid and colloid resuscitation on hemodynamic response and lung water following thermal injury. Ann. Surg., 197:520, 1983.
31. Gottschlich, M. M., and Alexander, J. W.: Fat kinetics and recommended dietary intake in burns. J. Parenteral Enteral Nutr., 11:80, 1987.
32. Gough, D. B., Moss, N. M., Jordan, A., et al.: Recombinant interleukin-2 (rIL-2) improves immune response and host resistance to septic challenge in thermally injured mice. Surgery, 104:292, 1988.
33. Greco, R. J., Hartford, C. E., Haith, L. R., Jr., et al.: Hydrofluoric acid-induced hypocalcemia. J. Trauma, 28:1593, 1988.
34. Hakim, A. A.: An immunosuppressive factor from serum of thermally traumatized patients. J. Trauma, 17:908, 1977.
35. Hales, C. A., Barkin, P., Jung, W., et al.: Bronchial artery ligation modifies pulmonary edema after exposure to smoke with acrolein. J. Appl. Physiol., 67:1001, 1989.
36. Hammarqvist, F., Wernerman, J., Ali, R., et al.: Addition of glutamine to total parenteral nutrition after elective abdominal surgery spares free glutamine in muscle, counteracts the fall in muscle protein synthesis and improves nitrogen balance. Ann. Surg., 209:455, 1989.
37. Hansbrough, J. F., Boyce, S. T., Cooper, M. L., et al.: Burn wound closure with cultured autologous keratinocytes and fibroblasts attached to a collagen-glycosaminoglycan substrate. J.A.M.A., 262:2125, 1989.
38. Harms, A., Bodai, B. I., Kramer, G. C., et al.: Microvascular fluid and protein flux in pulmonary and systemic circulations after thermal injury. Microvasc. Res., 23:77, 1982.
39. Heggers, J. P., Robson, M. C., Manavalen, K., et al.: Experimental and clinical observations on frostbite. Ann. Emerg. Med., 16:1056, 1987.
40. Heimbach, D., Luterman, A., Burke, J., et al.: Artificial dermis for major burns: A multi-center randomized clinical trial. Ann. Surg., 208:313, 1988.
41. Herndon, D. N., Barrow, R. E., Linares, H. A., et al.: Inhalation injury in burned patients: Effects and treatment. Burns, 14:349, 1988.
42. Horton, J. W., Baxter, C. R., and White, D. J.: Differences in cardiac responses to resuscitation from burn shock. Surg. Gynecol. Obstet., 168:201, 1989.
43. Horton, J. W., White, J., and Baxter, C. R.: The role of oxygen-derived free radicals in burn-induced myocardial contractile depression. J. Burn Care Rehabil., 9:589, 1988.
44. Huang, Y., Li, A., and Yang, Z.: Effect of smoke inhalation injury on thromboxane levels and platelet counts. Burns, 14:440, 1988.
45. Jin, L. J., Lalonde, C., and Demling, R. H.: Lung dysfunction after thermal injury in relation to prostanoid and oxygen radical release. J. Appl. Physiol., 61:103, 1986.
46. Kalaja, E.: Acute excision or exposure treatment? Secondary reconstructions and functional results. Scand. J. Plast. Reconstr. Surg., 18:95, 1984.
47. Katz, A., Ryan, P., Lalonde, C., et al.: Topical ibuprofen decreases thrombox-

ane release from the endotoxin-stimulated burn wound. J. Trauma, 26:157, 1986.

48. Lund, T., and Reed, R. K.: Microvascular fluid exchange following thermal skin injury in the rat: Changes in extravascular colloid osmotic pressure, albumin mass, and water content. Circ. Shock, 20:91, 1986.

49. Lund, T., Wiig, H., and Reed, R. K.: Acute postburn edema: Role of strongly negative interstitial fluid pressure. Am. J. Physiol., 255:H1069, 1988.

50. Maresca, L., and Vasko, J. S.: Treatment of hypothermia by extracorporeal circulation and internal rewarming. J. Trauma, 27:89, 1987.

51. Mazur, P.: Freezing of living cells: Mechanisms and implications. Am. J. Physiol., 247:C125, 1984.

52. McIrvine, A. J., O'Mahony, J. B., Saporoschetz, I., et al.: Depressed immune response in burn patients: Use of monoclonal antibodies and functional assays to define the role of suppressor cells. Ann. Surg., 196:297, 1982.

53. McManus, A. T.: Pseudomonas aeruginosa: A controlled burn pathogen? Antibiot. Chemother., 42:103, 1989.

54. McManus, A. T., Kim, S. H., McManus, W. F., et al.: Comparison of quantitative microbiology and histopathology in divided burn-wound biopsy specimens. Arch. Surg., 122:74, 1987.

55. Melikian, V., Laverson, S., and Zawacki, B.: Oxygen-derived free radical inhibition in the healing of experimental zone-of-stasis burns. J. Trauma, 27:151, 1987.

56. Moore, D. B., Rainey, W. C., Caldwell, F. T., Jr., et al.: The effect of rapid resuscitation upon cardiac index following thermal trauma in a porcine model. J. Trauma, 27:141, 1987.

57. Morganroth, M. L., Till, G. O., Schoeneich, S., et al.: Eicosanoids are involved in the permeability changes but not the pulmonary hypertension after systemic activation of complement. Lab. Invest., 58:316, 1988.

58. Moss, N. M., Gough, D. B., Jordan, A. L., et al.: Temporal correlation of impaired immune response after thermal injury with susceptibility to infection in a murine model. Surgery, 104:882, 1988.

59. Mozingo, D. W., Smith, A. A., McManus, W. F., et al.: Chemical burns. J. Trauma, 28:642, 1988.

60. Mueller, M., Sartorelli, K., DeMeules, J. E., et al.: Effects of fluid resuscitation on cardiac dysfunction following thermal injury. J. Surg. Res., 44:745, 1988.

61. Munster, A. M., Winchurch, R. A., Birmingham, W. J., et al.: Longitudinal assay of lymphocyte responsiveness in patients with major burns. Ann. Surg., 192:772, 1980.

62. Nagasaka, T., Hirata, K., Mano, T., et al.: Heat-induced finger vasoconstriction controlled by skin sympathetic nerve activity. J. Appl. Physiol., 68:71, 1990.

63. Nieman, G. F., Clark, W. R., Jr., Goyette, D., et al.: Wood smoke inhalation increases pulmonary microvascular permeability. Surgery, 105:481, 1989.

64. Nieman, G. F., Clark, W. R., Jr., Wax, S. D., et al.: The effect of smoke inhalation on pulmonary surfactant. Ann. Surg., 191:171, 1980.

65. Novick, M., Gard, D. A., Hardy, S. B., et al.: Burn scar carcinoma: A review and analysis of 46 cases. J. Trauma, 17:809, 1977.

66. Oluwasanmi, J., and Chvapil, M.: A comparative study of four materials in local burn care in a rabbit model. J. Trauma, 16:348, 1976.

67. Ozkan, A. N., Hoyt, D. B., and Ninnemann, J. L.: Generation and activity of suppressor peptides following traumatic injury. J. Burn Care Rehabil., 8:527, 1987.

68. Peterson, M. W.: Neutrophil cathepsin G increases transendothelial albumin flux. J. Lab. Clin. Med., 113:297, 1989.

69. Pitt, R. M., Parker, J. C., Jurkovich, G. J., et al.: Analysis of altered capillary pressure and permeability after thermal injury. J. Surg. Res., 42:693, 1987.

70. Prien, T., Linares, H. A., Traber, L. D., et al.: Lack of hematogenous mediated pulmonary injury with smoke inhalation. J. Burn Care Rehabil., 9:462, 1988.

71. Prien, T., Strohmaier, W., Gasser, H., et al.: Normal phosphatidylcholine composition of lung surfactant 24 hours after inhalation injury. J. Burn Care Rehabil., 10:38, 1989.

72. Pruitt, B. A., Jr.: Discussion of Caldwell, F. T., and Bowser, B. H.: Critical evaluation of hypertonic and hypotonic solutions to resuscitate severely burned children: A prospective study. Ann. Surg., 189:551, 1979.

73. Pruitt, B. A., Jr.: Phycomycotic infections. In Alexander, J. W. (Ed.): Problems in General Surgery. Difficult Surgical Infections (Series). Vol. I, No. 4, 1984, pp. 664–678.

74. Pruitt, B. A., Jr.: The diagnosis and treatment of infection in the burn patient. Burns, 11:79, 1984.

75. Pruitt, B. A., Jr.: The universal trauma model. Bull. Am. Coll. Surg., 70:2, 1985.

76. Pruitt, B. A., Jr., and Goodwin, C. W., Jr.: Stress ulcer disease in the burned patient. World J. Surg., 5:209, 1981.

77. Pruitt, B. A., Jr., and Levine, N. S.: Characteristics and uses of biologic dressings and skin substitutes. Arch. Surg., 119:312, 1984.

78. Pruitt, B. A., Jr., Mason, A. D., Jr., and Goodwin, C. W.: Epidemiology of burn injury and demography of burn care facilities. In Gann, D. S. (Ed.): Problems in General Surgery. Vol. 7. Philadelphia, J. B. Lippincott Company, 1990, pp. 235–251.

79. Pruitt, B. A., Jr., Mason, A. D., Jr., and Moncrief, J. A.: Hemodynamic changes in the early postburn patient: The influence of fluid administration and of a vasodilator (Hydralazine). J. Trauma, 11:36, 1971.

80. Rubinsky, B., Pegg, D. E.: A mathematical model for the freezing process in biological tissue. Proc. Soc. Lond. (Biol.), 234:343, 1988.

81. Sakai, H., Daniels, J. C., Beathard, G. A., et al.: Mixed lymphocyte culture reaction in patients with acute thermal burns. J. Trauma, 14:53, 1974.

82. Schreiber, M. M.: Exposure to sunlight: Effects on the skin. Compr. Ther., 12:38, 1986.

83. Shirani, K. Z., Pruitt, B. A., Jr., and Mason, A. D., Jr.: The influence of inhalation injury and pneumonia on burn mortality. Ann. Surg., 205:82, 1987.

84. Tchervenkov, J. I., Epstein, M. D., Silberstein, E. B., et al.: Early burn wound excision and skin grafting postburn trauma restores in vivo neutrophil delivery to inflammatory lesions. Arch. Surg., 123:1477, 1988.

85. Teodorczyk-Injeyan, J. A., Sparkes, B. G., Mills, G. B., et al.: Impaired expression of interleukin-2 receptor (IL 2R) in the immunosuppressed burn patient: Reversal by exogenous IL 2. J. Trauma, 27:180, 1987.

86. Teodorczyk-Injeyan, J. A., Sparkes, B. G., Mills, G. B., et al.: Increase of serum interleukin 2 receptor level in thermally injured patients. Clin. Immunol. Immunopathol., 51:205, 1989.

87. Till, G. O., Beauchamp, C., Menapace, D., et al.: Oxygen radical dependent lung damage following thermal injury of rat skin. J. Trauma, 23:269, 1983.

88. Till, G. O., Guilds, L. S., Mahrougui, M., et al.: Role of xanthine oxidase in thermal injury of skin. Am. J. Pathol., 135:195, 1989.

89. Urschel, J. D.: Frostbite: Predisposing factors and predictors of poor outcome. J. Trauma, 30:340, 1990.

90. Vaughan, G. M., Becker, R. A., Unger, R. H., et al.: Nonthyroidal control of metabolism after burn injury: Possible role of glucagon. Metabolism, 34:637, 1985.

91. Warden, G. D.: Burn-related humoral immunosuppressants. In Proceedings of the 40th Anniversary Symposium, U.S. Army Institute of Surgical Research, Fort Sam Houston, Texas, 1989, p. 134.

92. Waxman, K., Holness, R., Tominaga, G., et al.: Hemodynamic and oxygen transport effects of pentastarch in burn resuscitation. Ann. Surg., 209:341, 1989.

93. Wilmore, D. W., Goodwin, C. W., Aulick, L. H., et al.: Effect of injury and infection on visceral metabolism and circulation. Ann. Surg., 192:491, 1980.

94. Wilmore, D. W., Long, J. M., Mason, A. D., Jr., et al.: Catecholamines: Mediator of the hypermetabolic response to thermal injury. Ann. Surg., 180:653, 1974.

95. Wood, J. J., Rodrick, M. L., O'Mahony, J. B., et al.: Inadequate interleukin 2 production: A fundamental immunological deficiency in patients with major burns. Ann. Surg., 200:311, 1984.

96. Xiao, G. X., Chopra, R. K., Adler, W. H., et al.: Altered expression of lymphocyte Il-2 receptors in burned patients. J. Trauma, 28:1669, 1988.

97. Yurt, R. W., Mason, A. D., Jr., and Pruitt, B. A., Jr.: Evidence against participation of mast cell histamine in formation of burn wound edema. Surg. Forum, 33:71, 1982.

98. Yurt, R. W., and Pruitt, B. A., Jr.: Decreased wound neutrophils and indiscrete margination in the pathogenesis of wound infections. Surgery, 98:191, 1985.

99. Zacarian, S. A., Stone, D., and Clater, M.: Effects of cryogenic temperatures on microcirculation in the golden hamster cheek pouch. Cryobiology, 7:27, 1970.

12

PRINCIPLES OF OPERATIVE SURGERY

Antisepsis, Technique, Sutures, and Drains

Julio Hochberg, M.D., and Gordon F. Murray, M.D.

> Many surgeons have genius without industry; others have industry without genius; while many who have both are still deficient in judgment.
>
> *John Abernethy*

It is the wisdom of a nineteenth century surgeon that directs this revision of Principles of Operative Surgery toward the next 100 years of technical advances in surgical therapy. Brilliant development of surgical skills and instrumentation have provided a precise understanding of an operative intervention. Today, most surgical procedures are assessed by rigorous scientific methods, and such procedures become reproducible and predictable. Elaborate algorithms are available to calculate the requirement to replace or repair, to lengthen or shorten, ablate or enhance, to drain or not. However, traditional axioms are often contravened. Urgent operations and foreign body insertion are undertaken when one is confronted with acute sepsis; adhesives and staples are substituted for sutures; balloons challenge the bypass, and lasers the scalpel. The essence of the modern surgeon is now, more than ever before, that quality called "judgment"—the ability to know what to use, when to use it and for how long.

ANTISEPSIS AND ASEPSIS

The development of antisepsis in the late nineteenth and early twentieth centuries revolutionized health care.[24] The word *antisepsis* translates from the Greek, "against putrefaction." In present use, *antisepsis* refers to the use of antimicrobial chemicals on human tissue, whereas disinfection applies to the employment of these agents on inanimate objects. Hygienic handwashing, preoperative preparation of the patient's skin, gloving and sterile draping during operative procedures, isolation precautions, autoclaving of instruments, and proper waste disposal are all examples of practices that are standard in modern medical institutions—the aseptic technique. Nevertheless, nosocomial infection continues to be one of the major preventable, iatrogenic complications of hospitalization. Affecting at least 5 per cent of discharged patients, nosocomial infection costs acute care facilities alone more than $4 billion annually.

HISTORICAL ASPECTS. In the latter half of the eighteenth century and early nineteenth century the status of surgery as a specialty was bleak. Serious infections among hospitalized patients were rampant, and the morbidity and mortality were astounding. Nearly all traumatic and surgical wound healing was accompanied by inflammation and suppuration. Primary closure of wounds was infrequently performed, in anticipation of "laudable pus." The concepts of antisepsis arose from separate sources at about the same time in the mid nineteenth century. In America, Oliver Wendell Holmes and, in Vienna, Ignaz Philipp Semmelweiss independently made the observation of high mortality among women hospitalized with puerperal fever. Both observed the death of a fellow physician who had been infected during participation in the autopsy of an infected subject. The experience brought attention to the fact that infection was being transmitted directly, and both urged washing of hands and changing of clothing. These policies caused a reduction in maternal mortality from 11.4 per cent in 1846 to 1.3 per cent in 1848. Subsequently, Pasteur's discovery of bacteria prompted Lister to recognize their implication in development of wound infections. Lister published his first descriptions of the "antiseptic principles" in 1867. Later progress by German physicians enabled Kocher to report a 2.3 per cent infection rate in clean wounds by 1899. This accomplishment remains an enviable standard for modern surgeons.

ASEPTIC PROCEDURES

THE OPERATING ROOM. The operating room (OR) should provide an environment that is as free of bacterial contamination as possible. The minimum size recommended for an OR is usually 20 by 20 feet, which should allow space for gowning of the operative team, draping of the patient, and movement of other personnel without contamination of sterile areas.[19] The concept of separating clean traffic from dirty traffic is theoretically sound but has not been shown to lower wound infection rates. Studies suggest that the redispersal of bacteria from the OR floor into the air is very low. Appropriate ventilation rapidly clears bacteria from the air, and the degree of floor contamination should not contribute to increased infection rates. The very low concentrations of airborne particulate matter and bacteria in most ORs are achieved by changing room air 20 to 25 times each hour and passing the inflow air through a high-efficiency particulate air (HEPA) filter, which efficiently removes bacteria and fungi but not viruses. The pattern of air inflow is designed to decrease turbulence at the operating table and prevent entrainment of air from the periphery. All OR doors should remain closed except as needed for passage of equipment, personnel, and the patient. Also, the pressure in the OR should be positive relative to the outside corridor for preventing particles and bacteria from entering the room. Only infrequently is the OR air implicated as a possible source of infection. Although viable organisms, including staphylococci, streptococci, and bacterial spores, are certainly present in the air of an occupied OR and bacteria are regularly recovered from surgical wounds, organisms recovered from air often are not those that cause wound infection.

The absence of measurable benefit following efforts to diminish environmental sources of infection is probably related to the fact that the primary source of perioperative infection is the *patient,* and the secondary source is the OR *team.*

THE PATIENT. The most important source of contamination in the OR is the patient. Infections that develop from operations classified as clean-contaminated, contaminated, or dirty are primarily caused by bacteria already present in the operative field as a result of disease or the procedure performed.[22] Wound infections that occur in clean operations are often caused by staphylococci or other bacteria from a source in the patient such as the skin or nares. The danger is especially evident in operations in which prosthetic devices are implanted. Preparation of the patient's skin before an incision is one of the most important methods of decreasing infection.[13] It is effective to have the patient shower with an antibacterial preparation the night before elective procedures. Hair removal should be employed only when it is anticipated that hair interferes with performance of the procedure. Shaving the patient with a razor the night before the operation has been associated with a relatively high wound infection rate.[34] The infection risk is decreased by shaving the patient in the OR immediately before the procedure or in the same setting by using a depilatory cream or electric clippers.[9] The most commonly used antimicrobial agents for intact antisepsis are iodophors (Betadine).[13] Iodine is recognized as a broad-spectrum antimicrobial with activity against fungi, viruses, and gram-positive and gram-negative bacteria. Highly complexed iodine compounds are very stable, do not stain, have no odor, and are considerably less irritating to tissues than tincture of iodine. After contact with the skin, such complexes release iodine slowly, causing prolonged activity. The most commonly accepted technique in cleansing the patient's skin is to begin with the area where the incision is to be made and to consider this as the cleanest portion of the area of operation. The contaminated sponge stick should never be returned to the cleansing solution. The skin is cleansed in ever-widening circles, and the surgeon never returns the cleansing sponge to the incision site from the periphery.[34]

Intact skin can withstand very strong disinfecting agents, whereas cells of a fresh surgical wound are very susceptible to further damage.[6] Solutions containing iodophors and hexachlorophene are not safe for use in surgical wounds. Contaminated experimental wounds subjected to a topical treatment with these scrub solutions developed more infections than wounds subjected to 0.9 per cent saline. In heavily contaminated wounds, high pressure irrigation can be of benefit to decrease the number of bacteria and to clean the wound of small particulate matter and soil. High pressure irrigation can be accomplished inexpensively with a 19-gauge needle, a 35-ml. syringe, and a sterile electrolyte solution. The tip of the needle is placed perpendicular and as close as possible to the surface of the wound (Fig. 1).

The patient has another role in the bacterial versus host relationship, and that is the intrinsic resistance to withstand contamination.[29] A complete history and comprehensive physical examination often define the risks of infection with which the patient enters the hospital, and these risks may be independent of the technical ability to prevent infection. Age, obesity, diabetes, cirrhosis, uremia, and connective tissue disorders as well as hereditary or induced immune deficiency states have all been associated with increased infection rates. The general state of nutrition and nutritional effects on cell-mediated immunity are clearly linked to the rate of infection and mortality of patients undergoing surgical procedures. Hunt[17] has emphasized that the remaining strides in reducing the incidence of wound infection probably relate to an increasing knowledge of the complexities of the immune system and to the ability to adjust and enhance them.

THE OR TEAM. The preparation and conduct of the OR team is of paramount importance in the aseptic treatment of the sur-

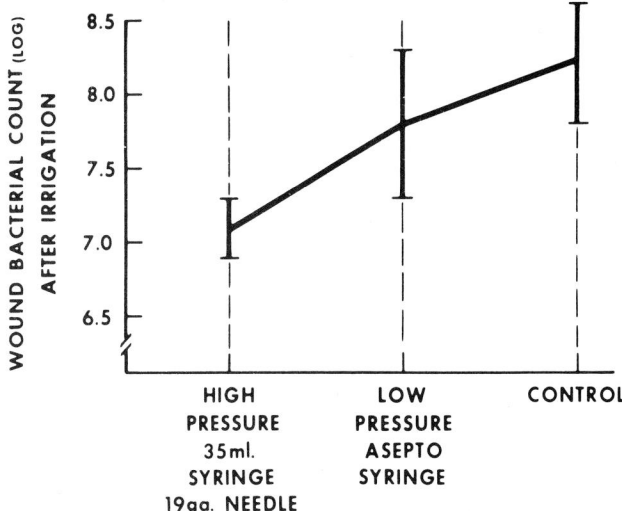

Figure 1. Bacterial removal efficiency of fluids delivered by an Asepto syringe or by a 35 ml. syringe via a 19-gauge needle. (From Stevenson, T. R., Thacker, J. G., Rodeheaver, G. T., Bacchetta, C., Edgerton, M. T., and Edlich, R. F.: Cleansing the traumatic wound by high pressure syringe irrigation. J.A.C.E.P., 5:17, 1976.)

gical patient. Contamination is directly related to the number of people in the room, to activity in the room, and to the amount of conversation. The OR team should scrub their hands and arms to the elbows with an antiseptic solution before each operation. Agents such as iodophors and chlorhexidine combined with a detergent have proved effective, and no significant difference in wound infection rate has been demonstrated between these agents.[9] In addition, no difference in wound infection rate has been noted between scrub times of 3 to 5 minutes and longer times, or between use of a sponge and use of a brush for scrubbing. Sensitization to either the antiseptic or the detergent may develop in some personnel, and continued use may cause dermatitis. In this case, desquamation of inflamed skin with high bacterial counts may increase the risk of contaminating the patient.[42]

During operative procedures, a face mask should cover the mouth and nose comfortably, yet snugly enough to alter the projectile effect introduced by talking and breathing.[35] Up to 40 per cent of surgical personnel carry *Staphylococcus aureus* in their nasal and oral cavities, and escaped droplets could, in theory, transfer bacteria to the patient. It is of interest that recent studies have questioned the utility of wearing a mask at all. A prospective randomized study from Sweden[48] found no difference in wound infection rates when masks were eliminated (except for personnel with respiratory infection). The overall infection was 4.8 per cent with masks and 3.6 per cent without masks. No similar published studies have evaluated the efficacy of wearing gloves. It should be appreciated that gloves perform a dual function: They protect the patient from the hands of the surgeon and protect the surgeon from potentially contaminated blood. A major current concern to the surgical team members is the acquired immunodeficiency syndrome (AIDS), which can be transmitted in ways similar to those in which hepatitis B can be transmitted.[50]

A sterile gown contains the skin flakes constantly shed by each member of the surgical team and thereby functions as a barrier preventing the transmission of bacteria to the patient. The most important aspect of gown material is impermeability to moisture, because the wicklike effect of a wet gown transmits bacteria from one side of the material to the other. Studies of bacterial penetration of gown materials have shown that contamination is highest with cloth, less with paper, and least with plastic. Use of disposable gowns has been associated with a significant decrease in the number of wound infections. Although shoe covers do not influence the risk of wound infection, they may protect the shoes from spills and soilage.

The primary function of the sterile drapes is to define and preserve the sterile field during operative procedures. Drapes, as well as gowns, used in the OR should be made of reusable or disposable fabrics that have been shown to be nearly impermeable to bacteria, even when wet.[4] In the draping process, the material should be held above waist level, in a compact position, draping from the operative site to the periphery. When placing drapes, the gloved hand should be protected by cuffing draping material over the hands. Once placed in position, sterile drapes should not be moved or lifted. The sterile field should be constantly monitored and maintained. Every team member should observe for events that may compromise the sterile field and initiate corrective action. All personnel moving within or around a sterile field should do so in a manner to maintain its integrity. Scrubbed surgical team members may move from sterile area to sterile area. If they must change positions, they should turn back to back or face to face while maintaining a safe distance between each other. All cables, lines, and tubing for equipment should be secured onto the sterile field with a nonperforating clamp. Nonsterile equipment brought onto the field should be draped in a sterile envelope.

Instruments and equipment to be used at the operating table can be sterilized by steam heat, chemical solutions, dry heat, or gas methods. The method chosen is usually dependent on the characteristics of the material being sterilized. Autoclaves are often used in the operating suite to sterilize instruments that have become contaminated and are needed again quickly. Chemical sterilization is an appropriate technique for disinfecting equipment that is not suitable for exposure to steam heat but can tolerate moisture. Two per cent aqueous solutions of glutaraldehyde is often used for disinfection of urologic equipment, such as catheters, and can be used with almost any form of rubber or plastic. Items that can tolerate heat but not moisture or that are not penetrated well by steam can be sterilized with dry heat. Gas methods are critical for sterilization of delicate instruments that might corrode and plastic or other nonmetal items that may melt. Gas sterilization combined with nonporous wrappers also provides the advantage of significantly longer shelf life for some instruments.

As soon as the sterile surgical pack is opened, the instruments should be arranged in a predetermined, standard configuration. Instruments should be passed deliberately so they arrive securely in the surgeon's hand in a functional position. When the maneuver is finished, the assistant should return the instrument to its proper place on the stand for future use. Instruments left on the drapes surrounding the operative site are difficult to locate or may be dropped to the floor.

SURGICAL TECHNIQUE

Surgeons must be very careful when they take the knife!
Underneath their fine incisions stirs the culprit life!

The poignant poetry of Emily Dickinson eloquently emphasizes the primacy of the surgical operative event. Whereas the surgeon must exhibit a capacity for compassionate interest and concern in all that illness implies to the patient and his family, he must also devise an objective pattern for decision making in the most impersonal aspect of the operative procedure. The discipline is properly named. *Surgery* is derived from its earlier name *chirurgery*, which means "hand work." Halstedian teaching emphasized gentle handling of the tissues, careful hemostasis, and appropriate irrigation of the wounds to enhance healing and prevent infection. These principles remain valid today.

INCISIONS. The principles of selecting an incision are simple and include assurance of adequate exposure and good healing with an acceptable scar.[12] An incision should be properly planned as to shape, direction, and size. In general, incisions are made along the normal skin lines. In reoperations, every attempt should be made to use the original incision. Countertraction, if properly applied, allows the surgeon to make a clean, precise scalpel incision. Skin incisions should be made with the stainless steel surgical scalpel, and care should be taken to ensure that the cutting edge does not drag or crush as it cuts. Often incisions are made with the No. 15 blade on a flat surface. Cutting with the tip of a blade makes it more difficult to control the depth of the incision. Incision of the skin should be perpendicular to the epidermal surface. If the wound is made at an oblique angle, it may cause a "trapdoor" appearance. An incision should be beveled only to preserve the integrity of hair follicles. Present studies indicate that the old surgical practice of discarding the skin knife before making the deep incision can be abandoned without increasing the risk of infection.[18]

ATRAUMATIC HANDLING. Skin margins should be handled gently to minimize necrosis that may promote infection or delay healing.[37] Adson tooth forceps are the preferred forceps for this purpose. Skin hooks are the least traumatizing instruments with which to hold or pull back skin borders. The two-pronged hook is especially useful in fixing the skin for placement of a suture, because the needle may be passed between the two prongs.

DISSECTION. The least amount of trauma is accomplished in dissecting natural tissue planes. The surgeon's index finger will readily dissect many lightly adherent normal tissue planes leading to a more bloodless division of the structures. Sometimes the tissue density and adherence require the use of a dampened gauze sponge or gauze instrument (Küttner pledget). Blunt-tipped scissors are excellent for opening tissue planes that are too dense for finger or sponge dissection. A sharp knife is needed for dissection whenever tissue is heavily scarred or very dense. Countertraction is one of the most important features of dextrous and smooth surgical dissection.[37] If the edge of the scalpel is held stationary and gently pressed downward without stroking, it easily separates any encountered collagen fibers that are under tension.

DÉBRIDEMENT. Débridement is the most important single factor in the management of the contaminated wound.[46] Débridement removes tissue heavily contaminated by bacteria or foreign bodies and protects the patient from the threat of invasive infection. In heavily contaminated wounds, high-pressure irrigation can be of benefit to decrease the number of and to clean the wound of small particulate matter and soil. Determination of the exact limits of devitalized tissue in wounds may be difficult. Color is of doubtful value in determining the viability of muscle; muscle is viable if it contracts after being stimulated. The viability of skin is usually easier to judge than that of muscle. Tissues such as dura, fascia, and tendon may survive without living cells if immediately covered by healthy vascularized flaps. In general, they should be left in the wound.

HEMOSTASIS. The objectives of hemostasis are to minimize blood loss during and after operation and to prevent hematoma.[33] Hematomas constitute a nidus for infection and prevent fibroblast migration and capillary formation. It is also imperative to maintain a clear, bloodless field during incision and dissection. A rhythm can be established whereby the assistant alternately blots the field and the surgeon dissects. If digital pressure is maintained for 15 to 20 seconds, small clots usually form in the ends of smaller vessels that have been divided, and no further bleeding occurs. Compression can be accomplished by instrument, sponge or stick-sponge packing, or bidigital pressure on the vessel (pinch method).[12] Definitive hemostasis of larger vessels is obtained by ligatures, suture ligatures, or metal clips. It must be appreciated that unnecessary ligatures may cause excessive devitalization of living tissue with resultant poor healing or infection. Carefully selected alternatives for hemostasis include vasoconstricting drugs, clotting agents, systemic hypotension, intra-arterial embolism, and intravascular balloon tamponade. The surgeon should never resort to hot (150° F. or 55° C.) wet sponges for hemostasis. This treatment causes hyperthermic injury to tissue that potentiates the development of infection.

WOUND CLOSURE. The relationship between the number of viable bacteria in an open wound and the ability to successfully close that wound has been clearly demonstrated.[9] Wounds containing less than 10^5 bacterial organisms per gram of tissue nearly always heal primarily following closure, unless specific factors that impair host resistance are present. These quantitative wound relationships have been defined for almost all organisms but do not apply to the more virulent beta-hemolytic streptococci. A wound containing greater than 10^5 bacterial organisms per gram of tissue cannot be reliably closed, because the incidence of wound infection that follows is 50 to 100 per cent. When the wound is contaminated by exceedingly large numbers of organisms (greater than 10^9), primary closure of the wound should be avoided. This circumstance is encountered when the wound surface is contacted by feces. Delayed primary closure should be considered only on or after the fourth day after wounding, at which time the wound has gained considerable resistance to infection. One effective method for delayed wound closure uses initial temporary skin grafting to provide a closed, sterile wound for subsequent definitive flap reconstruction. When wounds involve vital structures that may be destroyed by exposure, however, flaps must be transposed immediately.[46] Only well-vascularized flaps, such as muscle and myocutaneous flaps, are chosen. In wounds following irradiation-induced ischemic ulceration, closure can be accomplished only with pedicled flaps that bring in a new blood supply. Dead space in wounds allows fluid collections to form and should be avoided. The collapse of such spaces should be achieved by physiologic methods such as relaxing incisions, rotation of flaps, and splinting. The closure of dead space by sutures produces localized areas of wound ischemia and necrosis, and the presence of additional suture material potentiates the development of infection.[13]

SUTURING. Simple interrupted sutures are the most useful finishing stitches. They coat the wound edges and correct any intervening gaps in the suture line or discrepancies in height between the two sides. The skin stitches are made to extend as little as possible from the wound edges. The passage of the needle should include deep dermis that is further removed from the cut margin of the skin.[17] The result is a slight elevation of the skin edges that is beneficial to postoperative healing (Fig. 2). Closely placed, fine stitches create a stronger suture line than widely spaced heavy sutures. Subcuticular sutures are an excellent choice when good cosmetic results are desired. They lower the tension on the skin margins and allow earlier removal to avoid hatchmarking. Subcuticular sutures should not be placed in the superficial dermis.

Running intradermal pull-out suture is most valuable in closing skin. It may be placed in the dermis close to the skin surface,

since it is removed postoperatively. The suture material used must be strong and smooth, such as polypropylene or nylon.

Running cuticular suture is an easy and rapid method of skin closure, and readily removed postoperatively. However, it does not approximate skin as accurately as interrupted sutures and tends to cause ischemia of the skin margins. If a single knot unties, or if the suture breaks, the entire suture line undergoes dehiscence. If the suture remains in place too long, an unsightly scar may result.

Mattress sutures are frequently used to close abdominal or chest wall incisions. Vertical mattress sutures are intended to gain both a secure grasp of tissue and a good approximation of the skin margins. Unfortunately, permanent hatchmark scars result if the sutures are left in place for over 5 to 7 days. Horizontal mattress sutures have even less to recommend them than vertical mattress sutures. Partial necrosis of the skin margin is not uncommon in the postoperative period.

Retention sutures are utilized when one is closing wounds under tension and there is a risk of fascial dehiscence. Bolsters are frequently used to distribute the tension forces of horizontal mattress sutures over a large skin area to prevent pressure or ischemic necrosis. Plain plastic buttons, red rubber catheters, or folded pieces of Telfa are ideal for this use.

DRESSING. Wound dressing constitutes a major part of wound care and has a direct influence on the course of healing.[13] Ideally, a dressing should protect wounds against mechanical trauma and bacterial invasion. Sterile dressings should be applied before surgical drapes are removed to avoid contamination of the incision. During the early postoperative period (48 hours), the fresh incision should be protected by dry dressings until epithelization is completed. A nonstick dressing (Telfa) is preferred. Draining and infected wounds require dressings that can absorb exudate and remove necrotic tissue remnants after surgical debridement. Wide-mesh cotton gauze applied to the wound surface traps necrotic debris and exudate, and these are removed when the dressing is changed. When skin loss is extensive, biological dressings are helpful in achieving wound coverage and protection against bacterial invasion and evaporative loss. Allografts, xenografts, and various skin substitutes have been used.

IMMOBILIZATION. When the site of any injury is immobilized, lymphatic flow is reduced, thereby minimizing the spread of the wound microflora.[13] Moreover, immobilized tissue demonstrates more resistance to the growth of bacteria than nonimmobilized tissue. Elevation of the injured site limits the accumulation of fluid in the wound interstitial spaces. The wound with little edema proceeds more rapidly to complete rehabilitation. Whenever possible, the site of injury should be elevated above the patient's heart.

SUTURE REMOVAL. One important factor that influences the timing of suture removal is the eventual cosmetic result. Percutaneous sutures create a sinus tract; and, with time, an epithelial-lined tract through the dermis remains after suture removal. Some of the cells may form keratin and inclusion cysts, or a puncture scar. A typical railroad track appearance is the final result. In general, early suture removal (4 to 5 days) is possible in those areas with excellent blood supply (Table 1).

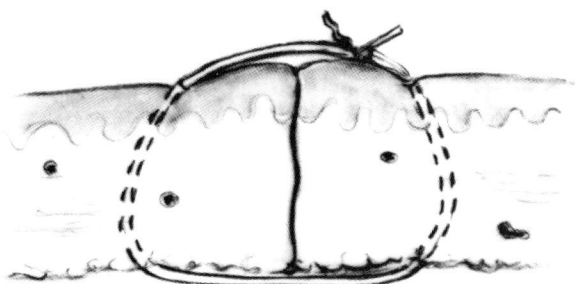

Figure 2. Whenever a skin edge is sutured with a simple full-thickness cuticular suture, the passage of the needle should include deep dermis that is further removed from the cut margin of the skin than is the entrance or exit point of the suture through the epidermis. The mild vertical lifting of the entire suture line that results is sometimes called the "Halsted roll." (From Edgerton, M. T.: The Art of Surgical Technique. Baltimore, Williams & Wilkins, 1988. © Williams & Wilkins, 1988.)

TABLE 1. Guidelines for Suture Removal

Anatomic Location	Removal Day(s)
Eyelid	2–3
Face	4–5
Neck	3–5
Scalp	7
Trunk	6–14
Extremities	10–21
Joints	14

Another determinant of the timing of suture removal is the amount of tension on the wound edges. For example, distraction of the wound edges is greater with vertical incisions on the back and with large elliptical excisions on the extremity. Other factors that determine the timing of suture removal include nutritional status, prior radiation therapy, concurrent chemotherapy, exogenous steroid administration, and the presence of sepsis.

Utmost care is needed in removing sutures. One must remember that dehiscence is likely to occur with injudicious provocation. Gently cleansing with hydrogen peroxide to remove crusted blood allows better visualization. The knot should be grasped with the forceps and the scissor tip used to cut the suture. Gentle pulling on the knot toward the incision line frees the suture.

PROPHYLACTIC ANTIBIOTICS. Prophylactic antibiotics are defined as those administered in the absence of or before infection and are distinguished from therapeutic antibiotics used to treat an established infection. Prophylactic antibiotics are recommended for operations that are associated with a high risk of infection—most alimentary tract operations, cesarean sections, hysterectomies, and selected biliary tract operations—and operations associated with life-threatening consequences if infection occurs—neurosurgical, cardiovascular, and operations involving implantable devices.[34] Parenteral antibiotic prophylaxis should be started within 2 hours before the operation. In cesarean sections, prophylaxis is usually given intraoperatively after the umbilical cord is clamped. They should not be continued for more than 48 hours. Prophylactic orally administered antibiotics do not decrease the incidence of infection in patients with suture closure of simple lacerations.[45]

ELECTROCAUTERY

Bovie discovered that high-frequency alternating current could be used to incise or coagulate tissue to obtain hemostasis. The technique was popularized by Cushing in the performance of neurosurgical procedures and subsequently extended to other operations.

A *unipolar* electrosurgical unit is used both for surgical dissection and for hemostasis.[13] When undamped high-frequency electrical current is passed through tissue, the active electrode functions as a bloodless knife, and the cells at the edges of the wound disintegrate. A mild thermal injury occurs away from the plane of cutting, and blood vessels thrombose. When the oscillations are dampened, hemostasis is accomplished without cutting. The cells experience a rapid dehydration, and the vessels within the tissue coagulate. The damage to adjacent tissue may be extensive. The precise tip of the divided vessel is all that requires coagulation, and the power of the unit should be set at the lowest level possible.

The cutting cautery may be of significant value in saving operative time and diminishing blood loss during massive excisional surgery or when large flaps of skin or muscle are elevated. However, compared with cold knife dissection, there is an increased susceptibility to infection and seromas. The grounding plate must be well secured at some appropriate point under the patient and kept as large as possible for dispersing the energy. If the ground plate becomes detached, energy leaves the patient through any available portal, such as electrocardiographic leads. Because these leads are much smaller points of exit, burns of the skin may occur with serious consequences to the patient.

A *bipolar* cautery is more precise and confines the damage to the tissues between the tips of the cauterizing forceps. Notably, the bipolar instrument can be used in a wet environment. It is indicated for controlling bleeding in microvascular and microneural surgery.

Finally, the *hemostatic scalpel,* developed by Shaw,[12] combines the advantages of a sharp knife with a heated blade for dissection. Heat seals small blood vessels as they are divided, and blood loss is minimized.

MEDICAL LASERS

The laser was first successfully operated in 1960. The term is an acronym for *L*ight *A*mplification by *S*timulated *E*mission of *R*adiation. The concept of light as a source of energy is realized in medical lasers.[3] Surgeons can now employ energy from light as a scalpel. Such energy consists of photons that are both waves and particles. The wavelength is expressed in nanometers. Laser radiation is coherent, both temporally and spatially. The light is monochromatic which permits selective optical absorption and consequent selective tissue heating, thereby providing a new approach to the damage or removal of tissue. It must be noted that, despite technologic advances, laser surgery remains cumbersome and not without complications.[14] The most common problems are endotracheal explosions and facial burns. In the hands of well-trained practitioners, the complication rate should be less than 1 per cent.

ARGON LASER. Argon lasers used in surgical procedures obtain their energy from rotation and vibration of electrons of argon with resultant emission of a monochromatic beam of blue-green light (488 to 514 nm.) that has the ability to be highly focused.[3] The energy is absorbed by red cell hemoglobin, transformed to heat, and superficial thermal injury results. Argon lasers have for years been the mainstay of ophthalmologic treatment and prevention of intraocular hemorrhage. Extensive experimental efforts support the potential benefits of laser fusion of tissue. The proposed advantages include speed, improved healing without the foreign body reaction associated with sutures, and reduction of intimal hyperplasia that is often seen in the region of sutured anastomoses. Exciting preliminary results have concluded that argon laser vascular tissue fusion is possible in humans when reliable primary sealing of the vascular anastomosis is achieved.[49] In addition, laser thermal arterial recanalization may become an effective adjunct or alternative to balloon angioplasty.

CO_2 LASER. This energy source is now being used by some surgeons to cut tissue. The CO_2 laser produces its effect as a result of instantaneous heating of intracellular water to boiling, exploding cells in its pathway. Further heating generates steam and carbonization of tissues. The laser creates a 0.1-mm. zone of histologic necrosis, which is equivalent to that of the scalpel. The superior hemostatic effect of the laser scalpel makes it especially suitable for massive surgical excision; electrosurgical excision has 1.67 times the blood loss of laser excision.[13] Unfortunately, experimental wounds made by a laser are approximately tenfold more susceptible to infection than those made by electrocautery. This infection-potentiating effect of the laser scalpel militates against its use in incisional surgery.

Nd:YAG LASER. Forward penetration of the laser beam is least with the argon laser, intermediate with the CO_2 laser, and deepest with the neodymium:yttrium-aluminum-garnet (Nd:YAG) laser, the latter laser energy (1060 nm.) providing destructive coagulation effects on tissues. The Nd:YAG laser is capable of directing light energy via a flexible quartz fiber, permitting the use of fiberoptic endoscopes in the paranasal sinuses and tracheobronchial tree.

TUNABLE DYE LASER. The modern tunable dye laser (577 nm.) has recently provided excellent results in the difficult treatment of port-wine stains.[31]

CUSA KNIFE

The CUSA knife (Cavitron ultrasonic surgical aspirator) is an ultrasound probe that functions as an acoustic vibrator. The instrument selectively fragments and aspirates tissue of high water and low collagen content, i.e., tumors, sparing other tissues such as blood vessels and nerves.[1]

The Cavitron was introduced into clinical use in 1967 for phacoemulsification of cataracts, and a more powerful version was approved for use in neurosurgery in 1976. The ability to remove a tumor without causing adjacent brain tissue trauma due to suctioning, coagulation, or manipulation has been greatly augmented with the development of the Cavitron. Advantages of reduced blood loss, reduced tissue injury, and improved visibility, compared with the scalpel or cautery, have been demonstrated for hepatic, splenic, and renal resection. Ultrasonic fragmentation appears to be useful either as the primary technique for mucosal proctectomy in difficult cases, or as an adjunct to manual dissection to decrease the incidence of residual mucosa.[20]

Application in cardiovascular surgery is also being explored. In coronary bypass surgery, the ultrasonic aspiration permits confirmation of the location and exposure of an embedded coronary artery prior to the institution of cardiopulmonary bypass.[30] It is further suggested that dissection of the internal mammary artery may be performed with shorter harvesting time and less bleeding.[44]

SUTURES AND NEEDLES

HISTORICAL ASPECTS. The act of sewing is probably older than *Homo sapiens,* since Neanderthal man wore some sort of clothing. However, the overall priority for stitching probably should be credited to the *ants,* who had the idea long before man. *Oecophylla smaragdina* discovered a way to sew leaves with a triple combination of clamping, stitching, and gluing.[27] Stitching of wounds among primitive man is exceptional. An ancient Egyptian scroll (3500 B.C.) alludes to sutures and suturing of wounds. Perhaps the world's oldest suture was placed by an embalmer on the belly of a twenty-first dynasty mummy about 1100 B.C. In Sustruta's Samhita (600 B.C.) there is mention of suture material made from animal sinews, braided horsehair, leather strips, and vegetable fibers. *Suture* means "to sew" or "seam" and Hippocrates used the word in this sense circa 400 B.C. Celsus wrote about sutures in the treatise De Medicina, describing the suturing of soft tissue with human hair. Galen, who was physician to Roman Gladiators in the second century A.D., recommended the use of silk and hemp ligatures for hemostasis. Andreas Vesalius first advocated the suturing of all fresh wounds as well as severed tendons and nerves.[41]

During the Middle Ages, surgery regressed and sutures were forgotten until revived by Ambroise Paré (1510–1590). Paré revolutionized the treatment of wounds by substituting the ligation of blood vessels for cauterization. John Hunter (1728–1793) and Philip Syng Physick (1768–1837) were the early English and American exponents, respectively, of sutures and their routine use in surgery. Physick, first Professor of Surgery at the University of Pennsylvania, has been credited with the development in 1806 of absorbable ligatures using kid and buckskin. Joseph Lister (1827–1912) discovered that bacteria present in the suture strands and not the suture itself caused wound infection. He obtained good results with wound healing by disinfection of the sutures with carbolic acid. Lister's utilization of sterile sutures made possible the use of buried sutures in clean wounds without infection.

SELECTION OF SUTURE MATERIAL. A wide choice of suture materials and suture/needle combinations are available today. The choice of suture for a particular procedure should logically be based on the known physical and biologic characteristics of the suture material and the healing properties of the sutured tissues. Adequate suture tensile strength is required for wound closure, but the finest suture that holds the tissues together safely should be used. A suture need be no stronger than the sutured tissues, and it is unwise to implant more foreign

materials than is necessary. Unsecured knots allow slippage, a phenomenon that occurs to some degree with all knots. Factors that influence knot security are the material coefficient, length of the cut ends, and the structural configuration.[43] Regardless of the material employed, meticulous superimposition of squared knots is far superior to any other configuration. Multifilament or braided sutures are easier to handle and have better knot holding properties. Monofilament materials glide through tissue easily and are less reactive. However, they are more difficult to handle or knot and are more likely to cut through tissue. Coating of a multifilament suture with silicon or Teflon renders it serum-proof, with improved gliding characteristics. Unhappily, the superior knotting quality of the suture is lost. All sutures should be avoided in dirty, contaminated, or infected wounds whenever possible. All sutures, as foreign bodies, have clearly been shown to impair the wound's ability to resist infection. When suture use is necessary in this setting, synthetic monofilament nonabsorbable sutures are recommended.

NEEDLE SELECTION. Needle selection is determined by the type of tissue to be sutured, the tissue's accessibility, and the diameter of the suture material. Surgical needles are composed of three anatomic parts: the eye, the body, and the point. The needle eye may be open, closed, or swaged. The open–French eye needle is easy to load with sutures of varying caliber but has additional bulk. Similarly, the eye of the closed-eye needle is wider than the needle body itself and has a tendency to spread the tissue. This disadvantage is resolved by the "swaged-on" needle, in which the suture is placed within the end of the needle. The body of the needle is fashioned from high quality stainless steel and may be straight or curved. In cross-section, the needle may be round, triangular, or flattened and available in varying sizes and gauges. The needle point may be cutting, tapered, or blunt. The cutting point is used to cut through tough tissues, such as skin.[47] The tapered point is used on soft, vulnerable tissue; and the blunt point is used in suturing friable tissues or in cannulating. The endothelial trauma at the site of microsurgical repairs has been minimized with the development of extremely fine needles (50 to 75 μ).[25] In contrast, arthroscopic meniscus repair has been made possible by the development of high quality needles with the strength, sharpness, length (2 to 10 inches), and flexibility to pass smoothly through instruments and tissue.[32]

Surgical needles are designed to lead suture material through tissue with minimal injury. Available types of suture to be guided by surgical needles include a wide variety of materials. They may be absorbable or nonabsorbable, natural or synthetic, braided or monofilament, and clear or colored.

ABSORBABLE SUTURES

The term *absorbable suture* implies absorption and eventual disappearance of the suture from the tissue implantation site. The rate of absorption depends on the type of material used. Selecting a specific absorbable suture requires assessment of the length of time the material is maintained and the strength it has over that time. For example, plain catgut should not be used for major fascial repair with collagen deposition and maturation occurring at 7 to 42 days.

CATGUT. The origin of the name *catgut* or *kittegut* is from a very delicate musical instrument called a kitte—a type of fiddle that required fine gut for its strings. At present, catgut is made from the intestines of cattle or sheep. The absorption rate of plain catgut is about 10 days. Chromic catgut has been treated with a chromium salt to retard its absorption by conditioning the surgical gut to resist digestion by the body. Absorption of the treated catgut is delayed up to 20 days. Catgut acts as an active foreign body in the tissue and may interfere with wound healing. Plain catgut usually evokes a greater inflammatory reaction than chromic catgut. There is no evidence that catgut can produce an allergic response.[7] Catgut is useful for tying off subcutaneous bleeding vessels and for closing the skin of the scrotum and perineum.

POLYGLYCOLIC ACID. An absorbable, braided, synthetic suture material, polyglycolic acid (Dexon), has a higher tensile strength than catgut. Total reabsorption by hydrolysis during wound healing occurs at 60 to 90 days postoperatively. Dexon contains no collagenous protein, no antigens, and no pyrogens, therefore causing minimal tissue reaction. It should not be used for suturing heart valves and vascular prostheses, which depend on a permanent tissue bond. Dexon is useful in muscle, fascia, capsule, tendon, and subcuticular skin closure. Generally, braided suture, absorbable or nonabsorbable, adversely influences bacterial growth. Bacteria may be carried into the interstices of braided sutures and escape phagocytosis, thus causing chronic suture infection, granulomas, and sinuses. Any braided material passed through the skin has a high propensity to form abscesses at the skin-suture interface. Of the foregoing absorbable sutures, Dexon evokes the least inflammatory response and has significantly lower infection rates than either plain or chromic gut sutures.[28]

POLYGLACTIC ACID. Polyglactic acid (Vicryl) is a braided synthetic suture that is similar to Dexon in many respects. The tensile strength is very high (second to that of Dexon), and it is completely absorbed in 60 days[41] (Fig. 3). Vicryl may be purchased as either clear or violet-colored. It is extremely useful as a completely buried suture to approximate wound edges until the wound has gained enough strength to keep the edges from separating. As noted above, these braided sutures may induce bacterial infection, and percutaneous sutures are contraindicated.

POLYDIOXANONE. The synthetic polymer of poly-para-dioxanone (PDS) is a suture that has the distinct advantage of being a monofilament absorbable suture with a long duration of absorbability and an extremely high tensile strength. It is, however, somewhat stiff and difficult to handle and knot. PDS may be either undyed or violet-colored. The low reactive suture is capable of maintaining its integrity in the presence of bacterial infection and represents a major advance when used in closure of abdominal wounds.[39] Another singular advantage of this suture material is that it can be extruded into various forms such as absorbable clips and staples. Importantly, the nonmetallic polymer avoids distortion when seen by computed tomography and nuclear magnetic resonance scanning.

NONABSORBABLE SUTURES

SILK. Silk is a protein filament obtained from the silkworm larva. The silk is dyed, treated with polybutylate, and braided.

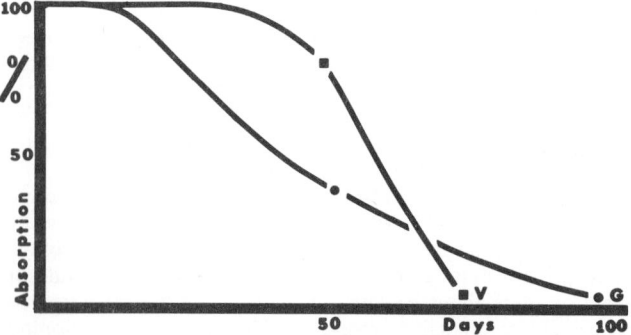

Figure 3. Absorption profile of chromic surgical gut (G) and synthetic absorbable polyglactin 910 (Vicryl) suture (V). Size 4-0 sutures were implanted in rat gluteal muscle and absorption calculated from cross-sectional area remaining. Absorption of surgical gut is seen by 14 days, and synthetic absorbable suture shows evidence of absorption at about 35 days but is more rapid thereafter. (From Salthouse, T. N.: Biologic Response to Sutures. Otolaryngol. Head Neck Surg., *88*:658, 1980.)

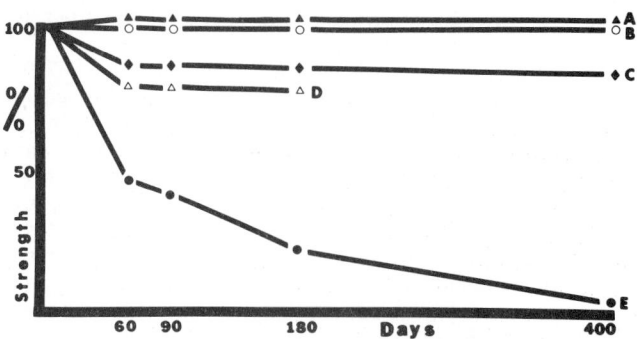

Figure 4. Nonabsorbable sutures, percentage strength remaining. Polyester (Ethibond and Mersilene) sutures (A) and polypropylene (Prolene) sutures (B) retained 100 per cent of original breaking strength after 400 days. Monofilament nylon (Ethilon) sutures (C) retained about 80 per cent. Multifilament nylon (D) lost slightly more of its original strength than the monofilament suture. Silk sutures (E) degrade and lose strength more rapidly, with usually less than 50 per cent of the original strength remaining at 2 months. Data shown are from size 2-0 and 4-0 sutures implanted in rat subcutaneous sites. (From Salthouse, T. N.: Biologic Response to Sutures. Otolaryngol. Head Neck Surg., *88*:658, 1980.)

The suture has good tensile strength, is easy to handle, and has excellent knot characteristics. Although classified as nonabsorbable, silk does degrade at a variable rate in tissue and loses its tensile strength. Silk is a very comfortable suture for the patient when used as a permucosal suture in the mouth.

COTTON. Processed from braided cotton fibers, cotton suture material is strong and pliable. Wetness makes the material stronger and the knot firmer, a property not associated with any other material. It is essentially identical to silk with regard to its reactivity and infection-carrying capacity. Cotton should not be used in wounds known to be or suspected of being contaminated.

POLYESTER. Constructed of polyester fibers (Dacron), these braided sutures have superior strength and durability, which make them an excellent choice for fascial closure (Fig. 4). The uncoated suture (Mersilene) tends to cut slightly when pulled through tissue; thus, Teflon (Tevdek), silicone (Tri-Cron), and polybutilate (Ethibond) have all been employed in its manufacture. The material requires a minimum of five throw knots for knot security, as compared with two throw knots for steel and three for silk, cotton, polyglactic, or polyglycolic acid sutures. The knotting characteristics and the fact that it is braided and cannot be used in the presence of infection or contamination constitute its only disadvantages. *Polibutester* is a special type of polyester suture (Novafil). A monofilamentous suture, it is slippery and plastic like polypropylene, but ties like polyester. Novafil may be blue or clear and induces very little inflammatory reaction when buried in tissue.

NYLON. A synthetic polyamide polymer, nylon is available in both monofilament and multifilament forms. It is very strong and smooth, but extra care must be taken in tying to prevent knot slippage. Nylon may be black, green, or clear color. The suture is degraded and absorbed in about 2 years; thus, its tensile strength decreases significantly with time. Its smooth monofilament composition ensures facile passage through tissue and minimal reaction. Nylon sutures are the most commonly used sutures in cutaneous surgery—both percutaneous and subcuticular.[16]

POLYPROPYLENE. A monofilament suture material, polypropylene (Prolene) provides smooth passage through tissues and minimal tissue reaction. Prolene may be clear or blue in color. A special manufacturing process tapers the end of the suture, which allows it to be swaged to a needle of similar diameter, providing a hemostatic advantage for vascular anastomoses. Prolene sutures retrieved from vascular grafts at 2 to 6 years have shown no loss of tensile strength.[10] Easy removability renders it an ideal suture for a running intradermal stitch, and it is a superior suture for fascial closure in the presence of contamination or infection. In fine-caliber sizes, Prolene is invaluable for microvascular surgery.

STAINLESS STEEL. Stainless steel wire, made from low-carbon iron alloy, can be monofilament or multifilament. Wire is the strongest and least reactive suture. However, its handling characteristics are very poor, and great care must be taken to prevent kinking and cutting through tissue. Wire is used mainly in ligament, tendon, and bone surgery. Although excellent in strength, wire is not particularly durable; and fatigue and fracture of the wire with time is not uncommon. Two considerable disadvantages of metal suture material are the linear artifacts caused by high-atomic-number substances on computer-assisted tomography images, and possible movement of metal sutures during nuclear magnetic resonance studies.

STAPLES

HISTORICAL ASPECTS. Surgical stapling was developed in 1908 by Humer Hultl in Austria.[26] The original instrument was massive by today's standards, weighing 7½ pounds. Modifications performed by Von Petz provided a lighter and simpler stapling device, and in 1934 Friedrich of Ulm designed an instrument that resembled the modern linear stapler. The next and most major advances came from Russia after World War II. In 1958, the instruments were brought to the United States by Ravitch, who through research and development, refined the instruments to their current state and widespread use today. The most significant recent modification has been the introduction of absorbable staples (Lactomer). When used in gynecologic operations, morbidity related to infections, granulomas, and chronic dyspareunia has been diminished.

Cox[8] has appropriately cautioned that mechanical stapling instruments do not absolve the surgeon from respecting the rules of operative surgery, such as clean, sharp, atraumatic dissection; careful hemostasis; and respect for tissue viability and blood supply. As do any surgical instruments, stapling devices have the risk of faulty use. Therefore, considerable attention to detail with this instrument, as with any other, is imperative for the successful outcome of any operation.

Contemporary devices include a great variety of skin and internal stapling instruments: TA30, TA55, TA90, GIA, EEA, LDS, and skin and fascia staplers.

TA INSTRUMENTS. The TA instruments place a linear everting (mucosa to mucosa) double line of staggered staples 30, 55, and 90 mm. long. Two staple sizes are available, 3.5 and 4.8 mm., depending on the thickness of the tissue stapled. The TA30 has, in addition, a special vascular cartridge (3.2 mm.) with closely spaced staples for closing vessels in procedures such as lobectomy and pneumonectomy (Fig. 5).

GIA INSTRUMENT. The GIA instrument places two double-staggered rows of staples and in the same operation divides the tissues between these pairs of staggered rows. The instrument was initially employed to form side-to-side intestinal anastomoses with serosal apposition. It is now used as an instrument for resection as well as other forms of anastomosis. Stapling of internal organs is faster than traditional hand sewn efforts, causing reduced operation and anesthesia time, tissue trauma, blood loss, and eventual hospital stay.

EEA INSTRUMENT. The EEA instrument is employed for end-to-end and end-to-side minimally inverting anastomoses. The ends of the bowel to be anastomosed are secured with pursestring sutures about the central rod, the instrument is tightened, the central rings of tissue are stamped out by a circular knife, and the staples are applied in an encircling anastomosis. The EEA instrument and proximate ILS (Ethicon intraluminal stapling device) have become most popular in esophageal and rectal anastomoses. The ability to achieve a lower resection and end-to-end anastomosis of the bowel than previously possible has led to more sphincter-saving resections for rectal carcinoma and an improved quality of life.

LDS INSTRUMENT. The LDS instrument places two metal clips of stainless steel on either side of a dividing blade. The instrument can be used in the simultaneous ligation and division of mesenteric, gastric, and omental vessels. The totally disposable powered instrument represents a quantum improvement over its relatively clumsy metal predecessor. Disposable skin and fascial staplers have also been devised.

SKIN TAPES

Ambroise Paré, the French military surgeon, introduced the use of stitched strips of linen adhesives to close saber wounds. Modern skin tapes are manufactured so that they are relatively nonocclusive and yet have excellent adhesive characteristics.[5] The microporous surgical tapes with a backing of viscous rayon fibers coated with an adhesive copolymer are pervious to sweat but not to blood or purulent material. The advantage of using tapes to hold wound edges together is that puncture of the skin surface is avoided. This practice maintains the integrity of the epidermis, lessens the likelihood of tissue strangulation and wound infection, and avoids suture marks. Skin tapes may be used in conjunction with subcuticular sutures and to secure skin grafts; and to decrease skin tension on a sutured skin wound in areas of motion. If percutaneous sutures or staples are initially used, skin tapes are commonly applied to the wound at the time of suture or staple removal to give support to the wound edges. Application of the skin tapes minimizes the opportunity for wound dehiscence and allows earlier suture or staple removal. In addition, skin tapes may be reapplied to the wound for long periods of time to provide continuous support to the wound edges and may discourage scar expansion. In children, selection of skin tapes avoids the ordeal of suture placement and removal. To be noted is that skin tapes do not effectively evert the edges of the wound and readily loosen when wet by blood or serum.

SURGICAL ADHESIVES

AUTOLOGOUS FIBRIN GLUE. Autologous fibrin glue is a biological adhesive consisting of fibrinogen, factor XIII, fibronectin, thrombin, apoprotinin, and calcium chloride. The mechanism by which fibrin glue works as an adhesive is by emulation of the exudative phase of wound healing. Animal and clinical studies have demonstrated its efficacy in stabilizing esophagogastric, small intestinal, and nerve anastomoses. It is also effective in obtaining hemostasis at skin graft donor sites. Fixation of skin grafts with excellent take and without the requirement of any sutures or pressure dressings is achieved.[38] The preparation of the glue is easy and can be done on the morning of operation

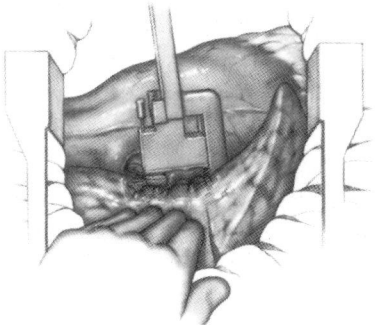

Figure 5. TA stapling instruments create a linear everting staple line. Pulmonary vessels are safely and securely closed with TA30 (3.2 mm.) vascular staples. (From Steichen, F. M. and Ravitch, M. M.: Contemporary stapling instruments and basic mechanical suture techniques. Surg. Clin. North Am., *64*:425, 1984.)

with approximately 200 ml. of autologous blood. The autologous fibrin glue is prepared from single donor human plasma, eliminating the danger of multidonor pools.

FIBRIN SEAL ADHESIVE. Fibrin seal adhesive is a two-component system (Tissucol) derived from whole blood. When mixed, the elements reproduce the final pathway of blood coagulation to form a viscous adhesive that maintains tissue approximation. The sealant, which is produced commercially only in Austria, is used both clinically and experimentally in Europe. In the United States, fibrin seal is currently available only for experimental use. Because fibrin seal is a blood product, there is a possibility that its use may be associated with the transmission of acquired immunodeficiency syndrome (AIDS) or hepatitis, although this has not been substantiated.

CYANOACRILATE. Numerous encouraging experimental and clinical reports advocate the use of cyanoacrilate tissue adhesives for repair of organs, or as hemostatic agents in emergency situations. However when cyanoacrilate is applied to skin closure, the polymer acts as a barrier, prevents wound apposition, delays healing, and increases the infection rate. The adhesive has proved useful in the fixation of the articulating surface of artificial joints of the hip; but some problems exist, especially loosening of the adhesive over a period of time.

MUSSEL ADHESIVE PROTEIN. Mussel adhesive protein (MAP) is a promising new tissue adhesive obtained from the blue mussel, *Mytilus edulis*.[15] It has unique properties, including adhesion in a saline environment, which make it well-suited to surgical and dental applications. MAP is in an experimental phase but has shown few intraocular inflammatory reactions or toxic effects. MAP may be significant in the attachment of appropriate tissue to metal in total joint replacement surgery.

DRAINS

HISTORICAL ASPECTS. The use of drainage systems dates back to Hippocrates and may be divided into passive and active categories. Metal tubes, glass tubes, bone, gauze, wicking, and combinations of gauze and rubber were the initial means of providing *passive* drainage. The tapered lead and bronze tubes placed into the abdominal cavity by Celsus in the first century A.D. are the earliest examples of gravity drainage. Capillary attraction in small-bore tubes, the basis of all passive methods, was observed by Leonardo daVinci, although the laws of hydrostatics explaining this phenomenon would only be elucidated 3 centuries later (1805) by Thomas Young, a physician and physicist. Such was still the state of the art when the familiar Penrose wick (1890) and later the cigarette drain (1897) were described. Heaton (1889) discovered air-vent suction, or *active*, drainage. Subsequently, Yates, in his 1905 classic article, concluded that "drainage of the general peritoneal cavity is physically and physiologically impossible"; and the concept has not been seriously challenged.

PRINCIPLES OF WOUND DRAINAGE. It is probable that in the abdominal cavity drains can serve only two purposes. The first is the provision of egress for loculated pus or intestinal contents. Second is the prophylactic removal of any fluids within the peritoneal cavity, such as bile and pancreatic juices, before their presence can lead to complications. However, the use of prophylactic drains for peritoneal contamination has been abandoned. Abdominal drains are quickly surrounded by omentum and bowel, which isolate the drains as ineffective sinus tracts. Soft tissue drains may help coapt tissue and prevent the collection of serum or blood underneath large undermined areas. However, drains must not be considered a substitute for hemostasis or as a replacement for meticulous technique.[36] For either prophylactic or therapeutic indications, the surgeon should select the form of drainage, either passive or active, that is best suited for the purpose intended. The drain must be appropriate to the demands of the viscosity or the volume of the

expected drainage. In general, prophylactic drainage may be best accomplished by the use of closed-wound suction drainage. As the volume or complexity of drainage increases and therapeutic drainage is indicated, passive and sump drains are more efficacious. Decreased drainage or the absence of drainage usually indicates that the drain may be withdrawn. The material of which the drain is made is of utmost concern: it should be soft, to avoid injury; nonirritating to the tissue, firm, to remain in intended place; resistant to decomposition; and smooth, to allow easy removal. Three types of drains are used primarily: (1) the Penrose drain, (2) the closed suction drain, and (3) the sump drain. Percutaneous catheter drainage represents a new method that is proving to be exceedingly valuable.

PENROSE DRAIN. The Penrose drain is a soft, flexible latex rubber wick ranging from 1/4 to 1 inch in diameter, and is usually employed to drain purulent material, blood, or serum from a body cavity. Intra-abdominal drains should optimally be brought out through a stab wound in the flank and not the abdominal incision itself. A drain tract coming through the suture line increases the risk of infection and is a potential source of weakness that may lead to a ventral hernia. The drain tract incisions should be placed lateral to the rectus muscle beyond the epigastric vessels, and the tract wounds wide enough to enable the surgeon's finger to pass easily from within the abdominal cavity through to the skin. The use of two drains is advantageous in allowing egress of fluid along the planes between the drains. The drains should be anchored to the skin with a nonabsorbable suture, and placement of a sterile safety pin will prevent retraction of the drains into the wound. Management of the drains consists of either completely removing them or cracking and gradually withdrawing them several centimeters a day. The theory behind the latter technique is that the development of a fluid collection or abscess cavity deep to the drains is prevented. The length of time a Penrose is left in place varies with the initial indication for drainage, the presence of a foreign body, and the patient's overall status. Drain tract sinography can be useful in determining the proper timing of intra-abdominal drain removal and may avoid the septic complication of drain removal in cases of residual intra-abdominal sepsis or undiagnosed enterocutaneous fistula.[11]

CLOSED SUCTION DRAIN. Closed suction drains are firm, multiholed catheters made of polyvinyl chloride or silicone. The silicone material is softer, less irritating to the tissues, and less likely to cause infection. These drains are particularly effective under large skin flaps, such as those encountered after radical neck or breast dissections. Closed-suction drainage decreases the incidence of infection occurring secondary to contamination of the drain itself and is mandatory in the presence of a foreign body. When drainage diminishes, the tube may be removed directly, preferably within 24 to 72 hours.

SUMP DRAIN. Sump drains are available with double or triple lumens that allow irrigation and aspiration. Pressure in the catheter is maintained at atmospheric levels, and tissue occlusion of the drain is less likely. The sump drain is most useful in the management of established enteric fistulas with high volumes.

CATHETER DRAIN. Through modern radiologic techniques, diagnosis of localized accumulations of fluid in different areas of the body can be made much earlier than in the past and confirmed by aspiration. In many instances adequate treatment can be instituted by means of percutaneous catheters inserted by radiologists guided by computed axial tomographic scanning or, less reliably, ultrasonography. Antibiotics are considered to be essential for success. It is recognized that unilocular abscesses that contain thin fluid can be treated simply and expeditiously by catheter drainage. However, open drainage may be a more appropriate, even lifesaving, alternative approach.[2]

CONTROVERSY. The continued use of drains in circumstances where experimental evidence suggests that they do no good or are detrimental is presumably a counsel of caution, rather than perfection: "When in doubt, drain," and "It is better to have it and not need it than to need it and not have it." These concepts apparently are based on the assumption that there are no complications related to the use of drains. Drains left *in situ* are not innocuous: they may erode into the intestine or the blood vessels and thus promote the development of adhesions leading to intestinal obstruction. Avoidance of technical complications, such as hematoma, retraction of the drain into the wound, or herniation through the stab wound have been mentioned. Sutures can be inadvertently placed around or through drains, and drains may break off inside the body. Careful record keeping related to the number, type, and length of drains inserted and removed may avert the disastrous consequences of retained drains. For the benefit of wound drainage, the surgeon must consider the risk of contaminating the wound and increasing the incidence of infection. Accumulated wound fluids have been shown to contain decreased levels of opsonizing proteins, making these fluids especially vulnerable to infection. It has been clearly documented that placing a drain in patients undergoing routine splenectomy increases the morbidity of the procedure. Similarly, researchers have demonstrated that children in whom Penrose drains were placed at operation for perforated appendicitis averaged nearly 4 more hospital days than those without drains. Additional reports indicate lower morbidity and shorter hospital stays in series of cholecystectomy patients where nondrainage or selective drainage is practiced.[23] Numerous experiments constitute good evidence for the harmful effects if peritoneal drains are placed close to bowel suture lines.[40] The decision to drain a doubtful anastomosis is fraught with hazards. A recent controlled trial has reported no significant differences in anastomotic dehiscence between colonic anastomoses that were and those that were not drained.[21] However, in two overt leaks the drain did not discharge pus or feces. To drain or not, which drain, and for how long all remain unanswered questions; but the diversity of answers suggests that no single policy is necessarily correct.

SELECTED REFERENCES

Edgerton, M. T.: The Art of Surgical Technique. Baltimore, Md., Williams & Wilkins Company, 1988.
A refreshing and detailed focus on "how to do it." A plastic surgeon with years of experience in the broadest realms of reconstructive surgery, Edgerton is a master of the art of surgical technique. He provides a simple and basic description of operative techniques, the principles and details of which apply to all of surgical procedures.

Edlich, R. F., Rodeheaver, G., Thacker, J. G., and Edgerton, M. T.: Fundamentals of Wound Management in Surgery. South Plainfield, N.J., Chirurgecom, Inc., 1977.
An extensive and excellent review of the scientific basis of surgical techniques. Experimental data relating to antisepsis, debridement, drains, and a host of other factors in the creation and care of the operative wound are presented.

Polk, H. C., Jr., Simpson, C. J., Simmons, B. P., and Alexander, J. W.: Guidelines for prevention of surgical wound infection. Arch. Surg., 118:1213, 1983.
At the request of the Centers for Disease Control, these authors formulated current guidelines for prevention of surgical wound infections. The specific factors addressed in these recommendations included surveillance and classification, patient preparation, preparation of the surgical team, ventilation and air quality in the operating room, cleaning and culturing, operative technique, wound care, prophylactic antibiotics, and topical antibiotics.

Steichen, F. M., and Ravitch, M. M.: Stapling in Surgery. Chicago, Year Book Medical Publishers, 1984.
This superbly illustrated text is written by two pioneers in the field of operative stapling. The text reviews the history and experimental background of suturing with staples and gives a thorough assessment of their current use.

Wilmore, D. W., Brennan, M. F., Harken, A. H., Holcroft, J. W., and Meakins, J. L.: American College of Surgeons: Care of the Surgical Patient. Vol. 2, Elective Care. New York, Scientific American, Inc., 1989.
Care of the Surgical Patient is sponsored by the Pre- and Postoperative Care Committee of the American College of Surgeons and is written by individuals who are recognized experts. The text represents their approaches to clinical problems and to other important issues in surgical practice. The content includes initial evaluation for elective surgery, perioperative care, and infection.

REFERENCES

1. Adelson, M. D., Baggish, M. D., Seifer, D. B., Cassell, S. L., and Thompson, M. A.: Cytoreduction of ovarian cancer with the cavitron ultrasonic surgical aspirator. Obstet. Gynecol., 75:140, 1988.
2. Aeder, M. I., Wellman, J. L., Haaga, J. R., and Hau, T.: Role of surgical and percutaneous drainage in the treatment of abdominal abscesses. Arch. Surg., 118:273, 1983.
3. Arndt, K. A., Noe, J. M., Northam, D. B. C., and Itzkan, I.: Laser therapy: Basic concepts and nomenclature. J. Am. Acad. Dermatol., 5:649, 1981.
4. Beck, W. C.: Aseptic barriers in surgery: Their present status. Arch. Surg., 116:240, 1981.
5. Bennett, R. G.: Selection of wound closure materials. J. Am. Acad. Dermat., 18:619, 1988.
6. Branemark, P. I., Albrektsson, B., Lindstrom, F., and Lundborg, G.: Local tissue effects of wound disinfectants. Acta. Chir. Scand. (Suppl.), 357:166, 1966.
7. Carroll, R. E.: Surgical catgut: The myth of allergy. The J. Hand Surg., 14B:218, 1989.
8. Cox, C. E.: Principles of operative surgery: Antisepsis, technique, sutures, and drains. In Sabiston, D. C. (Ed.): Textbook of Surgery: The Biological Basis of Modern Surgical Practice. Philadelphia, W. B. Saunders Company, 1986, p. 244.
9. Cruse, P. J., and Foord, R.: The epidemiology of wound infection: A 10 year prospective study of 62,939 wounds. Surg. Clin. North Am., 60:27, 1980.
10. Dobrin, P. B.: Surgical manipulation and the tensile strength of polypropylene sutures. Arch. Surg., 124:665, 1989.
11. Dougherty, S. H., and Simmons, R. L.: The drain-tract sinogram: Guide to the removal of drains and the diagnosis of postoperative abdominal sepsis. Am. Surg., 49:511, 1983.
12. Edgerton, M. T.: The Art of Surgical Technique. Baltimore, Williams & Wilkins Company, 1988.
13. Edlich, R. F., Rodeheaver, G., Thacker, J. G., and Edgerton, M. T.: Technical factors in wound management. In Fundamentals of Wound Management of Surgery. South Plainfield, Chirurgecom, Inc., 1977, p. 364.
14. Fried, M. P.: A survey of complications of laser laryngoscopy. Arch. Otolaryngol., 110:31, 1984.
15. Fulkerson, J. P., and Massicotte, J. M.: Mussel adhesive protein from *Mytilus edulis*: Applications in orthopaedic research and surgery. Biol. Bull., 171:500, 1986.
16. Goulbourne, I. A., Nixon, S. J., Naylor, A. R., and Varma, J. S.: Comparison of polyglactin 910 and nylon in skin closure. Br. J. Surg., 75:586, 1988.
17. Hunt, T.: Surgical wound infections: An overview. Am. J. Med., 76:717, 1981.
18. Hasselgren, P. O., Hagberg, E., Malmer, H., Saljo, A., and Seeman, T.: One instead of two knives for surgical incision. Arch. Surg., 119:917, 1984.
19. Health and Human Services: Requirements of construction and equipment for hospitals and medical facilities. Publication No. HR5-M-HF-84-1. Rockville, Md., United States Department of Health and Human Services, 1984.
20. Heimann, T. M., Slater, G., Kurtz, R. J., Szporn, A., and Greenstein, A. J.: Ultrasonic mucosal protectomy in patients with ulcerative colitis. Ann. Surg., 210:787, 1989.
21. Hoffman, J., Hosein, S. A. M., Damm, P., and Jensen, R.: A prospective controlled study of prophylactic drainage after colonic anastomosis. Dis. Colon Rectum, 30:449, 1987.
22. Howard, J. M., Barker, W. F., Culbertson, W. R., Grotzinger, P. J., Iovine, V. M., Keehn, R. J., and Radvin, R. G.: Factors influencing the incidence of wound infection. Ann. Surg. Suppl., 160:32, 1964.
23. Irwin, S. T., Moorehead, R. J., and Parks, T. G.: Effect of drainage on subhepatic collections and respiratory function after elective cholecystectomy. Br. J. Surg., 75:476, 1988.
24. Larson, E.: Innovations in health care: Antisepsis as a case study. Am. J. Publ. Health, 79:92, 1989.
25. Lourie, G. M., Seaber, A. V., and Urbaniak, J. R.: Microanastomotic Response to Needle and Suture Size. J. Reconstr. Microsurg., 1:135, 1984.
26. MacIntyre, I.: A history of surgical stapling. Nat. News, 25:15, 1988.
27. Majno, G.: The Healing Hand—Man and Wound in the Ancient World. Cambridge, Harvard University Press, 1975:93, 307.
28. Mcgeehan, D., Hunt, D., Chaudhuri, A., and Rutter, P.: An experimental study of the relationship between synergistic wound sepsis and suture materials. Br. J. Surg., 67:636, 1980.
29. Meakins, J. L.: Host defense mechanisms, wound healing and infection. In Fundamentals of Wound Management of Surgery. South Plainfield, N.J., Chirurgecom, Inc., 1977, p. 242.
30. Mitsui, T., Onizuka, M., Ijima, H., Maeta, H., Okamura, K., Sakai, A., Tsutsui, T., Mitsui, K., and Hori, M.: Ultrasonic aspiration in coronary artery surgery. Ann. Thorac. Surg., 40:199, 1985.
31. Morelli, J. G., Tan, O. T., Garden, J., Margolis, R., Seki, Y., Boll, J., Anderson, R. R., Furumoto, H., and Parrish, J. A.: Tunable dye laser (577 mm) treatment of port wine stains. Lasers Surg. Med., 6:94, 1986.
32. Morgan, C. D., and Casscells, S. W.: Arthroscopic meniscus repair: A safe approach to the posterior horns. Arthroscopy, 2:3, 1986.
33. Mulliken, J. B., and Healey, N. A.: Pathogenesis of skin flap necrosis from an underlying hematoma. Plast. Reconstr. Surg., 63:540, 1979.
34. Polk, H., Simpson, C. J., Simmons, B. P., and Alexander, J. W.: Guidelines for prevention of surgical wound infection. Arch. Surg., 118:1213, 1983.
35. Ritter, M. A., Eitzen, H., French, M. L. V., and Hart, J. B.: The operating room

environment as affected by people and the surgical face mask. Clin. Orthop., 11:147, 1975.

36. Robinson, J. O.: Surgical drainage: An historical perspective. Br. J. Surg., 73:422, 1986.

37. Salasche, S. J., Winton, G. B., and Adnot, J.: Surgical pearls. Dermatol. Clin. 7:75, 1989.

38. Saltz, R., Dimick, A., Grotting, J. C., Psillakis, J., and Vasconez, L. O.: Application of Autologous Fibrin Glue in Burn Wounds. J. Burn Care Rehabil., 10:504, 1989.

39. Schoetz, D. J., Coller, J. A., and Veidenheimer, M. C.: Closure of abdominal wounds with polydioxanone. Arch. Surg., 123:72, 1988.

40. Smith, S. R. G., Connolly, J. C., Crane, P. W., and Gilmore, O. J. A.: The effect of surgical drainage materials on colonic healing. Br. J. Surg., 69:153, 1982.

41. Snyder, C. C.: On the history of the suture. Plast. Reconstr. Surg., 58:401, 1976.

42. Steere, A. C., and Mallison, G. F.: Handwashing practices for the prevention of nosocomial infections. Ann. Intern. Med., 83:683, 1975.

43. Stone, I. K.: Suture materials. Clin. Obstet. Gynecol., 31:712, 1988.

44. Summa, H., Fukumoto, H., and Takeuchi, A.: Application of ultrasonic aspirator for dissection of the internal mammary artery in coronary artery bypass grafting. Ann. Thorac. Surg., 43:676, 1987.

45. Thirlby, R. C., Blair, J., and Thal, E. R.: The value of prophylactic antibiotics for simple lacerations. Surg. Gynecol. Obstet., 156:212, 1983.

46. Tobin, G. R.: Closure of contaminated wounds: Biological and technical considerations. Surg. Clin. North Am., 64:639, 1984.

47. Towler, M. A., McGregor, W., Rodeheaver, G. T., Cutler, P. V., Bond, R. F., Phung, D., Morgan, R. G., Thacker, J. G., and Edlich, R. F.: Influence of cutting edge configuration on surgical needle penetration forces. J. Emerg. Med., 6:475, 1988.

48. Tuneval, T. G.: Surgical face mask: With or without? Presented at the 32nd World Congress of Surgery, Sydney, Australia, September 28, 1987.

49. White, R. A., White, G. H., Fujitani, R. M., Vlasak, J. W., Donayre, C. E., Kopchok, G. E., and Peng, S-K.: Initial human evaluation of argon laser-assisted vascular anastomosis. J. Vasc. Surg., 9:542, 1989.

50. Wilmore, D. W., Breman, M. F., Harken, A. H., and Holcroft, J. W.: Preparing the operating room. In American College of Surgeons: Care of the Surgical Patient, Vol. 2. Elective Care. New York, Scientific American, Inc., 1989.

13

SURGICAL INFECTIONS

I

SURGICAL INFECTIONS AND CHOICE OF ANTIBIOTICS

J. Wesley Alexander, M.D., Sc.D., and E. Patchen Dellinger, M.D.

At the time anesthesia was introduced by Morton in 1846, numerous operations had been performed, including lithotomy for bladder calculus, amputation for compound fractures or gangrene, gastrointestinal resections, ligation of aneurysms, rhinoplasty, mastectomy, ovariectomy, repair of vesicovaginal fistula, extraction of cataracts, bone resections, and others. However, even after anesthesia was widely employed and surgeons could operate more deliberately, elective operations remained an unacceptable alternative for most patients with surgical diseases, because almost all operative wounds became infected and almost half of patients who underwent a major operation died as a result of infection. The most frequent complications of wounds were erysipelas, hospital gangrene (presumably necrotizing streptococcal infection and/or mixed synergistic infections), septicemia, and tetanus. Infection was so common in wounds that it was thought by many to be an important part of the normal healing process. In fact, many surgeons fervently hoped for the development of "laudable pus" in their wounds (presumably caused by staphylococcal infection) instead of the all too frequent rapidly fatal hospital gangrene. This was perhaps a classic example of the clinical application of bacterial antagonism. In above-knee amputation for compound fracture, survival was often less than 10 per cent; and when patients did survive, it was usually after a protracted course of infection.

Lister has been generally recognized as the founder of the antiseptic principle in surgery, and his paper "On the Antiseptic Principle in the Practice of Surgery," published in 1867, was instrumental in revolutionizing the practice of surgery; the infection rate in elective operations dropped from 90 per cent or more to 10 per cent or less with the application of Listerian principles. Lister's work came at a crucial and opportune time. He was guided and stimulated by the work of Pasteur on the nature of fermentation and putrefaction, and his contributions related well to the observations and work of many such as Oliver Wendell Holmes, Ignaz Semmelweis, and Theodor Kocher. Even though many others preceding Lister contributed, Lister's concepts and techniques met widespread disbelief during the latter part of the nineteenth century and were resisted. However, the superior results could not be ignored, and the concepts of asepsis as pioneered by Semmelweis in 1847 and antisepsis by Lister in 1867 were gradually amalgamated so that aseptic-antiseptic principles were almost completely developed by 1900 and have been without change in concept during this century.

These basic principles of infection control set forth primarily in the 33 years between 1867 and 1900 changed surgical therapy from a dreaded event, with infection almost universal and death expected, to one that now provides an enormous alleviation of suffering and prolongation of life with near universal success when carefully performed. Today, wound infections are expected to occur in less than 1.5 per cent of clean cases, less than 3 per cent of clean-contaminated cases, and less than 5 per cent of contaminated cases (Table 1). Infection should be determined at 30 days postoperatively, rather than at discharge, because more than half occur after discharge. It has been demonstrated that simple monitoring of surgical specific infections with feedback to the surgeon reduces the incidence by approximately 50 per cent. In monitoring infections, an unbiased observer is required, and infection should be diagnosed whenever there is discharge of any purulent material from the wound. For patients in whom infection develops, there is not only an increased morbidity but also significant mortality. The cost of the care of postoperative wound infections alone in the United States is still enormous, totaling several billion dollars every year. For any type of operation, the development of a wound infection approximately doubles the cost of hospitalization.

With the introduction of antibiotic therapy, it was hoped that serious infections complicating surgical practice would be eliminated. Unfortunately, this has not occurred. Not only has the problem of postoperative wound and hospital-acquired infections continued, but widespread antibiotic therapy has often made prevention and control of surgical infections more difficult. In this regard has been the emergence of increasing numbers of serious infections related to a complex combination of factors, including the performance of more complicated and longer operations; an increase in the number of geriatric patients with accompanying chronic or debilitating diseases; many new surgical procedures with implants of foreign materials, including artificial hearts, joints, and vessels; a rapidly expanding number of organ transplants requiring the use of immunosuppressive agents; and increased utilization of diagnostic and treatment modalities that cause greater bacterial exposures or the suppression of normal host resistance. Unfortunately, many infections continue to follow laxity in aseptic technique, disregard for established surgical principles, and unwarranted reliance upon prophylactic antibiotic therapy. Not only are these infections of medical significance, but they represent important medicolegal problems. Today surgeons must accept the responsibility of coping with infections and realize that knowledge of many aspects of microbiology, immunology, and pharmacology is essential to complement surgical skills. Basic understanding of the body's defense against infection is essential to a rational application of surgical and other therapeutic principles to the control of infection.

TABLE 1. Classification of Surgical Wounds According to Risk of Infection

Type	Definition	Unacceptable Infection Rate* at 30 Days
Clean	Nontraumatic No break in technique Respiratory, alimentary, or genitourinary (GU) tract not entered	>1.5%
Clean-contaminated	Gastrointestinal (GI) or respiratory tract entered without significant spillage Oropharynx, vagina, or noninfected GU or biliary tract entered Minor break in technique	>3%
Contaminated	Major break in technique Traumatic wound Gross spillage from GI tract Entrance into GU or biliary tracts in presence of infected urine or bile	>5%

* Defined as discharge of *any* purulent material.

CAUSES OF WOUND INFECTION

Simply stated, infections of surgical wounds occur whenever the microbial inoculum in the wound is sufficient to overcome the local host defense mechanisms and establish progressive growth. The host defense interaction with potential pathogens is an extremely complex process beyond the scope of this presentation. However, certain factors should be emphasized.

Bacterial Factors

The deposition and growth of bacteria within wounds is an obvious prerequisite for the development of infection, and the type and numbers of bacteria contribute significantly to the establishment of overt infection, or the lack of it. Several bacterial species have surface components that contribute to their pathogenicity by inhibiting phagocytosis (e.g., the capsules of *Klebsiella* and pneumococci). Other bacteria, notably the enterobacteria, have surface components (endotoxin) that are toxic, and still others, such as certain strains of *Clostridium* and *Streptococcus*, produce powerful exotoxins. The development of infection is thus somewhat dependent upon the toxins produced by the organism and the organism's ability to resist phagocytosis and intracellular destruction. With highly virulent and pathogenic organisms, such as *Streptococcus pyogenes* group A or *Pasteurella pestis*, relatively few may be required to establish an infection.

Careful studies of the bacterial flora of surgical wounds obtained at the time of closure have demonstrated that one or more types of organisms can be cultured from most wounds. In wounds classified as clean, there are usually skin bacteria such as *Staphylococcus epidermidis* or diphtheroids. In traumatic wounds, the most likely organisms are *Staphylococcus aureus* and *S. pyogenes*. When a body viscus is entered, the natural or disturbed resident flora become the expected potential pathogen(s). Because devitalized tissues and foreign materials are invariably present, far fewer organisms are necessary to cause infection in wounds than in normal tissues. However, overt infection is unusual unless cardinal surgical principles are violated or exceptionally large numbers of organisms were introduced into the wound. Studies of traumatic wounds in healthy subjects have demonstrated that bacterial contamination with

greater than 10^5 organisms frequently causes infection, whereas contamination with less than 10^5 usually does not. The normal defense mechanisms, therefore, are of great importance in the prevention of infection, but it is easily recognized that wound infection is inevitable if the bacterial inoculum is sufficiently large.

Local Wound Factors

In daily practice, inhibition of local defense mechanisms for clearing bacteria is perhaps the most important cause of wound infections. Nearly anything that interferes with the ability of phagocytic cells to directly contact and kill bacteria potentiates wound infection. Such factors include the presence of foreign bodies, including sutures, lack of accurate approximation of tissues, strangulation of the tissues with sutures that are too tight, and the presence of any dead tissue, hematomas, or seromas. Fortunately, most of these factors can be minimized by good surgical technique.

Patient Factors

Wound infections are more common in the very young and the very old, perhaps most prominently because of immature or senescent resistance mechanisms. Anything that causes reduction of blood flow to the surgical incision as may be found in vascular occlusive states, hypovolemic shock, or the use of vasopressors or vasoconstrictors locally or systemically increases the incidence of infection. In addition, all conditions that reduce vascular reactivity as may be found in uremia, old age, or the use of high doses of steroids and other drugs cause an increased susceptibility to infection. More complex problems leading to increased infection include cancer and trauma, both of which may be associated with complement activation and the generation of both tissue-derived and complement split product–derived inhibitors of cellular function, which influence both T-cell and phagocytic cell function. In many patients, these factors are thought to be primarily responsible for a decreased reactivity to delayed hypersensitivity antigens, causing an anergic state that has been demonstrated to be associated with an increased incidence of infectious complications.

PREVENTION OF WOUND INFECTION

Prevention of infectious complications is far more practical than treatment when they are established. Fortunately, strict adherence to the principles of wound care and application of knowledge concerning the pathogenesis of wound infections prevent the majority of infectious complications in surgical practice. One of the most important factors in preventing wound infection is constant vigilance of the operating team (Table 2).

TABLE 2. Important Factors in Preventing Wound Infection

Preoperative antimicrobial shower.
Hair removed by clipping, not shaving, immediately before operation.
Vigilance for breaks in aseptic technique by O.R. team.
Use of antimicrobial incise drape after short alcohol or tincture of iodine scrub without soap.
Preventive antibiotics with therapeutic levels during entire operative procedure.
Limited use of electrocautery for dissection.
Limited suture and ligatures. Continuous suture closure preferred.
Use of monofilament sutures.
Closed suction rather than open drainage.
Meticulous skin closure.
High postoperative inspired O_2.
Surveillance of wound infection.

Avoidance of Bacterial Contamination

ENVIRONMENTAL FACTORS. Engineering and architectural advances have helped to limit airborne contamination in modern operating rooms to very low levels, but these have not been followed by substantial reductions in wound infections because the two greatest sources of significant microbial contamination of operative wounds are exogenous contact from breaks in technique by the operating team and endogenous contamination from the patient's skin and various bacteria-containing tracts. Of the two, endogenous contamination is responsible for a greater number of infections in all types of wounds except those classified as "clean" (see Table 1). The use of ultraviolet light for decontamination of the operating room and laminar flow ventilation systems may be helpful in certain situations, such as insertion of prostheses for orthopedic reconstruction. Such techniques may be especially valuable in older style operating rooms that do not have the benefit of high-flow terminal filtration air systems. Perhaps as important are limitation of traffic into and out of the operating room, provision of positive pressure in the operating room, and limitation of activity and talking within the operating room. It appears self-evident that with an increasing number of personnel at the operating table there is increased opportunity for breaks in sterile technique.

In addition to the considerations for management of air, there must be strict monitoring of sterilization techniques.

PREOPERATIVE PREPARATION OF THE PATIENT. Many patients who are in the hospital for prolonged periods or who have substantial illness have increased numbers of resident organisms on the skin, especially in the groin and intertriginous areas. For these and perhaps all patients, it is advisable to require a preoperative shower (whenever the patient is able) the night before operation with an antibacterial soap such as chlorhexidine or povidone-iodine. Chlorhexidine appears to be the preferred material for reduction of residual bacteria for a prolonged period. Whenever possible, all cutaneous infections should be controlled or cleared before the time of an elective operation.

HAIR REMOVAL. Skin bacteria become especially important when the operative area is shaved because the injury of shaving may promote bacterial growth. In fact, hair removal by shaving regularly increases the infection rate approximately 100 per cent when compared with removing the hair by clippers or no hair removal at all. Because of this, the practice of shaving the patient before an operation should be abandoned.

SKIN PREPARATION. The skin is an important source of organisms contaminating surgical wounds. There are basically two methods that can be recommended for prevention of skin organisms from entering the wound. The first and time-honored technique is to scrub the entire operative area of the patient for 5 to 7 minutes with a germicidal solution and paint the region with an antimicrobial solution of either tincture of iodine, povidone-iodine, or chlorhexidine. When the skin incision has been made, the wound edges and exposed skin should be covered immediately with cloth towels held in position to the wound edges with towel clips or sutures. An alternative method of isolation of the skin from the wound is to use an antimicrobial incision drape applied to the entire operative area with the incision made through the plastic. Before application of the incision drape, the skin should be scrubbed for 1 minute with a 70 per cent solution of alcohol or a solution of 2 per cent iodine in 90 per cent alcohol to kill surface bacteria. It is important to realize that when using the incise drape the skin should not be scrubbed with a detergent solution because it interferes with the ability of the drape to adhere to the skin. When incise drapes are used, their effectiveness is lost when the drape lifts from the skin at the incision site. Thus, a technique of drape application

that includes cleansing of surface fat and debris from the skin and application only to a dry surface becomes important for its success.

The Operating Room Team and Discipline

It appears obvious that contamination can occur easily from the operating room team and this is, as an aggregate, one of the most important sources of organisms causing infection in clean cases. The operating team should be garbed in clean scrub suits, wear caps that do not shed lint and completely cover the hair, and wear masks that effectively filter the exhaled air. Before each operation, thorough cleansing and scrubbing of the hands and forearms should be done with an antimicrobial soap for at least 5 minutes for the first case or after any contaminated case, and for 3 minutes for second cases. The most popular antimicrobial scrubs at present are chlorhexidine and povidone-iodine. Careful gowning and gloving techniques should be employed, and special attention should be rendered to avoid contamination when the patient is draped. It is perhaps during the gowning/gloving procedure and draping of the patient that the most breaks in technique occur in the modern operating room environment. Another frequent source of contamination is sterile light handles, which become contaminated by the headgear of the operating team.

As many as 90 per cent of the members of an operative team puncture or tear their gloves at some time during a prolonged operation. These gloves must be changed immediately to avoid bacterial contamination of the wound, because the hands can never be sterilized by scrubbing. Although the numbers of organisms present after a surgical scrub are low, they tend to increase with the length of the operation, and the numbers of organisms inside gloves at puncture sites increase remarkably when blood has gained entrance. These minor infringements must not go unnoticed and should receive immediate attention, just as major breaks in technique do. Gowns worn by the operating room team may also be an important source of contamination, and the "contact areas," i.e., the sleeves and the front of the gown, should be impervious to bacteria and fluids whether the gowns are disposable or reusable.

Endogenous Contamination

Another very important but not always heeded source of bacterial contamination of the surgical wound is endogenous contamination at the time of transection of the gastrointestinal, respiratory, or genitourinary tract. Bacterial contamination occurs to varying degrees any time a hollow viscus is transected, but exceptional efforts to minimize the amount of contamination produce a gratifyingly low occurrence of bacterial infection. Before a hollow viscus is entered, the operative area should be carefully isolated from the remainder of the operative field. A completely different set of instruments should be used for that portion of the operation until the hollow viscus is closed. At closure of the hollow viscus, all instruments, towels, and sponges that may have come into contact with the contaminated area must be removed from the operative field, and the gowns and gloves of the operative team should be changed. By strict observance of aseptic technique in clean-contaminated cases, the incidence of operative infections can be markedly reduced.

When contamination of the operative site has occurred, topical antibiotics can be used effectively to reduce the bacterial inoculum. Liberal irrigation of the wound with a saline solution containing 1.0 gm. of kanamycin per liter has been an effective adjunct for preventing infections.

The Importance of Surgical Technique

As previously emphasized, infections in wounds associated with injury or planned operative procedures have a profound effect on morbidity and mortality. Every patient deserves meticulous wound care, but this is particularly important in those instances in which there may be an impairment of host defense, since nearly every wound transecting the gastrointestinal tract and even a large percentage of "clean" surgical wounds are contaminated by viable and potentially pathogenic bacteria. Gentle care of the tissues to minimize local damage is one of the most important factors in preventing wound infection.

All devitalized tissues and foreign bodies should be removed from traumatic wounds. When complete débridement is not possible, the wound should not be closed, because foreign bodies left in a wound may decrease the minimal infective dose of a bacterial inoculum 10,000-fold or more. More than a million viable staphylococci are necessary to produce a clinical infection when injected subcutaneously or intradermally into normal tissue, but when these same organisms are introduced on a piece of silk suture material, as few as 100 can produce a significant infection. Similar results have been demonstrated with the enhancement of clostridial infections by devitalized muscle and sterile foreign bodies. It is understandable that in grossly contaminated wounds, not only must all contaminated foreign bodies be removed, but careful consideration must also be given to the introduction of new foreign bodies such as prostheses, grafts, and suture materials. In contaminated wounds, experimental studies have demonstrated that monofilament suture materials are preferable to multifilament materials. Thus, silk should never be used to tie or repair large blood vessels where there is a high potential for infection, because infection involving the suture often causes rupture of the vessel and fatal hemorrhage. This disastrous complication is much less frequent when polypropylene sutures and ligatures are employed. At present, the best nonabsorbable sutures for use in contaminated wounds are polypropylene and nylon. Absorbable materials should not be used for fascial or bowel closure in infected or highly contaminated wounds. The technique of closure is also important. For fascial closures, the use of running sutures is preferable in most instances when the wound has been heavily contaminated.

The presence of hematomas, seromas, or dead space favors bacterial localization and growth and prevents the delivery of phagocytic cells to such bacterial foci. One mistake frequently encountered in closing contaminated wounds is leaving a dead space between the layers. Where a large potential dead space occurs in an operative wound that is potentially contaminated but not yet infected and is not obliterated by fascial and dermal sutures, the best method for preventing fluid collection and infection is to provide a system of closed suction drainage. In contrast, open drainage of wounds increases, rather than decreases, the degree of contamination and the incidence of infection. Because of this, a Penrose type of drain should not be used for drainage of any wound that is not already infected.

In heavily contaminated wounds or in wounds in which all the foreign bodies or devitalized tissues cannot be satisfactorily removed, delayed primary closure, in most instances, minimizes the development of serious infection. With this technique, the subcutaneous tissues and skin are left open and "packed" loosely with gauze after fascial closure. The number of phagocytic cells at the wound edges progressively increases to reach a peak approximately 5 days after injury. Capillary budding is intense at this time, and closure may usually be accomplished successfully even when there is heavy bacterial contamination since phagocytic cells can be delivered to the site in large numbers. It has been demonstrated experimentally that the number of organisms required to initiate an infection in a surgical incision progressively increases as the interval of healing increases, up to the fifth postoperative day.

For heavily contaminated wounds, the authors have used an alternative method of treatment that greatly reduces the incidence of infection. After fascial closure, a closed suction catheter is brought into the length of the wound through a separate stab wound. A watertight skin closure is accomplished using a running polypropylene or nylon suture; and a solution of topical kanamycin (as previously described) is instilled through the catheter, sufficient to fill the wound cavity. The tubing is clamped for 2 hours, holding the solution in the wound, and the drain is then placed on suction to remove the fluid and close the dead space. The catheter is removed in 48 hours.

In patients for whom sutures must be left for a prolonged time, dressings should be used to prevent suture line infection. Skin closure should be accomplished to prevent skin overlap, which predisposes to infection, especially if the wound needs to be reopened.

Systemic Factors

Host resistance has been found to be abnormal in a variety of systemic conditions and diseases, including leukemia, diabetes mellitus, uremia, prematurity, burn or traumatic injury, advanced malignancy, old age, obesity, malnutrition, several diseases of inherited immunodeficiency, acquired immunodeficiency, and immunosuppression. When treating surgical patients with these or similar problems, extraordinary precautions should be taken to prevent the development of wound infections. These should include correction or control of the underlying defect whenever possible.

Recent studies have indicated that malnutrition, even when subclinical, can cause a significant impairment of host defense mechanisms. Many surgical patients have some degree of malnutrition, especially when there is stress leading to hypermetabolism. This type of "insidious" malnutrition is probably the most important cause of acquired immunologic deficiencies leading to serious infection in surgical patients. Thus, one of the most important measures in preventing infection is to correct any underlying malnutrition before surgical therapy or as soon thereafter as possible. Alimentation by the oral route is clearly preferable, when possible. In stressed patients, recent evidence indicates an increased requirement for protein and arginine.

Perhaps of even more importance is avoiding disturbances of the circulation during the intraoperative and immediate postoperative period. Anything that reduces blood flow to the incision decreases the delivery of phagocytic cells and increases the incidence of infection. Therefore, it is important not only to keep the blood pressure within normal range but also to prevent reduction of cutaneous blood flow, which often occurs with the use of vasopressors. Oxygen delivery to the incision is an important factor in prevention of wound infection. It has been suggested by some investigators that oxygen tension in the wound may be as important as antibiotics in the prevention of growth of bacteria. Because of this, a relatively high inspired fraction of oxygen ($FIo_2 \geq 40$ per cent) during the immediate postoperative period is recommended for nearly all patients.

The administration of many drugs, including steroids, antimetabolites, and anticancer agents, has been found to be associated with an increased incidence of septic complications. Unnecessary use of these drugs is to be avoided in the surgical patient. The role of antibiotics in opportunistic infections is discussed later.

Social Considerations

Several studies have shown that accurate and continued surveillance for wound infection with communication to the surgeon reduces the incidence of wound infection by approximately 50 per cent. This simple technique may be a powerful method in controlling wound infection, because nearly every surgeon will increase efforts to control infectious complications if they are perceived to be a problem.

Immunotherapy

Active and passive immunization procedures for the prevention of surgical infections have merit in only a few specific instances. Tetanus is one condition in which the use of immunotherapy has had outstanding success in prevention of the disease. After a full course of active immunization, most individuals are protected against the development of tetanus for years, and many for a lifetime. In such individuals, a booster injection of toxoid invariably elicits protective levels of antibody for up to 20 years after active immunization, and the administration of antitoxin for the prophylaxis of tetanus in these patients is not indicated except in unusual circumstances. It is important for those individuals who have not been actively immunized against tetanus before the time of penetrating injury to receive tetanus antitoxin. At the time of injury, 250 to 500 units of human tetanus antitoxin should be administered intramuscularly, the dose depending upon the severity of the injury. If the patient is observed more than 24 hours after injury, the dose should be increased. Simultaneous administration of the initial injection of tetanus toxoid for active immunization is indicated in every case. A careful follow-up is necessary to ensure completion of the course of active immunization. Tetanus antitoxin does not prevent infection with *Clostridium tetani*, but it does inactivate the toxin produced. Therefore, careful surgical débridement with removal of all devitalized tissue is clearly the most important means of prevention. The administration of systemic antibiotics has been recommended in the past for the prevention of tetanus, but this is of secondary importance and usually unnecessary.

Passive immunization for rabies is also highly effective in preventing the disease in exposed patients or those thought to be exposed. The use of pooled human gamma globulin for the prevention of bacterial infections or treatment of bacterial infections in surgical patients is not warranted unless they have agammaglobulinemia or dysgammaglobulinemia.

Reducing the Bacterial Load by Prophylactic Chemotherapy

The use of systemic prophylactic chemotherapeutic and antibiotic agents has continued to be controversial, primarily because of a lack of understanding of the basic principles involved. Experience has proven that the effectiveness of antibiotic treatment depends upon the observance and practice of these principles. If they are ignored, the results are haphazard failures. There is little doubt that the administration of therapeutic doses of antimicrobial agents is capable of preventing infection in wounds contaminated by specific bacteria highly sensitive to the agents. The decision for the use of prophylactic antibiotic therapy, however, must be based on the weight of evidence for possible benefit against the weight of evidence for possible adverse effects. Indiscriminate or blind use of antibiotics is discouraged because it may lead to secondary or superimposed infection with antibiotic-resistant strains of organisms, serious hypersensitivity reactions, and postponement of indicated surgical treatment. Their use may also mask the signs and symptoms of established infections, making diagnosis more difficult. An equal or even greater problem caused by the frequent use of antibiotics is the development of antibiotic-resistant strains within the hospital environment.

Prophylactic systemic antibiotics are clearly not indicated in the management of most patients undergoing clean surgical operations in which no obvious bacterial contamination or insertion of a foreign body has occurred. The incidence of wound infections in elective clean operations such as herniorrhaphy and thyroidectomy is less than 1 per cent when careful, gentle, meticulous, aseptic technique is practiced. When infections do occur, they can usually be traced to poor surgical technique or errors in aseptic technique. Prophylactic antibiotic therapy is no substitute for careful surgical technique based on established surgical principles, and its indiscriminate or general use is not in the best interest of the patient. Experience has added emphasis to the fact that antibiotic agents can be used effectively only as adjuvants to adequate surgical therapy.

There are several clinical situations in which the administration of prophylactic systemic antibiotic therapy is usually of benefit. In principle, these situations usually involve a brief period of contamination by species of organisms that can be predicted with reasonable accuracy. As examples, prophylactic systemic antibiotics are usually recommended in the following circumstances:

1. Accidental wounds with heavy contamination and tissue damage. In such instances, the antibiotic should be given by the intravenous route as soon as possible after injury.

2. Accidental wounds requiring surgical therapy in which treatment is unavoidably delayed.

3. Injuries in which adequate débridement cannot be accomplished and contaminated or devitalized tissue must remain of necessity.

4. When known gross bacterial contamination has occurred in any wound.

5. Penetrating injuries of a hollow intra-abdominal viscus.

6. Resection and anastomosis of the colon or small intestine. The administration of oral nonabsorbable antibiotics for the suppression of growth of both aerobic and anaerobic intestinal bacteria has been successful in controlled trials, but some regimens, especially those without activity against anaerobic bacteria, are detrimental. If oral antibiotics are administered as preparation for colon surgery, neomycin plus erythromycin administered only on the day before operation is the most well-established combination at present. The authors' experience has led to the conclusion that thorough mechanical cleansing of the intestinal tract is critically important and is equally efficacious, provided systemically administered antibiotic therapy is given immediately before, during, and after operation. For this purpose, the authors have effectively used cefoxitin, cefotetan, or a combination of gentamicin and clindamycin. These drugs should be administered for no longer than 24 hours. Many authorities believe a combination of oral nonabsorbable and intravenous antibiotics is preferable, but this practice has not been confirmed by controlled studies.

7. In operative procedures categorized as "clean-contaminated," when there is transection or resection of a hollow viscus of the gastrointestinal tract, biliary tract, respiratory tract, or genitourinary tract, with varying degrees of bacterial contamination, the decision for the use of antibiotic therapy must be based on careful consideration of the evidence for and against its effectiveness. Evaluation should include an estimate of the degree of contamination, the length and severity of the operation, and the status of nonspecific host resistance, including the age of the patient, underlying disease conditions, and associated drug therapy. Each patient must be evaluated individually. Examples of "clean-contaminated" operations for which prophylactic systemic antibiotics should be used routinely include common bile duct exploration for the presence of calculi and gastrectomy for carcinoma or bleeding.

8. When emergency operation is indicated in patients with pre-existing or recently active infection.

9. When pre-existing valvular heart damage is present in a patient, in order to prevent the development of bacterial endocarditis.

10. Vaginal or abdominal hysterectomy.

11. Cardiovascular surgery with placement of a prosthesis.

12. Amputation of an extremity with impaired blood supply, particularly in the presence of a current or recent ulcer.

13. Operations entering the oral pharyngeal cavity in continuity with neck dissections.

14. Injuries prone to clostridial infection because of extensive devitalization of muscle, heavy contamination, and/or impairment of blood supply.

15. In patients with open fractures, penetrating joint injuries, and joint prostheses or other devices.

Prophylactic antibiotic therapy is clearly more effective when initiated preoperatively and continued through the intraoperative period with the aim of achieving therapeutic blood levels throughout the operative period. This produces therapeutic levels of the antibiotic agents at the operative site in any seromas and hematomas that may develop. Antibiotics initiated as late as 1 to 2 hours after bacterial contamination are markedly less effective, and they are completely without value for prophylaxis after wound closure. Failure of the effectiveness of prophylactic antibiotic agents has resulted in part from a lack of recognition of the importance of the timing and dosage of these agents, which are critical determinants. For most patients with elective surgery, the first dose of prophylactic antibiotics should be given intravenously at the time of the induction of anesthesia. It is unnecessary to initiate them more than 1 hour preoperatively, and it is unnecessary to continue them after the patient leaves the operating room. A single dose, depending upon the drug employed and the length of the operation, is often sufficient. Administering prophylactic antibiotics for more than 12 hours for a planned operation is seldom indicated.

Prophylactic antibiotic therapy is generally ineffective in those clinical situations in which continuing contamination is apt to occur. Examples are as follows:

1. In patients with tracheostomies or tracheal intubation to prevent pulmonary infections.

2. In patients with indwelling urinary catheters.

3. In patients with indwelling central venous lines.

4. In most open wounds, including burn wounds.

5. In immunologically deficient patients or those receiving immunosuppressive therapy unless there are other indications for systemic antibiotic therapy.

The use of topical antibiotics has proved to be effective in many instances in diminishing the incidence of infection in contaminated wounds. Topical antibiotics should be considered as an alternative to the use of systemic prophylactic antibiotics, especially when it is desirable to avoid the latter, and as a complement to their use when heavy contamination has occurred. They may be particularly useful in those situations in which the indications for systemic prophylactic antibiotics are marginal, such as clean wounds. The most popular antibiotics for topical irrigation are kanamycin or a first-generation cephalosporin. The use of other topical agents such as the iodophors for wounds that are to be closed is seldom indicated. Topical agents for burn wounds (discussed elsewhere) may be used in large open wounds in selected patients.

THE NATURE, DIAGNOSIS, AND TREATMENT OF SURGICAL INFECTIONS

Surgical infections are distinguished from medical infections by the presence of an anatomic or mechanical problem that must be resolved by operation or other invasive procedure to cure the infection. Such procedures include, but are not limited to, incision and drainage of an abscess, opening an infected wound, removing an infected foreign body, repairing or diverting a bowel leak, or draining an intra-abdominal abscess with a percutaneous catheter. Antibiotic treatment of a surgical infection without this mechanical solution does not resolve the infection. The most important aspect of the initial approach to a surgical infection is the recognition that operative intervention is required.

Some broad generalizations can be made concerning typical differences between surgical and medical infections. In community-acquired medical infections, such as primary pneumonia, general host defenses are usually intact, although in certain conditions such as chronic granulomatous disease, specific congenital, enzyme-specific defects may create susceptibility to specific infectious agents. Some exceptions to intact host defenses are in patients undergoing systemic treatment for malignancy or for transplant rejection and patients with human immunodeficiency virus Type 1 (HIV-1) infection. Most surgical infections, in contrast, are the result of damaged host defenses, especially injury to the epithelial barrier that normally protects the sterile internal environment from endogenous and exogenous bacteria. Immunologic defects may be acquired, due either to trauma (accidental or surgical) or to tumor. Nonmechanical host defense defects are global, caused by nutritional deficiency and/or the systemic effects of trauma.

The pathogens found in medical infections usually are single and aerobic. They are derived from exogenous sources or are present only in a minority of asymptomatic normal hosts. Typically, they possess virulence properties, allowing them to establish invasive infection despite an intact epithelial barrier. Examples include beta-hemolytic streptococci, *Streptococcus pneumoniae*, and enteric pathogens such as *Shigella*, *Salmonella*, and *Vibrio cholerae*. The pathogens causing surgical infections, in contrast, are frequently mixed, involving aerobes and anaerobes, and usually originate from the patient's own endogenous flora. These pathogens are opportunistic, often depending upon an acquired epithelial defect to cause infection.

Soft Tissue Infections

The distinction between surgical and medical infections in superficial tissues depends upon the recognition of dead tissue in surgical infections. The most obvious example of a surgical infection is a subcutaneous abscess, an infectious process characterized by a necrotic center without a blood supply, composed of debris from local tissues, dead and dying white cells, components of blood and plasma, and bacteria. This semiliquid central portion (pus) is surrounded by a vascularized zone of inflamed tissue. Such an abscess does not resolve without drainage and evacuation of the pus. It is recognized clinically as a localized swelling with signs of inflammation and tenderness. An abscess must be distinguished from cellulitis, which is a soft tissue infection with intact blood supply and viable tissue, marked by an acute inflammatory response with small vessel engorgement and stasis, endothelial leakage with interstitial edema, and polymorphonuclear leukocyte infiltration. Cellulitis resolves with appropriate antibiotic therapy alone if treatment is initiated before tissue death occurs.

An abscess may be mistaken for cellulitis when the central necrotic portion is located deeply beneath overlying tissue layers and cannot be readily detected by physical examination. It may also be disguised in anatomic locations where fibrous septa join skin and fascia, dividing subcutaneous tissue into compartments that limit the local expression of fluctuance, while leading to high pressures that promote early tissue death. Examples of such infections include perirectal abscesses, breast abscesses, carbuncles on the posterior neck and upper back, and infections in the distal phalanx of the finger (felon).

Knowledge of the local anatomy and pathophysiology of these special abscesses aids in providing optimal treatment. A perirectal abscess is often associated with a fistula communicating with the anus at a crypt. A fistula should be sought and, if found, unroofed at the time a perirectal abscess is drained. If a fistula is not found acutely, the surgeon should be alert for its occurrence in the postoperative period. A breast abscess is preferably drained by a circumferential incision in natural skin lines. Drainage of a felon should be made through a lateral incision to avoid a painful scar on the pressure-bearing distal pulp. At the time of incision and drainage for a felon, all fibrous septa in the infected pulp must be broken to achieve resolution of the infection.

Superficial abscesses on the trunk and head and neck are most commonly caused by *Staphylococcus aureus,* often combined with streptococci. Abscesses in the axillae often have a prominent gram-negative component. Abscesses below the waist, especially on the perineum, are frequently found to harbor a mixed aerobic and anaerobic gram-negative flora.

Necrotizing Soft Tissue Infections

Necrotizing soft tissue infections, both clostridial and nonclostridial, are less common than subcutaneous abscesses and cellulitis but much more serious conditions the severity of which initially may be unrecognized. These infections are marked by the absence of clear local boundaries or palpable limits. This lack of clear boundaries is responsible both for their severity and for the frequent delay in recognizing their surgical nature. Anatomically, these infections are marked by a layer of necrotic tissue, which is not walled off by a surrounding inflammatory reaction and thus does not present a clear boundary. In addition, the overlying skin has a relatively normal appearance in the early stages of infection, and the visible degree of involvement is substantially less than that of the underlying tissues. A clostridial infection classically involves underlying muscle, and is termed clostridial myonecrosis or gas gangrene. Most nonclostridial and some clostridial necrotizing infections spread in the subcutaneous fascia between the skin and the deep muscular fascia. These infections have been described under a variety of labels but are most commonly termed necrotizing fasciitis (Table 3).

Rapid progression of a soft tissue infection, a marked hemodynamic response to infection, or the failure to respond to conventional nonoperative therapy may be the earliest sign of a necrotizing soft tissue infection. An apparent cellulitis with ecchymoses, bullae, any dermal gangrene, or crepitus suggests an underlying necrotizing infection and mandates operative exploration to confirm the diagnosis and perform definitive treatment. The critical step in diagnosis is to recognize the nonlocalized, necrotizing nature of the infection and the need for operative treatment. This is more important than applying a very specific diagnostic label to the process. Operative treatment requires excision of involved tissues for clostridial myonecrosis; on an extremity this may mean amputation. Nonclostridial infections can often be managed by wide incision and débridement and do not usually require amputation. In either case, all areas of necrotic tissue must be unroofed and débrided, and this often causes large, disfiguring wounds.

The most common organisms associated with clostridial infections are *Clostridium perfringens, C. novyi,* and *C. septicum.* Other bacteria are commonly found in association with the clostridial organisms. The only bacterium commonly reported as the sole cause of nonclostridial necrotizing soft tissue infections is the beta-hemolytic streptococcus, *Streptococcus pyogenes.* This is the most common pathogen recovered when there has not been a prior injury or operation as the cause of infection. Postoperative and postinjury cases of necrotizing soft tissue infection are most commonly caused by mixed bacterial species, including aerobic and anaerobic pathogens, both gram-positive and gram-negative, a very similar spectrum to that observed in intra-abdominal infections.

TABLE 3. Comparison of Clostridial and Nonclostridial Infections

	Clostridial Myonecrosis	Nonclostridial Necrotizing Infections
Erythema	Usually absent	Present, often mild
Swelling/edema	Mild to moderate	Moderate
Exudate	Thin	"Dishwater" to purulent
White cells	Usually absent	Present
Bacteria	GPR* ± others	Mixed ± GPR
		May be GPC† alone
Advanced signs	Hypesthesia	Hypesthesia
	Bronze discoloration	Ecchymoses
	Hemorrhagic bullae	Bullae
	Dermal gangrene	Dermal gangrene
	Crepitus	Crepitus
Deep involvement	Muscle > skin	Subcutaneous tissue ± fascia ± muscle (uncommon) > skin
Histology	Minimal or no inflammation	Acute inflammation
	Muscle necrosis	Microabscesses
		Viable muscle
Physiology	Rapid onset of tachycardia, hypotension, volume deficit ± intravascular hemolysis	Variable—minimal to tachycardia, hypotension, and volume deficit
Treatment		
General	Aggressive cardiopulmonary resuscitation	Aggressive cardiopulmonary resuscitation
Antibiotics	Penicillin G plus broad spectrum	Cefotaxime + metronidazole
Hyperbaric O$_2$	If it does not delay other treatment	No
Surgery	Aggressive removal of infected tissue; amputation of extremity often required	Débridement and exposure; not much removal required; usually no amputation
Antitoxin	No	No

* GPR, gram-positive rods.
† GPC, gram-positive cocci.
Adapted from Dellinger, E. P.: Crepitus and gangrene. *In* Platt, R., and Kass, E. H. (Eds.): Current Therapy in Infectious Diseases—3. Toronto, B. C. Decker, 1990.

Intra-abdominal and Retroperitoneal Infections

The majority of serious intra-abdominal infections require surgical intervention for resolution. In this context, the term *surgical intervention* includes percutaneous drainage of intra-abdominal abscesses. The specific exceptions to this include pyelonephritis, salpingitis, amebic liver abscess, enteritis (*Shigella, Yersinia,* etc.), spontaneous bacterial peritonitis, and some cases of diverticulitis and cholangitis. However, all of these "exceptions" can be diagnosed presumptively with a rapid initial evaluation. If the diagnosis of one of these exceptions cannot be made, a patient with fever and abdominal pain should not be given antibiotics without a plan leading to operation or another drainage procedure. The administration of antibiotics in this setting prior to diagnosis may obscure subsequent findings and delay diagnosis and certainly delay definitive operative management. If the patient is too ill without antibiotic therapy, he is also too ill to avoid operative intervention and definitive diagnosis and treatment.

Despite modern antibiotics and intensive care, mortality from serious intra-abdominal or retroperitoneal infection remains high (5 to 50 per cent) and morbidity is substantial. The systemic response to intra-abdominal or retroperitoneal infection is accompanied by fluid shifts similar to those observed in patients with major burns. Fever, tachycardia, and hypotension are common; and a severe hypermetabolic, catabolic response is universal. If corrective surgery and effective antibiotics are not employed promptly, the sequence of events termed multiple organ failure syndrome may ensue, with death of the patient even after the primary focus of infection has been controlled. Regardless of the initial antibiotic choice and operative procedure, there is a significant likelihood that a change in antibiotics may be required and that a reoperation may be necessary. The physician caring for a patient with intra-abdominal infection must be alert to these possibilities and diligent in following and re-examining the patient in order to make this decision at the earliest possible time. Outcome is improved by early diagnosis and treatment. The risk of death and complications increases with increased age, pre-existing serious underlying diseases, and malnutrition. The risk of death or failure to control the abdominal source of infection can also be demonstrated to relate to the normal homeostatic balance of the patient at the time of diagnosis and initiation of definitive therapy. This balance can be measured by a number of scales designed to quantitate the number of physical findings and laboratory tests that are abnormal. One of the most widely used scales is the Acute Physiology and Chronic Health Evaluation (APACHE) scoring system. The higher the score, the more abnormal tests and findings are present, and the greater the risk of death.

When a patient is diagnosed with intra-abdominal infection, initial treatment consists of cardiorespiratory support, antibiotic therapy, and operative intervention. In most patients, the responsible bacterium is not known for at least 24 hours and sensitivity information is not available for 48 to 72 hours after cultures are obtained during the operative procedure. Since most intra-abdominal infections yield three to five different aerobic and anaerobic pathogens, specific, targeted antibiotic therapy is not possible at first and the initial choice must be empiric, designed to cover a range of possible organisms. The antibiotic combination with the greatest experience and published information is an aminoglycoside combined with clindamycin or metronidazole. In recent years, a host of new antibiotics has widened the available choices. For infections acquired in the community with a small likelihood of resistant gram-negative rods and for a patient who is not severely ill, empiric therapy can be initiated with cefoxitin or cefotetan. For a more severely ill patient or a patient who has been hospitalized or has recently been treated with antibiotics, more comprehensive treatment is required. This could be imipenem or a combination chosen from Table 4, a selection of one antibiotic from the aerobic column and one from the anaerobic column (see below for discussion of specific antibiotics.) Empiric antibiotic choice for other serious infections with a similar spectrum of pathogens, such as the necrotizing soft tissue infections, is the same.

OPERATIVE INTERVENTION FOR INTRA-ABDOMINAL OR RETROPERITONEAL INFECTION. The goal of operative intervention in patients with intra-abdominal infection is to correct the underlying anatomic problem that either caused the infection or perpetuates it. An obstructed organ (appendix, bowel, common bile duct) must be rendered free of obstruction (bowel, bile duct) or removed (appendix). A perforated bowel must be closed (perforated ulcer), resected (appendix, most cases of diverticulitis), bypassed, or defunctionalized (low rectal perforation, unresectable acute diverticulitis). Foreign material in the peritoneal cavity that inhibits white blood cell function and promotes bacterial growth (feces, food, bile, mucin, blood) must be removed. Large deposits of fibrin that entrap bacteria, allowing bacterial growth and preventing phagocytosis, should be removed. Attempts to perform "radical débridement" of the peritoneal cavity, removing all infected material, are thought by some, but not all authorities, to improve results in the treatment of diffuse but not localized peritonitis.

An intra-abdominal or retroperitoneal abscess requires drainage. In prior years this usually required an open operation. Recently, computed tomographic (CT) scans have provided precise localization of intra-abdominal abscesses, permitting selected abscesses to be drained percutaneously under radiologic or ultrasound guidance. If the abscess is single and has a straight path to the abdominal wall that does not transgress bowel (Fig. 1A), it will be amenable to percutaneous drainage. This is accomplished by needle puncture with aspiration of a small sample of pus to confirm the location and diagnosis. Subsequently a floppy guide wire is passed through the needle and is then removed. The guide wire allows dilation of the tract, followed by placement of a drainage catheter. The progress of abscess closure can be followed by plain radiographs after instillation of contrast materials (Fig. 1B).

When a patient has multiple abscesses or abscesses combined with underlying disease that requires operative correction or when a safe percutaneous route to the abscess is not present, open operative drainage may be required. A single abscess in the subphrenic or subhepatic position may be drained by an extraperitoneal subcostal or posterior twelfth-rib approach, which provides open drainage without exposing the entire peritoneal cavity to the abscess contents. Similarly, most retroperitoneal abscesses should be drained with a retroperitoneal approach. However, most pancreatic "abscesses," which, in reality, more often consist of diffusely infected, necrotic, peripancreatic retroperitoneal tissue, require transabdominal operation and débridement. A pelvic abscess may be amenable to transrectal or transvaginal drainage. Retroperitoneal phlegmon

TABLE 4. Antibiotics with Predominantly Aerobic or Anaerobic Broad-Spectrum Activity

Aerobic Coverage	Anaerobic Coverage
Gentamicin	Clindamycin
Tobramycin	Metronidazole
Amikacin	Chloramphenicol
Netilmicin	
Cefotaxime	
Ceftizoxime	
Ceftriaxone	
Ceftazidime	
Aztreonam	
Ciprofloxacin	

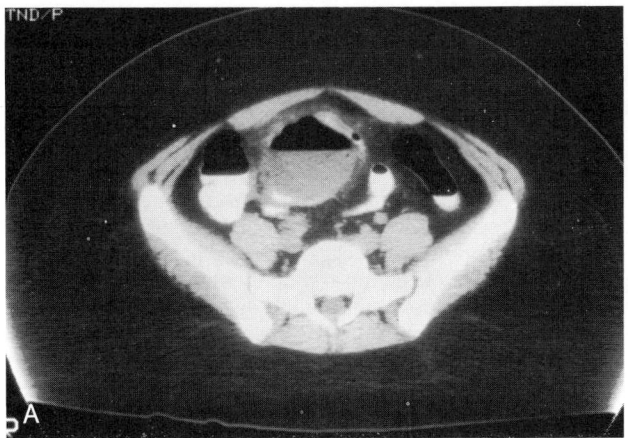 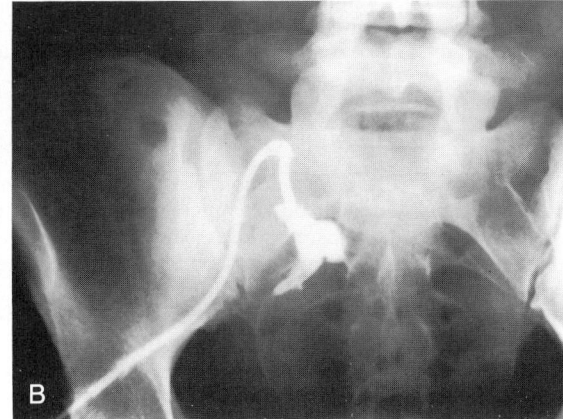

Figure 1. *A,* CT scan demonstrating a right lower quadrant abscess containing gas, fluid, and barium in a young woman with 3 days of abdominal pain and fever and right lower quadrant tenderness. A mass was not palpable, probably because of marked obesity. *B,* A sinogram obtained after contrast injection into a percutaneous catheter placed 7 days earlier in the same patient.

(necrotizing cellulitis) is a rare condition, usually associated with extravasation of infected urine, which requires extensive débridement similar to that used to treat necrotizing fasciitis.

POSTOPERATIVE FEVER. Approximately 2 per cent of all primary laparotomies are followed by an operation for intra-abdominal infection, and approximately 50 per cent of all serious intra-abdominal infections are postoperative. Wound infections are more common but less serious. Postoperative fever occurs frequently and may be a source of concern to the physician and patient. Fever is associated with infection, and the empiric prescription of antibiotics is a common response to this phenomenon. However, the majority of febrile postoperative patients are not infected, and, indeed, a significant proportion of infected patients may not be febrile, depending on the definition of *fever.* Because fever is common in the absence of infection, it is important to consider causes of postoperative fever other than infection and to make a presumptive diagnosis prior to the insitution of antibiotic treatment.

The most common nonsurgical causes of postoperative infection and fever—urinary tract infection, respiratory tract infection, and intravenous catheter-associated infection—are all readily diagnosed. The other important causes of postoperative infection and fever—wound infection and intra-abdominal infection—require operative treatment and are not properly managed with antibiotics in the absence of operative treatment. The most sensitive test for suspecting infection and determining its location continues to be a conscientious physician utilizing the time-honored skills of history and physical examination. Supportive laboratory and radiographic evaluation, including white blood cell count, blood cultures, and computerized tomography, can be quite useful in supplementing the physical examination. Fever in the first 3 days after operation is most likely to have a noninfectious etiology. However, when the fever begins 5 or more days postoperatively, the incidence of wound infections exceeds the incidence of undiagnosed fevers. Neither the prolongation of perioperative prophylactic antibiotics nor the initiation of empiric therapeutic antibiotics is indicated without a presumptive clinical diagnosis and a plan for operative intervention when indicated.

Only two important infectious causes of fever are likely in the first 36 hours after a laparotomy. Both can be diagnosed readily if they are suspected and appropriate examinations are made. The first is an injury to bowel with an intraperitoneal leak. This is characterized by marked hemodynamic changes, first tachycardia and then hypotension and a falling urinary output. Fluid requirements are large, and physical examination reveals diffuse abdominal tenderness. The other early cause of fever and infection is an invasive soft tissue infection, beginning in the wound, caused either by beta-hemolytic streptococci or by clos-

tridial species (most commonly *C. perfringens*). The diagnosis of this event is made by inspection of the wound and Gram's stain of wound fluid, which demonstrates either gram-positive cocci or gram-positive rods. White cells are usually present with streptococcal infections but may be absent in clostridial infection.

Nonsurgical Infections in Surgical Patients

Postoperative patients are at increased risk for a variety of nonsurgical postoperative nosocomial infections. The most common of these is urinary tract infection. Any patient who has had an indwelling urinary catheter as part of operative management is at increased risk for a urinary tract infection. Despite the benign course of most urinary tract infections, the occurrence of one in a surgical patient is associated with a threefold increase in deaths occurring during hospitalization. The best prevention is to use urinary catheters sparingly and for specific indications and to employ strict closed drainage techniques for those that are employed.

Lower respiratory tract infections are another common cause of nosocomial infection in surgical patients and are the leading cause of death due to nosocomial infection. Diagnosis is usually relatively straightforward in a patient who is breathing spontaneously. However, a patient who is intubated and being ventilated because of the adult respiratory distress syndrome (ARDS) presents an extremely difficult diagnostic problem. Patients with ARDS commonly have abnormal chest film findings, abnormal blood gas levels, and elevated temperatures and white blood cell counts even in the absence of infection. Both false-positive and false-negative diagnosis of pneumonia is common. A surgeon confronted with a postoperative patient with fever frequently considers pneumonia or atelectasis in the differential diagnosis. It should be remembered, however, that after an abdominal operation one of the most common causes of lower lung field atelectasis and/or pleural effusion is an inflammatory process below the diaphragm.

Prosthetic Device–Associated Infections

As the ability to replace parts of the body has increased, so has the potential for infectious complications associated with these replacements. Some of the most significant complications associated with vascular grafts, cardiac valves, pacemakers, and artificial joints are caused by infections at the site of implantation. The presence of the foreign material (the prosthetic device) impairs local host defenses, especially polymorphonuclear leukocyte function. Accordingly, most such infections resist treatment short of removing the offending device. Morbidity and mortality associated with infection are high. Some success can be obtained by intensive antibiotic therapy, removal of the device under antibiotic cover, and replacement with a new device, followed by prolonged antibiotic treatment. This approach is warranted when the device is life-sustaining, as in the case of a cardiac valve.

PATHOGENS IN SURGICAL INFECTIONS

This discussion of pathogens commonly responsible for surgical infection is not intended to be a complete review. Rather, it focuses on some broad distinctions and classifications that have been found helpful in organizing the vast body of data available concerning the usual bacterial flora of different surgical infections and the antibiotic susceptibility patterns of these pathogens. Bacteria important in surgical infection are broadly divided into aerobic and facultative bacteria in one group and anaerobic bacteria in the other; into gram-positive and gram-negative bacteria; and into bacilli (rods) and cocci.

Gram-Positive Cocci

Gram-positive cocci of importance to surgeons include staphylococci and streptococci. Staphylococci are divided into coagulase-positive and coagulase-negative strains. Coagulase-positive staphylococcus are *Staphylococcus aureus* and are the most common pathogen associated with infections in wounds and incisions not subject to endogenous contamination. In the 1990s most coagulase-positive staphylococci should be assumed resistant to penicillin and require treatment by a penicillinase-resistant antibiotic. Extensive use of penicillinase-resistant beta-lactam antibiotics during the past 2 decades has encouraged the emergence of methicillin-resistant *Staphylococcus aureus* (MRSA). These organisms do not appear to have intrinsic pathogenicity greater than that of other staphylococci, but they are more difficult to treat because of antibiotic resistance. The prevalence of MRSA varies considerably by geographic region. They are especially common in cases of endocarditis associated with intravenous drug use. Methicillin-resistant staphylococci must be treated with vancomycin or a similar agent.

Coagulase-negative staphylococci were considered contaminants and skin flora incapable of causing serious disease for many years. However, it has become increasingly clear that in the correct clinical setting coagulase-negative staphylococci can cause serious disease. This is most common in patients who have been compromised by trauma, extensive surgical procedures, or metabolic disease, and who have invasive vascular devices in place. Coagulase-negative staphylococci are the most common organisms recovered in nosocomial bacteremia and are frequently associated with clinically significant infections of intravascular devices. Coagulase-negative staphylococci are also found in endocarditis, prosthetic joint infections, vascular graft infections, and postsurgical mediastinitis. The majority of coagulase-negative staphylococci are methicillin-resistant. While most intravascular device–associated coagulase-negative staphylococcus infections are cured simply by removing the device, if empiric antibiotic therapy is indicated, it should be with vancomycin.

The streptococcal species include beta-hemolytic streptococci, *Streptococcus pneumoniae*, other alpha-hemolytic streptococci, and enterococci. The first three species are uniformly sensitive to penicillin G and almost all other beta-lactam antibiotics. The beta-hemolytic streptococci, while not commonly recovered from soft tissue wounds, are capable of causing life-threatening infections alone. *S. pneumoniae* is a common cause of community-acquired pneumonia but is a less common pathogen in hospitalized surgical patients. The other alpha-hemolytic streptococci or viridans streptococci are rarely significant pathogens in a surgical setting. They are commonly found on mucous membranes and skin and may be recovered from the peritoneal cavity after upper gastrointestinal perforations but are rarely found as the sole cause of significant surgical infections.

The precise significance of enterococci in surgical infections is controversial. Enterococci are commonly recovered as part of a mixed flora in intra-abdominal infections. It is rare to recover enterococci alone from a surgical infection. In animal models of infection, enterococci clearly can increase the virulence of other bacteria. Enterococcal bacteremia in association with a surgical infection has a grave prognosis. It is likely that the occurrence of the bacteremia itself signals a profound compromise of host defenses. Enterococci clearly cause significant disease in the urinary and biliary tracts and probably contribute to morbidity and mortality from intra-abdominal infections in high-risk patients with serious underlying diseases or protracted illnesses with impairment of host defenses. The stimulus for discussing the pathogenic significance of enterococci derives from the relative resistance of these species to antibiotic therapy. No single antibiotic is reliably effective for eradicating deep-seated infections or bacteremia. The most effective antibiotic combination for treating enterococcal infections is gentamicin combined with either ampicillin (or another advanced-generation penicillin) or vancomycin.

Aerobic and Facultative Gram-Negative Rods

A great variety of gram-negative rods are associated with surgical infections. The greatest number of these are included in the family Enterobacteriaceae. These are all facultative anaerobic bacteria and include the familiar genera, *Escherichia, Proteus,* and *Klebsiella*. These three genera ("easy" gram-negative rods) are considered together because they are relatively common in mixed surgical infections and because they tend to be relatively sensitive to a broad variety of antibiotics, especially first- and second-generation cephalosporins. Other genera within the Enterobacteriaceae that are also common in surgical infections include *Enterobacter, Morganella, Providencia,* and *Serratia*. These genera ("difficult" gram-negative rods) commonly exhibit greater intrinsic antimicrobial resistance. Empiric antibiotic therapy directed at these organisms requires a third-generation cephalosporin, one of the expanded spectrum penicillins, a monobactam, carbapenem, quinolone, or aminoglycoside. These organisms are more common in hospital-acquired and postoperative surgical infections. Infection by gram-negative rods recovered from infections originating in the community, such as uncomplicated appendicitis, is less likely to involve antibiotic-resistant strains.

Obligate aerobic gram-negative rods often found in surgical infections include *Pseudomonas* species and *Acinetobacter* species. These organisms are most commonly found in hospital-associated pneumonias in surgical patients but may also be recovered from the peritoneal cavity or severe soft tissue infections. These species are often antibiotic-resistant and require treatment with specific antipseudomonal antibiotics such as ceftazidime, aztreonam, imipenem, ciprofloxacin, an acylureido-penicillin, or an aminoglycoside. A significant proportion of these species exhibit strains resistant to even the most effective antibiotics, and patients with such pathogens are probably best treated empirically with two antibiotics prior to availability of *in vitro* susceptibility testing. Even after susceptibility data are known, critically ill patients may benefit from treatment with two effective agents. Bacteria from both of these genera have a tendency to develop resistance to antibiotics during therapy. While use of two agents cannot demonstrate reduction of this process, it leaves the patient with at least one effective drug when it occurs.

Anaerobes

Anaerobic bacteria are the most numerous inhabitants of the normal gastrointestinal tract, including the mouth. The most common anaerobic isolate from surgical infections is *Bacteroides fragilis*. *Bacteroides fragilis* and *Bacteroides thetaiotaomicron* are two common anaerobic species with significant resistance to many beta-lactam antibiotics. The most effective antibiotics against these species are metronidazole, clindamycin, chloramphenicol, imipenem, and the combination ticarcillin/clavulanate. Other anaerobic species commonly recovered from surgical infections but with less significant bacterial resistance patterns include *Bacteroides melaninogenicus* and most of the anaerobic cocci.

The other important genus of anaerobic bacteria found in surgical infections is *Clostridium,* previously mentioned under necrotizing soft tissue infections. While they can survive for variable periods exposed to oxygen, they require an anaerobic environment for growth and invasion and for elaboration of the toxins which represent their dramatic virulence in soft tissue infections. The *Clostridium* species are all gram-positive, spore-forming rods. However, when present in human infections they do not form spores; therefore, gram-stained material from a soft tissue infection demonstrates gram-positive rods without spores. *Clostridium tetani* is the member of this genus responsible for tetanus. The prevention of tetanus is accomplished solely through active and passive immunization and not through antibiotic administration.

Anaerobic bacteria have a special significance in relation to surgical infections. These strains grow only in settings with a low oxidation reduction potential that is incompatible with the survival of mammalian tissue. Thus, the recovery of anaerobes from a soft tissue infection or from the blood implies their growth and multiplication in a focus of dead tissue. The predominant source of anaerobic bacteria is the gastrointestinal tract; and thus, an anaerobic infection implies a defect in the anatomic integrity of the gastrointestinal tract. Both of these conditions require surgical correction; and thus, the great majority of anaerobic infections (other than lung abscess) require surgical intervention. Certainly an anaerobic bacteremia should always prompt a search for an abscess or for an enteric lesion that requires surgical intervention.

Fungi

Fungi are infrequently the primary pathogens in deep-seated surgical infections. Pathogens of the *Candida* genus, however, may be observed frequently as opportunistic invaders in patients with serious surgical infections who have received broad-spectrum antibiotic treatment suppressing normal endogenous flora. These infections are best avoided through judicious use of systemic broad-spectrum antibiotics and prophylaxis with oral nystatin or ketoconazole when broad-spectrum antibacterial therapy is required. *Candida* species recovered from open wounds usually represent contamination and not true invasion. Recovery of *Candida* species from peptic ulcer perforations also does not usually require treatment; however, recovery of *Candida* from an established intra-abdominal abscess or from urine and sputum in an otherwise compromised patient may warrant therapy. Intra-abdominal *Candida* infections are more common in association with infections following severe pancreatitis. Therapy for *Candida* infections in this setting is commonly successful with lower doses of amphotericin than are the doses used for systemic medical fungal infections with pathogens such as *Cryptococcus, Blastomyces,* or *Histoplasma.* Surgical patients with fungal colonization of multiple sites or with fungi in well-drained abscesses have been managed successfully with total doses of amphotericin, 3 to 5 mg./kg. administered over 10 to 14 days. There are few data available regarding the efficacy of ketoconazole in this setting.

Viruses

Viruses do not cause any infections that require operative intervention for resolution and thus are not discussed in any detail in this chapter. As a result of immune suppression for the prevention of rejection, transplant patients are at significant risk of viral infection, especially with cytomegalovirus. The viral infections of most relevance to routine surgical patients are the blood-borne viruses, which may be transmitted as a result of blood transfusion. These are the hepatitis B virus (HBV), the hepatitis C virus (HBC, formerly included in non-A, non-B), and the human immunodeficiency virus (HIV). Currently transmission of HBV and HIV is unusual because of the use of accurate tests for screening infected units of blood. At this time, HBC is one of the most common viruses transmitted by transfusion in the medical setting. A new test for this virus should greatly reduce that risk. Cytomegalovirus is also commonly transmitted by transfusions. It is quite likely, however, that other blood-borne viruses (including hepatitis non-A, non-B, non-C?) will be described in the future. For this reason, it is consistent with good medical practice to limit blood transfusion to circumstances clearly requiring it.

ANTIBIOTICS

The discussion of antibiotics that follows is not intended to be exhaustive. Rather, it focuses on those antibiotics that are most commonly indicated in the treatment of patients with surgical infections. Antibiotics with their relative half-lives, important toxicities, and general antibacterial spectra are listed in Table 5. Several references exist that provide more detailed information regarding all commercially available antibiotics, doses and dose ranges, pharmacokinetic data, sensitivity patterns, incompatibilities, excretion data, and other information.

One of the largest and most versatile classes of antibiotics is the beta-lactam group. Penicillin G was the prototype of this group, which now includes the penicillins, the cephalosporins, the carbapenems, and the monobactams. All of these antibiotics possess the four-member beta-lactam ring (Fig. 2). All but the monobactams have another ring attached, and all have various side chains that determine their antibacterial activity, enzyme stability, and pharmacokinetic characteristics (see Fig. 2). All of this group act on bacteria by binding to one of several penicillin-binding proteins and interfering with bacterial cell wall synthesis.

PENICILLINS. The penicillins are broadly divided into those that are stable against staphylococcal penicillinase and all others. The antistaphylococcal penicillins are active against methicillin-susceptible staphylococcal species but have reduced activity against streptococcal species and essentially no activity against gram-negative rods or anaerobic bacteria. All the remaining penicillins are readily hydrolyzed by staphylococcal penicillinase and are therefore unreliable for treating staphylococcal infections. They all have excellent activity against other gram-positive cocci with the exception of enterococci, which are variably resistant. The major difference among these penicillins is in their spectrum of aerobic and facultative gram-negative rod activity. The more advanced acylureido-penicillins are very active against this group, including the "difficult" gram-negative rods.

Recently, various penicillins have been combined with one of the beta-lactamase inhibitors, clavulanic acid or sulbactam. These combinations provide antibiotic compounds that retain their broad gram-negative activity while also providing activity against methicillin-sensitive staphylococci and anaerobes, facultative species, and aerobic bacteria that are resistant to the penicillins by virtue of beta-lactamase production. The beta-lactamases produced by some *Escherichia coli,* and by *Pseudomonas* species, *Enterobacter* species, *Citrobacter* species, and *Serratia* species, however, are not susceptible to these inhibitors; and so these organisms are not susceptible to the antibiotic combinations that rely on clavulanic acid or sulbactam unless they are susceptible to the antibiotic alone.

CEPHALOSPORINS. The cephalosporin class is currently the largest and most frequently used group of antibiotics. It is commonly divided into three "generations," but there are also important differences between members within each generation. The first-generation cephalosporins have excellent activity against methicillin-susceptible staphylococci and all streptococ-

TABLE 5. Antibiotics Commonly Used in Surgical Practice

Drug Class and Name	Comment	Half-life	Toxicity	Antibacterial Spectrum
Penicillins Penicillin G	Prototype. Hydrolyzed by all beta-lactamases.	Short	Low, but rarely allergic reaction may be life-threatening.	Streptococcal species except enterococcus; *Neisseria* species, except lactamase-producing gonococci.
Antistaphylococcal Methicillin	First antistaphylococcal drug.	Short	Interstitial nephritis.	Staphylococcal species (methicillin-sensitive) and streptococcal species except *Enterococcus*.
Oxacillin		Short	Same	
Nafcillin		Short	Same	Narrow spectrum: usually used for staphylococcal infections only.

"Easy" gram-negative
  Ampicillin
  Amoxicillin
	Hydrolyzed by all beta-lactamases.	Low
		Medium
			Diarrhea and rashes.
			Same
				Streptococcal species including enterococcus, *Neisseria* species (non–lactamase-producing), *Haemophilus influenzae* (non–lactamase-producing), some *E. coli* and *Proteus mirabilis*.

Expanded spectrum Carbenicillin	Hydrolyzed by all beta-lactamases.	Short	High sodium load. Inhibition of platelet aggregation.	Greatly expanded gram-negative spectrum while still active against streptococcal species including *Enterococcus*.
Ticarcillin	Same	Short		Moderate antianaerobe activity. May not be reliable as sole agent for established gram-negative rod infections.

Very advanced spectrum
  Mezlocillin
  Piperacillin
	Hydrolyzed by all beta-lactamases.	Short
		Short
			Low
			Low
				Same as expanded-spectrum penicillins with more activity against *Pseudomonas, Acinetobacter,* and *Serratia* species.

Beta-lactamase inhibitor combinations			Low; same as constituent beta-lactam.	

Clavulanic acid plus
  Ticarcillin
  Amoxicillin
	
	Oral only.
		
		Short
		Medium
				Same as ticarcillin or amoxicillin plus staphylococcus (methicillin-sensitive), lactamase-positive *H. influenzae*, and some lactamase-producing gram-negative rods and anaerobes.

Sulbactam plus Ampicillin	IV only.	Short		Similar to cefoxitin with activity against enterococcus.

Cephalosporins
  "First" Generation
  Short half-life
   Cephalothin
   Cephapirin
	
	Prototype of class.
		
		Short
		Short
			
			Low
			Low
				Streptococcal species except *Enterococcus*, staphylococcal species (methicillin-sensitive), and "easy" gram-negative rods.

Longer half-life Cefazolin		Medium	Low	

"Second" generation
  Poor anaerobic activity
  Shorter half-life
   Cefamandole
   Cefuroxime
		
		Short
		Medium
			
			Low
			Low
				Same as first-generation cephalosporins with expanded gram-negative activity *not* including *Pseudomonas, Acinetobacter,* or *Serratia*.

Longer half-life
   Ceforanide
   Cefonicid
	
	Reduced antistaphylococcal activity.
		Long
		Long
			Low
			Low	

Good anaerobic activity
  Short half-life
   Cefoxitin
		
		Short
			
			Low
				Same as above plus most anaerobes.

Longer half-life Cefotetan		Long	Prolonged prothrombin times.	

"Third" generation
  Poor *Pseudomonas* activity
  Short half-life
   Cefotaxime
   Ceftizoxime
		
		Short
		Medium
			
			Low
			Low
				Very active against most gram-negative rods except *Pseudomonas, Acinetobacter,* and *Serratia*. Poor against anaerobes.
				
				Less activity against streptococcal and staphylococcal species than first- and second-generation cephalosporins.

Long half-life Ceftriaxone		Long	Low	Same as above plus activity against many *pseudomonas, Acinetobacter,* and *Serratia* species.

Good *Pseudomonas* activity
   Cefoperazone
   Ceftazidime
		Medium
		Medium
			Low
			Low	

Monobactams Aztreonam	Safe for most patients	Short	Low	Excellent activity against most gram-negatives,

TABLE 5. Antibiotics Commonly Used in Surgical Practice *Continued*

Drug Class and Name	Comment	Half-life	Toxicity	Antibacterial Spectrum
	with penicillin allergy.			including *Pseudomonas* and *Serratia*. Inactive against gram-positive cocci, anaerobes, and most *Acinetobacter* strains.
Carbapenems				
Imipenem	Provided combined with cilastatin to prevent renal breakdown and renal toxicity.	Short	Low. Seizures in certain high-risk patients.	Extremely broad gram-positive and gram-negative aerobic and anaerobic. Modest activity against *Enterococcus*. Inactive against *Xanthomonas maltophilia*.
Quinolones				
Norfloxacin	Oral only; urine levels only.		Low	Very broad gram-negative activity.
Ciprofloxacin	Oral only; IV in the near future.	Long	Interaction leads to accumulation of theophylline.	Gram-positive and very broad gram-negative activity including *Pseudomonas*, *Acinetobacter*, and *Serratia*.
Aminoglycosides	All have low ratio of therapeutic/toxic levels. All are frequently underdosed. All exhibit significant postantibiotic effect.*	Medium	Nephrotoxicity and VIII nerve toxicity, both auditory and vestibular.	Extremely broad coverage of gram-negative rods. Poor activity against streptococci. Some synergism with penicillins or vancomycin against enterococci. No activity against anaerobes.
Gentamicin	See above.	Medium	See above.	Most active against enterococci and serratia.
Tobramycin	See above.	Medium	Statistically but questionably clinically significant decrease in nephrotoxicity.	More active against *Pseudomonas*.
Amikacin	See above.	Medium	See above (aminoglycosides).	Active against a significant number of gentamicin- and tobramycin-resistant organisms.
Netilmicin	See above.	Medium	See above (aminoglycosides).	See above (aminoglycosides).
Other				
Antianaerobes				
Chloramphenicol	Oral or IV.	Long†	Dose-dependent, reversible bone marrow suppression. Rare (1/25,000–40,000) irreversible bone-marrow aplasia.	Many gram-positive and easy gram-negative rods, *H. influenzae*, most anaerobes.
Clindamycin	Oral or IV.	Long†		Streptococcal species except enterococci, staphylococci, most anaerobes. Inactive against gram-negative rods.
Metronidazole	Oral or IV.	Long†	Disulfiram-type (Antabuse) reaction. Peripheral neuropathy with prolonged use.	Very active against most anaerobes. Inactive against facultative and aerobic bacteria. Active against protozoa (*Amoeba* and *Giardia*).
Glocypeptides				
Vancomycin		Long	Hypertension and histamine release phenomena (Redman syndrome) during infusion. Nephrotoxicity and ototoxicity.	Streptococcal species, including many enterococci, staphylococci (including methicillin-resistant strains), clostridium species. No activity against gram-negative rods.
Macrolides				
Erythromycin	Oral or IV.	Medium	Cholestasis with estolate (IV) form.	Most gram-positive, *Neisseria*, *Campylobacter*, *Mycoplasma*, *Chlamydia*, *Rickettsia*, *Legionella*.
Tetracyclines				
Tetracycline	Oral or IV.	Long	Stains teeth of children.	Many gram-positive, easy gram-negative rods, some anaerobes, *Rickettsia*, *Chlamydia*, *Mycoplasma*.
Doxycycline	Oral or IV.	Very long		
Antifungal				
Amphotericin		Very long	Nephrotoxicity, fever and chills.	Most fungi.
Ketoconazole	Oral only.	Long		Many fungi.

Drugs have been grouped into those with short, medium, and long half-lives. Short half-life drugs usually have a half-life of 1 hour or less and are commonly administered every 3 to 6 hours, depending on the severity of the infection and the sensitivity of the pathogen. Medium half-life drugs usually have half-lives of 1 to 2 hours and are administered every 6 to 12 hours, most commonly every 8 hours. Long half-life drugs have half-lives longer than 2 hours and are usually administered every 12 to 24 hours. Amphotericin with a half-life of approximately 24 hours can be administered every other day.

* The postantibiotic effect is the effect of certain antibiotics which results in inhibition of bacterial growth for several hours *after* the antibiotic levels have fallen below the minimal inhibitory concentration.

† Chloramphenicol, clindamycin, and metronidazole all have half-lives greater than 2 hours but traditionally have been administered at 6- to 8-hour intervals.

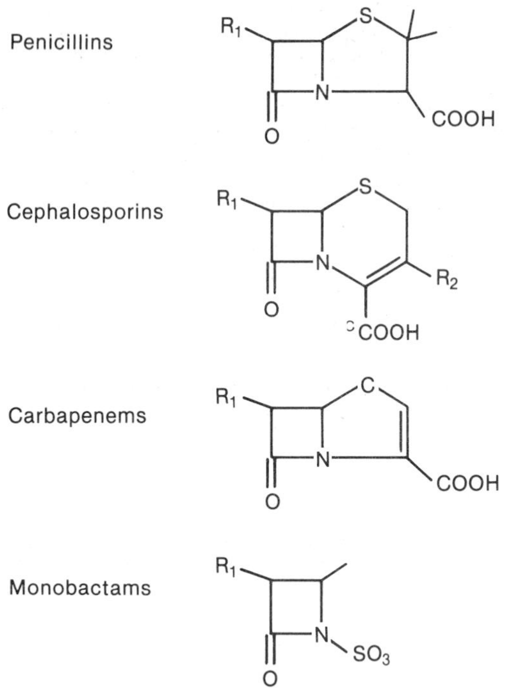

Penicillins

Cephalosporins

Carbapenems

Monobactams

Figure 2. The four-member beta-lactam ring. R_1, R_2, side chains.

cal species except enterococci. No cephalosporin in any generation has reliable activity against enterococci, and indeed many cephalosporins appear to encourage enterococcal overgrowth. The first-generation cephalosporins also have modest activity against the "easy" Enterobacteriaceae such as *E. coli*, *Proteus mirabilis*, and many *Klebsiella* species. The only important difference between members of the first generation is in half-life. Cefazolin, with its longer half-life, can be administered every 8 hours, rather than 4 to 6 hours, and maintains more reliable serum and tissue levels when used for prophylaxis when compared with the other members of this class.

The second-generation cephalosporins have expanded gram-negative activity when compared with the first generation but still lack activity against many gram-negative rods. They can be employed when susceptibility patterns are known or when community-acquired infections with a low probability of antibiotic-resistant bacteria are being treated. This class of antibiotics is not reliable for empiric treatment of hospital-acquired gram-negative rod infections. The most important distinction within the second generation is between those antibiotics with good activity against anaerobes (cefoxitin and cefotetan) and those without important anaerobic activity (cefamandole, ceforanide, and cefonicid). Within each of these groups are antibiotics with relatively short half-lives (cefamandole and cefoxitin) and with relatively long half-lives (cefotetan, ceforanide, and cefonicid).

The third-generation cephalosporins have greatly expanded activity against gram-negative rods, including many resistant strains, and rival the aminoglycosides in their coverage while having a much more favorable safety profile. In exchange for this gram-negative coverage, most members of this group have significantly less activity against staphylococci and streptococcal species than first- and second-generation cephalosporins. Anaerobic coverage is, in general, rather poor as well. The important distinction in the third-generation cephalosporins is between those with significant activity against *Pseudomonas* species (cefoperazone and ceftazidime) and those without (cefotaxime, ceftizoxime, and ceftriaxone).

MONOBACTAMS. Aztreonam is the only currently available member of the class of monobactams. It has gram-negative coverage, including most *Pseudomonas* species, similar to the aminoglycosides, and, like the aminoglycosides, lacks signifi-

cant activity against gram-positive cocci and anaerobes. It has the safety profile of other beta-lactam antibiotics but does not cross-react in patients who are allergic to penicillins or cephalosporins.

CARBAPENEMS. Imipenem is the first representative of the class of carbapenems. It has probably the broadest spectrum of antibacterial activity of any antibiotic currently available. It has excellent activity against all gram-positive cocci, with the exception of methicillin-resistant staphylococci and only modest activity against enterococci. It is very active against all anaerobic bacteria. It has broad activity against gram-negative rods, including most *Pseudomonas* species, but it is inactive against *Pseudomonas cepacia* and *Xanthomonas maltophilia* (formerly *Pseudomonas maltophilia*), and strains of indole-positive *Proteus* are often resistant. As with all other antibiotics, *Pseudomonas* species have an unfortunate propensity to develop resistance during treatment. Imipenem is provided only in combination with the enzyme inhibitor, cilastatin, which prevents its hydrolysis in the kidneys and resultant nephrotoxicity.

QUINOLONES. The quinolone class of antibiotics was long represented solely by nalidixic acid, useful only for urinary tract infections. More recently, a large number of quinolone antibiotics are in development; two are currently available. As a class, the quinolones are marked by extremely broad activity against gram-negative rods, including *Pseudomonas* species. Most also have relatively broad activity against gram-positive cocci, including some methicillin-resistant staphylococci, although there is insufficient clinical information to recommend their routine use against methicillin-resistant staphylococci. Activity against anaerobes is mixed but generally not impressive. The currently available members of this class are norfloxacin, which has useful levels only in the urine, and ciprofloxacin, which is effective against sensitive pathogens throughout the body. Ciprofloxacin is currently available only as an oral drug, but a parenteral form should be available soon.

AMINOGLYCOSIDES. For many years the aminoglycoside class of antibiotics was the only reliable class of drugs for the empiric treatment of serious gram-negative infections. In recent years, the availability of third-generation cephalosporins, advanced generation penicillins, monobactams, carbapenems, and now quinolones has greatly reduced instances in which aminoglycosides must be employed. As a class, aminoglycosides have very broad activity against aerobic and facultative gram-negative rods. They have relatively indifferent activity against gram-positive cocci but are an important component of synergistic therapy against enterococci when combined with a penicillin or vancomycin. Aminoglycosides have no activity against anaerobes or against facultative bacteria in an anaerobic environment.

Clinically aminoglycosides are difficult to use because the ratio of therapeutic levels to toxic levels is low, approximately 2 to 3. The primary toxicities are nephrotoxicity and eighth nerve damage, both auditory and vestibular. Aminoglycosides distribute in interstitial fluid, a body compartment that tends to vary significantly with disease and is greatly enlarged in patients with life-threatening infections. For this reason aminoglycoside doses and intervals of administration need to be individualized, and the results must be confirmed by determination of serum levels. No nomogram or dosing scheme is sufficiently reliable to be recommended without this testing. In routine clinical practice, it is far more common to find inadequate levels of aminoglycosides than toxic levels. Because of these difficulties, many clinicians now reserve aminoglycosides for specific therapy of known resistant organisms or as part of a synergistic combination to treat serious enterococcal infections or certain gram-negative rod infections.

ANTI-ANAEROBES. The antibiotics with important anti-anaerobic activity are not logically grouped except by this characteristic. The oldest effective anti-anaerobe drug is chloramphenicol. It is still very active against most anaerobic pathogens by *in vitro* testing but is uncommonly used because of its potential for bone marrow toxicity. Clindamycin possesses excellent activity against more anaerobic bacteria as well as most gram-positive bacteria. Its complete lack of activity against gram-negative aerobic and facultative rods implies that it must always be used essentially in combination with another antibiotic to cover these pathogens, which commonly accompany anaerobes in clinical infections.

Metronidazole is the antibiotic that currently possesses the most complete activity against all anaerobic pathogens. It has, however, no activity against any aerobic or facultative pathogen, either gram-negative or gram-positive. Accordingly, it must always be combined with another antibiotic for complete coverage. Because it has no activity against the gram-positive cocci as clindamycin does, its combination with an aminoglycoside in the treatment of mixed aerobic and anaerobic infections leaves this potentially important group of pathogens uncovered. For this reason, metronidazole is theoretically better combined with a third-generation cephalosporin. No actual trials confirm the importance of this recommendation. Other antibiotics with important anti-anaerobic activity, including cefoxitin, cefotetan, ticarcillin/clavulanate, and imipenem are discussed elsewhere.

MACROLIDES. Erythromycin is a macrolide antibiotic with only modest anti-anaerobic activity in the concentrations that can be achieved systemically. It has found widespread use, however, as an oral agent (erythromycin base) used in combination with an aminoglycoside for reduction of numbers of bacteria in the lumen of the bowel prior to operations on the colon. In the concentrations achieved within the lumen of the colon, it achieves marked suppression of anaerobic growth. Erythromycin is also active against most gram-positive cocci and the *Neisseria* species. For this reason, it is sometimes used as an alternate agent for patients allergic to penicillins. In addition, it has significant activity against mycoplasmas, *Chlamydia*, *Legionella* species, and *Rickettsia*. It is also an effective antibiotic against *Campylobacter jejuni*.

TETRACYCLINES. Two decades ago tetracyclines were an important class of antibiotics with significant anti-anaerobic activity. In addition to activity against anaerobes, tetracyclines possess modest activity against easy gram-negative rods and many gram-positive cocci. In the 1990s, other agents are preferable as first and second choices for the overwhelming majority of surgical infections.

GLYCOPEPTIDES. Vancomycin is currently the only glycopeptide antibiotic available, but another (teicoplanin) is currently undergoing clinical testing. Vancomycin is active against essentially all gram-positive cocci, especially the methicillin-resistant staphylococci, for which it is currently the only reliable antibiotic. It also has moderate activity against enterococci. Vancomycin is active against most *Clostridium* species, especially *C. difficile*, the primary pathogen responsible for antibiotic-associated diarrhea.

General Principles

Whichever antibiotics are employed, the goal of therapy is to achieve levels of antibiotics at the site of infection that exceed the minimal inhibitory concentration for the pathogens present. For mild infections, including most that can be managed on an outpatient basis, this may be achievable with oral antibiotics when appropriate choices are available. For severe surgical infections, however, the systemic response to infection may make gastrointestinal absorption of antibiotics unpredictable and thus antibiotic levels unreliable. In addition, for intra-abdominal infections, there is often direct impairment of gastrointestinal function. For this reason, most initial antibiotic therapy of surgical infections is initiated intravenously.

Each patient with a serious infection should be evaluated daily or more frequently to assess response to treatment. If obvious improvement is not observed within 2 to 3 days, one often hears the question, "Which antibiotic should be added/switched to?" That question is appropriate, however, only after the following question has been addressed: Why is the patient failing to improve? Likely answers include the following:

1. The initial operative procedure was not adequate.
2. The initial procedure was adequate, but a complication has occurred.
3. A superinfection has developed at a new site.
4. The drug choice is correct but not sufficiently administered.
5. Another/a different drug is needed.

The choice of antibiotics is not the most common cause for failure unless the original choice was clearly inappropriate, such as failing to provide coverage for anaerobes in an intra-abdominal infection.

As the patient improves, a decision must be made to discontinue antibiotics. For most surgical infections, there is not a specific duration of antibiotics known to be ideal. Antibiotics generally serve to support local host defenses until the local responses are sufficient to limit further infection. When an abscess is drained, the antibiotics prevent invasive bacterial infection in the fresh tissue planes opened in the course of drainage. After 3 to 5 days, the local responses of new capillary formation and inflammatory infiltrate provide a competent local defense. For deep-seated or poorly localized infections, longer treatment may be required. A good guideline is to continue antibiotics until the patient has demonstrated an obvious clinical improvement based on clinical examination with a normal temperature for 48 hours or more. Signs of improvement include improved mental status, return of bowel function, and spontaneous diuresis.

The white blood cell count has not always returned to normal when antibiotics are discontinued. If the white blood cell count is normal, the likelihood of further infectious problems is minor. If the white blood cell count is elevated, further infections may be detected; but in most cases they are not prevented by continuing antibiotics. Rather, a new infection requires drainage or different antibiotics for a new, resistant pathogen in a different location. In this case, the best approach is to discontinue the existing drugs and observe the patient closely for subsequent developments.

SUPERINFECTION. A superinfection is defined as a new infection that develops during antibiotic treatment for the original infection. Whenever antibiotics are used, they exert a selective pressure on the endogenous flora of the patient and on exogenous bacteria that colonize sites at risk. Bacteria that remain are resistant to the antibiotics employed and become the pathogens in superinfection. Respiratory tract infections are common superinfections that occur during the treatment of intra-abdominal infection. The greater the severity of the abdominal infection and the greater the risk of poor outcome from it, the greater the risk of pneumonia as well.

Careful surveillance of hospitalized patients reveals superinfections in 2 to 10 per cent of antibiotic-treated patients, depending on the underlying risk factors. The best preventive action is limiting the dose and duration of antibiotic treatment to that obviously required and being alert to the possibility of superinfections. The use of increasingly powerful and broad-spectrum antibiotics during the past 2 decades has also led to an increasing incidence of fungal superinfections.

Antibiotic-associated colitis is another significant superinfection that can occur in hospitalized patients with mild to serious illness. The entity is caused by the enteric pathogen, *Clostridium difficile*, and has been reported after treatment with every antibiotic except vancomycin. *C. difficile* colitis can vary from a mild, self-limited disease to a rapidly progressive septic process culminating in death. The most important aspect of treating this disease is suspecting it. Diagnosis is by endoscopy, revealing the typical mucosal changes with inflammation, ulceration, and plaque formation, stool assay for the characteristic toxin, and stool culture to recover *C. difficile.* Treatment is supportive with fluid and electrolytes, withdrawal of the offending antibiotic if possible, and oral vancomycin or metronidazole to treat the superinfection.

SELECTED REFERENCES

Alexander, J. W.: The contributions of infection control to a century of surgical process. Ann. Surg., 201:423, 1985.
The role of infection control in the development of surgical practice is highlighted.

Alexander, J. W., Aerni, S., and Plettner, J. P.: Development of a safe and effective one-minute preoperative skin preparation. Arch. Surg., 120:1357, 1985.
Report of a controlled clinical trial of the use of a 1-minute preparation and an incise drape, compared with a standard scrub with antimicrobial soap and the use of wound towels.

Alexander, J. W., Fischer, J. E., Boyajian, M., Palmquist, J., and Morris, M. J.: The influence of hair-removal methods on wound infections. Arch. Surg., 118:347, 1983.
The adverse effect of shaving to remove hair is demonstrated in this prospective controlled study.

Altemeier, W. A., Burke, J. F., Pruitt, B. A., Jr., and Sandusky, W.: Control of surgical infection of the Committee on Pre- and Postoperative Care, American College of Surgeons, 2nd ed. Philadelphia, J. B. Lippincott Company, 1984.
This is a manual used by all personnel who have an interest in the control of surgical infection. It is an official publication of the American College of Surgeons and a summary of reports and discussions of worldwide authorities in the field of surgical infections.

Bennett, J. V., and Brachman, P. (Eds.): Nosocomial Infections. Boston, Little, Brown and Company, 1986.
This multiauthored text provides a cross section and compilation of data related to hospital-acquired infections. It is highly recommended for an understanding of these complications.

Burke, J. F.: The effective period of preventing antibiotic action in experimental incisions and dermal lesions. Surgery, 50:161, 1961.
This classic study demonstrates the importance of the definitive short period during which developing staphylococcal dermal or incisional wound infection may be suppressed by antibiotics. It emphasizes the fact that antibiotics give maximal suppression if given before bacteria gain access to the tissues.

Cruse, P. J. E., and Foord, R.: A five year prospective study of 23,649 surgical wounds. Arch. Surg., 107:206, 1973
This retrospective analysis provides remarkably clear insight into the factors which predispose to wound infections.

Dellinger, E. P.: Severe necrotizing soft-tissue infections: Multiple disease entities requiring a common approach. J.A.M.A., 246:1717, 1981.
This paper discusses, compares, and contrasts the various forms of necrotizing soft tissue infection. It illustrates the differences between clostridial and nonclostridial infections and the common elements of treatment for all necrotizing soft tissue infections.

Dellinger, E. P.: Use of scoring systems to assess patients with surgical sepsis. Surg. Clin. North Am., 6:123, 1988.
This paper compares and contrasts a variety of scoring systems that have been used to assess surgical infections.

Dellinger, E. P.: Approach to the patient with post-operative fever. *In* Gorbach, S. L., Bartlett, J. G., and Blacklow, N. R. (Eds.): Infectious Diseases in Medicine and Surgery. Philadelphia, W. B. Saunders Co., 1990.
This paper discusses the incidence of postoperative fever, its various causes, and the approach to diagnosis and management of postoperative fevers.

Dellinger, E. P., Wertz, M. J., Meakins, J. L., et al.: Surgical infection stratification (SIS) system for intraabdominal infection: Multicenter trial. Arch. Surg., 120:21, 1985.
This paper describes the application of an infection severity scoring system to 187 patients operated on for peritonitis or an intra-abdominal abscess.

Finegold, S. M.: Anaerobic Bacteria in Human Disease. New York, Academic Press, 1977.
This is a clinically oriented text on infections caused by anaerobic bacteria. It is an excellent reference and a practical guide that is useful for students, residents, and surgeons in the diagnosis and treatment of many anaerobic bacterial diseases.

Garibaldi, R. A.: Prevention of intraoperative wound contamination with chlorhexidine shower and scrub. J. Hosp. Infect. 11(Suppl. B):5, 1988.
One of several articles demonstrating the benefit of a preoperative shower with an antimicrobial agent.

Hau, T., Ahrenholz, D. H., and Simmons, R. L.: Secondary bacterial peritonitis: the biologic basis of treatment. Curr. Prob. Surg., 16:1, 1979.
This now classic monograph explores the pathophysiology of peritonitis and the scientific rationale for currently employed treatment approaches.

Hau, T., Haaga, J. R., and Aeder, M. I.: Pathophysiology, diagnosis, and treatment of abdominal abscesses. Curr. Prob. Surg., 21:1, 1984.
This comprehensive monograph examines in detail the diagnosis and treatment of intra-abdominal abscesses.

Knighton, D. R., Fiegel, V. D., Halverson, T., Schneider, S., Brown, T., and Wells, C. L.: Oxygen as an antibiotic. The effect of inspired oxygen on bacterial clearance. Arch. Surg., 125:97, 1990.
The rather profound effect of adequate oxygenation is reviewed in this article.

Laufman, H.: Current use of skin and wound cleansers and antiseptics. Am. J. Surg., 157:359, 1989.
A recent review of antiseptics for skin preparation.

Moylan, J. A., Fitzpatrick, K. T., and Davenport, K. E.: Reducing wound infections. Improved gown and drape barrier performance. Arch. Surg., 122:152, 1987.
Reduction of infection rates is related to gown and drape performance.

Pechere, J. C., Acar, J., Armengaud, M., Grenier, B., Moellering, R., Jr., Sande, M., Waldvogel, E., Zinner, S., and Cherubin, C.: Infections: Recognition, understanding, treatment. Philadelphia, Lea & Febiger, 1984.
This multiauthored text provides a review of infections in general including many nonsurgical infections. Its design is geared toward the practicing clinician, and the concepts are well presented.

Polk, H. C., and Ausobsky, J. R.: The role of antibiotics in surgical infections. Adv. Surg., 216:225, 1983.
A good review integrating physiology and antimicrobial considerations.

Polk, H. C., Jr., and Fry, D. E.: Radical peritoneal debridement for established peritonitis: The result of a prospective randomized clinical trial. Ann. Surg., 192:350, 1980.
A well-conducted trial addressing an important question in a complex area.

Roote, R. D., Trunkey, D. D., and Saunde, M. A. (Eds.): New surgical and medical approaches in infectious diseases. New York, Churchill Livingstone, 1987.
This multiauthor book explores a variety of infectious disease areas of interest to surgeons.

Sanford, J. P.: Guide to antimicrobial therapy—1989. West Bethesda, Antimicrobial Therapy, Inc., 1989.
This pocket-sized guide lists every available antibiotic, its usual spectrum of activity, half-life, dosing recommendations, usual indications, and side effects. It is updated yearly.

Simmons, R. L., and Howard, R. J. (Eds.): Surgical Infectious Disease. East Norwalk, Connecticut, Appleton and Lange, 1988.
This important text is devoted entirely to the problem of surgical infections. It is a well-written and comprehensive review of the entire field.

Tobin, G. R.: Closure of contaminated wounds. Biologic and technical considerations. Surg. Clin. North Am., 64:639, 1984.
This is a condensed review of the basic principles involved.

Wilmore, D. W., Brennan, M. F., Harken, A. H., Holcroft, J. W., and Meakins, J. D. (Eds.): American College of Surgeons: Care of the Surgical Patient, Section IX: Infection. New York, Scientific American, Inc., 1989.
This section of a larger text, which is a publication of the Committee on Pre- and Postoperative Care of the American College of Surgeons, contains nine chapters exploring various aspects of infection important to the surgical patient. It is a loose-leaf text that is updated periodically as new developments become available.

II ―――――――――――――――――――――――――――――――――

SURGICAL ASPECTS OF THE ACQUIRED IMMUNODEFICIENCY SYNDROME

Douglas S. Tyler, M.D., and H. Kim Lyerly, M.D.

The acquired immunodeficiency syndrome (AIDS) features profound defects in cellular immunity, leading to opportunistic infections and unusual neoplasms and was first recognized in homosexual men in 1981.[72,131,172] It was subsequently described in intravenous drug users, Haitian immigrants, recipients of factor VIII concentrates, blood transfusion recipients, and children and sexual partners of AIDS patients.[17,18,41] Gallo, at the National Institutes of Health, and Montagnier, at the Pasteur Institute, share credit for discovering the human retrovirus that is the causative agent of AIDS and was subsequently termed human immunodeficiency virus Type 1 (HIV-1).[11,64]

HIV-1 is a single-strand RNA virus, approximately 100 nm. in diameter, with a characteristic cylindrical nucleoid core containing core proteins, genomic RNA, and the RNA-dependent DNA polymerase, reverse transcriptase. The core is surrounded by a viral envelope derived from the membrane of the host cell and is studded by the viral envelope glycoproteins GP 120 and GP 41.[71,155]

HIV-1 has a unique tropism for the CD4 molecule found on T-helper/inducer cells and monocytes/macrophages, although a number of other cells can be infected. The HIV-1 replication cycle begins by the binding of the virion to the target cell by a specific interaction between the viral envelope and the host cell membrane. This specificity is due to the high-affinity binding of the GP 120 studded in the viral envelope and the target cell CD4 molecule.[43,100,109,124]

After virus adsorption and internalization of the viral core components, reverse transcription of the viral RNA genome leads to a double-strand copy of the viral genome that can be incorporated into the host DNA. It is this step that is terminated by zidovudine (AZT), a thymidine analog that undergoes intracellular triphosphorylation and acts as a chain terminator for the reverse transcriptase-driven elongation of HIV-1 DNA.[135] However, when the viral genome is incorporated into the host genome, AZT cannot halt expression of the viral DNA, which is controlled by viral and host regulatory elements and leads to the production of infectious progeny.[8,180] Release of infectious progeny may lead to the destruction or dysfunction of the infected cell.

Because the CD4-expressing T helper/inducer cell has a key role in the host cellular immune system by orchestrating the proliferation of natural killer cells and cytotoxic T cells, any disturbance in T-helper/inducer cell number or function has dire consequences for the host.[12,52,108] The development of AIDS in a patient infected with HIV-1 reflects the presence of profound damage to the cellular immune system caused by years of HIV-1–induced T-helper/inducer cell depletion or dysfunction; however the exact pathogenesis of the immune defects observed in patients with HIV-1 infection is not completely understood at present.

The current understanding of the natural history of clinical HIV-1 infection is incomplete. Acute infection with HIV-1 may cause a mononucleosis-like syndrome, but after the acute infection a variable asymptomatic period may occur.[182] This period may be influenced by factors such as the inoculum of HIV-1 received or the immune status of the host and may last as long as 7 to 10 years.[118] After infection, the patient usually responds

with specific anti–HIV-1 antibodies, which are usually detectable within 6 to 8 weeks; however, periods as long as years may pass before antibodies can be detected in infected individuals.[4,63,153,194] In patients who are infected but are seronegative the infection is not detected by routine testing, which relies on antibody detection, but is detected by determining the presence of specific viral antigens or nucleic acids.[92]

The asymptomatic period may be followed by symptomatic disease consisting of constitutional signs such as weight loss, fever, night sweats, or infections that do not meet the criteria for the complete syndrome known as AIDS-related complex (ARC).[25] Other manifestations of progressive HIV-1 infection include immune thrombocytopenia and neurologic disease.[88,90,121,136] AIDS represents the most severe manifestation of infection with HIV-1; however, it appears that although a wide spectrum of syndromes may exist after HIV-1 infection, most, if not all, of those infected develop AIDS within a mean period of 8 years.[118]

AIDS as defined by CDC criteria (Table 1) is characterized by a progressive lymphopenia, predominantly of T-helper/inducer cells, that is clinically manifested threatening opportunistic infections and malignancies. When an individual has been diagnosed with AIDS, a clinical course characterized by recurrent infections and/or neoplasms is anticipated for the remaining lifetime. Life expectancy is estimated to be less than 1 year without specific anti–HIV-1 therapy.[126,163] Although great strides have been made in managing the infectious and neoplastic complications of AIDS, the severity and current irreversibility of the immune defects associated with AIDS lead to perpetual susceptibility to infections. Despite recent studies with anti–HIV-1 chemotherapy that have demonstrated some progress, no curative therapy is currently available. The use of AZT has led to an improvement in the quality and length of life for patients with AIDS and has been demonstrated to decrease the number and severity of opportunistic infections in AIDS patients.[39,58,203]

There are two fundamental methods of testing for HIV-1 infection: (1) by the identification of anti–HIV-1 specific antibodies and (2) by the detection of HIV-1 itself or specific antigens or nucleic acids. Because most HIV-1 infected individuals have specific antibodies against HIV-1, HIV-1 infection is defined as a clearly positive HIV-1 antibody test, usually an enzyme-linked immunosorbent assay (ELISA). This is followed by confirmation of specific anti–HIV-1 antibodies by the Western blot test, which allows demonstration of antibodies against the envelope and/or core proteins or the full array of HIV-1 proteins.[15,23,91,123,147,200]

It is possible for an individual to be infected but not have antibodies to HIV-1 for weeks to years.[77,92,153] They can be documented to be infected only by the direct detection of HIV. Direct detection of HIV-1 infection is not routinely determined, but can be done by viral culture, the identification of HIV-1 specific proteins in body fluids, or the detection of specific nucleic acid sequences in cellular material.[73,74,79,167] Recent work with the polymerase chain reaction (PCR) may allow its use in detecting minute levels of HIV-1 nucleic acids in infected cells of individuals.[54,80,103,106,119,139,146,162]

TABLE 1. CDC and WHO Definitions of AIDS

AIDS-Surveillance Definition of the Centers for Disease Control

The occurrence of a disease that is at least moderately predictive of a defect in cell-mediated immunity, occurring in a person with no known cause for diminished resistance to that disease. These diseases include:
- Kaposi's sarcoma (in patients less than 60 years of age)
- Primary lymphoma of the central nervous system
- *Pneumocystis carinii* pneumonia
- Unusually extensive mucocutaneous herpes simplex of more than 5 weeks' duration
- *Cryptosporidium* enterocolitis of more than 4 weeks' duration
- Esophagitis due to *Candida albicans,* cytomegalovirus, or herpes simplex virus
- Progressive multifocal leukoencephalopathy
- Pneumonia, meningitis, or encephalitis due to one or more of the following:
  - *Aspergillus, C. albicans, Cryptococcus neoformans,* cytomegalovirus
  - *Nocardia, Strongyloides, Toxoplasma gondii, Zygomycosis,* or atypical
  - *Mycobacterium* species (not tuberculosis or lepra)

In the absence of the above opportunistic infections, any of the following diseases if the patient has a positive serologic or virologic test for HTLV-III/LAV:
- Disseminated histoplasmosis
- Isosporiasis, causing diarrhea for over 1 month
- Bronchial or pulmonary candidiasis
- Non-Hodgkin's lymphoma of high grade pathologic type and of B cell or unknown phenotype
- Kaposi's sarcoma (in patients over 60 years of age)

Patients who have a lymphoreticular malignancy diagnosed over 3 months after the diagnosis of an opportunistic disease used as a marker for AIDS will not be excluded. Patients will be excluded if they have a negative result on testing for serum antibody to HTLV-III/LAV, have no other type of HTLV-III/LAV test with a positive result, and do not have a low number of T helper cells or a low T-helper/T-suppressor ratio.

Pediatric AIDS-Provisional Surveillance Definition of the Centers for Disease Control

Same as AIDS in adults, with the following provisions:
A. Congenital infections that must be excluded are
  1. *T. gondii* in patients less than 1 month of age
  2. Herpes simplex virus in patients less than 1 month of age
  3. Cytomegalovirus in patients less than 6 months of age
B. Specific conditions that must be excluded in children are
  1. Primary immunodeficiency diseases, severe combined immunodeficiency, Di George syndrome. Wiskott-Aldrich syndrome, ataxiatelangiectasis, graft-versus-host disease, neutropenia, neutrophia function abnormality, agammaglobulinemia, or hypoglobulinemia with raised IgM
  2. Secondary immunodeficiency associated with immunosuppressive therapy, lymphoreticular malignancy, or starvation
C. Histologically confirmed diagnosis of chronic lymphoid interstitial pneumonitis in a child, unless tests for HTLV-III/LAV are negative

AIDS-Related Complex (ARC)

Any Two Clinical Features	Plus	Any Two Laboratory Abnormalities
Fever over 100° F. (37.8° C.) for 3 months or longer		Helper T cells less than 400/mm.
Weight loss over 10% or 15 pounds		Helper:suppressor ratio less than 1.0
Lymphadenopathy over 3 months		Leukothrombocytopenia, anemia
Diarrhea		Elevated serum globulins
Fatigue		Depressed blastogenesis
Night sweats		Anergy to skin test

From Lyerly, H. K., Weinhold, K. J., and Bolognesi, D. P.: Surgical aspects of viral hepatitis and the acquired immune deficiency syndrome (AIDS). *In* Sabiston, D. C., Jr. (Ed.): Essentials of Surgery. Philadelphia, W. B. Saunders Co., 1987.

EPIDEMIOLOGY

HIV-1 infection is a global epidemic with cases reported in Europe, Africa, the Caribbean, Asia, Australia, and Latin America.[3,13,16,69,70,128] In the United States, since the first patients were reported in 1981, over 100,000 cases of AIDS have been reported.[29] In the affected adults, 61 per cent have been in homosexual or bisexual males, 21 per cent in intravenous drug users, 7 per cent in males who are both homosexual and intravenous drug users, 1 per cent in hemophiliacs, 2 per cent in recipients of blood or blood products, 5 per cent in heterosexual partners of infected patients, and 3 per cent in those with undetermined exposure. Of the affected women (constituting 10,369 patients or 9 per cent of the total adult population affected), 52 per cent have been intravenous drug users, 31 per cent heterosexual partners of infected patients, 10 per cent recipients of blood or blood products, and 7 per cent patients with undetermined exposure. In the pediatric population, 81 per cent have had a parent with or at risk for AIDS, 11 per cent have been recipients

of blood or blood components, 5 per cent have been hemophiliacs, and 3 per cent have had undetermined exposure.[29]

The extent of HIV-1 infection is estimated to be 0.5 to 3 million in the United States.[24,145,157,174,186] High seropositivity rates are found in populations of homosexual men, 12 to 70 per cent being seropositive, and intravenous drug users, 0 to 50 per cent being seropositive.[5,32,37,42,78,93,133,137,160,175,196] Because of transfusion of HIV-1 contaminated clotting factors, approximately 80 per cent of treated hemophilia A patients and 50 per cent of hemophilia B patients are antibody-positive.[51,69,76] As of July 1989, 5 per cent (1044 of 20,000) of hemophiliacs in the United States have developed AIDS.

Transmission of HIV-1 is through sexual contact with infected partners, direct exposure to contaminated blood or blood products, and perinatal transmission from infected mothers to their offspring.[22] HIV-1 can be isolated in almost all body fluids, including semen, saliva, tears, cerebrospinal fluid, breast milk, amniotic fluid, urine, vaginal/cervical secretions, and bronchioalveolar fluid.[46,62,75,87,88,89,90,115,116,121,138,150,173,181,188,189,202,204]

Other fluids that have not yet been systematically studied include aqueous and vitreous humor, gastrointestinal secretions, and sweat. The source of the virus in fluids other than blood has usually been demonstrated to be lymphocytes, although extracellular virus has been demonstrated, most notably in cerebrospinal fluid. Although the virus is theoretically transmissible through these fluids, no case of HIV-1 transmission by external body fluid other than semen has been documented.

Although not the first human retrovirus identified, the recognition of HIV-1 as the human pathogen with profound clinical manifestations has led to an increased awareness of related human retroviruses as potential pathogens. Human T-cell leukemia/lymphoma virus Type I (HTLV-I) was isolated prior to the isolation of HIV-1 and has been associated with a variety of clinical syndromes including an asymptomatic carrier state, neurologic disease (tropical spastic paraparesis, myelopathy), cutaneous lesions, lymphadenopathy, hepatosplenomegaly, hypercalcemia, and adult T-cell leukemia and lymphoma.[99,111,134] Epidemiologic data from endemic areas such as Japan and the Caribbean indicate a long latency period (10 to 30 years) between infection and clinical illness. Transmission is associated with sexual contact, intravenous drug use, *in utero* exposure, and receipt of cellular blood products.[49] HTLV-II is a human retrovirus, the amino acid sequence homology and immunologic cross-reactivity of which link it closely to HTLV-I. HTLV-II was originally isolated from patients with hairy cell leukemia, but has been only rarely associated with human malignancy. Little is known about its long-term effects or geographic origin. A significant proportion of intravenous drug users appear to be infected.[112] HTLV-II is probably transmitted by contaminated needles shared during intravenous drug use. Other viruses related to HIV-1 include HIV-2, which is a closely related virus found predominantly in western Africa. Infection, which may cause less fulminant disease than HIV-1, is rarely reported in the United States, although occasional cases have been reported in Europe.

Occupational Risk of Health Care Workers

Viruses other than HIV-1, with similar modes of transmission, such as hepatitis B virus, are known to be transmitted to health care workers through occupational exposure. Over 4000 health care workers have been enrolled in studies and tested for evidence of HIV infection, including more than 1200 subjects who have sustained accidental parenteral exposures. Five documented cases of occupational transmission have been demonstrated in study subjects.[27,59,65,66,67,81,85,94,101,105,122,125,129,178,195] Case reports of occupational HIV-1 infection demonstrate that the risk for HIV-1 transmission occurs in the health care workplace; however, these reports provide limited insight into the magnitude of risk for occupational exposure. Several prospective studies of health care workers who deliver care to HIV-1 infected patients provide the best available evidence regarding the magnitude of risk for occupational exposure.[87] Combining data from 10 prospective studies, the risk for HIV-1 transmission from a single parenteral exposure is 0.37 per cent. Eight studies evaluated the risk for occupational infection among health care workers, reporting mucous membrane exposure to blood or body fluids from an HIV-1–infected patient.[82] No infection occurred in these studies, suggesting the risk of transmission associated with a single mucous membrane exposure to be less than that following parenteral exposure.

Prevention of occupational infection with HIV-1 has primarily focused on preventing occupational exposure by universal blood and body fluid precautions.[6,20,21] Current recommendations from the American College of Surgeons and the Society of Thoracic Surgeons are listed in Table 2.[120,177] Whereas the implementation of universal precautions may reduce the incidence of occupational exposure, use of these precautions does not entirely eliminate the risk of occupational HIV-1 infection, because accidental exposures occasionally occur.

TABLE 2. Precautions for Health Care Workers in Prevention of AIDS

1. Place AIDS patients on blood/body fluid precautions with appropriate identification of the disease on the patient, room, and chart.
2. Sharp items (needles, scalpel blades, and other sharp instruments) should be considered potentially infectious and handled and disposed of with extraordinary care.
3. Protective clothing and coverings should be used to prevent exposure to blood, body fluids contaminated with blood, semen, and aerosols or droplets during patient care or procedures. Hands should be washed thoroughly and immediately if they become contaminated.
4. Clearly label, double bag in impermeable bags, and use gown and gloves when handling AIDS specimens.
5. Notify operating room and laboratory personnel prior to planned procedures on AIDS patients.
6. All nondisposable items and work surfaces should be decontaminated with freshly prepared 1:5 dilution of 5.25% sodium hypochlorite (household bleach).

From Lyerly, H. K., Weinhold, K. J., and Bolognesi, D. P.: Surgical aspects of viral hepatitis and the acquired immune deficiency syndrome (AIDS). *In* Sabiston, D. C., Jr. (Ed.): Essentials of Surgery. Philadelphia, W. B. Saunders Co., 1987.

Although the risk of infection following exposure is minimal, methods to further reduce the risk of HIV-1 infection after exposure are being investigated because no curative therapy is currently available. The course of some retroviral illnesses in animals has been demonstrated to be altered by the postexposure administration of AZT. Both Ruprecht and associates and Tavares and associates have demonstrated that AZT administered immediately after exposure to Rauscher murine leukemia virus (RLV) and feline leukemia virus (FLV) alters the course of these animal retroviral infections.[165,179] RLV and FLV are only distantly related to HIV-1, and the natural histories of these retroviral infections appear to be disparate from the natural history of human HIV-1 infection. Nonetheless, postexposure chemoprophylaxis with AZT has been advocated for health care workers exposed to HIV-1.

AZT acts to terminate viral DNA elongation by reverse transcriptase, which prevents susceptible cells from *de novo* infection but has no effect when the viral genome is incorporated into the host cell's genome. Ruprecht and associates demonstrated suppression of viremia when AZT was administered 4 hours after inoculation with RLV. They noted that after AZT was discontinued late recurrences may occur. Tavares and co-workers assessed the efficacy of AZT administered at various intervals after the infection of cats with FLV.[179] Administration of AZT within 1 hour of infection in this study led to the prevention of FLV viremia. AZT postexposure chemoprophylaxis is consequently thought to require rapid administration after exposure.

Chemoprophylaxis programs at San Francisco General Hospital/University of California, San Francisco (SFGH/UCSF) and at the National Institutes of Health (NIH) recommend AZT on the basis of the severity of exposure.[83,107] AZT is recommended for massive exposure (injections or transfusions of HIV-1 containing blood), is endorsed for serious parenteral exposures (deep needle sticks), and is available but not encouraged for less severe exposures.

Dosage and duration of AZT administration at the NIH is 200 mg. of AZT every 4 hours for 42 days; whereas at SFGH/UCSF the same dose is administered, but the 4 A.M. dose is omitted, and the duration of therapy is 28 days. No data are available to suggest that one approach is more effective than the other. All employees receive appropriate follow-up care for monitoring toxicity.

The primary toxicities of AZT observed have been hematologic and dose-related, but toxicity related to other organ systems has been identified.[159] Up to 75 per cent of treated patients develop macrocytosis, although most are not anemic. Severe anemia, neutropenia, and thrombocytopenia rarely occur during the first 4 weeks of therapy. Other adverse effects include headache, fatigue, myalgias, insomnia, nausea, myositis, paresthesias, hepatitis, and possible mutagenesis and teratogenesis. Toxicity to AZT with short-course therapy in otherwise healthy individuals is rarely severe; however, subjective complaints, which include a flulike syndrome, profound fatigue, and insomnia, are common. Exclusion criteria for entry into AZT prophylaxis include pregnancy, and relative contraindications include renal or hepatic insufficiency.

Because of the potential toxicity of AZT, its administration is based on the serologic status of the source. For some, the serologic status of the source may be unknown; and for some, it may be impossible to ascertain if the patient has been discharged or has died. Alternatives for individuals exposed to potentially seropositive sources include assessment of the serologic status of the source prior to initiating therapy or beginning chemoprophylaxis immediately, later terminating the treatment if the serologic status of the source is determined to be negative.[55,84,98,152,187]

Transfusion-Associated AIDS

Transmission of HIV-1 has been documented after transfusion of the following single-donor blood and blood components: whole blood, packed red blood cells, fresh frozen plasma, cryoprecipitate, and platelets.[2,48] Plasma-derived blood products manufactured from plasma pooled from 2000 to 30,000 donors can transmit HIV-1, depending upon the production process. Currently, 3 per cent of adult cases and 12 per cent of pediatric cases of AIDS were caused by HIV-1–contaminated transfusions.[29] Almost all were due to blood transfused before HIV-1 antibody testing became available in March 1985. Ninety per cent of recipients transfused with HIV-1 antibody–positive blood become antibody-positive at follow-up.[47] There are an estimated 12,000 living transfusion recipients, many unaware that they are infected.[149] HIV-1 antibody testing should be considered by all individuals who underwent a transfusion between 1978 and March 1985.

Transfusion-transmitted HIV-1 has become rare since the beginning of voluntary deferral of donors at risk for HIV-1 infection and the routine testing of all donations. Despite these measures, there is an estimated risk of acquiring HIV-1 ranging from 1 in 36,000 to 1 in 100,000 per unit of blood transfused.[36,102,194]

Blood bank screening by the detection of anti–HIV-1 antibodies fails when at-risk individuals are not excluded from donation. Although laboratory screening is more than 99 per cent sensitive, it may fail because of technical errors or the inability to detect infected individuals who have not yet developed anti–HIV-1 antibodies.

Other human retroviruses, such as HIV-2, HTLV-I, and HTLV-II, may also be transmitted by blood transfusion. Current ELISA tests for HIV-1 antibodies detect 42 to 92 per cent of HIV-2 infections.[38,164] Serologic screening can detect both HTLV-I and HTLV-II without distinguishing between them, so they are collectively designated HTLV-I/II. Since July 1989, blood donations in the United States have also been screened for HTLV-I/II.[112] One in 1000 to 1 in 4000 donors are positive for HTLV-1.[183]

HIV-1 has been transmitted via kidney, liver, heart, pancreas, bone, and possibly skin transplants.[26,28,34,40,50,87,141,158,176,204] It has also been transmitted through artificial insemination. The current risk of HIV-1 infection from organ transplantation is unknown, but is thought to be comparable to the risk in blood transfusion.

CLINICAL FEATURES

The majority of the morbidity and mortality observed in AIDS patients is related to overwhelming infection. Clinical syndromes that occur frequently include diffuse pneumonia, fever, diarrhea, central nervous system disorders, generalized lymphadenopathy, and esophagitis. The opportunistic infections most commonly observed in HIV-1–infected individuals are listed in Table 3. Although infectious complications are a prominent feature of AIDS patients, unusual neoplasms are also encountered in a large number. These include Kaposi's sarcoma and non-Hodgkin's lymphoma.

Kaposi's sarcoma (KS) was first described in 1872 by Moritz Kaposi. In its classic form, the disease usually occurs in older individuals of European or Jewish origin.[35,166] The epidemic form of KS is usually encountered in AIDS patients and is characterized by the sudden onset and often widespread appearance of lesions involving not only the skin but the oral mucosa, lymph nodes, and visceral organs.[191] The average survival of patients is 18 months.[113] The presence or absence of lymph

TABLE 3. Opportunistic Infections in AIDS

Organisms	Clinical Syndrome
Protozoa	
Pneumocystis carinii	Pneumonia
Toxoplasma gondii	Encephalitis
	Chorioretinitis
	Lymphadenopathy
Cryptosporidium	Enterocolitis
Fungi	
Candida species	Stomatitis
	Esophagitis
	Enterocolitis
	Gastrointestinal bleeding
Cryptococcus neoformans	Meningitis
	Peritonitis
	Dissemination
Histoplasma capsulatum	Hepatosplenomegaly
Mycobacteria	
Mycobacterium avium-intracellulare	Hepatosplenomegaly
	Lymphadenopathy
	Enterocolitis
	Pneumonitis
	Debilitation
Mycobacterium tuberculosis	Pneumonia
	Draining lesions
Bacteria	
Salmonella	Proctocolitis
Shigella	
Campylobacter	
Neisseria gonorrhoeae	
Treponema pallidum	
Other microorganisms	
Giardia lamblia	Proctocolitis
Entamoeba histolytica	
Chlamydia	
Viruses	
Cytomegalovirus (CMV)	Gastrointestinal bleeding
	Gastrointestinal perforation
	Diarrhea
	Proctocolitis
	Chorioretinitis
	Hepatitis
	Lymphadenopathy
Ebstein-Barr virus	Lymphadenopathy
Hepatitis B, C	Hepatitis
Herpes simplex	Skin lesions
	Esophagitis
Herpes zoster	Disseminated skin lesions

node involvement appears to have no effect on prognosis; however, visceral involvement does imply a poor prognosis.[190] The lung, as well as the gastrointestinal tract, liver, and spleen, may be involved.[95] Patients with gastrointestinal involvement have a reduced survival, whereas patients with pulmonary KS have a median survival of 2 months. It has not been demonstrated that local or systemic therapy for KS alters the ultimate course of the disease. Small localized lesions may be satisfactorily treated by electrodessication and currettage or by surgical excision. KS tumors are generally responsive to local radiation, and excellent palliation has been obtained with doses of 200 cGy.[33,142]

Most AIDS-related lymphomas have been B-cell tumors of high pathologic grade.[19] Most of these patients present with systemic symptoms, including fever, night sweats, and weight loss. A distinctive feature is the frequency of extranodal disease. As many as 63 per cent may present with Stage IV disease. The therapy of choice for AIDS-related lymphoma is unknown. The patients usually have high-grade disease, mandating the use of intensive multiagent chemotherapy. However, because of underlying HIV-1–induced immunosuppression, multiagent chemotherapy may worsen the patient's immune dysfunction and susceptibility to infection. Median survival of patients with AIDS-related lymphoma is less than 1 year.

SURGICAL CONSIDERATIONS IN HIV-1–INFECTED INDIVIDUALS

HIV-1–infected individuals are susceptible not only to routine conditions and surgical disorders but may also tolerate surgical interventions differently from nonimmunosuppressed individuals as well as being susceptible to a variety of unique conditions that frequently require surgical intervention. As the number of HIV-1–infected individuals increases, it becomes important for surgeons not only to understand the surgical problems associated with HIV-1 infection but also to appreciate how HIV-1 infected patients tolerate surgical procedures.

Evaluation by Organ System

ESOPHAGUS. Diffuse esophagitis is the most common esophageal lesion observed in HIV-1–infected individuals. While *Candida albicans* is probably the most frequent etiologic agent, other causes include herpesvirus and cytomegalovirus (CMV).[127] Because the presenting symptoms are usually dysphagia and retrosternal discomfort, this syndrome can easily be confused with reflux esophagitis. If oral thrush is present, *Candida* esophagitis is the most likely diagnosis. If oral lesions appear as shallow ulcerations, herpes simplex esophagitis becomes more likely. Most clinicians attempt empiric therapy with ketoconazole and acyclovir for suspected *Candida* and herpesvirus esophagitis, respectively, without initial endoscopy. If empiric therapy is unsuccessful, endoscopy and biopsy are performed to differentiate lesions. Specimens should be sent for fungal and viral cultures, and the pathologist should be aware of the need for viral and fungal immunofluorescent stains on biopsy samples. Other lesions involving the esophagus include esophageal ulcers, which are thought to be secondary to an as yet undefined virus, and KS. KS lesions can not only bleed but in rare instances can cause pharyngeal obstruction and thus require excision.[148]

STOMACH AND DUODENUM. Lesions related to HIV-1 infection that most commonly affect the stomach and duodenum are KS, non-Hodgkin's lymphoma, and cytomegalovirus (CMV) infections. Although gastrointestinal KS lesions are usually asymptomatic, they are the most common cause of upper GI bleeding in HIV-1 infected individuals and can occasionally cause gastric outlet obstruction.[30,127] In these situations, radiotherapy, chemotherapy, and immunotherapy have had mixed results; and surgical therapy is occasionally required. Non-Hodgkin's lymphoma of the stomach usually presents with signs of hemorrhage, but obstruction and perforation can

occur.[61] Diagnosis can be made with endoscopy and biopsy. Surgical excision is frequently performed before treatment with chemotherapy as cases of intestinal perforation secondary to extensive tumor lysis after chemotherapy have been reported.[61] CMV involvement of the stomach and duodenum is usually in the form of ulcerating lesions. CMV inclusions in the endothelium of biopsy specimens is diagnostic. Free perforation can occur and requires surgical intervention. Despite operation, morbidity and mortality following perforation secondary to CMV are high.[104,185]

LIVER. The liver can be affected by both infectious and neoplastic complications of HIV-1 infection, but rarely is operation required as a therapeutic intervention. Approximately 95 per cent of patients have serologic evidence of previous hepatitis B infection, between 10 and 30 per cent having detectable circulating surface antigen.[170] Interestingly, no cases of primary hepatocellular carcinoma have been reported in an AIDS patient to date.[170] The other types of viral hepatitis (A, C, and Delta agent) all appear common in HIV-1–infected individuals. Several HIV-1–related opportunistic infections, including those caused by *Mycobacterium avium-intracellulare*, *Mycobacterium tuberculosis*, cytomegalovirus, *Cryptococcus neoformans*, *Histoplasma capsulatum*, *Candida albicans*, and *Coccidioides immitus*, can involve the liver as can non-Hodgkin's lymphoma and Kaposi's sarcoma. Clinical characteristics of liver involvement include constitutional symptoms such as fever, malaise, and weight loss along with hepatomegaly. Liver function tests reveal mild to moderate elevations. Alkaline phosphatase can be markedly elevated when granulomata or abscesses are present.[169] Lymphoma usually causes a marked increase in the serum bilirubin.[61] Diagnostic work-up usually involves a computed tomographic (CT) scan and/or a liver biopsy. Although most abscesses can be drained with percutaneous CT scan–guided needle aspiration, surgical therapy is occasionally required.

GALLBLADDER AND BILIARY TRACT. Biliary complications related to HIV-1 infection are being reported with increasing frequency. Because HIV-1–infected individuals are usually young, cases of cholecystitis secondary to gallstones are relatively uncommon. Interestingly, however, numerous cases of acute acalculous cholecystitis have been documented.[10,14,161,201] Cryptosporidiosis and cytomegalovirus (CMV) appear to be the most common inciting organisms, although cases secondary to *Campylobacter* and *Candida* have occurred.[10] Patients usually present with fever, fatigue, diarrhea, and right upper quadrant pain. Ultrasound, the diagnostic test of choice, often demonstrates a thickened gallbladder wall, pericholecystic fluid, and a positive transducer-induced Murphy's sign. Despite the absence of stones, radionuclide scintigraphy is usually positive. Cholecystectomy is the preferred treatment and is usually well tolerated in asymptomatic HIV-1–infected individuals.[10] The morbidity and mortality of cholecystectomy in AIDS patients, however, is much higher.[110]

Papillary stenosis and sclerosing cholangitis are also observed with surprising frequency in HIV-1–infected individuals. The etiology of these changes appears related to either cryptosporidiosis or CMV infections involving the bile ducts.[130] Presenting symptoms include fever, nausea, vomiting, diarrhea, and right upper quadrant pain. Jaundice is only occasionally observed, because biliary tract obstruction is rarely complete. Laboratory studies reveal a markedly elevated alkaline phosphatase level, a mildly elevated bilirubin level, and frequently normal transaminase levels.[170] Initial screening is usually performed with ultrasound and/or CT scanning in an attempt to exclude extrinsic compression of the bile ducts secondary to Kaposi's sarcoma lesions, lymphadenopathy, or lymphoma. Endoscopic retrograde cholangiopancreatography (ERCP) is preferable to transhepatic cholangiography and can help to further define the anatomy of the intrahepatic and extrahepatic bile ducts. In patients with papillary stenosis, prompt relief is usually obtained when endoscopic sphincterotomy is performed.[169] Patients with sclerosing cholangitis are best treated with balloon dilatation and stenting, especially when areas of localized stricture are present.[170] Surgical intervention is best reserved for lesions causing extrinsic compression and for patients in whom endoscopic sphincterotomy fails.

PANCREAS. The effect of HIV-1 infection on pancreatic function is not well studied to date. Pancreatitis unrelated to alcohol, gallstones, or hyperlipidemia is not an uncommon finding in HIV-1–infected individuals. Although some reports demonstrate that this can occur secondary to pancreatic involvement by opportunistic infections (CMV, *Mycobacterium avium-intracellulare*) or neoplasms (KS, lymphoma), the majority of these cases have no clear cause.[104] One report, examining pancreatitis in a simian immunodeficiency model, offers a possible explanation for this finding by suggesting that HIV-1 infection may lead to the reactivation of other pancreatitis-causing viruses such as adenoviruses that are latent within the host.[114] In addition, certain drugs that are used to treat AIDS-related illnesses, such as pentamidine, may cause pancreatitis.[9]

INTESTINE. HIV-1–related lesions affecting the intestine are both neoplastic and infectious in nature. Non-Hodgkin's lymphoma and Kaposi's sarcoma (KS) are the most common neoplasms affecting the intestine. Usually, the lymphomas are symptomatic, presenting with signs of pain, fever, night sweats, weight loss, jaundice, ascites, obstruction, bleeding, and/or perforation. Usually, the diagnosis of lymphoma can be made with CT scanning, and therefore it is the test of choice.[127] Occasionally, additional information can be obtained from barium studies. Surgical therapy is usually required in cases that present with obstruction, hemorrhage, or perforation. Because several cases of perforation secondary to postchemotherapy tumor lysis have been reported, resection of localized lesions prior to chemotherapy has also been advocated.[61] Intestinal KS lesions are present in between 40 to 50 per cent of patients with cutaneous KS lesions but are usually asymptomatic.[61] Rarely, they present with bleeding or obstruction requiring surgical intervention. In general, the prognosis is poor for patients with intestinal KS, and treatment is directed more toward the underlying HIV-1 infection.

Infections involving the small intestine can also cause surgical problems. There are numerous reports of intestinal perforation secondary to cytomegalovirus infection.[60,110,201] Despite surgical exploration and segmental bowel resection, morbidity and mortality remain high because of the lack of appropriate systemic anti-viral therapy.[185,201] Several organisms can cause an inflammatory response in the terminal ileum mimicking regional enteritis or appendicitis and lead to surgical exploration. The most common of these organisms are *Yersinia*, *Campylobacter*, *Shigella*, *Salmonella*, and *Mycobacterium avium-intracellulare*.[10,151] Diagnosis can be difficult because the presence of these organisms in the patient's stool does not always imply that they are the cause of the abdominal pain.

APPENDIX. While appendicitis occurs in HIV-1–infected individuals via the same mechanisms through which it occurs in seronegative individuals, there are several reports that appendiceal obstruction may also follow AIDS-related neoplasms such as Kaposi's sarcoma and lymphoma.[10] In addition, because these patients frequently have chronic abdominal complaints, appendicitis is often more difficult to diagnose. This is borne out by anecdotal reports suggesting that an HIV-1–infected individual, especially one with AIDS, is more likely to have a perforated appendix at the time of exploration.[10,143] On the basis of one report, the most common presenting symptoms of appendicitis in AIDS patients are increasing abdominal pain and diarrhea. Because they found fever and leukocytosis to be unreliable, this group recommended the aggressive use of ultrasound in the evaluation of this problem.[127]

COLON. Lesions affecting the colon in HIV-1–infected individuals are predominantly infectious in nature. CMV infection

TABLE 4. Infectious Etiologies of Abdominal Pain in AIDS

Bacterial	Nonbacterial
Salmonella	*Entamoeba histolytica*
Shigella	*Giardia lamblia*
Campylobacter	*Cryptosporidium*
Neisseria gonorrhoeae	*Isospora belli*
Treponema pallidum	*Candida albicans*
Mycobacterium avium-intracellulare	*Cryptococcus neoformans*
Mycobacterium tuberculosis	*Histoplasma capsulatum*
Listeria monocytogenes	Cytomegalovirus
	Herpes simplex

of the colon can lead to perforation requiring surgical intervention.[171] In addition, a number of bacterial and parasitic organisms (Table 4) can cause a severe colitis, which usually presents with abdominal pain and diarrhea. Occasionally, the colitis caused by these organisms is so severe that diagnostic surgical exploration is performed because of the presence of peritoneal signs.

ANUS AND RECTUM. Anorectal complaints are common in HIV-1 infected individuals, especially homosexuals and AIDS patients. Symptoms of anorectal problems include pain, discharge, incontinence, bleeding, mass and/or tenesmus. A wide variety of infections, anorectal lesions and tumors, as listed in Table 5, can cause these symptoms. Recent studies would indicate that the frequency of these lesions in AIDS patients increases their risk of developing anal and rectal carcinoma.[44,45] When one is evaluating anorectal lesions, therefore, it is important that anoscopy and/or sigmoidoscopy be performed along with rectal swabbing for ova and parasites, bacteria, and viruses. Biopsies of any suspicious lesion or mass should be obtained.

Treatment of the various anorectal lesions is as conservative as possible based upon two studies which demonstrate that AIDS patients heal poorly after attempted surgical therapy. One of the studies reviewed 73 anorectal procedures (23 biopsies, 16 cases of incision and drainage, 14 fistulotomies, 8 sphincterotomies, 8 excisions, 3 colostomies, and 1 hemorrhoidectomy) in 52 patients with AIDS and found an 88 per cent incidence of poor wound healing and an 18 per cent perioperative mortality rate.[197] Although a similar perioperative mortality (16 per cent) was present in the second study of 18 anorectal procedures in 17 AIDS patients, in most, the wounds healed uneventfully.[10] Al-

TABLE 5. Infections and Lesions of the Anorectum in AIDS

Infections	Lesions
Neisseria gonorrhoeae	Anal fissures
Syphilis	Anal fistulas
Lymphogranuloma venereum	Perirectal abscess
Chlamydia trachomatis	Hemorrhoids
Herpes simplex Type II	Lymphoma
Herpes zoster	Kaposi's sarcoma
Campylobacter	Condylomata acuminata
Cytomegalovirus	Trauma-induced
Mycobacterium tuberculosis	Squamous cell carcinoma
Mycobacterium avium-intracellulare	
Histoplasma	
Giardia lamblia	
Shigella	
Isospora belli	
Cryptosporidium	
Entamoeba histolytica	
Clostridium difficile	
Candida albicans	
Vibrio parahemolyteus	

though caution is recommended for most anorectal problems, certain lesions should be regarded as emergencies (i.e., perirectal abscesses), and expedient definitive therapy should be performed in the operating room.

Evaluation by Clinical Signs or Symptoms

ABDOMINAL PAIN. Although it is difficult to estimate the percentage of HIV-1–infected individuals who develop abdominal pain, most large group studies suggest that abdominal pain requiring surgical intervention is uncommon.[9,10] As shown in Table 6, only 115 abdominal operations were reported in the seven largest published series of AIDS patients followed over a prolonged period of time. An examination of the various operations reported in each series suggests that patient populations differed in each study. Despite the variation, three broad categories of abdominal pain have been found in this patient population: abdominal pain secondary to standard surgical problems, abdominal pain secondary to AIDS-related surgical problems, and nonsurgical abdominal pain.

Abdominal pain secondary to standard surgical problems occurs in HIV-1–infected individuals, as it does in the uninfected population. Cases of appendicitis, cholecystitis, perforated gastric or duodenal ulcer, diverticulitis, adhesive small bowel obstruction, and incarcerated hernias have all been reported in the above studies. Interestingly, most cases of appendicitis and cholecystitis appeared to have an AIDS-related inciting factor as discussed in the previous section. This finding has led one group to speculate that the HIV-1–infected patient may be more prone to infections of the appendix and gallbladder because these structures are supplied by predominantly terminal arteries.[110] In general, the more immunocompromised the HIV-1–infected individual, the more often an atypical presentation and poor outcome can be expected. This is borne out by the finding that of 12 AIDS patients who were explored and found to have appendicitis, 4 died in the postoperative period.[9,10]

Most patients reported in the above studies had surgical conditions that could be directly related to their HIV-1 infection. AIDS-related neoplasms such as KS and non-Hodgkin's lymphoma have been described as causing gastrointestinal bleeding, intestinal obstruction, intestinal perforation, and retroperitoneal adenopathy, all leading to surgical intervention. AIDS-related infections, most notably those secondary to CMV, can also lead to a number of surgical conditions. CMV is a member of the herpesvirus family and is found in almost all HIV-1–infected individuals. Enterocolitis and colitis are two manifestations of CMV infection that occur when the virus infects the endothelial cells of the intestine or colon, leading to inflammation and ulceration. The presence of CMV inclusions in endothelial cells with surrounding vasculitis on biopsy specimens confirms the role of CMV as the etiologic agent.[60,132] Common symptoms include abdominal pain, bleeding, and diarrhea. Surgical intervention is required when free perforation, uncontrollable hemorrhage, or toxic megacolon occurs. A perioperative mortality of 40 per cent can be expected, primarily because of the immunosuppressed condition of the patient and the lack of an effective anti-CMV chemotherapy regimen.[30,185,201] The most promising agent currently under investigation is ganciclovir, but its effectiveness remains to be determined.[31]

The majority of HIV-1–infected patients who have abdominal pain do not require surgical intervention.[9,10] Most often the etiology of the abdominal pain is related to some infectious etiology that can be treated medically. The various infectious agents that can cause abdominal pain are listed in Table 4. The evaluation of these problems involves a number of diagnostic studies, such as endoscopy with biopsy and culture; stool examination for enteric pathogens, ova and parasites; and CT. Occasionally, laparotomy is required when the diagnosis remains

TABLE 6. Abdominal Operations in AIDS

Author	Hospital, AIDS Patients, Years of Study	Abd oper	Apy	Chol	Perf	Hem	Sple	LN Bx	Obs	Oth
LaRaja[110]	Cabrini Medical Center (904 AIDS patients), NY, 1985–1988	38	7	12	5	1	7	—	2	4
Ferguson[56]	Crawford Long Hospital (79 AIDS patients), GA, 1982–1987	14	—	1	2	—	6	4	—	1
Barone[9]	St. Vincent's Hospital and Medical Center (235 AIDS patients), NY, 1982–1985	5	—	—	1	2	—	—	—	2
Nugent[143]	Kaiser Permanente Medical Center (110 AIDS patients), LA, 1984–1985	5	1	1	1	—	1	—	—	1
Wilson[201]	8 Southern California Hospitals (3500 beds) 1984–1988	36	1	3	10	3	6	6	6	1
Burack[14]	Montefiore Medical Center and Affiliated Hospitals, NY, 1984–1987	10	3	2	4	—	—	—	1	—
Robinson[161]	Harbor/UCLA Medical Center, Torrance and UCLA Medical Center, LA, 1982—1985	7	—	2	2	—	—	1	1	1

Abd oper, abdominal operations; Chol, cholecystectomy; Hem, uncontrolled hemorrhage; LN Bx, lymph node biopsy; Oth, other; Apy, appendectomy; Perf, perforated viscus; Sple, splenectomy; Obs, intestinal obstruction.

elusive, an abdominal mass is present, and/or the patient's condition deteriorates.

THROMBOCYTOPENIA. Thrombocytopenic purpura is a common hematologic problem in HIV-1–infected individuals, approximately 11 per cent of patients having platelet counts of less than 100,000 per cu. mm.[162] Cases for which no obvious etiology can be determined other than coexisting HIV-1 infection have been diagnosed as HIV-1–associated thrombocytopenia (HAT). HAT is thought to be secondary to either high levels of platelet-bound IgG and circulating immune complexes or a specific antiplatelet antibody.[96,140,192] The failure to find a unifying mechanism for all cases of HAT suggests that this syndrome may have several different etiologies.

Clinically, HAT is a syndrome that does not appear to be associated with progression of HIV-1 infection to ARC or AIDS and is characterized by a spontaneous remission rate of between 10 and 30 per cent.[192] Interestingly, although platelet counts may frequently drop below 20,000 cu. mm., episodes of life-threatening bleeding have rarely been reported.[57,184] Because of its relatively indolent course, high spontaneous remission rate, and the undefined mechanisms, no unified consensus has emerged concerning the most effective treatment for HAT.

Steroids were initially the treatment of choice in managing HAT because they led to an increase in the platelet count in 60 to 90 per cent of patients in whom they were tried.[1,193] Enthusiasm for steroids has diminished, however, because increases in platelet counts are rarely maintained when steroids are withdrawn. Not wanting to chronically immunosuppress individuals whose underlying problem is immunodeficiency, physicians have tried other treatments. More recently, marked short-term improvement in patient platelet counts after splenectomy has led some to propose this operation as a first line of therapy.[57,156] However, although approximately 75 per cent of patients still have counts above 100,000 per cu. mm. 1 year after splenectomy, platelet counts continue to fluctuate markedly.[184] Continued debate as to the long-term effectiveness of splenectomy and its possible role in accelerating HIV-1 infection have diminished enthusiasm for this procedure.

There are now several reports, including prospective placebo-controlled studies, of increases in circulating platelet counts following treatment of HAT with zidovudine (AZT).[86,144] In patients who respond, platelet counts begin to rise within the first week and often are over 100,000 per cu. mm. by the end of the first month. The reason for the increase in patient platelet counts and the duration of effect is unclear; but because there are fewer theoretical risks for an individual taking zidovudine, as compared with steroids, this medication has become acceptable therapy for HAT. Steroids and splenectomy are reserved for those individuals who are refractory to or cannot tolerate zidovudine. The algorithm currently in use at Duke University Medical Center for the treatment of HAT is shown in Figure 1.

GI BLEEDING. Gastrointestinal (GI) bleeding is an unusual occurrence in HIV-1–infected individuals. A study from San Francisco General Hospital evaluated 37 AIDS cases over a 35-month period between 1985 and 1987 with this problem.[30] Interestingly, most lesions causing the GI bleeding were directly related to the HIV-1 infection. Thirteen of the 37 patients presented with *upper* GI bleeding; 4 were found to be bleeding from KS lesions, 2 from gastric lymphoma, and 2 from CMV-induced ulcerations. Non–AIDS-associated lesions were found in the remaining 5 patients. Evaluation of the 24 patients who presented with lower GI bleeding revealed most to have distal rectal lesions, again frequently related to their underlying HIV-1 infection. The most common of these lesions was a localized colitis found in 14 patients, the cause of which included CMV (5), bacteria (4), idiopathic ulcerative disease (2), and herpes simplex virus (2). Other lesions responsible for lower GI bleeding in this group included idiopathic proctitis (2), hemorrhoids (4), and KS (2). This study concluded that GI bleeding

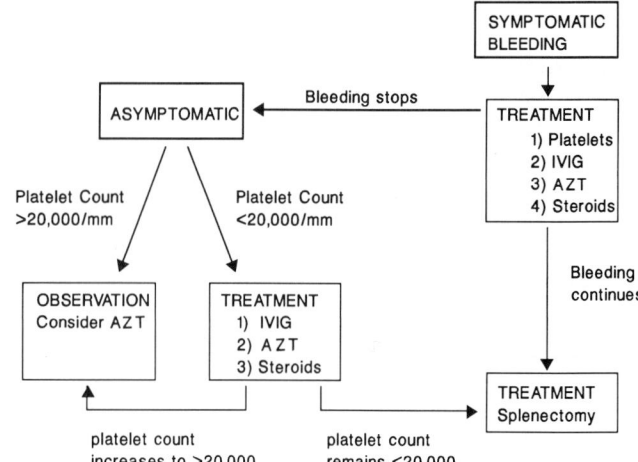

Figure 1. Algorithm used at Duke University Medical Center for the treatment of HAT.

should be treated aggressively in HIV-1–infected individuals who are not terminally ill, because frequently treatable lesions are found. Evaluation of GI bleeding in AIDS patients usually begins with endoscopy. If bleeding is too brisk, nuclear scintigraphy and/or angiography may be required.

LYMPHADENOPATHY. Generalized lymphadenopathy is a relatively common finding in patients with HIV-1 infection. Before the recognition that HIV-1 was the etiologic agent of AIDS, lymph node biopsy was frequently utilized in an attempt to diagnose this syndrome. Although there are no characteristic histologic patterns pathognomonic of AIDS, the finding of KS, B-cell lymphoma, or specific opportunistic infections can be diagnostic.

With the development of accurate serologic tests for antibodies to HIV-1 toward the end of 1985, the role of lymph node biopsy in HIV-1–infected individuals became unclear. Three prospective studies examining lymph node biopsies in HIV-1–infected individuals with persistent generalized lymphadenopathy (PGL) found that biopsy results altered clinical management in only 2 of 71 patients.[53,68,154,171] All three studies suggested that the routine use of lymph node biopsy in HIV-1–infected individuals with uncomplicated PGL was unnecessary. Instead, they concluded that lymph node biopsy be reserved for those individuals who have lymphadenopathy in the setting of constitutional symptoms, splenomegaly, cytopenia, oral candidiasis, or hilar adenopathy. In addition, a solitary lymph node enlarged disproportionately in relation to other lymph nodes should be removed for examination.[117] This selective use of lymph node biopsy would increase the likelihood of diagnosing a specific infection, lymphoma, or another disease process that could alter the clinical management of the patient.

Other Considerations

POSTOPERATIVE COURSE. The postoperative morbidity and mortality in HIV-1–infected individuals appear to be related to the patient's underlying immunocompetence and the nature of the underlying illness requiring surgery. Asymptomatic HIV-1–infected individuals undergoing elective surgical procedures do not exhibit significantly more problems with wound healing and infection than their uninfected counterparts.[127] Debate continues regarding the healing ability of patients with AIDS after elective procedures. One study reviewing elective anorectal surgical procedures in patients with AIDS and ARC described a high incidence of complications and poor wound healing.[197] Other studies suggest that AIDS patients appear to tolerate elective abdominal operations reasonably well, especially if surgical therapy is for an illness unrelated to HIV-1 infection.[201] Surgical intervention in this patient population, however, has been reported to occasionally exacerbate underlying HIV-1 infection.[56] Extremely high morbidity and mortality have been reported in two recent studies examining emergent abdominal operations in AIDS patients, attesting to the serious nature of surgical infections in immunocompromised hosts.[14,110,161]

TRAUMA. Another area where surgeons frequently encounter HIV-1 infection unknowingly is in managing trauma victims. In 1987, a report from Johns Hopkins Hospital revealed that 3 per cent of 203 severely injured or critically ill patients initially evaluated in the emergency department were seropositive for HIV-1.[7] Interestingly, all seropositive individuals in this study (n = 6) were trauma victims between the ages of 25 to 34 years and represented 16 per cent of this age group. Of more concern was the finding that all 6 patients were actively bleeding at the time of presentation and all required multiple invasive procedures in the emergency room.

A follow-up study, done by the same group, of all patients presenting to the Johns Hopkins Hospital emergency room who had blood drawn during a 6-week period in 1987 found that 4 per cent (92/2275) had unrecognized HIV-1 infection.[97] The highest seroprevalence in the study was 11.4 per cent, found among black males between 30 to 34 years old. Interestingly, the only clinical presentation associated with an increased seroprevalence (13.6 per cent), independent of other known predictors of infection, was penetrating trauma.

These studies emphasize the need for surgeons managing trauma patients to be knowledgeable about HIV-1 infection. Unfortunately, as these two studies have demonstrated, there is no clinical indicator that allows identification of seropositive individuals with any certainty. Although rapid determination tests for detection of antibodies to HIV-1 within 5 minutes exist, their use has been restricted by HIV-1 testing laws.[98] As a result, a policy of universal blood and body precautions should be followed by all health care workers regardless of whether the HIV-1 status is known or not. Utilizing universal blood and body fluid precautions should help to keep the already small risk of occupationally acquired HIV-1 infection as low as possible.

SELECTED REFERENCES

AIDS and Surgery

Gastroenterology Clinics of North America. Vol. 17, No. 3, September 1988.
The entire volume is devoted to the gastrointestinal manifestations of AIDS and contains several excellent articles written by both gastroenterologists and surgeons. The articles are all extensively referenced.

LaRaja, R. D., Rothenberg, R. E., Odom, J. W., and Mueller S. The incidence of intra-abdominal surgery in acquired immunodeficiency syndrome: A statistical review of 904 patients. Surgery 105:175–179, 1989.
These authors reviewed 38 abdominal operations in HIV-1 infected individuals over a 3 year period in the New York area. Being the largest review to date, it provides a good overview of the types of surgical procedures performed in this population.

Wilson, S. E., Robinson, G., Williams, R. A., and Stabile, B. L. Acquired immunodeficiency syndrome: Indications for abdominal surgery, pathology and outcome. Ann. Surg., 1990, **210**, 428–433, 1989.
This is the second largest review of abdominal procedures in HIV-1 infected individuals and most recent. It too provides an excellent overview of surgical procedures and outcome in HIV-1 infected patients.

Centers for Disease Control: Update: Acquired immunodeficiency syndrome and human immunodeficiency virus infection among health care workers. MMWR. 37:229–239, 1988.
Provides the most up-to-date summary of occupationally acquired HIV-1 infection among health care workers.

Centers for Disease Control:Supplement. Recommendations for prevention of HIV transmission in health-care settings. MMWR. 36:1S–18S.
Provides an excellent discussion of current tests for HIV-1 and what is implied by a positive result. A thorough discussion of the risk of infection to health care workers and methods for preventing occupationally acquired infection are also presented.

Kelen, G. D., Fritz, S., Qaqish, B., et al. Unrecognized human immunodeficiency virus infection in emergency department patients. NEJM 318:1645–1650.
This study is a 6-week survey of patients presenting to the Johns Hopkins Hospital

emergency room. It found that 4% of all emergency room patients had unrecognized HIV-1 infection and that penetrating trauma was the only clinical presentation associated with an increased seroprevalence rate. This paper should be reviewed by all surgeons who work in the emergency room or intensive care setting.

DeVita Jr., V. T., Hellman, S., and Rosenberg, S. A. (Eds.): AIDS: Etiology, Diagnosis, Treatment, and Prevention. 2nd Edition. J. B. Lippincott Co. 1989.
This 500-page reference book discusses all aspects of HIV-1 infection by the authoritative figures in the field. It is concise, well illustrated, and extensively referenced.

REFERENCES

1. Abrams, D. I., Kiprov, D. D., Goerdert, J. J., Sarngadharan, M. G., Gallo, R. C., and Volberding, P. A.: Antibodies to human T-lymphotropic virus type III and development of the acquired immunodeficiency syndrome in homosexual men presenting with immune thrombocytopenia. Ann. Intern. Med., 104:47, 1986.
2. AIDS-Hemophilia French Study Group: Natural history of primary infection with LAV in multitransfused patients. Blood, 68:89, 1986.
3. AIDS Surveillance in Europe. Paris: World Health Organization Collaborating Centre on AIDS, 1987, Vol. 13, pp. 1–26.
4. Allain, J. P., Paul, D. A., Laurian, Y., et al.: Serological markers in early stages of human immunodeficiency virus infection in haemophiliacs. Lancet, 2:1233, 1986.
5. Anderson, R. E., and Levy, J. A.: Prevalence of antibodies to AIDS associated retrovirus in single men in San Francisco. Lancet, 1:217, 1985.
6. Arden, J.: Anesthetic management of patients with AIDS. Anesthesiology, 64:660, 1986.
7. Baker, J. L., Kelen, G. D., Sivertson, K. T., et al.: Unsuspected human immunodeficiency virus in critically ill emergency patients. J.A.M.A., 257:2609, 1987.
8. Baltimore, D.: RNA-dependent DNA polymerase in virions of RNA tumor viruses. Nature, 226:1209, 1970.
9. Barone, J. E., Gingold, B. S., Nealon, T. F., et al.: Abdominal pain in patients with acquired immune deficiency syndrome. Ann. Surg., 204:619, 1986.
10. Barone, J. E., Wolkomir, A. F., Muakkassa, F. F., et al.: Abdominal pain and anorectal disease in AIDS. Gastroenterol. Clin. North Am. 17:631, 1988.
11. Barre-Sinoussi, F., Chermann, J. C., Rey, F., et al.: Isolation of a T lymphotropic retrovirus from a patient at risk for acquired immunodeficiency syndrome (AIDS). Science, 220:868, 1983.
12. Biggar, R. J., Melbye, M., Ebbesen, P., et al.: Low T-lymphocyte ratios in homosexual men. J.A.M.A., 251:1441, 1984.
13. Biggar, R. J.: The AIDS problem in Africa. Lancet, 1:79, 1986.
14. Burack, J. H., Mandel, M. S., and Bizer, L. S.: Emergency abdominal operations in the patient with acquired immunodeficiency syndrome. Arch. Surg., 124:285, 1989.
15. Burke, D. S., Brundage, J. F., Redfield, R. R., et al.: Measurement of the false positive rate in a screening program for human immunodeficiency virus infections. N. Engl. J. Med., 319:961, 1988.
16. Bygbjerg, I. C.: AIDS in a Danish surgeon (Zaire, 1976). Lancet, 1:925, 1983.
17. Centers for Disease Control: Pneumocystis carinii pneumonia among persons with hemophilia A. M.M.W.R., 31:365, 1982.
18. Centers for Disease Control: Possible transfusion associated acquired immunodeficiency syndrome (AIDS)-California. M.M.W.R., 31:652, 1982.
19. Centers for Disease Control: Revision of the case definition of acquired immunodeficiency syndrome for national reporting—United States. Ann. Intern. Med., 103:402, 1985.
20. Centers for Disease Control: Recommendations for preventing transmission of infection with human T-lymphotropic virus type III/lymphadenopathy-associated virus in the workplace. M.M.W.R., 34(45):681, 691, 1985.
21. Centers for Disease Control: Recommendations for preventing transmission of infection with human T-lymphotropic virus type III/lymphadenopathy-associated virus during invasive procedures. M.M.W.R., 35(14):221, 1986.
22. Centers for Disease Control: AIDS Weekly Surveillance Report—United States, August 10, 1987.
23. Centers for Disease Control: Public Health Service guidelines for counseling and antibody testing to prevent HIV infection and AIDS. M.M.W.R., 36:509, 1987.
24. Centers for Disease Control. Human immunodeficiency virus infection in the United States: A review of current knowledge. M.M.W.R., 36(Suppl 6):1, 1987.
25. Centers for Disease Control: Revision of the CDC surveillance case definition for acquired immunodeficiency syndrome. M.M.W.R., 36(Suppl 1S):3S, 1987.
26. Centers for Disease Control: Human immunodeficiency virus infection transmitted from an organ donor screened for HIV antibody—North Carolina. M.M.W.R., 36:306, 1987.
27. Centers for Disease Control: Update: Acquired immunodeficiency syndrome and human immunodeficiency virus infection among health-care workers. M.M.W.R., 37:229, 239, 1988.
28. Centers for Disease Control: Transmission of HIV through bone transplantation: Case report and public health recommendations. M.M.W.R., 37:597, 1988.
29. Centers for Disease Control: Acquired Immunodeficiency Syndrome Weekly

Surveillance Report—United States AIDS Program. August 18, 1989, pp. 1–5.

30. Cello, J. P., and Wilcox, C. M. Evaluation and treatment of gastrointestinal hemorrhage in patients with AIDS. Gastroenterol. Clin. North Am. 17:639, 1988.

31. Chachoua, A., Dietrich, D., Krasinski, K., et al.: 9-(1,3-dihydroxy-2-propoxymethyl) guanine (Ganciclovir) in the treatment of cytomegalovirus gastrointestinal disease with acquired immunodeficiency syndrome. Ann. Intern. Med., 107:133, 1987.

32. Chaisson, R. E., Moss, A. K., Onishi, R., et al.: Human immunodeficiency virus infection in heterosexual intravenous drug users in San Francisco. Am. J. Public Health, 77:169, 1987.

33. Chak, L. Y., Gill, P. S., Levine, A. M., et al.: Radiation therapy for acquired immunodeficiency syndrome-related Kaposi's sarcoma. J. Clin. Oncol., 6:863, 1988.

34. Clarke, J. A.: HIV transmission and skin grafts (letter). Lancet, 1:983, 1987.

35. Classics in Oncology: Kaposi, M., Idiopathic multiple pigmented sarcoma of the skin. Cancer, 32:342, 1982.

36. Cohen, N. D., Munoz, A., Reitz, B. A., et al.: Transmission of retroviruses by transfusion of screened blood in patients undergoing cardiac surgery. N. Engl. J. Med., 320:1172, 1989.

37. Collier, A. C., Barnes, R. C., and Handsfield, H. H.: Prevalence of antibody to LAV/HTLV-III among homosexual men in Seattle. Am. J. Public Health, 76:564, 1986.

38. Courouce, A. M.: HIV-2 in blood donors and in different risk groups in France (Letter). Lancet, 1:1151, 1987.

39. Creagh-Kirk, T., Doi P., Andrews, E., et al.: Survival experience among patients with AIDS receiving zidovudine: Follow-up of patients in a compassionate plea program. J.A.M.A., 260:3009, 1988.

40. Curie-Cohen, M., Luttrell, L., and Shapiro, S.: Current practice of artificial insemination by donor in the United States. N. Engl. J. Med., 300:585, 1979.

41. Currin, J. W., Lawrence, D. N., Jaffe, H., et al.: Acquired immunodeficiency syndrome (AIDS) associated with transfusions. N. Engl. J. Med., 30:69, 1984.

42. D'Aguilla, R., Williams, A. B., Kleber, H. D., et al.: Prevalence of HTLV III infection among New Haven, Connecticut, parenteral drug abusers in 1982–983 (Letter). N. Engl. J. Med., 314:117, 1986.

43. Dalgleish, A. G., Beverly, P. C. L., Clapham, P. R., et al.: The CD4 (T4) antigen is an essential component of the receptor for the AIDS retrovirus. Nature, 312:763, 1984.

44. Daling, J. R., Weiss, N. S., Klopfenstein, L. L., Cochran, L. E., Chow, W. H., and Daifuku, R.: Correlates of homosexual behavior and the incidence of anal cancer. J.A.M.A., 247:1988, 1982.

45. Daling, J. R., Weiss, N. S., Hislop, T. G., Maden, C., Coates, R. J., Sherman, K. J., Ashley, R. L., Beagrie, M., Ryan, J. A., and Corey, L.: Sexual practices, sexually transmitted diseases, and the incidence of anal cancer. N. Engl. J. Med., 317:973, 1987.

46. Dean, N. C., Golden, J. A., Evans, L. A., et al.: Human immunodeficiency virus recovery from bronchoalveolar lavage fluid in patients with AIDS. Chest, 93:1176, 1988.

47. Donegan, E., and Transfusion Safety Study Group: Course of HIV infection in transfusion recipients. IV International Conference on AIDS. Stockholm, 1988, Vol. 2, p. 7710.

48. Donegan, E., and Transfusion Safety Study Group: Comparison of HTLV-I/II with HIV-1 transmission by component type and shelf storage before administration. Presented at the American Association of Blood Banks 42nd Annual Meeting, New Orleans, October 21–26, 1989.

49. Ehrlich, G. D., and Poiesz, B. J.: Clinical and molecular parameters of HTLV-I infection (Review). Clin. Lab. Med., 8:65, 1988.

50. Erice, A., Rahme, F., Sullivan, C., et al.: Human immunodeficiency virus (HIV) infection in organ transplant recipients (OTRS) (Abstract). IV International Conference on AIDS. Stockholm, 1988, p. 7756.

51. Eyster, M. E., Goedert, J. J., Sarngadharan, M. G., et al.: Development and early natural history of HTLV-III antibodies in patients with hemophilia. J.A.M.A., 253:2219, 1985.

52. Fahey, J. L., Prince, H., Weaver, M., et al.: Quantitative changes in the T helper or T suppressor/cytotoxic lymphocyte subsets that distinguish acquired immunodeficiency syndrome form other immune subset disorders. Am. J. Med., 76:95, 1984.

53. Farthing, C. F., Henry, K., Shanson, D. C., et al.: Clinical investigations of lymphadenopathy, including lymph node biopsies, in 24 homosexual men with antibody to the human T-cell lymphocytotropic virus type III (HTLV-III) Br. J. Surg., 73:180, 1986.

54. Farzadegan, H., Polis, M. A., Wolinsky, S. M., et al.: Loss of human immunodeficiency virus type 1 (HIV-1) antibodies with evidence of viral infection in asymptomatic homosexual man: A report from the multicenter AIDS cohort study. Ann. Intern. Med., 108:785, 1988.

55. FDA: 5-Minute DNA test for HIV-1 antibodies. FDA Drug Bulletin 1989;19(February):7–8.

56. Ferguson, C. M.: Surgical complications of human immunodeficiency virus infection. Am. Surg., 54:4, 1988.

57. Ferguson, C. M.: Splenectomy for immune thrombocytopenia related to human immunodeficiency virus. Surg. Gynecol. Obstet., 167:300, 1988.

58. Fischel, M. A., Richman, D. D., Grieco, M. H., et al.: The efficacy of azidothymidine (AZT) in the treatment of AIDS or AIDS-related complex. N. Engl. J. Med., 317:185, 1987.

59. Flynn, N. M., Pollet, S. M., Van Horne, J. R., et al.: Absence of HIV antibody

among dental professionals exposed to infected patients. West. J. Med., 146:439, 1987.

60. Frank, D., and Raicht, R. F.: Intestinal perforation associated with cytomegalovirus infection in patients with acquired immune deficiency syndrome. Am. J. Gastroenterol., 79:201, 1984.

61. Friedman, S. L.: Gastrointestinal and hepatobiliary neoplasms in AIDS. Gastroenterol. Clin. North Am. 17:465, 1988.

62. Fujikawa, L. S., Palestine, A. G., Nussenblatt, R. B., et al.: Isolation of human T-lymphotropic virus type III from the tears of a patient with the acquired immunodeficiency syndrome. Lancet, 2:529, 1985.

63. Gaines, H., Sonnerborg, A., Czajkowski, J., et al.: Antibody response in primary immunodeficiency virus infection. Lancet, 1:1249, 1987.

64. Gallo, R. C., Salahuddin, S. Z., Popovic, M., et al.: Frequent detection and isolation of cytopathic retroviruses (HTLV-III) from patients with AIDS and at risk for AIDS. Science, 224:500, 1984.

65. Gerberding, J. L., Nelson, K., Greenspan, D., et al.: Risk to dentists from occupational immunodeficiency virus (HIV): Followup (Abstract). Washington, D.C.: Twenty-seventh Interscience Conference on Antimicrobial Agents and Chemotherapy. American Society for Microbiology, 1987.

66. Gerberding, J. L., Bryant-LeBlanc, C. E., Nelson, K., et al.: Risk of transmitting the human immunodeficiency virus, hepatitis B virus, and cytomegalovirus to health-care workers exposed to patients with AIDS and AIDS-related conditions. J. Infect. Dis. 156:1, 1987.

67. Gerberding, J. L., Henderson, D. K.: Design of rational infection control policies for human immunodeficiency virus infection. J. Infect. Dis. 156:861, 1987.

68. Godley, M. J.: AIDS and lymphadenopathy. Br. J. Surg., 73:170, 1986.

69. Goedert, J. J., Sarngadharan, M. G., Eyster, M. E., et al.: Antibodies reactive with human T cell leukemia viruses (HTLV-III) in the serum of hemophiliacs receiving factor VIII concentrate. Blood, 65:492, 1985.

70. Goedert, J. J., Blattner, W. A.: The epidemiology of AIDS and related conditions. In DeVita, V. T., Hellman, S., Rosenberg, S. A. (Eds.): AIDS: Etiology, diagnosis, treatment, and prevention. Philadelphia, J. B. Lippincott Company, 1985.

71. Gonda, M. A., Braun, M. J., Clements, J. E., et al.: Human T-cell lymphotropic virus type III shares sequence homology with a family of pathogenic lentiviruses. Proc. Natl. Acad. Sci. USA, 83:4007, 1986.

72. Gottlieb, M. S., Schroff, R., Schanker, H. M., et al.: Pneumocystis carinii pneumonias and mucosal candidiasis in previously healthy homosexual men: Evidence of a new acquired immunodeficiency. N. Engl. J. Med., 305:1425, 1981.

73. Goudsmit, J., De Wolf, F., Lange, J. M. A.: Expression of human immunodeficiency virus antigen (HIV-Ag) in serum and cerebrospinal fluid during acute and chronic infection. Lancet, 2:177, 1986.

74. Goudsmit, J., Lange, J. M. A., Paul, D. A., Dawson, G. J.: Antigenemia and antibody titers to core and envelope antigens in AIDS, AIDS-related complex, and subclinical human immunodeficiency virus infection. J. Infect. Dis., 155:558, 1987.

75. Groopman, J. E., Salahuddin, S. Z., Sarngadharan, M. G., et al.: HTLV-III in saliva of people with AIDS-related complex and healthy homosexual men at risk for AIDS. Science, 226:447, 1984.

76. Gurtler, L. G., Wernicke, D., Eberle, J., et al.: Increase in prevalence of anti-HTLV-III in haemophiliacs (Letter). Lancet, 2:1275, 1984.

77. Haseltine, W. A.: Silent HIV infections (Editorial). N. Engl. J. Med., 320:1487, 1989.

78. Hardy, A. M., Allen, J. R., Morgan, W. M., et al.: The incidence rate of acquired immunodeficiency syndrome in selected populations. J.A.M.A. 253:215, 1985.

79. Harper, M. E., Marselle, L. M., Gallo, R. C., Wong Staal, F.: Detection of lymphocytes expressing human T lymphotropic virus type III in lymph nodes and peripheral blood from infected individuals by in situ hybridization. Proc. Natl. Acad. Sci. 83:772, 1986.

80. Hart, C., Schochetman, G., Spira, T., et al.: Direct detection of HIV RNA expression in seropositive subjects. Lancet, 2:596, 1988.

81. Henderson, D. K., Saah, A. J., Zak, B. J., et al.: Risk of nosocomial infection with human T cell lymphotropic virus type III/lymphadenopathy associated virus in a large cohort of intensively exposed health care workers. Ann. Intern. Med., 104:644, 1986.

82. Henderson, D. K.: HIV-1 in the health care setting. In Mandell, G. F., Douglas, R. G., Jr., Bennett, J. E. (Eds.): Principles and practice of infectious diseases, 3rd ed. New York, John Wiley & Sons, 1989.

83. Henderson, D. K., and Gelberding, J. L.: Prophylactic zidovudine after occupational exposure to the human immunodeficiency virus: An interim analysis. J. Infect. Dis., 160:321, 1989.

84. Heyward, W. L., Curran, J. W.: Rapid screening tests for HIV infection (Editorial). J.A.M.A., 260:542, 1988.

85. Hirsch, M. S., Wormser, G. P., Schooley, R. T., et al.: Risk of nosocomial infection with human T cell lymphotropic virus III (HTLV-III). N. Engl. J. Med., 312:1, 1985.

86. Hirschel, B., Glauser, M., Chave, D., Tauber, M., and Swiss Group for Clinical Studies on the Acquired Immunodeficiency Syndrome: Zidovudine for the treatment of thrombocytopenia associated with the human immunodeficiency virus. Ann. Intern. Med., 109:718, 1988.

87. Ho, D. D., Schooley, R. T., Rota, T. R., et al.: HTLV-III in the semen and blood of a healthy homosexual man. Science, 226:447, 1984.

88. Ho, D. D., Rota, T. R., Schooley, R. T., et al.: Isolation of HTLV-III from

cerebrospinal fluid and neural tissues of patients with neurologic syndromes related to the acquired immunodeficiency syndrome. N. Engl. J. Med., 313:1493, 1985.

89. Ho, D. D., Byington, R., Schooley, R. T., et al.: Infrequency of isolation of HTLV-III virus from saliva in AIDS. N. Engl. J. Med., 313:1606, 1985.

90. Hollander, H., Levy, J. A.: Neurologic abnormalities and recovery of human immunodeficiency virus from cerebrospinal fluid. Ann. Intern. Med., 106:692, 1987.

91. HTLV-III antibody ELISA results(Letter).Lancet 1:1222, 1985.

92. Imagawa, D. T., Lee, M. H., Wolinsky, S. M., et al.: Human immunodeficiency virus type 1 infection in homosexual men who remain seronegative for prolonged periods. N. Engl. J. Med., 320:1458, 1989.

93. Jaffe, H. W., Darrow, W. W., Echenberg, D. F., et al.: The acquired immunodeficiency syndrome in a cohort of homosexual men: A six year follow-up study. Ann. Intern. Med., 103:210, 1985.

94. Joline, C., Wormser, G. P.: Update on a prospective study of health care workers exposed to blood and body fluids of acquired immunodeficiency syndrome patients. Am. J. Infect. Control. 15:86, 1987.

95. Kaplan, L. D., Hoopewell, P. C., Jaffe, H., et al.: Kaposi's sarcoma involving the lung in the acquired immunodeficiency syndrome. J. Acquir. Immune Defic. Syndr. 1:23, 1988.

96. Karpatkin, S., Nardi, M., Lennette, E. T., Byrne, B., and Poiesz, B.: Antihuman immunodeficiency virus type 1 antibody complexes on platelets of seropositive thrombocytopenic homosexuals and narcotic addicts. Proc. Natl. Acad. Sci., 85:9763, 1988.

97. Kelen, G. D., Fritz, S., Qaqish, B., et al.: Unrecognized human immunodeficiency virus infection in emergency department patients. N. Engl. J. Med., 318:1645, 1988.

98. Kemp, B. E., Rylatt, D. B., Bundensen, P. G., et al.: Autologous red cell agglutination assay for HIV-1 antibodies: Simplified test with whole blood. Science, 241:1352, 1988.

99. Kim, J. H., Durack, D. T.: Manifestations of human T-lymphotropic virus type I infection. Am. J. Med., 84:919, 1988.

100. Klatzmann, D., Champagne, E., Chamaret, S., et al.: T-lymphocyte T4 molecule behaves as the receptor for human retrovirus LAV. Nature, 312:767, 1984.

101. Klein, R. S., Phelan, J., Friedland, G. H., et al. Prevalence of antibodies to HTLV-III/LAV among dental professionals (Abstract). American Society for Microbiology, Twenty-sixth Interscience Congress on Antimicrobial Agents and Chemotherapy, New Orleans, 1986, p. 283.

102. Kleinman, S., Secord, K.: Risk of human immunodeficiency virus (HIV) transmission by anti-HIV negative blood: Estimates using the lookback methodology. Transfusion, 28:499, 1988.

103. Klotman, M. E., DeRossi, A., Buchbinder, A., Wong-Staal, F.: RNA splicing events detected in early in vitro HIV infection using the polymerase chain reaction (PCR) (Abstract). V International Conference on AIDS. Montreal, 1989.

104. Kotler, D. P.: Intestinal and hepatic manifestations of AIDS. Adv. Intern. Med., 34:43, 1989.

105. Kuhls, T. L., Viker, S., Parris, N. B., et al.: Occupational risk of HIV, HBV, and HSV-2 infections in health care personnel caring for AIDS patients. Am. J. Public Health 77:1306, 1987.

106. Kwok, S., Mack, D. H., Mullis, K. B., et al.: Identification of human immunodeficiency virus sequences by using in vitro enzymatic amplification and oligomer cleavage detection. J. Virol. 61:1690, 1987.

107. LaFon, S. W., Nusinoff-Lehrman, S., Barry, D. W.: Prophylactically administered Retrovir in health care workers potentially exposed to the human immunodeficiency virus (Letter). J. Infect. Dis. 158:503, 1988.

108. Lane, H. C., Masur, H., Gelmann, E. P., et al.: Correlation between immunologic function and clinical subpopulations of patients with the acquired immune deficiency syndrome. Am. J. Med., 78:417, 1985.

109. Lasky, L. A., Nakamura, G., Smith, D. H., et al.: Delineation of a region of the human immunodeficiency virus type 1 gp120 glycoprotein critical for the interaction with the CD4 receptor. Cell, 50:975, 1987.

110. LaRaja, R. D., Rothenberg, R. E., Odom, J. W., et al.: The incidence of intra-abdominal surgery in acquired immunodeficiency syndrome: A statistical review of 904 patients. Surgery, 105:175, 1989.

111. Larson, C. J., Taswell, H. F.: Human T-cell leukemia virus type I (HTLV-I) and blood transfusion. Mayo Clin. Proc. 63:869, 1988.

112. Lee, H., Swanson, P., Shorty, V. S., et al.: High rate of HTLV-II infection in seropositive i.v. drug abusers in New Orleans. Science, 244:471, 1989.

113. Lemlich, G., Schwam, L., Lebwohl, M.: Kaposi's sarcoma and acquired immunodeficiency syndrome: Post-mortem findings in 24 cases. J. Am. Acad. Dermatol. 16:319, 1987.

114. Letvin, N. L., Eaton, K. A., and Aldrich, W. R.: Acquired immunodeficiency syndrome in a colony of macaque monkeys. Proc. Natl. Acad. Sci. USA, 80:2178, 1983.

115. Levy, J. A., Shimabukuro, J., Hollander, H., et al.: Isolation of AIDS-associated retroviruses from cerebrospinal fluid and brain of patients with neurological symptoms. Lancet, 2:586, 1985.

116. Levy, J. A., Kaminsky, L. S., Morrow, W. J. W., et al.: Infection by the retrovirus associated with the acquired immunodeficiency syndrome: Clinical, biological, and molecular features. Ann. Intern. Med., 103:694, 1985.

117. Lipsett, P., and Allo, M. D.: AIDS and the surgeon. Surg. Clin. of North America, 68:73, 1988.

118. Liu, K. J., Darrow, W. W., and Rutherford, G. W.: A model based estimated for the mean incubation period for AIDS in homosexual men. Science, 240:1333, 1988.

119. Loche, M., and Mach, B.: Identification of HIV-infected seronegative individuals by a direct diagnostic test based on hybridisation to amplified viral DNA. Lancet, 2:418, 1988.

120. Lotze, M. T.: AIDS: A surgeon's responsibility. ACS Bull., 70:6, 1985.

121. McArthur, J. C.: Neurologic manifestations of AIDS (Review). Medicine (Baltimore) 66:407, 1987.

122. McCray, E., and Cooperative Needlestick Group: Occupational risk of the acquired immunodeficiency syndrome among health care workers. N. Engl. J. Med., 314:1127, 1986.

123. MacDonald, K. L., Jackson, J. B., Bowman, R. J., et al.: Performance characteristics of serologic tests for human immunodeficiency virus type 1 (HIV-1) antibody among Minnesota blood donors. Public health and clinical implications. Ann. Intern. Med., 110:617, 1989.

124. McDougal, J. S., Kennedy, M. S., Sligh, J. M., et al.: Binding of HTLV-III/LAV to T4+ T cells by a complex of the 110K viral protein and the T4 molecule. Science, 231:382, 1986.

125. McEvoy, M., Porter, K., Mortimer, P., et al.: Prospective study of clinical, laboratory, and ancillary staff with accidental exposures to blood or body fluids from patients infected with HIV. Br. Med. J. 294:1595, 1987.

126. McGrady, G. A., Jason, J. M., and Evatt, B. L.: The course of the acquired immune deficiency syndrome in the United States hemophilia population. Am. J. Epidemiol., 126:25, 1987.

127. Macho, J. R.: Gastrointestinal surgery in the AIDS patient. Gastroenterol. Clin. North Am. 17:563, 1988.

128. Mann, J. M., Chin, J., Piot, P., Quinn, T. C.: The international epidemiology of AIDS. Scientific American 259:82, 1988.

129. Marcus R. Surveillance of health care workers exposed to blood from patients infected with the human immunodeficiency virus. N. Engl. J. Med., 319:1118, 1988.

130. Margulis, S. J., Honig, C. L., Soave, R., et al.: Biliary tract obstruction in the acquired immunodeficiency syndrome. Ann. Intern. Med., 105:207, 1986.

131. Masur, H., Michelis, M. A., Greene, J. B., et al.: An outbreak of community acquired Pneumocystis carinii pneumonia: Initial manifestations of cellular dysfunction. N. Engl. J. Med., 305:1431, 1981.

132. Meiselman, M. S., Cello, J. P., and Margaretten, W.: Cytomegalovirus Colitis: A report of the clinical, endoscopic, and pathologic findings in two patients with the acquired immune deficiency syndrome. Gastroenterology, 88:171, 1985.

133. Melbye, M., Biggar, R. J., Chermann, J. C., et al.: High prevalence of lymphadenopathy virus (LAV) in European hemophiliacs. Lancet 2:40, 1984.

134. Minamoto, G. Y., Gold, J. W. M., Scheinberg, D. A., et al.: Infection with human T-cell leukemia virus type 1 in patients with leukemia. N. Engl. J. Med., 318:219, 1988.

135. Mitsuya, H., Weinhold, K. J., Furman, P. A., et al.: 3'-Azido-3'-deoxythymidine (BWA 509U): An antiviral agent that inhibits the infectivity and cytopathic effects of human T-lympho-cytotropic virus type III/lymphadenopathy associated virus in-vitro. Proc. Natl. Acad. Sci. USA, 82:1333, 1985.

136. Morris, L., Distenfeld, A., Amorosi, E., Karpatkin, S.: Autoimmune thrombocytopenic purpura in homosexual men. Ann. Intern. Med., 96:714, 1982.

137. Mortimer, P. P., Vandervelde, E. M., Jesson, W. J., et al.: HTLV-III antibody in Swiss and English intravenous drug abusers. Lancet 2:449, 1985.

138. Mundy, D. C., Schinazi, R. F., Gerber, A. R., et al.: Human immunodeficiency virus isolated from amniotic fluid (Letter). Lancet 2:459, 1987.

139. Murakawa, G. J., Zaia, J. A., Spallone, P. A., et al.: Direct detection of HIV-1 RNA from AIDS and ARC patient samples. DNA 7:287, 1988.

140. Murphy, M. F., Metcalfe, P., Waters, A. H., Carne, C. A., Weller, I. V. D., Linch, D. C., and Smith, A.: Incidence and mechanism of neutropenia and thrombocytopenia in patients with human immunodeficiency virus infection. Br. J. Haematol., 66:337, 1987.

141. Neumayer, H. H., Fassbinder, W., Kresse, S., Wagner, K.: Human T-lymphotropic virus III antibody screening in kidney transplant recipients and patients receiving maintenance hemodialysis. Transplant Proc. 19:2169, 1987.

142. Nobler, M. P., Leddy, M. E., Huh, S. H.: The impact of palliative irradiation on the management of patients with acquired immune deficiency syndrome. J. Clin. Oncol., 5(1):107–112, 1987.

143. Nugent, P., and O'Connell, T. X.: The surgeon's role in treating acquired immunodeficiency syndrome. Arch. Surg., 121:1117, 1986.

144. Oksenhendler, E., Bierling, P., Ferchal, F., Chauvel, J. P., and Seligmann, M.: Zidovudine for thrombocytopenic purpura related to human immunodeficiency virus (HIV) infection. Ann. Intern. Med., 110:365, 1989.

145. Osmond, D., Moss, A. R.: The prevalence of HIV infection in the United States: A reappraisal of the Public Health Service estimate. In Volberding, P., Jacobson, M.: 1989 Clinical AIDS Review. New York, Marcel Dekker, 1990.

146. Ou, C., Kwok, S., Mitchell, S. W., et al.: DNA amplification for direct detection of HIV-1 in DNA of peripheral blood mononuclear cells. Science, 239:295, 1988.

147. Pan, L.-Z., Chang-Mayer, C., Levy, J. A.: Patterns of antibody response in individuals infected with the human immunodeficiency virus. J. Infect. Dis., 155:626, 1987.

148. Patow, C. A., Stark, T. W., Findlay, P. A., Steis, R., Longo, D. L., Masur, H., and Macher, A. M.: Pharyngeal obstruction by Kaposi's sarcoma in a homosexual male with acquired immune deficiency syndrome. Otolaryngol. Head Neck Surg., 92:713, 1984.

149. Peterman, T. A., Lui, K. J., Lawrence, D. N., Allen, J. R.: Estimating the risk of

transfusion-associated acquired immune deficiency syndrome and human immunodeficiency virus infection. Transfusion 27:371, 1987.

150. Petito, C. K., Bradford, A. N., Cho, E. S., et al.: Vacuolar myelopathy pathologically resembling subacute combined degeneration in patients with the acquired immunodeficiency syndrome. N. Engl. J. Med., 312:874, 1985.

151. Potter, D. A., Danforth, D. N., Macher, A. M., et al.: Evaluation of abdominal pain in the AIDS patient. Ann. Surg., 199:332, 1984.

152. Quinn, T. C., Riggin, C. H., Kline, R. L., et al.: Rapid latex agglutination assay using recombinant envelope polypeptide for the detection of antibody to the HIV. J.A.M.A. 260:510, 1988.

153. Ranki, A., Valle, S.-L., Krohn, M., et al.: Long latency precedes overt seroconversion in sexually transmitted human-immunodeficiency-virus infection. Lancet, 2:589, 1987.

154. Rashleigh-Belcher, H. J. C., Carne, C. A., Weller, I. V. D., et al.: Surgical biopsy for persistent generalized lymphadenopathy. Br. J. Surg., 73:183, 1986.

155. Ratner, L., Haseltine, W., Patarca, R., et al.: Complete nucleotide sequence of the AIDS virus, HTLV-III. Nature, 313:217, 1985.

156. Ravikumar, T. S., Allen, J. D., Bothe, A., and Steele, G.: Splenectomy: The treatment of choice for human immunodeficiency virus-related immune thrombocytopenia? Arch. Surg., 124:625, 1989.

157. Rees, M.: The sombre view of AIDS. Nature, 326:343, 1987.

158. Rekart, M.: HIV transmission by artificial insemination (Abstract). IV International Conference on AIDS. Stockholm, 1988, p. 4026.

159. Richman, D. D., Fischl, M. A., Grieco, M. H., et al.: The toxicity of azidothymide (AZT) in the treatment of patients with AIDS and AIDS-related complex: A double-blind, placebo-controlled trial. N. Engl. J. Med., 317:192, 1987.

160. Robertson, J. R., Bucknall, A. B., Welsby, P. D., et al.: Epidemic of AIDS related virus (HTLV-III/LAV) infection among intravenous drug abusers. Br. Med. J., 292:527, 1986.

161. Robinson, G., Wilson, S. E., and Williams, R. A.: Surgery in patients with acquired immunodeficiency syndrome. Arch. Surg., 122:170, 1987.

162. Rogers, M. F., Ou, C.-Y., Rayfield, M., et al.: Use of the polymerase chain reaction for early detection of the proviral sequences of human immunodeficiency virus in infants born to seropositive mothers. N. Engl. J. Med., 320:1649, 1989.

162a. Rossi, G., Gorla, R., Stellini, R., et al.: Prevalence, clinical, and laboratory features of thrombocytopenia among HIV-infected individuals. AIDS Research and Human Retroviruses, 6:261, 1990.

163. Rothenberg, R., Woelfel, M., Stoneburner, R., et al.: Survival with the acquired immune deficiency syndrome. N. Engl. J. Med., 317:1297, 1987.

164. Routes of HIV-2 transmission in western Europe (Letter). Lancet, 1:1150, 1987.

165. Ruprecht, R. M., O'Brien, L. G., Rossoni, R. D., Nusinoff-Lehrman, S.:Suppression of mouse viraemia and retroviral disease by 3'-azido-3'-deoxythymidine (Letter). Nature, 323:467, 1986.

166. Safai, B., Good, R. A.: Kaposi's sarcoma: A review and recent developments. Cancer, 32:2, 1981.

167. Salahudden, S. Z., Markham, P. D., Popovic, M., et al.: Isolation of human T leukemia virus type III (HTLV-III) from patients with acquired immunodeficiency syndrome (AIDS) or AIDS-related complex (ARC) and from healthy carriers: A study of risk groups and tissue sources. Proc. Natl. Acad. Sci. USA, 254:5530, 1985.

168. Schneider, P. A., Abrams, D. I., Rayner, A. A., et al.: Immunodeficiency-associated thrombocytopenia purpura (IDTP). Arch. Surg., 122:1175, 1987.

169. Schneiderman, D. J., Arenson, D. M., Cello, J. P., Margaretten W., and Weber, T. E.: Hepatic disease in patients with the acquired immune deficiency syndrome (AIDS). Hepatology, 7:925, 1987.

170. Schneiderman, D. J.: Hepatobiliary abnormalities of AIDS. Gastroenterol. Clin. North Am. 17:615, 1988.

171. Scott, H. J., Glynn, M. J., Lane, I. F., et al.: Strategy for lymph node biopsy in homosexual men suspected of having LAV/HTLV-III related disease. Br. J. Surg., 73:186, 1986.

172. Seigel, F. P., Lopez, C., Hammer, G. S., et al.: Severe acquired immunodeficiency in male homosexuals, manifested by chronic perianal ulcerative herpes simplex lesions. N. Engl. J. Med., 305:1439, 1981.

173. Shaw, G. M., Harper, M. E., Hahn, B. H., et al.: HTLV-III infection in brains of children and adults with AIDS encephalopathy. Science, 227:177, 1985.

174. Sivak, S. L., Wormser, G. P.: How common is HTLV-III infection in the United States? (Letter). N. Engl. J. Med., 313:1352, 1985.

175. Spira, T. J., Des Jarlais, D. C., Marmor, M., et al.: Prevalence of antibody to lymphadenopathy-associated virus among drug detoxification patients in New York. N. Engl. J. Med., 311:467, 1984.

176. Stewart, G. J., Cunningham, A. L., Driscoll, G. L., et al.: Transmission of human T-cell lymphotropic virus type III (HTLV-III) by artificial insemination by donor. Lancet, 2:581, 1985.

177. Stiles, Q. R., Carey, J. S., Clark, R. E., et al.: The Society of Thoracic Surgeons Ad Hoc Committee on AIDS: Report to the membership. Ann. Thorac. Surg., 47:946, 1989.

178. Stricof, R. L., Morse, D. L.: HTLV-III/LAV seroconversion following a deep intramuscular needlestick injury (Letter). N. Engl. J. Med., 314:1115, 1986.

179. Tavares, L., Roneker, C., Johnston, K., et al.: 3'-azido-3'-deoxythymidine in feline leukemia virus-infected cats: A model for therapy and prophylaxis of AIDS. Cancer Res., 47:3190, 1987.

180. Temin, H. M., Mitzutani, S.: RNA directed DNA polymerase in virions of Rous sarcoma virus. Nature, 226:1211, 1970.

181. Thiry, L., Sprecher-Goldberger, S., Jonckheer, T., et al.: Isolation of AIDS virus from cell-free breast milk of three healthy virus carriers. Lancet, 2:891, 1985.

182. Tindall, B., Barker, S., Donovan, B., et al.: Characterization of the acute illness associated with human immunodeficiency virus infection. Arch. Int. Med., 148:945, 1988.

183. Transfusion Safety Study Group: Antibody to HTLV-I/II among blood donors in four cities of the United States. V International Conference on AIDS. Montreal, 1989. Mosley, JW: Abstract, p. 146.

184. Tyler, D. S., Shaunak, S., Bartlett J. A., et al.: HIV-1 associated thrombocytopenia: The role of splenectomy. Ann. Surg., 211:211, 1990.

185. Tyms, A. S., Taylor, D. L., and Parkin, J. M.: Cytomegalovirus and the acquired immunodeficiency syndrome. J. Antimicrob. Chemother., 23 (Suppl. A):89, 1989.

186. U.S. Department of Health and Human Services, Public Health Service. Coolfont report: A PHS plan for prevention and control of AIDS and AIDS virus. Pub. Health Rep., 101:341, 1986.

187. Van de Perre, P., Nzaramba, D., Allen, S., et al.: Comparison of six serological assays for human immunodeficiency virus antibody detection in developing countries. J. Clin. Microbiol., 26:552, 1988.

188. Vogt, M. W., Craven, D. E., Crawford, D. F., et al.: Isolation of HTLV-III/LAV from cervical secretions of women at risk for AIDS. Lancet, 1:525, 1986.

189. Vogt, M. W., Witt, D. J., Craven, D. E.: Isolation patterns of the human immunodeficiency virus from cervical secretions during the menstrual cycle of women at risk for the acquired immunodeficiency syndrome. Ann. Intern. Med., 106:380, 1987.

190. Volberding, P. A., Kaslow, K., Bilk, M., et al.: Prognostic factors in staging Kaposi's sarcoma in the acquired immunodeficiency syndrome (Abstract). Proc. Am. Soc. Clin. Oncol. 3:51, 1984.

191. Volberding, P. A.: Kaposi's sarcoma in AIDS. Med. Clin. North Am., 70:665, 1986.

192. Walsh, C. M., Nardi, M. A., and Karpatkin, S.: On the mechanism of thrombocytopenic purpura in sexually active homosexual men. N. Engl. J. Med., 311:635, 1984.

193. Walsh, C. M., Krigel, R., Lennette, E., and Karpatkin, S.: Thrombocytopenia in homosexual patients: Prognosis, response to therapy, and prevalence of antibody to the retrovirus associated with the acquired immunodeficiency syndrome. Ann. Intern. Med., 103:542, 1985.

194. Ward, J. W., Holmberg, S. D., Allen, J. R., et al.: Transmission of human immunodeficiency virus (HIV) by blood transfusions screened as negative for HIV antibody. N. Engl. J. Med., 318:473, 1988.

195. Weiss, S. H., Saxinger, W. C., Rechtman, D., et al.: HTLV-III infection among health care workers: Association with needlestick injuries. J.A.M.A., 254:2089, 1985.

196. Weiss, S. H., Ginzburg, H. M., Goedert, J. J., et al.: Risk for HTLV-III exposure and AIDS among parenteral drug abusers in New Jersey (Abstract). In The International Conference on Acquired Immunodeficiency Syndrome: Abstracts. Philadelphia, The American College of Physicians, 1985.

197. Wexner, S. D., Smithy, W. B., Milson, J. W., et al.: The surgical management of anorectal diseases in AIDS and pre-AIDS patients. Dis. Colon. Rectum, 29:719, 1986.

200. Wilber, J. C.: Serologic testing of human immunodeficiency virus infection (Review). Clin. Lab. Med., 7:777, 1987.

201. Wilson, S. E., Robinson, G., Williams, R. A., et al.: Acquired immunodeficiency syndrome: Indications for abdominal surgery, pathology and outcome. Ann. Surg. 210:4, 1989.

202. Wofsy, C. B., Cohen, J. B., Hauer, L. B., et al.: Isolation of AIDS associated retrovirus from genital secretions of women with antibodies to the virus. Lancet, 1:527, 1986.

203. Yarchoan, R., Klecker, R. W., Weinhold, K. J., et al.: Administration of 3'-azido-3'-deoxythymidine: An inhibitor of HTLV-III/LAV replication, to patients with AIDS or AIDS-related complex. Lancet, 1:575, 1986.

204. Zagury, D., Bernard, J., Leibowitch, J., et al.: HTLV-III in cells cultured from semen of two patients with AIDS. Science, 226:449, 1984.

14

BITES AND STINGS

Kenneth P. Ramming, M.D.

SNAKEBITE

Incidence

The World Health Organization estimates that as many as 300,000 snakebites occur throughout the world each year, causing perhaps 30,000 to 40,000 deaths. The largest number of fatal snakebites occur in Southeast Asia (approximately 25,000). The mortality in South America is 3000 to 4000 annually.[14] In the United States, approximately 45,000 snakebites are reported each year, of which some 7000 are treated as venomous. Only 14 to 15 deaths occur annually in this country.[46,59]

At least one venomous snake species is indigenous to every state in the United States except Maine, Alaska, and Hawaii. The largest number of snakebites occur in Texas. States having the highest incidence per 100,000 population are, in order, North Carolina, Arkansas, Texas, Georgia, West Virginia, Mississippi, Louisiana, and Oklahoma. Few bites are reported in New England. More than 90 per cent of all snakebites occur from April through October.[14,46,59] Males between the ages of 5 and 19 are most often afflicted.

Approximately 10 per cent of snakes in the United States are poisonous. Pit vipers, including rattlesnakes, copperheads, and cottonmouths, constitute 99 per cent of all venomous bites. The diagnosis and management of bites from this group are essentially the same. Coral snakes and snakes from other areas of the world in captivity in the United States are responsible for the remainder of venomous bites.[14]

Identification of venomous snakes in the United States is relatively simple. As depicted in Figure 1, pit vipers have a characteristic pit located between the eye and the nostril on each side of the head. They also have elliptical pupils, two well-developed fangs that protrude from the maxilla, and single subcaudal plates. Harmless snakes have round pupils, no pits, no fangs, and double subcaudal plates. The one exception is the coral snake, an indigenous poisonous snake with round eyes and no fangs. It has brightly colored bands of red, yellow, and black and is the only snake to have adjacent red and yellow bands ("red touching yellow means a dangerous fellow"). Information on venomous snakes in the United States is summarized briefly in Table 1.

Biology

The fangs of pit vipers are long, hollow tubes set forward in the maxilla, ideal for delivery of venom. Pit vipers can control the position of the fangs and the amount of venom injected, and this may represent some variability in the toxic effects of different bites. The fangs of the coral snake are fixed. Large snakes produce more venom than small ones.[11,47,56]

Snake venoms are complex mixtures of polypeptides with diverse pharmacologic effects. Enzymes such as phospholipase A, hyaluronidase, adenosine triphosphatase (ATPase), 5-nucleotidase, and NAD are found in venom. Phospholipase A is the most potent contributor to toxicity, converting lecithin to lysolecithin, a substance very destructive to human tissues. Local tissue damage, neurotoxicity, hemolysis, histamine release, and possibly anaphylaxis have been attributed to this enzyme. Hyaluronidase aids in spreading venom by lysis of ground substance. ATPase and 5-nucleotidase depress metabolism and contribute to shock. Other enzymes isolated from some venoms are cholinesterase, L-amino acid oxidase, protease, phosphomonoesterase, RNAase, and DNAase. Also present in venoms are polypeptide elements that have a direct toxic effect on cells. Crotoxin, for example, has been implicated in causing hemolysis, paralysis, bradykinin release, and direct toxicity to cardiac muscle. Collectively, snake venoms have effects on every organ system. In most cases, however, the deleterious effects are directed toward the blood and also the cardiovascular, nervous, and respiratory systems.[11,14,57]

Clinical Manifestations

In *Crotalus* (pit viper) bites, there is an almost immediate, intense destruction of local tissue. Edema and erythema result, provoking a subjective sensation of intense pain. Permeability of blood vessels is altered and extravasation of plasma and blood into tissues causes ecchymosis and bulla formation. Sloughing of tissues often occurs at the wound site.

When large amounts of venom are injected, severe systemic effects ensue. Often massive tissue necrosis and edema of an entire extremity result. Red blood cells respond by swelling and becoming spherical, and some are lysed. The hematocrit falls, and the number of platelets can be markedly reduced. Bleeding, coagulation, and prothrombin times are increased. Hematuria, melena, hematemesis, epistaxis, and hemoptysis may result. Blood vessel walls are altered, and there is increased resistance in postcapillary veins, causing pooling of blood in the lungs and chest. Pulmonary edema may ensue, and bleeding may occur in the peritoneum or pericardium. All these, together with direct toxic effects on the myocardial cells, contribute to the clinical presentation of peripheral vascular collapse.

The renal lesion of crotalid envenomation is glomerulonephritis, often accompanied by progressive, proliferative endarteritis and cortical necrosis. Necrosis of the tubular epithelium appears to be a direct local effect of the toxin.[15] This, along with profound circulatory collapse and intravascular hemolysis, is responsible for the occurrence of acute renal failure frequently observed in rattlesnake bite. A systemic anaphylaxis has also been described.[14,56]

Elapidae *(coral snake)* venoms cause less tissue damage and far greater neuromuscular changes. Reaction around the bite is frequently absent, pain is minimal, and symptoms are systemic, such as numbness, nausea, vomiting, euphoria, salivation, paresthesia, ptosis, weakness, abnormal reflexes, depression, dyspnea, and respiratory arrest. In most experimental preparations, the first changes in electrical conduction induced by crude venom occur at the neuromuscular junction, but with low doses, changes of varying degree occur. The ultimate clinical catastrophe acutely presenting is total respiratory paralysis.[49,56]

Some 200 strains of bacteria have been isolated from snake venom. Ledbetter found *Clostridia* in 48 of 100 venoms cultured and in 43 of 50 fangs, but coagulase-positive *Staphylococcus* was

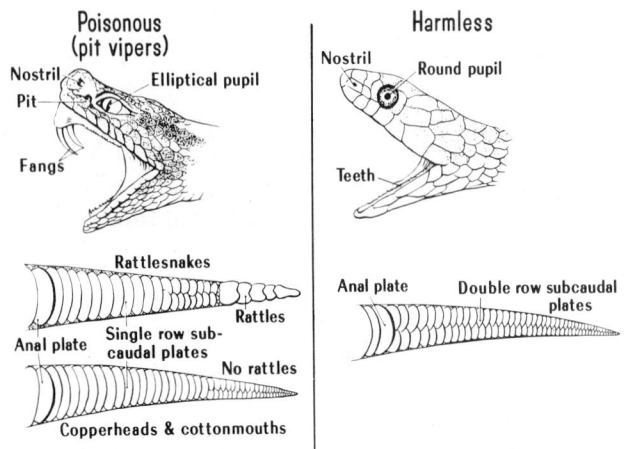

Figure 1. Characteristics that differentiate poisonous pit vipers from nonpoisonous snakes. (From Parrish, H. M.: Incidence of treated snakebites in the United States. Public Health Rep., *81*:269, 1966.)

not found. The most prevalent gram-negative organisms were *Aerobacter, Proteus,* and *Pseudomonas.*[40]

Management

Therapy for snakebite must be initiated early. The single most important aspect of treatment of snakebite is transporting the patient to a hospital facility as rapidly as possible. Prompt hospital treatment, more than any other factor, minimizes the morbidity of snakebite.

Correct diagnosis is essential. Pit vipers usually leave characteristic paired puncture wounds made by fangs, whereas bites of nonpoisonous snakes often leave tooth marks in a U shape. Bites by poisonous snakes usually cause immediate and intense pain. A convenient classification for bites by pit vipers is that of Wood and associates as modified by Parrish[46,57]:

Grade 0—no venenation: Fang or tooth marks; minimal pain; edema and erythema of less than 1 inch in 12 hours; usually no systemic involvement.

Grade 1—minimal venenation: Fang or tooth marks; severe pain; 1 to 5 inches of surrounding edema in first 12 hours; usually no systemic involvement.

Grade 2—moderate venenation: Fang or tooth marks; severe pain; 6 to 12 inches of surrounding edema and erythema in first 12 hours; systemic involvement sometimes present, such as neurotoxic symptoms, nausea, giddiness, shock, palpable regional lymph nodes.

Grade 3—severe venenation: Fang or tooth marks; severe pain; more than 12 inches of surrounding edema and erythema; systemic symptoms such as hypotension, generalized petechiae and ecchymosis, shock.

Grade 4—very severe venenation: Fang or tooth marks, multiple; local edema may be present beyond involved extremity to ipsilateral trunk; systemic symptoms always present and may include renal failure, coma, blood-tinged secretions.

In Parrish's nationwide survey, 27 per cent of venomous snakebites were classified Grade 0; 37 per cent were Grade 1; 22 per cent were Grade 2; and 14 per cent were Grades 3 and 4.[46]

The management of snakebites should follow a rational sequence. The following are suggested as guidelines.

1. *Retard absorption of the venom.* A tourniquet should be applied several inches above the bite. It must be emphasized that the tourniquet should occlude venous and lymphatic return but not arterial flow. Snyder has demonstrated that a tourniquet reduces the uptake of I-labeled venom in animals by two thirds. Loosening the tourniquet every 15 minutes actually increases the spread of venom, and it should be left in place for up to 2 hours without release. Immobilization of the bitten extremity aids in slowing the spread of venom.[46,47] The oral administration of alcohol, a vasodilator, should be avoided. Immersion of the bitten extremity in ice would theoretically appear to be beneficial by inducing vasoconstriction. However, the mortality and morbidity in experimental animals have been increased by prolonged exposure to ice. In addition, the application of ice has led to numerous tragic excesses of therapy, including many cases of limb loss when the bite was not even envenomated. *Therefore, the use of cryotherapy is absolutely contraindicated.*[24,46,47,49,64]

2. *Remove as much venom as possible from the wound.* Not everyone has the ability or temperament to make incisions over the fang marks; however, this has long been advised for re-

TABLE 1. Classification of Poisonous Snakes Indigenous to the United States

Family	Genus	Common Name	Identification	Characteristics
Crotalidae	Crotalus	Large rattlesnake (diamondback, mojave, timber, sidewinder, pacific, prairie)	Broad head, many coloration patterns, light belly; often has diamond markings. Rattles; up to 6 feet in length.	Can strike long distance. Potent cytotoxic venom. Accounts for most severe bites and fatalities.
	Sistrurus	Small rattlesnake (pigmy, massasauga)	Less than 3 feet in length.	Rattlers often small and audible only at close range. Bites cause severe pain, swelling, few fatalities.
	Ancistrodon	Copperhead	Pink, russet, or orange-brown with dark brown or reddish crossbands. Head is triangular, yellow to copper with pale sides. Two to 3 feet in length.	Accounts for most bites in eastern United States. Fatalities almost unknown.
		Cottonmouth	Olive or brown with wide black crossbands. Yellow belly marked with gray. White interior of mouth (cottonmouth). Around 4 feet in length.	Semiaquatic. Belligerent, aggressive behavior. Rare fatalities, but severe tissue destruction by venom.
Elapidae	Micrurus	Coral snake	Complete rings of yellow, black, red, and sometimes white with red and yellow adjacent. Less than 4 feet in length.	Frequently bites are not envenomated. Little local reaction at bite site, but neurotoxin-induced respiratory paralysis in several hours is usually fatal.

moval of the venom and as emergency field therapy in remote areas probably still is advisable. This maneuver should not impede the rapidity of getting the patient to a hospital facility.

Small incisions ¼ inch long and ⅛ to ¼ inch deep are made over the bite, and mechanical suction is employed. Cruciate incisions heal poorly and are not required. Suction by mouth may be used if necessary. Venom is not absorbed through intact oral mucosa, but is absorbed through any mucosal laceration. Digestive juices neutralize any swallowed venom. Over 50 per cent of venom can be removed in 15 minutes by this measure.[58]

If possible, direct surgical excision of the bitten area is probably the best immediate treatment. Huang and associates noted that much of the injected venom remains in the adjacent subcutaneous tissue compartment following envenomation. In a series of 54 patients observed in the hospital within 2 hours of the snakebite, wide excision of the bitten area was performed. Skin flaps were elevated, and the ecchymotic subcutaneous tissue was removed. This greatly reduced systemic toxicity (no antivenin was necessary in this series), and the clinical judgment as to whether fasciotomy would be necessary was facilitated.[34,35] Snyder, Glass, and others have also advocated excision of the bitten area.[27,60]

3. *Neutralize the venom.* Administration of polyvalent antivenin to neutralize the venom has traditionally been advocated. However, there are recent series that bring the advisability of using antivenin into question. Burch and associates reported the care of 81 patients with crotalin envenomation using the usual supportive methods, but without antivenin administration. The results were comparable to those of any series using antivenin.[12] One disadvantage of antivenin is that it causes serum sickness almost uniformly if more than two ampules are administered. However, the main objection centers about its lack of efficacy. In experimental animal studies, the therapeutic effect of antivenin is relatively weak. Administered prior to experimental envenomation, it is moderately effective in reducing and neutralizing the toxicity. However, when administered late, usually an interval of 30 to 60 minutes after envenomation, which more closely parallels the situation in human snakebite, it is essentially ineffective. A randomized, prospective study of antivenin use in humans has never been and may never be conducted. However, it is clear that the benefits of antivenin appear to be much less than formerly thought; and with the exception of use in patients with heavy envenomation from large rattlesnakes, who are observed early after envenomation, its routine use is not encouraged.[12,37]

The guidelines for the use of antivenin were established in the past and are as follows: Polyvalent antivenin (Wyeth) is administered intravenously, or intra-arterially, not intramuscularly or locally at the wound site. A useful guide for administration is no antivenin for Grade 0; 10 ml. (one ampule) for Grade 1; 30 to 40 ml. for Grade 2; and 50 ml. or more for Grades 3 and 4. A form of antivenin was developed in horses by Calmette in 1848, and the material used today is still an equine serum. In sensitive patients skin tests should be done first, but in severe cases withholding the antivenin may be more dangerous than administering it. The incidence of serum sickness in recipients of more than two ampules of antivenin is significant.[47,49,59,64]

4. *Prevent or reduce the effects of the venom.* Appropriate infusions of saline, plasma, blood, and vasopressor drugs should be instituted to prevent shock. Blood coagulation studies should be obtained, and fibrinogen replacement may be required. Fasciotomy may become necessary to prevent ischemic necrosis in a grossly edematous limb. This relatively simple surgical procedure must be constantly borne in mind during the management of severe bites, because the massive edema induced by the venom can lead to necrosis of tissue confined to normal nonexpansible fascial compartments of the extremity.[42]

Previous studies have demonstrated that small to moderate doses of corticosteroids may prolong life but do not affect mortality. However, Glass has recommended massive doses of hydrocortisone (1 gm. intravenously every 4 hours) at the first sign of systemic toxicity. With this regimen, coupled with early wide wound incision and fasciotomy, he has achieved good functional limb salvage, particularly in patients with known sensitivity to antivenin.[26,27] However, the routine use of massive corticosteroids has not gained universal acceptance.

5. *Prevent complications.* Broad-spectrum antibiotics are given to combat infection, and tetanus toxoid or tetanus immune globulin is administered. Vomiting, excessive salivation, and convulsions are treated symptomatically. Assisted ventilation may be necessary, and renal function must be monitored. Patients bitten by coral snakes should be admitted to the hospital for careful observation for at least 48 hours, because the effects of this venom characteristically develop slowly. The wound should be carefully cleansed because small amounts of the highly toxic venom may remain on the skin. The only commercially available coral snake antivenin is Soro Anticlapidico, manufactured by the Instituto Butantan, São Paulo, Brazil, and is available from most zoos and reptile houses in the United States. Twenty milliliters should be given at once, and 120 ml. or more should be administered if signs of venenation develop. If respiratory paralysis develops, intubation and assisted respiration is required. Intravenous fluid maintenance, a urinary catheter, a Levin tube, antibiotics, and tetanus prophylaxis are required. It is encouraging that some patients with respiratory paralysis from coral snake venom have recovered completely after variable periods of total respiratory support.[49]

RABIES

Rabies has been considered an invariably fatal, terrifying disease for centuries. As early as the first century A.D., Celsus recognized the infectivity of the bite of a mad dog and recommended cauterization of such wounds. Since the classic work of Pasteur in the 1880s and the development of the first rabies vaccine, the incidence of this disease has declined appreciably. Yet the persistent incidence of rabies virus in wildlife reservoirs and the dread complications of the clinical syndrome in humans continue to keep rabies an ever-present menace to mankind.

Incidence

Approximately 2 million people are bitten by animals annually, 500,000 by dogs. The incidence of rabies in humans has declined markedly in recent years (9 cases being reported in the United States from 1963 through 1968 in contrast to 230 cases between 1946 and 1963). This is the result of an intensive vaccination program for pets, primarily dogs and cats.

In the United States, rabies in humans has decreased from an average of 22 cases per year in 1946 to 1950 to zero to 5 cases per year since 1960. The number of rabies cases among domestic animals has decreased similarly. In 1946, more than 8000 rabies cases were reported among dogs; 153 cases were reported in 1982. Thus, the likelihood of human exposure to rabies in domestic animals has decreased greatly, although bites by dogs and cats continue to be the principal reasons given for antirabies treatments.[38,43]

The disease in wildlife, especially skunks, foxes, raccoons, and bats, has become more prevalent in recent years, representing approximately 85 per cent of all reported cases of animal rabies annually since 1976. Wild animals now constitute the most important potential source of infection for both humans and domestic animals in the United States. Rabies among animals is present throughout the United States; only Hawaii remains consistently rabies-free.

Four of the six rabies fatalities in United States citizens occurring between 1980 and 1983 were related to exposure to rabid dogs outside the United States. In much of the world, including

most of Asia and all of Africa and Latin America, the dog remains the major source of human exposure.

Although dogs and cats represent only 20 per cent of animal
rabies in the United States, bites by these animals are responsible for most of the approximately 30,000 postexposure rabies
prophylactic treatments administered annually.[38,65] The cost of
animal bites to society, in terms of funds expended and man-
hours lost, is substantial.[8]

Biology

The rabies virus is a large, nonfilterable particle that measures
75 by 180 μ. Infected nervous tissue or salivary gland tissue is
the best source of the virus. At refrigerator temperature the
virus may remain active for several weeks, and at subfreezing
temperature for 1 or more years. Rabies virus is inactivated by
exposure to a temperature of 56° C. for an hour or less. It is
rapidly destroyed by sunlight or ultraviolet radiation and is
readily inactivated by formalin, bichloride of mercury, strong
acids, and quaternary ammonium compounds. It is not affected
by any antibiotics or common bacteriostatic agents.[68]

The virus is usually transmitted through a break in the skin or
by direct contact with the mucous membrane. Airborne infection is possible, has been reported clinically in humans exploring in areas inhabited by rabid bats, and has been responsible
for the death of 1 laboratory technician handling infected tissue.[69] A patient who died of a Guillain-Barré–like syndrome,
found to be undiagnosed rabies at autopsy, transmitted the disease to the recipient of his corneal transplants.[33] The virus may
persist in the inoculation site for several days. Progression of the
virus occurs passively through the nerve-associated spaces. In
the central nervous system, the virus is found in the gray matter
and appears to multiply in the neurons. The incubation period is
usually 3 to 6 weeks but has been reported at 6 days to 23
months. Because the virus travels in association with nervous
structures, those areas rich in nerve endings (the fingers and
face) provide rapid access for the rabies virus, and multiple
facial or finger bites have the shortest incubation periods.[68]

The human disease is characterized by three phases: a prodromal phase, an acute excitement phase, and a paralytic phase.
The prodromal phase is nonspecific and may be manifested by
fever, headache, malaise, anorexia, and sore throat. The most
notable clinical symptom of rabies is related to swallowing, with
violent and painful contractions of the muscles of deglutition.
The excitement phase is marked by increasing nervousness, insomnia, anxiety, and apprehension. Convulsive seizures are
common, and unusual behavior patterns may appear. If the
patient survives, the paralytic phase (due to neuronal death)
follows. Depressive or paralytic symptoms may predominate
any time during the course of the disease. Hypoxia, cardiac
arrhythmias, hemiparesis, and coma are usually present. Although the almost invariable outcome is death, the actual cause
of death has never been clearly established. Patients usually die
within 4 to 10 days, but delayed clinical courses of up to 133
days have been observed.[9]

At autopsy, dark inclusion bodies (Negri bodies) are found in
the brain in the area of the thalamus and lentiform nucleus.
False-negative results of tests to demonstrate these bodies in
animals have occurred, and a human death has been ascribed to
this error. The fluorescent antibody test as described by Goldwasser and associates is currently used, and a diagnosis may be
obtained in a few hours.[52,66] Inoculation of mice and demonstration of the virus or Negri bodies in their nervous tissue is still a
valuable diagnostic test.

Therapy

The management of dog and other animal bites involves the
application of the usual surgical principles in the care of soft
tissue injury (cleansing, antisepsis, and, if necessary in severe

bites, débridement of necrotic tissue). The most pressing medical decision is whether or not to treat the bitten patient for
rabies. In patients in whom the biting animal is known and
confined, this problem is resolved, because therapy can be deferred during an observation period during which the animal
will die or survive. Rabies virus must be demonstrated in the
animal's saliva or glands during this time. However, when the
animal has not been captured, this decision must be made on
the basis of the incidence of rabies in that species in the locale
and especially on the behavior of the animal.

Animal rabies can be classified as furious or dumb. In furious
rabies, animals show a prolonged excitation phase, becoming
increasingly apprehensive and nervous. This is the most dangerous phase, because a dog may demonstrate no recognition of
its master and exhibit only an insane desire to bite. In wild
animals, the daytime appearance of abnormal behavior (loss of
fear of humans and attacks on livestock or man) should induce a
high order of suspicion. In dumb rabies there is a very short
excitation phase, after which the animal becomes apathetic,
appears to seek solitude, and eventually dies of progressive
paralysis, coma, and death.

Rabies is not endemic in rodents. Bites by rats, mice, chip-
munks, squirrels, rabbits, or other rodents have never been
proved to produce human rabies, and postexposure prophylaxis
is currently not indicated. However, rabies is endemic in bats in
every state except Hawaii, and all individuals bitten by a bat
that escapes should receive postexposure prophylaxis. The rationale for treatment is based on the severity and location of the
attack, the immune status of the attacking animal, the clinical
status of the attacking animal, and occasionally on the immune
status of the victim.[3,65] Therapy should be instituted promptly
according to the guidelines for postexposure prophylaxis in
Table 2.

LOCAL TREATMENT. Repeated swabbing and flushing
with soap and water reduce rabies in the wound site. This provides significant protection up to 12 hours after the bite. Fuming
nitric acid cauterization should be avoided. The infiltration of
antirabies serum under the wound itself has been effective in
animals and should be administered in severe bites. A minimum
of 5 ml. of serum should be injected.

SYSTEMIC TREATMENT. Rabies virus is poorly antigenic. In
clinical infection, it appears that the virus must reach the brain
before high antirabies antibody levels are achieved. Although
the virus may be eliminated ("autosterilization") by this immune response, the course of the disease is unfortunately not
altered. The rationale for postexposure prophylaxis is therefore
to administer vaccine to induce an immune response against
rabies and to administer antiserum (passive transfer) to effect
elevated antibody levels immediately while the body produces
its own immune response to the vaccine.[9,14,65]

Prior to 1980, duck embryo vaccine was the only licensed
vaccine available in the United States. However, human diploid
cell rabies vaccine is now approved and widely available. This
vaccine, derived from human cells in culture, has the significant
advantages of being more immunogenic and not causing toxicity (pain, fever, erythema, allergic reactions, anaphylaxis associated with duck embryo vaccine) and is now the treatment of
choice. Hyperimmune rabies immune globulin (HRIG) obtained from human volunteers is now available. The recommended dose of HRIG is 20 I.U. per kg.[3,7,16,17,19,29,44,45,52,54,59]

A well-documented complete recovery from clinical rabies in
an 8-year-old boy bitten by an infected bat has been accomplished.[27] The success of this treatment followed the anticipation of complications in the natural course of the disease, such
as hypoxia, convulsions, elevated intracranial pressure, arrhythmias, and aspiration, followed by aggressive treatment of
each as they occurred. Other cases of survival following proven
rabies infection have been recorded.[51] These landmark cases
dispel the absolute finality of this dreaded disease and at long

TABLE 2. Postexposure Antirabies Treatment Guide

Animal Species	Condition of Animal at Time of Attack	Treatment of Exposed Individual*
Domestic		
Dog and cat	Healthy and available for 10 days of observation.	None, unless animal develops rabies.†
	Rabid or suspected rabid.	RIG and HDCV.‡
	Unknown (escaped).	Consult public health officials. If treatment is indicated, give RIG and HDCV.‡
Wild		
Skunk, bat, fox, coyote, raccoon, bobcat, and other carnivores	Regard as rabid unless proven negative by laboratory tests.§	RIG and HDCV.‡
Other		
Livestock, rodents, and lagomorphs (rabbits and hares)	Consider individually. Local and state public health officials should be consulted on questions about the need for rabies prophylaxis. Bites of squirrels, hamsters, guinea pigs, gerbils, chipmunks, rats, mice, other rodents, rabbits, and hares seldom require antirabies prophylaxis.	

* All bites and wounds should immediately be thoroughly cleansed with soap and water. If antirabies treatment is indicated, both rabies immune globulin (RIG) and human diploid cell rabies vaccine (HDCV) should be administered as soon as possible, regardless of the interval from exposure. Local reactions to vaccines are common and do not contraindicate continuing treatment.

† Begin human rabies immune globulin and human diploid cell rabies vaccine at first sign of rabies in biting dog or cat during holding period (10 days).

‡ Vaccine antibody, human rabies immune globulin (RIG), is administered only once, at the beginning of antirabies therapy. The recommended dose is 20 I.U. per kg. Up to half the dose should be infiltrated around the wound and the rest administered intramuscularly in the buttocks. Five 1-ml. doses of human diploid cell rabies vaccine (HDCV) are given, one as soon as possible after exposure along with human rabies immune globulin. Subsequent injections of HDVC are given at 3, 7, 14, and 28 days after the first dose. Discontinue vaccine if fluorescent antibody tests of the animal killed at the time of attack are negative.

§ The animal should be killed and tested as soon as possible. Holding for observation is not recommended.

Adapted from Advisory Committee on Immunization Practices: Rabies prophylaxis. M.M.W.R., 33(28), 1984.

last lend hope to both the victim of rabies and the physicians treating him.

HUMAN BITES

Human bites are relatively rare, but can constitute serious clinical problems. There are three types: (1) a genuine bite in which the assailant sinks his teeth into the victim, producing puncture wounds, lacerations, or avulsion of tissue (particularly of the tip of the nose, the earlobe, or the tongue); (2) abrasion and laceration of the knuckles and hand, which occur from the clenched fist striking the victim's mouth and teeth; and (3) a self-inflicted bite, usually of the tongue or lip, occurring often after falls or seizures.

Bacteriology

Infection is the most severe complication of human bites. The human mouth contains many more pathogenic organisms than those of most animals and can be a reservoir for *Staphylococcus*, *Streptococcus*, anaerobic streptococci, gonococci, Vincent's bacillus, fusiform bacilli, spirochetes, tetanus bacilli, gas gangrene bacilli, *Treponema pallidum*, and others. Heavy contamination of the wound should be assumed and treatment directed toward its eradication.

Therapy

All wounds should be cultured, thoroughly scrubbed with bacteriostatic soap, and liberally irrigated with sterile saline.

Examination of damage to deep structures should be made and tendon injury noted. Damaged tissues should be débrided. Severed tendons and nerves should not be sutured primarily.

Despite the potential for infection, with the immediate administration of antibiotic therapy, soft tissue wounds of the head and face area, properly cleansed and débrided, can usually be sutured primarily when observed within 6 hours of injury. This applies even when cartilage of the nose or ear is exposed. Good cosmetic effects usually result. All other wounds should be left open. Attempts to reattach totally avulsed segments of ear or nose rarely are successful. Broad-spectrum antibiotics in therapeutic dosage are routinely administered systemically and are modified subsequently on the basis of the organism cultured. Tetanus toxoid is administered.

All patients should be observed carefully for signs of cellulitis or gangrene, especially in bites of the fingers. Wounds observed late with cellulitis and secondary infections require hospitalization for massive antibiotic therapy, immobilization, and débridement. Avulsed wound defects require plastic surgery repair after infection subsides.[10,18,41,50]

SPIDER BITES

Black Widow Spider Bite

The black widow spider *(Latrodectus mactans)* is found everywhere in the United States except Alaska. The female is distinguished by a shiny black globular body with a red hourglass mark on the abdomen (Fig. 2). These spiders prefer dry, dimly

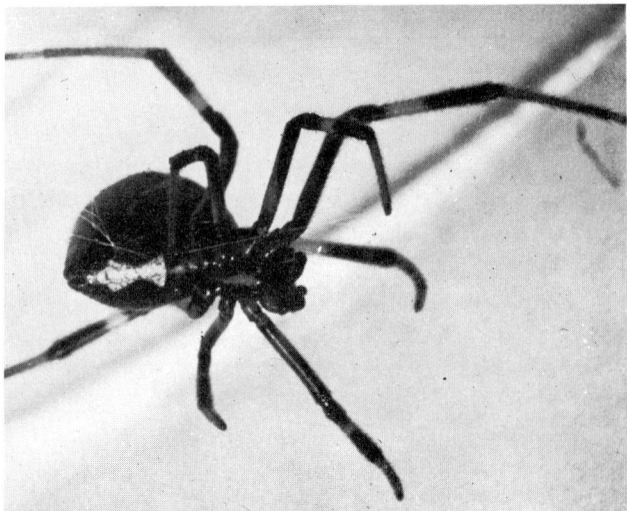

Figure 2. The female black widow spider has a shiny, black, globular body with a red hourglass mark on the abdomen. (From Paton, B. C.: Bites—human, dog, spider, and snake. Surg. Clin. North Am., *43:*537, 1963.)

lighted places and are most commonly found around houses and buildings, under stones and lumber piles, between cracks and crevices, and in debris. Sixty-three deaths occurred in the United States between 1950 and 1960 from the bite of this spider.

Frequently a definite history of bite cannot be obtained. The venom is primarily neurotoxic and centers in the spinal cord. A victim may recall a pinprick sensation followed by dull and somewhat numbing pain. Slight local swelling and tiny red fang marks may be found. In a severe bite, pain in the chest soon follows upper extremity bites, and abdominal rigidity follows lower extremity bites. Spasms soon appear in all major muscle groups, and abdominal rigidity occurs, suggesting an acute abdominal emergency, although it is usually nontender. Intense pain and spasms continue, usually resolving in 24 to 48 hours. Ptosis, dizziness, conjunctivitis, respiratory distress, nausea, and skin rash may occur. A burning sensation in the soles of the feet may be present during convalescence. Mortality is 4 per cent, usually following shock or respiratory arrest.

THERAPY. Therapy in adults consists of narcotics for relief of the agonizing pain and muscle relaxants to relieve muscle spasms. In children under 6 years, in debilitated or aged adults, or in cases of severe envenomation, antivenin (Lyovac) is administered. One ampule in 50 ml. of saline is usually sufficient. Intense supportive therapy, including intravenous fluids, may be necessary.[21,22,28,57,63]

Brown Recluse Spider Bite

The brown recluse spider (*Loxosceles reclusa*) is widely disseminated through the southern and central United States, and its range is increasing. Rocks, barks, and woodpiles are the common habitats in the southern states, while in cooler climates the spiders have moved indoors and are found in closets, cellars, and used clothing. They are 10 to 15 mm. long, light tan to dark brown in color, and have flat bodies with a species-specific, dark, violin-shaped band over the dorsal cephalothorax (Fig. 3.)[20,21]

BIOLOGY. The venom is necrotizing and hemolytic and contains a spreading factor (probably hyaluronidase). Shortly after inoculation of venom into guinea pigs, capillary dilation and pooling of blood occur, followed by the presence of hyalinized thrombi at 24 hours and coagulation necrosis and subcutaneous abscesses by 72 hours. In humans, edema and thickening of vascular endothelium are observed at 18 hours, followed by

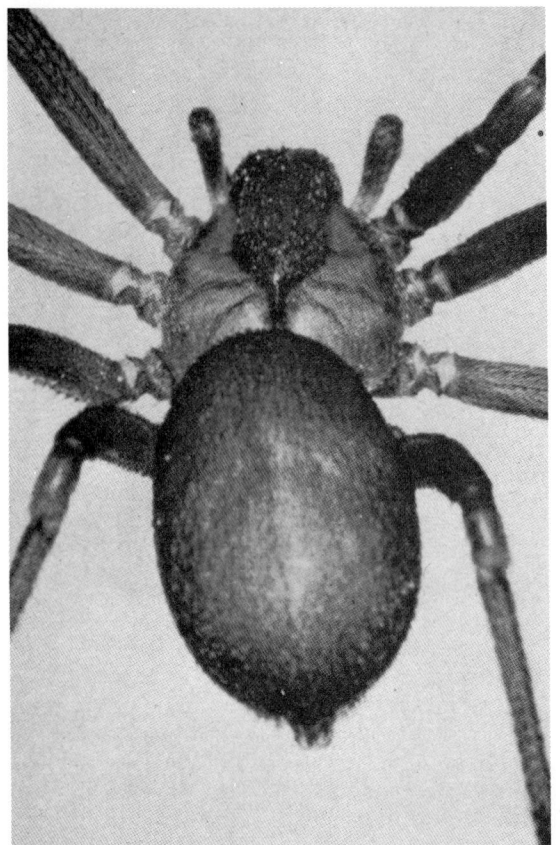

Figure 3. The brown recluse spider is 10 to 15 mm. long, is light tan to dark brown in color, and has a species-specific dorsal, dark, violin-shaped band. (From Dillaha, C. J., Jansen, G. T., Honeycutt, W. M., and Hayden, C. R.: Surgical treatment of brown spider bites. J.A.M.A., *188:*33, 1964. Copyright 1964, American Medical Association.)

progressive endothelial thickening and occlusion. Sludging with perivascular infiltrate occurs at the periphery of the lesion. Hemolysis, hemoglobinuria, hemolytic anemia, and renal failure can develop.[20,21,57]

The patient may or may not have severe pain at the time of the bite, which frequently occurs in bed. After several hours a painful red area appears with a pale, mottled, cyanotic center, which may blister. A zone of hemorrhage with induration and a surrounding halo of erythema, which may be very extensive, develop. Pain is severe. A central black eschar forms by 6 or 7 days, and soon there is a slough, leaving an open ulcer that may continue to enlarge. Deep and wide necrosis of fat undermining the skin around the eschar is a characteristic finding in this lesion, as shown in Figure 4.[1,2,20,22]

Severe systemic symptoms may occur, especially in small children, with fever, malaise, weakness, nausea, vomiting, and petechiae developing early. Fatalities have been reported.

THERAPY. Severe systemic symptoms must receive supportive therapy as appropriate, including intravenous fluids, analgesics, and other supportive measures as required. Antibiotics are always administered. No specific antivenin exists.

The administration of steroids has not halted the progression of necrotic lesions in animal studies, and they should not be used for this purpose in humans. Steroids have been given to ameliorate systemic toxicity, although absolute guidelines for their use do not exist. Antihistamines, low-molecular-weight dextran, heparin, EDTA, and ε-aminocaproic acid are not agents of proven benefit, and their use at this time is not recommended.[2,4-6] The administration of dapsone, an oral drug used to reduce the inflammation induced in leprosy and pyoderma, may be of value in reducing tissue necrosis.[39] This medi-

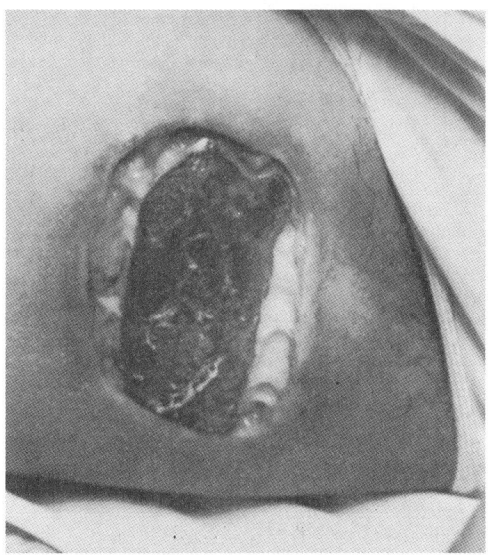

Figure 4. A central black eschar surrounded by deep necrosis of fat which undermines the skin is seen about 7 days after a brown recluse spider bite. (From Hershey, H. R., and Aulenbacker, C. E.: North American loxoscelism. Ann. Surg., 170:300, 1969.)

cation has proved to have some beneficial effect in experimentally induced brown recluse spider bites in animals. However, its routine use is not advised, because the preparation is toxic and hemolysis and agranulocytosis can occur after only a few days of treatment.[70]

The primary surgical treatment of the brown recluse spider is based on the concept that the toxin can be physically removed if treated early, thereby eliminating the area of necrosis. Although early surgical excision has been used successfully by some authors, the results have not been uniformly good. Early excision may be inadequate, because normal-appearing tissue can already be envenomated but not necrotic. Conversely, tissue appearing destined to cause full-thickness loss can occasionally make a remarkable recovery, making excision unnecessary. Janson and associates demonstrated that healing in animals treated by early excision and grafting was inferior to that in animals treated without excision.

Therefore, it would appear reasonable to withhold surgical débridement until the necrosis is well demarcated. This constitutes the cornerstone of secondary treatment of the local wound. Other aims of treatment include prevention of secondary infection with local antibiotics such as Silvadene cream, tetanus prophylactics, and possibly systemic antibiotics.

Rare, systemic complications related to exposure to the toxin can include hemolysis, renal failure, and disseminated intravascular coagulation (DIC). Appropriate clinical laboratory examinations for diagnosing and treating these complications occasionally are indicated.[32,67,70]

BITES OF BEES, WASPS, HORNETS, AND OTHER INSECTS

Incidence

Arthropods of the order Hymenoptera include the honeybee, bumblebee, wasp, yellow jacket, yellow and black hornet, ant, and sawfly. Probably more than 100,000 species of this order exist, and more bites and stings are inflicted upon man by these creatures than by any other venomous group. Their venom is just as toxic as that of the rattlesnake, and more deaths result from insect bites in the United States yearly than from all snakebites. Less venom is injected in insect bites, and severe allergic

reactions rather than direct toxic effects of the venom represent most fatalities. Bees, wasps, hornets, and ants constitute 65 per cent of deaths; spiders, 31 per cent; and scorpions, 4 per cent.

Biology

All insects of the order Hymenoptera, except the bee, retain their sting and can sting repeatedly, injecting a portion of the venom sac contents each time. The barbed stinging apparatus of the honeybee cannot be withdrawn; and as the bee attempts to escape, it is disemboweled. The remaining anchored sting is driven farther into the skin by rhythmically contracting muscles attached to it, and venom from the sac can be injected for as long as 20 minutes.

Insect venoms, like those of snakes, contain a mixture of proteinlike substances of varying antigenicity, kinins, histamine, and serotonin. Humans vary greatly in their reaction to insect bites, and these characteristics govern therapy. In general, the more rapid the onset of symptoms, the more severe the reaction is likely to be. Stings of the head, face, and neck tend to cause more serious effects. A transient, painless papule may result, or violent, diffuse burning pain can occur together with itching, paresthesias, areas of anesthesia, and headache. Urticaria, edema, erythema, and intense angioneurotic edema may appear as histamine is liberated by the toxin. The site of the sting can swell and may become septic or gangrenous. Muscular weakness, spasm, twitching, and paralysis may be seen. Respiratory distress, cyanosis, dysphagia, ocular palsies, apprehension, fever, nausea, bradycardia or tachycardia, and shock occur in severe cases. A delayed hypersensitivity reaction resembling serum sickness may occur 10 to 14 days after injury.

Therapy

In 50 cases of fatal anaphylaxis following insect bites over a 10-year period, 62 per cent of the patients were dead in the first hour because of inadequate treatment or none at all. In a similar survey of 100 nonfatal cases of severe anaphylaxis, 87 per cent of the patients received treatment in the first hour after the bite. The most frequent types of systemic reactions in these survivors were general urticaria (74 per cent), syncope (65 per cent), and respiratory tract obstruction (38 per cent).

LOCAL CARE. The retained sting shaft, if present, should be scraped off with a blade. The wound is washed with soap and water. Cellulitis or gangrene may require débridement. Local injection of lidocaine (Xylocaine) in uncomplicated cases has relieved persistent pain.

TOXIC REACTIONS. In multiple bites, the total amount of injected toxin may be sufficient to cause severe systemic symptoms, principally diarrhea, vomiting, fainting, edema, muscle spasms, or convulsions. Supportive therapy such as sedation, intravenous fluids, antibiotics, and antihistamines may be necessary. The toxic effects of the venom can be counteracted by calcium gluconate infusion.

ALLERGIC REACTIONS. Immediate treatment is the key to success. Epinephrine, 1:1000, 0.3 to 0.5 ml. for adults, is given subcutaneously. This is short-acting, and the dose may have to be repeated at 15- to 20-minute intervals. An antihistamine is also injected immediately. In severe cases, intravenous fluids, pressor agents, plasma expanders, and respiratory assistance may be required.

PREVENTION. All patients with a history of severe reaction to insect bites should be desensitized according to the directives of the Insect Allergy Committee of the American Academy of Allergy. The use of specific venom skin tests is probably the most accurate way to determine insect hypersensitivity.[13,36,61] Desensitization should be instituted 14 days after a severe bite. Sensitive patients should wear long-sleeved clothing, avoid obvious hazards, and carry a kit containing 10-mg. isoproterenol tablets for sublingual use, epinephrine aerosol for inhalation, and tweezers for removing the sting shaft.[14,21,23,57,62]

SELECTED REFERENCES

Burch, J. M., Agarwal, R., Mattox, K. L., Feliciano, D. V., and Jordan, G. L.: The treatment of crotalid envenomation without antivenin. J. Trauma, 28:35, 1988.
This landmark paper reports 81 patients treated for crotalid envenomation without using antivenin. The historical evolution of antivenin is discussed, along with animal experiments that support the authors' treatise that antivenin has limited use in the treatment of most snakebites. The discussion of this paper by other experts in the field is also of great interest.

Christy, N. P.: Poisoning by venomous animals. Am. J. Med., 42:107, 1967.
This monograph presents a lucid review of the biochemical composition and physiologic effects in humans of animal venoms. Currect aspects of therapy are clearly presented. The historical development of clinical treatment is of particular interest.

Edmonds, C.: Dangerous marine animals. Aust. Fam. Physician, 5:381, 1976.
This is a practical and concise guide to the first aid, local care, and systemic treatment of the more commonly observed injuries induced by marine animals, including stingrays, sea snakes, fish, sharks, coelenterates, and catfish. The recommendations for first aid and waterside management are particularly useful.

Frazier, C. A.: Insect Allergy. St. Louis, Warren H. Green, Inc., 1969.
This thorough and factual book contains detailed information about the toxicology, physiology, and therapy associated with insect allergy in humans. Complete and containing many references, this well-illustrated volume is probably the definitive work on insect allergy for clinicians.

Halstead, B. W.: Poisonous and Venomous Marine Animals of the World. Princeton, Darwin Press, 1978.
This current comprehensive, encyclopedic volume contains plates for the identification of marine animals that can be dangerous to man and includes information on the pharmacology of their toxins and therapy for the unique clinical problems associated with the bite of these creatures. It is probably as complete a reference work on marine trauma as exists in one volume.

Russell, F. E.: Venomous animal injuries. Curr. Probl. Pediatr., 3:1, 1972.
This is a very complete, detailed, yet practical overview of the pharmacology and therapy of bites from all classes of venomous animals. The section on marine animals, often not included in similar presentations, is particularly useful.

United States Department of the Navy, Bureau of Medicine and Surgery: Poisonous Snakes of the World. Washington, D.C., U.S. Government Printing Office, 1968.
Concise and practical, this monograph presents in outline form information about the identification, habits, and habitats of poisonous snakes throughout the world. The plates, many in color, are excellent. Treatment from first aid to surgical therapy is thoroughly covered.

United States Public Health Service Advisory Committee on Immunization Practices: Rabies Prophylaxis. M.M.W.R., 23:28, 1984.
In this concise monograph, the development of human diploid cell rabies vaccine and human rabies immune globulin is discussed. The data concerning the incidence of rabies in wildlife reservoirs, dogs and cats, and humans in the past decade is presented. Specific pre- and postexposure treatment regimens are presented.

REFERENCES

1. Arnold, R. E.: Brown recluse spider bites: Five cases with a review of the literature. J. Am. Coll. Emerg. Phys., 5:262, 1976.
2. Auer, A. I., and Hershey, F. B.: Surgery for necrotic bites of the brown spider. Arch. Surg., 108:612, 1974.
3. Baer, G. M.: Advances in post-exposure rabies vaccination. A review. Am. J. Clin. Pathol., 70 (Suppl. 1):185, 1978.
4. Barnard, J. H.: Studies of 400 Hymenoptera sting deaths in the United States. J. Allergy Clin. Immunol., 52:259, 1973.
5. Berger, R. S.: A critical look at therapy for brown recluse spider bite. Arch. Dermatol., 107:298, 1973.
6. Berger, R. S., Millikan, L. E., and Conway, F.: An in vitro test for Loxosceles reclusa spider bites. Toxicon, 11:467, 1973.
7. Bernard, K. W., Mallonee, J., Wright, J. C., Reid, F. L., Makintubee, S., Parker, R. A., Dwyer, D. M., and Winkler, W. G.: Pre-exposure immunization with intradermal human diploid cell rabies vaccine. J.A.M.A., 257(8):1059, 1987.
8. Berzon, D. R., and DeHoff, J. B.: Medical costs and other aspects of dog bites in Baltimore. Public Health Rep., 89:377, 1974.
9. Bhatt, D. R., Hazttwick, M., Gerdsen, R., Emmons, R. W., and Johnson, H. N.: Human rabies. Am. J. Dis. Child., 127:862, 1974.
10. Brandt, F. W.: Human bites of the ear. Plast. Reconstr. Surg., 43:130, 1969.
11. Buckerl, W., Buckley, E., and Deulofeu, V. (Eds.): Venomous Animals and Their Venoms. New York, Academic Press, 1968.
12. Burch, J. M., Agarwal, R., Mattox, K. L., Feliciano, D. V., and Jordan, G. L.: The treatment of crotalid envenomation without antivenin. J. Trauma, 28:35, 1988.
13. Busse, W. W., and Yunginger, J. W.: The use of the radioallergo-sorbent test in the diagnosis of Hymenoptera anaphylaxis. Clin. Allergy, 8:471, 1978.
14. Christy, N. P. (Ed.): Poisoning by venomous animals. Am. J. Med., 42:107, 1967.
15. Chugh, K. S., Aikat, B. K., Sharma, B. K., Dash, S. C., Matthew, M. T., and Das, K. C.: Acute renal failure following snakebite. Am. J. Trop. Dis. Hyg., 24:692, 1975.
16. Corey, L, and Hattwick, M. A.: Treatment of persons exposed to rabies. J.A.M.A., 232:272, 1975.
17. Crick, J., and Brown, F.: Efficacy of rabies vaccine prepared from virus grown in duck embryo. Lancet, 1:1106, 1970.
18. Curtin, J. W., and Greely, P. W.: Human bites of the face. Plast. Reconstr. Surg., 28:394, 1961.
19. Ellenbogen, C., and Slugg, P.: Rabies neutralizing antibody: Inadequate response to equine antiserum and duck-embryo vaccine. J. Infect. Dis., 127:433, 1973.
20. Fordon, D. W., Wingo, C. W., Robinson, D. W., and Masten, F. W.: The treatment of brown spider bite. Plast. Reconstr. Surg., 40:482, 1967.
21. Frazier, C. A.: Diagnosis and treatment of insect bites. Clin. Sympos., 20:75, 1968.
22. Frazier, C. A.: Insect Allergy. St. Louis, Warren H. Green, Inc., 1969.
23. Gephardt, D.: Anaphylaxis from insect stings. J. Emergency Nurs., 4(3):19, 1978.
24. Gill, K. A.: The evaluation of cryotherapy in the treatment of snake envenomization. South. Med. J., 63:552, 1970.
25. Girard, K. F.: Rabies in Massachusetts: Eleven years in retrospect. N. Engl. J. Med., 288:319, 1973.
26. Glass, T. G.: Snakebite. Hosp. Med., 1971, p. 31.
27. Glass, T. G.: Early debridement in pit viper bites. J.A.M.A., 235:2513, 1976.
28. Harves, A. D., and Millikan, L. E.: Current concepts of therapy and pathophysiology in arthropod bites and stings. II. Insects. Int. J. Dermatol., 14:621, 1975.
29. Hattwick, M. A. W., Corey, L, and Creech, W. B.: Clinical use of human globulin immune to rabies virus. J. Infect. Dis., 133(Suppl. A):266, 1976.
30. Hattwick, M. A. W., Rubin, R. H., Music, S., Sikes, R. K., Smith, J. S., and Gregg, M. B.: Postexposure rabies prophylaxis with human rabies immune globulin. J.A.M.A., 227:409, 1974.
31. Hattwick, M. A. W., Weis, T. T., Stechschulte, C. J., Baer, G. M., and Gregg, M. B.: Recovery from rabies. Ann. Intern. Med., 76:931, 1972.
32. Hollabaugh, R. S., and Fernandes, E. T.: Management of the Brown Recluse Spider Bite. Grune & Stratton, 1989.
33. Houff, S. A.: Neurological victims: questionable donors. U.S. Med., 15:7, 2, 1979.
34. Huang, T. T., Blackwell, S. J., and Lewis, S. R.: Hand deformities in patients with snakebite. Plast. Reconstr. Surg., 62:32, 1978.
35. Huang, T. T., Lynch, J. B., Larson, D. L., and Lewis, S. R.: The use of excisional therapy in the management of snakebite. Ann. Surg., 179:598, 1974.
36. Hunt, K. J., Valentine, M. D., Sobotka, A. K., and Lichtenstein, L. M.: Diagnosis of allergy to stinging insects by skin testing with Hymenoptera venoms. Ann. Intern. Med., 85:56, 1976.
37. Jurkovich, G. J., Luterman, A., McCullar, K., Ramenofsky, M. L., and Curreri, P. W.: Complications of Crotalidae antivenin therapy. J. Trauma, 28:1032, 1988.
38. Kauffman, F. H., and Goldmann, B. J.: Rabies. Am. J. Emerg. Med., 4(6):525, 1986.
39. King, L. E., and Rees, R.: Dapsone treatment of a brown recluse spider bite. J.A.M.A., 250:648, 1983.
40. Ledbetter, E. O., and Kutscher, A. E.: Aerobic and anaerobic flora of rattlesnake fangs and venom. Arch. Environ. Health, 19:770, 1969.
41. Mann, R. J., Hoffeld, T. A., and Farmer, C. B.: Human bites of the hand: Twenty years of experience. J. Hand Surg., 2:97, 1977.
42. Marten, E.: The surgical treatment of snake bites. Toxicon (Suppl.), 1:471, 1978.
43. Miller, A., and Nathanson, N.: Rabies: Recent advances in pathogenesis and control. Ann. Neurol., 2:511, 1977.
44. Morrison, A. J., Hunt, E. H., Nuzhet, O. A., Schwartzman, J. D., and Wenzel, R. P.: Rabies pre-exposure prophylaxis using intradermal human diploid cell vaccine: Immunologic efficacy and cost-effectiveness in a university medical center and a review of selected literature. Am. J. Med. Sci., 293:293, 1987.
45. Nicholson, K. G., and Turner, G. S.: Studies with human diploid cell strain rabies vaccine and human antirabies immunoglobulin in man. Dev. Biol. Stand., 40:115, 1978.
46. Parrish, H. M.: Incidence of treated snakebites in the United States. Public Health Rep., 81:269, 1966.
47. Parrish, H. M., and Carr, C. A.: Bites of copperheads (Ancistrodon contortrix) in the United States. J.A.M.A., 201:927, 1967.
48. Parrish, H. M., and Dannell, H. D., Jr.: Bites by cottonmouths. (Ancistrodon piscivorus) in the United States. South. Med. J., 60:42, 1967.
49. Parrish, H. M., and Kahn, M.S.: Bites by coral snakes: Report of 11 representative cases. Am. J. Med. Sci., 253:561, 1967.
50. Paton, B. C.: Bites—human, dog, spider, and snake. Surg. Clin. North Am., 43:537, 1963.
51. Porras, C., Barboza, J. J., Fuenzalida, E., Adaros, H. L., Oviedo, A. M., and Furst, J.: Recovery from rabies in man. Ann. Intern. Med., 85:44, 1976.
52. Plotkin, S. A.: Rabies vaccination in the 1980s. Hosp. Pract., 11:63, 1980.
53. Rubin, R. H., Hattwick, M. A. W., Jones, S., Gregg, M. B., and Schwartz, V. D.:

Adverse reactions to duck embryo rabies vaccine. Ann. Intern. Med., 78:643, 1973.

54. Rubin, R. H., Sikes, R. K., and Gregg, M. B.: Human rabies immune globulin. J.A.M.A., 224:871, 1973.

55. Russell, F. E.: Pharmacology of animal venoms. Clin. Pharmacol. Ther., 8:849, 1967.

56. Russell, F. E.: Clinical aspects of snake venom poisoning in North America. Toxicon, 7:33, 1969.

57. Russell, F. E.: Venomous animal injuries. Curr. Probl. Pediatr., 3:1, 1973.

58. Snyder, C. C., and Knowles, R. P.: Snakebites: Guidelines for practical management. Postgrad. Med., 83:52, 1988.

59. Snyder, C. C., Pickins, J. E., Knowles, R. P., Emerson, J. L., and Hines, W. A.: A definitive study of snakebite. J. Fla. Med. Assoc., 55:330, 1968.

60. Snyder, C. C., Straight, R., and Glenn, J.: The snakebitten hands. Plast. Reconstr. Surg., 49:275, 1972.

61. Sobotka, A. K.: Diagnosis of insect hypersensitivity. J. Allergy Clin. Immunol., 60:213, 1977.

62. Sobotka, A. K., Valentine, M. D., Benton, A. W., and Lichtenstein, L. M.: Allergy to insect stings. J. Allergy Clin. Immunol., 53:170, 1974.

63. Sutherland, S. K., and Trinca, J. C.: Survey of 2144 cases of red-back spider bites: Australia and New Zealand, 1963–1976. Med. J. Aust., 2:620, 1978.

64. United States Department of the Navy, Bureau of Medicine and Surgery: Poisonous Snakes of the World. Washington, D.C., U.S. Government Printing Office, 1968.

65. United States Public Health Service Advisory Committee on Immunization Practices: Rabies prophylaxis. M.M.W.R., 33:28, 1984.

66. Vella, E. E.: Research into rabies. Ann. Intern. Med., 86:462, 1977.

67. Wasserman, G. S.: Wound care of spider and snake envenomations. Ann. Emerg. Med., 17:1331, 1988.

68. White, D. L.: Rabies 1970. N.Y. J. Med., 70:2456, 1970.

69. Winkler, W. C., Fashinell, T. R., Feffingwell, L., Howard, P., and Conomy, J. P.: Airborne rabies transmission in a laboratory worker. J.A.M.A., 226:1219, 1973.

70. Young, V. L., and Pin, P.: The brown recluse spider bite. Ann. Plast. Surg., 20:447, 1988.

15

TRAUMA

Management of Acute Injuries

Gregory J. Jurkovich, M.D., and C. James Carrico, M.D.

The trauma surgeon is the critical component of modern trauma care systems. This pivotal role mandates a working knowledge of all components of trauma care, including prevention, prehospital care, emergency room care, and rehabilitation, in addition to directing and providing acute surgical care. The provision of acute care is likewise not solely limited to recognition of injuries and operative repair. Acute care of the trauma patient encompasses all of the physiologic problems of shock, fluid resuscitation, blood transfusion, electrolyte imbalance, infections, pulmonary support, nutritional supplementation, and gastrointestinal problems unique to the surgical patient. Many of these topics are covered in other sections of this general surgery text. This chapter will focus on the acute management of specific injuries and the development of trauma care systems.

HISTORICAL PERSPECTIVE

The *Edwin Smith Surgical Papyrus* is not only the oldest known surgical text but also the oldest available scientific document of any kind. This Egyptian papyrus was written about 1600 B.C. and is probably a copy of a much older text (3000–2500 B.C.) originally authored by Imhotep, the physician and architect who is credited with designing the famous pyramids at Gizeh. Forty-four of the scroll's 48 cases deal with adult trauma cases, including head and spine injuries, facial wounds, and upper extremity injuries; no abdominal or thoracic wounds are mentioned. Each case consists of a title, examination, diagnosis, treatment recommendations, prognosis, and commentaries by subsequent ancient readers. It is arranged in the order that later was to become the traditional one, *a capite ad calcem,* that is, from head to foot. The text is unique in that it is a surgical treatise of actual cases and emphasizes rational surgical judgment, rather than folklore or magical recipes.[158]

The surgeon's role in providing care to the injured has been documented throughout recorded history. According to Majno, the first mention of organized battlefield care was in Homer's *Iliad,* composed about 1000 B.C.[77] The wounded were removed from the battlefield and cared for in barracks (klisiai) or in nearby ships. In the *Iliad,* 147 wounds are specifically mentioned, with an overall mortality of 77 per cent. The oldest pictorial representation of bandaging and wound management was also inspired from the *Iliad.*[115] This scene is Achilles bandaging his cousin and intimate friend Patroclus. The pictoral was originally found on a kylix, a Greek drinking vessel, dating from about 490 B.C. This illustration is now also found on medallions of several modern surgical societies.

The Romans also had considerable experience with care of the wounded. As early as 480 B.C., the wounded were assigned to the care of the patricians. In the first and second centuries A.D., the Romans established hospitals along the borders of the Roman Empire to care for the wounded. Archaeologists have identified at least 25 of these hospitals.

Baron Larrey, Napoleon's chief surgeon, developed two concepts to improve the care of the wounded that extend to modern times.[101] The first was the "flying ambulance," which reduced the time required to provide definitive care to the injured. Prior to the invention of these ambulances, the injured often remained on the battlefields for periods of 24 to 36 hours. Larrey's second innovation was to concentrate the casualties in one area and to operate on them as close to the front lines as possible.

Throughout the ensuing two centuries these two concepts have been embraced and further developed. During the American Civil War transportation times were measured in days, and the overall war mortality was 14 per cent. During World War I, the time from injury to surgery was between 12 and 18 hours. This time was reduced during World War II to between 6 and 12 hours. One of the most dramatic reductions in the time lag from injury to definitive care occurred during the Korean conflict. The United States Army Medical Corps decided to bypass the battalion aid station and take the injured soldiers directly from the field to the mobile army surgical hospital (MASH). The average time from injury to definitive care was reduced to 2 to 4 hours during the Korean conflict, and the overall mortality was reduced to 2.4 per cent (Fig. 1). This tactic was improved upon during the Vietnam conflict, when casualties were directly airlifted from the battlefield to the Corps Surgical Hospital, bypassing both the battalion aid station and MASH. Studies in Vietnam showed that the average time from injury to emergency care was 65 minutes, and the overall mortality was a remarkably low 1.8 per cent, statistics civilian urban trauma centers often have difficulty reproducing. This military experience of rapid transportation to definitive centralized care centers has been an incentive and a model for the development of civilian regional trauma systems. (See Trauma Care System.)

INITIAL MANAGEMENT OF THE ACUTELY INJURED PATIENT

Priorities

Initial care of the injured patient necessitates two assumptions. The first is that the patient may have more than one injury; the second is that the obvious injury is not necessarily the most important one. Successful resuscitation requires an approach predicated on prioritizing injuries. A simple method of prioritization includes the following schema and examples. It identifies four categories of injury:

1. Exigent: the most life-threatening conditions, requiring instantaneous intervention (e.g., laryngeal fracture with complete upper airway obstruction)
2. Emergency: those conditions requiring immediate intervention over a period of a few minutes (e.g., tension pneumothorax)
3. Urgent: those conditions requiring intervention within the

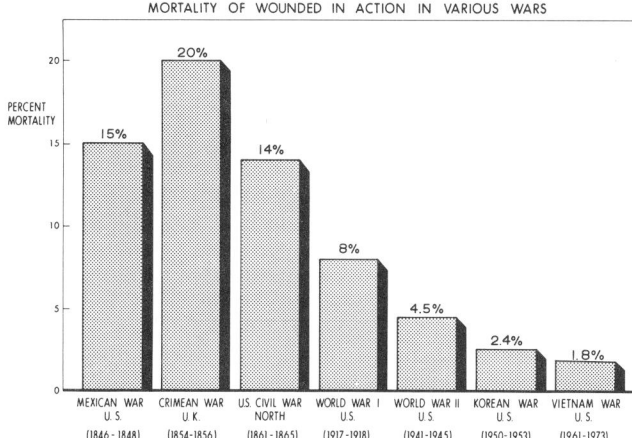

Figure 1. Mortality of soldiers wounded in action in various wars.

first hour (e.g., hemoperitoneum due to continued intra-abdominal bleeding)

4. Deferrable: those conditions that may or may not be immediately apparent but will subsequently require treatment (e.g., urethral disruption)

Utilization of this scheme requires a deliberate and regimented approach to resuscitation with the flexibility of resetting priorities depending upon the diagnostic disclosures that arise during resuscitation. It is maintenance of this balance between a structured resuscitation protocol and the need to properly change directions that generates the necessity for one person to be in charge of the entire resuscitation procedure.

Steps in Initial Resuscitation

AIRWAY. The crucial first step in the management of injured patient is the securing of an adequate airway. The mechanical removal of debris and the "chin lift" or "jaw thrust" maneuvers, both of which pull the tongue and oral musculature forward from the pharynx, are often useful in clearing the airway of less severely injured patients. However, when there is any question about the adequacy of the airway, when there is evidence of severe head injury, or when the patient is in profound shock, more definitive airway control is appropriate. In most patients this involves endotracheal intubation. Unfortunately, control of the airway is sometimes more complex than simply placing an endotracheal tube. The occurrence of cervical spine injury in the unconscious patient is always a possibility, and injudicious movement of the neck in the process of endotracheal intubation can result in devastating consequences. One approach to selecting the optimal airway control in these patients is outlined in Figure 2.

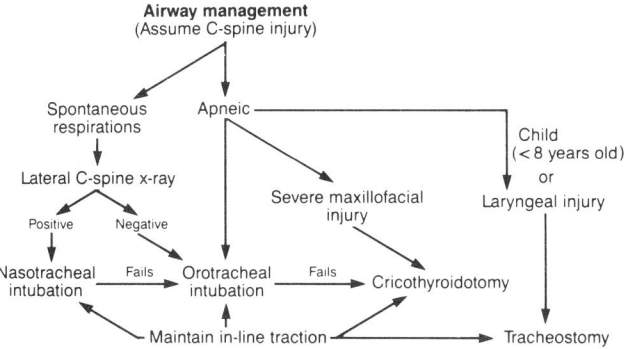

Figure 2. Algorithm for airway management in the trauma patient. (From Maier, R. V.: Airway management. *In* Moore, E. E. (Ed.): Early Care of the Injured Patient, 4th ed. Toronto, B. C. Decker, Inc., 1990.)

The most direct method for establishing an airway is endotracheal intubation. This requires that the head and neck be held in a neutral position to avoid exacerbation of potential cervical spine injury and that the spine be stabilized until an injury has been definitively excluded. When the patient has no evidence of soft tissue or bony injury to the midface and is breathing spontaneously, *naso*tracheal intubation is an acceptable alternative to *oro*tracheal intubation. In a few patients, a surgical airway may be required. While classical tracheostomy may be indicated in select patients, such as those with laryngeal injuries, cricothyroidotomy is generally the preferable emergency procedure. These surgical procedures may be preceded by needle cricothyroidotomy with jet insufflation to improve oxygenation and allow the surgical procedure to be performed in a more orderly fashion.[129]

BREATHING. If there is decreased respiratory drive or an unstable chest wall, assisted ventilation is usually necessary. The three most common reasons for ineffective ventilation following successful placement of an airway are malposition of the endotracheal tube, pneumothorax, and hemothorax. Therefore, palpation and auscultation of the chest are necessary diagnostic adjuncts at this point. A supine anteroposterior (AP) chest film can validate the physical examination and better define chest wall and pleural abnormalities. Although there generally is time to obtain a chest radiograph prior to invasive therapeutic procedures, in the patient with profound hemodynamic instability and a probable tension pneumothorax, a needle catheter decompression can be both diagnostic and therapeutic. Under these circumstances decompression of the chest prior to the radiograph is appropriate.

CIRCULATION. When possible, control of the hemorrhage precedes placement of the intravenous lines. This may be as simple as a compressive dressing over a bleeding wound or large vessel or may require broader compression, such as the application of the pneumatic antishock garment in the patient who has an obvious pelvic fracture. Intravenous cannulas are usually placed percutaneously in the arm or groin. They should be large-bore, and a minimum of two should be placed. Lines should not be inserted distal to extremity wounds with potential vascular injury. Alternatives are a cut-down by either the antecubital or the saphenous route or the intraosseus route in children under the age of three.[76] With the exception of the use of the large (No. 8 French) introducer catheter, subclavian venipuncture is not a rapid route for fluid administration and is best reserved for monitoring response to fluid therapy. Fluid resuscitation begins with a 1000-ml. bolus of lactated Ringer's solution in an adult, or 20 ml. per kg. in a child. Response to therapy is monitored by skin perfusion, urinary output, and central venous pressure readings when that line has been placed.

DISABILITY/NEUROLOGIC ASSESSMENT. At this juncture, a brief examination to determine level of consciousness, pupillary response, and movement of extremities is a necessary prelude to the determination of severity of neurologic injury. In addition, this information becomes initial data in the computation of the Glasgow Coma Scale, which is a method of both following the evolution of neurologic disability and prognosticating future recovery (Table 1).[83] It is worth noting that pupillary response can still be assessed in the paralyzed patient. In recording the Glasgow Coma Scale in intubated and paralyzed patients, the authors have added the modifiers *T* and *P* (intubated/paralyzed) to signify that the score may be inaccurate.

EXPOSURE FOR COMPLETE EXAMINATION. By this time, most injuries that are either exigent or emergencies have been recognized and treated. The next step is to re-examine the patient completely, but expeditiously, for the purpose of diagnosing other injuries. Complete physical examination is typically done in a head-to-toe manner and includes ordering and collecting data from appropriate laboratory and radiologic tests. Data accumulated can then be used to reset priorities. This time

TABLE 1. The Glasgow Coma Scale

Eyes open	Never	1
	To pain	2
	To verbal stimuli	3
	Spontaneously	4
Best verbal response	No response	1
	Incomprehensible sounds	2
	Inappropriate words	3
	Disoriented and converses	4
	Oriented and converses	5
Best motor response	No response	1
	Extension (decerebrate rigidity)	2
	Flexion abnormal (decorticate rigidity)	3
	Flexion withdrawal	4
	Localizes pain	5
	Obeys	6
Total		3–15

period also allows for the placement of additional lines, catheters (nasogastric, Foley), and monitoring devices. When the patient is oxygenating, ventilating, and perfusing adequately, a priority plan should be established for subsequent treatment.

The following section deals with the management of specific injuries and is organized to reflect, in general, the probability that these specific injuries will impact negatively on airway, breathing, and circulation. As such, thoracic and abdominal injuries are first, followed by the head and central nervous system, the neck, the face, and finally the extremities.

RECOGNITION AND MANAGEMENT OF SPECIFIC INJURIES

THORAX

One quarter of civilian trauma deaths are caused by thoracic trauma, and two thirds of these deaths occur after the patient reaches the hospital. The mortality of hospitalized patients with an isolated chest injury ranges from 4 to 8 per cent and increases from 10 to 50 per cent when one other organ system is involved, rising to 35 per cent when multiple additional organ systems are involved.[38] Many of these deaths can be prevented with prompt diagnosis and correct management. Despite these high mortality rates, most thoracic injuries do not require a thoracotomy, but rather simple life-saving maneuvers of airway control and tube thoracostomy.

MECHANISM OF INJURY

The life-threatening injuries incurred in penetrating trauma are distinctly different from those of blunt injuries. The initial care of patients with thoracic trauma must focus on the mechanism of injury and evaluate the patient's conditions accordingly for respective life-threatening injuries. Penetrating injuries include stab wounds, gunshot wounds, and impalement on a foreign body. All penetrating injuries that enter or traverse the mediastinum must be evaluated for potential cardiac, great vessel, or esophageal injury. Peripheral lung injuries frequently produce both hemothorax and pneumothorax. More than 80 per cent of all penetrating chest wounds cause hemothorax, and nearly all cause pneumothorax.[93]

Blunt trauma can induce injury by three distinct mechanisms: a direct blow (e.g., rib fracture) to the chest, deceleration injury (e.g., pulmonary or cardiac contusion, aortic tear), and compression injury (e.g., cardiac rupture, diaphragm rupture). Rib fracture is the most common sign of blunt thoracic trauma. The less common scapular, sternal, or first-rib fracture suggests massive force of injury and should invoke a thorough search for

multisystem injury.[142,182] In adults the bony thoracic cage absorbs much of the shock of blunt trauma. In children, the flexible cartilaginous thoracic structures allow the transmission of blunt force to the intrathoracic structures, which results in a higher incidence of pulmonary contusion than of rib fractures.

PATHOPHYSIOLOGY

The thorax is responsible for the vital delivery of oxygenated blood to metabolically active tissues. Three pathologic consequences of thoracic injury, either alone or in combination, are responsible for inadequate oxygen delivery: hypoxemia, hypervolemia, and myocardial failure.[93] Hypoxemia can follow such divergent etiologies as airway obstruction, pneumothorax, flail chest, pulmonary contusion, tracheobronchial injury, and diaphragm rupture. Each of these injuries limits the physiologic function of air exchange. Hypovolemia from intrathoracic hemorrhage is second only to rib fractures as a sequel of thoracic trauma. As much as 40 per cent of the circulating blood can accumulate in a hemothorax, and thoracic bleeding most frequently occurs from injuries to the lung parenchyma or intercostal vessels. Cardiac pump failure may follow both blunt or penetrating thoracic injuries. Cardiac contusion is estimated to occur in 20 per cent of patients with major thoracic trauma, although many cardiac contusions go unrecognized because the clinical manifestations are subtle and the diagnosis is imprecise.[87] Penetrating injuries following direct cardiac injury and pericardial tamponade may rapidly compromise cardiac function. Other rare causes of cardiac pump failure include rupture of the ventricular septum and valvular muscle and coronary air embolus. The initial management of patients with thoracic trauma must focus on both the mechanisms of injury and the pathologic consequences responsible for inadequate oxygen delivery.

INITIAL TREATMENT

The initial approach to the thoracic trauma patient follows the basic tenants of resuscitation of all critically injured patients. The primary goal is to provide oxygen to vital organs. Airway control and maintenance of adequate ventilation are top priorities. Rapid control of external bleeding and replenishment of intravascular volume are the next concern. Persistent shock despite adequate oxygenation in volume restoration suggests cardiogenic shock from tension pneumothorax, myocardial contusion or infarction, cardiac tamponade, or coronary air embolism. Maximal attention should be given these immediate life-threatening problems.

The next priority is assessment of the patient's overall condition and recognition of other potentially lethal injuries. Some specific features of the initial management of thoracic trauma patients bear emphasis. Patency of the airway and adequate ventilation are the first priority. Restlessness, confusion, and anxiety are the first signs of hypoxemia. Stridor and supraclavicular and intercostal retraction suggest airway obstruction. The airway is manually cleared of debris and secretions are suctioned. Active airway control (endotracheal intubation or tracheostomy) may be required. In blunt trauma or gunshot wounds to the neck, cervical spine injury must be assumed until it is excluded.

Venting a major hemothorax or pneumothorax in the thoracic patient in extremis is an integral part of establishing adequate ventilation and should not await radiologic confirmation. Rapid tube thoracostomy re-expands the collapsed lung and tamponades lung parenchymal injuries against the chest wall and allows the monitoring of ongoing blood loss. Large-bore needle insertion may elevate a tension pneumothorax and obviate the need for "crash" intubation. Tube thoracostomy should follow.

Airway control and assurance of adequate ventilation and oxygenation, restitution of intravascular volume, and control of overt external hemorrhage are the next treatment priorities.

With chest trauma, persistent hypotension secondary to intrathoracic bleeding is assumed until disproven by tube thoracostomy and radiologic confirmation. The patient with thoracic trauma who remains hypotensive despite adequate oxygenation and fluid resuscitation must be evaluated for cardiogenic shock. Causes include tamponade, myocardial contusion, and coronary air embolism. Tension pneumothorax can mimic these causes of cardiac dysfunction by limiting cardiac preload. Jugular venous distention or elevated central venous pressures may help in differentiating the diagnosis. The diagnosis of cardiac tamponade is based on clinical findings or in association with a high-risk wound and unexplained hypotension. The majority follow penetrating mediastinal injuries. Only one third of patients have the classic triad of tamponade: hypotension, distant or muffled heart sounds, and distended neck veins. Confirmation of the diagnosis by needle pericardiocentesis or emergency cardiac ultrasound is required. Volume resuscitation will transiently improve cardiac output and can be used as a temporizing maneuver. After the initial and rapid treatment of life-threatening injuries, a complete assessment and search for associated injuries is required. The treatment of other specific thoracic injuries is detailed below.

TREATMENT OF SPECIFIC INJURIES

Chest Wall

RIB FRACTURES. Fracture of the ribs is the most common thoracic injury (Fig. 3). With simple fractures, pain on inspiration is the principal symptom. Localized pain, tenderness, and occasionally crepitus confirm the diagnosis. A chest film should be obtained to exclude other intrathoracic injuries and not necessarily to identify rib fractures. Narcotics in small amounts, intercostal nerve blocks, and muscle relaxants are usually adequate. Hospital admission for pain relief, cough assistance, and endotracheal suction may be necessary for several days, particularly in elderly patients. Rib belts and adhesive taping, although once popular, should be avoided because the limitation

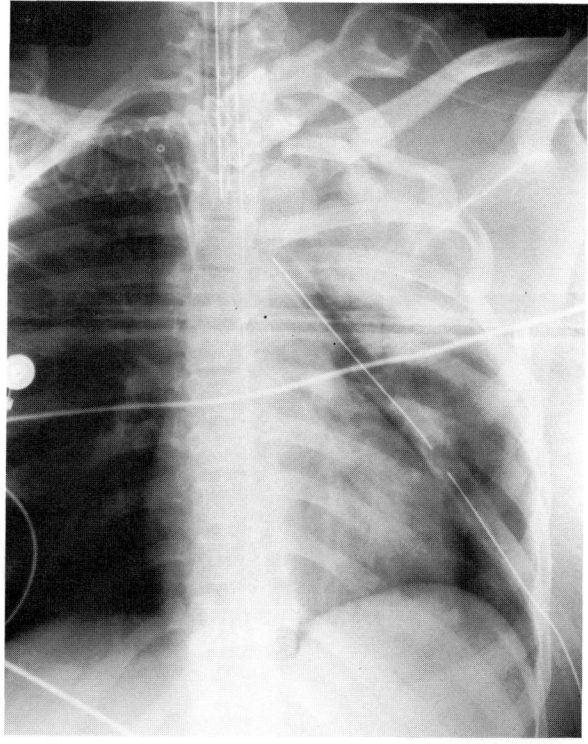

Figure 3. Flail chest over left upper thoracic and shoulder girdle region. Fracture displacement of ribs 1 through 4. Underlying pulmonary contusion is evident. No associated major vascular injury occurred.

in motion increases the incidence of retained secretions and atelectasis. Fracture of the upper ribs (first to third), clavicle, or scapula implies significant trauma, and associated major vascular injury must be suspected.[142,182] One report cites a 14 per cent incidence of vascular injury in patients sustaining first-rib fractures, but all had an associated absent pulse, a brachial plexus injury, or a displaced fracture, implying that angiography may be selectively employed in this group of patients.[142]

FLAIL CHEST. Unilateral fracture of four or more ribs anteriorly and posteriorly or bilateral anterior or costochondral fracture of four or five ribs will produce enough instability that paradoxical respiratory motion results in hypoventilation of an unacceptable degree (see Fig. 3). Although usually visually apparent in the unconscious patient, because of splinting, the flail segment may not be readily apparent in the conscious patient. If it is severe and untreated, atelectasis, hypercapnia, hypoxia, accumulation of secretions, and ineffective cough occur. The pathophysiologic effects may be present immediately or may progress over several hours and present as late respiratory decompensation.

Many methods have been improvised to stabilize the chest wall with variable results. If spontaneous respirations prove inadequate, endotracheal intubation with the use of a volume respirator has largely supplanted attempts at stabilization of the chest wall. A respiratory rate of greater than 40 breaths per minute and a Po_2 of less than 60 mm. Hg on 60 per cent Fio_2 are indications for intubation and mechanical ventilation. In addition, pre-existing chronic lung disease, a depressed level of consciousness, and concomitant intra-abdominal injuries are relative indications. Once the patient has been ventilated, the use of serial intercostal rib blocks or even a segmental epidural anesthetic may be helpful in reducing pain and hypoventilation. Only rarely are sternal fracture displacement and rib overlap and displacement severe enough to warrant open reduction and fixation.

Respiratory difficulty in flail chest injury is invariably aggravated by an underlying pulmonary contusion (see Fig. 3). Trinkle and co-workers and Shackford and associates have in fact concluded that the major respiratory problem is the underlying pulmonary injury and that paradoxical movement is a minor factor.[162,186] These reports demonstrate a reduced need for mechanical ventilation if care is exercised in avoiding fluid overresuscitation. If intubation is required, positive end-expiratory pressure (PEEP) may be helpful in restoring functional residual capacity and reducing intrapulmonary shunts. Mechanical ventilation and a better understanding of the underlying pulmonary contusion has reduced the mortality of flail chest from 50 to less than 5 per cent.

OPEN PNEUMOTHORAX. A defect in the chest wall provides a direct communication of the pleural space with the environment. A wound of sufficient size to exceed the laryngeal cross-sectional area will provide an alternative air pathway with less resistance than that of the normal tracheobronchial tree. Inability to generate negative intrathoracic pressure results in lung collapse and marked paroxysmal shifting of the mediastinum with each respiratory effort. The resultant hypoventilation and diminished cardiac output can become immediately life-threatening. Diagnosis is readily apparent as each inspiration draws air into the intrapleural space, causing the characteristic "sucking chest wound." Treatment consists of prompt closure of the defect with a sterile dressing followed by venting of the chest with either a flutter valve or chest tube to treat the possible resultant tension pneumothorax.

Lungs

PULMONARY CONTUSION. Pulmonary contusion occurs in most patients with flail chest but can also appear without any evidence of rib fracture. It must be remembered that critical intrathoracic trauma may be present in the absence of skeletal

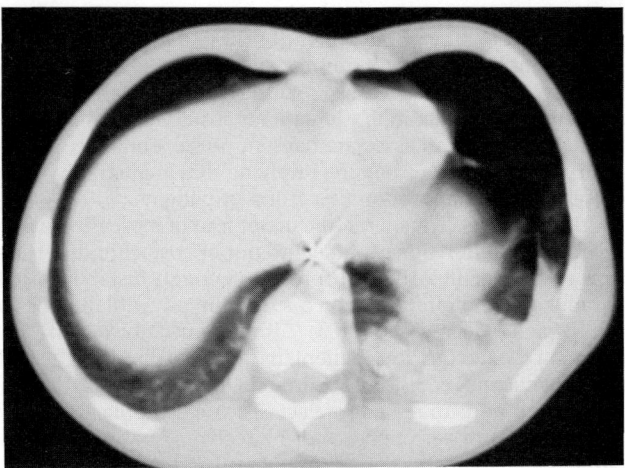

Figure 4. Chest computed tomographic scan of a 10-year-old patient after blunt chest trauma. There is evidence of significant pulmonary contusion.

injury, particularly in children, because of the marked elasticity of the rib cage. Fluid and blood from ruptured vessels enter the alveoli, interstitial spaces, and bronchi and produce localized airway obstruction. As this process progresses, pulmonary compliance decreases and ventilation becomes more difficult. Pulmonary contusions are contrasted to localized lung hematomas, which are the result of local parenchymal injury and hemorrhage (Fig. 4). Most hematomas resolve adequately with expectant treatment. Pulmonary contusion may be confused with the adult respiratory distress syndrome (ARDS) or may even be associated with it. Physical examination is usually unrewarding. In contrast, radiographic examination eventually demonstrates patchy consolidation, from minimal to lobar. Chest films showing parenchymal consolidation immediately following injury are suggestive of pulmonary contusion (see Fig. 3). In children, the relative elasticity of the thoracic cage makes pulmonary contusion likely even in the absence of rib fractures (Fig. 5).

Management involves careful pulmonary support and clearing of secretions, with ventilatory support if arterial blood gas values cannot be maintained in a physiologic range. Fluid overload should be assiduously avoided. The use of albumin to maintain plasma oncotic pressure in this clinical setting is controversial. The hemorrhage and edema are self-limited and clear if infection or other problems do not intervene. Although pulmonary contusion is usually a localized parenchymal defect, positive end-expiratory pressure (PEEP) may be a useful adjunct in the management of those patients requiring ventilation, particularly if they have more generalized infiltration on chest x-ray examination.

PNEUMOTHORAX. Pneumothorax occurs as a result of lacerations of the chest wall or lung, or rupture of alveoli ("paper bag effect"), and can be caused by either penetrating or blunt trauma. Tension pneumothorax develops when a flap valve leak allows air to enter the pleural space but prevents its escape. Intrapleural pressure rises, causing total lung collapse and a shift of the mediastinum to the opposite side (Fig. 6). This pressure must be relieved immediately so that interference with ventilation in the opposite lung and impairment of cardiac function from impediment of venous return can be avoided. Tension pneumothorax is a true surgical emergency, requiring immediate diagnosis and chest tube insertion. The presence of subcutaneous emphysema, absent breath sounds, mediastinal shift, and acute respiratory distress warrants chest tube insertion without waiting for a chest film to be taken. In contrast, a simple pneumothorax (without tension) of traumatic origin should also be managed by chest tube insertion but only after documentation by chest x-ray examination. In many circumstances, 15 to 20 cm. water seal suction is all that is necessary. The temptation to observe a minimal pneumothorax should be resisted. Delayed increase in the volume of the pneumothorax may occur and become life-threatening after the patient has been transferred from the critical care area. This is more apt to occur when the patient requires anesthesia, intubation, and a positive pressure breathing system or when assisted mechanical ventilation is otherwise required.

HEMOTHORAX. Hemorrhage into the pleural space occurs in some quantity in almost every patient with a diagnosable chest injury.[92] Blood loss may vary from slight to extensive. Although an upright chest film can show an intrathoracic accumulation of more than 200 ml. of blood, a supine film may miss collections of up to 1 liter. Bleeding may be from any intrathoracic structure, although massive hemothorax generally signals a systemic arterial or major pulmonary vascular injury. Because the lung itself is a low-pressure system with an average pulmonary artery pressure of 15 mm. Hg, spontaneous hemostasis

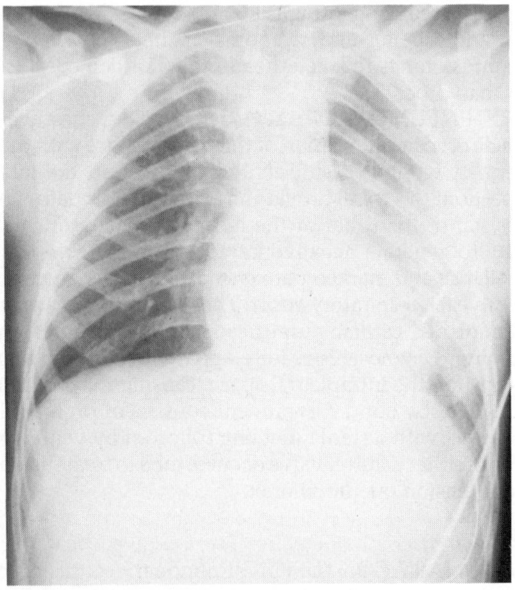

Figure 5. Chest AP radiograph of the 10-year-old boy, shown in Figure 4, involved in a motor vehicle accident. Despite the lack of rib fractures, significant pulmonary contusion is apparent.

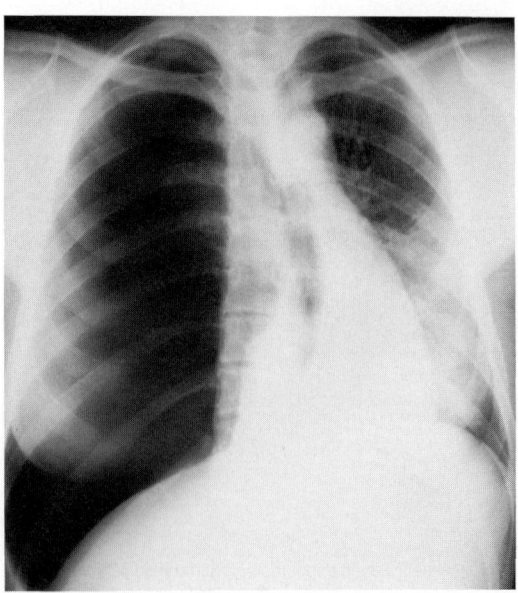

Figure 6. Right tension pneumothorax following a stab wound to the chest.

occurs for all but central injuries. Most often significant, persistent hemothorax is from intercostal arteries; and in penetrating wounds, a bleeding internal mammary artery is often the source (Fig. 7). Tube thoracostomy with a No. 32 to 36 French chest tube placed in the sixth or seventh intercostal space at the midaxillary line should be promptly performed.[92] Note that this insertion point is somewhat lower than is required for pneumothorax, to permit better sulcus drainage. Needle aspiration is not adequate. Early tube thoracostomy prevents clotted hemothorax or subsequent fibrothorax in most instances. When massive hemothorax is present, preparation for collection of the blood for autotransfusion should be made prior to insertion of the tube. A sodium citrate solution can be added to the blood collection device to ensure anticoagulation and permit autotransfusion.

In 85 per cent of patients, tube thoracostomy is the only treatment required. Unrelenting hemorrhage following either penetrating or blunt thoracic trauma is an indication for immediate thoracotomy. An initial thoracic blood loss greater than 1500 ml. (30 per cent blood volume) or an ongoing loss of 250 ml. (5 per cent blood volume) for 3 consecutive hours serves only as a practical guideline. The clinical situation and overall condition of the patient are the most influential factors. A study by Rene and associates has demonstrated that an acute hemothorax of 1500 ml. following penetrating trauma causes a surgically correctable lesion 85 per cent of the time.[148] With blunt trauma thoracotomy is less likely to demonstrate a discrete source of hemorrhage.

TRACHEAL AND BRONCHIAL INJURIES. Blunt tracheal or bronchial injuries are often due to compression of the airway between the sternum and the vertebral column in decelerating "steering wheel" accidents with resultant shearing of the right main stem bronchus from the carina or transverse lacerations of the trachea. Alternatively, a rupture of the membranous trachea may occur during chest wall compression with a closed glottis. Patients with tracheal injuries may present with mediastinal and deep cervical emphysema or pneumothorax with a massive air leak. Hemoptysis, hemopneumothorax, subcutaneous crepitance, and respiratory distress are frequent. When accompanied by acute airway obstruction, the immediate priority is establishment of an effective airway. If possible, this should be preceded by endoscopic evaluation of the injury prior to blind endotracheal intubation. Emergency treatment consists of inserting the endotracheal tube beyond the injury to facilitate ventilation and prevent aspiration of blood. Tube thoracostomy is clearly indicated in the presence of a hemothorax or pneumothorax. If endotracheal intubation is not possible or if the anatomy is

significantly distorted, surgical entry into the trachea for placement of a tracheostomy tube may be necessary.

The definitive diagnosis of tracheal or bronchial injury usually requires confirmation by bronchoscopy. When early diagnosis is made, the contralateral bronchus is intubated and primary repair is performed. Although small lesions may be managed initially without operation, delayed healing invites stricture formation, resulting in recurrent atelectasis, infection, and bronchiectasis, and parenchymal destruction will finally occur. For an early stricture, either resection or a bronchoplastic procedure may be performed. After permanent parenchymal damage, pulmonary resection should be performed.

Heart and Aorta

CONTUSION AND CARDIAC RUPTURE. Cardiac contusion occurs in 20 per cent of patients with blunt chest injuries and in an estimated 70 per cent of multisystem trauma patients admitted to an intensive care unit.[93] Fifty per cent of autopsies performed on victims of fatal automobile accidents demonstrate significant trauma to the pericardium and heart.[96] The injury varies from a localized contusion to complete cardiac rupture, with the right ventricle most frequently involved because of its proximity to the sternum (Fig. 8). Although most patients with rupture of the atrial or ventricular chambers do not reach a medical facility, survivors have been reported if vital signs can be maintained during transport.

Myocardial contusion may vary from superficial epicardial petechiae to transmural damage. Delayed ventricular rupture can occur months after a seemingly incidental myocardial contusion, with the resultant development of an acute left-to-right shunt. Injury and thrombosis of the coronary vessels can also result from this type of trauma. The major difficulty in treatment is early recognition. The correct diagnosis is made only pathologically, with findings of myocardial wall bruise or hematoma. There are no specific and practical laboratory findings, and many cardiac contusions are probably not recognized. Suspicious clinical findings include new arrhythmias, friction rubs, chest pain, murmurs, and evidence of low cardiac output or right heart dysfunction (elevated central venous pressure). Electrocardiograms (ECGs) may show nonspecific ST-T wave changes. Intensive care unit monitoring for 24 hours is indicated when ECG abnormalities are present or when a major contusion is suspected.[116] In addition, immediate echocardiography may be helpful in diagnosing dysfunction of the ventricular wall and in detecting blood in the pericardium. The management of myocardial contusion is supportive and similar to that for acute myocardial infarction.

TAMPONADE. Cardiac tamponade is most frequently caused by penetrating thoracic injuries, but occasionally it is observed in blunt thoracic trauma from myocardial rupture, coronary artery laceration, or ascending dissection of an aortic tear. Accumulation of as little as 150 ml. of blood in the pericardium may impair diastolic filling sufficiently to produce distended neck veins, shock, and cyanosis. Beck's classic triad of distended neck veins, muffled heart sounds, and hypotension is present in only one third of patients with tamponade and pulsus paradoxus is even less frequently discernible.[165] Immediate treatment consists of pericardiocentesis with an 18-gauge needle, which also provides the diagnosis. However, approximately 15 per cent of pericardiocenteses give false-negative results because of a clotted hemopericardium.[17] Therefore, echocardiography prior to needle aspiration is advisable if promptly obtainable. A subxiphoid pericardial window is an alternative, but it is best performed in the operating room. If the patient is *in extremis,* emergency thoracotomy with pericardiotomy and cardiac repair should be performed. Reports of successful emergency cardiorrhaphy for stab wounds vary from 15 to 80 per cent. Most patients with penetrating cardiac trauma do not require cardiopulmonary bypass. The presence of a postin-

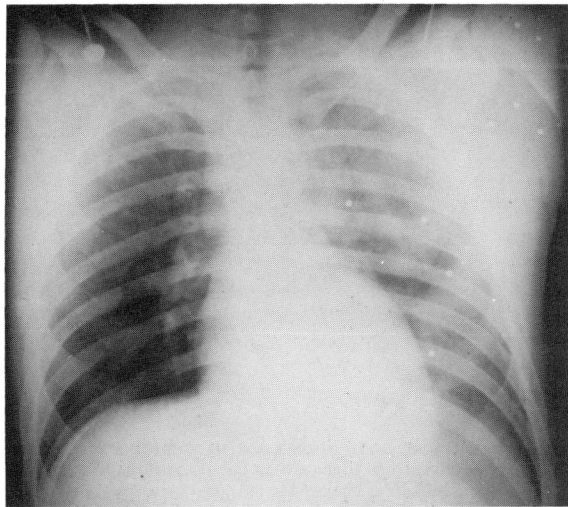

Figure 7. Massive hemothorax from a gunshot wound to the left chest.

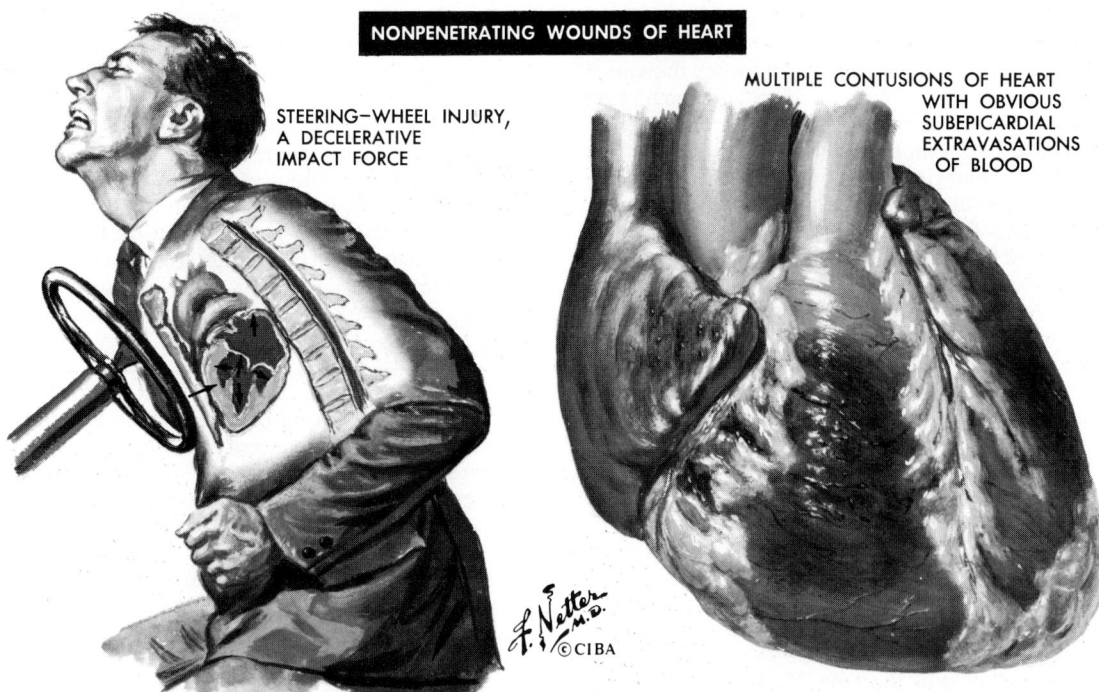

NONPENETRATING WOUNDS OF HEART

STEERING—WHEEL INJURY,
A DECELERATIVE
IMPACT FORCE

MULTIPLE CONTUSIONS OF HEART
WITH OBVIOUS
SUBEPICARDIAL
EXTRAVASATIONS
OF BLOOD

Figure 8. Mechanism for development of myocardial contusion with compression of the heart between the sternum and vertebral column. (Courtesy of CIBA Pharmaceuticals.)

jury cardiac murmur, suggesting valvular insufficiency or septal defect, should be an indication for echocardiography, cardiac catheterization, or angiography. Repair of these lesions may involve valve replacement or repair or patch closure of septal lesions.

AORTA. Rupture of the thoracic aorta is the most lethal injury following blunt chest trauma and causes 15 to 40 per cent of fatalities in motor vehicle accidents.[38,66] The exact mechanism of injury is not fully understood, but it is thought that the aortic arch at the descending aorta undergoes flexion or torsion, disrupting the aortic wall at the ligamentum arteriosum immediately distal to the left subclavian artery. Occasionally, the ascending aorta at the root of the heart may be injured. Injuries to the innominate artery or the subclavian artery at the origin have also been reported. In addition, the descending thoracic aorta may be avulsed from one or several intercostal arteries.

Most patients with aortic rupture die immediately of exsanguination. However, in approximately 20 per cent of these patients, the periaortic tissues in the pleura contain the intravascular pressure and produce a traumatic aneurysm. When this occurs, the aneurysm is usually located in the aortic isthmus. Typically, there is partial or complete circumferential tearing of the aortic wall, and the two ends retract from 1 to 2 cm. Survival is dependent on retention of the hematoma in the aortal adventitia until definitive repair can be performed. Therefore, time is of the essence. Historical data show that of those patients with a torn thoracic aorta who survive 1 hour, 15 per cent will die of exsanguination within 6 hours and 25 per cent, within 24 hours.[139] The few who survive the initial period develop a false aneurysm that slowly enlarges over a period of months to years. Calcification in the aneurysm wall usually appears, and aneurysms of this type may span periods of 20 years or more.

There may be no symptoms or findings to suggest aortic injury in those patients who do not undergo exsanguination immediately. Other lesions, such as intracranial trauma, chest wall injury, or a ruptured spleen or liver, explain most of the clinical findings. The most common abnormality is a widening of the mediastinal shadow on x-ray examination, although only 20 to 43 per cent of patients with a widened mediastinum have aortic

injury (Fig. 9).[69] Kirsh and Sloan have described the following 10 signs of aortic injury: (1) a mediastinum greater than 10 cm., (2) a loss of aortic contour, (3) a shift of the endotracheal tube and trachea to the right, (4) an elevation of the left main stem bronchus, (5) depression of the right main stem bronchus, (6) a shift of the nasogastric tube to the left, (7) apical capping, (8) first-rib fracture, (9) acute left-sided hemothorax, and (10) retrocardiac density.[98,168]

Aortography is indicated if aortic injury is suspected on the basis of the mechanism of injury and any of these suggestive findings (Fig. 10). Although computed tomographic (CT) scanning has been evaluated as a possible means for early diagnosis, retrograde aortography remains the standard of diagnosis.

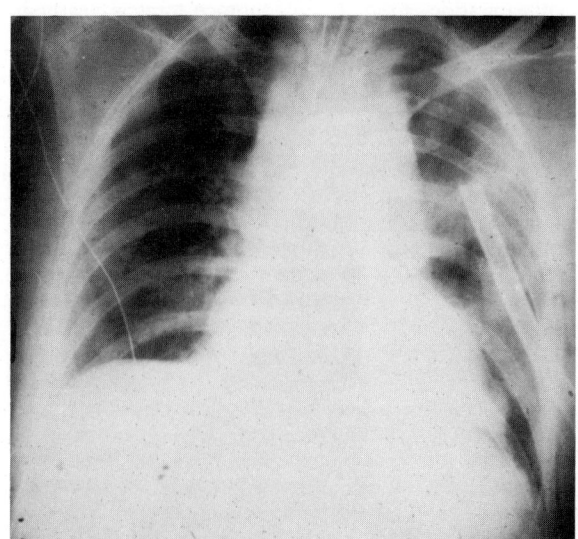

Figure 9. Chest film status after a high-speed motor vehicle accident. Note that the mediastinum is greater than 10 cm. across, there is loss of contour of the aortic knob, the endotracheal tube is displaced to the right, there is left apical capping, and there is left hemothorax. These signs are all highly suggestive of aortic disruption.

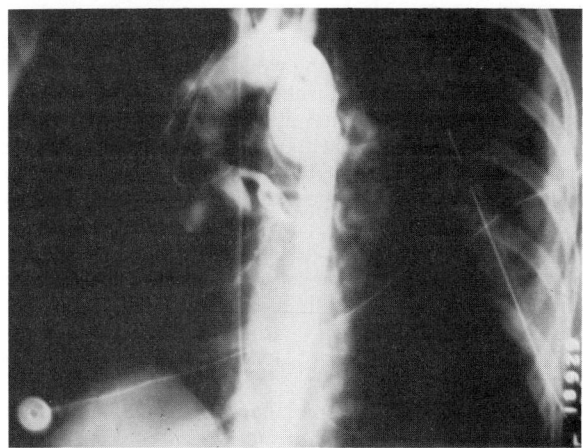

Figure 10. Aortogram of the patient in Figure 9 demonstrating rupture of the thoracic aorta to the left subclavian artery.

Surgical repair should be performed immediately because of the risk of fatal hemorrhage. Several methods of partial bypass have been advocated and successfully used and are discussed in Chapter 52. Partial atrioarterial bypass employing a nonheparinized centrifugal pump is the current preferred technique. Although the mandatory use of a shunt or bypass is controversial, its main advantage is to protect the spinal cord from ischemia. End-to-end suture is occasionally feasible, but usually a short segment of woven Dacron graft must be interposed.

Other Injuries

DIAPHRAGM. Penetrating lacerations of the diaphragm outnumber blunt ruptures at least four to one, and both may result in herniation through the diaphragm. Therefore, both require therapy. Herniation has been reported years after an initial small stab wound. Most blunt diaphragmatic ruptures result from motor vehicle accidents (Fig. 11). Rupture of the diaphragm may be either small or large and may involve almost any part of the diaphragm but is usually radial in location. Herniation of the viscera may not occur immediately, delaying the diagnosis for an indefinite period of time. The diagnosis is often incidentally made at time of laparotomy, since 85 per cent of patients with left diaphragmatic rupture have associated intra-abdominal injuries. With right-sided diaphragmatic rupture, this is less likely, and chest films may be normal in 30 per cent of the patients. Although classically it has been observed that left-sided diaphragm injuries are more common than right-sided, the more frequent use of CT scans and an awareness of the likelihood of this injury may explain the recent observations of a more equal distribution.[194] If the diagnosis is made early, an abdominal approach is usually indicated to exclude associated injuries. If the diagnosis has been substantially delayed to exclude intra-abdominal injuries, repair may be preferred via a thoracic approach, particularly for right-sided injuries.

ESOPHAGUS. Blunt injury of the esophagus is rare, and penetrating injuries are rarely isolated. The most common symptom of esophageal perforation is extreme pain with the slow evolution of fever several hours later. Regurgitation of blood, hoarseness, dysphagia, or respiratory distress may also be present because of injuries to the trachea. Suspicious radiographic findings are mediastinal air and widening or presence of a foreign body. Pleural effusion or hydropneumothorax is frequently seen. All mediastinal traversing gunshot wounds or stab wounds near the posterior midline should be evaluated for possible esophageal injury. Both endoscopy and esophagography have reported sensitivities that vary from 50 to 90 per cent.[60,198] Improvement of this accuracy can be obtained if the initial water-soluble contrast films are followed by barium studies. Endoscopy and esophagography should be considered complimentary studies. Esophageal injury requires immediate debridement, suture closure, and drainage. Delays of 12 to 24 hours may preclude primary repair and mandate proximal diversion and distal feeding access.

ABDOMEN: MECHANISMS AND DIAGNOSIS OF INJURY

The abdomen is the third most commonly injured region, with injuries requiring operation occurring in about 20 per cent of civilian trauma victims. Abdominal injuries can be particularly dangerous, because it is often difficult to assess intra-abdominal pathology in the multiply injured victim. *Blunt trauma* continues to be the most common mechanism of injury to the abdomen. This is in part related to the consequences of motor vehicle accidents, although falls, assaults, and industrial accidents contribute significantly. In children, automobile and pedestrian accidents, recreational activities (bicycling, falls), and child abuse are the leading causes of abdominal injury. In the urban setting, *penetrating trauma* is often more frequent than blunt abdominal injuries. Knife wounds are more common than gunshot wounds and generally less lethal (Fig. 12). After several decades of a generally accepted mandatory exploration policy for any penetrating abdominal wound, several large urban trauma centers have again advocated a more selective approach to the management of penetrating wounds, particularly stab injuries.[112,123] This is due in part to the large number of penetrating wounds evaluated at these institutions but also to improved accuracy and availability of diagnostic techniques.

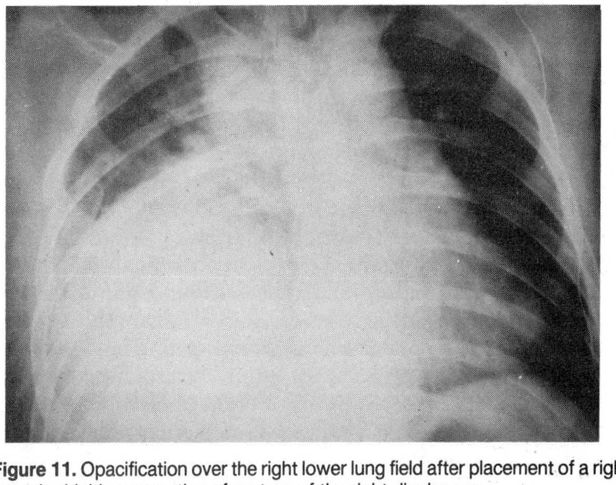

Figure 11. Opacification over the right lower lung field after placement of a right chest tube highly suggestive of rupture of the right diaphragm.

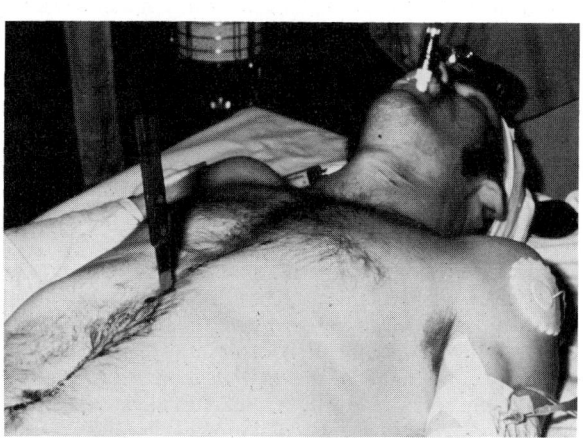

Figure 12. Butcher knife impaled in the epigastrium.

CURRENT DIAGNOSTIC TECHNIQUES

In the awake, alert, responsive patient with isolated abdominal injury, the physical examination and history are very helpful in predicting the presence of significant visceral injury. For this reason, additional laboratory, radiographic, and invasive procedures have a limited role as adjuncts to the physical examination in the patient with *isolated* abdominal injuries. However, in the multiply injured patient with brain involvement, an impaired ability to recognize abdominal pain, or hypotension not attributable to other injuries, additional diagnostic modalities may be of significant benefit. Two highly accurate diagnostic modalities—diagnostic peritoneal lavage (DPL) and CT—have greatly assisted the surgeon in assessing abdominal injury. Nuclear magnetic resonance, while providing detailed anatomic reconstructions, has yet to be clinically adopted in abdominal trauma.

In the early 1960s, needle pericentesis was incorporated as a method of determining intraperitoneal hemorrhage in comatose patients. When positive, the test was highly predictive of significant intra-abdominal injury. Unfortunately, most of the early studies demonstrated a false-negative rate averaging 9.4 per cent, but ranging as high as 36 to 40 per cent.[146,154] Accordingly, in 1965 Root and associates attempted to improve these results by adding an infusion of one liter of normal saline to the technique of paracentesis, then retrieving and sampling the effluent.[154] In Powell's review of 31 collected series involving 10,358 patients in whom diagnostic peritoneal lavage was used in evaluating blunt trauma to the abdomen, the false-positive and false-negative rates were 1.4 per cent and 1.3 per cent, respectively.[146] Many other large reviews have confirmed an overall sensitivity of 95 per cent, specificity of 98 to 99 per cent, and accuracy of 97 per cent for this technique.[51,173] As a result, DPL remains the mainstay for diagnosis of intraperitoneal hemorrhage in the patient who is not awake, alert, or responsive. An additional indication for its use is the patient in whom sequential abdominal examinations will be impossible, for example, a patient undergoing extensive operative procedures such as multiple fracture fixations. In that circumstance, peritoneal lavage may be helpful in excluding the possibility of intraperitoneal injury. Several retrospective studies have demonstrated the greater safety of the open technique versus the percutaneous technique. The expected complication rate with the former should be less than 2 per cent.

CT was added to the surgeon's diagnostic armamentarium for blunt abdominal trauma in 1981.[45] The accuracy of CT scans in abdominal trauma has improved with experience and an understanding of what constitutes abnormal findings.[45,189] It has proven extremely valuable in assessing the retroperitoneum, an anatomic area of injury for which DPL is not helpful but should not be performed in the unstable patient, because such patients are best evaluated by exploratory laparotomy or diagnostic peritoneal lavage. Peitzman and colleagues have provided five indications for abdominal CT scans in trauma victims: (1) hemodynamic stability with an equivocal abdominal examination; (2) closed head injury; (3) spinal cord injury; (4) hematuria in the stable patient; and (5) pelvic fractures and significant bleeding.[140] These are generally accepted; and if the patient is truly hemodynamically stable, the time required to perform CT does not delay surgical procedures, and experienced personnel are available for immediate interpretation of the results.

Controversy continues regarding the use of adjunctive diagnostic measures for patients who have penetration of the anterior abdominal wall fascia. A prospective study evaluated the role of physical examination, local wound exploration, and quantitative peritoneal lavage in the management of stab wounds to the abdomen.[132] In the patient who is awake, alert, and responsive, physical examination with positive findings is 99 per cent predictive of intra-abdominal injury. The most common physical findings in patients with stab wounds to the abdomen are shock, peritonitis, and evisceration. When the physical examination is negative, the wound is explored under local anesthesia with direct visualization for possible penetration of the fascia. If there is no penetration of the anterior fascia, the incidence of intra-abdominal injury is zero. In a patient who has benign abdominal findings but positive fascial penetration, quantitative peritoneal lavage is helpful in reducing the incidence of negative laparotomies while avoiding overlooked significant injuries. With a lavage effluent count of greater than 1000 red blood cells per mm. as an indication for exploratory laparotomy, the overlooked injury rate is reduced to zero and the negative laparotomy rate is reduced to 10 per cent. Others have advocated a less stringent lavage red cell count cutoff but sacrifice sensitivity.[46]

Although certain investigators have suggested the use of lavage or even observation for gunshot wounds of the abdomen, the most current opinion is that because 94 per cent of the time there is intra-abdominal injury in association with gunshot wounds to the abdomen, mandatory exploration is the preferred approach for diagnosis.

Penetrating wounds of the back and flank present significant management dilemmas. Because neither physical examination nor peritoneal lavage is initially helpful in determining retroperitoneal colon, duodenal, renal, or pancreatic injuries, many surgeons favor mandatory exploratory laparotomy for any penetrating wound to the back or flank. However, the incidence of significant intra-abdominal injury varies from only a 5 to 10 per cent for stab wounds to 50 to 75 per cent for gunshot wounds.[191] Contrast-enhanced CT has been suggested as a method of non-invasively evaluating these patients, but the utility and accuracy of this technique needs to be confirmed.[143]

Other investigators have been accurate in both diagnosis and treatment of solid organ injury with the use of visceral arteriography. In a large prospective study of patients who were hemodynamically stable but who still had hemoperitoneum, arteriography was 95 per cent diagnostic and 80 per cent accurate.[8] However, because of the time and expense involved with arteriography and because of the lower false-positive and false-negative rates with peritoneal lavage, arteriography is not an alternative to peritoneal lavage at this time, but rather more useful for specific diagnostic and therapeutic procedures.

INTRAPERITONEAL INJURIES

Spleen

The spleen is the most commonly injured intra-abdominal organ. Splenic injury must therefore be suspected in any patient with blunt abdominal trauma, particularly if associated with left lower rib fractures. The diagnosis is often suspected on physical examination, but generally confirmed by diagnostic peritoneal lavage or abdominal CT scan. Although splenectomy has long been considered the only option for splenic injuries, trauma surgeons must now also consider splenic repair or nonoperative management as viable options in selected patients. These new options have been fostered by the recognition of the rare but highly lethal syndrome of overwhelming postsplenectomy sepsis.

OVERWHELMING POSTSPLENECTOMY SEPSIS. The immunologic function of the spleen has been reviewed by Llende and associates and by others.[105] In brief, asplenic individuals have impaired capacity for clearance of blood-borne particles, depressed phagocytic activity of alveolar macrophages, decreased antibody response to specific antigens, decreased levels of circulating opsins, and altered levels of circulating immunoglobins, such as decreased levels of immunoglobulin M. Many of these immunologic alterations in asplenic individuals are transient; yet the risk of increased susceptibility to sepsis appears to be indefinite.

In 1952, King and Schumacher reported a postsplenectomy syndrome of severe, sometimes fatal meningitis and sepsis in 4 out of 5 children splenectomized before the age of 6 months for congenital hemolytic anemia.[97] The term *overwhelming postsplenectomy infection* was suggested by Diamond in 1969 in a report in which he "incidentally" discounted the risk of infection after splenectomy for trauma.[41] This syndrome of overwhelming postsplenectomy sepsis (OPSS) is unlike fulminating bacteremias and septicemias in individuals with normal splenic function. Rarely does a patient with bacteremia deteriorate from good health to death in less than 24 hours, whereas the overwhelming postsplenectomy infection syndrome constitutes a distinct entity that often lasts only 12 to 18 hours. The onset is sudden, with nausea, vomiting, headache and confusion, leading to coma; the infecting organism is *Pneumococcus* in just over half the patients. *Escherichia coli, Hemophilus influenzae, Meningococcus, Staphylococcus,* and *Streptococcus* organisms are found with decreasing frequency. Disseminated intravascular coagulation is common. Severe hypoglycemia, electrolyte imbalance, and shock are often present. Of particular interest is the occasional presence of diplococci on peripheral blood smears. Blood cultures in these patients indicate that there may be as many as 10^6 organisms per cu. mm., which clearly separates this syndrome from the bacteremia accompanying pneumonia and other ordinary infections.

Rapidity of course from onset until death with failure of antibiotic therapy is characteristic. The overall mortality rate has generally been reported to be as high as 50 per cent and even up to 80 per cent for pneumococcal infections. However, a recent review reported a much lower, 7 per cent, mortality for postsplenectomy sepsis.[64] This discrepancy may be attributable to the universal use of polyvalent pneumococcal vaccine and close follow-up after trauma splenectomy in their patients.

The true incidence of overwhelming postsplenectomy sepsis is not well defined. In 1973, Singer, in his often quoted survey of his and 23 other reported series of infection following splenectomy, attempted to establish the incidence of sepsis following splenectomy in nine categories of disease.[166] With specific reference to trauma, Singer reviewed the courses of 688 patients (388 children, 300 adults) who underwent splenectomy for injury to the spleen. Among these were 10 patients with sepsis, 4 of whom died, resulting in a mortality of 0.58 per cent. When combined with four deaths from sepsis following splenectomy for trauma in a series of 342 children reported by Eraklis and Filler the incidence rate of mortality from sepsis is 0.78 per cent, for a total of 78 times the expected rate as calculated by Singer in the general population.[44] Green and colleagues in the report cited above estimate the risk of postsplenectomy septicemia, pneumonia, and meningitis to be 8.3 per cent in trauma patients, or 166 times the 0.05 per cent rate expected in the general population. Only one patient of the 144 (0.7 per cent) followed in that series died from a pneumococcal infection, and that single episode occurred 3 years after splenectomy. The longest follow-up of splenectomy patients is data compiled by Robinette involving 740 World War II veterans who underwent splenectomy between 1939 and 1945.[153] Six patients in this group (0.8 per cent) died from pneumonia, whereas none of the 740 matched control patients had succumbed to this disease. Most trauma surgeons recommend that splenectomy patients receive the most currently available polyvalent pneumococcal vaccine soon after splenectomy. The timing and use of prophylactic antibiotics in asplenic patients is unresolved.

SPLENORRHAPHY OR PARTIAL RESECTION. The recognition of the important immunologic function of the spleen has renewed interest in splenic salvage; the segmental anatomy and blood supply of the spleen make splenic salvage a possibility. The splenic artery, which delivers 4 per cent of the circulating blood volume per minute, divides into several segmental branches in the hilum, entering the spleen surrounded by the

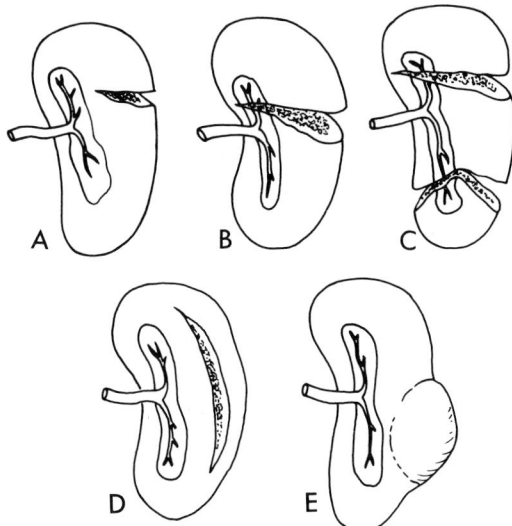

Figure 13. Common patterns of splenic injury. *A,* Simple laceration that involves both the capsule and the parenchyma. *B,* Laceration that involves the splenic pedicle. *C,* Fragmentation with complete devascularization of a portion of the spleen. *D,* Laceration along the dome. *E,* Subcapsular hematoma.

white pulp, where they are known as central arteries. Leaving the white pulp, the blood passes through an ill-defined vascular space called the *marginal zone* before entering the venous sinuses of the red pulp. Most spleen injuries result in various degrees of transverse rupture of the spleen following the trabeculae and segmental blood supply (Fig. 13). Attempts have been made to *grade* the severity of splenic injury, generally in an effort to predict which spleens can be safely repaired or nonoperatively managed (Table 2).[31,161]

Reports of surgical procedures less than total splenectomy in the management of patients with splenic injury have appeared in the literature since the sixteenth century. A rent in the capsule may be conveniently treated by a mattress suture; this is also true of a puncture or stab wound. An absorbable suture is preferable and must be inserted with gentleness and tied with caution over cotton or Teflon pledgets (Fig. 14). For a laceration that

TABLE 2. Splenic Organ Injury Scale

Class I	Nonexpanding subcapsular hematoma <10% surface area.
	Nonbleeding capsular laceration with <1 cm. deep parenchymal involvement.
Class II	Nonexpanding subcapsular hematoma 10–50% surface area.
	Nonexpanding intraparenchymal hematoma <2 cm. in diameter.
	Bleeding capsular tear or parenchymal laceration 1–3 cm. deep without trabecular vessel involvement.
Class III	Expanding subcapsular or intraparenchymal hematoma.
	Bleeding subcapsular hematoma or subcapsular hematoma >50% surface area.
	Intraparenchymal hematoma >2 cm. in diameter.
	Parenchymal laceration >3 cm. deep or involving trabecular vessels.
Class IV	Ruptured intraparenchymal hematoma with active bleeding.
	Laceration involving segmental or hilar vessels producing major (>25% splenic volume) devascularization.
Class V	Completely shattered or avulsed spleen.
	Hilar laceration that devascularizes entire spleen.

Adapted from Cogbill, T. H., Moore, E. E., Jurkovich, G. J., Morris, H. A., Mucha, P., and Shackford, S. R.: Nonoperative management of blunt splenic trauma: A multi-center experience. J. Trauma, 29:1312, 1989. © by Williams & Wilkins, 1989.

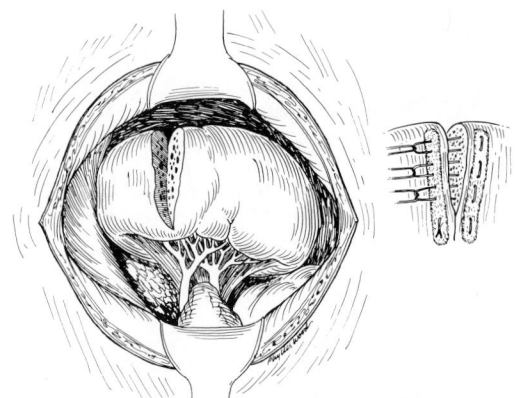

Figure 14. In order to perform a splenorrhaphy, the spleen must be properly mobilized into the operative field. The sutures are placed through the cotton pledgets so that when they are tied down, approximation of the parenchyma and capsule can occur without the sutures tearing through, as depicted in the inset.

does not involve the hilum of the spleen and that has adequate blood supply to all segments, the laceration is reapproximated with application of transverse mattress sutures over cut pledgets to reappose the cut surface of the spleen. More significant injuries may require partial resection. Successful splenorrhaphy requires complete mobilization of the spleen. The splenic pedicle is approached through the gastrosplenic ligament, and the vessels in the hilus of the spleen supplying the injured portion of the spleen are ligated. Demarcation of the devascularized segment then becomes apparent, allowing accurate segmental resection of the injured tissue. Mattress sutures placed parallel to the cut surface of the spleen may be required to control bleeding. Alternatively, ligation of the individual bleeding points and the application of topical hemostatic agents may suffice. Other adjuncts useful in obtaining splenic hemostasis include microfibrillar collagen, thrombin, fibrin biologic glues, absorbable mesh, and new electrocautery devices such as the argon beam coagulator. Although the reported success of splenic repair varies, most large urban trauma centers report splenic salvage rates of between 40 and 60 per cent of all splenic injuries managed.[144,161] Reoperation for continued or delayed bleeding following suture repair or splenorrhaphy is infrequent.[178,185]

TOTAL SPLENECTOMY. Despite the segmental arrangement of the splenic arterial supply, the friability of the spleen often renders repair or partial resection impossible. The primary indications for splenectomy following trauma are hilar vascular injury, massive subcapsular hematoma, extensive fragmentation, or total avulsion of the spleen; severe associated injuries requiring prompt attention; and continued bleeding after attempted splenic repair. In patients with multiple intra-abdominal injuries or extensive peritoneal contamination from visceral perforation, it is good surgical judgment to weigh the benefits of splenic salvage against the safer course of splenectomy. Most reserve splenic repair for patients in whom it is an isolated organ injury, who are normotensive and do not have other bodily injuries of greater priority. In addition, splenic salvage is probably not warranted if only 50 per cent or less of the splenic substance is to be preserved.

NONOPERATIVE MANAGEMENT. The safety and effectiveness of nonoperative management of selected pediatric patients with isolated splenic injuries has been confirmed by numerous reports. However, application of this technique to the management of splenic injuries in adults has been subject to controversy. The long-term outcome of the nonoperative management is not fully known, but the incidence of delayed splenic rupture in these patients appears to be extremely small. In addition, controversy exists with respect to the incidence of associated injuries; some have reported incidences as high as 12 to 20 per cent.[185] These figures are probably related to the mechanism of injury and are lower in the groups reporting satisfactory results from nonoperative management. A recent multicenter retrospective review of 832 blunt splenic trauma patients reported that 112 splenic injuries (13 per cent) were intentionally managed nonoperatively.[31] Patients were considered candidates for nonoperative management if they were hemodynamically stable, there were no serious associated abdominal organ injuries, and no extra-abdominal injuries precluded assessment of the abdomen. Approximately two thirds of the patients were adults. In this select group of patients, nonoperative management was successful in 98 per cent of the children and 83 per cent of the adults. These authors suggested that patients with isolated splenic injuries of Class I, II, or III (see Table 2) who meet the above criteria are candidates for nonoperative management. It would appear that although nonoperative management can be successful in highly selective patients, its injudicious administration to the generalized population could have unfavorable consequences. The long-term risk of splenectomy for isolated spleen injury (including the operative mortality and the long-term risk of overwhelming postsplenectomy sepsis) is probably a maximum of 1.5 per cent. It seems rational that any alternative to splenectomy for isolated splenic injury must not exceed this long-term risk.

An additional factor to be considered in weighing the risk of nonoperative management versus splenorrhaphy or splenectomy is the need for blood transfusion. Luna and Dellinger report a statistical analysis comparing the risk of postsplenectomy sepsis with the risk of blood transfusion–related infections.[109] They suggest that because of the additional blood requirements of nonoperative management, the conditional probability of death in both children and adults managed nonoperatively is higher than it is when immediate operation and splenectomy or repair are performed. Although this analysis is subject to statistical manipulation and reinterpretation, a policy of abandoning nonoperative management if the observed patient requires any blood transfusion because of splenic injury is a wise one.

Liver and Biliary Tree

LIVER. The liver is the second most commonly injured organ following blunt trauma and is the most commonly injured organ following penetrating trauma. Liver trauma is increasing in frequency with the incidence of motor vehicle and recreational accidents, but in many circumstances, the injury *per se* is insignificant and is easily managed. In fact, 50 per cent of all liver injuries are nonbleeding at the time of initial exploration, and an additional 20 per cent can be managed either by direct suture or by hemostatic agents such as microfibrillar collagen. Nonetheless, severe liver injuries are difficult to manage and are responsible for the high overall liver injury mortality of 11 per cent and an overall morbidity rate of 22 per cent.[48] There are seven basic techniques that are useful in operative management: (1) suture, (2) drainage, (3) inflow occlusion, (4) resection, (5) hepatic artery ligation, (6) packing, and (7) atriocaval shunting. The anatomy of the liver and the distribution of injuries permit separation of the roles of these approaches.

When the liver is the only organ injured, half of the lacerations are nonbleeding and do not require suture. In most of those that are bleeding, the source is within the substance of the liver and control can be obtained by direct ligation. After obtaining adequate exposure, the depth of the wound can be explored in detail and significant vessels and biliary radicals individually suture-ligated or secured with hemoclips. Digital compression and direct ligation are preferred over parallel vertical mattress sutures (which may be used if the entire cut surface of the liver is bleeding extensively). Topical hemostatic agents, biologic fibrin glue, and electrocautery are occasionally useful adjuncts but not substitutes for direct ligation of bleeding structures. If these measures are successful, closed drainage is established to control bile leakage.

With deeper lacerations, bleeding may initially be so significant as to prevent adequate exposure. Under these conditions, the next maneuver is that of inflow occlusion (Pringle maneuver) by placing a noncrushing clamp across the hepatoduodenal ligament, with occlusion of the common hepatic artery and the portal vein. Often this method provides adequate exposure of the wound (including mobilization of the ventral attachments of the liver) to allow for direct ligation of vessels and biliary radicals. Liver lacerations should not be sutured closed. This predisposes to liver abscesses and hemobilia. Some authors have advocated local hepatic hypothermia and systemic steroids if hepatic inflow occlusion is used, although intentional hypothermia in the trauma victim may be ill-advised.[91,136] Although the exact length of warm ischemic time tolerated by the human liver is not known, inflow occlusion for at least 20 minutes, and perhaps up to 1 hour, appears to be well tolerated.[48,78]

If inflow occlusion is unsuccessful, it is presumed that the patient has a retrohepatic inferior vena cava injury, hepatic vein injury, or juxtacaval intraparenchymal hepatic vein injury. In that circumstance, the liver injury is tightly packed, a median sternotomy is performed, and the diaphragm is divided. This allows further mobilization of the liver so that the vena cava can be isolated superiorly within the pericardium and inferiorily above the renal veins. With combined application of inflow occlusion and outflow occlusion, the hepatic vein or inferior vena cava can then be repaired or, occasionally, in the case of the hepatic veins, ligated. In less than 1 per cent of all liver injuries, atriocaval shunting may be considered (Fig. 15). This occurs when vena caval occlusion has already been obtained and the patient cannot be restored to a normovolemic state. The authors have used this procedure only in circumstances of hepatic vein or suprarenal caval injuries. Despite this technique, mortality for retrohepatic caval and intraparenchymal hepatic vein injuries exceeds 50 per cent. After a brief period of enthusiasm for selective ligation of the right or left hepatic artery, it is now believed that it should be reserved for the occasional stab wound or the gunshot wound involving one lobe where exposure to the wound will require extensive incision of the liver. This should be necessary in less than 1 per cent of all liver injuries.[30] The proper hepatic artery must never be ligated, and injudicious hepatic artery ligation may result in liver infarction (Fig. 16).

Resection of hepatic parenchyma is unusual following liver injuries. In a 5-year review of 1335 liver injuries treated at six trauma centers, hepatic resectional débridement was performed in only 36 patients (2.6 per cent), hepatotomy and vessel ligation in 50 patients (3.7 per cent), and segmentectomy in 18 patients (1.3 per cent).[30] Formal hepatic lobectomy was performed in only 12 patients (0.9 per cent). In most circumstances, resection is performed to débride a segment or lobe that has been completely fractured or devitalized. Less commonly, resection is performed for vascular control of large stellate lacerations extending deep into the parenchyma and involving more than one segment. In conjunction with resection, the gallbladder must often be removed because of loss of blood supply from the cystic artery. Extensive drainage is indicated for all major hepatic resections. An 8 per cent incidence of biliary fistula was noted in the 210 patients with significant injuries (Classes III, IV, and V) reported in the above review.

The resurgence of *perihepatic packing* has been a significant advance in the management of complex liver trauma. A number of recent reports have reconfirmed the value of temporary packing with delayed reoperation in a selected group of patients.[49,180] When used as an adjunct in the presence of coagulopathy after completion of hepatic repair, one group reports a 34 per cent survival in 41 patients. In contrast, there were no survivors if perihepatic packing was used as a final desperation technique in the setting of massive injury. When the patient has a devastating injury or bilobular involvement and there is some question of the availability of blood resources, liver packing seems to be a reasonable alternative. Packing does not appear to be as effective for actively bleeding hepatic vein or retrohepatic caval injuries. Arteriography and therapeutic embolization of hepatic arterial injury may be of benefit prior to re-exploration.

A preferred method of packing involves the use of gauze laparotomy pads either alone or in combination with a sterile plastic drape at the liver surface to prevent tight adherence of the lap pad to the exposed liver surface. Packs are removed in the operating room when the patient is rewarmed, the coagulopathy corrected, and fluid requirements stabilized. This generally occurs 24 to 72 hours after injury. Débridement of necrotic liver tissue and suture ligation of specific bleeding points

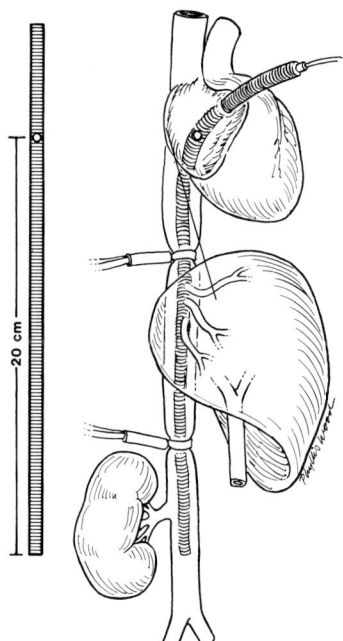

Figure 15. The atriocaval shunt placed through the auricular appendage. It has been guided to a position below the renal veins but above the iliac veins. In addition, as depicted, the retrohepatic vena cava has been isolated. A side hole has been cut to allow blood return to the right atrium. This allows total isolation of the venous outflow of the liver, so that when combined with inflow occlusion (clamping the porta hepatis), repair of hepatic veins can be obtained or the retrohepatic inferior vena cava can be properly exposed.

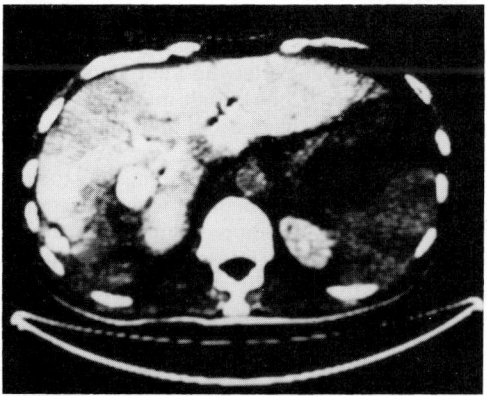

Figure 16. Computed tomographic scan demonstrating infarction of both segments of the right lobe and part of the medial segment of the left lobe, with specific demarcation between infarcted and normal liver. In addition, the administration of intravenous contrast material has shown a connection between the arterial and biliary tree (hemobilia). The fracture site is evident along the posterior lateral aspect of the right lobe of the liver.

are occasionally necessary. Closed suction drains are always inserted when the packing is removed. The incidence of intra-abdominal abscess in survivors of liver packing is generally less than 15 per cent.

PORTA HEPATIS. Isolated penetrating or blunt injuries to the porta hepatis are uncommon. They usually occur in association with injury to the liver, duodenum, or other upper abdominal organs. As a rule, combination injuries of the common bile duct, portal vein, and hepatic artery are involved. It is unusual to see only one of these portal triad structures injured. Porta hepatis injuries pose difficult problems in management. Life-threatening hemorrhage and associated organ injury characterize the immediate concern, and delayed stricture of the common bile duct is the major factor in determining morbidity. Since most patients present to the emergency room in shock, the indication for operation is immediately established.

Unless there are associated injuries to the aorta and inferior vena cava (which take priority) at laparotomy, an immediate Pringle maneuver will frequently allow isolation of the structures in the porta hepatis and allow determination of whether the injury involves the portal vein, hepatic arteries, or common bile duct. Repair of vascular injuries takes precedence over that of biliary structures.

Injuries to the portal vein are most likely to cause fatality, and combined series report a 50 per cent mortality. The portal vein supplies 80 per cent of the total hepatic blood flow and 50 per cent of the oxygen delivery. Techniques of portal vein repair are varied, but lateral venorrhaphy with 5-0 polypropylene suture is preferred. Alternatives are ligation, resection with end-to-end anastomosis, interposition grafting, and portal-systemic shunting. Although management of the portal vein injury by simple ligation alone is an attractive alternative, there is considerable controversy concerning this decision. Recent reports have demonstrated that ligation is compatible with survival, but the surgeon must anticipate mesenteric venous congestion and massive fluid requirements.[136,176] A "second-look" operation in 24 hours is advisable. Ligation in a patient with massive liver injury, hypotension, and multiple blood transfusions has an unacceptably high mortality. Interposition grafting with autogenous vein (jugular, splenic) is preferred, but a Gortex vascular graft may provide a temporary conduit. Portosystemic shunt is generally not an advisable alternative because, in a healthy patient with normal hepatic flow, it usually results in severe encephalopathy.

If injury to the porta hepatis involves only the common hepatic artery and the repair is not easily accomplished, ligation should be performed. However, in those patients with cirrhosis or severe pre-existing liver disease or even with prolonged periods of hypotension, hepatic artery ligation has been reported to result in hepatic infarction. In such patients, efforts should be made to repair the hepatic artery. When the patient has a combined injury of the hepatic artery and portal vein, after hemostasis has been obtained by the Pringle maneuver, it is advisable that the injured artery be ligated and that attempts be made at portal vein repair.

The most important factor in determining how to manage the common bile duct injury is whether the duct is completely or incompletely transected. Attempts at primary repair or duct-to-duct anastomosis of complete transections or injuries involving more than 50 per cent of the circumference of the bile duct wall cause a late stricture rate of over 50 per cent.[21,81] The late stricture rate drops to about 5 per cent if biliary-enteric anastomosis is performed for similar injuries. If the duct has been only perforated or incompletely divided (less than 50 per cent), primary repair can be successfully performed and is typically done over a T-tube or ureteral catheter stent. The T-tube should not be brought out through the repaired suture line. External drainage is provided in all circumstances. In an unstable patient, T-tube drainage of the duct and perihepatic drainage are carried out

with definitive repair of the ductal injury performed at a later date.

Injury to the gallbladder has been reported following both penetrating and blunt trauma. Cholecystostomy is indicated in only a few patients and should be regarded as a temporary procedure. The experience of Soderstrom and colleagues suggests that even with minimal injury the gallbladder is nonfunctional and becomes inflamed unless it is removed.[174] Cholecystectomy is the procedure of choice for severe contusion, avulsion, or perforating injuries to the gallbladder.

Stomach

Most full-thickness gastric injuries are caused by penetrating trauma. Gastric rupture secondary to blunt trauma is rare; Yajko and colleagues documented only 35 cases in the literature from 1930 to 1972.[202] Vigorous ventilation with an endotracheal tube misplaced in the esophagus, however, can cause iatrogenic gastric rupture in the trauma patient.

When vomitus or gastric aspirate is bloody, an injury to the stomach should be suspected. However, it is not unusual for small amounts of blood to be found in the gastric aspirate, even though laparotomy reveals no grossly apparent lesion. At laparotomy, if there is any reason to suspect a gastric injury, the gastrocolic omentum must be widely opened so that the entire posterior surface of the stomach may be completely inspected. If there is any blood in the gastrohepatic ligament, the lesser curvature of the stomach must be closely examined.

Most gastric injuries can be treated simply with débridement and closure in layers. The healthy blood supply of the stomach allows gastric healing to occur readily but also predisposes gastric wounds to postoperative bleeding. Bleeding from the gastric submucosal vessels is more likely to occur postoperatively than from small bowel or colonic submucosal vessels, and it is especially important to repair gastric perforations with an inner row of continuous 3-0 Dexon or Vicryl suture and an outer seromuscular row of interrupted silk. If prolonged gastric decompression seems necessary and there is a strong likelihood that the patient will develop respiratory complications, a gastrostomy should be considered. Gastric diversion or resection is rarely necessary unless the amount of tissue destruction is extensive, such as with high-velocity gunshot or shotgun wounds.

Small Intestine

The incidence of small bowel injury secondary to blunt trauma varies from 5 to 15 per cent and approaches 50 per cent for all penetrating abdominal injuries.[39] Injuries to the small intestine following blunt trauma are due to three mechanisms: (1) crush injury between the vertebrae and the anterior abdominal wall; (2) sudden increase in the intraluminal pressure; and (3) tears at the junction of a mobile and a fixed segment of bowel. Motor vehicle accidents, child abuse, bicycle accidents, and assorted falls represent the majority of these injuries. The sudden deceleration causes the mobile portion of the bowel to move away from its point of fixation (ligament of Treitz, ileocecal junction, sites of adhesions) causing a tangential tear. Rarely, adhesions involve a portion of the bowel in such a manner that during sudden compression of the abdomen a closed-loop phenomenon is created with a resultant blowout of the area. Occasionally, direct trauma from a blow or seat belt may be responsible for the damage that occurs at the point of impact. The association of the Chance type of lumbar compression fracture with intestinal injuries in children and adults wearing only a lap belt restraining device has now been recognized with sufficient frequency as to require exclusion.[152]

Most patients with a perforated small intestine exhibit some evidence of peritoneal irritation and may have frank abdominal rigidity. Lacerations of the lower small bowel may be particularly deceptive, however, because surrounding loops may cover the damaged area quickly and efficiently. In such cases, the patient may appear surprisingly well for days, demonstrating only mild localized tenderness. Free air may not be visible radiographically, and bowel sounds may persist. Such patients may eat and have bowel movements for a week or more before fever and other signs of intraperitoneal sepsis appear. Occasionally, damage may occur to the mesentery without involving the bowel. Minor tears are of little significance, but large hematomas may ultimately compress the adjacent mesenteric vessels and cause intestinal ischemia with later perforation.

Diagnostic peritoneal lavage is 95 per cent accurate in identifying small bowel injury. Diagnostic errors are generally due to small intestinal perforations with minimal bleeding that develop delayed signs of peritonitis. CT is less precise and requires both oral and intravenous contrast and careful inspection for the presence of bowel wall thickening, mesenteric hematoma, or fluid of nonblood density pooling in the pelvis. The presence of any of these signs, particularly when combined with abdominal tenderness or absent bowel sounds, warrants further emergency evaluation or surgical exploration.

During any laparotomy for possible intra-abdominal injuries, the entire small bowel should be meticulously examined. Each tear, as it is encountered, should be clamped or quickly sutured for prevention of further leakage and contamination of the peritoneal cavity during the remainder of the exploration. The wounds of entrance and exit on the abdominal wall cannot be used for predicting the likely site of a small bowel injury, because of the mobility of the small intestine and the variability of the patient's position at the time of injury.

Simple lacerations of the small bowel are sutured with a single layer of interrupted nonabsorbable Lembert sutures after removal of any tissue even questionably nonviable. Patients who have multiple additional injuries, shock, dilated small bowel, or a coagulopathy may benefit from a two-layer closure to ensure hemostasis. Care is taken to avoid excessive narrowing of the bowel by repair. Where damage to the bowel wall is extensive or where multiple tears are situated fairly close to one another, resection of the involved segment, rather than repair of the individual perforations, is preferred. Removal of the extensively damaged intestine is generally safer, provided that a sufficient length of viable bowel remains to permit adequate absorption of food.

Colon and Rectum

The colon is second only to the small bowel in frequency of abdominal organs in gunshot wounds, and is third (liver, small bowel) in abdominal stab wounds. In most contemporary series, the infectious morbidity is 25 to 35 per cent, and the mortality is 3 to 12 per cent. Major injuries to the rectum cause an even higher mortality, 4 to 22 per cent. Most of the infectious morbidity following abdominal injury occurs as a consequence of delayed diagnosis or inadequate therapy for colon injuries.[75]

The importance of early diagnosis and treatment of colon wounds is dramatically illustrated by the results of a recent report documenting no mortality and an 11 per cent infection rate in colon wounds diagnosed and treated within 2 hours of injury.[133] Because most colon injuries can only be definitively recognized at laparotomy, an aggressive approach to the management of penetrating abdominal trauma is generally warranted. As previously stated, gunshot wounds to the abdomen generally require exploratory laparotomy. DPL can be beneficial in diagnosing intra-abdominal injury following stab wounds to the anterior abdomen. However, because considerable portions of the colon are retroperitoneal, DPL has limited value in identifying such injuries when the stab is to the flank or back. Many surgeons therefore advocate a policy of routine abdominal exploration for any penetrating wound to the back or flank, although recently some have suggested using intravenous, oral, and rectal contrast-enhanced CT to evaluate back and flanks penetrating wounds.[143]

In an effort to minimize the infectious wound complications, all individuals who sustain penetrating trauma to the abdomen who are at risk for a colon injury should receive preoperative antibiotics in the emergency department. In most patients with proven colon injuries requiring colon resection, primary closure of the skin and subcutaneous tissues is also avoided.

When a colon injury has been identified, a decision regarding management must be made. Because of concern about infection following primary repairs, it has long been believed that the safest practice is to divert the fecal stream and anticipate a delayed colostomy closure. This concept has dominated modern management of colon wounds and dates to the experience of World War II surgeons, where colostomy was credited with reducing the mortality from colonic injury to 37 per cent, down from the World War I mortality of 60 per cent for colon injuries treated by primary repair.[181] However, the need for uniform colostomy in civilian colon trauma has been challenged, the premise being that unlike war injuries, most civilian colon wounds are due to low-velocity handgun shootings or stabbings. As a consequence, many trauma surgeons maintain that more than half of all civilian colon injuries can be treated by primary repair instead of exteriorization or colostomy. This change in practice has been documented by Nance, who has reviewed published reports from major trauma centers in the United States demonstrating the increasing incidence of primary repair versus colostomy for colon wounds during the past two decades (Table 3).[122]

While the controversy between proponents of primary suture and colostomy continues, it is important to emphasize that neither suggests that all colon injuries should be managed by one single technique. Instead, there appears to be agreement among most trauma surgeons that four techniques currently have a place in the management of colon injuries: primary repair, resection and primary anastomosis, exteriorization of repair, and colostomy. Exteriorization of primary repair, with subsequent delayed return of the repaired colon to its intra-abdominal location, has been proposed as an alternative to colostomy or primary repair. This technique supposedly represents an intermediate between the two extremes of repair and colostomy. The injured bowel is repaired but is exteriorized on the anterior abdominal wall to be returned to the abdomen in approximately 1 week. Several reports document an approximately 50 per cent failure rate with this technique, which requires attentive nursing care and occasionally causes colon obstruction.[20,183]

The available data indicate that primary closure of colon wounds without decompressive proximal colostomy can be performed selectively, using a number of criteria to determine in individual patients which type of surgical treatment should be performed. General guidelines that must be met to consider primary repair of a colon wound instead of a colostomy include the following: operation within 4 to 6 hours of injury; less than six units of blood transfusion; no evidence of prolonged shock or hemodynamic instability; minimal soilage of the peritoneal cavity; injury limited to one aspect of the colon; no associated colonic vascular injury; no loss of abdominal wall or need for synthetic mesh repair. In addition, some would not perform primary repair when there is associated renal pelvic or pancreatic injury, or when two of more other intra-abdominal organs have been injured.[163] With these selective criteria, primary repair of either the right or left colon can be accomplished with minimal morbidity and mortality.

Although all these techniques are applicable to any segment of the colon, most surgeons treat the various anatomic components of the colon with unique distinction. This is emphasized in a recent large review (727 patients) of colon trauma by Burch and colleagues from the Ben Taub Medical Center in Houston.[20] Ninety-seven per cent of the injuries were from penetrating wounds, and distribution between right, transverse, and descending colon was approximately equal. Primary repair was

TABLE 3. Collected Series of Colon Repair Techniques

Reporting Institution	Colostomy		Primary Repair: No Colostomy	
	No. (%)	Mortality (%)	No. (%)	Mortality (%)
Charity Hospital, New Orleans, 1988 (347 patients)	202 (58)	16	145 (42)	6
Jefferson Davis (Ben Taub) Hospital, 1962 (272 patients)	52 (19)	33	220 (82)	6
Ben Taub Hospital, 1971 406 patients)	182 (45)	21	224 (55)	8
Denver General Hospital, 1985 (228 patients)	83 (36)	2	110 (48)	1
Harlem Hospital, 1972 (138 patients)	49 (36)	18	85 (64)	5
Grady Memorial, 1979 (268 patients)	201 (75)	10	67 (25)	1
San Francisco General Hospital, 1977 (129 patients)	91 (71)	0	38 (29)	11
Total	860 (49)	13.7	890 (51)	5.6

Adapted from Nance, F. C.: Injuries to the colon and rectum. *In* Mattox, K. L., Moore, E. E., and Feliciano, D. V. (Eds.): Trauma. Norwalk, Conn., Appleton & Lange, 1988, p. 495.

performed in 51.7 per cent of the patients, colostomy in 32.5 per cent, exteriorization in 14.4 per cent, and resection anastomosis in 1.4 per cent. This experience demonstrates the general trend to primarily repair *right* colon injuries and *stab* wounds or *low-velocity* gunshot wounds. The right colon was primarily repaired in 78 per cent of the injuries, the transverse colon in 62 per cent, and the left colon in only 32 per cent. Seventy per cent of stab wounds were primarily repaired versus 47 per cent of gunshot wounds and 28 per cent of blunt injuries.

The added morbidity of closing a colostomy is often considered in the operative decision to perform colostomy versus primary repair or exteriorization. Some series have reported significant morbidity related to the creation of stomas; and, rarely, the required closure of the stoma has caused death. Parks and Hastings' report and review of colostomy closures documented an overall complication rate of 9 to 49 per cent; intra-abdominal complications occurred in 2 to 23 per cent.[137] In this report, complications were less likely if the interval to colostomy closure was greater than 90 days. Thal and Yeary reviewed 137 patients who had colostomy closure following colostomies for trauma.[181] Of those patients, 14 had postoperative complications, for an overall morbidity of 10.2 per cent. There were no deaths in this series. Morbidity was lowest (4.8 per cent) in those patients undergoing colostomy closure between 4 and 8 weeks after injury. They also concluded that colostomy closure in trauma patients appeared to be safer than in patients in whom colostomy was constructed for nontraumatic reasons.

Based on the above discussion, the authors' general management plan for colon wounds is as follows. Small stab wounds or low-velocity gunshot wounds to the right colon may undergo primary repair by adhering to the general guidelines outlined above. More significant penetrating injuries and most blunt injuries to the right colon are managed by right colectomy. Primary reconstruction via ileotransverse colostomy may be performed in a stable patient in whom there is an isolated injury with no evidence of shock or gross fecal contamination. Otherwise, a right colectomy is accompanied by the creation of an ileostomy and mucous fistula. The same guiding principles for primary repair of minor wounds are followed for the left colon, although resection with primary anastomosis is generally not recommended because of the different vascularity, fecal consistency, and bacterial load. More extensive left colon injuries are generally treated by resection with proximal end colostomy and distal mucous fistula or Hartmann's pouch. Stab wounds

and low-velocity gunshot wounds of the transverse colon are considered for primary repair or exteriorized as loop colostomies. Major injuries, including most blunt injuries, are resected with the creation of an end colostomy and a mucous fistula.

RECTUM. The same diagnostic modalities previously discussed for intraperitoneal colon injuries are used for rectal injuries, with the addition of two other procedures. Abdominal radiographs are obtained for determination of retroperitoneal air, and proctosigmoidoscopy is performed for direct visualization of the injury or for evidence of hemorrhage. Primary closure is not used without colostomy if the wound is full-thickness and occurs above the dentate line. The value of proximal diverting colostomy following rectal trauma was established during World War II, but subsequent civilian reports have occasionally advocated primary closure without fecal diversion. The resultant mortality has been higher than 20 per cent. In contrast, Trunkey and co-workers reviewed the management plan outlined below for rectal trauma, with only 1 death in 54 patients.[190] For wounds occurring below the dentate line, the plan of management was débridement accompanied by appropriate drainage. Colon diversion was not performed routinely. For wounds above the levators with penetration of the pelvirectal space, the treatment included (1) closure, if possible, (2) proximal *diverting* colostomy, (3) presacral (retrorectal) drains, and (4) irrigation of the rectal stump with Betadine. Although some have questioned the advisability of rectal stump irrigation, recent evidence suggests it decreases the incidence of pelvic abscess, rectal fistulas, and sepsis.[164]

RETROPERITONEAL INJURIES

Duodenum

Approximately three quarters of duodenal injuries are the result of penetrating trauma, and one quarter are the result of blunt injuries. The most common mechanism producing blunt injury is a steering wheel blow to the abdomen in an unrestrained automobile driver. Penetrating injuries are usually readily diagnosed at operation, but the insidious nature of many blunt duodenal injuries makes the initial diagnosis difficult. In reviewing their experience with duodenal injury, Lucas and Ledgerwood documented a delay in diagnosis of greater than 12 hours in 53 per cent of their patients and a delay of greater than 24 hours in 28 per cent.[106] This delay markedly increases morbidity and mortality. Their reported mortality was 40 per cent among the patients in whom the diagnosis was delayed more than 24 hours versus an 11 per cent mortality in those patients operated upon in less than 24 hours.

In addition to maintaining a high index of suspicion with regard to patients with an appropriate injury mechanism, in patients with blunt abdominal trauma, serum amylase should be measured initially. If the level is elevated, the test should be repeated at 6-hour intervals. Although hyperamylasemia can be diagnostically confusing (see Pancreas), a persistently elevated or rising amylase may indicate pancreatic or duodenal injury and mandates further evaluation or operative exploration. The radiologic signs of duodenal injury on the initial plain abdominal or upright chest radiograph are subtle, seen only as mild scoliosis, obliteration of the right psoas muscle, or retroperitoneal air that is difficult to distinguish from the overlying transverse colon. An early suspicion of retroperitoneal duodenal rupture is best confirmed (or excluded) by a Gastrografin upper gastrointestinal series or abdominal CT scan with oral and intravenous contrast enhancement. DPL is unreliable in detecting duodenal and other retroperitoneal injuries. Nevertheless, DPL may be useful in patients with duodenal injuries, since approximately 40 per cent have associated intra-abdominal injuries that would cause a positive peritoneal lavage and subsequent surgical exploration.

Factors that influence the morbidity and mortality following duodenal trauma have also been reviewed by Snyder and colleagues.[172] In their review of 247 patients sustaining duodenal trauma, they reported an overall duodenal fistula rate of 7 per cent and an overall 10 per cent mortality. These authors thought that five factors listed in Table 4 most significantly correlate with the severity of duodenal injury and subsequent morbidity and mortality. Snyder and colleagues demonstrated that patients with "mild" duodenal trauma had a 0 per cent mortality and 2 per cent duodenal fistula rate, as compared with a 6 per cent mortality and 10 per cent fistula rate among those with "severe" duodenal injuries (see Table 4).

According to this classification system, approximately 80 to 85 per cent of duodenal wounds can be primarily repaired safely. Approximately 15 to 20 per cent are "severe" injuries that require more complex procedures. Débridement or segmental resection and primary anastomosis may be attempted in all but the second portion of the duodenum for wounds that involve the near total circumference. An alternative is a Roux-en-Y jejunal limb anastomosis to the duodenal injury. Pancreatoduodenectomy is rarely required for duodenal injuries unless uncontrollable pancreatic hemorrhage or combined duodenal, ampullary, and/or intrapancreatic bile duct injury is present.

Protection of a tenuous duodenal repair may be aided by the diversion of gastric contents. This may be accomplished by a Berne duodenal "diverticulization" or by the pyloric exclusion

and gastrojejunostomy advocated by Vaughan and others (Fig. 17).[9,192] An alternative to gastric diversion is lateral tube duodenostomy or duodenal drainage via a retrograde jejunostomy. Hasson and colleagues recently reviewed the literature on duodenal trauma and tube duodenostomy and reported that the overall mortality with any type of tube decompression was 9 per cent, compared with 19.4 per cent without decompression.[74] The morbidity of duodenal fistula occurred in 2.3 per cent of patients undergoing adjuvant tube duodenostomy, compared with 11.8 per cent without decompression. They concluded that duodenal tube drainage should be performed via either stomach or retrograde jejunostomy, because these methods had the lowest fistula rate and less overall mortality than lateral tube duodenostomy. Stone and Fabian also appear to support this conclusion, reporting a duodenal fistula in only 1 of 232 patients with a variety of duodenal injuries all treated by retrograde jejunostomy.[175] It should be noted, however, that there has been no prospective or controlled analysis of the efficacy of either type of tube duodenal drainage or gastric diversion techniques in the management of duodenal wounds. On balance, the most effective and least morbid adjunctive procedure for *major* injuries is the Vaughan pyloric exclusion.

Duodenal hematoma usually does not require operative intervention. It can be diagnosed either by contrast-enhanced CT scan or upper gastrointestinal study. The initial Gastrografin examination should be followed by barium studies to provide greater detail needed to detect the "coiled spring" or "stacked coin" sign. Although characteristic of intramural duodenal hematoma, this finding is present in only approximately one quarter of patients with hematoma. Associated injuries should be excluded with particular attention directed to the potential for pancreatic injuries. Continuous nasogastric suction should be employed and total parenteral nutrition initiated. The patient should be re-evaluated with upper gastrointestinal contrast studies at 5- to 7-day intervals. Operative exploration and evacuation of the hematoma may be considered after 2 weeks of conservative therapy.[184]

Pancreas

Pancreatic trauma is relatively uncommon, representing less than 10 per cent of all abdominal injuries. Although the pancreas is relatively protected in the retroperitoneum, the increasing frequency of high-speed motor vehicle accidents and large-caliber, high-velocity civilian gunshot wounds contribute to an increasing incidence of pancreatic injury. Several large series

TABLE 4. Determinants of Duodenal Injury Severity

	Mild	Severe
Determinants of Injury Severity		
Agent	Stab	Blunt or missile
Size	<75% wall	>75% wall
Duodenal site	3, 4	1, 2
Injury-repair interval (hours)	<24	>24
Adjacent injury	No CBD	CBD
Outcome		
Mortality (%)	6%	16%
Duodenal morbidity (%)	6%	14%

CBD, common bile duct.
Adapted from Snyder, W. H. III, Weigelt, J. A., Watkins, W. L., and Bietz, D. S.: The surgical management of duodenal trauma. Precepts based on a review of 247 cases. Arch. Surg., 115:422, 1980. Copyright 1980, American Medical Association.

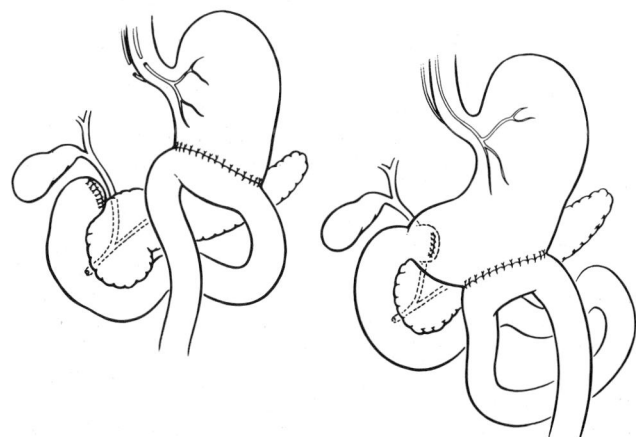

Figure 17. Illustration of Berne's "duodenal diverticulization" (left) and Vaughan's "pyloric exclusion" procedure (right) utilized as adjuncts to repair of severe duodenal or combined duodenopancreatic injury. Note that the Berne diverticulization includes vagotomy and antrectomy, whereas the Vaughan pyloroplasty is intended to be a temporary duodenal bypass. (From Jurkovich, G. J., and Carrico, C. J.: Management of Pancreatic Trauma. Surg. Clin. North Am., 70:575, 1990.)

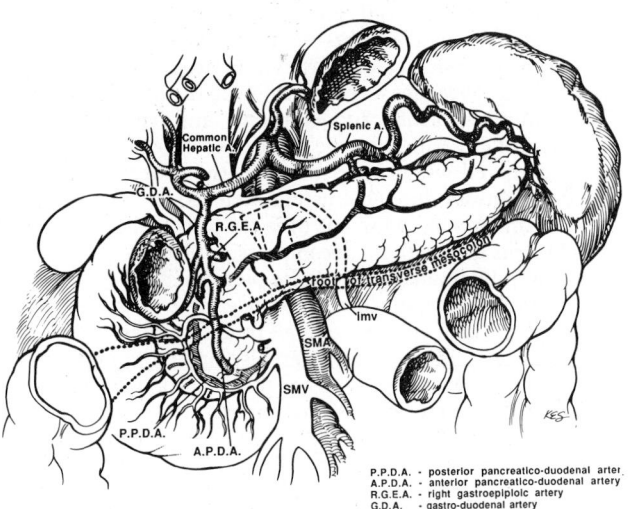

Figure 18. The blood supply to the pancreas and the pancreatic relational anatomy to other intra-abdominal organs. (From Jurkovich, G. J., and Carrico, C. J.: Management of Pancreatic Trauma. Surg. Clin. North Am., 70:575, 1990.)

P.P.D.A. - posterior pancreatico-duodenal artery
A.P.D.A. - anterior pancreatico-duodenal artery
R.G.E.A. - right gastroepiploic artery
G.D.A. - gastro-duodenal artery

from urban trauma centers report that penetrating injuries represent 70 to 80 per cent of pancreatic wounds. The mortality rates from several large series of pancreatic trauma patients are 10 to 25 per cent; major complications such as pseudocysts, abscesses, hemorrhage or pancreatic fistulas develop in 30 to 40 per cent of patients surviving their initial injury.[90] This combined mortality and morbidity of approximately 50 per cent emphasizes the significance of pancreatic injuries.

Because the pancreas is surrounded by major abdominal organs and blood vessels, associated injuries are common (Fig. 18). Overall, 90 per cent of patients with pancreatic injuries have at least one associated injury, with an average of 3.5 associated intra-abdominal injuries per patient. The aorta, portal vein, or vena cava is injured in over 75 per cent of cases of penetrating pancreatic trauma; and injuries to the liver, spleen, or hollow viscus of the gastrointestinal tract are equally common in blunt trauma. The significance of the associated injuries is highlighted by morbidity and mortality statistics. Intra-abdominal vascular injuries are responsible for one half of the

overall mortality and nearly all of the immediate deaths.[86] Infection and multiple organ failure are responsible for the majority of the late deaths. Approximately 10 per cent of deaths are directly attributable to the pancreatic injury.[169] The key determinant of long-term outcome is the presence or absence of pancreatic duct injury, since most postoperative complications can be attributed to inadequate control of major duct disruption.[10] The implication of these observations is that the first priority in managing pancreatic trauma should be control of hemorrhage and repair of intestinal injuries to limit bacterial contamination. A diligent search for potential pancreatic injury should follow.

PREOPERATIVE EVALUATION. The preoperative evaluation and management of patients with penetrating abdominal wounds and possible pancreatic injury is relatively straightforward. Unless injury to the intraperitoneal or retroperitoneal abdominal contents can be definitively excluded, abdominal exploration is warranted. No further diagnostic test for pancreatic injury is required, because thorough intraoperative evaluation must be performed.

The evaluation of patients with possible blunt pancreatic injury is more complex and requires evaluation based on injury mechanism (e.g., steering wheel injury) and associated injuries. Since a significant proportion of pancreatic trauma patients have associated intra-abdominal injuries, clear-cut indications for laparotomy frequently exist (e.g., peritonitis, intra-abdominal hemorrhage, positive diagnostic peritoneal lavage). These patients require no further preoperative evaluation to identify a possible pancreatic injury because a thorough, direct intraoperative pancreatic examination can be performed. In contrast, identifying a pancreatic injury in the absence of other indications for laparotomy is challenging. Patients with complete ductal transection have been reported to be asymptomatic for weeks to months following the initial injury, although the more typical presentation is increasing abdominal pain with time.[10,169] Early identification of a subtle pancreatic injury therefore requires a high index of suspicion, a thoughtful diagnostic approach, and serial physical examinations.

Serum amylase determination has limited sensitivity or specificity for pancreatic injury. In Jones' review of pancreatic trauma, the serum amylase level was elevated in only 16 per cent of the patients with penetrating pancreatic injuries and in only 61 per cent of those with blunt pancreatic trauma. Even with complete transection of the pancreas, only 65 per cent of

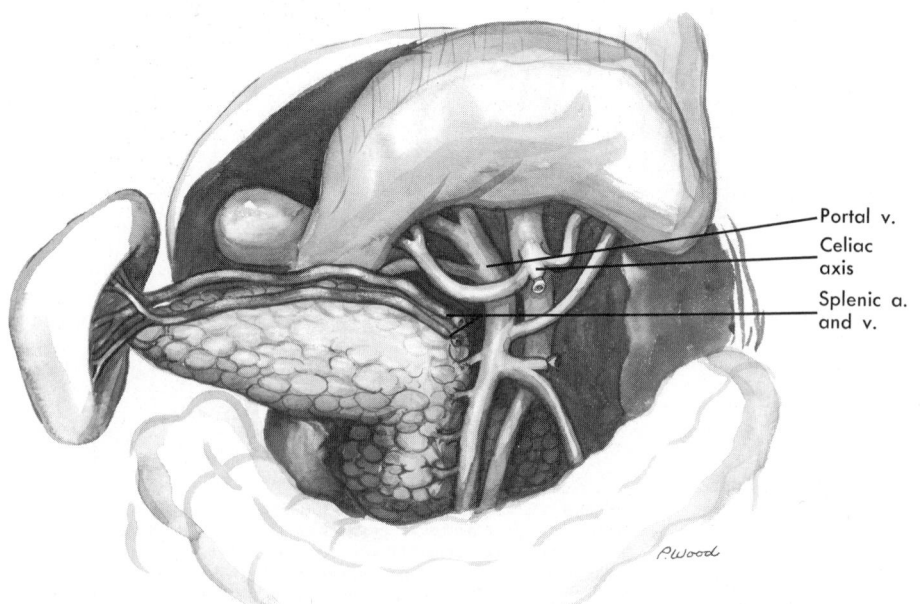

Portal v.
Celiac axis
Splenic a. and v.

Figure 19. The spleen and pancreas have been dissected from the retroperitoneum and transferred in the right upper quadrant. Adequate mobility of the pancreas is essential for assessment of potential posterior pancreatic injuries.

the patients had elevated serum amylase levels.[86] Other reports have documented that as few as 8 per cent of blunt abdominal injuries with hyperamylasemia involved pancreatic injury.[201] Isoamylase differentiation, initially hailed as an advance in diagnosing pancreatic injury, unfortunately has not increased the test's accuracy.[14] Nonetheless, an elevated serum or peritoneal lavage effluent amylase raises concern about pancreatic injury and mandates further evaluation. Persistent elevation and the development of abdominal symptoms are indications for further evaluation or surgical exploration.

CT can be helpful in diagnosing pancreatic injury. Abdominal CT scans are currently reported as having sensitivity and specificity in excess of 80 per cent, although the accuracy of this examination varies with interpreter experience and the quality of the scanner.[82]

INTRAOPERATIVE EVALUATION. Even at operation, the diagnosis of significant pancreatic injury may be difficult. A Kocher maneuver should be performed, with mobilization of the hepatic flexure and the third portion of the duodenum to the superior mesenteric vessels. This allows adequate inspection of the C loop of the duodenum and the posterior head of the pancreas. Inspection is continued by opening the lesser sac, allowing examination of the medial aspect of the duodenum and anterior surface of the pancreas, including its superior and inferior margins. When posterior injuries of the pancreas are suspected, mobilization of the spleen with elevation of the spleen and tail of the pancreas allows inspection of the posterior pancreas (Fig. 19).

The majority (95 per cent) of pancreatic injuries can be diagnosed by careful inspection following adequate exposure. The remaining 5 per cent of injuries may require more elaborate investigative techniques to diagnose ductal injury. Intraoperative ultrasound and intraoperative endoscopic studies have been suggested as a possible means of identifying major ductal injuries. To date, the applicability and accuracy of these approaches have not been validated. The authors continue to use contrast studies through the biliary tree, ampulla, or tail of the pancreas when there is major concern about the integrity of the main pancreatic duct (Figs. 20 to 22). Skilled endoscopists may be of assistance in performing intraoperative endoscopic retrograde pancreatography if the surgeon is reluctant to perform a duodenostomy or distal pancreatectomy. Routine performance of intraoperative pancreatography when proximal duct injury is

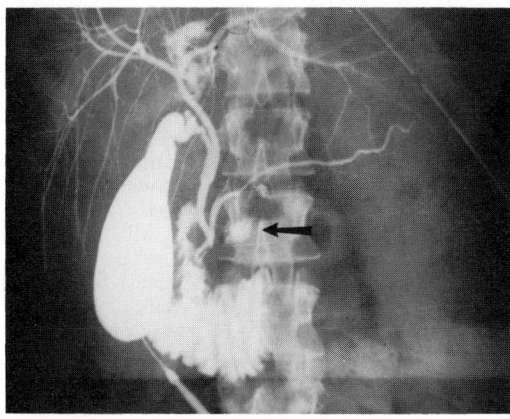

Figure 21. A cystocholangiogram demonstrating filling of the pancreatic duct, with extravasation in the proximal pancreatic duct (arrow).

strongly suspected decreased postoperative morbidity from 55 per cent to 15 per cent at the authors' institution.[10]

CLASSIFICATION AND TREATMENT. The classification system and management guidelines favored are outlined in Table 5. This system addresses the key issues of parenchymal disruption and major pancreatic duct status by focusing on the anatomic location of the injury rather than the degree of injury itself. Although there is no anatomic distinction within the gland itself, the superior mesenteric vessels pass behind the pancreas at the junction of the pancreatic head and body; the pancreas to the patient's left is considered distal. The principles of managing pancreatic injuries are to control hemorrhage, débride devitalized pancreatic tissue, provide adequate drainage of injuries or resections, and preserve as much functional pancreatic tissue as possible. The difficult decisions in managing pancreatic trauma involve patients with parenchymal disruption and major duct injury. By focusing on the anatomic location of the duct and parenchymal injury (proximal versus distal), the proposed system provides a useful management guide.

Type I pancreatic injuries (no major duct involved) are the most common (80 per cent) and generally require only hemostasis and drainage. Type II pancreatic injuries (distal major duct injury) are best treated by distal pancreatectomy with or without splenectomy. If there is concern regarding the status of the remaining proximal duct, intraoperative pancreatography can be performed through the open end of the proximal ducts (see Fig. 41). If the remaining proximal duct is normal, the transected

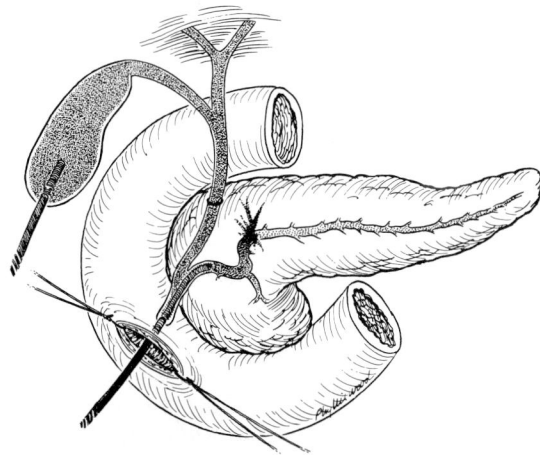

Figure 20. Opening of the duodenum at the level of the papilla of Vater, with direct cannulation of the pancreatic duct. This is best done following the administration of 70 units of secretin intravenously so that the pancreatic sphincter will relax and the tube will preferentially move into the pancreatic duct instead of the common bile duct. Two to 4 ml. of contrast material is injected by gravity flow only, demonstrating extravasation of the proximal pancreatic duct. Prior to the duodenotomy, the gallbladder is cannulated and a cholecystocholangiogram is always performed so that if reflux into the pancreatic duct occurs, a duodenotomy can be avoided.

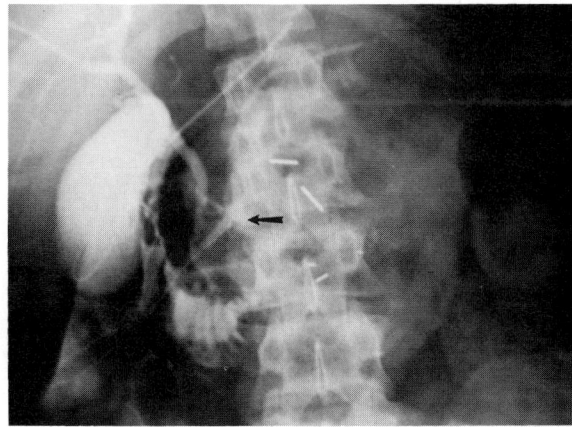

Figure 22. Simultaneous cholecystocholangiogram and cannulation of the pancreatic duct through a duodenotomy. The injection demonstrates extravasation in the proximal pancreatic duct at a position in such proximity to the common bile duct that had a subtotal pancreatectomy been performed, the common bile duct would probably have been injured. This use of intraoperative pancreatography demonstrated the need for a Whipple resection.

TABLE 5. Classification of Pancreatic Injuries

Injury Type	Injury Definition	Treatment*
I	Contusion and laceration *without* duct injury	External drainage Infrequent distal pancreatectomy
II	*Distal* transection and/or parenchymal injury with duct injury	Distal pancreatectomy
III	*Proximal* transection or parenchymal injury with probable duct injury	Distal pancreatectomy or Roux-en-Y pancreaticojejunostomy (see text)
IV	*Combined* pancreatic and duodenal injury Ampulla/blood supply intact	Repair/exclude duodenum (see text) Treat pancreas as per I, II, III
	Massive injury: ampulla destroyed; devascularization	Pancreaticoduodenectomy

* External drainage is necessary following any pancreatic resection, débridement, or repair.

duct and gland parenchyma are sutured closed and external drainage is provided. Type III pancreatic injuries (proximal duct injury) require pancreatectomy distal to the duct injury, subtotal removal of the gland. If there is concern that the residual pancreatic tissue is inadequate to provide endocrine or exocrine function, preservation of the body and tail using a Roux-en-Y pancreaticojejunostomy is an option. If complete duct transection is not apparent clinically, confirmation by intraoperative pancreatography should be performed prior to performing the formidable subtotal pancreatic resection. If the duct is spared, wide external drainage is generally adequate treatment.

The management of Type IV pancreatic injuries remains problematic. Because of the large number of combinations of injuries to the pancreas and duodenum that may occur, no one form of therapy is appropriate for all patients. In Feliciano and associates' review of 129 cases of combined pancreatoduodenal injuries, 24 per cent of the patients were treated with simple repair and drainage, 50 per cent underwent repair and pyloric exclusion, and only 10 per cent required a Whipple procedure.[48] Selection of the best treatment option for these combined injuries is dependent upon the integrity of the distal common bile duct and the ampulla and the severity of the duodenal injury. For that reason, any patient with a combined pancreatoduodenal injury requires a cholangiogram, a pancreatogram, and evaluation of the ampulla.

When the common bile duct and ampulla are intact (as is the situation in the majority of the cases), the duodenum can be closed primarily and the pancreatic injury treated as previously described. If there is concern about the integrity of the duodenal closure, adjunctive techniques described in the previous section on duodenal injuries may be considered (see Fig. 17).

Rarely, in very massive injuries of the proximal duodenum and head of the pancreas, destruction of the ampulla and proximal pancreatic duct or distal common bile duct may preclude reconstruction. In this situation, a pancreaticoduodenectomy may be required (Fig. 23). The authors' experience suggests that if confined to strict criteria pancreaticoduodenectomy is a viable option and can be performed for injury with less morbidity and mortality than described in resections done for cancer.[86,131]

POSTOPERATIVE CARE. Although complications are frequent following pancreatic injury, some reports indicate that up to one half of the postoperative complications can be avoided with careful inspection of the pancreas and accurate determination of the status of the main pancreatic duct.[86,90,169] Pancreatic fistula occurs in up to 35 per cent of patients with significant pancreatic injuries, but the majority resolve spontaneously if adequate external drainage has been provided. Intra-abdominal abscess and wound infection are nearly as frequent, but a true pancreatic abscess occurs in less than 5 per cent of patients. Unlike controlled external fistulas, pancreatic abscesses require prompt surgical débridement and drainage. Pseudocyst formation and postoperative pancreatitis are less frequent complications, but can greatly prolong the recovery time. Adequate nutritional support is essential throughout the postinjury period. Placement of a feeding jejunostomy (needle catheter or small feeding tube) at the time of laparotomy for pancreatic trauma often proves useful in supplying enteral nutrients in the early postoperative period. The low-fat, higher pH elemental feeding formulas appear to cause less pancreatic stimulation than standard enteral formulas and should be tried prior to committing the patient to total parenteral nutrition.

Major Abdominal Vessels

The mortality from abdominal vascular trauma is still 30 to 60 per cent despite improvements in emergency resuscitation, transport, and trauma system development. As expected, most deaths are due to exsanguination. One third of patients with abdominal vascular trauma come to the emergency room in shock. Rapid control of the injury is the primary management goal, and since most injuries are due to penetrating wounds, immediate triage to the operating room is simplified and must be encouraged. The importance of arresting hemorrhage is illustrated by Ekbom and colleagues' review demonstrating that persistent hypotension despite intravascular volume replacement occurred in 55 per cent of the fatal abdominal vascular injuries, whereas hypotension was prolonged in only 10 per cent of the survivors.[43]

Fully 40 per cent of intra-abdominal vascular injuries involve

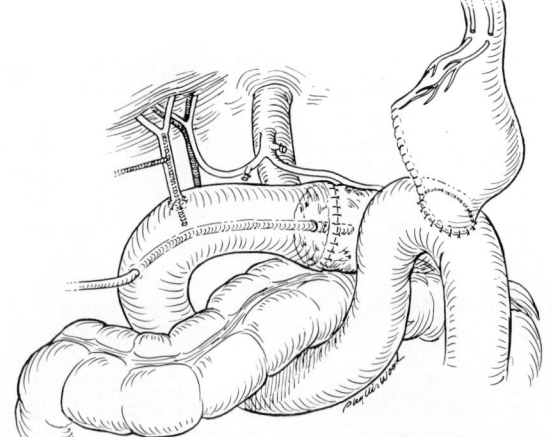

Figure 23. Surgical reconstruction following a pancreaticoduodenectomy for trauma. The pancreaticojejunostomy is an end-to-end two-layer anastomosis over an indwelling stint. The choledochojejunostomy is an end-to-side anastomosis in a single layer with a dwelling stint depending upon the size of the common bile duct. The gastrojejunostomy is an end-to-side two-layer anastomosis. The pancreatic and bile duct stints are brought out through separate stab wounds on the abdominal wall.

two or more major vascular structures. Mortality is directly related to the number of vascular structures injured, the site of injury, and the mechanism of injury. Aortic wounds have a 40 to 80 per cent mortality, highest from shotgun and gunshot wounds and highest with injuries in the suprarenal location. Vena cava injuries have a lower (10 to 40 per cent) mortality, suprarenal wounds again being the most difficult to repair. Iliac artery and vein injuries incur 15 to 40 per cent and 10 to 25 per cent mortality, respectively. Superior mesenteric artery and vein injuries both have a 30 to 40 per cent mortality.[139,156,167]

When the diagnosis is uncertain, peritoneal lavage may reveal intraperitoneal bleeding and present clear indications for exploration. Alternatively, CT in the hemodynamically stable patient may reveal an initially unsuspected mesenteric or retroperitoneal hematoma. If the patient is stable and uncertainty exists as to the need for exploration (as may be seen in a patient with a stab wound or following blunt trauma), arteriography can confirm the diagnosis. Diagnostic studies, however, should never delay surgical exploration of the patient in shock. Absence of distal pulses and limb ischemia are difficult to interpret in hypotensive patients, and massive retroperitoneal bleeding may occur without being obvious.

INITIAL MANAGEMENT. Operative control of major vessel hemorrhage can be challenging. At the time of exploration, any retroperitoneal hematoma should suggest the possibility of associated vascular injury. Central hematomas above the renal vessels suggest suprarenal aortic–vena caval injuries or injury to the celiac axis or superior mesenteric artery or vein. Inferior central hematomas imply distal aortic or vena caval wounds. A lateral hematoma suggests renal artery or vein injury. Pelvic hematoma suggests iliac artery or vein injury.

The approach to the operative management of the patient with a suspected major intra-abdominal vascular injury is different from that of the stable patient with penetrating or blunt abdominal injury. It is recommended that the approach be similar to that of managing a patient with a suspected ruptured aortic aneurysm; that is, these hemodynamically unstable patients are taken immediately to the operating room and preparations for operation completed as necessary; diagnostic maneuvers are interpreted, and additional lines are placed. The patient is prepared from chin to mid thigh. Warming blankets and blood warmers should be in place, as well as an autotransfusion device. The operating team is scrubbed and ready to intervene if there is sudden collapse. Anesthesia is not initiated until just before the incision is made. With initiation of anesthesia, the blood pressure may fall suddenly as abdominal muscular relaxation occurs; then fluid and blood replacement must be accomplished rapidly while bleeding is being controlled.

If a major arterial wound is suspected because of hypotension, a distended abdomen, or combined chest and abdominal penetration, some surgeons recommend entering the chest through the seventh interspace and obtaining control of the aorta before the distended abdomen is explored.[103,139] This has not been the authors' standard approach, because in most circumstances it has been found that the abdominal aorta can be controlled at the level of the diaphragm.[193] However, this approach is advocated for the hypotensive patient in whom suprarenal aortic injuries are suspected by mechanism or projectile pathway. A retroperitoneal hematoma in this location obscures the gastrohepatic ligament and the diaphragmatic hiatus, making visual exposure of the abdominal aorta impossible.

If active hemorrhage is encountered upon opening the peritoneum, it must be controlled before any other intraoperative maneuvers are performed. Injuries to solid organs with bleeding are usually rapidly packed, and standard techniques of vascular control are used to control the active hemorrhage. Proximal and distal control is needed for any major abdominal arterial injury. Direct digital or sponge compression at the site of injury is often required in obtaining such control. Major venous injuries, however, are often not amenable to proximal and distal clamping. Direct digital compression or use of a sponge stick may secure venous vascular control adequate for repair of tangential wounds with 4-0 or 5-0 polypropylene. If the patient has a contained retroperitoneal hematoma, the surgeon may rapidly clamp or repair bowel injuries and thereby limit contamination. Specific approaches to individual intra-abdominal vessels depend on the location of the surrounding hematoma.

EXPOSURE AND TREATMENT OF SPECIFIC INJURIES. *Midline suprarenal hemorrhage* is perhaps the most difficult to control, since the aorta, celiac axis, mesenteric vessels, or vena cava may be responsible. In addition, with the usual penetrating wound, associated gastric, duodenal, or pancreatic injuries are likely. Proximal aortic control may be attempted via direct aortic compression through the gastrohepatic ligament, although a left anterolateral thoracotomy and thoracic aortic clamping may be necessary.[103,193] Rotation of the colon, spleen, pancreas, and left kidney to the mid-line allows complete exposure of the aorta from the hiatus to the aortic bifurcation. The left diaphragmatic crux may be divided to provide even more proximal exposure. When control has been obtained and the aortic wound exposed, it is recommended that exploration be completed and resuscitation initiated before definitive repairs are begun. In patients who have already experienced massive hemorrhage, continued bleeding, even at relatively low rates, from uncontrolled sources can cause significant blood loss. Autotransfusion can have a significant role in the resuscitation of these patients. In patients sustaining mesenteric vascular injuries, intestinal viability must be assured at completion of the operation. A "second-look" procedure may be advisable in selected patients.[167]

Suprarenal vena caval injuries are approached with an extended Kocher maneuver, rotating the right colon and duodenum to midline and retracting the liver superiorly. Retrohepatic vena caval injuries are extremely difficult to control, and subsequently a retrohepatic caval shunt (Schrock shunt) has been developed (see Fig. 15).[159] Modifications of this shunt allow its insertion through the saphenofemoral junction or, more commonly, through the cardiac atrial appendage.[145] Survival even with early use of this technique remains dismal.

Midline infrarenal hematomas can usually be approached directly through the retroperitoneum or the base of the mesentery, and direct control with vascular clamps can be accomplished. The maneuvers utilized are similar to those used in approaching abdominal aortic aneurysms.

Lateral hematomas may be due to renal parenchymal or vascular injury. If they are the result of blunt abdominal trauma, it is helpful if the preoperative evaluation includes an assessment of renal function. If the kidney is well perfused and the hematoma nonexpanding, with no urine leak, no further exposure is required (see kidney section). In penetrating trauma, however, all lateral hematomas should be explored and the path of injury meticulously followed. Renal vascular control should first be obtained prior to opening Gerota's fascia. This step, although often unnecessary, clearly decreases the incidence of nephrectomy. The left renal vessels can generally be looped through direct exposure at the base of the mesocolon. The right renal vein, however, is more readily exposed after mobilizing the duodenum and unroofing the venal cava at its junction with the renal veins.

The approach to *pelvic hematomas* again depends on mechanism of injury. As discussed in the pelvic fracture section, blunt pelvic trauma can cause massive retroperitoneal pelvic hematomas. Approximately 15 per cent of these hematomas are the result of arterial injuries. Pelvic bone fixation and angiography with embolization have a role in managing these injuries, but direct operative exploration of the hematoma does not. Penetrating pelvic wounds, however, require exploration of the projectile or stab pathway. Direct compression of active bleeding or an expanding hematoma precedes proximal and distal control.

Proximal control of either the distal aorta or common iliac artery is obtained by eviscerating the small bowel and incising the retroperitoneum over the aortic bifurcation. Distal control is obtained just proximal to the inguinal ligament. Control of the internal iliac vessels is more problematic. Direct digital or sponge stick compression may be most efficacious while vascular loops are placed about the common iliac bifurcation. Injuries to the common or external iliac artery should be repaired if at all possible. In contrast, injuries to the internal iliac artery can be ligated with impunity, even if they occur bilaterally.[139,156]

The general principles of vascular repair apply in abdominal vascular injuries. Débridement of devitalized tissue, tension-free anastomosis, and the preferential use of autogenous tissue to bridge extensive gaps are applicable to all vascular repairs. Lateral repair of the aorta or vena cava is often possible, even after local débridement. Removal of all damaged tissue is important, however, and should not be ignored in order to simplify the subsequent repair. If a lateral repair without vessel narrowing is not possible, patch graft angioplasty can be done. Occasionally, a limited resection and anastomosis can be performed, but mobility of the aorta and vena cava is not great, and it is better to interpose a graft than to compromise the repair by constructing it under excess tension.

Wounds to the inferior vena cava below the renal veins or involving the iliac veins are generally easier to control than aortic wounds. If the laceration involves only one wall, a partial occluding clamp such as a Satinsky may be properly positioned for doing the repair. Through-and-through injuries of the vena cava can be repaired by enlarging the anterior wound so that the posterior injury can be sutured through the anterior wound. If greater mobility of the vena cava is required, a few lumbar veins or the gonadal vein may be ligated to allow rotation, although this is a more dangerous maneuver.

If the cava is severely lacerated and requires complicated repairs or graft interposition, or if repair poses a prohibitive risk in a patient with multiple injuries who is unstable, ligation of the infrarenal cava should be considered. If performed, it is important to maintain adequate intravascular volume and to keep both legs elevated for 5 to 7 days postoperatively wrapped with elastic compression dressings. Ligation of the suprarenal vena cava is not performed unless early reconstruction is planned. Although this maneuver has been supported by Allen and Blaisdell, in a large review by Graham and associates, it was necessary in less than 10 per cent of the patients.[2,63] Alternatively, inferior vena caval repair by interposing a vascular prosthesis (PTFE) graft has been successful.[37] Another option is the use of a segment of iliac or jugular vein to restore continuity. In most cases, construction of venous grafts for restoration of continuity is not required, and the time and effort necessary to perform such repairs may unnecessarily increase the operative morbidity and mortality.

Urinary Tract

Unless the patient has gross hematuria, urologic injury is usually initially unsuspected. Since urologic injuries are frequently associated with life-threatening emergencies, their diagnosis may be delayed for hours or even days until the patient is stabilized. A key tenet to be applied in diagnosing urologic trauma is to suspect injury by assessing the mechanism and forces involved. Urologic injury is particularly likely when there has been a crush injury of the upper abdomen or pelvis, when there has been a direct forceful blow to the back or flank, or when the patient has sustained a severe accelerating or decelerating injury, such as in a fall from a height or in an automobile or automobile-pedestrian accident. Signs of forceful injury include femur fracture, fracture of the pelvis, crush injury of the chest, severe bruising of the abdomen, and severe head trauma.

Specific signs of upper urologic tract injury include either gross or microscopic hematuria, fracture of the lower rib cage, or fracture of a lumbar process. The most positive signs of a lower urinary tract injury include the presence of blood at the urinary meatus, a "high riding" or misplaced prostate that cannot be palpated on rectal examination, and urinary retention, bladder distention, and the desire to void with inability to empty the bladder. The clinical signs of urinary tract injury may be initially absent, particularly in the rapidly transported multitrauma victim. Evaluation of possible urologic trauma must therefore often be based on the mechanism and associated injuries.

INITIAL EVALUATION. On presentation to the emergency room, every trauma patient should be asked immediately to produce a urine specimen. If he or she is unable to do so, catheterization may be necessary, particularly if the patient has suffered severe trauma. Under no circumstances should the patient be catheterized prior to urethrography if blood is present at the meatus of the penis or if the mechanism of injury suggests urethral injury. If there is resistance to catheterization, all efforts to catheterize the patient should cease, and urologic consultation should be obtained. Inability to easily pass a Foley catheter into the bladder supports the possibility of a posterior urethral disruption, particularly when the patient has an associated pelvic fracture. If possible, the Foley catheter should never be passed until a rectal examination has been done. Inability to palpate the prostate in a male is highly suggestive of complete urethral transection (Fig. 24).

If upper or lower urinary tract injury is suspected, the initial evaluation depends in part on the patient's associated injuries and hemodynamic stability. If the patient requires emergent operation, a limited "one-shot" intravenous pyelogram may be performed in the emergency room or on the operating room table by the rapid intravenous injections of 60 ml. of high-density contrast medium followed by a flat plate radiograph of the abdomen and pelvis in 1 to 5 minutes. This study generally identifies the presence or absence of functioning kidneys but is extremely limited and may fail to identify a renal outline in the presence of shock. In patients sustaining penetrating trauma, the entrance and exit wounds of the missile are marked with steel clips for determining the path of the bullet. The presence of pelvic crush injuries or blood at the urinary meatus suggests the need to obtain a retrograde cystourethrogram. Cystography is performed by filling the bladder to capacity with 200 to 300 ml. of contrast medium to distend the bladder lumen maximally. Films are obtained with the bladder distended and emptied to demonstrate extravasation (Fig. 25).

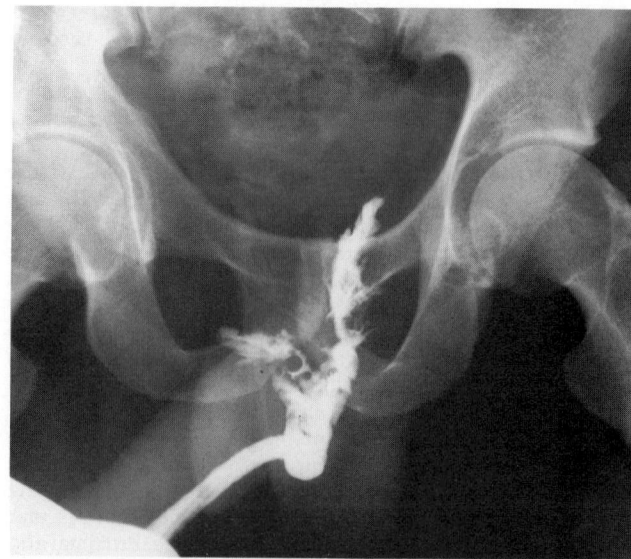

Figure 24. A retrograde cystourethrogram demonstrating complete disruption of the posterior urethra with extravasation of dye. Subsequent evaluation identified the tear just distal to the membranous urethra.

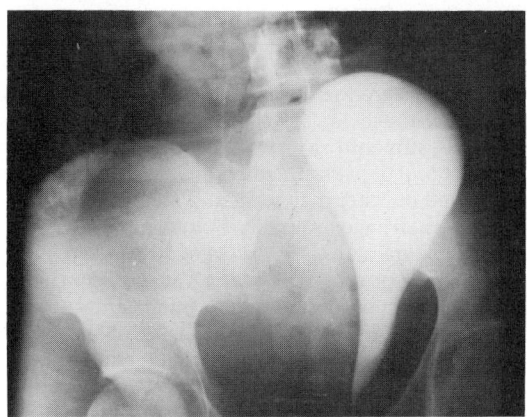

Figure 25. Cystogram demonstrating lateral displacement of the bladder secondary to a large pelvic hematoma.

The greatest diagnostic problem in blunt urologic trauma is recognition of renal pedicle injury. A high degree of suspicion is frequently the only mechanism to prevent the surgeon from overlooking this injury. There is no absolute amount of microscopic hematuria that accurately predicts significant urinary tract injury. At the authors' institution, all patients with gross hematuria or any degree of microscopic hematuria combined with associated abdominal injuries, shock, or a mechanism that suggests renal trauma, undergo an evaluation to exclude the possibility of renal pedicle injury. In addition, all patients with penetrating wounds near the urinary tract system are operatively explored or undergo radiographic evaluation.

Intravenous pyelography (IVP) and CT with intravenous contrast are effective methods for evaluating the urinary tract, although CT scans provide more detailed information about the urologic injury and the potential associated intra-abdominal and retroperitoneal injuries. IVP is also less accurate in the unprepared patient, and the dynamic phase of the CT scan provides additional information regarding renal function. The degree of renal parenchymal injury identified on CT scans is also useful in classifying the injury and defining a management plan.[18] Demonstration by either CT scan or IVP of the apparent presence of a solitary kidney or a lack of function of a segment of the kidney is an indication for immediate arteriography.

KIDNEYS. Penetrating injury to the kidney may be secondary to a gunshot wound, a stab wound, or impalement. Parenchymal injury caused by a low-velocity weapon is usually not life-threatening and is generally easily treated with débridement and primary repair of the kidney, with dependent drainage. Occasionally, a partial nephrectomy may be necessary when the wound is in a polar position. High-velocity bullet wounds are different. Many nephrectomies and partial nephrectomies are done in patients with high-velocity penetrating injury because of inability to control hemorrhage and accurately define the extent of the injury. In addition, injudicious rapid incision of Gerota's capsule with an extensive injury to the kidney may cause unnecessary nephrectomy. Preoperative arteriography is helpful in defining vascular disruption and may be therapeutic if embolization can be performed. Unfortunately, most patients are too unstable because of other intra-abdominal injuries to warrant this time-consuming maneuver. A key operative technique is the proximal control of the renal pedicle prior to opening Gerota's fascia in any kidney trauma. If the injury involves the hilum of the kidney, repair may be attempted in an isolated renal injury; but salvage of renal function is minimal in most circumstances, and associated organ injuries may take precedence. Any injury to the collecting system should be débrided and sutured in a watertight manner. Preservation of as much renal parenchyma as possible is mandatory.

Although nearly all penetrating renal trauma patients are explored because of the high incidence of associated intra-abdominal injuries (90 to 100 per cent for gun shot wounds, 60 to 75 per cent for stab wounds), many blunt renal trauma patients can be managed nonoperatively.[25,67,157] Selection of patients for operative treatment of the renal lesion should be based on the overall clinical status of the patient and the necessity of surgical repair or resection, which is based on the natural history of the lesion.[18,25,67]

A classification system used by the authors to differentiate patients who have suffered minor renal trauma from those who have suffered major renal trauma is based on the principles illustrated in Figure 26. The key components of the classification system are (1) the presence and extent of nonfunctioning renal segments, (2) the extent of perinephric hematoma, and (3) the degree of contrast extravasation. Eighty-five per cent of patients have minor renal injuries that can be managed expectantly. Patients with minor renal injuries have few serious sequelae. Approximately 10 per cent of patients have immediately life-threatening renal injuries consisting of a shattered kidney, renal pedicle injury, or cortical laceration with disrupted fragments and extensive extravasation. These patients undergo surgical exploration and repair or resection, since the natural history of these lesions is such that the incidence of secondary nephrectomy, hypertension, abscess, and late bleeding in those managed nonoperatively is quite high. Additionally, approximately 15 per cent of these patients have significant injury to other abdominal viscera.

Only approximately 5 per cent of patients appear to have an intermediate degree of renal injury. Management may be nonsurgical or surgical, depending upon the clinical status of the patient and the need for treatment of other associated injuries. Major cortical laceration with undisplaced fragments held in

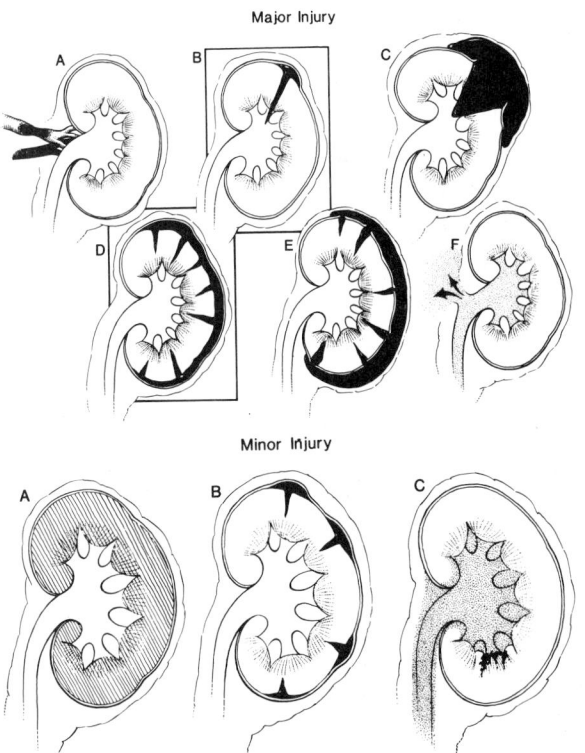

Figure 26. A system for classifying renal trauma. Six types of major injury are (A) renal pedicle injury, (B) deep parenchymal injury with an intact capsule, (C) deep parenchymal injury with a disrupted capsule, (D) shattered kidney with an intact capsule, (E) shattered kidney with a disrupted capsule, and (F) ureteral or renal pelvis injury. Minor injury can be classified as (A) contusion, (B) shallow cortical laceration, and (C) forniceal disruption. (From Guerriero, W. G.: Trauma to the kidneys, ureters, bladder, and urethra. Surg. Clin. North Am., 62:1047, 1982.)

place by an intact renal capsule with minimal or no extravasation and the shattered functioning kidney with contained fragments are examples of this type. CT has been particularly helpful in identifying the extent of these injuries. If a significant hematoma is also demonstrated, angiographic evaluation and embolization can be successfully employed. In most cases, the kidney heals, but sequelae such as hypertension are common.[117]

URETERS. Injury to the ureter usually follows penetrating trauma. Fistula and stricture formation are the inevitable sequelae of undetected ureteral injury. Early detection and operative repair are preferred with a ureteral transection in which the blood supply of the ureter has not been injured and the injury is not far below the pelvic brim. The principles of ureteral repair are adequate débridement, tension-free repair, spatulated anastomosis, watertight closure, ureteral stenting, and drainage. Injuries in the upper and middle thirds of the ureter can usually be managed by primary ureteroureterostomy. Injuries to the distal third of the ureter should be treated with ureteroneocystostomy. The ureter should be stented with an indwelling polyvinyl Silastic catheter if there is associated vascular injury or if damage to the ureteral blood supply is suspected. Injury to the upper ureter may be stented with a concomitant nephrostomy in order to drain urine from the site of the injury. If primary repair is not immediately possible due to shock, associated injuries, or long segmental ureteral damage, diversion of the distal fistula with a percutaneous nephrostomy and secondary repair is the method of management. Alternatives to immediate diversion when there is extensive ureteral injury in the stable patient are transureteroureterostomy and autotransplantation.[68]

BLADDER. The bladder is the most commonly injured organ in association with pelvic fractures (see Fig. 25). In Brosman and Paul's series, 72 per cent of patients with trauma to the bladder had associated pelvic fracture.[19] The bladder may be contused, penetrated, or ruptured intraperitoneally or extraperitoneally. Large defects can be present despite a negative cystogram, particularly if the cystogram is obtained at a date later than the patient's initial examination, because blood clot, tissue, or peritoneal contents can fill the defect. False-negative cystograms are common with penetrating injuries to the bladder. A postevacuation cystogram should always be obtained for determining whether extravasation has occurred on the oblique or lateral projections. CT cystograms are helpful in evaluating the more subtle bladder injury.

Treatment of bladder injuries is usually straightforward. Isolated extraperitoneal bladder ruptures can be treated with 10 days of Foley catheter drainage if no other operative intervention is planned.[33] However, most of the extraperitoneal bladder ruptures are associated with pelvic fracture in which the anterior wall of the bladder has been perforated by a spicule of bone. The fracture should be reduced and stabilized away from the bladder, and the bladder wound should be débrided and closed in two layers. After the repair, the bladder should be tested for integrity by being filled with saline to capacity of 400 ml. If the bladder can be made watertight, and if the patient's other injuries are minimal, Foley drainage is adequate. If prolonged bed rest is expected or if there is a question of the integrity of bladder closure, a suprapubic catheter should be used.

Intraperitoneal rupture occurs in the posterior bladder wall when the patient has a compression injury of the abdomen with a full bladder, or it may be due to the penetrating trauma. Injuries of this type are repaired by developing the edge of the wound to mobilize the peritoneum off the ragged bladder tear and to permit a three-layer closure. Catheterization of ureteral orifices may help to protect the ureter during the closure of the bladder. The bladder should be inspected for water-tightness, and a Foley catheter or suprapubic tube should be left in for drainage according to the principles just mentioned.

PELVIS AND PERINEUM

Pelvic Fractures

Pelvic fractures are the third most common injury sustained in motor vehicle accidents. Whereas the majority constitute rather simple, straightforward orthopedic problems, approximately 20 per cent of pelvic fractures are complex injuries with a high likelihood of other major organ system trauma or significant pelvic hemorrhage. Mortality from complex crush injuries and open pelvic fractures is in excess of 50 per cent, with morbidity 30 to 74 per cent. The major cause of morbidity and mortality is associated organ system injury and uncontrolled blood loss. In one review of 538 consecutive pelvic fracture patients, 92 patients (17 per cent) required greater than 6 units of blood.[118] Twenty-six per cent of this group died, half of associated injuries and half of recalcitrant bleeding or delayed pelvic sepsis. If injuries to the iliac or femoral vessels are present, mortality in excess of 80 per cent has been reported. This contrasts with the overall reported mortality from pelvic fractures of approximately 5 per cent, with 80 per cent of deaths due to associated injuries and only 20 per cent directly attributable to the pelvic fracture. Mucha and Farnell's recent review of 534 patients with pelvic fractures documented an overall mortality of 6.4 per cent, although the pelvic fracture was directly responsible for less than 1 per cent mortality and the remainder were due to associated head and torso injuries.[120]

The initial approach to the patient with a pelvic fracture should first follow the basic principles of resuscitation outlined earlier. Associated injuries should be sought and treated as their emergent nature mandates. Immobilization of the patient on a back board is indicated while pelvic and spinal stability is assessed. The pneumatic anti-shock garment (PASG) has been recommended to stabilize pelvic fractures and tamponade pelvic bleeding. Although there have been no prospective randomized or cross-over studies to assess its efficacy, several uncontrolled studies have supported its utility.

Examination of the pelvis begins by applying anteroposterior and lateral compression to assess for instability and pain. All patients should receive a digital rectal and vaginal examination to assess for blood, bony fragments, and mucosal lacerations. In the male, particular attention should be directed to identifying the location of the prostate gland, because a "high-riding" or misplaced prostate indicates urethral disruption. Direct inspection of the urethral meatus is mandatory prior to insertion of a Foley catheter. The presence of meatal blood mandates retrograde urethrography prior to Foley insertion in the male, because of the length of the urethra and the possibility of converting a partial urethral tear into a complete disruption and false passage (see Fig. 24). The initial radiographic examination should include an AP plain film of the pelvis. As time and the patient's condition allows, more select views may be indicated. CT is particularly helpful in delineating complex pelvic and acetabular fractures, often providing additional anatomic information. Pelvic bone CT scanning is time-consuming and does not take precedence over the search for associated injuries.

The description of pelvic fractures should include each fracture line and the aspect of pelvic bone anatomy involved. A number of attempts have been made to classify pelvic fracture patterns. Pennal and others have championed a classification based on vectors of force: anteroposterior compression, lateral compression, vertical shear, and combined mechanical injury.[36,141] Alternatively, an anatomic classification commonly applied is Kane's modification of the Key and Conwell classification as outlined in Table 6.[95] The usefulness of any classification system is in its ability to help direct treatment or predict morbidity. In Mucha and Farnell's review of pelvic fracture management, Type 3 and 4 fractures had a significantly higher incidence of associated injuries, morbidity, and mortality.[120]

TABLE 6. Kane's Modification of Key and Conwell's Pelvic Fracture Classification

Type 1	*Individual bones not involving the pelvic ring.* Includes avulsion fractures of a single ramus and isolated fractures of the iliac wing.
Type 2	*Single breaks of the pelvic ring.* Fractures occurring through (1) two ipsilateral rami or (2) one sacroiliac joint (rare) or (3) subluxation of the symphysis and pubis.
Type 3	*Double breaks in the pelvic ring.* Fractures include three subsets: (1) the Malgaigne variants, also called the double vertical or dimetric fractures; (2) bilateral double ramus fractures, referred to as either straddle fractures or butterfly fractures; and (3) severe multiple or crushing fractures.
Type 4	*Acetabular fractures.* There are three types: (1) rim fractures; (2) central acetabular fractures; and (3) ischioacetabular fractures.

Modified from Kane, W. J.: Fractures of the pelvis. *In* Rockwood, C., and Green, D. P., (Eds.): Fractures. Philadelphia, J. B. Lippincott Company, 1975, p. 923.

Cryer and colleagues suggest that "unstable" fractures correlate well with higher blood loss.[34] Posterior pelvic fractures appear to have more associated injuries and complications, require more resuscitation fluid, and have a higher rate of mortality than anterior fractures.[59]

The management objectives in a patient with a pelvic fracture are control of hemorrhage, skeletal fixation, and treatment of associated injuries. The initial objective is control of exsanguinating blood loss. Massive hemorrhage (up to 20 units) can occur into the retroperitoneal space, where it may be difficult to diagnose and control. Experimental evidence suggests the pelvic retroperitoneal space can contain up to 4000 ml. of blood under pressure equal to or lower than the pressure in the pelvic vessels.[55] The source of such significant blood loss can occur from pelvic arteries, veins, or the fracture line. Extensive collateralization, difficult exposure, and release of the tamponade effect of the posterior peritoneum make surgical exploration of pelvic hematomas generally frustrating and fruitless. Application of the PSAG is recommended as a temporizing agent, pending either immediate skeletal fixation or arteriographic evaluation and embolization. Some studies have suggested that if pelvic hematoma-related blood requirements exceed 6 units, angiographic intervention is indicated.[53] However, since most of the bleeding associated with pelvic fractures is venous in origin, angiographic control may not be possible. Immediate fixation of the unstable fracture may be more helpful in this situation. Some centers advocate early open reduction and internal fixation of the unstable pelvic fracture, maintaining that bulky external fixaters or spica casts limit ambulation and invite all the complications associated with prolonged immobilization.[61] No comparative data are available on the basis of which one can determine which method or approach is superior.

The search for associated intra-abdominal injuries in the hemodynamically stable patient with a pelvic fracture may require CT scan of the abdomen or DPL. Peritoneal lavage should be performed in the supraumbilical location in patients with significant pelvic fractures so that the potentially blood-filled anterior abdominal preperitoneal space, an extension of Retzius' space between the bladder and the symphysis pubis is not entered. False-positive peritoneal lavage rates vary from 16 to 50 per cent if lavage is performed in the standard infraumbilical location, although it must be remembered that approximately 25 per cent of pelvic fracture victims have associated intra-abdominal injury.[53,118] Gross blood on the initial aspirate is an indication for immediate exploratory celiotomy.

The patient with a positive peritoneal lavage or CT scan evidence of intra-abdominal injury and combined pelvic fracture and hematoma presents the trauma surgeon with a difficult challenge. The authors have generally adopted the following management guidelines. A hemodynamically unstable patient with grossly positive peritoneal lavage undergoes immediate exploratory celiotomy. After repair of associated intra-abdominal injuries, angiographic evaluation and embolization or skeletal fixation is performed, depending on the likelihood of an arterial source of the pelvic bleeding. If exploratory celiotomy is not required, immediate angiography or skeletal fixation is conducted if transfusion of 6 or more units of blood has been required for pelvic hemorrhage or if the presenting hematocrit is low (less than 25 per cent) and blood loss is localized to the pelvis. If angiography is performed first, skeletal fixation follows. The sequence of intervention commonly depends on the expertise and availability of support personnel. Although it is difficult to predict which individual patient is at risk for significant hemorrhage, the presence of posterior element fracture or "unstable open book" pelvic fracture appears to correlate with increased blood loss from an arterial source.

Perineal Wounds

Massive soft tissue injury of the perineum may occur in association with some pelvic fractures, but this injury can occur without bony pelvic injury. It is frequently advisable to divert the fecal stream away from these injuries via a descending colostomy. Early débridement and operative inspection of the wound is required. No attempt should be made to initially close the wound. Undermined skin flaps should be excised, necrotic muscle débrided, and deep space infections or pockets eradicated. Repeat operating room inspections, débridement, and pulse irrigations should be planned on a daily basis.[100] Eventual closure often requires skin grafting or rotational flaps.

VAGINAL INJURIES. Vaginal lacerations in association with pelvic fractures are less common (3.5 per cent) but should be suspected when vaginal bleeding occurs in association with pelvic injury. The laceration should be carefully cleansed, débrided as necessary, and primarily closed if recognized early.[128]

CENTRAL NERVOUS SYSTEM

Cranium and Brain

Although injury to the head may cause damage to the scalp, skull, face, and subcranial structures, it is often the presence of brain injury alone or in combination with other injuries that is the major determinant of survival or functional outcome. Since the initial care of the patient with a head injury is usually rendered by a physician who is not specially trained in neurosurgery, the purpose of this section is to develop a clinical approach to the emergency diagnosis and management of serious head injuries.

The two guiding principles of initial care of the patient with severe head injuries are assessment of the severity of injury and protection of the brain from further injury until a definitive diagnosis and therapy can be determined. The treatment plan depends on identifying the two fundamental varieties of head injury, focal and diffuse. Focal injuries consist of mass lesions that cause neurologic dysfunction, largely by brain compression, and often require surgical evacuation. Diffuse brain injuries are equally frequent and cause prolonged coma without intracranial masses. These do not require surgical therapy but can be as devastating as focal injuries.

INITIAL MANAGEMENT. The ultimate outcome of brain injury is as much dependent on the early establishment of an airway, ventilation, control of hemorrhage, and restoration of perfusion as is that of injury of any other organ, if not more so.

The previous protocol proposed for resuscitation of the multiply injured patient is equally applicable to the patient who has isolated brain injury. The airway should be secured immediately, and care should be taken to remember that spinal cord injury is present in as many as 10 per cent of patients with head injuries. Although brain injury *per se* rarely causes hypotension during the early period following trauma, its disturbed tissue matrix is most susceptible to lowered perfusion states during this period; consequently, it is critical that adequate arterial pressure, blood volume, and oxygenation be maintained in such patients. Appropriate fluid and blood replacement should be undertaken and carefully monitored so that perfusion is maintained and volume overload avoided.

ASSESSMENT OF SEVERITY OF INJURY. The severity of brain injury can be estimated in less than 1 minute by evaluating three factors: *level of consciousness, pupillary function,* and *lateralized weakness of the extremities.*

Level of consciousness is best assessed by the Glasgow Coma Scale (GCS), a system that evaluates eye opening, best motor response, and verbal response (see Table 1). The GCS is determined by taking the best response in each category and totaling the responses; it ranges from 3 to 15.[83] Because of its repeatability, a difference of 2 signals a change in neurologic status; a decrease of 3 usually indicates an enlarging hematoma and demands prompt treatment. *Pupillary function* is assessed by the size, equality, and response to bright light. Whether or not there has been ocular injury, any pupillary asymmetry greater than 1 mm. must be attributed to intracranial injury unless proved otherwise. With few exceptions, the largest pupil is on the side of the mass lesion. The *lateralized extremity weakness* is detected by testing motor power in patients able to cooperate or by observing symmetry of movement in response to painful stimulus. As the severity of injury worsens, lateralized weakness is more difficult to appreciate, and small differences may be important.

The Glasgow coma score should be assessed in the field or by the first responders, then reassessed after specific treatment interventions. Because intubation and paralyzing agents alter the ability to assess the components of the GCS, the authors have noted the presence of an endotracheal tube or the recent administration of paralytic agents by the modifiers *T* and *P*, respectively, when computing the GCS score.

The presence of any of the following criteria suggest serious injury: (1) a GCS score of less than 10; (2) a decrease in the GCS score by 3 or more regardless of the initial GCS score; (3) pupillary inequality greater than 1 mm. regardless of the GCS score; (4) lateralized extremity weakness regardless of the GCS score; (5) markedly depressed skull fractures; and (6) open cranial wounds with brain exposed.[16]

PROTECTION FROM FURTHER INSULT. Cerebral ischemia is present in more than 90 per cent of patients who die of head trauma and is the most preventable complication. Most ischemic complications occur soon after injury, are much more common when multisystem trauma is present, and can be reversed in the early phases of care. In ischemia, fewer nutrients are reaching the brain than its metabolism demands, which can be compensated by maximizing oxygen and glucose delivery to the brain. This requires ample blood flow to the brain and adequate concentration of oxygen and glucose in the blood. However, excess fluid resuscitation or blood pressure elevation must be avoided, because the cerebral vessels do not react normally after injury; they fail to constrict if subjected to elevated blood pressure. Invasive monitoring devices such as Swan-Ganz catheterization of the right side of the heart may be necessary for determining the appropriate fluid requirements.

For sufficient oxygen delivery to the brain, the arterial oxygen content must be optimized, which is best done by supplying supplemental oxygen and ensuring adequate ventilation. Adequate ventilation can be accomplished by treating systemic or local causes of ventilatory insufficiency (e.g., airway obstruc-

tion, pneumothorax) and by assisted ventilation if necessary. Endotracheal intubation is often required for definitive treatment of head injuries. If urgent intubation is required, the same techniques that are used in the operating room should be applied. Failure to use paralytic agents, pharyngeal anesthesia, and barbiturate induction invites massive elevation of intracranial pressure (ICP) during intubation.

Even after relatively short periods of ischemia, the brain may respond to reperfusion in a pathologic manner with prompt and severe brain swelling and marked increases in ICP.[57] Elevated ICP can best be managed in the early phases of injury by decreasing the intravascular cerebral blood volume. Intravascular cerebral blood volume is best decreased by controlled hyperventilation, because the arterial carbon dioxide concentration is the most potent known regulator of cerebral vessel size. For extremely serious head injuries, hyperventilation to Pco_2 values in the low 20s may be necessary. Decreasing brain water may also be beneficial and is accomplished with diuretics or hyperosmotic agents, the latter being more rapid.

DEFINITIVE CARE. Definitive care begins with a definitive diagnosis, which is established exclusively by CT. Cranial CT has a high priority in the evaluation of a patient with altered level of consciousness or lateralizing neurologic signs. It should be performed as soon as cardiorespiratory stability has been achieved and a lateral cervical spine roentgenogram demonstrates no fracture or dislocation. Seriously injured patients who are intubated should receive neuromuscular blockage during the study. A good quality CT scan identifies focal mass lesions and allows the diagnosis of the presence of diffuse brain injury. Focal injuries with significant mass effect require surgical evacuation; patients with these injuries go directly to the operating room. Patients with diffuse brain injury are managed in the intensive care unit. Monitoring devices for ICP are placed for on-line management of intracranial hypertension in both groups. Definitive care continues, with the principal effort directed toward controlling intracranial hypertension in order to keep the ICP within normal limits. Therapy is added as necessary to achieve this goal as follows: moderate hyperventilation (Pco_2, 20 to 30), diuretics (furosemide, 20 to 40 mg. three times a day), and hyperosmolar therapy (20 per cent mannitol to keep serum osmolality 305 to 315 mOsm. per kg.). Although both barbiturates and glucocorticoids have been advocated in the management of severe head injury, recent clinical evidence does not support their use.[40,195] Systemic support must be vigorous to ensure continued cerebral oxygenation and to prevent infectious complication of prolonged coma.

Vertebrae and Spinal Cord

The incidence of spinal cord injury in the United States is approximately 50 cases per 1 million population per year. Motor vehicle accidents alone involve over 500 quadriplegics per year.[155] Approximately 6 per cent of all injury hospitalizations are due to vertebrae injuries, and 1 per cent are from spinal cord injuries.[149] While these injuries represent a small proportion of the total injury-related hospitalizations, they cause significant physical and psychologic changes, often requiring long-term and expensive medical treatment and rehabilitation. The average hospital charge for a quadriplegic survivor was $50,000 in 1988.[155] Although brain and spinal cord injuries are the primary determinants of long-term disability, many spinal cord injuries are incomplete and, given proper care, may have a remarkable capacity for recovery. Many of the acute problems and complications that the patient with spinal cord injury confronts have been identified, and there are effective procedures for preventing or limiting these problems. Rehabilitation programs for patients with spinal cord injuries have also been developed that help the patient attain the highest possible functional level of recovery.

Bohlman, in a review of 300 acute cervical fractures and dislocations, reports that motor vehicle accidents (one third), falls (one third), and athletic injuries or missile wounds are the usual causes of injury to the cervical spine.[12] Other reports suggest that motor vehicle accidents are responsible for up to 60 per cent of spinal cord injuries, falls for 20 to 30 per cent, and diving accidents for 5 to 10 per cent.[149] In Bohlman's series, the condition of one third of the patients was not diagnosed when they were first seen in the emergency room. Bohlman identified the following four specific categories of patients whose diagnoses were likely to be delayed: (1) patients with head injuries; (2) patients with multiple injuries, including fractures elsewhere; (3) patients with brain injuries and impaired consciousness; and (4) intoxicated patients. Careful follow-up examinations must be made during a traumatized patient's hospitalization when he complains of pain in the back or neck; when weakness, numbness, or loss of control of extremities or sphincters develops; or when only screening radiographs were obtained during admission evaluation.

INITIAL CARE. Proper care of the potentially unstable spine begins at the scene of injury and continues until the spine has been proved stable. Adequate help is essential. Gentle manual traction stabilizes the head, which can be turned to the mid-line if necessary to protect the airway and to correct gross deformity. The neck should be placed and maintained in a position of minimal extension and taped to a padded spine board or similar support during transportation. The lower spine is protected by taping the patient to the backboard above and below major joints. Sandbags on each side of the head in addition to a cervical collar provide additional stability when the patient is transported from one location to another. The forehead should be taped to the backboard.

The history should include information determining the site and duration of any pain. Transient or persistent numbness, tingling, and weakness or other neurologic problems must be noted, as should any prior injuries or other difficulties involving the spine or spinal cord.

Physical examination should include notation of abrasions or contusions anywhere on the head or trunk. They provide clues to the mechanism of injury. Spinal deformity can occasionally be seen, but palpation of the spine processes is frequently more rewarding. The patient should be log-rolled and the dorsal spine palpated and inspected for localized tenderness, swelling, rotational deformity or the presence of a gap between the spinous processes (indicative of a rupture of the posterior ligaments with resultant instability).

If a neurologic deficit is present, the examination focuses on defining the neurologic level of injury and on determining whether or not there is sparing of some spinal cord function across this level. The patient with incomplete spinal cord injury has motor or sensory function below the injury level. Sacral sparing may be the only evidence that paralysis is not complete. Therefore, sensation in the perineum, voluntary sphincter contraction, and toe flexion must be carefully examined. Most incomplete spinal cord injuries exhibit mixed motor and sensory sparing rather than a classic pattern of partial injury. The natural course of incomplete cord injuries is improvement. Well-documented evidence of deterioration is rare. If deterioration is observed, emergency diagnostic and surgical treatment may be warranted. A patient with complete spinal cord injury has no distal motor or sensory function. It is essential that neurologic function be accurately recorded in the prehospital and emergency room notes to allow later comparison.

Immediately after a spinal cord injury there is a transient period of disordered function termed *spinal shock*. During this time, no reflex or voluntary activity can be elicited distal to the level of the injury. When some reflex activity has returned, the spinal cord lesion can be deemed complete if there is no distal sensation or voluntary motor control. The normal sacral reflexes are the earliest to recover from spinal shock, usually within the

first 24 hours. One such reflex is the bulbocavernosus reflex, contraction of the anal sphincter produced by compression of the glans or clitoris or by tugging gently on the Foley catheter. The other is the anal wink, or contraction of the anal sphincter in response to a pinprick adjacent to it. By following these reflexes during the early stages of spinal cord injury, valuable prognostic information can be obtained.

Good quality roentgenograms are as essential as the history and physical examination in the thorough evaluation of the patient with spinal injury. Radiologic examination of the cervical spine must be accomplished before moving the neck in all patients with blunt trauma, particularly those who are unconscious, obtunded, or complaining of neck pain. The initial screening view is a cross-table lateral view of the supine patient, taken with the film just lateral to one shoulder, with both shoulders actively or passively depressed so the entire cervical spine is visualized from the occiput to the top of T1 (Fig. 27). It is important to note that the head is stabilized during this maneuver and not actively distracted away from the body, which can be disastrous in a severe C1–2 ligamentous injury. Formal AP, lateral, and odontoid views should be obtained before the cervical spine is "cleared," but flexion and extension radiograms are rarely indicated when the preliminary films have shown no sign of instability and the patient is conscious and cooperative. The signs of impending spinal cord damage may be subtle. A small bony avulsion or slight malalignment of vertebrae may be the only suggestion of gross ligamentous instability. The physician who is seeking only fractures may ignore subluxations and even dislocations.

New-generation CT scanners greatly facilitate the evaluation of spinal trauma. Sagittal reconstructions can provide excellent portrayals of alignment, without the risk of positioning often required by conventional tomography or flexion and extension films. Retropulsion of bone fragments and occasionally of disc material can be demonstrated, clearly showing the amount of canal narrowing that results. Magnetic resonance imaging (MRI) can beautifully demonstrate detailed neuropathology, disc herniation, and ligamentous injuries noninvasively and will probably have an increasing role in the evaluation of spinal trauma.

TREATMENT OF SPECIFIC INJURIES. The authors recommend that the injured spinal cord be treated by prompt reduc-

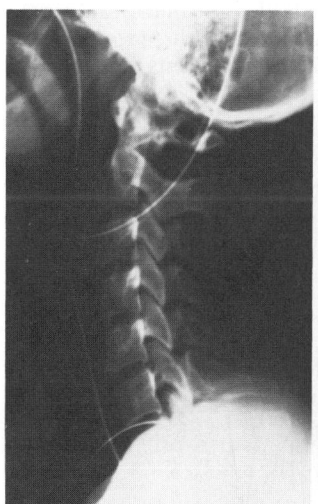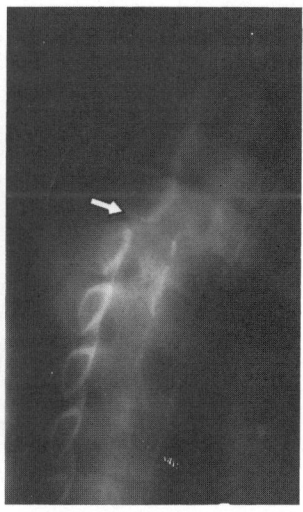

Figure 27. The importance of completely visualizing all seven cervical vertebrae in a cross-table lateral cervical spine radiograph is illustrated in these two photoradiographs. Inadequate cross-table lateral cervical spine radiograph (C7 not visualized) following blunt neck trauma. Tomography was required for evaluation of the entire cervical spine of C7 on T1 (arrow). (From Jurkovich, G. J.: The neck. In Moore, E. E. (Ed.): Early Care of the Injured Patient, 4th ed., Toronto, B. C. Decker, Inc., 1990, p. 129.)

tion of any dislocation or angular deformity that compromises the spinal canal. Effective splinting of the spine and spinal cord can prevent recurrent deformity or excessive mobility that might jeopardize the local microcirculation. This can usually be achieved with traction and the appropriate positioning of the patient. In patients with cervical spine injuries, skeletal traction may be applied readily with Gardner-Wells tongs or a cranial halo. Frequent radiographs and neurologic monitoring are necessary for identifying deterioration, overdistraction, or loss of alignment during reduction and when gradually increasing distraction weight is applied. If closed means are not effective in restoring the spinal canal or if an incomplete spinal cord lesion is deteriorating, emergency surgical treatment, either open reduction or an anterior decompression and fusion, may be necessary. Experience with incomplete thoracic level paraplegia suggests that an aggressive posture of immediate posterior Harrington distraction instrumentation or anterior transthoracic decompression and fusion is preferable to postural reduction or late anterior decompression with improved neurologic function demonstrated in 90 per cent of patients so treated.[99]

NECK

The neck is a unique trauma organ with multiple vital structures concentrated in a small anatomic area, yet generally unprotected by bone or dense muscular covering. Although most significant neck injuries are the result of penetrating trauma, blunt neck trauma occurs and can be particularly difficult to manage, since it often involves the airway, the first priority in trauma care. In addition, major blood vessel injury of the neck can occur as a consequence of cervical spine hyperextension, even in the absence of bony injury. Although the frequency of neck trauma is small (5 to 10 per cent of all injuries), the consequences are great. Fatality rates for penetrating neck trauma extend from 2 per cent for stab wounds to 50 per cent for rifle or shotgun blasts. It is estimated that one half of these deaths are preventable with appropriate early care.[94]

The neck is classically divided into a number of anatomic triangles (Fig. 28). Two large triangles are important in discussing penetrating neck trauma. Penetrating wounds that enter through the sternocleidomastoid muscle or anterior triangle have a high likelihood of significant vascular, airway, or esophageal injury. In contrast, wounds to the posterior triangle rarely involve the esophagus, airway, or major vascular structures, although if directed inferiorly intrathoracic injury can occur.

The anterior neck is further divided into three zones defined by horizontal planes (Fig. 29). Zone I represents the base of the

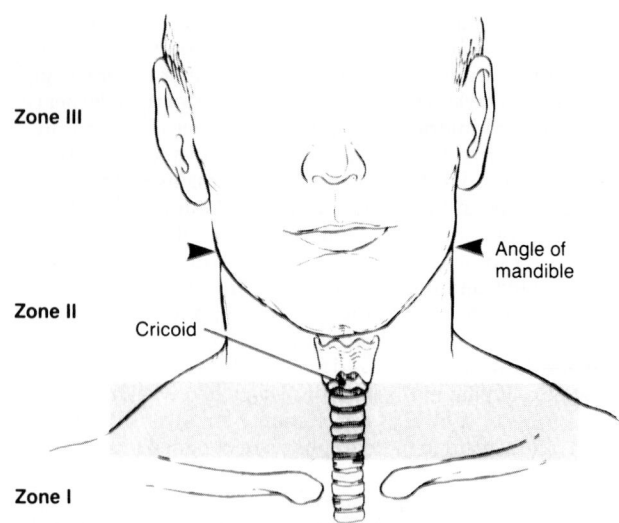

Figure 29. Zones of the neck. The junction of Zone I and Zone II is usually described as the cricoid cartilage or alternatively, the top of the clavicles. (From Jurkovich, G. J.: The neck. *In* Moore, E. E. (Ed.): Early Care of the Injured Patient, 4th ed. Toronto, B. C. Decker, Inc., 1990, p. 127.)

neck and thoracic outlet. Injuries here have the highest mortality because of the risk of major vascular and intrathoracic injury. Zone II represents the largest portion, or midbody of the neck. Because of its relative size, Zone II injuries are most common but have the lowest mortality. Significant injury is generally apparent, and exposure of vital structures is readily accomplished. Zone III is that part of the neck above the angle of mandible. The risk of injury to the distal carotid artery, salivary glands, and pharynx is greatest in this zone, and exposure can be particularly difficult.

The other major anatomic landmark in the neck is the platysma muscle. This thin, broad muscle lies just beneath the skin and covers the entire anterior triangle and anteroinferior aspect of the posterior triangle. Wounds that fail to penetrate the platysma are considered superficial and do not warrant extensive evaluation. Wounds that do penetrate the platysma mandate hospital admission and further evaluation.

Selective Versus Mandatory Exploration

Controversy continues regarding management of neck wounds that penetrate the platysma muscle.[23] There are two management regimens on this subject, one advocating mandatory surgical exploration of all such wounds[11] and one favoring a more selective approach.[1,94] Those favoring routine exploration justify their position by emphasizing the disastrous complications of overlooked injuries and the relative safety and short hospital course of a negative exploration. Authors favoring a more selective approach berate the high incidence of negative explorations and the fact that some injuries are overlooked despite a formal exploration. Merion and associates analyzed 27 series reported in the literature in which the clinical course of over 4000 patients with penetrating neck trauma had been documented[114] (Table 7). This review emphasizes the similar outcomes with these two approaches and argues that either approach can be justified.

Perhaps more significant than this controversy are the areas of uniform agreement. All patients with clinical signs of significant injury require prompt exploration (Table 8). All other patients (clinically silent) with wounds that penetrate the platysma should at least be admitted to the hospital and observed. The disagreement is whether patients without positive clinical findings should routinely undergo a surgical neck exploration or alternatively undergo extensive diagnostic evaluation.[23] At Harborview Medical Center in Seattle, the authors continue to

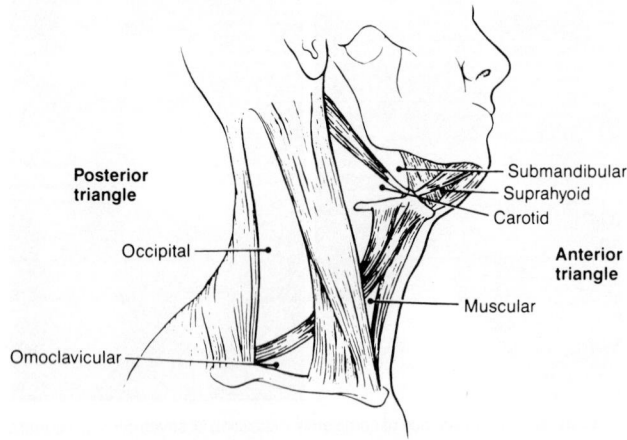

Figure 28. Anatomic triangles of the neck. The large *posterior triangle* is composed of the smaller occipital and omoclavicular triangles; the large *anterior triangle* is composed of the smaller suprahyoid, submandibular, carotid, and muscular triangles. (From Jurkovich, G. J.: The neck. *In* Moore, E. E. (Ed.): Early Care of the Injured Patient, 4th ed. Toronto, B. C. Decker, Inc., 1990, p. 127.)

TABLE 7. Summary of 27 Collected Series of Mandatory Exploration Versus Selective Observation Policy for Penetrating Neck Trauma

	Selective Observation Policy (13 Series, 2659 Patients)	Mandatory Exploration Policy (14 Series, 1777 Patients)
Immediate operation	52.4%	88.7%
Injury requiring repair	67.0%	61.3%
Observed	47.6%	11.3%
Delayed operation/missed injury	2.4%	7.8%
Mortality		
Immediate operation group	9.2%	8.3%
Initially observed group	1.7%	4.1%
Delayed operation group	16.7%	13.3%

Adapted from Carducci, B., Lowe, R. A., and Dalsey, W.: Penetrating neck trauma: Consensus and controversies. Ann. Emerg. Med., 15:208, 1986; and from Merion, R. M., Harness, J. K., Ramsburgh, S. R., et al.: Selective management of penetrating neck trauma: Cost implications. Arch. Surg., 116:691, 1981. Copyright 1981, American Medical Association.

explore the majority of neck wounds that penetrate the platysma. More specifically, injuries to the base of the skull and thoracic outlet (Zones III and I) require angiography prior to, and occasionally in lieu of, exploration. Injuries to the midneck (Zone II) are generally managed by exploration without prior invasive diagnostic studies.

Initial Management

Active airway management is critical in the patient with a serious neck wound and takes precedence over all other aspects of evaluation and resuscitation. Emergency intubation is necessary when spontaneous respirations are inadequate, when blood or vomit obstructs the airway, or when progressive cervical swelling from hemorrhage threatens to occlude the airway. Procrastination converts a simple intubation into a difficult, bloody emergency tracheostomy. If the airway is not jeopardized, nasogastric and endotracheal intubation may be deferred so that endoscopic evaluation of the larynx and hypopharynx is made possible. The remainder of the initial therapy follows the guidelines previously outlined, with particular attention directed toward excluding cervical spine injury, providing adequate ventilation, and evaluating neurologic status.

After initial resuscitation, a complete physical examination is performed to detect associated injuries and to better define the extent of neck trauma. The clinical signs that mandate neck

TABLE 8. Clinical Signs of Significant Injury in Penetrating Neck Trauma

Vascular

Shock
Expanding hematoma
External hemorrhage
Diminished carotid pulse

Digestive Tract

Subcutaneous air
Hemoptysis
Dysphagia/odynophagia

Airway

Stridor
Hoarseness
Dysphonia/voice change

Neurologic

Lateralized neurologic deficit
Altered state of consciousness
Brachial plexus injury

exploration should be sought (see Table 8). All patients should have a chest radiograph to exclude thoracic trauma. Stable patients should undergo soft tissue neck films for detecting retropharyngeal hematoma, tracheal narrowing or deviation, retained missile fragments and pathways, and subcutaneous or retropharyngeal air. Neck CT is particularly helpful in blunt trauma for evaluating laryngeal structures.[71] Patients who sustain blunt neck trauma, with a neurologic examination inconsistent with findings on head CT scan, should undergo four-vessel angiography.

As previously mentioned, the need for further diagnostic testing (angiography, panendoscopy, esophagography) versus immediate operative neck exploration is controversial. The authors believe preoperative angiography is indicated in the hemodynamically stable patient with multiple wounds or penetrating wounds to Zone III (because of the possible inaccessibility of internal carotid artery lesions) and Zone I (to identify injuries to the thoracic outlet vessels). Symptomatic isolated injuries to the midneck (Zone II) are generally explored without the aid of arteriography. Endoscopy is usually performed intraoperatively when pharyngeal or esophageal injury is suspected but cannot be found and routinely when a nonoperative policy is selected. The sensitivity of endoscopy for esophageal injuries is reported to be 29 to 83 per cent.[60,94,198] The addition of esophagography increases the accuracy and should be considered a complementary procedure.

Exploration should be performed in the operating room under general endotracheal anesthesia. A nasogastric tube is usually passed to assure an empty stomach. Preparation and draping of the patient prior to induction of anesthesia allows control of hemorrhage if the patient starts to gag at the time of placement of the endotracheal tube. The chest is also auscultated before operation, and a chest film is routinely obtained. Wounds at the base of the neck (Zone I) may follow a downward path with pleural penetration. A pneumothorax may not develop until positive pressure ventilation is applied and may initially present as unexplained hypotension during anesthesia. The incision is planned to allow full exposure of the tract of the injury. Proximal and distal control of the major vessels must also be considered in the length and position of the incision, and the patient is always prepared for a possible median sternotomy. An oblique incision along the anterior border of the sternocleidomastoid muscle usually provides access to the vessels and other important cervical structures. If bilateral exposure is required, a transverse "collar" incision may be preferable. The tract of the injury is followed to its depth, with systematic examination of each structure in or near the tract.

Management of Specific Injuries

BLOOD VESSELS. Blood vessels are the most commonly injured structures in the neck, with major arterial injuries occurring in 18 per cent of penetrating neck wounds and major venous injuries in 26 per cent.[23] The patient with the carotid artery injury can rapidly present with exsanguinating hemorrhage. The principles of operative repair of vascular structures in the neck are the same as those for other major blood vessels discussed later in the text. The topic of management of carotid artery injury and neurologic deficits has received considerable attention. Shock, coma, and neurologic deficit are adverse prognostic indicators but not contraindications to carotid repair. Patients without a neurologic deficit and a carotid injury should have restoration of vascular continuity with little expected morbidity or mortality. Patients with all grades of neurologic deficits except coma should also have primary vascular repair, since neurologic outcome and survival are improved with arterial reconstruction.[197] In comatose patients, neither repair nor ligation appears to influence a poor prognosis. The impact of prolonged ischemia and potential revascularization injury is not well defined. Ligation of the carotid artery is indicated in the comatose patient with no prograde flow, in the presence of uncontrollable hemorrhage, and when technical reasons prohibit repair. The role of extracranial-intracranial bypass in the patient requiring carotid artery ligation is evolving.

TRACHEA AND LARYNX. Penetrating injuries to the trachea and larynx are usually readily apparent and dramatic in their clinical presentation. Rapid endotracheal intubation by field paramedics may, however, mask a high tracheal injury. Primary surgical repair is always indicated and generally involves débridement of devitalized cartilage, mucosal coverage of exposed cartilage, and closure of tracheal defects. Tracheostomy is not always required, but is useful if extensive edema or prolonged airway compression is anticipated.

Blunt laryngotracheal injuries are not always obvious and are easily overlooked in the multiple trauma victim. The patients may initially appear deceptively normal, only to suddenly develop severe respiratory distress. Physical examination, flexible fiberoptic endoscopy, and computed tomography may be helpful in assessing the neck for blunt laryngotracheal injury (Fig. 30). If an emergency airway is required, direct endotracheal intubation may be performed when the laryngeal structures are well visualized, particularly when the endotracheal tube can be passed over a flexible endoscope. However, even in the most experienced hands this may be impossible and risks worsening the tracheal injury. Equipment for emergency tracheostomy must always be ready. If an emergency airway is required following blunt laryngotracheal injuries, tracheostomy is generally recommended initially, even though it also carries the risk of further injury.[71]

The basic principles of repairing tracheal injuries are primary closure of mucosal lacerations and reduction of cartilaginous fractures. Mucosal repairs should be performed with fine absorbable suture. Simple lacerations of the subglottic trachea can generally be primarily repaired with simple non-absorbable sutures. If the defect cannot be primarily closed, tracheal mobilization may bridge a gap of several tracheal rings. Controversial areas in the surgical care of patients with laryngotracheal trauma include the timing of operation, the role of laryngeal stints, the use of steroids, indications for skin grafting, and the techniques of operative exposure of the larynx.[70]

PHARYNX AND ESOPHAGUS. Injuries to the esophagus are most difficult to diagnose. The sensitivity of esophagography in detecting esophageal injury varies from approximately 50 to 90 per cent; the sensitivity of endoscopy varies from 29 to 83 per cent.[60,198] These modalities should be considered complementary; when combined, they have an accuracy of nearly 100 per cent. Operative exposure of the esophagus can be difficult. The morbidity and mortality of an overlooked esophageal injury demand a high index of suspicion, since nearly all reported deaths from cervical esophageal injuries are the result of a delayed or missed diagnosis. When injured, the structures may be repaired primarily in two layers with absorbable and nonabsorbable suture. It is important to drain all such wounds because infection or salivary fistula is not an infrequent complication. If there is massive loss of tissue as with a shotgun blast, it may be necessary to perform a cutaneous esophagostomy for feeding purposes and a cutaneous pharyngostomy for salivary drainage. A secondary reconstructive procedure is then required after the initial healing is complete. Most surgeons advocate primary repair of all esophageal injuries if accomplished early. Delays of greater than 12 hours significantly increase the risk of repair dehiscence, wound abscess, and death. Neck esophageal injuries diagnosed more than 24 to 48 hours after injury are best managed initially by diversion and drainage.

NERVES. A preoperative neurologic examination should be performed whenever possible. Brachial plexus, deep cervical plexus, phrenic nerve, and cranial nerves are systematically tested. The vagus nerve can be observed by examination of the vocal cords. A hypoglossal or spinal accessory nerve injury is particularly easy to overlook unless a preoperative neurologic examination is performed. An associated head injury or drug intoxication frequently complicates the neurologic evaluation. Primary débridement and repair of all severed or lacerated nerves is preferred, with the use of fine interrupted nonabsorbable suture on the perineurium. If a motor nerve deficit is apparent, an expendable sensory nerve such as the great auricular nerve may be interposed as a nerve graft to allow anatomosis without tension.

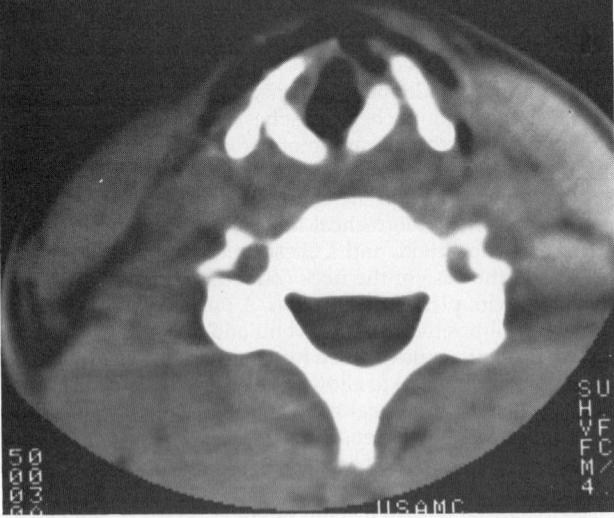

Figure 30. Computed tomography following blunt neck trauma. Subcutaneous emphysema, midline fracture and diastasis of the thyroid cartilage, and postero-lateral displacement of the right cricoarytenoid complex are demonstrated. (From Jurkovich, G. J.: The neck. *In* Moore, E. E. (Ed.): Early Care of the Injured Patient, 4th ed. Toronto, B. C. Decker, Inc., 1990, p. 126.)

MAXILLOFACIAL INJURIES

General Considerations

Maxillofacial injuries are among the most frequent injuries seen in the emergency room and have a special significance to the patient. The significance of injuries to the human face stems from its conspicuous location, aesthetic importance, and the psychologic image of "self." In addition, the face is the site of the senses of sight, smell, and taste and is the center for the vital functions of speech and mastication. Optimal management of such injuries requires a skilled approach for establishing both the nature and extent of injuries, assessing associated injuries, and initiating the appropriate treatment.

DIAGNOSTIC TECHNIQUES. CT has become an invaluable tool in the evaluation of significant maxillofacial trauma. The accuracy of defining specific fracture patterns is unsurpassed with CT scanning when compared with plain radiographs or tomograms.[50,111] CT scans are also helpful in diagnosing occult injuries that might otherwise have become apparent only during later stages of recovery and healing. In particular, the evaluation of injuries to the paranasal sinuses, orbits, and mandibular condylar heads is enhanced by the use of CT scanning. Fine-cut axial CT images with coronal reconstructions or direct fine-cut coronal scans can accurately define the extent of injuries, comminution of bony fragments, and degree of displacement (Fig. 31). In addition, specific soft tissue involvement such as medial or inferior herniation of the orbital contents through fracture lines can be accurately diagnosed only by CT scanning. This information can be extremely useful to the surgeon in directing a treatment plan.

AIRWAY COMPROMISE. Preserving sight and speech and minimizing deformity are important goals, but they have relatively low priority in the care of the multiply injured patient. Rather, the maxillofacial trauma frequently associated with upper airway compromise mandates early attention in the resuscitation of the trauma victim. The initial approach to a patient with maxillofacial trauma is no different from the assessment of any patient with multiple trauma. Respiratory obstruction is often due to the accumulation of blood, broken teeth, or other foreign substances. Certain constellations of facial and mandibular fractures are particularly prone to cause respiratory obstruction. Pulling the tongue or intact mandible anteriorly, suctioning the posterior pharynx, and passing an oro- or nasopharyngeal or endotracheal tube often is necessary to re-establish the airway. In addition, laryngeal injuries should be suspected in all patients sustaining blunt facial trauma (see neck section).

The initial management of patients with combined facial trauma and a compromised airway is critical. Transoral endotracheal intubation is sometimes complicated by the possibility of cervical spine injury. Nasotracheal intubation is hazardous in patients with mid-face fractures due to the disruption of the ethmoid plate and the potential for injury to the base of the brain. In addition, derangement of the larynx may cause a misdirected submucosal intubation and complete airway obstruction. Tracheostomy or cricothyroidotomy is therefore often required to secure the airway of a patient with significant facial injuries.[70,71]

HEMORRHAGE. Severe hemorrhage in conjunction with a facial fracture usually occurs from the nasal or oral cavity and can usually be controlled by fracture reduction combined with pressure and packing. Bleeding from nasoethmoid and/or maxillary fractures may require placement of posterior nasopharyngeal packing in addition to anterior nasal packs. Substantial hemorrhage in a patient with severe midface fractures that is not controlled by a standard nasal packing technique should arouse suspicion of laceration of one or both internal maxillary arteries, or basilar skull fracture with internal carotid artery involvement. If anatomic stabilization combined with anterior and posterior nasal and oropharyngeal packing fails to control hemorrhage, immediate angiographic evaluation and embolization are indicated and generally preferred to operative attempts at external carotid artery or selective branch ligation.

Treatment of Specific Injuries

EYES. The reported frequency of intraocular trauma in patients with facial fractures varies widely, reflecting the occult nature of some ocular injuries. Luce defined an incidence of major injury (globe rupture, laceration, a loss of sight) of 2.5 per cent.[107] The importance of visual function and the potential occult nature of ocular injuries mandates eye examinations in any patient with upper facial trauma. Assessment of visual acuity by a standard eye chart, testing of the ocular muscles and their associated cranial nerve supply, and direct visualization of the cornea, anterior chamber, and retina should be routine. A more detailed ophthalmologic and slit-lamp examination may be indicated as directed by the severity of injury. As part of the initial assessment, intraocular injury must be suspected in patients with periorbital ecchymosis, edema, or lid lacerations. Frequently, the edema is sufficiently severe to make direct examination of the eye difficult. Injuries such as anterior hyphema (blood in the anterior chamber), soft globe, loss of light perception, foreign bodies, and scleral laceration can be detected on an initial eye examination, which should be performed by all trauma surgeons.

UPPER THIRD OF THE FACE. Fractures of the upper third of the face may be accompanied by ocular or central nervous system (CNS) complications as well as by facial deformity. The facial bones are suspended from the base of the skull, and fractures of the superior facial region (e.g., the ethmoid sinuses) may readily extend into the cranial vault. Pertinent facial fractures in this region are those of the supraorbital ridge, orbital roof, frontal sinus, and nasoethmoid or orbital area. Fractures of the orbital roof are frequently associated with frontal sinus and nasoethmoid fractures but may occur as an isolated injury or as

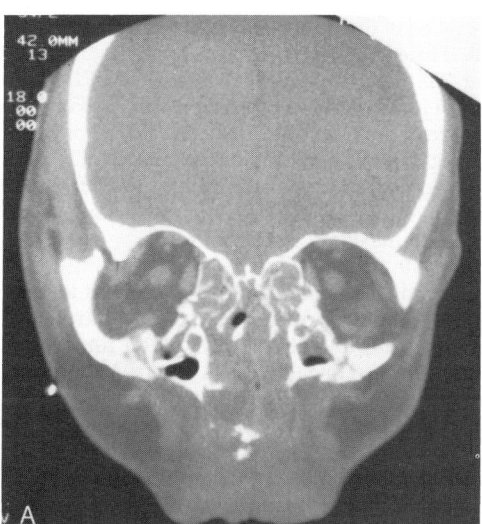

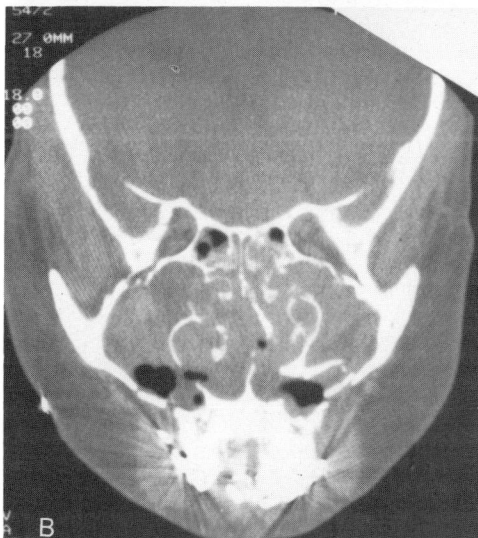

Figure 31. Computed tomography of the face. Coronal views (15-mm. separation) demonstrate the presence of a Le Fort III fracture of the right and a Le Fort II fracture of the left.

an extension of a low frontal skull fracture. The loss of upward gaze in association with this fracture indicates involvement of the superior rectus muscle and possibly superior oblique muscles. However, the most common cause of loss of upward gaze is due to orbital floor injury and associated entrapment or injury of the inferior rectus muscle. Occasionally, a fracture of the orbital roof may be so comminuted as to defy repair, and débridement with primary or delayed bone grafting may be necessary.

MIDDLE THIRD OF THE FACE. Patients with fractures of the middle third of the face may have aesthetic, CNS, ocular, and dental complications. The middle third of the face includes the maxilla, zygomas, orbits, and nose. In 1901 Le Fort published the results of his monumental experiments on human cadavers to determine the lines of least resistance in fractures of the face.[102] The classification system proposed by Le Fort has great utility in describing the most common types of traumatic mid-face fractures. In a *Le Fort I fracture* (also known as Guérin's fracture, or dentoalveolar dysjunction), the fracture lines are transverse through the pyriform aperture above the alveolar ridge and course posteriorly to the pterygoid region (Fig. 32). The dental alveolar supporting bone and palate of the maxilla are involved as a single detached block. In addition, segmental fractures of the alveolar ridge and palate can also occur. The diagnosis of Le Fort I fracture may be suggested by the presence of upper lip lacerations, complaints from the patient of malocclusion, and mobility of the fracture fragment on digital manipulation of the incisor teeth by the examiner's thumb and index finger. Required treatment varies from closed reduction with arch bars and intermaxillary fixation to open reduction with internal fixation and often bone grafting (e.g., intraosseous wiring or small plate osteosynthesis).

In *Le Fort II fractures* (pyramidal fracture of midface), the superior fracture lines are transverse through the nasal bones or through the articulation of the maxillary and nasal bones with the frontal bones. The fracture line extends laterally from that superior point into the medial orbital wall, through the lacrimal and ethmoid bones, and exits the orbital floor anteriorly at the medial to middle portions of the infraorbital rim (see Fig. 32). Occasionally, the right and left sides of the maxilla are completely separated at the midline of the hard palate, with each unit containing maxillary and palatal bones. This fracture line, or "palatal split," may splay the maxillary alveolar ridge laterally and outside the occlusal arch of the mandible. The diagnosis is established by digital manipulation of the anterior max-illa and observation for mobility of the central triangle, consisting of the maxilla and the nose. Treatment involves reduction of the maxilla, repair of any nasoethmoid component, and fixation in the proper position—to the cranial base above and to the mandible below.

The *Le Fort III fractures* (craniofacial dysjunction) represent the highest level of maxillary injuries. The central third of the face is literally displaced from its attachments to the cranial base. The transverse superior fracture line is similar to that of the Le Fort II fracture, but at the medial orbital wall it extends posteriorly or laterally, rather than anteriorly, and continues across the orbital floor to the inferior orbital fissure (see Fig. 32). From that point, the lines course through the lateral orbital wall and rim to the pterygoid fossa, zygomatic arch, and pterygoid process. An important component is a fracture line through the septum and the perpendicular plate of the ethmoid. This fracture may extend into the cribriform plate of the anterior cranial fossa and produce cerebrospinal fluid rhinorrhea, a finding that is deceptively common in patients with Le Fort II, Le Fort III, and nasoethmoid fractures.

The clinical diagnosis of Le Fort III fractures is not difficult. Massive facial edema and ecchymosis, an elongated face without normal projection, and mobility of the entire middle third of the face on digital manipulation of the maxilla establish the diagnosis. Management of Le Fort III fractures is usually deferred for stabilization and treatment of other injuries. Repairs and extensions of the principles outlined for the treatment of Le Fort I and II fractures, namely, reduction and stabilization of the midfacial complex between the cranial base and mandible, and treatment of associated fractures still apply. Le Fort III fractures often require open reduction and internal fixation with interosseous wiring or plating of the frontal bone medially at the nasal root and laterally at the orbital rim, repair of the associated nasoethmoid-orbital component, suspension to the frontal bone, and intermaxillary fixation.

The *zygoma* is also considered a structure of the middle third of the face, and its position and contour render it vulnerable to fracture. The zygoma tends to fracture at four main articulations. The fracture line at the infraorbital rim is through the infraorbital foramen or more laterally at the zygomaticomaxillary suture and then continues laterally across the orbital floor at the juncture of the zygoma with the sphenoid bone and through the lateral orbital rim at the frontozygomatic suture line. Disruption of the orbital floor may allow prolapse and herniation of the orbital contents into the maxillary antrum. The

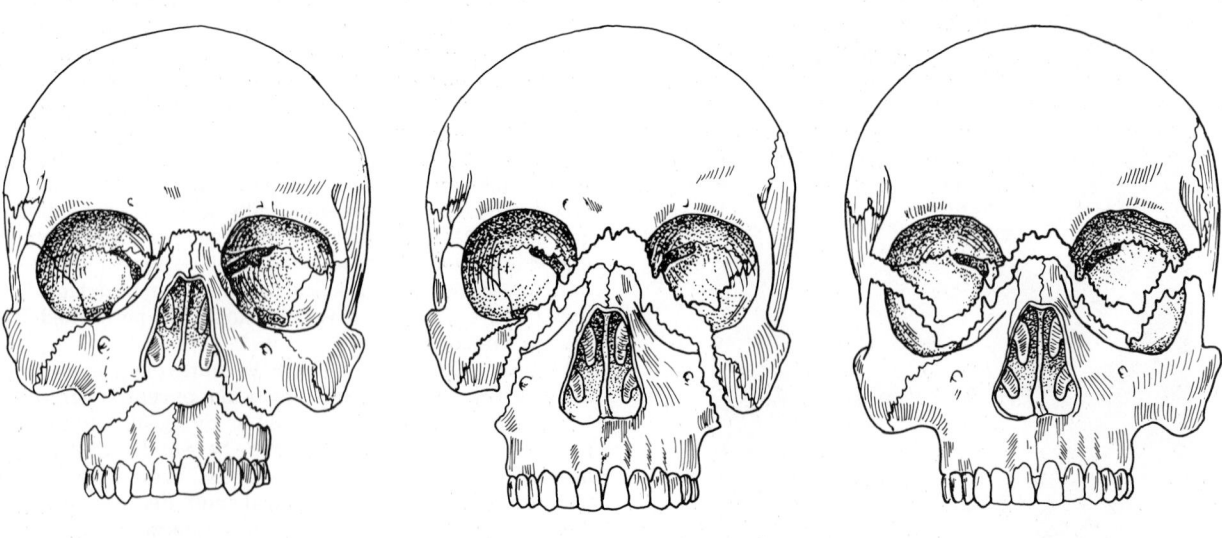

Le Fort type I   Le Fort type II   Le Fort type III

Figure 32. Le Fort I, II, and III fracture lines as seen in the frontal view.

loss of orbital fat and/or increase in orbital volume may produce a shrunken or hollow appearance to the eye or an inferior displacement of the globe, again often obscured by early postinjury edema. Of particular importance is the simultaneous herniation of the inferior rectus and oblique muscles of extraocular motion. Incarceration or entrapment of these two muscles may prevent the eye from rotating downward and outward but more commonly acts as an impediment to upward rotation by the action of the superior rectus. This loss of upward gaze should be evident on examination and produces diplopia. Unilateral pain on closing the mandible may suggest depression of the zygomatic arch component. Medial displacement of the arch fragments readily impinges on the coronoid process of the mandible and temporalis muscle and can prevent normal motion. The fourth articulation involved with the fracture is at the maxillary buttress. This can be very easily palpated intraorally at the maxillary buccal vestibule. Loss of sensation over the cheek, side of the nose, upper lip, gum, and teeth on the ipsilateral side of the fracture is a common finding in zygomatic fractures. Damage to the infraorbital nerve from a direct blow or impingement at the infraorbital foramen and as the nerve traverses the orbital floor by bone fragments is responsible. The authors have generally adopted an aggressive treatment plan for zygomatic fractures that incorporates traditional orthopedic principles of open, direct reduction and internal fixation.

LOWER THIRD OF THE FACE. The lower third of the face contains a single facial bone, the mandible. After the nasal bones, the mandible is the second most commonly fractured facial bone. The mandible does not articulate directly with the other facial bones but is suspended from the base of the skull at the temporomandibular joints. The location and direction of the fracture line are of critical importance in the degree of displacement of the fracture fragments and the success of maintenance of reduction. The sites of mandibular fractures are most commonly grouped anatomically: the regions of the coronoid process, the condyle, ramus, angle, body, parasymphysis, and symphysis (Fig. 33).

Patients may have little evidence of injury if they have sustained a single closed fracture of the condyle, although swelling, edema, and some pain on motion of the mandible are almost invariable with any fracture. Intraoral examination should focus on the occlusion, the presence of lacerations, displaced mandibular fragments, and ecchymosis of the floor of mouth. The mandible may be gently manipulated bimanually for detection of false motion or palpable fracture lines. The region of the condyles can be assessed by insertion of the examiner's finger into each external auditory canal during movement of the mandible for detection of asymmetry and absence of the normally palpable condylar head. The clinical suspicion of the fractured mandible can be confirmed on radiographic examination.

Reduction and fixation of mandibular fractures should be accomplished as precisely and expeditiously as possible, because malocclusion is a major long-term complication.[130] The risk of osteomyelitis and nonunion is enhanced by an extended period after injury without reduction and fixation. If a fracture line comminutes intraorally, bacterial colonization of the bone continues until the fragments are reduced. For these reasons,

antibiotics with coverage of common oral microflora are used in the interim between injury and reduction of the fractures.

The timing of operative repair of other facial fractures is somewhat controversial. Advocates of "early" reduction and fixation recommend that repair within 24 hours of injury is readily accomplished because of minimal edema formation and subsequently a shorter hospital stay and less patient discomfort. Proponents of a "staged" approach prefer to wait for resolution of facial edema, utilizing the time for preoperative planning, more detailed radiographic analysis, and the production of operative aids such as acrylic interocclusal splints. In addition, many of these patients have significant associated injuries that require stabilization and treatment, and the facial fractures have a lower overall priority. The ideal window for staged facial fracture repair is generally between 3 and 14 days, depending on the facial edema, associated injuries, and general status of the patient.

EXTREMITIES AND PERIPHERAL VASCULAR INJURIES

Early Fracture Stabilization

Hemorrhage due to massive disruption or transection of major blood vessels constitutes the only situation in which extremity injuries are immediately life-threatening. However, multiple long-bone fractures have recently been recognized as having a strikingly adverse impact on overall survival following injury. While specific treatment of fractures is not addressed in this chapter, the crucial role of early fracture fixation in the care of the multiply injured victim cannot be overemphasized. Early fixation of long bone fractures decreases the incidence of adult respiratory distress syndrome, fat embolization syndrome, and subsequent development of sepsis and multiple organ failure.[85,160] The exact mechanism of this beneficial effect remains unknown but appears to be related to the *early* fracture stabilization with subsequent diminished inflammatory response and an ability to rapidly mobilize the patient and initiate early feedings. Early discharge of the patient from the intensive care unit undoubtedly has additive beneficial effects.

Soft Tissue Injuries

Rarely immediately life-threatening, extensive soft tissue wounds present a difficult therapeutic challenge with significant morbidity and mortality, even with optimal treatment. The principles of management of soft tissue injuries are débridement of devitalized tissue, restoration of adequate blood supply, and adequate coverage of vital structures, including nerves, blood vessels, tendons, and other soft tissues subject to desiccation.

All lacerations and penetrating injuries of the extremities should be cleansed and meticulously débrided. No maneuver contributes as much to the prevention of tetanus or gas gangrene infection as *complete débridement of all devitalized tissue*. Following initial débridement, if there is question regarding the viability of remaining muscle or other soft tissue, re-exploration under anesthesia should be scheduled within the ensuing 24 hours. Rapidly spreading cellulitis, crepitus, erythema, or unexplained pain in an extremity is an indication for immediate surgical exploration and débridement.

Restoration of blood supply to an injured extremity receives high priority, since a few hours of ischemia may cause tissue necrosis and subsequent amputation. The classic signs of vascular compromise include *pain, palor,* and *pulselessness,* although more subtle findings, such as delayed capillary refill and venous congestion, are signs of vascular compromise that jeopardize healing of soft tissue wounds and invite secondary infection.

Adequate soft tissue coverage of exposed vital structures is essential to preventing desiccation, secondary infection, and vascular suture disruption. Although primary closure of native

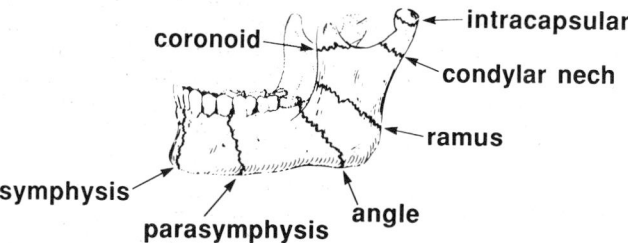

Figure 33. Anatomy of the mandible and common lines of fracture.

soft tissue is ideal, this is often impossible because of the presence of ischemic tissue, infection, or large area soft tissue defects. Early closure with auto-, allo-, or xenografts of skin provides temporary coverage pending more elaborate soft tissue reconstructive maneuvers such as free muscle flaps or combined muscle and skin rotational flaps.

PRIMARY AMPUTATION. The decision to perform primary amputation of an injured extremity is predicated on the futility of attempted limb salvage. The combination of crush or avulsion soft tissue defects with complex bony fractures and neurovascular disruption, particularly avulsion or transection of nerves to weight bearing or sensation surfaces, makes the extremity nonsalvageable. Early amputation of such mangled extremities spares the patient the morbidity and expense of a long hospital stay with multiple surgical procedures, recurrent infections, pain, and delayed rehabilitation due to a useless appendage. Extremities with less severe combined injuries represent a more difficult challenge to the surgeon's judgment; and age, associated medical problems, and concurrent injuries must also be considered.[73]

TETANUS. Tetanus is caused by the anaerobic organism *Clostridium tetani* and its toxins and is characterized by local convulsive spasm of the voluntary muscles and a tendency toward episodes of respiratory arrest. It may occur as a complication of large or small wounds, including lacerations, open fractures, burns, abrasions, or even hypodermic injections. Regardless of the active immunization status of the patient, meticulous surgical care, including removal of all devitalized tissue and foreign bodies, should be provided immediately for all wounds. Such care is as essential for the prevention of tetanus as it is for the prevention of other types of wound infection. However, the fact that approximately one third of patients seen with active tetanus either have no obvious wound or have wounds considered to be insignificant emphasizes the problem of tetanus prophylaxis following unknown or minimal wounds and suggests that the disease is not eliminated until universal active immunization has been achieved. The recommended prophylaxis schedule is outlined in Table 9.

The value of antibiotic agents in the prophylaxis of tetanus remains questionable. There is no doubt that *tetani* is sensitive *in vitro* to penicillin and tetracycline, as well as other antibiotics, but there appears to be some difficulty in delivering an adequate

dose of antibiotics to the susceptible bacteria before they liberate toxin. The tetanus-prone wound characteristically has a decreased blood supply and contains necrotic tissue that may prevent high antibiotic levels from reaching the infecting bacteria. It is recommended that antibiotic therapy not be relied upon as adequate prophylactic therapy in place of immunization. For patients with extensive necrotic wounds, particularly those in whom débridement has been delayed or compromised, penicillin and tetracycline have often been used as prophylaxis against other types of wound infection that occur as well as for prophylactic action against tetanus.

Peripheral Vascular Injuries

Penetration, perforation, transection, and lateral lacerations are the usual forms of injury among patients with penetrating wounds, whereas fracture of the intima with obstruction and thrombosis is the usual type of arterial injury following blunt trauma. Both mechanisms may also induce significant arterial spasm in the vicinity of the injury, which diminishes extremity blood flow but will improve spontaneously. Because of the possibility of hidden lacerations or the delayed development of aneurysm or arteriovenous fistulas, injuries *near* all major blood vessels should be thoroughly explored or arteriography performed (Fig. 34). Although some authors have advocated only observation of wounds in proximity to blood vessels without major signs of vascular injury, these very reports contain case studies of delayed diagnoses and overlooked injuries.[56] Although this particular issue remains controversial, current consensus favors angiographic evaluation for wounds in proximity to major vessels.

Although most cases of penetrating extremity trauma do not present a diagnostic dilemma, it may be helpful to obtain an

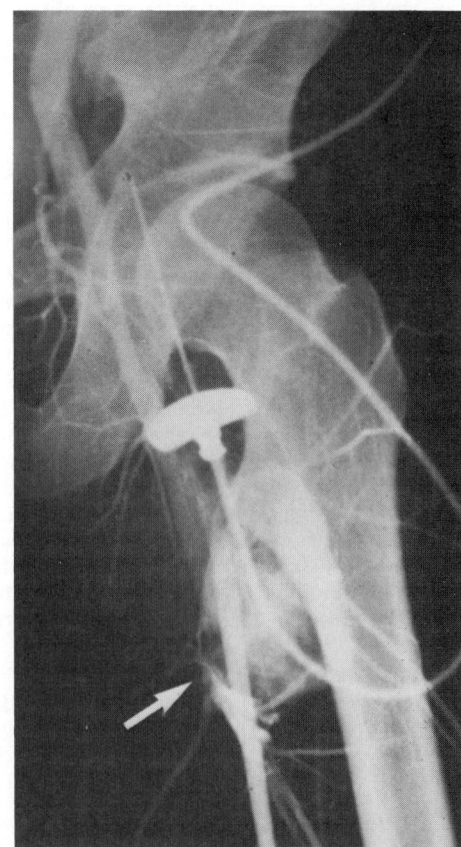

Figure 34. Penetrating wounds of the thigh can injure the profunda femoris artery, and there may be few signs except bleeding. This arteriogram reveals leakage of contrast medium (arrow) from such a wound. (From Perry, M. O.: The Management of Acute Vascular Injuries. Baltimore, Williams & Wilkins, 1981.)

TABLE 9. Immunization Schedule

Verify a history of tetanus immunization from medical records so that appropriate tetanus prophylaxis can be accomplished.

Td: Tetanus and diphtheria toxoids adsorbed (for adult use)
TIG: Tetanus immune globulin (human)

History of Adsorbed Tetanus Toxoid (Doses)	Tetanus-Prone Wounds		Nontetanus-Prone Wounds	
	*Td**	*TIG*	*Td**	*TIG*
Unknown or fewer than 3	Yes	Yes	Yes	No
3 or more†	No‡	No	No§	No

* For children less than seven years old: DTP (DT, if pertussis vaccine is contraindicated) is preferable to tetanus toxoid alone. For persons seven years old and older, Td is preferable to tetanus toxoid alone.

† If only three doses of fluid toxoid have been received, a fourth dose of toxoid, preferably an adsorbed toxoid, should be given.

‡ Yes, if more than 10 years since last dose.

§ Yes, if more than 5 years since last dose. (More frequent boosters are not needed and can accentuate side effects.)

From Advanced Trauma Life Support Course Manual. Chicago, American College of Surgeons, 1989.

arteriogram in order to ascertain the extent of damage, especially if multiple vascular injuries may be involved. Additionally, if it is believed that the proposed exploration may not allow complete visualization of the vulnerable portions of the artery and vein, arteriogram may be helpful in planning the operative approach. If severe hemorrhage has occurred, it is often prudent to perform such studies in the operating room, where resuscitation is usually easier. Spontaneous cessation of bleeding is often only temporary, and the sudden recurrence of severe hemorrhage is likely.

In the distal part of the leg, vascular injuries are more commonly associated with long-bone fractures. More extensive diagnostic studies are often required in patients with these injuries. In particular, fracture dislocation at the level of the knee is often associated with combined popliteal artery and vein injury, and arteriography should be routinely considered with a "free-floating" or posterior knee dislocation (Fig. 35). Popliteal vascular trauma is particularly devastating, requiring amputation more often than any other arterial injury. In one report, 32 per cent of patients with knee dislocations had arterial injuries, and the amputation rate was 86 per cent in those limbs that were not revascularized within 8 hours.[65] When treated by simple ligation in World War II, 73 per cent of these injuries required amputation; and despite rapid transport and improved vascular techniques, the amputation rate remained approximately 30 per cent in Vietnam and remains above 10 per cent after civilian trauma.[171]

For fracture dislocations at the knee, a coordinated approach is necessary to allow early rigid fixation of the bony injury and restoration of perfusion as early as possible. The authors have used temporary intraluminal plastic shunts positioned in the popliteal artery (and vein, if necessary) to restore perfusion and to allow the orthopedic surgeons the time necessary for reduc-

tion and fixation of the bone.[84] After this, primary repair of the blood vessel is often possible. This approach is most applicable where there is extensive soft tissue and bony injury and where immediate débridement and extensive extremity manipulation are required prior to bony fixation.

The principles of operative treatment of vascular injuries of the extremity are identical to those described in Chapter 52 for elective vascular repair. However, fasciotomy is perhaps more often used in the trauma setting. Fasciotomy is almost always necessary in situations in which there are combined popliteal artery and vein injuries, when the patient has extensive bony and muscular injury, after prolonged shock, or after several hours of ischemia. Current techniques allow routine and frequent measurements of compartment pressures and accurately indicate those patients requiring fasciotomy. Matsen and Krugmire concluded that when compartmental pressure exceeds 45 mm. Hg, cell damage is more likely and decompression may be needed, regardless of distal arterial pressure.[110] When fasciotomy is performed in this setting with these measurements, there is usually a prompt decrease in pressure followed by a return of neuromuscular function. The authors do not perform a percutaneous fasciotomy but, rather, prefer a double-incision, four-compartment fasciotomy with full incision of the skin.[119]

Whether venous injuries are best treated by repair or by ligation is still controversial. Data compiled by the Vietnam Vascular Registry revealed a significant reduction in the morbid sequelae of lower extremity venous injuries treated by repair instead of ligation, especially when associated arterial injuries were present.[150] Civilian trauma experience supports this observation, and most trauma surgeons favor simple venorrhaphy repair of major unpaired venous lacerations in the stable patient. The controversy relates to complex venous reconstruction in seriously injured patients who require extensive procedures for other injuries. In addition, the incidence of postrepair thrombosis is high, prompting the employment of a number of adjunctive techniques to maintain patency.[151] The sequelae of ligation or early thrombosis includes diminished venous outflow and hence compromised arterial inflow, extremity edema, venous stasis, and postphlebitic syndrome. Even transient patency of the venous repair allows time for the development of collateral circulation and improves arterial reperfusion. If ligation is performed, prolonged postoperative elevation and elastic extremity wrapping are suggested to reduce edema and decrease late morbidity.[121]

TRAUMA CARE SYSTEMS

Trauma is the leading cause of death in children and adults up to the age of 44 years, and injuries kill more Americans aged 1 to 34 years than all diseases combined. Because trauma is often a problem of the young, it is responsible for more productive years of life lost than cancer and all cardiovascular diseases combined. Each year, more than 140,000 Americans die of injuries, and 1 individual in 3 suffers a nonfatal injury.[127] One of every eight hospital beds is occupied by an injured patient. The cost of caring for these injuries is staggering. Direct and indirect health costs for trauma care in 1989 were an estimated $100 billion and continue to rise.

Such statistics have earned trauma the infamous recognition as the "last major plague" of the young. In 1966 the National Research Council (NRC) presented a landmark report entitled "Accidental Death and Disability: The Neglected Disease of Modern Society," documenting how little progress had been made in explicating the scientific aspect of injury control and applying what was known.[126] In 1985, the National Research Council again reported the status of trauma care in the United States in the report "Injury in America: A Continuing Health Problem."[127] Injury was again identified as "the principal public health problem in America today," highlighted by the fact that

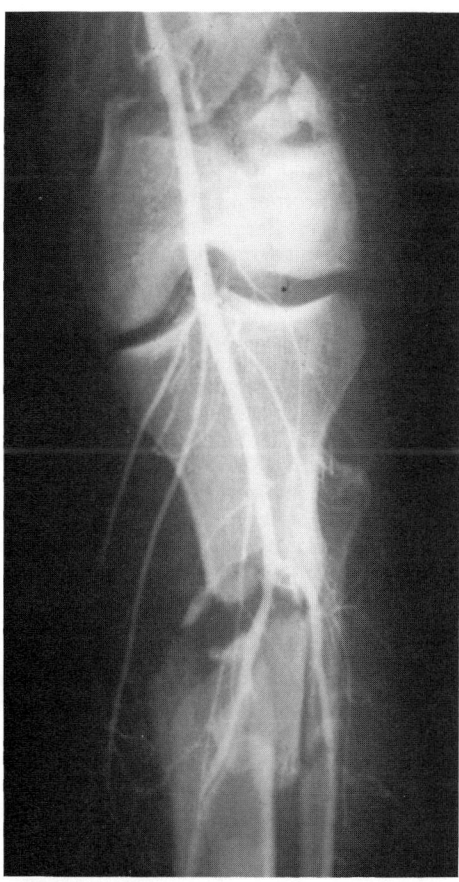

Figure 35. Vascular trifurcation injury in a patient with a "free-floating" knee from distal femur and proximal tibia-fibular fractures.

over 2.5 million Americans had died from injuries since the 1966 report. These two sentinel reports acknowledged the absence of a coordinated national approach to trauma care and suggested that special emphasis be directed to six specific topics: data collection, injury prevention, biomechanics research, prehospital and hospital care, and rehabilitation. Regionalized trauma centers, integrated with public education, injury prevention, prehospital care, quality assurance, and rehabilitation, form the basis for a systems approach to trauma care.

PREVENTION AND INJURY CONTROL

Over 50 per cent of trauma deaths occur within seconds or minutes of injury; and essentially no organized trauma care system, no matter how sophisticated, can prevent these deaths. Most, however, could be prevented.[187] Over half of the motor vehicle–related deaths in the United States involved intoxicated drivers; a staggering 80 per cent of intentional penetrating trauma deaths occur in intoxicated individuals.[127] Cities and countries with fewer handguns have a significantly lower homicide rate.[168] The mandatory use of seat belts in Australia effected a 27 per cent reduction in motor vehicle fatalities.[188] Each of these statistics represents a potential area of injury control.

The field of injury control has moved from the traditional focus on "accident prevention" to an examination of potential methods of limiting the extent of damage, i.e., the injury, to the individual.[72] The injury itself should be considered to follow energy transfer to the individual that exceeds the threshold for tissue damage. This damage can be controlled by preventing occurrence of the event (e.g., the motor vehicle crash), lessening the energy transfer to the individual (e.g., using seat belts and air bags) or by limiting the extent of the injury when it has occurred (e.g., prompt EMS and trauma center care).

Concurrent with this broadening of the scope of injury control is the shift from active to passive approaches to prevention. Active strategies are those that require active, continued cooperation on the part of the individual. In contrast, passive strategies are effective without requiring any special response from the individual. Passive approaches and combinations of passive and active strategies have proven much more successful in reducing the toll from injuries than has sole reliance on active strategies.[147] Motor vehicle occupant injuries can be prevented by the use of seat belts or air bags. The latter is a much more effective option, particularly for teenagers and intoxicated drivers because they work automatically, without requiring action by the individual user. Tap water scalds in young children can be prevented by constant and close parental supervision for the first 5 years of the child's life; alternatively, the water heater temperature setting can be lowered to 125 degrees, or, better yet, preset to this temperature at the factory.

Legislation has also been used successfully in injury control. Motorcycle helmet laws are remarkably successful in increasing helmet use from approximately 50 per cent to more than 95 per cent.[196] All 50 states have mandatory child seat restraint legislation, and more than one half have mandatory seat belt use laws for drivers and other passengers. These laws have increased seat restraint use more than 60 per cent nationwide[125] with 9 to 12 per cent reduction in occupant fatalities.[147] Many states have legislation requiring water heaters to preset at 120 to 125 degrees, eliminating the risk of this type of burn in those states.

Many problems remain, however. The politically sensitive topic of handgun control is also one of the most glaring public health and trauma problems. Each year, more than 30,000 people lose their lives from gunshot wounds, either accidentally or as a result of suicide or homicide.[5] Approximately 10-fold more are injured and require hospital and surgical care. The majority of firearm misuse is related to handguns. Substance abuse, particularly alcohol, also makes an enormous contribution to the injury toll. Although the proportion of motor vehicle fatalities involving alcohol decreased from 56 to 52 per cent between 1981 and 1986, 77 per cent of nighttime fatal crashes involve intoxicated drivers.[124] The recent Surgeon General's Workshop on Drunk Driving prepared a clear agenda for combating the problem, including administrative revocation of licenses, random breath testing, mandatory jail sentences, increased excise taxes, and lowered legal blood alcohol concentration limits.[179]

REGIONAL ORGANIZATION OF TRAUMA CARE

The goal of a trauma care system is to decrease mortality and minimize disability and morbidity following injury. Trunkey and others have suggested that trauma deaths follow a trimodal distribution: immediate, early, and late.[187] With the exception of a few patients injured in urban areas with rapid transport, most immediate deaths (severe head injury, transected aorta) can be prevented only by public education and new insights into injury control. Those patients dying an early death most often have a severe, yet correctable, injury such as epidural or subdural hematoma, hemopneumothorax, spleen or liver fracture, or blood loss from fractures and multiple injuries. The interval between injury and treatment and the quality of treatment are particularly critical in these patients. Trauma Center hospitals and coordinated prehospital care have the most direct impact on these patients. Those trauma victims who now die late generally succumb to infection, sepsis, and multiple organ failure, often as a consequence complications of initial management. It is maintained that these patients, too, will benefit from regionalized trauma care, by concentrating the most difficult patients in centers specially equipped and staffed.

The concept of regionalization of medical care is neither new nor unique to trauma care. Luft and colleagues have presented data on twelve complex general surgical procedures that demonstrate decreasing mortality with increasing volume, arguing for concentration of resources.[108] The decreasing mortality of war victims over the past century can also be directly attributable to "regionalization" of care, as discussed in the historical introduction to this chapter (see Fig. 1). West Germany studied the battlefield care in Vietnam and adopted a regionalized trauma care system along their major autobahns in 1970. Integral to this system is rapid prehospital transport, primarily by helicopters but also incorporating ground ambulances, such that 90 per cent of all West German citizens are no more than 15 minutes from a designated trauma center. This regionalized trauma care system is credited with reducing motor vehicle mortality by 25 per cent.[188] In the United States, several studies have now demonstrated the value of regionalized civilian trauma care by focusing on the concept of a "preventable" trauma death.[22] Notably, these studies from diverse geographic and demographic areas report a similar 25 to 35 per cent incidence of preventable deaths with a well-functioning trauma system.

Incorporation of regionalized trauma care throughout the United States involves immense cooperation between governments, insurance agencies, hospitals, physicians, and other health care providers. Proof that such a drastic alteration in the current practice of trauma care is truly beneficial is required prior to the wholesale commitment of resources. Data such as that provided by a number of currently functioning regional trauma care systems that clearly show a decrease in mortality and morbidity at a reasonable cost and applicable to other areas are needed.

Regionalized trauma care ideally should incorporate all three phases of trauma care: prehospital, hospital, and rehabilitation.[42] The vital components of prehospital care include a committed medical control, established lines of communication, tested triage criteria, effective transportation, and a cadre of prehospital providers well trained in specific field interventions. Hospital care consists of care provided in the emergency room, operating room, and acute care wards. Rehabilitation, too frequently ignored in regionalization concepts, has an integral role in returning the patient to a productive life-style.

Prehospital Care

Although hospitals were first developed by the Romans for care of the military legions, prehospital or field care of the injured victim can be traced to the *Edwin Smith Papyrus* (3000–1600 B.C.), and undoubtedly was provided in prehistoric times. Most of the ancient history of medicine involves the field care of the injured patient, consisting primarily of "first aid." The beginning of modern emergency medical services (EMS) can perhaps be traced to 1962, when the Chicago Committee on Trauma and the Chicago Fire Department collaborated to develop a prehospital trauma school. In 1966 the National Highway Safety Act authorized the Department of Transportation to fund ambulance services, communication systems, and training programs to address the need of the trauma victim prior to reaching the hospital. In 1969 the United States Department of Transportation published the first manual for Emergency Medical Technician-Ambulance (EMT-A) training, based on the Chicago trauma school program, to which has subsequently been added training for paramedics (EMT-P). Although emergency medical technicians now provide emergency care for nearly all aspects of medicine, trauma care clearly provided the impetus for the development of this system.

MEDICAL CONTROL. An integral component of an EMS system is active physician involvement in establishing, directing, and monitoring emergency medical care. The 1973 Emergency Medical Services Systems (EMSS) Act authorized federal funding for EMS systems that regionalized prehospital emergency care into a series of interrelated components and identified physician involvement as an essential element of this EMS system. State and local governments have since assumed responsibility for EMS development and its medical control with variable enthusiasm and effectiveness. As a result, there is wide regional variability in the policies, procedures, and authority of medical control of EMS systems. Nonetheless, the basic premise of medical control of an EMS system remains the physician-directed assurance of quality emergency medical care. In caring for the trauma patient, such assurance requires that surgeons and other physicians involved and interested in and committed to quality trauma care be knowledgeable and active participants in the medical control of EMS systems.

McSwain and others have suggested that medical control consists of three phases: prospective, immediate, and retrospective.[113] The prospective phase consists of writing treatment protocols and policies, training and certification of prehospital care providers, establishing communication, transfer and transport networks, and defining operational guidelines for record keeping and data collection.

The immediate, or "on-line," phase consists of supervision of EMS units on the scene, usually by base-hospital monitoring of communications or by the supervising physician in contact with field providers via a portable radio. The concept of immediate medical control is controversial. Some authorities believe that direct physician contact assists in triage and monitoring field times.[89] Others believe that pre-established protocols, i.e., "standing orders," expedite care and shorten field times.[79] The training and experience of prehospital providers varies widely, and the utility of pre-established treatment protocols must consider this variability. In some rural areas, direct contact with medical control may not even be immediately possible, because of long distances or adverse terrain. Nonetheless, the constant availability of physician medical control for prehospital care is essential, since the medical control physician is medically and legally responsible for the care rendered by the prehospital providers.

The retrospective phase of medical control consists of a routine review of field run sheets and emergency room care, with the goal of identifying errors in individual care or inadequacies in system policies. It is essential that data collection and record keeping be accurate and up-to-date for effective quality assurance. The development of continuing education programs is also a component of the retrospective phase of medical control. Trauma surgeons can be particularly effective educators in updating prehospital providers on individual cases and new treatment modalities. Surgeons must further continue to be involved and provide the leadership in directing and reviewing prehospital trauma care as an integral component of the trauma care system.

TRIAGE. The term *triage* is derived from the French word *trier*, meaning "to sort" or "to cull out," originally used to describe the practice of sorting wool into various categories, depending on its quality. Military triage involves prioritizing victims according to the severity of injury, likelihood of survival, and urgency of care. The goal of civilian prehospital triage in modern trauma systems is the rapid and accurate field identification of high-risk injured patients who would benefit from treatment in a trauma center. Since only 5 to 10 per cent of all injured patients are thought to require high-level trauma center care, a second consideration of civilian triage is to limit the transport of the less severely injured victims to trauma centers, thereby preventing overburdening and involving local or community hospitals in the care of the less severely injured trauma victims.[42]

The accurate field identification of a patient with high risk of major injury is problematic. Assessment often must be made quickly, often under adverse conditions with very limited resources. In addition, current schemes for identifying such high-risk patients are of limited accuracy. Many patients with severe injuries and at risk of dying can be identified at the scene of the accident by their abnormal physiology. A far more difficult problem in triage is the identification of high-risk patients whose physiologic status is normal at initial evaluation. A number of scoring systems, check lists, and criteria have been recommended to assist the EMS providers in this task of field triage[27,62,200] and to aid hospitals and trauma systems in comparing outcomes.[6,15] Perhaps the most useful currently available system is that advocated by the Committee on Trauma of the American College of Surgeons, which assesses four components: physiologic response; injury anatomy; injury biomechanics; and co-morbid factors (Fig. 36).[4]

Since the goal of a trauma system is to prevent unnecessary death, a certain degree of "over-triage" can be accepted, if trauma center care can decrease the morbidity and mortality of injury, as compared with non-trauma center care. "Under-triage" is therefore less desirable, implying that an injured patient who would have benefited from trauma center care was misclassified and sent to a non-trauma center. Studies have suggested that an over-triage rate of up to 50 per cent may be required to maintain a minimal level of under-triage. That is, 50 per cent of patients brought to the trauma center did not constitute "major trauma victims." The absolute number of patients over-triaged is small. A 1-year review of Orange County, California trauma center triage documented a 60 per cent over-triage rate based on a definition of a major trauma victim as a patient with an Injury Severity Score of 16 or greater; yet only 5.5 per cent of all paramedic transports of trauma patients during that same year went to trauma centers.[199]

FIELD INTERVENTIONS. The principles of field treatment of the trauma victim include (1) securing the area and preventing further injury, (2) determining the need for emergency treatment, (3) initiating treatment according to protocols or medical control direction, (4) communication with medical control, and (5) rapid transport of the patient to the appropriate trauma facility. The treatment rendered at the scene varies, depending on patient injury, local medical practices (as determined by medical control), and the training and experience of prehospital providers. In general, the prehospital care and hospital destination of the trauma patient is much different from

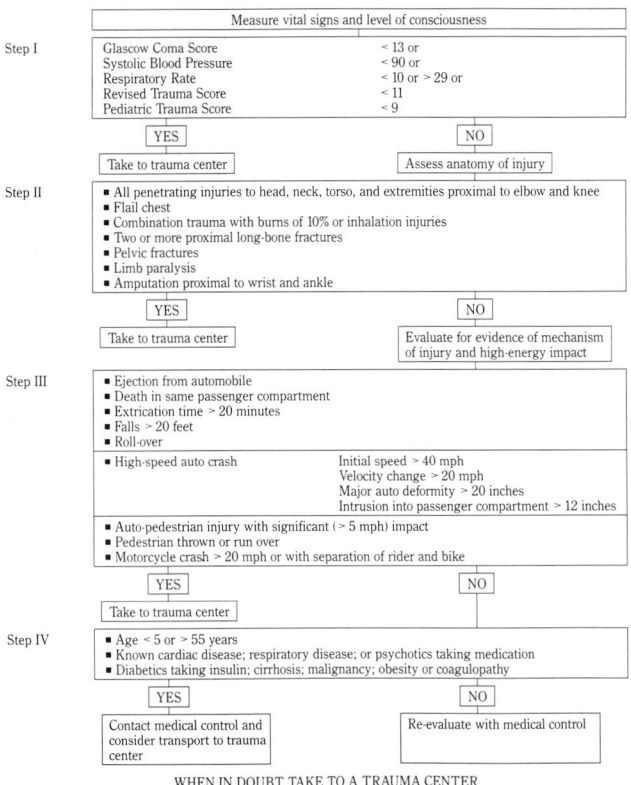

Measure vital signs and level of consciousness	

Step I

Glascow Coma Score	< 13 or
Systolic Blood Pressure	< 90 or
Respiratory Rate	< 10 or > 29 or
Revised Trauma Score	< 11
Pediatric Trauma Score	< 9

YES	NO
Take to trauma center	Assess anatomy of injury

Step II

- All penetrating injuries to head, neck, torso, and extremities proximal to elbow and knee
- Flail chest
- Combination trauma with burns of 10% or inhalation injuries
- Two or more proximal long-bone fractures
- Pelvic fractures
- Limb paralysis
- Amputation proximal to wrist and ankle

YES	NO
Take to trauma center	Evaluate for evidence of mechanism of injury and high-energy impact

Step III

- Ejection from automobile
- Death in same passenger compartment
- Extrication time > 20 minutes
- Falls > 20 feet
- Roll-over
- High-speed auto crash

  Initial speed > 40 mph
  Velocity change > 20 mph
  Major auto deformity > 20 inches
  Intrusion into passenger compartment > 12 inches

- Auto-pedestrian injury with significant (> 5 mph) impact
- Pedestrian thrown or run over
- Motorcycle crash > 20 mph or with separation of rider and bike

YES	NO
Take to trauma center	

Step IV

- Age < 5 or > 55 years
- Known cardiac disease; respiratory disease; or psychotics taking medication
- Diabetics taking insulin; cirrhosis; malignancy; obesity or coagulopathy

YES	NO
Contact medical control and consider transport to trauma center	Re-evaluate with medical control

WHEN IN DOUBT TAKE TO A TRAUMA CENTER

Figure 36. An example of a field triage decision scheme, as advocated by the Committee on Trauma of the American College of Surgeons. Note the four-step assessment of physiologic response, anatomic location, injury mechanism, and co-morbid factors. (From American College of Surgeons Committee on Trauma: Field categorization of trauma patients (field triage). *In* Resources for Optimal Care of the Injured Patient. Chicago, 1990, p. 17.)

that of the medical arrest victim. While advanced cardiac life support measures at the scene clearly improve survival for cardiac victims, the goal in prehospital trauma care is to deliver the patient to a hospital where definitive operative capabilities exist.

The role of advanced life support (ALS) interventions in the trauma victim is a topic of considerable debate, centering around the efficacy of immediate evacuation ("scoop and run") versus scene resuscitation ("stay and play").[13] Regions with highly trained and experienced paramedics often support the judicious use of prehospital ALS skills such as intravenous access and fluid administration, endotracheal intubation, and needle thoracentesis.[35,54,134] Others contend that such interventions merely prolong field times and delay the definitive operative intervention that is required. Gervin and Fischer and Ivatury and associates have shown that delayed transport time due to paramedic field interventions decreases survival in patients with penetrating cardiac injuries.[58,81] Smith and associates have termed prehospital resuscitation of the trauma victim a "failed concept," suggesting that in the urban setting the time required to establish an intravenous line is often longer than transport times.[170] Utilizing a physiologic computer model, Lewis demonstrated that intravenous fluid resuscitation in the field cannot be beneficial unless the bleeding rate is initially 25 to 100 ml. per minute, prehospital time exceeded 30 minutes, and intravenous infusion rate equaled the bleeding rate.[104]

In contrast, few would dispute that establishment of an effective airway and control of external hemorrhage are beneficial prehospital maneuvers.[134] In some systems, the field resuscitation can mimic the emergency room maneuvers, short of diagnostic steps, and save emergency room time while not delaying transport. Over a 3-year period, the Seattle Medic One paramedic EMS system transported 5761 injured patients to the same

trauma center.[32] One hundred thirty-one of these patients required cardiopulmonary resuscitation. Thirty of the 131 patients survived. An endotracheal tube was successfully placed in 29 of 30 survivors, and two intravenous lines were successfully placed in all the survivors. Twenty-two hundred milliliters of lactated Ringer's solution was administered, and the transport time averaged 22 minutes. Such interventions were interpreted as effective in resuscitating the trauma victim, as evidenced by a statistically significant increase in blood pressure from the field to the trauma center. The Denver paramedic experience is similar.[35]

TRANSPORTATION. The concept of rapid transport of injured patients to a medical facility was probably originated by Dominique Jean Larrey, the chief surgeon of Napolean's French Army. Larrey is credited with developing horse-drawn carts, or "flying ambulances," to transport the wounded as quickly as possible to medical care behind the battle lines. Until that time, the wounded were left on the battlefield until combat had ceased. By World War I the horse-drawn ambulance carts had been replaced by motorized vehicles, although the first civilian use of a motorized ambulance was during the 1906 San Francisco earthquake, when trucks and milk wagons were pressed into service to help transport the injured. The Korean Conflict introduced helicopter transportation of the wounded, a technique that was expanded and refined during the Vietnam War. Civilian aeromedical transport has been possible via military helicopters in the MAST (Military Assistance to Safety and Traffic) program since 1970, and the first hospital-based aeromedical transport program in the United States was established in Denver in 1972.[24,29] However, the explosion of hospital-based aeromedical transport programs did not occur in the United States until the early 1980s. According to the Association of Air Medical Services, in 1990 there were 180 hospital-based helicopter programs in the United States (personal communication).

The preferred method of transportation of the injured victim depends on the patient's condition, the distance to the regional trauma center, accessibility of the scene, and weather conditions. In the urban setting, ground ambulances usually afford the most efficient means of delivering the injured patient to a capable trauma center, although urban sprawl, traffic congestion, and natural barriers such as rivers may influence the decision to utilize helicopter transport.[52] In rural areas, however, the time and distance to a regional trauma center may be long, and the prehospital care provider may be confronted with the decision to transport to a closer non-trauma center or call for a remote aeromedical helicopter. Developing clear transportation guidelines is an integral component of regionalized trauma care. Such guidelines must consider regional variabilities in personnel, facilities, and geography. In general, helicopter transport may be beneficial when 15 to 20 minutes of prehospital time can be saved or when the distance to the nearest trauma center is greater than 20 to 30 miles. If transport distances exceed 100 to 150 miles, fixed-winged aircraft are more useful.[7]

The American College of Surgeons Committee on Trauma, among other organizations, has developed a list of useful and required equipment and personnel training for ambulances, ALS (paramedic-staffed) units, and aeromedical transporters.[3] The number of ambulances, ALS units or medical helicopters in any region is a function of system design, required response times, and geography. Regional medical control, supported by professional medical societies (county or state medical societies) must exercise judgment and direction to avoid inappropriate use of expensive and limited resources and prevent potential political and turf protection battles at the expense of sound patient care.

Hospital and Emergency Room Care

TRAUMA TEAM CONCEPT. Trauma care is complex, with many confusing facets; a successful patient outcome demands concise thinking and practiced execution. The care of the multi-injured victim is best suited to a team approach, with help from nurses, aides, medical technicians, and consulting physicians. The importance of predesignated team members and preassigned duties cannot be overemphasized. Of equally vital importance is the predetermined selection of a single individual as the "team leader" or "captain". It is critical that the team captain is willing to accept the responsibility of leadership and that other team members acknowledge and accept this individual as the team captain. Ideally, the team captain is the most senior trauma surgeon available, although in some institutions an emergency physician assumes this role until the surgeon is available. Overall patient assessment and all management decisions are made by the team captain; but when possible, technical procedures should be delegated to other team members. This allows the team captain to continually oversee the resuscitation, ensuring that no details are neglected or overlooked, and that the resuscitation is appropriately focused.

Other physician team members may include surgical house staff, emergency physicians, anesthesiologists, or primary care physicians experienced in trauma resuscitation. The available manpower clearly depends on the type of medical institution (i.e., community hospital versus university teaching hospital) and its resources, but sufficient personnel must be preassigned and available for trauma resuscitation. The primary role of the physician team members is to execute the therapeutic and diagnostic maneuvers ordered by the team captain, and they must refrain from independent clinical decision making. Emergency department nurses are also invaluable in trauma resuscitation. Their primary responsibilities include measuring and reporting vital signs, providing resuscitation fluids, and assisting in procedures, although a myriad of related activities are dependent on nursing organization and preparation. Documentation of resuscitation activities is an essential component of care and may require a single individual's attention. The organized response and duties of aides, technicians, (laboratory, radiology, respiratory) and assistants should add efficiency, not chaos, noise, or confusion.

The emergency room is the portal of entry into the hospital's services, not the site of definitive care. Definitive care in trauma victims often requires a surgical operation, and considerable judgment must be exercised by the team captain in not delaying essential operative procedures by minor therapeutic efforts and nonessential diagnostic maneuvers.

TRAUMA REGISTRY AND QUALITY ASSURANCE. The assurance of quality of care implies a documentation of the care delivered, an assessment of outcome, and implementation of change as a result of the assessment. Minimal operative standards of care have not been defined for trauma centers, but it has been estimated that a trauma surgeon should perform at least 50 trauma-related operations per year and that an institution should see and treat at least 500 to 1000 major trauma victims per year. Eastman and colleagues have further calculated that a single trauma center can serve approximately 1 million people.[42]

The classic method of a weekly surgical morbidity and mortality review is well suited to trauma care assessment. In addition, the periodic or ongoing audit of critical measures of quality of care such as response times, emergency room to operating room times, unplanned repeat operations, length of time to perform diagnostic maneuvers, and other similar criteria can be defined internally and should be monitored on a regular basis. The trauma registry has become an essential component of the trauma center, serving as a catalog of patients and procedures unique to trauma care.

Rehabilitation

Care of the disabled patient perhaps represents the most significant deficiency in trauma care in the United States today. For each trauma-related death, 2 to 3 patients suffer associated per-manent or partial disabilities, annually involving 350,000 patients. However, only 1 in 10 newly disabled patients will use rehabilitation facilities. The cost of disability is staggering, representing an estimated annual $35 billion in lost wages and 570 million recuperating days off work.[149] Yet for every dollar spent on rehabilitation, several dollars are saved by state and federal governments in long-term support. The relatively low incidence and prevalence of neurologic, multiple orthopedic, and burn injuries fail to show how important and costly the resulting problems can be. Unfortunately, there are no aggregate statistics on the lifetime impact of these conditions.

With the exception of a few excellent spinal cord rehabilitation centers, insignificant effort has been expended on incorporating rehabilitation into regionalized trauma care systems. However, the efficacy of rehabilitation has been well documented, at least for spinal cord injuries. Rehabilitation can provide deinstitutionalization for 85 per cent of spinal cord center patients and decrease the incidence of complications and subsequent hospitalization while costing less than one-tenth the cost of custodial care and repeated hospitalizations.[127] The spinal cord rehabilitation system should serve as a model example of incorporating regionalized rehabilitation into the global trauma care system.

RESEARCH AND EDUCATION

Identifying future directions in trauma care and injury research is also a requirement of regional centers. Research and education remain the mainstay of medical advances, and trauma care is no exception. Training providers of trauma care has historically been the province of surgery departments, with little emphasis placed on research into the epidemiology, biomechanics, rehabilitation, or prevention aspects of trauma care. Calls for improving trauma research expenditures have produced the formation of the Center for Injury Control (CIC) as a section of the Centers for Disease Control and an increased focus on trauma care as a health and social issue. Support of research in the academic setting has been a goal of the CIC and will indirectly contribute to the care rendered and the training of future researchers. Adequate funding remains problematic in a time of restricted resources and multiple major federal commitments.

In summary, idealized trauma care involves what has come to be known as "the systems approach" to trauma care. The key components of an idealized, well-functioning trauma care system begin with public education and injury prevention. Significant improvements in prehospital, hospital, and rehabilitative care can be accomplished by thoughtful organization and concentration of scarce and expensive resources. Many leaders in the field of trauma care contend that regionalization of care, increased funding for research, education, and prevention, and an equitable method of providing health care for the uncompensated or uninsured trauma victim are desperately required at this time.

REFERENCES

1. Adolfo, A. M., Kaledzi, Y. L., Parsa, M. H., and Freeman, H. P.: Penetrating neck wounds: Mandatory versus selective exploration. Ann. Surg., 202:563, 1985.
2. Allen, R. E., and Blaisdell, F. W.: Injuries to the inferior vena cava. Surg. Clin. North Am., 52:699, 1972.
3. American College of Surgeons Critical Care Air Ambulance Service. Committee on Trauma: In Resources for Optimal Care of the Injured Patient. Chicago, 1990, p. 21.
4. American College of Surgeons Critical Care Air Ambulance Service. Committee on Trauma: Field categorization of trauma patients (field triage). In Resources for Optimal Care of the Injured Patient. Chicago, 1990, p. 15.
5. American Medical Association Council on Scientific Affairs: Firearm injuries and deaths: A critical public health issue. Public Health Rep., 104:111, 1989.

6. Baker, S. P., O'Neill, B., Haddon, W., et al.: The injury severity score: A method for describing patients with multiple injuries and evaluating emergency care. J. Trauma, 14:187, 1974.

7. Baxt, W. G., and Moody, P.: The impact of rotocraft aeromedical emergency care service on trauma mortality. J.A.M.A., 249:3047, 1983.

8. Ben-Menachem, Y.: Angiography in Trauma: A Work Atlas. Philadelphia, W. B. Saunders Company, 1981.

9. Berne, C. J., Donovan, A. J., White, A. J., and Yellin, A. E.: Duodenal "diverticulization" for duodenal and pancreatic injury. Am. J. Surg., 127:503, 1974.

10. Berni, G. A., Bandyk, D. F., Oreskovich, M. R., et al.: Role of intra-operative pancreatography in patients with injury to the pancreas. Am. J. Surg., 143:602, 1982.

11. Bishara, R. A., Pasch, A. R., Douglas, D. D., Schuler, J. J., Lim, L. T., and Flanigan, D. P.: The necessity of mandatory exploration of penetrating zone II neck injuries. Surgery, 100:655, 1986.

12. Bohlman, H. H.: Acute fractures and dislocations of the cervical spine. J. Bone Joint Surg., 61A:119, 1979.

13. Border, J. R., Lewis, F. R., Aprathamian, C., Haller, J. A., Jacobs, L. M., and Luterman, A.: Prehospital patient care: Stabilize a scoop and run. J. Trauma, 23:708, 1983.

14. Bouwman, D. L., Weaver, D. W., and Walt, A. J.: Serum amylase and its isoenzymes: A clarification of their implication in trauma. J. Trauma, 24:573, 1984.

15. Boyd, C. R., Tolson, M. A., and Copes, W. S.: Evaluating trauma care: The TRISS method: trauma score and injury severity score. J. Trauma, 27:370, 1987.

16. Braakman, R.: Systematic selection of prognostic features in patients with severe head injury. Neurosurgery, 6:362-370, 1980.

17. Breaux, E. D., Dupont, J. B., Albert, H. M., et al.: Cardiac tamponade following penetrating mediastinal injuries-improved survival with early pericardiocentesis. J. Trauma, 19:461, 1979.

18. Bretan, P. N., Jr., McAninich, J. W., Federle, M. P., and Jeffrey, R. B., Jr.: Computerized tomographic staging of renal trauma: 85 consecutive cases. J. Urol., 136:561, 1986.

19. Brosman, S. A., and Paul, J. G.: Trauma of the bladder. Surg. Gynecol. Obstet., 143:605, 1976.

20. Burch, J. M., Brock, J. C., Gevirtzman, L., Feliciano, D. V., Mattox, K. L., Jordan, G. L., and DeBakey, M. E.: The injured colon. Ann. Surg., 203:701, 1986.

21. Busuttil, R. W.: Management of blunt and penetrating trauma to the portal hepatis. Ann. Surg., 191:641, 1980.

22. Cales, R. H., and Trunkey, D. D.: Preventable trauma deaths: A review of trauma care systems development. J.A.M.A., 254:1059, 1985.

23. Carducci, B., Lowe, R. A., and Dalsey, W.: Penetrating neck trauma: Consensus and controversies. Ann. Emerg. Med., 15:208, 1986.

24. Carraway, R. P., Brener, M. E., Lewis, B. R., Shaw, R. A., Ferry, R. W., and Watson, L.: Lifesaver: A complete team approval incorporated into a hospital-based program. Am. Surg., 50:173, 1984.

25. Cass, A. S., and Luxenberg, M.: Which renal lacerations will heal satisfactorily with nonsurgical management? Urology, 33:367, 1989.

26. Champion, H. R., Gainer, P. S., and Yackee, E.: A Progress report on the trauma score in predicting a fatal outcome. J. Trauma, 26:927, 1986.

27. Champion, H. R., Sacco, W. L.: Trauma scoring. In Mattox, K. L., Moore, E. E., and Feliciano, F. V. (Eds.): Trauma. Norwalk, Conn., Appleton & Lange, 1988, p. 63.

28. Champion, H. R., Sacco, W. J., Gainer, P. S., et al.: The effect of medical direction on trauma triage. J. Trauma, 28:235, 1988.

29. Cleveland, H. C., Bigelow, D. B., Dracon, D., et al.: A Civilian air emergency service: A report of its development, technical aspects, and experience. J. Trauma, 16:452, 1976.

30. Cogbill, T. H., Moore, E. E., Jurkovich, G. J., Feliciano, D. V., Morris, J. A., and Mucha, P.: Severe hepatic trauma: A multi-center experience with 1335 liver injuries. J. Trauma, 28:1433, 1988.

31. Cogbill, T. H., Moore, E. E., Jurkovich, G. J., Morris, H. A., Mucha, P., and Shackford, S. R.: Nonoperative management of blunt splenic trauma: A multi-center experience. J. Trauma, 29:1312, 1989.

32. Copass, M. K., Oreskovich, M. R., Bladergren, M., and Carrico, C. J.: Prehospital cardiopulmonary resuscitation of the critically injured patient. Am. J. Surg., 148:20, 1984.

33. Corriere, J. N., Jr., Sandler, C. M.: Management of the ruptured bladder: 7 years of experience with 111 cases. J. Trauma, 26:830, 1986.

34. Cryer, H. M., Miller, F. B., Evers, B. M., Rouben, L. R., and Seligson, D. L.: Pelvic fracture classification: Correlation with hemorrhage. J. Trauma, 28:973, 1988.

35. Cwinn, A. A., Pons, P. T., Moore, E. E., Marx, J. A., Honigman, B., and Dinerman, N.: Prehospital advanced life support for critical blunt trauma victims. Ann. Emerg. Med., 16:399, 1987.

36. Dalal, S. A., Burgess, A. R., Siegel, J. H., Young, J. W., Brumback, R. J., Poka, A., Dunham, C. M., Gens, D., and Bathon, H.: Pelvic fracture in multiple trauma: Classification by mechanism is key to pattern of organ injury, resuscitative requirements, and outcome. J. Trauma, 29:981, 1989.

37. Dale, W. A., Harris, J., and Terry, R. B.: Polytetrafluoroethylene reconstruction of the inferior vena cava. Surgery, 95:625, 1984.

38. Daughtry, D. C.: Thoracic Trauma. Boston, Little, Brown & Company, 1980.

39. Dauterive, A. H., Flancbaum, L., and Cox, E. F.: Blunt intestinal trauma: A modern-day review. Ann. Surg., 201:198, 1985.

40. Dearden, N. M., Gibson, J. S., McDowall, D. G., Gibson, R. M., and Cameron, M. M.: Effect of high-dose dexamethasone on outcome from severe head injury. J. Neurosurg., 64:81, 1986.

41. Diamond, L. K.: Splenectomy in childhood and the hazard of overwhelming infection. Pediatrics, 43:886, 1969.

42. Eastman, A. B., Lewis, F. R., Jr., Champion, H. R., and Mattox, K. L.: Regional trauma system design: Critical concepts. Am. J. Surg., 154:79, 1987.

43. Ekbom, G. A., Towne, J. B., Jajewski, J. T., and Woods, J. H.: Intra-abdominal vascular trauma: A need for prompt operation. J. Trauma, 21:1040, 1981.

44. Eraklis, A. J., and Filler, R. M.: Splenectomy in childhood: A review of 1413 cases. J. Pediatr. Surg., 4:382, 1972.

45. Federle, M. P., Goldberg, H. I., Kaiser, J. A., Moss, A. A., Jeffrey, R. B., Jr., Mall, J. C.: Evaluation of abdominal trauma by computed tomography. Radiology, 138:637, 1981.

46. Feliciano, D. V., Bitondo, C. G., Steed, G., Mattox, K. L., Burch, J. M., and Jordan, G. L., Jr.: Five hundred open taps of lavages in patients with abdominal stab wounds. Am. J. Surg., 148:772, 1984.

47. Feliciano, D. V., Jordan, G. L., Bitondo, C. G., Mattox, K. L., Burch, J. M., and Cruse, P. A.: Management of 1000 consecutive cases of hepatic trauma (1979–1984). Ann. Surg., 204:438, 1986.

48. Feliciano, D. V., Martin, T. D., Cruse, P. A., et al.: Management of combined pancreatoduodenal injuries. Ann. Surg., 205:673, 1987.

49. Feliciano, D. V., Mattox, K. L., Burch, J. M., et al.: Packing for control of hepatic hemorrhage. J. Trauma, 26:738, 1986.

50. Finkle, D. R., Ringler, S. L., Luttenton, C. R., Beernink, J. H., Peterson, N. T., and Dean, R. E.: Comparison of the diagnostic methods used in maxillofacial trauma. Plast. Reconstr. Surg., 75:32, 1985.

51. Fischer, R. P., Beverlin, B. C., Engrav, L. H., Benjamin, C., and Perry, J. F., Jr.: Diagnostic peritoneal lavage: Fourteen years and 2586 patients later. Am. J. Surg., 136:701, 1978.

52. Fischer, R. P., Flynn, T. C., Miller, P. W., et al.: Urban helicopter response to the scene of injury. J. Trauma, 24:946, 1984.

53. Flint, L. M., Blown, A., Richardson, J. D., and Polk, H. C.: Definitive control of bleeding from severe pelvic fractures. Ann. Surg., 189:709, 1979.

54. Fortner, G. S., Oreskovich, M. R., Copass, M. K., and Carrico, C. J.: The effects of prehospital trauma care on survival from a 50-meter fall. J. Trauma, 23:976, 1983.

55. Fox, M. A., and Fabian, T. C.: The Pelvis. In Moore, E. E. (Ed.): Early Care of the Injured Patient, 4th ed. Toronto, B. C. Becker, 1990, p. 176.

56. Frykberg, E. R., Crump, J. M., Vines, F. S., McLellan, G. L., Dennis, J. W., Brunner, R. G., and Alexander, R. H.: A reassessment of the role of arteriography in penetrating proximity extremity trauma: A prospective study. J. Trauma, 29:1041, 1989.

57. Garcia, J. H.: Morphology of global cerebral ischemia. Crit. Care Med., 16:979, 1988.

58. Gervin, A. S., and Fischer, R. P.: The importance of prompt transport in salvage of patients with penetrating heart wounds. J. Trauma, 22:443, 1982.

59. Gilliland, M. D., Ward, R. E., Barton, R. M., Miller, P. W., and Derke, J. H.: Factors affecting mortality in pelvic fractures. J. Trauma, 22:691, 1982.

60. Glatterer, M. S., Toon, R. S., Ellestad, C., et al.: Management of blunt and penetrating external esophageal trauma. J. Trauma, 25:784, 1985.

61. Goldstein, A., Phillips, T., Scalafani, S. J., et al.: Early open reduction and internal fixation for the disrupted pelvic ring. J. Trauma, 26:325, 1986.

62. Gormican, S.: CRAMS scale: Field triage of trauma victims. Ann. Emerg. Med., 11:132, 1982.

63. Graham, J. M., Mattox, K. L., Beall, A. C., Jr., and DeBakey, M. E.: Traumatic injuries of the inferior venal cava. Arch. Surg., 113:413, 1978.

64. Green, J. B., Shackford, S. R., Sise, M. J., and Fridlund, P.: Late septic complications in adults following splenectomy for trauma: a prospective analysis in 144 patients. J. Trauma, 26:999, 1986.

65. Green, N. E., and Allen, B. L.: Vascular injuries associated with dislocation of the knee. J. Bone Joint Surg., 59A:236, 1977.

66. Greendyke, R. M.: Traumatic rupture of aorta. Special reference to automobile accidents. J.A.M.A., 195:527, 1966.

67. Guerriero, W. G.: Trauma to the kidney, ureters, bladder, and urethra. Surg. Clin. North Am., 62:1047, 1982.

68. Guerriero, W. G.: Ureteral trauma. In McAninch, J. W. (Ed.): Trauma Management. Vol. 2, Urogenital trauma. New York, Thieme-Stratton, 1985, p. 50.

69. Gundry, S. R., Williams, S., et al.: Indications for aortography in blunt thoracic trauma: A reassessment. J. Trauma, 22:664, 1982.

70. Gussack, G. S., and Jurkovich, G. J.: Treatment dilemmas in laryngotracheal trauma. J. Trauma, 28:1439, 1988.

71. Gussack, G. S., Jurkovich, G. J., and Luterman, A.: Laryngotracheal trauma: A protocol approach to a rare injury. Laryngoscope, 96:660, 1986.

72. Haddon, W., Jr.: Advances in the epidemiology of injuries as a basis of public policy. Public Health Rep., 95:411, 1980.

73. Hansen, S. T., Jr.: Overview of the severely traumatized lower limb: Reconstruction versus amputation. Clin. Orthop., 243:17, 1989.

74. Hasson, J. E., Stern, D., and Moss, G. S.: Penetrating duodenal trauma. J. Trauma, 24:471, 1984.

75. Haygood, F. D., and Polk, H. C.: Gunshot wounds of the colon: a review of 100 consecutive patients with emphasis on complications and their causes. Am. J. Surg., 131:213, 1976.

76. Hodge, D.: Intraosseous infusions: A review. Pediatr. Emerg. Care, 1:215, 1985.

77. Homer, The Iliad, Book XVI. In Homer's Poetical Works, translated by Alexander Pope. New York, Leavitt and Allen, 1870.
78. Huguet, C., Nordlinger, B., and Bloch, P.: Tolerance of human liver to prolonged normothermic ischemia. Arch. Surg., 113:1448, 1978.
79. Hunt, R. C., Bass, R. R., Graham, R. G., et al.: Standing orders vs. voice control. J. Emergency Med. Serv., 7:26, 1982.
80. Ivatury, R. R., Nallathambi, M. N., Roberge, R. J., et al.: Penetrating thoracic injuries: In-field stabilization vs. prompt transport. J. Trauma, 27:1066, 1987.
81. Ivatury, R. R., Rohman, M., and Nallathambi, M.: The morbidity of injuries of the extra-hepatic biliary system. J. Trauma, 25:967, 1985.
82. Jeffrey, R. B., Federle, M. P., and Crass, R. A.: Computed tomography of pancreatic trauma. Radiology, 147:491, 1983.
83. Jennett, B.: Prognosis of patients with severe head injury. Neurosurgery, 4:243, 289, 1979.
84. Johansen, K. H., Bandyk, D., Thiele, B., and Hansen, S. T.: Temporary intraluminal shunts: resolution of a management dilemma in complex vascular injuries. J. Trauma, 22:395, 1982.
85. Johnson, K. D., Cadambi, A., and Seibert, G. B.: Incidence of adult respiratory distress syndrome in patients with multiple musculoskeletal injuries: Effect of early operative stabilization of fractures. J. Trauma, 25:375, 1985.
86. Jones, R. C.: Management of pancreatic trauma. Am. J. Surg., 150:698, 1985.
87. Jones, J. W., Hewitt, R. L., and Drapana, P.: Cardiac contusion: A capricious syndrome. Ann. Surg., 181:567, 1975.
88. Jurkovich, G. J.: The Neck. In Moore, E. E. (Ed.): Early Care of the Injured Patient, 4th ed. Toronto, B. C. Becker, 1990, p. 126.
89. Jurkovich, G. J., Campbell, D., Padrta, J., et al.: Paramedic perception of elapsed field time. J. Trauma, 27:892, 1987.
90. Jurkovich, G. J., and Carrico, C. J.: Management of pancreatic injuries. Surg. Clin. North Am., 70:575, 1990.
91. Jurkovich, G. J., Greiser, W. B., Luterman, A., and Curreri, P. W.: Hypothermia in trauma patients: An ominous predictor of survival. J. Trauma, 27:1019, 1987.
92. Jurkovich, G. J., and Moore, E. E.: Hemothorax. In Edlich, R. F. (Ed.): Emergency Medical Therapy—1984. Norwalk, Conn. Appleton-Century Crofts, 1984.
93. Jurkovich, G. J., and Moore, E. E.: Thoracic trauma. Trauma Q., 1:37, 1984.
94. Jurkovich, G. J., Zingarelli, W., Wallace, J., and Curreri, P. W.: Penetrating neck trauma: Diagnostic studies in the asymptomatic patient. J. Trauma, 25:819, 1985.
95. Kane, W. J.: Fractures of the pelvis. In Rockwood, C. A., Green, D. P. (Eds.): Fractures. Philadelphia, J. B. Lippincott Company, 1975, p. 923.
96. Kemmerer, W. J., Eckert, W. G., and Gathright, J. B.: Patterns of thoracic injuries and fatal traffic accidents. J. Trauma, 1:595, 1961.
97. King, H. K., and Schumacher, H. B.: Splenic studies. I. Susceptibility to infection after splenectomy performed in infancy. Ann. Surg., 136:239, 1952.
98. Kirsh, M. M., and Sloan, H.: Blunt Chest Trauma: General Principles of Management. Boston, Little, Brown & Company, 1977.
99. Krengel, W. F., Anderson, P. A., and Henley, M. B.: Neurologic recovery in patients with incomplete paraplegia due to thoracic level spinal cord injury. Presented at American Academy of Orthopedic Surgeons Annual Meeting, New Orleans, February 1990.
100. Kudsk, K. A., Voeller, G. R., McQueen, M., Mangiante, E. C., and Fabian, T. C.: Management of complex perineal soft-tissue injuries. Presented at the American Association for the Surgery of Trauma, Chicago, October 1989.
101. Larrey, D. J., Wilmott, R. (Trans.): Memoirs of a Military Surgeon. Birmingham, Ala., Classics of Surgery Library, 1985.
102. Le Fort, R.: Experimental study of fractures of the upper jaw. Rev. Chir. Paris, 23:208, 360, 479, 1901. Translated by Tessier, P. Classic Reprint: Experimental study of fractures of the upper jaw. Plast. Reconstr. Surg., 50:497; 600, 1972.
103. Ledgerwood, A. M., Kazmers, M., and Lucas, C. E.: The role of thoracic aortic occlusion for massive hemoperitoneum. J. Trauma, 16:610, 1976.
104. Lewis, F. R., Jr.: Prehospital intravenous fluid therapy: Physiologic computer modeling. J. Trauma, 26:804, 1986.
105. Llende, M., Santiago-Delpin, E. A., and Lavergne, J.: Immunobiological consequences of splenectomy: A review. J. Surg. Res., 149:716, 1985.
106. Lucas, C. E., and Ledgerwood, A. M.: Factors influencing outcome after blunt duodenal injury. J. Trauma, 15:839, 1975.
107. Luce, E. A., Tubb, T. D., and Moore, A. M.: Review of 1000 major facial fractures and associated injuries. Plast. Reconstr. Surg., 63:26, 1978.
108. Luft, H. S., Bunker, J. P., and Enthoven, A. C.: Should operations be regionalized? The empirical relation between surgical volume and mortality. N. Engl. J. Med., 301:1364, 1979.
109. Luna, G. K., and Dellinger, E. P.: Nonoperative observation therapy for splenic injuries: A safe therapeutic option? Am. J. Surg., 153:462, 1987.
110. Matsen, F. A., and Krugmire, R. B.: Compartmental syndromes. Surg. Gynecol. Obstet., 147:943, 1978.
111. Mayer, J. S., Wainesright, D. J., Yearley, J. W., Lee, K. F., Harris, J. H., and Kulkarni, M.: The role of three-dimensional tomography in the management of malliofacial trauma. J. Trauma, 28:1043, 1988.
112. McAlvanah, M. J., and Shaftan, G. W.: Selective conservatism in penetrating abdominal wounds: A continuing appraisal. J. Trauma, 18:296, 1978.
113. McSwain, N. J.: Medical control of prehospital care. J. Trauma, 24:172, 1984.
114. Merion, R. M., Harness, J. K., Ramsburgh, S. R., et al.: Selective management of penetrating neck trauma: Cost implications. Arch. Surg., 116:691, 1981.
115. Meuller, C. B.: Achilles bandaging Patroclus. Surgery, 106:589, 1989.
116. Miller, F. B., Shumate, C. R., and Richardson, J. D.: Myocardial contusion. When can the diagnosis be eliminated? Arch. Surg., 124:805, 1989.
117. Monstrey, J. J. M., Bierthuizen, G. I., VanderWerken, C., Delruyne, F. M. J., and Gopix, R. J. A.: Received treatment and hypertension. J. Trauma, 29:65, 1989.
118. Moreno, C., Moore, E. E., Majure, J. A., et al.: Hemorrhage associated with major pelvic fractures: A multispecialty challenge. J. Trauma, 26:821, 1986.
119. Mubarak, S. J., and Owen, C. A.: Double-incision fasciotomy of the leg for decompression in compartment syndromes. J. Bone Joint Surg., 59A:134, 1977.
120. Mucha, P. Jr., Farnell, M. B.: Analysis of pelvic fracture management. J. Trauma, 24:379, 1984.
121. Mullins, R. J., Lucas, C. E., and Ledgerwood, A. M.: The natural history following venous ligation for civilian injuries. J. Trauma, 20:737, 1980.
122. Nance, F. C.: Injuries to the colon and rectum. In Mattox, K. L., Moore, E. E., and Feliciano, D. V. (Eds.): Trauma. Norwalk, Conn., Appleton & Lange, 1988, p. 495.
123. Nance, F. C., Wennar, M. H., Johnson, L. W., Ingram, J. C., and Cohn, I., Jr.: Surgical judgement in the management of penetrating wounds of the abdomen: experience with 2212 patients. Ann. Surg., 179:639, 1974.
124. National Highway Traffic Safety Administration: Fatal Accident Reporting System, 1988. DOT HS 807 245, March 1988.
125. National Highway Traffic Safety Administration: Traffic Status Report, 1989.
126. National Research Council—National Academy of Sciences: Accidental Death and Disability: The Neglected Disease of Modern Society. Washington, D.C., 1966.
127. National Research Council: Injury in America: A Continuing Public Health Problem. National Academy Press, Washington, D.C., 1985.
128. Niemi, T. A., and Norton, L. W.: Vaginal injuries in patients with pelvic fractures. J. Trauma, 25:547, 1985.
129. Neff, C. C., Pfister, R. C., and VanSonnenberg, E.: Percutaneous transtracheal ventilation: Experimental and practical aspects. J. Trauma, 23:84, 1983.
130. Olson, R. A.: Fractures of the mandible: a review of 580 cases. J. Oral Maxillofac. Surg., 40:23, 1982.
131. Oreskovich, M. R., and Carrico, C. J.: Pancreaticoduodenectomy for trauma: A viable option? Am. J. Surg., 147:618, 1984.
132. Oreskovich, M. R., and Carrico, C. J.: Stab wounds of the anterior abdomen: Analysis of a management plan using local wound exploration and quantitative peritoneal lavage. Ann. Surg., 198:411, 1983.
133. Oreskovich, M. R., Dellinger, E. P., Lennard, E. S., Wertz, M., Carrico, C. J., and Minshew, B. H.: Duration of preventive antibiotic administration for penetrating abdominal trauma. Arch. Surg., 117:200, 1980.
134. Ornato, J. P., Craren, E. J., Nelson, N. M., et al.: Impact of improved emergency medical services and emergency trauma care on the reduction in mortality from trauma. J. Trauma, 25:575, 1985.
135. Pachter, H. L., Drager, S., Godfrey, N., et al.: Traumatic injuries of the portal vein: Role of acute ligation. Ann. Surg., 189:383, 1979.
136. Pachter, H. L., Lian, H. G., and Hofsteffer, S. R.: Injury to the liver and biliary tract. In Mattox, K. L., Moore, E. E., and Feliciano, D. V. (Eds.): Trauma. Norwalk, Conn., Appleton & Lange, 1988, p. 429.
137. Parks, S. E., and Hastings, P. R.: Complications of colostomy closure. Am. J. Surg., 149:672, 1985.
138. Parmley, L. F., Mattingly, T. W., et al.: Non-penetrating traumatic injury of the aorta. Circulation, 17:1086, 1958.
139. Patel, K. R., Kulkarni, S., Semel, L., Babu, S., and Clauss, R. H.: Abdominal vascular trauma. Contemp. Surg., 30:13, 1987.
140. Peitzman, A. B., Makaroun, M. S., Slasky, B. S., and Ritter, P.: Prospective study of computed tomography in initial management of blunt abdominal trauma. J. Trauma, 26:585, 1986.
141. Pennal, G. F., Tile, M., Waddell, J. P., and Garside, H.: Pelvic disruption: Assessment and classification. Clin. Orthop., 151:12, 1980.
142. Phillips, E. H., Rogers, W. F., and Gaspar, M. R.: First rib fractures: incidence of vascular injury and indications for angiography. Surgery, 89:42, 1981.
143. Phillips, T., Sclafani, S. J. A., Goldstein, A., Scalea, T., Panetta, T., and Shaftan, G.: Use of contrast-enhanced CT enema in the management of penetrating trauma to the flank and back. J. Trauma, 26:593, 1986.
144. Pickhardt, B., Moore, E. E., Moore, F. A., McCroskey, B. L., and Moore, G. E.: Operative splenic salvage in adults: A decade perspective. J. Trauma, 29:1386, 1989.
145. Pilcher, D. B., Harmon, P. K., and Moore, E. E.: Retrohepatic venal cava balloon shunt introduced via the saphenofemoral junction. J. Trauma, 17:837, 1977.
146. Powell, D. C., Bivins, B. A., and Bell, R. M.: Diagnostic peritoneal lavage. Surg. Gynecol. Obstet., 155:257, 1982.
147. Pruesser, D. F., Lund, A. K., Williams, A. F., and Blomberg, R. D.: Belt use by high risk drivers before and after New York's seat belt use law. Accid. Anal. Prev., 20:245, 1988.
148. Rene, G. J., Mattox, K. L., and Beall, A. C.: Recent advances in operative management of massive chest trauma. Ann. Thorac. Surg., 16:52, 1973.
149. Rice, D. P., MacKenzie, E. J., et al.: Cost of injury in the United States: A report to congress. San Francisco, Institute for Health and Aging, University of California, and Injury Prevention Center, The Johns Hopkins University, 1989, p. 7.
150. Rich, N. M., Hughes, C. W., Baugh, J. H.: Management of venous injuries. Ann. Surg., 171:724, 1970.

151. Richardson, J. B., Jurkovich, G. J., Walker, G. T., Nenstiel, R., and Bone, E. G.: A temporary arteriovenous shunt (Scribner) in the management of traumatic venous injuries of the lower extremity. J. Trauma, 26:503, 1986.

152. Rivara, F. P., Anderson, P. P., Maier, R. V., and Drake, C.: The epidemiology of seat belt associated injuries. J. Trauma, 1991. In press.

153. Robinette, C. D.: Splenectomy and subsequent mortality in veterans of the 1939 to 1945 war. Lancet, 2:127, 1977.

154. Root, H. D., Houser, C. W., McKinley, C. R., et al.: Diagnostic peritoneal lavage. Surgery, 57:633, 1965.

155. Roye, W. P., Dunn, E. L., and Moody, J. A.: Cervical spinal cord injury: A public catastrophy. J. Trauma, 28:1260, 1988.

156. Ryan, W., Snyder, W. III, Bell, T., and Hunt, J.: Penetrating injuries of the iliac vessels: Early recognition and management. Am. J. Surg., 144:642, 1982.

157. Sagalowsky, A. I., McConnell, J. D., and Peters, P. C.: Renal trauma requiring surgery: An analysis of 185 cases. J. Trauma, 23:128, 1983.

158. Salander, J. M., Rich, N. M., Collins, G. J., Youkey, J. R., Elliott, B. M., and Donohue, H. J.: The Edwin Smith Surgical Papyrus. Presented at the 44th Annual Meeting of the American Association for the Surgery of Trauma, New Orleans, Sept., 1984.

159. Schrock, T., Blaisdell, F. W., and Mathewson, C.: Management of blunt trauma to the liver and hepatic veins. Arch. Surg., 96:698, 1968.

160. Seibel, R., LaDuca, J., Hassett, J. M., Babikian, G., Mills, B., Border, D. O., and Border, J. R.: Blunt multiple trauma (ISS 36), femur traction, and the pulmonary failure-spetic state. Ann. Surg., 202:283, 1985.

161. Shackford, S. R., Sise, M. J., Virgilio, R. W., et al.: Evaluation of splenorrhaphy: A grading system for splenic trauma. J. Trauma, 21:538, 1981.

162. Shackford, S. R., Virgilio, R. W., and Peters, R. M.: Selective use of ventilator therapy in flail chest injury. J. Thorac. Cardiovasc. Surg., 81:194, 1981.

163. Shannon, F. L., and Moore, E. E.: Primary repair of the colon: when is it a safe alternative? Surgery, 98:851, 1985.

164. Shannon, F. L., Moore, E. E., Moore, F. A., and McCroskey, B. L.: Value of distal colon washout in civilian rectal trauma-reducing gut bacterial translocation. J. Trauma, 28:989, 1988.

165. Shoemaker, W. C., Carey, J. S., Yae, S. T., et al.: Hemodynamic monitoring for physiologic evaluation, diagnosis and therapy of acute hemopericardial tamponade from penetrating wounds. J. Trauma, 13:36, 1979.

166. Singer, D. B.: Post-splenectomy sepsis. Perspect. Pediatr. Pathol., 1:285, 1973.

167. Sirinek, K. R., and Levine, B. A.: Traumatic injury to the proximal superior mesenteric vessels. Surgery, 98:831, 1985.

168. Sloan, J. H., Kellerman, A. L., Reay, D. T., Ferris, J. A., Koepsell, T., Rivara, F. P., Rice, C., Gray, L., and LoGerfo, J.: Handgun regulations, crimes, assaults, and homicide: A tale of two cities. N. Engl. J. Med., 319:1256, 1988.

169. Smego, D. R., Richardson, J. D., Flint, L. M.: Determinants of outcome in pancreatic trauma. J. Trauma, 25:771, 1985.

170. Smith, J. P., Bodai, B. I., Hill, A. S., et al.: Prehospital stabilization of critically injured patients: A failed concept. J. Trauma, 25:65, 1985.

171. Snyder, W. H., III, Thal, E. R., and Perry, M. O.: Peripheral and abdominal vascular injuries. In Rutherford, R. B., (Ed.): Vascular Surgery. Philadelphia, W. B. Saunders Company, 1984, p. 460.

172. Snyder, W. H. III, Weigelt, J. A., Watkins, W. L., and Bietz, D. S.: The surgical management of duodenal trauma: Precepts based on a review of 247 cases. Arch. Surg., 115:422, 1980.

173. Soderstrom, C. A., DuPriest, W., and Cowley, R. A.: Pitfalls for peritoneal lavage in blunt abdominal trauma. Surg. Gynecol. Obstet., 151:513, 1980.

174. Soderstrom, C. A., Naekawa, K., and DuPriest, R. W., Jr.: Gallbladder injuries resulting from blunt abdominal trauma. Ann. Surg., 193:60, 1981.

175. Stone, H. H., and Fabian, T. C.: Management of duodenal wounds. J. Trauma, 19:334, 1979.

176. Stone, H. H., Fabian, T. C., and Turkleson, M. L.: Wounds of the portal venous system. World J. Surg., 6:335, 1982.

177. Stone, H. H., and Fabian, T. C.: Management of perforating colon trauma: Randomization between primary closure and exteriorization. Ann. Surg., 190:430, 1979.

178. Strauch, G. O.: Preservation of splenic function in adults and children with injured spleens. Am. J. Surg., 137:478, 1979.

179. Surgeon General's Workshop on Drunk Driving: Recommendations. Department of Health and Human Services, Rockville, Md., 1988.

180. Svoboda, J. A., Peter, E. T., Dang, C. V., et al.: Severe liver trauma in the face of coagulopathy: A case for temporary packing and early re-exploration. Am. J. Surg., 144:717, 1982.

181. Thal, E. R., and Yeary, E. C.: Morbidity of colostomy closure following colon trauma. J. Trauma, 20:287, 1980.

182. Thompson, D. A., Flynn, T. C., Miller, P. W., and Fischer, R. P.: The significance of scapular fracture. J. Trauma, 25:974, 1985.

183. Thompson, J., Moore, E. E.: Factors affecting the outcome of exteriorized colon repairs. J. Trauma, 22:403, 1982.

184. Touloukian, R. J.: Protocol for the nonoperative treatment of obstructing intramural duodenal hematoma during childhood. Am. J. Surg., 145:330, 1983.

185. Traub, A. C., and Perry, J. F.: Splenic preservation following splenic trauma. J. Trauma, 22:496, 1982.

186. Trinkle, J. K., Richardson, R. D., Franz, J. L., Grover, F. L., Arom, K. V., and Holmstrom, F. M. G.: Management of flail chest without mechanical ventilator. Ann. Thorac. Surg., 19:355, 1975.

187. Trunkey, D. D.: Trauma. Sci. Am., 249:28, 1983.

188. Trunkey, D. D.: Issues in Trauma Care. In Davis, J. H. (Ed.): Clinical Surgery, St. Louis, C. V. Mosby Co., 1987, p. 2759.

189. Trunkey, D. D., and Federle, M. P.: Computed tomography in perspective. J. Trauma, 26:660, 1986.

190. Trunkey, D. D., Hays, R. J., and Shires, G. R.: Management of rectal trauma. J. Trauma, 13:411, 1973.

191. VanderZee, J., Christenberry, P., and Jurkovich, G. J.: Penetrating trauma to the back and flank: A reassessment of mandatory celiotomy. Am. Surg., 53:220, 1987.

192. Vaughan, G. D., Frazier, O. H., Graham, D. Y., Mattox, K. L., Petmecky, F. F., and Jordan, G. L.: The use of pyloric exclusion in the management of severe duodenal injuries. Am. J. Surg., 134:785, 1977.

193. Veith, F. J., Gupta, S., and Daly, V.: Technique for occluding the supraceliac aorta through the abdomen. Surg. Gynecol. Obstet., 151:427, 1980.

194. Waldschmidt, M. L., and Laws, H. L.: Injuries of the diaphragm. J. Trauma, 20:587, 1980.

195. Ward, J. D., Becker, D. P., Miller, J. K, Choi, S. C., Marmarou, A., Wood, C., Newlon, P. G., and Keenan, R.: Failure of prophylactic barbiturate coma in the treatment of severe head injury. J. Neurosurg., 62:383, 1985.

196. Watson, G. F., Zador, P. L., and Wilks, A.: The repeal of motorcycle helmet use laws and increased motorcyclist mortality in the United States, 1975–1978. Am. J. Public Health, 70:579, 1980.

197. Weaver, F. A., Yellin, A. E., Wagner, W. H., Brooks, S. H., Weaver, A. A., and Milford, M. A.: The role of arterial reconstruction in penetrating carotid injuries. Arch. Surg., 123:1106, 1988.

198. Weigelt, J. A., Thal, E. R., Snyder, W. H., et al.: Diagnosis of penetrating cervical esophageal injuries. Am. J. Surg., 154:619, 1987.

199. West, J. G., and Eastman, A. B.: Field triage. In Mattox, K. L., Moore, E. E., and Feliciano, F. V. (Eds.): Trauma. Norwalk, Conn., Appleton & Lange, 1988, p. 79.

200. West, J. G., Murdock, N., Baldwin, N., et al.: A method for evaluating field triage criteria. J. Trauma, 26:655, 1986.

201. White, P. H., and Benfield, J. R.: Amylase in the management of pancreatic trauma. Arch. Surg., 105:158, 1972.

202. Yajko, R. D., Seydel, F., and Trimble, C.: Rupture of the stomach from blunt abdominal trauma. J. Trauma, 15:177, 1975.

16

SURGICAL COMPLICATIONS

A. R. Moossa, M.D., F.R.C.S., A. David Mayer, M.S., F.R.C.S.,
and M. Lavelle-Jones, M.D., F.R.C.S.

Any deviation from the expected steady recovery after a surgical operation is defined as a complication. In general, most surgical complications can be traced to the operating room and are often related to the general health of the patient and to the magnitude of the operation. Each type of surgical procedure may present special problems. Some complications may be unavoidable, particularly after emergency operations, when time does not permit optimal preoperative preparation and investigation. When planning a surgical procedure, it is a wise dictum to "strive for the best but be prepared for the worst." Good perioperative care of surgical patients is designed to minimize the incidence and severity of complications:

Preoperatively: Review all surgical and anesthetic options and the associated hazards. Anticipate potential complications in each patient. Protect patients at risk with antibiotic and thromboembolic prophylaxis, and so forth.

Intraoperatively: Monitor vital functions. Use meticulous surgical technique with attention to detail. Avoid excessive operating time.

Postoperatively: Monitor to detect and correct abnormalities early. Prevent complications with physiotherapy, early ambulation, nutritional support, and so forth.

POSTOPERATIVE FEVER AND INFECTION

An elevated temperature often occurs during routine observation of the postoperative patient but does not necessarily signal a serious complication or necessarily warrant an extensive diagnostic work-up. A specific cause is identified in less than 20 per cent of patients with pyrexia during the initial 24 hours; in the remainder it may be regarded as a normal response to surgical trauma. A comprehensive clinical examination is essential in the initial assessment of postoperative fever, although the timing and pattern of pyrexia may provide a clue to its origin.

Infective Causes of Postoperative Fever

The origin of contamination that leads to clinical infection directly influences subsequent prevention and treatment efforts. Community-acquired infections are initiated before a patient's contact with the hospital environment. Such pathogens tend to pose less difficult management problems because they have not been exposed to the chronic selective pressures created by the antibiotic-laden atmosphere and to the concentration of critically ill patients in the hospital.

The majority of postoperative infections follow contamination at the time of operation, at the operation site itself, via the airway during the general anesthesia, or from cannulas and catheters inserted in the operating room. Many are caused by hospital-acquired pathogens, which have often evolved through generations of antibiotic exposure and may have developed resistance to chemotherapeutic agents.

Local and systemic factors may compromise the ability of the host defense mechanisms to cope with contamination. The most important local factor is the adequacy of the blood supply. In devitalized tissue, necrotic areas provide an ideal environment for bacteria, where they are protected from circulating host defenses. Foreign bodies serve in a similar role, as do hematomas, in which hemoglobin is an additional potent adjuvant to bacterial proliferation.

Reduction in morbidity and mortality in patients with postoperative infection can be achieved only by a thorough understanding of prevention, early diagnosis, and definitive therapeutic intervention.

Since the mid nineteenth century, a host of independent observations and studies has broadened understanding of the infection process. Semmelweis noted that contagion that passed from the physician to the patient was responsible for the dreaded childhood fever and for subsequent septic deaths of postpartum patients. Pasteur and Koch recognized bacteria as pathogens in human infection. Lister demonstrated the usefulness of antisepsis, which led to the evolution of asepsis, and emphasized the need for even more sophisticated efforts to control infection, which remains the most persistent enemy of the surgeon.

Clinical manifestations of postoperative infection generally cause either local or systemic signs and symptoms. Local signs of postoperative infection include the traditional cardinal signs of inflammation—namely, calor, dolor, rubor, and tumor. These signs, respectively, represent clinical evidence of the nonspecific inflammatory response (heat, pain, redness, and presence of mass) in surgical patients and should serve as significant indicators of emerging infection.

Systemic manifestations of postoperative infection are usually consequences of the host febrile response. Chills, rigors, and elevated core body temperature all represent systemic manifestations of the febrile response. A specific series of pathophysiologic events triggers this response. Agents that provoke fever are referred to as endogenous or exogenous pyrogens. In patients with postoperative fever, the exogenous pyrogens are usually bacterial organisms.

A variety of systemic factors have been noted to increase vulnerability to infection. Neonates have inadequately developed host defenses, and elderly patients often experience a progressive decline in immunocompetence. The immune system may also be compromised in malnutrition, diabetes, hepatic disease and disseminated malignancy and, of course, by immunosuppressant therapy, including corticosteroids.

Obesity increases the likelihood of infection, particularly in surgical and traumatic wounds, probably due to the relatively poor blood supply of large reservoirs of subcutaneous adipose tissue. Similarly, it appears that chronic or acute severe malnutrition predisposes to infection.

Many systemic illnesses are identified with increased rates of infection. Patients with disseminated malignancy are at increased risk, at least in part, owing to the cachectic influences of the primary neoplasm and the immunosuppressive influences of systemic chemotherapy. In addition, there is increasing evidence that the patient with an active infection is at increased risk of development of a second remote septic focus.

Moreover, selected medications and drugs contribute to increased frequency and severity of infection. Acute and chronic alcohol ingestion also appears to have an immunoinhibitory effect.

Diagnostic and therapeutic efforts in the patient with postoperative fever should be directed toward recognition and eradication of the primary source of exogenous pyrogens. Characteristics of the postoperative fever may be significant in definition of the primary cause. Fever that begins within 24 hours after operation usually suggests atelectasis. Wound infections and, more rarely, abdominal abscesses are usually not identifiable until the fifth to tenth postoperative day or even later, although these patients often have fever beginning early in the postoperative course. Abscesses commonly have a recurrent, spiking pattern. Infections arising from environmental contamination during the postoperative period commonly show an antecedent period of no fever prior to temperature elevation. Foley catheter and intravenous cannula–associated infections are commonly of this type.

A comprehensive physical examination is essential in the initial assessment of postoperative fever. Specific attention should be focused on identifying signs of inflammation, such as unusual wound tenderness. Rhonchi or rales on auscultation of the chest in the early postoperative period may point to a pulmonary cause of the fever.

Pulmonary infections are common in postoperative patients. Atelectasis frequently follows general anesthesia, and aspiration or, more rarely, contaminated ventilation equipment contributes to chest infections in the immediate postoperative period. Smokers and patients with nasogastric tubes are at particular risk. Urinary tract infections are usually associated with indwelling catheters, bladder outflow obstruction, or anorectal or urologic operations.

Postoperative suppurative parotitis is now a rare complication but is still occasionally observed in elderly or debilitated patients. Parotitis is associated with dehydration and poor oral hygiene; the time of onset is usually within 2 weeks of operation and the organism is usually staphylococcus aureus.

The operative site must always be considered a potential source of sepsis. The patient often has a fever beginning early in the postoperative course, although wound infections and intraabdominal and intrathoracic abscesses are usually not identifiable clinically until at least the fifth postoperative day. Abscesses are typically associated with a recurrent, spiking fever. The pelvis and subphrenic spaces are the most common sites for intra-abdominal sepsis.

A rectal examination to exclude a pelvic collection is an essential part of any clinical examination in the febrile patient. Subphrenic collections may be associated with shoulder tip pain, tenderness on palpation of the subcostal region, or signs of a sympathetic pleural effusion with elevation of the diaphragm on clinical examination and chest films. However, there may be no localizing clinical features; and when intraperitoneal soiling is followed by a septic course, the subphrenic space should always be suspected.

Intravenous lines must also be considered as a possible site of infection, especially if blood cultures are positive. Infection at a peripheral cannulation site is usually obvious, with local cellulitis, which may be accompanied by inflammation along the course of the vein, or by lymphangitis and regional lymphadenopathy. Central line sepsis, in contrast, is often clinically occult because it is usually due to an infected thrombus at the catheter tip, rather than to sepsis at the site of skin puncture. Catheter-related sepsis is best diagnosed by culturing blood drawn through the line or the tip of the catheter following its removal.

Miscellaneous Causes of Postoperative Fever

THROMBOPHLEBITIS. Noninfective thrombophlebitis at an intravenous infusion site is a relatively common occurrence in patients receiving prolonged intravenous fluids or locally noxious drugs. Occasionally, bacterial contamination may be superimposed upon these primary chemical processes, causing suppurative infection within the vessel lumen. Unfortunately, unlike chemical thrombophlebitis, septic thrombophlebitis requires more treatment than simple removal of the intravenous catheter. Phlebitis is one of the most common causes of fever after the third postoperative day. Venous catheters should be removed at the first sign of redness, induration, or edema. Phlebitis is most frequent with cannulation of lower limb veins; thus, this route should be used only when upper extremity veins are unavailable. With suppurative phlebitis, the patient appears ill and, in addition to the local signs of inflammation, pus may be expressed from the venipuncture site. High fever and positive blood cultures are common. Treatment consists of excising the affected vein.

POSTOPERATIVE PAROTITIS. Normal saliva from healthy patients has intrinsic bacteriostatic activity. This property makes spontaneous salivary gland infection very unusual in the absence of salivary duct obstruction except in elderly and debilitated patients. Predisposing factors include poor oral hygiene, old age, avitaminosis, malnutrition, and malignancy. The time of onset is usually within 2 weeks after a major operation; the initiating factors are usually dehydration and poor oral hygiene. The infection is usually staphylococcal in origin. The diagnosis is usually evident by palpation of the swollen tender parotid gland, and a drop of pus may be observed at the intraoral opening of Stensen's duct; there is normally a high fever and a leukocytosis. Prevention requires attention to those factors that predispose the patient to these infections, such as adequate oral hygiene, avoidance of dehydration, and attention to use of anticholinergic drugs. When signs of acute parotitis appear, fluid from Stensen's duct should be cultured and an appropriate antibiotic administered. If the disease progresses, incision and drainage become necessary, care being taken to avoid damage to the facial nerve.

Noninfective Causes of Postoperative Fever

Postoperative pyrexia is not necessarily infective in origin. It may be a manifestation of the underlying disease, as in the patient with disseminated malignancy. Transfusion or drug reactions may induce fever in the early postoperative period. A hematoma may elicit a mild febrile response, or fever may originate from inflammation around an intravenous catheter after the administration of irritant fluids or drugs. Deep vein thrombosis, with the risk of pulmonary embolism, may be associated with a mild pyrexia and usually presents after the fifth postoperative day.

Postoperative acute pancreatitis is an occasional complication after upper abdominal surgery, especially operations on the biliary tract and stomach. It probably occurs more often than the quoted 3 per cent incidence because mild attacks are difficult to detect. Severe episodes have a high mortality and present with persistent postoperative fever, abdominal pain, and distention due to ileus and may progress to multisystem failure. Serum amylase and lipase are usually elevated but are not diagnostic in the postoperative patient, and computed tomographic (CT) scanning is required to establish the diagnosis. There is no specific treatment other than intensive supportive care, although pancreatitic collections and areas of necrosis may subsequently require drainage and debridement.

Metabolic causes of postoperative fever are rare but are life-threatening if untreated. Thyroid storm is an extreme manifestation of thyrotoxicosis with hyperpyrexia, tachycardia, arrhythmias, hypotension, and sweating precipitated by the stress of surgical intervention in a patient with unrecognized hyperthyroidism or thyroidectomy in an inadequately prepared patient with thyrotoxicosis. The immediate danger is tachyarrhythmia, and propranolol should be administered to control the heart rate. If still in progress, the operation should be terminated as soon as possible, and appropriate antithyroid therapy administered to block thyroid hormone synthesis.

Pheochromocytoma, a tumor derived from the adrenal medulla that produces catecholamines, may also be revealed by the stress of operation or anesthesia. It may present with fever associated with extremely labile hypertension and tachycardia, flushing, headaches, nausea, and vomiting. Treatment is to control the effects of catecholamine release with beta and alpha blockers, supplemented with a sodium nitroprusside infusion to control excessive fluctuations in blood pressure.

Malignant hyperthermia is a rare complication following the administration of muscle relaxants such as succinylcholine and inhalation general anesthetics and amide local anesthetics. It is due to a genetically determined defect in calcium release from the sarcoplasm of skeletal muscles and is manifest in approximately 1:50,000 adults but more common in children. Blood creatinine phosphokinase is elevated in 70 per cent of patients, but muscle biopsy is required to establish the diagnosis. It usually presents with high fever, tachycardia, rigidity, skin mottling, and cyanosis, usually within 30 minutes after induction of anesthesia, but occasionally with a delay of several hours. There is an associated metabolic acidosis and hyperkalemia. Treatment is to administer dantrolene, which blocks calcium release from the sarcoplasmic reticulum; to infuse sodium bicarbonate and dextrose and insulin to combat potentially lethal hyperkalemia; and to actively cool the patient. Early recognition and prompt treatment is essential in this condition, which is associated with mortality in excess of 30 per cent.

WOUND COMPLICATIONS

All surgeons must be adept in managing the problem of wound complications. The incidence depends upon the type of operation, the patient's disease and condition, and the technical proficiency and judgment of the surgeon. Most surgical services have an infection rate of 2 to 4 per cent in clean wounds. Other complications such as dehiscence, hernias, and hematoma raise the complication rate in clean wounds to approximately 5 per cent. In contaminated cases and in trauma surgery, the complication rate is higher. In emergency operations on unprepared bowel or an infected urinary tract, the rate of wound complications in reported series is as high as 50 to 60 per cent. However, as noted by several investigators, these figures are higher than they should be for all categories.

With perfect foresight, serious wound complications would be rare, because techniques for their prevention are known. Wound healing is an exceptionally complicated process; however, there are four basic phases: inflammation, epithelialization, contraction, and collagen metabolism. These four phenomena occur in an ordered sequence and are interdependent. They may be altered by a number of factors that can ultimately lead to abnormal wound healing.

Hematoma and Seroma

A hematoma is a collection of blood in the wound, usually due to inadequate hemostasis. Patients being administered low-dose heparin or aspirin have a slightly higher risk, greater still in those who are fully anticoagulated or who have a coagulation disorder. Hypotension may cause vessel spasm during operation, and the wound may appear dry at the time of closure, only to develop a hematoma a few hours later when normal blood pressure is restored.

Hematomas cause fluctuant swelling and discomfort in the wound, and there may be local bruising or discharge between sutures. Large hematomas may collect after operations such as mastectomy where the surrounding skin has been extensively undermined. Blood loss may be sufficient to cause tachycardia, hypotension, and a subsequent fall in hematocrit. Small hematomas may resorb, but they increase the incidence of wound infection. Treatment of larger collections requires evacuation of the clot under sterile conditions, ligation of bleeding vessels, and re-closure of the wound.

A seroma is a collection of fluid other than pus or blood. In small wounds, it usually follows liquefaction of necrotic fat. Large seromas are associated with operations that involve elevation of skin flaps and division of numerous lymphatic channels (e.g., mastectomy and axillary clearance or groin dissection). They can usually be prevented by placing closed suction drains beneath the flaps. Like hematomas, they provide an excellent culture medium for bacteria. Treatment consists of aspiration; if they reaccumulate, it may be necessary to insert more drains.

Wound Infection

A wound infection is a collection of pus in the wound. If there is no systemic disturbance and the complication is completely resolved by simple aspiration or discharge of pus, it can be considered a minor wound infection. A major wound infection is defined as one that makes the patient ill or delays discharge from hospital.

The infection may be primary, when the initial collection is pus, or secondary, when a sterile hematoma, seroma, or area of fat necrosis is subsequently colonized by bacteria from the blood (bacteremia) or from the environment. An infection is endogenous if the source of the bacterial inoculum is from the patient and exogenous if the source is the environment.

As previously mentioned, modern surgical therapy was made possible by the work of Pasteur, who realized that sepsis was due to microorganisms, and Lister, who introduced the concept of antisepsis. Previously, surgical procedures were generally complicated by exogenous infection with streptococci and staphylococci. Today, with the important exceptions of trauma and burns, exogenous infection is uncommon and usually indicates a break in aseptic technique or an excessively lengthy procedure. Most wound infections are endogenous, predominately caused by enteric organisms.

Wound infection follows proliferation of microorganisms in the wound. This requires

1. Inoculation of the wound with the microorganism. Experimental data indicate that an inoculum of a million or more viable staphylococci is required to produce a subcutaneous abscess in normal individuals. Almost all surgical wounds are contaminated with some microbes, but small numbers of microorganisms can be eliminated by leukocytes and antimicrobials from the bloodstream.

2. A favorable environment for bacterial proliferation such as blood or serous fluid, avascular or necrotic tissue, or foreign material that incites a tissue reaction. A wound hematoma provides an excellent culture medium for bacteria. Ischemia limits the access of host defenses from the blood, and bacteria can proliferate without hindrance if there is avascular necrotic tissue, clot, or foreign material in the wound. Wound infections develop in the subcutaneous adipose tissue, which has poor blood supply and is easily strangulated by sutures. Fat necrosis can also be caused by imprecise use of the diathermy coagulator. Many surgeons attempt to eliminate a potential dead space with fat sutures. This may be counterproductive. Skillful surgical technique, which minimizes tissue trauma, maintains the blood supply, produces good hemostasis with negligible local

necrosis, and avoids foreign material (including sutures) in the adipose layer, yields the lowest incidence of wound infections.

If bacterial swabs are obtained from the viscera at the operation's site during operation and from the wound before skin closure, wounds can be graded as *clean* if there is no growth from either swab, or *potentially contaminated* if the visceral swab is positive, or *contaminated* if the wound swab is positive.

Clean wounds rarely become infected. Occasionally, a sterile collection or area of necrotic tissue becomes secondarily infected. In contrast, in 30 per cent of contaminated wounds a wound infection develops, even if prophylactic antibiotics are administered during the operation. Wounds that are only potentially contaminated have a much lower incidence of infection (approximately 10 per cent), which suggests that direct inoculation of the wound during operation, rather than bacteremia, is the most important cause of wound infection.

Potentially contaminated wounds are usually associated with operations that involve opening a hollow viscus, and wound infection rates correlate with the bacterial load in the viscus. Thus, the greatest risk is in colonic operations, especially those involving the left colon and rectum. The bacterial count can be reduced by mechanical preparation with purgatives or enemas, but the colon cannot be completely sterilized even if nonabsorbable antibiotics are administered orally. Indeed, the efficacy of prophylactic oral antibiotics has been questioned, because they may merely lead to colonization of the bowel by resistant organisms.

The crucial element in the prevention of wound infection is a scrupulous surgical technique that avoids contamination of the wound. Occasionally, contamination is unavoidable, as in emergency laparotomy for generalized peritonitis. Wounds that are recognized as contaminated at the time of operation should be treated as infected from the outset and left open. If the wound is clean after at least 24 hours, a delayed primary closure can then be performed. Serious infections have resulted after failure to observe this important surgical principle.

The judicious use of prophylactic antibiotics has been demonstrated to reduce the incidence of wound infection in contaminated and potentially contaminated wounds. The principle is to have a high concentration of an appropriate antibiotic in the tissues and blood at the time of operation in order to eliminate any bacteria released into the operative field or bloodstream during the procedure. A single dose of antibiotic is probably sufficient unless the operation is prolonged, although two additional doses are frequently given postoperatively. Inappropriately extended administration of antibiotics intended for prophylaxis is condemned because it leads to the development of bacterial resistance. Similarly, prophylactic antibiotics should not be used as a remedy for poor aseptic technique in clean operations. It is important to distinguish prophylactic from therapeutic indications for antibiotics, because this will not only influence duration of administration, but may influence antibiotic selection. Appropriate antibiotics for these two distinct indications should be administered.

Unexplained fever in a postoperative patient always requires inspection of the wound, which may be painful and appear swollen, red, and indurated. A deep wound infection in an obese patient may not become evident for several days. The temperature usually subsides when pus is discharged.

The initial approach to an area of possible wound infection is to obtain a sample of pus or exudate for bacterial culture by needle aspiration using aseptic technique. The only definitive treatment for an infected wound is to drain it. Antibiotics are indicated only as an adjunct to surgical drainage if there is evidence of systemic infection. When wound infection is confirmed, the area should be opened to allow free drainage. Sutures or staples may need to be removed, and necrotic tissue in the wound may need to be débrided. Some irrigate the area with antiseptics to sterilize it, others pack it with gauze to keep it from closing, and others merely cover it with a pad to absorb the exudate. There is no evidence that any one of these measures is superior, provided free drainage is achieved.

Wound Failure

Wound failure is defined as partial or total disruption of any or all layers of the operative wound. There are two types of wound failure: (1) early (wound dehiscence) and (2) late (incisional hernia).

Dehiscence of chest wounds is rare; but when it occurs, it usually follows median sternotomy. Rupture of all layers of the abdominal wall with extrusion of the viscera is termed evisceration ("burst abdomen"). Evisceration occurs in approximately 1 per cent of laparotomy wounds and is associated with a mortality of approximately 20 per cent. Infection is associated with more than half of wounds that rupture.

Factors that appear to interfere with wound healing and are associated with wound failure include malnutrition, sepsis, anemia, uremia, liver failure, diabetes, and corticosteroid therapy. Obesity, heavy coughing or retching, and the accumulation of ascites, which strain the wound during the postoperative period, also predispose to failure. However, even in these patients, dehiscence is an avoidable complication if the wound is closed securely.

The strength of a wound lies in the musculoaponeurotic layer (or bony layer in the case of a median sternotomy). In the early postoperative period, it depends upon the sutures employed to close this layer of the wound. Wound dehiscence occurs because sutures break, stretch, or cut out of the tissues, because knots slip or because an insufficient number of sutures are inserted. Thus, in closing a wound, the following factors must be considered:

1. *The tensile strength of the suture material.* Suture materials may be absorbable or nonabsorbable, monofilament or braided, reactive or inert. Most surgeons use nonabsorbable sutures for wound closure because they retain tensile strength. Their disadvantage is that they persist as a foreign body in the wound and may provide a focus for infection and sinus formation, especially if made of a braided and reactive material such as silk. Absorbable sutures weaken with time, and the use of catgut, which is rapidly degraded, is associated with an unacceptable incidence of dehiscence in laparotomy wounds. The newer, relatively inert, longer-lasting absorbable materials, such as polydioxane, retain their strength during the initial weeks of wound healing and appear to be a satisfactory alternative to nonabsorbable materials.

2. *The stretching and knotting characteristics of the sutures.* Braided materials, such as silk, have little plastic or elastic stretch and are easy to knot securely. However, they may predispose to wound infection because bacteria can lie harbored in the interstices of the material, which are difficult for leukocytes to penetrate. Monofilament materials, such as nylon, require careful handling and knotting. They may stretch and lose strength if they are kinked or crushed with instruments. Some materials have "memory," so that the loops used when knotting tend to straighten, causing a knot to slip. However, secure knots can be formed when a sufficient number of "throws" are used, when the knots are squared, and when friction knots or fishermen's knots are employed.

3. *The depth of bite and number of sutures used.* A suture will cut out if the fascia being sutured is weak, especially in patients with conditions associated with poor wound healing. Sutures should be placed at least 1 cm. from the wound edge. They should be tied sufficiently tightly to obtain secure apposition of the cut edges, but not so tightly as to cause strangulation. They should be placed no more than 1 cm. apart to prevent herniation of viscera between sutures. It is useful to use at least four times as much suture as the length of the wound. Continuous suture

technique is frequently employed because of ease in performance. However, if the material should fail or cut out at a single point, the entire wound may be compromised. Interrupted suturing is more tedious to perform but is more reliable, particularly in the septic or debilitated patient.

4. *The site of the incision.* After a midline laparotomy incision, the linea alba can be closed as a single layer with secure deep bite sutures (mass closure). This is associated with a lower incidence of wound dehiscence than the standard paramedian incision, which requires separate suturing of the anterior and posterior rectus sheath with shallower bites to avoid strangulating the rectus muscles. Incisional hernia appears to be more common after mass closure, perhaps because the longer lengths of the individual sutures stretch more and because apposition of the layers of the cut edges is less precise. A "near-far, far-near" technique may remedy this problem. A secure closure can be obtained with a lateral paramedian incision. This ensures wide separation of the incisions in the anterior and posterior sheaths with the rectus muscle, which reinforces the wound. However, unless a long incision is made, access to the abdomen may be impaired. Transverse incisions, which can be closed either by a mass or a layered technique, also have a good reputation for secure closure.

In wounds that are mending securely, a healing ridge (in the form of a palpable thickening about 0.5 cm. on each side of the incision) normally appears near the end of the first week after operation. This ridge is invariably absent from wounds that rupture. Usually, the first sign of the impending problem is a discharge of serosanguinous fluid from the wound, but in some cases dehiscence presents as a sudden evisceration following an episode of coughing or retching (Table 1).

Evisceration is a harrowing experience for the patient. Immediate measures include calm reassurance, adequate analgesia, and covering of the viscera with a sterile moist towel. The wound can then be explored under general anesthesia. Devitalized tissues are excised and the wound closed with strong, nonabsorbable, nonreactive, interrupted sutures, taking deep bites into healthy tissue. "Near-far, far-near" placement prevents long intraperitoneal bridges of suture that would threaten to erode into the viscera. If the wound has dehisced but not eviscerated, an alternative in the patient who might not tolerate a further anesthetic is to pack the wound, provide external support with a binder, and accept the hernia that inevitably follows.

Hernia formation is a relatively common complication of abdominal and flank wounds. Its incidence after primary healing is approximately 1 per cent, rising to 10 per cent for infected wounds and 30 per cent after dehiscence and reclosure. Although there is evidence that fascial separation occurs in the early postoperative period in patients in whom incisional hernias develop, the defect may not become apparent for months or even years after the operation. Small abdominal hernias are often not noticed unless the patient increases intra-abdominal pressure by sitting up or coughing. Hernias with narrow necks may present acutely with incarceration, intestinal obstruction, or, if the blood supply is obstructed, strangulation.

Incisional hernias can be difficult to repair, with recurrence rates up to 40 per cent. If possible, the repair should be delayed

TABLE 1. Causes of Abdominal Wound Dehiscence

Imperfect technical closure
Increased intra-abdominal pressure from bowel distention, ascites, coughing, vomiting, or straining
Hematoma with or without infection
Infection
Metabolic diseases such as diabetes mellitus, uremia, Cushing's disease, and malignant disease with starvation
Tissues inadequate for strong closure

until the wound has healed, that is, for at least 6 months. Grossly obese patients rarely undergo successful repair unless they lose their excess weight.

RESPIRATORY COMPLICATIONS

Despite improvements in surgical and anesthetic techniques, pulmonary disorders remain the most frequent postoperative problem encountered in the surgical patient. They are cited as the principal cause of death in 25 per cent of surgical fatalities and as significant contributory factors in an additional 25 per cent. Morbidity reported for chest complications depends upon the diligence with which it is investigated. Research studies that subject all patients to postoperative blood gas analysis and chest radiographs reveal imperfections in lung function in over 50 per cent of patients after general anesthesia for cholecystectomy. However, less than 20 per cent have abnormal clinical signs, and perhaps 10 per cent are considered to have a clinically significant chest complication.

Several factors militate against normal respiratory function in the early postoperative period:

1. Effects of general anesthesia, mechanical ventilation, and postoperative analgesia, which depress the respiratory system and suppress reflexes such as coughing, which clears secretions, and periodic deep breathing and yawning, which expand collapsed alveoli
2. Depression of the immune system by trauma or sepsis
3. Progressive reduction in vital capacity by 50 to 70 per cent during the initial 12 to 18 hours after thoracotomy and laparotomy[6,9]

Even with a 70 per cent reduction in vital capacity, ventilatory reserve should be adequate to allow deep breathing and coughing unless a complication supervenes. Factors that predispose to chest complications include chronic restrictive or obstructive chest disease, smoking, obesity, prolonged general anesthesia, and the presence of a nasogastric tube.

Respiratory complications that occur in the postoperative patient can be separated into two general categories: (1) atelectasis/pneumonia and (2) acute respiratory failure.

Atelectasis and Pneumonia

The terms *atelectasis* and *collapse* are often used synonymously; but strictly, atelectasis implies that the lung tissue has never expanded. It has, however, been used to describe the postoperative condition in which small airways and alveoli lose their patency and collapse. Atelectasis is the most common complication of operations performed under general anesthesia, with radiologic evidence in up to 70 per cent of patients after thoracotomy and laparotomy.

If air passages are occluded by secretions, perhaps in association with bronchospasm, alveolar air is absorbed and the alveoli collapse. This is the most likely explanation for collapse that involves the entire segment or lobe of a lung, especially if the patient has thick, tenacious secretions. However, atelectasis is often patchy and diffuse, appearing as plates of collapsed tissue on chest films. Even during normal breathing, some alveoli collapse at the end of expiration but re-expand on inspiration. Re-expansion is facilitated by periodic deep breaths. Alveoli are able to re-expand because of surfactant, the release of which is stimulated by deep breathing, and which reduces surface tension as alveolar volume diminishes. Postoperatively, low tidal volumes and lack of periodic deep breaths inhibit release of surfactant and prevent the alveoli from re-expanding.

Therapy is directed toward prevention and early treatment. Smoking, bronchitis, prolonged general anesthesia, and nasogastric tubes all predispose to atelectasis; the incidence can be reduced if careful consideration is given these risk factors. Smokers should be urged to abstain at their initial consultation, because at least 4 days are required for any benefit. Elective operations should be delayed so that intensive preoperative physiotherapy is allowed in patients with bronchitis. The incidence of chest complications is considerably reduced in such patients if operations such as hernia repair are performed under local anesthesia. Nasogastric tubes should be removed as soon as they are no longer required.

Radiologic signs of atelectasis ("plate atelectasis") may occur in the absence of clinical evidence. Stasis in the airways is accompanied by an accumulation of secretions that are prone to infection, especially at the lung bases. Thus, the first clinical signs of atelectasis are rales, diminished breath sounds, and bronchial breathing, often accompanied by fever, tachycardia, and radiologic evidence of consolidation due to the associated pneumonia.

Treatment is directed toward clearing the secretions and re-expanding the alveoli. Physiotherapy with postural drainage and encouragement to expectorate is often effective in removing secretions. Suction is useful in patients unable to expectorate by coughing, either by the endotracheal route or via a thin, plastic cannula inserted percutaneously into the trachea ("mini-tracheostomy"). In patients with collapse of an entire lung segment or lobe, bronchoscopy may be required for visualizing and removing thick mucus obstructions from first- and second-degree bronchi.

Nebulized bronchodilators (e.g., salbutamol) should be used if there are wheezes characteristic of bronchospasm, and patients with thick secretions may also be helped by nebulized mucolytic agents (e.g., acetylcysteine). Antibiotics should be reserved for those patients with evidence of an established infection. The choice of antibiotic depends upon sputum bacteriology.

When the airway has been cleared, re-expansion often follows with deep breathing exercises and early ambulation. Mechanical intermittent positive pressure breathing (IPPB) may be effective in the delivery of nebulized inhalations, but its ability to reinflate alveoli is countered by the possibility that secretions may be propelled into more distal air passages. On balance, it is not usually recommended.

Selection of the appropriate regimen of analgesia is crucial in patients with shallow breathing. Postoperative pain is one of the major causes of decreased tidal volume, but it is important to titrate the dose of analgesia to avoid depressing the respiratory center. Atelectasis is exacerbated by shallow respirations; and if the patient demonstrates evidence of respiratory insufficiency despite the measures outlined above, endotracheal intubation and intermittent mechanical ventilation (IMV), with positive end-expiratory pressure (PEEP) to reinflate the lung, are necessary, combined with frequent endotracheal suction.

Pulmonary Aspiration

Aspiration of material from the alimentary tract into the airway can lead to two distinct complications: *aspiration pneumonitis*, which is due to the chemical composition of the aspirate; and *aspiration pneumonia*, which is due to its bacterial content. The two can coexist, with aspiration pneumonia as a complication of aspiration pneumonitis.

ASPIRATION PNEUMONITIS. Aspiration pneumonitis is caused by the aspiration of gastric contents, which are normally sterile. The consequences depend upon the nature of the aspirated material. If the pH of the aspirate is less than 2.5, it can cause a chemical burn to the airways. The syndrome was first described by Mendelson [11] in 1946 as a devastating complication of obstetric anesthesia. In addition to the effects of gastric acid, tiny particles of food cause an intense inflammatory reaction if they reach the distal air passages. Larger particles obstruct the airway, leading to collapse, and can rapidly cause hypoxic cardiac arrest if the trachea or main bronchi are occluded and not cleared rapidly.

Preventative measures minimize the risk of aspiration. The patient should take nothing orally for at least 6 hours prior to operation or, in the urgent situation, have had nasogastric drainage. As soon as muscle relaxants are administered during induction of anesthesia, the airway should be protected by cricoid pressure, followed by rapid intubation and inflation of a cuffed endotracheal tube. The development of Mendelson's syndrome may be reduced by pretreatment with antacids and H_2-antagonists.

The clinical features of dyspnea, cyanosis, and tachycardia usually appear within half an hour of aspiration, with rales and expiratory wheezes on auscultation. Chest films reveal interstitial pulmonary edema. Arterial blood gases demonstrate hypoxia and hypercapnia. The condition may rapidly deteriorate into respiratory failure and is associated with high mortality.

The supine posture and the absence of normal protective reflexes during general anesthesia predispose the surgical patient to pulmonary aspiration. The risk is increased during pregnancy, in the elderly, in the obese, and in those with hiatal hernia, full stomach, or intestinal obstruction. Because the right main bronchus is more in line with the trachea than the left, the right lung is more often affected.

Aspiration usually occurs at the time of induction, when passive regurgitation occurs during the interim between administration of muscle relaxant and intubation, and following extubation, when active vomiting may occur as a side effect of narcotic analgesia.

ASPIRATION PNEUMONIA. Aspiration pneumonia is usually due to inhalation of contents from the oropharynx that are normally at physiologic pH but contain bacteria, particularly anaerobes. It is a common cause of postoperative pneumonia and is particularly associated with poor oral hygiene and the prolonged use of nasogastric and endotracheal tubes. The risk is also increased in patients with neurologic impairment and those with compromised upper airway defenses, including smokers, the elderly, and those with a chemically induced aspiration pneumonitis. It also has a predilection for the right lung. Unlike aspiration pneumonitis, however, the episode of aspiration is usually not observed and clinical signs of pneumonia develop gradually, with fever, productive cough, rales, decreased breath sounds, and bronchial breathing. It may present as a lung abscess, which is classically associated with aspiration of purulent material and blood during dental extraction or tonsillectomy. A lung abscess presents with the production of large amounts of foul-smelling sputum or a characteristic cavity with a fluid level on chest films.

Pulmonary Edema

Pulmonary edema in the postoperative patient may be due to left ventricular failure following cardiac complications or to injury to the alveolar membrane as a result of sepsis, oxygen toxicity, and so forth, but is generally the result of circulatory overload following excessive administration of intravenous fluids. Circulatory overload may also follow absorption of fluids used for irrigation of the peritoneum or hollow viscera such as the bladder or may occur during mechanical bowel preparation, especially in those with a history of cardiac disease.

Ordinarily, plasma oncotic pressure is sufficient to retain fluid in the capillaries during alveolar gas exchange; any fluid that escapes into the interstitial space is removed by lymphatic absorption. If capillary hydrostatic pressure rises after circulatory overload or left heart failure, fluid leaks out of the capillaries, overwhelms the lymphatic drainage, and enters the alveolar lumen. The situation is exacerbated if the plasma oncotic pressure is low, for example, following massive infusions of crystalloids, or when alveolar membrane permeability increases to permit the egress of plasma proteins with the edema fluid. Edema fluid predominates at the most dependent part of the lung, where hydrostatic pressure is greatest. Therefore, the typical clinical features include orthopnea and basal crepitations. As the condition progresses, the airways fill with pink, frothy fluid, which induces bronchospasm, and the patient becomes increasingly hypoxic.

Postoperative pulmonary edema can be avoided by careful attention to fluid balance, especially in patients with a history of cardiac problems. Auscultation of the chest and observation of the jugular venous pressure remain invaluable indicators of circulatory overload in the postoperative patient receiving fluid therapy. If large fluid infusions are anticipated, a central venous or pulmonary artery line should be inserted preoperatively for monitoring the effects of fluid therapy.

Patients in the supine position are at particular risk of drowning in their edema fluid, and the immediate treatment of severe pulmonary edema is upright positioning of the patient, discontinuance of intravenous fluids, and provision of oxygen. An electrocardiogram (ECG) may demonstrate evidence of myocardial infarction or an arrhythmia requiring urgent treatment. Drug therapy includes diuretics to reduce circulatory volume, digoxin to increase cardiac output, and morphine which is known to be effective, although the mechanism is unclear. If the condition is refractory to these measures, mechanical ventilation may be necessary for treating respiratory failure and phlebotomy or hemofiltration for correcting fluid overload.

Immediate Postoperative Respiratory Depression

Respiratory depression immediately following operation is usually due to the persistent effects of narcotic analgesia used during anesthesia, or to the sustained action of muscle relaxants. Narcotics depress the respiratory center in the brain stem and can usually be reversed by antagonists such as naloxone. Patients with emphysema who rely upon an elevated $Paco_2$ to drive their respiratory center are particularly sensitive to narcotics, and respiratory efficiency may also be compromised by muscle weakness in elderly, malnourished, and septic patients.

Nondepolarizing muscle relaxants such as curare are relatively long acting. Their efforts can be potentiated by large doses of aminoglycoside antibiotics, particularly intraperitoneal irrigation with neomycin, which is readily absorbed. They can sometimes be reversed by an anticholinesterase such as neostigmine, administered in combination with atropine to prevent cholinergic bradycardia. Muscle relaxation with depolarizing agents such as neostigmine usually dissipates within about 10 minutes. The effects may be prolonged in patients taking anticholinesterase therapy for glaucoma and, more often, in those with atypical plasma cholinesterase. This is a congenital disorder with homozygous inheritance that affects 0.05 per cent of the population. It may be suspected from the family history and can be confirmed by measuring the plasma cholinesterase activity.

If respiratory depression is refractory to pharmacologic intervention outlined above, mechanical ventilation must be continued until the effects of the offending anesthetic agent disappear. It is important to be aware, however, that respiration may also be compromised in the immediate postoperative period because of aspiration, laryngeal edema, bronchospasm, massive atelectasis, pneumothorax (especially following insertion of a central venous cannula), pulmonary edema, and hypothermia. These must be sought separately and treated expeditiously because they may not respond to, and may be exacerbated by, mechanical ventilation.

Acute Respiratory Failure

Acute respiratory failure is defined as a direct, life-threatening inability to maintain adequate gas exchange in the lungs.[15] Acute respiratory insufficiency is defined as a condition in which gas exchange in the lungs can be maintained at an acceptable level only at the expense of significantly increased work of the cardiopulmonary system.[1] The increased work cannot be maintained indefinitely, so that unless the situation is improved, respiratory failure ensues. Although criteria for instituting mechanical ventilation require an assessment of arterial blood gases, ventilation, dead space, and muscle strength, in practice, respiratory failure is considered to be imminent if arterial partial pressure of oxygen (Pao_2) is less than 60 mm. Hg when one is breathing room air, or the arterial partial pressure of carbon dioxide ($Paco_2$) is greater than 60 mm. Hg in the absence of metabolic alkalosis.[12]

Postoperative respiratory failure can be caused by one, or a combination, of pulmonary defects: (1) hypoventilation, (2) imbalance between ventilation and perfusion, and (3) diminished alveolar oxygen diffusion. In addition, it may be aggravated by factors such as decreased cardiac output, anemia, and impaired oxygen-hemoglobin dissociation, which restricts oxygen delivery from the lungs to the tissues, or by sepsis, severe trauma, burns, and some formulations of intravenous nutrition that increase oxygen demand and carbon dioxide output.

Numerous etiologic features have been implicated in association with acute respiratory failure following trauma and surgical procedures (Table 2). A number of associated syndromes have been described, many of which are synonymous, including acute respiratory distress syndrome, adult respiratory distress syndrome (ARDS), Da Nang lung, and shock lung. Essentially, however, they all refer to a lung injury that causes arterial hypoxemia and hypercarbia. Mechanisms suggested for the pathogenesis of the injury in the various syndromes described include bacterial injury, endotoxin, complement activation, autoimmunity, microemboli, ischemia, and oxygen toxicity.

Although the pathogenesis of the lesion is unclear, the site of injury in all these syndromes is at the interface between the alveoli and the pulmonary capillaries. Initially, inflammatory cells and edema accumulate in the interstitial space; but as the lesion progresses, protein-rich fluid enters the alveoli. This leads to pulmonary edema and the development of hyaline membrane, which acts as a barrier to gas diffusion. Pulmonary vascular resistance increases with a consequent rise in pulmonary artery pressure. The injury also leads to loss of Type II alveolar cells, which produce surfactant. Surfactant regulates surface tension in the alveolar membranes; without it, alveoli that collapse at the end of expiration are unable to re-expand, and compliance diminishes (the lungs become stiffer).

In terms of ventilatory parameters, the pathophysiology of acute respiratory insufficiency is characterized by a decrease in functional residual capacity of the lung, indicating that the amount of air within the lungs at the end of normal respiration is reduced. As the expiratory lung volume diminishes, an increasing number of small airways collapse at the end of normal tidal respiration. This leads to progressive atelectasis with a

TABLE 2. Etiologic Factors Associated with Acute Respiratory Failure

Via the Airway
Aspiration
Oxygen toxicity
Smoke inhalation
Diffuse pneumonia
Lung contusion

Via the Blood
Sepsis
Transfusion
Fat embolism
Acute pancreatitis

Other
Head injury
Massive trauma
Radiation

diminished ventilation-perfusion ratio (intrapulmonary shunt), and a reduction in lung compliance.

The onset of acute respiratory insufficiency may be insidious. Clinically, there is a progressive increase in respiratory rate and effort due to a combination of hypoxemia and decreased lung compliance. Hyperventilation may initially induce a fall in $Paco_2$.

In the early stages of the process, some patients may respond to an increased inspired concentration of oxygen delivered by a face mask. However, the mainstay of treatment is to provide ventilatory support with IMV and to reinflate collapsed alveoli with PEEP. It is important to understand that patients with hypoxemia are not improved by mechanical ventilation alone because without PEEP alveolar collapse occurs with each expiratory phase of the respiratory cycle. PEEP also permits the inspired oxygen concentration to be reduced, which is important in the context of oxygen toxicity.

The role of ventilatory support in these patients has altered the primary concern from one of providing adequate oxygenation to one of reducing the work in breathing. The rationale for IMV is to provide an intermediate support between 100 per cent mechanical ventilation and spontaneous respiration that is tailored to the individual patient's requirement. The overall goal in postoperative respiratory failure is to provide early intervention with PEEP and IMV when hypoxemia and hypercarbia are detected, in order to avoid using continuous mechanical ventilation in the exhausted patient with noncompliant lungs and carbon dioxide retention.

Theoretically, PEEP should be administered in stepwise increments until adequate oxygenation, 70 mm. Hg, is obtained. There are, however, specific complications of PEEP therapy. Alveolar rupture, with the development of tension pneumothorax, occasionally occurs. More frequently, PEEP reduces cardiac output because intrathoracic pressure remains positive throughout the ventilatory cycle, inhibiting venous return to the heart. This is an indication for pulmonary artery catheterization and measurement of cardiac output in order to optimize the myocardial performance and to exclude other causes of diminished cardiac output.

Continuous positive airway pressure (CPAP) administered to the spontaneously breathing patient by a tight-fitting mask has been used as an alternative to PEEP therapy in patients who require intervention for hypoxemia, without hypercarbia or ventilatory insufficiency. CPAP has two advantages over PEEP: (1) there is less effect on cardiac output because negative intrathoracic pressures continue to be generated during spontaneous inspiration; (2) peak inspiratory pressures are lower, reducing the risk of pneumothorax. The disadvantage is that the patient is not relieved of the work of breathing, which increases oxygen consumption. Thus, a higher concentration of inspired oxygen must be delivered, which may exacerbate the lung lesion. This problem can be countered by delivering CPAP in conjunction with IMV to a spontaneously breathing but intubated patient.

Because of the contribution of pulmonary edema to the disease process, careful attention must be given to fluid balance, with particular care to avoid fluid overload and maintain colloid osmotic pressure. Pulmonary edema may be ameliorated by diuretics, but they should be used judiciously, because decreased vascular volume may aggravate the effect of PEEP on cardiac output.

In addition to ventilatory support, a careful search for an underlying disorder such as sepsis should be sought and treated appropriately.

SHOCK

Acute circulatory failure, commonly termed *shock*, may be defined as a life-threatening inability of the cardiovascular system to maintain adequate tissue perfusion. It is caused by a reduction in blood volume, a deterioration in cardiac output, or a combination of both. Shock can be classified into three categories according to etiology: (1) hypovolemic, (2) cardiogenic, and (3) septic.

Hypovolemic Shock

Hypovolemic shock is due to a fall in circulating blood volume and is the most frequent cause of postoperative shock. Seventy percent of circulating blood volume is in the venous system, with major venous reservoirs in the cutaneous, hepatic, and pulmonary vascular beds. An acute loss of approximately 30 per cent of blood volume can be temporarily accommodated by compensatory mechanisms:

1. Catecholamine release activated by baroreceptors in the carotid sinus and aortic arch that stimulate the sympathetic nervous system and the adrenal medulla and inhibit vagal tone. This has a positive inotropic effect on the heart, accompanied by tachycardia, arterial vasoconstriction, and increased venomotor tone, causing a relative redistribution of blood from the venous system to the arterial system and from the skin, muscle, pulmonary, splanchnic and renal beds to the heart and brain.
2. Fluid shift from the extravascular compartment into the circulation due to the reduction in hydrostatic pressure in the capillaries.
3. Increased sodium and water reabsorption from the kidneys mediated via the renin-angiotensin-aldosterone response and vasopressin release from the pituitary.

If acute blood loss exceeds approximately 40 per cent, or if shock is prolonged, there may be irreversible consequences:

1. Coronary hypoperfusion with the risk of infarction, leading to cardiac failure and secondary cardiogenic shock.
2. Renal ischemia, causing acute tubular necrosis.
3. Metabolic acidosis due to a combination of deficient renal excretion of hydrogen ions and increased anaerobic metabolism with lactate production by the tissues, which may further depress the myocardium.
4. Cerebral hypoperfusion, which is aggravated by the reduction in $Paco_2$ associated with metabolic acidosis.
5. An initial increase in blood coagulability, which may progress to disseminated intravascular coagulation. Subsequently, clotting factors are diminished, both as a result of consumption and because of hepatic ischemia.
6. Depression of the reticuloendothelial system, in particular the Kupffer cells in the liver, which detoxify portal blood from the bowel. This predisposes to the added insult of endotoxemia.
7. Ischemic injury to vascular endothelium following prolonged vasospasm, which increases capillary permeability, leading to generalized edema and *shock lung*.

Hypovolemia may reflect an uncorrected preoperative volume deficit, unreplaced blood or other fluid losses during the operation, or an inadequate postoperative fluid regimen. Continuing hemorrhage in the postoperative period must always be considered.

Tachycardia is the earliest sign of hypovolemia, followed by hypotension when compensatory mechanisms are overwhelmed. The mucus membranes are dry, there is loss of cutaneous elasticity, and the skin is pale, cold, and sweaty in response to catecholamine release. The respiratory rate increases in response to catecholamine release, baroreceptor reflexes, tissue hypoxia, and metabolic acidosis. Confusion is a sign of compromised cerebral blood flow.

Treatment is by rapid replacement of the volume deficit with intravenous fluids through one or more large caliber intravenous cannulas, and should be monitored by measurement of pulse rate, arterial and central venous or pulmonary artery pressures, urinary output, and return of skin blood flow (core-peripheral temperature). The choice of fluid used to correct hypovolemia is controversial and depends upon the cause. Blood and colloid solutions may be used to maintain circulating volume during active hemorrhage but are not adequate to resuscitate the patient with a large extracellular or "third space" loss. Exteriorization of the viscera and extensive dissection of tissue planes are associated with loss of extracellular fluid through evaporation. Postoperatively, there is a redistribution of tissue fluids due to interstitial edema, and sequestration into the bowel. Optimal replacement is provided by fluids that are evenly distributed throughout the extracellular space, limiting the value of colloids and plasma expanders such as dextran, which are retained in the intravascular compartment alone. Maximal benefit is obtained with a combination of packed red cells to replace the red cell volume loss, together with a balanced electrolyte solution such as Hartmann's or Ringer's lactate to replace the extracellular fluid.

Resuscitation is adequate when the systolic blood pressure has returned to the preoperative level, with a central venous pressure (CVP) between 5 and 10 cm. H_2O or a pulmonary artery (PA) wedge pressure between 10 and 15 mm. Hg. The urinary output should exceed 30 ml. per hour. If this cannot be achieved or sustained, the likelihood of continuing hemorrhage must be considered. This may be obvious if copious amounts of blood appear from drainage tubes. However, bleeding from the operative site may be difficult to detect, especially after an abdominal operation even when drains are present.

Hemorrhage in the immediate postoperative period (reactionary hemorrhage) is usually due to a single bleeding vessel, whereas delayed (secondary) hemorrhage is often associated with diffuse bleeding from an infected operative site. When a major transfusion has been required, a coagulation profile may reveal a hemorrhagic diathesis, which requires specific treatment with coagulation factors and platelets.

Cardiogenic Shock

Cardiogenic shock is usually secondary to myocardial ischemia or infarction with left ventricular failure or arrhythmia, causing inadequate cardiac output. Cardiac failure due to tamponade, mediastinal distortion or compression can occur following cardiothoracic surgery. Cardiac failure may also complicate severe hypovolemic or septic shock and, conversely, may be induced by fluid overload, especially in the elderly or those with pre-existing heart disease.

Accurate diagnosis is essential because treatment regimens for cardiogenic and hypovolemic shock are quite different. Even in the absence of ECG changes, cardiogenic shock is suggested on clinical examination by an elevated jugular venous pressure, gallop rhythm, and bilateral chest crepitations due to pulmonary edema, in addition to the features of poor peripheral perfusion.

Accurate evaluation and optimal therapy require invasive monitoring in an intensive care unit (ICU). The assessment of cardiac performance by CVP measurement is limited. The normal range of CVP is from 2 to 10 cm. H_2O, and values exceeding this range suggest a fluid overload or primary cardiac failure, as does an increase greater than 2 cm. H_2O above the control level in response to a 250-ml. fluid challenge. Pulmonary artery pressure measurements by means of a Swan-Ganz catheter allow more clear discrimination between inappropriate fluid replacement and pump failure. This balloon-tipped catheter, when wedged in a distal pulmonary artery, accurately reflects the left ventricular filling pressure and provides a sensitive guide to fluid loading when myocardial function is compromised. A pressure in excess of 15 mm. Hg indicates fluid overload, and a pressure below 10 mm. Hg suggests hypovolemia. In addition, cardiac output can be computed by means of thermodilution techniques if a thermistor-tipped catheter is used.

The accurate monitoring of fluid status and cardiac performance achieved by these methods allows fluid status to be carefully controlled to optimize filling of the heart (ventricular preload) in accordance with Starling's law, and then to direct attention to optimizing myocardial efficiency by means of inotropic vasoactive drugs.

A positive inotropic agent increases the force of myocardial contraction without increasing the heart rate. Conversely, some drugs (e.g., beta blockers) and metabolic abnormalities, especially hypoxia and acidosis, have a negative inotropic effect, and their correction may be of paramount importance. Cardiac glycosides such as digoxin increase myocardial contractility and may improve cardiac output in cardiac failure, especially if there is associated cardiomegaly. However, their use is controversial because they increase myocardial oxygen requirements, which may precipitate ischemia; they can induce serious arrhythmias; and digitalis toxicity is potentiated by electrolyte disturbances (hypokalemia and hypomagnesemia) and hypoxia in the metabolically unstable patient and by some anesthetic agents.

Catecholamines exert a positive inotropic effect through beta$_1$ receptors in the myocardium. In addition, vasoactivity may be mediated through alpha (vasoconstriction) and beta$_2$ (vasodilatation) receptors and renal dilatation through dopaminergic receptors. Epinephrine is the most potent inotrope, but its use is associated with a high incidence of arrhythmias; it increases myocardial oxygen consumption, and vasoactive effects redistribute blood to skeletal muscle and decrease diastolic pressure, which may reduce coronary blood flow. Norepinephrine, a powerful vasoconstrictor, has similar disadvantages and markedly increases heart rate (positive chronotropic effect) but can be beneficial in patients with bradycardia.

Dopamine and dobutamine are the two most frequently used catecholamines. Although similar to epinephrine at high doses (more than 5 μg. per kg. per minute), at lower dosages dopamine increases cardiac output without incurring the unwanted alpha-adrenergic effects that lead to peripheral vasoconstriction and decreased renal perfusion, and improves renal function by stimulating dopamine receptors. Dobutamine is less potent as an inotrope, but it has the least effect on heart rate and arrhythmias and induces vasodilation without vasoconstriction, increasing myocardial blood flow. It is thus the agent of choice following myocardial infarction and is frequently used in combination with dopamine in patients in shock with poor renal perfusion.

If cardiac output remains inadequate despite optimal ventricular preload and contractility, vasodilators may help to reduce ventricular afterload (peripheral resistance). They are indicated for severe hypertension, especially after cardiac surgery, and when there is poor peripheral perfusion due to high peripheral resistance. They may also relieve pulmonary edema associated with left ventricular failure or mitral incompetence. However, they can all cause profound hypotension and should not be used if blood pressure drops below approximately 90 mm. Hg. Sodium nitroprusside has a very rapid onset and offset of action, allowing fine control. It dilates venules as well as arterioles, reducing both preload and afterload. Hydralazine has a longer duration of action, but its effects are limited to the arterioles. Nifedipine is a calcium channel blocker, causing arteriolar dilatation.

If pharmacologic measures fail, an intra-aortic counterpulsation balloon pump may be considered. This is introduced via the femoral artery into the thoracic aorta just distal to the left subclavian artery. It is synchronized with the ECG and used to augment coronary flow by inflation during diastole and deflation during systole. The principal indications are to support patients after cardiac surgery until myocardial function is recovered and after myocardial infarction while consideration is given to coronary artery bypass.

Septic Shock

While small numbers (less than 10^3) of bacteria are commonly found in the blood (bacteremia) after minor procedures such as dental extraction, septicemia is defined as the proliferation of bacteria in the bloodstream. This is accompanied by systemic manifestations of sepsis including rigors, fever or hypothermia (characteristic of gram-negative septicemia with endotoxemia), leukocytosis or leukopenia (characteristic of profound septicemia or viremia), and tachycardia or circulatory collapse. Septicemia may be a direct complication of the surgical procedure (e.g., anastomotic leak), a complication of invasive investigations or monitors (e.g., infected CVP line), or secondary to another infective complication (e.g., chest or urinary tract infection). It may also complicate the late stages of hypovolemic shock due to intestinal ischemia and Kupffer cell failure.

The increasing incidence of septic shock may reflect the increasing numbers of patients who survive major operations and severe trauma, the development of antibiotic-resistant hospital organisms, or the more frequent use of invasive techniques. Elderly, malnourished, and immunocompromised patients are at particular risk, as are those with a septic focus underlying their original disease. Any organism, including bacteria, fungi, rickettsiae, and viruses may be involved, but gram-negative bacteria that produce endotoxin predominate. Improvements in culture techniques have yielded an increasing association with anaerobe infection.

Septic shock follows a combination of loss of vasomotor tone, increased capillary permeability, and myocardial depression. The pathogenesis of these lesions is still not completely clear. Platelets and white blood cells appear to be consumed in the process, and the vascular lesions may originate from an uncontrolled response of normal defense mechanisms to bacteria within the bloodstream, with dissemination of powerful vasoactive substances such as histamine, serotonin, and prostaglandins, which also increase capillary permeability. Complement activation causes white cell aggregates, and factors involved in phagocytosis by leukocytes, such as lysosomal enzymes and oxygen-derived free radicals, may be released, damaging capillary endothelium.

Gram-negative infections have a much worse prognosis than gram-positive infections, possibly because of an associated endotoxemia. However, the role of endotoxin, a complex lipopolysaccharide found in the cell wall of gram-negative bacteria, is unclear, because although it causes fatal shock in experimental animals, gram-positive bacteria can produce a similar syndrome.

Myocardial depression may also be due to the release of toxins from bacteria or phagocytic cells, or it may be secondary to lactic acid released from hypoxic cells. Pancreatic ischemia causes the release of a specific "myocardial depressant factor."

Clinically, there are two patterns of septic shock:

1. *Warm shock* is characterized by tachypnea, rigors, fever spikes, and a hyperdynamic circulation. The periphery is warm to the touch and appears well perfused because of diffuse peripheral dilatation. The veins are dilated, which increases vascular capacitance and causes a reduction in effective blood volume.[10]

2. *Cold shock*, however, is characterized by peripheral vasoconstriction and is associated with hypovolemia, occurring most frequently in patients who have extensive extracellular fluid losses following burns, peritonitis, or intestinal obstruction. A transition from the warm to the cold type may occur if circulating volume diminishes.

Uncontrolled sepsis leads to the development of multiple organ failure, with acute pulmonary failure (ARDS), acute renal failure, hepatic failure, gastrointestinal ulceration and hemorrhage, adrenal failure, and cerebral failure as potential additional manifestations. Disseminated intravascular coagulation (DIC) is precipitated by the release of thromboplastin from damaged tissue into the circulation and consumption of clotting factors and platelets in the microcirculation. In addition, both cell-mediated immunity and antibody production are impaired, together with depression of the reticuloendothelial system. The

patient is thus deprived of the essential mechanisms to combat the underlying sepsis and exposed to the added complication of opportunistic infection.

Therapy is directed toward supporting the cardiovascular and other compromised systems while the underlying septic focus is identified and treated aggressively.

Volume replacement is vital for prevention of the transition of warm shock to cold shock with its attendant high mortality. In severe sepsis, CVP correlates poorly with pulmonary wedge and left ventricular filling pressure, especially when there is an associated ARDS, and Swan-Ganz pressure monitoring is required. Under these conditions, optimal fluid replacement and inotropic and vasoactive support may be administered. Ideally, the choice of solution for volume expansion should reflect the underlying pathophysiologic abnormality. The relative hypovolemia due to increased vascular capacitance in warm shock requires volume supplementation with colloid. However, if increased capillary permeability is the prime concern, as in cold shock, infusion of large amounts of protein-rich fluid can aggravate fluid sequestration and protein accumulation in the interstitial space. This is of particular importance in the lungs, where colloidal solutions may enhance pulmonary edema and contribute to ARDS. Thus, some clinicians would maintain that it is more appropriate to expand volume with a crystalloid such as a lactated Ringer's solution. Others maintain that crystalloids leak out of the circulation more rapidly than colloids, and the large volumes required produce osmotic abnormalities. Both have merit; and, in practice, a compromise is expedient, with infusion of crystalloid as the principal component for volume replacement, together with sufficient colloid to maintain plasma oncotic pressure.

It may be impossible to optimize ventricular filling or even to maintain a sufficient cardiac output to prevent renal failure without precipitating severe pulmonary edema. In these circumstances, it is essential to establish priorities. Acute renal failure is usually reversible, and a period of dialysis may have to be endured to allow optimal treatment of the life-threatening pulmonary complication. When renal failure develops, pulmonary edema is refractory to diuretics, but excess fluid can be removed by means of hemofiltration. In the hemofilter, arterial blood, flowing from an arterial cannula, passes over a membrane that is permeable to water and electrolytes but not to protein or cells, before being returned to the circulation by way of a venous cannula. The rate at which fluid is removed can be adjusted to optimize fluid balance. Hemofiltration is extremely useful in patients in renal failure who require precise control of fluid status and yet require intravenous nutrition—a mandatory requirement in severely septic patients.

The source of sepsis must be urgently sought and treated. Collections of pus or anastomotic leaks cannot be remedied by antibiotics and require surgical intervention. A localized accumulation of pus in a suitable anatomic location may be more appropriately drained by nonsurgical means with interventional radiologic techniques. Where possible, blood and other specimen cultures should be obtained before antibiotic therapy. Until the offending organisms have been identified, broad spectrum antibiotics active against common gram-positive and gram-negative bacteria and anaerobes should be administered. The antibiotic regimen is subsequently adjusted on the basis of bacteriologic reports, and unnecessary drugs must then be omitted for limiting the development of resistant strains, opportunistic fungal infection, and pseudomembranous colitis.

The emergence of multiorgan system failure in the postoperative period has served as a clinical indicator of continued intraabdominal infection; but, ideally, the clinical situation should not be allowed to reach this advanced stage. Drainage is the only effective treatment for an abdominal abscess. Only by complete evacuation of the intra-abdominal purulence can clinical resolution be achieved. The most frequent site of major pus collections in the abdomen are the subdiaphragmatic spaces, the pelvis, and the liver. The lateral gutters and pockets among adherent loops of bowel represent other sites.

The methods for drainage of abdominal abscess continue to be controversial, particularly in the current era of aggressive interventional radiologists. A limited abdominal exploration may be justified in the patient whose abscess is well localized by preoperative evaluation and who also tolerates the clinical infection with relatively little difficulty. This limited approach prevents complications of inadvertent enterotomy and subsequent fistula formation. In the situation of a well-localized abscess, particularly if it is in the liver, there is good reason for insertion of a catheter under radiologic guidance by an experienced radiologist.

However, the patient without preoperative localization of the abscess cavity or the patient who is not tolerating the systemic manifestations of sepsis should have a complete exploratory operation of the abdomen. This approach avoids the possibility of overlooking multiple abscesses or inadequately drained established abscesses.

Subphrenic Abscess

The most common site of intra-abdominal abscess formation is beneath the diaphragm. Unfortunately, a large collection of pus may exist in either the right or left subphrenic space with few localizing symptoms. However, when intraperitoneal soiling is followed by a septic course, and especially if lung infection or pelvic abscess has been nearly excluded, the subphrenic space should always be suspected. Hence the surgical dictum: "Pus somewhere; pus nowhere; pus under the diaphragm."

RENAL FAILURE

Acute renal failure (ARF) is defined as an abrupt reduction in excretion of waste products by the kidney that leads to a progressive rise in plasma creatinine and urea (azotemia). The onset is usually associated with oliguria, defined as a urinary output of less than 0.5 ml. per kg. per hour, which is equivalent to 35 ml. per hour for a 70-kg. man.

Acute renal insufficiency must be considered in any patient with oliguria after an operation. However, it must be remembered that operative procedures during anesthesia cause large increases in plasma vasopressin concentration, [8] and this may be potentiated by postoperative pain and by some narcotics. The antidiuretic effect of vasopressin is to reduce the flow and increase osmolality, whereas in ARF concentrating ability is lost. Therefore, urine concentration as well as flow must be considered during the immediate postoperative period.

The cause of ARF can be grouped into three categories: (1) prerenal, (2) renal, and (3) postrenal.

Prerenal failure implies an inadequate renal blood flow and is usually a direct result of diminished circulating blood volume. Cardiac failure, due either to inadequate cardiac output or to vasoactive drugs, such as epinephrine used to support the failing myocardium, is occasionally responsible. In the hypovolemic patient, the catecholamine response to maintain systemic blood pressure constricts the renal arterioles. Arterial blood pressure may not, therefore, accurately reflect circulating blood volume or renal perfusion. Clinically, the patient may appear "dry," but clinical assessment alone provides only an approximate guide to fluid status. If the urinary output does not rapidly improve after an intravenous fluid challenge with 500 to 1000 ml. of an isotonic saline solution administered over 30 to 60 minutes, a central venous or pulmonary artery catheter should be inserted so that fluid requirements can be accurately assessed.

Acute parenchymal renal failure usually follows uncorrected prerenal failure. The condition is frequently referred to as *acute tubular necrosis*, because this is the predominant lesion observed histologically. However, necrosis of renal tubules is a very variable feature and may not be present. Thus, some nephrologists prefer the terms *vasomotor nephropathy* or *acute reversible intrinsic renal failure* (ARIRF), which defines the clinical condition more precisely. Although ischemic injury confined to the renal medulla usually recovers with appropriate therapy, cortical necrosis, which can be diagnosed only on biopsy, is more serious because it is irreversible.

Direct injury to the renal parenchyma can be caused by nephrotoxic drugs, in particular, aminoglycosides and intravenous radiocontrast agents; incompatible blood transfusions causing acute hemolysis and hemoglobinuria; and severe muscle injury with myoglobinuria. Renal failure may ensue, especially in dehydrated patients and those with previously compromised renal function. ARF is also observed postoperatively in jaundiced patients with hepatic edema. In these circumstances, it is essential to establish priorities. ARF is usually reversible and prevented by ensuring adequate hydration and diuresis throughout the perioperative period. The pathogenesis is unclear, but endotoxin has been implicated because the patient can be protected by measures to eliminate gram-negative bacteria, including antibiotics and mechanical bowel preparation using mannitol.

Postrenal failure is caused by obstruction of the urinary tract and usually presents with acute anuria. Obstruction should always be considered in the postoperative patient with poor or absent urinary output. It is most common in elderly male patients with prostatic enlargement and in patients with an obstructed urinary catheter. A more serious complication is accidental ligation of both ureters during abdominal or gynecologic surgery.

Accurate identification of the cause of postoperative renal failure is obviously important. Elementary problems such as bladder outflow obstruction and catheter blockage can easily be remedied. Prerenal failure and parenchymal renal failure are usually differentiated on the basis of clinical and laboratory features. Volume status, when assessed, should be rapidly corrected with appropriate intravenous fluid therapy. If adequate urinary output (more than 40 ml. per hour) is not achieved, an intravenous infusion of mannitol, 25 mg.; furosemide, 250 mg. over 20 minutes; or a low-dose infusion of dopamine (2 to 5 μg. per kg. per hour) may be considered.

The use of diuretics is controversial, because clinical trials have failed to demonstrate their efficacy in preventing or reversing ARF[4] and, theoretically, they may aggravate the situation. Diuretics should never be administered to the oliguric patient until fluid status has been assessed and corrected, because although they may induce a reassuring diuresis, they only aggravate dehydration in the hypovolemic patient. Mannitol is an osmotic diuretic that is not metabolized and if not excreted in the urine, can increase the osmolarity of the extracellular fluid as well as the blood, which could precipitate pulmonary edema. Therefore, if a single dose fails to produce a diuresis, it should not be repeated. Furosemide is a powerful loop diuretic that also increases cortical blood flow; but there is some evidence that it potentiates nephrotoxicity, at least in combination with some antibiotics. Dopamine may be a more effective alternative. In addition to its beta$_1$ receptor–mediated inotropic action on the heart, at low doses it improves renal perfusion via dopaminergic receptors in the renal arteries. The patient requires careful monitoring, however, because the effective renal dose may be near the higher dose that induces tachycardia, arrhythmias, and alpha receptor–mediated vasoconstriction.

Lack of response to the measures outlined suggests acute renal parenchymal or postrenal failure. The ratio of urine to plasma sodium, urea and osmolality, and the relative elevations in plasma urea (uremia) and creatinine concentrations may further differentiate renal from prerenal failure. If plasma sodium concentration is within the normal range, a urinary sodium of less than 20 mmol. per liter indicates increased renal conservation of sodium in association with reduced renal perfusion, whereas values greater than 40 mmol. per liter are consistent with acute parenchymal renal failure. Similarly, a urinary osmolality of greater than 500 mOsm. per liter indicates that the kidney is still able to concentrate urine, while formation of urine with a low specific gravity (approximately 1.010) and osmolality of less than 400 mOsm. per liter is evidence of a parenchymal injury. In prerenal failure, sodium conservation is associated with an increased renal reabsorption of urea, decreasing the urine-blood urea ratio from a normal 30:1 to less than 20:1. Creatinine, however, is not reabsorbed; and thus the rise in blood urea to plasma creatinine concentration is usually less than 10.

Before instituting an ARF regimen, the possibility of postrenal failure must be excluded. The index of suspicion varies with the operative procedure and is obviously highest following operations involving a retroperitoneal or pelvic dissection. Unilateral ureteric ligation is usually silent because the remaining kidney can compensate for the loss. In contrast, bilateral ligation causes anuria. Obstruction to the outflow tract usually leads to hydronephrosis, which can be identified on ultrasound scan. If the kidney is able to excrete some urine, either because the ureters have been damaged but not ligated or because of bladder outflow obstruction, the anatomic site of the injury can be demonstrated on intravenous pyelography (IVP). Otherwise, cystography and retrograde pyelography are required. Renal isotope scans (renograms) may also be useful. Dynamic imaging with technetium-labeled diethylene tetramine pentacetic acid (DTPA) can be used to assess glomerular filtration by each kidney. Failure of renal concentration indicates renal ischemia, while progressive increase in renal concentration over 30 minutes indicates obstruction. Static imaging using technetium-labeled dimercaptosuccinic acid (DMSA) is useful in identifying and quantifying parenchymal damage, because DMSA is concentrated only by functioning renal tissue.

Untreated, acute renal failure leads to progressive electrolyte disturbance and metabolic acidosis, terminating in cardiac arrest from hyperkalemia. In postoperative patients, it is usually reversible, although it may require a prolonged period of support with dialysis. However, it is associated with a mortality of approximately 50 per cent because of the underlying disorder, usually hypovolemic or septic shock.

Close attention to fluid balance is paramount. Initially, fluids are usually administered to optimize cardiac output, and thus renal perfusion, by increasing central venous or left atrial pressures. When it is clear that renal failure has become established, however, it is crucial to abandon aggressive fluid replenishment in order to avoid serious overload and to discontinue potassium. Changes in the patient's weight provide a useful guide to fluid balance and should be recorded daily. Fluid intake can be titrated to central venous or Swan-Ganz pressure, but an approximate guide to fluid intake is to replace urinary output and other measured losses plus approximately 500 ml., replace insensible losses (which increase with pyrexia and tachypnea), and to adjust these in accordance with changes in weight and clinical signs of fluid overload (elevated JVP, dependent edema, chest crepitations), or dehydration (dry skin and mucus membranes). Most postoperative patients with renal failure are in a highly catabolic state; and parenteral nutrition with glucose and essential amino acids or, if possible, a high-calorie, low-potassium diet, provides optimal protein sparing. If the requirement for fluids associated with nutrition exceeds that dictated by fluid balance, hemofiltration or dialysis may be required.

The choice between hemodialysis and peritoneal dialysis depends upon the feasibility of peritoneal dialysis, the availability of hemodialysis, the cardiovascular stability of the patient, and local preferences. The indications for dialysis include the following:

1. Plasma potassium greater than 6.5 mmol. per liter
2. Volume overload
3. Plasma urea greater than 35 mmol. per liter
4. Plasma creatinine greater than 900 μmol. per liter
5. Severe metabolic acidosis

Careful monitoring should allow severe electrolyte and acid-base disturbances to be anticipated and dialysis instituted to prevent, rather than correct, complications of renal failure. Hyperkalemic cardiac arrest is the most dangerous complication. In the urgent situation, dextrose and insulin or a calcium ion exchange resin can be used to rapidly reduce plasma potassium concentration.

If the underlying problem can be corrected, postoperative renal failure often resolves. Resolution is frequently heralded by polyuria, indicating the diuretic phase of acute renal failure. Again, this must be anticipated and may require frequent adjustments to the volume and electrolyte content of fluid regimens.

DEEP VEIN THROMBOSIS AND PULMONARY EMBOLISM

Thrombosis in the veins draining the lower limbs is an important cause of morbidity in the surgical patient, both because of its frequency and because of the potentially fatal consequences should the clot become detached from the vein wall and embolize in the pulmonary arteries. Studies using radioactive fibrinogen scans indicate a prevalence of deep vein thrombosis (DVT) in excess of 40 per cent in postoperative patients. One per cent of general surgical patients die from pulmonary embolism (PE).

Clinically, the classic features of DVT are calf swelling and tenderness, elevated temperature, and a positive Homans' sign (calf pain on dorsiflexion of the foot). Phlegmasia cerulea dolens (painful blue leg) represents the extreme situation caused by massive thrombosis involving the iliac veins and extending into the most distal venules in the leg; it is usually associated with an underlying malignancy (e.g., pancreatic cancer). However, clinical diagnosis of DVT is notoriously unreliable; only 50 per cent of patients with evidence of DVT on venography have any clinical sign. Moreover, the majority of patients suffering fatal pulmonary embolism have no clinical features of venous thrombosis prior to sudden cardiovascular collapse.

The risk of DVT and pulmonary embolism is increased with age, obesity, oral contraception, cardiovascular disease, malignancy, leg trauma, and immobility. In addition, patients undergoing pelvic surgery or orthopedic operations on the hip are at increased risk. Immobility, preoperatively, during a lengthy operation, or postoperatively, is an important contributory factor.

Venous thrombosis begins in areas of stasis, particularly in the small calf veins or behind venous valve cusps. Hypercoagulability due to surgical stress and trauma, the effects of pooling and low venous flow in hypotonic limb muscles during anesthesia, and local vascular damage from extrinsic compression of the calf increase the risk of thrombosis.

Flanc and associates have demonstrated that of the thrombi formed, spontaneous lysis occurs in one third.[3] Of the remaining two thirds, half of the emboli are localized in the calf, and the remainder move into the popliteal and femoral veins and may embolize. The clinical signs of DVT correlate poorly with the extent of the thrombosis.

Venography is the standard means of diagnostic investigation and is the assessment against which all new techniques are compared. Venography does not aggravate pre-existing thrombosis, nor does it predispose to embolization. The major disadvantages are the expense, invasive nature, and need to move the postoperative patient to a radiology suite for examination. Current interest centers on those procedures that may be performed expeditiously at the bedside, such as (1) Doppler ultrasonography, (2) ^{125}I-fibrinogen studies, and (3) plethysmography. All have the advantage of being noninvasive and may be performed without moving the patient. Doppler ultrasonography provides an audible signal in response to blood flow. The normal venous flow is phasic with respiration and is augmented by calf compression; a Doppler sonogram detects any alteration in this pattern. Although its accuracy depends upon the skill of the examiner, a sensitivity and specificity in excess of 90 per cent can be achieved. The technique is most proficient in detecting major venous thrombosis and is least able to localize small vein thrombi.

^{125}I-fibrinogen leg scanning measures local fibrinogen isotope activity as a percentage of the background cardiac fibrinogen activity. It is specific for fresh or recently formed thrombi and differentiates them from previous venous thrombosis. The technique is most effective in detecting small calf thrombi but lacks sensitivity above the midthigh level. Currently, its expense and time-consuming nature restrict its widespread application.

Plethysmography detects changes in limb volume in response to heartbeat or after the temporary occlusion of venous return. Various methods, including strain gauge, air or impedance plethysmography, have been employed. Like ultrasonography, it is better designed to determine major venous thrombosis than small calf vein thrombi.

Prophylaxis

Prophylactic measures directed to prevention of deep vein thrombosis and, more important, fatal pulmonary embolism, may be divided into mechanical devices that prevent venous pooling and stasis in the lower limbs and drugs that inhibit blood coagulation. The former group includes leg elevation, elastic compression or pneumatic stockings, and electrical stimulation of the calf muscles. However, with the possible exception of pneumatic calf compression devices, their efficacy has not been substantiated.

Anticoagulant drugs such as heparin, warfarin, and low-molecular-weight dextran and platelet inhibitors such as aspirin have been extensively studied, but all remain quite controversial. The objective is to prevent clotting in blood pooled in the lower limb veins without increasing the risk of perioperative hemorrhage. Low-dose heparin has been used as a prophylactic drug in general surgical patients but is flawed by the risk of sensitizing the patient to heparin and the development of DIC. Radiolabeled fibrinogen studies demonstrate a reduction in the incidence of deep vein thrombosis to below 10 per cent,[7] and a subcutaneous regimen of 5000 units preoperatively and 12 hourly thereafter until the patient is mobile does not appear to cause excessive bleeding. However, the subject remains controversial because heparin prophylaxis has not been conclusively proven to decrease the incidence of *fatal* pulmonary embolism. The treatment is reviewed in Chapter 51.

PULMONARY EMBOLISM

In the United States, many deaths per year may be attributed to pulmonary embolism. Of every 200 patients who undergo a major operative procedure 1 dies from a massive pulmonary embolus. Although data clearly indicate that low-dose heparin prophylaxis reduces the incidence of postoperative venous thrombosis, evidence that fatal pulmonary embolism is reduced is less clear. In several large trials, although fewer deaths due to pulmonary emboli occurred in the heparin-treated patients, the percentages were of debatable statistical significance and probably reflect the difficulties inherent in obtaining a sufficiently large patient population for study. Undoubtedly, certain groups are at greater risk. Ten per cent of elderly patients who undergo repair of a fractured hip suffer a pulmonary embolus, compared with an incidence of 0.2 per cent of the general surgical population older than 40 years of age. Currently, research is being directed toward development of an index that may define the high-risk group. Details of diagnosis and management of pulmonary emboli are discussed in Chapter 51.

FAT EMBOLISM

Approximately 5 per cent of trauma patients suffer fat embolism, especially after long-bone fracture. Orthopedic patients are also at risk. Fat emboli probably originate from the bone marrow and enter the circulation through torn venules at the fracture site. Although direct occlusion of small blood vessels in the lungs, brain, and skin by fat droplets may cause ischemic injury, the pathogenesis of the syndrome probably involves generation of toxic free fatty acids by lipase in the lungs or platelet aggregation around the fat droplets, with release of vasoactive mediators such as serotonin.

The classic triad of the fat embolism syndrome consists of respiratory insufficiency, neurologic signs, and a petechial rash, although many patients exhibit only one or two of these features. Respiratory insufficiency is associated with dyspnea, inspiratory crepitations, and hypoxemia. Neurologic disturbance ranges from mild confusion to severe impairment of consciousness, which may be accompanied by focal neurologic signs. The petechial rash characteristically occurs in the distribution of the carotid and subclavian arteries, affecting skin, mucous membranes, and conjunctiva. Pyrexia, tachycardia, retinopathy, and oliguria due to renal embolization are additional features.

Laboratory investigations may reveal fat droplets in the blood, urine, or sputum; increased serum lipase and free fatty acid levels; decreased serum albumin and calcium levels; and decreased platelet count. However, none of these tests is specific for fat embolism syndrome, and a combination of clinical and laboratory features is required to establish the diagnosis.

No specific treatment is of proven benefit after fat embolism. Heparin, low-molecular-weight dextran, aprotonin, and alcohol have all been suggested on theoretic grounds, but may add more risks than benefits. There is anecdotal evidence that high dose steroids, which stabilize membranes and reduce the inflammatory response, may limit the pulmonary injury. Early immobilization of fractures is a logical preventative measure, and internal fixation may be the most effective method. Measures directed to early identification and correction of hypoxia and avoidance of hypercarbia, which may exacerbate the neurologic injury, are currently the mainstay of treatment.

FLUID, ELECTROLYTE, AND pH IMBALANCE

Isotonic or hypertonic dehydration is common in patients requiring emergency abdominal operations and in those who undergo major surgical therapy without adequate fluid therapy. Special problems are encountered in patients with renal insufficiency who are liable to fluid overload and hyperkalemia and those with hepatic insufficiency who are unable to achieve sodium homeostasis because aldosterone metabolism is impaired.

Several factors may contribute to a fluid deficit in surgical patients:

1. Preoperative fluid depletion, especially in patients with intestinal obstruction, diarrhea, or vomiting.

2. Intraoperative fluid loss. Considerable amounts of water may be lost by evaporation during laparotomy and thoracotomy because of the exposure of large areas of moist mesothelium.

3. Postoperative fluid loss. Fluid loss from nasogastric aspirates, drains, and fistulas can be measured. In addition, several liters of fluid may be sequestered into the "third space" comprising the interstitial space, peritoneal or pleural cavities, and bowel lumen. Insensible fluid loss, principally via the respiratory tract, must also be considered and may contribute up to 1 liter per day in the hypermetabolic postoperative patient.

Clinical assessment can provide a guide to fluid status. Dry mucous membranes and loss of skin turgor are cardinal signs of dehydration, whereas an elevated jugular venous pressure and crepitations at the lung bases suggest fluid overload. However, in the patient at risk of severe fluid imbalance, the central venous or left atrial pressure must be measured.

Wherever possible, half of the estimated fluid deficit should be replaced during the first 2 hours, the balance being corrected over the following 6 to 12 hours. Water lost by evaporation from mesothelial surfaces and as insensible loss from the lungs is best replaced with 5 per cent dextrose in water (DW). Fluid from drains, nasogastric aspirates and fistulas, and third-space losses contain electrolyte concentrations similar to plasma and should be replaced with a balanced electrolyte solution such as Ringer's lactate. Urinary output must also be considered; a good, sustained urinary output of 1000 to 1500 ml. per day (40 to 60 ml. per hour) is required for excretion of the solute load created by the catabolic state.

Hyponatremia in the early postoperative period is frequently due to a stress-induced increase in antidiuretic hormone causing retention of water in excess of sodium. Catabolism also aggravates hyponatremia by the release of water from glycogen, fat, or protein breakdown. Both of these effects resolve spontaneously. However, erroneous replacement of gastrointestinal losses with sodium-free fluids leads to dilutional hyponatremia requiring correction. Patients with dilutional hyponatremia may become waterlogged and are best treated with fluid restriction and diuresis until excess water has been eliminated by the kidneys, followed by careful sodium replenishment with isotonic saline. Severe cases, in which sodium levels may fall below 115 mmol. per liter, are often accompanied by neurologic disturbances, with confusion, headaches, and paroxysms. However, rapid correction with hypertonic saline solutions is potentially hazardous because of large alterations in the osmotic gradient across neuronal cell membranes.

Hypernatremia, which is an excess of sodium relative to water, is less common in the postoperative period. Most frequently it is iatrogenic, induced by sodium-rich parenteral alimentation or prolonged infusion of isotonic saline. Less often, hypernatremia may arise after inadequate replacement of insensible loss, which is hypotonic with respect to plasma. Correction should be made by infusion of balanced saline solutions. As in hypernatremia, no attempt should be made to obtain rapid correction with salt-poor solutions because this causes rapid movement of water into the intracellular compartment, leading to cell edema.

Potassium Imbalance

Hypokalemia in postoperative patients is most commonly associated with fluid loss from the gastrointestinal tract. This may be due to direct loss of potassium, as in diarrhea, or secondary to the metabolic alkalosis caused by vomiting or prolonged nasogastric aspiration, which promotes the renal excretion of potassium. Hypokalemia may also be induced by diuretic therapy. Muscle contractility and nerve conduction depend upon the ratio of intracellular to extracellular potassium concentrations. Hypokalemia affects skeletal muscle, causing weakness and diminished tendon reflexes; smooth muscle, causing paralytic ileus; and cardiac muscle. A serum potassium below 2.5 mmol. per liter may be associated with U waves and flattened T waves on the ECG. Patients on digitalis derivatives are at a particular risk of ventricular ectopic beats and tachyarrhythmias.

Hyperkalemia is most frequently observed in patients with renal insufficiency, and particular care must be taken with potassium intake in postoperative patients with poor urinary output. Potassium is the principal intracellular cation, and plasma levels may be elevated after extensive tissue damage, particularly in trauma patients who have suffered a crush injury. Massive blood transfusion is another cause, due to release of potassium into the plasma from stored red cells. Hyperkalemia can induce spasm in the smooth muscle of the gastrointestinal tract, causing abdominal pain, diarrhea and vomiting, peaked T waves on the ECG, and the danger of cardiac arrest. A serum potassium level above 7 mmol. per liter constitutes a surgical emergency requiring aggressive treatment with intravenous glucose and insulin (100 ml. of 50 per cent dextrose and 20 units of insulin), together with ion exchange resins (calcium resonium, 30 to 60 gm. orally or rectally). Diuretics combined with intravenous saline infusion promote potassium excretion in patients with normal kidneys, but dialysis may be needed in those with compromised renal function.

Acid-Base Imbalance

Acid-base imbalance in the postoperative patient is usually associated with respiratory insufficiency, renal impairment, or net loss of hydrogen ions or bicarbonate from the gastrointestinal tract. Marked deviations in blood pH compromise cellular metabolism, and the heart is especially vulnerable. Acidosis reduces myocardial contractility, while alkalosis is associated with decreases in serum potassium and ionized calcium that increase myocardial irritability. Cerebral vascular resistance is also dependent on blood pH as well as carbon dioxide content. Acidosis increases cerebral blood flow, and exacerbates cerebral edema associated with head injury.

A pure respiratory acidosis reflects inadequate pulmonary ventilation, with an increase in blood pH secondary to carbon dioxide retention. Diminished tissue oxygenation induces anaerobic glycolysis, increasing lactic acid production and creating a metabolic component to the acidosis. Abnormal bicarbonate losses in diarrhea, or from biliary or pancreatic fistulas, or an increase in ketone or lactate production associated with diabetes or starvation can produce a metabolic acidosis without any respiratory component. Any disturbance in blood pH stimulates compensatory responses. In respiratory acidosis, bicarbonate is retained by the kidneys; in metabolic acidosis, the respiratory rate rises, increasing carbon dioxide excretion.

Respiratory acidosis usually responds to improved ventilation, whereas metabolic acidosis may require correction with sodium bicarbonate infusion. Correction of a severe metabolic acidosis may lead to fluid overload and should be staged, directed initially toward one-half correction, followed by reassessment of the acid-base and fluid balance. Dialysis may be required in patients with renal insufficiency.

Respiratory alkalosis in the postoperative period, due either to spontaneous hyperventilation (frequently in response to pain) or to excessive mechanical ventilation, usually responds to appropriate analgesia or readjustment of the ventilator settings. A metabolic alkalosis reflects depletion of extracellular hydrogen and potassium ions and is observed in gastric outlet obstruction or prolonged nasogastric aspiration. Fluid and potassium replacement usually enables the kidneys to restore normal pH through bicarbonate excretion. Acidifying agents such as arginine monohydrochloride or dilute hydrochloric acid are rarely, if ever, required.

ALIMENTARY TRACT DYSFUNCTION

After laparotomy, the normal propulsive activity of the gastrointestinal tract is temporarily depressed, a condition termed *postoperative ileus*. It probably follows trauma to the intestine if a laparotomy was performed or, in other procedures, increased sympathetic discharge from splanchnic nerves. The term "ileus" is misleading because small bowel motility rapidly returns, and feeding through a tube jejunostomy is often initiated within 24 hours. Gastric peristalsis returns 24 to 48 hours after operation, and colonic activity usually returns after 48 hours, beginning at the cecum and progressing caudally. This postoperative ileus leads to mild abdominal distention (primarily from a distended colon) and absent bowel sounds in the first 48 to 72 hours. Return of normal peristaltic activity is often noted by mild cramps, passage of flatus, and return of appetite.

Acute Gastric Dilatation

Acute gastric dilatation follows massive overfilling of the stomach by fluids and gas. It is more common in malnourished and chronically immobilized patients. Gastric outlet obstruction may cause gross distention of the stomach. Acute gastric dilatation is occasionally observed in asthmatics and young children in whom oxygen masks are used in the immediate postoperative period, which suggests excessive air swallowing as an initiating event. Gastric dilatation may also follow forceful insufflation of air during emergency resuscitation or during endoscopy. Surgical procedures in the vicinity of the stomach, such as fundoplication and splenectomy, may inhibit the intrinsic pacemaker of the stomach, and this is also the presumed mechanism in diabetics (diabetic gastroparesis).

As the stomach distends, it descends across the duodenum, producing a mechanical obstruction that exacerbates the problem. Increased intragastric pressure produces venous engorgement of the mucosa, causing fluid secretion and mucosal hemorrhage. If this is allowed to continue, ischemic necrosis and perforation result. The distended stomach pushes the diaphragm upward, causing collapse of the lower lobe of the left lung, rotation of the heart, and obstruction of the inferior vena cava. The acutely dilated stomach is also prone to gastric volvulus.

Clinically, the patient has severe pain and dyspnea, suggesting myocardial infarction. Frequently, however, the onset is insidious, the patient appearing ill, with sweating and hiccups, and dehydrated, with a hypochloremic metabolic alkalosis due to fluid and electrolyte loss into the stomach. The abdomen is distended, and the cardinal sign is a gastric splash.

Treatment consists of gastric decompression with a nasogastric tube and appropriate fluid replacement. In the late stages, gastric necrosis may necessitate gastrectomy.

Gastroduodenal Muscosal Hemorrhage

Hemorrhage from acute shallow ulcers in the stomach and duodenum is a well-recognized complication in severely ill and septic postoperative patients. It is associated with failure of multiple organ systems and is probably due to a defect in the protective gastric mucus layer, rendering the mucosa susceptible to acid injury. Histamine receptor antagonists have been recommended as prophylaxis in high-risk patients. Endoscopy usually reveals multiple erosions in the stomach or duodenum. Treatment with histamine receptor antagonists and antacids is usually effective, and surgical therapy, which may entail total gastrectomy, is now required infrequently.

Intestinal Obstruction

Intestinal obstruction in the early postoperative period may be the result of paralytic ileus or mechanical obstruction. Ileus may be prolonged in patients with metabolic disturbances (hypokalemia, uremia, diabetes), intraperitoneal or retroperitoneal inflammation or hematomas, and mesenteric vascular insufficiency and those taking tricyclic antidepressant drugs. Acute colonic pseudo-obstruction (Ogilvie's syndrome) is a localized form of paralytic ileus affecting the large bowel, most frequently the proximal colon. It is observed in patients who have undergone surgical procedures not involving the abdomen, in particular, major orthopedic operations, when colonic activity appears to be impaired. Increasing abdominal distention develops with risk of cecal perforation. Treatment is by colono-

scopic decompression or, if this fails, laparotomy and tube cecostomy.

Mechanical intestinal obstruction is most often caused by postoperative adhesions or an internal hernia. The diagnosis may be difficult because the symptoms may first be attributed to paralytic ileus. The majority of postoperative patients with mechanical obstruction experience a short period of apparently normal recovery of intestinal function before manifestations of obstruction supervene. If plain films of the abdomen demonstrate air-fluid levels in loops of small bowel, mechanical obstruction is the likely diagnosis. Strangulation is uncommon because the adhesive bands are broader and more pliable than in the case of late small bowel obstruction. Thus, initial treatment is conservative, with nasogastric decompression and careful observation. If the obstruction does not resolve spontaneously within 48 hours, or if tachycardia or increasing abdominal signs develop, laparotomy should be performed.

Postoperative Fecal Impaction

Fecal impaction after operative procedures is usually the result of colonic ileus and impaired rectal sensation. It is principally a disease of the elderly but may occur in younger patients who have predisposing conditions such as paraplegia. The use of opiate analgesics and anticholinergic drugs may be aggravating factors. Patients who have undergone anal surgery such as hemorrhoidectomy may also be inhibited because of pain. Some patients complain of constipation, abdominal pain, distention, and anorexia; but diarrhea due to overflow of liquid feces around the impacted solid material is also a common presentation. In advanced cases, mechanical obstruction occurs and may progress to colonic perforation. The diagnosis is established by rectal examination. The impaction is manually removed, if necessary under general anesthesia, and enemas are given. A high-fiber diet together with increased oral fluids should then be encouraged.

Constipation affecting principally the right colon often follows hardening of barium from an enema performed before operation, which is more difficult to clear than fecal impaction. Treatment is with laxatives and enemas.

Colitis

Return of bowel function following an abdominal operation is frequently heralded by the passage of liquid feces. Persistent postoperative diarrhea is occasionally due to pathogenic organisms such as *Shigella*, *Salmonella*, or *Campylobacter*, which should be identified from a fecal specimen. Patients treated with antibiotics are at risk of bacterial overgrowth with resistant staphylococci in the bowel, but a more serious consequence of antibiotic therapy is pseudomembranous colitis.

Pseudomembranous colitis is associated with *Clostridium difficile*, an anaerobic bacterium that releases a toxin. The condition can be induced by a variety of antibiotics, especially clindamycin and lincomycin. In addition to diarrhea, which may be the only symptom in mild cases, systemic illness with abdominal pain and fever may develop. Severe cases lead to colonic dilatation and perforation. Sigmoidoscopy reveals a characteristic yellow pseudomembrane associated with a friable rectal mucosa, and the diagnosis is confirmed by demonstrating the organism or its toxin in the feces or a rectal biopsy.

Anastomotic Leak

Anastomotic leakage is usually a technical complication. The cardinal principles of any gastrointestinal anastomosis are as follows:

1. Avoid tension across the anastomosis.
2. Ensure good blood supply to both ends of the bowel.
3. Achieve accurate and watertight apposition of the cut

edges with inversion of the bowel edges to obtain serosa-to-serosa apposition.

  4. Prevent sepsis or gross contamination.
  5. Prevent distal obstruction.

Studies with radiographic contrast material following colorectal procedures indicate that most large bowel anastomotic leaks are well localized, and only a minority have any clinical sequelae. A pericolic abscess may form at the site of the leak, causing pyrexia, which resolves when the abscess discharges back into the bowel. This is frequently accompanied by an episode of diarrhea.

An enterocutaneous fistula results if the anastomotic leak discharges through the abdominal wound. If there is no persistent distal obstruction and the anastomosis was performed between healthy tissue, such fistulas heal, but a period of parenteral alimentation may be indicated to reduce the flow through the fistula.

Diffuse peritonitis is the most serious consequence of anastomotic disruption. The patient requires rapid resuscitation with intravenous fluids and nasogastric aspiration, followed by laparotomy. Because of their more tenuous blood supply, large bowel anastomoses are at greatest risk of leakage; and because of the associated contamination, initial surgical management is to exteriorize both ends of the anastomosis. Leaks from proximal gastrointestinal anastomoses are less common and can often be managed by primary reconstruction of the anastomosis, preventing the substantial fluid losses that can follow a high gastrointestinal stoma or fistula.

Hepatobiliary Complications and Jaundice

Hepatic dysfunction leading to an elevated serum bilirubin follows 1 per cent of surgical procedures performed under general anesthesia. As expected, the incidence of hepatobiliary complications is greatest after operations on the liver, biliary tract, and pancreas. Postoperative hyperbilirubinemia may be categorized as prehepatic, hepatocellular, or extrahepatic (obstructive).

Prehepatic jaundice is due to bilirubin overload, most often from hemolysis or the reabsorption of hematomas. Transfusion reactions, drugs, sepsis, and hypoxia in patients with hemoglobinopathies are common causes.

Hepatocellular insufficiency follows hepatic cell necrosis or extensive hepatic resection. Drugs, hypoxia, hypotension, and sepsis are among the injurious factors. Anesthetic agents, particularly halothane, have been implicated as a cause of potentially fatal postoperative hepatitis, especially after re-exposure to the same agent. Posttransfusion hepatitis with hepatitis B, cytomegalovirus, and, in particular, hepatitis C has been reported in up to 10 per cent of patients receiving blood transfusions. Although this usually has a long latent period, it may develop as early as the third postoperative week.

Extrahepatic obstruction is caused by direct surgical injury to the bile ducts, retained common bile duct stones, tumors, or pancreatitis. Acute acalculous cholecystitis is associated with jaundice in one third of cases. It is a disease largely confined to the patient who has a prolonged stay in the ICU, often requiring respiratory and other supports, including prolonged intravenous nutrition. Other associations include prolonged ileus and prolonged morphine administration. The pathogenesis appears to be gallbladder distention following deficient release of endogenous cholecystokinin-pancreozymin. Secondary mucosal injury and vascular thrombosis often lead to transmural necrosis and perforation of the gallbladder.

The diagnosis is often delayed, and an emergency cholecystectomy has a high mortality. Acute acalculous cholecystitis should always be suspected in the critically ill patient in whom an *unexpected septic pattern* develops. Ultrasonography of the gallbladder usually demonstrates a dilated gallbladder, with an edematous gallbladder wall, containing biliary sludge. In the early stage a percutaneous cholecystostomy may be attempted. Generally, direct visualization of the gallbladder, accomplished through a small abdominal incision under local anesthesia, may be required to totally exclude or confirm the diagnosis. If the gallbladder appears normal, the mini-incision is closed. If the gallbladder appears inflamed and is surrounded by omentum, a standard cholecystectomy under general anesthesia is essential.

NEUROLOGIC COMPLICATIONS

Focal lesions in the central nervous system may occur as a direct result of operative trauma during operations on the brain or spinal cord, as a complication of spinal or epidural anesthesia, or as a consequence of focal ischemia, usually embolic in origin. Septic emboli may cause a brain abscess.

Peripheral nerves may also be inadvertently damaged during operative procedures. Examples include injury to the recurrent laryngeal nerve during thyroid or parathyroid surgery, to the facial nerve during parotidectomy, to the ilioinguinal nerve during inguinal hernia repair, and to the sciatic nerve during operations on the hip. Ischemic injury may also occur during prolonged use of a tourniquet used to obtain a bloodless field during orthopedic operations.

Prolonged Alteration of Consciousness

Patients subjected to general anesthesia undergo an induced loss of consciousness. Usually, this rapidly reverses after cessation of anesthesia. If the patient reacts to painful stimuli and all reflexes are present, with pupils that are of equal size and react to light, the prognosis for a rapid and complete recovery is favorable. Unfortunately, there are some patients who do not recover promptly, if at all.

The most common cause of delayed recovery is the excess or prolonged effect of the anesthetic agent. Elderly patients may be especially sensitive to anesthetic drugs, especially opiate analgesics; these can be specifically reversed with naloxone. Renal and hepatic insufficiency pose special problems for drug metabolism and elimination, and obese patients can absorb large amounts of a fat-soluble anesthetic agent that is slowly released from fat deposits postoperatively.

The major concern in patients who fail to recover consciousness after anesthesia is that they have suffered irreversible brain injury. In the patient with diabetes, this may be due to profound hypoglycemia following insulin therapy in a starved patient during anesthesia. However, the most devastating complication of general anesthesia is a hypoxic brain injury. Cerebral hypoxia may follow restricted oxygen supply during anesthesia (a complication modern anesthetic monitoring equipment is designed to prevent), overdosage of narcotics in the postoperative period, various types of pulmonary insufficiency, or the reduced oxygen carrying capacity of the blood.

Brain damage may also be caused by diminished cerebral perfusion after a period of reduced cardiac output and hypotension during the operation or may follow a cerebrovascular accident. Cerebrovascular accidents occur most frequently in elderly patients with atherosclerosis who become hypotensive during operation. Severe hypertension, such as experienced by patients with thyrotoxicosis or pheochromocytoma, and embolism from atherosclerotic plaques, blood clots, fat, or air are additional possible causes.

Prompt recognition and correction of the underlying cause is, of course, vital in hypoxic, hypotensive, or hypoglycemic patients. Individuals who sustain a mild brain injury may remain obtunded for 72 hours and then rapidly regain a normal state of consciousness without apparent sequelae. In contrast, those who sustain a severe brain injury commonly have abnormal limb reflexes, posture, and pupil size and may have convulsions or decerebrate rigidity. Although the prognosis is usually poor, even these severe manifestations of hypoxic damage are sometimes reversible if cerebral edema can be controlled with hyperventilation, mannitol, and steroids. Barbiturate therapy has also been advocated to protect the brain from further hypoxic damage.

Strokes occur in 1 to 3 per cent of patients after carotid endarterectomy or other reconstructive operations on the extracranial portion of the carotid system. The outcome following perioperative strokes is as widely variable as it is in nonoperative stroke situations, ranging from complete recovery to serious or even fatal sequelae.

Convulsions

The previously mentioned cerebral injuries are capable of producing convulsions. Epilepsy or metabolic derangements may also lead to convulsions in the postoperative period. For unknown reasons, patients with complications of ulcerative colitis and Crohn's disease are particularly susceptible to convulsions with loss of consciousness in the postoperative period.

Therapy for convulsions in the postoperative period is not different from that for seizures in general. Close observation with maintenance of an adequate airway and oxygen administration is essential, because hypoxia may have an important part in the cause of this disorder. Moreover, because of residual anesthesia, reintubation and ventilation assistance may be required. Intravenous diazepam, barbiturates, or phenytoin may be required if the convulsions do not abate spontaneously. Complete laboratory analysis should be ordered immediately; and abnormalities such as hypoxia, hypomagnesemia, hypocalcemia, hypokalemia, and hypernatremia should be corrected appropriately. Excessive fluid overload should be treated by cautious diuresis and a reduction in maintenance fluids.

When the patient's condition is stable, a routine examination for epilepsy may be indicated. A decision can then be made as to whether maintenance therapy with phenytoin and phenobarbital is indicated to prevent the likelihood of further convulsions.

Postoperative Psychosis and Delirium

Anxiety and fear are normal in patients who undergo surgical procedures. Confusion is common in elderly patients who awaken in strange surroundings in pain or under the influence of anesthetic and analgesic agents. Sleep deprivation, which is especially common in patients in intensive care units, may cause disorientation and hallucinations. Alteration in body image is a major cause of morbidity in patients requiring a stoma, a mastectomy, or amputation. The ability to manage these stresses is largely determined by the patient's psychic strength. The boundary between these normal manifestations of stress and postoperative psychosis may be difficult to establish.

The incidence of postoperative psychosis is approximately 0.2 per cent for general surgical patients but is much higher following open heart surgery, where postcardiotomy delirium is a well-recognized syndrome. Five specific criteria are necessary for the diagnosis of delirium (American Psychiatric Association, 1980)[2]:

1. Diminished consciousness
2. Disturbance of perception, speech, sleep, or psychomotor activity
3. Disorientation and memory impairment
4. Rapid onset and fluctuating course of the illness
5. Identification of a specific organic factor related to the mental disturbance

Delirium in surgical patients was described in the nineteeth century as *interval psychosis*, referring to the lucid postoperative interval of days that may precede the onset of delirium.

A variety of factors predispose to postoperative delirium. Preoperative factors include age; chronic alcohol abuse; drug dependency; dementia; brain lesions such as tumors and infections; metabolic abnormalities, including uremia and hepatic insufficiency; and a previous history of delirium. Intraoperative and postoperative factors include hypotension, hypoxia, metabolic derangements, sepsis, and drugs. The duration of cardiopulmonary bypass may be related to the development of postcardiotomy delirium.

In general, psychiatric problems should be anticipated by the surgeon and the nursing staff in the elderly with chronic disease or in patients with other risk factors. Most overt psychiatric problems are observed after the third postoperative day. Some severe disturbances may be avoided by appropriate preoperative counseling of the patient by the surgeon.

Characteristically, delirium has a rapid onset, and symptoms may appear simultaneously in many areas of psychologic functioning. Typically, the patient is disorientated with respect to time, place, or person; but the severity of the disorientation may vary. The patient may show impaired perception, misidentifying shadows, sounds, and smells in a terrifying way. Hallucinations are characteristically visual and are exacerbated at night. Delirious patients who are agitated and combative may hurl themselves out of bed to escape imaginary assailants.

The distress and panic following disordered perception and thought require immediate symptomatic treatment until the delirium clears. Haloperidol, 1 to 5 mg. intramuscularly, is the drug of choice. Phenothiazines such as chlorpromazine are also effective and cause sedation but may cause hypotension. Benzodiazepines are, in general, contraindicated because they overly sedate the patient, are short-lived, and may not affect the psychotic symptoms. They may even aggravate the agitation and confusion. Fortunately, most psychiatric postoperative problems are of short duration and leave the patient without permanent disability.

SELECTED REFERENCES

Carey, L. (Ed.): Surg. Clin. North Am., Vol. 63, December 1983.
This issue reviews the complications of the most common general surgical operations in a comprehensive manner.

Greenfield, L. J. (Ed.): Complications in Surgery in Trauma. Philadelphia, J. B. Lippincott Company, 1984.
In this text, 67 authorities have contributed to all aspects of the complications of surgical therapy and trauma and their management.

Hardy, J. D. (Ed.): Complications in Surgery and Their Management, 4th ed. Philadelphia, W. B. Saunders Company, 1981.
This extensive survey of surgical complications contains a wealth of information regarding the underlying pathophysiology and the appropriate treatment.

Moossa, A. R. (Ed.): Tumors of the Pancreas. Baltimore, Williams & Wilkins, 1980.
This monograph provides the details of complications associated with pancreatic surgery and invasive investigations of the pancreas.

Moossa, A. R., Robson, M. C., and Schimpff, S. C. (Eds.): Comprehensive Textbook of Onocology, 2nd ed. Baltimore, Williams & Wilkins, 1990.
This text contains in detail all aspects, including complications of the multidisciplinary approaches of the diagnosis and treatment of cancer.

REFERENCES

1. Braunwald, E., et al.: Principles of Internal Medicine, 11th ed. New York, McGraw-Hill Book Company, 1977.
2. Diagnostic and Statistical Manual of Mental Disorders, 3rd ed. Washington, D. C., American Psychiatric Association, 1980.
3. Flanc, C., Kakkar, V. V., and Clarke, M. B.: Postoperative deep vein thrombosis–effect and intensive prophylaxis. Lancet, 1:477, 1969.
4. Ganeval, D., Kleinknecht, D., and Gonzales-Duque, L. A.: High-dose furosemide in renal failure. Br. Med. J., 1:244, 1974.
5. Greenfield, L. J.: Intraluminal techniques for vena caval interruption and pulmonary embolectomy. World J. Surg., 2:4559, 1978.
6. Hamilton, W. K., et al.: Postoperative respiratory complications. Anesthesiology, 25:607, 1964.

7. Kakkar, V. V., Corrigan, T. P., and Fossard, D. P.: International multicentre trial. Prevention of fatal postoperative embolism by low doses of heparin. Lancet, 2:45, 1975.
8. Korde, M., and Warde B. E. Serum potassium concentrations after succinylcholine patients with renal failure. Anesthesiology, 36:142, 1972.
9. Lee, A. B., et al.: Effects of abdominal operation on ventilation and gas exchange. J. Natl. Med. Assoc., 61:164, 1969.
10. MacLean, L. D., Mulligan, W. B., MacLean, A. P. H., and Duff, J. H.: Patterns of septic shock in man: A detailed study of 56 patients. Ann. Surg., 166:543, 1967.
11. Mendelson, C.: Aspiration of stomach contents during obstetric anesthesia. Am. J. Obstet. Gynecol., 52:191, 1946.
12. Pontoppidan, H.: Treatment of respiratory failure in nonthoracic trauma. J. Trauma, 8:938, 1968.
13. Strandness, D. E., Jr., and Summer, D. E.: Ultrasonic velocity detector in the diagnosis of thrombophlebitis. Arch. Surg., 104:180, 1972.
14. Urokinase-streptokinase embolism trial and phase 2 results: A cooperative study. J. A. M. A. 229:1606, 1974.
15. Wilson, R., et al.: Acute respiratory failure: Diagnostic and therapeutic criteria. Crit. Care Med., 2:293, 1974.
16. Wiren, F. E., Janson, L., and Hellekant, C.: Respiratory complications after upper abdominal surgery. Acta Chir. Scand., 147:623, 1981.

17

ACUTE RENAL FAILURE IN SURGICAL PATIENTS

Prevention and Treatment

R. Randal Bollinger, M.D., Ph.D., and Steve J. Schwab, M.D.

Acute renal failure (ARF) is a potentially lethal complication. Despite recent advances in dialysis and intensive care, almost half of patients in whom ARF develops in the postoperative period succumb. The severity of the trauma, the magnitude of the surgical procedure, the gravity of underlying medical conditions that predispose to ARF, and the high incidence of sepsis all contribute to multiorgan failure, which causes the high mortality. Prompt and effective treatment of each component of the multifaceted etiology of ARF can prevent the syndrome and offers the surgical patient the best likelihood of survival.

Acute renal failure is defined as an abrupt decline in renal function sufficient to cause retention of nitrogenous waste.[3] This definition of ARF does not depend upon the urinary output of the patient. The emphasis is on the quality of the urine, rather than the quantity, because nonoliguric forms of ARF occur quite frequently.[4] Whether or not oliguria is present, a progressive rise in blood urea nitrogen and serum creatinine concentration in the posttrauma or postoperative period should suggest the presence of ARF. Because ARF represents one of the few incidences of completely reversible severe organ failure, early intensive and continuing treatment is indicated.

THE LESSONS OF WAR

During World War I the problem of hypovolemic shock was observed among injured soldiers and civilians. The acute anuria that accompanied the hypovolemia responded to fluid replacement. Those patients with persistent ARF uniformly died. However, it was not until World War II that Bywaters and Beall described the new syndrome of renal shutdown following extensive crush injuries, particularly of the extremities.[21,22] After the introduction by Kolff of the artificial kidney in the late 1940s, it was realized that the human kidney could recover from such a severe injury. Using the new technology of hemodialysis, Swan and Merrill of Boston achieved a 54 per cent survival rate in 85 patients.[92] Both the incidence of ARF and the outcome were favorably affected by this improved treatment.

The first widespread application of the new dialysis technology occurred in the Korean War. The incidence of ARF among critically wounded soldiers decreased slightly from 42 per cent to 35 per cent. However, the mortality after combat injuries causing ARF declined from 90 per cent in World War II to 53 per cent in the later years of the Korean War.[90,94] Better management of shock was largely responsible for this improvement, although dialysis became available near the end of the war. The Vietnam War experience demonstrated a significant beneficial effect of early dialysis. Conger reported in 1975 in a prospective trial of prophylactic dialysis in posttraumatic ARF among United States combat casualties that rates of various septic, hemorrhagic, and neurologic complications tended to be less in

the more vigorously dialyzed patients. Survival was threefold better in those patients receiving more intensive dialysis.[26] Because of efficient evacuation by helicopter and rapid resuscitation, the incidence of acute renal failure declined to 0.17 per cent during the Vietnam War, but the mortality for those few patients in whom renal failure developed remained excessively high, at 77 per cent.[37] The clear lesson from the recent war experience is that prevention of acute renal failure in the surgical patient is much more effective than any treatment available.

CLASSIFICATION

When renal failure, defined as a decline in renal function sufficient to cause retention of nitrogenous waste, occurs abruptly, *acute* renal failure is present. When the azotemia develops gradually over many weeks or months, the renal failure is termed *chronic*. If a patient in renal failure presents with asymptomatic azotemia, the differentiation of acute from chronic disease may be difficult. Several aspects of the history and radiologic examination, particularly the presence of small *end-stage* kidneys, correctly classify the patient's disease as discussed subsequently.

Renal failure is termed *oliguric* if less than 400 ml. of urine is produced in 24 hours. Patients with *nonoliguric* renal failure void large volumes of isosthenuric urine but are unable to clear nitrogenous waste from their systems. Diuretic therapy may convert the oliguric form to the more easily managed nonoliguric form of renal failure.

Acute renal failure is conveniently classified according to its cause as prerenal, renal, or postrenal (Table 1). Each of these types may present in either the oliguric or nonoliguric form, and all are associated with a rising blood urea nitrogen (BUN) and serum creatinine. All of the conditions that may impair renal function must be considered in the differential diagnosis of postoperative ARF. Foremost among the *prerenal* causes are volume depletion, heart failure, and abnormalities in the renal vasculature. Volume depletion may be due to blood loss either internally or externally, dehydration, or third-space sequestration in the GI tract or other extravascular fluid spaces. Renal artery stenosis, renal artery emboli, and renal vascular thrombosis, although much less common than volume depletion, all can produce prerenal azotemia. The treatment for all prerenal conditions is correction of the internal environment toward the normal state by replacing the lost volume, improving cardiac function, removing sources of sepsis, and correcting abnormalities in the renal vasculature.

The intrinsic renal causes of ARF commonly observed in postoperative and posttrauma patients are acute tubular necrosis, pigment nephropathy from free myoglobin or hemoglobin, nephrotoxicity from drugs or radiographic contrast material,

TABLE 1. Common Causes of Surgical Acute Renal Failure

Prerenal
    Hypotension
    Hypovolemia
    Arterial occlusion or stenosis
    Cardiac failure

Intrarenal
    Toxins (radiographic contrast, endotoxin)
    Drugs (aminoglycosides, cyclosporine, amphotericin B, nonsteroidal
        antiinflammatory drugs)
    Pigment nephropathy(myoglobin, hemoglobin)

Postrenal
    Ureteral obstruction or tear (stones, trauma, surgical injury)
    Bladder dysfunction (anesthetic, nerve injury, drugs)
    Urethral obstruction (trauma, BPH, malignancy)

sepsis, and acute interstitial nephritis. The common cause of acute tubular necrosis is shock, although any of the prerenal conditions already listed, as well as prolonged obstructive uropathy, may produce necrosis of the tubular lining. When ischemia becomes severe or prolonged, actual cortical necrosis, an irreversible condition, may develop. There are, of course, many other intrinsic renal diseases that may produce renal failure but are more closely associated with medical disease states than with the postoperative surgical patient and are not discussed in this chapter. Therapy for intrinsic renal causes of ARF is directed to support of the patient with hemodialysis or peritoneal dialysis until recovery of native renal function occurs.

Postrenal causes of ARF are obstructive uropathy and urinary extravasation. The obstruction can occur in the renal pelvis or ureter as the result of a stone, tumor, or clot. Injury to the ureter, sometimes iatrogenic, should be suspected when anuria develops after pelvic or retroperitoneal surgery or trauma. More distal obstruction in the urethra can be due to a bladder stone, stricture, or benign prostatic hypertrophy. A common but easily corrected cause of obstructive uropathy in the postoperative period is an improperly placed or blocked Foley catheter. Urinary extravasation usually follows trauma that injures the bladder or urethra or, postoperatively, disruption of a cystotomy incision. Therapy for postrenal causes of ARF is directed to relief of the obstruction or repair of the urinary leak.

The difficult problem posed by surgical patients is distinguishing a normal kidney attempting to function in an abnormal internal environment (prerenal failure) from a kidney that is no longer able to maintain the internal environment (renal failure). In order to differentiate the large number of possible disorders posed by a postoperative patient with diminished renal function, and to arrive at the correct conclusion and treatment, one must have knowledge of the physiology of acute renal failure.

PHYSIOLOGY OF ACUTE RENAL FAILURE

Normal Renal Physiology

The kidneys are paired organs that lie retroperitoneally along each side of the vertebral column between the twelfth thoracic and third lumbar vertebrae. Each kidney is supplied by a single renal artery that originates from the aorta at the level of the first lumbar vertebra. Occasionally, however, a single kidney is supplied by two or more main renal arteries that serve overlapping regions of the renal parenchyma. As the main renal artery enters the renal midsection, it divides into the progressively smaller interlobar, arcuate, and interlobular arteries that branch into the

afferent arterioles that supply each glomerulus. The glomerulus is a network of capillaries that are arranged around a mesangial matrix to form glomerular capillary tufts. After looping out and turning back on themselves, the capillaries rejoin to form an efferent arteriole, which exits the glomerulus at the vascular pole. After a short distance the efferent arteriole branches into another capillary bed that surrounds the renal tubules. These capillaries eventually coalesce to form venules, which ultimately join together as exiting renal veins. Functionally, therefore, the renal circulation is characterized by a number of progressively smaller arteries and two capillary beds in series — the glomerular capillary bed and the peritubular capillary bed. The afferent and efferent arterioles of the glomerulus are extremely active as variable resistance vessels and thus are important in autoregulating renal blood flow (RBF) and the glomerular filtration rate (GFR). This anatomic configuration of the individual nephron with its distinctive blood supply forms the basis of the current understanding of renal function and pathogenesis of vasomotor ischemic tubular injury (Fig. 1).

The glomerular capillary network is surrounded by a relatively impermeable epithelial capsule (Bowman's capsule), which forms a space that communicates directly with the lumen of the contiguous proximal tubule. Formation of urine begins with the filtration of plasma across the glomerular capillary wall and basement membrane into the lumen of Bowman's capsule. The passage of fluid across this filtration barrier depends primarily upon the difference between the hydrostatic pressure within the capillary and the hydrostatic pressure that is in the surrounding Bowman's space. The hydrostatic pressure in Bowman's space is normally vented through the renal proximal tubule, so the variable that is normally responsible for the quantity of glomerular filtrate is the positive hydrostatic pressure within the glomerular capillary. Fixed oncotic forces owing to plasma proteins in the capillary oppose filtration as do the glomerular basement membrane and its cellular accoutrement. Ischemic or chemical injury may decrease the formation of ultrafiltrate.[27]

The hydrostatic pressure in the glomerular capillaries depends upon the difference in vascular resistance and pressure of the afferent and the efferent arterioles. Modulation of the afferent arteriolar resistance appears to be an intrinsic property of the arteriolar wall itself and is significantly influenced as well by renal sympathetic nerves, circulating catecholamines, angiotensin, and vasoactive prostaglandins and kinins.[9,30,73] Resistance of the efferent arteriole appears to be modulated primarily by angiotensin and norepinephrine but may be significantly influenced by prostaglandins and kinins under certain circumstances. Adjustments in these two resistances can maintain glomerular capillary pressure at a relatively constant level despite wide fluctuations in systemic and renal arterial pressure. For example, when systemic arterial blood pressure falls, glomerular capillary filtration pressure is still maintained by coordinated decreased resistance in the afferent arteriole and increased resistance in the efferent arteriole. The consequence of these changes in vascular resistance is to aid delivery of blood to the glomerular capillary system and hydrostatically force a greater fraction of the total glomerular blood flow per unit time across the capillary wall as filtrate. However, if the mean arterial blood pressure falls below a critical level, even this compensatory mechanism fails to maintain glomerular filtration rate. A corollary consequence of efficient arteriole vasoconstriction is reduction in peritubular blood supply; this relationship is depicted in Figure 2.

The principal functions of the kidney are to maintain the volume and ionic composition of the extracellular fluid (ECF) and to excrete the metabolic nitrogenous waste products. Maintenance of ECF volume and composition is accomplished by tubular regulation of the secretion and reabsorption of solutes

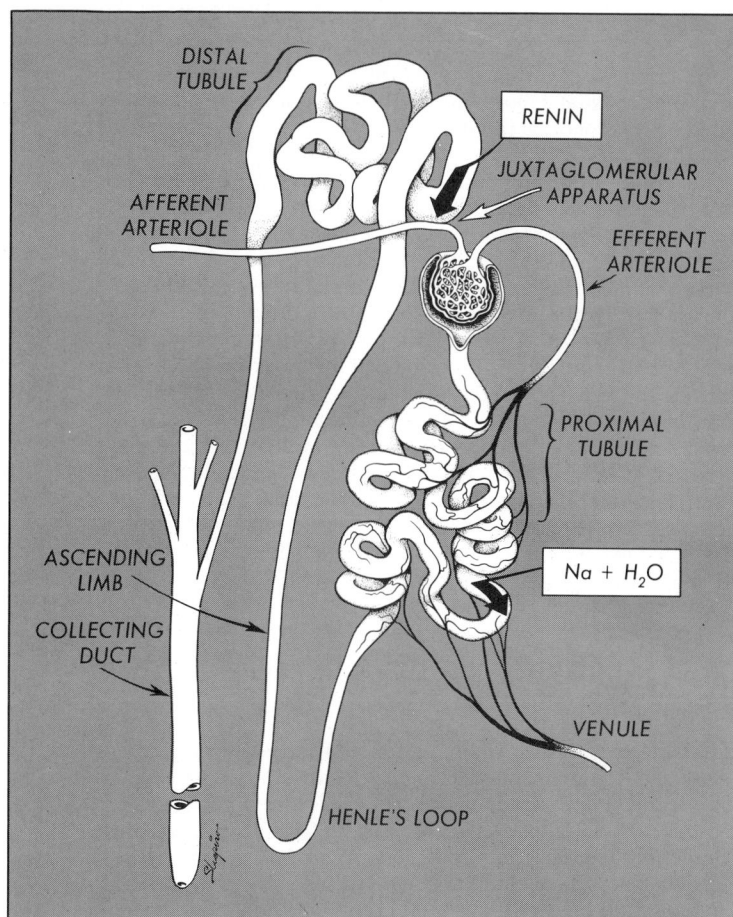

Figure 1. Principal structural features of the nephron and its blood supply. Blood enters the glomerulus through the afferent arteriole and exits through the efferent arteriole. Active dilation and constriction of these muscular vessels significantly modulate glomerular filtration. The tubule receives its blood supply primarily from the efferent arteriole. Renin is secreted by the juxtaglomerular apparatus in response to afferent blood flow and distal nephron urinary flow and composition.

and water as the plasma filtrate flows through the renal tubule. The proximal tubule serves primarily to reclaim the bulk of glomerular filtrate, which is more than 150 liters of fluid per day. Thus, in the proximal nephron, large amounts of filtered sodium, chloride, potassium, calcium, bicarbonate, and phosphate are reabsorbed isotonically, together with glucose, amino acids, and other filtered solutes. Along the distal nephron and collecting duct, the chemical composition of the passing luminal fluid is more finely regulated. It is here that potassium secretion

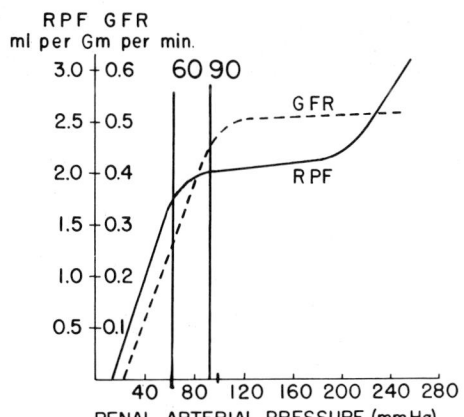

Figure 2. Autoregulation of renal plasma flow (RPF) and glomerular filtration rate (GFR) with varying arterial mean pressure. GFR and RPF are well maintained until mean pressure falls below 90 mm. Hg. GFR is reduced by approximately one half when pressure reaches 60 mm. Hg. (Adapted from Ochwadt, B.: The relation of renal blood supply to diuresis. Prog. Cardiovasc. Dis., 3:501, 1961.)

is modulated, acid is secreted, new bicarbonate is generated and delivered back into peritubular blood, sodium excretion is finely modulated, and water can be conserved or excreted. Proper performance of each of these precisely regulated functions requires sufficient blood flow to the glomeruli, sufficient filtration pressure, structurally intact tubules with operational metabolic systems, adequate flow of filtrate throughout the nephron, and adequate peritubular circulation. Disturbance or disruption of any one or all of these factors can cause tubular dysfunction and homeostatic failure in the chemical balance of the body fluids.

Excretion of nitrogenous wastes depends primarily on renal blood flow and the rate of glomerular filtration. Urea is passively distributed across cellular membranes, so that its entry and passage through the nephron and excretion in the urine is entirely dependent upon the GFR and the rate of urinary flow through the nephron. Creatinine is removed from the body primarily by filtration, and its accumulation in the blood is a reasonable reflection of glomerular filtration function. Other nitrogenous products such as uric acid are eliminated mainly through tubular secretion, which is dependent on blood flow.

Alterations in Acute Renal Failure

Acute renal failure with rapid deterioration of renal function and azotemia not due to extrarenal factors connotes acute tubular necrosis (ATN), which is actually a histologic diagnosis but represents the final common denominator in most forms of acute intrinsic renal failure. Acute suppression of urine formation (oliguria or anuria) generally occurs, but nonoliguric forms of renal failure are increasingly recognized where there is a marked disturbance in renal homeostatic and excretory function but a relatively high output of urine persists. *Azotemia* is a term that simply reflects the abnormal retention of nitrogen products in the blood; it is characterized by elevated serum concentrations of urea. Urea itself, however, is not a toxic compound and is not responsible for the symptoms of illness that accompany renal failure, although it serves as a reasonably good marker for other more toxic metabolites that are difficult to measure.[15]

Regardless of the initiating event or events that cause tubular injury, a number of factors function to perpetuate nephron dysfunction and delay renal recovery.[91] Thus, pathogenetic factors in ARF can be divided into those that initiate renal failure and those that maintain renal failure. The initiating event is a hemodynamic or nephrotoxic insult that causes tubular cellular injury. The extent of the tubular injury depends upon various counterbalancing factors that obtain at the time of insult. These include the status of extracellular fluid volume and cardiac output, intrarenal blood flow and baseline renal vascular resistance, and urinary flow rate. Following tubular cell injury, a series of events are activated that maintain the renal dysfunction: (1) intratubular obstruction by cellular debris, (2) persistent renal vasoconstriction, (3) back-leakage of luminal fluid across the damaged tubular epithelia, and (4) possible alterations in glomerular membrane permeability.[45,92]

INITIATION OF TUBULAR INJURY

Ischemia

As effective arterial volume or pressure declines, renal arterial blood flow is maintained through the vasomotor process of autoregulation, whereby afferent arteriolar tone diminishes and efferent arteriolar tone slightly increases. This process sustains glomerular filtration rate, but does so at the expense of decreased peritubular blood delivery. As mean systemic arterial pressure falls below 90 mm. Hg, hormonal and autonomic responses are evoked which cause the RBF and GFR to fall progressively, and intense renal vasoconstriction is demonstrated. The principal event is constriction of the afferent arteriole[27] probably mediated by the combined action of circulating and sympathetically released norepinephrine and perhaps angiotensin.[45] These two agents probably couple to further increase efferent arteriole vasoconstriction. The result is a sharp reduction in glomerular and tubular blood flow and cellular hypoxia. The extent of cellular necrosis depends upon the severity of blood flow restriction and the duration of ischemia.

Toxins

Tubular injury from nephrotoxins is initiated through different mechanisms, although there appears to be an element of vasoconstriction with each of the commonly encountered nephrotoxins.[45] With aminoglycosides, at least three mechanisms appear to be operative in the evolution of renal injury. Renal vasoconstriction is a dose-dependent feature that can be documented after a single dose as well as after chronic administration. Alterations in glomerular capillary permeability (K_f) and direct tubular cell disruption, presumably from the intracellular accumulation of the drug, are also consistently observed.[83] Loss of luminal brush border membranes and intracellular vacuolization are observed histologically.[79] Myoglobinuric renal failure is accompanied by early vasoconstriction, accumulation of pigment casts in the proximal tubular lumen, and accumulation of hematin in the cells, which is directly toxic to the cell when present in large amounts.[38] Dissociation of hematin from the pigment molecule is a pH-dependent event, which explains why injury is more likely in circumstances of acid urine pH. The almost immediate precipitation of myoglobin in the proximal tubule forms an obstruction that directly blocks filtration. Radiocontrast agents also are directly toxic to tubular cells and additionally induce prolonged vasoconstriction.[20,70]

MAINTENANCE OF TUBULAR INJURY

In a number of experimental models of ARF there is evidence that intraluminal obstruction by cellular edema and accumulation of sloughed cellular debris and proteinaceous casts is an important factor in sustaining renal dysfunction.[91] Renal histology demonstrates edematous cells and intraluminal casts with obliteration of tubular lumens. Dilation of some proximal tubular lumens is an additional prominent histologic feature that is considered evidence of distal tubular obstruction (Fig. 3). Increased intratubular pressure in obstructed tubules is transmitted retrograde and opposes glomerular filtration.[91] This factor is considered critically important in the evolution of ischemic renal failure. Persistent intrarenal vasoconstriction is another important factor in the maintenance of acute tubular necrosis.[45]

Numerous experimental studies have also demonstrated that back-leakage of luminal fluid across damaged tubular epithelium may occur. Evidence supporting this hypothesis centers largely on observations in animals that a normally impermeable material, horseradish perioxidase, can pass paracellularly in areas of definite anatomic disruption of tubules; and observations in humans suffering from postsurgical ARF show that abnormal permeability to inulin exists.[29,71] Back-leakage of filtrate is thus considered an important factor contributing to the sustained renal dysfunction observed in ischemic ARF. In addition, carefully performed micropuncture studies have documented that the glomerular barrier to filtration is directly altered by ischemic and aminoglycoside injury such that fluid filtration is impaired.[27,83] The mechanism of this change is unknown.

Acute renal failure is most commonly initiated by a critical underperfusion of the kidney with consequent intense arteriolar vasoconstriction that causes ischemic tubular injury. In other circumstances, direct tubular cell damage is sustained from a toxin such as aminoglycoside or amphotericin. Myoglobin or hemoglobin pigment may cause direct tubular injury and intratubular obstruction when proteins coagulate. Iodinated contrast and nonsteroidal anti-inflammatory drugs may also be cellular toxins but are also powerful mediators of intrarenal vasoconstriction. When tubular damage is sustained, a number of factors converge to maintain the renal failure. These include back-leakage of filtrate across disrupted tubular barriers, intraluminal obstruction from cell swelling and sloughing, persistent vasoconstriction that might serve to perpetuate cellular ischemia, and changes in glomerular capillary membrane permeability (Fig. 4). Even in apparently intact renal tubular cells, the intracellular metabolism that supports the transport functions of the cell appears to be severely disturbed by hypoxia, free oxygen radical accumulation, and high levels of free ionized cytoplasmic calcium. The result is failure in the homeostatic maintenance of the extracellular fluid and failure to excrete accumulating toxic metabolic wastes.

BIOCHEMICAL ABERRATIONS IN ACUTE RENAL FAILURE

Retention of Nitrogenous Compounds

The progression of azotemia in ATN occurs at a rate that is largely determined by the degree of tissue catabolism and protein breakdown. In the acutely ill patient who is hypercatabolic because of recent surgical intervention, trauma, or burn injury, the plasma urea nitrogen concentration may increase by as much as 40 mg. per dl. per day. In patients who are not excessively catabolic, the plasma urea nitrogen level may rise by only 10 to 20 mg. per dl. per day. Therefore, the rate of rise of urea can be used as an indication of severity of catabolism. It is important to bear in mind that for any specific level of plasma urea nitrogen or creatinine in the setting of ARF, the severity of clinical illness generally is more pronounced than that usually observed with comparable levels of azotemia in a patient with

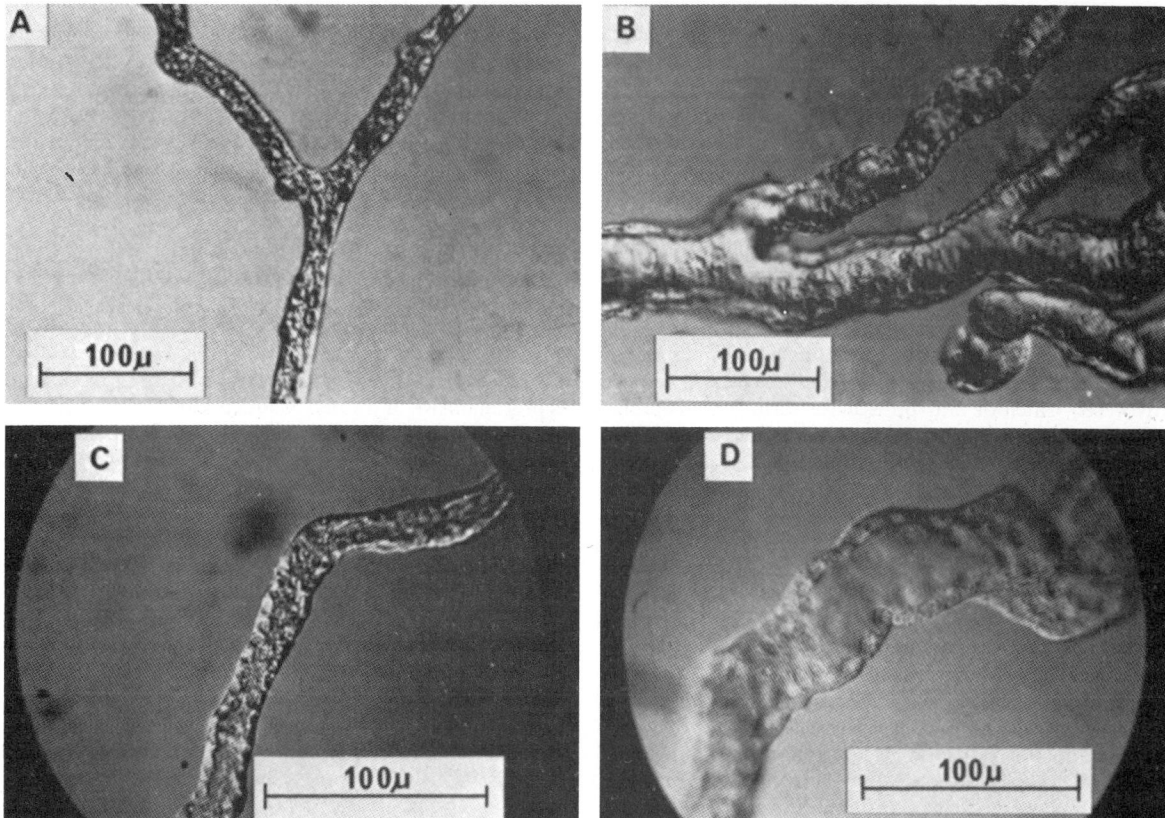

Figure 3. Microdissected tubules from ischemia-damaged kidneys showing tubular obstruction. *A,* Collecting and distal tubules from normal kidney. *B,* Collecting and distal tubules from kidney 1 day after temporary ischemia. Tubule lumens are distended and filled by a hyaline cast. Cells are swollen. *C,* Distal convoluted tubule from normal kidney. *D,* Distal convoluted tubule from kidney 5 hours after release of temporary artery occlusion. The lumen is distended and filled with material. Cells are swollen. (From Tanner, G. A., and Sophasan, S.: Kidney pressures after temporary renal artery occlusion in the rat. Am. J. Physiol., *230(4):*1173, 1976.)

chronic renal insufficiency. This difference in the severity of the uremic state is probably related to the rapidity with which the abnormalities of fluid composition evolve in ARF. In the patient with chronic renal failure, adaptive responses that attenuate the chemical derangements have had time to develop. In addition, in the setting of acute postoperative renal failure, tissue injury and cellular disintegration cause rapid liberation of intracellular products and their metabolites into the circulation; their accumulation is acute. In general, therefore, the severity of the acute uremia is closely correlated with the extent of associated catabolism, which is largely influenced by concurrent illness. Assessment of uremic symptoms and complications relies more on the clinical examination of the patient than on chemical indices.

Metabolic Acidosis

Plasma pH is maintained within extremely narrow limits by the concerted action of three mechanisms: (1) chemical buffer-

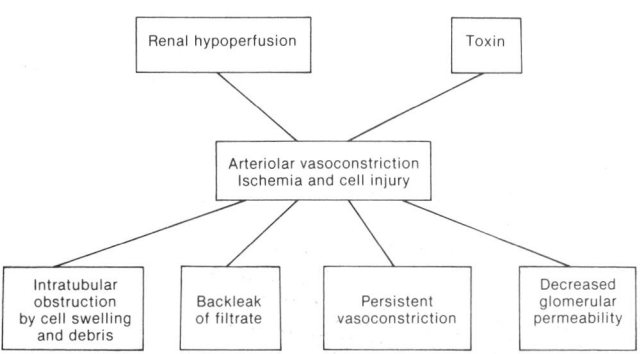

Figure 4. Evolution of acute renal failure.

ing, which is provided by plasma bicarbonate, cellular membrane proteins, intracellular compounds such as hemoglobin, cytosolic proteins, and phosphates, and bone buffers; (2) respiratory compensation, which is accomplished by altering arterial P_{CO_2}; and (3) renal excretion of fixed acids and tubular regeneration of new bicarbonate. In postoperative patients with ARF, acid production is substantially increased from cellular catabolism and release of fixed acid equivalents such as sulfate, phosphate, and a number of organic compounds into the circulation. Chemical buffering occurs instantaneously and is manifested by a steady decline of plasma bicarbonate. The inability of the kidneys to excrete the accumulating acid load and regenerate new bicarbonate, however, causes a severe metabolic acidosis, for which respiratory compensation is usually inadequate.

Hyperkalemia

Serum potassium is also rigidly maintained within extremely narrow limits by precisely regulated secretion into the distal nephron. Acute reductions in renal blood flow and acute tubular injury severely compromise potassium transport and its elimination. Moreover, because body tissues contain large quantities of potassium ions intracellularly (approximately 155 mEq. per liter), substantial amounts of potassium are liberated into the circulation if tissues are injured or necrotic. Because of oliguria or tubular injury, potassium released from the injured tissue cannot be effectively excreted into the urine, and dangerous hyperkalemia may evolve. Hyperkalemia is also a consequence of systemic acidosis because of redistribution of potassium ions from intracellular water to the extracellular fluid.

Hyponatremia

Hyponatremia is another commonly observed electrolyte disturbance in patients with acute oliguric renal failure. It is usually ascribable to the intravenous administration of salt-free water at rates that exceed the renal capacity for excretion. Metabolic water production from metabolism of nutrients and the liberation of intracellular water from tissue breakdown also contribute to the excess of free water. Undesirable consequences of hyponatremia include mental aberrations, convulsions, and cerebral edema.

Hyperphosphatemia and Hypocalcemia

Hyperphosphatemia evolves in patients with posttraumatic ARF because of inadequate excretion and excessive release from injured tissue. In patients with rhabdomyolysis, serum phosphate levels may exceed 12 mg. per 100 ml.[40,62]

The untoward consequence of acute hyperphosphatemia is hypocalcemia, which tends to be especially severe in major rhabdomyolysis. Calcium and phosphate form an insoluble precipitate when the product of their respective serum concentrations exceeds 55 mg. per 100 ml. Injured tissue is usually the site of calcium phosphate deposition, but there is evidence that normal tissue can accumulate free calcium in the cytosol causing cellular necrosis following activation of certain proteolytic enzymes.

Hypermagnesemia

The kidney is a major regulatory organ for magnesium balance. In renal failure, magnesium can accumulate rapidly owing to dietary intake and to the use of magnesium-containing antacids or cathartics. Symptomatic hypermagnesemia probably occurs only when patients with ARF are administered large amounts of these magnesium-containing antacids. For this reason, the clinician should choose aluminum hydroxide or aluminum carbonate when antacids are prescribed.

SURGICAL AND MEDICAL CONDITIONS THAT PREDISPOSE TO ACUTE RENAL FAILURE

Acute renal failure is a frequent complication of surgical procedures. The most common cause of ARF is acute tubular necrosis. Of the approximately 30 patients per year per million population who require dialysis for ARF, 20 have ATN, three quarters of these as a complication of surgical intervention.[51] Many factors cause this high incidence of ARF in the postoperative period. An important factor is the severity of underlying diseases, both medical conditions pre-existing in the patient before surgical therapy and the trauma or illness associated with the surgical procedure. Moreover, exposure to anesthetic agents and the risk of incompatible blood transfusion, both possible causes of ARF, are high in the operative group. The most important factor, however, is hypovolemia from preoperative fluid restriction, surgical fluid loss, surgical blood loss, and gastric tube drainage of fluids.[5] The already ischemic kidney in the hypovolemic patient may be injured easily by nephrotoxic antibiotics and other drugs. The combination of toxic and ischemic damage to tubular epithelium is the direct cause of postoperative ARF. Prevention of this often fatal complication depends upon recognition of predisposing conditions and correction of the physiologic disturbances for timely preservation of the sensitive renal tubular cells. The general physiologic disturbances confronted by many surgical patients are well illustrated by the trauma victim.

Trauma

Posttraumatic ARF was first described by Bywaters and Beall in the victims of crushing injuries during World War II.[21] They observed that hemorrhagic hypotension alone was rarely, if ever, associated with renal failure, whereas the combination of hypotension and crushing injuries frequently caused renal shutdown. The victim of severe trauma usually suffers from some degree of hypovolemia. In addition to external acute blood loss, the patient may have internal hemorrhage, occult gastrointestinal bleeding, and gross hematuria. Extrarenal fluid loss in the form of vomiting and nasogastric suction contributes to volume depletion. Renal loss and excessive sweating with hyperpyrexia may further aggravate the hypovolemia. In the most severe case, the burn victim has a massive leak of fluid from the vascular bed into the wound during the first 6 to 8 hours after injury due to dilatation and increased permeability of the damaged skin capillaries.

The kidney can normally withstand wide variations in renal perfusion pressure by the process of renal autoregulation, which maintains the RBF and GFR nearly unchanged. However, below a blood pressure of approximately 90 mm. Hg, the RBF is reduced and GFR decreases. Early in the course, the result is prerenal ARF. If trauma produces hemorrhage and other fluid losses sufficient to lower the blood pressure below the limit for autoregulation, immediate blood transfusion and fluid infusion are indicated before the ischemic injury progresses to acute tubular necrosis or, in the most severe and prolonged cases, acute cortical necrosis, which is irreversible. Rhabdomyolysis and myoglobinuria commonly accompany crush injury. Myoglobin pigment is prone to precipitate in the tubules during hypovolemic shock.

The requirement to transfuse the trauma and surgical patient has additional risks for acute renal failure if mismatched blood is transfused. After transfusion of small amounts of incompatible blood, readily reversible ARF occurs as a consequence of intravascular hemolysis and hemoglobinuria. When 200 to 500 ml. has been transfused, ATN and a life-threatening hemorrhagic diathesis attributed to disseminated intravascular coagulation (DIC) may develop.

The trauma victim who requires surgical intervention is further subjected to the nephrotoxicity of anesthetic agents. Premedications, induction agents, and inhalational anesthetics may all impair renal function. For example, morphine may cause a reduction in urinary output and in solute excretion, as well as a reversible fall in the GFR and RBF. Urine volume, RBF, and the GFR fall transiently after barbiturate induction of anesthesia. It is likely this reflects vasorelaxation and vascular pooling. The commonly used fluorinated inhalational anesthetic agents have been responsible for many cases of ARF following operation. Methoxyflurane has been particularly troublesome; toxicity from this agent is usually mild and consists of a transient decrease in the GFR and a concentrating defect. However, patients with more severe toxicity have been reported with a clinical course typical of ATN. It is generally thought that the fluoride ion, which is liberated from the fluorinated ether by the liver, is the true toxic metabolite. Fewer problems occur with enfluorane and isofluorane; and the most commonly used agent, halothane, is an extremely uncommon cause of renal damage even after prolonged anesthesia.[5,25]

The trauma victim who survives the initial resuscitation and anesthesia must still encounter several challenges to renal function. Severe plasma volume depletion may occur during the course of prolonged ileus. Peritonitis or acute posttraumatic pancreatitis causes the loss of additional fluid into the peritoneal cavity. The resulting severe hypovolemia may be further aggravated by the endotoxemia of sepsis, causing shock, ARF, and sometimes death.

Sepsis

When gram-negative bacteria invade the bloodstream, they produce the syndrome of septic shock. Common sources include urinary tract infections, biliary or intraperitoneal sepsis, colon surgery, and severe trauma, although the source is not always evident. The patient develops fever, chills, dyspnea, confusion, and hypotension. A frequent consequence is acute renal failure. The offending agent for the multiple deleterious effects is lipid A, which is a fatty acid liberated from within the gram-negative bacterial wall. Endotoxin has numerous effects on cells throughout the body, the primary targets being the lung (shock lung), the liver (reticuloendothelial system blockade), the gastrointestinal tract (ulcers), and the kidneys (ARF).[97] Hypovolemic shock due to reduced cardiac output and capillary leaks, as well as diffuse intravascular coagulation, further damage the kidneys. The prerenal ARF induced by mild endotoxemia is readily reversed by improving renal perfusion.[5] Larger amounts of endotoxin cause severe vasoconstriction, local coagulation, and endothelial damage, which cause ATN. These patients create a therapeutic dilemma because nephrotoxic bactericidal antibiotics are used to treat gram-negative sepsis. It is sometimes impossible to know whether ARF is produced by the antibiotic or the massive release of endotoxin from killed bacteria, or both.[98]

Cardiopulmonary Bypass

In addition to the general risk of surgical procedures because of anesthesia, hypotension, blood transfusion, and the administration of numerous drugs, open heart surgery has an added risk for ARF. As many as 25 per cent of patients undergoing open heart surgery experience nonoliguric ARF, and another 5 per cent have oliguric ARF.[2,13,100] While cardiac function is poor, prerenal ARF may develop from hypoperfusion of the kidneys. This condition is readily reversible if the cardiac output is increased by successful surgical therapy, but it progresses to ATN if allowed to continue for a protracted period. The kidneys are perfused at a volume of 200 to 500 ml. per minute during cardiopulmonary bypass. This relative underperfusion produces a markedly decreased glomerular filtration rate, which returns to normal in most patients with satisfactory cardiac output when the operation is completed.[5] Some patients, however, have persistent postoperative prerenal ARF continuing for several days. These patients have a low GFR following poor left ventricular function, low systemic blood pressure, and associated decreased renal blood flow. The fall in GFR is disproportionately greater than the decrease in RBF. Myers and associates[72] have suggested that serum creatinine be monitored in these patients when vasodilator agents are used to reduce systemic vascular resistance, because a fall in blood pressure below the autoregulatory range may greatly reduce the GFR, causing a rise in creatinine. When the impairment in hemodynamics is prolonged and severe, ischemic ATN with back-leakage of glomerular filtrate through the damaged tubular epithelium occurs. Regeneration of the renal tubular lining requires days to weeks and may prolong the patient's recovery time.

Renal Transplantation

When a kidney transplant fails to function in the early postoperative period, several possible causes of ARF should be considered. A technical problem with the renal artery or renal vein may cause thrombosis in the vessels. Urinary flow may be obstructed by edema, clot, stenosis, or kinking of the ureter. Low intravascular volume may impair glomerular filtration. A lymphocele, hematoma, or urinoma may compress the kidney and its collecting system. Acute tubular necrosis may be present because of ischemia in the donor prior to organ procurement prolonged warm ischemia during the donor nephrectomy, or inadequate preservation during transportation of the kidney. In addition, hyperacute rejection, an uncommon but devastating complication causing nonfunction and destruction of the kidney, may be present. Pre-existing circulating humoral antibody is the usual cause of hyperacute rejection. If the kidney fails to become pink and have normal turgor despite a strong pulse and good renal vein outflow, biopsy should be undertaken at the time of operation. If thrombosis has occurred within the renal vessels and leukocytes are present in the interstitium and glomerular capillaries, immediate nephrectomy is indicated.

Measurements of central venous pressure and hematocrit suggest whether hypovolemia from bleeding is the cause of posttransplantation ARF. Early re-exploration to control the bleeding, relieve renal compression, and restore blood volume usually cause prompt return of renal function. Radionuclide renal scans and arteriography are helpful in the differential diagnosis of early posttransplantation ARF (discussed under radiographic studies). If the graft implantation site and ipsilateral leg become swollen and tender, iliac vein compression or thrombosis should be considered. A sonogram indicates whether a collection of blood, lymph, or urine is compressing the kidney and vein and whether dilatation of the collecting system indicative of ureteral obstruction is present. A more precise diagnosis can be made by needle aspiration or open exploration of the transplant wound. If the fluid collection proves on chemical analysis to be urine, immediate drainage is indicated. A Foley catheter prevents extravasation from a bladder or ureteroneocystostomy leak. If ureteral necrosis is suspected, the wound should be re-explored and a new ureteroneocystostomy, pyeloureterostomy, pyelocystostomy, or nephrostomy performed. Urine allowed to remain in and around the kidney usually becomes infected and leads to devastating complications, including death.

The differential diagnosis of acute tubular necrosis and rejection may be difficult in the early postoperative period. Acute tubular necrosis should be suspected whenever there is prolonged hypotension in the donor, extensive warm ischemia time during the harvest procedure, or very long cold preservation times. Since all cadaveric kidneys experience these problems to some extent, they are more susceptible to acute tubular necrosis from additional minor insults than are normally functioning native kidneys. Acute tubular necrosis usually appears immediately or within 24 hours of transplantation and resolves within 3 weeks in most cases, although up to 3 months may be required. If renal failure develops later after grafting, the likelihood of rejection increases. Oliguria, decreased creatinine clearance, and impaired function by renogram are evident. Graft tenderness, fever, edema, increase in weight, and hypertension may develop. On palpation, the graft may be swollen and tender. When ATN cannot be clearly differentiated from rejection, percutaneous needle biopsy of the kidney should be considered to establish the diagnosis, prognosis, and plan of immunosuppressive therapy. Biopsy is especially helpful in managing transplant patients receiving the effective but nephrotoxic drug cyclosporine. In conjunction with cyclosporine serum levels and measures of renal function, the degree and type of cellular infiltrate observed in the renal biopsy help differentiate ARF due to rejection from that due to drug toxicity.

Urologic Surgery

Most of surgically associated renal failure is due to ATN after trauma, sepsis, or gastrointestinal and cardiovascular surgery. Urologic procedures pose additional, special problems because of postrenal ARF produced by obstruction. Of 685 patients with ARF in one hospital series, 5 per cent had urinary obstruction as the primary diagnosis.[51] Although obstruction is one of the most frequent causes of chronic renal failure, it is a relatively uncommon cause of ARF, because urinary flow must be suddenly and bilaterally interrupted for renal function to cease.[23] Postrenal ARF from obstruction is more likely to occur when only a single kidney is present due to nephrectomy, congenital absence of a kidney, or more commonly, transplantation. Another important example that should never be overlooked is the patient with stable but moderately advanced intrinsic renal insufficiency. In these patients, a single renal stone, the most common cause of obstructive uropathy in the general population, or papillary necrosis may cause postrenal ARF. In patients with two functioning kidneys, bladder stones, bladder or urethal tumors, and commonly benign prostatic hypertrophy in the male may cause postrenal ARF. Urethral obstruction in females may be caused by a retroverted gravid uterus, fibroids, ovarian cysts, obstetrical trauma, or neoplasms of the pelvic organs. In children, congenital problems such as urethral valves or urethral atresia can produce renal failure. A history of excruciating, colicky pain in the flank with radiation to the abdomen, passage of stones, hematuria, dysuria, or persistent backache suggests ureteric obstruction as the cause of oliguria. Infravesicular obstruction is suggested by decreased force of the urinary stream, frequency, urgency, postvoid dribbling, and overflow incontinence preceding anuria. Obstruction must be suspected any time anuria develops after surgical intervention or trauma to the pelvis or retroperitoneum. Numerous other causes of postrenal failure have been described.[23]

Persistent urinary obstruction eventually causes changes in renal morphology and metabolism. Reduced renal blood flow and ischemia develop, and progressive interstitial fibrosis and tubular damage ensue which, after approximately 2 to 3 weeks of obstruction, become increasingly irreversible. Prompt diagnosis and treatment of the cause of obstruction lead to a rapid recovery of renal function. Postrenal failure should be considered whenever complete anuria develops suddenly or whenever intermittent oliguria occurs. It cannot be differentiated from other types of ARF by means of laboratory tests, but radiologic studies, including a plain film of the abdomen, sonograms, computed tomography, renograms, and intravenous pyelography, may be quite helpful.

Liver Failure

Austin Flint observed in 1863 that some patients with cirrhosis and hydroperitoneum developed severe oliguria and died. In 1932 the term *hepatorenal syndrome* (HRS) was introduced to designate unexplained renal failure following biliary tract surgery.[76] The term is now used to define any renal failure occurring in patients with parenchymal liver disease when no other known cause of renal failure can be found. In 1960 Kiley reported that the single most common operative procedure in civilian practice associated with acute postoperative renal failure was a complicated operation on the biliary tract.[54] The functional renal failure associated with icteric liver disease is indistinguishable from prerenal azotemia early in its course, except that it is only transiently responsive to volume expansion. In some patients there is progression to acute tubular necrosis, whereas in 10 to 20 per cent of patients spontaneous remission occurs with improvement of liver function. Interestingly, the kidney from an HRS patient functions normally when transplanted to an individual without liver disease,[55] and successful transplantation of the liver in an HRS patient also corrects the kidney failure.[47] In this syndrome, renal function is determined by the hepatic environment.

Patients with obstructive jaundice have a definite predilection to develop ATN. When renal failure occurs after biliary tract procedures, the possibility of an hepatorenal syndrome exists, but ATN occurs much more often. Other conditions observed in surgical patients which can mimic HRS are infections (sepsis, hepatitis-B), shock, toxins, and pharmacologic agents (methoxyfluorane, halothane, tetracycline, streptomycin, sulfonamides, etc.) and metastatic neoplasms such as renal cell carcinoma. In these situations, injury occurs simultaneously to both the liver and kidney causing failure of both organs. These conditions should be distinguished from the hepatorenal syndrome so that treatment is efficiently directed to the underlying cause.

In the United States most patients who develop the hepatorenal syndrome have established alcoholic cirrhosis, but postnecrotic and idiopathic cirrhosis may also cause kidney failure.[99] In the patient with cirrhosis, kidney failure may be precipitated by surgical intervention, gastrointestinal bleeding, abdominal paracentesis, induced diuresis, or progression of jaundice, although no precipitating event is apparent in some patients.[12] The kidneys of these patients are perfectly normal without any evidence of identifiable primary renal disease by histology. However, the patient with fulminant hepatic failure, rather than cirrhosis, is likely to demonstrate ATN on microscopic examination of the kidneys. There is little evidence that bilirubin directly damages the kidney. However, bilirubin or bile acids may make the kidney more sensitive to ischemia, and jaundiced serum may contain materials other than bilirubin that increase vascular responsiveness to vasoconstrictor stimuli. In the early stages of HRS all of the renal functional characteristics of a hypoperfused kidney are present, including a concentrated urine and low urine sodium concentration. Further impairment of effective renal perfusion ultimately leads to ATN and renal failure. Treatment before and after surgical therapy should be directed to expansion of effective plasma volume, both to differentiate HRS from prerenal azotemia and as the most effective treatment for the renal functional impairment accompanying liver failure.

Vascular Disease

Grafting of an abdominal aortic aneurysm is a procedure early recognized to have substantial risk of renal failure performed on an elective or on an emergency basis.[54] The common factor in both is the placement of a clamp across the aorta just distal to the renal arteries. The probability that renal failure would occur postoperatively increases with the length of time that the aortic clamp remained in place. Acute tubular necrosis occurs in 30 per cent of patients when the aortic clamp was left in place for 100 minutes or more. Occasionally, the aneurysm extends above the level of the renal arteries, necessitating total interruption of flow to the kidney for a portion of the grafting procedure. If the period is less than an hour and the patient does not have pre-existing renal ischemia or other renal disease, renal failure usually does not occur. Longer periods of interrupted renal blood flow require preservation using hypothermia or temporary shunting of blood to the distal renal artery if acute renal failure is to be prevented.

The operative manipulation required to mobilize and clamp the aorta stimulates the rich plexis of autonomic nerves surrounding the origin of the renal arteries causing vasoconstriction and ischemia. Pharmacologic blockade of these nerves has offered significant protection to the kidneys in experimental studies. Atheromatous emboli to the kidneys may also follow manipulation and cross-clamping of the diseased aorta. The already ischemic kidneys are further damaged by washout acidosis as the lower body is reperfused.[95]

Atherosclerotic vascular disease not only produces aneurysms, but also stenoses of the renal arteries. When a stenosis is high grade, renal ischemia results and ARF may occur with levels of hypotension that would be tolerated by individuals with normal renal arteries. The stenosis may progress to renal arterial thrombosis and loss of functioning renal tissue. The kidney may also be destroyed by renal vein thrombosis which may also cause renal arterial thrombosis. These events may be silent unless the patient has a solitary kidney or has already sustained a similar injury to the other kidney, in which case abrupt anuria and progressive azotemia occurs.

Bilateral ureteral obstruction has been reported after aortic or iliac bypass surgery.[23] The renal failure may occur weeks or even months after the operation because of obstruction produced by an organizing hematoma around the vascular anastomoses or ureteral strictures at sites of ureteric devascularization. Another complication of abdominal vascular injury or surgical intervention that can lead to ARF is postoperative hemorrhage. Even if intravascular volume is maintained, the rise in intra-abdominal pressure can lead to renal failure.[80] Polyuria and resolution of the ARF occur in response to operative decompression of the abdomen.

Hypotension and Hypovolemia

Mild hypovolemia and hypotension evoke a number of vasoactive responses in the kidney to maintain renal blood flow and glomerular filtration.[88] Autoregulatory decrease in afferent arteriolar tone coupled with an increase in efferent arteriolar tone preserves glomerular flow and glomerular filtration rate. Intrarenal prostaglandin activity also increases, which mediates further vasodilation.[30] However, these preservative mechanisms are counterbalanced by vasoconstricting activities of circulating catecholamines and circulating angiotensin, which uphold central mean arterial pressure. A relative redistribution of renal blood flow from outer cortical nephrons to inner cortical and juxtamedullary nephrons during mild hypotension also occurs. This redistribution of renal blood flow is believed to follow vasoconstriction of the blood supply to the outer cortical nephrons and a relative vasodilation of the blood supply to the inner cortical nephrons, which is mediated by prostaglandin activity.[31] The renal tubular functional response is to conserve sodium and water. Because of diminished urinary flow rates, azotemia evolves. In this state, the kidney is particularly susceptible to further reduction in perfusion pressure or interference with the adaptive mechanisms. As long as the intrarenal adaptive mechanisms remain intact and the humoral vasoconstrictive responses to the hypotension do not override the autoregulatory capacity of the kidney, this condition does not in itself lead to ATN. However, persistence of hypovolemia makes the kidney quite vulnerable to other factors which might eventuate in renal damage, such as myoglobinuria, hemoglobinuria, radiocontrast material, nephrotoxic antibiotics, and nonsteroidal anti-inflammatory drugs, which can severely compromise the intrarenal vasodilatary adaptation by interfering with vasodilating prostaglandin synthesis. In this clinical setting, there is a period of time in which restitution of effective extracellular fluid volume and elevation of blood pressure can prevent secondary insults and progression to ischemic tubular necrosis.

Cardiac Failure

Acute renal failure as a consequence of myocardial infarction and cardiogenic shock is rare, perhaps because survival is limited because of the usually massive cardiac injury. Nevertheless, in the patient with mild or moderate congestive heart failure, there is reduction in renal blood flow, elevated serum renin and angiotensin levels, and increases in circulating catecholamines and intrarenal vasodilating prostaglandin compounds.[89] Like the kidney that is underperfused because of hypovolemia or hypotension, intrarenal blood flow and the GFR are precariously balanced. A further decrease in effective arterial volume and renal perfusion pressure from either overdiuresis or worsening congestive heart failure can cause further intrarenal vasoconstriction and ischemic renal damage. The tubule in this setting is again more likely to sustain toxic injury from pigment, drugs, or radiocontrast.

Pre-existent Renal Disease

When the serum creatinine is greater than 2 mg. per 100 ml. at baseline, there has already been an approximately 75 per cent loss of nephron function. Whether the kidney is diseased because of diabetes mellitus and nephrosclerosis, chronic glomerulonephritis, or chronic tubular interstitial nephritis, it is predisposed to development of ARF from a variety of insults.[12] Autoregulatory capacity is compromised; so decreases in renal perfusion pressure can have a dramatic impact on the GFR and peritubular blood flow. Numerous prospective and retrospective studies have documented that pre-existent renal insufficiency is a major risk factor for radiocontrast-induced renal failure and nephrotoxic injury.[44,96] Awareness of the predisposition for tubular injury in this setting is the primary requirement for successful prophylaxis. Dosages of antimicrobial agents must be altered and volume status carefully maintained. If a radiocontrast study is required, adequate hydration prior to the study and following the administration of the contrast material is essential. Nonsteroidal anti-inflammatory drugs should probably be avoided in patients with renal insufficiency.

Radiographic Contrast Agents

Acute renal failure following the administration of radiocontrast agents occurs frequently.[10] It may range in severity from a nonoliguric, asymptomatic, and transient decline in renal function to fulminant oliguric renal failure requiring dialysis. The exact pathogenesis of the mechanism of renal injury is not well defined. A number of possibilities have been proposed, including prolonged vasoconstriction, direct cellular toxicity due to the iodinated compound with consequent degeneration and sloughing of cells, tubule obstruction by proteinaceous casts of cell debris and mucoprotein, and uric acid precipitates.[10] The incidence in patients without the well-recognized risk factor of pre-existent renal insufficiency appears to be very low.[20,28,44,77,85,96] Available data indicate that the greater the level of pre-existing renal impairment, the greater the likelihood of nephrotoxicity from radiocontrast, regardless of underlying illness. It is generally agreed that susceptible patients who are at greater risk of developing radiocontrast-induced ARF should be adequately hydrated prior to the administration of the contrast. Advanced age, diabetes mellitus, congestive heart failure, and the amount of contrast agent administered are probably additional risk factors. Non-ionic low osmolar contrast agents have fewer systemic side effects but have equal propensity to cause renal toxicity and should therefore also be used with caution.[28,85]

Pigment Nephropathy

Acute renal failure associated with both myoglobinuria and hemoglobinuria has been recognized for many years. However, numerous studies indicate that neither myoglobin nor hemoglobin is a direct cellular toxin.[38] Only when the myoglobin and hemoglobin molecules are dissociated into ferrihemate (hematin) and the specific globin moiety of the macromolecule can tubular toxicity be demonstrated. This dissociation occurs at or below a urine pH of 5.6. There is now evidence that hematin is probably the toxic component of these globin pigments.[38] Many investigators believe that intratubular obstruction by the local precipitation of these pigments is a more important mechanism in pigment nephropathy. Thus, pigment-induced nephropathy appears to be a more severe problem during ECF volume depletion with low urinary flow and with acid urine. These observations have provided the basis for a therapeutic approach to the prevention and treatment of myoglobin- or hemoglobin-associated ARF. When myoglobinuria from rhabdomyolysis or hemoglobinuria from intravascular hemolysis occurs, it is recommended that the clinician (1) infuse saline or Ringer's solution with or without mannitol to enhance urinary flow, thereby flushing out the pigment and precluding its intratubular precipitation and (2) infuse sodium bicarbonate to limit the generation of free hematin in acid urine (attempt urine pH > 7). The clinician must be alert for the development of oliguric ARF. When this occurs, fluid infusion must be curtailed.

Drugs

Aminoglycosides are well known for their nephrotoxic potential. Even with carefully monitored serum levels in the therapeutic range, aminoglycosides are concentrated in the renal cortex and cause histologically noticeable cellular damage.[10,79] Under the best of circumstances, the incidence of aminoglycoside nephrotoxicity is on average approximately 10 per cent and occurs more frequently with gentamicin than tobramycin.[50,58,82] The duration of therapy, the daily quantity of drug administered, and the dosage schedule all influence aminoglycoside toxicity. Extracellular volume contraction, metabolic acidosis, and constant blood levels, rather than high peaks and low valleys, also predispose to nephrotoxicity. Amphotericin B and cyclosporine A are also dose-dependent agents that cause tubular damage.[19,68] Appropriate treatment is always reduction in the dose.[11]

Nonsteroidal anti-inflammatory drugs operate by inhibiting prostaglandin synthesis. In the kidney that is hypoperfused, locally produced vasodilating prostaglandin hormones function critically to preserve intrarenal blood flow. Administration of a nonsteroidal anti-inflammatory drug in this context can precipitate acute renal insufficiency by interference with the prostaglandin-dependent vasodilatory adaptive response.[16] Conversely, in a patient already receiving nonsteroidal anti-inflammatory medication, evolution of mild volume depletion might abruptly induce acute renal insufficiency because prostaglandin-mediated vasodilation is inoperative.

PREVENTION OF ACUTE RENAL FAILURE

Current knowledge of the pathophysiology of acute renal failure and reflection upon the surgical and medical conditions that predispose to it suggest several steps that help to prevent ARF (Table 2). Any postrenal problem that is allowed to persist may lead to acute tubular necrosis. Postoperative and trauma patients with a sudden onset of anuria should be considered to have mechanical obstruction of the ureters or lower urinary tract until this possibility has been excluded. Operative or traumatic injury of the urinary tract in the retroperitoneal or pelvic areas should be excluded whenever absolute anuria develops, because total anuria is rarely seen in the intrinsic renal and prerenal forms of ARF. The diagnosis can be established by

TABLE 2. Practical Guide to the Prevention of Postoperative Acute Renal Failure

Principle	Method
Monitor renal function	Serum creatinine Serum BUN Urinary output
Assess volume status	Physical examination Serial body weights Central venous pressure Pulmonary capillary wedge pressure
Control blood pressure	Intra-arterial monitoring Avoid hypotension (dopamine, isoproterenol) Reverse severe hypertension (nitroprusside)
Optimize cardiac function	Monitor cardiac output Afterload reduction Inotropic agents
Relieve urinary obstruction	Prompt radiographic diagnosis Catheter drainage Surgical correction
Avoid nephrotoxins	Limit radiologic contrast, aminoglycosides, etc. Adjust drug dosages
Prevent sepsis	Catheter care Abscess drainage Isolation techniques Antibiotics
Consider diuresis	Mannitol Furosemide Dopamine

cystoscopy, retrograde catheterization of the ureters, and radiographic techniques including ultrasound, intravenous pyelography, and computed tomographic (CT) scan of the abdomen.

The cystogram and urethrogram demonstrate traumatic rupture of the bladder and disruption of the urethra, respectively. These causes of acute postrenal ARF should be suspected in cases of pelvic fracture, particularly if the rectal examination reveals displacement of the prostate gland. Prompt recognition of the postrenal problem and surgical correction of the obstruction lead to complete recovery, whereas delayed recognition causes ARF.

Prerenal causes of ARF are prevented by optimizing volume status, cardiac function, and blood pressure, while avoiding nephrotoxins and infections. Extracellular volume can be estimated by physical examination in many cases. When it cannot be judged accurately, central venous pressure or pulmonary capillary wedge pressure must be measured. One of the most important means of evaluating the volume status in an oliguric patient is by fluid challenge. The intravascular volume is increased by infusing crystalloid or colloid until the wedge pressure is raised to 15 to 18 cm. H_2O. A brisk diuresis suggests a prerenal cause for the oliguria. If oliguria persists, an intrinsic renal problem is suspected.

The mean arterial blood pressure must be restored to normal levels and vasoconstriction reversed to maintain the GFR above 60 ml. per minute and avoid activation of the renin-angiotensin system. In patients who are oliguric after hypotension, the blood pressure should be monitored by means of an intra-arterial cannula. Blood pressure should be restored to a mean pressure of 80 mm. Hg and maintained at that level by adequate volume replacement. The extracellular volume replacement is adequate if urinary output is 40 ml. or more per hour and the central venous pressure is normal. If hypotension, oliguria, and renal vasoconstriction have persisted for more than a few hours, the kidney becomes progressively less responsive to volume replacement. During this stage of functional renal failure, the administration of furosemide or mannitol may facilitate the partial return of renal function in association with adequate volume replacement.

Treatment with a loop diuretic such as furosemide or an osmotic agent such as mannitol may reverse early ARF by flushing the tubules and reducing distal tubal oxygen consumption. This treatment may convert oliguric renal failure to the nonoliguric form, but it does not alter the course of acute tubular necrosis. High-output renal failure is easier to manage clinically and may have a better prognosis for survival.[3,4] Although loop diuretics such as ethacrynic acid and furosemide are effective agents for increasing urinary flow in postoperative and posttrauma patients, they should not be used until the extracellular fluid volume has been restored to normal. Because furosemide is such an effective diuretic, it may induce a large urinary loss in a patient already volume depleted and whose oliguria is a normal response to the physiologic condition. Furosemide may convert homeostatic oliguria to ARF. To guard against the indiscriminate and dangerous use of loop diuretics, measurement of central venous or left atrial pressure should be made before administering these agents to an oliguric patient. When the extracellular fluid volume is proven normal, up to 200 mg. of furosemide or a single dose of 12.5 gm. of mannitol may be given intravenously for determining their efficacy. Alternatively, 5 μg. per kg. per min. of dopamine, a nonpressor dose, may be administered to increase renal blood flow directly. If these measures fail to reverse the acute oliguria, further diuretic therapy does not help, and dialysis should be instituted as metabolic abnormalities or uremic symptoms develop.[36,95] In cases of hemorrhagic or septic shock, diuretic therapy may be administered as part of the resuscitation. If the pulmonary capillary wedge pressure is normal or low, mannitol is an appropriate agent. If the wedge pressure is high, furosemide is better choice. Dopamine should be given with either regimen; but regardless which agent is chosen, diuretic therapy is no substitute for adequate volume replacement. In fact, even dopamine administered alone can dehydrate critically ill patients.[36]

Specific disease states require specific steps to prevent ARF in the perioperative period. For example, when liver failure is present, most data indicate that the effective circulating volume of the patient is reduced. In order to prevent ARF under these circumstances, the vascular space should be cautiously expanded to achieve a central venous pressure of greater than 8 cm. H_2O. Moreover, any reduction in volume that reduces renal perfusion should be avoided. Diuretics must be used cautiously so that diuresis is slow and gradual (no more than 0.5 kg. daily). Paracentesis should be used only for essential diagnosis and therapy. Nephrotoxic drugs, radiographic contrast, and nonsteroidal anti-inflammatory agents are particularly dangerous in the setting of kidneys prone to underperfusion and should be used only for clear and pressing indications.[75,76]

DIAGNOSIS OF ACUTE RENAL FAILURE

Deterioration of renal function in the postoperative setting usually attracts attention because of oliguria and rising creatinine concentrations. A systematic approach to such a patient is of great importance. The physician must first consider and evaluate prerenal and postrenal causes of the deteriorating renal function before concluding that intrinsic renal tubular damage has occurred. Often, the distinction between prerenal failure and ischemic tubular necrosis is unclear. In these instances, assessing the patient's response to careful volume expansion and optimization of cardiac performance are essential. In the absence of a premorbid serum BUN or creatinine, as is often the case in the emergency patient admitted for reparative operation, it is essential to consider the possibility that volume contraction, or compromised cardiac output, or some toxic insult is superimposed upon pre-existing chronic renal insufficiency. In this situation as well, the most important diagnostic test may be volume restitution and improving the cardiac performance. In addition, the surgeon is commonly confronted with critically ill patients whose multiple clinical problems and recent tissue injury provide reason for considering not only acute ischemic tubular necrosis but the concomitant presence of prerenal and postrenal compromises. Indeed, acute azotemia in the postoperative setting is commonly associated with combinations of volume depletion, third-spacing of body fluids, heart failure, and intrinsic tubular injury from ischemia and toxins and perhaps even an element of urinary tract obstruction. Failure to systematically consider and reasonably evaluate each of these possibilities for the declining renal function delays specific effective therapy and jeopardizes renal recovery.

Clinical Assessment

Evaluation should begin with a careful consideration of the clinical context, a review of the clinical course, and a physical examination with attention to blood pressure, heart rate, orthostatic changes if possible, and serial changes in body weight. Prerenal azotemia arises from inadequate perfusion of the kidneys. This must be considered in the patient with hemorrhage, an antecedent clinical history of congestive heart failure, a rapid diuresis induced by potent diuretic therapy, and loss of fluid by exudation from burned or otherwise traumatized tissue or by redistribution of intravascular fluid to a third space, such as in the patient with ascites, pleural effusions, or chest tube drainage. Detailed examination of intake and output is essential. Nasogastric fluid losses, diarrheal fluid losses, and fluid losses from drains all need to be counted in addition to the urinary output. Fluid intake should match these fluid losses both in quantity and in quality. For example, if blood losses or exudated fluid losses are replaced solely by protein-free crystalloid solutions, intravascular volume contraction evolves because only a fraction of administered pure crystalloid is retained in the intra-

vascular space. Intravascular volume depletion can be suspected by the detection of orthostatic changes in blood pressure and heart rate and mucous membrane dryness. Heart failure is apparent by the finding of rales, distended jugular veins, and S3 gallop, or sacral or lower extremity edema.

Specific clinical signs can aid in the diagnosis of obstructive ARF as well. Acute distention of the renal capsule causes flank pain, but this symptom is nonspecific and is also produced by pyelonephritis or renal infarction. Flank pain that radiates toward the groin may reflect ischemic necrosis and sloughing of renal papillae with obstruction or the presence of a stone. Disorders predisposing to renal papillary necrosis include chronic urinary tract obstruction with infection, diabetes mellitus, sickle cell disease, and analgesic overuse. Acute obstruction from nephrolithiasis is an unusual event, but demands consideration in the patient who has known renal stones and is experiencing a deterioration in renal function. Obstruction of the ureter or the urethra from blood clots may occur in patients with urogenital trauma and gross hematuria or in patients who have recently undergone retrograde instrumentation as a diagnostic procedure. Edema and spasm at the ureterovesicle junction is another complication from instrumentation that can impair urinary outflow. Finally, forced bed rest often eventuates in inadequate bladder emptying and urinary retention, particularly in the elderly individual who might have an enlarged prostate or relaxed pelvic musculature. The complaint of suprapubic discomfort and the percussion of a distended tender bladder are signs of this problem. Simply inserting a Foley catheter and draining a large volume of retained urine can be a very valuable diagnostic and therapeutic maneuver.

Acute tubular injury is suspected when the clinical history and examination allow exclusion of prerenal and postrenal causes of ARF and include data such as periods of hypotension, recent crush injury, or exposure to nephrotoxins. The patient may be in shock; with mottled cool skin and poor mentation, or may show signs of fluid overload and cardiac failure because of excessive fluid administration at a time when renal function is severely compromised. More specific diagnostic data are derived from laboratory studies.

The quantity of urine is helpful in the differential diagnosis. A twenty-four urine volume less than 100 ml. is most often associated with complete urinary tract obstruction, bilateral renal cortical necrosis from prolonged shock, or bilateral renal artery occlusion. If there is fluctuation in urinary flow from oliguria to polyuria, the physician should consider intermittent urinary tract obstruction. Prerenal states are most often associated with diminished urinary flows, since the kidney is hypoperfused and is attempting to maximally conserve salt and water. Acute tubular necrosis, however, may present with oliguria or polyuria. Nonoliguric ARF from acute tubular injury is increasingly recognized and is thought to reflect a less severe form of tubular injury.

LABORATORY STUDIES

Urinalysis

Examination of the urine is an essential diagnostic test. A grossly cloudy urine suggests infection or crystalluria. Pink or red urine suggests the presence of either red cells, myoglobin, or free hemoglobin. A positive urine test for blood on the dip stick in the absence of red cells on microscopic examination is consistent with free hemoglobin or myoglobin. In patients with prerenal azotemia, the urine is usually concentrated and there may be numerous hyaline and finely granular casts. In patients with ATN, sloughed tubular cells, brown tubular cell casts, and numerous granular casts are common. In patients with urinary obstruction, the urine sediment is frequently unremarkable but may contain fragments of tissue, mucus, red blood cells, or numerous crystals of urate or calcium oxalate. Papillary necrosis is often associated with numerous red and white blood cells and

TABLE 3. Urine Diagnostic Indices*

	Prerenal Azotemia	Tubular Injury	Obstruction
Urine osmolality	>500	<350	Variable
U/P osmolality	>1.25	<1.1	Variable
U/P urea	>8	<3	Variable
U/P creatinine	>40	<20	<20
Urine sodium	<20	>40	>40
FE sodium	<1	>3	>3

* U/P, urea to plasma ratio; FE, fractional excretion.

small fragments of recognizable papillary tissue. In patients who have allergic interstitial nephritis from a drug reaction, leukocyturia and eosinophiluria are frequently noted. A number of diagnostic indices derived from urinary and serum chemistries have been developed to differentiate prerenal ARF from ATN. These are listed in Table 3 and are easily derived from simultaneously obtained spot urine and blood samples. Sodium, creatinine, urea, and osmolality should be measured on each sample.

Urine Osmolality

The urine in ATN is *isosthenuric*—that is, the urine osmolality is very close to that of plasma. Thus, oliguric patients with a urinary osmolality near 300 mOsm. per liter are likely to have ATN, whereas patients with prerenal azotemia are likely to have a more concentrated urine with osmolality greater than 500 mOsm. per liter. However, in actuality, many patients in either group have values between 300 and 500 mOsm. per liter, so that urine osmolality values do not provide precise discriminatory information. The ratio of urine to plasma osmolality, however, has been shown to be more discriminating than urinary values alone. Urine to plasma osmolality ratios less than 1.10 are consistent with ATN, whereas ratios greater than 1.25 are more consistently found in prerenal states.

Urinary Urea and Creatinine

Urine-to-plasma urea and urine-to-plasma creatinine ratios are more useful and widely used than osmolality ratios. A urine-to-plasma creatinine ratio below 20 is indicative of ATN, whereas a urine-to-plasma creatinine ratio above 40 indicates prerenal azotemia; values between 20 and 40 are nondiscriminatory. Likewise, a urine-to-plasma urea ratio less than 3 reflects tubular injury and a value greater than 8 is held to reflect prerenal azotemia. Again, values between 3 and 8 are nondiscriminatory. In patients with obstructive renal failure, decreased urine-to-plasma creatinine urea and ratios are found, but these tests are not helpful in this category of patient and can be misleading.

Urine Sodium

Much has been written concerning the usefulness of the urinary sodium concentration and the fractional excretion of sodium (FE$_{Na}$) as more precise diagnostic indices of the etiology of oliguria.[18,32,33,74] The hypoperfused kidney is sodium avid and a low urinary sodium concentration is characteristic of prerenal azotemia. However, when actual tubular injury has occurred, there is diminished renal sodium reabsorption. Thus, patients with established ATN or prolonged urinary obstruction usually have a higher urine sodium—specifically above 40 mEq. per liter. Urinary sodium values between 20 and 40 mEq. per liter are nondiscriminatory and may reflect evolving tubular injury from a prolonged prerenal state. Because so many patients appear to be in the nondiagnostic zone, the urinary sodium concentration has not provided confident diagnostic discrimination between the two most frequently encountered causes of ARF, prerenal failure, and ATN. Therefore, the fractional excretion of sodium, which is that percentage of filtered sodium that escapes

reabsorption, has been held as a more precise index of renal sodium handling and is generally believed to more effectively discriminate acute tubular injury from prerenal azotemia.[69] Calculation of the fractional excretion of sodium (FE$_{Na}$) requires simultaneous measurement of serum sodium and creatinine and urine sodium and creatinine. As shown in the following formulas, urine volume is not pertinent; therefore, the spot urine sample is sufficient.

$$FE_{Na} = \frac{\text{Excreted Na}}{\text{Filtered Na}}$$

$$FE_{Na} = \frac{U_{Na}V}{P_{Na} \times GFR}$$

$$FE_{Na} = \frac{U_{Na}V}{P_{Na}} \times \frac{Pcreat}{UcreatV}$$

$$FE_{Na} = \frac{U_{Na} \times Pcreat}{P_{Na} \times Ucreat}$$

Under normal circumstances the fractional excretion of sodium is less than 1 per cent of the filtered load. Acute renal failure from established tubular injury or obstruction is associated with FE$_{Na}$ values above 3 per cent. While the FE$_{Na}$ has become a widely used and credible diagnostic guide to the nature of the ARF, two exceptions to these rules have been well-documented: (1) radiocontrast-induced ATN is often associated with FE$_{Na}$ values below 1 per cent,[34] and (2) occasional patients whose clinical course suggests the diagnosis of ATN have initial urine sodium values and FE$_{Na}$ less than 10 mEq. per liter and 1 per cent, respectively, but later become higher.[101] It is thought that these patients sustain tubular injury from prolonged hypotension or multiple episodes of such, so that they initially have less sodium in their urine. Additionally, diuretics administered within 12 hours prior to the test may alter these values.

Each of these diagnostic indices is useful and should routinely be employed; together, they can provide highly accurate diagnostic information. However, each test has known exceptions and should not be interpreted rigidly, particularly if it counters clinical judgment. Most important, regardless of the values of these renal failure indices, the patient should be examined carefully, and efforts should be directed toward improving circulatory hemodynamics, treating infection, relieving obstruction, and removing nephrotoxins. Following the clinical course while making these improvements may prove to be the most important diagnostic maneuver.

RADIOGRAPHIC STUDIES

The cause of ARF can usually be ascertained after eliciting a careful history, performing a thorough physical examination, and obtaining blood and urine tests as outlined. When the diagnosis is not clear after these steps, more sophisticated radiographic studies may be necessary. Radiologic techniques detect hydronephrosis, impairments in renal arterial or venous blood flow, abnormalities of size, shape or location of the kidney, and certain abnormalities of the collecting system.

Plain Film of the Abdomen

The plain film of the kidneys, ureter, and bladder (KUB) or tomography of the kidney is a simple and safe approach in demonstrating renal size and the presence of radiopaque stones. Longitudinal calcifications may suggest the presence of an abdominal aortic aneurysm.

Ultrasonography

In any patient with ARF, the possibility of obstruction should be considered. A safe and effective method of evaluating this possibility is provided by renal ultrasonography. The presence of the kidneys, their size, and the morphology of the collecting system can be defined. This completely noninvasive technique detects small renal calculi by their strong acoustic reflection at the surface of the stone and distal accoustic shadowing. Obstruction produces hydronephrosis, which is observed on the sonogram as a sonolucent "fluid-filled" area representing the dilated calices and renal pelvis surrounded by the echogenic renal parenchyma.

Radionuclide Scan

Radioisotopic renograms have been used to study both the perfusion and function of kidneys in ARF patients.[8,23,87] The primary value of renal scans is to crudely assess perfusion of the kidneys. These examinations are most useful after major aneurysm repair and renal transplantation to assess patency of vessels. They are also useful in the evaluation of urine extravasation after pelvic trauma. Although the GFR can be calculated following injection of ^{99m}Tc-sodium pertechnetate or DTPA (diethylene-triamine-penta-acetic acid), the two most commonly used radiopharmaceuticals, this is rarely of clinical benefit in the acute evaluation of ARF.

Indiscriminate use of this expensive test should be discouraged. When assessment of renal perfusion is important, however, these remain useful. Arteriography is usually preferred to determine the cause and extent of most anatomic vascular obstruction and is essential if operation is being considered.

Intravenous Pyelography (IVP)

In ARF, the need for a contrast study must be weighed carefully against the known risk of contrast-related nephrotoxicity and allergy. Twenty to 60 gm. of elemental iodine is commonly used in evaluating adults with azotemia.[8] The contrast agents are excreted by glomerular filtration; enter the tubules of the renal cortex to produce the nephrogram phase; and then are eventually excreted into the calices, pelvis, and ureter to produce the pyelogram phase. IVP is particularly valuable in the recognition of obstructive ARF because the level of obstruction may be identified. In fact, the absence of a diagnostic pyelogram suggests that obstruction is not the etiology of the ARF. Patients with partial urinary tract obstruction filter the contrast and then reabsorb it in the tubules, thus speeding the development of the nephrogram and making it increasingly more dense. In obstructed patients with slow excretion into the collecting system, delayed films 12 to 24 hours after injection may be necessary to demonstrate the site of blockage. An immediate, dense, and persistent nephrogram is also characteristic of ATN. Retrograde pyelography is rarely used because it is painful, risks infection, and traumatizes the urinary tract, and the information it provides can now be obtained by less invasive techniques under most circumstances.[23]

Computed Tomography

CT scanning is a noninvasive, accurate procedure that can define kidney location and size as well as diagnose obstruction. The dilated renal collecting system can be visualized clearly without contrast media. In most cases of ARF, a sonogram or a intravenous pyelogram provides sufficient diagnostic data without need of the more expensive CT scan. However, when an aortic aneurysm, retroperitoneal fibrosis, or retroperitoneal malignancy is suspected as the cause of postrenal ARF, the CT not only discloses the obstruction but may also define the cause.

Arteriography

Arteriography is useful in selected patients when one suspects renal artery embolism (e.g., atrial fibrillation with history of mural thrombus), arteriosclerotic renal artery occlusion, abdominal aorta or renal artery aneurysm, or a systemic vasculitis affecting the kidneys (e.g., polyarteritis nodosa). Radionuclide scans of the kidney can exclude renal artery thrombosis but cannot document the degree of renal artery stenosis. Digital subtraction arteriograms demonstrate the renal arteries while

minimizing the exposure of the kidney to nephrotoxic contrast material. ARF due to bilateral renal vein thrombosis in dehydrated children is diagnosed with venography.[8]

BIOPSY

Biopsy is reserved for those cases of ARF where the diagnosis of acute tubular necrosis appears doubtful and where one or more intrinsic renal etiologies may be present, such as acute glomerular nephritis, acute interstitial nephritis, or acute vasculitis. When postrenal and prerenal causes of ARF have been excluded in surgical patients, most have ATN, and so renal biopsy has a *very* limited role in their management. An exception is the renal transplant patient with ARF where biopsy has an important part in differentiating acute rejection from acute tubular necrosis, drug toxicity, and recurrent primary disease. Percutaneous needle biopsy of the kidney has some risk (e.g., a 9 per cent complication rate in one series); therefore, it should be performed only for clear indications such as prolonged renal failure beyond 3 weeks and is contraindicated in the presence of bleeding diathesis or uncontrolled hypertension.[8,56]

MANAGEMENT OF THE PATIENT WITH ESTABLISHED ACUTE RENAL FAILURE

When oliguria and/or a rise in BUN and creatinine supervene in the postoperative patient, the clinician should be alert to the possibility of evolving acute renal failure. The clinician's attention at this time should be directed toward considering, seeking, and excluding specific reversible causes of the apparent deterioration of renal function. When the reversible factors have been corrected and the urinary indices have established tubular injury, a program of therapy should be immediately undertaken. The principles of therapy center on (1) anticipating the electrolyte and fluid balance problems that are known to be associated with ARF; (2) anticipating the consequences of various tests and fluid prescriptions so as to prevent electrolyte and volume disturbances from evolving; (3) correcting any existing biochemical and fluid balance aberrations; (4) preventing late systemic complications from the hypercatabolic state and uremia; and (5) adjusting the dosage of administered drugs to compensate for their impaired elimination (Table 4).

FLUID AND ELECTROLYTE MANAGEMENT

Hyperkalemia

Early attention must be given the fluid and electrolyte status of the patient, even while diagnostic information is being obtained. Of all the electrolyte abnormalities that might be en-

TABLE 4. Management Priorities in the Patient with Acute Renal Failure

Initial
1. Review clinical setting, examine patient
2. Exclude/correct prerenal and postrenal factors
3. Analyze blood and urine for electrolyte emergencies, renal failure indices, sediment
4. Correct hyperkalemia, acidosis, volume

Ongoing
1. Monitor chemistries, fluid intake, output, daily weight
2. Match intake to output plus insensible losses
3. Initiate dialysis early, anticipate complications, individualize the prescription
4. Anticipate infection, sepsis, bleeding, volume problems
5. Initiate nutritional support early
6. Alter drug therapy
7. Anticipate and prevent additional injury

countered in ARF, hyperkalemia is the most serious and must be treated rapidly. The threat of hyperkalemia is cardiac arrest. The severity of hyperkalemia can be judged by the electrocardiographic (ECG) changes, which include peaked T waves, prolongation of PR intervals, loss of P waves, and widening of the QRS complex. These changes indicate diminished cardiac excitability and imminent cardiac standstill.

When significant ECG changes are apparent, emergent therapy is indicated. First, a calcium infusion with 1 to 3 ampules of 10 per cent calcium gluconate should be administered over 5 to 15 minutes to stabilize the cardiac membranes and reverse the toxic effects of hyperkalemia. This membrane-stabilizing action of calcium is immediate in onset but is relatively short-lived. It is often lifesaving, but other therapy must be instituted to actually lower the serum potassium and remove the excess potassium from the body. These therapies include the administration of concentrated glucose and insulin and intravenous sodium bicarbonate therapy.

Glucose and insulin therapy is best administered as a 10 per cent glucose solution with 20 to 30 units of regular insulin per liter. The rate of intravenous administration should be titrated according to serial serum potassium values but may be administered as rapidly as 500 ml. per hour. The clinician might choose to initiate glucose-insulin therapy with a bolus of 50 per cent glucose plus 10 units of regular insulin intravenously, followed by the drip infusion. The action of glucose and insulin begins with 10 minutes and may persist for as long as the drip is continued.

Sodium bicarbonate can be administered either as a bolus over 5 to 10 minutes or diluted in 5 to 10 per cent glucose in water and infused slowly. Both forms of therapy lower the serum potassium level by driving potassium into cells, rather than removing it from the body. Ultimately, therefore, enteral administration of cation-exchange resins such as sodium polystyrene sulfonate (Kayexelate) or dialytic therapy must be employed to remove the potassium from the body.

Each type of therapy has its limitations. With glucose-insulin infusion, water overload with progressive hyponatremia is a concern; and with large amounts of sodium bicarbonate, volume overload, pulmonary congestion, and hypernatremia are problems. Cation-exchange resins are most effective if administered orally with sorbitol. The presence of an ileus or intestinal injury precludes this mode of administration and the less effective but still useful rectal route of administration is employed. In addition, precipitous reduction in serum potassium via hemodialysis can be associated with complex ventricular arrhythmias, particularly if other electrolyte disturbances coexist. Continuous ECG monitoring is mandatory.

Fluid Volume

Volume overload is another concern in the patient with acute renal failure. Careful monitoring of fluid intake and output along with daily weights can prevent this undesirable situation. If the patient is oliguric, excessive salt and water input cause hypertension and pulmonary edema with their attendant complications. The clinician should restrict fluid intake to match actual fluid losses plus 500 to 700 ml. per day of insensible loss and 200 ml. per day per degree of fever. It is important that frequent regular quantitation of all fluid losses be assessed, because nasogastric drainage, wound drainages, stool losses, or urine flow vary from hour to hour. It is best that standing orders for a fixed amount of fluid per day not be written, because fluid administration must match fluctuating losses and represent necessary administration of blood products, antibiotics, nutrition, etc. Volume overload in the oliguric patient can be treated successfully only with phlebotomy or some mode of dialysis.

Hyponatremia

Evolution of hyponatremia indicates that free water intake is exceeding free water elimination. Severe hyponatremia is often

a contributing factor to the encephalopathy and propensity to convulsions that complicate acute renal failure. This most often obtains when administered intravenous fluid is excessive and hypotonic. When hyponatremia begins to evolve, free water restriction must be prescribed. If the serum sodium concentration falls below 120 mEq. per liter, convulsions are imminent. Dialysis is the only maneuver that can correct the hyponatremia in this situation; hypertonic NaCl should not be administered in the oliguric patient with severe hyponatremia, because this patient is nearly always already fluid overloaded. Hyponatremia is best managed by an awareness of how it might evolve and preventing it.

Metabolic Acidosis

Metabolic acidosis often accompanies acute renal failure, especially in association with major surgical therapy, traumatic injury, or sepsis. In the hypercatabolic patient, acid production is substantially increased, and the markedly reduced renal function allows no means for excretion of the accumulating acid nor the regeneration of consumed bicarbonate. There are a number of potentially harmful effects from the progressive metabolic acidosis. These include nausea, vomiting, and cerebral dysfunction, as well as cardiac depression, insulin resistance, and impaired cellular metabolism. Acidosis is also an important factor contributing to hyperkalemia. Metabolic acidosis is treated with oral administration of Shohl's solution, intravenous or oral sodium bicarbonate, or dialysis. Enough alkali must be administered to not only repair the already existing acidosis but to maintain arterial pH and bicarbonate reserves at a level that matches the daily endogenous acid production from catabolism. In the average resting adult, daily acid production is approximately 1 mEq. per kg. per day. Therefore, 70 to 100 mEq. of alkali would maintain acid base balance. However, in the hypercatabolic patient who has tissue injury, has undergone a recent surgical procedure, or has sepsis, endogenous acid production can be two to three times this amount, which would require equal alkali administration. Care must be taken with administration of such large amounts of sodium bicarbonate. It expands extracellular volume, may precipitate pulmonary edema, and is often associated with hypernatremia because it is packaged as a hypertonic solution. If large amounts of sodium bicarbonate are required to maintain arterial pH, dialytic therapy must be initiated.

Hypocalcemia and Hyperphosphatemia

In an occasional patient, hypocalcemia and hyperphosphatemia may evolve. This occurrence is most common in the patient who has experienced tissue necrosis from a crush injury or a burn. When the serum phosphate exceeds 6 mg. per 100 ml., magnesium-free phosphate-binding antacids should be prescribed with meals to minimize elevations in the calcium-phosphate product and attenuate soft tissue deposition of calcium-phosphate crystals. Ionized calcium in acute renal failure is usually near normal, owing to acidosis, uremic state, and hypoalbuminemia. Infusion of calcium is therefore unnecessary unless carpopedal spasm or tetany develops. If phosphate is not lowered, infusion of calcium causes soft tissue precipitation of calcium-phosphate. Ultimately dialysis may be required to control phosphate and calcium balance.

Use of Diuretics

The therapeutic value of diuretics in the patient with acute tubular necrosis has been extensively investigated, but there is no general agreement as to whether their use can influence the recovery of renal function or requirement for dialysis.[36,61] Thus, at this time, it appears that high-dose diuretic use in patients with established ATN may increase the patient's urinary output and ease problems with fluid management. There is no certainty that it enhances renal recovery or diminishes the need for dialysis. It is generally agreed that diuretic use has no statistical influ-

TABLE 5. Indications for Dialysis

TABLE 5. Indications for Dialysis

Absolute indications (when unresponsive to conservative management)
1. Volume overload
2. Electrolyte abnormalities
3. Acidosis
4. Uremic signs and symptoms

Relative indications (when needed for improved patient management)
1. BUN >100 mg/dl in patient with ARF
2. Need for enteral or hyperalimentation in patient with ARF
3. Need for multiple transfusions in patient with ARF
4. Hemorrhagic complications in patient with ARF
5. Drug intoxication with hemodialyzable substance

ence on ultimate patient outcome or mortality. Multiple large doses of loop-blocking diuretics may cause transient or permanent nerve deafness and seizures in patients with renal impairment.

One cannot predict *a priori* which patient might be better served by a nonoliguric state. Higher urinary flow might obviate pulmonary congestion, ease blood product administration, and permit greater volumes of hyperalimentation solutions. Although these benefits might not be statistically quantifiable, they could be pivotal in an individual patient. Mortality in ARF is determined not so much by the renal failure itself but by supervening complications such as malnutrition, susceptibility to infection, bleeding, and cardiovascular events. To the extent that higher urinary flow might permit better management of these issues, then benefit from diuretic conversion to a nonoliguric state might accrue. Simultaneously, one must be aware of the ototoxic potential of the loop diuretics and of the necessity to follow any ensuing diuresis with appropriate volume replacement to avoid extracellular fluid volume contraction.

USE OF DIALYSIS IN ACUTE RENAL FAILURE

Dialysis should be initiated when there is life-threatening hyperkalemia, severe acidosis, volume overload, uremic encephalopathy, or uremic pericarditis (Table 5). It should be borne in mind, however, that dialysis is best initiated prophylactically before the occurrence of any of these life-threatening complications of ARF, rather than as an urgent procedure.

The goals of dialysis therefore are (1) to remove uremic nitrogenous metabolites and amelioration of the uremic state, (2) to correct metabolic acidosis, (3) to remove excess fluid, (4) to normalize serum electrolyte concentrations, (5) to improve platelet and leukocyte function, and (6) to permit effective hyperalimentation.

There are currently three forms of renal replacement therapy available for patients suffering from ARF. Hemodialysis, peritoneal dialysis, and hemofiltration are each available for use in a series of modifications. Each mode of therapy has its own advantages and disadvantages (Table 6). Usually one form of therapy is best for an individual patient. Consultation with a nephrologist to select and initiate renal replacement therapy is usually the best course of action.

HEMODIALYSIS

For the hypercatabolic patient, hemodialysis is usually the treatment of choice because of its extreme efficiency. Early initiation of dialysis is now the practiced rule, because the demonstration that prophylactic dialysis initiated before the creatinine exceeds 8 to 10 mg. per 100 ml. and BUN exceeds 100 ml. per 100 ml. improves patient outcome. The frequency of dialysis depends upon the severity of catabolism, the severity of uremia, the urgency of volume overload and serum electrolyte control, and certain accompanying clinical complications such as bleeding or sepsis. The dialysis prescription must be individualized and is best devised in cooperation with the consulting nephrologist.

In some postoperative patients, 4 to 5 hours of daily dialysis may be required to attenuate hypercatabolism and uremia; in others, a dialysis session 3 or 4 times per week may suffice. The degree of catabolism may be gauged by the interdialytic rise of BUN and fall in serum HCO_3. In general, dialyzing to maintain the BUN below 100 mg. per 100 ml. is a reasonable goal in this context.

It is important that the administration of blood products be coordinated with the dialysis treatments. Removal of fluid by ultrafiltration during dialysis is controllable and can be increased to create the necessary "space" for the blood products. Banked blood often is a source of free potassium, owing to leakage from within the erythrocytes. Administration during dialysis can provide an exit for this exogenous potassium load. As a practical consideration, it is particularly stressful and expensive to the patient to undergo a 4-hour treatment in the morning, only to return to dialysis that night because of transfusions given in the day that caused pulmonary edema or hyperkalemia.

Hemodialysis efficiently clears certain antibiotics from the circulation. Aminoglycosides undergo approximately 50 per cent clearance with a 4-hour dialysis, so their administration should be specifically ordered after each treatment, and the dose should be gauged according to measured serum concentrations. Penicillins and cephalosporins also have high clearances, and their administration should coincide with the end of dialysis.

TABLE 6. Renal Replacement Therapy for ARF

Modality	Hemodialysis	Peritoneal Dialysis	Hemofiltration
Efficiency	High for toxin and electrolyte removal	Moderate for toxin and electrolyte removal	Moderate for toxin and electrolyte removal
Frequency	Intermittent 3–4 hr./day	Continuous 24 hr./day	Continuous 24 hr./day
Access	Venous catheter required	Abdominal catheter required	Venous and arterial catheters required
Cardiovascular strain	Significant	Limited	Limited
Anticoagulation	Not usually needed*	Not needed	Needed

* "No heparin" or citrate regional anticoagulation.

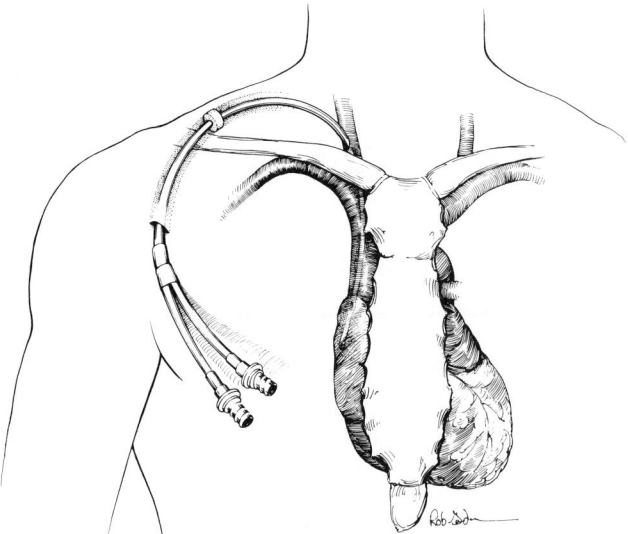

Figure 5. A Permcath hemodialysis catheter inserted in the right internal jugular position. The felt cuff and subcutaneous tunnel reduce the frequency of catheter-mediated bacteremia. It has a longer use-life than standard subclavian dialysis catheters for treatment of acute renal failure. (From Schwab, S. J., et al.: Prospective evaluation of a Dacron cuffed hemodialysis catheter for prolonged use. Am. J. Kidney Dis., *21:*166, 1988.)

Vascular access for hemodialysis is usually provided by double lumen venous dialysis catheters inserted percutaneously at the bedside in the jugular, subclavian, or femoral position. The continuous blood path made possible by the double lumen design allows highly efficient toxin clearances and "no heparin" dialysis techniques. The life of these catheters varies from 3 days for femoral insertion to 2 weeks for jugular and subclavian positions.[86] When dialysis dependence is prolonged, surgically inserted felt-cuffed dialysis catheters allow a longer use[86] (Fig. 5). Regardless of the catheter or site chosen, strict aseptic tech-

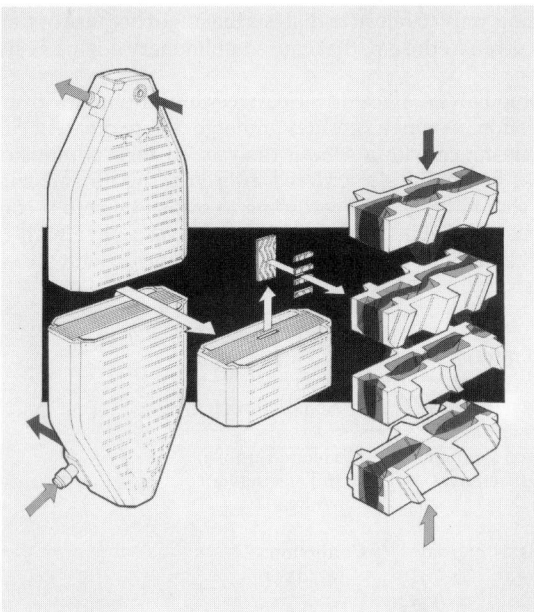

Figure 6. A cross-sectional view of one type of modern counter-current flow dialyzer. Blood enters the dialyzer at the top through a central inlet, where it is evenly and symmetrically distributed to a number of parallel channels between pairs of membranes, and is then discharged at the bottom after treatment. The dialysis fluid flows against the current of the blood from bottom to top on the other side of the membranes, in order to provide maximal gradients for solute diffusion. Constant changes in microchannel geometry create optimal conditions for solute transfer. (Diagram provided by Gambro AB, Lund, Sweden.)

nique must be observed and regular maintenance care must be performed. These indwelling foreign bodies can be a source of secondary bacteremia and sepsis.

The advantages of hemodialysis rest almost exclusively with its highly efficient clearance of toxins and fluids. It remains the most efficient form of therapy readily available. New techniques and technology applied to hemodialysis have dramatically broadened the number of patients who can receive this therapy (Fig. 6). Hemodialysis can now be safely provided for the majority of unstable patients. Techniques for "no heparin" dialysis[24,81,84] and citrate regional anticoagulation[41,78] have eliminated the mandatory need for anticoagulation, minimizing dialysis associated bleeding. Nonetheless, some significant disadvantages or complications remain; these also relate to the efficiency of the treatment.

Complications of Hemodialysis

HYPOTENSION. Hypotension frequently accompanies acute hemodialysis in the critically ill patient.[60] It arises from a number of factors. First, there is an obligate extracorporeal blood volume of approximately 125 to 175 ml. This may be sufficient intravascular depletion to cause a fall in blood pressure, particularly since coexistent acidosis, uremia, hypoxemia, and hyperkalemia may impair the cardiovascular reflex responses that might otherwise attenuate the hypotension. Routinely priming the patient with albumin, saline, or Ringer's solution should mitigate this problem. Secondly, as the dialysis proceeds, extracellular water and sodium are removed by ultrafiltration at a rate determined by dialyzer characteristics and transmembrane hydrostatic pressures. Hypotension caused by ultrafiltration or vascular unresponsiveness can be minimized by saline or blood product administration and modulation of the transmembrane pressures. The change in osmolarity of the blood as urea is removed is another important cause of hypotension because this is associated with shifts of plasma water into the intracellular compartment; it can be particularly troublesome if the patient already has low plasma oncotic pressure from hypoalbuminemia. Using high sodium dialysate (140 to 144 mEq. per liter) and volumetric fluid removal or sequential ultrafiltration minimizes these problems. Use of acetate as the dialysate buffer is also associated with hypotension, particularly in the unstable patient, because of its action as a vasodilator. For this reason, bicarbonate is now used as the dialysate buffer in unstable patients. Blood oxygen saturation frequently decreases 5 to 10 torr in patients undergoing dialysis.[43] This can be hazardous in the marginal patient; therefore, oxygen should be administered or FIO_2 increased in borderline hypoxic patients.

In summary, significant advances in dialysis technology have minimized hypotension so that this therapy can be offered to unstable patients from whom it was previously withheld. Nonetheless, hypotension remains a significant complication that must be respected and anticipated.

BLEEDING. Despite the development of techniques for "no heparin" dialysis[24,81,84,93] and new methods of regional anticoagulation using citrate,[39,78] postoperative patients in whom ARF develops are at risk of bleeding for many reasons. The incision has exposed many tiny vessels, which are apt to bleed if coagulation is not intact. Additionally, uremia is accompanied by a platelet defect that prolongs bleeding time and impairs clot formation. Blood loss and multiple transfusion might have depleted coagulation factors and impaired their cascade interaction because of the accompanying citrate, which complexes calcium ions. The convergence of these problems explains why hemorrhage is a major cause of death in postoperative patients with ARF. Effective dialysis improves the platelet defect. Administration of plasma or cryoprecipitate can restore coagulation factors with sometimes dramatic effectiveness. Administration of desmopressin acetate (DDAVP) and cryoprecipitate and intravenous administration of estrogens help correct the platelet defect of uremia.[48,63,64]

DYSEQUILIBRIUM SYNDROME. The dysequilibrium syndrome is a constellation of symptoms and signs experienced by intensively dialyzed individuals that consists of nausea, vomiting, muscle twitching, lethargy, and confusion and may progress to coma and convulsions. It follows the rapid removal of solutes from extracellular fluid, paradoxical cerebrospinal fluid (CSF) acidosis, and cerebral edema. The best management is prevention. The intensity of a dialysis session must be reduced at the first sign that dysequilibrium is evolving; extracorporeal blood flow should be slowed, and the dialysis session should be shortened. Infusion of mannitol may effectively attenuate the osmolarity changes. Because of the problems that dysequilibrium can create, initial dialysis sessions are usually conducted with slower blood flow rates and shorter durations. This may mandate more frequent sessions and is one principal reason for initiating dialysis early in the course of ARF.

ARRHYTHMIAS. Cardiac rhythm disturbances are not infrequent in patients with ARF undergoing hemodialysis. They have the risk of causing sudden death. Acute changes in serum potassium, calcium, pH, and perhaps sodium as well as the hypoxemia, hypocapnia, and release of catecholamines that accompany hemodialysis explain the risk. For this reason, continuous ECG monitoring is essential in the acutely uremic patient with electrolyte aberrations. Further into the course of renal failure, when serum electrolytes are stable between dialysis sessions, a more casual posture regarding continuous monitoring is permissible.

PERITONEAL DIALYSIS

In a patient with severe coronary artery disease, acute myocardial infarction, advanced cardiac failure, and hypotension, or known cerebrovascular disease, hemodialysis may be deemed too hazardous. Similarly, a patient with dramatic or recurrent bleeding or multiple severe electrolyte abnormalities and advanced uremia may be harmed by the vigor of hemodialysis. In these situations, peritoneal dialysis may be safer than hemodialysis.

Peritoneal dialysis (PD) can accomplish removal of toxic metabolites, correction of electrolyte disturbances, and fluid removal by ultrafiltration at approximately one fifth the efficiency of hemodialysis. However, PD is a 24-hour continuous therapy; so the apparent inefficiency is not as prohibitive as it appears initially. It is precisely for this reason that it might be preferable in the above-mentioned circumstances. For the patient with a fragile cardiovascular system, hypotension is avoided because fluid shifts are slower and there is no extracorporeal blood circulation. Solute shifts are also slower with PD than with hemodialysis, which reduces the problems of disequilibrium and cardiac and neuromuscular irritability from rapid electrolyte changes. In addition, anticoagulants are not required for PD.

In treating acute renal failure with peritoneal dialysis, a small-lumen rigid *acute* catheter inserted by direct puncture may be used. The dialysis provided by this catheter is satisfactory, but peritonitis is an expected complication after more than 72 hours of use. The advantage of the acute catheter is that higher volumes (2 liters) of exchange are usually possible without leakage. Alternatively, a single-cuff Tenckhoff catheter can be placed either at the bedside or in the operating room. Sterile technique is essential, and a tunnel should be constructed to minimize fluid leaks and the likelihood of infection. Utilizing a modern titanium tubing adaptor and single-bag technique that is employed for outpatient ambulatory dialysis, the dialysis procedure can be accomplished easily and aseptically. The Tenckhoff catheter is suitable for prolonged use, but initially lower volumes (1 liter per exchange) are required to minimize leaking around the catheter. When leaking occurs, volume of exchange should be reduced. If leaking continues, PD should be temporarily discontinued to prevent peritonitis. PD should be performed with fluid continuously present in the abdomen and one to two hourly exchanges of the fluid with 1000 to 2000 ml. of dialysate. The larger the volume of dialysate and the more frequent the exchange of fluid, the more efficient is the dialysis. The higher the glucose concentration, the more efficient the ultrafiltration.

One contraindication to PD is the hypercatabolic patient. When the rate of ureagenesis is high, PD may simply be inadequate. Peritoneal sclerosis, multiple intra-abdominal adhesions, and compartmentalization of the peritoneal cavity may preclude catheter insertion and cause inadequate fluid flow. Although PD can be done in the postoperative abdomen, protruding drains, leaking incisions, and the presence of an enterostomy make this technique extremely hazardous in terms of infection and incomplete healing. Fresh vascular grafts in the abdomen are a relative contraindication to PD because of the risk that peritonitis would lead to graft infection. Respiratory complications are not infrequent. The presence of 1.5 to 2 liters of fluid in the abdomen impairs ventilation and can cause hypoxia, atelectasis, and pneumonia. Communications between the pleural and peritoneal cavities are sometimes present, either congenital or acquired, and instilled peritoneal fluid may accumulate within the pleural space.

HEMOFILTRATION

Hemofiltration is a technique of renal replacement therapy that uses the patient's own blood pressure to provide blood flow through a highly permeable artificial kidney (hemofilter). This technique requires a large-bore arterial line (usually femoral) and a large-bore venous return line (usually femoral). The higher the blood pressure, the better the blood flow; therefore effectiveness improves. In cases of adequate blood pressure, a Scribner shunt can provide vascular access. When ultrafiltration alone is desired, the technique is termed slow continuous ultrafiltration (SCUF). When ultrafiltrate is steadily replaced with a replacement fluid, the technique is termed continuous arteriovenous hemofiltration (CAVH). When dialysate is dripped in a counter current manner as in hemodialysis, the technique is termed continuous arteriovenous hemodiafiltration (CAVHD).[7,41,42,49,57,59,65]

The advantages of this technique are similar to those of peritoneal dialysis. This technique provides smooth, continuous, moderately effective therapy. Demands on the cardiovascular system are minimal, hypotension is limited, and continuous fluid removal is allowed. The disadvantages include some form of continuous anticoagulation, because flows are not rapid enough for "no heparin" techniques and 24 hours of citrate regional anticoagulation is very difficult. In addition, a large bore arterial line is required in most instances. It is, however, an excellent mode of therapy in patients after abdominal surgery, when circulatory instability or the need for continuous fluid therapy makes hemodialysis less desirable. The effectiveness of this therapy is similar to that of peritoneal dialysis, and this makes it less desirable in highly catabolic and hyperkalemic patients. In some instances, hemofiltration and hemodialysis are used in combination to achieve the goal of continuous fluid removal and effective solute removal.

MANAGEMENT OF THE LATE COMPLICATIONS OF ACUTE RENAL FAILURE

Probably the one factor that determines patient survival in ARF more than any other single factor is the nature and severity of the associated illnesses. Nevertheless, in examining the primary causes of death in patients with ARF, it is apparent that the evolution of complications during the course of renal failure has

TABLE 7. Complications of Acute Renal Failure

Early Complications	Late Complications
Hyperkalemia	Bleeding
Hyponatremia	Localized infections
Acidosis	Sepsis
Hypocalcemia, hyperphosphatemia	Malnutrition
Volume overload, pulmonary edema	Poor healing
Pericarditis	Cardiac failure
Arrhythmias	Somnolence, coma
Nausea, vomiting	
Convulsions, coma	

a dramatic impact on patient prognosis. Today, more than 50 per cent of patients who die of ARF do so because of sepsis and pulmonary infections. Respiratory and cardiac failure represents another 25 per cent, and severe bleeding is responsible for 10 to 15 per cent of patient deaths. Malnutrition is a frequent concomitant and is probably a primary permissive factor. Therefore, when the postoperative patient with ARF is stabilized with regard to acute fluid and electrolyte complications and the intensity of the uremia is under control by an individualized dialysis prescription, attention must be directed toward preventing and managing these late complications (Table 7).

Nutrition

Adequate nutrition is a daily concern in any postoperative patient; in the context of acute renal failure it assumes even greater importance. Acute uremia is a catabolic condition. The postoperative or trauma patient who cannot eat is also catabolic. Tissue catabolism in these patients releases potassium, acids, water, phosphorus, and nitrogenous products into the extracellular fluid. Such hypercatabolism not only contributes to the uremic problems that the patient is encountering but delays tissue healing, reduces immunity to infection, and weakens mucosal-epithelial barriers. Tissue breakdown and catabolic processes may be delayed by the administration of adequate calories and protein. However, the optimal amounts of calories and protein have not yet been precisely defined. Certainly, this varies in patients and is determined in part by age, body size, and associated illness and stress. The basal metabolic energy requirement for an adult is approximately 25 kcal. per kg. per day. When major surgical procedures, trauma, or renal failure supervenes, the number of calories required to neutralize tissue breakdown rises to approximately 40 to 50 kcal. per kg. per day.[54] The severely burned patient may require 60 to 75 kcal. per kg. per day. The relatively simple maneuver of supplying sufficient calories can markedly reduce endogenous protein catabolism and delay urea appearance in ARF, as was documented in 1949 and has since become the cornerstone of nutritional support.[17,67] The other major thrust in nutritional support has been the use of high-quality protein feeding. Excessive protein intake simply increases the nitrogen load and ureagenesis. However, a limited high quality protein intake can further improve nitrogen balance and net urea production over that achieved with carbohydrate support alone.[14] This observation has been documented and confirmed with elemental enteral feeding, as well as with elemental parenteral amino acid administration.[1,35]

Accordingly, the following guidelines aid formulation of a nutritional plan for the surgical patient with acute renal failure: (1) Supplement nutrition should be initiated as early as possible to attenuate catabolism, support healing, and decrease uremia. (2) Approximately 30 to 50 kcal. per kg. per day should be administered either enterally or parenterally, or both. Three quarters of the calories should be derived from carbohydrates. (3) Approximately 20 to 40 gm. of high-quality protein should

be supplied daily; it does not appear to be critical whether this is administered orally or parenterally. Patients receiving peritoneal dialysis or daily hemodialysis may require 10 to 15 gm. more per day to replace dialysis losses. (4) A minimal volume of water should be used to administer these supplements to avoid volume overload and hyponatremia. (5) It is preferable to increase the frequency and intensity of dialysis so as to allow hyperalimentation rather than to spare its prescription if volume considerations become critical. (6) Insulin should be added to manage hyperglycemia; and potassium, sodium, chloride, calcium, magnesium, and phosphorus levels should be carefully monitored and their administration individualized to avoid electrolyte aberrations.

Infection

Infection is the most common late complication of established acute renal failure and is estimated to occur in up to 90 per cent of surgical or trauma patients with ARF.[46,53,66] Pulmonary infections and septicemia represent the majority of cases. The primary reason for the high incidence of infection is the fact that the resistance of these patients is severely compromised. Uremia is associated with impaired white cell function, and the usual mechanical barriers to pathogen invasion are generally breached by indwelling venous and arterial catheters, arteriovenous shunts, endotracheal tubes, wounds, drains, and Foley catheters. To the extent possible, vascular lines should be minimized and eliminated, and those that are essential should be cleaned and dressed aseptically on a daily basis. At the first sign of cutaneous inflammation or infection, the line should be removed and the tip and skin area cultured. Foley catheters should be removed if the patient is oliguric. Routine use of prophylactic antibiotics in these patients is not indicated. No salutary effect has been demonstrated, and their use may even lead to an increased frequency of infection with resistant strains of bacteria. Infection surveillance should be a daily routine, and identified infections should be treated promptly with specifically directed antimicrobial therapy.

Bleeding

Gastrointestinal bleeding has been a particularly morbid complication in postoperative patients with ARF and may contribute to 20 per cent of deaths.[53,66] With early aggressive prophylactic dialysis and the common use of antacids and H_2 histamine blockers, the incidence and severity have decreased.[66] Bleeding follows a number of factors, including irritated mucosa from nasogastric tubes, stress ulcerations, inadequate nutrition, depletion of coagulation factors from repeated transfusions, and a platelet defect associated with uremia. Management priorities include adequate dialysis with minimal heparin or "no heparin" techniques or via the peritoneal route, maintenance of a neutral gastric pH, inclusion of fresh frozen plasma when numerous transfusions are being administered, and minimizing nasogastric tube suctioning. If bleeding is a threat or is not easily controlled, fresh cryoprecipitate may be beneficial. The platelet defect of uremia may be treated with DDAVP, cryoprecipitate, or conjugated estrogen.[48,63,64]

Drug Administration

Patients suffering from acute renal failure frequently require medications that are normally excreted by the kidneys. Digitalis and the penicillin, cephalosporin, and aminoglycoside families of antibiotics are common examples. Awareness of which drugs require dosage modifications is important in the management of these patients. The clinician should assume that each drug might require alteration in dosage and should consult the hospital pharmacist, nephrologist, infectious disease consultant, or appropriate literature references before prescribing potentially hazardous medication.[11]

PROGNOSIS OF ACUTE RENAL FAILURE

Untreated acute renal failure in surgical patients rapidly causes death from fluid overload or hyperkalemia. When early resuscitation efforts are successful, infection becomes the overwhelming concern. Among published series reviewing mortality in patients with ARF, 50 to 80 per cent of deaths are due to infections. In the Brigham Hospital series, for example, bronchopneumonia represented 27.5 per cent and gram-negative septicemia 25 per cent of deaths in patients with ARF.[95] Infections may arise from necrotic tissue in the operative site or from undetected abscess cavities. Particularly common are infections of the urinary tract and lungs, especially in patients with urethral catheters, endotracheal tubes, and intravenous lines. Anesthesia, surgical procedures, and uremia produce immune defects that contribute to this high incidence of infection. Renal transplant patients with ARF and drug immunosuppression might be expected to have an especially high mortality. The low mortality actually observed is probably due to the careful isolation techniques routinely employed in their care.

Despite advances in dialysis and nutrition, the mortality among surgical and trauma patients with ARF remains higher than that among medical patients, primarily because of their differing underlying diseases. Otherwise healthy patients in whom medical causes of ARF develop have only 3 per cent mortality.[6] Patients who have severe, multisystem trauma, ruptured abdominal aortic aneurysms, or major surgical procedures for advanced cancer, abdominal catastrophes, or cardiovascular circulatory failure in addition to ARF have mortality greater than 50 per cent in nearly every reported series.[95] The rate has decreased only modestly in the past 15 years, which emphasize again the lesson of the wartime experience: Mortality due to ARF has been lowered primarily by a decrease in the incidence of ARF (42 per cent in World War II versus 0.17 per cent in Vietnam) after trauma and surgical therapy, rather than by improvements in the treatment of established ARF (90 per cent fatality in World War II versus 77 per cent fatality in Vietnam). An alternate explanation for the high mortality in surgical ARF is that patients with a higher percentage of multiorgan failure are surviving because of improved emergency room and intensive care unit support. Therefore, a much higher percentage of patients with multiorgan failure are surviving and thus subject to the development of ARF.

Recovery from Acute Tubular Necrosis

With early, aggressive, repeated dialysis to prevent the metabolic derangements associated with ARF and successful management of the late complications of bleeding, sepsis, and drug intoxication, most patients recover renal function after postoperative ARF. Among 353 patients who survived acute tubular necrosis, a spectrum of results was observed[52]: 30 to 40 per cent of patients had normal renal function, 40 to 50 per cent of patients had complete clinical recovery but persistent defects in glomerular or tubular function, 10 per cent required medical management, and the remaining 10 to 20 per cent required dialysis. Other studies demonstrate still lower likelihood of dialysis dependence in patients who survive ARF. Even after prolonged dialysis dependence (less than 1 month), recovery of renal function is the usual course. The regenerating tubular epithelium is particularly susceptible to further insult from ischemia, sepsis, and nephrotoxic drugs. Careful fluid management, not only during dialysis, but also as urinary flow returns, is necessary to prevent volume depletion, hypotension, and return to another period of acute renal failure. Accurate daily measurements of urine volume, electrolyte concentration, and patient weight with meticulous replacement of all fluid losses can prevent this frequently fatal complication. Initial recovery is indicated by an increase in urinary flow. However, dialysis must be continued for a period of a few days to weeks until the nephrons regain their concentrating and excretory capabilities. Until the GFR and clearance return to normal and the kidneys can again maintain the integrity of the internal environment, the physician must continue to protect the patient from all of the insults that might reinjure the recovering kidneys. Even during the recovery phase, *prevention* of acute renal failure is much easier, more cost-effective, and more successful than its treatment.

SELECTED REFERENCES

Bennett, W. M., Muther, R. S., Parker, R. A., Feig, P., Morrison, G., Golper, T. A., and Singer, I.: Drug therapy in renal failure: dosing guidelines for adults. Ann. Int. Med., *93*:62, 286, 1980.
This lengthy review provides important information on drug dosage modifications in the patient with renal failure. It is an essential reference for anyone caring for patients with impaired renal function.

Brenner, B. M., and Lazarus, J. B. (Eds.): Acute Renal Failure, 2nd ed. Philadelphia, W. B. Saunders Company, 1988.
This comprehensive monograph provides a complete review of medical and surgical aspects of acute renal failure. The section on differential diagnosis by Rudnick and associates is especially useful.

Drukker, W., Parsons, F. M., and Maher, J. F. (Eds.): Replacement of renal function by dialysis, 2nd ed. Boston, Martinus Nijhoff, 1983.
This text on dialysis provides extensive information on hemodialysis and peritoneal dialysis including their complications and a chapter by Kjellstrand and associates on the dialytic management of acute renal failure.

Tilney, N. L., Morgan, A. P., and Lazarus, J. M.: Acute renal failure in surgical patients. In Tilney, N. L., and Lazarus, J. M. (Eds.): Surgical Care of the Patient with Renal Failure. Philadelphia, W. B. Saunders Company, 1982.
Diagnosis and care of previously healthy individuals in whom renal failure develops during the course of operation, trauma, or other catastrophes are admirably discussed according to clinical patterns of presentation.

REFERENCES

1. Abel, R. M., Beck, C. H., Abbott, W. M., Ryan, J. A., Barnett, G. O., and Fischer, J. E.: Improved survival from acute renal failure after treatment with intravenous essential L-amino acids and glucose. N. Engl. J. Med., *288*:695, 1973.
2. Abel, R., Buckley, J., Austen, W., Barnett, G., Beck, G., and Fischer, J.: Etiology, incidence and prognosis of renal failure following cardiac operations. J. Thorac. Cardiovasc. Surg., *71*:323, 1976.
3. Anderson, R. J., and Schrier, R. W.: Clinical spectrum of oliguric and non-oliguric acute renal failure. In Brenner, B. M., and Stein, J. H. (Eds.): Acute Renal Failure. New York Churchill Livingstone, 1980.
4. Anderson, R. J., Linas, S. L., Berns, A. S., Hinrich, W. L., Miller, T. R., Gabow, P. A., and Schrier, R. W.: Non-oliguric acute renal failure. N. Engl. J. Med., *296*:1134, 1977.
5. Andreucci, V.: Different forms of ischemic/toxic acute renal failure in humans. In Andreucci, V. (Ed.): Acute Renal Failure. Boston, Martinus Nijhoff, 1984.
6. Balslov, J. T., and Jorgensen, H. E.: A survey of 499 patients with acute anuric renal insufficiency: Causes, treatment, complications and mortality. Am. J. Med., *34*:753, 1963.
7. Bartlett, R. H., Mault, J. R., Dechert, R. E., Palmer, J., Swartz, R. D., and Port, F. K.: Continuous arteriovenous hemofiltration: Improved survival in surgical acute renal failure. Surgery, *100*:400, 1986.
8. Bast, C. P., Rudnick, M. E., and Narins, R. G.: Diagnostic approaches to acute renal failure. In Brenner, B. M., and Stein, J. H.: Acute Renal Failure. New York, Churchill Livingstone, 1980.
9. Baylis, C., and Brenner, B. M.: The physiologic determinants of glomerular ultrafiltration. Rev. Physiol. Biochem. Pharm., *80*:1, 1978.
10. Bennett, W. M., Luft, F., and Porter, G. A.: Pathogenesis of renal failure due to aminoglycosides and contrast media used in roentgenography. Am. J. Med., *69*:767, 1980.
11. Bennett, W. M., Muther, R. S., Parker, R. A., Feig, P., Morrison, G., Golper, T. A., and Singer, I.: Drug therapy in renal failure: dosing guidelines for adults. Ann. Intern. Med., *93*:62, 286, 1980 (Parts I and II).
12. Better, O. S., and Berl, T.: Jaundice and the Kidney. In Suki, W. N., and Eknoyan (Eds.): The Kidney in Systemic Disease, 2nd ed. New York, John Wiley, 1981.
13. Bhat, J. G., Gluck, M. C., Lowenstein, J., and Baldwin, D. S.: Renal failure after open heart surgery. Ann. Intern. Med., *84*:677, 1976.
14. Blagg, C. R., Parsons, F. M., and Young, G. A.: Effect of dietary glucose and protein in ARF. Lancet, *1*:608, 1962.
15. Brenner, B. M., and Lazarus, J. M.: Acute Renal Failure. Philadelphia, W. B. Saunders Company, 1983.

16. Brezin, J. H., Katz, S. M., Schwartz, A. B., and Chinitz, J. L.: Reversible renal failure and nephrotic syndrome associated with non-steroidal anti-inflammatory drugs. N. Engl. J. Med., 301:1271, 1979.

17. Bull, G. M., Joekes, A. M., and Lowe, K. G.: Conservative treatment of anuric uraemia. Lancet 2:229, 1949.

18. Bull, G. M., Joekes, A. M., and Lowe, K. G.: Renal function studies in acute tubular necrosis. Clin. Sci., 9:379, 1950.

19. Butler, W. T., Bennett, J. E., Alling, D. W., Wertlake, P. T., Utz, J. P., and Hill, G. J., II: Nephrotoxicity of amphotericin B: Early and late effects in 81 patients. Ann. Intern. Med., 64:175, 1964.

20. Byrd, L., and Sherman, R. L.: Radiocontrast induced acute renal failure: A clinical and pathophysiologic review. Medicine, 58:270, 1979.

21. Bywaters, E. G. L., and Beall, D.: Crush injuries with impairment of renal function. Br. Med. J., 1:427, 1941.

22. Bywaters, E. G. L.: Ischemic muscle necrosis. J.A.M.A., 124:1103, 1944.

23. Canton, A. D., and Andreucci, V. E.: Acute obstructive renal failure (postrenal failure). In Andreucci, V. E. (Ed.): Acute Renal Failure. Boston, Martinus Nijhoff, 1984.

24. Casati S., Moia, M., Graziani, G., et al.: Hemodialysis without anticoagulants. Int. J. Artif. Organs, 5:233, 1982.

25. Coggins, C. H., and Fang, L. S. T.: Acute renal failure associated with antibiotics, anesthetic agents, and radiographic contrast agents. In Brenner, B. M., and Lazarus, J. M. (Eds.): Acute Renal Failure. Philadelphia, W. B. Saunders Company, 1983, p. 283.

26. Conger, J. D.: A controlled evaluation of prophylactic dialysis in post-traumatic acute renal failure. J. Trauma, 15:1056, 1975.

27. Daughtry, T. M., Ueki, I. F., Mercer, P. F., and Brenner, B. M.: Dynamics of glomerular ultrafiltration in the rat. V. Response to ischemic injury. J. Clin. Invest., 53:105, 1974.

28. Davidson, C., Hlatky, M., Morris, K., Schwab, S., and Bashore, T.: Cardiovascular and renal toxicity of non-ionic radiographic contrast following cardiac catheterization: A prospective trial. Ann. Intern. Med., 110:119, 1989.

29. Donohoe, J. F., Venkatachalam, M. A., Bernard, D. B., and Levinsky, N. G.: Tubular leakage and obstruction after renal ischemia: structural-functional relationships. Kidney Int., 13:208, 1978.

30. Dunn, M. J., and Hood, V. L.: Prostaglandins in the kidney. Am. J. Physiol., 233:F169, 1977.

31. Dunn, M. J., and Zambraski, E. J.: Renal effects of drugs that inhibit prostaglandin synthesis. Kidney Int., 18:609, 1980.

32. Espinel, C. H.: The FE_Na Test: Use in the differential diagnosis of acute renal failure. J.A.M.A., 236:579, 1976.

33. Espinel, C. H., and Gregory, A. W.: Differential diagnosis of acute renal failure. Clin. Nephrol., 13:73, 1980.

34. Fang, L. S. T., Sirota, R. A., Ebert, T. H., and Lichtenstein, N. S.: Low fractional excretion of sodium with contrast media induced acute renal failure. Arch. Intern. Med., 140:531, 1980.

35. Feinstein, E. I., Blumenkrantz, M. J., Healy, M., Koffler, A., Silberman, H., Massry, S. G., and Kopple, J. D.: Clinical and metabolic responses to parenteral nutrition in acute renal failure. Medicine, 60:124, 1981.

36. Fink, M. Are diuretics useful in the treatment or prevention of acute renal failure? So. Med. J., 75:239, 1982.

37. Fischer, R. P.: High mortality of post-traumatic renal insufficiency in Vietnam: A review of 96 cases. Am. Surg., 40:172, 1974.

38. Flamenbaum, W., Gehr, M., Gross, M., Kaufman, J., and Hamburger, R.: Acute renal failure associated with myoglobinuria and hemoglobinuria. In Brenner, B. M., and Lazarus, J. M. (Eds.): Acute Renal Failure. Philadelphia, W. B. Saunders Company, 1983, p. 269.

39. Flanigan, M. J., VonBrecht, J., Freeman, R. M., and Lim V. S.: Reducing the hemorrhagic complications of hemodialysis: A controlled comparison of low-dose heparin and citrate anticoagulation. Am. J. Kidney Dis., 9:147, 1987.

40. Gabow, P. A., Kaehny, W. D., and Kelleher, S. P.: The spectrum of rhabdomyolysis. Medicine, 61:141, 1982.

41. Geronemus, R., and Schneider, N.: Continuous arteriovenous hemodialysis: A new modality for treatment of acute renal failure. Trans. Am. Soc. Artif. Intern. Organs, 30:610, 1984.

42. Golper, T. A., Ronco, C., and Kaplan, A.: Continuous arteriovenous hemofiltration: Improvements, modifications and future directions. Am. J. Kid. Dis., 1:50, 1988.

43. Garella, S., and Chang, C. S.: Hemodialysis-associated hypoxemia. Am. J. Nephrol., 4:263, 1984.

44. Harkonen, S., and Kjellstrand, C.: Contrast nephropathy. Am. J. Nephrol., 7:69, 1987.

45. Hofstetter, T. H., Wilkes, B. M., and Brenner, B. M.: Renal circulatory and nephron function in experimental acute renal failure. In Brenner, B. M., and Lazarus, J. M. (Eds.): Acute Renal Failure. Philadelphia, W. B. Saunders Company, 1983, p. 99.

46. Hou, S. H., Bushinsky, D. A., Wish, J. B., Cohen, J. J., and Harrington, J. T.: Hospital acquired renal insufficiency: A prospective study. Am. J. Med., 74:243, 1983.

47. Iwatsuki, S., Popoutzer, M. D., Corman, J. L., Ishikawa, M., Putnam, C. W., Katz, F. H., and Starzl, T. E.: Recovery from "hepatorenal syndrome" after orthotopic liver transplantation. N. Engl. J. Med., 289:1155, 1973.

48. Janson, P., Jubelirer, S., Weinstein, M., and Deykin, D.: Treatment of the bleeding tendency in uremia with cryoprecipitate. N. Engl. J. Med., 303:1318, 1980.

49. Kaplan, A. A., Longnecker, R. E., and Folkert, V. W.: Continuous arteriovenous hemofiltration. Ann. Int. Med., 100:358, 1984.

50. Kaloyanides, G. J., and Pastoriza-Munoz, E.: Aminoglycoside nephrotoxicity. Kidney Int., 18:571, 1980.

51. Kasiske, B. L., and Kjellstrand, C. M.: Perioperative management of patients with chronic renal failure and postoperative acute renal failure. Urol. Clin. North Am., 10:35, 1983.

52. Kennedy, A. C.: Long term follow-up of renal function after recovery from acute tubular necrosis. In Andreucci, V. (Ed.): Acute Renal Failure. Boston, Martinus Nijhoff, 1984.

53. Kennedy, A. O., Burton, J. A., Luke, R. G., Briggs, J. O., Lindsay, R. M., Allison, M. E. M., Edward, N., and Dargie, H. J.: Factors affecting the prognosis in acute renal failure. Quart. J. Med., 42:73, 1973.

54. Kiley, J. E., Powers, S. R., and Beebe, R. J.: Acute renal failure. Eighty cases of renal tubular necrosis. N. Engl. J. Med., 262:481, 1960.

55. Koppel, M. H., Coburn, J. W., Mims, M. M., Goldstein, H., Boyle, O. D., and Rubini, M. E.: Transplantation of cadaveric kidneys from patients with hepatorenal syndrome: Evidence for the functional nature of renal failure in advanced liver disease. N. Engl. J. Med., 280:1367, 1969.

56. Kourilsky, O., Morel-Maroger, L, and Richet, G.: Renal biopsy in acute renal failure: Its indications and usefulness. In Andreucci, V. (Ed.): Acute Renal Failure. Boston, Martinus Nijhoff, 1984.

57. Kramer, P., Wigger, W., Rieger, J., Matthaei D., and Scheler, F.: Arteriovenous haemofiltration: A new and simple method for treatment of overhydrated patients resistent to diuretics. Klin. Wochenschr., 55:1121, 1977.

58. Kumin, G. D.: Clinical nephrotoxicity of tobramycin and gentamicin: A prospective study. J.A.M.A., 249:1808, 1980.

59. Lauer, A., Sacaggi, A., Ronco, C., Belledonne, M., Glabman, S., and Bosch, J. P.: Continuous arteriovenous hemofiltration in critically ill patients. Ann. Int. Med., 99:455, 1983.

60. Lazarus, J. M.: Complications in hemodialysis: An overview. Kidney Int., 148:783, 1980.

61. Kevinsky, N. G., Bernard, D. B., and Johnston, P. A.: Mannitol and loop diuretics in acute renal failure. In Brenner, B. M., and Lazarus, J. M. (Eds.): Acute Renal Failure. Philadelphia, W. B. Saunders Company, 1983, p. 712.

62. Llach, F., Felsenfeld, A. J., and Haussler, M. E.: The pathophysiology of altered calcium metabolism in rhabdomyolysis-induced acute renal failure: Interactions of parathyroid hormone, 25-hydroxycholecalciferol, and 1,25-dihydroxycholecalciferol. N. Engl. J. Med., 305:117, 1981.

63. Liuio, M., Mannuccio, P., Vigano, G., Mingardi, G., Lombardi, R., Mecca, G., and Remuzzi, G.: Conjugated estrogens for the management of bleeding associated with renal failure. N. Engl. J. Med., 315:1106, 1986.

64. Mannucci, P., Remmuzzi, G., Pusiweri, F., Lombardi, R., Valsechi, C., Mecca, G., Zimmerman, T.: Deamino-8-D-arginine vasopressin shortens the bleeding time in uremia. N. Engl. J. Med., 308:8, 1983.

65. Mault, J. R., Dechert, R. E., Lees, P., Swartz, R. D., Port, F. K., and Bartlett, R. H. Continuous arteriovenous filtration: An effective treatment for surgical acute renal failure. Surgery, 101:478, 1987.

66. McMurray, S. D., Luft, F. C., Maxwell, D. R., Hamburger, R. J., Futty, D., Szwed, J. J., Lavelle, K. J., and Kleit, S. A.: Prevailing patterns and predictor variables in patients with acute tubular necrosis. Arch. Int. Med., 138:950, 1978.

67. Michel, L., Serrano, A., and Matt, R. A.: Nutritional support for hospitalized patients. N. Engl. J. Med., 304:1147, 1981.

68. Mihatsch, M. J., Thiel, G., Basler, V., Ryffel, B., Landmann, J., von Overbeck, J., and Zollinger, H. U.: Morphological patterns in cyclosporine-treated renal transplant recipients. Transplant. Proc., 17:101, 1985.

69. Miller, T. R., Anderson, R. J., Linas, S. L., Henrich, W. L., Berns, A. S., Gabow, P. A., and Schrier, R. W.: Urinary diagnostic indices in acute renal failure: A prospective study. Ann. Int. Med., 89:47, 1978.

70. Mudge, G. H.: Nephrotoxicity of urographic contrast drugs. Kidney Int., 18:540, 1980.

71. Myers, B. D., Carrie, B. J., Yee, R. R., Hilberman, M., and Michaels, A. S.: Pathophysiology of hemodynamically mediated acute renal failure in man. Kidney Int., 18:495, 1980.

72. Myers, B. D., Hilberman, M., Carne, B. J., Spencer, R. J., Stinson, E. B., and Robertson, C. R.: Dynamics of glomerular ultrafiltration following open heart surgery. Kidney Int., 20:366, 1981.

73. Navar, L. G., Rosivall, L.: Contribution of the renin-angiotensin system to the control of intrarenal hemodynamics. Kidney Int., 25:857, 1984.

74. Oken, D. E.: On the differential diagnosis of acute renal failure. Am. J. Med., 71:916, 1981.

75. Papper, S.: Hepatorenal syndrome. Contrib. Nephrol., 23:55, 1980.

76. Papper, S.: Hepatorenal syndrome. In Andreucci, V. (Ed.): Acute Renal Failure. Boston, Martinus Nijhoff, 1984.

77. Parfrey, P. S., Griffiths, S., Barrett, B., Paul, M., George, M., Withers, J., Farid, N., and McManamon, P.: Contrast material induced renal failure in patients with diabetes mellitus, renal insufficiency or both. N. Engl. J. Med., 320:143, 1989.

78. Pinnick, R. V., Wiegmann, T. B., and Diederich, D. A.: Regional citrate anticoagulation for hemodialysis in the patient at high risk for bleeding. N. Engl. J. Med., 308:258, 1983.

79. Porter, G. A., and Bennett, W. M.: Nephrotoxic acute renal failure due to common drugs. Am. J. Physiol., 241:F1, 1981.

80. Richards, W. O., Scovill, W., Shin, B., and Reed, W.: Acute renal failure

associated with increased intra-abdominal pressure. Ann. Surg., *197*:183, 1983.

81. Sander, P.W., Taylor, H., and Curtis, J. J.: Hemodialysis without anticoagulation. Am. J. Kidney Dis., *5*:32, 1985.

82. Schentag, J. J., Plaut, M. E., and Cerra, F. B.: Comparative nephrotoxicity of gentamicin and tobramycin: Pharmacokinetic and clinical studies in 201 patients. Antimicrob. Agents Chemother., *19*:859, 1981.

83. Schor, N., Ichikawa, I., Rennke, H., and Brenner, B. M.: Pathophysiologies of ultraglomerular function in aminoglycoside-treated rats. Kidney Int., *19*:288, 1981.

84. Schwab, S., Onorato, J., Sharar, L., and Dennis, P.: Hemodialysis without anticoagulation: Results of a one year prospective trial in hospitalized patients at risk for bleeding. Am. J. Med., *83*:405, 1987.

85. Schwab, S., Hlatky, M., Pieper, K., Morris, K., Davidson, C., and Bashore, T.: Contrast nephrotoxicity: A prospective randomized trial of a nonionic vs. an ionic radiographic contrast agent. N. Engl. J. Med., *320*:149, 1989.

86. Schwab, S., Buller, G., McCann, R., Bollinger, R., and Stickel, D.: Evaluation of a dacron cuffed jugular venous hemodialysis catheter for prolonged use. Am. J. Kidney Dis., *11*:166, 1988.

87. Sherman, R. A., and Byun, K. J.: Nuclear medicine in acute and chronic renal failure. Semin. Nucl. Med., *12*(3):265, 1982.

88. Skorecki, K. L., and Brenner, B. M.: Body fluid homeostasis in man: A contemporary overview. Am. J. Med., *70*:77, 1981.

89. Skorecki, K. L., and Brenner, B. M.: Body fluid homeostasis in congestive heart failure and cirrhosis with ascites. Am. J. Med., *72*:323, 1982.

90. Smith, L. H., Jr., Post, R. S., Teschan, P. E., Abernathy, R. S., Davis, J. H., Gray, D. M., Howard, J. M., Johnson, K. E., Klopp, E., Mundy, R. L., O'Meara, M. P., and Rush, B. F., Jr.: Posttraumatic renal insufficiency in military cas-

ualties. II. Management, use of an artificial kidney, prognosis. Am. J. Med., *18*:187, 1955.

91. Stein, J. H., Lifschitz, M. D., and Barnes, L. D.: Current concepts on the pathophysiology of acute renal failure. Am. J. Physiol., *234*:F171, 1978.

92. Swan, R. C., and Merrill, J. P.: Clinical course of acute renal failure. Medicine, *32*:215, 1953.

93. Swartz, R. D., and Port, F. K.: Preventing hemorrhage in high-risk hemodialysis: Regional versus low-dose heparin. Kidney Int., *16*:513, 1979.

94. Teschan, P. E.,Post, R. S., Smith, L. H. Jr., Abernathy, R. S., Davis, J. H., Gray, D. M., Howard, J. M., Johnson, K. E., Klopp, E., Mundy, R. L., O'Meara, M. P., and Rush, B. F., Jr.: Posttraumatic renal insufficiency in military casualties. I. Clinical characteristics. Am. J. Med., *18*:172, 1955.

95. Tilney, N. L., Morgan, A. P., and Lazarus, J. M.: Acute renal failure in surgical patients. *In* Tilney, N. L., and Lazarus, J. M. (Eds.): Surgical Care of the Patient with Renal Failure. Philadelphia, W. B. Saunders Company, 1982.

96. Van Zee, B. E., How, W. E., Talley, T. E., and Jaenike, J. R.: Renal injury associated with intravenous pyelography in nondiabetic and diabetic patients. Ann. Int. Med., *89*:51, 1978.

97. Wardle, E. N.: Endotoxin and acute renal failure: A review. Nephron., *14*:321, 1975.

98. Wardle, N.: Acute renal failure in the 1980's: The importance of septic shock and of endotoxemia. Nephron, *30*:193, 1982.

99. Wong, P. Y.: The hepatorenal syndrome. Gastroenterology, *77*:1326, 1979.

100. Yeboah, E. D., Petrie, A., and Pead, J. L.: Acute renal failure and open heart surgery. Br. Med. J., *1*:415, 1972.

101. Zarich, S., Fang, L. S. T., and Diamond, J. R.: Fractional excretion of sodium: exceptions to its diagnostic value. Arch. Int. Med., *145*:108, 1985.

18

TRANSPLANTATION

I

HISTORICAL ASPECTS

R. Randal Bollinger, M.D., Ph.D., and Delford L. Stickel, M.D.

ANCIENT ACCOUNTS OF TRANSPLANTATION

Transplantation, the removal or partial detachment of a part of the body and its implantation to the body of the same or a different individual, has fascinated mankind for centuries. Legends of transplantation are recorded in the early written histories of both Eastern and Western cultures. Homer in his *Iliad* describes the monstrous Chimaera, a remarkable creature of transplanted animal parts created by the gods. This mythical hybrid animal had the heads of a lion, a goat, and a serpent. All three of its heads breathed fire.[34] The term *chimaera* is now used in transplantation to describe individuals who possess hybrid characteristics such as the circulating cells of both donor and recipient after bone marrow transplantation.

A Chinese document written in approximately 300 B.C. contains this legendary account of transplantation: "One day two men, Lu and Chao, called on the surgeon Pien Ch'iao. He gave them a toxic drink and they were unconscious for three days. Pien Ch'iao operated and opened their stomachs and explored the heart; after removing and interchanging their organs he gave a wonderful drug and the two men went home recovered."[61]

The legend of Cosmas and Damian describes transplantation as one of the miraculous feats of these two medical martyrs. Born in Arabia in the third century A.D. and trained in medicine in Syria, Cosmas the physician and Damian the surgeon performed numerous miraculous healings until their martyrdom in 287 A.D. by decapitation. The miracle of the black leg is said to have occurred posthumously in approximately 348 A.D. While an elderly parishioner with a gangrenous, cancerous leg lay sleeping in the Basilica of Cosmas and Damian, the Saints came to him and removed the diseased leg with a saw. They replaced the destroyed tissue with the fresh leg of a Moor buried that same day in the cemetery of Saint Peter. The new leg was attached at the thigh and ointment applied to the site. The parishioner awoke to find himself free of pain and able to walk on his new healthy black leg.[36] Attempts at transplantation during the Middle Ages did not always end so successfully. Tragically, in 1492 two boys were bled to death in a vain attempt to save the life of Pope Innocent VIII by means of transfusion of young blood.[61]

The oldest evidence of grafting that could have been of some therapeutic benefit is observed in the remains of trephined prehistoric skulls. The trephine holes were usually small, but in a Bronze Age skull, a rather large defect evidently was filled by reimplanting the removed fragment.[29] In this specimen, the cut margin showed no sign of healing, so the operation may have been fatal. Recovery from primitive skull trephination is well documented, however, both archeologically and in studies of primitive peoples in modern times, and it is conceivable that such trephination was sometimes therapeutically effective.

Ancient Hindu surgeons described methods for repairing defects of the nose and ears using techniques of grafting similar to those used in modern times. The following technique for nasal reconstruction is quoted from a translation of the *Suśruta Samhitá*, a document written about 700 B.C.[6]

Now I shall deal with the process of affixing an artificial nose. First the leaf of creeper, long and broad enough to fully cover the hole or the severed or clipped off part should be gathered; and a patch of living flesh equal in dimension of the preceding leaf, should be sliced off from down upward from the region of the cheek and, after scarifying it with a knife, swiftly adhered to the severed nose. Then the cool-headed physician should steadily tie it up with a bandage decent to look at and perfectly suited to the end for which it has been employed. The physician should make sure that the adhesion of the severed parts has been fully effected and then insert two small pipes into the nostrils to facilitate respiration and to prevent the adhesioned flesh from hanging down. After that the adhesion part should be dusted with the powders of sappanwood, licorice-root and bayberry pulverized together; and the nose should be enveloped in cotton and several times sprinkled over with a refined oil of pure sesamum. . . . As soon as the skin has grown together with the nose, he cuts through the connection with the cheek.

This *Indian method* was lost to Western medicine until 1794 when English surgeons stationed in India described nasal reconstruction as they had seen it performed by an Indian surgeon, the technique quite similar to that described more than 1000 years earlier.[60]

A new Western tradition of transplantation surgery arose during the Renaissance in Bologna. The sixteenth century anatomist and surgeon Gasparo Tagliacozzi developed his technique for reconstruction using a flap of skin from the inner aspect of the upper arm. He carved the flap of skin in the shape of the patient's nose and then stitched it to the forehead and inner surface of the cheek, leaving a slender attachment to the arm to maintain blood supply until circulation was re-established from the face. Following this painful procedure, the patient had to sit upright with the arm alongside the face and the head turned toward the arm for the next 3 weeks of healing; then the attachment to the arm was severed. Tagliacozzi was successful in replacing noses cut off in combat or for punishment or destroyed by syphilis. The technique is still in use, known as the tagliacotian flap, or the *Italian method.*[18] In considering but discarding the idea of grafting tissue donated by another individual, Tagliacozzi made the following remarkable statement:

The singular character of the individual entirely dissuades us from attempting this work on another person. For such is the force and the power of individuality, that if anyone should believe that he could accelerate and increase the beauty of union, nay more, achieve even the least part of the operation, we consider him plainly superstitious and badly grounded in the physical sciences.[55]

EARLY EXPERIMENTS IN TRANSPLANTATION

The Scottish surgeon John Hunter (1728–1793) is known as the father of experimental surgery because of his pioneering research. Several of his experimental procedures involved transplantation, and some of his specimens are still preserved in the Hunterian Museum in London. One of Hunter's famous autografts wherein a cock's claw was transplanted to its comb is depicted in Figure 1. The claw not only survived autografting but grew circularly toward the beak of the animal. John Hunter revived the practice of transplanting teeth, which had been utilized in ancient Egypt, Greece, Rome, Arabia, and pre-Columbian America, as well as by Ambroise Paré of Paris in the sixteenth century.[45] In the xenograft experiment shown in Figure 2, Hunter transplanted a tooth to the comb of a cock. With his crude techniques of transplanting tissues without primary revascularization and without antisepsis, John Hunter was unable to distinguish allografts from autografts on the basis of graft survival. About this operation he wrote:

> Success of this operation is founded on the disposition of all living substances to unite when brought in contact with one another, although they are of different structure and even though the circulation is carried in one of them.[9]

In other animal experiments he successfully autografted and allografted chicken testes and observed that the ends of severed Achilles tendons grew together after suturing. A variety of connective tissue transplant procedures were performed successfully for the first time during the eighteenth and nineteenth centuries. Foremost among these were skin grafts and corneal transplants.

SKIN GRAFTS. The first well-documented report of successful free autografts of skin was in 1804 by Baronio, who experimented with sheep, although free autografts of human skin may have been used successfully centuries before.[9,18,45,60] In 1822, Bunger reported successful use of a free full-thickness human skin autograft to repair a nasal defect. In 1870 Reverdin reported the observation that small grafts of epidermis on a granulating surface increased in size and grew out to coalesce with adjacent grafts. In 1886 Thiersch in Germany described the resurfacing of wounds with large sheets of split-thickness skin. Such grafts are still sometimes termed Thiersch's grafts,

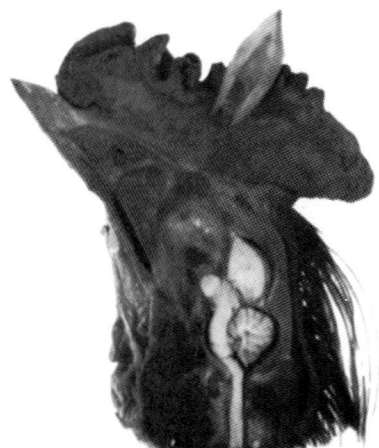

Figure 2. Tooth transplanted to the comb of a cock. The eighteenth century experimental surgeon John Hunter revived the ancient practice of transplanting teeth. This specimen from one of his xenograft experiments is preserved in the Hunterian Museum, London.

although essentially the same procedure was reported 14 years earlier by Ollier in France.

In 1863 Paul Bert, a student of Claude Bernard, reported that autografts, allografts, and xenografts behaved differently.[18,60] The significance of these observations received little attention, however; nineteenth century authors (including Baronio and Reverdin) generally failed to observe that the results of allografts and autografts of skin were different. Skin allografts were used to some extent clinically, as illustrated in a story by Winston Churchill of his donating a small piece of skin to a wounded fellow officer in 1898.[18] There appear to have been three reasons for the mistaken belief that skin allografts grew permanently, a belief still widely held as late as the third decade of the twentieth century: (1) for a week or more skin allografts are indistinguishable from autografts; (2) it is difficult to distinguish between permanent survival of a small skin graft and ingrowth of adjacent host skin to cover the area of a sloughed graft; and (3) corneal allografts survive permanently.

CORNEAL TRANSPLANTS. Corneal xenografts attempted early in the nineteenth century were unsuccessful. A successful corneal allograft between two gazelles was reported by Bigger in 1835[45,60]; but the necessity of using a cornea from the same species was not recognized until the period 1872 to 1880, when successful corneal allografts were reported in animals and in man. Refinements of operative techniques, methods of preservation of grafts, and systems of graft procurement were subsequently developed. During the period 1925 to 1945 corneal transplantation emerged as a widespread and generally accepted therapeutic practice.[18,45,60]

TRANSPLANTATION IN THE TWENTIETH CENTURY

Although important developments in the last half of the nineteenth century such as the use of ether and other general anesthetics and the acceptance of Lister's principles of antiseptic surgery were important in the progress of transplantation, organ replacement is a development of the twentieth century. Transplantation of vascularized organs, including the kidney, liver, heart, lung, pancreas, and intestine, was first made possible when techniques for vascular anastomosis were developed.

The first long-functioning renal transplant was reported by Emerich Ullmann in March 1902. He transplanted kidneys in dogs using magnesium tube stents and ligatures to make the vascular anastomoses.[57] That same year the French surgeon Alexis Carrel reported his new technique of suturing blood vessels together using triangulation and fine silk suture material

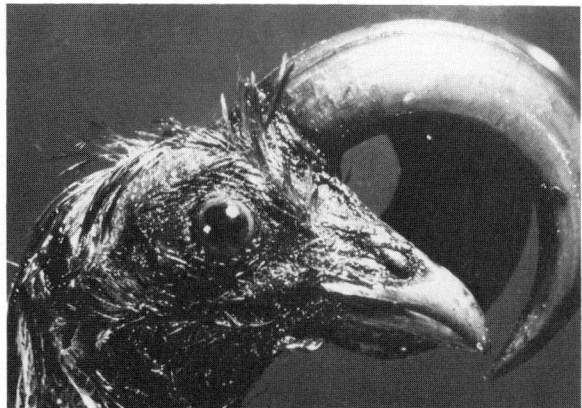

Figure 1. Autograft of a cock's claw to its comb. John Hunter (1728–1793) is considered the father of experimental surgery because of his pioneering operations. This specimen is preserved in the Hunterian Museum, London.

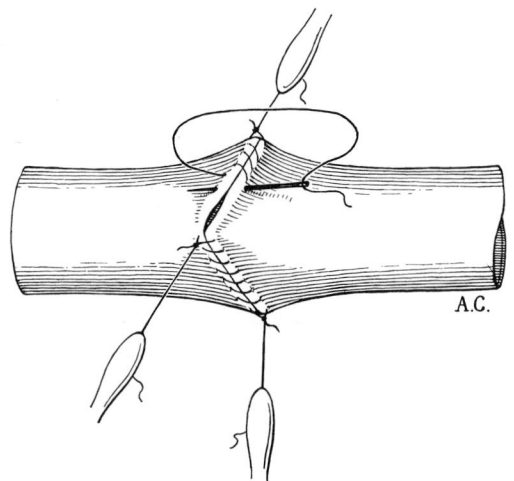

Figure 3. Carrel's technique of vascular anastomosis. Shortly after Alexis Carrel reported his new technique of suturing blood vessels together using triangulation and fine silk suture material, he applied the method to the transplantation of blood vessels, hearts, spleens, kidneys, and extremities. (From Carrel, A.: La techique opératoire des anastomoses vasculaires et la transplantation des viscères. Lyon Med., *98:*859, 1902.)

(Fig. 3).[11] His revolutionary technique was rapidly applied to the problems of organ transplantation. Between 1902 and 1912, Carrel and Guthrie of Chicago performed a large series of animal transplantation experiments including the transfer of blood vessels, kidneys, hearts, spleens, ovaries, thyroids, extremities, and even the head and neck. In 1905 in his preliminary communication entitled "The Transplantation of Organs" Carrel stated:

This operation consists of extirpating an organ with its vessels, of putting it in another region, and of uniting its vessels to a neighboring artery and vein. If the organ is replaced in the same animal from which it was removed the operation is called an *autotransplantation.* If it is placed in another animal of the same species it is called a *homotransplantation,* while if it is placed into an animal of a different species, the operation is called a *heterotransplantation.*[12]

TERMINOLOGY. Although the terms defined by Carrel are still used occasionally, the preferred nomenclature is now *allotransplantation* (allograft) for transplants between nonidentical members of the same species and *xenotransplantation* (xenograft) for transplants between members of different species (Table 1). *Graft* is commonly used as a synonym for transplant and *host* as a synonym for recipient. The prefix *iso-* is ambiguous because it is used with two distinctly different meanings, as discussed by Gorer.[26] The term *isograft* as shown in Table 1 derives from geneticists' use of the term *isogeneic* in referring to genetically *identical* individuals, whereas for over 70 years immunologists have used *iso-* to refer to immunity to antigens of blood and tissues of genetically *dissimilar* individuals of the same species (isoimmune, isoantigen, isoantibody, etc.). De-

TABLE 1. Transplantation Terminology

Recent Nomenclature	Older Nomenclature	Relationship of Donor and Recipient of Graft
Syngeneic (isogeneic) graft	Autograft Isograft	Same individual Same species and genetically identical
Allogeneic graft	Homograft	Same species but not genetically identical
Xenogeneic graft	Heterograft	Different species

pending upon the site of implantation, grafts are termed *orthotopic* if surrounded by the same type of tissues or located in the same part of the body after transplantation as previously; otherwise they are termed *heterotopic.* Heterotopic grafts are sometimes implanted into *privileged sites,* i.e., locations that protect the graft from rejection (e.g., the anterior chamber of the eye, the brain, the testes, or in a diffusion chamber).

PROBLEM OF REJECTION. Alexis Carrel did not understand the biologic basis for differences in graft outcome among the various types of grafts he attempted, although by 1910 he recognized the problem of rejection:

Should an organ, extirpated from an animal and replanted into its owner by a certain technique, continue to functionate normally, and should it cease to functionate when transplanted into another animal by the same technique, the physiological disturbance could not be considered as brought about by the surgical factors. The changes undergone by the organ would be due to the influence of the host, that is, the biological factors.

Elucidation of the biologic factors hypothesized by Carrel required several decades and is in fact continuing today. A few of the milestones in transplantation immunology are cited.

Although the immunity theory of graft rejection was postulated by several authors during the first decade of the century, a number of other theories were held by prominent authorities such as Loeb. The immunity theory was questioned largely because there was no direct evidence that circulating antibody—the traditional hallmark of immunity—was involved in the rejection process. Antibodies had been demonstrated in response to allografts of tumor but not allografts of normal tissues, and attempts to confer allograft immunity passively with serum were unsuccessful. The discovery of cellular immunity, histocompatibility antigens, and immunologic tolerance were important steps in the understanding of transplant rejection.

CELLULAR IMMUNITY. In 1914, Murphy reported lymphocytic infiltrates in host tissues surrounding rejecting transplanted tumors.[18,60] He postulated that the small lymphocyte was responsible for that rejection, and he used radiation and treatment with benzene to modify the process. The role of *cellular immunity* (lymphocytes), as distinguishable from *humoral immunity* (circulating antibody), was not firmly established, however, until experiments were performed in which certain forms of immunity were observed to be transferable to an unimmunized subject by lymphoid cells and not by serum.[60] By 1954, these "adoptive transfer" experiments were performed by Potter and then Mitchison for tumor allograft immunity in mice and by Landsteiner and Chase for delayed-type hypersensitivity reactions in man. In 1954, Billingham, Brent, and Medawar reported the use of lymphoid cells to transfer immunity to skin and other tissue grafts in mice. Only viable cells were capable of transferring the immunity, a phenomenon designated "adoptively acquired immunity" to distinguish it from passive immunity produced by injections of antibody.

THE SECOND-SET PHENOMENON. In 1903, Jensen observed that a second graft did not survive as long as the first when a mouse received two grafts of a tumor separated by an interval of several days, and he suggested that immunity was responsible for the difference. This effect of more rapid rejection of a second graft was not always observed with transplants of tumor, however. Under certain conditions survival of the second graft was prolonged. Casey, in 1932, termed the latter phenomenon *"enhancement,"* and Kaliss in 1953 reported that enhancement is transferable to normal animals by injections of serum.[60] The effect was subsequently demonstrated to be due to an immunoglobulin, and enhancing or blocking antibodies have been used experimentally to prolong the survival of nonneoplastic as well as neoplastic tissues.

The second-set phenomenon in human skin graft recipients was observed by Holman while treating burn patients at the

Johns Hopkins Hospital. He reported in 1924 that a second group of pinch grafts from the same donor was rejected more rapidly than the first and that "the destroying agency is specific for each set of grafts." [33] He postulated that each group of grafts developed its own antibody. In 1932, Shinoyi in Japan described the specificity of the second-set phenomenon. Gibson and Medawar, working in England in 1943, reported similar observations with burn patients, and use of the term *second set* dates to this report.[9,18,41,60] In subsequent controlled experiments with rabbits, Medawar demonstrated the immunologic specificity of the phenomenon, which was observed uniformly only when the same donor was used for both the first set and the second set of grafts. Medawar also contrasted the histologic characteristics of first- and second-set rejections, the first-set rejection being predominantly a cellular event, whereas both cellular and humoral mechanisms are involved in the rejection of the second set of grafts.

TRANSPLANTATION ANTIGENS. When immunity, both cellular and humoral, had been established as the cause of graft rejection, study was focused on the antigens that both stimulated graft rejection and were the targets of the ensuing immune response. The antigens responsible for graft rejection and the genetic control of these antigens have been most extensively studied in the mouse. The influence of genetic factors was documented by Jensen, Tyzzer, and Little in the first 2 decades of the century.[45,60] In 1948, Gorer, Lyman, and Snell described H-2 as a genetic locus controlling strong histocompatibility antigens in the mouse. Subsequently this locus and numerous minor histocompatibility loci were characterized in great detail.

The definition of the major histocompatibility locus of man, HLA, is intertwined with the evolution of typing and crossmatching for human blood donor selection. The work of Landsteiner during the first 4 decades of this century with erythrocyte ABO and RH antigens was necessary for blood banking and transfusion, which became extensively used during and after World War II. The development of blood transfusion contributed to progress with the problem of graft rejection in three respects. First, the A and B erythrocyte antigens are widely distributed in tissues and are transplantation antigens that must be considered in the selection of tissue and organ donors. Second, by analogy with typing and crossmatching for blood donor selection, one of the major approaches to the problem of graft rejection has been tissue compatibility testing. Third, the sera of patients who have received multiple blood transfusions frequently contain antibodies to human leukocytes. It is now known that these are HLA antibodies, and sera from such patients were a principal source of antibodies in early studies of the HLA system.

The serologic identification of transplantation antigens began in 1952 when Dausset discovered a leukocyte antigen responsible for transfusion reactions.[10] Payne found in 1958 that antileukocyte antibodies were frequent in the sera of multiparous women, thus establishing a rich source of reagents for tissue typing. The new system of tissue matching was first used to select appropriate donors and recipients by Hamburger of Paris.[30] In 1964, Payne reported the first clear evidence that these leukocyte antigens segregated in families as a genetic system. Whereas the original serologic identification of transplantation antigens was done by leukoagglutination, Terasaki in 1964 introduced a much more sensitive and specific microlymphocytotoxicity test.[56] Definition of the HLA system, the major histocompatibility gene complex of man, has followed a series of international workshops, the first of which was organized in 1964 by Amos at Duke University. A major advance that same year was the discovery that lymphocytes from potential donors and recipients, when mixed together in tissue culture, undergo a vigorous proliferative response. This reaction, termed a mixed lymphocyte culture (MLC), became, along with microlymphocytotoxicity, a major approach for histocompatibility testing.[10]

IMMUNOLOGIC TOLERANCE. The chimaera, an organism carrying living tissues of two or more genetically different individuals, exists not only as a creature of Greek mythology but also naturally in dizygotic cattle twins. Owen in 1945 reported that each of such twins has two different types of erythrocytes, and he postulated that the marrow of each individual had become populated by cells of both *in utero* when the circulation of the two placentas was mixed.[44] Owen successfully exchanged skin grafts between the cattle twins, and in 1955 Simonson reported that kidneys as well as skin could be readily transplanted between them. In 1953, Dunsford discovered a human twin carrying both A and O erythrocytes, but the other member of the pair died in infancy. In 1959, Woodruff and Lennox reported successful exchange of skin grafts from dizygotic human twins showing blood chimaerism with types A and O.[41,60] Allografts on a chimaera from donors other than the chimaeric mate were rejected in the normal manner. Thus, a natural chimaera is specifically nonreactive to the tissue antigens of its chimaeric mate. Such nonreactivity specifically limited to particular antigens is termed *immunologic tolerance*. In contrast, *immunosuppression* is nonspecific suppression of immune responses to antigens generally. The most common example of naturally occurring tolerance is the normal state of nonreactivity to self antigens, i.e., to the antigens of one's own body. Autoimmune diseases are the consequence of abnormal reactivity to self antigens. Burnet conceived recognition of self antigens as one of the aspects of embryologic maturation of the immunologic system.[41,60]

The creation of states of *acquired tolerance*, i.e., induced specific immunologic tolerance, has been achieved largely by exposure of embryonic, fetal, or early postnatal hosts to grafts that the normal adult animal would reject. Before tolerance was defined immunologically, Murphy, in 1912, observed that rat sarcomas grew on chicken embryos but not in mature chickens, and he observed that the chick acquired the adult capacity to reject the tumor approximately 5 days after completion of shell life.[18,60] In 1929, Danforth and Foster reported successful skin grafts between newly hatched Rhode Island red and Plymouth Rock chicks (Fig. 4).[41] In 1950, Cannon and Longmire reported similar observations, but they noted additionally that the percentage of take was only 1 per cent if the grafts were performed on chicks 3 days old and was nil at the age of 14 days.[41,60] A landmark article in the understanding of transplantation immunology appeared on October 3, 1953, when Billingham, Brent, and Medawar reported their experiments on "actively acquired tolerance of foreign cells."[7] They systematically studied the phenomenon of actively acquired tolerance between inbred strains of mice of various ages before and after birth. It became clear that the barrier between self and non-self could be overcome if the exposure to alloantigens occurred in the neonatal period. Grafts established on the fetus survived permanently and the host was tolerant of other grafts from the donor strain; grafts performed more than 1 or 2 days after birth were rejected, and the rejection of subsequent grafts from the donor strain was accelerated. These authors also reported "breaking" tolerance, i.e., reversing tolerance and terminating the chimaeric state, by injecting lymphoid cells of normal adult host–strain mice into tolerant animals. The reversal of the tolerant state in these experiments was marked by the sloughing of long-established grafts of skin and other tissues from the donor strain.

Animals rendered tolerant prenatally or neonatally were normal except for being chimaeras and for being specifically nonreactive to antigens of the donor. Many subsequent studies have been directed toward the objective of inducing tolerance in the adult by methods that would be applicable to therapeutic transplantation in man. Lasting tolerance has been produced in adult mice that were temporarily immunosuppressed at the time of initial exposure to donor antigens, but tolerance is readily produced by this means only if the donor-recipient incom-

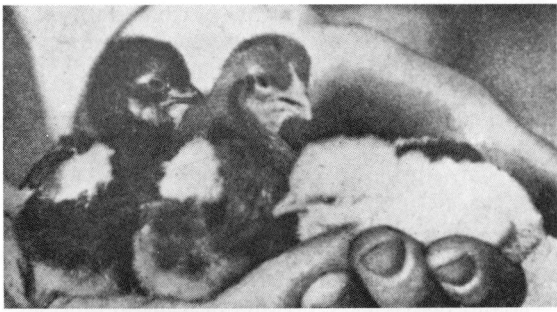

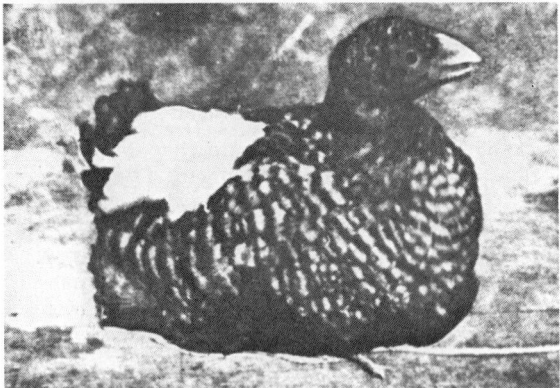

Figure 4. Tolerant chickens. In 1929 Danforth and Foster successfully transplanted skin between newly hatched Plymouth Rock (light) and Rhode Island red (dark) chickens. Such grafts take shortly after birth, but not 2 weeks later, an example of actively acquired tolerance. (From Moore, F. D.: Give and Take: The Development of Tissue Transplantation. Philadelphia, W. B. Saunders Company, 1964.)

patibility is weak. Immunity, not tolerance, usually results if the incompatibility is strong. Since an effective method of producing acquired tolerance to transplantation antigens in adult animals and humans has not yet been discovered, the progress of transplantation has depended upon the development of methods of immunosuppression.

IMMUNOSUPPRESSION. Total-body irradiation had been used extensively to prevent rejection of grafts in experimental animals before it was used in the first successful human allografts from living, related donors in Paris and in Boston.[41] However, in the 4 years between March 1958 and March 1962, of 12 potential recipients at the Peter Bent Brigham Hospital who were subjected to total-body x-irradiation with or without marrow infusion, only 1 survived. Although the one patient with a successful allograft lived for 25 years, irradiation therapy as an immunosuppressive agent was judged "too blunt, nonspecific and unpredictable."[42] Schwartz and Dameshek reported in 1959 that 6-mercaptopurine blocked the capacity of rabbits to form antibody.[49] The animals could still react with proteins administered before or after the period of 6-mercaptopurine treatment, suggesting an element of specificity in the suppression. Calne and Zukoski independently used the drug successfully for canine renal transplants, and Hitchings and associates developed an imidazole derivative, azathioprine, in 1961 that could be administered conveniently and safely in an oral form. Murray, Hume, and Starzl reported clinical successes with the new drug that same year, thus initiating the modern era of transplantation.[42]

In the 1950s, numerous authors reported the efficiency of adrenocortical steroids in reversing the manifestations of various immunopathologic disease states. In 1963, Starzl reported that prednisone added to azathioprine produced good results in most patients. The following year Marchioro and associates reported the successful use of prednisone to reverse established manifestations of renal allograft rejection. Anti-lymphocyte

serum was demonstrated by Woodruff and Anderson in 1963 to prolong skin allograft survival in rats and was used clinically in 1966 by Starzl.[9,42] The immunosuppressive properties of cyclosporine were discovered by Borel in 1972, used by him in animal studies in 1974, and utilized clinically by Calne in kidney transplantation trials in 1978.[8] Whereas the indiscriminate use of immunosuppression in the 1950s and 1960s utilized modalities that affected cells and tissues in addition to the immunocompetent cells responsible for allograft rejection, cyclosporine and, subsequently, monoclonal antibodies allowed modulation of more defined populations of the involved cells. Although alloantigen-specific immunosuppression remained an elusive goal of transplantation research, cyclosporine markedly improved the results of liver, heart, and heart-lung transplantation, making them for the first time broadly applicable as therapies for end-stage organ failure.

THE ERA OF ORGAN REPLACEMENT

With the advent of chemical immunosuppression, the brief but exciting history of clinical transplantation began. For the first time, several vascularized organs were transplanted with regular success. Foremost among these was the kidney.

KIDNEY TRANSPLANTATION. The technical barriers to kidney transplantation were overcome early in the twentieth century by Ullmann[57] and Carrel.[13] In 1908 Carrel wrote:

It is to be concluded that an animal which has undergone a double nephrectomy in the grafting of both kidneys from another animal can secrete almost normal urine with his new organs, and live in good health at least for a few weeks. This demonstrates that it is possible to re-establish sufficiently functions of transplanted kidneys.

In 1906, Jaboulay attempted two kidney xenografts from a pig and a goat to the extremities of patients with chronic renal failure. The kidneys failed after only 1 hour. In 1909, Unger attempted a monkey-to-human kidney transplant to save a girl dying in renal failure. The kidney was sutured to her thigh vessels, but no urine was produced.[31] The first human kidney allograft was performed in 1933 in the Ukraine by Voronoy. He transplanted a human kidney donated from a head injury victim to a patient with acute renal failure from mercuric chloride poisoning. Six hours were required to transplant the kidney to the recipient thigh vessels under local anesthesia, and the transplanted organ never functioned. Voronoy reported six unsuccessful human renal allograft attempts between 1933 and 1949. A kidney allograft to the arm vessels was performed by Hufnagel, Hume, and Landsteiner in Boston in 1946. The transplanted kidney functioned transiently until the patient's own kidneys recovered, and she eventually left the hospital fully recovered.[41] Between 1950 and 1953, human kidney allografts were attempted without immunosuppression in Paris and Boston.[31,40] Most of these kidneys failed immediately, but one transplant recipient of Hume had life-sustaining renal function for several months. Living-related transplantation commenced in 1953 when Michon of Paris transplanted a kidney from a mother to her son, whose solitary kidney had been damaged in a road accident. The kidney functioned for 22 days before it was rejected.[31] In 1954, Murray performed the first renal transplant between monozygotic twins and achieved excellent, long-term function.[42] In March 1958, Murray, in Boston, and Hamburger, in Paris, each performed a series of human kidney allografts using total-body irradiation for immunosuppression.[31] The modern era of immunosuppression had begun, and the subsequent history of renal transplantation paralleled the development of immunosuppressive drugs.

LIVER TRANSPLANTATION. Canine liver grafts were shown to function after transplantation to the pelvis by Welch in 1955. Orthotopic liver transplantation in dogs was attempted by Cannon in 1956 and performed successfully by Moore in

1959. The first attempt at liver allotransplantation in man was made by Starzl at the University of Colorado on March 1, 1963.[51] The 3-year-old recipient with extrahepatic biliary atresia died of hemorrhage on the day of transplantation. Ensuing attempts in Denver, Boston, and Paris were unsuccessful until 1967, when the first extended survival of a human liver allograft recipient was achieved by Starzl. The addition of cyclosporine immunosuppression by Calne in 1978 and then combination therapy with cyclosporine and prednisone by Starzl in 1980, as well as better liver preservation and surgical techniques, improved the prospects for clinical liver transplantation.

HEART TRANSPLANTATION. Carrel and Guthrie performed the first heart transplant in 1905 at the University of Chicago.[15] They transplanted a canine heart to the neck of another dog and observed rhythmic contraction for 2 hours until coagulation occurred in the cavities of the heart. Mann and associates, in 1933, transplanted canine hearts to the neck with more success. One of their dogs survived 8 days, allowing them to be the first to recognize cardiac allograft rejection.[39] The first clinical heart transplant was performed by Hardy in Jackson, Mississippi, in January 1964.[32] A 68-year-old patient in cardiogenic shock received a chimpanzee heart when the prospective human donor became unsuitable. The small animal heart proved inadequate to take the patient's venous return, and the recipient died after 1 hour. The first successful clinical transplant was performed on December 3, 1967, when Dr. Christian Barnard, at the University of Cape Town, transplanted the heart of a young man to a 54-year-old patient with a heart irreparably damaged by repeated myocardial infarction.[4] The recipient lived 18 days before dying of gram-negative pneumonia. The historical foundations of heart transplantation are reviewed by Griepp and Ergin.[27]

LUNG TRANSPLANTATION. In contrast to the success of cardiac allografts, clinical lung transplantation proved much more difficult.[59] The first human lung transplant was performed by Hardy on June 11, 1963, in a patient with chronic lung disease and carcinoma of the left lung. The patient survived 18 days before dying of renal insufficiency. Because of the difficulty of finding suitable donors, bronchial anastomotic complications, and allograft rejection, only 38 lung transplants were performed in the first 15 years of clinical experience.[58] The longest survivor was a 23-year-old sandblaster with micronodular silicosis who lived 10 months after lung allotransplantation.[20] The tracheobronchial anastomotic complications were overcome by simultaneous transplantation of the lungs and heart, a procedure first performed by Reitz and associates at Stanford in 1981.[48]

PANCREAS TRANSPLANTATION. The first clinical pancreatic transplant was performed on December 20, 1893, in Bristol, England, by Williams. His patient, a 15-year-old boy, died in coma 3 days later.[22] Work in this area was sporadic and unsuccessful until 1922, when Banting and associates corrected the hyperglycemia of human diabetes mellitus by injection of bovine pancreatic extract.[3] However, clinical application of whole pancreas transplantation in a systematic manner was not to occur for more than 40 years. In 1970, Lillehei published the first cases in the extensive University of Minnesota series of clinical pancreatic allotransplants which began in 1966.[38] In the original 14 cases of pancreaticoduodenal transplantation, four patients and one graft survived more than 1 year, and one recipient was still alive in 1984. The same institution reported the first large series of human islet allografts in 1977. However, none of 20 islet allografts led to insulin independence, and only 3 of 10 islet autografts for chronic pancreatitis led to insulin independence.[43] The historical development of pancreatic islet transplantation is reviewed by Downing.[22]

During the short history of clinical pancreas transplantation, the difficult problem of eliminating or draining the pancreatic exocrine secretions was managed in several ways. Gliedman and associates attempted to anastomose the pancreatic duct to the ureter.[25] Duct ligation was attempted by the same group as well as by Groth in 1976.[28] The technique of injecting the pancreatic duct with a synthetic polymer to block exocrine function was reported by Dubernard and associates in 1978.[23] Free drainage of the duct into the peritoneal cavity was investigated by Sutherland and reported in 1979.[53] However, intractable ascites occurred in some patients and an overall technical complication rate of 50% mandated reinvestigation of enteric drainage.[52] Bladder drainage as popularized by Sollinger and associates[50] produced improved results with combined kidney-pancreas transplants. Using the segmental technique and a pancreaticojejunostomy, living-related donor pancreas transplantation began in 1979.[54]

INTESTINE TRANSPLANTATION. Although *auto*transplantation of the bowel is among the most frequently used and successful forms of organ transplantation (see Part XII), intestinal *allo*transplantation has been generally unsuccessful. Clinical small intestinal allografting was attempted in several patients after 1967 for bowel infarction,[37] repeated sepsis on total parenteral nutrition,[1] and Gardner's syndrome with recurrent desmoid tumors of the bowel.[24] Even in the case of the HLA-identical graft, which survived 76 days, minimal useful bowel function was observed. Rejection, graft-versus-host disease, infection, and high operative mortality historically diminished surgical enthusiasm for intestinal transplantation. The advent of cyclosporine immunosuppression reawakened interest in the field.[19,21,46]

XENOTRANSPLANTATION. When the techniques of vascular anastomosis were sufficiently well known to permit successful auto- and allotransplantation, a number of human xenogeneic transplants were attempted. Between 1905 and 1910, several workers, including Jaboulay in France and Unger in Germany, performed xenografts but did not document graft function.[31] When the immunologic basis of rejection was established, renewal of interest in clinical xenotransplantation awaited the development of new immunosuppressive measures. After the efficacy of chemical immunosuppression with azathioprine, prednisone, and mitomycin-C was established, Reemtsma and associates, in 1963 and 1964, undertook xenografts in patients in renal failure using kidneys from nonhuman primates.[47] Several of these cases showed satisfactory immediate function, but all were eventually rejected within a few months. When cyclosporine became available for clinical use, human xenografting was again attempted in 1984.[2] A baboon heart was transplanted to a child born with a severe congenital malformation of the heart. Despite intensive immunosuppression, rejection developed and the infant died within weeks of transplantation.

TISSUE AND ORGAN PRESERVATION. Along with the improved capability of transplanting tissues and organs, interest in preservation and storage of living tissue developed. The structural integrity and the viability of the graft had to be maintained during the interval from removal to implantation. Basically, two approaches were available: (1) methods that reduced or brought to a reversible standstill the need for oxygen and other metabolic requirements and (2) systems that supported active metabolism. Of the several methods that were tried to achieve long-term preservation, including freezing, only hypothermia and organ perfusion are in general use today. In addition, chemical inhibition of metabolism in the form of cardioplegia solution was utilized for cardiac transplantation and many other open heart surgical procedures as discussed in Chapter 56.

In 1908 Carrel removed an artery from one animal, preserved it with hypothermia for days, and then successfully transplanted it to another animal.[14] The numerous other contributions of Carrel to tissue culture and ultimately organ perfusion were reviewed by Humphries and Dennis in their ''Historical

Developments in Preservation."[35] Using his newly developed media and culture techniques, Carrel was able to maintain chick embryo fibroblasts in continuous culture for more than 25 years! His attempts at organ culture were less successful. Using a pump and perfusion apparatus designed by Charles Lindbergh, organs were perfused for 20 to 40 days with normothermic serum. Although some cells remained viable, reimplantation of the organs was not undertaken to test the effectiveness of the preservation system. Maximal preservation of kidneys was approximately 2 days.[16]

A variety of solutions were used for continuous perfusion of organs. Humphries achieved 24-hour dog kidney preservation using continuous perfusion with dilute blood at 10° C. Plasma protein fraction, cryoprecipitated plasma, silicone-gel fraction of plasma, and albumin were all added to electrolyte solutions to improve preservation. Belzer and associates, in 1967, introduced a new pump and perfusate containing lipoprotein-free serum for continuous pulsatile perfusion at 10° C. that enabled him to consistently preserve kidneys for 72 hours.[5]

HYPOTHERMIA. At temperatures of 0° to 4° C., tissues remain viable in the absence of circulation 10 or more times longer than at normal body temperature. The simple method of hypothermia proved useful in preserving skin, cornea, kidney, liver, heart, pancreas, and blood. Flushing an organ with a cold perfusate, usually a balanced electrolyte solution, was used widely as a means of rapid cooling, within seconds, to temperatures that by surface cooling were achieved only after a number of minutes and at the expense of loss of viability. In 1960, Lapchinsky, of Moscow, reported successful reimplantation of dog kidneys and hind limbs after 24 to 28 hours of preservation using cold storage. He perfused the kidney or limb for 1 hour with cooled whole blood, then kept the organ cold at 2° to 4° C. until 1 hour before reimplantation, when he perfused the tissue again for 1 hour, this time with warm blood.[35] Collins and associates, in 1969, developed a flushing solution that mimicked intracellular fluid.[17] With this hyperkalemic and hyperosmolar solution, they flushed kidneys, kept them cold on ice, and obtained excellent function after 30 hours of iced storage. By removing the magnesium from Collins' solution, the Euro-Collins solution, widely used by European transplant centers, was developed in 1976. Euro-Collins and Sacks' solution, developed in 1978, successfully preserved human kidneys for 50 hours or more.[35] The use of preservation solutions to flush grafts and reduce their metabolism through hypothermia, hyperkalemia, hyponatremia, and hypocalcemia before cold storage should be distinguished from perfusion methods designed to support metabolism by simulating as fully as possible the normothermic internal environment of the organ. However, elements of the two approaches were often combined in the form of continuous perfusion at 4° to 10° C.

ORGAN-SHARING NETWORKS. A natural outgrowth of the capabilities for organ preservation and tissue matching was the development of networks for sharing kidneys on the basis of histocompatibility. For example, in 1968, Hume, at the Medical College of Virginia, in cooperation with Amos, of Duke University, developed an organ-sharing plan to enlarge the potential recipient pool for each new kidney that became available so that better tissue matches between donor and recipient could be obtained. The resulting organization, termed the South-Eastern Organ Procurement Foundation (SEOPF), shared kidneys among nine institutions based on computer-assisted matching of all potential recipients in that region. The SEOPF network expanded to include 46 transplanting institutions and led in 1984 to the incorporation of the United Network for Organ Sharing (UNOS), to facilitate organ placement throughout the United States. Similar organ-sharing networks were developed in Europe, Scandinavia, the United Kingdom, and elsewhere. These regional networks began to cooperate in the sharing of human organs and tissues on an international scale.

SELECTED REFERENCES

Converse, J. M., and Casson, P. R.: The historical background of transplantation. *In* Rapaport, F. T., and Dausset, J. (Eds.): Human Transplantation. New York, Grune & Stratton, 1968.
The authors present a history of the principal developments in transplantation from ancient to modern times, and they include some details not included in the other histories cited.

Griepp, R. B., and Ergin, M. D.: The history of experimental heart transplantation. Heart Transplant., 3:145, 1984.
The authors present a brief, interesting, and well-illustrated summary of the development of heart transplantation.

Hamilton, D.: Kidney transplantation: A history. *In* Morris, P. J. (Ed.): Kidney transplantation principles and practice. London, Grune & Stratton, 1984.
In this new chapter written for the second edition of Kidney Transplantation, the author presents an interesting account of the evolution of human kidney transplantation from early European experiments to the modern era.

Moore, F. D.: Give and Take. Philadelphia, W. B. Saunders Company, 1964.
In this volume is presented a concise review of developments in basic biology and in medicine and surgery that apply to therapeutic renal transplantation. Interesting aspects of historic renal transplants in Boston are described by the author, who was there at the time and has communicated personally with scientists there and elsewhere who have made notable contributions. For the student, this book is an informative introduction to the subject of transplantation, and for the lay reader, a readily understood account of some interesting developments in biology and medicine.

Starzl, T. E., Iwatsuki, S., Van Thiel, D. H., Gartner, J. C., Zitelli, B. J., Malatack, J. J., Schade, R. R., Shaw, B. W., Jr., Hakala, T. R., Rosenthal, J. T., and Porter, K. A.: Evolution of liver transplantation. Hepatology, 2:614, 1982.
The researcher, physician, and author who has contributed the most to the development of liver transplantation provides an authoritative account of the development of the field.

Worshofsky, F.: The Rebuilt Man. New York, Thomas Y. Crowell Company, 1965.
This book is a brief historical review of the development of transplantation from ancient to modern times. Written by a science writer for lay readers, the discussion is well documented by references to and quotations from the scientific literature.

REFERENCES

1. Alican, F., Hardy, J. D., Cayirli, M., Varner, J. E., Moynihan, P. C., Turner, M. D., and Anas, P.: Intestinal transplantation: Laboratory experience and report of a clinical case. Am. J. Surg., 121:150, 1971.
2. Bailey, L. L., Nehlsen-Cannarell, S. L., Concepcion, W., and Jolley, W. B.: Baboon-to-human cardiac xenotransplantation in a neonate. J.A.M.A., 254:3321, 1985.
3. Banting, F., Best, C., Gollip, J., Campbell, W., and Fletcher, A.: Pancreas extracts in the treatment of diabetes mellitus. Can. Med. Assoc. J., 12:141, 1922.
4. Barnard, C. N.: A human cardiac transplant: An interim report of a successful operation performed at Groote Schuur Hospital, Cape Town. S. Afr. Med. J., 41:1271, 1967.
5. Belzer, F. O., Ashby, B. S., and Dunphy, J. F.: 24-hour and 72-hour preservation of canine kidneys. Lancet, 2:536, 1967.
6. Bhisragratna, K. K.: The Sushruta Sanhita. An English translation based on the original Sanscrit text. Calcutta, 1907.
7. Billingham, R. E., Brent, L., and Medawar, P. B.: Actively acquired tolerance of foreign cells. Nature, 172:603, 1953.
8. Borel, J. F.: Cyclosporine: Historical perspectives. Transplant. Proc., 15(4) Suppl. 1):2219, 1983.
9. Calne, R. Y.: Renal Transplantation. London, Edward Arnold, 1967.
10. Carpenter, C. B.: Clinical histocompatibility testing: A brief historical perspective. Transplant. Proc., 13(1)(Suppl. 1):55, 1981.
11. Carrel, A.: La Technique operatoire des anastomoses vasculaires et la transplantation des viscères. Lyon Med., 98:859, 1902.
12. Carrel, A.: The transplantation of organs: A preliminary communication. J.A.M.A., 45:1645, 1905.
13. Carrel, A.: Transplantation in mass of the kidney. J. Exp. Med., 10:140, 1908.
14. Carrel, A.: Results of the transplantation of blood vessels, organs and limbs. J. Am. Med. Assoc., 51:1662, 1908.
15. Carrel, A., and Guthrie, C. C.: The transplantation of veins and organs. Am. Med., 10:1101, 1905.
16. Carrel, A., and Linbergh, C. A.: The Culture of Organs. New York, Paul B. Hoeber, 1938.
17. Collins, G. M., Bravo-Shugarman, M., and Terasaki, P. I.: Kidney preservation for transportation. Lancet, 2:1219, 1969.
18. Converse, J. M., and Casson, P. R.: The historical background of transplantation. *In* Rapaport, F. T., and Dausset, J. (Eds.): Human Transplantation. New York, Grune & Stratton, 1968.
19. Craddock, G. N., Nordgren, S. R., Reznick, R. K., Gilas, T., Lossing, A. G., Cohen, Z., Stiller, C. R., Cullen, J. B., and Langer, B.: Small bowel transplantation in the dog using cyclosporine. Transplantation, 35:284, 1983.
20. Dermon, F., Barbier, F., Ringoir, S., Versieck, J., Rolly, G., Berzsenyi, G.,

Vermeire, P., and Vrints, L.: Ten-month survival after lung homotransplantation in man. J. Thorac. Cardiovasc. Surg., 61:835, 1971.

21. Diliz-Perez, H. S., McClure, J., Bedetti, C., Hong, H., de Santibanes, E., Shaw B. W., Jr., Van Thiel, D., Iwatsuki, S., and Starzl, T. E.: Successful small bowel allotransplantation in dogs with cyclosporine and prednisone. Transplantation, 37:126, 1984.

22. Downing, R.: Historical review of pancreatic islet transplantation. World J. Surg., 8:137, 1984.

23. Dubernard, J. M., Traeger, J., Neyra, P., Touraine, J. L., Tranchant, D., and Blanc-Bruant, N.: A new method of preparation of segmental pancreatic grafts for transplantation: Trials in dogs and in man. Surgery, 84:633, 1978.

24. Fortner, J. G., Sichuk, G., Litwin, S. D., and Beattie, E. J., Jr.: Immunological responses to an intestinal allograft with HL-A-identical donor-recipient. Transplantation, 14:531, 1972.

25. Gliedman, M. L., Gold, M., Whittaker, J., Rifkin, H., Soberman, R., Freed, S., Tellis, V., and Veith, F. J.: Pancreatic duct to ureter anastomosis in pancreas transplantation. Am. J. Surg., 125:245, 1973.

26. Gorer, P. A.: Transplantese. Ann. N.Y. Acad. Sci., 87:604, 1960.

27. Griepp, R. B., and Ergin, M. A.: The history of experimental heart transplantation. Heart Transplant., 3:145, 1984.

28. Groth, C., Lundgren, G., Arner, P., Collste, H., Hardstedt, C., Lewander, R., and Ostman, J.: Rejection of isolated pancreatic allografts in patients with diabetes. Surg. Gynecol. Obstet., 143:933, 1976.

29. Guthrie, D.: A History of Medicine. Philadelphia, J. B. Lippincott Company, 1946, p. 12.

30. Hamburger, J., Vaysse, J., Crosnier, J., Auver, J., Lalanne, M., and Hopper, J., Jr.: Renal homotransplantation in man after radiation of the recipient. Am. J. Med., 32:854, 1962.

31. Hamilton, D.: Kidney transplantation: A history. In Morris, P. J. (Ed.): Kidney Transplantation Principles and Practice. London, Grune & Stratton, 1984.

32. Hardy, J. D., Chavez, C. M., Kurrus, F. D., Neely, W. A., Eraslan, S., Turner, M. D., Fabian, L. W., and Labeckiz, T.: Heart transplantation in man: Developmental studies and report of a case. J.A.M.A., 188:1132, 1964.

33. Holman, E.: Protein sensitization in isoskingrafting. Surg. Gynecol. Obstet., 38:100, 1924.

34. Homer: The Iliad, Book 6.

35. Humphries, A. L., and Dennis, A. J., Jr.: Historical Developments in Preservation. In Toledo-Pereyra, L. H. (Ed.): Basic Concepts of Organ Procurement, Perfusion and Preservation for Transplantation. New York, Academic Press, 1982, p. 1.

36. Kahan, B. D.: Cosmas and Damian revisited. Transplant. Proc., 15:2211, 1983.

37. Lillehei, R. C., Idezuki, Y., Feemster, J. A., Dietzman, R. H., Kelly, W. D., Merkel, F. K., Goetz, F. C., Lyons, G. W., and Manax, W. G.: Transplantation of stomach, intestine, and pancreas: Experimental and clinical observations. Surgery, 62:721, 1967.

38. Lillehei, R. C., Simmons, R. L., Najarian, J. S., Weil, R., Uchida, H., Ruiz, J. O., Kjellstrand, C. M., and Goetz, F. C.: Pancreaticoduodenal allotransplantation: Experimental and clinical experience. Ann. Surg., 172:405, 1970.

39. Mann, F. C., Priestley, J. T., Markowitz, J., and Yater, W. M.: Transplantation of the intact mammalian heart. Arch. Surg., 26:219, 1933.

40. Merrill, J. P.: Early days of the artificial kidney and transplantation. Transplant. Proc., 13(Suppl. 1):4, 1981.

41. Moore, F. D.: Give and Take: The Development of Tissue Transplantation. Philadelphia, W. B. Saunders Company, 1964.

42. Murray, J. E.: Remembrances of the early days of renal transplantation. Transplant. Proc., 13(Suppl. 1):9, 1981.

43. Najarian, J. S., Sutherland, D. E. R., Matas, A. J., Steffes, M. W., Simmons, R. L., and Goetz, F. C.: Human islet transplantation: a preliminary experience. Transplant. Proc., 9:233, 1977.

44. Owen, R. D.: Immunogenetic consequences of vascular anastomoses between bovine twins. Science, 102:400, 1945.

45. Peer, L. A.: Transplantation of Tissues. Baltimore, Williams & Wilkins, 1955.

46. Raju, S., Didlake, R. H., Gayirli, M., Turner, M. D., Grogan, J. B., and Achord, J.: Experimental small bowel transplantation utilizing cyclosporine. Transplantation, 38:561, 1984.

47. Reemtsma, K., McCracken, B. H., Schlegel, J. U., and Pearl, M.: Heterotransplantation of the kidney: Two clinical experiences. Science, 143:700, 1964.

48. Reitz, B. A., Wallwork, J. L., Hunt, S. A., Pennock, J. L., Billingham, M. E., Oyer, P. E., Stinson, E. B., and Shumway, N. E.: Heart-lung transplantation: Successful therapy for patients with pulmonary vascular disease. N. Engl. J. Med., 306:557, 1982.

49. Schwartz, R., and Dameshek, W.: Drug-induced immunological tolerance. Nature, 183:1682, 1959.

50. Sollinger, H. W., Pirsch, J. D., D'Alessandro, A. M., Kalayoglu, M., and Belzer, F. O.: Advantages of bladder drainage in pancreas transplantation: A personal view. Clin. Transplant., 4:32, 1990.

51. Starzl, T. E., Iwatsuki, S., Van Thiel, D. H., Gartner, J. C., Zitelli, B. J., Malatack, J. J., Schade, R. R., Shaw, B. W., Jr., Hakala, T. R., Rosenthal, J. T., and Porter, K. A.: Evolution of liver transplantation. Hepatology, 2:614, 1982.

52. Sutherland, D. E. R., Goetz, F. C., Elick, B. A., and Najarian, J. S.: Experiments with 49 segmental pancreatic transplants in 45 diabetic patients. Transplantation, 34:330, 1982.

53. Sutherland, D. E. R., Goetz, F. C., and Najarian, J. S.: Intraperitoneal transplantation of immediate vascularized segmental grafts without duct ligation: A clinical trial. Transplantation, 28:485, 1979.

54. Sutherland, D. E. R., Goetz, F. C., and Najarian, J. S.: Living-related donor segmental pancreatectomy for transplantation. Transplant Proc., 12(Suppl. 2):19, 1980.

55. Tagliacozzi, G.: De curtorum chirurgia per insitioneum. Venice, 1597, p. 61.

56. Terasaki, P. I., and McClelland, J. D.: Microdroplet assay of human serum cytotoxins. Nature, 204:998, 1964.

57. Ullmann, E.: Experimentelle nierentransplantation. Wien. Klin. Wochenschr., 15:281, 1902.

58. Veith, F. J.: Lung transplantation. Surg. Clin. North Am., 58:357, 1978.

59. Veith, F. J., Kamholz, S. L., Mollenkopf, F. P., and Montefusco, C. M.: Lung transplantation 1983. Transplantation, 35:271, 1983.

60. Woodruff, M. F. A.: The Transplantation of Tissues and Organs. Springfield, Ill., Charles C Thomas, 1960.

61. Worshofsky, F.: The Rebuilt Man. New York, Thomas Y. Crowell, 1965.

II

THE IMMUNOLOGY OF TRANSPLANT ANTIGENS

D. Bernard Amos, M.D., and Fred Sanfilippo, M.D., Ph.D.

The major histocompatibility complex (MHC) was so named because of its influence on transplant survival. This distinction between the MHC and minor histocompatibility antigens was established in 1948 through experimental grafts between different strains of inbred mice.[25] It was established in the 1960s for man through test skin grafts and kidney grafts exchanged between members of families. Since these pioneering transplant experiments, other studies have shown that the MHC is essential for the differentiation of self from many forms of non-self and altered self. MHC interactions are involved in nearly every type of immune response; there is presumptive evidence that many other cell-cell interactions, e.g., those occurring during growth and inflammation are also MHC-regulated.

Although the term *MHC* is a cumbersome designation for this array of genes, it is an appropriate one; *major*, because it is the most powerful and ubiquitous recognition system; *histocompatibility*, because it recognizes individual tissue differences; and *complex*, because it is a gene complex consisting of a variety of different but closely linked genes of astonishing polymorphism. Indeed, this polymorphism is so great that it is difficult for many to grasp just how extensive it is; a comparison of the well-known individuality of fingerprint patterns to that of the less well known MHC would not be inappropriate.

This chapter primarily concerns the nature and biologic function of the human MHC, termed *HLA*, in the recognition of self and non-self and in allograft survival. Although most human transplants now come from cadaveric donors and few are from living donors—usually from close relatives, the fundamental properties of HLA in transplantation have been most clearly established through a comparison of HLA identical sibling grafts with grafts involving other donor recipient pairs. In this and in the succeeding chapter the immunologic and genetic factors involved in graft rejection, are reviewed, the measures that attempt to minimize alloimmune responses while preserving intact the normal immunologic defenses are examined, and some perspectives of current and future trends are presented. Those who believe that the objectives of the transplant surgeon can be met by the administration of even more potent immunosuppressive agents must consider that despite the magnificent advances of the past 40 years, grafts as well as patients are too often lost to infection or to rejection. Even more grafts are slowly losing function consequent to the insidious effects of chronic rejection despite immunosuppression. Thus, although pride can be taken in the achievements to date, there remains much to be learned and applied.

HISTORICAL ASPECTS

THE EXPERIMENTS OF MEDAWAR: DEMONSTRATION OF INDIVIDUALITY. Some of the earliest studies yielding significant information about transplantation immunology were conducted during World War II by Sir Peter Medawar,[37] who was asked by the British government to determine why skin grafts from cadavers used to treat burned fighter pilots were rejected. The objective was to prevent this rejection process. The animal experiments he devised were of classic design and simplicity, and clearly demonstrated the three basic characteristics of immune responsiveness: recognition of non-self, memory, and specificity. First, rabbit skin was cut into squares. The squares were then grafted in a checkerboard manner so that animals received patches of their own skin (autografts) alternating with patches of skin from another rabbit (allografts). Within a few days all grafts had healed and become well vascularized. By about the tenth day, however, although the autografts were still in excellent condition, the adjacent allografts became darker and eventually necrotic, demonstrating host recognition of foreign (non-self) tissue. Following complete rejection of the allografts as a "first-set," or primary, reaction, fresh grafts from the same donor were given to the same recipient. In this case, a much more vigorous and rapid rejection response was seen almost immediately following vascularization of the graft (usually within 5 to 6 days), demonstrating immunologic memory. (Fig.1).

The supposition that the accelerated rejection of a second graft involved specific sensitization of the recipient against the donor was confirmed by double-grafting experiments. After a typical first-set rejection of an allograft from one donor rabbit, a second graft was transplanted from the same donor rabbit along with an additional graft from a different donor. In this case, the repeat graft was rejected quickly as a second-set response, while the graft from the different rabbit survived longer and showed only first-set rejection, demonstrating the specificity of host recognition. These few basic experiments demonstrated the fundamental features of immune responsiveness, and indicated the immunologic nature of allograft rejection.

Medawar also examined the histology of rejection.[38] The finding of vascular degeneration with an intense infiltration of small mononuclear cells into the graft and graft bed led him to suggest that the mononuclear cell (lymphocyte) had an important part in allograft destruction, and to propose that the process was similar to one that had been previously described for the delayed hypersensitivity response to tuberculin. The suggestion that graft rejection was due to cellular-mediated immunity was strengthened by the subsequent work of Mitchison.[40] Using a system now referred to as adoptive transfer, he transferred lym-

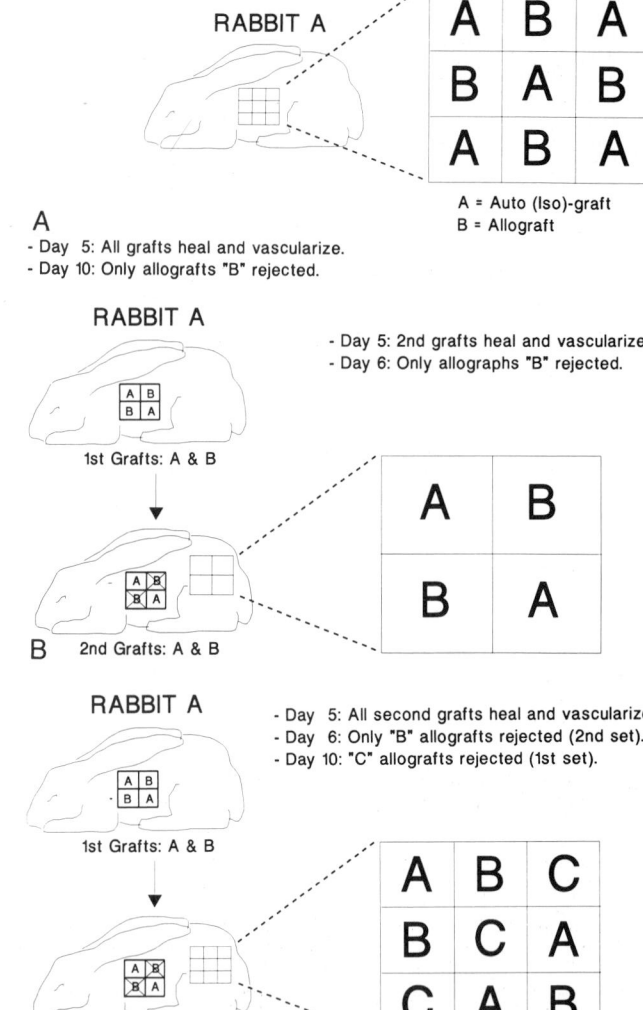

RABBIT A

A	B	A
B	A	B
A	B	A

A = Auto (Iso)-graft
B = Allograft

A
- Day 5: All grafts heal and vascularize.
- Day 10: Only allografts "B" rejected.

RABBIT A

- Day 5: 2nd grafts heal and vascularize.
- Day 6: Only allographs "B" rejected.

1st Grafts: A & B

| A | B |
| B | A |

B   2nd Grafts: A & B

RABBIT A

- Day 5: All second grafts heal and vascularize.
- Day 6: Only "B" allografts rejected (2nd set).
- Day 10: "C" allografts rejected (1st set).

1st Grafts: A & B

A	B	C
B	C	A
C	A	B

C   2nd Grafts: A,B,C

Figure 1. A, First-set rejection. The individuality of tissues is shown by a simple exchange of skin. A graft from an unrelated individual (allograft) is rejected while a graft taken elsewhere from the same (recipient) rabbit persists indefinitely. B, Second-set rejection. A second graft from the original (sensitizing) donor is more rapidly rejected (second-set reaction) than the original allograft. Autografts are not rejected. C, Mixed rejection. Fine specificity is shown by including a graft from a third party. The timing is the same as for B. Grafts from the sensitizing donor are rejected in second set fashion, while grafts from the third party donor are rejected as first-set grafts and the autografts are not rejected at all.

phocytes from previously sensitized recipients into nonimmunized animals. Mitchison's experiments demonstrated that specific immunity could be transferred with cells from lymph nodes draining the grafted tissue but not from the contralateral side, and that the development of immunity was time-dependent. Lymphoid cells transferred during the first 3 or 4 days after sensitization did not influence graft rejection in the recipient; cells harvested at the peak of rejection (about the fifth to seventh day in Mitchison's system) were most effective, whereas activity waned by about the tenth day after rejection. Other investigators later reported a second wave of reactivity 3 to 4 weeks after the initial exposure to alloantigens. A refinement of Mitchison's procedure was introduced by Winn.[64] In the Winn assay, the effector lymphocytes are administered together with the target cells. This assay allows the effector population to be manipulated or modified; certain subsets of cells can be depleted or enriched, can be antibody treated, or can be taken from various sites at various times and combined according to the wishes of the investigator.

THE EXPERIMENTS OF GORER: IDENTIFICATION OF

THE MHC. While Medawar's experiments demonstrated individual specificity, they were not informative about the antigens recognized. For this, Peter Gorer, who demonstrated that transplantation antigens could be identified on the blood cells of inbred mice, is credited. For most of his experiments he relied on transplantable tumors, thus demonstrating that a variety of tissues shared the same antigens. From antibodies made between inbred strains Gorer was able to identify individual specific histocompatibility (H) antigens termed H-2 antigens. By using hybrid animals in which the H-2 antigens segregated, Gorer, with Lyman and Snell, demonstrated that the H-2 antigens provided the major stimulus for rejection.[25] Gorer and colleagues later demonstrated that there were at least two separate but closely linked antigens in H-2 and that antibodies were regularly produced during graft rejection.[3]

OTHER OBSERVATIONS. A special type of response known as the "white graft" was observed when a second graft was applied at a critical time after sensitization.[23] In man, this is usually approximately 10 days after rejection of an initial skin graft. This (third) type of reaction (also known as "hyperacute rejection") has a distinctive histologic pattern with an absence of lymphocyte infiltration into the graft; instead, a dense band of acute inflammatory cells, especially neutrophils, is present at the graft border. These grafts never become vascularized; hence their white color. A fourth histologic pattern has been noted when rejection is very indolent, the "blue graft." Termed *blue* because of its gross appearance on a routine hematoxylin and eosin–stained section, such grafts have diffuse lymphocytic infiltrates with little evidence of vascular damage. Often the epidermal layer and skin appendages remain intact despite the very heavy infiltration. Although less commonly observed, these last two forms of rejection are important because they indicate that lymphocyte infiltration *per se* is not always necessary or sufficient for allograft destruction.

The cell type and architecture of a transplanted organ or tissue, its vascularization, and its physical relationship to elements of the immune system are important in determining the type of host immune response generated. The importance of some of these features has been demonstrated in several ways. Gorer recognized three different histologic patterns of graft rejection, depending on the type of tumor used.[24] The first was observed when lymphomas were transplanted to an incompatible, allogeneic host (allograft). Rejection of these tumors was associated with increased vascular permeability and collagen degeneration; host cellular reactivity was minimal until the end of the reaction and then was largely histiocytic. The histology of the rejection of transplanted carcinomas resembled that of the skin graft response, with lymphoid infiltration and vascular damage. A third pattern was noted when sarcomas were transplanted. Histiocytes began to proliferate at the margin of the graft about 5 days after transplantation, often advancing as a syncytial mass. Frequently both the histiocytes and the tumor cells would die, especially in preimmunized animals. These early experiments on the histology of tumor rejection are relevant to organ transplantation, because they indicate that histologic changes other than the classic mononuclear cell infiltration noted by Medawar may occur.

Rejection of organs receiving their blood supply from a major artery differs greatly from graft rejection of organs or tissues with substantial lymphatic connections, especially when the highly vascularized graft has poor lymphatic connections. If a graft is placed on an extremity and then removed, systemic immunity can still develop. The importance of the draining lymph can be demonstrated by removing the regional lymph nodes together with the graft. If ablation is performed early (within 48 hours), immunity does not develop. Dependence upon lymphatic connections was demonstrated by Barker and Billingham,[11] who prepared skin pedicles by raising skin flaps that were connected only by a bundle of vessels. Some of the vascular connections were comprised of artery, vein, and lymphatics; whereas others consisted of only artery and vein. When an allogeneic skin graft was placed on a skin flap having a lymphatic connection, the graft was rejected normally. In graft beds with no lymphatic connection, the graft persisted in a fully viable state for the life of the pedicle. However, if animals carrying a viable graft on a flap without lymphatic connections were given another graft from the same donor at the site with lymphatic connections, both grafts were rejected.

Taken together, the fundamental experiments described above suggest a minimum of three components in the response to a transplant: an afferent arc, by which antigenic material is transported to the regional node; a central component in which immunity is developed, generally in draining lymph nodes but also in the spleen for grafts having major venous connections; and an efferent arc, which the Barker and Billingham experiments showed to be the blood supply. These descriptive studies provided a basis for subsequent work which examined the mechanisms involved in allograft recognition and response. Other fundamental studies further established that some of the antigens present on tissues were much more potent than others in stimulating immunity to a transplant and thus helped to identify the special role of the antigens of the major histocompatibility complex.[53]

THE MAJOR HISTOCOMPATIBILITY COMPLEX

GENERAL FEATURES. The most important factor leading to rejection of nearly any tissue in all higher species (from reptile or bird to man) is incompatibility at the major histocompatibility complex (MHC). The human MHC is known as the HLA system, and its gene complex occupies part of the short arm of the sixth chromosome. This segment of chromosome is also termed the HLA haplotype. The MHC of many other species is similarly named and has analogous features; thus, *RhLA* for Rhesus, *SLA* for swine, *DLA* for dog, etc. Terminological exceptions are *H-2 of the mouse* and *RT1 of the rat.* Details of the organization of the MHC in different species may differ, but the Class I and Class II components of the MHC haplotype are almost identical. This is true even in the chicken: even though the MHC of fowls is located on a microchromosome, a new Class I–like molecule is present (B-G) and the complement genes are elsewhere.[30]

The MHC haplotype consists of a series of gene families that probably arose early in vertebrate evolution from immunoglobulin-like genes. These were reduplicated and modified by mutation. The integral parts of this interactive system include genes for the so-called Class I antigens, glycoproteins expressed on most types of cells; genes for Class II antigens, another set of glycoproteins that are regulated differently and with restricted cell expression; and genes for some of the components of complement, sometimes referred to as Class III gene products. Included in the haplotype or adjacent to it are genes for other cell surface glycoproteins and for enzymes that have (as yet) no known relevance to the function of the MHC. The MHC also includes regulatory genes referred to above that are not fully defined and are the focus of intense investigation.

THE CLASS I ANTIGENS. The Class I antigens are by far the best known component of the HLA system, mainly for historical reasons. Because the many alleles were identified by the reactions of readily available antisera and are found on most tissues, their elucidation proceeded rapidly. The definition of these antigens was until recently (and unfortunately) based exclusively on the reactions of selected sera. The DNA sequences of the genes, the amino acid sequences of the antigens, and functional assays are all providing fresh insights leading to new definitions of the antigens.

The heavy chain of a Class I antigen is a 44,000-dalton transmembranous glycoprotein that has a domain structure similar to that of immunoglobulin.[43] The C terminus is cytoplasmic and typically has several half-cysteines that may be phosphorylated. Conformation of the three extracellular domains α_1, α_2, and α_3 of the heavy chain is stabilized in part by its noncovalent binding to the light chain, which consists of a second, smaller, glycoprotein known as β_2.microglobulin(β_2m). Mutant cells that lack β_2m and molecules from which β_2m has been stripped fail to bind the appropriate alloantisera against Class I molecules. Conversely, antibody to β_2m can compete with some monoclonal antibodies directed against antigenic determinants (epitopes) present on the Class I antigen. From a variety of competitive binding studies of this type, it is known that a single HLA Class I molecule carries at least four antibody combining sites (epitopes), two or more of which are alloantigens and vary from person to person; whereas two or more appear to be invariant and characteristic of the species.[44] Four epitopes represent a minimal estimate; Parham and colleagues have compared 39 different Class I sequences. There were 71 positions at which amino acid substitutions had occurred; 6 were locus-specific, 10 were frequently ($\geq$5 per cent) variable for HLA-A, and 5 were specific for HLA-B. Interestingly, although there was little variability in the α_3 domain, that which did occur was mainly in HLA-A.

The structure of HLA-A2, a typical Class I molecule, is shown schematically in Figure 2. The three identifiable Class I products expressed on the human cell surface (i.e., HLA-A, HLA-B, HLA-C) are described in detail below and correspond to the H-2D, H-2K, and H-2L antigens of the mouse. HLA-A and HLA-B are expressed on most tissues; HLA-C is more variable. There is indirect evidence that other Class I antigens may be transiently expressed during activation or differentiation. Approximately 36 DNA sequences resembling those of the typical heavy chain Class I genes have been detected on the sixth chromosome of man, the majority coding for molecules other than HLA-A,-B, or -C or representing pseudogenes. Three of the additional genes have recently been identified and are desig-

nated HLA-E, -F, and -G; but the clinical relevance of these molecules has not been established.[15,63] It also appears likely that HLA-C is feebly immunogenic.

A peculiarity of HLA-B is that each molecule carries, in addition to the subtypic specificity such as HLA-B44, a second (supertypic) specificity designated Bw4 or Bw6. Originally termed 4a and 4b by van Rood, this diallelic system of antigens presented many technical difficulties; they could be precisely identified by very few clinical laboratories.[61] The technical problems of recognizing Bw4 and Bw6 have now been overcome by the use of monoclonal antibodies, and these antigens are now regularly identified. A multiplicity of other supertypic specificities can be found with alloantisera and with monoclonal antibodies; these have not yet been classified. Some investigators believe the broadly distributed, supertypic antigens to be functionally important in antigen presentation and in clinical transplantation.

MIXED LYMPHOCYTE REACTIONS AND HLA-D. Bach, Bain, and colleagues independently found that lymphocytes from one individual would, with very rare exceptions, stimulate lymphocytes from an unrelated individual when the two lymphocyte populations were cultured together in the mixed leukocyte reaction, or MLR.[9,10] Ceppellini demonstrated that cells from family members were sometimes stimulatory and sometimes not,[19] and Bach and Amos demonstrated by inheritance studies that the ability to stimulate segregated with HLA.[8] Family members who differed at one or both haplotypes usually stimulated while siblings who were HLA identical failed to stimulate. Occasional exceptional families, however, indicated that the ability to stimulate was not due to HLA (Class I) antigens alone; the existence of a distinct stimulatory (MLR-S) locus was postulated.[45] Inheritance of the MLR-S characteristic could be readily studied in families; but because nearly all unrelated individuals stimulated each other, there was no way in which MLR-S could be analyzed in the hospital population and especially in unrelated donor-recipient pairs. A solution to this unsatisfactory situation emerged when Jorgensen and co-workers identified a child of a consanguineous marriage, "J," who inherited both HLA haplotypes from one great-grandparent; they found that cells from J would not stimulate a response from the parents or from other family members inheriting this haplotype.[28] They also demonstrated that cells from this subject failed to stimulate responses from some unrelated subjects, so that in effect, cells from J could be used to identify unrelated individuals or family members with the same MLR-S allele as J. J had inherited two copies of one haplotype passed down from the great-grandfather and was the first homozygote for HLA to be recognized.

These studies on the responses of an HLA homozygous individual made the cellular typing of unrelated subjects possible, and this stimulator "locus" has now been designated HLA-D. However, no tangible product of an HLA-D locus has as yet been detected. The identification of the alleles of HLA-D is therefore dependent upon functional tests using special stimulators, similar to J, and termed homozygous typing cells (HTCs). Because the alleles of HLA-D could not be given a definitive serologic or biochemical identification, they have retained their provisional "workshop" designation (w) as Dw1, Dw2, etc. Lymphocytes from two subjects who might have the same HLA-D characteristics gave different degrees of stimulation. Responses to the same stimulators could also differ greatly at different times or between different subjects while HTCs appearing to define the same allele would, not infrequently, stimulate each other. For these and other technical reasons, the MLR test is now frequently replaced by an assay performed with responder cells (that can be stored frozen) that have been previously primed by a known stimulator cell: primed lymphocyte typing (PLT). Use of the PLT assay has also revealed that pairs of individuals (including rare pairs of HLA identical siblings)

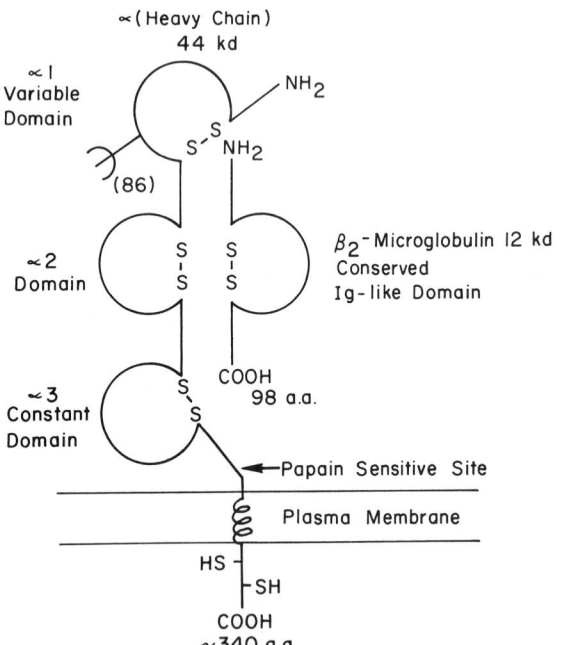

Figure 2. Schematic diagram of a Class I HLA antigen. The domain structure of the heavy chain (44,000 daltons) is stabilized by internal disulfide bonds. Conformation of the molecule is maintained by the noncovalently bound β_2-microglobulin molecule. Antigenic properties are conferred by amino acid substitutions, predominantly in α_1 and α_2, and at least two variable antibody binding sites are present. On the HLA-B molecule one serologically identified site represents Bw4 or Bw6 supertypic determinants and a second site represents "subtypic" or "private" specificities. The papain-sensitive site is indicated external to the hydrophobic β pleated transmembrane sequence. The C terminal cytoplasmic tail has half cysteines, which may be phosphorylated and interact with the cytoskeleton.

who fail to stimulate in MLR occasionally stimulate in PLT. Based on these and other findings, Mawas, Shaw, and colleagues independently proposed the existence of a locus closely linked to but separated from HLA-A, -B, -C and -D, which was originally designated the SB locus and has now been redesignated DP.[31] It is now established that several HLA loci, including DR and DP in the D region, contribute to MLR and PLT stimulation; HLA-D responses are, in fact, compound.

HLA-D, MIXED LYMPHOCYTE REACTIONS, AND CLASS II ANTIGENS. The DR antigens were the first Class II antigens to be detected serologically and were at first thought to be identical to HLA-D. Van Rood and associates demonstrated by indirect fluorescence that alloantibodies which could specifically block a specific MLR would bind to the B cells used as stimulators.[60] Antibodies that would block the reactions due to the Dw1 allele were said to react with products of a D-related (DR) allele DR1. Dw1 and DR1 segregate together in most families; but when populations are tested, some individuals who type as Dw1 are not DR1, and conversely not all DR1 individuals type as Dw1. Sera blocking the HLA-D alleles Dw1 to Dw8 were soon identified. DR alleles DR1 to DR8 are, by definition, frequently associated with the corresponding Dw1 to DR8 specificities in Caucasians. However, there may be little or no correspondence in non-Caucasians. Attempts to continue with a simple correspondence between DR and Dw alleles was abandoned as newer alleles of each were identified.[15,63]

Although the first antibodies to Class II antigens were identified in sera which blocked MLR, blocking tests were too cumbersome for clinical purposes, and a cytotoxic reaction similar to that used for the detection of Class I antigens was soon developed. Anti–Class II antibodies were found in pregnancy sera; they also occurred after transfusion and transplant rejection. While a few of the sera defined the subtypic antigens DR1 to DR8, the majority appeared to recognize two series of supertypic specificities. These were initially termed the MB and MT antigens. The MB antigens were found to reside on a new class of molecule resembling DR but different from DR. Now known as DQ, these are the products of a separate cluster of genes closely linked to DR. The MT antigens are epitopes on beta chains of the DR cluster (β_2 and β_3) and are designated DRw52 and DRw53. Antibodies to the members of the DP series of antigens are usually weak and are often overshadowed by the more reactive antibodies to DR and DQ in the same sera. DN/DO, a new cluster, is not defined serologically but is identified by DNA probes.

BIOCHEMISTRY AND GENERAL PROPERTIES OF CLASS II AND CLASS III PRODUCTS. Class II antigens are noncovalently bound heterodimers that differ greatly in their genetics, biochemistry, and function from Class I. The Class II genes occur in clusters, in which an alpha (heavy) chain gene is found in association with one or more beta (light) chain genes, for a total of seven light chain genes. (Also, see Class II genes below.) A DRα chain can apparently associate with any β from its own cluster but not with the β from a different cluster. However, DQα1 may also combine with a β_1 from the other haplotype (trans-pairing). Not all the β chains are expressed in every individual or on every tissue. Translation occurs progressively and there is an increase in the number of Class II antigens as the cell differentiates. As with Class I antigens, the chains of the heterodimers are not covalently bound, but the attraction between the α and the β chains is very strong, and heat as well as pH change is required for their dissociation. Clusters identified to date have received official designations DP, DQ, DR, and DO/DN.[15,63] In each case the heavy chain α gene codes for a transmembrane acidic glycoprotein of approximately 33,000 daltons and the light chain β gene for a basic transmembrane glycoprotein of 27,000 daltons (Fig. 3).

During assembly and intracellular processing, the α and β chains of a Class II molecule are transiently associated with a

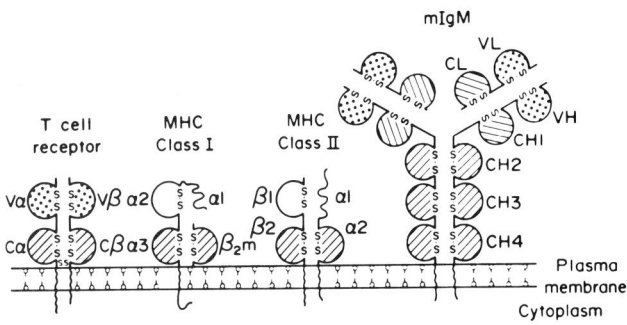

Figure 3. Schematic of immunoglobulin-like products, which include the Class I and Class II MHC antigens. Note the domain structure of the Class II glycoprotein. (From Strominger, J. L.: Biology of the human histocompatibility leukocyte antigen (HLA) system and a hypothesis regarding the generation of autoimmune diseases. J. Clin. Invest., 77:1411, 1986, by copyright permission of the American Society of Clinical Investigation.)

third or invariant (I) chain. The complex of α chain, β chain, and I chain can be traced through the Golgi to the cell surface where the I chain dissociates, leaving the α and β chains in apposition.[36] Most of the alloantigenicity is exhibited by the β chain, the exception being the α chain of the DQ antigens, which has a slight degree of polymorphism.[6] In contrast to the Class I antigens, the Class II antigens have a limited tissue distribution. They are found predominantly on B cells, on some macrophages, on cells of the endothelial and lymphoreticular system, or on parenchymal cells and T cells that have been activated, most often by lymphokines released by inflammation or by mitogen stimulation.[62]

Class III may not be an entirely appropriate term for the third designated set of products of the MHC haplotype because they are very heterogeneous. Their common link is that they are related to the complement cascade. Class III products include C2, C4a, C4b, and Factor B (Bf).[17] Of these the most complex are C4a and C4b which are both identified as a series of electrophoretic variants; Bf can be characterized by electrophoretic mobility into two fast and two slow forms. C2, which appears to be invariant, was mapped to the haplotype by demonstrating that C2 deficiency segregated with HLA in families.

Other genes in close association with the MHC haplotype are the enzymes glyoxylase and 21-hydroxylase in the human, and neuraminidase, phosphoglycerokinase-2, and kidney catalase-2 in the mouse. A gene implicated in the pathogenesis of hemochromatosis is also closely linked to the HLA haplotype.[32] Tumor necrosis factor (TNF) genes, TNFα, and TNFβ are closely linked to HLA-B.[42]

REGULATION OF MHC ANTIGENS. Although remaining relatively constant throughout life, wide variations may occur in the level of expression of both Class I and Class II antigens. Extreme depression of Class I or Class II antigens, or both, is found in the condition known as *bare lymphocyte syndrome*. The basis for this rare disease is not known. Because it can affect several members of the same family, it was originally believed to be a genetic abnormality; but studies demonstrated that lymphocytes from patients with bare lymphocyte syndrome expressed normal levels of Class II antigens after cultivation *in vitro*. A regulatory defect appears likely.

To a limited extent, Class I antigen expression—and, to a much greater extent, Class II expression—increases after activation with a variety of stimuli, including plant lectins and exposure to allogeneic cells.[33] This increased expression of antigens is believed to be important in transplantation and is discussed in the succeeding chapter. Cells and tissues that express only low levels of Class II antigens in the resting state become strong expressers during, for example, inflammation or rapid cell division. The histiocytic and lymphoid cells escaping from a graft (passenger leukocytes) may be activated by lymphokines and then become highly immunogenic and trigger a strong host antigraft reaction.[34] Increased expression of HLA antigens is also believed to contribute to the sudden episodes of acute rejection that may threaten a long tolerated transplant following a mild intercurrent infection. Increased antibody levels to HLA have been observed after therapeutic immunization of an immune subject.

Down-regulation of Class II antigens has been observed after treatment of cells *in vitro* with vitamin D_3 analogs.[18] This offers one empirical approach to manipulation of a transplant. Other approaches can be anticipated as the genes affecting the expression of the antigens become better known. At present it is known that there are at least two loci affecting Class II expression, one of which is closely linked to HLA and one of which is not.[22,65] In T-cell–B-cell hybrids, the HLA genes of the T-cell partner become expressed even if the HLA of the B-cell partner is deleted during mutagenesis. The transacting stimulator is clearly outside the deleted HLA haplotype of the B cell. Additional information about the regulator genes is urgently needed for control of the biological effects of cytokines such as interferon-γ, TNF, and interleukin-1 (IL-1) in promoting immune responses.

THE HLA ANTIGENS IN CLINICAL TYPING. Class I antigens serve as the major targets for antibody and cell-mediated cytolysis and thus are prime targets for allograft reactions against transplanted cells and tissues. As stated earlier, these antigens were originally detected and defined by the reactions of alloantisera. These sera were obtained from subjects immunized by transfusion, lymphocyte infusion, kidney graft rejection, or pregnancy. Such allogeneic antisera have been of major clinical importance for HLA typing but are now gradually being supplanted by monoclonal antibodies produced in rodents and occasionally in human heterokaryons formed by the fusion of a myeloma cell with an antibody-secreting lymphocyte.[46]

The most widely used assay for detecting the expression of Class I antigens on cells is the microlymphocytotoxicity test.[56] A small volume of antiserum is incubated with a suspension of lymphocytes (prepared from blood, lymph node, or spleen), and the sensitized cells are then lysed by the addition of complement, usually from rabbit serum. This procedure, introduced over 20 years ago, remains the most widely used test in clinical transplantation despite many attempts at automation. The microcytotoxicity test requires few cells (as few as 200 per determination), very little serum (as little as 0.5 μl), no radioisotopes, and a skilled technician who can record the outcome of each serum reaction in 3 seconds or less. The sensitivity of the test is increased and the likelihood of false-negative reactions is decreased if the sensitized cells are washed before complement is added.[2]

HLA-A, -B, and, to a lesser extent, HLA-C are highly polymorphic; that is, they exist in many alternative or allelic forms, as indicated in Table 1. Although it is becoming apparent that the present serologic classification is inadequate, because other properties, including proliferative and cytotoxic reactivity, nucleic acid sequence, and the charge on the molecule, as measured by isoelectric focusing, give different indications of fine reactivity, identification of the different HLA-A, -B, and -C antigens, or "specificities," is still performed serologically by clinical laboratories. Sera collected by laboratories around the world are tested against cells of various unrelated subjects and family members. When general agreement is reached that a set of sera recognizes a new specificity, a designation of that specificity, or antigen, is then made.

The first international meeting to unify antigen assignment and to standardize procedures was held in Durham, North Carolina, in 1964. This first workshop has been followed at 2 to 3 year intervals by other International Histocompatibility Workshops at which new sera and cells are tested and new specificities are defined. The results are transmitted to the World Health

TABLE 1. HLA Specificities (1987)

A	B	C	D	DR	DQ	DP
A1	B5	Cw1	Dw1	DR1	DQw1	DPw1
A2	B7	Cw2	Dw2	DR2	DQw2	DPw2
A3	B8	Cw3	Dw3	DR3	DQw3	DPw3
A9	B12	Cw4	Dw4	DR4	DQw4	DPw4
A10	B13	Cw5	Dw5	DR5		DPw5
A11	B14	Cw6	Dw6	DRw6		DPw6
Aw19	B15	Cw7	Dw7	DR7		
A28	B16	Cw8	Dw8	DRw8		
	B17		Dw9	DR9		
	B18		Dw10	DRw10		
	B21	Cw11				
	Bw22		Dw12			
	B27		Dw13			
	B35		Dw14			
	B37		Dw15			
			Dw16			
	B40					
Aw36	Bw41					
Aw43	Bw42		Dw20	DRw52		
			Dw21			
			Dw22	DRw53		
	Bw46		Dw23			
	Bw47		Dw24			
	Bw48		Dw25			
			Dw26			
	Bw53					
	Bw59					
	Bw67					
	Bw70					
	Bw73					
	Bw4					
	Bw6					

Specificity in parenthesis after a narrow specificity, e.g., HLA-A23(9) is optional. The following is a listing of these specificities that arose as clear-cut splits of the broad specificities.

Original Broad Specificities	Splits
A9	A23,A24
A10	A25,A26,Aw34,Aw66
Aw19	A29,A30,A31,A32,Aw33,Aw74
A28	Aw68,Aw69
B5	B51,Bw52
B12	B44,B45
B14	Bw64,Bw65
B15	Bw62,Bw63,Bw75,Bw76,Bw77
B16	B38,B39
B17	Bw57,Bw58
B21	B49,Bw50
Bw22	Bw54,Bw55,Bw56
B40	Bw60,Bw61
Bw70	Bw71,Bw72
Cw3	Cw9,Cw10
DR2	DRw15,DRw16
DR3	DRw17,DRw18
DR5	DRw11,DRw12
DRw6	DRw13,DRw14
DQw1	DQw5,DQw6
DQw3	DQw7,DQw8,DQw9
Dw6	Dw18,Dw19
Dw7	Dw11,Dw17
Bw4?	
Bw6?	

Adapted from the WHO report of 1987.[63]

Organization (WHO) and have formed the basis for a number of summary reports.[1] Because many of the sera initially encountered are weak, are in short supply, or are contaminated with other HLA antibodies, the initial recognition of specificities is usually tentative. New specificities are therefore assigned the suffix w (workshop). These w, or provisional, designations are deleted when sufficient agreement as to their characterization is reached; thus the antigen once called HLA-Bw16 is now designated HLA-B16. Definitions of HLA antigens are also subject to frequent revision and subdivision. For the example cited above, new antisera were later identified that reacted with lymphocytes from only a proportion of subjects originally classified as HLA-B16. Two subgroups were identified; one was designated B38; the other, B39. Most tissue typing laboratories can identify B16, but fewer have the reagents (sera) to make the distinction between B38 and B39. Tissue typing laboratories normally report the finest subdivision obtained (usually termed a "subtypic" specificity or "split") and indicate the broader ("typic" or "supertypic") antigen in parentheses, e.g., B38(16). These splits are identified in a separate section of Table 1. Exceptions to the deletion of the provisional or w designation occur in the HLA-C and HLA-D series. The w is retained for HLA-C to avoid confusion with the complement component nomenclature; it is retained for HLA-D because HLA-D is not a gene product, but a functional definition.

THE CLINICAL RELEVANCE OF THE HLA HAPLOTYPE. Each individual inherits a single sixth chromosome from each parent and therefore has two HLA haplotypes, the haplotype being defined as that stretch of chromosome carrying all of the major structural genes of the MHC. The expression of HLA antigens is co-dominant, so that an individual normally expresses two specificities for each locus. A typical HLA profile, or phenotype, would be HLA-A1,A2;B12,B8;Cw1,Cw3,DR3, DR4 and the haplotypes that delineate the genotype of that individual would probably be identified through family segregation patterns as HLA-A1,B8,Cw1,DR3 and A2,B12,Cw3,DR4. Segregation analysis is illustrated in Figure 4. Occasionally only one specificity is found at a specific locus, indicating either that an individual has two identical copies of the gene and is homozygous for that antigen (e.g., HLA-A1,A1) or that the panel of typing sera did not include antibodies that could detect a second specificity. The individual would then be HLA-A1,AX, where X is an unknown antigen. Unknown or untyped antigens are especially likely in non-Caucasians, because there are great racial variations in HLA antigen specificities; the antigens of many ethnic groups have not yet been adequately characterized. Segregation analysis (Fig. 4) allows the genetic relationship between family members to be defined and allows the haplotypes to be precisely characterized.

Several thousand molecules of each HLA-A and -B specificity are expressed on most nucleated cells, and each cell expresses all

of the phenotypically defined antigens encoded by the genome. There is also quantitative variation of HLA-A and -B expression between tissues. Cells of the lymphoid system have abundant Class I antigens, whereas parenchymal cells (e.g., kidney) often have less, and other cells such as erythrocytes have virtually none. Thymus cells express relatively low levels, and tumor cells can vary greatly in their expression of HLA. Cells other than lymphoid cells and platelets may be difficult to type; this is especially true of tumor cells. The expression of antigen usually increases with activation following transformation in culture. The change in phenotype following manipulation is sometimes erroneously reported as evidence for neoantigens on tumors.

The complexity (polymorphism) of the HLA system is demonstrated to some extent in Table 1. By 1987, there was recognition of 22 alleles of HLA-A, 52 of HLA-B, and 11 of HLA-C. The official list of antigens was again updated in 1989.[63] Certain of the newer antigens are restricted to particular ethnic groups and there are even marked differences in the frequencies of many antigens that are shared among populations.[4] There are also differences in the ease with which an antigenic specificity can be detected. Generally, the antigens that were easiest to detect were the first to be identified and thus tend to have low numbers (e.g., A1, A2, A3, B5, B7). Antigens that have more recently been recognized, e.g., Bw62, may be more difficult to identify, especially when the typing laboratory has access to only a limited set of typing sera.

The transplant surgeon needs to be aware of the divergence between the classification of antigens being developed by leading research laboratories and the routine clinical laboratories. The HLA antigens recognized in 1987 are listed in Table 1. Table 2 is abstracted from the current (1989) WHO list and details some variants of HLA-A2, HLA B27, and HLA-DR4. For a complete listing the reader is referred to the original publications.[15,63] Even from the abbreviated lists presented in Tables 1 and 2 it is obvious that two subjects classified as serologically identical (six-antigen match) and therefore assumed to be functionally identical may have very different fine-structural forms of these antigens. Although the differences may be due to as

TABLE 2. Designations of HLA-A2, -B27, and -DR4 Alleles and Specificities

Some Class I Alleles		
HLA Allele	**HLA Specificity**	**Previous Equivalents**
A*0201	A2	A2.1
A*0202	A2	A2.2f
A*0206	A2	A2.4a
A*0209	A2	A2-02B
B*2701	B27	27f
B*2702	B27	27e 27K B27.2
B*2705	B27	27a 27w B27.1
B*2706	B27	27D B27.4

Some Class II Alleles			
HLA Allele	**HLA Specificity**	**HLA-D Associated**	**Previous Equivalents**
		(T-cell–defined specifities)	
DRB1*0401	DR4	Dw4	
DRB1*0402	DR4	Dw10	
DRB1*0403	DR4	Dw13	DR4 Dw13a
DRB1*0404	DR4	Dw14	14.1

This abbreviated table lists 4 alleles each of HLA-A2, -B27, and -DR4. The 1990 report from which these data come[15] lists 10 alleles of HLA-A2, 6 of -B27, and 8 of -DR4.

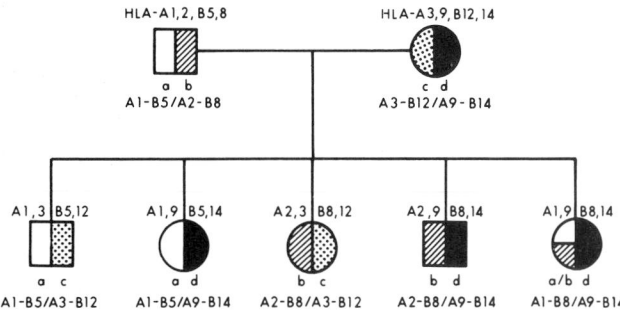

Figure 4. Inheritance pattern of HLA in a family. Code letters a, b, c, and d represent haplotypes, and the four possible combinations usually seen are represented. A crossover of parental haplotypes can result in a recombinant offspring, such as is seen here in the last sibling (a/bd), who received part of the haplotype (A1) and part of the b haplotype (B8) from the ab parent.

little as a substitution of a single amino acid, the biologic implications may be profound. An experimental observation from the authors' laboratory serves as an eloquent example. The mouse strain C57BL6 is H-2^b; a mutant, H-2^{ba}, differs from it by only two amino acids; and this mutation, like several others, cannot be detected by routine serologic tests. Each rapidly rejects the other's skin. In mixed lymphocyte culture, strong proliferative responses are observed between these strains, and H-2^{ba} readily produces cytotoxic cells lytic for an H-2^b tumor. The occasional strong rejection episodes observed against "phenotypically identical" or "six-antigen matched" grafts in man (HLA-A, -B, and -DR) may be due to such apparently inconsequential genetic and biochemical differences.

Details of the procedures used for the complete identification of DR, DQ, DP, and DO alleles is beyond the scope of this chapter. The elucidation of their specificities requires a battery of techniques, including serologic testing, DNA sequencing, restriction fragment length polymorphism comparisons, and determination of electrophoretic mobility. For example, clinical laboratories may recognize few, if any, DQ antigens; yet over a dozen alleles of DQβ are now recognized by specialized laboratories. Recognition of the numerous alleles is technically difficult because of the limited substitutions distinguishing the variants of each chain and the extensive cross-reactivity that is commonly encountered in serotyping similar alleles.[16] Fortunately, the strong linkage disequilibrium between DR and DQ alleles (see below) can be used to help separate some of the DQ variants. In addition to any impact on the transplant, another point of great clinical importance of these subtle differences is that different alleles may be associated with different diseases.

MOLECULAR GENETICS

CLASS I GENES. As explained in other sections of this chapter, the genes that constitute the HLA haplotype are closely linked and are carried on the short arm of the sixth chromosome. Some of the structural genes are tightly clustered; others are separated by other gene clusters, including those for the complement components C2, C4 and Bf.

The Class I genes are the most distal. Scattered along the subregion of the haplotype are numerous pseudogenes. These are not translated, but they can contribute to the genetic reserve of the individual, because parts of their sequences can be "read" through the process known as gene conversion.[39] Gene conversion can be regarded as a way in which a short sequence of DNA is moved from one gene to another gene, usually on the same chromosome. The result is the formation of a mutant gene in a somewhat controlled manner. It may be compared with the rearrangement that occurs during B-cell or T-cell differentiation. Gene conversion usually leads to the substitution of very few codons, but the mutation affects germ line genes and is inherited in a mendelian manner. Although gene conversion is a rare event, it is important in the generation of the extraordinary polymorphism of HLA.

The Class I genes (heavy chain genes) consist of a leader sequence, exons for the α_1, α_2, and α_3 domains, an exon for the transmembrane portion, and three exons for the short intracytoplasmic portion. During intracellular processing, the molecule becomes glycosylated at position 85 and associates noncovalently with a second molecule, β_2m, which is coded for on chromosome 15. The heavy chain–light chain dimer is then integrated into the membrane through the hydrophobic transmembraneous sequence. The light chain of β_2m, which is invariant in man and which is highly conserved in different species, is encoded by a cluster of four exons. The β_2m molecule may facilitate insertion into the membrane. Although there is some controversy on this point, there is general agreement that β_2m is essential for the proper conformation of the functional Class I molecule.

The three-dimensional structure of Class I molecules has been deduced through x-ray crystallography.[13,14] Its outstanding feature is a cleft that is bounded at the sides by α helical sequences of the α_1 and α_2 domains, with a floor composed of β pleated sheets. In the intact molecule, this cleft is probably occupied by a peptide. Variability and specificity of binding to the T-cell receptor follows amino acid substitutions in the α_1 and α_2 domains lining the cleft.

Although it is easy to visualize the binding of a peptide to charged residues in the cleft, there are several unanswered questions. It is apparent that binding of T cells to allogeneic targets uses some portions of the structure described above, but the specificity of T-cell binding is not the same as the specificity of antibody binding; there is no simple way of equating these two specificities. Also, the identity of the peptides occupying the cleft is not fully known. For Class I antigens it is believed that endogenous fragments, for example, mitochondrial peptides, can be bound (or trapped—it is not yet certan which) during the formation of the HLA molecule. The T-cell receptor appears to recognize both the bound peptide and adjacent molecular groupings on the HLA molecule. The effect of an amino acid substitution in one position on adjacent epitopes on the molecule may need to be elucidated. Position effects of the type alluded to have been investigated for several "model" antigens, including cytochrome C[27] and sperm whale myoglobulin[12]; differences between subtypic epitopes may provide the molecular basis for the observed differences in the binding of supertypic Bw4 and Bw6 and other cross-reactive antibodies.

CLASS II GENES. Understanding of the complexities of Class II genes and their products has been greatly simplified by the development of the procedure termed the polymerase chain reaction (PCR).[5] Oligonucleotide probes have been constructed for the variable portion of many Class II alleles. DNA from the unknown sample is heated for separation of the strands and is then annealed to two primers, one on each side of the gene, in the presence of TAQ polymerase, which is heat-stable.[41] The PCR allows the rapid and continuous replication of targeted sequences. Nucleotide sequence analysis is then attainable even from minute quantities of DNA. The introduction of this procedure has been invaluable in the analysis of Class II genes.

The Class II genes are arranged on the haplotype so that an α chain gene and one or more β chain genes are grouped in the same subregion. Typically, the first of the five exons of the Class II α chain gene encodes the 5' untranslated region, together with a leader sequence and the first few amino acids of the α_1 domain. The second and third exons code for the remainder of the extracytoplasmic portion of the molecule. The transmembrane portion and the cytoplasmic tail are, with a connecting piece, encoded by the fourth exon, whereas the fifth exon is for the 3' untranslated region. The β chain gene is typically arranged in the opposite sense and has an additional exon.[54].

The DRα genes sequenced to date have been invariant, and there is only one per haplotype. DRβ genes are more complex. The number of DRβ genes varies between individuals; so the sequences of the various β chain genes also vary from individual to individual and from gene to gene. The subtypic specificities of DR are largely coded for by the β_1 chain gene. Sequence analysis of the DRβ gene region has revealed an astonishing degree of complexity. For example, the DR3 and DR4 haplotypes have been compared by a procedure known as cosmid mapping.[48] DRα and DRβ were isolated on overlapping clones spanning 130 kb and lie in opposite transcriptional orientation. Sequence differences between different DRβ chains are dispersed across the molecule. Two of the remaining β chains (e.g., β_2, β_3) code for DRw52 and DRw53. A lesser degree of sequence variability has been found in these genes. It is probable that the flexibility of immune responses to alloantigens and to nominal antigens resides partially in the T-cell receptor and partially in the DRβ chain.

The DQα genes resemble DRα, but sequence variability is occasionally found in the DQα₁ chain gene.[47] A second gene, DQα₂, is not translated. There are two DQβ genes, which diverge from each other. DQβ₁ shows considerable allelic diversity, especially in the first domain.[57] DQβ₂, like its companion, DQα₂, is not expressed. All of these genes and their products, however, show considerable sequence homology.

HLA-DNα resembles the other α chain genes, but the DOβ with which it is associated has additional base pair substitutions, especially in positions 46 to 65.[35] Conserved sequences are shared between all D region β chain genes as well as between mouse IAβ and IEβ chain genes. Truncated (pseudo) genes are common in the Class II segments. The HLA-DP region also contains two sets of genes (DPα₁,DPα₂; DPβ₁,DPβ₂) and again, only one pair (DPα₁β₁) is expressed.[26] Variability has been observed between DPα₁ alleles as well as in DPβ₂; but since only six alleles of DP are known, the degree of polymorphism appears to be less than that for DR and DQ. The organization of this subregion differs from that of the other Class II genes, and DP presents many interesting theoretic challenges.

THE IMMUNOBIOLOGY OF HLA

Supergene, gene family, and *gene complex* are all terms that have been applied to the MHC. They all emphasize the proximity of a series of closely related genes on the haplotype. Although their identities are now revealed by molecular genetic probing, the individuality of the genes was first demonstrated by observing the formation of a recombinant haplotype in offspring within a nuclear family. Segregation analysis is a classic tool of mendelian genetics. Extensively used to investigate inheritance patterns in simpler organisms such as *Drosophila* or moths in which the bands associated with some genes could be seen, the relationship between linear distance and frequency of recombination was for many years regarded as constant; the greater the distance between two genes, the more frequently they would recombine. From this it was an easy step to calculate distances between genes by counting recombinants. It is now known that several factors can modify this simple relationship. A segment of chromosome can become inverted. When this occurs, recombination between the abnormal haplotype carrying the inversion and a normal haplotype is greatly reduced; conversely, the frequency of recombination in subjects carrying two abnormal haplotypes of this type appears to be increased. Extensively explored in the Tt series of developmental abnormalities of mice, it has been proposed as a mechanism to explain some situations in which certain gene combinations occur more frequently than expected in man. These are the so-called extended haplotypes described by Yunis and colleagues.[7] Many of the extended haplotypes are marked by a deletion of one of the genes for the C4 component of complement. Extended haplotypes have been reported from a variety of disease states.

While this interesting hypothesis still awaits proof, it is one facet of a rather nebulous, but very important, relationship between haplotype and genetic fitness of the individual. It is likely that the constitution of the haplotype, rather than the presence of any allele, determines the manner in which the individual responds to the environment. Response, in this context, has a very broad meaning; it can extend from the propensity of an individual to develop autoimmune diseases, to resist infection, to conceive and bear children successfully, and to accept or reject an organ transplant.

In order that this topic be understood, it is necessary to elaborate briefly on some of the original observations about the haplotype and its products. These include linkage disequilibrium, recombinational hot spots, discrimination between self and non-self, the contributions of unconventional pairing of antigen chains, gene conversion, the polymorphism of the MHC genes and haplotypes, and the role of these genes and haplotypes in antigen presentation.

LINKAGE DISEQUILIBRIUM. Certain combinations of alleles at different loci of the MHC are found much more frequently than would be expected, if one assumes that recombination is a random event. For example, HLA-A1 is found in approximately 17 per cent of European haplotypes, and HLA-B8 is found on about 11 per cent of these haplotypes. The two alleles would be expected to be found on the same haplotype in 1.87 per cent (17 per cent × 11 per cent) of cases, whereas the observed coincidence of these alleles is approximately 9 per cent. The difference between the observed and expected haplotype frequencies is termed the delta value; it is a measure of linkage disequilibrium. In the illustration provided here, the observed occurrence is five times as high as would be expected. High deltas have been observed in nearly all populations studied, although the cause of these high levels of association is controversial. The cause may be trivial: it may simply reflect the sudden expansion of a previously small and somewhat homogeneous population, as occurred following the Industrial Revolution. However, it may signify a biologic advantage of individuals in the population carrying the relevant haplotype. In favor of the former explanation is the finding that the high delta values observed in almost all of the world's populations involve different combinations of alleles; in favor of the latter is the finding that different regions of the same haplotype may have very different delta values; thus some segments of the haplotype appear to be differentially favored.[21]

The finding of high delta values has two practical applications. The segment of haplotype with high deltas may include disease-associated genes; for example, the DR3,DQw2 haplotype may be associated with insulin-dependent diabetes mellitus.[57] Alternatively, the recognition of a well-identified allele at one locus may aid in the identification of a less easily defined allele at a second locus; this is especially valuable in assigning some DQ specificities when DR is known and has also been of value in assigning HLA-C alleles when B is known. Obviously a "hitchhiker" gene such as TNF will be in strong linkage disequilibrium if the flanking HLA genes are also in strong linkage disequilibrium.

RECOMBINATIONAL HOT SPOTS. As mentioned above, it was assumed that recombination was a random event occurring at any point along the haplotype; this is certainly not true for the H-2 haplotype of the mouse. Early observations were that recombination tended to occur more often in the progeny of recombinants and that hybrids formed between some pairs of mouse strains (e.g., H-2ᵈ × H-2ᵇ) were more likely to provide recombinant offspring than others (H-2ᵏ × H-2ᵇ). Multiple recombinants were also encountered in certain human families, for example, a kindred with multiple members affected with rheumatic diseases.[49] The siblings of leukemic children had recombinant HLA haplotypes more often than expected. Unfortunately, these were all anecdotal examples. Experimentally, a hybrid mating has now been tested that gives a greater than expected frequency of recombination and the molecular basis is known. When wild *Mus casteneus* is hybridized with different strains of laboratory mice (*Mus musculus*), three hot spots of frequent recombination are found.[59] These lie in the IA subregion of H-2, one near the αβ₃ gene, another between αβ₃ and αβ₂, and one close to Eβ. The DNA in these regions appears normal, with no evidence for unequal crossing over or deletion, but the affected sequences have high homology to the chi sequences of bacteriophage lambda and to a sequence in human satellite DNA. Chi was so named because of its association with chiasma formation. Chi sequences are also believed to be responsible for gene conversion. These observations are of great value to the geneticist investigating gene interactions and to the physician investigating HLA-linked diseases. To the surgeon they may explain why some transplants between HLA identical siblings fail unexpectedly; one sibling might be an undetected recombinant.

DISCRIMINATION BETWEEN SELF AND NON-SELF. That the MHC was responsible for the recognition of self and the elimination of unwanted variants was proposed as part of the network hypothesis of Jerne to explain the extraordinary numbers of thymic cells constantly being destroyed as well as for the extreme polymorphism of the MHC.[50] An extension of Jerne's hypothesis forms the basis for speculation about the manner in which T cells "learn" to distinguish self from non-self in the thymus. It is generally believed that positive selection involves the recognition by a subset of T cells of those MHC molecules expressed in the thymus. In transgenic mice, the precursors of mature T cells are cells that can bind to polymorphic regions of MHC molecules expressed in the thymus of the animal from which they were derived. These cells would mature and then pass from the thymus. Cells that did not bind would not mature, would not leave the thymus, and would die.[29]

The thymus appears to be the organ in which tolerance to self antigens is acquired. Briefly, the reasoning is that because the generation of T-cell diversity leads to the somewhat haphazard union of many hypervariable T-cell receptor sequences to one of 12 random D sequences and to a random J sequence, at least tens of thousands of specificities are possible. Many of these must, by chance, bind to autologous structures and thus be autoreactive. A clone of cells having strong reactivity for determinants on the mouse Class II molecule I-E–negative are found at high (10 per cent) frequency in I-E–negative strains.[29] Similar cells are present among the precursor T cells of I-E–positive strains but only in negligible numbers among the mature thymic or peripheral T cells. Most of the autoreactive T cells have, therefore, been deleted. Deletion of other autoreactive clones undoubtedly occurs at the same time.

The derivation of mature T cells depends upon their ability to recognize some attribute of the MHC. From other lines of evidence, it is known that the T cell recognizes processed, rather than intact, antigen. Similar considerations apply to the recognition of nominal antigen during MHC-restricted immune responses. Most T-cell responses are of this type; a response occurs only if antigen is presented in close relationship to (in the context of) those MHC molecules it identifies as self.[20] How this is achieved is still speculation. The speculation centers around the peptide fragments which are believed to lie within the cleft in the Class I and, by analogy, to a similar structure in the Class II molecule. Some peptides are believed to be a polymorphic fragment of the MHC. Recognition is thought to be of the certain groupings on the peptide together with residues from the MHC molecule surrounding the peptide. T cells expressing CD8 on their surface respond best to MHC Class I stimulators, and T cells (helpers) respond best to MHC Class II molecules, as explained in the following chapter. It is believed that several types of cells can present antigen; the common denominator is that they all express Class II molecules. Dendritic cells, macrophages and monocytes, endothelial cells, B cells, and, in the human, activated T cells are all candidates for antigen presentation.[51] Their availability and thus the immunogenicity of the tissue varies greatly from organ to organ and undoubtedly correlates inversely with the severity of rejection of the transplant.

THE ROLE OF THE MHC IN IMMUNE RESPONSES. The causes of the extraordinary polymorphism of the HLA and H-2 systems have been repeatedly debated. At issue have been the large number of genes and of alleles of these genes in the HLA gene family and the peculiar finding that most of the alleles are present with high frequency; many genes of other systems have multiple alleles, but most of these alleles are rare. Recent evidence suggests that coincidence of multiple genes and multiple common alleles of these genes is retained because of their adaptive advantage. Recognition of the central role of the MHC came from several laboratories; the response to several antigens in-

volved the recognition of self plus the recognition of the antigen. Zinkernagel and Doherty, for example, demonstrated that the effector cytotoxic T lymphocytes (CTLs) generated in response to virally infected cells recognize the viral antigen only in association with a serologically defined (Class I) MHC antigen of that infected host.[66] Thus, virus-infected cells of one mouse strain could not be destroyed by CTLs from a strain with a different H-2 haplotype or Class I recombinant; i.e., T-effector cell function is restricted by Class I MHC antigens. This finding has been confirmed in other species and with chemically as well as virally modified antigens.[52] It is now known that CTLs possess specific receptors recognizing both nominal, e.g., viral or chemical, antigens and MHC antigens together. Two signals, one of which is provided by the MHC, are required for many forms of lymphocyte interaction.

This finding is consistent with much of our basic understanding of the immune system. A primary function of the immune system is to provide defense against infectious organisms. The vast diversity of bacteria, viruses, fungi, protozoa, metazoa, and other agents challenging man and most other mammals has led to strong evolutionary pressures to develop diverse means of countering these infectious agents. Extracellular organisms are usually eliminated by antibody in concert with complement and phagocytes. Parasites such as fungi and intracellular bacteria are controlled primarily by macrophages activated by T-cell lymphokines in the context of granulomatous inflammation. The first line of immune defense against viruses is usually humoral, at the level of epithelial or endothelial cell contact. However, in the absence of sensitization, or upon establishment of viral infection, host defense is primarily cellular and often mediated by CTL destruction of host cells harboring reproducing virus. The presence of CTL receptors for a viral-host MHC antigen complex thus provides a means for recognizing virally infected cells and inhibits effector cell neutralization or distraction by circulating virus or viral antigens. In addition, because each cell expresses each of its coded MHC antigens, there are multiple virus-MHC targets (some of which are now known to be more effective targets than others for specific viruses) that can be recognized by host cytotoxic T cells. Experiments with influenza A virus–infected human cells[58] have demonstrated that the level of T-lymphocyte–mediated cytotoxicity is a function of the individual MHC allele and of the viral antigen. This observation was used to demonstrate the existence of multiple variants of the HLA-A2 specificity, subdivisions confirmed by DNA sequence analysis.

There appears to be a selective advantage for the individual as well as the species to have a high degree of polymorphism at several Class I loci, because the constant mutation of many infective viruses undoubtedly leads to variations of the effective interaction between any one tissue antigen and the constantly changing viral antigens. This point has special relevance to the clinician concerned with the postoperative care of the transplant patient, because infections with viruses and fungi are frequently complications of immunosuppressive therapy directed to reducing the immune response to the alloantigens of the transplant. Because immunosuppressive agents depress cellular immunity in a relatively nonspecific manner, it is not surprising that antifungal and antiviral immunity decreases in transplant recipients. Bacterial immunity, however, is often dependent upon opsonization by preformed antibody and subsequent phagocytosis by granulocytes. Immunosuppressive drugs normally exert only a minor effect upon pre-existing antibody responses. This is fortunate as far as antimicrobial defenses are concerned, but unfortunate in that preformed cytotoxic antibodies to HLA that are reactive against an allograft tend to persist despite immunosuppressive therapy.

The role of Class II antigens in immune responsiveness has also been better defined in the past few years. In a manner perhaps analogous to that of T-effector cells, the nature of T-helper–cell activation by antigen appears dependent upon proper processing and presentation (by the macrophage, B cell or other cell types) in association with Class II antigens.[49] Similarly, certain interactions between T-helper and T-effector or B cells is restricted by the expression of appropriate Class II antigens.

An elegant experiment by Sprent and Schaffer illustrated the differing functions of Class I and Class II antigens in stimulating proliferation of Class I and Class II restricted T cells.[55] Responder T cells from C57B16 mice were exposed to stimulators from two mutant strains, bm1, with mutant Class I antigen, and bm12, with a mutant Class II antigen. The response to bm12 was almost exclusively by T cells with the CD4 (helper) phenotype and to bm1 by T cells with the CD8 (cytotoxic-suppressor) phenotype.

FUTURE STUDIES

Despite all of the advances made since the discovery of HLA in 1965, the full complexity of the HLA system has not yet been revealed. The haplotype contains many genes that are not normally expressed. The existence of some of these genes has been most clearly established in the rodent. Lying close to H-2 but generally regarded as outside the H-2 region are numerous Class I–like genes of the Qa-T1 complex. It is believed that at least some of these genes are activated during embryonic development. The haplotype also includes many incomplete sequences for Class I–like or Class II–like antigens that cannot be expressed. These are potentially useful for maintaining the diversity or polymorphism of HLA, because short segments of DNA may be incorporated into a normal gene by gene conversion. Several mutants have been identified in which a sequence occurring only in an untranslated gene is incorporated in the appropriate position in the mutant gene. Many of the mutants that have been identified in mice are undetectable serologically and are recognized only through transplant rejection. Although undetected by antisera, they are readily detected by T cells in proliferation assays or cytotoxicity tests. Through such mutants the epitopes recognized by T cells are becoming known. Much of the future of transplantation and of the immunobiology of the MHC depends upon the proper identification of these important epitopes.

At present only one epitope is designated on most HLA molecules. Still to come is a classification of the second and third epitopes, which *are* detectable serologically such as Bw4 and Bw6 for HLA-B. There are undoubtedly other epitopes on HLA-A. Not knowing these epitopes, presently two subjects are classified as having the same subtypic antigen, e.g., HLA-A2. While this characterization is correct, there are at least two additional epitopes on the molecule that are currently uncharacterized and consequently ignored. These are the epitopes recognized by T cells directed against the influenza-A2 epitope and the other by monoclonal antibodies cross-reactive with A2 and certain HLA-B epitopes. Because there are at least two more epitopes on each HLA molecule that are not currently characterized, HLA phenotyping is far from complete. Indeed, it is surprising that phenotyping for transplantation is as successful as it is. Almost certainly this is because of the linkage disequilibrium between epitopes on the same molecule.

SELECTIVE REFERENCES

Bjorkman, P. J., Saper, M. A., Samraoui, B., et al: Structure of the human class I histocompatibility antigen, HLA-A2.Nature, 329:506, 1987.
The structure and function of the HLA Class I molecule has been debated for many years. This report ended most of the speculation about the molecular structure. The paper presents the crystallographic analysis of a purified HLA-A2 molecule at 3.5Å resolution. The most notable feature is a cleft running across the molecule. The cleft contains a less well defined peptide believed to be a fragment of an HLA molecule. T cells bind to this region of the HLA molecule.

Bjorkman, P. J., Saper, M. A., Samraoui, B. et al.: The foreign antigen binding site and T cell recognition regions of class I histocompatibility antigens. Nature, 329:512, 1987.
This companion to the preceding paper delineates some of the functional properties of the Class I histocompatibility antigen. The carbon backbone of the α_1 and α_2 domains of the molecule is represented graphically. Featured are the conserved or invariant parts of the structure. The report identifies some of the amino acids that contribute to receptor binding.

Pease, L. R., Schulze, D. H., Pfaffenbach, G. M., et al.: Spontaneous H-2 mutants provide evidence that a copy mechanism analogous to gene conversion generates polymorphism in the major histocompatibility complex. Proc. Natl. Acad. Sci USA, 80:242, 1983.
The mutational process known as gene conversion is accepted as contributing extensively to the great polymorphism of the major histocompatibility complex genes. The participation of what was previously regarded as a specialized process giving genetic variability to lower forms was deduced by a comparison of the amino acid sequences of a number of spontaneous mutants of H-2 Class I genes of the mouse. It is now accepted as the most likely mechanism for the generation of genetic variation in HLA.

Robinson, M. A., and Kindt, T. J.: Major histocompatibility complex antigens and genes. In Paul, W. J.: Fundamental Immunology, 2nd ed. New York, Raven Press, 1989, pp. 489–539.
This is a beautifully crafted and comprehensive review of the genes and antigens of the MHC. The emphasis is on HLA but evidence from the mouse is also presented when relevant. This review details how the MHC genes are arranged on the chromosome and how they are translated into the Class I and Class II proteins. It is especially valuable to the nonspecialist because of the large number of clear illustrations but is rewarding to the molecular biologist and immunologist, too, because it provides sufficient detail to support the assumptions made.

Seigler, H. F., Amos, D. B., Ward, F. E., et al.: Immunogenetics of consanguineous allografts in man. I. Histocompatibility testing and skin allografts. Ann. Surg. 172:151, 1970.
This is a cornerstone paper linking serology to function of HLA; the inheritance of HLA haplotypes can be determined by serologic testing of leukocytes of family members. Siblings inheriting the same pair of HLA haplotypes retain skin grafts for 23 days; sibs inheriting two different haplotypes reject them in 11 days. This study, which was followed by a companion article dealing with intrafamilial kidney grafts proves that HLA is the major histocompatibility system of man; other histocompatibility antigens exist but are much weaker.

Shearer, G. M., Rhen, T. G., and Garbarino, C. A.: Cell mediated lympholysis of trinitrophenyl-modified autologous lymphocytes: Effector cell specificity to modified cell surface components controlled by the H-2K and H-2D serological regions of the murine major histocompatibility complex. J. Exp. Med., 141:1348, 1975.
In the mid 1970s several laboratories demonstrated that the target for cell-mediated immunity was compound. In this report the targets were chemically modified autologous lymphocytes. The important principle, now universally accepted, is that the immune system recognizes modified autologous or self-antigens and thus discriminates against non-self.

Zinkernagel, R. M., and Doherty, P. C.: Restriction of in vitro T cell-mediated cytotoxicity in lymphocytic choriomeningitis within a syngeneic or semiallogeneic system. Nature, 248:701, 1974.
One of the focal points of contemporary immunology is the ability to discriminate between self and non-self. The previous reference relates how chemical modification can be detected. In this equally important and often cited paper, lymphocytic choriomeningitis virus was the trigger. The immune system can distinguish between self and virally modified self.

REFERENCES

1. Albert, E. D., et al.: Nomenclature for factors of the HLA system. In Albert, E. D., Baur, M. P., and Mayr, W. R. (Eds.): Histocompatibility Testing 1984. Berlin, Springer-Verlag, 1984.
2. Amos, D. B., Bashir, H., Boyle, W., MacQueen, M., and Tiilikainen, A.: A simple microcytotoxicity test. Transplantation, 7:220, 1969.
3. Amos, D. B., Gorer, P. A. and Mikulska, Z. B.: The antigenic structure and genetic behavior of a transplanted leukosis. Br. J. Cancer, 9:209, 1955.
4. Amos, D. B., and Ward, F. E.: Immunogenetics of the HL-A system. Physiol. Rev., 55:206, 1975.
5. Andersson, G., Larhammar, D., Widmark, E., et al.: Class II genes of the human major histocompatibility complex: Organization and evolutionary relationship of the DR β genes. J. Biol. Chem., 262:8748, 1987.
6. Auffray, C., and Strominger, J. L.: Molecular genetics of the human major histocompatibility complex. Adv. Hum. Genet., 15:197, 1986.
7. Awdeh, Z. L., Raum, D., Yunis, E. J., and Alper, C. A.: Extended HLA/complement allele haplotypes: Evidence for a T/t-like complex in man. Proc. Natl. Acad. Sci. USA, 80:259, 1983.
8. Bach, F. H., and Amos, D. B.: Hu-1: major histocompatibility locus in man. Science, 156:1506, 1967.
9. Bach, F., and Hirschhorn, K.: Lymphocyte interaction: a potential histocompatibility test in vitro. Science, 143:813, 1964.

10. Bain, B., Vas, M. R., and Lowenstein, L.: The development of large immature mononuclear cells in mixed leukocyte culture. Blood, 23:108, 1964.

11. Barker, C. F., and Billingham, R. E.: The role of regional lymphatics in the skin homograft response. Transplantation, 5:962, 1967.

12. Berzofsky, J. A., Buckenmeyer, G. K., Hicks, G., et al.: Topographic antigenic determinants recognized by monoclonal antibodies to sperm whale myoglobin. J. Biol. Chem., 257:3189, 1982.

13. Bjorkman, P. J., Saper, M. A., Samraoui, B., et al.: Structure of the human class I histocompatibility antigen, HLA-A2. Nature, 329:506, 1987.

14. Bjorkman, P. J., Saper, M. A., Samraoui, B., et al.: The foreign antigen binding site and T cell recognition regions of Class I histocompatibility antigens. Nature, 329:512, 1987.

15. Bodmer, J. G., Marsh, S. G. E., Parham, P., et al.: Nomenclature for factors of the HLA system. Human Immunol., 28:326, 1990.

16. Brodsky, F. M., and Parham, P.: Monomorphic anti-HLA, B, C monoclonal antibodies detecting molecular subunit and combinatorial determinants. J Immunol., 128:129, 1982.

17. Campbell, R. D., Lau, S. K. A., Reid, K. B. M., et al.: Structure organization and regulation of the complement genes. Ann. Rev. Immunol., 6:161, 1988.

18. Carrington, M. N., Tharp-Hiltbold, B., Knoth, J. and Ward, F. E.: 1,25-Dihydroxyvitamin D_3 decreases expression of HLA class II molecules in a melanoma cell line. J. Immunol., 140:4013, 1988

19. Ceppellini, R., Curtoni, E. S., Leigheb, G., et al.: An Experimental Approach to Genetic Analysis of Histocompatibility in Man. In Balmer, H., Cleton, F. J., and Feinisse, J. G. (Eds.): Histocompatibility Testing 1965. Copenhagen, Munksgaard, 1965, pp. 13–23.

20. Davis, M. M., and Bjorkman, P. J.: T-cell antigen receptor genes and T-cell recognition. Nature, 334:395, 1988.

21. Dawkins, R. L., Leaver, A., Cameron, P. U., et al.: Some disease-associated ancestral haplotypes carry a polymorphism of TNF. Human Immunol., 26:91, 1989.

22. DeMars, R., Chang, C. C., Shaw, S., et al.: Homozygous deletions that simultaneously eliminate expressions of class I and class II antigens of EBV-transformed B-lymphoblastoid cells: Reduced proliferative responses of autologous and allogenic T cells to mutant cells that have decreased expression of class II antigens. Hum. Immunol., 11:77, 1984.

23. Eichwald, E. J., Wetzel, B., and Lustgraff, E. C.: Genetic aspects of second set skin grafts in mice. Transplantation, 4:260, 1966.

24. Gorer, P. A., and Kaliss, N.: The effect of isoantibodies in vivo on three different transplantable neoplasms in mice. Cancer Res., 19:824, 1959.

25. Gorer, P. A., Lyman, S. and Snell, G. D.: Studies on the genetic and antigenic basis of tumour transplantation: Linkage between a histocompatibility gene and "fused" in mice. Proc. Soc. Lond. [Biol.], 135:499, 1948.

26. Gustafsson, K., Widmark, E., Jonsson, A. K., et al.: Class II genes of the human major histocompatibility complex. Evolution of the DP region as deduced from nucleotide sequences of the four genes. J. Biol. Chem., 262:8778, 1987.

27. Jemmerson, R., Margoliash, E.: Topographic antigenic determinants on cytochrome c: Immunoadsorbent separation of the rabbit antibody populations directed against horse cytochrome c. J. Biol. Chem., 254:12706, 1979.

28. Jorgensen, F., Lamm, L. U., and Kismeyer-Nielson, F.: Three LD (MLC) determinants: A Danish population study. Tissue Antigens, 4:419, 1974.

29. Kappler, J. W., Roehm, N., and Marrack, P.: T cell tolerance by clonal elimination in the thymus. Cell, 49:273, 1987.

30. Kaufman, J., Skjoedt, K., and Salomondsen, J.: The MHC Molecules of Nonmammalian Vertebrates. Immunol. Rev. 113:1-35, 1990.

31. Kelly, A., and Trowsdale, J.: Complete nucleotide sequence of a functional HLA-DP β gene and the region between the DPβ1 and DPα1 genes: Comparison of the 5' ends of HLA class II genes. Nucleic Acids Res., 13:1607, 1985.

32. Kravitz, K., Skolnick, M., Cannings, C., et al.: Genetic linkage between hereditary hemochromatosis and HLA. Am. J. Hum. Genet., 31:601, 1979.

33. Ko, S. S., Fu, S. M., and Winchester, R. J.: Ia determinants on stimulated human T lymphocytes: Occurrence on mitogen and antigen-activated T cells. J. Exp. Med., 150:246, 1979.

34. Lafferty, K., Prowse, S., Simeonovic, C., and Warren, H. S.: Immunobiology of tissue transplantation: A return to the passenger leukocyte concept. In Paul, W. E., Fathman, C. G. (Eds.): Annual Review of Immunology. Palo Alto, Annual Reviews, 1983, pp. 143–173.

35. Long, E. O., Rosen-Bronson, S., Jacobson, S., et al.: Isotypic diversity and function of HLA class II antigens. In Silver, J. (Ed.): Molecular Biology of HLA Class II Antigens. Boca Raton, CRC Press, (In press).

36. Machamer, C. E., and Cresswell, P.: Monensin prevents terminal glycosylation of the N- and O-linked oligosaccharides of the HLA-DR-associated invariant chain and inhibits its dissociation from the α-β chain complex. Proc. Natl. Acad. Sci., U.S.A., 81:1287, 1984.

37. Medawar, P. B.: The behaviour and fate of skin autografts and skin homografts in rabbits. J. Anat., 78:176, 1944.

38. Medawar, P. B.: The immunology of transplantation. Harvey Lectures, Series 52, 1956–1957, 52:144–176, 1958.

39. Mengle-Gaw, L., Conner, S., McDevitt, H. O., et al.: Gene conversion between murine class II major histocompatibility complex loci. J. Exp. Med., 160:1184, 1984.

40. Mitchison, N. A.: Passive transfer of transplantation immunity. Proc. R. Soc. Lond. [Biol.], 142:72, 1954.

41. Mullis, K., Faloona, F., Schraf, S., et al.: Specific enzymatic amplification of DNA in vitro: The polymerase chain reaction. Cold Spring Harbor Symposium, Quant. Biol., 51:263, 1986.

42. Nedwin, G. W., Naylor, S. L., Sakaguchi, A. Y., et al.: Human lymphotoxin and tumor necrosis factor genes: Structure homology and chromosomal location. Nucleic Acid Res. 13:6361, 1985.

43. Orr, H. T., Lancet, D., Robb, R. J., et al.: The heavy chain of human histocompatibility antigen HLA-B7 contains an immunoglobulin-like region. Nature, 282:266, 1979.

44. Parham, P., Lomen, C. E., Lawlor, D. A., et al.: Nature of polymorphism in HLA-A, -B, and -C molecules. Proc. Natl. Acad. Sci. USA, 85:4005, 1988.

45. Plate, J. M., Ward, F. E., and Amos, D. B.: The mixed leucocyte culture reaction between HLA identical siblings. In Terasaki, P. I. (Ed.): Histocompatibility Testing. Copenhagen, Munksgaard, 1970, p. 531.

46. Radka, S. F., Kostyu, D. D., and Amos, D. B.: A monoclonal antibody directed against the HLA-Bw6 epitope. J. Immunol. 128:2804, 1982.

47. Robinson, M. A., and Kindt, T. J.: Major histocompatibility complex antigens and genes. In Paul, W. J.: Fundamental Immunology, 2nd ed. New York, Raven Press, 1989, pp. 489–539.

48. Rollini, P., Mach, B., and Gortski, J.: Linkage map of three HLA-DR β chain genes: Evidence for a recent duplication event. Proc. Natl. Acad. Sci. USA, 82:7197, 1985.

49. Rossen, R. D., Brewer, E. J., Sharp, R. M., et al.: Familial rheumatoid arthritis: A kindred identified through a proband with seronegative juvenile arthritis includes members with seropositive, adult-onset disease. Hum. Immunol. 4:183, 1982.

50. Sha, W. C., Nelson, C. A., Newberry, R. D., et al.: Positive and negative selection of an antigen receptor on T cells in transgenic mice. Nature, 336:73, 1988.

51. Shastri, N., Malissen, B., and Hood, L.: Ta transfected cell fibroblasts present a lysosomal peptide but not the native protein to lysozyme-specific T cells. Proc. Natl. Acad. Sci. USA, 82:5885, 1985.

52. Shearer, G. M.: Cell-mediated cytoxicity to trinitrophenyl-modified syngeneic lymphocytes. Eur. J. Immunol., 4:527, 1974.

53. Silvers, W. K., Wilson, D. B., and Palm, J.: Typing and immunosuppression in rats. Transplantation, 5:1053, 1967.

54. Spies, T., Sorrentino, R., Boss, J. M., et al.: Structural organization of the DR subregion of the human major histocompatibility complex. Proc. Natl. Acad. Sci. USA, 82:5165, 1985.

55. Sprent, J., and Schaeffer, M.: Antigen presenting cells for unprimed T cells. Immunology Today, 10:17, 1989.

56. Terasaki, P. I., and McClelland, J. D.: Microdroplet assay of human serum cytotoxins. Nature, 204:998, 1964.

57. Todd, J. A., Bell, J. I., and McDevitt, H. O.: HLA-DQ β gene contributes to susceptibility and resistance to insulin-dependent diabetes mellitus. Nature, 329:599, 1987.

58. Townsend, A., and Bodmer, H.: Antigen recognition by class I-restricted T lymphocytes. Am. Rev. Immunol., 7:601, 1989.

59. Uematsu, Y., Fischer L. K., and Steinmetz, M.: The same MHC recombinational hot spots are active in crossing-over between wild/wild and wild/inbred mouse chromosomes. Immunogenetics, 27:96, 1988.

60. Van Rood, J. J., van Leeuwen, A., and Pleom, J. S.: A method to detect simultaneously two cell populations by two colour fluorescence. Nature, 262:795, 1976.

61. Van Rood, J. J., van Leeuwen, A., and Zweerus, R.: The 4a and 4b antigens: Do they or don't they? In Terasaki, P. (Ed.): Histocompatibility Testing. Copenhagen, Munksgaard, 1970, pp. 93–104.

62. Weiss, A.: T Lymphocyte Activation. In Paul, W. (Ed.): Fundamental Immunology, 2nd ed., New York, 1989, Raven Press, pp. 359–384.

63. WHO Nomenclature Committee: Nomenclature for factors of the HLA system, 1987. Vox Sang., 55:119, 1988.

64. Winn, H. J.: Immune mechanisms in monotransplantation, II. Quantitative assay of the immunologic activity of lymphoid cells stimulated by tumor homografts. J. Immunol., 86:228, 1961.

65. Yang, Z., Accolla, R. S., Pious, D., et al.: Two distinct genetic loci regulating class II gene expression are defective in human mutant and patient cell lines. EMBO J., 7:1965, 1988.

66. Zinkernagel, R. M., and Doherty, P. C.: Immunological surveillance against altered self components by sensitised T lymphocytes in lymphocytic choriomeningitis. Nature, 251:547, 1974.

III ———————————————————————————————————

MECHANISMS AND CHARACTERISTICS OF ALLOGRAFT REJECTION

Fred Sanfilippo, M.D., Ph.D., and D. Bernard Amos, M.D.

HISTORICAL ASPECTS

During the past 3 decades knowledge about the immune mechanisms involved in allograft responses has increased dramatically. This has led to many of the advances in immunosuppressive manipulation, surgical techniques, donor organ preservation, recipient monitoring, and histocompatibility testing that have been applied to clinical organ transplantation; these advances also have significantly improved the outcome of patients receiving solid organ allografts, especially during the past 5 years. Reports from the organ procurement and transplant network of the United States, the United Network for Organ Sharing (UNOS), reveal excellent early graft survival for primary kidney and heart transplants performed during 1987 and 1988, and good results for primary heart/lung, liver, and pancreas transplants (Table 1).[5] Similar results have also been reported from other regions of the world.[140] Nevertheless, allograft rejection and complications of the immunosuppressive therapy required to prevent or treat rejection constitute the major causes of morbidity and mortality for organ allograft recipients. In particular, patients sensitized to HLA antigens, especially because of prior graft rejection, demonstrate substantially poorer outcome in the United States (see Table 1) and throughout the world,[5,140] indicating the continued importance of host immunity to disparate histocompatibility antigens as a risk factor for rejection.[88] Moreover, the necessity for maintaining continuous immunosuppression following transplantation emphasizes the ever present risk of rejection for allograft recipients. Thus, the primary goal of transplantation research is still unreached, that is, finding a means of avoiding or overcoming host immune responsiveness to alloantigens of potential graft donors without impairing immunity to other foreign (especially microbial) antigens.

Histocompatibility Testing

Antigens of the major histocompatibility complex (MHC) have a singular role in acting as major stimulants and targets of allograft rejection reactions. Historically, this was well documented by experimental animal studies that led to the identification of the MHC and its gene products as being primarily responsible for allograft rejection.[50,131] Subsequent observations in clinical kidney transplantation also demonstrated a strong correlation between the risk of rejection and the degree of donor-recipient disparity at the human MHC: the HLA complex.[91,143] Transplants between genetically identical monozygotic twins were not rejected, whereas dizygotic twins or siblings sharing both HLA chromosomal segments (haplotypes) had better graft survival than those sharing only one haplotype, who had a better outcome than those sharing neither. Moreover, with unrelated cadaveric donor grafts, the risk of rejection was associated with the number of mismatched donor antigens. Even with the improved results achieved in recent years, there remains a significant relationship between rejection and HLA disparity in kidney transplantation[87,124,142,144] and suggested effects for transplantation of other organs.[72,135]

The role of histocompatibility testing in clinical transplantation has progressed significantly since its first application to organ transplantation. Initially, HLA compatibility with potential family kidney donors was determined by comparing reaction patterns given by lymphocytes from donors and recipients tested with relatively poorly characterized antisera, usually obtained from multiparous females. While this approach usually allowed discrimination among HLA identical, one-haplotype identical, and fully mismatched family members, the inability to accurately determine HLA phenotypes was a significant problem in selecting the most compatible recipients for unrelated cadaveric donors throughout the 1960s. However, as a result of International Histocompatibility Workshops, which have been held every 2 to 3 years since the first in 1964 at Duke University, general agreement has been reached among laboratories on what HLA specificities are being recognized by various typing sera. By the early 1970s many of the Class I HLA-A and -B locus antigens were serologically well defined and could be identified at most transplant institutions; by the early 1980s serologic phenotyping had progressed to the point where almost all patients in well-studied Caucasian populations could be fully characterized for HLA-A and HLA-B.

The identification of other MHC loci beyond HLA-A and HLA-B was postulated in the early 1970s[98,153] largely based on studies utilizing the mixed lymphocyte reaction (MLR). The finding in 1964 that lymphocytes from different individuals would usually stimulate each other in culture[9,10] led to inheritance studies in families demonstrating that MLR stimulation was associated with certain types of HLA disparity.[8] In a manner analogous to the assignment of serologic Class I HLA-A and -B specificities based on consensus agreement at workshops, the Class II HLA-D locus was designated by functional assays,[78] with "alleles" defined by responsiveness to specific stimulator cells. The finding by van Rood and co-workers in 1973 that certain alloantibodies could block specific stimulator cells in MLR[147] provided the first serologic correlation with this functionally defined locus, and led to the designation of the Class II HLA-DR (D-related) locus. Other loci closely linked to HLA-DR were subsequently identified by functional and serologic means in the early 1980s and eventually were designated as HLA-DP and DQ at later international workshops.

The development of human T cell clones and molecular genetic techniques for identifying cellular defined HLA molecular determinants and the genes encoding expressed HLA molecules has led to a more complete understanding of the HLA complex (see Chapter 18, Part II). Thus, characterization of donor-recipient compatibility for HLA has evolved in 20 years from the simple serologic identification of only common Class I HLA-A and -B antigens to extensive characterization of the multiple Class II loci using serologic, functional, and molecular genetic methodologies.

The other important aspect of histocompatibility testing for transplantation has involved identification of host presensitization to potential donor HLA antigens, which has also progressed dramatically over the past 20 years. The occurrence of hyperacute rejection in some renal allograft recipients was found to be associated with the presence of preformed antibodies to donor HLA antigens in the late 1960s.[64,92,150] This rapidly led to the routine use of pretransplant leukocyte crossmatching

TABLE 1. Results of Organ Transplantation in the U.S. 1987–88

Organ	Six-Month Actuarial Graft Survival (Number of Transplants)	
	First Transplants	Repeat Transplants
Kidney		
Cadaveric	82% (5828)	73% (1101)
Live donor		
2-Haplotype	96% (183)	90% (20)
1-Haplotype	93% (508)	95% (44)
0-Haplotype	94% (68)	100% (6)
Heart	85% (1473)	59% (54)
Heart and lung	75% (58)	— (4)
Lung	46% (19)	— (1)
Liver	74% (1267)	40% (273)
Pancreas	71% (137)	25% (61)

From Annual Report of the United Network for Organ Sharing, Richmond, Virginia, 1989.

of recipient sera with donor cells in the 1970s to avoid hyperacute rejection of renal allografts. Similarly, the screening of patient sera for the presence of anti-HLA antibodies to identify unacceptable HLA antigens for particular recipients rapidly became a standard procedure at most centers to optimize cadaver donor allocation.

Significant developments have also occurred in the tests used for crossmatching and anti-HLA antibody screening. Complement-dependent microcytotoxicity assays initially utilized unseparated donor lymphocyte populations for crossmatch testing.[141] This was extended at some centers in the 1970s to include testing of patient sera with more sensitive methods, and by using separated donor T and B cells at different temperatures, since some reactions were not thought to adversely effect graft survival. In the early 1980s, it was further determined that patients who lost preformed antibodies to donor HLA antigens could often be successfully transplanted,[24,126] providing greater access to donors for such individuals. Since the mid-1980s, the development of more sensitive and specific crossmatching techniques, such as flow cytometry, have further refined pretransplant screening and crossmatch testing for potential transplant recipients.[11,21]

Allograft Rejection

Understanding of the basic mechanisms involved in allograft rejection has developed slowly over the past half century. The classic experiments of Medawar[77] in the 1940s, and subsequent studies described in the previous chapter, initially suggested a predominant role for cellular immunity in graft rejection. However, other reactions (especially in presensitized animals) indicated that alternative mechanisms leading to more acute inflammatory reactions predominated by neutrophils could also occur. Early clinical observations in human renal transplantation documented that the variable histologic manifestations of rejection previously described in animals with different presensitization,[40] or receiving different types of allograft tissue,[49] could also be seen in man.

The initial classification of renal allograft rejection by Porter[100] in 1967 drew a correlation between the clinical-temporal characteristics of rejection and the histopathologic reaction seen within the graft (Table 2). *Hyperacute rejection* was identified as a very rapid loss of graft function which usually occurred immediately after transplantation, and was characterized by acute inflammation with predominantly vascular injury, leading to hemorrhage and necrosis. *Acute rejection* was described as typically occurring within weeks after transplantation; being rapid in onset; and associated with mononuclear cell infiltration throughout the interstitium, often accompanied by some degree of vascular involvement. *Chronic rejection* was described as the indolent type of rejection generally seen months after transplantation. This reaction was characterized by gradual graft dysfunction, nonresponsiveness to treatment, and a histologic appearance of interstitial fibrosis and vascular sclerosis with a relatively mild infiltration of mononuclear cells.

Although the mechanism of hyperacute rejection has become fairly well understood, the *in situ* processes whereby acute and chronic types of rejection lead to graft dysfunction remain unclear. In particular, the basis for the extreme immunogenicity of allografts has been only recently understood at the cellular and molecular level since the finding in the mid 1970s that T cells recognize antigen in association with MHC molecules.[154] Subsequent studies demonstrated that a high frequency of host T cells that recognize specific antigens in association with self MHC molecules also react directly with particular allogeneic MHC molecules, thus accounting in part for the strength and predisposition of cellular responses against allografts.

While these key findings have helped explain the long-puz-

TABLE 2. General Criteria Used to Classify Allograft Rejection

Clinical		Immunopathologic		
Classification	Kinetics	Target	Response	Reactions
Hyperacute	Very rapid onset, minutes to hours after transplantation	Vessels: large, small	Humoral	Granulocytic infiltrates, vasculitis, hemorrhage
Acute	Rapid onset, usually early after transplant			
Interstitial		Parenchyma, small vessels	Cellular ≥ humoral	Interstitial edema, mononuclear mixed cell inflammation
Vascular		Vessels: large, intermediate	Humoral > cellular	Vasculitis, granulocyte mixed cell infiltrates
Chronic	Slow onset, usually late after transplant			
Interstitial		Parenchyma	Cellular > humoral	Interstitial fibrosis, mononuclear cell infiltrates
Vascular		Vessels: large, intermediate	Humoral ≥ cellular	Sclerotic vascular changes, secondary ischemic injury

zling observation that allografts (which do not normally occur in nature) generally evoke the most vigorous immune response of a host to any antigenic challenge, many fundamental issues remain unresolved. In particular, there is not yet a firm understanding of what alloantigen determinants are recognized by the host, although studies of the past 2 years strongly suggest that the peptide fragments bound to MHC molecules have an important role in recognition by alloreactive T cells. The expanded understanding of the cellular and molecular aspects of immune responsiveness has clearly increased awareness of the complexity of host interactions with organ and tissue allografts and how this leads to their dysfunction and rejection.

IMMUNE MECHANISMS OF ALLOGRAFT REJECTION

Inflammatory Cells and Molecular Mediators

A wide range of cells can participate in inflammatory responses such as those seen in allograft rejection, with lymphocytes, macrophages, and granulocytes having the most dominant role. However, other cells such as vascular endothelial cells, platelets, basophils, and mast cells can also be involved, especially in the production of inflammatory molecules. This section provides a brief review of the major characteristics of inflammatory cells with emphasis on antigen recognition, chemotaxis, activation, effector function, and the inflammatory mediators they elaborate.

Although antigen-specific recognition is the hallmark of immune responses, all of the cells in the immune system express various antigen-nonspecific receptors that are capable of triggering or modifying immune responses. These include receptors for cytokines (e.g., interleukin-1 [IL-1], IL-2, interferon-γ [IFN-γ]), the constant regions of immunoglobulin (e.g., IgM, IgG or IgE, Fc domains), and complement breakdown products (e.g., C3b, C3dg). Some immunocompetent cells (especially lymphocytes) can also be activated by antigen-nonspecific molecules such as microbial products and plant lectins. As discussed in the previous chapter, immune responses are usually initiated by antigen-presenting cells (APCs), which typically are Class II MHC antigen-positive macrophages, B cells, or dendritic cells of the mononuclear-phagocyte system. These cells are able to recognize a wide range of potentially antigenic molecules using a variety of surface proteins and receptors, with the Class II antigens themselves having an important direct role in antigen binding. When large antigenic molecules are processed by different types of macrophages, various portions or conformations of the molecule may be preferentially presented and thus alter the antigenic determinant to which a response is directed. Different APCs also express different levels of self Class II MHC antigens (as well as Class I MHC antigens and other receptors), which may affect their ability to bind antigen and present it in an immunogenic manner.

In contrast to all other cells involved in inflammation, lymphocytes alone express receptors that have antigen specificity; B cells directly recognize antigenic determinants by means of surface IgM as a receptor, whereas T cells utilize a clonotypic T-cell receptor (TcR) that recognizes antigen in association with Class I or Class II MHC molecules. While polymorphonuclear leukocytes (PMNs) express neither antigen-specific receptors (as do lymphocytes) nor Class II MHC molecules (as do macrophages and APCs), they can recognize antigen indirectly by receptors for immunoglobulin or complement products that may be bound to antigens.

The migration and accumulation of inflammatory cells at sites of antigen deposition are central to the inflammatory process and are characterized by a variety of chemotactic factors and adhesion molecules that promote local reactions. Macrophages and PMNs are motile and can perceive gradients of chemoattractant molecules such as C5a and leukotriene B$_4$ (LTB$_4$) by means of surface receptors, whereas the migration of lymphocytes is largely directed by interactions with adhesion molecules expressed on vascular endothelium.[39] The interaction between LFA-1 (CD11a) on lymphocytes and its ligand ICAM-1 (CD54) on other cells appears to have an important role in promoting lymphocyte interactions. Other adhesion molecules such as the C3bi receptor (CD11b) and gp150/95 (CD11c) are similarly involved in cell-cell interactions, and their expression can be regulated by inflammatory mediators such as IFN-γ. T-cell subsets also express receptors for monomorphic (invariant) determinants of Class I and Class II molecules (CD8 and CD4, respectively), which act to stabilize binding interactions of these T cells with other cells expressing the appropriate MHC molecule. Thus, these receptors usually reflect the nature of MHC-associated antigen recognition (restriction) of the TcR of a particular T cell; CD4$^+$ T cells typically exhibit Class II restriction; and CD8$^+$ T cells, Class I restriction.

Activation of inflammatory cells involves complex interactions that are highly dependent upon soluble factors. The activation of lymphocytes generally involves a two-signal mechanism, the first provided by antigen binding to the antigen-specific receptor (surface IgM for B cells, TcR for T cells) and the second by a cytokine (e.g., IL-1 for T-helper [Th] cells, IL-2 for T-cytotoxic cells, IL-4 for B cells). Upon activation, lymphocytes express a variety of functions and cytokines (Table 3) that contribute to further leukocyte activation, differentiation, and production of inflammatory mediators. At least two subsets of CD4$^+$ T cells have been recently characterized in terms of lymphokine production and apparent helper function.[19] Upon activation, the Th1 subset secretes IL-2, IL-3, IFN-γ, and tumor necrosis factor (TNF)-β, preferentially stimulating T cell and macrophage cellular responses. The Th2 subset secretes IL-4, which preferentially drives B-cell activation and differentiation into antibody-producing plasma cells. After activation, these two subsets also appear to be largely regulated by their own cytokines (IL-2 and IL-4, respectively). Some of these stimulatory lymphokines are counterbalanced by suppressive factors also produced by T lymphocytes, e.g., transforming growth factor (TGF)-β. Recent evidence suggests that prior to stimulation, CD4$^+$ T cells appear to express an isoform (CD45RA) of a family of T-200 molecules that is lost upon activation of the two T-helper subsets. However, a third CD4$^+$ T-cell subset may retain CD45RA and function as a suppressor cell population that is regulated by IL-6 (and perhaps IL-1), but not IL-2 or IL-4.[23]

Upon activation, various lymphocytes can exhibit cytotoxic activity mediated by several mechanisms,[152] including secretion of cytokines (e.g., perforin, TNF-β) and serine esterases. Cytotoxic T lymphocytes (CTLs) typically express CD8 and utilize an antigen specific TcR comprised of a rearranged α,β heterodimer (α,β TcR) in association with the CD3 T-cell antigen complex. Some CTLs appear to express CD3, but not CD8 (or CD4) molecules, and utilize a rearranged γ,δ TcR that appears fully capable of recognizing specific HLA class I determinants.[30] Natural killer (NK) cells are not restricted by Class I or II MHC antigens, do not appear to utilize an antigen-specific TcR,[107] and do not express CD3, CD4, or CD8 T-cell markers. They express various other markers (e.g., NKH1) and can spontaneously kill tumor or virus-infected cells directly. Killer (K) cells also do not express T-cell markers or either type of TcR, but recognize antigen specific targets via a receptor for Fc determinants of IgG (CD16) to mediate antibody-dependent cellular cytotoxicity (ADCC).

Activation of macrophages occurs as a result of interaction with components of complement, microbial products, or lymphokines such as IFN-γ, IL-2, and TNF-β. In addition to having increased phagocytic activity, activated macrophages secrete an

TABLE 3. Immune Cell Products That Mediate Inflammation

Cellular Source	Mediator	Activity
Monocyte/ macrophage	Complement components	Cell injury, opsonization, chemotaxis
	Interleukin-1 (IL-1)	Pleotropic; lymphocyte and endothelial cell activation
	Tumor necrosis factor-α (TNF-α)	Pleotropic IL-1– like activity, cytostatic
	Leukotrienes	Chemotaxis, vasopermeability, smooth muscle contraction
	Thromboxanes	Vasoconstriction, coagulation
	Prostaglandins	Vasodilation
	Transforming growth factor-β (TGF-β)	Fibrosis, angiogenesis; inhibition of lymphocyte proliferation
	Colony-stimulating factor (CSF)	Leukocyte activation, chemotaxis; hematopoiesis
	Lysosomal enzymes	Proteolysis, tissue injury
T lymphocytes	Interleukins (IL-2 to 8)	Stimulate activity and differentiation of various leukocytes
	Interferon-γ (IFN-γ)	Stimulates macrophages, lymphocytes, endothelial cells; induces acute phase proteins, fever; enhances MHC expression
	Lymphotoxin (TNF-β)	Similar to IL-1 activity, cytolytic
	Perforin	Cytolysis, cell injury
Mast cells, basophils	Histamine	Increased vascular permeability, smooth muscle contraction
	Chemotaxic factors	Eosinophil, neutrophil chemotaxis
	Heparin	Anticoagulant
	Leukotrienes, thromboxanes, prostaglandins	See above
Neutrophils	H_2O_2, myeloperoxidase	Generation of toxic oxygen radicals
	Lysosomal enzymes	Proteolysis, tissue injury

array of biologically and immunologically active products (see Table 3), including arachidonic acid metabolites (e.g., prostaglandins, thromboxanes, leukotrienes), complement components, lysosomal enzymes, and cytokines (e.g., IL-1, TNF-α). Granulocytes are activated via receptors for IgG and complement (C3a, C5a, C3b, C3bi), whereas mast cells, basophils, and eosinophils have Fc receptors for IgE that upon cross-linking with bound antigen lead to release of preformed and newly synthesized inflammatory mediators (see Table 3). Some of the important molecular mediators involved in causing tissue injury or organ dysfunction are grouped as follows:

LIPID MEDIATORS. Phospholipids are major constituents of cell membranes (including those of leukocytes and platelets) and are subject to degradation during inflammatory conditions. Cleavage of phospholipids leads to the release of arachidonic acid, which can be further metabolized into a number of biologically potent mediators and modulators of inflammation. The cyclo-oxygenase pathway of arachidonic acid metabolism yields prostaglandins (PGE_2, PGF_{2a}), thromboxanes, or prostacyclins, depending on the isomerase enzymes present in the particular tissue. Thromboxanes are vasoconstrictors, whereas prostacyclins are potent vasodilators. PGE_2 can enhance vascular permeability, is pyrogenic, can upregulate IFN-γ receptors on T cells, and increases sensitivity to pain. PGE_2 also stimulates the formation of cyclic adenosine monophosphate (cAMP) in many types of inflammatory cells and thereby suppresses a number of immunologic responses, including lymphocyte proliferation, lymphocyte-mediated cytotoxicity, and the release of mediators from mast cells. An important source of PGE_2 in immunologic reactions is the macrophage. The hydroxyeicosatetraenoic acids (HETEs) and the derivatives of 5-hydroperoxyeicosatetraenoic acid (leukotrienes) are products of the lipoxygenase pathway of arachidonic acid metabolism and are synthesized by granulocytes, macrophages, and basophils. 5,12-HETE, also termed LTB_4, is a potent chemotactic factor, whereas LTC_4 and LTD_4 stimulate smooth muscle contraction. LTC_4 and 5-HETE also can stimulate IFN-γ production by T-helper cells. Platelet-activating factors (PAFs) are a group of acetyl-alkyl-glycerol ether analogs of aklyl-phosphatidylcholine, which cause platelet aggregation and are potent leukocyte activators and metabolites; PAFs are produced by leukocytes and vascular endothelium after stimulation by inflammatory mediators.

COMPLEMENT COMPONENTS. Complement components function as important amplifiers of inflammatory reactions; are produced by a variety of cells, including macrophages and vascular endothelium; and can be activated by bound immunoglobulins or mechanisms such as the release of hydrolytic enzymes from injured cells or leukocytes. The complement cleavage products C3a and C5a mediate a number of biologic responses, including smooth muscle contraction, enhanced vascular permeability, degranulation of mast cells and basophils, and secretion of lysosomal enzymes by leukocytes. They also have various immunoregulatory effects; C3a suppresses, whereas C5a enhances, humoral immune responses *in vitro* by affecting T lymphocytes. In addition, C5a is an extremely potent chemoattractant for polymorphonuclear leukocytes, monocytes, and macrophages. Complement components (e.g., C3b) bound to target antigens can also enhance phagocytosis (opsonization) by interaction with specific complement receptors expressed by phagocytic cells.

CYTOKINES. Cytokines are immunoregulatory molecules synthesized by mononuclear leukocytes.[12] Some of these proteins are termed interleukins (ILs), whereas others are designated for their biologic activity. Stimulation of macrophages by antigens as well as by factors from lymphocytes initiates the secretion of IL-1, a 15-kd. peptide with diverse biologic activities, including T-cell activation. TNF-α, a 19-kd. monokine, has many of the biologic activities of IL-1 and is also directly cytotoxic for many types of tumor cells. T cells produce a wide range of lymphokines with diverse activities that can amplify and regulate humoral and cellular immune responses. Th1 cells produce IL-2 as an autocrine and paracrine, a 15-kd. polypeptide that stimulates effector T cells and macrophages. Stimulated T cells also produce IL-3, a B-cell differentiation factor; IL-4, a Th2 (autocrine and paracrine) and B-cell activation factor; IL-5, which stimulates eosinophils and B cells (in mice); TGF-β, which has numerous immunosuppressive activities, can modulate MHC expression, and may promote tissue repair; IFN-γ, a cytokine with a wide range of effects, including activation of macrophages, B cells, and endothelial cells, upregulation of MHC and adhesion molecule expression, and cytostatic activity; and lymphotoxin (TNF-β), a pluripotential factor with many of the properties of IFN-γ. Many cytokines are labile and effective in truly minute amounts, so their detection is difficult; nevertheless, it is certain that more will be identified in the near future.

Types of Inflammatory Immune Responses

While a fundamental purpose of the immune system is host protection, certain immune mechanisms are pathologic to the host and can lead to various types of tissue damage.[18] Coombs and Gell have classified four types of immune reactions[34] that are associated with particular forms of tissue damage as outlined in Table 4. This classification, although oversimplified, is useful when considering tissue transplantation, since at least two of the four reactions characterize the major types of allograft rejection and provide some indication of underlying immune mechanisms.

TYPE I REACTIONS. These involve the cytotropic binding (via the Fc fragment) of reaginic antibodies (primarily IgE) to cells such as mast cells, basophils, and platelets. Cross-linking of the cytotropic antibody upon re-exposure to antigen can induce the release of products (see Table 3) that can have a variety of effects, especially on hemostasis, vascular tone, and function of the organ involved. Although the role of Type I reactions in allograft rejection is unclear, vasoactive products typically released during such reactions (e.g., thromboxanes, leukotrienes, prostaglandins, histamine), are being increasingly recognized as involved in graft dysfunction during rejection reactions. Moreover, the presence of eosinophil infiltration is a very poor prognostic indicator during allograft rejection,[46,139] suggesting the possible involvement of Type I reactions, since they are commonly associated with eosinophil chemotaxis and infiltration.

TYPE II REACTIONS. These are directed by antibody and most often amplified by complement activation and release of chemotaxins (e.g., C5a). A pattern of acute exudative inflammation is typically seen with congestion, edema, PMN infiltrates, and fibrinoid necrosis. Thus, host antibodies directed against donor alloantigens expressed on vessel walls can lead to significant organ injury, with necrosis, hemorrhage and infarction similar to that seen with severe vasculitis.

TYPE III REACTIONS. These involve immune complexes usually composed of antibody and antigen. The classic examples used to describe immune complex disorders are the Arthus and serum sickness reactions. The Arthus reaction is due to localized tissue interactions of antigen and antibody, leading to severe inflammation usually involving adjacent small vessels. Serum sickness follows an analogous reaction between circulating antibody and antigen in which the complexes are formed, and deposited or trapped in various vascular beds, depending upon the size and charge of the complex. In the transplant recipient, immune complex–mediated damage can be seen in a variety of settings, including *de novo* membranous glomerulonephritis in renal allograft recipients, and as reactions to heterologous (e.g., horse, rabbit, or mouse) anti–T-cell or lymphocyte antibodies, which are used prophylactically for immunosuppression or in treating rejection episodes. Since the acute inflammatory reactions observed with Type III reactions are similar to those of Type II (i.e., secondary to complement binding by antibody-antigen complexes), it is often clinically difficult to determine whether certain changes in allograft function (especially kidney) are the result of rejection or antirejection therapy with heterologous antibodies. Although severe Type III reactions are much less common after treatment with mouse monoclonal antibodies than after treatment with polyclonal horse or rabbit antibodies, the detection of circulating antibody to the heterologous serum, or direct identification of complexes within a transplant biopsy, may be needed for a definitive diagnosis.

TYPE IV REACTIONS. These involve cellular immune responses as the cause of tissue damage and typically are expressed as mononuclear inflammatory cell infiltration. The antigen-specific effector cells of Type IV reactions are T cells, which can act directly or indirectly to injure target cells. The classic model of Type IV reactions is delayed type hypersensitivity (DTH) of the tuberculin type, in which sensitized T-helper cells produce lymphokines (e.g., IFN-γ, IL-2, TNF-β) that activate local macrophages. This combination of activated macrophages and sensitized T lymphocytes leads to severe local damage and histologically appears as chronic or granulomatous inflammation. The enzymes and proteases released by activated macrophages (see Table 3) can cause significant tissue destruction. Jones-Mote or Dienes hypersensitivity is clinically similar to DTH hypersensitivity but occurs in individuals with antibodies reactive against the relevant antigens and is associated with the appearance of mast cells. Cell-mediated responses are clinically the most common form of allograft injury and can involve large vessels, parenchyma, or both.

Stimulation of Allogeneic Responses

Although it has been long recognized that allografts provoke an immunologic response that is generally stronger than that to any naturally occurring stimulus, it has been only in the last 10 to 15 years that the underlying basis for this phenomenon has been well understood. Host responses to typical foreign (nominal) antigens initially involve their processing and/or presentation on host antigen presenting cells (APCs) such as monocytes, tissue macrophages, B cells, or dendritic cells, all of which express Class II MHC antigens and secrete cytokines that can provide a second signal (e.g., IL-1) for T-helper–cell activation. The antigen specific T-cell receptor (TcR) is able to recognize only nominal antigens that are associated with self Class I or II MHC molecules[53,61] as a result of positive selection by the thymus during T-cell ontogeny. Typically, the frequency of T-cell clones in a host capable of recognizing any particular MHC restricted antigen is relatively small (less than 1 per cent of the approximately 10^8 different clones present), and the stimulation of such clones is generally limited to an interaction with an APC expressing the corresponding nominal antigen and self MHC molecule. Thus, the initial stimulus of an antigen specific immune response generally involves an interaction between an APC presenting a specific antigen and a T-helper cell that recognizes that antigen plus self Class II MHC (i.e., Class II–restricted). Such MHC Class II–restricted helper T cells usually express the CD4 receptor, which strengthens their binding interaction via the Class II MHC on APCs.

The relatively high frequency of host T-cell clones found capable of recognizing alloantigens initially suggested that such clones had "cross-reactive" recognition of allo-MHC by utilizing the same TcR specific for an unrelated nominal antigen plus

TABLE 4. Types of Inflammatory Immunopathologic Reactions

Type of Inflammation	Antigen Recognition	Inflammatory Mediators	Inflammatory Response
I. Immediate hypersensitivity	IgE	Histamine, granulocyte chemotaxins, heparin, prostaglandins	Edema, vasodilation, eosinophil and neutrophil infiltrates
II. Antibody mediated	IgG, IgM, IgA	Complement activity and products	Lysis/phagocytosis, acute inflammation
III. Immune complex	IgG, IgM, IgA	Complement activity and products	Acute inflammation
IV. Delayed-type hypersensitivity	T-cell receptor	Lymphokines, monokines	Chronic inflammation, mononuclear cell infiltration

self MHC. Indeed, during the past 5 years it has been demonstrated that a very high frequency (usually more than 50 per cent) of T cell clones generated against specific nominal antigens (e.g., natural or synthetic peptides) in association with specific self-MHC antigens can also be stimulated directly with various allogeneic APCs.[7] The distribution of allogeneic APCs that could stimulate nominal antigen specific T-cell clones in these studies also suggests that such cross-reactive recognition is often of "public," rather than "private," MHC determinants. This provides a unique means by which allografts may stimulate host responses, since a relatively high percentage of T-cell clones in the host express TcRs capable of directly recognizing intact allogeneic MHC antigens (allo-MHC) on the APCs of the donor graft. Thus, as shown in Figure 1, allografts appear to stimulate different clones of host helper T cells by two distinct mechanisms: (1) direct activation of host clones recognizing intact allo-MHC on donor APCs and (2) activation of host clones recognizing processed allo-MHC peptide fragments presented on host APCs as nominal antigens.[129]

The implications of these findings clearly are profound in helping to explain many of the phenomena observed in clinical transplantation: (1) They explain why MHC disparity is so strongly associated with allograft rejection, since a high percentage of normal host T cells specific for various antigens are also capable of responding to allo-MHC and can be stimulated directly by donor APCs. (2) The relative strength and clonal diversity of allo-MHC stimulation also explains why attempts to inhibit allograft rejection often require immunosuppressive therapy so great as to compromise host responses to nominal antigens of infectious organisms and thus provide a high risk for infectious complications. (3) The greater propensity for certain tissues and organs (e.g., lung, bowel) to elicit strong rejection reactions is presumably related to the greater number and types of donor APCs (e.g., monocytes, B cells) within such grafts. (4) It suggests why an infection or inflammatory reaction occurring in an otherwise stable allograft recipient may lead to a rejection reaction, since certain viral or other antigen-specific T-cell clones activated by infection may also recognize alloantigen[151]

and promote rejection. In addition, inflammatory reactions unrelated to rejection (e.g., infection, drug reaction) may locally lead to the increased production of cytokines (e.g., IFN-γ), which can enhance Class II MHC antigen expression and activation of local donor APCs to provoke a rejection reaction. (5) It suggests that certain forms of injury associated with organ recovery or preservation might promote allograft rejection. Indeed, ischemic or physiologic injury to donor organ tissues can lead to the release of inflammatory mediators that might amplify the immunogenicity of donor APCs as a result of their increased activation, MHC expression, or proliferation. Moreover, the release of chemotaxins and the enhanced adhesion of leukocytes to injured/activated vessels can lead to an increased influx of host inflammatory cells following engraftment, which may cause rejection reactions as described above.

In addition to the important contribution of donor APCs and passenger lymphoid cells in stimulating host responses to the allograft, the role of donor vascular endothelial cells (VECs) has also become increasingly appreciated in recent years. In particular, human VECs fulfill all of the criteria for APCs in that they constitutively express Class II MHC molecules, elaborate cytokines (e.g., IL-1) that can act as second signals for T cells, and express adhesion molecules that can promote T-cell interactions leading to their activation.[71] As the component of an organ allograft that is first encountered by circulating leukocytes of the host, the potential role of VECs in stimulating and acting as targets (see below) for allograft rejection must not be underrated. Indeed, removal of VECs from vessel allografts has been shown to inhibit their rejection.[47] Paradoxically, VECs may also be important in promoting allograft acceptance. Sinusoidal VECs of the liver are unable to stimulate unprimed T cells,[112] which may in part be responsible for the apparent lower immunogenicity of this organ. In addition, total lymphoid irradiation (TLI), which is known to promote allograft acceptance, causes changes in VECs that affect leukocyte adhesion, which may contribute to this phenomenon.

After the initial activation of helper T cells either directly by donor APCs, or indirectly by self APCs with processed alloanti-

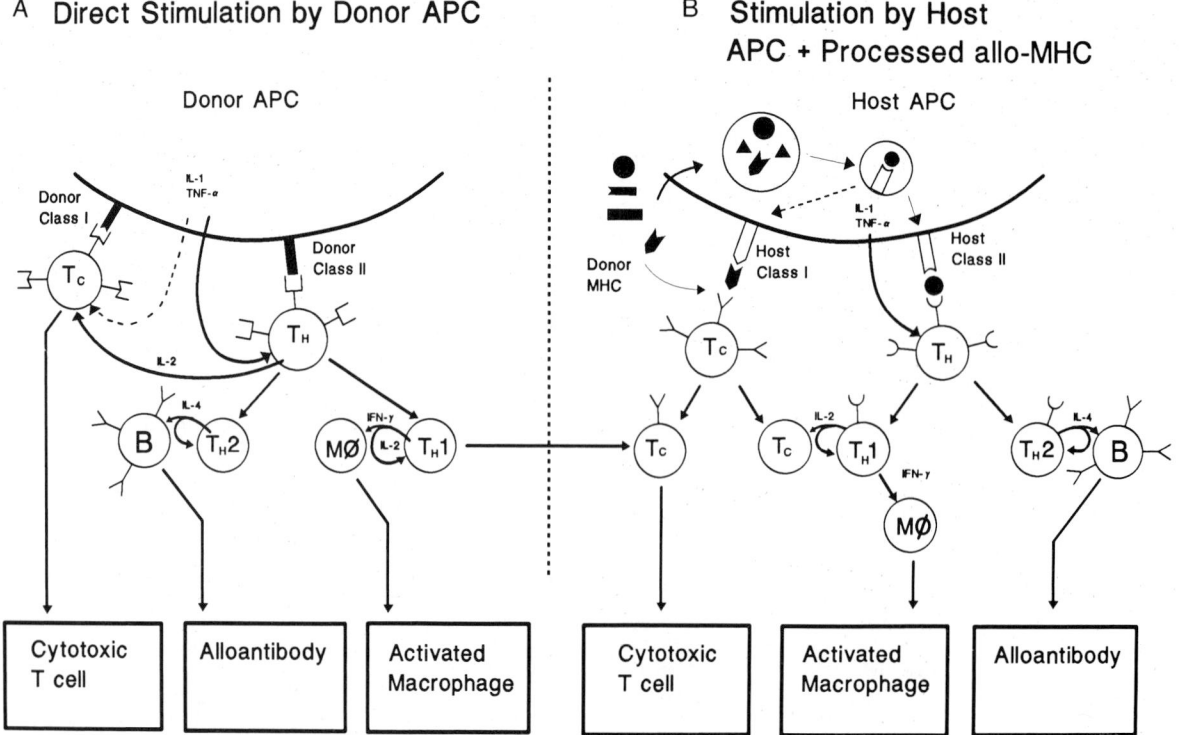

Figure 1. Dual means of host immune responsiveness to an allograft (see text).

gen, a wide variety of immune responses can occur. Preferential stimulation of Th1 can promote the development of cell-mediated (Type IV) responses, characterized by the presence of cytotoxic T cells and activated macrophages as effector populations. The repertoire of allospecific cytotoxic T cells predominantly involves populations that recognize allogeneic MHC Class I determinants and are Class I MHC restricted. Although most cytotoxic T cells are Class I MHC restricted and express the CD8 monomorphic Class I MHC binding receptor, alloreactive cytotoxic T cells of the CD4 phenotype have also been identified, which normally are specific for Class II alloantigens. In addition, cytotoxic T cells that do not express CD8 or CD4 and appear to utilize the γ,δ-TcR have been found to recognize specific Class I HLA alloantigens.[30]

Although not well appreciated in early studies of transplantation, humoral responses are known to have an important role in allograft rejection. B cells recognizing alloantigens by their surface immunoglobulin receptor can be stimulated by second signals from activated Th2 cells leading to specific alloantibody production. The class and subclass of antibody produced can have a significant effect on the resulting inflammatory reaction, since antibodies have differential activities in fixing complement, stimulating antibody-dependent cellular cytotoxicity, and acting as ligands for different leukocyte receptors.

Targets of Allogeneic Responses

NON-MHC ANTIGENS. A variety of antigens and molecules expressed on donor tissue can act as targets of host immune responses. In addition to molecules encoded by genes of the MHC complex, the products of nearly any polymorphic gene system expressed on accessible donor cell surfaces have the potential to be targets of an allogeneic response. However, since most cell surface molecules are highly conserved within a species and are not commonly allelic, there appear to be only a limited number of antigen systems of relevance to clinical transplantation.

The greatest non-MHC antigen system of clinical importance in transplantation is the ABO blood group. Others, such as the VEC antigen system,[27] the human monocyte antigen (HMA) system,[57] Lewis blood group antigens, certain tissue specific antigens,and allelic or polymorphic forms of certain cell receptors or enzymes, are of unclear importance. ABO blood group antigens were clearly identified as targets of hyperacute or accelerated acute antibody-mediated rejections in the 1960s. The presence of a high titer of IgM isohemagglutinins against A or B blood group antigens normally expressed on the vasculature of a donor organ could often lead to Type II inflammatory reactions. The ability of Lewis blood group antigens to adhere to vascular endothelium in secretor-positive patients has also been suggested to stimulate rejection reactions in renal allograft recipients,[134] although this association remains unclear at present. In occasional cases of renal and cardiac transplantation, otherwise unexplained severe allograft rejection reactions have been associated with the presence of antibodies against antigens expressed on donor VECs, monocytes, or both.[20,26,28] Recent evidence suggests that a non–HLA-linked human monocyte antigen (HMA) system exists in man with at least two alleles expressed,[57,58] but the role of such antigens in allograft rejection is unclear. The potential role of tissue specific non-HLA antigen acting as a stimulus or target for allograft rejection has been demonstrated for skin-specific antigens in mice[127] and has been suggested for renal tubular epithelium in man.[60,93] Although sex-linked antigens have been suggested as targets in human bone marrow transplantation,[51] they have not been associated with the rejection of solid organ transplants in man. Disparity for non-MHC or non-ABO antigens, although not associated with early or severe acute rejections, may contribute to the poorly understood process of chronic allograft rejection.

CLASS I VERSUS CLASS II MHC ANTIGENS. The molecular basis for recognition of specific Class I versus Class II MHC antigens in rejection reactions has received considerable attention during the past decade. Using allospecific T-cell clones, monoclonal and polyclonal anti-HLA antibodies, and molecular genetic mapping techniques, it has been well demonstrated that many epitopes on Class II HLA molecules (especially HLA-DP and -DQ) recognized by the TcR are not recognized by antibody, which suggests that effector responses to donor Class II antigens may be more often cellular than humoral. Moreover, host alloantibody responses to organ grafts tend to be frequently directed at public (shared) HLA Class I determinants, often leading to broad humoral sensitization following allograft rejection and removal. The expression of Class I MHC on nearly all parenchymal cells (versus the generally restricted expression of Class II) might also suggest a greater risk with Class I–directed responses. It could therefore follow that rejection reactions against Class II MHC should be more easily reversed than those against Class I antigens, since immunosuppressive therapy is generally less effective against antibody responses. However, such differences in risk have not yet been demonstrated clinically. A recent evaluation of Class I (HLA-A, B) versus Class II (HLA-DR) disparity in human renal kidney transplantation shows an equivalent risk of rejection for each in cyclosporine-treated patients.[124] Other studies have suggested that disparity for HLA-B and -DR is associated more with outcome than with disparity for HLA-A in kidney transplantation.[86]

Both Class I and Class II MHC differences are clearly capable of provoking rejection reactions. Although experimental models have demonstrated a greater ease in promoting allograft acceptance in rats and pigs exhibiting only Class I MHC differences,[94,114] limited amino acid substitutions for Class I or Class II MHC antigens can lead to brisk skin graft rejection in rodents.[14,84] Recent evidence indicates that Class I–restricted helper T cells can also be involved in anti-Class I allogeneic responses[109,110] and can potentially be stimulated by the Class I MHC disparate APCs directly.[18] Even without direct stimulation by APCs, processed allogeneic Class I molecules presented on host APCs are capable of stimulating an anti–Class I host response.

ALLO-MHC RECOGNITION. The basis by which the T-cell receptor recognizes antigen plus MHC[17] has received considerable attention since the actual structure of the HLA-A2 molecule was determined by crystallographic studies in 1987.[16] It now appears that the peptide bound in the antigen groove of MHC molecules has an important role in TcR recognition of Class I and Class II alloantigens. Several models of the interaction between TcR and allo-MHC have been proposed, as depicted in Figure 2. The traditional concept of allo-MHC recognition is shown in Figure 2A, simply involving recognition of allo-MHC structural determinants by the variable regions of the TcR. This model would correlate with the recognition and binding of allotypic determinants of the allo-MHC α-helices that form the lateral (outside) walls of the antigen binding groove by variable sequences of the α, β-heterodimer of the clonotypic TcR. However, the presence of a peptide fragment in the MHC binding groove raises the question of to what extent the TcR binds to epitopes on the peptide versus the MHC molecule itself. Two extreme possibilities are (1) that allospecific TcRs do not recognize peptide at all (Fig. 2A) and (2) that they recognize determinants on the peptide alone (Fig. 2B). However, neither is likely, because TcR recognition of nominal antigen peptides involves self-MHC restriction, and allo-MHC recognition is likely to be similar, based upon the cross-reactive recognition of allo-MHC and nominal antigen plus self MHC by most TcRs. Indeed, results from several recent studies indicate that the interaction between MHC and peptide has a crucial role in the ability of allospecific T cells to recognize allo-MHC.[73,97,148] The effect of specific amino acid substitutions at different sites of allo-MHC molecules on the reactivity of allogeneic T-cell clones

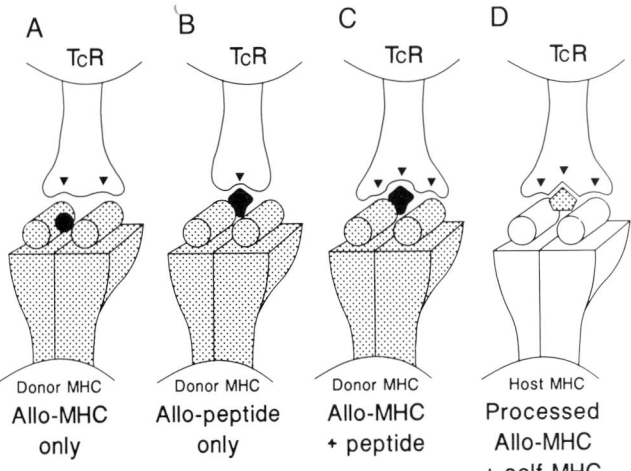

Figure 2. Proposed mechanisms of host T-cell receptor (TcR) interaction with alloantigens. *A*, Recognition of intact donor MHC molecule alone. *B*, Recognition of only the allogeneic peptide (non-MHC) fragment bound to an intact donor MHC molecule. *C*, Recognition of determinants on both donor MHC molecule and its bound (non-MHC) peptide. *D*, Recognition of a processed donor MHC fragment presented on a host MHC molecule. The stippled structures indicate donor MHC.

suggests that changes in areas likely to affect peptide binding (e.g., the β sheet floor and medial walls of the α-helixes) have a greater effect on allo-MHC recognition than those in direct contact with the TcR (e.g., lateral walls of α-helixes). Thus, the immunogenicity of intact allo-MHC on donor APCs is likely to be affected by the peptide bound, as depicted in Figure 2C, in a manner analogous to TcR recognition of processed allo-MHC peptides bound to host APCs (Fig. 2D). However, the nature of interactions between bound peptide, allo-MHC, and the TcR remain to be fully elucidated.

Regulation of Allogeneic Responses

Although only partially understood, a variety of immune mechanisms are involved in regulating the type and extent of effector responses against allografts. Clearly, factors such as the degree and type (e.g., Class I versus Class II) of MHC disparity between a donor and recipient may affect the number and subclass of T cells initially stimulated by the allograft. Also of critical importance is the architecture of the transplanted organ, especially in terms of the number and location of donor APC or passenger leukocytes, the degree of vascularization, and the extent of MHC expression on parenchymal cells. For example, the relatively high level of Class I expression seen on renal tubular epithelium, in contrast to a lower expression on cardiac myocytes and liver hepatocytes, may in part be responsible for the apparent greater immunogenicity of the former. Similarly, highly vascularized tissues with abundant dendritic cells (e.g., skin) or lymphoid tissue (e.g., lung, bowel) are likely to be more immunogenic than tissues without significant vascularization or APC (e.g., cornea). Indeed, the risk of human cornea allograft rejection is significantly associated with vascularization,[74] and the role of donor HLA disparity in provoking corneal rejection has been most clearly demonstrated in recipients with vascularized corneal beds or those who previously rejected a graft.[121]

The repertoire of host T cells that can potentially react with an antigen is presumed to have a considerable effect on the strength and nature of host responses to that antigen. Recent studies examining the functional basis for observed differences between mouse strains in their response to particular antigens suggest that "high responder" animals may have an increased repertoire of T cells able to recognize immunodominant epitopes formed by the association of antigen plus self-MHC.[65] In addition, the same antigen bound to different Class II MHC

molecules can regulate the functional response of host cells.[83] One extrapolation of these findings to allo-MHC recognition would suggest that those individuals with an expanded repertoire of T cells reactive against particular immunodominant allo-MHC epitopes on either allogeneic cells (donor APCs) or processed allo-MHC determinants on host APCs may be patients with a high response to particular allografts. Some evidence supports this possibility, including the clinical observation that the frequency and strength of rejection may correlate with the precursor frequency of alloreactive T cells in the circulation,[55] and that during rejection reactions predominant alloreactive clones may be preferentially involved, even during sequential rejection episodes.[79,80]

The inflammatory reaction that follows the initiation of rejection can itself promote the rejection process. In particular, the release of IFN-γ by activated T cells can activate donor APCs and up-regulate MHC expression on the graft, providing further stimulation and potential targets for host allogeneic responses. However, immune regulatory mechanisms may also reduce reactions against allografts when they are maintained for a period of time in the host. The replacement of donor APCs by those of the host has been demonstrated in several animal models of induced allograft tolerance; this has also been observed clinically in liver transplantation with the replacement of donor by host Kupffer cells.[52] However, this has not been demonstrated for other transplanted human organs.[111] Long-term human allograft acceptance has also been associated with a diminished circulation of donor-specific alloreactive T cells.[33,55]

The role of regulatory immune responses in promoting allograft acceptance remains poorly understood. A variety of T suppressor cell populations have been identified in the circulation of stable allograft recipients[25,104] and have been directly isolated from human kidney and liver allografts.[41,42] The presence of anti-idiotypic antibodies directed against donor-specific alloantibodies has also been associated with improved renal graft outcome in patients with a history of sensitization to particular donor HLA antigens.[96,99,105] Immune regulation may also occur at the level of inflammatory mediator production to promote allograft acceptance. Several studies have demonstrated that the presence of a high frequency of functionally active alloreactive T cells within rat kidney[6,36,113] or liver[115] allografts does not necessarily lead to rejection. Indeed, in such models immunohistopathologic evaluation demonstrates a pattern of severe rejection, yet graft function is not impaired. Although the basis for this phenomenon remains unclear, the role of suppressor T cells[103] and anti-idiotypic antibodies[38] has been suggested, and the production, release, or activity of certain inflammatory mediators (e.g., thromboxane, IL-2) appears to be reduced.[35,113]

CLINICAL ASPECTS OF ALLOGRAFT REJECTION

Classification of Rejection

Allograft rejection can be categorized by immunologic, histopathologic, or clinical criteria. The value of any type of classification scheme is, of course, dependent upon its use and purpose. For the immunologist, the point of classifying allograft rejection is to identify differences in immune mechanisms; for the pathologist, it is to characterize differences in the type and degree of tissue damage; for the clinician, it is to provide information regarding the potential response to treatment and ultimately to predict outcome.

Clinical signs and symptoms of rejection are highly dependent upon the organ or tissue transplanted; their classification is discussed in detail in the appropriate parts of subsequent chapters. In general, the clinical changes associated with graft rejection for each type of organ transplant are the result of similar immune processes leading to comparable types of tissue damage. As discussed earlier, Type II (antibody-mediated) and Type IV (cell-mediated) immunopathologic reactions are those most commonly associated with allograft rejection. Because systemic posttransplant monitoring of immune function has not yet provided consistent or accurate methods for predicting or assessing graft rejection, the most useful means of classification still rely on clinical signs and symptoms as well as the immunopathologic changes observed in the graft tissue itself.

The hallmark of all types of graft rejection is inflammation. Both clinical and pathologic changes associated with rejection are influenced by the intensity, pattern, and type of inflammation affecting the graft. Therefore, proper and accurate classification is generally dependent upon these factors. In addition, the time after transplant at which rejection occurs and the speed of development are often useful indicators of the type of rejection process involved, although the terminology used can be misleading. For example, when rejection occurs later than 6 or 12 months following kidney transplantation, it is usually considered "chronic" and generally is slow and indolent in progression. However, in some patients a fulminant rejection can develop very quickly in a well-functioning graft years after transplant, often having been precipitated by patient noncompliance with therapy or some other host inflammatory process such as infection. Clearly, classifying this second type of process as "chronic" rejection may be misleading, because it has an "acute" onset.

Use of the terms *chronic* and *acute* may not only suggest the time after transplant or the speed of onset but can also imply the nature of the inflammatory reaction. Chronic inflammation suggests a predominantly cellular response (Type IV reaction), whereas acute inflammation suggests an antibody-mediated process (Type II or III reactions). The pathologic pattern of acute or chronic inflammation tends to correlate more with the speed of onset than with the time after transplant, but neither correlation is absolute; therefore, these terms must be qualified when used. A generalized scheme for correlating the temporal or clinical presentation of renal allograft rejection with immunologic and pathologic characteristics is depicted in Table 2.

HYPERACUTE REJECTION. As noted previously, hyperacute rejection is typically seen very soon after perfusion of the transplanted organ with host blood. Histologically, severe vascular damage is present and includes thrombosis, congestion, inflammation, and necrosis. There is extensive PMN infiltration, especially in and around vessels. The presumptive etiology of hyperacute rejection is humoral presensitization to donor ABO or HLA antigens; and although it is mediated by a Type II reaction, the analogy to an Arthus reaction is compelling. By means of immunofluorescence, deposits of immunoglobulin, complement, and fibrin are often observed in vessel walls, presenting a pattern very similar to that of a necrotizing vasculitis.

ACUTE REJECTION. Several subtypes of acute rejection have been proposed in attempts to separate cellular from humoral immune mechanisms or to differentiate interstitial from vascular damage (see Table 2). Acute rejection usually occurs within the first few weeks or months after transplantation and is of rapid onset. Early signs include fever, graft tenderness, edema, and decreased function. The variety of histologic patterns presumably reflects varying contributions from cellular and humoral immune mechanisms. One form of acute rejection, termed acute *humoral-vascular rejection,* is characterized by acute fibrinoid inflammation of arteries and arterioles with little cellular infiltration. This type of damage appears similar to that seen in hyperacute rejection, is associated with complement activation, and may also be analogous to a Type III serum sickness reaction, because the arterial system is primarily affected. However, while circulating immune complexes are often seen

after transplantation, they have no apparent correlation with rejection. Acute rejection reactions against vascular endothelium can also damage arteries as well as capillaries and other vessels that express MHC or other transplantation antigens and can be the result of cellular or ADCC-mediated reactions.[81] It is often difficult to obtain a direct assessment of the *in vivo* role of antibodies in acute rejection reactions, because anti-HLA as well as other antibodies can sometimes be eluted from the organ but not detected in the serum until the organ is removed.[76] Antibody could thus be causal, contributory, or secondary to these types of rejection.

A more common histologic pattern seen in acute rejection involves predominantly mononuclear cellular infiltrates in the interstitium *(interstitial-cellular rejection),* vessels, or both, leading to subsequent parenchymal and vascular damage. In some cases, significant reactions may be directed against epithelial cells, such as on renal tubules or hepatic bile ducts. These types of histologic and clinical reactions may represent a first-set (primary) response or a mixed first- and second-set (anamnestic) response that is delayed in onset by immunosuppression. A combination of antibody and cellular reactions is the most likely mechanism in this type of response, and the analogy to the Jones-Mote form of hypersensitivity appears close.

CHRONIC REJECTION. The most common pattern of chronic rejection is similar to that of a "cellular" rejection with pronounced mononuclear cell infiltration of the interstitium, vessels, or both. Because of the more indolent course of this process, a significant degree of scarring, often with chronic ischemic changes, is present. Classical delayed-type hypersensitivity (Type IV) and Jones-Mote reactions are both likely candidates for this rejection process. The difference in timing of onset may occur because of more adequate immunosuppression or because the reaction is against weaker histocompatibility disparities than in acute rejection. Recent studies also have suggested an association between chronic vascular rejection and increased dendritic cells in the walls of affected vessels.[85]

One additional form of allograft rejection should be mentioned, although it actually represents an attempt by cells in the graft to reject the host, i.e., the graft-versus-host (GVH) response. While GVH-mediated disease is most commonly seen in bone marrow transplantation when an immunoincompetent recipient differs from the donor at the HLA Class II region, the risk of GVH disease following lung or bowel transplantation is also significant because of the presence of abundant passenger lymphocytes in these organs. In addition, donor lymphocytes may produce antibodies against various antigens, leading to false-positive serologic results in the recipient[45] or hemolytic reactions when the donor and host are not ABO blood group–identical.[132]

DIAGNOSIS OF REJECTION. The presence of allograft rejection is typically indicated by graft dysfunction. However, because specific noninvasive means for documenting most causes of dysfunction are lacking, tissue biopsy of kidney, heart, and liver allografts has been routinely utilized to discriminate rejection from other processes, and to provide a qualitative and quantitative measure of any rejection reaction present to guide therapy. Routine serial biopsies of heart and liver allografts have proved to be an important means of predicting and assessing rejection; the value of renal allograft biopsy in cases of acute dysfunction has also been well documented.[117] Biopsy changes in the early posttransplant period are often helpful in distinguishing ischemic injury during donor organ recovery and preservation from humoral-vascular–mediated rejection or early aggressive acute cellular types of rejection. In clinically suspected cases of acute rejection at any time after transplantation, the presence of humorally mediated or severe vascular injury is usually a poor prognostic sign. The exclusion of other factors such as infection, drug toxicity, and *de novo* or recurrent disease is also very important in determining what therapy should be implemented. In cases of suspected chronic rejection, biopsy is often helpful in determining the extent and type of injury to guide future therapy.

Immune Risk Factors

PRESENSITIZATION AND PRIOR GRAFT FAILURE. Immune presensitization to donor alloantigens (especially ABO or HLA) provides a significant risk of rejection in renal and cardiac transplantation, and recently has been shown to be detrimental in liver transplantation.[37,48] Preformed antibodies to other donor antigens expressed on vascular endothelial cells have also been associated with renal and cardiac rejection, and their presence may therefore be considered a contraindication to transplantation.[20,28] Attempts to identify the risks associated with antibodies of different classes against different target alloantigens have involved a variety of analytic techniques utilizing different target cells, as summarized in Table 5. Unfortunately, most of these conclusions have been drawn by necessity from retrospective analyses of sera from patients undergoing rejection.

Sensitization to HLA antigens is most frequently the result of prior graft rejection, especially of poorly matched organs.[120] Pregnancy and blood transfusion also cause sensitization, but at somewhat lower rates and with a less detrimental effect on graft outcome.[125] It is now thought that preformed IgG antibodies against donor HLA Class I antigens present at any time prior to transplantation are a strong contraindication, whereas loss of IgM anti-donor HLA antibodies prior to transplantation may be safe, especially for primary graft recipients.[138] Actively reducing the titer of isohemagglutinins has permitted renal transplantation of ABO incompatible family members with good success.[2] The common presence of anti-A (A$_1$) blood group antibodies in patients who are of a different A blood group subtype (e.g., A$_2$) has also led to the practice of transplanting such patients with grafts from O blood group donors. Reciprocally, A$_2$ blood group donor organs have been successfully transplanted into O recipients.

For largely technical reasons, the evaluation of host presensitization to potential donor alloantigens has generally focused on humoral presensitization. However, it is clear that cellular presensitization exists and can potentially be measured by available *in vitro* assays. In this regard an association between humoral sensitization following donor specific blood transfusion and elevated anti-donor MLR activity has been reported.[119] Moreover, the MLR and assays of donor-specific cell-mediated lympholysis (CML) have been useful in assessing the potential for rejection (and graft-versus-host disease) in allogeneic bone marrow transplantation. Finally, limiting dilution analyses to quantitate the precursor frequency of cytotoxic or proliferative T-cell responses against donor alloantigens have been used clinically and experimentally in posttransplant monitoring but have not yet provided a consistent prediction of graft rejection when assessed prior to transplantation. The significant amount of time (days) needed for performance of such cellular assays makes their clinical application, at least for cadaveric transplantation, impractical.

Prior rejection of an organ allograft commonly leads to sensitization and has been consistently associated with poorer outcome of a subsequent graft, although the reasons for this remain unclear. One explanation involves the concept that such patients are "high responders" to alloantigens, so that first graft rejection is simply an indicator of their greater propensity to exhibit allogeneic responses. Related to this is the common finding that patients who have rejected a graft frequently develop alloantibodies of relatively broad specificity that are reactive with public epitopes. Thus, the risk associated with prior graft rejection may also be due to the presence of undetected presensitization to donor alloantigens not shared with the initial donor. The observation that very good HLA matching has a more profound effect in reducing rejection of retransplanted and highly sensitized patients[88,95] supports both of these possibilities.

HLA MISMATCHING. The importance of HLA mismatching between donor and recipient remains controversial, based on the perception by some that current immunosuppressive regimens can fully obviate the underlying risk of donor HLA disparity. Several single center and a few large multicenter studies[43,69] have suggested no significant risk with HLA mismatching for first kidney transplant recipients. However, in all of these studies the number of well-matched patients included was too small to permit valid statistical conclusions that HLA matching provided no benefit. In addition, these studies generally have considered only short-term (less than 3 years) outcome, a period during which the full impact of the risk of HLA mismatching on chronic rejection cannot be evaluated. Nearly all large studies involving a sufficient number of good and poorly HLA-matched patients for valid statistical comparisons have consistently demonstrated that poorly matched kidney transplant patients remain at a higher risk for graft rejection even with the excellent results seen over the past 5 years.[5,87,88,140,142,144] Because the degree of HLA matching is associated with a variety of potentially confounding factors (e.g., presensitization, transplant number, donor/recipient race, use of local versus shared organs), appropriately stratified studies are necessary and multivariate analysis desirable to clearly identify the relative risk of HLA mismatching. One such study of almost 6000 renal transplants between 1983 and 1988 from

---

TABLE 5. Evaluation of Preformed Antidonor Antibodies

Target Specificity	Additional Tests	Interpretation
T cell	Historic versus current	IgG anti-donor HLA Class I a contraindication in current or historic samples. IgM anti-HLA Class I may be acceptable in historic samples.
B cell	Identify isotype, temperature reactivity, target	Warm-reactive, IgG or high titer IgM anti-donor HLA Class II a contraindication. IgM anti-Class II acceptable if in historic samples only.
Autologous lymphocytes	Autoabsorption; test chronic lymphocytic leukemia cells (negative)	Often IgM, cold-reactive, B-cell-reactive, with low avidity. Not a contraindication for transplantation.
ABO blood group	Subgroup (e.g., A$_2$) identification	A$_1$ donor to A$_2$ recipient may be contraindicated; A$_2$ donor may be acceptable for O recipient.
Monocyte	Screen for vascular endothelial cell (VEC) reactivity	Non-HLA or VEC reactive (e.g., anti-HMA) not a contraindication.
Vascular endothelial cell (VEC)	VEC panel screening	Suggested association with renal, cardiac rejection with donor-specific reactivity.

TABLE 6. The Significance and Relative Risk of Factors Associated with Renal Allograft Failure

Variable*	Level	P Value	Relative Risk†
Delayed function	Yes	$<10^{-5}$	1.98
CsA use	No	$<10^{-5}$	1.73
Presensitization (PRA)	>60%	$<10^{-5}$	1.45
Diabetes	Yes	<0.003	1.39
Race	Black	<0.0008	1.23
Prior failure	Yes	<0.005	2.80
Donor source	Shared	NS	1.07
Age	≤14	$<10^{-5}$	1.81
HLA-A,- B, -DR match	0 vs. 6	<0.0002	3.13
HLA-A, -B match	0 vs. 4	$<10^{-5}$	1.62
HLA-DR match	0 vs. 2	<0.0002	1.32

* Other variables included but not shown are nephrectomy; splenectomy; antilymphocyte serum use; year of transplant; recipient age 15 to 25, 25 to 44, 45 to 54, sex, and center identification.

† Relative risk determined by the Cox proportional hazards model for all 5954 patients who underwent transplantation at SEOPF centers between November 1983 and May 1987.

Data abstracted from Sanfilippo et al.[124]

the 50 centers of the South-Eastern Organ Procurement Foundation (SEOPF) in the United States demonstrated significant and independent risks for mismatching HLA-A, HLA-B, and HLA-DR antigens upon multivariate analyses that included many other risk factors.[124] As shown in Table 6, the relative risk for a 0 HLA-A, -B, -DR antigen match (compared with a 6 HLA antigen match) transplant recipient was found to be greater than that of any other risk factor identified. These results also demonstrate the significant risk of prior graft failure and broad humoral presensitization as measured by panel-reactive antibody (PRA, see below).

OTHER FACTORS. Two other important immunologic factors associated with graft outcome are donor graft injury and pretransplant blood transfusions. As mentioned above, inflammatory reactions in a graft due to ischemia, drug reaction, infection, or other factors may promote a rejection reaction by affecting the immunogenicity of the graft (by stimulating donor APCs, up-regulating donor MHC antigens, or causing the release of inflammatory mediators), or by the attraction of activated T cells directed against viral or other antigens that crossreact with donor MHC. Pretransplant blood transfusions have been long associated with improved allograft survival in experimental models and clinical practice, and will be discussed in detail below. A summary of immune risk factors is depicted in Table 7.

Immunologic Testing

Histocompatibility testing prior to transplant surgery has proven to be very useful in optimizing donor selection for individual patients by identifying organs that should be either (1) excluded because of presensitization or unacceptable incompatibility or (2) preferentially utilized because of an excellent HLA match. Histocompatibility testing of prospective transplant recipients typically involves several types of studies, including HLA typing of both donor and recipient, crossmatching of various serum samples from the recipient against donor lymphocytes, and prescreening serum samples from the recipient for anti-HLA antibodies.

HLA TYPING. While several methods are available for identifying HLA genes or their products,[108] the approaches used clinically in evaluating potential transplant recipients and donors are based largely on technical and practical considerations. The relatively short time available for HLA testing of cadaveric organ donors generally allows only microlymphocytotoxicity testing to identify serologically defined HLA-A, HLA-B, and HLA-DR antigens. Thus, the more time consuming (and costly) cellular and molecular genetic techniques used to better characterize HLA (especially Class II) specificities are not routinely applied at present for potential recipients of cadaver organs. Logistical difficulties also preclude HLA phenotyping the biologic relatives of cadaveric donors to identify haplotypes or homozygous (versus unidentified or blank) alleles. These constraints lead to a limited ability to match donors with recipients and prevent the identification of certain mismatched antigens. For example, if only one HLA-DR antigen is serologically identified upon HLA typing of a donor, it is quite possible that the donor is not homozygous for that antigen and expresses a second HLA-DR (mismatched) antigen that is not detected for technical reasons. Even if serologic identity is established for a donor and recipient at HLA-DR, this does not ensure their identity for all T-cell (or antibody) defined epitopes of HLA-DR. Moreover, identity at HLA-DR does not ensure identity for other Class II HLA antigens (DP, DQ), which are less frequently identified. Thus, the current practice of identifying up to six serologically defined HLA-A, -B, and -DR antigens for matching organ donors and recipients grossly underestimates the large number of potentially disparate cellular and serologically defined specificities that are expressed by these six molecules, as well as products of other untyped HLA loci.

In addition to technical problems in fully characterizing the HLA types of cadaveric donors, the tremendous polymorphism of the HLA system creates practical problems in identifying well-matched recipients for each donor. However, by placing patients from many centers on pooled computer lists, well-matched recipients can be more frequently transplanted by sharing of donor organs among centers, as has been the practice for many years in regions of the United States and Europe. Efforts to overcome these various technical and logistical difficulties in order to transplant cadaveric donor kidneys into well matched recipients has been largely justified by reducing the risk of rejection, lowering the rate of sensitization following graft failure, and increasing the transplant rate for highly sensitized patients.[89,120,124,136,142,144]

In cases where organ or tissue donation from a willing live-related donor is possible (i.e., kidney, bone marrow, segmental pancreas, or liver), HLA typing of the immediate family is usually performed (genotyping) to define the patient's haplotypes as well as to identify the best-matched prospective donor. This situation also provides sufficient time to apply additional cellular or molecular genetic procedures to identify any subtle HLA incompatibilities that may exist between potential donors and a related recipient. Although 1- to 3-year graft survival of HLA-identical sibling renal transplants is now only modestly greater

TABLE 7. Immune Factors Associated with Outcome in Organ Transplantation

Factor	Proposed Associations
Presensitization/prior graft rejection	"High responder" status; undetected (pretransplant) anti-donor immunity
ABO mismatch	Preformed/immune isohemagglutins leading to humoral rejection
HLA mismatch	Increased host stimulation, target antigens
Donor graft injury: inflammatory/ischemic	Increased donor organ immunogenicity
Pretransplant blood transfusion	Negative selection due to sensitization; induced unresponsiveness (?)

than 1 or 0 haplotype-matched transplants,[62,101,123] the recipient of a non–HLA-identical live-donor transplant is generally subject to an increased risk of graft rejection and therefore is usually placed on a protocol involving stronger immunosuppression or pretransplant transfusion.

HLA typing has also been proposed to be of clinical value in identifying any HLA allele or combination of antigens on the haplotype that may be more immunogenic than others. Immune response genes identified in the mouse have been directly associated with the level of host reactivity to particular antigens, and many of these are located in the mouse MHC. In the human, profound differences in immune responses to certain specific antigens have been demonstrated *in vivo* and *in vitro*, but detailed attempts to compare systematically the immunogenicity of HLA haplotypes have been unsuccessful even when family members tested were HLA-identical to the recipient but not available as organ donors.[3] Studies suggesting that HLA-DRw6 in renal allograft recipients is associated with a higher rate of rejection if mismatched[54] await confirmation and further analysis, because the serologically defined DRw6 antigen actually identifies a complex set of multiple alleles.

CROSSMATCHING. To identify the presence of donor-specific anti-HLA antibodies in a potential organ recipient, patient serum is tested against donor lymphocytes usually by microlymphocytotoxicity assay. A positive crossmatch reaction has been known for over 20 years to be associated with an increased risk of hyperacute kidney graft rejection, and the risks for heart and more recently liver transplants have been well recognized. Because presensitized patients are at the highest risk for a positive crossmatch, a fundamental conflict arises in trying to determine the best approach to crossmatch testing. Attempts to increase biologic sensitivity (i.e., decrease the rate of false-negative tests) generally decreases biologic specificity (i.e., increase the rate of false-positive tests). Thus, simply increasing the analytic sensitivity of the crossmatch assay may reduce the incidence of overall rejection in transplant recipients, but at a cost of inappropriately excluding potential donors for highly sensitized patients in whom transplantation is difficult. It should also be remembered that vascular endothelium (the primary target cell in this reaction) expresses various antigens other than HLA that may also function as potential targets for preformed antibodies that are not detected by routine testing. Crossmatch tests may therefore appear negative if the relevant donor antigens are not expressed on the cells tested[28,59] or if the assay tests an *in vitro* antibody function (e.g., complement-mediated lysis of donor cells) different from that of potential *in vivo* relevance (e.g., ADCC) to the particular host.[81] Because the association between rejection and a positive crossmatch by even the least sensitive method is not absolute,[92] selecting an assay of appropriate sensitivity and specificity, especially for sensitized patients urgently needing a transplant, remains a difficult problem.

Several studies and observations have helped to address these questions. Modifications of the standard microlymphocytotoxicity test have been employed to better characterize crossmatch reactions, and include adding wash steps, extending incubation times, or adding antiglobulin reagents to increase sensitivity; using isolated target populations (T cells, B cells, monocytes, vascular endothelial cells), testing at different temperatures, and adding IgM reducing agents to improve specificity; and absorbing test sera with autologous cells to remove autoreactive or nonspecific antibodies. In addition, flow cytometry and other binding or labeling procedures have been used to better characterize host antibody reactions against donor cells.[22,66,137]

The current status of crossmatch testing has been best evaluated for renal transplantation: the standard microcytotoxicity test against unseparated lymphocytes generally identifies the presence of IgG or IgM anti–donor Class I antibodies, which are a contraindication if present at the time of transplant. Although some reactions may be false-positive because of autoantibody or non-HLA antibodies, these can usually be identified by appropriate absorption. The use of donor B cells as targets can improve sensitivity, because they express higher levels of Class I HLA than T cells, but can diminish specificity, because of increased reactions by non-HLA antibodies, especially with the surface IgM receptor of B cells. B cells also express class II HLA and may therefore identify anti-donor Class II HLA antibodies, which can be detrimental, especially if at high titer. The presence of cold reactive or IgM anti-donor lymphocyte antibodies usually indicates acceptable non-HLA antibodies, although this is not always the case; simply inhibiting IgM reactions by adding reducing agents may occasionally eliminate important IgM anti-HLA antibodies and yield false-negative results.

Of particular clinical value has been the suggestion that patients who have lost donor-reactive alloantibody (i.e., have a positive crossmatch with historical but not current serum samples) should not necessarily be excluded as recipients of organs from such donors,[24,126] and may exhibit anti-idiotypic antibodies that have been associated with a reduced risk of graft rejection.[96,99,105] Because most current assays for anti-idiotypic antibody usually involve inhibition of specific alloantibody–mediated lysis of target cells, the presence of immune complexes (with donor HLA molecules) or other serum factors that may cause such reactions must be excluded before one can confirm the presence of such anti-idiotypic antibodies. Moreover, more recent studies indicate that the loss of some anti-HLA antibodies (e.g., IgG anti-Class I) may not substantially reduce the risk of rejection, especially in retransplanted patients who do not develop anti-idiotypic antibodies.[96,99,105,106,138,145]

ANTIBODY SCREENING. Patient sera are routinely tested prior to transplantation by microlymphocytotoxicity assay against a panel of lymphocytes from 30 to 100 HLA-typed volunteers for identification of the presence of preformed anti-HLA antibodies. The percentage of reactive panel cells indicates the degree of panel-reactive antibody (PRA), which approximately reflects the likelihood of a positive crossmatch with a random donor. For example, if a patient serum reacts with all 100 panel cells (PRA, 100 per cent), it is likely that cells from any potential donor will also react and yield a positive crossmatch. Conversely, a patient with a PRA of 0 per cent is likely to have a negative crossmatch with most donors. However, since not all HLA specificities are usually expressed on a screening panel, a patient with a 0 per cent PRA may have a positive crossmatch against some donors, just as a patient with a 100 per cent PRA may have a negative crossmatch with some very well matched donors. A very high PRA usually indicates the presence of multiple anti-HLA antibodies, antibodies against common (public) HLA specificities, or other (non-HLA) lymphocytotoxic antibodies such as autoantibodies. The reactivity pattern of panel cells often indicates the specificities of anti-HLA antibodies in the patient serum. Thus, if only panel cells expressing HLA-A1 are lysed by a patient serum, this antigen can be identified as "unacceptable," and donors expressing HLA-A1 are automatically excluded for this patient on computerized matching programs.

Unfortunately for many patients with a high PRA, specific unacceptable antigens cannot be identified, making it very difficult to find appropriate donors for them. Two approaches have been recently developed to address this problem: (1) sharing patient sera among many centers to test against multiple donors[67] and (2) testing patient sera against large extended panels to identify any disparate (non-self) HLA antigens that are acceptable.[31] The success of these and other approaches in transplanting highly sensitized patients clearly requires cooperation among many centers to share donor organs for such patients to increase the available donor pool. The sharing of very well matched organs for highly sensitized patients is of importance in reducing both the risk of a positive crossmatch and the risk of rejection if the patient undergoes transplantation.

POSTTRANSPLANTATION MONITORING. Although the diversity of immunologic assays that have been examined over the past 20 years for potential use in evaluating transplant recipients is impressive, nearly all have proved of limited value or impractical for general application. Highly sensitive assays employing antibody-dependent cellular cytotoxicity, radiolabeled targets, or labeled antibody techniques to identify circulating antibodies directed against donor-specific or non–donor-specific alloantigens have been used with variable success but frequently give false-negative results. In addition, testing of host cell-mediated alloimmunity using stimulation assays (such as MLR or mitogen responsiveness), effector function assays (such as cell-mediated cytotoxicity), regulatory cell assays (such as autologous MLR), or limiting dilution assays (to determine alloreactive T cell precursor frequencies) may yield useful data but generally require extensive time and expense that limit their utility. Technically simple tests such as phenotypic evaluation of circulating lymphocytes have generally not had a high predictive value for discriminating graft rejection from infection or other factors and probably are best suited for identifying severe depression of host immunity. A frequent problem with these and other assays utilizing peripheral blood lymphocytes or serum is the variable expression of rejection (humoral versus cellular). It is also clear that the most important reactions occur in the graft itself and are not necessarily manifested systemically.

Immune Manipulation

A major goal of research in transplantation has been to develop a means of promoting allograft acceptance by the host immune system; a partial list of approaches and methods directed toward this goal is presented in Table 8. Work in this area has involved manipulation of all three limbs of immune responsiveness (i.e., afferent, central, and efferent components) by attempting to (1) reduce host immune recognition or stimulation, (2) induce suppressive host immune regulatory responses, or (3) inhibit host immune effector reactions. Although several experimental approaches have focused on manipulating a particular limb of the immune system, the two methods most commonly employed in clinical transplantation are immunosuppressive therapy and pretransplant blood transfusion. Both have developed empirically and exhibit a variety of complex effects on all components of the immune system.

IMMUNOSUPPRESSIVE THERAPY. The goal of immunosuppressive therapy in the transplant recipient is to selectively reduce or eliminate donor-specific alloreactivity while preserving the remaining functions of the immune system to provide host defenses, especially against infection. Unfortunately, present therapeutic modalities are largely nonspecific in their effect on the immune system. Immunosuppressive therapy is often able to provide long-term graft survival or reverse rejection episodes, but at the expense of subjecting the patient to numerous complications and side effects, which most frequently involve infection, drug reactions, and lymphoproliferative disorders.

Current methods for preventing or treating graft rejection are diverse and include physical, pharmacologic, and immunologic means of eliminating immunocompetent cells or interfering with their activity. Physical techniques have included surgical therapy to remove thoracic duct lymphocytes by drainage or to excise other lymphoid and accessory tissue (e.g., spleen, thymus), irradiation to destroy or deplete lymphoid tissue, and pheresis to remove circulating leukocytes and/or antibodies. Drug therapy includes various immunosuppressive, anti-inflammatory, and cytotoxic agents that interfere with or prevent normal immune responsiveness, the most important of which are currently cyclosporine, glucocorticoids, and azathioprine. Immune therapy includes the use of heterologous (e.g., rabbit, horse) anti-thymocyte globulin (ATG) or anti-lymphocyte serum (ALS), and more recently mouse monoclonal antibodies against T cells (e.g., OKT3). The clinical application and mechanisms of action of these and several new, more potent agents are discussed in later sections.

THE TRANSFUSION EFFECT. Pretransplant blood transfusions were initially considered detrimental to graft survival because they were associated with recipient sensitization and thus increased the risk of hyperacute rejection. However, transfusion was often needed to treat the anemia seen with end-stage renal disease, and observations by the mid 1970s suggested that transfused recipients of crossmatch-negative renal grafts had substantially improved graft survival.[90] Although controversial, this finding was soon confirmed by numerous clinical studies and led to the general use of blood transfusion prior to cadaver donor renal transplantation. Based on these clinical observations and experimental studies in various animal models, the use of pretransplantation donor specific blood transfusions (DSBTs) was evaluated in one haplotype-identical living-related donor transplantation. Although a significant number of patients became sensitized to transfusions from their potential donor (leading to donor exclusion), there was a marked increase

TABLE 8. Immune Manipulations Prior to Transplant That May Promote Allograft Acceptance

Approach/Method	Immune Effects	Current Status
Transfusion enhancement: pretransplant donor or random blood	Presensitization (negative selection); stimulate anti-idiotypic Ab(?)	Commonly used in renal transplantation
Thoracic duct drainage	Host T-cell depletion, reduced immune responsiveness	Previously used in renal transplantation
Total lymphoid irradiation (TLI)	Reduced immune responsiveness, active tolerance induction (?)	Occasional use in renal transplantation
Depletion of specific T cell populations with monoclonal antibody (mAb)	Reduced responsiveness; promotes tolerance (?)	Extensive experimental work in animal models
Ab removal by plasmapheresis, absorption (± drug therapy)	Reduced Ab titer in presensitized patients; inhibited humoral rejection	Occasional use for ABO incompatible live donors of presensitized recipients
Induced chimerism: immune depletion plus donor (± host) bone marrow cells	Donor-specific tolerance	Extensive work in animals; occasional clinical application
Enhancement: passive transfer of anti-donor Ab	Reduced host anti-donor responsiveness	Experimental in animals
Active immunization with host anti-donor Ab or cells	Stimulated regulatory anti-idiotypic Ab or T cells	Experimental in animals
Tolerance induction to donor alloantigens (solubilized ± immunosuppression)	Specific unresponsiveness to donor	Experimental in animals
Donor organ treatment: ultraviolet radiation, mAb, prolonged culture, hyperbaric O$_2$	Depleted antigen-presenting cells, passenger cells in graft; reduced immunogenicity	Experimental for pancreatic islets and cornea grafting; some preliminary clinical application (islets)

in graft survival (for those patients not forming antibodies) to a level indistinguishable from that of HLA-identical siblings.[116] Pretransplant DSBT has also been used in patients with HLA mismatched living-unrelated (usually spouse) donors with remarkable success indicated from initial reports.[133] However, recent multicenter studies suggest that random blood transfusions are as effective as donor-specific transfusions for 1-haplotype and 0-haplotype matched live-donor renal transplants.[123]

Despite extensive examination, the mechanisms of transfusion enhancement remain unclear. Negative donor selection due to preferential transfusion-induced sensitization of patients at a higher risk of rejection (i.e., potential high responders) probably represents some but not all of the benefit associated with transfusion. The finding that transfusions provide some benefit when given at the time of transplant (i.e., after crossmatching) cannot be explained by selection.[56,122] In addition, reducing the degree of sensitization from DSBT by either storage of blood[68,149] or concurrent administration of low-dose azathioprine[4] has apparently not affected the observed increase in graft survival and also questions selection. Several clinical studies suggest that blood transfusions can suppress host immunity in a variety of ways. Random donor transfusions in potential cadaveric graft recipients have been associated with nonspecific suppression of cellular immunity by some investigators,[1,13,44] and others have identified the development of antibodies that suppress host immunity by inhibiting the Fc receptor of B cells[70] or demonstrating anti-idiotypic activity against alloantibody and allospecific T cells as discussed above. Surprisingly, only a few studies have examined the influence of transfusions on acute or chronic phase serum reactants in terms of potential allograft protection. Indeed, factors such as the serum protease inhibitor alpha$_2$-macroglobulin, which may have a role in protecting the fetus from maternal immunity, may also be affected by blood transfusion.

Recent detailed experiments in rats have demonstrated that DSBT does not inhibit the generation of alloreactive T-cell infiltration in kidney allografts.[6,36,113] However, in contrast to controls, rats given DSBTs have been reported to demonstrate normal renal graft function, and no elevation in allograft thromboxane[113] or IL-2 production[35] as observed in controls. In addition, DSBT alone appears to induce T-suppressor cells[103] as well as an anti-idiotypic antibody response that is accelerated following transplantation and associated with reduced IgG alloantibody production and graft deposition.[38] While not necessarily analogous to the situation in humans, these findings demonstrate the complexity of a phenomenon that has been studied for almost 2 decades in animals and utilized for over 10 years in clinical renal transplantation.

ALLOGRAFT ENHANCEMENT AND TOLERANCE. In seeking potential methods to immunologically enhance allograft survival, manipulations at the early recognition or regulation phases of responsiveness have been usually considered more likely to provide a complete and long-term effect than manipulation at the effector stage. The most direct way of blocking host immune stimulation by an allograft would be to functionally mask or delete the molecules (allo-MHC) or the major cells (donor APC) that stimulate host allograft responses. Several methods have been used in an attempt to reduce the immunogenicity of allografts, and in particular to deplete or inactivate donor APC. Most of these approaches are limited technically to relatively small tissue allografts (e.g., pancreatic islets, cornea, skin) because they involve manipulations of the graft in culture, such as using high oxygen tension, prolonged incubation, low temperature, or exposure to ultraviolet radiation. Each of these treatments can inhibit donor APC viability, function, or the expression of MHC antigens in a variety of ways and have been demonstrated to enhance allograft acceptance in numerous animal models.

For technical reasons, manipulation of large vascularized organs has been mainly limited to pretreatment with anti-inflammatory agents or monoclonal antibodies directed against donor APCs, with only limited success in reducing immunogenicity. Although some agents and media extend the preservation time of human organs and reduce ischemic or inflammatory injury, attempts to diminish immunogenicity by these methods has been disappointing to date. Even if donor MHC alloantigens could be completely blocked from stimulating a host response, the occasional rejection of HLA-identical sibling renal allografts demonstrates that other minor histocompatibility antigens not linked to the MHC cannot be ignored.

An alternative means of preventing host immunity to specific alloantigens is to selectively delete potential alloreactive clones prior to transplantation. Experiments in the mid 1970s provided some optimism for this approach. Donor-specific alloreactive cells from recipient rat strains were used to immunize other syngeneic (identical) recipient animals, which responded by deleting their own alloreactive clones, allowing marked prolongation of grafts from the donor strain.[15] Similar experiments using passively transferred antisera directed against allospecific receptors (idiotypes) gave comparable results. Unfortunately, these techniques were found to improve graft survival only in certain animal species and strain combinations, and in other cases anti-idiotypic reactions were found to stimulate, rather than suppress, host responses.

Other approaches for inducing enhanced graft survival have been directed to different regulatory stages of allogeneic responsiveness. Various experiments have shown that specific unresponsiveness or tolerance can be induced when certain alloantigens or allogeneic cells are presented in a particular manner, such as in soluble or membrane preparations (with cyclosporine or monoclonal anti–T-cell antibodies), or by exposure via portal vein inoculation. Specific allograft tolerance has also been induced in rats by treatment of graft recipients with hyperimmune antisera against donor alloantigens, a procedure demonstrated to induce T-suppressor cells in the host. The ability to generate human T-suppressor cells in vitro against autologous alloreactive T cells[82] has been demonstrated by means of peripheral blood T cells from transplant recipients,[42] raising the possibility of adoptively transferring autologous T-suppressor cells generated in vitro to promote tolerance, as recently described in the rat.[146] Host manipulation by total lymphoid irradiation (TLI) has yielded transplant tolerance in experimental models and apparent tolerance to renal allografts in limited clinical trials.[29] The effects of TLI are multifactoral but predominantly involve the inhibition of effector cell generation, migration, and function. Of particular interest have been experiments in which animals are given lethal or sublethal preconditioning regimens of irradiation,[128] chemotherapy,[75] or anti–T-cell monoclonal antibodies,[102] followed by reconstitution with donor (with or without host) bone marrow cells. This procedure leads to stable mixed chimerism, allowing specific allograft tolerance without further immunosuppressive treatment.

An additional means of promoting allograft acceptance has been directed toward inhibiting the production, activity, or utilization of inflammatory mediators released during rejection reactions. Preliminary studies utilizing this approach have been reported and have focused on using monoclonal antibodies directed to particular cytokines (e.g., IFN-γ) or their receptors (e.g., IL-2 receptor) or using synthetic analogs (e.g., thromboxane synthetase inhibitors) to block inflammatory reactions.[32,63,130] Clearly, this is an area of tremendous potential, and rapid advancements are possible as the key regulatory and effector molecules responsible for graft dysfunction due to rejection are identified. Attempts to functionally block inflammatory mediators or their cellular receptors at the molecular and genetic levels have already been initiated and are likely to yield interesting and important new data of potentially great clinical relevance in the very near future.

SELECTED REFERENCES

Ashwell, J. D., Chen, C., and Schwartz, R. H.: High frequency and nonrandom distribution of alloreactivity in T cell clones selected for recognition of foreign antigen in association with self class II molecules. J. Immunol., *136*:389, 1986.
This important paper effectively demonstrates that a high percentage of T-cell clones that recognize specific antigens plus host-MHC also recognize allogeneic APCs directly. A large series of T-cell clones were generated in a particular mouse strain (B10.A) against three different antigens (GAT, pigeon cytochrome c, sheep insulin). Clones specifically reactive with these antigens plus host-MHC determinants were examined for reactivity against allogeneic APCs of various haplotypes. Of the 62 clones identified, 38 (61 per cent) were reactive against allogeneic APCs, the majority of which demonstrated patterns of reactivity suggesting the recognition of "public" allodeterminants.

Braun, W. M.: Laboratory and clinical management of the highly sensitized organ transplant recipient. Hum. Immunol., *26*:245, 1989.
This article reviews the current status of presensitization in potential organ allograft recipients from both clinical and immunologic perspectives. Substantial information is provided on the interpretation of different crossmatch testing procedures. In particular, common misconceptions regarding test interpretation are provided. This review also examines the recent literature considering associations between certain types of positive serologic crossmatches and graft outcome and is important reading for those involved in clinical transplantation.

Kojima, M., Cease, K. B., Buckenmeyer, G. K., and Berzofsky, J. A.: Limiting dilution comparison of the repertoires of high and low responder MHC-restricted T cells. J. Exp. Med., *167*:1100, 1988.
This study examines the potential basis for high and low responder host status to particular antigens at the level of T-cell recognition. The reported findings support the concept that high responder status is associated with an increased repertoire of T cells that recognize immunodominant epitopes in the context of specific MHC restriction elements. Although the basis for immunodominance of particular epitopes is unclear and alternative explanations for the results of these experiments are provided, this paper provides a stimulating discussion of these fundamental concepts at the genetic, molecular, and cellular levels.

Mattson, D. H., Shimojo, N., Cowan, E. P., Baskin, J. J., Turner, R. V., Shvetsky, B. D., Coligan, J. E., Maloy, W. L., and Biddison, W. E.: Differential effects of amino acid substitutions in the β-sheet floor and α-2 helix of HLA-A2 on recognition by alloreactive viral peptide-specific cytotoxic T lymphocytes. J. Immunol., *143*:1101, 1989.
This is one of several recent studies examining the potential contributions of specific MHC determinants and bound peptide to T-cell receptor interactions. Using human alloreactive cytotoxic T lymphocytes and target cells with specific amino acid substitutions for HLA-A2, it was found that changes in areas presumed to affect peptide binding had the greatest effect on allorecognition. Although the nature of interactions among different sites on the MHC molecule, its bound peptide, and the T-cell receptor remain unclear, this paper provides a valuable framework for considering these issues.

Murray, J. S., Madri, J., Tite, J., Carding, S. R., and Bottomly K.: MHC control of CD4⁺ T cell subset activation. J. Exp. Med., *170*:2135, 1989.
This study examines the potential role of specific MHC Class II haplotypes in affecting the nature of host responsiveness via stimulation of different T-helper cell subsets. Responsiveness by different inbred strains of mice to collagen Type IV antigen demonstrated preferential activation of IL-2/IFN-γ–producing Th1 cells, whereas responses to the same antigen in a strain differing only for one MHC Class II gene led to activation of IL-4–producing (Th2) cells. These findings raise important issues as to the role of specific MHC haplotypes in controlling the nature (cellular versus humoral) of host responses to particular antigens.

Rosenberg, A. S., Mizvoch, T., Sharrow, S. O., and Singer, A.: Phenotype, specificity, and function of T cells subsets and T cell interactions involved in skin allograft rejection. J. Exp. Med., *165*:1296, 1987.
This study examines in detail the characteristics and interactions of T-cell subsets involved in rejecting mouse skin grafts. Several basic findings are of general importance. In particular, the data presented strongly support the concept that graft rejection (at least in this model) requires the in vivo interaction of functionally distinct T-cell subsets expressing helper and effector activities. Interestingly, these functionally distinct T-cell populations can express the same or different phenotype (CD4, CD8) and may even exhibit specificity for different alloantigens. Thus, assumptions of T-cell function based only on phenotype (CD4, CD8) or MHC specificity may be misleading.

Sanfilippo, F., Vaughn, W. K., Alexander, J. W., LeFor, W. M., Lucas, B. A., and Pfaff, W. W.: Organ sharing for good HLA-A, B, and DR matching improves cadaver renal graft survival in SEOPF: Retrospective and prospective studies considering delayed graft function, race, center effects, cyclosporine, and other factors. *In* Terasaki, P. I. (Ed.): Clinical Transplants 1988. Los Angeles, UCLA Tissue Typing Laboratory, 1988, pp. 211–223.
This report describes two multicenter studies from the same group of centers and examines the effect of HLA matching in renal transplantation, considering a large number of potentially confounding factors. An observational study using multivariate analysis documented the significant and independent benefits of HLA-A, HLA-B, and HLA-DR matching on overall graft outcome for patients undergoing transplantation at these centers. A prospective study also demonstrated that centers agreeing to share donor kidneys for well-matched recipients at a high frequency, beginning in 1986, had a significant increase in graft survival within 2 *years to a level greater than that of control centers, which showed no improvement during the study period.*

REFERENCES

1. Agostino, G. J., Kahan B. D., and Kerman, R. H.: Suppression of mixed leukocyte culture using leukocytes from normal individuals, uremic patients and allograft recipients. Transplantation, *34*:367, 1982.
2. Alexandre, G. P. J., Squifflet, J. P., DeBruyere, M., et al.: Present experiences in a series of 26 ABO-incompatible living donor renal allografts. Transplant. Proc., *9*:4538, 1987.
3. Amos, D. B., Ward, F. E., Zmijewski, C. M., et al.: Graft donor selection based upon single locus (haplotype) analysis within families. Transplantation, *6*:524, 1968.
4. Anderson, C. B., Sicard, G. A., and Etheridge, E. E.: Pretreatment of renal allograft recipients with azathioprine and donor-specific blood products. Surgery, *92*:315, 1982.
5. Annual Report of the United Network for Organ Sharing, Richmond, Virginia, 1989.
6. Armstrong, H. E., Bolton, E. M., McMillan, I., Spencer, S. C., and Bradley, J. A.: Prolonged survival of actively enhanced rat renal allografts despite accelerated cellular infiltration and rapid induction of both class I and class II MHC antigens. J. Exp. Med., *164*:891, 1987.
7. Ashwell, J. D., Chen, C., and Schwartz, R. H.: High frequency and nonrandom distribution of alloreactivity in T cell clones selected for recognition of foreign antigen in association with self class II molecules. J. Immunol., *136*:389, 1986.
8. Bach, F. H., and Amos, D. B.: Hu-1: Major histocompatibility locus in man. Science, *156*:1506, 1967.
9. Bach, F., and Hirschhorn, K.: Lymphocytic interaction: A potential histocompatibility test in vitro. Science, *143*:813, 1964.
10. Bain, B., Vas, M. R., and Lowerstein, L.: The development of large immature mononuclear cells in mixed leukocyte cultures. Blood, *23*:108, 1964.
11. Baldwin, W. M., III, and Sanfilippo, F.: Antibodies and graft rejection. Transplant. Proc., *21*:605, 1989.
12. Balkwill, F. R., and Burke, F.: The cytokine network. Immunology Today, *10*:299, 1989.
13. Bensussan, A., Klatzmann, D., Gluckerman, J. C., Kalil, J., Dausset, J., and Sasportes, M.: Probable role of suppressor cells and factors in kidney graft survival. Transplant. Proc., *14*:584, 1982.
14. Bill, J., Yague, J., Appel, V. B., White, J., Horn, G., Erlich, H. A., and Palmer, E.: Molecular genetic analysis of 178 I-Abm12-reactive T cells. J. Exp. Med., *169*:115, 1989.
15. Binz, H., and Wigzell, H.: Specific transplantation tolerance induced by autoimmunization against the individual's own naturally occurring idiotypic, antigen-binding receptors. J. Exp. Med., *144*:1438, 1976.
16. Bjorkman, P. J., Saper, M. A., Samraoui, B., Bennet, W. S., Strominger, J. L., and Wiley, D. C.: Structure of the human class I histocompatibility antigen, HLA-A2. Nature, *329*:506, 1987.
17. Bjorkman, P. J., Saper, M. A., Samraoui, B., Bennet, W. S., Strominger, J. L., and Wiley D. C.: The foreign antigen binding site and T cell recognition regions of class I histocompatibility antigens. Nature, *329*:512, 1987.
18. Boog, C. J. P., Boes, J., and Melief, C. J. M.: Role of dendritic cells in the regulation of class I restricted cytotoxic T lymphocyte responses. J. Immunol., *140*:3331, 1988.
19. Bottomly, K.: A functional dichotomy in CD4⁺ T lymphocytes. Immunol. Today, *9*:268, 1988.
20. Brasile, L., Rabin, B., Clarke, J., Abrams, A., and Cerilli, J.: The identification of antibody to vascular endothelial cells (VEC) in patients undergoing cardiac transplantation. Transplantation, *40*:672, 1985.
21. Braun, W. M.: Laboratory and clinical management of the highly sensitized organ transplant recipient. Hum. Immunol., *26*:245, 1989.
22. Bray, R. A., Lebeck, L. K., and Gebel, H. M.: The flow cytometric crossmatch. Transplantation, *48*:834, 1989.
23. Brod, S. A., Rudd, C. E., Purvee, M., and Hafler D. A.: Lymphokine regulation of CD45R expression on human T cell clones. J. Exp. Med., *170*:2147, 1989.
24. Cardella, C. J., and Falk, J. A.: Graft outcome in patients with antibodies reactive with donor T and B cells. Transplant. Proc., *15*:1142, 1983.
25. Carpenter, B. M., Lang, P., Martin, B., and Fries, D.: Specific recipient-donor unresponsiveness mediated by a suppressor cell system in human kidney allograft tolerance. Transplantation, *33*:470, 1982.
26. Cerilli, J., Brasile, L., Clarke, J., et al.: The vascular endothelial cell-specific antigen system: three years' experience in monocyte crossmatching. Transplant. Proc., *17*:567, 1985.
27. Cerilli, J., Brasile, L., Galouzis, T., et al.: The vascular endothelial cell antigen system. Transplantation, *39*:286, 1985.
28. Cerilli, J., Clarke, J., Doolin, T., Cerilli, G., and Brasile, L.: The significance of a donor-specific vessel crossmatch in renal transplantation. Transplantation, *46*:359, 1988.
29. Chow, D., Saper, V., and Strober, S.: Renal transplant patients treated with total lymphoid irradiation show specific unresponsiveness to donor antigens in the mixed leukocyte reaction (MLR). J. Immunol., *138*:3746, 1987.
30. Ciccone, E., Viale, O., Pende, D., et al.: Specificity of human T lymphocytes expressing a γ/δ T cell antigen receptor: Recognition of a polymorphic determinant of HLA class I molecules by a γ/δ clone. Eur. J. Immunol., *19*:1267, 1989.

31. Claas, F. H. J., and van Rood, J. J.: The hyperimmunized patient: From sensitization toward transplantation. Transplant Int., 1:53, 1988.

32. Coffman, T. M., Ruiz, P., Sanfilippo, F., and Klotman, P. E.: Chronic thromboxane inhibition preserves function of rejecting rat renal allografts. Kidney Int., 35:24, 1989.

33. Cohen, D. J., Lee, H. M., and Mohanakumar, T.: Mechanisms of CML hyporesponsiveness in long-term renal allograft recipients. Hum. Immunol., 14:279, 1985.

34. Coombs, R. R. A., and Gell, P. G. H.: Classification of allergic reactions responsible for clinical hypersensitivity and disease. In Gell, P., et al.: (Eds.): Clinical Aspects of Immunology. Oxford, Blackwell, 1975, p. 761.

35. Dallman, M. J., Wood, K. J., and Morris, P. J.: Recombinant interleukin-2 (IL-2) can reverse the blood transfusion effect. Transplant. Proc., 21:1165, 1989.

36. Dallman, M. J., Wood, K. J., and Morris, P. J.: Specific cytotoxic T cells are found in the nonrejected kidneys of blood-transfused rats. J. Exp. Med., 165:566, 1987.

37. Demetris, A. J., Jaffe, R., Tzakis, A., et al.: Antibody-mediated rejection of human orthotopic liver allografts: A study of liver transplantation across ABO blood group barriers. Am. J. Pathol. 132:489, 1988.

38. Downey, W. E., III, Baldwin, W. M., III, and Sanfilippo, F.: Association of donor specific blood transfusion enhancement of rat renal allografts with accelerated development of anti-idiotypic antibodies and reduced alloantibody responses. Transplantation, 49:160, 1990.

39. Duijvestijn, A., and Hamann, A.: Mechanisms and regulation of lymphocyte migration. Immunol. Today, 10:23, 1989.

40. Eichwald, E. J., Wetzel, B., and Lustgraff, E. C.: Genetic aspects of second set skin grafts in mice. Transplantation, 4:260, 1966.

41. Emara, M., Finn, O. J., and Sanfilippo, F.: Characteristics of a human liver allograft-derived T-cell line that exhibits suppressor activity. Hum. Immunol. 26:364, 1989.

42. Emara, M., Miceli, M. C., Finn, O. J., and Sanfilippo, F.: Human suppressor T cells induced in vitro with an autologous renal allograft-derived T cell line. I. Suppressor cell induction, function, and specificity. Hum. Immunol., 23:223, 1988.

43. Ferguson, R. M.: A multicenter experience with sequential ALB/cyclosporine therapy in renal transplantation. Clin. Transplant., 2:285, 1988.

44. Fischer, E., Lenhard, V., Siefert, P., Kluge, A., and Johannsen, R.: Blood transfusion-induced suppression of cellular immunity in man. Hum. Immunol., 3:187, 1980.

45. Flesland, O., Solheim, B. G., Gaustad, P., et al.: Antibody production by donor lymphocytes in transplant patients. Transplantation, 48:883, 1989.

46. Foster, P. R., Sankary, H. D., Hart, M., Ashmann, M., and Williams, J. W.: Blood and graft eosinophilia as predictors of rejection in human liver transplantation. Transplantation, 47:72, 1989.

47. Galumback, M. A., Sanfilippo, F., Hagen, P-O. F., Seaber, A. V., and Urbanick, J. R.: Inhibition of vessel allograft rejection by endothelial removal. Ann. Surg., 206:757, 1987.

48. Gordon, R. D., Fung, J. J., Markus, B., et al.: The antibody crossmatch in liver transplantation. Surgery, 100:705, 1986.

49. Gorer, D. A., and Kaliss, N.: The effect of isoantibodies in vivo on three different transplantable neoplasms in mice. Cancer Res., 19:824, 1959.

50. Gorer, P. A., Lyman, S., and Snell, D. G.: Studies on the genetic and antigenic basis of tumor transplantation. Linkage between a histocompatibility gene and "fused" in mice. Proc. R. Soc. Lond., 135:499, 1948.

51. Goulmy, B., Termijtelen, A., Bradley, B. A., et al.: Y-antigen killing by T-cells of women is restricted by HLA. Nature (London), 266:544, 1977.

52. Gouw, A. S. H., Houthoff, H. J., Huitema, S., Beelen, J. M., Gips, C. H., and Poppema, S.: Expression of major histocompatibility complex antigens and replacement of donor cells by recipient ones in human liver grafts. Transplantation, 43:291, 1987.

53. Haas, W., Mathur-Rochat, J., Kisielow, P., et al.: Cytolytic T cell hybridomas. III. The antigen specificity and the restriction of cytolytic T cells do not phenotypically mix. Eur. J. Immunol., 15:963, 1985.

54. Hendricks, G. F. J., Schreuder, G. M. Th., D'Amaro, J., and van Rood, J. J.: The regulatory role of HLA-DRw6 in renal transplantation. Tissue Antigens, 27:121, 1986.

55. Herzog, W.-R., Zanker, B., Irschick, E., Huber, C., Franz, H. E., Wagner, H., and Kabelitz, D.: Selective reduction of donor-specific cytotoxic T lymphocyte precursors in patients with a well-functioning kidney allograft. Transplantation, 43:384, 1987.

56. Hunsicker, L. G., Oei, L. S., Freeman, R. M., Thompson, J. S., and Corry, R. J.: Transfusion and renal allograft survival: Beneficial effect of transfusion given on the day of transplant. Arch. Surg., 115:737, 1980.

57. Jager, M. J., Class, F. H. J., D'Amaro, J., et al.: Two alloantigens on human monocytes: A diallelic system? Hum. Immunol., 19:215, 1987.

58. Jager, M. J., Claas, F. H. J., Schot, D. L., Gratama, W., de Lange, G., and van Rood, J. J.: Genetics of two human monocyte antigens. Hum. Immunol., 22:163, 1988.

59. Jordan, S. C., Yap, H. K., Sakai, R. S., et al.: Hyperacute allograft rejection mediated by anti-vascular endothelial cell antibodies with a negative monocyte crossmatch. Transplantation, 46:585, 1988.

60. Joyce, S., Flye, M. W., and Mohanakumar, T.: Characterization of kidney cell-specific, non-major histocompatibility complex alloantigen using antibodies eluted from rejected human renal allografts. Transplantation,46:362, 1988.

61. Kappler, J., Skidmore, B., White, J., et al.: Antigen inducible, H-2 restricted, interleukin-2 producing T cell hybridomas: Lack of independent antigens and H-2 recognition. J. Exp. Med., 153:1198, 1981.

62. Kaufman, D. B., Sutherland, D. E. R., Noreen, H., Najarian, J. S., and Fyrd, D. S.: Renal transplantation between living-related siblings pairs matched for zero-HLA haplotypes. Transplantation, 47:113, 1989.

63. Kirkman, R. L., Bacha, P., Barrett, L. V., Forte, S., Murphy, J. R., and Strom, T. B.: Prolongation of cardiac allograft survival in murine recipients treated with a diphtheria toxin-related interleukin-2 fusion protein. Transplantation, 47:327, 1989.

64. Kissmeyer-Nielsen, F., Olsen, S., Petersen, V. P., and Fjeldborg, O.: Hyperacute rejection of kidney allografts associated with pre-existing humoral antibodies against donor cells. Lancet, 1:662, 1966.

65. Kojima, M., Cease, K. B., Buckenmeyer, G. K., and Berzofsky, J. A.: Limiting dilution comparison of the repertoires of high and low responder MHC-restricted T cells. J Exp. Med., 167:1100, 1988.

66. Lazada, V. A., Pollak, R., Mozes, M. F., and Jonasson, O.: The relationship between flow cytometer crossmatch results and subsequent rejection episodes in cadaver renal allograft recipients. Transplantation, 45:562, 1988.

67. LeFor, W. M., Tardif, G. N., Niblack, G. D., and Sanfilippo, F.: Use of SEOPF regional crossmatch trays to share kidneys for presensitized patients: Local experience of three centers. Transplantation, 40:637, 1985.

68. Light, J. A., Metz, S., Oddenine, K., et al.: Donor-specific transfusion with diminished sensitization. Transplantation, 34:352, 1982.

69. Lungren, G., Gorth, C. G., Albrechtsen, D., et al.: HLA matching in cyclosporine treated renal transplant patients: a prospective Swedish-Norwegian multicenter study. In Terasaki, P. I. (Ed.): Clinical Transplants 1986. Los Angeles, UCLA Tissue Typing Laboratory, 1986, p. 79.

70. MacLeod, A. M., Mason, R. J., Stewart, K. N., et al.: Association of Fc receptor-blocking antibodies and human renal transplant survival. Transplantation, 34:273, 1982.

71. Mantovani, A., and Dejana, E.: Cytokines as communication signals between leukocytes and endothelial cells. Immunol. Today, 10:370, 1989.

72. Markus, B. H., Duquesnoy, R. J., Gordon, R. D., Fung, J. J., Vanek, M., Klintmalm, G., Bryan, C., Thiel, D. V., and Starzl, T. E.: Histocompatibility and liver transplant outcome. Transplantation, 46:372, 1988.

73. Mattson, D. H., Shimojo, N., Cowan, E. P., Baskin, J. J., Turner, R. V., Shvetsky, B. D., Coligan, J. E., Maloy, W. L., and Biddison, W. E.: Differential effects of amino acid substitutions in the β-sheet floor and α-2 helix of HLA-A2 on recognition by alloreactive viral peptide-specific cytotoxic T lymphocytes. J. Immunol., 143:1101, 1989.

74. Maumenee, A. E.: The influence of donor-recipient sensitization on corneal grafts. Am. J. Ophthalmol., 34:142, 1951.

75. Mayumi, H., and Good, R. A.: Long-lasting skin allograft tolerance in adult mice induced across fully allogeneic (multimajor H-2 plus multiminor histocompatibility) antigen barriers by a tolerance-inducing method using cyclophosphamide. J. Exp. Med., 169:213, 1989.

76. McCarty, G. A., King, L. B., and Sanfilippo, F.: Autoantibodies to nuclear, cytoplasmic and cytoskeletal antigens in renal allograft rejection. Transplantation, 37:446, 1984.

77. Medawar, P. B.: The behavior and fate of skin autografts and skin homografts in rabbits. J. Anat., 78:176, 1944.

78. Mempel, W., Albert, E., and Berger, A.: Further evidence for a separate MLC locus. Tissue Antigens, 2:250, 1972.

79. Miceli, M. C., and Finn, O. J.: T cell receptor β-chain selection in human allograft rejection. J. Immunol., 142:81, 1989.

80. Miceli, M. C., Barry, T. S., and Finn, O. J.: Human allograft-derived T-cell lines: Donor class I and class II-directed cytotoxicity and repertoire stability in sequential biopsies. Hum. Immunol., 22:185, 1988.

81. Miltenburg, A. M. M., Meijer-Paape, M. E., Weening, J. J., Daha, M. R., van Ex, L. A., and van der Woude, F. J.: Induction of antibody-dependent cellular cytotoxicity against endothelial cells by renal transplantation. Transplantation, 48:681, 1989.

82. Mohagheghpour, N., Damle, N. K., Takada, S., and Engleman, E. G.: Generation of antigen receptor-specific suppressor T cell lines in man. J. Exp. Med., 164:950, 1986.

83. Murray, J. S., Madri, J., Tite, J., Carding, S. R., and Bottomly K.: MHC control of CD4+ T cell subset activation. J. Exp. Med., 170:2135, 1989.

84. Nathenson, S. G., Giliebter, J., Pfaffenbach, G. M., and Zeff, R. A.: Murine major histocompatibility complex class I mutants: molecular analysis and structure function implications. Annu. Rev. Immunol., 4:471, 1986.

85. Oguma, S., Zerbe, T., Banner, B., Starzl, T., and Demetris, A. J.: Participation of dendritic cells in vascular lesions of chronic rejection of human allografts. Lancet, 2:933, 1988.

86. Opelz, G.: Correlation of HLA matching with kidney graft survival in patients with or without cyclosporine treatment. Transplantation, 40:240, 1985.

87. Opelz, G.: Effect of HLA matching in 10,000 cyclosporine-treated cadaveric kidney transplants. Transplant. Proc., 19:641, 1987.

88. Opelz, G.: Influence of HLA matching on survival of second kidney transplants in cyclosporine-treated recipients. Transplantation, 47:823, 1989.

89. Opelz, G.: The benefit of exchanging donor kidneys among transplant centers. N. Engl. J. Med., 318:1289, 1988.

90. Opelz, G., Mickey, M. R., Sengar, D. P. S., and Terasaki, P. I.: Effect of blood transfusions on subsequent kidney transplants. Transplant. Proc., 5:253, 1973.

91. Opelz, G., Mickey, M. R., and Terasaki, P. I.: Calculations on long-term graft and patient survival in human kidney transplantation. Transplant. Proc., 9:27, 1977.

92. Patel, R., and Terasaki, P. I.: Significance of a positive cross-match test in kidney transplantation. N. Engl. J. Med., 288:735, 1969.

93. Paul, L. C., Baldwin, W. M., and Van Es, L. A.: Transplantation antigens on renal endothelium. Neth. J. Med., 25:208, 1982.

94. Pescovitz, M. D., Thistlethwaite, J. R., Anchunclass, H., et al.: Effect of class II antigen matching on renal allograft survival in miniature swine. J. Exp. Med., 160:1495, 1984.

95. Pfaff, W. W., Vaughn, W. K., and Sanfilippo, F.: The effect of class I HLA matching on graft survival in sensitized patients. Transplant. Proc., 19:716, 1987.

96. Phelan, D. L., Rodey, G. E., and Anderson, C. B.: The development and specificity of antiidiotypic antibodies in renal transplant recipients receiving single-donor blood transfusions. Transplantation, 48:57, 1989.

97. Pierres, M., Marchetto, S., Naquet, P., Landais, D., Peccoud, J., Benoist, C., and Mathis, D.: I-Aα polymorphic residues that determine alloreactive T cell recognition. J. Exp. Med., 169:1655, 1989.

98. Plate, J. M., Ward, F. E., and Amos, D. B.: The mixed leukocyte culture reaction between HLA identical siblings. In Terasaki, P. I. (Ed.): Histocompatibility Testing. Copenhagen, Munksgaard, 1970, p. 531.

99. Pohanka, E., Manfro, R. C., Oto, C., et al.: "Anti-idiotypic" antibodies to HLA in transiently sensitized DSBT patients. Hum. Immunol., 26:17, 1989.

100. Porter, K. A.: Rejection in treated renal allografts. J. Clin. Pathol., 20:518, 1967.

101. Prisch, J. D., Sollinger, H. W., and Kalayoglu, M.: Living-related renal transplantation: Results in 40 patients. Am. J. Kidney Dis., 12:499, 1988.

102. Qin, S., Cobbold, S., Benjamin, R., and Waldmann, H.: Induction of classical transplantation tolerance in the adult. J. Exp. Med., 169:779, 1989.

103. Quigley, R. L., Wood, K. J., and Morris, P. J.: Mediation of antigen-induced suppression of renal allograft rejection by a CD4 (W3/25+) T cell. Transplantation, 47:684, 1989.

104. Ramos, E. L., Turka, L. A., Leggat, J. E., Wood, I. G., Milford, E. L., and Carpenter, C. B.: Decrease in phenotypically defined T helper inducer cells (T4+4B4+) and increase in T suppressor effector cells (T8+2H4+) in stable renal allograft recipients. Transplantation, 47:465, 1989.

105. Reed, E., Hardy, M., Benvenisty, A., et al.: Effect of antiidiotypic antibodies to HLA on graft survival in renal allograft recipients. N. Engl. J. Med., 316:1450, 1987.

106. Rodey, G. E., and Phelan, D. L.: Association of antiidiotypic antibody with successful second transplant of a kidney sharing HLA antigens with the previous hyperacutely rejected first kidney. Transplantation, 48:54, 1989.

107. Roman-Roman, S., Baixeras, E., Genevee, C., Hercend, T., and Triebel, F.: The T-cell receptor Vδ genes predominantly used by human peripheral γ/δ+ T lymphocytes are not rearranged in CD3- natural killer cells. Hum. Immunol., 26:75, 1989.

108. Rose, N. R., Friedman, H., and Fabey, J. L., (Eds.): Manual of clinical laboratory immunology, 3rd ed. Washington, D. C., American Society for Microbiology, 1986.

109. Rosenberg, A. S., Mizvoch, T., Sharrow, S. O., and Singer, A.: Phenotype, specificity, and function of T cells subsets and T cell interactions involved in skin allograft rejection. J. Exp. Med., 165:1296, 1987.

110. Rosenberg, A. S., Mizuochi, T., and Singer, A.: Evidence for involvement of dual-function T cells in rejection of MHC class I disparate skin grafts. J. Exp. Med., 168:33, 1988.

111. Rose, M., Navarette, C., Yacoub, M., and Festenstein, H.: Persistence of donor-specific class II antigens in allografted human heart two years after transplantation. Hum. Immunol., 23:179, 1988.

112. Rubinstein, D., Roska, A. K., and Lipsky, P. E.: Liver sinusoidal lining cells express class II major histocompatibility antigens but are poor stimulators of fresh allogeneic T lymphocytes. J. Immunol., 137:1803, 1986.

113. Ruiz, P., Coffman, T. M., Howell, D. N., Straznickas, J., et al.: Pretransplant donor blood transfusion prevents rat renal allograft dysfunction but not the in situ cellular alloimmune or morphologic manifestations of rejection. Transplantation, 45:1, 1988.

114. Ruiz, P., Fuller, J., and Sanfilippo, F.: Donor-specific cellular immunity in rejecting and long-term surviving class I disparate rat renal allograft recipients. Transplantation, 49:175, 1990.

115. Ruiz, P., Harland, R., Yamaguchi, Y., et al.: In situ and systemic cellular immunity associated with orthotopic rat liver allograft acceptance or rejection. Transplant. Proc., 21:416, 1989.

116. Salvatierra, I., Vincenit, F., Amend, W., et al.: Deliberate donor-specific blood transfusions prior to living related transplantation: A new approach. Ann. Surg., 192:543, 1980.

117. Sanfilippo, F.: Kidney Transplantation. In Sale, G. E. (Ed.): Pathology of Clinical Transplantation. London, Butterworths, 1990, p. 51.

118. Sanfilippo, F., Baldwin, W. M., and Snyderman, R.: Immunopathology. In Joklik, W. K., Willet, H. P., Amos, D. B., and Wilfert, K. (Eds.): Zinsser Microbiology, 19th ed. New York, Appleton-Lange, 1988, p. 265.

119. Sanfilippo, F., Crawford, J., Ness, G., Geier, S., and Bollinger, R. R.: Influence of donor specific blood transfusions on host cellular immune responsiveness. Transplant. Proc., 18:692, 1986.

120. Sanfilippo, F., Goeken, N., Niblack, G., et al.: The effect of first cadaver renal transplant HLA-A, B match on sensitization levels and retransplantation rates following graft failure. Transplantation, 43:240, 1987.

121. Sanfilippo, F., MacQueen, J. M., Vaughn, W. K. et al.: Reduced graft rejection with good HLA-A and HLA-B matching in high-risk corneal transplantation. N. Engl. J. Med., 315:29, 1986.

122. Sanfilippo, F., Spees, E. K., and Vaughn, W. K.: The timing of pretransplant transfusions and renal allograft survival. Transplantation, 37:344, 1984.

123. Sanfilippo, F., Spees, E. K., and Vaughn, W. K.: Living-donor renal transplantation in SEOPF: The impact of histocompatibility, transfusions and cyclosporine on outcome. Transplantation, 49:25, 1990.

124. Sanfilippo, F., Vaughn, W. K., Alexander, J. W., LeFor, W. M., Lucas, B. A., and Pfaff, W. W.: Organ sharing for good HLA-A,B, and DR matching improves cadaver renal graft survival in SEOPF: Retrospective and prospective studies considering delayed graft function, race, center effects, cyclosporine, and other factors. In Terasaki, P. I. (Ed.): Clinical Transplants 1988. Los Angeles, UCLA Tissue Typing Laboratory, 1988, p. 211.

125. Sanfilippo, F., Vaughn, W. K., Bollinger, R. R., et al.: The comparative effects of pregnancy, transfusion and prior graft rejection on sensitization and renal transplant results. Transplantation, 34:360, 1982.

126. Sanfilippo, F., Vaughn, W. K., Spees, E. K., and Bollinger, R. R.: Cadaver renal transplantation ignoring peak reactive sera in patients with markedly decreasing pretransplant sensitization. Transplantation, 39:151, 1984.

127. Scheid, M., Bovse, E. A., Carswell, E. A., et al.: Serologically demonstrable alloantigens of mouse epidermal cells. J. Exp. Med., 135:938, 1972.

128. Sharabi, Y., and Sachs, D. H.: Mixed chimerism and permanent specific transplantation tolerance induced by a nonlethal preparative regimen. J. Exp. Med., 169:493, 1989.

129. Sherwood, R. A., Brent, L., and Rayfield, L. S.: Presentation of alloantigens by host cells. Eur. J. Immunol., 16:569, 1986.

130. Skoglund, C., Scheynius, A., Holmdahl, R., and VanDerMeide, P. H.: Enhancement of DTH reaction and inhibition of the expression of class II transplantation antigens by in vivo treatment with antibodies against γ-interferon. Clin. Exp. Immunol., 71:428, 1988.

131. Snell, G. D.: Methods for the study of histocompatibility genes. J. Genetics, 49:87, 1948.

132. Solheim, B. G., Albrechtsen, D. A., Berg, K. J., et al: Hemolytic anemia in cyclosporine-treated recipients of kidney or heart grafts from donors with minor incompatibility for ABO antigens. Transplant. Proc., 19:4236, 1987.

133. Sollinger, H. W., Burlingham, W. J., Sparks, E. M., Glass, N. R., and Belzer, F. O.: Donor-specific transfusions in unrelated and related HLA-mismatched donor-recipient combinations. Transplantation, 38:612, 1984.

134. Spetainik, S., Pfaff, W., Cowles, J., et al.: Correlation of humoral immunity to Lewis blood group antigens with renal transplant rejection. Transplantation, 37:265, 1984.

135. Sutherland, D. E. R., Chow, S. Y., and Moudry-Munns, K. C.: International Pancreas Transplant Registry Report - 1988. Clin. Transplant., 3:129, 1989.

136. Takiff, H., Iwaki, Y., Cecka, M., and Terasaki, P. I.: The benefit and underutilization of sharing kidneys for better histocompatibility. Transplantation, 47:102, 1989.

137. Talbot, D., Givan, A. L., Shenton, B. K., et al.: The relevance of a more sensitive crossmatch assay to renal transplantation. Transplantation, 47:552, 1989.

138. Taylor, C. J., Chapman, J. R., Ting, A., and Morris, P. J.: Characterization of lymphocytotoxic antibodies causing a positive crossmatch in renal transplantation. Relationship to primary and regraft outcome. Transplantation, 48:953, 1989.

139. Ten, R. M., Gleich, G. J., Holley, K. E., Perkins, J. D., and Torres, V. E.: Eosinophil granule major basic protein in acute renal allograft rejection. Transplantation, 47:959, 1989.

140. Terasaki, P. I. (Ed.): Clinical Transplants 1988. Los Angeles, UCLA Tissue Typing Laboratory, 1988.

141. Terasaki, P. I., and McClelland, J. D.: Microdroplet assay of human serum cytotoxins. Nature, 204:988, 1964.

142. Terasaki, P. I., Takemoto, S., and Mickey, M. R.: A report on 123 six-antigen matched cadaver kidney transplants. Clin. Transplant., 3:301, 1989.

143. Terasaki, P. I., Vredevoe, D. L., Mickey, M. R., et al.: Serotyping for homotransplantation. VII. Selection of kidney donors for thirty-two recipients. Ann. N. Y. Acad. Sci., 129:500, 1966.

144. Thorogood, J., van Houwelingen, J. C., van Rood J. J., and Persijn, G. G.: Time trend in annual kidney graft survival. Transplantation, 46:686, 1988.

145. Turka, L. A., Goguen, J. E., Gagne, J. E., and Milford, E. L.: Presensitization and the renal allograft recipient. Transplantation,47:234, 1989.

146. Turka, L. A., Tanaka, K., Kupiec-Weglinski, J. W., et al.: In vivo activity of mixed lymphocyte response-generated suppressor cells and ability to prolong cardiac allograft survival in rats. Transplantation, 47:388, 1989.

147. Van Leeuwen, A., Schuit, H. R. E., and van Rood, J. J.: Typing for MLD (LD). II. The selection of non-stimulator cells by MLC inhibition tests using SD-identical stimulator cells (Misis) and fluorescent antibody studies. Transplant. Proc., 5:1539, 1973.

148. Vogel, J. M., Davis, A. C., McKinney, D. M., McMillan, M., Martin, W. J., and Goodenow, R. S.: Molecular characterization of the C3HfB/HeN H-2Kkm2 mutation: Implications for the molecular basis of alloreactivity. J. Exp. Med., 168:1781, 1988.

149. Welchel, J. S., Shaw, J. F., Curtis, J. J., Luke, R. G., and Diethelm, D. G.: Effect of pretransplant stored donor-specific blood transfusion on early renal allo-

graft survival in one-haplotype living-related transplants. Transplantation, 34:326, 1982.

150. Williams, G. M., Hume, D. M., Hudson, R. P., Morris, P. J., Kano, K., and Milgram, F.: "Hyperacute" renal-homograft rejection in man. N. Engl. J. Med., 279:611, 1968.

151. Yang, H., and Welsh, R. M.: Induction of alloreactive cytotoxic T cells by acute virus infection of mice. J. Immunol., 136:1186, 1986.

152. Young, J. D.-E., and Liu, C. C.: Multiple mechanisms of lymphocyte-mediated killing. Immunol. Today, 9:140, 1988.

153. Yunis, E. J., and Amos, D. B.: Three closely linked systems relevant to transplantation. Proc. Natl. Acad. Sci., 68:118, 1971.

154. Zinkernagel, R. M., and Doherty, P. C.: H-2 compatibility requirement for T-cell-mediated lysis of target cells infected with lymphocytic choriomeningitis virus: Different cytotoxic T-cell specificities are associated with structures encoded for in H-2K or H-2D. J. Exp. Med., 141:1427, 1975.

IV ————————————————————————

RENAL TRANSPLANTATION

Clyde F. Barker, M.D., Ali Naji, M.D., Ph.D., Donald C. Dafoe, M.D., and Leonard J. Perloff, M.D.

HISTORICAL ASPECTS

Although the first unsuccessful attempts at kidney transplantation were reported in 1902, the therapeutic possibilities of the procedure were defined in a series of animal experiments by Alexis Carrel between 1904 and 1910. Carrel successfully transplanted kidneys, hearts, and other organs into animals, devising at the same time the technique of modern blood vessel surgery. This brilliant work performed in Chicago and New York by the French surgeon led to a Nobel Prize in 1912 but proved to be four decades ahead of its time (Table 1). Not until the early 1950s did Medawar's description of rejection and his discovery with Billingham and Brent that it could be prevented by tolerance stimulate surgeons to resume experimental renal transplantation. Clinical trials were also undertaken during this period, but of 36 human renal allografts attempted without benefit of immunosuppression, only one significantly prolonged life. It became clear that failures were the result of rejection, since a concomitant series of identical twin transplants by Murray in Boston were successful. In the late 1950s, rejection was first circumvented in a few patients by Murray in Boston and Hamburger in Paris by the use of whole-body irradiation. The concurrent development of dialysis facilitated more extensive trials of transplantation, and in the early 1960s, transplant surgeons demonstrated that newly discovered immunosuppressive drugs could frequently prolong allograft survival. During the next 25 years, progress in immunogenetics, immunosuppressive therapy, and organ preservation, as well as accumulation of clinical experience, have all contributed to the present status of transplantation, which allows successful long-term management of previously fatal renal disease in most of the 9000 patients per year who now receive renal allografts.[37]

RECIPIENT SELECTION AND MANAGEMENT

Indications

The ideal recipient is an otherwise healthy young individual whose renal failure is not due to urinary outlet abnormalities or a systemic disease likely to damage the transplanted kidney. The most common diseases leading to eventual need for transplantation are glomerulonephritis, diabetes mellitus, hypertension, and pyelonephritis.

The presence of infection or malignancy that cannot be eradicated is an absolute contraindication to transplantation, because immunosuppression encourages both microbial and tumor growth. Noncompliance is also a contraindication, because careful adherence to immunosuppression is necessary. Advanced age (over 65 years) and severe cardiovascular disease

such as unreconstructable coronary artery or aortoiliac disease are also deterrents. However, in such patients, the long-term cumulative risks of dialysis are at least as great as those of transplantation. Therefore, with improvements in perioperative care and immunosuppression, many conditions once considered contraindications to transplantation because of inordinate risk have been removed. For example, diabetics, formerly considered poor candidates, clearly do better with transplantation than with dialysis.[40] Even diseases in which the transplanted kidney may eventually be damaged by recurrent disease (e.g., lupus erythematosus, cystinosis, amyloidosis, diabetes, and some forms of glomerulonephritis) are often better palliated by transplantation than by dialysis. Indeed, the improved results of transplantation over the last decade mandate serious consideration of this therapy in nearly any patient with terminal renal disease. Not only is the quality of life far better with transplantation than with dialysis, but because the mortality in the first year after transplantation is less than 5 per cent, survival is also superior. Unfortunately, an insufficient supply of kidneys and a lack of full appreciation of the present excellent results of transplantation keep some appropriate transplant candidates on chronic dialysis.

Recipient Evaluation and Preparation

The medical evaluation of all transplant candidates should include a history, a physical examination, a complete blood count, urinalysis, urine culture, a cytomegalovirus antibody titer, measurement of creatinine clearance, measurement of serum electrolytes, a serologic assay for syphilis, assays for human immunodeficiency virus and hepatitis B, evaluation of parathyroid status, chest films, an electrocardiogram (ECG), a coagulation profile, a Papanicolaou test, ABO and histocompatibility typing, urologic evaluation (including a voiding cystourethrogram in selected patients to assess outlet obstruction and reflux), gastrointestinal (GI) evaluation (as warranted by history of ulcer, diverticulitis, or other symptoms), and a psychiatric evaluation.

The proper timing of transplantation is a delicate decision, because the progression of renal dysfunction is variable and premature imposition of the risks of transplantation is not justified. However, dialysis and/or transplantation should not be withheld until advanced uremic symptoms ensue, such as pericarditis, cardiac failure, severe anemia, osteodystrophy, and neuropathy, because some of these complications may become irreversible (e.g., neuropathy). Pretransplant dialysis is often necessary, at least briefly, to optimize the patient's general condition (nutrition, electrolyte balance, coagulation status). Because cardiovascular complications are second only to infection

TABLE 1. Important Events in the Development of Kidney Transplantation

1902	First experimental kidney transplant (Ullman)
1906	First human kidney transplant (Jabouloy)
1904–10	Perfection of experimental kidney transplantation and vascular anastomoses (Carrel)
1946	Establishment of the principles of immunologic rejection (Medawar)
1950–53	Revived interest in experimental kidney transplants and the systematic study of their rejection (Simonsen, Dempster).
1953	Experimental demonstration of actively acquired tolerance of allografts (Billingham, Brent, and Medawar)
1950–53	Unsuccessful attempts of human kidney transplants without immunosuppression (Kuss and associates, Servelle and associates)
1954–58	Successful identical twin transplants (Murray)
1959–62	First attempts at immunosuppression for renal allografts by whole-body irradiation (Murray, Hamburger, Kuss)
1959	First experimental immunosuppression with a drug 6-mercaptopurine (Schwartz and Demeshek)
1960	Practicality of maintenance dialysis by development of lasting vascular access (Scribner)
1960–62	6-Mercaptopurine and azathioprine shown to prolong dog kidney allograft survival (Calne, Zukowski and Hume, Hitchings)
1963	Immunosuppressive effects of antilymphocytic serum described (Woodruff and Anderson)
1963	Consistent success of kidney allografts achieved with use of living related donors, azathioprine, and steroids (Starzl, Hume, Murray)
1962–66	Introduction of tissue typing to select donors, recognition of importance of crossmatch test (Hamberger, Dansch, Terasaki, Kissmeyer-Nielson, Starzl).
1963	Twelve-hour preservation of kidneys by surface cooling (Calne)
1967	Preservation of kidneys for 3 days by continuous perfusion (Belzer)
1978	Introduction of cyclosporine (Borel, Calne)
1981	Clinical use of monoclonal antibody OKT3 for antirejection therapy (Cosimi)

as a cause of posttransplantation mortality, the patient's cardiovascular status should be optimized. In older patients and diabetics, this may require stress testing or even pretransplant coronary artery bypass. Careful attention must be paid to eradication of all infections, including those of the urinary tract, lungs, and skin (especially at the site of the planned incision).

Dialysis Access

The use of external arteriovenous cannulas for hemodialysis has been replaced by internal shunting, which allows greater comfort and convenience and less likelihood of infection or thrombosis. If only a brief period of dialysis is contemplated, this may be accomplished via an indwelling double-lumen catheter placed in the subclavian or jugular vein. For chronic hemodialysis, the preferred vascular access is the arteriovenous fistula, which is an anastomosis of the radial artery to the cephalic vein at the wrist. This causes arterialization of the superficial arm veins, which can then be punctured percutaneously. If these vessels are diseased, have been used, or fail to generate adequate flow, a subcutaneously tunneled polytetrafluoroethylene (PTFE) graft between the radial artery and antecubital vein or the brachial artery and axillary vein is the procedure of choice. Arteriovenous grafts in the lower extremities are less satisfactory because of their propensity for infection and/or precipitation of limb-threatening ischemia.

Peritoneal dialysis is preferable to hemodialysis in some patients, e.g., those with inadequate peripheral vessels, repeatedly infected vascular access sites, or unstable cardiovascular status. Other patients simply prefer the greater convenience of home

dialysis achieved by continuous ambulatory peritoneal dialysis (CAPD). It is crucial that the time of the transplant operation not coincide with an episode of peritonitis or infection at the site of the indwelling peritoneal catheter.

Histocompatibility Typing and Crossmatching

Although opinions vary regarding the significance of histocompatibility testing for selection of unrelated donors, its importance is unquestionable for selection of the optimal donor within a family. Regardless of the donor source, compatibility for ABO blood groups and a negative leukocyte crossmatch are mandatory.

ABO BLOOD GROUPS. Because the major blood group antigens are not expressed by human leukocytes, it was initially assumed that they might be unimportant in transplant rejection. However, experimental and clinical evidence soon indicated that ABO antigens function as important histocompatibility antigens, probably because they are expressed on vascular endothelium.[5] Rapaport and Dausset demonstrated experimentally that prior exposure to erythrocytes from ABO-incompatible donors provoked accelerated rejection of skin grafts from donors of the same blood group. In the early days of renal transplantation, it was noted that ABO incompatibility often led to acute or hyperacute rejection, a finding which led to adherence to the rule of blood group compatibility. Recently, because of the donor organ shortage and reports of success with ABO incompatible liver and heart allografts, attempts have been made to breach the ABO barrier for kidney allografts. In 1982, Brynger and associates reported successful transplantation in blood group O recipients of kidneys from A_2 donors (who have a lower number of A antigenic determinants on their cells than A_1 donors). Successful ABO-incompatible transplants have also been reported in recipients whose ABO isoagglutinins have been removed by plasmapheresis or immunoadsorption. Because isoagglutinins eventually reappear and the long-term outcome of these transplants remains to be assessed, most centers have yet to employ this strategy. However, it is an attractive approach, especially for allowing utilization of HLA identical but ABO-incompatible family donors.

LYMPHOCYTOTOXIC CROSSMATCHING. Sensitization to human leukocyte antigen (HLA), as indicated by the presence of lymphocytotoxic antibodies in the recipient's serum, may occur as a result of pregnancy, blood transfusions, or renal transplantation. Presence of donor-reactive antibodies, detected by incubation of recipient serum with donor cells in the presence of complement (a positive "crossmatch"), is considered a contraindication to renal transplantation because of its strong association (80 per cent) with hyperacute renal allograft rejection. Serum from patients awaiting cadaveric renal transplantation is periodically screened against a panel of randomly selected HLA-typed lymphocyte donors. Nonreactivity of a patient's serum to the panel cells indicates a high likelihood of obtaining a crossmatch-compatible donor, whereas uniform reactivity of a patient's serum with panel cells greatly reduces this probability. The number of highly sensitized patients on most transplant waiting lists is increasing as less-sensitized patients receive transplants, whereas sensitized individuals remain on the list and those with failed renal allografts (frequently sensitized) are returned to the list.

Recently it was noted that successful transplantation can often be achieved despite the positivity of certain types of crossmatches, a finding that should allow transplantation of many apparently sensitized patients.[63] For example, lymphocytotoxic autoantibodies do not cause rejection. In some patients the titer of bona fide lymphocytotoxic antibodies declines or disappears with time. In the past, it was a common practice to store serum from the period of peak sensitization for later use in crossmatching; and if it was found positive, transplantation was denied, even if current serum was negative. Several reports now indicate that a positive crossmatch using peak serum may be disregarded with only a minimal risk of hyperacute rejection, provided that current serum test results are negative. The conditions that allow transplantation in a patient with a "historic" positive but current negative crossmatch are not yet clearly defined. Most centers require a certain interval (1 to 12 months) between the last positive serum test results and transplantation.

There is controversy as to whether the most sensitive crossmatching methods, such as antiglobulin and flow cytometry techniques, should be used, because they may exclude donors whose kidneys might have been used successfully. In addition, the clinical relevance of positive crossmatches to B lymphocytes (especially if performed in the cold) and those caused only by IgM antibodies are questionable. Attempts have also been made to define the role of antibodies against non-HLA specificities. Cerilli has presented evidence that the presence of antibodies reacting with endothelial cells (but not with T cells) is often associated with early or severe rejection, although most centers have not employed this test.[15]

When patients are unequivocally and persistently sensitized to the Class I HLA antigens present on T cells, several methods of removing cytotoxic antibody are being evaluated to shorten waiting time and avoid accelerated rejection, including thoracic duct drainage, plasmapheresis, and total lymphoid irradiation. After extracorporeal immunoadsorption with staphylococcal protein A was used for removal of anti-HLA antibodies in 10 highly sensitized patients, 7 were able to obtain transplants, only 1 of which was rejected.[46] Because none of these maneuvers has yet gained wide acceptance, the increasingly large sensitized patient pool remains a formidable problem.

Pretransplant Blood Transfusions

The use of blood transfusions to condition prospective renal allograft recipients is controversial. For many years transfusions were scrupulously avoided to minimize possible formation of lymphocytotoxic antibodies. However, in 1973, Opelz and Terasaki[44] made the surprising observation that this policy was misguided, because renal allograft survival was, in fact, 10 to 15 per cent better in transfused than in nontransfused recipients. The worldwide policy of deliberate pretransplantation blood transfusions that followed this report was credited with the greatest improvement in the outcome of renal transplantation since the introduction of azathioprine.

The reason for the beneficial effect of transfusion is unclear.[64] It has been theorized that exposure of potential recipients to HLA antigens on leukocytes from various blood donors merely excludes "responder" patients, who, because they develop antibodies following transfusion, become ineligible for transplantation on the basis of positive crossmatches. Meanwhile, those transfused patients who remain crossmatch-negative despite transfusions are termed "nonresponders" and are likely to undergo successful transplantation sooner than the responder population. Another possible explanation of improved results is that transfusions have a true immunosuppressive effect, mediated through induction of suppressor T lymphocytes and/or enhancing alloantibodies. According to yet another theory, the kidney transplant acts as a secondary stimulus to an initial immune response elicited by transfusion, leading to proliferation of clones of cells reactive to antigens shared by the blood and kidney donors. These responsive clones, because of their activated status, are especially vulnerable and are deleted by high doses of immunosuppression used in the early posttransplant period.

Deliberate transfusions of blood from a prospective living related donor have also been used with considerable success, presumably on the basis of a mechanism similar to that of random transfusions. Salvatierra thereby improved the 2-year graft survival of one haplotype–matched related recipients from 56 to 91 per cent.[56] However, transfusion was associated with a 30

per cent risk of inciting cytotoxic antibodies, thus precluding transplantation from the selected related donor. In order to decrease the rate of sensitization, Anderson and associates advocate concomitant use of azathioprine at the time of donor-specific transfusions, reporting a sensitization rate of only 8 per cent while maintaining a graft survival of more than 90 per cent.[2]

With the improvement in graft survival attributed to the widespread use of cyclosporine immunosuppression since 1984, it has become unclear whether either random or donor specific blood transfusions should be employed. Opelz's analysis of data from a large collaborative study indicated that by 1985 the transfusion effect had nearly disappeared.[43] In contrast, Terasaki's large multicenter registry indicated that a strong transfusion effect remained evident during the same period.[66] Further analysis of single-center and multiple-center studies has failed to resolve these contradictory reports. If the transfusion effect has indeed been "lost," this loss is not attributable to a decline of graft survival in transfused patients, but rather to improved graft outcome in nontransfused recipients. Moreover, the observed change cannot be explained solely by the introduction of cyclosporine, because improvement in graft survival has been noted even in patients treated only with azathioprine and prednisone.

Although it appears likely that some transfusion effect remains, many authorities believe that whatever benefit might still be achieved is outweighed by the risk of disease transmission and sensitization associated with deliberate transfusion. The availability of recombinant erythropoietin now obviates the previous need for transfusion during prolonged dialysis. The fear of transmission of infection (HIV and hepatitis) is a major factor in patient nonacceptance of transfusions even if they are advised. Thus, although some centers continue to study the effects of donor-specific transfusions, deliberate preconditioning of transplant recipients with random transfusions is no longer recommended by most groups.

The transfusion effect remains a fascinating phenomenon, and its eventual explanation is not only of theoretic interest but great practical importance, because promotion of a permanent state of unresponsiveness by preconditioning with donor blood (or donor bone marrow as reported by Barber and associates) may prove superior to the chronic use of toxic immunosuppressive agents such as cyclosporine.[6]

Pretransplant Operations

Any necessary urinary tract reconstructions must be accomplished prior to transplantation (e.g., lysis of posterior urethral valves, transurethral resection for obstructing prostatic hypertrophy). Every effort should be made to utilize the patient's own bladder for ureteroneocystostomy even if this necessitates bladder reconstruction or augmentation of a small bladder by ileocecocystoplasty. Careful intermittent catheterization of a neurogenic bladder three to four times daily after transplantation is preferable to the use of an intestinal conduit. In the absence of an alternative strategy, ileal conduits should be constructed at least 6 weeks prior to the transplant operation.

Bilateral nephrectomy of the recipient was once routine, the rationale being that even if current urine was sterile, pyelonephritic kidneys would remain a dangerous focus of infection and that retained glomerulonephritic kidneys might be a stimulus for autoimmune destruction of the allograft. Because evidence to support these hypotheses was not forthcoming, bilateral nephrectomy is now performed only for special indications such as recalcitrant urinary tract infections (especially in the presence of stones, reflux, or obstruction), uncontrollable hypertension, massive proteinuria, bilateral renal tumors, and large polycystic kidneys, especially if they are bleeding or infected.

Splenectomy was at one time widely practiced for its nonspecific immunosuppressive effect even though conclusive evidence of its value was lacking. A large randomized study indicated that pretransplantation splenectomy modestly improved early, but not late, graft survival[62]; and other studies actually demonstrated a detrimental effect on patient survival.[1] During the precyclosporine era, a rationale used for splenectomy was the resultant increase in the white blood cell count, which allowed larger maintenance doses of azathioprine without leukopenia. Because cyclosporine does not cause leukopenia, there is now general agreement that splenectomy is rarely, if ever, indicated.

SELECTION AND MANAGEMENT OF LIVING DONORS

For the prospective recipient, there are major advantages to obtaining a related donor, obviating the discomfort, expense, and risks of prolonged dialysis during the waiting for a cadaver kidney. Posttransplantation morbidity is also minimized by decreasing the likelihood of acute tubular necrosis (ATN) or early rejection crises. Since the advent of cyclosporine therapy, short-term results of cadaveric transplantation in some centers now approach those with living related donors. Nevertheless, because of better histocompatibility, long-term results of related donor transplantation remain superior to those of cadaveric grafts. Thus, most authorities believe the use of living donors is still justified, and in the United States they are used for approximately 25 per cent of kidney transplants.

Histocompatibility Considerations in Living Donor Selection

The HLA antigens are gene products of alleles at a number of closely linked loci on the short arm of chromosome 6 in humans. At least six (A, B, C, DQ, DP, DR) have been defined, and the existence of several others has been deduced from family studies and immunochemical findings. The extreme polymorphism of the HLA system, which is the basis of infinite genetic variability of the human species, has a pivotal role in regulation of the immune response. The gene products of the HLA-A, -B, and -C loci are referred to as Class I major histocompatibility (MHC) antigens, and the products of the D region are Class II MHC antigens. MHC Class I antigens are expressed on all nucleated cells and can be readily detected serologically by using lymphocytotoxicity assays. Class II MHC antigens are important in antigen presentation and are expressed on B lymphocytes, dendritic cells, endothelium, and activated T cells.

HLA antigens are inherited as co-dominant alleles; and because of the relatively low recombinant frequency, the HLA genes are usually inherited en bloc from each parent. In immediate families inheritance of the HLA antigens, which is of overriding importance in determining transplant outcome, can be determined serologically and forms four different combinations of haplotypes. Any two siblings have a 25 per cent likelihood of being HLA-identical, i.e., having inherited the same chromosome 6 (haplotype) from each parent; a 50 per cent likelihood of sharing one haplotype; and a 25 per cent likelihood of sharing neither haplotype. Parent-to-child donation always involves a one-haplotype identity.

The importance of matching HLA antigens in the selection of living related donors for renal transplantation is well established. Excellent long-term graft survival (more than 90 per cent) can be expected when a related donor and recipient are HLA-identical. There is a progressively lower graft survival associated with one or zero haplotype match. The results of the two haplotype mismatched related donor grafts are not very much better than those that may be achieved with cadaveric grafts, causing reluctance at some transplant centers to use such donors. The shortage of cadaver donors may be the most compelling reason for use of totally mismatched related donors.

However, both donor specific blood transfusions and cyclosporine have dramatically improved the survival of haploidentical and totally mismatched living donor grafts.

Risks to the Living Donor

Despite the major advantages of related donors, their use can only be justified because the risks are minimal. Nevertheless, it is important to present these risks frankly to the donor. In addition to discomfort and the morbidity associated with any operation, there is an operative mortality of approximately 0.05 per cent. Concern for even a low mortality has led to a traditional policy of accepting as donors only individuals between 18 and 55 years of age and in nearly perfect health. As age limits are being extended in the modern era, it is important to exercise even greater care to avoid unacceptable risks.

Obviously, the donor must have two normal kidneys, as confirmed by standard renal function tests, intravenous pyelography, and arteriography. Despite the fact that unilateral nephrectomy for other reasons is known to be followed by compensatory hypertrophy of the remaining kidney, near normal renal function, and normal life expectancy, there has been recent re-examination of the long-term status of living donors. This concern is based on Brenner's finding that ablation of renal tissue in the rat leads to hyperfiltration by the remaining kidney tissue and eventual functional deterioration due to sclerosis.[10] Hakim and associates reported that after 10 years some human donors exhibited proteinuria and hypertension, but larger studies failed to confirm this.[25,74] Perhaps the most reassuring evidence that long-term sequelae are unlikely is that 98 per cent of insurance companies require no increase in life insurance premiums for otherwise healthy individuals after kidney donation.

The identification of a donor from a family group is preferably based on histocompatibility factors, although selection of a less well matched donor by a well-informed family must be respected. It is important that potential candidates be protected from pressure to donate against their will, especially if they are minors. However, most family members willingly donate and the psychologic benefits of doing so are often profound.

Living Unrelated Donors

Until recently, unrelated volunteers were generally excluded from donation, because the results were not sufficiently advantageous, compared with cadaver grafts, to warrant the risk. The improvement in unrelated kidney allograft survival with cyclosporine and the shortage of cadaver donors has provoked re-examination of this issue. Although the use of paid donors is unlawful, genetically unrelated but emotionally related donors (especially spouses) are now considered acceptable by many centers, and excellent results have been reported.[33] There has also been an interest in donor-specific transfusions in this group. Interestingly, the rate of sensitization by transfusion is much higher (60 per cent) with husband-to-wife than with wife-to-husband (11 per cent) transplantation, presumably because of previous pregnancies.

Techniques of Living Donor Nephrectomy

The left kidney is chosen if possible, because the renal vein is longer, facilitating the recipient operation. However, if the arteriogram shows multiple renal arteries on one side, the kidney with a single artery is usually selected to facilitate the anastomosis. A flank incision is used. After incision of Gerota's fascia, the greater curvature of the kidney and upper pole are mobilized, and the hilar structures are exposed. On the left side, the adrenal and gonadal veins are ligated, so that the full length of the renal vein can be utilized. Traction on the renal artery should be avoided because it causes spasm and decreased kidney perfusion. The ureter should be mobilized along with its blood supply and a generous amount of periureteric tissue. It is divided close to the bladder after ligation of the distal end. If the donor is well hydrated, urine should be observed issuing from the proximal end of the divided ureter. Mannitol and furosemide are useful in promoting a diuresis. At this stage attention is given to coordination with the recipient operation (which is performed simultaneously by a separate team). When the recipient iliac vessels and bladder have been prepared, the donor renal artery and vein are clamped and divided in that order. Blood is flushed from the kidney via the renal artery with 4° C. heparinized preservative solution; the kidney is immersed in a basin of the same solution and taken to the recipient operating room. The donor vessels are oversewn, and the incision closed without drainage.

SELECTION AND MANAGEMENT OF CADAVER DONORS

In the absence of a family donor, cadaveric renal transplantation is a satisfactory alternative. In most countries, acceptance of the concept of brain death allows removal of viable organs from donors whose hearts are beating, and cadaveric kidneys represent about 75 per cent of transplants. Should the results of cadaveric transplants continue to improve because of better immunosuppression, the shortage of cadaver kidneys may eventually be the only justification for use of living donors. At present the results (especially long-term results) remain better with a family donor.

The donor shortage is an important limitation. Although the Uniform Anatomical Gift Act has been adopted in all 50 states, few cadaver kidneys are actually obtained on the basis of donor cards alone without permission of the next of kin. Public opinion polls have shown that the majority of United States citizens would consent to donation of organs from deceased relatives, but organs are in fact recovered from fewer than 20 percent of potentially acceptable donors. Although it has been estimated that approximately 20,000 brain dead patients per year are acceptable donors, only 4500 have their kidneys recovered for transplantation.[18] The impact of required request legislation, passed in several states mandating that transplantation be discussed with families of all potential donors, remains to be determined. It is the responsibility (unfortunately not always fulfilled) of primary physicians, neurosurgeons, or intensive care nurses to identify potential donors. Procurement personnel (usually part of a regional team) can then help in obtaining permission from the family and coordinate removal and distribution of viable organs.

Cadaver donors should be previously healthy subjects between 3 and 65 years of age who have sustained fatal head injuries or cerebral vascular accidents. A careful history, a physical examination, and laboratory surveys should be performed for detecting contraindications to organ donation, such as the presence of generalized infections (including those that are occult, such as HIV or hepatitis B infections), malignancy other than nonmetastasizing brain tumors, and known renal disease, hypertension, and advanced arteriosclerosis. Donors over 65 may also sometimes be suitable, but the likelihood of vascular disease makes them less so. The use of kidneys from infants is also possible, but technical aspects are exacting and both kidneys may need to be implanted in a single recipient, a procedure associated with an increased incidence of technical complications.

The use of cadaver donors raises the ethical and legal problems of defining brain death. Consideration of transplantation should never be allowed to influence the definition or declaration of death, which must always be the responsibility of the patient's primary physician and/or of a neurologic consultant, with the full understanding and permission of the family. To avoid any conflict of interest, the transplant team must never be involved with care of the donor or with decisions regarding prognosis or therapy. Current criteria for brain death at the authors' hospital require two in-hospital examinations at least 12 hours apart by a neurologist or a neurosurgeon documenting loss of function of the entire brain. The interval between examinations must be extended to 24 hours in the case of anoxic-ischemic brain injury. Loss of cerebral function is documented by a lack of response to painful stimuli or movement except for spinal reflexes. The loss of brain stem function is documented by fixed pupils; absence of corneal, oculovestibular, and oculocephalic reflexes; loss of gag reflex; and absence of movement or spontaneous respiration off the respirator for 3 minutes, a test that is done only after other criteria indicate no brain function. The declaration of brain death may be accelerated by 6 hours if a confirmatory test is obtained, such as a flat electroencephalogram (EEG) or absence of cerebral blood flow on arteriography. Strict adherence to these criteria is not always possible. For example, EEG confirmation is not required for declaration of brain death in the presence of angiographic evidence for complete lack of blood flow to the brain, which may occur with severe brain swelling. The diagnosis of brain death should not be made in the presence of severe hypothermia, marked hypovolemia, or toxic levels of depressant drugs such as barbiturates, because these factors can produce an isoelectric EEG pattern that is reversible.

Donor Pretreatment

An interesting procedure that has been recommended but not widely accepted is donor pretreatment with immunosuppressive drugs, a strategy that could be employed only for cadaver donors.[24] The rationale is that interstitial cells of hematopoietic origin normally present in the transplant organ ("passenger" cells) contribute importantly to graft immunogenicity and that their removal is beneficial. Conflicting results with pretreatment of donors with such agents as methylprednisolone, cyclophosphamide, and cyclosporine emphasize that circulating passenger cells are not the only source of transplantation antigens within kidney allografts. Interstitial dendritic cells and vascular endothelial cells, which cannot be removed with present techniques, are probably also important in antigen presentation. Nevertheless, it is conceivable that more thorough eradication of passenger cells by vigorous prolonged treatment of donors or treatment of the *ex vivo* kidney might be more beneficial.[11]

HLA Considerations in Cadaver Donor Selection

Although the benefit of matching for HLA-A and -B antigens in selection of family donors is well established, its value for cadaveric grafts remains controversial. Reports from European centers have generally indicated that matching has a beneficial effect.[50] Not only was there a significant difference between grafts fully matched and totally mismatched for HLA-A and -B, but graded improvements in outcome could be related to the extent of the match (although the later phenomenon has become less clear in recent reports). The value of HLA-A and -B typing has been confirmed by some reports from North America but not by others. The benefit of matching is more apparent in long-term, rather than short-term, results.[57] Several possible explanations have been proposed for differences in American and European results, such as the greater genetic heterogeneity of the United States population and the uniformity of tissue typing, which in Europe is performed only in the select and highly experienced laboratories of Eurotransplant.

Both in Europe and the United States, Class II (HLA-DR) matching appears to be of greater benefit than Class I matching. Moreover, most studies indicate that this effect is even more pronounced if there is also HLA-B and HLA-DR identity.

Some authors believe that the improved survival of kidney allografts observed with cyclosporine overrides other previously considered important factors such as blood transfusions and HLA matching. Single-center and multicenter analyses can be found to both support and refute this claim. Perhaps the most convincing data are those of a collaborative study by Opelz in 1987 of over 10,000 cyclosporine-treated patients. This indicated that HLA-A/B, DR, and B/DR matching all remain significantly correlated with improved graft survival.[41]

The perception that cyclosporine overrides the effects of HLA mismatching has been used to argue that prompt local use of poorly matched kidneys is preferable to transplantation into better-matched recipients when this can be achieved only by their transportation to distant centers, thus incurring increased preservation time. The additive effects of cyclosporine toxicity and ischemic damage are additional concerns. Nevertheless, in comparing 9369 transplants done in the same center with 5553 exchanged between centers, Opelz found that in both groups HLA matching improved graft survival (85 per cent with local kidney and 86 per cent with exchanged kidneys).[42] Moreover, well-matched exchanged kidneys fared better than those poorly matched and transplanted locally.

Operative Technique for Cadaveric Donors

After declaration of brain death, the donor is brought to the operating room, and optimal respiration and circulation are maintained during the procedure. Before and during the operation, it is often necessary to administer large volumes of intravenous fluids because of diabetes insipidus or to restore blood volume, which may have been depleted during the premortem attempts to decrease brain swelling and achieve neurologic recovery.

Prior to the widespread application of extrarenal transplantation, the technique of cadaver nephrectomy was similar to that described for related donors. As multiorgan recovery has become routine, rather than the exception, the following technique of *in situ* perfusion and *en bloc* dissection has evolved as the standard (Fig. 1). The peritoneal cavity is entered through a midline incision usually extended to the suprasternal notch to facilitate heart, lung, and liver donation. After exploration for unsuspected neoplasia or infection, the small bowel is retracted and the posterior peritoneum incised in the midline up through the ligament of Treitz to expose the aorta and inferior vena cava. The peritoneal reflections around the cecum are incised and continued cephalad, allowing visualization of retroperitoneum. By retraction of the duodenum and pancreas superiorly, the proximal aorta and vena cava are exposed. Following dissection of the vascular structures of extrarenal organs to be concomi-

tantly harvested (liver, pancreas, heart, lung), the aorta and vena cava are divided just above their bifurcations after proximal insertion of large bore cannulas for retrograde *in situ* perfusion. Anticoagulation is achieved with intravenous heparin, and the aorta is clamped proximally (at the aortic arch for cardiac recovery, above the celiac axis for liver and pancreas, and just above the renal arteries if only the kidneys are to be removed), and infusion of cold (4° C.) preservation solution via the aortic cannula is initiated along with simultaneous decompression via the caval cannula. The kidneys rapidly become pale and cold and are mobilized while damage to the hilar structures and ureters is avoided. The divided distal aorta and vena cava are mobilized cephalad by securing the lumbar vessels between clips, and the aorta is divided above the renal arteries. The entire bloc of kidneys, ureters, aorta, and vena cava are transferred to a basin of cold solution where careful dissection of the renal vessels is performed. The kidneys are then separated by division of the vena cava and aorta and packaged for cold storage to allow time for recipient selection, tissue typing, and transportation.

Preservation of Cadaveric Kidneys

Two methods of preservation (simple cooling and continuous pulsatile perfusion) have become relatively standardized. Both allow sufficient time for transportation of kidneys to distant transplant centers. Simple cooling is achieved by flushing the allograft with a cold iso-osmolar or hyperosmolar buffered solution followed by storage at 4 to 10° C. Additives to the solutions include various ratios of K^+, Na^+, Cl^-, citrate, PO_4^-, SO_4^-, glucose, sucrose, mannitol, bicarbonate, and magnesium. These solutions are used for short-term (less than 48 hours) preservation. Although some disagreement exists, it is generally held that if longer preservation of organs is necessary (48 to 72 hours), it is best achieved by the use of a pulsatile perfusion apparatus that circulates through the kidney either cryoprecipitated homologous plasma, a saline-based electrolyte perfusate containing albumin, Plasmanate or silica gel fractionated plasma, or a preservation solution recently developed by Belzer (see further).

Controversy is unresolved over the best preservation method. However, in the late 1970s there was a trend away from machine pulsatile preservation (which previously was used by about two thirds of centers) toward simple cooling, which is now employed at most centers. Responsible for the

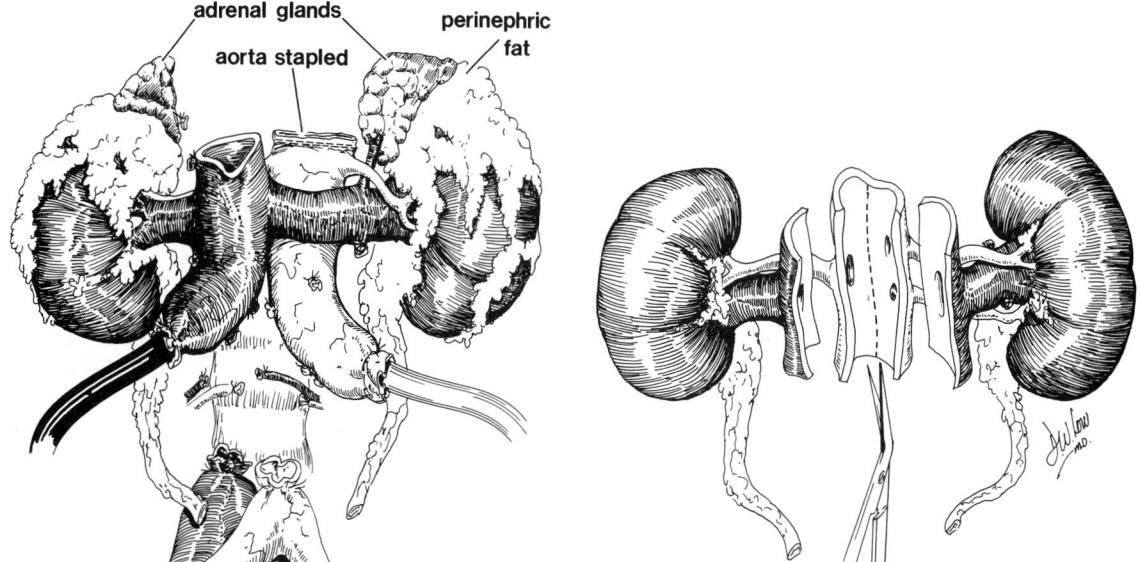

Figure 1. Dissection for cadaver kidney donation is depicted. Cannulas are placed in the aorta and vena cava for hypothermic perfusion to protect the kidneys during the terminal phases of the operation and for short-term storage. Segments of aorta and vena cava are left intact when the kidneys are separated. The use of a Carrel patch of aorta is especially helpful when there are multiple renal arteries.

change were the greater costs and inconvenience of machine perfusion, including the need for a trained attendant during transportation to distant centers. In addition, it was demonstrated that for short preservation times (less than 24 hours) pulsatile perfusion probably had little if any advantage. In 1987, Belzer introduced a solution (University of Wisconsin, or UW, solution) containing several new components (lactobionate, raffinose, hydroxethyl starch) that proved to substantially extend the period of storage possible for liver and pancreas to 24 hours.[7] Although the solution is in wide use by others for simple cold storage of kidneys, it has been used by Belzer with excellent results as a perfusate for machine preservation. Since even with improved preservation solutions simple cooling has a finite time limit it appears likely that major progress in preservation can come only from advances in perfusion techniques. Several groups that resisted the trend toward simple cooling and that continue to use machine perfusion have reported an extremely low incidence of ATN. The additive adverse effects of ischemia and cyclosporine nephrotoxicity may eventually provoke a general return to pulsatile preservation.

XENOGENEIC (INTERSPECIES) GRAFTS

In the early 1960s, subhuman primate kidneys were transplanted into 20 human patients who were immunosuppressed with azathioprine and steroids. Although several grafts functioned briefly and one for as long as 9 months, results were clearly inferior to those obtained at that time with human donors.[51] Therefore, no further human kidney xenografts have since been reported, although it is likely that somewhat better results could now be obtained with improved immunosuppression. The famous Baby Fae heart transplant that functioned for 4 weeks is the only human xenograft in which cyclosporine was used. The shortage in most parts of the world of prospective primate donors, the difficulty of breeding these animals in captivity, concern over simian pathogens, and the possible ethical question of their use are additional major deterrents to this approach, which at present make it quite impractical.

Some of these deterrents would not apply to nonprimate animal donors such as pigs or cows, but the even greater degree of histoincompatibility of such donors would be a major disadvantage. Before clinical trials of this type are attempted, much more should be learned about the process of xenograft rejection.[3] Although it is clear that the preformed antibodies naturally present in humans against most other species would cause immediate destruction of discordant xenografts, relatively little is known about the cellular immune response which would follow if methods were developed to avoid hyperacute rejection.

THE RECIPIENT OPERATION

General anesthesia is preferred by most transplant surgeons, although spinal anesthesia is also satisfactory. Good relaxation is important during the vascular and ureteral anastomosis, but excessive use of muscle relaxants (especially succinyl choline) must be avoided because low cholinesterase levels in dialysis patients may otherwise lead to prolonged apnea. The muscle relaxant atracurium can be used safely because this agent has a short half-life and its degradation is independent of renal and hepatic metabolism.

The iliac vessels are exposed retroperitoneally through an oblique incision just above the inguinal ligament (Fig. 2). The dissection is slightly easier on the right, but a more important consideration in selecting the appropriate side is avoiding sites of previous transplants, other operations (e.g., appendectomy, herniorrhaphy, bladder or ureteral operations), or peritoneal dialysis catheters. The least possible dissection is done to accomplish adequate exposure of planned anastomotic sites.

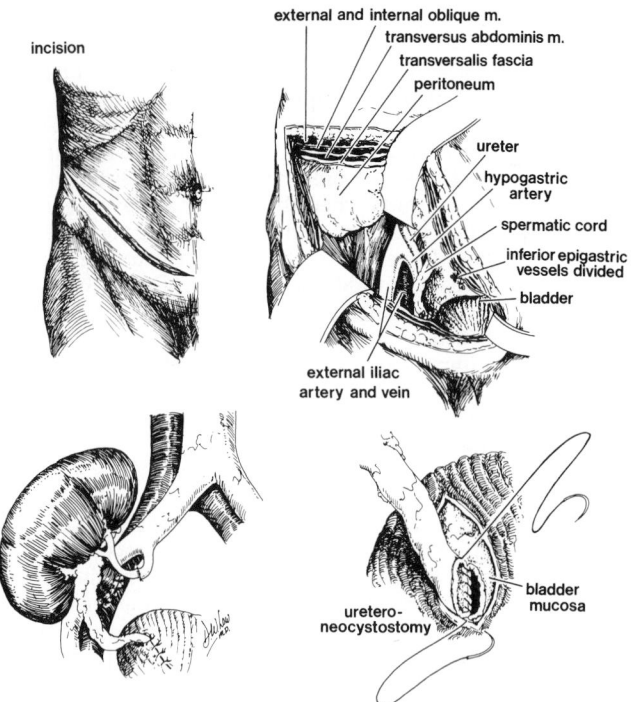

Figure 2. The recipient operation is done through a retroperitoneal incision using the iliac vessels to revascularize the kidney and a ureteroneocystostomy to establish urinary continuity.

Lymphatics which must be divided to expose the iliac vessels are ligated to prevent prolonged lymph drainage or lymphocele formation. Exposure of the bladder is facilitated by dividing the inferior epigastric vessels and, in females, the round ligament. Division of the spermatic cord should be avoided, because this may cause epidydimitis, testicular ischemia, and atrophy.

Traditionally, vascular anastomoses are performed between the end of the donor renal artery and the proximal end of the recipient's divided internal iliac artery and between the end of the donor renal vein and the side of the external iliac vein. More commonly an end-to-side anastomosis of renal artery to external iliac artery is now used, especially when there is significant atheromatous disease in the internal iliac artery, as there often is in older or diabetic recipients, or when the contralateral internal iliac artery has been ligated during a previous transplant operation. Many transplant surgeons routinely favor the end-to-side procedure, because exposure of the external iliac artery requires less dissection and because stenosis at the anastomosis may be less likely, especially when a Carrel patch of donor aorta is used (as is usually the case for cadaveric, but not living, donors).

If there are multiple donor renal arteries that are not on an aortic cuff, the authors favor anastomosis of the end of the smaller renal arteries to the side of the largest renal artery. These anastomoses can be performed deliberately under magnification while the *ex vivo* kidney is protected by immersion in a basin of cold saline (Fig. 3). Revascularization in the recipient can then be accomplished rapidly by a single anastomosis. The sacrifice of even small accessory donor renal arteries should be avoided, because occlusion of these end arteries causes renal infarcts. Preservation of accessory arteries to the lower portion of the kidney is especially important, because they may constitute the blood supply of a segment of collecting system or ureter and their ligation may lead to necrosis and urinary fistula. In 470 living related donors studied at the University of Pennsylvania, multiple renal arteries were present in one kidney in 30 per cent and bilaterally in 9 per cent.[53] In 42 patients in whom the type of *ex vivo* anastomosis described above was performed for multiple arteries, only one kidney was lost because of a

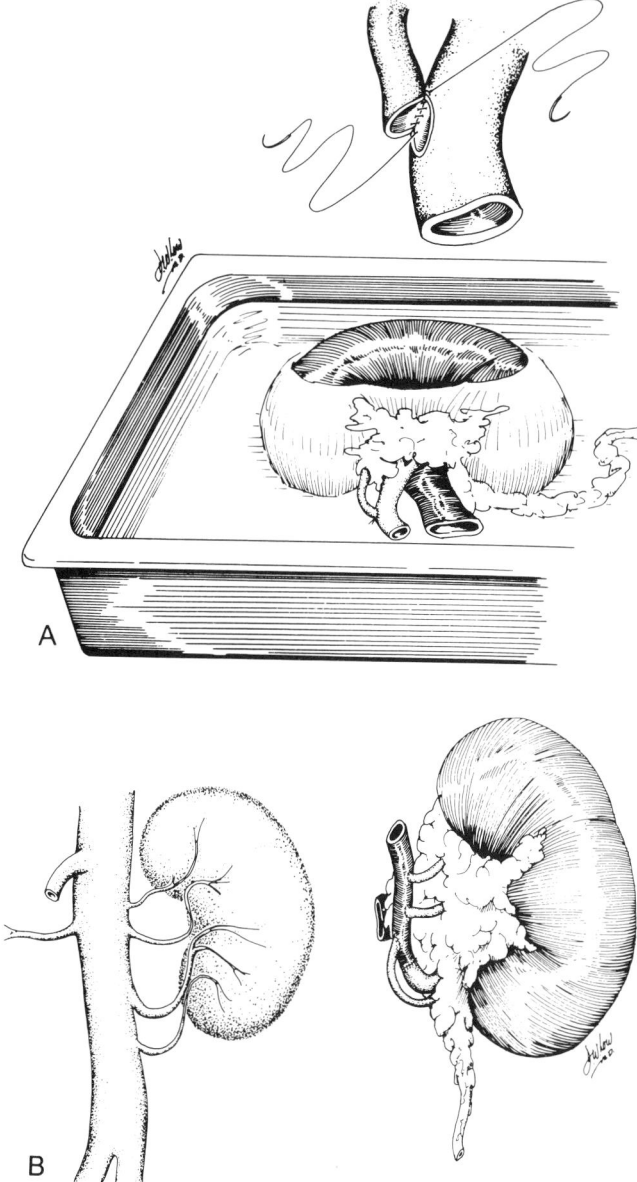

Figure 3. *A,* The smaller of two renal arteries is anastomosed to the larger one in an end-to-side manner while the *ex vivo* kidney is protected by submersion in cold (4° C.) electrolyte solution. *B,* With magnification and hypothermic protection, even complex *ex vivo* microvascular reconstructions can be performed safely. This donor kidney had four small renal arteries arising from the aorta. A short segment of autogenous saphenous vein was removed and under *ex vivo* hypothermia each of the four renal arteries was anastomosed separately into the vein. Revascularization in the recipient was then accomplished with only one anastomoses between the end of the saphenous vein graft and the recipient iliac artery.

technical complication, and the 1-year survival of 76 per cent was no different from that of single-artery kidneys in the precyclosporine period. Venous collateral circulation is generally adequate, so that in instances of multiple renal veins (which are even more common than multiple arteries), only one large vein need be saved for anastomosis.

If a large adult kidney is to be transplanted into a small child, a transperitoneal approach is used to provide adequate room for the kidney, which is revascularized via the aorta and vena cava.

Urinary tract continuity is usually established by ureteroneocystostomy. The ureter should pass beneath the spermatic cord to avoid obstruction. Ureteropyelostomy (anastomosis of the recipient's ureter to the pelvis of the donor kidney) is an alternative procedure that should be used in instances of transplant ureteral devascularization or injury. A few surgeons prefer this

procedure to ureteroneocystostomy, but it is associated with a higher incidence of urinary fistula.

Meticulous technique and hemostasis are particularly important because of the coagulopathy and susceptibility to infection of uremic immunosuppressed patients. The authors prefer to close the wound without drains; but if hemostasis is suboptimal, closed suction catheters may be used.

POSTTRANSPLANT MANAGEMENT

If the transplanted kidney has not suffered ischemic damage, a brisk diuresis is likely to begin within minutes of revascularization. Responsible for the diuresis (which may reach 1000 ml. per hour) are (1) osmotic factors secondary to uremia or high glucose concentrations in intravenous fluids; (2) total body fluid and electrolyte overload secondary to chronic uremia, and (3) mild proximal tubular damage following allograft ischemia. Early in the postoperative period mild diuresis is reassuring and should be encouraged by replacement of urine volumes and, if necessary, by diuretics. Initial inadequate replacement of fluid may lead to oliguria or impaired transplant function, interfering with diagnosis of vascular occlusion, urinary obstruction, or early rejection. Severe dehydration may follow inadequate replacement of losses during massive diuresis, especially in children. During the first few days there may also be a need for colloid or blood replacement because of losses into the wound.

Serious problems may also result from overreplacement of volume, especially if the transplant is not producing urine. Hyperkalemia is particularly dangerous in this setting and may necessitate administration of an ion-exchange resin (Kayexalate, 25 to 50 gm. orally or by enema). In more emergent circumstances, administration of intravenous glucose and insulin or prompt dialysis may be necessary to control hyperkalemia. Suggested replacement fluids include 0.45 per cent saline solution with or without isotonic glucose, sodium bicarbonate (30 mEq. per liter), and potassium (10 to 15 mEq. per liter), depending on the status of the serum electrolytes and blood glucose. If diuresis continues, fluid replacement should not exceed the urinary output, allowing gradual return to normal urine volumes over the next 12 to 24 hours.

Because of the retroperitoneal approach, the transplant operation is relatively nondisruptive to intestinal function, and medications and fluids can usually be given by mouth within 12 to 24 hours. Ambulation on the first postoperative day is beneficial. The Foley catheter can be removed within the first few days. Hypertension, which is common, should be managed conventionally with pharmacologic agents such as hydralazine, beta-blockers, calcium channel blockers, or angiotensin converting enzyme inhibitors. Antacids are given to prevent ulcers and nystatin for prophylaxis against monilial infections. Perioperative antibiotics (which should be given for no more than 48 hours) decrease the incidence of wound infection. Trimethoprim and sulfamethoxazole are used routinely by most centers for prophylaxis against urinary tract infections and *Pneumocystis carinii.* If rejection and other postoperative complications do not occur, the subsequent care is relatively simple, because the restoration of renal function is associated with a rapid return to normal health in patients who previously suffered from single organ system failure.

Immunosuppression

AZATHIOPRINE AND STEROIDS. In the late 1950s, rejection of human renal allografts was first prevented by subjecting patients to whole body irradiation, a profoundly immunosuppressive procedure. Although one of these irradiated patients retained his renal allograft for 25 years without ever receiving immunosuppressive drugs, 11 others developed lethal infections because of the generalized immunodepression.[38] In 1959, Schwartz and Dameshek reported that the antimetabolite

6-mercaptopurine inhibited humoral immunity in rabbits and shortly thereafter Calne and associates and Zukowski and co-workers succeeded in prolonging kidney allograft survival in dogs.[37,38] This drug and its derivative azathioprine had more predictable, reversible, and safer action than radiation and were soon found to circumvent rejection of human renal transplants.

The previously known immunosuppressive effects of adrenal corticosteroids were not sufficient in themselves to prevent rejection, but proved to be synergistic with those of azathioprine. The combination of azathioprine and steroids became standard therapy, although every institution appeared to have a somewhat different protocol for their use. Brief courses of high-dose steroid therapy could sometimes abort rejection, which usually ensued despite baseline immunosuppression. Thus, rejection was recognized to be an episodic and potentially quite reversible process.[61]

ANTILYMPHOCYTE ANTIBODIES. In the 1960s Woodruff, Medawar, Monaco, and others studied a new immunosuppressive agent, antilymphocyte serum (ALS), which appeared to be a more potent and more specific immunosuppressant than azathioprine.[75] ALS contained xenoantibody raised by repeated immunization of heterologous animals (e.g., rabbits, horses) with human lymphoid cells. In rodents, small doses of ALS strikingly reduced the number of circulating lymphocytes and prevented rejection of skin allografts. Although it was soon demonstrated that ALS was also a potent immunosuppressant in man, several problems diminished its usefulness.[60] Even the purified globulin fraction (ALG) sometimes provoked allergic reactions, leukopenia, and thrombocytopenia. The therapeutic window was small and large doses or prolonged therapy often led to serious infections, especially viral infections. In addition, patients formed antibodies to the heterologous protein, which diminished the effectiveness of prolonged or repeated courses. Thus, ALS could be given only for a limited time, at marginal doses, and only as an adjunct to "conventional" immunosuppressive agents. Some authorities reported that "prophylactic" use of ALS to delay rejection by a few weeks improved results, but others remained unconvinced of its usefulness, and randomized studies failed to demonstrate statistical benefits.[39,70] Subsequently, ALS was found to be very effective in reversing rejection crises, even those resistant to high-dose steroid therapy, and this became its most common indication.[27]

The effectiveness of ALS in reversing rejection was the rationale for the introduction by Cosimi and associates of monoclonal anti–T-cell antibodies for the same purpose.[17] Monoclonal anti–T-cell antibodies induce rapid depletion of T lymphocytes from peripheral blood while having little detrimental effect on other populations such as red blood cells, platelets, or granulocytes, all of which are affected by cross-reacting antibodies present in polyclonal ALS preparation. Because of greater availability, specificity, and ease of standardization, monoclonal pan–T-cell antibodies such as OKT3 have largely replaced ALS and ALG. The structure recognized by OKT3 is linked to the T-cell antigen receptor, which is critical for the activation of human T cells. *In vivo* depletion of T cells is believed to be mediated by mechanisms such as complement-mediated lympholysis or opsonization of cells. Multi-institutional randomized prospective trials revealed its efficacy in reversal of acute rejection in 94 per cent of cadaveric renal allograft rejections — a figure significantly better than the 75 per cent obtained with conventional steroid treatment.[45]

Side effects associated with OKT3 therapy (particularly the initial dose) include fever, shaking chills, headache, nausea, vomiting, diarrhea, wheezing, and pulmonary edema (probably due to release of cytokines) and can often be ameliorated by pretreatment with methylprednisolone, acetaminophen, and antihistamines. As with polyclonal ALG, the use of monoclonal antibody OKT3 induces rapid sensitization to mouse antibody, which commonly leads to the neutralization of OKT3 and reappearance in the peripheral blood of CD3$^+$ cells. Concomitant administration of azathioprine and steroids may delay the production of anti-OKT3 antibody and prolong its immunosuppressive effect. It is recommended that *in vivo* efficacy of OKT3 be monitored by sequential analyses of the CD3$^+$ T-cell populations in the peripheral blood and measurement of human antibodies to the murine immunoglobulin.

CYCLOSPORINE. Cyclosporine is credited with revolutionizing transplantation by facilitating successful extrarenal transplants and with improving cadaver kidney graft survival by as much as 20 per cent. Some of the improvement in results that occurred in the 1980s concurrently with the introduction of this new drug was probably attributable to concomitant progress in other aspects of transplantation, but cyclosporine was undoubtedly a major factor. Cyclosporine is a fungal derivative first noted by Borel in 1974 to have immunosuppressive qualities.[9] It appears to block T-lymphocyte production of the lymphokine IL-2 through inhibition of its messenger RNA. Like azathioprine and unlike OKT3 and ALS, cyclosporine is most useful for prophylaxis, rather than reversal of rejection. Calne, using it for single drug immunosuppression in 1979, reported promising results but found the agent quite toxic and its administration associated with infections, tumors, and renal failure.[12] By reducing the dose of cyclosporine and combining it with small doses of prednisone, Starzl subsequently reported spectacular improvement in the outcome of liver and kidney allografts (up to 90 per cent survival of cadaver kidney allografts).[52] Similarly, improved results were soon reported by others and confirmed by multicenter randomized studies in both Canada and Europe. Since its release for general use in 1983, cyclosporine has been adopted by nearly all centers as the basis of contemporary immunosuppressive protocols.[13]

Cyclosporine has the major advantage over azathioprine of lacking bone marrow toxicity, but it has the disadvantage of nephrotoxicity, which is its major side effect. Nephrotoxicity may be manifest as a delay in function of a newly transplanted kidney or impaired function of a well-established renal allograft. Although maintenance of blood levels in the therapeutic range is helpful, it does not eliminate the possibility of nephrotoxicity, which may occur even at "subtherapeutic" levels.[29] Even after prolonged stable low dose cyclosporine, elevated blood levels of the agent and toxicity may appear, especially during concurrent use of certain drugs which increase bioavailability (such as erythromycin, cimetidine, diltiazem, and ketoconazole). However, decreased blood levels may follow patient noncompliance or interactions of drugs such as phenobarbital, phenytoin, and trimethoprim-sulfamethoxazole, which activate the hepatic P-450 cytochrome system. In addition to nephrotoxicity, other side effects attributable to cyclosporine include hypertension, hepatotoxicity, seizures, tremor, hypertrichosis, nausea, vomiting, and diarrhea.

Delayed renal allograft function from ischemia, which is commonly encountered in cadaver kidneys, may be accentuated by nephrotoxic drugs. Therefore, many centers avoid the use of cyclosporine until ATN has resolved. A prophylactic course of ALG or OKT3 is advocated by some along with steroids and azathioprine to delay rejection until graft function allows institution of cyclosporine therapy. Even without initial ischemic renal damage, patients on cyclosporine tend to have persistently higher serum creatinine levels than patients treated with azathioprine (1.7 to 2.3 versus 1.4) and histologic changes of interstitial fibrosis in the kidney. Because of uncertainty regarding the risk of permanent renal damage from long-term cyclosporine therapy, some centers use minimal initial doses of cyclosporine in combination with azathioprine and prednisone (triple therapy). To avoid chronic nephrotoxicity, others eventually discontinue cyclosporine altogether and utilize only azathioprine and prednisone after stable graft function is established. This may precipitate an acute rejection episode, but these are usually responsive to steroids. Most clinicians, however, believe that the risks of chronic renal damage are outweighed by the substantial advantages of cyclosporine, including the possibility that in selected patients treated with cyclosporine, steroid therapy could eventually be completely withdrawn.

A typical "triple drug" regimen currently used at the University of Pennsylvania consists of intraoperative methylprednisolone (1 gm.) and azathioprine (10 mg. per kg.) intravenously (Fig. 4). Daily doses of prednisone are begun at 1.5 mg. per kg. and tapered to 30 mg. by the end of the first week and eventually to a maintenance dose of 10 mg. per day. Azathioprine is given at 1 mg. per kg. per day. Patients whose transplants function promptly receive oral cyclosporine 14 mg. per kg. per day on the first postoperative day and subsequent daily doses are determined by trough levels in whole blood, which are maintained at 100 to 200 ngm. per ml. (as determined by high performance liquid chromatography). This regimen leads to a lower incidence of nephrotoxicity than encountered in the early cyclosporine era, when higher doses were utilized without azathioprine.

Patient survival has also been improved by the introduction of cyclosporine, probably because of a decrease in incidence and severity of infections. Especially benefited are older patients, recipients of multiple transplants, and those with high immune responses. Many believe that histocompatibility matching is less important than it is when cyclosporine is not employed although this is controversial.[14,30] This may also be true of pretransplant transfusions, especially since highly sensitized patients appear to have a poor prognosis whether treated with cyclosporine or azathioprine. Disappointingly, there is no clear evidence that cyclosporine has the same favorable impact on long-term results as it does on early results. Both U. S. and European multicenter reports indicate a continuing attrition in late graft survival most likely due to chronic rejection, which apparently is not influenced by cyclosporine. It is even possible that the chronic nephrotoxicity of cyclosporine is additive to the effects of chronic rejection. Despite new problems associated with cyclosporine and uncertainty over its ultimate benefit, the introduction of the agent represents a major advance. New agents such as FK506 and monoclonal antibodies against T-cell subsets, receptors, or lymphokines may be anticipated to effect further improvements in the near future.

REJECTION

Considerable effort has been made to correlate allograft morphology with the clinical course of rejection. Histologic study of a kidney biopsy provides only a narrowly focused "snapshot" of the target of a complex systemic process, which is in continuous evolution while also being modified by immunosuppression. Rejection is conveniently categorized as hyperacute, acute, or chronic; but there are overlapping features and transitions between these categories.

Hyperacute Rejection

In the 1960s several instances were noted in which kidneys were rejected "hyperacutely." This phenomenon was observed within minutes of kidney revascularization and was evidenced by bluish discoloration of the kidney, deterioration of perfusion, and then sudden cessation of function. Histologically observed were extensive intravascular deposits of fibrin and platelets and intraglomerular accumulation of polymorphonuclear leukocytes, fibrin, platelets, and red blood cells along with accumulation of polymorphonuclear cells (PMNs) in the peritubular and glomerular capillaries (Fig. 5A).[31] This process proved refractory to immunosuppressive or anticoagulant therapy and inevitably led to rapid destruction of the kidney. It soon became evident that the occurrence of hyperacute rejection was usually correlated with the presence of preformed circulating antibodies against donor antigens which could be identified by a pretransplant crossmatch. The classic form of hyperacute rejection has become rare since transplants are no longer performed when the crossmatch is positive. Occasionally, a more subtle form of the pattern is observed in which the transplanted kidney initially appears normal and produces urine but within 24 to 48 hours undergoes abrupt rejection.

Acute Cellular Rejection

This type of rejection most commonly becomes evident during the early days or weeks after transplantation, although it may occasionally occur after months or years. Prompt diagnosis of rejection and initiation of appropriate antirejection treatment should be undertaken, because it can often prevent irreversible damage and reverse the entire process. The diagnosis of acute rejection is based on a constellation of findings that include clinical signs and symptoms, laboratory assays of blood and urine, radioisotope studies, and allograft biopsies. Classic signs and symptoms are malaise, fever, tenderness, and swelling of the wound (due to allograft edema pressing against the peritoneum), oliguria, and hypertension. However, most of these symptoms are rarely seen in patients receiving cyclosporine.

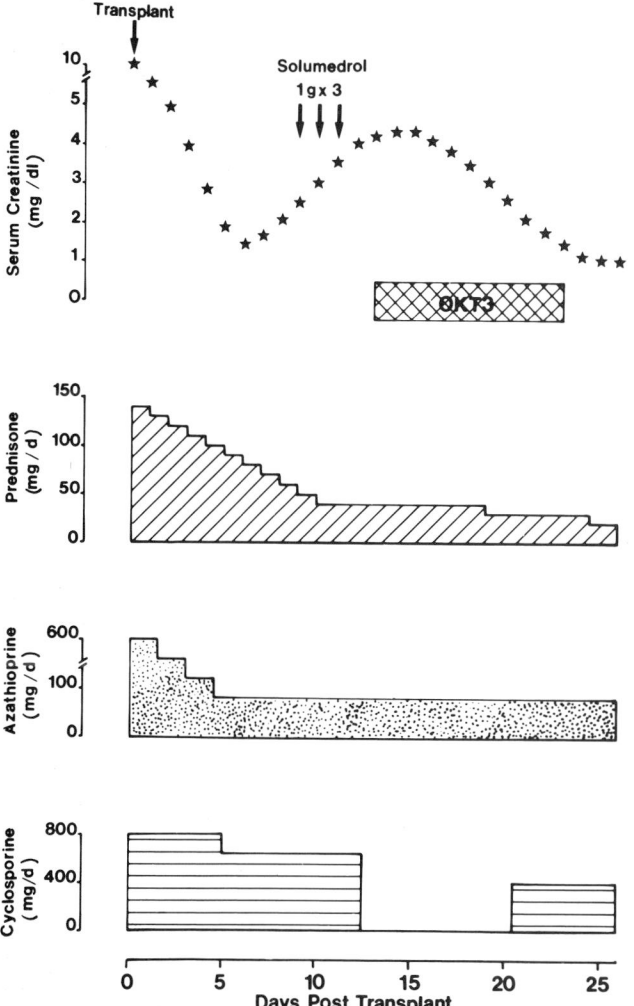

Figure 4. Clinical course of a renal allograft recipient under triple-drug immunosuppressive therapy. Rejection was ushered by a rising serum creatinine level that did not improve after high-dose steroid treatment. Because of the steroid "resistant" nature of rejection, "rescue" treatment consisting of a 10-day course of monoclonal antibody OKT3 was employed. This was followed by complete resolution of the rejection crisis and a normal creatinine level. Note that cyclosporine was discontinued during OKT3 treatment so that excessive immunosuppression could be avoided.

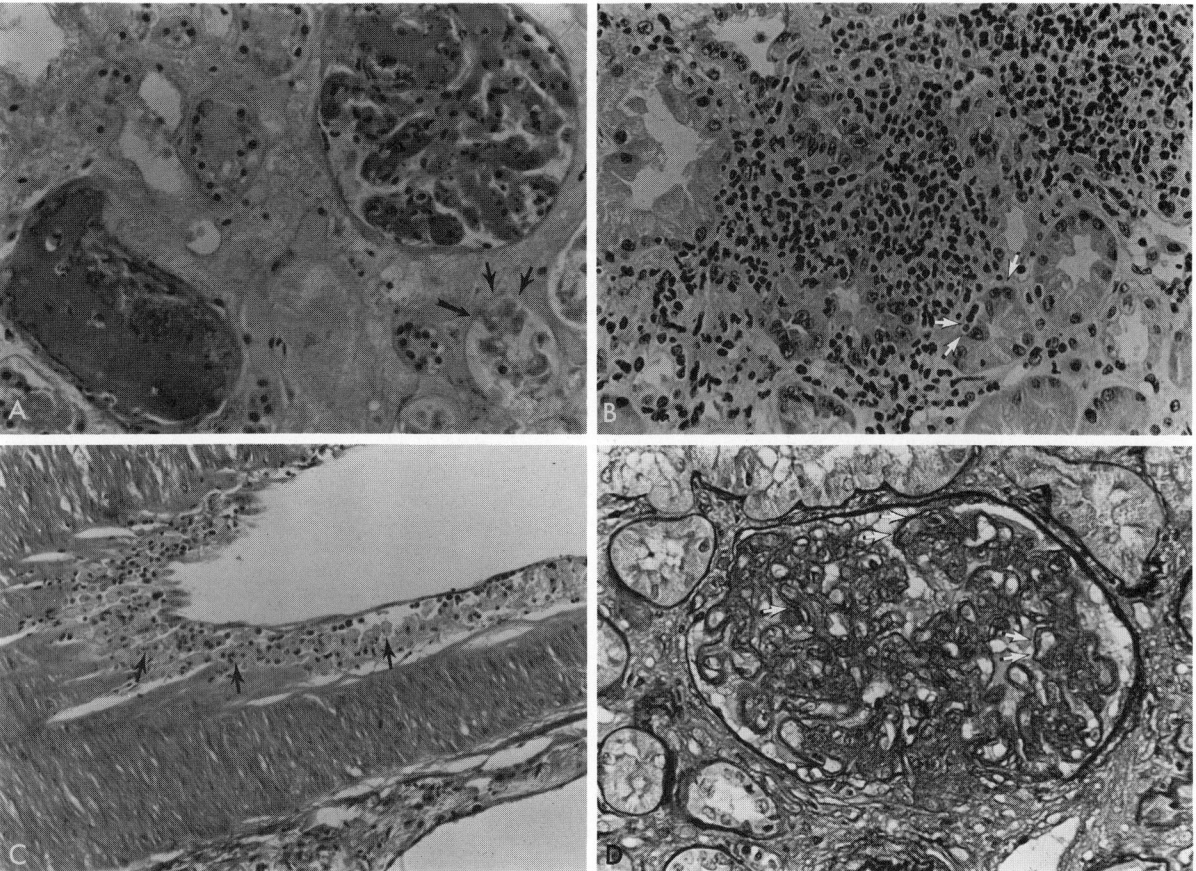

Figure 5. *A,* Allograft nephrectomy showing hyperacute rejection. Glomerulus and small arteries demonstrating massive occlusion by fresh thrombus and polymorphonuclear cells. Interstitium demonstrates edema, and tubules appear necrotic (arrows). Hematoxylin and eosin, ×1000. *B,* Renal allograft biopsy demonstrating predominantly acute cellular rejection with dense interstitial lymphocytic inflammatory infiltrate and tubulitis (arrows). Hematoxylin and eosin, ×1000. *C,* Allograft biopsy demonstrating early acute humoral rejection. Arcuate size artery with lifting of endothelium and subendothelial accumulation of inflammatory cells and foamy macrophages (arrows). Hematoxylin and eosin, ×1000. *D,* Posttransplant glomerulopathy with changes consistent with chronic humoral-mediated rejection. This glomerulus has a mesangiocapillary pattern with extensive double contours (arrows). Trichrome–methenamine silver, ×1000. (Courtesy of John E. Tomaszewski, M.D., Department of Pathology and Laboratory Medicine, University of Pennsylvania, Philadelphia.)

Under the influence of this agent, rejection assumes a more subtle clinical pattern in which fever and allograft swelling are absent and impaired renal function may be the only signal.

Under these circumstances, the authors usually obtain a radioisotopic renal perfusion scan, a test that cannot provide specific evidence of rejection, but helps to exclude several other conditions that can cause impaired renal function, such as vascular occlusion, ureteric obstruction, and urinary fistula.

Since the diagnosis of rejection on clinical grounds alone may be difficult, some transplant surgeons perform a biopsy whenever rejection is suspected. This procedure may be performed transcutaneously with little risk. Early microscopic signs of acute rejection include the adherence of lymphocytes to the endothelium of peritubular capillaries and venules, which then progresses to disruption of these vessels, tubular necrosis, and interstitial infiltrates. Cellular infiltration, which is the hallmark of rejection, is comprised initially of small lymphocytes and later consists of variable types of cells such as large lymphocytes and macrophages (Fig. 5*B*). As rejection proceeds toward irreversibility, there is greater involvement of the vascular elements of the graft. Swelling of the intima and focal fibrinoid necrosis of the media ensue (Fig. 5*C*), followed by endothelial cell proliferation and obliteration of the lumina of small arteries by fibrin, platelets, and lymphoid cells.

Total reliance cannot be placed on a biopsy as the standard for diagnosing acute rejection. Not only are biopsies subject to sampling error, but lymphocytic infiltration in itself does not represent conclusive evidence of rejection, since for obscure reasons even perfectly functioning renal allografts often exhibit some degree of mononuclear infiltration.

Distinguishing impairment of renal function due to rejection from cyclosporine nephrotoxicity is a challenging problem. Some authorities believe that biopsies can discriminate between these two entities, whereas others do not. In cyclosporine nephrotoxic states, variable degrees of lymphocytic infiltration in the interstitium of the kidney have been observed.[71] Careful attention to trends and fluctuations of cyclosporine blood levels may aid in decision making. Cyclosporine nephrotoxicity characteristically causes smaller increments in serum creatinine than rejection does, and these are usually reversible within a few days following dose reduction.

A particularly challenging clinical problem is the diagnosis of rejection in the setting of ATN. Under this circumstance, a biopsy may be the only aid to diagnosis. Unfortunately, however, even a skilled pathologist cannot always distinguish the histologic pattern of rejection from that of ATN (or cyclosporine toxicity). Therefore, enthusiasm for repeated biopsies varies, some transplant surgeons being content in most instances to rely on their clinical judgment. At times empiric antirejection therapy is employed as a diagnostic test for suspected rejection. In the presence of acute rejection (and the absence of ATN), this usually lowers the creatinine promptly.

If the diagnosis of acute rejection can be made with certainty (or even high probability), prompt institution of antirejection therapy (steroids, ALS, OKT3) is necessary to prevent permanent damage to the allograft. This treatment is usually capable of reversing the process, although recurrent acute rejection may ensue. Intravenous high-dose steroids (0.5 to 1.0 gm. methylprednisolone) are used as first-line therapy for rejection at most centers. The authors find that approximately 65 per cent of acute rejections respond to 3 to 5 doses. Steroid-resistant rejection may respond to ALG or OKT3 in an additional 30 per cent of cases.

It is important that antirejection therapy not be employed needlessly or for a prolonged period, since this is the cause of most morbidity and mortality. During the 1970s (prior to the introduction of cyclosporine), a progressive improvement in patient survival occurred in most centers.[68] This was the result of realization that overly intense immunosuppression and repeated courses of antirejection therapy were unwise and dangerous and that better long-term results were accomplished by more conservative therapy. Many groups adopted the policy of refusing to treat aggressively more than two episodes of acute rejection. Experience taught the important lesson that eventual loss of some grafts could not be avoided. Early recognition and acceptance of this eventuality, transplant nephrectomy, reinstitution of dialysis, and the likelihood of a later successful transplant were obviously preferable to employing heavy immunosuppression to the point of serious infection and death. Employment of this philosophy has allowed the reduction of the 1-year mortality of cadaveric transplantation to less than 5 per cent at the University of Pennsylvania in the last 5 years.

Immunologic Monitoring

Because the clinical diagnosis of rejection is so frequently uncertain, and always late if based on damage of the target organ, attempts have been made to assay the recipient's immune status to obtain an early diagnosis or even a prediction of rejection. Two types of assays have been used, those defining the level of specific antidonor activity and those reflecting the general level of immunosuppression and thus, presumably, the risk of rejection.

Assays of cellular and humoral immunity to donor antigens such as donor-specific cytotoxic T lymphocytes, antibody-dependent cellular cytotoxicity, complement-dependent cytotoxicity, and donor-specific anti–B-cell antibodies have been evaluated, but none is reliably correlated with early rejection. Enthusiasm has also declined for utilizing monoclonal antibody–determined circulating T-lymphocyte subset ratio as an index of adequate immunosuppression or impending rejection.[17] Unfortunately, a number of confounding factors such as generalized lymphopenia and lymphocyte subset variations associated with bacterial and viral infections limit the specificity and usefulness of such assays.

Study of the phenotypic composition of the interstitial cellular infiltrate obtained directly from the allograft by means of fine-needle aspiration has failed to gain popularity.[28] Currently, the value of serial determination in serum or urine of anti–IL-2 receptor or tumor necrosis factor as predictors of rejection is being investigated.[16]

Chronic Rejection

Chronic rejection is the usual cause of late deterioration of renal allografts, although other causes such as renal artery stenosis should be considered. The typical course of chronic rejection is gradual, progressive loss of renal function. It may begin after years of stable function but is more often observed in patients who have had multiple early and incompletely reversible episodes of acute rejection. Protracted humoral injury (thought to be a more important factor in this condition than in acute cellular rejection) is manifested histologically by intimal fibroproliferative arterial lesions. These intimal lesions probably stem from repetitive cycles of chronic immune injury to the endothelium with focal thrombosis and incorporation of thrombus into the arterial wall. Also observed in chronic rejec-

tion are glomerular changes (Fig. 5D). Histologically, increased mesangial matrix and mesangial proliferation are observed. The glomerular basement membrane is thickened; and focal deposition of IgM, IgG, and complement may be identified along capillary walls and within the mesangium. Clinically, these are manifested by proteinuria, microscopic hematuria, and slowly deteriorating function.

In the presence of these morphologic vascular and glomerular changes, antirejection therapy is ineffective. Employment of high-dose steroid or ALS or OKT3 therapy in the hope of reversing the process should never be risked, because this is of no benefit and may lead to opportunistic infection or other serious sequelae. However, abrupt cessation of immunosuppression is also unwarranted early in the course of chronic rejection because its progression may be slow and significant periods of useful, although diminishing, transplant function are possible. Some nephrologists believe that angiotensin converting enzyme inhibitors and restriction of dietary protein reduce the progression of renal insufficiency. Generally, immunosuppression should be reduced as renal failure progresses, because the additive immunodepressive effects of uremia and immunosuppressive drugs are particularly dangerous.

It is important to remember that acute cellular rejection is also occasionally encountered after years of stable transplant function, sometimes as the result of discontinuation of immunosuppression by the careless or noncompliant patient. This must be distinguished from chronic rejection if possible, although a timely diagnosis of late acute rejection is usually fortuitous since symptoms are uncommon. A prompt biopsy is warranted in cases of unexpected or precipitous deterioration in stable function, because late cellular rejection (unlike chronic rejection) can often be reversed if treated before severe damage occurs.

RECURRENT DISEASE IN TRANSPLANTED KIDNEYS

Because transplantation does not modify the underlying etiology of the renal disease, it is not surprising that the transplanted kidney is sometimes regarded by the host as an appropriate new target for destruction by the original disease process, especially in autoimmune diseases such as glomerulonephritis or in metabolic abnormalities such as diabetes, oxalosis, or cystinosis.

Glomerulonephritis

In the 1950s Murray diagnosed recurrent glomerulonephritic damage in transplants from monozygotic twin donors within a few months.[38] Late follow-up of this series of 30 twin grafts indicated that 8 failed from recurrent glomerulonephritis, leading some authorities to advocate the use of mild immunosuppression even in recipients of twin grafts.[69]

In allografts, the incidence of recurrent glomerulonephritis is more difficult to assess, since clinical manifestations and even histologic changes may be easily confused with those of chronic rejection. Membranoproliferative glomerulonephritis appears to be a form of the disease especially likely to recur, the crescentic and lobular types appearing earlier and progressing more rapidly than the electron-dense deposit type. Focal glomerular sclerosis also has a propensity for recurrence, as do IgA nephropathy and antiglomerular basement membrane nephritis. The importance of diagnosing recurrent glomerulonephritis is to distinguish it from acute rejection, which, unlike recurrent glomerulonephritis, can often be successfully treated.

Collagen Diseases

Collagen diseases, such as lupus erythematosus, are possible but unlikely causes of recurrent damage and are often well palliated by transplantation.

Metabolic Diseases

Cystinosis is a disorder which causes intracellular deposition of cystine crystals in various organs, usually leading to end-stage renal disease by age 10. Although extra-renal manifestations are not influenced by successful transplantation and eventual recurrent renal disease is inevitable, useful temporary palliation is expected following transplantation.

Oxalosis is likely to reappear in transplanted kidneys so rapidly (sometimes within a month) that it is not generally considered an indication for transplantation. However, hepatic transplantation reverses the metabolic defect and should be considered, especially in patients with renal and other systemic damage (neuropathy, cardiac conduction defects), because concomitant transplantation of the liver and kidney has been dramatically successful.[73]

Diabetes, when it causes end-stage nephropathy, has become one of the most common indications for renal transplantation. Although diabetics have an increased risk, their long-term survival is superior after renal transplantation to that associated with maintenance on dialysis. Diabetic nephropathy is thought to be caused by protracted abnormal glucose homeostasis which is not improved by renal transplantation. Indeed, steroid therapy is likely to aggravate hyperglycemia or even precipitate diabetes in previously normoglycemic patients. Thus, in diabetic patients it is not surprising that Kimmelstiel-Wilson lesions may be found on biopsies of the transplanted kidney within 2 years, although 10 to 20 years might be required for functional deterioration. Interestingly, pancreatic transplantation when performed concomitantly with renal transplantation has been demonstrated to prevent the early morphologic changes of diabetes in the transplanted kidney.[8]

COMPLICATIONS OF RENAL TRANSPLANTATION

Technical Complications

Complications occurring in the first few hours or days after transplantation are commonly related to technical problems in establishing vascular and urinary continuity or to damage which occurs during donor nephrectomy or preservation. Since rejection may also be an early event, its differentiation from various other causes of poor function may be difficult.

VASCULAR COMPLICATIONS. Arterial obstruction, although less common than ATN or urinary tract complications as a cause of early postoperative oliguria or anuria, should be considered promptly if an established diuresis suddenly ceases. A diseased hypogastric artery may thrombose and should never be used to vascularize the transplant. Instead, the usually more normal common or external iliac artery should be used in such instances. Partial occlusion of the transplant vessels may be caused by kinking from improper positioning of the kidney. Radioisotopic scanning and arteriography confirm suspected vascular occlusion, but immediate reoperation without delay for diagnostic studies allows the only likelihood of salvaging such a graft, since only a few minutes of total ischemia can be tolerated before damage becomes irreversible.

HEMORRHAGE. Imperfect operative hemostasis in the setting of uremic coagulopathy or anticoagulation during hemodialysis is the usual cause of early postoperative bleeding. Fracture or frank rupture of the transplanted kidney are unusual causes of bleeding, but may occur from rapid swelling of the transplant during acute rejection. Rupture is more common in kidneys from infant or child donors, in which the small organ is sometimes unable to tolerate adult levels of blood pressure and flow.

Bleeding from the arterial suture line, except in the early hours postoperatively, should bring to mind the strong possibility of infection. Resuturing of an infected suture line is futile, and recurrent disruption is nearly assured. The kidney should be removed, and the hypogastric artery securely ligated. If the anastomosis is in the common or external iliac artery, the problem is more serious. Even removal of the kidney necessitates a suture line to close the iliac arteriotomy. This then becomes a potential site of arterial disruption. Ligation of the iliac artery and extra-anatomic bypass (femorofemoral or axillofemoral) may be necessary.

RENAL TRANSPLANT ARTERY STENOSIS (RTAS). This condition may be confused with rejection, because both may lead to hypertension and diminished renal function. Although RTAS is a relatively unusual cause of decreased renal function, which is more commonly the result of rejection or cyclosporine toxicity, a high index of suspicion should be maintained, because it is correctable. The true incidence of RTAS is not known, but in patients in whom on clinical grounds renal artery stenosis is suspected, confirmation of the diagnosis by biplanar arteriography occurs in 4 to 12 per cent. However, when 100 consecutive transplant patients were subjected to routine postoperative arteriography by Lacombe, a surprising prevalence of stenosis was found (23 per cent).[32]

The cause of RTAS is usually technical, i.e., improper anastomosis, injury of the intima of the renal artery during washout or perfusion, or kinking at the anastomotic site from redundancy or twisting of the arteries. Arteriosclerotic lesions of the donor or recipient vessels may be a contributing factor. An immunologic pathogenesis has also been invoked, since intimal proliferation and subintimal fibrotic changes observed in RTAS are similar to small vessel changes caused by rejection. About 70 per cent of the lesions are at the anastomotic site, but 20 per cent are beyond the anastomosis in the transplant renal artery proper. Thus, even the use of a Carrel patch does not always prevent this complication.

Not all instances of RTAS are clinically relevant. Since the incidence of at least mild hypertension is as high as 50 per cent in transplant patients, RTAS is by no means always its cause. Thus its correction cannot always be expected to be followed by normotension. A trial of angiotensin converting enzyme inhibitors may be useful in identifying those patients whose hypertension may respond to correction of the stenosis, since these patients often respond to these drugs with a sudden rise in creatinine and a dramatic fall in blood pressure.

The authors presently advocate percutaneous transluminal angioplasty (PTA) in most instances of RTAS. Of 547 consecutive renal allograft recipients between 1979 and 1985, 39 thought to have RTAS because of refractory hypertension had the diagnosis confirmed by arteriography and underwent balloon dilation.[23] In this largest reported series, 76 per cent of PTAs were successful, whereas only one graft was lost. In three patients initially treated successfully recurrent stenosis developed, which was corrected operatively by patch angioplasty. Although some groups favor operation over PTA, the surgical treatment is difficult and not always successful. In seven instances of RTAS in 369 renal grafts prior to 1979, the authors found operative treatment to be successful in only four patients. The long-term results of PTA and surgical therapy are probably approximately comparable; but because of simplicity and patient acceptability, most surgeons advocate PTA as the initial approach with surgical therapy reserved for persistent or recurrent stenosis.[19]

VENOUS THROMBOSIS. Occlusion of the transplant renal vein, although rare, can follow technical anastomotic errors, kinking, or compression. Iliofemoral thrombosis occasionally follows renal transplantation, presumably because of clamping of the vein or compression by the transplant. The thrombus rarely extends into the renal vein, and standard anticoagulant treatment is generally effective. If pulmonary embolism occurs, despite adequate anticoagulation, caval interruption should be performed by standard techniques, such as a Greenfield filter, and rarely compromises transplant function.

URINARY TRACT COMPLICATIONS. The most common

cause of sudden cessation of urinary output in the immediate postoperative period is presence of a blood clot in the bladder or urethral catheter, which can be relieved by irrigation. Other more serious causes of urinary obstruction are unusual (2 to 5 per cent in most series) and should be investigated simultaneously with consideration of vascular occlusion, acute tubular necrosis, or rejection.[34] A ureteroneocystostomy may become occluded by a hematoma at the site of the submucosal tunnel in the bladder or by a technically unsatisfactory anastomosis. An adynamic ureter or edema at the orifice in the bladder can also cause temporary partial obstruction.

Devascularization of the ureter during donor nephrectomy is a more serious problem that may lead to ureteral necrosis and fistula within the first few days or weeks. Mild ureteral ischemia is the probable cause of an occasional late distal ureteral stenosis, which may lead to partial or total occlusion (Fig. 6). Fluid obtained from wound drains or needle aspiration can be identified as urine by its urea content, which is several times higher than that of serum or lymph. Ultrasound studies (for fluid collections), radioactive scans, and cystograms (which via reflux may visualize the ureter) are other helpful studies. However, ureterography is usually necessary to define the status of the ureter and is best accomplished by percutaneous fine-needle puncture of the kidney and antegrade catheterization of the pelvis and ureter. Treatment must be individualized and may consist either of reconstruction of the ureteroneocystostomy (if it is not ischemic) or of ureteropyelostomy using the patient's own ureter.

ACUTE TUBULAR NECROSIS. Ischemia occasionally precipitates ATN in a related donor transplant, but in cadaver transplants the incidence is much higher. Despite the fact that nearly all such kidneys are from cadavers with beating hearts, ATN occurs in 5 to 30 per cent, probably due to ischemic damage during preservation. Therefore, in the absence of vascular or ureteral problems, initially nonfunctional cadaver kidneys may be assumed to have ATN, especially if ^{131}I-technetium and iodohippurate scans demonstrate good blood flow and poor tubular function. At times, however, a kidney briefly has adequate urinary output and then lapses into ATN. Estimating the true output of the transplanted kidney may be difficult if the patient's own kidneys are producing substantial amounts of urine.

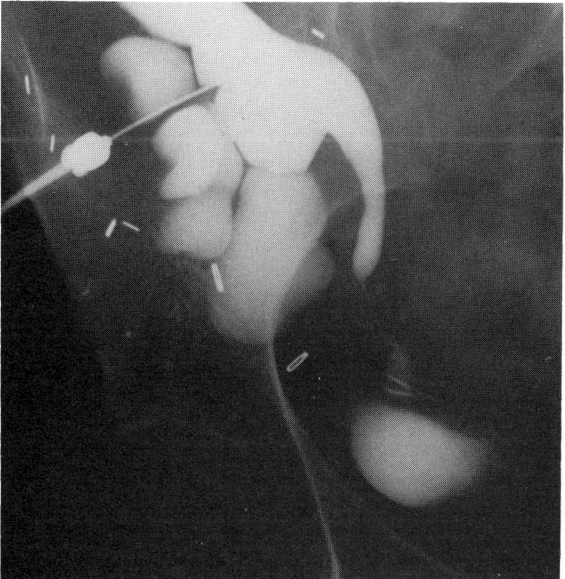

Figure 6. An antegrade percutaneous pyelogram of a renal allograft demonstrating obstruction of the distal ureter as it enters the bladder. Calyces are widely dilated and clubbed. (Courtesy of Mark Banner, M.D., Department of Radiology, University of Pennsylvania, Philadelphia.)

Oliguria in the early transplant period should be treated with aliquots of fluid and colloid to exclude hypovolemia, while care is taken not to fluid overload the patient. Mannitol, 12.5 to 25 gm., and furosemide, 100 to 200 mg., intravenously in divided doses may be used to increase the output but are unlikely to alter the course of true ATN. Although mild ATN *per se* does not significantly worsen the prognosis for eventual transplant success, the overall impact of ATN is definitely an adverse one.

Some kidneys which never produce urine (termed "primary nonfunction") are no doubt lost because potentially reversible damage from ATN is compounded by undiagnosed rejection before function returns, with the result that antirejection therapy is delayed until immunologic damage progresses to an irreversible stage. In an attempt to avoid this sequence, some centers employ ALG or monoclonal anti-T cell antibodies prophylactically in all instances of ATN. Since there is no specific treatment for ATN, the return of function (usually within 1 to 4 weeks) must be patiently awaited while adequate but safe immunosuppression and good general condition are maintained, if necessary by dialysis. If there is reasonable clinical confidence in the diagnosis of ATN, it is best to minimize the use of invasive studies such as cystoscopy, arteriography, or biopsy, none of which provide positive evidence of ATN. Serial renal scans to identify decreases in blood flow may be helpful in making the difficult diagnosis of rejection during ATN, but biopsy is often necessary for confirmation. Even in the absence of rejection, management of immunosuppression is difficult during ATN. The nephrotoxic potential of cyclosporine is particularly disturbing when renal function cannot be assessed. Blood levels of this agent should be carefully monitored during ATN. As noted, many centers avoid cyclosporine entirely during ATN because of the additive damage of ischemia and cyclosporine toxicity.

LYMPHOCELES. Failure to ligate lymphatics crossing the iliac vessels may cause lymphoceles, which have a variable reported incidence (0.6 to 18 per cent). Possible manifestations, which can occur weeks or months postoperatively, are swelling of the wound, edema of the scrotum, labia, and lower extremity, and urinary obstruction due to pressure on the collecting system or ureter. Ultrasound examination for identifying a fluid-filled mass is the most useful diagnostic study. Aspiration of the cyst is of only temporary benefit, because lymph rapidly reaccumulates. External drainage should be avoided, because this places the kidney and vascular suture line at risk from infection. The authors have successfully treated 12 patients with lymphoceles by marsupialization of the cyst into the peritoneal cavity. This is generally considered to be the treatment of choice, but recently a nonoperative treatment has been employed with success several times. Percutaneous drainage followed by repeated instillation of tetracycline or povidone iodine was successful in sclerosing and obliterating these cysts.

Nontechnical Complications

INFECTIONS. Factors predisposing to infection of transplant recipients include a major surgical operation involving the urinary tract, infection from the donor, indwelling catheters in the bladder, bloodstream, and peritoneal cavity. Because of these and the immunodepression associated with uremia and antirejection therapy, 30 to 60 per cent of patients suffer some type of infection during the first transplant year, and in half of the deaths that occur during the first year infection is an important contributing feature. More cautious use of immunosuppression over the last decade and the recent introduction of cyclosporine have reduced the magnitude of this problem, but infection remains the most common and most lethal complication of renal transplantation.

BACTERIAL INFECTIONS. During the first month after transplantation, conventional bacterial infections are the most common; and the urinary tract, respiratory system, and wound are the most prevalent sites.[54] These infections usually respond to prompt, vigorous conventional antibiotic therapy. Acute bacterial infections may have a clinical presentation that can be confused with rejection, i.e., fever, malaise, swelling, and tenderness of the wound, or even rising creatinine in the case of a urinary tract infection. It is especially important to exclude the possibility of infection prior to antirejection therapy, since during infection immunosuppression should be decreased, rather than intensified, even though this action may lead to acute rejection. The incidence of wound infections (reported to be 1 to 10 per cent) can probably be reduced by preoperative or intraoperative prophylaxis with a cephalosporine that should not be continued for more than 24 to 48 hours. Even more important, however, is meticulous surgical technique to avoid hematoma, urinary fistula, and lymphocele. Transplant recipients are subject to the usual respiratory infections that occur in normal or hospitalized individuals, and acute bacterial pneumonitis is a potentially lethal infection in these patients. Urinary tract infections, which are the most common bacterial infections in transplant recipients, can be decreased 50 per cent by using trimethoprim-sulfa antibiotics for the first 6 months after transplantation. This is also helpful in decreasing the incidence of *Pneumocystis carinii.*

OPPORTUNISTIC INFECTIONS. The period between 30 and 180 days after transplantation, usually the time of most intense immunosuppression, is most common for infection with opportunistic organisms, which in normal individuals rarely cause significant illness. In recent years, it has become evident that viral infections are more important than bacterial infection, in terms of prevalence, diagnostic and therapeutic difficulty, and immunologic and neoplastic ramifications. This epidemiologic change is probably due to cyclosporine therapy, which allows lower doses of azathioprine and steroids and has decreased the incidence of bacterial infections. Simultaneously, the use of antibodies against T lymphocytes, which cause seriously impaired antiviral defenses, has increased. Cytomegalovirus (CMV), a member of the herpesvirus family, is the most important viral pathogen. This ubiquitous agent infects most normal individuals at some point in their lives. In otherwise healthy individuals, CMV infections are either clinically silent or mild, although the presence of the latent virus and seropositivity persist for life. Following renal transplantation, previously seropositive patients usually excrete CMV and exhibit elevations of antibody titer, on the basis of either reactivation of latent virus during immunosuppression or transmission of virus latent in the donor tissues. Under these circumstances, symptomatic illness occurs infrequently (20 per cent) and is usually mild, supporting the hypothesis that previous exposure and immunity to the virus confers protection.[59] However, seronegative recipients who receive a kidney from a seropositive donor are subject to a three times greater incidence of symptomatic illness; and of affected patients, one fourth have severe disease. CMV "disease" (as distinguished from asymptomatic seroconversion) varies in severity from mild fever and malaise to a debilitating syndrome marked by leukopenia, hepatitis, interstitial pneumonia, arthritis, CNS changes including coma, GI ulceration and bleeding, renal insufficiency, bacterial or fungal infection, and even death.

Distinguishing CMV disease, which has its usual onset 4 to 6 weeks after transplantation, from rejection can be especially difficult, because the viral infection can cause renal insufficiency. Seroconversion may not occur for an additional 3 to 6 weeks, and viral cultures also require several weeks. Possible causes of renal malfunction during CMV infection include direct damage from the virus ("glomerulopathy") and triggering of rejection.[55] This is a dilemma, because delay in institution of antirejection therapy may lead to irreversible renal damage but intensification of immunosuppression may lead to lethal superinfection. In cases of decreasing renal function, a decision for or against antirejection therapy must often be based on clinical

grounds, but biopsy should probably be done first if CMV is suspected, because it may distinguish rejection from CMV. At some centers, a diagnosis can be made in 48 hours by an indirect immunofluorescence test utilizing a monoclonal antibody directed at an early CMV antigen.

Because CMV disease has an adverse impact on morbidity, mortality, and graft loss, it is important to avoid it. One obvious partial solution would be to avoid transplantation of all kidneys from seropositive donors to seronegative recipients. It has been estimated this might improve graft survival by 20 per cent in seronegative recipients. However, it would have the disadvantage of greatly reducing the donor pool for seronegative recipients, because most adult donors are CMV-seropositive. Another possibility would be active immunization for CMV, because the most severe disease occurs in seronegative recipients. A live attenuated CMV vaccine has been studied at the University of Pennsylvania. It is well tolerated, is not excreted, does not become latent, and produces serologic and cellular evidence of immunity. The vaccine does not totally prevent infection after transplantation, but the incidence of symptomatic and severe illness is reduced.[59] At the University of Minnesota, passive immunization with immune globulin has been found to be similarly effective in decreasing the severity of CMV disease.[4]

Fortunately, both the incidence and the severity of CMV disease appear to be diminished in cyclosporine-treated patients. There is impressive evidence that prophylactic acyclovir decreases the incidence of CMV, although prolonged administration of large doses is necessary.[4] In established CMV disease, neither adenine arabinoside nor acyclovir has been effective, although both, and especially the latter agent, are effective for herpes zoster and herpes simplex. Recently it has been demonstrated that gancyclovir (DHPG) is quite effective even in established severe CMV infections.[21]

Other opportunistic infections such as aspergillosis, blastomycosis, nocardiosis, toxoplasmosis, and cryptococcosis are particularly likely to occur in transplant patients. The protozoan *Pneumocystis carinii,* which has infected most individuals by age 10, is a pulmonary pathogen only in immunodepressed patients. It is the organism that most often causes fatal pneumonia in this group. A prompt diagnosis by aggressive measures such as bronchoscopic alveolar lavage and brushing and percutaneous transbronchoscopic or open lung biopsy is important in cases of *Pneumocystis carinii* infection, because effective treatment (trimethoprim and sulfamethoxazole) exists. Mycobacterial infections are also observed (5 in 565 transplant patients in 15 years at the Hospital of the University of Pennsylvania). Although the prevalence of these infectious complications is declining because of less dangerous immunosuppressive protocols, their potential lethality mandates constant vigilance.

HYPERGLYCEMIA. For reasons not entirely clear, but generally attributed to intensive or persistent steroid administration, previously normoglycemic patients may become diabetic in the posttransplant period. Requirement for insulin therapy may persist even when steroid doses are decreased or discontinued. Uncontrolled hyperglycemia may cause "pseudorejection" on the basis of interference with the laboratory determination for creatinine and increased serum osmolality with resultant intracellular and extracellular dehydration and impaired renal function.[35] In this condition, control of the blood glucose promptly leads to correction of the elevated creatinine level.

GASTROINTESTINAL COMPLICATIONS. Ulceration and perforation of the stomach, duodenum, and small and large intestine are relatively common following transplantation. The colon is especially vulnerable to ischemia and perforation, and in immunosuppressed patients abdominal pain or signs of peritoneal irritation merit very close attention if not immediate laparotomy.[48] Pancreatitis is also a recognized complication of both azathioprine and steroid therapy in transplant patients, in whom its course is frequently fulminating and fatal. Infectious

GI complications such as *Candida* stomatitis and esophagitis, pseudomembranous colitis, and CMV ulceration are also common. Symptoms and signs of these conditions may be masked by steroid therapy.

HYPERPARATHYROIDISM. Secondary hyperparathyroidism from chronic renal failure usually subsides after a successful transplant. However, its persistence ("tertiary hyperparathyroidism") has been reported in 2.6 to 70 per cent of patients, with the smaller number representing the true incidence. In cases in which significant hypercalcemia and elevated parathyroid hormone levels persist for more than 12 months after transplantation despite normal renal function, the authors advocate total parathyroidectomy and autotransplantation of fragments from a portion of one gland into the muscle of the forearm, where they are easily accessible for further resection without neck exploration should hypertrophy persist and recurrent hypercalcemia ensue. The sequelae of hyperparathyroidism, such as renal calculi, bone pain, and muscle weakness, are usually avoided by this procedure. The authors have observed a devastating complication of persistent hyperparathyroidism in four patients who developed diffuse cutaneous vascular calcification leading to extensive ulceration and gangrene.[49] Despite total parathyroidectomy, ischemic ulcers did not heal in three of these patients, which eventually led to sepsis and death. Common to these patients were persistent posttransplant elevation of the serum calcium level and radiographic evidence on xerography of extensive small and medium vessel calcification. Confronted with nonhealing ulceration occurring in unusual areas such as the upper extremities, elevation of serum calcium level, and increased parathyroid hormone levels, one should entertain this diagnosis.

TUMORS. In the early days of transplantation it was found that utilization of apparently uninvolved kidneys from donors with known cancer was likely to lead to transmission of the malignancy. Since then, in occasional instances, tumors have inadvertently been transplanted from donors with unrecognized cancer. If this complication is recognized early, cessation of immunosuppression is sometimes followed by rejection not only of the transplanted kidney but also of the allogeneic tumor. However, when the transplanted tumor becomes well established, it may continue to flourish and cause death even in the absence of immunosuppression, especially when the recipient is severely immunodepressed or when donor-recipient histocompatibility is close.

It has been known for many years that both naturally occurring and iatrogenic states of immune deficiency are accompanied by an increased risk of neoplasia.[47] Uremia *per se* is such a state, although the incidence of cancer in dialysis patients is only approximately twice that of the general population. In transplanted patients, the reported United States incidence of 6 per cent *de novo* malignant neoplasms represents a risk approximately 100 times greater than that in normal age-matched populations. The most common neoplasms are squamous cell carcinomas of skin and lip, which are especially prevalent in sunny areas, such as Australia and New Zealand, where patients who survive 15 years after transplantation have a striking 44 per cent incidence of skin cancer. In transplant patients, these tumors behave in an unusually aggressive manner and require early vigorous treatment.

Transplant recipients in all parts of the world have a disproportionately high incidence of lymphomas, which comprise 20 per cent of all tumors in this population. The risk of lymphoma in immunosuppressed patients is approximately 350 times normal and appears related to the degree of immunosuppression, rather than the agent used, although there is some evidence that cyclosporine may further increase the risk. Many of these tumors are in the central nervous system—an unusual site for lymphomas. A hypothesis for explaining the prevalence of malignancies in immunosuppressed patients is that a breakdown of normal immunologic surveillance mechanisms occurs that allows persistence of mutant malignant cells that would be recognized and destroyed by an intact immune system. It is theorized that such "forbidden clones" are particularly likely to go unrecognized in the brain, an immunologically privileged site. Other etiologic possibilities for the increased neoplasia are chronic immunologic stimulation of the lymphorecticular system by the transplant, direct carcinogenic action of immunosuppressive drugs, and oncogenesis by the viral pathogens the growth of which is encouraged by immunosuppression. The latter possibility is supported by the finding that tumors in which a viral pathogenesis appears likely (lymphoma, skin, lip, and uterine cervix cancers) are especially prevalent in transplant patients.

Recently, the interesting possibility has been raised that *de novo* lymphomas may begin as lymphoproliferative lesions induced by viruses. Compelling evidence of this is the finding of Epstein-Barr virus (EBV) incorporated into the genome of lymphoma cells. These patients often have a syndrome resembling mononucleosis, with fever, pharyngitis, and diffuse lymphadenopathy. Polyclonal B-cell proliferation, rather than true malignancy, is the finding in these early lesions of a diversity of cellular immunoglobulins.[26] During the stage of polyclonality, cessation of immunosuppression may allow regression of the lesions. The use of the antiviral agent acyclovir, which blocks EBV-inhibited oropharyngeal shedding of the virus, has also been reported to contribute to remissions. Tumors that are initially polyclonal may eventually undergo a cytogenetic alteration leading to malignant transformation and the monoclonality characteristic of true B-cell lymphomas. Monoclonal tumors do not regress after cessation of immunosuppression or acyclovir therapy. They are aggressive malignancies that can be treated only by surgical therapy and irradiation, neither of which is very effective.

RESULTS OF RENAL TRANSPLANTATION

Each human renal transplant is a unique clinical experiment, the outcome of which depends on many complex and interrelated variables. There is continuous controversy over the relative importance of each variable; over the last 30 years each has been the subject of multiple (frequently contradictory) reports. Only histocompatibility is a consistently crucial factor, perhaps not surprisingly, since rejection remains the chief deterrent to success. This was clear even in the earliest days of transplantation, when the success of HLA-identical sibling donor grafts (90 per cent) was noted to be twice that of cadaveric transplants (Fig. 7).[65] Although the short-term results of cadaveric grafts have improved greatly since then, the importance of histocompatibility remains obvious when long-term survival is examined. Even with cyclosporine immunosuppression, only 35 to 40 per cent of cadaveric grafts can be expected to survive after 10 years (Fig. 8), as compared with 80 per cent or more of HLA-identical sibling grafts.[66]

Although a well-matched family donor is the most important variable, other factors are also influential, some of them being more easily controlled than the type of donor. On the positive side these include (1) optimal immunosuppression, inclusion of cyclosporine being paramount; (2) previous blood transfusions, especially if from the kidney donor, although there is also a risk of sensitizing the recipient; (3) a well-matched donor, especially for HLA-DR, although this is far less important for unrelated than for related donors; (4) a youthful donor; (5) a youthful recipient; (6) a short preservation time and prompt transplant function, rather than ATN. Negatively influential variables include (1) a previously failed transplant, especially if rejection was early and vigorous; (2) a black donor or recipient, for unclear reasons, possibly including prevalence of hypertension or center effects; (3) associated diseases such as diabetes, lupus,

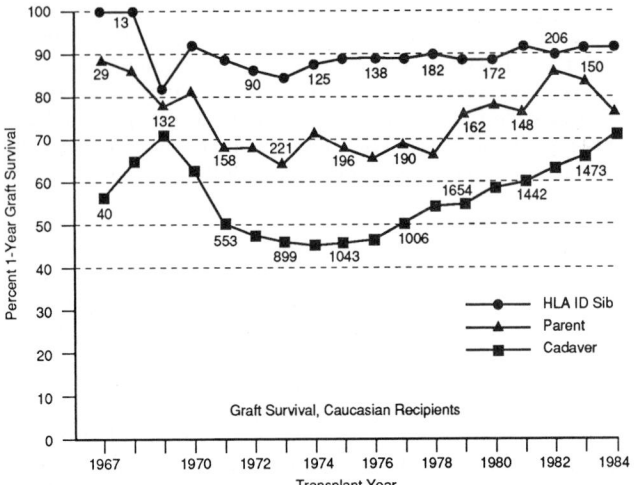

Figure 7. Note that 1-year survival of HLA-identical sibling grafts has been in the 90 per cent range for more than 25 years. A decrease in the success of parenteral and cadaveric grafts noted in the early 1970s has been attributed to withholding transfusions during that era. Subsequently, as deliberate transfusions were adopted, 1-year graft survival improved substantially. (From Terasaki, P. (Ed.): Clinical Kidney Transplants 1985. Overview. UCLA Tissue Typing Laboratory, Los Angeles, California.)

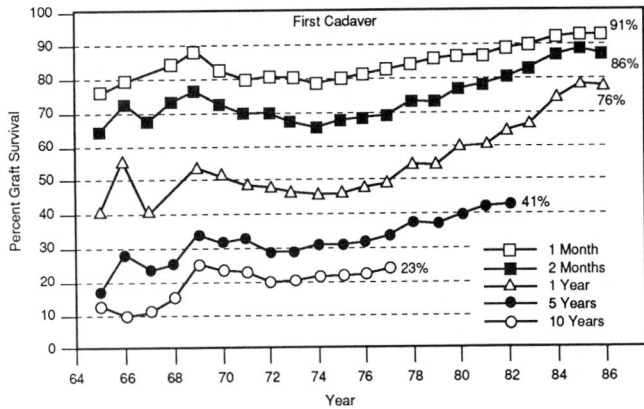

Figure 9. During the last 20 years the 1-year survival of first cadaver grafts has steadily improved. The 20 per cent improvement observed between 1973 and 1983 was probably attributable to deliberate transfusions, and since that time an additional 10 per cent improvement has been due to cyclosporine. (From Terasaki, P. (Ed.): Clinical Transplants 1987. Overview. UCLA Tissue Typing Laboratory, Los Angeles, California.)

Fabry's disease, or oxalosis; (4) concomitant generalized illness such as heart disease or hypertension.

An additional important variable is the "center effect," which is probably more influential than any single factor other than histocompatibility. Prior to cyclosporine, the best and poorest results reported by various centers differed by about 18 per cent; and since cyclosporine, by only 7 per cent. The center effect is probably the sum of several factors, such as patient selection, operative technique, and postoperative management. This factor is responsible for the extremely good results sometimes reported by particular centers, which are substantially better than the combined reports of the multicenter registries that exist in the United States, Britain, and Europe.

A multicenter registry maintained at the University of California, Los Angeles (UCLA) by Terasaki provides the most comprehensive overview of present United States results and is the basis of this summary. Results are most commonly reported as 1-year graft or patient survival. For HLA-identical sibling donors, better than 90 per cent 1-year graft survival has been reported for more than 25 years.[65] The 1-year graft survival of parental or one-haplotype sibling transplants has steadily improved during the last 20 years from about 70 per cent to the current 85 to 90 per cent.[66] During this same period the 1-year survival of cadaveric grafts has gradually improved from 50 per cent to 75 to 80 per cent (Fig. 9).[67] The 20 per cent improvement that occurred between 1973 and 1984 was probably due to the policy of deliberate pretransplant blood transfusions. The additional 10 per cent improvement since 1983 is attributed to cyclosporine. Cumulative experience and improvements in the art and science of transplantation undoubtedly also had a role in these progressively better short-term results.

One-year survival of recipients of cadaveric grafts has improved even more dramatically than graft survival and now closely approaches that observed for recipients of related donor grafts at greater than 90 per cent (Fig. 10).[65]

One disappointing aspect of the results is evident from examining long-term graft survival. Although as noted, both patient survival and short-term graft survival have dramatically improved over the last 2 decades, the rate of attrition of cadaveric grafts after 1 year has remained almost constant (about 7 per cent per year) even since the introduction of cyclosporine. Because of this, patients receiving cadaveric grafts in 1967 had a 10-year graft survival of 23 per cent, and those being performed

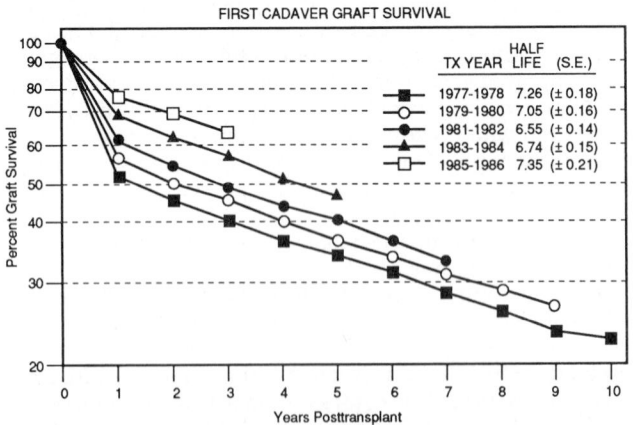

Figure 8. Cadaver donor kidney graft survival since 1977 showing a striking improvement in 1-year survival rates. However, the subsequent loss rate of transplants has not been affected. When plotted on a natural logarithmic scale, the survival curves 1-year after transplantation were essentially linear. The half-life of 7.26 in 1977/78 does not differ from the 7.35 half-life of transplants performed in 1985/86. Cyclosporine (CsA), used in about 90 per cent of the transplants during the latter period, did not influence long-term survival. (From Terasaki, P. (Ed.): Clinical Transplants 1988. Overview. UCLA Tissue Typing Laboratory, Los Angeles, California.)

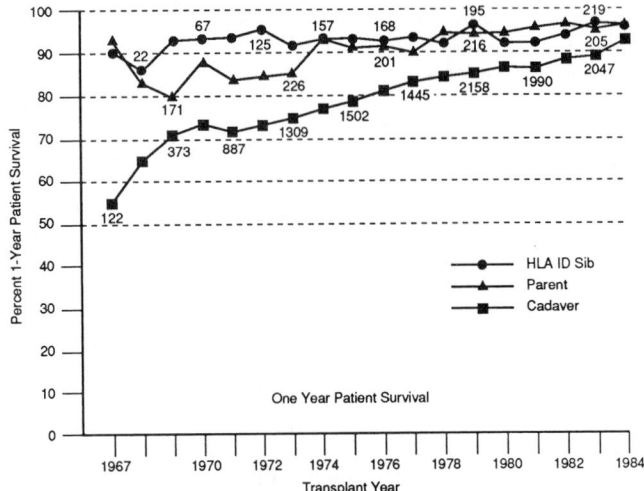

Figure 10. A progressive overall improvement in patient survival rates can be noted for all categories of kidney donors. Patient survival rates after cadaver donor transplants have increased markedly. (From Terasaki, P. (Ed.): Clinical Transplants 1985. Overview. UCLA Tissue Typing Laboratory, Los Angeles, California.)

today are not expected to have a better than 40 per cent 10-year graft survival, which emphasizes the need for further improvement (see Fig. 8).[66]

SOCIOECONOMIC CONSIDERATIONS IN TREATMENT OF END-STAGE RENAL DISEASE

Because the annual cost of funding the care of end-stage renal disease patients approaches $3 billion, it is important to note that transplantation is a more cost-effective treatment than chronic dialysis. Transplantation costs are $36,000 to $38,000 for the first year and, if successful, about $4000 per year thereafter.[58] Despite this high initial cost, the lower lifetime expense incurred by patients with functioning transplants compares so favorably with that of maintenance hemodialysis ($20,000 per year for life) that the costs of transplantation (including failed grafts) are recovered in about 3 years. In addition to cost-effectiveness and better survival (Fig. 11), transplantation is superior to dialysis because it returns 75 per cent of patients to work (as compared with 25 to 60 per cent of dialysis patients), with substantial consequent saving in expenses of dialysis and welfare payments and benefit to patients' families.[22,72]

For many years, more new patients were being added to dialysis lists than were undergoing transplantation. Recognition of the better survival and other advantages of transplantation by the public and by nephrologists appears to have had an impact, so that from 1978 to 1985 the number of patients enrolled for dialysis increased at an annual rate of only 11.2 per cent per year, whereas the number obtaining functioning grafts increased 20.6 per cent per year. Older patients continue to be treated by dialysis, rather than transplantation, but the number of patients younger than 25 years on dialysis is actually decreasing, while the number of transplants being performed is increasing and appears to be limited only by donor availability.[20]

Public interest in the field during the 1980s led to appointment of a task force to address issues such as the donor shortage, establishment of standards, and provision of transplant services to all citizens. As a result, the National Organ Transplant Act was passed by Congress, which mandated a National Organ Procurement and Transplantation Network (OPTN).[36] In 1986,

a government contract to provide these services was awarded to United Network for Organ Sharing (UNOS), a private nonprofit organization that had been formed by representatives of the majority of transplant centers in anticipation of these governmental actions.

The UNOS Board of Directors includes representatives of 11 regions that have been established in the United States and is composed of transplant surgeons and physicians, nurses, representatives of voluntary health organizations, transplant recipient families, lawyers, ethicists, theologians, and health care financing representatives. Criteria have been established for accreditation of transplantation surgeons and centers, histocompatibility laboratories, and local organ procurement organizations. All patients awaiting transplants must now be registered with UNOS. A central computer and a point system based on medical criteria determine the assignment of kidneys, which local organ procurement organizations distribute first locally, then regionally, and then nationally. Because hospitals performing transplantation must be members of UNOS to be eligible for Medicare funding, the organization has assumed a powerful role. Some ambivalence has been expressed regarding federal control of transplantation; but because transplant professionals have had a major role in the development and leadership of the OPTN, most believe that the organization holds promise for achieving standardization, equity for patients, and general progress in the field.

The evolution of renal transplantation from an experimental curiosity to a highly successful clinical therapy represents one of the remarkable medical achievements of the century. Terminal renal disease, an entity that 30 years ago was uniformly fatal, can now be treated with greater success than most cancers. The primary goal should be successful transplantation. Dialysis should be reserved for maintenance of patients awaiting a transplant or as a primary treatment of those patients unsuitable for transplantation because of age or other serious illness. Because most victims of end-stage renal disease are relatively young, the achievement of a successful transplant in this group is one of the most gratifying of all surgical therapies.

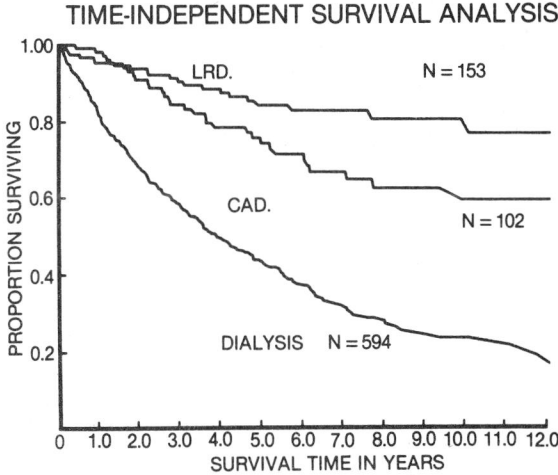

TIME-INDEPENDENT SURVIVAL ANALYSIS

LRD. N = 153

CAD. N = 102

DIALYSIS N = 594

Figure 11. The probability of survival for 849 patients with primary renal disease receiving transplants from living related donors (LRD) or cadaveric donors (CAD) or being treated with dialysis only. Estimates were obtained by using the method of Kaplan and Meier. This type of analysis is somewhat misleading, in that the dialysis results represent only patients who never received transplants, often the poorest risk group. When adjustments are made to give credit for dialysis time prior to transplantation, much more similar survival curves are seen for cadaveric transplantation and dialysis. However, the superiority of rehabilitation allowed by transplantation is unequivocal. (From Vollmer, W. M., Wahl, P. W., and Blagg, C. R.: Survival with dialysis and transplantation in patients with end-stage renal disease. N. Engl. J. Med., *308*:1553, 1983.)

SELECTED REFERENCES

Bruggemann, M., Winter, G., Waldmann, H., and Neuberger, M.S.: The immunogenicity of chimeric antibodies. J. Exp. Med., *170*:2153, 1989.
Rejection crisis resistant to initial intensification of immunosuppression is common, and rescue therapy has relied heavily on second-line agents such as antilymphocyte antibodies. A major complication in the use of polyclonal or monoclonal antibodies has been the antiglobulin response that xenogeneic antibodies elicit. Strategies to mitigate such responses include induction of tolerance to xenogeneic monoclonal antibody or use of human or chimeric antibodies. Efforts at minimizing the immunogenicity of antibodies and the implications of immunotherapy are discussed in this paper.

Kahan, B. D.: Cyclosporine. N. Engl. J. Med., *321*:1725, 1989.
When cyclosporine was released for general use in 1983, it was the first new immunosuppressive drug in 20 years and was credited with revolutionizing transplantation. The author, a foremost authority in experimental and clinical use of the agent, provides a comprehensive up-to-date review of its pharmacokinetics, mechanism of action, complications, and therapeutic effects.

Lagaaij, E. L., Hennemann, P. H., Ruigrok, M., DeHann, M. W., et al.: Effect of one-HLA-DR-antigen-matched and completely HLA-DR-mismatched blood transfusions on survival of heart and kidney allografts. N. Engl. J. Med., *321*:701, 1989.
Although induction of donor-specific tolerance in humans is the Holy Grail of transplantation, it is unlikely that this will be achieved in clinical transplantation in the near future. Immunologic preconditioning of recipients by HLA-DR–matched blood transfusions is attractive and practical. The results in this paper, if confirmed, may have a major impact in improving graft survival.

Morris, P. J. (Ed.): Kidney Transplantation. Philadelphia, W. B. Saunders Company, 1988.
The expanded third edition has 30 chapters by international experts that review history, recent developments, immunobiology, surgical techniques, pre- and postoperative management, histocompatibility testing, immunosuppression, histopathology of rejection, complications, and results. This text has become a modern standard in the field.

Pierce, G. A.: Legislative perspectives on the development of the end-stage renal disease network and the national organ procurement and transplantation network. *In* Flye, M. W. (Ed.): Principles of Organ Transplantation. Philadelphia, W. B. Saunders Company, 1989.

Described by the executive director of UNOS are recent events leading to governmental support and regulation of transplantation: the task force, legislation, government contract to implement a national organ procurement network, standards for membership and organ distribution, and development of a national registry. Government involvement, although unpopular with some, will be important in further development of the field and, if professional transplanters maintain leadership, can be a positive influence.

Terasaki, P. I. (Ed.): Clinical Transplants. Los Angeles, UCLA Tissue Typing Laboratory, 1988.

For the past 20 years this pioneer in histocompatibility testing has maintained a multi-institutional registry at UCLA, collecting data from more than 150 transplant centers from around the world. For 5 years he has published an annual volume correlating with graft survival multiple variables including matching, age, race, sex, antibody status, immunosuppressive protocols, transfusions, etc. Data on more than 50,000 patients are graphically presented. Examples of some of the pertinent illustrations are included in this chapter.

REFERENCES

1. Alexander, J. W., First, M. R., Majeski, J. A., Munda, R., Fidler, J. P., Morris, M. J., and Suttman, P.: The late adverse effect of splenectomy on patient survival following cadaveric renal transplantation. Transplantation, 37:467, 1984.
2. Anderson, C. B., Sicard, G. A., and Etheredge, E. E.: Pretreatment of renal allograft recipients with azathioprine and donor-specific blood products. Surgery, 92:315, 1982.
3. Auchincloss, H.: Xenogeneic transplantation. Transplantation, 46:1, 1988.
4. Balfour, H. H., Chace, B. A., Stapleton, J. T., Simmons, R. L., and Fryd, D. S.: A randomized, placebo-controlled trial of oral acyclovir for the prevention of cytomegalovirus disease in recipients of renal allografts. N. Engl. J. Med., 320:1381, 1989.
5. Bannett, A., Brynger, H., McAlack, R. F., Breimer, M., and Samuelson, B. (Eds.): ABO Incompatibility and Transplantation. New York, Grune & Stratton, 1987.
6. Barber, W. H., Diethelm, A. G., Laskow, D. A., Deierhoi, M. H., Julian, B. A., and Curtis, J. J.: Use of cryopreserved donor bone marrow in cadaver kidney allograft recipients. Transplantation, 47:66, 1989.
7. Belzer, F. O., and Southard, J. H.: Principles of solid organ preservation by cold storage. Transplantation, 45:673, 1988.
8. Bilous, R. W., Mauer, S. M., Sutherland, D. E. R., Najarian, J. S., et al.: The effects of pancreas transplantation on the glomerular structure of renal allografts in patients with insulin-dependent diabetes. N. Engl. J. Med., 321:80, 1989.
9. Borel, J. F., Feurer, C., Gubler, H. U., and Stahelin, H.: Biological effects of cyclosporin A: A new antilymphocyte agent. Agents Actions, 6:468, 1976.
10. Brenner, B. M., Meyer, T. W., and Hostetter, T. H.: Dietary protein intake and the progressive nature of kidney disease: The role of hemodynamically mediated glomerular injury in the pathogenesis of progressive glomerular sclerosis in aging, renal ablation and intrinsic renal disease. N. Engl. J. Med., 307:652, 1982.
11. Brewer, Y., Taube, D., Bewick, M., Hale, G., et al.: Effect of graft perfusion with two CD45 monoclonal antibodies on incidence of kidney allograft rejection. Lancet, 2:936, 1989.
12. Calne, R. Y., Rolles, K., White, D. J., Thiru, S., Evans, D. B., McMaster, P., Dunn, D. C., Craddock, G. N., Henderson, R. G., Azis, S., and Lewis, P.: Cyclosporin A initially as the immunosuppressant in 34 recipients of cadaveric organs: 32 kidneys, 2 pancreas, and 2 livers. Lancet, 2:1033, 1979.
13. Canadian multicentre transplant study group: A randomized clinical trial of cyclosporine in cadaveric renal transplantation: Analysis at three years. N. Engl. J. Med., 314:1219, 1986.
14. Cats, S., Terasaki, P., Perdue, S., and Mickey, M. R.: Effect of HLA typing and transfusions on cyclosporine treated renal allograft recipients. N. Engl. J. Med., 311:675, 1984.
15. Cerilli, J. G, and Brasile, L.: Tissue-specific antigens—A role in organ transplantation. *In* Cerilli, J. G. (Ed.): Organ Transplantation. Philadelphia, J. B. Lippincott Company, 1988, p. 208.
16. Colvin, R. B., Preffer, F. I., Fuller, T. C., Brown, M. C., et al.: A critical analysis of serum and urine interleukin-2 receptor assays in renal allograft recipients. Transplantation, 48:800, 1989.
17. Cosimi, A. B., Robert, B. C., Burton, R. C., Rubin, R. H., Goldstein, G., Kung, P. C., Hansen, W. P., Delmonico, F. L., and Russell, P. S.: Use of monoclonal antibodies to T-cell subsets for immunologic monitoring and treatment in recipients of renal allografts. N. Engl. J. Med., 305:308, 1981.
18. Darby, J. M., Stein, K., Grenvik, A., and Stuart, S. A.: Approach to management of the heartbeating "brain dead" organ donor. J. A. M. A., 261:2222, 1989.
19. DeMeyer, M., Pirson, Y., Dautrebande, J., Squifflet, J. P., et al.: Treatment of renal graft artery stenosis. Transplantation, 47:784, 1989.
20. Eggers, P. W.: Effect of transplantation on the Medicare end-stage renal disease program. N. Engl. J. Med., 318:223, 1988.
21. Erice, A., Jordon, C., Chace, B. A., Fletcher, C., et al.: Ganciclovir treatment of cytomegalovirus disease in transplant recipients and other immunocompromised hosts. J.A.M.A., 257:3082, 1987.
22. Evans, R. W., Manninen, D. L., Garrison, L. J., et al.: The quality of life of patients with end-stage renal disease. N. Engl. J. Med., 312:553, 1985.
23. Greenstein, S. M., Verstandig, J., McLean, G. K., Dafoe, D. C., et al.: Percutaneous transluminal angioplasty (PTA): The procedure of choice in the hypertensive renal allograft recipient with renal artery stenosis. Transplantation, 43:29, 1987.
24. Guttmann, R. D., Morehouse, D. D., Meakins, J. L., Milne, C. A., and Knaack, J.: Donor pretreatment as an adjunct to cadaveric renal transplantation—Update 1979. Transplant. Proc., 12:341, 1980.
25. Hakim, R. H., Goldszer, R. C., and Brenner, B. M.: Hypertension and proteinuria: Long term sequelae of uninephrectomy in humans. Kidney Int., 25:930, 1984.
26. Hanto, D. W., Gajl-Peczalska, K. J., Frizzera, G., Arthur, D. C., Balfour, H. H., McClain, K., Simmons, R. L., and Najarian, J. S.: Epstein-Barr virus (EBV) induced polyclonal and monoclonal B-cell lymphoproliferative diseases occurring after renal transplantation. Ann. Surg., 198:356, 1983.
27. Hardy, M. A., Nowygrod, R., Elberg, A., Appel, G.: Use of ATG in treatment of steroid-resistant rejection. Transplantation, 29:162, 1980.
28. Hayry, P., and von Willebrand, E.: Transplant aspiration cytology. Transplantation, 38:7, 1984.
29. Kahan, B. D.: Cyclosporine. N. Engl. J. Med., 321:1725, 1989.
30. Kahan, B. D., VanBuren, C. T., Flechner, S. M., Payne, W. D., Boileau, M., and Kerman, R. H.: Cyclosporine immunosuppression mitigates immunologic risk factors in renal allotransplantation. Transplant. Proc., 15:2469, 1983.
31. Kissmeyer-Nielson, F., Olsen, S., Petersen, V. P., and Fjeldborg, O.: Hyperacute rejection of kidney allografts, associated with preexisting humoral antibodies against donor cells. Lancet, 2:662, 1966.
32. Lacombe, M.: Arterial stenosis complicating renal allotransplantation in man. Ann. Surg., 181:283, 1975.
33. Levey, A. S., Hou, S., and Bush, H. L.: Kidney transplantation from unrelated living donors. N. Engl. J. Med., 314:914, 1986.
34. Loughlin, K. R., Tilney, N. L., and Richie, J. P.: Urologic complications in 718 renal transplant patients. Surgery, 95:297, 1984.
35. Matas, A. J., Simmons, R. L., Kjellstrand, C. M., and Najarian, J. S.: Pseudorejection: Factors mimicking rejection in renal allograft recipients. Ann. Surg., 186:51, 1977.
36. McDonald, J. C.: The national organ procurement and transplantation network. J.A.M.A., 259:725, 1988.
37. Moore, F. D. (Ed.): Transplant: The give and take of tissue transplantation. New York, Simon and Schuster, 1972.
38. Murray, J. E.: Reminiscences on renal transplantation. *In* Chatterjee, S. N. (Ed.): Organ Transplantation. John Wright, P. S., Inc., 1982, pp. 1–13.
39. Najarian, J. S., Simmons, R. L., Condie, R. M., Thompson, E. J., Fryd, D. S., Howard, R. J., Matas, A. J., Sutherland, D. E. R., Ferguson, R. M., and Schmidtke, J. R.: Seven years' experience with antilymphoblast globulin for renal transplantation from cadaver donors. Ann. Surg., 184:352, 1976.
40. Najarian, J. S., Sutherland, D. E. R., Simmons, R. L., et al.: Ten year experience with renal transplantation in juvenile onset diabetes. Ann. Surg., 190:487, 1979.
41. Opelz, G.: Effect of HLA matching in 10,000 cyclosporine-treated cadaver kidney transplants. Transplant. Proc., 19:641, 1987.
42. Opelz, G.: The benefit of exchanging donor kidneys among transplant centers. N. Engl. J. Med., 318:1289, 1988.
43. Opelz, G.: To transfuse or not before transplantation. *In* Morris, P. J., and Tilney, N. L. (Eds.): Transplantation Reviews. Philadelphia, W. B. Saunders Company, 1988.
44. Opelz, G., Dharmendra, P. S., Sengar, D. P. S., Mickey, M. R., and Terasaki, P. I.: Effect of blood transfusions on subsequent kidney transplants. Transplant. Proc., 4:253, 1973.
45. Ortho Multicenter Transplant Study Group: A randomized clinical trial of OKT3 monoclonal antibody for acute rejection of cadaveric renal transplants. N. Engl. J. Med., 313:337, 1985.
46. Palmer, A., Taube, D., Welsh, K., Bewick, M., Gjorstrup, P., and Thick, M.: Removal of anti-HLA antibodies by extracorporeal immunoabsorption to enable renal transplantation. Lancet, 1:10, 1989.
47. Penn, I.: Cancers following cyclosporine therapy. Transplantation, 43:32, 1987.
48. Perloff, L. J., Chon, H., Petrella, E. J., Grossman, R. A., and Barker, C. F.: Acute colitis in the renal allograft recipient. Ann. Surg., 183:77, 1976.
49. Perloff, L. J., Spence, R. K., Grossman, R. A., and Barker, C. F.: Lethal posttransplantation calcinosis. Transplantation, 27:21, 1979.
50. Persijn, G. G., Cohen, B., Lansbergen, Q., D'Amaro, J., Selwood, N., Wing, A., and VanRood, J. J.: Effect of HLA-A and HLA-B matching on survival of grafts and recipients after renal transplantation. N. Engl. J. Med., 307:905:1982.
51. Reemstma, K.: Heterotransplantation. *In* Rapaport, F. T., and Dausset, J. (Eds.): Human Transplantation. New York, Grune & Stratton, 1968, pp. 357–366.
52. Rosenthal, J. T., Hakala, T. R., Iwatsuki, S., Shaw, B. W., and Starzl, T. E.: Cadaveric renal transplantation under cyclosporine-steroid therapy. Surg. Gynecol. Obstet., 157:309, 1983.
53. Roza, A., Perloff, L. J., Naji, A., Grossman, R. A., and Barker, C. F.: Living-related donors with bilateral multiple renal arteries: A twenty year experience. Transplantation, 47:397, 1989.

54. Rubin, R. H., Wolfson, J. S., Cosimi, A. B., and Tolkoff-Rubin, N. E.: Infection in the renal transplant recipient. Am. J. Med., 70:405, 1981.
55. Rubin, R. H., Cosimi, B., Tolkoff-Rubin, N. E., Russell, P. S., and Hirsch, M. S.: Infectious disease syndromes attributable to cytomegalovirus and their significance among renal transplant recipients. Transplantation, 24:458, 1977.
56. Salvatierra, O., Flavio, V., Amend, W. J. C., Garovoyk, M. R., Potter, D., and Feduska, N. J.: The role of blood transfusions in renal transplantation. Urol. Clin. North Am., 10:243, 1983.
57. Sanfilippo, F., Vaughn, W. K., Spees, E. K., Light, J. A., and LeFor, W. M.: Benefits of HLA and HLA-B matching on graft and patient outcome after cadaveric-donor renal transplantation. N. Engl. J. Med., 311:358, 1984.
58. Showstack, J., Katz, P., Amend, W., Bernstein, L., et al.: The effect of cyclosporine on the use of hospital resources for kidney transplantation. N. Engl. J. Med., 321:1086, 1989.
59. Smiley, M. L., Wlodaver, C. G., Grossman, R. A., Barker, C. F., Perloff, L. J., Tustin, N. B., Starr, S. E., Plotkin, S. A., and Friedman, H. M.: The role of pretransplant immunity in protection from cytomegalovirus disease following renal transplantation. Transplantation, 40:157, 1985.
60. Starzl, T. E., Marchioro, T. L., Porter, K. A., Iwasaki, Y., and Cerilli, G. J.: The use of heterologous antilymphoid agents in canine renal and liver homotransplantation and in human renal homotransplantation. Surg. Gynecol. Obstet., 124:301, 1967.
61. Starzl, T. E., Marchioro, T. L., and Waddell, W. R.: The reversal of rejection in human renal homografts with subsequent development of homograft tolerance. Surg. Gynecol. Obstet., 117:385, 1963.
62. Sutherland, D. E. R., Fryd, D. S., So, S. K. S., Bentley, F. R., Ascher, N. L., Simmons, R. L., and Najarian, J. S.: Long-term effect of splenectomy versus no splenectomy in renal transplant patients. Transplantation, 38:619, 1984.
63. Taylor, C. J., Chapman, J. R., Ting, A., and Morris, P. J.: Characterization of lymphocytotoxic antibodies causing a positive crossmatch in renal transplantation. Transplantation, 48:953, 1989.
64. Terasaki, P. I.: The beneficial transfusion effect on kidney graft survival attributed to clonal deletion. Transplantation, 37:119, 1984.
65. Terasaki, P. I.: Patient graft and functional survival rates: An overview. In Clinical Kidney Transplants. Los Angeles, UCLA Tissue Typing Laboratory, 1985, pp. 1–26.
66. Terasaki, P. I., Cecka, J. M., Takemoto, S., Yuge, J., et al.: Overview. In Clinical Kidney Transplants. Los Angeles, UCLA Tissue Typing Laboratory, 1988, pp. 409–434.
67. Terasaki, P. I., Mickey, M. R., Cecka, M., et al.: Overview. In Clinical Transplants. Los Angeles, UCLA Tissue Typing Laboratory, 1987, pp. 467–490.
68. Terasaki, P. I., Perdue, S. T., Sasaki, N., Mickey, M. R., and Whitby, L.: Improving success rates of kidney transplantation. J.A.M.A., 250:1065, 1983.
69. Tilney, N. L.: Renal transplantation between identical twins: A review. World J. Surg. 10:381, 1986.
70. Turcotte, J. G., Reduska, N. J., Haines, R. F., Freier, D. T., Gikas, P. W., McDonald, F. D., Johnson, A. G., Morrell, R. M., and Thompson, N. W.: A clinical trial of antithymocyte globulin in renal transplant recipients. Arch. Surg., 106:484, 1973.
71. Verani, R. R., Flechner, S. M., vanBuren, C., Kahan, B. D.: Acute cellular rejection or cyclosporine A nephrotoxicity? A review of transplant renal biopsies. Am J. Kidney Dis., 4:185, 1983.
72. Vollmer, W. M., Wahl, P. W., and Blagg, C. R.: Survival with dialysis and transplantation in patients with end-stage renal disease. N. Engl. J. Med., 308:1553, 1983.
73. Watts, R. W. E., Calne, R. Y., Rolles, K., et al.: Successful treatment of primary hyperoxaluria type I by combined hepatic and renal transplantation. Lancet, 2:474, 1987.
74. Weiland, D., Sutherland, D. E. R., Chavers, B., Simmons, R. L., Ascher, N. J., and Najarian, J. S.: Information on 628 living related kidney donors at a single institution with long-term followup in 472 cases. Transplant. Proc., 16:5, 1984.
75. Wolstenholme, G. E. W., and O'Connor, M. (Eds.): Antilymphocytic Serum. Boston, Little, Brown and Company, 1968.

V

VASCULAR ACCESS PROCEDURES FOR RENAL DIALYSIS (INCLUDING PERITONEAL DIALYSIS)

Carl E. Haisch, M.D., and James Cerilli, M.D.

VASCULAR ACCESS

Historical Aspects

Without adequate hemoaccess the development of hemodialysis would not have been possible. The concept of dialysis is in part due to work of a chemist, Thomas Graham, who discovered the semipermeable membrane. The first major attempt to solve the problem of vascular access was performed in rabbits by means of siliconized glass tubes and heparin.[1] Other attempts to gain chronic access to the circulation led to major difficulties caused by septicemia, clotting, or pulmonary emboli. When it was found that glass tubes would not provide successful long-term access in humans, Quinton, Dillard, and Scribner utilized Teflon tubing as the conduit material.[25] However, there were still problems with thrombosis and infection. The development of the natural arteriovenous fistula in 1966 by Brescia and colleagues was a major breakthrough and allowed numerous patients to have chronic dialysis. The anastomosis of the radial artery to the cephalic vein at the wrist led to a high-flow system that could be repeatedly punctured.[5] This largely eliminated the problems of the external shunt and is still considered the standard against which all other access is measured. Many patients did not have a patent superficial cephalic vein and required some other means of vascular access. In 1969, May used a subcutaneous autogenous loop of saphenous vein between the brachial artery and vein in the forearm. This was discontinued because of aneurysm formation and a high incidence of thrombosis. A subcutaneous bovine heterograft also was used for access in the early 1970s.[25] This also caused significant problems with infection and patency rates. At the present time, the most common material used as a graft between an artery and vein is polytetrafluoroethylene (PTFE).

Indications

Hemoaccess via an arteriovenous fistula or a jump graft is appropriate when (1) frequent access to the vascular system is required, (2) a high-flow system is needed, (3) the ability to withstand multiple needle punctures is required, and (4) highly sclerotic solutions are administered intravenously. The most common uses of arteriovenous shunts or fistulas are hemodialysis for acute and chronic renal failure, administration of chemotherapeutic agents and other drugs,[21,47] and hyperalimentation.[68] Patients with hemophilia may also require a fistula for repeated infusions of factor VIII.[21]

Types of Angioaccess

EXTERNAL SHUNTS. The first successful shunt for repeated hemodialysis was the Scribner shunt, which employed a Teflon tip inserted into both the artery and the vein. Silastic tubing attached to the Teflon tip was placed through the skin, both ends were connected, and continuous blood flow was established (Fig. 1). These shunts are most commonly placed in the

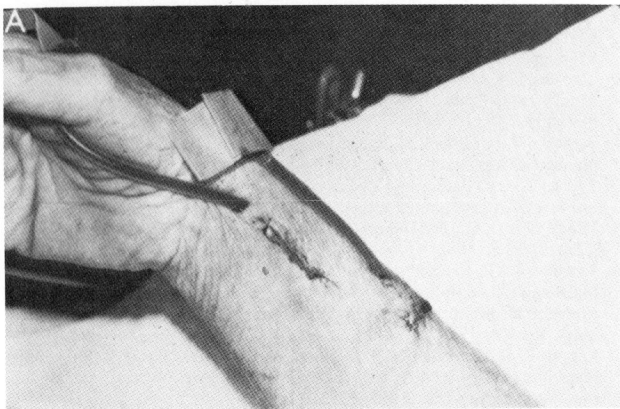

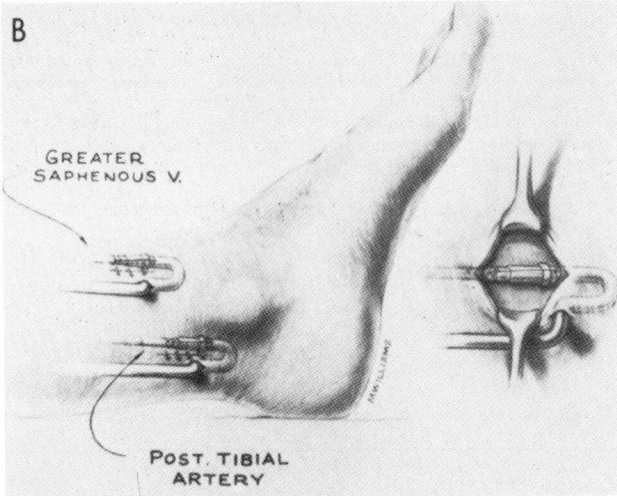

GREATER
SAPHENOUS V.

POST. TIBIAL
ARTERY

Figure 1. *A,* Shunt positioned in the forearm. *B,* The shunt is placed in the posterior tibial artery and the saphenous vein of the ankle. (From Ozeran, R. S.: Construction and care of external arteriovenous shunts. *In* Wilson, S. E., and Owens, M. L.: Vascular Access Surgery. Chicago, Year Book Medical Publishers, 1980.)

nondominant arm by use of the radial artery and an easily accessible (usually cephalic) vein. They are also inserted into the leg by means of the posterior tibial artery and the saphenous vein. If the radial artery is used, blood flow via the ulnar artery must be adequate. However, hand or finger ischemia is unusual following use of the radial artery for prosthetic shunts.

The major complications of these shunts are thrombosis, infection, bleeding, erosion of the skin, and dislodgement. Acute thrombosis is a major complication, particularly when there is injury to the vessel intima. Thrombosis occurs more often in patients with small or diseased arteries, i.e., small women, children, diabetics, and those with poor venous outflow, usually secondary to multiple prior intravenous punctures. Dislodgement can lead to death from exsanguination; these shunts have been used for suicide. Infection occurs with an incidence of 1 per 6.9 patient months to 1 per 35 patient months at the site of the Silastic tubing exiting the skin.[12,50] This is usually caused by *Staphylococcus aureus* or *Staphylococcus epidermitis* and can be minimized by aggressive and appropriate sterile techniques.[50]

The Thomas shunt is also occasionally used. It is a shunt in which the device is attached to the side of the femoral artery and vein. This can occasionally be used when other access has failed.[61]

The patency of external shunts is approximately 2 to 14 months.[28,30] Maintaining patients on low-dose aspirin (160 mg. per day) decreased the number of thromboses with an external shunt from 72 per cent in a placebo-treated group to 32 per cent in an aspirin-treated group over a 5-month period.[24] Sodium

warfarin (Coumadin) therapy (prothrombin time, 1.5 times normal) decreased the thrombosis rate from 1 per 3.6 patient months to 1 per 13 patient months.[12]

Short-term angioaccess for hemodialysis may be obtained by insertion of catheters in the subclavian or femoral vein or artery. The use of single-lumen subclavian and femoral catheters by means of the Seldinger technique provides a higher percentage of recirculation of blood, compared with use of the double-lumen catheter. Single- and double-lumen subclavian catheters have an infection rate one-fifth that of external shunts such as the Scribner. Because subclavian catheters do not utilize peripheral vessels, a higher construction rate of autogenous fistulas (71 per cent) is possible than that in patients who have the external shunts (46 per cent).[14] However, these percutaneously placed catheters may make construction of an autogenous or internal arteriovenous fistula more difficult when subclavian vein stenosis occurs, which is quite common.[13] This complication may not be apparent clinically because of collateral circulation, but a high-flow system such as a fistula makes this quite evident. The patient has a swollen arm or the fistula clots soon after placement. There may also be high venous pressures on dialysis. The Shiley femoral catheters are placed in the femoral veins at the bedside; after dialysis they are removed. Repeated use of these catheters may lead to iliofemoral thrombosis, local bleeding, or arterial puncture and injury.[48] However, the technique of multiple punctures, rather than the use of a continuous external shunt, does decrease the incidence of catheter thrombosis and blood-borne infections.

Additional experience has been gained with dual-lumen, silicone rubber catheters. These are usually placed via a cut down in the external jugular or internal jugular vein. These have a low percentage of recirculation (8 to 12 per cent); and no major complications have occurred, such as arterial injury or patient death. There is an incidence of thrombosis (4 per cent) and of infection (35 per cent).[16,35] However, these catheters can be of major use in a group of patients who have no place for an internal shunt or are awaiting placement or maturation of an internal fistula. Another advantage of the subclavian and jugular catheter is that it can be left in place and allows patient ambulation, which is not possible with the femoral catheter in place.[64]

INTERNAL ARTERIOVENOUS FISTULAS. Prosthetic material, regardless of type, has a greater tendency toward thrombosis than autogenous tissue. For this reason, the development of arteriovenous fistulas by direct anastomosis without the use of intervening prosthetic material represents one of the major advances in the management of patients with end-stage renal disease who are on hemodialysis. The most frequent fistula utilized and the standard with which all other fistulas are compared is the Brescia-Cimino fistula, which is an anastomosis between the radial artery and cephalic vein at the wrist.[5] An Allen test should be performed prior to operation to assure adequate collateral flow from the ulnar artery to minimize the problem of hand ischemia. The artery and vein are isolated through a longitudinal incision, care being taken to avoid the superficial branch of the radial nerve.[3] The artery and vein can be anastomosed in a number of ways including: side to side, end artery to side vein, side artery to end vein, or end artery to end vein (Fig. 2). The anastomosis can be made larger with more options for blood flow in a side-to-side anastomosis.[10] This can lead to the problem of venous hypertension in the hand, which can be solved by ligation of the vein distal to the anastomosis. The end-to-end anastomosis appears to be accompanied by a somewhat higher initial thrombosis rate because there are fewer collateral channels. Dilatation of the artery and vein at the time of creation of the fistula by insertion of Fogarty balloon catheters appears to diminish the initial thrombosis rate of these anastomoses.

TYPES OF ARTERIOVENOUS FISTULAS. There are several different

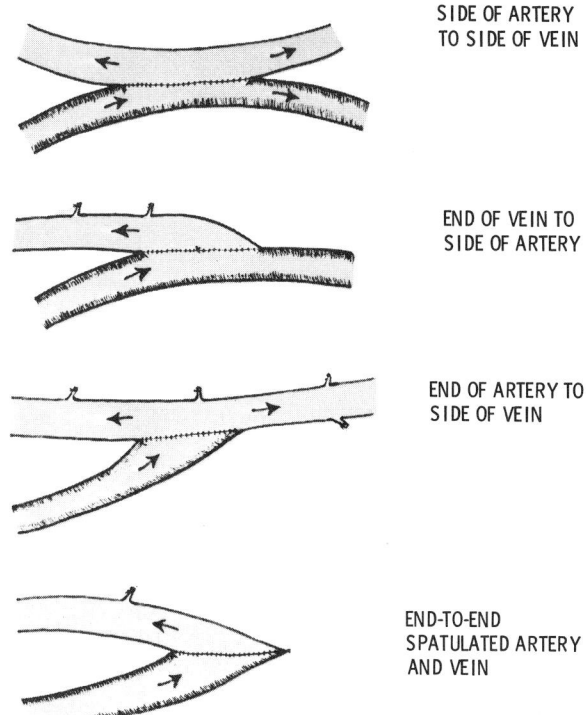

SIDE OF ARTERY
TO SIDE OF VEIN

END OF VEIN TO
SIDE OF ARTERY

END OF ARTERY TO
SIDE OF VEIN

END-TO-END
SPATULATED ARTERY
AND VEIN

Figure 2. Four different anastomoses commonly constructed between the radial artery and the cephalic vein. (From Ozeran, R. S.: Construction and care of external arteriovenous shunts. *In* Wilson, S. E., and Owens, M. L.: Vascular Access Surgery. Chicago, Year Book Medical Publishers, 1980.)

anastomotic possibilities for arteriovenous fistulas. In addition to the wrist fistula, other anastomoses include the snuff-box fistula, the fistula from the ulnar artery to the basilic vein (seldom used), the fistula from the antecubital vein to the brachial artery, and the brachiobasilic fistula. The latter requires dissecting the basilic vein and moving it to a superficial position on the medial portion of the upper extremity[33] (Fig. 3). If at all possible, the above options should be exhausted before nonautogenous material is considered for dialysis access. The patency of these shunts depends upon the anatomic type. The Brescia-Cimino arteriovenous wrist fistula has a patency at 2 years of between 55 and 89 per cent.[17,25] One analysis combined a collective series of over 1400 Brescia-Cimino fistulas and found an overall patency rate of 65 per cent at 1 year.[33] There is an early failure rate of 10 to 15 per cent caused by poor vessels, poor venous outflow, or excessive dehydration or hypotension. Patency rates for brachiocephalic fistulas are approximately 80 per cent.[17] In the combined series cited above, a 70 per cent patency rate at 1 year was found.[33] One arm should always be guarded in a potential dialysis patient to preserve veins for future fistula placement.

COMPLICATIONS OF INTERNAL FISTULAS. A number of complications occur with arteriovenous fistulas. The most common complication is stenosis at the proximal venous limb (48 per cent). Aneurysms (7 per cent) and thrombosis (9 per cent) are the next most common complications.[36] Aneurysms from repeated needle punctures are more likely to occur when venous access is obtained in the same location, leading to localized weakening of the vessel wall. Heart failure can occur in those patients with a marginal cardiac reserve and a fistula flow rate of more than 500 ml. per minute. The placement of a Teflon band around the outflow track of the fistula until the blood flow is decreased below 500 ml. per minute may reverse the cardiac failure; occasionally, the fistula requires ligation.[2] The arterial steal syndrome and its ischemia occur in approximately 1.6 per cent of patients with arteriovenous fistulas. This problem is unusual in

wrist fistulas (0.25 per cent) but is relatively common in the more proximal large brachiocephalic fistulas (approximately 30 per cent).[23] The steal syndrome is caused by blood flowing from the anastomosed artery to the low-resistance vein with additional blood flowing retrograde from the hand (approximately 30 per cent) into the fistula. This causes decreased blood flow to the hand and therefore ischemia. The complication of venous hypertension distal to the fistula follows high-pressure arterial blood flowing into the low-pressure venous system, causing venous hypertension with distal tissue swelling, hyperpigmentation, skin induration, and eventual skin ulceration similar to that observed in the legs of patients with venous stasis.[23] Both the steal syndrome and distal venous hypertension appear to occur more frequently with side-to-side anastomosis. Ligation of the distal limb of a side-to-side shunt corrects the problem, but this often leads to shunt occlusion because the proximal vein is usually at least partially occluded, causing redirection of blood through the distal limb of the venous anastomosis. This anatomic problem can be detected clinically by balloting the proximal vein to palpate a transmitted pulse wave or by using duplex scanning to map the veins of the arm.[49,63] Infection of a Brescia-Cimino arteriovenous fistula rarely occurs (less than 3 per cent).[26] Occasionally neurovascular problems develop, characterized by pain, weakness, paresthesias, and muscle atrophy. These can be reversed by closure of the fistula.[34]

PROSTHETIC GRAFTS FOR VASCULAR ACCESS. The construction of vascular access by means of subcutaneously placed prosthetic material joining an artery to a vein is becoming increasingly necessary in patients with poor peripheral veins or previously failed arteriovenous fistulas. The material ideally should be easy to handle and suture, allow graft-host biocompatibility, and be minimally thrombogenic. It should be inexpensive, seal after repeated needle punctures, and allow tissue ingrowth.[18] One of the initial materials used for the "jump" graft was the saphenous vein. Because of the extensive dissection required, the high incidence of stenosis, a 50 per cent thrombosis rate at 1 year, and possible need for the saphenous vein in subsequent coronary artery bypass surgery, other materials were tried.[19]

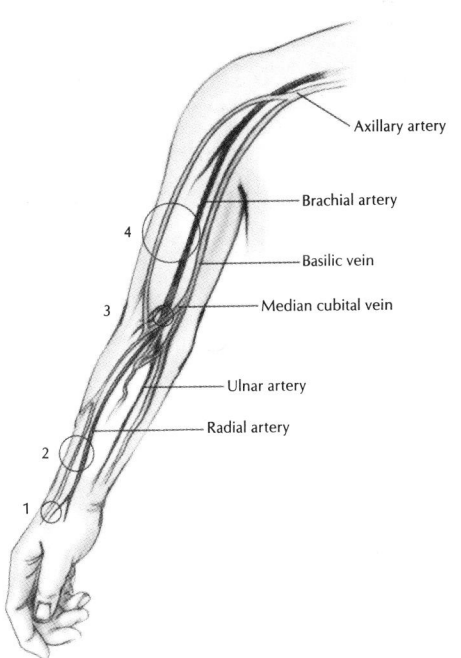

Axillary artery

Brachial artery

Basilic vein

Median cubital vein

Ulnar artery

Radial artery

Figure 3. Four possible anastomotic sites for arteriovenous fistulas in the upper extremity. (Redrawn from Tilney, N. L., and Lazarus, J. M. (Eds.): Surgical Care of the Patient with Renal Failure. Philadelphia, W. B. Saunders Company, 1982. (As shown in Haisch, C. E.: Chronic vascular and peritoneal access. *In* Davis, J. H., et al. (Eds.): Clinical Surgery. St. Louis, C. V. Mosby Company, 1987.)

Dacron is used only occasionally. The Sparks-Mandril graft, which creates a tube of autogenous tissue by implanting a prosthetic material with very loose interstices in the subcutaneous space, was initially used but has now been abandoned because it requires several weeks for the "tube" to be suitable for anastomosis. Bovine grafts obtained from the carotid artery of the cow have a propensity toward infection and, in particular, toward aneurysm formation.[39] Infected bovine grafts have a tendency to disintegrate, causing massive hemorrhage.[4]

Several different prosthetic materials have been used for "jump" grafts. Polytetrafluoroethylene (PTFE) is a material that permits ingrowth of tissue through the interstices of the graft, thus incorporating the graft in viable tissue. A neointima is formed in the graft, presumably lessening the likelihood of thrombosis. PTFE has a lower incidence of aneurysm formation than bovine grafts and does not always have to be removed when it becomes infected.

TECHNIQUE OF ARTERIOVENOUS JUMP GRAFTS. Successful creation of vascular access using prosthetic material requires good arterial inflow and venous outflow. As previously mentioned, duplex scanning can help to outline the arterial and venous vasculature.[52,63] Also, assessing digital pressures and comparing these with the brachial pressure provide information regarding the adequacy of small vessel inflow to the hand. The radial artery, especially in diabetic females, may be too small to provide good inflow necessary to maintain patency of a jump graft. Also, patients who have had multiple venous punctures and subsequent venous stenosis must have the site of the venous anastomosis chosen carefully so that it is proximal to these areas of obstruction. Rotation or pinching of the graft in its tunnel must be avoided. The graft must be large enough to readily permit needle puncture. A 6-mm. graft or a rapid taper 4- to 7-mm. graft is usually used. The latter provides approximately 20 per cent of the maximal flow that the straight 6-mm. graft offers at the same pressure and length.[27] Dialysis can usually be performed relatively promptly after the graft has been placed; however, hematoma formation from bleeding at the puncture site is a serious complication because of the propensity for infection and pressure occlusion of the graft. Allowing the graft to mature for 1 to 2 weeks minimizes this problem by permitting tissue ingrowth, which facilitates sealing of the graft at the needle puncture site.

Several graft configurations have been developed for dialysis. The nondominant arm should be used first, and an attempt should be made to use the forearm position first. A graft between the radial artery at the wrist and the cephalic vein just below the elbow accomplishes this. This graft has the lowest patency of any of the configurations because of the low flow through the radial artery. A forearm loop is easily constructed, joining the brachial artery to the cephalic vein or the brachial vein at the elbow. In the upper arm, a brachial artery to the axillary vein approach may be used. A loop between the axillary artery and axillary vein is also possible (Fig. 4). These upper arm grafts have a very high flow rate and a low incidence of thrombosis. However, they do tend to have a higher incidence of ischemia in the hand, compared with other grafts, because of preferential flow of arterial blood through the graft, rather than to the peripheral circulation (Fig. 5). After placement, swelling is frequently observed secondary to surgical trauma and changes in venous outflow. Both usually resolve with elevation and time.

Interposition grafts in the lower extremity are utilized for patients without available access in the upper extremities. A loop graft in the thigh (superficial femoral artery to saphenous vein) and a jump graft between the popliteal artery and the femoral vein are the two most common configurations. However, both of these grafts are associated with a high incidence of infection. They are an especially poor choice for diabetics and elderly patients who frequently have peripheral arterial insufficiency. A high mortality and amputation rate occur in patients in whom femoral triangle sepsis develops.[37]

In patients in whom all previously described sites have been exhausted, other sites can be utilized for the creation of an arteriovenous jump graft. These possibilities include a graft from axillary artery to axillary vein across the chest, a loop on the anterior chest, a graft from axillary artery to iliac vein, or an artery-to-artery graft (Fig. 6). The latter requires narrowing the artery between the anastomoses with the prosthesis to allow adequate flow through the graft itself.[22]

COMPLICATIONS. Early hemorrhage can occur at the anastomotic site, whereas late hemorrhage is usually secondary to needle puncture of the graft and bleeding into the perigraft space. Early thrombosis usually occurs for technical reasons, i.e., narrowing of inflow or outflow, whereas later thrombosis is secondary to venous intimal hyperplasia at or distal to the anastomosis.[8,9] Outflow stenosis or occlusion may be repaired by a patch graft, balloon dilatation of the strictured area, or a graft bypass of the obstruction. There have been a number of reports of the use of streptokinase to dissolve the clot in the graft and then balloon dilatation to repair the venous outflow obstruction. The results have been mixed; however, a recent article reported a satisfactory success rate with balloon dilatation with

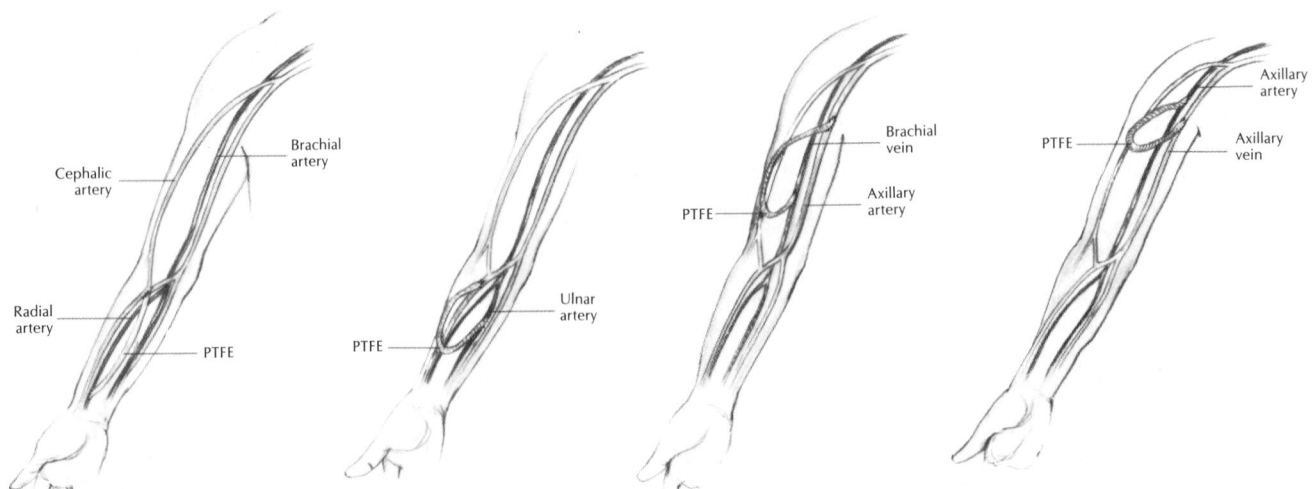

Figure 4. Four most common sites for placement of a jump graft in the upper extremity. (From Haisch, C. E.: Chronic vascular and peritoneal access. *In* Davis, J. H., et al. (Eds.): Clinical Surgery. St. Louis, C. V. Mosby Company, 1987.)

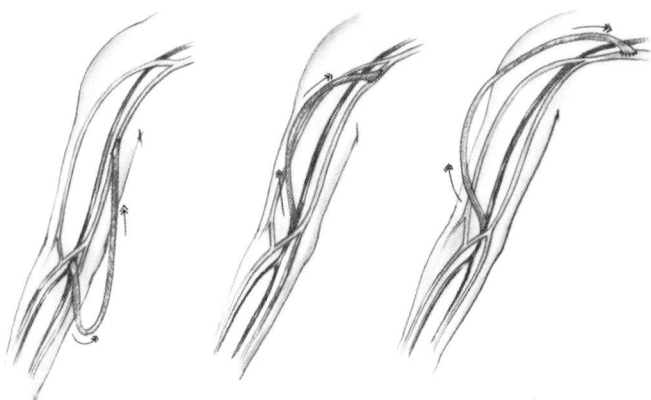

Figure 5. Three possible graft configurations for jump grafts in which standard sites have been used. (Redrawn from Tilney, N. L., and Lazarus, J. M. (Eds.): Surgical Care of the Patient with Renal Failure. Philadelphia, W. B. Saunders Company, 1982. As shown in Haisch, C. E.: Chronic vascular and peritoneal access. In Davis, J. H., et al. (Eds.): Clinical Surgery. St. Louis, C. V. Mosby Company, 1987.)

17 atmospheres of pressure in the balloon.[6,56] Low blood pressure or excessive external pressure applied to the graft can contribute to the incidence of thrombosis. Thrombosis unaccompanied by narrowing of either inflow or outflow is often corrected by simple thrombectomy of the graft. There is no reason relating to anatomy or blood pressure for a patient to have recurrent episodes of thrombosis. These patients may benefit from chronic aspirin use.[24] The use of Coumadin in these patients is still being considered.[53]

Infection is a major problem with prosthetic jump grafts. Local drainage and wound care may resolve the problem in a number of grafts if the suture line is not involved. In some cases, the infected area may be bypassed with a small local bypass or covered with a flap.[35,38] The major reasons for removal are involvement of the suture line, tunnel infection, clotted graft, or lack of success with conservative therapy. The salvage rate of infected grafts is low, 25 to 50 per cent.[46]

PTFE and other prosthetic materials are also associated with false aneurysms, usually secondary to laceration of the graft material with the dialysis needle; these can be excised and bypassed. The hemodynamic complications of venous hypertension, congestive heart failure, vascular steal, and vascular access neuropathy may occur with jump grafts, as they do with natural fistulas. The complications can be decreased with a rapid taper 4- to 7-mm. graft. This decreases the flow rate in the graft and has been used in elderly and diabetic patients.[27,51] The steal syndrome is more likely to occur in upper arm fistulas, compared with forearm fistulas.

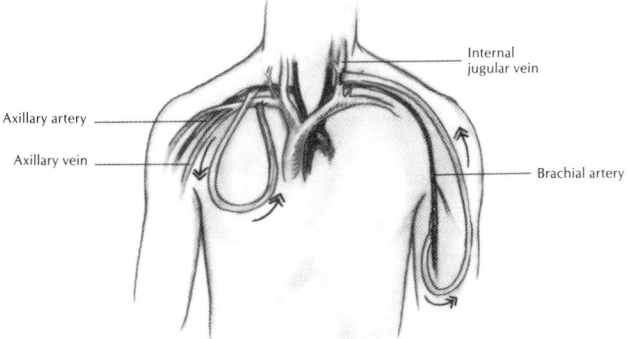

Figure 6. A graft from axillary artery to axillary vein with a loop on the chest. (Redrawn from Haimov, M.: Vascular access for hemodialysis: New modifications for the difficult patient. Surgery, 92:109, 1982. As shown in Haisch, C. E.: Chronic vascular and peritoneal access. In Davis, J. H., et al. (Eds.): Clinical Surgery. St. Louis, C. V. Mosby Company, 1987.)

PATENCY. The patency rate of jump grafts is less than that of autogenous arteriovenous fistulas. The patency rates of bovine grafts vary from 21 to 70 per cent at 12 months.[43] Raju has reported a 93 per cent patency rate for PTFE at 1 year and a 77 per cent patency rate at 2 years.[49] Munda and associates have analyzed their experience with PTFE and demonstrated that the location of the graft affects patency rates. In an upper arm location, the patency rate was 60 per cent at 12 months; a straight forearm graft had a 35 per cent patency rate at 12 months, compared with a 78 per cent patency rate for a forearm loop.[39] Wilson and Owens report a 12-month patency rate of 80 per cent for grafts in the thigh.[66] There are also some preliminary data to indicate that the 4- to 7-mm. taper graft may decrease the amount of intimal hyperplasia at the venous end, thus leading to a better long-term patency rate. Overall, the patency rate appears to be related to the magnitude of arterial inflow and the size and distensibility of the venous outflow system.[29,46,62] These factors are critical in choosing the initial site for vascular access.

Physiology

The physiologic consequences of arteriovenous fistulas depend upon the size of the proximal and distal arteries and veins, the collateral flow around the fistula, and the diameter of the fistula. The diameter of the fistula influences the flow very little when it is diminished to less than 20 per cent of the arterial diameter or enlarged to more than 75 per cent of the arterial diameter. Between these two values, however, small changes in the size of the fistula can change the flow dramatically. Most clinical fistulas are constructed to make the fistula greater in size than the arterial diameter, thus allowing some margin for error for subsequent stenosis.[15] Blood flow through a side-to-side or end vein-to-side artery wrist fistula is contributed by both the proximal and distal arteries, with as much as a third of the flow coming from the distal artery.[3]

A large functioning arteriovenous fistula may cause a fall in both systolic and diastolic blood pressure, an increase in cardiac output, an increase in venous blood pressure both proximal and distal to the fistula, an increase in pulse rate, and a slight increase in the size of the heart. There are also increases in blood volume in patients with chronic arteriovenous fistulas. These changes are reversible with closure of the fistula.[15]

Platelets and fibrin may accumulate in a chronic fistula with eventual closure of the lumen. With a larger fistula, there is usually progressive lengthening and dilatation of both the proximal artery and the outflow vein. The proximal artery elongates and dilates, and smooth muscle hypertrophy occurs. Eventually smooth muscle atrophy develops, and additional elongation and dilatation occur. This leads to aneurysmal dilatation and a tortuous vessel. The outflow vein develops an increase in smooth muscle, fibrous tissue, and collagen and also enlarges significantly. There is increased blood flow around the fistula and a corresponding increase in temperature. However, blood flow distal to the fistula may be decreased, with resulting cool temperatures, particularly in the hand.[15,66]

Summary

The development of convenient vascular access revolutionized and made possible chronic long-term hemodialysis. Clearly, the three major improvements in the development of adequate vascular access were (1) the development of the external shunt with prosthetic material penetrating the skin, (2) the development of the arteriovenous wrist fistula, and (3) the utilization of a subcutaneous prosthetic material to connect the artery and the vein. These techniques have been associated with increasing success and decreasing morbidity. However, there remain some patients in whom hemodialysis is not clinically appropriate. For patients with these and other indications, peritoneal dialysis is now widely used.

PERITONEAL DIALYSIS

HISTORICAL ASPECTS. The physiology of the peritoneal cavity was studied in the late 1800s by Wegner, who demonstrated that concentrated sugar solutions increased in volume while in the peritoneal cavity.[65] This work was extended in 1894 by Starling and Tubby, who demonstrated urinary excretion of methylene blue dye after introduction into the peritoneum.[57]

In 1923, Ganter treated a patient with acute uremia secondary to ureteral obstruction. He noted slight improvement after peritoneal dialysis. From 1946 to 1948, nephrologists in Boston were able to demonstrate successful use of peritoneal dialysis in azotemic patients. The procedure was still considered experimental in the early 1950s. After improvements in catheters and dialysate, the first patient to be chronically dialyzed was treated in 1960. This was done for 6 months, after which the patient refused further treatment and died.[41]

PHYSIOLOGY. The exact surface through which the exchange occurs is not known. The peritoneal surface approximates the total body surface area. However, the visceral peritoneum appears more crucial, although there are more capillaries in the parietal peritoneum. The exact route and mechanism by which solutes cross the peritoneal cell membrane are also unknown. Middle molecules (500 to 5000 daltons) such as vitamin B_{12} are cleared more rapidly in chronic ambulatory peritoneal dialysis (CAPD) than in hemodialysis, i.e., the equivalent of 50 liters of serum are cleared of vitamin B_{12} per week for CAPD, compared with 30 liters per week for hemodialysis (1008 liters per week for normal kidneys). This is not true for smaller molecules such as urea, the clearance rate of which is much lower in CAPD than in hemodialysis, i.e., 84 liters per week of urea clearance for CAPD, compared with 135 liters per week for hemodialysis (604 liters per week for normal kidneys). These rates can be increased by increasing the volume of fluid exchange; however, this has certain practical limitations. Dialysis flow required for a urea clearance of 40 ml. per minute is 18 liters per hour.[41]

The evidence that peritoneal capillary blood flow is the major source of fluid and solute exchange is indirect and is based on the following: (1) vasoconstrictors can decrease peritoneal clearance, (2) vasodilators increase peritoneal clearance, and (3) inflammation increases dialysate white cell counts. Peritoneal cavity clearance is not totally dependent on capillary blood flow. Peritoneal dialysis can be used even when blood pressure is low. A urea clearance of 70 per cent of normal levels can be obtained with patients in shock.

INDICATIONS. Short-term peritoneal dialysis is usually used (1) for acute renal failure until recovery is complete, (2) while a hemoaccess site is maturing, (3) when a patient with chronic renal failure has had an acute exacerbation, or (4) for insertion of chemotherapeutic agents in abdominal or hepatic malignancy.[59]

Chronic ambulatory peritoneal dialysis (CAPD) is indicated in patients (1) desiring home dialysis, (2) with no available sites for vascular access, (3) with repeated infections of vascular access sites, (4) with an unstable cardiovascular system, (5) with diabetes who would benefit from a constant insulin infusion from the peritoneal cavity, (6) above 65 years of age, (7) with bleeding problems (e.g., duodenal ulcer), (8) who wish to avoid blood transfusions, (9) with AIDS, and (10) who are small children. CAPD is frequently recommended and enthusiastically accepted by patients who wish to avoid the restriction of activity associated with hemodialysis.[45,60]

The number of absolute contraindications for the use of CAPD is few. When there is an obliterated peritoneal space from previous surgical procedures or infection, CAPD cannot be employed. When there is poor peritoneal clearance or lack of diaphragmatic integrity, CAPD cannot be used.[42] In the latter

case, this anatomic defect allows dialysate to move into the chest cavity, thereby causing pulmonary and cardiac compromise.

There are a number of relative contraindications, including (1) respiratory insufficiency, because the increased abdominal volume compromises respiratory function; (2) a diffuse peritoneal malignancy; (3) a large hernia; and (4) low back pain caused by degenerative disc disease.[41]

TECHNICAL PROCEDURES. Several types of catheters are available for use in peritoneal dialysis today. The Tenckhoff catheter has been used for percutaneous bedside insertion as well as for surgical insertion. The percutaneous route is used for acute dialysis, and the catheter usually has a single Dacron cuff. It is inserted aseptically below the umbilicus under local anesthesia and directed toward the pelvis.[54] The catheter exits through a subcutaneous tunnel to the side of the insertion site with the Dacron cuff placed in the tunnel at least 1 inch from the skin surface.

With local anesthesia, the Tenckhoff or Toronto Western catheter is placed by making a paramedian incision below the umbilicus longitudinally through the anterior rectus sheath and muscle and exposing the posterior fascia and peritoneum (Fig. 7). A pursestring suture is placed and the catheter directed toward the pelvis with a metal guide. Care is taken to avoid bowel or bladder injury. The deep Dacron cuff is left in the muscle just above the posterior fascia and is sutured into place with the pursestring suture. The anterior fascia is closed, and the cuff is placed in the subcutaneous tunnel with the catheter exiting distally. If necessary, placement and fixation of the catheter

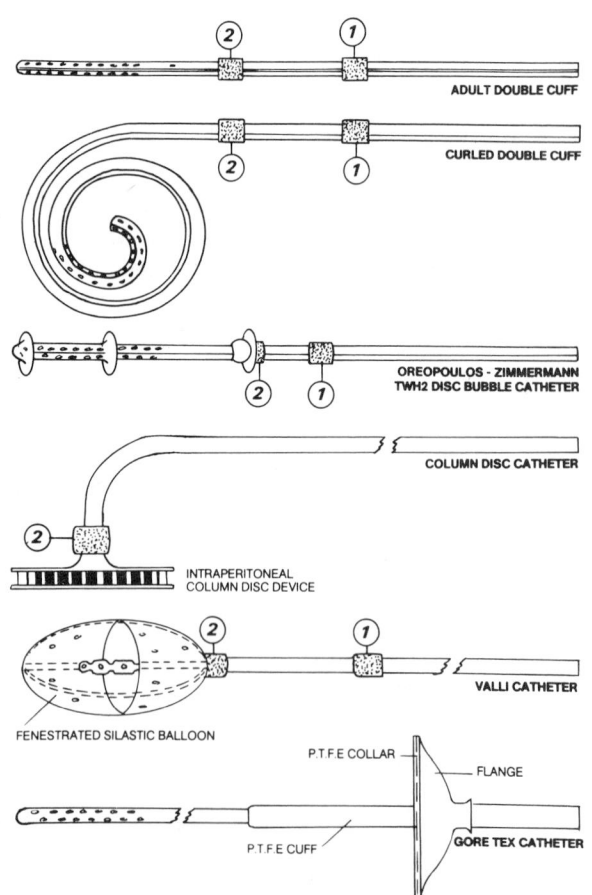

Figure 7. Main types of peritoneal catheters. *Adult double cuff* refers to the standard double-cuff Tenckhoff catheter. (From Mion, C.: Practical use of peritoneal dialysis. *In* Maher, J. F. (Ed.): Replacement of Renal Function by Dialysis, 3rd ed. Dordrecht/Boston/Lancaster, Kluwer Academic Publishers, 1989.)

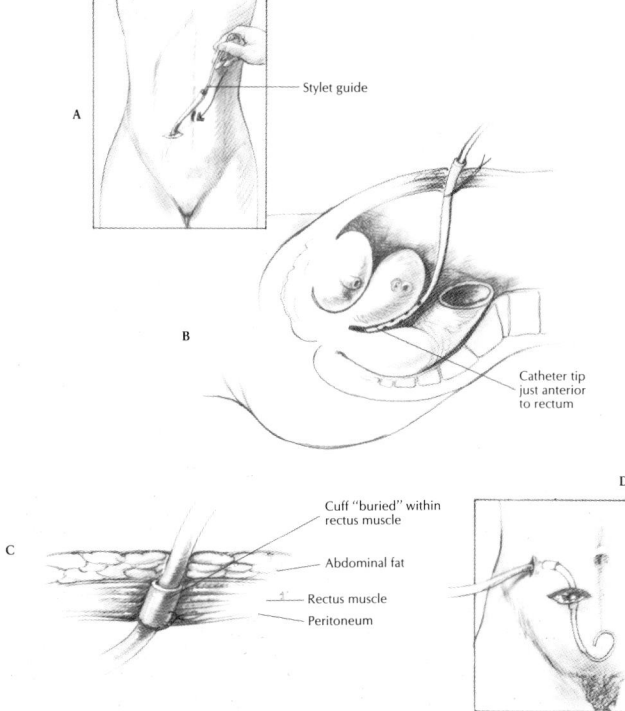

Figure 8. Location of the chronic ambulatory peritoneal dialysis catheter (CAPD). A, Location of the surgical incision. B, Location of the catheter in the pelvis. C, Dacron cuff at the level of the posterior rectus sheath. D, Exit site shown with final placement. (Redrawn from Simmons, R. L., et al (Eds.): Manual of Vascular Access, Organ Donation and Transplantation. New York, Springer-Verlag, 1984. As shown in Haisch, C. E.: Chronic vascular and peritoneal access. *In* Davis, J. H., et al. (Eds.): Clinical Surgery. St. Louis, C. V. Mosby Company, 1987.)

in the pelvis under direct vision decreases the incidence of nonfunctioning catheters (Fig. 8). Omentectomy may be necessary in some instances.[11,44]

DIALYSIS FLUIDS. The dialysate fluids vary in dextrose concentration. The lowest concentration, 1.5 per cent, causes very little ultrafiltration of fluid to occur (200 ml. per 2-liter exchange); the greatest concentration, 4.5 per cent, treats or prevents fluid overload (800 ml. per 2-liter exchange). The sodium and chloride concentrations approximate those in serum (Na, 132 mEq. per liter; Cl, 102 mEq. per liter). Lactate (35 mEq. per liter) is added along with calcium and magnesium at low concentrations (Ca, 3.5 mEq. per liter; Mg, 1.5 mEq. per liter); potassium is added only if needed. The pH of these solutions is approximately 5.2 to 6.2. In diabetics, insulin can be added. A typical exchange per day for CAPD is 2 liters four times a day. In some centers, this has been changed to 3 liters three times a day. This leads to better exchange for the patient and thus better overall results.[67] The exchange of acute peritoneal dialysis may be higher, depending on the needs of the patient. The technique of CAPD allows the patient to be at home and working, with minimal disruption of normal daily activities. In one study, 55 per cent of the patients on CAPD were able to pursue normal daily activities. This percentage was only 38 per cent for diabetics.[67]

This approach to the management of chronic renal failure is gaining popularity because of the decreasing incidence of catheter infections, fewer cardiac complications, less anemia, and greater convenience in comparison with hemodialysis. However, excellent patient compliance is necessary.

COMPLICATIONS. Complications may be divided into those related to surgical placement of the catheter and those occurring after placement. Those related to placement include (1) leakage of dialysate, (2) intraperitoneal bleeding, (3) bowel

or bladder perforation, (4) subcutaneous bleeding with hematoma formation from tunnel construction, and (5) ileus.[20,41] All of these, except ileus, can be prevented by close attention to technical details. Reflex ileus will gradually resolve, and most patients can eat within 24 hours.

Peritoneal infection is the leading complication after catheter placement, occurring approximately once every 16 to 18 months[40] (compared with every 6 to 8 months in the early experience).[31] There are five routes of infection: (1) through the dialysis tubing and peritoneal catheter, (2) through tissues around the catheter, (3) through fecal contamination, such as diverticulitis, (4) through blood-borne infections, and (5) through ascending infection from the fallopian tubes in women.[67] Grampositive organisms represent approximately 75 per cent of the infections, with gram-negative organisms causing approximately 20 per cent. *S. epidermidis* is the most common cause of gram-positive infections, with *S. aureus* the second most common. These two organisms together are responsible for over 90 per cent of the gram-positive infections. Uncommon causes of peritonitis are tuberculosis and fungi.[41] These infections are treated with peritoneal and parenteral antibiotics appropriate for the isolated organisms. The antibiotics should be bactericidal and administered in doses large enough to exceed the minimal inhibitory concentration by 2 to 4 times. If the infection does not resolve after a full course of antibiotics or the Dacron cuff is involved, the catheter must be removed.[54] Prevention of infection is critical and requires meticulous catheter maintenance and flawless technique in changing the bags and administering medications. Erosion and prolapse of the catheter cuff are caused by placement of the Dacron cuff too near the skin exit site. This leads to pressure necrosis of the skin with extrusion of the cuff causing infection of the catheter tunnel.

Catheter malfunction may be caused by a number of factors and is manifested by poor inflow or total obstruction. Poor inflow is caused by displacement, omental wrapping, or partial blockage of the catheter holes. Total obstruction is caused by kinking of the catheter, blockage of all catheter holes, or omental wrapping of the entire intra-abdominal portion of the catheter. Kinking of the catheter is rare and is prevented by attention to technical details during catheter insertion. Flipping of the catheter out of the pelvis can be minimized by the creation of a peritoneal tunnel for the catheter deep in the pelvis. Other complications include hernia formation at the point of peritoneal entry, which can be minimized by using a paramedian approach, and rupture of the subcutaneous Silastic tube segment by a sudden external force.

CATHETER LONGEVITY. The January 1984 report of the National CAPD Registry indicates that 85 per cent of catheters function for 1 year. This figure decreases significantly at the end of 2 years, when only 50 per cent of the original catheters function. The report also indicates that the probability of requiring three or more catheter placements during this time interval is very small.[58] Gloor and associates reported slightly better results with a 60 per cent patency rate in 85 catheters in patients whose cases were followed for 30 months.[20] The permeability of the peritoneal cavity can change over time. Also, patients with systemic vascular disease, scleroderma, malignant hypertension, and collagen vascular disease show a decrease in peritoneal permeability.[42] As new catheters and techniques are developed, these longevity rates may improve.

COST COMPARISONS. In-center hemodialysis costs approximately the same as does CAPD, but multiple hospitalizations for peritonitis can increase the cost of CAPD.[7,32] More centers are therefore treating peritonitis on an outpatient basis. Hemodialysis, exclusive of vascular access, costs about $30,000 per year, as compared with $25,000 per year for CAPD. It is clear that the cost of either form of dialysis significantly exceeds that of successful renal transplantation.

SELECTED REFERENCES

Brescia, M. J., Cimino, J. E., Appel, D., and Harwich, B. J.: Chronic hemodialysis using venipuncture and a surgically created arteriovenous fistula. N. Engl. J. Med., 275:1089, 1966.
This article is the original description of the wrist fistula, which revolutionized dialysis and allowed patients long-term vascular access with fewer complications than occurred with external shunts. The article describes the fistula by which all other methods of vascular access for dialysis are assessed.

Butt, K. M. H., Friedman, E. A., and Koutz, S. L.: Angioaccess. Curr. Probl. Surg., 131, 1976.
This is an overview that provides the state of the art and includes an overview of external shunts, fistulas, and jump grafts. The technical aspects, complications, and longevity of the types of grafts are presented.

Haimov, M. Baez, A., Neff, M., and Slifkin, R.: Complications of arteriovenous fistulas for hemodialysis. Arch. Surg., 110:708, 1975.
A group of over 400 patients with slightly over 500 arteriovenous fistulas are reported. The 30 vascular complications are examined. Complications including ischemia, steal, gangrene, aneurysm, and venous hypertension are outlined; and their incidence is noted. The therapy and outcome are outlined for these complications.

Hertizer, N. R.: Circulatory access for hemodialysis. *In* Rutherford, R. B. (Ed.): Vascular Surgery. Philadelphia, W. B. Saunders Company, 1984.
This chapter provides a good overview of hemoaccess. The article is technically oriented but has excellent overviews of complications and longevity of the various types of vascular access requiring surgical construction.

Marx, A. B., Landmann, J., and Harder, F. H.: Surgery for vascular access. Curr. Probl. Surg., 27:1, 1990.
A recommended overview of vascular access surgery for nonuremic patients as well as those requiring dialysis. Appropriate diagrams and a good overview of results for both acute and chronic hemodialysis are included.

Mennes, P. A., Gilula, L. A., Anderson, C. B., Etheredge, E. E., Weerts, C., and Harter, H. R.: Complications associated with arteriovenous fistulas in patients undergoing chronic hemodialysis. Arch. Intern. Med., 138:1117, 1978.
A review of the complications of these fistulas.

Nolph, K. D.: Peritoneal anatomy and transport physiology; and Mion, C. M.: Practical use of peritoneal dialysis. *In* Drukker, W., Parsons, F. M., and Maher, J. F. (Eds.): Replacement of Renal Function by Dialysis. Boston, Martinus Nijhoff, 1983.
These two chapters provide excellent overviews of peritoneal physiology and anatomy and the practical uses and limitations of peritoneal dialysis. The chapter on physiology compares peritoneal dialysis with hemodialysis and cites its limitations. The chapter on the use of peritoneal dialysis includes sections on solutions and catheter insertion, complications, and catheter longevity.

Somner, B. G., and Henry, M. L. (Eds.): Vascular Access for Hemodialysis. Chicago, W. L. Gore and Associates, Inc., and Pluribus Press, Inc., 1989.
Results of a meeting on dialysis access held in 1988, this is a review of some of the historical insights, physiologic changes, anesthetic techniques, and various types of access that can be used for patients with end-stage renal disease.

Wilson, S. E., and Owens, M. D. (Eds.): Vascular Access Surgery. Chicago, Year Book Medical Publishers, 1980.
The major portion of this book concerns access for hemodialysis. It includes sections on the physiology of shunts and fistulas, care of external shunts, and radiologic diagnosis of surgical problems with fistulas and shunts. The text also includes data on vascular access for nutrition. The last five chapters are devoted to complications that occur in vascular access procedures.

REFERENCES

1. Alwall, N., Bersten, B. W. B., Gedda, P. O., Norvitt, L., and Steins, A. M.: On the artificial kidney. IV. The technique on animal experiments. Acta Med. Scand., 132:392, 1949.
2. Anderson, C. B., Codd, J. R., Graff, R. A., Groce, M. A., Harter, H. R., and Newton, W. T.: Cardiac failure and upper extremity arteriovenous dialysis fistulas. Case reports and a review of the literature. Arch. Intern. Med., 136:292, 1976.
3. Anderson, C. B., Etheredge, E. E., Harter, H. R., Graff, R. J., Codd, J. E., and Newton, W. T.: Local blood flow characteristics of arteriovenous fistulas in the forearm for dialysis. Surg. Gynecol. Obstet., 144:531, 1977.
4. Bone, G. E., and Pomajzl, M. J.: Prospective comparison of polytetrafluoroethylene and bovine grafts for dialysis. J. Surg. Res., 29:223, 1980.
5. Brescia, M. J., Cimino, J. E., Appel, K., and Harwich, B. J.: Chronic hemodialysis using venipuncture and a surgically created arteriovenous fistula. N. Engl. J. Med., 275:1089, 1966.
6. Brooks, J. L., Sigley, R. D., May, K. J., Jr., and Mack, R. M.: Transluminal angioplasty versus surgical repair for stenosis of hemodialysis grafts: A randomized study. Am. J. Surg., 153:530, 1987.
7. Bulgin, R. H.: Comparative costs of various dialysis treatments. Peritoneal Dial. Bull., 1:88, 1981.
8. Butt, K. M. H.: Bovine heterograft for arteriovenous fistulas. *In* Sawyer, P. N.,

and Kplitt, M. J. (Eds.): Vascular Grafts. New York, Appleton-Century-Crofts, 1978.
9. Butt, K. M. H., Friedman, E. A., and Kountz, S. L.: Angioaccess. Curr. Probl. Surg., 13:1, 1976.
10. Cerilli, J., and Limbert, J. G.: Technique and results of the construction of arteriovenous fistulas for hemodialysis. Surg. Gynecol. Obstet., 137:922, 1973.
11. Cerilli, J., Walker, J., and Bay, W.: A new technique for placement of catheters for peritoneal dialysis. Surg. Gynecol. Obstet., 156:663, 1983.
12. Curtis, J., Eastwood, J., Smith, E., Storey, J. M., Veroust, P. T., et al.: Maintenance hemodialysis. Q. J. Med., 38:49, 1969.
13. Davis, D., Petersen, J., Feldman, R., Cho, D., and Stevick, C. A.: Subclavian venous stenosis. J.A.M.A., 252:3404, 1984.
14. Dorner, D. B., Stubbs, D. H., Shader, C. A., and Flynn, C. T.: Percutaneous subclavian vein catheter hemodialysis: Impact on vascular access surgery. Surgery, 91:712, 1982.
15. Dow, P., and Hamilton, W. F.: Handbook of Physiology. Section 2, Circulation, Vol. III. Washington, D. C., American Physiological Society, 1965.
16. Dunn, J., Nylander, W., and Richie, R.: Central venous dialysis access: Experience with a dual-lumen, silicone rubber catheter. Surgery, 102:784, 1987.
17. Friedman, E. A., Butt, K. M. H., Pascua, L. J., Hardy, M. A., Lawton, R. L., and Udall, P. R.: Vascular access update. Trans. Am. Soc. Artif. Intern. Organs, 25:526, 1979.
18. Garvin, P. J., Costaneda, M. A., and Codd, J. E.: Etiology and management of bovine graft aneurysms. Arch. Surg., 117:281, 1982.
19. Girandet, R. E., Hackett, R. E., Goodwin, N. J., and Friedman, E. A.: Thirteen months experience with the saphenous vein graft arteriovenous fistula for maintenance hemodialysis. Trans. Am. Soc. Artif. Intern. Organs, 16:285, 1970.
20. Gloor, H. J., Nichols, W. K., Sorkin, M. I., Provout, B. F., et al.: Peritoneal access and related complications in continuous ambulatory peritoneal dialysis. Am. J. Med., 74:593, 1983.
21. Goldenberg, H. S., Goldberg, E. M., and Kerstein, M. D.: The arteriovenous fistula: Its construction in the management of hemophilia. Arch. Surg., 115:857, 1980.
22. Haimov, M: Vascular access for hemodialysis: New modifications for the difficult patient. Surgery, 92:109, 1982.
23. Haimov, M., Baez, A., Neff, M., and Slifkin, R.: Complications of arteriovenous fistulas for hemodialysis. Arch. Surg., 110:708, 1975.
24. Harter, H. R., Burch, J. W., Majerus, P. W., Standord, N., Delmez, J. A., et al.: Prevention of thrombosis in patients on hemodialysis by low-dose aspirin. N. Engl. J. Med., 301:577, 1979.
25. Hertzer, N. R.: Circulatory access for hemodialysis. *In* Rutherford, R. B. (Ed.): Vascular Surgery. Philadelphia, W. B. Saunders Company, 1984.
26. Higgins, M. R., Grace, M., Bettcher, K. B., Silverberg, D. S., and Dossetor, J. B.: Blood access in hemodialysis. Clin. Nephrol., 6:473, 1976.
27. Hinsdale, J. C., Lipkowitz, G. S., and Hoover, E. L.: Vascular access for hemodialysis in the elderly: Results and perspectives in a geriatric population. Dial. Transplant., 14:560, 1985.
28. Ishihara, A. M., and Myers, C. H.: Longevity of arterio-venous shunts for hemodialysis. Ann. Surg., 168:281, 1968.
29. Jenkins, A. M., Burst, T. A. S., and Glover, S. D.: Medium-term follow-up of forty autogenous vein and polytetrafluoroethylene (Gore-Tex) grafts for vascular access. Surgery, 88:667, 1980.
30. Ku, G., and Moorhead, J. F.: The present status of hemodialysis. Practitioner, 207:622, 1971.
31. Kurtz, S. B., Wong, V. H., Anderson, C. F., Vogel, J. P., et al.: Continuous ambulatory peritoneal dialysis: Three years' experience at the Mayo Clinic. Mayo Clin. Proc., 58:633, 1983.
32. Luvin, M., McGoldric., M. D., and McCoy, G. C.: Charges for in-hospital treatment of peritonitis in continuous ambulatory peritoneal dialysis. Clin. Res., 31:300A, 1983.
33. Marx, A. B., Landmann, J., and Harder, F. H.: Surgery for vascular access. Curr. Probl. Surg., 27:1, 1990.
34. Matolo, N., Kostagiv, B., Stevens, L. E., Chrysanthakopoulos, S., et al.: Neurovascular complications of brachial arteriovenous fistula. Am. J. Surg., 121:716, 1971.
35. McKenna, P. J., and Leadbetter, M. G.: Salvage of chronically exposed Gore-Tex vascular access graft in the hemodialysis patient. Plast. Reconstr. Surg., 82:1046, 1988.
36. Mennes, P. A., Gilula, L. A., Anderson, C. B., Etheredge, E. E., et al.: Complications associated with arteriovenous fistulas in patients undergoing chronic hemodialysis. Arch. Intern. Med., 138:1117, 1978.
37. Morgan, A. P., Knight, D. C., Tilney, N. L., and Lazarus, J. M.: Femoral triangle sepsis in dialysis patients: Frequency, management and outcome. Ann. Surg., 191:460, 1980.
38. Moosa, H. H., Peitzman, A. B., Thompson, B. R., Webster, M. W., and Steed, D. L.: Salvage of exposed arteriovenous hemodialysis fistulas. J. Vasc. Surg., 2:610, 1985.
39. Munda, R., First, M. R., Alexander, J. W., Linneman, C. C., Fidler, J. P., and Kittler, D.: Polytetrafluoroethylene graft survival in hemodialysis. J.A.M.A., 249:219, 1983.
40. National CAPD Registry, National Institute of Diabetes and Digestive and Kidney Diseases, July 1988.
41. Nolph, K. D.: Peritoneal anatomy and transport physiology; and Mion, C. M.: Practical use of peritoneal dialysis. *In:* Drukker, W., Parsons, F. M., and

Maher, J. F. (Eds.): Replacement of Renal Function by Dialysis. Boston, Martinus Nijhoff Publishers, 1983.

42. Nolph, K. D., Miller, L., Husted, F. C., and Hirszel, P., Peritoneal clearances in scleroderma and diabetes mellitus: Effects of intraperitoneal isoproterenol. Int. Urol. Nephrol., 8:161, 1976.

43. Nordling, J., Lynggaard, F., Poulsen, L. R., Hansen, R. I., and Rasmussen, F.: Experience with bovine heterografts and polytetrafluoroethylene (Impra®) grafts for vascular access in chronic hemodialysis. Scand. J. Urol. Nephrol., 16:69, 1982.

44. Olcott, C., Feldman, C. A., Coplon, N. S., Oppenheimer, M. L., and Mehigan, J. T.: Continuous ambulatory peritoneal dialysis: Technique of catheter insertion and management of associated surgical complications. Am. J. Surg., 146:98, 1983.

45. Oreopoulos, D. G.: Chronic peritoneal dialysis. Clin. Nephrol., 9:165, 1978.

46. Palder, S. B., Kirkman, R. L., Whittemore, A. D., Hakim, R. M., Lazarus, J. M., and Tilney, N. L.: Vascular access for hemodialysis: Patency rate and results of revision. Ann. Surg., 202:235, 1985.

47. Raaf, J. H.: Vascular access grafts for chemotherapy use in forty patients at M. D. Anderson Hospital. Ann. Surg., 182:614, 1975.

48. Raja, R. M., Kramer, M. S., Fernandez, M., Rosenbaum, J. L., and Barber, K.: Subclavian vein and femoral vein catheterization for hemodialysis: one year comparison. Trans. Am. Soc. Artif. Intern. Organs, 28:58, 1982.

49. Raju, S.: PTFE grafts for hemodialysis access. Ann. Surg., 206:666, 1987.

50. Ralston, A. J., Harlow, G. R., Jones, D. M., and Davis, P.: Infections of Scribner and Brescia arteriovenous shunts. Br. Med. J., 3:408, 1971.

51. Rosenthal, J. J., Bell, D. D., Gaspar, M. R., Movius, H. J., and Lemire, G. G.: Prevention of high flow problems of arteriovenous grafts: Development of a new tapered graft. Am. J. Surg., 140:231, 1980.

52. Rittgers, S. E., Garcia-Valdez, C., McCormick, J. T., and Posner, M. P.: Noninvasive blood flow measurement in expanded polytetrafluoroethylene grafts for hemodialysis access. J. Vasc. Surg., 3:635, 1986.

53. Rizzuti, R. P., Hale, J. C., and Burkart, T. E.: Extended patency of expanded polytetrafluoroethylene grafts for vascular access using optimal configuration and revisions. Surg. Gynecol. Obstet., 166:23, 1988.

54. Rubin, J., Adair, C. M., Raju, S., and Bower, J. D.: The Tenckhoff catheter for peritoneal dialysis—An appraisal. Nephron, 32:370, 1982.

55. Schauzer, H., Kaplan, S., Bosch, J., Glabman, S., and Burrows, L.: Double-lumen silicone rubber, in dwelling venous catheters: A new modality for angioaccess. Arch. Surg., 121:229, 1986.

56. Schwab, S. J., Saeed, M., Sussman, S. K., McCann, R. L., and Stickel, D. L.: Transluminal angioplasty of venous stenoses in polytetrafluoroethylene vascular access grafts. Kidney Int., 32:395, 1987.

57. Starling, E. H., and Tubby, E. H.: On absorption from and secretion into the serous cavities. J. Physiol. (Lond.), 16:140, 1894.

58. Steinberg, S. M., Cutler, S. J., and Novak, J. W.: Report of the National CAPD Registry of the National Institutes of Health, January 1984.

59. Tenckhoff, H.: Peritoneal dialysis today: A new look. Nephron, 12:420, 1974.

60. Tenckhoff, H.: Home peritoneal dialysis. In Massry, S. G., and Sellers, A. L. (Eds.): Clinical Aspects of Anemia and Dialysis. Springfield, Ill., Charles C Thomas, 1976.

61. Thomas, G. I.: A large vessel applique A-V shunt for hemodialysis. Trans. Am. Soc. Artif. Intern. Organs, 15:288, 1969.

62. Tilney, N. L., Kirkman, R. L., Whittemore, A. D., and Osteen, R. T.: Vascular access for dialysis and cancer chemotherapy. In Mannick, J. A., Cameron, J. L., Jordan, G. L., et al. (Eds.): Adv. Surg., 19:221, 1986.

63. Tordoir, J. H. M., de Bruin, H. G., Hoeneveld, H., Eikelboom, B. C., and Kitslaar, P. J. E. H. M.: Duplex ultrasound scanning in the assessment of arteriovenous fistulas created for hemodialysis access: Comparison with digital subtraction angiography. J. Vasc. Surg., 10:122, 1989.

64. Uldall, P. R., Joy, C., and Merchant, N.: Further experience with a double-lumen subclavian cannula for hemodialysis. Trans. Am. Soc. Artif. Intern. Organs, 28:71, 1982.

65. Wegner, G.: Chirurgische Bermerkungen über die Peritonealhöhle mit Berucksichtigung der Ovcariotomie (Surgical considerations regarding the peritoneal cavity with special attention to ovariotomy). Langenbecks Arch. Chir., 20:51, 1877 (in German).

66. Wilson, S. E., and Owens, M. D. (Eds.): Vascular Access Surgery. Chicago, Year Book Medical Publishers, 1980.

67. Wu, G., Khanna, R., Vas, S. I., Digenis, G., and Oreopoulos, D. G.: Continuous ambulatory peritoneal dialysis: No longer experimental. Can. Med. Assoc. J., 130:699, 1984.

68. Zincke, H., Hirsche, B. L., Amomoo, D. G., Woods, J. F., and Andersen, R. C.: The use of bovine carotid grafts for hemodialysis and hyperalimentation. Surg. Gynecol. Obstet., 130:350, 1974.

VI

PRINCIPLES OF IMMUNOSUPPRESSION

Suzanne T. Ildstad, M.D., Richard L. Simmons, M.D., and John S. Najarian, M.D.

Transplantation of solid organs has become an accepted therapy for end-stage renal, hepatic, cardiac and pulmonary disease.[9] The field of transplantation has progressed rapidly in the past two decades primarily as a result of advances in immunosuppressive agents. After Alexis Carrel described the technique for vascular anastomosis in 1902, technical challenges for transplanting kidneys and other solid organ allografts were for the most part resolved. Subsequent advances that allowed solid organ transplantation to become clinically feasible were due to the development of immunosuppressive agents, which could control or prevent the rejection reaction.[2,9] Continued improvements involving manipulation of rejection are possible but require an understanding of the complexity of the immune system and the cells and other factors involved in the rejection response. Because this varies with the type of organ transplanted, organ-specific and recipient-specific immunosuppression depends upon an understanding of the response of the recipient to a specific organ graft.

APPROACHES FOR IMMUNOSUPPRESSION

Lymphocytes comprise the center of the immune system. The rejection reaction begins when these cells recognize foreign antigens present on cells of the transplanted tissue.[11] The foreign cell or antigen may or may not be first processed by macrophages, a predominant antigen-presenting cell. However, the immunologic specificity to differentiate self from non-self resides in the lymphocytes, which are activated by recognition of major histocompatibility complex (MHC) locus or transplantation antigen differences. Early in the development of the immune system, groups or clones of lymphocytes are formed that have rather discrete target specificities. A lymphocyte, therefore, can recognize only one or a few closely related antigens. The range of possible antigen configurations is matched by a panoply of lymphocyte clones arrayed against them. Immune specificity is acquired during early development, and it is postulated that fully competent clones of small lymphocytes are resting and waiting to respond to foreign antigens (Fig. 1).

Stimulation of a resting lymphocyte by the antigen for which it is specific causes it to transform into a large active cell that secretes signal substances called lymphokines (Table 1) effective across short distances that, in turn, amplify the response and activate other cells.[7,17] Before the antigen is disposed of, however, a myriad of cellular and subcellular events ensue. Manipulation of this complex of events offers many opportunities for immunosuppression to attempt to halt or prevent the rejection response.[1] For the transplant patient, the lymphocyte-antigen encounter is the first point of possible immunosuppressive attack. The earlier developmental steps leading to the quiescent small lymphocyte have taken place for the most part *in utero* and are no longer susceptible to inhibition. By birth the individual has full immunologic competence and has clearly

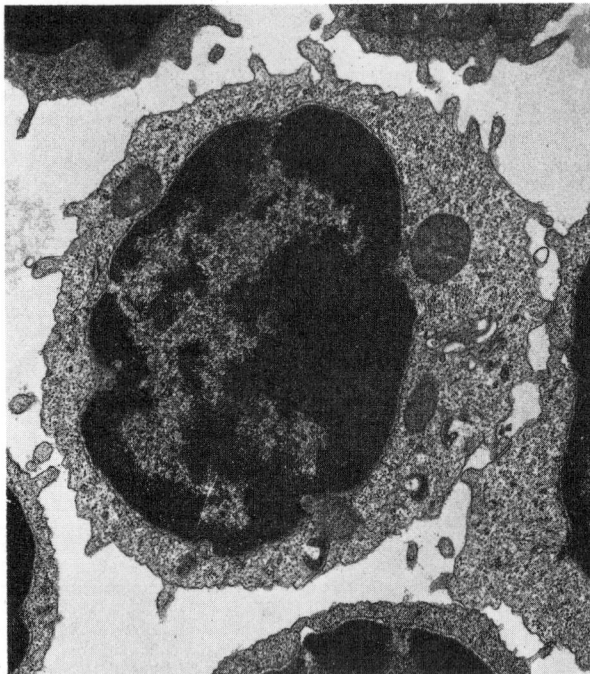

Figure 1. The morphology of these mouse small lymphocytes is typical of mammalian peripheral small lymphocytes from the blood, thoracic duct, lymph nodes, or spleen. The dense, inactive nucleus occupies much of the intracellular volume. The rim of cytoplasm contains ribosomes, a few inclusion bodies, and occasional mitochondria. The small lymphocytes are resting cells, awaiting immunologic stimulation that transforms them into large active cells ($\times$ 12,000).

defined self versus non-self.[11] The peripheral lymphoid tissues are established, and specificity and maturation of lymphocytes cannot be successfully impeded. This is an oversimplification, because cellular renewal follows and opens the possibility of blocking an earlier maturational step. What this step may be, however, remains unknown and awaits a better understanding of lymphocyte development and replenishment.

Immunosuppression is less effective after the lymphocyte has responded to the foreign antigen, and the immune response is far more difficult to control after activation.[9] Specific effectors, such as preformed antibodies and activated killer (cytotoxic) lymphocytes, in association with antigen-presenting cells or macrophages, as well as nonspecific agents such as platelets, neutrophils, complement, and coagulation factors, are difficult to suppress. Many cells and molecules are involved. The suppression of only one or two effectors is ineffective.[9]

In the early days of transplantation, the major problem was to suppress allograft rejection. This can now be achieved, but its consequences and dangers are apparent. Current immunosuppressive agents act in a nonspecific manner to suppress the entire immune response. Because of their mechanism of action, they have associated toxicities and side effects such as an increase in opportunistic infections and an increase in the rate of malignancy. Effective general immunosuppression may allow the graft to survive but may also cripple the host response to infections or prevent other proliferating cells, such as bone marrow and intestinal mucosal cells, from maintaining an adequate population. Infections with agents such as cytomegalovirus and *Pneumocystis carinii*, which do not present a life-threatening problem to the normal patient, frequently become lethal to the transplant patient.[1,9]

At present, clinical immunosuppression relies on two general approaches. The first is to simply reduce the number of peripheral lymphocytes by destroying them with corticosteroids or antiserum.[9] The second uses a variety of metabolic inhibitors to interrupt the antigen-induced lymphocyte proliferation and

differentiation that is required for graft rejection. These agents are biochemically specific but do not distinguish between dividing lymphocytes and other proliferating cells.[9]

Future progress in immunosuppression will involve a more selective approach in which the goal will be to induce donor-specific tolerance in the host with full preservation of immunocompetence.[1,17] As the complexities of the immune response become better understood, more direct and specific manipulation of it will become possible. The recent progress in transplantation has saved many lives. Despite its present benefit to patients, the full promise of transplantation will not be fulfilled until graft rejection can be specifically prevented while the integrity of the remaining immune system is maintained. Tolerance of the recipient to the transplanted organ without the requirement for nonspecific immunosuppression is the ultimate goal for transplantation.[1,17]

THE BIOLOGY OF GRAFT IMMUNITY

The development of the lymphoid system begins with a pluripotential stem cell in the liver and bone marrow of the fetus.[11] With maturation of the fetus toward term, the bone marrow becomes the primary site for lymphopoiesis. The thymus is the primary lymphoid organ in which one lymphocyte subpopulation, called the T lymphocyte (CD3+), is matured, or "educated," and released to stock the peripheral lymphoid tissues, such as lymph nodes, the spleen, and the gut. It is in the thymus that T lymphocytes (CD3+) acquire their subset differentiation markers (CD4+, CD8+, etc.), which in turn influence their ultimate functional role in the immune system.[4,13,15] Another subpopulation that descends from the stem cell is the B-cell line.[6] The primary lymphoid organ that produces B cells in mammals is unknown; in birds it is the bursa of Fabricius. Evidence suggests that the fetal liver or bone marrow may be the bursal equivalent in mammals.[6] Macrophages, which also have an integral role in the immune response, are derived from the same pluripotential stem cell, as are the intraepithelial cells, such as keratinocytes and tissue macrophages. They function to process antigen and present it to lymphocytes and to produce soluble factors (*monokines*) that amplify the immune response.[12]

There is evidence that the thymus produces a hormone-like substance (thymosin) that is necessary for full functional capacity of the peripheral T-cell system. The maturation of T cells and migration from bone marrow, through thymus, and on to the peripheral lymphoid tissues occur *in utero*, and humans are fully immunocompetent for T-cell function before birth. Although the human thymus begins to atrophy before puberty, T-cell function is well established in the periphery and remains self-perpetuating. Only slight deterioration comes with age. The mechanism responsible for the self-renewal of T lymphocytes after atrophy of the thymus is not understood.[9]

The ontogeny of B-cell immunocompetence in mammals is also poorly understood, but it is postulated that a humoral factor similar to that secreted by the thymus may have an integral role in the maturation and self-renewal of the population of immunocompetent B cells. Interleukin-4, interleukin-5 and interleukin-6 have been recently identified as lymphokines that stimulate the maturation and proliferation of primed B cells.[6,11]

There is a behavioral difference between B and T cells that reflects their functional abilities. B cells are relatively sessile within lymph nodes and the spleen. They secrete antibodies, which are mobile, soluble factors able to interact with foreign antigens at distant sites.[1] The T cells responsible for cell-mediated immunity are of necessity more peripatetic and must migrate to the periphery to eliminate or neutralize foreign antigens. From the peripheral blood, T cells enter the lymph nodes or spleen via highly specialized regions in the postcapillary venules. The T cells then percolate through the thoracic duct and return to the blood to begin recirculation in quest of an antigen.[11] When an organ is transplanted into a patient, activation of both T and B cells occurs in the lymph nodes, which filter out graft antigens.[4,6]

The T cells, B cells, and macrophages have unique roles in orchestrating the immune response. It is a very tightly con-

trolled network, the majority of communication mediated by soluble factors (lymphokines and cytokines). B cells synthesize antibody, and the subpopulations of T cells have several different activities. Certain T-effector cells can directly lyse a foreign cell, while others become killer (cytotoxic CD8$^+$) cells. In addi-

TABLE 1. Properties of Some Human Cytokines*

Cytokine	Alternative Name	Source	Target Cell Type	Action
IFN-α and IFN-β	—	Activated T cells, endothelial cells, macrophages, fibroblasts	Activated T and B, NK, LAK	Induces antiviral state; antitumor activity; induces fever; increases Class I and II MHC expression; stimulates activated B-cell differentiation and proliferation and NK activity; inhibits T and LAK cell activity
IFN-γ	—	Activated T cells, LAK cells	Activated and resting B, plasma, NK, endothelial, LAK, macrophage	Induces antiviral state; antitumor activity; induces fever; increases Class I and II MHC expression; stimulates activated B-cell differentiation and proliferation and NK and LAK activity; activates macrophages and endothelial cells; stimulates IgG2a isotype switch
TNF	—	Activated T cells, LAK cells, macrophages	Resting T, activated T and B, plasma, stem, endothelial, eosinophil, fibroblast, macrophage	Induces antiviral state; antitumor activity; induces fever; increases Class I MHC expression; activates macrophages, granulocytes, eosinophils, endothelial cells; chemotactic and angiogenic activity
IL-1	Endogenous pyrogen	Activated T and B cells, LAK cells, endothelial cells, macrophages, fibroblasts	Resting T and B, activated T and B, plasma, stem, endothelial, eosinophil, fibroblast, macrophage	Induces antiviral state; antitumor activity; induces fever; stimulates activated B-cell differentiation and proliferation; activates and stimulates proliferation of T cells; activates granulocytes and endothelial cells; stimulates hematopoesis
IL-2	T-cell growth factor	Activated T cells, LAK cells	Activated T, activated and resting B, NK, LAK, macrophage	Activates macrophages, T, NK, and LAK cells; stimulates differentiation of activated B cells; stimulates proliferation of activated B and T cells; induces fever
IL-3	Multi-CSF	Activated T cells	Stem, activated B, eosinophil	Stimulates hematopoesis, activated B cell proliferation, and eosinophil activity
IL-4	B-cell stimulating factor 1	Activated T cells	Activated T, activated and resting B, plasma, LAK, macrophage	Activates macrophages, T and B cells; stimulates differentiation of activated B cells; stimulates proliferation of activated B and T cells; induces IgE receptors on B cells; stimulates IgE and IgG1 isotype switch
IL-5	B-cell growth factor 2	Activated T cells	Activated and resting B, plasma, eosinophil	Stimulates IgA isotype switch and eosinophil activity
IL-6	B-cell stimulating factor 2, B-cell differentiating factor, interferon-β_2	Activated T cells, endothelial cells, fibroblasts, macrophages	Activated T, resting B, stem	Activates T cells; stimulates activated B-cell differentiation, activated T- and B-cell proliferation
IL-7	—	Activated T cells	Activated T and resting B	Stimulates activated T- and resting B-cell proliferation
IL-8	—	Activated T cells	Granulocytes	Stimulates granulocyte activity, chemotactic activity
G-CSF	—	Endothelial cells, fibroblasts, macrophages	Granulocytes	Stimulates granulocyte activity, hematopoesis
M-CSF	—	Macrophages	Macrophages	Activates macrophages
GM-CSF	—	Endothelial cells, fibroblasts, activated T cells	Stem, granulocyte, macrophage, eosinophil	Activates macrophages; stimulates granulocyte and eosinophil activity, hematopoesis

Cytokines are secreted polypeptides that mediate autocrine and paracrine cellular communication but do not bind antigen. They include those compounds previously termed interleukins and lymphokines. IFN, interferon; TNF, tumor necrosis factor; IL, interleukin; G, granulocyte; M, macrophage; CSF, colony-stimulating factor; NK, natural killer; LAK, lymphokine-activated killer.

*Based on the consensus cytokine chart of the British Cytokine Group.

From Balkwill, F. R., Burke, F.: The cytokine network. Immunol. Today, *10*:299, 1989.

tion, there are T-helper (CD4$^+$) and T-suppressor (CD8$^+$) cells that function to activate or suppress, respectively, the response to a given antigen.[11,15] Because each of these T-cell subpopulations expresses both the T-cell (CD3$^+$) receptor plus its own unique receptor antigen (CD4$^+$ or CD8$^+$), individual subpopulations can be depleted, enriched, or modulated by the use of antiserum or monoclonal antibody immunotherapy. OKT3, a monoclonal antibody directed against the T-cell receptor, is used clinically in episodes of acute solid organ graft rejection. The helper T cell has a central role in response to alloantigen. In response to antigen that has been processed and presented to it by the macrophage, the T-helper cell (CD4$^+$) proliferates. In addition, it produces lymphokines, or soluble factors, which amplify the immune response. Through lymphokines and direct effects, the T-helper cell functions to (1) stimulate B cells to produce antibody, (2) assist T precytotoxic cells to develop into mature effectors, and (3) stimulate macrophages to effect a nonspecific, delayed-type inflammatory response (see Table 1).[7,17] Some transformation may also occur within the graft by circulating T lymphocytes enticed to remain there. The result is an assault on the graft by a variety of sensitized cells and antibodies.

CELL-TO-CELL INTERACTIONS

Once confronted with an antigen, the response of the lymphocytes is complex (Fig. 2). Multiple cell-to-cell interactions are required to produce the final immune response.[4,8,9,11] T cells, B cells, macrophages, and cytokines all have a role. Critical to this response are macrophages, which act in a nonspecific manner to bind antigen and present it to T and B cells. Certain complex antigens may need to first be partially digested by phagocytic cells before the antigenic information can be presented to the lymphocyte for self and non-self recognition. In addition, the activated macrophages produce and secrete IL-1 (interleukin-1), a lymphokine that functions to further amplify

the response and stimulate T-lymphocyte and B-lymphocyte activation.[11,12]

Even the recognition of foreign cells is a complex process. One class of antigens on the surface of the graft cells stimulates certain T cells to divide.[11,15] The proliferating cells do not destroy the graft; rather, they activate another group of T cells (cytotoxic), which in turn damage the graft. The first group of T cells is called "helper" cells (CD4$^+$) because their proliferative response is necessary for the development of cell-mediated and antibody-mediated cytolytic activity in a less frequently dividing T-cell population. T-helper–cell proliferation is an important step mediating amplification of the immune response, and these actively dividing cells are particularly vulnerable to antimetabolites. The activities of the helper T cells are one of the major targets of clinical immunosuppression.[2,9] The details of the antigens involved are beyond the scope of this discussion, but the T cell–to–T cell interactions are among the types of cellular cooperation required to develop transplantation immunity (see Fig. 2).

While CD4$^+$ helper T cells function to augment the response of other T cells, another type is able to suppress the immune response. This type of T cell, the suppressor cell, a subset of the CD8$^+$ population of T cells, probably helps to regulate the immune response and prevent an overreaction to a given immunologic stimulus. Suppressor cells are currently the subject of much investigation and have been identified in a number of models of allograft tolerance.[1,9,11,13] Lymphocytes that apparently suppress antibody production have been generated experimentally both *in vivo* and *in vitro*. That suppressor cells might be able to inhibit the development of the immune response may open an avenue for clinical application in transplantation. Stimulating an abundance of specific suppressor lymphocytes would theoretically be a way to produce effective immunosuppression without toxicity.[1,2,9]

Although the T- and B-cell systems have been presented as independent of each other, they cooperate to enhance immunity against antigen. T cells develop "cellular immunity" in

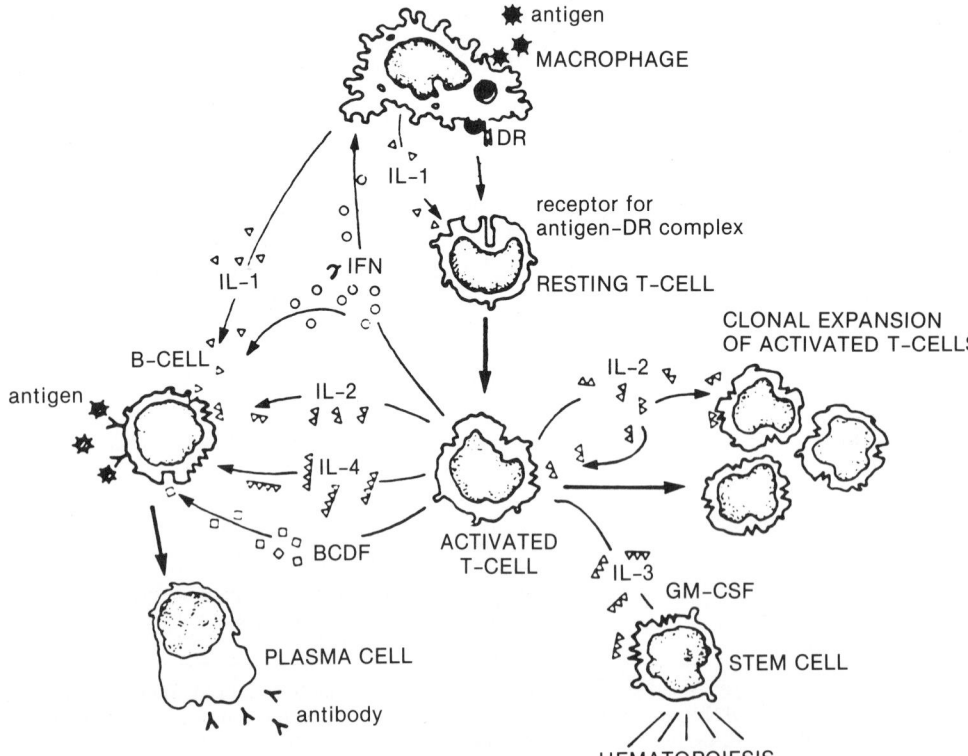

Figure 2. The roles of various lymphokines produced during antigenic challenge. Beginning with the uptake of antigen by the macrophage, processed antigen is presented to the resting T cell with the histocompatibilty molecule (DR) and interleukin-1 (IL-1). The T cell becomes an activated T cell, producing interferon (IFN-γ), interleukin-2, interleukin-3, interleukin-4, and interleukin-6, which is B-cell differentiating factor (BCDF). The antigen also activates B cells through surface antibodies, and under the influence of INF-γ, interleukins 1, 2, and 4, and B-cell differentiating factors, these cells become antibody-secreting plasma cells. Activated T cells also undergo clonal expansion under the influence of interleukin-2. Interleukin-3 and granulocyte-macrophage colony-stimulating factor (GM-CSF), produced by the activated T cell, induce hematopoiesis by stimulating the marrow stem cells. (From Dinarello, C. A., Mier, J. W.: Lymphokines. N. Engl. J. Med., *317*:940, 1987.)

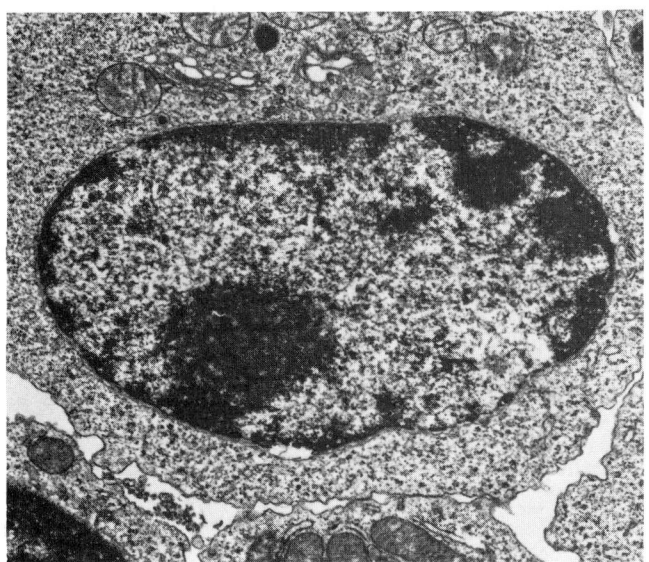

Figure 3. The transformed lymphocyte, 24 hours after stimulation, is a much larger, more active cell. The open nucleus is the site of increased RNA synthesis, and the enlarged cytoplasm contains abundant polysomes and mitochondria. Many subcellular changes take place in the conversion from resting to active lymphocytes. These biosynthetic events are vulnerable to the antimetabolites used to prevent allograft rejection. In addition, these cells begin to synthesize DNA at this time, increasing their susceptibility to antimetabolites, alkylating agents, and radiation (× 12,000).

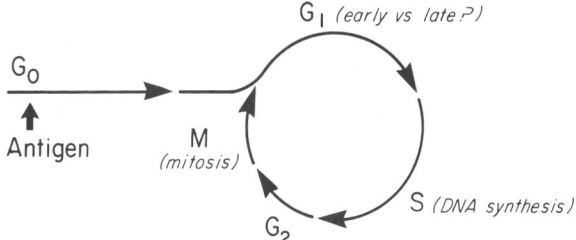

Figure 4. The phases of the cell cycle are depicted in this diagram. After stimulation by an antigen or another type of mitogen, small lymphocytes are activated. They are converted from the resting G_0 phase to the active G_1 phase. The G_1 phase lasts 10 hours or longer before DNA synthesis (S phase) begins. The S phase lasts about 10 hours and is followed by a short (2 to 4 hours) G_2 phase before mitosis (M phase). M phase is relatively brief, usually less than 2 to 3 hours, after which the cells are returned to the G_1 phase. The susceptibility of the cell to the immunosuppressive agents used in transplantation varies with the phase of the cycle. Periods of intense nucleic acid synthesis, particularly S phase, are most vulnerable to the antimetabolites. As discussed in the text, the resting, G_0, lymphocyte is also susceptible to several of the clinically used immunosuppressive agents.

response to transplantation antigens; in addition, helper T cells assist clones of B cells to produce specific antibody against the graft antigens. Finally, some T cells act as suppressors for antibody formation.[11] After immunity has been acquired, additional cellular cooperation contributes to the destruction of the graft during the rejection episode.

As the details of the cellular interactions in rejection are better defined, immunosuppression can potentially be tailored to interface with these interactions and influence the development of transplantation immunity. At the present time, clinical immunosuppression depends upon daily interference with the subcellular biochemical events in lymphocyte metabolism.

Subcellular Events

Mature small lymphocytes, both T and B cells, appear to be in a resting but immunologically ready state.[6,15] Antigenic stimulation of a clone of these cells triggers a remarkable cellular transformation. Gene activation is followed by a rapid increase in RNA and protein synthesis. A host of membrane, cytoplasmic, and nuclear changes are included in the many subcellular events that occur within the first 2 hours. Over the succeeding hours, the small lymphocyte is transformed into a large, active cell, bulging with polysomes and organelles (Fig. 3). Included in the activation are the complex cellular changes of further differentiation and proliferation. Two aspects of these changes are of the greatest importance: (1) the helper T cells secrete *lymphokines*, which function as intercellular mediators to aid the maturation of effector T cells and B cells; and (2) both T cells and B cells begin to proliferate in response to the lymphokines. It is at this point that the lymphocyte becomes most vulnerable to several of the commonly used immunosuppressive agents.

As lymphocytes transform from resting to dividing cells, they pass through distinct phases common to all cells (Fig. 4). Although the present subdivisions of the cell cycle are oversimplified, it has been found that susceptibility to the commonly used immunosuppressive agents varies over the different cell phases. The small lymphocyte is in a resting or G_0 phase. Antigenic stimulation activates the cell and moves it into the first gap or phase (G_1) of the proliferative cycle. The complex G_1 phase

includes the commitment to cell division, but whether this occurs early or late in G_1 is not known. After the cell becomes committed to divide, DNA synthesis (S phase) occurs. The gap (G_2) between S phase and the final mitosis (M phase) is relatively short. After mitosis has occurred, the cells enter into the G_1 phase again, and the cell cycle is complete.

Differentiation appears to progress with cell division; and, with each successive cycle, the cells become more and more capable of eliminating the activating antigen. After successive divisions, B cells become plasma cells, which are the most efficient producers of specific antibody. A similar progression occurs among T cells. T-cell activation occurs through the T-cell receptor complex (CD3), IL-2, and the IL-2 receptor.[12] Briefly, activated T cells secrete IL-2, a lymphokine that functions as a T-cell growth factor. The IL-2 then binds to the IL-2 receptor (IL-2R) on resting T cells and stimulates cell mitosis and DNA synthesis via activation of the inositol phosphate pathway with protein kinase C (Fig. 5). When the antigenic stimulus is no longer present, IL-2 is no longer produced and T-cell activation and proliferation cease. The continued presence of antigen causes an amplification of the T-cell response through the lymphokine IL-2. The presence of the IL-2 receptor for activation suggests a hormone-receptor system with negative feedback

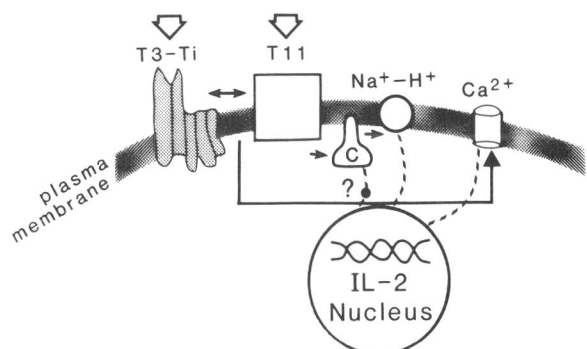

Figure 5. Circuitry of T-lymphocyte activation. Ligands bind to the T3-Ti receptors, the T11 receptors, or both, leading to synergistic signaling by means of both structures. Protein kinase C (C) moves to the inner leaflet of the plasma membrane as a consequence of activation of the inositol phosphate pathway. The protein kinase in turn activates the sodium-hydrogen antiporter. T3-Ti or T11 triggering also facilitates opening of a membrane calcium channel, partly by means of inositol triphosphate as a second messenger. Subsequently, these modifications (broken lines) activate the nuclear genes. Note that the circle and question mark suggest the possibility of a hypothetical transactivating transcriptional regulatory factor that is modified by calcium, protein kinase, or other variables to turn on the genes. (Redrawn from Roger, H. D., Reinherz, E. L.:T lymphocytes: Ontogeny, function and relevance to clinical disorders. N. Engl. J. Med., 317:1136, 1987.)

control (Fig. 6).[14] An understanding of the process of the activation of the T cell via its receptor pathway allows a more focused approach for immunosuppression.

Much of the susceptibility of lymphocytes to immunosuppression follows the vast cellular changes produced by immune stimulation. The many biosynthetic events that occur make the lymphocytes vulnerable to mistakes and inhibitions caused by structural analogs, termed *antimetabolites*.[2,9] Alkylating agents and radiation produce cross-linkages and breaks in DNA strands which interfere with cell differentiation and division. The subcellular actions of steroids are also complex. The actions of the individual immunosuppressive agents are discussed in more detail in subsequent sections. The inhibitory effects of these agents, with the exception of cyclosporine, OKT3, and antilymphocyte globulin, are not specific for lymphocytes, and similar consequences can be expected for other differentiating and dividing cells.

Graft Rejection

Graft rejection follows the participation of various combinations of immunologically specific and nonspecific cells. Three types of graft rejection are encountered. *Acute rejection* is the most common. It is mediated primarily by T lymphocytes and first occurs between 1 and 3 weeks following transplantation of a solid organ. *Hyperacute rejection* occurs during the first 1 to 2 days following transplantation and is primarily mediated by preformed antibody. *Chronic rejection* occurs over months and is probably caused by both T-cell and B-cell–mediated responses.

T cells have the major role in most graft rejection.[1,4,9,11] T cells can (1) be directly cytotoxic to graft cells, (2) be armed with specific antibodies and act as killer cells, (3) help B cells to produce antigraft antibody, and (4) recruit destructive activated macrophages. The helper T lymphocyte has a central role in the activation of other cells via the production of lymphokines. The graft is infiltrated with a variety of inflammatory cells, including sensitized helper T cells, cytotoxic T cells, noncommitted lymphocytes, sensitized and nonsensitized B lymphocytes, macrophages, and polymorphonuclear lymphocytes. B cells produce antigraft antibodies, which attach to the graft cells. Damage follows the activation of the complement, coagulation, and kinin pathways triggered by the antigen-antibody complexes. Vasoactive peptides, chemotactic factors, and thrombus formation then directly produce the damage by occluding small vessels, causing microinfarcts in the parenchyma. Neutrophils, platelets, and macrophages are called to the scene and release their many proteolytic enzymes. Antibody-mediated damage appears to be particularly important to the arteritis and proliferative occlusion observed in the arteries of grafted organs.

The preceding abbreviated description of the development of

allograft immunity reveals many vulnerable processes that may potentially be manipulated to suppress the immune response: (1) destroying the immunocompetent cells reactive to donor antigen prior to transplantation; (2) making the antigen unrecognizable or even toxic to the reactive lymphocyte clones; (3) interfering with antigen processing by the recipient cells; (4) inhibiting lymphocyte transformation and proliferation; (5) inhibiting production or release of the signal substances or interleukins (IL-1, IL-2, IL-3, IL-4, IL-5, IL-6, IL-7) involved with modifying lymphocyte differentiation to cytotoxic or antibody-synthesizing cells; (6) activating sufficient numbers of suppressor lymphocytes; (7) inhibiting destruction of graft cells by cytotoxic lymphocytes; (8) interfering with the binding of immunoglobulins to graft target antigens; (9) preventing tissue damage by the nonspecific cells and molecules that are activated by sensitized cells or antigen-antibody complexes; and (10) inducting donor-specific transplantation tolerance.[1,2,17]

At the present time, clinically useful immunosuppression primarily depends upon inhibition of the differentiation and proliferation of sensitized cells and destruction or elimination of the immunocompetent cells. Methods to induce specific transplantation tolerance have not yet been clinically successful. Moreover, it is more difficult to inhibit the immune response after sensitization has occurred. To be effective, immunosuppression must be present at the time of transplantation, or even before. Nevertheless, some success can be achieved in reversing the episodes of acute rejection observed in clinical transplantation.

Clinical Immunosuppression

Until recently, clinical immunosuppression has relied primarily upon agents or procedures with antiproliferative activity.[1,2,9,17] These include the antimetabolites, alkylating agents, toxic antibiotics, and irradiation, all of which are used in cancer chemotherapy. In the past, the only clinical immunosuppressive agents for transplantation included azathioprine, steroids, radiation, and antilymphocyte serum.[2,9] Recently, the introduction of cyclosporine and OKT3 has radically changed the principles of immunosuppression.

Antiproliferative Agents

Antiproliferative agents inhibit the full expression of the immune response by preventing the differentiation and division of the immunocompetent lymphocyte after it encounters antigen.[2] The plethora of investigational immunosuppressive drugs has been reduced to a few for clinical use. All of them, however, can be grouped into one of two broad mechanistic categories. They either structurally resemble needed metabolites or combine with certain cellular components, such as DNA, and thereby interfere with function.

The former group, the antimetabolites, have a structural similarity to cell metabolites and either inhibit enzymes of that metabolic pathway or are incorporated during synthesis to produce faulty molecules. The antimetabolites include purine, pyrimidine, and folic acid analogs that are most effective against proliferating and differentiating cells. They are given at the time of transplantation when the immunocompetent cells are first stimulated and then for the life of the graft to interfere with the continuing stimulus to the immune system.

Alkylating agents and certain antibiotics include those compounds that combine with DNA and other cellular components. Although these agents would be useful in the pretransplant period to reduce the number of effective immunocompetent cells in the recipients, and thereafter to prevent proliferation, their use has been limited to bone marrow transplantation and occasional substitution for azathioprine.

PURINE ANALOGS. Until recently, the purine analog azathioprine (Imuran) was the most widely used immunosuppressive drug in clinical organ transplantation. Azathioprine is 6-mercaptopurine (6-MP) plus a side chain to protect the labile

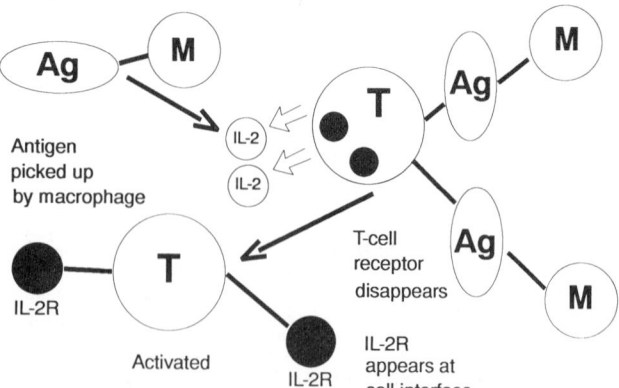

Figure 6. Steps in T-cell activation. T cells activated through antigen binding to the T-cell receptor secrete IL-2. The IL-2 binds to the IL-2 receptor (IL-2R) present on resting T cells to stimulate cell division. When the antigenic stimulus is no longer present, IL-2 is no longer produced, and T-cell activation and proliferation cease.

sulfhydryl group. In the liver, the side chain is split off to form the active compound 6-MP. The mechanism of action would appear to be similar for these two compounds; however, azathioprine appears to have the advantage of slightly lower toxicity.[2,9]

Full metabolic activity occurs in the cell with the addition of ribose-5-phosphate from phosphoribosyl pyrophosphate to form 6-MP ribonucleotide. The structural resemblance of this molecule to inosine monophosphate is obvious, and 6-MP ribonucleotide inhibits the enzymes that begin to convert inosine nucleotide to adenosine and guanosine monophosphate (Fig. 7). In addition, the presence of 6-MP ribonucleotides slows the entire purine biosynthetic pathway by fraudulent feedback inhibition of an early step. The steric similarity to either adenosine or guanine nucleotides is not sufficient to allow significant incorporation into DNA or RNA and synthesis of faulty molecules. The result of inhibiting these several enzymes, however, is to block the synthesis of cellular RNA, DNA, certain co-factors, and other active nucleotides.

The biologic activity of azathioprine and 6-MP is greatest when nucleic acid synthesis is most required.[2,9] They will inhibit the development of both humoral and cellular primary immunity by interfering with the differentiation and proliferation of the responding lymphocytes. The inhibition of nucleic acid synthesis by azathioprine is most effective in these rapidly replicating cells. When expansion of fully immunocompetent cells has been completed, nucleic acid synthesis is less important and the drug is less effective. The benefit of azathioprine may also follow a reduction of neutrophil production and macrophage activation. These effects would reduce the nonspecific inflammatory aspects of the immune reaction.

The toxicity of azathioprine follows the same mechanisms.[2,9] The primary toxic effect of azathioprine is bone marrow suppression, leading to leukopenia. Again, it is the antiproliferative effect of inhibiting nucleic acid synthesis that affects this rapidly dividing cell population. Liver toxicity can also occur, possibly because of the high rate of RNA synthesis by these cells; but because hepatic dysfunction does not appear to be dose-related, the mechanism is unclear.

PYRIMIDINE ANALOGS. Although pyrimidine analogs have been studied extensively as immunosuppressants in the laboratory, they have had only limited clinical use. The pyrimidine analog cytosine arabinoside inhibits DNA synthesis and, therefore, the proliferative phase of the immune response. This molecule has an altered sugar moiety and can be mistaken for cytosine riboside. Experimentally, the immunosuppressive effect of cytosine arabinoside has been more easily demonstrated

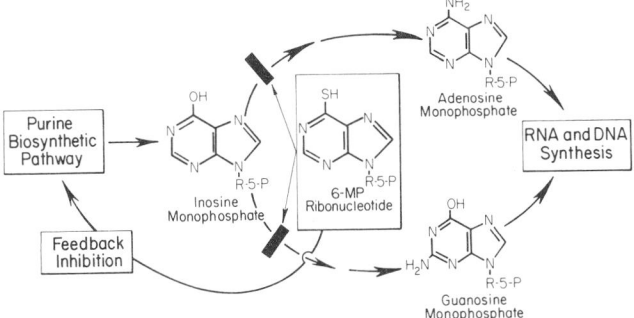

Figure 7. The mechanisms of action of the antimetabolites 6-mercaptopurine (6-MP) and azathioprine are similar. These molecules are converted in the cell to 6-MP ribonucleotide, which resembles inosine ribonucleotide in its steric configuration. Consequently, there is competition between these molecules in the pathways to adenosine monophosphate and guanosine monophosphate. Although 6-MP ribonucleotide is not extensively incorporated, it effectively inhibits the enzymes of these pathways, which reduces the precursors available for incorporation into RNA and DNA. In addition, 6-MP slows the purine biosynthetic pathway by feedback inhibition. The net effect of 6-MP and azathioprine is to greatly reduce DNA and RNA synthesis by their competitive activity.

in inhibition of primary antibody responses than in cell-mediated reactions. Clinically it is used in preparing leukemic recipients for bone marrow transplantation.[2,9]

FOLIC ACID ANTAGONISTS. The immunosuppressive effect of a diet deficient in pteroylglutamic acid was originally noted by Little and led to the use of the folic acid antagonists aminopterin and methotrexate. Both drugs inhibit the enzyme dihydrofolate reductase and prevent the conversion of folic acid to tetrahydrofolic acid. This step is necessary for the synthesis of DNA, RNA, and certain coenzymes.[2,9]

The ratio of immunosuppression to toxicity has not justified their use in clinical solid organ transplantation. The immune reactions that accompany bone marrow transplantation are more difficult to control, and methotrexate is used both to prevent and to reverse the severe graft-versus-host (GVH) reactions that occur. The toxic effects of methotrexate can be difficult to identify. Megaloblastic hematopoiesis, mucosal breakdown with severe gastrointestinal bleeding, and liver damage appear to be related to methotrexate therapy. These effects, even with high dosages of methotrexate, can usually be prevented by folinic acid (citrovorum rescue). Obviously, depression of the transplanted marrow may also follow the activity of methotrexate, although assigning the cause may be difficult in the complex clinical situation. In bone marrow transplantation, a combination of methotrexate with cyclosporine has afforded superior control of GVH disease with lower dosages of each drug. As a result, the toxicities have also been reduced.

ALKYLATING AGENTS. The alkylating agents have highly reactive rings as part of the molecular structure. These unstable rings have electron-seeking points that combine with electron-rich nucleophilic groups such as the tertiary nitrogens in purines and pyrimidines, or with $-NH_2$, $-COOH$, $-SH$, and $-PO_3H_2$ groups on a variety of molecules. The high-energy rings of alkylating agents break and combine with these constituents to form stable covalent bonds.[2,9] Obviously, many cell components have such groups, including DNA, RNA, and the enzymatic and structural proteins. Alkylation of DNA is probably the most detrimental. If the DNA strands are not repaired, chromosomal replication will be faulty in proliferating cells. Both DNA and RNA can be alkylated at several points, but a common site appears to be N-7 of the guanine ring (Fig. 8). Mispairing of DNA during replication may be caused by the presence of the alkylating agent itself, the clipping out of the alkylated guanine residue, or the cleavage of an alkylated guanine ring. Also, chain breaks and cross-linkages frequently interfere with chain replication.[2,9]

The damage to DNA can be repaired; so these effects are apparently time-dependent. Consequently, the administration of alkylating agents just before and during stimulation by the antigen would most interfere with the ability of the immunocompetent cells to respond to that antigen. Continued use of alkylating agents would also suppress the proliferative response of these cells in the presence of a persistent stimulus. There are differences, however, in the response of T and B cells. The B cell appears to be more susceptible to cyclophosphamide than the T cell. This drug is a potent inhibitor of antibody formation, but its effect on skin or kidney allograft rejection is much less spectacular. The reason for this apparent difference is unknown.[2,9]

The usefulness of alkylating agents, which include nitrogen mustard, phenylalanine mustard, busulfan, and cyclophosphamide, is limited by their toxicity. However, cyclophosphamide has been used with good results in renal transplantation when liver toxicity prohibited the use of azathioprine. Cyclophosphamide is frequently used in clinical bone marrow transplantation to prepare recipients for transplantation. In this setting, it potentiates the effects of radiation and enhances the disruption of DNA. When cyclophosphamide is used, lower doses of radiation are required to deplete the recipient bone marrow popula-

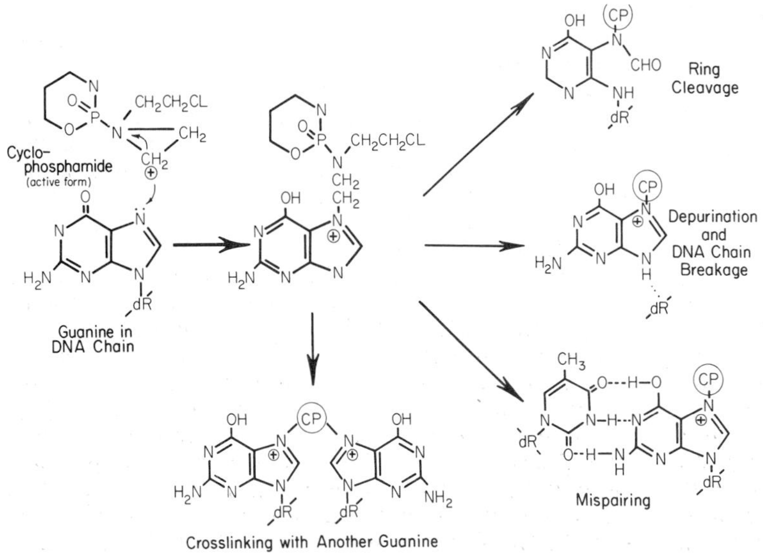

Figure 8. The alkylating agents have reactive rings that can combine with electron-rich points of a variety of molecules. The effect of the alkylating agents appears to be related to their DNA binding. Cyclophosphamide (CP), as an example, binds extensively to guanine molecules within the DNA chain. The guanine-CP complex has several possible consequences for the DNA strand. The ultimate effect of the four examples shown is to interfere with accurate base pairing and DNA replication.

tion and provide space for donor cells. When leukemia is the indication for bone marrow transplantation, cyclophosphamide also aids in the destruction of leukemic cells. More recently, cyclophosphamide has been used experimentally in the generation of suppressor cell–like activity to alloantigens and is most effective when given 2 to 4 days after antigenic exposure. If given earlier, it has the opposite effect and enhances the immune response.

Toxicity is high, however; and predictable reactions occur, principally to rapidly replicating cell populations. Stomatitis, nausea, vomiting, diarrhea, skin rash, anemia, and alopecia are all common reactions. The more specific effects of cyclophosphamide administration are prompt fluid retention, occasionally severe hemorrhagic cystitis, and cardiac toxicity. The cardiac and edema problems suggest that even nonreplicating cell populations are adversely affected by this drug.

ANTIBIOTICS. The immunosuppressive antibiotics include inhibitors of nucleic acid synthesis and chloramphenicol and puromycin, which interfere with cellular protein synthesis.[2,9] Actinomycin D binds to the guanine residue of DNA, thereby sterically interfering with RNA polymerase and consequently with DNA-directed RNA synthesis. This potentially effective means of suppressing the development of immunity led to its use in reversing acute rejection of kidney grafts. The toxicity of actinomycin D has limited its overall clinical benefit, however, and it has been used less and less frequently.

Mitomycin C combines with cellular DNA and hinders replication. This compound would also be useful in inhibiting allograft immunity, but its toxicity has precluded clinical use.

Puromycin structurally resembles an amino acid–charged transfer RNA molecule and is accepted into the ribosome. There is no amino acid to be donated, however; and the peptide chain is prematurely terminated. Although protein synthesis is obviously central to immunologic expression, it is so general a requirement for other cells that toxicity is widespread. Chloramphenicol has also been investigated experimentally. It is most potent in prokaryotic (bacterial) cell systems, and its effects on mammalian cells may be due to inhibition of mitochondrial synthesis. Unfortunately, it is only weakly immunosuppressive, and potentially severe bone marrow toxicity precludes its use.

CYCLOSPORINE. The discovery of cyclosporine in 1972 contributed significantly to the field of transplantation, especially for that of livers and hearts.[3] It represents a completely new class of clinically important immunosuppressive agents. Many of its suppressive effects on T cells appear to be related to the inhibition of T-cell receptor–mediated activation events. It

also inhibits lymphokine production by helper T cells *in vitro* and arrests development of mature CD8[+] and CD4[+] T cells in the thymus. Cyclosporine is a cyclic peptide (11 amino acids) produced by a fungus. It is nearly insoluble in aqueous solutions, and absorption from the gastrointestinal tract is slow and incomplete. Peak blood concentrations occur 2 to 4 hours after oral administration. There is a well-characterized enterohepatic cycle, and the excretion of the drug is primarily through the bile. About 40 per cent of the oral dose is absorbed, and 30 per cent undergoes first pass hepatic metabolism. Its half-life is variable, and the therapeutic range is poorly defined. Cyclosporine can be measured both in plasma and whole blood samples by radioimmunoassay (RIA) or high-pressure liquid chromatography (HPLC). RIA values are higher because the antibody also detects cyclosporine metabolites, but the clinical importance of these metabolites is not known. The release of cyclosporine from protein-binding sites as the sample temperature decreases from body to room temperature poses a disadvantage for determining plasma concentrations. The whole blood cyclosporine concentrations are usually twice that measured in plasma at room temperature.[3]

Cyclosporine was discovered to be immunosuppressive by its ability to suppress antibody production in mice during a screening of fungal extracts. Other *in vivo* immunosuppressive properties include inhibition of (1) plaque-forming colonies, (2) GVH disease, (3) skin graft rejection, (4) delayed solid organ allograft rejection, (5) delayed-type hypersensitivity reactions, and (6) natural killer cell (NK) activity. The lack of myelosuppression was a major advance over other immunosuppressive agents and indicated that the mechanism of action was relatively specific for lymphocytes.[1,3,17] Other inflammatory cells are much less sensitive to its immunosuppressive effects. Clinically, prophylactic administration of cyclosporine is suppressive of allograft rejection and GVH disease.

Assays of mitogen-induced proliferation and mixed lymphocyte reaction *in vitro* have shown that T lymphocytes are highly sensitive to cyclosporine inhibition. Memory cells were found to be especially sensitive. A series of elegant experiments outlining cyclosporine's effect on T-lymphocyte subset interaction have shown (1) inhibition of both IL-2–producing T lymphocytes and cytotoxic T lymphocytes, (2) inhibition of IL-2 release by activated T lymphocytes, (3) no inhibition of activated T lymphocytes in response to exogenous IL-2, (4) inhibition of resting T-lymphocyte activation in response to alloantigen and exogenous lymphokine, (5) inhibition of IL-1 production, and (6) inhibition of mitogen (concanavalin A) activation of IL-2–producing T lymphocytes. The above T-lymphocyte responses involve both CD4[+] (T-helper) and/or CD8[+] (T-cytotoxic/suppressor) lymphocytes, and the inhibition appears to occur at the level of activation, and perhaps even maturation, of the resting T cell. Recent data have indicated that maturation of T cells in mice, which occurs in the thymus, is significantly suppressed by cyclosporine, thus enriching a population of immature and less responsive T cells.[3]

A number of kidney and other solid organ transplantation trials have shown that cyclosporine induces potent immunosuppression without myelosuppression. The addition of steroids to cyclosporine has led to a lowering of the cyclosporine dosage and decreased nephrotoxicity. The introduction of cyclosporine has led to a substantial improvement in the outcome of cadaveric renal transplantation, with an average 1-year graft survival in the United States of 73 per cent. Similar beneficial results have been seen in heart and liver grafting.

The adverse effects of cyclosporine include hirsutism, tremor and other neurotoxicities, hypertension, hyperkalemia, nephrotoxicity, and hepatotoxicity. The principal toxic effect is nephrotoxicity. Cyclosporine appears to seriously aggravate any other nephrotoxic event. Although cyclosporine has made patient management more complex, transplantation of all solid organs has benefited from its use.

In summary, cyclosporine selectively inhibits activated T lymphocytes and prevents these cells from manufacturing and/or releasing IL-2.[3] In addition, resting T-lymphocyte activation by IL-2 is blocked by cyclosporine. Since IL-2 is necessary for the expansion of activated clones of T cells, cyclosporine effectively inhibits the immune responses to grafted antigens without eliminating any of the clonal repertoire.

FK506. FK506 is a potent new immunosuppressive agent isolated in Japan from *Streptomyces tsukubaensis*. Its immunosuppressive effects are approximately 500 times greater than those of cyclosporine. The molecular weight is 822 daltons. FK506 functions to (1) inhibit IL-2 production; (2) inhibit mouse mixed lymphocyte culture cellular proliferation, which is mediated by helper T cells; (3) inhibit the generation of murine cytotoxic T-cells; and (4) inhibit the appearance of IL-2 receptors on human lymphocytes. *In vivo*, FK506 has been demonstrated to prolong the survival of MHC-disparate skin, cardiac, renal, hepatic, and small bowel allografts. It is currently in use in clinical trials as an immunosuppressive agent for liver and renal allograft recipients.

LYMPHOCYTE DEPLETION MEASURES

A number of clinically important agents for immunosuppression are effective because they deplete the host of lymphocytes. As the mechanism of action of these agents is better understood, a more sophisticated classification system may evolve; but for the present, antilymphocyte globulin, radiation, and monoclonal antibody therapy appear to act by a relatively nonselective lymphocyte depletion or inactivation.[2,9]

ANTILYMPHOCYTE GLOBULIN (ALG). In 1899, Metchnikoff reported the ability of an antiserum to destroy white blood cells. After guinea pigs were stimulated with lymph node or spleen cells from either rats or rabbits, their serum would agglutinate and kill polymorphonuclear leukocytes of the donor species. In the same era, Flexner found that lymphoid depletion occurred in animals treated with anti-lymph node serum. Certain immunologic reactions such as tuberculin sensitivity and allograft rejection were found to be depressed. Monaco and Russell induced potent antisera which were effective in prolonging skin grafts with strong histocompatibility differences, including xenografts. Starzl was the first to use antilymphocyte globulin in the clinical setting for kidney transplantation, and subsequently these preparations have been widely used.

ALGs are produced when lymphocytes are injected into animals of a different species. The addition of adjuvants, usually

Freund's complete adjuvant, enhances the immunogenicity of the foreign lymphocytes and produces sera that are more immunosuppressive. The rabbit, goat, and horse are commonly used to produce antisera for clinical transplantation.[9]

The action of ALG appears to be directed mainly against the T cell, and the use of thymocytes therefore results in the most potent sera. The suppression produced by ALG can at least partially be reversed by T cells, but not by bone marrow cells. Thymectomy enhances the effect of ALG, and ALG decreases the number of circulating T cells. Even *in vitro*, ALG reduces the number of T cells. As would be expected, ALG administration interferes most with the cell-mediated reactions—allograft rejection, tuberculin sensitivity, and the GVH reaction. ALG can abolish pre-existing delayed hypersensitivity reactions, and larger doses prolong the survival of some xenografts. ALG has a definite, but lesser, effect on T-cell–dependent antibody production.

Lymphocytes coated with ALG share the fate of erythrocytes coated with antibody. They are either lysed or cleared from the blood by reticuloendothelial cells in the liver and spleen.

Antilymphocyte globulin is widely used in clinical transplantation. ALG can be administered prophylactically during the early posttransplantation period and is also effective in reversing ongoing rejection. Favorable results depend upon potent ALG and prolonged administration, rather than a single dose.

The use of ALG is not confined clinically to kidney transplantation, and beneficial results have also been reported in bone marrow and liver transplantation. In bone marrow transplantation, studies have suggested that ALG pretreatment of the recipient is of value in suppressing the response to the donor cells and for enlarging the marrow space. In addition, it appears that ALG may be useful in preventing the GVH reactions that arise in these patients.

The toxicity of any heterologous serum prepared against human tissue depends upon two factors: (1) its cross-reactivity with other tissue antigens and (2) the ability of the patient to make antibodies against the protein itself. Anemia and thrombocytopenia can occur and presumably are caused by a reaction between ALG and host erythrocytes and platelets. Although prior absorption with human platelets and red cell stroma reduces the severity, some cross-reactivity to these cells persists in all ALG preparations.

Allergic reactions to the antiserum itself are the most common clinical problem associated with the use of ALG. Urticaria, anaphylactoid reactions, and serum sickness, including joint pain, fever, and malaise, all follow immunity development by the patient to the heterologous globulin. These reactions are reduced in the presence of the other immunosuppressive drugs used in renal transplantation.

The major problem in the production of a standardized antihuman ALG is the inability to develop a method of assaying its *in vitro* immunosuppressive potency. Other immunosuppressive drugs are available in measurable quantities; therefore, the response is more predictable. Unfortunately, individual laboratories make their own ALG preparations, and a standard method of assay has not been developed. Cytotoxic assays, the formation of cellular rosettes by antibody-coated cells, and animal assays for immunosuppressive activity have been employed, but a consistent test has not emerged. A suitable assay is necessary for identifying the better ALG preparations and making their use increasingly beneficial.

MONOCLONAL ANTIBODY THERAPY. In 1975 Kohler and Milstein developed the technology for somatic cell hybridization (*hybridoma formation*), which could establish immortalized cultures of cell lines that each secrete a single, or *monoclonal, antibody* in limitless supply.[11] Subsequently, a number of monoclonal antibodies have been generated that react with T cells in general (OKT3, anti-CD3) and various T-cell subsets (OKT4, anti-CD4; OKT8, anti-CD8). OKT3 has become the most useful clinically. It is used to halt episodes of acute graft rejection in kidney, liver, heart, and heart-lung transplantation. OKT3 binds to a site associated with the T-cell receptor (CD3) and functions to modulate the receptor and inactivate T-cell function (Fig. 9).[10]

By engaging the T-cell receptor complex, OKT3 blocks not only the function of T cells but also the function of established cytotoxic T cells, thereby blocking cell-mediated cytotoxicity. OKT3 has been shown to block the T-cell effector functions involved in allograft rejection. After intravenous administration, OKT3 opsonizes or binds to T cells. These are then removed by the reticuloendothelial cells that reside in liver and spleen. The presence of circulating T cells therefore decreases abruptly after administration. Once OKT3 is stopped, the CD3+ cells rapidly return to their normal levels.[10]

The major limitation to use of OKT3 is that all antibodies are immunogenic and can therefore elicit immune reactions against themselves. After prolonged use, therefore, their action becomes less effective as antibody against the monoclonal antibody is produced, thus binding to and effecting removal of the circulating OKT3.

RADIATION. The concept of using total lymphoid irradiation (TLI) is based upon the profound immunosuppressive effects observed after TLI for treatment of Hodgkin's disease.[1,11] Preoperative TLI of allograft recipients has been shown to be immunosuppressive when used alone or together with chemical immunosuppression. Immunologic monitoring after TLI and transplantation has confirmed a sustained and uniform reduction in helper T cells (CD4+) and in the proliferative responses of these cells to mitogenic and allogeneic lymphoid stimulation during the first year after grafting. Other studies have shown an increase in numbers of cytotoxic/suppressor cells (CD8+) in these patients, and some postulate that the immunosuppression observed follows the generation of endogenous suppressor cells. B cells probably have a role in this effect as well, since they are relatively radiosensitive and are also affected by the radiation.

Radiation was probably the first agent used clinically to produce immunosuppression.[2,9] Ionizing radiation (x-rays, alpha rays, beta rays) affects both cellular proteins and nucleic acids. Despite the fact that relatively small doses of irradiation may disrupt the secondary protein structure formed by hydrogen bonding and the tertiary conformation that results, biologically significant alterations of protein function appear to require very high dosages. Consequently, most of the immunosuppressive effects of x-radiation are caused by changes produced in nucleic acids. DNA is particularly vulnerable; therefore, so is cellular replication. The most important of the several modes of damage is the production of scattered breaks in the deoxyribose-phosphate backbone of DNA. Disruption of either the carbon-to-carbon bonds of the deoxyribotides or the bonds involving the phosphate groups produces breaks in one of the DNA strands. Occasionally both strands are broken at the same point. Other sites of damage, such as the bases themselves, are even less frequent.

Repair mechanisms exist to mend the breaks, but insufficient time may be available in the dividing cell. Therefore, the effectiveness of radiation is dependent upon the phase of the cell cycle in which the cell is found. Cells in the M or G_2 phase are most sensitive to irradiation. Presumably, DNA breaks that occur during these phases cannot be repaired rapidly enough, and the synthetic events and precise apportionment of the cellular components that occur during mitosis may become scrambled (Fig. 10). Conversely, the early G_1 phase and the latter part of the S phase are the most resistant portions of the cell cycle. Although irradiation is, in general, most effective just prior to or during mitosis, lymphocytes represent a special case. For reasons that are not known, these cells are also sensitive in their resting, or G_0, phase and lysis of lymphocytes follows radiation of sufficient doses.[2,9]

Despite the complexity of the subcellular mechanism, the effect of irradiation on the immune response is predictable and depends greatly on its timing with relation to antigen exposure. The possibilities are best seen when a relatively simple response, antibody production against a defined antigen, is measured. When the antigen is given soon after irradiation, the immune response is inhibited because there is insufficient time for the immunocompetent cell population to recover before the antigen is encountered. If radiation is given during the time of maximal proliferation of the immunocompetent population to an antigen (soon after antigen administration), the response is strongly inhibited. However, if antigenic stimulation is delayed sufficiently for the precursor cells to recover from the radiation,

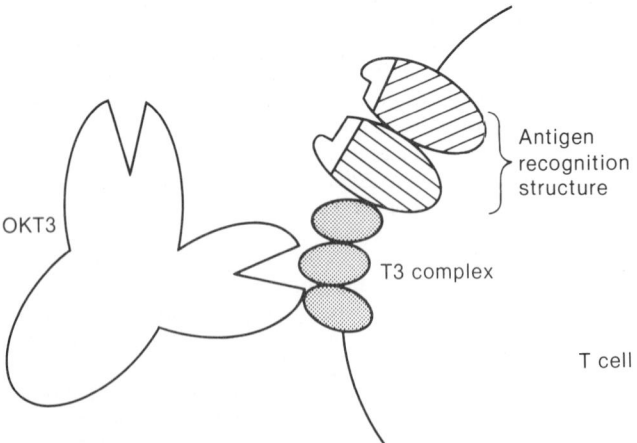

Figure 9. Diagrammatic representation of the T-cell receptor complex. OKT3 binds to a site on the complex, adjacent to the site which recognizes antigen and blocks T-cell effector functions involved in allograft rejections. (Redrawn from Goldstein, G.: Overview of the development of orthoclone OKT3: Monoclonal antibody for therapeutic use in transplantation. Transplant. Proc. 19:1, 1987.)

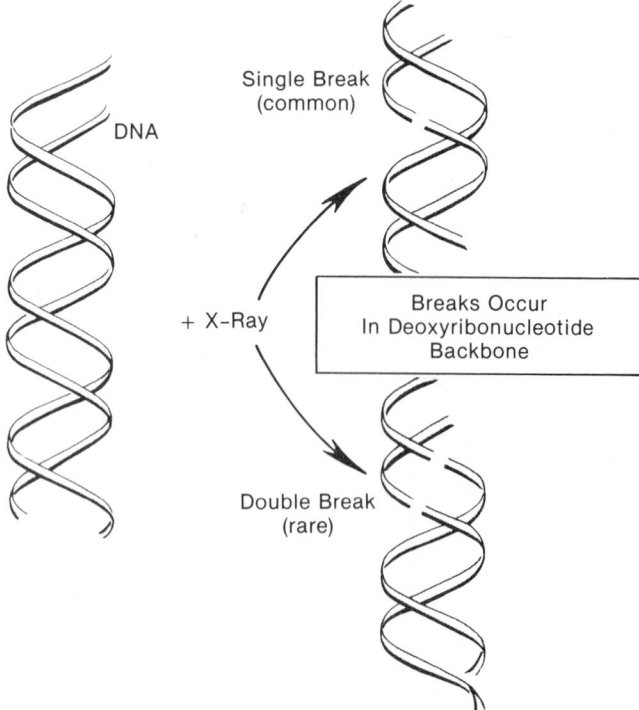

Figure 10. Roentgenologic induced damage of DNA molecules frequently induces single breaks in the deoxyribonucleotide backbone of the DNA double helix. More rarely, irradiation induces double breaks within the backbone. These breaks can be repaired if sufficient time exists before mitosis.

a slight augmentation of the response ensues. Radiation is also effective if initiated long after the antigen, when the mature population of antibody-synthesizing cells has been formed. Fully differentiated plasma cells, and presumably cytotoxic lymphocytes, are radioresistant. The timing of radiation must be carefully planned for the greatest immunosuppressive effect.

X-radiation has had limited use in clinical transplantation. After transplantation, radiation of the graft may damage invading cells as well as produce nonspecific anti-inflammatory effects. Although proof of the benefit is lacking, some centers irradiate the kidney graft at the onset of a rejection reaction.

Other methods of using radiation have been tried. Selective irradiation of circulating lymphocytes has been done experimentally by diverting blood via a shunt through an extracorporeal radiation source. The circulating lymphocytes are depleted, and immunocompetence is reduced. Selected irradiation has advantages in that the neutrophils remain active in clearing infection and protein loss is avoided. The inefficiencies of the system, however, and the need for nearly continuous irradiation make this technique impractical for clinical use.

Total-body radiation is used to prepare patients for bone marrow transplantation. In theory, the radiation treatment creates "space" in the bone marrow to allow the grafting of new cells. The toxicity is predictable. The rapidly replicating cells in the skin and the gastrointestinal tract are universally affected; and nausea, vomiting, diarrhea, and skin changes occur. Late problems are also probably attributable to damage to the cellular genetic apparatus: growth retardation, vertebral deformities, sterility, cataracts, and an increased incidence of cancer.

TOTAL LYMPHOID IRRADIATION (TLI) PLUS BONE MARROW TRANSPLANTATION. This technique combines the use of radiation and bone marrow transplantation to promote acceptance of kidney or other organ grafts.[1,2,17] It has generated a great deal of interest but is still highly experimental. Potential graft recipients are given a course of approximately 3000 rads to the lymphoid-bearing areas with shielding of the skull, ribs, lungs, and legs to preserve the bone marrow. After completion of the radiation, both a bone marrow transplant and an organ graft are performed. Proliferation of the donor bone marrow cells causes a partial chimeric state that facilitates acceptance of the organ graft. By a process not yet well understood, the donor and host bone marrow cells both repopulate the periphery, producing a form of tolerance. Experimentally, the tolerant state is stable and may be due in part to the generation of large numbers of suppressor cells. In contrast to the situation following total-body irradiation, the bone marrow following TLI does not as readily cause GVH disease. Experimental success has prompted a few clinical trials. TLI without bone marrow cells has been employed in highly sensitized recipients of second and third renal grafts at the University of Minnesota and Stanford University with fair success. However, without the concomitant transplantation of bone marrow, the tolerant state induced is less stable. In addition, the logistical difficulty of radiation administration and the uncertain interval between discontinuing the radiation and performing cadaveric transplantation reduce the attractiveness of the procedure.

ADRENAL CORTICOSTEROIDS. Adrenal corticosteroids are the immunosuppressive agents most commonly used in clinical practice.[2,3,5,9] They are effective in a variety of situations from transplantation to the treatment of lupus erythematosus, childhood nephrotic syndrome, and asthma. Glucocorticoids have many anti-inflammatory actions, which make them potent immunosuppressants (Fig. 11). A profound decrease in the blood lymphocyte count occurs within the first 6 hours of steroid administration. In humans, the decrease in peripheral blood lymphocytes reflects a redistribution of these cells out of the intravascular space into lymphoid depots. Recirculating lymphocytes (approximately two thirds of all lymphocytes) are mainly T cells, which travel back and forth between the intra-

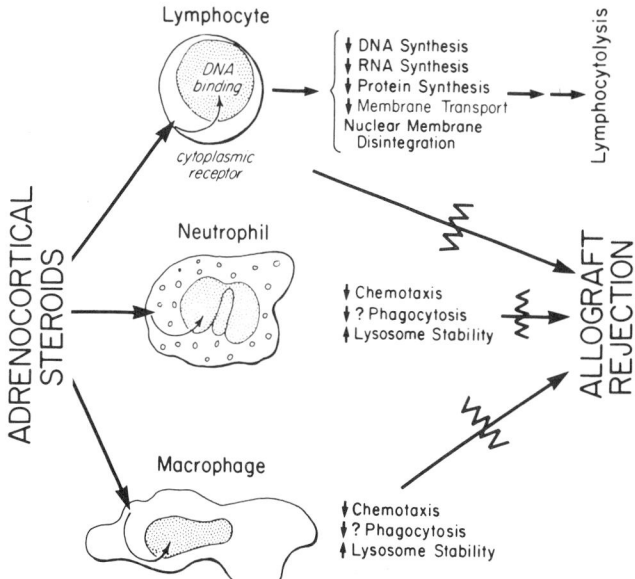

Figure 11. Adrenocortical steroids have an important role in clinical allograft immunosuppression. Many apparent sites of action have been located experimentally. These compounds bind to cytoplasmic receptors, and this complex combines with DNA. How this relates to the many functional consequences of steroids presented in this diagram is unclear. In the complex clinical transplantation setting, it is not possible to determine whether the primary suppression of lymphocytes is more important than the anti-inflammatory effects on neutrophils and macrophages in the suppression of allograft rejection. Nevertheless, steroids produce a significant portion of the immunosuppressive effect of current clinical therapy.

vascular compartment and lymphoid tissues such as the spleen, bone marrow, thoracic duct, and lymph nodes. Sessile lymphocytes, including some T and most B cells, stay within the vascular compartment. Glucocorticoids cause emigration of the recirculating T cells from the intravascular compartment to the lymphoid tissues, with less effect on the distribution of B cells. The mechanism of lymphocyte distribution is probably a cell surface alteration, making cells more or less "sticky" to vascular endothelium.[3,5,9]

Steroids also inhibit the production and the effect of T-cell lymphokines, which amplify the responses of the lymphocytes and macrophages. For example, interleukin-2 (IL-2) made by activated T-helper cells is an amplifier and promotes blast transformation, proliferation, and maturation of other T cells. Interleukin-2 production is severely impaired by glucocorticoids. Moreover, the ability of macrophages to respond to lymphocyte-derived signals such as migration inhibition factor (MIF) and macrophage activation factor (MAF) is also blocked by steroids. This may underlie the marked inhibition of the delayed-type hypersensitivity reactivity observed with steroids. Steroids have little net effect on antibody production.

The mechanisms by which glucocorticoids exert their effect have recently been elucidated. Much activity is initiated at the subcellular level by means of hormone receptors. Unlike insulin or other polypeptide hormones with receptors on the cell surface, steroids act on receptors in the cytoplasm. Glucocorticoids move freely through the cell membrane to bind receptors in the cytoplasm, producing a steroid-receptor complex. This complex then moves into the nucleus, where it attaches to the DNA, derepresses part of the genome, and causes transcription of specific messenger RNA. The RNA then directs production of new specific proteins that presumably are the effectors of glucocorticoid action.

Specific intracytoplasmic receptors for glucocorticoids have been identified in normal human lymphocytes, monocytes, neutrophils, and eosinophils. In addition, varying degrees of receptor density have been demonstrated in different lymphoid cell subpopulations. Presumably the sensitivity of a particular subpopulation of lymphocytes relates to the relative density of the intracytoplasmic receptors for the steroids. These messengers can act to inhibit DNA, RNA, and protein synthesis. Glucose and amino acid transport can also be affected.

The effectiveness of cortisone in suppressing allograft rejection was first recognized by its prolongation of skin graft survival in rabbits. Increased skin graft survival was subsequently shown in mice and guinea pigs, but the results were not as conclusive in pigs, dogs, monkeys, and human beings when cortisone was used alone. In experimental kidney allografts, steroids have not been convincingly effective by themselves, but are valuable in combination with such agents as azathioprine, nitrogen mustard, and antilymphocyte globulin. Similarly, steroids alone cannot prevent clinical allograft rejection, but together with other compounds are potent in both preventing and reversing rejection reactions.

Steroid toxicity of some degree is frequent and commonly includes a Cushingoid appearance. Other characteristic problems from steroid therapy are hypertension, weight gain, peptic ulcers and gastrointestinal bleeding, euphoric personality changes, cataract formation, hyperglycemia that may progress to steroid diabetes, pancreatitis, and osteoporosis with avascular necrosis of the femoral head and other bones. The appearance and severity of these complications vary considerably, but all too frequently they are life-threatening. Clinical transplantation will be improved tremendously when more specific means of immunosuppression are developed and present steroid dosages can be reduced.

THYMECTOMY. There is some evidence that the adult mammalian thymus continues to have a role, albeit a diminished one, in maintaining the immunologic responsiveness of the animal.[2,3,9] Its extirpation, therefore, may enhance the effects of immunosuppressive agents or irradiation. Unfortunately, it has not proved to be of use in clinical transplantation. In the early days of renal transplantation, Starzl performed thymectomy in a number of patients but had little improvement in results.

LYMPHOID EXTIRPATION. Immunity rapidly becomes systemic[2,9]; confinement to the regional lymph nodes or to a single major lymphoid organ such as the spleen is limited. Experimentally, the acquisition of immunity can be delayed for only brief periods by interrupting the lymphatic channels, by placing grafts in sites with poor lymphatic drainage, or by excising local lymphoid tissue. In one of the earliest clinical experiments, transplanted kidneys were placed in plastic bags after completion of vascular anastomoses. This approach failed, because vascularized organ grafts do not require lymphatic drainage to disseminate the antigen to awaiting lymphocytes. Excision of locally draining lymph nodes or the spleen is also ineffective as an immunosuppressive technique.

THORACIC DUCT DRAINAGE. Cannulation and drainage of the thoracic duct can successfully deplete the body of a large proportion of its circulating T lymphocytes.[2,9] Such depletion leads to prolongation of allograft survival and to decreases in the capacity for antibody synthesis. Thoracic duct cannulation has been successfully employed clinically to deplete lymphocytes and to prolong allograft survival but is no longer utilized. Cannula use is limited because its patency is difficult to maintain and prolonged hospitalization is required.

OTHER IMMUNOSUPPRESSIVE APPROACHES

BLOOD TRANSFUSION. Many studies have shown that blood transfusions prior to kidney transplantation improve kidney graft survival, and some form of transfusion protocol has become part of the preparative regimen for most patients in renal failure who are awaiting a graft.[1,5,9,11] The salutary effect of transfusion is also evident in nonrenal solid organ grafts. A recent retrospective analysis of cardiac transplant recipients showed a 13 per cent improvement in 1-year graft survival. There is growing evidence that transfusions from the donor induce a degree of specific immunologic hyporeactivity against graft antigens if administered several weeks prior to placement of the graft. However, 30 per cent of uremic individuals and nearly all nonuremic patients receiving deliberate transfusions become allosensitized. To circumvent this problem, azathioprine administered at the time of transfusion reduces the rate of sensitization to 5 per cent. The exact mechanism by which transfusions exert a beneficial effect is unknown, but evidence suggests a possible suppressor cell phenomenon.

Antibody, especially anti-idiotypic antibodies, may have a role in the generation of T-suppressor cells. The macrophage may also have a role by decreasing the production of IL-1 and tumor necrosis factor, lymphokines involved in allograft rejection. Induction of suppressor cells requires macrophages, mitogen, and T-helper (CD4+) cells. Therefore, a complex set of events is probably activated by blood transfusion to render the effect observed.

POTENTIAL NEW DIRECTIONS TO PREVENT REJECTION

THE INTERLEUKIN-2 (IL-2) RECEPTOR. The initial trigger for proliferation of most cells appears to be the interaction of exogenous growth factors (*cytokines* and *lymphokines*) with a cell surface growth factor receptor. For lymphocytes, one such factor is *IL-2*, formerly called T-cell growth factor (TCGF).[14,16] The IL-2 receptor on T cells has been characterized as a glycoprotein heterodimer. A low-affinity beta chain (55 kd.) combines with a constitutively expressed, medium-affinity alpha chain (70 to 75 kd.) during T-cell activation. Together they form a high-affinity receptor that mediates the proliferative effect of IL-2. IL-2 itself does *not* induce IL-2 receptor expression on resting lymphocytes in the absence of foreign antigen, but has been shown to increase IL-2R expression once activation has occurred. IL-2 exerts its effect via a hormone-receptor interaction. The immune response is up-regulated by IL-2R synthesis and expression. Down-regulation occurs within 1 to 2 hours of IL-2 receptor occupancy via internalization of the high-affinity receptor.[14,16]

It has recently been found that monoclonal antibodies against the IL-2R cause specific immune suppression GVH reactions, allograft rejection, and experimentally induced autoimmunity. Potential applications to the clinical setting may offer a new approach to more selective immunosuppressive therapy.

To date, the use of monoclonal antibodies that are broadly reactive against differentiation antigens on T lymphocytes does not solve the problem of side effects caused by general immunosuppression. Theoretically, the ideal therapeutic agent should eliminate not whole subsets of lymphocytes, but only those clones responding to a particular antigenic challenge.

SPECIFIC TRANSPLANTATION TOLERANCE

Bone marrow transplantation has been used in experimental animals to induce donor-specific transplantation tolerance, without the use of nonspecific immunosuppressive agents. In some models, the immunocompetence of the recipient is preserved as well as full reactivity to third party. The potential application of this method clinically remains to be determined.[1,17]

CLINICAL KIDNEY TRANSPLANTATION

Prior to the introduction of cyclosporine for clinical immunosuppression in 1978, most transplant surgeons used a combination of azathioprine and prednisone with or without ALG.[2,9] At the present time, at most transplant centers, recipients of cadaveric and living related donor kidneys (except HLA-identical recipients) receive cyclosporine and prednisone. Azathioprine is begun postoperatively and tapered to a dose adjusted according to peripheral white blood cell counts, platelet levels, and renal function. Recipients of HLA-identical antigen matches receive prednisone plus azathioprine. At some centers, ALG is given intravenously early postoperatively. The dosage is reduced if the platelet level is less than or equal to 150,000 per cu. mm. Treatment is continued for 2 weeks or until sensitivity to ALG appears.[2,9]

First rejection episodes in patients receiving conventional immunosuppression are treated with increased steroids (2 mg. per kg.) with a subsequent rapid taper in dosage. In addition, ALG and/or OKT3 may be added. Subsequent rejection episodes are treated with increased steroids alone. Increasing steroids is also the method of treatment in patients receiving cyclosporine immunosuppression.[2,9]

An important but unanswered question is how long immunosuppression therapy should be continued when the kidney functions well with no sign of rejection. Isolated successful instances of discontinuing medication have been reported, suggesting that some host-to-graft accommodation may occur. Rejection reactions do occur, however; and although there is some disagreement, it appears they are more numerous or intense than those that occur during therapy. Until more information is available, immunosuppressive therapy should therefore be considered a lifelong necessity.

CONSEQUENCES OF IMMUNOSUPPRESSION

In addition to the many specific immunologic and toxic effects of immunosuppressive drugs, there are several interesting and clinically important consequences of immunosuppression that must be considered.

PARAMETERS OF IMMUNOSUPPRESSION. The ability to diagnose or predict early allograft rejection is always a challenge to those caring for the transplant recipient. Accurate monitoring would be of value in regulating the amount of immunosuppression required and avoiding the dangers of over- or undertreatment. However, the complexity of the rejection reaction has so far defeated attempts to find a simple, clinically valuable measure of level of immunosuppression. Dosages at present are regulated primarily by the toxicity produced and by biopsy results. Although cyclosporine levels can be measured, they are subject to rapid fluctuations and at times do not correlate well with clinical toxicity.

INFECTION

BACTERIAL. Because of its nonspecific method of action, immunosuppression understandably increases the risk of infection; but the consequences may offer some surprises.[2,9] The routine posttransplantation immunosuppression regimen does not necessarily lead to a higher bacterial infection rate. At the University of Minnesota, the postoperative wound infection incidence is 0.7 per cent. These patients appear to cope satisfactorily with the inevitable contamination during the operation despite the increased immunosuppressive therapy used at the time. When there are no severe rejection reactions and the graft maintains good function, the day-to-day bacterial challenge to the recipient is managed. Although urinary tract infections are frequent, they are usually mild and easily controlled by antibiotics. Occasionally, unexplained septic arthritis develops in these patients. In addition, overwhelming pneumococcal sepsis has occurred in transplant patients without spleens.

It is not implied that bacterial infection is an insignificant problem for transplantation patients. On the contrary, infection is still the most common complication of immunosuppression,

and overall it is the most common cause of death in transplant recipients. However, increasing experience in prevention has both lowered the incidence of serious infection and delayed its occurrence.

Rejection of a kidney graft should not be fatal, because the patient can be maintained on hemodialysis. The difficulties appear to arise with the treatment of rejection. Rejection causes decreased kidney function, which further potentiates the increased immunosuppression required to combat the rejection episode. The consequence is usually a severely immunodepressed patient, often with very few circulating polymorphonuclear leukocytes, who is highly susceptible to infection. In this setting, particularly if it is prolonged, severe bacterial infections and generalized sepsis can still occur.

Most of the deaths early in the history of kidney transplantation occurred in the first few posttransplantation months caused by highly pathogenic bacterial infections. For example, pneumococcal pneumonia has been reported to be the most common type of pneumonia in kidney recipients. More recently, improved antibiotics and greater skill in immunosuppression therapy have shifted the spectrum of organisms. There has been a relative increase in lethal infection caused by opportunistic organisms that are normally weakly pathogenic. Antibiotics will eradicate the more aggressive bacteria, but they leave opportunistic organisms free to colonize the susceptible transplant patient.

FUNGAL AND PROTOZOAL. The opportunistic organisms, which are normally eliminated by cellular mechanisms, can now proliferate in the environment of the relative T-cell depression. Fungi are prominent opportunists, and they can cause urinary tract and pulmonary infections, skin lesions, and central nervous system involvement, as well as generalized sepsis.[2,9] *Candida albicans* infections are probably the most common. The inevitable mucosal candidiasis can be satisfactorily prevented by oral mycostatin. *Candida* organisms can become more deepseated, and the pneumonia, usually part of mixed infection, can be lethal. Characteristically, it produces soft, bulky infiltrates, although invasion of pulmonary arteries can lead to infarction and wedge-shaped peripheral infiltrates. *Candida* sepsis is most often associated with indwelling catheters, but it can assume a more entrenched systemic form.

Aspergillus species are probably the second most common cause of fungal infection and typically produce upper lobe pulmonary cavities. *Rhizopus oryzae, Histoplasma capsulatum,* and *Cryptococcus neoformans* also invade the lung, and the latter occasionally causes meningitis. The indolent bacterium *Nocardia asteroides* occasionally infects, producing nodular pulmonary lesions. The protozoan *Pneumocystis carinii,* more commonly seen in patients undergoing cancer chemotherapy, usually causes an alveolar infiltrate with disproportionate dyspnea and cyanosis.

Standard patient isolation precautions are useless against these organisms, and prophylactic antibiotics are not available for most of them. Prevention is dependent upon avoiding excessive doses of immunosuppressive agents in a futile attempt to prolong the function of a rejected graft.

VIRAL. Viral infections appear to be almost ubiquitous in kidney transplant recipients.[2,9] The herpes group of DNA viruses is most commonly present. Infection or antibody response to cytomegalovirus (CMV) is found in up to 90 per cent of patients after renal transplantation. Herpes simplex infection occurs in about 25 per cent and herpes zoster in 10 per cent of graft recipients. Reports from England have shown that the Epstein-Barr virus commonly infects transplant patients, but the clinical significance of this is unclear. Antigenic evidence for hepatitis B virus infection can be detected in 15 per cent of transplant patients. It appears almost certain that as detection methods improve, evidence of other types of viral infections in these transplantation patients will be demonstrated.

Several questions are raised by the recognition of viral infections in kidney recipients. Are these infections of clinical relevance? The case of the hepatitis B (HB) virus is particularly interesting. Transplantation and hemodialysis patients who have circulating HB antigen, paradoxically, usually have no symptoms of hepatitis. The reason that the disease is apparently much milder in these patients is unknown but intriguing. It appears likely that liver damage is mediated by an immune reaction against viral antigens on the cell surface, and this may be reduced in these immunodepressed patients.

The situation with CMV infection appears to be slightly clearer but no less intriguing. Most evidence suggests that CMV infection usually produces a clinical illness characterized by fever, neutropenia, and frequently a decrease in kidney function and apparent rejection. The virus may be newly acquired from blood transfusions or from the foreign graft itself.

Frequently, viral infection has been reported to coincide with acute rejection episodes. In these patients it remains unclear whether the infection causes the rejection or the rejection encourages viral activation. Rejection reactions are initiated by bursts of lymphocyte proliferation. Cell division is known to activate latent viruses experimentally; the most immunosuppressive agents are mutagenic. Viral infections, however, can be associated with either an augmented or a depressed immune response. If the patient is able to produce antibody against virus, graft rejection is also enhanced. In preimmunized individuals, viruses appear to act as immunologic adjuvants and to enhance the response to both virus and graft. When no antibody response accompanies the viral infection, a generalized immunodepression is usually present. At the present time it can be stated only that viral infections and rejection reactions are clearly linked; which initiates and which follows is usually unknown.

A special case of CMV infection is worthy of note. The typical CMV infection is a mild febrile illness, followed by an antibody response and regression of viral symptoms. A rejection episode usually accompanies the viral infection and raises the controversy discussed in the previous paragraph. These patients remain asymptomatic but may continue to excrete CMV in the urine or saliva despite the presence of antibodies to CMV. In certain patients, however, there is no antibody response or apparent rejection, and the infection can be lethal. The virus proliferates in many types of cells. Viral inclusion bodies have been found, for example, in the cells that rim the diffuse gastrointestinal ulcerations that can develop in these patients. The stomach and cecum are particularly vulnerable, but the ulcerations can be widespread. Viral infestation of the lungs and liver can cause a fulminant interstitial pneumonitis and hepatitis. Bone marrow involvement is manifested by leukopenia and thrombocytopenia. This group of severely immunosuppressed patients is at the mercy of this usually innocuous virus, which would suggest that rejection is not essential for viral activation. Certainly the ability of the patient to respond to the virus is very important to survival.

The other herpesviruses appear to behave in a similar manner. Transplant patients also have infections typical of herpes simplex and zoster. The infections may be more severe than in otherwise healthy patients; and although the lesions may be localized, the viruses are systemic and can be recovered in the urine. Fever, neutropenia, and allograft rejection may accompany the infection, and antibody responses to the virus appear to be important for the patient.

It is not certain when the viral infections occur in relation to the clinical symptoms. With the exception of hepatitis infection, these may represent activation of a normal intracellular viral flora, rather than recent infection. In transplant patients, studies suggest that cytomegalovirus "infection" occurs about the time of transplantation, when the mutagenic antirejection drugs are administered at high levels. Recent data indicate that the incidence of severe CMV infection is far lower in patients treated with cyclosporine and prednisone, compared with those treated with azathioprine and steroids.

MALIGNANCY

The incidence of malignancy is increased in recipients of transplants; the rate is not high enough, however, to contraindicate the transplant procedure. Tumors in kidney recipients originate from two general sources. Some unfortunately have been transplanted from cadaver donors in whom the cancer was unsuspected.[1,2,9] These tumors usually can be treated simply by halting immunosuppression therapy and allowing rejection of the tumor tissue, as well as the kidney, to occur. The more common cancers are the primary tumors that appear in the immunosuppressed recipient. The data are still accumulating on these primary tumors, and precise frequencies are not yet available. It would appear, however, that the rate of development of malignancy in patients surviving renal transplantation may be as high as 30 times that of a similar normal population.

Only certain tumors grow more readily in immunosuppressed patients.[2,9] Seventy-five per cent of the spontaneous cancers are either lymphoid or epithelial in origin. Carcinoma in situ of the cervix, carcinoma of the lip, and squamous or basal cell carcinomas constitute approximately half of this group, whereas lymphomas, predominantly reticulum cell sarcomas, represent the remainder. Recently, polyclonal and monoclonal B-cell lymphoproliferative disease, which is probably triggered by Epstein-Barr virus infection, has become an emerging entity. Up to 10 per cent of pediatric liver transplant recipients have been reported to develop this disease if followed long-term. The incidence is much lower in the adult, and the overall rate appears to be influenced by the cyclosporine level. It has been estimated that the risks to the transplant recipient of developing skin cancer, lymphoma, or reticulum cell sarcoma are increased by 4, 40, and 350 times, respectively. The lymphomas are unusual in both their frequency and behavior. Almost 50 per cent of the immunosuppressed patients with lymphomas have brain involvement, which occurs in only 1 per cent of non–transplant-related causes of lymphoma. These lymphomas, moreover, are difficult to treat and have led to death in almost all patients. The superficial malignant lesions of the lip, skin, and cervix are usually successfully treated by standard operative techniques. There is no need to jeopardize the allografts by reducing the immunosuppressive therapy.

It is not known why transplant patients have an increased risk for cancer in general and for epithelial and lymphoid cancers in particular. It has been postulated that the surveillance and elimination by lymphocytes of tumor cells as they arise are important natural defenses of humans against cancer. Certainly, this function would be depressed in transplant patients who are immunosuppressed by antirejection therapy. Despite this, two observations argue that this explanation is incomplete. First, only a few types of cancer are increased in these patients. Second, and perhaps more significant, is the finding that patients receiving hemodialysis have an increased risk of cancer, but the tumors arise with the usual spectrum and frequency distribution. Dialysis patients have decreased immunologic competence. Perhaps the inhibition of a surveillance mechanism contributes to their increased risk.

Transplant patients, however, must have additional factors that contribute to the development of cancer. They are immunosuppressed, which may be important, but the presence of the mutagen azathioprine is a more certain factor. Azathioprine, theoretically, could act as a primary mutagen on dividing lymphocytes and epithelial cells or could contribute to the activation of viruses and their transformation of normal cells into tumor cells.

Recently, a strong association has been identified between Epstein-Barr virus infection and the development of posttransplantation lymphoma. A viral etiologic source may be an important link in understanding the pathogenesis of cancer.

It would seem possible that the most important effect the immunosuppressive agents have on tumor development is to encourage viral transformation of normal cells into cancer cells. Cancers of the epithelium, for example, may be a consequence of herpesvirus transformation. This group of viruses is carcinogenic in animals, and circumstantial evidence exists for a role in human cervical cancer. Herpesviruses are usually dormant, but the stress of transplantation or the action of antimetabolites may activate them. The viruses might then either proliferate and cause a clinical viral illness or produce cellular transformation into cancer cells.

GROWTH

The antiproliferative effects of immunosuppressive drugs would appear to make satisfactory growth in children unlikely after transplantation.[2,9] Chronic renal failure itself inhibits development; so these children are usually far behind their peers in size. After successful transplantation, their growth response is highly variable and may depend on age, previous growth rate, renal function, and the immunosuppressive drug regimen. Although many children return to a normal growth rate, growth lost during the original illness is not regained; so these children will always be smaller than their peers.

Wound healing is a specific case in this category and is, to all outward appearances, normal. It is apparent clinically, however, that wound healing is severely affected when debilitation, chronic renal failure, and high steroid levels are present.

PREGNANCY

Many questions can be raised regarding the likelihood of a successful pregnancy and the birth of a normal child when one parent has received a kidney graft. Excessive steroid levels, the antigrowth and mutagenic effects of the immunosuppressive agents, and viral activation and infection all should be detrimental to the fetus. As usual, however, the situation is more complicated.[2,9]

The Human Renal Transplant Registry by 1975 had reported on 132 graft recipients who had become parents. The experience at the University of Minnesota has been examined in detail and appears to be representative. In that series, 17 patients became pregnant after transplantation, and 12 children were born. Only one spontaneous abortion occurred. The children had a normal size distribution, and no congenital defects were found. There is no doubt, however, that azathioprine and probably steroids are mutagenic and that the risk of congenital abnormalities is real. Multiple defects have been reported in the child of a male transplant recipient. From the overall experience, the risk is not high, but the incidence is still unknown. Steroids also cause their own peculiar problems, and a few cases of severe neonatal adrenocortical insufficiency, as well as lymphopenia, have been reported.

Transplant recipients who are pregnant are often beset with medical problems. Toxemia has occurred in over half of the pregnancies, and bacterial and viral infections, particularly of the urinary tract, are common. Both of these factors may contribute to the higher incidence of premature labor that has been reported in these patients. Another important medical concern is the effect of the pregnancy on renal function. Although the data are insufficient for judging whether or not pregnancy is deleterious to kidney function, each series has apparent examples that show that this may be true. An indication for the termination of pregnancy is the compromise of graft function. The increased risk of cancer, particularly of the cervix, in transplant patients has already been discussed. The effect of pregnancy on this tendency is unknown. Another important prob-

lem that must be faced is the decreased life expectancy of transplant recipients. Parenthood is a long-term obligation, and counseling of transplant patients should include a discussion of these considerations.

TOLERANCE

Many kidneys survive for years in their new host. The literature suggests that this survival represents an acquired tolerance, a specific nonreactivity to the graft antigens that is hoped for in immunosuppressive therapy. The question of tolerance has been raised earlier in this chapter, and the possible means of achieving it are discussed in the following section of experimental immunosuppression. At this time, acquired tolerance appears rarely, if ever, to occur. Reduction of immunosuppression, even after long accommodation of graft and host, almost invariably leads to rejection. Some adaptation must occur, however; and long-term graft survival can be achieved at immunosuppressive dosages that do not immunologically cripple the recipient or produce other severe toxic consequences.

EXPERIMENTAL IMMUNOSUPPRESSION

The currently available immunosuppressive agents have revolutionized the field of transplantation. However, because they act in a nonspecific manner to suppress all aspects of immune function, associated toxicities result.[1,2,9,17] Therefore, investigative efforts have been directed to finding an improved, more specific method of immunosuppression. The complexity of the immune response raises the hope that many potential points of vulnerability in activation and deployment of the cells responsible for the rejection reaction exist. New approaches are constantly being tried and old ones refined to produce better immunosuppressive therapy.

IMMUNOSUPPRESSION BY SPECIFIC ANTIGENS. The complications of immunosuppression constantly reinforce the importance of developing modes of immunosuppression that will be specific for the incompatible graft antigens. The immunosuppressive drugs and antilymphocyte globulin all act by suppressing the capacity of the immunocompetent cell to respond to any antigen. Thus, even ALG, with its predilection for cellular immunity, cannot select between T cells destined to reject an allograft and T cells necessary for immunity against viruses and tumors. The ability to produce a state of tolerance would obviously be of enormous benefit to the field of transplantation. Experimentally, a functional state of tolerance has been produced in two general ways: (1) by manipulation of the stimulating antigens or (2) by infusion of specific antibodies, which has been successful with soluble factors or infusion of cells.[1,2,9,17]

A variety of conditions have been shown to predispose to the induction of tolerance, rather than immunity, on exposure to antigen. The best example of antigen-directed immunologic unresponsiveness is the tolerance of animals to their own body constituents. This apparently develops early, during maturation of the immune mechanism, and is usually maintained throughout life. Burnet, as part of his clonal selection hypothesis, considered this unresponsive state to follow direct contact between "self" antigens and the individual's own lymphocytes. The clones of lymphocytes reactive to self are eliminated in the thymus, and tolerance ensues. This is referred to as *clonal deletion*.[11] He further predicted that specific unresponsiveness could be induced to foreign antigens if they were administered very early in life. Experimental proof by Billingham, Brent, and Medawar followed in 1953, demonstrating tolerance to major histocompatibility antigens after neonatal injection of allogeneic lymphoid cells.[11]

Obviously this opportunity has passed for transplant patients, but under certain carefully controlled conditions, tolerance has been produced experimentally in adult animals.[1,11,17] Thus, hope exists for future progress in this area, and several techniques have yielded limited but encouraging results. Repeated injection of small, subimmunogenic doses of antigen (low-zone antigen tolerance) or the use of very large amounts of antigen preparations (high-zone antigen tolerance) has produced unresponsiveness. Certain antigens (such as serum proteins) are endowed with properties that are particularly favorable for the induction of immunologic unresponsiveness, i.e., the ability to persist in the circulation and equilibrate within the extravascular spaces, thereby coming in contact with antigen-reactive cells in effective concentration. Whether or not this leads to deletion of the antigen-reactive lymphocytes, however, is unknown. The tolerant state induced by soluble antigen injection is a tenuous one and can be reversed, and clinical application of this modality holds limited promise.[2,9,11]

Unfortunately, viral and bacterial antigens and transplantation antigens do not have these properties and, in addition, possess multiple antigenic specificities. A diminished response to transplantation antigens can be induced in adult animals; but the antigen dose, physical state of the antigen, and route of injection all must be carefully chosen for avoidance of immunization. Tolerance is more easily induced in weak antigens; therefore, close histocompatibility matching is desirable. Irradiation, chemical immunosuppression, and antilymphocyte globulins have been used to inhibit the immune response and potentiate the emergence of a relatively unresponsive state. Although only modest successes have been achieved by these approaches, careful control of the conditions of antigen presentation may yet be important in the induction of tolerance.

In summary, the induction of tolerance by manipulating the presentation of the incompatible antigens is an attractive concept. Thus far, success in prolongation of allografts has not been achieved, but it remains a potentially promising pathway.[11]

The induction of specific unresponsiveness using cells, such as bone marrow, rather than isolated antigens, has also been explored.[1,17] In both adult and neonatal animal models, donor-specific transplantation tolerance has been achieved with the use of fully allogeneic bone marrow transplantation (A to B). Animals accept donor-specific skin and solid organ allografts and yet reject third-party grafts. Improved immunocompetence has been reported with mixed allogeneic reconstitution when a mixture of self-type (syngeneic) plus allogeneic bone marrow cells is transplanted (A + B to A). These models may have promise for clinical application in the future. This tolerant state is much more difficult to disrupt.[1,17]

IMMUNOSUPPRESSION BY SPECIFIC ANTIBODIES. Tolerance is not easily defined.[11] A simplistic definition of tolerance is the lack of reactivity toward self. However, this can occur at a number of different levels. Understanding the subcellular mechanisms involved is far more difficult, and they are just beginning to be understood. Tolerance may follow the absence or deletion of the reactive clone of lymphocytes. This could be explained by active suppression of anti-self reactivity through suppressor cells or by clonal deletion in which any lymphocyte which has anti-self reactivity is deleted from the repertoire during development. As a third explanation, tolerance could be due to an antibody that interferes with the development of immunity through blocking further activity. Although experimentally the immune response can be suppressed by passive transfer of specific antibody prior to or shortly after administration of antigen, this is probably not the mechanism responsible for true transplantation tolerance.

Two general mechanisms for this phenomenon have been proposed. The first states that the antibodies formed are inactive and do not trigger the effector mechanisms, such as complement. These blocking antibodies have been best demonstrated in tumor immunology, where they have been shown to enhance the growth of transplanted tumors and prevent rejection. The

second explanation is that the antibodies produce a negative feedback effect. The most striking example of this is the prevention of erythroblastosis fetalis in newborns by the administration of an Rh factor antiserum to the pregnant mother. The anti-Rh antibodies suppress the synthesis of antibodies in response to the foreign Rh antigens. Both of these mechanisms for production of tolerance require the presence of antibody to the antigen. While the appropriate antibodies cannot always be detected in animals after the induction of tolerance, they are often present. Moreover, antibodies are frequently detected in patients with well-functioning, long-term kidney allografts. Graft function is thought to be prolonged by the presence of a specific antibody that inhibits the development of truly effective anti-graft immunity. If immunosuppression is reduced, however, the balance is tipped, and the common result of graft rejection is observed. Consequently, the apparently paradoxical hypothesis that tolerance to an antigen requires the presence of antibodies to that antigen may yet be valid.

IMMUNOSUPPRESSION BY SUPPRESSOR CELLS

As previously mentioned, the ability to induce a sufficient number of specific suppressor T cells could effectively block graft rejection.[2,9] A further requirement, of course, would be that the suppressor cells be antigen-specific, to suppress only the rejection response, or general immunosuppression would result.

Additional leverage on the immune response may be gained by manipulating the genes that govern the response to histocompatibility antigens. Not all individuals respond in the same manner to different histocompatibility antigens, and part of this difference may be ascribable to a specific genetic locus. Matching the immune response governing loci in a similar manner to aligning histocompatibility antigens may yield improved results.

INTERFERENCE WITH NONSPECIFIC EFFECTORS

The combination of sensitized cells or antibodies with the foreign antigens marks the beginning of the active effort to reject the graft. The complex of sensitized cells, or antibodies, with the antigens activates the recruitment of a multitude of effector systems. The cascading enzyme system, the complement, clotting, and kinin pathways as well as the cellular mediators, lymphocytes, macrophages, platelets, and polymorphonuclear leukocytes have been discussed. These are enlisted both by the specific immunologic reaction itself and subsequent events. All have an active role in rejecting the allograft.[2,9]

It is conceivable that the effect of an immune response could be reduced by (1) interfering with the complement, clotting, and kinin cascades that are activated by antigen-antibody complexes; (2) destroying or blocking the factors secreted by activated cells (lymphokines and cytokines); or (3) neutralizing the vascular permeability factors, lysosomal enzymes, and lymphotoxins.[2,9]

A number of agents or combinations of agents that interfere with the expression of immunity have been tested. For example, anticomplement drugs (vitamin A, cobra venom factor) either are ineffective or, if potent, are short-acting and are not clinically useful. Antimacrophage globulin, carrageenan, and silica all destroy macrophages but are weak transplant immunosuppressants. Antibodies to lymphotoxins or migration inhibitory factors and other effector molecules are still in very early experimental states of evaluation. Anticoagulants (heparin), agents that interfere with platelet aggregation (dipyridamole, aspirin), and fibrinolytic agents have been employed to interfere with the thrombosis of graft vessels and the production of arterial narrowing, which often limit survival; the results have been discussed previously.

The limited success with these agents reinforces the difficulty in attempting to interfere with the immune response after antibody has been synthesized, and large numbers of immunologically committed effector cells have been mobilized. In fact, it is difficult to inhibit the secondary or anamnestic response of any immune reaction. Successful interference with the effector mechanism of graft rejection is prohibited by both the complexity and the interdependence of the reaction. Many pathways and cellular participants need to be blocked. In addition, there are points of cross-activation between these pathways that make it difficult to inhibit any or all of them effectively. If true immunosuppression is to be achieved, with respect to a certain antigen, interference probably must occur during the early phases of the primary immune response.[1,2,9,17]

MODIFICATION OF ANTIGEN-PRESENTING CELLS AND ANTIGENICITY BY DONOR AND/OR GRAFT PRETREATMENT

In an attempt to eliminate or reduce the requirement for chronic immunosuppression, modulation of donor organ immunogenicity through pretreatment of the donor or the allograft prior to transplantation has been investigated. Irradiation, cyclophosphamide, antilymphocyte globulin, and monoclonal antibody pretreatment have all been reported to decrease immunogenicity of grafts in laboratory animals. However, clinical trials have not demonstrated a significantly better outcome for renal grafts, and further laboratory studies are required before this technique is considered for clinical application. Without continuous treatment, regeneration of major histocompatibility complex alloantigens occurs and the immunogenicity of the graft returns.

Recent data have demonstrated that antigen-presenting cells of donor origin within grafts contribute to the immunogenicity of the graft. Efforts to remove these cells from grafts prior to transplantation using monoclonal antibody therapy have demonstrated a decrease in early immunogenicity. This approach may prove to be of value in clinical solid organ transplantation.[1,2,9,17]

THE EICOSANOIDS

The *eicosanoids* are the largest class of lipid mediators.[11] They are produced by all human cells except lymphocytes and possess a wide variety of biologic activities. The term includes the oxygenation products of long-chain polyunsaturated fatty acids such as arachidonic acid and linolenic acid, "essential" fatty acids, and the compounds such as prostaglandins into which they are incorporated for synthesis. The first recognition of prostaglandins as modulators of the immune system was made by Franks in 1971. Since that time, numerous other agents have been identified within this group. The immunomodulatory effects of the eicosanoids are mediated by direct actions on cells and also by indirect influences on the release of platelet activating factor, monokines, lymphokines, and other substances.[8,13]

The anti-rejection eicosanoids (prostaglandin [PG] E_2 and PGD_2) inhibit T-cell proliferation by inhibition of IL-1, IL-2, and Class II antigen expression on macrophages. Other prorejection eicosanoids (thromboxane A_2; leukotriene [LT] B_4 (LTB_4); LTC_4; and LTD_4) enhance T-cell proliferation. Investigations are preliminary but promising, and potential clinical applications to control or prevent rejection by manipulating these agents await further study.[8,13]

The above modalities may hold promise for potential future clinical application. However, until further investigation is pursued in the laboratory, the transplant surgeon must rely upon chronic, nonspecific immunosuppressive agents to prevent graft rejection.

SELECTED REFERENCES

Bach, F. H., and Sachs, D. H.: Transplantation immunology. N. Engl. J. Med., 317:489, 1987.
  The authors review the field of transplantation immunology. They include historical perspective and current immunosuppressive regimens used and discuss future directions.

Cooper, M. D.: B lymphocytes: Normal development and function. N. Engl. J. Med., 317:1452, 1987.
  This is a concise, state of the art review of lymphocyte function and activation as they pertain to the immune response.

Dinarello, C. A., and Mier, J. W.: Lymphokines. N. Engl. J. Med. 317:940, 1987.
  This is an excellent review of lymphokines as they relate to the immune response.

Golub, E. S. Immunology: A synthesis. Sunderland, Mass., Sinauer Associates, 1987.
  This is a complete review of immunology, including transplantation biology, in a format enjoyable to both immunologists and those new to the area.

Johnson, R. B.: Immunology: Monocytes and macrophages. N. Engl. J. Med., 318:747, 1988.
  This is a concise review of the monocyte and macrophage subpopulations and how they relate to the immune response.

Roger, H. D., and Reinherz, E. L.: T lymphocytes: Ontogeny, function and relevance to clinical disorders. N. Engl. J. Med., 317:1136, 1987.
  This is an excellent review of the T cell as it has been characterized to date. The nature of the T-cell receptor and how it relates to T-cell activation and the immune response are well presented.

REFERENCES

1. Bach, J. F.: The Mode of Action of Immunosuppressive Agents. Series of Frontiers of Biology, Vol. 41. New York, American Elsevier Publishing Company, 1975.
2. Bach, F. H., and Sachs, D. H.: Transplantation immunology. N. Engl. J. Med., 317:489, 1987.
3. Canafax, D., and Ascher, N. L.: Cyclosporine immunosuppression. Clin. Pharmacol., 2:515, 1983.
4. Chess, L., and Schlossman, S. F.: Human lymphocyte subpopulations. Adv. Immunol., 29:213, 1977.
5. Claman, H. N.: Glucocorticosterids. I. The anti-inflammatory mechanism. Hosp. Pract., July 1983, p. 123.
6. Cooper, M. D.: B lymphocytes: Normal development and function. N. Engl. J. Med., 317:1452, 1987.
7. Dinarello, C. A., and Mier, J. W.: Lymphokines. N. Engl. J. Med., 317:940, 1987.
8. Fawcett, D.: The Cell. Philadelphia, W. B. Saunders Company, 1981.
9. Foker, J. E., Simmons, R. L., and Najarian, J. S.: Allograft rejection. In Najarian, J. S., and Simmons, R. L. (Eds.): Transplantation. Philadelphia, Lea & Febiger, 1972, pp. 63–145.
10. Goldstein, G.: Overview of the development of orthoclone OKT3: Monoclonal antibody for therapeutic use in transplantation. Transpl. Proc., 19:1, 1987.
11. Golub, E. S.: Immunology: A Synthesis. Sunderland, Mass., Sinauer Associates, 1987.
12. Johnson, R. B.: Immunology: Monocytes and macrophages. N. Engl. J. Med., 318:747, 1988.
13. Kaplan, J. G. (Ed.): Molecular Basis of Immune Cell Function. Amsterdam, Elsevier–North Holland, 1979.
14. Osawa, H., and Diamantstein, T.: The interleukin-2 receptor, its physiology, and a new approach to a selective immunosuppressive therapy by anti-interleukin-2 receptor monoclonal antibodies. Immunol. Rev., 92:5, 1986.
15. Roger, H. D., and Reinherz, E. L.: T Lymphocytes: Ontogeny, function and relevance to clinical disorders. N. Engl. J. Med., 317:1136, 1987.
16. Rosenberg, A. S., Lotze, M. T., and Muul, L. M.: Observations on the systemic administration of autologous lymphokine-activated killer cells and recombinant interleukin-2 to patients with metastatic cancer. N. Engl. J. Med. 313:1485, 1985.
17. Sachs, D. H.: Antigen-specific transplantation tolerance. Clin. Transplant., 4:78–81, 1990.

VII ————————————————————————————

ORGAN PRESERVATION

Folkert O. Belzer, M.D., and James H. Southard, Ph.D.

Increasing reliance on organ transplantation as the treatment of choice for end-stage organ failure has necessitated continual improvements in methods of organ procurement and preservation. Large numbers of cadaveric donor organs are needed if organ transplantation is to be available to all suitable patients. Currently, there is a shortage of donor organs, and this situation will improve only with increased public and professional awareness of the need for organ donation and with the development of methods that make full use of all available organs.

The optimal use of available donor organs depends on effective methods for (1) managing brain-dead donors and (2) preserving organs, *ex vivo*, sufficiently long to allow them to be transported to the recipient hospital. By current standards, 24 to 40 hours of preservation are needed to optimally use most donor organs. Today, suitable preservation methods are available for the liver, kidney, and pancreas, but not for the heart or other transplantable organs (lungs, intestines).

The purpose of preservation is to maintain the viability of the donor organ until it can be transplanted. Organ preservation begins at the time the patient is declared brain dead and becomes a potential organ donor, and while the organ is still perfused with blood. (Donor management and its relationship to the success of organ preservation are not well understood and are not the subject of this chapter; interested readers should refer to the reviews by Cecka[6] and Calne.[3] The harvesting technique and the method of vascular flushing can greatly influence the outcome of preservation, and thus experienced harvesting teams can minimize the waste of valuable organs. The success of preservation is highly dependent on the method of preservation used (simple cold storage vs. continuous machine perfusion, temperature, type of preservation solution, and duration of storage). Finally, the outcome of a transplant operation may depend on how the recipient is managed, particularly on the effort made to minimize reperfusion injury to the organ. The extent of damage caused by reperfusion is affected by the composition of the reperfusion solution, for example, by the inclusion of Ca channel blockers,[24] O_2-free radical scavengers,[10] and agents that alter the interaction of blood components with the preserved organ.[29] This chapter discusses the use of different methods of preservation and the different types of preservation solutions.

HISTORICAL OVERVIEW

When successful living-related renal transplantation was demonstrated, an interest in transplantation of cadaveric organs began in the 1960s. It was recognized that to utilize these organs, methods to preserve the viability of the organ *ex vivo* were necessary to allow time to transport the organ to the recipient hospital. When removed from the donor, the organ is exposed to a period of ischemia (no blood flow, no oxygen or nutrients); earlier studies demonstrated that the tolerance to ischemia could be extended by cooling the organs.[16,17] Methods to cool the kidney included surface cooling or vascular flushout with cold saline or blood. These methods increased the time of safe preservation but only to about 4 to 8 hours.

In 1967, Belzer and associates[1] reported successful 3-day preservation of the canine kidney by continuous machine per-

fusion. This group found that low-flow (0.6 to 1.0 ml. per min.) and low-pressure (40 to 60 mm. Hg) pulsatile perfusion of the kidney with a perfusate consisting of cryoprecipitated plasma (CPP) was effective. The plasma, frozen prior to use, was thawed, and the precipitate of lipid materials was removed by ultrafiltration. In the cold, lipoproteins and other lipids were unstable and coalesced, thus obstructing the glomerular capillaries. Removal of these materials prior to continuous machine perfusion was essential for successful preservation. This method rapidly became assimilated into renal preservation and remains in use today, although with a different perfusion solution. The original perfusion machine was large and difficult to transport; subsequently a smaller version of the perfusion machine (Fig. 1) was developed that could be easily transported on aircraft and was battery operated.

In 1969, Collins and associates[7] demonstrated successful 30-hour preservation of the canine kidney by a method of simple cold storage. The kidney was flushed out with a solution (Collins' solution) that contained a high concentration of K (115 mmol. per liter), a low concentraton of Na (10 mmol. per liter), phosphate (57.5 mmol. per liter), and a large concentration of glucose (140 mmol. per liter). This solution became known as an intracellular cold storage solution because the high concentration of K resembled the high intracellular concentration of this cation in the kidney. The high concentration of glucose was necessary to raise the osmolality of the solution and was a primary reason why this solution was effective. Glucose is relatively impermeable across the renal cell membranes and suppresses hypothermia-induced cell swelling. This method of preservation quickly became favored among renal transplant surgeons because of its simplicity: a machine was not needed, nor was a trained technician. This method did not allow the quality or duration of preservation equivalent to machine per-

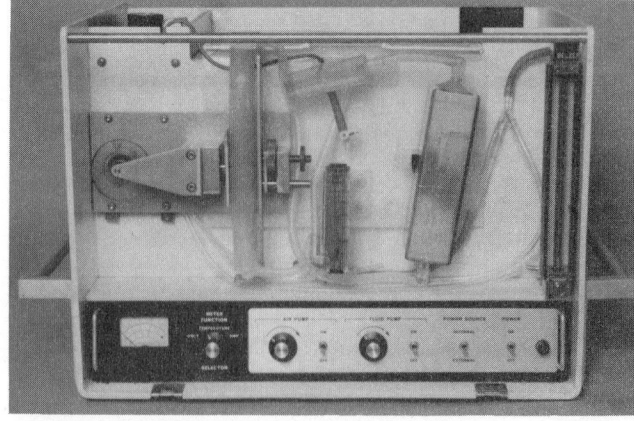

Figure 1. The mini-Belzer perfusion machine. Two kidneys could be preserved simultaneously and were kept in a plastic cassette placed in the machine and surrounded by an ice-water mixture. A pulsatile pump (60 beats per minute) compressed a pump head with one-way valves, and the force of the pump was regulated to deliver about 40 to 60 mm. Hg pressure to the kidney. The perfusate passed through a flowmeter and membrane oxygenator that was gassed with a mixture of oxygen–carbon dioxide regulated by a gas flowmeter. The machine weighed about 60 pounds and could be operated by enclosed batteries or electrically.

fusion, but because most kidneys could be transplanted within about 24 hours, this method became favored by transplant centers.

These methods of renal preservation were not particularly effective for preservation of other organs. However, in the early 1970s the long-term survival of liver, pancreas, and heart transplantation was not particularly favorable and there was not a great interest in transplanting these organs. In the early 1980s cyclosporine for immunosuppression became clinically available and changed organ transplantation. Now the liver, pancreas, and heart could be successfully transplanted with survival results nearly identical to those obtained with kidney transplantation.

METHODS OF ORGAN PRESERVATION

The general process of organ preservation is quite simple. Ideally, the time between the cessation of blood flow to the organ and the start of cooling by vascular flushing should be short. In multi-organ harvesting, the organs are usually cooled before they are removed. The cold-preservation solution is used to flush blood from the organ and to cool the organ to the preservation temperature (0 to 5° C.). The organ is stored in the preservation solution and kept at 0 to 5° C. Organs are preserved by either refrigeration storage (simple cold storage) or continuous machine perfusion.

HYPOTHERMIA AND CELL SWELLING

Two critical components of successful organ preservation are the maintenance of organ hypothermia (0 to 8° C.) and the suppression of cell swelling. Hypothermia is induced by flushing the vasculature of the organ with a cold solution (usually about 4° C.) that lowers the temperature of the organ to 4° C. within 5 to 15 minutes. The organ is then either stored at 0 to 4° C. on ice or machine perfused at 4 to 8°C. The value of hypothermia stems from the effect of temperature on metabolism (i.e., on enzyme activity). Arrhenius and van't Hoff showed that, in general, a 10° C. change in temperature produces about a twofold (1.5 to 2.5) change in enzyme activity.[17] An equation devised by van't Hoff shows that a decrease in temperature from 37° C. (normothermia) to an organ-storage temperature of 4° C. would theoretically decrease enzyme activity (metabolism) by 12 to 13 times. For a more concrete example, consider that a kidney can tolerate about 1 hour of warm ischemia (37° C.) before being irreversibly damaged, but if the kidney is flushed with cold blood (4° C.), tolerance to ischemia is increased to about 12 hours.[17] The tolerance of other organs to ischemia is also increased by cold, although not always to the same extent as are kidneys. Clearly, then, hypothermia increases the time an organ can be preserved.

The effect of hypothermia on metabolic rate suggests that one mechanism by which ischemia damages organs is related to rates of enzymatically catalyzed changes in the tissue (i.e., to degenerative changes in structural components [membranes] or to the loss of essential metabolites). The primary benefit of hypothermia is therefore the reduction of metabolism, including the requirements for a continual supply of nutrients, O_2, and energy (in the form of adenine nucleotides) and the suppression of hydrolytic enzymes (phospholipases, lysosomal enzymes, and proteases). Hypothermia is also beneficial because it suppresses the growth of microorganisms and provides the surgeon time to transplant the organ.

Hypothermia is essential for successful organ storage, but it also causes metabolic changes that cause cell swelling. Hypothermia-induced cell swelling (Fig. 2) follows a decrease in the activity of membrane-bound ion pumps (particularly the Na-K-ATPase pump) and from a decrease in the rate of ATP turnover; it is ATP that provides the energy for ion pump activity and for

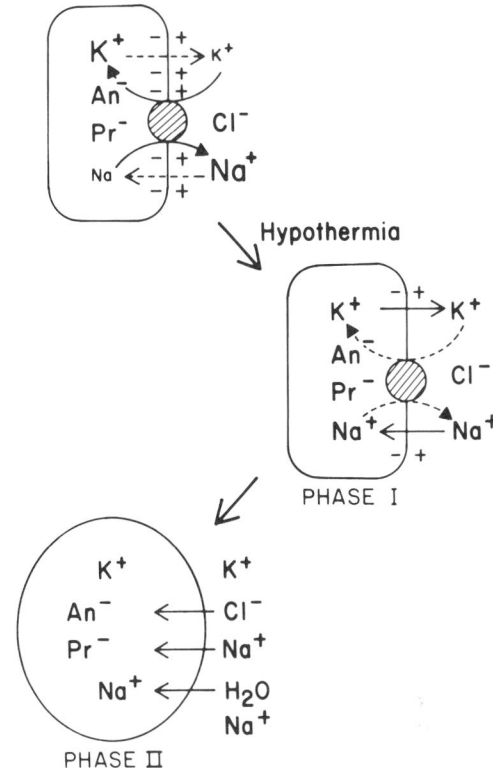

Figure 2. Schematic representation of hypothermia-induced cell swelling. A cell at normothermia *(top)* utilizes the Na pump (hatched circle) to maintain a high intracellular K and pump Na out of the cell. This makes Na an effective impermeant, which counteracts the oncotic pressure inside the cell derived from impermeable anions (An) and proteins (Pr). The Na pump also generates a membrane potential (negative inside relative to the outside of the cell). When cooled *(middle)*, the Na pump activity decreases and there is a stoichiometric exchange of K and Na derived by their chemical potentials (Phase I). This equilibration of cations is stoichiometric and does not cause the cell to gain water. However (Phase II, *bottom*), in the absence of a membrane potential, chloride diffuses down its concentration gradient and the increased osmotic activity inside the cell (as well as the presence of impermeable colloids) pulls water into the cell, causing cell swelling.

the control of cell volume. Normally the cell is bathed in a fluid that contains high concentrations of Na and chloride, while the inside of the cell contains a high concentration of K and impermeants (proteins and anions) that have a high relative molecular mass. The cell must expend considerable energy (ATP) to keep Na and Cl outside the cell wall. If the cell lacks sufficient energy, Na diffuses down its concentration gradient and is exchanged with K. This exchange is not lethal to the cell, and when normal metabolism is re-established Na is pumped back out of the cell in exchange for K. However, when ion pump activity is suppressed for long periods, the membrane potential is lost and chloride diffuses down its concentration gradient. Furthermore, the colloids in the cell exert a colloidal osmotic pressure that pulls water into the cell. The result is cell swelling, organelle swelling, a disruption of the architecture of the cell (cytoskeleton), and a dilution of the intracellular milieu. Cell swelling can be tolerated for short periods, but eventually it causes irreversible damage.

Successful organ preservation has, therefore, depended on the development of methods to safely and effectively suppress hypothermia-induced cell swelling. Agents that suppress cell swelling are termed impermeants (i.e., they are relatively unable to cross the plasma membrane). These impermeants exert sufficient osmotic force to counter the intracellular colloidal osmotic force. In general, cell swelling can be suppressed in cells that are metabolically depressed (due to hypothermia or the chemical inhibition of energy production) by including about 100 to 140 mmol. per liter of impermeant in a saline-based solution (140 mmol. per liter) that increases the osmotic strength of the solution from 300 mOsm. per liter to 400 to 440 mOsm. per liter. Saccharides (glucose, mannitol, sucrose, and raffinose) commonly serve as impermeants, and other agents that can also suppress cell swelling include impermeant anions (phosphate, sulfate, glycerophosphate, gluconate, lactobionate, and citrate). It is the cell membrane's limited permeability to these substances that determines their effectiveness. The permeability properties of cell membranes are a function of the type of organ, and impermeants effective for some organs are not effective for others. For example, glucose and mannitol suppress cell swelling in the kidney, but they are not as effective for the liver, pancreas, and heart.

Organs can be well preserved for relatively long periods with preservation solutions that suppress cell swelling. However, even if cell swelling is prevented, organs and tissues stored at hypothermia eventually lose viability. Some other mechanisms must therefore also cause cell death during organ storage. Exactly what these mechanisms are is unclear, but some evidence indicates that O_2-free radical injury, Ca-induced toxicity, the loss of energy-producing capabilities (mitochondrial injury, the loss of precursors to ATP resynthesis), the loss of phospholipids, and the activation of hydrolytic enzymes are involved in preservation injury. It is likely that several of these mechanisms are involved in the loss of organ viability during the long-term storage of organs.

KIDNEY PRESERVATION

The methods of preserving kidneys that were developed during the late 1960s by Collins[7] and Belzer[1] were quickly adopted for clinical use and had enormous impact on kidney transplantation. Successful storage methods greatly increased the number of cadaveric kidneys that were transplanted and the number of hospitals that performed kidney transplantations; they also eased the urgency of performing transplant operations and allowed time for tissue matching between donors and recipients. The success of these preservation methods is reflected in the fact that they have remained in use, essentially unchanged, for 30 years.

Collins and associates developed the method of simple cold storage for kidneys. Their preservation solution (Collins' solution; Table 1) was designed to mimic the intracellular milieu of the kidney and thus contains a high concentration of K and Mg, phosphate as a hydrogen ion buffer, and glucose to raise the osmolality to that of kidney cells. Glucose, the primary impermeant in Collins' solution, suppresses cell swelling in the kidney. This solution successfully preserved dog kidneys for as long as 30 hours after simple vascular flushing and storage at 0 to 4° C. Collins' solution preserves ideally harvested kidneys for as long as 48 hours, and the modified version, EuroCollins' solution (without Mg) is equally effective. EuroCollins' solution is currently used more than the original Collins' solution because Mg forms an insoluble precipitate with phosphate.

Because cold storage is so simple, many transplant centers

TABLE 1. Composition of Collins' C2 Solution

Component	gm./L.	mmol./L.
KH_2PO_4	2.05	15.0
K_2HPO_4 $3H_2O$	9.7	42.5
KCl	1.12	15.0
$NaHCO_3$	0.84	10.0
Glucose	25.0	139.0
$MgSO_4$ $7H_2O$	7.38	30.0

Na^+ = 10 mmol./L.; K^+ = 115 mmol./L.; PO_4 = 57.5 mmol./L.
Osmolality, 320 mOsm./L.; pH = 7.2.

TABLE 2. Composition of Citrate Solutions

Component	Hypertonic		Isotonic	
	gm./L.	mmol./L.	gm./L.	mmol./L.
K citrate	8.6	80	8.6	80
Na citrate	8.2	80	8.2	80
HCl (2 M.)	0.26	—	0.26	—
Mannitol	33.8	188	17.0	95
$MgSO_4$	10.0	35	10.0	35

Osmolality, 400 mOsm./L.; pH = 7.1 (hypertonic).
Na = 80 mmol./L.; K = 80 mmol./L.
Citrate = 55 mM.
Osmolality, 300 mOsm./L (isotonic).

have favored this method over the more complex method of continuous machine perfusion (see later). Several types of cold storage solution have been tested, and the most successful and widely accepted, other than the Collins' solution, is the Ross-Marshall solution (Table 2). This solution uses citrate as an impermeant; although poorly buffered (hydrogen ions), it has preserved kidneys for 3 days.[23] Other cold storage solutions include Sacks' solution, which contains a high concentration of mannitol for osmotic support, and a phosphate-buffered sucrose solution that has recently preserved dog kidneys for 3 days (Table 3).[13]

A second method of preserving kidneys is continuous hypothermic perfusion. This method was developed by Belzer and associates, who discovered that cryoprecipitated plasma is a good perfusion fluid for the 3-day preservation of dog kidneys. The plasma is frozen, thawed, and filtered to remove lipoproteins that accumulate in the capillaries of the kidney and block effective perfusion. The perfusate is pumped through the renal artery at a pressure of 40 to 60 mm. Hg with a pulsatile pump (60 beats per minute) that produces a flow rate of 0.6 to 1.0 ml. per minute. This low pressure prevents the perfusion-induced vascular damage that occurs at higher perfusion pressures. The initial experiments were performed with the perfusate continuously oxygenated (membrane oxygenator), but subsequent work showed that continuous oxygenation is not necessary and that the perfusate contains sufficient O_2 (from equilibration with room air) to support low-level aerobic metabolism in the kidney at 4 to 10° C.

Other perfusates have been developed, including a silica gel–filtered fraction of plasma.[26] Silica gel removes lipid material from plasma, and this perfusate is about as effective as cryoprecipitated plasma. Saline-based solutions containing human serum albumin also successfully preserve kidneys for about 48 hours.

Both simple cold storage and machine perfusion have been used clinically, and during the early history of kidney preservation and transplantation there was debate over which method was most effective. Continuous machine perfusion has consistently provided longer and better quality kidney preservation, both in the laboratory and in the clinic. However, most kidneys are transplanted within 20 to 30 hours after they are harvested, and a comparison of short- and long-term graft survival shows

TABLE 3. Composition of Phosphate-Buffered Sucrose

Component	gm./L.	mmol./L.
NaH_2PO_4	2.16	15.7
$NaHPO_4$	7.41	52.2
Sucrose	51.3	140.0

Osmolality, 320 mOsm./L.; pH = 7.2.

that the two preservation methods are equally effective. One difference, however, is that 15 to 50 per cent of kidneys preserved by cold storage need dialysis compared with 5 to 15 per cent of kidneys preserved by continuous machine perfusion.

Although simple cold storage and continuous perfusion were effective for kidney preservation, they were not particularly effective for the long-term preservation (more than 24 hours) of other organs. Moreover, neither method afforded successful preservation of kidneys for longer than about 3 days.

In the late 1970s and early 1980s, the authors' group studied methods of improving kidney preservation and developed a synthetic kidney perfusion fluid (Table 4). This solution contained hydroxyethyl starch as a colloid, replacing serum albumin. There is evidence that albumin causes endothelial injury during machine perfusion, and the search for effective colloids led to the discovery that hydroxyethyl starch is the most effective. Other colloids, such as Haemaccel,[18] may also be acceptable.

A colloid is essential with continuous machine perfusion to counteract the hydrostatic pressure produced by the perfusion pump. In addition to hydroxyethyl starch, the new perfusate contained gluconate as an impermeant anion to suppress cell swelling, adenosine and phosphate to stimulate ATP synthesis, glutathione to suppress damage due to lipid peroxidation and O_2-free radicals, and other agents. This solution preserved dog kidneys for 3 days, and it has proved successful for the clinical preservation of kidneys. Recently, this perfusate was modified by replacing the adenosine with adenine and ribose as precursors of ATP synthesis. Adenosine is catabolized during kidney perfusion and loses its ability to stimulate ATP synthesis. Adenine and ribose are not severely degraded during machine perfusion and consequently are able to keep ATP concentrations near normal during 5 days of preservation. It was also found that by including 0.5 mM. of Ca, kidneys could be successfully preserved for 5 days by machine perfusion.[15] This modified perfusion fluid is now being used in the clinic with excellent results.

PANCREAS PRESERVATION

Methods developed for kidney preservation proved unsuccessful for long-term pancreas preservation. The pancreas was difficult to preserve by continuous perfusion because it became edematous; so attention was turned to simple cold storage. Wahlberg and associates[28] experimented with different versions of the kidney perfusion solution that contained hydroxyethyl starch and found that a solution containing lactobionate prevented pancreatic edema during preservation and when the organ was reperfused. Lactobionic acid is the acid of the saccharide lactose (milk sugar), and it has a relatively large MW (358

daltons) compared with chloride (58 daltons) and gluconate (180 daltons). The combination of lactobionate and raffinose (100 mmol. per liter and 30 mmol. per liter, respectively) provided a preservation solution that effectively suppressed hypothermia-induced pancreas cell swelling. Wahlberg[27] used this solution for segmental pancreatic preservation in the autotransplant dog model; the results were consistent 3-day organ preservation and long-term animal survival. This solution (the University of Wisconsin (UW) solution) is very similar to the kidney perfusion solution described previously; its composition is shown in Table 5.

The UW solution has provided excellent clinical pancreas transplantation and has extended pancreas preservation from about 6 hours to more than 29 hours.[8] This solution also appears to preserve the pancreas sufficiently well so that islets can be isolated and used for islet cell transplantation.[32] While the UW solution was being developed, the Minnesota group obtained reasonably good pancreas preservation with a silica gel fraction of plasma that is similar to a kidney perfusate.[9] Both solutions appear to be clinically useful for preserving pancreases, but the silica gel fraction of plasma does not appear to be acceptable for the simple cold storage of livers and kidneys.

LIVER PRESERVATION

The two methods developed for kidney preservation were not as effective for long-term liver preservation. Collins' solution preserved dog livers for about 18 hours, but its safe clinical application was limited to only 6 to 10 hours. A plasma protein fraction also preserved dog kidneys for longer than 12 hours, but it too was considered clinically safe for only about 6 to 10 hours of liver preservation. Early work on liver preservation has been reviewed elsewhere.[4]

Shortly after Wahlberg developed the method for successfully preserving pancreases, Jamieson and Sundberg and associates[11] used the same UW solution for 48-hour preservation in the orthotopic dog liver transplant model. Dog livers flushed with the UW solution and stored for 48 hours were 100 per cent viable and showed a return of normal liver functions (bilirubin, serum enzymes, clotting factors) within about 2 to 3 days after transplantation. These studies prompted the clinical use of the UW solution for liver transplantation at the University of Wisconsin[12] and at other centers[25]; preservation times have been as long as 35 hours, and the results have been excellent.

Livers can be successfully preserved with simple cold storage, but recently an even better preservation of dog livers has been achieved with continuous machine perfusion.[20] A modified version of the UW kidney perfusion solution was used to preserve livers for 3 days. The modifications included reversing the ratio of cations (high K, low Na) and adding Ca, 1.0 mmol. per liter. Although it is an excellent method of preserving livers, continuous perfusion has not been used in the clinic.

TABLE 4. Composition of UW
Machine Perfusion Solution

Component	gm./L.	mmol./L.
Na gluconate	17.45	80
KH$_2$PO$_4$	3.4	25
Mg gluconate	1.04	5
Adenine	0.68	5
Ribose	0.75	5
Glutathione	0.922	3
CaCl$_2$	0.068	0.5
HEPES	2.38	10
Glucose	1.8	10
Mannitol	5.4	30
Penta starch	50	—

Na$^+$ = 100 mmol./L.; K$^+$ = 25 mmol./L.
Osmolality, 310 mOsm./L.; pH = 7.4.

TABLE 5. Composition of UW Solution

Component	gm./L.	mmol./L.
Penta starch (HES)	50	—
Lactobionic acid	35.83	100
KH$_2$PO$_4$	3.4	25
MgSO$_4$ 7H$_2$O	1.23	5
Raffinose	17.83	30
Adenosine	1.34	5
Glutathione	0.92	3
Allopurinol	0.136	1

Neutralized to pH 7.4 with NaOH:KOH.
Na$^+$ = 20 mmol./L.; K$^+$ = 140 mmol./L.
Osmolality, 320 mOsm./L.

Not only is the UW solution effective for the simple cold storage of pancreases and livers, but it is also effective for the simple cold storage of kidneys. Ploeg and associates[22] used the UW solution to preserve dog kidneys for 3 days, and a recent report describes its clinical use for kidney preservation.[2] In a prospective, randomized European trial to compare the UW solution with EuroCollins' solution in kidney preservation, kidneys preserved with the UW solution functioned, initially, better than those preserved with EuroCollins' solution.[21] The UW solution therefore appears to be close to a universal preservation solution for all intra-abdominal organs.

HEART PRESERVATION

Currently, hearts can be preserved for only about 4 hours before being transplanted. The solutions used vary among transplant centers, but they are similar to those developed by the groups at Stanford and St. Thomas Hospital. The heart, unlike other organs, must rapidly regain its maximal work capacity to support life and therefore must be optimally preserved. No heart has been optimally preserved for longer than about 10 hours by simple cold storage, as tested in an orthotopic transplant model, and consequently heart surgeons understandably have a sense of urgency when performing a heart transplantation.

The UW solution, or some modification of it, may be effective for preserving hearts. Recent studies have shown superior results in laboratory models of heart preservation and transplantation when the UW solution is compared with other solutions.[30] Exactly what additions or subtractions must be made to the UW solution to produce ideal heart preservation is not yet known.

Although simple cold storage is a convenient method of organ preservation, successful heart preservation may necessitate continuous perfusion, as suggested by the work of Collins and associates[31] and others. The longest successful preservation of hearts has been with continuous perfusion. Much additional work is needed to develop the optimal perfusate fluid and methods of perfusing the heart before these methods become clinically acceptable.

STATUS OF CLINICAL ORGAN PRESERVATION

Organs are preserved in the United States by simple cold storage, using either Collins' solution or the UW solution. Collins' solution is primarily used for kidneys, and the UW solution for kidneys, livers, and pancreases. Because of an increase in multi-organ donors and *in situ* vascular flushing, more organs are available now than in the past. Also, the longer preservation time provided by the UW solution allows organs to be more easily shipped between transplant centers, allows transplant surgery to be performed on an elective basis, and improves the quality of organs available for transplantation.

The main problems yet to be solved are (1) how to prevent primary nonfunction in transplanted livers and kidneys and (2) how to reduce the incidence of delayed graft function. Solutions to these problems may demand the development of a still better preservation solution and a greater understanding of the relationship between donor status and preservation quality. However, current methods of organ preservation appear satisfactory for most organs that are transplanted (except the heart, lungs, and intestine).

The goal of organ preservation research is to provide preservation of unlimited duration. This end may be accomplished only by cryopreservation (freezing), which recently has been discussed elsewhere.[31] In all probability, methods of hypothermic preservation (above freezing) have limits, but it is unlikely that those limits have been reached. The ability to preserve all organs for at least 1 week would make organ banks a reality. Organs could be transplanted on the basis of the best immunologic match and could be conveniently shipped throughout the world, and far fewer would be wasted. Long-term preservation may allow the immunoalteration of organs, reduce the recipient need for immunosuppressive drugs, and reduce the incidence of graft rejection. If livers could be preserved for longer than 1 week, they would be available for recipients who developed primary nonfunction and needed immediate retransplantation. Improved and long-term preservation will, however, necessitate an understanding of the mechanisms of tissue damage caused by hypothermic preservation. When these mechanisms are understood, a rational approach to therapeutic intervention can be defined, and better quality and long-term organ preservation will become a reality.

SELECTED REFERENCES

Cerilli, G. J. (Ed.): Organ Transplantation and Replacement. Philadelphia, J. B. Lippincott Company, 1988.
This book covers many aspects of organ transplantation. Noteworthy are two chapters, "Kidney Preservation by Perfusion" and "Kidney Preservation by Cold Storage," that discuss the current state of the art of preservation of these two organs.

Karow, A. M. Jr., and Pegg, D.E. (Eds.): Organ Preservation for Transplantation. New York, Marcel Dekker, 1981.
An excellent book that reviews many aspects of organ preservation from both a basic and clinical point of view. Chapters are written by well-known investigators in the fields of the biology of cell survival, viability analysis, hypothermia, and organ freezing; there are individual chapters on the many types of tissues, cells, and organs used in transplantation. Although about 9 years old, many of the principles discussed are current, and this book provides an excellent starting point for a review of organ preservation.

Southard, J. H.: Temperature effects and cooling. In Zelerock, G. B. (Ed.): Clinical Ischemic Syndromes: Mechanisms and Consequences of Tissue Injury. St. Louis, C. V. Mosby Company, 1989, pp. 303–326.
This article reviews the use of hypothermia in organ preservation, the mechanism of protection of cell viability during hypothermia, how hypothermia is injurious to cells, and the development of the University of Wisconsin solution for organ preservation.

REFERENCES

1. Belzer, F. O., Ashby, B. S., and Dumphy, J. E.: 24- and 72-hour preservation for transplantation: Initial perfusion and 30 hour ice storage. Lancet, 2:536, 1967.
2. Benoit, G., Moukarzel, M., Bitker, M., Bensadoun, H., Hiesse, C., Charpentier, B., Jardin, A., and Fries, D.: Intert de la solution UW dans la preservation renale en vue de transplantation. Presse Med., 27:1076, 1989.
3. Calne, R. Y.: Liver Transplantation. New York, Grune & Stratton, 1983.
4. Calne, R. Y.: Preservation of the liver. In Calne, R. Y. (Ed.): Liver Transplantation. New York, Grune & Stratton, 1983, pp. 17–24.
5. Calne, R. Y., Pegg, D. E., Pryse-Davies, J., and Leigh-Brown, F.: Renal preservation by ice cooling. Br. Med. J., 651, 1963.
6. Cecka, M. J.: Donor and preservation factors. In Terasaki, P. I. (Ed.): Clinical Transplants. Los Angeles, UCLA Tissue Typing Lab, 1989, pp. 399–408.
7. Collins, G. M., Bravo-Shugarman, M. B., and Terasaki, P. I.: Kidney preservation for transplantation: Initial perfusion and 30 hour ice storage. Lancet, 2:1219, 1969.
8. D'Alessandro, A. M., Stratta, R. J., Sollinger, H. W., Kalayoglu, M., Pirsch, J. D., and Belzer, F. O.: Use of UW solution in pancreas transplantation. Diabetes, 38(Suppl. 1):7, 1989.
9. Florack, G., Sutherland, D. E. R., Heil, J., Squifflet, J. P., and Marjarian, J. S.: Preservation of canine segmental allografts: Cold storage versus pulsatile machine perfusion. J. Surg. Res., 34:443, 1983.
10. Hernandez, L. A., and Granger, N. D.: Role of antioxidants in organ preservation and transplantation. Crit. Care Med., 16:543, 1988.
11. Jamieson, N. V., Sundberg, R., Lindell, S., Southard, J. H., and Belzer, F. O.: Preservation of the canine liver for 24–48 hours using simple cold storage with UW solution. Transplantation, 46:517, 1988.
12. Kalayoglu, M., Sollinger, H. W., Stratta, R. J., D'Alessandro, A. M., Hoffman, R. M., Pirsch, J. D., and Belzer, F. O.: Extended preservation of the liver for clinical transplantation. Lancet, 2:617, 1988.
13. Lam, F. T., Mavor, A. I. D., Potts, D. J., and Giles, G. R.: Improved 72 hour renal preservation with phosphate buffered sucrose. Transplantation, 47:767, 1989.
14. Lokkegaard, H., and Bilde, T.: Preselection and pretreatment of donor kidneys. In Marberger, M., and Dreikorn, K. (Eds.): Renal Preservation. Baltimore, Williams and Wilkins, 1983, pp. 165–176.

15. McAnulty, J. F., Ploeg, R. J., Southard, J. H., and Belzer, F. O.: Successful five day perfusion preservation of the canine kidney. Transplantation, 47:37, 1989.
16. Owens, T. C., Preuedel, A. E., and Swan, H.: Prolonged experimental occlusion of thoracic aorta during hypothermia. Arch. Surg. 70:95, 1955.
17. Pegg, D. E.: The biology of cell survival in vitro. In Karrow, A. M. Jr., and Pegg, D. E. (Eds.): Organ Preservation for Transplantation. New York, Marcel Dekker, 1981, pp. 31–52.
18. Pegg, D. E., and Green, C. J.: Renal preservation by hypothermic perfusion. 4. The use of gelatin polypeptide as the sole colloid. Cryobiology, 15:27, 1978.
19. Pegg, D. E., and Karow, A. M. Jr. (Eds.): The Biophysics of Organ Cryopreservation. Nato ASI Series, vol. 147. New York, Plenum Press, 1987.
20. Pienaar, B. H., Lindell, S. L., van Gulik, T., Southard, J. H., and Belzer, F. O.: 72 hour preservation of the canine liver by machine perfusion. Transplantation, 49:258, 1990.
21. Ploeg, R. J.: A clinical trial of the UW solution in organ preservation. Transplantation, (in press), 1990.
22. Ploeg, R. J., Goossens, D., McAnulty, J. F., Southard, J. H., and Belzer F. O.: Successful 72-hour cold storage of dog kidneys with UW solution. Transplantation, 46:191, 1988.
23. Ross, H., Marshall, V. C., and Escott, M. L.: 72-hour canine kidney preservation without continuous perfusion. Transplantation, 21:498, 1978.
24. Schrier, R. W., Arnoud, P. F., Van Putten, V. J., and Burke, T. J.: Cellular calcium in ischemic acute renal failure: Role of carcinoma entry blockers. Kidney Int., 82:313, 1987.
25. Todo, S., Nery, J., Yanaga, K., Podesta, R., Gordon, R., and Starzl, T. E.: Extended preservation of human liver grafts with UW solution. J.A.M.A., 261:711, 1989.
26. Toledo-Pereyra, L. H., Condie, R. M., Malmberg, R., Simmons, R. L., and Najarian, J. S.: A fibrinogen-free perfusate for preservation of kidneys for one hundred and twenty hours. Surg. Gynecol. Obstet., 138:901, 1974.
27. Wahlberg, J. A., Love, R., Landegaard, L., Southard, J. H., and Belzer, F. O.: 72-hour preservation of the canine pancreas. Transplantation, 43:5, 1987.
28. Wahlberg, J. A., Southard, J. H., and Belzer, F. O.: Development of a cold storage solution for pancreas preservation. Cryobiology, 23:477, 1986.
29. Weiss, S. J., and LoBuglio, A. F.: Phagocyte-generated oxygen metabolites and cellular injury. Lab. Invest., 47:5, 1982.
30. Wicomb, W. N., Collins, G. M., Wood, J. and Hill, J. D.: Improved cardioplegia using new perfusates. Transplant. Proc., 21:1357, 1989.
31. Wicomb, W. N., Hill, J. D., Avery, J., and Collins, G. M.: Comparison of cardioplegic and UW solutions for short-term rabbit heart preservation. Transplantation, 47:733, 1989.
32. Zucker, P. F., Bloom, A. D., Strasser, S., and Alyandro, R.: Successful cold storage preservation of canine pancreas with UW-solution prior to islet isolation. Transplantation, 48:168, 1989.

VIII

LIVER TRANSPLANTATION

Thomas E. Starzl, M.D., Ph.D., Robert D. Gordon, M.D.,
Andreas G. Tzakis, M.D., and Satoru Todo, M.D.

The liver has a far more complicated metabolism than other transplanted organs and malfunction leads to more complex physiologic derangements. Patients with liver disease are further handicapped by the lack of satisfactory means of artificial support comparable to renal dialysis. The transplanted liver must function efficiently from the time of anastomosis, or the patient may be lost. Despite these and other difficulties, the therapeutic power and appeal of liver transplantation has had a pervasive impact on hepatology and liver surgery. Today, it is difficult to envision a hepatology center without the capability for transplantation. Almost all victims of nonneoplastic chronic liver disease can at least be considered for liver transplantation, and even some of those with malignant hepatic tumors may be benefited. Acute liver disease was rarely suggested as a reason to consider liver transplantation until the mid 1980s, but now the rescue by this means of patients with fulminant hepatitis is common. Human survival of more than 20 years after liver transplantation has been achieved.

There are two general approaches to transplantation of the liver. With the first method, the host liver is removed and replaced with a homograft (orthotopic transplantation) (Fig. 1). The alternative technique is the insertion of an extra liver (auxiliary homotransplantation) at an ectopic site (Fig. 2). Both procedures were developed in dogs and later studied in other species, including rats, pigs, monkeys, and humans. The most encouraging results have been with orthotopic transplantation, for which reason this chapter is concerned primarily with this replacement operation. However, long survival has also been accomplished with auxiliary hepatic transplantation, and this option is briefly considered in a special section.

IMMUNOLOGIC CONSIDERATIONS

Is the liver a privileged graft? When liver replacement was first successfully performed in dogs, immunosuppression was discontinued after 4 months. A surprising number of animals continued to thrive either with no signs of rejection or with remittent rejection episodes.[9] One such dog lived in the authors' laboratory for more than 11 years after transplantation. The phenomenon of "graft acceptance" has been noted in dogs with renal transplants, although less frequently. The apparently immunologic advantage of the liver has been more clearly noted in pigs, some of which can survive chronically with no immunosuppressive therapy, despite the fact that the pigs regularly reject skin and kidney grafts.

In later years, numerous studies in inbred rats with known

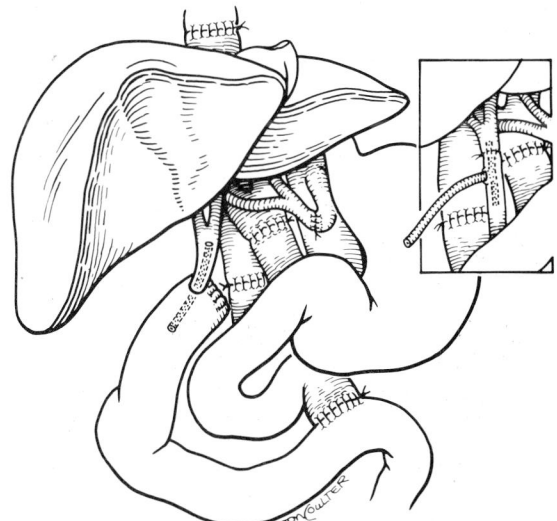

Figure 1. Orthotopic liver transplantation (liver replacement). Biliary tract reconstruction is usually done with choledochojejunostomy (to a Roux limb) or (inset) with a choledochocholedochostomy, which is stented with a T-tube. (From Starzl, T. E., Demetris, A. J., and Van Thiel, D. H.: Medical progress: Liver transplantation. N. Engl. J. Med., 321:1014, 1989.)

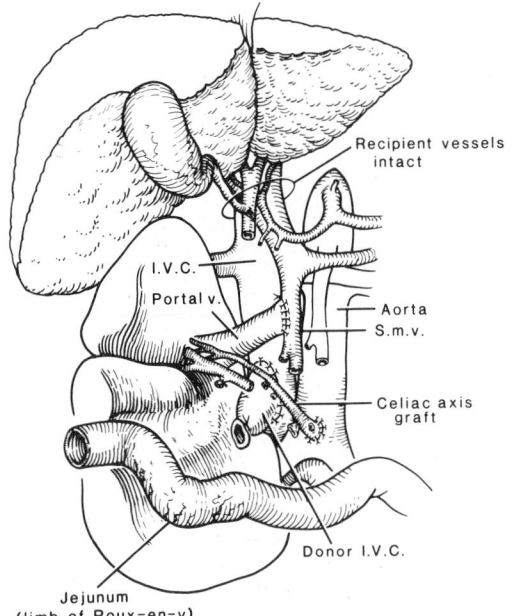

Figure 2. Auxiliary liver transplantation with a technique that provided an adequate blood supply for the homograft. Note that the transplant is given a double blood supply and that the venous component is from the nonhepatic splanchnic bed. Biliary drainage can be with a Roux-en-Y cholecystojejunostomy.

histocompatibility barriers have confirmed that the liver is more resistant to rejection than any other major organ. Permanent acceptance can be routinely induced in rats across major histocompatibility barriers with only 3 or 4 injections of immunosuppressive drugs during the early postoperative period.[8] Nearly a year later, the recipient animals retain an intact immunologic apparatus including the ability to vigorously reject skin from the original donor species. This kind of graft acceptance of hearts, kidneys, and other organs is much more difficult to achieve.

Another important advantage of the liver is resistance to antibody-mediated (humoral) rejection. Whereas kidneys and hearts usually are destroyed by hyperacute rejection in patients whose serum contains cytotoxic antibodies of the IgG class which are directed against HLA and other antigens in the donor, livers are spared this fate in most cases. The pathogenesis of hyperacute rejection includes obstruction of the microvasculature of nonhepatic grafts with clotting products and formed blood elements. This process usually does not occur in liver grafts, and what can be expected clinically is an unusually vigorous cellular rejection that can be treated with aggressive conventional immunosuppression. The practical implication is that a negative cytotoxic crossmatch that is a necessary condition for transplantation of other organs is not required for successful liver transplantation. Moreover, it has been established that the liver can provide a protective screen for otherwise vulnerable kidneys in highly sensitized recipients who need both a liver and a kidney. In such patients who receive a liver first, the titer of antidonor antibodies is drastically reduced during the first few hours after hepatic revascularization, making it possible then to insert a kidney from the liver donor without peril.[3]

The reasons the liver has these advantages are not understood. Whatever the explanation, overstatement of the case for the liver's privileged status could lead to erroneous conclusions about the practical requirements for immunosuppressive therapy following hepatic transplantation in man. In humans, control of hepatic rejection may be difficult or impossible despite very heavy immunosuppressive therapy.[10] When routine biopsies are obtained in patients after orthotopic liver transplantation, histopathologic evidence of rejection can be found in more than two thirds of patients. Effective management of this complication is the key to successful transplantation.

REJECTION REVERSAL

Rather than being unique, it is probable that liver homografts differ from other organs only by the degree of the host immunologic response they evoke. This has been demonstrated with genetically standardized inbred rat strains, and exceptionally clearly in mouse models in which knowledge of the major histocompatibility complex is even more complete. In this context, two key observations initially made with kidneys have been extended to the liver. The first is the reversibility of rejection. Reversal usually requires intensification of treatment, but it has sometimes been noted without any change in the pre-existing therapy, which suggests that such recoveries had an element of spontaneity. Long survival has been achieved in many, and possibly even most, patients without complete control of rejection. The grafts of such patients develop characteristic lesions of the intrahepatic portal triads in which the small bile ducts appear to be selectively and progressively damaged. Small numbers of lymphocytes are found in the vicinity of, or lifting up and destroying, ductal epithelial cells. This leads to the "disappearing bile duct syndrome." Studies of the antigenicity of the ducts and other constituents of liver grafts have demonstrated changing expression of Class 2 HLA antigens during rejection and have demonstrated that the areas of greatest injury are in vessels and ducts where dendritic cells of the macrophage system are heavily concentrated. These dendritic cells are important for efficient antigen presentation. The practical consequence is that patients with slowly rejecting liver grafts can have intrahepatic biliary obstruction (with jaundice), arteriopathy, and even graft cirrhosis while retaining good synthetic and other functions of the hepatocytes.[9,10] Such patients eventually become prime candidates for late retransplantation.

GRAFT ACCEPTANCE

The second observation of overriding practical and theoretic interest concerns what has already been referred to as graft acceptance. In many of the human kidney and liver recipients treated years ago, it was demonstrated that disappearance of host resistance to the homograft occurred surprisingly early after transplantation, sometimes following an acute rejection crisis. This was manifested by eventual declines in the doses of immunosuppressive agents necessary to retain stable graft function. In many patients, the level of chronic immunosuppression has proved to be less than that which at the outset failed to prevent the onset of a severe rejection. The ultimate step of cessation of all treatment has been too dangerous to attempt deliberately, but at least a dozen of the authors' liver recipients have for religious, noncompliance, or other reasons discontinued all therapy 5 to 10 years ago or longer with no subsequent problems.

The degree to which graft acceptance develops is a prime determinant of the long-term prognosis. More than one immunologic pathway may be involved.[8,9] One possibility is that there is a selective loss of responsiveness to antigens. It might be envisioned that specific lymphocyte clones, induced to replicate by the graft antigens, are thereby rendered more vulnerable to the killing effect of immunosuppressive agents than the remainder of the lymphocyte population (Fig. 3). Inasmuch as the maintenance of such activated cell lines appears to be thymus-dependent even in adult life, it is reasonable to be curious about the effect of thymectomy as an adjuvant immunosuppressive measure. The results of thymectomy in a series of the authors' human renal transplants compiled more than 25 years ago were inconclusive.

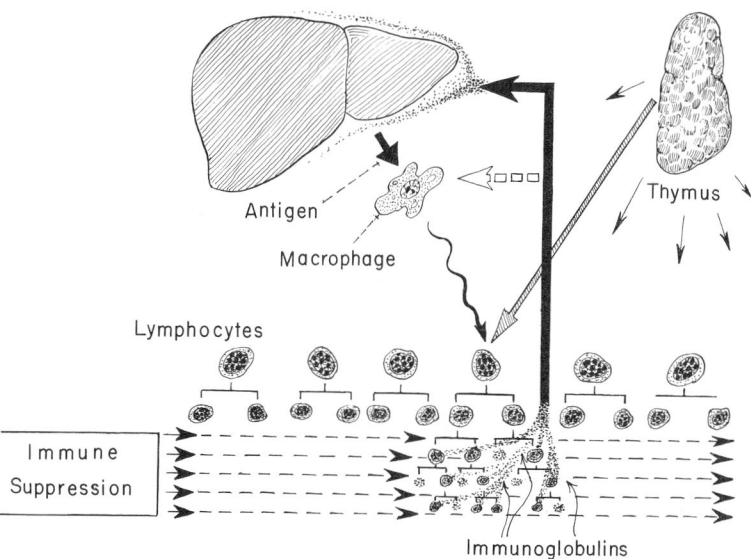

Figure 3. Hypothetical mechanisms by which nonspecific immunosuppression may lead to selective abrogation of the host immune response. Special susceptibility to these agents of a fraction of the lymphoid population could lead to exhaustion of a clone and, therefore, tolerance. Because maintenance of such cell lines even in adult life is apparently thymic-dependent in experimental animals, thymectomy would be expected to aid the process; this appears to be true in rodents, but such an effect of thymus removal has not been proved in dogs or humans. A possible protective role of immunoglobulins elaborated by the replicating cells is also demonstrated.

The concept of specific, differential tolerance through "clone stripping" can partially explain the characteristic cycle of rejection and reversal occurring after whole organ transplantation both in treated animals and in man as well as the weak and self-resolving crises in the untreated pig. Moreover, it is consistent with the fact that a wide variety of agents that are capable of general immunologic crippling can also provide specificity of action under the stipulated conditions of immunosuppressive treatment during presence of the antigen. However, classic immunologic tolerance cannot be demonstrated in most patients who have chronically functioning whole organ grafts.

These findings do not disprove tolerance through clonal deletion so much as they suggest that other mechanisms can be contributory. One mechanism, termed *passive enhancement,* has been envisioned as a process in which immunoglobins synthesized by the activated lymphoid tissues circulate to the target tissue and coat or protect it in some way that is not yet understood (see Fig. 3). The even more ambiguous term *active enhancement* describes a hypothesis that antibodies cause a central donor specific immunosuppression of the recipient immune apparatus.

During the last decade, techniques have been developed which allow the detailed identification of cells, cytokines, and other components of the immune response. When these methods were used in the study of rats that bore permanently accepted liver grafts almost a year after discontinuing all immunosuppression, the findings were surprising.[8] There were no alterations of lymphocyte subset distribution, no changes in suppressor cells, and no qualitative changes in anti-donor alloreactivity as measured *in vitro* with mixed lymphocyte culture techniques and *in vivo* by skin grafting from the donor species. There also was evidence of low level graft-versus-host activity, which presumably came from "carrier lymphocytes" still viable in the liver grafts. It was as if a symbiotic relationship had been established between the host and the graft, each without hazard to the other. This was not classic tolerance.

The hypothesis shown in Figure 3 is multifactorial. The observations cited above leave open the possibility of changes in the graft itself or functions that it performs that decrease its vulnerability to rejection. In humans, the macrophage (Kupffer) system is replaced entirely by differentiating host monocytes within 100 days after transplantation, an alteration that does not occur in the vascular endothelial cells or hepatocytes.[9] In addition, the liver graft permanently secretes significant amounts of soluble donor HLA antigens, enough to confer new HLA types to the recipient.[1] The role of these events in promoting graft acceptance is speculative.

TISSUE TYPING

ABO blood types of donor and recipient ideally should be the same; failing this, they should be compatible (example: O to A). In kidney transplantation, standard HLA typing has not been a precise method of selecting biologically suitable cadaveric donors. Even if these techniques were more reliable as an instrument of donor selection, it is unlikely that seeking well-matched livers would be possible. The need for transplantation has been so pressing in appropriate candidates that it often has been obligatory to proceed with the first available organ. Thus, most of the matches for liver transplantation worldwide have been poor ones. Puzzling reports have been published from two large centers (Pittsburgh and Cambridge) that survival after liver transplantation is actually inversely related to the quality of HLA matching.[10] This would be such a violation of an important biologic principle that much verifying data are required before indulging in speculation about what may prove to be a sampling error.

PROCUREMENT AND PRESERVATION OF ORGANS

In contrast to typing, the procurement of a fresh, functioning, nonischemic liver is of paramount advantage. Unquestionably, one of the most important advances that has been made in transplantation has been social in nature, i.e., acceptance by the public of the concept of cadaveric organ removal. The interval of normothermic ischemic injury was nearly eliminated, since the organ usually could be dissected free in the presence of an intact and effective circulation. Suitable donors usually are victims of head trauma or of asphyxia that has caused brain death.

During the last few years, the need for the procurement of multiple organs from the same donor has sharply increased. Exclusive of the pancreas, the most common combinations have been kidneys and liver; kidneys, liver, and heart; and kidneys and heart, in that order. Techniques have been developed that permit such removal without jeopardy to any of the individual grafts. The guiding principle is avoidance of warm ischemia in all organs. This is achieved by carefully timed and controlled *in situ* infusion of cold solutions into anatomic regions, the limits of which are defined by preliminary dissection.[12]

Until late 1987, the safe outer limit for human liver preservation was set at 6 or 8 hours. The Cambridge-King's College team in England and many European teams had used a plasma solution for cold infusion of the homografts. The alternative was a preservation fluid (Collin's solution) with a composition similar to that found in cells. In dogs, the two approaches yielded comparable results. These techniques permitted the shipment of livers from city to city. It was learned that excessive ischemia or bile left within the ducts could cause autolysis and facilitated delayed mucosal sloughing and cast formation.

The situation was dramatically improved with the introduction by Belzer, Jamieson, and Kalayoglu of the University of Wisconsin (UW) solution.[4,6] Although this solution has more than a dozen constituents, the essential ingredients are thought to be two sugars, lactobionate and raffinose, which are impermeants that prevent water imbibition by the cells. In addition to protecting the hepatocytes, there is much evidence that the microvasculature also is benefited. After perfusion with UW solution, cadaveric human livers can be stored safely for at least 18 hours. Beyond this time, there is a slowly increasing incidence of primary nonfunction, which reaches unacceptable levels after 24 hours.[16]

The gains in the effectiveness of organ procurement and distribution made possible by the UW solution have been large. All parts of North America have been placed within the range of all others. Even intercontinental sharing is now practical although infrequently practiced. Even with short periods of preservation, the quality of grafts is better when they are preserved with the UW solution versus the Collin's solutions, and the incidence of hepatic artery thrombosis is reduced. The UW solution is thought to be a generic advance applicable to all solid organs.

The next step in liver preservation probably is continuous perfusion techniques, using either blood or asanguineous fluids. This approach was demonstrated to be feasible more than 20 years ago, but the equipment was too cumbersome to be practical.

SURGICAL TECHNIQUES OF ORTHOTOPIC TRANSPLANTATION

THE BYPASS QUESTION. With removal of the host liver, it is necessary to temporarily cross-clamp the great veins draining the intestines (portal vein) and the lower half of the body (inferior vena cava). Dogs die promptly if the distal venous pools are not decompressed. In contrast, humans with liver disease often have tolerated this venous obstruction surprisingly well. The tolerance to portal and inferior vena caval cross-clamping was explained by man's inherently richer network of potential collateral channels for the return of blood to the right heart and by the presumed increase in the size and ramifications of these veins in consequence of the underlying liver disease. The authors were able to develop liver transplantation to an acceptable service level without decompressing the obstructed venous systems, and some surgeons continue to believe that this expedient usually is unnecessary.

However, the fact that most patients can recover from portal and inferior vena caval cross-clamping created a false impression about the safety of this practice. Venous hypertension of the obstructed venous beds contributes significantly to the bleeding of the anhepatic phase. Usually, there is gross swelling of the intestine during the period of occlusion. Subsequently, many patients suffer from third space fluid sequestration and postoperative renal failure.

The extent to which these complex physiologic events can contribute to the high perioperative mortality has become increasingly evident. The authors now perform venous bypasses in all adults and in most children weighing more than 15 kg. Cannulas are placed into the inferior vena cava through an iliac or femoral vein and into the portal system through the open end of the transected portal vein. During the anhepatic phase, the blood is pumped to a large vein in the neck or arm with equipment that does not require total body heparinization (Fig. 4).

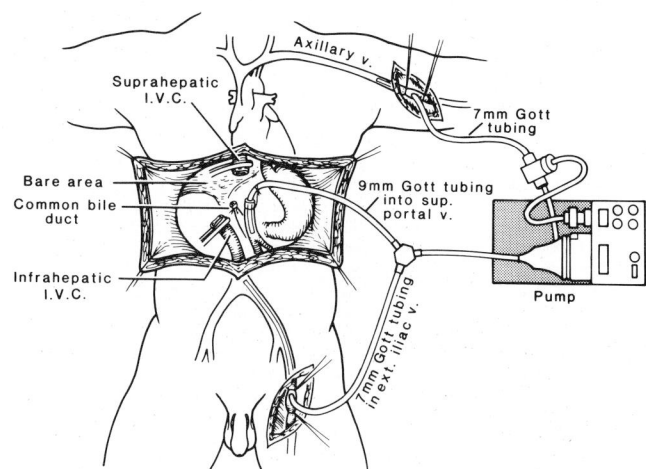

Figure 4. Venovenous bypass developed for use during the anhepatic phase of liver transplantation during which the new liver is connected to recipient vessels. By using coagulation-resistant tubing and an atraumatic pump, it has been possible to bypass large volumes of blood without using any heparin. The venovenous bypass has a revolutionary effect on the ease of liver transplantation in adults. (From Griffith, B. P., Shaw, B. W., Jr., Hardesty, R. L., et al.: Veno-venous bypass without systemic anticoagulation for transplantation of the human liver. Surg. Gynecol. Obstet., *160*:270, 1985.)

The safety of liver transplantation in adults has been greatly improved with this technique.

HEMORRHAGE

Other problems during and after operation may be caused by derangements in the coagulation mechanism, which may lead to hemorrhage or thrombosis. The nature of the underlying hepatic pathologic process produces portal hypertension in nearly every patient, and the nature of the operation tends to exaggerate it if bypasses are not used. The usual consequence is mechanical bleeding that in some cases can assume formidable proportions during the procedure. Many of the normal coagulation factors that might help control hemorrhage are dependent on the liver and are therefore defective. In addition, fibrinolysis can cause or complicate the coagulopathy in many cases. If the homograft does not function properly, hemostasis may be impossible to achieve.

When hemorrhage occurs, the surgeon's challenge is to use all available hemostatic tactics — ligatures, sutures, and cautery — until the revascularized homograft can participate in what is hoped is appropriate coagulation function. If hemorrhage cannot be controlled, fresh frozen plasma, platelets, and antithrombolytic agents such as ε-aminocaproic acid (EACA) may be required. With earlier patients, whose homografts were often of less than optimal quality, an attempt was made to treat bleeding problems by administering massive amounts of thrombogenic agents. However, hypercoagulability was caused in some instances with consequent thrombosis of the graft vessels. Ironically, the better the condition of the recipient and of the grafts, the greater the risk of unwanted coagulation if clot promoting therapy is used. Almost every series of liver transplants has had examples of thrombosis. Effective management of coagulation has been a special contribution of the anesthesiologists.[7]

AIR EMBOLI AND NEUROLOGIC DAMAGE

Eventually lethal neurologic invalidism was observed in 9 of the first 98 patients undergoing liver replacement. The complications occurred during or shortly after operation. Several of these patients awakened from anesthesia but then had a secondary decrease in consciousness, seizures, and other crippling abnormalities, including brain stem syndromes such as akinetic mutism. They died within a few days to 2 months. It ultimately was realized that air emboli from the homografts were responsible for some, although not all, of these cerebral or brain stem catastrophes.[13] The ease with which air passed to the systemic circulation was explicable by the right-to-left venous-arterial shunts that are common in chronic liver disease. Air released into the pulmonary circulation apparently passed through these collaterals to the systemic circulation, including the arterial supply to the brain.

With the delineation of this cause for the neurologic complications, measures were instituted to prevent it. During revascularization of the liver, electrolyte solution was slowly infused through a portal vein cannula. While the vena caval anastomoses were performed, air bubbles could escape from the graft vessels before a blood supply was restored (Fig. 5). Since the institution of this simple preventive measure, the incidence of neurologic complications has been reduced.

However, despite all efforts, neurologic complications can destroy an apparently perfect liver transplantation because of pre-existing abnormalities in the brain that can be the basis for perioperative or postoperative tragedies. Pathologic changes can almost always be found in the central nervous system of nontransplant patients who die of chronic liver disease. These include Alzheimer (proliferative) changes in the glial tissue, depletion of the myelin in the pons (central pontine myelinolysis) or elsewhere in the brain stem or higher brain (extrapontine myelinolysis), cortical atrophy, and edema. Alzheimer changes and central pontine myelinolysis can be produced reliably in rats and subhuman primates by portacaval shunt even though the animals appear well clinically. More recently, a role of perioperative hypernatremia in aggravating such lesions has been suggested.

VASCULAR ANOMALIES

In planning liver transplantation, the surgeon must be prepared for a high incidence of anatomic variations in either the graft or the host structures. These have been encountered in almost 40 per cent of the authors' patients. Multiple arteries have been the most frequent anomalies. If these are in the donor, the guiding principle is to convert these by back table anastomoses to a single vessel for anastomosis to a single recipient vessel (Fig. 6). If there are multiple recipient vessels, it may be possible to dissect back to a common trunk, or even to the celiac axis, for an anastomotic site. However, the best solution may be to place a donor iliac graft, which should always be brought back with the liver, from the infrarenal recipient aorta into the hilum (Fig. 7).

Thrombosis of the portal vein was formerly thought to be a contraindication to orthotopic liver transplantation. All that is necessary in such cases is to find an open segment in the superior mesenteric vein and to interpose a segment of donor iliac vein into the hilum. The vein graft is passed anterior to the pancreas and beneath the pylorus (Fig. 8). Retrieving a liver without the iliac artery and vein grafts may be responsible for the recipient's death, since the need for these vascular grafts is sometimes completely unexpected.

BILIARY TRACT PROBLEMS

Obstruction or bile fistula formation leads to repeated bacterial contamination, with resulting cholangitis and consequent systemic infection. An acceptable method of biliary reconstruction is choledochocholedochostomy, using a T-tube stent (see Fig. 1, inset) that is left in place for about 2 months. After the T-tube is removed, periodic retrograde cholangiography via the duodenum can be performed in such recipients.

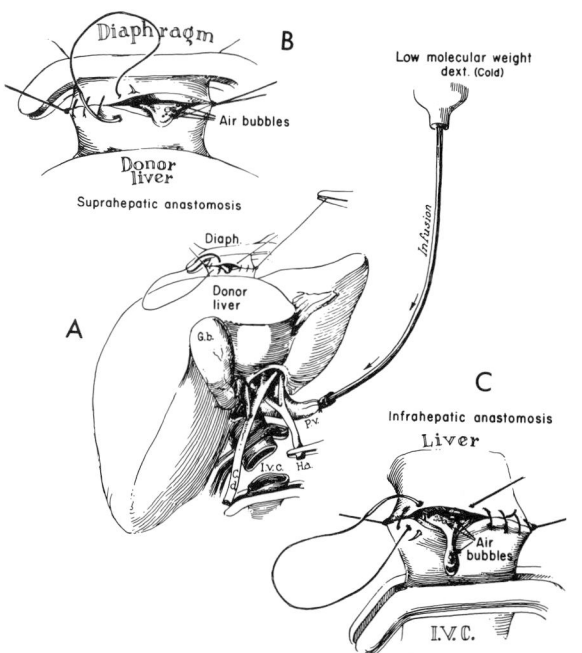

Figure 5. Technique to prevent air embolism from orthotopic liver homografts. *A*, Continuous perfusion of solution through the portal vein as vena caval anastomoses are constructed. *B* and *C*, Escape of air bubbles as the anastomoses are completed. (From Starzl, T. E., et al.: Acute neurological complications after liver transplantation with particular reference to intraoperative air embolus. Ann. Surg., *187*:236, 1978.)

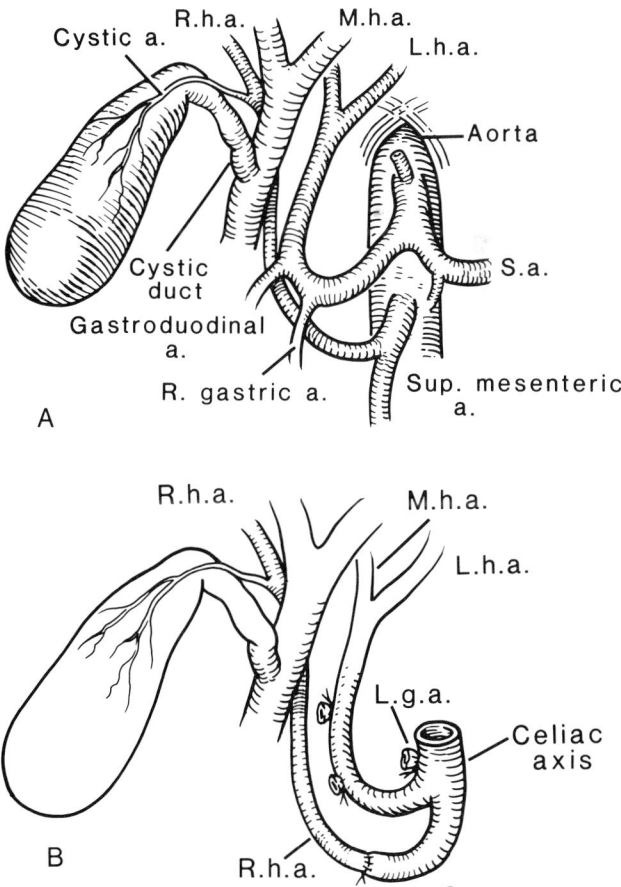

Figure 6. *A*, A common anomaly in which a right hepatic artery originates from the superior mesenteric artery. This right artery always is posterior to the portal vein. *B*, With the anomaly shown in *A*, the splenic artery can be anastomosed to the anomalous right hepatic artery, thereby converting the origin of the blood supply to a single vessel based on the celiac axis.

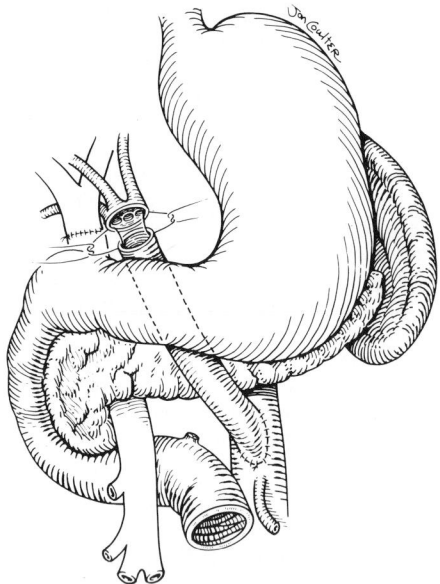

Figure 7. An antepancreatic route for a vascular graft placed onto the infrarenal abdominal aorta. The graft is brought either to the right or left of the middle colic vessels, anterior to the pancreas, and beneath the pylorus. Note the homograft anomaly in which a right, middle and left hepatic artery arise separately from the donor aorta. All three vessels were included in a Carrel patch, which was anastomosed as a cap onto the end of the iliac artery graft. (From Tzakis, A. G., Todo, S., and Starzl, T. E.: The arterial route for arterial graft in liver transplantation. Transpl. Int., 2:121, 1989.)

Choledochocholedochostomy often is not feasible, as for example in children with biliary atresia. Choledochojejunostomy (Fig. 1) to a Roux limb of jejunum is a highly satisfactory option and should be chosen if there is the slightest question about the quality of duct-to-duct repair.

With the simple techniques demonstrated in Figure 1, the descriptive term *Achilles heel of liver transplantation*, which formerly was applied to biliary tract reconstruction, no longer pertains. Nevertheless, the possibility of duct obstruction must be entertained in the postoperative management of liver trans-

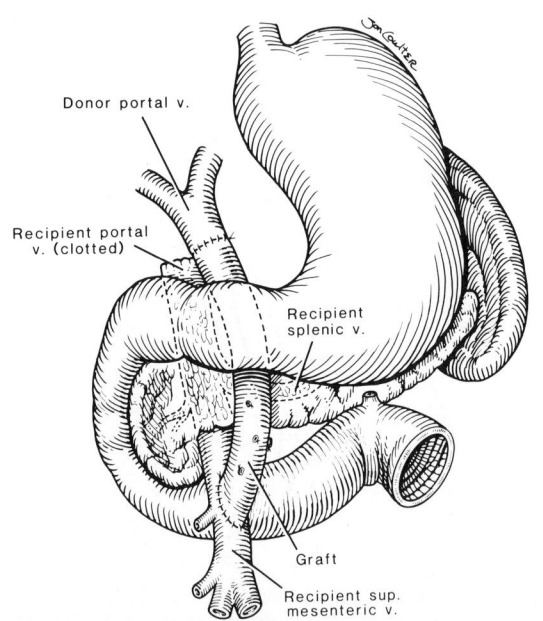

Figure 8. The use of antepancreatic iliac vein graft from the superior mesenteric vein circumvents portal vein thrombosis as a contraindication to transplantation, providing a good superior mesenteric vein is still open. (From Tzakis, A. G., Todo, S., Stieber, A., and Starzl, T. E.: Venous jump grafts in patients with portal vein thrombosis. Transplantation, 48:530, 1989.)

plantation whatever the method of reconstruction. Until the last few years, postoperative hepatic dysfunction was too readily ascribed to rejection, when, in fact, obstruction or cholangitis, or both, was frequently responsible. Even in the absence of a biliary tract problem, rejection may not be responsible. Hepatitis associated with hepatitis B surface antigen (HBsAg), cytomegalovirus (CMV), C virus, and other viruses has been observed as well as drug toxicity.[10] At the present time, the development of jaundice after transplantation is a signal for cholangiography and usually for liver biopsy. The histopathologic findings in the biopsy tissue may not provide an unequivocal answer. Then, the diagnosis of rejection must be made by exclusion.

ANESTHESIA

During operation there are metabolic abnormalities other than those concerned with coagulation that contribute to the complexity of anesthetic management. Not only is the procedure long and difficult, but, even more important, it is an operation on the primary organ involved in the metabolism and detoxification of most common anesthetics. At any point during the operation, the liver is inherently impaired, absent, or untried in its new setting. Therefore, the task of the anesthesiologist is to correctly administer pharmacologic agents that, first, are not hepatotoxic and, second, do not depend primarily on the liver for their degradation. In the authors' early cases, reliance was placed primarily on combinations of volatile agents in nonexplosive concentrations. Such management permitted use of electrocautery, gave flexibility in lightening or deepening anesthesia, and allowed anesthesia to be abruptly discontinued if required by changing physiologic circumstances. Recently, less effort has been made to use volatile anesthetics.

IMMUNOSUPPRESSION

The immunosuppressive regimens used and the year of their first clinical applications are summarized in Table 1. The movement through the years was toward increasing specificity of the immunologic target, culminating in the introduction of cyclosporine. The use of cyclosporine with steroids, and later the use of these two drugs with azathioprine and antilymphoid globulins, had an immediate impact on the transplantation of all organs, but especially of the liver.[5] The 1-year patient survival, which had been approximately 35 per cent before 1980, doubled (Fig. 9) or, in the case of low-risk patients, nearly tripled.

During the 1980s transplantation developed as a highly defined multidisciplinary special branch of medicine. In addition to the impetus provided by cyclosporine, the improvements in organ storage and the establishment of organ distribution systems that linked all parts of the United States and Canada were crucial pragmatic improvements.

Collateral developments in an understanding of the mechanisms of rejection and better understanding of how these are effected by immunosuppression have facilitated what may be even more important advances during the next decade. Cyclosporine inhibits the activation of T lymphocytes and depresses the production and expression of multiple cytokines of which interleukin-2 and interferon-γ have been most extensively studied.[5] The cyclosporine binding site is a low-molecular-weight cytosolic protein (cyclophilin) that is probably only one of a family of binding sites that participate in a broad range of physiologic effects.

It was realized at the outset that nephrotoxicity was the principal and dose-limiting side effect of cyclosporine; even when serum creatinine remains normal, hypertension and decreases in glomerular filtration occur. The remarkable spectrum of cyclosporine's actions can be demonstrated by other side effects, including gingival hyperplasia and hirsutism. Subtle changes in carbohydrate metabolism occur. Insulin secretion by the pancreatic islets is depressed with increased peripheral insulin re-

TABLE 1. Immunosuppressive Drug Regimens Used Clinically for Whole-Organ Transplantation

Agents	Year Described and Reported	Place	Deficiencies
Azathioprine	1962	Boston	Ineffective, dangerous
Azathioprine, steroids	1963	Denver	Suboptimal
ALG as adjunct to 2	1966	Denver	High incidence of infection
Cyclophosphamide substitute for azathioprine	1970	Denver	No advantage except for patients with azathioprine toxicity
Cyclosporine	1978–1979	Cambridge	Suboptimal
Cyclosporine, steroids with or without other adjuncts*	1980	Denver	Nephrotoxicity limits dose: rejection not always controlled
Monoclonal OKT3	1981	Boston	High incidence of infection
FK 506, steroids	1989	Pittsburgh	Being evaluated

*Lymphoid depletion with thoracic duct drainage, antilymphocyte globulin (ALG), OKT3, and/or azathioprine.

sistance. Other metabolic changes caused by cyclosporine include hypercholesterolemia and hyperuricacidemia. In addition, neurotoxicity is a pervasive finding in almost all patients. Although serious neurotoxicity occurs in about 20 per cent of patients, more subtle manifestations are trembling, sensitivity to light, paresthesias, mood changes, and insomnia.

These manifold effects of cyclosporine were not completely recognized until after more than 10 years of clinical use. It was assumed that the side effects of cyclosporine were largely idiosyncratic and not related to the desired effects on the immune system. The possibility that this may be an incorrect assumption has been raised by clinical observations with another agent called FK 506, which has a molecular structure completely different from that of cyclosporine.[11] Its binding site is distinct from cyclophilin, without cross-immunoreactivity to specific monoclonal antibodies, although both drugs have a *cis-trans* peptidyl-prolyl isomerase backbone.

Weight for weight, FK 506 is 100 times or more potent than

cyclosporine. Insofar as it has been determined, its effect on the lymphocyte population and cytokines is similar to, if not identical to, that of cyclosporine. The side effects are similar to those of cyclosporine, although there are important differences. FK 506 is less nephrotoxic, does not cause hypertension, causes a decline instead of an increase in cholesterol, and does not produce gingival hyperplasia. Instead of causing hirsutism, FK 506 may even cause hair loss. Thus, these two drugs affect the same clinically significant end points, but not to the same extent and sometimes not even in the same direction.

The molecular basis for these effects is not known. An unlikely possibility is that there is immune modulation of the diverse functions that are affected. Far more likely is an effect on secondary messenger systems, including but not limited to peptidyl-prolyl isomerase, which could modulate the amount or expression of hormones and other biologically active compounds. A better understanding of such details could provide a pathway for searching for other immunosuppressive drugs.

In the meanwhile, extensive clinical trials with FK 506 have been initiated in the United States and Europe. At the University of Pittsburgh, more than 350 patients have been administered this drug for primary therapy or for the rescue of failing liver grafts under cyclosporine regimens.

COMPLICATIONS OF IMMUNOSUPPRESSION

RISKS WITH ALL ORGANS. The most obvious penalty of a depressed immune system is heightened susceptibility to infection. It has also become obvious that chronically immunosuppressed patients have an increased vulnerability to *de novo* malignancies. This complication is presumably due to failure of the depressed immunologic surveillance mechanisms to identify the tumor tissues as alien and to eliminate them or restrict their growth.

EXTRA RISKS FOR LIVER RECIPIENTS. There are some special risks for the candidate for liver transplantation. One is the fact that hepatic injury in all types of organ recipients has commonly been produced by the agents, individually or in combination, of the therapeutic regimen. In some instances, viral hepatitis, apparently made chronic by the partial immunologic invalidism of the host, has been a plausible explanation. Lethal hepatitis due to adenovirus, cytomegalovirus, and herpes simplex and herpes zoster viruses has been recorded.[10] In other patients, hepatotoxicity of the drugs was probably responsible. With liver malfunction, dose control of some of the agents may become difficult, since the liver participates in their pathways of action or degradation. These hepatic factors are obviously important in any situation requiring immunosuppression, but they have heightened significance for a traumatized liver transplanted to a new and hostile environment.

In the liver recipient, postoperative bacterial sepsis of the graft itself has proved to be a special problem, undoubtedly in

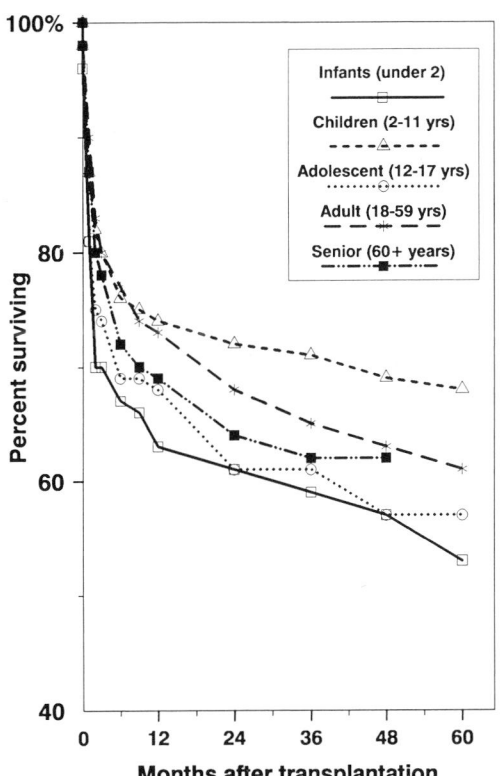

Figure 9. Actuarial (life-table method) patient survival rates for different age groups after liver transplantation under cyclosporine and low-dose prednisone. Based on 1565 patients receiving liver transplants at the University of Pittsburgh between 1981 and 1989.

part because of the anatomic location of the orthotopically placed organ interposed between the intestinal tract and the heart. Bacteria from the bowel, particularly of the gram-negative type, can be brought into contact with the transplanted liver via the intestinal veins draining into the portal vein or, far more important, by retrograde spread up the duct system after passage through the biliary anastomosis. In either event, the presence of nonviable hepatic tissues provides a perfect medium for bacterial growth. Eventually, abscesses or partial gangrene of the transplant can occur, with characteristic unvisualized areas of liver scans, gram-negative bacteremia, and all the findings of generalized sepsis.

AVOIDANCE OF HOMOGRAFT SEPSIS. Antibiotics are administered intraoperatively for the first several postoperative days. The authors' prophylactic protocol includes agents effective against gram-negative bacteria. The most important surgical technical step in reducing homograft sepsis has been to use biliary reconstructive techniques that prevent systematic contamination by gastrointestinal contents (see Fig. 1). All such efforts are futile if rejection with consequent tissue necrosis is allowed to occur. The paradox is that the immunosuppressive agents that weaken natural immune defenses against infection must be considered the foremost weapon in maintaining the tissue barrier against infection.

Until 1980, infection was the primary, or an important, contributory cause of most deaths. Moreover, the development of almost any type of intra-abdominal or intrathoracic complication could lead quickly to untreatable sepsis. The situation was dramatically improved when therapy with cyclosporine and low doses of prednisone was introduced in early 1980. The relative ease with which infections could now be controlled while preventing irreversible rejection was responsible for the improved results. In addition, the antiviral agents acyclovir and gancyclovir became available to treat or prevent infections by viruses of the herpes family, including, above all, CMV.

INDICATIONS FOR LIVER REPLACEMENT

Liver transplantation is being performed for a wide variety of indications. Under cyclosporine/steroid-based immunosuppression, over 1500 patients have received liver transplants since the program transferred from the University of Colorado to the University of Pittsburgh in 1981. High survival rates have been achieved, even in higher-risk patients such as infants and adults over the age of 60 (see Fig. 9).

INFANTS AND CHILDREN. The most common cause of conjugated hyperbilirubinemia persisting beyond the first 2 weeks of life is congenital biliary atresia, and more than half of the liver transplantations performed in infants are done for this indication. Portal decompression by portoenterostomy (Kasai operation) is possible in 20 to 30 per cent of patients but must be performed within 60 to 90 days after birth to be successful. Even with a successful Kasai operation, biliary cirrhosis is nearly certain to develop later in life. Recurrent cholangitis is the most common late complication after a Kasai operation. Although successful portoenterostomy can gain valuable time and permit growth of the patient, the possibility of making transplantation the first operation for biliary atresia has been discussed more openly in recent years now that techniques have been developed for using partial liver fragments from larger donors. If Kasai operations are used, it is important to avoid reoperation after an initial portoenterostomy, because these are usually fruitless, except for repair of minor technical faults or for relief of obstructions due to biliary stones. Multiple operations can seriously jeopardize a subsequent transplant procedure. Neonatal (giant cell) hepatitis is another important but much less common cause of persistent jaundice in infants. It is also an excellent indication for liver transplantation.

Liver transplantation in children has also been performed in patients with a wide variety of inherited inborn errors of metabolism such as alpha$_1$-antitrypsin deficiency, tyrosinemia, glycogen storage disease, Type II familial hypercholesterolemia (FH), protein-C deficiency, and some forms of hemophilia. The growing list of inborn errors which can be palliated with liver transplantation is given elsewhere.[10] The first survivor of a simultaneous heart-liver transplant was a 6-year-old child with FH who had a normal-appearing liver but had devastating coronary artery disease caused by a metabolic abnormality based in the liver. Replacement of a normal-appearing liver from this nonjaundiced child was necessary to prevent recurrence of disease in the transplanted heart.

Patients with inborn errors should undergo liver transplantation before developing irreversible sequelae such as neurologic injury (Wilson's disease, urea cycle enzyme deficiency), advanced pulmonary disease (alpha$_1$-antitrypsin deficiency), or hepatocellular cancer (tyrosinemia). In many of these disorders, the genetic defect is well understood, and cure by liver transplantation can be anticipated. For example, patients with alpha$_1$-antitrypsin deficiency assume the Pi (protease inhibitor) type of their donors and the low serum values of the deficient alpha globulin are promptly and permanently restored to normal. The abnormal amino acid pattern characteristic of tyrosinemia is almost completely rectified within hours. The same holds true for the aberrations caused by Type I glycogen storage disease (glucose-6-phosphatase deficiency), as exemplified by the ability of these patients to fast for 1 or 2 days after transplantation without the hypoglycemia that previously occurs within hours. Some of these inborn errors are known to be caused by a specific enzyme deficiency, whereas the pathogenesis of others, such as Wilson's disease, is not understood. Nevertheless, liver transplantation appears to be equally effective in the treatment of Wilson's disease, and recurrence has not been demonstrated for as long as 18 years after liver transplantation.

Other indications for liver transplantation in children have included postnecrotic cirrhosis, familial cholestasis, fulminant hepatic failure (viral or drug induced), secondary biliary cirrhosis, Budd-Chiari syndrome, and primary hepatobiliary cancers. As in adults, there is a high recurrence rate after liver transplantation for most hepatocellular or bile duct cancers. However, long-term survival has been achieved after liver transplantation for hepatoblastoma.

ADULTS. The most common indication for liver transplantation in adults is postnecrotic cirrhosis. Most of these patients have cryptogenic cirrhosis or non-A, non-B chronic aggressive hepatitis (hepatitis C). The true incidence of hepatitis C in this population is not yet known, but will become better defined in the next few years with the introduction of a specific test for detecting serum antibody to this agent. Also, it should be possible to determine the risk of reinfection with hepatitis C after liver transplantation.

In some regions of the third world, infection with the hepatitis B virus (HBV) is endemic and is the most common cause of advanced liver disease. It is also associated with an increased incidence of hepatoma. Recurrence of infection in HBsAg$^+$ patients after liver transplantation is high. More than 80 per cent of such patients remain carriers after transplantation, but the frequency and severity of reinfection is unpredictable and can be well tolerated by a significant proportion of patients. Although efforts to reduce the incidence and severity of reinfection with interferon and active and passive immunization have been disappointing, the value of transplantation has not been vitiated.

Alcoholic cirrhosis, the most common cause of chronic liver failure in Western society, has been a controversial indication for liver transplantation because of the social stigmata associated with the disease, fear of recidivism, and the poor medical condition of many of these patients. However, recent experience with a series of over 100 patients receiving liver transplants for this disease at the University of Pittsburgh has demonstrated excellent survival rates with follow-up to 4 years. Behavior modification through participation in a rehabilitation program for chemical dependency is an important part of the postoperative care of these patients.

Cholestatic liver diseases, including primary biliary cirrhosis and primary sclerosing cholangitis, are excellent indications for liver replacement. Previous surgical forays into the hepatic hilum in patients with sclerosing cholangitis can complicate eventual liver transplantation; and as a consequence, these operations are no longer employed.

Both before and after the introduction of cyclosporine, efforts were made to utilize liver transplantation for patients with primary hepatic malignancies that could not be managed by subtotal hepatic resection. Although some patients have had prolonged periods of effective palliation, recurrence of tumor within 3 to 18 months of transplantation is common and has limited the effectiveness of this approach. More radical operations, including the upper abdominal exenterations, in addition to transplantation and aggressive adjuvant chemotherapy are currently under investigation.

Fulminant hepatic failure may require emergency liver transplantation. It is unusual for patients with hepatitis A to require liver transplantation. Many patients with acute acetaminophen intoxication can recover despite alarming abnormalities of hepatocellular enzymes and prothrombin time. Approximately 40 per cent of patients with fulminant HBV infection recover with skilled medical care. However, it may be necessary to explore some of these patients with a new liver available and to determine by intraoperative biopsy of the native liver whether or not liver replacement is advisable. Fulminant non-A, non-B hepatitis has a poor prognosis, and liver transplantation is an important consideration early in the management of patients with this disease.

Regardless of etiology, the prognosis after liver transplantation for fulminant hepatic failure is influenced by renal failure, metabolic acidosis, and central nervous system deterioration. Early consultation with a liver transplant program is an important part of the modern management of the patient with fulminant hepatic failure.

As in children, there are many other conditions for which liver transplantation has been successfully performed in adults, including, but not limited to, congenital hepatic fibrosis, inborn errors of metabolism, Budd-Chiari syndrome, secondary biliary cirrhosis, massive hepatic trauma, cystic fibrosis, and polycystic liver disease.

RESULTS AND COMPLICATIONS

Improvements in operative technique and the routine use of the venovenous bypass in adults and large children have reduced intraoperative mortality to less than 1 per cent and perioperative (30-day) mortality to under 10 per cent for most groups of patients.

The life-table survival rates for major diagnostic groups after liver transplantation under cyclosporine and prednisone in 1565 patients at the University of Pittsburgh between 1981 and 1989 are summarized in Figure 10. Most of the mortality occurs within the first 6 months after transplantation. After transplantation for cholestatic liver disease, chronic active hepatitis (except HBsAg⁺), and alcoholic cirrhosis, 1-year patient survival is near 80 per cent and remains above 70 per cent or better at 5 years. Similar survival rates are seen after liver transplantation for most other causes of nonmalignant chronic liver disease.

Despite the significant risk of recurrent infection, survival at 5 years after liver transplantation for HBsAg⁺ cirrhosis is 50 per cent. Significant salvage has also been achieved for fulminant hepatic failure, and this may improve further with more aggressive referral of patients to transplant centers before irreversible

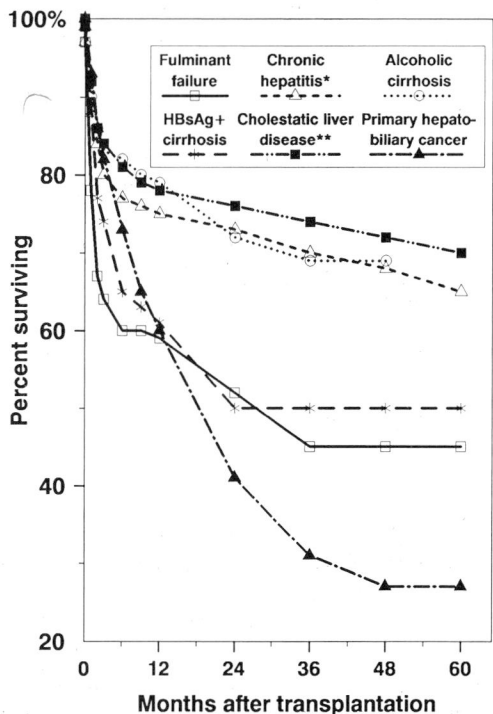

*excluding alcoholic or HBsAg+ cirrhosis
**includes primary biliary cirrhosis and
    primary sclerosing cholangitis.

Figure 10. Actuarial (life-table method) survival rates after liver transplantation for major diagnostic classes. HBsAg + cirrhosis = end stage cirrhosis in patients positive for the hepatitis B surface antigen. Based on 1565 patients receiving liver transplants at the University of Pittsburgh between 1981 and 1989.

medical complications occur. The poor long-term survival after transplantation for primary tumors reflects the high rate of recurrent disease for most tumors.

Approximately 20 per cent of patients require one or more retransplantations for primary graft nonfunction, rejection, technical complications (most often hepatic artery thrombosis), infections (viral hepatitis), or recurrent disease. Approximately 8 per cent of grafts fail to function within the first few days after transplantation. Some of these failures may be mediated by immunologic events that have yet to be completely delineated, and others are failures of preservation. Survival after retransplantation for chronic rejection is over 70 per cent. The outcome after retransplantation for technical failure or recurrent disease is dependent upon etiology.

Hepatic arterial thrombosis may cause acute hepatic gangrene; biliary tract necrosis with hepatic abscess formation; or relatively asymptomatic bacteremia, which may respond well to intravenous antibiotic therapy. Dearterialization must be suspected in any patient with fever and gram-negative sepsis or a biliary leak after liver transplantation. Because of the variable clinical presentation, not all patients require early retransplantation, and a few have not required it at all. However, the majority of patients who do not develop hepatic necrosis or abscess eventually develop intrahepatic biliary strictures that necessitate replacement of the graft.

Portal vein and vena caval thrombosis after liver transplantation are both uncommon but usually require replacement of the graft. Some patients with late portal vein thrombosis have been managed by performing distal splenorenal shunts. Biliary tract complications have been previously discussed. Ampullary dysfunction with generalized dilatation of the biliary system is the most frequent complication after duct-to-duct reconstruction over a T-tube stent. It is best treated by revision to a Roux-en-Y

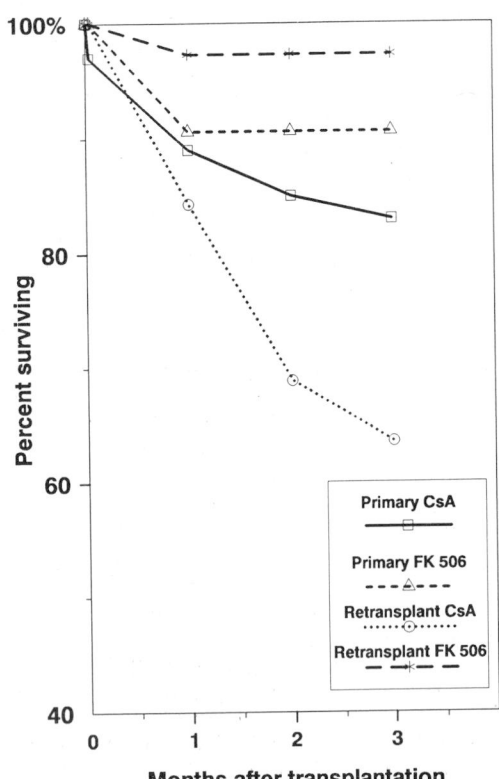

Figure 11. A comparison of early patient survival after primary liver transplantation and retransplantation under immunosuppression with cyclosporine or FK 506. The FK 506 results were in 76 patients treated during Phase 1 clinical trials of FK 506, conducted at the University of Pittsburgh during 1989, compared with the historical experience with cyclosporine from 1981 to 1989.

choledochojejunostomy, although some centers have managed this complication by endoscopic papillotomy.

The most common cause of death after liver transplantation is infection complicating immunosuppressive therapy. Sulfazoxasole-trimethoprim (Bactrim) prophylaxis has dramatically reduced the incidence of *Pneumocystis carinii* pneumonia in transplant recipients. Treatment with gancyclovir has also significantly reduced the morbidity and mortality of posttransplantation CMV infections.

With the use of FK 506, the early death rate after liver transplantation may have been influenced favorably. In Figure 11 is shown the 3-month survival after primary transplantation under FK 506/steroid treatment versus the historical record with the use of cyclosporine regimens. These hopeful but preliminary observations require extension, as well as confirmation by other workers.

AUXILIARY LIVER TRANSPLANTATION

The alternative to hepatic replacement is to leave the native liver in place and to transplant an extra liver that is in some ectopic site, such as the splenic bed, the right or left paravertebral gutter, or the pelvis. The main theoretic advantage of auxiliary transplantation is that the recipient is not at the outset placed totally at the mercy of homograft function. A second possible advantage would be avoidance of the technical hazards of recipient hepatectomy.

The provision of splanchnic venous inflow is critical for optimal graft function because this blood contains "hepatotrophic factors" of which insulin is the most important.[14] The condition of providing a splanchnic venous inflow to the auxiliary graft

has been met in almost all clinical trials, which by 1978 numbered more than 50.[2]

Auxiliary liver transplantation with real prolongation of life was first achieved at the New York Memorial Hospital on December 13, 1972.[2] The recipient, who had biliary atresia, is still alive more than 16 years later (personal communication, J. G. Fortner, April 1989). In 1980, a 29-month survival of an adult was reported from Paris. The patient, who had hepatitis B, died of a hepatocellular carcinoma in his host liver 8 years after transplantation (personal communication, H. Bismuth, January 1989).

With the increased success of orthotopic liver transplantation, interest in auxiliary transplantation waned. However, there has been a recent report of the transplantation of whole livers or liver fragments to the right paravertebral gutter of six adult recipients, by essentially the same operation as that tried earlier.[15] At the time of reporting, with follow-up of 5 to 23 months, all six recipients were alive. Cautious further trials undoubtedly can be expected.

SELECTED REFERENCES

Calne, R. Y. (Ed.): Liver Transplantation: The Cambridge-King's College Hospital Experience, 2nd ed. Orlando, Grune & Stratton, 1987, pp. 1–571.
This text is an updated account of what now is a 20-year experience with liver transplantation at Cambridge University and King's College Hospital, London. It summarizes briefly what has been accomplished in other centers as well, and annotates the wide-ranging basic and clinically oriented animal and bench research that has been a collateral theme throughout the entire time. The book provides information on the specific topic of liver transplantation that no new group can afford to ignore. More important, it provides insight into the intellectual processes of Calne, who ranks as one of the supreme surgeon-scientists of this or any era. Cyclosporine was introduced into clinical medicine by Calne, and the consequences of this major contribution can be traced through the pages of his book.

Kahan, B. D.: Cyclosporine. N. Engl. J. Med., 321:1725, 1989.
This scholarly account summarizes the world experience with cyclosporine over the first 10 years of its use. Although it is not specifically concerned with liver transplantation, all of the information is relevant. There has been no better description of the fundamental mechanisms of cyclosporine, its therapeutic powers, and its side effects.

Maddrey, W. C. (Ed.): Transplantation of the liver. New York, Elsevier, 1988, pp. 1–352.
The collection of chapters including contributions from experienced guest authors was largely an exercise of preparation for the addition of liver transplantation to the treatment armamentarium at the hepatology center at Thomas Jefferson University, Philadelphia. The perspective of the text was therefore different from the other recommended texts. The value of Maddrey's approach has been illustrated by the subsequent success of his program and its many contributions to the growth and policies of the field.

Starzl, T. E., and Demetris, A. J. (Eds.): Liver Transplantation. Chicago, Mosby–Year Book Inc., 1990, pp. 1–194.
A three-part modern day account of liver transplantation published in Current Problems in Surgery was converted to this textbook. The vast literature of the topic was summarized through the end of 1989, including the advances made possible with the UW preservation solution, and the first trials with the new immunosuppressive agent FK 506. An extensive update is included about developments in liver transplantation pathology.

Starzl, T. E., Porter, K. A., and Francavilla, A.: The Eck fistula in animals and humans. Curr. Probl. Surg., 20(11):687, 1983.
This monograph describes knowledge of the so-called hepatotrophic substances found in portal venous blood and describes the specific effects of venous blood from nonhepatic splanchnic organs in regulating liver structure and function. Hepatotropic physiology was developed as a consequence of research in auxiliary liver transplantation, and the resulting background is essential to an understanding of the physiology and vascularization requirements if auxiliary liver grafts are to be used.

Williams, J. W. (Ed.): Hepatic Transplantation. Philadelphia, W. B. Saunders Company, 1990, pp. 1–245.
In the late 1970s, Williams established at the University of Tennessee the second successful liver transplant program in the United States. He moved in 1984 to his present location at the Rush Presbyterian–St. Luke's Medical Center in Chicago. This book reflects Williams' passion for this kind of treatment, not only now when it is respectable, but at an earlier time when it was not. Williams' contributions to the field have been many, and perhaps less well recognized than their uniformly high quality and common sense merit.

REFERENCES

1. Davies, H. F. F. S., Pollard, S. G., and Calne, R. Y.: Soluble HLA antigens in the circulation of liver graft recipients. Transplantation, 47:524, 1989.
2. Fortner, J. G., Yeh, S. D. J., Kim, D. K., Shiu, M. H., and Kinne, D. W.: The case for and technique of heterotopic liver grafting. Transplant. Proc., 11:269, 1979.
3. Fung, J., Griffin, M., Duquesnoy, R., Tzakis, A., and Starzl, T.: Successful sequential liver-kidney transplantation in patients with preformed lymphocytoxic antibodies. Clin. Transplant. 1:187, 1987.
4. Jamieson, N. V., Sundberg, R., Lindell, S., Laravuso, R., Kalayoglu, M., Southard, J. H., and Belzer, F. O.: Successful 24 to 30 hour preservation of the canine liver: A preliminary report. Transplant. Proc., 20(Suppl. 1): 945, 1988.
5. Kahan, B. D.: Cyclosporine. N. Engl. J. Med., 321:1725, 1989.
6. Kalayoglu, M., Sollinger, W. H., Stratta, R. J., D'Alessandro, A. M., Hoffman, R. M., Pirsch, J. D., and Belzer, F. O.: Extended preservation of the liver for clinical transplantation. Lancet, 1:617, 1988.
7. Kang, Y. G., Martin, D. J., Marquez, J., Lewis, J. H., Bontempo, F. A., Shaw, B. W., Jr., Starzl, T. E., and Winter, P. M.: Intraoperative changes in blood coagulation and thrombelastographic monitoring liver transplantation. Anesth. Analg., 64:888, 1985.
8. Murase, N., Kim, D. G., Todo, S., Cramer, D. V., Fung, J. J., and Starzl, T. E.: FK 506 suppression of heart and liver allograft rejection II: The induction of graft acceptance in rats. Transplantation (in press).
9. Starzl, T. E. (with the assistance of C. W. Putnam): Experience in Hepatic Transplantation. Philadelphia, W. B. Saunders Company, 1969.
10. Starzl, T. E., Demetris, A. J., and Van Thiel, D. H.: Medical progress: Liver transplantation. N. Engl. J. Med., 321:1014; 1092, 1989.
11. Starzl, T. E., Fung, J. J., and Todo, S.: Contempo 90: transplantation. J.A.M.A., 263:2686–2687, 1990.
12. Starzl, T. E., Hakala, T. R., Shaw, B. W., Jr., Hardesty, R. L., Rosenthal, T. J., Griffith, B. P., Iwatsuki, S., and Bahnson, H. T.: A flexible procedure for multiple cadaveric organ procurement. Surg. Gynecol. Obstet., 158:223, 1984.
13. Starzl, T. E., Schneck, S. A., Mazzoni, G., Aldrete, J. A., Porter, K. A., Schroter, G. P. J., Koep, L. J., and Putnam, C. W.: Acute neurological complications after liver transplantation with particular reference to intraoperative cerebral air embolus. Ann. Surg., 187:236, 1978.
14. Starzl, T. E., Watanabe, K., Porter, K. A., and Putnam, C. W.: Effects of insulin, glucagon, and insulin/glucagon infusions on liver morphology and cell division after complete portacaval shunt in dogs. Lancet, 1:821, 1976.
15. Terpstra, O. T., Schalm, S. W., Weimar, W., Willemse, P. J. A., Baumgartner, D., Groenland, T. H. N., Ten Kate, P. W. J., Porte, R. J., De Rave, S., Reurers, C. B., Stibbe, J., and Terpstra, J. L.: Auxiliary partial liver transplantation for end-stage chronic liver diseases. N. Engl. J. Med., 319:1507, 1988.
16. Todo, S., Podesta, L., Ueda, Y., Imventarza, O., Casavilla, A., Oks, A., Okuda, K., Nalesnik, M., Vendataramanan, R., and Starzl, T. E.: A comparison of UW with other solutions for liver preservation in dogs. Clin. Transplant., 3:253, 1989.

IX

PANCREAS TRANSPLANTATION

Hans W. Sollinger, M.D., Ph.D., and Mark Stegall, M.D.

HISTORICAL ASPECTS

According to Erich Lexer, the first surgical step in treating Type I diabetes mellitus by transplantation of the pancreas was in 1891, 30 years before the discovery of insulin. An English surgeon, Williams, transplanted extracts of sheep pancreas into the abdominal wall of a comatose diabetic patient and his early trial demonstrates that the concept of replacing nonfunctioning islets by means of transplantation of vital endocrine tissue is a very old one. The first clinical pancreas transplant was performed by Kelly and Lillehei on December 17, 1966.[8] The type of transplant was a segmental graft transplanted to the iliac fossa with the pancreatic duct ligated. In 1973, Gliedman and associates[6] suggested for the first time the use of the urinary tract for exocrine pancreatic drainage. Merkel and colleagues[9] reported end-to-side anastomosis of the pancreatic duct to the ureter, with the belief that this would obviate the need for native nephrectomy when transplantation is performed in a non-uremic patient. In the mid 1970s the Stockholm group, headed by Groth, embarked on a larger series of enterically drained grafts.[7] A new method of handling exocrine secretions was suggested by Dubernard and associates.[5] They thought exocrine secretions could be obliterated by injecting the pancreatic duct with a polymer. In 1982, Cook and Sollinger, from the University of Wisconsin, suggested channeling of the exocrine secretions to the urinary bladder. In their initial clinical experience, the pancreatic duct of a segmental graft was sutured to the bladder mucosa. They later turned to whole pancreatic grafts, using the duodenal button technique, and, more recently, to the duodenal segment method as described by Nghiem and associates.[11] Other techniques of managing exocrine pancreatic secretions are enterically drained pancreaticoduodenal grafts, paratopic grafting with exocrine drainage into the stomach[4], and a variety of modifications of the bladder technique such as skeletonizing the pancreatic duct prior to implantation into the bladder, by the Göteborg group,[14] or implanting the entire cut edge of the pancreas end-to-side into the bladder.

INDICATIONS

The indications for transplantation of the pancreas remain controversial. It can be performed in three settings: alone in the preuremic patient; after successful kidney grafting; and simultaneously with a kidney transplant. Clearly, pancreas transplantation should be performed before the patient develops end-stage secondary complications such as advanced retinopathy leading to blindness, disabling neuropathy, end-stage nephropathy, or extensive macrovascular and microvascular disease. In the authors' view, pancreas transplantation in the preuremic patient is justified only in a setting in which careful long-term monitoring of its potential effect on secondary complications can be performed. These studies must include extensive investigation and monitoring of the progression of retinopathy and nephropathy. Transplantation of the pancreas after successful transplantation of the kidney has the advantage that the patient is already on immunosuppressive therapy. Unfortunately, the results of preuremia and sequential grafting are significantly worse than the results in combined transplantation of kidney and pancreas. For this reason, the majority of pancreas transplants in the past years have been combined transplants. In this setting, only one surgical procedure is required, and the patient receives an immunosuppressive regimen similar to that of a patient undergoing a kidney transplant alone. Absolute contraindications for pancreas transplantation are similar to the contraindications for kidney transplantation. They include the presence of malignancy and active infection. Patients with advanced cardiovascular disease, major amputations, blindness, and inability to understand the investigational nature of the procedure are excluded in the authors' program. Of major importance is the evaluation of the patient's cardiac status, because many diabetic patients, as a result of neuropathy, do not present with the classic symptoms of angina, even in the presence of advanced coronary artery disease. Therefore, preoperative evaluation requires thallium stress testing in all patients over the age of 30. If the thallium stress test is suggestive of coronary artery disease, patients must undergo coronary angiography.

DONOR SELECTION, ORGAN PROCUREMENT, AND PANCREAS PRESERVATION

Donor selection and organ procurement are of paramount importance to the success of pancreas transplantation. Age limits for donors range from 3 to 55 years. In older donors, the presence of significant atherosclerosis involving the celiac axis must be excluded. Absolute contraindications to pancreas donation include intra-abdominal contamination, acute pancreatitis, injury to the pancreas, and a history of diabetes in the donor. Donor blood glucose values and serum amylase levels do not reflect the quality of the graft. Procurement of the pancreas can be performed either as combined liver and pancreas procurement or pancreas procurement alone. Many teams in the United States now routinely perform combined liver and pancreas procurement, thus eliminating the controversy and competition between liver and pancreas transplant teams.[13] During the combined procurement of liver and pancreas, it is important that the portal vein is vented during the *in situ* flush so that the pressure in the splenic vein does not become elevated, which could lead to significant pancreatic edema (Fig. 1). After removal of both organs, the pancreas and liver are separated and prepared for transplantation. In most instances, pancreatic arterial blood supply has to be restored with an iliac artery Y graft (Fig. 2). Safe preservation times for the pancreas with either University of Wisconsin solution (Viaspan) or Minnesota SGF solution are between 20 and 30 hours. The average preservation time for pancreatic grafts at the authors' center is 18 hours.

SURGICAL ASPECTS

Since transplantation of the pancreas was first performed in December 1966, a number of technical procedures have been used, and only in the past 2 years have sufficient data been gathered on national and international level for the merits and disadvantages of these techniques to be evaluated. The pancreas can be transplanted as a whole graft, or a segment of the pancreas consisting of the tail and body can be transplanted as

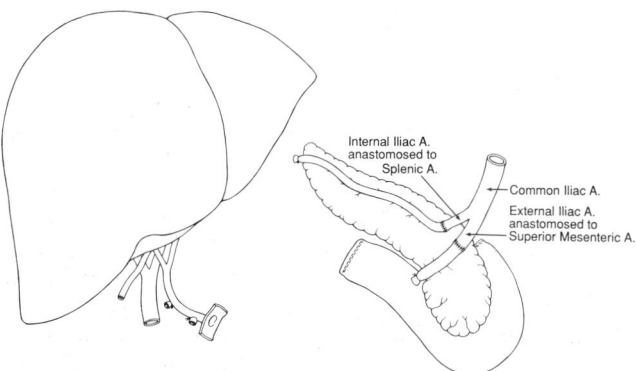

Figure 2. Reconstruction of the arterial blood supply of the pancreas after combined liver-pancreas procurement.

segmental grafts. Major controversy has surrounded the optimal management of exocrine pancreatic secretions. Possible approaches for managing the pancreatic duct include ligation of the pancreatic duct, leaving the pancreatic duct open, with drainage of exocrine pancreatic secretions into the peritoneal cavity; duct injection with polymers; enteric drainage into a Roux-en-Y loop; and anastomosis of the pancreatic duct to the bladder. When whole pancreas transplants are used, the duodenal segment can be sutured side-to-side to the bladder (Fig. 3), or side-to-side anastomosis to the small bowel can be performed. The most frequently used drainage procedures are duct injection, enteric drainage, and bladder drainage. The number of centers using bladder drainage has been increasing since 1984, while the use of enteric drainage or duct injection is declining, as demonstrated in Figure 4.

Duct injection with neoprine or prolamine has been championed by several European groups. In all cases a segmental pancreatic graft was used. Although the surgical procedure is rather simple, because no anastomosis to the draining organ is required, the results of duct injection in the leading centers have remained inferior to the best results reported for enteric drainage and bladder drainage. A leading cause of graft loss with segmental grafts using duct injection is venous thrombosis, which occurs in 15 to 20 per cent of all transplants (Table 1). In addition, fistula formation leading to peripancreatic infection is more common in grafts with duct injection than in other drainage procedures. Segmental pancreas transplantation with drainage of the pancreas into a Roux-en-Y loop was extensively used by the Stockholm group. The surgical complications of enteric segmental drainage versus bladder drainage are com-

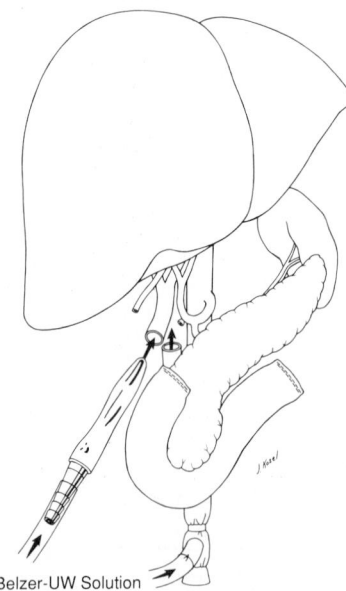

Figure 1. Technique of combined liver-pancreas procurement. The portal vein is divided before the *in situ* flush is started. This maneuver prevents pancreatic edema.

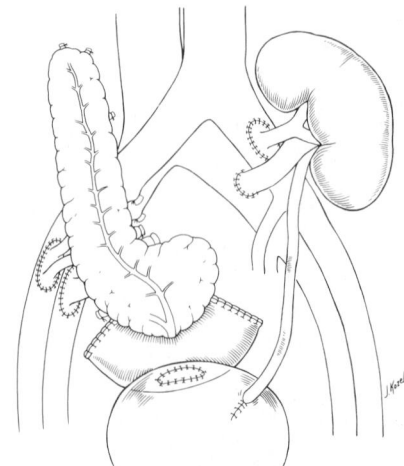

Figure 3. Pancreas transplantation with the duodenal segment technique.

Number of Centers
Duct Management Technique

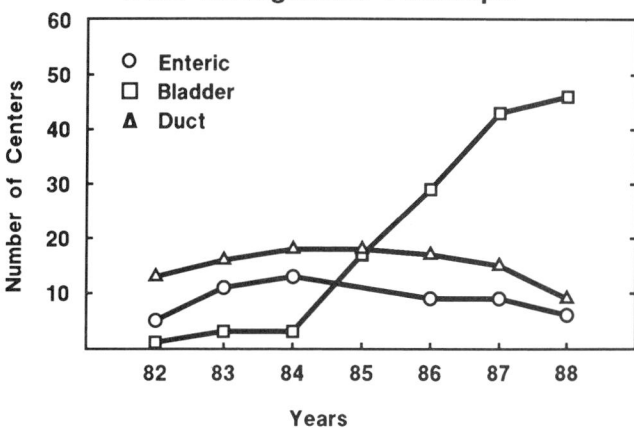

Figure 4. Number of centers using bladder drainage versus centers using enteric drainage or duct injection.

TABLE 2. Number of Patients Requiring Laparotomy After Pancreas Transplantation

Indication	Enteric Segmental n = 43 (Stockholm)	Bladder n = 55 (Madison)
Intra-abdominal infection	7 (16.2%)	1 (1.8%)
Bowel obstruction	6 (13.9%)	2 (3.6%)
Pancreatitis	5 (11.6%)	0
Leakage	4 (9.3%)	2 (3.6%)
Thrombosis	1 (2.3%)	0
Bleeding	2 (4.6%)	
Ureteral leak	0 (0%)	1 (1.8%)
Renal artery thrombosis	0 (0%)	
Negative findings	3 (6.9%)	0
Total	28 (65.1%)	6 (10.9%)

pared in Table 2, and it is obvious that the number of major surgical complications is significantly higher in the enteric segmental drainage group. Most recently, instead of a segmental graft, the whole pancreatic graft with the duodenal segment anastomosed side-to-side to the small bowel has been used for enteric drainage. Preliminary reports by the Stockholm group and the authors' experience demonstrate that this method is far safer than drainage of a segmental graft into a Roux-en-Y loop. The complication rate with the use of the whole pancreas and duodenal segment has been significantly reduced. Bladder drainage, at present the most popular technique, has the advantage of being technically simple and associated with a low infection rate. As exocrine pancreatic secretions can be determined by measuring urinary amylase, this technique has the advantage of facilitating the diagnosis of rejection, which is particularly important in sequential or isolated pancreatic grafting. The disadvantages of the bladder technique include metabolic acidosis caused by bicarbonate loss into the urine, urinary problems such as hematuria, urethral stricture, or frequent urinary tract infections, and reflux pancreatitis. Nevertheless, graft loss from technical complications with the use of bladder technique has become a rare exception at the authors' center.

DIAGNOSIS OF PANCREATIC ALLOGRAFT REJECTION

Rejection is the major cause of graft loss at present, representing approximately 40 per cent of graft failures, according to the International Pancreas Transplant Registry. The timely diagnosis and treatment of rejection currently represents a major obstacle to successful pancreas transplantation. These difficulties are due to the histologic sequence in which the rejection process occurs. Extensive studies by the Minnesota group have demonstrated that, in the initial phase of rejection, mononu-

TABLE 1. Duct Injection with Prolamine: Reasons for Graft Loss — University of Munich

Venous thrombosis	8 (15%)
Infected fistula	6 (12%)
Bleeding	1 (2%)
Rejection	8 (16%)
Death	1 (2%)

From Illner, W. D., Abendroth, D., Landgraf, R., and Land, W.: Pancreatic transplantation using the duct occlusion technique. *In* Terasaki, P. I. (Ed.): Clinical Transplants. UCLA Tissue Typing Laboratory, Los Angeles, California, 1988, pp. 65–72.

clear cell infiltration predominantly involves the acinar tissues and vasculitis may occur prior to any islet cell changes. Only in the later stages of advanced rejection has infiltration of islets and islet damage been observed. Therefore, elevation of serum glucose may occur at an already irreversible stage of rejection. Fortunately, in combined kidney-pancreas transplantation, almost in all instances renal allograft rejection and a rise in serum creatinine precedes pancreatic rejection. This setting may indeed be the most sensitive marker for pancreatic allograft rejection. Isolated rejection of a pancreas transplant without kidney rejection is a rare event. In isolated or sequential pancreatic grafting, where the kidney cannot serve as a monitor, the early diagnosis of pancreatic allograft rejection remains difficult. Urinary amylase monitoring has been demonstrated to be clinically the most useful test. This explains the superiority of urinary-drained grafts over duct-injected and enteric grafts for nonsimultaneous transplants. Other clinically useful methods include technetium-DTPA perfusion scanning. Characteristics of rejection include graft swelling, haziness of the pancreatic borders, and diminished visualization, especially in the tail of the pancreas. Ultrasound and MRI imaging have not been uniformly accepted as reliable techniques for the detection of pancreatic allograft rejection. In bladder-drained grafts, the pancreas and duodenum can be biopsied using cystoscopy; however, this requires general anesthesia and cannot be performed on a frequent basis. Percutaneous needle biopsy of the pancreas has recently been reported by Allen and associates[2] and, surprisingly, was associated with only minimal morbidity. If this experience can be confirmed by other centers in a larger series of patients, percutaneous needle biopsy might indeed become the standard for the diagnosis of pancreatic allograft rejection and the value of all other methods can be correlated with the biopsy result.

IMMUNOSUPPRESSION AND POSTOPERATIVE MANAGEMENT

Despite a diversity of immunosuppressive protocols, the results of clinical pancreas transplantation are remarkably similar. Current immunosuppressive strategies have evolved with an extrapolation of the experience gained with standard regimens in clinical renal transplantation (Table 3). Conventional immunosuppression (prednisone and azathioprine) has met with limited success in pancreas transplantation and has led to early trials of cyclosporine. Cyclosporine has been demonstrated to have modest immunosuppressive effects in an allogeneic pancreas transplant system in a number of species. However, cyclosporine is not nearly as successful in preventing rejection of pancreatic allografts as it is with other organs. The majority of North American transplant centers recently adopted the use of

TABLE 3. Immunosuppressive Protocol in Pancreas Transplantation

Days 1–14:	ALG 20 mg./kg. IV/day
	Prednisone 30 mg./day
	Cyclosporine 6–12 mg./kg./day
	Azathioprine 1–2 mg./kg./day
Days 15–60:	Prednisone 20–30 mg./day
	Cyclosporine 4–10 mg./kg./day
	Azathioprine 1–2 mg./kg./day

OKT3 may be used instead of ALG for induction therapy. Rejection episodes are treated with a steroid bolus or OKT3.

quadruple immunosuppressive therapy. This includes the administration of antilymphocyte globulin (ALG) for 7 to 14 days after transplantation; and maintenance therapy includes cyclosporine, prednisone, and azathioprine. In a recent trial at the authors' institution, substitution of OKT3 for antilymphocyte globulin in the induction period demonstrated no difference in 1- and 2-year graft survival; however, a higher incidence of viral infections was noted in the OKT3 group. Rejection episodes were slightly more frequent in the ALG induction group; however, more than 95 per cent of all rejection episodes can be successfully reversed with high-dose steroids, ALG, or OKT3 retreatment.

The general guidelines for the postoperative management of the recipient of a pancreas or combined pancreas-kidney transplant follow the rules established in kidney transplantation. However, two considerations specific for pancreas transplant recipients must be considered. As pancreas transplant recipients have a high thrombosis rate, many centers prefer to use anticoagulation, with either heparin or a combination of heparin and dextran. In the authors' experience, this regimen has not been found useful in preventing pancreatic allograft thrombosis and, in addition, has led to a significantly higher incidence of postoperative bleeding episodes. Antibiotic coverage after pancreas transplantation must be broad-spectrum, for aerobic, anaerobic, and fungal organisms. In whole pancreas transplantation with the duodenal segment, the content of the duodenal segment is cultured at the time of transplantation, and antibiotics are adjusted on the basis of culture result.

An infrequent but potentially fatal complication is the rapid development of adult respiratory distress syndrome after pancreas transplantation. This might be the result of preservation-induced pancreatitis, and patients experiencing this syndrome usually require intubation and maintainence on mechanical ventilation. Unfortunately, pulmonary damage is frequently extensive, and superimposed infections contribute greatly to long-term morbidity or patient death. If this syndrome occurs, consideration should be given to the immediate removal of the pancreas transplant.

Peripancreatic fluid collections as visualized by ultrasonography and computed tomographic scan are frequent and need only be addressed if there is a suspicion of infection. Fine-needle aspiration of the fluid collections and culture of the fluid aid in making the diagnosis. If a peripancreatic abscess is diagnosed, catheter drainage or open drainage should be performed. Constant awareness of the possibility that the vascular anastomosis may be eroded by the infectious process is of paramount importance. If there is any suspicion that this is the case, such as an unexpected drop in hematocrit or blood from the fistula, immediate removal of the pancreas is mandatory.

EFFECT ON SECONDARY DIABETIC COMPLICATIONS

Following successful pancreas transplantation, normalization of carbohydrate metabolism occurs. Although freedom from insulin injections undoubtedly improves the patient's quality of life, it is not in itself the purpose of the procedure, since instead of insulin, the patient is exposed to prolonged immunosuppressive therapy. The purpose of pancreas transplantation is to reverse or arrest secondary diabetic complications. The first evidence of the potential beneficial influence of pancreas transplantation on diabetic nephropathy was the observation that patients who receive a combined kidney-pancreas transplant do not develop diabetic nephropathy in their transplanted kidney.[3] These initial findings have most recently been confirmed by the Minnesota group, who demonstrated a significant difference between mesangial volume of the transplanted kidney in patients who receive a kidney transplant alone versus patients who receive a combined kidney-pancreas transplant. Many patients undergoing pancreas transplantation subjectively indicate improvement in neuropathy. Preliminary data from various centers indicate improvement in motor nerve conduction velocity in the upper and lower extremities, and in some patients, sensory conduction velocity.[15] With the use of thermography, muscle oxygen tension measurements, and laser Doppler determination, a beneficial effect of pancreas transplantation on microcirculation can be demonstrated.[1] The influence of pancreatic transplantation on diabetic retinopathy remains controversial. In an initial report, the Minnesota group did not find any improvement in diabetic retinopathy within the first 2 years after pancreas transplantation in preuremic patients.[12] More recently, however, the same group reported that during a longer follow-up of between 3 and 4 years, a trend in favor of pancreas transplantation is now being observed. In the authors' experience, improvement in retinopathy occurs primarily in patients with early lesions. When diabetic retinopathy is advanced and patients have received laser treatments or vitrectomy, little improvement can be expected. Quality of life assessments after combined kidney-pancreas transplantation have been investigated by several centers in Europe.[10] Patients receiving a combined kidney-pancreas transplant require less sickness pension than patients with a kidney transplant alone, more patients have full-term employment, and there is a 44 per cent reduction in lost work days.

TRANSPLANTATION OF PANCREATIC ISLETS AND FETAL PANCREAS

Transplantation of isolated pancreatic islets and fetal pancreas offers the possibility of restoring normoglycemia without the patient's undergoing a surgical procedure. In addition, in animal experiments, reduction of the immunogenicity of islets has been accomplished. Thus, it would be theoretically possible to transplant islets or fetal pancreatic tissue without the need for immunosuppressive therapy. Unfortunately, clinical transplantation of fetal pancreas and islets of Langerhans have met with very limited success. The problems associated with the transplantation of islets of Langerhans are related to the difficulty in isolating a sufficient number of islets from one single adult pancreas in order to restore normoglycemia in the recipient. Numerous investigators during the past 20 years have suggested a number of digestion and isolation procedures, and only recently have selected groups been successful in isolating a sufficient number of islets (300,000 to 500,000). The standard islet isolation techniques generally include mechanical separation of the gland, combined with partial digestion using collagenase to dissociate the islets from the endocrine tissue. The islets are then separated from the exocrine tissue by density gradient centrifugation. Islets can be implanted beneath the renal subcapsular space, into the splenic parenchyma, or they can be injected into the portal vein for engraftment in the liver. Recently, reports have been published for the first time, demonstrating significant levels of C-peptides in patients undergoing injection of pancreatic islets into the portal vein. These patients also received a kidney allograft from the same donor and underwent conventional immunosuppression. Unfortunately, islet function was demonstrated only for a few weeks, and no patient ever became totally insulin-independent. Therefore, it is necessary to develop a better immunosuppressive strategy to ensure long-term graft survival of pancreatic islets. In addition, with the increasing number of pancreas transplants performed in the United States, pancreatic grafts suitable for islet isolation will be more difficult to obtain. Moreover, because only a few thousand pancreata are available in the United States each year for islet isolation; and since at least one pancreas is necessary to obtain a sufficient number of islets, this approach, even if successful, will, like whole pancreas transplantation, be available only for a very small number of diabetic patients. Therefore, at least theoretically, the use of human fetal pancreas offers much more promise for the future. The typical fetal pancreas used for transplantation is from a 16- to 20-week-old human fetus and is approximately 0.5 cm. long and weighs 10 to 20 mg. A pancreas this size contains more than 50 per cent endocrine tissue in isolated immature beta cells and very little exocrine tissue. The immature beta cells release insulin in response to glucagon and theophylline but not to increased glucose concentrations. Nevertheless, human fetal pancreata grow and mature after transplantation and release a sufficient amount of insulin within 10 to 15 weeks after transplantation to cure a diabetic animal. There have been over 200 fetal pancreatic allografts performed worldwide; but, again, success has been limited. Very few grafts ever demonstrated any evidence of function, either by increasing the C-peptide levels or by reducing or abolishing exogenous insulin requirements. Clinical trials currently under way using multiple donors and cultured fetal pancreata may provide more information about the effectiveness of this form of islet transplantation. Ethical questions surrounding the use of fetal pancreatic tissue for transplantation, however, remain.

SELECTED REFERENCES

Groth, C. G. (Ed.): Pancreatic Transplantation. Philadelphia, W. B. Saunders Company, 1988.
This is the first book entirely dedicated to the topic, and it covers a wide range of all aspects. More than 30 nationally and internationally renowned authorities in the field discuss technical aspects, indications, patient selection, and pathologic aspects of pancreatic graft rejection. Several chapters are dedicated to metabolic control after pancreas transplantation as well as its effect on the secondary complications of diabetes.

Stratta, R. J., Perlman, S. B., Kalayoglu, M., Belzer, F. O., and Sollinger, H. W.: The diagnosis of rejection and immunosuppressive strategies in vascularized pancreas transplantation. *In* Reinout Van Schilfgaarde, R., and Hardy, M. (Eds.): Transplantation of the Endocrine Pancreas in Diabetes Mellitus. New York, Elsevier Science Publishers, 1988, pp. 251–266.
This chapter describes in a comprehensive manner experimental and clinical studies directed to the diagnosis of pancreatic allograft rejection. It is a most useful reference source, because it provides a complete overview of the current status of the diagnosis of pancreatic allograft rejection.

Sutherland, D. E. R., Dunn, D. L., Goetz, F. C., et al.: A 10-year experience with 290 pancreas transplants at a single institution. Ann. Surg., *210*:274, 1989.

The Minneapolis group not only has performed the first pancreas transplant but also has the largest experience in pancreas transplantation worldwide. This group has applied every technique of transplantation of the pancreas in their own institution and is eminently qualified to compare these techniques. In addition, the Minneapolis group has championed the long-term follow-up of patients receiving a transplant and has reported extensively on the effect of transplantation of the pancreas on diabetic retinopathy, neuropathy, and the influence of a pancreatic graft on diabetic nephropathy.

Sutherland, D. E. R., and Moudry, K.: Report of the International Pancreas and Islet Transplant Registry.
Sutherland has been responsible for collecting and analyzing the results of all pancreas transplants performed worldwide since 1966. This is the most comprehensive organ transplant registry in existence today. The report of the International Pancreas Transplant Registry are published at regular intervals in Clinical Transplantation *and are presented at major national and international meetings.*

Van Schilfgaarde, R., and Hardy, M. (Eds.): Transplantation of the Endocrine Pancreas in Diabetes Mellitus. New York, Elsevier Science Publishers, 1988.
This book is dedicated to the field of pancreas and islet transplantation. In addition to the surgical aspects, other aspects are covered in detail by the foremost authorities in the field, such as the isolation of pancreatic islets, immunomodulation, and the autoimmune etiology of diabetes mellitus.

REFERENCES

1. Abendroth, D., Illhmer, V. D., Landgraf, R., et al.: Are late diabetic complications reversible after pancreas transplantation? A new method of follow-up of microcirculatory changes. Transplant. Proc., *19*:23, 1987.
2. Allen, R. D. M., Chapman, J. R., Deane, S. A., et al.: Combined pancreas and kidney transplantation: A pilot study. Transplant. Proc., *21*:3784, 1989.
3. Bohman, S. O., Wilczek, H., Tyden, G., et al.: Recurrent diabetic nephropathy in renal allografts placed in diabetic patients and protective effect of simultaneous pancreatic transplantation. Transplant. Proc., *19*:2290, 1987.
4. Calne, R. Y., McMaster, P., Rolles, K., et al.: Technical observations in segmental pancreas allografting: observations on pancreatic blood flow. Transplant. Proc., *12*:51, 1980.
5. Dubernard, J. M., Traeger, J., Neyra, P., et al.: New method of preparation of a segmental pancreatic graft for transplantation: Trials in dogs and in man. Surgery, *84*:634, 1978.
6. Gliedman, M. L., Gold, M., Whittaker, J., et al.: Pancreatic duct to ureter anastomosis for exocrine drainage in pancreatic transplantation. Am. J. Surg., *125*:245, 1973.
7. Groth, C. G., Collste, H., Lundgren, G., et al.: Successful outcome of segmental human pancreatic transplantation with enteric exocrine diversion after modifications in technique. Lancet, *2*:522, 1982.
8. Kelly, W. D., Lillehei, R. C., Merkel, F. K., et al.: Allotransplantation of the pancreas and duodenum along with the kidney in diabetic nephropathy. Surgery, *61*:827, 1967.
9. Merkel, F. K., Ryan, W. G., Armbruster, K., et al.: Pancreatic transplantation for diabetes mellitus. Illinois Med., *144*:477, 1973.
10. Nakache, R., Tyden, G., Groth, C. G.: Quality of life in diabetic patients after combined pancreas-kidney or kidney transplantation. Diabetes, *38* (Suppl. 1):40, 1989.
11. Ngheim, D. D., Bentel, W. D.: Duodenocystostomy for exocrine drainage in total pancreatic transplantation. Transplant. Proc., *18*:1753, 1986.
12. Ramsay, R. C., Goetz, F. C., Sutherland, D. E. R., et al.: Progression of diabetic retinopathy after pancreas transplantation for insulin-dependent diabetes mellitus. N. Engl. J. Med., *318*:208, 1988.
13. Sollinger, H. W., Vernon, W. B., D'Alessandro, A. M., et al.: Combined liver and pancreas procurement with Belzer-UW solution. Surgery, *106*:685, 1989.
14. Tao, L., Sutherland, D. E. R., Cavallini, M., et al.: Duct drainage in the bladder for management of exocrine secretions of segmental pancreas grafts in dogs. Surg. Forum, *24*:376, 1983.
15. Van der Vliet, J. A., Navarro, X., Kennedy, W. R., et al.: The effect of pancreas transplantation on diabetic polyneuropathy. Transplantation, *45*:368, 1988.

X

CARDIAC AND CARDIOPULMONARY HOMOTRANSPLANTS

R. Morton Bolman III, M.D.

HISTORICAL ASPECTS

The evolution of heart and heart-lung transplantation has been an exemplary combination of progress in clinical and basic science. On the basis of his original work in the techniques of vascular suturing, Carrel, with Guthrie, in 1905 performed the first experimental heterotopic canine heart transplant in the neck. This preliminary demonstration of technical feasibility nurtured subsequent investigators in the field of organ transplantation.[10] Demikhov, a brilliant Russian investigator, performed a series of heterotopic canine cardiac and cardiopulmonary transplants. He was the first to demonstrate the ability of the donor heart to sustain the body circulation independently.[12]

Cardiac transplantation as a clinical reality was dependent on the development of techniques to perform open heart surgery and also to demonstrate the feasibility of human organ allotransplantation. Lillehei and co-workers, first with the technique of parental cross-circulation, subsequently with the "biological oxygenator" (canine lungs), and then with the demonstration by Gibbon of the feasibility of extracorporeal circulation, performed a series of open heart operations in children with congenital heart disease in whom early death was inevitable. These accomplishments stand among the greatest achievements in the history of surgery, distinguished equally by the ingenuity of conception and the courage of execution.[31]

Lower and Shumway published landmark work in 1960, reporting successful canine orthotopic cardiac transplantation. Based on the concept of safe, reliable cardiopulmonary bypass, these investigators described several techniques that are currently employed in the performance of these procedures. These include anastomosis of atrial cuffs as opposed to individual pulmonary and systemic venous anastomoses and the use of topical hypothermia during implantation of the heart.[18]

Technically, this provided the foundation for the performance of cardiac transplantation in man. Only the demonstration of the feasibility of organ allotransplantation in man as the stimulus for the first human heart transplant was lacking. In the 1950s and 1960s, the first successful human kidney transplants were performed; Barnard performed the first human heart transplant in December 1967. The patient died of pulmonary infection less than 3 weeks postoperatively, but the operation stimulated great interest worldwide.[3] His second patient survived 20 months. Shumway and associates, prepared by long-standing interest and laboratory investigation, performed their first transplant within weeks of Barnard's operation and, despite waning worldwide interest following the initial activity, maintained an ongoing and slowly growing program. With refinements, including improved recipient and donor selection criteria, the introduction of endomyocardial biopsy for rejection monitoring, and improvements in immunosuppression, surgical technique, and postoperative care, patient survival by the late 1970s was nearly identical to that being appreciated by recipients of cadaver kidney transplants.[25] This rekindled interest in cardiac transplantation in a few centers. Introduction of cyclosporine into clinical use in 1981 at Stanford and in 1982 at the University of Minnesota and its release for general use in 1984 have been associated with stimulation of activity in cardiac transplantation.[24] Currently, there are over 150 hospitals in the United States alone performing cardiac transplants.

Concomitant with the increase in hospitals performing transplantation has been a rapid rise in the numbers of procedures performed. From a few hundred per year in the early 1980s, activity has reached a level of over 1500 transplants annually in each of the past 3 years in the United States.[16]

Cardiopulmonary transplantation stimulated the interest of a number of investigators in the field of thoracic organ transplantation. Demikhov, utilizing an ingenious technique of serially anastomosing vessels such that donor/recipient perfusion might be maintained during orthotopic heart-lung transplantation, achieved a survivor of 6 days in 1951. The work of this Russian investigator went largely unnoticed in the Western world.[12] Work reported simultaneously by Neptune and associates from Hahnemann Medical College in Philadelphia and Marcus and associates from Chicago Medical School in 1953 demonstrated initial experimental efforts at heart-lung transplantation in the United States. Neptune and colleagues reported the first successful replacement of the heart and both lungs using hypothermia and circulatory arrest.[21] Marcus and associates described heterotopic heart-lung transplantation to the abdominal position. This heterotopic graft was functional, and the authors reported a method of open intracardiac surgery using a donor heart and lungs as the pump oxygenator.[19] The mechanical pump oxygenator was first employed to perform heart-lung transplantation in dogs by Webb and Howard in 1957. They noted that although all the cardiac function was sufficient following transplantation, the animals were unable to breathe spontaneously.[30] This and other work suggested that cardiopulmonary denervation was not well tolerated by dogs. Bleeding was also significant in early experiments. Haglin and associates suggested that there was a species difference in ability to tolerate denervation of both lungs with return of spontaneous respiration. These investigators found that primates resumed spontaneous respiration whereas dogs did not.[15] This work was verified in 1972 with the report by Castaneda and associates at the University of Minnesota. This group avoided allograft rejection by performing autotransplants and attempted to avoid respiratory difficulties by operating on primates. They achieved technical success and 6 of 40 baboons survived for more than a month, with several surviving more than a year after operation. With careful examination of pulmonary ventilation and perfusion and circulatory hemodynamics, these animals were found in all respects to be normal, and this study predicted that heart-lung transplantation would be successful in human patients.[11] Reitz and colleagues initiated their primate studies at Stanford University in 1978. Cyclosporine was being studied in several laboratories as a novel immunosuppressive agent. The drug was available for study in the Stanford laboratory and was successfully applied to monkeys undergoing heart-lung allotransplantation, comprising the first application of cyclosporine to experimental lung transplantation. Several animals survived for periods of greater than a year after heart-lung allotransplantation and some lived well over 5 years, demonstrating that normal hemodynamic and respiratory function could be anticipated following heart-lung allotransplantation.[26]

Clinically there were three early attempts at heart-lung transplantation that occurred at the time of initial enthusiasm over heart transplantation in the late 1960s. These attempts by Cooley, Lillehei, and Barnard between 1968 and 1971 did not achieve long-term success, but Lillehei's patient was extubated on the first postoperative day breathing spontaneously. This demonstration that heart-lung denervation in man did not prevent spontaneous breathing provided great hope for the future application of this procedure.[17]

The first planned program in clinical heart-lung transplantation was initiated at Stanford by Reitz and colleagues in 1981. The first patient, a 45-year-old woman with end-stage primary pulmonary hypertension, underwent transplantation and subsequently did well for more than 5 years after transplantation. A second patient had Eisenmenger's syndrome due to a ventricular septal defect and was transplanted several months later with long-term survival.[27] Additional problems occurred, including chronic rejection in the form of bronchiolitis obliterans and insufficient donors to meet the clinical need.

This chapter on the history of transplantation demonstrates dramatically the interdigitation of clinical and basic investigation in the search for a solution to an apparently unsolvable problem. The concept of heart and heart-lung replacement, once the realm of science fiction, is now an established reality since these procedures have demonstrated their feasibility in the therapeutic armamentarium of diseases of the heart and lungs.

CLINICAL CARDIAC TRANSPLANTATION

Recipient Selection

Criteria for candidate selection for cardiac transplantation have evolved as a result of improvements in techniques and outcomes. The acceptable age for transplant candidacy has expanded and now includes individuals from newborn age up to age 60 years routinely and age 65 years in unusual circumstances. Patients selected must experience symptoms that place them in Class IV of the New York Heart Association classification or must have angina pectoris that is severely limiting their life-style in a setting where revascularization is not an option. Certain individuals can be considered for transplantation prior to experiencing Class IV symptoms if they have life-threatening cardiac arrhythmias refractory to medical and surgical therapies. Patients undergo a careful screening process to ensure suitable extracardiac and psychosocial health status. Fixed, irreversible deficits in extracardiac organ function contraindicate transplantation, since they would not be expected to be corrected by improved cardiac function. Psychosocial screening is important to assure a proper support structure for the patient and strict compliance with prescribed medical regimens both before and after transplantation.

Patients must have end-stage heart disease not amenable to conventional medical or surgical therapies. From a hemodynamic standpoint, the most critical predictor of operative risk at the time of transplantation is the pulmonary vascular resistance, defined as the difference between the mean pulmonary artery pressure and the pulmonary capillary wedge pressure, divided by the cardiac output (PVR = mean PAP − mean $PCWP$ ÷ C.O.). If the pulmonary vascular resistance is greater than 5 to 6 Wood units and cannot be pharmacologically reversed with manipulations in the catheterization laboratory that could be duplicated at the time of transplantation, orthotopic transplantation would pose a substantial risk. Other options can be considered in this setting as appropriate, including heterotopic transplantation to preserve the recipient right ventricle. Deter-

TABLE 1. Recipient Selection Criteria for Heart Transplantation

Age newborn to 60 years
Irremediable cardiac disease — Class IV NYHA
Normal function or reversible dysfunction of kidneys, liver, lungs, central nervous system
Pulmonary vascular resistance less than 6–8 Wood units or pharmacologically reversible
Absence of:
    Active malignancy or infection
    Recent pulmonary infarction
    Severe peripheral or cerebrovascular disease

minations and decisions involving the pulmonary vascular resistance are among the most difficult in the area of heart transplantation. In children, these values must be indexed to body size to allow rational decisions to be reached.

There must be no active malignancy or infection in a potential recipient. Active peptic ulcer is a contraindication, at least in programs in which corticosteroids form a part of the immunosuppressive regimen. Severe peripheral or cerebral vascular disease may pose a relative contraindication as does insulin-dependent diabetes mellitus, although the author's program and others have demonstrated that these patients can undergo successful transplantation (Table 1).

Patients who underwent transplantation at the University of Minnesota and their diagnoses are shown in Table 2. Among 163 patients, approximately equal numbers had coronary artery disease and idiopathic cardiomyopathy as their underlying cardiac diagnosis. These two diagnostic categories constitute the most frequent indications for cardiac transplantation. Approximately 40 per cent of the author's transplant patients have had at least one previous cardiac operation, usually for coronary revascularization. Of note is the category of allograft coronary artery disease. Two patients in this series have required retransplantation for this problem, and in time this number is expected to increase.

Donor Selection

The donor should be a young individual who has sustained brain death either through accidental or natural causes. Cardiac retrieval is performed as part of a multiple-organ retrieval and requires careful coordination for a successful result. Criteria for donor selection are outlined in Table 3. Individuals up to 55 and occasionally 60 years of age, with demonstrable normal function of the heart and absence of severe coronary disease, can be suitable donors. These individuals should be on low-dose pressor support (less than or equal to 10 μg. per kg. per minute of dopamine or an equivalent dose of dobutamine). They should have a negative cardiac history and, of course, negative serologic tests for hepatitis and human immunodeficiency virus (HIV) infection. Useful screening tests include electrocardiography and echocardiography. The latter can be obtained in nearly

TABLE 2. Indications for Cardiac Transplantation at the University of Minnesota

Cause of Cardiomyopathy	Number of Patients (%)
Ischemic	75 (46)
Idiopathic	73 (45)
Rheumatic	8 (5)
Congenital	4 (2)
Others	3 (2)
Total	163

TABLE 3. Donor Selection Criteria for Heart Transplantation

Age less than 60 years
Minimal pressor support
Negative cardiac history
Normal electrocardiogram
Normal echocardiogram
ABO compatibility
Size within 20%–50% of recipient
Negative T-cell crossmatch if panel reactive antibodies 10% or greater
Negative serologic tests for hepatitis, HIV infection

all hospitals and provides a readily available assessment of anatomic features and functional status and should be obtained whenever possible. Donor and recipient in all cases need to be ABO-compatible, and a prospective crossmatch is not necessary provided the recipient is reactive to 10 per cent or less of a panel of randomly selected HLA types (panel reactive antibodies less than 10 per cent). Donor and recipient weight should be matched within 20 to 50 per cent, depending on the pulmonary vascular resistance level in the recipient. Individuals with high pulmonary vascular resistance require transplantation with the heart of a donor of at least equal size to provide a large right ventricular mass necessary to cope with the elevated pulmonary resistance.

Distant graft procurement is now routine, and approximately 80 per cent of donor hearts are currently retrieved at a distance.[29] In the author's program, as far as 2020 kilometers (1300 miles) have been traveled with successful graft function. The limiting factor, of course, is ischemic time of the graft; with careful preservation, up to 4 hours of *ex vivo* ischemia is well tolerated. Donor hearts are preserved with 1 liter of crystalloid cardioplegia coupled with copious topical cooling.

Operative Technique

Coordination of the retrieval and implantation portions of the transplant procedure is critical to minimize cardiopulmonary bypass time and graft ischemia time and to optimize function of the graft. When the surgeon has visually inspected the donor heart, preparation of the recipient may proceed. The recipient is cannulated for cardiopulmonary bypass with an aortic cannula in the usual position and right-angle venous cannulas far posterior in the right atrium. In cases with one or more previous cardiac procedures, it is advisable to have a femoral artery and vein exposed such that expeditious femoral-femoral bypass can be instituted in the event of a misadventure upon reopening the sternum or in mobilizing the recipient heart. The necessary dissection is completed such that the recipient heart can be removed expeditiously. The right atrium is divided at a level several centimeters anterior to the cannulas. The left atrium is entered just behind the aorta and the interatrial septum divided adjacent to the atrioventricular valves. The left atrium is transected in the plane of the coronary sinus and the left atrial appendage is excised, leaving a generous cuff of left atrium about the left pulmonary veins. The great vessels are transected at the level of the semilunar valves, and the aorta and pulmonary artery are separated using electrocautery. This completes preparation of the recipient mediastinum (Fig. 1A).

The donor heart is removed from its preservation container and tailored for implantation. The posterior wall of the left atrium is excised by connecting incisions in the pulmonary veins. The right atrium is excised from the inferior vena caval orifice to the right atrial appendage, avoiding the sinoatrial node. Implantation begins with anastomosis of donor and recipient left atria. The anastomosis begins at the level of the left pulmonary veins and is completed at the level of the interatrial septum (Fig. 1B). Timing of individual anastomoses at this point is determined by the elapsed ischemic time of the donor heart and the pulmonary vascular resistance of the recipient. Ideally,

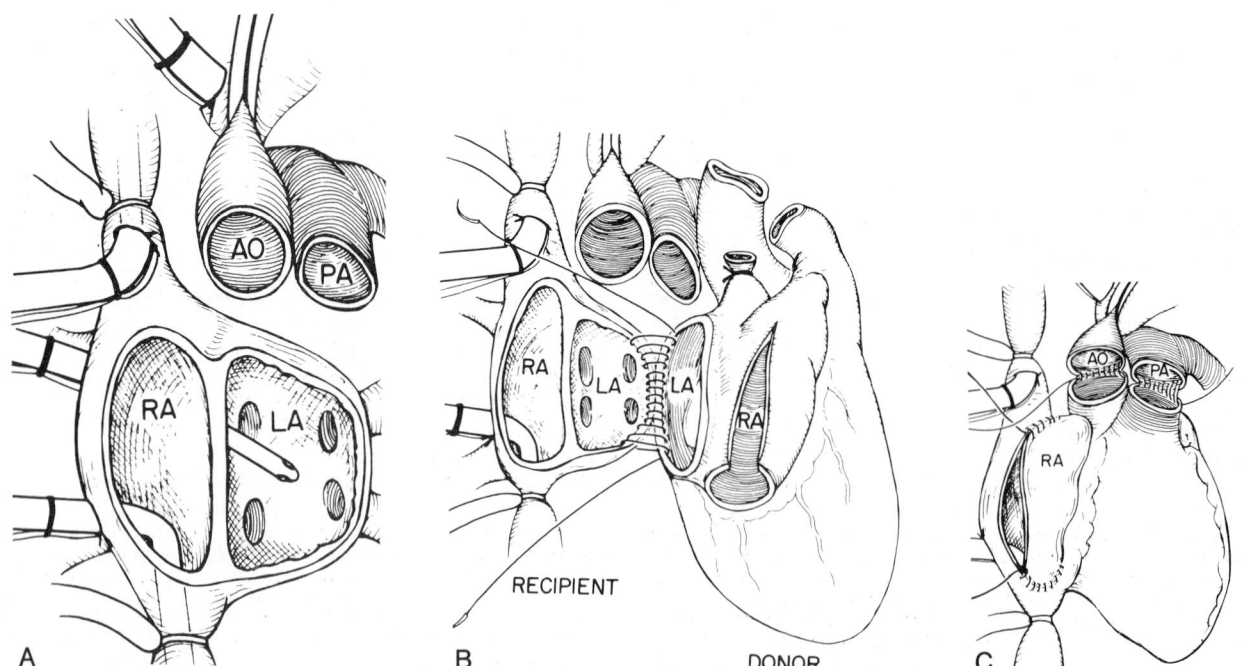

Figure 1. *A*, Appearance of the recipient mediastinum following excision of the diseased recipient heart. One can see the position of the arterial and venous cannulas for cardiopulmonary bypass as well as the left ventricular vent catheter passing via the right superior pulmonary vein. Posterior cuffs of left and right atria, aorta, and pulmonary artery have been fashioned. *B*, The donor heart has been lowered into the operative field, and the lateral wall of the left atrial anastomosis is being fashioned. *C*, The medial aspect of the right atrial anastomosis has been completed, and the methods of the anastomosis of the aorta and pulmonary artery are illustrated. The inset demonstrates the technique of venting air from the ascending aorta as the aortic cross-clamp is released, restoring perfusion to the donor heart. (From Bolman, R. M.: Cardiac transplantation: The operative technique. *In* Thompson, M. E. (Ed.): Cardiac Transplantation. Philadelphia, F. A. Davis, 1990, pp. 136–144.)

the order of anastomoses is left atrium, pulmonary artery, right atrium, aorta. However, in cases in which the ischemic time is already long and there is concern regarding donor right ventricular function because of elevated pulmonary vascular resistance in the recipient, it is prudent to perform the aortic anastomosis immediately following the left atrial anastomosis such that the cross-clamp can be released, thereby shortening the ischemic time and allowing earlier reperfusion of the donor heart (Fig. 1C). A principle to be observed in anastomosing the great vessels is that the aorta should be left long and the pulmonary artery should be trimmed short so that there is no redundancy with resumption of cardiac dynamics. Following at least 30 minutes of perfusion, during which hemostasis can be secured along the suture lines, the donor heart assumes the circulation. All patients receive an infusion of isoproterenol, and temporary atrial and ventricular pacing wires are routine. The chest is copiously irrigated with antibiotic solution and closed only when hemostasis is secured.[5]

In cases in which orthotopic transplantation is not feasible, a "piggyback" or heterotopic transplantation can be considered. Such instances include (1) a recipient with elevation of pulmonary vascular resistance that is fixed and cannot be reversed pharmacologically and (2) a small donor heart available for a large recipient who is critically ill. The completed procedure of heterotopic transplantation is depicted in Figure 2. Donor cardiectomy is similar to that for orthotopic transplantation with the exception that the entire superior vena cava is removed. In addition, a longer segment of aorta is retrieved to include the arch with ligated brachiocephalic vessels. The left-sided pulmonary venous orifices are opened widely and united in preparation for anastomosis with the left atrium of the recipient. The right-sided pulmonary veins are oversewn. The inferior vena cava is closed at its atrial junction and the superior vena cava is ligated distally. An incision is made into the posterior portion of the superior vena cava with the venotomy extended 3 to 4 cm. onto the right atrial surface. The incision is positioned posteriorly to minimize risk of injury to the sinus node.

The recipient is placed on cardiopulmonary bypass, and the left atrium of the recipient is incised just posterior to the interatrial groove, similar to the approach for mitral valve surgery. The donor heart is positioned in the right chest anterior to the

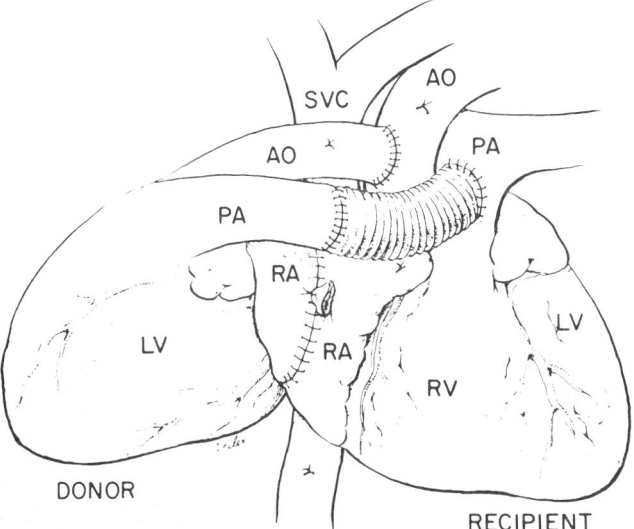

Figure 2. The completed procedure of heterotopic transplantation. The donor aorta is anastomosed directly to the side of the recipient ascending aorta. The donor pulmonary artery and recipient pulmonary artery have been joined with an interposed Dacron graft. Alternatively, this may be accomplished with interposition of a segment of donor descending aorta. The right atrial suture line is visible, as is the final orientation of donor and recipient hearts. (From Bolman, R. M.: Cardiac transplantation: The operative technique. In Thompson, M. E. (Ed.): Cardiac Transplantation. Philadelphia, F. A. Davis, 1990, pp. 136–144.)

lung, and the common orifice to the left pulmonary veins is anastomosed to the recipient left atrium. A right lateral atriotomy is created in the recipient heart, and a continuous anastomosis is created between the cavoatrial opening in the donor and the atriotomy in the recipient. Donor aorta is anastomosed end-to-side to the recipient ascending aorta, which is controlled with a side-biting vascular clamp. The main pulmonary artery of the donor is generally of insufficient length to reach the recipient pulmonary artery. This gap can be bridged with the right pulmonary artery of the donor or a segment of donor aorta or prosthetic graft that has been preclotted. Donor and recipient pulmonary arteries are then joined. The patient is allowed to return to normal temperature and is separated from cardiopulmonary bypass.[14] The operative procedure of cardiac transplantation, whether orthotopic or heterotopic, must be performed with meticulous attention to technical detail and hemostasis. The morbidity following technical and bleeding complications is apt to be high.

Immunosuppression

Prophylaxis against allograft rejection is currently performed using one of two protocols in most programs. Triple therapy, introduced by the author and colleagues in 1983, consists of the combination of cyclosporine, azathioprine, and prednisone and remains the mainstay of immunosuppressive management in this program. Patients receive cyclosporine 4 to 10 mg. per kg. as a preoperative dose, and azathioprine 2 to 3 mg. per kg. preoperatively. Perioperative methylprednisolone sodium succinate is administered 0.875 gm. in the 24 hours surrounding the procedure, and then prednisone is administered on day 2 at 1 mg. per kg. per day in divided doses. Cyclosporine is targeted to a 12-hour trough level of 200 to 300 ng. per ml. and azathioprine to a white blood cell count of 4000 to 5000 per cu. mm. Prednisone is tapered to a level of 5 to 10 mg. per day by 3 to 6 months. This regimen has been associated with the lowest reported incidence of cardiac rejection and has yielded excellent rates of survival and a low incidence of infection.[6–8]

The other major protocol is one in which the monoclonal antibody OKT3 is used in conjunction with triple therapy (the "induction" regimen). This innovative approach, introduced by Bristow and associates, involves the administration of OKT3 for 2 weeks beginning on day 2, during which time patients receive corticosteroid therapy and azathioprine. Cyclosporine is initiated just prior to the discontinuation of OKT3 and is titrated to therapeutic levels when OKT3 is discontinued. Patients are then maintained on cyclosporine and azathioprine, and prednisone is tapered off over a 2-week period in patients who do not reject. This regimen has been associated with a significant portion of patients being able to successfully discontinue steroid therapy, although the use of OKT3 has been associated with significant side effects.[9] Gay and colleagues report excellent results in 102 patients with this regimen,[13] but now believe it enhances development of coronary arteriosclerosis in the graft.

COMPLICATIONS

Allograft Rejection

The diagnosis of cardiac rejection depends on an index of suspicion associated with new-onset cardiac arrhythmia, hypotension, or fever. Associated symptoms may include fatigue, malaise, and shortness of breath. The electrocardiogram is not routinely useful in the diagnosis of rejection, and confirmation depends on the endomyocardial biopsy. A useful adjunct is radionuclide ventriculography, which, if performed as a baseline study in all patients shortly after transplant, can constitute a very helpful study to follow both grade and severity of rejection hemodynamically and its course with treatment. The histologic diagnosis of rejection depends on the finding of a diffuse amount of infiltrate apparent on most or all of the several specimens obtained.[28] The presence or absence of myocyte necrosis has not proved critical to the author's ability to diagnose allograft rejection.

Infection

Several measures of prophylaxis against infection have proved highly useful in the management of these postoperative transplant recipients. All patients who are seronegative for cytomegalovirus (CMV) prior to transplantation receive exclusively CMV-negative blood and blood products postoperatively. All patients receive nystatin orally and high-dose acyclovir (800 mg. four times a day) for 3 months and trimethoprim-sulfamethoxazole indefinitely following transplant. Perioperative wound prophylaxis consists of a second-generation cephalosporin and vancomycin coupled with copious intraoperative irrigation with a vancomycin solution. This regimen, coupled with the low incidence of rejection experienced as a result of triple therapy, has caused a very low incidence of serious infection, and none of the author's patients has had mediastinitis or a sternal wound infection.[1]

Transplant Coronary Artery Disease

A dreaded sequela of cardiac transplantation is that of transplant coronary artery disease. This entity continues to plague cardiac transplant recipients and is expected to become an increasing problem in time and with the increasing numbers of patients being transplanted. Olivari reported the experience at the University of Minnesota with this problem. When coronary artery disease is defined by any decrease in luminal diameter, 8 per cent at 1 year and 24 per cent at 2 years demonstrated findings of transplant coronary artery disease.[22] This incidence can be expected to increase with time. It is thought to represent a manifestation of chronic rejection in the form of immune complex disease directed at the intima of the major epicardial coronary vessels. Close surveillance is required, and some cases have been treated with percutaneous transluminal coronary angioplasty. If the problem becomes severe and/or associated with significant or multiple myocardial infarctions, retransplantation may be the only option available.

RESULTS

The results of transplantation in 163 patients transplanted at the University of Minnesota since 1983 (the introduction of triple therapy) are depicted in Figure 3. Actuarial patient survival of 78 per cent at 5 years posttransplant is demonstrated and documents the efficacy of the methods of recipient and donor selection, operative management, and immunosuppression outlined previously. These rates of survival contrast sharply with the life expectancy of individuals with end-stage heart failure who do not receive a heart transplant.

Rates of rejection, expressed as rejection-free survival, are demonstrated in Figure 4. Eighty-six per cent of patients are free of rejection at 1 year after transplantation when treated with triple therapy immunosuppression.[23] There is a very low incidence of serious and life-threatening infections in patients treated with this regimen. Since fewer patients require treatment for rejection, the total amount of immunosuppression received is less, and this is reflected in a decreased rate of infection. The routine administration of trimethoprim-sulfamethoxazole has proved very beneficial, as there have been no cases of *Pneumocystis* or *Nocardia* infection in these heart transplant recipients.[1]

SUMMARY

Since its inception in 1967, cardiac transplantation has progressed steadily. Today this procedure represents an established

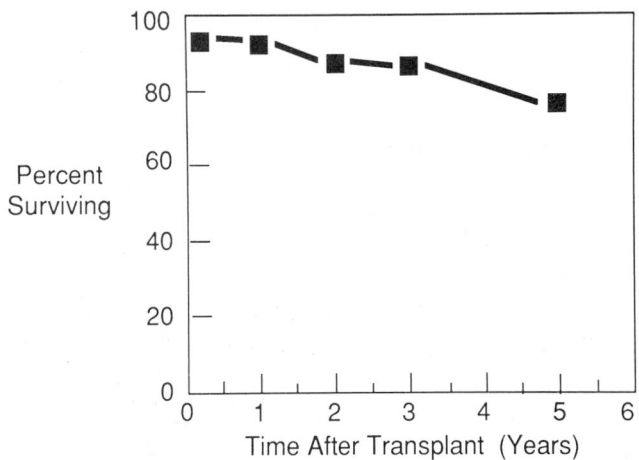

Figure 3. Actuarial survival in 163 patients transplanted at the University of Minnesota since the inception of triple-drug immunosuppression in 1983. Five-year survival is 78 per cent.

treatment for end-stage heart disease. Improved patient selection and effective, safe immunosuppressive strategies have restored health to patients formerly destined for premature death. Serious problems remaining to be solved include a shortage of donor organs and the problem of transplant coronary artery disease, which currently is the number one factor limiting long-term survival.

CARDIOPULMONARY TRANSPLANTATION

Recipient Selection

Certain individuals have disease of the heart and lungs that requires replacement of these organs. The dramatic advent of successful cardiopulmonary transplantation, introduced by Reitz and colleagues, has made this procedure a clinical reality.[27] Recipient selection criteria are outlined in Table 4. The most common indications for this procedure have been primary pulmonary hypertension and Eisenmenger's syndrome. Other less frequent diagnoses necessitating *en bloc* heart-lung replacement are cystic fibrosis, obstructive lung disease with cor pulmonale, and other end-stage lung diseases associated with severe right ventricular decompensation. With the development of successful lung transplantation, there is much interest in the application of single or bilateral lung transplantation to diseases

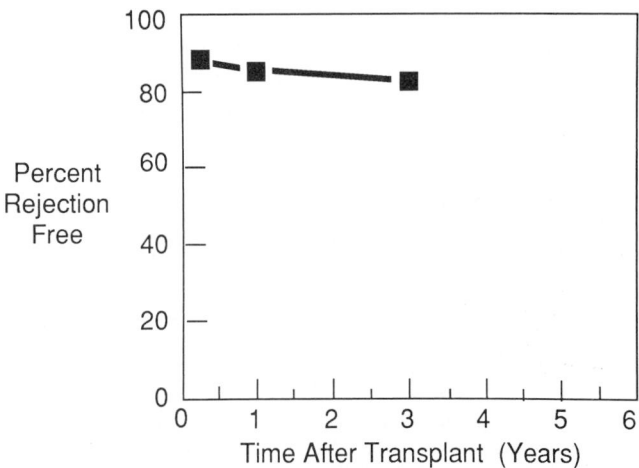

Figure 4. The incidence of acute allograft rejection in patients transplanted at the University of Minnesota since the inception of triple-drug immunosuppression in 1983.

TABLE 4. Recipient Selection Criteria for
Cardiopulmonary Transplantation

Age less than 50 years
End-stage pulmonary vascular or parenchymal disease associated with severe right ventricular compromise and/or severe tricuspid regurgitation
Absence of:
Other nonreversible organ dysfunction or disease
Major prior thoracotomy or sternotomy
High-dose steroid therapy

formerly thought appropriate for heart-lung transplantation. Certain examples would be patients with primary pulmonary hypertension before the onset of severe right ventricular failure and also those with Eisenmenger's syndrome with relatively straightforward congenital heart defects (atrial septal defect, patent ductus arteriosus, and so on). These individuals could undergo single lung transplantation combined with repair of the congenital cardiac defect. Such procedures, if feasible, increase the number of patients who can receive transplants. Donor hearts can be utilized for patients in need of heart transplantation, and donor lungs for patients with parenchymal lung disease or pulmonary vascular disease (primary or secondary) with adequate preservation of cardiac function.

Patients should be severely limited by their disease, unable to work or attend school, and most are on supplemental oxygen therapy. Because of the marked scarcity of suitable donors, individuals should be considered for transplantation only when their life-style is seriously impaired and it is believed that they are in the final 6 to 12 months of natural life. These individuals must fulfill all the other criteria for transplantation as outlined in the section on heart transplantation; namely, they must demonstrate normal extrathoracic organ function and must possess sufficient psychosocial stability and support to withstand the rigors of the procedure and postoperative period.

Donor Selection

A small percentage of donors suitable for heart donation also have lungs that can be transplanted (10 to 20 per cent). Increased awareness of the need as well as improved donor management can increase this percentage; however, lack of suitable donors continues to severely restrict the number of these procedures that can be performed. Criteria for suitable cardiopulmonary donors are depicted in Table 5. In addition to normal heart function, the heart-lung donor must have normal gas exchanges with a Pao_2 greater than 400 mm. Hg on 100 per cent inspired oxygen with peak airway pressures of 30 mm. Hg or less. The chest film should be normal and pulmonary secretions minimal. The presence of fungus in any amount or gram-negative bacteria in large numbers heralds increased risk of serious infection following transplantation and should contraindicate donation.

Donor and recipient are matched according to ABO type as well as on the basis of results of an HLA antibody screen. Size-matching is also important, and comparison of measurements made from standard portable roentgenograms is helpful in determining size compatibility. Donor and recipient height and

TABLE 5. Donor Selection Criteria for Cardiopulmonary
Transplantation

Close size match—donor smaller than or same size as recipient
Satisfactory gas exchange—arterial Po_2 > 400 mm. Hg on FIO_2 of 1.0
Normal lung compliance—peak airway pressure of 30 mm. Hg with normal tidal volume
Clear chest radiograph
Absence of purulent pulmonary secretions

weight should approximate one another; however, height is a better indicator of relative lung size than is weight.

Scrupulous attention to fluid management in the donor both before and during organ harvest is critical to avoid overload and compromise of suitability for transplantation. The donor should be maintained as dry as possible consistent with adequate function of the other organs being retrieved, and a central venous pressure of 5 cm. H_2O or less is desirable. Successful organ function has been repeatedly demonstrated following up to 4 hours of ex vivo preservation by means of either of two main techniques. The donor can be placed on cardiopulmonary bypass using a portable heart-lung machine. With this technique, the donor is cooled uniformly to a temperature of 15° to 18° C. and the heart-lung block is removed after the abdominal viscera are mobilized.[4] The other main technique in use is that of cardioplegic arrest of the heart, combined with pulmonary artery flushing with a modified Euro-Collins solution in the amount of 50 to 100 ml. per kg. donor weight. Copious topical cooling with 4° C. saline is also employed, and the donor is ventilated with small tidal volumes of room air while the flush solution is being delivered. This method is preferred by most groups because of its simplicity and the fact that it is somewhat cumbersome to transport a cardiopulmonary bypass circuit to a distant donor hospital.[2]

Operative Technique

As with heart transplantation, careful coordination between donor retrieval and recipient preparation is essential for a satisfactory outcome. The recipient is brought to the operating room and lines are placed, such that the surgical procedure can begin immediately upon receiving word that the donor organs are suitable for transplantation. Through a midline sternotomy, both pleural spaces are explored and any adhesions lysed prior to heparinization. This allows achievement of optimal hemostasis in the pleural spaces prior to the institution of cardiopulmonary bypass. The pericardium is then opened and the patient cannulated for bypass with standard aortic cannulation and bicaval cannulation via the posterior right atrium. Cardiopulmonary bypass is instituted and the heart is removed much as described for heart transplantation. Employing the electrocautery, an incision is made several centimeters behind the phrenic nerve bilaterally from the level of the pulmonary artery to the diaphragm to create a window for passage of the donor lungs into the recipient pleural spaces. Care must be taken to avoid injury to the phrenic nerves, and the recurrent laryngeal nerve can be damaged if the dissection is carried above the pulmonary artery on the left. The lungs are removed individually. The inferior pulmonary ligaments are divided, and the respective pulmonary hila are stapled with a TA90 surgical stapler. The lungs are then removed. This technique has greatly simplified this portion of the operation and improves hemostasis. It is then necessary to incise the posterior left atrium vertically in order to allow the donor lung to pass posterior to the right atrium and phrenic pedicle. The mediastinum with the heart removed, the left atrial incision, and the left pulmonary hilum being readied for the TA90 stapler are depicted in Figure 5. The trachea is then mobilized between the aorta and superior vena cava, taking care to avoid devascularizing the supracarinal portion. The main stem bronchi are mobilized and the trachea is transected just above the carina. With the thoracic organs removed, meticulous hemostasis should be achieved, since the posterior mediastinum is very difficult to visualize following implantation of the donor heart-lung block. The donor heart-lung block is placed into the chest with each lung placed into its respective hemithorax.

The transplant procedure begins with anastomosis of donor and recipient tracheas using a running suture technique with 3-0 monofilament suture. The donor trachea is transected two tracheal rings above the carina. When the tracheal anastomosis

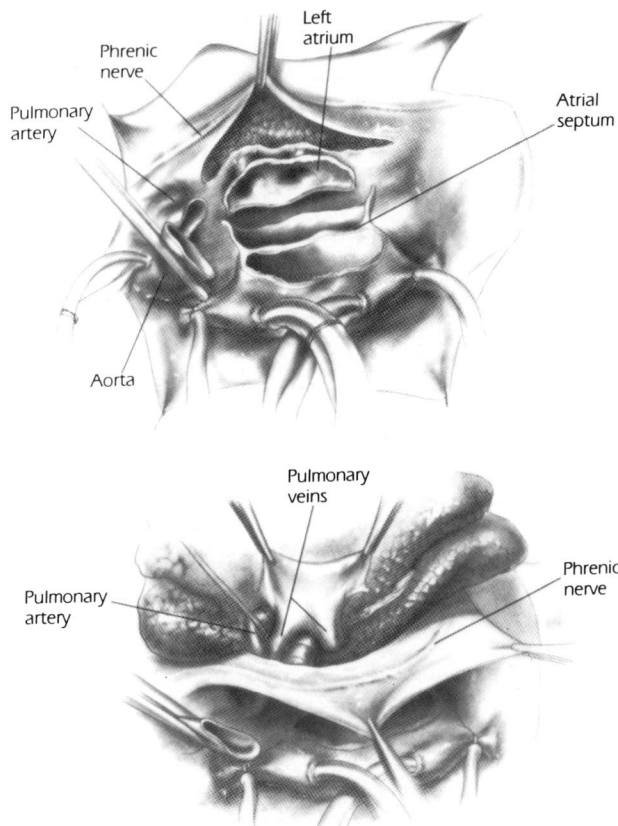

Figure 5. The upper figure depicts the recipient mediastinum after removal of the heart. The left atrium has been incised vertically to create a pathway for the donor right lung to enter the right pleural cavity behind the right atrium and phrenic nerve. In the lower figure, the left phrenic nerve has been isolated on a pedicle of pericardium and the left pulmonary hilum is being readied for excision by application of the TA90 stapler. (From Doty, D. B. (Ed.): Cardiac Surgery. Chicago, Year Book Medical Publishers, 1985, p. 15.)

is completed, ventilation with low tidal volume and room air is initiated. Donor and recipient aorta and right atria are then anastomosed, completing the procedure.

Another option is the "domino" heart-lung transplant procedure. This operation has been performed on two occasions at the author's institution. In this procedure, the recipient heart, which must be demonstrated to be suitable for transplantation, is removed and sent for implantation either in an adjacent operating room or in another transplant center. Individual caval anastomoses are necessary at the time of heart-lung implantation because the entire recipient right atrium is removed. Otherwise, the implant procedure is identical to that described in the preceding.

Immunosuppression

Recipients of heart-lung allografts receive cyclosporine and azathioprine perioperatively. Corticosteroids are administered intraoperatively and for the first 24 hours, and then are withheld for the next 2 weeks because of their deleterious effect on airway healing. Antilymphocyte globulin is administered for 3 to 5 days, during which time low levels of cyclosporine are maintained. This allows renal function to remain unaltered, thereby facilitating diuresis and early extubation. After 14 days, prednisone is begun at a low dosage. Maintenance therapy consists of cyclosporine, azathioprine, and prednisone.

COMPLICATIONS

Rejection

Most recipients experience an episode of rejection within the first 2 weeks. Heart and lungs do not necessarily reject synchro-

nously; therefore, heart biopsy is not a reliable means of monitoring lung rejection. The diagnosis of lung rejection depends on clinical grounds, although recent experience with the transbronchial biopsy suggests that this procedure is very useful if coupled with a careful assessment of the patient's clinical status. Signs of graft rejection include a decrease in oxygenation, a new radiographic infiltrate, fever, and auscultatory findings of basilar rales. Symptoms may include breathlessness, malaise, and a feeling of anxiety. Treatment is with pulse corticosteroid therapy for a period of 3 days followed by reassessment.

Infection

Infection prophylaxis in the heart-lung recipient is identical to that described for the heart transplant recipient. Most infections following heart-lung transplantation are in fact pulmonary. Any new radiographic abnormality, especially in the presence of fever, must be urgently evaluated by bronchoscopy with lavage. Broad-spectrum antibiotics are administered until specific culture data are available; at that time, all unnecessary antibiotics are discontinued. The use of trimethoprim-sulfamethoxazole routinely in patients has prevented infections caused by *Pneumocystis* and *Nocardia* organisms in the author's heart and heart-lung population.

Bronchiolitis Obliterans

One of the most serious complications in recipients of these procedures is that of bronchiolitis obliterans. This entity is thought to represent a form of chronic rejection analogous to transplant coronary artery disease in recipients of heart allografts. Indeed, in some autopsies of heart-lung recipients, both processes have been identified in the same patient. Often appearing without any obvious radiographic abnormality, bronchiolitis obliterans is an insidious process, initially causing a decrement in the midexpiratory flow measurement (forced expiratory flow, 25 to 75 per cent). There is then progression to breathlessness, and eventually the individual becomes severely limited. This occurs in 30 to 50 per cent of heart-lung recipients and may appear any time after the first several months following transplant. Attempts to reverse the course of this process in most cases prove futile, although in some cases the patient can be stabilized, albeit at a lower level of function. Approaches to treatment primarily involve increased immunosuppression.

CLINICAL OUTCOMES

The main impediment to progress in the field of cardiopulmonary transplantation has been the severe limitation in the numbers of available donors. Only a few centers in the United States have accrued a significant experience. Since the pioneering work of Reitz, subsequent investigators at Stanford have continued to develop the techniques of cardiopulmonary transplantation, including refined patient selection and improved posttransplant management. Comparing 30 patients transplanted between March 1981 and February 1986 with 32 patients transplanted subsequent to that period, this group was able to demonstrate improved in-hospital and long-term survival with a decreased incidence of bronchiolitis obliterans in the later group. Perioperative mortality decreased from 35 per cent to 16 per cent, 3-year survival improved from 43 per cent to 65 per cent, and the incidence of bronchiolitis obliterans decreased from 63 per cent to 20 per cent among hospital survivors. Survival at 3 years in the more recent group has paralleled that in heart transplants performed at Stanford during the same time span. The improved results are attributed to the routine employment of triple-drug immunosuppression and more aggressive surveillance for rejection and infection, including the routine application of bronchoscopy with bronchoalveolar lavage and transbronchial biopsy.[20]

Since 1986 at the University of Minnesota, there have been 18 heart-lung transplants performed in patients ranging from 6 to

TABLE 6. Indications for Heart-Lung Transplantation at the University of Minnesota 1986–1990

Diagnosis	Number of Patients
Primary pulmonary hypertension	9
Eisenmenger's syndrome	5
Alpha$_1$-antitrypsin deficiency	2
Lymphocytic interstitial pneumonitis	1
Cystic fibrosis	1
Total	18

54 years of age. Two of these were "domino" procedures with the recipient heart being transplanted in another individual. The diagnoses for which these patients underwent heart-lung transplantation are listed in Table 6. Despite prolonged, complicated hospital courses in some of these patients, there has been no perioperative mortality. Three patients have expired late after transplantation from bronchiolitis obliterans and a fourth is awaiting single lung transplantation for this disorder. Those not afflicted with bronchiolitis obliterans have enjoyed an excellent return to health.

SUMMARY

Owing to severe restrictions in donor availability, small numbers of these procedures have been performed in the United States each year.[16] Despite this, the gratifying results achieved in the individuals who do well have inspired further efforts in this field. Cardiopulmonary transplantation remains a therapeutic option for selected individuals for whom no other conventional or transplant alternative is available. Intensive research continues in the area of chronic rejection of the heart-lung allograft. This remains the single greatest impediment to long-term survival in these patients.

SELECTED REFERENCES

Demikhov, V. P.: Experimental Transplantation of Vital Organs. New York, Consultants Bureau, 1962.
This work by a brilliant Russian investigator antedated many of the current techniques in cardiothoracic surgery. He first performed mammary artery implants, and his descriptions of techniques of transplantation of heart and heart-lung blocks before the availability of cardiopulmonary bypass were innovative. He performed experimental transplants of many other vital organs but his work was overlooked for many years. Only recently has the importance of his work been realized.

Gay, W. A., O'Connell, J. G., Burton, N. A., et al.: OKT3 monoclonal antibody in cardiac transplantation: Experience with 102 patients. Ann. Surg., 208:287, 1988.
Experience with 102 patients undergoing cardiac transplantation under treatment with OKT3 monoclonal antibody is reported in this article. The results of this regimen are equal to those reported previously in cardiac transplantation in terms of survival, and the concept of steroid withdrawal was made possible by this regimen. This pioneered the application of this "induction" regimen utilizing OKT3, and this is an excellent immunosuppressive regimen.

McCarthy, P. M., Starnes, V. A., Theodore, J., et al.: Improved survival after heart-lung transplantation. J. Thorac. Cardiovasc. Surg., 99:54, 1990.
With the somewhat discouraging results experienced by many early in heart-lung transplantation, this excellent summary of two eras in heart-lung transplantation at Stanford provides encouragement for continuing application in selected circumstances. The authors demonstrate an improved survival and decreased incidence of chronic rejection in the form of bronchiolitis obliterans. The improvements are attributed to the routine employment of triple-drug immunosuppression and aggressive posttransplant monitoring with frequent bronchoscopy, bronchoalveolar lavage, and transbronchial biopsy for diagnosis of infection and rejection.

Oyer, P. E., et al.: One year experience with cyclosporin A in clinical heart transplantation. Heart Transplant, 1:285, 1982.
The Stanford group reports the initial experience with cyclosporine in heart transplantation. The increment in survival and decrease in serious infection reported in this paper served as inspiration to many programs in cardiac transplantation.

Reitz, B. A., Burton, N. A., Jamieson, S. W., et al.: Heart and lung transplantation, autotransplantation and allotransplantation in primates with extended survival. J. Thorac. Cardiovasc. Surg., 80:360, 1980.

This excellent article reports successful transplantation of heart and lungs in primates with long-term survival. This work clearly was the impetus for human clinical heart-lung transplantation. This study demonstrated conclusively that the denervated heart and lungs could function normally for long periods of time and support an entirely normal quality of life.

Reitz, B. A., Wallwork, J. L., Hunt, S. A., et al.: Heart-lung transplantation. Successful therapy for patients with pulmonary vascular disease. N. Engl. J. Med., 306:557, 1982.
This landmark report of the first successful human heart-lung transplants is one of the most significant contributions in vital organ transplantation as well as cardiothoracic surgery. Successful laboratory investigations, made clinical heart-lung transplantation a reality and served as an impetus for many future developments in this area, including single and double lung transplantation. This was the first demonstration that the transplanted airway could heal effectively.

REFERENCES

1. Andreone, P. A., Olivari, M. T., Elick, B., Arentzen, C. A., Bolman, R. M., Simmons, R. L., and Ring, W. S.: Reduction of infectious complications following cardiac transplantation. J. Heart Transplant, 5:13, 1986.
2. Baldwin, J. C., Frist, W. H., Starkey, T. D., et al.: Distant graft procurement for combined heart and lung transplantation using pulmonary artery flush and simple topical hypothermia for graft preservation. Ann. Thorac. Surg., 43:670, 1987.
3. Barnard, C. N.: A human cardiac transplant: An interim report of a successful operation performed at Groote Schuur Hospital, Capetown. S. Afr. Med. J., 41:1271, 1967.
4. Baumgartner, W. A., Williams, G. M., Frazer, C. D., et al.: Cardiopulmonary bypass with profound hypothermia: An optimal preservation method for multi-organ procurement. Transplantation, 47:123, 1989.
5. Bolman, R. M.: Cardiac transplantation: The operative technique. Cardiovasc. Clin., 20:133, 1990.
6. Bolman, R. M., Cance, C., Spray, T., et al.: The changing face of cardiac transplantation: Washington University program 1985–1987. Ann. Thorac. Surg., 45:192, 1987.
7. Bolman, R. M., Elick, B., Olivari, M. T., et al.: Improved immunosuppression for cardiac transplantation. J. Heart Transplant, 4:315, 1985.
8. Bolman, R. M., Olivari, M. T., Sibley, R., et al.: Current results with triple therapy for heart transplantation. Transplant Proc., 19:2490, 1987.
9. Bristow, M. R., Gilbert, E. M., Renlund, D. G., et al.: Use of OKT3 monoclonal antibody in cardiac transplantation: Review of the initial experience. J. Heart Transplant, 7:1, 1988.
10. Carrel, A., and Guthrie, C. C.: The transplantation of veins and organs. Am. J. Med., 10:1101, 1905.
11. Castaneda, A. R., Arnar, O., Schmidt-Habelmann, P., et al.: Cardiopulmonary autotransplantation in primates. J. Cardiovasc. Surg., 37:523, 1972.
12. Demikhov, V. P.: Experimental Transplantation of Vital Organs. New York, Consultants Bureau, 1962.
13. Gay, W. A., O'Connell, J. G., Burton, N. A., et al.: OKT3 monoclonal antibody in cardiac transplantation: Experience with 102 patients. Ann. Surg., 208:287, 1988.
14. Griffith, B. P., Kormos, R. L., and Hardesty, R. L.: Heterotopic cardiac transplantation: Current status. J. Cardiac Surg., 2:283, 1987.
15. Haglin, J., Telander, R. I., Muzzall, R. E., et al.: Comparison of lung autotransplantation in the primate and dog. Surg. Forum, 14:196, 1963.
16. Heck, C. F., Shumway, S. J., and Kaye, M. P.: The Registry of the International Society for Heart Transplantation: Sixth Official Report—1989. J. Heart Transplant, 8:271, 1989.
17. Lillehei, C. W.: Discussion of Wildevuur, C. R. H., and Benfield, J. R.: A review of 23 human lung transplantations by 20 surgeons. Ann. Thorac. Surg., 9:489, 1970.
18. Lower, R. R., and Shumway, N. E.: Studies on the orthotopic homotransplantation of the canine heart. Surg. Forum, 11:18, 1960.
19. Marcus, E., Wong, S. N. T., and Luisada, A. A.: Homologous heart grafts: Transplantation of the heart in dogs. Surg. Forum, 2:212, 1951.
20. McCarthy, P. M., Starnes, V. A., Theodore, J., et al.: Improved survival after heart-lung transplantation. J. Thorac. Cardiovasc. Surg., 99:54, 1990.
21. Neptune, W. B., Cookson, B. A., Bailey, C. P., et al.: Complete homologous heart transplantation. Arch. Surg., 66:174, 1953.
22. Olivari, M. T., Homans, D. C., Wilson, R. F., et al.: Coronary artery disease in cardiac transplant patients receiving triple-drug immunosuppressive therapy. Circulation Suppl. III:III–111, 1989.
23. Olivari, M. T., Kubo, S. H., Braunlin, E. A., Bolman, R. M., and Ring, W. S.: Five-year experience with triple-drug immunosuppressive therapy in cardiac transplantation. Circulation Suppl. IV:276, November 1990.
24. Oyer, P. E., et al.: One year experience with cyclosporin A in clinical heart transplantation. Heart Transplant, 1:285, 1982.
25. Reitz, B. A.: The history of heart and heart-lung transplantation. In Baumgartner, W. A., Reitz, B. A., and Achuff, S. C. (Eds.): Heart and Heart-Lung Transplantation. Philadelphia, W. B. Saunders Company, 1990, pp. 1–14.
26. Reitz, B. A., Burton, N. A., Jamieson, S. W., et al.: Heart and lung transplantation, autotransplantation and allotransplantation in primates with extended survival. J. Thorac. Cardiovasc. Surg., 80:360, 1980.

27. Reitz, B. A., Wallwork, J. L., Hunt, S. A., et al.: Heart-lung transplantation. Successful therapy for patients with pulmonary vascular disease. N. Engl. J. Med., *306*:557, 1982.
28. Sibley, R. K., Olivari, M. T., Ring, S. W., and Bolman, R. M.: Endomyocardial biopsy in the cardiac allograft recipient: A review of 570 biopsies. Ann. Surg., *203*:177, 1986.
29. Thomas, F. T., Szentpetery, S. S., Mammana, R. E., et al.: Long-distance transportation of human hearts for transplantation. Ann. Thorac. Surg., *26*:344, 1978.
30. Webb, W. R., and Howard, H. S.: Cardiopulmonary transplantation. Surg. Forum, *8*:313, 1957.
31. Wilson, L. G.: The development of cardiac surgery in Minnesota 1940–1960. *In* Wilson, B. A. (Ed.): Medical Revolution in Minnesota: A History of the University of Minnesota Medical School. St. Paul, Minn., Midewiwin Press, 1989, pp. 481–528.

XI

LUNG TRANSPLANTATION

Donald E. Low, M.D., F.R.C.S.(C), and Joel D. Cooper, M.D.

Progress with transplantation of the lung has lagged behind that of other organs, notwithstanding considerable interest and research activity in this field for several decades. Several problems unique to the lung have retarded progress both experimentally and clinically. The lung is a very fragile organ with intimate approximation of the air spaces and the capillaries such that even a relatively minor insult can cause significant malfunction. Such malfunction can jeopardize the survival of the lung transplant recipient who is dependent on the immediate function of the organ. The systemic arterial supply to the lung, the fine network of bronchial vessels, is interrupted and usually not restored at the time of transplantation, and the bronchial anastomosis is thus rendered ischemic. The lung is exposed to the atmosphere, which increases the susceptibility to infection, the risk of which is all the greater due to the immunosuppression necessary to prevent rejection.

Metras,[17] in France in 1950, and Hardin and Kittle,[12] in the United States in 1954, demonstrated the technical feasibility of lung transplantation in dogs, utilizing an approach that has not changed substantially. Most experimental work has been conducted in dogs with either a reimplantation model in which the lung is severed and reattached or allotransplantation of a lung from another dog. Reimplantation has been used for eliminating factors relating to rejection and in studying those factors associated with the technical aspects of the procedure as well as the effects of lymphatic, neural, and bronchial artery interruption. Early experiments suggested that there was a significant increase in pulmonary vascular resistance in the transplanted lung. Subsequently, it was demonstrated that with meticulous anastomotic technique for the pulmonary arterial and venous attachments the vascular resistance of the transplanted organ behaved almost normally.[1,3,7,27,28] Similarly, it has become apparent that interruption of the lymphatic connections, the vagal nerves, and the bronchial arteries does not cause any significant physiologic derangement. Progress in lung transplantation has been impeded in part by the lack of a suitable experimental model analogous to the usual clinical situation. With unilateral lung transplantation in the dog, the function of the remaining native lung is sufficient to sustain the animal, and physiologic malfunction of the transplanted lung may not be apparent. However, unilateral transplantation with immediate ligation of the contralateral pulmonary artery, or contralateral pneumonectomy, requires the transplanted lung to immediately accept the entire cardiac output, which is not analogous to the clinical situation. Pulmonary edema may develop in the immediate posttransplantation period, especially if lung preservation is not optimal.

Early malfunction of a transplanted lung has often been attributed to the "reimplantation response." This response is var-iably attributed to the effects of lymphatic, neural, or bronchial artery interruption along with possible effects of ischemia and reperfusion. With increasing clinical experience, it has become evident that such a response is not inevitable and is probably due primarily to ischemic and/or reperfusion injury. Accurate diagnosis of lung rejection remains elusive; and in the absence of reliable diagnostic criteria, excessive immunosuppression may be utilized with resultant increased risk of infectious complications. The combination of exposure to bacterial contamination from the atmosphere and ischemia of the donor airway due to interruption of the bronchial circulation, along with the need for immunosuppression, has, not surprisingly, created significant problems with pulmonary sepsis and poor healing of the airway anastomosis.

In addition, the effects of organ ischemia on posttransplantation function have been difficult to gauge. Thus, the period of safe ischemic time between extraction of the lung and restoration of its circulation has been difficult to ascertain. In summary, early malfunction of the transplanted lung may be attributed to numerous factors; and this, together with the lack of a clinically relevant animal model, has contributed to the slow pace of progress made with lung transplants, compared with other organ transplants.

HUMAN LUNG TRANSPLANTATION

In 1963, Dr. James Hardy[13] and co-workers reported the first human lung transplant. The recipient survived for 18 days and died of renal failure. This experience demonstrated the technical feasibility of lung transplantation and stimulated worldwide interest in the field. During the subsequent 20 years, approximately 40 lung or lobe transplants were performed worldwide with little clinical success. Only one recipient survived to be discharged from the hospital, a 23-year old man who underwent right lung transplant for advanced silicosis.[9] The patient was discharged from hospital 8 months after transplantation and died 2 months later of chronic rejection and pulmonary sepsis.

The report of a successful combined heart and lung transplant by the Stanford Group[22] in 1981 provided an important stimulus for further efforts in lung transplantation. This report confirmed that an individual can function satisfactorily solely on transplanted lung tissue, as previously suggested by the 10-month survival of Derom's patient.[9] The combined heart and lung transplant had been initially attempted by Cooley and associates[4] and subsequently by Lillehei[15] and by Barnard[12] all without success. However, subsequent attempts by the Stanford group utilizing cyclosporine as the primary immunosuppressive agent yielded repeated clinical success with the heart-lung transplant procedure in patients with right heart failure and pulmonary hypertension.

The authors' initial experience with unilateral lung transplant was in 1978, when a right lung transplant was performed for a ventilator-dependent patient with inhalation burns.[19] The recipient died in the third week of disruption of the bronchial anastomosis. Review of world experience to that date revealed that only nine patients had survived more than 2 weeks after unilateral lung transplantation, and six of these nine, including the authors' patient, died within the first month of bronchial anastomotic disruption. Following this experience, a laboratory program was undertaken for evaluation of factors affecting bronchial anastomotic healing after lung transplantation. The initial experiments involved canine lung autotransplantation, with severing and immediate reattachment of the lung. Half of the animals received no postoperative immunosuppressants; the other half received standard immunosuppression with azathioprine and prednisone. The treated animals exhibited significant bronchial anastomotic complications, including ischemia, necrosis, and disruption of the anastomosis, similar to previously reported complications following human lung transplantation.[16] The untreated animals exhibited primary healing of the bronchial anastomosis, although a degree of narrowing of the bronchus distal to the anastomosis was a frequent occurrence. It was concluded that the distal stenosis of the bronchial tree was most likely to be ischemic in origin.

Subsequent experiments suggested that adverse effects on bronchial healing in the immunosuppressed animals related entirely to the prednisone and that the use of azathioprine did not prejudice bronchial healing.[11] Experiments utilizing cyclosporine instead of prednisone indicated that the bronchial healing was not significantly different from that seen in the untreated animals. In an attempt to rapidly restore bronchial arterial blood supply after transplantation, a pedicle of omentum with its blood supply intact was brought into the chest. This was wrapped around the bronchial anastomosis after completion of the bronchial anastomosis. Subsequent studies of the omental pedicles confirmed rapid restoration of bronchial blood supply by means of omental collaterals with improved anastomotic healing following transplantation.[10,18]

Organization of a Transplant Program for End-Stage Lung Disease

Development of a program for transplantation of end-stage lung disease requires individuals with expertise in pulmonary medicine, cardiology, rehabilitation, physiotherapy, hematology, immunology, infectious disease, nutrition, intensive care, psychiatry, and nursing. The surgical team requires expertise in all aspects of pulmonary and airway surgery, cardiac surgery, respiratory care, and intensive care.

Selection of Recipients for Lung Transplantation

The authors' initial experience consisted of unilateral lung replacement in patients with end-stage pulmonary fibrosis.[25] These patients were thought to be particularly suited for single lung transplantation because the poor compliance and increased vascular resistance of the native lung ensured that both ventilation and perfusion would be preferentially diverted to the transplanted lung. However, during the past several years indications for single lung transplantation have been extended to include patients over 50 years of age with emphysema, patients with other obstructive pulmonary disorders such as lymphangioleiomyomatosis and eosinophilic granuloma, and patients with primary pulmonary hypertension, or Eisenmenger's syndrome. Initially there was concern that unilateral transplantation for emphysema might be problematic because of the potential for hyperexpansion and air trapping in the contralateral native lung producing a shift of the mediastinum and restriction of ventilation to the transplant. In the past year, however, single

lung transplants have been performed on 12 patients with emphysema. To date, all have demonstrated a successful outcome, which has included the elimination of the need for oxygen therapy and significant improvement in activity levels. Despite the fact that the native lung continues to receive a significant portion of the ventilation, postoperative exercise capacity has been measurably increased. Long-term follow-up studies are necessary before the role of unilateral lung transplantation for emphysema can be properly evaluated. During the past year, six single lung transplants for patients with primary pulmonary hypertension, or Eisenmenger's syndrome, have been performed. These procedures were successful in restoring normal pulmonary artery pressure and cardiac function, even in patients who showed a significant impairment in right heart function preoperatively.

Patients with bilateral pulmonary sepsis, either acute or chronic, are poorly suited for unilateral lung transplantation, because the remaining infected lung would not only contaminate the transplanted lung but would serve as a focus for systemic infection in the immunosuppressed patient. The philosophy has also been adopted that relatively young patients (under 50 years of age) with emphysema might benefit from the greater functional improvement associated with double lung transplantation.

The authors' initial experience with the double lung procedure involved the *en bloc* replacement of both lungs in association with total cardiopulmonary bypass and ischemic arrest of the heart. This approach, although initially successful in some patients, was associated with significant complications in patients with widespread vascular pleural adhesions and those with significant right ventricular dysfunction. In response to these problems, the *en bloc* double lung operation has been redesigned to a bilateral single lung transplant in which each lung is sequentially replaced with a bilateral transverse thoracosternotomy incision. This new procedure is associated with several distinct advantages: total cardiopulmonary bypass and ischemic arrest of the heart are avoided (partial bypass has been employed in 25 per cent cases), the bronchial anastomotic healing is much more satisfactory than healing of the tracheal anastomosis employed for the *en bloc* double lung transplant, and the absence of extensive mediastinal dissection eliminates the cardiac denervation frequently observed after the double lung procedure. This approach has been applied in 12 consecutive patients without a death or serious postoperative morbidity.

Because of recent success with the bilateral single lung transplant, the authors believe there is no further indication for use of the old *en bloc* double procedure. Significant advantages of the bilateral transplant procedure over heart-lung transplantation have also been identified. These advantages include a significantly shortened potential waiting period (2 versus 18 months) for patients undergoing lung transplantation, avoidance of unnecessary replacement of the recipient's heart, and utilization of the donor heart for a cardiac recipient.

Preoperative assessment of all potential lung transplant recipients begins with a 5-day hospital admission during which time tests documenting respiratory impairment and cardiac function are performed. Appropriate patients must demonstrate no history of recent cigarette use or evidence of alcohol or other substance abuse. They must have normal hepatic and renal function, be no more than 20 per cent above their ideal body weight, and have a negative serologic profile for hepatitis B virus and human immunodeficiency virus (HIV). They must also demonstrate the ability to move to our center and maintain themselves and a support individual for the 1- to 6-month preoperative waiting period and the 3-month posttransplant period of rehabilitation and careful surveillance.

Because of the experimental evidence indicating the adverse effects of routine prednisone administration in the early postoperative period, the authors have historically required that all transplant recipients be weaned entirely from steroids for at least 1 month before transplantation. Most patients with end-stage pulmonary fibrosis in need of a transplant have inactive disease, and for this reason such patients can generally be weaned without difficulty. Discontinuation of steroid medication in the emphysemic population, however, has frequently been more difficult; and in some cases recipients will now be considered when the daily prednisone dose has been lowered to 10 mg. or less.

Because of the severe shortage of suitable donor lungs, it has been necessary to adopt somewhat arbitrary guidelines for the selection of recipients. Thus, individuals over the age of 60, individuals who are ventilator-dependent, and those who have a history of previous malignancy have been excluded. An attempt is made to identify recipients who are likely to die of their disease within 12 to 18 months of evaluation. Such individuals are usually oxygen-dependent and demonstrate deterioration in pulmonary function with increasing oxygen requirements. Noninvasive monitoring of oxygen saturation during standardized exercise protocol has proven useful in documenting progression of the disease. Patients with end-stage pulmonary fibrosis generally have excellent respiratory muscle strength due

to the chronic workload of ventilating the fibrotic lungs. Such patients have some degree of pulmonary hypertension, but this is usually moderate, such that cor pulmonale is not present. The same is true for most patients with emphysema. Right ventricular function is evaluated noninvasively using echocardiography and nuclear angiography. All patients over the age of 40 also undergo cardiac catheterization and coronary angiography.

Prospective transplant recipients undergo extensive psychological testing to exclude the presence of psychosocial problems. The exclusion of these patients is important because of the considerable stress that the preoperative assessment, long waiting period, and postoperative recovery impose. Moreover, information regarding the patient's previous level of compliance with medical personnel is reviewed because of the importance of continued cooperation in producing a satisfactory long-term result.

Donor Selection

The lack of suitable donor lungs is a major obstacle to more widespread application of lung transplantation and impedes progress, which depends upon concentrated experience. Lungs are more difficult to obtain than other organs because of their

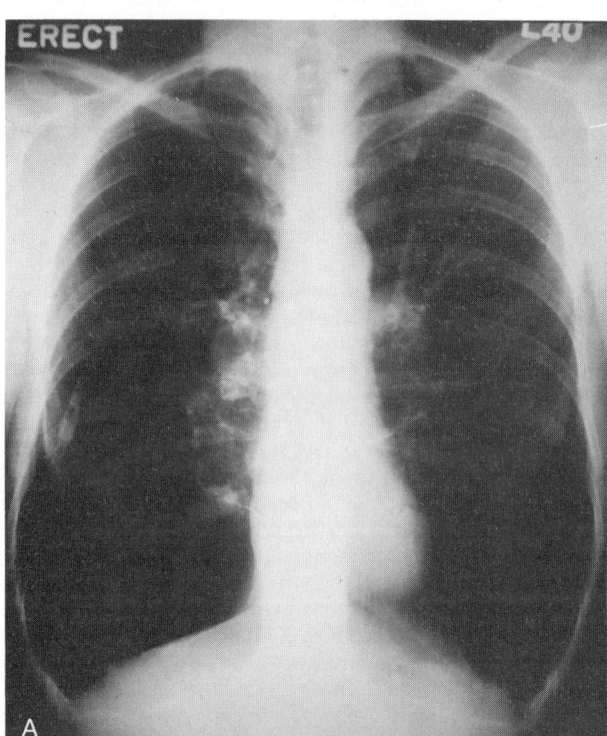

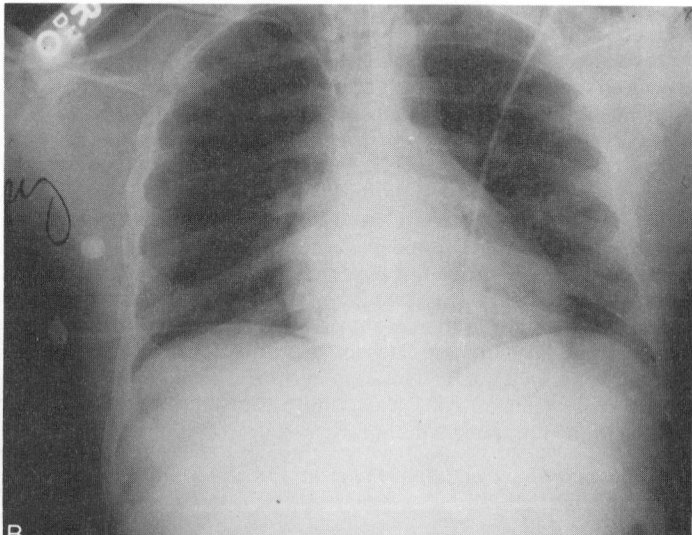

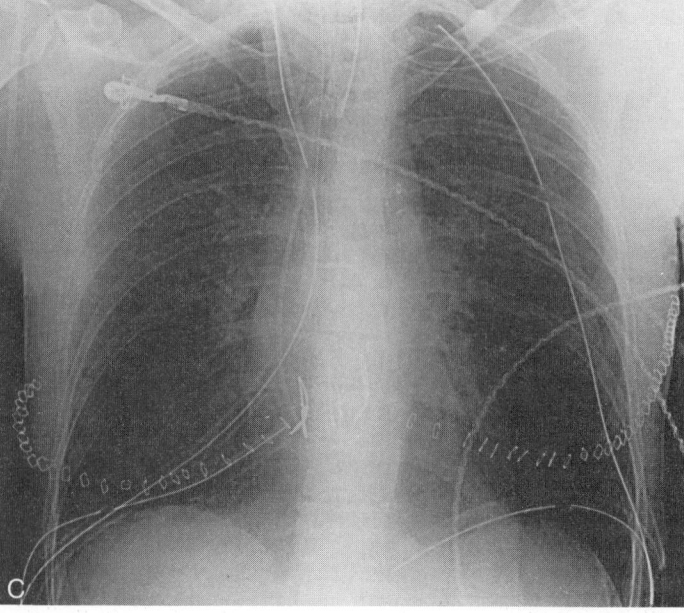

Figure 1. A, Preoperative chest film. B, Donor chest film. C, Immediate postoperative chest film. The total lung capacity (TLC) of the recipient was 11 liters. The estimated (predicted) TLC of the donor was 6.2 liters. However, despite the discrepancy, the postoperative chest film demonstrates good filling of both hemithoraces.

susceptibility to infection and edema, especially in the presence of brain death. Requirements include that the donor chest film be entirely clear, arterial oxygen tension exceed 300 mm.Hg with an FIO₂ of 100 per cent and 5 cm. of positive end-expiratory pressure, and bronchoscopy reveal no gross purulent secretions or suggestion of aspiration.

Initially a simple immersion of the extracted lung in cold solution was used for purposes of preservation, and satisfactory graft function was achieved for ischemic periods up to 5 hours. More recently, preservation has been by means of a cold flush of the pulmonary circulation consisting of 3 liters of Euro-Collins solution to which has been added 65 ml. of 50 per cent glucose and 2 ml. of 50 per cent MgSo₄ per liter. This flush is preceded by an injection of 500 μg. of prostaglandin E₁ into the pulmonary artery. With this method, satisfactory graft function for ischemic periods up to 9½ hours has been achieved. In the animal laboratory, a low-potassium dextran-containing solution has been employed with consistently excellent preservation for ischemic periods up to 12 hours.[14]

For the purpose of size matching, the vertical and transverse radiologic dimensions of the chest are used. Because lateral films are generally not available for the donor, the dimensions from the portable film must be utilized. Together with the radiographic dimensions, the sex, body weight, height, and chest circumference of the donor and recipient are compared in an attempt to assess the suitability of the match. Initially, the authors sought a donor lung of approximately the same size as the recipient chest but later realized that it would be more appropriate to select the lung on the basis of the "predicted normal for the height and weight of the recipient." For example, with pulmonary fibrosis, the recipient's chest is contracted because of the fibrotic, "shrunken" lungs. Chest dimensions are observed to return to a more normal configuration when a larger lung is inserted. With emphysema, however, the recipient's chest is grossly overexpanded. Insertion of a normal-sized lung is followed by elevation of the diaphragm to a more normal position and restoration of a more normal thoracic configuration (Fig. 1).

Lung transplantation can readily be performed on either side. With the single lung procedure, the side to undergo transplantation is determined primarily from the quantitative lung V/Q scan. In the majority of cases, the lung that demonstrates the most impaired function is replaced to reduce the likelihood of requiring cardiopulmonary bypass. This approach also maintains the greatest degree of pulmonary reserve should the function of the transplanted lung be temporarily impaired. In the case of primary pulmonary hypertension, the authors prefer to transplant the right lung because of the ease of cannulating the right atrium for cardiopulmonary bypass. In patients with Eisenmenger's complex with atrial septal defect, the right-sided approach is mandatory.

Currently donor matching is done on the basis of ABO compatibility and body size. Histocompatibility matching is done only in retrospect because the effect of such matching remains uncertain and the delay in obtaining prospective cross-matching will jeopardize the use of lungs from many unstable donors. In addition, cytomegalovirus (CMV)-negative recipients are provided organs from CMV-negative donors whenever possible.

Donor Preparation

Currently, most donor lungs are extracted in conjunction with multiple organ removal for transplantation. A method for removing the heart for cardiac transplantation without jeopardizing the use of the lungs has been developed.[24] The authors currently extract both lungs for transplantation either using each lung for separate recipients or using the two lungs for bilateral lung transplant, which is employed for cystic fibrosis, bronchiectasis, and a portion of patients with emphysema. The

heart is removed before the lungs, which leaves a cuff of left atrium containing the four pulmonary veins. To facilitate this, dissection of the interatrial groove is performed before cardiac extraction to increase the distance between the right pulmonary veins and atrial septum, which allows adequate left atrial cuff for both the heart and lung specimens.

Immediately prior to cross-clamping, 500 μg. of prostaglandin E₁ is given as a bolus injection into the pulmonary artery. After occlusion of the vena cava and aortic cross-clamping, cardioplegia is administered through an aortic cannula, and the lungs are flushed with 3 liters of cold Euro-Collins solution through a catheter placed in the common pulmonary artery. The cardioplegia is vented from the cardiac end of the divided inferior vena cava, and the pulmonary flush is vented by excision of the tip of the left atrial appendage. The superior and inferior vena cava, the ascending aorta, and the common pulmonary artery are then divided. Careful division of the left atrium is then accomplished to leave an adequate cuff on the heart as well as surrounding the four pulmonary veins (Fig. 2A). Separate excision of the heart requires only a few minutes more than is ordinarily required for cardiac excision without the use of the lungs. After removal of the heart, the trachea is doubly stapled at its midpoint and divided. The esophagus is stapled at the same level as the trachea and at a second point just above the diaphragmatic hiatus. This facilitates the *en bloc* removal of the entire contents of the mediastinum, including the esophagus and descending aorta, at the time of lung extraction. This method provides a safe but expeditious double lung extraction, producing minimal delay for the abdominal organ retrieval teams.

The double lung bloc is immersed in a bag containing ice-cold modified Euro-Collins solution, and the bag is placed in ice for transportation. If the two lungs are to be transported to separate transplant centers, then the lungs are separated at the donor institution. Otherwise, the two lungs are transported *en bloc* and prepared for right and left lung transplant at the authors' institution either for transplants into separate recipients or for bilateral lung transplantation.

At the time of separation, the stapled esophageal remnant as well as the remainder of the descending aorta and aortic arch are removed from the posterior aspects of the specimen. Each pulmonary artery is divided at its origin from the common pulmonary artery. The left atrium is split vertically in the midline, with a suitable cuff of left atrium preserved around the right and left pulmonary veins. Each donor bronchus is divided, with no more than two rings left proximal to the respective upper lobe bronchus (Fig. 2B). This step is thought to be particularly important because the short residual stump of donor bronchus minimizes the likelihood of posttransplant ischemia of the anastomosis.

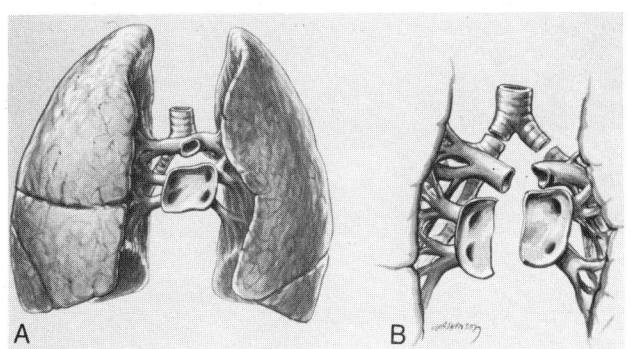

Figure 2. *A*, Double lung graft showing the two lungs together with the trachea, common pulmonary artery, and back wall of the left atrium containing the four pulmonary veins. *B*, Division of the common pulmonary artery, left atrial back wall, and sectioning of the main stem bronchus to produce the two separate lung grafts.

Recipient Procedure for Single Lung Transplant

Both right and left single lung transplants are performed with the air of one lung anesthesia utilizing a left-sided double-lumen endotracheal tube. Cardiopulmonary bypass is always available on a standby basis. It is routinely employed in the case of primary pulmonary hypertension and has been required for approximately 25 per cent of cases of pulmonary fibrosis. Bypass is usually not required for performing single lung transplant for emphysema.

The patient is positioned in the lateral thoracotomy position. The chest, abdomen, and ipsilateral groin are prepared and draped. Upon entering the chest, adhesions are divided by cautery wherever possible. The pulmonary artery is encircled intrapericardially; and on the left side, the ligamentum arteriosum is often divided for facilitating subsequent proximal clamping of the pulmonary artery. The pulmonary artery is temporarily clamped for determination of whether the transplantation procedure can be performed without the need of bypass. Cardiopulmonary bypass can be avoided if systemic blood pressure remains stable, arterial blood gases remain satisfactory, and contralateral pulmonary artery pressure does not rise too significantly during this period of temporary pulmonary artery occlusion. Monitoring of right ventricular function by means of transesophageal echocardiography is especially useful at this point. The pulmonary veins are isolated lateral to the pericardium; and during right lung transplantation, the interatrial groove is usually dissected for a short distance for facilitating subsequent clamping of the left atrium proximal to the right pulmonary veins. One mobilizes the main stem bronchi just proximal to the upper lobe bronchus, being careful to avoid unnecessary dissection around the recipient main bronchus. After preliminary thoracic dissection is accomplished, the omentum is mobilized through a small upper midline abdominal incision. Sufficient length is obtained to allow the apex of the omentum to easily reach the hilum of the lung. This generally requires nothing more than mobilization of the omentum from the transverse colon. A retrosternal tunnel is then created, and the omental pedicle is positioned in the anterior mediastinum for later withdrawal into the chest cavity.

If a trial of one lung anesthesia indicates the likely need for cardiopulmonary bypass, the femoral vessels on the side of the transplant are then prepared for cannulation. For primary pulmonary hypertension, cardiopulmonary bypass is required in all cases; and a right thoracotomy utilizing a single right atrial cannula for venous drainage and the right femoral artery for the return is favored. After complete hilar mobilization, the first branch of the pulmonary artery is divided between ligatures, and the remainder of the pulmonary artery is divided between staple lines just distal to this point, providing additional length as well as a somewhat reduced caliber, especially if the recipient pulmonary artery is large. In addition, the divided first branch of the pulmonary artery helps maintain orientation at the time of the pulmonary artery anastomosis. The two pulmonary veins are ligated extrapericardially and divided between ligatures or staples. The bronchus is divided just proximal to the upper lobe bronchus.

After removal of the recipient lung, the donor lung is oriented in the chest and packed with sponges and ice. The bronchial anastomosis is done initially with a continuous 4-0 monofilament absorbable suture of the posterior membranous wall, followed by interrupted 4-0 absorbable sutures with the knots placed exteriorly for the cartilaginous portion (Fig. 3). It has been found that starting with the bronchial anastomosis makes the procedure easier because of its posterior position; in addition, it provides an increased degree of stability during the subsequent vascular anastomoses. With completion of the bronchial anastomosis, the omentum is retrieved from its retrosternal position and brought inferior to the other hilar structures to completely encircle the bronchial anastomotic suture line. The omentum is tacked to itself as well as to surrounding mediastinal tissues for avoidance of displacement.

The donor and recipient pulmonary arteries are then trimmed, and the stump of the first branch of the recipient pulmonary artery is aligned with the first branch of the donor pulmonary artery for correct orientation. The pulmonary artery anastomosis is performed using continuous 5-0 polypropylene suture. Before the atrial anastomosis, the pericardium is opened circumferentially around the stumps of the pulmonary veins, and a Satinsky clamp is placed as centrally as possible on the left atrium without impinging on the contralateral pulmonary veins. On the right side, this maneuver is greatly facilitated by the previously described dissection in the interatrial groove. The ligatures on the pulmonary vein stumps are then removed, and an incision is made between the two veins to create a suitable atrial cuff. This cuff is then tailored to match the size of donor

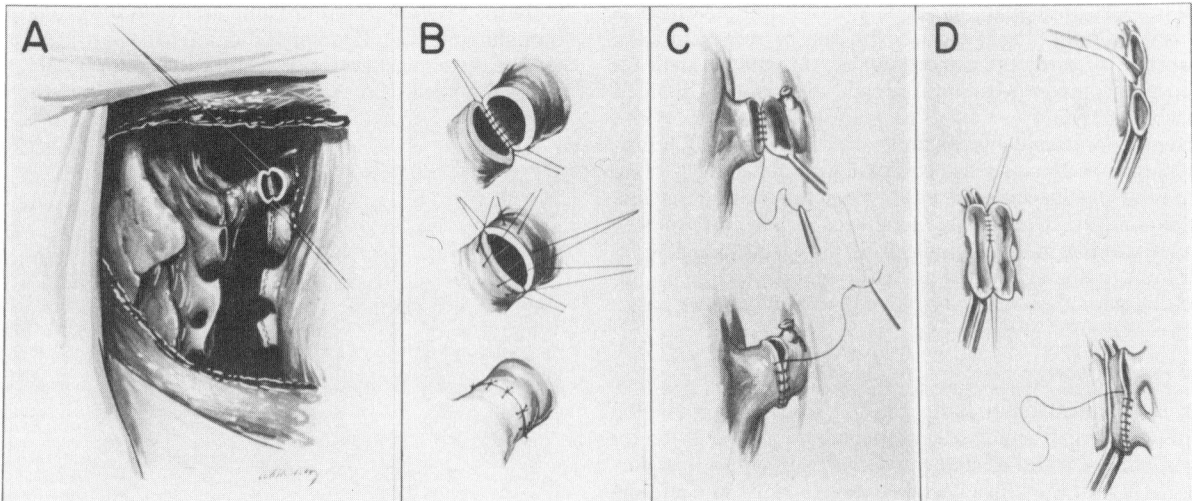

Figure 3. A, The bronchial anastomosis is completed first to give the transplanted lung stability within the chest. B, Bronchial anastomosis is done with a continuous suture on the membranous wall with interrupted sutures on the cartilaginous portion. C, Anastomosis of the pulmonary artery is performed with continuous nonabsorbable monofilament suture; the ligated first branch of the artery can be used for orientation. D, The recipient pulmonary veins are opened to produce a suitable cuff for anastomosis with continuous 4.0 polypropylene sutures.

atrial cuff. The back wall is anastomosed with a continuous 3-0 polypropylene suture; then similar sutures are placed anteriorly from the end points of the anastomosis to meet in the midline. The final suture is not secured to facilitate venting of the pulmonary circulation for elimination of air. This is accomplished by partial release of the pulmonary artery clamp, which allows controlled reperfusion of the pulmonary circulation. The ties on the atrial anastomosis are completed when blood is observed to flow freely through the anastomotic defect. After this, the clamps on the pulmonary artery and left atrium are removed for restoration of circulation to the transplanted lung, and the lung is immediately ventilated for avoidance of hypoxemia due to shunting.

Two chest tubes are placed, and the chest is closed in a standard manner. The average blood loss for this procedure has been less than one unit of blood. Even when cardiopulmonary bypass is required, bleeding has not been a problem because complete dissection of the recipient lung can usually be done prior to the administration of heparin. The double lumen endotracheal tube is replaced by a single lumen tube because most patients require ventilation for 24 to 48 hours postoperatively. All patients undergo endoscopic examination of the bronchial anastomosis prior to leaving the operating room.

Recipient Procedure for Bilateral Single Lung Transplant

The authors currently recommend bilateral lung replacement in all patients with pulmonary sepsis, specifically those with cystic fibrosis and bronchiectasis and, in addition, are now offering the operation to the majority of patients who present with end-stage emphysema under the age of 50. Historically, the authors' initial efforts at bilateral lung transplantation involved a procedure for simultaneous *en bloc* bilateral replacement, a procedure analogous to the combined heart-lung transplant without the need to transplant the heart. The concept of simultaneous *en bloc* bilateral pulmonary transplant was demonstrated in dogs by Vanderhoeft and co-workers in 1972.[26] That procedure, however, performed through a right thoracotomy is not suitable for use in humans. The technique initially employed utilized a median sternotomy, bilateral pneumonectomy, and implantation of the double lung block with three anastomoses, namely, the trachea, the common pulmonary artery, and a cuff of donor left atrium containing the pulmonary veins.[8,20]

Eight of the first nine double lung transplant procedures were successful,[5] with one fatality secondary to ischemia of the donor trachea. With further experience, the incidence of this complication rose to approximately 25 per cent.[21] Utilization of bilateral bronchial anastomosis, rather than tracheal anastomosis, significantly reduced the incidence of ischemic airway complications. Nonetheless, the double lung transplant as initally employed continued to have significant disadvantages, including the fact that the procedure itself is very complicated and difficult to teach. Extraction of the lungs through the median sternotomy can be technically difficult when the pleural spaces are fused with vascular adhesions secondary to cystic fibrosis. Postoperative cardiac dysfunction was a not uncommon sequela due to the prolonged period of total cardiopulmonary bypass and the need for ischemic arrest of the heart during this procedure. In addition, cardiac denervation was found to be present in a significant number of recipients after this procedure.

Recognizing the limitations of the original double lung transplant operation, the authors have changed their technique of double lung replacement to a double sequential single lung transplant or "bilateral lung transplant." Rather than being done via a median sternotomy, the bilateral lung transplant is done through a transverse inframammary thoracosternotomy that extends from one midaxillary line to the other, producing a

bilateral fourth or fifth interspace thoracotomy, preserving the latissimus dorsi and connected by a transverse sternotomy. The exposure offered by this incision permits excellent access for mobilization of intrapleural adhesions and hilar dissection without the routine need for cardiopulmonary bypass. The omentum is harvested in exactly the same manner as that used for the single lung transplant except that it is routinely divided into two pedicles, one for each bronchial anastomosis. The recipient is maintained with ventilation of the least impaired lung (as determined by quantitative V/Q scan) while the initial lung is excised and replaced exactly as for single lung transplantation. When the insertion of the initial lung is completed, the patient is then maintained on the newly transplanted lung while the second lung is excised and replaced. An important technical point when one is performing transplantation in patients with emphysema is to avoid opening the second hemithorax before transplantation of the initial lung is complete. It was found that opening both hemithoraces simultaneously resulted in overexpansion of the second lung out of the chest incision, which significantly complicated anesthetic management. This can be avoided by leaving the intercostal muscles intact until replacement of the first lung is completed.

If cardiopulmonary bypass is required during replacement of either lung, the aortic arch is cannulated in a standard manner, and a single right atrial drain is placed. The authors utilize a perfusion flow rate of approximately 1.5 liters per minute, adjusting the flow to maintain systolic pulmonary artery pressure below 30 mm.Hg. In several of the most recent cases, it has been found that systolic pulmonary artery pressures during insertion of the second lung have risen as high as 60 mm.Hg. This has not been an indication to initiate cardiopulmonary bypass if right heart function is preserved. Monitoring with transesophageal echocardiography has been most helpful in making this decision. It has been documented that there is no significant difference postoperatively in the function of the initially transplanted lung, which has sustained these elevated pulmonary artery pressures for the 1 to 2 hours required for insertion of the second lung.

One disadvantage of the sequential bilateral transplant is the extended period of ischemia for the second lung. This was extended to 8 hours in one case and 9½ hours in another, both of which were associated with excellent postoperative lung function and uncomplicated postoperative management. All patients undergo bronchoscopy prior to being transferred to the intensive care unit, where they remain intubated and ventilated in the initial postoperative period. In most recipients, pain control is managed with a constant infusion of epidural narcotics. Quantitative lung perfusion scans are obtained within 2 to 3 hours postoperatively to verify adequate blood flow to the new grafts. Inspired oxygen concentrations are rapidly decreased, maintaining an oxygen saturation greater than 90 per cent. Typically, patients can be decreased to an FIO_2 of 30 to 35 per cent within 12 to 24 hours. Ventilator settings include the maintenance of 5 cm. H_2O positive end-expiratory pressure to minimize intrapulmonary fluid extravasation; and after single lung transplantation, patients are nursed with the transplant side up.

Although intraoperative blood loss is usually in the range of 1 unit, most patients leave the operating room with a positive fluid balance of 5 to 10 liters. As a result, low filling pressures are not routinely used as an indication for fluid replacement. Inotropes are used to support blood pressure, and urinary output is maintained with a combination of blood or colloid infusion, loop diuretics, and low-dose dopamine infusion. Maintaining an adequate urinary output postoperatively is important because many of the medications given to transplant patients postoperatively are nephrotoxic.

Weaning from the ventilator is begun approximately 12 hours postoperatively, and 80 per cent of the patients are extubated between 24 and 48 hours. Apical chest drains are usually removed in the first 24 hours as long as there is no demonstrable air leak. Basal chest drains are routinely left in for 7 to 10 days because of previous experience with recurrent pleural effusions in this population, especially in the bilateral transplant group.

Immunosuppression

As a result of early laboratory studies which suggest an adverse effect of daily prednisone on bronchial healing, the authors currently attempt to avoid routine steroid administration for the initial 5 postoperative days unless treatment for suspected rejection is required.

IMMUNOSUPPRESSION REGIMEN

Preoperatively, azathioprine, a 2 mg. per kg. intravenous bolus, is given 1 to 2 hours prior to induction of anesthesia.

Postoperatively, antilymphocyte globulin (Minnesota Equine) is given in a 15 mg. per kg. intravenous infusion over 24 hours for 2 to 3 days, then over 6 hours for a total of 5 to 7 days. Infusion should be discontinued for an absolute lymphocyte count of less than 4000 per cu. mm. Azathioprine is also used in a dose of 2 mg. per kg. intravenously or orally. Note that one should reduce the dosage for a leukocyte count of less than 5000 per cu. mm. Cyclosporine is given as a constant intravenous infusion of 3 to 4 mg. per hour. Oral dosage should be initiated as soon as it can be tolerated and the dosage adjusted according to serum cyclosporine levels (target levels in first month, 400 to 500 ng. per ml. radioimmunoassay on whole blood). The dosage should be reduced for rising serum creatinine levels. No "routine" steroids should be used for the first 5 days. On day 5, prednisone, 10 mg. by mouth every morning, should be begun. The dosage should be increased to 0.5 mg. per kg. per day by 3 weeks. At 3 months one should begin tapering down to 0.15 mg. per kg. per day. At 1 year the dose should be at 15 mg. every other day.

Infection Prophylaxis

BACTERIAL. All patients undergo preoperative sputum cultures and unless otherwise indicated are given 1 gm. of cefazolin at the time of induction of anesthesia, which is continued for 1 week postoperatively. This bacterial coverage is modified if cultures of the donor and recipient bronchus obtained at the time of transplantation demonstrate organisms resistant to cefazolin.

PNEUMOCYSTIS CARINII. Double-strength trimethoprim/sulfamethoxazole is started twice a day on Monday, Wednesday, and Friday beginning at the end of the first week. If the patient has an allergy to sulfa medication, aerosolized pentamidine is given once a month.

VIRAL. As soon as oral medications can be tolerated, acyclovir, 200 mg. every 12 hours, is begun. In the case of a CMV mismatch (i.e., CMV-positive organ to CMV-negative recipient), the acyclovir dosage is increased to 800 mg. every 6 hours. Weekly serum buffy coat analysis and bronchial alveolar lavage performed at 2 weeks comprise the routine CMV screening in these postoperative patients. Biopsy-proven CMV infection is treated with intravenous gancyclovir.

FUNGUS. Oral Candida prophylaxis consists of oral nystatin, 500,000 units "swish and swallow," given each morning.

Physical Rehabilitation

Patients with end-stage lung disease and oxygen dependency have very limited physical reserve and tend to desaturate quickly with exercise. A sedentary existence follows with further progressive deterioration of muscle strength. A program of graded exercise and muscular training should begin prior to operation and include treadmill walking, cycling, and weight training, all with careful monitoring of pulse and oxygen saturation. Such monitoring ensures that the patients are exercising within safe limits and that adequate oxygen flow is being ad-

ministered. The authors have observed a significant improvement in exercise performance preoperatively in patients undergoing such rehabilitation and believe that this is reflected in an accelerated postoperative recovery.

An active exercise program is generally reinstituted 3 to 4 weeks after transplantation and maintained for a minimum of 3 months. Improvement in overall performance can be expected during the next 6 to 12 months, and most recipients are able to return to regular employment 4 to 6 months after transplantation. The 6-minute walk test is a convenient index of overall performance both preoperatively and postoperatively. For this test, patients are instructed to walk as quickly and comfortably as possible on a level course for 6 minutes. The patients are allowed to rest if necessary; and when required, oxygen is administered with a lightweight portable tank. The frequency of rests, the total distance covered, and the pulse and respiratory rate before and after the walk are recorded. In the authors' experience to date, the mean distance covered in 6-minute walk tests has increased from 346 meters preoperatively (with oxygen administration) to 462 meters at 1 month (no oxygen) and 649 meters (no oxygen) at 3 months after transplantation.

Bronchoscopic Surveillance

All patients undergo initial bronchoscopic evaluation before leaving the operating room. The next routine examination occurs within 12 to 48 hours at the time the patient is extubated, when the anastomoses are reinspected, repeat bronchial washings are taken for culture, and vocal cord function is assessed. In the third postoperative week, usually just prior to discharge from the hospital, patients undergo repeat bronchoscopy under local anesthesia. This examination usually coincides with the timing of increasing the oral prednisone to maximal levels (0.5 mg. per kg. per day); however, the timing of repeat bronchoscopy is often modified because of earlier suspicion of episodes of rejection or infection. At the time of the predischarge-bronchoscopy, transbronchial biopsy and bronchoalveolar lavage are performed.

After discharge, bronchoscopies are scheduled whenever indicated to help with the differential diagnosis between acute rejection and cytomegalovirus infection. Routine transbronchial biopsies are obtained at 3-, 6-, and 12-month evaluations.

Transplantation Results

The authors' most recent review of transplantation results involves the period between July 1989 and June 1990. During that period, 36 lung transplants were performed in 35 patients

TABLE 1. Diagnoses and Type of All Transplants Performed Between July 1, 1989, and June 30, 1990

Chronic Obstructive Pulmonary Disease	Single	Bilateral
Emphysema	9	2
Alpha$_1$-antitrypsin deficiency emphysema	3	6
Cystic fibrosis	0	3
Lymphangioleiomyomatosis*	1	0
Eosinophilic granuloma	1	0
Retransplant (obliterative bronchiolitis)	0	1
Retransplant (graft failure)	1	0
Chronic Restrictive Pulmonary Disease		
Idiopathic pulmonary fibrosis	2	1
Pulmonary Hypertension		
Primary pulmonary hypertension	5	0
Atrial septal defect/Eisenmenger's	1	0

* This patient also had Wolff-Parkinson-White syndrome and underwent coincident division of a left free wall accessory pathway by the epicardial approach at the time of left single lung transplant.

TABLE 2. Mean Forced Expiratory Volume in 1 Second for Transplant Patients with COPD at the Time of Evaluation and at 1, 3, and 6 Months Postoperatively

| | Number | FEV₁ (liters) | | |
		Total	Single	Bilateral
		n = 24	n = 14	n = 10
Evaluation	24	0.52	0.50	0.54
1 month	24	1.84*	1.29*	2.68*
3 months	18	1.91*	1.37*	3.04*
6 months	10	1.52*	1.21*	3.37*

Two patients have been excluded from this table. One died perioperatively, and in one the procedure was a retransplant.

* $p < 0.05$, compared with evaluation measurement.

(mean age, 44 years; range, 21 to 60 years). On eight occasions donor lungs were shared between 2 recipients; 4 of these 16 lungs were used concurrently in other institutions. In this group of 35 patients, 1 underwent *en bloc* double lung transplant, 12 had bilateral single transplants, and 23 single lung transplants were performed in 22 patients. Within this patient group there were two deaths, one in the hospital (the last use of the double lung procedure) and one late death, which translates into a 94.3 per cent absolute survival rate. The stay in the intensive care unit ranged from 1 to 36 days, with a median of 4 days. Hospital stay ranged from 15 to 66 days, with a median of 24 days. No patient currently requires supplemental oxygen, and satisfactory oxygen concentration on room air (Pao₂ greater than 60 mm. Hg) was obtained at a median of 7 days postoperatively (range, 2 to 40 days).

The primary diagnoses as well as the type of transplant performed in all the patients in this group are listed in Table 1. Currently, the most common indication for bilateral lung transplantation is in patients with either emphysema or cystic fibrosis. The improvement in FEV₁ in all patients with chronic obstructive pulmonary disease is demonstrated in Table 2. As shown, it was not unusual for patients undergoing bilateral lung transplantation to demonstrate quantitative improvement in FEV₁ on the order of 700 per cent. The long-term results of single lung transplant for pulmonary fibrosis have been published previously.[25] The authors embarked on the series of single lung transplants for pulmonary hypertension with a degree of caution and uncertainty. Follow-up right heart catheterization studies and radionuclide ventriculograms have been obtained in all patients, and it has been extremely gratifying thus far to see all six of the current patients demonstrate the re-establishment of normal pulmonary artery pressures and right ventricular ejection fractions within weeks of single lung transplant (Fig. 4).

Six-minute walk assessments demonstrated a significant improvement when measured 3 months postoperatively, with improvement in results reaching a plateau at 6 months. Supplemental oxygen was required to maintain saturations above 90 per cent in 89.3 per cent of patients at evaluation, 95.5 per cent of patients just prior to transplantation, and 22.2 per cent and 0 per cent of patients 2 weeks and 12 weeks postoperatively.

Morbidity and Mortality

As shown in Table 3, the incidence of complications in posttransplant patients is not insignificant. For this reason, it is essential that the personnel responsible for the immediate postoperative care of these patients be aware of the diverse nature of these problems so that their occurrence can be recognized and managed in the early stages. Not unexpectedly, pulmonary complications were the most commonly encountered postoperative problems. Eighteen patients (51 per cent) have had 21 biopsy-proven episodes of CMV disease (17 pneumonitis, with 3 recurrences and 1 hepatitis). No CMV deaths occurred, but in a patient who expired after a fatal airway hemorrhage, CMV pneumonitis was identified at the time of autopsy. When CMV infection is documented by biopsy or suspected on the basis of conventional culture or shell-vial assay of bronchoalveolar lavage fluid or serum buffy coats, it is treated with gancyclovir, 5 mg. per kg. every 12 hours intravenously for 2 to 3 weeks. No patient who was initially CMV-negative and received a CMV-negative organ had any evidence of CMV infection.

Eleven patients (31.4 per cent) required specific antibiotic treatment for microbiologically proven pulmonary infection. Five of these infections were due to organisms that had originally been present in donor bronchial washings. In three additional patients culture-proven evidence of fungal pulmonary infection developed. *Aspergillus fumigatus* was grown in one and *Torulopsis glabrata* was isolated in two additional patients. All three patients responded to intravenous amphotericin B therapy.

Problems with airway healing were detected in six patients. In three of these patients these problems were of clinical significance. In the other three, the problem consisted of noncircumferential areas of anastomotic necrosis and slough, which were detected on routine bronchoscopy in asymptomatic patients. As previously mentioned, one patient died after discharge as a result of a fatal bronchus to pulmonary artery fistula. Two additional patients were found to have significant bronchial anastomotic dehiscence that required stenting.[27] It has been found that in approximately 14 per cent of patients anastomotic defects will develop, most of which have no clinical significance. Bron-

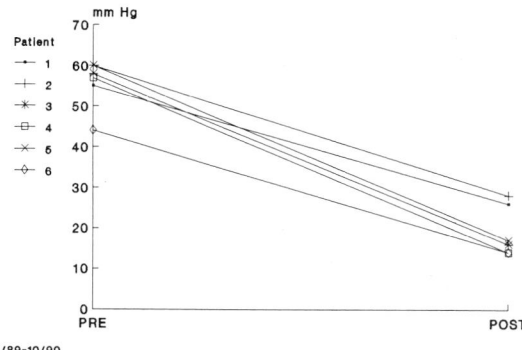

CHANGE IN MEAN PA PRESSURE
SINGLE LUNG FOR PULMONARY HTN

11/89–10/90

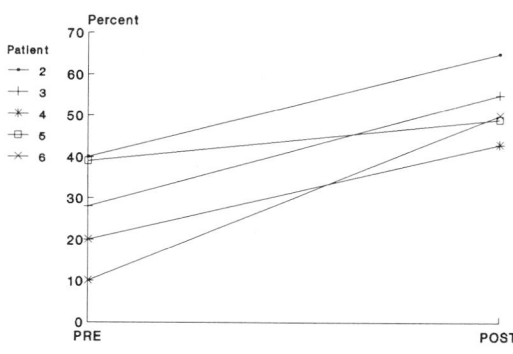

CHANGE IN RVEF
SINGLE LUNG FOR PULMONARY HTN

11/89–10/90

Figure 4. Patients with pulmonary hypertension are observed to re-establish normal mean pulmonary artery pressures and right ventricular ejection fractions when measured 1 to 2 months after single lung transplant.

TABLE 3. Incidence of Posttransplant Complications in 36 Consecutive Transplants

Pulmonary

Biopsy confirmed CMV infection	18
Bacterial pneumonia	11
Airway healing defects	6

Cardiac Complications

Supraventricular arrhythmias	9
Cardiopulmonary arrest	3
Myocardial infarction	2

Neurologic Complications

Grand mal seizures	2
Phrenic nerve palsy	2
Recurrent laryngeal nerve palsy	2

Gastrointestinal Complications

Clostridia difficile infection	7
Prolonged ileus	6
Herpetic pharyngitis	1
Acute cholecystitis	1

Hematologic Complications

Hemolytic anemia	4

Wound Complications 2

choscopy and thin slice computed tomographic (CT) scanning are invaluable for detection and follow-up of these defects. The majority of these lesions can be managed conservatively. However, in the authors' experience, 8 per cent have required stenting, and airway complication was the cause of death in 2 per cent of patients.[23]

Nine patients (25.7 per cent) experienced either atrial flutter or atrial fibrillation; only one required electrical cardioversion. Three patients suffered cardiac arrest in the postoperative period. Two of the three had undergone single lung transplant for pulmonary hypertension. All three patients were successfully resuscitated, but one required a prolonged episode of open cardiac massage. This patient developed diffuse transplant lung injury and required tracheostomy and mechanical ventilation for a month. This patient has subsequently completely recovered and has returned to work.

Four patients received lungs from donors of nonidentical blood groups (three group A recipients and one group B recipient received organs from group O donors). Three of these patients developed anemia associated with a positive direct Coombs' test, low haptoglobin, and the presence of ABO-directed antibodies in the blood between 1 and 3 weeks postoperatively. This immune-mediated phenomenon was presumed to be secondary to a production of ABO antibodies by the lymphocytes transplanted in the donor lung. Washed red cells were transfused from group O donors, and continued evidence of this problem disappeared after the third postoperative week.

One hospital and one late death occurred. The one in-hospital death involved the last of the original *en bloc* double lung transplants. This patient had an intraoperative myocardial infarction and died from cardiac failure 3 days postoperatively. The late death occurred after a single lung transplant in a 55-year-old man with alpha$_1$-antitrypsin emphysema. This patient was discharged well on the twenty-fifth postoperative day but died at home 3 weeks later because of a fistula between the right pulmonary artery and bronchial anastomosis. At the time of autopsy, the tips of the interrupted monofilament sutures used to complete the bronchial anastomosis were found to have caused small microperforations in the adjoining pulmonary artery. This occurred despite the fact that all bronchial anastomoses are wrapped with omentum.

Diagnosis of Rejection

The diagnosis of rejection remains imprecise and is based on a combination of suggestive signs and symptoms, including deterioration in arterial oxygenation, pyrexia, decreased exercise tolerance, decreased oxygen saturation with exercise, increased fatigability, and development of a radiologic infiltrate or hilar flair, together with the absence of any alternative cause of deterioration such as fluid overload or infection. Sequential quantitative lung perfusion scans are of assistance in diagnosing rejection after single lung transplant. A relative decrease in perfusion to the transplanted lung has frequently been observed in association with rejection episodes and reverses within hours following bolus steroids. The single most useful diagnostic method for the diagnosis of rejection is response to a pulse dose of intravenous methylprednisolone. Improvement in oxygenation, reduction in temperature, and improvement in exercise tolerance occur within hours. Radiologic alterations, if present, generally improve over a 12- to 24-hour period.

Most recipients undergo two or three significant rejection episodes in the first 3 to 4 weeks. The first episode commonly occurs at 4 to 7 days but may occur as early as 48 hours after transplantation. Essentially, all episodes of acute rejection occur within the first 6 weeks. Chronic rejection, however, has developed in some patients within the first year.

In patients with single lung transplant, the transplanted lung improves gradually over the initial 3 weeks, and this improvement is paralleled by an increase in perfusion. At 7 days, perfusion of the transplanted lung has been 47 to 87 per cent of the total pulmonary flow. This figure varies with the status of the transplanted lung and the pulmonary vascular resistance of the native lung. At 3 weeks, perfusion to the transplanted lung of between 64 and 90 per cent has been demonstrated. These figures usually increase further in the 3 months after transplantation. When single lung transplantation has been performed for primary pulmonary hypertension, quantitative perfusion scans performed immediately after the transplant have demonstrated 95 per cent of flow going to the transplanted lung. This has not been associated with the development of posttransplant edema or pulmonary dysfunction. Long-term function of the transplanted lung has generally been excellent, with little or no deterioration during follow-up periods, which currently exceed 6 years.[25]

International Lung Transplant Registry

In 1988, a registry for lung transplantation was established in St. Louis. The registry currently receives data from 52 registered transplant centers in the United States and 17 international centers. As of October 1990, the registry contained data on 432 lung transplants (302 singles, 130 doubles). Although the number of active lung transplantation centers has remained fairly constant, the incidence of lung transplantation has shown exponential growth. The most common indications worldwide for single lung transplantation include idiopathic pulmonary fibrosis (42 per cent), emphysema (34 per cent), and primary pulmonary hypertension (10 per cent). Patients with emphysema (48 per cent) and cystic fibrosis (35 per cent) form the largest two groups undergoing double lung replacement.

Analysis of these initial 432 cases dating back to 1983 has shown that 64 per cent of both single and double lung transplant patients are currently alive. It is clear from these survival curves that mortality is highest in the initial postoperative period, mortality in the first 2 weeks and 2 months being 16 and 26 per cent, respectively. These data suggest that survival beyond 2 months provides the potential for long-term survival. It is important to appreciate when one is examining lung transplantation survival data at this early point in its evolution that it will contain the learning periods of all the 69 currently registered centers. Further analysis has demonstrated a significant improvement in especially early, but also late, mortality during the last 2 years. This undoubtedly reflects not only increasing experience throughout the world with the technical aspects of transplantation but also improvement in graft preservation and immunosuppression protocols.

SUMMARY

Transplantation for end-stage lung disease remains at an early stage, but recent success suggests that transplantation for end-stage interstitial lung disease can achieve the same degree of success demonstrated with the transplantation of other organs. However, the solutions to many problems remain. These include improved means of immunosuppression, the ability to accurately diagnose rejection, and the securing of more transplantable lungs from the available donor population. These solutions require improved means of donor maintenance to avoid deterioration of the lung both before and after declaration of brain death and the ability to preserve lungs for 12 hours or more to allow transplantation of suitable lungs from greater distances.

Currently, the authors favor the use of single lung transplantation for pulmonary fibrosis, primary pulmonary hypertension, and for emphysema in patients over the age of 50. The bilateral lung transplant is employed for patients with cystic fibrosis and for younger patients with emphysema. Success with lung transplantation has been achieved with the experimental and clinical contributions of numerous investigators over a 40-year period. The demonstration of clinical success with the various types of lung transplants should provide additional stimulus for rapid advances in the future.

REFERENCES

1. Alican, F., et al.: Left lung replantation with immediate pulmonary artery ligation. Ann. Surg., *174*:34, 1971.
2. Barnard, C. N., and Cooper, D. K. C.: Clinical transplantation of the heart: a review of 13 years' personal experience. J. R. Soc. Med., *74*:670, 1981.
3. Benfield, J. R., and Coon, R.: The role of the left atrial anastomosis in pulmonary replantation. J. Thorac. Cardiovasc. Surg., *61*:847, 1971.
4. Cooley, D. A., et al.: Organ transplantation for advanced cardiopulmonary disease. Ann. Thorac. Surg., *8*:30, 1969.
5. Cooper, J. D., Patterson, G. A., Grosman, R., Maurer, J., and the Toronto Lung Transplant Group: Double lung transplant for advanced chronic obstructive lung disease. Am. Rev. Resp. Dis., *139*:303, 1989.
6. Cooper, J. D., Pearson, F. G., Patterson, G. A., Todd, T. R. J., Ginsberg, R. J., Goldberg, M., and Waters, P.: Use of silicone stents in the management of airway problems. Ann. Thorac. Surg., *47*:371, 1989.
7. Daicoff, G. R., Allen, P. D., and Streck, C. J.: Pulmonary vascular resistance following lung reimplantation and transplantation. Ann. Thorac. Surg., *9*:569, 1970.
8. Dark, J. H., Patterson, G. A., Al-Jilaihawi, A. N., Hsu, H., Egan T., and Cooper J. D.: Experimental en-bloc double-lung transplantation. Ann. Thorac. Surg., *42*:394, 1986.
9. Derom, F., Barbier, F., Ringoir, S., et al.: Ten month survival after lung homotransplantation in man. J. Thorac. Cardiovasc. Surg., *61*:835, 1971.
10. Dubois, P., Choiniere, L., and Cooper, J. D.: Bronchial omentopexy in canine lung allotransplantation. Ann. Thorac. Surg., *38*:211, 1984.
11. Goldberg, M., Lima, O., Morgan, E., et al.: A comparison between cyclosporin A and methylprednisolone plus azathioprine on bronchial healing following canine lung allotransplantation. J. Thorac. Cardiovasc. Surg., *85*:821, 1983.
12. Hardin, C. A., and Kittle, C. F.: Experiences with transplantation of the lung. Science., *119*:97, 1954.
13. Hardy, J. D., Webb, W. R., Dalton, M. L., and Walker, G. R.: Lung homotransplantation in man. J.A.M.A., *186*:1065, 1963.
14. Keshavjee, S. H., Yamazaki, F., Cardoso, P. E., McRitchie, D. I., Patterson, G. A., and Cooper, J. D.: A method for safe twelve-hour pulmonary preservation. J. Thorac. Cardiovasc. Surg., *98*:529, 1989.
15. Lillehei, C. W.: Discussion of Wildevuur, C. R. H., and Benfield, J. R.: A review of 23 human lung transplantations by 20 surgeons. Ann. Thorac. Surg., *9*:489, 1970.
16. Lima, O., Cooper, J. D., Peters, W. J., et al.: Effects of methylprednisolone and azathioprine on bronchial healing following lung autotransplantation. J. Thorac. Cardiovasc. Surg., *82*:211, 1981.
17. Metras, H.: Note preliminaire sur la graffe totale du poumon chez le chien. Fr. Acad. Sci., 1176, October 30, 1950.
18. Morgan, W. E., Lima, O., Goldberg, M., Ayabe, H., Ferdman, A., and Cooper, J. D.: Improved bronchial healing in canine left lung reimplantation using omental pedicle wrap. J. Thorac. Cardiovasc. Surg., *85*:139, 1983.
19. Nelems, J. M., Rebuck, A. S., Cooper, J. D., Goldberg, M., Halloran, P. F., and Vellend, H.: Human lung transplantation. Chest, *78*:569, 1980.
20. Patterson, G. A., Cooper, J. D., Goldman, B., Weisel, R. D., Pearson, F. G., Waters, P. F., Todd, T. R., Scully, H., Goldberg, M., and Ginsberg, R. J.: Technique of successful clinical double lung transplantation. Ann. Thorac. Surg., *44*:626, 1988.
21. Patterson, G. A., Todd, T. R., Cooper, J. D., Pearson, F. G., Winton, T. L., Maurer, J., and the Toronto Lung Transplant Group: Airway complications following double lung transplantation. J. Thorac. Cardiovasc. Surg., *99*:14, 1990.
22. Reitz, B. A., Wallwork, J. L., Hunt, S. A., et al.: Heart-lung transplantation: Successful therapy for patients with pulmonary vascular disease. N. Engl. J. Med., *3067*:557, 1982.
23. Schafers, H. J., Haydock, D. A., and Cooper, J. D.: The incidence and management of bronchial anastomotic complications in lung transplantation. J. Thorac. Cardiovasc. Surg., In press.
24. Todd, T. R., Goldberg, M., Koshal, A., Menkis, A., Boychuk, J., Patterson, G. A., and Cooper, J. D.: Separate extraction of cardiac and pulmonary grafts from a single organ donor. Ann. Thorac. Surg., *46*:3, 1988.
25. The Toronto Lung Transplant Group (including Cooper, J. D.): Experience with single lung transplantation for pulmonary fibrosis. J.A.M.A., *259*:2258, 1988.
26. Vanderhoeft, P., Dubois, A., Lauvan, N., de Francquen, P. H., Carpentier, Y., Rocmans, P., Nelson, R., Kaufman, S., Brickman, L., Gyhra, A., and Ectars, P.: Block allotransplantation of both lungs with pulmonary trunk and left atrium in dogs. Thorax, *278*:415, 1972.
27. Veith, F. J., and Richards, K.: Lung transplantation with simultaneous contralateral pulmonary artery ligation. Surg. Gynecol. Obstet., *129*:768, 1969.
28. Waldhausen, J. A., et al.: Physiologic changes associated with autotransplantation of the lung. Ann. Surg., *165*:580, 1967.

XII

AUTOTRANSPLANTATION

R. Randal Bollinger, M.D., Ph.D.

Autotransplantation is the transfer of an organ, part of an organ, a tissue, or cells from one place to another in the same individual. Autotransplantation has several practical advantages over *allotransplantation* (transfer between individuals of the same species) or *xenotransplantation* (transfer between individuals of different species). Immunologic rejection does not occur, the donor is at all times readily available, and prolonged preservation is usually unnecessary in the case of autotransplants. Because of these advantages, autotransplantation was used earlier, more successfully, and more widely by all surgical specialties than other forms of transplantation.

The first well-documented autografting technique was the transfer of skin and subcutaneous tissue from the forearm to the face to form a new nose (Fig. 1). The staged tubular pedicle graft technique was described in 1587 by Gasparo Tagliacozzi in his landmark textbook on plastic surgery, *De Cutorum Chirurgia per Insitionem (On the Surgery of Mutilation by Grafting)*. However, the earliest record of autogenous pedicled grafts antedates Tag-

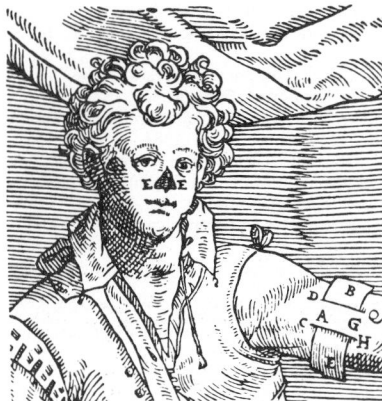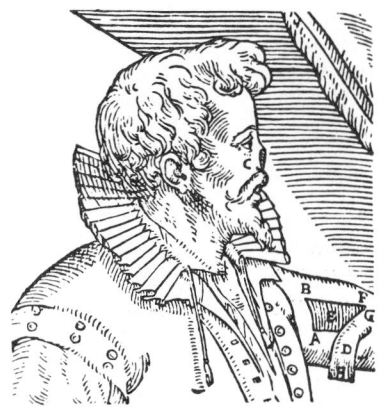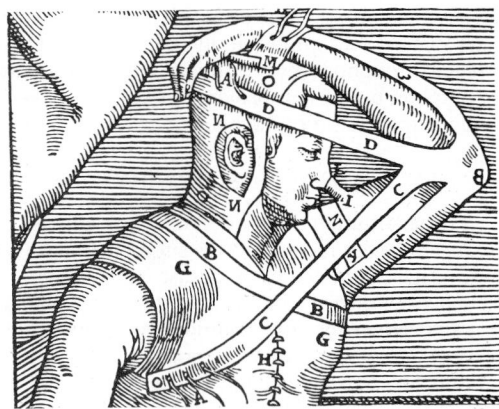

Figure 1. Reconstruction of the nose with a staged tubular pedicle graft. (From Tagliacozzi, G.: De Cutorum Chirurgia per Insitionem, 1587.)

liacozzi by more than 1000 years. The Sanskrit text of India, the *Súshruta Samhitá,* describes restoration of mutilations of the nose, ear, and lip using pedicled grafts from the forehead, neck, and cheeks.[60] From its origin in the transfer of skin for reconstructive surgery, autotransplantation has grown to include muscle, bone, joint, nerve, artery, vein, composite tissue, endocrine gland, bone marrow, kidney, ureter, bladder, and intestinal transfers.

SKIN AUTOGRAFTS

Skin grafts are used to cover wounds where insufficient skin is available to permit immediate (primary) or delayed (secondary) suture closure. All successful skin grafting was done on pedicles until 1804, when Giuseppe Baronio of Milan published the results of his experiments in sheep involving successful free transplantation of large pieces of skin from one site to another. The pinch graft introduced by Jacques Louis Reverdin in 1869 was followed by thin split-thickness grafts introduced by Louis Ollier and more carefully studied and described by Carl Thiersch.[60] The modern, thicker split-thickness grafts were popularized by Brown and McDowell.[8]

Prior to the advent of free skin grafting, surgeons had no alternative to allowing open wounds to heal by contraction and epithelialization. Unfortunately, the epithelium that migrates from the cutaneous perimeter of the wound across the granulating surface develops no firm attachment to the underlying connective tissue. The rete pegs, which are closely interlocking ridges of dermis and epidermis found in normal skin, do not develop. The new epidermis is easily torn from the underlying tissue, causing such re-epithelialized wounds to break down frequently. In addition, wound contraction during natural healing can cause contractures at joints and distortion of facial features. These unsatisfactory consequences of natural healing can be prevented by skin grafting.

A pedicle graft or one of several different types of free skin grafts may be selected, depending on the size of the site to be covered, the functional and cosmetic requirements of the recipient site, and the availability of donor sites. A *pedicle graft* is never separated from its blood supply, since revascularization at the recipient site is allowed to develop before the original blood supply is finally severed. Pedicle flaps, which include subcutaneous fat as well as skin, provide padding that prevents ulceration and so are useful for wounds, such as decubitus ulcers, that sustain frequent trauma. Pedicle flaps should be used to cover wounds requiring later reoperation (e.g., for bone, tendon, or nerve repair) and in some cases in which appearance is an important consideration. Pedicle grafts can be *advanced* or moved to recipient sites far from their place or origin. The graft in the form of a flap is first created by making skin and subcutaneous incisions along three sides, leaving intact the side with the best blood supply. The flap is undermined and may then be sutured immediately to an adjacent area requiring the graft or may be *delayed,* that is, allowed to remain in its primary bed until its new blood supply is better established. In the form of a flap or a tube, the pedicle may be *walked* through a series of repeated divisions and reattachments until a distant recipient site is reached. The donor site may be closed by primary suturing or by covering with a split-thickness skin graft.

A *free graft* is completely separated from its vascular, nervous, and lymphatic connections during the transplantation procedure. A *full-thickness* skin graft is a free graft including the entire epidermis and dermis, whereas a *partial* or *split-thickness* graft includes all of the epidermis and a variable part of the dermis. *Anastomosed free grafts,* in which the small arteries and veins supplying a graft are reanastomosed to small vessels at the recipient site, have gained in popularity as microsurgical techniques have improved. Anastomosed free grafts are discussed further in the section on composite tissue autotransplantation.

Full-thickness skin grafts are used when pigment matching, resistance to contraction, or growth of a child are important considerations in the outcome of wound healing. Full-thickness grafts require a better blood supply for survival than do split-thickness grafts because the graft vessels are cut below the level of their dermal branching. Relatively fewer cut vessels are available to absorb nutrients from the wound bed to meet the relatively greater nutritional needs of the thicker graft. Other disadvantages of full-thickness grafts include the limited area that can be covered, the need to surgically close the donor site, and the poor resistance to infection, which generally precludes use of these grafts on contaminated wounds. Full-thickness skin is best harvested from locations where the skin is thin, such as the eyelids, postauricular area, and supraclavicular area, or loose and redundant, such as the flexor creases of the elbow, buttock, or groin. The grafts are cut freehand, using a template pattern made of the defect, and must be completely free of subcutaneous fat in order to be successful.

Split-thickness skin grafts are able to survive on compromised surfaces, such as granulating wounds contaminated with bacteria, because split-thickness skin is more richly supplied with open blood vessels on its underside. Split-thickness skin is used to cover wounds with precarious circulation and those with large areas of skin loss from burns or other traumatic injuries, as well as to cover large full-thickness skin donor sites. The skin is cut through a preselected level of the dermis. The dermis is approximately 20 times thicker than the epidermis in most areas of the body, permitting a wide latitude in graft thicknesses. Average grafts are between 12/1000 and 18/1000 of an inch thick (0.30 to 0.45 mm.), but thinner grafts must be taken from children, from the aged, and from certain areas of the face where the skin is thinner. Since only a part of the dermis is taken, the donor site heals spontaneously by epithelial outgrowth from the remaining epithelial islands, sweat glands, and hair follicles.[59]

Split-thickness grafts are cut using freehand knives, hand-driven drum dermatomes, or power dermatomes. Before the introduction of power and drum dermatomes, all skin grafts were cut with hand-held knives. Since much skill and experience are required to cut grafts of uniform thickness, the freehand technique is now used primarily for covering small wounds requiring limited quantities of skin. The Goulian knife, which incorporates a guard, allows cutting of small split grafts that are far superior to the irregular, unsightly "pinch graft." The Padgett and Reese instruments are drum dermatomes. Both require the skin to be fixed to the drum with an adhesive. When the drum and adherent skin are elevated, the calibrated knife blade slides back and forth on an axle to cut a long, wide graft of uniform thickness. The dermatome most often used to harvest split-thickness skin is the power-driven Brown. The rapidly vibrating knife (similar to barber's clippers) is driven by an electric motor or gas turbine. The cutting width and depth are adjustable, much like a wood planer. The skin to be cut must be clean, well-lubricated with mineral oil, and locally anesthetized if the patient is not under general anesthesia. After the graft is cut, the donor site is dressed with fine mesh gauze and kept dry (e.g., with a hair dryer) until re-epithelialization is complete. The practical details of use for each type of dermatome are concisely described and clearly illustrated in the monograph by Rudolph and associates.[59]

Color match, texture, and scar visibility must be considered in choosing the donor skin, since grafted skin always maintains the epidermal specificity of its donor site. Split-thickness grafts are taken from broad flat areas such as the abdomen, thigh, buttock, medial arm, or chest. However, in difficult cases, such as extensively burned patients, any available skin can be used, and healed donor sites may be reused as often as necessary until coverage is complete. Split-thickness skin may be harvested from traumatically or surgically amputated tissue in order to close huge defects. Extra skin may be stored at 4° C. in normal saline with antibiotics for up to 4 weeks, then utilized in the same manner as fresh split-thickness skin.

A rich vascular supply is essential for support of a split-thickness graft. Skin does not survive when placed directly on bone, cartilage, or bare tendon. However, muscle, fascia, peritoneum, pleura, meninges, and vascularized fat, as well as bone debrided of its outer cortex to permit proliferation of granulation tissue, all support skin grafts. Exposed cartilage is best removed before grafting, and tendons are best covered by full-thickness flaps. The wound to be skin grafted must be clean and free from bleeding. Surgical debridement and frequent dressing changes are employed to remove necrotic tissues, exudate, and all foreign material from the recipient site. When healthy granulation tissue, appearing pink or beefy-red from its many blood vessels, fills the wound and epithelial ingrowth begins from the margins, the wound is ready for grafting. The granulating bed with its rich supply of phagocytic cells is resistant to infection but is not sterile. Skin grafts will generally survive when placed over beds containing less than 10^5 organisms per gram of tissue[58] unless the organisms are streptococci, which can rapidly dissolve transplanted skin. Further surgical debridement, administration of systemic antibiotics (e.g., penicillin) and topical antibacterials (e.g., silver sulfadiazine), and placement of pigskin xenografts or amnion allografts eliminate recipient site infections and promote healthy granulation tissue.

Hemostasis after debridement and at the time of grafting may be obtained by conservative electrocautery, temporary clamping, fine absorbable sutures, or direct pressure for 5 to 7 minutes. Topical hemostatic substances, such as oxidized cellulose or absorbable gelatin sponge, which create a diffusion barrier between the skin graft and its vascular bed, should be avoided. Meshing or perforation of the graft prevents serum accumula-tion beneath it. If the recipient site is free of debris and if bleeding is controlled and motion between the graft and its bed is prevented, the approximation necessary for fibrin adhesion and subsequent capillary invasion is achieved. A stable, firm pressure dressing or even splinting in plaster may be necessary to completely immobilize the graft.

NERVE AUTOGRAFTS

Nerve autografts are used to repair unsuturable defects in major peripheral nerves. Wallerian degeneration occurs in the distal damaged nerve and the donor graft before reinnervation. The Schwann cells, endoneural tubes, and connective tissue survive in the form of conduits through which the axons may regenerate to reach viable end-organs. Axon regeneration progresses at a rate of 1 mm. per day in free grafts and 1.5 mm. per day in revascularized nerve grafts. As with autografted skin, one key to success is adequacy of the residual or acquired blood supply. Since free grafts of thick nerves usually undergo central ischemic necrosis, thin nerves are usually employed alone or in groups known as *cable grafts*. The grafted and recipient nerves must be of similar diameter and the ends carefully approximated. Microneural interfascicular reconstruction improves results.[42] The sural, brachial cutaneous, superficial radial, or lateral femoral cutaneous nerves can be used. The greater auricular nerve has been autotransplanted to replace the facial nerve in cases of facial paralysis. When the nerve gap is large, when the recipient bed is scarred, or when a thick nerve is needed, conventional nerve grafts frequently fail owing to ischemia. Free vascularized nerve grafts of superficial radial nerve and the adjacent radial artery to supply blood have been utilized successfully in these adverse circumstances.[73] The combination of microneural and microvascular anastomoses provides hope for the future in an area of autotransplantation in which success is currently partial and unpredictable. Human muscle autografts that can provide long, large parallel arrays of basement membrane tubes to bridge large peripheral nerve gaps may also offer significant advantages over conventional techniques.[48]

MUSCULOSKELETAL AUTOGRAFTS

MUSCLE. Nonvascularized muscle transplants rapidly undergo ischemic necrosis, resorption, and replacement by fibrous tissue. Transfer of an entire muscle group without division of its neurovascular supply has been used to restore function in the distribution of an adjacent damaged nerve, for example, radial nerve and muscle transfer for ulnar palsy. Microneurovascular free muscle transplantation of gracilis muscle from the leg to the forearm to re-establish finger flexion in a patient with severe Volkmann's ischemic contracture has been reported.[71] Free grafts of latissimus dorsi, gracilis, or extensor digitorum brevis muscle have been used to treat facial paralysis. Transplanted whole muscle can survive and be reinnervated 5 months after microneurovascular anastomosis. Muscle is frequently a component of composite tissue autografts, as described in a subsequent section.

BONE. Autografts of bone in the form of trephine defects with reinserted bone plugs have been found in a Bronze Age skull. In 1809 Merrem reported the healing of autotransplanted dog skull. Subsequent experiments have demonstrated that the bulk of the bone implanted as a conventional free autograft does not survive transplantation.[53] All but the most superficial cells of cortical grafts die of ischemia, causing bone resorption and replacement in a process termed creeping substitution. Larger numbers of cells survive in the case of cancellous bone, which has an open structure that facilitates diffusion of nutrients and ingrowth of osteoclasts and osteoblasts.[7] Local blood supply and recipient bed conditions are crucial to the success of conventional bone grafts. Broad contact with recipient bone and complete immobilization contribute to success. Infection, scarring, and irradiation of the tissues usually cause failure.

Bone grafts are used for the reconstruction of major skeletal defects produced by trauma, disease, or congenital malformation. The open reduction and internal fixation of some fresh fractures is supplemented with cancellous implants to promote healing. Barrel-stave autografts are used to achieve bony union in cases of pseudarthrosis or delayed healing of fractures. Cortical bone is used to supplement joint arthrodesis, and cancellous bone to fill cavities in other bones, such as the defect left after curettement of a unicameral bone cyst. Reconstruction of the jaw and face after radical cancer surgery or severe trauma often utilizes combined bone and other tissue grafts to re-establish function and contour.

Cancellous bone is usually obtained from the iliac crest, although it is also available from the metaphyseal ends of long bones. Cortical grafts are derived from the ribs, the central and proximal portions of the fibula, and the diaphysis of long bones. Vascularized, "living" bone grafts, in which the primary blood supply to the bone is preserved or immediately reconstituted, avoid resorption and maintain their original size and structural strength.[50] Vascularized grafts of ribs, fibula, and ilium are discussed in the section on composite tissue autografts.

CARTILAGE. Autotransplantation of cartilage has been used primarily in reconstructive surgery to rebuild nasal contours, to repair the pinna of the ear, and to fill defects in the bones of the face and skull. The cartilage graft heals to adjacent tissue by formation of a fibrous or fibrocartilaginous scar. Grafts from adults do not grow in their new position, and portions of the graft frequently undergo slow resorption. Most grafts are taken from the costochondral junction of the ribs, but nasal septum and articular cartilage have also been used. Interestingly, because of its avascular structure, few cells, and large amounts of uniform, amorphous collagenous matrix, cartilage is an immunologically privileged tissue.[21] Although all cartilage grafts tend to degenerate in time, allografts of cartilage last nearly as long as autografts.

TENDON. Autografts of tendon are used to replace damaged or destroyed tendons in the hands and feet in order to restore motion and strength. Free tendon grafts are taken from the palmaris longus, the flexor digitorum superficialis of the ring finger, the triceps, the plantaris, or the extensor digitorum communis tendons of the toes. A more detailed discussion of tendon grafting is contained in Chapter 42, Part X.

OTHER CONNECTIVE TISSUE. Fascia lata from the thigh has been autografted to the groin to reinforce a hernia repair, to the neck to cover the carotid artery after neck dissection, and to heart valves to replace damaged leaflets.[2]

Hemijoints and whole joints have been autografted in animals and humans, with good early function but gradual destruction of the cartilaginous surface.[16] When small joints are transplanted on vascular pedicles, degenerative changes do not occur.[9]

COMPOSITE TISSUE AUTOGRAFTS. Composite tissue transplantation involves the transfer of entire functional units rather than individual components of the musculoskeletal or other systems. Toe-digital transfers and the iliac rib or fibular osteocutaneous neurosensory flaps are examples of composite tissue autografts.[64] Successful one-stage hallux-to-thumb transplantation was first performed in humans by Cobbett in 1969.[35] In addition to fixation of the bone autograft with intermedullary wires and suturing of the flexor and extensor tendon autografts, the toe-digital arteries, dorsal veins, and digital nerves are all anastomosed to their hand counterparts to achieve a fully functional thumb. Osteocutaneous transplantation allows simultaneous reconstruction of both bone and skin defects with provision of sensation in the transplanted skin. Conventional groin flap skin and subcutaneous tissue may be transplanted together with a segment of the underlying iliac bone, the origin of the sartorius and tensor fascia lata muscles, the superficial circumflex iliac artery and vein, and the lateral femoral cutaneous nerve.[72] This composite autograft can achieve a one-stage repair of bone, subcutaneous tissue, skin, and sensory defects following severe trauma. Similar grafts may be created from autogenous rib and fibula for reconstruction of the face and extremities, as described by Serafin and Buncke.[64] Objective monitoring of blood flow to the composite graft in the perioperative period is possible with laser Doppler flowmetry.[32]

VASCULAR AUTOGRAFTS

ARTERIAL REPLACEMENT. Both autogenous arteries and veins are used to replace destroyed or obstructed sections of major arteries. Veins were the first to be used successfully, experimentally by Carrel in 1905 and clinically by Goyanes in 1906, and are currently the most commonly used substitutes for peripheral arteries.[12] Although femoral, popliteal, upper extremity, and neck veins have been used, the greater saphenous vein has proved to be the most satisfactory arterial replacement. The wall is sufficiently strong to withstand arterial pressures without becoming dilated or aneurysmal, yet is flexible and easily sutured. The diameter is sufficiently great (minimum of 4 mm.) to avoid thrombosis, and nourishment is provided by the intraluminal blood flow. Saphenous vein is ordinarily harvested from the same leg for femoropopliteal bypass and from the opposite leg for repair of vascular trauma to the lower extremity. A groin incision over the saphenofemoral junction and one or more small longitudinal incisions over the course of the vein for ligation of tributaries permit removal of the vein as a continuous conduit. Alternatively, a single longitudinal incision may be used to remove the required length of saphenous vein. The vein segment is flushed with heparinized saline so that any leaks can be identified and repaired. Care is taken to avoid intimal damage, which would promote thrombosis. The vein is reversed to prevent obstruction by the valves and is sutured end-to-end for arterial replacement or end-to-side for arterial bypass. In cases of *in situ* saphenous vein bypass, the vein may be left in its bed, all branches ligated, all valves internally disrupted, and flow reversed by suturing the vein proximally to the femoral artery and distally to a tibial or peroneal artery.[34]

Autogenous saphenous vein is the material of choice for peripheral bypass procedures because it is the most resistant to clotting and infection. The smooth, natural endothelial lining is less thrombogenic than any known synthetic surface, particularly when placed across joints. Moreover, the lining surface heals itself and may sequester white cells to fight infection, unlike Dacron grafts, which provide a haven for infecting organisms in the interstices of their synthetic fibers. Autografts heal even when placed into the infected bed of a previous synthetic graft.

The versatility and ease of harvesting of greater saphenous vein grafts have led to their use in many locations. The subcutaneous crossover graft from a patent right femoral artery to an obstructed left femoral artery was performed in preference to an intra-abdominal aortofemoral bypass because of the patient's age and associated diseases. Saphenous vein is frequently used to bypass superficial femoral artery obstruction, by grafting from the proximal common femoral artery to either the popliteal artery or one of the smaller tibial arteries in the lower leg.[11] Visceral and cerebral ischemia has also been treated with saphenous vein bypasses from the thoracic or abdominal aorta. Patients with atherosclerotic coronary artery disease may have segmental occlusions bypassed with reversed saphenous vein grafts, a technique popularized by Favaloro in 1967.[49] Coronary artery bypass grafting is discussed more extensively in Chapter 56, Part XV.

Saphenous vein is also used to create vascular patches for

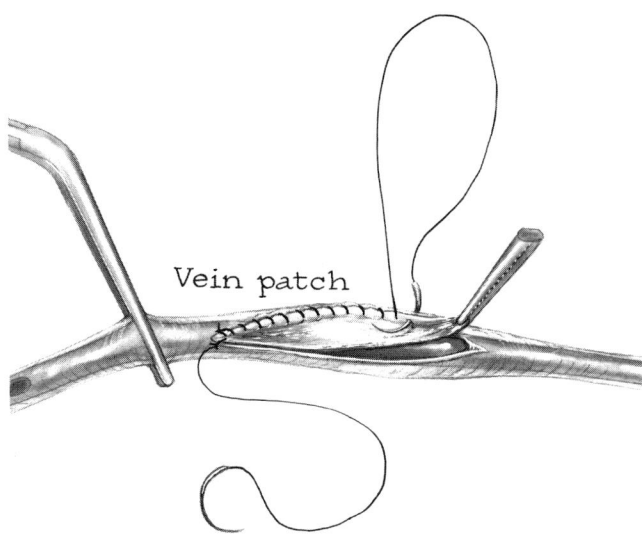

Figure 2. Application of a vein patch in closing an arteriotomy to avoid narrowing at the suture line. (From Wylie, E. J., Binkley, F. M., and Albo, R. J.: Femoropopliteal endarterectomy. Am. J. Surg., *108:*215, 1964.)

widening diseased arteries.[81] In order to prevent constriction at the site of a longitudinal arteriotomy, a diamond-shaped piece of vein may be inserted into the closure (Fig. 2). Whether used as a patch or as a tube graft, saphenous vein placed into the high-pressure, pulsatile arterial system undergoes a variety of pathologic changes, which are described and illustrated in Chapter 52.

Intimal hyperplasia occurs in both autografted arteries and veins, but stenosis due to fibrosis of venous valve cusps could be avoided if other arteries were used for replacement of the diseased arteries. Unfortunately, it is uncommon to find a long uninvolved segment of artery in patients with atherosclerosis severe enough to require autografting. Few dispensable large-diameter arteries are available, and more complicated operations than vein harvesting are required to obtain them. A variety of graft shapes may be created from the common, internal, and external iliac arteries. Certain dispensable arteries are anatomically situated in positions that allow relatively easy direct diversion to bypass obstructing lesions in more critical arteries. The internal mammary artery has been used increasingly as a preferred source of blood for partially occluded coronary arteries, and the splenic artery may be rotated down to the left renal artery to bypass proximal renal artery stenosis. In the Duke University renovascular hypertension clinical series, splenorenal arterial bypass has achieved durable control of hypertension in 91 per cent of patients.

Arterial autografts have been recommended for use in repairing fibromuscular dysplastic lesions of the renal artery and aneurysms of peripheral, renal, and visceral arteries. Arterial grafts are stronger and more flexible than synthetic grafts and are therefore especially useful in areas of extreme motion.[68] Infected prostheses, mycotic aneurysms, and infected arterial repairs can be successfully managed by excision and replacement with arterial autografts. Arterial and venous autografts are discussed further in Chapter 52, Part IV.

VENOUS REPLACEMENT. Autografting for repair of diseased or damaged veins has been much less successful than arterial replacement, primarily because of early graft thrombosis in low-pressure, low-flow venous systems. Autogenous vein remains the best replacement material, since no synthetic graft has consistently remained open except in the superior vena cava position.[30] The Vietnamese War experience demonstrated that acute venous hypertension following interruption of major lower extremity veins increased the rate of amputation but was preventable if autogenous vein interposition grafts were used.[57]

Edema was eliminated without production of thrombophlebitis or pulmonary embolism. During the 1- to 2-week period after grafting when a neointima is being formed, a distal arteriovenous fistula to increase flow through the graft and anticoagulation to diminish thrombosis may improve patency.[30]

ENDOCRINE AUTOGRAFTS

Autotransplantation of endocrine glands has had an indispensable role in the evolution of endocrinology. Berthold is acknowledged to be the father of experimental endocrinology for his studies in 1849 demonstrating that autotransplanted testes caused secondary sexual characteristics in castrated cocks.[33] Literally every endocrine gland has been experimentally autotransplanted, with identification of several technical requirements for success: delicate handling of the tissues, prevention of ischemia by cooling or placement in an appropriate medium, and implantation of small fragments. The oxygen and nutrients in interstitial fluid around a subcutaneous, intramuscular, or renal capsular implant maintain an endocrine graft until revascularization occurs if the fragments are no more than 1 mm. thick. Although thyroid,[70] pituitary,[33] ovary,[80] adrenal, testis, pancreas, and parathyroid have all been autografted in humans, only the last four are often transplanted therapeutically today. Excellent synthetic hormone replacement is available for thyroid, adrenal, and gonadal deficiency states.

TESTIS. Autotransplantation is the treatment of choice for an undescended testis.[22] The cryptorchid or ectopic testis must be removed from the abdomen and placed in a cooler location prior to age 6, and preferably at 1 year of age, for normal spermatogenesis to occur. Orchidopexy and repair of any associated hernia are performed as described in Chapter 38.

PANCREAS. Pancreatic autotransplantation has been performed both as segmental grafts and as isolated islet cells. Whereas it is clear that diabetes can be prevented when either type of graft is successful, each approach has its special problems that have limited its clinical usefulness. Segmental pancreas autografts contain large amounts of exocrine tissue with secretions that are difficult to manage. Despite occlusion of the pancreatic ductules by neoprene injection, all three autograft recipients in one series developed pancreatic fistulas but eventually recovered.[75] The tendency for venous thrombosis that causes ischemia and death of the tissue has been only partially relieved by creating a distal arteriovenous fistula between the splenic artery and vein.[39] Islets for autotransplantation have proved difficult to isolate in sufficient quantities from the fibrotic adult pancreas, particularly after chronic pancreatitis, and have often not prevented diabetes over the long term.[10,45] Moreover, when dispersed islets are injected directly into the human portal vein, they have occasionally produced untoward effects such as disseminated intravascular coagulation, portal hypertension, and hepatic necrosis.[10,74]

Pancreatic autotransplantation has been attempted most frequently in cases of total pancreatectomy for relief of the pain of chronic pancreatitis, but has also been used after a modified pancreaticoduodenectomy for carcinoma of the head of the pancreas.[39] A report from the International Pancreas and Islet Transplant Registry[69] reveals that 13 of 17 segmental or total autograft recipients and approximately half of 79 islet autograft recipients do not require insulin. However, in cases in which less than a 95 per cent pancreatectomy is performed, it is difficult to assess how much insulin is contributed by the pancreas left *in situ.*

PARATHYROID. Survival of parathyroid autotransplants in humans was demonstrated histologically (Fig. 3) and biochemically by Wells in 1975.[78] Since parathyroid hormone replacement is not available and medical therapy for hypoparathyroidism is complicated, preservation and autografting of parathyroid tissue is essential to prevent the deficiency symp-

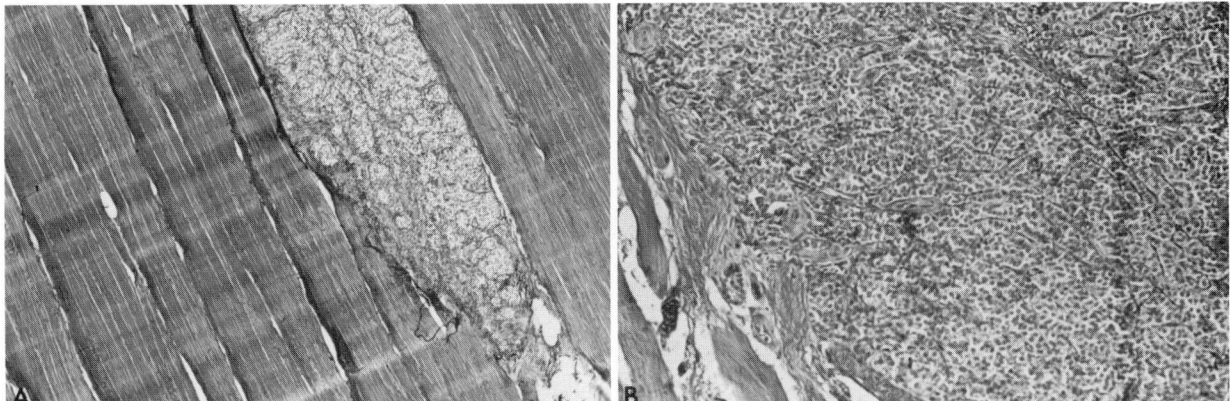

Figure 3. Histologic section of a parathyroid graft within a muscle bed at magnification of 41× (A) and 100× (B). (Courtesy of Samuel A. Wells, Jr., M.D.)

toms of tetany, psychologic disturbances, convulsions, coma, and death. Parathyroid glands removed during thyroid surgery should be cut into 1-mm. pieces and reimplanted into pockets in the sternocleidomastoid muscle.[38] When all glands are removed for diffuse parathyroid hyperplasia, implantation of fragments into the forearm muscles facilitates subsequent removal of more tissue under local anesthesia if hyperparathyroidism persists.[79] Parathyroid tissue that has been cryopreserved functions normally when autografted to treat hypoparathyroidism. Parathyroid autografting is discussed more extensively in Chapter 25.

ADRENAL. Hyperplastic human adrenal tissue has been successfully autotransplanted for many years.[14] Whole gland autotransplantation with vascular anastomosis to the inferior epigastric vessels has been used to treat Cushing's disease.[82] The report in 1987 of open microsurgical autotransplantation of adrenal medulla to the caudate nucleus of the brain for treatment of intractable Parkinson's disease awakened great interest in the topic.[36,37] Subsequent multicenter trials have demonstrated improvement, but not cure, of the disease and had substantial postoperative morbidity so the technique was not recommended for widespread use.[23]

BONE MARROW AUTOGRAFTS

High-dose irradiation or intensive chemotherapy can produce severe bone marrow depression leading to anemia, thrombocytopenic bleeding, and infection. Since 1956 it has been known that intravenous injection of bone marrow cells can restore hematopoiesis.[19] The responsible cells are hematopoietic stem cells, which occur at the low frequency of 4 per 1000 bone marrow cells, but which are capable of rapid replication and differentiation into myeloid, erythroid, megakaryocytic, and lymphoid cell series.[13] Bone marrow transplants are used to reconstitute the marrow of patients with acute leukemia and to speed bone marrow recovery in patients receiving high-dose myelosuppressive therapy for solid tumors.[26]

When marrow autografts are used, neither graft rejection nor the graft-versus-host reaction is a factor in transplantation success. Rather, outcome is determined by the number of leukemia cells in the remission marrow graft, the effectiveness of the antitumor therapy, and the number of stem cells that survive frozen storage. The hematopoietic marrow, obtained from a leukemia patient in remission or a patient with a solid tumor not involving the marrow, is harvested from the iliac crest and sternum by needle aspiration. The cells are mixed with a cryopreservative and cooled stepwise until frozen at −192° C. The patient is given intensive, high-dose chemotherapy or "lethal" doses of irradiation, which destroy not only the malignancy but also the remaining marrow. The preserved marrow is then thawed and infused intravenously to reconstitute the hematopoietic system. This procedure has proved helpful in the treat-

ment of non-Hodgkin's and Burkitt's lymphomas, ovarian cancer, and Stage IV melanoma as well as acute leukemia.[13]

URINARY AUTOGRAFTS

KIDNEY. Renal autotransplantation and extracorporeal reconstruction permit salvage of some kidneys that cannot be repaired by conventional *in situ* operative techniques.[67] The approach was originally reported by Hardy, who used autotransplantation of the kidney to manage a very proximal ureteral injury.[29] Belzer added hypothermic pulsatile perfusion to improve preservation and permit *ex vivo*, or "work bench," microvascular surgery on the kidney before reimplantation.[5] The kidney may be returned to its original site or grafted to the iliac vessels using the allotransplantation technique. The ureter may be reimplanted into the bladder or preserved intact during the autografting (Fig. 4).

In the case of a large high abdominal aortic aneurysm associated with a horseshoe kidney, hypothermic preservation and autografting to the Dacron aortic graft and vena cava were used to preserve renal function.[41] *Ex vivo* surgery or renal autografting has been employed for extensive renovascular disease from fibrous dysplasia, atherosclerotic disease, or abdominal aortic aneurysms; for repair of traumatic arterial injuries; for excision of renal cell carcinoma involving both kidneys or a solitary kidney; and for kidneys with diseased or damaged ureters too short for reimplantation.[55] Renovascular hypertension not amenable to correction by conventional surgical procedures responded to autotransplantation with normalization of blood pressure and creatinine.[65] A remnant of renal pelvis may be anastomosed directly to the bladder following resection and autotransplantation for renal pelvic and high ureteric tumors.[52] Long-term renal function after autotransplantation with direct pyelocystostomy has been excellent.[56]

URETER AND BLADDER. Synthetic prostheses and free grafts have generally failed as ureteral substitutes. Autotransplantation of the bladder in the form of a vesicopsoas hitch or a bladder flap is the treatment of choice for injury or disease in the distal third of the ureter.[6] Up to 18 cm. of distal ureter can be replaced with bladder by combining a tubular pedicle graft of bladder and the superior suturing (hitch) of posterior bladder to psoas tendon with chromic catgut. In cases in which a more proximal segment of ureter is lost or the entire bladder must be removed, autotransplantation of a segment of ileum currently provides the most successful replacement conduit (see Chapter 46). Alternative reconstructions include suturing one ureter to the other ureter (transureteroureterostomy), the skin (cutaneous ureterostomy), or the sigmoid colon (ureterosigmoidostomy). A contracted bladder from interstitial cystitis or partial resection can be enlarged successfully by autotransplantation of a seg-

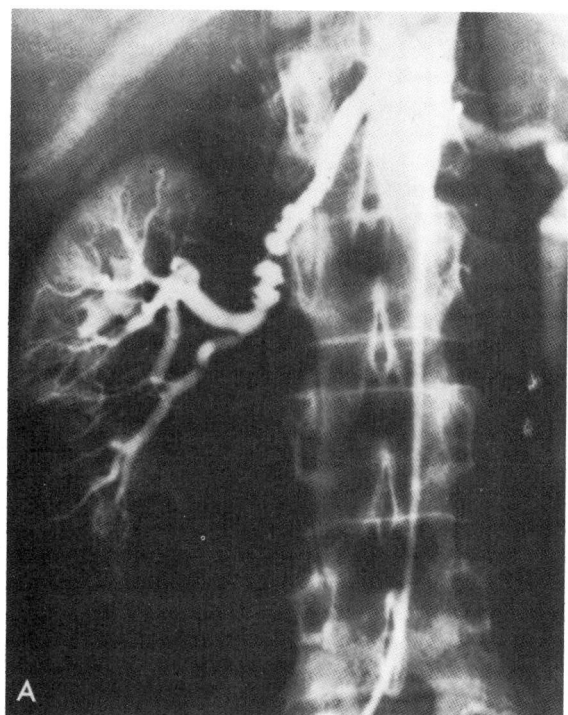
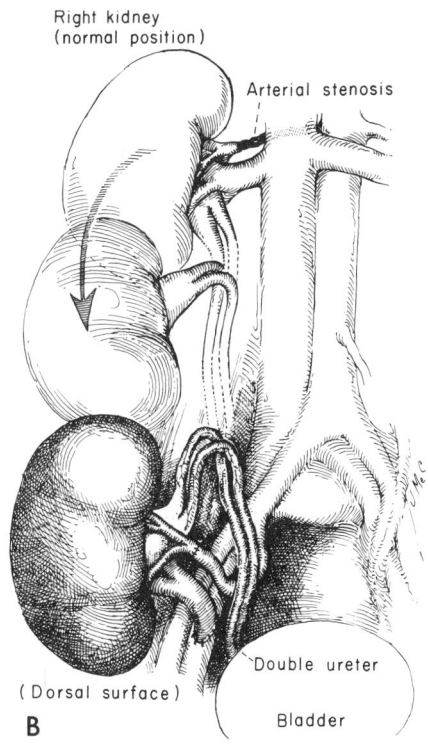

Figure 4. Ipsilateral renal autotransplant. A preoperative excretory urogram revealed a right complete ureteropelvic duplication, and an arteriogram *(A)* demonstrated medial fibroplasia involving the entire length of the right renal artery. The kidney was perfused extracorporeally while the renal artery was dissected. The organ was then rotated down into the iliac fossa *(B)* and rearterialized using the hypogastric artery without dividing the double collecting system. (From Corman, J. L., et al.: Surg. Gynecol. Obstet., *137:*659, 1973.)

ment of ileum and cecum, an augmentation ileocecocystoplasty.[83]

GASTROINTESTINAL AUTOGRAFTS

The gastrointestinal tract is ideally suited for autotransplantation. The mesentery provides a long, natural vascular pedicle for attached grafts, and the vascular arcades provide easily anastomosed arteries and veins for free grafts. Small intestinal autografts are widely used to replace the colon after proctocolectomy for inflammatory bowel disease.[25] The principles of gastrointestinal autografting are well demonstrated by the replacement of the hypopharynx and esophagus with transplanted stomach, jejunum, colon, or free intestinal segments. These operations are performed most commonly following extirpation of carcinomas of the larynx, pharynx, or esophagus but may also be used to reconstruct strictures following ingestion of caustic substances and defects from severe trauma to the face and neck.

STOMACH. Adams and Phemister reported the successful replacement of the lower esophagus with stomach after resection of an esophageal carcinoma in 1938.[1] To perform esophagogastrostomy, the stomach is mobilized by dividing all of its ligamentous, nervous, and vascular attachments except the right gastric artery. After performance of a pyloroplasty or pyloromyomectomy to ensure drainage from the distal stomach, the stomach is passed through the esophageal hiatus and anastomosed to the proximal esophageal remnant in the chest. The stomach may even be transposed into the neck and sutured to the pharynx at the base of the tongue for reconstruction after pharyngolaryngectomy.[3] Problems associated with esophagogastrostomy include acid regurgitation esophagitis, intrathoracic gastric distention, distal graft ischemia, and the dumping syndrome characterized by diarrhea, colicky pain, and a rapid transit time for ingested food. Despite these shortcomings, stomach remains the most frequently used autograft for esoph-

ageal reconstruction after extirpative surgery.[44] The procedure can be performed at low risk as a single-stage operation and achieve satisfactory long-term relief of dysphagia in at least 90 per cent of patients.[15] The greater curvature of the stomach may also be formed into an isoperistaltic tube, as described by Beck and Carrel in 1905, or an antiperistaltic one, popularized by Gavriliu and Heimlich, of sufficient length to reconstruct the entire esophagus. Gastric tubes, reviewed by Postlethwait,[54] have the advantages of a mucosal lining, a serosal covering, a natural opening into the stomach, and an excellent blood supply based on the gastroepiploic vessels.

JEJUNUM. Sections of jejunum with intact blood supply are most useful for replacing relatively short segments of the lower esophagus.[27] If a long graft is necessary, the jejunal arterial inflow and venous drainage may be tenuous at the proximal esophageal anastomosis. Careful section and positioning of the vascular pedicle (Fig. 5) are essential to success. The autograft is brought behind the transverse colon and stomach, through the esophageal hiatus, and into the posterior thorax without tension. A pyloroplasty and temporary gastrostomy should be performed. If there is any question of jejunal viability, the proximal end may be left exposed in the neck for several days of observation before the cervical anastomosis is completed. Alternatively, the jejunal graft may be abandoned and replaced with a segment of large bowel.

COLON. The right colon, transverse colon, left colon, and ileocolon have all been used for autografts. The ileocecal valve continues to function as a partially competent valve after transplantation, thus preventing reflux up the ileal component of the graft. However, the left colon has a better diameter, a more muscular and less distensible wall, and a more dependable blood supply for total esophageal replacement than has any other segment of large bowel.[28] Whether based on the left colic artery to produce an isoperistaltic graft or based on the middle colic artery to produce an antiperistaltic tube, the large marginal artery assures adequate perfusion (Fig. 6). The colon may be

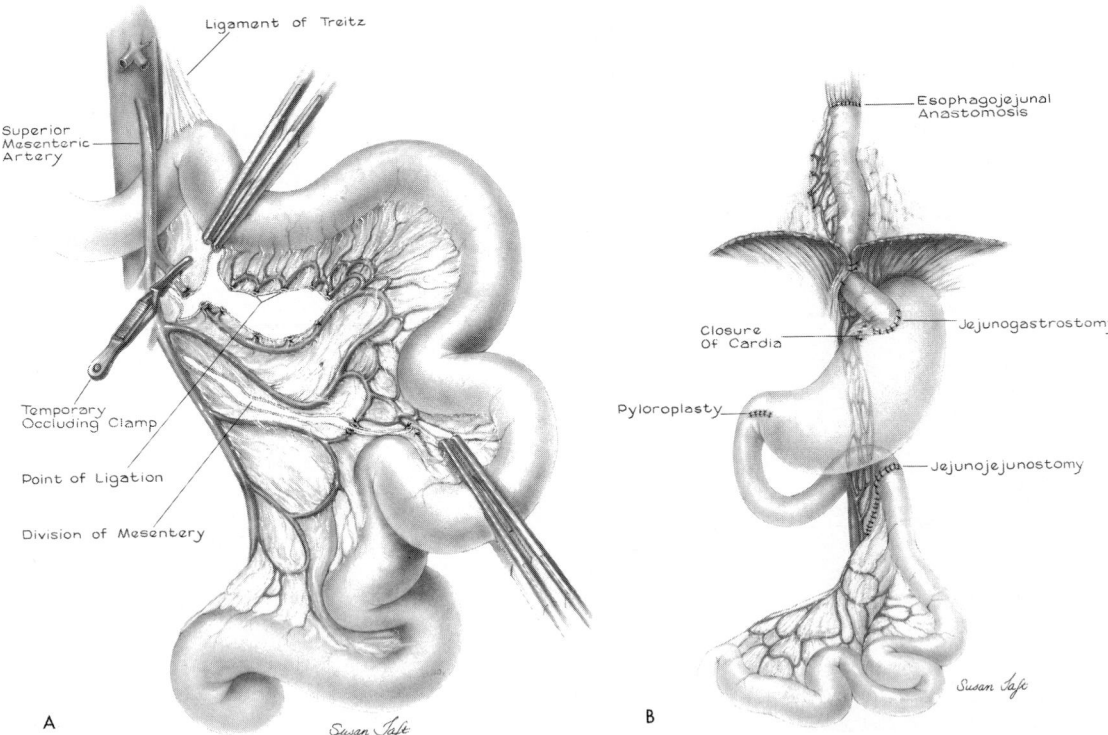

Figure 5. *A*, Preparation of the jejunal segment for interposition. The second artery in the jejunal mesentery has been divided after its temporary occlusion to ensure that the one remaining artery in the pedicle can adequately nourish the segment. *B*, The position of the jejunal transplant at completion of the procedure. During reconstruction of the esophageal hiatus, care is taken to avoid pressure on the vascular pedicle of the jejunal graft. (From Grimes, O. F.: Surgical reconstruction of the diseased esophagus. I. Interposition of the jejunum. Surgery, *61:325*, 1967.)

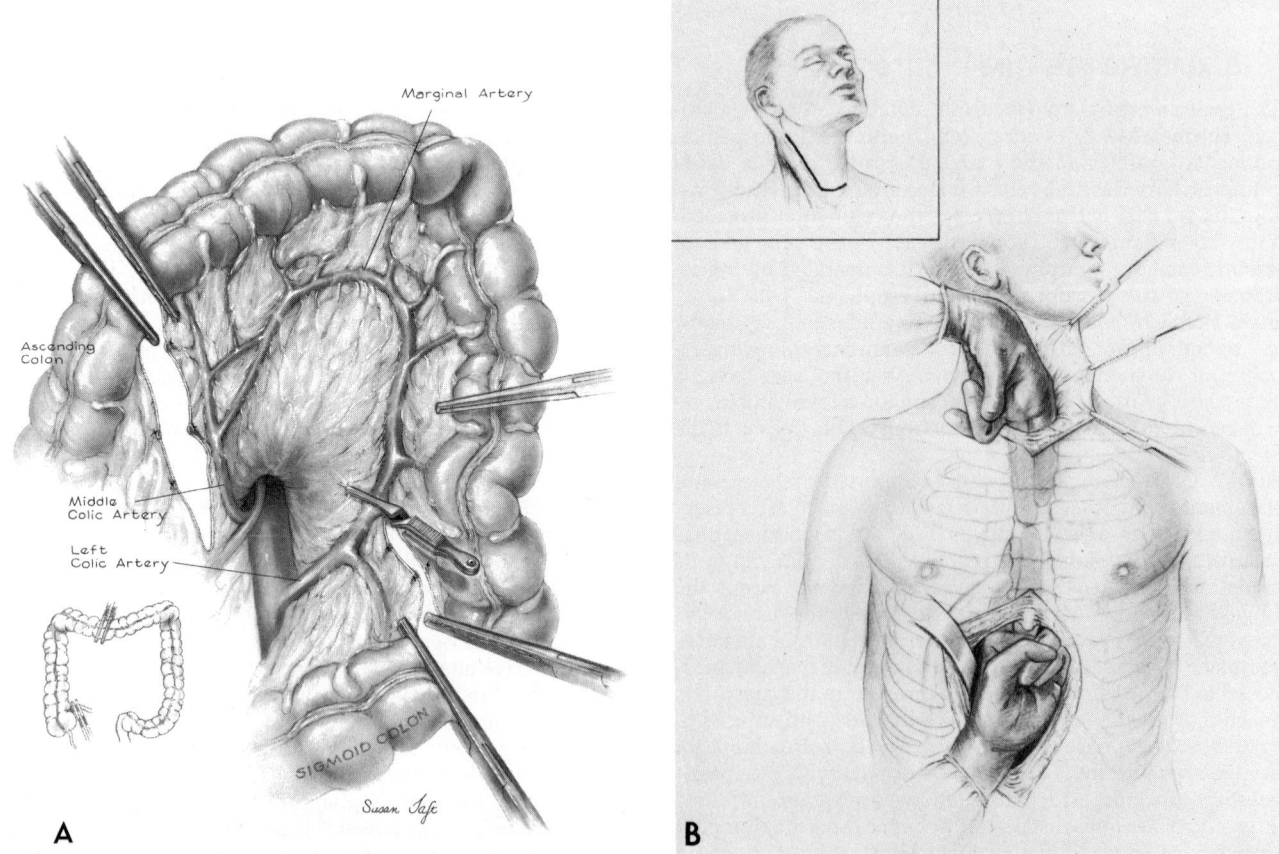

Figure 6. *A*, The middle colic or left colic artery used for blood supply to a left colon transplant. Note the rich collateral circulation via the marginal artery. *B*, A substernal tunnel is created by blunt dissection through which the colon transplant can be passed to the neck. (From Grimes, O. F.: Surgical reconstruction of the diseased esophagus. II. Interposition of the ileocolon and colon. Surgery, *61:487*, 1967.)

placed through a posterior mediastinal, substernal, or subcutaneous tunnel to reach the neck. The last two routes are especially useful for bypassing nonresectable carcinomas in debilitated patients. A pyloroplasty and temporary gastrostomy should be performed, particularly if the vagus nerves are resected.

FREE JEJUNAL AUTOGRAFTS. The first successful free intestinal autograft was reported by Seidenberg in 1959.[63] Although stomach, ileum, and colon have all been transplanted using microvascular techniques to re-establish their blood supply,[46] the jejunum just distal to the ligament of Treitz is currently the most frequently employed free graft.[39,40] This segment of bowel has the largest vasculature and best matches the size of the hypopharynx and cervical esophagus. After an initial tracheostomy, laryngopharyngoesophagectomy is performed with care to preserve the superior thyroid artery and a suitable vein as recipient vessels for the autograft.[18] If the parathyroid glands can be identified and safely separated from tumor, they may be transplanted as described in the section on parathyroid autografts. An appropriate length of proximal jejunum is then resected after careful delineation of its vascular pedicle. The graft is cooled by perfusion with cold saline or Ringer's or Sack's solution and insertion of an intraluminal cooling tube or ice slush–filled condom. The vascular anastomoses are completed under the operating microscope. When graft color, peristalsis, and bleeding are normal, the double-layer visceral anastomoses are formed. Unlike the colon transplants, which act merely as conduits without peristalsis, manometric studies of free jejunal grafts from many patients in the Duke University series show coordinated waves of peristalsis passing through the implants. Equal success has been reported using the transverse colon as a free intestinal autograft for pharyngoesophageal reconstruction.[43]

OTHER AUTOGRAFTS

Many other tissues have found limited but effective use as autotransplants. The greater omentum was transferred as a vascularized graft to reconstruct the scalp after massive skin and subcutaneous tissue loss,[31] as a pedicle graft to relieve chronic lymphedema of the extremities,[24] and as a free graft to relieve the pain of constrictive, radiation-induced brachial plexus paralysis.[76] However, free fat autografts are of questionable value because of unpredictable results due to variable graft survival with wide variations in the final bulk of the autograft.[4] A combination of well-vascularized omentum and pectoralis major muscle flaps permitted successful reconstruction of infected median sternotomy incisions with reduction of mortality from 10 per cent to zero.[51] Hair was transferred to the scalp as punch grafts, even through split-thickness skin grafts.[47] Tongue was autotransplanted to reconstruct defects of the lips,[17] and teeth were successfully autografted.[20] Bowel smooth muscle was autotransplanted as a sphincter replacement to create a continent colostomy.[62] Following pulmonary valve autograft replacement of diseased aortic valves, 40 of 43 patients in one series were reported to be well 2½ to 5 years after autotransplantation.[66] The entire heart was autotransplanted to permit removal of a large myxoma.[61]

Autotransplantation has proved to be a valuable research technique in experimental surgery. John Hunter successfully transplanted testis to the peritoneal cavity of an animal in 1771, and Berthold used autotransplantation in 1849 to demonstrate the endocrine function of cock testis.[33] Autotransplantation continues to be used experimentally today to study organ preservation, to develop and test new surgical techniques, and to evaluate the physiologic changes produced by denervation of organs, for example, erythropoietin production by the transplanted kidney and pulmonary blood flow in the transplanted lung. Single-lung autografts in dogs were demonstrated to provide adequate total respiratory function while carrying the entire pulmonary blood flow at tolerable arterial pressures without evidence of functional deterioration over more than 5 years.[77] Experimental autotransplantation studies such as these have preceded and supported the ultimate feasibility of many allotransplantation procedures currently in clinical use.

SELECTED REFERENCES

Grimes, O. F.: Surgical reconstruction of the diseased esophagus. I. Interposition of the jejunum. II. Interposition of the ileocolon and colon. Surgery, 61:325, 487, 1967.
The important surgical considerations in the selection and use of an intestinal autograft as a substitute for the esophagus are reviewed in these two well-written articles.

Ochsner, J. L., and Mills, N. L.: Coronary Artery Surgery. Philadelphia, Lea & Febiger, 1978.
The most common thoracic autograft, the saphenous vein coronary artery bypass, is discussed in a concise and practical manner. The pathophysiology of coronary artery disease is related to angiographic findings to permit selection of the appropriate bypass procedure.

Rudolph, R., Fisher, J. C. and Ninnemann, J. L.: Skin Grafting. Boston, Little, Brown & Company, 1979.
This book is a clearly written account of the biology and technique of modern skin grafting. The test progresses chronologically through the successive steps in skin grafting and is beautifully and profusely illustrated.

Serafin, D., and Buncke, H. J., Jr.: Microsurgical Composite Tissue Transplantation. St. Louis, C. V. Mosby, 1979.
This comprehensive monograph reviews the entire field of microsurgical composite tissue transplantation. Autografting of skin, various subcutaneous tissue flaps, muscle, omentum, intestine, and bone are covered.

REFERENCES

1. Adams, W. E., and Phemister, D. B.: Carcinoma of the lower thoracic esophagus: Report of a successful resection and esophagogastrostomy. J. Thorac. Surg., 7:621, 1938.
2. Bailey, C. P., Zimmerman, J., Hirose, T. T., Folk, F. S., and Bakst, A. A.: Reconstruction of cardiac valves with autologous tissue. Vasc. Surg., 10:99, 1976.
3. Baines, M. S., and Spiro, R. H.: Pharyngolaryngectomy, total extrathoracic esophagectomy and gastric transposition. Surg. Gynecol. Obstet., 149:693, 1979.
4. Billings, E., and May, J. W.: Historical review and present status of free fat graft autotransplantation in plastic and reconstructive surgery. Plast. Reconstr. Surg., February, 1989.
5. Belzer, F. O., Salvatierra, O., Palumbinskas, A., and Stoney, R. J.: Ex vivo renal artery reconstruction. Ann. Surg., 182:456, 1975.
6. Boxer, R. J., Johnson, S. F., and Ehrlich, R. M.: Ureteral substitution. Urology, 12:299, 1978.
7. Boyne, P. J.: Autogenous cancellous bone and marrow transplants. Clin. Orthop., 73:199, 1970.
8. Brown, J. B., and McDowell, F.: Skin Grafting, 3rd ed. Philadelphia, J. B. Lippincott Company, 1958.
9. Buncke, H. J., Jr., Daniller, A. E., Schulz, W. P., and Chase, R. A.: The fate of autogenous whole joints transplanted by microvascular anastomoses. Plast. Reconstr. Surg., 39:333, 1967.
10. Cameron, J. L., Mehigan, D. G., Broe, P. J., and Zuidema, G. D.: Distal pancreatectomy and islet autotransplantation for chronic pancreatitis. Ann. Surg., 193:312, 1981.
11. Darling, R. C.: Peripheral arterial surgery. N. Engl. J. Med., 280:26, 84, 141, 1969.
12. Darling, R. C., Linton, R. R., and Razzuk, M. A.: Saphenous vein bypass grafts for femoropopliteal occlusive disease: A reappraisal. Surgery, 61:31, 1967.
13. Dicke, K. A., Lotzova, E., Spitzer, G., and McCredie, K. B.: Immunobiology of bone marrow transplantation. Semin. Hematol., 15:263, 1978.
14. Drucker, W. D., Localio, S. A., Becker, M. H., and Berman, B.: Autotransplantation of hyperplastic human adrenal tissue. Arch. Intern. Med., 120:185, 1967.
15. Ellis, H. F., Jr., and Gibb, P. S.: Esophagogastrectomy for carcinoma. Ann. Surg., 190:699, 1979.
16. Entin, M. A., Daniel, G., and Kahn, P.: Transplantation of autogenous half-joints. Arch. Surg., 96:359, 1968.
17. Esser, E., Austermann, K. H., and Schmallenbach, H. J.: Lippenrotersatz durch gestielte Zungenlappen. Fortschr. Kiefer Gesichtschir., 23:31, 1978.
18. Flynn, M. B., and Acland, R. D.: Free intestinal autografts for reconstruction following pharyngolaryngoesophagectomy. Surg. Gynecol. Obstet., 149:858, 1979.
19. Ford, C. F., Hamerton, J. L., Barnes, D. W. H., and Loutit, J. F.: Cytological identification of radiation chimeras. Nature, 177:452, 1956.

20. Gardiner, G. T.: The autogenous transplantation of maxillary canine teeth. A review of 100 consecutive cases. Br. Dent. J., 146:382, 1979.

21. Gibson, T., Davis, W. B., and Curran, R. C.: The long term survival of cartilage homografts in man. Br. J. Plast. Surg., 11:177, 1958.

22. Glenn, J. F., and Boyce, W. H. (Eds.): Urologic Surgery, 2nd ed. New York, Harper & Row, 1975.

23. Goetz, C. G., Olanow, C. W., Koller, W. C., Penn, R. D., Cahill, D., Morantz, R., Stebbins, G., Tanner, C. M., Klawans, H. L., Shannon, K. M., Comella, C. L., Witt, T., Cox, C., Waxman, M., and Gauger, L.: Multicenter study of autologous adrenal medullary transplantation to the corpus striatum in patients with advanced Parkinson's disease. N. Engl. J. Med., 320:337, 1989.

24. Goldsmith, H. S., De los Santos, R., and Beattie, E. J., Jr.: Relief of chronic lymphedema by omental transposition. Ann. Surg., 166:573, 1967.

25. Goligher, J. C. (Ed.): Progress Symposium: Surgical treatment of inflammatory bowel disease. World J. Surg., 12:139, 1988.

26. Graze, R. R., and Gale, R. P.: Autotransplantation for leukemia and solid tumors. Transplant. Proc., 10:177, 1978.

27. Grimes, O. F.: Surgical reconstruction of the diseased esophagus. I. Interposition of the jejunum. Surgery, 61:325, 1967.

28. Grimes, O. F.: Surgical reconstruction of the diseased esophagus. II. Interposition of the ileocolon and colon. Surgery, 61:487, 1967.

29. Hardy, J. D.: High ureteral injury: Management by autotransplantation of the kidney. J.A.M.A., 184:97, 1963.

30. Hiratzka, L. F., and Wright, C. B.: Experimental and clinical results of grafts in the venous system. J. Surg. Res., 25:542, 1978.

31. Ikuta, Y.: Omental transplantation. In Serafin, D., and Buncke, H. J., Jr. (Eds.): Microsurgical Composite Tissue Transplantation. St. Louis, C. V. Mosby, 1979.

32. Jenkins, S., Sepka, R., and Barwick, W. J.: Routine use of laser doppler flowmetry for monitoring autologous tissue transplants. Ann. Plast. Surg., 21:423, 1988.

33. Krohn, P. L.: Transplantation of endocrine glands. In Peer, L. A. (Ed.): Transplantation of Tissues. Vol. II. Baltimore, Williams & Wilkins, 1959, p. 401.

34. Leather, R. P., Shah, D. M., Corson, J. D., and Karmody, A. M.: Instrumental evolution of the valve incision method of in situ saphenous vein bypass. J. Vasc. Surg., 1:113, 1984.

35. Littler, J. W.: On making a thumb — one hundred years of surgical effort. J. Hand Surg., 1:35, 1976.

36. Madrazo, I., Drucker-Colin, R., Diaz, V., et al.: Open microsurgical autograft of adrenal medulla to the right caudate nucleus in two patients with intractable Parkinson's disease. N. Engl. J. Med., 316:831, 1987.

37. Madrazo, I., Drucker-Colin, R., Leon, V., and Torres, C.: Adrenal medulla transplanted to caudate nucleus for treatment of Parkinson's disease: Report of 10 cases. Surg. Forum, 38:510, 1987.

38. Matsuura, H., Sako, K., and Marchetta, F. C.: Successful reimplantation of autogenous parathyroid tissue. Am. J. Surg., 118:779, 1969.

39. McDonald, J. C., Rohr, M. S., and Tucker, W. Y.: Recent experiences with autotransplantation of the kidney, jejunum, and pancreas. Ann. Surg., 197:678, 1983.

40. McKee, D. M., and Peters, C. R.: Reconstruction of the hypopharynx and cervical esophagus with a microvascular jejunal transplant. In Serafin, D., and Buncke, H. J., Jr. (Eds.): Microsurgical Composite Transplantation. St. Louis, C. V. Mosby, 1979.

41. McLoughlin, M. D., Williams, G. M., and Stonesifer, G. L., Jr.: Ex vivo surgical dissection: Autotransplantation in renal disease. J.A.M.A., 235:1705, 1976.

42. Millesi, H., Meissl, G., and Berger, A.: The interfasicular nerve grafting of the median and ulnar nerves. J. Bone Joint Surg., 54A:727, 1972.

43. Modica, L. A., and de Koos, P. T.: Free bowel autografts in pharyngoesophageal reconstruction: Colon revisited. Orolaryngol. Head Neck Surg., 9:73, 1988.

44. Mullen, D. C., Young, W. G., Jr., and Sealy, W. C.: Results of twenty years' experience with esophageal replacement for benign disorders. Ann. Thorac. Surg., 5:481, 1968.

45. Najarian, J. S., Sutherland, D. E. R., Baumgartner, D., Burke, B., Rynasiewicz, J. J., Matas, A. A., and Goetz, F. G.: Total or near total pancreatectomy and islet autotransplantation for treatment of chronic pancreatitis. Ann. Surg., 192:526, 1980.

46. Nakayama, K., Yamamoto, K., Tamiya, T., Makino, H., Odaka, M., Ohwada, M., and Takahashi, H.: Experience with free autografts of bowel with new venous anastomosis apparatus. Surgery, 55:798, 1964.

47. Nordstrom, R. E.: Punch hair grafting under split skin grafts on scalps. Plast. Reconstr. Surg., 64:9, 1979.

48. Norris, R. W., Glasby, M. A., Gattuso, J. M., and Bowden, R. E. M.: Peripheral nerve repair in humans using muscle autografts: A new technique. J. Bone Joint Surg., 70:530, 1988.

49. Ochsner, J. L., and Mills, N. L.: Coronary Artery Surgery. Philadelphia, Lea & Febiger, 1978.

50. Ostrup, L. T., and Frederickson, J. M.: Distant transfer of a free living bone graft by microvascular anastomoses: An experimental study. Plast. Reconstr. Surg., 54:274, 1974.

51. Pearl, S. N., and Dibbell, D. G.: Reconstruction after median sternotomy infection. Surg. Gynecol. Obstet., 159:47, 1984.

52. Pettersson, S., Brynger, H., Henriksson, C., Johansson, S., Nilson, A. E., and Ranch, T.: Autotransplantation with direct pyelovesical anastomosis in renal pelvic and ureteric tumors, a new approach. Scand. J. Urol. Nephrol. (Suppl.), 60:45, 1981.

53. Phemister, D. B.: The fate of transplanted bone and regenerative power of its various constituents. Surg. Gynecol. Obstet., 19:303, 1914.

54. Postlethwait, R. W.: Surgery of the Esophagus. New York, Appleton-Century-Crofts, 1979.

55. Putnam, C. W.: Renal autotransplantation and "bench work" surgery: Techniques and applications. In Rutherford, R. B. (Ed.): Vascular Surgery. Philadelphia, W. B. Saunders Company, 1977.

56. Ranch, T., Granerus, G., Henricksson, C., and Pettersson, S.: Renal function after autotransplantation with direct pyelocystostomy. Long-term follow-up. Br. J. Urol., 63:233, 1989.

57. Rich, N. M., Collins, G. J., Andersen, C. A., and McDonald, P. T.: Autogenous venous interposition grafts in repair of major venous injuries. J. Trauma, 17:512, 1977.

58. Robson, M. C., and Krizek, T. J.: Predicting skin graft survival. J. Trauma, 13:213, 1973.

59. Rudolph, R., Fisher, J. C., and Ninnemann, J. L.: Skin Grafting. Boston, Little, Brown & Company, 1979.

60. Saunders, J. B. de D. M.: A conceptual history of transplantation. In Najarian, J. S., and Simmons, R. L. (Eds.): Transplantation. Philadelphia, Lea & Febiger, 1972.

61. Scheld, H. H., Nestle, H. W., Kling, D., Stertmann, W. A., Langebartels, H., and Hehrlein, F. W.: Resection of a heart tumor using autotransplantation. Thorac. Cardiovasc. Surg., 36:40, 1987.

62. Schmidt, E., Bruch, H. P., Greulich, M., Rothhammer, A., and Romen, W.: Kontinente Colostomie durch freie Transplantation Autologer Dickdarmmuskulatur. Chirurg, 50:96, 1979.

63. Seidenberg, B., Rosenak, S., Surwitt, E. S., and Som, M. L.: Immediate reconstruction of the cervical esophagus by a revascularized isolated jejunal segment. Ann. Surg., 149:162, 1959.

64. Serafin, D., and Buncke, H. J., Jr. (Eds.): Microsurgical Composite Tissue Transplantation. St. Louis, C. V. Mosby, 1979.

65. Sicard, G. A., Valentin, L. I., Freeman, M. D., Allen, B. T., and Anderson, C. B.: Renal autotransplantation: An alternative to standard renal revascularization procedures. Surgery, 104:624, 1988.

66. Somerville, J., Ross, D., Sachs, G., Emanuel, R., and McDonald, L.: Long term results of pulmonary autograft replacement for aortic valve disease. Lancet, 2:730, 1972.

67. Stewart, B. H., Banowsky, L. H., Hewitt, C. B., and Straffon, R. A.: Renal autotransplantation: Current perspectives. J. Urol., 118:363, 1977.

68. Stoney, R. J., and Wylie, E. J.: Arterial autografts. Surgery, 67:18, 1970.

69. Sutherland, D. E. R.: Pancreas and Islet Transplant Registry statistics. Transplant. Proc., 16:593, 1984.

70. Swan, H., Harper, F., and Christensen, S. P.: Autotransplantation of thyroid tissue in the treatment of lingual thyroid. Surgery, 32:293, 1952.

71. Tamai, S.: Experimental neuromuscular transplantation. In Serafin, D., and Buncke, H. J., Jr. (Eds.): Microsurgical Composite Tissue Transplantation. St. Louis, C. V. Mosby, 1979.

72. Tamai, S.: Osteocutaneous transplantation. In Serafin, D., and Buncke, H. J., Jr. (Eds.): Microsurgical Composite Tissue Transplantation. St. Louis, C. V. Mosby, 1979.

73. Taylor, G. I.: Vascularized nerve transfer. In Serafin D., and Buncke, H. J., Jr. (Eds.): Microsurgical Composite Tissue Transplantation. St. Louis, C. V. Mosby, 1979.

74. Toledo-Pereyra, L. H., Rowlett, A. L., Cain, W., Rosenberg, J. C., Gordon, P. A., and MacKenzie, G. H.: Hepatic infarction following intraportal islet cell autotransplantation after near-total pancreatectomy. Transplantation, 38:88, 1984.

75. Tosati, E., Valente, U., Campisi, C., Barabino, C., and Pozzati, A.: Segmental pancreas autotransplantation in man following total or near total pancreatectomy for serious recurrent chronic pancreatitis. Transplant. Proc., 12:15, 1980.

76. Uhlschmid, G., and Clodius, L.: Eine neue Anwendung des frei transplantierten Omentums. Chirurg, 49:714, 1978.

77. Veith, F. J., and Montefusco, C. M.: Long term fate of lung autografts charged with providing total pulmonary function. Ann. Surg., 190:654, 1979.

78. Wells, S. A., Jr., Gunnells, J. C., Shelburne, J. D., Schneider, A. B., and Sherwood, L. M.: Transplantation of the parathyroid glands in man: Clinical indications and results. Surgery, 78:34, 1975.

79. Wells, S. A., Ross, A. J., Dale, J. K., and Gray, R. S.: Transplantation of the parathyroid glands: Current status. Surg. Clin. North Am., 59:167, 1979.

80. Woodruff, M. F. A.: The transplantation of tissues and organs. Springfield, Ill., Charles C Thomas, 1960.

81. Wylie, E. J., Binkley, F. M., and Albo, R. J.: Femoropopliteal endarterectomy. Am. J. Surg., 108:215, 1964.

82. Xu, Y., Qiao, Y., Wu, P., Chen, Z., and Jin, N.: Adrenal autotransplantation with attached blood vessels for treatment of Cushing's disease. J. Urol., 141:6, 1988.

83. Zinman, L., and Libertino, J. A.: Technique of augmentation cecocystoplasty. Surg. Clin. North Am., 60:703, 1980.

19

THE ROLE OF PROSTAGLANDINS, THROMBOXANE, AND LEUKOTRIENES IN SURGERY

Bernard M. Jaffe, M.D.

Historical Aspects

Prostaglandins were first recognized in 1933, when Goldblatt and von Euler independently identified a component of seminal fluid that had a differential effect on uterine musculature depending on the time in the menstrual cycle from which it was derived. The term *prostaglandin* was selected because it was presumed that these chemical agents were synthesized by the prostate. Despite the interest generated by these compounds, it was not until the early 1960s that the structures were identified (primarily by Samuelsson and associates) as substituted 20-carbon fatty acids, and the compounds were purified from seminal fluid and synthesized *de novo*. During the late 1960s and into the 1980s, additional groups of prostaglandins and related compounds were identified and characterized. A monumental discovery by Vane and colleagues in 1973 demonstrated that the mode of action of nonsteroidal anti-inflammatory agents, notably aspirin and indomethacin, was inhibition of prostaglandin biosynthesis. Recognition of the inhibitory effects of glucocorticoids followed shortly thereafter. From the pharmacologic point of view, the major recent advance has been the development of synthetic prostaglandin analogs with specific biologic actions, which initiated the era of prostaglandins as therapeutic agents.

Prostaglandin Biosynthesis

Since prostaglandins are nearly ubiquitous, the biosynthetic components are common to an enormous spectrum of cells and cell types. Because of the ready availability of precursors and inducible enzymes, the synthesis of these compounds is an extremely rapid process. The synthesis of all prostaglandins is a three-step process, as demonstrated in Figure 1. In response to appropriate stimuli, phospholipase is activated, permitting the cleavage from phospholipids of the major precursor fatty acid, arachidonic acid; as the final step, arachidonate is cyclized to form biologically active prostaglandins. Both glucocorticosteroids and nonsteroidal anti-inflammatory agents (aspirin, indomethacin, phenylbutazone, and so forth) have been recognized as potent inhibitors of prostaglandin synthesis, but they act on different steps. Glucocorticosteroids induce an enzyme, lipocortin, which interferes with activation of phospholipase and thus prevents the release of precursor fatty acids; this inhibition can be overcome by the addition of arachidonate and is ineffective in high arachidonate milieus. In contrast, the nonsteroidal anti-inflammatory agents inhibit the oxidative cyclization step; the arachidonic acid generated is either bound to albumin as a carrier or diverted through other related pathways, including lipoxygenase, which is discussed later.

Characteristics of the Natural Prostaglandins

A simplified synthetic scheme of prostaglandins is shown in Figure 2. As can be inferred, the prostaglandins constitute a substantial family of related compounds that share a number of general characteristics. They are all rapidly synthesized. The action of each prostaglandin counteracts the stimulus, and thus this action is controlled by feedback inhibition. Each of the compounds acts locally; when large amounts are synthesized, they have access to the bloodstream and function as hormones. In addition, these agents are extremely rapidly inactivated, with biologic half-lives of less than 20 seconds. An overall assessment would support the contention that the prostaglandins are delicate modulators of host defense mechanisms.

The complicated nomenclature for prostaglandins warrants comment. Prostaglandins are characterized by a cyclopentane ring (derivatives of which determine the group, i. e., PGE, PGF, and so on) and two aliphatic side chains; the subscripts (1, 2α, β, for example) represent the number of unsaturated side-chain bonds and the orientation of the H bond. For nearly all cases, the subscripts confer little specificity and can largely be disregarded. In man, the major prostaglandins are those of the 2 series (see Table 1 for actions).

Prostaglandin Analogs and Their Function

For most prostaglandins, the 15 position is critical to biologic function. Oxidation of the hydroxyl at this position to a keto group leads to total inactivation; conversely, protection or substitution at this position drastically curtails pulmonary and renal metabolism. As a result, a number of methylated (at or around the 15 position) analogs have been synthesized and utilized clinically. These analogs have actions nearly identical to those of the native prostaglandins, have half-lives of up to 6 to 8 hours, are active at extremely low doses, and are absorbable from the gastrointestinal tract (whereas natural prostaglandins are inactivated by gastric acid). They thus offer the clinician effective and available pharmaceuticals to reproduce the biologic actions of the natural prostaglandins.

Clinical Uses of Prostaglandins and Inhibitors of Prostaglandin Biosynthesis

CARDIOVASCULAR USES. The ductus arteriosus is quite sensitive to the vasodilatory effects of PGE compounds. This action has been exploited in the treatment of neonates with ductus-dependent cyanotic congenital heart disease. Infants with pulmonary valvular atresia or severe stenosis are totally dependent on pulmonary blood flow from the ductus, and dila-

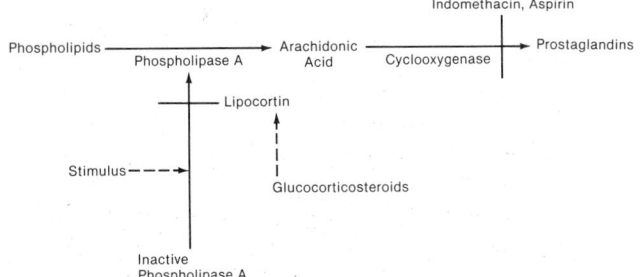

Figure 1. Scheme of prostaglandin synthetic pathways.

tion of the ductus leads to dramatic improvement in oxygenation and hemodynamics. A number of such cyanotic newborns (as well as other neonates with severe coarctation or interruption of the aortic arch) have been so treated with great success, with mean oxygen saturation levels raised from 50 per cent to an average of 80 per cent or higher without deleterious effects from the PGE_1 itself. These infusions have enabled the survival of such critically ill babies long enough to prepare them for surgical creation of aorticopulmonary shunts.

Coceani and associates have proposed that PGE compounds maintain the patency of the ductus *in utero*. This hypothesis is based on recognition of the vasodilatory effects of PGE compounds, the PGE biosynthetic ability of the umbilical vessels, and the long-term survival of circulating PGEs in the absence of pulmonary blood flow. This concept suggests that, at the time of delivery, initiation of pulmonary blood flow causes inactivation of circulating prostaglandin and abrogation of the stimulus for maintenance of ductal patency. In a small but substantial number of premature infants, this mechanism fails, and the ductus arteriosus remains patent after birth. In this circumstance, indomethacin-induced inhibition of prostaglandin biosynthesis has led to ductal closure in more than 85 per cent of treated babies.

It has long been recognized that myocardial blood supply automatically self-adjusts to meet the metabolic demands of the heart muscle tissue. More recent evidence suggests that the vasodilatory prostaglandins have a major role in this autoregulation. Occlusion of the coronary vasculature leads to synthesis of substantial amounts of PGI_2 and PGE_2; these prostaglandins augment myocardial blood flow and are important protective mechanisms. Indomethacin has a suppressive effect on basal coronary arterial flow and markedly inhibits the vasodilatory response to hypoxemia. The short-acting natural prostaglandins, particularly PGE_2 and PGI_2, have been shown to augment coronary arterial flow to hypoxic myocardium, but this effect is not clinically useful because of the short half-lives of these agents. The use of long-acting synthetic prostaglandin analogs has enormous promise for the treatment of myocardial hypoxia.

The low incidence of atherosclerosis in Greenland Eskimos has been correlated with the high concentration of Ω-3 polyunsaturated fatty acids, eicosopentaenoic acid (EPA) and docosahexaenoic acid, in their diet. Supplementation of Western diets

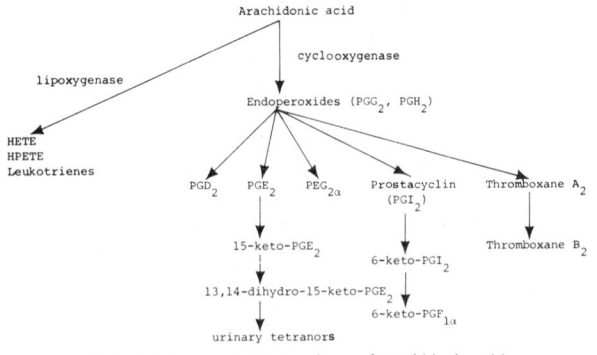

Figure 2. Prostaglandin products of arachidonic acid.

TABLE 1. Biologic Action of Principal Human Prostaglandins

Prostaglandin	Biologic Action
$PGF_{2\alpha}$	Contracts nonvascular smooth muscle
PGE_2	Contracts nonvascular smooth muscle
	Dilates vascular smooth muscle
	Inhibits gastric acid secretion
	Inhibits platelet aggregation
	Inhibits tumor cell replication
	Modulates humoral and cellular immunity
	Causes bone resorption
Thromboxane A_2	Enhances platelet aggregation
	Induces vasoconstriction
PGI_2	Inhibits platelet aggregation
	Dilates vascular smooth muscle
Leukotriene C_4	Modulates immune response
	Contracts nonvascular smooth muscle
	Induces chemotaxis
Lipoxin A_4	Produces superoxides
	Induces leukocytosis
	Causes local vasodilation

with these two fatty acids (in cod liver oil) produces a pronounced shift from doubly to triply unsaturated prostaglandins. In terms of their antiaggregatory and vasodilatory actions, PGI_3 and PGE_3 are at least as potent as PGI_2 and PGE_2. However, thromboxane A_3 is far less proaggregatory than thromboxane A_2. Thus, a diet rich in Ω-3 fatty acids lowers blood pressure, inhibits platelet aggregation, prolongs bleeding time, leads to a more favorable fatty acid profile, and protects against induction of myocardial and cerebral infarction. These simple dietary alterations may provide an important new approach to the prevention and/or treatment of atherosclerosis.

Endotoxemia is associated with a number of specific hemodynamic abnormalities, including hypotension, increased pulmonary arterial pressure, decreased cardiac output, and ultimately, increased peripheral vascular resistance. Endotoxemia and severe burns are also associated with substantial elevations in the levels of the vasoconstrictor prostaglandins, notably $PGF_{2\alpha}$ and thromboxane A_2. Indomethacin and, experimentally, imidazole and picotramide, selective thromboxane synthesis inhibitors, have demonstrated improvement in both hemodynamic parameters and survival. Similarly, leukotriene synthesis is increased during sepsis, and a lipoxygenase inhibitor has recently been shown to mitigate the changes associated with endotoxemia. Although the use of steroids in endotoxic shock is still controversial, the doses utilized are sufficient to suppress prostaglandin biosynthesis.

PERIPHERAL VASCULAR USES. Intra-arterial administration of PGE may be useful in the treatment of ischemic peripheral vascular disease. Relatively small doses of PGE_1 (1 to 10 ng. per kg. per minute) administered for 10 minutes per hour cause substantial increases in blood flow and skin temperature. The mechanism of this action is not clear, since the effects last for weeks and allow healing of chronic ischemic ulcers. Although experience with this therapeutic modality is relatively limited, in several studies, it has already been proved extremely effective. One specific application is the preservation of viability of severely ischemic extremities in preparation for bypass surgery.

CONTROL OF PLATELET FUNCTION. The platelet abnormality induced by aspirin attests to the importance of prostaglandins in the normal coagulation scheme. The specific prostaglandin responsible for normal clotting is thromboxane A_2. As outlined in Table 2, thromboxane A_2 is synthesized by platelets and serves to counteract the effects of injury by causing vasoconstriction and inducing platelet aggregation (mediated by calcium fluxes). The effects of thromboxane are opposed by those of prostacyclin (PGI_2). This prostaglandin, synthesized by endothelial cells, is the most potent vasodilator known and, in

TABLE 2. Comparative Effects of Thromboxane A_2 and PGI_2

Thromboxane A_2	PGI_2
Platelets	Endothelial cells
Aggregator	Antiaggregator
Vasoconstrictor	Vasodilator
Inhibits adenyl cyclase	Stimulates adenyl cyclase
Injury	Homeostasis

addition, is a very effective inhibitor of platelet aggregation. PGI_2 thus serves to maintain vascular homeostasis. The balance between these two agents, thromboxane A_2 and PGI_2, is responsible for the moment-to-moment control of blood flow. Although aspirin has been widely utilized as an antiplatelet drug in the long-term management of patients with coronary and cerebrovascular disease, there was until recently little evidence for the efficacy of this regimen. However, the Physicians' Health Study recently reported that this aspirin dose reduced the risk of myocardial infarction by 44 per cent.

This recent innovation in the use of low-dose aspirin therapy (325 mg. per day) is based on the presumption that thromboxane synthesis is significantly more sensitive to the effects of acetylsalicylic acid than is the synthesis of PGI_2. If correct, use of aspirin in this manner would lead to inhibition of thromboxane A_2 synthesis but would not affect the production of the antiaggregating and vasodilatory PGI_2. Unfortunately, it appears that this presumption may be incorrect and that aspirin may be equally effective in inhibiting the biosynthesis of both thromboxane A_2 and prostacyclin.

An extremely exciting recent observation is that these prostaglandins may be abnormal in atherosclerosis. Atherosclerotic vessels have decreased prostacyclin biosynthetic ability. Nicotine has been shown to inhibit prostacyclin generation. Compared with low cholesterol diets, solutions high in cholesterol are associated with significantly higher platelet levels of thromboxane A_2. The exact role of thromboxane and prostacyclin in atherogenesis is unclear but is being extensively studied.

Based on their antiaggregatory effects, both PGE_1 and PGI_2 have been utilized in extracorporeal circulations experimentally and clinically. In cardiopulmonary bypass, these prostaglandins (with or without heparin) prevent platelet aggregation, which is manifested by the prevention of thrombocytopenia, absence of microaggregates on the filters, and appropriate anti-coagulation. PGE_1 has one substantial advantage over PGI_2; as a result of pulmonary inactivation of PGE_1, at the conclusion of bypass when pulmonary blood flow is restored, coagulation parameters spontaneously return to normal.

PULMONARY DYSFUNCTION. Respiratory distress syndromes are characterized by interstitial edema, constriction of the pulmonary microvasculature, and loss of capillary integrity leading to transendothelial fluid leakage. Although the pathogenetic mechanisms in the syndromes are not known, eicosanoids are clearly involved. The leukotrienes and thromboxane A_2 induce platelet aggregation, vasoconstriction, and capillary leak; their effects in the lung are thought to have a significant role in the development of adult respiratory distress syndrome (ARDS) and persistent pulmonary hypertension of the newborn, as well as the pattern of injury induced by oleic and other fatty acids. The vasodilatory prostaglandins are protective. In fact, there is ample evidence that PGE treatment of patients with ARDS leads to better pulmonary function and improved survival. Manipulation of endogenous eicosanoid synthesis may thus allow prevention of both neonatal and adult respiratory distress symptoms.

GASTROINTESTINAL USES. The methyl analogs of PGE and PGA, particularly 15(R)- and 15(S)-methyl-PGE_2 and 16,16-dimethyl-PGE_2, have been used extensively as inhibitors of acid secretion in patients with peptic ulceration. They have been shown to hasten the healing of both duodenal and gastric ulcers. In hypersecreting patients with duodenal ulceration, this effect is presumably due to the ability of PGE and PGA compounds to inhibit gastric secretion of acid and pepsin and stimulate secretion of gastric mucus. Since most individuals with gastric ulcers are hyposecretors, another action must be responsible for the improvement in these patients. In this event, the effect is "cytoprotection," which implies that the gastric mucosa requires substantial amounts of prostaglandins to maintain its functional integrity. Cytoprotection may be mediated by secretion of bicarbonate ion, stimulation of mucus production, increased gastric mucosal blood flow, strengthening of the mucosal barrier, or accentuation of the sodium pump. Good documentation of the need for prostaglandin in the gastric mucosa is provided by the fact that aspirin suppositories and intravenous indomethacin can cause gastric ulceration. Steroid-induced gastric ulcers have been successfully treated with methyl prostaglandin analogs in patients who otherwise would have been candidates for surgical therapy. The effects of prostaglandins on gastric secretion are totally independent of H_2 receptors; thus, prostaglandins and H_2 receptor antagonists can be used concurrently in patients with massive hypersecretion.

Prostaglandins have been implicated in the pathogenesis of cholesterol gallstone formation. Prairie dogs fed a diet high in cholesterol routinely develop cholelithiasis. In this model, increasing biliary concentrations of cholesterol stimulate the secretion of PGE_2 and PGI_2, which augment mucus secretion by the gallbladder epithelium. The intraluminal mucin serves as a nidus for the formation of gallstones. Inhibitors of prostaglandin synthetase both curtail the secretion of mucus and prevent the development of stones. Eicosanoids have also been implicated in the pathogenesis of cholecystitis. In addition to their effects on mucus secretion and nidation, the prostaglandins inhibit biliary absorption of fluid and electrolytes and stimulate gallbladder motility, actions that induce some of the manifestations of cholecystitis. During inflammation, the gallbladder wall synthesizes several times more PGI_2 and PGE_2 than normal. In randomized prospective trials, prostaglandin synthetase inhibitors decreased the severity of cholecystitis and of biliary colic.

Patients with inflammatory bowel disease are known to have elevated mucosal and luminal concentrations of prostaglandins. Interleukin-1 has a significant role in augmenting the prostaglandin release. Because the prostaglandins increase intestinal motility, they may contribute to the diarrhea in these syndromes. Recently, Sharon and Stinson demonstrated that mucosa from patients with inflammatory bowel disease synthesizes excessive amounts of the lipoxygenase derivative leukotriene B_4. Inhibition of leukotriene synthesis by steroids and sulfasalazine may explain the beneficial effect of these drugs in inflammatory bowel disease.

When PGF and PGE compounds were initially used in the induction of abortion, a major side effect was diarrhea. The diarrhea is caused by a combination of motility and secretory effects. PGE and PGF cause contraction of nonvascular smooth muscle, leading to reduced intestinal transit times. In addition, PGE causes intestinal secretion (rather than absorption) of water and electrolytes. These effects are characteristic of a number of endocrine diarrheogenic states. As demonstrated in Table 3, a large number of patients with watery diarrhea, hypokalemia, achlorhydria (WDHA) and carcinoid syndromes and medullary carcinoma of the thyroid have elevated plasma levels of PGE and, to a lesser degree, of PGF. Treatment of these patients with indomethacin, as illustrated by a typical patient course (Fig. 3), leads to resolution of the diarrhea. This modality has been extremely useful in preparing patients for resection of diarrheogenic tumors as well as in the long-term management of patients with metastatic disease.

RENAL USES. Infusion of PGE_1 and PGE_2 into the renal artery decreases renal vascular resistance, increases renal blood flow, augments sodium and water excretion, contracts the ex-

TABLE 3. PGE Levels in Endocrine
Diarrheogenic Syndromes

Syndromes	Number of Patients	PGE (pg./ml.)
WDHA	26	935 ± 355
Medullary carcinoma of thyroid	20	1922 ± 541
Carcinoid	22	1367 ± 245
Controls		
Normal	61	272 ± 18
Nonendocrine diarrhea	34	353 ± 25
Zollinger-Ellison syndrome with diarrhea	26	338 ± 32

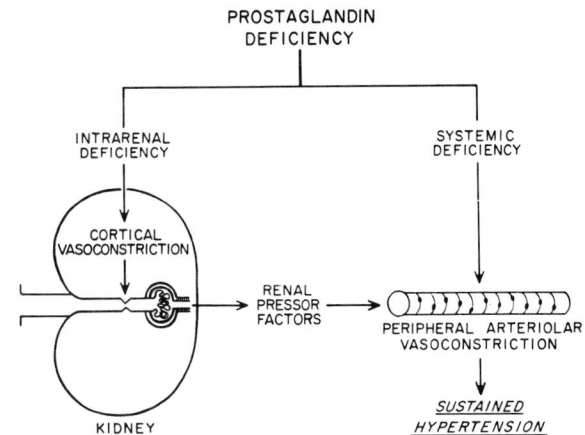

Figure 4. Schematic representation of the hypothesis implicating a prostaglandin deficiency in the genesis of essential hypertension.

tracellular fluid volume, and leads to a hypotensive effect. Since the PGE compounds dilate vascular muscle, the primary effect is on intrarenal resistance. It would be difficult to improve upon these characteristics, because they constitute the ideal properties of an antihypertensive diuretic agent. It is not necessary, however, to use PGE compounds directly in order to achieve these effects. It has become clear that the most common diuretic utilized in clinical practice, furosemide (Lasix), induces diuresis by stimulating endogenous prostaglandin synthesis. Consequently, addition of steroids or indomethacin to a regimen including furosemide markedly diminishes the diuretic effect of this drug. The prostaglandin-stimulating action of furosemide is not limited to the kidney. This biosynthetic effect presumably is responsible for the improvement in pulmonary ventilation and hemodynamics in patients with the adult respiratory distress syndrome associated with trauma; in this syndrome, furosemide induces its effect almost immediately, whereas diruesis reaches its maximum only at 1 to 1½ hours after injection. In addition, the vasodilatory effects of furosemide on the heart are presumably mediated by stimulation of endogenous PGE by endocardium and/or endothelium.

Bartter's syndrome is the result of juxtaglomerular hyperplasia. Clinically, the syndrome is manifested by hypokalemia, increased plasma renin activity, aldosteronism, and normal blood pressure. This relatively uncommon cause of hypokalemia is due to hypersecretion of PGE2 and PGI2 by the kidney. Consequently, the diagnosis can be easily established by measuring urinary levels of prostaglandins. More important, however, the disease responds to therapeutic doses of indomethacin, which has been used with nearly uniform success.

The final implication of prostaglandins in renal disease is the possibility that a prostaglandin deficiency has some role in the development of essential hypertension. Decreased renal synthesis of PGE2 would lead to unopposed vasoconstrictor mechanisms and allow for systemic hypertension (Fig. 4). Although there is no firm substantiation of this hypothesis, it is clear that

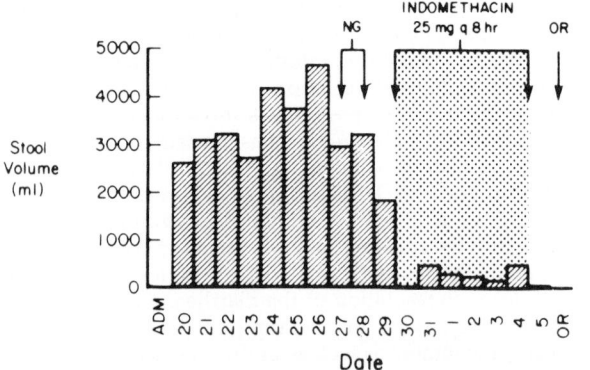

Figure 3. The effect of indomethacin on diarrhea in a patient with the WDHA syndrome associated with a prostaglandin-producing islet cell tumor of the pancreas.

kidneys from patients with essential hypertension have lower levels of PGE and that the same tissues have an impaired ability to convert precursor arachidonic acid to the native prostaglandins.

IMPLICATIONS IN TUMOR BIOLOGY AND VIROLOGY. Prostaglandins have been implicated in the pathogenesis of tumor-induced hypercalcemia. In approximately one third of patients harboring malignancies (most frequently renal cell carcinomas), hypercalcemia and hypophosphatemia (a parathyroid hormone–like syndrome) follow hyperprostaglandinemia due to excessive production of PGE2 by the tumors. Raisz and colleagues have demonstrated that prostaglandins induce bone resorption by mobilizing osteoclasts. In hyperprostaglandinemic patients without bone metastases, indomethacin has consistently normalized the serum calcium level. In contrast, in similar patients with bone metastases, indomethacin has proved relatively ineffective. This difference suggests that prostaglandins may have a role in the genesis of osseous metastases. This hypothesis was given substantial credence by the studies of Powles and associates using the VX2 rabbit adenocarcinoma. When these investigators inoculated rabbits in the muscle with this tumor, as little as 2 weeks later osteoclast numbers increased markedly in the corresponding femur, an event that was prevented by treatment with indomethacin. When the same experiment was continued for 4 weeks, the corresponding femur was destroyed by tumor; this pattern of metastases was similarly prevented by indomethacin. Since breast adenocarcinoma frequently metastasizes to bone, this malignancy has been studied most carefully. In the studies of Powles and colleagues and Bennett and associates, breast tumors that produced large amounts of prostaglandins were associated with a high frequency of metastasis to bones. Tumors that synthesized only small amounts of PGE2, however, rarely involved the bones. On the basis of these observations, there are now large-scale trials on breast cancer patients using inhibitors of prostaglandin biosynthesis in an effort to prevent osseous dissemination of tumor.

A, D, and J prostaglandins have been shown to potently inhibit viral replication. These naturally occurring prostaglandins interfere with DNA replication and/or cause a specific transcription block. There is also a clear relationship between PGA compounds and interferon. Both inhibit viral replication, elicit differentiation, induce the same cell membrane enzymes, stimulate macrophage function, and so on. Most important, prostaglandin synthesis inhibitors suppress the inhibitory actions of interferon. The interaction between prostaglandins and interferon is being extensively studied in an effort to exploit their possible clinical utility.

TRANSPLANTATION AND IMMUNOBIOLOGY. PGE2

and PGI_2 levels in tissue, plasma, and urine increase dramatically at the time of rejection of human and animal skin, kidney, and heart allografts. The released prostaglandins protect against rejection and maintain renal cortical blood flow, urinary output, and renal function. Long-acting prostaglandin analogs have been successfully utilized in animal models and are currently being evaluated as part of immunosuppressive regimens in clinical trials. In contrast, thromboxane A_2 released during rejection may mediate some of the vasoconstrictive effects. A thromboxane synthesis inhibitor has recently been shown to improve experimental renal allograft function.

It has recently been postulated that eicosanoids are involved as mediators of cyclosporine (CSA) nephrotoxicity. Administration of CSA constricts the renal vasculature, decreases the glomerular filtration rate, and releases prostaglandins. Preliminary data suggest that the use of a long-acting analog (Misoprostol) counters the deleterious effects of CSA on renal function.

Prostaglandins have long been recognized as mediators of inflammation. The recent identification of the leukotriene derivatives of arachidonate via the lipoxygenase pathway has increased understanding of the inflammatory process. Leukotrienes induce chemotaxis, produce edema, cause local vasoconstriction, and stimulate bronchoconstriction. It is now clear that leukotrienes mediate allergic reactions such as those to ragweed and drugs. A second more recently recognized group of lipoxygenase products, the lipoxins, are also proinflammatory. Lipoxin A_4, for example, activates protein kinase C, stimulates leukocytes, releases thromboxane A_2, contracts the bronchus, releases superoxides, and causes local vasodilation. These lipoxygenase-mediated effects are sensitive to steroids that prevent the release of the arachidonic acid precursor of these derivatives.

The synthesis of interleukin-1 (IL-1) by monocytes and macrophages is initiated by stimuli such as microbial, toxic, and immunologic substances during the acute phase response. Leukotriene B_4 (LTB_4) enhances IL-1 production, whereas PGE_2 leads to suppression of macrophage IL-1 production. IL-1 may be responsible for the initiation of the inflammatory response. It has multiple biologic actions, including induction of leukocytosis, stimulation of T-cell proliferation, and eicosanoid release. IL-1 stimulates the synthesis of PGI_2 and PGE_2 in endothelial cells and the release of thromboxane from neutrophils, leading to vasodilation and platelet aggregation, respectively. IL-2, produced by helper T cells and induced by IL-1, has an essential role in the cell-mediated immune response. By inhibiting the production of IL-2, PGE_2 is involved in the endogenous feedback regulation of interleukin synthesis and activity.

SELECTED REFERENCES

General

Flower, R. J.: Drugs which inhibit prostaglandin biosynthesis. Pharmacol. Rev., 26:33, 1974.
This is a major pharmacologic review of the efficacy of prostaglandin inhibitors. It comprises a discussion of the specificity and mechanism of action and includes an excellent description of the routes of prostaglandin biosynthesis.

Piper, P. J., Vane, J. R., and Wyllie, J. H.: Inactivation of prostaglandins by the lungs. Nature, 225:600, 1970.

Roth, G. J., Stanford, N., and Majerus, P. W.: Acetylation of prostaglandin synthetase by aspirin. Proc. Natl. Acad. Sci. USA., 72:3073, 1975.

Vane, J. R.: Inhibition of prostaglandin synthesis as a mechanism of action for aspirin-like drugs. Nature, 231:232, 1971.
This is the vitally important initial report that aspirin and other anti-inflammatory drugs inhibit prostaglandin biosynthesis. As such, it represents one of the classic articles in the archives of medicine.

Wong, P. Y-K., Sun, F. F., and McGiff, J. C.: Metabolism of prostacyclin in blood vessels. J. Biol. Chem., 253:5555, 1978.

Cardiovascular

Afonso, S., Barnow, G. T., and Rowe, G. G.: Indomethacin and the prostaglandin hypothesis of coronary blood flow regulation. J. Physiol., 241:299, 1974.

Alster, P., and Wennmalin, A.: Effect of nicotine on prostacyclin formation in rat aorta. Eur. J. Pharmacol., 86:441, 1983.
This article suggests a mechanism for the pathogenic effects of nicotine, decreasing the synthesis of PGIs by competitive inhibition of cyclo-oxygenase.

Dzau, V. J., Parker, M., Lilly, L. S., Swartz, S. L., Hollenberg, N. K., and Williams, G. H.: Prostaglandins in severe congestive heart failure. N. Engl. J. Med., 310:347, 1984.

Friedman, P. L., Brown, E. J. Jr., Gunther, S., Alexander, R. W., Barry, W. H., Mudge, E. H. Jr., and Grossman, W.: Coronary vasoconstrictor effect of indomethacin in patients with coronary-artery disease. N. Engl. J. Med., 305:1171, 1981.

Friedman, W. F., Hirschklau, M. J., Printz, M. P., Pitlick, P. T., and Kirkpatrick, S. E.: Pharmacologic closure of patent ductus arteriosus in the premature infant. N. Engl. J. Med., 295:525, 1976.

Graham, T. P. Jr., Atwood, G. F., and Boucek, R. J. Jr.: Pharmacologic dilation of the ductus arteriosus with prostaglandin E_1 in infants with congenital heart disease. South. Med. J., 71:1238, 1978.

Herndon, D. N., Abston, S., and Stein, M. D.: Increased thromboxane B_2 levels in the plasma of burned and septic burned patients. Surg. Gynecol. Obstet., 159:210, 1984.

Heymann, M. A., Rudolph, A. M., and Silverman, N. H.: Closure of the ductus arteriosus in premature infants by inhibition of prostaglandin synthesis. N. Engl. J. Med., 295:530, 1976.
The initial description of the use of indomethacin in the closure of the ductus arteriosus explores the appropriate doses and techniques for administration. The hemodynamic parameters for assessing ductal closure are discussed, and the uses and complications of indomethacin therapy in this series of 18 neonates are described.

Matera, G., Cook, J. A., Hennigar, R. A., Tempel, G. E., Wise, W. C., and Halushka, P. V.: Beneficial effects of a 5-lipoxygenase inhibitor in endotoxic shock in the rat. J. Pharmacol. Exp. Ther., 247:363, 1988.

Neutze, J. M., Starling, M. B., Elliott, R. B., and Barratt-Boyes, B. G.: Palliation of cyanotic congenital heart disease in infancy with E-type prostaglandins. Circulation, 55:238, 1977.
This is an excellent article describing the use of PGE to dilate the ductus arteriosus in infants with cyanotic congenital heart disease. The clinical features and hemodynamic parameters are carefully correlated. Although this represents an early trial, it carefully outlines the indications for and the successes of the use of PGEs in this clinical situation.

Peripheral Vascular

Nielson, P. E., Nielsen, S. L., Holstein, P., Poulsen, H. H., Hansen, E. H., and Lassen, N. A.: Intra-arterial infusion of prostaglandin E_1 in normal subjects and patients with peripheral arterial disease. Scand. J. Clin. Lab. Invest., 36:633, 1976.
This article explores the mechanism of the effect of intra-arterial PGE. After measurements of changes in isotope clearance, plethysmography, arterial pressure, and skin temperature, the data suggested that blood flow increased only in the proximal arterial tree. There was no correlation between changes in hemodynamics and symptomatic improvement.

Platelets

Chang, W-C., Fukuda, S., and Tai, H-H.: Cigarette smoking stimulates lipoxygenase but not cyclooxygenase pathway in platelets. Biochem. Biophys. Res. Commun., 115:499, 1983.

Fitzgerald, G. A., Oates, J. A., Havinger, J., Mass, R. L., Roberts, L. J., II, Lawson, J. A., and Brash, A. R.: Endogenous biosynthesis of prostacyclin and thromboxane and platelet function during chronic administration of aspirin in man. J. Clin. Invest., 71:676, 1983.

Hamburg, M., Svensson, J., and Samuelsson, B.: Thromboxanes: A new group of biologically active compounds derived from prostaglandin endoperoxides. Proc. Natl. Acad. Sci. USA, 72:2994, 1975.

Hennekens, C. H., et al.: Final report on the aspirin component of the ongoing Physicians' Health Study. N. Engl. J. Med., 321:129, 1989.
The results of a controlled, randomized trial demonstrated that at 60.2 months, 325 mg. per day of aspirin reduced the risk of myocardial infarction and had no significant effect on risk of stroke or on cardiovascular mortality.

Kappa, J. R., Musial, J., Fisher, C. A., and Addonizio, V. P., Jr.: Quantitation of platelet preservation with prostanoids during simulated bypass. J. Surg. Res., 42:10, 1987.

Longmore, D. B., Gueirrara, D., Bennett, G., Smith, M., Bunting, S., Reed, P., Moncada, S., Read, N. G., and Vane, J. R.: Prostacyclin: A solution to some problems of extracorporeal circulation. Lancet, 1:1002, 1979.

Needleman, P., Minkes, M., and Raz, A.: Thromboxanes: selective biosynthesis and distinct biological properties. Science, 193:163, 1976.
The role of thromboxanes in the coagulation mechanism is clearly defined in this study. The article defines platelet and vascular receptors and dissociates the vasoconstrictor and aggregating properties. It is a superb article that places thromboxanes in perspective.

Stuart, M. J., Gerrard, J. M., and White, J. G.: Effect of cholesterol on production of thromboxane B_2 by platelets in vitro. N. Engl. J. Med., 302:6, 1980.
This important study relates high-cholesterol diets with platelet aggregation and

vasoconstriction by demonstrating that cholesterol-enriched platelets synthesize substantially more thromboxane than do cholesterol-depleted platelets. This is a fundamental concept in the pathogenesis of vascular disease.

Vargas, J. R., Radomski, M., and Moncada, S.: The use of prostacyclin in the separation from plasma and washing of human platelets. Prostaglandins, 23:929, 1982.

Renal

Craven, P. H., and DeRubertis, F. R.: Calcium-dependent synthesis of renal medullary prostaglandin synthesis by furosemide. J. Pharmacol. Exp. Ther., 222:306, 1982.

Gill, J. R. Jr., Frolich, J. C., Bowden, R. E., Taylor, A. A. Keiser, H. R., Seyberth, H. W., Oates, J. A., and Bartter, F. C.: Bartter's syndrome: a disorder characterized by high urinary prostaglandins and a dependence of hyperreninemia on prostaglandin synthesis. Am. J. Med., 61:43, 1976.
This paper describes 4 patients with this illness, correlating the disturbances in physiology with rates of urinary excretion of prostaglandins. The pathophysiology of the illness is clearly characterized and the objectives of the therapy outlined.

Gross, J. B., and Bartter, F. C.: Effects of prostaglandins E_1, A_1 and $F_{2\alpha}$ on renal handling of salt and water. Am. J. Physiol., 225:218, 1973.
Although an animal study, this report clearly delineates the renal effects of prostaglandins. The conclusion is that prostaglandins decrease sodium and water resorption in the proximal tubule and increase renal blood flow without altering management of cyclic nucleotides.

Halushka, P. V., Wohltmann, H., Privatera, P. J., Hurwitz, G., and Margolius, H. S.: Bartter's syndrome: Urinary prostaglandin E-like material and kallikrein; indomethacin effects. Ann. Intern. Med., 87:281, 1977.

Herbaczynska-Cedro, K., and Vane, J. R.: Contribution of intrarenal generation of prostaglandin to autoregulation of renal blood flow in the dog. Circ. Res., 33:428, 1973.

Johnston, H. H., Herzog, J. P., and Lauler, D. P.: Effect of prostaglandin E_1 on renal hemodynamics, sodium and water excretion. Am. J. Physiol., 213:939, 1967.

Patak, R. B., Mookerjee, B. K., Bentzel, C. J., Hysert, P. E., Babej, M., and Lee, J. B.: Antagonism of the effects of furosemide by indomethacin in normal and hypersensitive man. Prostaglandins, 10:649, 1975.

Zipser, R. D., Speckart, P.F., Zia, P. K., Hahn, J. A., Boswell, W. P., and Horton, R.: Release of immuno-assayable prostaglandin E by the human kidney. J. Clin. Endocrinol. Metab., 47:914, 1978.

Pulmonary

Holcroft, J. W., Vassar, M. J., and Weber, C. J.: Prostaglandin E_1 and survival in patients with adult respiratory distress syndrome. Ann. Surg., 203:371, 1986.
This randomized prospective trial demonstrated that, as compared with placebo, PGE_1 infusion improved both pulmonary function and survival in patients with ARDS.

Shoemaker, W. C., and Appel, P. L.: Effects of prostaglandin E_1 in adult respiratory distress syndrome. Surgery, 99:275, 1986.

Gastrointestinal

Dozois, R. R., Kim, J. K., and Dousa, T. P.: Interactions of prostaglandins with gastric mucosal adenylate cyclase-cyclic AMP system. Am. J. Physiol., 235:E546, 1978.

Hunt, J. N., Smith, J. L., Jiang, C. L., and Kessler, L.: Effect of synthetic prostaglandin E_1 analog on aspirin-induced gastric bleeding and secretion. Dig. Dis. Sci., 28:897, 1983.

Jaffe, B. M., and Condon, S.: Prostaglandins E and F in endocrine diarrheagenic syndromes. Ann. Surg., 184:516, 1976.
This study documents elevated plasma prostaglandin levels in a large series of patients with the WDHA, carcinoid, and medullary thyroid carcinoma syndromes. Normal levels were found in controls, including normal individuals, and in patients with inflammatory bowel disease and Zollinger-Ellison syndrome with diarrhea. Diagnostic and therapeutic implications are discussed.

Jaffe, B. M., Kopen, D. F., DeSchryver-Kecskemeti, K., Gingerich, R. L., and Greider, M.: Indomethacin-responsive pancreatic cholera. N. Engl. J. Med., 297:817, 1977.

Kaminsky, D. L., Deshpande, Y. E., Watfall, S., and Herbold, D.: Evaluation of prostaglandin formation by human gallbladder. Arch. Surg., 124:277, 1989.

Lundstrom, S., Ivarsson, L., Lindblad, L., and Kral, J. E.: Treatment of biliary pain by prostaglandin synthetase inhibition with diclofenac sodium. Curr. Ther. Res., 57:435, 1985.

Miller, T. A., and Jacobsen, E. D.: Progress report: Gastrointestinal cytoprotection by prostaglandins. Gut, 20:75, 1979.

Robert, A.: Cytoprotection by prostaglandins. Gastroenterology, 77:761, 1979.
These two excellent review articles summarize the protective effects of prostaglandins on gastric mucosa. The mechanism of development of aspirin- and steroid-induced ulcers is discussed in detail, and the pertinent clinical implications are described with regard to management of these lesions.

Sharon, P., and Stenson, W. F.: Enhanced synthesis of leukotriene by colonic mucosa in inflammatory bowel disease. Gastroenterology, 86:453, 1984.

Wilson, D. E., Quertermus, J., Raiser, M., Curran, J., and Robert A.: Inhibition of stimulated gastric secretion by an orally administered prostaglandin capsule: A study in normal man. Ann. Intern. Med., 84:688, 1976.

Tumor Biology and Virology

Bennett, A., Simpson, J. S., McDonald, A. M., and Stamford, I. F.: Breast cancer, prostaglandins, and bone metastases. Lancet, 1:1218, 1975.

Demers, L. M., Allegra, J. C., Harvey, H. A., Lipton, A., Luderer, J. R., Mortel, R., and Brenner, D. E.: Plasma prostaglandins in hypercalcemic patients with neoplastic disease. Cancer, 39:1559, 1977.

Fukushima, M., Kato, T., Narumiya, S., Mizushima, Y., Sasaki, H., Terashima, Y., Nishiyama, Y., and Santoro, M. G.: Prostaglandin A and J: Antitumor and antiviral prostaglandins. Adv. Prostaglandin Thromboxane Leukotriene Res., 19:415, 1989.

Josse, R. G., Wilson, D. R., Heersche, J. N. M., Mills, J. R. F., and Murray, T. M.: Hypercalcemia with ovarian carcinoma. Cancer, 48:1233, 1981.

Seyberth, H. Segre, G. V., Morgan, J. L., Sweetman, B. J., Potts, J. T., Jr., and Oates, J. A.: Prostaglandins as mediators of hypercalcemia associated with certain types of cancer. N. Engl. J. Med., 293:1278, 1975.
This clinical study evaluated the effects of prostaglandin synthesis inhibitors in the treatment of tumor-induced hypercalcemia. The biochemical parameters related to calcium and phosphorus metabolism are well discussed in relation to prostaglandins. This report places the role of prostaglandins in hypercalcemia in perspective.

Transplantation and Immunology

Creticos, P. S., Peters, S. P., Adkinson, N. F. Jr., Naclerio, R. M., Hayes, E. C., Norman, P.S., and Lichtenstein, L. M.: Peptide leukotriene release after antigen challenge in patients sensitive to ragweed. N. Engl. J. Med., 310:1626, 1984.

Dahlen, S-E.: Pharmacological activities of lipoxins and related compounds. Adv. Prostaglandin Thromboxane Leukotriene Res., 19:122, 1989.

Kunkel, S. L., Chensue, S. W., and Phan, S. H.: Prostaglandins as endogenous mediators of interleukin production. J. Immunol., 136:186, 1986.

Paller, M. S.: Effects of the prostaglandin E_1 analog Misoprostol on cyclosporine nephrotoxicity. Transplantation, 45:1126, 1988.

Rankin, J. A., Hitchcock, M., Merrill, W. W., Huang, S. S., Brashler, J. R., Bach, M. K., and Askenase, P. W.: IgE immune complexes induce immediate and prolonged release of leukotriene C_4 from rat alveolar macrophages. J. Immunol., 132:1993, 1984.

Ruiz, P., Coffman, T. M., Klotman, P. E., and Sanfilippo, F.: Association of chronic thromboxane inhibition with reduced in situ cytotoxic T cell activity in rejecting rat renal allografts. Transplantation, 48:660, 1989.

Tannenbaum, J. S., Anderson, C. B., Sicard, G. A., McKeal, D.W., and Etheridge, E. E.:Prostaglandin synthesis associated with renal allograft rejection in the dog. Transplantation, 37:438, 1984.

20

IMMUNOBIOLOGY AND IMMUNOTHERAPY OF NEOPLASTIC DISEASE; MELANOMA; SOFT TISSUE SARCOMAS; TUMOR MARKERS

I

IMMUNOBIOLOGY AND IMMUNOTHERAPY OF NEOPLASTIC DISEASE

H. F. Seigler, M.D.

TUMOR-ASSOCIATED ANTIGENS

All mammalian species are afflicted with neoplastic diseases. Both animal and human studies have demonstrated that malignant cells express antigens that either are absent or are in low concentration on normal cells. Human tumor cells express both Class I and Class II major histocompatibility antigens on their cell surfaces. Additionally, antigens that are individually restricted to the patient's own tumor cells are also expressed. Certain other tumor-associated antigens are shared and are present on both autologous as well as allogeneic tumors. Other antigens are also expressed that are widely cross-reacting and have been detected on fetal cells, normal human cells, and malignant cells. The relative immunogenicity of tumor-associated antigens has yet to be defined. The immune response to tumor-associated antigens appears to be genetically controlled. Experimental animal data have suggested that if a host reacts to tumor-associated antigens, there must be compatibility for major histocompatibility antigens of the host and the tumor. In man, this has been described as cell killing restricted by compatibility for Class I histocompatibility antigens. Obvious benefit would be evident if increased immunogenicity of tumor cells could be accomplished by alteration of tumor antigen expression or increased host response to these antigens. Experimental animals immunized with intact tumor cells, or tumor antigen extracts, demonstrate either protection against subsequent tumor challenge or delay in growth of the tumor if a degree of immunity has been stimulated. Low levels of immunity are usually associated with humoral or cell-mediated immunity in *in vitro* assays but little or no protection against tumor growth *in vivo*.

Normal tissue cells express a variety of antigens that are membrane-associated. These antigens include isoantigens controlled by the genes included in the major histocompatibility complex (MHC). Blood group antigens, species-specific antigens, organ-specific antigens, and certain fetal antigens are also expressed. If a tumor is virus-associated, viral antigens are also expressed. As the cell is transformed from normal to malignant, the virus becomes incorporated into the cell genome, and antigens common for the virus are expressed as a membrane component. Antigens that are the gene product of oncogenes are expressed as nuclear, cytosol, and occasionally membrane components. Many malignant cells have high concentrations of fetal antigens present on their surfaces. Mutant cells often have different pathways of cell metabolism or, indeed, alteration of cell division that leads to differing levels of antigen concentration in both the cell cytosol and on the cell membrane. Glycoprotein, glycolipid, and gangliosides have been demonstrated on the cell membrane of neoplastic cells and can serve as distinguishing cell markers. In both animal and human experimental systems, viruses have been demonstrated to cause malignant transformation. As the virus becomes incorporated into the cell DNA, there is virus replication that leads to transcription and translocation, with resultant expression of antigens and protein products of these viral genes. The question then arises as to whether these gene protein products are recognized by the host as foreign and whether they are immunogenic. If indeed they are immunogenic, immunity is realized only if the host response to these antigens is adequate. Thymic-dependent cell (T-cell) receptors for these antigens must be present, and generated T-cell killing must be provoked. Certain chemicals have also demonstrated oncogenicity. Whereas virally transformed malignant cells express antigens that are cross-reactive and common to the virus-evoking transformation, chemically induced transformation more commonly induces individually specific antigens. These antigens are membrane-associated and, as such, act as tumor-specific transplantation antigens. Phenotypic differences are somewhat more common in metastatic deposits than in the primary lesion. The host response to the primary tumor and metastatic lesions is somewhat different. The host response includes circulating antibody, antigen-dependent cell killing (ADCC), natural killer (NK) cell activity, and T-cell and macrophage activity. All of these cellular responses are more effective against tumor cells of the primary lesion than those of the metastasis. *In vitro* cell killing studies require 40 times greater cell concentration to destroy tumor cell colonies grown from metastatic lesions than from primary lesions. Glycoproteins, glycolipids, mucins, and gangliosides have been detected on the membrane of human tumor cells. Monoclonal antibodies have been raised against these tumor-associated antigens, and this technology has permitted characterization of the membrane-associated antigens present on many human tumor cell types. Increasing the immunogenicity of tumor-associated antigens has been investigated as a possible approach for augmenting the ability of a host to develop stronger immune resistance to tumors. Heterogenization of tumors by viruses has been one approach to augmentation of tumor-associated antigens. Both influenza and vaccinia viral oncolysates have been demonstrated to augment host immune response and resultant tumor resistance in both animal and human studies. Glycoproteins, glycolipids, mucins, and gangliosides have been demonstrated to be immunogenic in primates immunized with human tumor cells and their extracts.[19-21] Human subjects serially immunized with human tumor cells have also demonstrated an immune response to human tumor-associated antigens.[12,13,17]

MONOCLONAL ANTIBODY UTILIZATION

In 1975, Kohler and Milstein reported a procedure for production of monoclonal antibodies to single antigen epitopes.[9] Monoclonal antibodies can be produced in large quantities and in reproducible lots, thus allowing large-scale manufacturing. The unique feature of monoclonal antibodies arises from their ability to recognize single antigenic determinants in a complex mixture of molecules. Cell hybridization techniques have improved dramatically during the past few years. Hybridoma cell lines are capable of producing monoclonal antibodies that react with a number of antigenic specificities present on human malignant cells. Initially, mice were immunized with fresh tumor cells and later with solubilized purified tumor antigen extracts. Sensitized murine lymphocytes were fused with mouse myeloma cells, and these hybrids produced murine monoclonal antibodies of different isotypes. More recently, monkeys, chimpanzees, and man have been serially immunized with intact tumor cells, membrane fractions, and purified solubilized tumor antigen preparations. Murine myeloma cell lines, human myelomas, and hybridized murine-human myeloma lines have been developed for fusion with sensitized lymphocytes obtained from immune rodents, primates, and man. Human-mouse, primate-mouse, primate-human, and human-human fusions have been accomplished. Thus, it is now feasible to raise monoclonal antibodies reactive with human tumor-associated antigens that are of human origin. These antibodies recognize distinct antigenic determinants that are expressed on human tumor cells. Clinical uses for these antibodies are depicted in Table 1. The epitopes that are recognized may be lipid, protein, or carbohydrate. At the present time, monoclonal antibodies are employed in immunopathology, immunochemistry, immuno-

scintigraphy, and immunotherapy. Pathologists now employ a panel of monoclonal antibodies to characterize the type of leukemia or lymphoma that more accurately guides selected therapeutic regimens. Cell markers present on the surface of leukemia and lymphoma cells serve as distinctive targets for monoclonal antibodies, and cell marker analyses have become standard in most pathology departments. Immunoperoxidase staining of tissue sections obtained from surgical specimens now permits specific diagnosis, whereas formerly the only determination was malignant cells of undetermined type. Circulating tumor antigen or antigen-antibody complexes in body fluids have been detected by using monoclonal antibodies in radioimmunoassay or immunoabsorbent assays. These serologic studies have led to both early diagnosis and documentation of recurrent disease prior to appearance of a measurable neoplastic lesion.

A major limitation of diagnostic radionuclide scanning is lack of specificity. An attractive feature of radiolabeled monoclonal antibodies is that they have the capability of specifically binding to target tumor cells. Imaging studies using isotopes of technetium, iodine, and indium have been evaluated,[2,3,10] as well as whole antibody and antibody fragments. With present technology, imaging with monoclonal antibodies is now feasible and provides a single test that can survey the entire body simultaneously. Areas of isotope localization can then be further evaluated by means of computerized tomography (CT) or magnetic resonance imaging (MRI).

Monoclonal antibodies continue to be evaluated in different therapeutic regimens. They have been administered intravenously, directly into body cavities, intralesional injection, and as immunoconjugates. Patients with cutaneous T-cell lymphoma experienced tumor regression in approximately half of the patients receiving intravenous monoclonal antibody. Unfortunately, most of the responses were of brief duration. A more innovative approach has been to use monoclonal antibodies specific for the individual tumor surface immunoglobulin idiotype. B-cell lymphomas have demonstrated the most dramatic regressions with this unique approach. Patients with acute leukemia experienced a reduction of cell counts; however, the response was of short duration. Patients with solid tumors, including ovarian carcinoma, colon carcinoma, and melanoma, have realized partial responses; but, again, the effect was temporary. Finally, a more innovative approach might well include monoclonal antibody arming of effector cells. Both *in vitro* and *in vivo* studies have demonstrated that membrane-associated tumor antigens serve as a target for immune destruction. Tumor cell cytolysis can be achieved using monoclonal antibodies alone. The additional ability of such antibodies to arm and direct effector cells was reported in an experimental animal model using human tumor xenografts in athymic nude mice.[7] In this report, cell-mediated killing following co-incubation with monoclonal antibody reactive with the tumor-associated antigen caused a highly efficient destruction of measurable tumor deposits.

HUMAN IMMUNE RESPONSE GENES

Both *in vitro* and *in vivo* studies have demonstrated that immune reactivity is controlled by immune response (IR) genes in the MHC in man. These data have increased the basic understanding of cellular interactions required for immune response. Much of the investigative background concerning immune response genes follows studies in the mouse. The IR region in the mouse is located on chromosome 17. Gene products following this chromosomal region are responsible for cell reactivity. These immune response–associated molecules are present on the surface of B cells, macrophages, some T cells, dendritic cells, and Langerhans cells. The human MHC region is on chromosome 6. There are three defined regions that encode molecules

TABLE 1. Potential Clinical Uses for Monoclonal Antibodies

Antibody for immunodiagnosis
    Development of radioimmunoassays
    Specific radionuclide scans
Antibody for detection of tumor antigen as a clinical management aid for following the course of the cancer
Antibody as a research method for characterizing the molecular characteristics of the antigen
Antibody as a possible agent for cancer therapy
    Antibody alone (serotherapy)
    Conjugates
        Antibody-drug
        Antibody-toxin
        Antibody-isotope

resembling murine IR gene products. These are referred to as DS, DR, and SB. These molecules are present on macrophages, B cells, some T cells, dendritic cells, and Langerhans cells. They serve as stimulating determinants in the mixed lymphocyte culture reaction and have a structure similar to that of the murine-defined analogs. IR gene function in man is difficult to determine because of experimental restriction. To date, much of immune responsiveness in man is inferred from murine studies. As T cells develop within the thymus, they contact IR gene products present on the surface of stromal cells. This contact causes immigration of only T cells, which can recognize self-IR molecules in conjunction with other conventional antigens. Activation of peripheral T cells requires that they recognize not only determinants inherent in conventional antigens but also determinants inherent in IR molecules displayed by antigen-presenting cells. It is evident, therefore, that products of IR genes are involved in determining antigen-reactive T cells that exit from the thymus and are necessary for antigen presentation to reactive T cells, thus dictating interactions involved in regulating immune reactivity. Available studies also suggest that human IR genes are important in determining the relative activity of helper versus suppressor cells in controlling specific immune reactivity.

IMMUNE RESPONSES TO TUMOR ANTIGENS

The host response to tumor includes a concert of cellular events. T-cell subsets may primarily serve a recognition function, with the actual rejection or tumor destruction conveyed by macrophages and NK cells. Triggered T cells elicit a factor that activates both cells and macrophages. It appears that spontaneous tumors in man are of questionable immunogenicity. If immunotherapy is to be effective, it is calculated that *in vitro* tests of tumor destruction should render 2 to 3 logs of cell killing. Attempts should be made to activate the entire cascade of cell-mediated responses. The ultimate success depends upon a small tumor burden in the affected host. Greater efficiency might be realized if the immunogenicity of the tumor cells could be increased. A number of manipulations have been studied. Physical alteration using x-irradiation, chemical treatment with compounds such as neuraminidase, and a variety of proteases suggests that host reactivity can be augmented. Biologic alterations of the tumor by means of techniques such as viral oncolysates have also dramatically increased the immunogenicity of tumor cell vaccines. In experimental animal models, the host response can be measured by (1) evaluation of the resultant antibody response, (2) delayed cutaneous hypersensitivity to the tumor vaccine, (3) provocation of a secondary antibody response, and (4) decrease in the growth rate or response of a tumor challenge.

EFFECTOR CELLS OF THE IMMUNE RESPONSE

The effector cells include cells of T-cell lineage, NK cells, and macrophages. T-cell subsets are characterized by their phenotypes (Fig. 1). The T-cell lineage includes inducer cells, helper cells, cytotoxic cells, and suppressor cells. T-cell–directed lysis is complement independent.[1] T-cell function requires both antigen recognition and processing; this is a highly specific activity that is stimulated by Class I MHC antigens. T-cell killing is HLA-restricted, and, in order to occur, cell-to-cell contact is necessary and eventual lysis depends upon effector cell-target cell contact. This activity is independent of both DNA and protein synthesis. T-cell subsets can be cloned and their growth generated with the T-cell growth factor interleukin-2 (IL-2). This technology permits selecting cytotoxic T-cell as well as suppressor or helper cell activity. The effector cell–target cell reaction requires antigen binding with resultant ionic changes

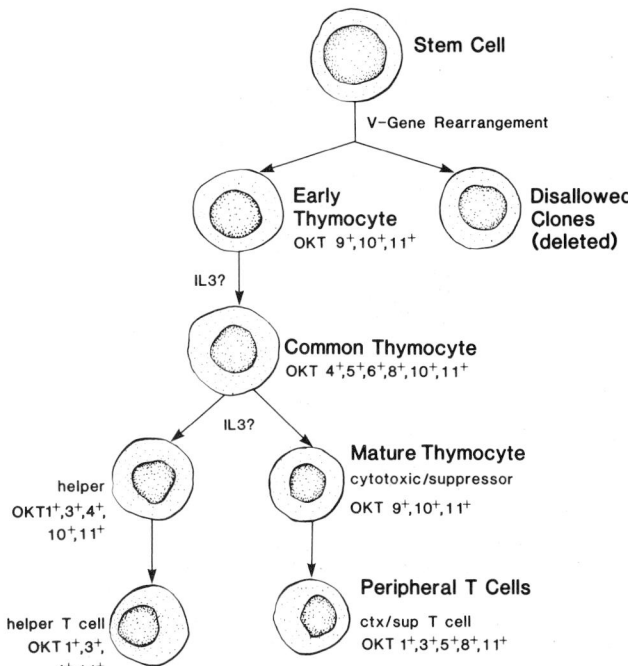

Figure 1. T-cell subsets express different phenotypes. These phenotypes are characterized by means of specific monoclonal antibodies.

that lead to increased cell membrane permeability. The cells then swell and respond to different osmotic conditions, finally causing membrane disruption and eventual cell death. If killer T cells are adoptively transferred, a secondary tumor immune response can be realized, and this results in a classic cell-mediated pathologic response in the target tumor with resultant tumor regression or death. Resting precursor T cells can be activated by tumor-associated or tumor-specific antigens (Fig. 2). They then respond to interleukin-1 (IL-1) and during this process gain IL-2 receptors. The initial IL-1 response is markedly accentuated by the response to IL-2. These two lymphokines generate marked cell growth, and thus the increased cell population of cytotoxic T cells can react to tumor-associated antigens with the potential for tumor destruction.

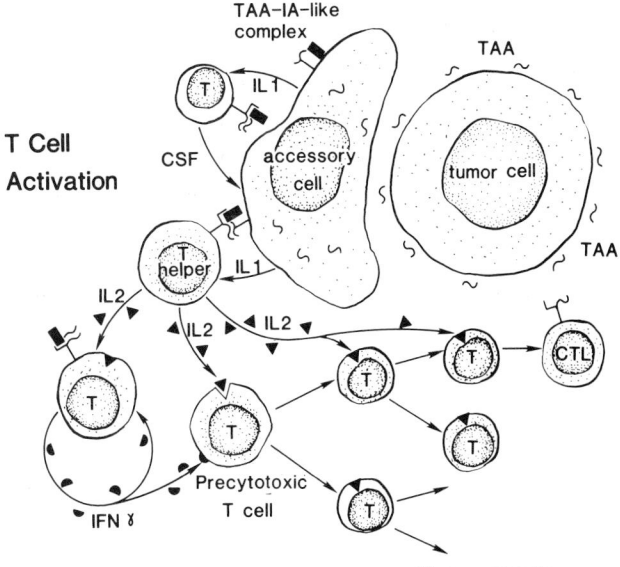

Figure 2. T-cell activation and lymphokine response to tumor-associated antigen are outlined.

Human macrophages have both effector and helper cell functions. Effector functions include both cytostasis and cytotoxicity. Macrophage-directed cell killing is an antigen-independent, antibody-dependent activity. Macrophage phagocytosis follows antigen processing, followed by mediator production and secretion. Interferon-γ (IFN-γ) is a prime macrophage-activating factor. IFN-α and IFN-β have similar but less effective activities. When human macrophages are activated by IFN, tumor-associated antigens can be a specific trigger leading to cell killing. A similar effect can be realized by arming macrophages with monoclonal antibodies.

Natural cell-mediated cytotoxicity is orchestrated by NK cells that have spontaneous reactivity to tumor cells. Human cells that are infected with certain viruses are destroyed by NK activity. NK reactivity is not MHC-restricted, as is T-cell function. NK activity is augmented by both IFN-α and IFN-γ as well as by IL-2. NK cells kill by a mechanism of lipophilic protein incorporation into the target-cell membrane, thus causing increased permeability, cell swelling, and, finally, destruction. NK cells appear to have a role in decreasing the incidence as well as the number of metastases in the tumor-bearing host. NK cells are also important as producers of cytokines. Cytokines produced by NK cells include IFN-α, IFN-γ, IL-1, IL-2, B-cell growth factor, lymphotoxin, and NK cytotoxic factors.

THE IMMUNE RESPONSE TO TUMOR CELLS

Animal studies as well as early human data would suggest that regulation of the immune response to tumor cells is dependent upon T-cell interactions as well as the host response to idiotypes and lymphokines. Suppressor T cells and subpopulations of macrophages can interfere with the host response to both spontaneous and induced tumors. Studies of host response to tumor challenge in animal systems would suggest that there is initially little or no immunity. This is followed by an interim short-term phase of cytotoxic T-cell predominance and host control. As the tumor grows, the cytotoxic T-cell predominance is replaced by suppressor T cells, and thus, immunity is overcome and tumor growth is enhanced. Experimental animal data have indicated that if suppressor T cells are preferentially destroyed with cytotoxic drugs and the animal is specifically immunized against the tumor, host immunity can be provoked. It appears that spontaneous human tumors have antigens that act as minor histocompatibility antigens, provoking little humoral immunoglobulin G (IgG) response. Instead, IgM is present on the surface of tumor cells, and this may prevent IgG binding and eventual cell destruction. Human tumor cells express histocompatibility antigens as well as oncofetal antigens. Oncofetal antigens are expressed on fetal cells and tumor cells, but not on neonatal or adult normal cells. Oncofetal antigens have been demonstrated to induce tumor transplantation resistance in experimental rodent models. Monoclonal antibodies have permitted definition of cell membrane antigenic profiles of human tumor cells. The use of serial immunization as a potential for therapy was suggested following reports of host anti-tumor immune reactivity and the demonstration of effectiveness of such therapy in selected animal models. Critical for this approach is the expression of tumor-associated antigens against which the host is able to respond immunologically to produce tumor cell destruction.

IDIOTYPES AND ANTI-IDIOTYPIC ANTIBODIES

The role of cell idiotypes and anti-idiotypes in host immunity to tumors continues to be investigated. An idiotype is defined as antigen determinants present in the variable region of immunoglobulins. Antibodies to the idiotype (anti-idiotype) can suppress or augment host response to different antigens. Indeed, idiotypic determinants may act as tumor-associated antigens. This phenomenon is plausible because immunoglobulin is present on the surface of most tumor cells. The potential for using anti-idiotypic antibodies for human neoplastic diseases was initially studied in patients with B-cell lymphoma. This particular tumor was ideal for this study because each B-cell tumor expresses a unique cell surface immunoglobulin. The idiotype of the tumor cell surface immunoglobulin thus represents a tumor specific antigen. Anti-idiotypic antibodies to the idiotype produced rather dramatic anti-tumor effects. These data stimulated experiments addressing adenocarcinoma, melanoma, and sarcoma tumor cell types. These studies suggest that utilization of anti-idiotypic antibodies can be of benefit and should continue to be explored.

IMMUNOTHERAPY

Scientists continue to search for ways to enhance the host response against malignant cells. Efforts have included immunologic techniques designed to potentiate a cancer patient's immune system against the growth of cancer cells. Immunotherapeutic techniques can be passive, active, immunorestorative, or adoptive (Table 2).

The advent of monoclonal antibody technology has provided tremendous impetus to passive immunotherapy. Hybridoma cells can now be maintained in culture with the capability of producing large volumes of monoclonal antibodies that can be used for serotherapy or conjugated to cytotoxic drugs, toxins, or isotopes. Monoclonal antibodies have also been used successfully to arm effector cells, thus enhancing cell-mediated tumor cell killing. The most straightforward application of monoclonal antibodies for therapeutic use is administration of the monoclonal antibody alone. With this approach, antibodies may directly react with target tumor cells and mediate tumor destruction by either binding complement or by effector cells that demonstrate antibody-dependent cell cytotoxicity. Experimental animal studies have demonstrated that specific monoclonal antibodies reactive with tumor-associated antigens are capable of destroying metastatic tumor deposits in liver. Additionally, selected monoclonal antibodies are able to mediate antibody-dependent cell-mediated cytotoxicity reactive against tumor cell targets; and this phenomenon can be enhanced by the administration of lymphokines. Murine monoclonal antibodies have been demonstrated to give strong ADCC when tested against human melanoma xenografts in nude mice. Conjugation of monoclonal antibodies to radioisotopes in an effort to enhance cell-killing capability continues to undergo intensive investigation. Monoclonal antibody conjugated to ^{131}I has been demonstrated to produce tumor regressions approximating 90 per cent in athymic nude mice transplanted with human neuroblastoma tumor.

TABLE 2. Immunotherapy

Passive
  Serotherapy
  Antibody-drug
  Antibody-toxin
  Antibody-isotope
  Antibody armed effector cells
Immunorestorative
  Thymic hormones
  Levamisole
  Prostaglandin antagonists
  Cytotoxic agents
Adoptive
  Cell transfer
  Bone marrow transplant
  Transfer factor, immune RNA
  Thymic hormones
  Lymphokines
Active
  Nonspecific
  Specific

Experimental animals administered low-dose ^{131}I-immunoconjugates experienced delay in tumor growth, while animals receiving up to 4200 cGy. had complete tumor inhibition.[4] Phase I clinical trials utilizing ^{131}I-monoclonal antibodies administered intrathecally into patients with carcinomatous meningitis have realized objective treatment responses.[11] The A fragment of both diphtheria toxin and ricin have proved highly toxic to target tumor cells both *in vitro* and *in vivo*. Tumor size and vascular supply are important if conjugate administration is to be effective for tumor cell destruction. Radionuclide scans have demonstrated that immunoconjugates consisting of monoclonal antibodies conjugated to chemotherapeutic agents and toxins localize *in vivo* into the tumor. Data generated by means of cell sorting after administration of antibody conjugates have permitted quantitation of the amount and percentage of tumor cells that bind the administered conjugates. Ricin is a potent plant toxin isolated from castor beans. The A chain of ricin is responsible for the enzymatic inactivation of protein synthesis. *In vitro* studies have demonstrated that ricin A-chain immunoconjugates reactive with tumor-associated antigen cause target-cell destruction.[18]

A number of animal studies have demonstrated that specific active immunotherapy, using intact tumor cells as the immunizing antigen, viral oncolysates of tumor cells, or purified tumor-associated antigen preparations, causes decreased tumor response and growth. The anti-tumor effect is augmented if host suppressor-cell activity is mitigated by the use of low doses of cyclophosphamide combined with administration of IL-2. It appears that IL-2 promotes cytotoxic T-cell growth and enhances NK and macrophage function. Specific active immunotherapy trials in man have demonstrated significant promise in patients with both melanoma and colorectal carcinoma. Patients with melanoma have been immunized with intact autochthonous or allogeneic cells or with a viral oncolysate prepared from such cells.[16,22] The results of these studies suggest that a statistically significant therapeutic benefit can be realized in high-risk Stage I and Stage II patients treated in the adjuvant mode. Human subjects with high-risk Stage I colorectal carcinoma and those with Stage II disease have also been immunized with irradiated autochthonous tumor cells. Again, the early data suggest that both improvement of the disease-free interval and ultimate survival are realized in immunized patients when compared with controls.[8]

Adoptive cellular immunotherapy requires transfer of either activated NK cells or specific cytotoxic T cells. Both primary tumor and metastatic disease in animal models can be reversed by the passive transfer of these cell populations when combined with lymphokines. The most pronounced effects have been realized in animal models that utilized T cells grown in the presence of IL-2 after *in vitro* modification. Preclinical studies demonstrated that lymphokine-activated killer cells administered with IL-2 produced a profound anti-tumor effect. These studies were followed by clinical trials using lymphokine-activated killer cells and IL-2 at variable concentration. Both complete and partial responses were realized in the study patients and duration of response was of significant magnitude to warrant continued study.[15] Lymphokine-activated killer cells targeted by monoclonal antibodies to gangliosides present on the surface of tumor cells have been demonstrated to specifically lyse human tumor xenografts growing in athymic nude mice. Such targeting of activated human effector cells may provide future directions for study of adoptive transfer as an effective immunotherapeutic regimen. More recently a subpopulation of T cells has been obtained from growing tumors, collectively termed tumor-infiltrating lymphocytes (TILs). When TILs are adoptively transferred in experimental animal models, they have been highly effective against both subcutaneous tumors as well as pulmonary metastases. When compared with lymphokine activated killer cells, the TILs are approximately 50 times more potent in mediating destruction of established micrometastases.

The simultaneous administration of IL-2 enhances the *in vivo* therapeutic efficacy. A Phase I clinical trial in patients with metastatic melanoma receiving adoptively transferred tumor infiltrating lymphocytes and IL-2 has demonstrated objective regression of the cancer in approximately 60 per cent of the patients under study.[14] Autologous tumor specific cytotoxic T cells can be generated by specific stimulation with autologous tumor and expanded in recombinant IL-2. The cell-mediated killing is MHC-restricted. These cytotoxic T cells appear to recognize a common tumor-associated antigen in the presence of HLA Class I determinants. These studies suggested that allogeneic tumors that express the restricting HLA-A region antigen could substitute for autologous tumor in the generation of the specific cytotoxic T cell population. This cell population is composed of both helper cells and cytotoxic cells. The cell-mediated cytolytic activity is predominantly from the cytotoxic T-cell population. The fact that cytotoxic T cells can be generated from peripheral blood, lymph node cells, and surgical specimen means that there is a renewable source of cells for therapeutic use. Because established HLA-compatible tumor cells can be used in the absence of autologous tumor, clinical trials appear to be both indicated and feasible.[5] Nude mice growing human tumor xenografts demonstrated a profound therapeutic benefit with adoptive transfer of cytotoxic T cells in conjunction with recombinant IL-2.[6] The therapeutic efficacy exceeded 90 per cent, and these animal studies support future clinical trials.

Interferon

Interferons were first described in 1957. These induced animal proteins were initially thought to have specific antiviral activity, much as immunoglobulins have similar activity against bacteria. Genetic engineering techniques have permitted production of very pure interferons, and characterization of these agents has been advanced by monoclonal antibody technology. Different human cells have the capability of producing interferons. Both T and B lymphocytes as well as non-T and non-B cells produce IFN-α. Macrophages and fibroblasts can be induced to produce both IFN-α and IFN-β. The third type of human interferon, IFN-γ, has been referred to as immune interferon. Generally, IFN-γ is produced by human T cells. Single genes are responsible for the production of IFN-β and IFN-γ, whereas 14 allelic genes are responsible for the production of human IFN-α. IFN-β is restricted in its activity to species specificity, whereas human IFN-α has activity in both human and animal cell cultures. INF-γ is produced by T lymphocytes in response to different immunogens. The response is dependent upon prior antigen exposure, and thus IFN-γ appears to be a lymphokine with a significant role in regulation of the human immune response in terms of antitumor effect. IFN-α has been demonstrated to have antitumor effects in humans, although benefits are often of short duration. Recombinant interferons have been reported to have therapeutic efficacy in approximately 15 per cent of patients with selected solid tumors. The antitumor effects of interferon remain unclear. IFN-γ continues to be evaluated in both experimental animal models as well as in human clinical trials. IFN-γ promotes both monocyte and macrophage function as well as HLA Class II antigen expression on both lymphocytes and target tumor cells. Recombinant IFN-γ appears to have a greater antiproliferative effect than either IFN-α or IFN-β. Early clinical trials have produced measurable antitumor responses, and intensive investigation continues with either IFN-γ alone or IFN-γ in combination with other lymphokines.

Cytokines

Cytokines are a broad class of cell regulators that are important in the human immune response. They regulate cell growth and are activated by a variety of stimuli. Generally, these proteins are low molecular weight polypeptides that affect cells that produce them or cells adjacent to the producing cell. Cytokines appear to be involved in the regulation of the amplitude and duration of the immune response. Interferons, tumor necrosis factor (TNF), interleukins, colony-stimulating factors, and transforming B-cell growth factors have been characterized and can now be produced in pure forms using recombinant DNA technology. Tumor necrosis factor genes are located on chromosome 6 and mapped within the MHC region. Recombinant TNF alone does not predictably have an antitumor effect; however, in combination with other cytokines, it has produced positive responses. Monoclonal antibody, recombinant IFN-γ, and TNF administered to nude mice bearing human melanoma xenografts have produced striking antitumor responses. Injection of TNF directly into the tumor induces migration of macrophages into the tumor and enhances tumor-cell killing. The interleukins are part of a complex cytokine network and are produced by more than one cell type. The interleukins can either stimulate or inhibit the production of other cytokines. As they are characterized, the interleukins are designated according to their biologic properties, and to date, six interleukins have been sequenced. IL-2 has been extensively studied and evaluated as a useful substance for immunotherapeutic trial. IL-2 is a T-cell growth factor and is capable of activating NK cells to become highly cytotoxic but nonspecific in their action. IL-2 is coded for by a single gene and is not related to the interferons or other interleukins. Resting T lymphocytes do not respond to IL-2 because they do not express IL-2 receptors. When the T cells have been antigen-activated, they initiate secretion of IL-2 and express IL-2 receptors.

Four human colony-stimulating factors have been identified and all are glycoproteins. The colony-stimulating factors each have distinct cell receptors and do not cross-compete. These compounds appear to have their major action on stem cells. They promote both growth and differentiation. It is doubtful that they will demonstrate an antitumor effect, but they will be important as factors that accelerate bone marrow recovery and will be used clinically to reduce the toxicity of high-dose chemotherapy.

ONCOGENIC VIRUSES AND ONCOGENES

Both DNA viruses and RNA viruses can cause neoplasms in animals. Adenoviruses, papovaviruses, herpesviruses and hepatitis viruses are DNA viruses that do not cause animal tumors in their natural state and species. However, if these criteria are violated, malignant transformation can occur. RNA viruses that are oncogenic are referred to as retroviruses. By means of the enzyme reverse transcriptase, these RNA viruses are copied into DNA. Retroviruses replicate and produce a viral envelope that is immunogenic. These viruses are incorporated into the cell genome and code for a cell membrane–associated antigen that is immunogenic to the host. Murine leukemia virus, mouse mammary tumor virus, and feline leukemia virus are examples of retroviruses that have a vaccine-induced immunity. Herpes-induced chicken lymphoma and New World monkey lymphoma have also been prevented by specific vaccination.

Accumulating data suggest that neoplasia can follow heritable changes that permit unrestrained growth of cells associated with altered expression of "cancer genes," or oncogenes. These genes have normal cellular counterparts that regulate both normal cell proliferation and differentiation and are referred to as proto-oncogenes. If genetic alterations, including point mutations, chromosomal translocation, or gene amplification, occur, activation of cellular oncogenes results, which in turn contributes to cell neoplastic transformation. Approximately 20 oncogenes carried by acute transforming retroviruses have been described. Human T-cell leukemia and B-cell lymphoma both appear to have a viral etiology. Human T-cell lymphotrophic viruses (HTLV-I and -II) and Epstein-Barr virus (causing a translocation of the *myc* gene) appear to be the oncogenic origin

of these malignancies. Hepatitis B virus also is oncogenic in man. Epidemiologic studies have revealed that in less than 2 per cent of non-hepatitis carriers does hepatocellular carcinoma develop, whereas, in approximately 60 per cent of carriers this malignancy eventually develops. Specific protein products of the viral oncogenes have been identified. The expression of these proteins should permit specific immunizations for both immunoprophylaxis and immunotherapy of these virally produced tumors. Monoclonal antibodies generated against oncogenes could well have an immunotherapeutic application as well as possibly serve as an immunoregulator, thus preventing actual malignant cell transformation.

SELECTED REFERENCES

Crowley, N. J., Slingluff, C. L., Darrow, T. L., and Seigler, H. F.: Autologous tumor-specific cytotoxic T-cells: Generation using HLA-A2 matched allogeneic melanomas. Cancer Res., 50:492, 1990.
Autologous tumor-specific cytotoxic T cells were generated with HLA-A2 region matched allogeneic melanomas for stimulation. The cytotoxic T cells demonstrated specific cell killing, and the data suggest they may be useful for adoptive immunotherapy of human melanoma.

Rosenberg, S. A., Packard, B. S., Aebersold, P. M., et al.: Use of tumor-infiltrating lymphocytes and interleukin-2 in the immunotherapy of patients with metastatic melanoma. N. Eng. J. Med., 319:1676, 1988.
Twenty patients with metastatic melanoma were administered tumor-infiltrating lymphocytes and interleukin-2. Regression was realized in 60 per cent of the treated patients.

Seigler, H. F., Wallack, M. K., Vervaert, C. E., et al.: Melanoma patient antibody responses to melanoma tumor-associated antigens defined by murine monoclonal antibodies. J. Biol. Resp. Mod., 8:37, 1988.
Patients immunized with specific melanoma vaccines produced seroantibodies reactive with both glycoproteins and gangliosides present on the surface of human tumor cells. This demonstrated antibody response to tumor-associated antigens suggests possible immunotherapeutic trials.

Wallack, M. K., Bash, J. A., Leftheriotis, E., Seigler, H. F., et al.: Positive relationship of clinical and serologic responses to vaccinia melanoma oncolysate. Arch. Surg., 122:1460, 1987.
High-risk patients with melanoma were immunized serially with a vaccinia melanoma oncolysate. The immunized patients realized a significant increase in disease-free survival when compared with the control population.

REFERENCES

1. Bodenham, D. C.: A study of 650 observed malignant melanomas in the southwest region. Ann. R. Coll. Surg., 43:218, 1968.
2. Carrasquillo, J. A., Abrams, P. G., Chroff, R. W., et al.: Effect of In-111 9.2.27 monoclonal antibody dose on the imaging of metastatic melanoma. J. Nucl. Med. (In press.)
3. Carrasquillo, J. A., Bunn, P. A., Jr., Keenan, A. M., et al.: Radioimmunotherapy of cutaneous T-cell lymphoma with In-111–labeled T101 monoclonal antibody. N. Eng. J. Med., 315:673, 1985.
4. Cheung, N. K., Landmeier, B., et al.: Complete tumor ablation with iodine-131 radiolabeled diasialoganglioside GD2 specific monoclonal antibody against a human neuroblastoma xenografted in nude mice. JNCI, 77(3):739-744, 1986.
5. Crowley, N. J., Slingluff, C. L., Darrow, T. L., and Seigler, H. F.: Autologous tumor-specific cytotoxic T-cells: Generation using HLA-A2 matched allogeneic melanomas. Cancer Res., 50: 492, 1990.
6. Crowley, N. J., Slingluff, C. L., Darrow, T. L., and Seigler, H. F.: Inhibition of the growth of human melanoma xenografts in nude mice by human tumor-specific cytotoxic T-cells. J. Surg. Oncol., 43:67, 1990.
7. Honsik, C. J., Gundram, J., and Reisfeld, R. A.: Lymphokine-activated killer cells targeted by monoclonal antibodies to the disialogangliosides GD2 and GD3 specifically lyse human tumor cells of neuroectodermal origin. Proc. Natl. Acad. Sci., 83:7893, 1986.
8. Hoover, H. C., Surdzke, M., Danzel, R. B., et al.: Prospectively randomized trial of adjusted active specific immunotherapy for human colorectal cancer. Cancer, 55:1236, 1985.
9. Kohler, G., Milstein, C.: Continuous cultures of fused cells secreting antibody of predefined specificity. Nature, 256:495, 1975.
10. Larson, S. M., Carrasquillo, J. A., Krohn, D. A., et al.: Localization of ^{131}I labeled P97 specific Fab fragments in human melanoma as a basis for radiotherapy. J. Clin. Invest., 72:2101, 1983.
11. Lashford, L. S., Davies, G., et al: A pilot study of ^{131}I monoclonal antibodies in the therapy of leptomeningeal tumors. Cancer, 61:857, 1988.
12. Livingston, P. O., Takeyama, H., Pollack, M. S., et al.: Serological responses of melanoma patients to vaccines derived from allogeneic cultured melanoma cells. Int. J. Cancer, 31:567, 1983.
13. Livingston, P. O., Watanabe, T., Shiku, H., et al.: Serological response of

melanoma patients receiving melanoma cell vaccines. I. Autologous cultured melanoma cells. Int. J. Cancer, *30:* 413, 1982.

14. Rosenberg, S. A., Packard, B. S., Aebersold, P. M., et al.: Use of tumor-infiltrating lymphocytes and interleukin-2 in the immunotherapy of patients with metastatic melanoma. N. Engl. J. Med., *319:*1676, 1988.

15. Rosenberg, S. A., Spiess, P., Lafreniere, R.: A new approach to the adoptive immunotherapy of cancer with tumor-infiltrating lymphocytes. Science, *233:*1318, 1986.

16. Seigler, H. F., Cox, E., Mutzner, L. S., et al.: Specific active immunotherapy for melanoma. Ann. Surg., *190:*366, 1979.

17. Seigler, H. F., Wallack, M. K., Vervaert, C. E., et al.: Melanoma patient antibody responses to melanoma tumor-associated antigens defined by murine monoclonal antibodies. J. Biol. Resp. Mod., *8:* 37, 1988.

18. Spitler, L. E., del Rio, M., Khentigan, A., et al.: Therapy of patients with

malignant melanoma using a monoclonal antimelanoma antibody-ricin A chain immunotoxin. Cancer Res., *47:*1717, 1987.

19. Stuhlmiller, G., Darrow, T. L., Haupt, D. M., and Seigler, H. F.: Immune response of chimpanzee to purified melanoma 250 kilodalton tumor-associated antigen. Cancer Immunol. Immunother., *25:* 193, 1987.

20. Stuhlmiller, G., Roberson, K. M., and Seigler, H. F.: Serological response of non-human primates to human melanoma disialoganglioside GD3. Cancer Immunol. Immunother., *29:*205, 1989.

21. Stuhlmiller, G., and Seigler, H. F.: Characterization of a chimpanzee anti-human melanoma antiserum. Cancer Res., *35:* 2132, 1975.

22. Wallack, M. K., Bash, J. A., Leftheriotis, E., Seigler, H. F., et al.: Positive relationship of clinical and serologic responses to vaccinia melanoma oncolysate. Arch. of Surg., *122:*1460, 1987.

II

MELANOMA

H. F. Seigler, M.D.

Melanoma is a neoplastic disorder produced by malignant transformation of the normal melanocyte. Melanocytes are the cells responsible for the production of the pigment melanin. During the first trimester of fetal life, precursor melanocytes arise in the neural crest. As the fetus develops, these cells migrate to areas including the skin, meninges, mucous membranes, upper esophagus, and eyes. In each of these locations, melanocytes have demonstrated a potential for malignant transformation. Historically, melanoma represented approximately 4 to 5 per cent of all skin malignancies and 3 per cent of cancers in general.[1] Despite general physician awareness and excellent public education, this malignancy has an approximate 50 per cent mortality in the United States. The actual incidence of melanoma is increasing more rapidly than that of any other malignancy. Over the past decade, this rise has exceeded 90 per cent.[38] In the early part of this century, the lifetime risk of a Caucasian's developing malignant melanoma was approximately 1 in 1500. Currently, this risk has increased to 1 in 128.

PRECURSOR FACTORS

Melanocytes in the skin of man divide approximately once in a 12-month cycle. Melanoma cells have been observed to divide as often as once in 24 hours. The transformed malignant cell obviously has a drastically altered cell cycle as well as cell function. The presence of a pre-existing mole at the site of primary cutaneous melanoma has been reported to be as low as 25 per cent and as high as 75 per cent. One must, therefore, focus on precursor pigmented lesions that have a high potential for malignant transformation if early diagnosis and appropriate therapy are to be meaningful. Rhodes and Melsky have reported a cumulative risk of melanoma for individuals with small congenital nevi to be as high as 5 per cent.[37] Spitz nevi are commonly confused with melanoma.[53] This nevus usually demonstrates a rapid growth pattern with differing pigmentation. The lesion is well circumscribed, is raised, and may vary in color from pink to dark brown to black or to blue-black. This lesion is most common in young adults. Simple but complete excision of the Spitz nevus is recommended. Giant congenital nevi occur in approximately 1 in 20,000 newborns. The consensus suggests that the risk of melanoma in these lesions is approximately 5 to 8 per cent.[53] Malignant transformation may be observed during early childhood; therefore, it is recommended that these lesions be prophylactically excised if possible. Although excision may re-

quire multiple procedures, the overall benefits usually outweigh the risks.

Melanoma may occur as a familial disease. Over 150 different kindreds have been reported in the literature, with an average of three cases per family. Half of the families report an affected parent and one or more affected siblings. The kindred reported by Anderson and associates had 15 affected individuals.[2] All reported kindreds were of Caucasian descent, with Celtic extraction being the most prevalent. Clark and co-workers were the first to describe the B-K mole syndrome.[10] The clinical features of this syndrome are characterized by diffuse distribution of large atypical, pigmented lesions. The B-K mole is irregular in both outline and pigmentation. There is usually a palpable dermal component with a cluster distribution on the upper back, chest, and arms. On histologic examination, atypical melanocytic hyperplasia or melanocytic dysplasia is evident. The greater risk for malignant transformation in this disorder requires that histologic confirmation be obtained and that active changes within the mole mandate prompt excision.

CLINICOPATHOLOGIC FEATURES

Melanoma is subdivided into four histopathologic types. The four groups include (1) lentigo maligna melanoma, (2) superficial spreading melanoma, (3) acral lentiginous melanoma, and (4) nodular melanoma. The first three groups have a junctional component, whereas nodular melanoma is entirely subjunctional. Junctional melanomas proliferate in a horizontal direction initially, and this is referred to as the radial growth phase. In time, vertical growth appears, and this progression may be associated with both invasive features and metastatic capabilities. Subjunctional melanomas usually demonstrate a predominant vertical growth phase and, therefore, have a very early metastatic potential.

Lentigo maligna melanoma (Fig. 1) is more commonly seen in individuals in their sixth, seventh, or eighth decade of life. On histologic examination (Fig. 2), most of the spindle-shaped malignant cells are junctional in location. The lesion has prominent solar elastosis with very atrophic epidermis. Pagetoid cells are usually not seen with this lesion.

Superficial spreading melanoma occurs on both sun-exposed and nonexposed areas of the body. Initially, the lesion demonstrates a radial growth phase, and, from a clinical standpoint, irregular margins with differing pigmentation are common (Fig.

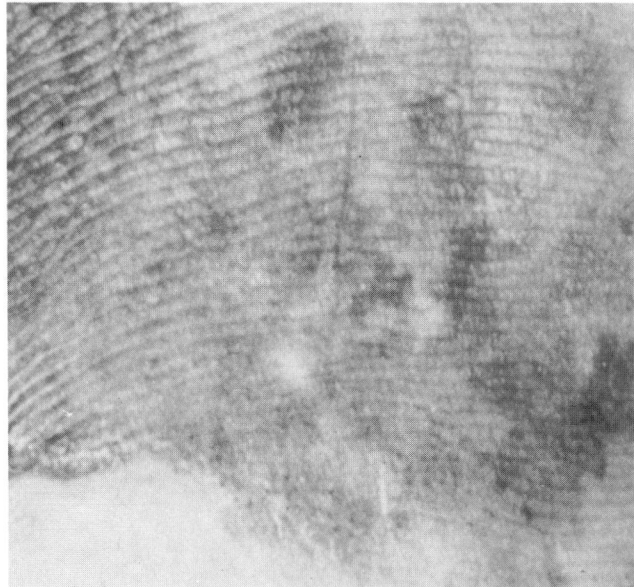

Figure 1. Clinical appearance of lentigo maligna melanoma.

3). In time, although radial growth continues, a vertical growth phase usually appears. This lesion is characterized histologically by pagetoid cells with both junctional activity and upward growth that causes bulging of the epidermis. Solar elastosis is not a dominant feature. The epidermis is not atrophic; rather, it may demonstrate hyperplastic characteristics (Fig. 4).

Acral lentiginous melanoma is most commonly seen on the palms, soles, subungual areas, and mucous membranes. Mucous membrane presentation is most commonly seen on the vulva; however, the vagina, clitoris, penis, anus, nasopharynx, sinuses, and oral cavity are other sites of involvement. Acral lentiginous melanomas in these distinctive sites are generally associated with a very poor clinical prognosis (Figs. 5 to 8). These lesions are devoid of pagetoid cells on histologic examination (Fig. 9). There is marked junctional proliferation with large atypical melanocytes with long dendritic processes. Both atrophic epidermal changes and solar elastosis are absent in this lesion.

Nodular melanoma does not express a junctional component;

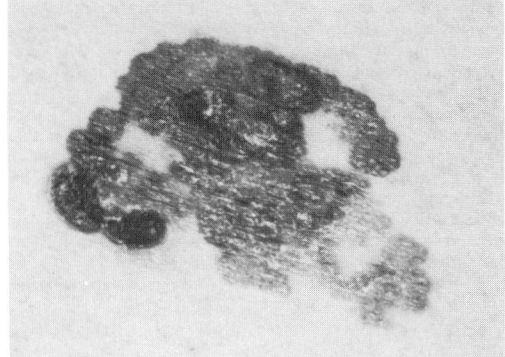

Figure 3. Superficial spreading melanoma with irregular borders, differing pigmentation, and nodular degeneration.

vertical growth predominates. The borders are usually well circumscribed, and pigmentation is generally uniform (Fig. 10). A variant of nodular melanoma is the polypoid lesion. This exophytic lesion has a characteristic appearance (Fig. 11). The histologic demonstration of upward growth and absence of an intraepithelial component is characteristic (Fig. 12).

EPIDEMIOLOGY

As previously stated, the incidence of melanoma is increasing. Since 1900 the lifetime risk for melanoma has increased from 1 in 1500 to a projected 1 in 90 by the year 2000. Lee has reported that the death rate from melanoma is rising for patients in the younger age groups.[20] Individuals with Celtic ancestry appear to have the highest predilection for the development of the disease. Population studies indicate that Celts have a higher incidence of melanoma than does the general population, even populations in Ireland, Northern Europe, and Scandinavia. As Celtic people migrate to more temperate climates, the incidence of melanoma increases and exceeds that of non-Celtic subjects living in a similar area.[21,27]

The role of ultraviolet light as an etiologic factor in melanoma remains unresolved. Malignant transformation is thought to require initiation of DNA damage, promoting factors, and altered stimulation for cell growth. Ultraviolet radiation is suspected to have a role in the development of basal cell cancer and squamous cell cancer as well as melanoma. Electromagnetic

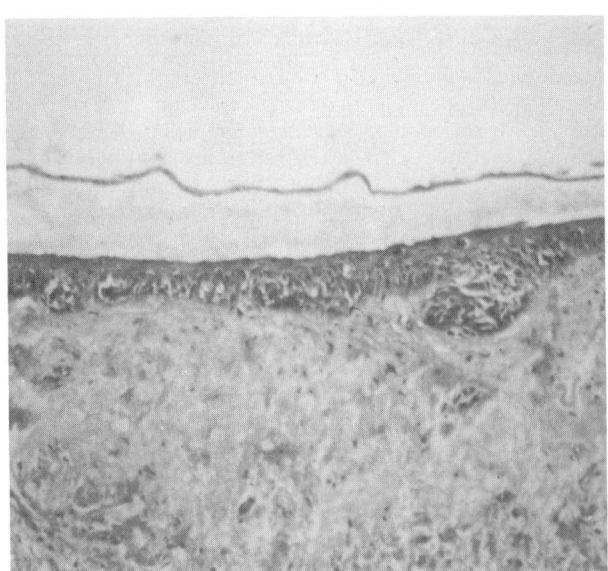

Figure 2. Histopathologic pattern of lentigo maligna melanoma.

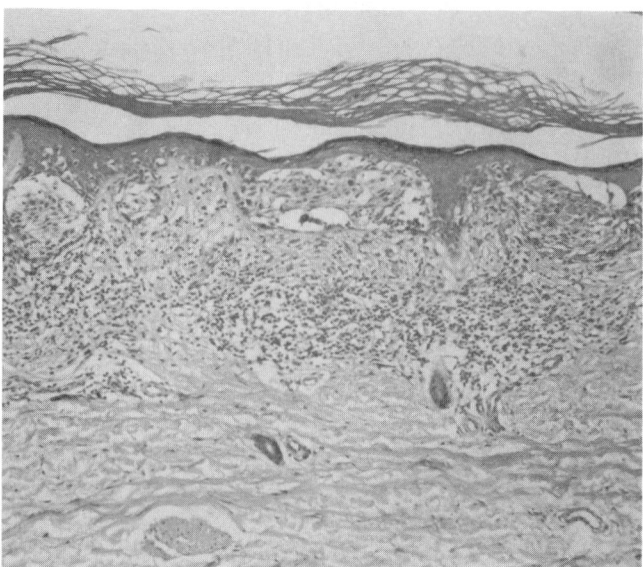

Figure 4. Histopathologic pattern of superficial spreading melanoma.

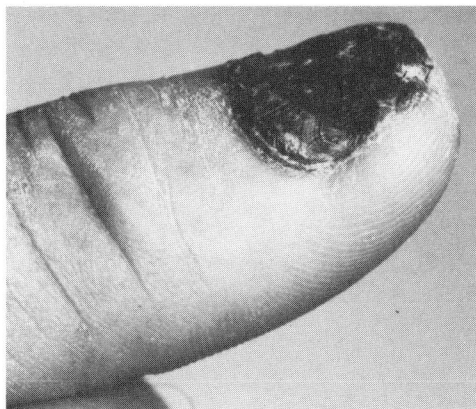

Figure 5. Subungual melanoma.

energy from the sun is divided into spectra according to the wavelength of the radiation. UVC (200 to 290 nm.), UVB (290 to 320 nm.), and UVA (320 to 400 nm.) comprise ultraviolet rays. UVC is most probably completely absorbed by the ozone layer. UVB radiation is responsible for sunburn and for inducing melanin production in skin, causing tanning. UVA penetrates more deeply into the dermis and most probably is responsible for most of the sun-induced changes of dermal connective tissue and loss of elasticity that characterizes the aging process and skin wrinkling. It is thought that both UVA and UVB radiation can be carcinogenic. Bodenham has suggested that both the incidence of melanoma and the subsequent mortality can be correlated with the degree of sunlight exposure.[4] Other reports are controversial. It is more likely that a number of factors are important in producing malignant transformation of the melanocyte. Age, hormonal status, genetic predisposition, environmental factors, and injury must be considered to fully comprehend the activation of the melanocytic oncogene. It is extremely rare for melanoma to occur prior to puberty. Pratt and coworkers reviewed 44 patients with prepubertal melanoma and discussed 31 of their patients diagnosed before 21 years of age.[29] Less than half of their series was composed of patients prior to puberty.

Melanoma is far more common in Caucasians than in the black population. Reintgen and associates have recently reviewed the literature and suggest that a ratio of whites to blacks for melanoma is 20 : 1.[31] The 10-year survival for black patients with melanoma is approximately 10 per cent.[31] Reasons for differences between these populations from all aspects remain unexplained.

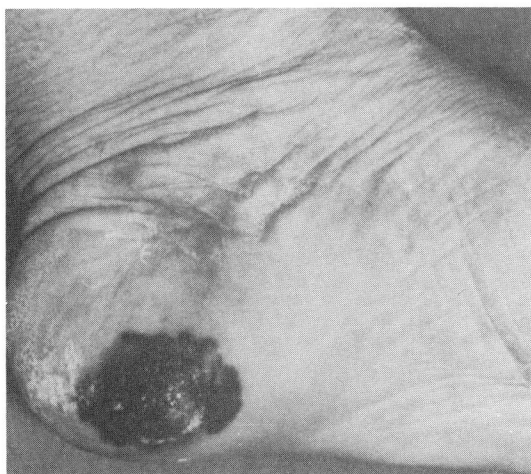

Figure 7. Plantar acral lentiginous melanoma.

PROGNOSTIC FACTORS

In melanoma, as in other neoplastic diseases, the extent of malignancy at the time of diagnosis is the most important prognostic indicator. Patients with Stage I disease (involving only the skin) have a better prognosis than patients with Stage II disease (including first-order lymph nodes or tissue locations between the primary site and first-order lymph nodes). When nodal disease has been realized, the ultimate prognosis is predicted by the number of lymph nodes involved. Patients with Stage III disease involving visceral organs, the skeleton, or the central nervous system have a very grave prognosis.

Identification of both clinical and pathologic features that accurately predict the biologic capability of the disease is an important concept. Many of these prognostic factors have been identified for mucocutaneous melanoma. The original paper by Clark and associates in 1969 documenting the different histologic types of melanoma and the importance of the level of invasion extends today as a major contribution to understanding of melanoma.[9] The levels of tumor invasion as described can be used for planning surgical management as well as any adjuvant regimen. Clark's criteria for levels of tumor invasion are

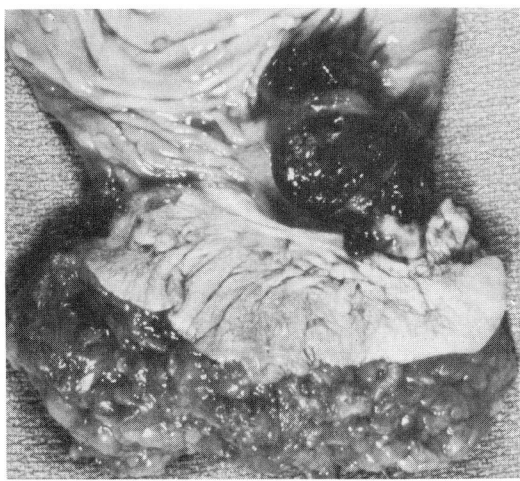

Figure 6. Anorectal melanoma.

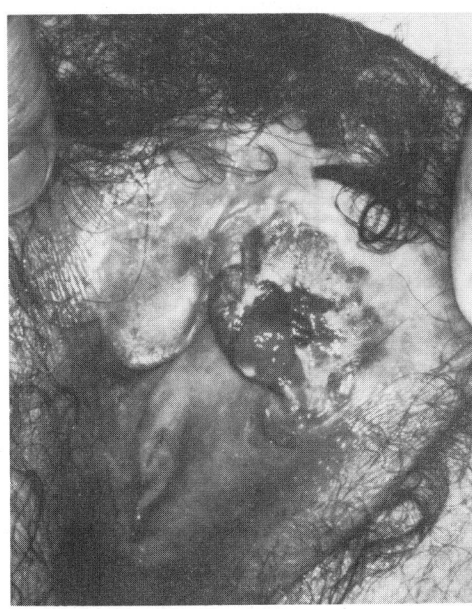

Figure 8. Acral lentiginous melanoma of the mucous membrane of labia majora.

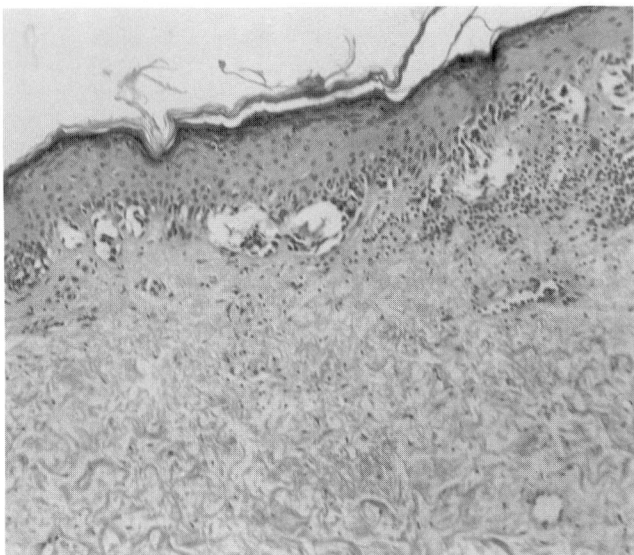

Figure 9. Histopathologic pattern of acral lentiginous primary lesion.

outlined in Table 1. The importance of tumor thickness in terms of predicting the biologic behavior of mucocutaneous melanoma was reported by Breslow.[6] Recent statistical analyses of large groups of patients suggest that tumor thickness is perhaps the most significant prognostic indicator. In Figure 13, a schematic reflection of both the determination of tumor thickness and its correlation with patient survival is depicted. Patients with tumor thickness less than 1.0 mm. are at relatively low risk for the development of secondary disease. Slingluff and associates reported an experience with lethal thin malignant melanoma.[45] Their prognostic model was designed to identify patients with potentially lethal thin primary lesions. The prognostic model was designed using two clinical risk factors (actual primary site and male sex) and two histologic risk factors (Clark's Level IV and histologic regression). Patients with both clinical risk factors or one clinical risk factor and one histologic risk factor were identified as high-risk patients with thin primary lesions. Balch and associates reported a multifactorial analysis of more than 4000 patients with cutaneous melanoma.[3] Their data suggest that thin melanomas measuring less than 0.76 mm. are associated with local disease only and a better than 90 per cent cure with simple excision alone. Patients with intermediate-thickness melanoma measuring 0.76 to 4.0 mm. had an increasing risk (up to 80 per cent) of subsequently developing regional and/or distant disease, whereas those with thick melanomas measuring greater than 4 mm. had at least an 80 per cent risk of having occult disease at the time of initial presentation.

Patients presenting with metastatic disease with an unknown

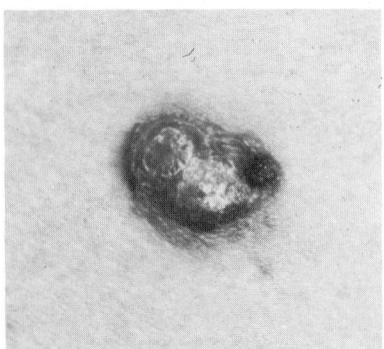

Figure 10. Clinical appearance of a nodular melanoma. The borders are well circumscribed, and the growth is in a vertical direction.

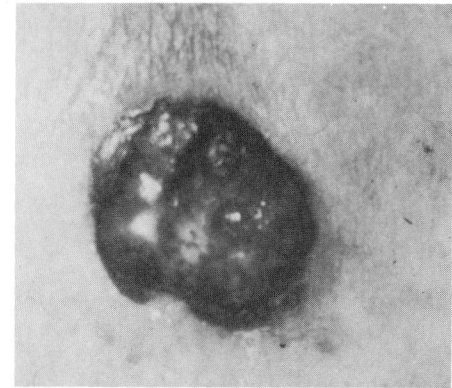

Figure 11. Polypoid variant of nodular melanoma. Surface is typically ulcerated.

primary site continue to pose both diagnostic and therapeutic dilemmas for the physician. Lopez and associates indicate that approximately 8 per cent of all patients with melanoma present with an unknown primary site.[22] Their data suggest that ultimate survival in this group is not greatly different from that in Stage II patients with a known primary site. With surgical management followed by adjuvant therapy, reasonable patient survival can be predicted.[32] The Duke series reports an approximate 5 per cent incidence of patients with unknown primary lesions. Regional lymph node disease was the most common presentation (two thirds of the patients), whereas patients who demonstrated hematogenous disease at the time of presentation had a poor ultimate prognosis.[11]

CLINICAL MANAGEMENT — CHOICE OF BIOPSY

A comprehensive treatment plan for melanoma is dependent on an accurate diagnosis and complete assessment of the histologic features that comprise the prognostic indicators. If the primary lesion is small, an excisional biopsy including subcutaneous fat should be performed. When the pathologist has the entire skin thickness and underlying adipose tissue, Breslow's and Clark's determinations can be utilized as well as evaluation of tumor ulceration, mitotic index, and microscopic satellitosis. If the lesion is greater than 2.0 cm. or is on an area of the body that may cause either functional or cosmetic problems, incisional biopsy can be completed. If incisional biopsy is chosen, the area of greatest tumor involvement, including the vertical

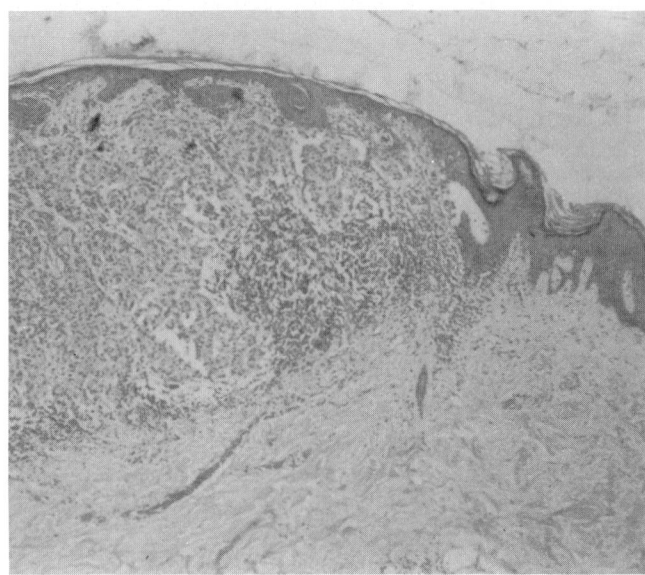

Figure 12. Histopathologic pattern of nodular melanoma.

TABLE 1. Clark's Levels of Tumor Invasion

Level	Description
1	All tumor cells above basement membrane
2	Invasion into loose connective tissue of papillary dermis
3	Tumor cells at junction of papillary and reticular dermis
4	Invasion into reticular dermis
5	Invasion into subcutaneous fat

growth phase, should be selected for biopsy. Shave biopsies, curettage, and electrocoagulation should not be considered for primary lesions suspected of being mucocutaneous melanoma.

SURGICAL MANAGEMENT OF THE PRIMARY LESION

When the diagnosis has been established, the amount of grossly normal tissue around the primary lesion is of prime concern. A number of studies have concerned the surgical margins. Numerous recent studies have led to the consensus that 2.0 cm. of normal tissue around the primary site is adequate for local control. This type of surgical excision permits primary wound closure in most areas of the body. The excision can be accomplished on an outpatient basis using local anesthesia, thus lowering cost, morbidity, and significant cosmetic deformity. Truncal melanomas can, almost without exception, be closed by primary intention. Only the very large lesions or those with macroscopic satellites require skin grafting. Melanomas of the extremities are treated in a manner similar to those on the trunk. Head and neck melanomas pose a more difficult problem for both the surgical oncologist and the reconstructive surgeon. Primary melanomas involving the mucous membranes, palmar

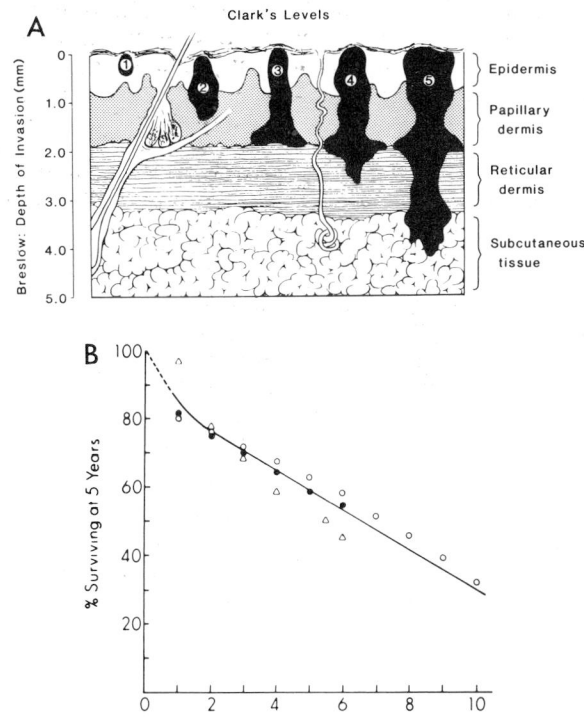

Figure 13. Schematic representation reflecting both the determination of tumor thickness (A) and its correlation to patient survival (B).

and plantar surfaces, nail bed, and anorectal junction require special expertise. Patients with mucosal melanomas usually have rather extensive primary disease, and local recurrence is the most common initial cause of failure in the majority. The nasopharynx and sinus primary sites usually present with epistaxis and obstructive symptoms. Both local and systemic recurrences are common because of the obscure site of the primary. Patients with genital and anorectal melanoma have a very low survival as documented by numerous reports in the literature. Only those patients with small thin primaries are salvaged by only simple surgical excision. Slingluff and associates recently reported 24 patients with anorectal melanoma with no survival beyond 6 years. Abdominal perineal resection decreased locoregional recurrence but did not alter ultimate patient survival.[46] The diagnosis of subungual melanoma is delayed in approximately 40 per cent of patients.[28] No attempt at local excision should be made. These patients require amputation at the distal interphalangeal joint for finger primaries and the interphalangeal joint for thumb primaries. This permits opposition and excellent functional characteristics. Krementz and associates report an overall 5-year survival of approximately 60 per cent for patients with subungual lesions.[18]

SURGICAL MANAGEMENT OF REGIONAL DISEASE

The role of elective lymphadenectomy continues to be an area of interest. Both Clark's level of invasion and Breslow's measurement of tumor thickness are the prime indicators for predicting the presence or absence of metastatic disease involving first-order lymph nodes. These prognostic factors have been used by a number of institutions and have proved to have excellent clinical application. Reintgen and associates have recently reported the probability of recurrent disease for patients with Stage I melanoma.[36] These authors reviewed 4185 patients with Stage I cutaneous melanoma. Approximately one third of the patients suffered recurrent disease. Patients with truncal, head and neck area, and extremity primaries, realized a 38 per cent, 46 per cent, and 30 per cent incidence of recurrent disease, respectively. The most common site of recurrence was the first-order lymph nodes. Two thirds of the recurrences were noted within the first 3 years. Balch and colleagues reported that those patients with tumor thickness between 1.0 and 4.0 mm. profited from surgical removal of their first-order lymph nodes on an elective basis. A similar experience was realized by Seigler and associates in a study of 613 patients demonstrating statistical significance of elective node dissection for patients with intermediate-thickness primary lesions.[30] Presently, there is general agreement that patients with primary tumor thickness less than 1.5 mm. have a low incidence of positive lymph nodes and have little to benefit from elective node dissection. There is also a consensus that patients with thick primary lesions exceeding 4.0 mm. have an approximate 70 per cent probability of systemic disease and thus have little benefit from regional therapy including elective removal of first-order lymph nodes. Patients with unknown primary lesions presenting with positive lymph nodes should be treated with standard surgical lymphadenectomy, unless disease can be documented beyond the lymph node group. Such patients comprise approximately 5 per cent of all patients with melanoma. The ultimate prognosis of this patient group is no less favorable than that of patients with lymph node metastasis from a known primary site and should be treated in a comparable manner.[32]

Regional disease involving the first-order lymph nodes constitutes approximately 80 per cent of tumor recurrences in patients with mucocutaneous melanoma. On certain areas of the body, the clinician can easily predict the lymphatic drainage, whereas in other areas this is quite ambiguous. Primary lesions involving the head and neck can drain to either the anterior cervical or posterior cervical chain. Extremity lesions can drain to the groin or axillae and may even involve popliteal or antecubital lymph nodes. Truncal primaries can be above or below Sappey's line and involve either ipsilateral or contralateral axillary, groin, or supraclavicular lymph nodes. Lymphoscintigraphy has been shown to have potential clinical application in patients with cutaneous melanoma arising on obscure sites of the body. This technique has been popularized by Reintgen and colleagues.[34] The isotope technetium is placed on antimony sulfur colloid and is injected into the skin in the four quadrants around the primary lesion. Serial lymphoscintigrams then demonstrate not only the lymphatic channels, but also the nodal group at risk for development of metastatic disease (Fig. 14). The technique is highly accurate, simple to perform, and associated with little or no patient morbidity. A number of authors have reported the efficacy of utilizing this technique preoperatively in patients whose first-order lymph node group is difficult to assess clinically.[12]

SURGICAL CONSIDERATIONS FOR DISTANT METASTATIC DISEASE

Locally recurrent disease is usually defined as those lesions occurring within 5 cm. of the primary site. These should be managed surgically. Whereas excision of primary lesions dictates 2-cm. margins, locally recurrent disease should, most probably, be managed in a more aggressive manner. Margins of 3.0 to 5.0 cm. are the usual recommendation. If the patient experiences in transit disease between the primary lesion and the first-order lymph nodes, this must be documented by complete surgical removal in preparation for a systemic treatment regimen. Amputation for extensive disease of the extremity is usually discouraged. Experience has supported the conclusion that hemipelvectomy and forequarter amputation for melanoma are rarely indicated. Such patients generally demonstrate systemic manifestations of their disease, negating any possibility of meaningful disease-free interval or prolongation of survival. Occasionally, partial amputation of an extremity for bulky or diffuse recurrent disease proves helpful. Approximately 20 per cent of the patients in this category experience an improved quality of life, with 5-year survival being reported.[49]

Metastatic disease to the lungs is all too frequent in patients with melanoma. Pulmonary involvement reflects hematogenous metastasis, and thus the long-term prognosis is quite poor. If computed tomographic examination of the chest fails to demonstrate hilar adenopathy but verifies the presence of a single metastatic lesion, surgical management may be considered. A

conservative approach should be outlined by both the surgical oncologist and medical oncologist working in concert. Such patients should be placed on a chemotherapeutic regimen and observed over a 40-day interval. If additional metastatic lesions are not evident and the tumor doubling time suggests that the biologic growth rate of the tumor is slow, removal of the metastatic lesion with continuation of postoperative chemotherapy is associated with both an increased disease-free interval and prolonged survival. Patients with multiple metastatic lesions in the lung are best managed by systemic therapy and are not significantly benefited by surgical removal of metastatic deposits.

Approximately 10 per cent of patients with melanoma experience metastatic disease to the skeleton. Most often the axial skeleton is involved. Bone pain is the usual presenting symptom and a bone scan is the most sensitive study in terms of diagnosis. Architectural changes are outlined by routine roentgenograms. If a pathologic fracture occurs, this can most often be successfully managed by conservative means. Irradiation and chemotherapy with external fixation followed by irradiation and chemotherapy are preferred. Occasionally, neurologic symptoms appear and can be improved by laminectomy. Because bone metastasis is indeed indicative of a grave prognosis with mean survival time of approximately 4 months, a conservative approach is recommended.[49] Unstable pathologic fractures of the long bones may require internal fixation and irradiation.

Hematogenous metastases from melanoma commonly affect the gastrointestinal tract. Reintgen and associates have reported this to be the most common malignancy to metastasize to the gastrointestinal tract.[35] In their series, the small intestine was involved in approximately one third of the patients with melanoma with bowel metastases, whereas the colon and stomach were less frequently involved. The polypoid masses involving the small intestine can cause occult bleeding as well as represent the focal point for an intussusception causing either intermittent or prolonged bowel obstruction. Ulcerating masses occasionally perforate. The endoscopic and radiographic findings are quite characteristic for this disorder. Although more than half of the patients with documented visceral metastases have other body sites affected, surgical intervention of symptomatic lesions should be considered. More than 90 per cent of patients gain relief of symptoms, and their overall survival and quality of life are improved.

Metastatic melanoma to the adrenal gland appears to be a favored site. Preoperative diagnosis was exceedingly rare prior to the development of computed tomographic scanning. Branum and colleagues have recently reported 26 patients with metastatic melanoma to the adrenal gland.[5] Twenty-three of the 26 patients had unilateral disease. Survival in the patients resected for cure was approximately 5 years, whereas survival in the group resected for palliation only was approximately 1 year. The authors indicate that patients with metastatic melanoma to the adrenal gland resected for cure clearly benefit from early detection and surgical intervention.

Metastatic melanoma involving the central nervous system occurs as a frequent complication in this disorder. Some authors have suggested that since melanoma has its embryologic origin from neural crest tissue, "homing" influence might explain the high frequency of this particular metastatic pattern. Involvement of the central nervous system occurs in approximately one third of patients. This can progress to more than 90 per cent involvement in autopsy series. Patients with a solitary brain metastasis managed by surgical extirpation experience a 1-year survival of approximately 45 per cent.[13] Bullard and associates have reported a very similar experience.[8] These authors, however, emphasize that multiple lesions of the central nervous system are present in approximately half of the patients. The present recommendation for metastatic disease involving the brain includes surgical removal of solitary lesions followed by

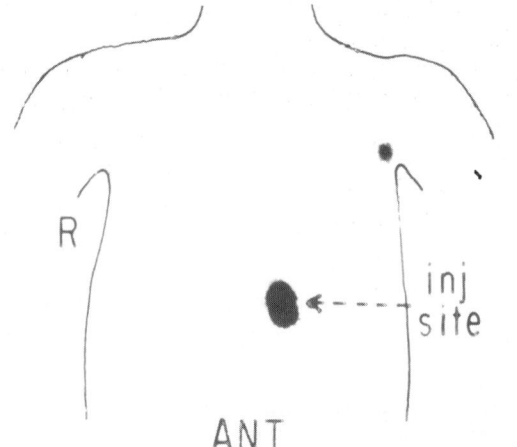

Figure 14. Lymphoscintigram showing the four quadrant injection of ⁹⁹ᵐTc-labeled antimony trisulfide and the first-order lymph node drainage localizing to the left axillary lymph nodes.

whole-brain irradiation and adjuvant systemic therapy if disease involving other organ sites is not self-limiting and indicative of restricted survival time. Patients with multiple metastases involving the central nervous system are best managed by irradiation, chemotherapy, and medication designed to control seizure activity. The development of magnetic resonance imaging has improved the diagnostic ability to document single or multiple lesions.

HORMONAL ASPECTS OF MELANOMA

Prognostic studies indicate that women have better survival with malignant melanoma. Multivariate analyses reveal that women have a higher survival rate than do men at each Clark's level of invasion and with each tumor thickness level.[43] Others have shown that women have a statistically significant longer survival than do men with Stage I disease. However, both male and female patients with Stage II and Stage III disease have similar survival, negating sex differences. A multivariate regression analysis confirms that gender remains a factor in the prognostic index after controlling for the input of factors such as histologic type, Clark's level, primary tumor thickness, and site of lesion.[33] These results suggest that there may indeed be a difference in the biologic behavior of melanoma in men and women.

The presence of estrogen receptors on malignant melanocytes has been evaluated extensively. Some groups have reported estrogen receptor binding as well as detection of these receptors using immunofluorescence techniques.[17,50] Others have questioned the presence of a true estrogen receptor in malignant melanoma. All tumors evaluated in which estradiol binding was observed were melanin-producing lesions. Purified tyrosinase appears to mimic the estrogen binding detected in melanoma cytosols. It appears that the estradiol-binding component in melanoma most likely represents an artifact and that true estrogen receptors are absent with this tumor.[25,55]

A very practical question concerns the importance of melanoma and pregnancy. Houghton's group reports a significantly poorer prognosis for patients whose melanoma developed during pregnancy compared with the control group.[15] Other authors have come to similar conclusions. Wong and associates have recently studied 66 patients with Stage I melanoma diagnosed during pregnancy.[54] These patients were compared with 619 nonpregnant female patients with melanoma. There was no significant difference between the pregnant population and control population with respect to location of the primary tumor, age at diagnosis, Clark's level, mean depth of invasion, and histologic type. These authors state that women diagnosed with melanoma during pregnancy fare no worse than do their nonpregnant counterparts. This experience has been questioned by Trapeznikov and associates.[51] These authors report a significantly lower 10-year survival in the pregnant patient population. Slingluff and associates studied 100 patients with melanoma arising during pregnancy.[44] The patients were compared with an age-matched group of 86 female patients who were not pregnant at the time of diagnosis. Among the pregnant group, there was an increased incidence of lymph node metastases during the first 7 years (13 per cent). There was a significantly shorter disease-free interval for the pregnant group with 45 per cent of pregnant patients and 60 per cent of control patients remaining disease-free at 10 years. The median disease-free interval for the pregnant population was 5.8 years and for the nonpregnant population 11.9 years. Multivariate analysis demonstrated that pregnancy at diagnosis was significantly associated with the development of metastatic disease, when controlling for all other factors. These authors suggest that patients who develop melanoma during pregnancy are at greater risk for metastatic disease than are those who are not pregnant when melanoma is diagnosed.

COMBINED MODALITY TREATMENT FOR MELANOMA

Systemic chemotherapy for melanoma must be considered only as a palliative measure and generally should be used only for disease beyond the first-order lymph nodes. The biologic growth rate and doubling time of malignant melanocytes suggests that this disease should be sensitive to chemotherapeutic agents. A multitude of clinical trials, however, reveals that single-drug response is approximately 20 per cent. Different combinations of drugs have been evaluated, and the most efficient appears to be multiple-drug regimens administered in a pulse-type manner. These regimens appear to be an effective palliative treatment for metastatic melanoma, with tumor response in approximately 40 per cent of the patients being observed.[26,41] A more direct technique for administration of a chemotherapeutic regimen is achieved by isolated limb perfusion. A number of investigators have reported therapeutic benefit using perfusion of the isolated extremity with either single or multiple-drug agents.[7,19] Prophylactic isolated perfusion as the primary therapy for invasive melanoma appears to be associated with both prolonged disease-free interval and increased patient survival.[24]

Response rates in patients with metastatic melanoma receiving interferon alone or interferon and tumor necrosis factor demonstrate benefit in only 15 to 20 per cent of patients evaluated. Monoclonal antibodies have been developed that react with melanoma tumor cells. Houghton and associates administered a murine monoclonal antibody reactive against gangliosides present on the surface of melanoma cells to 12 patients with metastatic disease. Tumor biopsies during and after treatment revealed lymphocyte and cell infiltration with clinical responses marked by significant tumor regression in 3 of the 12 patients studied.[16] Spitler and colleagues administered monoclonal antibodies conjugated to ricin-A chain and reported encouraging clinical results.[48]

High-dose recombinant interleukin-2, a T cell growth factor, has been utilized in the treatment of patients with metastatic melanoma. Partial tumor regressions have been reported.[23] Rosenberg and colleagues have utilized recombinant interleukin-2 and lymphokine-activated killer cells in patients with metastatic melanoma. Both partial and complete tumor regression have been reported by these authors.[39] More recently, this group has utilized recombinant interleukin-2 and tumor-infiltrating lymphocytes as an adoptive transfer for patients with metastatic melanoma. These authors state that patients with metastatic melanoma realize a clinical response rate greater than of those patients receiving recombinant interleukin-2 and lymphokine-activated killer cells.[40]

Seigler and associates have immunized patients in an adjuvant mode utilizing specific active immunotherapy. All of the immunogens utilized produced both a cellular and a humoral response that was enhanced with each booster immunization. Pre–immune cell–mediated and humoral responses were not reactive against the tumor-associated antigens present on the surface of melanoma cells. The induced cellular and humoral responses in the patients suggested that patients with melanoma can be immunized against tumor-associated antigens that are membrane-associated.[42] Patients with Stage II disease with greater than one lymph node positive for metastatic disease realized an approximate 20 per cent cell survival compared with the nonimmunized patient controls.[47] Both Hersey and colleagues and Wallack and associates have reported positive relationships of clinical and serologic responses to viral oncolysates administered to high-risk patients with melanoma.[14,52]

SELECTED REFERENCES

Breslow, A.: Thickness, cross sectional areas and depth of invasion in the prognosis of cutaneous melanoma. Ann. Surg., 172:902, 1970.

Tumor thickness is the most reproducible prognostic factor for mucocutaneous melanoma. Disease-free interval and ultimate patient survival are in a linear relationship with tumor thickness measured in millimeters.

McCarty, K. S., Jr., Wortman, J., Stowers, S., Lubahn, D. B., McCarty, K. S., Sr., and Seigler, H. F.: Sex steroid receptor analysis in human melanoma. Cancer, 46:1463, 1980.
Biochemical determination of estrogen receptors is detected as being positive for melanomas that are pigmented. The false-positive is predicted by reaction with a hydroxyl group on the molecule pyrosine. True estrogen receptors are absent for this tumor.

Reintgen, D. S., Cox, E. B., McCarty, K. S., Jr., Vollmer, R. T., and Seigler, H. F.: Efficacy of elective lymph node dissection in patients with intermediate thickness primary melanoma. Ann. Surg., 198:379, 1983.
Breslow's tumor thickness, ulceration, and elective lymph node dissection are statistically significant prognostic factors for patients with intermediate thickness melanomas. Multivariate analysis permits detection of the subset of patients who have the most to benefit from elective node dissection.

Rosenberg, S. A., Packard, B. S., Aebersold, P. M., Solomon, D., Topalian, S. L., Toy, S. T., Simon, P., Lotze, M. T., Yang, J. C., Seipp, C. A., Simpson, C., Carter, C., Bock, S., Schwartzentruber, D., Wei, J. P., and White, D. E.: Use of tumor-infiltrating lymphocytes expanded with recombinant interleukin-2 in the immunotherapy of patients with metastatic melanoma: A preliminary report. N. Engl. J. Med., 319:1676, 1988.
Administration of autologous tumor-infiltrating lymphocytes expanded with recombinant interleukin-2 and readministered to the patient as adoptive transfer is associated with an approximate 40 per cent response rate in patients with metastatic melanoma.

Seigler, H. F., Wallack, M. K., Vervaert, C. E., Bash, J. A., Roberson, K. M., and Stuhlmiller, G. M.: Melanoma patient antibody responses to melanoma tumor associated antigens defined by murine monoclonal antibodies. J. Biol. Response Mod., 8:37, 1989.
Patients immunized with x-irradiated melanoma cells produce a circulating antibody that reacts to the tumor-associated antigen present on more than 90 per cent of human melanoma cells. These data confirm that the high-molecular-weight glycoprotein is immunogenic in man.

REFERENCES

1. Adam, Y. G., and Efron, G.: Cutaneous malignant melanoma: Current views on pathogenesis, diagnosis, and surgical management. Surgery, 93:481, 1983.
2. Anderson, D. E., Smith, J. L., and McBride, C. M.: Hereditary aspects of malignant melanoma. J.A.M.A., 200:741, 1967.
3. Balch, C. M., Soong, S. J., Murad, T. M., Ingalls, A. L., and Maddox, W. L.: A multifactorial analysis of melanoma. II. Prognostic factors in patients with Stage I (localized) melanoma. Surgery, 86:343, 1979.
4. Bodenham, D. C.: A study of 650 observed malignant melanomas in the south-west region. Ann. R. Coll. Surg., 43:218, 1968.
5. Branum, G. D., Epstein, B. S., Leight, G. S., and Seigler, H. F.: The role of surgery in the management of melanoma to the adrenal. (Manuscript submitted.)
6. Breslow, A.: Thickness, cross sectional areas and depth of invasion in the prognosis of cutaneous melanoma. Ann. Surg., 172:902, 1970.
7. Brown, A. S., Wallack, M. K., Horstmann, J. T., Hamilton, R. W., Johnson, J. L., and Rosato, F. E.: Perfusion therapy for extremity melanoma. Arch. Surg., 111:961, 1976.
8. Bullard, D. E., Cox, E. B., and Seigler, H. F.: Central nervous system metastases in malignant melanoma. Neurosurgery, 8:26, 1981.
9. Clark, W. A., Jr., From, L., Bernardino, E. A., and Mihm, M. C.: The histogenesis and biologic behavior of primary human malignant melanomas of the skin. Cancer Res., 29:705, 1969.
10. Clark, W. H., Jr., Reimer, R. R., Greene, M., Ainsworth, A. M., and Mastrangelo, M. J.: Origin of familial malignant melanomas from heritable melanocytic lesions. "The B-K mole syndrome." Arch. Dermatol., 114:732, 1978.
11. Cox, E. B., Vollmer, R., and Seigler, H. F.: Melanoma in the Southeastern United States: Experience at the Duke Medical Center. *In* Balch, C. M., Milton, G. W., Shaw, H. M., and Soong, S.-J. (Eds.): Cutaneous Melanoma: Clinical Management and Treatment Results Worldwide. Philadelphia, J. B. Lippincott Company, 1985.
12. Fortner, J. G., MacLean, B., and Mulcare, R. J.: Treatment of recurrent malignant melanoma. *In* McCarthy, W. H. (Ed.): Melanoma and Skin Cancer. Sydney, VCN Blight, 1971, p. 453.
13. Galichich, J. H., Sundaresen, N., Arbit, E., and Passe, S.: Surgical treatment of single brain metastases: Factors associated with survival. Cancer, 45:381, 1980.
14. Hersey, P., Edwards, A., Coates, A., Shaw, H., McCarthy, W., and Milton, G.: Evidence that treatment with vaccinia melanoma cell lysates (VMCL) may improve survival of patients with Stage II melanoma. Cancer Immunol. Immunother., 25:257, 1987.
15. Houghton, A. N., Flannery, J., and Viola, M. U.: Malignant melanoma of the skin occurring during pregnancy. Cancer, 48:407, 1981.
16. Houghton, A. N., Mintzer, D., Cordon-Cardo, C., Welt, S., Fliegel, B., Vadhan, S., Carswell, E., Melamed, M. R., Oettgen, H. F., and Old, L. J.: Mouse mono-

clonal IGG3 antibody detecting GD3 ganglioside: A phase I trial in patients with malignant melanoma. Proc. Natl. Acad. Sci. U.S.A., 82:1242, 1985.
17. Karakousis, C. P., Lopez, R. E., Bhakoo, H. S., Rosen, F., Moore, R., and Carlson, M.: Estrogen and progesterone receptors and tamoxifen in malignant melanoma. Cancer Treat. Rep., 64:819, 1980.
18. Krementz, E. T., Reed, K. J., Coleman, W. P., Sutherland, C. N., Carter, D., and Campbell, M.: Acral lentiginous melanoma: A clinicopathologic entity. Ann. Surg., 195:632, 1982.
19. Krementz, E. T., and Ryan, R. F.: Chemotherapy of melanoma of the extremities by perfusion: Fourteen years clinical experience. Ann. Surg., 175:900, 1972.
20. Lee, J. A. H.: Current evidence about the causes of malignant melanoma. *In* Ariel, I. M. (Ed.): Clinical Cancer. New York, Grune & Stratton, 1977.
21. Lee, J. A. H., and Carter, A. P.: Secular trends in mortality from malignant melanoma. J. Natl. Cancer Inst., 45:91, 1970.
22. Lopez, R., Holtoke, E. D., Moore, R. H., and Karakousis, C. P.: Malignant melanoma with unknown primary site. J. Surg. Oncol., 19:151, 1982.
23. Lotze, M. T., Chang, A. E., Seipp, C. A., Simpson, C., Vetto, J. T., and Rosenberg, S. A.: High-dose recombinant interleukin-2 in the treatment of patients with disseminated cancer: Responses, treatment-related morbidity, and histologic findings. J.A.M.A., 256:3117, 1986.
24. McBride, C. M., Sugarbaker, E. V., and Hinkley, R. C.: Prophylactic isolation perfusion as the primary therapy for invasive malignant melanoma of the limbs. Ann. Surg., 182:316, 1975.
25. McCarty, K. S., Jr., Wortman, J., Stowers, S., Lubahn, D. B., McCarty, K. S., Sr., and Seigler, H. F.: Sex steroid receptor analysis in human melanoma. Cancer, 46:1463, 1980.
26. McClay, E. F., Mastrangelo, M. J., Sprandio, J. D., Bellett, R. E., and Berd, D.: The importance of tamoxifen to a cisplatin-containing regimen in the treatment of metastatic melanoma. Cancer, 63:1292, 1989.
27. McGovern, V. J., Lane Brown, M. M., and Sharpe, C.: Genetic predisposition to melanoma and other skin cancers in Australians. Med. J. Aust., 1:852, 1971.
28. Papachristou, D. N., and Fortner, J. G.: Melanoma arising under the nail. J. Surg. Oncol., 21:219, 1982.
29. Pratt, C. A., Palmer, M. K., Thatcher, N., and Crowther, D.: Malignant melanoma in children and adolescents. Cancer, 47:392, 1981.
30. Reintgen, D. S., Cox, E. B., McCarty, K. S., Jr., Vollmer, R., and Seigler, H. F.: Efficacy of elective lymph node dissection in patients with intermediate thickness primary melanoma. Ann. Surg., 198:379, 1983.
31. Reintgen, D. S., McCarty, K. S., Jr., Cox, E., and Seigler, H. F.: Malignant melanoma in the American black. Curr. Surg., 40:215, 1983.
32. Reintgen, D. S., McCarty, K. S., Jr., Woodard, B., Cox, E. B., and Seigler, H. F.: Metastatic malignant melanoma with an unknown primary. Surg. Gynecol. Obstet., 156:335, 1983.
33. Reintgen, D. S., Paull, D. E., Cox, E. B., McCarty, K. S., Jr., and Seigler, H. F.: Sex related survival differences in melanoma. Surg. Gynecol. Obstet., 159:367, 1984.
34. Reintgen, D. S., Sullivan, D., Coleman, E., Briner, W., Croker, B. P., and Seigler, H. F.: Lymphoscintigraphy for malignant melanoma. Surgical considerations. Am. Surg., 49:672, 1983.
35. Reintgen, D. S., Thompson, W., Garbutt, J., and Seigler, H. F.: Radiologic, endoscopic, and surgical considerations of melanoma metastatic to the gastrointestinal tract. Curr. Surg., March-April:87, 1984.
36. Reintgen, D. S., Vollmer, R., Tso, C. Y., and Seigler, H. F.: Prognosis for recurrent stage I malignant melanoma. Cancer, 122:1338, 1987.
37. Rhodes, A. R., and Melsky, J. W.: Small congenital nevocellular nevi and the risk of cutaneous melanoma. J. Pediatr., 100:219, 1982.
38. Rigel, D. S., Kopf, A. W., and Friedman, R. J.: The rate of malignant melanoma in the U.S.: Are we making an impact? J. Am. Acad. Dermatol., 17:1050, 1987.
39. Rosenberg, S. A., Lotze, M. T., Muul, L. M., Chang, A. E., Avis, F. P., Leitman, S., Linehan, W. M., Robertson, C. N., Lee, R. E., Rubin, J. T., Seipp, C. A., Simpson, C. G., and White, D. E.: A progress report on the treatment of 157 patients with advanced cancer using lymphokine-activated killer cells and interleukin-2 or high-dose interleukin-2 alone. N. Engl. J. Med., 315:889, 1987.
40. Rosenberg, S. A., Packard, B. S., Aebersold, P. M., Solomon, D., Topalian, S. L., Toy, S. T., Simon, P., Lotze, M. T., Yang, J. C., Seipp, C. A., Simpson, C., Carter, C., Bock, S., Schwartzentruber, D., Wei, J. P., and White, D. E.: Use of tumor-infiltrating lymphocytes and interleukin-2 in the immunotherapy of patients with metastatic melanoma: A preliminary report. N. Engl. J. Med., 319:1676, 1988.
41. Seigler, H. F., Lucas, V. S., Pickett, N. J., and Huang, A. T.: DTIC, CCNU, bleomycin, and vincristine (BOLD) in metastatic melanoma. Cancer, 46:2346, 1980.
42. Seigler, H. F., Wallack, M. K., Vervaert, C. E., Bash, J. A., Roberson, K. M., and Stuhlmiller, G. M.: Melanoma patient antibody responses to melanoma tumor associated antigens defined by murine monoclonal antibodies. J. Biol. Response Mod., 8:37, 1989.
43. Shaw, H. M., McGovern, V. J., Milton, G. W., Farago, G. A., and McCarthy, W. H.: Malignant melanoma: Influence of site of lesion and age of patient in female superiority in survival. Cancer, 46:2731, 1980.
44. Slingluff, C. L., Reintgen, D. S., Vollmer, R. T., and Seigler, H. F.: Malignant melanoma arising during pregnancy: A study of 100 patients. Ann. Surg. In press.
45. Slingluff, C. L., Vollmer, R., Reintgen, D. S., and Seigler, H. F.: Lethal "thin" malignant melanoma: Identifying patients at risk. Ann. Surg., 208:150, 1988.

46. Slingluff, C. L., Vollmer, R., and Seigler, H. F.: Anorectal melanoma: Clinical characteristics and results of surgical management of 24 patients. Surgery, 107:1, 1990.
47. Slingluff, C. L., Vollmer, R. T., and Seigler, H. F.: Stage II malignant melanoma: Presentation of a prognostic model and an assessment of specific active immunotherapy in 1,273 patients. J. Surg. Oncol., 39:139, 1988.
48. Spitler, L. E., del Rio, M., Khentigan, A., Wedel, N. I., Brophy, N. A., Miller, L. L., Harkonen, W. S., Rosendorf, L. L., Lee, H. M., Mischak, R. P., Kawahata, R. T., Stoudemire, J. B., Fradkin, L. B., Bautista, E. E., and Scannon, P. J.: Therapy of patients with malignant melanoma using a monoclonal antimelanoma antibody–ricin A chain immunotoxin. Cancer Res., 47:1717, 1987.
49. Stewart, W. R., Gilberman, R. H., Harrelson, J. M., and Seigler, H. F.: Skeletal metastases of melanoma. J. Bone Joint Surg., 60:645, 1978.
50. Thompson, A. J., Cook, M. G., and Gill, P. G.: Immunofluorescent detection of

hormone receptors in cutaneous melanocytic tumours. Br. J. Cancer, 43:644, 1981.
51. Trapeznikov, N. N., Khasanov, S. H., and Iavorskii, V. V.: Melanoma kozhi i beremennost [Melanoma of the skin and pregnancy]. Vopr. Onkkol., 33:40, 1987.
52. Wallack, M. K., Bash, J. A., Leftheriotis, E., Seigler, H. F., Bland, K., Wanebo, H., Balch, C., and Bartolucci, A. A.: Positive relationship of clinical and serologic responses to vaccinia melanoma oncolysate. Arch. Surg., 122:1460, 1987.
53. Weldon, D., and Little, J. H.: Spindle and epithelioid cell nevi in children and adults. Cancer, 40:217, 1977.
54. Wong, J. H., Sterns, E. E., Kopald, K. H., Nizze, J. A., and Morton, D. L.: Prognostic significance of pregnancy in Stage I melanoma. Arch. Surg., 124:1227, 1989.
55. Zava, D. T., and Goldhirsch, A.: Estrogen receptor in malignant melanoma: Fact or artifact? Eur. J. Cancer Clin. Oncol., 19:1151, 1983.

III

SOFT TISSUE SARCOMAS

LaSalle D. Leffall, Jr., M.D.

The soft tissues constitute nearly half of the body weight and thus represent the single greatest amount of tissue in the human body. Present in every organ of the body and primarily concerned with support and locomotion, they include the mass situated between the epidermis and the parenchymal organs. These consist of connective tissues and lymphatic vessels, smooth and striated muscle, fat, fascia, synovial structures, and reticuloendothelium.

Soft tissue sarcomas are relatively uncommon neoplasms, constituting only about 1 per cent of malignant tumors. These sarcomas differ widely in incidence and site and can be classified into many categories with different histopathologic charac-

TABLE 1. Classification of Soft Tissue Sarcomas

Cell of Origin	Type of Tumor	Subtypes
Fat cell	Liposarcoma Myxoid Round cell Pleomorphic	Well-differentiated
Fibroblast	Fibrosarcoma	Well-differentiated Poorly differentiated Dermatofibrosarcoma protuberans
Histiocyte	Malignant fibrous histiocytoma (fibroxanthosarcoma)	
Smooth muscle	Leiomyosarcoma	Leiomyoblastoma
Striated muscle	Rhabdomyosarcoma	Embryonal Botryoid Alveolar Pleomorphic
Osteoblast	Osteosarcoma	"Classic" Parosteal (juxtacortical)
Chondroblast	Chondrosarcoma	
Endothelium of blood vessels	(Hem) Angiosarcoma	Hemangioendothelioma (malignant) Hemangiopericytoma (malignant)
Endothelium of lymph vessels	Lymphangiosarcoma	
Synovial cells	Synovial sarcoma	
Pluripotential mesenchyme	Malignant mesenchymoma	
Ectoderm (peripheral nerve)	Malignant neurilemoma	
Uncertain	Alveolar soft tissue sarcoma Malignant granular cell tumor Kaposi's sarcoma Clear cell sarcoma of tendon sheath and aponeuroses Epithelioid sarcoma (acidophilic fascial sarcoma)	

Modified from Ackerman, L. V., and Rosai, J.: The pathology of tumors, part four: Grading, staging, and classification of neoplasms. CA, 21:373, 1971.

TABLE 2. Relative Incidence of Soft Tissue Sarcomas

Type	Percentage
Liposarcoma	20
Malignant fibrous histiocytoma	20
Fibrosarcoma	12
Rhabdomyosarcoma	10
Leiomyosarcoma	10
Synovial sarcoma	8
Mesenchymoma	4
Malignant neurilemoma	5
Kaposi's sarcoma	4
Angiosarcoma	2
Extraskeletal osteogenic sarcoma and chondrosarcoma	2
Other	3

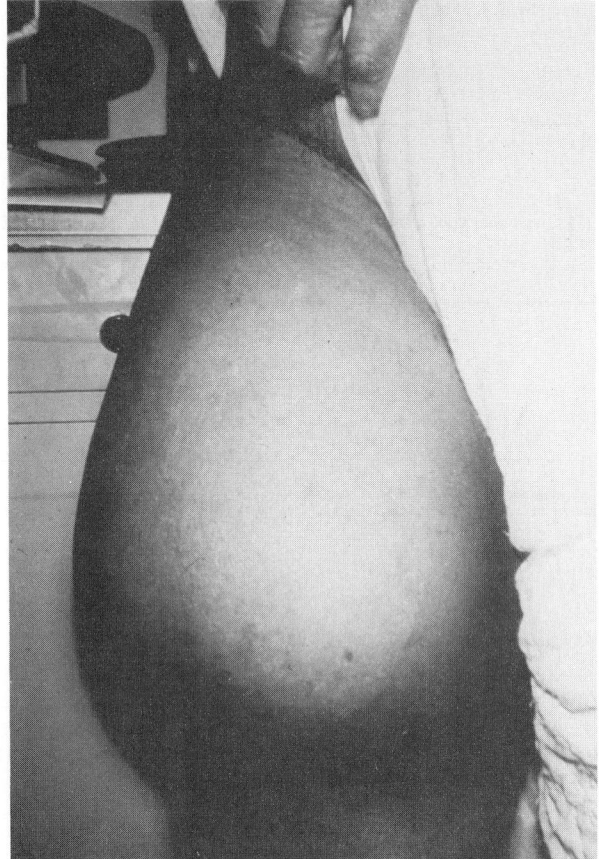

Figure 1. This huge mass in the right anterior thigh proved to be a liposarcoma.

teristics. There are more than 20 types of soft tissue sarcomas, each with distinguishing histologic and biologic behavior and varying tendencies for local infiltration and distant metastases.[45] A classification of these neoplasms is shown in Table 1. These tumors are derived from tissues arising from primitive mesenchyme. Although technically not soft tissue sarcomas, since they arise from ectoderm (peripheral nerves), malignant neurilemomas are included because they present as soft tissue tumors. Sarcomas that occur during childhood have great differences in histologic type, distribution, and response to therapy. In this age group, the two most common forms are rhabdomyosarcoma (43 per cent) and fibrosarcoma (20 per cent). In the adult population, liposarcomas, malignant fibrous histiocytomas, leiomyosarcomas, fibrosarcomas, and rhabdomyosarcomas occur most commonly (Table 2).[32,45,46]

Soft tissue sarcomas may develop at any site in the body. They are not encapsulated but possess a pseudocapsule of compressed malignant and normal cells. These tumors spread by direct local invasion, extending along fascial planes, muscle bundles, and nerve sheaths beyond the gross tumor. If local excision or simple enucleation is performed, local recurrence is high, up to 70 to 80 per cent.

Distant metastases occur frequently, most commonly to the lungs, by the hematogenous route. Some of these tumors, especially synovial sarcoma, embryonal rhabdomyosarcoma, epithelioid sarcoma, and malignant fibrous histiocytoma, may metastasize to regional lymph nodes in 10 to 20 per cent of patients, with the histiocytoma having the highest incidence of lymphatic spread in adults. However, early lymphatic spread of soft tissue sarcomas is quite uncommon. In a collected review over a 24-year period of 374 patients with a diagnosis of sarcoma, the study of incidence of lymph node metastases indicated that, in the 113 patients who had operations involving draining lymph nodes, only 3 (2.6 per cent) had evidence of sarcoma metastatic to draining lymph nodes. For this reason, prophylactic removal of draining lymph node areas in most adults with sarcoma is not recommended as part of surgical management.[50] However, lymph node dissection is indicated in children with embryonal rhabdomyosarcoma to provide information for staging. Chemotherapy is given to all children for 2 years, more intensive protocols being used for children with positive lymph nodes.

TYPES

MAJOR TYPES. Liposarcomas can become the largest of all soft tissue sarcomas, are among the most common neoplasms noted in most series, and are the most frequent sarcomas of the retroperitoneum (Fig. 1). Patients with well-differentiated liposarcoma may have 5-year survival rates of 70 to 80 per cent, whereas the 5-year survival rate of those with poorly differen-

tiated lesions is about 20 per cent. Liposarcomas are quite radioresponsive and are usually best treated by surgical therapy and irradiation.[13,25,34]

Malignant fibrous histiocytomas are among the most common soft tissue sarcomas of adults, occurring with almost the same frequency as liposarcomas. Located most often in the extremities and head and neck areas, they may also be associated with lymph node metastases (Fig. 2).[24]

Fibrosarcomas are seen less frequently now, because new histologic criteria classify some of them as malignant fibrous histiocytoma (Fig. 3). The histologic differentiation of fibrosarcomas from other lesions of fibrous tissue origin may be difficult, but it is important in order to determine proper treatment. Tumors of fibrous tissue origin appear most commonly in black patients.[5] Fibromatoses are connective tissue hyperplasias that infiltrate locally, do not metastasize, and tend to recur if not adequately excised.[37] They may be seen at any age, are circumscribed but not encapsulated, and usually arise from fascia. Some examples of fibromatoses are desmoids, nodular or pseudosarcomatous fasciitis, and plantar fibromatosis. The term *aggressive fibromatosis* is often used to better define the marked cellularity and aggressive local behavior of the lesion.[52] Adequate surgical excision is the treatment of choice.

Desmoids are usually located on the anterior abdominal wall, arising from the musculoaponeurosis of the rectus abdominis muscle and its sheath. They are more frequent in women in the childbearing years and may have their onset near the time of pregnancy. They may also arise in surgical scars. Extra-abdominal desmoids occur mainly in men in the third and fourth decades. Located most often in the region of the shoulders and thighs, they are more aggressive than those in the abdominal area (Fig. 4). Both abdominal and extra-abdominal desmoids are benign, do not metastasize to distant organs, and have a great

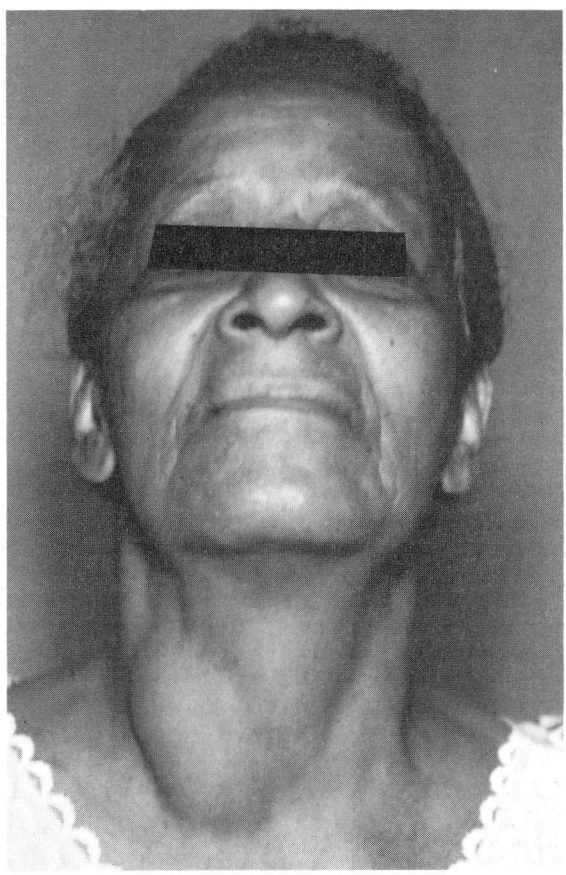

Figure 2. This slowly enlarging mass in the right lower neck proved on biopsy to be a malignant fibrous histiocytoma (fibroxanthosarcoma).

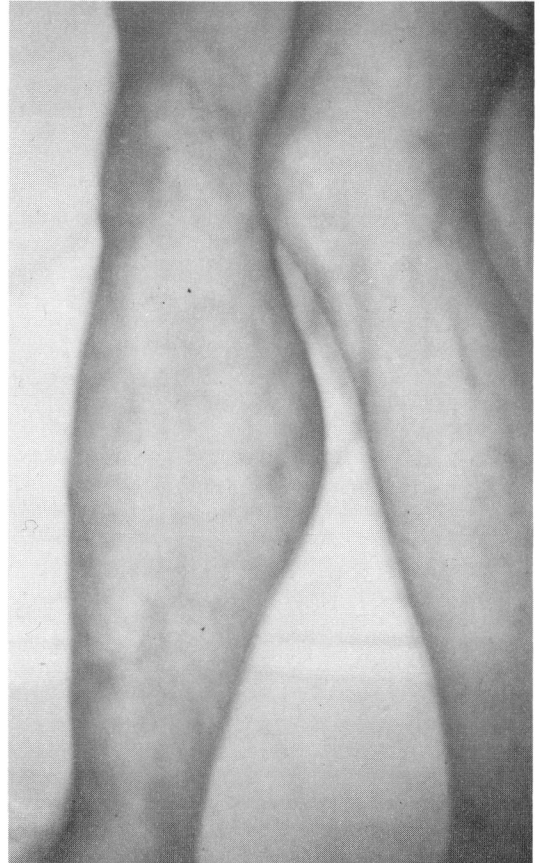

Figure 3. This tumor of the calf of the right leg represents a fibrosarcoma.

tendency for local recurrence. Wide excision is the treatment of choice. Large, nonresectable tumors may be controlled by irradiation or chemotherapy.[2,18,28,51]

Nodular (pseudosarcomatous) fasciitis originates from the fascia, affects middle-aged adults, and is most commonly located on the forearm.[6,36] It is a benign lesion of fibroblasts that may be incorrectly diagnosed and treated as sarcoma. Recurrences are rare after local excision.

Plantar fibromatosis is a benign lesion of fibrous tissue proliferation that characteristically replaces varying portions of the plantar aponeurosis, with eventual invasion of the overlying skin. Wide excision is essential to prevent recurrence.

Dermatofibrosarcoma protuberans (storiform fibrous histiocytoma) is considered to be a very low-grade fibrosarcoma.[30] It tends to recur locally but rarely metastasizes. The tumor develops as a protuberant lesion, most often arising from the skin of the trunk. The tumor involves the dermis, although it may invade the subcutaneous tissue. Histologically, the cartwheel or storiform arrangement of fibroblasts is quite characteristic of the lesion. Wide local excision is the treatment of choice.

Rhabdomyosarcoma is divided into four groups: (1) pleomorphic, (2) embryonal, (3) botryoidal, and (4) alveolar. The embryonal type may spread to lymph nodes in 10 per cent of cases. The pleomorphic type occurs most frequently and is usually found in patients over 35 years of age. Embryonal rhabdomyosarcoma is the most common soft tissue sarcoma in infants and children.[42]

Leiomyosarcomas are being reported with increasing frequency and are found most often in the viscera and retroperitoneum. They may arise in the smooth muscle of blood vessels.[23]

OTHER TYPES. Synovial sarcomas are the most common soft tissue sarcomas of the hands and feet and affect chiefly young adults. They occur in the vicinity of joints but seldom involve the synovial lining of the joint itself (Fig. 5). Lymph node metastases occur in 10 to 20 per cent of cases.

Malignant neurilemoma is uncommon, and metastases are slow but widespread.[19] About 50 per cent arise in patients with multiple neurofibromatosis (von Recklinghausen's disease). These tumors produce pain, tenderness, and paresthesias. Wide resection of the involved nerve is indicated.

Lymphangiosarcoma occurs rarely and may be secondary to postmastectomy lymphedema or to chronic congenital or idiopathic lymphedema.

Kaposi's sarcoma is a malignant blood vessel tumor and is

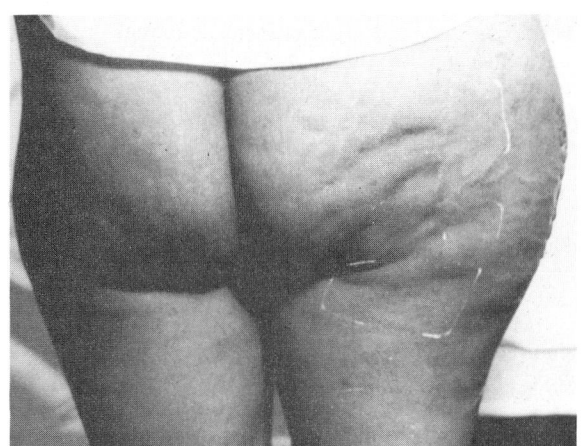

Figure 4. An extra-abdominal desmoid is responsible for the enlargement of the right lateral thigh.

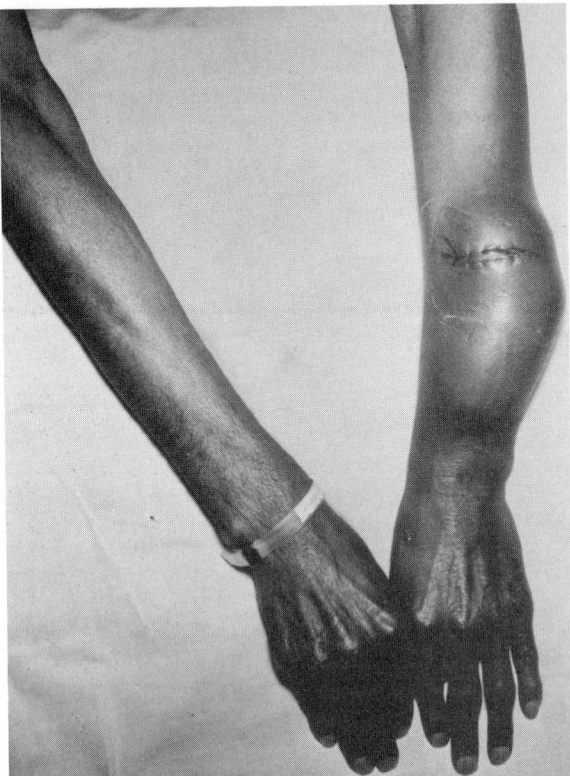

Figure 5. The tumor on the dorsal aspect of the left forearm represents a synovial sarcoma. The sutured transverse wound for incisional biopsy, although short, should have been placed in the longitudinal axis of the extremity.

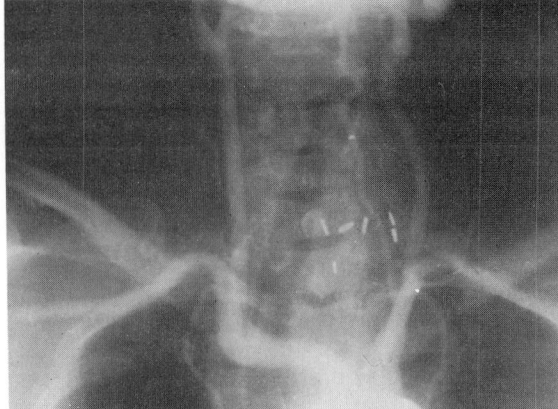

Figure 6. Retrograde aortogram reveals tortuosity and lateral displacement of the left common carotid artery secondary to a recurrent desmoid tumor that also displaces the trachea to the right and invades the superior mediastinum.

thought to be multicentric in origin.[8,40,43] It occurs predominantly in adult men and is greatly increased among homosexual men, recipients of renal allografts, and others receiving immunosuppressive therapy. In 75 to 85 per cent of cases, the primary tumor arises in the skin. Irradiation is the treatment of choice, although surgical therapy, chemotherapy, and interferon may be used in selected cases.[2]

CLINICAL MANIFESTATIONS

The most common presenting symptom of soft tissue sarcoma is a painless mass that gradually enlarges until it becomes painful or interferes with function. Pain alone without a palpable mass may be the earliest symptom. The pain usually persists despite rest. However, the growth rate of these tumors varies. Trauma may call attention to an unsuspected sarcoma but has not been proved to be an etiologic factor. Although uncommon, hypoglycemia has been described with some soft tissue sarcomas.[27,31] Physical examination usually reveals a firm, nontender tumor mass that may appear fairly well circumscribed because of its pseudocapsule. These neoplasms occur most often in the lower extremities, especially in the medial upper thigh, but may occur in other locations such as the upper extremities, trunk, retroperitoneum, head, and neck. There is a predilection for some types to originate in certain areas: (1) rhabdomyosarcomas in the upper thigh or arm in adults and in the extremity and genitourinary system in children; (2) liposarcomas in the thigh, shoulder, and retroperitoneum; (3) synovial sarcomas in the foot, hand, and knee; and (4) dermatofibrosarcoma protuberans in the trunk.[32]

DIAGNOSIS

Biopsy is essential to establish the diagnosis and institute proper therapy. Adequate tissue must be obtained for histo-

pathologic study. Excisional biopsy is used for lesions up to 3 cm in size; incisional or wedge biopsy is used for larger lesions. Biopsy incisions should be made along the longitudinal axis of the extremity so that the biopsy site may be included in the subsequent wide excision, if indicated, without sacrificing unnecessary overlying skin. Needle biopsy may be used, but often insufficient tissue is obtained to make a definitive diagnosis and incisional biopsy must be utilized. It is usually better not to rely on frozen section diagnosis but to await the results of permanent sections to afford the pathologist the best chance of making the correct diagnosis.[7] Accurate histologic diagnosis is mandatory before proper therapy can be given. The American Joint Commission has developed a staging system for soft tissue sarcoma that utilizes histologic grading as the primary determinant of stage. Thus, the staging system is based on four parameters: T, N, M, and G (referring to tumor size, regional node involvement, distant metastases, and grade).[4,46,48]

Chest films, tomograms, and/or computed tomographic scans are necessary to exclude pulmonary metastases. Soft tissue radiographs are of little value. Angiography may demonstrate tumor vessels characteristic of malignant tumors and can help determine relationships of the sarcomas to bone, nerves, and blood vessels but has been largely replaced by computed tomography (CT) and magnetic resonance imaging (MRI) (Fig. 6). Computed tomography is of great value in ascertaining spatial relationships of the sarcoma to normal structures (Fig. 7). Magnetic resonance imaging, which does not use ionizing radi-

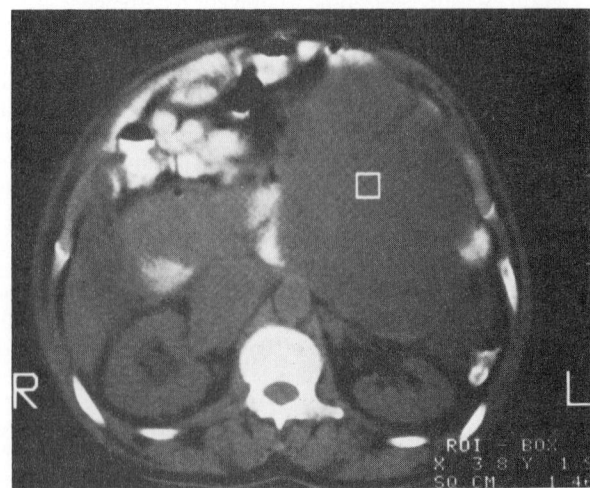

Figure 7. This computed tomographic scan reveals a large retroperitoneal tumor *(see marker)*, which is displacing the intestine and compressing the renal vasculature.

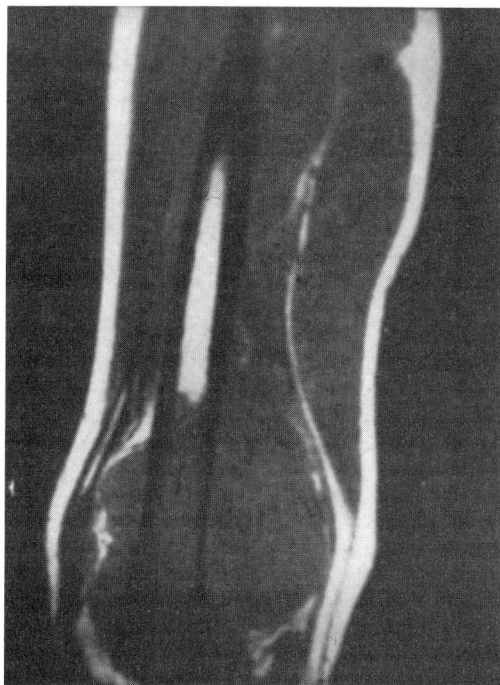

Figure 8. This magnetic resonance image reveals the relationship of a malignant fibrous histiocytoma of the lower thigh to normal structures.

ation, generally produces images superior to those of CT scanning (Fig. 8).[9]

MANAGEMENT

The treatment of choice for soft tissue sarcomas is adequate surgical resection in order to eradicate the disease and decrease the incidence of distant spread and local recurrence.[7,41] The following factors are important in helping determine the type of treatment: (1) histologic type, (2) histologic grade, (3) anatomic location, (4) status of tumor bed (primary or recurrent), (5) mode of spread, (6) size, and (7) mobility. Simple enucleation must be avoided, because this increases the chance for spread and decreases the chance for cure. Wide excision is essential, because these sarcomas spread by infiltration along muscle and fascia planes. Recurrent tumors behave in a more virulent manner than primary ones, and inadequate removal increases the likelihood of local recurrence. The surgical modalities are wide local excision, muscle group excision, and amputation. The wide excision must be three-dimensional in scope to obtain adequate margins in all directions around the tumor, if possible. Ideally, the surgeon should be incising through normal tissue at all times and should remove the sarcoma encompassed by normal tissue. In order to obtain good margins, major blood vessels may have to be sacrificed, with replacement by prosthetic or autologous grafts. Muscle group excision may be used for some sarcomas, requiring the removal of all involved muscles from their origin to insertion.

In a review of 38 patients with locally recurrent soft tissue sarcomas, various histologic types and grades (but without metastases) were evaluated. Preoperative doxorubicin (Adriamycin), radiation therapy, and wide resection of the recurrence were often recommended. A life-table analysis of these 38 patients shows an unexpectedly high predicted 5-year survival of 76 per cent (87 per cent for patients whose local recurrence could be completely resected). The investigators conclude that this highly positive response clearly justifies aggressive treatments for patients with recurrences alone and warrants attempts to salvage functional extremities.[15]

The decision to treat a patient by amputation is often very difficult. Generally, the amputation site is above the joint of the involved muscle groups. For sarcomas near the pelvic or shoulder girdle, hemipelvectomy or interscapulothoracic amputation may be indicated, whereas midhumeral or midthigh amputations are used for lesions below the elbow or knee. Adequate surgical resection of soft tissue sarcomas is often not technically feasible in lesions below the elbow or knee when the lesion is close to major neurovascular structures. Attempted wide surgical excision is often unsuccessful because the margin of normal tissue is very thin at one or more points, even though for most of the specimens the margin appears generous. Further adequacy of margin is difficult to assess for those tumors that are diffusely infiltrating. These factors account for a local recurrence rate of 25 to 30 per cent following wide surgical excision.[3] In such cases, amputation has historically been the recommended treatment of choice.

In recent years an alternative to amputation has become available. Radical high-dose precision radiation therapy (6000 to 7000 rads in 6 to 7 weeks), with or without limited surgical excision, has been effective in treating patients with early to moderately advanced soft tissue sarcomas.[11,26,29,33,47,54] The local recurrence rate following this type of treatment was reported to be 20 to 25 per cent, which compares favorably with the result reported following radical surgical excision (25 to 30 per cent). Amputation had been recommended in all the patients with lesions of the extremity. In addition, about 75 per cent of these patients retained a functional extremity free of pain and edema. Low-grade nonmetastasizing tumors such as desmoids, if not amenable to surgical resection (which is the treatment of choice), often can be treated successfully by radical dose irradiation. It has been shown that most soft tissue sarcomas, including well-differentiated tumors, are radioresponsive.

Limb-sparing surgical therapy should be considered in nearly all patients with extremity sarcomas. If limited resection and radical dose irradiation are used, amputation may be reserved for irradiation failures. In a recent series, multimodality management of high-grade soft tissue sarcomas of the extremity with preoperative intra-arterial doxorubicin and radiation therapy, radical surgical resection, and postoperative chemotherapy or chemoimmunotherapy resulted in preservation of a functional extremity in more than 90 per cent of patients. The results of the combined modality approach were significantly better in terms of both short-term, recurrence-free survival and salvage of a functional extremity than the results obtained in patients managed by surgical resection alone or by the combination of operation with another single therapeutic modality.[12,33,38,39]

The combination of selected surgical therapy, irradiation, and chemotherapy has produced marked improvement in the treatment of embryonal rhabdomyosarcoma in children.[10,17,20,35,53] With this regimen, amputations are rarely indicated for tumors of the extremities. When surgical treatment is not applicable, intensive irradiation and chemotherapy may produce local tumor control. The most effective chemotherapeutic combination is VAC (vincristine, actinomycin D, and cyclophosphamide) for a 1- to 2-year period. Current results indicate that children with completely resected localized disease experience an 83 per cent 5-year survival, whereas those with residual microscopic disease or involved regional lymph nodes experience a 70 per cent 5-year survival. Survival drops to 52 per cent for patients with gross residual disease, and only 25 per cent of patients with distant metastases at the time of diagnosis survive 5 years.

Hyperthermic perfusion with chemotherapeutic agents, combined with radiation therapy and surgical excision, may also be of value in the treatment of soft tissue sarcomas.[44] Recent studies have shown that the most active single agents in soft tissue sarcomas are doxorubicin (Adriamycin) and ifosfamide, whereas the most active chemotherapeutic combination is doxorubicin and dacarbazine (DTIC).[2]

Although irradiation and chemotherapy have added significantly to the therapeutic armamentarium, adequate surgical excision remains the treatment of choice and the most effective method of eradicating localized tumor. When total surgical excision of the sarcoma is not feasible, limited resections (tumor-debulking procedures) may be performed, to be followed by irradiation to the tumor bed and possibly by chemotherapy. Curative surgical resection should be considered in patients who have pulmonary metastases, even though lesions are multiple and bilateral.[21,22] In such patients, the primary lesion must be under control, and the lung must represent the only site of distant spread. The presence of a new primary cancer of the lung must also be kept in mind.

The survival rates for soft tissue sarcomas vary, depending on the type and grade of sarcoma. In the absence of distant metastasis, the most important factor affecting prognosis is the histopathologic grade of the tumor. Other significant factors are (1) tumor size, (2) depth or extent of invasion, and (3) whether the tumor is untreated or recurrent. Large tumors are those with a diameter greater than 5 cm.

Five-year survival rates have been shown to be inversely related to stage: 75 per cent, 50 per cent, 25 per cent, and 5 per cent for Stages I, II, III, and IV, respectively.[46] However, further improvement in survival can be expected with appropriate combination therapy using surgical therapy, irradiation, and chemotherapy. The role of immunotherapy has not yet been determined.[38]

SELECTED REFERENCES

Hayry, P., and Scheinin, T.: The Desmoid (Reitamo) Syndrome: Etiology, Manifestations, Pathogenesis and Treatment. Current Problems in Surgery, Vol. 25, No. 4, 1988.
This monograph from Finland is arguably the most authoritative source on the desmoid tumor. The authors describe with clarity the histologic and biologic characteristics of the tumor and the rationale of treatment. The relationship of the desmoid to Gardner's syndrome is explained in great detail. Broad discussion of all aspects of the desmoid tumor is included in this work.

Potter, D. A., Kinsella, T., Glatstein, E., Wesley, R., White, D. E., Seipp, C. A., Chang, A. E., Lack, E. E., Costa, J., and Rosenberg, S. A.: High-grade soft tissue sarcomas of the extremities. Cancer, 58:190–205, 1986.
Investigators at the National Cancer Institute report their treatment results with 211 patients with the diagnosis of soft tissue sarcoma of the extremities. Tumor site, histologic type, and microscopic margins of resection were not significant prognostic variables. There was no difference in disease-free or overall survival in patients undergoing amputation compared with those undergoing limb-sparing procedures plus postoperative radiotherapy. In a subset of 65 patients included in a prospective randomized trial evaluating the efficacy of adjuvant chemotherapy, a significant improvement in both disease-free and overall survival was seen in patients receiving chemotherapy.

Ryan, J. R., and Baker, L. O. (Eds.): Recent Concepts in Sarcoma Treatment. Dordrecht, Kluwer Academic Publishers, 1987.
This book, which contains chapters by different clinicians who have extensive experiences with soft tissue sarcomas, discusses in detail the role of limb-sparing surgical therapy combined with radiation and chemotherapy. The impressive results from multiple centers emphasize the merit of this treatment regimen in contrast to amputation. The information listed in this book documents with scientific accuracy the roles of different treatment modalities.

Shiu, M. H., and Brennan, M. F.: Surgical Management of Soft Tissue Sarcoma. Philadelphia, Lea and Febiger, 1989.
This comprehensive book represents the experience of a group of clinicians at one of our nation's leading cancer centers, who have dedicated themselves to the diagnosis and treatment of soft tissue sarcomas. Because of their relatively uncommon occurrence, these tumors are often treated inappropriately—all the more reason to consult this authoritative source. The authors emphasize the multidisciplinary approach essential to achieve the best results with these tumors. To provide the most current information concerning the various aspects of the overall management of these neoplasms, the two primary authors have chosen experts in the various disciplines. Progressing in an orderly manner from a discussion of concepts and principles to sarcomas in various locations and finally addressing multidisciplinary treatment, the contributors supply clinicians with detailed information to ensure the best treatment for their patients. With their vast experience at the Memorial Sloan-Kettering Cancer Center, these specialists give cogent reasons for their conclusions. The important roles of staging and diagnostic imaging techniques are discussed. Factors primarily responsible for prognosis are detailed in a scholarly manner. Although surgical resection is the treatment of choice for most of these tumors, proper emphasis is given to the role of radiation therapy and chemotherapy. The book is well written and well illustrated, with adequate documentation to support the views expressed. It is invaluable as a major reference for residents and other clinicians interested in soft tissue sarcomas.

Willett, C. G., Schiller, A. L., Suit, H. D., Mankin, H. J., and Rosenberg, A.: The histologic response of soft tissue sarcoma to radiation therapy. Cancer, 60:1500–1504, 1987.
The authors outline the role of preoperative radiotherapy combined with limb-sparing marginal surgical resection. Grade and size of soft tissue tumors were important predictors of response to radiotherapy, with higher grade and smaller tumors responding better. Preoperative twice daily radiotherapy may permit the conservative surgical excision of sarcomas of borderline resectability.

REFERENCES

1. Ackerman, L. V., and Rosai, J.: The pathology of tumors. 4. Grading, staging and classification of neoplasms. CA, 21:368, 1971.
2. Antman, K. H., and Elias, A. D.: Chemotherapy of advanced soft-tissue sarcomas. Semin. Surg. Oncol. 4:53, 1988.
3. Cantin, J., McNeer, G. P., Chu, F., and Booher, R. J.: The problem of local recurrence after treatment of soft tissue sarcoma. Ann. Surg., 168:47, 1968.
4. Costa, J., Wesley, R. A., Glatstein, E., and Rosenberg, S. A.: The grading of soft tissue sarcomas. Results in a clinicohistopathologic correlation in a series of 163 cases. Cancer, 53:530, 1984.
5. Crawford, M., Chung, E. B., Leffall, L. D., Jr., and White, J. E.: Soft part sarcomas in negroes. Cancer, 26:503, 1970.
6. Culberson, J. D., and Enterline, H. T.: Pseudosarcomatous fasciitis: A distinctive clinical-pathologic entity: Report of five cases. Ann. Surg., 151:235, 1960.
7. Das Gupta, T. K., and Brasfield, R. D.: Soft tissue tumors: Classification and principles of management. CA, 18:259, 1968.
8. Davis, J.: Kaposi's sarcoma. Present concept of clinical course and treatment. N. Y. State J. Med., 68:2067, 1968.
9. Demas, B. E., Heelan, R. T., Lane, J., Marcove, R., Hajdu, S., and Brennan, M. F.: Soft tissue sarcomas of the extremities: Comparison of MR and CT in determining the extent of disease. AJR, 150:615, 1988.
10. Donaldson, S. S., Castro, J. R., Wilber, J. R., and Jesse, R. H., Jr.: Rhabdomyosarcoma of head and neck in children: Combination treatment by surgery, irradiation, and chemotherapy. Cancer, 31:26, 1973.
11. Dritschilo, A., Weichselbaum, R., Cassady, J. R., Jaffe, N., Green, D., and Filler, R. M.: The role of radiation therapy in the treatment of soft tissue sarcomas of childhood. Cancer, 42:1192, 1978.
12. Eilber, F. R., Morton, D. L., Eckardt, J., Grant, T., and Weisenburger, T.: Limb salvage for skeletal and soft tissue sarcomas. Multidisciplinary preoperative therapy. Cancer, 53:2579, 1984.
13. Enterline, H. T., Culberson, J. D., Rochlin, D. B., and Brady, L. W.: Liposarcoma. A clinical and pathological study of 53 cases. Cancer, 13:932, 1960.
14. Fine, G., Hajdu, S. I., Morton, D. L., et al.: Soft tissue sarcomas. Classification and treatment. Pathol. Annu., 17:155, 1982.
15. Giuliano, A. E., Eilber, F. R., and Morton, D. L.: The management of locally recurrent soft-tissue sarcoma. Ann. Surg., 196:87, 1982.
16. Golding, S. J., and Husband, J. E.: The role of computed tomography in the management of soft tissue sarcomas. Br. J. Radiol., 55:740, 1982.
17. Grosfeld, J. L., Clatworthy, H. W., Jr., and Newton, W. A., Jr.: Combined therapy in childhood rhabdomyosarcomas: An analysis of 42 cases. J. Pediatr. Surg., 4:637, 1969.
18. Hill, D. R., Newman, H., and Phillips, T. L.: Radiation therapy of desmoid tumors. Am. J. Roentgenol., 117:84, 1973.
19. Jacobs, R. L., and Barmada, R.: Neurilemoma: A review of the literature with six case reports. Arch. Surg., 102:181, 1971.
20. Johnson, D. G.: Trends in surgery for childhood rhabdomyosarcoma. Cancer, 35(Suppl):916, 1975.
21. Joseph, W. L.: Criteria for resection of sarcoma metastatic to the lung. Cancer Chemother. Rep., 58:285, 1974.
22. Joseph, W. L., Morton, D. L., and Adkins, P. C.: Prognostic significance of tumor doubling time in evaluating operability in pulmonary metastatic disease. J. Thorac. Cardiovasc. Surg., 61:23, 1971.
23. Jurayj, M. N., Midell, A. I., Bederman, S., Gruen, J., and O'Brien, P. H.: Primary leiomyosarcomas of the inferior vena cava. Report of a case and review of the literature. Cancer, 26:1349, 1970.
24. Kempson, R. L., and Kyriakos, M.: Fibroxanthosarcoma of the soft tissues. A type of malignant fibrous histiocytoma. Cancer, 29:961, 1972.
25. Kinne, D. W., Chu, F. C., Huvos, A. G., Yagoda, A., and Fortner, J. G.: Treatment of primary and recurrent retroperitoneal liposarcoma. Twenty-five year experience at Memorial Hospital. Cancer, 31:53, 1973.
26. Lindberg, R. D., Martin, R. G., Romsdahl, M. M., et al.: Conservative surgery and postoperative radiotherapy in 300 adults with soft-tissue sarcomas. Cancer, 47:2391, 1981.
27. Mars, H., Schumacher, O. P., and McCormack, L. J.: Intraabdominal extrapancreatic neoplasm (leiomyosarcoma) associated with severe recurrent hypoglycemia. Cancer, 20:1155, 1967.
28. McKinnon, J. G., Neifeld, J. P., Kay, S., Parker, G. A., Foster, W. C., and Lawrence, W., Jr.: Management of desmoid tumors. Surg. Gynecol. Obstet., 169:104, 1989.

29. McNeer, G. P., Cantin, J., Chu, F., and Nickson, J. J.: Effectiveness of radiation therapy in the management of sarcoma of the soft somatic tissues. Cancer, 22:391, 1968.
30. McPeak, C. J., Cruz, T., and Nicastri, A. D.: Dermatofibrosarcoma protuberans: An analysis of 86 cases, five with metastasis. Ann. Surg., 166:803, 1967.
31. McPeak, C. J., and Papaioannou, A. N.: Nonpancreatic tumors associated with hypoglycemia. Arch. Surg., 93:1019, 1966.
32. Morton, D. L.: Soft tissue sarcomas. In Holland, J. F., and Frei, E., III (Eds.): Cancer Medicine. Philadelphia, Lea and Febiger, 1973, pp. 1845–1861.
33. Morton, D. L., Eilber, F. R., Townsend, C. M., Jr., Grant, T. T., Mirra, J., and Weisenburger, T. H.: Limb salvage from a multidisciplinary treatment approach for skeletal and soft tissue sarcomas of the extremity. Ann. Surg., 184:268, 1976.
34. Perry, H., and Chu, F.: Radiation therapy in the palliative management of soft tissue sarcomas. Cancer, 15:179, 1962.
35. Pratt, C. B., Hustu, H. O., Fleming, I. D., and Pinkel, C.: Coordinated treatment of childhood rhabdomyosarcoma with surgery, radiotherapy and combination chemotherapy. Cancer Res., 32:606, 1972.
36. Price, E. B., Silliphant, W. M., and Shuman, R.: Nodular fasciitis—a clinicopathologic analysis of 65 cases. Am. J. Clin. Pathol., 35:122, 1961.
37. Pritchard, D. J., Soule, E. H., Taylor, W. F., and Ivins, J. C.: Fibrosarcoma—a clinicopathologic and statistical study of 199 tumors of the soft tissues of the extremities and trunk. Cancer, 33:888, 1974.
38. Rosenberg, S. A., Kent, H., Costa, J., Webber, B. L., et al.: Prospective randomized evaluation of the role of limb sparing surgery, radiation therapy and adjuvant chemoimmunotherapy in the treatment of adult soft tissue sarcomas. Surgery, 84:62, 1979.
39. Rosenberg, S. A., Tepper, J., Glatstein, E., et al.: Prospective randomized evaluation of adjuvant chemotherapy in adults with soft tissue sarcomas of the extremities. Cancer, 52:424, 1983.
40. Schroff, R. W., Gottlieb, M. S., Prince, H. E., et al.: Immunological studies of homosexual men with immunodeficiency and Kaposi's sarcoma. Clin. Immunol. Immunopathol., 27:300, 1983.
41. Shiu, M. H., Castro, E. B., Hajdu, S. I., and Fortner, J. G.: Surgical treatment of 297 soft tissue sarcomas of the lower extremity. Ann. Surg., 182:597, 1975.
42. Soule, E. H., Mahour, G. H., Mills, S. D., and Lynn, H. B.: Soft tissue sarcomas of infants and children: A clinicopathologic study of 135 cases. Mayo Clin. Proc., 43:313, 1968.
43. Special Report: Epidemiologic aspects of the current outbreak of Kaposi's sarcoma and opportunistic infections. N. Engl. J. Med., 306:248, 1982.
44. Stehlin, J. S., de Ipolyi, P. D., Giovanella, B. C., Gutierrez, A. E., and Anderson, R. F.: Soft tissue sarcomas of the extremity—multidisciplinary therapy employing hyperthermic perfusion. Am. J. Surg., 130:643, 1975.
45. Stout, A. P., and Lattes, R.: Tumors of the soft tissues. Atlas of Tumor Pathology, Series 2, Fasc. I. Washington, D. C., Armed Forces Institute of Pathology, 1967.
46. Suit H. D.: Sarcoma of soft tissue. CA, 28:284, 1978.
47. Suit, H. D.: Soft tissue sarcomas: The role of radiation therapy. Hosp. Pract., 17:114, 1982.
48. Suit H. D., Russell W. O. and Martin R. G.: Sarcoma of soft tissue—clinical and histopathologic parameters and response to treatment. Cancer, 35:1478, 1975.
49. Torosian, M. H., Friedrich, C., Godbold, J., Hajdu, S. I., and Brennan, M. F.: Soft tissue sarcoma: Initial characteristics and prognostic factors in patients with and without metastatic disease. Semin. Surg. Oncol., 4:13, 1988.
50. Weingrad, D. N., and Rosenberg, S. A.: Early lymphatic spread of osteogenic and soft-tissue sarcomas. Surgery, 84:231, 1978.
51. Weiss, A. J., and Lackman, R. D.: Low-dose chemotherapy of desmoid tumors. Cancer, 64:1192, 1989.
52. Wilbur, J. R., Sutow, W. W., Sullivan, M. P., and Gottlieb, J. A.: Chemotherapy of sarcomas. Cancer, 36:765, 1975.
53. Wilkins, S. A., Jr., Waldron, C. A., Mathews, W. H., and Droulias, C. A.: Aggressive fibromatosis of the head and neck. Am. J. Surg., 130:412, 1975.
54. Wood, W. C., Suit, H. D., Mankin, H. J., et al.: Radiation and conservative surgery in the treatment of soft tissue sarcoma. Am. J. Surg., 147:537, 1984.

IV

TUMOR MARKERS

Jeffrey A. Norton, M.D., and Douglas L. Fraker, M.D.

HISTORICAL ASPECTS

In specific types of cancer, circulating markers have greatly facilitated the treatment of patients by early diagnosis and accurate reflection of residual microscopic disease. A clinically useful marker was first identified by Gutman and Gutman in 1938 when they detected elevated levels of the enzyme acid phosphatase in the serum of patients with metastatic prostate carcinoma.[37] Similarly, in 1965, Gold and Freedman showed that another fetal antigen (carcinoembryonic antigen [CEA]) was present in extracts of tumors from the gastrointestinal tract and fetal gut tissue, but not in extracts of adult intestinal tissue.[35] Subsequently, CEA was measured in the circulation of patients with cancer and not in the circulation of patients with nonmalignant conditions.

Several scientific advances during the past 20 years were instrumental in the development of clinically useful tumor markers. First, Yalow and Berson developed the technique of radioimmunoassay (RIA) for which they later received the Nobel prize. RIA allowed the reproducible, sensitive, and specific detection of minute amounts of substances in serum based on structural immunogenic characteristics of the marker as opposed to more cumbersome and less specific assays based on bioactivity. Second, the description of hybridomas that secrete monoclonal antibodies[57] has been applied to tumor antigens, which has greatly facilitated detection and characterization of new tumor markers. Finally, with recently developed molecular biology methods, tumor markers can be characterized at the gene level.[89,91]

USES OF AN "IDEAL" TUMOR MARKER

Successes and inadequacies of initial investigations with tumor markers help define the characteristics of an "ideal" tumor marker. First, markers must be specific; that is, false-positive tests in the normal population or in patients with benign conditions are rare. Second, a reliable tumor marker must have a low false-negative rate or a high degree of sensitivity. All patients with a particular histologic type of cancer should test positive for an ideal tumor marker with minimal tumor burden. Third, the circulating level of an ideal tumor marker should correlate directly with the amount of viable tumor present. A correlation between marker level and tumor burden augments the utility of a marker as a prognostic means and as a yardstick to measure the response to therapy. Finally, sensitive and specific assays for tumor markers must be reproducible and widely available at a reasonable cost.

The potential utility of an ideal tumor marker covers a broad array of clinical problems such as screening, diagnosis, prognosis, assessment of therapeutic efficacy, and detection of residual or recurrent disease. A successful screening test for the detection of cancer must have a high sensitivity for early lesions to detect disease in asymptomatic patients with small curable tumor burdens. In that situation, early diagnosis by tumor marker screening may translate into therapeutic cure. Currently, the performance of available tumor markers as screening tests for curable malignancies has been inadequate owing to reduced sensitivity and an inability to accurately detect small tumor burdens as well as the presence of numerous false-positive results. An exception to this generalization is patients who develop medullary thyroid carcinoma in familial settings who are detected by provocative testing and measurement of plasma calcitonin level.[93]

A second application for circulating tumor markers is as a diagnostic measure. The best examples of this application are the hormone markers of endocrine tumors. In these conditions, biological activity of the elevated circulating hormone levels defines the clinical syndrome (i.e., carcinoid syndrome), and the level of circulating hormone (serotonin) or hormone degradation products (urinary 5-HIAA) is the major diagnostic criterion for the disorder. The diagnosis is dependent on the measurement of the circulating marker or the staining of the tumor for the marker by immunohistochemistry.

A third application for measurement of tumor markers at the time of diagnosis is that some markers yield prognostic as well as diagnostic information. The presence or absence of a marker for a specific histologic type may be an independent prognostic variable. For example, patients with testicular cancer with normal serum marker levels respond better to therapy than do patients with markedly elevated ones.[15] In addition, the absolute serum level of tumor marker may predict outcome, as seen in patients with colorectal carcinoma whose prognosis worsens with greater serum elevations of preoperative CEA level.[85]

The final application for measurement of tumor markers and the area in which tumor markers appear to have the greatest clinical utility is as a reflection of treatment efficacy and in follow-up for recurrent disease. In these settings, alterations in tumor marker level may be the primary clinical variable influencing patient management decisions, such as continuing or discontinuing therapy or embarking on efforts to define the extent of disease by imaging studies or exploratory operation.

INADEQUACIES OF TESTING BY TUMOR MARKERS

Despite considerable technical advances and extensive clinical investigations, the actual benefits of any given tumor marker do not achieve the theoretical potential discussed. In other words, no ideal tumor marker exists at present. The characteristics of individual tumor markers such as specificity, sensitivity, and correlation of marker level with tumor burden define the actual clinical utility for each marker.

The measurement of tumor markers in serum must be integrated with other technical advances in medicine that relate to similar clinical questions. In this regard, the most important developments are the dramatic improvement in and availability of new radiologic imaging techniques, such as computed tomography (CT), high resolution ultrasound, and magnetic resonance imaging, which also advance initial diagnosis and detection of recurrent or metastatic disease. Data from measurement of serum markers must be interfaced with imaging results. For example, early studies evaluating serum CEA levels as a marker for recurrent colorectal cancer were done before the availability of CT scanners. Current strategy for the follow-up of patients with colorectal cancer should utilize both levels of CEA in serum as well as imaging techniques in a complementary manner. Another potential utility of the relationship between tumor markers and radiologic imaging techniques is their merging in tests to localize tumors not imaged by standard studies such as selective venous sampling for hormone levels or the use of radiolabeled antibody to tumor antigens.

Another reflection of the inadequacy of serum tumor markers is the overlap between different markers and different tumors, that is, many different types of tumors have elevations of two or more serum markers to variable extents, such as testicular tumors, which may produce elevations in serum levels of alpha-fetoprotein (AFP) and beta–human chorionic gonadotropin (β-HCG). Conversely, a given serum marker may be elevated in more than one tumor histology, such as AFP in both testicular tumors and hepatomas. This lack of specificity probably arises because many of the available tumor markers were developed from fetal tissue and not specific tumor tissues. As a reflection of the dichotomy, this chapter is divided into two sections. The first section is organized by tumor marker and describes the history, biochemistry, assay characteristics, and disease states in which individual markers are useful. The second section is organized by the type of neoplasm and describes the markers relating to that histologic type and the ways in which those markers are used.

TYPES OF TUMOR MARKERS

Circulating tumor markers can be categorized by functional and biochemical characteristics into tumor antigens, enzymes, hormones, and miscellaneous markers of tumor or host origin (Table 1).

Tumor antigens were identified and are defined by immunogenic structural characteristics. Enzymes and hormones are identified by bioactivity as catalysts of specific chemical reactions or effects from binding specific receptors, respectively. Although initially measured by bioassays utilizing these activities, immunoassays exist for essentially all enzymes and hormones used as tumor markers.

Tumor antigens can be subcategorized by historical, biochemical, and distributional features as *oncofetal antigens* and *polyclonal-* or *monoclonal-defined antigens*. Oncofetal antigens are compounds produced during normal development by the placental-fetal complex and are also produced by neoplastic tissue. This group contains the original and most prevalent tumor markers including CEA, AFP, and beta-HCG. A second and rapidly enlarging group of tumor markers are tumor-associated antigens detected by conventional immunologic techniques or by monoclonal antibodies directed against fresh tumor extracts or, more commonly, cell lines derived from human neoplasms. Tumor-associated antigens include the more recent serum markers such as CA 125, CA 19–9, and CA 15–3. As they are further characterized, these newer markers typically satisfy the criteria stated earlier for oncofetal antigens since they are present in specific fetal tissue as well as in neoplasms. The only real differences between these new cancer antigens (CA) and traditional oncofetal antigens is length of experience and familiarity with the markers.

Enzymes produced in excess amount by the tumor or by the tumor-bearing host constitute a third category of tumor markers and include neuron-specific enolase (NSE) and acid phosphatase. Hormones and hormone degradation products are specific and sensitive markers for a wide variety of endocrine tumors. A miscellaneous group of tumor markers includes host products that increase in response to tumors including serum ferritin levels, cytokine levels, and lipids.

CARCINOEMBRYONIC ANTIGEN

CEA is a glycoprotein (molecular weight, 180 kd.) consisting of a single polypeptide chain with a variable carbohydrate content.[41] Recent studies indicate that CEA is only one of a family of related molecules that share antigenic determinants.[89] Other glycoproteins in the CEA family include nonspecific cross-reacting antigen (NCA) and biliary glycoprotein.[82] Biliary glycoprotein is present in bile, and forms of NCA occur in normal lung, granulocytes, and epithelial cells. Differences in genetic and polypeptide sequences between CEA and related glycoproteins have been recently elucidated.[96] Description of this family of related compounds has led to the discovery of unique epitopes on CEA, which may enable development of a more specific assay by eliminating false-positive results because of shared epitopes with related glycoproteins in normal tissues.[96]

TABLE 1. Categorization of Tumor Markers

Type	Tumor Marker	Tumor Histologies
Tumor Antigen		
Oncofetal	Carcinoembryonic antigen (CEA)	Colorectal, pancreas, breast, lung, gastric
	Alpha-fetoprotein (AFP)	Hepatocellular carcinomas, testicular tumors
Polyclonal antibody–defined	Prostate-specific antigen (PSA)	Prostatic cancer
	Tissue polypeptide antigen (TPA)	Breast, gynecologic tumors
Monoclonal antibody– defined cancer antigens	CA 15–3	Breast
	CA 19–9	Colorectal, pancreas, gastric
	CA 50	Colorectal, pancreas, gastric
	CA 125	Ovarian, nonovarian gynecologic tumors
Enzymes		
	Neuron-specific enolase (NSE)	Neuroendocrine tumors (APUDomas) Small-cell lung cancer Medullary thyroid cancer Islet cell tumors, carcinoids
	Prostatic acid phosphatase (PAP)	Prostate
Hormones*		
	Beta–Human chorionic gonadotropin (β-HCG)	Testicular tumors, trophoblastic gestational tumors

* See Table 9 for additional hormones.

A variety of CEA immunoassay kits are commercially available. Normal serum values of CEA vary with different assays. In general, CEA serum levels less than 2.5 ng. per ml. are normal and CEA levels greater than 5.0 ng. per ml. are elevated. Serum levels beween 2.5 and 5.0 ng. per ml. are considered borderline. As with other tests, the normal range affects specificity and sensitivity of serum CEA determinations. If one attempts to increase sensitivity by indicating a lower level for normal CEA values, one loses specificity as a greater number of false-positive results are detected.

The serum half-life of CEA varies between 1 and 7 days dependent on hepatic function of the patient.[29] Large glycoproteins such as CEA are cleared mainly by Kupffer cells and hepatocytes. Therefore, both cholestatic and hepatocellular disorders prolong the half-life of CEA.[29]

CEA is a classic example of a tumor marker that, although widely used, is not an ideal marker because of low specificity and sensitivity. Both malignant and nonmalignant diseases may elevate serum CEA levels (Tables 2 and 3). Although CEA is primarily associated with colorectal cancer, serum levels may also be elevated in cancer of the pancreas, stomach, lung, breast, thyroid, and ovary (Table 3). The lack of specificity is further evidenced by nonmalignant conditions that also may elevate serum CEA levels (Table 2): gastrointestinal disorders (including peptic ulcer disease, gastritis, pancreatitis, and inflammatory bowel disease), hepatobiliary diseases (including cirrhosis, hepatitis, and obstructive jaundice), and nonmalignant pulmonary disease (bronchitis and emphysema) as well as benign prostatic hypertrophy and renal failure.

ALPHA-FETOPROTEIN

Alpha-fetoprotein was the first oncofetal antigen discovered and is currently a useful tumor marker for primary hepatocellular carcinoma and nonseminomatous germ-cell tumors of the testis. AFP is a single-chain glycoprotein (molecular weight, 70 Kd) with alpha-globulin electrophoretic mobility characteristics originally described as a predominant circulating species during fetal development. AFP is synthesized by fetal yolk sac, hepatic parenchymal cells, and other endodermally derived gastrointestinal tissue. Peak serum levels of AFP (3 mg. per ml.) occur during the twelfth week of gestation, then serum AFP levels decline to approximately 0.1 mg. per ml. at birth and continue to decrease to normal adult levels (<10 ng. per ml.) by 1 year of age.

In 1963, Abelev and colleagues first described the presence of an alpha$_1$-globulin immunochemically identical to AFP in the serum of adult mice with transplantable, chemically induced hepatomas.[1] The following year, AFP was measured in the serum of patients with hepatoma. Initially, investigators used low-sensitivity agar immunodiffusion assays (level of detection approximately 300 ng. per ml.) and were able to detect AFP in the serum of only 30 per cent of patients with hepatoma. Development of a radioimmunoassay for AFP improved the sensitivity of detection severalfold (10 ng. per ml.) and correspondingly improved the clinical utility of the marker.

Several commercially available immunoassays for AFP, both radiometric and enzyme-linked, are available today and reliably detect approximately 5 ng. per ml. of AFP in serum.[21] The half-life of circulating AFP in the serum of patients is 4 to 6 days.

Abnormal serum levels of AFP usually occur in malignant neoplasms but may occur in benign diseases of endodermally derived organs including hepatitis, inflammatory bowel disease, ataxia-telangiectasia, and hereditary tyrosinemia (Table 2). However, highly elevated serum levels of AFP (>500 ng. per ml.) are present almost exclusively in primary hepatocellular cancer and nonseminomatous testicular tumors. Patients with other malignant tumors can also have elevated serum levels of AFP. Twenty per cent of patients with gastric or pancreatic cancer and 5 per cent of patients with colorectal or lung cancer have significant elevations (>5 ng. per ml.) of serum AFP levels.

TABLE 2. Serum Levels of Markers in Healthy Normal Controls and Other Nonmalignant Conditions

Marker	Mean Level	Upper Limit Normal	Per Cent Controls with Abnormal Levels at Upper Limit Normal	Nonmalignant Conditions Associated with Elevated Levels
CEA	1.9 ng./ml.—nonsmokers	<2.5 ng./ml.	9–16	Hepatitis, cirrhosis, jaundice, COPD, peptic ulcer, pancreatitis, inflammatory bowel disease, renal failure
		<5.0 ng./ml.	1–5	
	3.1 ng./ml.—smokers	<10 ng./ml.	0–1	
AFP	1–10 ng./ml.	<10 ng./ml.	1–3	Chronic and active hepatitis, cirrhosis, pregnancy
		<40 ng./ml.	0	
β-HCG	<1 units/ml. men	<3 unit/ml.	<1	Pregnancy
	<3 units/ml. premenopausal women			
	3–4 units/ml. postmenopausal women	<8 unit/ml.	<1	
Prostate-specific antigen	1.1 ± 0.7 ng./ml.	<2.5 ng./ml.	1–3	Benign prostatic hypertrophy, prostatic massage or biopsy
Tissue polypeptide antigen	66 ± 16 units/L.	<100 unit/L.	5	
		<200 unit/L.	<1	
CA 15–3	13.3 ± 6 units/ml.	<22 unit/ml.	9	Acute and chronic hepatitis, cirrhosis, benign breast disease
		<25 unit/ml.	5	
		<30 unit/ml.	1.3	
CA 19–9	10.8 ± 7 units/ml.	<25 unit/ml.	1	Acute and chronic pancreatitis, cirrhosis, sclerosing cholangitis, other extrahepatic cholestatic diseases
		<37 unit/ml.	0–1	
CA 50	—	<17 unit/ml.	0–1	Pancreatitis, cirrhosis, ulcerative colitis, sclerosing cholangitis
CA 125	10–16 units/ml. (greater in women)	<35 unit/ml.	1	Pancreatitis, jaundice, pregnancy, menstruation, endometriosis, PID, renal failure
		<65 unit/ml.		
Neuron-specific enolase	4.7–9.3 ng./ml.	<13 ng./ml.	<1	
Prostatic acid phosphatase	Enzymatic assay: 0.1–0.5 unit/L.	<0.8 unit/L.	<1	Benign prostatic hypertrophy, hematologic disorders
	Immunoassay: 1.2 ± 0.5 ng./ml.	<2.1 ng./ml.	1–3	
Ferritin	27–96 ng./ml.	<300 ng./ml.	0–1	Alcoholism, hepatocellular disease, hematologic diseases, chronic inflammation

COPD, Chronic obstructive pulmonary disease; PID, pelvic inflammatory disease.

TABLE 3. Malignancies with Elevated Serum Carcinoembryonic Antigen (CEA) Levels

Tumor	Percentage of Patients with Elevated Serum Levels of CEA
Breast	
Local	0–2
Metastatic	41–71
Colorectal	
Dukes Stage A	3–5
Stage B	25
Stage C	33–45
Stage D	65–90
Gastric	30
Gynecologic	
Cervical	30–65
Endometrial	43–69
Ovarian	32–51
Vulvar	33–51
Lung	
Non–small-cell	15–25
Small-cell	23–59
Pancreas	
Local	71
Metastatic	87–100
Medullary thyroid carcinoma	80

and hepatocellular carcinomas because of the dramatic elevations of serum levels in these patients.

HUMAN CHORIONIC GONADOTROPIN

Human chorionic gonadotropin is a placental hormone that is also a tumor marker for gestational trophoblastic neoplasms and nonseminomatous testicular cancer. HCG is a glycoprotein consisting of two distinct noncovalently bound subunits. The alpha-subunit of HCG (molecular weight, 15 kd.) is identical to the alpha-subunit of the pituitary hormones luteinizing hormone (LH), follicle-stimulating hormone (FSH), and thyroid-stimulating hormone (TSH). The beta-subunit of these four glycoprotein hormones is distinct and defines the activity of each. In particular, the 29 amino acids on the carboxy-terminal end of the HCG beta-subunit are unique to that hormone, but there is an 82 per cent overall sequence homology between the beta-subunit of LH and HCG. Further evidence of the structural similarity between HCG and LH is that these two hormones bind to a common cell surface receptor on gonadal tissues.

Assays for levels of HCG in serum and urine have been available for 6 decades. Elevations of this hormone in women are diagnostic of pregnancy (Table 2). Initial bioassays for HCG were based on the appearance of hemorrhagic follicles or changes in ovarian weight. Owing to structural similarities to other glycoprotein hormones, initial immunoassays lacked specificity for HCG because antibodies to intact HCG cross-reacted with the alpha-subunit of TSH, FSH, or LH, and antibodies to the beta-subunit of HCG cross-reacted with the beta-subunit of LH. In 1972, Vaitukaitis and associates generated an antiserum, designated SB-6, that is highly specific against purified beta-subunit HCG and used it to develop an immunoassay specific for HCG.[90] Although this assay and many subsequently developed commercial assays are called beta-subunit HCG assays, they measure intact HCG as well as beta-subunit HCG. Recently, more specific assays indicate that HCG is present in three forms: intact HCG, β-HCG, and an 83–amino acid fragment of β-HCG termed the *beta core fragment*.[22] Although intact HCG is the predominant type present in pregnancy, the beta-subunit and the core fragment of the beta-subunit may be predominant in malignancies.[22] The serum half-life of beta HCG is 24 to 36 hours, and the serum half-life of the free beta-subunit is only 45 minutes.

Currently, there are many commercially available immunoassay kits for the measurement of HCG. The sensitivity of these assays is in the range of 1 unit per ml. or 0.2 ng. per ml. The upper limit of normal for circulating HCG is less than 5 to 8 units per ml. for women and less than 3 units per ml. for men.[25]

The application of HCG as a circulating tumor marker ranges from the prototype of an ideal tumor marker for gestational trophoblastic neoplasia[9] and a valuable aid in testicular cancer[6] to a less well defined role in other gynecologic malignancies,[22] uroepithelial tumors,[25] and a spectrum of other solid tumors. HCG is highly sensitive for the diagnosis of choriocarcinoma and the diagnosis of a trophoblastic neoplasm following evacuation of a molar pregnancy.[9] In testicular cancer, 70 to 75 per cent of nonseminomatous tumors and 10 per cent of pure seminomas are associated with elevated serum HCG levels. Serum HCG and AFP levels are very useful as markers to detect the response to therapy and for detection of persistent or recurrent testicular cancer. In addition, the serum levels of HCG are inversely proportional to outcome in patients with testicular cancer.[92]

Serum HCG elevations have been detected in a small proportion of patients with nontrophoblastic, nontesticular neoplasms (60 of 828, 7.2 per cent).[16] Specifically, 20 per cent of patients with bladder cancer,[25] between 13 and 36 per cent of patients with gynecologic cancers including cervical, endometrial, and vulvar cancer, and 5 per cent of patients with ovarian cancer[79] have elevated serum HCG levels. In addition, with newer techniques used to detect the free beta-subunit of HCG and the beta core fragment of HCG, 77 per cent of patients with ovarian and other gynecologic neoplasms have elevated serum HCG levels.[22]

TISSUE POLYPEPTIDE ANTIGEN

Tissue polypeptide antigen (TPA) is a proliferation antigen characterized by Bjorklund in 1957 and evaluated as a general circulating marker for all types of malignancy. TPA was identified by immunizing horses with pooled sera from cancer patients in an effort to locate a common cancer antigen. The horse anticancer serum was then absorbed with normal human tissue and normal sera. From these studies an antigenic determinant immunologically distinct from CEA, AFP, and other tumor markers was identified. Further study demonstrated that TPA was present in all autopsy specimens of malignant tissue regardless of histologic origin. TPA was also present in high concentrations in mature placentas and in fetal tissue including liver, kidney, gastrointestinal tract, and meconium.

The biochemical structure of TPA is not completely defined, but it is in part a 20-Kd protein that is located in the endoplasmic reticulum and plasma membrane of malignant cells.[68] In initial studies of TPA, a hemagglutination assay was used, and in recent work an RIA has been developed.

Abnormal serum levels of TPA (>90 ng. per ml.) have been reported in 50 to 90 per cent of patients with a wide variety of solid and hematologic malignancies (Table 1). Serum levels of TPA have been compared wth serum levels of CEA in patients with epithelial malignancies, and elevations of the two markers do not appear to correlate.[64] Other studies indicate that serum TPA levels offer no advantage over CEA in patients with breast cancer,[68] and serum TPA levels are nonspecific for differentiation of patients with gynecologic tumors.[51] Although used predominantly in Europe and Japan, serum TPA levels are not routinely used to monitor cancer patients in the United States because levels do not appear to offer any advantage over those of other tumor markers.

CA 125

CA 125 is a carbohydrate epitope on a glycoprotein carcinoma antigen that is useful as a serum marker for ovarian cancer. A murine monoclonal antibody was raised against a cultured cell line established from a patient with a serous papillary adenocarcinoma of the ovary.

CA 125 antigen is present in the fetus in derivatives of coelomic epithelium including peritoneum, pleura, pericardium, and amnion. In normal adults, immunohistochemical stains show CA 125 antigen to be present in the epithelium of the fallopian tubes, endometrium, and endocervix. Neither adult nor fetal ovarian epithelium expresses CA 125 activity. Immunoassay kits are available for measurement of CA 125, and normal serum levels are less than 35 units per ml. because only 1 per cent of normal subjects have a value greater than 35 units per ml. (Table 2).[10]

CA 125 antigen is abnormally elevated in the serum of 80 per cent of patients with nonmucinous epithelial ovarian carcinomas.[10] Serum levels of CA 125 correlate directly with tumor bulk. Elevated levels of CA 125 in the serum of patients with occult recurrent disease precedes other clinical signs of recurrent ovarian carcinoma.[69] Serum levels of CA 125 are also elevated in a high percentage of patients with fallopian, endometrial, and endocervical carcinoma.[70]

CA 19–9

CA 19–9 is a carbohydrate antigen that is identified by a monoclonal antibody raised against a colorectal cancer cell line. Serum from patients with colorectal, pancreatic, and gastric cancer can neutralize binding of this monoclonal antibody to its specific cell extracts, suggesting that CA 19–9 is present in the serum of these cancer patients. The antigen is present in normal fetal tissues, including salivary and lacrimal glands, conjunctivae, bronchi, pancreas, esophagus, stomach, small intestine, and gallbladder, but is absent from fetal colon.[73] The carbohydrate epitope may be present in the pancreas, salivary gland, endocervix, and gallbladder of normal adults.

Sensitive immunoassay kits are currently available for measurement of CA 19–9. A study of healthy subjects indicated that normal serum levels of CA 19–9 were less than 35 units per ml. (Table 2).[71] CA 19–9 is a serum marker for the management of patients with gastric, pancreatic, and colorectal cancer.[88] Patients with pancreatitis may also have an elevation of serum CA 19–9 levels. However, in patients with pancreatitis, the serum levels of CA 19–9 seldom exceed 100 units per ml., and patients with pancreatic cancer have higher levels of this marker (73 per cent have a value greater than 100 units per ml.).[40] In managing patients with gastric and colorectal cancer, serum CA 19–9 levels appear to offer no advantage over serum CEA levels.[71]

CA 50

CA 50 is a carbohydrate antigen closely related to CA 19–9 defined by monoclonal antibodies to a colorectal cancer cell line. CA 50 has the same determinants as CA 19–9, but it also has a unique carbohydrate moiety that lacks a fucose residue and is not associated with CA 19–9 activity. Serum levels of CA 50 can be detected in approximately 5 per cent of the population who are Lewis antigen–negative.[59] Serum levels of CA 50 less than 17 units per ml. are normal.

The utility of CA 50 parallels that of CA 19–9. CA 50 antigen is not detectable in normal tissue except the pancreas. CA 50 levels are not elevated in normal serum, but levels are increased in a few patients (less than 12 per cent) with benign liver disease and inflammatory bowel disease and patients with sclerosing cholangitis (Table 2).[38,49,59] Circulating CA 50 is elevated in a significant proportion of patients with colorectal, gastric, liver, biliary, prostatic, lung, and breast cancer.[38,49,59] The clinical utility of CA 50 and its comparison to other markers such as AFP, CEA, and CA 19–9 need further study.

CA 15–3

CA 15–3 is a glycoprotein antigen that serves as a marker for breast cancer. It is identified by two specific monoclonal antibodies that recognize different epitopes on an identical antigen.[45] CA 15–3 is both a differentiation antigen and a milk-related antigen because its production is increased during cell differentiation and it is present in breast milk.[83] The mean value of CA 15–3 in the serum of normal subjects is 13.3 ± 6 units per ml., and over 90 per cent of normal individuals have levels less than 22 units per ml. (Table 2).[45]

Initial clinical studies suggest that CA 15–3 serum levels may help in the management of patients with breast cancer.[45,78] The percentage of patients who have elevated serum levels of CA 15–3 increases with more advanced stage breast cancer. In addition, 66 per cent of patients with breast cancer who have normal serum levels of CEA will have elevated serum levels of CA 15–3.[78]

PROSTATE-SPECIFIC ANTIGEN

Prostate-specific antigen (PSA) is a glycoprotein specific for prostatic tissue with utility as a tumor marker for prostatic cancer. PSA was initially identified by immunizing rabbits with prostate extracts and absorbing the antiserum with normal female sera and nonprostatic tissues. Two immunologically distinct compounds were identified: prostatic acid phosphatase and prostate-specific antigen. PSA has also been used for semen detection during rape investigations.[36]

PSA is a glycoprotein with a molecular weight of 30 kd. that is found only in the cytoplasm of acinar and ductal epithelial cells of the prostate.[36] Functionally, PSA is a kallikrein with serine protease activity that acts primarily on seminal vesicle coagulum as a substrate.[63] A sensitive radioimmunoassay for PSA detects serum levels as low as 100 pg. per ml.[86] Male patients who have undergone radical prostatectomy and female patients have no detectable levels of serum PSA. Greater than 90 per cent of normal men have detectable serum levels of PSA (1.1 ± 0.7 ng. per ml.), and the normal range for men is less than 2.5 ng. per ml.[86]

PSA is a very sensitive marker for prostatic cancer since 96 per cent of patients with very early stage lesions (Stage A) and 100 per cent of patients with more advanced disease have elevated serum levels of PSA.[86] However, 86 per cent of patients with benign prostatic hypertrophy have moderate elevations of serum PSA levels, limiting its ability as a screening test for prostate cancer.[86] The level of the serum marker may also increase following prostatic massage, prostatic biopsy, and transurethral resection.[86]

PROSTATIC ACID PHOSPHATASE

Gutman and Gutman's report more than 50 years ago of elevated levels of acid phosphatase activity in the serum of patients with metastatic prostate cancer was the first identification of a circulating tumor marker.[37] Initial clinical applications were limited by the enzymatic assays used to measure serum acid phosphatase levels. Currently, a radioimmunoassay has improved the ability to measure low serum levels of specific prostatic acid phosphatase (PAP).[55] A recent study of healthy men reported a mean PAP serum level of 1.2 ± 0.5 ng. per ml. and a normal range of less than 2.1 ng. per ml.[86] Acid phosphatase activity detected by enzymatic assay ranges between 0.1 and 0.5 unit per liter in normal subjects with the upper limit of normal range less than 0.8 unit per liter (Table 2).[86]

Prostatic PAP is not a useful circulating tumor marker in patients with prostatic cancer. Although the initial studies using immunometric assays for PAP reported advantages over enzymatic assays, subsequent studies document limitations of serum acid phosphatase measurements using either an immunoassay or a biochemical assay. Specifically, serum PAP level is not useful as a screening test because elevations frequently occur in patients with benign prostatic hypertrophy, and serum levels are not usually elevated in patients with early prostatic cancer or small amounts of residual disease.

NEURON-SPECIFIC ENOLASE

Neuron-specific enolase (NSE) is an acidic isoenzyme of enolase. NSE was initially isolated from bovine brain and reported to be found exclusively in neural tissue. Subsequent studies indicated a high level of NSE in neuroendocrine tissues, the amine precursor uptake and decarboxylation (APUD) cells. NSE was then used as an immunohistochemical marker to identify and study the distribution and development of peripheral neuroendocrine cells.

The development of a specific radioimmunoassay enabled measurement of NSE in the serum of normal subjects and patients with malignant disease originating from neuroendocrine tissues.[20,24] Normal individuals have serum levels between 5 and 10 ng. per ml. (Table 2).[20,24] Study of patients with different neuroendocrine tumors demonstrated elevated serum levels of NSE in patients with pancreatic islet cell tumors, gut carcinoids, adrenal tumors, neuroblastomas, medullary cancer of the thyroid, and small-cell lung cancer. Because additional more specific and sensitive tumor markers exist for most patients with endocrine tumors, serum NSE levels do not help in the management of these patients. However, two recent studies suggest that circulating NSE levels may be a valuable marker for patients with small-cell lung cancer since other good alternative markers are not available.[20,24] Another potential application of serum NSE levels is for management of patients with seminomas because 73 per cent of patients have elevated levels.[60]

FERRITIN

Ferritin is a large storage protein (molecular weight, 450 kd.) composed of multiple identical subunits found in all tissues of the body, with highest concentrations in the liver, spleen, and bone marrow. Serum levels of ferritin directly correlate with total body iron stores. The normal range of serum ferritin levels is between 20 and 300 ng. per ml. with a mean level of 90 ng. per ml. (Table 2).[40] Serum ferritin levels are nonspecific and are elevated in a variety of malignant diseases including lymphoma, leukemia, and colorectal, breast, pancreas, and lung cancer. It is best utilized as a serum tumor marker in patients with hepatoma and reportedly is elevated in a high proportion of patients with normal serum levels of AFP.[67] Recent studies suggest that a related, more acidic tumor-derived ferritin is present in patients with hepatoma. This may explain why ferritin is a good serum marker in patients with hepatoma.[66]

ALPHA₁ – ACID GLYCOPROTEIN

Alpha₁–acid glycoprotein (AGP) is a member of the acute phase serum markers noted to be elevated in some patients with malignancies. AGP is limited as a useful tumor marker because of elevated serum levels in patients with non-neoplastic conditions. Nevertheless, reports using a radioimmunoassay to measure AGP suggest that this compound may be useful as a marker for colorectal cancer and lung cancer, but careful studies to evaluate its utility have not been done.

CYTOKINES

Recent investigations have identified a large number of endogenous peptides collectively known as cytokines that have diverse activities including immune effects, antimicrobial activity, antineoplastic activity, and metabolic effects.[26] Host cytokines may be secreted nonspecifically in response to neoplasms and may act as serum tumor markers. Recent studies suggest that serum levels of interferon[50] and tumor necrosis factor[7] are elevated in patients with cancer. However, these studies are preliminary and cytokines are not characterized well enough to be considered clinical tumor markers at the present time.

PROTON NUCLEAR MAGNETIC RESONANCE

Proton nuclear magnetic resonance (NMR) spectroscopy is a new technology being applied as an imaging technique for malignancies and other conditions.[31] A recent study evaluated NMR as a general blood screening test for the detection of cancer.[30] Proton NMR spectroscopy of serum reflects primarily water protons, but a water-suppressed proton NMR study is predominantly affected by aliphatic lipids of serum lipoproteins. A total of 331 people were studied with water-suppressed proton NMR, and a highly significant alteration in line-width was noted in cancer patients versus normal controls or non-cancer patients.[30] However, pregnant patients or men with benign prostatic hypertrophy had signals similar to patients with malignancies. The ability of this technique to reliably discriminate benign from malignant conditions remains to be defined, but initial studies are promising.

THE ROLE OF SERUM MARKERS IN SPECIFIC TUMORS

HEPATOMA

Hepatocellular carcinoma (HCC) is one of the most malignant and common cancers. The estimated annual world incidence of HCC is 0.3 to 1.2 million, with an apparent rise in frequency in many parts of the world.

One etiologic factor of HCC may be related to prior exposure to aflatoxin and other environmental and chemical agents, but the primary cause of the disease is chronic active liver infection with hepatitis B virus (HBV). In Taiwan, the chance of developing HCC in persons who are hepatitis B antigen (HBsAg)–positive is 233 times greater than in persons who are HBsAg-negative.[11] The use of alpha-fetoprotein as a specific diagnostic marker for HCC and as a means of monitoring response to therapy in patients with HCC has been well established. However, not all patients with HCC have elevated serum levels of AFP, and nearly 40 per cent of patients with HCC may have normal serum levels.[94]

Early Diagnosis

In 1983, a case report was published in the journal *Lancet* demonstrating the feasibility of screening a population at high risk for development of HCC with serial serum levels of alpha-fetoprotein.[46] High rates of primary HCC have been reported in Alaskan natives (Eskimos, Indians, Aleuts), the annual incidence being between 7.6 and 11.2 per 100,000 population. Sera from 24 members of a family with a strong history of HCC were screened every 6 months for HBV markers and AFP. The patient who eventually developed HCC was HBsAg-positive and on initial screening had normal serum levels of AFP (<25 ng. per ml.) (Fig. 1). Two years later serum levels of AFP rose to 104 ng. per ml., and 2 months later levels increased to 667 ng. per ml. Preoperative imaging studies including computed tomography, ultrasound, and selective arteriography failed to image the 2-cm. primary hepatocellular carcinoma that was subsequently removed from the left lobe of the liver. Serum AFP level at discharge from the hospital was 25 ng. per ml., and subsequent follow-up measurements demonstrated a further decline of AFP levels to 5 ng. per ml.[46] This report demonstrates the feasibility of screening populations at risk for development of HCC (patients who are chronic carriers of HBV). It also suggests that simple measurement of serum AFP level can be a sensitive and specific screening method for the early detection of HCC at a stage when surgical intervention can increase survival or provide cure.

Other investigators have tried to use serum AFP levels to detect HCC in at-risk populations with disappointing results. Serum AFP levels may be normal in 35 to 50 per cent of patients with biopsy proven HCC (Table 4).[21] In a minority of patients with HCC, serum levels of AFP will decline despite continued tumor growth, and other patients will have elevated levels of AFP and nonmalignant diseases of the liver (Table 4).

Because patients with cirrhosis of the liver are at risk for developing HCC, serum levels of AFP have been used in this group to diagnose HCC. Elevations of serum AFP levels are seen in approximately 85 per cent of patients who have HCC

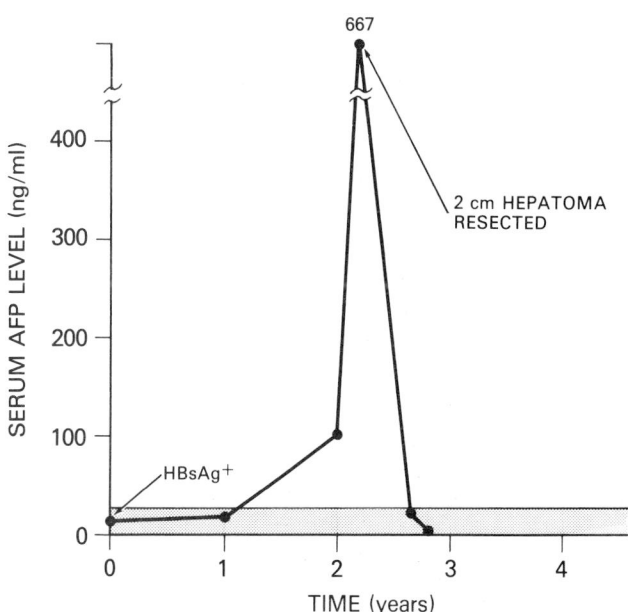

Figure 1. Alaskan native who was at risk for the development of hepatocellular carcinoma because of his family history and the fact that he was hepatitis B antigen (HBsAg) positive. He was followed with yearly serum alpha-fetoprotein (AFP) levels, which remained within the normal range (shaded area). After 2 years of follow-up, his serum AFP level was elevated at 104 ng. per ml.; repeat level 1 month later was further increased to 667 ng. per ml. Despite negative preoperative imaging, exploratory laparotomy demonstrated a 2-cm. hepatoma, which was resected. Postoperative serum levels of AFP declined to normal range.

TABLE 4. The Role of Serum Markers in the Management of Patients with Hepatocellular Carcinoma (HCC)

Marker	Screening and Early Diagnosis	Percentage of True Positives	Percentage of False-Negatives	Following Treatment	Comments
Alpha-fetoprotein (AFP)	Useful if positive but may have false-negatives	80 (60–90)	20 (10–40)	Correlates with tumor response but may decline falsely	Serum levels vary inversely with prognosis Patients with cirrhosis and active hepatitis may have falsely elevated AFP Levels >500 ng./ml. diagnostic False-negatives may approach 40%
PIVKA-II	Not useful	65	40	Correlates with tumor response	Elevated in some patients with HCC and normal serum AFP levels
Vitamin B_{12}–binding capacity	Not useful	55	50	Does not correlate with tumor response	May be useful only in fibrolamellar variant of HCC
CA 50	Not useful	64	40	No information	Experimental

within a cirrhotic liver. In patients with cirrhosis without hepatocellular carcinoma, only 5 per cent have elevated serum AFP levels, but in one series 40 per cent of patients with this diagnosis had elevated levels. These false-positive results usually occur in patients with cirrhosis and chronic active hepatitis, a condition in which the need for distinction from HCC seldom arises. In a recent prospective study of the ability to detect HCC in 450 patients with cirrhosis, the sensitivity and specificity of results were dependent on the definition of normal serum AFP level. If a serum AFP level greater than 10 ng. per ml. was chosen as abnormal, the sensitivity was 86 per cent and the specificity was 91 per cent. If the abnormal level was defined at greater than 500 ng. per ml., then sensitivity decreased to 62 per cent and specificity increased to 100 per cent. Thus, a serum AFP level greater than 500 ng. per ml. in the presence of cirrhosis was diagnostic for HCC.[52]

Prognosis

Serum levels of AFP in patients with HCC may be of prognostic value. The subgroup of patients who have HCC and normal serum levels of AFP appears to have a relatively good prognosis. In these patients, the primary factor predicting better prognosis may be the absence of cirrhosis. Normal serum AFP levels are more common in patients without underlying cirrhosis. A rapid AFP doubling time is also associated with a poorer prognosis (Table 4).

Tumor Recurrence

Resection of HCC in patients with HCC and cirrhosis has resulted in 2-year survival of 60 per cent and 5-year survival of 33 per cent.[53] Although the results after initial resection of patients with HCC are improving because of AFP-directed earlier tumor detection, the long-term survival after resection needs additional improvement because of tumor recurrence. In the management of 41 patients who underwent curative resection of HCC and developed recurrent HCC following resection, serial serum measurement of AFP levels was the best detector of recurrent disease. It was the first measured abnormality in 34 per cent, and imaging studies including ultrasound and CT were less sensitive than serum AFP level, 17 and 2 per cent respectively. However, in some patients who had elevated serum levels of AFP with their original HCC, postoperative levels of serum AFP were unreliable to detect recurrence because 5 of 41

patients (12 per cent) did not have elevated serum levels despite recurrent HCC.[54]

Serial measurement of serum AFP level can be helpful before and after presumably curative surgical therapy in patients with HCC. However, the serum levels of this tumor marker do not always show the presence of recurrent HCC. HCC may be recurrent despite normal serum AFP levels. There is variation in AFP synthesis in different parts of the same tumor. The ability of the tumor to secrete AFP may change with growth. It may be that tumor recurrences within the liver are really new primary tumors with different characteristics.[2]

Following Treatment Response

In the absence of effective anti-tumor therapy, serum AFP levels rise exponentially, the doubling time being approximately 40 days (the range is 6 to 120 days; poorer prognosis tumors have a more rapid AFP doubling time). Following complete resection of all hepatoma, AFP levels drop with a half-life of 4 days and should remain less than 10 ng. per ml. if all tumor has been removed (Fig. 1). Spontaneous regression of serum AFP level has been reported in some patients with HCC despite the persistence of tumor.[21] This event is unusual but did occur in 4 of 17 patients with metastatic HCC in whom serum AFP levels were carefully followed.[21] Serum AFP levels also decline with use of effective chemotherapy. This permits rapid *in vivo* testing of a particular chemotherapeutic regimen. If a given chemotherapy is effective, serum AFP levels fall continuously, indicating tumor regression and effective treatment. If serum AFP levels demonstrate a continued rise despite anti-tumor treatment, the tumor is resistant to the treatment and an alternative regimen should be used. Monitoring of serum AFP levels in patients with HCC avoids prolonged ineffective use of potentially toxic chemotherapy.

Serial estimation of serum AFP level in patients with metastatic or recurrent HCC is valuable in monitoring response to therapy (Table 4). However, some patients may have spontaneous regression of serum AFP levels without tumor imaging changes, and others—especially those without underlying cirrhosis—may have normal serum AFP levels despite disease. Another tumor marker that could be used to diagnose correctly and that would correlate with the extent of HCC would have value in some patients. AFP for HCC, like CEA for colon cancer, remains a good but not ideal marker.

Other Markers

Abnormal prothrombin, that is, protein induced by vitamin K absence or antagonist-II (PIVKA-II) is a tumor marker for hepatocellular carcinoma (Table 4). Patients with various liver diseases other than HCC had normal or slightly elevated levels of plasma PIVKA-II. In 63 patients with HCC, 52 of 63 (83 per cent) had elevated serum levels of AFP, whereas 41 of 63 (65 per cent) had elevated plasma levels of PIVKA-II. Some patients with HCC and normal serum AFP levels had elevated plasma PIVKA-II levels. Plasma PIVKA-II levels increased with disease progression and decreased after surgical resection of the tumor. Plasma PIVKA-II levels may be useful to diagnose and monitor therapy in patients with HCC and low serum AFP levels (Table 4).[33]

In patients with fibrolamellar hepatocellular carcinoma, serum levels of AFP may be normal and serum vitamin B_{12}-binding capacity levels may be markedly increased and mirror progressive or regressive disease following treatment. In a more recent study of patients with all types of HCC, 7 of 11 (64 per cent) patients had elevated serum AFP levels and 6 of 11 (55 per cent) patients had elevated serum B_{12} levels including elevated levels in 3 patients with normal AFP levels. However, in 4 patients with elevated serum B_{12} levels treated with chemotherapy, levels did not appear to reflect other parameters of disease status (Table 4).[17]

A similar nonspecific marker for HCC is serum ferritin level, which is elevated in 97 per cent of patients with HCC but is also elevated in 87 per cent of patients with uncomplicated cirrhosis. Serum ferritin levels rose in 85 per cent of patients who showed no clinical response to therapy and decreased in patients who responded to therapy. Serum ferritin levels do not appear to have a role in the differential diagnosis of HCC but may have a role in monitoring response to therapy of patients who are AFP-negative.

CA 50 is a carbohydrate antigen that is elevated in patients with cholangiocarcinomas, hepatocellular carcinomas, and metastatic carcinomas to the liver. In one recent study, circulating CA 50 levels were elevated in 14 of 22 (64 per cent) patients with HCC.[38] In a prospective comparison with AFP, serum levels of CA 50 antigen were elevated in 6 of 11 patients with HCC (55 per cent) whereas AFP levels were elevated in 9 of the same 11 patients (82 per cent).[59] AFP appears to be a better marker than CA 50 for HCC (Table 4).

COLORECTAL CANCER

Carcinoembryonic antigen has been studied as a marker of colorectal tumors for the past 2 decades. Although CEA is not colorectal tumor–specific, the highest concentrations in tissue and serum are found in patients with colorectal carcinoma. Tissue CEA concentrations and presumably CEA production vary in different tumors by up to 800-fold. Even when colorectal tumors have high concentrations of CEA, serum values are not always raised, possibly because of poor access from the tumor to the circulation or rapid clearance.[13]

Early Diagnosis

Serum CEA determinations are not useful in screening normal populations of adults for colorectal cancer (Table 5). Elevated CEA levels occur in only 5 per cent of patients with localized surgically curable colon cancer and 65 to 90 per cent of patients with either distant or locally advanced disease (Table 3), as well as some patients with noncancerous conditions produced by cigarette smoking or pulmonary inflammation (Table 2).[87] Therefore, serum CEA levels are only marginally useful in detecting early stage colon carcinomas, since benign unrelated conditions are the cause of most elevated CEA levels detected when serum CEA levels are used for screening.[13]

TABLE 5. Clinical Utility of Serum CEA Levels in Patients with Colorectal Cancer

Question	Answer	Comment
Early diagnosis?	No	Few patients (5%) with localized disease have elevated levels
Prognosis?	Yes	Higher levels have poorer prognosis
Detect recurrence?	Yes	67–79% of patients have elevated serum levels prior to or at the time of recurrence
Second-look procedures based on CEA?	Yes	All tumor can be removed in 60–70% of patients for an overall 5-year survival of 30% Radioimmunolocalization with CEA antibodies under investigation
Follow treatment response?	Yes	In 90% of patients serum CEA levels accurately reflect disease progression or regression

Screening of patients with conditions such as ulcerative colitis and polyposis coli that predispose to colorectal cancer has also been unsuccessful because these diseases may themselves produce elevated serum levels of CEA. Although benign polyps may cause slight elevations of serum CEA levels, levels exceeding five times normal are consistent with carcinoma. Measurement of serum CEA levels in a patient who presents with a suspicious polypoid lesion has been recommended by some clinicians, but most prefer colonoscopy and biopsy to obtain a definitive diagnosis.

Prognosis

Several reports have indicated that the preoperative serum CEA concentration prior to definitive resection of primary colorectal cancer is an independent prognostic parameter of subsequent survival, that is, the higher the serum CEA level, the poorer the prognosis of a given colorectal cancer (Fig. 2). The prognostic significance of the preoperative serum CEA level was still evident when selected subgroups were stratified for resectability and extent of local tumor involvement.[85] This information should be used when stratifying trials of adjuvant therapy after primary tumor resection, and when suggesting which individual patients may benefit from adjuvant therapy (Table 5).[13]

Tumor Recurrence

Surgical re-resection is the only method of treatment offering a significant chance of long-term survival to patients with recurrent colorectal cancer after apparently curative resection of the primary tumor.[6] Elevated serum CEA levels indicate recurrent colorectal cancer usually 4 to 6 months before it is clinically evident. In one study of 171 patients who developed proven or suggestive recurrence, 114 (67 per cent) had a prior rise in the serum CEA level, and in an additional 21 patients (total of 135 patients or 79 per cent) the serum CEA level rose simultaneously with recurrence (Table 5). The pattern of rise or the magnitude of rise of serum CEA level was of no practical value in distinguishing localized from distant disease.[48] It is important to note that in some studies some patients may have an elevation of serum CEA level on a single determination that subsequently returns to normal levels on another determination. Elevated serum CEA levels should be verified by repeating the analysis on a second or third occasion. In general, serum CEA level will be elevated in approximately 2 of 3 patients before any other evidence of recurrent colon or rectal cancer. Serum CEA levels need not have been raised preoperatively to be elevated postoperatively as a marker of tumor recurrence following resection.

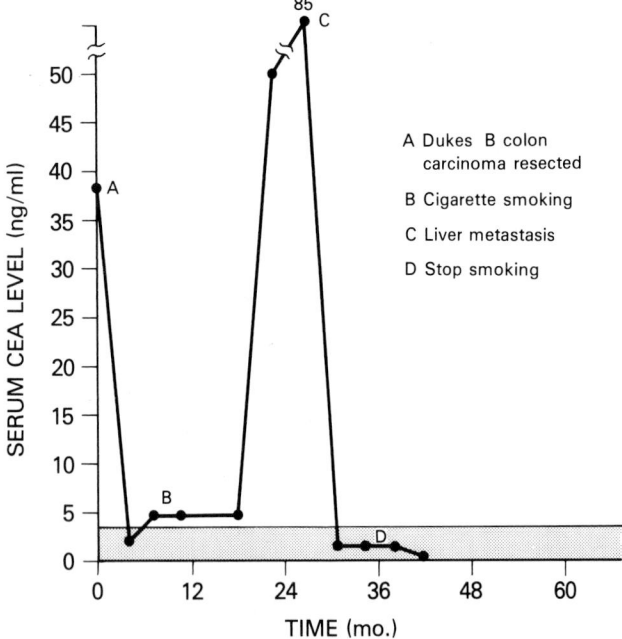

Figure 2. Patient who presented with a Dukes B colon carcinoma and an elevated serum level of carcinoembryonic antigen (CEA) (point A). The primary tumor was resected, and postoperative serum CEA levels dropped to the normal range (shaded area). The patient became a cigarette smoker and levels increased to minimally abnormal levels (point B). Approximately 2 years following his primary resection, the patient developed markedly elevated serum levels of CEA. Computed tomography of the chest and abdomen demonstrated a solitary liver metastasis (point C). This lesion was resected and the patient quit smoking. Postoperatively, serum CEA levels dropped to the normal range (point D).

If serial serum CEA levels rise following resection of primary colorectal carcinoma, the clinician is faced with a dilemma of how to treat tumor that is not clinically evident. One study of patients in this category randomized them to chemotherapy with 5-fluorouracil and methyl CCNU versus follow-up and therapy when clinical indications arose. Overall, there were no significant differences between the two groups with respect to disease-free interval and overall survival, indicating that CEA-initiated chemotherapy was of no benefit.[47] Because there is no dramatic effective therapy for nonimageable colorectal carcinoma, second-look exploratory operation with resection of recurrent disease has been used by many groups. Results of CEA-initiated second-look procedures vary among different groups with one group reporting ability to remove all tumor in 70 per cent of patients and others finding no benefit (Fig. 2). This strategy of reoperation can provide cure for a small percentage of patients (10 to 20 per cent) and document recurrent colorectal carcinoma in a majority of patients (80 per cent) who can then graduate to other therapies. In Martin and associates' large experience, second-look operation was initiated in approximately 20 per cent of patients with colorectal cancer who were followed postoperatively with serial serum CEA levels; in nearly 60 per cent of these patients, a complete surgical re-resection was possible and the 5-year survival in this group was over 30 per cent.[65] Others have performed second-look procedures based on elevated serum CEA levels and found that the actuarial 5-year survival rate was 33 per cent (Table 5).

Potential improvement in selection of patients and results for CEA-initiated second-look procedures may be achieved through better preoperative demonstration of the location and extent of disease. A new method is the use of radiolabeled antibody to CEA and external scintigraphy to detect the exact location and extent of recurrent tumor. Patients with localized, resectable recurrent disease can then be selected for second-look operation. In preliminary reports,[14] this method of radioimmunolocalization appears promising, and labeled monoclonal antibodies to tumor antigens are being developed to potentially image and treat tumor. Systemic preoperative imaging of patients with ¹¹¹In-labeled anti-CEA monoclonal antibody in one study detected 69 per cent of primary tumors and 42 per cent of liver metastases.[12] A more recent study showed increased sensitivity and ability to accurately image colorectal hepatic metastases; 80 per cent of lesions were imaged when 40 mg. of ¹¹¹In-anti-CEA monoclonal antibody was used.[75] Although these results probably represent the best possible current data for imaging with CEA-directed monoclonal antibodies, these data do not sufficiently establish this technique as standard in the management of patients with colorectal cancer. However, future methodologic improvements are likely to upgrade monoclonal antibody imaging of tumor antigens, making it sensitive, specific, and cost-effective.

Following Treatment Response

Serum CEA levels appear to correlate fairly well with disease extent in patients with colorectal cancer. Serum levels usually rise with progression and fall with disease regression, but once markedly elevated do not always correlate directly with tumor burden. Serum CEA levels have been used to follow the response to chemotherapy in patients with metastatic colorectal cancer. In patients with metastatic colorectal carcinoma who had elevated serum CEA levels and responded to chemotherapy, 89 per cent showed a decrease in serum CEA level. In patients who had progressive disease despite chemotherapy, 90 per cent had an increase in serum CEA level compared with pretreatment level (Table 5). The survival of patients with colorectal carcinoma who had a decrease in CEA level during chemotherapy was also significantly longer. In patients with other gastrointestinal cancers, changes in CEA levels do not correlate as well with clinical response as for patients with colorectal carcinoma.

Other Markers

Recently developed tumor antigens have been utilized to monitor tumor response in patients with colorectal carcinoma. These newer antigens include tissue polypeptide antigen, CA 19–9, and CA 125. In cancerous colon tissues, levels of both CEA and CA 19–9 antigens are significantly greater than levels in normal tissues; however, there are no differences in CA 125 levels (which has been primarily useful in epithelial ovarian cancers).[80] Direct comparison of these tumor markers in serum indicates that serum CEA levels are still the most useful clinical marker in patients with colorectal carcinoma. CEA has the greatest sensitivity to predict recurrent disease, and combinations of all markers do not increase sensitivity. Serum CEA level was the best individual predictor of recurrent colorectal cancer (sensitivity, 90 per cent) compared with TPA (sensitivity, 60 per cent) and CA 19–9 or CA 125 (sensitivity, 20 per cent). The specificity of serum CEA determinations was 78 per cent primarily because other benign and malignant processes (false-positives) can result in elevated serum CEA levels.[32] The commercial availability of CEA plus its sensitivity makes it the marker of choice to monitor response of disease to therapy in patients with colorectal carcinoma.

TESTICULAR GERM-CELL NEOPLASMS

Testicular cancers are relatively rare neoplasms with an incidence of 2.2 per 100,000 population and comprising only 2 per cent of malignant tumors in men.[4] These neoplasms do, however, affect young men in the prime of life, and testicular cancer is the most common cancer killer in men between the ages of 29 and 35.[4] The only known predisposing factor is a history of cryptorchidism, which increases the risk of developing testicular cancer from 10- to 1000-fold.[4]

Diagnosis and histologic classification of testicular germ-cell neoplasms have been advanced by the development of sensitive and specific assays to quantitatively measure elevated serum levels of the tumor markers alpha-fetoprotein and human chorionic gonadotropin, and immunohistochemical techniques to detect their presence in tissue specimens.

Diagnosis

Seventy-five of 101 patients (75 per cent) with proven nonseminomatous testicular germ-cell tumors had an increased serum AFP level (Table 6).[4] Most of these patients (75 per cent) had serum AFP levels greater than 40 ng. per ml. and less than 2000 ng. per ml. Seventy-three of these patients also had elevated serum HCG levels. More recent studies indicate that the incidence of elevated serum levels of beta-HCG in patients with nonseminomatous testicular neoplasms is lower, between 40 and 60 per cent. In addition, approximately 10 per cent of patients with pure seminoma also have elevated serum HCG levels.

If both markers are measured, 89 per cent of patients with nonseminomatous testicular cancer have an elevation of one or both serum markers.[4] The determination of both marker levels is very important, since nearly half of these tumors secrete only one substance. In addition to the high rate of marker positivity, there have been very few cases of spuriously elevated serum levels of HCG or AFP in patients with testicular cancer.

The value of preoperative serum HCG or AFP level to guide initial surgical therapy in a patient with a testicular mass lesion is limited. The presence of an elevated serum HCG and/or AFP level prior to orchiectomy makes the diagnosis of testicular cancer likely. However, most seminomas and nearly one third of other testicular tumors are marker-negative; therefore, the absence of elevated serum markers does not alter the necessity to perform a biopsy. In addition, patients who are marker-positive and become marker-negative following orchiectomy cannot be presumed to be disease-free, because a small percentage will have positive retroperitoneal lymph nodes at lymphadenectomy. The decision whether to perform lymphadenectomy should not be based solely on marker status, but serum marker status is helpful in following patients after operation both in detecting persistent or recurrent disease and in following response to therapy.

Neuron-specific enolase may be a useful serum marker in patients with seminoma (Table 6). Increased serum NSE activity was detected in 8 of 11 (73 per cent) patients with metastatic seminoma, whereas only 6 of 40 (15 per cent) patients with nonseminomatous testicular cancer had elevated levels.[60] NSE is a new marker for patients with metastatic seminoma, and because it is shed into the bloodstream as tumor cells are lysed, it may be able to monitor response to therapy in these patients.

Prognosis

Since specific tumor markers such as HCG and AFP are secreted by distinct clones of cells, serum tumor marker levels may be useful in identifying biologically distinct categories of morphologically similar tumors,[92] and marker levels may be a reflector of tumor virulence. This hypothesis was supported by examining the outcome of patients treated with similar regimens based on pretreatment serum levels of either AFP or HCG. Complete remissions occurred in 92 per cent of patients with both normal HCG and AFP levels, in 26 per cent of patients with elevated AFP only, in 46 per cent of patients with elevated HCG only, and in 35 per cent of patients (13 of 36) with elevations of both HCG and AFP. Patients with very high serum AFP or HCG levels responded very poorly to chemotherapy. It was noted that higher serum marker levels were seen in patients with larger tumor burdens, and the poor prognosis of elevated serum marker levels may simply represent extent of disease. Surgical therapy eliminated the correlation between the "poor prognostic factors" associated with specific marker elevations and could convert an incomplete response with chemotherapy alone to a complete response by resection of residual tumor.[92]

When patients are categorized by amount of advanced metastatic testicular cancer, the proportion of favorable responders is greater in patients with normal serum markers (99 per cent) compared with patients with markedly elevated serum markers (58 per cent). This finding in a separate group of patients stratified for extent and amount of disease also suggests that level of serum marker has a negative impact on prognosis.[15] Patients with similar tumor burdens and elevated serum HCG or AFP levels appear to do worse than patients with normal serum levels. This observation bears important prognostic information for individual patients and should be considered when clinical trials are designed. Therapeutic options in patients with testicular cancer should be modified based on tumor histology, extent of disease on imaging studies, and presence or absence of serum tumor markers.[81]

Tumor Recurrence and Following Treatment Response

The serial measurement of serum AFP and HCG level by radioimmunoassay appears to be very useful in monitoring the effectiveness of therapy in patients with nonseminomatous germ-cell tumors. In a small percentage of patients with metastatic testicular cancer, there is no response to chemotherapy, and the serum AFP and HCG levels progressively rise until death. In a larger percentage of patients, AFP and HCG serum levels drop into the normal range and remain in the normal range throughout the period of observation. These patients also have no tumor on imaging studies and HCG and AFP serum levels accurately predict no tumor recurrence. In a small group of patients (6 per cent), tumor masses do not regress during chemotherapy, but serum AFP and HCG levels decline to normal levels. Subsequent surgical resection of persistent mass lesions demonstrates tumor conversion to mature teratoma. The most interesting group is patients with no radiologic evidence of disease who have elevated serum levels of HCG or AFP. In one study, 28 of 34 patients had elevated serum marker levels following induction chemotherapy and no patient had any radiographic evidence of persistent disease. Each patient had clinically documented recurrent testicular cancer within a 2- to 14-month period of observation.[4] Although false-negative HCG or AFP estimations of testicular cancer occur between 10

TABLE 6. Serum Markers in the Diagnosis and Management of Testicular Cancer

Tissue Diagnosis	Percentage of Patients With				
	Elevated Serum HCG Level	Elevated Serum AFP Level	Elevated Serum AFP or HCG Level	Neither Elevated	Elevated Serum NSE Level
Nonseminomatous testicular cancer	40–60	75	89	10*	15
Seminoma	10	0	10	90	73

* Prognosis is better if neither serum HCG nor AFP is elevated.

and 15 per cent of the time, false-positive levels in patients followed with testicular cancer have not been noted. These studies indicate that serum levels of HCG and AFP are of great value in following the treatment of patients with testicular germ-cell neoplasms, especially patients without other evidence of disease. Newer urinary immunoassays for beta-HCG may further enhance the utility of this marker and its use in different cancerous diseases.[72]

Other Markers

The other markers for nonseminomatous testicular germ-cell neoplasms do not compare with HCG and AFP for sensitivity and specificity. In patients with known testicular cancer, 19 of 23 had elevated serum levels of either HCG or AFP or both, whereas only 6 of 20 had elevated serum neopterin levels.[61]

In patients with pure seminomas of the testis, measurement of serum HCG and AFP levels is not helpful. However, approximately 10 per cent of patients with seminoma have elevated serum levels of either HCG or AFP. If levels of these peptides are elevated, it indicates that the testicular tumor is not a pure seminoma. Serum neuron-specific enolase activity is abnormal in 73 per cent of patients with metastatic seminoma, and levels return to normal following successful therapy. Only 15 per cent of patients with metastatic nonseminomatous germ-cell neoplasms of the testis have elevated serum levels of NSE activity. Serum NSE activity is a new marker for patients with seminoma, and levels appear to accurately reflect response to therapy.[60]

GYNECOLOGIC CANCER

EPITHELIAL OVARIAN CANCER

Epithelial ovarian carcinomas are among the malignant diseases that respond to treatment with cytoreductive surgical therapy, radiotherapy, and cytotoxic chemotherapy. Monitoring the response to treatment has been difficult because these neoplasms often metastasize to peritoneal surfaces and form small metastatic nodules that cannot be detected by imaging studies. Medical oncologists have demanded restaging laparotomies that may be hazardous in the presence of tumor and multiple adhesions from prior surgical procedures. A glycoprotein antigen, CA 125, has been recognized that is associated with epithelial ovarian cancer and has been detected in the serum of patients with these neoplasms.[10]

Early Diagnosis

Elevated serum CA 125 levels (>35 units per ml.) were detected in 50 to 96 per cent of patients with nonmucinous epithelial ovarian carcinoma confined to the pelvis (Table 7).[19,56] A patient has been identified recently in whom serum CA 125 levels were elevated 12 months prior to the clinical diagnosis of Stage II ovarian cancer.[9] At diagnosis, 61 per cent of patients with Stage I or Stage II disease have serum levels greater than 35 units per ml. and 50 per cent have levels greater than 50 units per ml.[9] This finding suggests that measurement of CA 125 in the serum may be useful in the diagnosis of an ovarian mass lesion detected by physical examination or pelvic ultrasound. However, determination of CA 125 levels in the serum of patients with ovarian masses usually does not make the diagnosis of ovarian cancer.[8]

Ninety-nine per cent of normal subjects have serum levels of CA 125 less than 35 units per ml. Eighty-three per cent of patients with surgically proven ovarian cancer have elevated serum levels (Table 7). Elevations have also been found in the serum of patients with carcinomas of the endometrium, endocervix, fallopian tube, pancreas, stomach, liver, bile duct, lung, breast, and colon. Elevations of serum CA 125 levels also have been found in benign conditions including pregnancy, menstruation, endometriosis, pelvic inflammatory disease, pancreatitis, hepatitis, and renal failure (see Table 2).[9]

Following Treatment Response and Monitoring Recurrent Disease

Approximately 25 studies from different cancer centers have reported the use of serum CA 125 levels to monitor response of ovarian cancer to treatment and to detect recurrent disease following conclusion of treatment.[9] The newer studies have confirmed the original report[10] that serum CA 125 levels are elevated in approximately 80 to 85 per cent of patients with ovarian cancer. If abnormal, serum CA 125 levels have corre-

TABLE 7. New Promising Serum Markers that May Be Useful for the Diagnosis and Management of Cancer

Type of Malignancy	Marker	Percentage of Patients with Elevated Serum Levels	Comments
Ovarian cancer	CA 125	80–85	Changing levels correlate with tumor response Normalization of elevated levels does not allow discontinuation of therapy 40% of patients with Stage I disease have normal serum levels
Granulosa-cell tumors of the ovary	Inhibin	100	Granulosa-cell tumors produce inhibin Serum levels reflect size of tumor Useful as marker for primary as well as recurrent disease
Pancreatic cancer	CA 19–9	82–96	Able to distinguish benign from malignant diseases of the pancreas and biliary tree 78% sensitivity 75% specificity
Pancreatic cancer	CA 50	81	Able to distinguish benign from malignant diseases of the pancreas and biliary tree
Breast cancer	CA 15–3	73	Correlates with extent of disease Not specific for breast cancer Cannot distinguish whether localized breast disease is benign or malignant

lated with disease progression or regression in 80 to 95 per cent of cases.[9] New elevations of serum CA 125 levels have preceded clinical detection of recurrent ovarian cancer by a median time of 3 months. Elevation of serum CA 125 levels at the time of second-look procedures for ovarian cancer predicts that disease is present approximately 90 per cent of the time. However, CA 125 levels may return to normal and second-look operation still documents the presence of residual disease in 60 per cent of cases.[9] This finding of high false-negative rate indicates that one cannot withdraw chemotherapy based on a normal serum CA 125 level because over half of these patients still have persistent disease at laparotomy. If however, serum levels of CA 125 remain elevated during chemotherapy, there is a 90 per cent chance the patient has persistent disease, so additional therapy can be given without laparotomy.

CA 125 levels in peritoneal fluid washings may be more sensitive than serum levels and results may remain elevated with smaller amounts of residual disease. Therefore, if serum levels become normal during treatment, perhaps peritoneal fluid levels can distinguish the patients with persistent disease from those who are truly without disease.[3] Peritoneal fluid levels in normals were less than 200 units per ml., whereas most patients with ovarian cancer have levels greater than 200 units per ml.[3]

Another potential utility of CA 125 levels is the rate of decline of the antigen in the serum of patients with treated ovarian cancer. If all tumor is removed, serum CA 125 levels decline with a half-life of 4.5 days.[19] In patients with elevated serum levels of CA 125, levels should decline to less than 35 units per ml. within 3 months of the initiation of treatment. Of patients whose serum CA 125 levels failed to drop below 35 units per ml. after 3 months of treatment or remained persistently elevated despite treatment, nearly all had documented disease at laparotomy.[19]

Other Markers

Carcinoembryonic antigen, HCG, and tissue polypeptide antigen have also been used to predict disease extent or presence in patients with epithelial ovarian cancer. Serum levels of neither CEA nor HCG have any utility as tumor markers in ovarian carcinoma.[74] However, the utility of TPA and serum levels of CA 125 in monitoring ovarian cancer is confirmed. In one study, 86 per cent of patients with active ovarian cancer had an elevation of serum CA 125 levels and 76 per cent of patients had an elevation of TPA levels.[74] Moreover, for patients in clinical remission, the simultaneous measurement of TPA and CA 125 antigen in the serum revealed recurrent disease in more patients than either antigen alone, although CA 125 was the single better marker.[74]

Investigators have shown that a small population of subjects with nontrophoblastic gynecologic cancers have elevated serum levels of HCG, but only about 18 per cent of women with epithelial ovarian cancer have elevated levels. A recent study measuring urinary HCG fragments and subfragments in patients with gynecologic malignancies demonstrated that 73 per cent of patients with ovarian cancer had elevated levels of urinary gonadotropin fragments (UGF).[22] By stage, 50, 62, 75, 86, and 100 per cent of those patients with Stage I, II, III, or IV or recurrent disease, respectively, had elevated levels. The study suggests that UGF may be a promising new marker of ovarian and other gynecologic cancers.[22]

With the technology of monoclonal antibodies directed toward cancer antigens, two specific new antigens, TAG 72.3 and CA 15–3, have been developed that may add to the efficacy of determining CA 125 alone. In two independent studies of serum from patients with pelvic masses, determination of CA 125, TAG 72.3, and CA 15–3 in combination improved the sensitivity of CA 125 alone.[27,84] It may be that simultaneous measurements of multiple antigens in cancer patients will improve results compared with individual antigens alone. How-

ever, these results are preliminary, and, at present, CA 125 remains the marker of choice for epithelial ovarian cancer.

GRANULOSA-CELL TUMORS OF THE OVARY

Inhibin is a peptide hormone that is normally produced by ovarian granulosa cells. It can be detected at peak levels in the serum of women during the follicular phase of the menstrual cycle and it is undetectable in the serum of postmenopausal women. Peak serum levels in normal menstruating women are 770 units per liter. In patients with recurrent or persistent granulosa-cell tumor of the ovary, levels can exceed 3000 units per liter (Table 7).[62] It can become elevated in the serum prior to other clinical signs of detectable disease. After removal of tumor, serum inhibin levels become normal. Levels of inhibin are more sensitive for detection of disease than are levels of estradiol, the other proposed hormonal marker for these tumors. Serum inhibin levels accurately reflect the amount of tumor and can be used as a circulating marker for primary as well as recurrent disease.[62]

GESTATIONAL TROPHOBLASTIC NEOPLASIA AND GERM-CELL OVARIAN CANCER

With the rare exception of germ-cell tumors, HCG is generally produced by benign or cancerous trophoblastic cells. If pregnancy can be excluded, HCG is a specific and sensitive serum marker for trophoblastic tumors in women. Immunologic assays for β-HCG are very sensitive for the early detection of trophoblastic tumors. Only 10,000 tumor cells are required to produce a detectable level of HCG in serum.

Normalization of serum HCG levels has been used to confirm complete evacuation of benign gestational trophoblastic tumors including molar pregnancy. An increase or abnormal elevation of serum HCG levels following evacuation of an apparently benign tumor, an abortion, or a termination of a normal pregnancy can indicate the presence of a malignant trophoblastic tumor. Absolute serum levels of HCG distinguish good prognosis gestational cancers (<40,000 mIU per ml.) from poor prognosis cancers (>40,000 mIU per ml.).[9] Serum inhibin levels have also been suggested as a useful marker for hydatidiform mole. Serum inhibin levels are generally much higher in women with hydatidiform moles than in women with normal pregnancies.[95]

HCG is an excellent serum marker for diagnosis and detection of germ-cell ovarian cancers including choriocarcinomas and embryonal carcinomas. Sensitivity is approximately 50 per cent for these tumors and specificity nearly 100 per cent. Serum AFP levels may be elevated in ovarian embryonal carcinomas but will not be elevated in pure ovarian choriocarcinomas. Both serum AFP and HCG levels should be measured to document presence of tumor, to follow response to therapy, and to detect recurrence.[9]

Following Treatment Response

With effective treatment of malignant gestational trophoblastic cancer, the serum half-life of HCG is 36 hours, and the levels should decrease by 20 to 25 per cent following each treatment cycle.[42] Any plateau or increase in serum HCG level demands alternative therapy. Three consecutive serum HCG levels less than 5 mIU per ml. are diagnostic of complete remission. These levels should be obtained every month for 3 months before complete remission has been achieved.

The utility of HCG in the treatment of malignant gestational trophoblastic cancers is amplified because of the sensitivity of these tumors to aggressive chemotherapy. Recurrent elevations or plateau levels of serum HCG levels have prompted changing chemotherapeutic agents. The availability of a sensitive, specific marker as well as effective chemotherapy has provided an 80 to 100 per cent cure rate for patients with a previously uniformly fatal cancer.[42]

PANCREATIC CANCER

The incidence of pancreatic carcinoma is rising in the United States with an estimated 20,000 new cases each year. Early diagnosis of pancreatic cancer has been a major problem. Imaging studies such as computed tomography or endoscopic retrograde cholangiopancreatography have not improved detection of the disease. A specific blood marker could lead to earlier initiation of potentially curative treatment.[77]

CA 19–9 is a circulating marker that has sensitivity and specificity for pancreatic carcinoma. Initial work indicated that CA 19–9 was undetectable in the serum of normal subjects and patients with extragastrointestinal tumors or nonmalignant diseases. Patients with colorectal, stomach, and pancreatic cancer may have high levels of CA 19–9 in their serum.[58] Subsequently, studies indicate that the marker has its greatest utility in the diagnosis and management of patients with pancreatic cancer (Table 7).[5,77]

Diagnosis

Eighty-two per cent of patients with pancreatic cancer have elevated serum levels of CA 19–9, whereas few patients with pancreatitis, gallstones, or sclerosing cholangitis have elevated levels.[44] In addition, 89 per cent of patients with carcinoma of the gallbladder and 100 per cent of patients with carcinoma of the bile duct have elevated serum levels.[44] Another group demonstrated that serum levels of CA 19–9 were abnormally elevated in 5 of 121 patients with chronic pancreatitis (4 per cent), 7 of 30 patients with acute pancreatitis (23 per cent), and 82 of 99 patients with pancreatic cancer (85 per cent).[77] Measurement of the antigen in serum appears to reliably differentiate benign from malignant diseases of the pancreas and biliary tree.

In a direct comparison among CA 19–9, CA 125, and CEA as tumor markers for pancreatic cancer,[39] CA 19–9 had the greatest sensitivity (78 per cent) compared with approximately 50 per cent for CA 125 and CEA. Each had comparable specificity of 78 per cent. The addition of multiple tests (CA 19–9 and CA 125) increased the sensitivity by only 6 per cent.[39] From this and other comparisons,[44] it appears that serum CA 19–9 level currently is the best marker for pancreatic cancer.

However, serum CA 19–9 levels may be elevated in patients with other cancers including colorectal (15 per cent), stomach (5 per cent), bile ducts (95 per cent), hepatoma (7 per cent), lung (13 per cent), and ovary (2 per cent). In addition, it may be elevated in some patients with benign gastrointestinal diseases including pancreatitis (5 per cent), hepatitis (1 per cent), and cirrhosis (3 per cent).[5] Occurrence of these potential false-positive results explains why specificity of this marker is 75 per cent for the diagnosis of pancreatic cancer.

Following Treatment Response

Levels of the serum marker CA 19–9 in patients with pancreatic cancer do appear to correlate with amount of disease and therefore can be used to follow treatment response. In one series, 4 patients with known resected pancreatic cancer who were being followed without clinical evidence of disease had serum levels less than 17 IE per liter. Most patients with disease localized to the pancreas and without metastases had levels that were elevated (>120 IE per liter) but were not as elevated as those with documented metastatic disease.[44] Because presently there is no effective treatment for pancreatic carcinoma, evaluation of the serum marker's ability to reflect response to treatment is impossible. Although it appears that serum CA 19–9 levels do reflect extent of disease, better testing must await effective treatment modalities.

Monoclonal antibodies to the carbohydrate antigen CA 19–9 have been used to treat patients with pancreatic cancer. The trials are currently ongoing, but preliminary results indicate minimal efficacy.

Other Markers

CEA has been measured in patients with pancreatic cancer, and it is not a useful marker because it is elevated in only 45 to 65 per cent of patients with known cancer.[39,44] However, another recently identified carbohydrate antigen, CA 50, does show promise as a serum marker in patients with pancreatic cancer (Table 7). If the upper limit of normal for serum CA 50 level is defined as not exceeding 100 KU per liter, 81 per cent of patients with known pancreatic cancer have elevated levels and similar percentages of patients with biliary cancers have elevated serum levels. In addition, like CA 19–9, serum levels of CA 50 discriminate benign from malignant diseases of the pancreas and biliary tree, because patients with pancreatitis, gallstones, and/or sclerosing cholangitis have normal serum levels of CA 50.[44] Serum CA 50 levels show capability similar to that of serum CA 19–9 levels in diagnosis of pancreatic and biliary cancers. Both markers are still under investigation, but more studies with CA 19–9 have already been performed. That is why it appears to be the single best marker for pancreatic carcinoma. However, preliminary investigations and reports do demonstrate that CA 50 is comparable.[44]

BREAST CANCER

Breast cancer is the second leading cause of death from cancer in women, ranking below carcinoma of the lung. Each year approximately 120,000 newly diagnosed cases of breast cancer occur in the United States and nearly one third will be fatal. One in 10 women in this country will develop breast cancer. The mainstay of early diagnosis of breast cancer is self or physician examination and mammography. Serum markers are being developed, but their current clinical utility is limited.

Carcinoembryonic Antigen and Gross Cystic Disease Fluid Protein

CEA serum levels are normal in 98 per cent of patients with localized breast cancer and 60 per cent of patients with metastatic breast cancer. When serum levels are elevated and continue to rise on subsequent determination, nearly all (98 per cent) patients with breast cancer have metastatic disease. Serum CEA levels are elevated in only 20 per cent of patients with primary breast cancer, and the CEA-positive patients appear to have a significantly poorer prognosis. Serum levels of CEA and another marker called gross cystic disease fluid protein (CDP) can reflect increasing or decreasing tumor burden during therapy of metastatic breast cancer. Serum levels of CDP in patients with metastatic breast cancer are elevated in only 40 per cent of patients.

Neither serum CEA nor CDP levels are clinically useful markers for breast cancer. Neither can help with the early diagnosis of a breast mass. Because of widespread availability, CEA levels may be helpful in following treatment response in patients with metastatic breast carcinoma who have elevated serum levels.

CA 15–3

CA 15–3 is a recently described circulating antigen expressed by human breast carcinoma cells (Table 7). Recent studies have determined the percentage of patients with breast carcinoma with elevated serum levels of the antigen CA 15–3. Of 1050 normal subjects, serum from 99 (9 per cent) had CA 15–3 antigen levels greater than 22 units per ml. In contrast, 115 of 158 (73 per cent) patients with metastatic breast cancer had levels greater than 22 units per ml. Fifty per cent of patients with nodal metastases, 79 per cent of patients with bone metastases, and 83 per cent of patients with liver metastases had elevated serum levels of the antigen, so a greater percentage of patients with more advanced disease had elevated levels. Significantly, more patients in this population with breast cancer had elevated serum levels of CA 15–3 than of CEA. However, serum levels of CA 15–3 were elevated in some patients (20 per cent) with benign breast lesions and in some patients with other cancers (44 per cent of patients with gastrointestinal cancers, 71 per cent with lung cancer, and 66 per cent with epithelial ovarian cancer). Serum levels appear to correlate with and reflect either tumor progression or regression.[45] These results indicate that although nonspecific, CA 19–3 may have potential as a serum marker for diagnosing and evaluating treatment response in patients with metastatic breast carcinoma.

Another study using a greater serum level of CA 15–3 (40 units per ml.) to define the normal range had fewer false-positive results (0 per cent for control subjects, 1.5 per cent for patients with benign breast disease, and 6.5 per cent for other cancers) but, as expected, detected elevated circulating levels of the marker in fewer patients with localized disease (6 per cent of patients with Stage II disease) and all of 22 patients with Stage IV breast carcinoma. Following therapy, serum CA 15–3 levels were significantly different in patients without evidence of disease, patients with stable disease, and patients with progressive disease. However, in some individual patients, serum antigen levels did not appear to follow clinical response since 20 of 34 patients with objective responses had abnormally elevated serum levels including patients with complete response.[23] The results indicate that CA 15–3 serum levels do correlate with the stage of breast cancer and the response to therapy, but results in individual patients may be at variance with this general observation.

Finally, the most recent study by Pons-Anicet and associates corroborates the other two studies and identifies CA 15–3 as the most promising serum marker for patients with breast cancer.[78] This serum antigen was not useful for early diagnosis since only 16 per cent of patients with Stage I breast cancer had elevated serum levels (>25 units per ml.). As extent of disease progressed, more and more patients had elevated serum levels of CA 15–3: 54 per cent with Stage II disease, and 91 per cent with Stage III and IV disease. In addition, 70 of 100 women with metastatic breast cancer and normal serum levels of CEA had elevated serum levels of CA 15–3.[78]

The new marker CA 15–3 appears to be a promising recent advancement for the management of patients with breast cancer. Most patients with advanced or metastatic breast carcinoma have elevated serum levels, and in most patients serum levels accurately reflect response to therapy. However, it will not be useful for the early diagnosis of breast cancer in the normal population of women or women with breast masses, because few patients with localized breast cancer have elevated serum levels and a percentage of patients with benign breast disease have elevated serum levels. Finally, in some patients, despite documented metastatic breast carcinoma, serum levels of CA 15–3 are normal and in some patients serum levels do not accurately reflect disease response (or lack of it) to therapy.

LUNG CANCER

NON–SMALL-CELL LUNG CANCER

There are no clinically useful circulating markers for the management of patients with bronchogenic carcinoma. In a recent study of 100 patients with biopsy proven bronchogenic cancer, serum markers including CEA, TPA, CA 19–9, and combinations had less than 56 per cent sensitivity for the diagnosis of lung cancer. In addition, no marker had a diagnostic accuracy of 50 per cent.[18]

SMALL-CELL LUNG CANCER

Among the various histologic types of lung cancer, small-cell lung cancer (SCLC) has a number of unique characteristics. It is a very malignant tumor, rapidly proliferating with a clear tend-ency for early metastatic spread. Recent advances in chemotherapy and radiation therapy of SCLC have improved the outlook of patients with this tumor and dramatic responses have been documented during therapy. However, durable complete remissions are rare. Early diagnosis of persistent or recurrent disease is desirable to either alter or intensify therapeutic regimens. The need for reliable, sensitive serum markers for SCLC is apparent, since they can help guide therapeutic decisions.

Neuron-Specific Enolase

Serum levels of neuron-specific enolase, a glycolytic enzyme produced by neuroendocrine cells of the peripheral and central nervous system, have been shown to be elevated in newly diagnosed patients with SCLC. In the original report,[20] 15 of 38 (39 per cent) patients with limited disease and 49 of 56 (87 per cent) patients with extensive disease had elevated serum levels of NSE. Overall, 69 per cent of all patients with proven SCLC had elevated serum levels of NSE, and serial measurements in 23 patients receiving combination chemotherapy demonstrated an excellent correlation between serum NSE levels and clinical response. Cell lines established from 10 of the patients in the study each expressed high levels of NSE in the media.[20] Additional studies indicate that between 80 and 98 per cent of patients with extensive small-cell lung cancer have elevated levels of NSE in the serum, and approximately 55 per cent of patients with limited disease have elevated serum levels.[43] In addition, elevated levels of neuron-specific enolase in the cerebrospinal fluid (CSF) appear to indicate either parenchymal central nervous system metastases or meningeal carcinomatosis. CSF levels of NSE were elevated in 54 per cent of patients with brain parenchymal SCLC and 95 per cent of patients with meningeal carcinomatosis. The only other CSF marker with comparable percentages was ACTH, which was elevated in 85 per cent of patients with CNS metastases in one study.[43] Since as many as 50 per cent of patients with SCLC present with CNS disease, CSF levels of markers may be helpful in documenting extent of disease.

At present, serum neuron-specific enolase levels appear to be the best serum marker for patients with small-cell lung cancer. In comparison studies, it has the greatest sensitivity and specificity.[28] It is elevated in nearly all patients with progressive, metastatic SCLC and it appears to correlate well with response to therapy. However, its ability to establish with certainty no residual disease is poor because in some studies 50 to 70 per cent of patients with minimal disease have normal serum NSE levels. Therefore, one cannot withdraw therapy based on a normal serum NSE level, but one can fairly reliably document poor treatment response and alter therapy based on progressive serial elevations of serum NSE levels.

Other Markers

Many different hormonal peptides have been measured in the serum of patients with small-cell lung cancer. The most common hormone markers in these patients include calcitonin, adrenocorticotropic hormone (ACTH), antidiuretic hormone (ADH), melanocyte-stimulating hormone (MSH), oxytocin, parathyroid hormone (PTH), insulin, gastrin, glucagon, secretin, vasoactive intestinal peptide (VIP), growth hormone, and bombesin. The number of patients with small-cell lung cancer in whom serum levels of an individual hormone or marker were measured and the number who had elevated circulating levels is shown in Table 8. Serum calcitonin levels appear to be elevated in a significant percentage (59 per cent) of patients with SCLC. Calcitonin levels in these patients do not increase with provocative agents such as pentagastrin and/or calcium. Inappropriate ADH levels have been associated clinically with lung cancer, and 65 per cent of patients with small-cell lung cancer have elevated serum levels of ADH. Serum ACTH levels are important in these patients, because some patients present with

TABLE 8. Serum Markers and Hormones in Patients with Known Small-Cell Lung Cancer

Marker or Hormone	Total Number of Patients	Number of Patients with Elevated Serum Levels (%)
NSE	119	80(67)
Calcitonin	425	251(59)
ACTH	252	68(27)
ADH	103	67(65)
Oxytocin	61	18(30)
Gastrin	69	14(20)
MSH	43	8(19)
PTH	100	31(31)
Insulin	65	3(5)
Glucagon	46	5(11)
Secretin	46	0(0)
Growth hormone	46	4(9)
VIP	46	0(0)
Bombesin	28	2(7)
CEA	72	32(44)
TPA	22	12(55)
Ferritin	23	12(52)
AGP	60	54(90)
LDH	46	27(59)

Cushing's syndrome. These lung tumors are the most common cause of ectopic ACTH syndrome in most series, and 27 per cent of patients with SCLC have elevated serum ACTH levels.[43] In addition, it should be recognized that most radioimmunoassays for ACTH will cross-react with MSH and vice versa, and some patients with elevated MSH levels (19 per cent of patients with SCLC) may really have elevated ACTH levels. Finally, it is clear that because of the neuroendocrine origin of these tumors they may secrete any hormone, which may result in significant symptoms but, if recognized, also can result in a useful serum marker for a specific individual patient.

Other serum markers in patients with small-cell lung cancer include alpha$_1$–acid glycoprotein (AGP), carcinoembryonic antigen, and lactate dehydrogenase (LDH). These markers are not specific and therefore have not been used to establish the diagnosis of SCLC. They may be indicative of the presence of disease and have been used to follow treatment response. Of these serum markers, AGP is the best. It is elevated in 54 of 60 (90 per cent) patients with disease present, whereas CEA and LDH are elevated in only 52 and 59 per cent of patients, respectively.[34] In addition, the pair of serum markers (AGP and LDH) were used to correctly classify 37 patients in whom both serum measurements were obtained including 4 patients who were incorrectly classified with AGP alone. Each of the markers correctly tracked

TABLE 9. Serum and Urinary Markers for Diagnosis and Follow-up of Patients with Endocrine Neoplasms

Organ	Disease	Marker	Body Fluid	Special Test (stimulation or suppression)	Result	Diagnosis	Follow-up
Thyroid	Well-differentiated thyroid cancer	Thyroglobulin	Serum	None	Elevated levels indicate disease	Nonspecific but used to diagnose malignancy in patients with radiation exposure	Useful for follow-up of patients following thyroidectomy or radioactive iodine ablation
Thyroid	Medullary carcinoma[b,d]	Calcitonin	Serum	Pentagastrin/calcium test	CT levels increase	Sensitive, specific stimulation test	Sensitive, specific follow-up marker reflects tumor burden
Parathyroid	Hyperparathyroidism	Calcium, PTH, cAMP	Serum and urine	None	Elevated calcium and elevated PTH level and elevated UcAMP level	Sensitive Specific	Carcinoma is rare, but PTH and UcAMP are sensitive markers of persistent or recurrent disease
Adrenal cortex	Adrenal cancer	Cortisol[a]	Serum and urine	Dexamethasone suppression CRH stimulation	No change in cortisol levels	Sensitive but not specific for cancer; must rule out other causes of Cushing's syndrome	Urinary 17 OHCS and free cortisol usually reflects disease but some tumors dedifferentiate
Adrenal medulla	Pheochromocytoma[b,d]	Norepinephrine Epinephrine Catecholamines VMA, metanephrine	Serum and urine	Clonidine suppression	No change in serum epinephrine or norepinephrine with clonidine	Specific Sensitive	May be malignant; careful follow-up, urinary catecholamines important
Pancreatic islet cell	Gastrinoma (ZES)[b,c]	Gastrin	Serum Stomach acid	Secretin test	Increased gastrin level Elevated acid output	Specific Sensitive	Useful but may not accurately reflect tumor volume
	Insulinoma[b,c]	Insulin	Serum	Fast	Insulin levels still elevated with hypoglycemia	Sensitive Specific	Most benign, only 10% malignant
	Glucagonoma[b,c]	Glucagon	Serum	None	Elevated glucagon levels	Specific	Malignant
	VIPoma[b,c]	VIP	Serum	None	Elevated VIP levels	Specific	Malignant (note: any pancreatic islet cell tumor may secrete pancreatic polypeptide, which can be used for a marker)
Pancreas Testis Ovary Bronchus GI tract	Carcinoid[b,c,d]	Serotonin 5-HIAA (hydroxyindole acetic acid)	Urine	None	Elevated levels	73% sensitivity 100% specificity	Levels reflect tumor mass

[a] Adrenal cortical carcinomas may secrete androgens or aldosterone, which, if elevated, serve as marker substances. [b] Neuron-specific enolase is produced by nearly all neuroendocrine tumors and can be used as a serum marker. [c] Pancreatic polypeptide may be used as a serum marker in patients with pancreatic islet cell tumors but its sensitivity is only 45 per cent. [d] L-Dopa decarboxylase and/or chromogranin A have been measured in tissue extracts of these tumors and may be useful as a circulating marker, although studies are currently ongoing and not completed.

the clinical response to therapy in 2 of 3 patients in whom an individual marker was elevated at diagnosis.[34]

Detection of Central Nervous System Involvement

With an increase in the median survival of patients with SCLC, there is an increase in the frequency of CNS metastases. Despite careful neurologic evaluation, cytologic and biochemical evaluation of cerebrospinal fluid, and careful computed tomography or magnetic resonance imaging of the brain and spinal cord, 20 to 50 per cent of parenchymal and meningeal metastases are not diagnosed until death and autopsy.[76] Greater than 20 per cent of 2-year survivors with SCLC develop meningeal carcinomatosis that is difficult to diagnose because 50 per cent of patients with this disease have negative CSF cytologic findings for cancer cells.[76]

As previously mentioned, CSF levels of neuron-specific enolase is one proven method to document CNS involvement with SCLC since 71 per cent of individuals have elevated CSF levels. CSF levels of bombesin and calcitonin may also be helpful. CSF bombesin levels were detectable in 7 per cent of SCLC patients without CNS involvement, 21 per cent of patients with parenchymal involvement, and 78 per cent of patients with meningeal carcinomatosis.[76] In addition, 53 per cent of patients with meningeal carcinomatosis and 48 per cent with parenchymal SCLC had CSF calcitonin levels greater than 18 fmol. per ml., whereas only 7 per cent without CNS disease had these levels. Sixty-seven per cent of all patients with CNS involvement by SCLC had elevated CSF levels of either bombesin or calcitonin. Thus, in SCLC patients, an elevated CSF level of calcitonin or NSE suggests CNS metastases, and an elevated bombesin level suggests meningeal carcinomatosis.[76]

ENDOCRINE NEOPLASMS

In general, endocrine neoplasms secrete hormones that serve as serum markers of the tumor. The hormones secreted are measured in the serum or urine by radioimmunoassay, and elevated levels are diagnostic of specific tumors. A complete list of endocrine neoplasms and their marker serum hormones is given in Table 9. If an individual tumor is malignant and recurs or progresses, serum or urinary hormone levels reflect tumor burden and increase as tumor mass increases and decrease as tumor mass decreases. It is beyond the scope of this chapter to consider all endocrine tumors; rather the reader is referred to Table 9 and other chapters for specific serum or urinary markers.

SUMMARY

Serum markers have changed the diagnosis and management of patients with testicular, hepatocellular, trophoblastic, colonic, and endocrine neoplasms. New serum markers may have similar impact on patients with ovarian, pancreatic, breast, small-cell lung, and biliary cancer. Recent advances in technology may provide additional malignant tumor markers in the immediate future. This work updates the current status of available serum markers and provides the reader with the necessary background information to make decisions based on results of individual markers, in individual diseases and individual patients.

SELECTED REFERENCES

Anderson, T., Waldmann, T. A., Javadpour, N., and Glatstein, E.: Testicular germ-cell neoplasms: Recent advances in diagnosis and therapy. Ann. Intern. Med., *90*:373, 1979.
Although 12 years old, this paper describes the use of serum levels of alpha-feto-protein (AFP) and human chorionic gonadotropin HCG in the management of patients with testicular germ-cell neoplasms. The authors have a large experience in the management of these patients and they define the use of these serum markers

to make treatment decisions. Serum levels of HCG and/or AFP are elevated in 85 to 90 per cent of patients with nonseminomatous testicular cancer. Elevated serum levels reflect tumor presence and reliably indicate response to therapy. The reader who wants valuable information about the management of these patients should read this reference.

Begent, R. H.: The value of carcinoembryonic antigen in clinical practice. Br. J. Hosp. Med., April: 335, 1987.
This is an excellent article that carefully updates the potential of serum carcinoembryonic antigen levels in the management of patients with colorectal cancer. It especially suggests specific management questions in which serum CEA levels can be used in decision analysis. It also describes radioimmunolocalization of primary and metastatic tumor using isotopic scanning with radiolabeled CEA monoclonal antibodies.

Cole, L. A., Wang, Y., Elliott, M., Latif, M., Chambers, J. T., Chambers, S. K., and Shwartz, P. E.: Urinary human chorionic gonadotropin free β-subunit and β-core fragment: A new marker of gynecological cancers. Cancer Res., *48*:1356, 1988.
This article describes the use of urinary gonadotropin fragments (UGF) that include human chorionic gonadotropin (HCG), free β-subunit, and β-core fragment as serum markers for women with gynecologic cancers. In the past, only 13 to 36 per cent of patients with non-trophoblastic gynecologic cancers have had elevated serum levels of HCG, but in this study in which UGF fragments are measured, over 70 per cent of patients have elevated serum levels. These results are very promising and suggest that UGF is an important new marker of gynecologic cancer. Of course, the antigen CA 125 is the single best serum marker to document disease in patients with epithelial ovarian cancer.

Harmenberg, U., Wahren, B., and Wiechel, K. L.: Tumor markers carbohydrate antigens CA 19–9 and CA–50 and carcinoembryonic antigen in pancreatic cancer and benign diseases of the pancreaticobiliary tract. Cancer Res., *48*:1985, 1988.
This is a careful, comprehensive study of sera from patients with pancreatic and biliary diseases as well as healthy normal subjects. Importantly, serum levels of CA 19–9 and CA–50 can discriminate malignant from benign diseases of these organs. In general, the two tumor marker results are similar except in approximately 20 per cent of patients in whom the results may be complementary. In addition, serum levels of each antigen can also be used to follow response to therapy. The studies suggest that serum levels of CA 19–9 or CA–50 are useful circulating markers for pancreatic and biliary cancer.

Kanematsu, T., Matsumata, T., Takenaka, K., Yoshida, Y., Higashi, H., and Sugimachi, K.: Clinical management of recurrent hepatocellular carcinoma after primary resection. Br. J. Surg., *75*:203, 1988.
This article carefully documents the use of serum alpha-fetoprotein (AFP) levels to document recurrent hepatocellular carcinoma (HCC) following successful initial excision to remove the primary tumor in 121 patients wih primary HCC. Sixty-six per cent of 41 patients with documented recurrent HCC had elevated serum AFP levels at the time of detection of recurrent disease. However, 12 per cent of patients who had elevated serum AFP levels at the time of initial operation did not have elevated levels at the time of recurrence. Serum AFP levels will be helpful to detect recurrent tumor in most, but not all, patients with recurrent HCC.

REFERENCES

1. Abelev, G. I., Perova, S. D., Khramkova, N. I., et al.: Production of embryonal α-globulin by transplantable mouse hepatomas. Transplantation, *1*:174, 1963.
2. Ackerman, N. B., Nallathambi, M. N., Patel, K. R., et al.: Second hepatoma developing 13 years after resection of first tumor. Arch. Surg., *121*:726, 1986.
3. Allegra, C. J., Fine, R. L., Behrens, B. C., et al.: CA 125 antigen levels in peritoneal lavage fluid: A useful staging tool in ovarian carcinoma. Proc. Am. Soc. Clin. Oncol., *5*:118, 1986.
4. Anderson, T., Waldmann, T. A., Javadpour, N., and Glatstein, E.: Testicular germ-cell neoplasms: Recent advances in diagnosis and therapy. Ann. Intern. Med. *90*:373, 1979.
5. Andriulli, A., Gindro, T., Piantino, P., et al.: Prospective evaluation of the diagnostic efficacy of CA 19–9 assay as a marker for gastrointestinal cancers. Digestion, *33*:26, 1986.
6. August, D. A., Ottow, R. T., and Sugarbaker, P. H.: Clinical perspective of human colorectal cancer metastasis. Cancer Metastasis Rev., *3*:303, 1984.
7. Balkwill, F., Burke, F., Talbot, N., et al.: Evidence for tumor necrosis factor/cachectin production in cancer. Lancet 2:1229, 1987.
8. Barber, H. R.: Ovarian cancer: Cause, diagnosis and treatment. Comp. Ther., *13*:25, 1987.
9. Bast, R. C., Jr., Hunter, V., and Knapp, R. C.: Pros and cons of gynecologic tumor markers. Cancer, *60*:1984, 1987.
10. Bast, R. C., Jr., Klug, T. L., St. John, E., et al.: A radioimmunoassay using a monoclonal antibody to monitor the course of epithelial ovarian cancer. N. Engl. J. Med., *390*:883, 1983.
11. Beasley, R. P., Hwang, L. Y., Lin, C. C., et al.: Hepatocellular carcinoma and hepatitis B virus: A prospective study of 22,707 men in Taiwan. Lancet, 2:1129, 1981.
12. Beatty, J. D., Duda, R. B., and Williams, L. E.: Preoperative imaging of colorectal carcinoma with [III]In-labeled anticarcinoembryonic antigen monoclonal antibody. Cancer Res., *46*:6494, 1986.

13. Begent, R. H. J.: The value of carcinoembryonic antigen in clinical practice. Br. J. Hosp. Med., April: 335, 1987.
14. Begent, R. H. J., Keep, P. A., Searle, F., et al.: Radioimmunolocalisation and selection for surgery in recurrent colorectal cancer. Br. J. Surg., 73:64, 1986.
15. Birch, R., Williams, S., Cone, A., et al.: Prognostic factors for favorable outcome in disseminated germ cell tumors. J. Clin. Oncol., 4:400, 1987.
16. Braunstein, G. D., Vaitukaitis, J. L., Carbone, P. O., et al.: Ectopic production of human chorionic gonadotropin by neoplasms. Ann. Intern. Med., 78:39, 1973.
17. Buamah, P. K., James, O. F. W., Skillen, A. W., and Harris, A. L.: Serum vitamin B12 levels in patients with primary hepatocellular carcinoma during treatment with CB 3717. J. Surg. Oncol., 34:100, 1987.
18. Bucceri, G. F., Ferrigno, D., Sartoris, A. M., et al.: Tumor markers in bronchogenic carcinoma. Cancer, 60:42, 1987.
19. Canney, P. A., Moore, M., Wilkinson, P. M., and James, R. D.: Ovarian cancer antigen CA 125: A prospective clinical assessment of its role as a tumor marker. Br. J. Cancer, 50:765, 1984.
20. Carney, D. N., Ihde, D. C., Cohen, M. H., et al.: Serum neuron-specific enolase: A marker for disease extent and response to therapy in small-cell lung cancer. Lancet 1:583, 1982.
21. Chen, D. S., Juei-Low, S., Sheu, J. C., et al.: Serum α-fetoprotein in the early stage of human hepatocellular carcinoma. Gastroenterology, 86:1404, 1984.
22. Cole, L. A., Wang, Y., Elliott, M., et al.: Urinary human chorionic gonadotropin free B-subunit and B-core fragment: A new marker of gynecological cancer. Cancer Res 48:1356, 1988.
23. Colomer, R., Ruibal, A., Navarro, M., et al.: Circulating CA 15.3 levels in breast cancer. Our present experience. Int. J. Biol. Markers, 2:89, 1986.
24. Cooper, E. H., Splinter, T. A. W., Brown, D. A., et al.: Evaluation of a radioimmunoassay for neuron-specific enolase in small cell lung cancer. Br. J. Cancer, 52:333, 1985.
25. Dexeas, F., Logothetis, C., Hosson F., and Samuels M. L.: Carcinoembryonic antigen and beta-human chorionic gonadotropin as serum markers for advanced urothelial malignancies. J. Urol., 136:403, 1986.
26. Dinarello, C. A., and Mier, J. W.: Lymphokines. N. Engl. J. Med. 317:940, 1987.
27. Einhorn, N., Zurawaski, V. R., Knapp, R. C., and Bast, R. C. Jr.: Preoperative elevation of CA 125, CA 72 and 15–3 in patients with nonmucinous epithelial ovarian cancer. Proc. Am. Assoc. Can. Res., 28:357, 1987.
28. Fischbach, W., and Jany, B.: Neuron-specific enolase in the diagnosis and therapy monitoring of lung cancer: A comparison with CEA, TPA, ferritin and calcitonin. Int. J. Biol. Markers, 1:129, 1986.
29. Fletcher, R. H.: Carcinoembryonic antigen. Ann. Intern. Med., 104:66, 1986.
30. Fossel, E. T., Carr, J. M., and McDonagh, J.: Detection of malignant tumors: Water suppressed proton nuclear magnetic resonance spectroscopy of plasma. N. Engl. J. Med., 315:1369, 1986.
31. Fossel, E. T., Brodsky, G., DeLayre, J. L., et al.: Nuclear magnetic resonance for the differentiation of benign and malignant breast tissues and axillary lymph nodes. Ann. Surg. 198:541, 1983.
32. Fucini, C., Tommasi, S. M., Rosi, S., et al.: Follow-up of colorectal cancer resected for cure. Dis. Colon Rectum, 30:273, 1987.
33. Fujiyama, S., Morishita, T., Sagara, K., et al.: Clinical evaluation of plasma abnormal prothrombin (PIVKA–II) in patients with hepatocellular carcinoma. Hepatogastroenterology, 33:201, 1986.
34. Ganz, P. A., Ma, P. Y., Wang, H. J., and Elashoff, R. M.: Evaluation of three biochemical markers for serially monitoring the therapy of small-cell lung cancer J. Clin. Oncol., 5:472, 1987.
35. Gold, P., and Freedman, S. O.: Demonstration of tumor-specific antigens in human colonic carcinoma by imunological tolerance and absorption techniques. J. Exp. Med., 122:647, 1965.
36. Graves, H. C. B., Sensabaugh, G. F., and Blake, E. T.: Postcoital detection of a male specific semen protein. N. Engl. J. Med., 312:328, 1985.
37. Gutman, A. B., and Gutman, E. B.: An "acid" phosphatase occuring in the serum of patients with metastasizing carcinoma of the prostate gland. J. Clin. Invest., 17:473, 1938.
38. Habib, N. A., Hershman, M. J., Smudju, C., et al.: The use of CA–50 radioimmunoassay inhibition test in the differential diagnosis of benign and malignant liver diseases. Br. J. Surg., 73:758, 1986.
39. Haglund, C.: Tumour marker antigen CA 125 in pancreatic cancer: A comparison with CA 19–9 and CEA. Br. J. Cancer, 54:897, 1986.
40. Haglund, C., Roberts, P. J., Kuusela, P., et al.: Evaluation of CA 19–9 as a serum tumor marker in pancreatic cancer. Br. J. Cancer, 53:197, 1986.
41. Hammarstrom, S., Engvoll, E., Johansson, B. G., et al.: Nature of the tumor-associated determinants of carcinoembryonic antigen. Proc. Natl. Acad. Sci. USA, 72:1528, 1975.
42. Hammond, C. B., and Soper, J. T.: Poor-prognosis metastatic gestational trophoblastic neoplasia. Clin. Obstet. Gynecol. 27:228, 1984.
43. Hansen, M., and Pedersen, A. G.: Tumor markers in patients with lung cancer. Chest, 89:2195, 1986.
44. Harmenberg, U., Wahren, B., and Wiechel, K. L.: Tumor markers carbohydrate antigens CA 19–9 and CA–50 and carcinoembronic antigen in pancreatic cancer and benign diseases of the pancreaticobiliary tract. Cancer Res., 48:1985, 1988.
45. Hayes, D., Zurawski, V. R., and Kufe, D. W.: Comparison of circulating CA 15–3 and carcinoembryonic antigen levels in patients with breast cancer. J. Clin. Oncol., 4:1542, 1986.
46. Heyward, W. L., Lanier, A. P., Bender, T. R., et al.: Early detection of primary hepatocellular carcinoma by screening for alpha-fetoprotein in high-risk families. Lancet, 2:1161, 1983.
47. Hine, K. R., and Dykes, P. W.: Prospective randomized trial of early cytotoxic therapy for recurrent colorectal carcinoma detected by serum CEA. Gut 25:682, 1984.
48. Hine, K. R., and Dykes, P. W.: Serum CEA testing in the post-operative surveillance of colorectal carcinoma. Br. J. Cancer, 49:689, 1984.
49. Holmgren, J., Lindholm, L., Persson, B., et al.: Detection by monoclonal antibody of carbohydrate antigen CA 50 in serum of patients with carcinoma. Br. Med. J., 288:1479, 1984.
50. Horn, Y., Zeidman, J. L., Heller, A., et al.: Serum interferon as a biological marker in malignant tumors. Oncology, 42:164, 1985.
51. Inoue, M., Inoue, Y., Hiramatsu, K., and Ueda, G.: The clinical value of tissue polypeptide antigen in patients with gynecologic tumors. Cancer, 55:2618, 1985.
52. Johnson, P. J.: Tumour markers in the diagnosis and management of patients with hepatocellular carcinoma. Recent Results Cancer Res. 100:68, 1986.
53. Kanematsu, T., Takenaka, K., Matsumata, T., et al.: Limited hepatic resection effective for selected cirrhotic patients with primary liver cancer. Ann. Surg., 199:51, 1984.
54. Kanematsu, T., Matsumata, T., Takenaka, K., et al.: Clinical management of recurrent hepatocellular carcinoma after primary resection. Br. J. Surg., 75:203, 1988.
55. Killian, C. S., Emrich, L. J., Vargas, F. P., Yang, N., et al.: Relative reliability of five serially measured markers for prognosis of progression in prostate cancer. J. Natl. Cancer Inst., 76:179, 1986.
56. Kivinen, S., Kuoppala, T., Leppilampi, M., et al.: Tumor-associated antigen CA 125 before and during the treatment of ovarian carcinoma. Obstet. Gynecol. 67:468, 1986.
57. Kohler, G., and Milstein, C.: Continuous cultures of fused cells secreting antibodies of predicted specificity. Nature, 250:495, 1975.
58. Koprowski, H., Herlyn M., Steplewski, Z., and Sears, H. F.: Specific antigen in serum of patients with colon carcinoma. Science, 212:53, 1981.
59. Kuusela, P., Haglund, C., Roberts, P. J., and Jalanko, H.: Comparison of CA–50, a new tumour marker, with carcinoembryonic antigen (CEA) and alpha-fetoprotein (AFP) in patients with gastrointestinal diseases. Br. J. Cancer, 55:673, 1987.
60. Kuzmits, R., Schernthaner, G., and Krisch, K.: Serum neuron-specific enolase, a marker for response to therapy in seminoma. Cancer, 60:1017, 1987.
61. Kuzmits, R., Ludwig, H., Legenstein, E., et al.: Neopterin as tumour marker: Serum and urinary neopterin concentrations in malignant diseases. J. Clin. Chem. Clin. Biochem., 24:119, 1986.
62. Lappohn, R. E., Burger, H. G., Bouma, J., et al.: Inhibin as a marker for granulosa-cell tumors. N. Engl. J. Med., 321:790, 1989.
63. Lilja, H.: A kallikrein-like serum protease in prostatic fluid cleaves the predominant seminal vesicle protein. J. Clin. Invest., 76:1899, 1985.
64. Luthgens, M., and Schlegel, G.: Combined use of carcinoembryonic antigen in oncologic therapy and surveillance. Cancer Detect. Prev. 6:51, 1983.
65. Martin, E. W. Jr., Minton, J. P., and Carey, L. C.: CEA-directed second-look surgery in the asymptomatic patient after primary resection of colorectal carcinoma. Ann. Surg., 202:310, 1985.
66. Nagasue, N., Yukuya, H., Chang, Y., and Ogawa, Y.: Serum ferritin after resection of hepatocellular carcinoma. Cancer, 57:1820, 1986.
67. Nakano, S., Kumoda, T., Sugiyama, K., et al.: Clinical significance of serum ferritin determination for hepatocellular carcinoma. Am. J. Gastroenterol., 79:623, 1984.
68. Nemoto, T., Constantine, R., and Chu, T. M.: Human tissue polypeptide antigen in breast cancer. J. Natl. Cancer Inst., 63:1347, 1979.
69. Niloff, J. M., Bast, R. C., Schaetzl, E. M., and Knapp. R. C.: Predictive value of CA 125 antigen levels in second-look procedures for ovarian cancer. Am. J. Obstet. Gynecol., 151:981, 1985.
70. Niloff, J. M., Klug, T. L., Schaetzl, E., et al.: Elevation of serum CA 125 in carcinomas of the Fallopian tube, endometrium, and endocervix. Am. J. Obstet. Gynecol., 148:1057, 1984.
71. Novis, B. H., Gluck, E., Thomas, P. et al.: Serial levels of CA 19–9 and CEA in colonic cancer. J. Clin. Oncol., 4:987, 1986.
72. O'Connor, J. F., Schlatterer, J. P., Birken, S., et al.: Development of highly sensitive immunoassays to measure human chorionic gonadotropin, its β-subunit, and β-core fragment in the urine: Application to malignancies. Cancer Res., 48:1361, 1988.
73. Olding, L. B., Thuvin, J., Svalander, C., and Koprowski, H.: Expression of the gastrointestinal carcinoma-associated antigen (GICA) detected in human fetal tissues by monoclonal antibody NS–19–9. Int. J. Cancer, 34:187, 1985.
74. Panza, N., Pacilio, G., Campanella, L., et al.: Cancer antigen 125, tissue polypeptide antigen, carcinoembryonic antigen and beta-chain human chorionic gonadotropin as serum markers of epithelial ovarian carcinoma. Cancer, 61:76, 1988.
75. Patt, Y. Z., Lamki, L. M., Haynie, T. P., et al.: Improved tumor localization with increasing dose of indium-III-labeled anti-carcinoembryonic antigen monoclonal antibody ZCE–025 in metastatic colorectal cancer. J. Clin. Oncol., 6:1220, 1988.
76. Pedersen, A. G., Becker, K. L., Bach, F., et al.: Cerebrospinal fluid bombesin and calcitonin in patients with central nervous system metastases from small-cell lung cancer. J. Clin. Oncol., 4:1620, 1986.
77. Piantino, P., Andriulli, A., Gindro, T., et al.: CA 19–9 assay in differential diagnosis of pancreatic carcinoma from inflammatory pancreatic diseases. Am. J. Gastroenterol., 81:436, 1986.
78. Pons-Anicet, D. M. F., Krebs, B. P., Mira, R., and Namer, M.: Value of CA 15–3 in the follow-up of breast cancer patients. Br. J. Cancer, 55:567, 1987.

79. Punza, N., Pacilio, G., Campanella, L., et al.: Cancer antigen 125, tissue polypeptide antigen, carcinoembryonic antigen, and beta chain human chorionic gonadatropin as serum markers of epithelial ovarian carcinoma. Cancer, 61:76, 1988.

80. Quentmeier, A., Moller, P., Schwarz, V., et al.: Carcinoembryonic antigen, CA 19–9, and CA–125 in normal and carcinomatous human colorectal tissue. Cancer, 60:2261, 1987.

81. Richie, J. P., Sorinsky, M. A., Fung, C. Y., et al.: Management of patients with clinical stage I or II nonseminomatous germ cell tumors of the testis. Arch. Surg., 122:1443, 1987.

82. Rogers, G. T.: Carcinoembryonic antigens and related glycoproteins: Molecular aspects and specificity. Biochim. Biophys. Acta, 695:227, 1983.

83. Sekine, H., Ohno, T., and Kufe, D. W.: Purification and characterization of a high molecular weight glycoprotein detectable in human milk and breast carcinomas. J. Immunol., 135:3610, 1985.

84. Soper, J. T., Hunter, V., Tanner, M., et al.: Use of CA 125, CA 72 and CA 15–3 to discriminate malignant from benign pelvic masses. Proc. Am. Assoc. Cancer. Res., 28:205, 1987.

85. Staab, H. J., Anderer, F. A., and Brummendorf, T.: Prognostic value of preoperative serum CEA level compared to clinical staging of colorectal carcinoma. Br. J. Cancer, 44:652, 1981.

86. Stamey, T. A., Yang, N., Lay, A. R., et al.: Prostate-specific antigen as a serum marker for adenocarcinoma of the prostate. N. Engl. J. Med., 317:909, 1987.

87. Stockley, R. A., Shaw, J., Whitfield, A. G. W., et al.: Effect of cigarette smoking, pulmonary inflammation, and lung disease on concentrations of carcinoembryonic antigen in serum and secretions. Thorax, 41:17, 1986.

88. Szymendera, J. J.: Clinical usefulness of three monoclonal antibody-defined tumor markers: CA 19–9, CA 50, and CA 125. Tumour Biol., 7:333, 1986.

89. Thompson, J. A., Pande, H., Paxton, R. J., et al.: Molecular cloning of a gene belonging to the carcinoembryonic antigen gene family and discussion of a domain model. Proc. Natl. Acad. Sci. USA, 84:2965, 1987.

90. Vaitukaitis, J. L., Braunstein, G. D., and Ross, G. T.: A radioimmunoassay which specifically measures human chorionic gonadotropin in the presence of human luteinizing hormone. Am. J. Obstet. Gynecol., 113:751, 1972.

91. Viola, M. V., Fromowitz, F., Oravez, S., et al.: Expression of ras oncogene p 21 in prostate cancer. N. Engl. J. Med., 314:133, 1986.

92. Vugrin, D., Friedman, A., and Whitmore, W. F.: Correlation of serum tumor markers in advanced germ cell tumors with responses to chemotherapy and surgery. Cancer, 53:1440, 1984.

93. Wells, S. A. Jr., Baylin, S. B., Gann, D. S., et al. Medullary thyroid carcinoma: Relationship of method of diagnosis to pathologic staging. Ann. Surg., 188:377, 1978.

94. Yeh, Y. C., Tsae, J. F., Chuang, L. Y., et al.: Elevation of transforming growth factor alpha and its relationship to the epidermal growth factor and alpha-fetoprotein levels in patients with hepatocellular carcinoma. Cancer Res., 47:896, 1987.

95. Yohkaichiya, T., Fukaya, T., Hoshiai, H., et al.: Inhibin: A new circulating marker of hydatidiform mole? Br. Med. J., 298:1684, 1989.

96. Zimmerman, W., Weber, B., Ortlieb, B., et al.: Chromosomal localization of the carcinoembryonic antigen gene family and differential expression in various tumors. Cancer Res., 48:2550, 1988.

21

THE BREAST

J. Dirk Iglehart, M.D.

HISTORICAL ASPECTS

Diseases of the breast attracted medical interest as long ago as 3000 B.C. The Edwin Smith surgical papyrus, originating in the advanced civilization of Egypt during the Age of Pyramids (3000–2500 B.C.), described several cases of women with tumors of the breast. These included tumors that were hard and cool to the touch as well as abscesses and inflammations that were warm. It is probable that malignant tumors of the female breast were the first human cancers discovered and differentiated from other nonmalignant diseases. The Egyptian surgeons recognized that recovery was possible in cases of breast abscess and inflammation, but there was little that could be done to remedy "hard" tumors of the breast. It is not surprising that breast cancer should be considered today, 4000 years later, the best studied and understood of the solid tumors that afflict mankind.

The most influential physician of Greek antiquity was Hippocrates (460–370 B.C.), who is considered the founder of rational medicine based upon observation rather than upon supernatural intervention. He recognized the nature of malignant disease, which was called "karkinos" or "karkinoma," but he believed it was due to a systemic imbalance of the cardinal humours of the living body. Hippocrates considered these humours to be blood, yellow bile, black bile, and phlegm. He believed breast karkinos to be the result of cessation of menstrual flow, leading to imbalance and engorgement of the breast. Hippocrates was very skeptical of any medical intervention for cancers in the breast, saying that "It is better to give no treatment in cases of hidden cancer; treatment causes speedy death, but to omit treatment is to prolong life."

Celsus, living in the first century A.D., provided a description of stages of malignant growths and considered cancer a disease that "occurs mostly in the upper parts of the body, in the region of the face, nose, ears, lips, and in the breast of women. . . ." Celsus discouraged any treatment of cancer in its later stages and reserved intervention only for those early cases that would respond. In the same century, Leonidus gave a detailed description of operations on the breast, which were done by alternating sharp incision with the application of cauteries to stop bleeding. Very similar procedures were practiced 1500 years later during the Renaissance.

In the second century and for the next 1000 years, medical thinking was dominated by Galen (A.D. 130–203). Galen attributed cancer to an excess of black bile and, like Hippocrates earlier, to a systemic imbalance of the cardinal humours. He thought that the most common cancers arose in the female breast. Galen recommended complete excision of tumors of the breast "so as not to leave a single root. . . ." He likened cancer to the crab, with its central body and radiating growth and dilated veins.

Following the collapse of the Roman Empire in A.D. 576, medicine, along with other disciplines, entered the Dark Ages, which were characterized by the alienation of European communities. The Church was the strongest unifying force in this period of history. Medicine was practiced by monks, and surgery, so dependent upon an enlightened and scientific community, was further reduced to practice by empirics. During the Middle Ages, very little surgery was practiced or recorded with any regularity. Not until the Renaissance were Western scientists able to turn their attention to the study of anatomy and physiology and thus allow surgery again to advance.

During the sixteenth and seventeenth centuries, a resurgence of surgery occurred, owing in large measure to reintroduction of the study of human anatomy. In 1543, Andreas Vesalius, the father of modern anatomy, published his famous treatise *De Humani Corporis Fabrica*. Gabriele Falloppio, surgeon and anatomist at the renowned university in Padua, extensively discussed the nature of cancerous tumors. Although conservative in the application of surgery, a variety of techniques for removal of the breast were introduced during these 2 centuries. Vascular ligature was reintroduced as an alternative to cauterization by the famed surgeon to the French monarchy, Ambroise Paré. The study of normal anatomy naturally led to early concepts of pathophysiology. In the seventeenth century, Francois de le Boe Sylvius and Thomas Bartholin added to knowledge of the lymph system and placed great importance on its role in cancer initiation and spread. Also of seminal importance was the introduction of the microscope and microscopic anatomy in the late seventeenth and early eighteenth centuries. Although primitive, the early knowledge of anatomy and pathology set in motion a series of advancements in basic understanding that made application of surgery to the treatment of malignant disease possible. It is important for modern surgeons to appreciate how absolutely dependent the practice of this craft is on advancements in basic biology.

In 1757, Henry François LeDran offered a theory of the centrifugal spread of cancer from local to more distant sites. This was a fundamental break with the concept that cancer was a systemic disease of the body humours. LeDran's concept that if surgery could encompass the disease sufficiently a cure was possible held sway until the middle of the twentieth century. Bernard Peyrilhe advised removal of the entire breast, the pectoralis major muscle, and the axillary contents. Jean Louis Petit urged wide removal of the breast and axillary nodes and stressed avoidance of partial extirpation of the breast. Advances in science and medicine during the nineteenth century included the introduction of general anesthesia, histology, and appreciation of antisepsis. All these made the task of radical surgery more acceptable, improved the overall results, and afforded more credence to the concept of cancer as a curable local disease.

Charles Moore, of the Middlesex Hospital in London, went a step farther in arguing that inadequate operations for breast cancer led predictably to local failure. Clinical evidence was proffered that recurrences generally arose in surgical scars on the chest wall and were due to microscopic tumor fragments not encompassed by the surgical procedure. The basic tenents of mastectomy were clearly enunciated and included en bloc removal of the entire breast and axillary nodes. He also advised: "In the performance of the operation, it is desirable to avoid, not only cutting into the tumor, but also seeing it." These principles were adopted and extended by surgeons of Europe and America. Joseph Lister exposed the axilla by division of the pectoralis muscle and Samuel W. Gross, in the United States, advised removal of the pectoral fascia.

Strongly influenced by the work of the German histologists and surgeons, William Stewart Halsted of Baltimore presented a formal description of the "complete operation" for the surgical treatment of breast cancer in 1894. This operation ultimately became known as "radical mastectomy." Willie Meyer, Professor of Surgery at the New York Postgraduate Medical School, simultaneously published a description of a similar operation, differing only in the placement of the skin incision and by adding removal of the pectoralis minor muscle. To Halsted goes credit for his ability to synthesize the concepts of preceding generations and to present a unified treatment approach, including careful clinical description and documentation of outcome. In his now famous series of 50 patients, published in the *Johns Hopkins Hospital Reports* in 1894, Halsted meticulously documented a dramatic reduction to 6 per cent in the local recurrence rate of breast cancer, which contrasted with the recurrence rates of greater than 50 per cent routinely achieved by contemporary surgeons on both sides of the Atlantic. Physicians and surgeons were now free to attack problems of more fundamental nature, including control of metastatic disease, appreciation of the basic mechanisms of cancer initiation and spread, and control of disease through screening and prevention. These problems, which have dominated the attention of clinicians and scientists in the twentieth century, will be presented in this chapter.

ANATOMY

Knowledge of the anatomy and embryology of the breast and the chest structures beneath it is required not only for the performance of surgical procedures, but also in planning therapeutic radiation, predicting sites of locally recurrent disease, and assessing the adequacy of surgical procedures. Embryologically, the human breast develops in the thickened portion of ectodermal tissue known as the milk streak, coursing from the pubis to the axilla in early fetal life. Late in the first trimester, the milk streak atrophies, leaving only its pectoral portion, which continues to thicken and to form the nipple bud. The entire gland then forms as a dermally derived organ lying within the subcutaneous tissue, in a manner similar to that of sweat gland development. The ductal system develops from the nipple bud by invasion and downgrowth of primitive ectodermal cells from the nipple surface. The breast parenchyma lies cushioned in fat between the layers of superficial pectoral fascia (Fig. 1). Between the deep layer of the superficial fascia and the fascial investment of the pectoralis major muscle, the breast rests on a thin layer of loose areolar tissue, the retromammary space, containing lymphatics and small vessels. When one performs total mastectomy, the correct plane is found under the pectoral fascia and includes the retromammary space, as emphasized by Gross.

Deep to the pectoralis major muscle, the pectoralis minor muscle is enclosed in the clavipectoral fascia that envelops it and extends laterally to fuse with the axillary fascia. In a standard modified radical mastectomy, dissection along the lateral border of the pectoralis minor muscle divides the axillary fascia and exposes the contents of the axilla. Within the loose areolar fat of the axilla, one finds a variable number of lymph nodes grouped as shown in Figure 2. The number of lymph nodes found in the axillary space of patients undergoing mastectomy varies, depending on the extent of dissection and the diligence of methods used to identify these nodes. An upper limit is established by the work of Durkin and Haagensen using ethanol clearing.[60] These investigators found an average of 50 nodes in 100 specimens obtained in the course of a Halsted type of radical mastectomy. The current approach to less radical procedures has reduced the number of nodes retrieved.

To standardize the extent of axillary dissection, the axillary space is arbitrarily divided into three levels, shown in Figure 3.

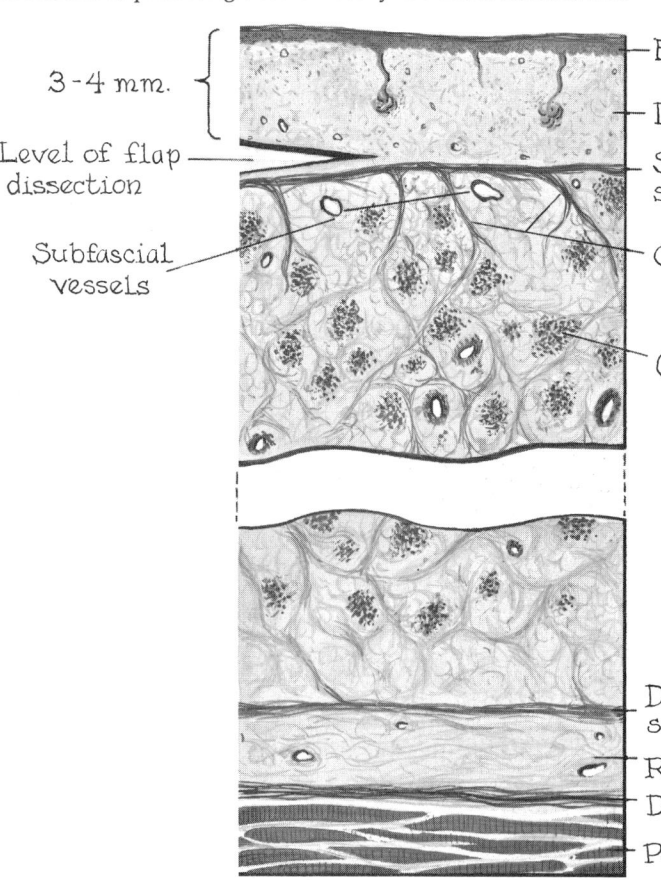

3 – 4 mm.

Level of flap dissection

Subfascial vessels

Epidermis

Dermis

Superficial layer of superficial fascia

Cooper's ligaments

Glandular tissue

Deep layer of superficial fascia

Retromammary space

Deep fascia

Pectoralis major m.

Figure 1. Diagrammatic cross-section of the breast showing its fascial relationships. Glandular tissue of the breast lies within a cushion of fat between the superficial and deep layers of the superficial pectoral fascia. Cooper's ligaments are fibrous continuations of the superficial fascia, which span the parenchyma of the breast coursing between the superficial and deep fascial layers. Dissection of the breast off the pectoralis major muscle usually includes the deep fascia. The clavipectoral fascia, not shown here, invests the pectoralis minor muscle and the undersurface of the pectoralis major muscle. (From Haagensen, C. D.: Diseases of the Breast, 3rd ed. Philadelphia, W. B. Saunders Company 1986, p. 15.)

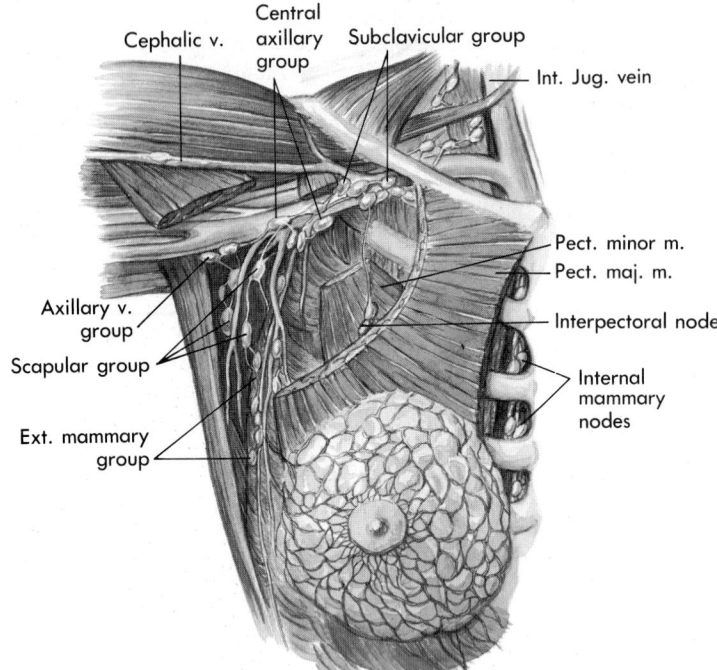

Figure 2. Contents of the axilla. Five named groups of lymph nodes are generally contained within a complete dissection of the axillary contents. These groups tend to follow the course of the major veins that are encountered within the axilla. Lymphatic afferent channels course under the deep layer of the superficial fascia in the retromammary space. The first node groups in the circuit are the external mammary, axillary, and central nodal groups. Scapular and subclavicular nodes are also contained in the axillary chain. However, lymphatic afferents drain directly to internal mammary nodes. In addition, more distal groups at risk for involvement in more advanced progression are the interpectoral nodes (Rotter's nodes), subclavicular nodes high along the axillary chain, and supraclavicular nodes above the ipsilateral clavicle. (Illustration from Donegan, W. L., and Spratt, J. S.: Cancer of the Breast, 3rd ed. Philadelphia, W. B. Saunders Company 1988, p. 19.)

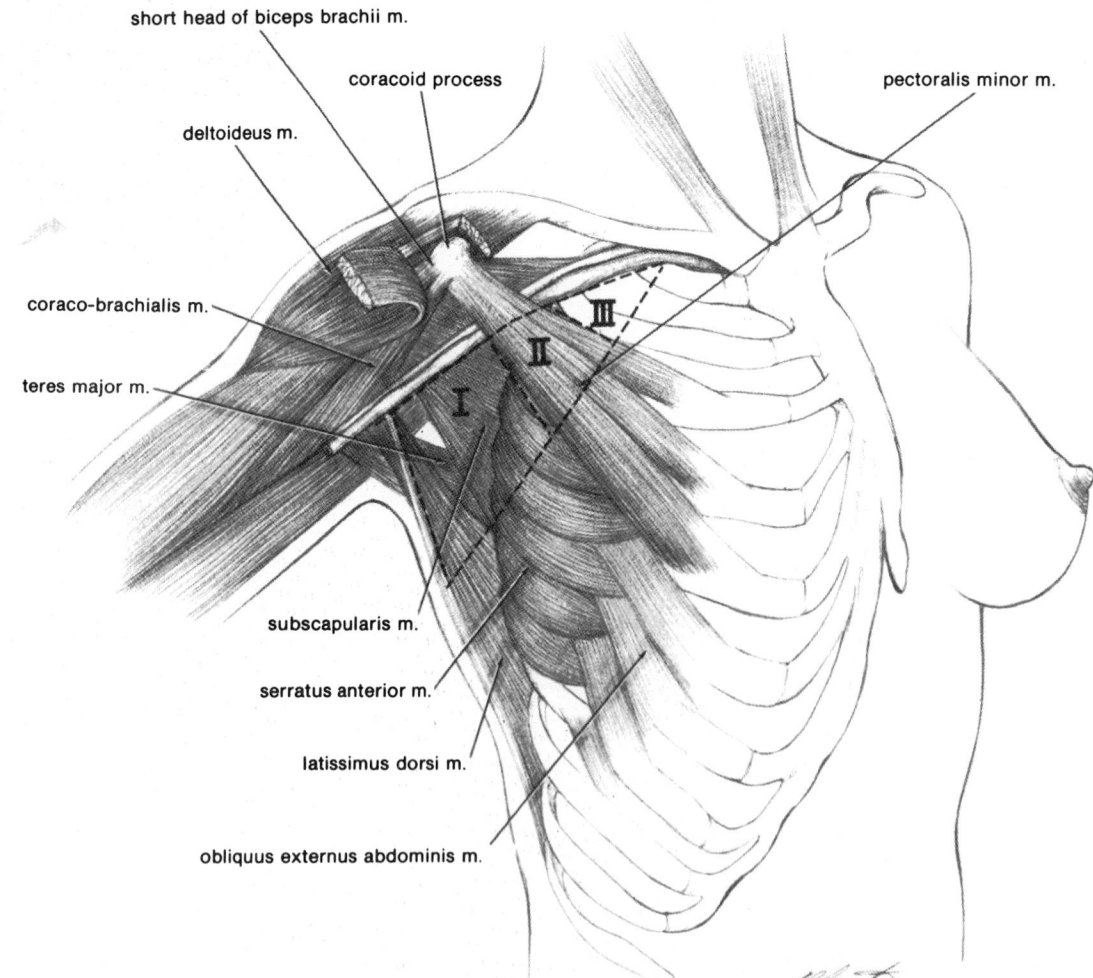

Figure 3. Standardized description of axillary nodal contents. The axillary nodes are divided into three groups defined by their position relative to the pectoralis minor muscle. Level I defines those nodes lateral to the pectoralis minor muscle. Level II nodes are those that lie under the pectoralis minor. The Level III nodes are located medial to the medial border of the minor muscle. In a normal patient, these nodes can be removed only after division or sacrifice of the minor muscle during a modified radical mastectomy or axillary dissection. They are routinely removed in a standard radical mastectomy. Operative notes should specify accurately the levels of axillary dissection. (From Donegan, W. L., and Spratt, J. S.: Cancer of the Breast, 3rd ed. Philadelphia, W. B. Saunders Company 1988, p. 425.)

Level I nodes are those in the external mammary, scapular, axillary vein, and central axillary groups, which lie lateral to the lateral border of the pectoralis minor muscle. Level II nodes are those in the central axillary group, which lie under the pectoralis minor muscle. Level III nodes are difficult to visualize and remove unless the pectoralis minor muscle is sacrificed or divided and include those subclavicular nodes medial to the minor muscle. The apex of the axilla is defined by the costoclavicular ligament (Halsted's ligament), at which point the axillary vein passes into the thorax and becomes the subclavian vein. Lymph nodes in the space between the pectoralis major and minor muscles are known as the interpectoral group, or Rotter's nodes, described by Grossman and Rotter. Unless this group is specifically exposed, they are not encompassed in surgical procedures that preserve the pectoral muscles.

The lymphatic drainage of the breast is rich, and appreciation of the major pathways allows one to predict the sites most commonly containing lymph-borne metastases. Lymphatic channels within the breast follow centrifugal pathways from the subareolar plexus along major lactiferous ducts and then along efferent veins to draining nodal beds. Three principal pathways are identified in Figure 2. The major site of drainage is to central axillary nodes. The internal mammary and interpectoral nodes, although primary routes of lymph flow, are rarely the sites of nodal metastasis from breast cancer in the absence of simultaneous axillary disease.[36,44,163,189] Secondarily, the lymphatic spread of cancer is into the high axillary nodes in the subclavicular chain and henceforth into the supraclavicular fossa.

As the surgeon endeavors to remove the lymph nodes of the axilla, a keen knowledge of the nerve structures in the axilla is required to avoid their sacrifice. Coursing close to the chest wall on the medial side of the axilla is the long thoracic nerve, or the external respiratory nerve of Bell, which innervates the serratus anterior muscle. This muscle is important in fixation of the scapula to the chest wall during adduction of the shoulder and extension of the arm, and its denervation results in the winged scapula deformity. For this reason, the long thoracic nerve is carefully preserved during standard axillary dissection. The second major nerve trunk encountered during axillary dissection is the thoracodorsal nerve to the latissimus dorsi muscle at the lateral border of the axilla. This nerve arises from the posterior cord of the brachial plexus and enters the axillary space under the axillary vein, close to the entrance of the long thoracic nerve, and then traverses the axilla to travel on the medial surface of the latissimus dorsi muscle. This nerve is usually preserved during dissection of axillary nodes, unless its sacrifice is required for complete removal of tumor-containing nodes.

Recently, innervation of the pectoralis major muscle has gained the attention of some who emphasize the advantage of protecting these nerves during modified radical mastectomy.[161,217,236] Loss of innervation results in a flaccid and atrophic muscle and a diminished tissue covering over the chest wall after amputation of the breast. These investigators have named the pectoral nerves according to their actual position as encountered during axillary dissection and preserve innervation to the lower third of the pectoralis major muscle.

The lateral pectoral nerve has a variable course, as depicted in Figure 4.[217] In the majority of patients, the lateral pectoral nerve travels around the lateral margin of the pectoralis minor muscle and is in a vulnerable position during the division of the clavipectoral fascia and exposure of the axillary space. If possible, this branch can be saved without compromising the dissection. The final nerves that are of interest to the surgeon are the large sensory intercostal brachial or brachial cutaneous nerves that span the axillary space and supply sensation to the undersurface of the upper arm and skin of the chest wall along the posterior margin of the axilla. Cutting these nerves, which is routinely done in removing the lymph node–containing tissues, causes cutaneous anesthesia in these areas. It is helpful to emphasize this to patients prior to operation. Denervation of the areas supplied by these sensory nerves can cause chronic and uncomfortable pain syndromes in a small percentage of patients.

MICROSCOPIC ANATOMY OF THE BREAST

The mature breast is composed of three principal tissue types: epithelium, fibrous stroma and supporting structures, and fat. The relative amounts tend to vary with age, but there is even greater variability among individual women. In youth, the predominant tissues are epithelium and stroma, replaced by fat in the breasts of older women. For this reason, mammography in women less than 30 years of age, whose breast tissue is dense

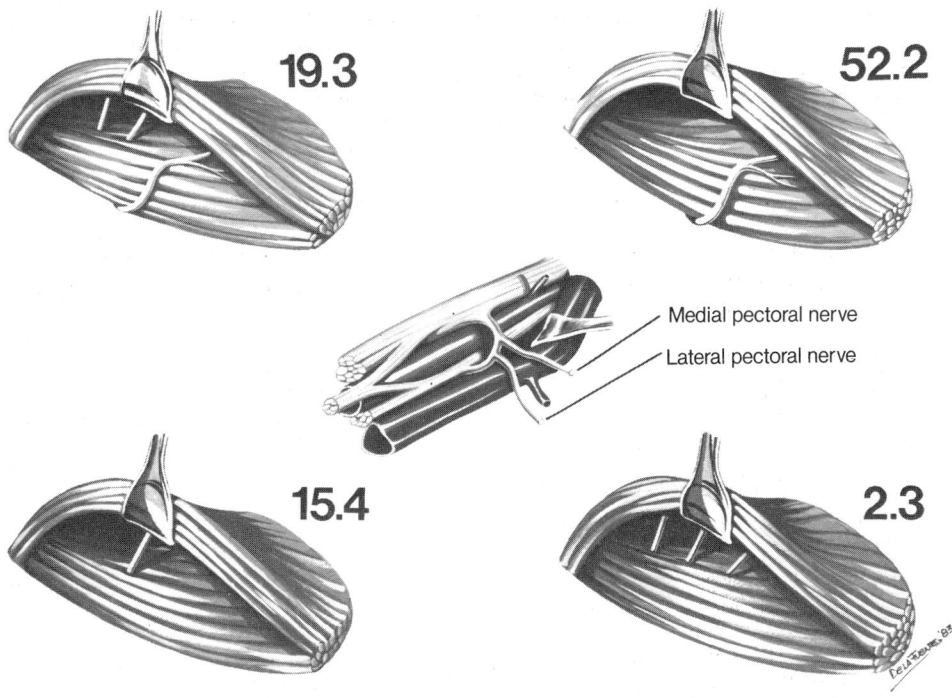

Figure 4. Variable relationship of the lateral pectoral nerve to the pectoralis minor muscle. The lateral pectoralis nerve is named for its anatomic location and is found either coursing around the lateral border of the pectoralis minor muscle, perforating the lateral half of the muscle belly, or splitting to lie in both locations. Its preservation during axillary dissection maintains innervation to the lower one third of the pectoralis major muscle. (Illustration from Serra, G. E., et al.: Lateral pectoralis nerve: The need to preserve it in the modified radical mastectomy. J. Surg. Oncol., 26:278, 1984. Reprinted with permission.)

Medial pectoral nerve
Lateral pectoral nerve

19.3

52.2

15.4

2.3

with stroma and epithelium, produces images without much definition that are rarely useful clinically. In contrast, fat absorbs relatively little radiation and provides a contrasting background, which favors detection of small density lesions in the older patient. Throughout the fat of the breast, coursing from the overlying skin to the underlying deep fascia, strands of dense connective tissue provide shape and hold the breast upward. These strands, devoid of epithelial elements, are called Cooper's ligaments (see Fig. 1). Because they are anchored into the skin, tethering of these ligaments by a small scirrhous carcinoma commonly produces a dimple or subtle deformity on the otherwise smooth surface of the breast (see Fig. 8).

The glandular apparatus of the breast is composed of a branching system of ducts, roughly organized in a radial pattern, which spread outward and downward from the nipple-areolar complex (Fig. 5.) These lactiferous ducts are so named because they carry the milk produced in the more distal lobular groupings. At the summit of the arborizing ductal system, the subareolar ducts widen to form the lactiferous sinuses, which then exit through 15 to 20 orifices on the nipple. These large ducts close to the nipple are lined with a low columnar or cuboidal epithelium that abruptly meets the squamous epithelium of the nipple surface, which invades the duct for a short distance. Awareness of this junction helps understand Paget's disease of the nipple, described later.

At the opposite end of the ductal system and after progressive generations of branching, the ducts end blindly in clusters of spaces that are called terminal ductules or acini. These are the milk-forming glands of the lactating breast and, together with their small efferent ducts or ductules, are known as the lobular units or lobules. As shown in Figure 6, the terminal ductules are invested in a specialized loose connective tissue that contains capillaries, lymphocytes, and other migratory mononuclear cells. This intralobular stroma is clearly distinguished from the denser and less cellular interlobular stroma and from the fat within the breast.

Under the luminal epithelium, the entire ductal system is surrounded by a specialized myoepithelial cell of ductal epithelial origin, which has contractile properties and serves to propel secretion of milk toward the nipple. Outside the epithelial and myoepithelial layers, the ducts of the breast are surrounded by a continuous basement membrane containing laminin, type IV collagen, and proteoglycans. The basement membrane layer is extremely important in differentiating in-situ from invasive breast cancer. Continuity of this layer around proliferations of ductal cells guarantees that progression to an invasive cancer has not yet occurred (Fig. 7).

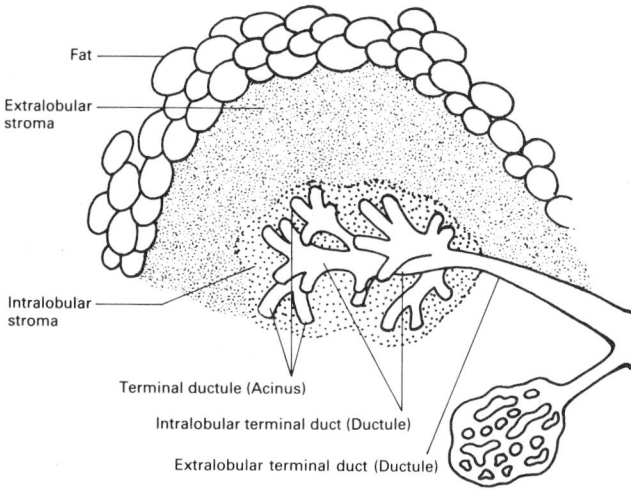

Figure 6. A mature resting lobular unit within the breast. The lobular unit consists of terminal ductules or acini surrounded by loose connective stroma and tiny efferent ductules referred to as extralobular terminal ducts. The surrounding intralobular stroma is denser and collagen-rich. The efferent ductules coalesce to form larger ducts that course up to the nipple-areola complex. (From Page, D. L., and Anderson, T. J.: Diagnostic Histopathology of the Breast. Edinburgh, Churchill Livingstone, 1987.)

BREAST DEVELOPMENT AND PHYSIOLOGY

In many mammalian species, full breast development requires the stimulation of copulation or pregnancy. Women do not require either of these two events to initiate and complete breast maturation. Appreciation of the stages of breast development is necessary to understand many benign and even malignant states that come to clinical attention. During adolescence, the breast is composed primarily of dense fibrous stroma and scattered ducts lined with epithelium. In the United States, puberty begins at about 12 years of age, during which time there is hormone-dependent maturation of the genital organs. In the breast, this process entails increased deposition of fat, formation of new ducts by branching and elongation, and the first appearance of lobular units. This process of growth entails cell division and is under the control of estrogen, progesterone, adrenal hor-

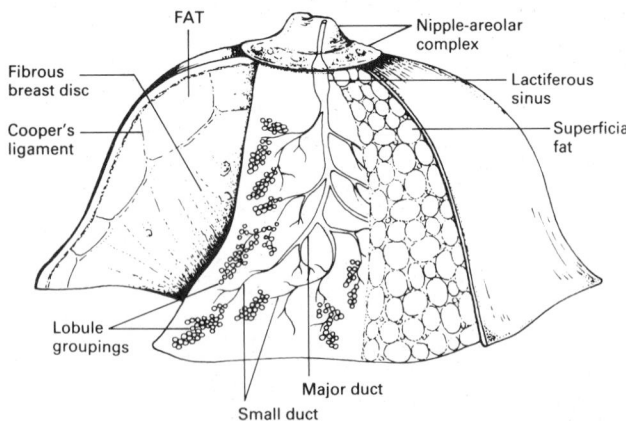

Figure 5. The mature breast, showing the organization of the ductal and lobular components and their relationship to the nipple-areola complex. (From Page, D. L., and Anderson, T. J.: Diagnostic Histopathology of the Breast. Edinburgh, Churchill Livingstone, 1987. Reprinted with permission.)

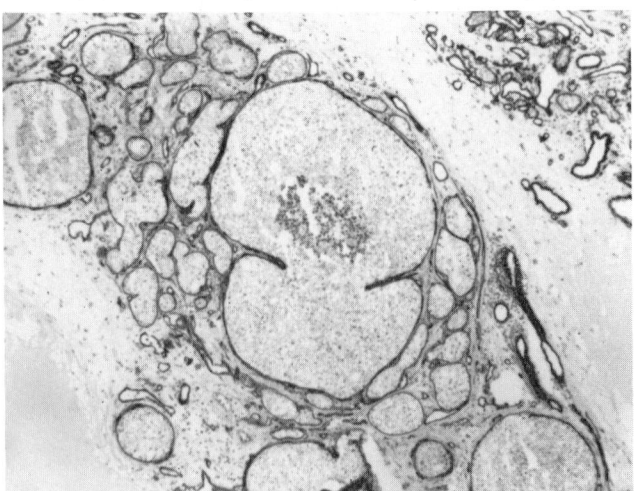

Figure 7. Integrity of the basement membrane around normal ducts and around intraductal neoplasm. Antibodies against collagen Type IV, a normal constituent of basement membrane, were reacted with fresh breast tissue from a case of *in situ* ductal carcinoma. Although greatly expanded and displaying central necrosis, the duct in the center of the illustration has an uninterrupted basement membrane highlighted by the immunohistochemical reaction. More normal ducts in the upper right are also contained by a continuous basement membrane.

mones, pituitary hormones, and trophic effects of insulin and thyroid hormone.[104,173] There is evidence that local growth factor networks are also important, including epidermal growth factor (EGF), which can replace estrogen as a developmental mammogen.[37] The exact timing of these events and the coordinated development of both breast buds may vary from the average in individual patients. The term *prepubertal gynecomastia* refers to the symmetrical enlargement and projection of the breast bud in a young girl before the average age of 12 years, unaccompanied by the other changes of puberty. This process, which may be unilateral, should not be confused with neoplastic growth and should not be biopsied.

The mature or "resting" breast contains fat, stroma, lactiferous ducts, and lobular units. During phases of the menstrual cycle or in response to exogenous hormones, the breast epithelium and lobular stroma undergo cyclic stimulation.[245] It appears that the dominant process is hypertrophy and alteration of morphology rather than hyperplasia. In the late luteal (premenstrual) phase, there is accumulation of fluid and intralobular edema, which appears to correspond to the clinical complaint of breast engorgement that may be painful. On physical examination, and even by mammography, this may lead to increased nodularity and even be mistaken for development of a dominant tumor. Accordingly, ill-defined masses in premenopausal women are correctly observed through the course of one or two menstrual cycles. Finally, any alteration in the periodicity of the menstrual cycle, such as anovulatory cycles, can cause accentuation of engorgement, pain, and nodularity.

With pregnancy, there is diminution of the fibrous stroma to accommodate the hyperplasia of the lobular units. This formation of many new acini or lobules is termed the *adenosis of pregnancy* and is influenced by high circulating levels of estrogen and progesterone, and levels of prolactin that steadily rise during gestation. After birth, there is sudden loss of the placental hormones and the high level of prolactin. This may be the principal trigger for lactation. The actual expulsion of milk is under hormonal control and is caused by the contraction of the myoepithelial cells that surround breast ducts and terminal ductules. There is no evidence for innervation of the myoepithelial cells; their contraction appears to be in response to the pituitary-derived peptide, oxytocin. Stimulation of the nipple appears to be the physiologic signal for continued pituitary secretion of prolactin and for the acute release of oxytocin.

When breast-feeding stops, there is a fall in prolactin and no stimulus for release of oxytocin. The breast then returns to a resting state and to the cyclic changes induced when menstruation begins again. With the approach of menopause, phases of the menstrual cycle may not be as symmetric and regular. This irregularity can induce functional nodularity and breast pain when there had been none in earlier years. Menopause is defined by a cessation in menstrual flow for a significant period of time (i.e., 6 months or more) and the variable appearance of constitutional systems such as diaphoresis, minor psychologic disturbances, or even clinical depression. For the breast, menopause results in involution and a general decrease in the epithelial elements of the resting breast. These changes include increased fat deposition, diminished connective tissue, and the virtual disappearance of the lobular units. The persistence of lobules, hyperplasia of the ductal epithelium, and even cyst formation can all occur under the influence of exogenous ovarian hormones. Most commonly, hormones are administered to relieve the symptoms of menopause, to prevent demineralization of bone, or to slow the appearance of atherosclerosis. The surgeon evaluating patients at any age for breast disease should inquire about the menstrual history, establish the cessation of menses in postmenopausal women, and record the use of any exogenous hormones. It is important that the pathologist who is examining biopsy material also have this information.

ABNORMAL PHYSIOLOGY AND DEVELOPMENT

GYNECOMASTIA. Hypertrophy of breast tissue in men is a common clinical entity for which there is frequently no identifiable cause. Haagensen distinguishes *puberal hypertrophy,* occurring in young boys between the ages of 13 and 17 years, from *senescent hypertrophy,* which occurs in men older than 50 years. The enlargement in teenage boys is very common and is frequently bilateral but may be unilateral. Unless it is unilateral or painful, it passes unnoticed and regresses with adulthood. Puberal hypertrophy is generally treated by reassurance and without operation. Surgical excision should be discussed only if the enlargement fails to regress and the breast is cosmetically unacceptable.

Hypertrophy in older men is also common and may regress spontaneously. It is frequently unilateral, although the contralateral breast may enlarge with the passage of time. The discoid mass is smooth, firm, and symmetrically distributed beneath the areola. It may be tender, and patients occasionally complain of breast discomfort. A number of commonly used medications, such as digoxin, thiazides, estrogens, phenothiazines, and theophylline, may exacerbate senescent gynecomastia. In addition, gynecomastia may be a systemic manifestation of hepatic cirrhosis, renal failure, and malnutrition. There should be little confusion with carcinoma occurring in the male breast. Carcinoma is usually not tender, is asymmetrically located either beneath or beside the areola, and may be fixed to the overlying dermis or to the deep fascia. As with puberal hypertrophy, gynecomastia in older men is usually left untreated. A dominant mass suspected of carcinoma should be biopsied or carefully followed.

NIPPLE DISCHARGE. The appearance of a discharge from the nipple of a nonlactating woman is frequently frightening to the patient and misunderstood by the physician. Nipple discharge is very common and rarely is associated with an underlying carcinoma. It is important to establish whether the discharge comes from one breast or from both breasts, whether it comes from multiple duct orifices or from just one, and whether the discharge is grossly bloody or contains blood. A milky discharge from both breasts is termed *galactorrhea.* In the absence of lactation or history of recent lactation, galactorrhea may be associated with increased production of prolactin. Radioimmunoassay for serum prolactin is diagnostic. However, true galactorrhea is very rare and is diagnosed only when the discharge is milky (contains lactose, fat, and milk-specific proteins).

Unilateral nonmilky discharge coming from one duct orifice is surgically significant and warrants special attention. However, the underlying cause is rarely a breast malignancy. In one review of 270 subareolar biopsy results of discharges coming from one identifiable duct and without an associated breast mass, carcinoma was found in only 16 patients (5.9 per cent). In each of these cases, the fluid was either grossly bloody or tested strongly positive for occult hemoglobin.[29] In another series of 249 patients, including both multi-duct and single-duct discharges, breast carcinoma was found in 10 (4 per cent).[48] In 8 of these patients, a mass lesion coexisted with the discharge. Among 67 patients with breast cancer presenting with nipple discharge and studied by Leis and colleagues, only 8 (12 per cent) had no palpable mass and 7 (10 per cent) had a negative mammogram.[140] To conclude, nipple discharge that comes from a single duct and contains blood must be investigated further. However, in the absence of a palpable mass or a suspicious mammogram, this symptom is usually not associated with cancer.

The most common cause of spontaneous nipple discharge from a single duct is a solitary intraductal papilloma in one of the large subareolar ducts directly under the nipple.[29,101,140] Fibrocystic change, or cystic mastopathy, typically produces multiduct discharge and is another commonly associated finding.[48] Subareolar duct ectasia, producing inflammation and dilatation of large collecting ducts under the nipple, is a common finding in the aging breast and usually produces multiduct discharge.[49] In summary, nipple discharge that is bilateral and comes from multiple ducts is usually not a surgical problem. Discharge from single ducts is not commonly associated with carcinoma in the absence of detectable blood or a palpable mass. Bloody discharge from a single duct requires surgical biopsy to establish diagnosis. Intraductal papilloma is found in the majority of cases. If an occult cancer is found, it invariably is an early intraductal lesion.[52]

BREAST PAIN. Painful breast tissue is an exceedingly common symptom but is usually of functional origin and very rarely a symptom of breast cancer. Haagensen carefully recorded the symptoms of women presenting with breast carcinoma and found pain as an unprompted symptom in only 5.4 per cent of patients.[100] Although not a symptom of cancer, breast pain is a common reason for patients to seek medical attention. Breast pain appears to be aggravated by abnormal menstrual cycles and may be seen in young women with menstrual irregularity, as a premenstrual symptom, or when exogenous ovarian hormones are administered during and after the menopause. In addition, fibrocystic change, in its severest forms, may cause disabling breast pain. Although many observers find that painful cystic mastopathy is aggravated by excessive intake of caffeine, nicotine, or commonly used antihistamines, other investigators disagree.[141,205]

FIBROCYSTIC CHANGE (CYSTIC MASTOPATHY, CYSTIC MASTITIS). Fibrocystic change, popularly referred to as "fibrocystic disease," represents a spectrum of clinical and histologic findings and describes a loose association of cyst formation, breast nodularity, stromal proliferation, and epithelial hyperplasia. Fibrocystic change appears to represent an exaggerated response of breast stroma and epithelium to a variety of circulating and locally produced hormones and growth factors. Clinically, patients with fibrocystic change have dense, firm breast tissue with palpable lumps that frequently contains gross cysts. This condition is commonly painful and tender to touch.

Histologically, the lesion recognized as fibrocystic complex contains macrocysts, microcysts, stromal fibrosis, adenosis, and a variable amount of epithelial metaplasia and hyperplasia. All these changes can occur alone or in combination and to a variable degree in the normal female breast. Autopsy studies have questioned whether any of these changes, except perhaps macrocysts, are abnormal. In fact, all these lesions occur commonly in the breasts of elderly patients and appear to have no particular pathologic potential.[49,136] Currently, it appears preferable to describe each of the lesions separately and comment about the extent and severity of the process. The term *fibrocystic disease* should be abandoned in the absence of any well-defined clinical and pathologic syndrome.[144]

As discussed later, there is no consistent association between fibrocystic complex and breast cancer.[144] It is well established that women who have undergone breast biopsy for any reason, regardless of the underlying pathology, have a slightly higher risk of developing subsequent breast cancer.[59,144] Moreover, the incidence of finding fibrocystic disease in autopsied breasts from women dying of causes other than breast cancer exceeds the incidence of these same changes in cancer-containing breasts.[144] For those patients with fibrocystic changes, higher risk appears to concentrate in those whose biopsy specimens show abnormal ductal and lobular hyperplasia[59,180] and, to a lesser extent, cyst formation. Therefore, the fibrocystic complex appears to be an exaggerated or abnormal response to otherwise physiologic stimuli in most patients and represents a health risk only in certain subsets.

GALACTOCELE. A galactocele is a milk-filled cyst which is round, well circumscribed, and easily movable within the breast. It usually occurs after the cessation of lactation or when feeding frequency has been curtailed significantly. Haagensen states that it may occur up to 6 to 10 months after breast feeding has stopped.[97] The pathogenesis of galactocele is not known for certain, but it is thought that inspissated milk within a large lactiferous duct is responsible. The tumor is usually located in the central portion of the breast or under the nipple. Needle aspiration produces thick, creamy material that may be tinged dark-green or brown. Although it appears purulent, the fluid is sterile. The treatment is needle aspiration. Withdrawal of thick, milky secretion confirms the diagnosis; operation is reserved for those cysts that cannot be aspirated or that become superinfected.

ABSENT OR ACCESSORY BREAST TISSUE. Absence of breast tissue (amastia) or absence of the nipple (athelia) are very rare anomalies. Unilateral rudimentary breast development is much more common, as is adolescent hypertrophy of one breast with more normal development of the other. In contrast, accessory breast tissue (polymastia) and accessory nipples (supernumerary nipples) are both quite common. Supernumerary nipples are usually rudimentary and occur along the milk line from the axilla to the pubis in both males and females. They may be mistaken by the patient for a small mole. However, accessory nipples are removed only for cosmetic reason. True polythelia refers to more than one nipple serving a single breast and is very rare.

Accessory breast tissue is commonly located above the breast in the axilla. Rudimentary nipple development may be present, and lactation is possible with more complete development. Accessory breast tissue, which may present as an enlarging mass in the axilla during pregnancy, is treated by surgical removal if it is large or cosmetically deforming, or to prevent enlargement during future pregnancy.

DIAGNOSIS OF BREAST DISEASE
HISTORY AND PHYSICAL EXAMINATION

HISTORY. For patients with benign breast conditions, the history is an exceedingly important part of the overall evaluation and frequently points to the underlying cause of the symptom or physical finding. For patients suspected of having cancer, the history directly aids in the approach to the patient and the ultimate treatment if cancer is confirmed and helps estimate the risk that cancer will be found. First, the examiner should determine the patient's age and obtain a careful menstrual history. The age of menarche, menstrual irregularities, and the age at menopause should be sought. Previous surgical procedures should be recorded, including hysterectomy and removal of the ovaries. Because hysterectomy is a common surgical procedure, accurate determination of menopause may be difficult. It is useful to inquire about menopausal symptoms in these patients. Determination of the menopausal status may be used as a deciding factor in recommending adjuvant therapy, and this information is required for entry into most therapeutic trials. In younger women, the history of pregnancy and lactation should be recorded. A careful accounting of drug use should pay particular attention to exogenous estrogen or progestins given for postmenopausal replacement or for contraception. As discussed later, the family history should be directed to cancer of the breast in primary relatives (mother, sisters, daughters).

In questioning the patient about the specific breast problem, it is worthwhile to inquire about breast pain, nipple discharge, and new masses in the breast. Obviously, if a mass is present, it helps to know how long it has been present, how it was found, and what has happened since its discovery. If cancer is likely, inquiry about constitutional symptoms, bone pain, weight loss, and similar clinical indications of metastatic disease may occasionally reveal unsuspected distant spread.

RISK FACTORS FOR BREAST CANCER. Identification of factors responsible for increasing an individual's chance of having breast cancer is important not only to the epidemiologist but also in common clinical practice. *Major* risk factors that are important in practice and *minor* risks that are less relevant clinically, although no less important to understanding mammary cancers, are listed in Table 1.

The age-adjusted incidence of breast cancer continues to increase with the advancing age of the population. Breast cancer is exceedingly rare under the age of 20 years and in women less than 30 years of age, it generally constitutes less than 2 per cent of the total cases in several reports.[99] Thereafter, the incidence rises to an annual frequency of greater than 300 cases per 100,000 in the eighth decade of life.

A personal history of mammary cancer in one breast increases the likelihood of a second primary cancer in the contralateral breast. In many studies, the relative risk (ratio of observed cases over expected cases) ranges between three and four.[15,114,125,181] The magnitude of relative risks depends on the age at diagnosis of the first primary cancer. For patients under age 45 years, the risk is five or six times that of the general population. In older patients, this decreases to a twofold or less increased risk. In absolute terms, the actual risk varies between 1 per cent per year in young patients to 0.2 per cent in older patients.

Many studies have evaluated the relation of family history and the risk of breast cancer.[3,16,146,172] These studies can be summarized as follows: (1) There is a two- to threefold excess risk of the disease in first-degree relatives (mothers, sisters, and daughters) of patients with breast cancer; (2) risk falls quickly with more distant affected relatives; (3) the risk is much higher if affected first-degree relatives had premenopausal onset or bilateral breast cancer. In families with bilateral premenopausal cancers, the absolute risk to first-degree relatives approaches 50 per cent, consistent with an autosomal dominant mode of inheritance in these particular pedigrees. An often difficult question posed by high-risk patients is that of prophylactic surgical therapy, either subcutaneous or a total mastectomy in the setting of a positive family history. Strong arguments can be made in favor of intervention for the young patient whose mother or sister(s) had bilateral cancer at an early age. In other situations, the recommendation is harder to justify. Useful tabulations of risk for various combinations of primary and secondary probands are now available to use in counseling families.[172]

It is well known that women with fibrocystic complex and those who have undergone breast biopsy are at increased risk of subsequent mammary carcinoma.[131] However, fibrocystic complex is a spectrum of pathologic changes that may include lobular and ductal epithelial proliferation, cyst formation, and stromal sclerosis. The excess risk of breast cancer in these patients concentrates in those whose biopsies show abnormal breast epithelial proliferation and, to a lesser extent, cyst formation.[98,131,144] Moreover, the addition of clinical features, such as history of breast cancer in first-degree relatives and age, produces additional risk.

Dupont and Page divide proliferative lesions into those with atypical epithelial hyperplasia and those without atypia.[59] The relative risk of cancer in women with atypical hyperplasia was 4.4 times the risk of developing breast cancer in a control population of women. The coexistence of a positive family history with atypia on biopsy increased the risk to nearly nine times the general population. These investigators have tabulated the cumulative effects of hyperplasia, age, family history, and calcification on the risk of breast cancer in a clinically useful manner. Breast biopsy is a common surgical procedure providing important prognostic information. Clinicians interpreting biopsy results for their patients should be familiar with the implications of the findings. Moreover, clinicians should request complete pathologic descriptions and not accept unqualified reports such as "fibrocystic disease" or "cystic mastitis."[144]

Noninvasive breast carcinoma is listed as a major risk factor in Table 1. The current management of lobular and ductal carcinomas *in situ* is discussed later in greater depth. However, many patients with lobular carcinoma *in situ* and certain patients with ductal *in situ* lesions are treated by biopsy only. These patients are subject to a considerable risk of subsequent invasive cancer and should be followed carefully if less aggressive surgical therapy has been recommended (see later).

PHYSICAL EXAMINATION. Breast examination should be done in a well-lighted room, preferably with an available indirect light source. Respect for privacy and patient comfort should always be considered. The examination begins with careful visual inspection for obvious masses, asymmetries, and skin changes. The nipples are inspected and compared for the presence of retraction, nipple inversion, or excoriation of the superficial epidermias in Paget's disease. Inspection should be done with the patient in the upright sitting position. The use of indirect lighting can unmask subtle dimpling of the skin or nipple caused by the scirrhous reaction of a carcinoma placing Cooper's ligaments under tension (Fig. 8). Simple maneuvers, such as stretching the arms high above the head, tensing the pectoralis muscles, or gently lifting the patient's breast, may accentuate asymmetries and dimpling. It is a misconception to equate skin dimpling with advanced cancer. This sign is *frequently* found in very small, scirrhous tumors that do not produce a large mass effect. If carefully sought, dimpling of the skin or nipple retraction is a sensitive and quite specific sign of underlying cancer.

Edema of the skin, frequently accompanied by erythema, produces a clinical sign known as peau d'orange (Fig. 9). When combined with tenderness and warmth, these signs and symptoms are the hallmark of inflammatory carcinoma and may be mistaken for acute mastitis. Although these clinical signs are often dramatic, they can be overlooked in dark-skinned people or if a careful examination with proper lighting is not performed. The inflammatory changes and edema are caused by obstruction of dermal lymphatic channels with emboli of carcinoma cells. Occasionally, a bulky tumor may produce obstruction of large lymph channels, which results in overlying skin edema. This is not, strictly speaking, an inflammatory carcinoma in which the visible signs are out of proportion to the palpable mass. In 40 patients with inflammatory carcinoma treated by Haagensen, all cases presented with erythema and edema of the skin; a palpable mass or localized induration was present in 19; and in 21 patients no localized tumor was present.[109]

Involvement of the nipple and areola is a common histologic finding in breasts removed for carcinoma. Direct involvement may accompany tumors originating in breast tissue under the areola and may result in retraction of the usually protruding nipple. Flattening or actual inversion of the nipple can be

TABLE 1. Risk Factors for Breast Cancer

Major	Minor
Sex (female ≫ male)	Early menarche
Age	Late menopause
Family history (mother, sister, or daughter with premenopausal or bilateral cancer)	Obesity
Personal history (of contralateral breast cancer)	Low-dose radiation
Noninvasive carcinoma (ductal or lobular CIS)	
Benign proliferative changes with atypia	

From Iglehart, J.D.: The diagnosis and management of breast cancers: An update. *In* Sabiston, D.C., Jr.: Textbook of Surgery. The Biological Basis of Modern Surgical Practice, Update 1. Philadelphia, W. B. Saunders Company, 1988.

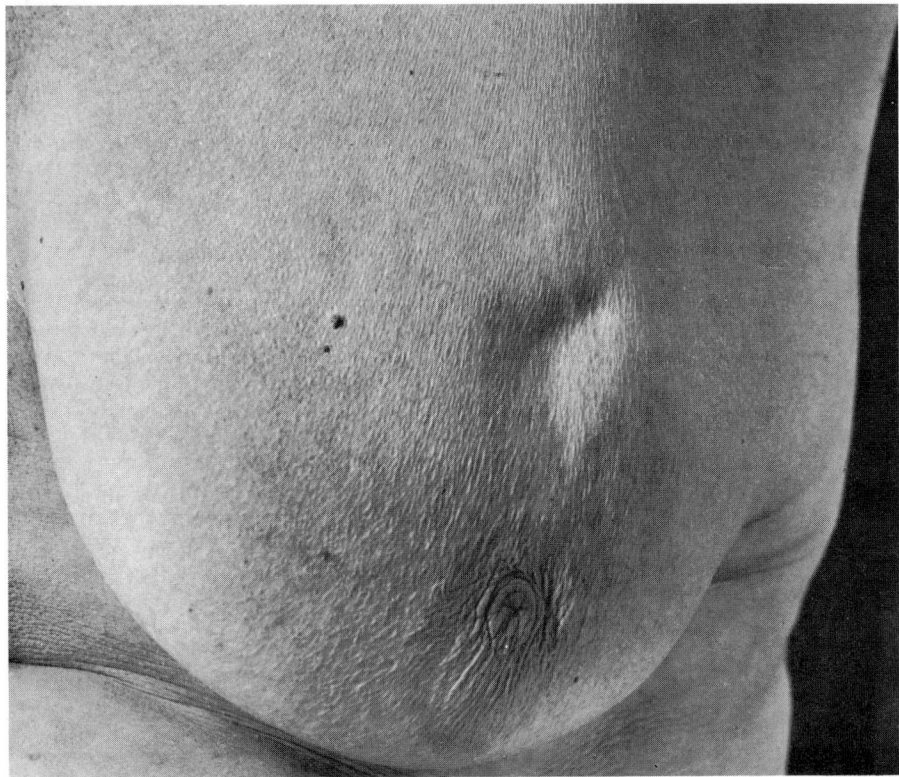

Figure 8. Dimple in the skin of the breast overlying a small carcinoma in the upper quadrant. The use of indirect lighting accentuates this subtle clinical finding, which might be overlooked if examined under poor lighting or without the subject sitting upright with the arm extended. (From Haagensen, C. D.: DIseases of the Breast, 3rd ed. Philadelphia, W. B. Saunders Company 1986, p. 521.)

caused by fibrosis in certain benign conditions, especially subareolar duct ectasia. In these cases, the finding is frequently bilateral, and the history confirms that the condition has been present for many years. Unilateral retraction or retraction developing over weeks or months is more suggestive of carcinoma. Centrally located tumors may directly invade and ulcerate the skin of the areola or nipple. More peripheral tumors may distort the normal symmetry of the nipples by traction on Cooper's ligaments.

A second clinical feature of carcinoma that directly involves the nipple was described by Sir James Paget in 1874 and named Paget's disease. Histologically, this disease is produced by intra-

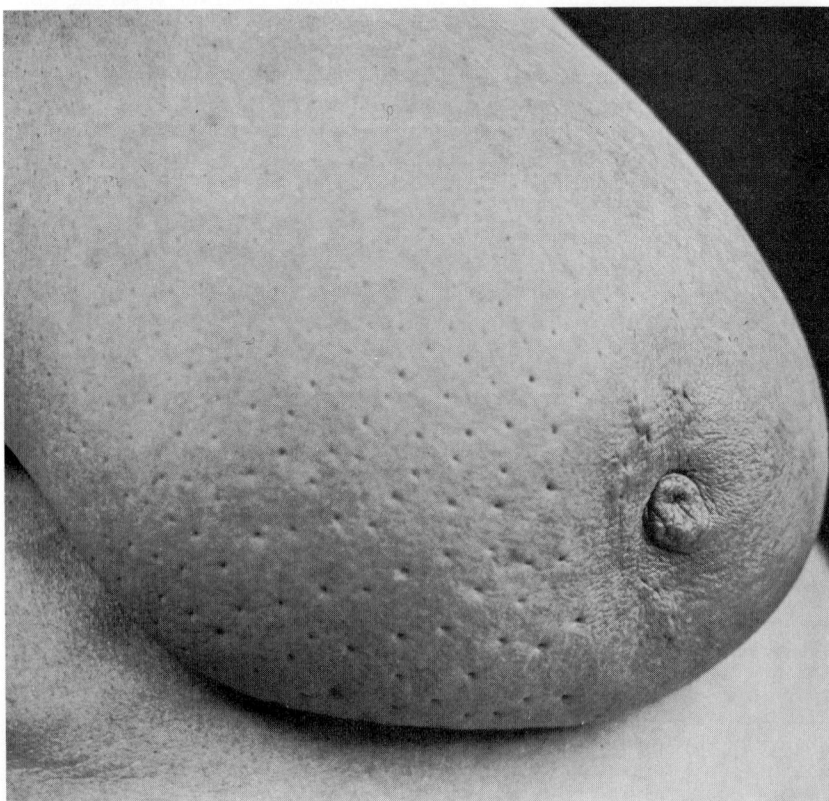

Figure 9. Edema of the skin in a breast with inflammatory carcinoma. Edema of the dermis produces the peau d'orange (orange peel) appearance of the skin. The pitting is caused by the tethering of the epidermis over the swollen dermis by small hair follicles. Erythema of the skin generally accompanies the peau d'orange change. (From Haagensen, C. D.: Diseases of the Breast, 3rd ed. Philadelphia, W. B. Saunders Company 1986, p. 521.)

ductal carcinoma occurring in the large sinuses just under the nipple. Carcinoma cells invade across the epidermal-epithelial junction and enter the epidermal layer of the skin of the nipple. Clinically, this histologic variant produces a dermatitis that may appear eczematoid and moist or dry and psoriatic. It is usually confined to the nipple, although it can spread to the skin of the areola. Haagensen points out that benign skin conditions frequently begin on the areola, whereas Paget's disease originates on the nipple and secondarily involves the areola.[108]

While the patient is still in the sitting position, the examiner supports the patient's arm and palpates each axilla to detect the presence of enlarged axillary lymph nodes. The supraclavicular space is similarly palpated for enlarged nodes. Palpation of the breast is always done with the patient lying supine on a solid examining surface and with the arm stretched above the head. Palpation of the breast while the patient is sitting is insensitive and inaccurate. The breast parenchyma is compressed against the chest wall, carefully palpating each quadrant and the tissue under the areola. Masses found during this examination are characterized according to their size, shape, consistency, and location. It is useful to remember that benign tumors, such as fibroadenomas and cysts, can be as firm as carcinoma. However, these tumors are usually quite distinct, well-circumscribed, and movable. Carcinoma is typically firm but less circumscribed, and its movement produces a drag of adjacent tissue. Neither benign nor malignant tumors are usually tender; tenderness is rarely a helpful diagnostic sign. Generally, 75 per cent of breast cancers produce palpable masses, and 75 per cent of palpable masses are discovered by patients during casual or intentional self-examination.

FINE-NEEDLE ASPIRATION. Fine-needle aspiration (FNA) has become a routine part of the physical diagnosis of breast masses. It can be done with a 22-gauge needle, an appropriate-size syringe, and an alcohol prep pad. Its main utility is the differentiation of solid from cystic masses, but it may be done whenever a new dominant, unexplained mass is found in the breast. This simple procedure is postponed only if mammography is necessary and there is worry that a small hematoma, resulting from needle puncture, might confuse the radiographic evaluation. In young women under 30 years of age, mammography is rarely used, and FNA is a quick and accurate way to diagnose a cyst and provide immediate reassurance. Cyst fluid is usually turbid dark green or amber in color and can be discarded if the mass totally disappears and the fluid is not bloody. By using FNA in the routine examination of the breast, unnecessary open biopsy of cystic change is avoided. As a result of adding FNA to the routine examination of breast masses, a restating of criteria for open biopsy is helpful. Carcinoma will not be missed if a formal biopsy is done when (1) needle aspiration produces no cyst fluid and a solid mass is diagnosed, (2) the cyst fluid produced is thick and blood tinged, (3) fluid is produced but the mass fails to resolve completely, and (4) the mass reappears in the same area after more than two aspirations. Donegan adds rapid accumulation of fluid after initial aspiration (less than 2 weeks) to this last criteria.[52]

If the mass is solid and the clinical situation is consistent with carcinoma, a cytologic examination of the aspirated material may be helpful. The needle is repeatedly inserted into the mass while constant negative pressure is applied to the syringe. Suction is released and the needle withdrawn. The scanty fluid and cellular material within the needle are submitted either in physiologically buffered saline (Normosol) or fixed immediately on slides in 95 per cent ethyl alcohol. Most authors would *not* recommend definitive treatment based only on a cytologic examination.[52] However, a positive result allows informed discussion with the patient, definite plans for treatment can be made, and appropriate consultations or second opinions can be obtained.

BREAST IMAGING

The goal of any technique that seeks to image the breast is to extend the capability of physical examination either to detect smaller abnormalities or to provide more information about palpable abnormalities. Currently, mammography is clearly the most sensitive and specific test that can be used to complement the physical examination of the breast. Mammography is used either as a diagnostic modality that seeks to answer specific questions about the health of the breast or as a screening test that seeks to find any abnormality within the breast. A variety of other methods have been used to generate useful images of the breast. Of these, ultrasonography is the only one in common usage today. Thermography, which images heat generated by the breast, was added to the Breast Cancer Detection Demonstration Project (BCDDP) to evaluate its usefulness as a screening tool. However, because of a low overall yield, thermography was dropped from the project. Other investigators have concluded that this modality has little to offer over high-quality mammography. Computed tomography (CT) has been used by some investigators with success, but it can require contrast enhancement, has limited ability to resolve small abnormalities, and requires a larger exposure to radiation.[135] CT appears to be the best way to image internal mammary nodes and to evaluate the chest and axilla following mastectomy.[133] Magnetic resonance imaging is a new technique, which requires expensive equipment and prohibitive time to construct a suitable image; currently, it has unproved efficacy for routine breast imaging.[133] Digital imaging is an evolving hybrid technology that has found application in chest radiography and may be used to store radiographic information in a digital format or to directly produce images.[223,225] This technology is improving and may have application in mammography.

DIAGNOSTIC MAMMOGRAPHY. Currently, two techniques are in popular use. Xeromammography (Xerox Corporation) uses a charged aluminum plate coated with selenium. Radiation passing through the breast is absorbed on the plate and causes a local reduction in charge. The plate is then sprayed with blue toner, transferred to paper, and heated to produce an image viewed in ambient reflected light. Film/screen mammography uses a combination of an enhancing screen that converts and amplifies a low energy radiation beam into high energy photons that, in turn, expose a standard x-ray film. In this technique, compression of the breast between Plexiglas plates enhances contrast. The image, like standard x-ray films, is viewed using transmitted light and is a negative image. Both techniques deliver a similar average glandular dose of radiation, which is less than 300 millirads (0.3 cGy. or 0.3 rad). Most current reviews suggest that there is little difference between the sensitivity and specificity of the Xerox and film/screen techniques.[133,165]

The mammographic features of malignancy can be broadly divided into density abnormalities (including masses, asymmetries, and architectural distortions) and microcalcifications. Each mammogram also should be assessed for the presence of abnormalities in the axillary nodes and for the presence of skin or nipple changes, such as thickening or retraction. Obviously, these mammographic features can coexist in any one abnormality and may exist in the presence or absence of physical findings. In fact, it is the integration of each of the radiographic features and the physical findings that leads to a prediction of malignancy. Moskowitz has attempted to quantify the predictive value of these signs in both the presence and absence of physical findings.[164] A fine atlas of mammographic abnormalities has been compiled recently by Kopans and includes excellent narrative descriptions and a general review of breast imaging.[133] Selected mammographic abnormalities are shown in Figures 10 and 11, which illustrate common findings of malignancy.

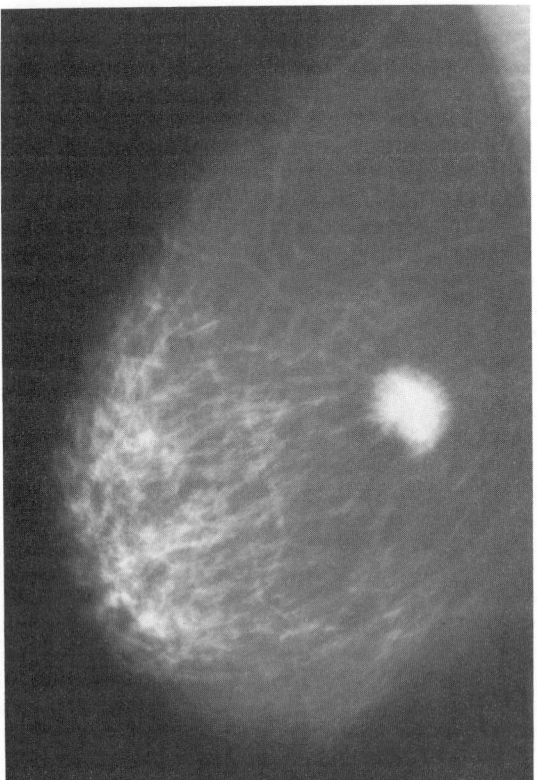

Figure 10. Mammographic features of malignancy: a stellate mass. The combination of a density, surrounding spiculations, and distortion of the breast architecture strongly suggest a malignancy in this mammogram.

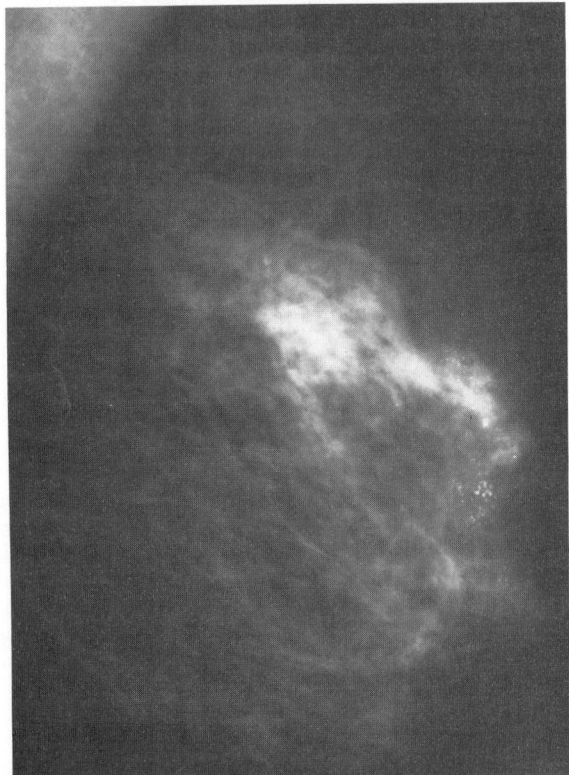

Figure 11. Mammographic features of malignancy: clustered microcalcifications. Fine, irregular, and branching forms suggest malignancy in this mammogram. Fine calcifications, less than 0.5 mm in size, are more often associated with cancer than larger, coarse calcifications.

NONPALPABLE MAMMOGRAPHIC ABNORMALITIES

Mammographic abnormalities that cannot be detected by physical examination are classified in three broad categories: lesions consisting of microcalcifications only, density lesions (masses, architectural distortions, and asymmetries), and those with both calcifications and density abnormalities. The incidence of malignancy after biopsy depends on the characteristics of the radiographic finding. The results of a recent review of 179 patients at Duke University are shown in Table 2. Overall, the incidence of malignancy was 24 per cent; this figure agreed with several similar studies reporting chances of malignancy of between 14 and 29 per cent.[221] Lesions with both microcalcifications and a mass effect, spiculated masses, and linear branching calcifications carry the highest probability of being malignant. However, even well-defined densities can be malignant. To be certain, not every abnormality should undergo biopsy, and recommendations must be made by the surgeon in consultation with an experienced radiologist. For those patients not undergoing biopsy, interval mammograms must be done to assure stability of the abnormality.

If a biopsy is performed, it is usually done after mammographic placement of a needle or hook wire.[134] Biopsy in the operating room with use of local anesthesia and sedation or general anesthesia is recommended. For lesions with calcification, a specimen radiograph must be done to confirm adequacy of the biopsy. For masses, gross examination or radiographs must be done to confirm success of the biopsy. Intraoperative cooperation of the pathologist, who should have access to the specimen radiograph, is required. After gross inspection, histologic examination is generally deferred until permanent sections are available. However, prior to fixation, it should be determined whether material needs to be retrieved for hormone receptor assays.

SCREENING MAMMOGRAPHY. The goals of screening mammography differ from those of diagnostic mammography. Screening studies seek to identify any abnormality, maximizing sensitivity and cost effectiveness. Results from six controlled

TABLE 2. Biopsy Results for Various Mammographic Features

Mammographic Feature*	Malignant	Benign	Per Cent Positive	
Asymmetric density†	6	25	19	
Architectural distortion	7	10	41	
Mass†	20	51	28	
Mass subtotals				
Stellate	6	2	75	
Irregularly defined	12	22	35	
Well-defined	2	27	6	
Number of calcifications				
>10	14	27	34	
≤10	8	44	15	p = 0.07
Size of calcifications				
≥0.4 mm.	13	41	24	
<0.4 mm.	9	30	23	p > 0.25
Distribution of calcifications‡				
Clustered	9	37	20	
Scattered	9	15	38	p = 0.15

*The radiographic features are considered independently (i.e., lesions having both a soft tissue lesion and calcifications are included twice).
†Lesions not associated with an architectural distortion.
‡Lesions having more than five calcifications.
From Skinner, M. A., Swain, M., Simmons, R., et al.: Nonpalpable breast lesions at biopsy. A detailed analysis of radiographic features. Ann. Surg., *208*:203, 1988.

trials and a single large uncontrolled study have demonstrated the value of screening mammography.[38,43,182,214,218,232,243] The Health Insurance Plan (HIP) of Greater New York randomized 62,000 women to a control group offered no sponsored screening and a study group who received annual mammograms and physical examinations for 4 years.[218] Overall, there was a 23 per cent reduction in mortality for the screened population at 18 years of follow-up. For women older than 50 years at entry, there was a greater than 50 per cent reduction in mortality. Similar results were reported from case-control trials in Sweden,[232] two cities in the Netherlands,[38,243] and in Florence.[182]

Following the lead of the HIP study, the American Cancer Society and the National Cancer Institute (NCI) joined in an uncontrolled project to demonstrate the feasibility of a population-based screening program. The Breast Cancer Detection Demonstration Project (BCDDP) screened 280,000 women in 29 centers throughout the United States. Each center offered free mammograms and a breast examination and taught breast self-examination. Five screening examinations were planned, and the last was completed in 1981. Survival data reported to 8 years of follow-up have been reviewed.[214] Since this was not a controlled trial, comparison has been made to national statistics compiled by the Surveillance, Epidemiology, and End Results (SEER) program within the NCI. Comparison of survival data 8 years after diagnosis of cancer in the BCDDP to corresponding data from the SEER program demonstrates improved survival in the screened population, which appears to be explained by a shift to earlier-stage disease in the BCDDP (Table 3).

As a result of these studies, guidelines from the American Cancer Society recommend annual mammograms for women 50 years and older. More controversial are recommendations for women under age 50 years. In these younger populations of women, most studies have failed to show a conclusive advantage for screening. A quantitative overview analysis of results from published studies has concluded that "mammography screening can detect some breast cancers before they are apparent by breast physical examination in women aged 40 through 49 years, and over the long run, mammography screening should be expected to reduce mortality. Mammography should be made available to women who understand the limits of its benefits, who understand its risks, and who are willing to pay its costs."[61]

BENIGN BREAST TUMORS AND RELATED DISEASES

BREAST CYSTS

Cysts within the breast are fluid filled, epithelial-lined cavities that may vary in size from microscopic to large, palpable masses containing as much as 20 to 30 ml. of fluid. As discussed, cysts are generally discovered by physical examination and confirmed by ultrasound or needle aspiration. At least 1 woman in every 14 will develop a palpable cyst, and 50 per cent of cysts are multiple or recurrent. Cysts occur as solitary abnormalities, called macrocysts or gross breast cysts, or as part of a generalized process of microscopic cyst formation. This latter disease process is frequently bilateral and the cystic transformation can be extensive. The pathogenesis of cystic formation is not well understood; however, cysts appear to arise from destruction and dilation of lobules and terminal ductules. Three-dimensional microscopic studies and extensive sectioning have shown that stricture and fibrosis at or near terminal branching of small ductules, combined with continued secretion by the distal lobule, result in expansion of a cavity containing fluid and lined by ductal epithelium.[233]

Cysts are unquestionably influenced by ovarian hormones, a fact that explains their sudden appearance during the menstrual cycle, their rapid growth, and their spontaneous regression with completion of the menses. Most women with new cyst formation present after the age of 35 years and rarely before the age of 25 years.[106] The incidence of cyst development steadily increases until the age of menopause and sharply declines after menopause (Fig. 12). Autopsy studies of women dying with clinically normal breasts generally confirm the age relationship of gross cyst development but do find that the breasts of older women can contain gross and microscopic cysts.[87] New cyst formation detected clinically in older women commonly is explained by the use of exogenous hormone replacement.

When encountered during operation, cysts are frequently dark in color. These are often referred to as "blue dome cysts," and they reflect the dark cyst fluid contained within. Grossly, they are usually unilocular and lined by a smooth and glistening surface, although larger cystic structures may be trabeculated and multiloculated. Histologically, cysts are frequently lined by

TABLE 3. Distribution by Stage and Survival Rates for Breast Cancer Detected by Screening in the BCDDP and SEER Programs

Stage	BCDDP Distribution by Stage (%)	BCDDP Survival at 8 yr. (%)	SEER Distribution by Stage (%)	SEER Survival at 8 yr. (%)
Noninvasive	17	97	NA	NA
Stage I	30	90	12	92
Stage II	37	76	57	72
Stage III	3	—	13	41
Stage IV	NA	NA	7	9
Unstaged	30	85	11	67
Total invasive cancers	100	81	100	65

Adapted from Seidman, H., Gelb, S.K., Silverberg, E., et al.: Survival experience in the Breast Cancer Detection Demonstration Project. CA, 37:258, 1987.

A lead time of 1 year was subtracted from follow-up in the BCDDP analysis.

BCDDP, Breast Cancer Detection Demonstration Project; SEER, Surveillance, Epidemiology, and End-Results Program (National Cancer Institute).

From Iglehart, J. D.: The diagnosis and management of breast cancer: An Update In Sabiston, O. C., Jr.; Textbook of Surgery: The Biological Basis of Surgical Practice, Update 1. Philadelphia W. B. Saunders Company, 1988.

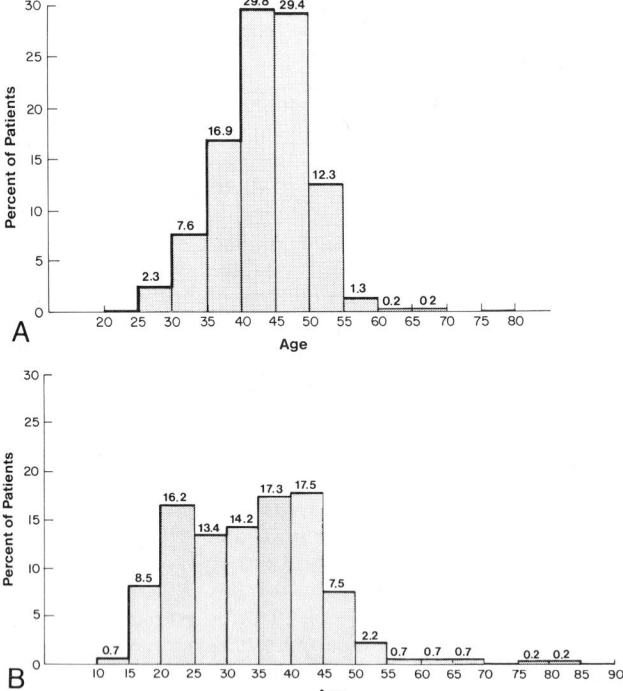

Figure 12. Age distribution of common benign breast tumors. In *A*, the age distribution of gross breast cysts is shown. The incidence is very low until the fourth decade of life, increases sharply until the age of menopause, and then declines sharply. In *B*, the age distribution of fibroadenoma is shown. In contrast to breast cysts, fibroadenoma can occur in young women after the menarche, but the incidence again declines sharply after menopause. (From Haagensen, C. D.: Diseases of the Breast, 3rd ed. Philadelphia, W. B. Saunders Company 1986, pp. 256 and 268.)

a flattened epithelium. However, the epithelial layer may display apocrine metaplasia or may have papillary features. Intracystic carcinoma is exceedingly rare. Rosemond was able to report only three examples in over 3000 cyst aspirations (0.1 per cent), and other investigators confirm this exceedingly low incidence.[1,199] Regarding the risk of developing cancer for women with cystic disease, no studies demonstrate an increased risk in women with small or microscopic cysts. For patients with large cysts, called gross cystic disease by Haagensen, there remains some controversy. Patey and Nurick found no increase in cancers subsequent to cyst aspiration. Of 810 patients with cancers treated by Patey, only 10 had a previous history of gross cysts.[186] Other recent reviews have emphasized that women with gross cysts have a risk of two- to fourfold that of age-matched women without cysts.[62] The studies of Page and associates[180] and Dupont and Page[59] do not show a significant increase in cancers after long-term follow-up of over 2000 women who underwent biopsy of palpable cysts when compared with the slight increase borne by women who have had breast biopsy alone.

FIBROADENOMA AND RELATED TUMORS

Fibroadenoma (adenofibroma) is a benign tumor composed of both stromal and epithelial elements in the breast. After carcinoma, fibroadenoma is the second most common solid tumor in the breast and is the most common tumor in women under the age of 30 years. The benign nature of this lesion was recognized in 1840 by Sir Astley Cooper, who referred to the lesions as "chronic mammary tumors." Clinically, they present as firm, solitary tumors that may increase in size over several months of observation. They may be lobulated but will slip easily under the examining fingers. At operation, fibroadenomas appear to be well-encapsulated masses that may easily detach from the

surrounding breast tissue. By history, fibroadenoma is favored over cyst in the adolescent or young adult (Fig. 12), and on examination, these tumors are distinguished from cysts by the needle aspiration that yields no fluid. Mammography is of little help in distinguishing between cysts and fibroadenomas; however, ultrasound usually clearly shows the cavity of a cyst.

The gross appearance and histopathology are distinctive of fibroadenoma. Grossly, the tumor appears well-encapsulated, with smooth borders that may be lobulated. Histologically, a variable proportion of epithelial and stromal proliferation is present, and the stroma may be quite cellular or replaced by acellular swirls of collagen. In older patients, the lesions may contain deposits of calcium within dense fibrosis. The epithelium can display the entire spectrum of proliferative changes seen elsewhere in the breast. Although fibroadenomas are not considered to have a malignant potential, the epithelial elements appear to be at risk for neoplasia just as epithelium elsewhere in the breast. More than 100 invasive and noninvasive carcinomas have been reported in pre-existing fibroadenomas since 1985.[174] Most of these (50 per cent) have been lobular carcinoma *in situ*; 35 per cent were infiltrating carcinomas; and 15 per cent were intraductal carcinoma. The risk of cancer in a newly discovered fibroadenoma found in the breast of a young woman is obviously exceedingly rare and is not an issue that influences treatment. A modest risk of subsequent carcinoma in women who have previously been treated for fibroadenoma has been reported, but the magnitude is about two times that of the general population. This is only slightly higher than the reported excess risk for all women who have had a breast biopsy.[59]

The treatment for fibroadenoma follows that for any unexplained solid mass within the breast. The great majority of patients should be treated by excisional biopsy to remove the tumor and establish the diagnosis. The approach to a young woman with a typical fibroadenoma on examination should be very different than that to an older woman with an indeterminate mass. Cosmetic incisions around the areola and a modest amount of tunneling to remove the lesion are commonly used techniques and are proper for the treatment of fibroadenoma. Emphasis should be placed on removing a minimal amount of breast tissue adjacent to a typical fibroadenoma. If the gross appearance is that of a fibroadenoma, frozen section is superfluous; the patient can be immediately reassured; and final diagnosis is established by inspecting permanent sections.

JUVENILE FIBROADENOMA, GIANT FIBROADENOMA. Clinicians treating breast masses should be aware of these two terms, which are sometimes confusing. Giant fibroadenoma is a descriptive term that applies to a fibroadenoma that attains an unusually large size, typically greater than 5 cm. Haagensen calls these lesions "massive adenofibromas in youth" to denote their common occurrence in adolescent women. Juvenile fibroadenoma refers to the occasional large fibroadenoma that occurs in adolescents and young adults and histologically is more cellular than the usual fibroadenoma. Both these lesions overlap, and both may display remarkably rapid growth within the breast. Although alarming to the patient and physician, prompt surgical removal is always curative. The term *benign cystosarcoma phyllodes* refers to a tumor that may be difficult to distinguish clearly from juvenile fibroadenoma. If the tumor has been completely removed, the diagnosis of "benign cystosarcoma" should reassure the surgeon and the patient that the risk of recurrence is low, particularly if the patient is an adolescent or a young adult.[174,190] Malignant cystosarcoma phyllodes is a distinctive and aggressive tumor, discussed later.

HAMARTOMA AND ADENOMA. Although probably not of the same histogenesis as fibroadenoma, these tumors are benign proliferations of variable amounts of epithelium and stromal supporting tissue. The hamartoma is a discrete nodule that contains closely packed lobules and prominent, ectatic extralobular ducts. By physical examination, mammography, and gross inspection, the hamartoma is indistinguishable from fibroadenoma. The nodule is entirely benign, and removal is curative. The mammary adenoma or tubular adenoma has been a more elusive entity to define. Page and Anderson describe this tumor as a cellular neoplasm of ductules packed closely together and forming a sheet of tiny glands without supporting stroma.[174] During pregnancy and lactation, these tumors may increase in size, and histologic examination shows secretory differentiation. Malignancy is not a feature of tubular adenoma or lactating adenoma, but biopsy is required to establish the diagnosis.

BREAST ABSCESS AND INFECTIONS

Breast abscess commonly occurs in the subareolar breast tissue and may be recurrent and difficult to treat. Although the exact cause is not known, subareolar duct ectasia and obstruction of major ducts may lead to proliferation of bacteria and subsequent abscess. Further destruction of the normal ductal openings leads to fistula formation and chronic recurrent abscess. Mammary duct ectasia, first named by Haagensen,[96] is an inflammatory condition that causes distortion and dilation of the lactiferous sinuses under the nipple. It is a common entity and is frequently responsible for nipple inversion in older women. In understanding subareolar abscess and probably mastitis in general, it is useful to remember that the nipple and areolar complex contain secretory ducts that are exposed to the environment. Chronic inflammation, duct dilation, and obstruction may combine at the nipple to produce circumstances that favor bacterial invasion.

The treatment of acute abscess of periareolar tissue should be conservative, if possible. Antibiotics with broad-spectrum coverage should be used initially. More severe infections may require hospitalization and intravenous antibiotics. Incision with drainage is avoided unless the process cannot be controlled by antibiotics alone. Needle aspiration may be attempted, but the abscess cavity is usually multiloculated. Recurrent infection is best treated by excision of the diseased subareolar ducts, as described by Haagensen and others.[107,140,145]

Mastitis describes a more generalized cellulitis of breast tissue that may involve a large area of the breast but may not form a true abscess. The etiology appears to be an ascending infection beginning in subareolar ducts and extending outward from the nipple. Occasionally, mastitis involves areas of cystic disease or complicates cyst aspiration. Mastitis presents with erythema of the overlying skin, pain, and tenderness to palpation. There is induration of the skin and underlying breast parenchyma. Especially in young women, an apparent mastitis may develop that is quite dramatic in its presentation and responds poorly to antibiotics but resolves spontaneously. The etiology is unknown but may be related to menstrual cycle irregularity. More commonly, mastitis complicates lactation, possibly due to inspissation of milk, obstruction, and secondary infection. Local measures such as application of heat, ice packs, or use of a mechanical breast pump on the affected side have all been recommended. If conservative measures are not effective, administration of broad-spectrum antibiotics is usually indicated.

In many situations, the differential diagnosis of acute mastitis includes inflammatory carcinoma. It is important to follow patients with mastitis and confirm that there has been a complete resolution of symptoms and signs. The erythema produced by an inflammatory carcinoma will not resolve with conservative measures and generally will worsen in a short period of follow-up.

PAPILLOMA AND RELATED DUCTAL TUMORS

Solitary intraductal papillomas are true polyps of epithelium-lined breast ducts. Solitary papillomas are located under the areola in the majority of cases. In contrast, certain patients have multiple intraductal papillomas, which Haagensen believes are more likely to be peripherally located and associated with an increased risk of cancer.[105] Solitary papillomas may be located in peripheral ducts and can grow to large size, presenting as a breast mass. When papillomas attain a large size, they may appear to arise within a cystic structure, probably representing a greatly expanded duct. In general, these lesions are less than 1 cm. in size but can grow to as large as 4 or 5 cm.

Tumors under the nipple and areolar complex often present with a bloody nipple discharge. Less frequently, they are discovered as a palpable mass under the areola or as a density lesion on the mammogram. Treatment is total excision through a circumareolar incision. The surgeon must keep in mind that one of the most difficult areas in differential diagnosis is between a papilloma and invasive papillary carcinoma. Because these lesions can infarct, scar, and even develop squamous metaplasia, they can appear quite bizarre and disordered. Most pathologists urge evaluation on permanent sections for the majority of papillary lesions before more extensive surgical therapy is undertaken.[145,175]

It is also important not to confuse the commonly used term *papillomatosis* with either solitary or multiple papillomas. Papillomatosis refers to epithelial hyperplasia, which commonly occurs in younger women or is associated with fibrocystic change. This lesion is not composed of true papillomas. Hyperplastic epithelium in papillomatosis may fill individual ducts like a true polyp but has no stalks of fibrovascular tissue nor the frondlike growth. Solitary papillomas are entirely benign and do not predispose to development of cancer in the patients who have them. Page and Anderson state that the degree of subsequent risk for breast cancer in patients with either papillomatosis or with true papillomas, either solitary or multiple, relates to the degree of atypical epithelial proliferation associated with them.[175]

SCLEROSING LESIONS

SCLEROSING ADENOSIS. Adenosis refers to an increased number of small terminal ductules, or acini. Adenosis is frequently associated with a proliferation of stromal tissue producing a histologic lesion, sclerosing adenosis, which can simulate carcinoma both grossly and histologically. There may be deposition of calcium, which can be seen on mammography in a pattern indistinguishable from that of microcalcifications in intraductal carcinoma. In fact, sclerosing adenosis was the most common pathologic diagnosis in patients undergoing needle-directed biopsy of microcalcifications at Duke University.[221] Skinner et al. Sclerosing adenosis is frequently listed as one of the component lesions of fibrocystic disease; it is very common and has no malignant potential.[145]

RADIAL SCAR. Radial scar belongs to a group of related abnormalities known as complex sclerosing lesions. They are important to the surgeon and pathologist because they can simulate carcinoma mammographically and on physical examination. These lesions contain microcysts, epithelial hyperplasia, adenosis, and a prominent display of central sclerosis. The gross abnormality is rarely more than 1 cm. in diameter. The larger lesions will form palpable tumors and appear as a spiculated mass with prominent architectural distortion on the mammogram. These tumors can even produce skin dimpling by traction on surrounding fibrous bands that become involved in the cicatrix. Biopsy is always recommended for tumors with these signs and symptoms. Apart from their confusing presentation, these lesions are benign.

FAT NECROSIS. As with the other sclerosing abnormalities, fat necrosis can mimic cancer by producing a mass, a density lesion on mammography that can calcify, and surrounding distortion of the normal breast architecture. Fat necrosis typically occurs in pendulous, fatty breasts, and although it may follow an episode of trauma, commonly there is no such history. Histologically, the lesion is composed of lipid-laden macrophages, scar tissue, and chronic inflammatory cells. This is not a lesion of epithelial tissue and has no malignant potential. It is usually biopsied because of the signs it produces.

MALIGNANT TUMORS OF THE BREAST

EPIDEMIOLOGY

Breast cancer is an exceedingly common disease. In 1985, the probability at birth of eventually developing an invasive breast cancer was close to 10 per cent for white females and 7.3 per cent for black females in the United States.[215] Overall, approximately 1 woman in 10 will contract breast cancer during her lifespan. Although carcinoma of the lung has recently overtaken breast cancer as the leading cause of cancer-related death in American women, breast cancer remains far more common. Of 490,000 new cases of cancer among women in 1989, 135,000 occurred in the breast whereas 52,000 arose in the lung.[219]

Several studies based upon cancer registries in the Surveillance, Epidemiology, and End Results (SEER) program of the NCI have reported an increasing attack rate for breast cancer in the United States.[126,157] In Washington State, there has been an annual estimated increase of 2.5 per cent. A greater increase was apparent among black and low-income women.[250] In the Connecticut Tumor Registry, the overall annual incidence rose from 53 cases per 100,000 women during the years 1935 to 1939 to an average annual rate of 86.4 per 100,000 women for the years 1975 to 1979. Data from other studies and from other Western countries confirm the recent increase in the incidence of breast cancer.[246] Risk factors that predispose to the development of breast cancer have been outlined earlier.

Despite the increased incidence, the age-adjusted death rate from carcinoma of the breast was stable until 1979 and may have decreased in the 5-year period between 1979 and 1984.[181,215] Although it is tempting to speculate that this is a real improvement attributable to early diagnosis or improved therapy, no direct proof can be cited.

THE PATHOLOGY OF BREAST CANCER

Modern classification of breast cancer attempts to recognize morphologic patterns that reflect both the histogenesis of the malignancy and its biologic behavior, or prognosis. As such, these classifications impose artificial divisions upon diseases that are fundamentally poorly understood. As advances are made in our understanding of breast malignancies, the classifications presented today will be improved upon by future generations of surgeons and pathologists. Malignancies of the breast are broadly divided into epithelial tumors of cells lining ducts and lobules and nonepithelial malignancies of the supporting stroma. A second important division of the epithelial tumors is between noninvasive and invasive cancers. The noninvasive malignancies are proliferations of either ductal or lobular cells confined by the basement membrane, illustrated in Figure 7. These are true carcinoma *in situ* (CIS). As in other organs, CIS of the breast commonly coexists with invasive cancer. In the breast, this association is very frequent and argues for the progression of cancer through stages of noninvasive proliferation, disruption of the basement membrane, and invasion of the supporting stroma.

Most pathologists utilize the classification scheme proposed

TABLE 4. The World Health Organization Classification of Breast Tumors

I. Epithelial Tumors		II. Mixed Connective Tissue and Epithelial Tumors	
A. *Benign*		A. *Fibroadenoma*	9010/0
1. Intraductal papilloma	8503/0*†	B. *Phyllodes Tumor (cystosarcoma phyllodes)*	9020/—†
2. Adenoma of the nipple	8506/0	C. *Carcinosarcoma*	8980/3
3. Adenoma	8140/0	**III. Miscellaneous Tumors**	
a. Tubular	8211/0	A. *Soft Tissue Tumors*	
b. Lactating‡		B. *Skin Tumors*	
B. *Malignant*		C. *Tumors of Hematopoietic and Lymphoid Tissues*	
1. Noninvasive		**IV. Unclassified Tumors**	8000/—†
a. Intraductal carcinoma	8500/2,	**V. Mammary Dysplasia/Fibrocystic Disease**	74320
b. Lobular carcinoma *in situ*	8520/2,	**VI. Tumor Like Lesions**	
2. Invasive		A. *Duct Ectasia*	32100
a. Invasive ductal carcinoma	8500/3	B. *Inflammatory Pseudotumors*	76820
b. Invasive ductal carcinoma with a		C. *Hamartoma*	75500
predominant intraductal	8500/3 and	D. *Gynecomastia*	71000
component	8500/2,	E. *Others*	
c. Invasive lobular carcinoma	8520/3		
d. Mucinous carcinoma	8480/3		
e. Medullary carcinoma	8510/3		
f. Papillary carcinoma	8503/3		
g. Tubular carcinoma	8211/3		
h. Adenoid cystic carcinoma	8200/3		
i. Secretory (juvenile) carcinoma	8502/3		
j. Apocrine carcinoma	8573/3		
k. Carcinoma with metaplasia			
i. Squamous type	8570/3		
ii. Spindle cell type	8572/3		
iii. Cartilaginous and osseous type	8571/3		
iv. Mixed type§			
l. Others			
3. Paget's disease of the nipple	8540/3¶		

* These code numbers correspond to ICD-O and SNOMED morphology fields.

† Code behavior: /0, benign; /1, uncertain whether benign or malignant; /3, malignant.

‡ No specific code available for lactating adenoma.

§ Code specific types.

¶ Paget's disease plus invasive carcinoma is coded 8541/3.

by the World Health Organization (WHO)[9,255] and outlined in the fascicles of the Armed Forces Institute of Pathology.[151] Historically, Foote and Stewart presented most of this material in 1945, including a recognition of noninvasive carcinoma and the differentiation between tumors originating in the breast lobule and those arising in the lactiferous ducts.[84] The WHO classification scheme, adding the approximate frequencies of the major histologic types, is shown in Table 4. Examples provided by WHO illustrating some of the common morphologies of invasive breast cancers are shown in Figure 13. The morphology of common noninvasive breast tumors from the WHO collection is shown in Figure 14.

DUCTAL CARCINOMA-IN-SITU, INTRADUCTAL CARCINOMA.[177] The concept of a purely noninvasive form of breast cancer and recognition of various subtypes have evolved slowly since the beginning of this century. Ductal carcinoma *in situ* (DCIS) was probably recognized first by surgeons who appreciated its favorable prognosis. Bloodgood at the Johns Hopkins Hospital, impressed by the tumor of an early patient of Halsted, recognized a disease he termed "pure comedo tumor" that had an extremely favorable prognosis. Pathologically, breast ducts become swollen with proliferating malignant epithelium. In the solid or comedo type, the ducts can expand to visible proportions 1 or 2 mm. in diameter. The term *pure intraductal carcinoma* refers to the absence of detectable invasion of the basement membrane, illustrated by special stains in Figure 7. Devoid of blood supply, the center of the lesion undergoes necrosis, and the intraductal spaces fill with necrotic cellular debris, as shown in Figure 14. The central detritus can undergo dystrophic calcification that is fine, focally clustered, and even

linear and branching when seen on high quality mammography (see Fig. 11). The process can produce a palpable mass locally if multiple ducts are involved.

Subtypes of DCIS are now well recognized and frequently reported pathologically. The solid or comedo type is most common and probably most virulent. This type, described above and illustrated in Figure 14, is characterized by the closely packed cells within ductal spaces that are susceptible to central necrosis. Papillary or cribriform DCIS is characterized by papillary projections of tumor cells into the ductal lumen or by the presence of a branching, cribriform pattern filling ducts (Fig. 14). These types are less likely to form palpable masses and uncommonly calcify to produce a mammographic abnormality. However, it is important to emphasize that these subtypes can coexist and that DCIS is best described by the pathologist in terms of its extent, multicentricity, and involvement of the surgical margin.

Confusion arises in a number of ways. First, the uninitiated may confuse the term *infiltrating ductal carcinoma* with the term *intraductal carcinoma*; the former is invasive disease and the latter, noninvasive disease. Second, these two stages of tumorigenesis usually coexist, particularly when they are carefully searched for in pathologic specimens. Finally, as discussed later, the treatment and outcome for patients with intraductal disease may depend on variables such as multifocality, multicentricity, and extent of disease in a way more demanding for the pathologists and surgeons than in the past.

LOBULAR CARCINOMA *IN SITU* OR LOBULAR NEOPLASIA. This disease of the breast lobules or acini was first clearly delineated by Foote and Stewart in 1941, who gave it the name

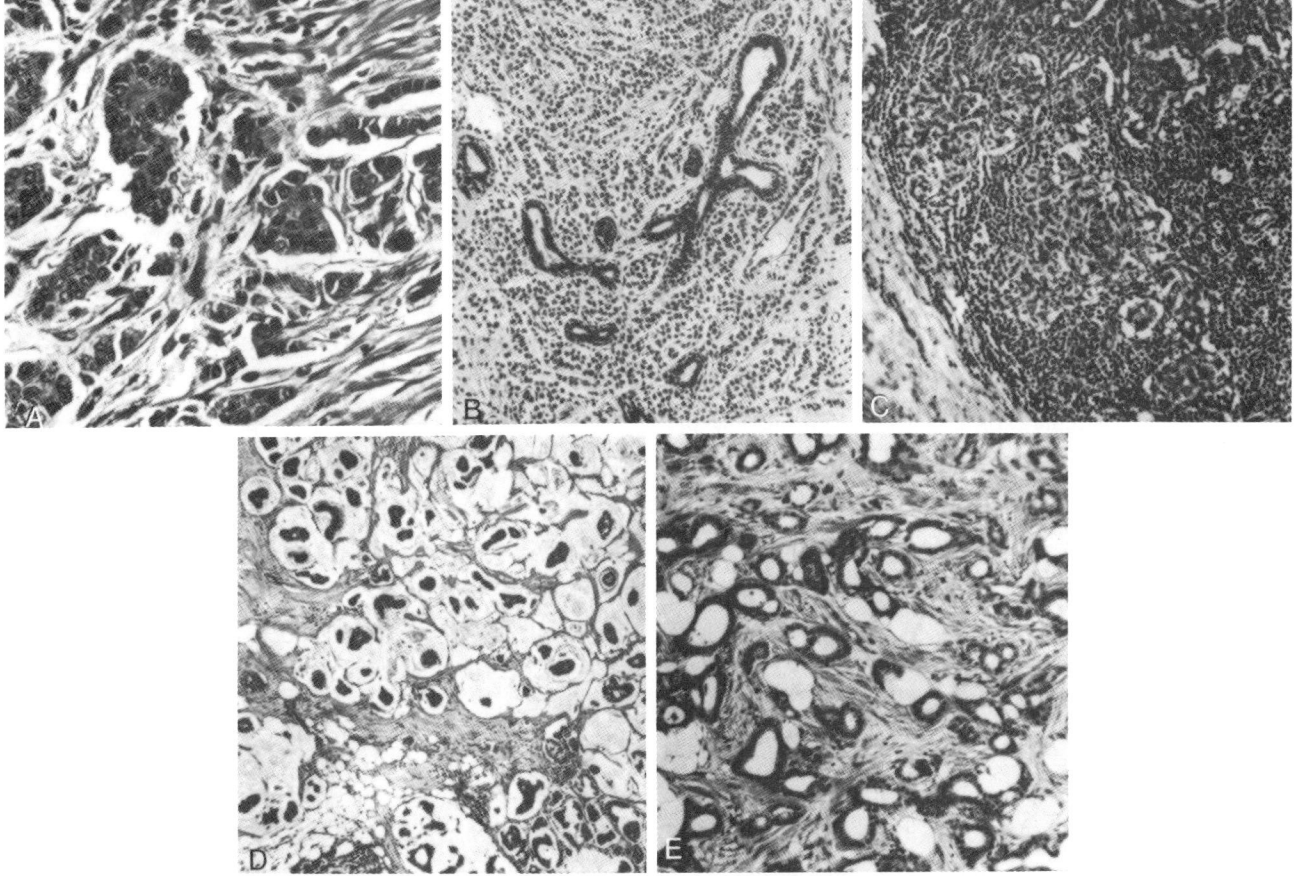

Figure 13. Histologic appearance of common breast tumors. *A*, Infiltrating ductal carcinoma, NOS. The tumor cells infiltrate the stroma without any distinctive morphologic pattern. *B*, Infiltrating lobular carcinoma. Small tumor cells infiltrate the stroma oriented in linear array known as an "Indian file" arrangement. *C*, Medullary carcinoma. Large and bizarre tumor cells are surrounded by a distinctive lymphocytic infiltrate. *D*, Mucinous carcinoma, also called colloid carcinoma. Well-differentiated tumor cells form islands within lakes of mucin. *E*, Tubular carcinoma. Small tubules are lined by well-differentiated, uniform tumor cells and infiltrate the stroma in a disorganized fashion. (Reprinted with permission from the World Health Organization, Geneva, Switzerland.)

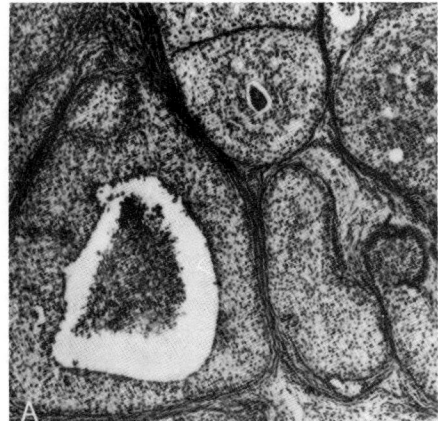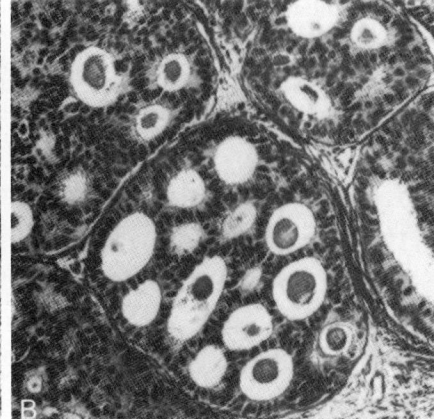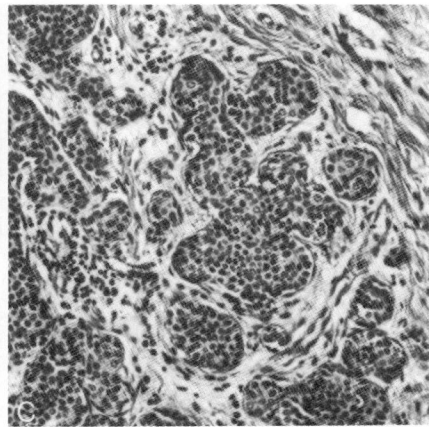

Figure 14. Noninvasive breast carcinoma or carcinoma *in situ* (CIS). *A,* Ductal carcinoma *in situ* (DCIS), solid or comedo growth pattern. Tumor cells fill and expand breast ducts and may undergo central necrosis. *B,* Ductal carcinoma *in situ* (DCIS), cribriform growth pattern. Papillary projections of tumor cells span the duct lumen to form a cribriform growth pattern. *C,* Lobular carcinoma *in situ* (LCIS). Tumor cells fill and distend the terminal ductules but preserve the architecture of the lobular unit.

lobular carcinoma in situ.[83] Haagensen first used the term *lobular neoplasia* to emphasize its more benign course.[112] Pathologically, it is a proliferation of small, round epithelial cells within lumens of multiple breast acini. The resulting presentation is multiple clusters of epithelial cells forming islands of neoplastic cells but maintaining a lobular architecture. Although the ducts expand with proliferating cells, they usually do not reach the large size seen with ductal carcinoma *in situ.* The typical lesion seen pathologically is shown in Figure 14.

Unlike DCIS, lobular carcinoma *in situ* never forms a palpable mass by itself and is therefore not recognized on physical examination. In addition, there are no mammographic findings in LCIS. It does not form a density and never calcifies, both of which are typical for DCIS. Therefore, this is a disease that is recognized incidentally after biopsy for another abnormality that is producing a clinical or mammographic finding. The treatment of this incidental pathologic entity still remains controversial and will be reviewed later.

INFILTRATING DUCTAL CARCINOMA. This is the most common malignant tumor in the breast recognized after biopsy. The term *ductal carcinoma* refers to its origin from ductal epithelium; infiltrating describes its growth pattern and distinguishes this lesion from noninvasive carcinoma. Some add the terms *not otherwise specified (NOS)* and *no special type (NST)* to emphasize that this disease is diagnosed after the other, more distinctive histologies have been eliminated. The tumor infiltrates into a variable amount of stroma as cords or islands of malignant epithelium (see Fig. 13). It may form primitive glandular forms, but not to the extent of a pure tubular carcinoma. As discussed, and as reflected in the WHO classification, many infiltrating carcinomas display an *in situ* component. This fact reflects its ductal origin and may be used to prove a mammary origin of the tumor. The stromal "reaction" may be intense and has led to the older term *scirrhous carcinoma* of the breast.

Clinically, most infiltrating ductal carcinomas present as a mass found on physical examination or as a density lesion on the mammogram. Microcalcifications seen mammographically are commonly found in the necrotic centers of the intraductal component but may be seen in the infiltrating component as well. The treatment of infiltrating carcinoma is discussed later, and the approach taken is generally the same, regardless of the morphologic appearance. However, the use of a general term to describe common breast cancer should not lull the student into thinking that these tumors are not further characterized.

Modern evaluation of breast cancer should always specify the tumor size, the status of the surgical margin, and the content of estrogen and progesterone receptors. In addition, the nuclear and histologic grade is frequently reported, and modern evalua-

tion may include measurement of DNA content and estimation of the proliferating fraction, or S-phase. Vascular invasion, tumor necrosis, and the extent of the intraductal component are all used to make decisions about the primary or adjuvant treatment of patients with operable breast cancer. The dedicated surgeon must be acquainted with all these parameters and their interpretation.

INVASIVE LOBULAR CARCINOMA. This disease probably originates in the breast lobule, a fact well studied by many surgeons and pathologists.[200] Invasive lobular carcinoma constitutes between 3 and 15 per cent of all invasive breast cancers, depending on the series consulted.[150] Histologically, the tumor is composed of small round cells that infiltrate surrounding stromal tissue in a peculiar "Indian file" fashion (see Fig. 13B). Lobular carcinoma presents in an identical fashion as ordinary infiltrating ductal carcinoma and produces no distinguishing mammographic features. The treatment of lobular carcinoma is the same as for the more common ductal carcinomas and may carry a better prognosis.[51] There may be a somewhat higher incidence of bilateral cancer or of second primaries in the contralateral breast.[50] However, this is rarely used to justify prophylactic procedures in the contralateral breast in the absence of synchronous disease.

LESS COMMON FORMS OF DUCTAL CARCINOMA. These tumors, although heterogeneous, are all morphologic variants of common ductal carcinoma. In general, these less common variants have improved prognosis, reflecting their more differentiated phenotype.[51,178] One exception to this rule is medullary carcinoma of the breast, which is pathologically characterized by bizarre and anaplastic tumor cells surrounded by a prominent lymphocytic infiltrate with a scant fibrous stroma (see Fig. 13C). Although the epithelial component is undifferentiated, this phenotype appears to enjoy a small but significant survival advantage when compared with infiltrating ductal carcinoma, NOS.[51,88,196] Mucinous carcinoma, also called colloid carcinoma, is characterized by well-differentiated epithelial cells surrounded by a large accumulation of extracellular and extraluminal mucin that is secreted by the carcinoma cells (see Fig. 13D). This histologic type enjoys a favorable prognosis in several published series.[34,51,88] Although there are no definite clinical or mammographic signs of mucinous and medullary carcinoma, these tumor types are suggested by a well-circumscribed density with smooth borders that tend to be softer on physical examination. The final major histologic type that is distinctive and well differentiated is tubular carcinoma. This tumor is characterized by infiltrating tubular structures, lined by one cell layer, and with an open central space (see Fig. 13E). The tumor is characteristically small and scirrhous and has an excellent prognosis after treatment.[51,88,187] The descriptions of these histologic variants refer to their predominant features. However, each may coexist with more undifferentiated infiltrating carcinoma of the usual type. In general, if the tumor is composed of definite infiltrating ductal carcinoma of poor differentiation, the final diagnosis reflects the poorest histologic pattern. Although these variants enjoy better prognosis after treatment, the primary treatment should be identical to that of usual ductal carcinoma as outlined later.

STAGING BREAST CANCER

The most widely used system for staging primary breast cancer has evolved from classifications proposed by the International Union Against Cancer (UICC) and the American Joint Committee on Cancer and is reproduced in Table 5. This modern system is based on the description of the primary tumor (T), the status of regional lymph nodes (N), and the presence of distant metastases (M). Reports may contain numerical codes

TABLE 5. 1986 TNM Classification

Measuring the Size of the Primary Cancer
The tumor size is a measure of the invasive component. If there is a large *in situ* component (e.g., 4.0 cm.) and a small invasive component (e.g., 0.5 cm.), the tumor is coded T_{1a}.

Multiple, Simultaneous Cancers
The following guidelines should be used when staging multiple, simultaneous primary (grossly measurable, infiltrating) cancers within the same breast. These criteria do not apply to multiple microscopic lesions (since they may represent intramammary spread).
    Use the largest primary cancer to stage the case.
    Enter on the record that the case is one of simultaneous, multiple primary cancers in one breast. These cases should be analyzed separately.
    Include in breast checklist (pathology) simultaneous, multiple, primary infiltrating cancers.
    Simultaneous *bilateral* breast cancers: Each should be staged independently.

Inflammatory Carcinoma
Inflammatory carcinoma of the breast is characterized by diffuse, brawny induration of the skin, with an erysipeloid edge, usually with no underlying palpable mass. The clinical presentation is due to tumor embolization of dermal lymphatics. The tumor of inflammatory carcinoma is coded T_{4d}.

Primary Tumor (T)
The size of the intact tumor should be measured before any tissue is removed for special studies, such as estrogen-binding studies.
T_x	The primary tumor cannot be assessed.
T_0	No evidence of primary tumor
TIS	Carcinoma *in situ*: intraductal carinoma, lobular carcinoma *in situ*, or Paget's disease of the nipple with no tumor. Paget's disease associated with a tumor is classified according to the size of the tumor.
T_1	Tumor is 2.0 cm. or smaller in greatest dimension.

	T_{1a}	0.5 cm. or smaller
	T_{1b}	Larger than 0.5 cm. but not larger than 1.0 cm.
	T_{1c}	Larger than 1.0 cm. but not larger than 2.0 cm.

T_2	Tumor is larger than 2.0 cm. but not larger than 5.0 cm. in greatest dimension.
T_3	Tumor is larger than 5.0 cm. in greatest dimension.
T_4	Tumor of any size with direct extension to chest wall or skin. (Chest wall includes ribs, intercostal muscles, and serratus anterior muscle, but not pectoral muscle.)
T_{4a}	Extension to chest wall.
T_{4b}	Edema (including peau d'orange), ulceration of the skin of the breast, or satellite skin nodules confined to the same breast.
T_{4c}	Both a and b, above.
T_{4d}*	Inflammatory carcinoma (as defined in introductory comments).

Note: Dimpling of the skin, nipple retraction, or other skin changes, except those in T_4, may occur in T_1, T_2, and T_3 without affecting the classification.

Regional Lymph Node Stations (N)
Axillary (ipsilateral) and *interpectoral* (Rotter's nodes): lymph nodes along the axillary vein and its tributaries, which may be divided into the following levels:
    Level I (low axilla): lymph nodes located lateral to the lateral border of the pectoralis major muscle.
    Level II (mid axilla): lymph nodes located between the medial and lateral borders of the pectoralis minor muscle and the interpectoral (Rotter's) lymph nodes.
    Level III (apical axilla): lymph nodes medial to the medial margin of the pectoralis minor, including those designated as the subclavicular, infraclavicular, or apical lymph nodes.
Intramammary lymph nodes are coded as axillary lymph nodes.
Internal mammary (ipsilateral): lymph nodes located in the intercostal spaces along the edge of the sternum in the endothoracic fascia.
All other lymph node metastases are coded as distant metastases (M_1), including supraclavicular, cervical, or contralateral internal mammary lymph nodes.
N—REGIONAL LYMPH NODES
N_x	The regional lymph nodes cannot be assessed (e.g., clinical staging: previously removed; pathologic staging: previously removed, or not removed for pathologic study).
N_0	No regional lymph node metastases.
N_1	Metastases in four or fewer ipsilateral axillary lymph nodes, none larger than 3.0 cm. in greatest dimension.

	N_{1a}	Only micrometastases (none larger than 0.2 cm.)
	N_{1b}	Metastases in 1–3 axillary lymph nodes, any one larger than 0.2 cm., but none larger than 3.0 cm.

N_2	Metastases in four or more ipsilateral axillary lymph nodes, and/or in any axillary lymph node larger than 3.0 cm., or in any ipsilateral internal mammary lymph node(s).
N_{2a}	Metastasis in five or more axillary lymph nodes, or any ipsilateral axillary metastasis larger than 3.0 cm.
N_{2b}	Metastasis in any ipsilateral internal mammary lymph node(s).

Distant Metastasis (M)
M_x	Distant metastasis cannot be assessed.
M_0	No distant metastasis.
M_1	Distant metastasis.

(continued)

TABLE 5. *(Continued)*

Clinical Staging

Clinical staging includes the following: physical examination, including careful inspection and palpation of the skin, the mammary glands, and the lymph nodes (axillary, supraclavicular, and cervical). Pathologic examination of the breast or other tissues to establish the diagnosis of breast cancer. The extent of tissues examined pathologically for clinical staging is less than that required for pathologic staging (see Pathologic Staging below). Appropriate operative findings are elements of clinical staging, including size and chest wall invasion of the primary cancer and the presence or absence of regional or distant metastasis.

Pathologic Staging

Pathologic staging includes the following:

All data used for clinical staging.

Surgical resection and pathologic examination of the primary cancer, including not less than excision of the primary carcinoma with no tumor in any margin of resection by *gross* pathologic examination. A case can be included in the pathologic stage if there is only microscopic, but not gross, involvement in a margin. If there is tumor in the margin of resection by gross examination, it is coded T_x.

Resection of at least 5 ipsilateral axillary lymph nodes.

Stage Groupings

Stage 0	TIS	N_0	M_0
Stage I	T_1	N_0	M_0
Stage II			
II_a	T_0	N_1	M_0
	T_1	N_1†	M_0
	T_2	N_0	M_0
II_b	T_2	N_1	M_0
	T_3	N_0	M_0
Stage III			
III_a	T_3	N_1	M_0
	T_1, T_2, T_3	N_2	M_0
III_b	T_4	Any N	M_0
Stage IV	Any T	Any N	M_1

* If the skin biopsy is negative and there is no localized, measurable primary cancer, the T category is pT, when pathologically staging a clinical inflammatory carcinoma, cT_{4d}.

† The prognosis of patients with N_{1a} is similar to that of patients with N_0.

From Lippman, M. E., Lichter, A. S., Danforth, D. N., Jr.: Diagnosis and Management of Breast Cancer. Philadelphia, W. B. Saunders Company, 1988.

behind each letter, such as $T_2N_1M_0$, which refers to a tumor greater than 2 cm. but less than 5 cm. (T_2), the presence of movable homolateral axillary nodes (N_1), and the absence of distant metastases (M_0). These designations may be combined as outlined in Table 5 to give a summary staging category, in this example Stage II. This system can be used to determine clinical stage, based on physical examination and radiographic findings, or to determine pathologic stage after operation and histologic evaluation of the surgical material.

Other systems of staging have been proposed and are used by their proponents for reporting end-results. The Columbia Clinical Classification system, used by Haagensen and others, contains four stages (A through D) and is based on clinical assessment of the primary and axillary nodes and on accumulation of "grave signs" in each case.[111] Any staging system seeks to provide information about the prognosis of patients after treatment and to allow comparison of results within and between clinical trials. It should be kept in mind that these divisions are imposed upon a spectrum of cancer presentations and are useful only if they are interpreted with knowledge of their limitations.

Very few studies of the natural history of untreated patients with breast cancer are available. Furthermore, the growth rate of breast cancer and its biologic behavior are very heterogeneous. The variability of growth rate and doubling time has recently been studied by Spratt based on sequential mammograms of untreated patients.[229] The ability of tumors to metastasize is a variable that cannot as yet be predicted and differs among individual patients and tumors. Haagensen has presented a well-documented patient with a tumor in the right breast that slowly grew for 30 years before the patient died. Bloom collected a remarkable series of 250 patients with untreated breast cancer from the Middlesex Hospital cancer charity ward between 1805 and 1933.[14] As shown in Figure 15, the median survival of these patients was 2.7 years, although 20 per cent survived more than 5 years from the time of presentation.

In the modern era of adjuvant therapy, it is helpful to review the natural history of patients with operable cancer treated with surgical therapy alone. In general, these are patients with Stage I or II breast cancer who underwent either radical or modified radical mastectomy before 1975, when adjuvant chemotherapy was first widely used. A cooperative Natural History Data Base was established at the National Cancer Institute in Milan, the Royal Marsden Hospital, and the M.D. Anderson Hospital, which included 1971 patients carefully staged and followed for at least 10 years.[160] Figure 16 displays the overall survival results by Kaplan-Meier estimation and shows the effect of tumor size

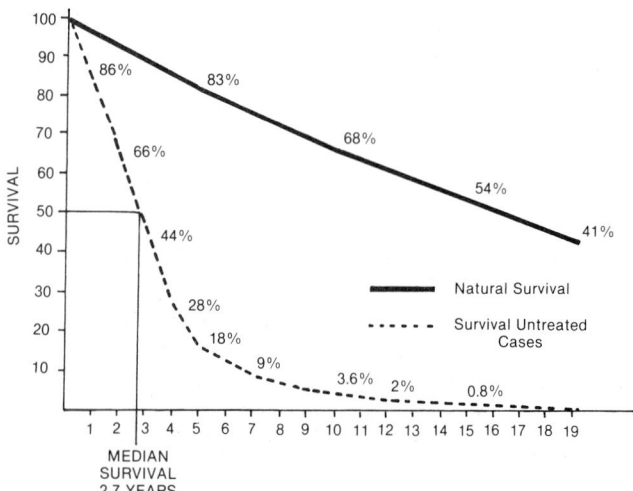

Figure 15. Length of survival in 250 patients with untreated breast cancer at the Middlesex Hospital between 1805 and 1933. (From Bloom, H. J. G., et al.: Natural history of untreated breast cancer (1805–1933). Br. Med. J., 2:213, 1962.)

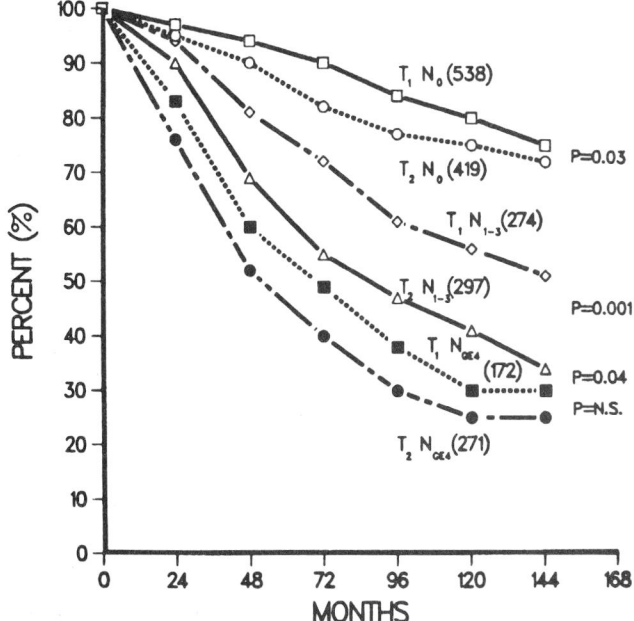

Figure 16. Survival by nodes and tumor size from a Natural History Data Base. The survival data from 1971 patients in whom follow-up was complete were collected from three hospitals to form a Natural History Data Base. These patients were treated by either radical or modified radical mastectomy; none of the patients received postoperative chemotherapy. (From Moon, T. E., et al.: Development of a natural history data base of breast cancer studies. *In* Jones, S. E., and Salmon, S. E. (Eds.): Adjuvant Therapy of Cancer IV. Orlando, Fla., Grune & Stratton, 1984.)

(T) and nodal status (N) divided into those with one to three and four or more nodes pathologically involved with cancer. As indicated by this analysis, the contribution of increasing nodal involvement is not reflected in the TNM staging system. This deficiency has been addressed in a national survey of the management and survival of female patients with breast cancer sponsored by the American College of Surgeons.[169] Five-year end-results of absolute survival and recurrence were tabulated in this survey, according to the number of pathologically positive axillary nodes, and revealed an almost linear decrement in survival with increasing nodal involvement (Table 6).

The survival of patients presenting with locally advanced or metastatic disease who are nonoperated, operated for palliation, or with recurrent cancer is heterogeneous but very poor. This group includes patients with Stage III and IV disease or with Stage C and D tumors defined by the Columbia Clinical Classification scheme. Certain patients with locally advanced Stage III disease have been operated for cure. Inclusion of these more favorable cases influences the reporting of results for this group. In general, no more than 20 per cent of patients presenting with locally advanced carcinoma will survive for 10 years. The median survival of patients with metastatic disease is in the range of 24 months from time of diagnosis but does vary according to the principal site of disease involvement.[54]

MODERN SURGICAL PROCEDURES FOR INVASIVE BREAST CANCER

The surgical treatment of breast cancer, for the most part, concerns the treatment of potentially curable cancer that is confined to the breast and regional lymph nodes. For early stages of breast cancer, surgical removal provides a reasonable chance for cure. Although the approach to operable breast cancer has changed dramatically over the past century, so too has the clinical presentation of breast tumors changed. In 1894, Halsted presented his first 50 patients treated by the "complete operation," which became the radical mastectomy.[113,155] Over the next 75 years, radical mastectomy was used to treat nearly every breast malignancy operated upon for cure in the United States.

Examination of Halsted's first cases found at least two thirds with locally advanced disease and 60 per cent with clinically evident axillary nodal metastases. By comparison, a 1980 survey by the American College of Surgeons found that 85 per cent of patients presented with Stage I or Stage II disease.[169] The frequency of cases with positive axillary lymph nodes was 40 per cent, and the average tumor presenting to physicians in the 1970s was 2 cm. or less in size. In addition to these fundamental changes, realization that 90 per cent of treatment failures will be systemic or visceral recurrences has led surgical oncologists to explore alternatives to radical mastectomy as an initial approach to operable breast cancer.

SURGICAL PROCEDURES PAST AND PRESENT

In 1982, the American College of Surgeons investigated surgical practice in cases of operable breast cancer and compared results with practice in earlier years (Fig. 17).[251] Clearly, a change in surgical practice occurred in the mid 1970s with an abrupt shift from radical mastectomy to modified radical mastectomy. Procedures that preserved the breast, as described later, were performed in only 7.2 per cent of cases in this survey. Current estimates of conservative breast procedures range between 20 and 40 per cent, and this procedure probably will continue to increase in popularity. The following paragraphs describe procedures in widespread use now and in the past.

RADICAL AND EXTENDED RADICAL MASTECTOMY

In the radical mastectomy, the breast and underlying pectoralis muscles are sacrificed, leaving a bare chest wall. Regional lymph nodes along the axillary vein up to the costoclavicular ligament (Halsted's ligament) are removed with the breast specimen. This procedure frequently requires a skin graft and uses incisions placed either vertically or obliquely. Prosthetic reconstruction is impossible unless muscle flaps are mobilized to cover the anterior chest defect. Cure of breast cancer can certainly be achieved by the application of this procedure alone, as shown earlier in Figure 16 from a natural history data base of surgically treated patients. Other studies document both the strengths and weaknesses of maximal local therapy represented by this procedure. The personal series of Haagensen reports results from treatment of 1036 patients; 727 patients with clinically negative nodes (Stage A, Columbia clinical staging) had a

TABLE 6. Five-Year End-Results (Absolute Survival, Cure, and Recurrence Rates) in 20,547 Patients with Breast Cancer According to Number of Pathologically Positive Axillary Nodes*

Number of Positive Axillary Lymph Nodes	Total Observed	Survival (%)	Cure (%)	Recurrence (%)
0	12,299	71.8	59.7	19.4
1	2012	63.1	48.4	32.9
2	1338	62.2	45.4	39.9
3	842	58.8	39.3	43.0
4	615	51.9	38.4	43.9
5	478	46.9	29.1	54.2
6–10	1261	40.7	23.0	63.4
11–15	562	29.4	14.8	71.5
16–20	301	28.9	13.3	75.1
21+	225	22.2	9.8	82.2
All nodes or some nodes positive	614	40.4	26.9	58.6
Total, positive nodes	8248	50.9	35.0	49.2

* Excluding cases with distant metastasis.
From Nemoto, T., Vana, J., Bedwani, R. N., et al.: Management and survival of female breast cancer: Results of a national survey by the American College of Surgeons. Cancer, 45:2917, 1980.

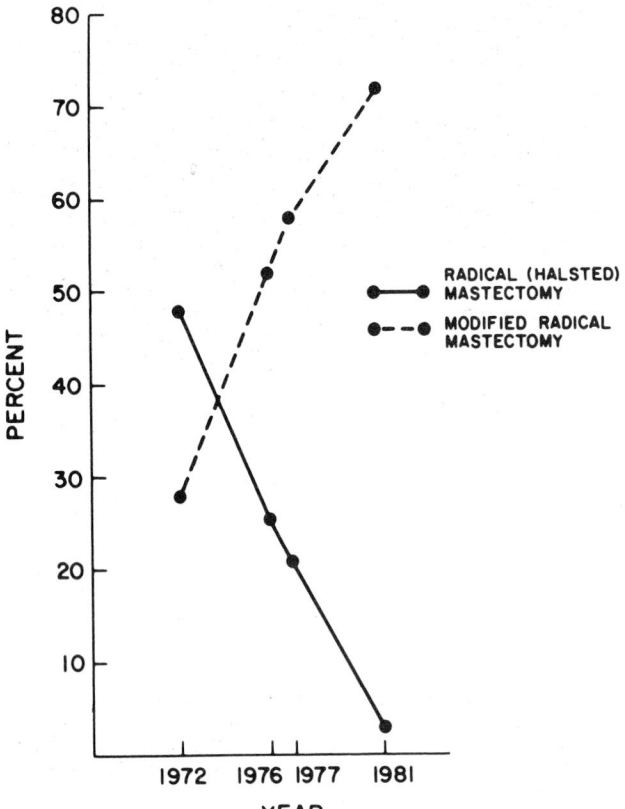

Figure 17. Trends in the procedures performed for operable breast cancer from 1972 to 1981. (From Wilson, R. E., et al.: The 1982 national survey of carcinoma of the breast in the United States by the American College of Surgeons. Surg. Gynecol. Obstet., *159:*309, 1984.)

survival of 72.4 per cent at 10 years. In contrast, only 42.3 per cent of clinically node-positive patients (Stage B) survived at 10 years.[102] These figures are confirmed by the National Surgical Adjuvant Breast and Bowel Project's (NSABP) early trial of adjuvant thiotepa.[75] By 10 years, 76 per cent of patients with histologically positive nodes suffered recurrence of breast cancer and one quarter of patients with negative nodes failed surgical treatment. In contrast, local failure rates have been extremely low since introduction of the Halsted radical mastectomy. Published figures are generally between 5 and 7 per cent and provide the standard against which newer procedures are judged.

The extended radical mastectomy is a standard radical mastectomy to which en bloc removal of internal mammary nodes is added. This procedure was popularized in the United States by Urban, who reported a 35.5 per cent 10-year survival in patients undergoing extended radical mastectomy.[239] Other studies have resulted in abandonment of the extended procedure. A large prospective trial[137] and several uncontrolled series[103,241] have failed to provide evidence of improved clinical outcome after extended radical mastectomy.

MODIFIED RADICAL MASTECTOMY

Modified radical mastectomy (MRM) refers to a procedure combining total mastectomy with removal of axillary lymph nodes in continuity with the mastectomy specimen. This is currently the most widely used procedure to treat operable breast cancer and is the alternative to breast-sparing procedures described later. Modified radical mastectomy leaves the pectoralis major muscle intact, providing a soft tissue covering over the chest wall and a normal-appearing junction of the shoulder with the anterior chest wall and avoiding the hollow defect inferior to the clavicle that accompanies the removal of the pectoralis muscle. The patient is left with intact musculature

around the shoulder and a situation well suited to prosthetic reconstruction (discussed in Chapter 23). Two forms of the procedure are currently in use by surgeons: the Patey procedure with modifications described by Scanlon, and the procedure described by Auchincloss.

David Patey, at the Middlesex Hospital in London, developed a procedure bearing his name that preserves the pectoralis major muscle and sacrifices the underlying pectoralis minor muscle in order to remove Levels I, II, and III lymph nodes in the axilla.[185] A large number of Patey procedures performed by Handley, who wrote extensively about this procedure, were reviewed independently and reported by Donegan and associates.[56] The survival of patients with negative axillary nodes was 82 per cent at 10 years, with a local recurrence rate of 5 per cent. For patients with positive nodes, the survival was 48 per cent, very similar to results with radical mastectomy. Thus, preservation of the pectoralis muscle did not appear to result in inferior results. Scanlon modified the Patey procedure by dividing but not removing the pectoralis minor muscle, allowing removal of apical (Level III) nodes and preservation of the lateral pectoral nerves to the major muscle.[209]

The procedure described by Auchincloss differs from the Patey procedure by not removing or dividing the pectoralis minor muscle.[8] This modification limits the complete removal of high axillary nodes but is justified by Auchincloss, who calculated that only 2 per cent of patients will potentially benefit by removal of the highest level nodes.[7] It is probable that the Auchincloss mastectomy was the most popular procedure for breast cancer in the United States during the past decade.

RADICAL VERSUS MODIFIED RADICAL MASTECTOMY

Radical mastectomy (RM) and MRM were directly tested in two randomized clinical trials in this country and in England. The first, from the Alabama Breast Cancer Project, was a community-based study that pre-randomized patients according to birth date to receive MRM or RM.[147] Stage I and II and operable Stage III tumors were included. Those with histologically positive axillary nodes were further randomized to receive two different adjuvant chemotherapy programs. A recent update reported 10-year results for 175 patients undergoing MRM and 136 patients treated with RM.[148] No significant difference in overall survival rates was demonstrated. However, there was a significantly higher local recurrence rate (p = 0.04) in patients undergoing MRM compared with RM. Moreover, patients with larger tumors and those with clinically positive nodes survived better after RM (p = 0.05). A university-based study in England randomized 534 patients to RM and MRM in a similar study design.[238] This study was limited to clinical Stage I and II patients. No significant differences in overall survival or event-free survival were seen. In addition, no consistent trends were seen in clinically or pathologically staged subgroups. These results, combined with the clear functional and cosmetic superiority of MRM, make this procedure the standard of care for nearly all patients with Stage I and II operable breast cancer.

WIDE LOCAL EXCISION AND PRIMARY RADIATION THERAPY

Excision of the primary tumor with preservation of the breast has been referred to by many terms, including partial mastectomy, segmentectomy, tylectomy, or lumpectomy. Wide local excision appears to be the most descriptive term for the procedure which removes the malignancy with a surrounding rim of grossly normal breast parenchyma. An even more aggressive local procedure designed to remove 1 to 2 cm. of adjacent breast and overlying skin is called quadrantectomy. In modern practice, these more limited surgical procedures are applied as part of a multidisciplinary approach to breast cancer and always include postoperative radiation therapy, giving at least 4500 cGy. to the whole breast and usually including a boost of radiation to the tumor bed. Axillary dissection is done through a separate incision in the majority of patients. Therefore, conservative breast surgery or breast preservation usually refers to wide local excision of the primary tumor, whole breast radiation, and a separate axillary dissection.

SURGICAL TRIALS OF LOCAL THERAPY FOR OPERABLE BREAST CANCER

The gradual change from radical surgical therapy toward preservation of the breast and soft tissues was influenced by the results of several large trials of lesser surgical procedures. The aforementioned Manchester and Alabama trials comparing radical with modified radical mastectomy were important in establishing the place of modified radical mastectomy as the standard surgical approach to patients with operable breast cancer. Other trials that should be mentioned include the Capetown Trial comparing radical mastectomy with simple mastectomy[120] and the Cardiff–St. Mary's Trial of modified radical mastectomy versus simple mastectomy with axillary node biopsy.[85] Although there are deficiencies in both trials, they generally support the concept that alternative strategies for the treatment of operable breast cancer do achieve acceptable survival results.

NSABP TRIAL B-04 COMPARING RADICAL MASTECTOMY WITH ALTERNATIVES

In 1971, the National Surgical Adjuvant Breast and Bowel Project (NSABP) initiated a large prospective trial to examine widely disparate approaches to the local and regional control of breast cancer. Protocol B-04 used radical mastectomy as its control arm and randomized patients with and without clinically positive axillary lymph nodes to receive alternative approaches to regional lymph nodes, as shown in Figure 18. Patients with clinically negative nodes were randomized to one of three treatment regimens: Halsted radical mastectomy (RM, 362 patients), total mastectomy with radiation treatment of the ipsilateral nodes (TM + XRT, 352 patients), and total mastectomy alone with delayed axillary dissection if nodes became enlarged (TM,

365 patients). Clinically node-positive patients were randomly allocated to receive radical mastectomy (RM, 292 patients) or total mastectomy with radiation of the enlarged nodes (TM + XRT, 294 patients). This study has been widely referred to for its contribution to understanding the significance of axillary and regional nodal metastases, the effect of local and regional therapy on recurrence, and the validity of anatomic principles in the treatment of breast cancer. First results of the landmark study were published in 1977,[68] and various aspects of the study have since been reported.[77,78,80]

A final update of Protocol B-04 was completed in 1985 and represents a complete 10-year follow-up.[71] No significant differences in overall survival or disease-free survival were noted for 1079 clinically node-negative patients treated by random allocation with RM, total mastectomy plus nodal radiation, or total mastectomy and delayed axillary dissection (Fig. 19). Likewise, for 586 clinically node-positive patients receiving either RM or total mastectomy and nodal radiation, survival and recurrence statistics were identical (Fig. 19). The only differences were local and regional failures experienced by clinically node-negative patients. Patients receiving radical mastectomy or total mastectomy plus regional radiation had local failures of less than 10 per cent, whereas those treated by mastectomy plus delayed nodal dissection experienced about a 15 per cent cumulative 10-year local recurrence rate. These survival statistics allow a number of conclusions:

1. Variations in local and regional treatments that involve total mastectomy do not alter the frequency or pattern of distant treatment failures. Although local treatment failures are influenced, overall survival was unaffected.

2. The mode and time of treatment of axillary nodes do not alter outcome, either disease-free survival or overall survival. Immediate removal, delayed removal, or radiation all produced equivalent results. Removal of lymph nodes provides the best indication of eventual relapse.

3. Results of breast cancer treatment trials can be assessed reliably at 5 years; the frequency of new events occurring in the second 5 years of Protocol B-04 was small and predictable. It is interesting that patients with positive nodes who were free of

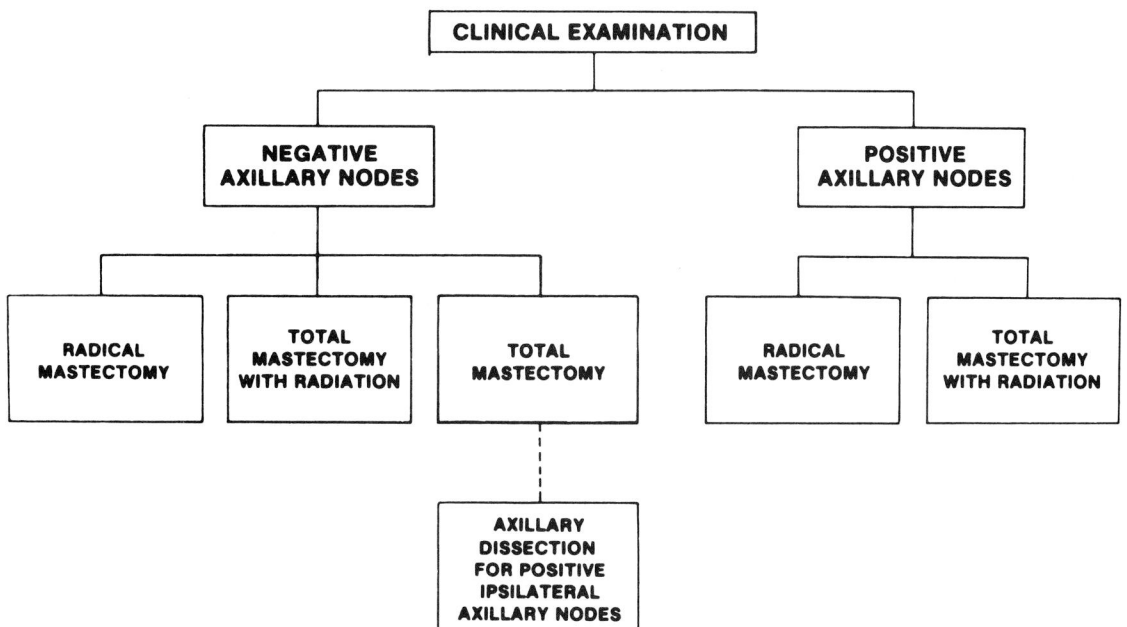

Figure 18. Randomization scheme for NSABP protocol B-04. Patients with clinically negative nodes were randomized to receive standard radical mastectomy, total mastectomy and radiation to undisturbed axillary nodes, or total mastectomy with axillary dissection reserved for patients developing delayed axillary node enlargement. Patients with clinically positive nodes were randomized to receive standard radical mastectomy versus total mastectomy with radiation to the involved nodes. (From Fisher, B., et al.: Findings from NSABP protocol No. B-04: Comparison of radical mastectomy with alternative treatments. II. The clinical and biologic significance of medial-central breast cancers. Cancer, 48:1863, 1981.)

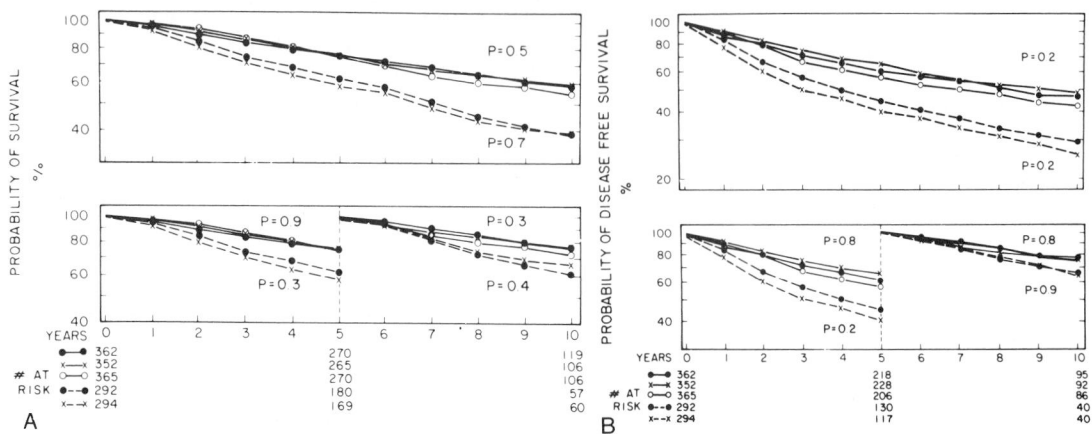

Figure 19. Tenth-year results of NSABP protocol B-04 comparing radical mastectomy with alternative treatments. Patients were randomly allocated to receive radical mastectomy (solid circle), total mastectomy and radiation to undisturbed axillary nodes (x), or total mastectomy alone with delayed axillary dissection only for patients developing clinically enlarged nodes (open circle). Patients with clinically negative nodes (solid line) and clinically positive nodes (broken line) were randomized. *A, Top,* Total survival of all groups through the tenth year. *Bottom left,* Survival through the fifth year. *Bottom right,* Survival during the next 5 years for all patients alive at the end of the first period. *B, Top,* Disease-free survival for the total study through 10 years. *Bottom left,* Survival free of disease during the first 5 years of study. *Bottom right,* Survival free of disease for patients free from disease at the end of the first period. (From Fisher, B., et al.: Ten-year results of a randomized clinical trial comparing radical mastectomy and total mastectomy with or without radiation. N. Engl. J. Med., *312:*674, 1985.)

disease at 5 years had about the same probability of remaining disease-free as did the negative-node group.

4. The location of the primary tumor in the breast does not influence outcome. Moreover, there was no justification for irradiation of internal mammary nodes in patients with medial quadrant lesions.

The results of the NSABP B-04 protocol address treatment alternatives that all use total mastectomy. The question of whether procedures substituting breast conservation for mastectomy can be safely applied to treatment of operable breast cancer was first addressed in uncontrolled trials in European centers,[27,228] by pioneering radiation therapists in the United States,[115,158,193] and finally by randomized prospective trials.[64,117,208,244]

CONSERVATIVE SURGERY FOR OPERABLE BREAST CANCER

Experimental arms in NSABP Protocol B-04 represented significant departures from local and regional treatment of operable breast cancer in the United States. As such, results of this study emphasized the overriding importance of distant disease as the cause of treatment failure in early-stage breast cancer. Moreover, the occurrence of distant disease was independent of local treatment over a wide range of approaches. As noted earlier, all arms in Protocol B-04 involved at least a conventional total mastectomy. It is instructive for students of modern techniques in surgical management to reflect on results obtained in older studies using strategies that depart from current practice. These studies were frequently retrospective but provided justification for the design of modern trials using the powerful methods of prospective randomization.

TRIALS USING TUMOR EXCISION ONLY OR RADIOTHERAPY ONLY

Most of the early noncontrolled trials of conservative surgical therapy combined wide local excision of the primary tumor with whole breast radiation. The use of radiation only, leaving the tumor *in situ,* was first reported by Keynes in 1928.[132] Satisfactory results were subsequently reported by several early investigators.[10,27] Calle and associates reported disease-free survival at 10 years of 43 per cent for patients with tumors 3 cm. or larger treated initially only by radiation.[27] However, 55 per cent of these patients required secondary surgical therapy for persistent or recurrent disease. There is little reason to recommend leaving

operable cancer in place, and no current clinical trials include a radiation-only arm.

Tumor excision alone has also been studied in retrospective as well as prospective clinical trials. Early reports from Cope and associates,[40] Crile and co-workers,[41] Adair,[2] and others[159,188] demonstrated the possibility that very limited treatment of certain breast cancers results in long-term cure. Further studies defined the local recurrence rate, which generally exceeded 20 per cent at intervals of 3 to 5 years.[89,138] In a series of more than 800 patients treated without mastectomy at the Princess Margaret Hospital between 1958 and 1980, 177 were treated by excision without radiation.[33] One hundred and four tumors treated in this manner were small T_1 (less than 2 cm.) lesions. Other groups treated included those receiving postsurgical radiation to the breast or to the breast and regional nodes. At 5 years, there was an 8.7 per cent relapse rate in the breast treated by excision plus radiation. With excision and no radiation, the local relapse rate was 24.9 per cent. By 10 years, local failure had occurred in 13.3 per cent and 28.3 per cent, respectively, despite the preponderance of smaller tumors in the excision-only group. Significantly, distant relapse and overall survival were unaffected by the choice of local therapy. The NSABP is currently randomizing patients with very small tumors to receive either excision alone, excision plus tamoxifen, or excision plus radiotherapy.

NONCONTROLLED TRIALS OF CONSERVATIVE SURGICAL THERAPY PLUS RADIATION THERAPY

Early work leading to the modern use of radiotherapy in the treatment of primary breast carcinoma began in European centers more than 40 years ago. Mustakallio was encouraged by favorable results in clinical Stage I patients and produced results comparable with radical mastectomy using tumor excision and radiotherapy.[166] Calle and colleagues reported similar favorable 10-year results at the Foundation Curie in Paris.[27] For patients with tumors less than 3 cm. in size and without clinical involvement of axillary nodes, excision plus radiotherapy produced absolute survival, free of disease, of 85 and 75 per cent at 5 and 10 years, respectively. Local recurrences occurred during the first 5 years in 16 (13 per cent) of 120 patients treated, three of which happened in axillary nodes.

American centers duplicated these results. Montague and associates treated patients at the M. D. Anderson Hospital between 1955 and 1980 and produced 10-year survivals in 80 per cent and 65 per cent of Stage I and Stage II patients, respectively.[158] Prosnitz and colleagues reported results from a cooperative study of breast preservation and radiotherapy in early stage breast cancer treated at four university hospitals in the Northeast.[193] Actuarial disease-free survival rates at 5 years were 91 and 60 per cent in Stage I and II disease. Similar results were reported from the Joint Center for Radiation Therapy at Harvard,[114] from Yale University,[194] from the Princess Margaret Hospital,[33] and from the University of Pennsylvania.[224] These studies were generally noncontrolled and retrospective; however, they provided sound evidence that tumor excision and modern radiotherapy offered an alternative treatment for certain patients with early stage breast cancer. Because of the inherent issue of patient selection that tends to include more favorable patients in alternative treatment approaches, randomized prospective trials were necessary to provide the remaining proof.

CONTROLLED TRIALS COMPARING BREAST PRESERVATION WITH MASTECTOMY

To date, nearly 3000 patients have been prospectively randomized to receive either mastectomy or wide local excision plus postoperative radiation therapy for treatment of operable Stage I or II breast carcinoma. These patients have participated in five separate clinical trials initiated in the United States and Europe.[63,64,117,208,244] These studies and summarized findings are listed in Table 7. Sufficient follow-up has not elapsed in all of these trials to make a blanket summary conclusion. However, when viewed in the context of the results from uncontrolled trials, conservative surgical therapy and radiation must be considered an alternative to mastectomy. Depending on many factors, including tumor size, breast size, tumor location, and patient preference, patients can safely be offered MRM, MRM with immediate or delayed reconstruction, or wide local excision and radiation. Currently, axillary dissection including at least level I and II nodes should accompany each of these procedures in all young patients who might be candidates for adjuvant chemotherapy (see later).

Certain comments should be made to assist the reader in interpreting results from the five prospective trials. The Guy's Hospital trials represent early experience and used admittedly inferior radiation techniques by modern standards.[117] Many of the treatment failures in radiation arms of the Guy's Hospital trials were local recurrences, particularly in the axilla, which was not dissected but received only 3000 rads postexcision. Overall survival and distant recurrences were similar in the two arms of the first trial that included both Stage I and II patients. Both the NSABP and Institut Gustave-Roussy report 5-year actuarial results, and the NSABP has recently published 3-year figures (see later).[64,208] The NSABP trial was by far the largest and randomized patients to receive mastectomy, tumor excision (segmental mastectomy) plus postoperative breast radiation, or tumor excision alone.[64,76] All patients underwent axillary dissection. The inferiority of excision alone was clearly demonstrated in 565 patients, 27.9 per cent of whom suffered an ipsilateral breast recurrence even though gross and histologically negative margins were required.

The NSABP trial allowed tumors as large as 4 cm. and included patients with movable but palpable axillary adenopathy (Stages I and II). In contrast, the Milan trial restricted enrollment to patients with tumors 2 cm. or less in diameter (T_1) and no clinically palpable adenopathy (N_0) (pure Stage I patients). The trial from the Institute Gustave-Roussy pursued an intermediate policy restricting study to 2-cm. primaries (T_1) but allowing movable axillary adenopathy (N_1). The NSABP trial specified local excision of the primary tumor and grossly negative surgical margins. This policy was quite different in the Milan trials, which practiced removal of the entire quadrant of breast tissue, including overlying skin. With the exception of the Guy's Hospital study, all modern randomized controlled trials of conservative surgical therapy have produced results that, to date, demonstrate the equivalence of conservative surgical therapy and mastectomy.[116]

The NSABP has recently updated results of protocol B-06 comparing total mastectomy with wide local excision (lumpectomy) with or without irradiation.[73] A total of 1855 women enrolled in this trial were eligible for comparison. As shown in Figure 20, breast irradiation after tumor excision significantly reduced the incidence of tumor recurrence in the ipsilateral breast from 39 per cent for those who received no irradiation to 10 per cent for patients treated by radiation after surgical excision. The effect was even more striking in positive-node patients but was significant in node-negative patients as well. The local recurrence rate following mastectomy, which cannot be analyzed with figures for breast recurrence, was 8.1 per cent overall. This study reaffirms the inadequacy of tumor excision alone for most patients with operable breast cancer. More than half of the first reported treatment failures were at distant sites, but all regional and distant failures were equally divided between the three treatment arms. Despite the higher rate of ipsilateral breast recurrence after tumor excision alone, distant disease-free survival rates were unaffected by assignment of local treatment. Finally, disease-free survival and overall actuarial survival rates were nearly identical in patients treated by tumor excision plus radiotherapy or by total mastectomy (Fig. 21). At the present time, patients with operable breast cancer may be offered either modified radical mastectomy or tumor excision to clear surgical margins and postoperative radiation therapy to the ipsilateral breast.

TREATMENT OF LOCALLY ADVANCED AND INFLAMMATORY BREAST CANCER

Locally advanced breast cancer is difficult to define precisely but generally refers to Stages IIIa and IIIb. Central to the concept is the belief that the disease is advanced on the chest wall

TABLE 7. Modern Prospective Studies Comparing Mastectomy with Conservative Surgery and Radiotherapy

Trial	No. of Patients		Actuarial Follow-up (Average in Years)	Local Recurrence (%)		Overall Survival (%)	
	Mastectomy	Radiation		Mastectomy	Radiation	Mastectomy	Radiation
Guy's Hospital Trials (II)	130*	122	11	8*	30 (p<0.001)	68	60 (p<0.002)
NSABP B-06	590	630	8	8.1	10†	71 ± 2.6	76 ± 2.1 (NS)
Gustave-Roussy	91	88	5	12	5 (NS)	91	95 (NS)
NCI–MILAN	349	352	5	<1	<1	90.1 ± 2.5	89.6 ± 2.6 (NS)
NCI–USA	95	102	NR	NR	NR	NR	NR

* The Guy's Hospital Trial compared radical mastectomy plus postoperative radiotherapy with wide local excision plus radiotherapy.

† Ten per cent of patients receiving postoperative radiotherapy had a breast recurrence but were not counted as a local failure; 8 per cent of patients receiving mastectomy had a chest wall recurrence and were counted as a local failure.

NS, not satistically significant; NR, not yet reported.

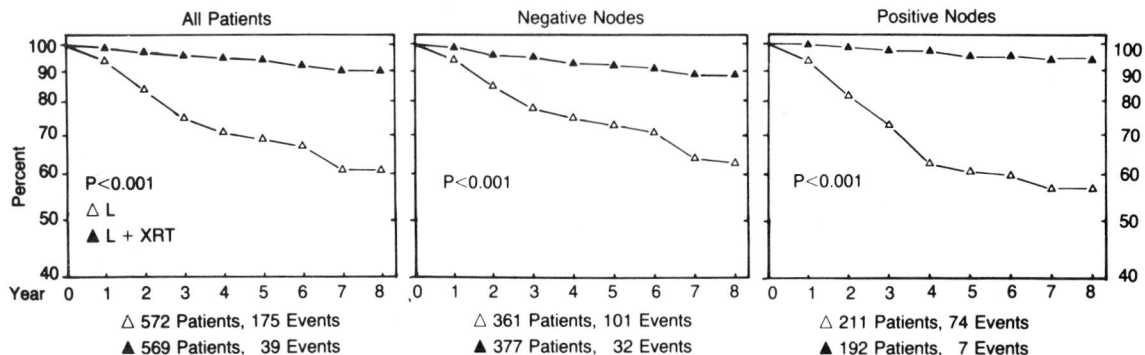

Figure 20. Life-table analysis showing the percentage of patients who remained free of tumor in the breast after lumpectomy (L) or after lumpectomy and breast irradiation (L + XRT). Results have been adjusted for the number of positive lymph nodes. For all patients, 90 per cent were free of tumor in the irradiated breast, compared with 61 per cent who were free of tumor after only lumpectomy. (From Fisher, B., et al.: Eight-year results of a randomized clinical trial comparing total mastectomy and lumpectomy with or without irradiation in the treatment of breast cancer. N. Engl. J. Med., 320:822, 1989.)

(any T_3 or T_4 tumor) and/or in regional nodes (N_2 or N_3 in the 1983 TNM system), but without evidence for distant metastases (M_0). In 1986, the AJCC specifically defined inflammatory carcinoma according to clinical criteria and assigned a new T code, T_{4d}, which falls under Stage IIIb disease. Confusion was compounded in older systems that placed inflammatory carcinoma in Stage IV and placed large T_3 tumors without nodal metastases in Stage III. The 1986 TNM system segregates the uncommon T_3N_0 case to Stage IIb, reflecting its more favorable prognosis after standard therapy. Moreover, metastasis to homolateral supraclavicular nodes now is coded as distant metastasis (M_1) and designated as Stage IV disease. This provides a more precise definition of locally advanced disease, which is composed of Stage III tumors in the 1986 AJCC TNM system and includes inflammatory carcinoma (see Table 5).

The treatment of noninflammatory, Stage III tumors has changed during the past 2 decades. The approaches were heterogeneous, and the results did not define the optimal therapy. However, if the cancers and regional nodes were technically removable, mastectomy appeared to be appropriate initial treatment. The use of breast-preserving procedures has not been specifically defined in these patients, but some investigators believe breast conservation may be appropriate in specific situations in which the tumor can be excised with clear surgical margins, leaving a cosmetically acceptable breast. When operative therapy is used alone, local relapse rates in the range of 30 to 50 per cent can be anticipated, and the long-term cure rates rarely exceed 30 per cent.[227] Similar results are reported when radiotherapy is the sole mode of local-regional treatment.[227] These poor results have motivated trials using multiagent chemotherapy, particularly combinations that include doxorubicin (Adriamycin). Investigators at the NCI in Milan pioneered the use of combination chemotherapy given prior to radio-

therapy or mastectomy; they reported 3- and 4-year survivals in the range of 50 per cent, which were better than historical controls.[46,47] Local control was similar in the mastectomy- and radiation-treated patients, in the range of 70 per cent. With combination chemotherapy before or after local treatment, improved survival and local control rates were reported by other groups.[94,143,226] Although the optimal approach has not been found, the modern approach to patients with large, locally aggressive breast cancer should include combination chemotherapy, given either before or after local treatment by mastectomy or intense radiotherapy.

INFLAMMATORY BREAST CARCINOMA. Inflammatory breast cancer presents as a dramatic clinical condition, described earlier. The pathologic hallmark, dermal lymphatic permeation by tumor cells, may be present. However, most investigators accept a clinical presentation of erythema and warmth that extends over a significant area of breast skin and may or may not be associated with a palpable mass. Diffuse invasion of lymphatic channels within the breast unifies the clinical presentation, with or without dermal lymphatic invasion. Axillary nodal metastases are almost always present, and distant disease should be sought using radiographic modalities such as bone scan and computed tomography. Recent treatment approaches emphasize the aggressive use of combined modality treatment, which can include combination chemotherapy, mastectomy, and radiotherapy.[25,210] The experience of investigators at the National Cancer Institute in Bethesda, using induction chemotherapy and hormonal synchronization has been reported recently.[231] Actuarial curves for both local control and overall survival from the NCI series of 45 patients with Stage IIIb inflammatory carcinoma of the breast are shown in Figure 22. Seven patients with inflammatory carcinoma in this series were randomized to high-dose melphalan chemotherapy with auto-

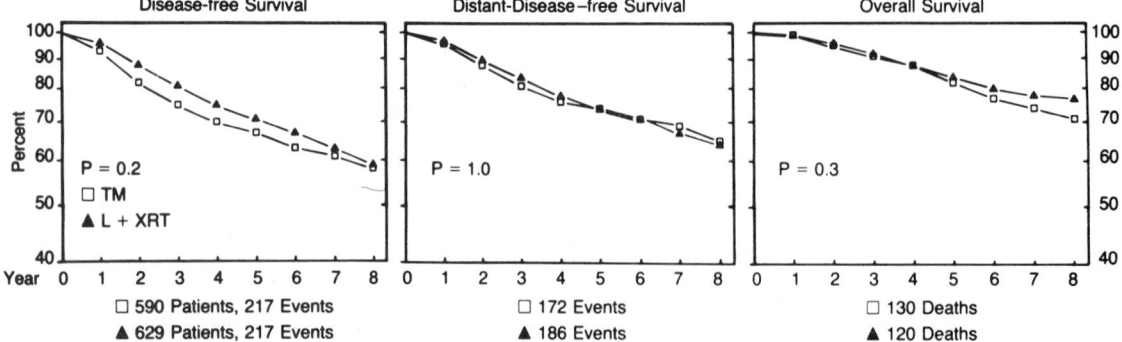

Figure 21. Life-table analysis showing the overall disease-free survival, distant disease-free survival, and overall survival of patients allocated to total mastectomy and axillary node dissection (TM) or to lumpectomy and breast irradiation (L + XRT). The results have been adjusted for the number of positive nodes. There are no significant differences between the two groups analyzed for either event-free survival or for overall survival at an average follow-up of 8 years. (From Fisher, B., et al.: Eight-year results of a randomized clinical trial comparing total mastectomy and lumpectomy with or without irradiation in the treatment of breast cancer. N. Engl. J. Med., 320:822, 1989.)

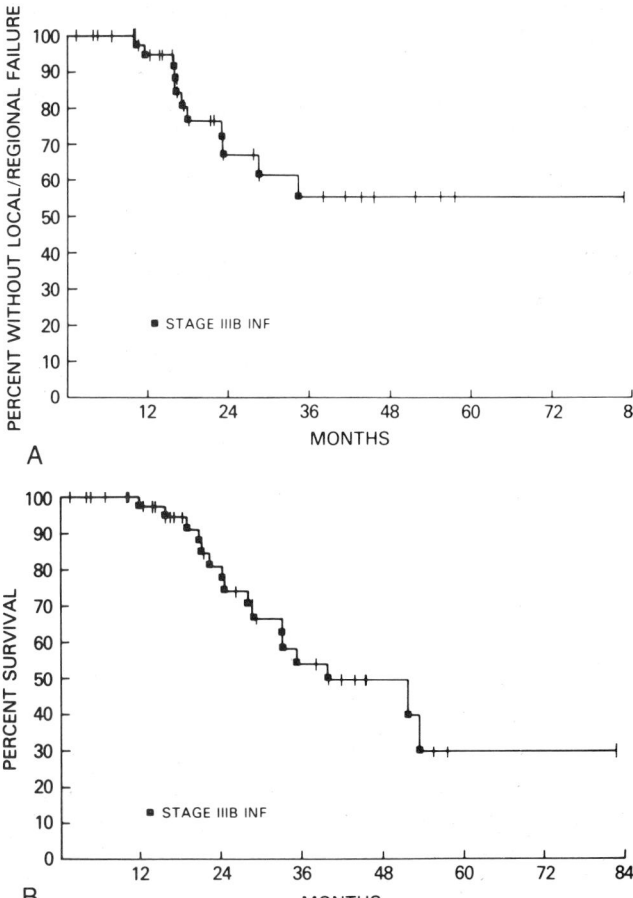

Figure 22. Results of treatment in patients with inflammatory carcinoma, using a multimodality approach at the National Cancer Institute. Patients were treated with combination chemotherapy to the point of maximal response with or without hormonal synchronization, followed by radiation in all patients and mastectomy for those not achieving a complete response. *A* displays the rate of local or regional failure. The 2-year actuarial local control rate was 67 per cent. *B* shows the overall survival. The median survival was 36 months. (From Swain, S. M., and Lippman, M. E.: Treatment of patients with inflammatory breast cancer. *In* DeVita, V. T., et al. (Eds.): Important Advances in Oncology 1989. Philadelphia, J. B. Lippincott Company, 1989.)

logous bone marrow transplantation and are being compared with a similar group receiving maintenance chemotherapy. Peters and colleagues at Duke University have one of the largest studies of bone marrow transplantation, randomizing patients with inflammatory carcinoma to receive aggressive standard chemotherapy or high-dose therapy and autologous marrow rescue followed by mastectomy and local radiation therapy. It is hoped that these newer approaches will improve the previously dismal outlook for patients with Stage III and inflammatory breast carcinoma.

MANAGEMENT OF NONINVASIVE (IN SITU) CARCINOMA

Special attention to the problem of *in situ* carcinoma is justified by the increasing frequency of its recognition and the controversy surrounding the proper treatment of noninvasive cancer of the breast. Treatment decisions require appreciation of the various types and stages of *in situ* disease and demand that the surgical oncologist understand this sometimes complicated disease process. Moreover, its relationship to invasive cancer is a fascinating biologic question. Understanding these early proliferative states should give investigators a clue to the underlying cause of breast cancer. Finally, finding early malignancy is the goal of population screening. It is hoped that the high cure

rate after treatment of noninvasive breast carcinoma will someday contribute to a decline in mortality from this malignancy.

DUCTAL CARCINOMA IN SITU (DCIS) OR INTRADUCTAL CARCINOMA

Prior to modern mammography, intraductal lesions presented as palpable tumors in 50 per cent or more of patients.[6,248] In the 1980s, more were recognized by the calcifications they produced and escaped physical detection. The comedo or solid form fills and expands small mammary ducts and is apt to undergo central necrosis. The central detritus within ducts undergoes dystrophic calcification, producing fine punctate and even linear calcification, which is seen first on mammography long before invasive disease develops into a palpable mass. Clearly, these are early lesions that can be approached in a different manner from that for usual invasive disease. Treatment recommendations for patients with intraductal carcinoma are based upon consideration of several issues, including (1) occult invasive cancer coexisting with the *in situ* lesion, (2) multicentricity of intraductal carcinoma, (3) the occurrence of disease in the contralateral breast, and (4) the natural history following diagnosis by biopsy.

The incidence and the significance of occult foci of invasive disease have been difficult to determine. Rosen found invasive disease in 12 (11 per cent) of 110 patients undergoing mastectomy for DCIS.[203] None of these patients had axillary nodal metastases. Carter and Smith examined mastectomy specimens from patients undergoing breast removal after a biopsy diagnosis of purely DCIS.[28] Seven patients (18 per cent) had residual invasive disease within the breast. Three patients with occult invasive disease had nodal metastases. Lagios and co-workers used specimen mammography and careful serial sectioning to examine breasts removed after a biopsy diagnosis of DCIS.[139] Overall, a 21 per cent incidence of residual invasive cancer was found. The study done by Lagios is summarized in Table 8 and will be discussed later. It is important to realize that axillary and distant metastases can come only from the invasive breast cancer within the tumor, which may or may not be found histologically.

Many workers who have written about intraductal carcinoma are influenced by the high incidence of multicentric, multifocal, and even bilateral disease. Multifocal is a term referring to disease within the vicinity or same quadrant as the dominant lesion. Multicentric refers to disease in distant sites or quadrants within the same breast. Bilateral implies the concurrent finding of disease in both breasts. The existence of multicentric disease has led many to favor mastectomy for the treatment of DCIS, and concerns about bilaterality have prompted the use of prophylactic procedures on the contralateral breast.

The most widely reported figure for the incidence of multicentric disease within the ipsilateral breast is 33 per cent, or one third of cases in which a biopsy discloses intraductal cancer as the predominant lesion. However, estimates vary, depending upon how extensively other quadrants of the breast are examined. For example, although a large review of NSABP material failed to find multicentric disease, only a single random section from remote quadrants was examined.[82] In contrast, Schwartz reported an incidence of approximately 37 per cent after examining four random sections from each remote quadrant and from under the areola.[212] Other estimates range between the results of these two studies.[23,139]

Using serial subgross examination and specimen mammography, the study of Lagios and associates provides useful clinical guidelines, as shown in Table 8.[139] The incidence of multicentricity, as well as unrecognized invasive disease and the presence of nodal metastases, is related to the size of the noninvasive lesion. Multicentric disease was found in only 2 of 24 (8 per cent) of patients whose principal lesion was less than 2 cm. in greatest diameter. In contrast, 100 per cent of patients with

TABLE 8. Relationship of Extent of DCIS to Frequency of Occult Invasion, Multicentricity, Nipple Involvement, Node
Metastases, and Local Recurrence, July 1, 1975 to December 31, 1980

Distribution	No. of Cases	Occult Invasion	Multicentric	Nipple	Node +	Recurrence
1 mm. or <	4	0	0	0	0	0
2–10 mm.	13	0	1	0	0	0
11–20 mm.	7	0	1	0	0	0
21–30 mm.	8	1	1	0	0	0
31–40 mm.	4	0	0	0	0	0
41–50 mm.	4	1	1	1	0	0
51–60 mm.	6	3	6	1	0	1
61 mm. or >	7	6	7	3	1	2
Total	53 (1.00)	11 (0.21)	17 (0.32)	5 (0.09)	1 (0.02)	3 (0.06)

From Lagios, M. D., Westdahl, P. R., Margolin, F. R., et al.: Duct carcinoma in situ. Relationship of extent of noninvasive disease to the frequency of occult invasion, multicentricity, lymph node metastases, and short-term treatment failures. Cancer, 50:1309, 1982.

lesions greater than 5 cm. had disease in remote quadrants of the ipsilateral breast. It is reasonable to conclude that DCIS is a heterogeneous disease that includes small lesions of low pathogenic potential and larger tumors that are more likely to be invasive or multicentric. The extent of the local in situ process is also an expression of multifocality; those lesions that are multifocal within the biopsy specimen are clearly more likely to be multicentric within the ipsilateral breast. Careful pathologic review of biopsies showing DCIS should include an estimate of the diameter of the process and a statement about multifocality within the specimen. This information will be useful to the surgeon in counseling patients and recommending treatment.

Treatment recommendations for DCIS are not easily made and are continually evolving (for a recent review, see reference 211). A number of clinical investigators recommending total mastectomy cite the high incidence of multicentricity.[6,23,212,240] Also cited are the long-term consequences after biopsy only of DCIS. In the studies of Betsill and colleagues[13] and Page and colleagues,[179] review of histologic sections from breast biopsies initially not showing carcinoma found unrecognized in situ ductal carcinomas that went untreated after biopsy. Betsill and colleagues estimated that at least 39 per cent of these patients with DCIS treated by biopsy alone subsequently developed clinically evident ipsilateral carcinoma, frequently invasive, with an average latent period of 10 years. Page and associates followed 25 women for at least 3 years and found 7 with invasive cancer, all in the same breast, after an average of 6.1 years. However, a national survey of noninvasive breast cancer by the American College of Surgeons found no difference in recurrence rates for patients treated by excision only compared with those treated by mastectomy, although follow-up averaged only 5 years.[204] Review of NSABP material from Protocol 6 found local recurrences in 14 per cent of patients treated by excision only, again with a short follow-up of only 16 months. Significantly, women treated by excision plus radiation therapy to the ipsilateral breast suffered a recurrence of 7 per cent, compared with 23 per cent in patients treated by excision only.[82]

The NSABP is accruing patients to Protocol 17, "A Clinical Trial to Evaluate Natural History and Treatment of Patients with Noninvasive Intraductal Adenocarcinoma and Lobular in-Situ Registry." Patients undergoing excision of pure DCIS and who have pathologically free margins are eligible for randomization to receive postbiopsy breast radiation or observation only. Patients with lobular carcinoma in situ are registered only and receive no further therapy. This study, which may answer several questions about the natural history of in situ carcinoma, is supported by the National Cancer Institute and has been joined by several other cooperative groups. However, certain recommendations for treatment of patients outside of a clinical trial can be made based upon previous studies. Patients with

small and unifocal DCIS—for example, those found as tiny clustered microcalcifications on mammography or those found incidentally adjacent to a benign lesion—can be offered careful observation as an alternative to further surgical therapy or radiation. Larger lesions may require re-excision to confirm that multifocal disease is not present and that margins are free of disease. Inability to achieve free margins or multifocal disease is an indication to recommend mastectomy, with or without low axillary dissection. Larger, localized lesions that are excised with free margins may be treated by breast radiation or by mastectomy. Again, the choice of axillary procedure is decided on a case-by-case basis. For extensive intraductal disease covering a large area of the breast, involving more than one quadrant, or manifested by diffuse microcalcifications, mastectomy with at least low axillary dissection is mandatory. From the data of Lagios and colleagues presented in Table 8, this more conservative approach should be followed when the intraductal disease is 5 cm. or more and considered for lesions greater than 2 cm. in total extent.

Recommendations for the contralateral breast are more difficult to support. Different from lobular carcinoma in situ, DCIS does not appear to carry an increased risk of subsequent contralateral breast cancer.[6,247] Weber studied cases submitted to the California and Connecticut tumor registries, reviewed cases of in situ cancer, and followed patients for an average of 9 years.[247] After excluding cases of concomitant contralateral breast cancer (3 cases in 116 studied), only one additional case developed in follow-up. The relative risk ratio of observed to expected cases of contralateral disease was 0.46 in this study. For the great majority of patients with DCIS, recommendations for procedures on the opposite breast are hard to support. Identification of patients with contralateral disease should be based upon careful follow-up and high-quality mammography for the majority of women with intraductal carcinoma.

LOBULAR CARCINOMA IN SITU

Lobular carcinoma in situ (LCIS) is a relatively uncommon disease that occurs predominantly in younger, premenopausal women. As noted earlier, this disease is rarely diagnosed prior to biopsy, does not form a palpable mass, and rarely calcifies. Haagensen has collected the largest series of patients, all of whom were identified by review of biopsy material.[112] In this review, LCIS was found in 3.6 per cent of more than 5000 biopsies done for benign disease. Haagensen prefers the term lobular neoplasia to emphasize that this pathologic entity predisposes to subsequent carcinoma after a long latency period. However, in a review of 297 patients with LCIS (lobular neoplasia) treated by biopsy and careful observation, Haagensen determined that the actuarial probability of developing carcinoma at the end of 35 years was 21.4 per cent. Compared with the Connecticut Tumor Registry data, a risk ratio (observed to expected cases) of 7 : 1 was calculated. Significantly, 40 per cent of the carcinomas that subsequently developed were purely *in situ* lesions, and one half of all subsequent carcinomas occurred in the contralateral breast. Haagensen prefers a practice of close observation after a biopsy diagnosis of LCIS. Similar data have led others to express doubts about the need for mastectomy.[79,249] These workers have recommended a conservative policy of close observation after a biopsy diagnosis of LCIS or lobular neoplasia.

A contrary position has been supported by Rosen and associates, who reviewed the experience of the Memorial Hospital Breast Service.[202] In a series of 99 patients with LCIS treated by biopsy alone, subsequent carcinomas developed in 37 per cent of patients followed for an average of 24 years. Consistent with Haagensen's data, recurrences were divided equally between the affected and the contralateral breast. Comparison with the Connecticut Tumor Registry produced a risk ratio for development of subsequent breast carcinoma of 9 : 1 in patients with a biopsy diagnosis of LCIS. Although similar in magnitude to the calculations of Haagensen, these investigators recommended total mastectomy with low axillary node dissection.

Although no direct survey of surgical practice has been done, a conservative approach to LCIS is probably more commonly practiced than mastectomy. Certainly, a policy of close observation is widely recognized as standard care. However, patients must be informed that LCIS predisposes to subsequent carcinoma, and that their risk is lifelong and increases over the passage of time. In selected patients, particularly young patients with a significant family history of invasive breast cancer, mastectomy may be an appropriate choice for a well-counseled patient to make. Since the risk of subsequent breast cancer is equal for both breasts, biopsy of the opposite breast will add little useful information. Subcutaneous mastectomy or glandular mastectomy, preserving the cosmetic appearance of the breast, would be an ideal procedure and could be done on both sides. Unfortunately, this procedure will not remove all tissue at risk and is an unproved method of cancer prevention. Total mastectomy remains the procedure of choice for those who elect surgical therapy in preference to observation; however, bilateral mastectomy is the only means to significantly diminish subsequent risk.

MALE BREAST CANCER

Breast cancer occurring in the mammary gland of males is infrequent, comprising no more than 1 per cent of the incidence in women.[55,110] It generally occurs at an older age; the average age at diagnosis is 10 years older in men than in women. Probably because the breast tissue is scant in men, breast tumors involve the pectoralis major muscle more commonly. Delay in diagnosis also must have a role in the more advanced presentation of male breast cancer.[55,257] Histologically, tumors of the male breast are most commonly infiltrating ductal carcinomas, similar in appearance to their counterparts in women. Lobular carcinoma, both invasive and noninvasive, is rarely seen in men. It is interesting that male breast cancer very often contains steroid hormone receptors. Gupta and colleagues found that 84 per cent of tumors arising in male mammary glands contain estrogen receptor,[95] and other studies support the high incidence of receptors and the frequent hormone sensitivity of male breast tumors.[184]

The treatment for carcinoma in the male breast depends upon the stage and local extent of the tumor. If the underlying pectoral muscle is involved, radical mastectomy is the procedure of choice. Alternatively, modified radical mastectomy with excision of the involved portion of muscle is adequate treatment. There appears to be little reason to practice breast preservation, but there are no studies to the contrary and no a priori reason for

excluding men from treatment by local excision and radiation if technically feasible and preferred by the patient. For smaller tumors that are movable across the chest wall, modified radical mastectomy appears to be the procedure of choice. Because of the local aggressiveness of these tumors, some workers have advocated the use of postoperative radiotherapy.[197]

The presence of nodal metastases appears to have at least the same prognostic power in men as in women. A large review of male breast cancer at Memorial Hospital reported survival in node-negative cancer similar to that in women. However, node-positive disease portended a worse prognosis in men than in women.[119] There is little experience with adjuvant chemo- or hormonal therapy in male breast cancer. Since the majority of these tumors are hormone sensitive, the use of adjuvant tamoxifen for node-positive and high-risk node-negative patients appears logical. Bagley and colleagues at the National Cancer Institute (NCI) have used CMF (cytoxan, methotrexate, 5-fluorouracil) combination chemotherapy in node-positive men according to the dose scheduling used in women.[11] The 5-year survival of more than 80 per cent of men treated with adjuvant therapy appeared to be a significant improvement over historical controls.

ADJUVANT CHEMOTHERAPY FOR OPERABLE BREAST CANCER

Perhaps no single aspect of modern cancer therapy has been so well studied as the use of adjuvant systemic treatment after definitive local therapy of breast cancer. Since 1980, 176 breast cancer treatment trials have opened with support from the NCI. In 1987, at least 2608 patients were entered into NCI-supported adjuvant trials.[58] The number of American trials conducted outside NCI auspices is harder to estimate, and trials in other countries, particularly in European centers, have registered thousands of patients. Many well-written recent reviews of adjuvant therapy are now available and summarize the best information available from randomized controlled trials.[91,123]

In 1985, the National Institutes of Health (NIH) sponsored a Consensus Development Conference on Adjuvant Therapy and Endocrine Therapy for Breast Cancer.[167,168] This conference brought together experts in the management of breast cancer who presented results of modern trials. A panel composed of representatives from medical oncology, surgery, biostatistics, nursing and other relevant basic and clinical disciplines agreed on a series of recommendations for the treatment of women with breast cancer outside of clinical trials. These recommendations have generally been accepted as standards of care and are summarized in Table 9.

Two trials that had the greatest influence on the NIH consensus panel were the NSABP Protocol B-05 comparison of L-phenylalanine mustard (L-PAM) and a placebo[65] and the NCI-Milan trial of combination cyclophosphamide, methotrexate, and 5-fluorouracil (CMF) versus no treatment.[17] Accrual to the NSABP trial was complete in 1974 and from Milan in 1975. Ten-year data on all patients were available in 1985[19,67] and 12-year results have since been presented.[21,74]

The design of these two trials is quite similar, allowing easy comparison of results. In the NSABP trial, all patients underwent RM as their only mode of local treatment. L-PAM or placebo was administered orally in 17 courses over 2 years to patients with histologically positive axillary nodes. Patients were stratified on the basis of age (less than age 50 years or 50 years and older). In common parlance, the younger group has been considered premenopausal and the older group postmenopausal. Cases were also stratified according to nodal status (greater than four nodes positive and one to three positive nodes). The Milan Cancer Institute used CMF combination therapy for node-positive women and stratified patients in essentially the same design used by the NSABP.

TABLE 9. 1985 NIH Consensus Development Conference Conclusion: Adjuvant Therapy of Stage I and II Breast Cancer

Menopausal Status	Axillary Nodes	Hormone Receptors	Recommended Treatment
Pre-	Positive	+ or −	Combination chemotherapy
Pre-	Negative	+ or −	Further clinical trials (combination chemotherapy considered)
Post-	Positive	+	Tamoxifen
Post-	Positive	−	Further clinical trials (combination chemotherapy considered)
Post-	Negative	+ or −	Further clinical trials

From Iglehart, J. D.: The diagnosis and management of breast cancer: An update. Sabiston, D. C., Jr.: Textbook of Surgery: The Biological Basis of Modern Surgical Practice, Update 1. Philadelphia, W. B. Saunders Company, 1988.

The results from these two trials are similar and convincingly positive for chemotherapy-treated women in certain subgroups. The greatest positive effect for chemotherapy is in women less than 50 years of age (premenopausal) with one to three lymph nodes containing metastatic cancer. In both studies, the magnitude of this difference was large and statistically significant. A trend toward prolongation of survival was seen in young women with four or more positive lymph nodes, but this group was obviously much more heterogeneous. In contrast to the positive effect of chemotherapy in younger patients, women greater than 50 years of age did not significantly benefit, as a whole, from the use of adjuvant cytotoxic chemotherapy. Ten-year results from the Milan trials using CMF compared with no-treatment controls is shown in Figure 23. Certain subsets of

postmenopausal women do, in fact, enjoy definite survival benefit from chemotherapy,[21] and the question of dose intensity in older women has also been addressed.[18] These types of detailed analyses are important both for understanding the mechanisms of action of adjuvant chemotherapy and for future study designs. Several subsequent randomized trials employing a no-treatment control arm have confirmed the results of the NSABP and Milan trials[92,234] (for review, see reference 123). Most authorities now believe no-treatment arms should be replaced by combination chemotherapy in future trials.

An overview analysis of 61 randomized trials involving 28,986 women with operable breast cancer receiving adjuvant cytotoxic or hormonal therapy has recently been published.[124] In this overview, results of 31 trials involving comparison of prolonged postoperative chemotherapy with no-treatment control arms were summarized. The reduction of the odds of death among patients of all ages receiving some form of chemotherapy was 14 (± 4) per cent. Since this overview was a composite analysis of many different regimens, it likely underestimated the benefit of application of the best agents in a well-managed individual case. For women less than 50 years of age who received CMF polychemotherapy, the reduction in odds of death was 37 (± 9) per cent. The estimated benefit of chemotherapy given as a postoperative adjuvant to women over the age of 50 years was statistically significant, but the confidence limit was wide, reflecting the variability of results from trials in these older women. Finally, the overview analysis confirmed the benefit of therapy using multiple agents when compared with single agents. The Milan Cancer Institute has shown the extremely low potential to induce second malignancies in women who receive CMF chemotherapy as an adjuvant.[242] Moreover, the same group has demonstrated the equivalent benefit of 6 months of therapy following mastectomy to its first 12-month trial.[20] Six months of CMF therapy, typically giving nine cycles of CMF, is a standard regimen that can be administered entirely in outpatient clinics. This appears to be the most widely prescribed adjuvant program given to women with node-positive breast cancer who are less than 50 years of age.

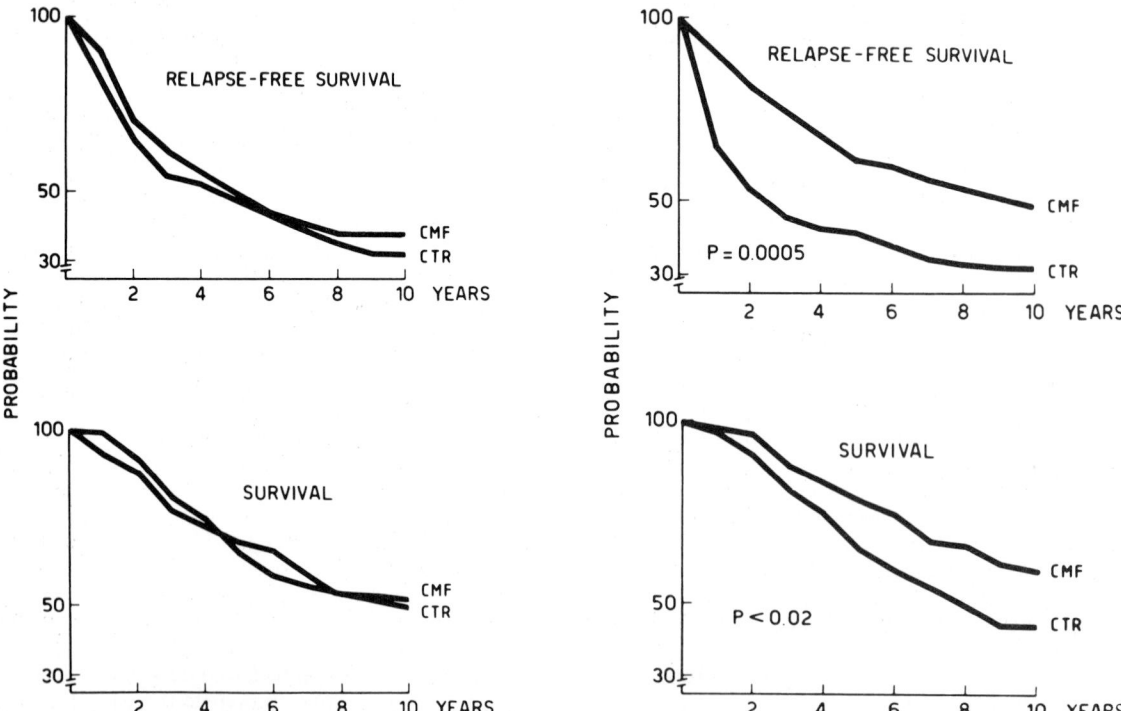

Figure 23. Ten-year actuarial relapse-free survival rates (upper panels) and overall survival rates (lower panels) for postmenopausal women (panels on the left) and premenopausal women (panels on the right) from the NCI Milan. (From Bonadonna, G., et al.: Ten-year experience with CMF-based adjuvant chemotherapy in resectable breast cancer. Breast Cancer Res. Treat., 5:95, 1985.)

ADJUVANT CHEMOTHERAPY IN NODE-NEGATIVE PATIENTS

Most chemotherapy trials that have reached mature follow-up have enrolled patients with positive axillary lymph nodes. However, at least one quarter of patients without axillary nodal involvement suffer relapse. A challenge for the next decade will be to reliably predict which of these patients harbor tumors that have a high incidence of recurrence. In these high-risk patients, adjuvant therapy can be selectively applied. Tumor size greater than 2 cm.,[169] poor histologic and nuclear grade,[81,39] absent hormone receptors,[32,235] high proliferative fraction (S-phase),[31,118,154,220] aneuploid DNA content,[31,118] overexpression of epidermal growth factor receptor (EGF-R),[206] and gene amplification and high-level overexpression of the receptor-like c-erbB-2 (HER-2, neu) product[222,256] have all been associated with a higher risk of relapse after treatment. Most studies of adjuvant chemotherapy in node-negative women have restricted enrollment to those patients with tumors possessing some markers of poor prognosis.

The results of published randomized trials of adjuvant chemotherapy in node-negative patients have been contradictory. Several trials have failed to show significant differences between patients receiving chemotherapy and controls treated only by operation. The largest and oldest trial, from the West Midlands Oncology Association, randomized 574 patients to receive oral 5-fluorouracil (5-FU), methotrexate, and chlorambucil or no treatment after operation.[162] At nearly 10 years of follow-up, there were no significant differences in relapse-free survival or overall survival, no matter how patients were divided into subgroups. Similar findings were reported from the OSAKO study in Eastern Switzerland using similar chemotherapy and bacille Calmette-Guerin (BCG) immunostimulation versus surgical controls.[216]

The Milan Cancer Institute randomized 90 node-negative and estrogen receptor–negative (ER⁻) patients to receive adjuvant CMF or to a surgical control group.[21] The results were conclusively in favor of the treated group, both for pre- and postmenopausal women. The control group in this study has experienced a higher than expected 5-year mortality of 35 per cent, and more than 50 per cent of patients relapsed by 5 years. Because of this incongruous observation and the small numbers in the trial, the Milan trial stands alone and is regarded cautiously by many investigators.

Since 1982, three large cooperative randomized trials in the United States and another international trial have been conducted to evaluate the value of adjuvant chemotherapy or hormonal therapy in node-negative breast cancer. Early results from the United States trials were summarized in May, 1988, by the NCI in the form of a Clinical Alert urging consideration of adjuvant systemic therapy in many node-negative patients.[35] Two of the trials from the NSABP, B-13 and B-14, concern ER⁻ and ER⁺ tumors, respectively. The third American trial (Int-0011) was an Intergroup trial contributed to by three cooperative trials groups and concerned either tumors larger than 3 cm. or ER⁻ tumors of any size. The last trial conducted by the Ludwig Breast Cancer Study Group used one perioperative course of CMF with leucovorin rescue immediately after operation and was compared with a surgical therapy only control group. The results of each of these studies were published jointly in 1989.[66,70,93,149] Actuarial relapse-free and overall survival rates are available only at 3 to 5 years of follow-up in these studies. In each study, advantage in disease-free survival was small but statistically significant; however, there were no significant differences in overall survival in any of the trials at the time of publication.

An important concept in the interpretation of these clinical trials was illustrated by the overview analysis of the treatment of early breast cancer referred to earlier.[124] Although the proportional reduction in mortality in node-negative patients may be of the same magnitude as the reduction in node-positive patients, the higher survival of node-negative patients makes the absolute differences very small and statistically insignificant. Caution in the interpretation of relative risk reporting and odds ratios was expressed in editorial response to the conclusions from the joint publication of the four clinical trials.[152] When considering cytotoxic or expensive treatment that is likely to benefit only a small number of patients, it is better to consider absolute survival data rather than normalized figures that obscure actual numbers. It is equally important to consider the number of patients who do not require treatment or who will not benefit from it. In the NSABP trial of methotrexate and flourouracil with leucovorin rescue, the disease-free survival (DFS) of treated patients was 80 per cent, whereas the DFS of untreated controls was 71 per cent, an absolute difference of 9 per cent. If all patients are treated, 20 per cent would relapse despite therapy, 71 per cent would not have required therapy, and only 9 per cent would benefit by a longer relapse-free survival. The cost of therapy, in terms of unnecessary exposure to cytotoxic drugs, would be borne by 91 per cent of treated patients.

Critics of the uniform treatment of node-negative patients also cite survival statistics from surgically treated series. Rosen and colleagues recently reviewed survival statistics from Memorial Sloan-Kettering for patients undergoing mastectomy without adjuvant treatment between 1964 and 1970.[201] For node-negative patients with tumors of 1 cm. or less, the likelihood of remaining disease free at 10 years was 91 per cent. For larger tumors, of between 1.1 and 2.0 cm., the chance of remaining disease free fell to 78 per cent. This series and others have identified unfavorable tumor characteristics, which include larger tumor size, the presence of vessel invasion within the tumor,[81] high proliferative fraction (S-phase),[31,118,154,220] and the absence of hormone receptors for estrogen and progesterone.[32,235] Adjuvant therapy may be worthwhile in these patients whose outlook is in an intermediate range similar to patients with less than four positive lymph nodes. Prospective or randomized studies have not yet addressed this question.

HORMONAL THERAPY OF BREAST CANCER

The effect of steroid hormones on sensitive tissues has been the subject of important basic and clinical efforts. Surgeons have participated in this research from its beginning. Beatson, surgeon to the Glasgow Cancer Hospital, was the first to demonstrate that bilateral oophorectomy, which deprives a woman of sex steroids, can lead to regression of metastatic breast cancer.[12] Surgical castration became the first effective means to control advanced breast cancer, producing a beneficial regression in 25 to 40 per cent of premenopausal patients.[230] Huggins and Bergenstal re-emphasized oophorectomy and demonstrated the effectiveness of adrenalectomy in the treatment of metastatic breast cancer.[127] Hypophysectomy, which deprives the patient of pituitary polypeptide hormones, results in palliative remissions of metastatic breast cancer in up to 40 per cent of patients.[86,252] This procedure, which carries an operative mortality of between 2 and 9 per cent and results in diabetes insipidus in a significant number of patients, is not widely used currently. In the last decade, endocrine organ ablation has been replaced by estrogen and antiestrogen therapy in the majority of patients. Oophorectomy has been compared with tamoxifen in two controlled clinical trials of patients with metastatic breast cancer.[24,128] Results are equivalent in both the surgically treated and drug-treated groups. Aminoglutethimide, which blocks a number of steroid hydroxylation steps in the adrenal gland and peripherally, appears capable of replacing adrenalectomy in the treatment of advanced disease.[207] Overall, tamoxifen is at least as effective as every form of endocrine ablative therapy with

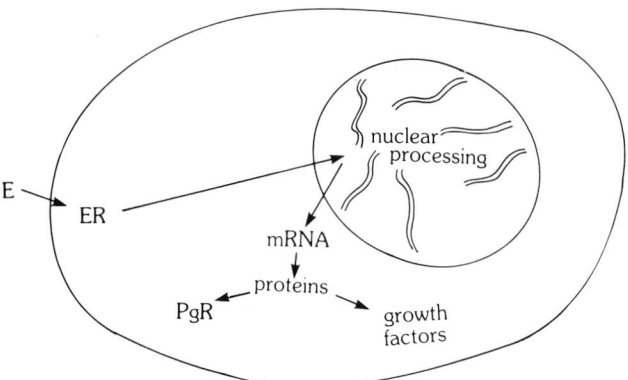

Figure 24. Mechanisms of estrogen action in breast cancer cells containing functional estrogen receptor. Lipid-soluble estrogen molecules (E) passively diffuse through the cell membrane where they bind to estrogen receptors (ER), most of which are located in the cell nucleus. The hormone-receptor complex interacts with specific sites on cellular DNA to stimulate transcription of mRNA and synthesis of cellular proteins. A predominant product in stimulated cells is the receptor for progesterone (PgR). Presence of PgR implies an intact estrogen-sensitive pathway. Cellular proliferation may depend on synthesis of certain polypeptide growth factors, such as the transforming growth factors (TGF-alpha and -beta) and insulin-like growth factors. By interacting with their specific receptors, these "second messengers" may close the loop and result in cellular division. (From Osborne, C. K.: Receptors. *In* Harris, J. R., et al. (Eds.): Breast Diseases. Philadelphia, J. B. Lippincott Company, 1987.)

which it has been compared.[121] Understanding the cellular and molecular mechanism underlying the trophic effect of estrogen and progesterone represents one of the major advances in the treatment of breast cancer and has allowed physicians to predict patient responses to hormone manipulation.

STEROID HORMONE RECEPTORS

Specific accumulation of estradiol in the reproductive organs of animals suggested the presence of receptors for sex steroids.[237] Availability of tritiated estradiol enabled investigators to demonstrate and measure specific, high-affinity protein receptors first for estrogen[90,129] and later for progesterone.[156,195] Numerous studies have demonstrated specific receptors for both estrogen and progesterone in tumor tissue from mammary origin.[153,195,253] These receptor proteins are probably located in the cell nucleus and are activated when occupied by their specific ligand. Activation of the estrogen receptor leads to the induction of numerous cellular genes, including those that may encode critical enzymes or secreted peptide growth factors[171] (Fig. 24). Clinically, the most important protein induced by the estrogen receptor (ER) is the receptor for progesterone (PgR).[171] Therefore, PgR may serve as an indicator for the presence of a functional ER. This relationship explains clinical observations that relate the presence of functional receptors to response to hormone manipulation.

The quantity of receptor is expressed as a binding capacity in femtomoles (10^{-15} moles) of labeled steroid bound per milligram of protein. In this assay format, levels of less than 3 fmol./mg. protein are considered negative and indicate a slim chance of hormone responsiveness. Levels above 10 fmol./mg. are clearly positive and indicate a high probability of hormone responsiveness. Newer assay formats are based on immunohistochemistry or enzyme-linked immunosorbent assays (ELISA) and are increasing in popularity. The majority of human breast tumors contain detectable amounts of either ER or PgR or both (Fig. 25). The content of measurable receptors may depend on the amount of circulating hormone. For example, high levels of estrogen may mask the presence of the ER when determined by ligand-binding assays.[254] Low levels of estrogen may fail to provide the stimulation necessary to express detectable levels of PgR.[254] As shown in Table 10, postmenopausal patients are more likely to have ER+ tumors than younger, premenopausal women. In contrast, the relationship between age and PgR is not as significant.[254]

The observation that the presence and the amount of ER was a positive marker for tumors likely to respond to endocrine therapy has been confirmed by many clinical investigators and

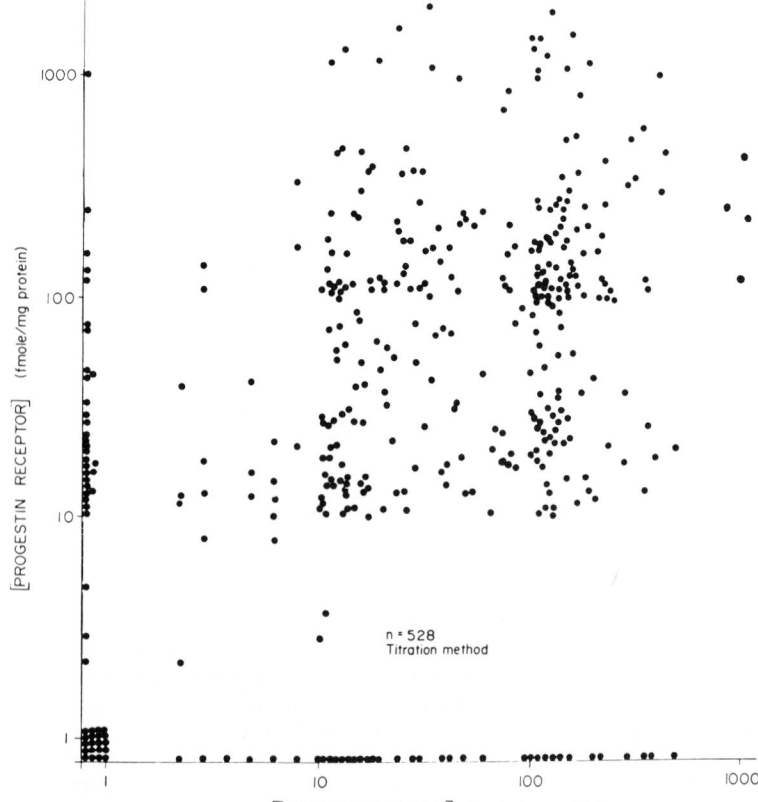

Figure 25. The content of estrogen and progesterone receptor proteins in human breast tumor tissues determined by titration analysis using radiolabeled ligands, expressed as fmol./mg. cytosol protein. (From Wittliff, J. L.: Steroid hormone receptors in breast cancer. Cancer, *53:*630, 1984.)

TABLE 10. Distribution of Steroid Receptors in Tumor Biopsies According to Patient Endocrine Status*

Receptor Status of Tumor Biopsy Specimen	Endocrine Status of Patient	
	Premenopausal (%)	Postmenopausal (%)
ER⁺, PgR⁺	222 (45)	520 (63)
ER⁺, PgR⁻	58 (12)	128 (15)
ER⁻, PgR⁻	136 (28)	137 (17)
ER⁻, PgR⁺	72 (15)	41 (5)
Total	488	826

* Fifty-five years of age was chosen as an age at which virtually every woman may be considered postmenopausal.

From Wittlift, J. L.: Steroid hormone receptors in breast cancer. Cancer, 53:630, 1984.

was summarized 15 years ago at an international meeting.[153] It was also recognized that the presence of ER predicted clinical response to all types of endocrine therapies, both additive and ablative. Furthermore, since PgR expression is induced by estrogen binding to ER, the presence of PgR also correlated with response to endocrine therapy. The presence of both receptors in a tumor is associated with an almost 80 per cent chance of favorably responding to hormone addition or blockade (Table 11).

Hormonal manipulation for the treatment of breast cancer has been simplified dramatically by the introduction of tamoxifen and related compounds.[121] Tamoxifen is a competitive antagonist of estrogen and will bind to estrogen receptors, preventing the binding of estrogen. However, other pathways appear to be active, including inhibition of growth factor production or production of inhibitory factors.[130] Regardless of its mode of action, tamoxifen can effectively replace oophorectomy in premenopausal women with metastatic cancer and is at least as effective as every form of endocrine therapy with which it has been compared.[121] The major toxicities of tamoxifen are few and include mild nausea, hot flashes, particularly in premenopausal women, and transient thrombocytopenia or leukopenia. Because of these facts, tamoxifen is widely considered the first drug to use when hormonal manipulation is chosen. Response rates in metastatic disease are approximately 50 per cent when ER or PgR is present and fall to 10 per cent for receptor-negative tumors.[153] It is no surprise that tamoxifen has been carefully tested as an adjuvant following surgical therapy or radiotherapy for primary breast cancer.

ADJUVANT HORMONAL THERAPY FOR OPERABLE BREAST CANCER

The first trial designed to test the use of adjuvant tamoxifen was begun in Copenhagen in 1975.[183] This study found benefit for postmenopausal women treated with tamoxifen compared

TABLE 11. Relationship Between Steroid Receptor (ER, PgR) Status of Breast Tumor and Patients' Objective Response to Endocrine Therapy

Steroid Receptor Status*			
ER⁺, PgR⁺	ER⁺, PgR⁻	ER⁻, PgR⁻	ER⁻, PgR⁺
135/174 (78%)	55/164 (34%)	17/165 (10%)	5/11 (45%)

* Number of patients responding to treatment/number of women with receptor status designated.

Based on the collective papers presented at the NIH Consensus Development Conference on Steroid Receptors in Breast Cancer (Proceedings of the NIH Consensus Development Conference, 1980).

From Donegan, W. L., and Spratt, J. S. (Eds.): Cancer of the Breast. Philadelphia, W. B. Saunders Company, 1988.

with placebo-treated controls. There have been several subsequent randomized trials comparing adjuvant tamoxifen with local therapy alone, as well as trials using chemotherapy with or without tamoxifen[22,42,69,72,92,170,192,234] (for review see reference 191).

The Nolvadex Adjuvant Trial Organization (NATO) entered 1285 patients aged 75 years or less into a two-arm study of tamoxifen versus no treatment.[170] Premenopausal women with positive axillary nodes and postmenopausal women with or without positive nodes were eligible. Treatment with tamoxifen was continued for 2 years or until relapse resulted in withdrawal from the study. Nearly one half (46 per cent) of tumors were assayed for ER content. Overall, 34 per cent fewer fatalities were observed in the treatment arm compared with the control group. Life-table analyses for the entire study are shown in Figure 26. When patients were stratified according to either menopausal, nodal, or receptor content, the beneficial effect of tamoxifen was felt equally in all treatment groups, compared with no-treatment arms. Only 25 (4 per cent) of patients receiving tamoxifen experienced side effects of treatment that resulted in withdrawal of the drug. Among patients with ER⁻ tumors, 104 received tamoxifen and 84 were randomized to no treatment. Deaths occurred in 19 (18 per cent) compared with 33 (39 per cent) of the two groups, respectively. The unexpected benefit of tamoxifen in cohorts of ER⁻ tumors prompted speculation about alternative effects of tamoxifen via pathways that bypass hormone receptors.

The second major trial of adjuvant tamoxifen in operable breast cancer was conducted in Scotland between 1978 and 1984; it randomized 1312 patients in a two-arm study similar to the NATO study.[22] The Scottish trial accepted patients 80 years of age or less who had negative lymph nodes or who were postmenopausal and had positive axillary nodes. The trial differed by using 5 years of adjuvant tamoxifen and by treatment of first relapses in the control arm with tamoxifen. More tumors (57 per cent) were analyzed for their ER content in the Scottish trial. When assessing survival data, it is necessary to remember that 93 per cent of patients suffering relapse in the control arm were treated with therapeutic tamoxifen. Therefore, the survival prolongation by use of adjuvant tamoxifen is determined by comparison with a policy of delayed tamoxifen after first relapse.

There were 157 recurrences in the tamoxifen-treated patients (24 per cent), compared with 250 recurrences (38 per cent) in the control arm. The distribution of recurrences was similar in node-positive and node-negative patients and in pre- and postmenopausal women. Although a trend in favor of improved disease-free survival for tamoxifen treatment was observed in patients with the highest ER levels, the data indicated benefit of adjuvant treatment at all levels of receptor content. This result was similar to findings in the NATO trial.

Overall survival analyses also show benefit of adjuvant tamoxifen given for a median of 47 months, compared with the use of tamoxifen for first recurrence. Eighteen per cent of patients in the adjuvant arm and 23 per cent in the control arm have died with breast cancer. Again, when patients are stratified by nodal and menopausal status and by ER content, cohorts receiving adjuvant treatment have a clear survival advantage.

The NATO and Scottish trials are both large and, to date, highly positive studies of adjuvant tamoxifen. Both studies have shown benefit in node-positive as well as node-negative patients. The benefit realized by node-negative patients was reiterated in the recent NCI Clinical Alert regarding adjuvant systemic treatment of patients with disease confined to the breast.[35] Although neither study directly compared adjuvant hormonal therapy in receptor-negative patients, subgroup analysis in both studies indicated total benefit of treatment. These results are hard to reconcile with data regarding the use of tamoxifen in patients with metastatic disease in whom receptor content is a potent predictor of response. Data from the control group in the

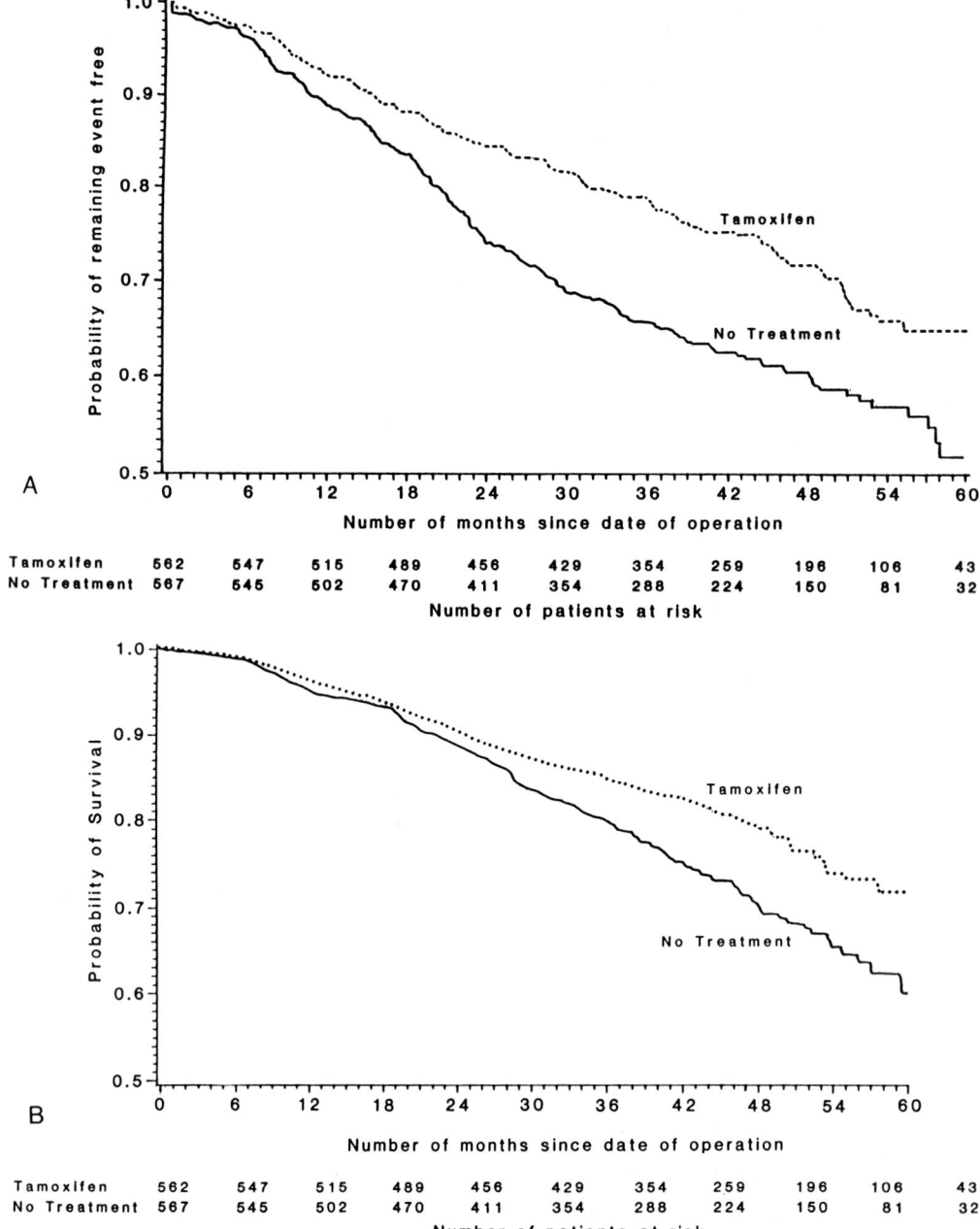

Tamoxifen   562   547   515   489   456   429   354   259   196   106   43
No Treatment 567   545   502   470   411   354   288   224   150   81   32

Number of patients at risk

Tamoxifen   562   547   515   489   456   429   354   259   196   106   43
No Treatment 567   545   502   470   411   354   288   224   150   81   32

Number of patients at risk

Figure 26. Fifth-year results of the Nolvadex Adjuvant Trial Organization. *A* presents disease-free survival through 5 years for the entire study. The benefit of tamoxifen (Nolvadex) was felt in pre- and postmenopausal patients, all nodal groups, and regardless of ER content. *B* shows a prolongation of survival in the tamoxifen-treated patients. (From Baum, M., et al.: Controlled trial of tamoxifen as single adjuvant agent in the management of early breast cancer: Analysis at six years by Nolvadex Adjuvant Trial Organization. Lancet, *1:*836, 1985.)

Scottish trial regarding the delayed use of tamoxifen after first recurrence should be informative. Moreover, exploration of alternate pathways of tamoxifen effects may uncover even more important means to influence the growth of breast epithelium.

In 1977, the NSABP initiated a study to compare the worth of adding tamoxifen to adjuvant chemotherapy in 1891 women with operable breast cancer (Protocol B-09).[69] Women of all ages and menopausal status with positive axillary lymph nodes were randomized to receive either L-phenylalanine mustard and 5-fluorouracil (PF) or PF plus tamoxifen (PFT) for a total of 2 years after operation. Considering all patients, there was a significant prolongation of the disease-free interval (but not overall survival) in the group receiving PFT. This benefit was restricted almost entirely to women over the age of 50 years and those with four or more positive lymph nodes. In this subgroup, there was a 66 per cent greater chance of remaining disease-free with PFT treatment, and there was a significant benefit in abso-

lute survival. In multivariate analyses, positive receptor content, particularly progesterone receptor, correlated best with the survival advantage in older patients receiving PFT. Younger patients, particularly with receptor-negative tumors, did not share in the benefits of adding tamoxifen. Although results from Protocol B-09 are complex, tamoxifen appears to provide additional benefit to cytotoxic chemotherapy in postmenopausal women with node-positive breast cancer. These results lend support to the opinion of some experts that tamoxifen be started after completion of chemotherapy in older women, particularly those whose tumors are ER+ or PgR+.

SUMMARY OF ADJUVANT CHEMOTHERAPY AND HORMONAL THERAPY

Based upon the low frequency of significant toxicity from adjuvant CMF and its ease of administration (nine separate cycles over 6 months), this combination appears to be the choice for treatment outside of clinical trials and has replaced the no-treatment arm in most clinical trials. It is definitely of benefit in premenopausal women and probably in high-risk cohorts of postmenopausal women who can tolerate 6 months of therapy. Node-positive patients are expected to experience a larger margin of benefit, but subsets of node-negative women may benefit also. Adjuvant hormonal therapy with tamoxifen is remarkably free from side effects in postmenopausal women and is standard therapy for postmenopausal node-positive patients. If chemotherapy is used, tamoxifen usually begins after completion of chemotherapy. Most authorities recommend that adjuvant tamoxifen continue for at least 2 years. Receptor-positive patients definitely benefit from treatment, but receptor-negative patients may be eligible for adjuvant hormonal therapy. One set of current recommendations for treatment outside of clinical trials is summarized in Table 12. Another NIH consensus conference is anticipated in 1990 to explore the extent of agreement about adjuvant treatment of node-negative and postmenopausal patients and the use of prognostic markers to assist in decision making. These recommendations are changing, and clinicians caring for patients with breast cancer must continue to seek new information and to utilize consultants with special knowledge in breast cancer management.

TREATMENT OF METASTATIC DISEASE

Once breast cancer has spread outside the confines of the breast and regional axillary lymph nodes, it is currently not curable. The median life expectancy of patients with newly diagnosed Stage IV breast cancer is about 24 months. However, although not curable, metastatic breast cancer can be controlled, and patients can be offered palliative therapy. Occasional patients, particularly those with skeletal disease or disease in soft tissues and those whose tumors are hormone sensitive, can survive many years with advanced disease. Newer therapies, such as autologous bone marrow transplantation after dose-intense chemotherapy, offer the chance for improvement in survival and perhaps, someday, long-term remission or cure.[5]

TABLE 12. Recommendations for Adjuvant Treatment Outside Clinical Trials

Menopausal Status	Axillary Nodes	Tumor Characteristics*	Recommended Treatment
Pre-	Positive	Favorable or unfavorable	Combination chemotherapy†
Pre-	Negative	Favorable	No data to support adjuvant therapy
Pre-	Negative	Unfavorable	Combination chemotherapy acceptable
Post-	Positive	Favorable	Tamoxifen ± chemotherapy
Post-	Positive	Unfavorable	Chemotherapy ± tamoxifen
Post-	Negative	Favorable	No data to support adjuvant therapy
Post-	Negative	Unfavorable	No data to support adjuvant therapy

* Favorable tumor characteristics include size < 2 cm., ER- or PgR-positive, nuclear and histologic grade good (1 or 2). Unfavorable tumor characteristics include size > 2 cm., ER- or PgR-negative, nuclear and histologic grade poor (3).

† Combination chemotherapy is usually CMF × 6 months (9 cycles).

Chemotherapy for Stage IV breast cancer is generally based upon the use of two drugs, cyclophosphamide and doxorubicin, frequently in combination with other agents. Some of the commonly encountered drug combinations used to treat metastatic breast cancer are listed in Table 13. Cyclophosphamide is a prototype alkylating agent that has been extensively studied in breast cancer and is used in the majority of combination programs. Doxorubicin is an anthracycline antibiotic that is the most active single agent in advanced breast cancer. Response rates in more than 50 per cent of patients who have not been previously treated have been reported. In the absence of investigational protocols, combinations of cyclophosphamide, fluorouracil, and methotrexate (CMF) or cyclophosphamide, doxorubicin (Adriamycin), and fluorouracil (CAF) offer response

TABLE 13. Commonly Used Combinations of Chemotherapy to Treat Advanced and Metastatic Breast Cancer

Cyclophosphamide-Based Regimens

CMFVP

C = Cyclophosphamide	2 mg./kg./day orally
M = Methotrexate	0.7 mg./kg./wk. intravenously × 8 wk.
F = 5-Fluorouracil	12 mg./kg./day × 4, then 500 mg./wk. intravenously
V = Vincristine	0.035 mg./kg./wk. intravenously
P = Prednisone	0.75 mg./kg./day orally

CMF

C = Cyclophosphamide	100 mg./sq. m./day orally on days 1–14
M = Methotrexate	30–40 mg./sq. m. intravenously on days 1 and 8 every 28 days
F = 5-Fluorouracil	400–600 mg./sq. m. intravenously on days 1 and 8 every 28 days

CFP

C = Cyclophosphamide	150 mg./sq. m./day orally × 5
F = 5-Fluorouracil	300 mg./sq. m./day intravenously × 5 q. 6 wk.
P = Prednisone	30 mg./day × 7

Doxorubicin-Based Regimens

FAC

F = 5-Fluorouracil	500 mg./sq. m. intravenously on days 1 and 8
A = Doxorubicin hydrochloride (Adriamycin)	50 mg./sq. m. intravenously on day 1 every 28 days
C = Cyclophosphamide	500 mg./sq. m. intravenously on day 1

ACMF

A = Adriamycin	40 mg./sq. m. on day 21
C = Cyclophosphamide	1000 mg./sq. m. on day 1
M = Methotrexate	30 mg./sq. m. on days 21, 28, and 35
F = 5-Fluorouracil	400–600 mg./sq. m. on days 21, 28, and 35. Repeat cycle q. 6 wk.

AC

A = Adriamycin	40 mg./sq. m.
C = Cyclophosphamide	200 mg./sq. m. on days 3 to 6. Repeat cycle q. 21 days.

This is an incomplete list of the many combinations of agents and dosage schedules used to treat metastatic breast cancer. The regimens listed here are commonly used and frequently quoted. They are taken from Cooper, R., Proc. AACR (Abstr.), 10:15, 1969; De Lena, M., Cancer, 35:1108, 1975; Broder and Tormey, Cancer Treat. Rev., 1:183, 1974; Blumenschein, G., Proc. ASCO (Abstr.), 15:193, 1974; Kennealey, G., Cancer, 42:27, 1978; and Salmon, S. E., and Jones, S. E.: Proc. AACR (Abstr.), 15:90, 1974.

Modified from Seeger, J., and Allegra, J. C.: Chemotherapy of breast cancer. In Donegan, W. L., and Spratt, J. S. (Eds.): Cancer of the Breast. Philadelphia, W. B. Saunders Company, 1988.

rates of up to 50 per cent. These combinations are standard care for patients after the first relapse of breast cancer.[45,122]

As discussed earlier, one of the most important discoveries that has improved the outlook for patients with breast cancer is the identification of hormone receptor in tumor tissue. Response rates to endocrine treatment in metastatic disease for patients whose tumors harbor hormone receptors are in excess of 50 per cent. The success rates for endocrine therapy of receptor-positive disease are at least as good as those reported for cytotoxic therapy. However, the time required for measurable response is frequently longer for hormone manipulation than for chemotherapy. Moreover, chemotherapy is more predictable and less dependent on the presence of hormone receptor content. In Figure 27, a series of clinical criteria and judgments are presented in algorithm format.[213] These judgments depend on knowledge of the estrogen and progesterone receptor status of the tumor, the age of the patient, menopausal status, overall health, and determination of how life-threatening the metastatic disease is at diagnosis. For patients with life-threatening metastases in visceral organs, for those whose tumors are ER⁻ and PgR⁻, and for those who are able to tolerate the side effects of cytotoxic drugs, combination chemotherapy is the first choice and a central entry in the algorithm. For older patients, patients with hormone-sensitive tumors, or those patients whose disease sites are in bone, soft tissues, or other nonthreatening locations, endocrine manipulation can be tried first. Tamoxifen appears to be the agent of first choice for most of these patients.

NONEPITHELIAL BREAST TUMORS

Cells comprising the connective tissue investments of the breast can give rise to both benign and malignant tumors. Generally, these tumors are sarcomas and can be categorized according to existing schemes describing sarcomas that originate in other body sites. An exception to this rule is the phyllodes tumor, or cystosarcoma phyllodes, which is peculiar to the mammary gland. Three principal tumor types are discussed under the category of nonepithelial tumors: angiosarcoma, cystosarcoma phyllodes, and other primary stromal sarcomas.

ANGIOSARCOMA. This exceedingly malignant tumor is perhaps related to benign hemangiomas that can occur in the breast. It generally presents as a spongy, ill-defined mass that is composed of numerous dilated vascular channels. If the tumor is located near the overlying skin, a characteristic bluish discoloration may be appreciated during visual inspection of the breast. Hemorrhage, either spontaneous or complicating biopsy, is not uncommon. Necrosis, which never occurs in hemangiomas, is characteristic of angiosarcoma. The tumor commonly achieves a large size by the time of presentation, usually larger than 5 cm., and the average age of patients with this malignancy is 10 to 15 years younger than for patients with usual ductal carcinomas. Metastases to regional nodes are extraordinarily rare; the usual mode of spread is hematogenous to the lungs, brain, bone, abdominal viscera, and even to the contralateral breast.

The treatment of angiosarcoma is total mastectomy in the great majority of cases. There appears to be agreement that axillary dissection is not necessary and should be reserved for those patients with clinically enlarged nodes.[30,53] Because radiotherapy is of benefit in the treatment of related sarcomas in other body sites, some workers recommend postoperative radiotherapy to the chest wall.[4] There are only anecdotal reports of chemotherapy in angiosarcoma. Most regimens reported to have activity in this tumor contain either actinomycin D or doxorubicin (Adriamycin). The role of adjuvant chemotherapy is even less well studied, but for high grade lesions it appears to be logical and offers the only chance to alter the natural history of this tumor.[4,57]

Survival appears to depend on the histologic grade of tumor.

High-grade lesions (Grade 3) are said to be the most lethal of all primary breast cancers[30,57] The survival rate of Grade 3 lesions was only 11 per cent of patients treated at Memorial Hospital. In contrast, low-grade lesions are more likely to be cured after total mastectomy. However, some of these lesions may be confused with benign hemangiomas. As emphasized by Page, size is a valuable means to differentiate benign hemangiomas from angiosarcoma. Benign lesions are frequently found histologically and are rarely large enough to form palpable lesions. In contrast, angiosarcomas are usually large, palpable masses that invade breast parenchyma. This fact, and the presence of mitoses and necrosis, usually differentiates the malignant vascular tumors from the benign ones.[176]

CYSTOSARCOMA PHYLLODES (PHYLLODES TUMOR). This tumor is the most common neoplasm of nonepithelial origin in the breast. It is also a unique neoplasm that occurs exclusively in the female breast and appears in no other site in the body. The term *phyllodes* comes from the Greek work *phyllon*, which means "leaf." This descriptive terminology refers to a bulky tumor whose cut surface is embossed with a leaflike appearance. The term *cystosarcoma* refers to the microscopic cyst-like spaces lined with a low epithelium, reminiscent of fibroadenoma. The inclusion of sarcoma in the terminology may be confusing, since the majority of these lesions are considered to be benign. For this reason, the World Health Organization classification of breast tumors uses the term *phyllodes* tumor, which carries no implication of biologic potential. A diagnosis of phyllodes tumor (or cystosarcoma) should be qualified by indication of its malignancy or benignity, or whether it has indeterminate characteristics, a so-called borderline lesion.

The majority of tumors are sharply demarcated and freely mobile, with a smooth contour. These tumors can be any size but frequently are large, with a median size of 4 to 5 cm.[176] They can occur in patients at any age, although the median age is generally in the fifth decade of life, at least a decade older than the average age of patients presenting with fibroadenoma. Mammographically, they present as round densities with a smooth border, which are indistinguishable from fibroadenoma. The diagnosis is suggested by their larger size, history of rapid growth, and occurrence in older patients. The diagnosis is usually made by excisional biopsy followed by careful pathologic review.

The clinical behavior of this tumor is difficult to predict with accuracy. Some low-grade tumors do have the potential to metastasize, a fact that dictates the surgical approach to most of these tumors. Wide local excision appears appropriate for those that appear "benign" histologically, but patients must be carefully followed because of the risk for local recurrence and metastases. If the diagnosis was not suspected preoperatively, as is frequently the case, pathologic review should be requested. If the tumor is low grade or named a *benign phyllodes tumor*, close follow-up may be advised. When the histologic appearance suggests malignancy or when the tumor is very large, total mastectomy appears to be warranted. In a review of seven series reporting 332 patients, axillary metastases were present in 3 (0.9 per cent) of the patients.[142] Formal axillary dissection appears to be unnecessary, but removal of low axillary lymph nodes cannot be criticized.

Most recurrences of phyllodes tumors are local recurrences in the site of excision. For these patients, total mastectomy is most appropriate. Metastatic disease is commonly seen in the lung, mediastinum, and skeleton. The optimal treatment of metastatic phyllodes tumors has not been found. Most investigators have used cyclophosphamide- or doxorubicin-containing combinations. Recently, three patients with metastatic tumors have been treated with cisplatin and etoposide combination chemotherapy. Effective palliation was achieved by this combination in two patients, and radiation to symptomatic metastases was helpful in all three. The tumors of two of these patients con-

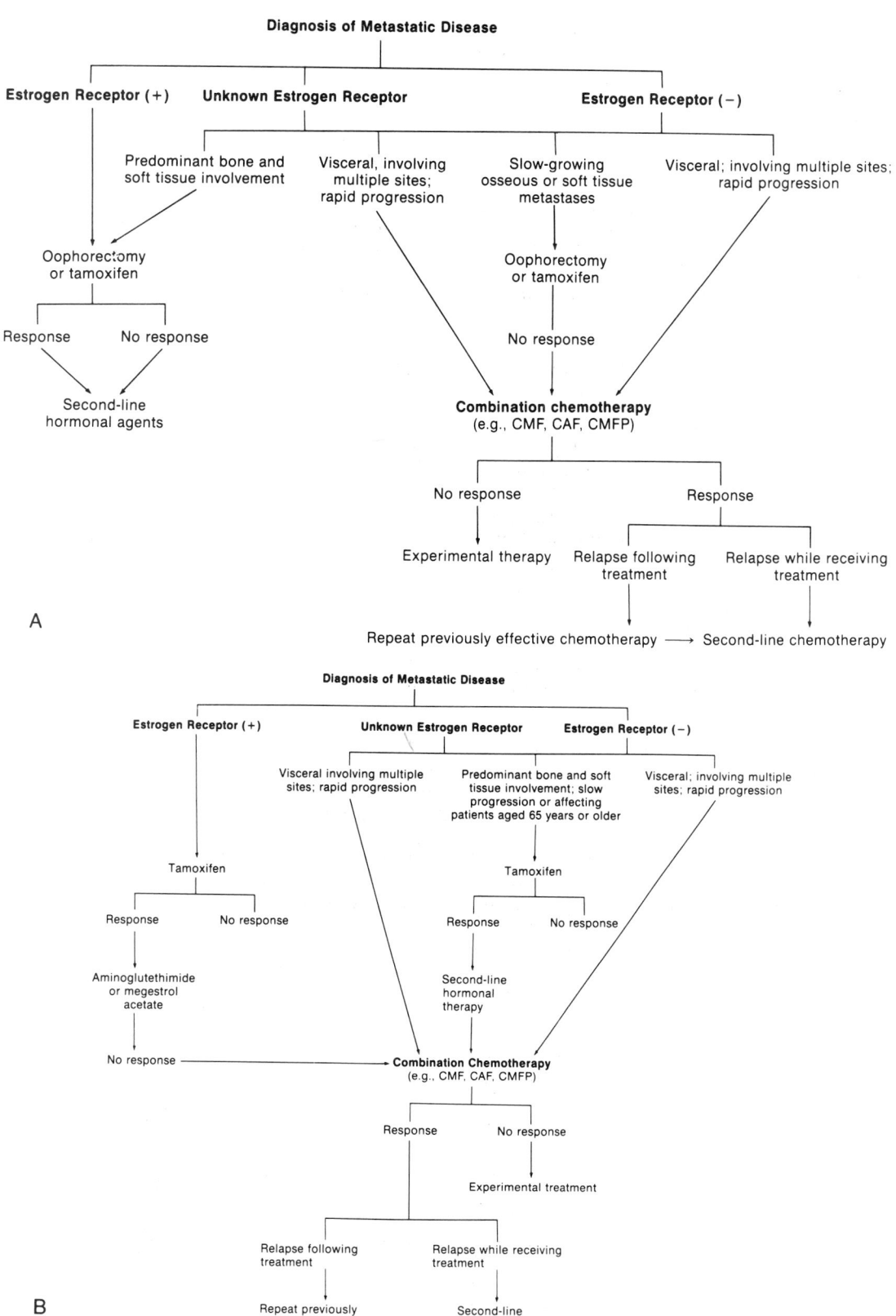

Figure 27. Decision-making algorithm for patients with metastatic breast cancer. In *A*, a decision tree for premenopausal patients with metastatic breast cancer is suggested. A major difference is the use of oophorectomy in young patients with hormone-sensitive tumors. *B* suggests a decision sequence for postmenopausal patients. Combination chemotherapy is central to both patient groups and is used for life-threatening disease, for hormone receptor–negative disease, or after failure of hormonal manipulation.

tained either estrogen or progesterone receptor, although hormone manipulation was ineffective.[26]

SELECTED REFERENCES

De Moulin, D.: A Short History of Breast Cancer. Boston, Martinus Nijhoff Publishers, 1983.
> *In just over 100 pages, Daniel De Moulin presents a history of breast cancer in an exhaustively referenced and very readable text. This monograph can be read in a matter of days and will give the student of history a complete view of the subject.*

Donegan, W. L., and Spratt, J. S., Jr.: Cancer of the Breast, 3rd ed. Philadelphia, W. B. Saunders Company, 1988.
> *This book, extensively expanded during the 9 years since publication of the second edition, represents one of the finest and most inclusive sources of information about breast diseases.*

Haagensen, C. D.: Diseases of the Breast. Philadelphia, W. B. Saunders Company, 1986.
> *In the third edition of this now classic monograph on all aspects of breast diseases, Dr. Haagensen reviews his personal experience with patients over the past 50 years. This experience has produced cohorts of patients with specific problems in breast diseases that have never been duplicated in their numbers, their follow-up, or the complete way they are presented and analyzed. This text is highly recommended. Dr. Haagensen takes his place with the handful of physicians and scientists who have made monumental contributions to the treatment of patients with breast disease.*

Harris, J. R., Hellman, S., Henderson, I. C., and Kinne, D. W.: Breast Diseases. Philadelphia, J. B. Lippincott Company, 1987.
> *Each of the editors and the contributors to this text are leading authorities on the subject of breast diseases and breast cancer. The text is readable and remarkably modern in its presentation of all aspects of breast disease. It is particularly useful for summaries of current treatment of breast malignancy.*

Kopans, D. B.: Breast Imaging. Philadelphia, J. B. Lippincott Company, 1989.
> *The author of this well-written and well-illustrated book is a recognized authority on all aspects of breast radiography. Dr. Kopans is a radiologist dedicated to breast diseases and his perspective includes an appreciation of clinical practice and of basic biology. The modern breast surgeon must be well acquainted with mammography and capable of interpreting breast radiographs with a high degree of confidence. This text is particularly oriented to the radiologist or surgical specialist in breast diseases.*

Lippman, M. E., Lichter, A. S., and Danforth, D. N., Jr.: Diagnosis and Management of Breast Cancer. Philadelphia, W. B. Saunders Company, 1988.
> *This modern textbook covers all aspects of breast malignancy. The sections dealing with chemotherapy, hormone receptors, and endocrine therapy, and the references to the basic science contributions of the senior editor, Dr. Lippman, make this a particularly up-to-date reference for the clinician dealing with breast cancer.*

Page, D. L., and Anderson, T. J.: Diagnostic Histopathology of the Breast. Edinburgh, Churchill Livingstone, 1987.
> *For those practitioners with a specialized interest in breast cancer, this book is a valuable resource for questions about breast pathology. All the histology is reproduced in black and white with remarkable clarity.*

REFERENCES

1. Abramson, D. J.: A clinical evaluation of aspiration of cysts of the breast. Surg. Gynecol. Obstet., 139:531, 1974.
2. Adair, F. E.: The role of surgery and irradiation in cancer of the breast. J.A.M.A., 121:553, 1943.
3. Anderson, D. E.: A genetic study of human breast cancer. J. Natl. Cancer Inst., 48:1029, 1972.
4. Antman, K. H., Corson, J., Greenberger, J., et al: Multimodality therapy in the management of angiosarcoma of the breast. Cancer, 50:2000, 1982.
5. Antman, K., and Gale, R. P.: Advanced breast cancer: High-dose chemotherapy and bone marrow autotransplant. Ann. Intern. Med., 108:570, 1988.
6. Ashikari, R., Hajdu, S. I., and Robbins, G. F.: Intraductal carcinoma of the breast (1960–1969). Cancer, 28:1182, 1971.
7. Auchincloss, H.: Significance of location and number of axillary metastases in carcinoma of the breast: A justification for a conservative operation. Ann. Surg., 158:37, 1963.
8. Auchincloss, H.: Modified radical mastectomy: Why not? Am. J. Surg., 119:506, 1970.
9. Azzopardi, J. G., Chepick, O. F., Hartmann, W. H., et al.: The World Health Organization Histological Typing of Breast Tumors–Second Edition. Am. J. Clin. Pathol., 78:806, 1982.
10. Baclesse, F.: Five year results in 431 breast cancers treated solely by roentgen therapy. Ann. Surg., 161:103, 1965.
11. Bagley, C. S., Wesley, M. N., Young, R. C., et al.: Adjuvant chemotherapy in males with cancer of the breast. Am. J. Clin. Oncol., 10:55, 1987.
12. Beatson, G. T.: On the treatment of inoperable cases of carcinoma of the mamma: Suggestions for a new method of treatment, with illustrative cases. Lancet, 2:104, 162, 1896.
13. Betsill, W. L., Jr., Rosen, P. P., Lieberman, P. H., et al.: Intraductal carcinoma. Long-term follow-up after treatment by biopsy alone. J.A.M.A., 239:1863, 1978.
14. Bloom, H. J. G.: The natural history of untreated breast cancer. Ann. N.Y. Acad. Sci., 114:747, 1964.
15. Bodian, C., and Haagensen, C. D.: Bilateral carcinoma of the breast. In Haagensen, C. D.: Diseases of the Breast. Philadelphia, W. B. Saunders Company, 1986, pp. 440–461.
16. Bodian, C., and Haagensen, C. D.: Family history of breast carcinoma predisposing to the disease. In Haagensen, C. D.: Diseases of the Breast, 3rd ed. Philadelphia, 1986, pp. 408–423.
17. Bonadonna, G., Brusamolino, E., Valagussa, P., et al.: Combination chemotherapy as an adjuvant treatment in operable breast cancer. N. Engl. J. Med., 294:405, 1976.
18. Bonadonna, G., and Valagussa, P.: Dose-response effect of adjuvant chemotherapy in breast cancer. N. Engl. J. Med., 304:10, 1981.
19. Bonadonna, G., Valagussa, P., Rossi, A., et al.: Ten-year experience with CMF-based adjuvant chemotherapy in resectable breast cancer. Breast Cancer Res. Treat., 5:95, 1985.
20. Bonadonna, G., Valagussa, P., Tancini, G., et al.: Current status of Milan adjuvant chemotherapy trials for node-positive and node-negative breast cancer. NCI Monogr., 1:45, 1986.
21. Bonadonna, G., Valagussa, P., Zambetti, M., et al.: Milan adjuvant trials for stage I-II breast cancer. In Jones, S. E., and Salmon, S. E. (Eds.): Adjuvant Therapy of Cancer V. Orlando, Fla., Grune and Stratton Company, 1987, pp. 211–221.
22. Breast Cancer Trials Committee, Scottish Cancer Trials Office (MRC), Edinburgh.: Adjuvant tamoxifen in the management of operable breast cancer: The Scottish trial. Lancet, 2:1–5, 1987.
23. Brown, P. W., Silverman, J., Owens, E., et al.: Intraductal "noninfiltrating" carcinoma of the breast. Arch. Surg., 111:1063, 1976.
24. Buchanan, R. B., Williams, C. J., Hall, V., et al.: Tamoxifen versus surgical oophorectomy in premenopausal women with advanced breast cancer. Proc. Am. Soc. Clin. Oncol., 4:59, 1985.
25. Burton, G. V., Cox, E. B., Leight, G. S., Jr., et al.: Inflammatory breast carcinoma: Effective multimodal approach. Arch. Surg., 122:1329, 1987.
26. Burton, G. V., Hart, L. L., Leight, G. S., et al.: Cystosarcoma phyllodes: Effective therapy with cisplatin and etoposide chemotherapy. Cancer, 63:2088, 1989.
27. Calle, R., Pilleron, J. P., Schlienger, P., et al.: Conservative management of operable breast cancer: Ten years' experience at the Foundation Curie. Cancer, 42:2045, 1978.
28. Carter, D., and Smith, R. R. L.: Carcinoma in situ of the breast. Cancer, 40:1189, 1977.
29. Chaudary, M. A., Millis, R. R., Davies, G. C., et al.: Nipple discharge. The diagnostic value of testing for occult blood. Ann. Surg., 196:651, 1982.
30. Chen, K. T. K., Kirkegaard, D. D., and Bocian, J. J.: Angiosarcoma of the breast. Cancer, 46:368, 1980.
31. Clark, G. M., Dressler, L. G., Owens, M. A., et al.: Prediction of relapse or survival in patients with node-negative breast cancer by DNA flow cytometry. N. Engl. J. Med., 320:627, 1989.
32. Clark, G. M., McGuire, W. L., Hubay, C. A., et al.: Progesterone receptors as a prognostic factor in stage II breast cancer. N. Engl. J. Med., 309:1343, 1983.
33. Clark, R. M.: Alternatives to mastectomy—The Princess Margaret Hospital experience. In Harris, J. R., Hellman, S., and Silen, W. (Eds.): Conservative Management of Breast Cancer: New Surgical and Radiotherapeutic Techniques. Philadelphia, J. B. Lippincott Company, 1983.
34. Clayton, F.: Pure mucinous carcinomas of breast: Morphologic features and prognostic correlates. Hum. Pathol., 17:34, 1986.
35. Clinical Alert from the National Cancer Institute. May 18, 1988.
36. Cody, H. S., III, Egeli, P. A., and Urban, J. A.: Rotter's node metastases. Therapeutic and prognostic considerations in early breast carcinoma. Ann. Surg., 199:266, 1984.
37. Coleman, S., Silberstine, G. B., and Daniel, C. W.: Ductal morphogenesis in the mouse mammary gland: Evidence supporting a role for epidermal growth factor. Dev. Biol., 127:304, 1988.
38. Collette, H. J. A., Day, N. E., Rombach, J. J., et al.: Evaluation of screening for breast cancer in a non-randomized study (the DOM project) by means of a case-control study. Lancet, 1:1224, 1984.
39. Contesso, G., Mouriesse, S., Friedman, S., et al.: The importance of histologic grade in long-term prognosis of breast cancer: A study of 1,010 patients, uniformly treated at the Institut Gustave-Roussy. J. Clin. Oncol., 5:1378, 1987.
40. Cope, O., Wang, C. A., Chu, A., et al.: Limited surgical excision as the basis of a comprehensive therapy for cancer of the breast. Am. J. Surg., 131:400, 1976.
41. Crile, G., Jr., Cooperman, A., Esselstyn, C. B., Jr., et al.: Results of partial mastectomy in 3 patients followed for five to ten years. Surg. Gynecol. Obstet., 150:563, 1980.
42. Cummings, F. J., Gray, R., Davis, T. E., et al.: Adjuvant tamoxifen treatment of elderly women with stage II breast cancer: A double-blind comparison with placebo. Ann. Intern. Med., 103:324, 1985.
43. Dales, L. G., Friedman, G. D., and Collen, M. F.: Evaluating periodic multiphasic health check-ups: A controlled trial. J. Chron. Dis., 32:385, 1979.
44. Danforth, D. N., Jr., Findlay, P. A., McDonald, H. D., et al.: Complete axillary lymph node dissection for stage I-II carcinoma of the breast. J. Clin. Oncol., 4:655, 1986.

45. Davidson, N. E., and Lippman, M. E.: Treatment of metastatic breast cancer. *In* Lippman, M. E., Lichter, A. S., and Danforth, D. N., Jr. (Eds): Diagnosis and Management of Breast Cancer. Philadelphia, W. B. Saunders Company, 1988.

46. De Lena, M., Viganotti, G., Varini, M., et al.: Multimodality treatment for locally advanced breast cancer. Result of chemotherapy-radiotherapy versus chemotherapy-surgery. Cancer Clin. Trials, 4:229, 1981.

47. De Lena, M., Zucali, R., Viganotti, G., et al.: Combined chemotherapy-radiotherapy approach in locally advanced (T3b-T4) breast cancer. Cancer Chemother. Pharmacol., 1:53, 1978.

48. Devitt, J. E.: Management of nipple discharge by clinical findings. Am. J. Surg., 149:789, 1985.

49. Devitt, J. E.: Benign disorders of the breast in older women. Surg. Gynecol. Obstet., 162:340, 1986.

50. Dixon, J. M., Anderson, T. J., Page, D. L., et al.: Infiltrating lobular carcinoma of the breast: An evaluation of the incidence and consequence of bilateral disease. Br. J. Surg., 70:513, 1983.

51. Dixon, J. M., Lee, D., Page, D. L., et al.: Long-term survivors after breast cancer. Br. J. Surg., 72:445, 1985.

52. Donegan, W. L.: Diagnosis. *In* Donegan, W. L., and Spratt, J. S. (Eds.): Cancer of the Breast, 3rd ed. Philadelphia, W. B. Saunders Company, 1988.

53. Donegan, W. L.: Sarcomas of the breast. *In* Donegan, W. L., and Spratt, J. S. Eds.): Cancer of the Breast, 3rd ed. Philadelphia, W. B. Saunders Company, 1988.

54. Donegan, W. L.: Staging and primary treatment. *In* Donegan, W. L., and Spratt, J. S. (Eds.): Cancer of the Breast. Philadelphia, W. B. Saunders Company, 1988.

55. Donegan, W. L., and Perez-Mesa, C.: Carcinoma of the male breast. Arch. Surg., 106:273, 1973.

56. Donegan, W. L., Sugarbaker, E. D., Handley, R. S., et al.: The management of primary operable breast cancer. A comparison of time-mortality factors after standard, extended, and modified radical mastectomy. Sixth National Cancer Conference Proceedings. Philadelphia, J. B. Lippincott Company, 1970.

57. Donnell, R. M., Rosen, P. P., Lieberman, P. H., et al.: Angiosarcoma and other vascular tumors of the breast. Pathologic analysis as a guide to prognosis. Am. J. Surg. Pathol., 5:629, 1981.

58. Dorr, A., Senior Investigator, Clinical Investigations Branch, Cancer Therapy Education Program, Division of Cancer Treatment, National Institutes of Health, National Cancer Institute, Bethesda, Md. (personal communications).

59. Dupont, W. D., and Page, D. L.: Risk factors for breast cancer in women with proliferative breast disease. N. Engl. J. Med., 312:146, 1985.

60. Durkin, K., and Haagensen, C. D.: An improved technique for the study of lymph nodes in surgical specimens. Ann. Surg., 191:419, 1980.

61. Eddy, D. M., Hasselblad, V., McGivney, W., et al.: The value of mammography screening in women under age 50 years. J.A.M.A., 259:1512, 1988.

62. Editorial.: Cystic disease of the breast. Lancet 2:253, 1985.

63. Findlay, P., Lippman, M., Danforth, D., et al.: A randomized trial comparing mastectomy to radiotherapy in the treatment of stage I-II breast cancer: A preliminary report. Proc. Am. Soc. Clin. Oncol., 4:60, 1985.

64. Fisher, B., Bauer, M., Margolese, R., et al.: Five-year results of a randomized clinical trial comparing total mastectomy and segmental mastectomy with or without radiation in the treatment of breast cancer. N. Engl. J. Med., 312:665, 1985.

65. Fisher, B., Carbone, P., Economou, S. G., et al.: 1-Phenylalanine mustard (L-PAM) in the management of primary breast cancer: A report of early findings. N. Engl. J. Med., 292:1, 1975.

66. Fisher, B., Costantino, J., Redmond, C., et al.: A randomized clinical trial evaluating tamoxifen in the treatment of patients with node-negative breast cancer who have estrogen-receptor-positive tumors. N. Engl. J. Med., 320:479, 1989.

67. Fisher, B., Fisher, E. R., Redmond, C., et al.: Ten-year results from the National Surgical Adjuvant Breast and Bowel Project (NSABP) clinical trial evaluating the use of L-phenylalanine mustard (L-PAM) in the management of primary breast cancer. J. Clin. Oncol., 4:929, 1986.

68. Fisher, B., Montague E., Redmond, C., et al.: Comparison of radical mastectomy with alternative treatments for primary breast cancer. A first report of results from a prospective randomized clinical trial. Cancer, 39:2827, 1977.

69. Fisher, B., Redmond, C., Brown, A., et al.: Adjuvant chemotherapy with and without tamoxifen in the treatment of primary breast cancer: 5-year results from the National Surgical Adjuvant Breast and Bowel Project trial. J. Clin. Oncol., 4:459, 1986.

70. Fisher, B., Redmond, C., Dimitrov, N. V., et al.: A randomized clinical trial evaluating sequential methotrexate and fluorouracil in the treatment of patients with node-negative breast cancer who have estrogen-receptor-negative tumors. N. Engl. J. Med., 320:473, 1989.

71. Fisher, B., Redmond, C., Fisher, E. R., et al.: Ten-year results of a randomized clinical trial comparing radical mastectomy and total mastectomy with or without radiation. N. Engl. J. Med., 312:674, 1985.

72. Fisher, B., Redmond, C., Fisher, E. R., et al.: Systemic adjuvant therapy in treatment of primary operable breast cancer: National Surgical Adjuvant Breast and Bowel Project experience. NCI Monogr., 1:35, 1986.

73. Fisher, B., Redmond, C., Poisson, R., et al.: Eight-year results of a randomized clinical trial comparing total mastectomy and lumpectomy with or without irradiation in the treatment of breast cancer. N. Engl. J. Med., 320:822, 1989.

74. Fisher, B., Redmond, C. K., Wolmark, N., et al.: Long term results from NSABP trials of adjuvant therapy for breast cancer. *In* Jones, S. E., and Salmon, S. E. (Eds.): Adjuvant Therapy of Cancer V. Orlando, Fla., Grune & Stratton Company, 1987, pp. 283–295.

75. Fisher, B., Slack, N., Katrych, D., et al.: Ten year follow-up results of patients with carcinoma of the breast in a co-operative clinical trial evaluating surgical adjuvant chemotherapy. Surg. Gynecol. Obstet. 140:528, 1975.

76. Fisher, B., and Wolmark, N.: Conservative surgery: The American experience. Semin. Oncol., 13:425, 1986.

77. Fisher, B., Wolmark, N., Bauer, M., et al.: The accuracy of clinical nodal staging and of limited axillary dissection as a determinant of histologic nodal status in carcinoma of the breast. Surg. Gynecol. Obstet., 152:765, 1981.

78. Fisher, B., Wolmark, N., Redmond, C., et al.: Findings from NSABP Protocol No. B-04: Comparison of radical mastectomy with alternative treatments. II. The clinical and biologic significance of medial-central breast cancers. Cancer, 48:1863, 1981.

79. Fisher, E. R., and Fisher, B.: Lobular carcinoma of the breast: An overview. Ann. Surg., 185:377, 1977.

80. Fisher, E. R., Gregorio, R., Redmond, C., et al.: Pathologic findings from the National Surgical Adjuvant Breast Project (Protocol No. 4): I. Observations concerning the multicentricity of mammary cancer. Cancer, 35:247, 1975.

81. Fisher, E. R., Sass, R., and Fisher, B.: Pathologic findings from the National Surgical Adjuvant Project for breast cancers (Protocol No. 4). X. Discriminants for tenth year treatment failure. Cancer, 53:712, 1984.

82. Fisher, E. R., Sass, R., Fisher, B., et al.: Pathologic findings from the National Surgical Adjuvant Breast Project (Protocol No. 6). I. Intraductal carcinoma (DCIS). Cancer, 57:197, 1986.

83. Foote, F. W., Jr., and Stewart, F. W.: Lobular carcinoma in situ: Am. J. Pathol., 17:491, 1941.

84. Foote, F. W., Jr., and Stewart, F. W.: A histological classification of carcinoma of the breast. Surgery, 19:74, 1946.

85. Forrest, A. P. M., Stewart, H. J., Roberts, M. M., et al.: Simple mastectomy and axillary node sampling (pectoral node biopsy) in the management of primary breast cancer. Ann. Surg., 196:371, 1982.

86. Fracchia, A. A., Farrow, J. H., Miller, T. R., et al.: Hypophysectomy as compared with adrenalectomy in the treatment of advanced carcinoma of the breast. Surg. Gynecol. Obstet., 140:528, 1975.

87. Frantz, V. K., Pickren, J. W., Melcher, G. W., and Auchincloss H., Jr.: Incidence of chronic cystic disease in so-called "normal breasts." A study based on 225 postmortem examinations. Cancer, 4:762, 1951.

88. Gallager, H. S.: Pathologic types of breast cancer: Their prognoses. Cancer, 53:623, 1984.

89. Ghossein, N. A., Vilcoq J., Stacey, P., et al.: Is it necessary to irradiate the breast after conservative surgery for localized cancer. Arch. Surg., 122:913, 1987.

90. Glascock, R. F., and Hoekstra, W. G.: Accumulation of tritium-labelled hexoestradiol by the reproductive organs of immature female goats and sheep. Biochem. J., 72:673, 1959.

91. Glick, J. H.: Meeting highlights: Adjuvant therapy for breast cancer. J. Natl. Cancer Inst., 80:471, 1988.

92. Goldhirsch, A., and Gelber, R.: Adjuvant treatment for early breast cancer: The Ludwig breast cancer studies. NCI Monogr., 1:55, 1986.

93. Goldhirsch, A., and the Ludwig Breast Cancer Study Group: Prolonged disease-free survival after one course of perioperative adjuvant chemotherapy for node-negative breast cancer. N. Engl. J. Med., 320:491, 1989.

94. Grohn, P., Heinonen, E., Klefstrom, P., et al.: Adjuvant postoperative radiotherapy, chemotherapy, and immunotherapy in stage III breast cancer. Cancer, 54:670, 1984.

95. Gupta, N., Cohen, J. L., and Rosenbaum, C.: Estrogen receptors in male breast cancer. Cancer, 46:81, 1980.

96. Haagensen, C. D.: Mammary-duct ectasia: A disease that may simulate carcinoma. Cancer 4:749, 1951.

97. Haagensen, C. D.: Diseases of the Breast, 3rd ed. Philadelphia, W. B. Saunders Company, 1986, p. 63.

98. Haagensen, C. D.: Diseases of the Breast, 3rd ed. Philadelphia, W. B. Saunders Company, 1986, pp. 259–266.

99. Haagensen, C. D.: Diseases of the Breast, 3rd ed. Philadelphia, W. B. Saunders Company, 1986, pp. 402–407.

100. Haagensen, C. D.: Diseases of the Breast, 3rd ed. Philadelphia, W. B. Saunders Company, 1986, p. 502.

101. Haagensen, C. D.: Diseases of the Breast, 3rd ed. Philadelphia, W. B. Saunders Company, 1986, pp. 503–504.

102. Haagensen, C. D.: Diseases of the Breast, 3rd ed. Philadelphia, W. B. Saunders Company, 1986, pp. 903–932.

103. Haagensen, C. D.: Diseases of the Breast, 3rd ed. Philadelphia, W. B. Saunders Company, 1986, pp. 939–941.

104. Haagensen, C. D.: Diseases of the Breast, 3rd ed. Philadelphia, W. B. Saunders Company, 1986, Chapter 2.

105. Haagensen, C. D.: Diseases of the Breast, 3rd ed. Philadelphia, W. B. Saunders Company, 1986, Chapter 13.

106. Haagensen, C. D.: Diseases of the Breast, 3rd ed. Philadelphia, W. B. Saunders Company, 1986, Chapter 16.

107. Haagensen, C. D.: Diseases of the Breast, 3rd ed. Philadelphia, W. B. Saunders Company, 1986, Chapter 21.

108. Haagensen, C. D.: Diseases of the Breast, 3rd ed. Philadelphia, W. B. Saunders Company, 1986, Chapter 44.

109. Haagensen, C. D.: Diseases of the Breast, 3rd ed. Philadelphia, W. B. Saunders Company, 1986, Chapter 48.

110. Haagensen, C. D.: Diseases of the Breast, 3rd ed. Philadelphia, W. B. Saunders Company, 1986, Chapter 64.

111. Haagensen, C. D., and Bodian, C.: A personal experience with Halsted's radical mastectomy. Ann. Surg., 199:143, 1984.

112. Haagensen, C. D., Lane, N., Lattes, R., et al.: Lobular neoplasia (so-called lobular carcinoma in situ) of the breast. Cancer, 42:737, 1978.

113. Halsted, W. S.: The results of operations for the cure of cancer of the breast performed at the Johns Hopkins Hospital from June, 1889 to January, 1894. Johns Hopkins Hosp. Bull., 4:297, 1894–1895.

114. Hankey, B. F., Curtis, R. E., Naughton, M. D., et al.: A retrospective cohort analysis of second breast cancer risk for primary breast cancer patients with an assessment of the effect of radiation therapy. J. Natl. Cancer Inst., 70:797, 1983.

115. Harris, J. R., and Hellman, S.: The results of primary radiation therapy for early breast cancer at the joint center for radiation therapy. In Harris, J. R., Hellman, S., and Silen, W. (Eds.): Conservative Management of Breast Cancer: New Surgical and Radiotherapeutic Techniques. Philadelphia, J. B. Lippincott Company, 1983, pp. 47–52.

116. Harris, J. R., Schnitt, S. J., Connolly, J. L., et al.: Conservative surgery and radiation therapy for early breast cancer (editorial). Arch. Surg., 122:754, 1987.

117. Hayward, J. L.: The Guy's Hospital trials on breast conservation. In Harris, J. R., Hellman, S., and Silen, W. (Eds.): Conservative Management of Breast Cancer: New Surgical and Radiotherapeutic Techniques. Philadelphia, J. B. Lippincott Company, 1983, pp. 77–90.

118. Hedley, D. W., Rugg, C. A., and Gelber, R. D.: Association of DNA index and S-phase fraction with prognosis of node positive early breast cancer. Cancer Res., 47:4729, 1987.

119. Heller, K. S., Rosen, P. P., and Schottenfeld, D.: Male breast cancer: A clinicopathologic study of 97 cases. Ann. Surg., 188:60, 1978.

120. Helman, P., Bennett, M. B., Louw, J. H., et al.: Interim report on trial of treatment for operable breast cancer. S. Afr. Med. J., 46:1374, 1972.

121. Henderson, I. C.: Endocrine therapy in metastatic breast cancer. In Harris, J. R., Hellman, S., Henderson, I. C., and Kinne, D. W. (Eds.): Breast Diseases. Philadelphia, J. B. Lippincott Company, 1987, pp. 398–424.

122. Henderson, I. C.: Chemotherapy for advanced disease. In Harris, J. R., Hellman, S., Henderson, I. C., and Kinne, D. W. (Eds): Breast Diseases. Philadelphia, J. B. Lippincott Company, 1988.

123. Henderson, I. C.: Adjuvant systemic therapy for early breast cancer. Curr. Probl. Cancer, 11:125, 1987.

124. Henderson, I. C., and the Early Breast Cancer Trialists' Collaborative Group: Effects of adjuvant tamoxifen and of cytotoxic therapy on mortality in early breast cancer. N. Engl. J. Med., 319:1681, 1988.

125. Hislop, T. G., Elwood, J. M., Coleman, A. J., et al.: Second primary cancers of the breast: Incidence and risk factors. Br. J. Cancer, 49:79, 1984.

126. Horm, J. W., Asire, A. J., Young, J. L., et al. (Eds.): Cancer Incidence and Mortality in the United States, 1973–81 (SEER Program). Biometry Branch, Division of Cancer Prevention and Control, National Cancer Institute, NIH Publication No. 85-1837, Bethesda, Md., 1984.

127. Huggins, C., and Bergenstal, D. M.: Inhibition of human mammary and prostatic cancer by adrenalectomy. Cancer Res., 43:413, 1952.

128. Ingle, J. N., Krook, J. E., Green, S. J., et al.: Randomized trial of bilateral oophorectomy versus tamoxifen in premenopausal women with metastatic breast cancer. J. Clin. Oncol., 4:8, 1986.

129. Jensen, E. V., and DeSombre, E. R.: Mechanism of action of the female sex hormones (review). Annu. Rev. Biochem., 41:203, 1972.

130. Jordan, V. C.: Laboratory models of breast cancer to aid the elucidation of anti-estrogen action. J. Lab. Clin. Med., 109:267, 1987.

131. Kelsey, J. L.: A review of the epidemiology of human breast cancer. Epidemiol. Rev., 1:74, 1979.

132. Keynes, G: Radium treatment of primary carcinoma of the breast. Lancet, 2:108, 1928.

133. Kopans, D. B.: Breast Imaging. Philadelphia, J. B. Lippincott Company, 1989.

134. Kopans, D. B., Lindfors, K., McCarty, K. A., et al.: Spring hookwire breast lesion localizer: Use with rigid compression mammographic systems. Radiology, 157:537, 1985.

135. Kopans, D. B., Meyer, J. E., and Sadowsky, N.: Breast imaging. N. Engl. J. Med., 310:960, 1984.

136. Kramer, W. M., and Rush, B. F., Jr.: Mammary duct proliferation in the elderly. A histopathologic study. Cancer, 31:130, 1973.

137. Lacour, J., Le, M. G., Hill, C., et al.: Is it useful to remove internal mammary nodes in operable breast cancer? Eur. J. Surg. Oncol., 13:309, 1987.

138. Lagios, M. D., Richards, V. E., Rose, M. R., et al.: Segmental mastectomy without radiotherapy: Short-term follow-up. Cancer, 52:23, 1983.

139. Lagios, M. D., Westdahl, P. R., Margolin, F. R., et al.: Duct carcinoma in situ. Relationship of extent of noninvasive disease to the frequency of occult invasion, multicentricity, lymph node metastases, and short-term treatment failures. Cancer, 50:1309, 1982.

140. Leis, H. P., Jr., Greene, F. L., Cammarata, A., et al.: Nipple discharge: Surgical significance. South. Med. J., 81:20, 1988.

141. Levinson, W., and Dunn, P. M.: Nonassociation of caffeine and fibrocystic breast disease. Arch. Intern. Med., 146:1773, 1986.

142. Lichter, A. S., and Lippman, M. E.: Special situations in the treatment of breast cancer. In Lippman, M. E., Lichter, A. S., and Danforth, D. N. (Eds.): Diagnosis and Management of Breast Cancer. Philadelphia, W. B. Saunders Company, 1988.

143. Loprinzi, C. L., Carbone, P. P., Tormey, D. C., et al.: Aggressive combined modality therapy for advanced local-regional breast carcinoma. J. Clin. Oncol., 2:157, 1984.

144. Love, S. M., Gelman, R. S., and Silen, W.: Fibrocystic "disease" of the breast —A nondisease? N. Engl. J. Med., 307:1010, 1982.

145. Love, S. M., Schnitt, S. J., Connolly, J. L., and Shirley, R. L.: Benign breast disorders. In Harris, J. R., Hellman, S., Henderson, I. C., and Kinne, D. W. (Eds): Breast Diseases. Philadelphia, J. B. Lippincott Company, 1987.

146. Lynch, H. T.: Genetics and Breast Cancer. New York, Van Nostrand Reinhold Company, 1981.

147. Maddox, W. A., Carpenter, J. T., Laws, H. L., et al.: A randomized prospective trial of radical (Halsted) mastectomy versus modified radical mastectomy in 311 breast cancer patients. Ann. Surg., 198:207, 1983.

148. Maddox, W. A., Carpenter, J. T., Laws, H. L., et al.: Does radical mastectomy still have a place in the treatment of primary operable breast cancer? Arch. Surg., 122:1320, 1987.

149. Mansour, E. G., Gray, R., Shatila, A. H., et al.: Efficacy of adjuvant chemotherapy in high-risk node-negative breast cancer. An intergroup study. N. Engl. J. Med., 320:485, 1989.

150. Martinez, V., and Azzopardi, J. G.: Invasive lobular carcinoma of the breast: Incidence and variants. Histopathology, 3:467, 1979.

151. McDivitt, R. W., Stewart, F. W., and Berg, J. W.: Tumors of the breast. Atlas of Tumor Pathology, second series, fascicle 2. Washington, D. C., Armed Forces Institute of Pathology, 1968.

152. McGuire, W. L.: Adjuvant therapy of node-negative breast cancer (editorial). N. Engl. J. Med., 320:525, 1989.

153. McGuire, W. L., Carbone, P. O., and Vollmer, E. P. (Eds): Estrogen Receptors in Human Breast Cancer. New York, Raven Press, 1975.

154. Meyer, J. S., Friedman, E., McCrate, M. M., et al.: Prediction of early course of breast carcinoma by thymidine labeling. Cancer, 51:1879, 1983.

155. Meyer, W.: An improved method of the radical operation for carcinoma of the breast. Med. Rec., 46:746, 1894.

156. Milgrom, E., Atger, M., Perrot, M., et al.: Progesterone in uterus and plasma: Uterine progesterone receptors during the estrous cycle and implantation in the guinea pig. Endocrinology, 90:104, 1972.

157. Miller, A. B.: Breast cancer epidemiology, etiology, and prevention. In Harris, J. R., Hellman, S., Henderson, I. C., and Kinne, D. W. (Eds.): Breast Diseases. Philadelphia, J. B. Lippincott Company, 1987, pp. 87–121.

158. Montague, E. D., Romsdahl, M. M., Schell, S. R., et al.: Conservation surgery and irradiation in clinically favorable breast cancer—the M. D. Anderson experience. In Harris, J. R., Hellman, S., and Silen, W. (Eds.): Conservative Management of Breast Cancer: New Surgical and Radiotherapeutic Techniques. Philadelphia, J. B. Lippincott Company, 1983, pp. 53–60.

159. Montgomery, A. C. V., Greening, W. P., and Levene, A. L.: Clinical study of recurrence rate and survival time of patients with carcinoma of the breast treated by biopsy excision without any other therapy. J. Roy. Soc. Med., 71:339, 1978.

160. Moon, T. E., Jones, S. E., Tong, T., et al.: Development of a natural history data base of breast cancer studies. In Jones, S. E., and Salmon, S. E. (Eds.): Adjuvant Therapy of Cancer IV. Orlando, Fla., Grune & Stratton, 1984.

161. Moosman, D. A.: Anatomy of the pectoral nerves and their preservation in modified mastectomy. Am. J. Surg., 139:883, 1980.

162. Morrison, J. M., Howell, A., Grieve, R. J., et al.: The West Midlands Oncology Association trials of adjuvant chemotherapy for operable breast cancer. In Salmon, S. E. (Ed.): Adjuvant Therapy of Cancer V. Orlando, Fla., Grune & Stratton, 1987.

163. Morrow, M., and Foster, R. S., Jr.: Staging of breast cancer. A new rationale for internal mammary node biopsy. Arch. Surg., 11:748, 1981.

164. Moskowitz, M.: The predictive value of certain mammographic signs in screening for breast cancer. Cancer, 51:1007, 1983.

165. Moskowitz, M.: Breast Imaging. In Donegan, W. L., and Spratt, J. S. (Eds.): Cancer of the Breast, 3rd ed. Philadelphia, W. B. Saunders Company, 1988.

166. Mustakallio, S.: Conservative treatment of breast carcinoma: Review of 25 years follow-up. Clin. Radiol., 23:110, 1972.

167. National Institutes of Health Consensus Conference: Adjuvant therapy for breast cancer. J.A.M.A., 254:3461, 1985.

168. National Institutes of Health Consensus Development Panel on Adjuvant Chemotherapy and Endocrine Therapy for Breast Cancer: Introduction and conclusions. NCI Monogr., 1:1, 1986.

169. Nemoto, T., Vana, J., Bedwani, R. N., et al.: Management and survival of female breast cancer: Results of a national survey by the American College of Surgeons. Cancer, 45:2917, 1980.

170. Nolvadex Adjuvant Trial Organization: Controlled trial of tamoxifen as single adjuvant agent in management of early breast cancer. Lancet, 1:836, 1985.

171. Osborne, C. K.: Receptors. In Harris, J. R., Hellman, S., Henderson, I. C., and Kinne, D. W. (Eds.): Breast Diseases. Philadelphia, J. B. Lippincott Company, 1987.

172. Ottman, R., Pike, M. C., King, M. C., et al.: Practical guide for estimating risk for familial breast cancer. Lancet, 2:556, 1983.

173. Page, D. L., Anderson, T. J. (Eds.): Diagnostic Histopathology of the Breast. Edinburgh, Churchill Livingstone, 1987, pp. 11–29.

174. Page, D. L., and Anderson, T. J. (Eds.): Diagnostic Histopathology of the Breast. Edinburgh, Churchill Livingstone, 1987.

175. Page, D. L., and Anderson, T. J.,: Papilloma and related lesions. In Page, D. L., and Anderson, T. J. (Eds.): Diagnostic Histopathology of the Breast. Edinburgh, Churchill Livingstone, 1987.

176. Page, D. L., Anderson, T. J., and Johnson, R. J.: Sarcomas of the breast. In Page, D. L., and Anderson, T. J. (Eds.): Diagnostic Histopathology of the Breast. Edinburgh, Churchill Livingstone, 1987.

177. Page, D. L., Anderson, T. J., and Rogers, L. W.: Carcinoma in situ (CIS). In Page, D. L., and Anderson, T. J. (Eds.): Diagnostic Histopathology of the Breast. Edinburgh, Churchill Livingstone, 1987.

178. Page, D. L., Anderson, T. J., and Sakamoto, G.: Infiltrating carcinoma: Major histological types. In Page, D. L. and Anderson, T. J. (Eds.): Diagnostic Histopathology of the Breast. Edinburgh, Churchill Livingstone, 1987.

179. Page, D. L., Dupont, W. D., Rogers, L. W., et al.: Intraductal carcinoma of the breast: Follow-up after biopsy only. Cancer, 49:751, 1982.

180. Page, D. L., Vander Zwaag, R., Rogers, L. W., et al.: Relation between component parts of fibrocystic disease complex and breast cancer. J. Natl. Cancer Inst., 61:1055, 1978.

181. Page, H. S., and Asire, A. J.: Cancer rates and risks. Washington, D.C., U.S. Department of Health and Human Services, NIH Publication No. 85-691, April, 1985.

182. Palli, D., Del Turco, M. R., Buiotti, E., et al.: A case-control study of the efficacy of a nonrandomized breast cancer screening program in Florence (Italy). Int. J. Cancer, 38:501, 1986.

183. Palshof, T., Mouridsen, H. T., and Daehnfeldt, J. L.: Adjuvant endocrine therapy of breast cancer—a controlled clinical trial of oestrogen and anti-oestrogen: Preliminary results of the Copenhagen breast cancer trials. Recent Results Cancer Res., 71:185, 1980.

184. Patel, J. K., Nemoto, T., and Dao, T. L.: Metastatic breast cancer in males. Assessment of endocrine therapy. Cancer, 53:1344, 1984.

185. Patey, D. H.: A review of 146 cases of carcinoma of the breast operated on between 1930 and 1943. Br. J. Cancer, 21:260, 1967.

186. Patey, D. H., and Nurick, A. W.: Natural history of cystic disease of the breast treated conservatively. Br. Med. J., 1:15, 1953.

187. Peters, G. N., Wolff, M., and Haagensen, C. D.: Tubular carcinoma of the breast. Clinical pathologic correlations based on 100 cases. Ann. Surg., 193:138, 1981.

188. Peters, M. V.: Wedge resection with or without radiation in early breast cancer. J. Radiat. Oncol. Biol. Phys., 2:1151, 1977.

189. Pigott, J., Nichols, R., Maddox, W. A., et al.: Metastasis to the upper levels of the axillary nodes in carcinoma of the breast and its implications for nodal sampling procedures. Surg. Gynecol. Obstet., 158:255, 1984.

190. Pike, A. M., and Oberman, H. A.: Juvenile (cellular) fibroadenoma. A clinicopathologic study. Am. J. Surg. Pathol., 9:730, 1985.

191. Pritchard, K. I.: Current status of adjuvant endocrine therapy for resectable breast cancer. Semin. Oncol., 14:23, 1987.

192. Pritchard, K. I., Meakin, J. W., Boyd, N. F., et al.: Adjuvant tamoxifen in postmenopausal women with axillary node positive breast cancer: An update. In Jones, S. E., and Salmon, S. E. (Eds.): Adjuvant therapy of cancer V. Orlando, Fla., Grune & Stratton, 1987, pp. 391–400.

193. Prosnitz, L. R., Goldenberg, I. S., Packard, R. A., et al.: Radiation therapy as initial treatment for early stage cancer of the breast without mastectomy. Cancer, 39:61, 1977.

194. Prosnitz, L. R., Goldenberg, I. S., Weshler, Z., et al.: Radiotherapy instead of mastectomy for breast cancer—the Yale experience. In Harris, J. R., Hellman, S., and Silen, W. (Eds.): Conservative Management of Breast Cancer: New Surgical and Radiotherapeutic Techniques. Philadelphia, J. B. Lippincott Company, 1983, pp. 61–70.

195. Rao, B. R., and Meyer, J. S.: Estrogen and progestin receptors in normal and cancer tissue. In McGuire, W. L., Raynaud, J. P., and Baulieu, E. E. (Eds.): Progesterone Receptors in Normal and Neoplastic Tissues (Progress in Cancer Research and Therapy, Vol. 4). New York, Raven Press, 1977.

196. Ridolfi, R. L., Rosen, P. P., Port, A., et al.: Medullary carcinoma of the breast. A clinicopathologic study with 10 year follow-up. Cancer, 40:1365, 1977.

197. Robinson, R., and Montague, E. D.: Treatment results in males with breast cancer. Cancer, 49:403, 1982.

198. Rose, C., and Mouridsen, H. T.: Treatment of advanced breast cancer with tamoxifen. Recent Results Cancer Res., 91:230, 1984.

199. Rosemond, G. P., Maier, W. P., and Brobyn, T. J.: Needle aspiration of breast cysts. Surg. Gynecol. Obstet., 128:351, 1969.

200. Rosen, P. P.: The pathology of breast carcinoma. In Harris, J. R., Hellman, S., Henderson, I. C., and Kinne, D. W. (Eds.): Breast Diseases. Philadelphia, J. B. Lippincott Company, 1987.

201. Rosen, P. P., Groshen, S., Saigo, P. E., et al.: A long-term follow-up study of survival in stage I (T1N0M0) and stage II (T1N1M0) breast carcinoma. J. Clin. Oncol., 7:355, 1989.

202. Rosen, P. P., Lieberman, P. H., Braun, D. W., Jr., et al.: Lobular carcinoma in situ of the breast: Detailed analysis of 99 patients with average follow-up of 24 years. Am. J. Surg. Pathol., 2:225, 1978.

203. Rosen, P. P., Senie, R., Schottenfeld, D., et al.: Noninvasive breast carcinoma: Frequency of unsuspected invasion and implications for treatment. Ann. Surg., 189:377, 1979.

204. Rosner, D., Bedwani, R. N., Vana, J., et al.: Noninvasive breast carcinoma: Results of a national survey by the American College of Surgeons. Ann. Surg., 192:139, 1980.

205. Russell, L. C.: Caffeine restriction as initial treatment for breast pain. Nurse Pract., 140:36, 1989.

206. Sainsbury, J. R. C., Farndon, J. R., Needham, G. K., et al.: Epidermal-growth-factor receptor status as predictor of early recurrence of and death from breast cancer. Lancet 1:1398, 1987.

207. Santen, R. J., Worgul, T. J., Samojlik, E., et al.: A randomized trial comparing surgical adrenalectomy with aminoglutethimide plus hydrocortisone in women with advanced breast cancer. N. Engl. J. Med., 305:545, 1981.

208. Sarrazin, D., Le, M., Rouesse, J., et al.: Conservative treatment versus mastectomy in breast cancer tumors with macroscopic diameter of 20 millimeters or less: The experience of the Institut Gustave-Roussy. Cancer, 53:1209, 1984.

209. Scanlon, E. F., and Caprini, J. A.: Modified radical mastectomy. Cancer, 35:710, 1975.

210. Schafer, P., Alberto, P., Forni, M., et al.: Surgery as part of a combined modality approach for inflammatory breast carcinoma. Cancer, 59:1063, 1987.

211. Schnitt, S. J., Silen, W., Sadowsky, N. L., et al.: Ductal carcinoma in situ (intraductal carcinoma) of the breast. N. Engl. J. Med., 318:898, 1988.

212. Schwartz, G. F., Patchefsky, A. S., Feig, S. A., et al.: Clinically occult breast cancer: Multicentricity and implications for treatment. Ann. Surg., 191:8, 1980.

213. Seeger, J., and Allegra, J. C.: Chemotherapy of breast cancer. In Donegan, W. L., and Spratt, J. S. (Eds.): Cancer of the Breast. Philadelphia, W. B. Saunders Company, 1988.

214. Seidman, H., Gelb, S. K., Silverberg, E., et al.: Survival experience in the Breast Cancer Detection Demonstration Project. CA, 37:258, 1987.

215. Seidman, H., Mushinski, M. H., Gelb, S. K., et al.: Probabilities of eventually developing or dying of cancer—United States, 1985. CA, 35:36, 1985.

216. Senn, H-J., and Barret-Mahler, R. (for the OSAKO and SAKK groups): Update of Swiss adjuvant trials with LMF and CMF in operable breast cancer. In Salmon, S. E. (Ed.): Adjuvant Therapy of Cancer V. Orlando, Fla., Grune & Stratton, 1987.

217. Serra, G. E., Maccarone, G. B., Ibarra, P. E., et al.: Lateral pectoralis nerve: The need to preserve it in the modified radical mastectomy. J. Surg. Oncol., 26:278, 1984.

218. Shapiro, S., Venet, W., Strax, P., et al.: Selection, follow-up, and analysis in the health insurance plan study: A randomized trial with breast cancer screening. NCI Monogr., 67:65, 1985.

219. Silverberg, E., and Lubera, J. A.: Cancer statistics, 1988. CA, 38:5, 1988.

220. Silvestrini, R., Daidone, M. G., and Gasparini, G.: Cell kinetics as a prognostic marker in node-negative breast cancer. Cancer, 56:1982, 1985.

221. Skinner, M. A., Swain, M., Simmons, R., et al.: Nonpalpable breast lesions at biopsy: A detailed analysis of radiographic features. Ann. Surg., 208:83, 1988.

222. Slamon, D. J., Godolphin, W., Jones, L. A., et al.: Studies of the HER-2/neu proto-oncogene in human breast and ovarian cancer. Science, 244:707, 1989.

223. Smathers, R. L., Bush, E., Drace, J., et al.: Mammographic microcalcifications: Detection with xerography, screen-film, and digitized film display. Radiology, 159:673, 1986.

224. Solin, L. J., Fowble, B., Martz, K. L., et al.: Definitive irradiation for early stage breast cancer: The University of Pennsylvania experience. Int. J. Radiat. Oncol. Biol. Physics, 14:235, 1988.

225. Sonoda, M., Takano, M., Miyahara, J, et al.: Computed radiography utilizing scanning laser stimulated luminescence. Radiology, 148:833, 1983.

226. Sorace, R. A., Bagley, C. S., Lichter, A. S., et al.: The management of non-metastatic, locally advanced breast cancer using primary induction chemotherapy with hormonal synchronization followed by radiation therapy with or without debulking surgery. World J. Surg., 9:775, 1985.

227. Sorace, R. A., and Lippman, M. E.: Locally advanced breast cancer. In Lippman, M. E., Lichter, A. S., and Danforth, D. N., Jr. (Eds.): Diagnosis and Management of Breast Cancer. Philadelphia, W. B. Saunders Company, 1988.

228. Spitalier, J. M., Gambarelli, J., Brandone, H., et al.: Breast-conserving surgery with radiation therapy for operable mammary carcinoma: A 25-year experience. World J. Surg., 10:1014, 1986.

229. Spratt, J. S., and Spratt, J. A.: Growth rates. In Donegan, W. L., and Spratt, J. S. (Eds.): Cancer of the Breast, 3rd ed. Philadelphia, W. B. Saunders Company, 1988.

230. Stoll, B. A.: Castration and oestrogen therapy. In Stoll, B. A. (Ed.): Endocrine Therapy in Malignant Disease. London, W. B. Saunders Company, 1972, pp. 139–163.

231. Swain, S. M., and Lippman, M. E.: Treatment of patients with inflammatory breast cancer. In DeVita, V. T., Hellman, S., and Rosenberg, S. A. (Eds.): Important Advances in Oncology 1989. Philadelphia, J. B. Lippincott Company, 1989.

232. Tabar, L., Fagerberg, C. J. G., Gad, A., et al.: Reduction in mortality from breast cancer after mass screening with mammography. Randomized trial from the breast cancer screening working group of the Swedish National Board of Health and Welfare. Lancet, 1:829, 1985.

233. Tanaka, Y., and Oota, K.: A stereomicroscopic study of the mastopathid human breast. II: Peripheral type of duct evolution and its relation to cystic disease. Virchows Arch. Pathol. Anat., 349:215, 1970.

234. Taylor, S. G., IV, Kalish, L. A., Olson, J. E., et al.: Adjuvant CMFP versus CMFP plus tamoxifen versus observation alone in postmenopausal, node-positive breast cancer patients: Three-year results of an Eastern Cooperative Oncology Group study. J. Clin. Oncol., 3:144, 1985.

235. Thorpe, S. M., Rose, C., Rasmussen, B. B., et al.: Prognostic value of steroid

hormone receptors: Multivariate analysis of systemically untreated patients with node negative primary breast cancer. Cancer Res., 47:6126, 1987.

236. Tobin, G. R.: Pectoralis major segmental anatomy and segmentally split pectoralis major flaps. Plast. Reconstr. Surg., 75:814, 1985.

237. Toft, D., and Gorski, J.: A receptor molecule for estrogens: Isolation from the rat uterus and preliminary characterization. Proc. Natl. Acad. Sci. USA, 55:1574, 1966.

238. Turner, L., Swindell, R., Bell, W. G. T., et al.: Radical versus modified radical mastectomy for breast cancer. Ann. R. Coll. Surg. Engl., 63:239, 1981.

239. Urban, J. A.: Management of operable breast cancer. Cancer, 42:2066, 1978.

240. Urban, J. A., and Castro, E. B.: Selecting variations in extent of surgical procedures for breast cancer. Cancer, 28:1615, 1971.

241. Valagussa, P., Bonadonna, G., and Veronesi, U.: Patterns of relapse and survival following radical mastectomy: Analysis of 716 consecutive patients. Cancer, 41:10, 1978.

242. Valagussa, P., Tancini, G., and Bonadonna, G.: Second malignancies after CMF for resectable breast cancer. J. Clin. Oncol., 5:1138, 1987.

243. Verbeek, A. L. M., Hendricks, J. H. C. L., Holland, R., et al.: Reduction of breast cancer mortality through mass screening with modern mammography. First results of the Nijmegen Project, 1975–1981. Lancet, 1:1222, 1984.

244. Veronesi, U., Saccozzi, R., Del Vecchio, M.: Comparing radical mastectomy with quadrantectomy, axillary dissection, and radiotherapy in patients with small cancers of the breast. N. Engl. J. Med., 305:6, 1981.

245. Vogel, P. M., Georgiade, H. G., Fetter, B. F., et al.: The correlation of histologic changes in the human breast with the menstrual cycle. Am. J. Pathol., 104:23, 1981.

246. Waterhouse, J., Shamugaratnam, K., Muir, C., et al. (Eds.): Cancer Incidence in Five Continents, Vol. IV. IARC Publications No. 42, Lyon, 1982.

247. Webber, B. L., Heise, H., Neifeld, J. P., et al.: Risk of subsequent contralateral breast carcinoma in a population of patients with in-situ breast carcinoma. Cancer, 47:2928, 1981.

248. Westbrook, K. C., and Gallager, H. S.: Intraductal carcinoma of the breast. A comparative study. Am. J. Surg., 130:667, 1975.

249. Wheeler, J. E., Enterlin, H. T., Roseman, J. M., et al.: Lobular carcinoma in situ of the breast: Long-term follow-up. Cancer, 34:554, 1974.

250. White, E., Daling, J. R., Norsted, T. L., et al.: Rising incidence of breast cancer among young women in Washington state. J. Natl. Cancer Inst., 79:239, 1987.

251. Wilson, R. E., Donegan, W. L., Mettlin, C., et al.: The 1982 national survey of carcinoma of the breast in the United States by the American College of Surgeons. Surg. Gynecol. Obstet., 159:309, 1984.

252. Wilson, R. E., Piro, A. S., Aliapoulos, M. A., et al.: Evaluation of adrenalectomy and hypophysectomy in treatment of metastatic cancer of the breast. Cancer, 24:1322, 1969.

253. Wittliff, J. L.: Specific receptor of the steroid hormones in breast cancer. Semin. Oncol., 1:109, 1974.

254. Wittliff, J. L.: Steroid receptor analyses, quality control, and clinical significance. In Donegan, W. L., and Spratt, J. S. (Eds.): Cancer of the Breast. Philadelphia, W. B. Saunders Company, 1988.

255. World Health Organization: Histological typing of breast tumors. Tumori, 68:181, 1982.

256. Wright, C., Angus, B., Nicholson, S., et al.: Expression of c-erbB-2 oncoprotein: A prognostic indicator in human breast cancer. Cancer Res., 49:2087, 1989.

257. Yap, H. Y., Tashima, C. K., Blumenschein, G. R.: Male breast cancer: A natural history study. Cancer, 44:748, 1979.

22

RECONSTRUCTIVE AND AESTHETIC BREAST SURGERY

Gregory S. Georgiade, M.D.

The introduction of newer improved surgical techniques and the constant improvement in the design and construction of mammary implants have allowed the surgeon to be increasingly innovative. This has produced continued improvement in the aesthetic result and patient satisfaction in breast surgery. Familial, congenital, and developmental breast abnormalities such as hypomastia, hypermastia, breast asymmetry, or breast ptosis all affect the patient's self-image and confidence. Desire for aesthetic surgery for suitable correction is ever present in patients with these deformities. The psychologic impact to the woman who has undergone ablative breast surgery for breast cancer cannot be underestimated. Reconstruction of the breast mound produces positive results in the patient's self-image by the restoration of a more normal body contour.

MAMMARY HYPERPLASIA

Breast hypertrophy in many patients limits physical activity and causes back, neck, and shoulder pain, accompanied by skin excoriations in the inframammary area. A reduction mammaplasty in this group of women can be performed at any age, many times on an outpatient basis or with a short hospitalization.

Reduction in breast volume and correction of the usually accompanying ptosis can be accomplished by a number of techniques. Many of the concepts in the management of the problem are predicated on the use of the nipple-areola and dermal pedicle flap (Fig. 1).[3,4,9,22,24,28,31,32]

The surgical design can be based on the resection of an inferior wedge of triangular breast tissue or the vertical excision of breast tissue.[25] A third concept, often utilized, involves maintenance of a central core of breast tissue with the associated nipple-areola complex and resection of the excess breast tissue in the medial, superior, and lateral positions.[1] The technique for minimizing the inferior areolar vertical scar and the inframammary scar should be incorporated in the reduction technique whenever possible.[21] In the author's experience, the most versatile of the techniques utilizes a pyramidal based breast flap with an inferior dermal nipple-areola pedicle.[9] A large reduction mammaplasty with resection of up to 3000 gm. of tissue from each breast can be achieved with this technique. Smaller breast reductions can also be done with this technique with excellent aesthetic results and improved functional aspects.

Massive breast hypertrophy of over 3000 gm. usually necessitates utilization of a breast amputation technique with immediate free nipple-areola grafting.[29]

HYPOMASTIA

The correction of hypomastia is designed to produce satisfactory volume, contour, and softness of the breast mound.

Prostheses

The prostheses utilized in breast augmentation consist of four basic types, all of which utilize a low-bleed, thin-walled Silastic shell with a composite construction to minimize gel bleed in a smooth, seamless Silastic envelope containing a viscous silicone gel or saline. A polyurethane covering can be incorporated on the outer layer of the Silastic envelope. A microtextured Silastic low-bleed envelope is also available. This new type of microtextured prosthesis appears to have the advantages of the polyurethane covered prosthesis in its ability to disrupt the linear scar formation that occurs around a smooth-walled prosthesis without the disadvantage of disintegration of the polyurethane covering. The use of these newer prostheses appears to produce a lower incidence of capsular contracture than that occurring with the smooth-walled prostheses.[6,16,23] The smooth wall and microtextured prostheses are available in many sizes and shapes designed to produce the desired contour.

The inflatable saline prostheses are available in various shapes and sizes and utilize a thicker Silastic envelope to prevent breakage with leakage of the saline from the prosthesis and the subsequent loss of the augmentation.

Surgical Techniques

Breast augmentation can be performed through a number of differently placed incisions. An inframammary incision approximately 5.5 cm. in length is the most popular surgical approach and perhaps the safest, although a small scar remains in the inframammary crease. Postoperatively, this is usually acceptable. A circumareolar incision or transareolar incision is also used frequently, particularly in patients with a large areola where the incision can be placed easily within the areola.[20] Often the size of the prosthesis used is limited with this approach, the exception being the saline-inflatable prosthesis, which can be inserted in a deflated condition and subsequently expanded by the insertion of saline. The axillary approach described by Hoehler[17] has the advantage of producing a breast augmentation without creating any visible scars on the breast. A 4-cm. incision is made in the anterior axillary line in the shadow of the pectoralis muscle. The dissection is then made either over the pectoral fascial plane or beneath the pectoralis major musculature. The dissection, using a urethral sound, produces a suitable pocket. A round prosthesis is inserted in the pocket so that prosthesis orientation is not necessary. Symmetry and adequate hemostasis are more difficult to achieve with the axillary technique.

Regardless of the surgical approach used for breast augmentation, a decision to place the prosthesis in the subpectoral position versus the submammary position must be weighed carefully, because there are several potential problems. The decision to place the prosthesis subpectorally is usually based on the clinical observation that the patient has a limited amount of breast tissue. In the subpectoral position, the appearance of the

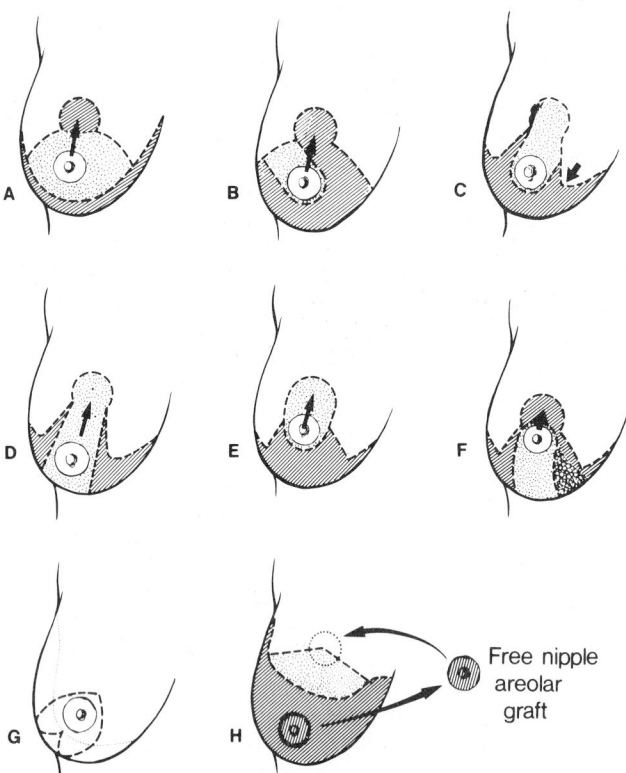

Figure 1. Multiple possible types of dermal flaps supporting the nipple areola. *A,* Horizontal (Strombeck, 1960). *B,* Lateral dermal pedicle (Skoog, 1963). *C,* Superior medial dermal (Orlando, 1975). *D,* Vertical bipedicle dermal (McKissock, 1972). *E,* Superior dermal (Cramer, 1971). *F,* Inferior dermal (Robbins, 1977). *G,* Oblique wedge (Dufourmentel, 1961). *H,* Amputation—dermal with free nipple areola graft (Rubin, 1976).

breast mound may be altered and often distorted by contracture of the pectoralis musculature in such positions as abduction of the arm in lifting weights.[2] Those patients who indulge in varied athletic pursuits should be advised of this possible undesirable effect.

Complications and Untoward Effects

Hematoma occurs infrequently, usually within the first 48 hours, although it can occur as late as 7 days postoperatively. The patient must always be advised to report sudden occurrence of "tightness" developing in the augmented breast postoperatively. Abstinence from aspirin products 10 days prior to operation should be the practice. When a hematoma is recognized, the prosthesis should be removed as soon as possible, and the hematoma should be carefully evacuated. All bleeding points should be identified and coagulated. The prosthesis can then be safely replaced and the operative incision carefully closed in layers. A supportive bulky dressing is then applied, and the patient is examined 24 hours later for further bleeding into the operative areas.

Extrusion of the breast prosthesis is encountered infrequently but can occur when too large a prosthesis has been inserted into too small a pocket, creating excessive tension on the surrounding tissues. Usually this can be remedied by removal of the prosthesis with subsequent creation of a larger pocket or with the insertion of a smaller prosthesis.

Capsular Contracture

The occurrence of a firm breast mound after an augmentation mammaplasty occurs with sufficient frequency (up to 25 per cent) to be of concern to the surgeon. Smooth-walled prostheses have been found to create a linear scar, which is more likely to

contract. Recent investigative and clinical observations have led to the development of polyurethane or microtextured outerwall prosthesis coverings that redirect the scar formation into an irregular contour, thus minimizing the possibility of linear scar contracture.[6,16,23]

Infection

Infection occurs infrequently; however, when it does occur, it should be treated vigorously with appropriate antibiotics determined by sensitivity tests. The prosthesis is usually removed, the infection controlled, and the prosthesis replaced 3 to 6 months later.

Severe capsular contracture can also occur secondary to *Staphylococcus epidermidis,* which causes a low-grade infection with an inflammatory response that produces excessive collagen scar formation. Removal of the prosthesis with resterilization and capsulectomy is necessary. This is followed by irrigation of the operative pocket with bacitracin and povidoneiodine solution, and the prosthesis can subsequently be replaced. The patient is then maintained on appropriate antibiotic therapy for at least 10 days.

BREAST PTOSIS

Ptosis of the breast is an aesthetic problem. The severity of the ptosis is determined by the relationship of the nipple to the inframammary line and listed as Stage A, B, or C ptosis, Stage C being the most severe. Depending on the degree of severity, ptosis can be corrected either by the insertion of a prosthesis alone in the minimally ptotic patient, or, more often, with a severe deformity, the combination of augmentation mammaplasty and elevation of the nipple-areola complex, performed simultaneously.[26] These procedures can usually be done under local anesthesia with intravenous sedation on an outpatient basis.

RECONSTRUCTION OF THE BREAST AFTER MASTECTOMY

Immediate

The feasibility of initiating reconstructive surgery at the time modified radical mastectomy is performed has been generally accepted as an excellent procedure since its introduction approximately 19 years ago.[2,7,11,18] If early reconstruction is considered, the feasibility of the procedure is determined by a team consisting of a surgical oncologist, a plastic surgeon, and a pathologist on the basis of clinical and pathologic evaluation of the size of the primary tumor, the tumor grade, lymph node status, and location. A thorough discussion with the patient as to her desires, expectations, and possible complications should follow. The expected number of operative procedures to fulfill these requirements is also discussed with the patient. The age of the patient is probably of minimal importance, because this procedure can be performed at any age.

When the decision to perform an immediate breast reconstruction has been made, incision planning should be a joint venture of the surgical oncologist and the plastic surgeon. A modified radical mastectomy with an *en bloc* removal of the axillary nodes is performed.

Reconstruction is initiated, using a 6-cm. horizontal slightly curved incision at the level of the sixth rib through the serratus muscle. A pocket is created beneath the serratus and pectoralis major muscles, extending medially to the perforating internal mammary vessels and inferiorly beneath the fascial insertion of the rectus abdominis muscle (Fig. 2). At this point, a determination is made whether to insert a gel-filled prosthesis or a tissue

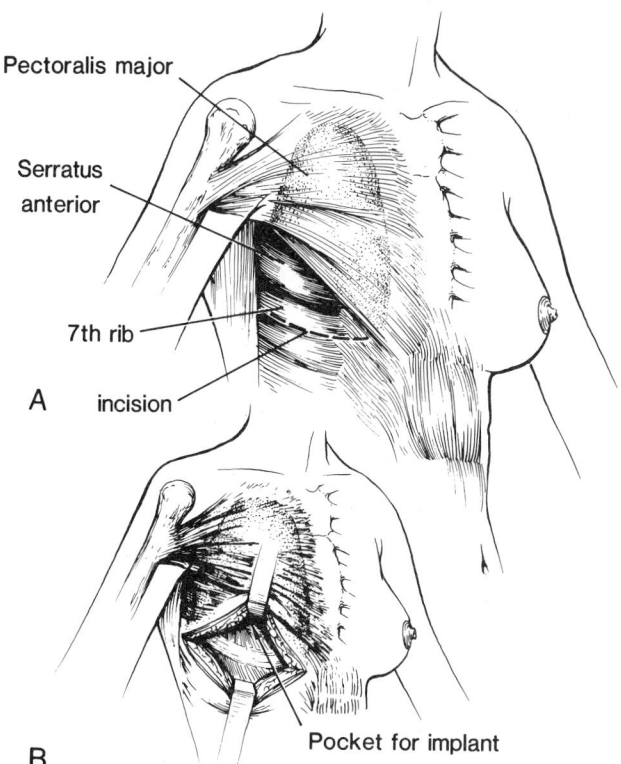

Figure 2. *A,* Location of the incision over the sixth or seventh rib. *B,* Undermining of the serratus anterior and pectoralis major muscles and, beneath, fascial insertion of the rectus abdominis muscle.

expander, to be filled with small increments of saline at a later date. The tightness of the skin closure and the desired eventual size of the mammary mound determines the type of prosthesis utilized. A suction drain is inserted into the subpectoral pocket and also into the axillary dissection area. The serratus muscle is closed with 4-0 nylon sutures, followed by 4-0 Vicryl and Dexon sutures in the dermis. A 4-0 Prolene subcuticular pullout suture is then inserted, followed by Steri-Strips for the skin closure.

If a tissue expander has been inserted, the subsequent expansion of the breast mound can be initiated approximately 3 weeks after the initial operation.[33] Up to 100 ml. of saline can usually be inserted in the prosthesis via the reservoir at one time. This procedure can be repeated at 2-week intervals until an overexpansion of approximately 150 ml. has been accomplished and maintained for 1 month. At this time, the expander can be removed, and the final gel-filled prosthesis can be inserted. The outer covering may be microtextured if desired to minimize the capsular contracture. The final procedure, nipple-areolar reconstruction, on an outpatient basis, involves the utilization of a full-thickness groin (inner thigh) skin graft to reconstruct the areola. Simultaneously, the nipple is reconstructed using either a portion of the opposite nipple as a composite graft or by elevation of a skin fat flap from the breast mound itself with subsequent tattooing of this new nipple at a later date. (Fig. 3).

In the author's experience, over the past 13 years, immediate breast reconstruction has had no adverse effect on the natural course of the patient's breast cancer. Psychologically, patient satisfaction has been extremely good in this series of over 350 patients who have undergone immediate breast reconstruction. Myocutaneous flaps, such as latissimus or rectus abdominis flaps, for immediate breast reconstruction have been used in a few selected patients when extensive skin or muscle resections have been done during ablative surgery. The use of a free microvascular rectus abdominis flap should also be considered when an extensive ablative procedure has been performed.

Delayed Breast Reconstruction

Reconstruction can be initiated postoperatively after the completion of adjuvant chemotherapy or radiation therapy. In this situation, it is not advisable to perform reconstructive surgery until this treatment phase has been completed and an adequate recovery period has been attained.[11]

The most commonly used procedure, when there is sufficient skin and pectoralis muscle present, is insertion of a prosthesis, either gel or expandable, into the subserratus-subpectoral pocket as previously described for immediate breast reconstruction.[2,7,11,33] If either the chest skin or the pectoralis major muscle is of insufficient quantity and quality, tissue must be brought into the area via remote skin and muscle flaps.

A latissimus dorsi musculocutaneous flap transferred on its blood supply via the thoracodorsal artery and vein is used commonly.[2,27] This yields a large composite flap of skin and muscle that is easily transferred from the back to allow the construction of the large breast mound augmented by a gel- or saline-filled prosthesis placed beneath the latissimus dorsi flap at the time of its insertion (Fig. 4). The nipple-areola reconstruction is performed at a later date when the breast mound is of stable size and contour in a manner similar to the reconstruction following immediate breast reconstruction.

Extensive postmastectomy defects necessitate the use of a larger musculocutaneous flap.[5,10,15,30] The use of a contralateral rectus abdominis musculocutaneous flap based on the superior epigastric vessels is the composite flap of choice (Fig. 5). In most situations, enough tissue can be transferred to obviate the necessity for a prosthesis. The use of the "free" rectus abdominis or other myocutaneous flaps have become increasingly popular. The thoracodorsal or anterior serratus vessels can usually be anastomosed to the inferior epigastric vessels of the rectus abdominis flap.[14]

Management of the Opposite Breast in Patients with Unilateral Breast Cancer

A subcutaneous mastectomy was performed on the opposite breast in over 300 patients. In this group, 12 per cent were found

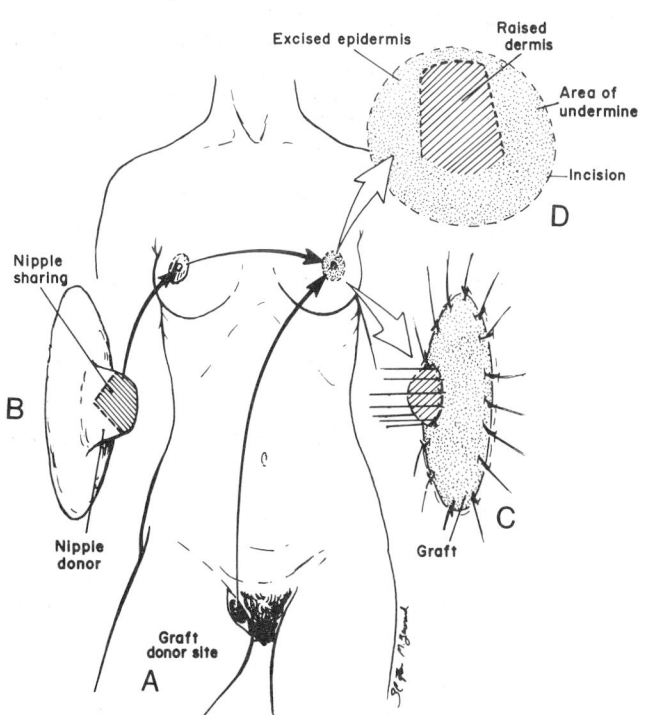

Figure 3. Possible sites and various techniques for constructing the nipple (*B* and *D*) and the areola (*A* and *C*).

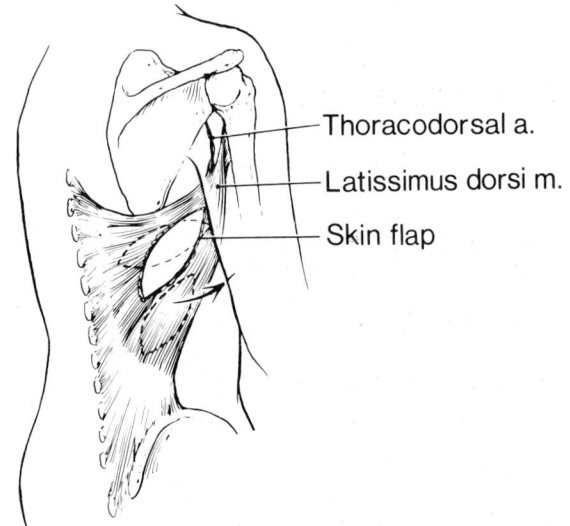

Figure 4. Various locations of the latissimus dorsi myocutaneous flap.

to have occult cancers present in the opposite breast. Another 40 per cent had epithelial hyperplasia of the acinar tissue with 18 per cent incidence of associated atypia. Preliminary studies at Duke University Medical Center with a 12-year follow-up of patients who have undergone subcutaneous mastectomy to the opposite breast appear to indicate a lower mortality in patients who had this prophylactic procedure performed within 3 years of the initial ablative surgery. Subcutaneous mastectomy in high-risk patients should be seriously considered as an optional treatment in situations where there is pathologic evidence of severe epithelial hyperplasia with atypia and a strong familial history of breast cancer.

Approximately 95 per cent of the breast tissue can be excised through an 8-cm. curvilinear submammary incision with subse-

quent preservation of the nipple-areola complex.[12,13,19] Breast mound reconstruction can be accomplished by simultaneously inserting an implant of suitable size in the subpectoral, subserratus position.

SUMMARY

Breast reconstruction initiated at the time of ablative surgery has increased in frequency until it now represents approximately 40 per cent of all breast reconstructions. The majority of patients reconstructed at present probably are best managed initially with the use of a mammary tissue expander, with gradual expansion to a suitable size followed by permanent prosthesis insertion. The opposite breast is treated on an individual basis. As the final step, the nipple-areola complex is constructed. Quite often, tattooing of the new nipple is necessary for appropriate nipple color matching.

SELECTED REFERENCES

Bohmert, H. H., Leis, H. P., and Jackson, I. T.: Breast Cancer: Conservative & Reconstructive Surgery. Stuttgart, New York, Georg Thieme Verlag, 1989.
This excellent textbook presents current information regarding treatment of breast cancer and reconstructive breast surgery by international authorities in the field.

Bostwick, J.: Aesthetic and Reconstructive Breast Surgery. St. Louis, C. V. Mosby Company, 1983.
This is an excellent textbook encompassing various aspects of aesthetic and reconstructive surgery.

Gallager, H. S., Leis, H. P., Jr., Synderman, R. K., and Urban, J. A.: The Breast. St. Louis, C. V. Mosby Company, 1978.
This book presents a comprehensive discussion of mammary cancer and the team approach to breast cancer management.

Georgiade, N. G. (Ed.): Aesthetic Breast Surgery. Baltimore, Williams & Wilkins, 1990.
This well-illustrated book is a compilation of the various current surgical procedures in all aspects of aesthetic breast surgery by the authorities in the field from many countries in the world.

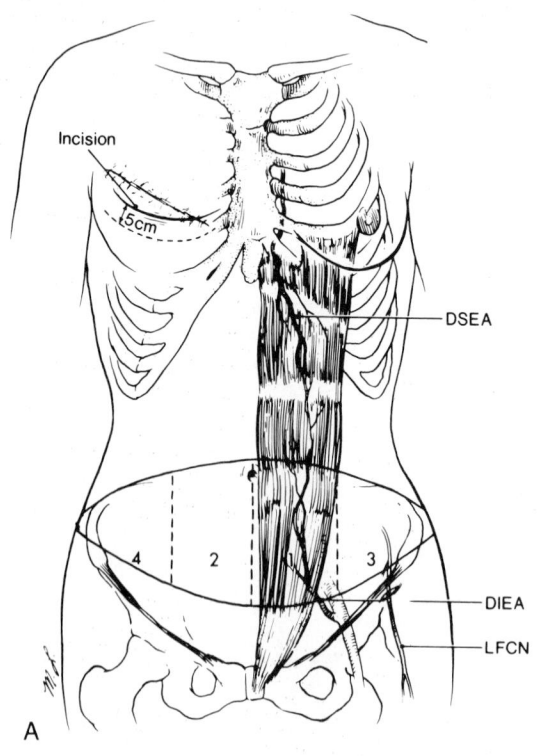

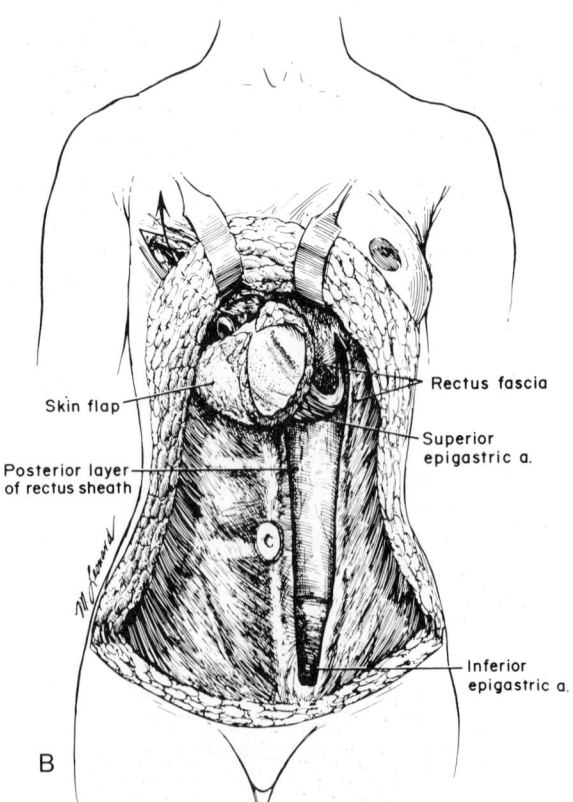

Figure 5. *A,* Location and design of the rectus abdominis myocutaneous flap utilizing the contralateral rectus flap. *B,* Rectus abdominis flap being transferred on the rectus muscle pedicle.

REFERENCES

1. Bolger, W., Seyfer, A., and Jackson, S.: Reduction mammaplasty using the inferior glandular "pyramid" pedicle. Plast. Reconstr. Surg., 80:75, 1987.
2. Bostwick, J.: Aesthetic and Reconstructive Breast Surgery. St. Louis, C. V. Mosby Co., 1983.
3. Cramer, L., and Chong, J.: Unipedicle cutaneous flap: Areola-nipple transposition or an end-bearing, superiorly based flap. In Georgiade, N. G. (Ed.), Reconstructive Breast Surgery, St. Louis, C. V. Mosby Company, 1976, p. 143.
4. Dufourmental, L., and Mouly, R.: Plastie mammairie par la methode oblique. Ann. Chir. Plast. 6:45, 1961.
5. Elliott, F., and Hartrampf, C.: Tailoring of the new breast using the transverse abdominal island flap. Plast. Reconstr. Surg. 72:887, 1983.
6. Ersek, R.: Progress in prostheses for breast augmentation. Travis County Med. Soc. J., 35:8, 1989.
7. Georgiade, G. S., Georgiade, N., McCarty, K., Jr., and Seigler, H.: Rationale for immediate reconstruction of the breast following modified radical mastectomy. Ann. Plast. Surg., 8:210, 1982.
8. Georgiade, G. S., Riefkohl, R., and Georgiade, N. G. To share or not to share. Ann. Plast. Surg., 14:180, 1985.
9. Georgiade, G., Riefkohl, R., and Georgiade, N.: Inferior pyramidal reduction mammaplasty: 10 years experience. Ann. Plast. Surg., 23:40, 1989.
10. Georgiade, G. S., Voci, V., Riefkohl, R., and Scheflan, M.: Potential problems with the transverse rectus abdominis myocutaneous flap in breast reconstruction and how to avoid them. Br. J. Plast. Surg., 37:121, 1984.
11. Georgiade, N. G. (Ed.): Breast Reconstruction Following Mastectomy. St. Louis, C. V. Mosby Company, 1979.
12. Georgiade, N. G., and Hyland, W.: Simultaneous correction for ptosis of the breast, subcutaneous mastectomy and augmentation mammaplasty. Plast. Reconstr. Surg., 56:121, 1975.
13. Georgiade, N., Serafin, D., Georgiade, G., and McCarty, K., Jr.: Subcutaneous mastectomy: An evolution of concept and technique. Ann. Plast. Surg., 8:8, 1982.
14. Grotting, J. C., Urist, M. M., Maddox, W. A., and Vasconez, L. O.: Conventional TRAM flap versus free microsurgical TRAM flap for immediate breast reconstruction. Plast. Reconstr. Surg., 83:828, 1989.
15. Hartrampf, C. R., Scheflan, M., and Black, P. W.: Breast reconstruction with a transverse abdominal island flap. Plast. Reconstr. Surg., 69:216, 1982.
16. Hester, T. R., Nahai, F., Bostwick, J., and Cukie, J.: A 5-year experience with polyurethane-covered mammary prostheses for treatment of capsular contracture, primary augmentation mammaplasty and breast reconstruction. Clin. Plast. Surg., 15:569, 1988.
17. Hoehler, H. Breast augmentation: The axillary approach. Br. J. Plast. Surg., 26:373, 1973.
18. Hueston, J., and McKenzie, G. P.: Breast reconstruction after radical mastectomy. Austr. N.Z. J. Surg., 39:367, 1970.
19. Jarrett, J. R., Cutler, R. G., and Teal, D. F.: Subcutaneous mastectomy in small, large or ptotic breasts with immediate submuscular placement of implants. Plast. Reconstr. Surg., 62:702, 1978.
20. Jones, F. R., and Tauras, A. A. P.: A periareolar incision for augmentation mammaplasty. Plast. Reconstr. Surg., 51:641, 1973.
21. Marchac, D., De Loarte, G.: Reduction mammaplasty and correction of ptosis with a short mammary scar. Plast. Reconstr. Surg., 69:45, 1982.
22. McKissock, P. K.: Reduction mammaplasty with a vertical dermal flap. Plast. Reconstr. Surg., 49:245, 1972.
23. Melmed, E. Polyurethane Implants: A 6-year review of 416 patients. Plast. Reconstr. Surg., 82:285, 1988.
24. Orlando, J., and Guthrie, R.: The superomedial dermal pedicle for nipple transposition. Br. J. Plast. Surg., 28:42, 1975.
25. Pitanguy, I.: Surgical treatment of breast hypertrophy. Br. J. Plast. Surg., 20:78, 1967.
26. Regnault, P.: Breast ptosis: Definition and treatment. Clin. Plast. Surg., 3:193, 1976.
27. Riefkohl, R., and Georgiade, N.: Latissimus dorsi musculocutaneous flap. In Georgiade, N. G. (Ed.): Breast Reconstruction Following Mastectomy. St. Louis, C. V. Mosby Company, 1979, p. 191.
28. Robbins, T.: A reduction mammaplasty with the nipple areola based on an inferior dermal pedicle. Plast. Reconstr. Surg., 55:64, 1977.
29. Rubin, L. R.: The surgical treatment of the massive hypertrophic breast. In Georgiade, N. G. (Ed.): Reconstructive Breast Surgery. St. Louis, C. V. Mosby Company, 1976.
30. Scheflan, M., Dinner, M. I.: The transverse abdominal island flap: indications, contraindications, results and complications. Ann. Plast. Surg., 10:24, 1983.
31. Skoog, T.: A technique of breast reduction: Transposition of the nipple on a cutaneous vascular pedicle. Acta Chir. Scand., 126:453, 1963.
32. Strombeck, J. O.: Mammaplasty: Report of a new technique based on the two pedicle procedure. Br. J. Plast. Surg., 13:79, 1960.
33. Ward, J., Cohen, I., Knaysi, G., and Brown, P.: Immediate breast reconstruction with tissue expanders. Plast. Reconstr. Surg., 80:559, 1987.

23

THE THYROID GLAND

I ———

HISTORICAL ASPECTS AND ANATOMY

H. Kim Lyerly, M.D.

HISTORICAL ASPECTS

Although thyroid surgery is now routinely performed for the treatment of thyroid neoplasm, multinodular goiter, and some forms of hyperthyroidism, it was formerly a perilous undertaking that even the world's greatest surgeons were reluctant to undertake and many in fact condemned. One need look no further than the past century to realize the many advances made toward the safe and effective methods of thyroid extirpation. These advances accurately reflect the development of the entire art and science of surgery. The first thyroidectomy was reportedly performed by a Moorish surgeon in A.D. 952 as described by Mandt:

I think it probable that Abul Casem Khalaf Ebn Abbas, usually named Albucasis, undertook about the year 330 a genuine extirpation of goitre. He lived in Bagdad, was a bold and, one may say, venturesome operator, and could the better hazard the operation because of the following experience: A "homo ignarus" had attempted a similar operation, and the patient having nearly bled to death from an injured artery Albucasis knew very well how to control the haemorrhage by ligature and the hot iron.[7]

Although extirpation of the thyroid gland was occasionally successfully performed, the early surgical literature is filled with reports of intraoperative catastrophe due to hemorrhage, as typified by the following cases reported by Fabric and Gooch, respectively:

In the year 1595 an empiric attempted to remove a goitre in the case of a 10-year-old girl. She died under the operation, and the surgeon was imprisoned.

After several fruitless attempts at ligation of the arteries, the severe hemorrhage was controlled by compression day and night during eight days by persons alternating with each other at the task.[7]

Even the most gifted surgeons of the era could not triumph over the technical obstacles of extirpation of the thyroid. Robert Liston's experience and teaching serve as a good example of the sentiments of the era. Liston, who taught anatomy with Syme, was the first to ligate the superior thyroidal artery and whose operative prowess was described in his obituary in the London Times by "the marvellous dexterity with which he used the surgeon's knife, and upon the profound knowledge of anatomy which enabled him to operate successfully in cases from which other surgeons shrank."[7] He poignantly stated in 1846:

You could not cut the thyroid gland out of the living body in its sound condition without risking the death of the patient from haemorrhage; and when that body has become hypertrophied to an immense extent, and all the veins and arteries are enormously enlarged, you can easily understand what dangers may arise from any attempt of the kind. It is a proceeding by no means to be thought of.[7]

Lister's discovery of antisepsis in 1867 and the development and use of hemostatic forceps in European clinics (*circa* 1870) heralded a new era of thyroid surgery. Into this arena entered the Professor of Surgery in Berne, Theodor Kocher. Switzerland has long been known for its high incidence of goiter, primarily due to iodine deficiency, especially in the mountainous regions. Kocher's first thyroidectomy was performed in 1872, the year following his appointment as professor of surgery at Berne. Within a short time he had done a large number of thyroidectomies for goiter with remarkable results. It is interesting that the operative mortality was originally 13 per cent, but by 1898 Kocher reported a series of 600 patients with only a single death. His near perfect results were achieved by careful attention to control of blood loss and protection of the parathyroid glands. He also emphasized avoidance of injury to the recurrent laryngeal nerves, which could lead to changes in the voice and, in its most severe form, to tracheal obstruction, especially if both recurrent nerves were injured. At the end of his career Kocher had performed more than 5000 thyroidectomies for goiter with the amazingly low mortality of only 1 per cent.

In addition to his contributions as a clinical surgeon, Kocher was also a distinguished physiologist. Quite early in his work on the thyroid he recognized that after thyroidectomy one third of his patients developed signs and symptoms of what was later to be described as thyroid insufficiency. He stated:

. . . the generalized use of surgery for goiter has to do with the physiological importance of the thyroid gland. Unfortunately, the physiologists know almost nothing about it, and this has probably been the main reason why surgeons have simply assumed that the thyroid gland has no function whatever. As soon as it had been learned that from the standpoint of technique total extirpation could be carried out successfully there was no longer reason to hesitate to remove the entire organ when both lobes were diseased.[12]

Nevertheless, Kocher was quick to recognize that problems could arise in patients upon whom he had operated and said in a postoperative follow-up:

Of the 18 patients with total excision who presented themselves for examination, only two show a state of health as good as or better than before the operation. The remaining 16 patients with total excision of the thyroid gland all show more or less severe disturbances in their general condition, the analysis of which has been drawn from precise records in each individual case. The time elapsed since the operation ranged from 3½ months to 9 years and 2 months, and the severity of the symptoms is far graver in the oldest cases. They are obviously progressive. All younger patients who were operated upon more than two years ago show these manifestations to a pronounced degree. As a rule, soon after discharge from the hospital, but in occasional cases not before the lapse of 4 or 5 months, the patients begin to complain of fatigue, and especially of weakness and heaviness in the extremities. The mental alertness decreases. This is particularly striking in children of school age, inasmuch as they drop in class standing, and that the teachers note a progressive diminution of their intellectual capabilities. In the majority of the cases, the swelling is a permanent puffiness of the face. Second only to the clumsiness, it is this which creates the impression among more distant acquaintances that the patient has become an idiot. If we are to give a name to this picture, we cannot fail to recognize its relation to idiocy and cretinism: the stunted growth, the large head, the swollen nose, thick lips, heavy body, the clumsiness of thought and speech, in the presence of well developed musculature undoubtedly point to a related evil. It is interesting that the individuals are not really stupid, which has often been emphasized by their families; they are fully conscious of the retardation of their mental capabilities and especially of the slowness of their comprehension, deliberation, and particularly, of their speech.

With this description Kocher had defined postoperative thyroid hormone insufficiency, or hypothyroidism.

This evolution of thyroid surgery can be no better summarized than by William S. Halsted, the first Professor of Surgery of the Johns Hopkins University School of Medicine, in his masterwork "Operative Story of Goitre," published in 1920.[7] Halsted, who patterned his training program after the great German university medical schools and was a great admirer of the careful surgical technique of Theodor Kocher, described his own method of thyroidectomy and the evolution of thyroidectomy: "In the story of the development of the operation for goitre the essential history of surgery is comprised."

In 1891 Murray, Gley, and Vassale demonstrated improvement in a myxedematous patient after the administration of a sheep thyroid extract. Baumann established the presence of a high iodine content in thyroid tissue in 1896. Oswald prepared iodothyroglobulin in 1904. Then in 1915 Kendall isolated thyroxin, and in 1927 Harrington and Barger synthesized it. Antithyroid medication made possible preoperative control of hyperthyroidism, thus greatly reducing the risks of thyroid operations for hyperthyroidism. With the surgical technique of thyroidectomy established, knowledge of the metabolic function and regulation of the thyroid provided the basis for further effective treatment of its disorders.

ANATOMY

EMBRYOLOGY. The thyroid gland is the first endocrine gland to appear in the fetus. The bulk of the gland develops in approximately the third to the fourth week from the entoderm of the floor of the pharynx, evaginating, then descending to emerge as a bilobed diverticulum connected to the pharynx by a narrow stalk known as the thyroglossal duct (Fig. 1). The thyroglossal duct is usually obliterated when the fetus is 8 weeks old and can be identified in the normal adult at its two ends: at its origin in the tongue, found as the *foramen cecum,* which is located in the midline of the tongue at the junction of its anterior two thirds and posterior one third, and at the thyroid end as a pyramidal lobe of the thyroid, found in 75 per cent of the population.[1] With further descent, the thyroid eventually reaches its definitive location in front of the hyoid bone and the laryngeal cartilages and assumes its fully developed configuration of two lateral lobes joined by a median isthmus. Failure of the embryologic process may cause a variety of midline abnormalities.

The developing thyroid meets and accommodates tissue from the ultimobrachial bodies, which develop from brachial pouches at the 5- to 6-week stage. The final coalescing occurs when the fetus is approximately 9 weeks old, and the ultimo-

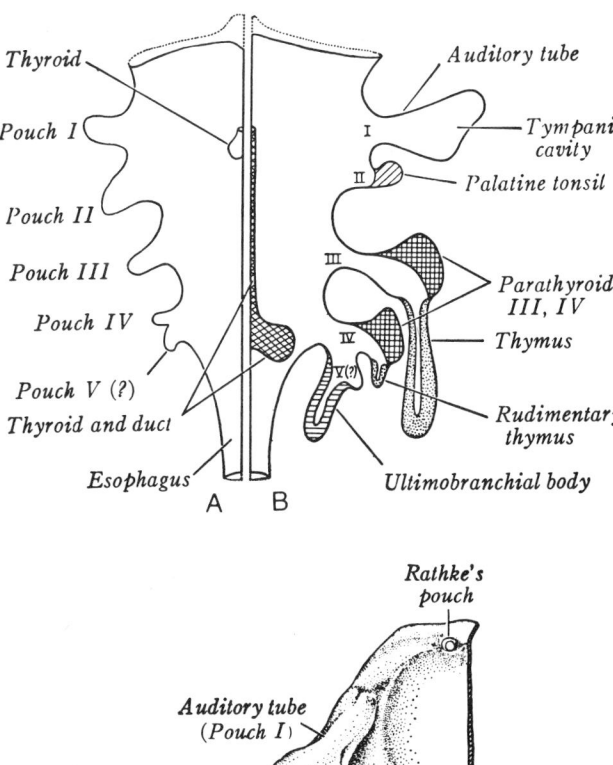

Figure 1. Derivative of the human pharynx. *A,* Right half in ventral outline, showing the entodermal pouches and the thyroid diverticulum in an embryo at 4 weeks. *B,* Left half of the pharynx in a 6-week embryo, illustrating the site of origin of tympanic, tonsillar, and glandular derivatives. *C,* Reconstruction (in dorsal view) of the left half of the pharynx of an embryo at 8 weeks. (From Arey, L. B.: Developmental Anatomy, 7th ed. Philadelphia, W. B. Saunders Company, 1974.)

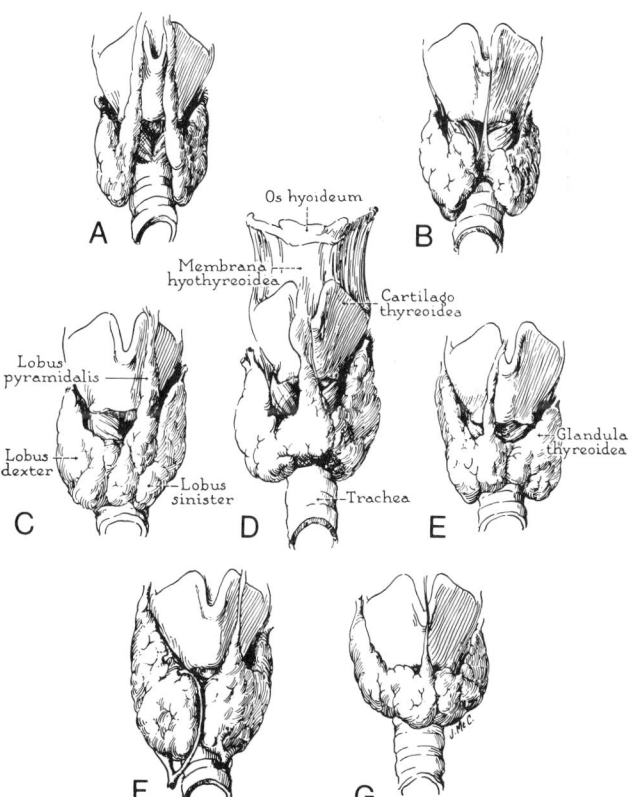

Figure 2. Thyroid gland. Variations in form and size. The gland may be disposed in two separate positions *(A).* The pyramidal lobe may lie in or near the median plane *(B, D,* and *G),* to either the right *(E)* or the left thereof *(C* and *F).* (From McVay, C. B.: Anson and McVay Surgical Anatomy, 6th ed. Philadelphia, W. B. Saunders Company, 1984.)

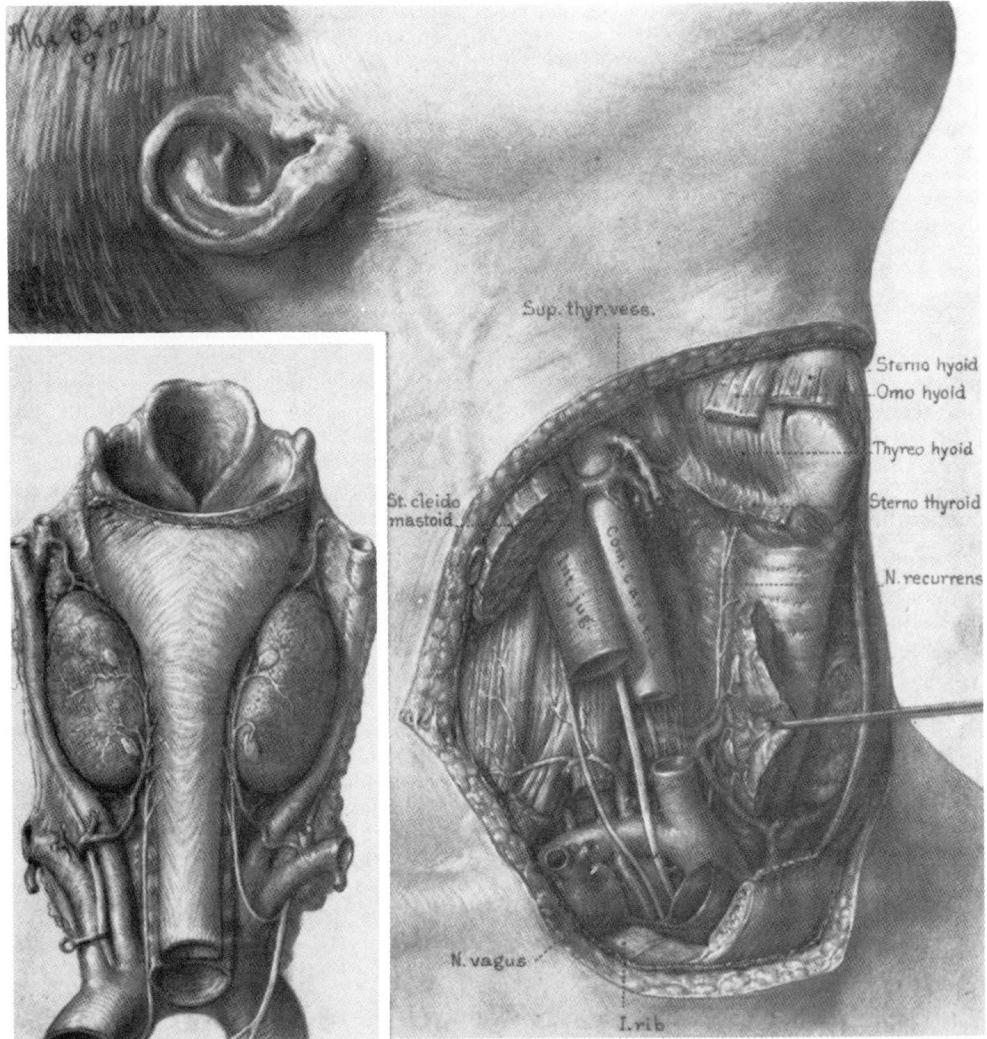

Figure 3. Dissection of the operative field. The right lobe of the thyroid gland has been removed in the typical manner, a slice having been left posteriorly in order to preserve the integrity of the parathyroid bodies and the recurrent laryngeal nerve. This slice is drawn toward the midline with a hook. The inset, slightly elaborated by Brödel, was drawn for the author by H. M. Evans in 1907 from one of many dissections made by the latter for his study of the arterial supply of the parathyroid glands. (Drawings from dissections made by Max Brödel for W. S. Halsted; original art in Brödel Collection. From Art As Applied to Medicine, The Johns Hopkins University School of Medicine.)

brachial cells—C cells, or parafollicular cells—reside within the basement membrane of follicles and form approximately 10 per cent of the adult thyroid.

At 7 to 10 weeks of fetal development, follicles containing colloid become visible, and the gland is able to accumulate iodine and probably begins to release thyroid hormone. From this time also the fetus secretes thyrotropin-stimulating hormone (TSH), to which the developing thyroid is sensitive. Parafollicular cells may be relatively quiescent in the fetus.

GROSS ANATOMY. The thyroid (from the Greek *thyreos,* a shield) in the newborn child weighs approximately 1.5 gm. The normal adult thyroid weighs approximately 15 to 20 gm. and has two lateral lobes, 4 cm. long and 2 cm. wide, found along the lower half of the lateral margins of the thyroid cartilage. The isthmus joins the two lobes, just below the crycoid cartilage, and usually obscures the second, third, and fourth tracheal rings anteriorly. There are many variations in the size, shape, and relative level of the gland (Fig. 2). A pyramidal lobe arises from the isthmus in approximately 75 per cent of patients.

The thyroid is surrounded by a thin fibrous capsule that is reinforced posteriorly to be attached to the trachea and larynx. This dense adherence to the trachea and larynx is responsible for the normal thyroid moving with the larynx during swallowing. The capsule also has septa that penetrate the gland, forming pseudolobules containing a variable number of follicles.

The immediate anterior relations of the gland are the sterno-

thyroid muscles and sternohyoid muscles. The sternothyroids lie on the thyroid capsule, meeting in the midline, and are innervated at their cranial ends by the descendens hypoglossi nerves and at the caudal end by the ansa hypoglossi. More superficial is the investing fascia of the neck, encasing the sternocleidomastoid muscles laterally, with the anterior jugular veins in between.

Laterally and posteriorly the lobes of the thyroid are related to the carotid artery, the internal jugular vein, the cervical sympathetic trunk, and the inferior thyroid artery. Posteriorly and medially are the parathyroid glands and the recurrent laryngeal nerves and the esophagus (Fig. 3).[8] The esophagus lies behind the trachea and larynx, and the recurrent laryngeal nerve ascends in the tracheoesohageal sulcus.[11,16-19,23]

HISTOLOGIC APPEARANCE. The microscopic appearance of the thyroid demonstrates numerous follicles (acini) filled with proteinaceous colloid. The wall of the acinus is composed of a single layer of cuboidal cells resting on a basement membrane richly supplied with capillaries. The acini are arranged in subunits of 20 to 40, demarcated by connective tissue to form lobules, each supplied by an individual artery. The height of the epithelial cells lining the follicles varies with the state of functional activity but normally is about 15 μm. The size of the follicles also varies, but approximates 200 μm. in diameter. In any microscopic section, the follicles vary widely in size as they are cut in different planes.[6,24]

MOLECULAR DETAILS. In the active, cuboidal follicle cell, the most prominent component of the cytoplasm is the rough endoplasmic reticulum (RER). This organelle occupies most of the space in the basal and paranuclear parts of the cell and gives the follicle cell a strong resemblance to exocrine glandular cells. The cisternae of the RER are fairly wide and contain a small granular material of low to moderate density. Most of the protein synthetic capacity of the RER is directed toward thyroglobulin synthesis.

As observed in the electron microscope, the follicular lumen is completely filled with a fine granular substance that appears homogeneous and moderately dense. Analysis of the protein composition of samples obtained by micro-puncture of follicles has demonstrated that practically all of the protein consists of thyroglobulin and larger iodoproteins.

ARTERIAL BLOOD SUPPLY. The blood flow to the thyroid is from 4 to 6 ml. per gm. per minute, or approximately 50 times as much blood per gram as in the body as a whole. The blood supply of the thyroid is primarily through the paired inferior thyroid arteries and the paired superior thyroid arteries. The inferior thyroid arteries, branches of the subclavian artery arising from the thyrocervical trunk, ascend the neck behind the carotid sheath, arch toward the gland, divide into upper and lower branches, and enter the thyroid. At some point in the last part of the course, the inferior thyroid artery is usually related to the recurrent laryngeal nerve. The nerve lies either in front of the artery, among its branches, or behind it. The superior arteries, usually arising as the first branches from the external carotid arteries, are closely related to the superior laryngeal nerves entering the superior poles of the thyroid to divide into anterior and posterior branches.[4,9,15] The thyroidea ima artery, a vestige of the embryonic aortic sac, varies in size from that of a minute vessel to that of the inferior thyroid artery and may originate from the innominate artery, the internal mammary artery, or the aortic arch. It courses upward anterior to the trachea to the inferior border of the thyroid and may be present in up to 12 per cent of the population.

VENOUS DRAINAGE. A venous plexus in the thyroid drains blood via three branches: the superior thyroid veins at the superior poles empty into the internal jugular or common facial veins; the middle thyroid veins, into the internal jugular veins; and the inferior thyroid veins, into the brachiocephalic veins.

LYMPHATIC DRAINAGE. The thyroid has a lymphatic capillary network that drains to lymph nodes on the larynx above the isthmus (Delphian node), the paratrachial nodes near the recurrent laryngeal nerve, and nodes on the anterior surface of the trachea. From these nodes, lymph drains to the cervical lymph chains.

INNERVATION. The thyroid receives sympathetic fibers originating in the cervical ganglia and reaching the gland along with the arteries.[14] There are also parasympathetic fibers, derived from the vagus, that enter the thyroid with branches of the superior laryngeal and recurrent laryngeal nerves. Within the gland, nerve fibers accompany the vessels and terminate close to both vessels and follicle cells. Cytochemical studies have shown that these nerves are both adrenergic and cholinergic.[20] In addition, neuropeptides have been demonstrated in thyroid nerve fibers. The nerves influence blood flow as well as follicle activity.

VARIANT ANATOMY. Complete or almost complete absence of the thyroid is said to occur in 1 of 10,000 live births and causes the infant to become a cretin.

Abnormalities in embryologic development cause a number of midline abnormalities. Proximity to the heart and aorta in the early phase of development explains why the lobules of glandular tissue may remain adherent to the aorta and its branches and why migration of thyroid tissue into the anterior mediastinum is not infrequent. Substernal goiter may develop in this location and often is continuous with the cervical thyroid. The thyroid remains within its capsule, and the arterial supply and

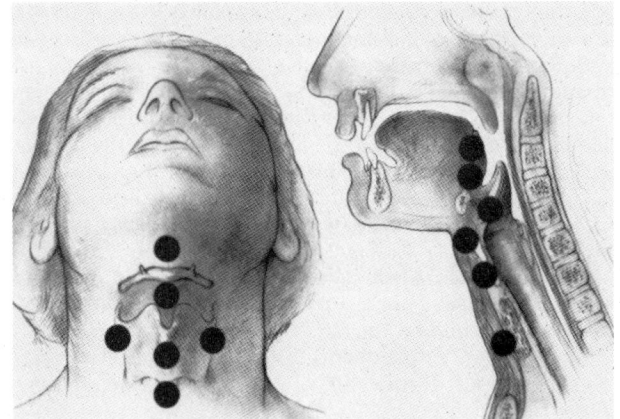

Figure 4. Various locations of cysts of the thyroglossal duct; frontal and lateral views of the neck. The cyst may be located in any of the following situations: below the chin (submental); below the hyoid bone (infrahyoid); to the side of the thyroid cartilage; through the center of the latter; or below it (infrahyoid, supersternal). (From Ward, P. H., Strahan, R. W., Acquarelli, M., et al.: The many faces of cysts of the thyroglossal duct. Trans. Am. Acad. Ophthalmol. Otolaryngol., 74:310, 1970.)

venous drainage of such a gland are by the normal routes. Extra vessels do not grow into the gland in the mediastinum, and the surgeon should not encounter abnormal bleeding while removing a retrosternal goiter from a neck incision as long as he works within the correct plane. Rarely, posterior mediastinal thyroid tissue is found, and from it may arise large goiters of the posterior mediastinum that are usually not continuous with the cervical thyroid gland. The entire gland may rarely descend into the thorax.

Other abnormalities include thyroid tissue in the duct between the tongue and the root of the neck and a lingual thyroid gland, a very rare abnormality in which the thyroid gland develops in the tongue and may represent the only thyroid tissue.[10] Thyroid tumors can occur in these tissues.[5] Patients usually present with swelling of the tongue, difficulty swallowing or breathing, or a change in speech. Surgical excision is sometimes required; however, total removal of a sublingual thyroid would be serious if the surgeon were not aware that it represented all of the thyroid tissue present. This can be determined by ^{131}I scan; and if it represents all thyroid tissue, autotransplantation of excised thyroid tissue is advocated by some.

Thyroglossal cysts and *fistulas* are conditions associated with a persistent thyroglossal duct.[3] The fistula may lie anterior or posterior to the hyoid bone or pass through the body of the hyoid bone. The cyst itself can occur anywhere from the foramen cecum to the supersternal notch. Thyroglossal duct cysts are most common in children at approximately the age of 5 years

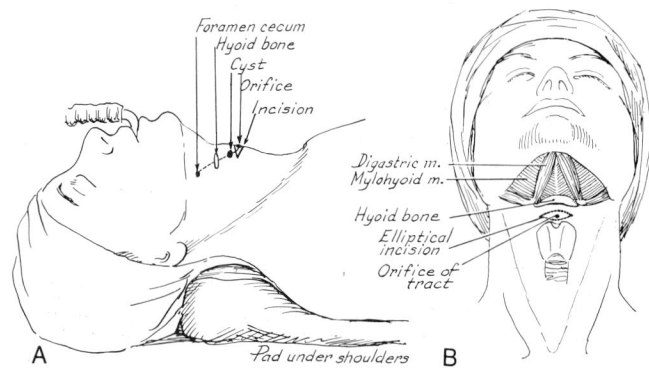

Figure 5. Thyroglossal duct. Surgical excision in relation to anatomic landmarks. *A*, The cyst of the duct, situated just caudal to the hyoid bone, is approached by a horizontal incision through the skin and platysma muscle. *B*, When a sinus tract is present, an elliptical transverse incision is made around the orifice of the duct. (From Converse, J. M.: Reconstructive Plastic Surgery, 2nd ed. Philadelphia, W. B. Saunders Company, 1977.)

and usually present as painless cystic swellings in the midline in the region of the hyoid bone (Fig. 4) and usually move with swallowing or protrusion of the tongue. Cysts frequently present with infection and are treated by incision and drainage of the cyst with excision of the fistula. The middle of the hyoid bone must be excised with the fistula because of the intimate relationship of the fistula with the middle of the hyoid bone (Fig. 5). Inadequate treatment can cause recurrence of the cyst, repeated infections, or the development of an external fistula or sinus.[2,3]

An important anatomic anomaly of the recurrent laryngeal nerve is the so-called nonrecurrent laryngeal nerve on the right side. It is not found on the left. The nerve runs directly to the larynx and does not pass beneath the right subclavian artery. This nerve is most at risk when the surgeon is seeking the right inferior thyroid artery.[22]

SELECTED REFERENCES

Deane, S. A., and Telander, R. L.: Surgery for thyroglossal duct and branchial cleft anomalies. Am. J. Surg., *136*:348, 1978.
  A recent review of thyroglossal duct abnormalities.

Ekholm, R.: Anatomy and development. *In* DeGroot, L. J. (Ed.): Endocrinology, 2nd ed. Philadelphia, W. B. Saunders Company, 1989.
  A concise review of the embryology and anatomy of the thyroid, with emphasis on cellular and molecular details.

Halsted, W. S.: The operative story of goiter. Johns Hopkins Hosp. Rep., *19*:71, 1920. Reprinted in Halsted, W. S.: Surgical Papers. Vol. II. Baltimore, The Johns Hopkins Press, 1928, p. 257.
  The definitive history of thyroid surgery. The author describes Halsted's operations on the thyroid gland.

Katz, A. D., and Zager, W. J.: The lingual thyroid. Its diagnosis and treatment. Arch. Surg., *102*:582, 1971.
  A concise review of lingual thyroid.

REFERENCES

1. Arey, L. B.: Developmental Anatomy, 7th ed. Philadelphia, W. B. Saunders Company, 1974.
2. Converse, J. M.: Reconstructive Plastic Surgery, 2nd ed. Philadelphia, W. B. Saunders Company, 1977.
3. Deane, S. A., and Telander, R. L.: Surgery for thyroglossal duct and branchial cleft anomalies. Am. J. Surg., *136*:348, 1978.
4. Durham, C. F., and Harrison, T. S.: The surgical anatomy of the superior laryngeal nerve. Surg. Gynecol. Obstet., *118*:38, 1964.
5. Fish, J., and Moore, R. M.: Ectopic thyroid tissue and ectopic thyroid carcinoma. Ann. Surg., *157*:212, 1963.
6. Fujita, H.: Fine structure of the thyroid gland. Int. Rev. Cytol., *10*:197, 1975.
7. Halsted, W. S.: The operative story of goiter. Johns Hopkins Hosp. Rep., *19*:71, 1920. Reprinted in Halsted, W. S.: Surgical Papers. Vol. II. Baltimore, Johns Hopkins Press, 1928, p. 257.
8. Halsted, W. S., and Evans, H. M.: The parathyroid glandules: Their blood supply and preservation in operations upon the thyroid gland. Ann. Surg., *46*:489, 1907.
9. Kark, A. F., Kissin, M. W., Auerbach, R., and Meikle, M.: Voice changes after thyroidectomy: Role of the external layngeal nerve. Br. Med. J., *289*:1412, 1984.
10. Katz, A. D., Zager, W. J.: The lingual thyroid. Its diagnosis and treatment. Arch. Surg., *102*:582, 1971.
11. Lahey, F. H.: Routine dissection and demonstration of recurrent laryngeal nerve in subtotal thyroidectomy. Surg. Gynecol. Obstet., *66*:775, 1938.
12. Lyerly, H. K., Sabiston, D. C., Jr.: Theodore Kocher. *In* Nobel Laureates in Surgery. In press.
13. McVay, C. B.: Anson and McVay Surgical Anatomy, 6th ed. Philadelphia, W. B. Saunders Company, 1984.
14. Melander, A., Ericson, L. E., Ljunggren, J.-G., et al.: Sympathetic innervation of the normal human thyroid. J. Clin. Endocrinol. Metab., *39*:713, 1974.
15. Moosman, D. A., DeWeese, M. S.: The external laryngeal nerve as related to thyroidectomy. Surg. Gynecol. Obstet., *127*:1011, 1968.
16. Peters, L. L., and Gardner, R. J.: Repair of recurrent laryngeal nerve injury. Surgery, *71*:865, 1972.
17. Riddell, V. H.: Injury to recurrent laryngeal nerves during thyroidectomy. Lancet, *2*:638, 1956.
18. Thompson, N. W., Harness, J. K.: Complications of total thyroidectomy for carcinoma. Surg. Gynecol. Obstet., *131*:861, 1970.
19. Thompson, N. W., Olsen, W. R., Hoffman, G. L.: The continuing development of the technique of thyroidectomy. Surgery, *73*:913, 1973.
20. Van Sande, J., Dumont, J. E., Melander, A., and Sundler, F.: Presence of influence of cholinergic nerves in the human thyroid. J. Clin. Endocrinol. Metab., *51*:500, 1989.
21. Ward, P. H., Strahan, R. W., Acquarelli, M., et al.: The many faces of cysts of the thyroglossal duct. Trans. Am. Acad. Ophthalmol. Otolaryngol., *74*:310, 1970.
22. Wijetilaka, S. E.: Non-recurrent laryngeal nerve. Br. J. Surg., *65*:179, 1978.
23. Williams, A. F.: Recurrent nerve lesions. Surgery, *43*:435, 1958.
24. Wollman, S. H.: Structure of the thyroid gland. *In* DeVisscher, M. (Ed.): The Thyroid Gland. New York, Raven Press, 1980, p. 1.

II

PHYSIOLOGY

H. Kim Lyerly, M. D.

The thyroid gland functions primarily to produce thyroid hormone for development and regulation of metabolism. A constant supply of thyroid hormone is necessary for growth, for brain development, and for maintaining metabolism and functional activity of most organs.

Thyroid hormone production is under the regulation of the anterior pituitary hormone thyrotropin, or thyroid-stimulating hormone (TSH), and by a system of autoregulation within the thyroid gland. The thyroid hormones are iodinated amino acids, thyroxine (T_4) and 3,5,3'-triiodothyronine (T_3). In the thyroid they are an integral part of thyroglobulin (Tg), in which they are synthesized and stored. In the plasma, they circulate as free amino acids in reversible equilibrium with the thyroid hormone–binding proteins; however, they have an effect on metabolism only when they are in the free form. Free thyroid hormones are able to penetrate cells to induce and stimulate oxygen consumption; increase body heat and the rates of me-

tabolism of carbohydrates, fats, and proteins; and stimulate the feedback mechanism with the pituitary gland.[31]

THYROID HORMONE SYNTHESIS

Iodine is necessary for the synthesis of thyroid hormones. In the normal American diet, about 200 to 500 μg. of iodine is ingested daily, mainly in drinking water, sea fish, salt, milk, and eggs. The inorganic iodine is reduced to iodide ion in the gut, where most is absorbed from the small intestine and is cleared from plasma by the thyroid to provide the normal thyroid requirement of 50 to 100 μg. or is excreted by the kidney. Approximately 150 to 500 mg. per day is excreted in the urine. Iodide clearance is dependent on the glomerular filtration rate (GFR) and increases and decreases with enhancement or reduction of GFR.

Thyroid hormone synthesis incorporates a complex sequence

of processes (Fig. 1).[52,63,74] The thyroid actively transports and concentrates iodide in the thyroid follicular cell and the colloid at a rate of about 2 μg. per hour. A concentration gradient of 20- to 40-fold is established that may be increased 20-fold by TSH stimulation, low dietary iodide, and pharmacologic interference with thyroid hormone formation.

Iodide remains free only briefly before being oxidized to a highly reactive form that binds to tyrosine residues in thyroglobulin. Thyroglobulin is a dimeric glycoprotein with a molecular weight of 660,000 and contains approximately 120 tyrosyl units, of which about 30 per cent undergo iodination. After its synthesis and intracellular transport, exophytic vesicles discharge their content into the follicle, and Tg accumulates in the lumen.[41,65] The colloid, which fills the follicle lumen, is almost exclusively composed of iodinated Tg. The iodination reaction of Tg is catalyzed by thyroid peroxidase (TPO). This is the step interrupted by the thiocarbamide group of drugs (such as propylthiouracil), which causes a large concentration of unbound iodide to remain in the thyroid.

After being bound to tyrosine residues in the thyroglobulin, iodide proceeds to be part of T_4 and T_3 via monoiodotyrosine (MIT) and diiodotyrosine (DIT). By this complex coupling mechanism, two molecules of DIT combine to form T_4, and one molecule of DIT plus one molecule of MIT form T_3.

Tg breakdown and thyroid hormone release occur when the colloid is engulfed by the apical pole, forming endocytotic vesicles that fuse with lysosomes and form phagolysosomes. Proteases within these vesicles then hydrolyze the thyroglobulin to iodothyronines, which are secreted. Free iodotyrosines formed by hydrolysates are deiodinated into tyrosine and iodide, which may be recycled to form new thyroid hormone molecules.[40] Some Tg molecules are not hydrolyzed and escape into the bloodstream.

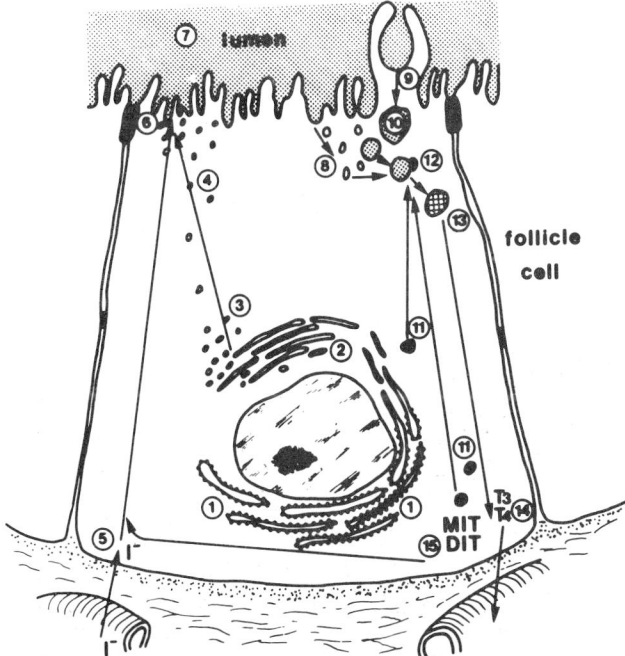

Figure 1. Diagrammatic scheme of thyroid hormone formation and secretion. 1, Thyroglobulin (Tg) and protein synthesis in the rough endoplasmic reticulum. 2, Coupling of the Tg carbohydrate units in the smooth endoplasmic reticulum and Golgi apparatus. 3, Formation of exocytotic vesicles. 4, Transport of exocytotic vesicles with noniodinated Tg to the apical surface of the follicle cell and into the follicular lumen. 5, Iodide transport at the basal cell membrane. 6, Iodide oxidation, Tg iodination, and coupling of iodotyrosyl to iodothyronyl residues. 7, Storage of iodinated Tg in the follicular lumen. 8, Endocytosis by micropinocytosis. 9, Endocytosis by macropinocytosis (pseudopods). 10, Colloid droplets. 11, Lysosomes migrating to the apical pole. 12, Fusion of lysosomes with colloid droplets. 13, Phagolysosomes with Tg hydrolysis. 14, T_3 and T_4 secretion. 15, MIT and DIT deiodination.

TABLE 1. Properties of Thyroid Binding Proteins

	Thyronine-Binding Globulin	Thyroxine-Binding Prealbumin	Albumin
Molecular weight	54,000	55,000	69,000
Structure	Monomer	Tetramer	Monomeric
Binding sites	1	2	5–6
Serum concentration	1.6 mg./dl.	25 mg./dl.	4000 mg./dl.
Relative distribution			
T_4	70%	25%	5%
T_3	70%	10%	20%
Half-life (days)	5	2	15

The normal thyroid contains approximately 8000 μg. of iodine, only about 1 per cent being inorganic iodide. T_4 constitutes approximately 35 per cent; T_3, 5 per cent; DIT, 25 per cent; and MIT, 25 per cent. Approximately 1 per cent of the hormone in the thyroid store is released to the circulation each day after being separated in the cell by acid proteases and peptide enzymes. Eighty to 100 μg. of T_4 and 26 to 39 μg. of T_3 are produced each day. T_4 has a half-life of 6 days, and T_3 has a half life of 1 to 3 days. The thyroid gland has a storage reserve of approximately 3 weeks.

The concentration of total thyroxine is 30 to 50 times the concentration of T_3. However, only 0.03 per cent of the total serum T_4 and 0.3 per cent of the total serum T_3 is present in the unbound or biologically active form. The major serum thyroid hormone–binding proteins are thyronine-binding globulin (TBG), thyroxine-binding prealbumin (TBPA), and albumin (ALB) (Table 1).

Hormone-binding proteins are the principal intravascular factors influencing total hormone concentration, which is normally maintained at a level appropriate for the concentration of carrier proteins in order to maintain a constant free hormone level. Various factors may cause changes in the concentration of TBG (Table 2).[2,4,8,25,43,44,53,57] Because alterations in TBG may alter the total hormone concentration independent of the metabolic status of the body, free hormone, rather than the total hormone, is a more accurate indicator of the thyroid hormone–dependent metabolic state (Fig. 2).[27,54]

Although T_4 is the principal secretory product of the thyroid gland, the principal active hormone in metabolic regulation is T_3. Under normal circumstances, most T_3 is produced in the liver, heart, and kidneys by peripheral conversion of T_4. The critical step in this pathway is T_4 5′-monodeiodination (Fig. 3). Because thyrotoxicosis can occur from elevations of T_3 when measured T_4 is within normal limits, it is sometimes an advantage to measure T_3 to diagnose T_3 thyrotoxicosis. Thyroxine is also metabolized to 3,3′,5′-triiodothyronine, reverse T_3, or rT_3, which is inactive.

Current concepts of thyroid hormone mechanisms generally consider the nucleus to be the site of initiation of hormone action. By control of the expression of genetic information, all other activities of the cell may be controlled. The diversity of thyroid hormone effects may be observed as the logical consequence of controlling the expression of specific sets of genetic information within the various tissue types, in concert with other regulatory factors. This regulation could also be dependent on the organism's development, thus explaining why certain effects are observed only when the hormone is administered or removed at certain times in the organism's developmental cycle. Thyroid hormone appears to have both generalized actions on RNA and protein synthesis and specific actions in the transcription of particular proteins.[18,50]

Thyroid hormones have numerous metabolic effects. Enhancement of the basal metabolic rate (BMR) as reflected by increased oxygen consumption is one of the classic actions of

TABLE 2. Conditions Associated with Alterations in TBG Concentration

	Increased	Decreased
Genetic	Inherited elevated TBG	Inherited absent or low TBG
Acquired diseases	Acute intermittent porphyia	Major illness
	Acute and chronic active viral hepatitis	Protein calorie malnutrition
	Primary biliary cirrhosis	Galactosemia
	Hepatocellular carcinoma	Nephrotic syndrome
	Myeloma	Hepatic cirrhosis
	Collagen disease	Acromegaly
	Hypothyroidism	Protein-losing enteropathy
		Hyperthyroidism
Drugs	Perphenazine	
	Heroin and methadone	
	Clofibrate	
	5-Fluorouracil	
Hormones	Estrogens	Androgens
	Hyperestrogenemic state (pregnancy, newborn, molar pregnancy, tumors)	Anabolic steroids
		Glucocorticoids
		L-asparaginase

thyroid hormone. An optimal amount is necessary for balanced growth and maturation, and many of the effects of thyroid hormones on carbohydrate metabolism appear permissive with respect to the effects of other hormones. They characteristically lower the level of serum cholesterol by enhanced excretion in the feces and conversion of cholesterol to bile acids. The generalized metabolic response increases the demand for vitamins and cofactors, and there is a magnified catecholamine effect produced by excess thyroid hormone.

MECHANISMS OF THYROID REGULATION

The principal regulatory mechanisms of the thyroid gland are the hypothalamic-pituitary-thyroid control system and the intrathyroidal autoregulatory system (Fig. 4). The former is represented by the pituitary thyrotropin TSH, which stimulates many aspects of thyroid activity, particularly thyroid hormone synthesis and secretion, and thyroid hormones inhibit the secretion of TSH by the pituitary.[19,37]

Thyroid-Stimulating Hormone

TSH is a glycoprotein hormone that, like luteinizing hormone (LH), follicle-stimulating hormone (FSH), and human chorionic gonadotropin (HCG), has alpha and beta subunits. The alpha subunits of these hormones are identical, and the beta subunits are responsible for their biologic and immunologic specificities.

TSH is required for the normal production and secretion of thyroid hormone; in its absence, the thyroid gland releases a reduced amount of thyroid hormone. TSH secretion is most profoundly influenced by tonic stimulation by hypothalamic thyrotropin-releasing hormone (TRH) and feedback inhibition by thyroid hormone.[24,68] The normal serum concentration of

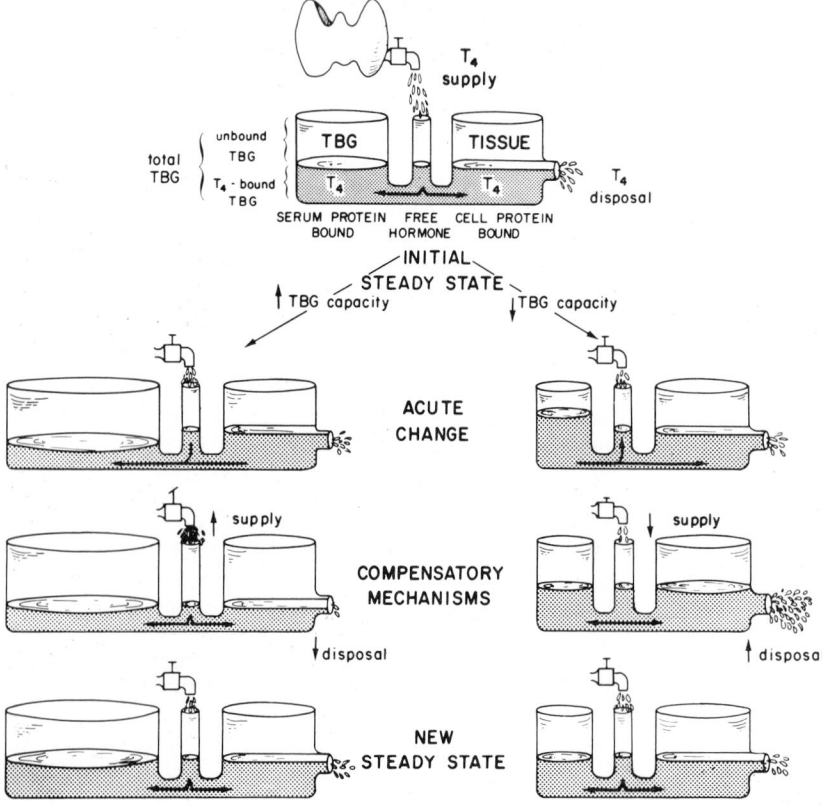

Figure 2. Graphic representation of the sequence of events following an acute change in serum TBG concentration in a subject with normal regulation of thyroid hormone secretion and metabolism. The communicating vessel principle is used for analogy. The width of the two large vessels represents available T_4 binding sites in serum (TBG) and in peripheral cells (tissue), which are partially saturated by T_4 (fluid level). The height of fluid in the small central vessel represents free T_4 concentration in equilibrium with bound T_4 in each of the large vessels. Free T_4 is proportional to the level of saturation of the binding sites in serum (TBG) and in cells (tissue). Thyroidal secretion (supply) of T_4 is represented by the input of fluid through the faucet, and hormone metabolism (disposal) by the overspill of the tissue reservoir. If TBG concentration is increased, the resulting increase in unoccupied binding sites produces a shift in the equilibrium between total and bound T_4, having as a net effect a diminution in the serum free T_4 concentration. The consequences are threefold. First, an equilibration of exchangeable T_4 occurs with a shift from tissues to blood; second, the resulting diminution in tissue supply of T_4 decreases its disposal; and third, activation of the hypothalamic-pituitary axis increases the thyroidal secretion of T_4. The last two compensatory mechanisms remain until a new steady state is reached in which the increased TBG concentration is associated with a higher concentration of total and bound T_4, compatible with a normal concentration of free T_4, a normal tissue supply of T_4, and a return to the same secretion and disposal rates as in the initial steady state. The converse sequence of events occurs during an acute decrease in TBG concentration.

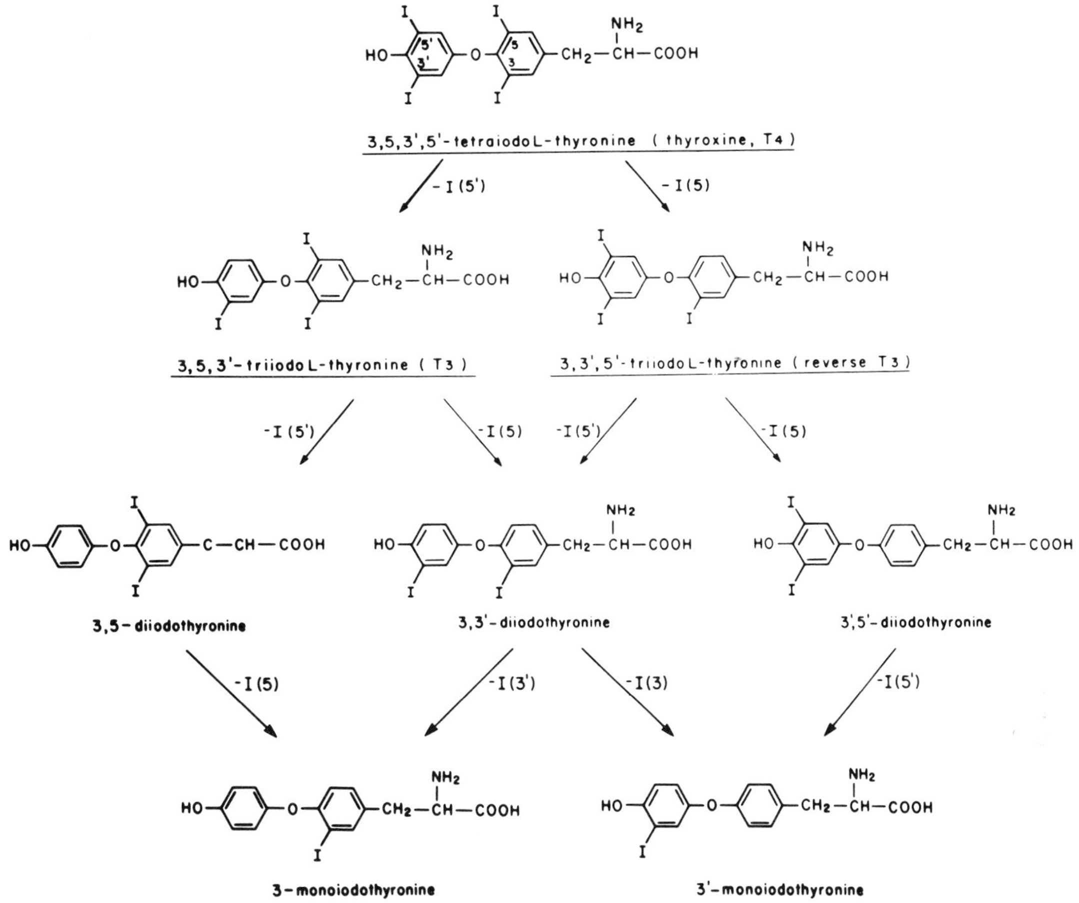

Figure 3. Products produced by the successive monodeiodination of thyroxine in the outer (5′) and inner (5) rings.

TSH is 0.5 to 4.5 μU. per ml. when assayed. The normal daily production and degradation is 40 to 150 μU. TSH secretion has a circadian rhythm, and the levels rise approximately 2 hours after sleep to peak between 2 and 4 A.M..[16]

An initial effect of TSH is in iodide transport, which is reflected by an acute increase in the efflux. Other effects of TSH include activation of iodide binding to thyroglobulins, increased coupling of monoiodotyrosine and diiodotyrosine to form T_3 and T_4, activation of exocytosis and transfer of protein in the lumen of the follicle, and secretion of thyroid hormone.

It is generally accepted that TSH has a major role in thyroid growth. Iodide deficiency and excessive treatment of hyperthyroidism with blockers of iodide binding to thyroglobulin lead to increased TSH secretion and thyroid enlargement. In situations in which TSH action is lacking, e.g., hypophysectomy or inactive TSH, the thyroid exhibits a decrease in size, whereas prolonged administration of TSH leads to an increase in thyroid weight. Chronic stimulation of the thyroid gland by TSH causes the proliferation of capillaries and fibroblasts, rather than follicle cells.

Thyrotropin-Releasing Hormone

TRH is a tripeptide (pyroglutamyl-histidylproline amide) and was the first hypothalamic hormone to be isolated. It is produced by the supraoptic and paraventricular nuclei of the hypothalamus and passes down their axons to the median eminence, where it is stored. Following secretion into the hypophyseal portal blood vessels, TRH travels to the pituitary and binds to specific receptor sites. TRH action on the pituicytes includes stimulation of TSH secretion and synthesis, as well as the stimulation of prolactin release and synthesis.[35,49,58]

The primary role of TRH appears to be tonic stimulation of TSH-producing cells within the pituitary, because the normal secretion of TSH and thyroid hormone is dependent on hypothalamic stimulation. The primary clinical use of this hormone is in the diagnosis of thyroid disease (Fig. 5). A dose-response relationship between TRH and TSH is found in humans with intravenous bolus doses between 6.5 and 400 μg. In hyperthy-

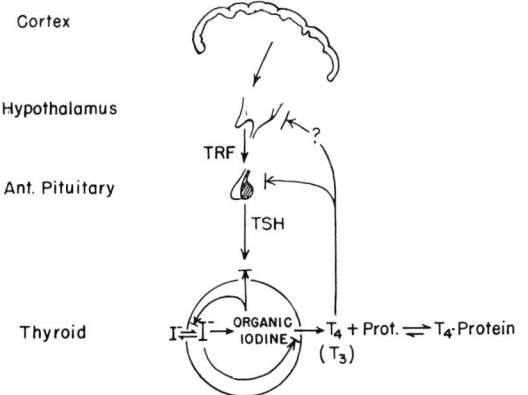

Figure 4. Schema of the homeostatic regulation of thyroid function. Secretion of thyroid-stimulating hormone (TSH) is regulated by a negative feedback system acting directly on the pituitary and is normally inversely related to the concentration of unbound hormone in the blood. Release of TSH is induced by the thyrotropin releasing factor (TRF), the secretion of which appears to set the level of pituitary feedback mechanism. Factors regulating secretion of TRF are uncertain but may include the free hormone, the blood, and stimuli from higher centers. Autoregulatory control of thyroid function is also shown. High concentrations of intrathyroid iodide decrease the rate of release of thyroid iodine. In addition, the magnitude of the organic iodine pool inversely influences the iodide transport mechanism and the response to TSH. (From Wilson, J. B., and Foster, D. W. (Eds.); Williams' Textbook of Endocrinology, 7th ed. Philadelphia, W. B. Saunders Company, 1985).

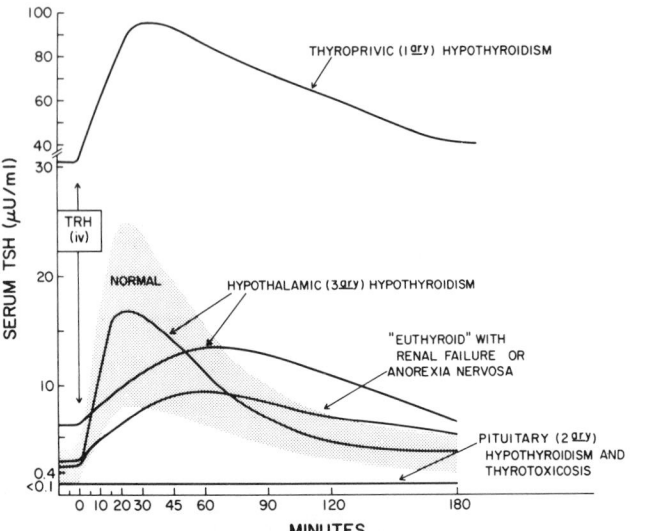

Figure 5. Typical TSH responses to the administration of a single intravenous 400-μg. bolus of TRH in various conditions. The normal response is represented by the shaded area. Data used for the figure are the average of several studies.

roid patients, there is no peak in TSH after TRH administration, because of autonomous thyroid function. There are other causes of a flat TRH response besides autonomous thyroid hyperfunction, including T_4 therapy, euthyroid ophthalmic Graves' disease, euthyroid multinodular goiter, and hypopituitarism.

In hypothyroidism due to primary thyroid disease, there is an exaggerated rise in TSH after TRH. In pituitary disease the TRH test is less useful, since a rise in TSH may still be observed in the presence of a low circulating thyroxine concentration.

Autoregulation of Thyroid Function

Although TSH is the primary regulator of the activity of the thyroid gland, the gland has intrinsic ability to alter the production and release of thyroid hormone. This autoregulatory ability is most prominent in adaptation to conditions of iodine deficiency or excess.

In humans, the Wolff-Chaikoff block (acute block of iodide binding) is induced by an elevation of the plasma iodide concentration to approximately 25 μg. per dl. As iodide levels in plasma increase, there is an increase in the amount taken up and bound by the thyroid gland. After a critical amount of iodide accumulates, there is a progressive inhibition of iodide binding to tyrosyl residues in thyroglobulin.

In addition to the Wolff-Chaikoff block, administration of potassium iodide to a patient with Graves' disease or a normal subject causes a prompt reduction in the release of iodine-containing compounds from the gland and a prompt decrease in serum thyroid hormone levels (Fig. 6). Moreover, there is a reduction of the hypervascularity and hyperplasia characteristic of Graves' disease. Conversely, exposure to large quantities of iodine can also induce hyperthyroidism. Although this was thought to occur in iodine deficient areas, it has also been recognized as responsible for nodular goiter in patients from iodine-sufficient areas.

Monovalent anions including thiocyanate, perchlorate, and nitrate inhibit iodide uptake. Thiocyanate and perchlorate both stimulate discharge of free iodide from the thyroid gland, and thiocyanate also inhibits iodide binding and iodotyrosine coupling. Lithium is concentrated in the thyroid by the same mechanisms as iodide and induces goiterous hypothyroidism in susceptible individuals.[7,60]

Thionamides such as methimazole and proplythiouracil are commonly used anti-thyroid medications. They impair the covalent binding of iodine to thyroglobulin and iodotyrosine coupling and appear to inhibit the thyroid iodide peroxidase.

Propylthiouracil and, to a lesser degree, methimazole also inhibit the peripheral tissue deiodination of T_4 to T_3.

Glucocorticoids influence thyroid function at multiple levels, including reducing the secretion of TSH. Estrogens may decrease serum TSH on an acute basis but chronically enhance the TSH response to TRH. They also increase the concentration of TBG and consequently increase total serum T_4 and T_3, although free T_4 and T_3 do not change. Similarly, pregnancy is associated with several important alterations in thyroid function.[44] During the first trimester, there is a doubling of the serum TBG concentration, leading to an increase in the total serum T_4 and T_3 levels but normal free thyroid hormone levels. TSH levels are normal or slightly elevated and have an exaggerated response to the administration of TRH.

In infants, the normal range for serum T_4 remains approximately 25 per cent higher than for adults but progressively declines during childhood.[21] In healthy, elderly men, the T_4 turnover rate is decreased, basal metabolic rates are lower, and the uptake of radioactive iodine by the thyroid gland is diminished.[59,73]

Multiple alterations in thyroid physiology have been noted in the presence of other disease. Whereas basal TSH levels and the response to TRH are increased by iodine administration to normal subjects, this alteration is reduced or absent in sick patients. In patients with reduced thyroid levels and severe illness, there has been observed a rise in TSH levels during the recovery period, followed by a later rise in serum T_4 levels.

THYROID FUNCTION TESTS AND EFFECTS OF DRUGS ON THYROID FUNCTION

The fundamental issues in the evaluation of thyroid disease are the metabolic status of the patient, the etiology of the disease process responsible for the hormonal imbalance, and the etiology of the thyroid gland abnormality in the euthyroid patient.

Tests of Thyroid Gland Activity and Hormone Synthesis

THYROIDAL RADIOIODIDE UPTAKE (RAIU). After oral ingestion of ^{123}I (which has a short half-life and is associated with minimal radiation, compared with ^{131}I), the thyroid uptake

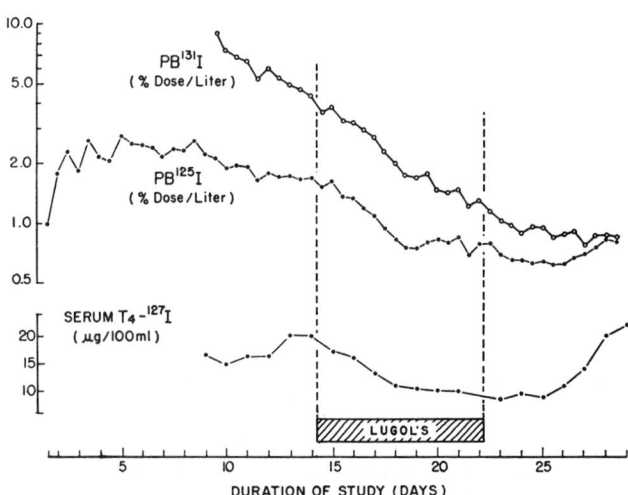

Figure 6. Iodide inhibition of thyroid hormone release. A patient with thyrotoxicosis was administered inorganic ^{125}I as a marker for newly synthesized iodoproteins and several days later was administered ^{131}I-T_4 to monitor the rate of clearance of thyroid hormone. Iodine was then administered in the form of Lugol's solution. Serum protein-bound ^{125}I (PB ^{125}I) and ^{131}I (PB ^{131}I) and nonradioactive T_4 (T_4-^{127}I) were measured serially. The decline in serum T_4 while peripheral ^{131}I-T_4 degradation remained stable indicates decreased release of hormone from the thyroid gland during iodine administration. (Redrawn from Wartofsky, L., Ransil, B. J., and Ingbar, S. H.: Inhibition by iodine of the release of thyroxine from the thyroid glands of patients with thyrotoxicosis. J. Clin. Invest., *49*:78, 1970, copyright by the American Society for Clinical Investigation.)

is near its peak at 24 hours.[48] A dose of 400 μCi. is usually administered orally, and the quantity accumulated by the thyroid gland at various intervals is measured by counting with a gamma scintillation counter. Normal values for 24-hour RAIU in most parts of the North America are approximately 15 to 30 per cent. Disease states leading to excessive production and release of thyroid hormone are most often associated with an increased thyroid RAIU, and those causing hormone underproduction are associated with a decreased RAIU.[26]

PERTECHNETATE-99M UPTAKE MEASUREMENT. Because thyroidal uptake in the very early period after administration of radioiodine reflects mainly trapping activity, ^{99m}Tc may be used to assay thyroid trapping. In euthyroid patients, thyroid trapping is maximal at about 20 minutes and is approximately 1 per cent of the administered dose.

Measurement of Thyroid Hormone and Other Compounds in Blood

Measurement of T_4 and T_3 in serum and the estimation of their free concentration have become the most commonly used tests for the evaluation of the thyroid hormone–dependent metabolic status. Although total levels do not reflect the metabolic state of the patient, the free T_4 index remains a popular indirect measure of free T_4.

TOTAL THYROXINE (TT_4). The usual concentration of TT_4 in adults ranges from 5 to 11.5 μg. per dl. TT_4 measures both the protein-bound and free T_4 and is not affected by iodine-containing drugs but can be altered by changes in TBG level.

TOTAL TRIIODOTHYRONINE (TT_3). Normal serum TT_3 concentrations in the adult are 80 to 190 ng. per dl. Measurement of TT_3 is useful in the diagnosis of T_3 toxicosis, where the T_4 level is normal and serum TSH is suppressed.[33,61] It is less appropriate for the diagnosis of hypothyroidism and is subject to the same abnormalities due to TBG as TT_4 measurement.

RESIN TRIIODOTHYRONINE UPTAKE (RT_3U). RT_3U measures the unoccupied thyroid hormone binding sites on TBG by measuring the competitive binding for radioactive T_3 between TBG and a resin and provides an indirect measure of free T_4. The radioactive T_3 added to the system is bound preferentially by the resin if the thyroid hormone binding sites on TBG are occupied by T_4. The resin uptake of T_3 is directly proportional to the fraction of free T_4 in the serum and inversely related to the unoccupied TBG binding sites. RT_3U is high in thyrotoxicosis and low in hypothyroid states. Depending on the method used, typical normal values of RT_3U are 25 to 35 per cent. The test serves as an indirect measurement of the unbound fraction of T_4 and is valuable because it is simpler to perform than other measurements of T_4.[62]

FREE THYROXINE AND T_3. The first and still standard method for estimation of the free T_4 and T_3 concentration employs equilibrium dialysis, which uses the proportion of the TT_4 and TT_3 capable of diffusing through a dialysis membrane. Direct measurements of the T_4 and T_3 can be interpreted without concern for the quantity of TBG in the blood and are not affected by conditions affecting TBG. Both can be measured most specifically and easily by radioimmunoassay.[38,76]

SERUM THYROGLOBULIN. Thyroglobulin is present in normal serum at a low concentration (5 to 10 ng. per ml.), which reflects normal thyroid secretion. Radioimmunoassay methods are now used routinely for measurement of Tg in serum. Elevated serum levels are present in patients with goiter, hyperthyroidism, thyroiditis, and thyroid tumors. Serum thyroglobulin is suppressed in factitious thyrotoxicosis, a feature that helps differentiate this condition from subacute thyroiditis.[45]

The major clinical application of serum thyroglobulin levels is in the management of thyroid carcinoma.[56,64] Because thyroglobulin levels are increased in both benign and malignant tumors, thyroglobulin determination cannot be used to differentiate these disorders; however, determination of serum thyroglobulin levels is helpful in following patients with thyroid cancer after thyroidectomy. Serum thyroglobulin levels should revert to normal or undetectable levels if metastatic disease is absent. Most patients who have a recurrence of a tumor or metastatic disease demonstrate an increase in serum thyroglobulin.[5,13]

SERUM CALCITONIN. Calcitonin is a hormone secreted by the parafollicular cells of the normal thyroid. It functions to reduce the resorption of calcium from bone, lowering serum calcium in opposition to parathormone. It is released in response to hypercalcemia, gastrin, and cholecystokinin but is not governed by the anterior pituitary. Radioimmunoassays are now available that distinguish the normal range of plasma calcitonin from elevated levels. Plasma calcitonin is elevated in association with a number of conditions. Clinically, the most important is medullary thyroid carcinoma (MTC).[70] Plasma calcitonin levels are elevated in the majority of patients with MTC. In some patients with MTC, the basal serum calcitonin level is normal. The diagnosis of MTC in these patients is made by documenting an increase in the serum calcitonin level in response to provocative testing with calcium or pentagastrin.[32]

Tests Assessing the Effects of Thyroid Hormone on Body Tissues

The basal metabolic rate (BMR) is a measure of oxygen consumption under basal conditions by allowing the individual to breathe into a closed system, under presumably basal conditions of overnight fasting and rest from mental and physical exertion. It can be estimated from the oxygen consumed over a timed interval by analysis of samples of expired air. In addition to BMR, deep tendon reflex time, cardiovascular function, and serum cholesterol can also be measured to reflect hypothyroidism and hyperthyroidism.[23,36,39,58]

Evaluation of the Hypothalamic Pituitary Thyroid Axis

THYROTROPIN (TSH). The development of radioimmunoassays for the routine measurement of TSH in serum and the availability of synthetic TRH have led to increased reliance on tests assessing the hypothalamic pituitary control of thyroid function (Fig. 7). Concentrations of TSH become elevated before there is any measurable reduction in serum T_4 or T_3, and the elevated TSH levels observed in primary hypothyroidism help confirm this diagnosis. Reliable detection of low levels of TSH is difficult, so that a true absence of the hormone is difficult to

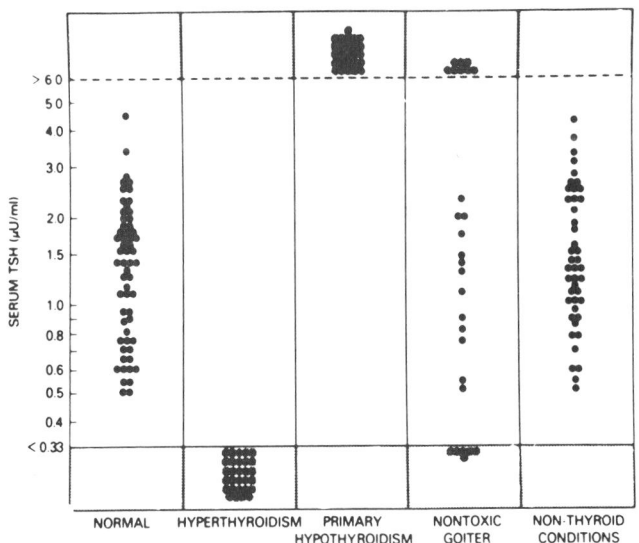

Figure 7. Serum TSH in thyroid disease. Serum TSH levels were measured by a sensitive assay in normal subjects and in patients with hyperthyroidism, primary hypothyroidism, nontoxic goiter, and various nonthyroid conditions. (From Wehman, R., Rubenstein, H. A., Pufeat, M. A., and Nisula, B. C.: Extended clinical utility of a sensitive and reliable radioimmunoassay of thyroid-stimulating hormone. South. Med. J., 76:969, 1983.)

TABLE 3. Classification of Hypothyroidism by Level of Lesion

	Hypothalamus	Primary Pituitary	Thyroid
Serum TSH	Low	Low	High
Serum TSH after TRH stimulation	Increase	No response	Exaggerated increase
Thyroid response to exogenous TSH*	Increase	Increase	No response

* In thyroid radioiodine uptake and serum thyroxin.

distinguish from a nondetectable level that may be observed in some normal individuals. However, a low or undetected TSH level in association with a low thyroxine concentration is indicative of pituitary or hypothalamic disease (Table 3).[51]

THYROTROPIN STIMULATION TEST. This test is employed to differentiate primary thyroid failure from thyroid hypofunction caused by inadequate TSH stimulation.[9] If an increase in radioactive iodine uptake of 10 per cent or more or a rise in T_4 of at least 2 μg. per 100 ml. can be demonstrated, it is likely that the thyroid can respond to exogenous TSH stimulation. Thyrotropin is administered in a dose of 5 to 10 units intramuscularly for assessment of primary thyroid insufficiency or diminished thyroid reserve. Increased amounts of TSH may be necessary in the presence of pituitary failure (see Table 3).

THYROID RELEASING HORMONE STIMULATION TEST. The TRH test measures the increase of pituitary TSH in serum in response to the administration of synthetic TRH. The magnitude of the TSH response to TRH is modulated by the thyrotrope response to active thyroid hormone and is thus inversely proportional to the concentration of free thyroid hormone in serum. The standard test dose is a single TRH dose of 400 μg. per 1.73 sq. m. of body surface area. Serum is collected at intervals, and in normal individuals there is a prompt increase in serum TSH, with a peak level at 20 to 40 min., which is on average five times the basal level. The test provides a unique method of distinguishing between secondary and tertiary hypothyroidism. A TSH response is indicative of a hypothalamic disorder, and a failure to respond is compatible with intrinsic pituitary dysfunction (see Fig. 5).

THYROID SUPPRESSION TEST. This test is based on the principle that the administration of thyroid hormone does not suppress the patient's thyroid function when normal homeostatic mechanisms are disrupted. After an initial radioactive iodine uptake test, T_3 is administered in a dose of 100 μg. daily for 7 days. Evidence for thyrotropin suppression is present if follow-up radioactive iodine uptake is less than 20 per cent. Values above 20 per cent in 24 hours indicate a disturbance of homeostatic control, which might be present in hyperthyroidism or in the presence of thyroid hormone–secreting tumors.

Anti-thyroid Antibodies

The primary indications for measuring anti-thyroid antibodies include diagnosis of Hashimoto's disease and identification of those patients with Graves' disease who, by having antibodies, are particularly susceptible to hypothyroidism after subtotal thyroidectomy. In Hashimoto's disease, antibodies may be detected against thyroglobulin, usually in a titer of more than 1 : 100, and to microsomes in the thyroid cell in a titer of more than 1 : 32. Other antibodies that may be detected include those against another colloid antigen (second colloid antigen), which is of no value in the diagnosis of Hashimoto's disease, those to cell surface antigen, which has an unestablished value, and those to TSH receptors on thyroid cells. The latter are thyroid-stimulating immunoglobulins (TSI), also called long-acting thyroid-stimulating substance protector (LATS-P), and are found in patients with Graves' disease and in patients with Graves' disease after thyroidectomy.

Factors Affecting Thyroid Function Tests

A large number of compounds may affect thyroid function and economy (Table 4).[22,34,46,72]

ANATOMIC AND TISSUE DIAGNOSIS

RADIOACTIVE SCANNING. This long-established test using ^{131}I or ^{99m}Tc remains useful. A ^{99m}Tc thyroid scan can be obtained almost immediately, and the dose required is quite small. An ^{131}I scan must be delayed for at least 24 hours and requires a larger dose. ^{131}I is useful for confirming the autonomy of a hyperactive nodule and for the surveillance and treatment of patients with thyroid cancer.

Radioactive scanning is very useful in distinguishing a solitary nodule from a multinodular goiter. In a multinodular goiter, the normal activity pattern is absent and uptake is distributed throughout the gland in a haphazard manner. When a solitary nodule is present, the basic thyroid pattern is normal: a solitary nodule may have a complete lack of uptake producing no activity (cold nodule), constitute the entire radioactive pattern if all uptake is confined to the nodule (hot nodule), or have no effect.[6] An intrathoracic or retrosternal goiter extends the haphazard uptake of a multinodular goiter down into the chest, but not all intrathoracic goiters appear to take up radioactive tracer. Radioactive scanning is useful in localizing aberrant thy-

TABLE 4. Agents That May Affect Thyroid Hormone Function or Measurement

Inhibit conversion of T_4 to T_3
PTU
Glucocorticoids
Propranolol
Iodinated contrast agents
Amiodarone
Clomipramine

Stimulate degradation or fecal excretion
Phenytoin
Carbamazepine
Phenobarbital
Cholestyramine
Soybeans

Interfere with binding to TBG
Salicylates
Furosemide
Dinitrophenol
Phenylbutazone
Fenclofenac
Monovalent anions
Phenytoin
Sulfonylureas
Free fatty acids
Halofenate
Orphenadrine
Thyroid analogs

Alter TBG concentration
See Table 2.

roid tissue in the tongue and in the line of the thyroid's descent in the midline of the neck.

FLUORESCENT SCANS. This technique allows thyroid scanning without the administration of radioisotopes. It involves the focal irradiation of the thyroid gland with a 60-keV. γ-ray derived from an ^{241}Am source. Its interaction with stable iodine (^{127}I) within the gland produces the emission of a characteristic 28.5-keV. K-α (fluorescent) x-ray that is picked up by a lithium-drifted silicone detector. The resulting scan demonstrates the distribution of stable iodine within the gland, and the content can be quantitated by the use of appropriate iodide standards.

ULTRASOUND SCANNING. Ultrasound can be used to distinguish between solid and cystic lesions, which is a distinction that cannot be made by radioactive scanning.[12,30,66] Although most cystic lesions are benign, ultrasound cannot distinguish between a solid benign lesion and a carcinoma. Papillary carcinoma is found in a cystic form very rarely.

COMPUTED TOMOGRAPHY (CT) AND MAGNETIC RESONANCE IMAGING (MRI). CT provides useful information on the location and architecture of the thyroid gland as well as its relationship to surrounding tissues. An important application is the assessment and delineation of mediastinal tumors. MRI may also be useful in the evaluation of mediastinal tumors. Both CT and MRI are also useful in the evaluation of exophthalmos to exclude retro-orbital mass lesions.

BIOPSY. Closed biopsy can be made by the Vim-Silverman or Tru-cut needle, which provides a core of tissue for histologic study.[14,15,67] Another technique is fine-needle aspiration, where cells are aspirated into a syringe barrel and then smeared onto a glass slide. These techniques can be helpful in diagnosing thyroiditis, anaplastic carcinoma, and malignant lymphoma.[1,20,29,42,47] Analysis of DNA content in aspirated cells may also be helpful in delineating benign from malignant lesions.[3]

SELECTED REFERENCES

Ingbar, S. H.: The thyroid gland. *In* Wilson, J. D., and Foster, D. W. (Eds.): Williams Textbook of Endocrinology, 7th ed. Philadelphia, W. B. Saunders Company, 1985.
This chapter in the standard textbook of endocrinology provides an excellent review of thyroid physiology.

Lissitzky, S., Torresani, J., Carayon, P., and Amr, S.: Physiology of the thyroid. *In* DeGroot, L. J. (Ed.): Endocrinology, 2nd ed. Philadelphia, W. B. Saunders Company, 1989.
This series of chapters in a multivolume text includes extensive reviews of the physiology and regulation of the thyroid. It includes clinical and experimental details as well as an extensive bibliography.

Larsen, P. R.: Thyroid-pituitary interaction: Feedback regulation of thyrotropin secretion by thyroid hormones. N. Engl. J. Med., 306:23, 1982.
This article reviews thyroid pituitary regulation.

Jackson, I. M. D.: Thyrotropin-releasing hormone. N. Engl. J. Med., 306:145, 1982.
This article reviews TRH and pituitary regulation and interaction.

Backdahl, M., Wallin, G., Lowhagen, T., Auer, G., and Granberg, P. O.: Fine-needle biopsy cytology and DNA analysis. Surg. Clin. North Am., 67:197, 1987.
This is a review of the uses of cytology and DNA analysis in the management of thyroid neoplasms.

REFERENCES

1. Al-Sayer, Z. M., Krukowski, Z. H., Williams, V. M. M., and Matheson, N. A.: Fine needle aspiration cytology in isolated thyroid swelling: A prospective two-year evaluation. Br. Med. J., 290:1490, 1985.
2. Azizi, F., Vagenakis, A. G., Portnay, G. I., et al.: Thyroxine transport and metabolism in methadone and heroin addicts. Ann. Intern. Med., 80:194, 1974.
3. Backdahl, M., Wallin, G., Lowhagen, T., et al.: Fine-needle biopsy cytology and DNA analysis. Surg. Clin. North Am., 67:197, 1987.
4. Barbosa, J., Seal, U. S., and Doe, R. P.: Effects of anabolic steroids on hormone-binding proteins, serum cortisol and serum nonprotein-bound cortisol. J. Clin. Endocrinol. Metab., 32:232, 1971.
5. Barsano, C. P., Skosey, C., DeGrott, L. J., Refetoff, S.: Serum thyroglobulin in the management of patients with thyroid cancer. Arch. Intern. Med., 142:763, 1982.
6. Beierwaltes, W. H.: Are thyroid scans of value in evaluating thyroid nodules? *In* Thompson, N. W., and Vinik, A. I. (Eds.): Endocrine Surgery Update. New York, Grune & Stratton, 1983, p. 18.
7. Bochm, T. M., Burman, K. D., Barnes, S., and Wartofsky, I.: Lithium and iodine combination therapy for thyrotoxicosis. Acta Endocrinol., 94:174, 1980.
8. Burgi, H., Wimpfheimer, C., Burger, A., et al.: Changes of cirulating thyroxine, triiodothyronine and reverse triiodothyronine after radiographic contrast agents. J. Clin. Endocrinol. Metab., 43:1203, 1976.
9. Burke, G.: The thyrotrophin stimulation test. Ann. Intern. Med., 69:1127, 1968.
10. Burr, W. A., Ramsden, D. B., and Hoffenberg, R.: Hereditary abnormalities of thyroxine-binding globulin concentration. Q. J. Med., 49:295, 1980.
11. Clark, D. E., Moe, R. H., and Adams, E. E.: The rate of conversion of administered inorganic radioactive iodine into protein-bound iodine of plasma as an aid in the evaluation of thyroid function. Surgery, 26:331, 1949.
12. Clark, O. H., Greenspan, F. S., Coggs, G. C., and Goldman, L.: Evaluation of solitary cold thyroid nodules by echography and thermography. Am. J. Surg., 130:206, 1975.
13. Colacchio, T. A., LoGerfo, P., Colacchio, D. A., and Feind, C.: Radioiodine total body scan versus serum thyroglobulin levels in follow-up of patients with thyroid cancer. Surgery, 91:42, 1982.
14. Crill, G., Jr.: The danger of surgical dissemination of papillary carcinoma of the thyroid. Surg. Gynecol. Obstet., 102:161, 1956.
15. Crill, G., Jr., Esselstyn, C. B., and Hawk, W. A.: Needle biopsy in the diagnosis of thyroid nodules appearing after radiation. N. Engl. J. Med., 301:997, 1979.
16. DeCostre, P., Buhler, U., DeGrott, L. J., and Refetoff, S.: Diurnal rhythm in total serum thyroxine levels. Metabolism, 20:782, 1971.
17. DeGroot, P.: Endocrinology. Philadelphia. W. B. Saunders Company, 1989.
18. DeGroot, I. J., Rue, P., Robertson, M., et al.: Triiodothyronine stimulates nuclear RNA synthesis. Endocrinology, 101:1690, 1977.
19. Dumont, J. E., and Lamy, F.: The regulation of thyroid cell metabolism, function, growth, and differentiation. *In* De Visscher, M., (Ed.): The Thyroid Gland. New York, Raven Press, 1980, p. 153.
20. Engzell, U., Espoti, P. L., and Rubio, C.: Investigation on tumour spread in connection with aspiration biopsy. Acta Radiol. (Stockh.), 10:385, 1971.
21. Fisher, D. A., and Klein, A. H.: Thyroid development and disorders of thyroid function in the newborn. N. Engl. J. Med., 304:702, 1981.
22. Franklyn, J. A., Davis, J. R., Gammage, M. D., et al.: Amiodarone and thyroid hormone action. Clin. Endocrinol., 22:257, 1985.
23. Friedman, M. J., Okada, R. D., Ewy, G. A., et al.: Left ventricular systolic and diastolic function in hyperthyroidism. Am. Heart J., 104:1303, 1982.
24. Furmaniak, J., Nakajima, Y., Hashim, F. A., et al.: The TSH receptor: Structure and interaction with autoantibodies in thyroid disease. Acta Endocrinol., 115 (Suppl. 281):166, 1987.
25. Garnick, M. B., and Larsen, P. R.: Acute deficiency of thyroxine-binding globulin during L-asparaginase therapy. N. Engl. J. Med., 301:252, 1979.
26. Gluck, F. B., Nusynowitz, M. L., and Plymate, S.: Chronic lymphocytic thyroiditis, thyrotoxicosis, and low radioactive iodine uptake: Report of four cases. N. Engl. J. Med., 293:624, 1975.
27. Gordon, A. H., Gross, J., O'Connor, D., Pitt-Rivers, R.: Nature of circulating thyroid hormone-plasma protein complex. Nature, 169:19, 1952.
28. Hamburger, B., et al.: Fine needle aspiration biopsy of thyroid nodules, impact on thyroid practice and cost of care. Am. J. Med., 73:381, 1982.
29. Harsoulis, P., Leontsini, M., Economou, A., Gerasimidis, T., and Smbarounts, C.: Fine needle aspiration biopsy cytology in the diagnosis of thyroid cancer: Comparative study of 213 operated patients. Br. J. Surg., 73:461, 1986.
30. Hegedus, L., Perrild, H., Poulsen, L. R., et al.: The determination of thyroid volume by ultrasound and its relationship to body weight, age, and sex in normal subjects. J. Clin. Endocrinol. Metab., 56:260, 1983.
31. Hennemann, G. (Ed.): Thyroid Hormone Metabolism. New York, Marcel Dekker, 1986.
32. Hennessy, J. F., et al.: A comparison of pentagastrin injection and calcium infusion as provocative agents for the detection of medullary carcinoma of the thyroid. J. Clin. Endocrinol. Metabol., 39:487, 1974.
33. Hollander, C. S., Stevenson, C., Mitsuma, T., et al.: T_3 toxicosis in an iodide-deficient area. Lancet, 2:1276, 1972.
34. How, A. S. M., Khir, A. N., Bewsher, P. D.: The effect of atenolol on serum thyroid hormones in hyperthyroid patients. Clin. Endocrinol., 13:299, 1980.
35. Jackson, I. M. D.: Thyrotropin-releasing hormone. N. Engl. J. Med., 306:145, 1982.
36. Klein, I., and Levey, G. S.: New perspectives on thyroid hormone, catecholamines, and the heart. Am. J. Med., 76:167, 1984.
37. Larsen, P. R.: Thyroid-pituitary interaction: Feedback regulation of thyrotropin secretion by thyroid hormones. N. Engl. J. Med., 306:23, 1982.
38. Lehotay, D. C., Weight, C. W., Seltman, H. J., et al.: Free thyroxin: A comparison of direct and indirect methods and their diagnostic usefulness in nonthyroidal illness. Clin. Chem., 28:1826, 1982.
39. Lewis, B. S., Ehrenfeld, E. N., Lewis, N., et al.: Echocardiographic LV function in thyrotoxicosis. Am. Heart J., 97:460, 1979.
40. Lissitzky, S: Deiodination of iodotyrosines. In Reinwein, D., and Klein, E. (Eds.): Diminished Thyroid Hormone Formation: Possible Causes and Clinical Aspects. Stuttgart, Schattauer Verlag, 1982, pp. 49–61.

41. Lissitzky, S.: Thyroglobulin entering into molecular biology. J. Endocrinol. Invest., 7:65, 1984.
42. Lowhagen, T., Willems, J. S., Lundell, G., Sundblad, R., and Granberg, P. O.: Aspiration biopsy cytology in diagnosis of thyroid carcinoma. World J. Surg., 5:61, 1981.
43. McKerron, C. G., Scott, R. L., Asper, S. P., Levy, R. I.: Effects of clofibrate (Altromid S) on the thyroxine-binding capacity of thyroxine-binding globulin and free thyroxine. J. Clin. Endocrinol. Metab., 29:957, 1969.
44. Malkasian, G. D., Mayberry, W. E.: Serum total and free thyroxine and thyrotropin in normal and pregnant women, neonates, and women receiving progestogens. Am. J. Obstet. Gynecol., 108:1234, 1970.
45. Mariotti, S., Martino, E., Cupini, C., et al.: Low serum thyroglobulin as a clue to the diagnosis of thyrotoxicosis factitia. N. Engl. J. Med., 307:410, 1982.
46. Martino, E., Safran, M., Aghini-Lombardi, F., et al.: Environmental iodine intake and thyroid dysfunction during chronic amiodarone therapy. Ann. Intern. Med., 101:28, 1984.
47. Miller, M. J., Hamburger, J. B., and Kini, S.: Diagnosis of thyroid nodules: Use of fine needle aspiration and needle biopsy. J.A.M.A., 241:4812, 1979.
48. MIRD: Dose estimate report no. 5: Summary of current radiation dose estimates to humans from ^{123}I, ^{130}I, ^{131}I, and ^{132}I as sodium iodide. J. Nucl. Med., 16:857, 1975.
49. Morley, J. E.: Neuroendocrine control of thyrotropin secretion. Endocrinol. Rev., 2:396, 1981.
50. Narayan, P., Liaw, C. W., and Towle, H. C.: Rapid induction of a specific nuclear mRNA precursor by thyroid hormone. Proc. Natl. Acad. Sci. USA, 81:4687, 1984.
51. Nelson, J. C., Johnson, D. E., and Odell, W. D.: Serum TSH levels and the thyroidal response to TSH stimulation in patients with thyroid disease. Ann. Intern. Med., 76:47, 1972.
52. Nunez, J.: Iodination and thyroid hormone synthesis in the thyroid gland. In De Visscher, M. (Ed.): The Thyroid Gland. New York, Raven Press, 1980, pp. 39–59.
53. Oltman, J. E., and Friedman, S.: Protein-bound iodine in patients receiving perphenazine. J.A.M.A., 185:726, 1963.
54. Oppenheimer, J. H.: Role of plasma proteins in the binding, distribution, and metabolism of the thyroid hormones. N. Engl. J. Med., 278:1153, 1968.
55. Parisi, A. F., Hamilton, B. P., Thomas, C. N., et al.: The short cardiac preejection period: An index to thyrotoxicosis. Circulation, 49:900, 1974.
56. Refetoff, S., and Lever, E. G.: The value of serum thyroglobulin measurement in clinical practice. J.A.M.A., 250:2352, 1983.
57. Ruiz, M., Rajatanavin, R., Young, R. A., et al.: Familial dysalbuminemic hyperthyroxinemia: A syndrome that can be confused with thyrotoxicosis. N. Engl. J. Med., 306:635, 1982.
58. Sachson, R., Rosen, S. W., Cuatrecasas, P., et al.: Prolactin stimulation by thyrotropin-releasing hormone in a patient with isolated thyrotropin deficiency. N. Engl. J. Med., 287:972, 1972.
59. Sawin, C. T., Chopra, D., Azizi, F., et al.: The aging thyroid: Increased prevalence of elevated serum thyrotropin levels in the elderly. J.A.M.A., 242:247, 1979.
60. Segal, R. L., Rosenblatt, S., Eliasoph, I.: Endocrine exophthalmos during lithium therapy of manic-depressive disease. N. Engl. J. Med., 289:136, 1973.
61. Sterling, K., Refetoff, S., and Selenkow, H. A.: T$_3$ toxicosis: Thyrotoxicosis due to elevated serum triiodothyronine levels. J.A.M.A., 213:571, 1970.
62. Sterling, K., and Tabachnick, M.: Resin uptake of ^{131}I-triiodothyronine as a test of thyroid function. J. Clin. Endocrinol. Metab., 21:456, 1961.
63. Van den Hove-Vandenbroucke, M. F.: Secretion of thyroid hormones. In De Visscher, M. (Ed.): The Thyroid Gland. New York, Raven Press, 1980, pp. 61–79.
64. Van Herle, A. J., and Uller, R. P.: Elevated serum thyroglobulin: A marker of metastases in differentiated thyroid carcinoma. J. Clin. Invest., 56:272, 1975.
65. Van Herle, A. J., Vassart, G., and Dumont, J. E.: Control of thyroglobulin synthesis and secretion (II). N. Engl. J. Med., 301:307, 1979.
66. Walfish, P. G., Hazani, E., et al.: Combined ultrasound and needle aspiration biopsy in the assessment of hypofunctioning thyroid nodule. Ann. Intern. Med., 87:270, 1977.
67. Wang, C., Vickery, A. L., Jr., Maloof, F.: Needle biopsy of the thyroid. Surg. Gynecol. Obstet., 143:365, 1976.
68. Wartofsky, L., Dimond, R. C., Noel, G. L., et al.: Effect of acute increases in serum triiodothyronine on TSH and prolactin responses to TRH, and estimates of pituitary stores of TSH and in normal subjects and in patients with primary hypothyroidism. J. Clin. Endocrinol. Metab., 42:443, 1976.
69. Wartofsky, L., Ransil, B. J., and Ingbar, S. H.: Inhibition by iodine of the release of thyroxine from the thyroid glands of patients with thyrotoxicosis. J. Clin. Invest., 49:78, 1970.
70. Wehman, R., Rubenstein, H. A., Pufeat, M. A., and Nisula, B. C.: Extended clinical utility of a sensitive and reliable radioimmunoassay of thyroid-stimulating hormone. South. Med. J., 76:969, 1983.
71. Wells, S. A., Williams, M. D., Dilley, W. G., et al.: Early diagnosis and treatment of medullary thyroid carcinoma. Arch. Intern. Med., 145:1248, 1985.
72. Wenzel, K. W.: Pharmacological interference with in vitro tests of thyroid function. Metabolism, 30:717, 1981.
73. Westgren, U., Burger, A., Ingemansson, S., et al.: Blood levels of 3,5,3'-triiodothyronine and thyroxine: Differences between children, adults, and elderly subjects. Acta Med. Scand., 200:493, 1976.
74. Westgren, U., Melander, A., Ingemansson, S., et al.: Secretion of thyroxine, 3,5,3'-triiodothyronine and 3,3',5'-triiodothyronine in euthyroid man. Acta Endocrinol., 84:281, 1977.
75. Wilson, J. B., and Foster, D. W. (Ed.): Williams' Textbook of Endocrinology, 7th ed. Philadelphia, W. B. Saunders Company, 1985.
76. Witherspoon, L. R., Suler, S. E., Garcia, M. M., Zollinger, L. A.: An assessment of methods for the measurement of free thyroxine. J. Nucl. Med., 21:529, 1980.

III _____

HYPERTHYROIDISM

H. Kim Lyerly, M.D.

Hyperthyroidism is caused by increased levels of thyroid hormone with a loss of the normal feedback mechanism controlling the secretion of thyroid hormone. Common types of hyperthyroidism, including diffuse toxic goiter (Graves' disease, named after the Dublin physician Robert Graves [1796–1853] who described it in 1835 but known since its original description by Parry in 1786 and described by von Basedow in 1840) and toxic adenoma or toxic multinodular goiter (Plummer's disease).[61,69] Uncommon causes include thyrotoxicosis factitia, functioning metastatic thyroid carcinoma, trophoblastic tumors that secrete human chorionic gonadotropin having thyroid-stimulating properties, inappropriate secretion of thyrotropin by pituitary tumors, struma ovarii, iodide-induced hyperfunction and thyroiditis.[2,37,43,75,80,81]

One must distinguish between hyperthyroidism due to Graves' disease or due to single or multiple adenomas of the thyroid. Graves' disease is a systemic autoimmune syndrome with variable expression that includes goiter with hyperthyroidism, exophthalmos, pretibial myxedema, and acropachy.[45] Any or all of these features may be present since Graves' disease reflects disturbances of immunity not yet clearly defined. In contrast, an adenoma may be viewed as benign neoplasia associated with excess secretion of thyroid hormone and is thus a localized disease.

GRAVES' DISEASE

Epidemiology

Investigators at the Mayo Clinic established the incidence of Graves' disease in Rochester, Minnesota, and its neighboring county for the years 1935 to 1967. Approximately 36 females and 8 males per 100,000 of female and male population developed Graves' disease annually during that period.[26] The relative incidence of adenomatous hyperthyroidism and Graves' disease varies geographically, although precise assessment is complicated by differing diagnostic criteria. In a retrospective study of patients with hyperthyroidism in two clinics—one in Cardiff and the other in Toronto—the incidence of Graves' disease was 70 per cent; toxic multinodular goiter and toxic adenoma occurred more frequently in Cardiff (25 per cent versus 8 per cent), whereas thyroiditis predominated in Toronto (17 per cent versus 1 per cent).[3,91,100]

Pathogenesis

A hereditary component of Graves' disease has been recognized; one of the first analyses was by Bartels.[4] Further evidence of genetic factors associated with Graves' disease include the increased incidence of clinical thyroid disorders and thyroid antibodies in families with Graves' disease.[38] Graves' disease may be found with other autoimmune conditions in the same individual and within families. These conditions include Type I diabetes mellitus, Addison's disease, pernicious anemia, myasthenia gravis, rheumatoid arthritis, Sjögren's syndrome, vitiligo, idiopathic thrombocytopenic purpura, and chronic hepatitis.[21] There are also several pairs of homozygous twins, one of whom has Graves' disease and the other, Hashimoto's disease. There is an increased frequency of specific HLA antigens associated with Graves' disease, including B8 and DR3 in Caucasian populations, Bw35 in Japanese populations, and Bw46 in Chinese populations.[14,68,83]

Graves' classic article described six patients, all of whom were recently pregnant women. In one patient, he noted, "the emotional disturbances preceded the onset of tachycardia by several weeks." His observation is of interest because clinicians describing the disease have been consistently impressed with the emotional component. Parry's original description included a "psychic trigger" to the illness. The precise cause-and-effect relationship between emotional disturbance and thyrotoxicosis is not always easy to establish.[36] Susceptibility to the development of thyrotoxicosis in response to emotional upheaval appears to vary widely. It has not been possible to predict such susceptibility, but there is little doubt that thyrotoxicosis does not develop in the majority of those who experience emotional upheavals pronounced enough to produce thyrotoxicosis in susceptible individuals.[11,67,93]

Consumption of iodide in excess of that normally available and use of thyroid hormone have also been implicated as activators of hyperthyroidism in various reports.

Although the origin of Graves' disease remains obscure, current evidence suggests it is an autoimmune disorder caused by thyroid-stimulating immunoglobulins (TSI) that have been produced against an antigen in the thyroid. These polyclonal immunoglobulins appear to be directed to thyroid-stimulating hormone (TSH) receptors and can be detected by sensitive and specific radioreceptor assays. Graves' disease may also follow defective immune surveillance.[76]

In 1956, Adams and Purves made the initial observation that led, during the next 8 years, to the recognition that in many instances of Graves' disease there is a circulating thyroid-stimulating immunoglobulin (IgG) that can be measured by an *in vivo* mouse bioassay; this is the substance known as the long-acting thyroid stimulator (LATS).[1,50] It is now known not to be the cause of Graves' disease. As assays were developed to detect and quantify TSI, two basic assay procedures were developed, involving either inhibition of the binding of ^{125}I-TSH to its receptor or the direct stimulation of a thyroid preparation. TSH-binding inhibition (TBI) is nonspecific, in that there are many recognized instances in which the IgG that inhibits TSH binding may not stimulate the thyroid gland. Thyroid-stimulating immunoglobulin (TSI) determination is specific for thyroid stimulation; and although not all laboratories report identical results, TSI is present in over 90 per cent of patients with active Graves' disease and is now considered to be the probable cause of Graves' disease.[63] TSI levels are sensitive and specific and correlate with the activity of hyperthyroidism, having been reported to decrease to normal in approximately 50 per cent of patients treated with antithyroid medications or radioactive iodine and in 83 per cent after successful subtotal thyroidectomy.[102]

The pathogenesis of ophthalmopathy is less well understood than that of hyperthyroidism. Possibilities include a pituitary exophthalmos-producing substance (EPS), circulating antibodies that bind specifically to eye muscle antigens, circulating lymphocytes sensitized to an antigen in the extraocular tissue, and a complex of thyroglobulin and antithyroglobulin antibody formed in the blood that is bound by the external orbital muscles.[40,46,95,101]

Clinical Features

The symptoms and signs of hyperthyroidism are well known and depicted in Table 1. Graves' disease is usually not difficult to diagnose clinically, because the history of irritability, weight loss, heat intolerance, and emotional instability is quite distinctive when joined with the physical findings of goiter, exophthalmos, and other eye signs.[24]

The eye features of Graves' disease include a continuum from mere stare and lid lag to complete visual loss from corneal or optic nerve involvement.[98] Diagnostic difficulty arises when the ophthalmopathic process occurs in a patient who is euthyroid or who has minimal or unrecognized symptoms or signs of hyperthyroidism, especially if the eye involvement is unilateral; the diagnosis then becomes one of exclusion of all other potential causes, particularly retrobulbar space–occupying lesions.

Laboratory examinations are now available to confirm the diagnosis; however, no single laboratory test is consistently superior to the others, because occasionally a test may yield results in the diagnostic range in one thyrotoxic patient but remain in the upper limit of normal in another.[82] Hyperthyroidism is usually confirmed by measuring circulating thyroid hormone concentrations of thyroxine (T_4). Resin uptake of ^{125}I-triiodothyronine (T_3) is concomitantly assessed for determining the free T_4 index, since the increased total T_4 may reflect a familial increase in TBG or be secondary to estrogen, as in pregnancy or the use of oral contraceptives. Free T_4 may also be directly determined. Serum concentration of T_3 is almost always enhanced in conjunction with an elevated T_4; however, the frequency of hyperthyroidism due to excess T_3 with a normal concentration of T_4 is sufficient to warrant measurement of T_3 in all those in whom clinical suspicion of hyperthyroidism remains despite a normal value of T_4.

Measurement of thyroid uptake of radioiodine is not routinely performed, but may be useful if the T_3 and the T_4 are at the upper limit of normal. If the radioactive iodine uptake (RAIU) is elevated, it may be diagnostic for hyperthyroidism; however, if the patient has been taking appreciable amounts of iodine, either in the diet or in medication, the RAIU may be capriciously low. A thyroid suppression test can then be used in diagnosing hyperthyroidism, because autonomously functioning thyroid should not be suppressible. However, this test is now rarely indicated; and when a more elaborate test is required to establish a diagnosis of Graves' disease, a TRH test is employed. Patients with Graves' disease should have a flat response to the TRH test. An increase in serum TSH within 15 to

TABLE 1. Symptoms and Signs of Hyperthyroidism

Symptoms	Signs
Irritability, emotional lability	Tremor
Sweating, heat intolerance	Warm, moist skin
Palpitations	Tachycardia, atrial fibrillation
Shortness of breath	Heart failure
Fatigue, muscle weakness	Myopathy
Prominent eyes	Lid retraction, lid lag
Increased appetite, weight loss	
Diarrhea	
Goiter with or without a bruit	
Hair loss and pruritis	
Menstrual irregularities	

30 minutes of the intravenous injection of 100 to 400 *μ*g. of TRH indicates that the pituitary thyrotrope is not receiving an excess of thyroid hormone; i.e., there is no hyperthyroidism at that time.

Treatment

Hyperthyroidism in Graves' disease is managed with a number of strategies. The thyroid hypersecretion can be controlled by reducing the functional mass of thyroid tissue by surgical removal of a large part of the gland or by destruction of most of the gland with radioiodine. Thyrotoxicosis can also be controlled with antithyroid drugs to reduce the secretion of thyroid hormone, and by drugs that block beta-adrenergic receptors. Most methods cause a reduction of the net secretion of thyroid hormone to euthyroid levels, and features of each are summarized in Table 2. Because each method has specific advantages and specific contraindications, the surgeon must choose the most appropriate treatment for each individual with Graves' disease.

ANTITHYROID DRUGS. Thyrotoxicosis is effectively controlled by antithyroid drugs, and trials with antithyroid drugs are used in most patients to control signs and symptoms. Unfortunately, these agents may succeed in inducing a permanent remission in only a small minority of adults and in approximately 20 per cent of children (Fig. 1).[78,94] In addition, prolonged use of these agents is limited due to toxic side effects such as rash, liver dysfunction, neuritis, arthralgia, myalgia, lymphadenopathy, psychosis, and the occasional development of irreversible agranulocytosis (1 in 200).[15] Therefore, antithyroid drugs are used primarily in patients in whom a remission is expected, such as younger patients with small goiters, and are administered for 18 to 24 months for maintaining a euthyroid state.[29] Factors predicting remission include a small toxic goiter, mild elevation of serum T_4 and T_3, rapid remission with antithyroid medication, and decrease in gland size following initiation of therapy.[54,71]

Beta-receptor blockade, while effectively controlling some of the major effects of thyrotoxicosis, has not been effective as a sole means of therapy.[48,55] Beta-receptor blockade improves cardiovascular and central nervous complications such as the pulse rate, tremor, and anxiety, but hypermetabolism, and weight loss continue. Important roles for beta-blockade in the treatment of hyperthyroidism include treatment of tachycardia that has not resolved with adequate antithyroid drug therapy and treatment in conjunction with iodide for the preoperative management of patients allergic or resistant to antithyroid drugs. Contraindications include (1) significant myocardial disease, because beta receptor blockade may precipitate heart failure; and (2) asthma.

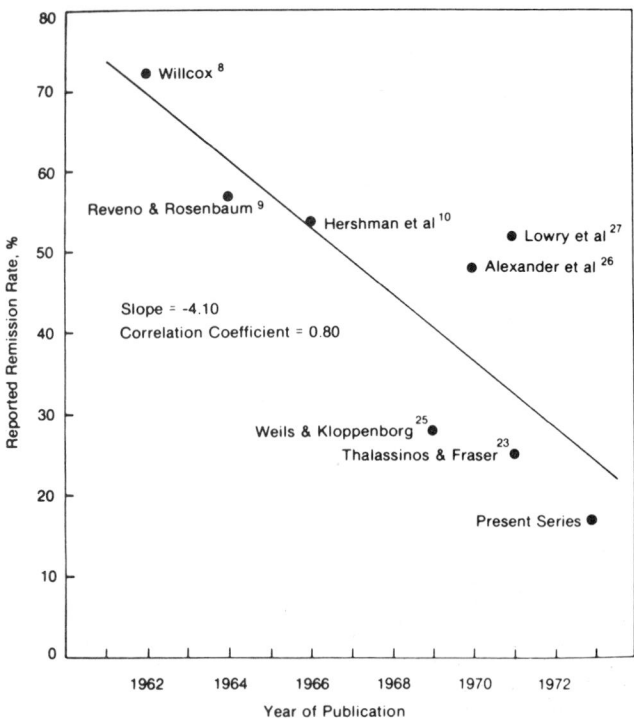

Figure 1. Declining incidence of remission rate as reported in publications from 1962 through 1973. (From Wartofsky, L.: Low remission after therapy for Graves' disease. Possible relation of dietary iodine with antithyroid therapy results. J.A.M.A., *226:*1083, 1973. Copyright 1973, American Medical Association, with permission. The superscript numbers in the figure identify the publications quoted in the article.)

RADIOIODINE. Radioiodine therapy may be considered as therapy for nearly all patients with thyrotoxicosis except newborns, pregnant females, or when it is precluded by a low iodine uptake.[58] Treatment is highly effective although hypothyroidism requiring thyroid replacement is common (Fig. 2). Potential complications of radiotherapy including thyroid carcinoma and congenital abnormalities in future offspring have not been demonstrated; however, there is still reluctance to treat children and women of childbearing age with radioiodine.[10,13,31,34,39,77,97]

SUBTOTAL THYROIDECTOMY. Although most patients with Graves' disease are treated with radioiodine or antithyroid drug therapy, a significant percentage of patients require surgical therapy. Indications for subtotal thyroidectomy for Graves' disease include (1) intolerance or noncompliance with antithyroid drug therapy and (2) contraindications to radioiodine therapy. Conditions in patients who undergo subtotal thyroidec-

TABLE 2. Management of Hyperthyroidism

	Antithyroid Drugs	Radioiodine	Subtotal Thyroidectomy
Success in control	Yes	Yes	Yes
Recurrence	Up to 72%	Up to 10%	Up to 10%
Side effects	Agranulocytosis Peripheral neuritis Hepatitis Arthralgia Myalgia Lymphadenopathy Psychosis	Permanent hypothyroidism in 40–70% at 10 years.	Postoperative hypothyroidism less than 15%. Rarely permanent hypoparathyroidism and damage to recurrent laryngeal nerve.
Contraindications	Allergy Toxicity	Pregnancy	

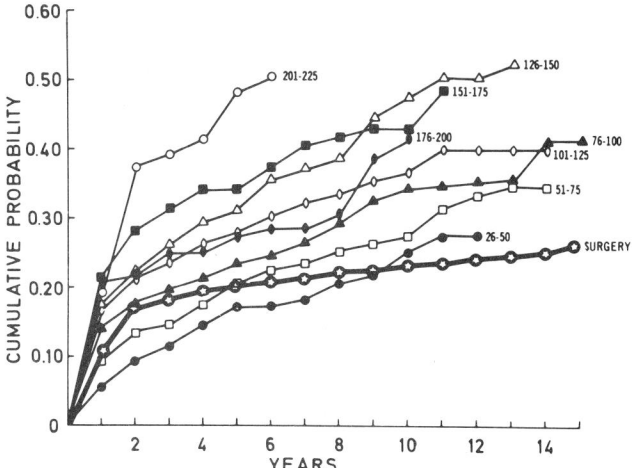

Figure 2. Experience of the Cooperative Thyrotoxicosis Therapy Follow-up Study initiated by the Bureau of Radiological Health of the United States Public Health Service. The 6000 patients included in this study had had no previous treatment for hyperthyroidism and received a single dose of ^{131}I; the number of patients in each dose category averaged 750. The cumulative probability of becoming hypothyroid is plotted on the ordinate and on the abscissa is the interval in years from the time of administration of [131]I. Radioiodine dosage is indicated on the chart from the lowest dose of 26 to 50 mCi. per estimated gram of thyroid to the highest dose of 201 to 225 mCi. per gm.; these assessments refer to millicuries of ^{131}I delivered to the thyroid and not to the oral dose. The heavy line shows the appearance of hypothyroidism following surgical treatment in 5200 patients. After the third year the probability of becoming hypothyroid if less than 125 mCi. per estimated gram of gland had been given was 2.3 per cent per year; from the second year after operation the average probability of becoming hypothyroid was 0.7 per cent. (From Becker, D. V., McConahey, W. M., Dobyns, B. M., et al.: The results of the Thyrotoxicosis Therapy Follow-up Study. *In* Fellinger, K., and Hofer, R. (Eds.): Further Advances in Thyroid Research. Vienna, Verlag der Wiener Medizinischen Akademie, 1971, p. 603.)

tomy include Graves' disease occurring in children and adolescents, in women who are potential mothers, in patients under the age of 20 unlikely to undergo remission because of a large goiter, and in those who do not experience a remission as indicated by persistent thyromegaly or the need for continued antithyroid medication beyond 1 or 2 years.[8,35,88]

Surgical management of hyperthyroidism is directed to removal of sufficient thyroid tissue to render the patient euthyroid and is accomplished in 95 to 97 per cent of patients. Control of hyperthyroidism is immediate, and the need for drug therapy and the genetic hazards associated with radioiodine therapy are avoided. Surgical risks are minimal but include recurrent laryngeal nerve injury, hypoparathyroidism, and permanent hypothyroidism.

PREOPERATIVE PREPARATION. Subtotal thyroidectomy should be performed after thyrotoxicosis is controlled medically. Restoration of euthyroidism improves nutritional status and provides the patient with normal homeostatic mechanisms and responses to the stress of operation. Propylthiouracil is used to inhibit thyroid hormone synthesis and limit peripheral conversion of T_4 to T_3. Absence of symptoms, a pulse below 100 beats per minute, and normal precordial activity indicate euthyroidism, which can be confirmed by a normal thyroid function test. The most common causes of failure to control hyperthyroidism are inadequate drug dose and lack of compliance; therefore, dosage should be adjusted if hyperthyroidism persists after 2 weeks of therapy. Agranulocytosis should be considered in patients with rash, fever, or sore throat, and a white blood count should be obtained. Drug therapy may be changed to methimazole if toxicity is present. Thyroidectomy performed immediately after control of thyrotoxicosis is associated with a risk of thyroid crisis, and it is preferable to wait approximately 2 months after a patient is euthyroid.

Thyrotoxic patients are usually treated with iodide and iodine, (Lugol's solution, which is a combination of potassium iodide, 10 mg. per 100 gm., and iodine, 5 gm. per 100 gm.), for 10 days before operation to decrease the vascularity of the gland.[52] Preoperative preparation with Lugol's solution without propylthiouracil to control the thyrotoxicosis is now uncommon, and operation must be scheduled before thyroid escape from iodine control occurs after 10 days of treatment. Thyroid hormone, rather than iodine, can also be used to reduce the vascularity of the gland treated with propylthiouracil, because adequate doses of thyroid hormone suppress the TSH increase associated with propylthiouracil and decrease the thyroid vascularity stimulated by that mechanism.

Beta-adrenergic blockade alone has been prescribed for preoperative preparation but is more commonly used as an adjunct to thioamides, particularly if the patient at the time of operation is not euthyroid. Propranolol may be used alone or in conjunction with Lugol's solution in the preparation of the patient who is intolerant of antithyroid drugs or is noncompliant.[22] Propranolol administered in conjunction with Lugol's solution allows a patient to be prepared for thyroidectomy within 10 to 14 days. Propranolol is continued throughout the operation and continued postoperatively for several days.

Preoperative evaluation of patients undergoing surgical treatment for thyrotoxicosis includes a thyroid scan and fine needle aspiration if there is asymmetry of the gland or reason to suspect neoplasm. Serum calcium and phosphorous levels are determined to indicate baseline parathyroid gland function. A chest film is helpful to evaluate possible mediastinal extension of the goiter. Laryngoscopy to assess vocal cord and recurrent laryngeal nerve function is advocated by some.

SURGICAL TECHNIQUE (Fig. 3). Knowledge of the anatomy of the thyroid gland and its surrounding structures is crucial for the surgeon performing thyroid procedures. The recurrent laryngeal nerve, the external motor branch of the superior laryngeal nerve, and the parathyroid glands are intimately located near the thyroidectomy dissection; therefore, awareness of the fine details of surgical anatomy is necessary if they are to be spared injury.

A curvilinear skin incision is made 2 cm. above the suprasternal notch and the clavicles, extending laterally to the sternocleidomastoid muscle. The platysma muscle is divided, and superior and inferior skin flaps are developed beneath it. The midline raphe between the strap muscles is divided longitudinally. The surgeon may elect to divide the strap muscles horizontally to improve surgical access in patients with large goiters. A plane is developed between the strap muscles and the capsule of the thyroid gland, avoiding the small branches of the thyroid veins present on the surface of the gland.

Subtotal resection is performed in cases of toxic multinodular goiter, nontoxic multinodular goiter, or Graves' disease. The principle of the resection is excision of the majority of each lobe, with division and ligation of the superior thyroid vessels, the middle thyroid vein, and the inferior thyroid vein. The anterolateral aspect of each lobe, the isthmus, and the pyramidal lobe, when present, are excised, and the thyroid remnant of each lobe should be approximately 3 to 4 gm. The inferior thyroid arteries, the recurrent laryngeal nerves, the external laryngeal branch of the superior laryngeal nerve, and the parathyroid glands are left intact.

The recurrent laryngeal nerve lies adjacent to the posteromedial aspect of the thyroid (Fig. 4). It contains the motor fibers innervating the abductor muscles of the true vocal cords. Immediate hoarseness occurs if it is divided unilaterally, and the voice never recovers it timbre and focus, even though effective phonation can eventually be achieved. Bilateral recurrent nerve injury with acute paralysis of both vocal cords may obstruct the airway and require emergency tracheostomy, since the true vocal cords are adducted. Permanent debilitating hoarseness follows bilateral recurrent nerve injury.

As important as sparing the recurrent laryngeal nerve from

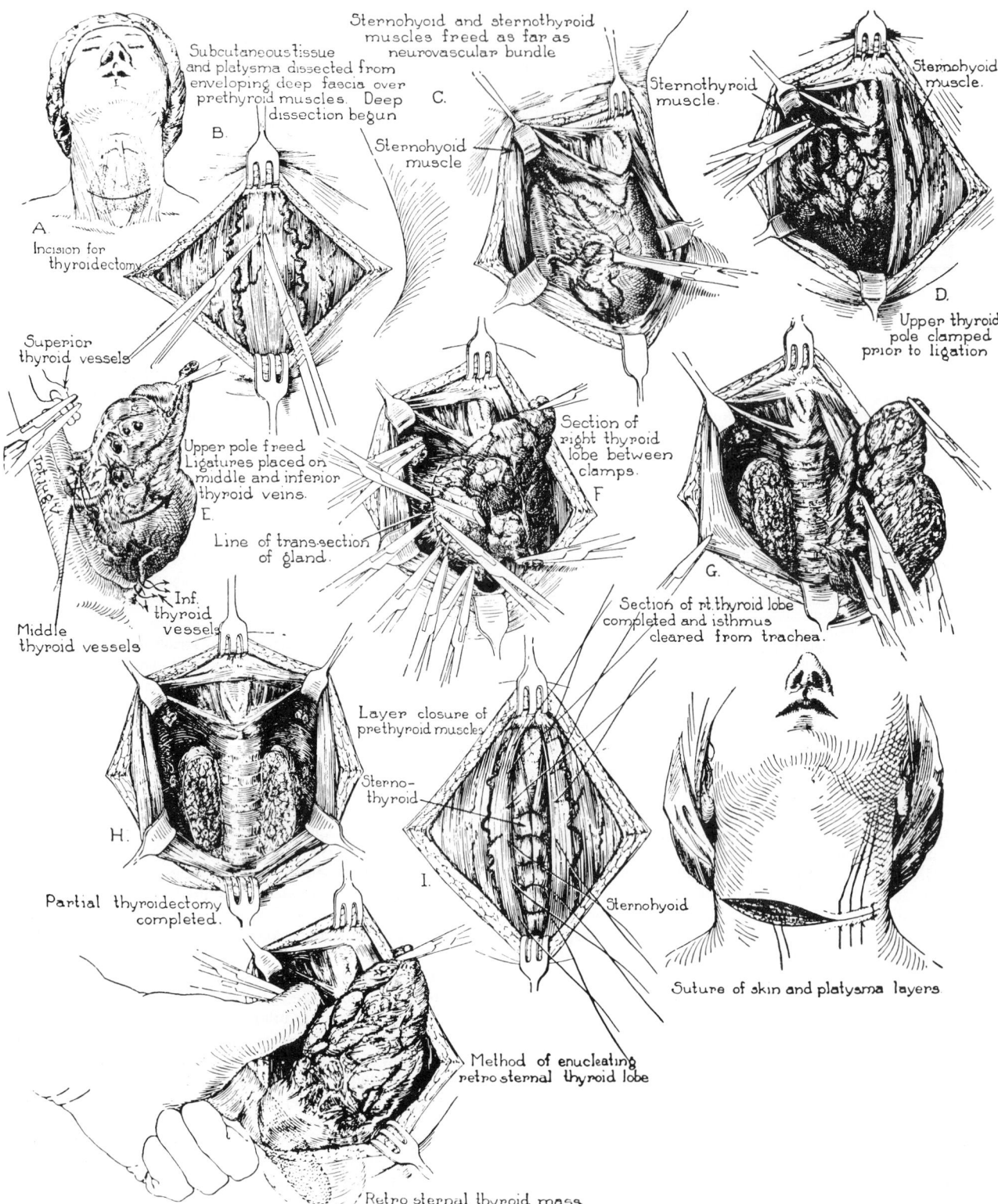

Figure 3. Subtotal thyroidectomy. (Modified from Mont Reid.) (From McVay, C. B.: Surgical Anatomy. 6th ed. Philadelphia, W. B. Saunders Company, 1984, p. 276.)

operative injury is preservation of the parathyroid glands. Normal parathyroid glands are a brownish yellow color, distinct from adjacent fat and from lymph node tissue, with which they are sometimes confused. Parathyroids and their blood supply are fragile and easily injured, and injury can lead to infarction of the glands.

The inferior parathyroids can usually be found by following the origin of their arterial blood supply from the inferior thyroid artery. There is less variability in the location of the superior parathyroids, which may be found posteromedial to the inferior portion of the superior pole of the thyroid gland. There are usually four parathyroid glands, but there may be as many as seven. The inferior parathyroids originate from the third pharyngeal pouch, from which the thymus also arises, and the inferior parathyroids may descend long distances into the anterior mediastinum, within or adjacent to the thymus gland.

The external branch of the superior laryngeal nerve is also vulnerable to injury during thyroidectomy. The consequences

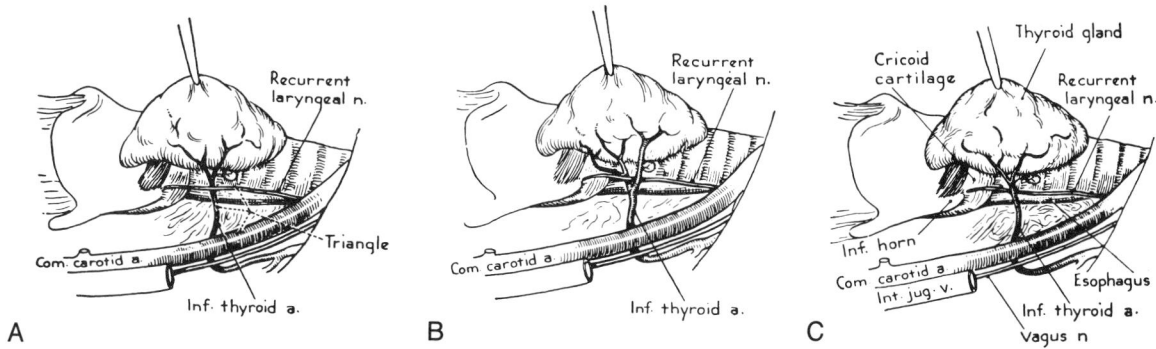

Figure 4. Relation of recurrent laryngeal nerve to the inferior thyroid artery in 86 dissections. *A*, Lateral, 15 times. *B*, Passing between arteries and branches, 6 times. *C*, Medial, 65 times. (From Simon, M. M.: Recurrent laryngeal nerve in thyroid surgery. Am. J. Surg., *60*:212, 1943.)

of superior laryngeal nerve injury are more subtle than those following recurrent laryngeal nerve injury. The external branch of the superior laryngeal nerve contains the motor fibers to the cricothyroid muscle, which functions to maintain the tone of the true vocal cord. When the cricothyroid is paralyzed, the voice loses its timbre and focus. Although many can compensate for such a tendency by spacing the conversational use of the voice, in some crucial situations such as in opera singers, this is not possible. Injuries to the superior laryngeal nerve have been overlooked in the past because voice fatigue and loss of timbre have been ascribed to tracheitis and chronic laryngitis following thyroidectomy.

Other complications of thyroid surgery include infection, bleeding, air embolism, and thyroid storm, which are rare in modern surgical practice.

RESULTS. Subtotal thyroidectomy effectively and immediately controls thyrotoxicosis. The incidence of recurrent disease is inversely related to the incidence of hypothyroidism and is 1 to 5 per cent.

Within 1 to 2 years, hypothyroidism may develop in 5 to 50 per cent of patients, with a slight additional increase in subsequent years. The incidence of hypothyroidism can be related to the estimated weight of the thyroid remnant. The incidence is 45 per cent or higher with a remnant weight of 2 to 4 gm., compared with an incidence of less than 20 per cent when a remnant of 8 to 10 gm. is left.[90] The autoimmune nature of the disease also influences the overall rate of hypothyroidism. Patients with high titers of antibodies and lymphocytic infiltration of the thyroid tissue are more likely to develop postoperative hypothyroidism. Postoperative hypothyroidism is effectively treated with thyroid replacement.

The mortality of the subtotal thyroidectomy with adequate preoperative preparation using modern anesthetic agents and performed by an experienced thyroid surgeon approaches zero. The associated morbidity, related primarily to damage to the recurrent laryngeal nerves and parathyroid glands, is estimated to be 0.5 to 3.0 per cent.[59] There is no reliable information concerning the incidence of damage to the external branch of the superior laryngeal nerve.

Thyroid Storm

An important feature of thyrotoxicosis treated by any modality is thyroid crisis or thyroid storm. Although it is usually milder with preoperative control of thyrotoxicosis, it continues to occur not only in patients after operation for thyrotoxicosis but also in those with undiscovered hyperthyroidism and in thyrotoxic patients with active infection.[19]

The manifestations of thyroid storm include hyperthermia, tachycardia, intense irritability, profuse sweating, hypertension, extreme anxiety, and eventual prostration, hypotension, and death—all of which are impressive adrenergic phenomena and each of which has been produced experimentally by either epinephrine or norepinephrine administration. It is pertinent that clinical hyperthyroidism and experimentally administered thyroid hormone excess both greatly augment many actions of catecholamines.

It is thought that thyroid storm is an acute adrenergic outburst in an organism tremendously sensitized to the effects of the adrenergic amines by thyroid hormone induction of additional myocardial catecholamine receptors. Sympatholytic treatment has been the most effective. Reserpine and guanethidine have been used to dissipate the thyroid crisis gently and effectively. Beta-adrenergic blockade is used to control the tachycardia, tremor, and anxiety.[16] Oxygen is delivered, as well as liberal amounts of intravenous glucose. Intravenous sodium or potassium iodide (1 to 2.5 gm.) is also recommended. Large doses of adrenal steroids have been advised, because cortisol breakdown is accentuated by excess thyroid hormone.

Ophthalmopathy

Although exophthalmos frequently occurs in hyperthyroidism, the majority of patients require no heroic measures for a condition that is self-limiting and one that to a variable degree regresses.[5,30] Treatment is directed to reducing periorbital swelling and safeguarding against infection. Malignant exophthalmos is fortunately rare, but sight may be endangered from optic nerve pressure or from corneal inflammatory involvement. Medical treatment includes high-dose systemic corticosteriod therapy or retrobulbar injection of a depot of corticosteroid.[85] Failure of medical therapy is a serious problem and is an indication for surgical intervention to relieve pressure on orbital contents.[18,65] Alternative therapy is irradiation of retro-orbital tissue, and radiotherapy combined with steroid administration may be especially useful. Rarely, cryosurgical destruction of the pituitary may be indicated.[93] Plasma exchange therapy and administration of immunosuppressive therapy such as cyclosporine or azathioprine have provided favorable results in some patients; however, these modalities must be considered investigational at present.[7,39,42,96] The infiltrative edema that occurs in the orbital tissues may also involve those in the periorbital region, and occasionally pretibial myxedema is an accompanying finding.

TOXIC ADENOMA

Hyperfunctioning adenomas are often first recognized on a thyroid scan, where they appear as hot nodules. Often the patient is still euthyroid, because even though the adenoma is hypersecreting independently of the pituitary feedback system, suppression of thyroid secretion from the normal gland maintains a physiologic net secretion rate of thyroid hormone. Only when the normal gland can no longer be suppressed and the adenoma continues to increase its secretion rate of thyroid hormone does laboratory or clinical evidence of hyperthyroidism appear.[73]

Clinical Features

The clinical features of hyperthyroidism due to toxic adenoma may be compared with those due to Graves' disease, and many points of difference are discernible. In adenomatous disease these include a slower rate of recognition of symptoms; the older age group affected, especially in multinodular disease; and the more common predominance of cardiac symptoms. However, the only clinical aspect that clearly differentiates one from the other is the presence of ophthalmopathy, pretibial myxedema, or acropachy in patients with Graves' disease. The correct diagnosis may rest with the character of the goiter. When there is a toxic adenoma, paranodular tissue and the contralateral lobe are functionally suppressed and are usually minimally, if at all, palpable. If the adenoma has developed in a multinodular goiter or if there are multiple adenomas, the clinical character of the goiter may be no different from that of the diffuse hyperplasia of Graves' disease being superimposed on preceding irregular enlargement. A diagnosis of toxic adenoma becomes unlikely if there is a family history of Hashimoto's or Graves' disease, extrathyroidal features of Graves' disease, or thyroid antibodies in the blood.

The diagnosis is suggested by thyroid scanning after administration of radioiodine; and when the diagnosis is in doubt, a suppression test can be useful. The autonomous nodule has persistent elevated RAIU, whereas normal thyroid tissue RAIU is suppressed. Confirmation of the diagnosis is commonly performed by a repeat uptake and scan after administration of TSH. In the presence of an autonomous nodule, TSH stimulates suppressed thyroid tissue to accumulate radioiodine, so that the entire thyroid, including the autonomous nodule, is visualized on the scan.

Treatment

There is no evidence that drugs such as propylthiouracil exert a direct, permanent effect on thyroid function so that cessation of therapy inevitably is followed by relapse. Ablation of the neoplasm or neoplasms is the only course to be offered these patients.[51] Thyroid nodules of various forms require a clear understanding for treatment, and these features are discussed in detail elsewhere. For purposes of control of hyperthyroidism, eventual or achieved, surgical excision of the thyroid lobe containing the hyperfunctioning adenoma is simple, safe, and effective. If the patient is clinically hyperthyroid, preoperative control with antithyroid drugs, using the same principles as previously discussed, is wise. With radioactive iodine therapy for hot nodules, there is an unacceptably high risk of permanent hypothyroidism. Whichever form of ablation is chosen, the para-adenoma tissue will become active and maintain the patient in an euthyroid state, at least for several years.

APATHETIC HYPERTHYROIDISM

Attention should be directed to various forms of hyperthyroidism in elderly patients in whom the diagnosis is not suspected because of the insidious onset of the disease, which can be quite atypical. Diffuse myopathy, myocardial failure, and cachexia without adequate explanation may all be found to have occult hyperthyroidism as their basis, especially in older patients. The various thyroid function tests may be invaluable in establishing the diagnosis. The principles of treatment are the same as in Graves' disease, and it is expected because of their age that more patients will be found suitable for radioactive iodine treatment.

HYPERTHYROIDISM IN PREGNANCY

There is an increase in thyroid-binding globulin in pregnancy, and for this reason, serum T_4 levels tend to be elevated.

Awareness of this and measurement of both serum T_3 and displacement of resin-bound T_3 are therefore most helpful in the establishment of the diagnosis of hyperthyroidism in the pregnant patient.[28] The management of such patients with hyperthyroidism is controversial. Radioactive iodine is absolutely contraindicated because destruction of the fetal thyroid would follow its use. Antithyroid drugs in conventional doses have a risk of development of fetal goiter that may obstruct the fetal airway at birth. Minimal-dose antithyroid drug therapy reduces this risk.[56] The cause-and-effect relationship of mental retardation in the newborn and antithyroid medication in the mother has been suggested but is difficult to substantiate.[12]

In the middle trimester of pregnancy, subtotal thyroidectomy after a short course of antithyroid drugs and propranolol has been effective. So far as can be determined, the risks to the mother and to the fetus from the operation are comparable to those of nonoperative treatment.

SELECTED REFERENCES

Burrow, T. N.: The management of thyrotoxicosis in pregnancy. N. Engl. J. Med., 313:562, 1985.
A recent review of the management of thyrotoxicosis in pregnancy.

Clark, O. H.: Surgical Endocrinology of the Thyroid and Parathyroid Glands. St. Louis, C. V. Mosby Company, 1985.
An outstanding text detailing preoperative evaluation as well as operative technique. It should be read by all serious students of thyroid surgery.

Cooper, D. S.: Antithyroid drugs. N. Engl. J. Med., 311:1353, 1984.
A review of antithyroid medications.

Harada, T., Shimaoka, K., Mimura, T., and Ito, K.: Current management of Graves' Disease. Surg. Clin. North Am., 67:299, 1987.
A recent review of the medical and surgical options in the management of Graves' disease. The entire volume is dedicated to endocrine surgery.

McKenzie, J. M., and Zakarija, M.: Hyperthyroidism. *In* DeGroot, L. J. (Ed.): Endocrinology, 2nd ed. Philadelphia, W. B. Saunders Company, 1989.
A chapter in a multivolume text concerning hyperthyroidism. It includes clinical and experimental details as well as an extensive bibliography.

Thomas, C. G., and Croom, R. D.: Current management of the patient with autonomously functioning nodular goiter. Surg. Clin. North Am., 67:315, 1987.
A review of the preoperative evaluation and therapy for autonomously functioning nodular goiter. Case reports illustrate specific management features.

REFERENCES

1. Adams, D. D., and Purvis, H. D.: Abnormal responses in the assays of thyrotrophin. Proc. Univ. Otago Med. Sch., 34:11, 1956.
2. Amir, S. M.: Human chorionic gonadotropin: A negligible human thyroid stimulator. *In* Ingbar, S. H., and Braverman, L. E. (Eds.): The Thyroid, 5th ed. Philadelphia, J. B. Lippincott Company, 1986, p. 1088.
3. Barker, D. J. P., and Phillips, D. I. W.: Current incidence of thyrotoxicosis and past prevalence of goitre in 12 British towns. Lancet, 2:567, 1984.
4. Bartels, E. D.: Heredity in Graves' Disease. Copenhagen, Monksgaard, 1941.
5. Beahrs, O. H., Ryan, R. F., et al.: Surgical thyroidectomy in the management of exophthalmic goiter. Arch. Surg., 96:512, 1968.
6. Becker, D. V., McConahey, W. M., Dobyns, B. M., et al.: The results of radioiodine treatment of hyperthyroidism: A preliminary report of the thyrotoxicosis therapy follow-up study. *In* Fellinger, K., and Hofer, R. (Eds.): Further Advances in Thyroid Research. Vienna, Verlag der Wiener Medizinischen Akademie, 1971, p. 603.
7. Brabant, G., Peter, H., Schwarzrock, R., et al.: Cyclosporin in infiltrative eye disease. Lancet, 1:515, 1984.
8. Bradley, E. I., DiGirolamo, M., and Tarcan, Y.: Modified subtotal thyroidectomy in the management of Graves' disease. Surgery, 87:623, 1980.
9. Braverman, L. E., Woeber, K. A., and Ingbar, S. H.: Induction of myxedema by iodide in patients euthyroid after radioiodine or surgical treatment of diffuse toxic goiter. N. Engl. J. Med., 281:816, 1969.
10. Bremner, W. F., McDougall, I. R., and Greig, W. R.: Results of treating 297 thyrotoxic patients with ^{125}I. Lancet, 2:281, 1973.
11. Burger, A., Dinichert, D., Nicod, P., et al.: Effects of amiodarone on serum triiodothyronine, reverse triiodothyronine, thyroxine and thyrotropin. J. Clin. Invest., 58:255, 1976.
12. Burrow, T. N.: The management of thyrotoxicosis in pregnancy. N. Engl. J. Med., 313:562, 1985.
13. Cevalos, J. L., Hagen, G. A., et al.: Low dosage ^{131}I therapy of thyrotoxicosis (diffuse goiters): A five-year follow-up study. N. Engl. J. Med., 290:141, 1974.
14. Chan, S. H., Yeo, P. P. B., Lui, K. F., et al.: HLA and thyrotoxicosis (Graves' disease) in Chinese. Tissue Antigens, 12:109, 1978.

15. Cooper, D. S.: Antithyroid drugs. N. Engl. J. Med., *311*:1353, 1984.
16. Das, G., and Krieger, M.: Treatment of thyrotoxic storm with intravenous administration of propranolol. Ann. Intern. Med., *70*:985, 1969.
17. DeGroot, L. J., and Paloyan, E.: Thyroid carcinoma and radiation: A Chicago endemic. J.A.M.A., *225*:487, 1973.
18. DeSanto, L. W.: Surgical palliation of ophthalmopathy of Graves' disease: Transantral approach. Mayo Clin. Proc., *47*:989, 1972.
19. Dobyns, B. M.: Prevention and management of hyperthyroid storm. World J. Surg., *2*:293, 1978.
20. Durham, C. F., and Harrison, T. S.: The surgical anatomy of the superior laryngeal nerve. Surg. Gynecol. Obstet., *118*:38, 1964.
21. Faird, N. R.: Immunogenetics of autoimmune thyroid disorders. Endocrinol. Metab. Clin. North Am., *16*:229, 1987.
22. Feek, C. M., Sawyers, J. S. A., Irvine, W. J., Beckett, G. J., Ratcliffe, W. A., and Toft, A. D.: Combination of potassium iodide and propranolol in preparation of patients with Graves' disease for thyroid surgery. N. Engl. J. Med., *302*:883, 1980.
23. Fish, L. H., Schwartz, H. L., Cavanaugh, M. D., et al.: Replacement dose, metabolism, and bioavailability of levothyroxine in the treatment of hypothyroidism. N. Engl. J. Med., *316*:764, 1987.
24. Forfar, J. C., and Toft, A. D.: Thyrotoxic atrial fibrillation: An underdiagnosed condition? Br. Med. J., *285*:909, 1982.
25. Friedman, M. J., Okada, R. D., Ewy, G. A., et al.: Left ventricular systolic and diastolic function in hyperthyroidism. Am. Heart J., *104*:1303, 1982.
26. Furszyfer, J., Kurland, L. T., McConahey, W. M., et al.: Epidemiologic aspects of Hashimoto's thyroiditis and Graves' disease in Rochester, Minnesota (1935–1967), with special reference to temporal trends. Metabolism, *21*:197, 1972.
27. Goldstein, R., Hart, I. R.: Follow-up of solitary autonomous thyroid nodules treated with ^{131}I. N. Engl. J. Med., *309*:1473, 1983.
28. Goluboff, L. G., Sisson, J. L., and Hamburger, J. I.: Hyperthyroidism associated with pregnancy. Obstet. Gynecol., *44*:107, 1974.
29. Greer, M. A., Kammer, H., and Bouman, D. J.: Short-term antithyroid drug therapy for the thyrotoxicosis of Graves' disease. N. Engl. J. Med., *297*:173, 1977.
30. Grove, A. S., Jr.: Evaluation of exophthalmos. N. Engl. J. Med., *292*:1005, 1975.
31. Halnan, K. E.: Risks from radioiodine treatment of thyrotoxicosis. Br. Med. J., *287*:1821, 1983.
32. Halsted, W. S.: The operative story of goiter. Johns Hopkins Hosp. Rep., *19*:71, 1920. Reprinted in Halsted, W. S.: Surgical Papers. Vol. II. Baltimore, The Johns Hopkins Press, 1928, p. 257.
33. Halsted, W. S., and Evans, H. M.: The parathyroid glandules: Their blood supply and preservation in operations upon the thyroid gland. Ann. Surg., *46*:489, 1907.
34. Hayek, A., Chapman, E. M., and Crawford, J. D.: Long term results of I-131 treatment of thyrotoxicosis in children. N. Engl. J. Med., *283*:949, 1970.
35. Heimann, P.: Should hyperthyroidism be treated by surgery? World J. Surg., *2*:281, 1978.
36. Hermann, H., and Quarton, G.: Psychological changes and psychogenesis in thyroid hormone disorders. J. Clin. Endocrinol. Metab., *25*:327, 1965.
37. Hershman, J. M., and Higgins, H. P.: Hydatidiform mole — A cause of clinical hyperthyroidism. N. Engl. J. Med., *284*:573, 1971.
38. Howell-Evans, A. W., Woodrow, J. C., McDougall, C. D. D., et al.: Antibodies in the families of thyrotoxic patients. Lancet, *1*:636, 1967.
39. Howlett, T. A., Lawton, N. F., Fells, P., et al.: Deterioration of severe Graves' ophthalmopathy during cyclosporin treatment. Lancet, *2*:1101, 1984.
40. Jacobson, D. H., and Gorman, C. A.: Endocrine ophthalmopathy: Current ideas concerning etiology, pathogenesis and treatment. Endocrinol. Rev., *5*:200, 1984.
41. Kark, A. F., Kissin, M. W., Auerbach, R., and Meikle, M.: Voice changes after thyroidectomy: Role of the external laryngeal nerve. Br. Med. J., *289*:1412, 1984.
42. Kelly, W., Longson, D., Smithand, D., et al.: An evaluation of plasma exchange for Graves' ophthalmopathy. Clin. Endocrinol., *18*:485, 1983.
43. Kempers, R. D., Dockerty, M. B., Hoffman, D. L., et al.: Struma ovarii — Ascitic, hyperthyroid and asymptomatic syndromes. Ann. Intern. Med., *72*:883, 1970.
44. Konno, N.: The relationship between the timing of the Korotkoff sound (QKd) and the serum thyroid hormone concentrations. Folia Endocrinol. Jpn., *52*:158, 1976.
45. Kriss, J. P.: Pathogenesis and treatment of pretibial myxedema. Endocrinol. Metab. Clin. North Am., *16*:409, 1987.
46. Kriss, J. P., Knoishi, J., and Herman, M.: Studies on the pathogenesis of Graves' ophthalmopathy (with some related observations regarding therapy). Recent Prog. Horm. Res., *31*:533, 1975.
47. Lahey, F. H.: Routine dissection and demonstration of recurrent laryngeal nerve in subtotal thyroidectomy. Surg. Gynecol. Obstet., *66*:775, 1938.
48. Lee, T. L., Coffey, R. J., Mackin, J., et al.: The use of propranolol in surgical treatment of thyrotoxic patients. Ann. Surg., *177*:643, 1975.
49. Lewis, B. S., Ehrenfeld, E. N., Lewis, N., et al.: Echocardiographic LV function in thyrotoxicosis. Am. Heart J., *76*:460, 1979.
50. Lipman, L. M., Green, D. E., Snyder, N. J., et al.: Relationship of long-acting thyroid stimulator to the clinical features and course of Graves' disease. Am. J. Med., *43*:486, 1967.
51. Livadas, D., Psarras, A., and Koutras, A.: Malignant cold thyroid nodules in hyperthyroidism. Br. J. Surg., *33*:726, 1976.
52. Marigold, J. H., Morgan, A. K., Earle, D. J., et al.: Lugol's iodine: Its effect on thyroid blood flow in patients with thyrotoxicosis. Br. J. Surg., *72*:45, 1985.
53. Martino, E., Aghini-Lombardi, F., Mariotti, S., et al.: Treatment of amiodarone associated thyrotoxicosis by simultaneous administration of potassium perchlorate and methimazole. J. Endocrinol. Invest., *9*:201, 1986.
54. McGregor, A. M., Rees-Smith, B., Hall, R., et al.: Prediction of relapse in hyperthyroid Graves' disease. Lancet, *1*:1101, 1980.
55. McLarty, D. G., Brownlie, B. E. W., Alexander, W. D., et al.: Remission of thyrotoxicosis during treatment with propranolol. Br. Med. J., *2*:332, 1973.
56. Momotani, N., Noh, J., Oyanagi, H., et al.: Antithyroid drug therapy for Graves disease during pregnancy: Optimal regimen for fetal thyroid status. N. Engl. J. Med., *315*:24, 1986.
57. Moosman, D. A., and DeWeese, M. S.: The external laryngeal nerve as related to thyroidectomy. Surg. Gynecol. Obstet., *127*:1011, 1968.
58. Nofal, M. M., Beierwaltes, W. H., and Patno, M. E.: Treatment of hyperthyroidism with sodium iodide I-131. J.A.M.A., *197*:605, 1966.
59. Parfitt, A. M.: The incidence of hypoparathyroidism tetany after thyroid operations: Relationship to age, extent of resection and surgical experience. Med. J. Aust., *1*:1103, 1971.
60. Parisi, A. F., Hamilton, B. P., Thomas, C. N., et al.: The short cardiac preejection period: An index to thyrotoxicosis. Circulation, *49*:900, 1974.
61. Parry, C. H.: Collections from the Unpublished Medical Papers of the Late Caleb Hillier Parry, M.D., F.R.S. Vol. 2. London, Underwoods, 1825, p. 111.
62. Peters, L. L., and Gardner, R. J.: Repair of recurrent laryngeal nerve injury. Surgery, *71*:865, 1972.
63. Rapoport, B., Greenspan, F. S., Filetti, S., et al.: Clinical experience with a human thyroid cell bioassay for thyroid stimulating immunoglobulin. J. Clin. Endocrinol. Metab., *58*:332, 1984.
64. Riddell, V. H.: Injury to recurrent laryngeal nerves during thyroidectomy. Lancet, *2*:638, 1956.
65. Riley, F. C.: Surgical management of ophthalmopathy in Graves' disease: Transfrontal orbital decompression. Mayo Clin. Proc., *47*:986, 1972.
66. Rodbard, D., Fujita, T., Rodbard, S.: Estimation of thyroid function by timing the arterial sounds. J.A.M.A., *201*:206, 1967.
67. Safran, M., Paul, T. L., Roti, E., and Braverman, L. E.: Environmental factors affecting autoimmune thyroid disease. Endocrinol. Metab. Clin. North Am., *16*:327, 1987.
68. Sasazuki, T., Kohno, Y., Iwamoro, L., et al.: HLA B-D haplotypes associated with autoimmune disease in Japanese populations. Tissue Antigens, *10*:218, 1977.
69. Sattler, H.: Basedow's Disease. New York, Grune & Stratton, 1952, p. 393.
70. Sawin, C. T., Surks, M. I., London, M., et al.: Oral thyroxine: Variation in biologic action and tablet content. Ann. Intern. Med., *100*:641, 1984.
71. Schernthaner, G., Schleurener, H., Kotulla, P., et al.: Prediction of relapse of long term remission in hyperthyroid Graves' disease. Lancet, *2*:323, 1981.
72. Shapiro, S. J., Friedman, N. B., et al.: Incidence of thyroid carcinoma in Graves' disease. Cancer, *26*:1261, 1970.
73. Silverstein, G. E., Burke, G., and Cogan, R.: The natural history of the autonomous hyperfunctioning thyroid nodule. Ann. Intern. Med., *67*:539, 1967.
74. Simon, M. M.: Recurrent laryngeal nerve in thyroid surgery. Am. J. Surg., *60*:212, 1943.
75. Smallridge, R. C., and Smith, C. E.: Hyperthyroidism due to thyrotropin-secreting pituitary tumors. Arch. Intern. Med., *143*:503, 1983.
76. Smith, B. R., and Hall, R.: Thyroid stimulating immunoglobulins in Graves' disease. Lancet, *2*:427, 1974.
77. Smith, R. N., Munro, D. S., and Wilson, G. M.: Two clinical trials of different doses of radio-iodine ^{131}I in the treatment of thyrotoxicosis. *In* Fellinger, K., and Hofer, R. (Eds.): Further Advances in Thyroid Research. Vienna, Verlag der Wiener Medizinischen Akademie, 1971, p. 611.
78. Solomon, B. L., Evaul, J. E., Burman, K. D., et al.: Remission rates with antithyroid drug therapy: Continuing influence of iodine intake. Ann. Intern. Med., *107*:510, 1987.
79. Spencer, C. A., Lai-Rosenfield, A. O., Guttler, R. B., et al.: Thyrotropin secretion in thyrotoxic and thyroxine-treated patients: Assessment by a sensitive immunoezymometric assay. J. Clin. Endocrinol. Metab., *63*:349, 1986.
80. Steigbigel, N. H., Oppenheim, J. J., Fishman, L. M., et al.: Metastatic embryonal carcinoma of the testis associated with elevated plasma TSH-like activity and hyperthyroidism. N. Engl. J. Med., *271*:345, 1964.
81. Sung, L. C., Cavalieri, R. R.: T_3 thyrotoxicosis due to metastatic thyroid carcinoma. J. Clin. Endocrinol. Metab., *36*:215, 1973.
82. Tamai, H., Nakagawa, T., Ohsako, N., et al.: Changes in thyroid functions in patients with euthyroid Graves' disease. J. Clin. Endocrinol. Metab., *50*:1089, 1980.
83. Tamai, H., Uno, H., Hirota, Y., et al.: Immunogenetics of Hashimoto's and Graves' diseases. J. Clin. Endocrinol. Metab., *60*:62, 1985.
84. Temple, R., Berman, M., Carlson, H. E., et al.: The use of lithium in Graves' disease. Mayo Clin. Proc., *47*:872, 1972.
85. Thomas, I. D., and Hart, J. K.: Retrobulbar repository corticosteroid therapy in thyroid ophthalmopathy. Med. J. Aust., *2*:484, 1974.
86. Thompson, N. W., and Harness, J. K.: Complications of total thyroidectomy for carcinoma. Surg. Gynecol. Obstet., *131*:861, 1970.
87. Thompson, N. W., Olsen, W. R., and Hoffman, G. L.: The continuing development of the technique of thyroidectomy. Surgery, *73*:913, 1973.
88. Toft, A. D.: Thyroid surgery for Graves' disease. Br. Med. J., *286*:740, 1983.
89. Toft, A. D.: Thyroid enlargement. Br. Med. J., *290*:1066, 1985.

90. Toft, A. D., Irvine, W. J., Sinclair, I., McIntosh, D., Seth J., and Cameron, E. H. D.: Thyroid function after surgical treatment of thyrotoxicosis. N. Engl. J. Med., *298*:643, 1978.
91. Tunbridge, W. M. G., Evered, D. C., Hall, R., et al.: The spectrum of thyroid disease in a community: The Whickham Survey. Clin. Endocrinol., *7*:481, 1977.
92. Vagenakis, A. G., Wang, C.-A., Burger, A., et al.: Iodide-induced thyrotoxicosis in Boston. N. Engl. J. Med., *287*:523, 1972.
93. Van Onwerkerk, B. M., Wijugaarde, R., Hennemann, G., et al.: Radiotherapy of severe ophthalmic Graves' disease. J. Endocrinol. Invest., *8*:241, 1985.
94. Wartofsky, L.: Low remission after therapy for Graves' disease: Possible relation to dietary iodine with antithyroid therapy results. J.A.M.A., *226*:1083, 1973.
95. Warthin, A. S.: The constitutional entity of exophthalmic goiter and so-called toxic adenoma. Ann. Intern. Med., *2*:553, 1928.

96. Weetman, A. P., McGregor, A. M., Ludgate, M., et al.: Cyclosporin improves Graves' ophthalmopathy. Lancet, *2*:486, 1983.
97. Weidinger, P., Johnson, P. M., Werner, S. C.: Five years' experience with iodine 125 therapy of Graves' disease. Lancet, *2*:74, 1974.
98. Werner, S. C.: Classification of the eye changes of Graves disease. J. Clin. Endocrinol. Metab., *29*:982, 1969.
99. Williams, A. F.: Recurrent nerve lesions. Surgery, *43*:435, 1958.
100. Williams, I., Ankrett, V. O., Lazarus, J. H., et al.: Aetiology of hyperthyroidism in Canada and Wales. J. Epidemiol. Commun. Health, *37*:245, 1983.
101. Winand, R. J., Kohn, L. D.: The binding of {3H} thyrotropin and a 3H-labeled exophthalmogenic factor by plasma membranes of retroorbital tissue. Proc. Natl. Acad. Sci. USA, *69*:1711, 1972.
102. Zakarija, M., McKenzie, J. M., Banovac, K.: Clinical significance of assay of thyroid-stimulating antibody in Graves' disease. Ann. Intern. Med., *93*:28, 1980.

IV

THYROIDITIS

H. Kim Lyerly, M.D.

The term *thyroiditis* refers to the infiltration of the thyroid gland by inflammatory cells, caused by a diverse group of infectious and inflammatory disorders. Inflammation of the thyroid may be organ-specific or part of a multisystem process and may be acute and self-limiting or chronic and progressive.

AUTOIMMUNE THYROIDITIS

The term *autoimmune thyroid disease* defines a group of conditions characterized by the presence of circulating thyroid antibodies and immunologically competent cells capable of reacting with certain thyroid constituents.[16] However, it does not imply that these antibodies or cells necessarily have any causal relationship to the thyroid disease. These autoimmune thyroid diseases are Hashimoto's disease (lymphocytic thyroiditis), primary myxedema, and juvenile, fibrous, focal, and painless varieties of thyroiditis.

Hashimoto's Disease (Lymphocytic Thyroiditis)

Hashimoto's disease was first described in Japan by Hawkin Hashimoto in 1912 and is the most well known of the immunologic thyroid diseases. It is the most common cause of goitrous hypothyroidism in adults and sporadic goiter in children.[25] The incidence is 0.3 to 1.5 cases per 1000 population per year and is 10 to 15 times more common in women than men, with the highest incidence in the age group of 30 to 50 years.[8]

In Hashimoto's disease, thyroid tissue damaged by immunologic factors is replaced by lymphocytes, plasma cells, and fibrosis.[5] Antithyroid antibodies in the serum of patients with Hashimoto's disease were first discovered in 1957 by Doniach and Roitt. These antibodies have subsequently been demonstrated to be directed against elements in the thyroid cell or colloid such as thyroglobulin, a second colloid antigen (other than thyroglobulin), microsomes, and perhaps to a cell surface antigen.[3,6,18,29] No antibodies to the TSH receptor of the cell surface (as seen in Graves' disease) have been associated with Hashimoto's disease.[20]

Patients with Hashimoto's disease usually have detectable antithyroid antibodies at some time in the course of their disease. The important cytotoxic effects of microsomal antibodies are increasingly recognized, and further studies on the exact prevalence of growth-modulating immunoglobulins will undoubtedly establish their role. T-cell-mediated factors may also be important, as it has been observed that lymphocytes from patients with Hashimoto's disease secrete lymphokines and undergo blast transformation when exposed to thyroid cells *in vitro*.[2,22]

The mechanism leading to antithyroid antibody formation and cell-mediated immune reactivity has not been fully established. Experiments in animal models point toward antibody-dependent cell-mediated cytotoxicity, antibody-dependent complement-mediated cytotoxicity, and direct T-cell killing as relevant mechanisms; however, their role in human disease is less clear.

CLINICAL FEATURES. Symptoms of hypothyroidism in association with a painless, firm goiter are frequent presenting complaints; however, patients may be euthyroid. The thyroid may be two to three times normal size, firm, and as the lobules become more prominent finely nodular on palpation. In some, the gland is frankly nodular, rather than diffusely enlarged. Tenderness is uncommon. Large goiters may be associated with pressure symptoms in the neck and rarely with superior vena caval obstruction.

The diagnosis of Hashimoto's begins by documenting hypothyroidism with thyroid function tests. Serum thyroid-stimulating hormone (TSH) is also measured as total thyroxine (T_4) and triiodothyronine (T_3) may be normal in patients with minor degrees of thyroid failure, but the serum TSH level is invariably raised. A normal serum TSH in the presence of low T_4 and T_3 levels excludes primary thyroid failure.

Although Hashimoto's disease is usually associated with hypothyroidism, thyroid function may change during the course of the disease.[9,26] Transient hyperthyroidism may be present when inflammatory changes cause disruption of follicles with leakage of thyroid hormone into the circulation. This is associated with a decreased radioactive iodine uptake, in contradistinction to Graves' disease, in which the hyperthyroidism is characterized by diffuse glandular hyperfunction and increased radioactive iodine uptake. In Hashimoto's disease, after a period of 2 to 8 weeks, the thyroid stores in the gland are depleted, and the thyroid function decreases to normal or hypothyroid levels.

Routine tests for thyroglobulin and microsomal antibodies should be performed to confirm the diagnosis of Hashimoto's disease, since the presence and the titer of these antibodies correlate with the severity and extent of the autoimmune process. The titer regarded as positive varies in different laboratories and with the particular method and reagents used.

Hypothyroidism associated with a goiter but negative thyroid antibodies suggests use of goitrogen, a dyshormonogenetic goiter, or an endemic goiter.

If thyroid neoplasia is suspected clinically due to asymmetry of the goiter, cervical lymphadenopathy, pressure symptoms, hoarseness, or enlargement of the goiter despite adequate thyroid replacement, fine-needle aspiration or open biopsy of the suspicious area should be performed. There is a strong relationship between thyroiditis and malignant thyroid lymphoma.[11] This tumor is rare, but the risk of thyroid lymphoma is greatly increased in patients with Hashimoto's disease, in comparison with the general population.

PATHOLOGY. The enlarged thyroid is pale and firm, with a finely nodular surface and a pale yellow color. Adjacent lymph nodes may be enlarged. Histologically, there is diffuse infiltration of the gland by lymphocytes and plasma cells, with formation of lymphoid follicles and germinal centers. The thyroid follicles are disrupted, and the follicular basement membrane is damaged. Some epithelial cells are enlarged and show a characteristic oxyphilic change in the cytoplasm (Askanazy cells)[14]

TREATMENT. There is no specific treatment for Hashimoto's disease. Patients are usually followed medically, and replacement therapy with T_4 is begun in patients with hypothyroidism that is symptomatic or associated with a goiter that is causing pressure symptoms. There is no indication for treating asymptomatic patients without goiter with T_4 because such treatment does not slow the progression of the thyroiditis.

Surgical reduction of goiter should be performed if severe pressure symptoms that have not responded to corticosteriod therapy are present.[17] This usually consists of subtotal thyroidectomy. Biopsy to exclude malignancy in nodules suspicious for thyroid carcinoma (usually papillary) or lymphoma is indicated.[12,13,17,24] If carcinoma is suspected, a lobectomy should be performed; and if frozen section demonstrates carcinoma, a subtotal or total thyroidectomy should be performed.[4]

Remission of hypothyroidism in patients with autoimmune thyroiditis has recently been suggested. In geographic areas of high iodine ingestion, prior to commencement on replacement therapy there may be an indication for a trial of iodine restriction in patients with a goiter and a high iodine uptake who are found to be hypothyroid.

Painless Thyroiditis

This syndrome, increasingly described over the past decade and referred to as silent or painless thyroiditis but most accurately as lymphocytic thyroiditis with spontaneous resolving hyperthyroidism, is now recognized as a distinct entity.[21,23,30] The differentiation from subacute thyroiditis (SAT) is important. Hyperthyroidism, which is usually self-limiting, develops abruptly in a patient in whom the thyroid is painless and only slightly enlarged, has low radioactive iodine uptake, and histologically demonstrates lymphocytic infiltration without the characteristic giant-cell and granulomatous changes seen in SAT. Differentiation from SAT appears worthwhile, because with long-term follow-up, it is clear that whereas few patients with SAT have a recurrence or progress to permanent thyroid disease, this is not the situation with the painless thyroiditis syndrome. In one series 26 of 54 patients with painless thyroiditis had persistent or progressive disease or recurrence of transient episodes of hyperthyroidism.

DE QUERVAIN'S (SUBACUTE OR GIANT-CELL) THYROIDITIS

SAT represents approximately 1 per cent of all cases of thyroid disease, is much less common than Hashimoto's thyroiditis, and has only one-eighth the incidence of Graves' disease. It is uncommon in children, being most frequent in the third to fifth decades, with a female-to-male ratio of 5:1. Although a causative agent is rarely demonstrated, it often follows upper respiratory tract infections, suggesting that it is due to a viral infection.[5,10,28]

CLINICAL FEATURES. Pain in the thyroid gland often develops rather suddenly, often with radiation to the jaw and ears and may be associated with marked tenderness and dysphagia. The gland is generally moderately enlarged. Hyperthyroidism is observed in the early stages of the disease and is due to the sudden disruption of the follicular structure with discharge of large quantities of thyroid hormone into the circulation. The syndrome lasts for several weeks to several months.

The general laboratory findings include an increased erythrocyte sedimentation rate (ESR), a generalized increase in immunoglobulins, and a neutrophil leukocytosis or lymphocytosis in some. The changes in thyroid function are quite characteristic, with an early thyrotoxic stage followed by hypothyroidism and usually euthyroidism.[15] In the thyrotoxic stage, there is a sudden discharge of T_4 and T_3 into the circulation. The thyroidal radioactive iodine uptake (RAIU) and TSH are characteristically reduced. Graves' disease and the thyrotoxic phase of SAT are differentiated by thyroid scan: patients with Graves' disease have diffuse increased uptake, whereas patients in the thyrotoxic phase of SAT demonstrate diffuse decreased uptake. SAT differs from Hashimoto's disease in that SAT is not consistently associated with antithyroid antibodies. Hypothyroidism may be observed after 2 to 4 weeks in those with SAT that progresses to thyroid failure. In addition, thyroid function returns to baseline after a period of months. Goiter associated with discrete nodularity of the gland is an indication for fine-needle aspiration or biopsy to differentiate SAT from colloid nodules or thyroid cancer.

PATHOLOGY. There is generally moderate thyroid enlargement, which may be asymmetric. The inflammatory reaction involving the thyroid may lead to adherence of the gland to the capsule and immediate extrathyroid tissues. Histologic features include desquamation of the follicular cells and disturbance and loss of colloid material. There is invasion of the thyroid by polymorphonuclear leukocytes, lymphocytes, and foreign body giant cells. The most characteristic feature is the granuloma, which consists of giant cells clustered around foci of degenerating thyroid follicles.[19]

TREATMENT. This condition remits spontaneously after a variable period from a few days to a few months and relapses occasionally before the disease remits permanently. The treatment consists of analgesics such as aspirin or ibuprofen in mild cases. Steroids are effective in controlling symptoms in the more severe cases. Prednisone is usually initiated and tapered over a period of months. A follow-up thyroid scan is indicated to document return of thyroidal RAIU to normal and recovery from the disease. Medical therapy for the transient thyrotoxic phase is indicated. However, spontaneous recovery is observed in over 90 per cent of patients; and therefore subtotal thyroidectomy is not indicated.

ACUTE SUPPURATIVE THYROIDITIS

This is a rare condition of the thyroid gland that is usually due to bacterial infection.[1,11] Common pathogens include Streptococcus, *Staphylococcus*, and *Pneumococcus*, and rarely *Salmonella* or *Bacteroides*. Other extremely rare causes of a more indolent infection include tuberculosis, actinomycoses, echinococcosis, aspergillosis, and syphilis. Normal thyroid glands are susceptible to infection, as are those with underlying disorders. Infections usually arise from adjacent structures such as the oropharynx or the lymph nodes or from congenital abnormalities such as a persistent thyroglossal duct or fistula; but infection can also occur via hematogenous spread or after direct trauma.

CLINICAL FEATURES. Symptoms occur with an acute onset and characteristically include tenderness, enlargement, warmth, erythema, and neck pain exacerbated by neck extension and swallowing. Septicemia or direct extension to the neck or chest may occur. The presence of blood-tinged sputum with the acute onset of symptoms suggests tracheal involvement. Thyroid function is usually normal, as is the RAIU although should an abscess develop, it will be observed as an area of decreased uptake on the thyroid scan. Transient hyperthyroidism may occur if thyroid hormone is released from inflamed follicles. Ultrasound may demonstrate a partially cystic mass within the thyroid. Fine-needle aspiration may be diagnostic when polymorphonuclear leukocytes and organisms are observed.

Although the clinical characteristics of acute suppurative thyroiditis are usually straightforward, differentiation from de Quervain's thyroiditis is important. The latter is characterized by less severe pain and lack of involvement of adjacent neck tissues, a markedly elevated (ESR), a markedly depressed RAIU, and a greater likelihood of transient hyperthyroidism.

Patients with chronic suppurative thyroiditis usually present with a slowly growing neck mass, which is suspected of being a cyst or adenoma; and only on biopsy or surgical exploration is the correct diagnosis made.

PATHOLOGY. Histologic examination of the gland reveals a marked polymorphonuclear leukocyte and lymphocytic infiltrate in the acute phase, which may be associated with frank thyroid necrosis and abscess formation. Fibrosis occurs with healing.

TREATMENT. Primary treatment of suppurative thyroiditis consists of appropriate antibiotics against the causative organism. Measurable improvement is usually observed within 48 to 72 hours and complete resolution in 2 to 4 weeks. Thyroid abscesses should be drained, and cysts communicating with the pyriform sinus or trachea recur and require excision.

RIEDEL'S THYROIDITIS

Riedel's thyroiditis is a very rare inflammatory condition, being reported in only 20 of 42,000 surgical specimens of the thyroid at the Mayo Clinic. The most common ages of presentation are 30 to 60 years, and females are more frequently affected than males.[8]

The etiology of invasive fibrous thyroiditis remains uncertain. There is little evidence to support the formerly popular view that this condition represents a late stage of either autoimmune thyroiditis or SAT. There are reports linking it to extracervical fibrosclerosis, which includes retroperitoneal and mediastinal fibrosis, fibrosing cholangitis, pseudotumor of the orbit, and fibrosis of the lacrimal gland. It appears likely that the invasive fibrous thyroiditis represents one aspect of a generalized process that is not specifically related to the thyroid gland.

CLINICAL FEATURES. The patient generally presents with a history of rapid increase in thyroid size, which is frequently associated with symptoms of tracheal and/or esophageal compression. The gland is often described as "woody" in texture, is generally uniformly enlarged, nontender, and strikingly hard on palpation; and is often mistaken for thyroid carcinoma. There are usually no other clinical features, although the disease may be associated with retroperitoneal fibrosis and other disorders.

There are no characteristic laboratory findings except that there are absent to low titers of antithyroid antibodies. In late stages of disease hypothyroidism may be present. The diagnosis can be confirmed only by biopsy.

PATHOLOGY. The gland is involved wholly or in part by a dense, invasive fibrosis that extends to involve the surrounding tissues, so that the capsule and anatomic margins of the gland cannot be precisely defined. There is no lymphocytic infiltrate in the tissue, but a lymphocytic perivasculitis is observed in most cases.

TREATMENT. Medical therapy includes thyroid replacement if hypothyroidism is present. Surgical treatment is indicated if pressure symptoms in the neck require relief, and partial thyroidectomy is required in the majority of these patients. The operation requires meticulous dissection because fibrosis may involve surrounding structures such as the trachea, the carotid sheath, and the recurrent laryngeal nerve. Although in most patients the fibrous process is confined to the neck and the disease is relatively benign, a minority of patients develop multifocal fibrosis up to 10 years later, which may be life-threatening.[27,31]

SELECTED REFERENCES

McGregor, A. M., and Hall, R.: Thyroiditis. In DeGroot, L. J. (Ed.): Endocrinology, 2nd ed. Philadelphia, W. B. Saunders Company, 1989.
    This chapter in a multivolume text concerning thyroiditis includes clinical and experimental details as well as an extensive bibliography.

Linden, M. C., Jr., and Clark, J. H.: Indications for surgery in thyroiditis. Am. J. Surg., 118:829, 1969.
    This article is a review of surgery for thyroiditis.

Clark, O. H., Greenspan, F. S., and Dunphy, J. E.: Hashimoto's thyroiditis in thyroid cancer. Indications for operation. Am. J. Surg., 140:665, 1980.

REFERENCES

1. Altemeier, W. A.: Acute pyogenic thyroiditis. Arch. Surg., 61:76, 1950.
2. Aoki, N., and DeGroot, L. J.: Lymphocyte blastogenic response to human thyroglobulin in Graves' disease: Hashimoto's thyroiditis and metastic thyroid cancer. Clin. Exp. Immunol., 38:523, 1979.
3. Burek, C. L., Hoffman, W. H., and Rose, N. R.: The presence of thyroid autoantibodies in children and adolescents with autoimmune thyroid disease and their parents. Clin. Immunol. Immunopathol., 25:395, 1982.
4. Crile, G., Jr., and Hazard, J. B.: Incidence of cancer in struma lymphomatosa. Surg. Gynecol. Obstet., 115:101, 1962.
5. de Quervain, F.: Die akute, nicht eiterige thyroiditis. Mitt. Grenzgeb. Med. Chir. 2(Suppl.):1, 1904.
6. Doniach, D., Hudson, R. V., and Roitt, I. M.: Human autoimmune thyroiditis: Clinical studies. Br. Med. J., 1:365, 1960.
7. Doniach, D., Bottazzo, G. F., and Russell, R. C. G.: Goitrous autoimmune thyroiditis (Hashimoto's disease). Clin. Endocrinol. Metab. 8:63, 1978.
8. Furszyfer, J., Kurland, L. T., and Woolner, L. B., et al.: Hashimoto's thyroiditis in Olmstead County, Minnesota, 1935–1967. Mayo Clin. Proc., 45:586, 1970.
9. Gluck, F. B., Nusynowitz, M. L., and Plymate, S.: Chronic lymphocytic thyroiditis, thyrotoxicosis, and low radioactive iodine uptake. N. Engl. J. Med., 293:634, 1975.
10. Greene, J. N.: Subacute thyroiditis. Am. J. Med., 51:97, 1971.
11. Hagan, A. D., Goffinet, J., and Davis, J. W.: Acute streptococcal thyroiditis. J.A.M.A., 202:829, 1969.
12. Hamberger, J. L., Miller, J. M., and Kini, S. R.: Lymphoma of the thyroid. Ann. Intern. Med., 99:685, 1983.
13. Holm, L. E., Blomgren, H., and Lowhagen, T.: Cancer risks in patients with chronic lymphocytic thyroiditis. N. Engl. J. Med., 312:601, 1985.
14. Knecht, H., and Hedinger, C. E.: Ultrastructural findings in Hashimoto's thyroiditis and focal lymphocytic thyroiditis with reference to giant cell formation. Histopathology, 6:511, 1982.
15. Larsen, P. R.: Serum triiodothyronine, thyroxine and thyrotropin during hyperthyroid, hypothyroid and recovery phases of subacute thyroiditis. Metabolism, 23:467, 1974.
16. Levine, S. N.: Current concepts of thyroiditis. Arch. Intern. Med., 143:1952, 1983.
17. Linden, M. C., Jr., and Clark, J. L. L: Indications for surgery in thyroiditis. Am. J. Surg., 118:829, 1969.
18. McLachlan, S. M., McGregor, A. M., Rees Smith, B., and Hall, R.: Thyroid-autoantibody synthesis by Hashimoto thyroid lymphocytes. Lancet, 1:162, 1979.
19. Mizukami, Y., Michigishi, T., Kawato, M., and Matsubara, F.: Immunohistochemical and ultrastructural study of subacute thyroiditis, with special reference to multinucleated giant cells. Hum. Pathol., 18:929, 1987.
20. Mulhern, I. M., Masi, A. T., Shulman, L. E.: Hashimoto's disease: A search for associated disorders in 170 clinically detected cases. Lancet, 2:508, 1966.
21. Nikolai, T. F., Brosseau, J., Kettrick, M. A., et al.: Lymphocytic thyroiditis with spontaneously resolving hyperthyroidism (silent thyroiditis). Arch. Intern. Med., 140:478, 1980.
22. Okita, N., Kidd, A., Row, V. V., and Volpe, R.: Sensitisation of T-lymphocytes in Graves' and Hashimoto's disease. J. Clin. Endocrinol. Metab., 51:316, 1980.
23. Papapertrou, P. D., and Jackson, I. M. D.: Thyrotoxicosis due to "silent" thyroiditis. Lancet, 1:361, 1975.

24. Rudman, I., Novota, O. J., and Keener, R. L.: Complications of Hashimoto thyroiditis surgery. Arch. Surg., 83:822, 1961.
25. Tunbridge, W. M. G., Evered, D. C., Hall, R., et al.: The spectrum of thyroid disease in a community: The Whickham survey. Clin. Endocrinol., 7:481, 1977.
26. Tunbridge, W. M. G., Brewis, M., French, J. M., et al.: Natural history of autoimmune thyroiditis. Br. Med. J., 1:258, 1981.
27. Turner-Warwick, R., Nabarro, J. D. N., and Doniach, D.: Riedel's thyroiditis and retroperitoneal fibrosis. Proc. R. Soc. Med., 59:596, 1966.
28. Volpe, R., Row, V. V., Ezrin, C.: Circulating viral and thyroid antibodies in subacute thyroiditis. J. Clin. Endocrinol. Metab., 27:1275, 1967.
29. Weetman, A. P., McGregor, A. M.: Autoimmune thyroid disease: Developments in our understanding. Endocrinol. Rev., 5:309, 1984.
30. Woolf, P. D., Daly, R.: Thyrotoxicosis with painless thyroiditis. Am. J. Med., 60:73, 1976.
31. Woolner, L. B., McConahey, W. M., and Beahrs, O. H.: Invasive fibrous thyroiditis. J. Clin. Endocrinol., 17:201, 1957.

V

NODULAR GOITER AND BENIGN AND MALIGNANT NEOPLASMS OF THE THYROID

George S. Leight, Jr., M.D.

The normal thyroid gland is a homogeneous structure that normally weighs approximately 20 gm. (Fig. 1). The commonly accepted definition of a goiter is a thyroid gland that is at least twice the normal size gland. Goiter can also be described as a diffuse enlargement of the thyroid gland (diffuse goiter) or enlargement by one or more nodules (nodular goiter). Goiter can be further classified as endemic, sporadic, or compensatory. The classification system for goiter of the American Thyroid Association is represented in Table 1.

NODULAR GOITER

INCIDENCE. On a worldwide basis, nodular goiter remains a problem of enormous magnitude, although the exact incidence is not available. The World Health Organization estimated in 1958 that goiter was present in 200 million individuals, which

TABLE 1. Classification of Nontoxic Goiter

Nontoxic diffuse goiter
 Endemic
  Iodine deficiency
  Iodine excess
  Dietary goitrogens
 Sporadic
  Congenital defect in thyroid hormone biosynthesis
  Chemical agents, e.g., lithium, thiocyanate, *p*-aminosalicylic acid
  Iodine deficiency
 Compensatory following subtotal thyroidectomy

Nontoxic nodular goiter due to causes listed above
 Uninodular or multinodular
 Functional, nonfunctional, or both

From Burrow, G. N.: Nontoxic goiter—diffuse and nodular. *In* Burrow, G. N., Oppenheimer, J. H., and Volpe, R. (Eds.): Thyroid Function and Disease. Philadelphia, W. B. Saunders Company, 1989. Modified from Werner, S. C.: J. Clin. Endocrinol. 29:860, 1969.

represented 7 per cent of the world's population at that time.[20] Endemic goiter refers to a situation in which more than 10 per cent of the local population have goiter, usually because of low iodine intake. In some areas, the incidence of goiter may exceed 85 per cent. Marine, in 1917, popularized the use of iodized salt in North America in order to prevent endemic goiter.[23] Since that time, the incidence of goiter throughout the United States has diminished sharply since adequate dietary iodine has become available in all geographic areas. Comprehensive population surveys have demonstrated that the prevalence of palpable thyroid nodules in the adult population of the United States is approximately 4 per cent. In the Framingham study, there was an overall 4.2 per cent incidence of nodular thyroid disease; the incidence was higher in females (6.4 per cent) than in males (1.5 per cent).[35] Nodular thyroid disease, however, is more prevalent than these studies would suggest, as is indicated by autopsy surveys that have demonstrated an even higher incidence of nodular goiter. In a thorough autopsy study of 821 patients whose thyroid glands had been considered normal clinically, 50 per cent were found to have nodules; 75 per cent of the glands were multinodular, and 25 per cent contained single nodules.[26] Recent ultrasonographic studies of the thyroid have revealed nodules in up to 50 per cent of the population over the age of 50 years.[17]

ETIOLOGY. The mechanisms by which the normal, homoge-

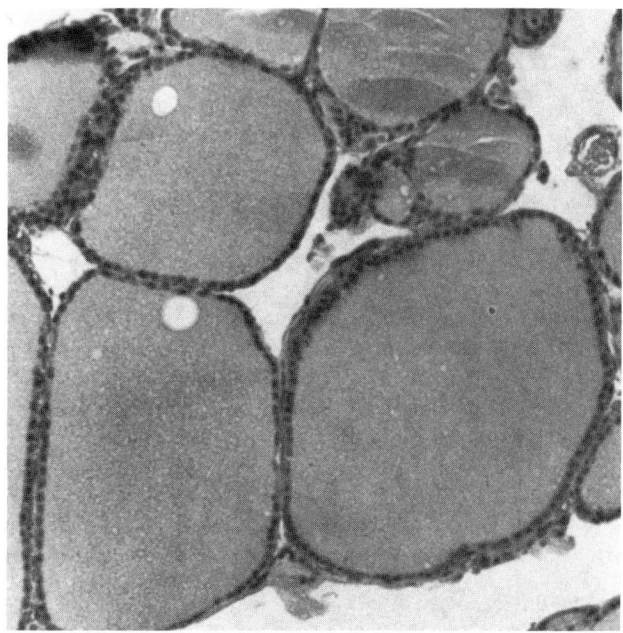

Figure 1. Photomicrograph (hematoxylin and eosin, ×100) of normal thyroid demonstrating follicles of uniform size replete with colloid. (From LiVolsi, V. A. (Ed.): Surgical Pathology of the Thyroid. Philadelphia, W. B. Saunders Company, 1990.)

neous thyroid gland changes to become the enlarged, nodular structure characteristic of multinodular goiter have for many years puzzled clinicians. Goiter can most simply be considered a compensatory mechanism for a deficiency in the production of thyroid hormone. The reason for this inadequate production may be a deficiency of iodine in the diet, the presence of substances in the diet or medications that impair the synthesis of thyroid hormone, a defect or absence of an enzyme essential for biosynthesis or secretion of thyroid hormone, or an immunologic cause (Hashimoto's thyroiditis) that damages follicular cells, impairing production of thyroid hormone. The final common pathway to goiter formation in each of these situations depends on the central role of thyroid-stimulating hormone (TSH) and its ability to promote thyroid growth. Although some studies have demonstrated no difference in serum TSH levels between goitrous and nongoitrous patients in endemic regions, this may be a function of the age of the patient population rather than the lack of a central role for TSH. Serum TSH levels are higher in early goiters and are higher during the early decades with a progressive decrease of TSH secretion and reserve with advancing age.[2] Thyroid growth is more rapid during the initial 4 decades of life and then regresses, although thyroid nodularity may increase with age.

More recently, there has been new information that growth factors other than TSH may have a role in goiter formation. Thyroid-stimulating immunoglobulins that promote growth of thyroid follicles have been found in patients with nontoxic goiters as well as in those with Graves' disease.[34] Epidermal growth factor as well as insulin-like growth factors I and II have been recognized as potent stimulators of thyroid cell growth.[12,37] The lack of negative growth control factors such as transforming growth factor beta may also cause a disequilibrium in thyroid cell homeostasis, permitting the development of nodular goiter.[15]

The mechanisms by which TSH and other growth factors actually produce nodular goiter have been best described by Studer and colleagues.[32] They have demonstrated heterogeneity in the function of thyroid follicular cells that may be responsible for the characteristic heterogeneity of shape and function among newly generated follicles arising during the process of transformation of a normal thyroid into a multinodular goiter. This explanation is based on the observations that (1) the follicular cells of a normal thyroid are not identical but have highly individualized metabolic capabilities and (2) daughter follicles produced during goitrogenesis arise from a few predestined follicular cells with the propensity to replicate at higher rates. Whenever the thyroid gland is forced to grow (produce new follicles), the daughter follicles may therefore differ significantly from the mother follicle with respect to growth, iodination and thyroglobulin synthesis, and endocytosis. Since the progenitor cells of the daughter follicles are different functionally, clusters of follicles of different size and function arise. The process would be accelerated by any type of growth stimulus such as TSH or thyroid-stimulating immunoglobulins, although the nature of the stimulus that produces follicular cell growth is of little importance. As long as a growth-enhancing agent is acting for a sufficient length of time on thyroid follicular cells with even slightly different growth rates, a nodular growth pattern is the ultimate outcome. During goiter growth, the function of cells with a high growth rate expands at the expense of slower growing cells, increasing the autonomous growth rate of the whole goiter. This may be an explanation why many goiters continue to grow even though the initial activating mechanism may no longer be present and why there is frequently a failure of nonendemic goiters to respond to TSH suppressive treatment. Other factors may also contribute to the growth characteristics and appearance of nodular goiters. The new follicles are supplied by a network of blood vessels. If the follicle grows

more rapidly than its blood supply, focal necrosis followed by scarring and an inelastic fibrous network within the goiter may result. The growth patterns of other follicles may then be altered by this network of scarring throughout the gland.

PATHOLOGY. The thyroid gland in patients with multinodular goiter may be slightly to massively enlarged and has a characteristic nodular external surface (Fig. 2). Cut section shows multiple nodules that vary in size and consistency from solid follicular lesions to colloid-rich nodules or degenerative cystic structures. Variable amounts of normal thyroid tissue, fibrous tissue, and calcification are observed interspersed among the nodules. Areas of hemorrhage and cysts are also often detected. On microscopic examination, normal to hyperplastic foci of thyroid tissue, large areas of colloid, hemorrhage, fibrosis, and calcification are observed in addition to variable amounts of lymphocytic infiltrate.

NATURAL HISTORY. The prevalence of nodular goiter in nonendemic areas (sporadic goiter) increases from 1 per cent in patients under 20 years old to approximately 5 per cent in patients over the age of 60.[24] The peak incidence of endemic goiter occurs at 10 to 50 years and decreases thereafter. A high incidence of childhood goiter in an area correlates with an increased likelihood that the goiter will persist into adult life with the eventual appearance of nodularity. In all age groups, there is a three- to sixfold higher incidence of thyroid dysfunction and goiter in females compared with males. The pattern of growth of nodular goiter is unpredictable, ranging from slow steady growth extending over decades to rapid growth of one or more nodules within a multinodular goiter.

With continued growth, nodular goiters come to clinical attention for a variety of reasons. Outside of areas in which goiter is endemic, nodular goiter is usually found during routine physical examination or is noticed by the patient as a neck mass. Patients are usually unaware of nodules smaller than 2 cm., although rapid growth or hemorrhage into the nodule that produces pain may bring the nodule to attention. Even though large multinodular goiters rarely cause symptoms, the enlarging goiter can cause compression of neck structures such as the trachea or esophagus, causing dysphagia, cough, respiratory compromise, or a feeling of fullness in the neck. Symptoms related to compression are more common with goiters located substernally because of the limited space for expansion and the

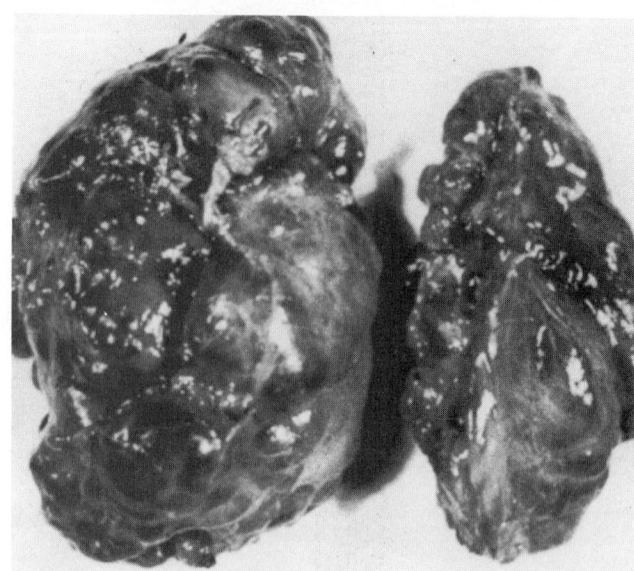

Figure 2. Multinodular goiter demonstrating asymmetric size of the two lobes and multiple nodules. (From LiVolsi, V. A. (Ed.): Surgical Pathology of the Thyroid. Philadelphia, W. B. Saunders Company, 1990.)

proximity of critical structures. Radiographs may show deviation and occasionally compression of the trachea by the enlarging goiter. This can be documented more precisely by computed tomographic scanning of the neck structures. Peak inspiratory and expiratory flow rates can be used to document the diminished flow rates diagnostic of upper airway obstruction. This is a situation that should be viewed with concern, since further airway compromise from a foreign body or tracheitis with edema could quickly produce a respiratory emergency or arrest. Other clinical problems presented by a goiter include hypothyroidism or the emergence of autonomous hyperfunctioning nodules with accompanying hyperthyroidism. Thyrotoxicosis may be difficult to recognize in the elderly, and periodic laboratory studies of thyroid function are mandatory in these patients.

The risk of underlying malignancy must also be considered in patients with nodular goiter. The presence of a multinodular goiter is usually considered to be associated with a low risk of malignancy of approximately 0.5 per cent; reports that indicate a 4 to 17 per cent incidence of carcinoma in surgically treated multinodular goiters are thought to be due to selection of these patients.[6] If there is a nodule within a multinodular gland that appears different from the other nodules or has undergone recent change or growth, the possibility of malignancy must be considered. Although fine-needle aspiration biopsy has been most useful in the management of single thyroid nodules, it can also be used effectively in the evaluation of specific nodules within a multinodular gland.

TREATMENT. Prophylaxis and treatment for endemic goiter can be managed by the administration of iodine. In most developed countries, this has been achieved by the addition of iodine to salt or its use as a preservative in bread. In the treatment of long-standing endemic goiter, iodine therapy may cause the goiter to diminish somewhat in size, but the large nodules usually remain without significant alteration in size. A possible complication of iodine therapy in these patients is thyrotoxicosis, although this is generally transient and self-limited.

Treatment of the other types of goiter is based on suppression of TSH secretion by administration of adequate amounts of exogenous thyroid hormone. Such replacement therapy with thyroxine (T_4) is considered to be successful if a 30 per cent reduction in goiter size is accomplished; a larger decrease in size is rarely achieved. Such a significant decrease in size of the multinodular goiter may initially be observed in approximately 50 per cent of patients, although this does not eliminate the possibility of later goiter growth because of the mechanisms reviewed in a previous section (see Etiology). Patients receiving replacement therapy with T_4 must be monitored carefully, since the addition of exogenous hormone to that produced endogenously may cause thyrotoxicosis. Although most multinodular goiters regress very little with T_4 therapy, if malignancy has been excluded and the goiter shrinks somewhat or remains stable, these patients may be comfortable and safe for many years on thyroid hormone replacement. Overall, however, the enthusiasm for medical treatment of nodular goiters in nonendemic areas is diminishing.[31]

Common indications for surgical therapy in patients with nodular goiter are the presence of obstructive symptoms or cosmetic problems related to the size of the goiter. When obstructive symptoms occur, medical therapy is extremely unlikely to produce an improvement. The goal of surgical therapy is to remove all of the abnormal, nodular thyroid tissue, since all nodules may contain autonomously growing cells with the potential to cause recurrence of the goiter. Such surgical treatment should correct the current problem and free the patient from the possibility of obstructive symptoms occurring later.

Nodules that grow despite adequate T_4 therapy are autonomous and are associated with a higher incidence of malignancy. Needle biopsy should be performed in this situation, and when

cytology is indicative of malignancy, surgical treatment should be employed. Recurrent cysts and toxic nodules in a large multinodular goiter are also considered to be indications for surgical management. If the lesion is larger than 3 cm., surgical removal may be indicated.

Substernal Goiter

Substernal goiter follows the downward growth of the enlarged thyroid gland through the thoracic inlet into the mediastinum. Because the goiter is growing in a confined space containing many critical structures, the potential for complications is significant. The same complications that can occur in all goiters, such as thyrotoxicosis or malignancy, can also occur in substernal goiters. The potential for significant tracheal deviation or obstruction is perhaps greater with substernal goiter because of the limited space for expansion of the goiter. Obstruction of the superior vena cava with resulting dilated cervical and facial veins is a complication limited to substernal goiter.

Because substernal goiter rarely regresses with thyroid hormone treatment and since tracheal compression can cause serious respiratory embarrassment, substernal extension of goiter is usually considered an indication for surgical removal. In patients who have not had prior thyroid operations, the majority of substernal goiters can be removed through a standard cervical incision. The arterial blood supply to the substernal goiter arises in the neck primarily from the inferior thyroid artery. After the arterial supply is controlled, the goiter is freed from the mediastinal structures by finger dissection and is delivered through the thoracic inlet. When substernal goiters obstruct venous return, significant venous bleeding may occur until the goiter can be delivered through the thoracic inlet, relieving the venous obstruction and bleeding. The recurrent laryngeal nerve and parathyroid glands are usually displaced posteriorly by the goiter; so they are not likely to be injured during delivery of the substernal goiter. If the recurrent nerve can be visualized prior to this step, it should be identified and protected during this time. In some instances when the size of the goiter prevents delivery through the thoracic inlet, the capsule of the goiter can be opened with removal of colloid and seminecrotic material, allowing delivery into the neck. Median sternotomy or thoracotomy is rarely necessary to remove a substernal goiter, although it is more often necessary in patients who have previously undergone thyroid operations.

BENIGN NEOPLASMS

Thyroid adenomas are benign neoplasms arising from follicular tissue. These lesions can be classified histologically as the more common follicular adenoma and the very rare papillary adenomas and teratomas (Table 2). Most papillary tumors are considered to be malignant, and the diagnosis of papillary adenoma should be made with great caution. Thyroid adenomas are usually considered to be distinct etiologically from the multiple adenomas that occur in multinodular goiter. Recently, it has been suggested that true adenomas may be the product of

TABLE 2. Benign Neoplasms of the Thyroid

Adenoma
  Follicular
    Colloid variant
    Embryonal
    Fetal
    Hürthle cell variant
  Papillary
  Atypical
Teratoma

clones of follicular cells with very high individual growth rates.[32]

Follicular adenomas are well circumscribed, solitary, homogeneous lesions that are usually surrounded by a capsule separating them from the adjacent normal thyroid tissue. Follicular adenomas are subdivided according to their architecture, cellularity, and amount of colloid into fetal (microfollicular), colloid (macrofollicular), embryonal (trabecular), and Hürthle (oxyphil) cell types. Colloid adenomas are similar histologically to the multiple nodules found in multinodular goiter. On microscopic examination these lesions have large colloid-filled follicles within an incomplete capsule (Fig. 3). These are classified by some pathologists as colloid nodules, suggesting a focal process that is different from the development of a true adenoma.

Fetal adenoma is composed entirely of small follicles, whereas embryonal adenomas are composed of cells arranged in solid cords. The individual cells in these lesions resemble those in normal thyroid tissue. Hürthle cell lesions contain cells that are markedly eosinophilic and the cytoplasm of which contains abundant mitochondria when examined by electron microscopy (Fig. 3). Some pathologists prefer the term *Hürthle cell tumor* because of the difficulty in establishing malignant potential of these lesions using histologic criteria.

Some pathologists classify all papillary lesions as malignant, although others consider selected papillary tumors to be benign adenomas. Teratomas of the thyroid are rare, and although most are benign, malignant teratomas may also occur.

CLINICAL FEATURES. Adenomas usually grow slowly, remain undetected for years, and are typically asymptomatic. They are usually discovered incidentally by the patient or physician; rarely they may present with local compressive symptoms or pain. Adenomas may undergo hemorrhagic necrosis, calcification, or cystic degeneration. Hemorrhage into the adenoma may cause pain, tenderness, and an increase in size, thus drawing attention to the nodule.

Approximately 70 per cent of adenomas do not accumulate radioactive iodine and are "cold" on scan; 20 per cent demonstrate uptake approximately equivalent to the remaining normal thyroid tissue and are designated "warm." Five to 10 per cent of adenomas are hyperfunctional and may produce thyrotoxicosis, particularly when the lesion exceeds 3 cm. in size.

Adenomas occasionally develop microinvasion, which is an indication of malignant degeneration. Colloid adenomas have no potential for microinvasion, but the cellular adenomas including those of microfollicular, Hürthle cell, and embryonal types do demonstrate the potential for microinvasion. Approximately 5 per cent of microfollicular and Hürthle cell tumors demonstrate capsular or vascular invasion, which is considered to be a definite indication of malignancy. The only method for differentiating these benign from malignant lesions is careful study of multiple tissue sections for evidence of capsular or vascular invasion.

TREATMENT. The most important factor in the management of the majority of thyroid adenomas is their differentiation from malignant thyroid lesions (see following discussion, Management of Thyroid Nodules). When it can be established by aspiration cytology or other biopsy techniques that a nodule is a benign adenoma, the patient is usually followed closely. In the past, most of these patients have been placed on thyroid hormone suppressive therapy, but this has remained controversial, and recent studies have demonstrated that suppressive therapy has no significant effect on nodule size.[13] Adenomas that continue to enlarge progressively, cause compressive symptoms, or cause thyrotoxicosis should be considered for surgical resection.

Management of Thyroid Nodules

Thyroid nodules are very common with an incidence in the adult population in the United States of approximately 4 per cent. Despite this high frequency of thyroid nodules in the general population, clinically evident thyroid carcinoma is rare, occurring at a rate of 39 cases per 1 million population.[7] It is thus a challenge to select from this large group of patients with thyroid nodules those who require further investigation and perhaps surgical therapy. Although there has been improvement in the diagnostic evaluation of thyroid nodules, especially with the more widespread use of needle aspiration biopsy, this remains a somewhat controversial clinical problem.

Most retrospective studies have demonstrated that cancers occur more often in solitary nodules than in multinodular goiters. Thus, these two separate entities are usually managed differently, although it must be remembered that this classification based on physical examination is neither accurate nor reliable. In addition, the finding of a multinodular goiter does not exclude the presence of coexisting cancer, and a dominant nodule in a multinodular gland must be considered with the same concern as a single nodule. Since the problem of multinodular disease has been discussed, this section is limited to solitary thyroid nodules.

A wide range of thyroid problems can present as a solitary thyroid nodule (Table 3). A careful history and physical examination may provide important information about the risk of malignancy. Thyroid nodules in children are usually regarded with increased suspicion, although studies that exclude children who have had irradiation report an incidence of cancer similar to that observed in adults.[18] In the elderly population, thyroid nodules are common and the proportion that are malignant is not different from that of the general population. Thyroid nodules are more common in adult women, but when they occur in men they are more likely to be malignant. Although a family

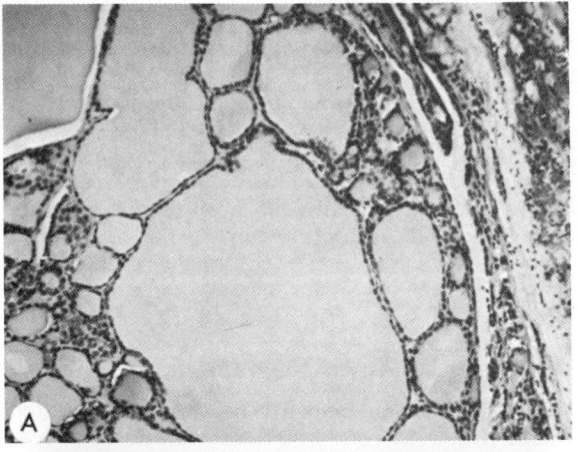
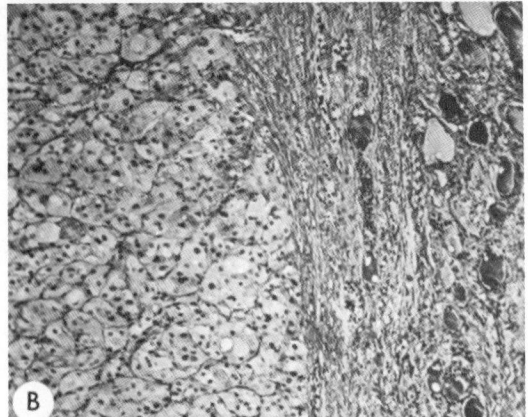

Figure 3. *A*, Colloid nodule demonstrating large follicles and minimal capsule. *B*, Hürthle cell adenoma. (From DeGroot, L. J., Larsen, P. R., Refetoff, S., and Stanbury, J. B.: The Thyroid and Its Diseases. New York, John Wiley & Sons, 1984.)

TABLE 3. Differential Diagnosis of a Solitary Thyroid Nodule

Cyst
    Simple cyst
    Mixed cystic-solid (complex)
Thyroid adenoma
    Autonomously functioning (hot)
    Non- or hypofunctional
Colloid nodule
Thyroiditis
Infection
    Granulomatous disease
    Abscess
Developmental abnormalities
    Unilateral lobe agenesis
    Cystic hygroma
    Dermoid
    Teratoma
Carcinoma
    Primary thyroid
    Metastatic to thyroid
Thyroid lymphoma

history of benign thyroid disease is reassuring, a history of thyroid carcinoma in other family members should raise concern about the possibility of medullary thyroid carcinoma or familial papillary thyroid carcinoma. Historical information concerning the pattern of growth of the nodule may be important. Presence of a stable nodule for many years is suggestive of a benign process, although a slowly growing malignancy cannot be excluded. A rapid, progressive pattern of growth raises the level of concern about malignancy; very sudden enlargement over a period of hours or days, however, is more frequently associated with hemorrhage into a benign tumor or cyst. Dyspnea, dysphagia, hoarseness, vocal cord paralysis, or Horner's syndrome may be indicative of local tissue invasion from a thyroid malignancy. It must also be remembered that all of these problems can be caused by benign thyroid lesions.[25] A history of exposure of the head and neck areas to ionizing radiation is associated with a higher incidence of thyroid nodules and a higher risk of malignancy in these nodules.

Physical examination characteristics of a nodule that are suggestive of malignancy include a firm texture, irregularity, fixation to surrounding structures, and enlarged ipsilateral cervical lymph nodes. The presence of clinically positive lymph nodes is the most reliable physical examination indicator of malignancy, since all the other findings can be associated with benign lesions. Consistency of the nodule is of limited diagnostic importance, since calcification of a benign adenoma may cause it to be quite hard, whereas soft nodules may occasionally be malignant. The most important function of physical examination, however, is the detection of the thyroid nodule rather than the determination of its benign or malignant status.

NONINVASIVE EVALUATION. Studies of thyroid function are of little value in establishing the benign or malignant nature of a thyroid nodule. Thyroid function is usually normal in patients with thyroid carcinoma. Serum thyroxine (T_4), triiodothyronine (T_3), and TSH can be used to detect thyrotoxicosis and hypothyroidism. Serum thyroglobulin assay is of no specific value in evaluating patients with thyroid nodules. Serum antithyroglobulin or antimicrosomal antibodies do not differentiate benign from malignant nodules. The likelihood of a solitary nodule being malignant in a patient with Hashimoto's thyroiditis is the same as in a patient whose thyroid gland is normal.[33] The only specific assay for the presence of thyroid carcinoma is the determination of thyrocalcitonin following provocative testing in patients with suspected medullary thyroid carcinoma (see Medullary Thyroid Carcinoma, Chapter 23, Part VI). Since

sporadic medullary carcinoma represents only 4 to 5 per cent of all thyroid carcinomas, the use of this test in the absence of a suggestive family history of other features of the multiple endocrine neoplastic Type II-A or Type II-B syndrome is not justified.

Because the thyroid gland occupies a superficial, accessible location, ultrasonography, which is a noninvasive, radiation-free procedure, is frequently used in the evaluation of thyroid nodules. Recent advances have provided the technology for the precise delineation of thyroid gland anatomy. Ultrasound thus permits the classification of a nodule as solid, cystic, or mixed solid and cystic. High-resolution ultrasonography can detect lesions as small as 1 mm. and has demonstrated multiple small nodules in as many as 40 per cent of patients with clinically solitary nodules.[30] Although ultrasonography demonstrates high sensitivity for detection of thyroid nodules, there are, unfortunately, no specific ultrasonographic criteria for malignancy. Ultrasound is therefore not usually considered essential in the evaluation of thyroid nodules, although it can be useful in detecting multinodularity, screening high-risk patients, and assessing response of nodules to therapy.[19]

Thyroid scintiscanning has been the most widely used screening procedure in the evaluation of thyroid nodules. The most commonly used isotopes are radioiodine (^{123}I, ^{131}I) and technetium (^{99m}Tc). Radioiodine is trapped and bound to thyroglobulin by the thyroid follicular cells whereas technetium is only trapped. Thyroid nodules are classified as cold (nonfunctional), warm (normal), or hot (hyperfunctioning). The rationale for scintiscanning is that malignant thyroid nodules usually do not bind iodine; hypofunctional nodules are thus more likely to be malignant than are functioning nodules. Hyperfunctioning nodules are very rarely found to be malignant. The main limitation of radionuclide scanning is that it does not clearly differentiate benign from malignant lesions. In most studies, 80 to 85 per cent of nodules are cold, 10 to 15 per cent are warm, and 5 per cent are hot. Malignancy is present in 10 to 15 per cent of cold nodules but is also reported in 9 per cent of warm nodules and 4 per cent of hot nodules.[36] Thus, although malignant nodules are usually cold on scan, most cold lesions are benign; conversely, the presence of a hot nodule reduces the risk of malignancy but does not totally exclude it. Other limitations of radionuclide scanning include inadequate visualization of nodules at the periphery or isthmus and cold nodules surrounded by normal thyroid tissue. Certain artifacts such as an asymmetric gland, agenesis of a lobe, or a tortuous carotid artery may distort a normal gland, producing an abnormal scan.[25]

For many years, clinicians have used thyroid hormone suppression in an attempt to distinguish benign from malignant nodules. The rationale has been that with suppression of TSH by exogenous thyroid hormone, benign nodules would decrease in size because of their dependency on TSH for maintaining growth whereas the autonomous growth of malignant nodules would continue. Although many trials have examined the utility of this approach, the interpretation of results has been limited by imprecise and subjective criteria for response and adequacy of suppression. In addition, malignant thyroid tissue has TSH receptors, and well-differentiated carcinomas occasionally demonstrate a slowing of growth with thyroid hormone suppression.[3] A randomized, prospective study of suppressive therapy for benign thyroid nodules has recently been reported.[13] Nodule size was documented by high-resolution ultrasonography, TSH suppression was documented by a thyrotropin-releasing hormone test, and patients were treated with levothyroxine for 6 months. The nodules were documented to be benign by needle biopsy. This study failed to demonstrate a significant decrease in size of the benign nodules in patients treated with levothyroxine. It is thought that the practice of selecting patients for surgical therapy on the basis of response to a trial of suppression is no longer considered valid.

NEEDLE BIOPSY. Needle biopsy is now accepted as the most precise diagnostic screening procedure for differentiating benign from malignant thyroid nodules (Fig. 4). Because it is safe, inexpensive, and accurate, needle aspiration biopsy is used routinely as the initial diagnostic technique in management of thyroid nodules. With experienced physicians performing needle biopsy and experienced cytopathologists interpreting the results, a reported accuracy of 95 to 97 per cent has been achieved.[14]

Several different techniques for performing needle biopsy have been described. Fine-needle aspiration biopsy (FNAB) using a 21- to 25-gauge needle provides a specimen for cytologic study. Large-needle biopsy and cutting-needle biopsy provide tissue for histologic study. The FNAB procedure has emerged as the most widely used technique, since it provides reliable information, has few complications, and is well tolerated by patients. The important factors for a satisfactory test include a representative specimen from the nodule and an experienced cytologist to interpret the findings. An unsatisfactory specimen, which occurs in 7 to 18 per cent of reported series, is a problem that decreases with the increasing experience of the individual performing the aspirate and with increasing the number of needle aspirations.[29] Sampling errors may occur with lesions larger than 4 cm., and lesions smaller than 1 cm. may be difficult to aspirate.

The accuracy of FNAB is dependent on the type of tumor being sampled. A correct diagnosis is achieved in over 90 per cent of undifferentiated, medullary, and papillary carcinomas; accuracy in follicular carcinoma is approximately 40 per cent

because of the difficulty in distinguishing benign from malignant follicular tumors by FNAB. The diagnosis of follicular carcinoma requires the identification of invasion into or through the capsule of the lesion or into vascular structures. A FNAB specimen from the center of a follicular lesion cannot provide the information necessary to make this diagnosis. Differentiation between benign and malignant lesions using morphologic analysis of the nuclei or studies of DNA content is not yet considered reliable enough for clinical use. When such a hypercellular aspirate preventing a clear distinction between benign and malignant is observed, most cytologists classify these as follicular tumors or suspicious for malignancy. Such lesions require surgical removal except for those which are hyperfunctioning on radionuclide scanning. Because the possibility of malignancy in hot nodules is low, thyroid scanning may be useful in the selection of these hypercellular lesions with suspicious cytology for surgical removal.

Nodules with suspicious or indeterminant cytology that are hypofunctioning by scan remain the most important problem with FNAB. Approximately 60 to 75 per cent of FNAB specimens are benign and approximately 5 per cent are malignant. The remaining 20 to 35 per cent are classified as being indeterminant, and at least 20 per cent of these are found to be thyroid carcinomas. Since there is no other method that consistently identifies the thyroid carcinomas in this group, surgical resection is required to confirm the diagnosis.

Although FNAB is currently the best method for diagnosing thyroid carcinoma, it does have an approximately 10 per cent false-negative diagnosis rate. It is therefore mandatory that patients with an initial benign FNAB be closely followed and repeat aspirations be performed in patients with persistent thyroid nodularity. Benign lesions continue to demonstrate consistently benign cytology; when identified, cytologically suspicious or indeterminant lesions should be removed surgically. Despite these limitations, the use of FNAB has reduced the number of patients requiring surgical therapy while increasing the incidence of malignancy in excised nodules. Another advantage of FNAB is the therapeutic aspiration of cystic thyroid nodules. The majority of cysts are benign, and aspiration alone is sufficient therapy for many cysts. Lesions that recur after repeated aspirations or have suspicious cytology should be surgically excised. A diagnostic approach for management of thyroid nodules based on FNAB is shown in Figure 5.

THYROID CARCINOMA

Thyroid carcinomas are a heterogeneous group of tumors that demonstrate considerable variability in biologic behavior, histologic appearance, and response to therapy (Table 4). Although benign thyroid nodules are common, clinically detectable thyroid carcinoma is rare, representing approximately 1 per cent of all malignancies. Thyroid carcinoma occurs with an incidence of

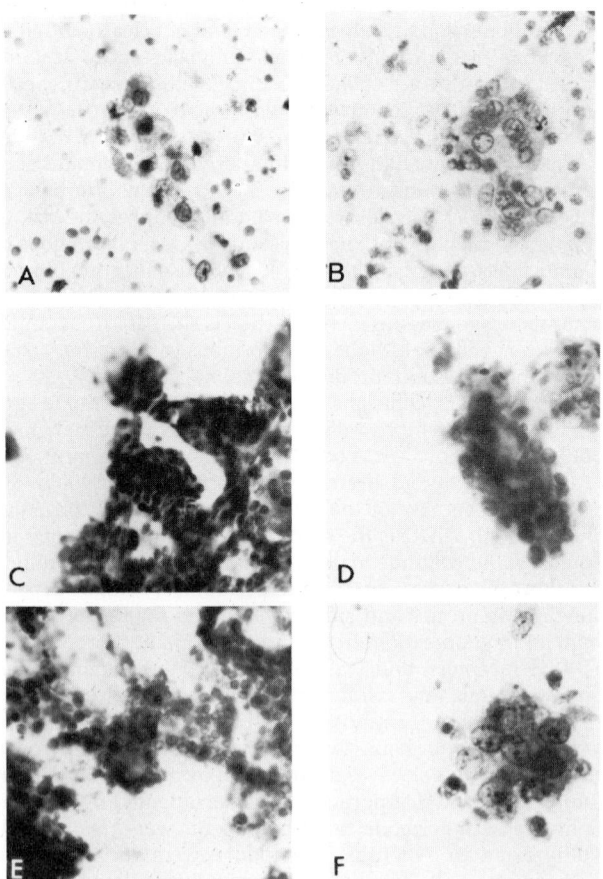

Figure 4. Cytologic patterns from fine-needle aspiration biopsy of thyroid nodules. *A*, Colloid nodule with benign-appearing thyroid epithelial cells and colloid. *B*, Hashimoto's thyroiditis with benign-appearing epithelial cells and lymphocytes. *C*, Follicular adenoma. *D*, Follicular carcinoma demonstrating a pattern similar to follicular adenoma. *E*, Papillary carcinoma demonstrating papillary projections of malignant cells. *F*, Anaplastic carcinoma.

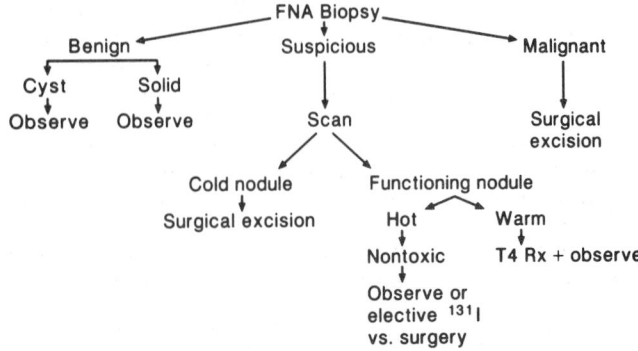

Figure 5. Management of thyroid nodule based on fine-needle aspiration biopsy as the initial diagnostic test. (From Gharib, H., and Goellner, J. R.: Evaluation of nodular thyroid disease. Endocrinol. Metab. Clin. North Am., *17*:511, 1988.)

TABLE 4. Malignant Thyroid Neoplasms

Well-differentiated neoplasms
  Papillary adenocarcinoma
    Mixed papillary-follicular carcinoma
    Follicular variant of papillary carcinoma
    Encapsulated variant
  Follicular adenocarcinoma
    Minimally invasive, encapsulated follicular carcinoma
    Widely invasive, angioinvasive follicular carcinoma
  Hürthle cell carcinoma
  Medullary carcinoma

Undifferentiated
  Spindle and giant cell carcinoma
  Small cell carcinoma

Miscellaneous
  Lymphoma
  Squamous cell carcinoma
  Microepidermoid carcinoma
  Teratoma
  Sarcoma
  Metastatic

approximately 36 to 60 cases per million population per year. These tumors are rare in children and increase in frequency with increasing age; a female:male ratio of 2.5:1 is reported, although an increasing incidence in males has been observed.[27] The autopsy incidence of thyroid carcinoma in the United States has been reported to be 0.9 to 13 per cent, depending on how extensively the thyroid glands were studied pathologically. It is likely that many thyroid carcinomas detected in these studies are not clinically significant and do not have a role in the clinical course of the patient. The annual mortality from thyroid carcinoma in the United States is only 6 individuals per million. This discrepancy between incidence and mortality presumably reflects the favorable prognosis for most thyroid carcinomas, although these tumors are capable of aggressive behavior with metastatic disease and ultimately death.

ETIOLOGY. Thyroid carcinomas can be induced in laboratory animals by exposing the thyroid gland to goitrogenic drugs, iodide deficiency, external radiation, radioactive iodide, or a combination of these factors. The carcinogenic effects of ionizing radiation are thought to occur by two different mechanisms. Radiation causes damage to cellular DNA, causing cellular injury with altered cell division and replication of nucleic acids. The radiation damage to the cell also decreases its capacity to produce thyroid hormone, thus subjecting the thyroid to chronic TSH stimulation.

The importance of irradiation as an etiologic factor in the development of thyroid carcinoma in humans is well documented. External radiation therapy was widely used from the 1920s through the 1950s for a variety of benign conditions of the head and neck region, predominantly in infants and children. Conditions such as enlarged thymus, tonsils, or adenoids as well as hemangiomas and acne were frequently managed with external radiation therapy. It was not until 1950 that Duffy and Fitzgerald[11] made the observation that many children with thyroid carcinoma had received external irradiation to the neck or mediastinum. It has subsequently been demonstrated unequivocally that exposure of the thyroid to external irradiation is directly related to the subsequent development of benign and malignant thyroid nodules. The threshold dose is thought to be very low, and an exposure of as little as 7 rads is reported to increase the incidence of cancer. The incidence of malignancy is proportional to the dose administered with a direct dose-response relationship through 1000 rads; this increased incidence diminishes with higher levels of radiation exposure, which may destroy the thyroid epithelium. With significant doses in the 200- to 500-rad range, thyroid nodules develop at the rate of 2 per cent per year, carcinoma develops in 0.5 per cent per year, and the overall risk of malignancy is approximately 5 per cent by 20 years after exposure.[8] The adult thyroid is also sensitive to the carcinogenic effects of irradiation, but the risk of carcinogenesis appears to be less than that observed in children. Benign nodules also develop at a high rate, occurring with perhaps ten times the frequency of cancers. The malignancies that develop typically begin to appear within 3 to 5 years after radiation exposure and reach a peak incidence at 15 to 25 years after exposure. How long the increased risk of developing thyroid malignancy persists is unknown. The types of thyroid cancer observed in this population are similar to those that develop in nonirradiated individuals of comparable age, with papillary or mixed papillary-follicular tumors predominating. A characteristic difference of the radiation-associated tumors is the presence of tumor multicentricity, which is found in up to 55 per cent of irradiated patients compared with only 22 per cent in the nonirradiated patients with thyroid malignancy. The natural history of radiation-associated thyroid carcinoma is basically the same as in nonirradiated patients in the same age group. Therapy also follows the same guidelines in the two groups,[8] with some exceptions noted in the section on treatment.

The administration of ^{131}I for the treatment of hyperthyroidism has not caused a subsequent increase in risk of thyroid carcinoma.[10] This may be because the treatment has been used primarily in older adults and the large radiation dose may effectively ablate the thyroid epithelium.

Factors Influencing Survival

The prognosis in most patients with well-differentiated thyroid cancer is quite favorable; however, the histologic type of tumor, size, stage, and age and sex of the patient are all factors that influence prognosis.

PATHOLOGY. Patients with papillary or mixed papillary-follicular carcinoma have the most favorable prognosis. Prognosis in follicular carcinoma is slightly less favorable than in papillary carcinoma. Prognosis is generally poorer in patients with medullary carcinoma and is least favorable in those with undifferentiated cancer. It has been reported that analysis of DNA content may be useful in predicting prognosis, since tumors with an aneuploid pattern tend to be aggressive whereas those that are euploid are less aggressive.[5]

STAGE OF TUMOR. Most treatment decisions are determined primarily by the clinical stage of the cancer as determined by preoperative findings, intraoperative findings, and final pathology. The staging system of DeGroot[9] has proved to be useful for clinical staging:

Stage I: Tumors with single or multiple intrathyroidal foci.
Stage II: Tumors with cervical metastases that are not fixed and without invasion.
Stage III: Thyroid tumors with local cervical invasion or fixed cervical metastases.
Stage IV: Lesions metastatic outside the neck.

Patients with Stage I differentiated carcinomas have a very good prognosis. The influence of nodal metastasis on prognosis is a controversial issue, but in general it can be stated that this finding represents a more extensive thyroid tumor and is associated with an increased recurrence rate and a poorer prognosis. Children with thyroid cancer have an 80 per cent incidence of clinically positive cervical nodes, but their prognosis is excellent. Palpable nodal metastases are present in only 10 to 20 per cent of adults. If age-matched patient groups are compared, however, the prognosis is better at any age for those patients without nodal metastases (Fig. 6). Patients with Stage III cancers with invasion into the adjacent neck structures have a poorer prognosis. The presence of distant metastases is likewise associated with the poorest prognosis.

AGE AND SEX. Age at the time of diagnosis has consistently

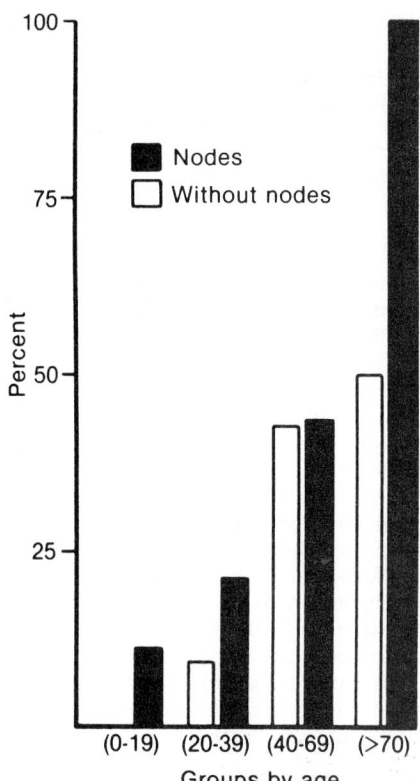

Figure 6. Comparison of deaths from all causes in patients with and without lymph node metastases with differentiated thyroid cancer. (From Horwood, J., Clark, O. H., and Dunphy, J. E.: Am. J. Surg., *136*:107, 1978.)

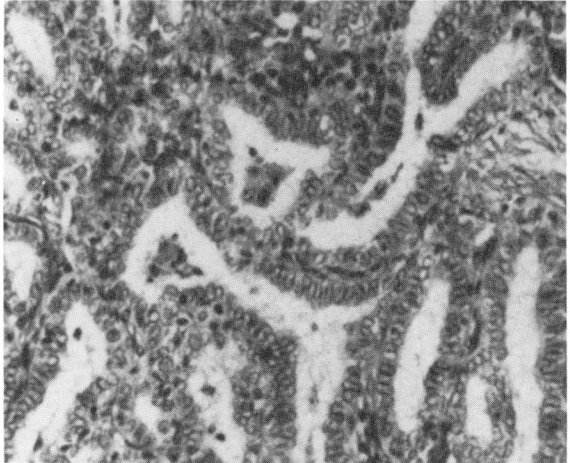

Figure 7. Papillary carcinoma. Photomicrograph (×160) demonstrates papillary carcinoma with branching papillary fronds, ground-glass nuclei, and glandular component. (From Kini, S. R. (Ed.): Guides to Clinical Aspiration Biopsy. Thyroid. New York, Igaku-Shinon, 1987.)

been demonstrated to have a profound influence on prognosis in patients with well-differentiated thyroid carcinomas. This has been most convincingly demonstrated in patients with papillary and mixed papillary-follicular carcinomas. Children and young adults have an excellent prognosis despite the fact that a high percentage have nodal metastases at the time of diagnosis. Patients under 40 years old have a better prognosis than do older patients in whom the disease is more aggressive. Mortality is higher in men and women over 50 years of age, increasing in one series from 2 per cent in patients under age 20 to 34 per cent in patients over 50 years old.[4] Age continues to be the most important single variable in the determination of prognosis. In addition, women appear to have a better prognosis than do men in most series, although this point has been debated.

Strategies in Treatment

PAPILLARY CARCINOMA. Although the primary management of papillary thyroid carcinoma is surgical excision, the extent of the resection and the indications for regional lymph node dissection remain controversial. In the absence of randomized, prospective studies, recommendations for therapy must be based on retrospective studies that have been conducted in an uncontrolled manner. Enthusiasm for radical surgical procedures must be tempered by the knowledge that the majority of patients do quite well when a conservative surgical approach is taken. However, 40 to 50 per cent of patients dying of papillary carcinoma do so because of local invasion.

Papillary carcinoma has its peak incidence in the third and fourth decades and the lesions that are frequently multicentric remain confined to the thyroid for extended periods of time (Fig. 7). When spread of disease occurs, it is usually to regional lymph nodes or by direct extension into extrathyroidal structures. Approximately 5 per cent of patients present with distant metastases. All these factors must be considered in developing a safe, effective treatment strategy for papillary thyroid carcinoma.

Most experienced surgeons agree that thyroid lobectomy and isthmusectomy is the appropriate initial procedure for a thyroid nodule that might be cancer (Fig. 8). Small anterior nodules or nodules at the isthmus may be locally resected with the anterior third of each lobe. If the nodule is found to be papillary carcinoma by frozen section, the surgeon has several options for management.

Surgical options include lobectomy, near-total thyroidectomy (ipsilateral total lobectomy and contralateral subtotal lobectomy), and total thyroidectomy. As the extent of thyroidectomy increases, the risk of complications such as recurrent nerve injury and hypoparathyroidism also increases. Each surgeon must select an approach that provides satisfactory results with low operative morbidity.

The extent of thyroidectomy is best determined by the extent to which the thyroid gland is involved with the tumor. Total thyroidectomy would be justified in patients with gross evidence of extensive bilateral carcinoma. Many surgeons believe this procedure should also be used in all patients whose tumors are larger than 1.5 cm. Several reasons have been advanced to support this position. Total thyroidectomy is associated with a lower rate of local recurrence than are less aggressive procedures, and approximately 50 per cent of the patients who develop recurrent thyroid cancer die from the disease. Long-term survival has been reported to be better after total thyroidectomy when compared with lesser procedures. Papillary carcinoma is frequently multifocal and bilateral, and malignant foci in residual thyroid tissue become clinically evident in 5 to 10 per cent of patients who then require completion thyroidectomy.[21] These reoperations are associated with a higher risk of complications. Total thyroidectomy also facilitates the use of ^{131}I total body scan for the detection of recurrent or distant disease and allows the most efficient use of ^{131}I for treatment of metastatic disease. Total thyroidectomy also increases the sensitivity of thyroglobulin measurements, which may be useful in detecting recurrent disease. Although total thyroidectomy is associated with a higher complication rate, it remains a safe operation with experienced surgeons. Several large series of total thyroidectomy have reported an incidence of recurrent laryngeal nerve injury of less than 1 per cent and permanent hypoparathyroidism in less than 3 per cent.[16] Total thyroidectomy is preferred in patients with a history of significant radiation therapy because of the higher incidence of multicentricity and bilaterality.

Many authors advocate thyroid lobectomy or near-total thyroidectomy for papillary carcinoma confined clinically to one lobe. They report that the more extensive total thyroidectomy

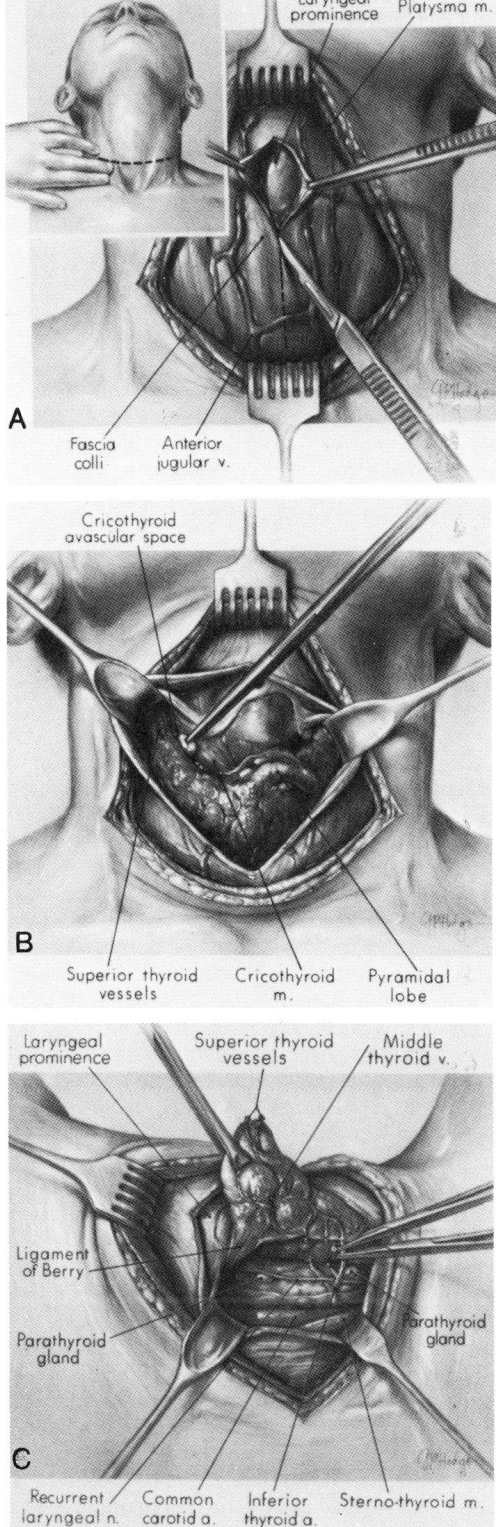

Figure 8. Technique of thyroidectomy. *A*, With the head extended, a curvilinear transverse incision is made approximately 3 cm. above the clavicular heads. After elevation of superior and inferior flaps, the cervical fascia is divided in the midline. *B*, The cricothyroid space is opened to allow exposure of the superior pole vessels. *C*, The thyroid gland is rotated anteriorly, exposing branches of the inferior thyroid artery, recurrent laryngeal nerve, and parathyroid glands. The terminal branches of the inferior thyroid artery are divided after the recurrent laryngeal nerve is identified and protected. Blood supply to the parathyroid glands should be preserved if possible. (From Thompson, N. W., Olsen, W. R., and Hoffman, G. L.: The continuing development of the technique of thyroidectomy. Surgery, *73*:913, 1973.)

does not improve survival but substantially increases the complication rate. The issue of whether total thyroidectomy leads to better survival in these patients cannot be resolved by the studies that are available at this time. Until more conclusive studies establishing the optimal surgical procedures for papillary carcinoma are available and since papillary carcinoma usually has an excellent prognosis, the more extensive operations should be performed only if they can be done with very low morbidity. These factors are related to the skill and experience of the individual surgeon. An alternative procedure when removal of all thyroid tissue is warranted is to follow near-total thyroidectomy with a dose of ^{131}I to destroy the thyroid remnant. For those tumors less than 1.5 cm., it is generally agreed that total thyroidectomy is not required.

Patients with papillary thyroid carcinoma frequently have metastatic involvement of regional lymph nodes. Occult nodal metastases have been reported in 21 to 82 per cent of patients with papillary carcinoma larger than 2 cm.; fortunately, only approximately 10 per cent of patients not undergoing node dissection develop clinically recurrent disease. Delay in removal of lymph nodes until they become palpable does not adversely affect survival, and there appears to be no place for routine prophylactic neck dissection in these patients. There is also no need for *en bloc* dissection, since lymph node metastases of these cancers seldom extend beyond the lymph node capsule. When total thyroidectomy is performed for papillary carcinoma, the central neck nodes including those in the ipsilateral tracheoesophageal groove, pretracheal area, along the recurrent laryngeal nerve and inferior thyroid veins, and in the anterior mediastinum are removed with the operative specimen. In patients with palpably enlarged lateral cervical nodes, most surgeons believe that their removal by modified neck dissection is indicated. Jugular nodes may also be sampled through the thyroidectomy incision, and the decision to proceed with node dissection can be based on histologic evaluation of these nodes. The procedure includes resection of the entire jugular chain and contents of the posterior triangle of the neck with preservation of the sternocleidomastoid muscle, jugular vein, and spinal accessory nerve. A suprahyoid dissection is usually not necessary, since nodes in this area rarely contain metastases. This procedure avoids the cosmetic and functional problems associated with standard radical neck dissection, and the results are essentially equivalent to those achieved with the radical procedure.

FOLLICULAR CARCINOMA. Follicular carcinoma represents 15 to 20 per cent of thyroid cancers and is more prevalent in iodide-deficient areas. These tumors occur in older patients with a peak incidence in the fifth decade of life. Follicular carcinoma usually presents as a solitary mass in the thyroid. This lesion has a marked propensity for vascular invasion but does not invade lymphatic channels, and lymph node metastases are much less common than in papillary carcinoma. Follicular carcinoma frequently disseminates hematogenously with bone, lungs, brain, and liver as the most frequent sites of metastases. These distant metastases portend an extremely grave prognosis. Pathologically, two types of follicular carcinoma are recognized, that is, the minimally invasive and widely invasive forms. The minimally invasive follicular carcinoma resembles a follicular adenoma with a well-defined capsule. The diagnosis is based on the microscopic demonstration of invasion of the capsule, invasion through the capsule, or invasion into veins in or beyond the capsule. These lesions are rarely multicentric, rarely metastasize, and in general are associated with an excellent prognosis. These well-differentiated follicular carcinomas can be safely managed by total lobectomy as long as they are confined to one lobe.

The widely invasive follicular carcinoma is the most aggressive of the well-differentiated thyroid cancers, frequently demonstrating extension through the thyroid capsule into surrounding structures. The prognosis in these patients is poor with one series reporting that 80 per cent of patients with widely invasive follicular carcinoma developed metastases and 20 per cent died of the tumor.[22] Because of these factors, patients who present with locally aggressive tumors or those with proven metastatic disease are best treated with near-total or total thyroidectomy, which optimizes the effectiveness of ^{131}I treatment for residual or distant disease. Node dissection is performed only in those rare situations when nodes are clinically involved.

HÜRTHLE CELL CARCINOMA. The Hürthle cell is derived from follicular epithelium and is characterized morphologically by its larger size and voluminous granular cytoplasm that is produced by numerous huge mitochondria filling the cell. These cells are found in a variety of conditions affecting the thyroid and are thought to represent a degenerative or metaplastic phenomenon of the follicular epithelium. The majority of nodules containing Hürthle cells are not neoplastic but represent Hürthle cell change of existing follicular adenomatous nodules in goiters or thyroiditis. These lesions must be distinguished from the true Hürthle cell neoplasms, which are solitary, encapsulated lesions composed of Hürthle cells in a follicular or solid pattern. When studies include only Hürthle cell neoplasms, the incidence of malignancy has been 5 to 67 per cent. Whether this tumor should be considered a subtype of follicular carcinoma or a separate, distinct entity remains controversial. The pathologic criteria for malignancy including vascular and capsular invasion are the same as for follicular carcinoma; in the absence of these changes, Hürthle cell tumors should be considered benign.

The biologic behavior of Hürthle cell tumors has been controversial because of reports that tumors that appeared to be benign histologically may produce metastatic disease. Most authors, however, have concluded that biologic behavior does correlate with histologic appearance and that lobectomy is adequate treatment for benign Hürthle cell tumors. Malignant Hürthle cell lesions are generally considered to be more aggressive than other well-differentiated thyroid carcinomas metastasizing to both regional lymph nodes and distant sites and demonstrating a high local recurrence rate after resection. Management usually requires total thyroidectomy with node sampling and neck dissection when there are metastases to cervical nodes.

MEDULLARY THYROID CARCINOMA. See discussion on medullary thyroid carcinoma, Chapter 23, Part VI.

UNDIFFERENTIATED THYROID CARCINOMA. Undifferentiated or anaplastic carcinomas occur predominantly in patients over age 50 with a peak incidence at approximately 65 years of age. This tumor, which is the most aggressive of all thyroid malignancies, fortunately comprises only 5 to 10 per cent of thyroid cancers. There is frequently a history of a long-standing goiter or nodular thyroid in affected patients. The tumor is more frequent in endemic goiter regions, and there are reports that external irradiation may have a role in development. The usual clinical presentation is rapid enlargement in a nodular thyroid accompanied by symptoms of local invasion such as dyspnea or dysphagia. At the time of diagnosis, the majority of undifferentiated carcinomas have spread locally to vital structures in the neck, precluding surgical resection. The small number of patients in whom operative resection is possible usually have evidence of disease of limited extent on physical examination. In patients with diffuse, infiltrative lesions, surgical resection or debulking is rarely indicated; therapy with external radiotherapy and chemotherapy may provide limited palliation. Tracheostomy may be required for maintenance of the airway because of the propensity for invasion of the trachea. Prognosis is predictably quite poor with a mean survival of 6 months and a 7 per cent 5-year survival rate reported.[1]

LYMPHOMA. Primary malignant lymphoma of the thyroid is a rare malignancy that typically presents as a rapidly enlarging, firm, painless mass in older women. This entity frequently arises in glands with evidence of chronic lymphocytic thyroiditis. The diagnosis can sometimes be made by fine-needle aspiration biopsy or cutting-needle biopsy, although surgical resection is frequently undertaken because the diagnosis cannot be established with certainty with needle biopsy techniques. It is critical that this lesion be distinguished from anaplastic carcinoma, which it frequently resembles in clinical presentation, since successful therapeutic options are available for lymphoma. Following diagnosis, appropriate staging should be performed to determine the extent of disease. Patients with local disease are treated with radiation therapy since this lesion is quite radiosensitive. In patients in whom lymphoma is discovered at the time of surgical therapy, survival is unaffected by the extent of operation even if only biopsy is obtained. When there is extrathyroidal extension, the surgical procedure should be limited to obtaining a diagnostic specimen, since more aggressive procedures may cause increased morbidity without improving survival. Patients with more extensive disease or those who relapse are treated with chemotherapy.

Postoperative Treatment

The role of radioiodine in the postoperative management of patients with well-differentiated thyroid cancer remains controversial in large part because mortality is so low in this disease. However, it must also be considered that numerous convincing studies have demonstrated that the lowest recurrence and death rates are found in patients who have received both radioiodine and thyroid hormone suppression. This survival advantage is observed primarily in patients with follicular and mixed papillary-follicular tumors; patients with papillary carcinoma whose tumors have a significant follicular component should thus benefit from radioiodine.[28] Most experts recommend that patients with well-differentiated thyroid cancers larger than 1.5 cm. receive postoperative radioiodine. Beneficial effects of radioiodine are less certain in patients under 40 years, and some authors do not routinely perform ablation in younger patients who have tumors less than 1.0 cm. unless there is a history of radiation exposure. Therapeutic radioiodine is useful in the treatment of microscopic or occult metastases and other forms of metastatic disease such as micronodular pulmonary metastases. In order for the radioiodine to be most effective, however, normal thyroid tissue must first be removed, since it accumulates the isotope more avidly than do thyroid cancers.

Postoperative ^{131}I scans are usually performed 2 to 3 months following operation for well-differentiated thyroid cancer. A 2-week period without thyroid hormone replacement should precede the scan in order to achieve maximal concentration of endogenous TSH, which stimulates uptake of ^{131}I by any remaining thyroid tissue and metastatic lesions. Optimally, TSH levels should be determined prior to the scan, and patients should be advised to restrict iodine intake in preparation for the scan. Patients with significant residual functioning tissue and those with metastatic disease are candidates for radioiodine ablation. Ablation of residual thyroid tissue can usually be accomplished with one dose of 30 mc. of ^{131}I; patients with metastatic deposits in the neck are given 75 to 100 mc. and those with distant metastases 150 to 200 mc. Radioiodine scan and treatment is then repeated at 6- to 9-month intervals until tumor uptake of the isotope is abolished or adverse effects of radioiodine are encountered. Female patients should always be carefully screened for pregnancy prior to radiation treatment, since damage to the fetus can occur.

Essentially all patients who undergo operations for well-differentiated thyroid carcinoma should receive thyroid hormone. This may be necessary to prevent hypothyroidism in many patients. In addition, there is abundant evidence that TSH can stimulate growth of differentiated thyroid carcinoma, and thyroid hormone given in adequate doses suppresses TSH. Recurrence rates of both papillary and follicular carcinoma are lower in patients treated postoperatively with thyroid hormone. Patients without known metastatic disease are then followed at 3- to 6-month intervals and ^{131}I scans are performed approximately 1 year after operation and then at 3 and 5 years. All patients receive thyroid hormone in doses that restore euthyroidism and maintain TSH suppression. Serum thyroglobulin measurements are helpful in determining the presence of recurrent disease in patients who have undergone ablative therapy of all thyroid tissue. Thyroglobulin is produced only by thyroid tissue, and increasing levels in these patients is suggestive of disease recurrence.

EXTERNAL RADIATION. External radiation has a limited role in the management of well-differentiated thyroid carcinoma since these tumors are relatively radioresistant. It may be useful for the palliative treatment of patients with unresectable cancers that do not take up radioiodine and has a primary role in the treatment of lymphoma and undifferentiated thyroid carcinomas.

CHEMOTHERAPY. Chemotherapy is the third line of therapy for those thyroid malignancies that are not adequately controlled by surgical therapy and radiation. Numerous chemotherapeutic agents have been tried, although the most widely used agents are doxorubicin, 5-fluorouracil, methotrexate, actinomycin D, and cyclophosphamide. Doxorubicin alone or in combination with other agents produces response rates of 30 to 40 per cent; a longer survival time is observed in patients whose tumors respond to chemotherapy. The usefulness of these single agents and multidrug combinations remains uncertain pending results of well-conducted studies comparing various drugs.

SELECTED REFERENCES

DeGroot, L. J.: Diagnostic approach and management of patients exposed to irradiation to the thyroid. J. Clin. Endocrinol. Metab., 69:925, 1989.
This concise article covers the salient features of management of patients subjected to radiation of the thyroid gland. The recommendations are based on the author's extensive experience with this problem on the Thyroid Study Unit at the University of Chicago. Excellent discussion of evaluation, surgical management, follow-up, and prophylaxis are included.

Kramer, J. B., and Wells, S. A.: Thyroid carcinoma. Adv. Surg., 72:195, 1989.
This comprehensive review article explores in depth the subject of thyroid carcinoma. Excellent sections on etiology, pathology, and clinical presentation are followed by a complete discussion of diagnostic evaluation. Each of the major types of thyroid carcinoma is then reviewed in depth with consideration of prognosis, surgical treatment, and postoperative management.

Mazzaferri, E. L., de los Santos, E. T., and Rofagha-Keyhani, S.: Solitary thyroid nodule: Diagnosis and management. Med. Clin. North Am., 72:1177, 1988.
This is a complete and authoritative review of the various modalities used in the evaluation of thyroid nodules. The subject of fine-needle aspiration biopsy (FNAB) is covered in particular detail. A detailed plan for the diagnostic approach to thyroid nodules based on FNAB is presented. The bibliography is particularly valuable because of its completeness.

Studer, H., Peter, H. J., and Gerber, H.: Natural heterogeneity of thyroid cells: The basis for understanding thyroid function and nodular goiter growth. Endocr. Rev., 10:125, 1989.
A noted expert in the field reviews current understanding of the development of nodular goiters. Many of the important advances in this area have come from this laboratory. Basic premises presented include the concepts that follicular thyroid cells are not identical but have highly individual metabolic potential and that new follicles produced during goitrogenesis arise from a few predestined follicular cells with a propensity to replicate at higher than average rates. This stimulating article provides insights that may be applicable to other organ systems and provides new understanding of nodular goiter formation.

van de Velde, C. J. H., et al.: International symposium on controversies in the management of differentiated thyroid carcinoma. Eur. J. Clin. Endocrinol., 24:287, 1988.
This symposium provides an excellent review and update of several important topics in the diagnosis and management of thyroid cancer. It includes excellent articles on evaluation of nodules, total thyroidectomy, modified neck dissection, survival analysis, and the use of radioactive iodine. There is also a consensus

report on the management of differentiated thyroid cancer in the Netherlands. Having so much valuable and current information available in one issue makes this an extremely valuable contribution.

REFERENCES

1. Aldinger, K. A., Samaan, N. A., Ibanez, M., et al.: Anaplastic carcinoma of the thyroid. A review of 84 cases of spindle giant cell carcinoma of the thyroid. Cancer, 41:2267, 1978.
2. Bachtarzi, H., and Benmiloud, M.: TSH-regulation and goitrogenesis in severe iodine deficiency. Acta Endocrinol., 103:21, 1983.
3. Balme, H. W.: Metastatic carcinoma of the thyroid successfully treated with thyroxine. Lancet, 1:812, 1954.
4. Cady, B., Sedgwick, C. E., Meissner, W. A., et al.: Changing clinical, pathologic, therapeutic, and survival patterns in differentiated thyroid carcinoma. Ann. Surg., 184:541, 1976.
5. Cohn, K. H., et al.: Prognostic value of nuclear DNA content in papillary thyroid carcinoma. World J. Surg., 8:474, 1984.
6. Cole, W. H., Majarahis, M. D., and Slaughter, D. P.: Incidence of carcinoma of the thyroid in nodular goiter. J. Clin. Endocrinol., 9:1007, 1949.
7. Cutler, S. J., and Young, J. L., Jr. (Eds.): Third National Cancer Survey: Incidence Data. National Cancer Institute Monograph 41, DHEW Publication No. (NIH) 75–787. Bethesda, National Cancer Institute, 1975, pp. 107–111.
8. DeGroot, L. J.: Diagnostic approach and management of patients exposed to irradiation to the thyroid. J. Clin. Endocrinol. Metab., 69:925, 1989.
9. DeGroot, L. J., and Sridama, V.: Thyroid neoplasia. In DeGroot, L. J. (Ed.): Endocrinology. Philadelphia, W. B. Saunders Company, 1989, p. 768.
10. Dobyns, B. M., Sheline, G. E., Workman, J. B., Tompkins, E. A., McConahey, W. M., and Becker, D. V.: Malignant and benign neoplasms of the thyroid in patients treated for hyperthyroidism: A report of the cooperative thyrotoxicosis therapy follow-up study. J. Clin. Endocrinol. Metab., 38:976, 1974.
11. Duffy, B. J., Jr., and Fitzgerald, P. J.: Cancer of thyroid in children: A report of twenty-eight cases. J. Clin. Endocrinol., 10:1296, 1950.
12. Eggo, M. C., Bachrach, L. K., Fayet, G., Errick, J., Cohen, M. F., Kudlow, J. E., and Burrow, G. N.: Effect of growth factors and serum on DNA synthesis and differentiation in thyroid cells in culture. Mol. Cell Endocrinol., 38:141, 1984.
13. Gharib, J., James, E. M., Charboneau, J. W., et al.: Suppressive therapy with levothyroxine for solitary thyroid nodules: A double-blind controlled clinical study. N. Engl. J. Med., 317:70, 1987.
14. Goellner, J. R., Gharib, H., Grant, C. S., et al.: Fine needle aspiration cytology of the thyroid, 1980 to 1986. Acta Cytol. (Baltimore), 31:587, 1987.
15. Grubeck-Loebenstein, B., Buchan, G., Sadeghi, R., Kissonerghis, M., Londei, M., Turner, M., Pirich, K., Roka, R., Niederle, B., Kassal, H., Waldhausl, W., and Feldmann, M.: Transforming growth factor beta regulates thyroid growth. Role in the pathogenesis of nontoxic goiter. J. Clin. Invest., 83:764, 1989.
16. Harness, J. K., Fung, L., Thompson, N. W., et al.: Total thyroidectomy: Complications and technique. World J. Surg., 10:781, 1986.
17. Horlocker, T. T., Hay, J. E., James, E. M., et al.: Prevalence of incidental nodular thyroid disease detected during high-resolution parathyroid ultrasonography. In Medeiros-Neto, G., and Gaitan, E. (Eds.): Frontiers in Thyroidology. New York, Plenum Medical Book Company, 1986, p. 1309.
18. Hung, W., August, G. P., Randolph, J. G., et al.: Solitary thyroid nodules in children and adolescents. J. Pediatr. Surg., 17:225, 1982.
19. James, E. M., and Charboneau, J. W.: High-frequency (10 MHz) thyroid ultrasonography. Semin. Ultrasound CT MR, 6:294, 1985.
20. Kelly, F. C., and Snedden, W. W.: Prevalence of distribution of endemic goiter. Bull. WHO, 18:5, 1958.
21. Kramer, J. B., and Wells, S. A.: Thyroid carcinoma. Adv. Surg., 22:195, 1989.
22. Lang, W., Choritz, H., and Hundeshagen, H.: Risk factors in follicular thyroid carcinomas. A retrospective followup study covering a 14 year period with emphasis on morphological findings. Am. J. Surg. Pathol., 10:246, 1986.
23. Marine, D.: Etiology and prevention of simple goiter. Medicine, 3:453, 1924.
24. Maxon, H. R., et al.: Ionizing irradiation and the induction of clinically significant disease of the human thyroid gland. Am. J. Med., 63:967, 1977.
25. Mazzaferri, E. L., de los Santos, E. T., and Rofagha-Keyhani, S.: Solitary thyroid nodule: Diagnosis and management. Med. Clin. North Am., 72:1177, 1988.
26. Mortensen, J. D., Woolner, L. B., and Bennett, W. A.: Gross and microscopic findings in clinically normal thyroid glands. J. Clin. Endocrinol. Metab., 15:1270, 1955.
27. Rossi, R. L., Cady, B., Silverman, M. L., et al.: Current results in conservative surgery for differentiated thyroid carcinoma. World J. Surg., 10:612, 1986.
28. Samaan, N. A., Maheshwari, Y. K., Nader, S., et al.: Impact of therapy for differentiated carcinoma of the thyroid: Analysis of 706 cases. J. Clin. Endocrinol. Metab., 56:1131, 1983.
29. Schmid, K. W., Hofstladter, F., Propst, A., Jr., et al.: A 14 year practice with the fine-needle aspiration biopsy of the thyroid in an endemic area. Pathol. Res. Pract., 181:308, 1986.
30. Solbiati, L., Volterrani, L., Rizzatto, G., et al.: The thyroid gland with low uptake lesions: Evaluation by ultrasound. Radiology, 155:187, 1985.
31. Studer, H., Gerber, H., and Peter, H. J.: Multinodular goiter. In DeGroot, L. J. (Ed.): Endocrinology. Philadelphia, W. B. Saunders Company, 1989, p. 722.

32. Studer, J., Peter, H. J., and Gerber, H.: Natural heterogeneity of thyroid cells: The basis for understanding thyroid function and nodular goiter growth. Endocr. Rev., *10*:125, 1989.

33. Thompson, N. W.: Editorial: Current diagnostic techniques for single thyroid nodules. Curr. Surg., *40*:255, 1983.

34. Valente, W. A., Vitti, P., Rotella, C. M., et al.: Antibodies that promote thyroid growth. A distinct population of thyroid-stimulating autoantibodies. N. Engl. J. Med., *309*:1028, 1983.

35. Vander, J. B., Gaston, E. A., and Dawber, T. R.: The significance of nontoxic thyroid nodules: Final report of a 15 year study of the incidence of thyroid malignancy. Ann. Intern. Med., *69*:537, 1968.

36. Van Herle, A. J., Rich, P., Ljung, B., et al.: The thyroid nodule. Ann. Intern. Med., *96*:221, 1982.

37. Westermark, K., Karlsson, F. A., and Westermark, B.: Epidermal growth factor modulates thyroid growth and function in culture. Endocrinology, *112*:1680, 1983.

VI

THE MULTIPLE ENDOCRINE NEOPLASIAS

Samuel A. Wells, Jr., M.D, and Terry C. Lairmore, M.D.

Tumors of the endocrine system most often develop within a single gland. There are genetic disorders, however, that are characterized by a predisposition to the development of neoplasms in multiple endocrine glands. In these diseases, which are usually familial, the endocrine tumors may be benign or malignant and develop either synchronously or metachronously. The pathologic change in affected glands is characteristically multicentric and may be expressed as hyperplasia, adenoma, or carcinoma.

The multiple endocrine neoplasia (MEN) syndromes are classified according to the pattern of involvement. In its full expression, MEN-I is characterized by the concurrence of parathyroid hyperplasia, pancreatic islet cell neoplasms, and adenomas of the anterior pituitary gland. MEN-IIa is characterized by the concurrence of medullary thyroid carcinoma (MTC), pheochromocytoma, and parathyroid hyperplasia; whereas MEN-IIb consists of MTC, pheochromocytoma, mucosal neuromas, and a distinctive "marfanoid" habitus. These syndromes are transmitted as mendelian autosomal dominant traits.

MULTIPLE ENDOCRINE NEOPLASIA TYPE I

Historical Aspects

The first description of associated endocrinopathies is believed to be Erdheim's report[6] in 1903 of an acromegalic patient who at necropsy was found to have a pituitary eosinophilic adenoma and four enlarged parathyroid glands. In 1927, Cushing and Davidoff[5] reported a patient with simultaneous neoplasms of the pituitary gland (eosinophilic adenoma), parathyroids (two adenomas), and endocrine pancreas (islet cell adenoma).

Shelburne and McLaughlin[19] in 1945 described the treatment of a patient with hypoglycemia, visual field defects, and nephrolithiasis. In 1954, Wermer[37] described the familial occurrence of tumors involving the pituitary gland, parathyroids, and pancreatic islets. The disease was subsequently termed multiple endocrine adenomatosis (MEA) and more recently has been designated multiple endocrine neoplasia type I (MEN-I). In the family studied by Wermer, the father and four of nine children were affected. Four of the five had pituitary tumors and peptic ulcer disease, and three had hypercalcemia and pancreatic adenomas. He proposed that the syndrome in this family was caused by an autosomal dominant gene with a high degree of penetrance.

The peptic ulcer diathesis frequently associated with MEN-I was often noted to be associated with a pancreatic neoplasm. In 1955, Zollinger and Ellison[42] reported two cases of severe recurrent peptic ulcer disease associated with pancreatic islet cell tumors. The ulcer disease was markedly resistant to standard operative treatment and was characterized by the secretion of hydrochloric acid in large volumes. These investigators proposed that the islet cell tumors of the pancreas were ulcerogenic. In 1960, Gregory and associates[7] demonstrated that an extract from a non–beta cell adenoma of the head of the pancreas excised from a patient with this disease stimulated acid secretion from a denervated gastric pouch. The extracted substance resembled neither histamine nor insulin, and these investigators concluded that the material was similar to antral gastrin in its chemical and physiologic properties. McGuigan[14] in 1968 demonstrated by immunofluorescence that gastrin was indeed the hormone produced by these pancreatic tumors. It was also subsequently demonstrated that a marked elevation in the serum gastrin concentration was associated with the Zollinger-Ellison (Z-E) syndrome.

Genetic Studies and Pathogenesis

The mendelian autosomal dominant inheritance pattern of the trait for MEN-I has been clearly established. Recent studies using DNA probes to detect linkage between restriction fragment length polymorphisms (RFLPs) and the disease locus have mapped the MEN-I gene to the long arm of chromosome 11.[11]

Previous theories have postulated that a primary defect in the pancreatic islet cells might cause excess production of insulin, gastrin, or glucagon and lead secondarily to stimulation and neoplastic development in the parathyroids and pituitary.[29] However, scientific support for these hypotheses is lacking. It appears most likely that the parathyroid, pancreatic islet, and pituitary derangements all result from a single mutated locus. Oncogenesis in the MEN syndromes may require two separate mutational events, as demonstrated for other inherited neoplasms (notably retinoblastoma). According to this model, the first mutation is inherited in the germ line and confers susceptibility to neoplastic change in the involved endocrine tissues. Elimination of the remaining normal allele through a second somatic mutational event, or "second hit" (such as a gene deletion), unmasks the inherited recessive mutation and causes the development of adenoma or carcinoma. The occurrence of multiple second hits would then cause multiple clones of neoplastic cells and the multicentric involvement characteristically observed in affected endocrine tissues.

In fact, the use of DNA probes that detect restriction fragment length polymorphisms for comparison of constitutional and tumor tissue genotypes from patients with MEN-I has demonstrated allelic deletions on chromosome 11.[11]

Clinical Features and Management

The clinical expression of MEN-I most often develops in the third or fourth decade, and the onset of symptoms is rare before age 10. Males and females are affected equally, as predicted by the autosomal dominant inheritance pattern. MEN-I has been described in many geographic regions and in many ethnic groups, and no racial predilection has been demonstrated.

The gene for MEN-I is transmitted with nearly 100 per cent penetrance, but with variable expressivity, such that each affected individual exhibits some but not necessarily all of the components of the syndrome. The most common abnormality in MEN-I is parathyroid hyperplasia, which occurs in nearly all affected individuals, followed by pancreatic islet cell neoplasms and pituitary adenomas. The distribution of endocrine involvement varies according to the method of study and the patient population, but approximately 90 to 97 per cent of patients have biochemical evidence of hyperparathyroidism, whereas pancreatic islet cell neoplasms are manifested in 30 to 80 per cent, and pituitary tumors occur in 15 to 50 percent.[3] If followed long enough, most affected individuals eventually develop involvement of several endocrine tissues, and one study of MEN-I patients at necropsy detected pathologic involvement in all three endocrine tissues in more than 90 per cent of patients.[12]

The clinical manifestations of patients with MEN-I depend on the endocrine tissue involved and, particularly in the case of the pancreatic islet and pituitary neoplasms, the overproduction of a specific hormone. Symptoms may also arise as a result of the tumor mass itself. In a classic review of 85 patients by Ballard and associates[1] in 1964, the most frequent mode of clinical presentation was peptic ulcer disease or its complications. Manifestations of hypoglycemia represented the second most common presenting feature, while symptoms of hyperparathyroidism or complaints referable to pituitary dysfunction (headaches, visual field defects, and secondary amenorrhea) least often led to the diagnosis. It is important to note, however, that the mode of clinical presentation did not actually indicate the incidence of involvement of the various endocrine tissues.

PARATHYROIDS. The most common endocrine abnormality in MEN-I is hyperparathyroidism, occurring in more than 90 per cent of patients. Most affected individuals exhibit generalized parathyroid hyperplasia with involvement of all four glands. In contrast, fewer than 20 per cent of patients with sporadic primary hyperparathyroidism have multiglandular involvement. Although there has been some debate among pathologists with respect to the occurrence of multiple adenoma versus asymmetrical or nodular hyperplasia in MEN-I, most agree that generalized chief cell hyperplasia is the characteristic pathologic lesion.

Hyperparathyroidism is usually the first biochemical abnormality detected in MEN-I and may precede the clinical onset of an islet cell or pituitary neoplasm by several years. The symptoms in the setting of MEN-I are similar to those of patients with sporadic primary hyperparathyroidism. Asymptomatic hypercalcemia may be present in many patients over a long period of observation. Symptomatic patients may develop renal or ureteral lithiasis and/or nephrocalcinosis. Skeletal manifestations of hyperparathyroidism occur but are uncommon. In general, hyperparathyroidism in MEN-I has an earlier age of onset and usually causes a milder hypercalcemia than that observed in primary sporadic hyperparathyroidism. The diagnosis is made by measurement of serum calcium, phosphate, and parathormone levels.

Patients with MEN-I and parathyroid hyperplasia have most often been managed by subtotal (3½-gland) parathyroidectomy in an attempt to render them normocalcemic. Unfortunately, the incidence of recurrent hyperparathyroidism postoperatively has been as high as 40 per cent,[17] whereas the incidence of permanent hypoparathyroidism has been approximately 25 per cent.[28] For these reasons, in patients with multiglandular hyperplasia, total parathyroidectomy with autotransplantation of parathyroid tissue into an ectopic site such as the forearm muscle has been advocated.[36] The potential advantages of this technique include a lower incidence of hypocalcemia and the feasibility of managing recurrent hyperparathyroidism should it develop by excision of a portion of the grafted parathyroid tissue under local anesthesia (obviating the morbidity of repeat neck exploration).

PANCREAS. The second most frequent expression of MEN-I is neoplasia of the pancreatic islet cells. The pathologic change is typically multicentric and diffuse hyperplasia and microadenoma formation may be present in areas of the gland distant from grossly evident tumor.

The most common pancreatic islet cell lesion in patients with MEN-I is gastrinoma. Clinically, patients present with a severe peptic ulcer diathesis following autonomous gastrin hypersecretion. Gastrinomas associated with MEN-I comprise 20 to 50 per cent of all cases of the Z-E syndrome.[30] The diagnosis of gastrinoma is made by the documentation of hyperacidity and associated abnormally elevated levels of serum gastrin (greater than 1000 pg. per ml.). In patients with minimal elevations of serum gastrin (250 to 1000 pg. per ml.), the intravenous administration of potent gastrin secretagogues such as calcium or secretin are useful in establishing the diagnosis. Generally, a 50 per cent increase of borderline elevated gastrin levels above basal or an absolute increase of basal levels by 250 pg. per ml. is strongly suggestive of a gastrinoma.

Gastrinomas that develop in patients with MEN-I are usually multicentric and malignant, as indicated by the presence of regional or distant metastases. Because of the multicentricity, these lesions cannot be localized by computed tomographic scanning, angiography, or portal venous sampling and measurement of plasma gastrin levels.

Previously, the accepted surgical therapy for this disease was total gastrectomy. However, H_2-receptor antagonists are often effective in controlling acid hypersecretion and its attendant complications and have largely replaced gastrectomy except in cases where the acid secretion is refractory or the patients are noncompliant. Resection of the islet cell tumors is rarely attempted in these patients, in contrast to patients with sporadic gastrinomas that are solitary and can be totally resected. Although the gastrinomas in patients with the MEN-I syndrome are malignant, the disease progression is indolent in many patients. With aggressive medical management, affected individuals may tolerate the malignancy well and enjoy relatively long survival.

The second most common pancreatic islet cell neoplasm in patients with MEN-I is insulinoma. The insulinomas are usually small (less than 1 cm.) and are usually multiple in contrast to those that occur sporadically, where approximately 80 per cent are solitary. Patients commonly present with recurrent symptoms of neuroglycopenia: sweating, dizziness, confusion, or syncope. The diagnosis of insulinoma is made by documenting hypoglycemia concomitant with inappropriately elevated plasma insulin levels during the fasting state. Symptoms of hypoglycemia may occur during the fast. Provocative testing with tolbutamide or leucine, although previously advocated, is rarely used today because of insensitivity and potential morbidity and even mortality. There is no suitable medical therapy for insulinoma; therefore, these lesions are generally treated surgically even though they are multicentric. Often patients become asymptomatic with normoglycemia after surgical resection or debulking. Approximately 10 per cent of insulinomas occurring in patients with MEN-I are malignant. Patients with disseminated or diffuse carcinomas may respond to treatment with streptozotocin, and some control of hypoglycemia may be achieved by the administration of diazoxide, an inhibitor of insulin secretion.

Other pancreatic islet cell neoplasms, such as glucagonoma, somatostatinoma, and tumors secreting vasoactive intestinal peptide or pancreatic polypeptide, occur rarely in association with MEN-I.

PITUITARY. Pituitary neoplasms occur in 15 to 50 per cent of patients. Most of these tumors were formerly thought to be nonfunctioning chromophobe adenomas. However, recent evidence indicates that prolactin-secreting microadenomas may be the most common abnormality. Pituitary tumors cause symptoms either by hypersecretion of hormones or compression of adjacent structures. Large adenomas may cause visual field defects by pressure on the optic chiasm or manifestations of hypopituitarism through compression of the adjacent normal gland. Prolactin-secreting tumors cause amenorrhea/galactorrhea in females or hypogonadism in males. Approximately 30 per cent of patients exhibit acromegaly following growth hormone overproduction.[1] Much less commonly, patients present with Cushing's disease as a result of excess adrenocorticotropin (ACTH) secretion.

Pituitary tumors, either functioning or nonfunctioning, may require ablation by surgical therapy or irradiation. Bromocriptine, a dopamine agonist and an inhibitor of prolactin secretion, has been used to treat prolactinomas medically.

OTHER TUMORS. Forty per cent of patients with MEN-I develop adrenocortical lesions, including adenomas and asymmetric or nodular hyperplasia. The neoplasms may arise *de novo* or as a result of an ACTH-secreting pituitary tumor, but adrenocortical hyperfunction is rare.

Follicular or papillary thyroid carcinomas or colloid nodules occur in up to 15 per cent of patients. Rarely, multiple subcutaneous or visceral lipomas and bronchial or gastrointestinal carcinoid tumors may occur in association with the MEN-I syndrome.

MULTIPLE ENDOCRINE NEOPLASIA TYPES IIA AND IIB

Historical Aspects

Medullary thyroid carcinoma, first described as a distinct clinicopathologic entity in 1959 by Hazard and associates,[8] was distinguished by its solid nonfollicular histologic pattern, a high incidence of lymph node metastases, and material in the stroma with the staining properties of amyloid. Sipple[21] in 1961 noted an association of thyroid carcinoma with pheochromocytoma, and Williams[39] observed in 1965 that this thyroid neoplasm was MTC. In 1966, Williams[40] correctly deduced that MTC is derived from the parafollicular or C cells, which were subsequently demonstrated to be the source of secretion of the polypeptide hormone calcitonin (CT).

The term *multiple endocrine neoplasia Type II* (MEN-II) was originally introduced by Steiner and associates[24] in 1968 to describe the familial occurrence of MTC, pheochromocytoma, and parathyroid hyperplasia. This syndrome is now known as MEN-IIa. In 1966, Williams and Pollack[41] described patients with MTC, pheochromocytoma, and multiple mucosal neuromas; and this pattern of endocrine involvement was recognized as a distinct entity by Schimke and co-workers[18] in 1968. Chong and associates[4] suggested that this syndrome be termed *MEN type IIb* (MEN-IIb) to distinguish it from MEN-IIa. The MEN-IIb syndrome has also been referred to as MEN-III.

Genetic Studies and Pathogenesis

Both MEN-IIa and MEN-IIb are inherited in an autosomal dominant pattern. Recent genetic linkage studies[13,20] have mapped the locus for MEN-IIa to the pericentromeric region of chromosome 10. Significantly, identification of more tightly linked markers to the MEN loci will allow presymptomatic genetic diagnosis of the trait with a high level of confidence.

A possible unifying explanation for the pathogenesis of the MEN syndromes, particularly MEN-IIa and MEN-IIb, is provided by embryologic and cytochemical studies. Elegant experiments by Pearse[16] have demonstrated that the thyroid C cells derive embryologically from the neural crest. These cells are members of a class of polypeptide producing cells termed APUD cells, an acronym for high Amine content, amine Precursor Uptake and amino acid Decarboxylation. These cytochemical attributes are shared by a dispersed family of endocrine cells. The chromaffin cells of the adrenal medulla are also derived from the neural crest and have APUD cell characteristics. The inheritance of simultaneous MTC and pheochromocytoma may follow a single defect or combination of defects in the development of neural crest tissue. The nature of this defect and whether it may arise from the inheritance of one disease locus has not been defined.

This explanation is particularly attractive in the case of MEN-IIb, which consists of MTC and pheochromocytoma developing in cells of neural crest origin and widespread involvement of peripheral nerves, all representing derangements of the neuroectoderm. A deficiency of this hypothesis in the case of MEN-IIa is the occurrence of hyperparathyroidism. Parathyroid cells are thought not to be derived from the neural crest and do not have the biochemical properties of APUD cells. It has been postulated that parathyroid hyperplasia might arise secondarily as a result of the chronic hypocalcemic effects of excess CT produced by MTC cells, but support for this view is lacking. In particular, patients with sporadic MTC and MEN-IIb do not have hyperparathyroidism. It appears that parathyroid hyperplasia is a primary feature of MEN-IIa, and its relationship to the other tumors is not well understood.

Clinical and Pathologic Features

The MEN-IIa and MEN-IIb syndromes are inherited in an autosomal dominant pattern; however, MEN-IIb in particular may occur sporadically or arise as a new mutation with autosomal dominant transmission in subsequent generations. As is the case for MEN-I, the traits for MEN-IIa and MEN-IIb are transmitted with near 100 per cent penetrance, but with variable expressivity. Bilateral MTC occurs in nearly every affected individual with MEN-IIa and MEN-IIb. In addition, patients with MEN-IIa may have associated pheochromocytoma (less than 50 per cent) or parathyroid hyperplasia (less than 50 per cent).

Medullary thyroid carcinoma occurs in the rarer MEN-IIb syndrome in association with pheochromocytoma, mucosal neuromas ("bumpy lips"), diffuse ganglioneuromas of the gastrointestinal tract, skeletal abnormalities, and a "marfanoid" habitus. Patients with MEN-IIb have a characteristic physical appearance (Fig. 1A to C), and affected individuals are often recognizable at birth or in early infancy. Significantly, the MTC in MEN-IIb occurs earlier (sometimes before 2 years of age) and is a much more aggressive neoplasm biologically, compared with its counterpart in patients with MEN-IIa. Patients with MEN-IIb may die from widespread metastatic MTC at an early age, which underscores the need for early biochemical diagnosis and total thyroidectomy in affected patients as soon as the trait is recognized. Owing to the aggressive nature of the disease, families with MEN-IIb are characteristically small, encompassing only two or three generations.

MEDULLARY THYROID CARCINOMA. Medullary thyroid carcinoma constitutes 5 to 10 per cent of all thyroid malignancies. Approximately 80 per cent of these represent sporadic cases of MTC. Twenty per cent of MTC cases occur in a familial setting, either in association with MEN-IIa or MEN-IIb or less commonly as familial MTC not associated with other endocrinopathies (FMTC).

Medullary thyroid carcinoma is usually the first abnormality expressed in both MEN-IIa and MEN-IIb, and in the majority of patients MTC is diagnosed either before or concurrently with pheochromocytoma. The peak incidence of MTC in the setting of MEN-IIa or MEN-IIb is in the second or third decade, compared with the fifth or sixth decade in patients with sporadic MTC.

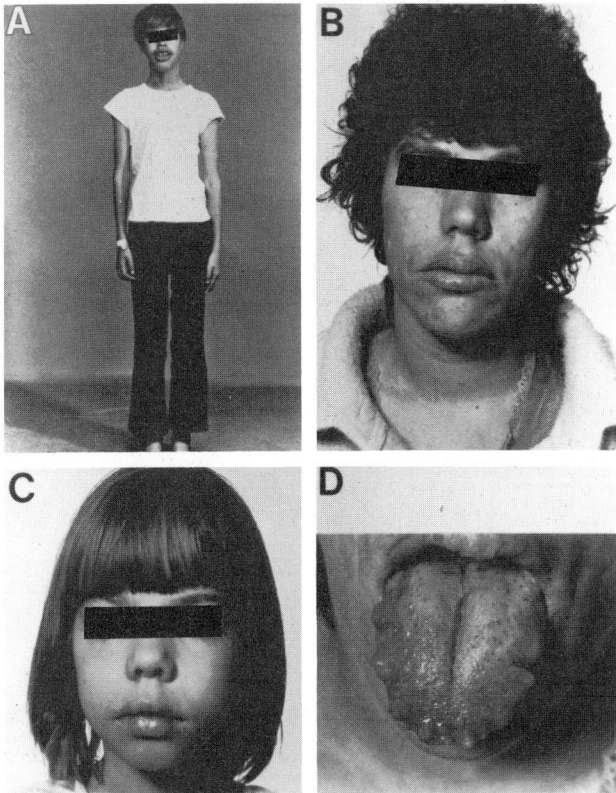

Figure 1. *A* to *C*, Characteristic phenotypic appearance of three patients with MEN-IIb. *D*, Multiple neuromas on the tongue and oral mucosa in a patient with MEN-IIb.

Sporadic MTC is nearly always unilateral. In patients with MEN-IIa or MEN-IIb, MTC nearly always occurs as bilateral, multicentric foci of tumor in the middle and upper portions of each thyroid lobe. A diffuse premalignant proliferation of C cells in the thyroid gland of patients with familial MTC has been described and termed C-cell hyperplasia (CCH). Parafollicular clusters of C cells represent the early manifestation of hyperplasia or microinvasive carcinoma which progresses to multifocal MTC. The presence of bilateral MTC or microscopic evidence of CCH in areas of the thyroid adjacent to macroscopic foci of MTC strongly suggests the presence of familial disease.

Medullary thyroid carcinoma usually appears grossly as a circumscribed, gritty, whitish-tan nodule.[2] Microscopically, it consists of nests or sheets of uniform round or polygonal cells separated by variable amounts of fibrovascular stroma. Less commonly, MTC may occur in a carcinoid-like trabecular pattern, or it may have a predominance of oval or spindle-shaped cells. Material with the staining properties of amyloid is frequently present in the stroma of MTC. This amyloid-like material has been demonstrated to be composed of an aggregate of a prohormone for CT synthesized by the tumor cells.[23] Although the presence of an amyloid-like material in a thyroid neoplasm constitutes a distinctive feature of MTC, it is not present in all tumors. Medullary thyroid carcinoma can be diagnosed immunohistochemically by demonstrating calcitonin within the MTC cells.

Medullary thyroid carcinoma cells are capable of great biosynthetic activity and have been reported to secrete (in addition to calcitonin) ACTH, prostaglandins, melanin, and serotonin. However, the most important product of MTC cells is calcitonin, which serves as a sensitive plasma tumor marker for the presence of the tumor whether in preoperative screening or postoperative evaluation. Although uncommon, patients with MTC may present with any of several paraneoplastic syndromes, in-

cluding Cushing's syndrome, or the carcinoid syndrome. Diarrhea occurs in up to 30 per cent of patients with MTC and is attributed to increased jejunal water and electrolyte secretion stimulated by very high plasma calcitonin levels.

Medullary thyroid carcinoma may be detected when it is clinically occult. Significantly, asymptomatic members of kindreds with MEN-IIa or FMTC may be diagnosed as having MTC by the detection of an elevated plasma calcitonin level either basally or after the administration of provocative agents. These patients are likely to have MTC confined to the thyroid gland, and nearly all are cured by total thyroidectomy. Patients with clinically evident MTC present with a palpable thyroid nodule or a multinodular thyroid gland. Enlarged, firm cervical lymph nodes suggest metastatic disease. Patients with locally advanced disease may present with hoarseness, dysphagia, or respiratory distress or with signs of distant metastases, most commonly to lung, liver, or bone.

Medullary thyroid carcinoma may also exhibit distinctive radiographic features. Plain films of the cervical region often reveal irregular dense calcifications, owing to the propensity of primary and metastatic MTC lesions to undergo degenerative calcification. Similarly, chest radiographs may reveal large calcified hilar or mediastinal nodes corresponding to calcified deposits of metastatic MTC.

PHEOCHROMOCYTOMA. The pheochromocytomas in patients with MEN-IIa and MEN-IIb are characterized by their tendency to appear in the second or third decade of life. Approximately 60 to 80 per cent are bilateral, compared with 10 per cent of sporadic pheochromocytomas. The majority of these tumors are diagnosed concurrently or a few years subsequent to the detection of MTC, and pheochromocytoma is infrequently the initial presenting feature. The pheochromocytomas are nearly always limited to the adrenal medulla, and they are nearly always benign. The histologic appearance of the tumor cells is similar to that observed in pheochromocytomas that occur in a nonfamilial setting.

Patients with MEN-IIa or MEN-IIb develop hyperplasia of the adrenal medulla prior to the development of pheochromocytomas. A spectrum of disease including nodular or asymmetric hyperplasia, multiple small pheochromocytomas, or a diffuse thickening of all adrenal medullary tissue may be observed. This pattern of adrenal involvement is comparable to the finding of C-cell hyperplasia in the thyroid of patients with MEN-IIa or MEN-IIb.

The pheochromocytomas in patients with MEN-IIa or MEN-IIb may be either clinically silent or associated with dramatic clinical symptoms such as severe pounding frontal headaches, episodic diaphoresis, palpitations, and vague feelings of anxiety. Hypertension, if present, may be sustained or episodic.

PARATHYROIDS. Hyperfunction of the parathyroid glands in patients with MEN-IIa is the most variable component of the syndrome. Many patients are asymptomatic, and recognition of the parathyroid lesions may stem from the finding of hypercalcemia during routine laboratory studies. However, it is not uncommon to find one or more enlarged parathyroid glands at the time of thyroidectomy for MTC in a patient who is normocalcemic. The most common symptom of altered calcium homeostasis in patients with MEN-IIa is the presence of asymptomatic or symptomatic renal stones. More advanced signs of hyperparathyroidism such as osteitis fibrosa cystica or nephrocalcinosis are unusual.

The parathyroid lesions in patients with MEN-IIa consist primarily of generalized chief cell hyperplasia, and typically there is multiple gland enlargement.

Although some investigators have reported equivocal histologic abnormalities or increased numbers of chief cells in the parathyroid glands of patients with MEN-IIb, hyperparathyroidism rarely if ever occurs in this syndrome.

NONENDOCRINE MANIFESTATIONS OF MEN-IIb. In

addition to MTC and pheochromocytoma, patients with MEN-IIb develop abnormalities of the musculoskeletal and nervous systems. Unlike patients with MEN-I or MEN-IIa, patients with MEN-IIb have a characteristic phenotype, including a tall, thin "marfanoid" body habitus (see Fig. 1A to C). Multiple neuromas develop on the lips, tongue, and oral mucosa and result in the appearance of thick, "bumpy" lips (see Fig. 1D). Slit lamp examination of the eyes often reveals hypertrophied corneal nerves. Patients may develop diffuse ganglioneuromatosis of the gastrointestinal tract, characterized microscopically by hypertrophy and nerve fiber disarray of the myenteric and submucosal plexuses. A history of chronic constipation or recurrent crampy abdominal pain may be present because of the disordered motility of the gut. Contrast studies may reveal evidence of colonic dilatation or megacolon. There is also a high incidence of skeletal anomalies, including congenital dislocation of the hip, pes planus or cavus, pectus excavatum, and kyphosis.

Diagnosis

It is unusual that one is able to accurately diagnose and treat cancer when it is clinically occult. It is possible to detect minimal elevations of CT in plasma by using very specific immunoassays. Because MTC occurs in nearly 100 per cent of patients with MEN-IIa and MEN-IIb, and is usually the first abnormality expressed, diagnosis of the disease in kindred members at risk is accomplished by screening for the presence of the thyroid tumor.

In 1970, Tashjian and associates[25] first described the measurement of human calcitonin by radioimmunoassay and documented that nearly all patients with clinically detectable MTC have elevated plasma CT levels. In normal individuals, basal plasma CT levels are either very low or less than 200 pg. per ml. Patients with clinically palpable MTC generally have plasma CT levels greater than 1000 pg. per ml. With extensive disease, basal plasma values may exceed several thousand picograms per milliliter.

Subsequently, Melvin and colleagues[15] documented that patients with clinically occult MTC may have minimally elevated plasma CT levels. These workers also demonstrated that such patients frequently have normal basal plasma CT levels that markedly increase after a calcium infusion (15 mg. per kg. over 4 hours). The presence of MTC was correctly diagnosed in 11 patients whose only indication of disease was an elevated plasma CT level either basally or after a calcium infusion. At thyroidectomy, these patients had small medullary carcinomas.

The peptide pentagastrin subsequently proved to be more potent than the standard 4-hour calcium infusion in stimulating CT secretion from MTC cells.[9] After a bolus intravenous injection of pentagastrin (0.5 μg. per kg. over 5 seconds), peak plasma CT levels were two to three times higher, and they occurred within 1 to 5 minutes after injection (Fig. 2).

Subsequently, it was demonstrated that the sequential intravenous administration of calcium gluconate (2 mg. per kg. over 1 minute), followed by a bolus injection of pentagastrin (0.5 μg. per kg. over 5 seconds), stimulated higher peak levels of plasma CT than did either agent alone (Fig. 3).[34] The importance of provocative testing in the early diagnosis of patients with familial MTC has recently been demonstrated.[33] Kindred members with clinically occult MEN-IIa whose MTC was diagnosed by provocative testing were younger, had smaller primary tumors, and had a lower incidence of MTC metastatic to regional lymph nodes and distant sites than did patients whose MTC was diagnosed by physical examination. Also, the number of patients cured by total thyroidectomy, a parameter easily determined by measuring stimulated plasma CT levels postoperatively (Fig. 4), was significantly higher in the former group than the latter.

The authors recommend that members of kindreds at risk for the development of MTC undergo annual calcium pentagastrin stimulation testing, beginning as early as age 5 years and con-

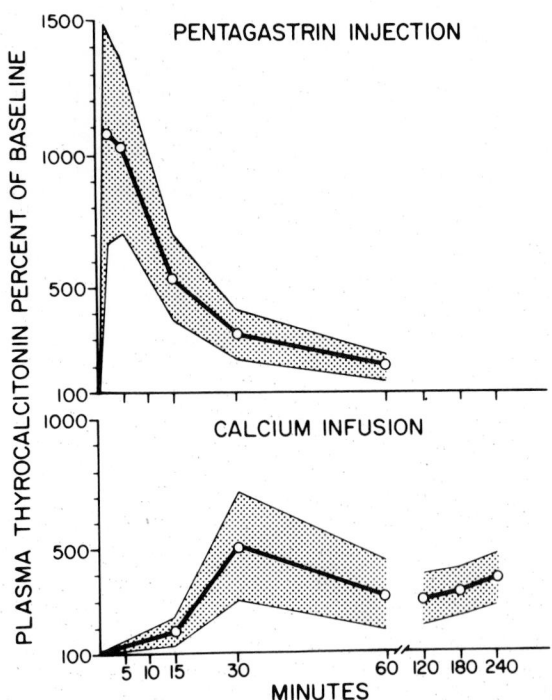

Figure 2. Combined responses of seven patients with elevated baseline levels of plasma calcitonin to pentagastrin injection and calcium infusion. Each patient received both tests on separate days, pentagastrin injection being the initial test in four of the patients and calcium infusion being the initial test in three. Open circles and solid lines represent the mean responses, and the shaded areas indicate the range of the standard errors. (From Hennessy, J. C., et al.: A comparison of pentagastrin injection and calcium infusion as provocative agents for the detection of medullary carcinoma of the thyroid. J. Clin. Endocrinol. Metabol., 39:487, 1974.)

tinuing until the age of 40 to 45 years. In families with MEN-IIa or FMTC, stimulated plasma CT levels greater than 300 pg. per ml. are highly suggestive of MTC. The diagnosis is virtually assured in patients with plasma CT levels exceeding 1000 pg. per ml. Occasionally, kindred members are found whose basal

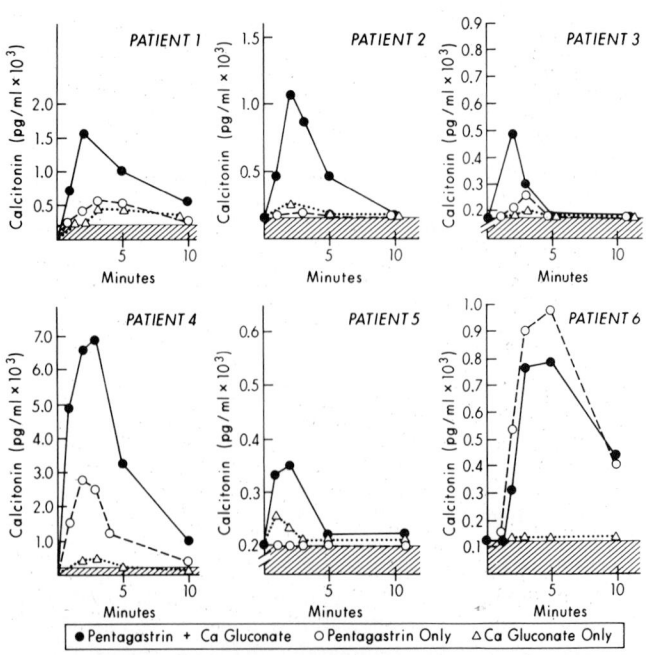

Figure 3. Plasma calcitonin levels following the administration of pentagastrin (0.5 μg. per kg. over 5 seconds), calcium gluconate (2 mg. per kg. over 1 minute), and a combination of the two in six patients with familial medullary thyroid carcinoma. (From Wells, S. A., Jr., et al.: Provocative agents and the diagnosis of medullary carcinoma of the thyroid gland. Ann. Surg., 188:139, 1978.)

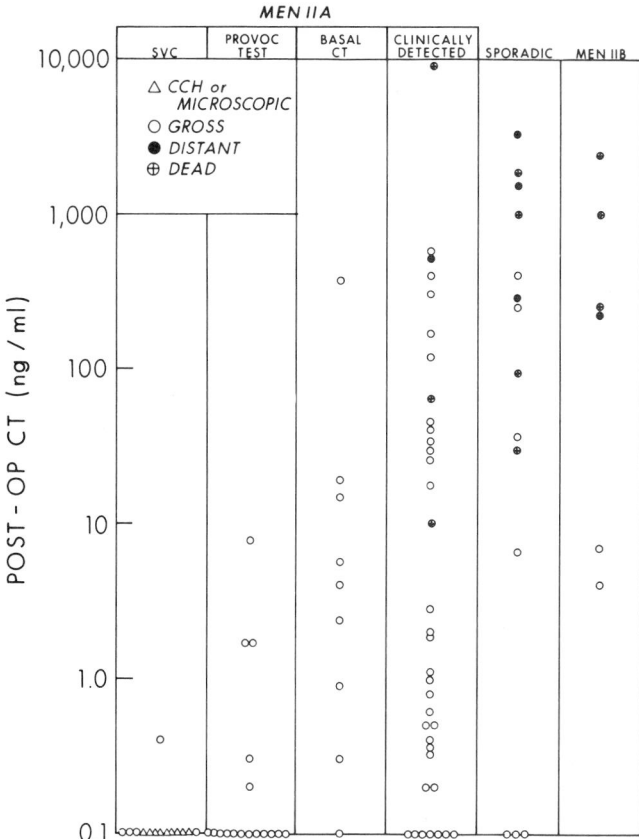

Figure 4. Postoperative stimulated plasma calcitonin (CT) levels in patients with MEN-IIa diagnosed by selective venous catheterization with provocative testing (SVC, n = 14); documentation of increased plasma CT levels in peripheral plasma following provocative testing (Provoc Test; n = 17); documentation of elevated basal CT in peripheral plasma (Basal CT; n = 9); and palpation of the neck (clinically detected, n = 36). Postoperative CT values are also shown in patients with sporadic MTC and those with MEN-IIb. The incidence of residual or recurrent MTC postoperatively (as indicated by an elevated plasma CT [> 300 pg. per ml.] after provocative testing) increases as the method of diagnosis becomes less sensitive; i.e., residual or recurrent disease is much lower in cases diagnosed by SVC than in those diagnosed by physical examination. Patients presenting with sporadic MTC or MEN-IIb are rarely cured by thyroidectomy regardless of the method of diagnosis. (From Wells, S. A., Jr., et al.: Early diagnosis and treatment of medullary thyroid carcinoma. Arch. Intern. Med., 145:1248, 1985. Copyright 1985, American Medical Association.)

plasma CT levels are undetectable but increase modestly (250 to 1000 pg. per ml.) after provocative testing. In these patients, selective thyroid venous catheterization and measurement of CT levels in blood collected after provocative testing have identified patients with early MTC and clearly separated them from subjects with non–C-cell disorders.[32] Patients identified by this technique usually have very early MTC, often evident only on microscopic examination. As might be expected in these patients, there are rarely metastases to regional lymph nodes or evidence of residual MTC postoperatively.

The diagnosis of pheochromocytoma in patients with MEN-IIa and MEN-IIb can be made biochemically by measurement of the urinary excretion of catecholamines and catecholamine metabolites. Patients with symptoms characteristic of pheochromocytoma should have a 24-hour urine collection for measurement of total urinary catecholamines, epinephrine, norepinephrine, metanephrines, and vanillylmandelic acid (VMA). It is imperative that patients with MEN-IIa and MEN-IIb have pheochromocytoma excluded prior to undergoing thyroidectomy. This is particularly important because the pheochromocytoma may be unsuspected clinically. If a patient with MTC is found to have a pheochromocytoma, adrenalectomy should be performed, followed by thyroidectomy in 1 to 2 weeks.

If the 24-hour urinary excretion rates of catecholamines and metabolites are equivocal and there is any question about the presence of a pheochromocytoma, computed tomography of the abdomen should be performed to exclude the presence of adrenal enlargement. Lesions 1 cm. or more in size can be identified, and rarely adrenal hyperplasia is suggested. Beierwaltes and associates[22,38] have utilized ^{131}I-metaiodobenzylguanidine (^{131}I-MIBG) scintigraphy in a large number of patients to localize pheochromocytomas. This agent is structurally similar to norepinephrine and is taken up and stored in adrenergic vesicles. The normal adrenal glands are not visualized at 24 to 48 hours. The ^{131}I-MIBG is very specific for pheochromocytomas, and positive identification has been possible in 90 per cent of patients. There have been less than 5 per cent false-positive tests. This technique provides functional and anatomic localization of hyperfunctioning chromaffin tissue and has been useful in demonstrating intra- and extra-adrenal pheochromocytomas as well as adrenal medullary hyperplasia. This agent has proved particularly useful in patients with ectopic pheochromocytomas that had not been found at prior operation.

The diagnosis of hyperparathyroidism in patients with MEN-IIa depends largely on serial measurements of the plasma calcium concentration. Peripheral plasma parathyroid hormone levels can be measured; but this may be misleading, because increased values have been reported in members of involved kindreds who have neither hypercalcemia nor MTC.

GENETIC SCREENING BY DNA POLYMORPHISM ANALYSIS. Screening members of families with MEN-IIa by provocative testing to detect the presence of MTC in its earliest stages has been the most sensitive method of identifying affected individuals. A significant contribution to the presymptomatic diagnosis of families with the MEN syndromes will undoubtedly be provided by the identification of chromosomal markers closely linked to the disease loci. Tight genetic linkage exists when two loci are closely situated on the same chromosome such that the probability of crossover between them is very low. In families with parents who are informative (heterozygous) for the marker used, inheritance of the disease can be predicted with a high level of confidence by demonstrating coinheritance with the marker. Preclinical diagnosis using DNA polymorphism analysis may eventually allow early identification of affected patients, who should then be followed closely for the development of MTC. The availability of this technology may lead to the performance of prophylactic thyroidectomy in patients identified as having the gene for the disease. It almost certainly will obviate endocrine testing in patients with a minimal likelihood of possessing the trait.

Surgical Management

PHEOCHROMOCYTOMA. If pheochromocytoma is detected, the patient should have a bilateral subcostal incision and exploration of both adrenal glands, the sympathetic chain, and the organ of Zückerkandl. Bilateral pheochromocytomas require bilateral adrenalectomy. Although a matter of some controversy, in patients with unilateral pheochromocytoma and a palpably normal contralateral gland, it is acceptable policy to perform a unilateral adrenalectomy. Such patients should be followed carefully at 6-month to yearly intervals for recurrence in the contralateral gland. It is recognized that adrenal medullary hyperplasia may often be present in the grossly normal gland, and that approximately 30 per cent of patients initially managed by unilateral adrenalectomy develop pheochromocytoma in the remaining gland.[26] However, bilateral adrenalectomy necessitates lifelong glucocorticoid and mineralocorticoid replacement therapy with the attendant risks of Addisonian crisis, and this must be considered when one plans removal of a grossly normal gland.

Preoperatively, patients with pheochromocytomas should be hospitalized to receive alpha adrenergic blockade with phenoxybenzamine. They should be expected to develop postural hypotension. Beta-adrenergic blackade may be necessary if tachycardia or arrhythmias develop after the administration of phenoxybenzamine. Beta-blockade without prior alpha-blockade is dangerous, because patients are subjected to unopposed vasoconstriction. Intraoperative control of hypertension, which frequently occurs with manipulation of the tumor, is most effectively achieved with sodium nitroprusside or phentolamine.

MEDULLARY THYROID CARCINOMA. The surgical treatment of familial or sporadic MTC is total thyroidectomy. Meticulous removal of all thyroid tissue should be undertaken at the initial operation, because MTC in the setting of MEN-IIa or MEN-IIb is nearly always multicentric and bilateral and may metastasize early to cervical lymph nodes. Dissection of the nodes in the central compartment of the neck (between the jugular veins and from the hyoid bone to the sternal notch) should be performed in all patients with either clinically evident or occult MTC. Patients with macroscopic regional lymph node metastases should undergo ipsilateral neck dissection in addition to total thyroidectomy. Postoperatively, residual or recurrent MTC can be readily detected by repeat calcium-pentagastrin stimulation and measurement of plasma CT levels.

Until recently, repeat neck exploration in an attempt to resect residual disease has infrequently caused normalization of elevated plasma CT levels. However, Tisell and colleagues[27] have reported 11 patients with MTC (7 sporadic, 4 familial) with persistently elevated plasma CT levels after total thyroidectomy and central zone lymphadenectomy. These patients underwent reoperation and meticulous superior mediastinal and bilateral lymph node dissection under magnification with the intent of removing all tumor in the neck. Stimulated postoperative plasma CT levels were normalized after reoperation in four of the patients who proved to have a few microscopic metastases.

HYPERPARATHYROIDISM. The characteristic parathyroid lesion in patients with MEN-IIa is hyperplasia with involvement of all four glands. In patients with documented hypercalcemia, one can expect to find enlarged parathyroid glands at operation. However, grossly enlarged parathyroid glands may be found during thyroidectomy for MTC in a patient in whom hyperparathyrodism has never been documented. Although some surgeons perform a subtotal (3½-gland) parathyroidectomy in patients with parathyroid hyperplasia and MEN-IIa, it has been the authors' policy to perform total parathyroidectomy with autograft of parathyroid tissue into the forearm musculature. In patients without hypercalemia undergoing thyroidectomy for MTC, grossly normal parathyroid glands should be left in place.

PROGNOSIS. The course of patients with MEN-IIa and MEN-IIb is essentially that of the thyroid lesion. Medullary thyroid carcinoma in general has an intermediate grade of malignancy, as compared with the more malignant anaplastic thyroid carcinomas or the less malignant papillary or follicular carcinomas. It should be emphasized, however, that MTC exhibits variable biologic aggressiveness within the different MEN syndromes and sometimes from kindred to kindred. The MTC in the setting of MEN-IIb is very aggressive, and patients may die at a young age. Medullary thyroid carcinoma in patients with MEN-IIa is usually indolent and progresses very slowly. In some patients the disease has a more aggressive course.

Bigner and associates[2] evaluated resected tissue from 72 patients with MEN-IIa who had undergone total thyroidectomy. They found that metastases to regional lymph nodes and residual MTC postoperatively, as indicated by increased plasma CT levels, were significantly higher in patients who had larger primary thyroid malignancies (greater than 1.5 cm. in diameter) than in patients who had smaller lesions (less than 0.5 cm. in diameter). Wells and associates[33] evaluated 92 patients with familial MTC to determine whether the preoperative stimulated CT level was of prognostic significance. Patients whose preop-

TABLE 1. Plasma Calcitonin Levels and Prognosis

Group	Preop. CT (pg./ml.)	RLNM* (%)	Postop. CT* (%) (>300 pg./ml.)	DM (%)	DTH (%)
1	250–1000 (n = 25)	1(4)	1(4)	0	0
2	1000–5000 (n = 36)	3(8.3)	6(16.7)	0	0
3	5000–10,000 (n = 8)	2(25)	1(12.5)	0	0
4	>10,000 (n = 23)	13(57)	14(61)	4(17)	2(8.7)

* Group 1 or Group 2 versus Group 4, p < 0.001.
Preop CT, preoperative stimulated plasma CT level; Postop CT, postoperative stimulated plasma CT level; RLNM, regional lymph node metastases; DM, distant metastases; DTH, death.

erative peak stimulated plasma CT levels were less than 1000 pg. per ml. had a much better prognosis than patients whose peak CT levels were greater than 10,000 pg. per ml. Specifically, metastases to regional lymph nodes, residual MTC postoperatively, distant metastases, and death were significantly less frequent in the former group than in the latter (Table 1).

Not surprisingly, it has been demonstrated that patients whose MTC is diagnosed biochemically have a more favorable pathologic stage than do patients whose tumor is diagnosed clinically. The authors' group[31] has divided patients into three categories: those with no clinical evidence of MTC and undetectable basal plasma CT levels that became elevated following provocative testing with calcium or pentagastrin (Group 1), patients with no clinical evidence of MTC but elevated basal plasma CT levels (Group 2), and patients with clinically evident MTC (Group 3). Regional lymph node metastases were present less frequently in cases diagnosed biochemically (5/28; Groups 1 and 2) than in those where there was clinically evident disease (15/24; Group 3, p < 0.02). In addition, the incidence of residual MTC after thyroidectomy, as evidenced by persistently elevated stimulated plasma CT levels postoperatively, was less frequent in cases diagnosed biochemically (6/34; Groups 1 and 2) than in those with clinically evident MTC (17/26; Group 3, p < 0.002).

Since Ishikawa and Hamada[10] demonstrated elevated plasma levels of carcinoembryonic antigen (CEA) in patients with MTC, several investigators have evaluated this glycoprotein as an additional tumor marker. Basal plasma CEA levels are rarely increased in patients with early MTC, and they do not increase after calcium or pentagastrin stimulation. However, in some patients the serial measurements of plasma CEA levels may provide a better index of tumor burden than plasma calcitonin levels, and the measurement of this marker may be useful in following patients with metastatic disease.

The ideal treatment of patients with nonresectable metastatic MTC is unclear. Medullary thyroid carcinoma is relatively resistant to radiation therapy, and various chemotherapeutic agents have infrequently demonstrated significant responsiveness. It is imperative that families with hereditary MTC be identified and managed by an aggressive screening program, because early diagnosis and thyroidectomy cures MTC in a large percentage of patients.

SELECTED REFERENCES

Ballard, H. S., Frame, B., and Hartsock, R. J.: Familial multiple endocrine adenoma-peptic ulcer complex. Medicine, 43:481, 1964.
This paper represents an extensive evaluation of patients with MEN-I. It covers all aspects of the disease, including clinical, genetic, and pathologic manifestations.

Brown, J. S., and Steiner, A. L.: Medullary thyroid carcinoma and the syndromes of multiple endocrine adenomas. Disease-a-Month, 28:1, 1982.

This monograph is primarily devoted to discussions of the familial medullary carcinoma syndromes, especially MEN-IIa and MEN-IIb.

Cance, W. G., and Wells, S. A., Jr.: Multiple endocrine neoplasia type IIa. Curr. Probl. Surg., 22:1, 1985.

This monograph is an extensive review of a series of 122 patients with MEN-IIa and covers the natural history, clinicopathologic manifestations, and methods of diagnosis and treatment

Welbourn, R. B., Manolas, K. J., Khan, O., and Galland, R. B.: Tumors of the neuroendocrine system (APUD cell tumors-apudomas). Curr. Probl. Surg., 21:1, 1984.

Welbourn's endocrine surgery group at Hammersmith Hospital in London has made many significant contributions to endocrine surgery. This monograph concerns APUDomas, especially neoplasms of the adrenal and pituitary glands. Also discussed are the familial endocrinopathies MEN-I, MEN-IIa, and MEN-IIb.

REFERENCES

1. Ballard, H. S., Frame, B., and Hartsock, R. J.: Familial multiple endocrine adenoma-peptic ulcer complex. Medicine,43:481, 1964.
2. Bigner, S. H., Mendelsohn, G., Wells, S. A., Jr., Cox, E. B., Baylin, S. B., and Eggleston, J. C.: Medullary carcinoma of the thyroid in the multiple endocrine neoplasia IIa syndrome. Am. J. Surg. Pathol., 5:459, 1981.
3. Brandi, M. L., Marx, S. J., Aurbach, G. D., and Fitzpatrick, L. A.: Familial multiple endocrine neoplasia type I: A new look at pathophysiology. Endocr. Rev., 8:391, 1987.
4. Chong, G. C., Beahrs, O. H., Sizemore, G. W., and Woolner, L. H.: Medullary carcinoma of the thyroid gland. Cancer, 35:695, 1975.
5. Cushing, H., and Davidoff, L. M.: The pathological findings in four autopsied cases of acromegaly with a discussion of their significance. Monograph 22. New York, The Rockefeller Institute for Medical Research, 1927.
6. Erdheim, J.: Zur normalen und pathologischen Histologie der Glandula thyreoidea, parathyreoidea, und hypophysis. Beitr. Pathol. Anat. Allg. Pathol., 33:158, 1903.
7. Gregory, R. A., Tracy, H. J., French, J. M., and Sircus, W.: Extraction of a gastrin-like substance from a pancreatic tumor in a case of Zollinger-Ellison syndrome. Lancet, 1:1045, 1960.
8. Hazard, J. B., Hawk, W. A., and Crile, G., Jr.: Medullary (solid) carcinoma of the thyroid: A clinico-pathologic entity. J. Clin. Endocrinol. Metab., 19:152, 1959.
9. Hennessy, J. F., Wells, S. A., Jr., Ontjes, D. A., and Cooper, C. W.: A comparison of pentagastrin injection and calcium infusion as provocative agents for the detection of medullary carcinoma of the thyroid. J. Clin. Endocrinol. Metab. 39:487, 1974.
10. Ishikawa, N., and Hamada, S.: Association of medullary carcinoma of the thyroid with carcinoembryonic antigen. Br. J. Cancer, 34:111, 1976.
11. Larsson, C., Skogseid, B., Oberg, K., Nakamura, Y., and Nordenskjold, M.: Multiple endocrine neoplasia type I gene maps to chromosome 11 and is lost in insulinoma. Nature, 332:85, 1988.
12. Majewski, J. T., and Wilson, S. D.: The MEA-I syndrome: An all or none phenomenon. Surgery, 86:475, 1979.
13. Mathew, C. G. P., Chin, K. S., Easton, D. F., Thorpe, K., Carter, C., Liou, G. I., Fong, S. L., Bridges, C. D. B., Haak, H., Nieuwenhuijzen Kruseman, A. C., Schifter, S., Hansen, H. H., Telenius, H., Telenius-Berg, M., and Ponder, B. A. J.: A linked genetic marker for multiple endocrine neoplasia type 2a on chromosome 10. Nature, 328:527, 1987.
14. McGuigan, J. E.: Gastric mucosal intracellular localization of gastrin by immunofluorescence. Gastroenterology, 55:315, 1968.
15. Melvin, K. E. W., Miller, H. H., and Tashjian, A. H., Jr.: Early diagnosis of medullary carcinoma of the thyroid gland by means of calcitonin assay. N. Engl. J. Med., 285:1115, 1971.
16. Pearse, A. G. E.: Common cytochemical and ultrastructural characteristics of cells producing polypeptide hormones (the APUD series) and their relevance to thyroid and ultimobranchial C-cells and calcitonin. Proc. R. Soc. Lond. [Biol.], 170:71, 1968.
17. Prinz, R. A., Gamvros, O. I., Sellu, D., and Lynn, J. A.: Subtotal parathyroidectomy for primary chief cell hyperplasia in the multiple endocrine neoplasia type I syndrome. Ann Surg, 193:26, 1981.
18. Schimke, R. N., Hartmann, W. H., Prout, T. E., and Rimoin, D. L.: Syndrome of bilateral pheochromocytoma, medullary thyroid carcinoma and multiple neuromas. N. Engl. J. Med., 279:1, 1968.
19. Shelburne, S. A., and McLaughlin, C. W.: Coincidental adenomas of islet-cells, parathyroid gland and pituitary gland. J. Clin Endocrinol. Metab., 5:232, 1945.
20. Simpson, N. E., Kidd, K. K., Goodfellow, P. J., McDermid, H., Myers, S., Kidd, J. R., Jackson, C. E., Duncan, A. M. V., Farrer, L. A., Brasch, K., Castiglione, C., Genel, M., Gertner, J., Greenberg, C. R., Gusella, J. F., Holden, J. J. A., and White, B. N.: Assignment of multiple endocrine neoplasia type 2a to chromosome 10 by linkage. Nature, 328:528, 1987.
21. Sipple, J. H.: The association of pheochromocytoma with carcinoma of the thyroid gland. Am. J. Med., 31:163, 1961.
22. Sisson, J. C., Frager, M. S., Valk, T. W., Gross, M. D., Swanson, D. P., Wieland, D. M., Tobes, M. C., Beierwaltes, W. H., and Thompson, N. W.: Scintigraphic localization of pheochromocytoma. N. Engl. J. Med., 305:12, 1981.
23. Sletten, K., Westermark, P., and Natvig, J. B.: Characterization of amyloid fibril proteins from medullary carcinoma of the thyroid. J. Exp. Med., 143:993, 1976.
24. Steiner, A. L., Goodman, A. D., and Powers, S. R.: Study of a kindred with pheochromocytoma, medullary thyroid carcinoma, hyperparathyroidism and Cushing's disease: Multiple endocrine neoplasia type 2. Medicine, 47:371, 1968.
25. Tashjian, A. H., Jr., Howland, B. G., Melvin, K. E. W., and Hill, C. S., Jr.: Immunoassay of human calcitonin: Clinical measurement, relation to serum calcium and studies in patients with medullary carcinoma. N. Engl. J. Med., 283:890, 1970.
26. Tibblin, S., Dymling, J. F., Ingemansson, S., and Telenius-Berg, M.: Unilateral versus bilateral adrenalectomy in multiple endocrine neoplasia IIa. World J. Surg., 7:201, 1983.
27. Tisell, L. E., Hansson, G., Jansson, S., and Salander, H.: Reoperation in the treatment of asymptomatic metastasizing medullary thyroid carcinoma. Surgery, 99:60, 1986.
28. van Heerden, J. A., Kent, R. B., Sizemore, G. W., Grant, C. S., and ReMine, W. M.: Primary hyperparathyroidism in patients with multiple endocrine neoplasia syndromes: Surgical experience. Arch. Surg., 118:533, 1983.
29. Vance, J. E., Stoll, R. W., Kitabchi, A. E., Buchanan, K. D., Hollander, D., and Williams, R. H.: Familial nesidioblastosis as the predominant manifestation of multiple endocrine adenomatosis. Am. J. Med., 52:211, 1972.
30. Vieto, R. J., Hickey, R. C., and Samaan, N. A.: Type I multiple endocrine neoplasias. Curr. Probl. Cancer, 7(5):1, 1982.
31. Wells, S. A., Jr., Baylin, S. B., Gann, D. S., Farrell, R. E., Dilley, W. G., Preissig, S. H., Linehan, W. M., and Cooper, C. W.: Medullary thyroid carcinoma: Relationship of method of diagnosis to pathologic staging. Ann. Surg. 188:377, 1978.
32. Wells, S. A., Jr., Baylin, S. B., Johnsrude, I. S., Harrington, D. P., Mendelsohn, G., Ontjes, D. J., and Cooper, C. W.: Thyroid venous catheterization in the early diagnosis of familial medullary thyroid carcinoma. Ann. Surg. 196:505, 1982.
33. Wells, S. A., Jr., Baylin, S. B., Leight, G. S., Dale, J. K., Dilley, W. G., and Farndon, J. R.: The importance of early diagnosis in patients with hereditary medullary thyroid carcinoma. Ann. Surg. 195:595, 1982.
34. Wells, S. A., Jr., Baylin, S. B., Linehan, W. M., Farrell, R. E., Cox, E. B., and Cooper, C. W.: Provocative agents and the diagnosis of medullary carcinoma of the thyroid gland. Ann. Surg. 188;139, 1978.
35. Wells, S. A., Jr., Dilley, W. G., Farndon, J. A., Leight, G. S., and Baylin, S. B.: Early diagnosis and treatment of medullary carcinoma of the thyroid. Arch. Intern. Med., 145:1248, 1985.
36. Wells, S. A., Jr., Farndon, J. R., Dale, J. K., Leight, G. S., and Dilley, W. G.: Long term evaluation of patients with primary parathyroid hyperplasia managed by total parathyroidectomy and heterotopic autotransplantation. Ann. Surg. 192:451, 1980.
37. Wermer, P.: Endocrine adenomatosis and peptic ulcer in a large kindred: Inherited multiple tumors and mosaic pleiotropism in man. Am. J. Med., 35:205, 1963.
38. Wieland, D. M., Wu, J., Brown, L. E., Mangner, T. J., Swanson, D. P., and Beierwalters, W. H.: Radiolabeled adrenergic neuron-blocking agents: adrenomedullary imaging with (131I) iodobenzylguanidine. J. Nucl. Med., 21:349, 1980.
39. Williams, E. D.: A review of 17 cases of carcinoma of the thyroid and phaeochromocytoma. J. Clin. Pathol., 18:288, 1965.
40. Williams, E. D.: Histogenesis of medullary carcinoma of the thyroid. J. Clin. Pathol., 19:114, 1966.
41. Williams, E. D., and Pollack, D. J.: Multiple mucosal neuromata with endocrine tumours: A syndrome allied to von Recklinghausen's disease. J. Pathol. Bacteriol., 91:71, 1966.
42. Zollinger, R. M., and Ellison, E. H.: Primary peptic ulceration of the jejunum associated with islet cell tumors of the pancreas. Ann. Surg., 142:709, 1955.

24

THE PARATHYROID GLANDS

Samuel A. Wells, Jr., M.D., and Stanley W. Ashley, M.D.

HISTORICAL ASPECTS

In 1880, a Swedish student, Ivar Sandström,[67] first described the parathyroid glands in several animals, including man. His discovery went unnoticed until 1891, when the glands were rediscovered by Gley,[30] who demonstrated that their removal led to tetany. MacCallum and Voegtlin[46] subsequently noted a decrease in blood calcium levels of thyroparathyroidectomized animals and found that the tetany that ensued could be corrected by the infusion of calcium salts.

In the same year as Gley's discovery, von Recklinghausen[77] described a characteristic disease of bone that later was found to be caused by hyperparathyroidism. The first to describe the association of bone disease and parathyroid neoplasia was Askanazy,[6] who in 1904 studied a woman with pain in the extremities and spontaneous fractures. At autopsy, she was found to have both the generalized osteitis fibrosa cystica described earlier by von Recklinghausen and an "incidental" tumor lateral to the thyroid gland. In 1907, Erdheim[25] studied several patients who had died of osteomalacia and correctly concluded that the marked parathyroid hyperplasia observed was secondary to the bone disease. Thereafter, the theory evolved that all parathyroid tumors, single as well as multiple, arose to compensate for various osseous abnormalities. Schlagenhaufer in 1915[69] argued that it was unlikely for compensatory hypertrophy to involve only a single gland and suggested that some parathyroid tumors were primary and caused secondary changes in the skeleton. Mandl[48] confirmed this hypothesis 10 years later when he excised an enlarged parathyroid gland from a Viennese streetcar conductor who was admitted to the hospital clinic with hypercalcemia, hypercalciuria, roentgenographic changes of von Recklinghausen's bone disease, and a broken leg. After surgical therapy, the calcium in the blood and urine decreased, the bones became more dense and pain-free, and the patient became ambulatory. Within 6 years, however, his disease recurred and became progressively worse, ultimately causing death. At the time of recurrence, he underwent a second neck exploration, but no abnormal parathyroid tissue was found then or at necropsy 3 years later.

The first parathyroid exploration in the United States was performed in 1926 at the Massachusetts General Hospital on a merchant marine with severe bone disease, Captain Charles Martell.[59] Unfortunately, the abnormal gland was not found until his seventh operation in 1932; and he subsequently died in tetany during a ureterolithotomy. The first successful parathyroidectomy was performed at Barnes Hospital in St. Louis in 1929 and was reported by Barr, Bulger, and Dixon.[8] They first proposed the term *hyperparathyroidism*. In 1934, Albright and colleagues[2] noted an association of osteitis fibrosa cystica with renal stones and subsequently identified a group of patients with hyperparathyroidism who had calculi or nephrocalcinosis but no bone disease.

Biologically active parathyroid extracts were first prepared by Collip in 1925.[18] Parathyroid hormone was isolated and purified by Rasmussen and Craig[60] and Aurbach[7] in 1959. In 1963, Berson and associates[9] developed a radioimmunoassay for parathyroid hormone.

EMBRYOLOGY

Phylogenetically, the parathyroids appear relatively late, being first seen in the Amphibia. In man, the superior parathyroids arise from the fourth pharyngeal pouch and the inferior parathyroids from the third (Fig. 1). During the branchial complex stage, the glands are intimately associated with the derivatives of their respective pouches—the inferior parathyroids with the thymus and the superior parathyroids with the lateral thyroid complex. As the embryo matures and the thymus cord descends, the inferior parathyroids migrate caudally. Typically, the separation of these glands from the thymus becomes complete when they lie posterior to the lower pole of the thyroid lobe. This migration is extremely variable; and as a result, the inferior glands are more likely to be found in an ectopic location than the superior. At one extreme the parathyroids may be found embedded in the pharyngeal mucosa or, at the other, they may be found in the thoracic cavity, usually adherent to the thymus gland. Rarely, the parathyroids become completely enclosed within the thyroid parenchyma during migration of the lateral thyroid complex.

ANATOMY

Typically, there are four parathyroid glands. In Alveryd's series of 354 adults studied at autopsy, 90.6 per cent had four glands, 3.7 per cent had five glands, 5.1 per cent had three glands, and 0.6 per cent had two glands.[4] In only 1 of Alveryd's 18 patients with three identified parathyroids was the combined weight of the glands sufficiently high to suggest that none had been overlooked.

Akerström and associates[1] performed autopsy studies on 503 cadavers and found four parathyroid glands in all but 18 (3 per cent). In 421 cases, there were four glands; however, more than four glands were detected in 64 cases (13 per cent). Most often, the supernumerary gland was located in the thymus. The anatomic location of the parathyroid glands demonstrated considerable constancy and is shown in Figure 2. In each of the two patients with renal osteodystrophy, eight parathyroid glands were identified.

In the 109 cases of Norris[53] and the 35 cases of Boyd,[12] in which parathyroids were identified by studying serial sections of embryos, at least four parathyroid glands were found in every specimen. Norris considered supernumerary glands the result of the separation of parathyroid remnants when the glands pulled away from the pouch structures during the branchial complex phase.

The vascular supply to the parathyroid glands is usually from the inferior thyroid artery, but it can arise from the superior thyroid artery, the thyroid ima artery, and arteries in the larynx, trachea, esophagus, or mediastinum or from anastomoses be-

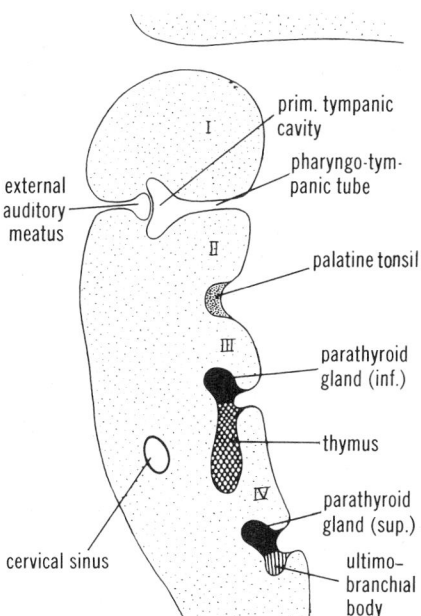

Figure 1. Schematic representation of the development of the pharyngeal pouches. The inferior parathyroid arises from the third pouch in conjunction with the thymus; the superior arises from the fourth in conjunction with the developing thyroid or ultimobranchial body. (From Langman, J.: Medical Embryology, 3rd ed. Baltimore, Williams & Wilkins Company, 1975, p. 266.)

tween these vessels. The inferior, middle, and superior thyroid veins drain the parathyroid glands.

About 50 per cent of all parathyroids are found adjacent to the area where the inferior thyroid artery enters the thyroid parenchyma. The superior parathyroid glands are usually embedded in fat and located on the posterior surface of the middle or upper portion of the thyroid lobe close to the point where the recurrent laryngeal nerve enters the larynx. The lower parathyroid glands are more ventral, close to the lower pole of the thyroid gland and the "thyrothymic ligament." In approximately 1 to 5 per cent of patients, an inferior parathyroid gland is located in the deep mediastinum. The normal glands tend to be flat and ovoid; but on enlargement, they become globular. Normally, they measure 5 to 7 mm. by 3 to 4 mm. by 0.5 to 2 mm. The combined weight of the parathyroid glands is 90 to

200 mg., and the upper glands generally are smaller than the lower. In adults, the parathyroids are usually red-brown to yellow, whereas in the newborn they are gray and semitransparent.

HISTOLOGY

The parathyroid glands consist of a parenchyma containing chief and oxyphil cells and a stroma composed primarily of adipocytes (Fig. 3). The chief and oxyphil cells are arranged in trabeculae or islands. The main cell of primate glands and the only cell of many lower species is the chief cell. Through infancy and early childhood the glands are composed almost entirely of chief cells. Normally present but few in number are the polygonal water-clear cells, glycogen-laden chief cells with little visible cytoplasm. Acidophilic, mitochondria-rich oxyphil cells appear near puberty and increase in number with age. The functional significance of the various cell types remains unclear. The water-clear and oxyphil cells are derived from chief cells and apparently remain capable of secreting parathyroid hormone.

PHYSIOLOGY

MINERAL METABOLISM

Calcium is a constituent of all animal fluids and is involved in a variety of physiologic processes, from blood coagulation and bone formation to milk production. It represents a major cellular messenger and is critical in both muscle contraction and membrane repolarization. It constitutes about 2 per cent of the adult body weight, and almost all is contained in the skeleton. Plasma calcium measures 9.0 to 10.5 mg. per 100 ml. (4.5 to 5.2 mEq. per liter) and is approximately equally divided between an ionized and a protein-bound phase. Five per cent is bound to organic anions. Approximately 80 per cent of the bound calcium is complexed to albumin. The amount of protein and the body fluid pH are the two most important factors regulating the distribution of calcium in plasma. Hydrogen ion competes with calcium for the same binding sites for all the calcium binding proteins in plasma. In general, for each gm. of alteration of the total protein there is a similar 0.8 mg. per 100 ml. change in the total serum calcium. Of greatest importance is the ionized calcium, which is the form most immediately related to the activity of the parathyroid glands.

Calcium, in the inorganic form, is absorbed in the upper small intestine. On a regular diet, approximately 1 gm. is ingested daily. The calcium in the extracellular fluid is constantly being exchanged with that in the exchangeable bone, the intracellular

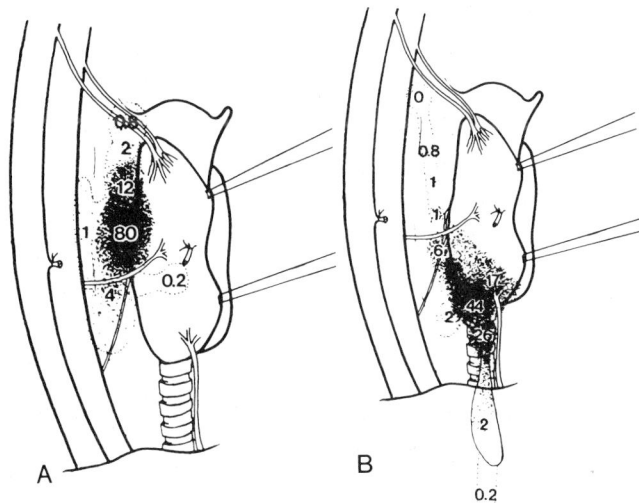

Figure 2. Locations of the superior (A) and inferior (B) parathyroid glands. The more common locations are indicated by the darker shading. The numbers represent the percentages of glands found at the different locations. (From Akerström, G., Malmaers, J., and Bergstrom, R.: Surgical anatomy of human parathyroid glands. Surgery, 95:17, 1984.)

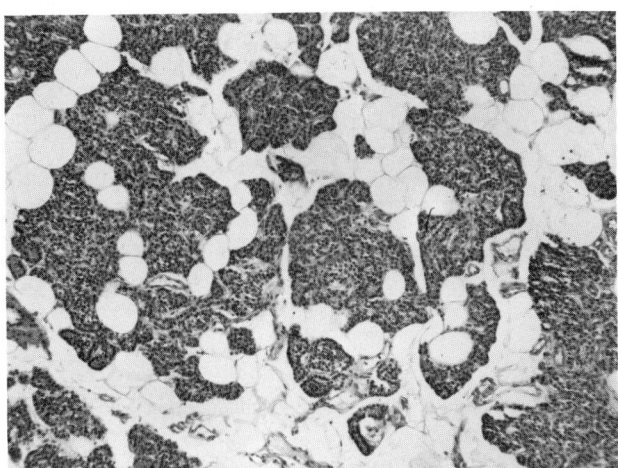

Figure 3. Normal adult parathyroid, composed of approximately 50 per cent parenchymal cells and 50 per cent stromal fat.

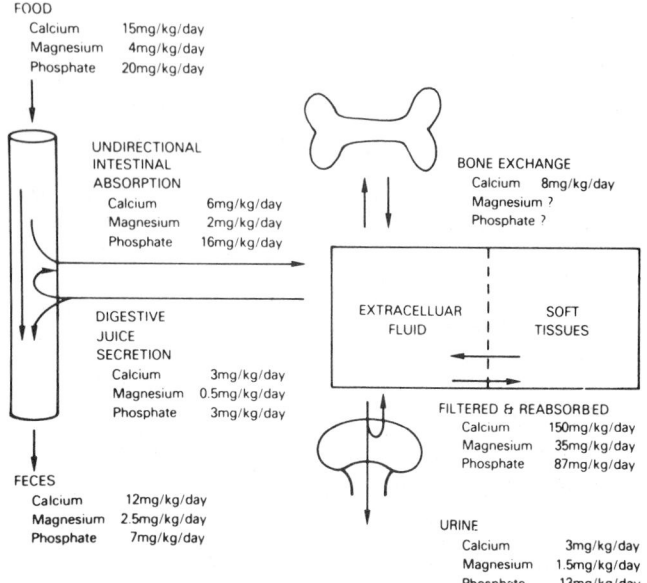

FOOD
Calcium   15mg/kg/day
Magnesium   4mg/kg/day
Phosphate   20mg/kg/day

UNDIRECTIONAL
INTESTINAL
ABSORPTION
Calcium   6mg/kg/day
Magnesium   2mg/kg/day
Phosphate   16mg/kg/day

BONE EXCHANGE
Calcium   8mg/kg/day
Magnesium   ?
Phosphate   ?

DIGESTIVE
JUICE
SECRETION
Calcium   3mg/kg/day
Magnesium   0.5mg/kg/day
Phosphate   3mg/kg/day

EXTRACELLUAR
FLUID   SOFT TISSUES

FILTERED & REABSORBED
Calcium   150mg/kg/day
Magnesium   35mg/kg/day
Phosphate   87mg/kg/day

FECES
Calcium   12mg/kg/day
Magnesium   2.5mg/kg/day
Phosphate   7mg/kg/day

URINE
Calcium   3mg/kg/day
Magnesium   1.5mg/kg/day
Phosphate   13mg/kg/day

Figure 4. Typical daily exchanges of calcium, magnesium, and phosphate among anatomic compartments in adults. (From Williams, R. H. (Ed.): Textbook of Endocrinology, 6th ed. Philadelphia, W. B. Saunders Company, 1981, p. 927.)

fluid, and the glomerular filtrate, 99 per cent of which is reabsorbed by the normal kidney.

The adult body contains about 700 gm. of phosphate, most being located in the bones and teeth. Plasma phosphate measures 2.5 to 4.3 mg. per 100 ml. The plasma levels of calcium and phosphate vary inversely with one another. Normally, the relationship is such that the product of plasma calcium and phosphate (measured in mg. per 100 ml.) is constant and between 30 and 40. On a regular diet, approximately 1500 mg. is ingested daily.

Magnesium, the fourth most abundant metal in mammals and the second most prevalent intracellular cation, is located primarily in the mineral phase of bone. Magnesium is important in the activation of enzymes necessary for intermediary metabolism and phosphorylation, in protein and nucleic acid synthesis, and in mitochondrial regulation. Approximately 300 mg. is ingested daily.

The daily exchanges of calcium, phosphate, and magnesium are shown in Figure 4.

Regulation of Calcium Metabolism

The primary agents responsible for regulation of calcium metabolism are parathyroid hormone, vitamin D, and calcitonin. Their major actions are summarized in Table 1.

PARATHYROID HORMONE. Parathyroid hormone (PTH) is synthesized within the parathyroid as a larger precursor, preproparathyroid hormone, which is cleaved in the parathyroid first to proparathyroid hormone and then to the final 84-amino acid PTH. The hormone is secreted and then metabolized in the liver into hormonally active N-terminal and inactive C-terminal fragments. Parathyroid hormone secretion is inversely related to the serum calcium and also to the levels of 1,25-dihydroxyvitamin D. It has direct effects on the kidney and skeleton and indirect effects on the gastrointestinal tract through vitamin D.

In the skeleton, parathyroid hormone promotes a release of calcium in two phases. The first is by an active transport process and the latter by a process that requires lysosomal enzymes and the synthesis of hydrolytic enzymes. Parathyroid hormone inhibits osteoblasts and stimulates osteoclasts.

In the kidney, parathyroid hormone causes a decrease in calcium clearance at any specific concentration of extracellular fluid calcium. Calcium is cleared linearly with sodium, and it appears that these two ions share a common transport mechanism. The hormone also causes an increased excretion of renal phosphate by inhibiting its reabsorption in the renal tubule. Enhanced bicarbonate secretion is also promoted by parathyroid hormone.

There is substantial evidence that parathyroid hormone stimulates hydroxylation of 25-hydroxyvitamin D to 1,25-dihydroxyvitamin D in the kidney, and it is the latter metabolite that then causes enhanced absorption of calcium from the intestine.

VITAMIN D. The major D vitamins are vitamin D_2 and vitamin D_3. The most important physiologically is vitamin D_3, which is derived from ultraviolet activation of 7-dehydrocholesterol in the skin. The bulk of commercially prepared vitamin D is vitamin D_2. It is derived from ergosterol and is the major form of vitamin D used clinically in the treatment of certain skeletal diseases. Vitamin D increases the intestinal absorption of calcium, and secondarily phosphate, and increases the mobilization of calcium and phosphate from bone to blood. Vitamin D appears to exert a growth-promoting effect that is not explained by mineral retention.

CALCITONIN. Calcitonin (CT) inhibits bone resorption and produces hypocalcemia when administered to experimental animals. The hormone also induces the urinary excretion of calcium and phosphate. Several secretagogues for calcitonin have been identified, including beta-adrenergic catecholamines, glucagon, and cholecystokinin, but the most potent appear to be calcium and pentagastrin.

The activity of parathyroid hormone and calcitonin appears to be mediated by cyclic 3'5'-adenosine monophosphate (cyclic AMP) produced through specific hormonal activation of the enzyme adenyl cyclase in bone and kidney. Calcitonin has not been demonstrated to be important in the control of serum calcium in man.

In summary, serum calcium is closely regulated by the action of parathyroid hormone. A reduction in serum ionized calcium increases secretion of parathyroid hormone which secondarily stimulates production of $1,25(OH)_2D_3$. Conversely, a rise in serum calcium inhibits both PTH secretion and the formation of active calciferol.

TABLE 1. Actions of Major Calcium-Regulating Hormones

	Bone	Kidney	Intestine
Parathyroid hormone	Stimulates resorption of calcium and phosphate	Stimulates reabsorption of calcium and conversion of $25(OH)D_3$ to $1,25(OH)_2D_3$; inhibits reabsorption of phosphate and bicarbonate	No direct effects
Vitamin D	Stimulates transport of calcium	Inhibits reabsorption of calcium	Stimulates absorption of calcium and phosphate
Calcitonin	Inhibits resorption of calcium and phosphate	Inhibits reabsorption of calcium and phosphate	No direct effects

DISORDERS OF THE PARATHYROID GLANDS

HYPERPARATHYROIDISM

The cause of spontaneous hyperfunction of the parathyroid glands is unknown; and, as with many endocrine neoplasms, overactivity is recognized not because of anatomic enlargement, but because of the peripheral effects of excess hormone. Primary hyperparathyroidism occurs when the normal feedback control by serum calcium is disturbed and there is increased production of parathyroid hormone. Secondary hyperparathyroidism occurs most commonly in patients with renal disease but also compensates for the true hypocalcemia associated with some diseases of the gastrointestinal tract, bone, or other endocrine organs. There is a defect in mineral homeostasis leading to a compensatory increase in parathyroid gland function and size. Occasionally with prolonged compensatory stimulation, a hyperplastic gland develops autonomous function. This state is referred to as tertiary hyperparathyroidism.

PRIMARY HYPERPARATHYROIDISM. Formerly thought to be a relatively rare condition associated with advanced renal or bone disease, primary hyperparathyroidism has been detected with increasing frequency in recent years, probably as a result of the widespread use of automated technology for determining serum calcium concentration.

The incidence of hyperparathyroidism is approximately 25 per 100,000 in the general population, and approximately 50,000 new cases occur annually. The incidence of the disease increases markedly with age, and it is especially common in postmenopausal women: in women over 65 years of age the incidence is 2.5 per 1000. The gender and age of 100 patients with primary hyperparathyroidism studied in the authors' clinic are shown in Figure 5. Christensson,[16] in a study of 15,903 individuals undergoing a "health checkup" in Sweden, found the prevalence of hyperparathyroidism to be 5 per 1000. No cause could be found for the substantially higher incidence in that country.

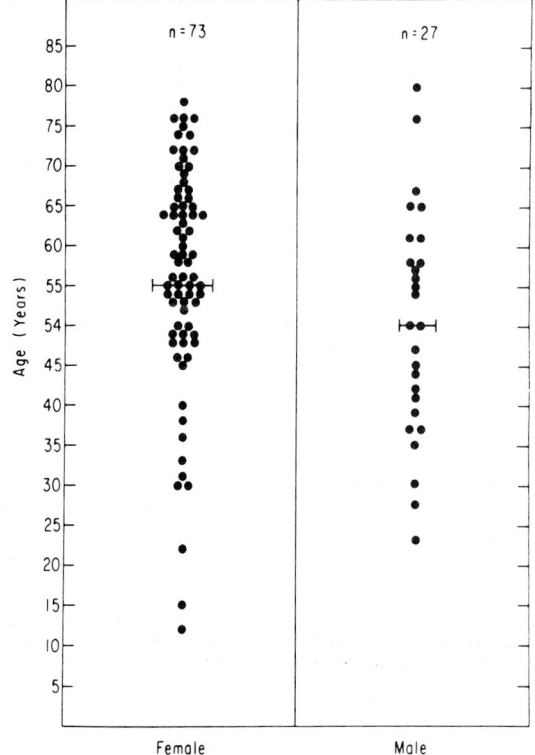

Figure 5. Age and sex distribution of 100 consecutive patients with surgically proven primary hyperparathyroidism. (From Wells, S. A., Jr., Leight, G. S., and Ross, A. J.: Primary hyperthyroidism. Curr. Probl. Surg., *17*:400, 1980.)

Etiology

The etiology of hyperparathyroidism is unknown and probably varies with the underlying pathologic condition. Single-gland or adenomatous disease is more consistent with a mechanism involving spontaneous hyperfunction, whereas multiglandular disease suggests the presence of some exogenous stimulus. Recent studies[38] have challenged the concept of complete parathyroid autonomy. An alteration in the set point, the sensitivity of the glands to suppression by calcium, appears more consistent with the present data. It has been proposed that a renal leak of calcium, if sufficient, may lead to hypocalcemia, thus stimulating parathyroid hormone secretion and ultimately hyperfunctional parathyroid glands. It has been demonstrated that loss of renal function with age is associated with increased plasma levels of parathyroid hormone as well as increases in nephrogenous cyclic AMP and decreases in renal phosphate clearance. This suggests increased biologic effects of parathyroid hormone. The role that either the renal calcium leak or the increased plasmic levels of parathyroid hormone with age has in the etiology of hyperparathyroidism is unclear.

Several investigators have reported an increased incidence of hyperparathyroidism in patients exposed to low-dose ionizing irradiation, usually in childhood. In the study of Christensson,[17] 8 (14 per cent) of 58 individuals found to have hyperparathyroidism had received ionizing irradiation to the neck at a young age. Nine of 58 normal subjects matched for age and sex had not been previously irradiated. Several other investigators have confirmed an association of radiation exposure to the neck and hyperparathyroidism.

Recent data on the etiology of hyperparathyroidism in multiple endocrine neoplasia Type I (MEN I), discussed in Chapter 24 in greater detail, may have significance for sporadic disease as well. Friedman and associates[29] have identified Chromosome 11 deletions, including a gene locus previously associated with MEN-I, in 10 of 16 parathyroid tumors in patients with known MEN-I. Similar losses were demonstrated in 11 of 34 sporadic adenomas. The implications of such genetic abnormalities are only beginning to be explored.

Clinical Presentation (Signs and Symptoms)

Since the advent of routine screening for calcium and phosphate, hyperparathyroidism has been detected with increasing frequency. Although in the past most patients presented with severe bone or renal disease, an increasing percentage of patients today are asymptomatic. For example, in a 1980 article from the Mayo Clinic,[34] only 49 per cent of patients had a serious complication that could directly be attributed to parathyroid disease. However, when carefully questioned, many of these patients describe symptoms or associated conditions that can be related to hyperparathyroidism; and their symptoms improve after parathyroidectomy.

The most frequent symptoms in 100 consecutive patients evaluated by the authors at the time of diagnosis are shown in Table 2. The usual symptomatic patient with hyperparathyroidism is in the chronic phase of disease with signs and symptoms from secondary changes in the genitourinary system and skeleton. The earliest complaints, such as muscle weakness, anorexia, nausea, constipation, polyuria, and polydipsia, occasionally cause the patient to seek medical advice; but often the examining physician does not suspect hyperparathyroidism.

RENAL COMPLICATIONS. Renal complications are generally the most severe clinical manifestations of hyperparathyroidism. Many patients have only frequency, nocturia, and polydipsia; but usually the presenting symptoms are related to nephrolithiasis, which occurs in approximately 30 per cent of cases; conversely, approximately 5 to 10 per cent of previously unscreened patients presenting with nephrolithiasis have hyperparathyroidism. Patients complain of back pain, hematuria,

TABLE 2. Presenting Symptoms in 100 Patients with Primary Hyperparathyroidism

Symptoms	Percentage of Population
Nephrolithiasis	30
Bone disease	2
Peptic ulcer disease	12
Psychiatric disorders	15
Muscle weakness	70
Constipation	32
Polyuria	28
Pancreatitis	1
Myalgia	54
Arthralgia	54

and the passing of renal calculi, most of which are composed of calcium phosphate or calcium oxalate. Nephrocalcinosis represents calcification within the parenchyma of one or both kidneys; it occurs in only 5 to 10 per cent of patients with primary hyperparathyroidism. It is very unusual for nephrolithiasis and nephrocalcinosis to occur simultaneously. Although renal stones can be removed surgically or treated with shock wave lithotripsy, there is little that can be done for nephrocalcinosis; and even after definitive treatment of hyperparathyroidism there is rarely improvement of this condition. Renal damage is much more common in patients with nephrocalcinosis, but it can occur in the absence of renal calcification. If renal impairment is severe preoperatively, it tends to remain unchanged or to become progressively worse postoperatively; mild degrees of renal damage are usually functional and reversible. Careful evaluation of renal function reveals some degree of abnormality in 80 to 90 per cent of patients with hyperparathyroidism.

The incidence of hypertension in patients with hyperparathyroidism was about 70 per cent in Hellstrom and Ivemark's series of 139 patients,[35] although other authors have reported a much less marked association. Hypertension, with its associated clinical complications (heart failure, cerebral hemorrhage, and renal insufficiency), was responsible for death in 30 per cent of the patients in whom it persisted after parathyroid surgery. Hellstrom's investigation demonstrated in a striking manner the importance of this complication in hyperparathyroidism and the urgency of early diagnosis and treatment if the late cardiovascular and renal sequelae are to be minimized. Various mechanisms have been proposed to explain this relationship of hyperparathyroidism with hypertension; it appears to be most closely correlated with the degree of renal impairment. Despite this, Diamond and associates[21] found that parathyroidectomy led to a substantial fall in both systolic and diastolic pressures in 54 per cent of hypertensive subjects unrelated to improvements in renal function. Unfortunately, such improvement does not always occur.

BONE DISEASE. Many of the first descriptions of hyperparathyroidism were of patients who had severe bone disease characterized by osteitis fibrosa cystica generalisata, a condition with a unique x-ray picture that is pathognomonic of hyperparathyroidism. Although the incidence of bone disease in patients with primary hyperparathyroidism reported in earlier studies was as high as 50 to 90 per cent, the reported incidence in more current series is 5 to 15 per cent.

Skeletal involvement is most readily demonstrated by industrial radiographs of the hands (Fig. 6). Subperiosteal resorption, pathognomonic of hyperparathyroidism, is usually evident on the radial aspect of the middle phalynx of the second or third fingers. In more advanced cases, cysts are present, and there is tufting of the distal phalanges. The skull is the second most commonly affected skeletal site and presents a mottled appear-

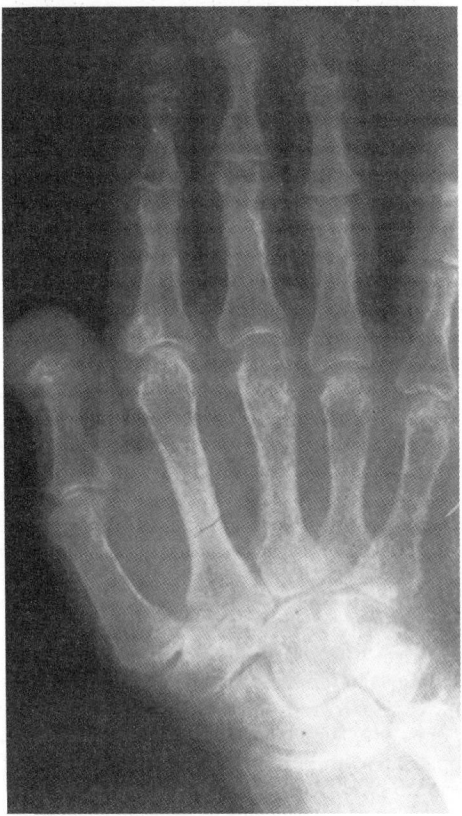

Figure 6. Hand radiograph. Note the uniform demineralization with concomitant soft tissue clubbing, severe erosion of distal phalanges, and cyst at base of middle phalanx, index finger. Subperiosteal cortical resorption is best shown along the metacarpal shaft of the fifth digit.

ance often associated with diffuse granularity and cystic lesions (Fig. 7A). Also, with advanced disease, osteoclastomas, or "brown tumors," may be present (Fig. 8). With the use of more sophisticated and sensitive technology, such as x-ray spectrophotometry and phosphate absorptiometric analysis, subtle derangements in bone density can be detected; and the incidence of "bone disease" in patients with hyperparathyroidism has been shown to be relatively common. Although the significance of subtle bone loss has been questioned, Kochensberger and associates[41] recently demonstrated an increased prevalence of vertebral fractures in patients undergoing parathyroidectomy, compared with an otherwise matched group of patients undergoing cholecystectomy.

Lloyd[44] evaluated 138 consecutive patients with primary hyperparathyroidism and classified them into three groups: those with bone disease only, those with kidney disease (stones) only, and those with neither bone disease nor kidney disease. Twelve with bone disease had previously suffered from renal stones, and were not classified. Comparing patients with bone disease only with those with kidney disease only, the mean plasma calcium was higher (13 mg. per 100 ml. versus 11.6 mg. per 100 ml.; p < 0.001), the mean tumor weight was greater (5.9 gm. versus 1.05 gm.; p < 0.001), and the duration of symptoms was shorter (3.6 years versus 6.8 years; p < 0.001). On the basis of this observation, he proposed that there were two different types of parathyroid tumors: one growing rapidly, being highly active, and causing overt bone disease; and the other growing slowly, being of low activity, and causing kidney stones. There was no characteristic tumor histology associated with either type of disease, and the basis for this clinical variability remains unexplained.

GASTROINTESTINAL MANIFESTATIONS. An increased incidence of peptic ulcer disease in patients with primary hyperparathyroidism was first reported by Rogers[63] in 1946. Most,

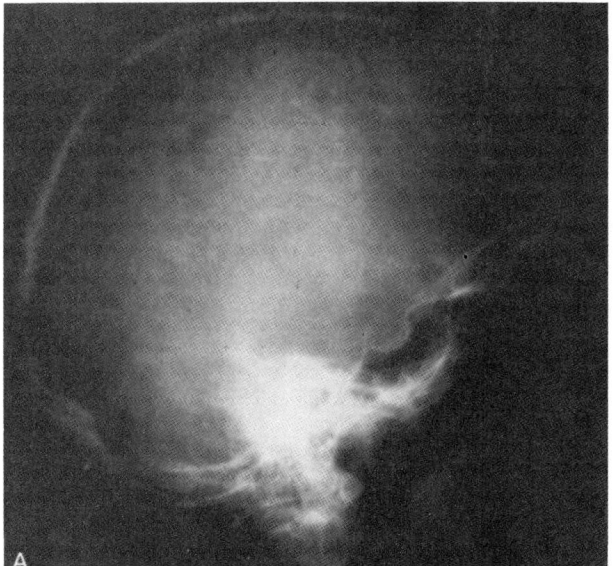

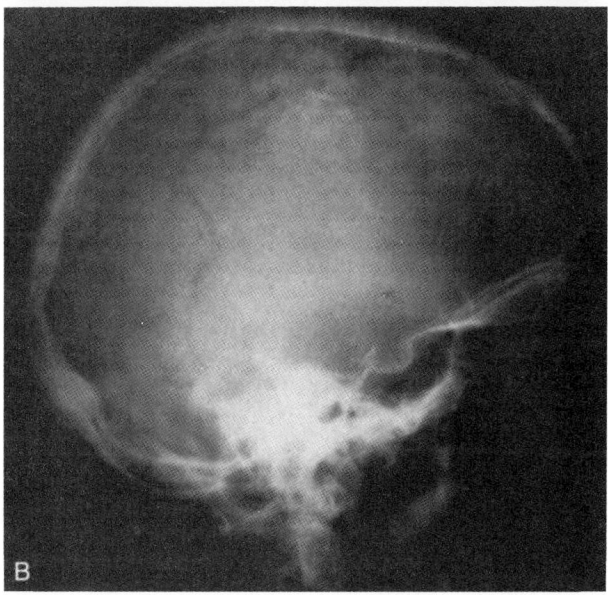

Figure 7. *A,* Skull film of a patient with hyperparathyroidism. There is demineralization imparting a salt-and-pepper texture to the calvarium with obliteration of the normal vascular grooves of the inner table. The cortex of the ascending ramus and alveolar ridge of the mandible are severely demineralized. *B,* Two years after removal of parathyroid adenoma, there is restoration of normal bone mineralization.

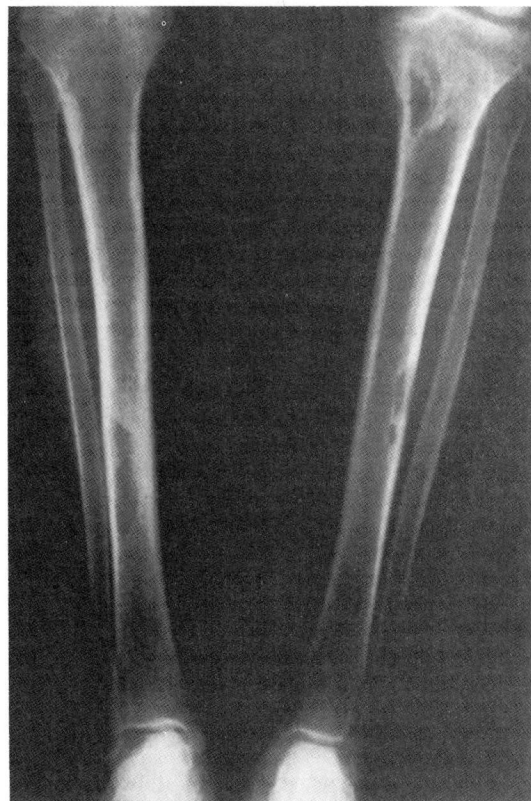

Figure 8. Lower leg radiograph. Multiple bone cysts (brown tumors) are present. The cortical location and sharp margins are characteristic.

but not all, subsequent studies have confirmed this association. The association appears logical, because the induction of hypercalcemia experimentally in normal subjects is associated with increased gastric acid secretion and hypergastrinemia. In an experimental animal model, Bolman and associates[11] clearly demonstrated that infusion of parathyroid hormone into the gastroepiploic artery supplying the gastric antrum caused hypergastrinemia, even though blood calcium levels were not increased, which demonstrated the effect of parathyroid hormone on gastric secretion. Although some investigators have demonstrated significant reductions in serum gastrin levels and gastric acid secretion following the surgical correction of hyperparathyroidism, others have not. At present, it appears that the relationship of hyperparathyroidism to peptic ulcer disease is unclear.

The association of pancreatitis and hyperparathyroidism was first reported by Smith and Cooke in 1940.[74] Even though an increased incidence of pancreatitis was reported from various clinics in the subsequent two decades, there were no carefully controlled studies evaluating the relationship. Between 1962 and 1972, Rosin[65] screened the records of 1000 patients with hyperparathyroidism from 26 hospitals in Great Britain and found pancreatitis in less than 1 per cent. A similar incidence was reported in the study of Bess and associates[10] in their analysis of 1153 cases. In the majority of the cases reported in the latter study, the presence of gallstone disease or alcoholism was also detected. In a more recent study, however, Reeve and Delbridge[62] evaluated the concentration of serum amylase in 86 patients undergoing neck exploration for hyperparathyroidism. Postoperative hyperamylasemia (> 300 I.U.) occurred in 35 per cent of the group and clinically significant pancreatitis (serum amylase of > 1000 I.U. associated with abdominal pain) occurred in 8 of the patients (10 per cent). Such as association has not been reported by other investigators and awaits confirmation. Pancreatitis also occurs in other conditions producing hypercalcemia.

There also appears to be an increased incidence (25 to 35 per cent) of cholelithiasis in patients with hyperparathyroidism. This is presumably due to a high concentration of calcium in the bile, which leads to the formation of calcium bilirubinate stones.

EMOTIONAL DISTURBANCES. Patients with hypercalcemia of any cause may develop neurologic or psychiatric disturbances ranging from depression or anxiety to psychosis or coma. Most of the mental derangements associated with hyperparathyroidism are subtle. Petersen[58] performed psychiatric examinations on 54 patients with hyperparathyroidism and detected mental disturbances in more than half of them. Four patients had acute organic psychosis that returned to normal after surgical therapy. Most often, however, such severe disturbances are not correctable by parathyroidectomy. Joborn and associates[39] recently examined monoamine metabolite levels in 48 such patients and found subnormal levels that improved after parathyroidectomy. Similar abnormalities have been associated with endogenous depression. Many patients after parathyroidectomy experience a sense of well-being and relief of fatigue and dullness that often was not fully appreciated preoperatively.

ARTICULAR AND SOFT TISSUE MANIFESTATIONS. There is an increased prevalence of chondrocalcinosis and pseudogout in patients with hyperparathyroidism, the incidence being 3 to 7 per cent. Characteristically, one can see radiographic evidence of calcium pyrophosphate deposition in the articular cartilages and menisci. Vascular and cardiac calcification, skin necrosis, and band keratopathy of the cornea have all been reported in patients with hyperparathyroidism. The latter usually occur, however, only in association with decreased renal function and hyperphosphatemia.

NEUROMUSCULAR COMPLICATIONS. It is well recognized that muscular weakness, fatigue, and even mental aberrations may occur in patients with hyperparathyroidism. Most commonly, the weakness is in the proximal muscle groups. In a study by Patten and associates,[57] 14 (87.5 per cent) of 16 patients with primary hyperparathyroidism demonstrated weakness, easy fatigability, and muscle atrophy. There were sensory abnormalities in 50 per cent of the patients, and muscle biopsies demonstrated atrophy of Type II muscle fibers most consistent with a neuropathic lesion and not a primary myopathy. The etiology of these findings remains unclear.

Physical Findings

The diseased parathyroid glands are rarely palpable in patients with hyperparathyroidism, and a palpable gland in the neck should suggest the presence of a thyroid nodule.

Laboratory Diagnosis

The diagnosis of hyperparathyroidism is dependent upon the documentation of an elevated serum calcium concentration usually in conjunction with an elevated serum parathyroid hormone.

Serum calcium is best determined by atomic absorption spectrophotometry, and each laboratory should determine its own normal range, but values usually are from 8.5 to 10.5 mg. per 100 ml. Theoretically, one should be concerned with the serum ionized or free fraction of serum calcium rather than that portion bound to protein or organic anions. The measurement of ionized calcium is possible by means of a calcium-sensitive flow-through electrode. In evaluating 19 patients with subtle hyperparathyroidism and intermittent, minimal elevations of serum calcium, McLeod and associates[45] obtained 151 concurrent preoperative measurements of total calcium and ionized calcium. Only 46 (30.5 per cent) of the total calcium measurements were elevated, whereas 134 (88.7 per cent) of the ionized calcium determinations were increased. Hyperparathyroidism was confirmed at operation, and postoperatively the values of total and ionized calcium returned to normal.

It might appear that the most efficient method of diagnosing hyperparathyroidism would be to document an increased concentration of parathyroid hormone in plasma. Berson and colleagues[9] first described a radioimmunoassay for parathyroid hormone in 1963. Owing to the heterogeneity of the circulating forms of parathyroid hormone, most of the early studies using radioimmunoassay techniques reported conflicting results. The methodology has been greatly refined, however, and currently has wide clinical use. It is important to remember that the finding of an elevated plasma level of parathyroid hormone does not in itself establish the diagnosis of hyperparathyroidism. One must evaluate the parathyroid hormone level as a function of the serum calcium concentration. Subjects with increased serum concentrations of both calcium and parathyroid hormone generally have hyperparathyroidism (Fig. 9).

Following secretion, parathyroid hormone is very rapidly

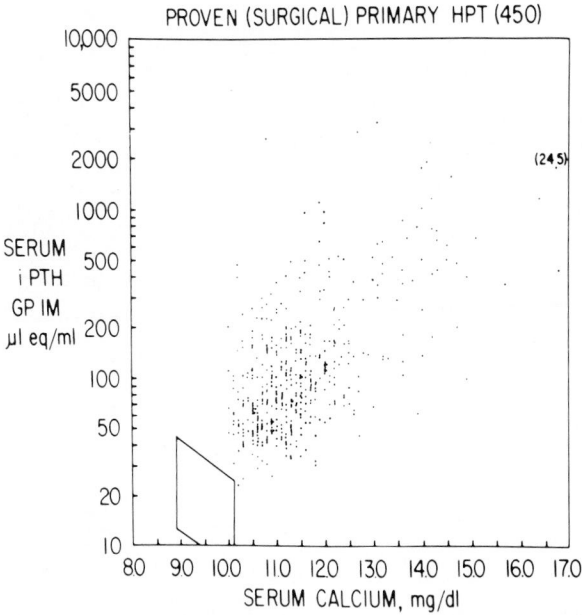

Figure 9. Serum iPTH values in 450 patients with surgically proven primary hyperparathyroidism as a function of serum calcium concentration. Serum iPTH was measured with a radioimmunoassay using GP Im antiserum. The area enclosed by the solid lines represents the normal range ± 2 SD for serum iPTH and serum calcium. Note that there is a 10 per cent overlap of serum iPTH with the normal range but that greater than 95 per cent of normal sera and all hyperparathyroid sera have measurable iPTH. Formal discriminative analysis of serum iPTH and serum calcium separates 100 per cent of hyperparathyroid patients from normal subjects (From Arnaud, C. D., et al.: Excerpta Medical International Congress Series, No. 270, 1973, p. 281.)

cleaved into an amino-terminal fragment and a carboxy-terminal fragment. The intact molecule and the biologically active amino-terminal fragment have half-lives of minutes, whereas the inactive carboxy-terminal fragment has a half-life of hours. Generally, antibodies directed against the carboxy-terminal fragment have been more useful in radioimmunoassay to establish the diagnosis of hyperparathyroidism.

The concentration of serum phosphate varies between 2.5 and 4.5 mg. per 100 ml. Approximately half the patients with primary hyperparathyroidism have hypophosphatemia. However, in the presence of significant renal impairment, levels may be considerably elevated.

The serum concentration of alkaline phosphatase is normally below 110 I.U. per 100 ml. Ten to 40 per cent of patients with hyperparathyroidism have increased levels. In such patients, there is almost always some degree of bone disease, and after surgical therapy, the serum calcium concentration may fall more rapidly to lower levels, compared with that of patients whose serum alkaline phosphatase levels are normal. Alkaline phosphatase level is not helpful in diagnosing hyperparathyroidism, because it is also very often elevated with other causes of hypercalcemia.

Because of the effect of PTH on bicarbonate excretion in the kidney, patients with hyperparathyroidism often have a hyperchloremic metabolic acidosis at the time of diagnosis. Palmer and associates[56] evaluated the serum concentration of chloride as a function of the concentration of phosphate in 25 patients with hyperparathyroidism. The Cl/PO_4 ratio was above 33 in 96 per cent of the patients. Conversely, in 27 patients with hypercalcemia with other causes, the ratio was less than 30 in 92 per cent of the patients. The Cl/PO_4 ratio may have value in patients in whom the differential diagnosis of hypercalcemia is difficult.

The serum concentration of magnesium is below normal in only 5 to 10 per cent of patients with hyperparathyroidism. If there is concomitant hypocalcemia and hypomagnesemia following parathyroidectomy, it is difficult to correct the hypocalcemia until the serum magnesium concentration has been returned to normal.

The serum concentrations of calcium, phosphate, alkaline phosphatase, and chloride, as well as the Cl/PO$_4$ ratio, in 100 consecutive patients with primary hyperparathyroidism studied in the authors' clinic are depicted in Figure 10.

NEPHROGENOUS CYCLIC AMP. The interaction of parathyroid hormone with specific receptors in the renal tubule causes activation of adenylate cyclase and an increase in cyclic AMP inside the cell. Because the cyclic AMP leaks into the tubular fluid, increased concentrations of cyclic AMP are present in the urine of patients with hyperparathyroidism. When measured as a function of creatinine clearance (nephrogenous cyclic AMP), it has been demonstrated that 90 per cent of patients with hyperparathyroidism have increased urinary levels. The measurement of nephrogenous cyclic AMP has been useful in the differential diagnosis of hyperparathyroidism, although it may be elevated in certain cases of malignancy-associated hypercalcemia.

URINARY CALCIUM. In hyperparathyroidism urinary calcium excretion is almost always elevated. This has assumed increasing importance in differentiating hyperparathyroidism from the recently recognized syndrome of familial hypercalcemic hypocalciuric hyperparathyroidism.

BONE BIOPSY AND DENSITOMETRY. Iliac crest bone biopsy and photon beam bone scanning can detect subtle changes when conventional radiographs are negative. These findings may help to establish the diagnosis in otherwise equivocal cases.

OTHER HORMONES. Primary hyperparathyroidism is a component of the multiple endocrine neoplasia syndromes (MEN) Type I and IIa. Farndon and associates[26] recently examined the utility of testing for other components of these syndromes in a group of 100 patients undergoing surgical therapy for primary hyperparathyroidism. Measuring serum gastrin, calcitonin, and prolactin both pre- and postoperatively, they did not identify any patient with either type of multiple endocrine neoplasia. They concluded that laboratory measurements are not indicated in the absence of a family history or other clinical indications.

Less Common Manifestations

FAMILIAL HYPERPARATHYROIDISM. The familial incidence of hyperparathyroidism is well established. In its simplest form, it occurs as a single disease with no associated abnormalities, whereas in its more complex form, it presents as a part of one of the multiple endocrinopathy syndromes. MEN Type I is characterized by the association of parathyroid hyperplasia, pituitary adenomas, pancreatic islet cell neoplasia, and, occasionally, tumors of the thyroid or adrenal cortex. MEN Type IIa is represented by medullary thyroid carcinoma, pheochromocytoma, and parathyroid hyperplasia.

In 1972, Foley and associates[28] described a syndrome characterized by the familial occurrence of hypercalcemia, hypocalciuria, and generalized parathyroid enlargement. These patients have little morbidity from the hyperparathyroidism, and the hyperparathyroidism is difficult to cure surgically. Even with aggressive therapy (three and one-half gland parathyroid-

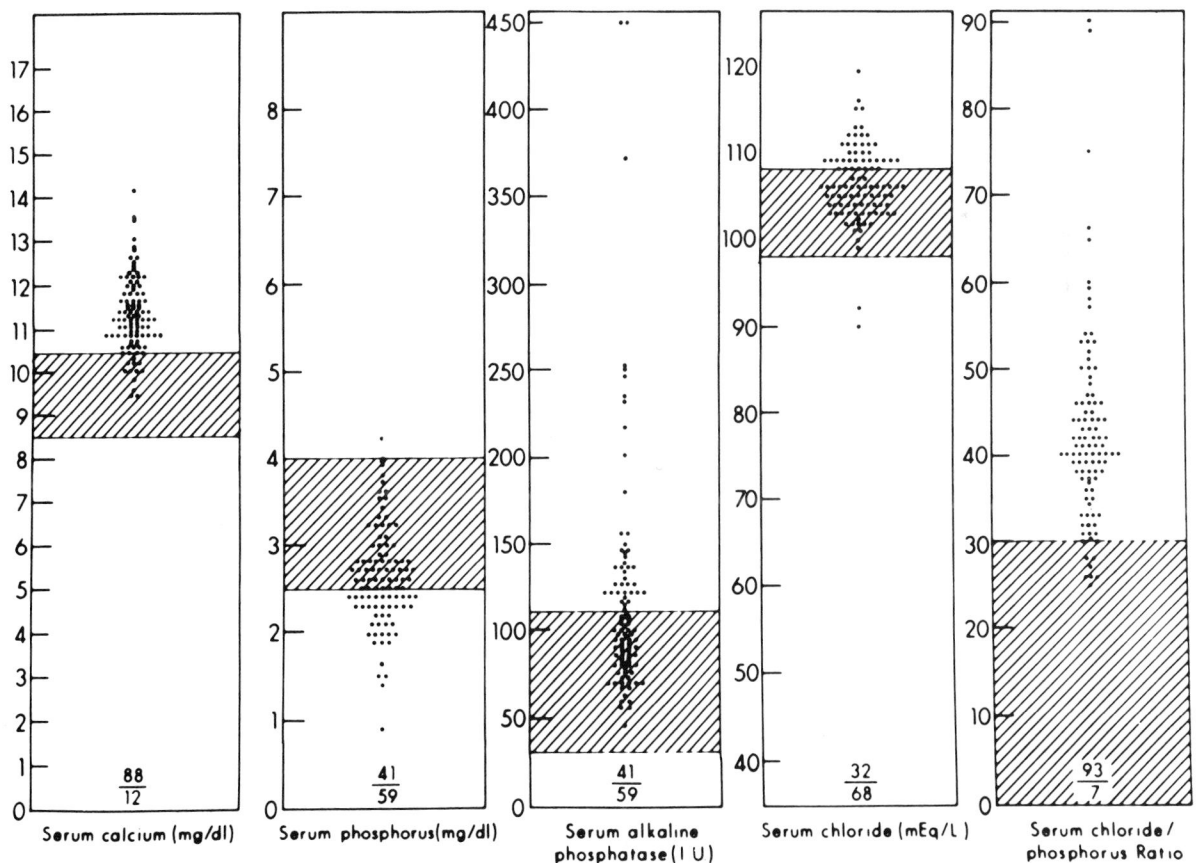

Figure 10. The serum concentrations of calcium, phosphorus, alkaline phosphatase, and chloride in 100 consecutive patients with surgically proven hyperparathyroidism. The ratio of serum chloride to phosphorus is also shown (extreme right). The fractions at the bottom of each bar represent the number of abnormal values over the number of normal values. The laboratory values shown represent the determinations made at the time of hospital admission for parathyroidectomy. Even though 12 patients had serum calcium concentrations in the normal range, all had been demonstrated to be hypercalcemic on several preoperative determinations. (From Wells, S. A., Jr., Leight, G. S., and Ross, A. J.: Primary hyperparathyroidism. Curr. Probl. Surg., 17:400, 1980.)

ectomy), there is a high incidence of persistent or recurrent hypercalcemia postoperatively.

Each of these syndromes is characterized by an autosomal dominant pattern of inheritance. The multiple endocrine neoplasia syndromes are discussed at greater length in Chapter 24.

HYPERPARATHYROIDISM IN PREGNANCY. Primary hyperparathyroidism in pregnancy is rare and is associated with neonatal tetany, stillbirth, and abortion.[42] The risk of fetal complications appears to be higher if the hyperparathyroidism is untreated. When the diagnosis is made, the mother should undergo operation, if possible during the second trimester.

NEONATAL PRIMARY HYPERPARATHYROIDISM. This rare condition is characterized by hypotonia, poor feeding, constipation, and respiratory distress.[33] At least a quarter of cases have occurred in families with familial hypocalciuric hypercalcemia. The 1-year survival in symptomatic untreated patients is less than 50 per cent, and total parathyroidectomy with autotransplantation has been recommended as the treatment of choice. A more conservative approach may be justified in the absence of symptoms.

PARATHYROID CARCINOMA. Parathyroid carcinoma is rare and probably represents less than 1 per cent of patients with hyperparathyroidism and increased PTH. Parathyroid carcinoma usually presents in a manner different from that of benign hyperparathyroidism (Table 3). The diagnosis is most accurately made on histologic examination when there is local invasion of surrounding tissues or metastases to regional lymph nodes or distant sites. However, some pathologists believe that the diagnosis can be made when there is histologic evidence of vascular invasion, frequent mitotic figures, and capsular invasion. Characteristically, the serum concentrations of calcium, PTH, and alkaline phosphatase are markedly increased, compared with concentrations in patients with benign hyperparathyroidism. In approximately 50 per cent of patients with parathyroid carcinoma, the involved parathyroid gland is palpable, a finding rarely observed in patients with benign hyperparathyroidism. Most patients with parathyroid carcinoma are symptomatic at the time of diagnosis and complain of nausea, vomiting, polyuria, generalized weakness, and weight loss. Moreover, both kidneys and skeleton are commonly affected in this disease, often in the same patient, a finding distinctly different from that observed in benign hyperparathyroidism.

It is important to recognize the disease at the initial neck exploration, because radical resection of the malignant parathyroid gland, the ipsilateral thyroid lobe, and involved adjacent soft tissue and regional lymph nodes offers the only possibility for cure. If the disease recurs, reoperation is indicated (including resection of pulmonary or liver metastases) because patients, if untreated, succumb to uncontrolled hypercalcemia. In a review by Holmes and associates,[36] the 5-year survival was 50 per cent; however, only 13 per cent of patients lived 10 years. Neither chemotherapy nor radiation therapy offers any benefit.

Hyperparathyroid Crisis

Most patients presenting with hyperparathyroidism are chronically ill with symptoms referable to the kidneys or the skeleton. Rarely, however, patients may become acutely ill with urgent symptoms that sometimes prove fatal. The terms *acute hyperparathyroidism* and *hyperparathyroid crisis* have been used to describe this clinical dilemma. The onset is usually characterized by rapidly developing muscular weakness, nausea and vomiting, weight loss, fatigue, drowsiness, and confusion. Males and females are affected equally. The serum calcium concentration is almost always elevated (16 to 20 mg. per 100 ml.), and azotemia is usually present. This clinical pattern not only is associated with hyperparathyroidism but also is observed in patients with acute hypercalcemia accompanying other diseases. The offending parathyroid gland(s) is usually large; and in about one third of the patients, a tumor is palpable in the neck preoperatively, which is not surprising, because larger parathyroid glands are usually associated with higher calcium values than are smaller ones. The genesis of the condition appears to involve uncontrolled PTH secretion followed by hypercalcemia, polyuria, dehydration, reduced renal function, and increasing hypercalcemia.[27]

Although the definitive therapy is resection of the hyperfunctioning parathyroid tissue, it is unwise to proceed with neck exploration until the patient has been prepared and the calcium concentration lowered, if possible. The cornerstone of therapy is diuresis, preferably with 0.9 per cent sodium chloride in sufficient amounts to maintain urinary output above 100 ml. per hour. When urinary output becomes satisfactory, potassium chloride should be administered. The diuretic furosemide increases the renal excretion of sodium and calcium and should not be used until the patient is well hydrated. If the serum calcium remains elevated with adequate sodium infusion and hydration, other agents that are known to lower the serum calcium concentration should be administered (Table 4). If a diagnosis of hyperparathyroidism is in doubt, an ultrasound examination or a computed tomographic (CT) scan of the neck may be useful in identifying an enlarged parathyroid gland. The disease can be dramatically reversed by surgical therapy. Masselly and associates[49] reported the successful surgical treatment of 10 comatose patients with hyperparathyroid crisis.

TABLE 3. Benign Primary Hyperparathyroidism vs. Parathyroid Carcinoma

	Primary Hyperparathyroidism		Parathyroid Carcinoma	
	Mallette et al.[47]	Heath et al.[34]	Holmes et al.[36]	Shane and Bilezikian[72]
Period of review	1965–1972	1974–1976	1933–1968	1968–1981
Number of cases	57	51	46	62
Female:male ratio	1.4:1	3.6:1	0.8:1	1.2:1
Average age (yr.)	51	62	44	48
Serum calcium (mg./100 ml.)	11.7	10.8*	15.9	15.5
Renal involvement	21 (37%)	2 (4%)	15 (32%)	37 (60%)
Skeletal involvement	8 (14%)	10 (20%)†	34 (73%)	34 (55%)
No symptoms	13 (23%)	26 (51%)		1 (2%)

* The normal range for serum calcium in this study was 8.9 to 10.1 mg. per 100 ml., lower than the range reported for the others (approximately 8.8 to 10.7.)

† This number included patients with osteoporosis.

From Shane E., and Bilezikian, J. P.: Parathyroid carcinoma. Endocrinol Rev., 3:218, 1982.

TABLE 4. Agents Used in the Treatment of Hypercalcemia

Agent	Dosage	Administration	Comment
Calcitonin	2–6 MRC units/kg. 10–20 MRC units	Subcutaneous, every 6–8 hr. Intravenous, hourly	Nausea and vomiting are side effects. Allergy is the only contraindication. Onset of calcium-lowering effect is rapid.
Mithramycin	25 μg./kg.	Intravenously over 1 hr. in 100 ml. 0.9% saline or 5% dextrose	Contraindications are renal or hepatic dysfunction. Calcium-lowering effect occurs within 24 hr. Drug is useful when diuretic and intravenous saline are contraindicated. Nausea and vomiting are side effects.
Glucocorticoids	Prednisone 40–50 mg./day Prednisolone phosphate 40 mg.	Oral Intramuscularly or intravenously every 8 hr.	Lag period may be 7–10 days. Glucocorticoids are safe for short-term use. Alternate-day oral program may be used for long-term use.
Orthophosphate	1–2 gm./24 hr.	Oral	Dosage must be adjusted for renal impairment. Soft tissue calcification may occur. Intravenous phosphate is not recommended.
Prostaglandin synthetase inhibitors	Indomethacin, 25–50 mg. 3 times a day	Oral	Unless increased prostaglandin secretion is measured, this drug should not be used alone.

From Purnell, D. C., and van Heerden, J. A.: Management of symptomatic hypercalcemia and hypocalcemia. World J. Surg., 6:702, 1982.

Secondary Hyperparathyroidism (Renal Osteodystrophy)

Since the initiation of maintenance dialysis and renal transplantation, the lives of patients with chronic renal failure (CRF) have been prolonged. Secondary hyperparathyroidism develops as a result of the metabolic alterations occurring in CRF. Phosphate retention and hyperphosphatemia in conjunction with a decrease in the renal production of 1,25(OH)$_2$ vitamin D$_3$ reduce the serum calcium producing secondary hyperparathyroidism. Also, aluminum present in the dialysate water and in oral phosphate binder medications accumulates in bone and contributes substantially to the osteomalacia component of the disease. The pathogenesis of renal osteodystrophy is depicted in Figure 11. Therapy should be directed toward controlling the serum phosphate by dietary restriction and phosphate gels, maintaining adequate calcium intake, administering vitamin D sterols, and reducing aluminum in the dialysate bath and the diet.

Differential Diagnosis

Many diseases are associated with hypercalcemia (Table 5). They must be excluded before subjecting a patient with suspected hyperparathyroidism to operation. Unfortunately, there is no single test, other than neck exploration, that with certainty establishes the diagnosis of hyperparathyroidism.

Of the more common causes, hyperthyroidism, the milk-alkali syndrome, hypervitaminosis D or A, and immobilization can be excluded by a careful history and physical examination. In patients with sarcoidosis or multiple myeloma, the serum

globulin levels are usually elevated and there are characteristic radiographic findings, as there are also in patients with Paget's disease of the bone. If patients with hypercalcemia are taking thiazide diuretics, the drug should be discontinued and, if this is responsible, the calcium returns to normal within a few weeks.

HYPERCALCEMIA AND MALIGNANCY. In hospitalized patients, malignancy rather than hyperparathyroidism is the most common cause of hypercalcemia; and, generally, patients can be divided into three groups: (1) those with hematologic malignancies (30 per cent), (2) those with solid tumors and lytic bone metastases (50 per cent), and (3) those with solid tumors without bone metastases (20 per cent).[52]

Patients in Group 1 usually have multiple myeloma, lymphosarcoma, or lymphoma. The bone lesions are lytic and histologically demonstrate increased osteoclast bone resorption adjacent to tumor cells. The cause of the hypercalcemia in these patients appears to be osteoclast-activating factor (OAF), a bone-resorbing lymphokine secreted by normal activated T and B lymphocytes and also by neoplastic lymphoid cells. Prostaglandin synthesis by monocytes appears to be important in regulating OAF production.

Patients in Group 2 most commonly have carcinoma of the breast, lung, kidney, or pancreas. In this setting, malignant cells shed from the tumor enter the bloodstream and lodge in distant organs, including bone. The exact mechanism of bone resorption is unclear but appears to involve primarily the tumor cell, but also OAF and prostaglandin secreted from lymphocytes and

TABLE 5. Diseases Causing Hypercalcemia

Hyperparathyroidism
Malignancy
   With skeletal metastases
   Without skeletal metastases
Hyperthyroidism
Multiple myeloma
Sarcoidosis and other granulomatous diseases
Milk-alkali syndrome
Vitamin D intoxication
Vitamin A intoxication
Paget's disease
Immobilization
Thiazide diuretics
Addisonian crisis
Familial hypocalciuric hypercalcemia
Idiopathic hypercalcemia of infancy

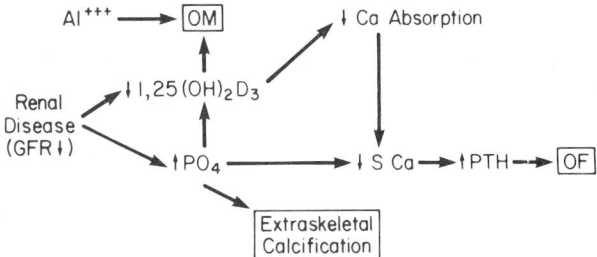

Figure 11. Scheme showing the proposed pathogenesis of secondary hyperparathyroidism and osteomalacia in renal failure. GFR, glomerular filtration rate; OM, osteomalacia; OF, osteitis fibrosa; SCa, serum calcium. (From Coburn, J. W.: Renal osteodystrophy. In Clinical Disorders of Bone and Mineral Metabolism. Amsterdam, Excerpta Medica, 1983, p. 250.)

monocytes drawn to the area as an immune response to the tumor cell.

Patients in Group 3 have perhaps proved the most interesting. The hypothesis that these tumors inappropriately secrete PTH is unlikely,[73] and it now appears that many are associated with a PTH-like peptide.[37] This peptide is found in normal tissue, but it appears to be expressed in abnormal amounts in some tumors.

Histologically, the skeleton from these patients shows increased osteoclast bone resorption and decreased bone formation. Although prostaglandins are known to be involved in bone resorption, as previously mentioned, they alone do not appear to be of major importance here, because no prostaglandin has sufficient potency to induce hypercalcemia.

Localization

Approximately 95 per cent of patients with primary hyperparathyroidism are cured at initial neck exploration performed by an experienced surgeon. This must be borne in mind in evaluating the need for methods to localize the site of hyperfunctioning parathyroid tissue. No study has yet demonstrated that preoperative localization reduces either the duration of the operation or the incidence of complications, and most surgeons believe these techniques should be reserved for the patient undergoing re-exploration after a failed initial procedure. In this situation, glands are frequently found in ectopic locations, and the normal tissue planes may be obscured. Generally, invasive techniques, such as arteriography and venography, have no place in localization prior to the initial operation for hyperparathyroidism. Older noninvasive techniques, such as barium cine-esophagography and parathyroid scanning with selenomethionine, are infrequently positive and of little use. Newer noninvasive methods with greater utility include high-resolution, real-time ultrasonography; CT; magnetic resonance imaging (MRI); and thallium-technetium subtraction scanning.

High-resolution, real-time ultrasonography differs from conventional ultrasound scanning in that the emitted sound waves are of higher frequency (10 MHz), permitting resolution of structures less than 1 mm. in size but limiting the depth of visualization to 4 or 5 cm. from the skin. In an evaluation of 100 consecutive patients undergoing neck exploration at the Mayo Clinic,[75] the radiologic accuracy was 76 per cent; however, the success rate of identifying the parathyroid lesion at operation was the same with (96 per cent) or without (97 per cent) the utilization of ultrasound. Similar results have been reported by others. The usefulness of this technique in patients with hypercalcemic crisis has previously been mentioned. Sonographically guided fine-needle aspiration with cytology and immunostaining for parathyroid hormone may be helpful in confirming the localization if necessary.[32]

In most recent studies, CT scanning appears to be equally as effective as ultrasound.[22] It is more expensive but is less operator-dependent than sonography. CT appears to be superior for identifying ectopically located glands, particularly those in the mediastinum. MRI appears to be equally sensitive.

Thallium-technetium subtraction scanning is a recently developed technique that depends on the uptake of thallium 201 by both the thyroid and parathyroid, whereas technetium 99m is taken up only by the thyroid.[55] The images are subtracted, leaving only the parathyroid image. This is a theoretically appealing technique that appears to have a sensitivity comparable to ultrasound and CT.

A recent study by Roses and associates[64] suggests that when these techniques are employed in centers without a particular interest in their development, the utility may be considerably less. In examining 36 patients with primary disease, the sensitivity of ultrasound was only 34 per cent, whereas CT and thallium-technetium scanning identified 41 and 49 per cent of abnormal glands, respectively. The precise role for noninvasive localization techniques remains to be determined.

Treatment

With the use of automated technology for determining the serum concentration of calcium, the diagnosis of hyperparathyroidism is made increasingly more often in asymptomatic patients. Whether all patients with hyperparathyroidism should undergo operation has been questioned, and some physicians have proposed that asymptomatic patients be followed intermittently without operative intervention. This at first may seem to be a reasonable proposal, because there appears to be little evidence that patients with mild hypercalcemia develop renal damage or are otherwise physically impaired by their abnormality. The major questions to be answered in this group of patients are: will they (and especially postmenopausal females) become progressively osteopenic with time? will they develop hyperparathyroid crisis? and will they be lost to follow-up?

Scholz and Purnell[70] in 1981 reported the results of a 10-year study in which 142 patients with a biochemical diagnosis of mild hyperparathyroidism were followed. Operative intervention was advised if patients developed a mean serum calcium concentration greater than 11 mg. per 100 ml., roentgenographic evidence of bone disease, decreased renal function, metabolically active or infected renal stones, or gastrointestinal complications. Neck exploration was also advised if prolonged observation became impractical. After 10 years, 33 patients (23 per cent) had undergone operation, 32 (23 per cent) had died of causes apparently unrelated to hyperparathyroidism, 19 (13 per cent) had been lost to follow-up or had declined follow-up, and 42 (29 per cent) had persistent or indeterminate disease. Sixteen patients (12 per cent) entered the study with persistent postoperative hypercalcemia, and follow-up data were available in 9, none of whom had undergone repeat operation.

Scholz and Purnell[70] found that they were unable to define criteria that would predict which patients with asymptomatic hyperparathyroidism would ultimately require surgical correction. Their final recommendation was that in patients whose laboratory studies supported the diagnosis of hyperparathyroidism surgical exploration by an experienced surgeon was indicated. The complication rate is less than 3 per cent in most series, and the cost of medical follow-up has been shown to exceed the cost of diagnosis and surgical therapy within 4 to 6 years.[34] Despite this, a number of authors have continued to advocate nonoperative management.[43,66] This approach has been stimulated by recent evidence that estrogen may be useful in postmenopausal women with mild hyperparathyroidism. Selby and Peacock[71] treated 17 patients with estrogen and found evidence of reduction in bone turnover and plasma calcium.

Resolution of this question requires a randomized, controlled trial, and until that time the only curative treatment for primary hyperparathyroidism is surgical therapy. Medical management is reserved for patients who are either extremely debilitated or have another life-threatening illness. Before subjecting a patient to operation, the surgeon should be confident of the diagnosis and have adequate experience to systematically explore the neck, recognizing in the process the normal and abnormal parathyroid glands. The patient should be made fully aware of the complications associated with the neck exploration, including potential damage to the superior and recurrent laryngeal nerves and the development of hypocalcemia with associated symptoms of tetany. In the asymptomatic patient, the alternative of nonoperative or medical management should be presented. The possibility of an unsuccessful parathyroid search should be mentioned, and the patient should be made aware that repeat operation, including a mediastinal exploration, may be required if the planned operation is unsuccessful. Although the likelihood of these complications is small, it is best to discuss them prior to the initial neck exploration.

A second exploration of the neck because of failure to locate the lesion at the initial procedure is very difficult and should be

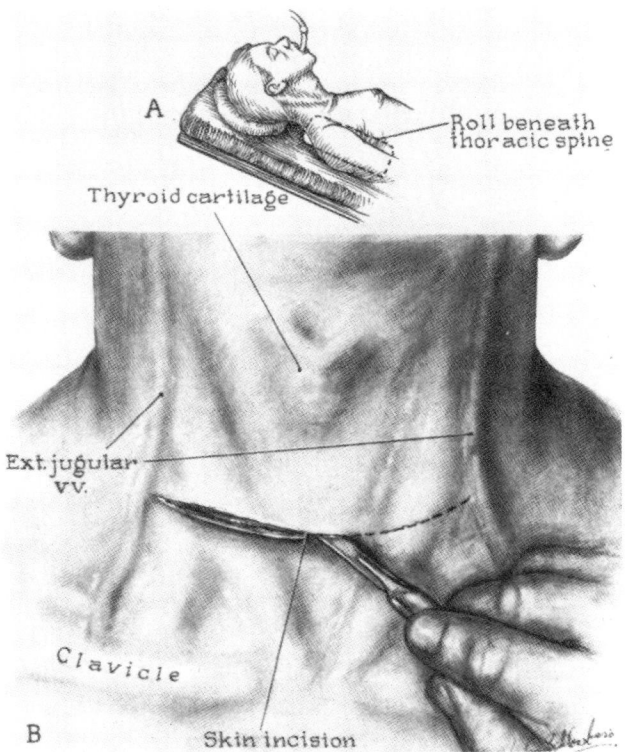

Figure 12. The cervical incision is usually made two fingerbreadths above the sternal notch. (From Wells, S. A., Jr., Leight, G. S., and Ross, A. J.: Primary hyperparathyroidism. Curr. Probl. Surg., *17*:400, 1980.)

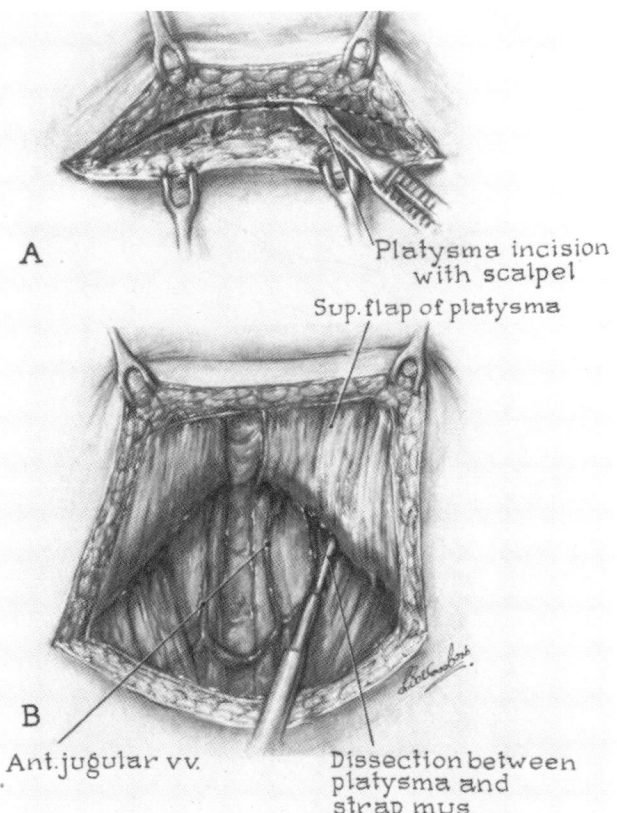

Figure 13. After incision of the platysma (A), superior and inferior flaps are developed (B). (From Wells, S. A., Jr., Leight, G. S., and Ross, A. J.: Primary hyperparathyroidism. Curr. Probl. Surg. *17*:400, 1980.)

avoided by an assiduous primary operation. If reoperation is required, not only is parathyroid tissue more difficult to identify, but damage to the recurrent laryngeal nerve is more likely.

General anesthesia is used, and the neck is opened through a transverse cervical incision (Figs. 12 and 13). After the strap muscles are separated in the midline (Fig. 14), a chosen lobe of the thyroid gland is elevated and rotated medially. The tissues inferior to the thyroid lobe are cleaned down to the trachea to expose the recurrent laryngeal nerve and the inferior thyroid artery. In most patients, the nerve lies in the tracheoesophageal groove; less commonly, lateral to the trachea; and rarely, anterolateral to the trachea, where it is especially vulnerable to injury. A laryngeal nerve may be given off directly in the neck without the usual looping around the right subclavian artery. The external branch of the superior laryngeal nerve is the most important tensor of the vocal cords, and it usually lies immediately adjacent and medial to the vascular pedicle of the superior thyroid lobe. With mobilization of the lobe, care must be taken not to injure this nerve. Four or more parathyroid glands may be present and abnormal, and the reconnaissance of the neck area requires great patience. The help of an experienced pathologist is required, because frozen-section identification of the parathyroid glands is helpful. The upper parathyroid glands are more easily found and are usually located far dorsally on the surface of the thyroid lobe at the level of the upper two thirds of the gland. The lower glands (Fig. 15A) are larger than the upper and less constant in location, being normally distributed from well above the upper half of the thyroid to well within the mediastinum. The lower glands are usually more anterior than the upper glands. If the upper glands are identified (Fig. 16) and normal but either of the lower glands cannot be found, the thymus pedicle on the side of the unfound gland should be carefully examined (Fig. 15B) and removed. Most parathyroid adenomas located in the mediastinum can be removed through the cervical incision.

Weller[78] termed the inferior parathyroid gland the "parathymus" to indicate the frequent association of the two structures. In approximately half of normal subjects, the inferior parathy-

roid gland is adherent to or embedded in the cord of the thymus that extends out of the mediastinum and thoracic inlet to the inferior pole of the thyroid gland, the "thyrothymic ligament." Edis and associates[23] emphasized the clinical importance of the variable descent of the inferior parathyroid gland in 7 patients with hyperparathyroidism, 6 of whom required a repeat neck operation for identification of the lesion (Fig. 17A and B).

If no parathyroid tissue is found after the thymus pedicle is removed, the surgeon should mobilize, examine, and palpate both lobes of the thyroid gland, because occasionally a parathyroid is completely encapsulated within the thyroid paren-

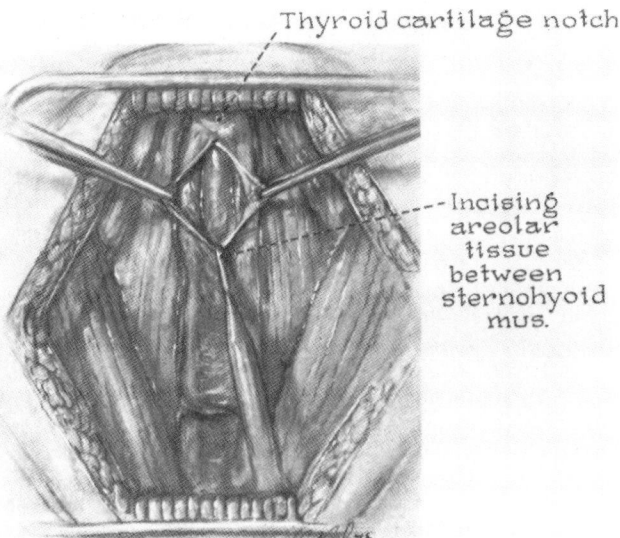

Figure 14. Separation of the pretracheal fascia and strap muscles in the midline. (From Wells, S. A., Jr., Leight, G. S., and Ross, A. J.: Primary hyperparathyroidism. Curr. Probl. Surg., *17*:400, 1980.)

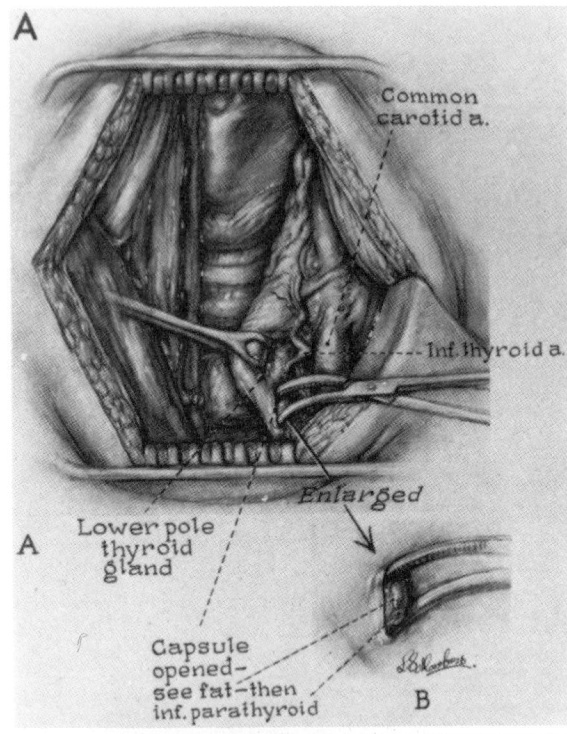

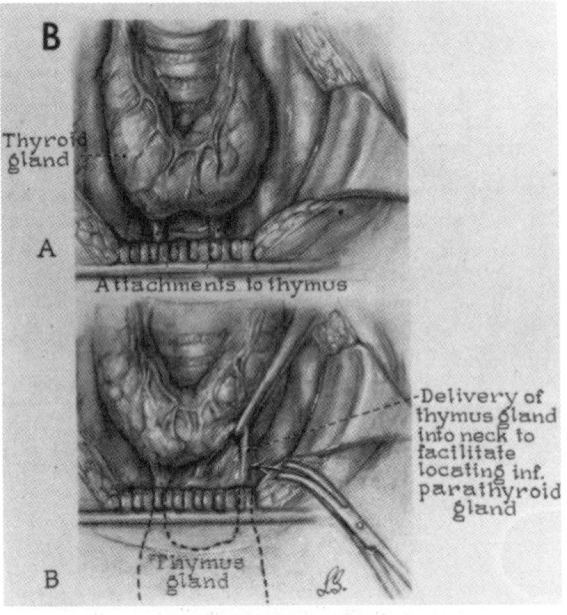

Figure 15. *A*, Identification of left lower parathyroid gland. *B*, Elevation of the thymus gland into the cervical incision. (From Wells, S. A., Jr., Leight, G. S., and Ross, A. J.: Primary hyperparathyroidism. Curr. Probl. Surg., *17*:400, 1980.)

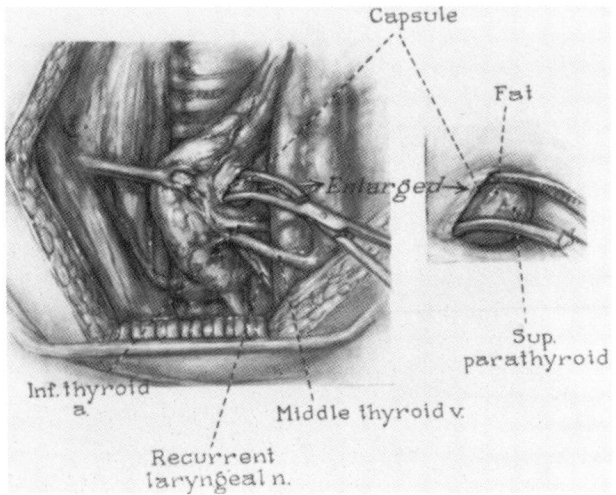

Figure 16. Identification of left superior parathyroid gland. (From Wells, S. A., Jr., Leight, G. S., and Ross, A. J.: Primary hyperparathyroidism. Curr. Probl. Surg., *17*:400, 1980.)

chyma. Removal of a thyroid lobe on the side where a parathyroid gland is not found is occasionally indicated as a last resort but should by no means substitute for a meticulous search for parathyroid tissue. It is also helpful to follow the branches of the inferior thyroid artery, especially if one is enlarged, because these often lead to an abnormal parathyroid gland or adenoma. Because of the possibility of multiple-gland involvement, every effort must be made to identify all four parathyroids. To ensure that one has actually identified parathyroid tissue, small biopsies of the suspected glands should be taken. The organs must be handled with extreme care, however, because they are delicate structures and their blood supply is easily damaged.

The operative management depends upon the number of enlarged parathyroid glands. The incidence of single and multi-

ple-gland enlargement in 100 consecutive patients with hyperparathyroidism is depicted in Table 6. If one gland is large and the remaining three are of normal size, resection of the enlarged gland is curative in nearly all patients. In the event that two or three parathyroid glands are enlarged, most surgeons resect them, leaving the normal-sized glands undisturbed except for a biopsy. The question of whether these represent multiple adenomas or primary hyperplasia has not been resolved. Of 76 patients treated in such a manner and followed for 12 to 140 months postoperatively, 8 (10.5 per cent) had recurrent hypercalcemia.[80] This recurrent disease tended to be mild, and it was concluded that the described management is generally acceptable. In patients with generalized (glandular) enlargement or parathyroid hyperplasia, the surgical management is much more difficult and the postoperative results less satisfactory.

PARATHYROID HYPERPLASIA (GENERALIZED [FOUR-GLAND] PARATHYROID ENLARGEMENT). This phenomenon occurs in two forms: water-clear cell hyperplasia and chief cell hyperplasia. Albright and associates[3] described water-clear cell hyperplasia in 1934. Clinically it is indistinguishable from the hyperparathyroidism associated with single-gland disease, but the gross appearance at operation is characteristic. All four glands are diffusely enlarged and dark brown with uneven surfaces and numerous pseudopods. The cut surface appears cystic. Microscopically the glands are composed almost entirely of water-clear cells.

Primary chief cell hyperplasia was first described by Cope and colleagues[19] in 1958. There may be a great difference in the size of the glands, the superior frequently being larger than the inferior. The glands are often nodular and red-brown and grossly are characterized by the presence of fibrous septa within the parenchyma. Histologically, chief cells predominate, but there are also nests of water-clear and oxyphil cells. In Cope's original series, several patients had associated endocrine disturbances, including insulin-producing and non–insulin-producing pancreatic islet cell adenomas, pituitary tumors, adrenal hyperplasia, and thyroid adenomas. It is now known that chief cell hyperplasia is the pathologic entity most commonly associated with familial hyperparathyroidism, particularly MEN Types I and IIa.

The standard therapy for patients with hyperparathyroidism and generalized parathyroid enlargement has been radical subtotal (three and one-half–gland) parathyroidectomy. Castleman and Cope[14] reported a 55 per cent incidence of recurrent hyperparathyroidism in patients undergoing this procedure for water-clear cell hyperplasia. Castleman and associates[15] re-

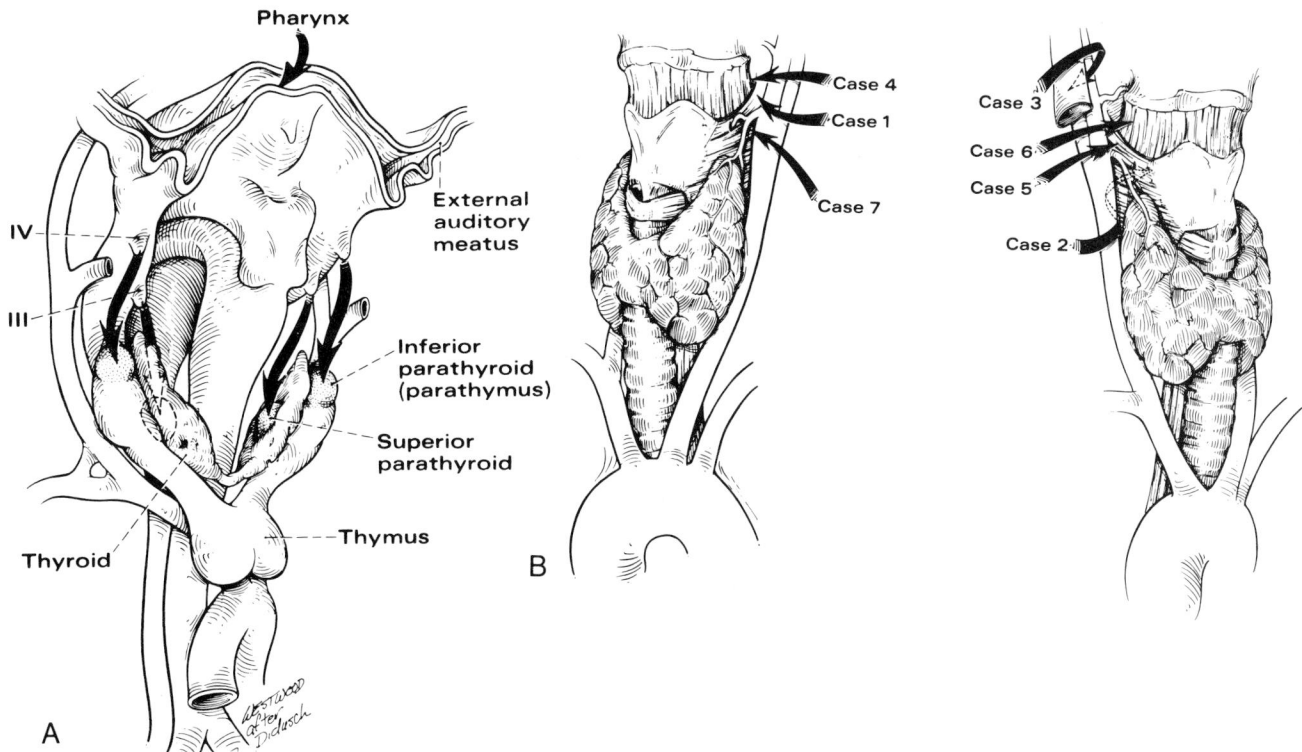

Figure 17. *A*, Inferior parathyroid glands and thymus have a common embryologic origin from the third branchial pouch and are closely related during caudal descent—hence the term *parathymus*. Arrested descent leads to undescended parathymus. Superior parathyroid glands arise from the fourth pouch and are thereafter more closely associated with thyroid. *B*, Locations of adenomas of undescended parathymus glands in 7 patients. (From Edis, A. J., Purnell, D. C., and van Heerden, J. A.: The undescended "parathymus." Ann. Surg., *190:*64, 1979.)

ported an 11 per cent incidence of recurrent hyperparathyroidism and a 15 per cent incidence of permanent hypoparathyroidism in patients with chief cell parathyroid hyperplasia who were treated by subtotal resection. Edis and associates[24] evaluated 55 patients with chief cell hyperplasia treated by three and one-half–gland parathyroidectomy. Persistent hypercalcemia was documented in 13 per cent and permanent hypoparathyroidism in 5 per cent. Transient hypoparathyroidism of up to 2 years' duration (average of 10 months) was noted in 27 per cent of the 55 patients.

Van Heerden and associates[76] reported surgical results in 45 patients with MEN Types I and IIa who had biochemically documented hyperparathyroidism. Sixty-nine per cent of the patients had hyperplasia and underwent subtotal parathyroidectomy. Ninety-three per cent were cured; however, 25 per cent developed permanent postoperative hypoparathyroidism.

Because of the relatively increased incidence of postoperative hypoparathyroidism and hyperparathyroidism in patients with

TABLE 6. Gland Enlargement in 100 Patients with Primary Hyperparathyroidism

Number of Glands Enlarged	Number of Patients
1	65
2	15
3	10
4	10

From Wells, S. A., Leight, G. S., and Ross, A. J.: Primary hyperparathyroidism. *In* Ravitch, M. M., et al. (Eds.): Current Problems in Surgery. Chicago, Year Book Medical Publishers, 1980.

"parathyroid hyperplasia," the authors have elected to manage them by total parathyroidectomy and heterotopic autotransplantation.

If after diligent search in the neck, including exploration of the upper mediastinum, retroesophageal area, carotid sheaths, and thyroid gland, no enlarged parathyroid gland has been found, a decision must be made regarding mediastinotomy. Most surgeons favor delay of this procedure, reasoning that the blood supply to the hyperfunctional gland may have been damaged during manipulation or that the pathologist may find the abnormal gland on further sectioning of the submitted tissues. Others have favored mediastinotomy at the time of the negative cervical exploration. Mediastinotomy is indicated in only about 1 to 2 per cent of patients. If this procedure is elected, it should probably be done 2 to 4 weeks after the neck operation, if serum calcium values remain elevated. In Hellstrom and Ivemark's series of parathyroid adenomas,[35] 15 patients required subsequent mediastinal exploration following negative exploration of the neck. Six of the 15 patients were found to have a parathyroid adenoma still confined to the neck. This emphasizes the importance of locating the offending parathyroid tissue at the initial exploration.

In mediastinal exploration, a vertical incision is made from the center of the cervical incision to the xiphoid. The sternum is completely divided in the midline and a retractor is inserted. The remaining thymus tissue is first isolated and examined, because an adenoma may be associated with this structure located in front of the great vessels. In parathyroid adenomas that are true mediastinal organs, the blood supply is often from the mediastinal vessels and not the inferior thyroid artery. If the anterior mediastinal exploration is negative, the posterior mediastinum is next examined, especially posterior and lateral to the trachea (Fig. 18).

Norton and associates[54] recently reported their experience with 33 patients who underwent mediastinotomy for primary

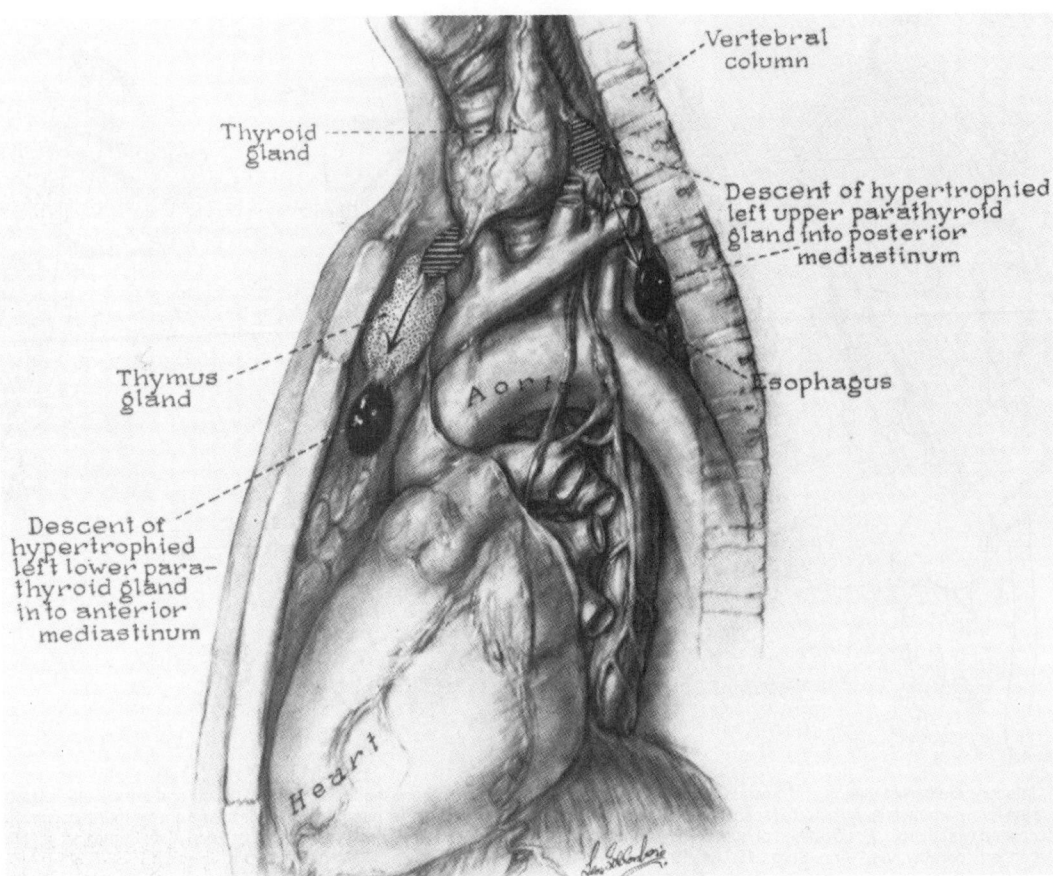

Figure 18. Ectopically located inferior parathyroid glands are most often located anteriorly in association with the thymus gland. Ectopically displaced superior parathyroid glands are usually located posteriorly in the tracheoesophageal groove or the posterior mediastinum. (From Wells, S. A., Jr., Leight, G. S., and Ross, A. J.: Primary hyperparathyroidism. Curr. Probl. Surg., 17:400, 1980.)

hyperparathyroidism. Nineteen of the abnormal glands were located within the thymus, 5 were posterior to the thymus along the aortic arch, and 4 were in the thyroid. One was in an undescended parathymus, and one was in the tracheoesophageal groove. Twenty-eight patients (85 per cent) were cured of their hypercalcemia, but 12 per cent suffered complications. Only one patient is presently hypoparathyroid.

It should be mentioned that although the pathologist can readily distinguish parathyroid tissue from other tissue by frozen section, it is often difficult to discriminate between parathyroid "adenomas" and "hyperplasia." In a recent study,[68] three pathologists were asked to review 50 slides of parathyroid tissue, and their diagnoses were compared with those made by the surgeon at the time of operation. A specific diagnosis of adenoma was correct in only 83 per cent of interpretations and of hyperplasia in only 60 per cent. The most reliable index of abnormality is the surgeon's determination of gland size by visual observation.

SURGERY FOR PERSISTENT OR RECURRENT HYPERPARATHYROIDISM. In the patients who remain hypercalcemic after neck exploration, approximately 60 per cent have a missed adenoma. Inadequately excised hyperplastic tissue is another common cause of recurrent disease. Rattner and associates[61] recently reported four patients with late recurrence as a result of tissue that had inadvertently spilled from a broken gland and implanted at the time of the initial operation. In most cases, review of the original operative notes and pathologic report provides clues as to the position of undetected glands. The location of parathyroids missed at the initial operation but found on subsequent exploration in one large series is shown in Figure 19.

In contrast with initial operations, most surgeons agree that

localization studies should be performed prior to re-exploration. A combination of the noninvasive studies described above should be utilized. If these are unsuccessful, selective angiography and venous sampling for parathyroid hormone have been utilized.

Miller and associates[50] recently reported that superselective digital subtraction angiography may be the most accurate technique, correctly localizing parathyroids in 62 per cent of 26 patients with negative noninvasive studies. This technique offers the additional potential for angiographic ablation of adenomas with ionic contrast. In one recent study,[51] ablation was successful in 85 per cent of patients in whom the catheter could be wedged into the feeding artery. A wider experience with this technique is required before its role can be clearly defined.

Venous sampling for PTH has been helpful in re-evaluating patients. However, interpretation can be complicated by the collateralization that occurs after venous ligation during the initial operative procedure. In Brennan's study[13] of 130 patients studied by venous sampling, 75 per cent had a parathyroid lesion localized. At subsequent operation, the site of their enlarged gland correlated with the localization data in only 46 per cent. He concluded that this relative nonspecificity makes venography of limited value.

Arteriography and venous sampling require a technical expertise that is not widely available. Significant complications of selective arteriography including transient cortical blindness, transverse myelitis, and cerebrovascular accidents and death have been reported by some investigators. This emphasizes the importance of having an experienced and skilled vascular radiologist to perform these invasive procedures.

Grant and associates[31] reported their 6-year experience with 157 patients undergoing re-exploration for persistent or recur-

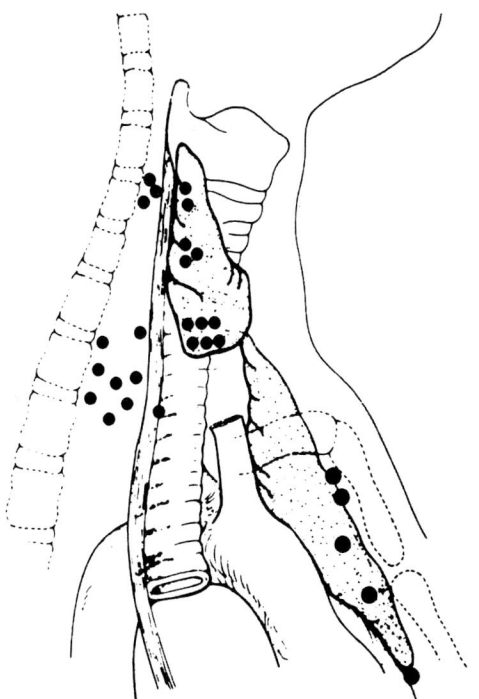

Figure 19. Location of parathyroids missed at initial operation but found on subsequent successful surgical re-exploration. (From Brennan, M. F., Doppman, J. L., Marx, S. J., Spiegel, A. M., Brown, E. M., Krudy, A., Costa, J., Saxe, A., and Aurbach, G.,: Reoperative parathyroid surgery for persistent hyperparathyroidism. Surgery, 83:669, 1978.)

rent hyperparathyroidism following 197 previous operations. These included 100 cervical explorations, 38 combined cervical and mediastinal explorations, and 9 mediastinal explorations. No invasive localizing studies were employed. Successful resolution of the hypercalcemia occurred in 89 per cent of patients. Permanent unilateral recurrent laryngeal nerve injury occurred in 4 per cent. Thirteen per cent of patients became permanently hypoparathyroid.

Two adjunctive techniques have recently been reported to be of use at the time of re-exploration. Kern[40] found that 76 per cent of abnormal glands could be visualized by intraoperative ultrasound, leading to a significant reduction in operative time. Darling and associates[20] measured urinary cyclic AMP intraoperatively to determine the adequacy and completeness of resection. Cyclic AMP levels fell in 21 of 25 patients in whom normocalcemia followed resection of an enlarged parathyroid.

MANAGEMENT OF SECONDARY HYPERPARATHYROIDISM. There are four indications for parathyroidectomy in patients with secondary hyperparathyroidism: (1) persistent and symptomatic hypercalcemia in prospective renal transplant patients; (2) bone pain or pathologic fractures; (3) ectopic calcification, and (4) intractable itching. These patients can be managed by subtotal (three and one-half–gland) parathyroidectomy or total parathyroidectomy with heterotopic (forearm) autotransplantation. Andress and associates[5] have recently demonstrated that parathyroidectomy can actually enhance aluminum deposition in the bone so that all aluminum excess should be corrected by chelation before operation.

PARATHYROID TRANSPLANTATION. There are certain clinical situations in patients with hyperparathyroidism in which it would be preferable to reduce the total parathyroid mass and still have a portion of parathyroid tissue to maintain the patient in normal calcium homeostasis. As previously mentioned, parathyroid hyperplasia, either primary or secondary, has been a malady most frequently treated by subtotal parathyroidectomy. If patients develop hypercalcemia after operation, a second neck exploration with all its attendant risks is usually

required. It was previously demonstrated in animals that parathyroid glands could be transplanted as autografts or as allografts if the host were immunosuppressed. The success of the transplantation depended upon the freshly removed parathyroid tissue being sliced into very small pieces for subsequent implantation into a muscle bed. This technique has been applied in patients with both primary and secondary parathyroid hyperplasia.[79] A total parathyroidectomy is performed, and approximately 20 to 25 parathyroid pieces are autografted to the forearm musculature. If the patient subsequently develops hypercalcemia from the grafted parathyroid tissue, a few of the pieces can be removed under local anesthesia. The fact that the transplanted parathyroid tissue functions is documented by the patient's maintaining normocalcemia with the grafted tissue as the only source of parathyroid hormone. Moreover, large concentrations of parathyroid hormone are detectable in the antecubital vein draining the graft bed, compared with normal parathyroid hormone levels in the contralateral antecubital vein.

It has also been demonstrated that parathyroid glands can be viably frozen in dimethyl sulfoxide and autologous serum for as long as 12 to 18 months. This capability offers the surgeon great versatility, because when there is uncertainty about the amount of parathyroid tissue in the neck following resection of hyperparathyroid tissue in a patient undergoing reoperation, a portion can be frozen viably to await the postoperative course. If the patient becomes hypocalcemic, parts of the frozen autologous parathyroid tissue can be reimplanted under local anesthesia.

HYPOPARATHYROIDISM

The most common cause of hypoparathyroidism is damage to the parathyroid glands during thyroid surgery, and it occurs more commonly with total thyroidectomy. It is not unusual for patients undergoing operative procedures on the thyroid gland to experience a drop in serum calcium following operation. This probably represents bruising or compromise of the blood supply of the parathyroids, and the hypocalcemia is transient. In patients with significant hyperparathyroidism and bone disease, there may be significant skeletal calcium deposition, so-called bone hunger. Serum calcium reaches its lowest level in about 48 to 72 hours and returns to normal 2 to 3 days thereafter. The sooner after operation the drop in serum calcium occurs and the longer it persists, the greater the likelihood that all parathyroid glands have been damaged and the poorer the prognosis for recovery. The major signs and symptoms of hypocalcemia are directly attributable to the reduction of plasma ionized calcium, which leads to increased neuromuscular excitability. Clinically, the earliest manifestations are numbness and tingling in the circumoral area, the fingers, and the toes. Mental symptoms are common, and patients are anxious, depressed, or occasionally confused. Tetany may develop, characterized by carpopedal spasms, tonic clonic convulsions, and laryngeal stridor, which may prove fatal. On physical examination, contraction of the facial muscles is elicited by tapping on the facial nerve anterior to the ear (Chvostek's sign). This sign is present in a small number of normal individuals. Trousseau's sign is elicited by occluding blood flow to the forearm for 3 minutes. The development of carpal spasm indicates hypocalcemia.

A far less common cause of hypoparathyroidism is idiopathic lack of function. There have been approximately 150 cases reported, most of which occurred in childhood and some of which appeared to be familial. Hypoparathyroidism in newborns frequently follows prenatal suppression of fetal parathyroid glands by the hyperparathyroid mother. In DiGeorge's syndrome, there is congenital absence of the parathyroid glands and the thymus. In addition to hypocalcemia, these children suffer from absence of the thymus-dependent lymphoid system.

The treatment of acute hypocalcemia is intravenous administration of calcium gluconate or calcium chloride. Vitamin D and oral calcium are used for long-term management.

SELECTED REFERENCES

Alveryd, A.: Parathyroid glands in thyroid surgery. Acta Chir. Scand. (Suppl.), 389:1, 1968.
This is a thorough monograph discussing the anatomically important relationships of the normal and abnormal parathyroid glands.

Frame, B., and Potts, J. T., Jr. (Eds.): Clinical Disorders of Bone and Mineral Metabolism. Amsterdam, Excerpta Medica, 1983.
This publication, from an international symposium, reviews bone and mineral disorders associated with parathyroid diseases. The sections on clinical application of parathyroid hormone immunoassays, primary hyperparathyroidism, renal osteodystrophy, and non-parathyroid hypercalcemia have particular clinical relevance.

Saxe, A.: Parathyroid Transplantation: A Review. Surgery, 95:507, 1984.
A concise review of the history and current status of parathyroid auto- and allotransplantation.

Wang, C.: Surgical Management of Primary Hyperparathyroidism. In Ravitch, M. M., et al. (Eds.): Curr. Probl. Surg., 22(11):1, 1985.
This monograph is a succinct review of the author's extensive experience with the management of primary hyperparathyroidism at the Massachusetts General Hospital. It presents the rationale and results of this controversial surgical approach utilizing unilateral neck exploration.

Wells, S. A., Jr., Leight, G. S., and Ross, A. J.: Primary hyperparathyroidism. Curr. Probl. Surg., 17(8):400, 1980.
This monograph reviews the pathophysiology and clinical manifestations of primary hyperparathyroidism. Methods of diagnosis and operative management are also discussed.

REFERENCES

1. Akerström, G., Malmaers, J., and Bergstrom, R.: Surgical anatomy of human parathyroid glands. Surgery, 95:14, 1984.
2. Albright, F., Baird, P. C., Cope, O., and Bloomberg, E.: Studies in the physiology of the parathyroid glands. IV. Renal complications of hyperparathyroidism. Am. J. Med. Sci., 197:49, 1934.
3. Albright, F., Bloomberg, E., Castleman, B., and Churchill, E. D.: Hyperparathyroidism due to diffuse hyperplasia of all parathyroid glands rather than adenoma of one. Clinical studies on three such cases. Arch. Intern. Med., 54:315, 1934.
4. Alveryd, A.: Parathyroid glands in thyroid surgery. Acta Chir. Scand. (Suppl.), 389:1, 1968.
5. Andress, D. L., Oh, S. M., Maloney, N. A., and Sherard, D. J.: Effect of parathyroidectomy on bone aluminum deposition in chronic renal failure. N. Engl. J. Med., 312:468, 1985.
6. Askanazy, M.: Über ostitis deformans ohne osteoides gewebe. Arb. Geb. Path. Anath. Inst. zu Tubingen (Leipzig), 4:398, 1903.
7. Aurbach, G. D.: Isolation of parathyroid hormone after extraction with phenol. J. Biol. Chem., 234:3179, 1959.
8. Barr, D. P., and Bulger, H. A.: The clinical syndrome of hyperparathyroidism. Am. J. Med. Sci., 179:449, 1930.
9. Berson, S. A., Yalow, R. S., Aurbach, G. D., and Potts, J. T.: Immunoassay of bovine and human parathyroid hormone. Proc. Natl. Acad. Sci., 49:613, 1963.
10. Bess, M. A., Edis, A. J., and van Heerden, J. A.: Hyperparathyroidism and pancreatitis: Chance or a causal association? JAMA, 243:246, 1980.
11. Bolman, R. M., Cooper, C. W., Garner, S. C., Munson, P. L., and Wells, S. A., Jr.: Stimulation of gastrin secretion in the pig by parathyroid hormone and its inhibition by thyrocalcitonin. Endocrinology, 100:1014, 1977.
12. Boyd, J. D.: Development of the thyroid and parathyroid glands and the thymus. Ann. R. Coll. Surg. Engl., 7:455, 1950.
13. Brennan, M. F., and Norton, J. F.: Reoperation for persistent and recurrent hyperparathyroidism. Surgery, 201:40, 1985.
14. Castleman, B., and Cope, O.: Primary parathyroid hyperplasia. Bull. Hosp. Joint Dis., 12:368, 1951.
15. Castleman, B., Schantz, A., and Roth, S. I.: Parathyroid hyperplasia in primary hyperparathyroidism. Cancer, 38:1668, 1976.
16. Christensson, T.: Familial hyperparathyroidism. Ann. Intern. Med., 85:614, 1976.
17. Christensson, T.: Hyperparathyroidism and radiation therapy. Ann. Intern. Med., 89:216, 1978.
18. Collip, J. B.: The extraction of a parathyroid hormone that will prevent or control parathyroid tetany and which regulates the level of blood calcium. J. Biol. Chem., 63:293, 1925.
19. Cope, O., Keynes, W. M., Roth, S. I., and Castleman, B.: Primary chief cell hyperplasia of the parathyroid glands: A new entity in the surgery of hyperparathyroidism. Ann. Surg., 148:375, 1958.
20. Darling, G. E., Marx, S. J., Spiegel, A. M., Aurbach, G. D., and Norton, J. A.: Prospective analysis of intraoperative and postoperative urinary cyclic adenosine 3',5'-monophosphate levels to predict outcome of patients undergoing reoperation for primary hyperparathyroidism. Surgery 104:1128, 1988.
21. Diamond, T. W., Both, J. R., Wing, J., Meyers, A. W., and Kalk, W. J.: Parathyroid hypertension: A reversible disorder. Arch. Intern. Med. 146:1709, 1986.
22. Duh, Q. Y., Sancho, J. J., and Clark, O. H.: Parathyroid localization. Acta. Chir. Scand., 153:241, 1987.
23. Edis, A. J., Purnell, D. C., and van Heerden, J. A.: The undescended "parathymus." Ann. Surg., 190:64, 1979.
24. Edis, A. J., van Heerden, J. A., and Scholz, D. A.: Results of subtotal parathyroidectomy for primary chief cell hyperplasia. Surgery, 86:462, 1979.
25. Erdheim, J.: Über epithelkörperchenbefunde bei osteomalacie. S. B. Akad. Wiss. Math. Naturw. Cl., 116:311, 1907.
26. Farndon, J. R., Geraghty, J. M., Dilley, W. G., Handwerger, S., and Leight, G. S.: Serum gastrin, calcitonin, and prolactin as markers of multiple endocrine neoplasia syndromes in patients with primary hyperparathyroidism. World J. Surg. 11:252, 1987.
27. Fitzpatrick, L. A., and Bilezikian, J. P.: Acute primary hyperparathyroidism. Am. J. Med. 82:275, 1987.
28. Foley, T. P., Jr., Harrison, H. C., Arnaud, C. D., and Harrison, H. E.: Familial benign hypercalcemia. J. Pediatr., 81:1060, 1972.
29. Friedman, E., Sakaguchi, K., Bale, A. E., Falchetti, A., Strecter, E., Zimering, M. B., Weinstein, L. S., McBride, W. O., Nakamura, Y., Brandi, M., Norton, J. A., Aurbach, G. D., Spiegel, A. M., and Marx, S. J.: Clonality of parathyroid tumors in familial multiple endocrine neoplasia type I. N. Engl. J. Med., 321:213, 1989.
30. Gley, E.: Sur les fonctions du corps thyroide. C. R. Soc. Biol., 43:841, 1891.
31. Grant, C. S., van Heerden, J. A., Charboneau, J. W., James, E. M., and Reading, C. C.: Clinical management of persistent and/or recurrent primary hyperparathyroidism. World. J. Surg., 10:555, 1986.
32. Gulekunst, R., Valesky, A., Borisch, B., Haufmann, W., Kiffner, E., Thies, E., Löhrs, U., and Scriba, P. C.: Parathyroid localization. J. Clin. Endocrinol. Metab., 63:1390, 1986.
33. Harris, S. S., and D'Ercole, A. J.: Neonatal hyperparathyroidism. The natural course in the absence of surgical intervention. Pediatrics, 83:53, 1989.
34. Heath, H., Hodgson, S. F., and Kennedy, M. A.: Primary hyperparathyroidism. N. Engl. J. Med., 302:189, 1980.
35. Hellstrom, J., and Ivemark, B. I.: Primary hyperparathyroidism. Acta Chir. Scand. (Suppl.), 194:1, 1962.
36. Holmes, E. C., Morton, D. L., and Ketcham, A. S.: Parathyroid carcinoma: A collective review. Ann. Surg., 169:631, 1969.
37. Ikeda, K., Weir, E. C., Maugin, M., Dannies, P. S., Kinder, B., Deftos, L. J., Braun, E. M., and Broadus, A. E.: Expression of messenger ribonucleic acids encoding a parathyroid hormone-like peptide in normal human and animal tissues with abnormal expression in human parathyroid adenomas. Mol. Endocrinol., 2:1230, 1988.
38. Insogna, K. L., Mitnick, M. E., Stewart, A. F., Bartis, W. J., Mallette, L. E., and Broadus, A. E.: Sensitivity of the parathyroid hormone--1,25-dihydroxy vitamin D axis to variations in calcium intake in patients with primary hyperparathyroidism. N. Engl. J. Med., 313:1126, 1985.
39. Joborn, C., Hetta, J., Johanson, H., Rastad, J., Ågren, H., Åkerstrom, G., and Ljunghall, S.: Psychiatric morbidity in primary hyperparathyroidism. World J. Surg., 12:476, 1988.
40. Kern, K. A., Shawker, T. H., Doppman, J. L., Miller, D. L., Marx, S. J., Spiegel, A. M., Aurbach, G. D., and Norton, J. H.: The use of high-resolution ultrasound to locate parathyroid tumors during reoperation for primary hyperparathyroidism. World J. Surg., 11:579, 1987.
41. Kochersberger, G., Buckley, N. J., Leight, G. S., Martinez, S., Studenski, S., Vogler, J., and Lyles K. W.: What is the clinical significance of bone loss in primary hyperparathyroidism? Arch. Intern. Med. 147:1951, 1987.
42. Kristofferson, A., Dahlgren, S., Lithmer, F., and Järhult, S.: Primary hyperparathyroidism in pregnancy. Surgery, 97:326, 1984.
43. Lafferty, I. W., and Hubay, C.: Primary hyperparathyroidism. Arch. Int. Med., 149:789, 1989.
44. Lloyd, H. M.: Primary hyperparathyroidism: An analysis of the role of the parathyroid tumor. Medicine, 47:53, 1986.
45. McLeod, M. K., Monchik, J. M., and Martin, H. F.: The role of ionized calcium in the diagnosis of subtle hypercalcemia in symptomatic primary hyperparathyroidism. Surgery, 95:667, 1984.
46. MacCallum, W. B., and Voegtlin, C.: On the relation of tetany to the parathyroid glands and to calcium metabolism. J. Exp. Med., 11:118, 1909.
47. Mallette, L. E., Bilezikian, J. P., Heath, D. A., and Aurbach, G. D.: Primary hyperparathyroidism: Clinical and biochemical features. Medicine, 53:127, 1974.
48. Mandl, F.: Therapeutischer Versuch bei einem Falle von Ostitis fibrosa generalisata mittels Exstirpation eines epithelkörperchen Tumors. Zentralbl. Chir., 5:260, 1926a.
49. Masselly, M. J., Lawrence, A. M., Brooks, M., Barhato, A., Braithwaite, S., Osalapas, R., and Paloyan, E.: Hyperparathyroid crisis: Successful treatment of 10 comatose patients. Surgery, 90:741, 1981.
50. Miller, D. L., Chang, R., Doppman, J. L., and Norton, J. A.: Localization of parathyroid adenomas: Superselective arterial DSA versus superselective conventional angiography. Radiology, 170:1003, 1989.
51. Miller, D. L., Doppman, J. L., Chang, R., Summons, J. T., O'Leary, T. J., Norton, J. A., Spiegel, A. M., and Marx, S. J.: Angiographic ablation of parathyroid adenomas.: Lessons from a 10-year experience. Radiology, 165:601, 1987.

52. Mundy, G. R., Ibbotson, K. J., D'Souza, S. M., Simpson, E. J., Jacobs, J. W., and Martin, T. J.: The hypercalcemia of malignancy: Clinical implications and pathogenic mechanisms. N. Engl. J. Med., 310:1718, 1984.
53. Norris, E. H.: The parathyroid glands and the lateral thyroid in man: Their morphogenesis, histogenesis, topographic anatomy, and prenatal growth. Contrib. Embryol., 26:247, 1937.
54. Norton, J. A., Schneider, P. D., and Brennan, M. F.: Median sternotomy in reoperation for primary hyperparathyroidism. World J. Surg., 9:807, 1985.
55. Okerlund, M. D., Sheldon, K., Cerpuz, S., O'Connell, W., Faulkner, D., Clark, O., and Galante, M.: A new method with high sensitivity and specificity for localization of abnormal parathyroid glands. Ann. Surg., 200:381, 1984.
56. Palmer, F. J., Nelson, J. C., and Bacchus, H.: The chloride-phosphate ratio in hypercalcemia. Ann. Intern. Med., 80:200, 1974.
57. Patten, B. M., Bilezikian, J. P., Mallette, L. E., Prince, A., Engel, W. K., and Aurbach, G. D.: Neuromuscular disease and primary hyperparathyroidism. Ann. Intern. Med., 80:182, 1974.
58. Petersen, P.: Psychiatric disorders in primary hyperparathyroidism. J. Clin. Endocrinol. Metab., 28:1491, 1968.
59. Richardson, E. P., Aub, J. C., and Bauer, W.: Parathyroidectomy in osteomalacia. Ann. Surg., 90:730, 1929.
60. Rasmussen, H., and Craig, L. C.: Purification of the parathyroid hormone by use of countercurrent distribution. J. Am. Chem. Soc., 81:5003, 1959.
61. Rattner, D. W., Marrone, G. L., Kasdon, E., and Silen, W.: Recurrent hyperparathyroidism due to implantation of parathyroid tissue. Am. J. Surg., 149:745, 1986.
62. Reeve, T. S., and Delbridge, L. W.: Pancreatitis following parathyroid surgery. Ann. Surg., 195:1581, 1982.
63. Rogers, H. M.: Parathyroid adenoma and hypertrophy of the parathyroid glands. J.A.M.A., 130:22, 1946.
64. Roses, D. F., Sudarsky, L. A., Sanger, J., Ragharendra, B. N., Reede, D. L., and Blum, M.: The use of preoperative localization of adenomas of the parathyroid glands by thallium-technetium subraction scintigraphy, high resolution ultrasonography and computed tomography. Surg. Gyn. Obst., 168:99, 1989.
65. Rosin, R. D.: Pancreatitis and hyperparathyroidism. Postgrad. Med. J., 52:95, 1976.
66. Sampson, M. J., Van 'T Hoff, W., and Bickwell, E. J.: The conservative management of primary hyperparathyroidism. Quart. J. of Med., 65:1009, 1987.
67. Sandström, I.: On a new gland in man and several mammals (glandulae parathyroeoideae). Upsala Läk.-Fören. Förh., 15:441, 1879–80.
68. Saxe, A., Raile, R., Tesluk, H., and Toreson, W.: The role of the pathologist in the surgical treatment of hyperparathyroidism. Surg. Gynecol. Obstet., 161:101, 1985.
69. Schlagenhaufer, F.: Zwei Fälle von Parathyreoideatumoren. Wien. Klin. Wochenschr., 28:1362, 1915.
70. Scholz, D. A., and Purnell, D. C.: Asymptomatic primary hyperparathyroidism: 10-year prospective study. Mayo Clin. Proc., 56:473, 1981.
71. Selby, P. L., and Peacock, M.: Ethinyl estradiol and norethindrone in the treatment of primary hyperparathyroidism in postmenopausal women. N. Engl. J. Med., 314:1481, 1986.
72. Shane, E., and Bilezikian, J. P.: Parathyroid carcinoma: A review of 62 patients. Endocrinol. Rev., 3:218, 1982.
73. Simpson, E. L., Mundy, G. R., D'Souza, S. M., Ibbetson, K. J., Beckman, R., and Jacobs, J. W.: Absence of parathyroid hormone messenger RNA in nonparathyroid tumors associated with hypercalcemia. N. Engl. J. Med., 309:325, 1983.
74. Smith, F. B., and Cooke, R. T.: Acute fatal hyperparathyroidism. Lancet, 2:650, 1940.
75. van Heerden, J. A., James, E. M., Karsell, P. R., Charboneau, J. W., Grant, C. S., and Darnell, D. C.: Small part ultrasonography in primary hyperparathyroidism: Initial experience. Ann. Surg., 195:774, 1982.
76. van Heerden, J. A., Kent, R. B., Sizemore, G. W., Grant, C. S., and Remine, W. H.: Primary hyperparathyroidism in patients with multiple endocrine neoplasia syndromes. Arch. Surg., 118:533, 1983.
77. von Recklinghausen, F. D.: Die Fibröse oder deformierte Ostitis, die Osteomalacie und die Osteoplastische carcinose in ihren gegenseitigen Beziehungen. Festschr. Rud. Virchow, Berlin, 1:89, 1891.
78. Weller, G. L.: Development of the thyroid, parathyroid and thymus glands in man. In Contributions to Embryology, No. 141, Vol. 24, Baltimore, Carnegie Institution of Washington, 1932, pp. 95–139.
79. Wells, S. A., Gunnells, J. C., Shelburne, J. D., Schneider, A. B., and Sherwood, L. M.: Transplantation of the parathyroid glands in man: Clinical indications and results. Surgery, 78:34, 1975.
80. Wells, S. A., Jr., Leight, G. S., Hensley, M., and Dilley, W. G.: Hyperparathyroidism associated with the enlargement of two or three parathyroid glands. Ann. Surg., 202:533, 1985.

25

THE PITUITARY AND ADRENAL GLANDS

Samuel A. Wells, Jr., M.D., and David I. Soybel, M.D.

PITUITARY

HISTORICAL ASPECTS

The word *hypophysis* arises from Greek roots meaning "undergrowth." According to Davey,[52] the word *pituitary* is traced to the Latin *pituita*, which means "phlegm." The anatomic term *pituitary* thus derives from an Aristotelian teaching, later modified by Galen, that structures in the base of the brain distilled vital spirits into animal spirits, which were then distributed via nerves to the body.[4,76] According to this concept, the waste product of this distillation, the *pituita*, was refined by the pituitary gland and passed to the nose and oropharynx for excretion.

In 1538, Vesalius[226] first described the anatomy of the pituitary fossa. Three hundred years later, in 1838, Rathke discovered the dual embryonic origin of this gland from a pouch of entoderm (Rathke's pouch) and from neuroectoderm.[180] Microscopic descriptions of the gland appeared at the turn of the century: Schönemann in 1892 described glandular cells which absorbed basic dyes (basophils), acid dyes (acidophils) or no dye (chromophobes).[198] Enlargement of the pituitary and hypertrophy of its cells were observed after castration by Tandler and Grosz[213] in 1907 and 1908 and during pregnancy by Erdheim and Stumme[66] in 1909.

Insight into pituitary function was gained during the early twentieth century from associations of pituitary tumors with obesity (Mohr, 1840),[155] acromegaly (Marie, 1886),[146] and sexual infantilism (Fröhlich, 1901).[74] Other investigators performed animal experiments that demonstrated that removal of the pituitary gland was not compatible with survival. Paulesco demonstrated that excision of the anterior lobe led to immediate death of the animal, while removal of the posterior lobe did not.[173]

With increasing awareness of the pituitary and its role in physiologic and pathologic processes, clinicians began to develop surgical approaches to the gland. In 1886, Horsely removed the pituitary of a dog and in 1889 that of a human, using a two-stage approach: an initial subtemporal decompression followed by tumor removal a few days later.[101] Harvey Cushing initially observed a pituitary tumor in conjunction with sexual infantilism in 1902 at the Johns Hopkins Hospital.[47] He failed to find a neoplasm during three craniotomies and detected the cystic neoplasm only at autopsy. After perfecting the technique of hypophysectomy experimentally in over 100 dogs, he successfully removed a pituitary tumor causing acromegaly in a 38-year-old South Dakota farmer. Using a transsphenoidal approach in 263 operations reported in 1927,[48,49] surgical mortality was 6.7 per cent and the incidence of early postoperative meningitis was 2.3 per cent. For the larger tumors that contributed to the bulk of his practice, Cushing later preferred a transfrontal approach, and in 91 patients so treated the operative mortality was 4.5 per cent and early postoperative meningitis nil, a remarkable achievement even by the standards of today's antibiotic era.

Treatment of pituitary tumors using external beam irradiation was first reported in the 1920s[52] with favorable results. With the advent of more sensitive imaging techniques and sophisticated staging, it is now possible to select combinations of radiation and surgical therapy for individual patients. The availability of replacement therapies using thyroxine, cortisone, and other hormones and the introduction of antibiotics and of newer microsurgical techniques have led to surgical approaches as primary therapy for many of these neoplasms.

ANATOMY

The major structure for orientation is the sella turcica, a fossa bordered anteriorly, posteriorly, and inferiorly by bone and laterally by the cavernous sinus. The floor of the sella forms the roof of the sphenoid sinus. The anterior (glandular) and posterior (neural) lobes of the pituitary reside in this fossa. The carotid arteries and cranial nerves III, IV, and VI traverse the cavernous sinus just lateral to the sella (Fig. 1). The diaphragma sellae, a thick reflection of dura mater, forms the roof of the sella. In 50 per cent of individuals, the diaphragma closely encircles the pituitary stalk and forms an anatomic barrier. In the remainder, the diaphragma does not tightly surround the stalk (40 per cent) or is thin (10 percent).[12] These latter variations may permit superior extension of pituitary tumors. Above the diaphragma sellae lies the suprasellar cistern, an anatomic space filled normally with fluid. In proximity are the optic nerves and chiasm, the mamillary body, and the median eminence. Contiguous and superior to these structures lies the hypothalamus.

The arterial supply to the hypothalamus-pituitary region derives from three sources. The inferior hypophyseal artery branches from the carotid artery within the cavernous sinus and supplies the posterior lobe of the pituitary. The superior hypophyseal arteries link the circle of Willis to the median eminence and surrounding area. The middle hypophyseal arteries, of variable origin, connect the carotid artery to the pituitary stalk. No direct arterial supply to the anterior pituitary has been documented. Capillary portions of the superior hypophyseal arteries drain from the hypothalamus, the median eminence, and the superior portions of the pituitary stalk. These vessels drain into the "primary plexus" of veins (Fig. 2) of the hypophyseal portal system. Long hypophyseal portal veins originate from the primary plexus, travel to the anterior pituitary lobe to form a secondary venous plexus, and drain ultimately to the cavernous sinus.[11,169] Additional vessels, the trabecular arteries, also originate from the superior hypophyseal arteries and drain separately to short hypophyseal veins (see Fig. 2).

The average dimensions of the adult pituitary are 10 mm. anterior to posterior, 15 mm. side to side, and 5 mm. superior to inferior. The gland fills approximately three-fourths of the sellar space. The average adult female gland is approximately 20 per cent larger than that of the average adult male. During pregnancy, the female gland also increases in size by about 10

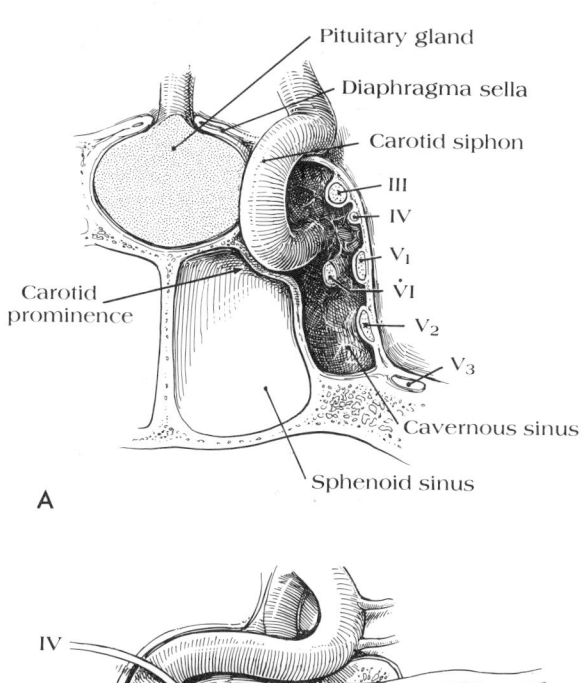

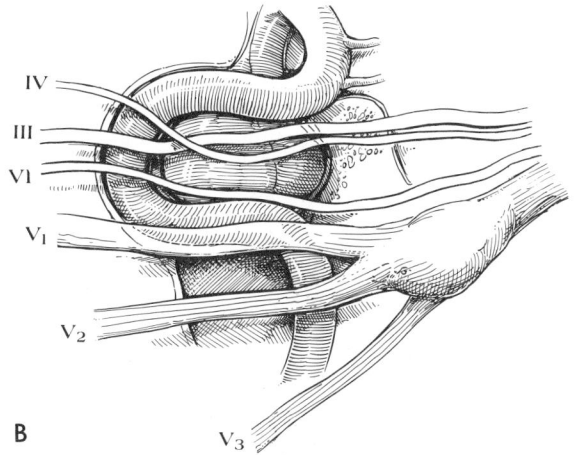

Figure 1. *A*, Schematic representation of the cranial nerves within the cavernous sinus from a coronal perspective. *B*, The carotid artery and cavernous sinus are viewed from the lateral perspective.

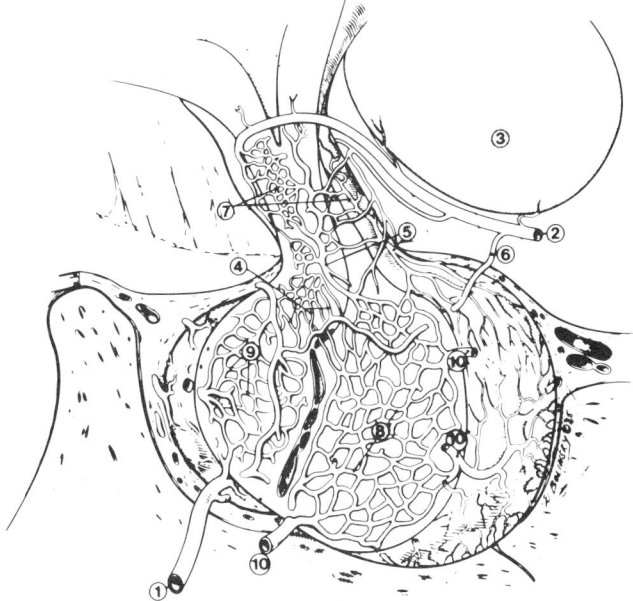

Figure 2. Blood supply of the pituitary gland: (1) inferior hypophysial artery, (2) superior hypophysial artery, (3) optic chiasm, (4) short hypophysial portal veins, (5) long hypophysial portal veins, (6) artery of trabecula, (7) primary plexus of the hypophysial portal system, (8) secondary plexus of the pituitary portal system, (9) capillary plexus of the infundibular process, (10) efferent veins to the dural sinuses. (From Sabshin, J. K.: The pituitary gland—Anatomy and physiology. *In* Goodrich, I., and Lee, K. J. (Eds.): The Pituitary. Amsterdam, Elsevier, 1987, p. 22.)

per cent because of hypertrophy of prolactin-secreting cells.[177] Histologically, the pituitary is divided into anterior and posterior lobes. According to more recent nomenclature,[11] the neurohypophysis is composed of the posterior lobe together with the pituitary stalk and the median eminence (Fig. 3). The posterior, or neural, lobe contains the terminal portions of axons originating in the supraoptic and paraventricular nuclei of the hypothalamus. Antidiuretic hormone (ADH) and oxytocin precursors are synthesized in these nuclei, transported via the axons to the posterior lobe where the active hormones are separated, and then released into the capillary circulation.

The anterior pituitary also consists of three portions: pars distalis, pars intermedia (vestigial in man), and pars tuberalis (Fig. 4). The pars tuberalis lies above the diaphragma sellae in proximity to the median eminence. The presence of glandular pituitary above the diaphragma may explain why residual secretion of adenohypophyseal hormone is sometimes observed following hypophysectomy.[95,130] The anterior lobe tissue is comprised of at least six different cell types. Previous nomenclature distinguished acidophil, basophil, and chromophobe cell types, based on reactions of fixed and sectioned specimens with dyes. Newer classifications identify glandular pituitary cells by their secretory products. Thus, cells are identified by immunochemical staining methods as somatotrophs (growth hormone [GH]), adrenocorticotrophs (adrenocorticotropic hormone [ACTH]), thyrotrophs (thyroid-stimulating hormone [TSH]), lactotrophs (prolactin [PRL]), gonadotrophs (follicle

stimulating hormone [FSH] and luteinizing hormone [LH]), and cells that produce melanocyte-stimulating hormone (MSH). Paradoxically, recent observations have indicated that chromophobes, which were formerly thought to be dormant, may in fact exhibit heightened rates of hormone secretion. Thus, absence of dye would appear to represent depletion of prohormone or hormone stores due to higher rates of secretion.[39,70,124]

Regulation of anterior pituitary hormone secretions is directed partly by cells residing within the parvicellular system of the hypothalamus (see Fig. 4). The very small cell bodies of neurons in this system are concentrated in the arcuate and other anterior nuclei of the hypothalamus. The axonal processes of these cells terminate in the median eminence, next to portal capillaries. Such axonal processes can release factors that are transported to inhibit or stimulate anterior pituitary hormone secretions. Generally, each pituitary cell type secretes one hormone. The gonadotroph is the only cell thus far identified that secretes two hormones, LH and FSH.

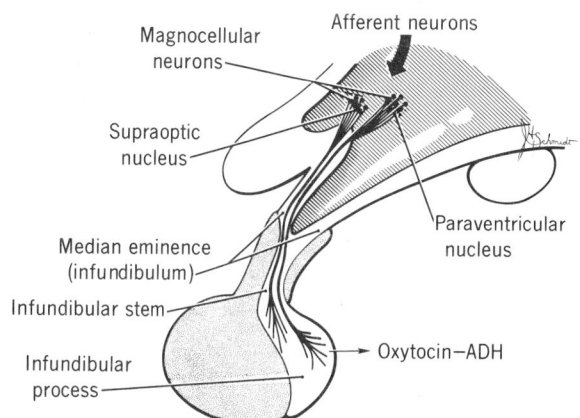

Figure 3. Diagrammatic representation of the neurohypophysis and its relationship to the hypothalamus. According to newer terminology, the neurohypophysis consists of the infundibular process (posterior pituitary), infundibular stem (pituitary stalk), and infundibulum (median eminence).

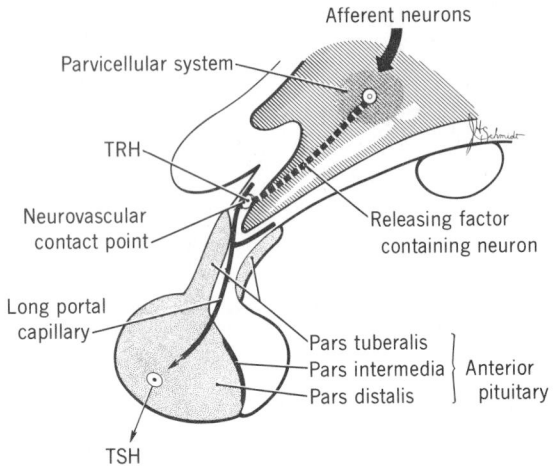

Figure 4. Diagrammatic representation of the adenohypophysis or anterior pituitary and its relationship to the hypothalamus. As a representative example, a neuron secreting TRH and a cell producing TSH are illustrated.

PHYSIOLOGY

Neurohypophysis

The two principal hormones secreted by the posterior lobe are vasopressin (VP, also known as ADH) and oxytocin. Both hormones contain nine residues, and both have a cys-cys bridge in the 1-6 position (Fig. 5). Both are derived from a common ancestor compound, vasotocin, the single neurohypophyseal hormone secreted by most vertebrates other than mammals.

Oxytocin and vasopressin are synthesized and released in conjunction with carrier proteins known as neurophysins. Oxytocin and its related neurophysin I are released via neural pathways, during distention of the vagina or uterus or suckling of the nipples. Oxytocin stimulates uterine contractions during labor and elicits milk ejection by myoepithelial cells of the mammary ducts. At physiologic serum levels, oxytocin does not markedly influence systemic blood pressure or water homeostasis.

ADH is synthesized and released in conjunction with neurophysin II. Stimuli to release of ADH to the circulation include increases in plasma osmolality above 285 mOsm. per liter and decreases in circulating blood volume by 5 per cent or more.[184] ADH may also be secreted in response to catecholamines, the renin-angiotensin hormone system, opiates, and other analgesics or anesthetic agents. Drugs such as phenytoin, alcohol, and lithium appear to suppress release of ADH.[127] The sensation of thirst is regulated by the same stimuli but does not appear to be directly influenced by circulating levels of ADH.

ADH binds to receptors in epithelial cells of the medullary thick ascending loop of Henle, causing increased rates of Na^+ and Cl^- reabsorption. In addition, ADH enhances permeability to water within the collecting ducts of the medulla. The effects of ADH on salt and water conservation can be diminished by local mechanisms within the kidney, particularly by increases in levels of prostaglandin E_2.[83,89] ADH actions at the cellular level and their modulation by prostaglandins appear to be mediated through cyclic adenosine monophosphate (cAMP)–dependent mechanisms.[83,89]

Adenohypophysis

The anterior pituitary secretes two functionally distinct classes of trophic hormones: The first group, including GH and prolactin (PRL), includes hormones that influence activity in more than one target tissue. The secretory products or metabolites that provide feedback to the pituicytes that secrete GH and PRL have not yet been identified (Fig. 6). The second group, including LH, FSH, TSH, and ACTH, influences rates of secretion by the gonads, thyroid, and adrenal, respectively. The secretions of these glands influence target tissues and exert feedback influences on pituitary function and on the trophic substances released by the hypothalamus (see Fig. 6).

LH AND FSH. The gonadotropic hormones are both glycoproteins, each consisting of an identical alpha subunit of 15,000 molecular weight and distinct beta subunits of 13,000 molecular weight (LH) and 25,000 molecular weight (FSH), respectively.[222] In the adult male, LH (formerly designated ICSH, or interstitial cell–stimulating hormone) stimulates Leydig cells to produce testosterone. FSH binds to receptors on the Sertoli cells to enhance spermatogenesis (Fig. 7). Testosterone, present in 100-fold greater concentrations in the testes than in the blood, also binds to cytoplasmic and nuclear receptors within the Sertoli cell.[84] These hormones thus influence the numbers of germ cells that may ultimately differentiate (early effects) as well as the rate at which they differentiate into mature sperm. In peripheral tissues, testosterone and its metabolite, dihydrotestosterone, stimulate the growth of the penis and scrotum and development of facial, axillary, and pubic hair, and influence appetitive states of libido and aggressiveness.

In the adult male, LH and FSH secretions are stimulated by hypothalamic release of the gonadotropic releasing hormone (LH-RH or Gn-RH). Inhibitory inputs on FSH and LH secretions arise from androgens that are synthesized by the testis in response to gonadotropin. One per cent of testosterone is converted into estradiol in peripheral tissues and in the hypothalamus. Estradiol independently suppresses LH release from the pituitary and Gn-RH from the hypothalamus. An additional peptide, inhibin,[68] appears to be released by the Sertoli cells and suppresses release of FSH but not LH. Thus, a number of hormones interact to provide regulatory inputs for FSH and LH secretion in the male.

In the adult female, LH and FSH regulate cyclic ovarian function. FSH stimulates maturation of the graafian follicle and its production of estradiol. The midcycle surge of LH causes follicular rupture, ovulation, and establishment of the corpus luteum. LH maintains luteal function until pregnancy or luteolysis. In general, sex steroids exert negative feedback effects on release of LH and FSH by the pituitary.[119,187] Just prior to ovula-

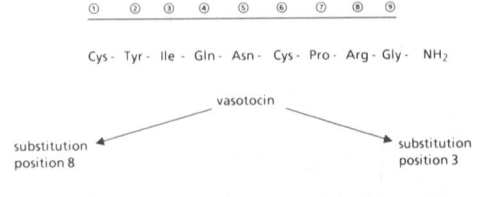

Cys - Tyr - Ile - Gln - Asn - Cys - Pro - Arg - Gly - NH₂

vasotocin

substitution　　　　　　　　　　　　　substitution
position 8　　　　　　　　　　　　　　position 3

Cys - Tyr - Ile - Gln - Asn - Cys - Pro - Leu - Gly - NH₂　　　Cys - Tyr - Phe - Gln - Asn - Cys - Pro - Arg - Gly - NH₂
oxytocin　　　　　　　　　　　　　　　　　　arginine-vasopressin

Figure 5. The neurohypophysial hormones.

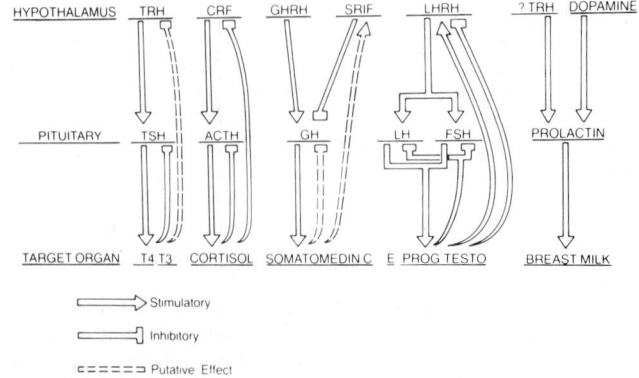

Figure 6. Hypothalamus–pituitary–target tissue interaction. (From Caldwell, B. V., and Kayne, R. D.: Normal endocrine function of the pituitary. *In* Goodrich, I., and Lee, K. J. (Eds.): The Pituitary. Amsterdam, Elsevier, 1987, p. 30.)

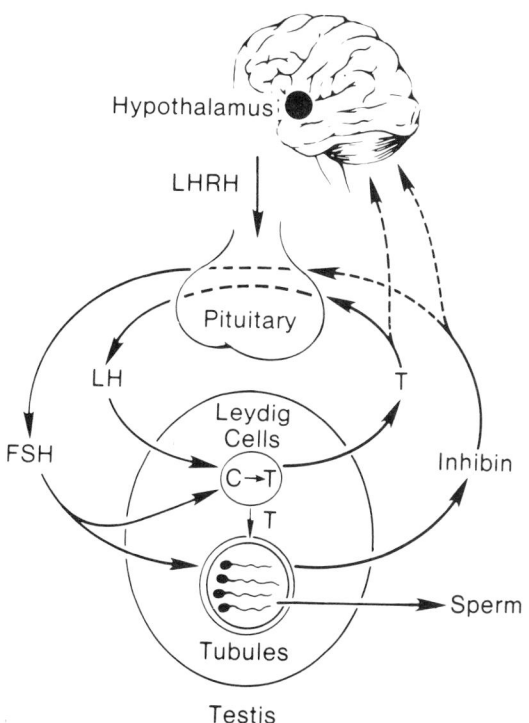

Figure 7. Hypothalamus–pituitary–testicle interrelationships. Schematic diagram to indicate feedback relationship to testosterone and inhibin produced by the testes on gonadotropin secretion by the hypothalamic-pituitary complex and the site of action of FSH and LH on the testis. C, cholesterol; T, testosterone; FSH, follicle stimulating hormone; LH, luteinizing hormone; LH-RH, gonadotropin-releasing hormone. (From Griffin, J. E., and Wilson, J. D.: Disorders of the testes and male reproductive tract. *In* Bondy, P. K., and Rosenberg, L. E. (Eds.): Metabolic Control and Disease. Philadelphia, W. B. Saunders Company, 1980, p. 1535.)

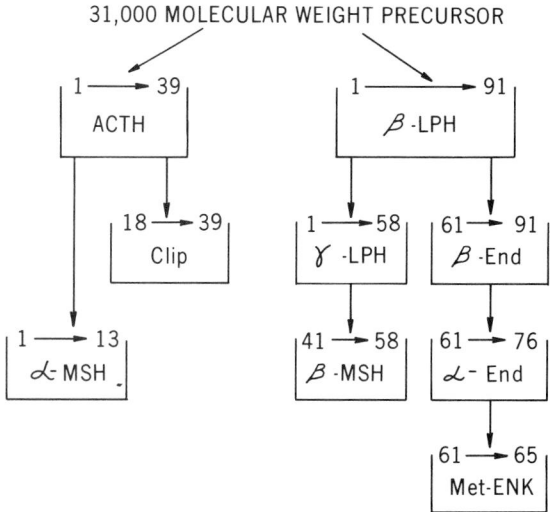

Figure 8. High-molecular-weight precursor of ACTH and several other peptides secreted by the anterior pituitary. Clip, Clip peptide; MSH, melanocyte-stimulating hormone; LPH, lipotropin; End, endorphin; Met-ENK, metencephalin.

tion, however, estradiol and progesterone transiently (i.e., over a 24- to 36-hour interval) stimulate LH secretion and, to a lesser extent, FSH secretion. A gradual increase in plasma estradiol to levels above 300 pg. per ml. for a duration of 5 to 7 days, followed by a rise in plasma progesterone from 0.5 to 1.5 ng. per ml., provides conditions for positive feedback stimulation and release of LH and FSH.[119]

TSH. TSH is a glycoprotein of 28,000 molecular weight. It contains an alpha subunit identical to that of FSH and LH and a unique beta subunit. TSH binds to receptors on the cell membrane of the thyroid epithelium, activating adenyl cyclase and increasing cytosol levels of cAMP. TSH stimulates increased rates of iodide transport, thyroglobulin synthesis, triiodothyronine (T_3) and thyroxine (T_4) formation, and T_3 and T_4 release. In addition, TSH elicits increases in the size and vascularity of the gland.

Negative feedback regulation of TSH release occurs at the level of the pituitary. Elevated circulating levels of T_4 and T_3 can inhibit response of the pituitary to the hypothalamic thyrotropin-releasing hormone (TRH).[120,132] Agents promoting release of TSH include TRH, and those suppressing it include somatostatin, also of hypothalamic origin. T_3 decreases binding of TRH to the pituitary cell membrane[107] but has not been demonstrated to influence TRH secretion from the hypothalamus.

ACTH. The corticotroph synthesizes a 31,000 molecular weight precursor (pro-opiomelanocortin [POMC]), which can be lysed into several biologically active polypeptides (Fig. 8).[128] These include ACTH (30 residues), β-lipotropin (β-LPH, 91 residues), and an incompletely characterized 78-residue fragment termed glycopeptide.[9] The biologic activity of ACTH resides in its initial 24-amino acid sequence, which has been synthesized and is available for clinical use. Synthesis of POMC and secretion of ACTH and endogenous opioid peptides by the pituitary are regulated by stimulatory influences, which include hypo-

thalamic corticotropin-releasing factor (CRF) and by negative feedback actions, which include circulating glucocorticoids.[215] In addition, ACTH and CRF secretions can be limited by circulating levels of ACTH.[214,215]

ACTH binds to receptors in the adrenal cortex, activating membrane-bound adenyl cyclase. With rises in cellular levels of cAMP, cholesterol is converted to androgen, estrogen, and corticosteroid precursors. Synthesis of mineralocorticoid (aldosterone) is not as completely directed by circulating levels of ACTH. Under normal circumstances, plasma ACTH and serum cortisol levels are lowest between 10:00 P.M. and 2:00 A.M. and highest at approximately 8:00 A.M.[51,214] This diurnal pattern of secretion can be altered during periods of stress, such as those arising from acute illnesses, trauma, fever, and hypoglycemia. Under these circumstances, 2- to 10-fold increases in corticosteroid secretions have been measured. An additional ultradian (less than 24 hours) rhythm has been observed. In this pattern, 8 to 10 pulses of ACTH and cortisol secretion occur during sleep and waking, superimposed on the more predictable diurnal rhythm.[51,214]

The endogenous opioids, β-endorphin and met-enkephalin, are contained within the β-LPH sequence. These opioids compete for receptors in brain and spinal cord that bind morphine and other opiates. The enkephalins and endorphins possess potent analgesic properties and influence release of pituitary hormones such as LH, PRL, and vasopressin. The endogenous opioids are released during periods of stress, shock, or hypoglycemia, presumably from many central nervous system (CNS) sites in addition to the hypophysis.[98a,231] Recent observations[51,63a,215] have suggested that a number of hypothalamic and hypophyseal polypeptides, including ACTH, CRF, TRH, endorphins, and enkephalins, help to integrate the somatic and central responses to stress. The relative contributions of the hypothalamus and hypophysis in the response to stress versus those of other CNS sites remain to be defined.

GH. GH, a polypeptide hormone containing 191 residues, is synthesized by somatotropic cells that constitute less than half of the pituitary cell population. The somatotrophs are more concentrated in lateral areas of the gland, just as GH-secreting adenomas tend to arise more frequently in these areas. GH elicits longitudinal growth of the skeleton, with increased sulfate uptake into the epiphyseal cartilage and higher rates of protein polysaccharide and DNA synthesis in cartilage and bone. In peripheral tissues, GH antagonizes the effects of insulin; but within the pancreas, GH stimulates insulin secretion. GH also produces direct stimulation of liver cell growth and adipocyte metabolism with increased serum levels of free fatty acid. Many of these actions are mediated by polypeptides, known as somatomedins, which are synthesized in the liver[73] and are structurally similar to proinsulin.

GH levels in the plasma of adults are generally low (less than 5 ng. per ml.) through most of the day. Bursts of secretion are consistently noted 3 to 4 hours after mealtime and during Stage III and IV sleep. Stress, exercise, hypoglycemia, protein depletion, administration of glucagon and L-dopa can stimulate secretion of GH. Acute hyperglycemia suppresses GH secretion. The hypothalamus elaborates two peptides that regulate pituitary GH release. GH-releasing hormone (GHRH) (somatocrinin) stimulates release, and somatostatin (SRIF) suppresses it. Glucocorticoids appear to enhance the secretory stimulation elicited by GHRH.[232] It is not clear whether there is a more classic feedback regulation of GH secretion by the activities or products of its target tissues.

PRL. PRL is a 23,000 molecular weight polypeptide secreted by the lactotroph, a cell also more prevalent in the lateral areas of the pituitary. PRL initiates and sustains lactation by the breast glands, which are prepared for this function by the gonadal and placental estrogens and progesterones of pregnancy. PRL may influence synthesis and release of progesterone by the ovary and testosterone by the testis.

PRL secretion is inhibited by dopamine released into the pituitary portal circulation.[136] The PRL-releasing hormone has not yet been identified, although thyrotropin releasing hormone (TRH) is a leading candidate. The main physiologic stimulus for PRL release is a centrally mediated response to suckling of the breast. The suckling stimulus and lactation inhibit release of gonadotropins and may provide a means of suppressing ovulation and thus of controlling birth rates.[205] Different medications, including metaclopramide, haloperidol, chlorpromazine, and reserpine enhance PRL secretion by interfering with release of dopamine into the pituitary portal circulation. L-dopa inhibits PRL secretion.

EVALUATION AND DIAGNOSIS OF PITUITARY DISEASE

Pituitary lesions produce structural and functional abnormalities. Structural abnormalities follow outgrowth of pituitary neoplasms to adjacent CNS regions. Lesions producing these abnormalities may be suspected by anatomically directed neuro-ophthalmologic evaluation and can be diagnosed by radiologic imaging. Lesions producing functional abnormalities are suspected by the history and physical examination and can be diagnosed by measurements of pituitary endocrine function.

Structural Abnormalities

SIGNS AND SYMPTOMS. Pituitary neoplasms enlarge in a superior direction and may first be suspected because of visual field changes. Bedside testing with confrontation detects gross field cuts only. Small field defects can be detected by formal visual field testing. A newer approach uses visually evoked responses of the electroencephalogram (EEG) and detects lesions causing small visual field cuts.[99] The characteristic defect involves bitemporal hemianopsia and is not always apparent to the patient. Fundoscopic examination may reveal pallor of the optic disc suggestive of early optic atrophy. Papilledema is most unusual in patients with pituitary adenomas. Examination of the extraocular muscle movements may detect encroachment on cranial nerves adjacent to the pituitary. Involvement of cranial nerves III, IV, and VI may occur in 5 to 10 per cent of patients with pituitary adenomas and would reflect compression or invasion of the cavernous sinus.[100] Spontaneous cerebral spinal fluid (CSF) rhinorrhea occurs rarely (0.5 per cent of patients), but a pituitary lesion is the tumor most likely to cause this symptom.[188,228]

Hemorrhage within pituitary neoplasms has been more commonly recognized than previously since the introduction of computed tomography (CT).[100,228,229] Symptomatic hemorrhage is observed in as many as 9 per cent of patients with pituitary adenomas and unrecognized hemorrhage detected at operation or autopsy in an additional 6 per cent of patients.[228,229] Pituitary apoplexy due to hemorrhage or infarct is characterized by severe headache, sudden visual loss, meningismus, decreased sensorium, and bloody CSF. Ocular palsy may be observed as well. The size of the tumor and its functional state do not clearly correlate with the incidence of hemorrhage.

DIAGNOSTIC IMAGING. Size and location of pituitary lesions can be determined using a number of imaging techniques. Available modalities include plain skull films, arteriography, CT scanning, and nuclear magnetic resonance imaging (MRI). Plain skull films, including a posteroanterior view at 0 degrees, provide measurements of the depth, length, and width of the sella turcica. The calculated volume of the sella (volume=length $\times$ width $\times$ depth $\div$ 2) correlates well with anatomic measurements in normal subjects.[56] In patients with pituitary tumors, it is important to note that sellar width may not reflect lateral extension of the tumor accurately. Radiologic signs of pituitary tumor include asymmetrical enlargement in one dimension, focal bony erosion, or a double floor. Elevation of the anterior clinoids and posterior displacement of the posterior clinoids indicate suprasellar extension. A uniformly enlarged sella ("empty sella"), however, can reflect pathologic processes other than pituitary tumor (Table 1). When the pituitary or hypothalamic areas contain calcifications, a craniopharyngioma should be suspected.

In the past, arteriography provided additional information about pituitary lesions. Such studies detect displacement of the posterior segment of the carotid siphon in the anteroposterior view, unwinding or opening of the siphon in the lateral view. In addition, stretching of segments of the circle of Willis can be observed with suprasellar extension of the tumor. Moreover, angiography has been useful in excluding lesions such as meningioma or cerebral aneurysm. The present role of arteriography in evaluation of pituitary tumors is controversial. Angiography, particularly when performed with digital subtraction techniques, can detect abnormal carotid siphon anatomy and identify the positions of segments of the circle of Willis. In the future, newer techniques utilizing CT and MRI may obviate the need for invasive studies.

Until recently, the CT scan has been the imaging modality of choice when a pituitary lesion has been suspected. CT has supplanted plain films, hypocycloidal tomography, and pneumoencephalography for the purpose of identifying sellar tumors. Optimal imaging involves use of intravenous contrast agents, with 1.5- to 2.0-mm. sections constructed in the coronal plane. The coronal image best demonstrates the relationships of the sella to surrounding structures, the dimensions of the sella, the contour of the diaphragma sellae, and the sellar floor. Some tumors defined easily by CT do not alter dimensions or contour

TABLE 1. Causes of Enlarged Sella

Common	Rare
Pituitary adenoma or other parasellar tumors	Vascular lesions
Empty sella syndrome	Aneurysms
Primary—not associated with identifiable causes	Ectatic internal carotid artery
Secondary	Long-standing target organ failure
Increased intracranial pressure	Hypothyroidism
Loss of pituitary mass, e.g., infarction of adenoma	Primary hypogonadism
	Cysts
	Familial causes

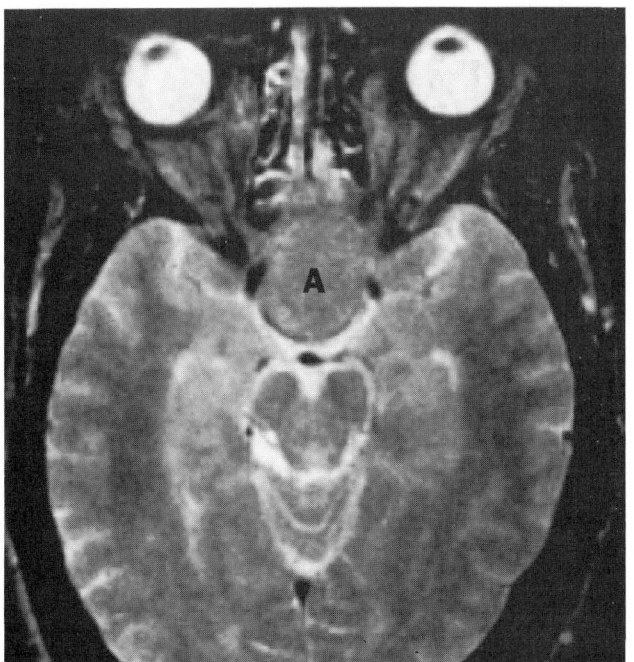

Figure 9. Axial spin echo T2-weighted MR image. A large pituitary adenoma (A) occupies the suprasellar cistern. (Courtesy of F. J. Wippold, M.D., Mallinckrodt Institute of Radiology, Washington University School of Medicine, St. Louis, Missouri.)

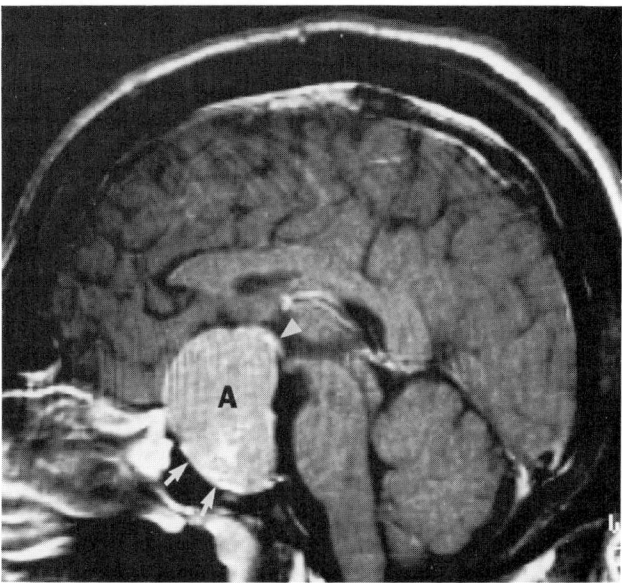

Figure 11. Sagittal spin echo T1-weighted MR image after Gd-DTPA enhancement. The enhancing adenoma (A) fills an expanded sella turcica (white arrows) and extends into the suprasellar cistern. The mass indents the third ventricle (white arrowhead). (Courtesy of F. J. Wippold, M.D., Mallinckrodt Institute of Radiology, Washington University School of Medicine, St. Louis, Missouri.)

of the borders of the sella.[56,216] With intravenous contrast enhancement, the carotid siphon and cranial nerves within the cavernous sinus can be identified.

The most characteristic appearance of a pituitary microadenoma includes a well-circumscribed, focal, nonmidline lesion, which may be hyper- or hypodense.[53] Midline abnormalities can reflect benign cystic lesions of the pars intermedia, which may be present in up to 20 per cent of autopsy specimens.[34] With erosion of the adjacent portion of the sella, the finding of a hypolucency greater than 2 mm. is highly suggestive of a

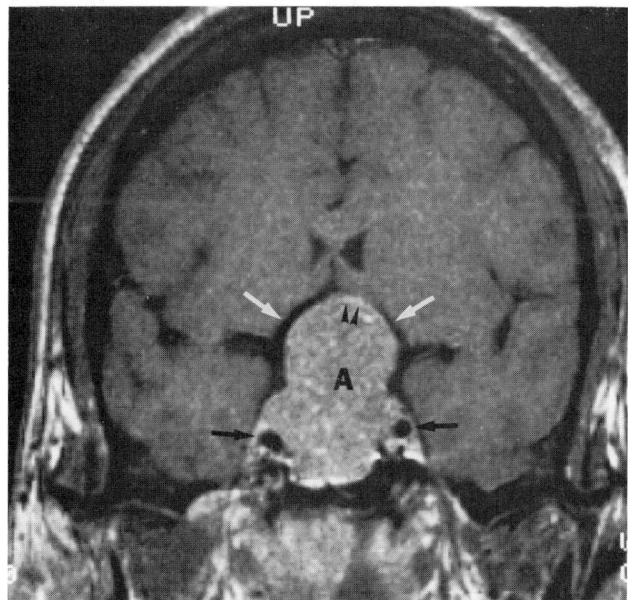

Figure 10. Coronal spin echo T1-weighted MR image after Gd-DTPA enhancement. The adenoma (A) enhances therefore increasing its signal. The tumor displaces the carotid arteries laterally (black arrows). Note that the A1 segments of the anterior cerebral arteries (white arrows) and the chiasm (arrowheads) drape over the mass. (Courtesy of F. J. Wippold, M.D., Mallinckrodt Institute of Radiology, Washington University School of Medicine, St. Louis, Missouri.)

tumor. It should be noted, however, that up to 40 per cent of microadenomas may be isodense with surrounding tissues, or not large enough to be resolved with present scanning techniques.[53]

In the future, MRI may supplant CT as the imaging modality most useful for pituitary lesions (Figs. 9 to 11), since ionizing radiation and intravenous or intrathecal contrast injection are not required. In addition, cavernous portions of the cranial nerves are visualized against signals from flowing blood in the carotid siphon and cavernous sinuses. MRI is as sensitive as CT in detecting tumors that enlarge the pituitary gland and is becoming as sensitive in identifying microadenomas within the gland.[114,134] MRI is superior to CT in providing measurements of the dimension of the sella and identifying pathology in juxtasellar regions.[114,134]

Functional Abnormalities

Detailed evaluation of pituitary function is now feasible because of the availability of radioimmunoassay for pituitary hormones. There are several reasons necessitating evaluation of endocrine function of the pituitary: to confirm a clinical suspicion of hypersecretion of one of the pituitary hormones or a diagnosis of panpituitary hypofunction, to provide follow-up on the adequacy of therapy for hypersecretory lesions, and to assess the degree of functional impairment of normal pituitary tissue before and after treatment of a focal pituitary lesion is instituted. Pituitary function can improve in some patients with excision of lesions that encroach on surrounding normal tissue.[160]

Assessment of anterior pituitary function includes measurement of plasma levels of a hormone under basal standard conditions and reserve function during provocation or suppression tests (Fig. 12). A convenient protocol utilizes insulin-induced hypoglycemia in combination with administration of L-dopa, TRH, and LH-RH to test reserves of prolactin, TSH, LH, FSH, and ACTH. Serial evaluations using this "battery" can be performed to follow the progress of pituitary function over time. Hypersecretory states may be evaluated by means of suppression tests, for example, inhibition of growth hormone release by hyperglycemia. Hypoglycemia is a potent stimulus that can raise plasma levels of GH and other anterior pituitary hor-

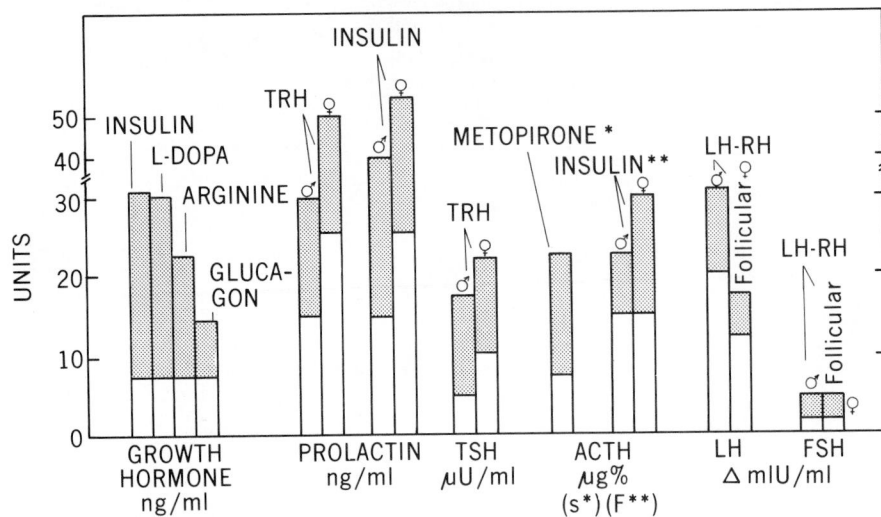

PROVOCATIVE TESTS OF ANTERIOR PITUITARY FUNCTION

STIMULATORY TESTS ☒ NORMAL RESPONSE
☐ BLUNTED RESPONSE

Figure 12. Overview of the tests available to stimulate various anterior pituitary hormones. The height of the shaded bars represents mean levels in normal subjects after provocative stimulation. The open bars reflect blunted responses. Growth hormone, prolactin, TSH, LH, and FSH are usually measured directly, whereas cortisol (compound F) or compound S (11-desoxycortisol) is used as an indirect marker of ACTH secretion. Note that sex differences must be considered in the interpretation of certain tests.

mones. In addition, the demonstration of nonsuppressibility is important in evaluating whether high plasma levels of hormone are due to autonomous hypersecretion by adenoma, rather than stress.

Posterior pituitary function can be evaluated indirectly.[152] The diagnosis of diabetes insipidus is suspected by high osmolality of the plasma and low osmolality of the urine during water deprivation. Correction of these parameters by exogenously administered ADH excludes renal causes of diabetes insipidus. Radioimmunoassays for ADH have recently become available and establish a diagnosis of ADH deficiency or the syndrome of inappropriate ADH secretion (SIADH). In questionable cases, measurement of plasma ADH levels during hypertonic saline infusion establish a diagnosis of nonsuppressible, inappropriate secretion of ADH.[152,185]

GENERAL APPROACH TO DIAGNOSIS AND MANAGEMENT OF PITUITARY DISORDERS

The differential diagnosis of sellar and parasellar tumors includes pituitary adenoma, craniopharyngioma, parasellar meningioma, and sarcoidosis. Rarely, metastatic lesions, gliomas, and other tumors are encountered. In the past, patients with pituitary lesions presented with well-characterized endocrine and neuro-ophthalmologic abnormalities, and tumors were large. Currently, most patients who present with syndromes of endocrine hypersecretion are recognized earlier and lesions may be less than 10 mm. in diameter. The typical sites of origin of pituitary tumors associated with different endocrine syndromes are listed in Figure 13. Nonfunctioning tumors are diagnosed when they cause symptoms from encroachment on adjacent structures. One third of these patients seek attention from an ophthalmologist for progressive loss of vision and bilateral hemianopsia. Tumors reaching 5 to 10 cm. can distort the third ventricle or reach the posterior fossa, causing hydrocephalus and fifth or sixth nerve palsies.

Evaluation of patients presenting with endocrine hyper- or hyposecretion, or suggestive neuro-ophthalmologic symptoms, should include a comprehensive neurologic examination, neuro-ophthalmologic evaluation, and formal testing of visual fields. Imaging studies should include plain skull films and either CT (contrast-enhanced) or MRI. Arteriography is performed to exclude aneurysms of the circle of Willis or to delineate anatomic distortion or anomalies of the carotid siphon.

Pituitary function is assessed by careful history and physical examination, followed by measurements of specific hormones and their releasing factors, under control conditions and during conditions of suppression and/or stimulation. A provocative battery to evaluate reserve pituitary function, as described earlier, is often helpful. Minimally, evaluation of reserve pituitary function includes measurement of morning plasma cortisol, free thyroxine, LH, FSH, TSH, and PRL.

Therapeutic alternatives for pituitary tumors differ, depending on the degree of endocrine dysfunction, encroachment on adjacent structures, and the general health of the patient. A classification of pituitary tumors is given in Table 2 and has been useful in directing therapy for individual patients.[92,93] In some settings, medical management has been advocated as primary or adjuvant therapy for tumors causing symptoms of endocrine hypersecretion. Indications for radiation as primary therapy have included small (Grade I), noncystic lesions with-

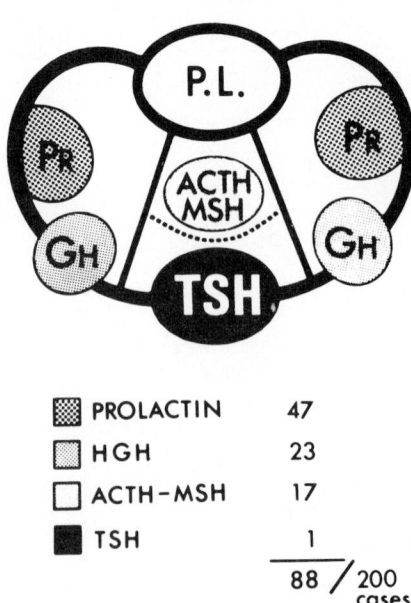

☒ PROLACTIN	47	
☒ HGH	23	
☐ ACTH–MSH	17	
■ TSH	1	
	88	/ 200 cases

Figure 13. Sites of various pituitary adenomas in Hardy's series. (From Hardy J.: Transsphenoidal surgery of hypersecreting pituitary tumors. *In* Kohler, P. O., and Ross, G. T. (Eds.): Diagnosis and Treatment of Pituitary Tumors. Amsterdam, Excerpta Medica, 1973, p. 179.)

TABLE 2. Pituitary Tumor Classification

I. Enclosed microadenoma—sella of normal size with focal asymmetry of the floor or normal sella
II. Enclosed adenoma—sella enlarged with an intact floor
III. Localized invasive adenoma—sella enlarged with localized erosion of the floor
IV. Diffuse invasive adenoma—entire floor of sella destroyed by tumor
    A. Small suprasellar extension filling only the suprachiasmatic cistern
    B. Large suprasellar extension deforming the anterior recesses of the third ventricle

Data according to Hardy, J. and Vezina, J. L.: Transsphenoidal neurosurgery of intracranial neoplasm. Adv. Neurol., 15:261, 1976, and Hardy, J., Somma, M., and Vezina, J. L.: Treatment of acromegaly: Radiation or Surgery? In Morley, T. P. (Ed.): Current Controversies in Neurosurgery. Philadelphia, W. B. Saunders Company, 1976, pp. 377–391.

TABLE 3. Complications of Radiation and Surgical Therapy in Management of Pituitary Tumors

Radiation	Surgical Therapy
Tumor necrosis and hemorrhage	Hemorrhage
Optic nerve degeneration	Air embolus
Malignant transformation of radiated tissue	Meningitis
Hypopituitarism	CSF rhinorrhea (transsphenoidal)
	Injury to optic nerves (transfrontal)
	Hypopituitarism

out suprasellar extension[85,86] or patients who are poor surgical risks. Radiation is also used as adjuvant therapy following surgical resection and for treatment of late recurrences.[85,86]

Neurosurgical techniques, particularly transsphenoidal hypophysectomy, have developed in parallel with improvements in diagnostic methods. Tumors as small as 2 mm. in diameter can now be excised with little morbidity and mortality. With the transsphenoidal approach, the neurosurgeon makes an incision on the gingival mucosa beneath the upper lip and then successively enters the nasal cavity, sphenoid sinus, and sella turcica. Intraoperative microscopy and image-intensification fluoroscopy facilitate maximal visualization of the operative field. The exposure provided by this approach allows selective removal of the tumor with preservation of normal pituitary tissue. As discussed earlier, the diaphragma sella offers a protective barrier of variable integrity above the lesion. In certain centers, tumors detected only by endocrine tests but not yet visible on radiographs are removed by the transsphenoidal approach. The many advantages of this technique, including low morbidity and mortality, hidden incision within the oral cavity, and excellent exposure, have made it the procedure of choice for the treatment of microadenomas.

Tumors greater than 1 cm. may remain within the sella turcica and cause symmetrical enlargement or ballooning (Grade II). Alternatively, they may grow superiorly into the suprasellar cistern or inferiorly into the sphenoid sinus (Grades III and IV, A and B). The transsphenoidal approach is preferred for tumors remaining predominantly in the sella or growing inferiorly (Grades I to III). Approaches to lesions with well-defined superior extension and a diameter of less than 2 cm. are individualized.[135] The transfrontal approach allows better visualization of tumors that have transgressed the diaphragma sellae into the subarachnoid space. Distortions of the neural and vascular structures from tumor growth into the suprasellar cistern are better approached transfrontally. In general, tumors with marked suprasellar extension, invasion through the diaphragma sellae, or large suprasellar dumbbell components are best managed by the transfrontal route. Under some circumstances, however, even these tumors may be initially treated by the transsphenoidal method.[135,239]

Complications of radiation therapy and surgical therapy used for treatment of pituitary lesions are outlined in Table 3. In properly selected cases, approximately 70 per cent of patients respond to radiation therapy. The full effects of radiation may not be realized for several years, and as many as 25 to 40 per cent of these patients develop panhypopituitarism. Other complications of radiation in properly selected patient series occur in 1 to 3 per cent of patients. Malignant degeneration of radiated tissues is a very rare complication of therapy. In contrast, surgical therapy, especially in conjunction with adjuvant radiation,

restores hormone levels with resolution of visual symptoms but also leads to higher rates of late recurrence.[85,86] Early postoperative complications of surgical therapy occur in approximately 2 per cent of operations for microadenoma and in 15 per cent of operations undertaken for macroadenoma.[135,239] Permanent panhypopituitarism, as reflected by unremitting diabetes insipidus, is observed in less than 0.1 per cent of operations performed for microadenoma and generally in about 1 to 2 per cent of operations for macroadenoma.[135,239] With these general considerations in view, it is useful to consider diagnostic and therapeutic approaches to specific disorders of the pituitary.

DIAGNOSIS AND MANAGEMENT OF SPECIFIC PITUITARY DISORDERS

PROLACTINOMA. These tumors constitute 30 to 60 per cent of pituitary neoplasms and are the most common cause of nonphysiologic hypersecretion of PRL.[161] Other causes of PRL excess include centrally acting antihypertensive agents (methyldopa), psychotropic drugs (phenothiazines, opiates, butyrophenones), estrogens and oral contraceptives, hypothalamic disorders, hypothyroidism, adrenocortical insufficiency, and stress. Eighty-five percent of pituitary prolactinomas are diagnosed in women, and symptoms of PRL excess include amenorrhea, galactorrhea, infertility, hot flashes, dyspareunia, and sometimes polycystic ovary syndrome. Prolactinoma should be suspected if amenorrhea and galactorrhea persist more than 6 months after discontinuing oral contraceptive use.[145,161] Two thirds of these lesions in women are diagnosed in the microadenoma stage (less than 1 cm.). Most men with prolactinomas present with macroadenomas (more than 1 cm.), and symptoms of a space-occupying lesion of the sella.[32] Only 15 per cent of men with prolactinomas, however, present with symptoms such as impotence, infertility, or gynecomastia.[32]

Plasma PRL measurements by radioimmunoassay are central to diagnosis of a PRL-secreting tumor. Basal plasma levels in normal women are usually below 30 ng. per ml. Basal levels above 200 ng. per ml. indicate a strong likelihood of prolactinoma. Most medications do not lead to plasma PRL levels above 100 ng. per ml., although higher levels are occasionally observed in patients receiving phenothiazines. Stimulation of PRL by TRH, insulin-induced hypoglycemia, or chlorpromazine and suppression by dopamine are not generally helpful in diagnosing PRL-secreting tumors.

Therapeutic goals in managing prolactinomas include (1) removal of the tumor or at least local control of growth and (2) remission of symptoms and restoration of fertility. In women with Grade I or II lesions and who wish to become pregnant, the preferred management includes removal of the tumor by the transsphenoidal approach. This operation, selective adenectomy, provides cure and restores menses in 80 per cent of patients.[3,145,178] Forty per cent of patients with microadenomas treated by this approach may be able to bear children.[91,145] Intermediate-range follow-up (4 to 5 years) has indicated that at least 15 to 20 per cent of patients with normal plasma PRL levels after surgical therapy may relapse.[135] In the event of a relapse, medical therapy with bromocriptine is initiated. Radiotherapy is not recommended for patients who wish to become pregnant, because PRL levels may correct only after 2 or 3 years following treatment. Recent studies have suggested that microadenomas do not enlarge significantly during pregnancy. Consequently, radiotherapy or surgical therapy is not mandatory if the patient is pregnant when the diagnosis of prolactinoma is made. Macroadenomas, however, enlarge during pregnancy and may cause visual disturbances.[60,161] Such lesions should be removed or debulked if pregnancy is desired.

Medical therapy alone has been advocated by a number of authors for treatment of prolactin-secreting microadenomas or Grade II macroadenomas.[186] Bromocriptine in divided doses totaling 5 to 15 mg. per day is sufficient to return PRL levels to normal in most patients. The effects of bromocriptine administration during pregnancy, e.g., teratogenicity, have not been well characterized. In addition, it is not clear whether the normalization of PRL levels and tumor shrinkage observed during bromocriptine therapy persist beyond the period of therapy. Optimal duration of therapy is also not yet established.[109,171]

When fertility is not a leading consideration or the tumor is Grade III or IV, the major goal of therapy is local control of tumor and cure or palliation of neuro-ophthalmologic symptoms. In such cases, rigorous reduction to normal PRL levels may not be necessary to control symptoms. Surgical excision or debulking is sometimes performed with a transsphenoidal approach but more ideally with a transfrontal approach. Long-term recurrence rates may exceed 50 per cent with a transsphenoidal approach to these larger lesions.[202] Bromocriptine has therefore been advocated as the initial therapy for large, invasive prolactinomas, since more than 90 per cent of these lesions may respond to this therapy.[156,230] In patients with symptoms of extrasellar extension, radiation may provide immediate improvement and diminish long-term recurrence rates.[36] The recommended approach to lesions not amenable to surgical extirpation thus would include bromocriptine in patients with minimal or no symptoms and radiation and bromocriptine in patients requiring tumor shrinkage to relieve symptoms. Surgical excision is advocated, unless absolutely contraindicated by the patient's medical condition, for patients requiring urgent debulking of tumor or for patients who have failed first-line therapies.[186]

SOMATOTROPIN-SECRETING TUMORS. Excess secretion of GH leads to the syndrome of acromegaly (Table 4). Symptoms and physical changes progress slowly. It is not unusual to make the diagnosis 10 or 15 years after the onset of symptoms, and at this point gross clinical features are present. The diagnosis can now be confirmed in the presence of milder symptoms, since sensitive radioimmunoassays for GH are available.

TABLE 4. Clinical Features in Acromegaly

Features	Prevalence (%)
Acral enlargement	98
Hyperhidrosis	70
Menstrual disturbance	69
Headache	59
Weakness	59
Glucose intolerance	40
Skin tags	38
Impotence	34
Visual field abnormality	28
Goiter	25
Hypertension	23

Modifed from Melmed, S., et al.: UCLA Conference: Pituitary tumors secreting growth hormone and prolactin. Ann. Intern. Med., 105:245, 1986.

Growth hormone influences a wide variety of tissues, including soft tissues, bone, gonads, myocardium, lungs, and the gastrointestinal tract. Thus, physical features[150] characteristic of acromegaly include coarsening of facial features, enlargement of hands, feet, and tongue, carpal tunnel syndromes from soft tissue growth, frontal bossing, protruding jaw, hypertrophic osteoarthropathy, and kyphosis. In addition, the liver, spleen, kidney, and heart enlarge with asymmetrical cardiac septal hypertrophy and left ventricular hypertrophy. Colon cancers are found more frequently in patients with acromegaly than in control populations.[106] Glucose intolerance is frequently observed, but only 10 to 15 per cent of patients with acromegaly are overtly diabetic.[150] Menstrual abnormalities in women with GH excess are frequently observed. In some cases, macroadenomas may be associated with these symptoms by compressing normal pituitary tissue and causing hyposecretion of FSH and TSH. In other cases, compression of the pituitary stalk may disrupt dopaminergic pathways, leading to disinhibition of the lactotrophs and hyperprolactinemia. In a third group, PRL and GH may be secreted together by mixed somatroph and lactotroph adenomas. Overall, 25 per cent of patients with acromegaly are found to have such tumors with mixed cell populations.[87]

The diagnosis of a GH-secreting tumor requires elevated levels of GH as measured by radioimmunoassay. Fasting growth hormone levels of at least 10 ng. per ml. are observed in 95 per cent of patients with the clinical syndrome of acromegaly.[150] To date, there are no tests of suppression or stimulation of GH secretion that are sufficiently sensitive to distinguish tumors from other causes of GH hypersecretion.[112] Somatomedin C (insulin-like growth factor I) is elevated in patients with acromegaly and correlates best with the clinical course of the patient.[183] Thus, current recommendations for evaluation of patients with a suspected GH hypersecretion syndrome include basal plasma GH level, basal plasma somatomedin C level, and measurement of GH during the oral glucose tolerance test.[150] If CT and MRI of the sella do not reveal a microadenoma or larger tumor, then ectopic sources of GH production in carcinoids or islet cell tumors should be sought by means of abdominal and chest CT scans. Plasma GH-releasing hormone (GH-RH) levels should be measured to exclude rare hypothalamic lesions or ectopic sources.[219]

Without treatment, patients with acromegaly die prematurely because of metabolic complications of GH excess.[237] Cardiovascular and respiratory complications represent the majority of deaths. Morbidity for this condition also arises from sleep apnea disorders, kidney stones, and osteoporosis.[28] The goals of therapy include preventing tumor enlargement; arresting physical disfigurement; and reversing cardiovascular, respiratory, and metabolic complications of GH excess. Reduction of GH levels is achieved most rapidly by excision of the adenoma, preferably by the transsphenoidal approach (Fig. 14). Eighty per cent of patients with acromegaly who have lesions localized to the sella and minimal signs of local invasion experience a fall in plasma GH below 10 ng. per ml.[133,142,239] Postoperative radiation may reduce the size of the tumor and diminish GH secretion in large lesions (Grades III and IV) that are not completely surgically excised.[133] Clinical improvement after radiation as a primary therapy may be realized only 2 or 3 years after treatment.[63,203] When surgical approaches and radiation have failed or are contraindicated, high doses of bromocriptine (up to 60 mg. per day) may suppress GH secretion to some extent. As primary therapy for acromegaly, high-dose bromocriptine suppresses GH levels to less than 5 ng. per ml. in less than 20 per cent of patients with acromegaly[15] and is not recommended. Criteria for cure include plasma GH levels less than 5 ng. per ml. and less than 2 ng. per ml. during oral glucose tolerance testing and normalization of somatomedin C levels in the plasma.[150] Recurrences are diagnosed with the use of similar criteria.

CORTICOTROPIN-SECRETING TUMORS. Presentation

ACROMEGALY—COMPARATIVE TREATMENT RESULTS

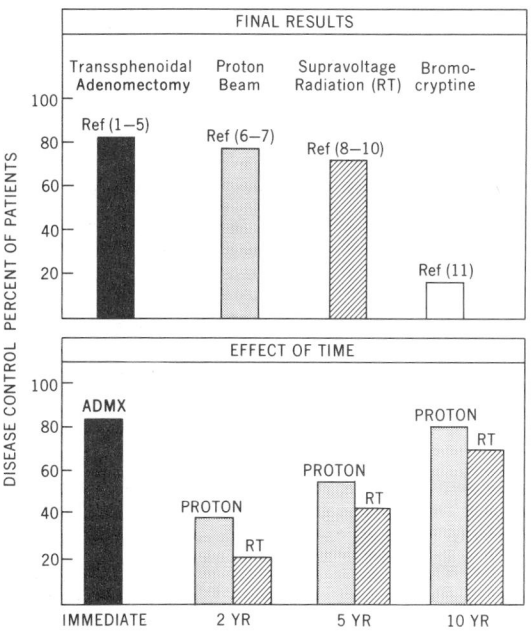

Figure 14. Comparative treatment results in acromegaly. *Top,* Percentage of patients with control of disease (i.e., growth hormone levels below 10 ng. per ml.) in response to various therapies. The data reflect the following series: (1) Laws et al. (1979); (2) Ludecke et al. (1976); (3) U et al. (1977); (4) Hardy et al. (1976); (5) Williams et al. (1975); (6) Linfoot et al. (1975, 1979); (7) Kjellberg et al. (1973); (8) Lawrence et al. (1971); (9) Sheline et al. (1973); (10) Eastman et al. (1979); (11) Besser et al. (1978). *Bottom,* The time required to achieve the final results observed from each therapy.

and diagnosis of patients with ACTH excess are discussed in the adrenal section of this chapter. Classically, it had been held that 10 to 20 per cent of cases of ACTH-dependent hypercortisolism (Cushing's disease) were attributable to pituitary adenomas. Recent re-evaluation has revealed that up to 80 per cent of patients with Cushing's disease (bilateral adrenocortical hyperplasia with elevated plasma ACTH levels) are found to harbor a pituitary microadenoma.[190,221,227] Preferred approaches to such microadenomas begin with transsphenoidal excision. Recent updates of clinical series suggest that 60 to 90 per cent of patients with microadenomas may undergo remission through surgical excision alone,[16,19,25,42,135,164] but among these patients recurrence rates may be as high as 10 to 15 per cent.[16,164] Preoperative imaging of a microadenoma as a cause of hypercortisolism can be difficult, because 50 per cent of such tumors may be less than 5 mm. in diameter.[135] Thus, when pituitary imaging studies do not reveal a sellar lesion, it is imperative to re-evaluate the patient for causes of hypercortisolism such as adrenal tumor or ectopic sources of ACTH such as oat cell tumor of the lung, bronchial carcinoid, or thymoma. When endocrine studies have indicated a high likelihood of a pituitary lesion and CT scans of the chest and abdomen reveal no likely source of ectopic ACTH production, exploration of the sella may be undertaken via a transsphenoidal approach.[19,135] If the lesion is not visible on the surface of the gland, a vertical and several horizontal incisions open the interior of the gland for inspection. Resection of the central portion or total excision of the gland may be required if the adenoma cannot be identified by these maneuvers.

Macroadenomas are much less commonly a source of Cushing's disease than are microadenomas. Complete removal by surgical approaches may be obtained in 50 per cent of patients,[19,135] with a recurrence rate of approximately 10 per cent. Patients in whom the tumor cannot be completely removed at operation may require additional radiation or heavy particle therapy with proton beam.[139] Up to 90 per cent of patients so

treated experience remission. After radiation, cortisol levels diminish over a period of 6 to 12 months, and medical suppression of cortisol secretion may be required until the full benefits of radiation appear. Medical therapies with cyproheptidine (4 to 20 mg. a day), an antiserotonergic and antihistaminic agent, may reduce ACTH secretion in one third of patients; however, improvement may not be observed until 3 to 5 weeks after therapy is initiated.[126] Therapies for reducing adrenocortical secretion by direct action on the adrenal gland are discussed in the adrenal section of this chapter. Criteria for cure, as defined by Orth and Liddle,[168] include (1) urinary 17-hydroxycorticosteroid levels to less than 7 mg. per gm. of creatinine, (2) normal serum cortisol, and (3) evening plasma cortisol less than 7 μg. per 100 ml. if diurnal rhythm reappears or less than 10 μg. per 100 ml. if diurnal rhythm remains absent. A normal plasma ACTH level, below 20 pg. per ml., is also expected after curative therapy.

GONADOTROPIN-SECRETING TUMORS. Patients with tumors secreting LH and FSH do not experience symptoms referable to hormone excess. Consequently, such patients present with signs and symptoms of an expanding sellar mass. Recent observations indicate that these tumors are not quite so rare as formerly thought and may constitute as many as 30 per cent of chromophobe adenomas previously thought to be hormonally inert.[207] Most of these tumors have been found in men, often with a previous history of hypogonadism. Elevation of FSH is observed more frequently than that of LH.[57,207] These tumors are managed, if possible, by a transsphenoidal surgical approach, or a frontal approach if necessary, and by radiation therapy if surgical excision is not feasible or medically contraindicated. Hormone levels in the plasma are used in follow-up of patients for evidence of cure or recurrence.

THYROTROPIN-SECRETING TUMORS. These tumors are the rarest of adenohypophyseal adenomas and produce a syndrome of hyperthyroidism with elevated TSH levels.[78] Some have been reported, however, in patients with a previous history of hypothyroidism.[78,194] These observations have suggested that autonomous thyrotropin-secreting tumors of the pituitary may arise, in some cases, because of the absence of feedback inhibition induced by the normal secretion of thyroid hormone. Treatment strategies are similar to those used for other pituitary tumors causing syndromes of hormone hypersecretion.

NONFUNCTIONING ADENOMA. Before the development of immunohistochemistry and sensitive hormone measurements, pituitary tumors were divided into those staining with basic dyes (basophilic), those staining with acid dyes (acidophilic), and nonstaining types (chromophobe). As noted above, approximately 30 per cent of chromophobe adenomas may secrete PRL, and others secrete FSH and TSH. There remains a significant proportion of these lesions in which hormone hypersecretion cannot be demonstrated. Patients with apparently nonsecretory tumors usually present with symptoms of the sequential loss of LH and FSH, TSH, and finally ACTH secretion. Impotence or amenorrhea is a common early symptom, whereas fatigue and cold intolerance related to hypothyroidism usually occur later. Visual field defects and headache caused by the growing mass are the presenting complaints in over one third of patients. These tumors are generally larger than those that present with a syndrome of hormone hypersecretion because the diagnosis is made later in the clinical course. Treatment is directed toward control of tumor mass effects. When no suprasellar extension is present, the preferred surgical approach is transsphenoidal. Postoperative irradiation is advocated by some authorities to prevent later recurrence. Selected patients in this group, particularly those without visual field defects, are treated with irradiation alone as a means of preventing further tumor growth. Patients with large tumors that cross the diaphragma sellae and who present with visual impairment are usually approached by the transfrontal route. Objective improvement in vision can be documented postoperatively in 75 per cent of these patients.[90,211] Postoperative irradiation is required in this group to prevent tumor regrowth. However, more patients with suprasellar tumors and visual field abnormalities are currently being operated on through the transsphenoidal approach.[236] These patients can also be expected to experience some postoperative improvement in vision.[96] A decision regarding the surgical technique depends upon tumor size, degree of invasion of the subarachnoid space, and presence or absence of cerebral dysfunction related to mass effects of tumor.

OTHER TUMORS. Craniopharyngioma presents at any age and arises from cells above or below the diaphragma sellae. Lesions may be cystic or solid and usually contain calcium. Patients with these tumors complain of visual loss, headache, symptoms of endocrine deficiency, or problems relating to mass effects of tumor on cerebral function. Total surgical excision is advocated as treatment by some authorities, whereas cyst drainage followed by radiation therapy is espoused by others.[113,118,125,212] Gliomas and metastatic tumors rarely may present as pituitary mass lesions and often are mistaken for other tumors. Meningiomas of the tuberculum sellae or intrasellar carotid aneurysms may closely mimic pituitary tumors.

PITUITARY APOPLEXY. Sudden hemorrhage into pituitary tumors (functioning or nonfunctioning) produces the syndrome of pituitary apoplexy.[225] Acute onset of headache, stiff neck, loss of vision, extraocular nerve palsies, syncope, adrenal insufficiency, and blood in the cerebrospinal fluid (CSF) characterizes this syndrome. Mass effects occur because of sudden expansion and upward encroachment due to blood within the tumor. Surgical decompression is necessary to restore vision that is acutely lost. In patients with an intact diaphragma sellae, oculomotor nerve palsy and panhypopituitarism may occur gradually or acutely without associated symptoms. Pituitary apoplexy often appears in association with radiation therapy of tumors, anticoagulation, or closed head trauma but may also occur spontaneously in 5 per cent of patients.

SHEEHAN'S SYNDROME. Pituitary apoplexy occurring during complicated parturition, particularly in the presence of massive blood loss, causes immediate or delayed hypopituitarism. Amenorrhea is followed by signs and symptoms of hypothyroidism. Hormone replacements are required.

EMPTY SELLA SYNDROME. An enlarged sella turcica, often with asymmetrical enlargement and thinning of the anterior and inferior portions, may occur in the absence of recognized pituitary tumor. The CT scan usually reveals fluid density within the confines of the sella. Metrizamide injection into the subarachnoid space may be used as contrast material to delineate the CSF-containing space within the sella. Two types of patients with empty sella have been described (see Table 1). The primary type presents in obese, hypertensive women who complain of headache but have no underlying neurologic disorders. Pituitary function is usually normal, but occasionally PRL is increased and GH reserve reduced. The secondary type is observed in patients with otherwise benign CSF hypertension and those with a loss of pituitary function due to apoplexy or surgical therapy. Hypersecretion of GH, PRL, or ACTH may persist in such patients. The pathogenesis of the primary and secondary syndromes is probably due to an incomplete diaphragma sella,[217] loss of pituitary mass, elevation of intracranial pressure, or a combination of factors. No treatment exists for the primary condition. For the secondary empty sella syndrome, correction of the inciting cause is usually warranted.

HYPOTHALAMIC LESIONS. Neoplasms of the hypothalamus are rare and produce symptoms due to hypothalamic dysfunction or endocrine abnormality. Disordered temperature regulation, rage reactions, and abnormalities of appetite, sleep control, and sympathetic function may be found. Disruption of releasing-factor secretion may produce endocrine deficiency.

Alternatively, interruption of inhibitory influences on gonadotropin secretion can cause precocious puberty.[191] Specific etiologies of hypothalamic disease include trauma, neoplasms, degenerative diseases, congenital cysts, hydrocephalus, inflammatory or infiltrating lesions, and vascular anomalies. Rarely, hamartomas of the hypothalamus appear to secrete LH-RH and produce precocious puberty.[110] Lesions of these areas are not usually curable by surgical treatment but may require exploration for diagnosis or shunt placement, or both.

OUTDATED INDICATIONS FOR PITUITARY SURGERY

BREAST CANCER. Total surgical ablation of the pituitary contents was previously advocated as treatment for certain patients with carcinoma of the breast. The rationale for this procedure is the reduction of pituitary factors that stimulate tumor growth. With careful operative technique, reduction of GH and PRL secretion to undetectable levels is readily achievable. However, it is difficult to reduce estrogen production totally with hypophysectomy.[95] The primary effect of hypophysectomy is considered to be the lowering of estrogen levels as a result of adrenal and ovarian atrophy. The stimulatory roles of PRL and GH on human breast cancer are not clearly established.

Alternative methods of reducing the stimulatory effects of estrogen on breast tumors now exist. Tamoxifen, an antiestrogen, blocks estrogen action at the cellular level. In postmenopausal women, the aromatase inhibitor aminoglutethimide blocks estrogen production. These two agents are now widely employed to replace surgical ablation of the pituitary as treatment of breast cancer.

PROSTATE CARCINOMA. Complete hypophysectomy has also been used in the treatment of carcinoma of the prostate for relief of bone pain. This procedure is used only after initial response or orchiectomy. The rationale is a reduction in adrenal androgen production. Objective responses are rarely observed, and subjective pain relief persists for less than 6 months to 1 year. Consequently, chemotherapy and supportive measures are used more commonly than hypophysectomy.[151]

DIABETIC RETINOPATHY. Hypophysectomy causes regression of diabetic retinopathy in highly selected patients with rapidly progressive disease.[80] The rationale for this procedure is largely empirical. Prior criteria for selection include rapid progressive neovascularization documented by serial photographs, impending blindness, sufficient compliance of the patient for rigid control of diabetes postsurgically, and absence of severe renal disease or orthostatic hypotension. Several controlled studies document the benefit of this procedure[121,122]; however, this technique has been largely replaced by use of laser photocoagulation and vitrectomy.

ADRENAL CORTEX

EMBRYOLOGY

The adrenal gland is comprised of a cortex and medulla, each having distinct embryologic, anatomic, histologic, and functional characteristics.[46] The adrenal cortex arises from mesodermal tissue in the fourth to sixth weeks of life. By the eighth week, it has differentiated into a thin outer neocortex and a thick inner "fetal zone." This fetal zone gradually involutes after birth but, during gestation, actively produces fetal steroids that are metabolized into estrogens by the placenta. In the fourth month of fetal life, the adrenals are three to four times larger than the kidneys, but they begin to decrease in size relative to the kidney thereafter and through the first year of life.

In the seventh week of gestation, ectodermal cells (pheochromoblasts) migrate from the neural crest toward the acidophilic cell mass of adrenal cortex and to the para-aortic and paraverte-

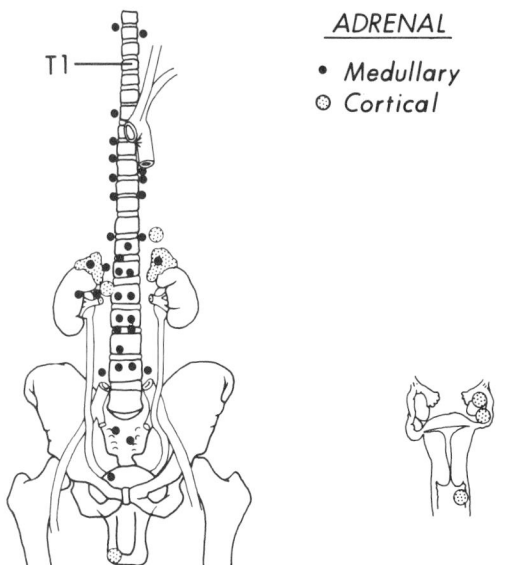

ADRENAL

• *Medullary*
⊙ *Cortical*

Figure 15. The sites of extra-adrenal chromaffin and medullary tissues.

bral regions. By the twentieth week, clusters of these cells are present in the center of the adrenal mass, but the adrenal medulla does not become a distinct structure until atrophy of the fetal zone in the cortex postnatally. Neuroblasts, also derived from neural crest, migrate to the medulla and ultimately differentiate into sympathetic ganglion cells.

Aberrant adrenal cortical tissue is now recognized more commonly than formerly thought: Graham[81] described accessory adrenal cortical tissue in one third of 100 autopsies, but such foci averaged less than 1 cm. in diameter. Such accessory tissue usually is found near the kidney or in the pelvis, along the path of migration of structures arising from the urogenital ridge.[81,193] Adrenocortical tissue may also be found in locations that are not explained by normal patterns of migration of fetal tissues.[81] The occurrence of extra-adrenal chromaffin tissue is commonly observed, as depicted in Figure 15.

ANATOMY

GROSS. Each adrenal gland weighs 4 gm. and is perched on the superior medial aspect of the upper pole of the kidney. The pyramid-shaped right adrenal lies close to the inferior vena cava and frequently abuts the diaphragm and the bare areas of the liver. The left adrenal is larger and flatter and is found between the kidney and aorta, near the tail of the pancreas and the splenic artery. The adrenal glands are firmer than surrounding perirenal fat and can be palpated as distinct structures. The normal adrenal cortex is bright yellow and thicker than the red-brown medulla. These glands are highly vascular, deriving their blood supply from the inferior phrenic artery superiorly, the aorta medially, and the renal artery inferiorly. The primary blood supply of the right adrenal is derived from superior and inferior adrenal arteries; the left adrenal is supplied primarily by the middle and inferior adrenal branches. Additionally, numerous smaller arterial branches enter the gland. The right adrenal gland venous effluent drains to the inferior vena cava through a wide but short central vein. The venous blood of the left adrenal gland empties primarily into the left renal vein but occasionally may drain directly to the vena cava.

Lymphatic plexuses within the subcapsular portion of the adrenal cortex and the adrenal medulla drain to the adjacent para-aortic subdiaphragmatic and renal lymph nodes. Neural fibers into the adrenal cortex have not been demonstrated. The adrenal medulla, however, is richly supplied by preganglionic sympathetic nerves coursing from the greater splanchnic nerve,

celiac ganglion, and other plexuses. Parasympathetic nerves to the medulla have not been characterized.

HISTOLOGY. In the adult, the adrenal cortex is comprised of three zones: an outer zona glomerulosa, a middle zona fasciculata, and an inner zona reticularis. Each zone has distinct features when examined by light and electron microscopy. Aldosterone is synthesized exclusively in the zona glomerulosa, whereas cortisol and androgens are produced in the fasciculata and reticularis layers. Under stimulation of ACTH, cells of the two inner zones enlarge with increased storage of lipid, proliferation of mitochondria and endoplasmic reticulum, and alteration of mitochondrial configuration.

The adrenal medulla contributes approximately 10 per cent of the total gland weight. Adrenal medullary cells are polyhedral and arranged in cords. They contain catecholamines and precipitate chromium salts that stain brown with hematoxylin and eosin. On electron microscopy, core vesicles containing epinephrine and norepinephrine are apparent.

The microvasculature of the adrenal gland integrates the functions of the cortex and medulla. As the major and minor arteries approach the gland, they tend to anastomose and form a plexus at the capsular surface. A number of small vessels pass through the cortex to the medulla, but most enter the cortical plexus. Within the zona fasciculata the capillaries enlarge; and in the zona reticularis there is an increase in branching and anastomosing of these vessels. Blood, now enriched with adrenocortical hormones, enters the medulla. There hormones induce synthesis and activation of the medullary enzyme (phenylethanolamine N-methyl transferase), which converts norepinephrine to epinephrine in the chromaffin cells.

PHYSIOLOGY

As discussed previously, ACTH is secreted by the corticotropin cells of the pituitary and stimulates synthesis and secretion of adrenocortical hormones. ACTH secretion is activated by hypothalamic corticotropin releasing factor (CRF) and is suppressed by the glucocorticoid hormone, cortisol (see Fig. 2). Adrenocortical hormones are synthesized from cholesterol, which is derived from plasma or manufactured locally within the cortex. By a series of enzymatic degradations within the cristae of the mitochondrion, cholesterol is cleaved to Δ-5 pregnenolone, the precursor for glucocorticoid hormone (cortisol), mineralocorticoid hormone (aldosterone), and sex steroid hormones (dehydroepiandrosterone). Biosynthetic pathways leading to these structures are summarized in Figure 16. After leaving the mitochondrion, pregnenolone enters the smooth endoplasmic reticulum (SER), where it is shunted to these divergent pathways. As discussed later, congenital absence of enzymes involved in one of these pathways shunts pregnenolone derivatives through unaffected pathways, causing specific clinical syndromes.

GLUCOCORTICOID PHYSIOLOGY. Pregnenolone is oxidized at C17 by 17α-hydroxylase to become 17-hydroxypregnenolone. Through the actions of 3β-hydroxydehydrogenase, Δ5, Δ4-isomerase, and 21-hydroxylase, 11-deoxycortisol is synthesized. Addition of a hydroxyl group at C11 (11β-hydroxylase) causes formation of cortisol. Corticosterone follows a parallel pathway in its biosynthesis but does not undergo the initial hydroxylation at C17.

Cortisol production remains constant as a function of body size (12 mg. per sq. mm. body surface area) during all phases of life. A normal adult secretes 10 to 30 mg. of cortisol each day. In plasma, approximately 75 per cent of cortisol is bound to transcortin, a corticosteroid binding globulin, 15 per cent is bound to albumin, and 10 to 15 per cent is unbound. Plasma transcortin levels are increased during pregnancy and by pharmacologic doses of estrogen. Alterations in transcortin or albumin levels in plasma can alter the total plasma cortisol concentration without altering its free concentration. The plasma half-life is approxi-

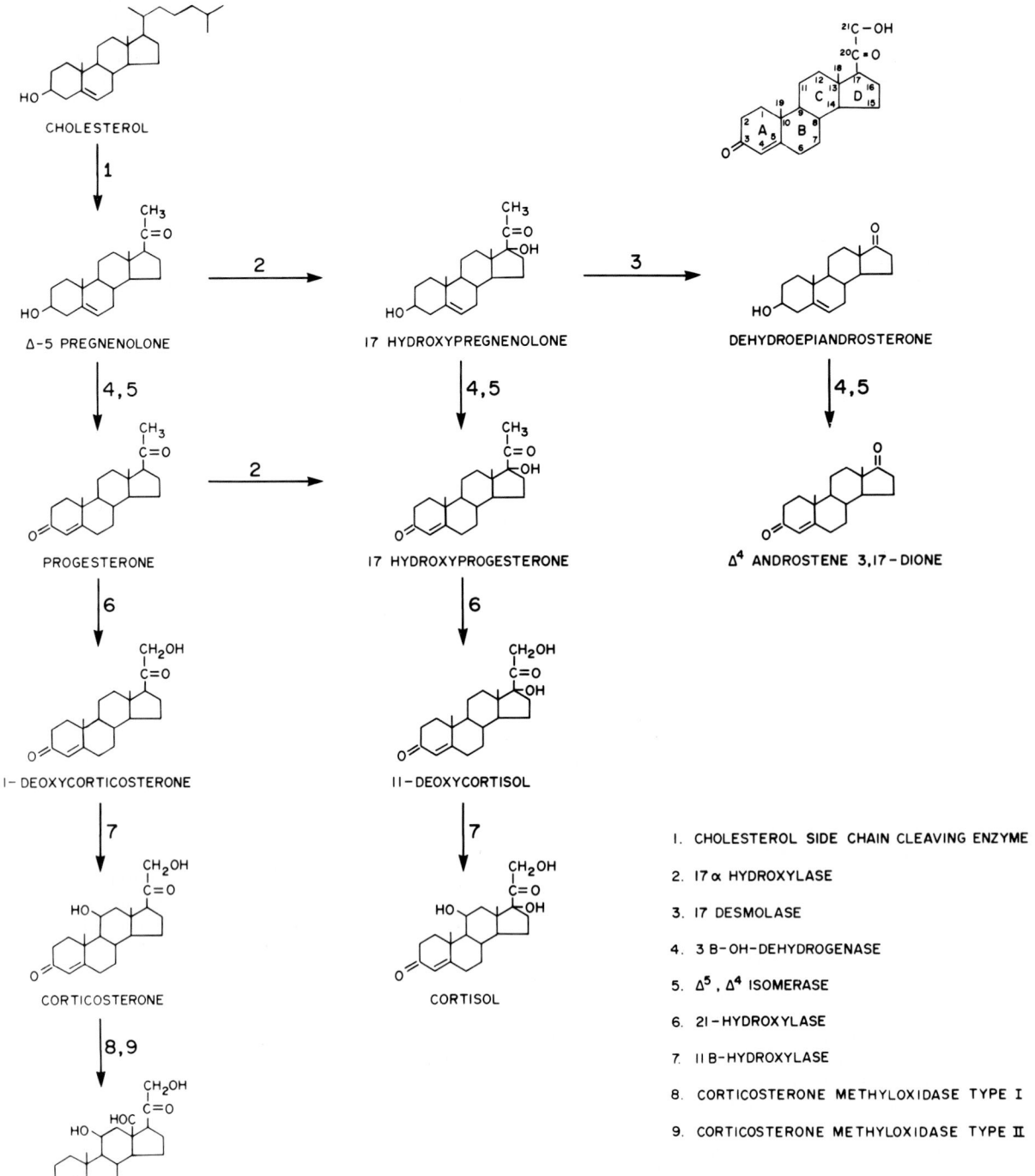

Figure 16. The biosynthetic pathways of adrenal corticosteroids.

mately 90 minutes. Cortisol is cleared, predominantly by the liver, transformed to inactive metabolites such as dihydrocortisol and tetrahydrocortisol, cortone, and cortolone. These compounds are conjugated with glucuronate and excreted in the urine, where they may be measured as 17-hydroxy- or 17-keto-steroids. A small fraction of unmetabolized cortisol can be measured in the urine as well.

Both cortisol and corticosterone influence carbohydrate metabolism, primarily by promoting gluconeogenesis and accumulation of glycogen in the liver. These glucocorticoids also may influence glucose metabolism indirectly by enhancing peripheral breakdown of white adipose tissue and of muscle, thereby increasing substrate delivery to the liver (Fig. 17). In

peripheral tissues, glucocorticoids antagonize actions of insulin, decreasing glucose uptake and utilization. Thus, glucocorticoids function anabolically in the liver, but catabolically in skin, muscle, lymphoid tissues, and fat cells. Prolonged administration of exogenous corticosteroids leads to a catabolic state, with negative nitrogen balance, proximal muscle weakness, and insulin-resistant diabetes mellitus. There is, in addition, a redistribution of body fat characterized by truncal obesity and peripheral depletion. The mechanisms underlying the centripetal accumulation of fat are unclear.

Glucocorticoids are also well recognized as anti-inflammatory and immunosuppressive agents.[149,172] Glucocorticoids suppress lymphocytic proliferation, induce cytolysis of T lympho-

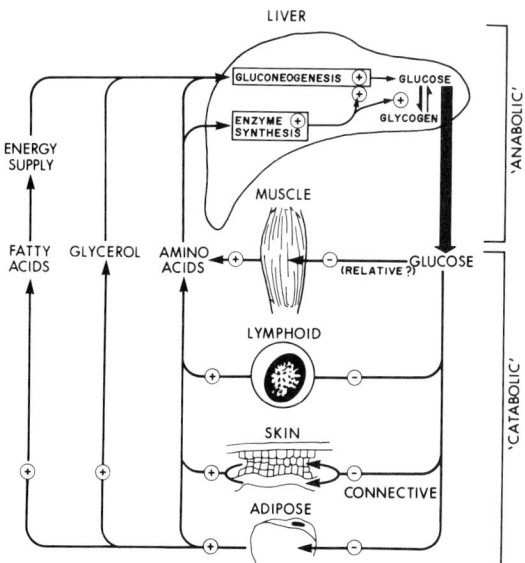

Figure 17. Glucocorticoid actions on carbohydrate, lipid, and protein metabolism. The plus signs indicate stimulation, and the minus signs indicate inhibition. (From Baxter, J. D., and Forsham, P. H.: Tissue effects of glucocorticoids. Am. J. Med., *53:*573, 1972.)

cytes, and inhibit circulation of monocytes and also their accumulation in areas of inflammation. By antagonizing the effects of migration inhibitory factor (MIF), glucocorticoids diminish recruitment of neutrophils and monocytes to areas of injury or infection. Cortisol inhibits histamine release by mast cells and histamine-induced release of lysosomal granules. Corticosteroids impair the process by which the hypothalamus induces fever. They also modulate antibody formation by inhibiting T-cell circulation and, at high doses, by directly inhibiting B-cell activities.

Glucocorticoids retard wound healing by impairing collagen formation and fibroblast activity. They also inhibit osteoblastic function and stimulate osteoclasts, thereby decreasing bone formation and increasing bone resorption. In addition, intestinal calcium absorption is impaired, leading to elevated parathyroid hormone secretion and bone turnover.[8] Other effects of chronic corticosteroid excess include emotional and psychologic disturbances, cataracts, and corneal ulcers. Glucocorticoids also retard growth and promote early closure of bone growth plates in children and adolescents.

PHYSIOLOGY OF ADRENAL SEX STEROIDS. After conversion of pregnenolone to 17-hydroxypregnenolone, 17-desmolase in the SER cleaves the link between carbons 17 and 20 to form dehydroepiandrosterone (DHEA). This is the major C19 sex steroid produced by the adrenal cortex, although the sulfated derivative of DHEA and Δ4-androstenedione are also produced. Only minute amounts of testosterone or estrone are synthesized under normal circumstances.

In fetal life, circulating androgens influence development of the male external genitalia, the male ductal structures such as the vas deferens, epididymus, and seminal vesicles, and the prostate. In the absence of androgens, female genitalia and a vagina develop. After birth, androgens stimulate growth of the phallus, muscle mass, and body hair. Estrogens influence growth and maturation of the breast tissue, uterus, and vagina. Normally, the major source of sex steroid production resides in the gonads. Disorders associated with excess adrenal production of these hormones are discussed.

PHYSIOLOGY OF THE MINERALOCORTICOIDS. In man, the major mineralocorticoid hormone is aldosterone, which is synthesized in the zona glomerulosa. This outer zone lacks 17α-hydroxylase, and therefore pregnenolone is converted to progesterone through the activity of 3-hydroxydehydrogenase and

isomerase enzymes. Subsequent 21-hydroxylation in the SER and 11β-hydroxylation in the mitochondrion cause formation of corticosterone. Aldosterone is derived from actions of corticosterone methyl oxidase Types I and II on corticosterone. In the zona fasciculata and zona reticularis, the presence of 17α-hydroxylase shunts pregnenolone and progesterone into the biosynthetic pathways for cortisol and androgens.

Approximately 100 to 150 mg. of aldosterone is secreted each day, and its plasma half-life is 15 minutes. Aldosterone binds loosely to plasma proteins and is cleared from the plasma in a single passage through the liver. Metabolic degradation occurs in the liver and kidney by enzymatic reduction and by conjugation with glucuronic acid. Only minute amounts of free aldosterone are excreted in the urine.[54]

The principal mechanisms that regulate aldosterone synthesis and secretion include ACTH, the renin-angiotensin system, and plasma levels of Na^+ and K^+. The ACTH secreted by the pituitary does not directly influence aldosterone production; in fact, the zona glomerulosa does not atrophy after hypophysectomy, unlike the zona reticularis and fasciculata.[54] Nevertheless, aldosterone secretion is greatly diminished in experimentally hypophysectomized rats.[170] Although hypophysectomy does not lower aldosterone levels acutely in man, it does blunt the response of aldosterone secretion in response to physiologic stimuli such as deprivation of dietary sodium.[235] Although ACTH administration may acutely stimulate aldosterone hypersecretion, prolonged administration of ACTH ultimately leads to diminished aldosterone secretion. These findings have suggested the presence of an additional pituitary-derived factor that might stimulate aldosterone production. Such an "aldosterone-stimulating factor" (ASF), a 26,000 dalton glycoprotein, has been purified from human urine and detected by immunocytochemical methods in the anterior pituitary of experimental animals.[30] Although ASF has been found in high concentrations of patients with aldosterone-secreting tumors, its role in physiologic regulation of aldosterone secretion remains unclear.

The major influence on aldosterone secretion is the renin-angiotensin system.[167] Renin, an enzyme formed in the kidney, acts on angiotensinogen to produce angiotensin I, which is altered by the angiotensin-coverting enzyme (ACE) in the lung to angiotensin II. Angiotensin II elicits marked increases in peripheral vascular resistance, arterial blood pressure, and aldosterone biosynthesis. A reduction in renal arterial blood pressure (e.g., from hypovolemia) or a decrease in serum Na^+ levels stimulates renin secretion from the juxtaglomerular cells of the kidney. With restoration of blood volume and pressure secondary to high aldosterone, production of renin and angiotensin is suppressed.

The K^+ ion also markedly influences aldosterone secretions.[77,98] Williams and associates[235] have demonstrated that an increase of serum K^+ levels by 0.2 mEq. per liter increases aldosterone secretion by almost 50 per cent, whereas a fall in serum K^+ levels decreases aldosterone secretion by 50 per cent. Hypokalemia blunts the aldosterone secretion that would otherwise be observed in a number of clinical settings. Restoration of serum K^+ levels restores the response. Serum K^+ has been shown to influence activity of a number of steps within the aldosterone biosynthetic pathway.

The mineralocorticoid hormones act on a variety of tissues to excrete potassium and to conserve sodium for the extracellular space. Aldosterone stimulates a variety of epithelia to absorb Na^+ and excrete K^+ and H^+. The target organ of greatest significance in this function is the renal tubule, particularly its distal segment, and the cortical collecting duct. Glucocorticoids also display mineralocorticoid activity. In addition, glucocorticoids appear to influence the glomerular filtration rate (GFR) independently through effects on the microvasculature of the nephron. Glucocorticoids also may be necessary for the kidney to maximally dilute and concentrate the urine.[199] Thus, aldosterone and the adrenal glucocorticoids act in concert to preserve

Na^+, K^+, and volume homeostasis of the extracellular and intravascular body spaces. High levels of circulating mineralocorticoid tend to expand these volumes and suppress renin production.

DISEASES OF THE ADRENAL CORTEX

Cushing's Syndrome

In 1932, Harvey Cushing[50] published his classic treatise on the clinical entity that would come to be known as Cushing's syndrome. He described eight patients with central obesity, glucose intolerance, hypertension, plethora, hirsutism, osteoporosis, nephrolithiasis, menstrual irregularity, muscle weakness, and emotional lability. Basophilic adenomas of the pituitary were noted in six of these patients, but the relationship to adrenocortical hyperplasia was not appreciated. It is now known that Cushing's syndrome is attributable to increased levels of plasma corticosteroid. Today many patients have this syndrome because of exogenous administration of corticosteroid. Causes of endogenously elevated levels of corticosteroid include autonomously hypersecreting adenomas or carcinomas of the adrenal glands or bilateral adrenal cortical hyperplasia. In addition, hypersecretion due to stimulation from ACTH-secreting tumors of the pituitary or ectopic sources has been observed. The first priority in evaluation of a patient with a clinical diagnosis of Cushing's syndrome is to establish the presence of high levels of plasma cortisol. Subsequent priorities include considering the differential diagnosis, defining the cause, and initiating therapy based on the anatomic site of the lesion.

CLINICAL PRESENTATION. Symptoms and signs of Cushing's syndrome and their frequency of occurrence are listed in Table 5.[103] In almost every patient, centripetal obesity and the "orange on toothpicks" habitus are present. Excessive accumulation of fat around the head and neck is responsible for the characteristic "moon facies" and "buffalo hump." Patients usually appear plethoric, and purple striae are most often observed on the abdomen and extremities. Purpura and easy bruisability

TABLE 5. Clinical Features of Cushing's Syndrome

Clinical Feature	Reported Incidence (%)*
Centripetal obesity	79–97
Weakness/proximal myopathy	29–90
Hypertension	74–87
Skin changes	
Thin skin/bruising	23–84
Acne, greasy skin	26–80
Hirsutism	64–81
Plethora	50–94
Abdominal striae	51–71
Infection (e.g., tinea versicolor)	30
Pigmentation	4–16
Psychiatric changes	31–86
Oligo/amenorrhea	55–80
Impotence	55–80
Osteoporosis	
Backache	40–50
Vertebral collapse	40–50
Pathologic fracture	40–50
Thirst/polyuria	25–44
Glucose intolerance	39–90
Ankle edema	28–60
Renal calculi	15–19
Exophthalmos	0–33
Headache	0–47
Abdominal pain	0–21

From Howlett, T. A.: Cushing's syndrome. Clin. Endocrinol. Metab., 14:916, 1985.

are often evident, and acne and superficial skin infections are common. Hirsutism is often a striking feature in women. Wound healing is frequently prolonged.

Menstrual abnormalities are present in most women, as is impotence in men. High blood pressure is common and usually moderate, although malignant hypertension has been observed. Volume expansion and sodium retention both contribute to elevation in diastolic blood pressure. In an older series,[175] Plotz and co-workers noted that hypertension and arteriosclerosis represented 40 per cent of deaths of their patients with Cushing's syndrome.

Muscle weakness and bone pain, particularly backache, are also common. The weakness is due in part to muscle wasting but also to hypokalemia. The bones demineralize, and pathologic fractures are observed in advanced cases. In adults, the demineralization usually persists even after removal of the lesion causing Cushing's syndrome. In children, it is reversible after cure of the lesion and, following restoration of normal plasma cortisol levels, a growth spurt and resolution of osteoporosis are observed. Neurologic symptoms, including headache, emotional lability, depression, and even schizophrenic symptoms may be observed.

Glucose intolerance is common in patients with Cushing's syndrome. The diabetic state can often be managed by alterations in diet alone, but insulin therapy may be required in 10 to 15 per cent of patients. In 50 per cent of patients, the white blood cell count is approximately 10,000 per cu. mm. and the red cell count is above 5,000,000 per cu. mm. Hypercalciuria may be present, but the serum calcium level is normal unless hyperparathyroidism and MEN Type I are present. Serum K^+ is often low because of the mineralocorticoid properties of cortisol and corticosterone.

LABORATORY DIAGNOSIS. The diagnosis of Cushing's syndrome requires a documentation of hypercortisolism. No single test is absolutely reliable, however, in establishing this diagnosis. The ranges of normal plasma and urinary values for adrenocortical hormones are provided in Table 6.

Cortisol is secreted episodically. With normal sleep-wake patterns, plasma levels peak between 4:00 A.M. and 8:00 A.M. and are lowest between 8:00 P.M. and 12:00 P.M. In adults, 10 to 30 mg. of cortisol are secreted by the adrenal cortex each day. Plasma cortisol levels may vary considerably due to diurnal variation (see Table 6). Patients with Cushing's syndrome do not exhibit this diurnal variation. Thus, comparison of 8:00 A.M. and 8:00 P.M. plasma cortisol levels may help in establishing the diagnosis. A more reliable screening evaluation, which eliminates sampling errors, measures free cortisol concentration in a 24-hour collection of urine. Obese individuals may be found to have elevated free urinary cortisol levels without having Cushing's syndrome, because cortisol production is proportional to body mass. A ratio comparing urinary steroid content to urine creatinine content may control such increases in urinary free cortisol excretion.

Plasma ACTH levels normally are between 10 and 100 pg. per ml., with diurnal variations preceding those of cortisol by 1 to 2 hours. Suppression of the absolute level of ACTH and its diurnal cycle is nearly diagnostic of adrenocortical neoplasms, which secrete cortisol and thus inhibit ACTH release by the pituitary. In patients with pituitary neoplasms leading to bilateral adrenocortical hyperplasia, ACTH levels may range from the upper limits of normal (less than 100 pg. per ml.) to 500 pg. per ml.[14,137] The highest plasma levels of ACTH (more than 1000 pg. per ml.) have been observed in patients with tumors in ectopic sites (e.g., small-cell lung carcinomas) that produce ACTH.[14,137] In most patients, the tumor is clinically evident. In others, the lesion is occult, and the cause of hypercortisolism may be deduced through other tests.

The dexamethasone suppression test, originally devised by Liddle,[137] is useful in establishing a diagnosis of hypercortisol-

TABLE 6. Laboratory Evaluation of Adrenal Function

Normal Values	Male	Female
Glucocorticoids		
Plasma cortisol μg./100 ml.		
A.M.	5–25	5–25
P.M.	1–10	1–10
Urinary free cortisol μg./24 hr.	15–100	15–100
Plasma 17-hydroxyprogesterone ng./100 ml.	30–210	10–80
		(follicular phase)
		30–290
		(luteal phase)
Androgens		
Plasma testosterone ng./100 ml.	300–1200	20–80
Plasma androstenedione ng./100 ml.	63–180	63–272
Plasma dehydroepiandrosterone sulfate (plasma 17-ketosteroids) ng./ml.	700–3500	700–3500
Estrogens		
Plasma estradiol pg./ml.	15–40	20–200
		(follicular phase)
		190–340
		(luteal phase)
Plasma estrone pg./ml.	40–65	40–200
		(follicular phase)
		60–200
		(luteal phase)
Mineralocorticoids		
Plasma aldosterone ng./100 ml.		
Upright	5–30	5–30
Supine	3–16	3–16
Saline infusion	<10	<10
Urine aldosterone μg./24 hr.		
Random	4–20	4–20
Low-salt diet	17–44	17–44
High-salt diet	1–4	1–4

ism and in distinguishing pituitary from adrenal causes. Dexamethasone, a synthetic glucocorticoid, is more potent than cortisol in suppressing ACTH release from the pituitary. In the overnight dexamethasone test,[45,165] the patient ingests 1 mg. of dexamethasone at 11:00 P.M., and plasma cortisol is obtained at 8:00 A.M. the following day. In normal individuals, the 8:00 A.M. plasma cortisol level is less than 5 μg. per 100 ml. Less than 2 per cent of individuals with Cushing's syndrome demonstrate normal suppression[45] of plasma cortisol to levels below 5 μg per 100 ml. False-positive tests can be observed in pregnant and very obese individuals and in patients taking oral estrogens or phenytoin.

Following the overnight study, additional information may be available from sequential low-dose and high-dose dexamethasone suppression tests. Twenty-four hour urine specimens are collected for 6 consecutive days. During the first 2 days, baseline urine samples are collected. Over the third and fourth days, patients receive 0.5 mg. of dexamethasone every 6 hours, and during the fifth and sixth days they receive 2.0 mg. of dexamethasone every 6 hours. Urine samples are assayed for urinary free cortisol or 17-hydroxycorticosteroid (17-OHCS). Under normal circumstances, on the fourth day the free urinary cortisol levels fall below 20 μg. per 24 hours and the 17-hydroxycorticosteroids fall below 2 mg. per gm. creatinine per 24 hours. Failure to suppress indicates hypercortisolism.[165] On the sixth day, patients with Cushing's disease (pituitary-dependent bilateral adrenocortical hyperplasia) display reduction of urinary 17-OHCS to 50 per cent of baseline values on days 1 and 2. Patients with adrenal tumors or ectopic production of ACTH do not suppress below 50 per cent. A variation on this 6-day study utilizes measurements of plasma cortisol and dehydroepiandrosterone sulfate.[5]

The metyrapone stimulation test is also useful in distinguishing subsets of patients with Cushing's syndrome.[103,138] Metyrapone inhibits, although not completely, the enzyme 11β-hydroxylase and thus conversion of 11-deoxycortisol to cortisol and 11-deoxycorticosterone to corticosterone and aldosterone. The compensatory rise in ACTH secretion by the pituitary stimulates the adrenal cortex to produce increased quantities of cortisol precursors, which are detected in the urine as increased levels of 17-OHCS. In this test, metyrapone is taken orally, 10 mg. per kg. every 4 hours for a total of 6 doses. In normal subjects, there is a two-fold or greater increase in total urinary 17-OHCS on that day and the subsequent day, as compared with baseline measurements on the previous days. An overnight test has also been devised[209] in which the individual takes a 30 mg. per kg. dose at 12:00 midnight and then has plasma 11-deoxycortisol and cortisol levels drawn at 8:00 A.M. on the following day. In normal subjects, plasma deoxycortisol levels between 7 and 20 μg. per 100 ml. and cortisol levels less than 10 μg. per 100 ml. are observed. In patients with hypothalamic pituitary-dependent Cushing's disease, a decrease in cortisol secretion is sensed, ACTH release increases, and serum deoxycortisol and urinary 17-OHCS levels rise. In hypercortisolism due to an adrenal lesion or to ectopic ACTH hyperproduction, the pituitary is suppressed and serum deoxycortisol and urinary 17-OHCS levels do not change.

The ACTH stimulation test is useful in diagnosis of adrenocortical insufficiency.[147,208] ACTH normally elicits a rise in adrenocortical steroid release within a few minutes after intravenous or intramuscular administration. In the rapid ACTH test, cosyntropin (0.25 mg.) is given intramuscularly or intravenously and plasma cortisol levels are obtained at 0 and 60 minutes. A normal rise in plasma cortisol of at least 7 μg. per 100 ml. excludes primary adrenal insufficiency. Short-term and long-term tests also have been described and distinguish patients who may have subnormal responses in the rapid screening study but in fact do not have adrenal insufficiency. These tests are also helpful in identifying individuals on chronic corticosteroid therapy who may require "stress doses" of steroid during major surgical procedures or after trauma.[116] There is no rationale for employing these tests to distinguish subgroups of patients with Cushing's disease.

To summarize the laboratory approach to the diagnosis of hypercortisolism, it is worthwhile to re-emphasize that a careful history and physical diagnosis provide the basis for suspecting this condition. Urinary free cortisol measurements provide the initial screening evidence for the diagnosis, and loss of diurnal variations with high levels of cortisol measured in the plasma confirm it. Metyrapone stimulation, dexamethasone suppression, and plasma ACTH measurements may provide information for identifying the source of excess cortisol production in the adrenal cortex, pituitary, or ectopic sites.

ETIOLOGIES OF HYPERCORTISOLISM

PITUITARY CAUSES. When Cushing described pituitary basophil tumors in 6 of 8 patients with bilateral adrenal hyperplasia and clinical findings of hypercortisolism, he assumed that the pituitary was responsible for the syndrome. In the strictest sense, hypercortisolism due to ACTH hypersecretion by the pituitary is termed Cushing's disease. In the 1970s, two technical advances permitted recognition of the pituitary-hypothalamic axis as the most common cause of hypercortisolism (excluding exogenous administration of corticosteroid). First, computerized tomography and magnetic resonance imaging have demonstrated lesions in the pituitary gland in 60 to 70 per cent of patients with Cushing's syndrome. Second, the transsphenoidal approach to surgical resection, originated by Schloffer[196] and used for a time by Cushing,[49] has been resurrected. Clinical applications of this approach using microsurgical techniques and the operating microscope enabled cure of Cushing's disease by selective resection of the adenoma without extirpation of the pituitary gland in most patients with bilateral adrenal cortical hyperplasia. The role of the hypothalamus in creating conditions favorable for pituitary adenomas is not known. A recent study[220] revealed that the corticotropin releasing factor (CRF) levels in the CSF are lower than normal in 13 of 14 patients with Cushing's disease. This observation suggests that hypothalamic hypersecretion of CRF does not usually contribute to the disease and that the primary defect lies in the pituitary.

ADRENOCORTICAL CAUSES. Ten to 20 per cent of patients with Cushing's syndrome are found to have adrenal adenomas. In 80 to 90 per cent, the neoplasms are solitary and associated with atrophy of adjacent and contralateral cortical tissue. In the remaining 10 to 20 per cent, nodular hyperplasia of the cortex is found in both glands. Although nodular hyperplasia represents a diffuse process, one or more distinct nodules may simulate adenomas. A small subset of patients with bilateral nodular hyperplasia may prove to have pituitary adenomas.[26] The majority of patients have lesions that are independent of pituitary function. The metyrapone stimulation test appears useful in identifying forms of nodular hyperplasia that are pituitary-dependent. These are recognized with increased levels of urinary 17-OHCS levels on day 1 or 2 following metyrapone, whereas nondependent forms are associated with no change in urinary 17-OHCS.[45,103]

ECTOPIC ACTH SYNDROME. Approximately 15 per cent of patients with Cushing's syndrome have a lesion secreting ACTH from a site other than the pituitary (Table 7). Ectopic sites of ACTH production have included small-cell carcinomas of the lung; carcinoid tumors in the bronchi, alimentary tract, and pancreas; and other epithelial tumors.[55] Ectopic production of CRF has been reported as a cause of Cushing's syndrome rarely.[43] Sources of ectopic and autonomous production of CRF have included carcinoma of C cells of the thyroid and carcinoma of the prostate. Patients with malignancies causing ectopic hypersecretion of ACTH, with or without CRF, do not

TABLE 7. Sources of Ectopic ACTH in 100 Cases

Tumor	Number
Carcinoma of lung	52
Carcinoma of pancreas (including carcinoid)	11
Thymoma	11
Benign bronchial adenoma (including carcinoid)	5
Pheochromocytoma	3
Carcinoma of thyroid	2
Carcinoma of liver	2
Carcinoma of prostate	2
Carcinoma of ovary	2
Undifferentiated carcinoma of mediastinum	2
Carcinoma of breast	1
Carcinoma of parotid gland	1
Carcinoma of esophagus	1
Paraganglioma	1
Ganglioma	1
Primary site uncertain	3

usually appear cushingoid, but present with signs of advanced malignancy such as weakness and weight loss. A severe metabolic alkalosis with hypokalemia is frequently present. A presumptive diagnosis of ectopic ACTH hypersecretion is made on the basis of (1) increased plasma cortisol levels, (2) increased urinary levels of 17-OHCS and 17-ketosteroids (17-KS) that fail to be suppressed after administration of dexamethasone, and (3) increased plasma ACTH. Treatment consists of removal of the primary lesion. With unresectable primary lesions or recurrences, debulking of the primary lesion with or without bilateral adrenalectomy may provide palliation. In some patients, metyrapone, aminoglutethimide, and mitotane (o, p'DDD) have been used to suppress production of corticosteroid.

ADRENOCORTICAL CARCINOMA. This is a rare but aggressive malignancy commonly presenting in the third to fifth decades of life. Women are affected twice as frequently as men. Approximately 60 per cent of these tumors synthesize bioactive steroids, and these patients may present with hypercortisolism, hyperaldosteronism, virilization or feminization, or various combinations of these syndromes. Nonfunctioning adrenocortical carcinomas present most commonly with abdominal pain, increased girth, weight loss, weakness, anorexia, nausea and headache. Approximately half of patients have a palpable abdominal mass, and 25 per cent have hepatomegaly. In 138 cases reviewed by Hutter and Kayhoe,[105] the right adrenal was as frequently the site of origin as the left. Spread to local structures (peritoneum, retroperitoneal space, lymph nodes) was evident in 65 per cent. Although there are exceptions, any adrenal neoplasm in excess of 50 gm. should be considered malignant.[97,117,140] Among patients with Cushing's syndrome, virilization and elevated levels of 17-KS and dehydroepiandrosterone-sulfate (DHEA-S) in the urine suggest the presence of carcinoma. Among tumors of the adrenal cortex found incidentally on CT scan obtained for other reasons, carcinoma is suggested by tumor diameter greater than 6 cm.[97,117,140] The management of these so-called "incidentalomas" is discussed below.

TREATMENT OF CUSHING'S SYNDROME. In the past 40 years, treatment of Cushing's syndrome has focused increasingly on removing the source of cortisol excess, whether a primary adrenal process or secondary to lesions in the pituitary-hypothalamic axis. Management of lesions arising in the hypothalamus-pituitary and producing corticotropin excess has been discussed previously. The transsphenoidal approach, used initially by Harvey Cushing but later abandoned in favor of the transfrontal approach, is again the preferred management for pituitary lesions 1 cm. or less in diameter. It is also the preferred approach when laboratory testing and absence of other adrenal or ectopic foci suggest the pituitary as a source of the stimulus to cortisol excess. Secretion of other pituitary hormones can be preserved if this approach is used and if the tumor has not replaced the whole sella volume. Transfrontal approaches are used for tumors invading structures outside the sella (see the previous section on the pituitary). Radiation and pharmaceutic approaches to pituitary ablation (cyproheptidine) have been used with some objective responses in patients with unresectable disease.

Formerly, bilateral adrenalectomy was performed in patients with pituitary lesions causing bilateral adrenocortical hypertrophy and hypercortisolism. Bilateral adrenalectomy is now rarely practiced as primary therapy for Cushing's disease. Adrenalectomy may be indicated for patients who fail to undergo remission after hypophysectomy. It may also be preferred in patients with severe forms of the disease as the surest means of reducing cortisol production. This operation has a 5 to 10 per cent perioperative mortality and morbidity and a serious long-term mortality.[117,144] Patients require lifetime replacement of glucocorticoid and mineralocorticoid. Some authors have advocated bilateral adrenalectomy and heterotopic autotransplantation of adrenocortical tissue.[71,94] Theoretically, recurrent disease could be treated by resecting portions of the implant.

Medical approaches to blocking cortisol production by the adrenal gland include agents such as metyrapone, mitotane, aminoglutethimide, and ketoconazole.[38,111,141] Metyrapone, as noted previously, blocks 11β-hydroxylation and reduces cortisol and corticosterone levels in the plasma. ACTH hypersecretion can override the effects of metyrapone, however, and metyrapone is best used in combination with other agents. The required daily doses of metyrapone may be as high as 4000 mg. per day. Gastrointestinal disturbances and accumulation of androgen with hirsutism are the major side effects. Mitotane selectively and reversibly destroys the zona fasciculata and reticularis, but not the zona glomerulosa.[111] Doses of 2 to 6 gm. per day lower circulating cortisol levels after several weeks. The drug is not appropriate if rapid reductions in cortisol are the goal of therapy. Side effects include nausea, ataxia, and other CNS disturbances. Aminoglutethimide inhibits conversion of cholesterol to pregnenolone, thus diminishing production of all adrenocortical hormones. Side effects of this latter drug include gastrointestinal disturbance, skin rash, and hypnotic effects. Combination of aminoglutethimide and metyrapone may offer long-term control of corticosteroid synthesis with minimization of side effects.[38] Ketoconazole inhibits steroid formation through several arms of the biosynthetic pathway.[141] It is emphasized that these latter pharmacologic approaches are used for short-term reduction of cortisol levels prior to or after surgical therapy fails to produce a response. They are only rarely indicated as primary therapy in Cushing's disease.

The primary approach to lesions arising in the adrenal gland requires removal of the affected gland. Adrenal adenomas are cured by adrenalectomy.[223] Adrenocortical carcinomas are frequently inoperable but may be resected in approximately 25 to 35 per cent of patients.[22,40,97] Hypercortisolemia occurs along or in combination with other syndromes in approximately 50 to 60 per cent of patients.[117] In cases not amenable to resection or in patients with recurrence of Cushing's syndrome due to adrenocortical carcinoma, mitotane is a first-line therapy. Clinical responses with decreased cortisol production and tumor size may be achieved in as many as 35 per cent of patients treated with mitotane, but lasting remission is nearly unknown.[117] Symptoms of cortisol excess may be treated with aminoglutethimide, metyrapone, mitotane, ketoconazole, or combinations of these agents.

A rare cause of Cushing's syndrome, nodular adrenal hyperplasia or dysplasia, has been recognized with increasing frequency.[108,131] This entity is distinguished as a primary adrenal process by the absence of cortisol suppression by dexamethasone. The condition is bilateral and is cured only by bilateral adrenalectomy. Pharmacologic approaches with adrenolytic agents such as mitotane or agents interfering with cortisol production are not presently recommended.[108,131]

CUSHING'S SYNDROME IN CHILDREN. The most common cause of hypercortisolism in children is adrenocortical neoplasia. Girls are affected three times as often as boys; and in patients younger than 15 years of age, the majority of lesions are malignant. Cushing's disease is relatively uncommon in children, and the ectopic production of ACTH from malignant neoplasms is rare.

As in adults, the predominant feature of Cushing's syndrome in children is obesity. However, reduced growth velocity in association with obesity in children provides an important clue to cortisol excess, because exogenous obesity causes accelerated rates of growth in children. Striae, plethora, headaches, hypertension, ecchymoses, osteoporosis, hypercalciuria, and impaired carbohydrate tolerance are also present. Virilization associated with hirsutism and acne is a frequent finding.

The treatment of choice for a child with adrenocortical neoplasm is surgical resection. Children with Cushing's disease may be managed by transsphenoidal resection of the microadenoma. Although pituitary irradiation is frequently beneficial, some endocrinologists have expressed concern regarding the long-term effects of irradiation in children.

Recently, Thomas and associates[217] reviewed 18 children ranging in age from 18 months to 18 years with Cushing's syndrome. Eight patients had adrenal neoplasms, including five adenomas and three carcinomas. One patient with adrenal carcinoma died of recurrent disease, but the other two were well 11 and 20 years after adrenalectomy. Eight other patients underwent bilateral adrenalectomy for hypercortisolism. Complications of adrenalectomy were common in this group; five of six who reached adult stature were significantly stunted, and four of six who had Cushing's disease developed Nelson's syndrome (see later discussion) at 2, 6, 10, and 12 years after surgical resection.

COMPLICATIONS OF BILATERAL ADRENALECTOMY: NELSON'S SYNDROME. Nelson and associates[162] described a patient who developed a pituitary tumor 3 years after bilateral adrenalectomy for Cushing's disease. The patient had progressively increasing skin pigmentation, amenorrhea, and visual field disturbances due to a functioning pituitary tumor. High concentrations of ACTH were demonstrated in plasma by bioassay. This phenomenon, termed Nelson's syndrome, occurs in approximately 10 per cent of patients who have undergone bilateral adrenalectomy for Cushing's disease. It has subsequently been confirmed by radioimmunoassay that high concentrations of ACTH and melanocyte-stimulating hormone (MSH) are present. Moore and associates[158] reviewed 120 patients with Cushing's disease who had been treated by bilateral adrenalectomy 2 to 20 years previously. Nine patients (8 per cent) developed this complication. Manolas and associates[144] reported 74 patients treated for pituitary-dependent Cushing's disease by total or near total adrenalectomy. Close long-term follow-up suggested that almost 50 per cent of patients might progress to Nelson's syndrome. Combined approaches using surgical therapy and/or radiation were successful in selected patients, but usually these tumors tended to be insensitive to radiation and to recur locally after transsphenoidal resection.

Conn's Syndrome (Hyperaldosteronism)

In 1955, Conn[41] described a 34-year-old woman who for 7 years had experienced generalized weakness and hypertension. She excreted approximately 4 liters of urine per day, and her plasma electrolyte levels included a depressed potassium level and elevated sodium and bicarbonate levels. Urinary 17-KS and 17-OHCS levels were normal. Exploration of the abdomen revealed an adenoma arising in the cortex of the right adrenal. All metabolic abnormalities corrected within 2½ weeks after operation, and the patient's blood pressure normalized. Conn hypothesized that these abnormalities were due to primary hypersecretion of aldosterone by the adenoma. Two years later, when assays for the hormone were available, this hypothesis was confirmed when stored urine samples from this patient were found to contain levels of the hormone 10- to 20-fold greater than normal.

PRIMARY HYPERALDOSTERONISM (LOW-RENIN HYPERALDOSTERONISM). In relatively unselected series[88] of patients with hypertension, surgically correctable forms (renovascular hypertension, endocrine causes, coarctation, etc.) comprise approximately 5 to 10 per cent of cases. Primary hyperaldosteronism, which suppresses endogenous renin production, has been observed in approximately 0.1 to 0.4 per cent of these unselected cases and in 1 to 2 per cent of patients with diastolic hypertension.[37] Curiously, as many as 20 per cent of patients with essential hypertension may have suppressed levels of plasma renin; thus, low plasma renins are necessary but not sufficient to make the diagnosis of primary hyperaldosteronism.

Signs and symptoms of low-renin hyperaldosteronism are mild and nonspecific. Grant and co-workers[82] reported 105 patients with well-documented primary hyperaldosteronism observed at the Mayo Clinic from 1969 to 1981. Headache, fatigue, and nocturia were the most prevalent symptoms; parasthesias and muscle cramps were not uncommon. The hypertension associated with mineralocorticoid excess is often not very severe. Among 80 patients treated at the Cleveland Clinic from 1970 to 1980,[21] diastolic pressures above 120 mm. Hg were recorded in 18 per cent, pressures between 110 to 120 mm. Hg were recorded in 30 per cent, and pressures between 100 and 110 mm. Hg were recorded in 42 per cent. Ten per cent of patients had diastolic pressures consistently below 100 mm. Hg. Significant retinopathy of hypertension is observed in less than

10 per cent of cases,[82] and the syndrome of malignant hypertension is rare.

Laboratory evaluations reveal hypokalemia (<3.5 mEq. per liter) in 75 per cent or more of patients not currently taking diuretic or other hypokalemic agents.[21,82,233] Conversely, it has been suggested that as many as 40 per cent of patients with hypertension and otherwise unexplained hypokalemia may have primary hyperaldosteronism.[123] Additional suggestive indicators include increased urinary K^+ excretion (more than 30 to 40 mEq. per day) and elevated plasma HCO_3 levels (more than 31 mEq. per liter), measured in the absence of diuretic therapy. These initial clinical and laboratory findings should suggest the possibility of primary hyperaldosteronism and can be followed by more definitive evaluations.

On the basis of measurements of plasma and urinary aldosterone and plasma renin levels obtained under controlled conditions, primary aldosteronism may be reliably diagnosed or excluded (Fig. 18).[238] Before these studies are performed, all medications should be discontinued for at least 2 weeks, estrogens and spironolactone for 6 weeks. For detection of hypokalemia and inappropriately elevated urinary K^+ excretion, the patient receives a high-Na^+ diet for 5 days before urine collections are begun. The 24-hour urinary excretions of aldosterone estimates endogenous production of the hormone and correlates inversely with urinary Na^+ excretion. Subjects with primary hyperaldosteronism do not demonstrate suppressibility after 5 days on a high-sodium diet. Severe hypokalemia, however, can suppress aldosterone production in some patients and these evaluations should be conducted following replacement of plasma K^+ levels to at least 3 mEq. per liter.

Intravenous saline infusions have also been used for establishing the diagnosis of primary aldosteronism. After several days of low-Na^+ diet (120 to 150 mEq. per day), 2 liters of normal saline are infused intravenously over 4 hours while the

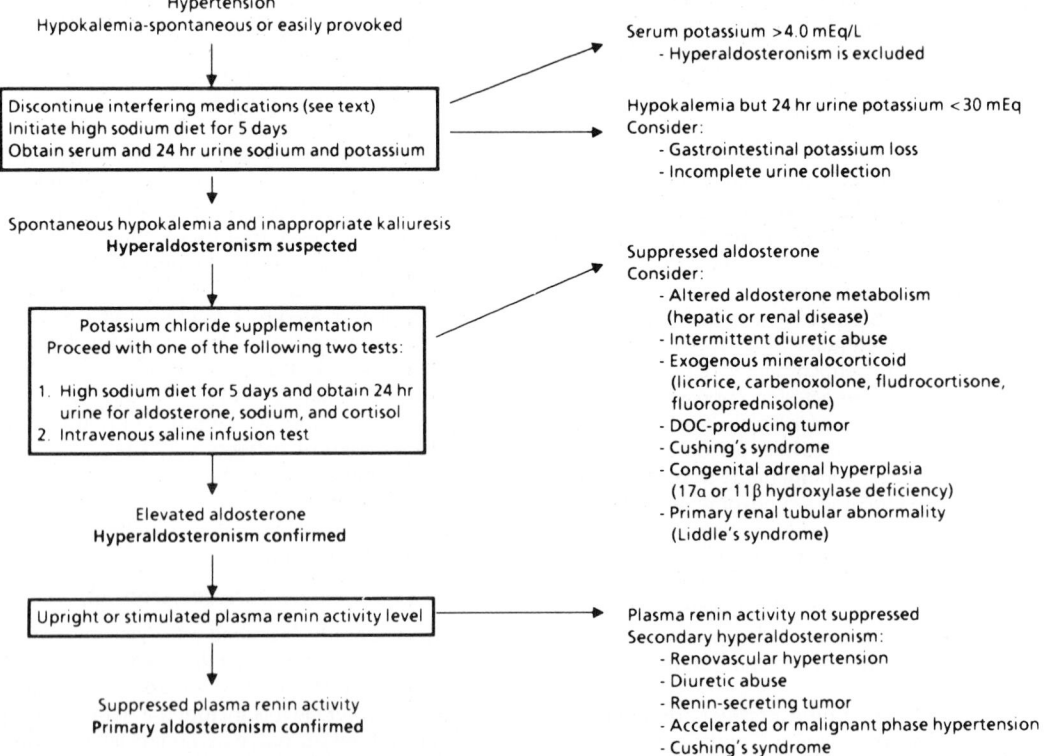

Figure 18. Algorithm for the diagnostic confirmation of primary aldosteronism. Details are discussed in the text. (Modified from Young, W. F., and Klee, G. C.: Primary aldosteronism. Endocrinol. Metab. Clin. North Am., 17:367, 1988.)

TABLE 8. Causes of Primary Aldosteronism

Adrenocortical adenoma
Bilateral adrenocortical hyperplasia (idiopathic aldosteronism or pseudoprimary aldosteronism)
Glucocorticoid-suppressible hyperaldosteronism
Adrenocortical carcinoma
Ovarian neoplasm producing excess aldosterone

patient is supine. In patients with primary hyperaldosteronism, plasma aldosterone does not decrease to levels below 10 ng. per ml., as they do in normal subjects undergoing the infusion. Measurements of 24-hour urinary excretion of aldosterone, as described above, provides almost 100 per cent sensitivity and above 90 per cent specificity in distinguishing patients with hyperaldosteronism from those with essential hypertension.[21,123,233,238] Measurements of plasma aldosterone suppressibility following saline infusion do not appear to be nearly as reliable in all forms of primary aldosteronism.[21,123,233,238]

The differential diagnosis of primary or low renin hyperaldosteronism includes five conditions (Table 8). Identification of the specific lesion involved is important, since adrenalectomy is indicated in some settings, whereas medical therapy may be more appropriate in others. An algorithm for distinguishing, by laboratory testing and computed tomography, these possibilities is depicted in Figure 19.

Approximately 80 per cent of cases are attributable to a solitary, unilateral adrenocortical adenoma (APA) curable by surgical excision. Fifteen percent of cases are associated with bilateral adrenocortical hyperplasia (IHA), which is cured perhaps 20 per cent of the time by surgical approaches, including bilateral adrenalectomy.[204] Hyperaldosteronism suppressible by administration of dexamethasone has an unknown etiology, is frequently familial, and is managed by administration of corticosteroids. Adrenocortical carcinomas producing aldosterone are also quite rare and are managed by surgical removal or debulk-

ing followed by chemotherapy. Ectopic production of aldosterone by ovarian neoplasms has also been reported and is amenable to surgical therapy followed by chemotherapy. Thus, the primary consideration in most cases of primary aldosteronism is to distinguish between APA and IHA lesions.

Two laboratory evaluations are useful in this regard. First, blood samples of aldosterone, cortisol, renin activity, and K^+ are collected at 8:00 A.M. on a morning following several days on a high-salt diet. The initial sample at 8:00 A.M. is collected after the patient has been recumbent overnight, and similar samples are collected 4 hours later, after the patient has been upright. Patients with APA demonstrate a diurnal variation in aldosterone levels, which is unaffected by standing erect. IHA is more sensitive to small changes in angiotensin II, and aldosterone is elevated by at least 33 per cent. If the physiologic nadir of circulating cortisol levels is not observed at 8:00 A.M., the test may not be valid.[204] Levels of 18-hydroxycorticosterone in the serum have also been useful in distinguishing these entities: patients with APA usually have supine 8:00 A.M. levels greater than 100 ng. per 100 ml., whereas those with IHA have levels less than 100 ng. per 100 ml. Each of these tests has an accuracy of more than 80 per cent in diagnosis of APA; it is unclear whether the accuracy of diagnosis improves with the combination of the two tests.

To these functional studies, imaging by CT, MRI, and NP-59 radionuclide scans may add definitive information. CT and MRI can resolve lesions within the adrenal or ovary as small as 1 cm. in diameter. They are usually reliable in distinguishing unilateral adenomas from bilateral nodules characteristic of hyperplasia. Functional lesions larger than 3 cm. must be suspected of harboring carcinoma. As is discussed in more detail, it is important to remember that approximately 1 to 2 per cent of body CT scans detect an incidental nonfunctioning adrenal lesion. The finding of a unilateral mass by CT scan in a patient with primary hyperaldosteronism does not by itself confirm a diagnosis of APA.

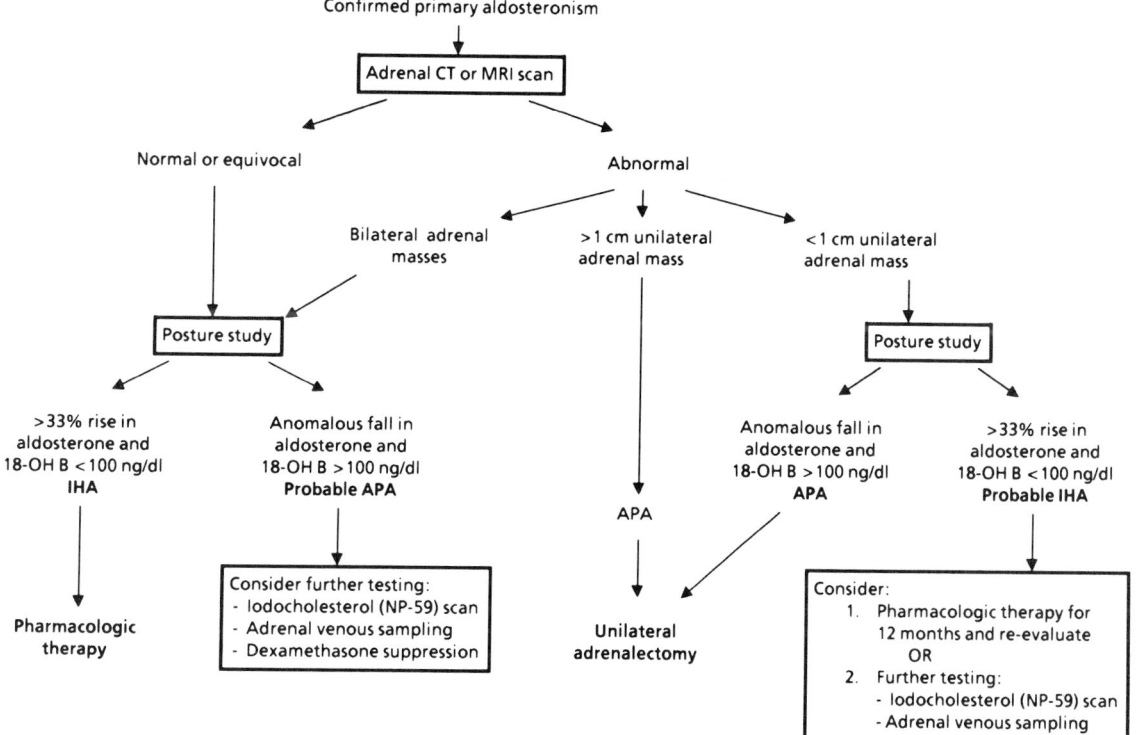

Figure 19. Algorithm for the diagnostic differentiation between aldosterone-producing adrenocortical adenoma (APA) and aldosterone-producing, idiopathic nodular hyperplasia of the adrenal cortex (IHA). The details are discussed in the text. 18-OH B, 18 hydroxycorticosterone; CT, computerized tomography; MRI, magnetic resonance imaging. (From Young, W. F., and Klee, G. C.: Primary aldosteronism. Endocrinol. Metab. Clin. North Am., *17*:367, 1988.)

NP-59 ([6β-^{131}I] iodomethyl-19-norcholesterol) scanning also distinguishes APA and IHA. Pretreatment with dexamethasone suppresses ACTH, and Lugol's iodine is also necessary to suppress thyroid uptake of the tracer. NP-59 uptake 3 to 5 days after injection is unilateral in APA and bilateral in IHA. If the abdominal CT has not provided evidence of adrenal abnormalities, however, the test is usually not helpful.

When doubts concerning unilateral or bilateral disease arise, selective sampling of adrenal vein effluents for aldosterone may be performed. The study is optimally performed during continuous intravenous infusion of ACTH. The ratio of aldosterone to cortisol from the affected side versus that from the contralateral side should be greater than 4 : 1 for a diagnosis of APA. In IHA, the ratio is generally less than 4. This test is technically difficult, and it may not be possible to obtain an adequate study in 25 per cent of patients.

MANAGEMENT OF PRIMARY HYPERALDOSTERONISM. In patients with adrenocortical adenomas, removal of the adrenal gland leads to cure or substantial improvement in over 90 per cent of patients.[7,23,204] Normokalemia is achieved in nearly all cases. Preoperatively, spironolactone and potassium are given to replete K$^+$ stores. Side effects of spironolactone include gynecomastia, impotence, gastric distress, and lassitude. Amiloride, a K$^+$-sparing diuretic, may be substituted if the side effects of spironolactone are not tolerated. Administration of spironolactone to individuals with primary hyperaldosteronism predicts outcome after operation. Brown and associates[23] administered 32 patients with this disorder 50 to 400 mg. of spironolactone daily for 4 weeks. Generally, a significant fall in blood pressure with spironolactone predicted a successful outcome after adrenalectomy. Response to adrenalectomy also may be influenced by the duration and severity of the hypertension and by the presence of histologic changes in the kidney.[154,233]

The preferred surgical technique for removal of an adrenal aldosteronoma involves a posterior approach. Morbidity and mortality are almost negligible.[7,204] Aldosterone-producing carcinomas are frequently too large to permit a posterior approach. Abdominal approaches are preferred for carcinoma, since they permit assessment of local extension and metastasis to the liver and other abdominal sites. Surgical therapy for glucocorticoid-suppressible forms is unnecessary. For idiopathic, bilateral nodular hyperplasia, surgical therapy is not beneficial in more than 20 or 30 per cent of cases. Medical management is preferred in IHA associated with aldosterone excess.

Medical therapy for glucocorticoid-suppressible forms includes dexamethasone, 0.5 to 1.0 mg. per day. Because Cushing's syndrome may follow this single drug regimen, combinations of spironolactone, triamterene, or other K$^+$-sparing diuretic regimens may be helpful in reducing corticosteroid requirements. Medical therapy for aldosterone-producing carcinomas includes K$^+$-sparing diuretic regimens. In addition, mitotane (2 to 6 gm. daily) is employed for its adrenolytic effects, with an overall response rate of 45 per cent.[40,97,117,220] Perioperative and postoperative corticosteroid and mineralocorticoid replacements are mandatory.

Additional medicines which may be useful in ameliorating effects of aldosterone excess include calcium-channel blockers such as nifedipine, which reduces blood pressure and plasma aldosterone in patients with APA or IHA. Angiotensin-converting enzyme inhibitors are useful in patients with IHA, but not APA, for reasons discussed above. Inhibitors of steroid production such as trilostane, aminoglutethimide, and ketoconazole are probably not as useful in patients with hyperaldosteronism as in those with certain forms of hypercortisolism.

The Adrenogenital Syndromes

These conditions arise from a deficiency of one or several of the enzymes necessary for synthesis of cortisol (Table 9). With diminished circulating levels of cortisol, ACTH production increases, stimulating hyperplasia of the adrenal cortex and the production of cortisol precursors. Shunting of these precursors into pathways for synthesis of androstenedione and testosterone leads to the associated virilizing signs and symptoms. In males, clinical manifestations of these disorders are not present at birth. By age 2 or 3, there may be hypertrophy of the phallus, of the muscle mass, and increase in body hair. In females, the inappropriately elevated androgen levels lead to hypertrophy of the clitoris, fusion of the labioscrotal folds, and a urogenital sinus that may appear as a phallic urethra. Internal female organs (ovaries, fallopian tubes, uterus) are not influenced by androgens and develop normally. With correction of the external anomalies and control of the endocrine defect, these females can ultimately bear children.[234] It is crucial to recognize this disease early in life and not rear the child psychosocially as a male. In females, this syndrome is classified under pseudohermaphroditism, and five grades of the disorder have been described.[176]

Postnatally, these disorders are characterized by rapid somatic growth, advanced bone age, early closure of epiphyses, and short stature. Males continue to have accelerated patterns of growth of body hair and secondary sexual attributes. Females may develop polycystic ovaries and irregular menses. Males may have alterations in fertility as well. Hyperpigmentation may occur from high levels of circulating fragments of proopiomelanocortin.

21-HYDROXYLASE DEFICIENCY. Most cases (94 per cent) of adrenogenital syndrome are attributable to a 21-hydroxylase deficiency in the steroidogenesis pathway, and the incidence in live births in the general white population varies between 1 in 5000 to 1 in 15,000. A much higher incidence (approximately 1 in 700) has been noted in certain Alaskan Eskimo populations. With this deficiency, progesterone and 17-hydroxyprogesterone cannot be converted to 11-deoxycorticosterone and 11-deoxycortisol, respectively. Levels of cortisol and aldosterone are decreased. Two forms are recognized, involving partial or complete absence of the enzyme. The complete form is characterized by androgen excess at birth, salt-wasting in the urine and stool, diarrhea, hypovolemia, hyponatremia, hyperkalemia, and hyperpigmentation. The partial form is characterized by virilization only, at birth or perhaps not appearing until late childhood or puberty. Because the defect is only partial, increased levels of ACTH may be capable of driving cortisol and aldosterone production into normal ranges. Thus, salt-wasting and hypovolemia may be mild or absent, and hyperpigmentation may also be mild.

Laboratory diagnosis of this deficiency is straightforward. Untreated patients with 21-hydroxylase deficiency may present with minimal or marked deficiencies in plasma cortisol and in 24-hour free urinary cortisol excretion. The most characteristic abnormality is elevation of 17-hydroxyprogesterone levels in the plasma and urine. Samples of blood should be obtained at 8:00 A.M. and 1 hour after infusions of ACTH or cosyntropin (ACTH 1–24). Complete forms of the disorder are distinguished by comparing baseline and stimulated levels of 17-hydroxyprogesterone.[234] Partial forms are difficult to distinguish from complete forms based on this test alone. However, salt-wasting forms can be distinguished by diminished aldosterone production and plasma and urinary electrolyte abnormalities.

Therapy consists of replacement of glucocorticoid and mineralocorticoid hormones. Adequacy of therapy is documented by correction of urinary 17-hydroxyprogesterone hyperexcretion. Female patients with ambiguity of the genitalia may require surgical correction (vaginoplasty and/or clitoral recession). These procedures are best undertaken early, between the second and eighteenth months of life.

Genetic studies[153,234] have suggested that various forms of 21-hydroxylase deficiency are attributable to a single gene locus, which appears closely linked to the HLA major histocompatability locus located on the short arm of chromosome 6. It is possible to predict which members of the patient's family have

TABLE 9. Defects of Adrenal Steroidogenesis*

Deficiency	Syndrome	Ambiguous Genitalia	Postnatal Virilization	Salt Metabolism	Steroids Increased	Steroids Decreased	Enzyme	Chromosome	Frequency†
Cholesterol desmolase	Lipoid hyperplasia	Males	No	Salt-wasting	None	All	P450scc	15	Rare
3β-OH-steroid dehydrogenase	Classic	Males and ? females	Yes	±Salt-wasting	DHEA, 17-OH-pregnenolone	Aldo, cortisol, T	3β-OH-steroid dehydrogenase	?	Rare
	Nonclassic	No	Yes	Normal	DHEA, 17-OH-pregnenolone	—	3β-OH-steroid dehydrogenase	?	? Frequent
17-Hydroxylase	—	Males	No	Hypertension	DOC, corticosterone	Cortisol, T	P450c17	10	Rare
17,20-Lyase	—	Males	No	Normal	—	DHEA, T, androstenedione	P450c17	10	Rare
21-Hydroxylase	Salt-wasting	Females	Yes	Salt-wasting	17-OHP, androstenedione	Aldo, cortisol	P450c21	6p (HLA)	1/10,000
	Simple virilizing	Females	Yes	Normal	17-OHP, androstenedione	Cortisol	P450c21	6p (HLA)	1/20,000
	Nonclassic	No	Yes	Normal	17-OHP, androstenedione	—	P450c21	6p (HLA)	0.1–1% (3% in European Jews)
11-Hydroxylase	Classic	Females	Yes	Hypertension	DOC, 11-deoxycortisol	Cortisol, ±aldo	P450c11	8q	1/100,000
	Nonclassic	No	Yes	Normal	11-deoxycortisol, ±DOC	—	P450c11	8q	? Frequent
Corticosterone methyl oxidase II	—	No	No	Salt-wasting	18-OH-corticosterone	Aldo	P450c11	8q	Rare (except in Iranian Jews)

*Deficiency of 17,20-lyase is expressed in the gonads but is included here because it apparently involves the same gene as 17-hydroxylase deficiency.
†"Rare" denotes a syndrome accounting for less than 1 percent of reported cases of congenital adrenal hyperplasia, which has an overall frequency of about 1 in 5000 births. "? Frequent" syndromes may occur at frequencies similar to that of nonclassic 21-hydroxylase deficiency, but prevalence data are not available.
DHEA, dehydroepiandrosterone; DOC, deoxycorticosterone; 17-OHP, 17-hydroxyprogesterone; Aldo, aldosterone; T, testosterone.
From White, P. C., New, M. I., and DuPont, B.: Congenital adrenal hyperplasia. N. Engl. J. Med., 316:1580, 1987.

the allele as a heterozygote with a normal allele. This can be performed by measuring urinary excretion of 17-hydroxyprogesterone as compared to excretion of free cortisol. It appears that heterozygotes who have the gene for salt-wasting forms may demonstrate a higher ratio than do normal individuals with virilizing forms only. An equally important implication of this technology is the feasibility of prenatal diagnosis of 21-hydroxylase deficiency through amniocentesis. Administration of corticosteroids to the mother can suppress the fetal hypothalamic-pituitary-adrenal axis and prevent virilization of the female fetus.[153,234] Chorionic villous sampling can also provide material for genetic analysis before the end of the first trimester.[234]

11β-HYDROXYLASE DEFICIENCY. This deficiency constitutes about 5 per cent of cases of congenital adrenal hyperplasia. Its incidence in the white population is approximately 1:100,000 live births. In this disorder, 11-deoxycorticosterone and 11-deoxycortisol cannot be converted to corticosterone or cortisol. As with 21-hydroxylase deficiency, cortisol levels are low. The mineralocorticoid properties of the large quantities of 11-deoxycorticosterone, however, may not only compensate for the lack of aldosterone but also lead to hypertension and hypokalemia. Virilization and hyperpigmentation are present, as they are in cases of 21-hydroxylase deficiency. Deficiency of 11β-hydroxylase is diagnosed by increased levels of urinary excretion of 17-hydroxyprogesterone, androgens (androstenedione, testosterone), and 17-ketosteroids. Treatment includes administration of glucocorticoids and surgical correction of external genitalia in affected female infants. The 11β-hydroxylase gene is not HLA-linked and is present on the long arm of chromosome 8. Prenatal diagnosis and corticosteroid therapy to the mother during pregnancy is possible.[153,234]

3-β-HYDROXYDEHYDROGENASE. This deficiency affects pathways of glucocorticoid, mineralocorticoid, and androgen synthesis; 17-hydroxypregnenolone and dehydroepiandrosterone, a weak androgen, accumulate. Females are mildly virilized. Males are incompletely virilized and are born with hypospadias. Marked salt-wasting is usually present, and infants often do not survive the first days of life. The responsible gene has not yet been mapped.

17-HYDROXYLASE DEFICIENCY. Also rare, this deficiency leads to decreased cortisol production and decreased androgen production. Aldosterone synthesis is not directly affected, and the rise in ACTH due to decreased cortisol can lead to accelerated rates of synthesis of aldosterone and deoxycorticosterone. Thus, hypertension and hypokalemia are prominent in patients with this deficiency, who present as incompletely masculinized males or infertile females. The responsible gene has not yet been mapped. Treatment, again, involves corticosteroid and androgen replacement.

CONGENITAL ADRENAL LIPOID HYPERPLASIA. This is due to a deficiency of cholesterol desmolase (side-chain cleaving enzyme). All adrenal and gonadal synthetic pathways for steroid biosynthesis are inhibited, and infants die of adrenal insufficiency despite replacement therapy. The gene for this disorder has been attributed to chromosome 15.

Adrenal Neoplasms Associated with Excess Sex Steroids

In children, premature secretion of sex steroids may produce the syndrome of sexual precocity. If the hormone secreted in excess is appropriate for the child's sex, the condition is called *isosexual precocity*; if inappropriate, it is termed *heterosexual precocity*. One type of sexual precocity follows excess gonadotropin secretion, as a result of CNS lesions or secondary to hepatomas or other tumors. In the second type, the sex steroids are produced by gonadal or adrenal tumors (Table 10). Testicular and ovarian neoplasms that secrete increased quantities of androgens or estrogens are usually palpable by the time sexual precocity is evident.

ADRENAL VIRILIZING TUMORS. Adrenal virilizing tumors

TABLE 10. Causes of Sexual Precocity*

Cause	Females (No.)	Males (No.)
Increased gonadotropin levels		
Cerebral	71	82
Idiopathic	507	126
Ectopic	4	1
Increased sex steroid levels		
Adrenal: virilizing	272†	69
Adrenal: feminizing	8	1
Ovarian	65	0
Testicular	0	9
Total	927	288

*Five collected series.
†Predominantly virilizing congenital adrenal hyperplasia.

are twice as common in females as in males; however, they rarely present in the first year of life. In young females, clitoral enlargement or the development of pubic hair may occur. Unlike females with congenital adrenal hyperplasia, no labial fusion is seen. In males, hirsutism and macrogenitosomia praecox develop, but the testes remain small and there may be inhibition of spermatogenesis. Affected children are well developed and may experience growth spurts with androgen excess. Early epiphyseal closure, however, causes short stature in adulthood. The development of an adrenal virilizing tumor in adult females causes hirsutism and masculinization. There may be a decrease in the size of the breasts and increased libido. Such tumors in the male may go unnoticed until signs and symptoms from tumor enlargement or distant metastases are detected.

These tumors secrete inordinately large amounts of the androgen precursor dehydroepiandrosterone, which can be measured either directly in plasma or in urine as a 17-ketosteroid. Characteristically, plasma levels of this hormone are not suppressed by dexamethasone administration. The treatment of patients with adrenal virilizing tumors is resection of the adrenal gland and the neoplasm, with care being taken not to damage the tumor capsule. Histologically, it may be difficult to determine whether a specific tumor is benign or malignant; the presence of either local invasion or distant metastases makes the diagnosis obvious. These neoplasms grow relatively slowly; however, only 3 of the 8 children reported by Burrington and Stephens[27] were alive 18, 3½, and 2 years after tumor resection. Recurrence of the neoplasm is usually evidenced by return of the signs and symptoms of virilization and by the detection of increased 17-ketosteroids in the urine. Aminoglutethimide or mitotane may be useful in controlling signs and symptoms in patients with metastatic disease.

FEMINIZING ADRENAL TUMORS. Feminizing adrenal neoplasms are extremely rare. In young males, gynecomastia is common but by no means pathognomonic, because it represents a normal physiologic pubertal change in approximately 90 per cent of males. The association in young males of bilateral gynecomastia with rapid growth and advanced bone age should suggest a feminizing adrenal tumor. Usually, urinary secretion of 17-ketosteroids and estrogens is elevated. Of the seven cases of feminizing adrenal tumors in young males reported by Howard and associates,[102] four were thought to be benign and three were diagnosed as carcinomas. Five of the 7 patients were alive with no evidence of recurrence at 14, 10, 5, 1, and 1 year following tumor extirpation. Most of these tumors, however, occur in adult males in the second through the fourth decades of life. Gynecomastia and testicular atrophy are frequently noted, and patients usually complain of impotence.

In young females who develop feminizing adrenal tumors,

TABLE 11. Causes of Addison's Disease

Autoimmune disease (idiopathic)
Tuberculosis
Trauma or surgical resection
Intra-adrenal hemorrhage
    Anticoagulation
    Waterhouse-Friderichsen syndrome secondary to bacterial infection
       (usually meningococcemia or systemic *Pseudomonas* infection)
Fungal infections
    Coccidioidomycosis
    Blastomycosis
    Histoplasmosis
Metastases to the adrenal glands
Prolonged adrenocortical therapy
Congenital adrenocortical unresponsiveness to ACTH
Familial
    Adrenoleukodystrophy

there is precocious puberty with breast enlargement, development of a female escutcheon, and onset of menses. In adult females, the detection of these neoplasms may be more difficult. Biochemically, the diagnosis depends upon the demonstration of elevated urinary levels of estrogens and 17-ketosteroids. Approximately 50 per cent of patients have a palpable abdominal mass at the time of diagnosis. The treatment of choice is surgical resection. Generally, patients with benign adenomas do well and experience a normal survival, whereas the prognosis is poor in patients with adrenal carcinoma.

Adrenocortical Insufficiency and Hypoaldosteronism

In 1855 Thomas Addison[1] described 11 patients with primary adrenal insufficiency, including 5 patients with tuberculous destruction of the adrenal glands. One year later, Brown-Sequard[24] demonstrated that removal of the adrenals from experimental animals uniformly caused death. Until recently, tuberculosis was the most common cause of bilateral cortical adrenal destruction, now designated Addison's disease, and still represents 20 per cent of cases.[163] Although the idiopathic form of Addison's disease is now the most prevalent, increasing numbers of cases are reported in association with tuberculous

and other mycotic infections associated with the human immunodeficiency virus (HIV). Carcinomas, especially those originating in the lung, may cause adrenal insufficiency.[33,181] Although overt adrenal insufficiency is not common, an insidious onset of symptoms and signs of Addison's disease may be present in approximately 20 to 30 per cent of patients with bilateral adrenal metastatic lesions detected by CT scan. These patients are recognized by their abnormally weak responses to stimulation by ACTH.[181] Various causes of Addison's disease are listed in Table 11.

The idiopathic form of Addison's disease is marked by a 2 : 1 predominance of females. The pathologic process of bilateral cortical destruction in this entity follows autoimmune mechanisms, leading to infiltration of the cortex by lymphocytes. Circulating antibodies to the cortex have been identified with this form of Addison's disease. Additional evidence that these patients have a more broad-based disturbance of autoimmune regulation is derived from the observation that patients with Addison's disease may also have higher than expected risks for hypothyroidism, diabetes mellitus, gonadal dysfunction, hypoparathyroidism, and pernicious anemia.[44]

CLINICAL PRESENTATION AND DIAGNOSIS. Addison's disease combines signs and symptoms of deficiencies of glucocorticoid and mineralocorticoid. The diverse clinical manifestations of this disease are outlined in Table 12. Most frequent complaints include fatigue (more than 90 per cent), weight loss (90 per cent), anorexia (85 per cent), nausea and vomiting (65 per cent), abdominal pain (28 per cent), and diarrhea (18 per cent). Hyperpigmentation of skin, especially of palmar creases, is observed in 40 per cent of patients and pigmentation of buccal or tongue mucous membranes in approximately 50 to 60 per cent. Hypertension, temperature disturbance (hyper- or hypothermia), vitiligo, and calcification of the pinnae are much less common signs.

Characteristic laboratory findings include hyponatremia in two thirds, hyperkalemia in half, azotemia in half, and fasting or reactive hypoglycemia in one fifth of patients. Hypercalcemia may also be present. The peripheral blood smear may demonstrate eosinophilia in 15 to 20 per cent of patients. Adrenal calcifications may be visible on plain abdominal radiographs in

TABLE 12. Major Signs and Symptoms of Addison's Disease

Glucocorticoid Deficiency-Related
    Gastrointestinal: anorexia, nausea, vomiting, hypochlorhydria, abdominal pain, weight loss
    Mental: diminished vigor, lethargy, apathy, confusion, psychosis
    Energy metabolism: impaired gluconeogenesis, impaired fat metabolization and utilization, liver glycogen depletion, fasting hypoglycemia
    Cardiovascular-renal: impaired ability to excrete "free water," impaired pressor responses to catecholamines, hypotension
    Pituitary: unrestrained secretion of ACTH and MSH, causing mucocutaneous hyperpigmentation
    Impaired tolerance to stress: any of the above manifestations might become more pronounced during trauma, infection, or fasting
Mineralocorticoid Deficiency-Related
    Inability to conserve sodium
        Decreased extracellular fluid volume
        Weight loss
        Hypovolemia
        Hypotension
        Decreased cardiac size
        Decreased cardiac output
        Decreased renal blood flow
        Prerenal azotemia
        Increased renin production
        Decreased pressor response to catecholamines
        Weakness
        Postural syncope
        Shock
    Impaired renal secretion of potassium and hydrogen ions
        Hyperkalemia
            Cardiac asystole
        Mild acidosis

From Liddle, G. W.: The adrenal cortex. *In* Williams, R. H. (Ed.): Textbook of Endocrinology, 5th ed. Philadelphia, W. B. Saunders Company, 1974, pp. 270–271.

15 per cent. Antibodies to parietal cells, thyroid microsomes, and sex-steroid or corticosteroid-secreting cells are not uncommon.[44]

The most direct test of adrenal insufficiency is the rapid ACTH test, described earlier. False-positive results have been observed with this type of evaluation, and positive tests should be confirmed by the standard, prolonged ACTH infusion test. A high plasma concentration of ACTH (more than 200 pg. per 100 ml.) associated with decreased plasma cortisol (less than 10 μg. per 100 ml.) is diagnostic of Addison's disease in a patient with characteristic symptoms and signs.

TREATMENT AND FOLLOW-UP. Acute adrenocortical insufficiency may arise from cessation of chronic corticosteroid therapy, from severe stress (infection or trauma) in a patient with minimal reserve, or from sudden adrenal hemorrhage, or destruction by infection. In addition, thyroid replacement in a patient with long-standing symptoms of myxedema may also precipitate such a crisis. Signs and symptoms of acute "addisonian crisis" are listed in Table 13. Management of the crisis includes high-dose corticosteroid treatment (hydrocortisone acetate, 100 mg. intravenously every 6 to 8 hours, or dexamethasone, 8 to 12 mg. per day in divided doses). In addition, volume replacement with normal or hypertonic saline and dextrose is essential. A rapid ACTH stimulation test may be performed after baseline plasma ACTH and cortisol samples are drawn in order to establish the diagnosis. Extreme states of hyponatremia should not be corrected too rapidly. Recognition and treatment of the underlying cause, particularly if it is infectious, usually resolves the crisis. CT or MRI scanning may be helpful in identifying hemorrhage within the adrenals.

Chronic adrenal insufficiency requires maintenance corticosteroid and mineralocorticoid therapy. In the average adult, daily doses of 30 to 40 mg. of cortisone acetate or its equivalent is administered in divided doses, along with 0.05 to 0.10 μg. of fluorohydrocortisone. During periods of stress, doses such as those used to treat episodes of crisis may be required. Measurements of pituitary ACTH secretion and adrenal responsiveness are employed for determining whether cortisol deficiency is primary (inability of the adrenal to respond) or secondary (lack of ACTH with normal adrenal responsiveness to exogenous ACTH).

Chronic mineralocorticoid deficiency, isolated from glucocorticoid deficiency, may follow primary alterations of the zona glomerulosa or deficiencies of renin. Hyporeninemic hypoaldosteronism is associated with diabetes, parenchymal renal disease, hypertension, use of cyclo-oxygenase inhibitors, and lead poisoning. Replacement therapy with fluorohydrocortisone

TABLE 13. Symptoms and Signs in Acute Adrenocortical Insufficiency ("Crisis")

Symptom/Signs (Clinical Deterioration Without Obvious Cause)	Prevalence (100%)
Fever	70%
Nausea and vomiting	64%
Abdominal pain	46%
Hypotension	36%
Abdominal distention	32%
Obtundation/lethargy	26%
Hyponatremia	45%
Hyperkalemia	25%

Modified from May, M. E., Vaughan, E. D., Jr., and Carey, R. M.: Adrenocortical insufficiency: Clinical aspects. In Vaughan, E. D., Jr., and Carey, R. M. (Eds.): Adrenal Disorders. Thieme Medical Publishers, Inc., 1989, p. 176.

and follow-up studies of plasma electrolytes are the principles of management.

ADRENAL MEDULLA

PHYSIOLOGY

The cells of the adrenal medulla secrete a number of biologically active amines, including the dihydroxylated phenolic amines: dopamine, norepinephrine, and epinephrine. These compounds, known as catecholamines, are synthesized in the brain, in nerve endings of sympathetic neurons, and in the chromaffin cells of the adrenal medulla, organ of Zuckerkandl, and other extra-adrenal tissues derived from neural crest. The pathway begins with tyrosine, derived either from diet or by endogenous conversion from phenylalanine. Four enzymes are involved: (1) tyrosine hydroxylase, which converts tyrosine to L-dihydroxyphenylalanine (dopa); (2) aromatic L-amino acid decarboxylase, which converts dopa to dopamine; (3) β-hydroxylase, which converts dopamine to L-norepinephrine; and (4) phenylethanolamine N-methyl transferase (PNMT), which completes the transformation to L-epinephrine. PNMT is localized exclusively in cells of the adrenal medulla and the organ of Zuckerkandl. With rare exceptions, epinephrine-secreting tumors arise only in these two tissues.

The conversion of tyrosine to dopa (step 1) requires tetrahydropteridine as a cofactor. This step is rate-limiting for synthesis of catecholamines and its activity is suppressed by excess of catecholamines, especially of norepinephrine. The conversion of dopa to dopamine (step 2) requires pyridoxal phosphate (vitamin B_6) and the conversion of dopamine to L-norepinephrine (step 3) requires oxygen, ascorbic acid (vitamin C), and fumarate. PNMT activity, which completes step 4, transfers the activated methyl group from S-adenosyl methionine (SAM) to the norepinephrine molecule. PNMT does not require cofactors. Steps 1 and 2 occur within the cytoplasm. Dopamine then enters the granulated cytoplasmic vesicles and is converted (step 3) to norepinephrine. Norepinephrine then re-enters the cytoplasm by unknown pathways to be converted by PNMT (step 4) to epinephrine. Approximately 80 per cent of the stored catecholamines in adrenal medulla consists of epinephrine; 20 per cent is norepinephrine; and a minute fraction, dopamine.

Synthesis of catecholamines is regulated by a number of factors. Most important is splanchnic nerve activation, which dramatically increases the rate of catecholamine synthesis in the adrenal medulla. The metabolic milieu greatly influences tyrosine hydroxylase activity: physpholipids, cyclic AMP, ATP, protein kinase, and Mg^{2+} increase the affinity of the enzyme for its cofactor and decrease the effectiveness of catecholamines as inhibitors of step 1. The activity of the final step, involving PNMT, is markedly enhanced in the presence of glucocorticoid, which does not increase the rate of PNMT synthesis, but rather stabilizes the enzyme from degradation.

The presence of cytoplasmic granules in cells of the adrenal medulla and sympathetic nerve endings was first described by Blaschko and Welch.[17] Excitation of these cells stimulates discharge of the granules with release of catecholamines into the circulation. These neurotransmitters profoundly alter the cardiovascular system, smooth and skeletal muscle activity, metabolism, and blood flow within the liver, spleen, lung, brain, and fatty tissues. Endocrine functions of several organs are altered as well. Adrenergic receptors present in the cells of the microcirculation and perhaps parenchymal cells of these organs mediate these effects.

The division between alpha and beta receptors for catecholamines was introduced by Ahlquist in 1948[2] (Table 14). These receptors were distinguished by their relative responsiveness to natural and artificial bioamines: alpha receptors had highest affinity for norepinephrine, less for epinephrine, and least for isoproterenol, whereas beta receptors were most responsive to

TABLE 14. Adrenergic Receptors

Alpha Receptor

		Alpha-2
Agonists	Epinephrine, norepinephrine, phenylephrine, isoproterenol	
Agonist potency	E ≥ NE > PE > I	
Antagonists	Phentolamine, phenoxybenzamine	
Subtypes	Alpha-1	Alpha-2
Selective agonists	Phenylephrine	Clonidine
	Methoxamine	Alpha-methyl-NE
Second messenger	Ca²⁺	cAMP
	Phosphatidylinositol turnover	
Representative responses	Vasoconstriction	Presynaptic NE release
	Intestinal relaxation	Platelet aggregation
	Uterine contraction	
	Pupillary dilatation	
Selective antagonists	Prazosin	Yohimbine

Beta Receptor

		Beta-2
Agonist potency	I > E ≥ NE > PE	
Antagonists	Propranolol, alprenolol, nadolol, timolol	
Subtypes	Beta-1	Beta-2
	(E = NE)	(E >> NE)
Selective agonists	Dobutamine	Metaproterenol
		Albuterol
		Terbutaline
		Isoetharine
Second messenger	cAMP	cAMP
Representative responses	Cardiac stimulation	Bronchodilatation
	Lipolysis	Vasodilation
	Intestinal relaxation	Uterine relaxation
		Presynaptic NE release
Selective antagonists	Metoprolol	
	Atenolol	

I, isoproterenol; E, epinephrine; NE, norepinephrine; PE, phenylephrine.
From Landsberg, L., and Young, J. P.: Catecholamines and the adrenal medulla. *In* Wilson, J. D., and Foster, D. W. (Eds.): Williams' Textbook of Endocrinology. Philadelphia, W. B. Saunders Company, 1985, p. 908.

isoproterenol and least to norepinephrine. In addition, specific antagonists were identified for each receptor class: alpha activities were antagonized by phentolamine and phenoxybenzamine, whereas beta effects were suppressed by propranolol. More recently, two classes of beta receptors have been identified: beta 1, present in cardiac muscle, adipose tissue, and small intestine, and beta 2, present in vascular, tracheal, and uterine smooth muscle, skeletal muscle, and liver. Alpha receptors are now also divided into alpha 1, which cause vasoconstriction, pupillary dilatation, and uterine contractions, and alpha 2, which mediates presynaptic norepinephrine release and platelet aggregation. Classes of receptors responsive to dopamine have also been identified. This catecholamine exerts inotropic and chronotropic effects on cardiac muscle and induces mild peripheral vasoconstriction. Dopamine also elicits dilatation of renal arterioles.

There are three pathways by which secreted catecholamines are removed from the circulation: first, these substances are taken up and retained by postganglionic neurons and sympathetic nerves. They may be recycled or degraded by various enzyme systems. A second mechanism involves nonspecific uptake and degradation in peripheral tissues. Finally, free catecholamines can be excreted in the urine, where they are measurable. Metabolism of catecholamines is mediated by two enzymes (Fig. 20). The first, monamine oxidase (MAO), is present in high concentrations in the liver, kidney, intestine, and stomach. MAO converts epinephrine or norepinephrine to the alcohol, 3,4-dihydroxyphenylglycol (DOPG), or the acid, 3,4-dihydroxymandelic acid (DOMA). The second enzyme, catechol-O-methyl transferase (COMT), transfers an O-methyl group to the meta position. S-adenosyl methionine (SAM) again provides the methyl group for transfer. COMT represents the primary inactivation step for catecholamines. In fact, MAO has

a higher affinity for the O-methylated metabolites as substrates, rather than the native catecholamines themselves. COMT is also found in high concentration in the liver and kidney. When inactivated by MAO and/or COMT, these compounds may be excreted free or as conjugates of glucuronide or sulfate. Thus, enzymatic degradation of catecholamines leads to excretion of normetanephrine, metanephrine, vanillylmandelic acid (VMA), and methoxyhydroxyphenylglycol (MHPG), which are measurable in the urine as well (see Fig. 20).

PHEOCHROMOCYTOMA

Of the surgically correctable causes of hypertension, none has a more variable clinical presentation or more volatile natural history than pheochromocytoma. This unique neoplasm, arising in the adrenal medulla or in certain extra-adrenal sites, takes its name from the Greek words *phaios* and *chroma*, or "dusky color." The term was introduced by Pick,[174] who noted that such tumors stained a deep rust color when exposed to chromium salts. The first description of a pheochromocytoma was by Frankel in 1886.[69] He reported bilateral adrenal tumors at autopsy in an 18-year-old woman who had died suddenly. In 1922, L'abbé and associates[129] reported a 28-year-old woman with paroxysmal hypertension; at autopsy she was found to have a pheochromocytoma. In 1926, Roux[189] successfully resected a pheochromocytoma. Mayo[148] reported the first successful removal of a pheochromocytoma in the United States in 1927. In the early 1950s, von Euler and associates[65,67] demonstrated large quantities of catecholamines in the urine of patients with these tumors. Subsequently, it was demonstrated that VMA and normetanephrine were excreted in the urine along with the parent epinephrine and norepinephrine compounds. Although this tumor occurs rarely, a sufficient experi-

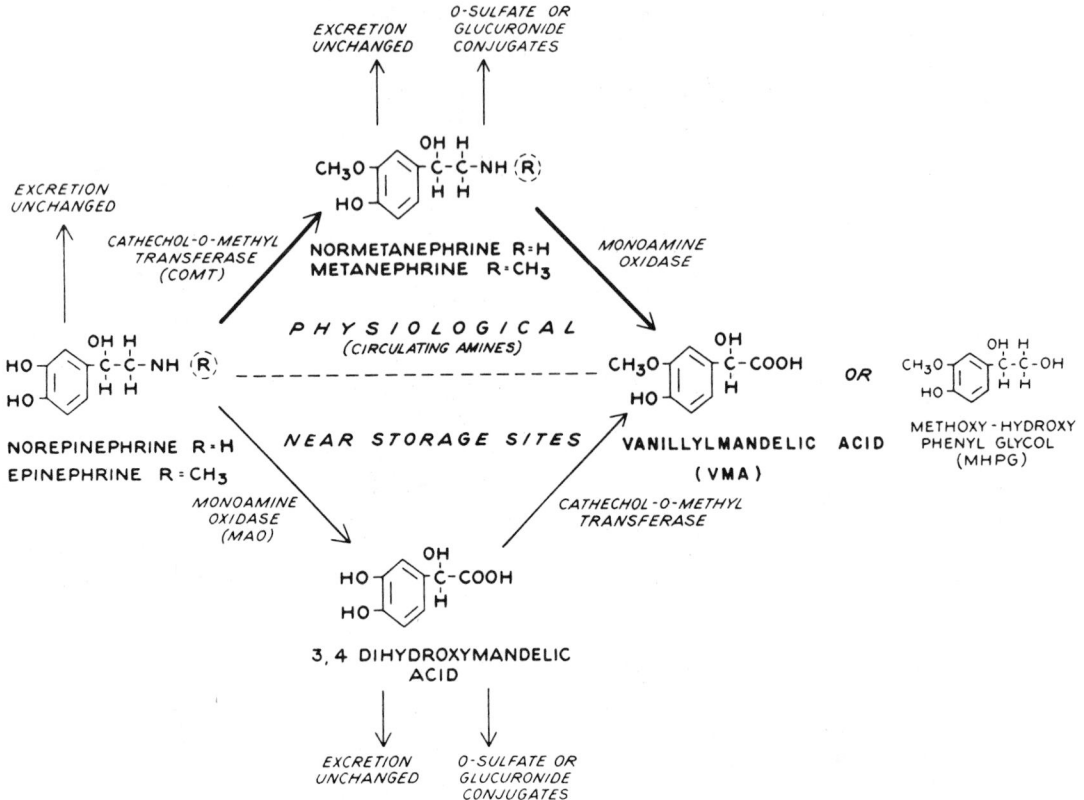

Figure 20. Biochemical pathways for catecholamine metabolism. (From Melmon, K. L.: Catecholamines and the adrenal medulla. *In* Williams, R. H. (Ed.): Textbook of Endocrinology, 6th ed. Philadelphia, W. B. Saunders Company, 1981.)

ence has been accumulated to permit general agreement regarding approaches to its diagnosis, preoperative preparation, and operative management.

Clinical Manifestations

The clinical presentation of a patient with pheochromocytoma is often dramatic. The patient may present in hypertensive crisis, with diaphoresis, headache, and palpitations. A myocardial infarction or stroke may be in evolution. Less spectacular presentations are diabetes or those mimicking hyperthyroidism. These tumors may also be detected during routine evaluation for diastolic hypertension. This is rare: only 0.1 to 0.2 per cent of patients with diastolic hypertension are found to have a pheochromocytoma.[88] These lesions may also be detected during screening studies of patients belonging to kindreds with specific familial syndromes.[29] The tumor occurs in children but is encountered usually in the third to fifth decade; there is no sex predilection.

Although hypertension is the most consistent sign of pheochromocytoma, only half of the patients with this lesion have sustained hypertension.[143,201,224] Paroxysmal hypertension, with or without underlying sustained elevations in blood pressure, has been reported in 50 to 70 per cent of patients. The frequency of paroxysms may vary widely among individuals, but 75 per cent of patients report at least one per week. Most paroxysms continue 15 to 30 minutes; factors that elicit paroxysms can often be identified, including physical exercise, sexual intercourse, micturition, laughing or coughing, even wearing of tight clothing. Foods high in tyramine can elicit increased frequency of paroxysms, including beer, wine, and cheese. Pharmacologic agents that may precipitate hypertensive crises include tyramine, histamine, nicotine, glucagon, succinylcholine, phenothiazines, ACTH, saralasin, and β-adrenergic antagonists such as propranolol.

Other signs and symptoms associated with these lesions are outlined in Table 15. As with hypertension, these accessory symptoms may be persistent or paroxysmal, and all are attributable to the excess of circulating catecholamine. Asymptomatic patients with functioning tumors are rare. Nonfunctioning tumors are also uncommon. Twenty-five per cent of patients

TABLE 15. Symptoms of Pheochromocytoma

	Approximate Percentage	
Symptom*	Paroxysmal (37 Patients)	Persistent (39 Patients)
Headaches (severe)	92	72
Excess sweating (generalized)	65	69
Palpitations ± tachycardia	73	51
Anxiety or nervousness (± fear of impending death; panic)	60	28
Tremulousness	51	26
Pain in chest and/or abdomen (usually epigastric) and or lumbar regions and/or lower abdomen and/or groin	48	28
Nausea ± vomiting	43	26
Weakness, fatigue, prostration	38	15
Weight loss (severe)	14	15
Dyspnea	11	18
Warmth ± heat intolerance	13	15
Visual disturbances	3	21
"Dizziness" or faintness	11	3
Constipation	0	13
Paresthesias or pain in arms	11	0
Bradycardia (noted by patient)	8	3
Grand mal	5	3

*Symptoms presumably due to excess catecholamines and/or hypertension.

From Manger, W. M., and Gifford, R. W.: Pheochromocytoma. New York, Springer-Verlag, 1977, p. 89.

may develop a myocarditis induced by excess circulating catecholamines.[143] In addition, gastrointestinal motility is depressed, leading to severe ileus, obstipation, and sometimes megacolon.[143] It is important to note that sudden death has been reported in patients with known or unsuspected pheochromocytomas who have undergone surgical procedures for other indications.

Conditions Associated with Pheochromocytoma

MULTIPLE ENDOCRINE NEOPLASIA TYPE II (MEN-II). The multiple endocrine neoplasia Type IIa syndrome is characterized by a hereditary, autosomal dominant predisposition to medullary carcinoma of the thyroid (MTC), pheochromocytoma, and parathyroid hyperplasia. Nearly all affected individuals develop MTC, whereas only half develop pheochromocytoma or parathyroid hyperplasia.[29] In these patients, the pheochromocytomas occur bilaterally and often are multiple (Figs. 21 and 22). As with MTC and C-cell hyperplasia, hyperplasia of the adrenal medulla is observed before the appearance of the neoplasm.[29,143] The MEN-IIb syndrome is much less common than MEN-IIa. Affected patients have MTC and pheochromocytoma. In addition, they may develop multiple mucosal neuromas, ganglioneuromatosis, and a characteristic facies and habitus. Patients with MEN-IIb rarely develop hyperparathyroidism. The MEN-IIb syndrome may occur sporadically or be inherited as an autosomal dominant trait. It is imperative that patients with MTC be screened for the presence of pheochromocytoma, especially if there is a family history of either lesion. Approximately 10 per cent of patients with MEN-IIa present with symptoms of pheochromocytoma before those of MTC.[29,143] Relatives of these patients should be screened for associated endocrinopathies even if they are asymptomatic. Screening strategies are more thoroughly discussed in the previous chapter on MEN syndromes.

NEUROECTODERMAL DYSPLASIAS. Neurofibromatosis (von Recklinghausen's disease) occurs in approximately 5 to 10 percent of patients with pheochromocytoma, although less than 1 per cent of patients with von Recklinghausen's disease develop pheochromocytoma. Other neuroectodermal dysplasia syndromes associated with pheochromocytomas include tuberous sclerosis, Sturge-Weber syndrome, and von Hippel-Lindau disease (retinal angiomatosis and hemangioblastoma of the cerebellum or spinal cord). In 1979, Atuk and associates[6] described a kindred of patients with von Hippel-Lindau disease, pheochromocytoma, and hypercalcemia. Curiously, surgical resection of the pheochromocytoma in 10 members of the

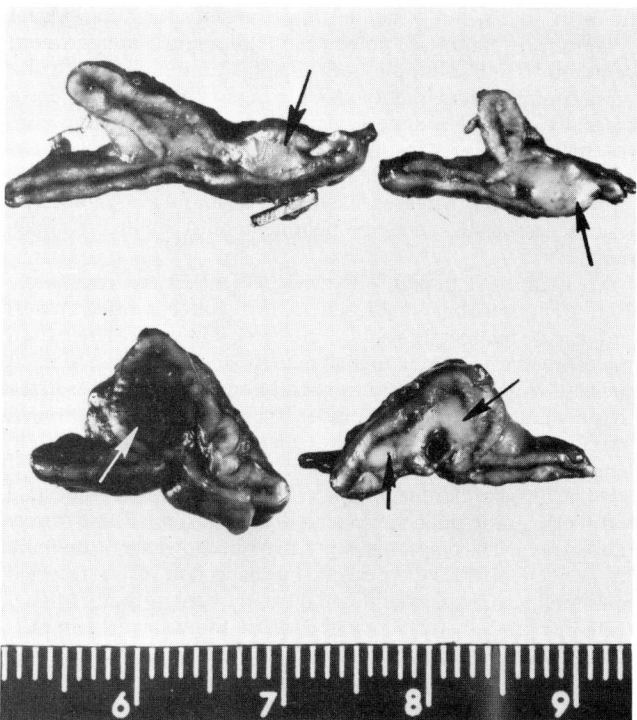

Figure 22. A small pheochromocytoma (arrow) and adrenal medullary hyperplasia (two arrows) are noted in the lower adrenal glands. Adrenal medullary hyperplasia (arrows) is demonstrated in the adrenal glands above.

kindred relieved the hypercalcemia. Ducatman[61] collected 10 cases of renal cell carcinoma associated with pheochromocytoma and suggested this association may reflect underlying von Hippel-Lindau disease. Vascular anomalies are also associated with these syndromes; aortic coarctation and renal artery aneurysm or stenosis may be present as well.

Unusual Manifestations of Pheochromocytoma

PHEOCHROMOCYTOMA IN PREGNANCY. Nearly 130 cases of pheochromocytoma requiring management during pregnancy have been reported.[64,75] This diagnosis is made, however, in less than half of the patients before delivery.[75,195] It has been emphasized that antenatal diagnosis reduces mortality at the time of delivery.[75,195] Shenker and Chowers,[195] reviewing 89 such cases, found that maternal mortality was 18 per cent if the lesion was detected antenatally and 58 per cent when the diagnosis was established postpartum or at postmortem examination. Fetal mortality was approximately 50 per cent.

Pheochromocytoma may be suspected in pregnant women under a variety of circumstances. The tumor may cause preeclampsia, paroxysmal hypertension, or other typical symptoms without hypertension. In addition, it can cause sudden shock and death at the time of anesthesia and delivery or it can cause unexplained hyperpyrexia after delivery. The period of greatest hazard occurs from the onset of labor until 48 hours *post partum*. If diagnosed during the first or second trimester, surgical resection is recommended as soon as antiadrenergic therapy has been established. In the third trimester, the patient may be managed medically and undergo combined cesarean section and removal of the pheochromocytoma.[75] There is no direct evidence that short-term use of anti-alpha-adrenergic therapy with phenoxybenzamine is harmful to the fetus, but the long-term effects of the drug are unclear.

PHEOCHROMOCYTOMA IN CHILDHOOD. Approximately 10 per cent of pheochromocytomas occur in individuals under 20 years of age. Among children, boys before the age of puberty are most commonly affected. Symptoms are similar to

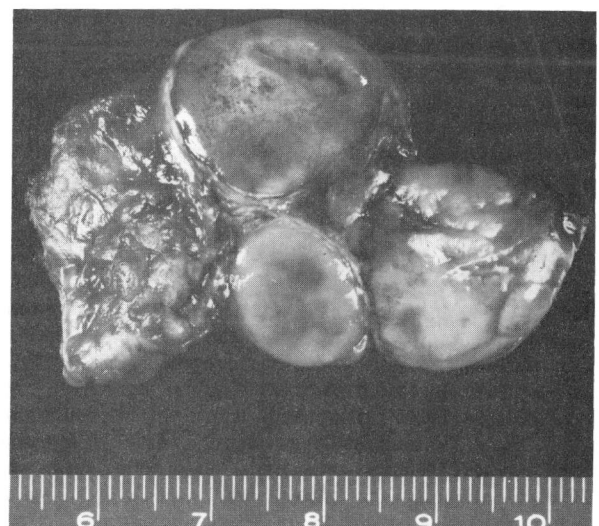

Figure 21. Multiple pheochromocytomas in a single adrenal gland resected from a patient with multiple endocrine neoplasia, Type IIa.

those in adults, but sustained hypertension, sweating, visual symptoms, weight loss, polydipsia, and polyuria appear more common.[18,115,210] Multiple and bilateral tumors appear to be more common than in adults, occurring in 40 per cent of these cases. Extra-adrenal tumors were much more common, occurring in one third of Stackpole's patients.[210] The recently updated 30-year experience at the Mayo Clinic emphasizes these observations and the increased likelihood of finding extra-adrenal lesions, associated endocrinopathies, and familial components.[115]

MALIGNANT PHEOCHROMOCYTOMAS. Approximately 10 to 20 per cent of sporadically occurring pheochromocytomas prove to be malignant. Females are three times more likely than males to harbor such a malignancy. It is controversial, at present, whether such lesions in children are more or less likely to be malignant than in adults.[18,31,104,115,210] There is much stronger evidence, however, that pheochromocytomas found in extra-adrenal sites are two to three times as likely to be malignant as those of adrenal origin.[182] The hypertension associated with malignant pheochromocytomas is sustained and rarely paroxysmal. The diagnosis of malignancy, however, is difficult, by both preoperative criteria or by inspection of the resected specimen. On gross examination, many benign tumors penetrate the capsule and may even invade the veins draining the gland. Microscopic examination of both benign and malignant lesions may reveal cellular pleomorphism, mitoses, and atypical nuclei. The diagnosis of malignancy, therefore, is established only by demonstrating invasion of adjacent structures or by documenting the presence of nodal or distant metastases. In Schonebeck's[197] report of 41 patients with malignant pheochromocytoma, metastases to bone occurred in 44 per cent, to liver in 37 per cent, to lymph nodes in 37 per cent, to lungs in 27 per cent, to the CNS in 10 per cent, to pleura in 10 per cent, to kidney in 5 per cent, to omentum in 2 per cent, and to pancreas in 2 per cent. Recurrences usually appear within 5 to 10 years after resection of the primary lesion[182,197] but may be detected as many as 20 years later. There are no clear differences in secretion rates of the different catecholamines to distinguish benign from malignant lesions.

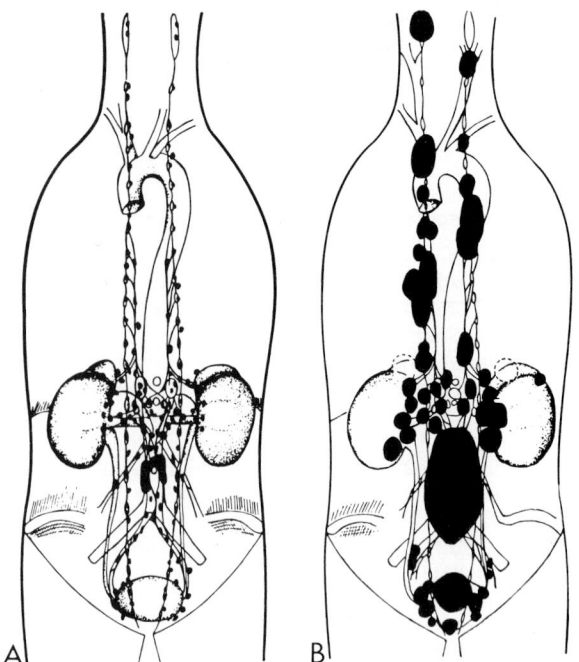

Figure 24. *A,* Distribution of extra-adrenal chromaffin tissue in the newborn. *B,* Distribution of extra-adrenal pheochromocytomas reported since 1965. (From Coupland, R.: The Natural History of the Chromaffin Cell. Essex, Longmans, Green and Company, 1965.)

EXTRA-ADRENAL PHEOCHROMOCYTOMAS. Approximately 98 per cent of pheochromocytomas arise within the abdomen (Fig. 23). Of these, 85 to 90 per cent originate in adrenal medullary tissue. Extra-adrenal pheochromocytomas occur and may be identified at any site where chromaffin tissue is located (Fig. 24). Such extra-adrenal lesions have been found in the paraganglia, the organ of Zuckerkandl, and the urinary bladder. Extra-abdominal pheochromocytomas have been identified near sites of the sympathetic ganglia in the posterior mediastinum, for example, in the carotid body ("chemodectomas"), or in the glomus jugulare body of the jugular bulb.[59]

Pheochromocytomas arising in the organ of Zuckerkandl may secrete both epinephrine and norepinephrine. This organ, a vestigial structure, is located in the region of the inferior mesenteric artery, anterior aorta, and aortic bifurcation. Pheochromocytomas arising from this structure may become large enough to press on adjacent vascular or genitourinary structures. They are quite vascular and may be difficult to resect.

Pheochromocytomas arising in the bladder are most frequently located in the wall of the bladder distant from the trigone,[166,179] although the trigone is the next most common site.[166] Hypertension, hematuria, and paroxysmal symptoms during micturition are the most characteristic clinical manifestations. Diagnosis is often established by cystoscopy; and, in fact, cystoscopy can elicit a paroxysm. Partial cystectomy is usually adequate treatment; 10 to 15 per cent are malignant.

Laboratory Diagnosis of Pheochromocytoma

The *sine qua non* for establishing a diagnosis of pheochromocytoma is measurement of increased excretion rates of urinary epinephrine and norepinephrine and of their metabolites, metanephrine, normetanephrine and vanillylmandelic acid. More than 90 per cent of patients with pheochromocytomas have distinctly elevated levels of norepinephrine and epinephrine in the urine. Normal ranges for 24-hour excretion rates of catecholamines and their metabolites are listed in Table 16. Sjoerdsma and associates[206] measured 24-hour excretion rates of free catecholamines, metanephrines, and VMA in 64 patients with proven pheochromocytoma (Fig. 25). The VMA assay may

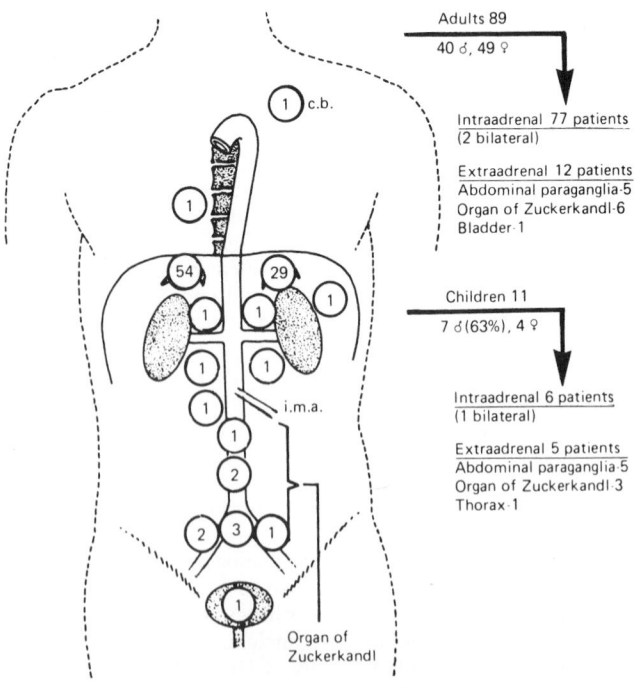

Adults 89
40 ♂, 49 ♀

Intraadrenal 77 patients
(2 bilateral)

Extraadrenal 12 patients
Abdominal paraganglia-5
Organ of Zuckerkandl-6
Bladder-1

Children 11
7 ♂ (63%), 4 ♀

Intraadrenal 6 patients
(1 bilateral)

Extraadrenal 5 patients
Abdominal paraganglia-5
Organ of Zuckerkandl-3
Thorax-1

Organ of Zuckerkandl

Figure 23. Locations of 107 pheochromocytomas in 100 patients. (From Manger, W. M., Gifford, R. W., and Melicow, M. M.: Pheochromocytoma. New York, Springer-Verlag, 1977, p. 45.)

TABLE 16. Normal Values for Urinary Catecholamines and Metabolites

Urine
  Catecholamines
    Norepinephrine: 10–70 μg./24 hr.
    Epinephrine: 0–20 μg./24 hr.
    Normetanephrine and metanephrine: <1.3 mg./24 hr.
    Vanillylmandelic acid: 1.8–9.0 mg./24 hr.
    Dopamine: <200 μg./24 hr.

From Melmon, K. L.: Catecholamines and the adrenal medulla. *In* Williams, R. H. (Ed.): Textbook of Endocrinology, 5th ed. Philadelphia, W. B. Saunders Company, 1974, p. 309.

be influenced by ingestion of coffee, tea, raw fruits or by drugs such as alpha-methyldopa; it therefore can lead to false-positive results under some circumstances. Under controlled conditions of collection, however, all three assays are highly sensitive.[20,206] Measurements of plasma catecholamines are not as useful in distinguishing patients with pheochromocytoma from those with essential hypertension, although they are usually elevated above levels observed in normotensive patients[26] (Fig. 26).

Because some patients with pheochromocytoma may not have urinary or plasma catecholamine levels distinct from those observed in essential hypertension, stimulation and suppression tests have been devised in order to establish a diagnosis in doubtful cases. Glucagon is used to stimulate catecholamine release only when the blood pressure is normal or nearly normal and when catecholamine levels in urine and serum are nearly normal. Glucagon has fewer side effects than other provocative agents such as tyramine or histamine and is administered as a 1.0- to 2.0-mg. bolus intravenously. A positive test requires at least a threefold increase in plasma catecholamines, or levels above 2000 pg. per ml., within 2 to 3 minutes after administration. In patients with elevated catecholamine levels but normal or nearly normal blood pressure, a clonidine suppression test

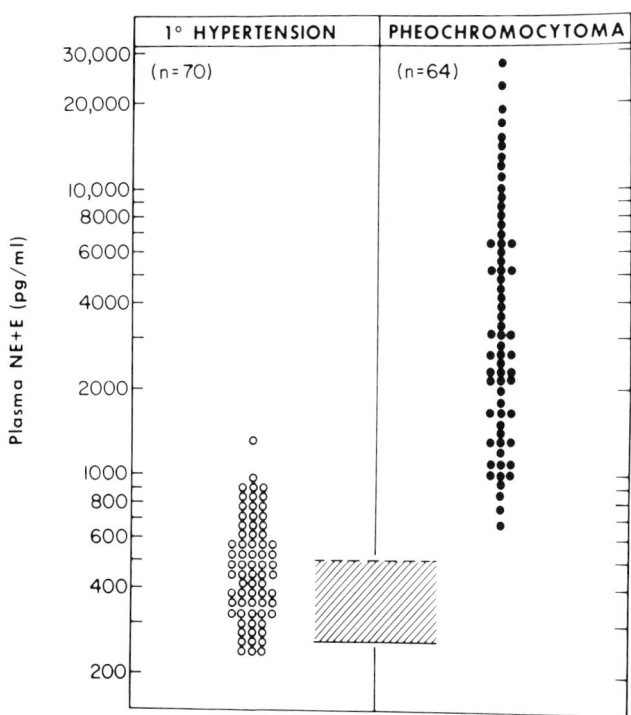

Figure 26. Supine resting plasma catecholamine values in patients with essential hypertension or pheochromocytoma. The cross-hatched area represents the mean (260 pg. per ml.) + 2 S.D. (500 pg. per ml.) of values in 47 normotensive healthy adults with an age and sex distribution similar to that of the two patient groups. For subjects with essential hypertension, the mean + 2 S.D. was 516+950 pg. per ml.; four patients with pheochromocytoma had levels that fell within the range of values in patients with essential hypertension. NE+E, norepinephrine plus epinephrine. (From Bravo, E. L., and Gifford, R. W.: Pheochromocytoma: Diagnosis, localization and management. N. Engl. J. Med., *311*:1298, 1984.)

may be used. Clonidine is a centrally acting alpha-adrenergic agonist that suppresses the neurogenically mediated release of catecholamines. In theory, the autonomous release of catecholamines by a pheochromocytoma would not be suppressed by clonidine. The test must be performed in well-hydrated patients and all β-adrenergic antagonists must be discontinued for at least 2 days before the test. Only assays which measure free, not conjugated, catecholamines should be used or false-positives may be encountered. Normal clonidine suppression occurs when the level of plasma norepinephrine and epinephrine together falls below 500 ng. per ml. 2 to 3 hours following an oral dose of 0.3 mg. clonidine (Fig. 27).

Surgical Treatment

PREOPERATIVE PREPARATION. When the diagnosis of pheochromocytoma has been established and localization studies have been completed, the patient must be prepared for surgery. A major point of controversy in patients undergoing abdominal exploration for pheochromocytoma is whether or not to administer alpha- and, in some cases, beta-adrenergic blocking agents during the preoperative period. Although there have been reports[58] of patients with pheochromocytomas who have been operated on without receiving alpha-adrenergic blockade, such a practice is unusual. In most patients, the authors administer alpha-blocking agents consisting of phenoxybenzamine in a dose of 1 mg. per kg. in divided doses to reduce gastrointestinal symptoms. The initial dose is 10 mg. twice a day; increments of 10 to 20 mg. per day are usually required to control clinical manifestations and reduce blood pressure to normal or nearly normal levels. The drug is usually administered for 1 to 3 weeks prior to operation. Alpha blockade may also be accomplished by the oral administration of phentolamine (50 mg. every 4 hours). However, there are appreciable gastrointestinal side effects as-

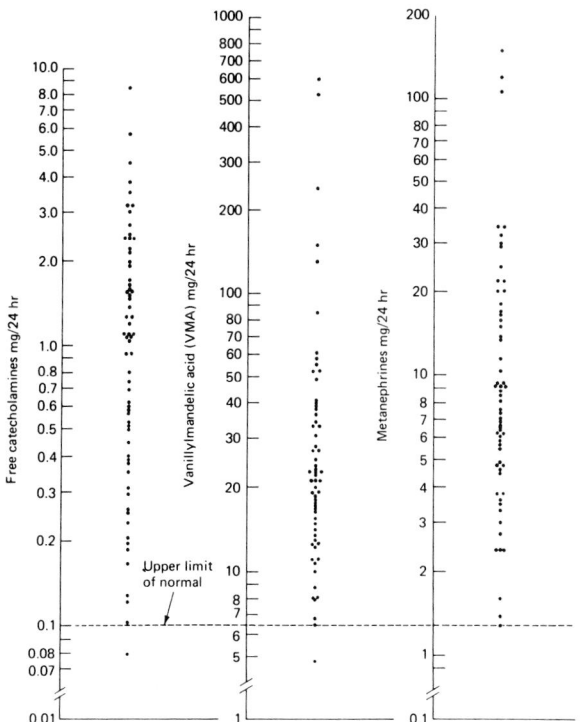

Figure 25. Levels of epinephrine, norepinephrine (free catecholamines), vanillylmandelic acid (VMA), and metanephrines in 24-hour urine samples obtained from 64 patients with proven pheochromocytoma. (From Sjoerdsma, A., et al.: Pheochromocytoma: Current concepts of diagnosis and treatment. Ann. Intern. Med., *65*:1306, 1966.)

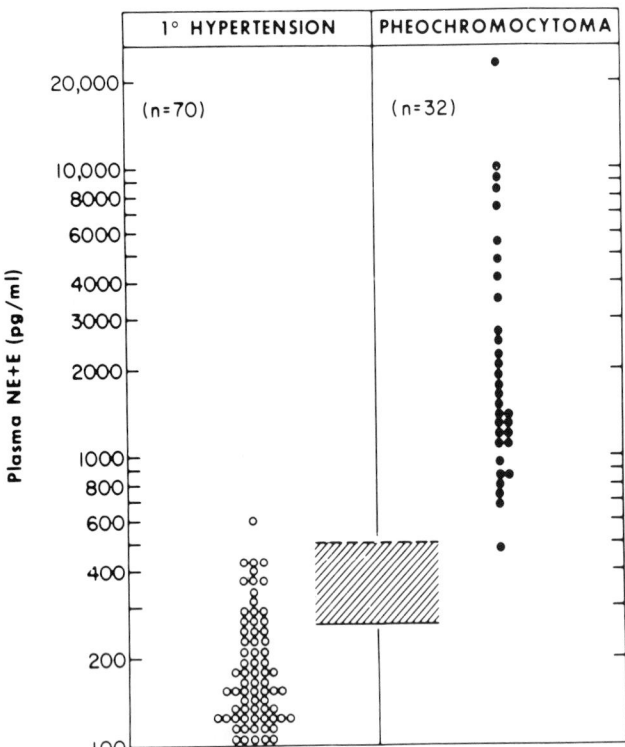

Figure 27. Effect of oral clonidine (0.3 mg.) on plasma catecholamine values in patients with essential hypertension or pheochromocytoma. Values shown represent the lowest levels reached (at either 2 or 3 hours) after administration of clonidine. The crosshatched area represents the mean + 2 S.D. of basal values in normotensive control subjects. All but one patient with pheochromocytoma had values above 500 pg. per ml. after clonidine administration. One patient with essential hypertension had a value above 500 pg. per ml. NE+E denotes norepinephrine plus epinephrine. (From Bravo, E. L., and Gifford, R. W.: Pheochromocytoma: Diagnosis, localization and management. N. Engl. J. Med., *311*:1298, 1984.)

sociated with this drug, and it is generally less satisfactory than phenoxybenzamine. The side effects of alpha blockade include postural hypotension, reflex tachycardia, nasal congestion, and inability to ejaculate. Preoperative blockade with phenoxybenzamine offers several advantages, the most notable being the reversal preoperatively of the relative hypovolemia that is usually present and the prevention of severe perturbations in blood pressure during intraoperative manipulation of the pheochromocytoma. The main disadvantage, although minor, to alpha blockade is that the intraoperative search for occult pheochromocytoma may be more difficult because the characteristic rise in blood pressure following manipulation of the tumor may be abolished. It might be wise to omit alpha-blocking agents in patients whose pheochromocytomas have not been localized preoperatively or in those in whom a small neoplasm is suspected. The administration of propranolol as a beta-adrenergic blocking agent is indicated in patients who have a heart rate greater than 140 beats per minute, who have any history of arrhythmia or persistent ventricular extrasystoles, or who harbor tumors that secrete primarily epinephrine. Propranolol should be withheld until alpha blockade has been established; otherwise the creation of beta blockade inhibits epinephrine-induced vasodilatation, thereby increasing hypertension and placing further strain on the heart. Also, propranolol may produce profound bradycardia and heart block and may precipitate congestive heart failure. Cardiac standstill and death following propranolol administration have been reported in patients with pheochromocytoma. Special caution must be exercised in administering propranolol to patients who are receiving cardiac glycosides.

Suitable surgical results have been obtained with or without

the administration of preoperative alpha- or beta-adrenergic blocking agents. The critical factors in a successful result depend more upon the expertise and experience of the internist, the surgeon, and the anesthesiologist than on whether or not the patient receives a specific antiadrenergic regimen preoperatively.

If alpha-adrenergic blockade is not employed before surgical resection, great care must be taken to monitor the blood volume intraoperatively, especially after resection of the pheochromocytoma, and for 48 hours postoperatively. Vasodilatation and relative hypovolemia following reduction of circulating norepinephrine levels may lead to tachycardia and hypotension, which must be aggressively managed by the intravenous administration of crystalloid and, occasionally, whole blood.

ANESTHETIC MANAGEMENT. Prior to leaving the ward, patients should receive diazepam, 10 mg. orally. In the operating room, an arterial line should be placed for careful monitoring of blood pressure on an oscillograph and for ready access for determination of arterial blood gases should it be needed. A central venous line is placed for venous pressure measurement. A bladder catheter is inserted so that urinary output can be quantitated during the operative procedure. Monitoring of the electrocardiogram (ECG) is also maintained throughout the procedure. Induction is performed with sodium thiopental in divided doses, followed by nitrous oxide, oxygen, and enflurane by face mask. After the patient is deeply anesthetized, a muscle relaxant, such as pancuronium, is administered. The trachea is then sprayed with 4 per cent lidocaine, and intubation is achieved. Anesthesia is maintained with enflurane, nitrous oxide, and oxygen. Lidocaine is also administered topically to the tracheal mucosa during the procedure.

The patient is placed into a slightly reversed Trendelenburg position, so that the lower extremities may be used as volume capacitors during the procedure. When the pheochromocytoma has been removed and vasodilatation occurs, the patient may be returned to the horizontal position for increasing the blood volume.

Hypertensive episodes may occur during handling of the pheochromocytoma; these are most effectively managed by administration of the peripheral blocker sodium nitroprusside. This material is sensitive to light; therefore, the bottle and tubing containing it must be wrapped in aluminum foil. The alpha-adrenergic blocker phentolamine may be used as an antihypertensive agent, rather than sodium nitroprusside. However, this drug is longer-acting, and control of hypertensive episodes is generally less precise.

Cardiac arrhythmias may occur, with sudden increases in catecholamine secretion. These can usually be effectively controlled by the intravenous administration of lidocaine. Some anesthesiologists prefer the administration of propranolol or a combination of propranolol and lidocaine to control arrhythmias.

The danger period does not end with resection of the pheochromocytoma. During the intraoperative and postoperative periods, these patients may develop profound hypotension as a result of the vasodilatation that occurs following tumor resection. Arterial blood pressure, venous pressure, and urinary output should be monitored continuously during the first 24 hours after operation, and confinement of patients to the recovery room or an acute care unit during the immediate postoperative period is indicated.

IMAGING OF ADRENAL TUMORS

Neoplasms of the cortex and medulla are rarely palpable unless they are malignant. Preoperative localization of functioning adrenal lesions has been considerably improved with CT and MRI. In addition, use of radionuclide markers, which are sequestered in the adrenal cortex or medulla, have permitted localization of primary adrenal tumors and metastases. Arteriographic techniques and venous sampling have been used under selected circumstances to help plan operative strategy in locating these tumors and determining a higher level of suspicion for bilateral or multiple tumors.

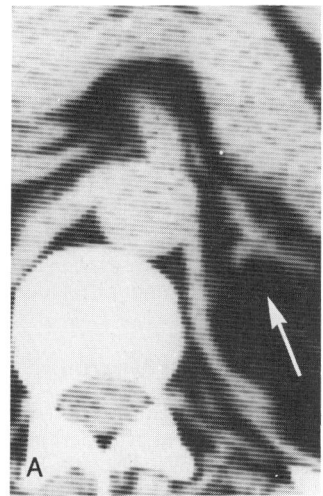

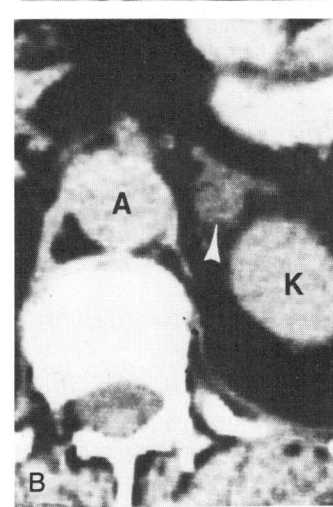

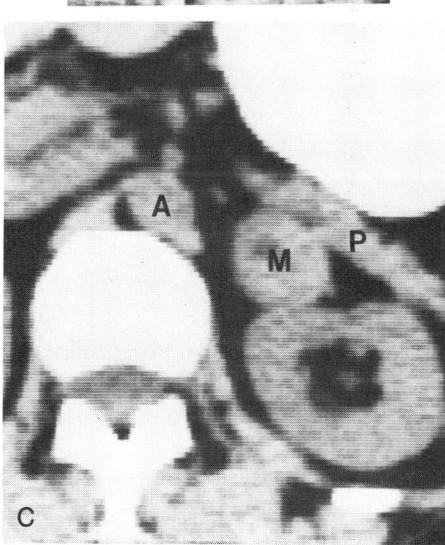

Figure 28. Computed tomography of the adrenal glands. A, Normal adrenal gland (arrow). B, Adrenal cortical adenoma 1.5 cm. in diameter (arrowhead) arising between the limbs of the left adrenal gland. A, aorta; K, upper pole of left kidney. C, Pheochromocytoma (M) 2.5 cm. in diameter in the left adrenal gland. A, aorta; P, tail of pancreas. (Courtesy of M. Korobkin, M.D., Duke University Medical Center, Durham, North Carolina.)

NONINVASIVE TECHNIQUES

Conventional urography may demonstrate downward displacement of the kidney if a large adrenal mass is present. It is difficult to detect masses less than 2 cm., and lesions such as extra-adrenal pheochromocytomas are not identified unless they displace the ureter or bladder. Although less than 50 per cent of adrenal lesions are visualized by this technique, valuable ancillary information can be gained and the functional integrity of both kidneys documented.

The employment of nephrotomography with intravenous pyelography enhances the likelihood of detecting suprarenal masses, although lesions less than 2 cm. in diameter are rarely detected.

ULTRASONOGRAPHY. Some reports[13] suggest that gray-scale ultrasonography is useful in detecting adrenal lesions. As with urography combined with nephrotomography, this technique rarely identifies adrenal neoplasms smaller than 2 to 3 cm. in size. Moreover, a high degree of technical expertise is required to obtain and interpret the images.

COMPUTED TOMOGRAPHY. CT has been used by various investigators[62,157] to identify adrenal lesions. The greatest advantage of this technique is its ability to detect lesions less than 2 cm. in size. Montagne and associates[157] were able to identify both adrenal glands in 78 per cent of 60 randomly evaluated normal patients. In a study by Dunnick and associates[62] of 26 patients with a variety of adrenal lesions, 23 (89 per cent) were identified by CT studies. Three lesions were overlooked because of small adrenal masses (less than 0.5 cm.) or lack of retroperitoneal fat. The smallest lesion identified was 1 cm. in diameter. This technique offers great promise in the identification of both primary and metastatic adrenal lesions. Adrenal neoplasms that are demonstrable by CT are presented in Figure 28.

MAGNETIC RESONANCE IMAGING. This is a relatively new diagnostic modality, and experience with adrenal imaging is limited. An important advantage of MRI is natural contrast between adrenal tissue and surrounding fatty and vascular structures. Ionizing radiation of conventional tomographic techniques is avoided, and intravenous contrast materials are unnecessary. In pregnant patients, this is a significant advantage. In addition, images can be weighted to provide greater anatomic detail between structures (T1-weighted), or they can be weighted to discriminate between normal and pathologic tissues (T2-weighted).[79] Extra-adrenal pheochromocytomas are easily detected. In some cases, it is possible to distinguish adre-

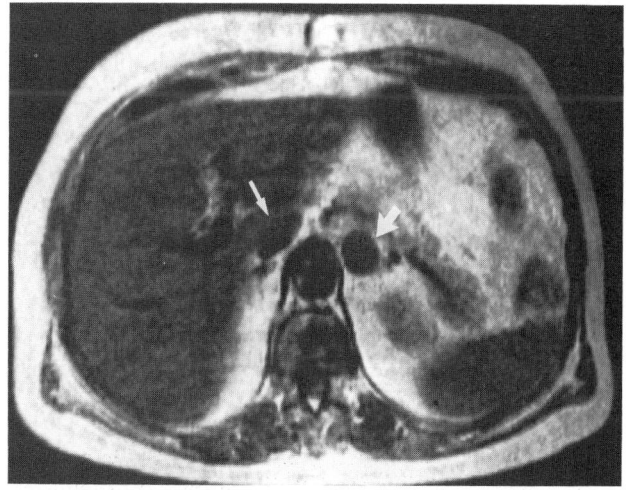

Figure 29. Magnetic resonance tomogram, T2-weighted image, of a left adrenal cortical adenoma (thick arrow). The vena cava is outlined on the right (thin arrow) just anterior to the normal right adrenal gland. The homogeneous nature of the adenoma is apparent. (Courtesy of J. Heiken, M.D., Mallinckrodt Institute of Radiology, Washington University School of Medicine, St. Louis, Missouri.)

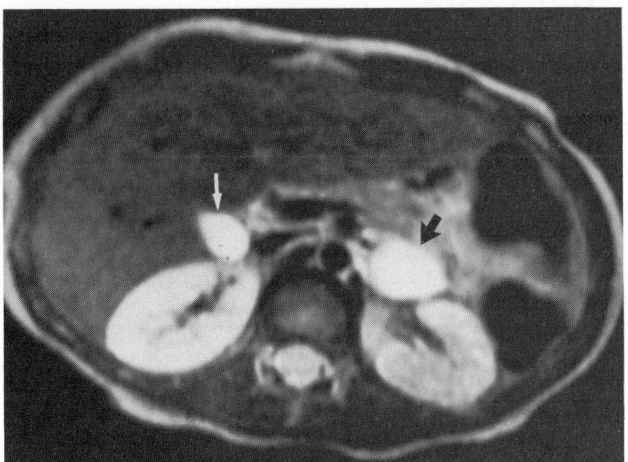

Figure 30. Magnetic resonance tomogram, T2-weighted image, of a left-sided pheochromocytoma (heavy arrow). The gallbladder (light arrow) has a high signal intensity, due to its high water content. Pheochromocytoma, adrenocortical carcinomas, and metastatic lesions to the adrenal demonstrate this high signal intensity, possibly because of their high water content. (Courtesy of J. Heiken, M.D., Mallinckrodt Institute of Radiology, Washington University School of Medicine, St. Louis, Missouri.)

nocortical adenomas, pheochromocytomas, and adrenal metastases of other tumors[35,79] (Figs. 29 and 30).

RADIONUCLIDE IMAGING. In 1971, Beierwaltes and associates[10] introduced the technique of adrenal scanning utilizing [131]I-19-iodocholesterol. It is possible to identify adrenal glands in some normal patients with this technique. Pheochromocytomas, however, are difficult to discern because the surrounding adrenal cortex is either markedly displaced or attenuated. Also, adrenocortical carcinomas frequently are not visualized, most likely because they do not efficiently concentrate the tracer. The main disadvantage of adrenal scintiscanning with [131]I-19-iodocholesterol is that repeat studies 4 to 19 days after injection are usually required for identifying adrenocortical tissue. A newer agent, [131]I-6B-iodomethyl-19-norcholesterol,[72] may obviate this problem. Adrenal scintiscanning should still be considered an experimental technique because it is used at only a few medical centers.

In 1984, Thompson and associates[218] reported the results of a 3-year study at the University of Michigan in which 95 patients with pheochromocytomas were evaluated with use of the adrenal scanning agent ^{131}I-metaiodobenzylguanidine (^{131}I-MIBG). Pheochromocytomas were visualized preoperatively in 85 patients. There were no false-positive results. Of 18 patients with extra-adrenal pheochromocytomas, 15 had lesions that were visualized by ^{131}I-MIBG.[218] Nine of these lesions were in the mediastinum, and five intracardiac lesions required cardiopulmonary bypass for excision. Ten patients with unresectable metastases for inoperable primary tumors that demonstrated ^{131}I-MIBG uptake were administered therapeutic doses of this agent (optimally 300 mCi. or 10,200 rads). Five patients demonstrated objective responses as determined by a 50 per cent decrease in tumor size or a significant decrease in urinary catecholamine levels. ^{131}I-MIBG scintigraphy represents an important advance both in the diagnosis and treatment of pheochromocytomas.

INVASIVE TECHNIQUES

ARTERIOGRAPHY. Although associated with some risk, aortography or selective adrenal arteriography is employed in localizing adrenal neoplasms, particularly pheochromocytomas, which are usually highly vascular and frequently bilateral and multiple. The contrast medium used in arteriography may stimulate release of catecholamines and induce a hypertensive crisis. Great caution must be exercised during this procedure, and, in most cases, adrenergic blockade with Dibenzyline is indicated before the study. Arteriography is not as helpful in the localization of adrenocortical lesions.

ADRENAL VENOGRAPHY. Catheterization of the adrenal vein serves a dual purpose in patients with functioning adrenal neoplasms; often a tumor can be identified by the injection of contrast material into a selectively catheterized adrenal vein, and lesions have been detected by phlebography when they were missed by other radiographic procedures, including arteriography. Although adrenal venography is a useful technique for localizing adrenal tumors, morbidity has accompanied its use.

Also useful is the selective catheterization and sampling of the adrenal venous effluent for measurement of corticosteroids

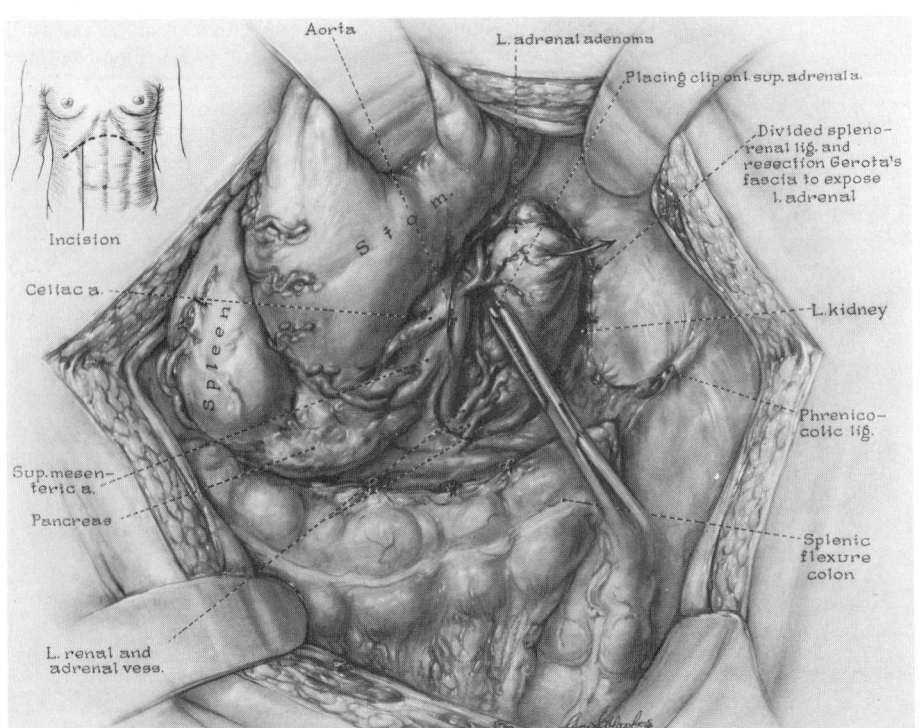

Figure 31. Transabdominal approach to the left adrenal gland.

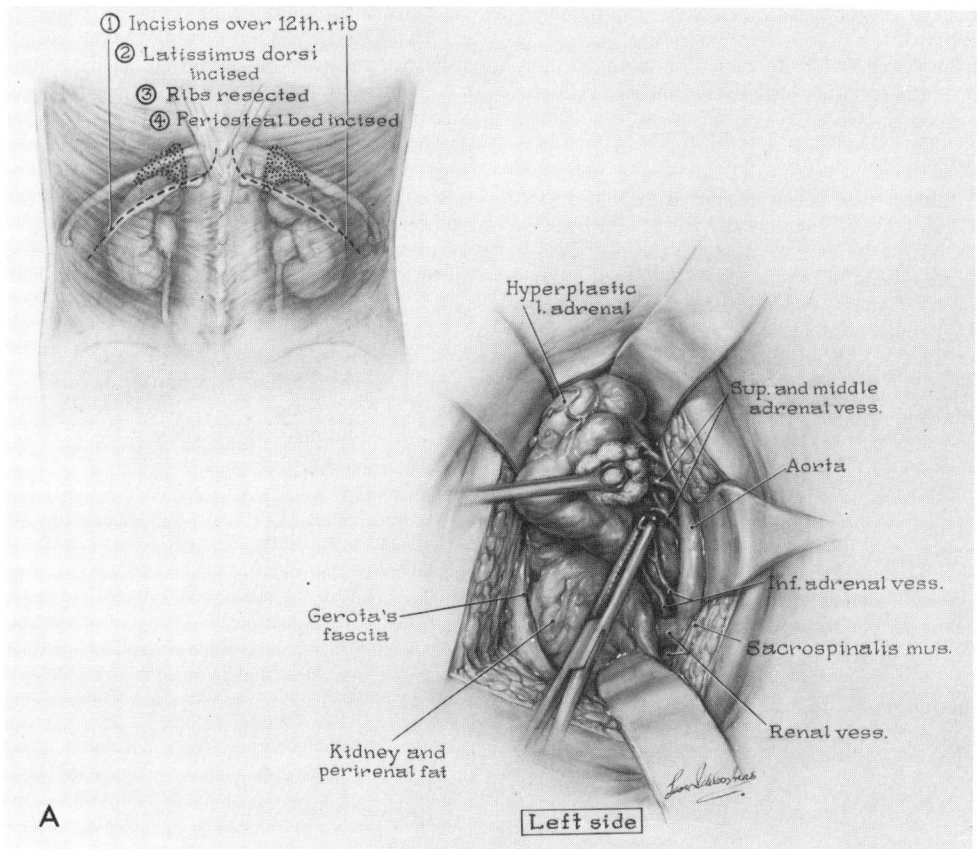

① Incisions over 12th. rib
② Latissimus dorsi incised
③ Ribs resected
④ Periosteal bed incised

Hyperplastic l. adrenal

Sup. and middle adrenal vess.

Aorta

Inf. adrenal vess.

Sacrospinalis mus.

Renal vess.

Gerota's fascia

Kidney and perirenal fat

A

Left side

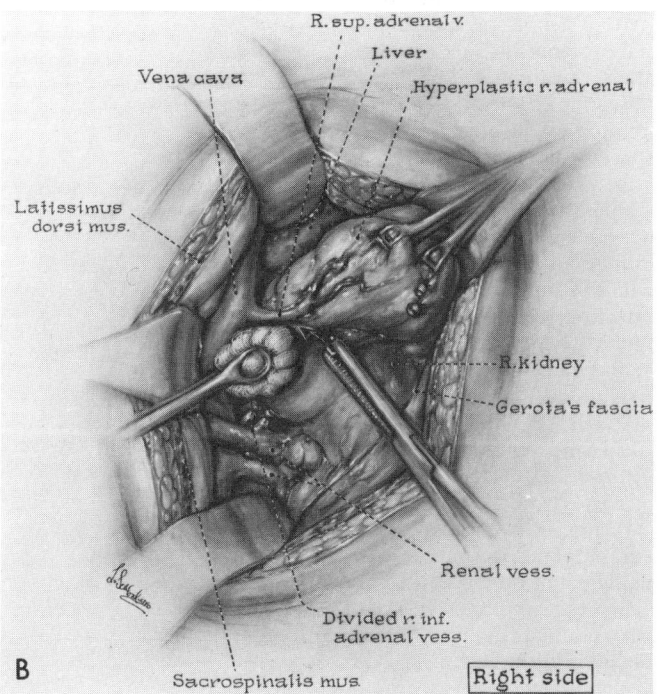

R. sup. adrenal v.

Liver

Hyperplastic r. adrenal

Vena cava

Latissimus dorsi mus.

R. kidney

Gerota's fascia

Renal vess.

Divided r. inf. adrenal vess.

Sacrospinalis mus.

B

Right side

Figure 32. Posterior approach to the adrenal gland. *A*, left side. *B*, right side.

or catecholamines to localize functioning adrenal cortical or medullary tumors that have not been detected by other radiographic techniques. This method depends upon the detection of a higher concentration of the secretory product (cortisol, aldosterone, or catecholamine) in one adrenal vein compared with the other, or, in the case of ectopic neoplasms, higher concentrations of the secretory product in the vena cava, abdominal veins, or pelvic veins. The use of this technique in the diagnosis

of aldosteronomas and the identification of unilateral adenomas from bilateral hyperplasia has already been mentioned. Abdominal venous sampling with determination of catecholamine levels has also been helpful in localizing occult pheochromocytomas. This procedure is especially useful when other localization procedures have failed and in patients with pheochromocytomas that remain undetected despite previous exploration.

Although each of the aforementioned radiographic techniques has special indications under certain circumstances, it is rare for the clinician to choose only one procedure. Rather, several localization studies, particularly those that are noninvasive, may be employed.

The Incidentally Discovered Adrenal Mass

With the wide utilization of CT scanning of the abdomen, adrenal masses are discovered incidentally. Most of these lesions are benign cortical adenomas. Copeland recently developed an algorithm for evaluating such lesions. Generally, large (more than 6 cm.) solid masses should be resected whether cystic or solid and whether hormonally hyperfunctional or nonfunctional. Obviously, patients should be prepared preoperatively if the lesions are hormonally active. Lesions less than 6 cm. may be followed nonoperatively if they are not hormonally hyperfunctional and if they do not increase in size on repeated study after 18 to 24 months.

SURGICAL MANAGEMENT OF ADRENAL LESIONS

Many surgeons advocate an anterior transabdominal approach for all adrenal neoplasms regardless of type. This technique is uniformly indicated in patients with intra-abdominal pheochromocytomas, because the incidence of either bilateral or extra-adrenal neoplasms is approximately 10 per cent. Not only must the obvious pheochromocytoma be resected, but the contralateral adrenal gland, the paraspinal area, the organ of Zuckerkandl, and the bladder must be carefully examined. Moreover, the tumors are often large, and it would be difficult to extract them through a posterior incision.

Conversely, most adrenocortical lesions can be resected from a posterior approach. In patients whose neoplasms are single and have been localized, a unilateral posterior incision may be performed. In patients with Cushing's syndrome and bilateral adrenal hyperplasia or in those who require bilateral adrenalectomy for palliation of metastatic carcinoma of the breast, a bilateral posterior approach should be used. Compared with transabdominal incisions, posterior incisions are generally tolerated better by the patient, and the postoperative convalescence is more rapid. The exposure is comparable during both procedures, although the operative field is smaller with a posterior incision. The one exception, in which a transabdominal approach is indicated for resection of an adrenocortical lesion, is in patients with adrenocortical carcinoma. These lesions are usually very large and highly vascular, and they may invade adjacent soft tissue and organs.

THE TRANSABDOMINAL APPROACH. For resecting pheochromocytomas or adrenocortical carcinomas, the authors usually prefer a bilateral subcostal approach. It is rarely necessary to extend this incision into the thorax, although such a modification may be indicated in patients with very large neoplasms. For exploration of the left adrenal gland, the left colon is reflected inferiorly, the splenocolic ligament divided and the spleen and pancreas reflected medially, the left kidney and adrenal gland thus exposed (Fig. 31). An alternate approach used by some surgeons consists of an entry into the lesser sac between the stomach and colon.

The right adrenal gland may be exposed by mobilizing the hepatic flexure of the colon inferiorly and reflecting the duodenum medially. The right kidney is retracted inferiorly, and the right adrenal gland is identified in the perinephric fat. In resection of adrenal tumors, silver clips are used to control the arteries and veins. Great care must be taken in securing the right adrenal vein, because it is wide but very short and empties directly into the vena cava.

In patients with Cushing's syndrome who have marked central abdominal obesity, the adrenal glands may be approached laterally through the flank, first exposing and resecting one adrenal gland and then turning the patient and making a separate incision to resect the other. Such a maneuver appears unnecessarily complicated and would be indicated only under rare circumstances.

The posterior approach to the adrenal gland is depicted in Figure 32A and B. The lumbodorsal fascia is incised, and the sacrospinalis muscle is retracted medially. The twelfth rib is resected, and the kidney is manually depressed. Great care must be taken to identify the pleura, which can usually be observed during respiration. If the pleura is entered, a small chest tube is placed and exited through the wound. It is removed on the second postoperative day.

If there is a likelihood that bilateral adrenalectomy will be required, corticosteroids should be administered preoperatively. The authors' policy has been to administer 50 mg. of cortisone acetate intramuscularly 48 and 24 hours prior to and on the morning of operation. During the operative procedure, the patient is administered 100 mg. of hydrocortisone sodium succinate when the adrenals are removed. An additional 100 mg. is administered intravenously 8 and 16 hours postoperatively and on the first and second postoperative days. Cortisone acetate is gradually reduced to a maintenance dose of 25 mg. in the morning and 12.5 mg. in the afternoon. By the second postoperative week, fludrocortisone acetate, 0.1 mg. twice a week, is added to the regimen.

SELECTED REFERENCES

Pituitary

Cushing, H.: The basophil adenomas of the pituitary body and their clinical manifestations. Bulletin of the Johns Hopkins Hospital, 50:137, 1932.
An elegant study using case histories of eight patients to catalogue the manifestations and natural history of the disease to which the author's name has been attached.

Goodrich, I., and Lee, K. J.: The Pituitary. Amsterdam, Elsevier, 1988.
A concise, well-written book covering history, presentation, diagnosis, and management of pituitary disorders.

Adrenal Gland

Addison, T.: On the constitutional and local effects of disease of the suprarenal capsules. London, Highley, 1885.
The original article describing manifestations of acute adrenocortical insufficiency. It is well worth the trouble to find this monograph.

Cance, W. G., and Wells, S. A., Jr.: Multiple endocrine neoplasia type IIa. Curr. Probl. Surg., 22:1, 1985.
This monograph details the senior author's experience in screening, diagnosis, and management of all components of this hereditary endocrinopathy, including pheochromocytoma.

Hutter, A. M., and Kayhoe, D. E.: Adrenal cortical carcinoma: Clinical features of 138 patients. Am. J. Med. 41:572, 1966.
An older study of presentation of this disease in the era prior to CT scan and providing evidence of the benefits of treating residual disease with mitotane.

Manger, W. M., and Gifford, R. W., Jr.: Pheochromocytoma. New York, Springer-Verlag, 1977.
A classic text in medicine, addressing history, pathology, pathophysiology, presentation, diagnosis, and management of pheochromocytoma. This monograph is recommended together with the subsequent review of Dr. Gifford's experiences (N. Engl. J. Med., 311:1298, 1984) in localization and management of these lesions.

Young, W. F., and Klee, G. C.: Primary aldosteronism. Endocrinol. Metab. Clin. North Am., 17:367, 1988.
An up-to-date review of presentation and diagnosis of this disorder. The entire issue in which this review appears is recommended to students interested in a concise and recent review of diagnosis and medical management of a number of endocrine tumors.

REFERENCES

1. Addison, T.: On the constitutional and local effects of disease of the suprarenal capsules. London, Highley, 1885.
2. Ahlquist, R. P.: A study of adrenotropic receptors. Am. J. Physiol., 153:586, 1948.
3. Arafah, B. M., Brodkey, J. S., and Pearson, O. H.: Prolactin secreting pituitary adenomas in women. In Santen, R. J., and Manni, A. (Eds.): Diagnosis and

Management of Endocrine-Related Tumors. Boston, Martinus Nijhoff Publishers, 1984, pp. 63–79.

4. Aristotle: On the Parts of Animals, Book II, Chapter 7, Berlin Nos. 652a, 24; 652b, 25–35; 653a, 1–5.

5. Ashcraft, M. W., Van Herle, A. J., Vener, S. L., and Geffner, D. L.: Serum cortisol levels in Cushing's syndrome after low- and high-dose dexamethasone suppression. Ann. Intern. Med., 97:21, 1982.

6. Atuk, N. O., McDonald, T., Wood, T., Carpenter, J. T., Walzak, M. P., Donaldson, M., and Gillenwater, J. W.: Familial pheochromocytoma, hypercalcemia, and von Hippel-Lindau disease. Medicine, 58:209, 1979.

7. Auda, S. P., Brennan, M. F., and Gill, J. G.: Evolution of the surgical management of primary aldosteronism. Ann. Surg., 191:1, 1980.

8. Avioli, L. V.: Effects of chronic corticosteroid therapy on mineral metabolism and calcium absorption. Adv. Exp. Med. Biol., 171:81, 1984.

9. Axelrod, J., and Reisine, T. D.: Stress hormones: Their interaction and regulation. Science, 224:452, 1984.

10. Beierwaltes, W. H., Lieberman, L. M., Ansari, A. N., and Nishiyama, H.: Visualization of human adrenal glands in vivo by scintillation scanning. J.A.M.A., 216:275, 1971.

11. Bergland, R. M., and Page, R. B.: Can the pituitary secrete directly to the brain? Affirmative anatomical evidence. Endocrinology, 102:1325, 1978.

12. Bergland, R. M., Ray, B. S., and Torack, R. M.: Anatomical variations in the pituitary gland and adjacent structures in 225 autopsy cases. J. Neurosurg., 28:93, 1968.

13. Bernardino, M. E., and Goldstein, G. B.: Gray scale ultrasonography of adrenal neoplasms. A.J.R., 130:741, 1978.

14. Besser, G. M., and Edwards, C. R. W.: Cushing's syndrome. Clin. Endocrinol. Metab., 1:451, 1972.

15. Besser, G. M., Wass, J. A. H., and Thorner, M. O.: Acromegaly: Results of long-term treatment with bromocriptine. Acta Endocrinol., 88:187, 1978.

16. Bigos, S. T., Somma, M., Rasio, E., Eastman, R. C., Lanthier, A., Johnston, H. H., and Hardy, J.: Cushing's disease: Management by transsphenoidal pituitary microsurgery. J. Clin. Endocrinol. Metab., 50:348, 1980.

17. Blaschko, H., and Welch, A. O.: Localization of adrenalin and cytoplasmic particles of the bovine adrenalmedulla. Arch. Exp. Pathol., 219:9, 1953.

18. Bloom, D. A., and Fonkalsrud, E. W.: Surgical management of pheochromocytoma in children. J. Pediatr. Surg., 9:179, 1974.

19. Boggan, J. E., Tyrell, J. B., and Wilson, C. B.: Transsphenoidal microsurgical management of Cushing's disease: Report of 100 cases. J. Neurosurg., 59:195, 1983.

20. Bravo, E. L., and Gifford, R. W., Jr.: Pheochromocytoma: Diagnosis, localization and management. N. Engl. J. Med., 311:1298, 1984.

21. Bravo, E. L., Tarazi, R. C., Duston, H. P., Fouad, F. M., Textor, S. C., Gifford, R. W., and Vidt, D. G.: The changing clinical spectrum of primary aldosteronism. Am. J. Med., 74:641, 1983.

22. Brennan, M. F.: Adrenocortical carcinoma. CA, 37:348, 1987.

23. Brown, J. J., Davies, D. L., Ferriss, J. B., Fraser, R., Haywood, E., Lever, A. F., and Robertson, J. I. S.: Comparison of surgery and prolonged spironolactone therapy in patients with hypertension, aldosterone excess, and low plasma renin. Br. Med. J., 2:729, 1972.

24. Brown-Sequard, E.: Ces capsules surrenates. Arch. Gen. Med., 8:385, 1856.

25. Burch, W.: A survey of results with transsphenoidal surgery in Cushing's disease. N. Engl. J. Med., 308:103, 1983.

26. Burke, C. W., and Beardwell, C. G.: Cushing's syndrome: An evaluation of the clinical usefulness of urinary free cortisol and other urinary steroid measurements in diagnosis. Q. J. Med., 42:175, 1973.

27. Burrington, J. D., and Stephens, C. A.: Virilizing tumors of the adrenal gland: Report of eight cases. J. Pediatr. Surg., 4:291, 1969.

28. Cadieux, R. J., Kales, A., Santen, R. J., Bixler, E., and Gordon, R.: Endoscopic findings in sleep apnea associated with acromegaly. J. Clin. Endocrinol. Metab., 55:18, 1982.

29. Cance, W. G., and Wells, S. A., Jr.: Multiple endocrine neoplasia type IIa. Curr. Prob. Surg., 22:1, 1985.

30. Carey, R. M., Sen, S., Dolan, L., Malchoff, C. D., and Bumpus, M. F.: Idiopathic hyperaldosteronism: A possible role for aldosterone stimulating factor. N. Engl. J. Med., 311:94, 1984.

31. Carney, J. A., Sizemore, G. W., and Tyre, G. M.: Adrenal medullary disease in multiple endocrine neoplasia, type 2: Pheochromocytoma and its precursor. Am. J. Clin. Pathol., 66:279, 1976.

32. Carter, J. N., Tyson, J. E., Tolis, G., Van Vliet, S., Faiman, C., and Friesen, H. G.: Prolactin-secreting tumors and hypogonadism in 22 men. N. Engl. J. Med., 299:847, 1978.

33. Cedermark, B. J., Blurenson, L. F., Pickren, J. W., Holyoke, D. E., and Elias, E. G.: The significance of metastases to the adrenal glands in adenocarcinoma of the colon and rectum. S.G.O., 144:537, 1977.

34. Chambers, E. F., Turski, P. A., LaMasters, D., and Newton, J. H.: Regions of low density in the contrast-enhanced pituitary gland: Normal and pathologic processes. Radiology, 144:109, 1982.

35. Chang, A., Glazer, H. S., Lee, J. K. T., Ling, D., and Heiken, J. P.: Adrenal gland: MR imaging. Radiology, 163:123, 1987.

36. Chang, C. H., and Pool, J. L.: The radiotherapy of pituitary chromophobe adenomas. Radiology, 89:1005, 1967.

37. Channick, B. J., Adlin, E. V., and Marks, A. D.: Suppressed plasma renin activity in hypertension. Arch. Intern. Med., 123:131, 1969.

38. Child, D. F., Burke, C. W., Burley, D. M., Rees, L. H., and Fraser, J. R.: Drug control of Cushing's syndrome. Acta Endocrinol. (Copenh.), 82:330, 1976.

39. Child, D. F., Nader, S., Mashiter, K., Kjeld, M., Banks, L., and Fraser, T. R.: Prolactin studies in "functionless" pituitary tumors. Br. Med. J., 1:604, 1975.

40. Cohn, K., Gottesman, L., and Brennan, M. F.: Adrenocortical carcinoma. Surgery, 100:1170, 1986.

41. Conn, J. W.: Presidential Address: 1) Painting background. 2) Primary aldosteronism. J. Lab. Clin. Med., 45:661, 1955.

42. Cook, D. M.: Pituitary tumors: Diagnosis and therapy. CA, 33:215, 1983.

43. Corey, R. M., Varma, S. K., Drake, C. R., Jr., Thorner, M. O., Kovacs, K., Rivier, J., and Vale, W.: Ectopic secretion of corticotropin-releasing factor as a cause of Cushing's syndrome. N. Engl. J. Med., 311:13, 1984.

44. Crabbé, J., and Vandeput, Y.: Associated endocrine disorders in the chronic form of pituitary adrenocortical failure. Horm. Res., 16:298, 1982.

45. Crapo, L.: Cushing's syndrome: A review of diagnostic tests. Metabolism, 28:955, 1979.

46. Crowder, R. E.: Development of adrenal gland in man, with special reference to origin and ultimate location of cell types, and evidence in favor of cell "migration" theory. Contrib. Embryol. Carnegie Inst., 36:193, 1957.

47. Cushing, H.: Sexual infantilism with optic atrophy in cases of tumor affecting the hypophysis cerebri. J. Nerv. Ment. Dis., 33:704, 1906.

48. Cushing, H.: Partial hypophysectomy for acromegaly. Ann. Surg., 50:1002, 1909.

49. Cushing, H.: Acromegaly from a surgical standpoint. Br. Med. J., 2:48, 1927.

50. Cushing, H.: The basophil adenomas of the pituitary body and their clinical manifestations (pituitary basophilism). Bull. Johns Hopkins Hosp., 50:137, 1932.

51. Daughaday, W. H.: The anterior pituitary. In: Wilson, J. D., and Foster, D. W. (Eds.): Textbook of Endocrinology. Philadelphia, W. B. Saunders Company, 1985, pp. 568–613.

52. Davey, L. M.: Early historical aspects of the pituitary gland. In: Goodrich, I., and Lee, K. J. (Eds.): The Pituitary. Amsterdam, Elsevier, 1988, pp. 1–17.

53. Davis, P. C., Hoffman, J. C., Jr., Tindall, G. T., and Braun, I. F.: Prolactin-secreting pituitary microadenomas: Inaccuracy of high resolution CT imaging. A.J.R., 144:151, 1985.

54. Deane, H. G.: The anatomy, chemistry, and physiology of adrenocortical tissue. Handbuch Exp. Pharmakol., 14:1, 1962.

55. DeBustro, S. A., and Baylin, S. B.: Hormone production by tumors: Biological and clinical agents. J. Clin. Endocrinol. Metab., 14:911, 1985.

56. DeChiro, G., and Nelson, K. B.: The volume of sella turcica. A.J.R., 87:989, 1962.

57. Demura, R., Kubo, O., Demura, H., et al.: FSH and LH secreting pituitary adenoma. J. Clin. Endocrinol. Metab., 45:653, 1977.

58. Desmonts, J. M., LeHoueller, J., Redmond, P., and Duvaldestin, P.: Anaesthetic management of patients with pheochromocytoma. Br. J. Anaesthesiol., 49:991, 1977.

59. Dial, P., Marks, C., and Bolton, J.: Current management of paraganglionoma. Surg. Gynecol. Obstet., 155:187, 1982.

60. Dommerholt, H. B., Assies, J., and Van der Werf, A. J.: Growth of a prolactinoma during pregnancy: Case report and review. Br. J. Obstet. Gynaecol., 88:62, 1981.

61. Ducatman, B. S., Schiethower, B. W., van Heerden, J. A., and Sheedy, P. F.: Simultaneous pheochromocytoma and renal cell carcinoma. Br. J. Surg., 70:415, 1983.

62. Dunnick, N. R., Schaner, E. G., Doppman, J. L., Strott, C. A., Gill, J. R., and Javadpour, N.: Computed tomography in adrenal tumors. A.J.R., 132:43, 1979.

63. Eastman, R. C., Gorden, P., and Roth, J.: Conventional supervoltage radiation is an effective treatment for acromegaly. J. Clin. Endocrinol. Metab., 48:931, 1979.

64. El-Manawi, M. F., Paulino, E., Cuesta, M., and Ceballos, J.: Pheochromocytoma masquerading as pre-eclamptic toxemia. Am. J. Obstet. Gynecol., 109:389, 1971.

65. Engel, A., and Euler, U. S., von: Diagnostic value of increased urinary output of noradrenalin and adrenalin in pheochromocytoma. Lancet, 2:387, 1950.

66. Erdheim, J., and Stumme, E.: Ueber die Schwanger Schaftsveranderung der Hypophyse. Beitr. Pathol. Anat. Allg. Pathol., 46:1, 1909.

67. Euler, U. S., von: Increased urinary excretion of noradrenalin and adrenalin in cases of pheochromocytoma. Ann. Surg., 134:929, 1951.

68. Franchimont, P., Demoulin, A., Bourguignon, J. P., and Santen, R.: Role of inhibin in the regulation of gonadotropin secretion in the male. Pediatr. Adolesc. Endocrinol., 6:47, 1979.

69. Frankel, F.: Ein Fall von doppelseitigem völlig latent verlaufenen Nebennierentumor und gleichzeitiger Nephritis mit Veränderungen am Circulationsapparat und Retinitis. Virchows Arch. [A], 103:244, 1886.

70. Franks, S., and Nabarro, J. D. N.: Prolactin secretion in patients with chromophobe adenomas of the pituitary: Incidence and presentation of hyperprolactinaemia: Results of surgical treatment. Ann. Clin. Res., 10:157, 1978.

71. Franksson, C., Birke, G., and Plantin, L. O.: Adrenal autotransplantation in Cushing's syndrome. Acta Chir. Scand., 117:409, 1959.

72. Freitas, J. E., Grekin, R. J. Thrall, J. H., Gross, M. D., Swanson, D. P., and Beierwaltes, W. H.: Adrenal imaging with iodomethyl-norcholesterol (I-131) in primary aldosterone. J. Nucl. Med., 20:7, 1979.

73. Froesch, E. R., Schmid, C., Schwander, J., and Zapf, J.: Actions of insulin-like growth factors. Annu. Rev. Physiol., 47:443, 1985.

74. Fröhlich, A.: Ein Fall von Tumor der Hypophysis cerebri ohne Acromegalie. Wien Klin. Rundsch., p. 47, 1901.

75. Fudge, T. L., McKinnon, W. M. P., and Geary, W. L.: Current surgical man-

agement of pheochromocytoma during pregnancy. Arch. Surg., 115:1224, 1980.

76. Galen: De Uso Partium, Book 9, Chapter 4. De Usu Partium, Chapter 2.

77. Gann, D. S., Delea, C. S., Gill, J. R., Jr., Thomas, J. P., and Bartter, F. C.: Control of aldosterone secretion by change of body potassium in normal man. Am. J. Physiol., 202:991, 1964.

78. Gharib, H., Carpenter, P. C., Scheithauer, B. W., and Service, F. J.: The spectrum of inappropriate pituitary thyrotropin secretion associated with hyperthyroidism. Mayo Clin. Proc., 57:556, 1982.

79. Glazer, G. M.: MR imaging of the liver, kidneys and adrenals. Radiology, 166:303, 1988.

80. Goldberg, M. F., and Fine, S. L. (Eds.): Symposium on the Treatment of Diabetic Retinopathy. U.S. Public Health Service Publication 1890. Washington, D.C., U.S. Government Printing Office, 1969.

81. Graham, L. S.: Celiac accessory adrenal glands. Cancer, 6:149, 1953.

82. Grant, C. S., Carpenter, P., van Heerden, J. A., and Hamberger, B.: Primary aldosteronism: Clinical management. Arch. Surg., 119:585, 1984.

83. Grantham, J. J., and Orloff, J.: Effect of prostaglandin E₁ on the permeability of the isolated collecting tubule to vasopressin, adenosine 3'-5' monophosphate and theophylline. J. Clin. Invest., 47:1154, 1968.

84. Griffin, J. E., and Wilson, J. D.: Disorders of the testes and male reproductive tract. In Wilson, J. D., and Foster, D. W. (Eds.): Textbook of Endocrinology. Philadelphia, W. B. Saunders Company, 1985, pp. 259–311.

85. Grigsby, P. W., Simpson, J. R., Emami, B. N., Fineberg, B. B., and Schwartz, H. G.: Prognostic factors and results of surgery and postoperative irradiation in the management of pituitary adenomas. Int. J. Radiat. Oncol. Biol. Phys., 16:1411, 1989.

86. Grigsby, P. W., Stokes, S., Marks, J. E., and Simpson, J. R.: Prognostic factors and results of radiotherapy alone in the management of pituitary adenomas. Int. J. Radiat. Oncol. Biol. Phys., 15:1103, 1988.

87. Guyda, H., Robert, F., Colle, E., and Hardy, J.: Histologic, ultrastructural and hormonal characterization of a pituitary tumor secreting both LGH and prolactin. J. Clin. Endocrinol. Metab., 36:531, 1973.

88. Hall, W. D., Wollam, G. L., and Tuttle, E. P., Jr.: Diagnostic evaluation of patient with hypertension. In Hurst, J. W., (Ed.): The Heart. New York, McGraw Hill Book Company, 1986, p. 1057.

89. Handler, J. S.: Vasopressin-prostaglandin interactions in the regulation of epithelial cell permeability to water. Kidney Int., 19:831, 1981.

90. Hankenson, J., and Banna, M.: Pituitary and Parapituitary Tumors. Philadelphia, W. B. Saunders Company, 1976.

91. Hardy, J.: Transsphenoidal microsurgical treatment of pituitary tumors. In Linfoot, J. A. (Ed.): Recent Advances in the Diagnosis and Treatment of Pituitary Tumors. New York, Raven Press, 1979, pp. 375–388.

92. Hardy, J., Somma, M., and Vezina, J. L.: Treatment of acromegaly: Radiation or surgery? In Morley, T. P. (Ed.): Current Controversies in Neurosurgery. Philadelphia, W. B. Saunders Company, 1976, pp. 377–391.

93. Hardy, J., and Vezina, J. L.: Transsphenoidal neurosurgery of intracranial neoplasm. Adv. Neurol., 15:261, 1976.

94. Hardy, J. D.: Surgical management of Cushing's syndrome with emphasis on adrenal autotransplantation. Ann. Surg., 188:290, 1978.

95. Harvey, H. A., Santen, R. J., Osterman, J., Samojlik, E., White, D. S., and Lipton, A. A.: A comparative trial of transsphenoidal hypophysectomy and estrogen suppression with aminoglutethimide in advanced breast cancer. Cancer, 43:2207, 1979.

96. Henderson, W. R.: The pituitary adenomata: A follow-up study of the surgical results in 338 cases. Br. J. Surg., 26:811, 1938.

97. Henley, D. J., van Heerden, J. A., Grant, C. S., et al.: Adrenal cortical carcinoma: A continuing challenge. Surgery, 94:926, 1983.

98. Himathongkam, T., Dluhy, R. G., and Williams, G. H.: Potassium-aldosterone renin interrelationships. J. Clin. Endocrinol. Metab., 41:153, 1975.

98a. Holaday, J. W., Long, J. B., Martinez-Arizala, A., Chen, H. S., Reynolds, D. G., and Gurll, N. J.: Effects of TRH in circulatory shock and central nervous system ischemia. Ann. N. Y. Acad. Sci., 553:370, 1989.

99. Holder, G. E.: The effects of chiasmal compression on the pattern visual evoked potential. Electroencephalogr. Clin. Neurophysiol., 45:278, 1978.

100. Hollenhorst, E. W., and Younge, B. R.: Ocular manifestations produced by adenomas of the pituitary gland: Analysis of 1000 cases. In Kohler, P. O., and Ross, G. T. (Eds.): Diagnosis and Treatment of Pituitary Tumors. Amsterdam, Excerpta Medica, 1973, p. 53.

101. Horsely, V.: On the technique of operations on the central nervous system. Br. Med. J., 2:411, 1906.

102. Howard, C. P., Takahashi, H., and Hayles, A. B.: Feminizing adrenal adenoma in a boy: Case report and review of the literature. Mayo Clin. Proc., 52:354, 1977.

103. Howlett, et al.: Cushing's syndrome. Clin. Endocrinol. Metab., 14:911, 1985.

104. Hume, D. M.: Pheochromocytoma in the adult and in the child. Am. J. Surg., 99:458, 1960.

105. Hutter, A. M., and Kayhoe, D. E.: Adrenal cortical carcinoma: Clinical features of 138 patients. Am. J. Med., 41:572, 1966.

106. Ituarte, E. A., Petrini, J., and Hershman, J. M.: Acromegaly and colon cancer. Ann. Intern. Med., 101:627, 1984.

107. Jackson, I. M. D.: Thyrotropin-releasing hormone. N. Engl. J. Med., 306:145, 1982.

108. Joffe, S. N., and Brown, C.: Nodular adrenal hyperplasia and Cushing's syndrome. Surgery, 94:919, 1983.

109. Johnston, D. G., Prescott, R. W., Kendall-Taylor, P., Hall, K., Crombie, A. L.,

110. Hall, R., McGregor, A., Watson, M. J., and Cook, D. B.: Hyperprolactinemia: Long-term effects of bromocriptine. Am. J. Med., 75:868, 1983.

110. Judge, D. M., Kulin, H. E., Page, R., Santen, R. J., and Trapukdi, S.: Hypothalamic hamartoma. N. Engl. J. Med., 296:7, 1977.

111. Kaminsky, N., Luse, S., and Hartroft, P.: Ultrastructure of adrenal cortex of the dog during treatment with DDD. J.N.C.I., 29:127, 1962.

112. Karpf, D. B., and Braunstein, G. D.: Current concepts in acromegaly: Etiology, diagnosis and treatment. Comp. Ther., 12:22, 1986.

113. Katz, E. L.: Late results of radical excision of craniopharyngiomas in children. J. Neurosurg., 42:86, 1975.

114. Kaufman, B.: Magnetic resonance imaging of the pituitary gland. Radiol. Clin. North Am., 22:795, 1984.

115. Kaufman, B., Telander, R. L., van Heerden, J. A., Zimmerman, D., Sheps, G. S., and Dawson, B.: Pheochromocytoma in pediatric age groups: Current status. J. Pediatr. Surg., 18:879, 1983.

116. Kehlet, H., and Binder, C.: Value of an ACTH test in assessing hypothalamic-pituitary-adrenocortical function in glucocorticoid treated patients. Br. Med. J., 2:142, 1973.

117. Kelly, W. F., MacFarlane, I. A., Longson, D., Davies, D., and Sutcliffe, H.: Cushing's disease treated by total adrenalectomy. Q. J. Med., 52:224, 1983.

118. Kjellberg, R. N.: Craniopharyngiomas. In Tindall, G. T., and Collins, W. F. (Eds.): Clinical Management of Pituitary Disorders. New York, Raven Press, 1979, pp. 373–388.

118a. Kjellberg, R. N., and Kliman, B.: A system for therapy of pituitary tumors. In Kohler, P. O., and Ross, G. T. (Eds.): Diagnosis and Treatment of Pituitary Tumors. Int. Congress Series 303. Amsterdam, Excerpta Medica, 1973, p. 234.

119. Knobil, E.: The neuroendocrine control of the menstrual cycle. Recent Prog. Horm. Res., 36:53, 1980.

120. Koenig, R. J., Leonard, J. L., Senator, D., Rappaport, N., Watson, A. Y., and Larsen, P. R.: Regulation of thyroxine 5'-deiodinase activity by 3,5,3'-triiodothyronine in cultured rat anterior pituitary cells. Endocrinology, 115,324, 1984.

121. Kohner, E. M., Dollery, C. T., Fraser, T. R., and Bulpitt, C. J.: The effect of pituitary ablation on diabetic retinopathy studied by fluorescein angiography. Diabetes, 19:703, 1970.

122. Kohner, E. M., Hamilton, A. M., and Joplin, G. F.: Florid diabetic retinopathy and its response to treatment by photocoagulation of pituitary ablation. Diabetes, 25:104, 1976.

123. Kotchen, T. A., Mulrow, P. J., Morrow, L. B., Shutkin, P. M., and Marieb, N.: Renin and aldosterone in essential hypertension. Clin. Sci., 41:321, 1971.

124. Kovacs, K., Corenblum, B., Sirek, A. M. T., Penz, G., and Ezrin, C.: Localization of prolactin in chromophobe pituitary adenomas: Study of human necropsy material by immunoperoxidase technique. J. Clin. Pathol., 29:250, 1976.

125. Kramer, S.: Craniopharyngioma: The best treatment is conservative surgery and postoperative radiation therapy. In Morley, T. P. (Ed.): Current Controversies in Neurosurgery. Philadelphia, W. B. Saunders Company, 1976, pp. 336–343.

126. Krieger, D. T.: Medical treatment of Cushing's disease. In Tolis, G., Labrie, F., Martin, J. B., and Naftolin, F. (Eds.): Clinical Neuroendocrinology: A Pathophysiological Approach. New York, Raven Press, 1979, pp. 423–427.

127. Krieger, D. T.: Neuroendocrine physiology. In Felig, P., Baxter, J. D., Broadus, A. E., and Frohman, L. A. (Eds.): Endocrinology and Metabolism, New York, McGraw-Hill Book Company, 1981, pp. 151–175.

128. Krieger, D. T.: The multiple faces of pro-opiomelanocortin, a prototype precursor molecule. Clin. Res., 31:342, 1983.

129. L'abbe, M., Tinel, J., and Doumer, E.: Crises solaires et hypertension paroxystique en rapport avec une tumeur surrenale. Bull. Soc. Med. Hop., 46:982, 1922.

130. LaRossa, J. T., Strong, M. S., and Melby, J. C.: Endocrinologically incomplete transethmoidal transsphenoidal hypophysectomy with relief of bone pain in breast cancer. N. Engl. J. Med., 298:1332, 1978.

131. Larsen, J. L., Cathey, W. J., and Odell, W. D.: Primary adrenocortical nodular dysplasia, a distinct subtype of Cushing's syndrome. Am. J. Med., 80:976, 1986.

132. Larsen, P. R.: Thyroid-pituitary interaction. N. Engl. J. Med., 306:23, 1982.

133. Laws, E. R., Jr., Piepgras, D. G., Randall, R. V., et al.: Neurosurgical management of acromegaly. J. Neurosurg., 50:454, 1979.

134. Lee, B. C. P., and Deck, M. D. F.: Sella and juxtasellar lesion detection with MRI. Radiology, 157:143, 1985.

135. Lee, K. J., Goodrich, I., and Pensak, M.: Pituitary surgery: Current status, including transsphenoidal surgery. Am. J. Otolaryngol., 5:138, 1984.

136. Leong, D. A., Frawley, L. S., and Neill, J. D.: Neuroendocrine control of prolactin secretion. Annu. Rev. Physiol., 45:109, 1983.

137. Liddle, G. W.: Tests of pituitary-adrenal suppressibility in the diagnosis of Cushing's syndrome. J. Clin. Endocrinol. Metab., 20:1539, 1960.

138. Liddle, G. W., Estep, H. L., Kendall, J. W., Jr., William, W. C., Jr., and Townes, A. W.: Clinical application of a new test of pituitary reserve. J. Clin. Endocrinol., 29:875, 1959.

139. Linfoot, J. A.: Heavy ion therapy: Alpha particle therapy of pituitary tumors. In Linfoot, J. A. (Ed.): Recent Advances in the Diagnosis and Treatment of Pituitary Tumors. New York, Raven Press, 1979, pp. 245–267.

139a. Linfoot, J. A., Nakagawa, J. S., Wiedemann, E., Lyman, J., Chong, C., Carcia, J., and Lawrence, J. H.: Heavy particle therapy: Pituitary tumors. L. A. Bull. Neurol. Soc., 42:175, 1975.

140. Lipsett, M. B.: Treatment of adrenal carcinoma. *In* Nelson, D. H. (Ed.): Modern Treatment. New York, Harper & Row, 1966, pp. 1377–1388.

141. Loli, P., Berselli, M. A., and Tagliaferri, M.: Use of ketoconazole in the treatment of Cushing's syndrome. J. Clin. Endocrinol. Metab., *63:*1365, 1986.

142. Ludecke, D., Kautzky, R., Saeger, W., and Schrader, D.: Selective removal of hypersecreting pituitary adenomas? An analysis of endocrine function, operative and microscopical findings in 101 cases. Acta Neurochir., *35:*27, 1976.

143. Manger, W. M., and Gifford, R. W., Jr.: Pheochromocytoma. New York, Springer-Verlag, 1977.

144. Manolas, K. J., Farmer, H. M., Wilson, H. K., et al.: The pituitary before and after adrenalectomy for Cushing's syndrome. World J. Surg., *8:*374, 1984.

145. March, C. M., Mishell, D. R., Kletsky, O. A., Israel, R., Davajan, V., and Nakamura, R. M.: Galactorrhea and pituitary tumors in postpill and non-postpill secondary amenorrhea. Am. J. Obstet. Gynecol., *134:*45, 1979.

146. Marie, P.: Sur deux cas d'acromegalie, hypertrophie singulière, non congenitale, des extrémités supérieures, inférieures, etc. céphalique. Rev. Med., *6:*297, 1886.

147. Mattingly, D., and Sheridan, P.: Simultaneous diagnosis and treatment of acute adrenal insufficiency. Lancet, *1:*432, 1976.

148. Mayo, C. H.: Paroxysmal hypertension with tumor of retroperitoneal nerve: Report of a case. J.A.M.A., *89:*1047, 1927.

149. McPartland, R. P.: Metabolic and pharmacologic actions of glucocoorticoids. *In* Mulrow, P. J. (Ed.): The Adrenal Gland. New York, Elsevier, 1986, pp. 85–116.

150. Melmed, S., et al.: Pituitary tumors secreting growth hormone and prolactin (UCLA Conference). Ann. Intern. Med., *105:*238, 1986.

151. Menon, M., and Walsh, P. C.: Hormonal therapy for prostatic cancer. *In* Murphy, G. P. (Ed.): Prostatic Cancer. Littleton, Mass., PSG Publishing Company, 1979, pp. 175–200.

152. Miller, M., Dalakos, T., Moses, A. M., Fellerman, H., and Streeten, D. H. P.: Recognition of partial defects in antidiuretic hormone secretion. Ann. Intern. Med., *73:*721, 1970.

153. Miller, W. M., and Levine, L. S.: Molecular and clinical advances in congenital adrenal hyperplasia. J. Pediatrics, *111:*1, 1987.

154. Milsom, S. R., Espiner, E. A., Nicholls, M. G., et al.: The blood pressure response to unilateral adrenalectomy in primary aldosteronism. Q. J. Med., *61:*1141, 1986.

155. Mohr, B.: Tumor of the pituitary body. Wochenschr. Ges. Heilk., Berlin, *6:*565, 1840.

156. Molitch, M. E., Elton, R. L., Blackwell, R. E., et al.: Bromocriptine as primary therapy for prolactin-secreting macroadenomas: Results of a prospective multicenter study. J. Clin. Endocrinol. Metab., *6:*698, 1985.

157. Montagne, J. P., Kressel, H. Y., Korobkin, M., and Moss, A. A.: Computed tomography of the normal adrenal glands. A.J.R., *130:*963, 1978.

158. Moore, T. J., Dluhy, R. G., Williams, G. H., and Cain, J. P.: Nelson's syndrome: Frequency, prognosis, and effect of prior pituitary irradiation. Ann. Intern. Med., *85:*731, 1976.

159. Murayama, T., Karvati, K., and Nijimon, T.: Relationship between postoperative blood pressure change and renal pathophysiology in primary aldosteronism. Urol. Int., *39:*364, 1984.

160. Murray, F. T., Osterman, J., Sulewski, J., Page, R., Bergland, R., and Hammand, J. M.: Pituitary function following surgery for prolactinomas. Obstet. Gynecol., *54:*65, 1979.

161. Nabarro, J. D. N.: Pituitary prolactinomas. Clin. Endocrinol., *17:*129, 1982.

162. Nelson, D. H., Meakin, J. W., and Thorn, G. W.: ACTH-producing pituitary tumors following adrenalectomy for Cushing's syndrome. Ann. Intern. Med., *52:*560, 1960.

163. Nerup, J.: Addison's disease — Clinical studies: A report of 108 cases. Acta Endocrinol., *76:*127, 1974.

164. Nolan, P. M., Sheeler, L. R., Hahn, J. F., et al.: Therapeutic problems with transsphenoidal pituitary surgery for Cushing's disease. Cleveland Clin. Q., *49:*199, 1982.

165. Nugent, C. A., Nichols, T., and Tyler, F. H.: Diagnosis of Cushing's syndrome: Single dose dexamethasone suppression test. Arch. Intern. Med., *116:*172, 1965.

166. Ochi, K., Yoshioka, S., Morita, M., and Takeuchi, M.: Pheochromocytoma of women. Urology, *17:*228, 1981.

167. Oparil, S., and Haber, E.: The renin angiotensin system. N. Engl. J. Med., *291:*389, 446, 1974.

168. Orth, D. N., and Liddle, G. W.: Results of treatment in 108 patients with Cushing's syndrome. N. Engl. J. Med., *285:*243, 1971.

169. Page, R. B., and Bergland, R. M.: The neurohypophyseal capillary bed. I. Anatomy and arterial supply. Am. J. Anat., *148:*345, 1977.

170. Palmore, W. P., and Mulrow, P. J.: Control of aldosterone secretion by the pituitary gland. Science, *158:*1482, 1967.

171. Parks, D.: Drug therapy: Bromocriptine. N. Engl. J. Med., *301:*873, 1979.

172. Parrillo, J. E., and Fauci, A. S.: Mechanisms of glucocorticoid action on immune processes. Ann. Rev. Pharmacol. Toxicol., *19:*179, 1979.

173. Paulesco, N. C.: L'hypophyse du cerveau. Paris, Vigot Frères, 1908.

174. Pick, L.: Das Ganglioma embryonale sympathicum (Sympathoma embryonale) eine Typsche bosartiga geshwuestform des sympathischen Nervensystems. Berl. Klin. Wochenschr., *49:*16, 1912.

175. Plotz, C. M., Knowlton, A. I., and Rogan, C.: The natural history of Cushing's syndrome. Am. J. Med., *13:*597, 1952.

176. Prader, A.: Die haufigkeit der kongenitalen adrenogenitalen syndroms. Helv. Paediatr. Acta, *13:*426, 1958.

177. Randall, R. V.: Neuroendocrinology. *In* Younan, R. S. (Ed.): Neurological Surgery. Vol. 12. Philadelphia, W. B. Saunders Company, 1977, pp. 931–988.

178. Randall, R. V., Laws, E. R., Jr., Abboud, C. F., et al.: Transsphenoidal microsurgical treatment of prolactin-producing pituitary adenomas. Mayo Clin. Proc., *58:*108, 1983.

179. Raper, A. J., Jessee, E. F., Texter, J. H., Giffler, R. F., and Hietala, S. O.: Pheochromocytoma of the urinary bladder: A broad clinical spectrum. Am. J. Cardiol., *40:*820, 1977.

180. Rathke, M. H.: Ueber die Entstehung der Glandula pituitar. Mullens Arch. Anat. Physiol. Wissensch. Med., *5:*482, 1838.

181. Redman, B. G., Pazdur, R., Zingas, N. P., and Loredo, R.: Prospective evaluation of adrenal insufficiency in patients with adrenal metastases. Cancer, *60:*103, 1987.

182. Remine, W. H., Chong, G. C., van Heerden, J. A., Sheps, S. G., and Harrison, E. G.: Current management of pheochromocytoma. Ann. Surg., *179:*740, 1974.

183. Rieu, M., Girard, F., Bricaire, H., and Binoux, M.: The importance of insulin-like growth factor (somatomedin) measurements in the diagnosis and surveillance of acromegaly. J. Clin. Endocrinol. Metab., *55:*147, 1982.

184. Robertson, G. L., and Athar, S.: The interaction of blood osmolality and blood volume in regulating plasma vasopressin in man. J. Clin. Endocrinol. Metab., *42:*613, 1976.

185. Robertson, G. L., Aycinena, P., and Zerbe, R. L.: Neurogenic disorders of osmoregulation. Am. J. Med., *72:*339, 1982.

186. Robinson, A. G., and Nelson, P. B.: Prolactinomas in women: Current therapies. Ann. Intern. Med., *99:*115, 1983.

187. Ross, G. T., Cargille, C. M., and Lipsett, M. B.: Pituitary and gonadal hormones in women during spontaneous and induced ovulatory cycles. Recent Prog. Horm. Res., *26:*1, 1970.

188. Rothrock, J. F., Laguna, J. F., and Reynolds, A. F.: CSF rhinorrhea from untreated pituitary adenoma. Arch. Neurol., *39:*442, 1982.

189. Roux: Thesis, Lousanne, 1926. Cited by Barbeau, A., Marc-Aurele, J., Brouillet, J., Vitye, B., Leboeuf, G., Cartier, P., Mignault, G., and Genest, J.: Le pheochromocytome bilateral: Presentation d'un cas et revue de literature. Union Med. Can., *87:*165, 1958.

190. Salassa, R. M., Laws, E. R., Jr., Carpenter, P. C., and Northcutt, R. C.: Transsphenoidal removal of pituitary microadenoma in Cushing's disease. Mayo Clin. Proc., *53:*24, 1978.

191. Santen, R. J., and Kulin, H. E.: The male reproductive system. *In* Kelley, V. C. (Ed.): Practice of Pediatrics. Vol. 1. New York, Harper & Row, 1976, pp. 1–44.

192. Santen, R. J., and Manni, A. (Eds.): Controversies in the treatment of endocrine tumors: Medical and surgical management of prolactinomas and thyroid cancer. *In:* Diagnosis and Management of Endocrine-Related Tumors. Boston, Martinus Nijhoff Publishers, 1984, pp. 419–437.

193. Schechter, D. C.: Aberrant adrenal tissue. Ann. Surg., *167:*421, 1968.

194. Scheithauer, B. W., Kovacs, K., Randall, R. V., and Ryan, N.: Pituitary gland in hypothyroidism. Arch. Pathol. Lab. Med., *109:*499, 1985.

195. Schenker, J. G., and Chowers, I.: Pheochromocytoma and pregnancy. Obstet. Gynecol. Surg., *26:*739, 1971.

196. Schloffer, H.: Erfolgreiche Operation eines Hypophysentumors auf Nasalem. Wege. Wein Klin. Wochenschr., *20:*621, 1907.

197. Schonebeck, J.: Malignant pheochromocytoma. Scand. J. Urol. Nephrol., *3:*64, 1969.

198. Schönemann, A.: Hypophysis und thyreoidea. Arch. Pathol. Anat., *129:*310, 1892.

199. Schrier, W., and Linas, S. L.: Mechanisms of the defect in the water excretion in adrenal insufficiency. Miner. Electrolyte Metab., *4:*1, 1980.

200. Schteingart, D. E., Motazedi, A., Noonan, R. A., et al.: Treatment of adrenal carcinomas. Arch. Surg., *117:*1142, 1982.

201. Scott, H. W., Jr., Oates, J. A., Nies, A. S., Burke, H., Page, D. L., and Rhany, R. K.: Pheochromocytoma: Presentation, diagnosis and management. Ann. Surg., *183:*587, 1976.

202. Serri, O., Rasio, E., Beauregard, H., Hardy, J., and Somma, M.: Recurrence of hyperprolactinemia after selective transsphenoidal adenomectomy in women with prolactinemia. N. Engl. J. Med., *309:*280, 1983.

202a. Sheline, G. E.: Treatment of chromophobe adenomas of the pituitary gland and acromegaly. *In* Kohler, P. O., and Ross, G. T. (Eds.): Diagnosis and Treatment of Pituitary Tumors. Amsterdam, Excerpta Medica, 1973, p. 201.

203. Sheline, G. R.: Radiation therapy of pituitary tumors. *In* Givens, J. R. (Ed.): Hormone-Secreting Pituitary Tumors. Chicago, Year Book Medical Publishers, 1982, pp. 121–143.

204. Shenker, Y.: Medical treatment of low-renin aldosteronism. Endocrinol. Metab. Clin. North Am., *18:*415, 1989.

205. Short, R. V.: Breast feeding. Sci. Am., *250:*35, 1984.

206. Sjoerdsma, A., Waldman, T. A., Cooperman, T. A., and Hammond, W. G.: Pheochromocytoma: Current concepts of diagnosis and treatment. Ann. Intern. Med., *65:*1302, 1966.

207. Snyder, P. J., Bigdeli, H., Gardner, D. F., Mihailovic, V., Rudenstein, R. S., Sterling, F. H., and Utiger, R. D.: Gonadal function in fifty men with untreated pituitary adenomas. J. Clin. Endocrinol. Metab., *48:*309, 1979.

208. Speckart, P. F., Nicoloff, J. T., and Bethone, J. E.: Screening for adrenocortical insufficiency with cosyntropin. Arch. Intern. Med., *128:*761, 1971.

209. Spiger, M., Jubiz, W., Meikle, A. W., West, C. D., and Tyler, H.: Single dose metyrapone test. Arch. Intern. Med., 135:698, 1975.
210. Stackpole, R. H., Melicow, M. M., and Uson, A. C.: Pheochromocytoma in children. J. Pediatr., 63:315, 1963.
211. Svien, H. J., Love, J. G., Kennedy, W. C., Colby, M. Y., and Kearns, T. P.: Status of vision following surgical treatment for pituitary chromophobe adenoma. J. Neurosurg., 22:47, 1965.
212. Sweet, W. H.: Radical surgical treatment of craniopharyngioma. In Schmidek, H. H., and Sweet, W. H. (Eds.): Current Techniques in Operative Neurosurgery. New York, Grune & Stratton, 1977, pp. 199–221.
213. Tandler, J., and Grosz, S.: Über den Einfluss der Kastration auf den Orangismus. Wien Klin. Wochenschr., 20:1596, 1907.
214. Tanoka, K., Nicholson, W. E., and Orth, D. N.: Diurnal rhythm and disappearance half-time of endogenous plasma immunoreactive βMSH (LPH) and ACTH in man. J. Clin. Endocrinol. Metab., 46:883, 1978.
215. Taylor, A. L., and Fishman, L. M.: Medical progress: Corticotropin-releasing hormone. N. Engl. J. Med., 319:213, 1988.
216. Taylor, S.: High resolution computerized tomography of the sella. Radiol. Clin. North Am., 20:207, 1982.
217. Thomas, C. G., Smith, A. T., Griffith, J. M., and Askin, F. B.: Hyperadrenalism in childhood and adolescence. Ann. Surg., 199:538, 1984.
218. Thompson, N. W., Allo, M. D., Shapiro, B., Sisson, J. C., and Beierwaltes, W. H.: Extra-adrenal and metastatic pheochromocytoma: The role of ^{131}I-meta-iodobenzylguanidine (^{131}I-MIGB) in localization and management. World J. Surg., 8:605, 1984.
219. Thorner, M. O., Frohman, L. A., Leong, D. A., et al.: Extrahypothalamic growth-hormone-releasing factor (GRF) levels in 177 acromegalic patients. J. Clin. Endocrinol. Metab., 59:846, 1984.
220. Tomori, N., Suda, T., Tozawa, F., Demura, H., Shizuma, K., and Mouri, T.: Immunoreactive corticotropin-releasing factor concentrations in cerebrospinal fluid from patients with hypothalamic pituitary adrenal disorders. J. Clin. Endocrinol. Metab., 57:1305, 1983.
221. Tyrell, M. B., Brooks, R. M., Fitzgerald, P. A., et al.: Cushing's disease: Selective transsphenoidal resection of pituitary microadenomas. N. Engl. J. Med., 298:753, 1978.
221a. U, H. S., Wilson, C. B., and Tyrrell, J. B.: Transsphenoidal microhypophysectomy in acromegaly. J. Neurosurg., 47:840, 1977.
222. Vaitukaitis, J. L., Ross, G. T., Braunstein, G. D., et al.: Gonadotropins and their subunits: Basic and clinical studies. Recent Prog. Horm. Res., 32:289, 1976.
223. Valimaki, M., Pelkonen, R., Porkka, L., Sivula, A., and Kahri, A.: Long-term results of adrenal surgery in patients with Cushing's syndrome due to adrenocortical adenoma. Clin. Endocrinol., 20:229, 1984.
224. Van Heerden, J. A., Steps, S. G., Hamberger, B., Sheedy, P. F., Poston, J. G., and Remine, W. H.: Pheochromocytoma: Current status and changing trends. Surgery, 91:367, 1982.

225. Veldhuis, J. D., and Hammond, J. M.: Endocrine function after spontaneous infarction of the human pituitary: Report, review and reappraisal. Endocrinol. Rev., 1:100, 1980.
226. Vesalius, A.: De Humani Corporis Fabrica. Basel, Ioannis Openini, 1543, p. 663.
227. Wajchenberg, B. L., Silveira, A. A., Goldman, J., Cesar, F. P., Marino, R., Jr., and Lima, S. S.: Evaluation of resection of pituitary microadenoma for the treatment of Cushing's disease in patients with radiologically normal sella turcica. Clin. Endocrinol., 11:323, 1979.
228. Wakai, S., Fukushima, T., Teramoto, A., and Sano, K.: Pituitary apoplexy: Its incidence and clinical significance. J. Neurosurg., 55:187, 1981.
229. Wakai, S., Yamakawa, K., Manaka, S., and Takakura, K.: Spontaneous intracranial hemorrhage caused by brain tumor: Its incidence and clinical significance. Neurosurgery, 10:437, 1982.
230. Wass, J. A. H., Williams, J., Charlesworth, M., et al.: Bromocriptine in management of large pituitary tumors. Br. Med. J., 284:1908, 1982.
231. Watson, J. D., Varley, J. G., Tomlin, S. J., Medbak, S., Rees, L. H., and Hinds, C. J.: Biochemical characterization of circulating met-enkephalins in canine endotoxin shock. J. Endocrinol., 111:329, 1986.
232. Wehrenberg, W. B., Baird, A., and Ling, N.: Potent interactions between glucocorticoids and growth hormone-releasing factor in vivo. Science, 221:556, 1983.
233. Weinberger, M. H., Grim, C. E., Hollifield, J. W., Kem, D. C., Ganguly, A., Kramer, N. J., Yune, H. Y., Wellman, H., and Donohue, J. P.: Primary aldosteronism. Diagnosis, localization and treatment: A clinical review. Ann. Intern. Med., 90:386, 1979.
234. White, P. C., New, M. I., and Dupont, B. O.: Congenital adrenal hyperplasia. N. Engl. J. Med., 316:1519, 1580, 1987.
235. Williams, G. H., Rose, L. I., Dluhy, R. G., Dingman, J. F., Lavier, D. P.: Aldosterone response to sodium restriction and ACTH stimulation in panhypopituitarism. J. Clin. Endocrinol. Metab., 32:27, 1971.
235a. Williams, R. A., Jacobs, H. S., Kurtz, A. B., Millar, J. G. B., Oakley, N. W., Spathias, G. S., Sulway, M. J., and Nabarro, J. D. N.: The treatment of acromegaly with special reference to transsphenoidal hypophysectomy. Q. J. Med., 44:79, 1975.
236. Wilson, C. B.: Neurosurgical management of large and invasive pituitary tumors. In Tindall, G. T., and Collins, W. F. (Eds.): Clinical Management of Pituitary Disorders. New York, Raven Press, 1979, pp. 335–342.
237. Wright, A. D., Hill, D. M., Lowy, C., and Fraser, T. R.: Mortality in acromegaly. Q. J. Med., 39:1, 1970.
238. Young, W. F., and Klee, G. C.: Primary aldosteronism. Endocrinol. Metab. Clin. North Am., 17:367, 1988.
239. Zervas, N. T.: Surgical results for pituitary adenomas: Results of an international survey. In Black, P. M., Zervas, N. T., Ridgeway, E. C., and Martin, J. B. (Eds.): Secretory Tumors of the Pituitary Gland: Progress in Endocrine Research and Therapy. New York, Raven Press, 1984, pp. 377–385.

26

THE ESOPHAGUS

I ——————————————————————————————————

HISTORICAL ASPECTS AND ANATOMY

Mark B. Orringer, M.D.

HISTORICAL ASPECTS

The modern surgical treatment of esophageal disease is the result of refinements in both anesthetic and operative techniques as well as methods of assessing normal and abnormal anatomy and physiology. The earliest esophageal operations were limited to cervical procedures, primarily for removal of foreign bodies. Semeleder (1863) used a forceps with spoon-shaped blades to view the upper esophagus.[23] Rigid esophagoscopy was first used successfully in 1868 by Waldenberg, who examined the cervical esophagus, and by Kussmaul, who in the same year used a modified urethroscope to diagnose a carcinoma of the thoracic esophagus. An esophagoscope with a distal electric light source was described by Mikulicz in 1881, and one fitted with an incandescent light was developed by Einhorn in 1902.[22] The same year, Killian reported the first removal of a foreign body through an esophagoscope. Subsequent refinements in the optical system used in rigid esophagoscopy, as well as the development of flexible fiberoptic esophagoscopy by Lo-Presti and Hilmi in 1964,[32] have provided a procedure that is now performed almost universally in the evaluation of patients with esophageal symptoms. The pioneering clinical work of Chevalier Jackson established guidelines for proper rigid endoscopic technique that remain valid after almost 50 years.[23,24]

Safe operations on the thoracic esophagus awaited the development of anesthetic techniques that would permit the chest to be opened. Resection of the cervical esophagus for carcinoma was first performed successfully by Billroth (1871)[6] and Czerny (1877).[10] Von Mikulicz first resected and reconstructed the cervical esophagus with a skin tube (1886).[56] Torek (1915) performed the first successful resection of the intrathoracic esophagus for carcinoma without esophageal reconstruction.[49] Janeway and Green (1910) first suggested a combined thoracoabdominal incision for carcinoma of the distal esophagus.[25]

Denk (1913) performed blunt transmediastinal esophagectomy without thoracotomy in cadavers and experimental animals using a vein stripper to avulse the esophagus from the posterior mediastinum.[12] The British surgeon Turner (1933) performed the first successful transmediastinal blunt esophagectomy for carcinoma and established continuity of the alimentary tract with an antethoracic skin tube at a second stage.[50] As endotracheal anesthesia became available, however, permitting transthoracic esophagectomy under direct vision, the technique of transhiatal esophagectomy without thoracotomy did not gain widespread use. Ohsawa (1933) performed the first successful transthoracic esophagectomy and esophagogastric anastomosis for esophageal carcinoma.[35] This feat was first accomplished in the United States by Marshall (1937)[33] and Adams and Phemister (1938).[1] Sweet (1945) and Garlock (1946), pioneers in American surgery, developed a number of techniques and principles

of esophageal surgery that are still used today.[16,46] Ivor Lewis (1946) popularized the right-sided transthoracic approach to carcinoma of the esophagus.[30,40] As methods of esophageal resection became refined, techniques of visceral esophageal substitution with stomach, jejunum, and colon were likewise developed.

Until relatively recently, surgical procedures for most benign esophageal disease have been empiric and directed toward abnormal anatomy, rather than deranged physiology. A pharyngoesophageal diverticulum was first resected successfully in 1886.[57] During the subsequent 5 to 6 decades, discussion centered upon the advisability of one-stage versus two-stage procedures for resection of these pouches, rather than upon the abnormal cricopharyngeal motor function responsible for their formation. Similarly, in discussing the treatment of pulsion diverticula of the thoracic esophagus, Allen and Clagget (1965) and Belsey (1966) emphasized the need to perform an esophagomyotomy at the time of resection of the pouch.[2,4] They emphasized that elimination of the cause of the diverticulum, i.e., the elevated intraesophageal pressure due to motor dysfunction, was more important than operating upon the diverticulum.

Thomas Willis (1674) used ordinary esophageal bougienage to treat achalasia.[13] Forceful dilation with disruption of the lower esophageal sphincter using pneumatic dilators,[7,29] hydrostatic dilators,[36] and expanding metal dilators[41] was subsequently reported. Although a number of operations on the distal esophagus were employed in the early 1900s to treat achalasia, the origin of the currently used esophagomyotomy is credited to Heller (1913).[18] The operation initially described by Heller consisted of two cardioesophagomyotomies, one on either side of the distal esophagus, performed transabdominally. Zaaijer (1923) modified the operation to a single esophageal incision,[58] and Ellis and associates established the merits of transthoracic esophagomyotomy in the treatment of achalasia.[13]

Early "hiatal hernia" surgery also emphasized anatomy, rather than physiology. Harrington (1928) reported 51 cases of diaphragmatic herniation, 27 of which had been repaired.[17] Included among these cases were traumatic diaphragmatic hernias as well as hernias through the esophageal hiatus. Emphasis was placed upon correction of the anatomic defect and closure of the diaphragmatic hiatus, and this approach influenced the surgical therapy of hiatal hernias for more than two decades. Although Allison (1951) first coined the term *reflux esophagitis* and clearly established gastroesophageal reflux as a cause for many of the symptoms experienced by patients with hiatal hernias,[3] he, too, emphasized anatomic correction of the hernia, rather than correction of the abnormal distal esophageal sphincter mechanism in these patients. Thus, several "hiatus hernia" operations were described over the next few years, culminating in the reports by Nissen[34] in Switzerland in 1961 and Skinner and Belsey[43] in England in 1967 of the use of fundoplication to create an intra-abdominal esophageal valve mechanism to control gastroesophageal reflux. These latter operations introduced the era of true "anti-reflux" operations designed to restore a functional lower esophageal sphincter mechanism.

In the past 40 to 50 years, a number of diagnostic studies have been refined to provide greater objectivity in the assessment of esophageal function. With the development of manometric techniques and the ability to document gastroesophageal reflux with the intraesophageal pH electrode, surgical therapy for esophageal motor disorders has become more of a science based on objective data. Cannon (1907) first reported use of intraesophageal balloons to record esophageal peristalsis.[8] Code and associates (1958),[9] Vantrappen and associates (1958),[54] Texter and colleagues (1957),[48] and Ingelfinger (1959),[21] refined esophageal manometric techniques and made substantial contributions to the understanding of normal and deranged esophageal physiology. Tuttle and Grossman (1958) developed the intraesophageal pH electrode for the direct intraluminal assessment of gastroesophageal reflux.[53] Tuttle and associates (1960) diagnosed "reflux" by slow withdrawal from the stomach of a pH electrode in 1-cm. increments and noting whether or not intraesophageal pH was 4 or less at least 4 cm. above the pressure inversion point.[52] Modification of intraesophageal pH reflux testing followed. Piccone and associates (1965) instilled acid into the stomach, fixed the pH probe 5 to 10 cm. above the esophageal hiatus, and tried to evoke reflux by having their subjects perform Valsalva maneuvers, touch their toes, and so forth.[39] Kantrowitz and associates (1969) performed provocative pH testing with the pH probe fixed 5 cm. above the lower esophageal sphincter.[27] Skinner and Booth (1970) further modified this test to what is now termed the standard acid reflux test (SART), which places 300 ml. of 0.1 N HCl into the stomach, fixes the pH electrode 5 cm. above the lower esophageal sphincter, and documents the number of pH drops below 4 with the patient supine, on the right side, on the left side, and in the Trendelenburg position while standardized reflux provocative maneuvers are performed.[44]

An effort to circumvent the relatively "artificial" nature of the standard acid reflux test was the basis for prolonged lower esophageal pH monitoring introduced by Spencer (1969)[45] and Pattrick (1970).[37] Johnson and DeMeester (1974) first used "normal" controls in their evaluation of patients with abnormal gastroesophageal reflux with 24-hour distal esophageal pH monitoring.[26] They subsequently classified their patients into upright, supine, and combined (upright and supine) refluxers.[11] Since then, 24-hour monitoring of distal esophageal pH has become the standard for objectively diagnosing gastroesophageal reflux.

The acid perfusion test developed by Bernstein and Baker (1958) was proposed as a simple test for differentiating patients with chest pain of cardiac origin from those with esophagitis.[5] Long experience with this test has indicated that a "positive Bernstein test" indicates *only* that the patient has an acid-sensitive esophagus, and *not* that there is esophagitis or gastroesophageal reflux present. Similarly, measurement of the potential difference of esophageal mucosa was initially thought to be of value in the assessment of patients with reflux disease.[19,51] This study, however, is technically difficult to perform and evaluate and has thus not gained widespread use.

Radionuclide scanning using ^{99m}Tc-sulfur colloid to detect gastroesophageal reflux was first reported by Fisher and associates (1976)[14]; and although the test is clearly more sensitive than either standard radiology or short-term pH monitoring in diagnosing reflux,[28,55] it is unlikely to replace 24-hour distal pH monitoring as the most valuable diagnostic method. Esophageal manometry and intraesophageal pH reflux testing have become basic in the preoperative assessment of most patients with benign esophageal disease and are now used extensively to assess objectively the operative results of procedures designed to treat abnormal gastroesophageal reflux and esophageal motor function.

ANATOMY

The esophagus is a hollow tube of muscle that is approximately 25 cm. (10 inches) in length and extends from the pharynx to the stomach. It is arbitrarily divided into four segments: pharyngoesophageal, cervical, thoracic, and abdominal. The length between the laryngopharynx and the cervical esophagus is the *pharyngoesophageal segment.* The pharyngeal musculature includes the superior, middle, and inferior constrictors, as well as the stylopharyngeus muscles. The inferior pharyngeal constrictor, or thyropharyngeus muscle, passes obliquely and superiorly from its origin on the thyroid cartilage to its posterior insertion in the median raphe (see Part IV, Fig. 1). The esophageal introitus, the cricopharyngeus muscle, or upper esophageal sphincter, is the most inferior portion of the inferior pharyngeal constrictor and is clearly identifiable by the transverse direction of its fibers. The transition between the oblique fibers of the thyropharyngeus muscle and the transverse fibers of the cricopharyngeus muscle creates a point of potential weakness in the pharyngoesophageal segment, which is the site of origin of pharyngoesophageal (Zenker's) diverticula as well as a common site of perforation during esophagoscopy (see Part V, Fig. 1). The cricopharyngeal sphincter is unique to the gastrointestinal tract, because it consists not of a circular ring of muscle, but rather of a "bow" of muscle connecting the two lateral borders of the cricoid cartilage. The cricopharyngeus muscle fibers blend into the longitudinal and circular muscle of the *cervical esophagus,* a 5- to 6-cm.-long segment that extends to the beginning of the first thoracic vertebra. Although the cervical esophagus is a midline structure positioned posteriorly to the trachea, it tends to course more to the left of the trachea and is therefore more readily approached cervically through a left neck incision (Fig. 1). The cervical esophagus lies just anterior to the prevertebral fascia and can normally be separated from its loose fibrous posterior attachments by blunt finger dissection of the prevertebral space. The *thoracic esophagus* passes into the posterior mediastinum, narrowing slightly behind the aortic arch and great vessels, and curving somewhat to the left of the trachea as it passes behind the left mainstem bronchus. It then deviates slightly to the right for several centimeters in the subcarinal area, gradually returning to the left of midline and anterior to the thoracic aorta as it proceeds behind the pericardium approximately to the level of the seventh thoracic vertebra. At this point, the esophagus deviates further to the left and anteriorly entering the esophageal diaphragmatic hiatus at the level of the eleventh thoracic vertebra. The lateral boundaries of the thoracic esophagus are the right and left parietal pleurae, which are easily injured during esophageal operations.

The diaphragmatic esophageal hiatus is a sling of muscle fibers that arises from the *right* crus in approximately 45 per cent of patients. At times, however, both the left and right crura contribute to the hiatus. The *abdominal esophagus* varies in length from one to several centimeters, extending from the esophageal hiatus to the point at which it joins the stomach, the "cardia," or esophagogastric junction. The precise location of the esophagogastric junction is a matter of considerable controversy, because this area has been defined in at least three different ways: (1) the junction of esophageal squamous and gastric columnar epithelium, (2) the point at which the tubular esophagus joins the gastric pouch, and (3) the junction of the esophageal circular muscle layer with the oblique sling fibers of the stomach (the loop of Willis or the collar of Helvetius). Each definition has its merit as well as its shortcomings. The squamocolumnar epithelial junction is normally recognizable by direct

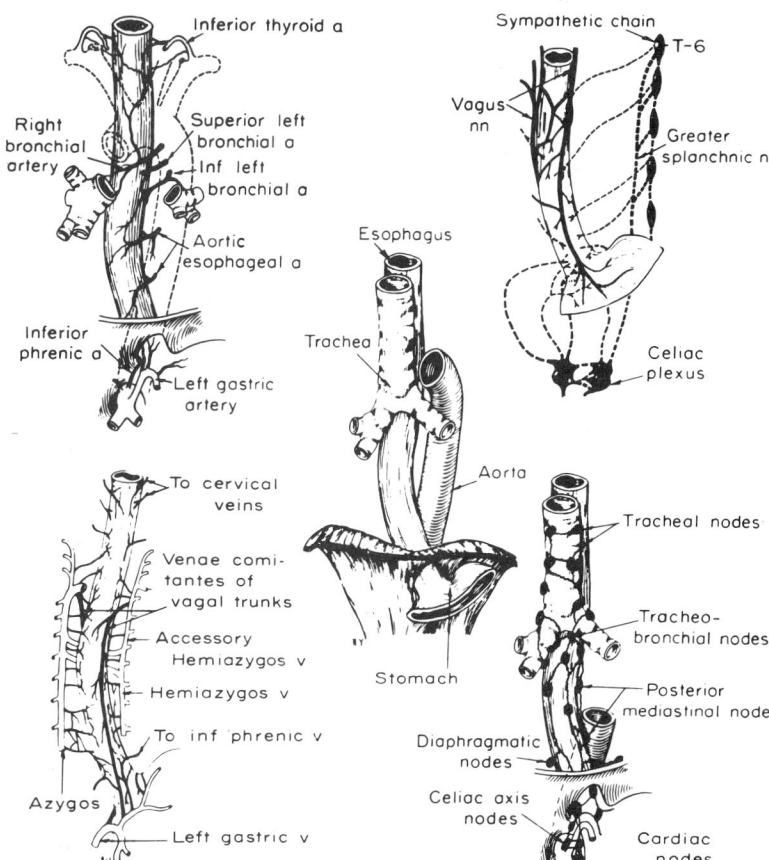

Figure 1. Anatomy of the esophagus. Arterial supply *(upper left)*, innervation *(upper right)*, lymphatic drainage *(lower right)*, and relationship of esophagus to trachea, aorta, and diaphragm.

vision and endoscopic biopsy, but junctional columnar epithelium may line the distal esophagus for 1 to 2 cm. The point at which the tubular esophagus joins the stomach may be very difficult to identify in the presence of a hiatal hernia or "patulous cardia." The junction of the inner layer of esophageal muscle with the gastric sling fibers is the most accurate and consistent definition of the gastroesophageal junction, but it is not readily identified without dissection. The squamocolumnar epithelial junction usually occurs at this point, and esophageal submucosal glands are not found distal to this area. However, this anatomic landmark may be obscured by the presence of a hiatal hernia, a patulous cardia, or reflux esophagitis. Clinically, however the squamocolumnar epithelial junction (the ora serrata or Z line), as identified endoscopically, is the most practical definition of the gastroesophageal junction, provided that the patient does not have a columnar-lined lower esophagus (Fig. 2). The *phrenoesophageal membrane* is a fibroelastic sheet of tissue that extends circumferentially from the muscular margins of the diaphragmatic hiatus to the esophagus. It is a misnomer to refer to this tissue as the phrenoesophageal "ligament," because such terminology erroneously implies strong fibrous bands that connect bones or supporting viscera. Most of the phrenoesophageal membrane arises from the endoabdominal fascia and inserts into the esophagus for a distance of 2 to 3 cm. above the hiatus and 3 to 5 cm. above the mucosal junction.[15,20,38] Fibrous strands from the upper surface of the diaphragm (fascia of Laimer) contribute to the phrenoesophageal membrane. The functional significance of the phrenoesophageal membrane remains undetermined. However, it is now clear that this tissue lacks sufficient strength to reliably anchor the esophagogastric junction in the abdomen in performing an anti-reflux operation.

The esophagus has three distinct areas of naturally occurring anatomic narrowing (Fig. 3). The *cervical constriction* occurs at the level of the cricopharyngeus sphincter, the narrowest point of the gastrointestinal tract, typically measuring 14 mm. in di-

ameter. The *bronchoaortic constriction* (15 to 17 mm.) is located at the level of the fourth thoracic vertebra behind the tracheal bifurcation where the left mainstem bronchus and aortic arch cross the esophagus. The *diaphragmatic constriction* (16 to

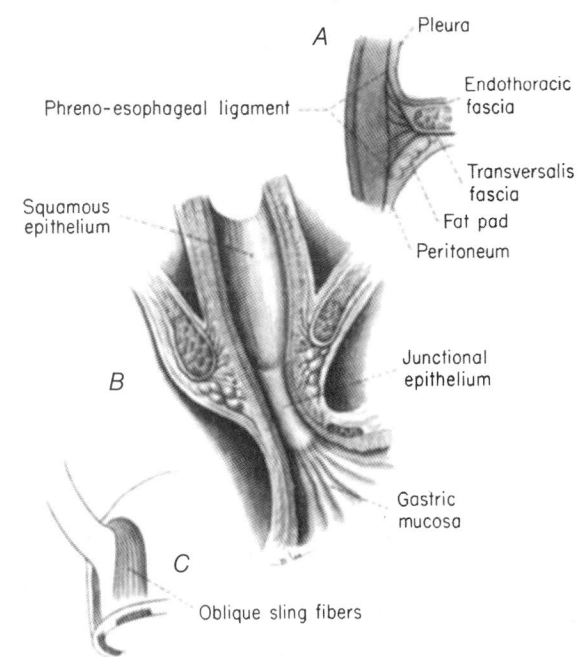

Figure 2. Gross anatomy of the esophagogastric junction area. *A*, Details of origin and insertion of phrenoesophageal membrane or ligament. *B*, Cross-section of distal esophagus and proximal stomach. *C*, Oblique gastric sling fibers. (From Pairolero, P., Trastek, V. F., and Payne, W. S.: Esophagus and diaphragmatic hernias. In Schwartz, S. I. (Ed.): Principles of Surgery, Vol. I, 5th ed. New York, McGraw-Hill Book Company, 1989, pp. 1103–1156.)

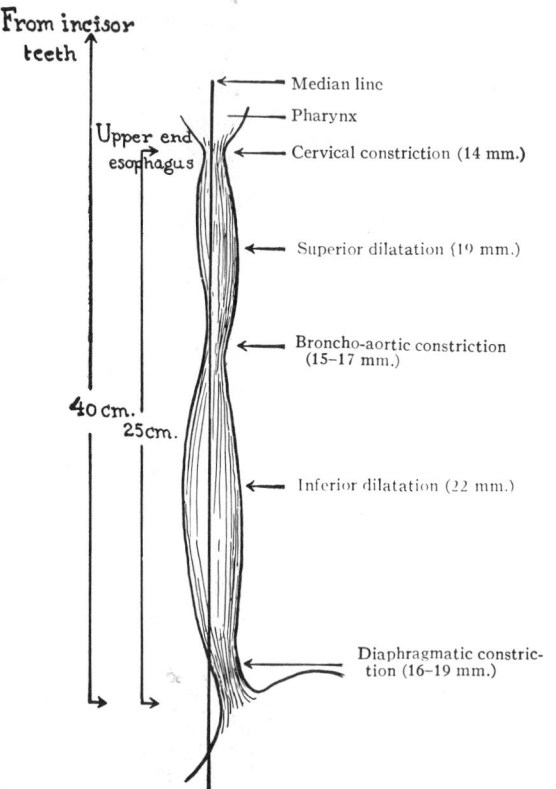

Figure 3. Normal esophageal constrictions, dilatations, and measurements. (From Shackelford, R. T.: Surgery of the Alimentary Tract, 2nd ed. Philadelphia, W. B. Saunders Company, 1978, p. 9.)

19 mm.) occurs where the esophagus traverses the diaphragm. The esophagus between these three areas of constriction has a wider caliber and is termed the *superior* and *inferior dilatation*, respectively. The normal adult thoracic esophagus has a maximal diameter of approximately 2.5 cm. on barium swallow examination.

The esophagus is a mucosa-lined muscular tube that lacks a serosa. It is surrounded by adventitia or mediastinal connective tissue, a layer of loose fibroareolar tissue. Beneath the adventitia is a coat of longitudinal muscle that overlies an inner layer of circular muscle. Between the two muscular layers is a thin, connective-tissue, intramuscular septum that contains fine blood vessels and ganglion cells of Meissner's and Auerbach's plexuses. Both the longitudinal and circular muscle layers of the upper third of the esophagus are striated, whereas in the lower two thirds they are nonstriated. The fatty and relatively thick submucosa permits considerable mobility of the esophageal mucosa, a point of particular importance in constructing anastomoses. The submucosa contains the mucous glands, blood vessels, Meissner's neural plexus, and an extensive lymphatic network. The esophageal mucosa consists of squamous epithelium except for the distal 1 to 2 cm., which are junctional columnar epithelium. Occasionally, islands of ectopic gastric mucosa may be found through the length of the esophagus.

The notorious "poor" blood supply of the esophagus is more of an excuse for complications of poor surgical technique than actual fact. Although it has a segmental blood supply, the esophagus is nourished by a number of arteries. The cervical esophagus receives blood from the superior thyroid artery as well as the inferior thyroid artery of the thyrocervical trunk, both sides communicating through collaterals. The major blood supply of the intrathoracic esophagus is from four to six aortic esophageal arteries, supplemented by collaterals with the inferior thyroid, intercostal and bronchial, inferior phrenic, and left gastric arteries. Recent anatomic studies of the aortic esophageal

arteries indicate that these vessels terminate in fine capillary networks before actually penetrating the esophageal muscle layer.[31] Therefore, if in the process of blunt esophageal mobilization, the dissection is kept close to the esophageal wall, the risk of serious hemorrhage from a sizable vessel is minimal. After penetrating and supplying the muscular layers of the esophagus, the esophageal capillary network courses longitudinally in the submucosa. The extensive venous drainage of the esophagus includes the hypopharyngeal, azygos, hemiazygos, intercostal, and gastric veins.

The esophagus has both sympathetic and parasympathetic innervation.[42] In the neck, the superior laryngeal nerves arise from the vagus nerves and divide into the external and internal laryngeal branches. The external laryngeal nerve innervates the cricothyroid muscle and also, in part, the inferior pharyngeal constrictor. The internal laryngeal nerve is the sensory nerve of the pharyngeal surface of the larynx and the base of the tongue. The recurrent laryngeal branches of the vagus nerves provide parasympathetic innervation to the cervical esophagus as well as innervation to the upper esophageal sphincter. Thus, injury to the recurrent laryngeal nerve may cause not only hoarseness but also upper esophageal sphincter dysfunction with secondary aspiration on swallowing. In the thorax, the vagus nerves send fibers to the striated muscle as well as parasympathetic preganglionic fibers to the smooth muscle. The sympathetic innervation consists of fibers to the cervical esophagus from the superior and inferior cervical sympathetic ganglia, to the thoracic esophagus from the upper thoracic and splanchnic nerves, and to the intra-abdominal esophagus from the celiac ganglion. In addition, Meissner's and Auerbach's plexuses provide an intrinsic autonomic nervous system within the esophageal wall. Meissner's plexus of nerves is located in the submucosa, whereas Auerbach's plexus is in the connective tissue between the circular and longitudinal muscle layers. The two vagus nerves lie along either side of the thoracic esophagus and form two large nerve plexuses supplying the esophagus and the lungs. Two to 6 cm. above the esophageal hiatus, the esophageal vagus plexuses coalesce and become single trunks, the left vagus coming to lie anterior to the esophagus, and the right vagus posterior at the diaphragmatic hiatus.

The esophagus has an extensive lymphatic drainage that consists of two lymphatic plexuses, one arising in the mucosa and the other in the muscular layer.[47] Mucosal lymphatic capillaries may pierce the muscular layer and drain to regional lymph nodes. Alternatively, these lymphatic capillaries may course longitudinally in the esophageal wall before exiting through the muscle into adjacent lymph nodes. In general, the flow of lymphatics of the upper two thirds of the esophagus tends to be upward, whereas that of the distal third tends to be downward. Thus, esophageal carcinomas may metastasize to internal jugular nodes in the neck; paratracheal nodes in the superior mediastinum; subcarinal nodes in the midchest; periesophageal nodes in the lower mediastinum, and inferior pulmonary ligaments, perigastric, and left gastric artery lymph nodes.

Thoracic Duct Anatomy

The proximity of the thoracic duct to the esophagus makes it vulnerable to injury during esophageal surgery. It is therefore appropriate to emphasize this relationship. The thoracic duct forms at the confluence of the cisterna chyli at a level between the twelfth thoracic and second lumbar vertebrae and to the right side of the abdominal aorta. The duct enters the posterior mediastinum through the aortic hiatus at the level of T10–T12 and continues cephalad on the anterior surface of the vertebral column between the aorta and the azygos vein and behind the esophagus. At the T4–T5 level, the duct crosses to the left of the spine, under the aortic arch, and continues along the left side of the esophagus, ascending into the neck posterior to the left subclavian artery. In the neck, the duct lies anterior to the vertebral artery and vein, thyrocervical trunk, and phrenic nerve, and it enters the venous system at the junction of the left subclavian and left internal jugular veins. Operations on the thoracic esophagus, particularly after previous surgical or radiation therapy that has produced periesophageal fibrosis, may cause chylothorax due to thoracic duct injury.

REFERENCES

1. Adams, W. E., and Phemister, D. B.: Carcinoma of the lower thoracic esophagus; report of successful resection and esophagogastrostomy. J. Thorac. Surg., 7:621, 1938.
2. Allen, T. H., and Clagget, O. T.: Changing concepts in the surgical treatment of pulsion diverticula of the lower esophagus. J. Thorac. Cardiovasc. Surg., 50:455, 1965.
3. Allison, P. R.: Reflux esophagitis, sliding hiatal hernia, and the anatomy of repair. Surg. Gynecol. Obstet., 92:149, 1951.
4. Belsey, R.: Functional diseases of the esophagus. J. Thorac. Cardiovasc. Surg., 52:164, 1966.
5. Bernstein, L. M., and Baker, L. A.: A clinical test for esophagitis. Gastroenterology, 34:760, 1958.
6. Billroth, T.: Ueber die Resection des Oesophagus. Arch. Klin. Chir., 13:65, 1871.
7. Browne, D. C., McHardy, G.: A new instrument for use in esophagospasm. J.A.M.A., 113:1963, 1939.
8. Cannon, W. B.: Esophageal peristalsis after bilateral vagotomy. Am. J. Physiol., 19:436, 1907.
9. Code, C. F., Creamer, B., Schlegel, J. F., et al.: An Atlas of Esophageal Motility in Health and Disease. Springfield, Ill., Charles C Thomas, 1958.
10. Czerny, J.: Neue Operationen: Vorlaufige Mittheilung. Abl. Chir., 4:433, 1877.
11. DeMeester, T. R., Johnson, L. F., Joseph, G. J., Toscano, M. S., Hall, A. W., and Skinner, D. B.: Patterns of gastroesophageal reflux in health and disease. Ann. Surg. 184:459, 1976.
12. Denk, W.: Zur Radikaloperation des Osophaguskarzinoms. Zentralbl. Chir., 40:1065, 1913.
13. Ellis, F. H., Jr., and Olsen, A. M.: Achalasia of the Esophagus. Major problems in Clinical Surgery. Vol. 9. Philadelphia, W. B. Saunders Company, 1969.
14. Fisher, R. S., Malmud, L. S., Roberts, G. S., and Lobis, I. F.: Gastroesophageal (GE) scintiscanning to detect and quantitate GE reflux. Gastroenterology, 70:301, 1976.
15. Friedland, G. W., Melcher, O. H., Berridge, F. R., et al.: Debatable points in the anatomy of the lower oesophagus. Thorax, 21:487, 1966.
16. Garlock, J. H.: Re-establishment of esophagogastric continuity following resection of esophagus for carcinoma of middle third. Surg. Gynecol. Obstet., 78:23, 1944.
17. Harrington, S. W. Diaphragmatic hernia. Arch. Surg. 16:386, 1928.
18. Heller, E.: Extramukose Cardiaplastik beim chronischen Cardiospasmus mit Dilatation des Oesophagus. Mitt. Grenzgeb. Med. Chir., 27:141, 1913.
19. Helm, W. J., Schlegel, J. F., Code, C. F., and Summerskill, W. H. J.: Identification of the gastroesophageal mucosal junction by transmural potential in healthy subjects and patients with hiatal hernia. Gastroenterology, 48:25, 1965.
20. Higgs, B., Shorter, R. G., and Ellis, F. H., Jr.: A study of the anatomy of the human esophagus with special reference to the gastroesophageal sphincter. J. Surg. Res., 5:503, 1965.
21. Ingelfinger, F. J.: Esophageal motility. Physiol. Rev., 38,533, 1959.
22. Jackson, C.: Tracheo-bronchoscopy, Esophagoscopy, and Gastroscopy. St. Louis, The Laryngoscope Company, 1907, pp. 13–14.
23. Jackson, C.: Difficulties and pitfalls in the insinuation of the esophagoscope. Am. Otol. 45:1109, 1936.
24. Jackson, C., and Jackson, C., Jr.: Bronchoesophagology. Philadelphia, W. B. Saunders Company, 1950.
25. Janeway, H. H., and Green, N. W.: Cancer of the oesophagus and cardia. Ann. Surg., 52:67, 1910.
26. Johnson, L. F., and DeMeester, T. R.: Twenty-four hour pH monitoring of the distal esophagus. Am. J. Gastroenterol., 62:325, 1974.
27. Kantrowitz, P. A., Corson, J. G., Fleischli, D. J., and Skinner, D. B.: Measurement of gastroesophageal reflux. Gastroenterology, 56:666, 1969.
28. Kaul, B., Peterson, H., Grettle, K., Erichsen, H., and Myrvold, H. E.: Scintigraphy, pH measurement and radiography in the evaluation of gastroesophageal reflux. Scand. J. Gastroenterol. 20:289, 1985.
29. Kurlander, D. J., Radkin, H. F., Kirsner, J. B., and Palmer, W. L.: Therapeutic value of the pneumatic dilator in achalasia of the esophagus: long-term results in sixty-two living patients. Gastroenterology, 45:604, 1963.
30. Lewis, I.: The surgical treatment of carcinoma of the esophagus: With special reference to a new operation for growths of the middle third. Br. J. Surg., 34:18, 1946.
31. Liebermann-Meffert, D. M. I., Luescher, U., Neft, V., Ruedi, T. P., and Allgower, M.: Esophagectomy without thoracotomy: is there a risk of intramediastinal bleeding. Ann. Surg., 206:184, 1987.
32. LoPresti, P. A., and Hilmi, A. M.: Clinical experience with a new foroblique fiberoptic esophagoscope. Am. J. Dig. Dis., 9:690, 1964.
33. Marshall, S. F.: Carcinoma of the esophagus: Successful resection of lower end of esophagus with re-establishment of esophageal gastric continuity. Surg. Clin. North Am., 18:643, 1938.
34. Nissen, R.: Gastropexy and fundoplication: in surgical treatment of hiatal hernia. Am. J. Dig. Dis., 6:954, 1961.
35. Ohsawa, T.: The surgery of the oesophagus. Arch. Jpn. Chir., 10:605, 1933.
36. Olsen, A. M., Harrington, S. W., Moersch, H. J., and Andersen, H. A.: The treatment of cardiospasm: analysis of a twelve-year experience. J. Thorac. Cardiovasc. Surg. 22:164, 1951.
37. Pattrick, F. G.: Investigation of gastroesophageal reflux in various positions with a two lumen pH electrode. Gut, 11:659, 1970.
38. Peters, P. M.: Closure mechanisms at the cardia with special reference to the diaphragmaticoesophageal elastic ligament. Thorax, 10:27, 1955.
39. Piccone, V. A., Gutelius, J. R., McCorriston, J. R.: A multiphase esophageal pH test for gastroesophageal reflux. Surgery, 57:638, 1965.
40. Postlethwait, R. W.: Resection and reconstruction of the esophagus. In Surgery of the Esophagus. Norwalk, Connecticut, Appleton-Century-Crofts, 1979, pp. 439–475.
41. Schindler, R.: Observations on cardiospasm and its treatment by brusque dilatation. Ann. Intern. Med. 45:207, 1956.
42. Shackelford, R. T.: Surgery of the Alimentary Tract, 2nd ed. Philadelphia, W. B. Saunders Company, 1978, pp. 16–19.
43. Skinner, D. B., and Belsey, R. H. R.: Surgical management of esophageal reflux and hiatus hernia. J. Thorac. Cardiovasc. Surg., 53:33, 1967.
44. Skinner, D. B., and Booth, D.: Assessment of distal esophageal function in patients with hiatus hernia and/or gastroesophageal reflux. Ann. Surg., 172:627, 1970.
45. Spencer, J.: Prolonged pH recording in the study of gastroesophageal reflux. Br. J. Surg., 54:912, 1969.
46. Sweet, R. H.: Transthoracic resection of esophagus and stomach for carcinoma: Analysis of postoperative complications, causes of death, and late results of operation. Ann. Surg., 121:272, 1945.
47. Terracol, J., and Sweet, R. H., Diseases of the Esophagus. Philadelphia, W. B. Saunders Company, 1958, p. 27.
48. Texter, E. C., Jr., Smith, H. W., Moeller, H. C., et al.: Intraluminal pressures from the upper gastrointestinal tract. I. Correlations with motor activity in normal subjects and patients with esophageal disorders. Gastroenterology, 32:1013, 1957.
49. Torek, F.: The operative treatment of carcinoma of the oesophagus. Ann. Surg., 61:385, 1915.
50. Turner, G. G.: Excision of thoracic esophagus for carcinoma with construction of extrathoracic gullet. Lancet, 2:1315, 1933.
51. Turner, K. S., Powell, D. W., Carney, C. N., Orlando, R. T. C., and Bozymski, E. M.: Transmural electrical potential difference in the mammalian esophagus in vivo. Gastroenterology, 75:286, 1978.
52. Tuttle, S. G.: Bettarello, A., and Grossman, M. I.: Esophageal acid perfusion test and a gastroesophageal reflux test in patients with esophagitis. Gastroenterology, 38:861, 1960.
53. Tuttle, S. G., and Grossman, M. I.: Detection of gastroesophageal reflux by simultaneous measurement of intraluminal pressures and pH. Proc. Soc. Exp. Biol. Med., 98:225, 1958.
54. Vantrappen, G., Liemer, M. D., Ikeya, J., et al.: Simultaneous fluorocinematography and intraluminal pressure measurements in the study of esophageal motility. Gastroenterology, 35:592, 1958.
55. Velasco, N., Pope, C. E., Gamnan, R. M., Roberts, P., Hill, L. D.: Measurement of esophageal reflux by scintigraphy. Dig. Dis. Sci., 29:977, 1984.
56. Von Mikulicz, J.: A case of resection of the esophagus with plastic reconstruction of the excised piece. Prag. Med. Wochenschr., 11:93, 1886. Cited by Saint: Arch. Surg., 19:53, 1929.
57. Wheeler, W. I.: Pharyngocele and dilatation of pharynx with existing diverticulum at lower portion of pharynx lying posterior to the esophagus, cured by pharyngotomy, being the first case of the kind recorded. Dublin J. Med. Sci., 82:349, 1886.
58. Zaaijer, J. H.: Cardiospasm in the aged. Ann. Surg., 77:615, 1923.

II

PHYSIOLOGY

Mark B. Orringer, M.D.

The esophagus is a muscular tube that begins proximally with the upper esophageal sphincter (UES) or cricopharyngeus muscle and ends distally with the lower esophageal sphincter (LES). Its basic function is to transport swallowed material from the pharynx into the stomach. Secondarily, retrograde flow of gastric contents into the esophagus is prevented by the lower sphincter, and entry of air into the esophagus with each inspiration is prevented by the upper sphincter, which normally remains closed as a result of tonic contraction of the cricopharyngeus muscle. Much of the current knowledge of esophageal physiology is the result of relatively recent developments in manometric techniques that permit recordings of intraesophageal pressure phenomena, such as the amplitude and length of the upper and lower sphincters, the extent and duration of relaxation of the sphincters with swallowing, and the characteristics of peristaltic activity in the body of the esophagus. As indicated above, the earliest esophageal manometric recordings were generated from small swallowed balloons.[3,17] After it was demonstrated that the size of the balloons influenced the pressure recordings,[14] small catheters bonded together with terminal openings at different levels and intermittently flushed to provide a constant column of liquid were soon replaced by constantly perfused systems, which proved to be more reliable in recording esophageal peristalsis and lower esophageal sphincter pressures.[12,21,22,24] Perfusion manometry was further refined with the introduction of constant, smaller volumes of water delivered through a noncompliant capillary system.[1] Concerned that variable sphincter pressure values were a function of movement proximal or distal to the recording orifice, Dent (1976) developed a 5 cm. long perfused sleeve that records the highest pressure at any point over its length and therefore more reliably reflects lower esophageal sphincter pressure despite movement of the gastroesophageal junction.[6] The advent of micropressure transducers allowed measurement of esophageal pressures more simply and without the need for a water-perfused system.[7,10] These microtransducers, fastened directly to the swallowed end of the recording catheters, are extremely accurate and more sensitive to pressure changes within the esophagus than the water-perfused system. However, the multitransducer catheters are very expensive and difficult to maintain and repair, and they have therefore not gained widespread popularity in clinical use.

The most common method of measuring intraluminal esophageal pressure currently in use involves the transmission of pressure changes through swallowed hollow tubes connected externally to transducers and a recording system. The standard motility catheter is a triple-lumen, constantly perfused system of polyethylene or polyvinyl tubing with either an open end or a lateral orifice (Fig. 1). Although esophageal motility studies have become a standard diagnostic tool in the evaluation of disorders of esophageal motor function, dysphagia, chest pain of undetermined origin, and gastroesophageal reflux, it must be realized that a multitude of factors affect the pressures recorded in individuals and from one laboratory to another. These variables include catheter size,[16,18,23] the character of the swallowed bolus (e.g., hot versus cold liquid, dry versus wet swallow), and resting time between swallows.[9,26] The inherent inaccuracies of these measurements have generated controversy as to the value of esophageal manometry as a clinical assessment.[19,23] It would appear most prudent, however, to recognize that the quantitative values obtained from esophageal manometry are *not* absolute and that this study provides additional corroborative information to be used in conjunction with the history, barium swallow, and endoscopic findings in the assessment of esophageal function.

Swallowing normally involves both voluntary and involuntary muscle function. It begins with voluntary movement of the tongue. This initiates an involuntary peristaltic wave that rapidly traverses the pharynx and reaches the UES, producing a brisk, coordinated relaxation that is followed by a postdeglutitive contraction (Fig. 2). The UES is usually 3 cm. in length and has a mean resting pressure of between 20 and 60 mm. Hg. Its duration of relaxation with swallowing is approximately 0.5 to 1 second. Contraction of the UES after the relaxation phase produces intraluminal pressures of 70 to 100 mm. Hg, which continues 2 to 4 seconds. As the swallowed bolus enters the esophagus, a *primary* peristaltic wave is activated, normally propelling the swallowed material from the pharynx into the stomach in 4 to 8 seconds in an orderly, progressive manner (Fig. 3). Normally a progressive peristaltic contraction (primary wave) follows 97 per cent of all swallows.[8] Pressure within the body of the esophagus is a reflection of negative intrathoracic pressure, being maximally negative (−5 to −10 mm. Hg) during deep inspiration, and highest (0 to 5 mm. Hg) during expiration. Esophageal peristaltic pressure is 20 to 100 mm. Hg, with a duration of contraction of between 2 and 4 seconds.[7,8,11,20,22] If the entire swallowed bolus of food does not empty from the esophagus into the stomach, *secondary* peristaltic waves are initiated. These contractions, like the primary waves, are progressive and sequential but begin in the smooth muscle segment of the esophagus (near the level of the aortic arch) and continue until retained intraesophageal contents are emptied into the stomach. Thus, unlike the primary wave, the secondary contraction is not initiated by a voluntary swallow but rather is initiated by local distention of the esophagus. *Tertiary* contractions are simultaneous, nonprogressive, nonperistaltic, mono-

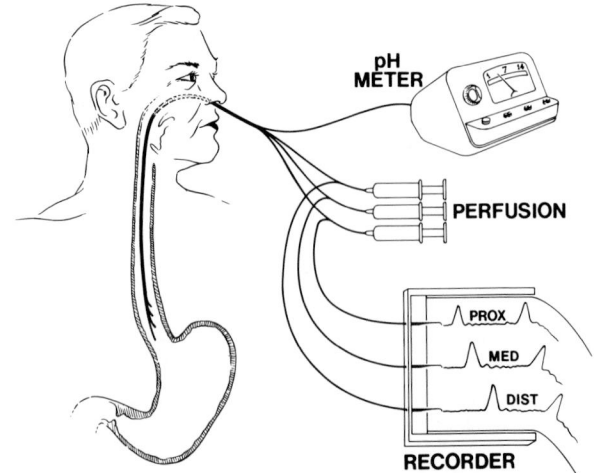

Figure 1. Schematic representation of combined manometric pH recording system used in the evaluation of esophageal function. The triple-lumen perfused recording catheter measures intraluminal pressures from three levels in the esophagus, each separated from the next by 5 cm. Measurements are made in terms of centimeters from the nostrils to the proximal opening of the recording catheter (PROX). The medial catheter (MED) records pressures 5 cm. distal to the proximal opening; and the distal catheter (DIST), 5 cm. below this. The intraesophageal pH electrode is used for documenting gastroesophageal reflux.

UPPER ESOPHAGEAL SPHINCTER-NORMAL

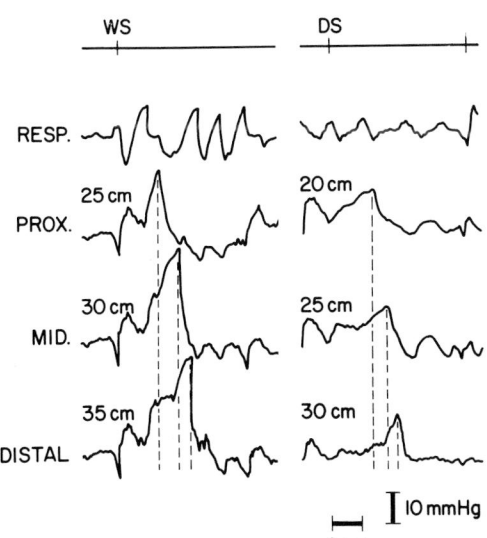

Figure 2. Motility tracing showing relaxation of the upper esophageal sphincter (U.E.S.). As the triple-lumen recording catheter is withdrawn through the upper esophagus, the most proximal recording port first passes through the upper esophageal high-pressure zone, which corresponds to the cricopharyngeal sphincter mechanism. Withdrawal of the catheter ceases when the middle port is within the U.E.S. Each time the patient swallows, pharyngeal contraction (proximal catheter), cricopharyngeal relaxation (middle catheter, arrows), and the peristaltic wave propagated by the swallow (distal catheter) are observed.

or multiphasic waves that can occur throughout the esophagus and represent uncoordinated contractions of the smooth muscle that are responsible for the classic "corkscrew" appearance of esophageal spasm on barium swallow examination. Increased resting pressures within the body of the esophagus and abnormal motor function are observed with obstruction, either mechanical or functional.

The term *lower esophageal sphincter* implies the presence of an anatomic sphincter such as the pylorus or the anus. Although no such *anatomic* lower esophageal sphincter has been demon-

strated, manometry has defined an elevated distal esophageal resting pressure 3 to 5 cm. in length, which serves as the barrier against abnormal regurgitation of gastric contents into the esophagus and represents a *functional* sphincter (Fig. 4). Thus, the LES is more accurately referred to as the LES *mechanism* or the *distal esophageal high pressure zone* (HPZ). The factors responsible for maintaining competence of the LES are poorly understood, but the presence of an intra-abdominal segment of distal esophagus, under the influence of positive intra-abdominal pressure, appears important to the success of most antireflux operations.

"Normal" resting pressure within the HPZ is 10 to 20 mm. Hg, but it should be emphasized that *no absolute HPZ value per se indicates either competence or incompetence of the LES mechanism.* Patients with no gastroesophageal reflux may have an extremely "low" HPZ amplitude on manometric recordings, whereas others with massive reflux may have seemingly high distal pressures. This inconsistency is a reflection of both HPZ variation due to individual body habitus as well as the radial asymmetry of the lower sphincter, which produces varied readings during "pull-through" determinations, depending upon the orientation of the catheter recording port. The Dent pressure recording sleeve allows more accurate LES pressure determinations.[6] HPZ pressures of 0 to 5 mm. Hg are more likely to be associated with incompetence of the LES and gastroesophageal reflux. Much more meaningful in the demonstration of abnormal gastroesophageal reflux, however, is the intraesophageal pH electrode, the use of which has been expanded from the standard pH reflux test[2] to 24-hour monitoring of distal esophageal pH.[5,15] Esophagoscopy, the barium swallow examination, and the acid perfusion (Bernstein) test remain poor and inconsistent indicators of gastroesophageal reflux.

The distal HPZ is located in the region of the diaphragmatic hiatus. With standard pull-through studies, the distal portion of

NORMAL HPZ

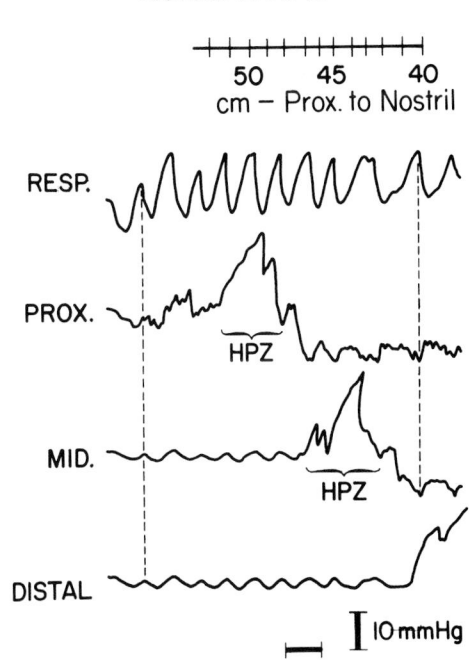

Figure 4. Motility tracing showing normal distal sphincter mechanism or HPZ. As the recording catheter is withdrawn from the stomach into the esophagus, the HPZ is identified sequentially in each catheter. Mean basal pressure within the thoracic esophagus is lower than that within the stomach (below the diaphragm). Below the diaphragm, within the stomach, a positive deflection is observed during respiratory excursions at the peak of inspiration (when the diaphragm is lowest). Conversely, in the esophagus, at the peak of inspiration, intrathoracic pressure is maximally negative, and a negative deflection during inspiration is observed (dotted lines).

PROGRESSIVE PERISTALSIS

Figure 3. Motility tracing showing normal peristalsis. With each swallow, a progressive esophageal contraction is generated, passing first by the proximal recording port, then the middle, and finally the distal port. WS, wet swallow; DS, dry swallow.

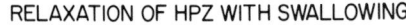

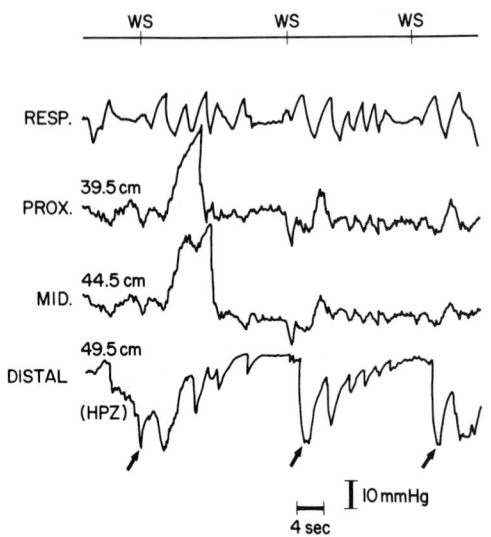

Figure 5. Motility tracing demonstrating normal relaxation of the distal HPZ with swallowing. The distal recording port is within the HPZ (49.5 cm. from the nostrils). Each swallow normally causes relaxation of the HPZ (arrows) followed by a sustained postdeglutitive contraction, after which pressure again returns to the basal level.

the sphincter demonstrates respiratory variations like those in the abdomen (increased pressure with inspiration, decreased pressure with expiration) (see Fig. 4). In the proximal portion of the HPZ, however, there is an intrathoracic pattern of respira-

tory variation: negative pressure with inspiration, positive pressure with expiration. The terms *point of respiratory reversal* or *pressure inversion point (PIP)* are used to designate the site at which this transition in respiratory pattern occurs on manometric tracings. In patients who totally lack a distal HPZ, the PIP is used as a reference point that is indicative of the cardia, 5 cm. above which the pH electrode can be positioned for acid-reflux testing (see Part III, Fig. 19). Within 1.5 to 2.5 seconds after a swallow is initiated, distal HPZ relaxation occurs, continuing for 4 to 6 seconds (Fig. 5). A postdeglutitive contraction then occurs, generating pressures of 25 to 35 mm. Hg for 7 to 10 seconds, after which HPZ tone returns to resting levels.

Distal HPZ pressure varies continually in individuals, being influenced by a host of neural, hormonal, myogenic, mechanical, and environmental factors (Table 1).[13]

REFERENCES

1. Arndorfer, R. C., Stef, J. J., Dodds, W. J., Lineham, J. H., and Hogan, W. J.: Improved infusion system for intraluminal esophageal manometry. Gastroenterology, 73:23, 1977.
2. Benz, L. J., Hootkin, L. A., Margolies, S., et al.: A comparison of clinical measurements of gastroesophageal reflux. Gastroenterology, 62:1, 1972.
3. Cannon, W. B.: Esophageal peristalsis after bilateral vagotomy. Am. J. Physiol., 19:436, 1907.
4. Code, C. F., Creamer, B., Schlegel, J. F., Olsen, A. M., Donoghnee, E. E., and Andersen, H. A.: An atlar of esophageal motility in health and disease. Springfield, Ill., Charles C Thomas, 1958.
5. DeMeester, T. R., Wang, C. I., Wernly, J. A., et al.: Technique, indications, and clinical use of 24 hour esophageal pH monitoring. J. Thorac. Cardiovasc. Surg., 79:656, 1980.
6. Dent, J.: A new technique for continuous sphincter pressure measurement. Gastroenterology, 71:263, 1976.
7. Dodds, W. J., Hogan, W. J., Lydons, S. B., Steward, E. T., Stef., J. J., and

TABLE 1. Factors Affecting Distal High Pressure Zone (HPZ) Tone

Factors	Increased HPZ Tone	Decreased HPZ Tone
Hormonal	Gastrin	Secretin
	Motilin	Cholecystokinin
	Prostaglandin $F_{2\alpha}$	Glucagon
	Bombesin	Progesterone
		Estrogen
		Prostaglandins E_1, E_2, A_2
Drugs	Caffeine	Alpha-adrenergic blockers
	Alpha-adrenergic agents	Phentolamine
	Norepinephrine	Anticholinergics
	Phenylephrine	Atropine
	Anticholinesterase	Theophylline
	Edrophonium	Beta-adrenergic blockers
	Cholinergic agents	Isoproterenol
	Bethanecol (Urecholine)	Ethanol
	Methacholine (Mecholyl)	Epinephrine
	Betazole	Nicotine
	Metoclopramide	Nitroglycerin
Foods	Protein meal	Fatty meal
		Chocolate
Myogenic	Normal resting muscle tone	? Aging
		? Diabetes mellitus
Mechanical	Anti-reflux operation	Hiatal hernia
		Abnormal phrenoesophageal ligament insertion
		Short or absent intra-abdominal distal esophageal segment
		Nasogastric tube
Miscellaneous	Gastric alkalinization	Gastric acidification
	Gastric distention	Gastrectomy
		Hypoglycemia
		Hypothyroidism
		Amyloidosis
		Pernicious anemia
		Epidermolysis bullosa

Modified from Hurwitz, A. L., Duranceau, A., and Haddad, J. K.: Disorders of Esophageal Motility. Philadelphia. W. B. Saunders Company, 1979, p. 120.

Arndorfer, R. C.: Quantitation of pharyngeal motor function in normal human subjects. J. Appl. Physiol., *39*:692, 1975.

8. Duranceau, A. C., DeVroede, G., Lafontaine, E., and Jamieson, G. G.: Esophageal motility in asymptomatic volunteers. Surg. Clin. North Am., *63*:777, 1983.

9. Funch-Jensen, P., and Jacobsen, E.: Esophageal peristalsis before, during, and after food intake in healthy people. Scand. J. Gastroenterol., *16*:209, 1981.

10. Gauer, O. H., and Gienapp, E.: A miniature pressure recording device. Science, *112*:404, 1950.

11. Henderson, R. D.: Normal esophageal motor activity: Function and control. *In* The Esophagus-Reflux and Primary Motor Disorders. Baltimore, Williams & Wilkins, 1980, pp. 11–21.

12. Hollis, J. B., and Castell, D. O.: Amplitude of esophageal peristalsis as determined by rapid infusion. Gastroenterology, *63*:417, 1972.

13. Hurwitz, A. L., Duranceau, A., Haddad, J. K., et al.: Normal esophageal motility. *In* Disorders of Esophageal Motility. Philadelphia, W. B. Saunders Company, 1979, pp. 14–26.

14. Ingelfinger, F. J.: Esophageal motility. Physiol. Rev., *38*:533, 1958.

15. Johnson, L. F., and DeMeester, T. R.: Twenty-four hour pH monitoring of the distal esophagus: A quantitative measurement of gastroesophageal reflux. Am. J. Gastroenterol., *62*:325, 1974.

16. Kaye, M. D., and Showalter, J. P.: Measurement of pressure in the lower esophageal sphincter: The influence of catheter diameter. Am. J. Dig. Dis., *19*:860, 1974.

17. Kronecker, H., and Meltzer, S. J.: Der Schulkmechanismus, seine Erregung und seine Hummung. Arch. P. F. Physiol. Leipz. (Suppl.), p. 338, 1883.

18. Lydon, S. B., Dodds, W. J., Hogan, W. J., and Arndorfer, R. C.: The effect of manometric assembly diameter on intraluminal esophageal pressure recording. Am. J. Dig. Dis., *20*:968, 1975.

19. Meyer, G. W., and Castell, D. O.: In support of the clinical usefulness of lower esophageal sphincter pressure determination. Dig. Dis. Sci., *26*:1028, 1981.

20. Nelson, J. L., Richter, G. E., Gohns, D. N., Castell, D. O., and Centola, G. M.: Esophageal contraction pressures are not affected by normal menstrual cycles. Gastroenterology, *87*:867, 1984.

21. Pope, C. E.: A dynamic test of sphincter strength: Its application to the lower esophageal sphincter. Gastroenterology, *52*:779, 1967.

22. Pope, C. E.: Effect of infusion on force of closure measurements in the esophagus. Gastroenterology, *58*:616, 1970.

23. Pope, C. E.: Is measurement of lower esophageal sphincter pressure clinically useful? Dig. Dis. Sci., *26*:1025, 1981.

24. Quigley, J. B., and Brody, D. A.: A physiologic and clinical consideration of the pressures developed in the digestive tract. Am. J. Med., *13*:397, 1959.

25. Stef, J. J., Dodds, W. J., Hogan, W. J., Lineham, J. H., and Stewart, E. T.: Intraluminal esophageal manometry: An analysis of variables affecting recording fidelity of peristaltic pressures. Gastroenterology, *67*:221, 1974.

26. Winship, D. H., Viegas de Andrade, S. R., and Zboralske, F. F.: Influence of bolus temperature on human esophageal motor function. Clin. Invest., *49*:243, 1970.

III

DISORDERS OF ESOPHAGEAL MOTILITY

Mark B. Orringer, M.D.

Functional disorders of the esophagus are those conditions that interfere with the normal act of swallowing or produce dysphagia without any associated intraluminal organic obstruction or extrinsic compression of the esophagus.[5] Among these disorders are the abnormalities of esophageal motility, most of which have now been precisely defined by esophageal manometry, a vital part of the evaluation of these patients. Although the cine-esophagogram and a skilled radiologist may diagnose disordered esophageal motility, the information obtained by the addition of esophageal manometry and acid reflux testing is more precise. Early achalasia and diffuse esophageal spasm, for example, may be indistinguishable radiologically, although each condition has its specific manometric characteristics. The differentiation is more than academic: a distal esophagomyotomy for achalasia may not relieve the symptoms of esophageal spasm. Generally, a barium swallow, esophagoscopy, and esophageal function tests, including manometry and intra-esophageal pH reflux testing, constitute the minimal evaluation of the patient with a suspected disorder of esophageal motility.

UPPER ESOPHAGEAL SPHINCTER DYSFUNCTION

Numerous terms have been used to define the symptom complex that follows abnormal function of the upper esophageal or cricopharyngeal sphincter. Such terms as *cricopharyngeal chalasia, achalasia,* and *spasm* have little more validity in these patients than the archaic diagnosis of globus hystericus, which was often applied to those who complained of a sensation of "a lump in the throat." In most patients, standard esophageal manometric techniques have been unable to demonstrate either true hypotonicity or hypertonicity of the upper esophageal sphincter (UES) or failure of the UES to relax with swallowing (achalasia). This is because of the limitations of existing equipment in recording the rapid sequence of events that occurs with normal deglutition in a unique asymmetrical sphincter that changes position with laryngeal excursions during swallowing,[106] another situation in which the Dent manometric sleeve

has applicability and advantages.[25] The terms *oropharyngeal dysphagia*[28] and *cricopharyngeal dysfunction*[75] perhaps best describe the symptom complex that results when there is difficulty propelling liquid or solid food from the oropharynx into the upper esophagus. The causes of this difficulty include abnormalities of the central and peripheral nervous systems, metabolic and inflammatory myopathy, gastroesophageal reflux, and other currently undefinable factors (Table 1).[28,55]

Other nonmotor causes of upper esophageal dysphagia, such as carcinoma, caustic stricture, cervical vertebral bone spurs, thyromegaly, and trauma, should always be excluded. The designation of "globus hystericus," indicating a purely psychologic basis for a patient's complaint of cervical dysphagia, is a diagnosis, made only after excluding significant esophageal disease. After careful evaluation, few patients complaining of cervical dysphagia should have their symptoms ascribed to "nerves."

Despite the variety of neurogenic and myogenic conditions involving the pharyngoesophageal junction, the resulting oropharyngeal dysphagia has a remarkably constant clinical presentation.[75] The patient complains of *cervical dysphagia,* which is localized between the thyroid cartilage and the suprasternal notch. There is a feeling of a "lump in the throat," a constriction around the neck, or occasionally pain radiating to the jaws and ears. *Expectoration of excessive saliva* is common in patients who are unable to swallow normally the 1 to 1½ liters of saliva produced in the mouth each day. The interesting occurrence of *intermittent hoarseness* further helps identify the patient with cricopharyngeal dysfunction. The inferior pharyngeal constrictor muscle, of which the cricopharyngeal sphincter is a part, may affect the vocal cords in two ways. First, contraction of the inferior pharyngeal constrictor adducts or approximates the alae of the thyroid cartilage, lengthening and tensing the vocal cords. Second, by pulling the cricoid cartilage posteriorly, the cricopharyngeal muscle acts with the lateral cricothyroid muscle to stretch the vocal cords. Thus, there is adequate physiologic explanation for the association between symptoms of cervical dysphagia and hoarseness in the patient with cricopharyngeal dysfunction; and in this author's experience, the

TABLE 1. Causes of Oropharyngeal Dysphagia

I. Neurogenic
  A. Central nervous system disease
    1. Neurologic disorders
      a. Amyotrophic lateral sclerosis
      b. Multiple sclerosis
      c. Spinocerebellar degeneration
      d. Syringobulbia
      e. Bullar poliomyelitis
      f. Progressive bulbar paralysis
      g. Parkinson's disease
      h. Huntington's chorea, Sydenham's chorea
      i. Tabes dorsalis
      j. Congenital and degenerative disorders
      k. Dysautonomia
    2. Vascular lesions
      a. Cerebrovascular accident
      b. Basilar artery thrombosis
      c. Aneurysm and brainstem compression
    3. Tumors
      a. Brainstem
      b. Base of the skull
    4. Operations
    5. Trauma
II. Myogenic
  A. Motor end-plate disease
    1. Myasthenia gravis
    2. Tetanus
  B. Skeletal muscle disease
    1. Muscular dystrophy
      a. Oculopharyngeal
      b. Myotonic
    2. Inflammatory
      a. Polymyositis
      b. Dermatomyositis
    3. Metabolic myopathy
      a. Thyrotoxicosis
      b. Hypothyroidism

III. Structural causes
  A. Idiopathic: without pharyngo-esophageal (Zenker's) diverticulum
  B. With pharyngoesophageal diverticulum
IV. Mechanical causes
  A. Endoluminal
    1. Inflammatory disease
    2. Foreign body
    3. Webs
    4. Benign tumors
    5. Malignant tumors
  B. Extraluminal
    1. Thyromegaly
    2. Lymphadenopathy
    3. Skeletal hyperostosis
    4. Cervical spine osteophytes (dysphagia psittaca)
    5. Cervical lordosis
    6. Congenital vascular abnormalities (dysphagia lusoria)
    7. Hypertrophied or tortuous aorta (dysphagia aortica)
    8. Heart disease
    9. Pericarditis and mediastinitis
V. Iatrogenic causes
  A. Neck surgery
    1. Laryngectomy
    2. Thyroidectomy
    3. Parathyroid exploration
    4. Tracheostomy
  B. Thoracic surgery: lung, mediastinal, or esophageal surgery with recurrent laryngeal nerve trauma
  C. Irradiation
VI. Gastroesophageal reflux

Modified from Duranceau, A. C., Lafontaine, E., and Taillefer, R.: Oropharyngeal dysphagia. *In* Jamieson, G. G. (Ed.): Surgery of the Oesophagus. Edinburgh, Churchill-Livingstone, 1988, pp. 416–417.

patient who has these two complaints is seldom malingering. *Weight loss* secondary to impaired caloric intake completes the diagnostic symptom complex of cricopharyngeal dysfunction. Symptoms of gastroesophageal reflux occur in 30 to 90 per cent of patients with cricopharyngeal dysfunction,[47,75] and it is unclear whether refluxed gastric acid is actually causing local irritation of the upper sphincter in these patients or whether distal esophageal reflux is activating reflex incoordination of the pharyngoesophageal junction.[9,51,54]

The barium esophagogram in patients with cricopharyngeal dysfunction may be normal, particularly in those with intermittent symptoms who are asymptomatic at the time of radiographic evaluation. Alternatively, hypertonicity of the upper sphincter, a typical posterior cricopharyngeal bar, or a pharyngoesophageal (Zenker's) diverticulum may be observed (Figs. 1 to 3). A *complete* esophagogram, not one that focuses solely on the cervical esophagus, should be obtained to exclude other significant esophageal pathology, particularly a hiatal hernia or gastroesophageal reflux, which may produce symptoms that are referred to the cervical esophagus. Similarly, although esophagoscopy may provide little helpful information, it excludes neoplasm and reflux esophagitis, both of which can cause cervical dysphagia.

Esophageal function studies (manometry and acid reflux testing) should be performed whenever possible. With standard perfused recording catheters, however, manometric abnormalities of the UES are detected in approximately only half of these patients. True spasm, hypotonicity, lack of UES relaxation (achalasia), or incoordinated cricopharyngeal relaxation have been documented in a minority of patients with oropharyngeal

dysphagia due to a number of causes.[27,56] Incoordination of the temporal relationship between pharyngeal contraction and cricopharyngeal relaxation has been reported to be responsible for the development of pharyngoesophageal diverticula.[30,37,54,59] Abnormalities of thoracic esophageal peristalsis may be found

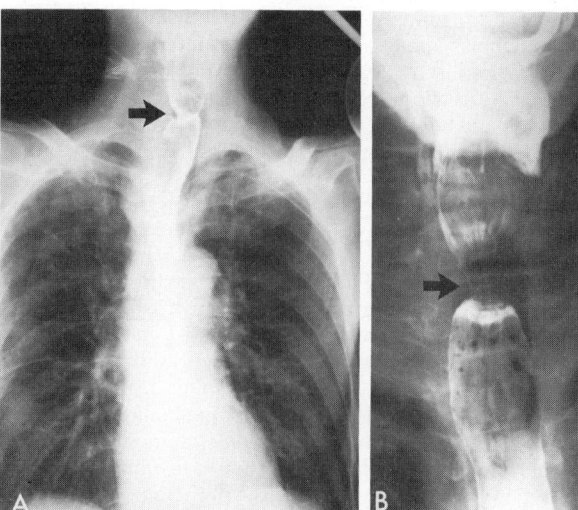

Figure 1. *A*, Prominence of the cricopharyngeal sphincter (arrow) in a patient with cervical dysphagia and symptomatic gastroesophageal reflux. *B*, Detail of cervical esophagus (arrow). (From Orringer, M. B.: Extended cervical esophagomyotomy for cricopharyngeal dysfunction. J. Thorac. Cardiovasc. Surg., *80*:669, 1980.)

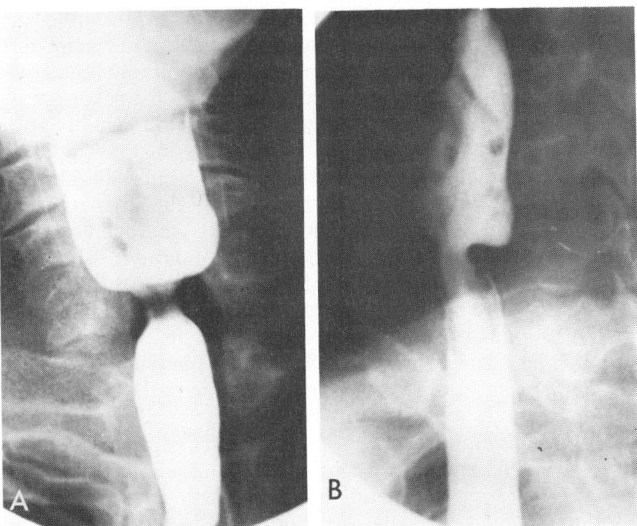

Figure 2. A, Typical appearance of hypertrophic cricopharyngeal sphincter (anteroposterior view). B, Lateral view showing posterior cricopharyngeal bar. (From Orringer, M. B.: Extended cervical esophagomyotomy for cricopharyngeal dysfunction. J. Thorac. Cardiovasc. Surg., 80:669, 1980.)

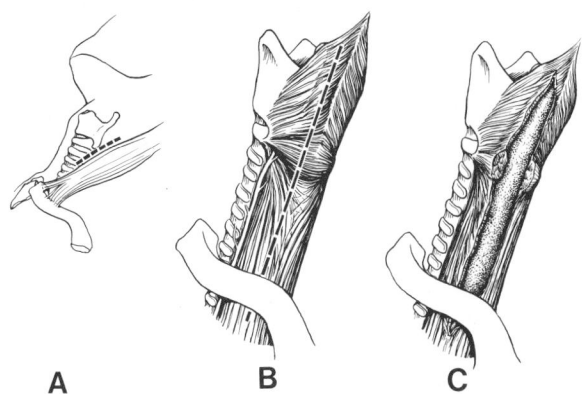

Figure 4. Cervical esophagomyotomy for cricopharyngeal dysfunction. A, A 5-cm. oblique skin incision anterior to the sternocleidomastoid muscle and centered over the cricoid cartilage. B, With a 40 French bougie within the esophagus, the esophagomyotomy is placed on the left posterolateral aspect of the esophagus to avoid injury to the recurrent laryngeal nerve, seen in the tracheoesophageal groove. C, Completed esophagomyotomy extends from the level of the superior cornu of the thyroid cartilage inferiorly to 1 to 2 cm. behind the clavicle. (From Orringer, M. B.: Extended cervical esophagomyotomy for cricopharyngeal dysfunction. J. Thorac. Cardiovasc. Surg., 80:669, 1980.)

in one third of patients with cricopharyngeal dysfunction, suggesting that the cervical esophageal complaints are only a manifestation of disordered esophageal motor function that is not limited to the pharyngoesophageal junction. Perhaps the most important information gained from esophageal function tests in these patients is the assessment with the intraesophageal pH electrode of distal high pressure zone (HPZ) competence. If a cervical esophagomyotomy for cricopharyngeal dysfunction is ultimately considered, the presence of massive gastroesophageal reflux through an incompetent lower esophageal sphincter (LES) might contraindicate the cervical procedure. Alternatively, if the LES is competent, the patient is not rendered liable to the hazards of tracheobronchial aspiration from gastroesophageal reflux by dividing the UES.

The treatment of cricopharyngeal motor dysfunction is as varied as the conditions with which it is associated and therefore must be individualized. Medical or surgical treatment of documented gastroesophageal reflux may eliminate secondary cervical complaints.[16,45,47,54] However, patients with severe cervical dysphagia and minimal or no reflux symptoms associated

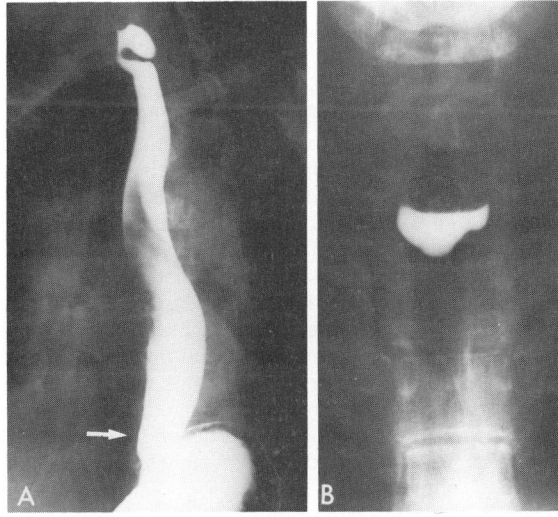

Figure 3. A, Zenker's diverticulum in a patient with an associated "patulous cardia" (arrow) and asymptomatic gastroesophageal reflux without esophagitis. B, Residual barium in the 2.5-cm. pouch (anteroposterior view). (From Orringer, M. B.: Extended cervical esophagomyotomy for cricopharyngeal dysfunction. J. Thorac. Cardiovasc. Surg., 80:669, 1980.)

with an incompetent LES may be treated successfully with a cervical esophagomyotomy and institution of upright posturing and medical therapy for reflux without the need for an anti-reflux operation.[48,75] When myasthenia gravis is under good medical control, dysphagia, a common presenting symptom,[13] is relieved. Intermittent outpatient esophageal bougienage with size 54 to 56 French dilators may produce dramatic temporary relief of incapacitating cervical dysphagia in the patient with polymyositis, Parkinson's disease, or the residua of a midbrain (basilar artery) cerebrovascular accident. Alternatively, in the presence of incapacitating cervical dysphagia and aspiration and a radiographically or manometrically documented abnormal UES, a cervical esophagomyotomy is a relatively low-risk operation that may produce gratifying relief.[63,69]

A cervical esophagomyotomy for cricopharyngeal dysfunction in the absence of a Zenker's diverticulum is performed through a 5- to 8-cm. oblique left cervical incision centered at the level of the cricoid cartilage and paralleling the anterior border of the sternocleidomastoid muscle (Fig. 4). The sternocleidomastoid muscle and carotid sheath and its contents are retracted laterally, and the trachea is retracted medially. Care is taken to avoid placement of retractors on the tracheoesophageal groove and subsequent injury to the recurrent laryngeal nerve. The dissection proceeds directly posteriorly through the cervical fascial layers to the prevertebral fascia. The esophagus is immediately anterior to the prevertebral fascia. With a 40 French bougie within the esophagus, the cervical esophagomyotomy is performed on the posterolateral esophageal wall. The incision extends from the level of the tip of the superior cornu of the thyroid cartilage inferiorly to 1 to 2 cm. behind the clavicle and is 7 to 10 cm. long. This extended cervical esophagomyotomy is recommended to ensure division of all incoordinated upper esophageal sphincter muscle fibers. A cervical esophagomyotomy is successful in relieving cervical dysphagia from cricopharyngeal motor dysfunction in 65 to 85 per cent of patients undergoing operation.[47,75]

MOTOR DISORDERS OF THE BODY OF THE ESOPHAGUS

The esophageal motor disorders are best viewed as a continuum, with hypomotility (achalasia) at one extreme and hypermotility (diffuse spasm) at the other.[19,104] Between these extremes are conditions such as vigorous achalasia, which has certain elements of both achalasia and esophageal spasm, as

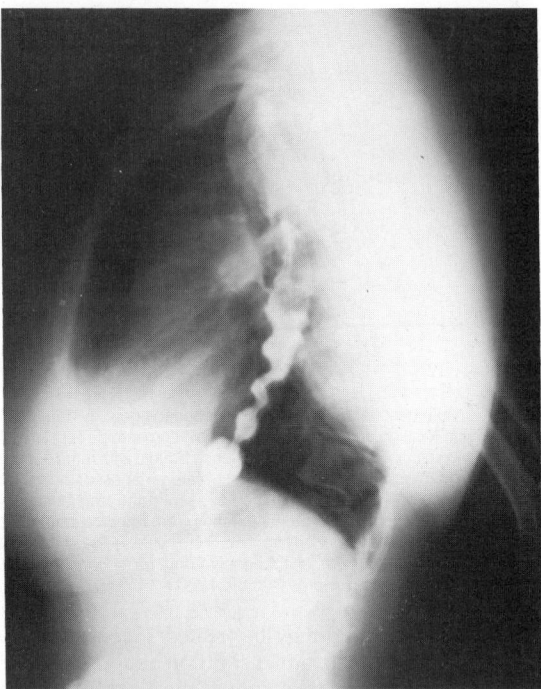

Figure 5. Esophagogram showing tertiary contractions of the circular muscle responsible for the characteristic "corkscrew" esophagus of diffuse esophageal spasm. This pattern may also be seen in totally asymptomatic individuals.

well as a number of less well-characterized examples of neuromotor dysfunction. One of these latter conditions, "curling," represents tertiary contractions of the esophagus that produce the "corkscrew" esophagus observed on barium swallow examination (Fig. 5). This pattern is often, but by no means always, observed in patients with diffuse esophageal spasm and can occur in totally asymptomatic individuals, particularly the elderly who have an associated small sliding hiatal hernia.

Neuromotor esophageal dysfunction, that is, loss of generally progressive peristalsis and the appearance to varying degrees of simultaneous, weak-to-absent esophageal contractions after swallowing, is present in numerous conditions, such as those characterized by peripheral neuropathy (diabetes, alcoholism), collagen vascular diseases (scleroderma, dermatomyositis), myasthenia gravis, multiple sclerosis, and amyotrophic lateral sclerosis. In none of these conditions is an absolutely diagnostic esophageal motor disturbance present, but rather an alteration of normal sequential peristaltic contractions with swallowing is often evident. As a muscular tube, the esophagus is limited in its response to these various neuromotor diseases. Thus, in the presence of distal obstruction from either tumor or a benign stricture, tertiary esophageal contractions may be observed in the body of the esophagus, both radiographically and with motility studies. It must be remembered, therefore, that despite the emphasis on the need for esophageal function tests in assessing patients with neuromotor disorders of the esophagus, esophageal motility studies are only *one* facet of the total evaluation, and they should be interpreted according to the particular clinical situation, as well as the barium swallow and endoscopic findings.

Achalasia

The term *achalasia* is of Greek derivation and literally means "failure or lack of relaxation." First coined by Hurst in 1915 as a reference to the failure of the LES in patients with this disease to relax normally with swallowing, the term *achalasia* focuses on the distal sphincter, when, in fact, this is a condition that involves the entire body of the esophagus. After its original description by Willis in 1674, the history of achalasia was chronicled by Ellis and Olsen in their classic review of the subject.[34]

The etiology of achalasia remains obscure, but the characteristic clinical, radiographic, and manometric findings have occurred following a variety of situations, including severe emotional stress; major physical trauma; Chagas' disease in South America[60]; and, in the author's experience, drastic weight reduction in some markedly obese dieting patients. In Chagas' disease, caused by parasitic infestation by the leishmanial forms of *Trypanosoma cruzi*, the ganglionic cells of Auerbach's plexus are destroyed, causing motor dysfunction and progressive dilation not only of the esophagus but also of the colon, ureters, and other viscera. Rake (1926) first reported the findings of disintegrated esophageal ganglionic cells in patients with achalasia unrelated to Chagas' disease.[34] Since then histologic studies of autopsy and surgical specimens of the esophageal wall obtained at the time of esophagomyotomy have documented the loss of ganglion cells in the myenteric plexus[21] and neuronal degeneration.[89] Various animal experiments indicate a relationship between either central or peripheral vagal nerve dysfunction and the development of achalasia. Experimentally, an achalasia-like pattern can be induced in dogs by vagal nerve injury and in cats by ablation of the dorsal motor nucleus of the vagus.[34] However, because in these animals the body of the esophagus contains striated muscle, an analogy to the human disease is inappropriate. Recent studies have demonstrated that in patients with achalasia, cholecystokinin octapeptide (CCK-OP) produces a paradoxical rise in LES pressure due to direct esophageal smooth muscle stimulation.[26] This suggests that the underlying pathophysiology in achalasia is loss of nonadrenergic, noncholinergic inhibitory nerves. Except in Chagas' disease, the exact cause of the denervation is unknown. A familial tendency has been reported in isolated instances.[97,109] Although the exact mechanism remains unclear, the multiple conditions, including infections and physical and emotional stress, that appear to "trigger" achalasia again suggest that the esophagus can respond in only a limited number of ways to a number of factors acting upon it—in the case of achalasia, conditions affecting either the central or peripheral vagal innervation of the esophagus or the ganglion cells of Auerbach's plexus.

The classic triad of presenting symptoms in achalasia includes dysphagia, regurgitation, and weight loss. Low retrosternal "hesitancy" or "sticking" of both solid and liquid foods is described. The sensation of dysphagia may at times be referred to the suprasternal notch. Stress or the ingestion of cold liquids may aggravate the symptoms. Patients with achalasia eat slowly and use large volumes of water to wash food into the stomach. They may contort their bodies, twisting the upper torso, elevating the chin and extending the neck, or walk about the room while eating in an effort to force down solid foods. As more water is swallowed, the weight of the fluid column in the esophagus increases, along with the sensation of retrosternal fullness, until the lower esophageal sphincter is forced open, and the patient feels sudden relief as the esophagus empties. Retrosternal pain on ingestion of food is not characteristic of achalasia, although occasionally in the early stages of the disease such discomfort occurs and may radiate to the jaw or the intrascapular region. Effortless regurgitation occurs shortly after eating, particularly if the patient bends forward or reclines, but there is usually no sour taste to the undigested food, in contrast to acid regurgitation in gastroesophageal reflux. When the esophagus has become markedly dilated, the patient may complain of regurgitation or eructation of the foul-smelling stagnating intraesophageal contents. Weight loss may be appreciable and is common.

A graphic example of the pulmonary complications of impaired swallowing, achalasia often causes recurrent respiratory symptoms due to aspiration pneumonitis, which may cause lung abscess, bronchiectasis, hemoptysis, or asthma (Fig. 6). At times, marked distention of the dilated esophagus may produce

ence this symptom have nocturnal tracheobronchial aspiration. Hematemesis in achalasia is rare. Occasionally, it is associated with retention esophagitis (to be discussed), but it is generally an ominous sign indicative of carcinoma. Achalasia is a premalignant lesion of the esophagus, with carcinoma developing as a late complication in approximately 1 to 10 per cent of patients who have this condition an average of 15 to 25 years.[58,87,105,107] This is most likely the result of mucosal irritation and subsequent metaplasia induced by the retention esophagitis. Esophageal carcinoma in achalasia tends to arise in the mid third of the organ, below the point at which the air-fluid level is most often seen on barium swallow examination and mucosal irritation is believed to be most pronounced. These tumors, usually squamous-cell histologically, generally grow to a large size, unnoticed by the patient with a dilated esophagus and chronic dysphagia, and are hopelessly incurable when discovered.

The radiographic appearance of achalasia varies with the extent of the disease, the barium esophagogram showing mild dilation in the early stages and massive dilation, tortuosity, and a sigmoid shape in the later stages. Retained intraesophageal contents are typically observed. Peristalsis is disordered in the early stages and totally lacking in the later stages. The roentgenographic hallmark of achalasia on barium swallow examination is the distal "bird beak" taper of the esophagogastric junction (Fig. 7). The characteristic appearance of a "double mediastinal stripe" throughout the length of the chest on a posteroanterior (PA) view of the standard chest roentgenogram and a posterior

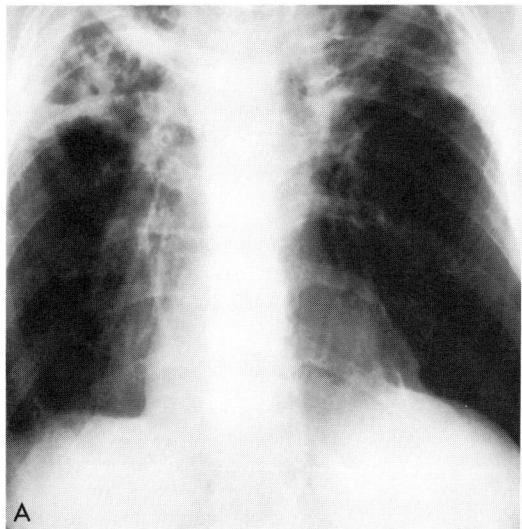

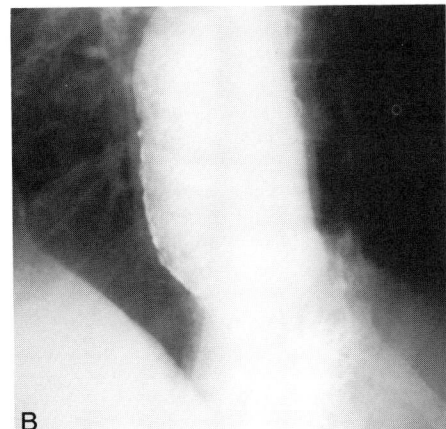

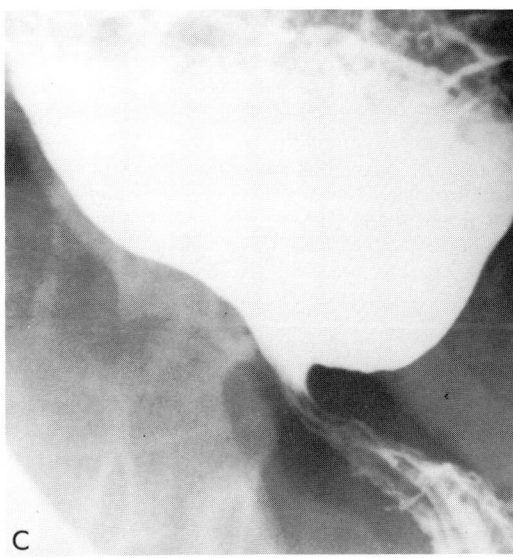

Figure 6. *A*, Chest roentgenogram of a 54-year-old woman with long-standing achalasia treated 13 years before with an esophagomyotomy. The patient had recurrent dysphagia and regurgitation as well as massive hemoptysis from aspiration pneumonia and secondary bilateral apical inflammatory lung disease. *B*, Esophagogram showing a megaesophagus with retained secretions in this patient. *C*, Detail of esophagogastric junction showing the characteristic "bird beak" taper of achalasia.

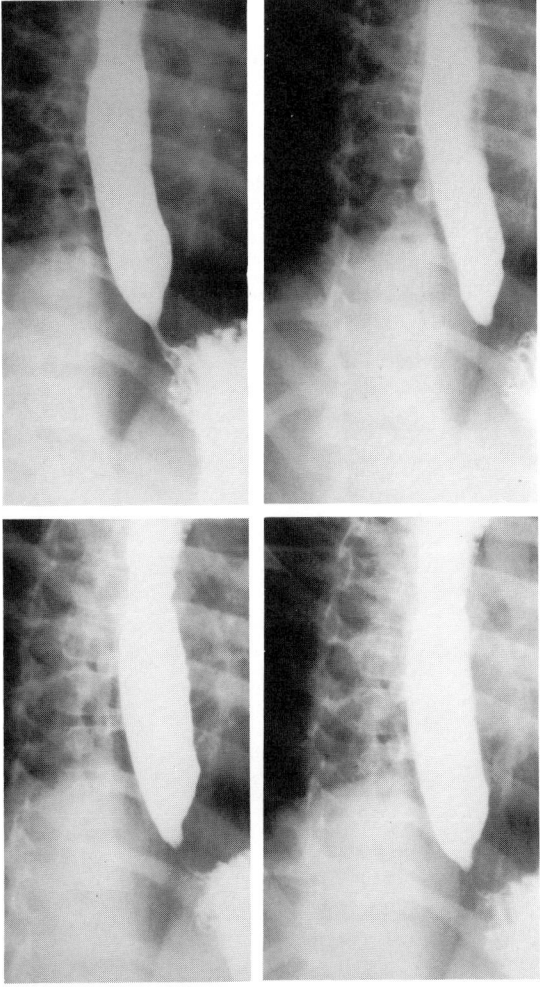

Figure 7. Multiple views in a cine esophagogram in a patient with early achalasia showing a persistent "bird beak" taper at the esophagogastric junction and impaired esophageal emptying.

pronounced shortness of breath and dyspnea owing to displacement of adjacent intrathoracic organs. The patient should be asked whether he soils his pillow at night with regurgitated intraesophageal contents, because most patients who experi-

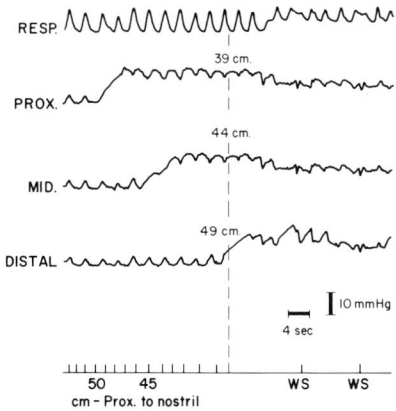

Figure 8. Motility tracing of the distal high pressure zone (HPZ) in achalasia. In contrast to the normal findings on withdrawing the recording catheter from the stomach into the esophagus (see Fig. 3), basal intraesophageal pressure is *greater* than that within the stomach. In addition, when the distal recording port is positioned in the HPZ and the patient swallows, there is neither reflex relaxation of the HPZ nor propagation of a progressive peristaltic contraction. WS, wet swallow.

mediastinal air-fluid level on a lateral view in a patient with typical symptoms are diagnostic of achalasia.

The manometric criteria of achalasia are failure of the LES to relax reflexively with swallowing and lack of progressive peristalsis throughout the length of the esophagus. As the manometric recording catheter is withdrawn from the stomach into the esophagus, often there is absence of the normal fall in mean intraesophageal pressure below mean intragastric pressure as the thorax is entered, the pressure in the esophagus being higher than that below the diaphragm (Fig. 8). In the early stages of achalasia, contractions after swallowing may be of normal amplitude, but they are synchronous and simultaneous (Fig. 9). Later, contractions are either totally absent or weak and simultaneous (Fig. 10). Distal esophageal HPZ pressure is generally normal or somewhat elevated, but the marked hypertonicity of the spastic esophagus is not seen. Thus, the term *cardiospasm* is totally inappropriate when referring to achalasia. With mild esophageal dilation on the esophagogram, it may be difficult to differentiate early achalasia from diffuse spasm or scleroderma. The mecholyl test, in which 5 to 10 mg. of methacholine —a vagomimetic drug—was initially used to help in diagnosing achalasia manometrically,[61] producing marked elevation of the intraesophageal pressure and increased amplitude and frequency of simultaneous esophageal contractions that correspond with the patient's complaints of chest pain. This response does not occur in scleroderma but is quite common

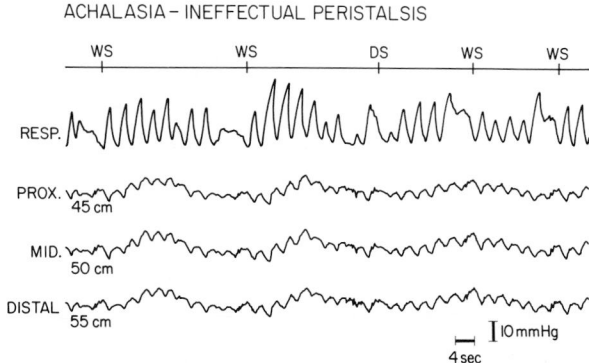

Figure 10. Motility tracing in advanced achalasia with megaesophagus on barium esophagogram. Essentially no esophageal contractions are generated by swallowing. DS, dry swallow; WS, wet swallow.

both in diffuse esophageal spasm and achalasia. Thus, it is not considered a diagnostic test. The patient with intermittent diffuse esophageal spasm, however, usually has some degree of progressive peristalsis on standard manometric evaluation, and the LES in diffuse esophageal spasm shows reflex relaxation with swallowing. In their early stages, therefore, these two conditions can be differentiated manometrically. Because of the rather severe systemic vagal effects methacholine may induce in the patient with either achalasia or diffuse esophageal spasm, bethanechol (Urecholine), a milder vagomimetic, is now generally substituted (Fig. 11).

Esophagoscopy is indicated in achalasia to assess the presence and extent of retention esophagitis, to exclude the possibility of associated carcinoma, and to determine whether there is a distal esophageal stricture from reflux esophagitis that may have followed prior forceful dilations or an esophagomyotomy that destroyed the LES mechanism. Retention esophagitis in advanced achalasia is quite different endoscopically from reflux esophagitis. With chronic esophagitis due to reflux, the distal esophagus often appears whitish and fibrotic, with superficial mucosal ulceration. When there is prolonged retention esophagitis associated with achalasia, however, the irritating effects of putrifying food on the esophageal mucosa may induce severe edema with red to purple discoloration and marked friability. When performing esophagoscopy in the evaluation of achalasia, the presence of retained fluid and food in the dilated esophagus, even after an overnight fast, complicates the procedure. The technique of esophagoscopy in the patient with achalasia is discussed in Part V. Patients with achalasia should be evaluated under general anesthesia, with the airway protected by an en-

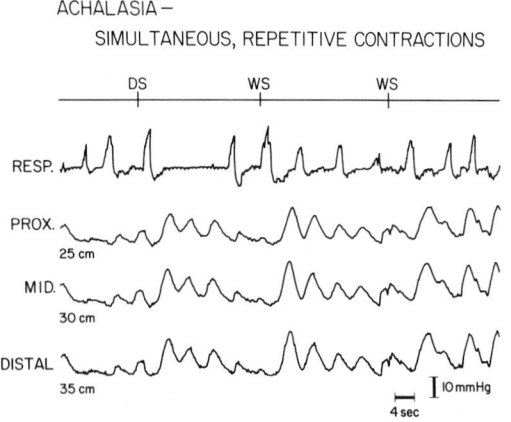

Figure 9. Motility tracing in early achalasia with minimal esophageal dilation on barium esophagogram. Esophageal contractions after swallowing are of normal amplitude, but they are simultaneous, multiphasic, and nonprogressive. DS, dry swallow; WS, wet swallow.

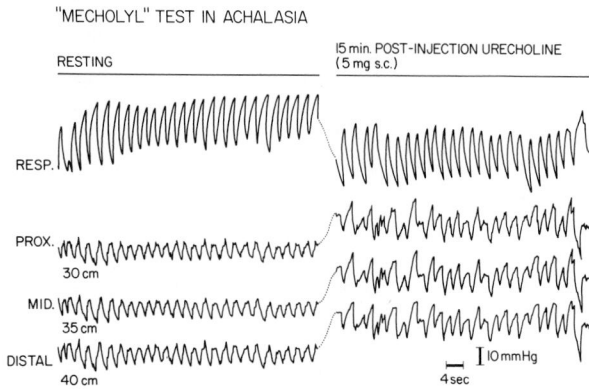

Figure 11. Motility tracing showing positive "mecholyl test" in achalasia. Administration of a vagomimetic drug (in this case, bethanechol, 10 mg. subcutaneously) causes elevation of the resting pressures in all recording catheters, as well as an increase in the frequency and amplitude of spontaneous simultaneous esophageal contractions. Chest pain and regurgitation may also be experienced by the patient with achalasia in response to these drugs. Both the symptoms and the manometric changes are reversed by administering atropine, 0.4 mg. intravenously.

dotracheal tube cuff, by means of the rigid esophagoscope, which permits evacuation of particulate esophageal contents and optimal visualization, and a flexible fiberoptic esophagoscope for assessing the esophagogastric junction. It is important to exclude a tumor of the cardia, which may mimic achalasia.[93] If severe retention esophagitis is detected in the patient with achalasia, esophageal decompression by an indwelling nasogastric tube may be required for several days before operation can be undertaken safely.

The treatment of achalasia is purely palliative, because this condition is incurable, and the derangement in esophageal motor function never returns to normal. This knowledge, as well as the extent of the disease when it is first diagnosed, must influence therapy. Both the nonsurgical and surgical forms of treatment of achalasia are directed toward relieving the obstruction caused by the nonrelaxing LES. In the early stages of the disease, before esophageal dilation occurs, sublingual nitroglycerin before or during meals, long-acting nitrates, and calcium-channel blocking agents improve swallowing.[3,39] These drugs are most useful in the short-term treatment of achalasia prior to more definitive therapy or in elderly patients who are not candidates for other methods of treatment. Passage of mercury-weighted bougies in the 48 to 54 French range may relieve the dysphagia for several days or weeks but is seldom a satisfactory long-term solution.

The two most widely used and analyzed methods of therapy of achalasia are forceful dilation, either pneumatic or hydrostatic, and thoracic esophagomyotomy. At the Mayo Clinic, both forms of therapy have been successful. The comparative results of esophagomyotomy versus forceful dilation for achalasia in 899 patients were reported by Okike and associates (Table 2).[73] Not only is esophagomyotomy safer than dilation (perforation occurs four times more often with dilation, 4 per cent versus 1 per cent), but it is also more reliable, providing good to excellent relief of dysphagia in 85 per cent of patients, compared with 65 per cent of patients treated with hydrostatic dilation. The late results of esophagomyotomy are also significantly better than those for forceful dilation. Of the patients treated by hydrostatic dilation, 82 per cent were treated once, 16 per cent required two dilations, and 2 per cent were dilated three times or more. Although the clearly superior results of esophagomyotomy make a compelling argument for this approach as the preferred treatment of achalasia, the fact that 65 per cent of patients undergoing hydrostatic dilation have a good or excellent result cannot be ignored, particularly because both approaches are palliative in nature, and the mortality for both is quite low. Gastroesophageal reflux secondary to disruption of the incoordinated lower esophageal sphincter is a potential

complication of both methods of treatment. The Mayo Clinic data indicate no increased morbidity in patients undergoing esophagomyotomy after prior hydrostatic dilations. Others have also substantiated the effectiveness of forceful balloon dilation in achalasia, reporting good or excellent results in 77 per cent of their patients so treated[102] and an incidence of perforation ranging from 1 to 5 per cent.[94] When a perforation does occur after balloon dilation, it can usually be managed by keeping the esophagus empty with tube aspiration, antibiotics, and parenteral nutrition.[103] Other significant complications of pneumatic dilation are infrequent, and late gastroesophageal reflux and esophagitis appear to occur in fewer than 1 per cent of patients. Relative contraindications to balloon dilation for achalasia include an extremely poor overall medical condition that would preclude repair if a perforation should occur, extremely young age (infants and small children), a tortuous sigmoid-shaped esophagus, a previous esophagomyotomy, and the presence of a concomitant sliding hiatal hernia. The list of "contraindications" is steadily being revised and shortened as greater experience with balloon dilation is obtained. Although more reliable and sustained relief of dysphagia may be achieved with an esophagomyotomy for achalasia,[22] pneumatic dilation by experienced personnel currently appears to be the most reasonable initial treatment, reserving esophagomyotomy for those who fail to respond to pneumatic dilation.

In the United States, distal esophagomyotomy for achalasia is generally performed through a left thoracotomy and involves a longitudinal incision 7 to 10 cm. in length through the esophageal musculature to approximately the level of the inferior pulmonary vein (Figs. 12 and 13). Transthoracic esophagomyotomy is a modification of the original operation for achalasia described by the German surgeon Heller in 1913.[46] Heller's procedure was performed transabdominally and involved an esophagomyotomy on both the anterior and posterior walls of the esophagogastric junction. Zaaijer (1923) popularized a variation in Heller's operation, performing the myotomy on only the anterior wall of the esophagus.[108] Distal esophagomyotomy for achalasia has subsequently been performed successfully through either the abdominal or the thoracic routes.

Unresolved technical questions concern the distal extent of the esophagomyotomy and the need for a concomitant antireflux procedure. The Mayo Clinic experience indicates only a 3 per cent incidence of late serious complications of gastroesophageal reflux in patients undergoing esophagomyotomy without the routine addition of an antireflux operation.[73] They advocate

TABLE 2. Comparison of Results of Hydrostatic Dilation and Esophagomyotomy (1949–1975)

Factors	Dilation (431 Patients)	Esophagomyotomy (468 Patients)
Mortality	2 (0.5%)	1 (0.2%)
Esophageal perforation	19 (4%)	5 (1%)
Requiring operation	10	3
Follow-up	311 (72%)	456 (97%)
Duration	1–18 yr.	1–17 yr.
Result		
Excellent	28 } 65*	50 } 85*
Good	37	35
Fair	16	9
Poor	19	6

*Significantly different (p < 0.001).

Modified from Okike, N., Payne, W. S., Neufeld, D. M., et al.: Esophagomyotomy versus forceful dilation for achalasia of the esophagus: Results in 899 patients. Ann. Thorac. Surg., *28*:119, 1979.

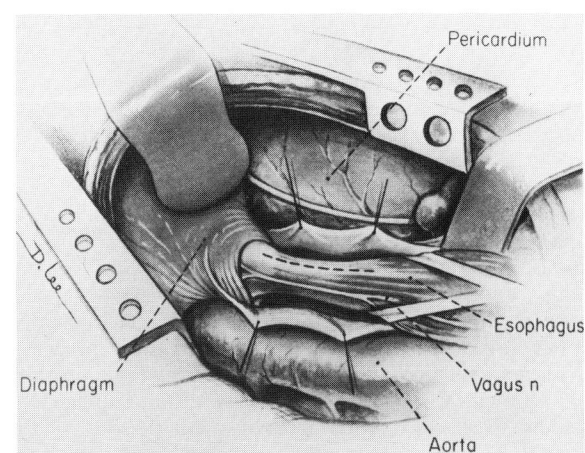

Figure 12. Transthoracic exposure of the distal esophagus for esophagomyotomy. After dividing the inferior pulmonary ligament and retracting the lung superiorly, the mediastinal pleura is opened, and the esophagus and vagus nerves are encircled with a rubber drain. (From Ellis, F. H., Jr., Kaiser, J. C., Schlegel, J. F., Earlam, R. J., McVey, J. L., and Olsen, A. M.: Esophagomyotomy for esophageal achalasia: Experimental, clinical, and manometric aspects. Ann. Surg., *166*:640, 1967.)

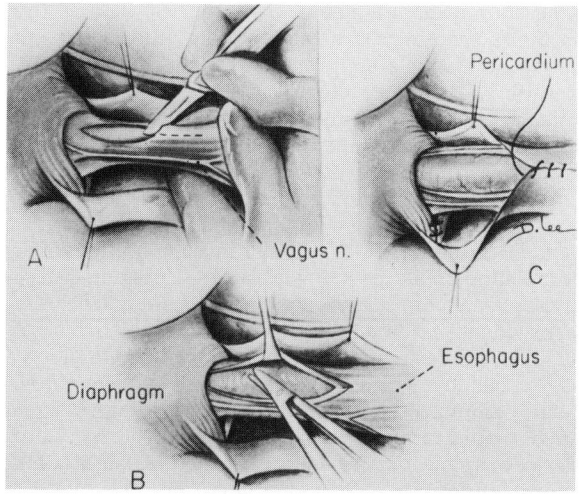

Figure 13. Technique of transthoracic esophagomyotomy. *A*, The longitudinal and circular esophageal muscle fibers are incised from beyond the esophagogastric junction to the level of the inferior pulmonary vein. *B*, The muscle layers of the esophagus are dissected away from the mucosa and submucosa for at least 50 per cent of the circumference. *C*, When the esophagomyotomy is completed, the esophagogastric junction is restored to an intra-abdominal location after addition of a modified Belsey fundoplication, and the crura are approximated posterior to the esophagus. (From Ellis, F. H., Jr., Kaiser, J. C., Schlegel, J. F., Earlam, R. J., McVey, J. L., and Olsen, A. M.: Esophagomyotomy for esophageal achalasia: Experimental, clinical, and manometric aspects. Ann. Surg., 166:640, 1967.)

extending the esophagomyotomy onto the stomach only far enough to ensure complete division of the distal esophageal musculature but not to induce incompetence of the LES mechanism. Ellis (1980) also does not recommend an antireflux procedure at the time of esophagomyotomy.[33] Others, however, believe that complete relief of the obstruction caused by the incoordinated LES can be achieved only by rendering it incompetent, that is, extending the esophagomyotomy onto the stomach for 1 to 2 cm.[4,95] The gastric extension of the myotomy required by this approach makes reconstruction of the esophagogastric junction compulsory to prevent reflux and its complications. This is supported by a 3 to 50 per cent reported incidence of reflux after esophagomyotomy in some series.[8,14,57,62,67,70,72]

Because the patient with achalasia has distal esophageal obstruction, unless the incoordinated lower sphincter fibers are completely divided, dysphagia may not be relieved. Thus, attempts by some to perform a "limited" esophagomyotomy without an antireflux procedure have an 8.3 per cent incidence of reflux and a 20.8 per cent incidence of inadequate correction of the distal esophageal obstruction.[86] Most surgeons now advocate a complete esophagocardiomyotomy for achalasia with some type of fundoplication to prevent the subsequent development of gastroesophageal reflux. Although some have advocated a very loose, short 360-degree Nissen fundoplication,[91] others have cautioned that the combination of a total fundoplication and an atonic esophagus may produce obstruction that becomes more evident with long-term follow-up.[29] A partial fundoplication of the Belsey[5] or Dor types[40,41,85,99] appears more satisfactory in controlling gastroesophageal reflux following an esophagomyotomy for achalasia, because these procedures provide good reflux control without producing too competent a lower esophageal sphincter and relative distal esophageal obstruction. Excellent long-term results with these procedures suggest that a distal esophagomyotomy combined with a partial fundoplication is the approach of choice in patients with achalasia requiring surgical therapy.

Patients with recurrent esophageal obstruction following a prior esophagomyotomy or a reflux-induced peptic stricture after either esophagomyotomy or forceful dilation pose a difficult dilemma for the surgeon. Ellis and associates have reported

that only two thirds of patients having a repeat esophagomyotomy benefited from the operation, and even poorer results occurred after a fundoplication for reflux symptoms.[32] A more reliable approach may be esophageal resection and visceral esophageal substitution, preferably with stomach, which provides definitive treatment of the esophageal abnormality and can be accomplished transhiatally without opening of the thorax. This approach is being used with increased frequency in patients with failed prior operations for achalasia or in those with advanced achalasia and a megaesophagus that may fail to empty adequately, even after an esophagomyotomy (see Fig. 7).[15,80,84]

Diffuse Esophageal Spasm and Related Hypermotility Disorders

Diffuse esophageal spasm (DES) is a poorly understood and equally poorly treated hypermotility disorder in which patients experience chest pain and/or dysphagia as a result of repetitive, simultaneous, high-amplitude esophageal contractions. The etiology of DES is unknown, and there is no consistent evidence that this condition is an early form of achalasia. The patient with DES is typically anxious and complains of chest pain inconsistently related to eating, exertion, and position. The character of the chest pain may mimic that of angina pectoris due to coronary artery disease, often being described as squeezing, oppressive, retrosternal pressure that has a variable intensity and radiates toward the jaw, down the arms, and frequently "straight through" to the intrascapular region of the back. Symptoms are often greatest during periods of emotional stress, but the occasional association of dysphagia with chest pain suggests an esophageal, rather than a cardiac, abnormality. Although patients may experience slow emptying of the esophagus, obstructive symptoms are uncommon, and regurgitation of food is unusual. Many patients, however, experience regurgitation of intraesophageal saliva ("phlegm" or "foam") during bouts of the esophageal colic. Ingestion of cold liquids or foods may aggravate DES, as can gastroesophageal reflux. Most patients with DES, however, do *not* have associated gastroesophageal reflux. A history of irritable bowel syndrome, pylorospasm, spastic colon, or other functional gastrointestinal complaints is common; and gallstones, peptic ulcer disease, and pancreatitis can all activate DES.

The initial evaluation of the patient with DES is essentially the same as that of the patient with chest pain of undetermined etiology: a chest roentgenogram and a standard electrocardiogram (ECG). In our "cardiac-oriented" Western society, despite a normal ECG, stress ECG, and dipyridamole thallium cardiac

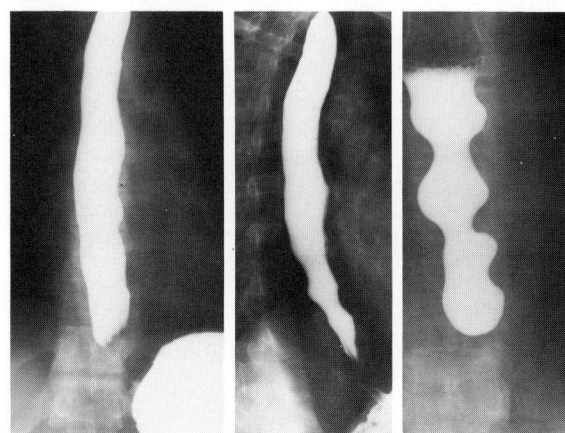

Figure 14. Three views from barium esophagograms in the same patient with intermittent diffuse esophageal spasm showing wide variability of roentgenographic findings in this condition, from a nearly normal appearance *(left)*, to a distal esophageal taper suggesting achalasia *(center)*, to a typical "corkscrew" esophagus *(right)*. Esophageal manometry is essential for establishing a diagnosis in such a patient.

scan in a patient with recurrent chest pain, cardiac catheterization in search of coronary artery disease is frequently considered before less invasive evaluation of the esophagus with a contrast study and esophageal function tests. By the time an esophageal evaluation is undertaken, significant coronary artery disease often has already been excluded with cardiac catheterization, or the patient has even undergone coronary artery bypass but still has persistent chest pain.

A careful history is among the most important aspects of the diagnosis of DES, and causative intra-abdominal pathology (e.g., gallstones, gastric or ulcer disease) should be excluded. The roentgenographic findings of DES are frustratingly variable (Fig. 14). At times, classic "curling" or "corkscrew" esophagus caused by segmental contractions of the circular muscle may be apparent; but not infrequently, little if any impairment of peristalsis or even a distal "beaklike taper" suggesting early achalasia is observed. An esophageal wall thickness of more than 5 mm. on a barium swallow examination suggests esophageal muscular hypertrophy in the patient with symptoms of DES. A hiatal hernia and/or gastroesophageal reflux may be revealed. The finding of an esophageal pulsion diverticulum, particularly in a patient with angina-like symptoms, is virtually diagnostic of DES. Esophagoscopy should be performed in the patient with DES, because a distal esophageal obstructing lesion may produce proximal tertiary esophageal contractions that are con-fused with DES on barium study, and an infiltrating tumor, esophageal fibrosis, or esophagitis causing radiographic distal esophageal narrowing should be excluded.

Traditionally, esophageal manometry has been considered the "ultimate test" in the diagnosis of DES. Unfortunately, however, this condition is typically characterized by *intermittent*" episodes of spasm; and unless the patient is experiencing spasm at the time of the manometric study, just as with the barium esophagogram, the results may be entirely normal. The evaluation of the patient with diffuse esophageal spasm is further complicated by the fact that some of the radiographic and manometric criteria of this disorder are observed in asymptomatic patients, and the factors responsible for producing esophageal pain in these patients have not been established. In addition, the problem has become more complicated by the inclusion of a number of related hypermotility disorders, e.g., "nutcracker esophagus," hypertensive LES, nonspecific esophageal motility disorders (NEMD), and vigorous achalasia under the generic heading "diffuse esophageal spasm." These conditions, however, are best defined by precise manometric criteria, an understanding of which provides an objective rationale for differentiating them in the evaluation of the patient with chest pain of esophageal origin (Table 3). The classic manometric criteria of DES are simultaneous, multiphasic, repetitive, often high-amplitude contractions that occur after a swallow and

TABLE 3. Manometric Criteria of Primary Esophageal Motility Disorders

Normal
1. LES pressure 15–25 mm. Hg (never >45 mm. Hg) with normal relaxation with swallowing
2. Mean amplitude of distal esophageal peristaltic wave 30–100 mm. Hg (never >190 mm. Hg)
3. Simultaneous contractions occurring after <10% of wet swallows
4. Monophasic wave forms (with not more than 2 peaks)
5. Duration of distal esophageal peristaltic wave: 2–6 seconds
6. No repetitive contractions

Primary Motility Disorders
Achalasia
1. Aperistalsis in esophageal body
2. Partial or absent LES relaxation with swallowing
3. LES pressure normal or >45 mm. Hg
4. Intraesophageal basal pressure > intragastric
Diffuse esophageal spasm (DES)
1. Simultaneous (nonperistaltic) contractions
   a. Repetitive (at least 3 peaks)
   b. Increased duration (>6 seconds)
2. Spontaneous contractions
3. Intermittent normal peristalsis
4. Contractions may be of increased amplitude
"Nutcracker esophagus"
1. Mean peristaltic amplitude (10 wet swallows) in distal esophagus >180 mm. Hg
2. Increased duration of contractions (>6 seconds) frequent
3. Normal peristaltic sequences
Hypertensive LES
1. LES pressures >45 mm. Hg but with normal relaxation
2. Normal esophageal peristalsis
Nonspecific esophageal motility disorders (NEMD)
1. No or decreased amplitude of peristalsis
   a. Normal LES pressure
   b. Normal LES relaxation
2. Abnormal peristalsis, including any of the following:
   a. Abnormal wave forms
   b. Isolated simultaneous contractions
   c. Isolated spontaneous contractions
   d. Normal peristalsis sequence maintained
   e. LES normal
Vigorous achalasia
1. Repetitive simultaneous contractions in body of esophagus (as with DES)
2. Partial or absent LES relaxation (as with achalasia)

Modified from Khan, A. A., and Castell, D. O.: Primary diffuse esophageal spasm and related disorders. *In* Jamieson, G. G. (Ed.): *Surgery of the Oesophagus.* Edinburgh, Churchill-Livingstone, 1988, pp. 483–488.

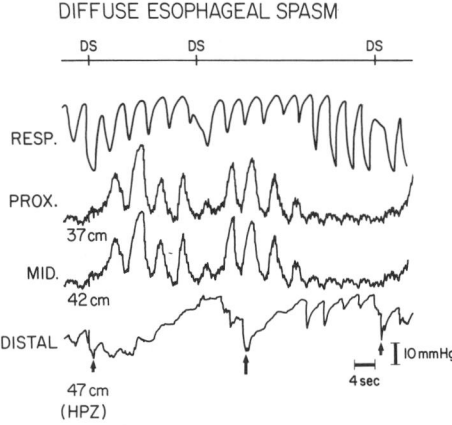

DIFFUSE ESOPHAGEAL SPASM

Figure 15. Motility tracing in diffuse esophageal spasm. This condition is characterized by simultaneous, nonprogressive, multiphasic esophageal contractions occurring both spontaneously and after swallowing. Unlike achalasia, however, reflex relaxation (arrows) of the distal sphincter with swallowing is still apparent. DS, dry swallow; WS, wet swallow; HPZ, distal high pressure zone.

spontaneously in the smooth muscle portion of the esophagus (Fig. 15). Occasional progressive peristalsis may be observed but is most often present in the upper third of the esophagus. Upper and lower sphincter resting pressures and relaxation with swallowing are usually normal, although a hypertensive LES with sustained contractions after swallowing may be seen. When standard manometry fails to demonstrate DES, evocative maneuvers using ice water[68] or hydrochloric acid,[7] intraesophageal infusions, or the administration of bethanechol,[66] pentagastrin,[74] or ergonovine[23] may induce the motility disorder. The diagnostic hallmark of DES is the correlation of subjective complaints with objective evidence of spasm on manometric tracings (Fig. 16). Unfortunately, as indicated above, normal asymptomatic individuals may occasionally demonstrate either radiographic or manometric esophageal spasm, whereas those with typical symptoms of DES may have entirely normal results of barium swallow examinations and motility studies when they are not experiencing symptoms.

Data from the University of Michigan Thoracic Surgery Esophageal Clinic illustrate the aforementioned points. Among 134 consecutive patients with chest pain evaluated with esophageal function studies, cardiac catheterizations had been performed in 75 (56 per cent). Significant coronary artery disease, however, was documented in only 23 per cent of these patients who had angiograms. One fourth of the patients had symptoms of gastroesophageal reflux. Sublingual nitroglycerin relieved the chest pain in 50 per cent of these patients (completely in 75 per cent and partially in 25 per cent), adding to the confusion

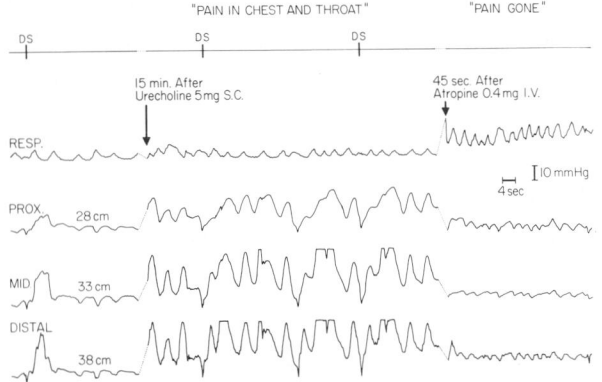

Figure 16. Motility tracing showing positive Urecholine test in diffuse esophageal spasm. The vagomimetic drug causes the development of both manometric and symptomatic esophageal spasm, both of which are eliminated within seconds of administering atropine, 0.4 mg. intravenously. DS, dry swallow.

with coronary artery disease. Barium swallow abnormalities included abnormal peristalsis (27 per cent), a hiatal hernia (18 per cent), gastroesophageal reflux (12 per cent), and esophageal pulsion diverticulum (2 per cent). Standard esophageal function tests in these patients demonstrated abnormal acid clearing ability in 66 per cent, abnormal peristalsis (but not diagnostic spasm) in 31 per cent, abnormal gastroesophageal reflux in 30 per cent, and a positive acid perfusion (Bernstein) test in 16 per cent. The response to a 10-mg. bethanechol challenge in these patients was an extremely useful diagnostic procedure, with 37 per cent (49 patients) experiencing subjective chest pain in association with typical manometric evidence for esophageal spasm. Both the symptoms and manometric abnormalities were eliminated within seconds of administering 0.4 mg. of atropine intravenously.

Because of the general lack of understanding of the etiology of this condition, it is not surprising that the treatment of DES is far from satisfactory. Many patients with esophageal spasm have an underlying psychiatric abnormality. The gut has long been known to be sensitive to emotional stimuli, and the striking clinical similarities between esophageal spasm and irritable bowel syndrome appear far from coincidental. Both the esophageal and colonic abnormalities, for example, are manifested by stress or reflex-induced spastic contractions, both occur predominantly in women, and both are associated with psychiatric disturbances. Documented psychiatric disorders, including depression, psychosomatic complaints, and anxiety, have been reported in more than 80 per cent with esophageal manometric contraction abnormalities.[17]

For many patients with DES, simply establishing an esophageal etiology for their previously unexplained chest pain and providing reassurance is therapeutic and a great source of relief. Those complaining of dysphagia should avoid stress during meals as well as "trigger" foods or drinks. Psychiatric family counseling may be useful. If symptoms of gastroesophageal reflux are present or if gastroesophageal reflux is documented with esophageal function tests, medical treatment of reflux should be instituted. Cimetidine may be very helpful in patients in the latter group. Antispasmodics are occasionally helpful. The response of DES to sublingual nitroglycerin is variable but may be dramatic. Patients in whom sublingual nitroglycerin administered prior to meals is effective for intermittent bouts of pain or dysphagia may find more sustained relief with long-acting nitrates. Calcium channel blockers (e.g., nifedipine and diltiazem)[90] have also demonstrated variable efficacy in these patients. Esophageal dilation with Hurst-Maloney bougies (50 to 60 French) may relieve dysphagia and chest pain from DES for weeks to months, and if this is the case, self-dilations at home should be considered. Although there are anecdotal reports of the efficacy of pneumatic dilation in patients with DES,[82,100,102] there is obvious concern that forceful dilation of a hypertonic, spastic esophagus may predispose to major esophageal disruption.

Although thoracic esophagomyotomy for DES has been advocated by some physicians,[31,36,38,102] the results are much less reliable and much less favorable than when used in the treatment of achalasia[35,81]—variable success being achieved in perhaps only 50 to 60 per cent of patients. Despite apparent improvement in the manometric and radiographic indicators of DES after esophagomyotomy, patients may continue to complain of chest pain and slow emptying of the esophagus. When the spasm is secondary to gastroesophageal reflux and LES competence is restored, relief of both reflux symptoms and those due to spasm may be gratifying. Unfortunately, however, *long-term* relief from the pain of DES is seldom achieved, and pain may persist despite a competent LES, multiple esophagomyotomies, and even total thoracic esophagectomy with visceral esophageal substitution.[78] Therefore, only in the most *extenuating circumstances,* when a patient is nearly incapacitated by chest pain or dysphagia or in the presence of a pulsion diverticulum of the intrathoracic esophagus (to be discussed), should an esophagomyotomy be performed for DES.

It is traditionally taught that a long esophagomyotomy should be performed for DES.[31] A longer esophagomyotomy is needed than that for achalasia, because it is desirable to divide all the spastic esophageal circular muscle fibers, usually at least those from the level of the aortic arch to the esophagogastric junction. Although it has been proposed that the proximal extent of the esophageal spasm on manometric evaluation dictates the cephalad extent of the esophagomyotomy at operation, it is impossible to extrapolate in the operating room to an exact location on the esophagus measurements made in the esophageal laboratory. Therefore, the thoracic esophagomyotomy should be extended as high as possible in these patients, if necessary, under the aortic arch and into the superior mediastinum to the level of the thoracic inlet. If only the distal two thirds of the esophageal circular muscle is divided, high retrosternal chest pain and dysphagia may persist because of residual spasm in the upper third of the esophagus.[50] Controversy exists regarding the need to extend the myotomy entirely through the LES and onto the stomach, rather than limiting its distal extent to avoid the development of subsequent gastroesophageal reflux. Although it is a noble endeavor to preserve the distal esophageal sphincter mechanism in the patient with DES who is undergoing an esophagomyotomy, so long as the distal circular esophageal muscle fibers remain undivided, the potential for bouts of uncorrected spasm and obstruction exists. The author therefore endorses Belsey's view that the incision should be extended onto the stomach for at least 1 cm. to ensure that all circular esophageal muscle fibers have been divided. The incompetent LES mechanism thereby created should then be reconstructed with a modified Belsey Mark IV operation.[5] A poorly contracting esophagus after an esophagomyotomy contraindicates a 360-degree fundoplication for reflux control in these patients, just as is the case with achalasia.

The *"nutcracker,"*[6] or *super-squeeze," esophagus*[11] is a hypermotility disorder characterized by extremely high amplitude (up to 225 to 430 mm. Hg) progressive peristaltic contractions, often of prolonged duration. Symptoms of chest pain, dysphagia, and odynophagia may be similar to those of DES. Some patients develop clinical and manometric findings of both achalasia and DES and are characterized as having *vigorous achalasia.*[10,92] As in patients with achalasia, dysphagia and regurgitation are common in patients with vigorous achalasia, but chest pain typical of DES also occurs. Segmental spasm, rather than esophageal dilation, is often observed on barium swallow examination. Esophageal manometry demonstrates failure of normal LES relaxation, which is frequently terminated by premature contractions. There is a lack of progressive peristalsis, and esophageal contractions after swallowing are powerful, simultaneous, and repetitive.

Scleroderma

Esophageal motor disturbances occur in several of the collagen vascular diseases, such as dermatomyositis, polymyositis, and lupus erythematosus, but particularly in scleroderma. Scleroderma, or systemic sclerosis, is a disease of unknown etiology that is characterized by induration of the skin, fibrous replacement of the smooth muscle of internal organs, and progressive loss of visceral and cutaneous function. Disruption of normal esophageal peristalsis is so common in scleroderma that it is recognized as a major diagnostic sign of the disease. This is particularly true in acrosclerosis, the type of scleroderma associated with Raynaud's phenomenon, even in the absence of the typical skin changes. As fibrous replacement of esophageal smooth muscle progresses, the distal esophageal HPZ loses its tone and normal response to swallowing, and gastroesophageal reflux occurs (Figs. 17 and 18). In the distal two thirds to three

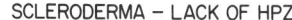

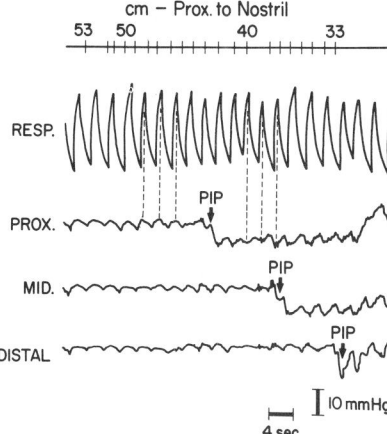

Figure 17. Motility tracing showing the resting-pressure profile of the gastroesophageal junction in scleroderma. As the recording catheter is withdrawn from the stomach into the esophagus, there is almost lack of a distal esophageal high pressure zone (HPZ). Distal to the pressure inversion point (PIP), there is an intraabdominal pressure pattern, with peak intraluminal pressures occurring at the height of inspiration. Proximal to this point, within the thorax, intraesophageal pressures are negative at the peak of inspiration. For subsequent acid reflux testing (see Fig. 18), the intraesophageal pH probe is positioned 5 cm. proximal to the PIP. (From Orringer, M. B., Dabich, L., Zarafonetis, C. J., and Sloan, H.: Gastroesophageal reflux in esophageal scleroderma: Diagnosis and implications. Ann. Thorac. Surg., 22:120, 1976.)

quarters of the thoracic esophagus, normal progressive peristalsis changes to weak, simultaneous, nonpropulsive contractions (Fig. 19). Thus, most patients with scleroderma with esophageal involvement initially complain of slow emptying of the esophagus, which requires that they use large amounts of water to wash food through the esophagus. More disturbing to them, however, are the severe heartburn and gastroesophageal reflux that they experience. The prolonged duration of contact between refluxed gastric acid and the esophageal mucosa that occurs because of the impaired ability of the atonic lower esophagus to clear refluxed gastric contents back into the stomach can cause progression from a nearly normal-appearing barium esophagogram to one demonstrating a distal stricture with proximal esophageal dilation within a period of only several years (Fig. 20).[77] The barium esophagogram is a relatively crude early indicator of esophageal pathology in these patients, occasionally appearing completely normal or showing a mild motility disturbance but frequently failing to demonstrate significant gastroesophageal reflux. Esophageal manometry and acid reflux testing with the intraesophageal pH electrode are the most sensitive means of defining both the motility disorder and abnormal gastroesophageal reflux in these patients.[77] At esophagoscopy, ulcerative distal esophagitis, with or without significant stricture formation, is common.

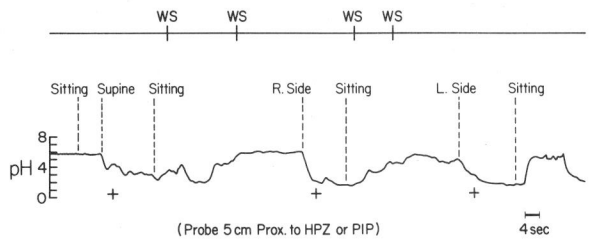

Figure 18. Strongly positive (3+) acid reflux test in the same patient with scleroderma as in Figure 17. Gastroesophageal reflux (+), indicated by drops in intraesophageal pH below 4, occurs whenever the patient assumes a supine position or lies on either side. WS, wet swallow; HPZ, high pressure zone; PIP, pressure inversion point. (From Orringer, M. B., Dabich, L., Zarafonetis, C. J., and Sloan, H.: Gastroesophageal reflux in esophageal scleroderma: Diagnosis and implications. Ann. Thorac. Surg., 22:120, 1976.)

SCLERODERMA – APERISTALSIS

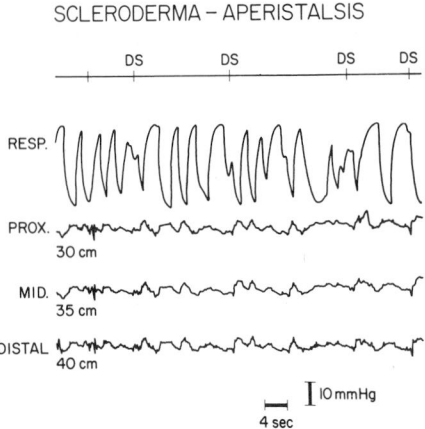

Figure 19. Motility tracing showing aperistalsis in esophageal scleroderma. There is a lack of effective peristalsis with swallowing in the distal esophagus. DS, dry swallow. (From Orringer, M. B., Dabich, L., Zarafonetis, C. J., and Sloan, H.: Gastroesophageal reflux in esophageal scleroderma: Diagnosis and implications. Ann. Thorac. Surg., 22:120, 1976).

Although death due to cardiac, renal, and pulmonary involvement is common, 5-year survival from the time of the initial diagnosis of scleroderma varies from 33 to 70 per cent.[65,101] Therefore, many of these patients require prolonged medical management. A standard medical anti-reflux regimen consisting of elevation of the head of the bed on 4- to 6-inch blocks, antacids after meals and at bedtime, and refraining from eating for several hours before retiring is often inadequate in controlling intractable reflux symptoms in these patients. The addition of H_2 inhibitors (e.g., cimetidine or ranitidine) at bedtime may be of great benefit. If severe symptoms of ulcerative esophagitis persist, however, surgical control of gastroesophageal reflux should be considered. Inferences about poor general wound healing in the patient with scleroderma are based on the well-known chronicity of fingertip ulcerations that so commonly occur in association with Raynaud's phenomenon, sclerodactyly, and poor peripheral circulation in these patients. In the author's experience, however, these considerations do not apply to the healing of thoracic and abdominal incisions in scleroderma; many of these patients can successfully undergo antireflux surgery without an increased rate of complications.[49,79] The pathophysiology of the disease has direct bearing on the operation of choice. The standard antireflux operations —Hill, Belsey, or Nissen—all rely on the restoration to the abdominal cavity of a 3- to 5-cm. segment of distal esophagus, wrapped to varying degrees by a fundoplication that further transmits positive intra-abdominal pressure. Lasting control of gastroesophageal reflux with these operations is jeopardized by the presence of esophagitis and stricture formation that both prevent a tension-free reduction of the distal esophagus below the diaphragm and require that sutures be placed into inflamed distal esophageal muscle and submucosa. In addition, in scleroderma, fibrinoid degeneration and atrophy of esophageal smooth muscle is most marked in the distal esophagus, where esophageal sutures used in the standard repairs are placed.

For these reasons, the combined Collis gastroplasty–Nissen fundoplication procedure has been advocated in patients with scleroderma with esophageal involvement and mild to moderate radiographic esophageal dilation.[79] The Collis gastroplasty is constructed over a 54 to 56 French bougie from the proximal stomach, that portion of the gastrointestinal tract that is least often involved in scleroderma (Fig. 21). This provides a healthy new "distal esophagus" around which to perform a short (2-cm.) loose fundoplication (over the same dilator used to construct the gastroplasty) without the need to suture to the inflamed abnormal esophagus (Figs. 22 and 23). Tension on the

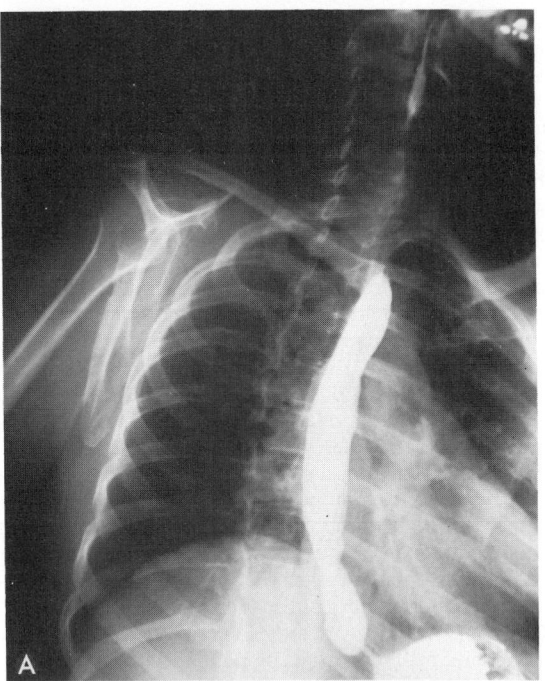

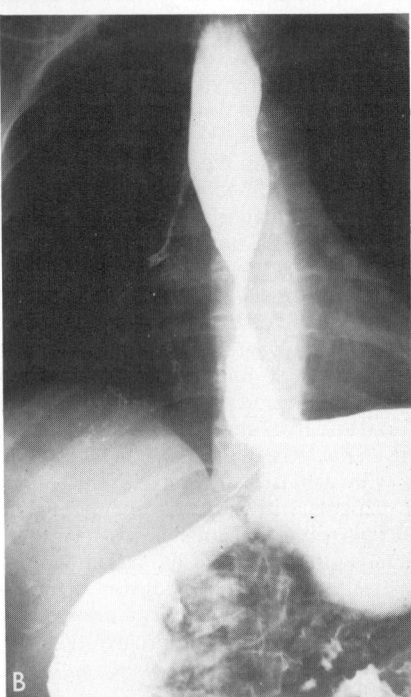

Figure 20. Progression of reflux esophagitis in scleroderma. *A*, Normal esophagogram at the time scleroderma was diagnosed (1969). *B*, Same patient (1974) with esophageal dilation proximal to a stricture and aspiration of barium in the right middle lobe secondary to the obstruction. (From Orringer, M. D., Dabich, L., Zarafonetis, C. J., and Sloan, H.: Gastroesophageal reflux in esophageal scleroderma: Diagnosis and implications. Ann. Thorac. Surg., 22:120, 1976.)

repair is eliminated because of the additional length provided by the gastroplasty tube. Unfortunately, long-term follow-up of patients with scleroderma undergoing the Collis-Nissen operation to control reflux esophagitis has yielded disappointing results, with unsatisfactory relief of reflux symptoms and/or dysphagia in 58 per cent.[96] In patients with advanced esophageal scleroderma manifested by pronounced roentgenographic dilation or a distal esophageal reflux stricture that is refractory to dilatation and medical therapy, transhiatal esophagectomy without thoracotomy and construction of a cervical esophago-

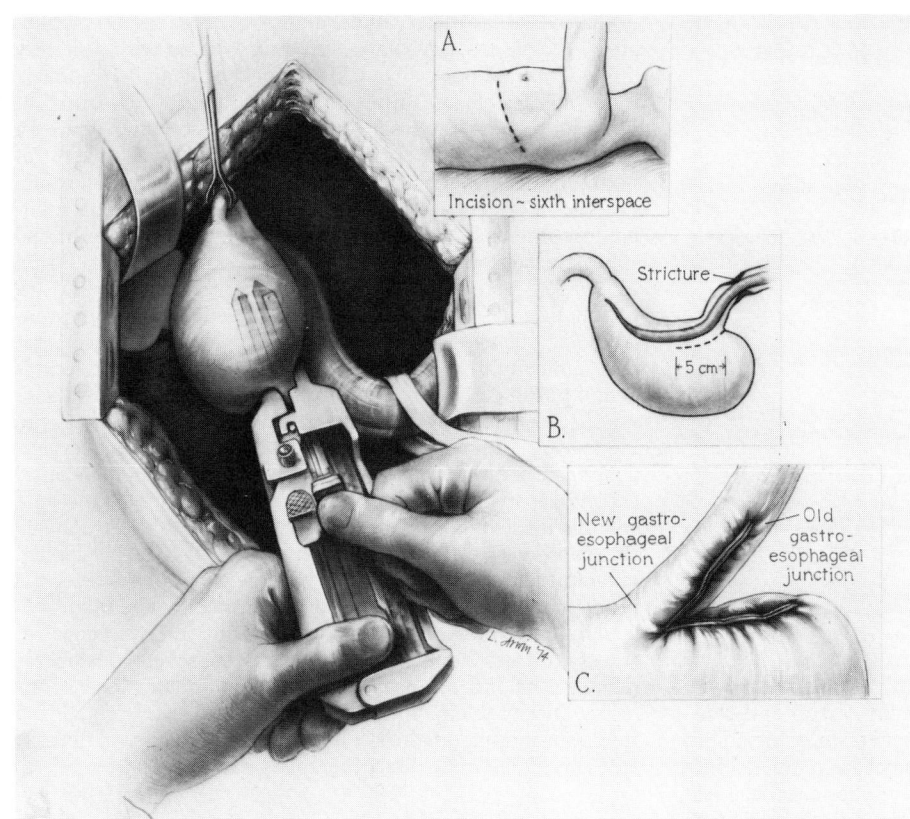

Figure 21. Construction of the Collis gastroplasty tube with the GIA surgical stapler. *A,* Mobilization of the esophagus and gastric fundus is performed through a lateral thoracotomy in the sixth or seventh left intercostal space. *B,* A 54 or 56 French Maloney dilator is passed through the esophagogastric junction and displaced against the lesser curvature of the stomach, and the stapler is applied. The knife assembly is advanced (main illustration), and the stapler is removed. The staple suture line is oversewn with a running 4-0 Prolene Lembert stitch. *C,* The result is a 5-cm. gastric tube extension into the esophagus. (From Orringer, M. B., and Sloan, H.: Collis-Belsey reconstruction of the esophagogastric junction: Indications, physiology, and technical considerations. J. Thorac. Cardiovasc. Surg., *71:*295, 1976.)

Figure 22. The combined Collis-Nissen reconstruction of the esophagogastric junction. The main drawing illustrates the elongated, narrowed gastric fundus available for fundoplication after completion of the Collis procedure. *Inset A* shows the placement of the left thoracotomy. *Insets B* and *C* show the gastric fundus being wrapped around the gastroplasty tube and adjacent stomach. The posterior crural sutures are placed but left untied until the fundoplication is reduced below the diaphragm. (From Orringer, M. B., and Sloan, H.: Combined Collis-Nissen reconstruction of the esophagogastric junction. Ann. Thorac. Surg., *25:*16, 1978.)

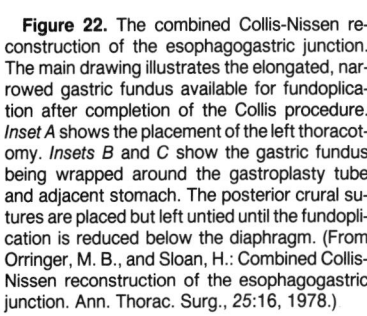

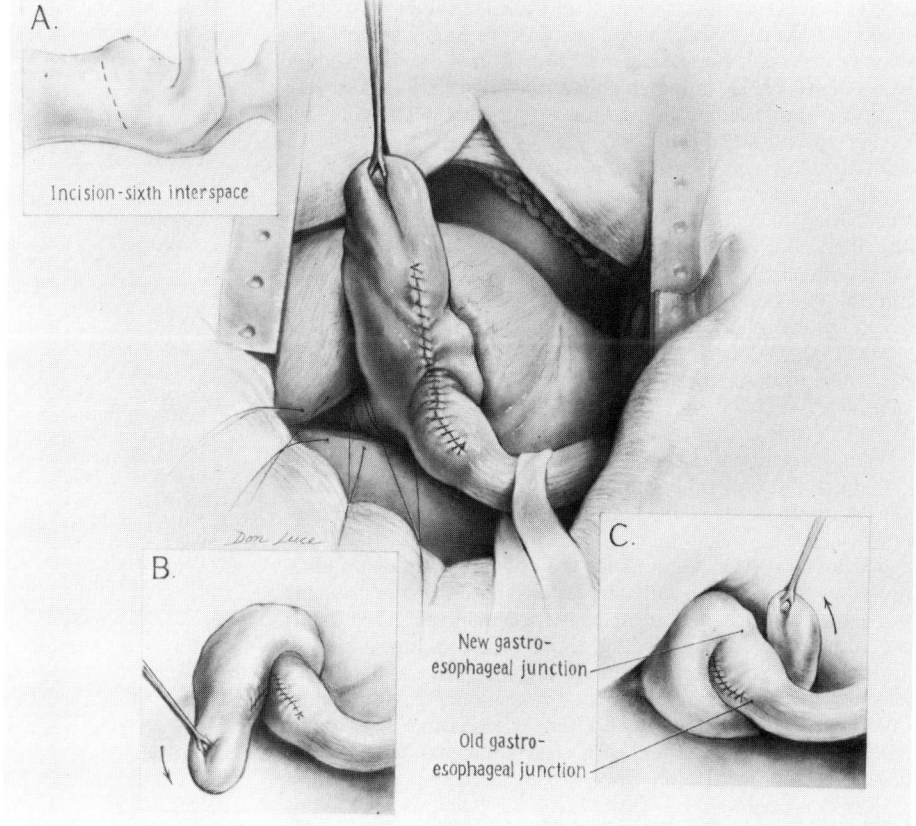

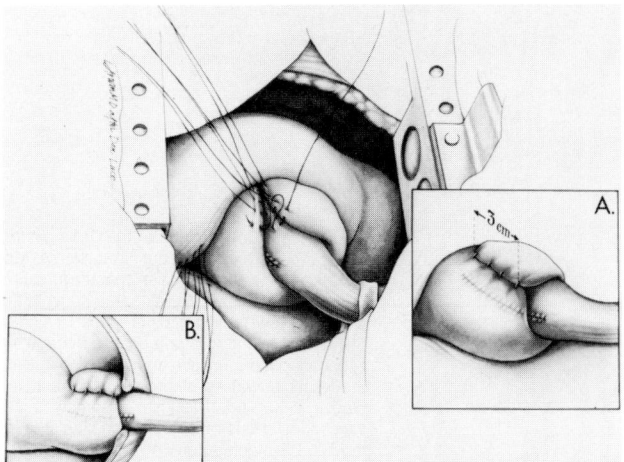

Figure 23. Completion of the combined Collis-Nissen procedure, with fundoplication limited to 3 cm. in length. *A,* Four seromuscular 2-0 silk sutures placed 1 cm. apart (main illustration) are used to construct the fundoplication around the gastroplasty tube. *B,* The fundoplication reduced beneath the diaphragm. In patients with scleroderma who have impaired esophageal motility, the fundoplication must be performed loosely to minimize postoperative obstructive symptoms. (From Stirling, M. C., Orringer, M. B.: The combined Collis-Nissen operation for esophageal reflux strictures. Ann. Thorac. Surg., *45:*148, 1988.)

gastric anastomosis eliminates the offending organ and clinically significant gastroesophageal reflux and restores the ability to swallow comfortably.[76] This approach has been utilized successfully by the author in patients with scleroderma whose systemic disease is not so advanced as to contraindicate major surgical therapy.

Miscellaneous Motor Disorders of the Lower Esophageal Sphincter

HYPERTENSIVE LOWER ESOPHAGEAL SPHINCTER. Some patients complain of low retrosternal chest pain, occasionally aggravated by swallowing, and are found to have unusually elevated, hypertensive LES pressures on manometric evaluation.[10,18,83] Manometry demonstrates elevated lower sphincter pressure, but normal relaxation with swallowing still occurs, and normal progressive peristalsis is preserved. Patients with the Zollinger-Ellison syndrome have normally relaxing hypertensive sphincters but usually no dysphagia. Because gastroesophageal reflux may induce intermittent LES hypertonicity, this condition should be excluded with pH reflux testing in these patients. Patients with a hypertensive LES may respond to intermittent bougienage but occasionally require esophagomyotomy for relief of symptoms.

HYPOTENSIVE LOWER ESOPHAGEAL SPHINCTER. It must be emphasized repeatedly that hiatal hernia and gastroesophageal reflux are not synonymous terms and that each may occur in the absence of the other. There are some patients who have an incompetent LES mechanism but no apparent associated hiatal hernia on barium esophagogram.[53] A patient with symptoms of gastroesophageal reflux but normal results on barium swallow examination merits further evaluation with esophageal function tests. Manometry may demonstrate distal HPZ pressures of less than 5 mm. Hg, but this finding *per se* does not prove the presence of abnormal gastroesophageal reflux. Using the intraesophageal pH electrode, acid reflux testing should be performed. An incompetent LES in the absence of a hiatal hernia may follow operations on the lower sphincter (esophagomyotomy, vagotomy) or may occur in scleroderma. Therapy of the hypotensive LES is that of gastroesophageal reflux and is discussed in Part VIII.

POSTVAGOTOMY DYSPHAGIA. Dysphagia following truncal vagotomy has been recognized for many years and occurs in 1 to 3.6 per cent of patients undergoing this operation,

primarily as a denervation injury of the distal esophagus.[20,24,42,44,71] Selective vagotomy is associated with a slightly higher (4 to 12 per cent) incidence of dysphagia.[2] Dysphagia following a Collis gastroplasty, which requires "clearing" of tissue along the high lesser curvature of the stomach, or after a standard hiatal hernia repair may therefore be a function of both the local denervation as well as too tight a fundoplication. Whereas in some patients with postvagotomy dysphagia, manometric studies have demonstrated a lack of distal esophageal sphincter relaxation with swallowing and abnormal distal esophageal peristalsis,[1,64] in others, acute periesophageal inflammation has been thought to be the etiology of the problem.[12,98] Patients with postvagotomy dysphagia usually experience difficulty in swallowing when oral intake of solid food is begun postoperatively. The barium esophagogram shows poor esophageal emptying and a tapered distal esophagus, suggesting spasm. At times, the patient experiences referred cervical dysphagia or hiccoughs as food passes slowly through the distal esophagus. In most patients, reassurance and maintenance of a soft diet for several days is adequate treatment. If the dysphagia still continues to be a problem, passage of 46 to 50 French tapered Maloney dilators at the bedside generally relieves the problem. No distal resistance to the passage of the dilators is usually encountered, and in most patients, the dysphagia resolves with 1 to 3 dilatations during the first several postoperative weeks.[43] If resistance to the passage of dilators is encountered, the problem is likely mechanical, e.g., too tight a fundoplication, too narrow a hiatus, or periesophageal fibrosis; and alternative more direct therapy is required.

REFERENCES

1. Anderson, H. A., Schlegel, J. F., and Olsen, A. M.: Post-vagotomy dysphagia. Gastrointest. Endosc., 12:13, 1966.
2. Andrup, E., Andersen, D., and Hostrup, H.: The Aarthus County vagotomy trial. I. An interim report on primary results and incidences of sequelae following parietal cell vagotomy and selective gastric vagotomy in 748 patients. World J. Surg., 2:85, 1978.
3. Becker, B. S., and Burakoff, R.: The effect of verapamil on the lower esophageal sphincter pressure in normal subjects and in achalasia. Am. J. Gastroenterol., 78:773, 1983.
4. Belsey, R.: In discussion of Tuttle, W. M., Crowley, R. T., and Barrett, R. J.: Achalasia of the esophagus: Further thoughts on surgical management. J. Thorac. Surg., 36:453, 1958.
5. Belsey, R.: Functional diseases of the esophagus. J. Thorac. Cardiovasc. Surg., 52:164, 1966.
6. Benjamin, S. B., Gerhardt, D. C., and Castell, D. O.: High amplitude peristaltic esophageal contraction associated with chest pain and/or dysphagia. Gastroenterology, 77:478, 1979.
7. Bernstein, L. M., and Baker, L. A.: A clinical test for esophagitis. Gastroenterology, 34:760, 1958.
8. Black, J., Vorbach, A. N., and Collis, J. L.: Results of Heller's operation for achalasia of the esophagus: The importance of hiatal hernia repair. Br. J. Surg., 63:949, 1976.
9. Bonavina, L., Khan, N. A., and DeMeester, T. R. Pharyngoesophageal dysfunctions: The role of cricopharyngeal myotomy. Arch. Surg., 120:541, 1985.
10. Bondi, J. L., Goodwin, D. H., and Garrett, J. M.: "Vigorous achalasia": Its clinical interpretation and significance. Am. J. Gastroenterol., 58:145, 1972.
11. Brand, D. L., Martin, D., and Pope, C. E., II.: Esophageal manometrics in patients with angina-like chest pain. Am. J. Dig. Dis., 22:300, 1977.
12. Bruce, J., and Small, W. P.: Dysphagia following vagotomy. J. R. Coll. Surg. Edinb., 4:170, 1959.
13. Carpenter, R. J., McDonald, T. J., and Howard, F. M. The otolaryngologic presentation of myasthenia gravis. Laryngoscope, 89:922, 1979.
14. Castrini, G., and Pappalardo, G.: Our experience in the surgical treatment of achalasia. *In* DeMeester, T. R., and Skinner, D. B. (Eds.): Esophageal Disorders: Pathophysiology and Therapy. New York, Raven Press, 1985, pp. 423–426.
15. Ceconello, I., DaRocha, J. M., Pollara, W., Zilberstein, B., and Pinotti, H. W. Long-term evaluation of gastroplasty in achalasia. *In* Siewart, J. R., and Holscher, A. H. (Eds.): Diseases of the Esophagus. Berlin, Springer-Verlag, 1988, pp. 975–979.
16. Cherry, J., Siegel, C. I., Margulies, S. I., and Donner, M.: Pharyngeal localization of symptoms of gastroesophageal reflux. Ann. Otorhinol. Laryngol., 79:912, 1970.
17. Clouse, R. E., and Lustman, P. J.: Psychiatric illness and contraction abnormalities of the esophagus. N. Engl. J. Med., 309:1337, 1983.

18. Code, C. F., Schlegel, J. F., Kelley, M. L., Jr., et al.: Hypertensive gastroesophageal sphincter. Proc. Staff Meet. Mayo Clinic, 35:391, 1960.

19. Cohn, S.: Motor disorders of the esophagus. N. Engl. J. Med., 301:184, 1979.

20. Cox, A. G., Spencer, J., and Tinker, J. Clinical results reviewed. In Williams, J. A., and Cox, A. G. (Eds.): After Vagotomy. New York, Appleton-Century-Crofts, 1969, pp. 119–130.

21. Csendes, A., Smok, G., Braghetto, I., Ramirez, C., Velasco, N., and Henriquez, A.: Gastroesophageal sphincter pressure and histological changes in distal esophagus in patients with achalasia of the esophagus. Dig. Dis. Sci., 30:941, 1985.

22. Csendes, A., Velasco, N., Braghetto, I., and Henriquez, A.: A prospective randomized study comparing forceful dilatation and esophagomyotomy in patients with achalasia of the esophagus. Gastroenterology, 80:789, 1981.

23. Davies, H. A., Kaye, M. D., Rhodes, J., Dart, A. M., and Henderson, A. N.: Diagnosis of esophageal spasm by ergometric provocation. Gut, 23:89, 1982.

24. Degradi, A. E., Stempien, S. J., Seifer, H. W., et al: Terminal esophageal (vestibular) spasm after vagotomy. Arch Surg., 85:955, 1962.

25. Dent, J.: A new technique for continuous sphincter pressure measurement. Gastroenterology, 71:263, 1976.

26. Dodds, W. J., Dent, J., Hogan, W. J., Patel, G. I. F., Toouli, J., and Arndorfer, R. C.: Paradoxical lower esophageal sphincter contraction induced by cholecystokinin-octapeptide in patients with achalasia. Gastroenterology, 80:327, 1981.

27. Duranceau, A., Beauchamp, G., Jamieson, G. G., and Barbeau, A.: Oropharyngeal dysphagia and oculopharyngeal muscular dystrophy. Surg. Clin. N. Am., 63:825, 1983.

28. Duranceau, A. C., Lafontaine, E., and Taillefer, R.: Orpharyngeal dysphagia. In Jamieson, G. G. (Ed.): Surgery of the Oesophagus. Churchill, Livingstone, Edinburgh, 1988, pp. 413–434.

29. Duranceau, A., LaFontaine, E., and Vallieres, B.: Effects of total fundoplication on function of the esophagus after myotomy for achalasia. Am. J. Surg., 143:22, 1982.

30. Duranceau, A., Rheault, M. J., and Jamieson, G. G.: Physiologic response to cricopharyngeal myotomy and diverticulum suspension. Surgery, 96:655, 1983.

31. Ellis, F. H., Jr., Code, C. F., and Olsen, A. M.: Long esophagomyotomy for diffuse spasm of the esophagus and hypertensive gastroesophageal sphincter. Surgery, 48:115, 1960.

32. Ellis, F. H., Jr., Crozier, R. E., and Gibb, S. P.: Reoperative achalasia surgery. J. Thorac. Cardiovasc. Surg., 92:859, 1986.

33. Ellis, F. H., Jr., Gibb, S. P., and Crozier, R. E.: Esophagomyotomy for achalasia of the esophagus. Ann. Surg., 192:157, 1980.

34. Ellis, F. H., Jr., and Olsen, A. M.: Achalasia of the esophagus. Philadelphia, W. B. Saunders Company, 1969.

35. Ellis, F. H., Jr., and Payne, W. S.: Motility disturbances of the esophagus and its inferior sphincter: Recent surgical advances. Adv. Surg., 1:179, 1965.

36. Ellis, F. H., Jr., Schlegel, J. F., Code, C. F., et al.: Surgical treatment of esophageal hypermotility disturbances. J.A.M.A., 188:862, 1964.

37. Ellis, F. H., Jr., Schlegel, J. F., Lynch, V. P., et al: Cricopharyngeal myotomy for pharyngoesophageal diverticulum. Ann. Surg., 170:340, 1969.

38. Flye, W. W., and Sealy, W. C.: Diffuse spasm of the esophagus. Ann. Thorac. Surg., 19:677, 1975.

39. Gelfand, M., Rozen, P., and Gilat, T.: Isosorbide dinitrate and nifedipine treatment of achalasia: A clinical, manometric, and radionuclide evaluation. Gastroenterol., 83:963, 1982.

40. Gerzic, A., Knezevic, J., Milicevic, M., Rakic, S., Dunjic, M., and Randjelovic, T.: Results of transabdominal cardiomyotomy with Dor partial fundoplication in the management of achalasia. In Siewart, J. R., and Holscher, A. H. (Eds.): Diseases of the Esophagus. Berlin, Springer-Verlag, 1988, pp. 970–974.

41. Gozzetti, G., Mattioli, S., Spangaro, M., Pilotti, V., Bassi, F., Felice, V., Conci, A., and Lerro, F.: Results of surgical therapy of achalasia with three different techniques. In Siewart, J. R., and Holscher, A. H. (Eds.): Diseases of the Esophagus. Berlin, Springer-Verlag, 1988, pp. 950–952.

42. Grimson, K. S., Baylin, G. J., Taylor, H. M., Hesser, F. H., and Rundles, R. W.: Transthoracic vagotomy. J.A.M.A., 134:925, 1947.

43. Guelrud, M., Zambrano-Rincones, V., Simon, C., et al.: Dysphagia and lower esophageal sphincter abnormalities after proximal gastric vagotomy. Am. J. Surg., 149:232, 1985.

44. Guillory, J. R., Jr., and Clagett, O. T.: Postvagotomy dysphagia. Surg. Clin. North. Am., 47:833, 1967.

45. Hallewell, J. D., and Cole, T. B.: Isolated head and neck symptoms due to hiatus hernia. Arch. Otolaryngol., 92:449, 1970.

46. Heller, E.: Extramucous cardioplasty in chronic cardiospasm with dilatation of the esophagus. [In German.] Mitt. Grenzgeb. Med. Chir., 27:141, 1913.

47. Henderson, R. D.: Disorders of the pharyngoesophageal junction. In The Esophagus: Reflux and Primary Motor Disorders. Baltimore, Williams & Wilkins, 1980, pp. 223–247.

48. Henderson, R. D., and Marryatt, G.: Cricopharyngeal myotomy as a method of treating cricopharyngeal dysphagia secondary to gastroesophageal reflux. J. Thorac. Cardiovasc. Surg., 74:271, 1977.

49. Henderson, R. D., and Pearson, F. G.: Surgical management of esophageal scleroderma. J. Thorac. Cardiovasc. Surg., 66:686, 1973.

50. Henderson, R. D., and Pearson, F. G.: Reflux control following extended myotomy in primary disordered motor activity (diffuse spasm) of the esophagus. Ann. Thorac. Surg., 22:278, 1976.

51. Henderson, R. D., Woolf, C., and Marryatt, G.: Pharyngoesophageal dysphagia and gastroesophageal reflux. Laryngoscope, 86:1531, 1976.

52. Hiebert, C. A.: Primary incompetence of the gastric cardia. Am. J. Surg., 119:365, 1970.

53. Hiebert, C. A.: Long-term follow-up of patients with achalasia treated by myotomy and partial fundoplication. In Siewart, J. R., and Holscher, A. H. (Eds.): Diseases of the Esophagus. Berlin, Springer-Verlag, 1988, pp. 962–965.

54. Hunt, P. S., Connell, A. M., and Smiley, T. B.: The cricopharyngeal sphincter in gastric reflux. Gut, 11:303, 1970.

55. Hurwitz, A. L., Duranceau, A., and Haddad, J. K.: Oropharyngeal dysphagia. In Disorders of Esophageal Motility. Vol. 16, Major Problems in Internal Medicine. Philadelphia, W. B. Saunders Company, 1979, pp. 67–84.

56. Hurwitz, A. L., Nelson, J. A., and Haddad, J. K.: Oropharyngeal dysphagia: Manometric and cine esophagographic findings. Am. J. Dig. Dis., 20:313, 1975.

57. Jara, F. M., Toledo-Pereyra, L. H., Lewis, J. W., and Magilligan, D. J.: Long-term results of esophagomyotomy for achalasia of the esophagus. Arch. Surg., 114:935, 1979.

58. Just-Viera, J. O., and Haight, C.: Achalasia and carcinoma of the esophagus. Surg. Gynecol. Obstet., 128:1081, 1969.

59. Knuff, T. E., Benjamin, S. B., and Castell, D. O.: Pharyngoesophageal (Zenker's) diverticulum: A re-appraisal. Gastroenterology, 82:734, 1982.

60. Koberle, F.: Enteromegaly and cardiomegaly in Chagas' disease. Gut, 4:399, 1963.

61. Kramer, P., and Ingelfinger, F. J.: Esophageal sensitivity to mecholyl in cardiospasm. Gastroenterology, 19:242, 1951.

62. Lobello, R., Edwards, D. A. W., and Gummer, J. W. P.: The antireflux mechanism after cardiomyotomy. Thorax, 33:569, 1978.

63. Loizou, L. A., Small, M., and Dalton, G. A.: Cricopharyngeal myotomy in motor neurone disease. J. Neurol. Neurosurg. Psychiatr., 43:42, 1980.

64. Mazur, J. M., Skinner, D. B., Jones, E. L., and Zuidema, G. D.: Effect of transabdominal vagotomy on the human gastroesophageal high pressure zone. Surgery, 73:818, 1973.

65. Medsger, T. A., Jr., Masi, A. T., Rodnan, G. P., et al.: Survival with systemic sclerosis (scleroderma): A life-table analysis of clinical and demographic factors in 309 patients. Ann. Intern. Med., 75:369, 1971.

66. Mellow, M.: Symptomatic diffuse esophageal spasm: Manometric follow-up and response to cholinergic stimulation and cholinesterase inhibition. Gastroenterology, 73:237, 1977.

67. Menguy, R.: Management of achalasia by transabdominal cardiomyotomy and fundoplication. Surg. Gynecol. Obstet., 133:482, 1971.

68. Meyer, G. W., and Castell, D. W.: Human esophageal response during chest pain induced by swallowing cold liquids. J.A.M.A., 246:2057, 1981.

69. Mills, C. P.: Dysphagia in pharyngeal paralysis treated by cricopharyngeal sphincterotomy. Lancet, 1:455, 1973.

70. Moraldi, A., Bruscoli, A., Schillaci, A., and Stipa, S.: Results of achalasia of the esophagus. In Stipa, S., Belsey, R. H. R., and Moraldi, A. (Eds.): Medical and Surgical Problems of the Esophagus. London, Academics, 1981, pp. 293–295.

71. Moses, W. R.: Critique on vagotomy. N. Engl. J. Med., 237:603, 1947.

72. Nemir, P., Jr., Fallahnejad, M., Bose, B., et al.: A study of the cause of failure of esophagocardiomyotomy for achalasia. Am. J. Surg., 121:143, 1971.

73. Okike, N., Payne, W. S., Neufeld, D. M., et al.: Esophagomyotomy versus forceful dilation for achalasia of the esophagus: Results in 899 patients. Ann. Thorac. Surg., 28:119, 1979.

74. Orlando, R. C., and Bozymski, E. M.: The effects of pentagastrin in achalasia and diffuse esophageal spasm. Gastroenterology, 77:474, 1979.

75. Orringer, M. B.: Extended cervical esophagomyotomy for cricopharyngeal dysfunction. J. Thorac. Cardiovasc. Surg., 80:669, 1980.

76. Orringer, M. B.: Transhiatal esophagectomy for benign disease. J. Thorac. Cardiovasc. Surg., 90:649, 1985.

77. Orringer, M. D., Dabich, L., Zarafonetis, C. J., et al: Gastroesophageal reflux in esophageal scleroderma: diagnosis and implications. Ann. Thorac. Surg., 22:120, 1976.

78. Orringer, M. B., and Orringer, J. S.: Esophagectomy: Definitive treatment for esophageal neuromotor dysfunction. Ann. Thorac. Surg., 24:237, 1982.

79. Orringer, M. B., Orringer, J. S., Dabich, L., et al.: Combined Collis-gastroplasty-fundoplication operations for scleroderma reflux esophagitis. Surgery, 90:624, 1981.

80. Orringer, M. B., and Stirling, M. C.: Esophageal resection for achalasia-indications and results. Ann. Thorac. Surg., 47:340, 1989.

81. Paris, F., Benages, A, Berenguer, J., et al.: Pre- and postoperative manometric studies in diffuse esophageal spasm. J. Thorac. Cardiovasc. Surg., 70:126, 1975.

82. Patterson, D. R.: Diffuse esophageal spasm in patients with undiagnosed chest pain. J. Clin. Gastroenterol., 4:415, 1982.

83. Pedersen, S. A., and Alstrup, P.: The hypertensive gastroesophageal sphincter. A manometric and clinical study. Scand J. Gastroenterol., 7:531, 1972.

84. Pinotti, H. W., Bettarello, A. Chagasic mega-oesophagus. In Jamieson, G. G., (Ed.): Surgery of the Oesophagus. Edinburgh, Churchill-Livingstone, 1988, pp. 471–481.

85. Pinotti, H. W., Nasi, A., Cecconello, I., Zilberstein, B., and Pollara, W.: Chagas' disease of the esophagus. Dis. Esoph., 1:65, 1988.

86. Possati, L., Bragaglia, S., Mattioli, M., Spangaro, M., Bortolotti, M., and Bassi,

F.: Surgical management of achalasia of the esophagus. *In* Stipa, S., Belsey, R.H.R., and Moradi, A. (Eds.): Medical and Surgical Problems of the Esophagus. London, Academic Press, 1981, pp. 279–280.

87. Postlethwait, R. W.: Surgery of the Esophagus. Norwalk, Conn., Appleton-Century-Crofts, 1979, p. 93.

88. Ibid., p. 541.

89. Qualman, S. J., Haupt, H. M., Yang, P., and Hamilton, S. R.: Esophageal Lewy bodies associated with ganglion cell loss in achalasia. Gastroenterol., 87:848, 1984.

90. Richter, J. E., Spurling, T. J., Cordova, C. M., Castell, D. O.: Effects of oral calcium blocker, diltiazem, on esophageal contraction: studies in volunteers and patients with "nutcracker esophagus". Am. J. Dig. Dis., 29:649, 1984.

91. Rossetti, M.: Esophagocardiomyotomy and fundoplication: A physiologic operation for cardiospasm and megaesophagus. [In German.] Schweiz. Med. Wochenschr., 93:925, 1963.

92. Sanderson, D. R., Ellis, F. H., Jr., Schlegel, J. F., et al.: Syndrome of vigorous achalasia: Clinical and physiologic observations. Dis. Chest, 52:508, 1967.

93. Sandler, R. S., Bopzymski, E. M., and Orlando, R. C.: Failure of clinical criteria to distinguish between primary achalasia and achalasia secondary to tumor. Dig. Dis. Sci., 27:209–213, 1982.

94. Slater, G., and Sicular, A.: Esophageal perforations after forceful dilatation in achalasia. Ann. Surg., 2:186, 1981.

95. Stipa, S., Thau, A., and Belsey, R.: Esophagomyotomy and antireflux operation for achalasia. Chir. Gastroenterol., 10:3, 1976.

96. Stirling, M. C., and Orringer, M. B.: Continued assessment of the combined Collis-Nissen operation. Ann. Thorac. Surg., 47:224, 1989.

97. Stoddard, D. J., and Johnson, A. G.: Achalasia in siblings. Br. J. Surg., 69:84, 1982.

98. Temple, T. G., and McFarland, J.: Gastro-oesophageal reflux complicating highly selective vagotomy. Br. Med. J., 2:168, 1975.

99. Torres, A. J., Suarez, A., Hernandez, F., Ruiz, A., Cuberes, R., Lapena, L., Fernandez, R., Villacorta, J., and Balibrea, J. L.: Importance of antireflux mechanism of typical achalasia of the cardia. *In* Siewart, J. R., and Holscher, A. H. (Eds.): Diseases of the Esophagus. Berlin, Springer-Verlag, 1988, pp. 936–941.

100. Traube, M., Lagarde, S., and McCallum, R. W.: Isolated hypertensive lower esophageal sphincter: Treatment of a resistant case by pneumatic dilatation. J. Clin. Gastroenterol., 6:139, 1984.

101. Tuffanelli, D. L., and Winkelman, R. K.: Systemic sclerosis: A clinical study of 727 cases. Arch. Dermatol., 84:349, 1961.

102. Vantrappen, G., and Hellemans, J.: Treatment of achalasia and related motor disorders. Gastroenterol., 79:144, 1980.

103. Vantrappen, G., and Janssens, J.: To dilate or operate? That is the question. Gut, 24:1013, 1983.

104. Vantrappen, G., Janssens, J., Hellemans, J., et al.: Achalasia diffuse esophageal spasm, and related motility disorders. Gastroenterology, 76:450, 1979.

105. Williams, J. L.: Carcinoma of the oesophagus as a complication of achalasia of the cardia. Thorax, 11:268, 1956.

106. Winans, C. S.: The pharyngoesophageal closure mechanism: a manometric study. Gastroenterology, 63:768, 1972.

107. Wychulis, A. R., Woolam, G. L., Andersen, H. A., et al.: Achalasia and carcinoma of the esophagus. J.A.M.A., 215:1638, 1971.

108. Zaaijer, J. H.: Cardiospasm in the aged. Ann. Surg., 77:615, 1923.

109. Zimmerman, F. H., and Rosensweig, N. S.: Achalasia in a father and son. Am. J. Gastroenterol., 79:506, 1984.

IV

DIVERTICULA AND MISCELLANEOUS CONDITIONS OF THE ESOPHAGUS

Mark B. Orringer, M.D.

DIVERTICULA

Esophageal diverticula are epithelial-lined mucosal pouches that protrude from the esophageal lumen. Almost all are acquired and occur predominantly in adults. Esophageal diverticula have been classified both according to location and to the extent of the esophageal wall thickness that accompanies them. They commonly occur at three separate sites and are designated as *pharyngoesophageal* when they occur at the junction of the pharynx and esophagus, *parabronchial* (midesophageal) when they are located near the tracheal bifurcation, and *epiphrenic* (supradiaphragmatic) when they arise from the distal 10 cm. of esophagus. A "true" diverticulum contains all layers of the normal esophageal wall, including mucosa, submucosa, and muscle; whereas a "false" diverticulum consists primarily of only mucosa and submucosa.

Esophageal diverticula are further categorized as being of either the pulsion or traction type, according to their presumed mechanism of formation. Pulsion diverticula arise because elevated intraluminal pressure forces the mucosa and submucosa to herniate through the esophageal musculature; therefore, they are "false" diverticula. Traction diverticula are the result of external inflammatory reaction in adjacent mediastinal lymph nodes that adhere to the esophagus and attract the entire wall toward them as they heal and contract; they are "true" diverticula. Pharyngoesophageal and epiphrenic diverticula are pulsion diverticula that typically arise as a result of abnormal esophageal motility. Parabronchial diverticula are generally of the traction type and include all layers of the esophageal wall.

PHARYNGOESOPHAGEAL DIVERTICULA. A pharyngoesophageal diverticulum was first described as an autopsy finding by Ludlow in 1764.[47] In 1878, Zenker and von Ziemssen reviewed 22 cases from the literature and added 5 of their own.[81] Zenker's name subsequently became associated with this entity. The pharyngoesophageal diverticulum is the most common esophageal diverticulum, generally occurring in patients between 30 and 50 years of age and therefore believed to be acquired. The diverticulum characteristically arises within the inferior pharyngeal constrictor, between the oblique fibers of the thyropharyngeus muscle and the more horizontal fibers of the cricopharyngeus muscle, the upper esophageal sphincter (UES) (Fig. 1). The transition in the direction of these muscle fibers (Killian's triangle) is believed to represent a point of potential weakness in the posterior pharynx and is the site of formation of the pharyngoesophageal diverticulum. Due to the unique characteristics of the UES and the speed with which neuromotor events in this area occur during deglutition, precise documentation of the exact abnormality in pharyngoesophageal motor function in patients with Zenker's diverticula is extremely difficult to obtain. Ellis and associates first reported manometric abnormalities of the UES in these patients, namely, incoordination in the swallowing mechanism, with pharyngeal contraction occurring after cricopharyngeal closure, and resting pressures *lower* than in controls.[21] As indicated previously (see Chapter 27, Part III), the unique anatomic configuration of the UES—its asymmetry and change in position with laryngeal excursions—makes its manometric assessment by means of standard esophageal recording equipment difficult. A modification of the Dent pressure sensor sleeve may prove most appropriate for recordings in this area.[17] However, given the limitations of existing standard recording equipment, it is not surprising that the manometric abnormalities of the UES in patients with pharyngoesophageal diverticula originally described by Ellis and later confirmed[20] have not been found consistently

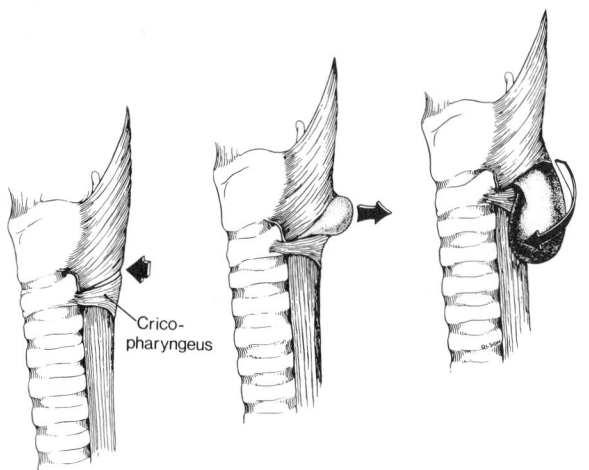

Figure 1. Formation of pharyngoesophageal (Zenker's) diverticulum. *Left,* Herniation of the pharyngeal mucosa and submucosa occurs at the point of transition (arrow) between the oblique fibers of the thyropharyngeus muscle and the more horizontal fibers of the cricopharyngeus muscle. *Center* and *right,* As the diverticulum enlarges, it dissects toward the left side and downward into the superior mediastinum in the prevertebral space.

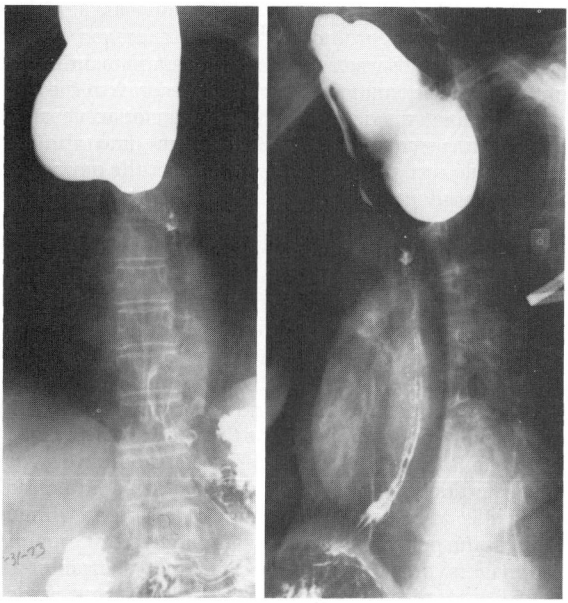

Figure 2. Posteroanterior *(left)* and oblique *(right)* views from barium esophagogram demonstrating a huge 15-cm. pharyngoesophageal diverticulum in an elderly woman who presented with cervical dysphagia, a 40-lb. weight loss, and a right superior mediastinal paratracheal "mass" (the diverticulum) on a standard chest roentgenogram and who was thought to have esophageal carcinoma. She was treated with diverticulectomy and cervical esophagomyotomy.

by other investigators. Hunt and associates reported that mean resting UES pressure was more than double that in their controls.[31] Pedersen and associates found no abnormality in either sphincter pressure or coordination.[59] Lichter confirmed Ellis' findings of premature relaxation of the UES in patients with Zenker's diverticula.[46] Two recent studies have reported lower than normal UES pressures in these patients, as originally described by Ellis, but they could not substantiate the finding of incoordination in swallowing.[15,39] Regardless of the limitations of existing recording equipment in defining the underlying motor abnormality in these patients, however, it is clear that a pulsion diverticulum would not occur unless there were *some* abnormality distal to it generating unusually elevated pharyngeal pressures. Thus the swallowed bolus exerts pressure within the pharynx, and mucosa and submucosa herniate through the anatomically weak area above the cricopharyngeus muscle. In time, the diverticulum enlarges, drapes over the cricopharyngeus, and dissects inferiorly in the prevertebral space behind the esophagus, occasionally into the superior mediastinum.

Pharyngoesophageal diverticula are usually associated with complaints of cervical dysphagia, effortless regurgitation of undigested particles of food or pills sometimes consumed hours earlier, a gurgling sensation in the neck on swallowing, choking, and recurrent aspiration. Weight loss and dysphagia suggesting an esophageal malignancy may occur when the pouch is enlarged greatly and the esophageal obstruction becomes severe (Fig. 2). The results of the barium esophagogram establish the diagnosis. Surgical therapy in symptomatic patients is indicated in most cases, regardless of the size of the pouch and, one hopes, before complications occur. A patient with a 5-mm. Zenker's diverticulum may be equally or even more symptomatic than a patient with a 3-cm. pouch. It is the degree of cricopharyngeal muscle dysfunction, not the absolute size of the diverticulum, that determines the relative severity of cervical dysphagia experienced by these patients. Therefore, the proper surgical treatment of the pharyngoesophageal diverticulum, like that of *every* pulsion diverticulum, must be directed toward the underlying motor abnormality responsible for formation of the pouch and not at the pouch *per se*.

The history of the surgical management of the pharyngoesophageal diverticulum includes a number of innovative operations. The earliest reports of resection of pharyngoesophageal diverticula were by Wheeler (1886), von Bergmann (1892), Kocher (1892), and Girard (1896).[35,61] The morbidity and mortality of these one-stage resections, however, were prohibitive, wound infection and sepsis from esophageal suture-line disruption being the primary complications. As a result, the concept of a two-stage procedure emerged. At the first operation, the pouch was isolated and suspended by suturing it to the skin so that it could empty through its now-dependent mouth and surrounding adhesions could develop, which would prevent later spreading cellulitis and mediastinitis. After 2 to 3 weeks, the pouch was resected at the second operation. This approach, first reported by Goldman (1909),[35] gained widespread popularity and was championed by Lahey, who subsequently reported a series of 365 patients with only 2 deaths and 12 recurrences.[41]

At the time the two-stage approach was being developed, Jackson attacked the problem of infection following one-stage diverticulum resection by first aspirating the contents of the pouch through an esophagoscope.[34] Others adopted this approach, and shortly after Lahey's 1954 report of his successful two-stage approach, Sweet (1956) reported 77 patients treated with one-stage resection with no deaths, one fistula, and one recurrence.[73] This approach was adopted at the Mayo Clinic, where 888 patients were treated from 1944 to 1978 with a 1.2 per cent mortality and a 3.6 per cent recurrence.[58] More recently, the Mayo Clinic group has added a cricopharyngeal myotomy to their operation.

Alternative surgical approaches to pharyngoesophageal diverticula have not gained as widespread use as the currently advocated cervical esophagomyotomy and resection. Diverticulopexy—simply mobilizing the pouch, inverting it, and suspending it from adjacent tissues so that the mouth is dependent—has a high recurrence rate[41] unless combined with a cricopharyngeal myotomy.[5,18] Invagination of the diverticulum has been utilized alone or combined with a cervical esophagomyotomy.[53] Endoscopic diversion of the common wall between the diverticulum and esophagus (internal pharyngo-oesophagotomy, the Dohlman procedure) has been utilized with success by a relatively small number of surgeons,[14,75] concern about the potential for mediastinitis from this procedure discouraging its widespread use. In one of the largest such series, vanOverbeck and Hoeksema (1982) reported 211 patients with good results in 91.5 per cent and a 5 per cent incidence of esophageal perforation.[75]

Regardless of the surgical approach, operations directed primarily to the diverticulum without consideration of the underlying incoordinated cricopharyngeal sphincter leave the potential for recurrence of the diverticulum and suture-line disruption, because the factor responsible for the development of the increased pharyngeal pressure and formation of the pouch has not been eliminated. Elevated pharyngeal pressure proximal to the cricopharyngeus cannot occur if this muscle is divided, and this is the basis for the most popular current surgical approach to the incoordinated UES.[54] The operation is performed through an oblique left cervical incision that parallels the anterior border of the sternocleidomastoid muscle or a transverse cervical incision centered over the cricoid cartilage. The sternocleidomastoid muscle and carotid sheath and its contents are retracted laterally, and the thyroid and the trachea are retracted medially. The diverticulum is consistently located beneath the inferior thyroid artery, an important anatomic landmark for this operation. With a 40 French bougie within the esophagus, the pouch is dissected to its base, and an extramucosal esophagomyotomy is performed in either vertical direction from the base of the pouch for several centimeters to ensure that all cricopharyngeal muscle fibers are divided (Fig. 3). Most pouches between 1 and 2 cm. in diameter simply "disappear" and blend into the bulging mucosa after the cervical esophagomyotomy. Larger pouches are excised with an automatic stapler. After completion of the myotomy and resection of the diverticulum, a nasogastric tube is inserted by the anesthetist and is gently guided into the upper esophagus. Air is insufflated, and the area of the esophagomyotomy is tested under saline for ensuring that no mucosal tear has occurred. Cricopharyngeal myotomy, with or without diverticulectomy, is an extremely effective means of treating cricopharyngeal muscle dysfunction in these patients and has a very low morbidity. Despite the lack of manometric evidence that cricopharyngeal motor dysfunction is an inevitable occurrence in the patient with a Zenker's diverticulum, cricopharyngeal myotomy adds little morbidity to the operation and appears justified empirically in all patients undergoing surgical therapy for this problem.

MIDESOPHAGEAL (TRACTION) DIVERTICULA. Traction diverticula of the midesophagus are invariably associated with mediastinal granulomatous disease (e.g., tuberculosis, histoplasmosis).[48] They are characteristically quite small, with a blunt tapered tip that points upward to the adjacent subcarinal and parabronchial lymph nodes to which they are adherent, quite different from the large, round, relatively narrow-mouthed pulsion diverticula (Fig. 4). These diverticula are usu-

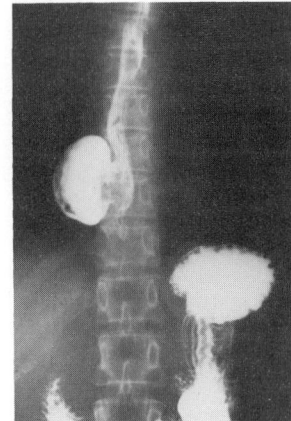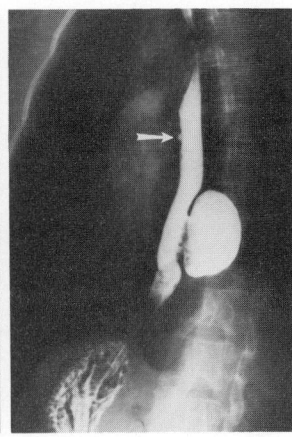

Figure 4. Posteroanterior (left) and oblique (right) views in barium esophagograms showing both a typical pulsion diverticulum of the junction of the mid and distal esophagus and a small traction diverticulum (arrow) of the mid esophagus.

ally seen as incidental findings on a barium esophagogram. They rarely cause symptoms and require no treatment. Occasionally, however, inflammatory necrosis of the granulomatous process causes a fistulous communication between the esophagus and the respiratory tract that requires division of the fistula and interposition of adjacent normal tissues.[3,8] Midesophageal traction diverticula are to be differentiated from pulsion diverticula occurring in this location (Fig. 4). The latter occur in association with neuromotor esophageal dysfunction,[7,36,64] as do the most common pulsion diverticula of the body of the esophagus, epiphrenic diverticula.

EPIPHRENIC DIVERTICULA. Epiphrenic or supradiaphragmatic diverticula generally occur within the distal 10 cm. of the thoracic esophagus and are pulsion diverticula that arise either because of esophageal motor dysfunction or a mechanical distal obstruction.[1,9,12,27,32] As with pharyngoesophageal diverticula, abnormally elevated intraluminal pressure is responsible for a "blowout" of mucosa and submucosa through the muscle of the esophagus. Many patients are asymptomatic when their epiphrenic diverticulum is diagnosed on barium esophagogram. In other patients, symptoms are difficult to differentiate from the frequently associated esophageal lesions—hiatal hernia, diffuse esophageal spasm, achalasia, reflux esophagitis, and carcinoma. Dysphagia and regurgitation are common symptoms, as is retrosternal pain from associated diffuse esophageal spasm. Although the diagnosis is readily apparent on barium esophagogram, esophageal function studies should be performed if possible to define the associated motor disturbance or the presence of an incompetent LES mechanism. Mildly symptomatic patients with pouches smaller than 3 cm. often require no treatment, whereas those with progressively severe dysphagia and chest pain or an anatomically dependent or enlarging pouch are surgical candidates. As with pharyngoesophageal diverticula, unless there is an associated distal esophageal stricture or tumor, it must be inferred that abnormally elevated intraesophageal pressure responsible for the pouch is caused by a motor disturbance, which can frequently be documented manometrically. Therefore, the operation, performed through a left thoracotomy, involves not only resection of the diverticulum but also a long extramucosal thoracic esophagomyotomy from beneath the aortic arch to the esophagogastric junction (Fig. 5). An associated hiatal hernia or incompetent LES should also be repaired during the same operation. As long as an esophagomyotomy is performed, suture-line disruption and recurrence following resection of the diverticulum are rare (Fig. 6). As is the case when an esophagomyotomy for achalasia is being performed, the question of the distal extent of the muscle incision and the need for a concomitant antireflux operation arises. Ellis has maintained that the lower esophageal sphincter should not

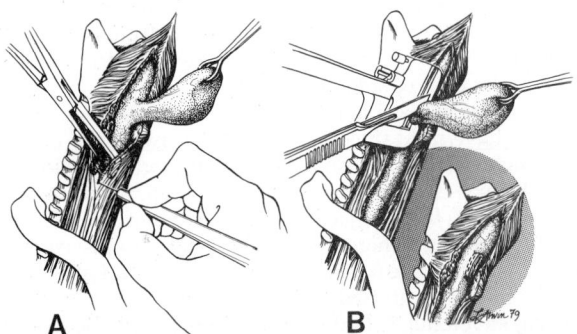

Figure 3. Cervical esophagomyotomy and concomitant resection of a pharyngoesophageal diverticulum. A, after mobilization of the diverticulum, the esophagomyotomy is performed in either direction from the base of the pouch for the same distance as described in Figure 4. B, After the esophagomyotomy is completed, the base of the diverticulum is crossed with a TA 30 stapler and amputated. (From Orringer, M. B.: Extended cervical esophagomyotomy for cricopharyngeal dysfunction. J. Thorac. Cardiovasc. Surg., 80:669, 1980.)

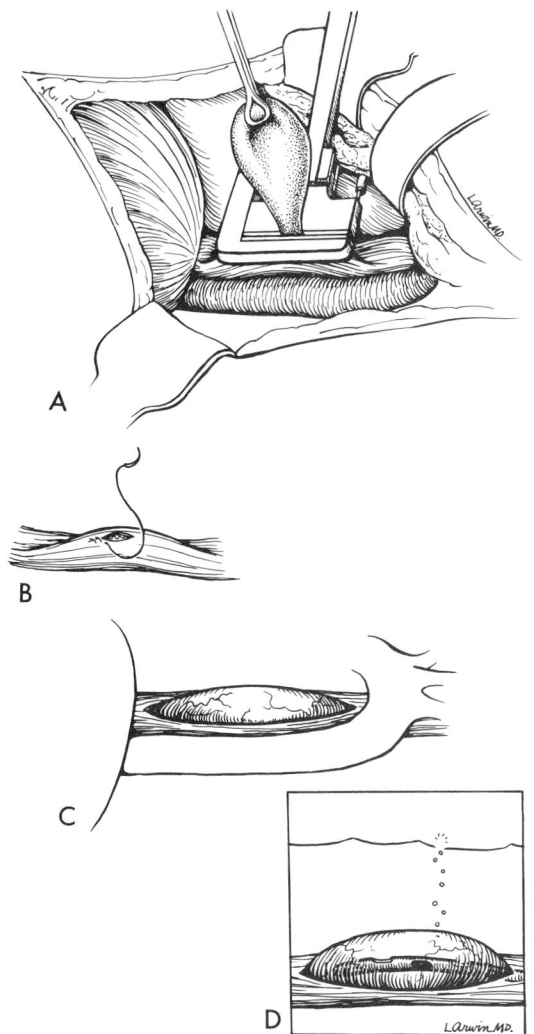

Figure 5. Technique of resection of epiphrenic diverticulum and concomitant thoracic esophagomyotomy. *A*, After the diverticulum is mobilized to its base, it is amputated with a TA 30 surgical stapler. *B*, The staple suture-line is oversewn by approximating adjacent muscle. *C*, A long esophagomyotomy from the esophagogastric junction to the aortic arch is performed on the opposite wall of the esophagus. *D*, Air is insufflated through an intraesophageal nasogastric tube with the esophagus immersed in saline so that any disruption of the mucosa can be identified and repaired. (From Orringer, M. B.: Complications of esophageal surgery and trauma. *In* Greenfield, L. J. (Ed.): Complications of Surgery and Trauma, 2nd ed. Philadelphia, J. B. Lippincott Company, 1990, pp. 302–325.)

be disturbed if preoperative esophageal function tests demonstrate that it is normal.[19] However, Belsey has emphasized the need to eliminate completely the distal esophageal obstruction and routinely divides the LES, extending the muscle incision 1.5 cm. onto the stomach.[5] When an antireflux procedure is being performed on a myotomized esophagus, a partial fundoplication of the Belsey type, rather than a 360-degree Nissen fundoplication, is less likely to produce functional obstruction on long-term follow-up.[16]

MISCELLANEOUS CONDITIONS OF THE ESOPHAGUS

SIDEROPENIC DYSPHAGIA (PLUMMER-VINSON OR PATTERSON-KELLY SYNDROME). Sideropenic dysphagia refers to the development of cervical dysphagia in patients with iron deficiency anemia. These patients are usually edentulous women over the age of 40 years. They have atrophic oral mucosa with glossitis and brittle spoon-shaped fingernails (koilonychia). The cause of the dysphagia is usually, but not always, a cervical esophageal web (Fig. 7). Treatment consists of esoph-

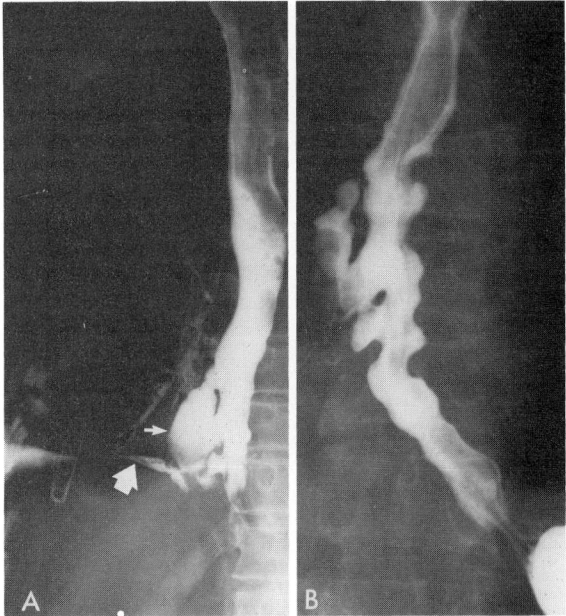

Figure 6. *A*, Esophagogram showing an esophagopleural cutaneous fistula (large arrow) and a recurrent epiphrenic diverticulum (small arrow) in a patient who had undergone prior resection of the diverticulum without an esophagomyotomy. *B*, The patient's underlying esophageal neuromotor problem is evident in this view from the same esophagogram, showing a typical "corkscrew" esophagus. The relative distal esophageal obstruction secondary to intermittent spasm had not been relieved when the diverticulum was resected; disruption of the suture-line with fistula formation and recurrence of the diverticulum followed. (From Orringer, M. B.: Complications of esophageal surgery and trauma. *In* Greenfield, L. J. (Ed.): Complications of Surgery and Trauma, 2nd ed. Philadelphia, J. B. Lippincott Company, 1990, pp. 302–325.)

ageal dilatation and correction of the nutritional deficiency. This syndrome has a high incidence in Scandinavia and Great Britain and is regarded as a premalignant lesion, because in approximately 10 per cent of patients so affected squamous cell carcinoma of the hypopharynx, oral cavity, or esophagus develops.[80] Kelly[37] and Patterson[57] described this condition in England in 1919. In the United States, the syndrome was reported by Plummer (1914) and Vinson (1922).[76]

DISTAL ESOPHAGEAL WEB (SCHATZKI'S RING). Distal esophageal webs are commonly observed radiographically at the esophagogastric junction in patients with a sliding hiatal hernia. They appear as annular strictures that project into the lumen at a right angle to the long axis of the lower esophagus (Fig. 8). Originally described by Templeton (1944),[74] Schatzki and Gary (1953)[67] and Ingelfinger and Kramer (1953)[33] were the first to attribute symptoms to the lesion. The incidence of Schatzki's ring is impossible to determine because most patients with this abnormality are asymptomatic. Intermittent dysphagia may occur when the ring size is 20 mm. or less, but the critical ring diameter at which dysphagia almost invariably occurs is 13 mm. or less. The etiology of the Schatzki ring has not been established. When it was in vogue to resect those rings that were associated with dysphagia, the web was typically found 1 to 2 cm. above the junction of the tubular esophagus and the saccular stomach and involved only the mucosa and submucosa, not the esophageal muscle. Microscopically, squamous epithelium covered the upper surface of the ring, and columnar epithelium covered the lower surface. There was only a slight amount of associated increased submucosal fibrosis.[60] Schatzki's ring, therefore, occurs precisely at the squamocolumnar epithelial junction and is observed radiographically on a barium esophagogram only because the squamocolumnar junction is above the diaphragm (i.e., because there is a hiatal hernia). The presence of a ring indicates that there is a hiatal hernia, but it does *not* indicate that there is either gastroesophageal

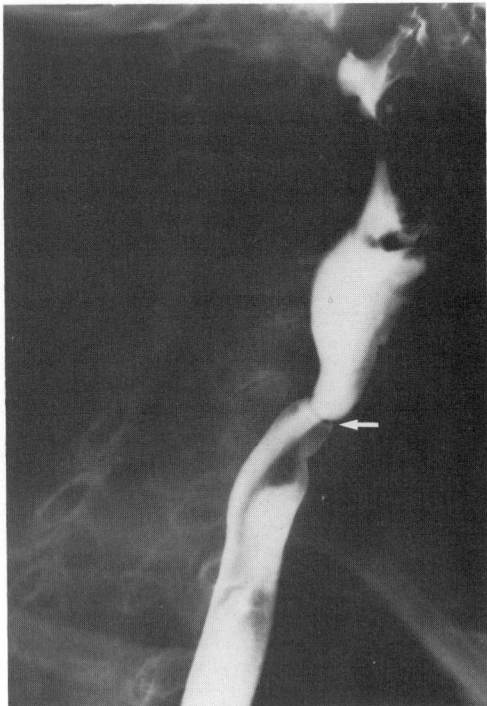

Figure 7. Esophagogram showing a cervical web (arrow), which is differentiated roentgenographically from a prominent cricopharyngeal sphincter by its location on the anterior esophageal wall.

reflux or esophagitis. Differentiation of this mucosal prominence at the esophagogastric junction from a localized peptic stricture owing to gastroesophageal reflux may be difficult. Many patients with symptomatic rings have no reflux symptoms and have an excellent response to intermittent esophageal bougienage. Others who have dysphagia as well as reflux symptoms may do well with periodic dilatations and an antireflux medical regimen. In those with refractory dysphagia or very symptomatic gastroesophageal reflux that fails to respond adequately to medical therapy, intraoperative dilatation in association with an antireflux procedure effectively relieves symptoms so long as reflux control is maintained by the operation. Resection of the ring alone, without repair of the associated hiatal hernia, should not be performed. A recent report by Ottinger and Wilkins (1980) suggests that there may be an inordi-

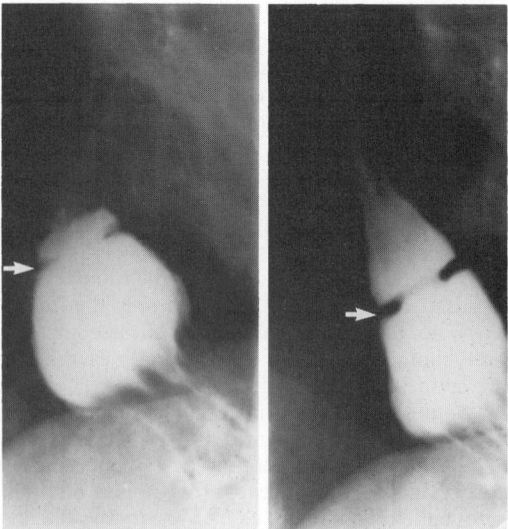

Figure 8. Esophagogram showing a distal esophageal (Schatzki) ring (arrows), which is always seen at the esophagogastric junction above a sliding hiatal hernia.

nately high incidence of recurrent hiatal hernia in patients undergoing dilatation of the ring and an antireflux procedure.[56]

MALLORY-WEISS SYNDROME (EMETOGENIC MUCOSAL LACERATION). During the act of extremely forceful emesis against the closed glottis, the rapid increase in intra-abdominal pressure is transmitted to the esophagus, where either a mucosal laceration at the esophagogastric junction (Mallory-Weiss syndrome) or a transmural esophageal tear (Boerhaave's syndrome) can occur. A history of emesis followed by either melena or hematemesis suggests the possibility of a Mallory-Weiss mucosal tear at the cardia.[49] However, the diagnosis may not be considered because of the clinical settings in which this condition may occur: alcoholism, pregnancy, peptic ulcer disease, cirrhosis, bowel obstruction, drug withdrawal, or food poisoning.[2,10,52,72] A barium contrast study is rarely diagnostic, although it may exclude other potential causes of bleeding. Selective celiac arteriography may at times demonstrate the site of bleeding if the volume of blood loss is brisk enough at the time of the study. Esophagoscopy may establish the diagnosis, but in this study, too, the site of bleeding is often not definitely seen. In more than 90 per cent of cases the bleeding ceases in response to nasogastric decompression, iced saline gastric lavage, and blood replacement.[38,66,77] If massive hemorrhage continues, however, the upper abdomen should be explored and a long proximal gastrotomy performed for inspection of the cardia. After evacuation of clots from the stomach, the mucosal tear is identified and oversewn.[4,23,30] The results of surgical treatment of Mallory-Weiss syndrome are excellent, and recurrence of bleeding is quite rare.

MONILIAL ESOPHAGITIS. *Candida albicans* is a fungus that is normally a commensal inhabitant of the human mouth, oropharynx, and gastrointestinal tract. The fungus may become pathogenic in severely debilitated or immunosuppressed patients. The incidence of monilial esophagitis is increasing because of the growing number of organ transplants, the use of chemotherapeutics in oncology and potent broad-spectrum antibiotics.[22,45,55,68,70] Typically, in acute monilial esophagitis with oropharyngeal involvement, the patient complains of painful swallowing. As the infection involves the thoracic esophagus, primary and secondary peristaltic waves are decreased in frequency and amplitude, and spasm may occur. With progression of the disease and before frank mucosal ulceration, as inflammation and edema of the submucosa occur, the "cobblestone" pattern of luminal nodularity is observed roentgenographically.[25] With advanced acute monilial esophagitis, ulceration of the mucosa and an irregular, shaggy-appearing, narrowed esophageal lumen due to mucosal and submucosal edema and pseudomembrane formation are apparent on barium swallow examination. At endoscopy the esophageal mucosa initially appears erythematous and nonulcerated, with an overlying whitish, cheesy exudate or pseudomembrane. As the disease progresses, the mucosa becomes more granular and friable as the inflammatory reaction extends into the wall of the esophagus, with fungal invasion of the mucosal, submucosal, and muscle layers. If such extensive panmural esophagitis can be controlled by antifungal therapy and if the patient survives the underlying disease, healing of the inflamed esophagus may cause a chronic stricture.[55,70] Strictures following monilial esophagitis tend to occur in the upper half of the thoracic esophagus, where the esophageal submucosal glands predominate. Inflammation of these glands from infection, stasis, or distal obstruction can produce dilation and outpouching, which have been termed "intramural esophageal pseudodiverticulosis," a pattern seen in many patients with monilial strictures[51,78] (Fig. 9).

Acute monilial esophagitis should be detected promptly in debilitated, postoperative, and immunosuppressed patients. Treatment with oral nystatin (Mycostatin), 500,000 to 1,000,000 units of the suspension every 6 hours, generally arrests the infection within 7 to 10 days. This therapy should be

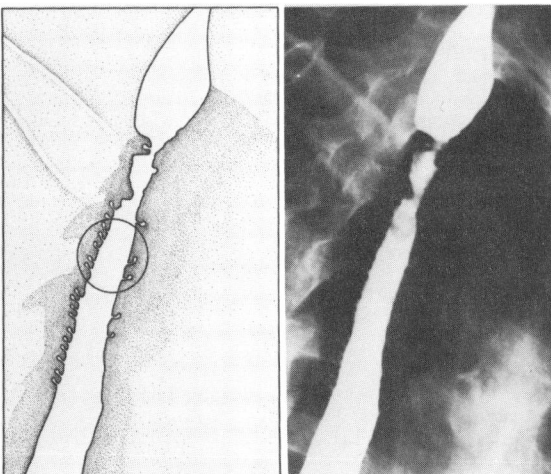

Figure 9. Esophagogram and line interpretation of irregular upper thoracic esophageal stricture from monilial esophagitis. The associated intramural pseudo-diverticulosis represents dilated submucosal esophageal glands. (From Orringer, M. B., and Sloan, H.: Monilial esophagitis: An increasingly frequent cause of esophageal stenosis? Ann. Thorac. Surg., 26:364, 1978.)

continued for 1 to 3 weeks. If the infection persists, intravenous amphotericin B, 1 to 10 mg. per day, for 7 to 10 days, or oral flucytosine, 50 to 150 mg. per kg. per day in divided doses for 4 to 6 weeks, is indicated.[26,40,68] Intravenous miconazole, 600 to 2000 mg. per day in divided doses, has also been used in treating esophageal candidiasis.[65] Because postinflammatory mural fibrosis can occur, patients recovering from severe acute monilial esophagitis should have several follow-up barium swallow examinations during the first year to ensure the earliest possible recognition of a developing stricture and institution of bougienage therapy.

RARE ESOPHAGEAL PATHOLOGY. Isolated cases of infectious esophagitis due to syphilis, tuberculosis, and herpes have been described. Crohn's disease of the esophagus has been reported as another rare cause of esophagitis. Various dermatologic conditions such as pemphigus vulgaris and epidermolysis bullosa may also involve the esophageal epithelium and produce dysphagia from esophagitis and stricture formation.[6,24,29,44,63,69,71] In certain situations, unusual causes of dysphagia may have to be considered in the differential diagnosis of patients with swallowing complaints. Dysphagia has been reported in patients with marked cardiac enlargement, hepatomegaly impinging the esophagus against the diaphragmatic hiatus, and tortuosity of the thoracic aorta.[13,28,42,43] Cervical dysphagia may also be caused by esophageal compression by thyroid or parathyroid tissue or by cervical vertebral body os-

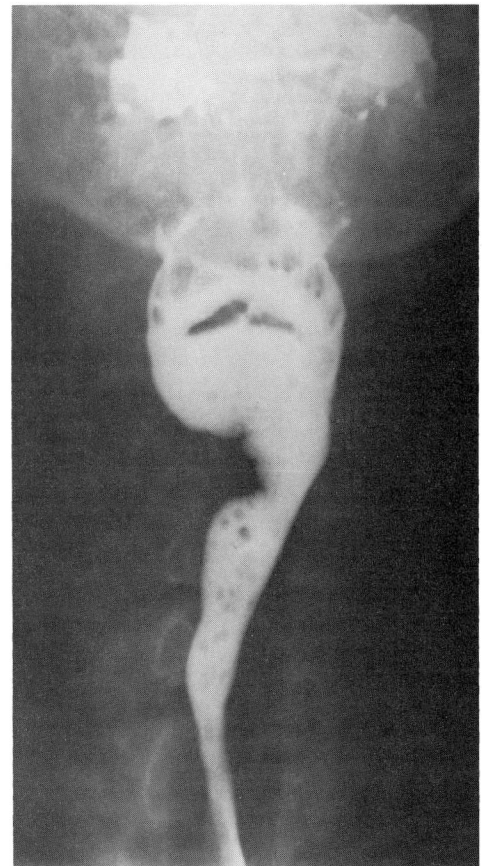

Figure 11. Cervical esophagogram showing an extrinsic right lateral mass. This patient with dysphagia had an aberrant location of the right lobe of the thyroid gland, which was found at operation to be posterolateral to the esophagus. A right thyroid lobectomy was performed and relieved the patient's dysphagia.

teophytic spurs (Figs. 10 and 11). Such exostoses typically involve the fifth, sixth, and seventh cervical vertebral interspaces and displace the esophagus from behind.[11,50,62] Esophagoscopy is obviously more dangerous in the presence of exostoses and should be performed with a pediatric flexible fiberoptic esophagoscope to exclude carcinoma in these patients with dysphagia. The flexible esophagoscope, however, does not eliminate the risk of esophageal perforation.[79] Although removal of osteophytes may relieve the dysphagia, associated cricopharyngeal motor dysfunction, which is more easily treated, should be excluded, and simple gentle dilation with a Maloney bougie may be therapeutic.

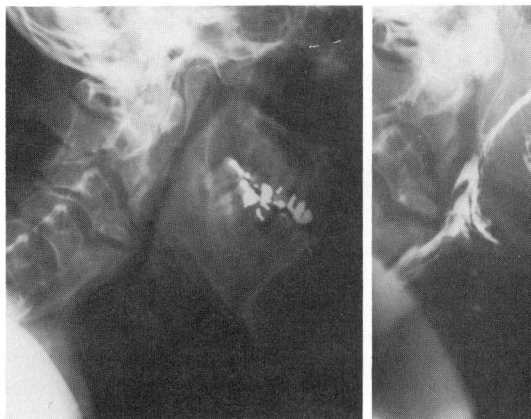

Figure 10. Cervical osteophytes displacing the esophagus anteriorly. *Left,* Soft tissue film of neck. *Right,* Displacement of the barium-filled esophagus.

REFERENCES

1. Allen, T. H., and Clagett, O. T.: Changing concepts in the surgical treatment of pulsion diverticula of the lower esophagus. J. Thorac. Cardiovasc. Surg., 50:455, 1965.
2. Atkinson, M., Bottrill, M. B., Edwards, A. T., Mitchell, W. M., Peet, B. G., and Williams, R. E.: Mucosal tears at the oesophagogastric junction (The Mallory-Weiss syndrome). Gut, 2:1, 1961.
3. Balthazar, E. M.: Esophagobronchial fistula secondary to ruptured traction diverticulum. Gastrointest. Radiol., 2:119, 1977.
4. Baue, A. E.: Bleeding from lacerations of the cardia: The Mallory-Weiss syndrome. J.A.M.A., 184:325, 1963.
5. Belsey, R.: Functional disease of the esophagus. J. Thorac. Cardiovasc. Surg., 52:164, 1966.
6. Benedict, E. B., and Lever, W. F.: Stenosis of the esophagus in benign mucous membrane pemphigus. Ann. Otol. Rhinol. Laryngol., 61:1120, 1952.
7. Borrie, J., and Wilson, R. L. K.: Oesophageal diverticula: principles of management and appraisal of classification. Thorax, 35:759, 1980.
8. Brian, J. E., and Stair, J. M.: Non colonic diverticular disease. Surg. Gynec. Obstet., 161:189, 1985.
9. Bruggeman, L. L., and Seman, W. B.: Epiphrenic diverticula. An analysis of 80 cases. Am. J. Roentgenol., 119:266, 1973.

10. Bubrick, M. P., Lundeen, J. W., Onstad, G. R., and Hitchcock, C. R.: Mallory-Weiss syndrome: analysis of 59 cases. Surgery, 88:400, 1980.

11. Carlson, M. J., Stauffer, R. N., Paynes, W. S.: Ankylosing vertebral hyperostosis causing dysphagia. Arch. Surg., 109:567, 1974.

12. Debas, H. T., Payne, W. S., Cameron, A. J., and Carlson, H. C.: Physiopathology of lower esophageal diverticulum and its implications for treatment. Surg. Gynecol. Obstet., 151:593, 1980.

13. Dines, D. E., and Anderson, M. W.: Giant left atrium as a cause of dysphagia. Ann. Int. Med., 65:759, 1966.

14. Dohlman, G., and Mattsson, O.: The endoscopic operation for hypopharyngeal diverticula: A roentgencematographic study. Arch. Otolaryngol., 77:744, 1960.

15. Duranceau, A., Beauchamp, G., and Jamieson, G. G.: The technique of cricopharyngeal myotomy: Esophageal surgery. Surg. Clin. N. Am., 63:833, 1983.

16. Duranceau, A., Cardin, J. L., and Taillefer, R.: Long-term effects of total fundoplication on the myotomized esophagus. In Siewert, J. R., and Holscher, A. H. (Ed.): Diseases of the Esophagus. Berlin, Springer-Verlag, 1988, pp. 1206–1209.

17. Duranceau, A., and Jamieson, G. G.: Recent advances in esophageal manometry. In DeMeester, T. R., and Matthews, H. R. (Eds.): International Trends in General Thoracic Surgery. Vol. 3, Benign Esophageal Disease. St. Louis, C. V. Mosby Company, 1987, pp. 42–54.

18. Duranceau, A., Rheault, M. J., and Jamieson, G. G.: Physiological response to cricopharyngeal myotomy and diverticulum suspension. Surgery, 94:655, 1983.

19. Ellis, F. H., Jr.: Surgical management of esophageal motility disturbances. Am. J. Surg., 139:752, 1980.

20. Ellis, F. H., and Crozier, R. E.: Cervical esophageal dysphagia: Indications for and results of cricopharyngeal myotomy. Ann. Surg., 194:279, 1981.

21. Ellis, F. H., Jr., Schlegel, J. F., Lynch, V. P., et al.: Cricopharyngeal myotomy for pharyngoesophageal diverticulum. Ann. Surg., 170:340, 1969.

22. Eros, P., Goldstein, M. S., and Sherlock, P.: Candida infection of the gastrointestinal tract. Medicine, 51:367, 1972.

23. Freeark, R. J., Norcross, W. J., Baker, R. J., et al.: The Mallory-Weiss syndrome. Arch. Surg., 88:882, 1964.

24. Gedde-Dahl, T., Jr.: Epidermolysis Bullosa: A Clinical, Genetic, and Epidemiological Study. Baltimore, The Johns Hopkins Press, 1971.

25. Goldberg, H. I., and Dodds, W. J.: Cobblestone esophagus due to monilial infection. Am. J. Roentgenol. Genol. Radium Ther. Nucl. Med., 104:608, 1968.

26. Gundry, S. R., Borkon, A. M., McIntosh, C. L., and Morrow, A. G.: Candida esophagitis following cardiac operations and short-term antibiotic prophylaxis. J. Thorac. Cardiovasc. Surg., 80:661, 1980.

27. Habein, H. C., Kirklin, J. W., Clagett, O. T., and Moersch, H. J.: Surgical treatment of lower esophageal pulsion diverticula. Arch. Surg., 72:1018, 1956.

28. Hanna, E. A., and Derrick, J. R.: Dysphagia caused by tortuosity of the thoracic aorta. J. Thorac. Cardiovasc. Surg., 57:134, 1969.

29. Hardy, K. M., Perry, H. O., Pingree, G. C., and Kirby, T. J., Jr.: Benign mucous membrane pemphigoid. Arch. Dermatol., 104:467, 1971.

30. Hinchey, E. J., and Hreno, A.: Postemetic gastroesophageal laceration with hemorrhage. Surg. Gynecol. Obstet., 126:324, 1968.

31. Hunt, P. S., Connell, A. M., and Smiley, T. B.: The cricopharyngeal sphincter in gastric reflux. Gut, 11:303, 1970.

32. Hurwitz, A. L., Way, L. W., and Haddad, J. K.: Epiphrenic diverticulum in association with an unusual motility disturbance: Report of surgical correction. Gastroenterology, 68:795, 1975.

33. Ingelfinger, J. F., and Kramer, P.: Dysphagia produced by contractile ring in lower esophagus. Gastroenterology, 23:419, 1953.

34. Jackson, C., and Shallow, T. A.: Diverticula of the esophagus, pulsion, traction, malignant and congenital. Ann. Surg., 83:1, 1926.

35. Jamieson, G. G., Duranceau, A. C., and Payne, W. S.: Pharyngo-oesophageal diverticulum. In Jamieson, G. G. (Ed.): Surgery of the Oesophagus. Edinburgh, Churchill-Livingstone, 1988, pp. 435–493.

36. Kaye, M. D.: Oesophageal motor dysfunction in patients with diverticula of the mid-thoracic oesophagus. Thorax, 29:666, 1974.

37. Kelly, A. B.: Spasm at entrance to oesophagus. J. Laryngol. Rhinol. Otol., 34:285, 1919.

38. Knauer, C. M.: Mallory-Weiss syndrome: Characterization of 75 Mallory-Weiss lacerations in 528 patients with upper gastrointestinal hemorrhage. Gastroenterology, 71:5, 1976.

39. Knuff, T. E., Benjamin, S. B., and Castell, D. O.: Pharyngoesophageal (Zenker's) diverticulum: A re-appraisal. Gastroenterology, 82:734, 1982.

40. Kodsi, B. E., Wickremesainghe, P. C., Kozinn, P. J., Iswara, K., and Goldberg, P. K.: Candida esophagitis—a prospective study of 27 cases. Gastroenterology, 71:715, 1976.

41. Lahey, F. H., and Warren, K. W.: Esophageal diverticula. Surg. Gynecol. Obstet., 98:1, 1954.

42. Lambert, A.: Surgical correction of esophageal obstruction due to tortuosity of the aorta. J. Thorac. Cardiovasc. Surg., 62:973, 1971.

43. LeRoux, B. T., and Williams, M. A.: Dysphagia megalatriensis. Thorax, 24:603, 1969.

44. Lever, W. F.: Pemphigous and Pemphigoid. Springfield, Ill., Charles C Thomas, 1965.

45. Lewicki, A. M., and Moore, F. P.: Esophageal moniliasis—a review of common and less frequent characteristics. A.J.R., 125:218, 1975.

46. Lichter, I.: Motor disorders in pharyngoesophageal pouch. J. Thorac. Cardiovasc. Surg., 76:273, 1978.

47. Ludlow, A.: Obstructed deglutition, from a preternatural dilatation of, and bag formed in, the pharynx. Med. Soc. Phys., 3:85, 1762–1767.

48. MacCarty, R. L., Dukes, R. J., Strimlan, C. V., Dines, D. E., and Payne, W. S.: Radiographic findings in patients with esophageal involvement by mediastinal granuloma. Gastrointest. Radiol., 4:11, 1979.

49. Mallory, G. K., and Weiss, S.: Haemorrhages from lacerations of the cardiac orifice of the stomach due to vomiting. Am. J. Med. Sci., 178:506, 1929.

50. Meeks, L. W., and Renshaw, T. S.: Vertebral osteophytes and dysphagia. Two case reports of the syndrome recently termed ankylosing hyperostosis. J. Bone Joint Surg., 55A:197, 1973.

51. Mendl, K., McKay, J. M., and Tanner, C. H.: Intramural diverticulosis of the esophagus and Rokitanski-Aschoff sinuses of the gallbladder. Br. J. Radiol., 33:496, 1960.

52. Michel, L., Serrano, A., and Malt, R. A.: Mallory-Weiss syndrome. Evolution of diagnostic and therapeutic patterns over two decades. Ann. Surg., 192:716, 1980.

53. Morton, R. P., and Giles, M. L.: Surgery for pharyngeal pouch. Aust. N.Z. J. Surg., 56:77, 1986.

54. Orringer, M. B.: Extended cervical esophagomyotomy for cricopharyngeal dysfunction. J. Thorac. Cardiovasc. Surg., 80:669, 1980.

55. Orringer, M. B., and Sloan, H.: Monilial esophagitis: An increasingly frequent cause of esophageal stenosis? Ann. Thorac. Surg., 26:364, 1978.

56. Ottinger, L. W., and Wilkins, E. W., Jr.: Late results in patients with Schatzki's ring undergoing destruction of the ring and hiatus herniorrhaphy. Am. J. Surg., 139:591, 1980.

57. Patterson, D. R.: A clinical type of dysphagia. J. Laryngol. Rhinol. Otol., 34:289, 1919.

58. Payne, S. W., King, R. M.: Pharyngoesophageal (Zenker's) diverticulum. S. Clin. N. Am., 63:815, 1983.

59. Pedersen, A. S., Hansen, J. B., and Alstrup, P.: Pharyngo-oesophageal diverticula: A manometric follow-up study of 10 cases treated by diverticulectomy. Scand. J. Thorac. Cardiovasc. Surg., 7:87, 1973.

60. Postlethwait, R. W.: Surgery of the Esophagus. Norwalk, Conn., Appleton-Century-Crofts, 1979, pp. 259–266.

61. Ibid., pp. 126–127.

62. Prince, D. S., Luna, R. F., Cohn, M. G., and Sabiston, W. R.: Osteophyte-induced dysphagia: Occurrence in ankylosing hyperostosis. J.A.M.A., 234:77, 1975.

63. Raque, C. J., Stein, K. M., and Samitz, M. H.: Pemphigus vulgaris involving the esophagus. Arch. Dermatol., 102:371, 1970.

64. Rivkin, L., Bremner, C. G., and Bremner, C. H.: Pathophysiology of mid-oesophageal and epiphrenic diverticula of the oesophagus. S. Afr. Med. J., 66:127, 1984.

65. Rutgeerts, L., and Verhaegen, H.: Intravenous miconazole in the treatment of chronic esophageal candidiasis. Gastroenterology, 72:316, 1977.

66. Saylor, J. L., and Tedesco, F. J.: Mallory-Weiss syndrome in perspective. Am. J. Dig. Dis., 20:1131, 1975.

67. Schatzki, R., and Gary, J. E.: Dysphagia due to diaphragm-like localized narrowing in lower esophagus (lower esophageal ring). Am. J. Roentgenol., 70:911, 1953.

68. Seelig, M. S., Speth, C. P., Kozinn, P. J., Toni, E. F., Taschdjian, C. L.: Candida endocarditis after cardiac surgery. Clues to earlier detection. J. Thorac. Cardiovasc. Surg., 65:583, 1973.

69. Shearman, D. J. C., and Finlayson, N. D. C.: Diseases of the Gastrointestinal Tract and Liver. Edinburgh, Churchill-Livingstone, 1982, p. 114.

70. Sheft, D. J., Shrago, G.: Esophageal moniliasis: the spectrum of the disease. J.A.M.A., 213:1859, 1972.

71. Shklar, G., McCarthy, P. L.: Oral lesions of mucous membrane pemphigoid: a study of 85 cases. Arch. Otolaryngol., 93:354, 1971.

72. Sugawa, C., Benishek, D., Walt, A. J.: Mallory-Weiss syndrome: A study of 224 patients. Am. J. Surg., 145:30, 1983.

73. Sweet, R. H.: Excision of diverticulum of the pharyngoesophageal junction and lower esophagus by means of the one-stage procedure. Ann. Surg., 143:433, 1956.

74. Templeton, F. E.: X-ray Examination of the Stomach: A Description of the Roentgenologic Anatomy, Physiology and Pathology of the Esophagus, Stomach, and Duodenum. Chicago, University of Chicago Press, 1944.

75. vanOverbeck, J. J. M., and Hoeksema, P. E.: Endoscopic treatment of the hypopharyngeal diverticulum: 211 cases. Laryngoscope, 92:88, 1982.

76. Vinson, P. P.: The Diagnosis and Treatment of Diseases of the Esophagus. Springfield, Ill. Charles C Thomas, 1940, pp. 136–145.

77. Weaver, D. H., Maxwell, J. G., and Castleton, K. B.: Mallory-Weiss syndrome. Am. J. Surg., 118:887, 1969.

78. Wightman, A. J. A., and Wright, E. A.: Intramural esophageal diverticulosis: A correlation of radiologic and pathologic findings. Br. J. Radiol., 47:496, 1974.

79. Wright, R.: Upper esophageal perforation with flexible endoscopy secondary to cervical osteophytes. Dig. Dis. Sci., 25:66, 1980.

80. Wynder, E. L., Hultberg, S., Jacobsson, F., et al.: Environmental factors in cancer of the upper alimentary tract: A Swedish study with special reference to Plummer-Vinson (Paterson-Kelly) syndrome. Cancer, 10:470, 1957.

81. Zenker, F. A., and von Ziemssen, H.: Diseases of the oesophagus. In Cyclopedia of the Practice of Medicine, Vol. 8. New York, William-Wood, 1878, pp. 1–214.

V

ESOPHAGOSCOPY

Mark B. Orringer, M.D.

Esophagoscopy, which permits direct evaluation of the interior of the esophagus, is among the most vital diagnostic tools in the assessment of the patient with esophageal symptoms from any cause. With technical advances in flexible fiberoptic esophagoscopy, the number of these procedures being performed on an outpatient basis has increased greatly. Unfortunately, as esophagoscopy has become a more commonly performed operation, a rather cavalier attitude toward this procedure has emerged. It should be borne in mind, however, that esophagoscopy, particularly with dilatation of a stricture, is one of the most dangerous operations performed, the horrendous complications of a perforation being all too familiar to those called upon to treat patients with esophageal disorders. Rigid adherence to basic principles of esophagoscopy is consistently rewarded by fewer complications.

INDICATIONS AND CONTRAINDICATIONS

Esophagoscopy is indicated in a variety of diagnostic and therapeutic situations.[2] Diagnostically, symptoms of dysphagia, heartburn, odynophagia, hematemesis, and atypical chest pain most often warrant esophagoscopy. Esophagoscopy is also useful in assessing established esophageal pathology — esophagitis, neuromotor dysfunction, caustic injury, or tumors. It is useful in defining and confirming radiologic abnormalities — stricture, hiatal hernia, suspected esophagitis, diverticula, varices, and extrinsic compression are common indications for esophagoscopy. Moreover, esophagoscopy is of great diagnostic value in the assessment of postoperative problems — anastomotic stricture, tumor recurrence, bleeding, dysphagia, or recurrent gastroesophageal reflux. From a therapeutic standpoint, dilation and biopsy of strictures, removal of foreign bodies, placement of endoluminal prostheses, sclerotherapy, endoscopic myotomy (Dohlman procedure), and laser photocoagulation for bleeding or tumor debulking are the usual indications for esophagoscopy.

Esophagoscopy is *not* a minor surgical procedure, as attested by the recognized disastrous implications of an esophageal perforation. It cannot be overemphasized that safe optimal esophagoscopy demands a well-trained endoscopist, properly functioning equipment, and resuscitative support in the event that a cardiorespiratory complication occurs. Esophagoscopy should not be performed in a struggling, uncooperative, agitated patient. Additional relative contraindications include a recent myocardial infarction, severe cervical spine deformities, and large thoracic aortic aneurysm.

GENERAL CONSIDERATIONS

The safe performance of esophagoscopy demands familiarity with normal esophageal anatomy, particularly the three areas of constriction and the course of the esophagus through the thorax (see Part I). Generally, an elective esophagoscopy should never be performed without a prior barium esophagogram, and these films ideally should be displayed in view of the endoscopist during the procedure. Knowledge of existing esophageal pathology that is readily visible on a barium esophagogram is extremely important. Perforating a pharyngoesophageal diverticulum, for example, cannot be condoned because the surgeon was unaware of its presence before esophagoscopy.

Before performing esophagoscopy, it is always helpful to relate pathology observed on the barium swallow examination to certain anatomic landmarks and then to extrapolate from this assessment the approximate level within the esophagus at which the abnormality should be seen. The cricopharyngeus sphincter, for example, is located on barium esophagogram at the level of the seventh cervical or first thoracic vertebral body, or approximately 15 cm. from the upper incisor teeth at esophagoscopy. Topographically, the angle of Louis (the sternomanubrial junction) on the anterior chest wall aligns with the tracheal bifurcation, which can usually be seen in most barium esophagograms at approximately the level of the fourth thoracic vertebra, and corresponds to a point 25 cm. from the incisors on esophagoscopy. The esophagogastric junction is typically seen endoscopically 40 cm. from the upper incisors at the level of the eleventh or twelfth thoracic vertebrae.

The choice of anesthesia for esophagoscopy must be individualized. Many patients tolerate the procedure with little sedation and only topical anesthesia of the posterior tongue and pharynx with 2 to 4 per cent lidocaine, tetracaine, or cocaine (2 to 3 ml. of a 5 per cent solution). Intravenous diazepam (Valium) sedation, 5 to 10 mg., provides excellent relaxation in apprehensive patients. The newer, more potent sedative midazolam (Versed), administered intravenously (1 to 5 mg.) is an excellent aid to comfortable endoscopy. It is foolhardy to persist with attempts at esophagoscopy in an anxious, combative, or uncooperative patient, and general anesthesia should be used in such cases. The *initial endoscopic evaluation* of a high-grade obstructing lesion requires prolonged manipulation of the esophagoscope, bougies, and forceps of various types. Such a procedure is not only painful for the patient but also requires the complete concentration of the surgeon on the operative field. General anesthesia is therefore preferred by the author when esophagoscopy is being performed to assess such obstructing lesions, regardless of the cause. There is little question that flexible fiberoptic esophagoscopy is an easier procedure for the patient than rigid esophagoscopy. However, there are definite situations in which rigid esophagoscopy has distinct advantages, and the endoscopist should therefore have at his disposal both the rigid and flexible instruments, which should be viewed as complementary, not mutually exclusive. The rigid esophagoscope is best for evaluating lesions at or just below the cricopharyngeal sphincter, for removing foreign bodies, for dilating of high-grade stenoses, and for obtaining larger and more adequate biopsies. Mucosal detail is best assessed with the flexible fiberoptic esophagoscope, which therefore has advantage in diagnosing reflux esophagitis and following Barrett's mucosa for progression or malignant degeneration.

TECHNIQUE

Rigid esophagoscopy is best performed with the patient under general anesthesia. After induction of anesthesia, the patient's eyes are padded, taped closed, and covered with a folded towel to prevent inadvertent injury during the procedure. The endotracheal tube is displaced to the left side of the mouth and secured with tape.

The lubricated rigid esophagoscope is introduced into the right side of the posterior pharynx, displacing the tongue and the endotracheal tube to the left. The epiglottis is elevated by the tip of the advancing esophagoscope, which is introduced into the esophagus behind the right arytenoid cartilage into the narrow opening seen between the larynx and the posterior wall of the pharynx. This is the most critical step of rigid esophagoscopy. Because of the natural "pull" of the cricopharyngeus muscle against the cricoid cartilage, making this the narrowest point of the gastrointestinal tract, unless upward displacement of the larynx by the advancing esophagoscope is maintained, a posterior perforation by the instrument can occur, typically just proximal to the sphincter (Fig. 1). This is the most common mechanism of endoscopic esophageal injury. The esophageal lumen must be kept in view at *all times.* If the opening of the upper sphincter is not readily apparent, gentle introduction of a 12 or 14 French gum-tipped Jackson dilator as a guide or "follower" through upper sphincter facilitates entry of the esophagoscope into the upper esophagus. Because introduction of the rigid esophagoscope is performed under direct vision, in contrast to flexible esophagoscopy, the posterior pharynx and esophageal introitus are routinely examined as part of the procedure.

As the thoracic esophagus is traversed, the patient's head should be turned, raised, or lowered as necessary so that the lumen remains in view at all times. When the tip of the esophagoscope is beyond the level of the aortic arch, the neck is extended and the head lowered and rotated gradually to the right as the instrument is advanced. This is particularly true as the distal esophagus is approached, since the esophagus normally deviates to the left and anteriorly as it leaves the thorax and joins the stomach. After visualization of the mucosa, measurement of the level of the esophageal pathology in centimeters from the upper incisors, biopsy, and obtaining brushings for cytologic evaluation, the esophagoscope is slowly withdrawn, again concentrating on maintaining the lumen within the center of the visual field at all times and manipulating the patient's head to achieve this as required.

The flexible fiberoptic esophagoscope is more easily passed into the esophagus and is therefore better tolerated by the patient with only topical anesthesia. With the patient in the sitting position for minimizing the risk of aspiration of regurgitated gastric contents, the instrument is advanced into the posterior pharynx and then the upper esophagus as the patient swallows. Introduction of the flexible esophagoscope through the posterior pharynx and cricopharyngeal sphincter is performed "blindly," and significant pathologic condition may be overlooked unless a concerted effort to evaluate these areas is made upon withdrawal of the instrument from the esophagus.

ENDOSCOPIC EVALUATION OF REFLUX ESOPHAGITIS

One of the most common indications for esophagoscopy is the assessment of the presence and extent of esophagitis associated with gastroesophageal reflux. The traditional designations of "mild," "moderate," and "severe" endoscopic esophagitis have inherent wide variations in meaning among various observers. The consistent use of a standardized grading system for endoscopic reflux esophagitis provides a more objective description of the gross pathologic changes seen and permits a more meaningful evaluation of patients at different times and by different endoscopists. Two such classifications of reflux esophagitis have been proposed, one by Skinner and Belsey (1967),[19] and the other by Savary and Miller (1978).[16]

Classification of Endoscopic Grades of Esophagitis

Skinner and Belsey's classification of esophagitis (1967) is as follows:

Grade I: Distal esophageal mucosal erythema (which may obscure the esophagogastric squamocolumnar junction).
Grade II: Mucosal erythema with superficial ulceration, typically linear and vertical, with an overlying fibrinous membranous exudate that is easily wiped away, leaving a bleeding surface (often misinterpreted as "scope trauma" by the inexperienced endoscopist).
Grade III: Mucosal erythema with superficial ulceration and associated submucosal fibrosis on biopsy—a dilatable early stricture.
Grade IV: Extensive ulceration and fibrous luminal stenosis—may represent irreversible panmural fibrosis.

Savary and Miller's classification (1978) is as follows:

Stage I: One or more non-confluent longitudinal mucosal erosions.
Stage II: Confluent ulcerations which do not cover the entire circumference.
Stage III: Erosive esophagitis with exudative lesions covering the entire esophageal circumference but without an associated stricture.
Stage IV: Chronic changes of reflux (stricture, ulcer formation, Barrett's mucosa).

Regardless of which classification is used, the endoscopist should have such an orderly method of defining the changes of reflux esophagitis observed at the time of esophagoscopy.

ENDOSCOPIC EVALUATION AND DILATION OF ESOPHAGEAL STRICTURES

Two questions must be answered concerning every esophageal stricture: is the stricture benign or malignant, and if benign, can the stricture be dilated? Both of these questions are answered by esophagoscopy, which is a mandatory part of the evaluation of *every* stricture. Dilation of an esophageal stricture is among the most dangerous operations performed, and a consistent, organized operative approach is mandatory before it is begun. As previously indicated, the *initial* endoscopic evaluation of a high-grade (i.e., very tight) esophageal stricture should be performed with a rigid esophagoscope and with the patient under general anesthesia for optimizing conditions for both the patient and the surgeon. The pliability and extent of the stenosis cannot be adequately assessed through a flexible fiberoptic esophagoscope. A mild stricture can be dilated directly with the rigid esophagoscope. A high-grade firm stenosis, however, re-

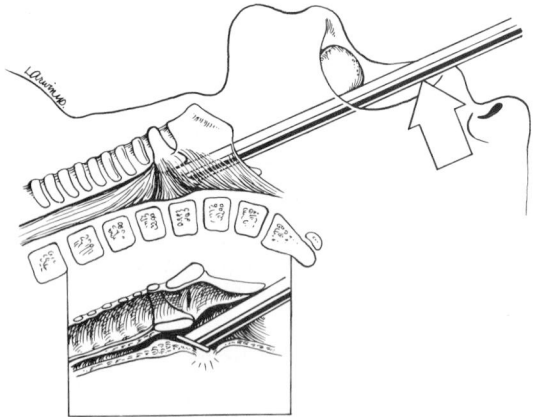

Figure 1. Mechanism of endoscopic cervical esophageal perforation. In performing rigid esophagoscopy, it is essential that a gentle, steady lifting force (arrow) be exerted for obtaining forward displacement of the larynx and cricoid cartilage. Failure to overcome the natural pull of the upper esophageal sphincter against the cricoid cartilage causes a typical posterior perforation *(inset).* (From Orringer, M. B.: Complications of esophageal surgery and trauma. *In* Greenfield, L. J. (Ed.): Complications of Surgery and Trauma, 2nd ed. Philadelphia, J. B. Lippincott Company, 1990, pp. 302–325.)

quires gentle probing and evaluation with gum-tipped bougies passed under direct vision through the stenosis. The largest such dilator that will pass through most rigid esophagoscopes is a 26 French dilator. If the stricture is pliable and if minimal resistance is encountered during this dilation, the esophagoscope is removed and the dilation is continued with tapered mercury-filled Maloney rubber dilators passed "blindly" through the mouth. Alternatively, if the initial evaluation of the stricture indicates that it is dense and rigid, a dilator passed blindly may "curl" proximal to the nonyielding stenosis, and a perforation may occur (Fig. 2). In such difficult cases, an alternative method of dilatation is needed. In the method used by the author, the standard rigid esophagoscope is removed and replaced by a special order 45-cm.-long rigid esophagoscope (Pilling Company), which accommodates up to a 50 French bougie. After introducing this esophagoscope to the level of the stricture, progressively larger dilators, beginning with a 28 French dilator, are passed *under direct vision* through the stenosis. To obtain comfortable swallowing, dilatation of the stricture to at least the size of a 46 French bougie is performed. After dilating the stricture, esophageal biopsies and brushings for cytologic evaluation are performed to exclude carcinoma. Nearly all reflux strictures that can be dilated either directly *per os* or through the esophagoscope to at least the size of a 40 French bougie can be dilated intraoperatively to the 56 to 60 French bougie range at the time of an antireflux operation. Those strictures that will not accept a 40 French bougie may represent advanced, irreversible panmural fibrosis, which requires esophageal resection for relief of the obstruction. Other techniques of esophageal dilation over a previously swallowed thread (Plummer dilator) or metal wire positioned fluoroscopically (Eder-Puestow dilator) or retrograde through a gastrostomy (Tucker dilators) are technically more difficult and generally less safe than the tapered mercury-filled Maloney bougies. The newer Savary-Gilliard bougies represent a major advance in esophageal dilators and appear safer and more effective than previously available instrumentation.[9] This system offers smooth, noncompressible tapered dilators that are flexible and are introduced over an improved metallic guide wire that minimizes the risk of perforation. This may prove to be the most superior available instrumentation for dilatation of difficult reflux strictures.

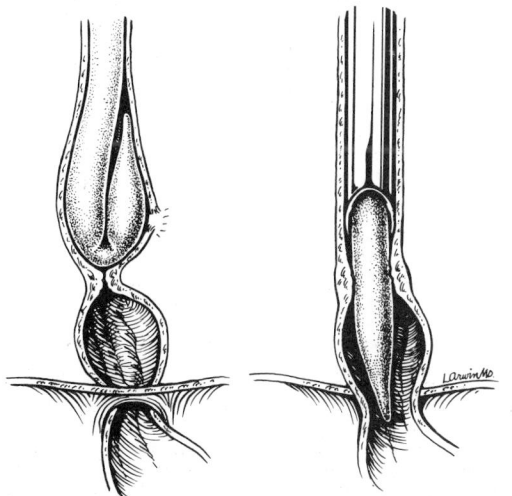

Figure 2. *Left,* Attempt to dilate a tight esophageal stricture by "blind" passage of a dilator has caused curling of the bougie proximal to the stenosis and disruption of the esophagus as the dilator is advanced. *Right,* By means of a special-order large esophagoscope that accommodates up to a 50 French dilator, the stricture can be visualized directly for dilation. (From Orringer, M. B.: Complications of esophageal surgery and trauma. *In* Greenfield, L. J. (Ed.): Complications of Surgery and Trauma, 2nd ed. Philadelphia, J. B. Lippincott Company, 1990, pp. 302–325.)

ESOPHAGOSCOPY IN ADVANCED ACHALASIA WITH MEGAESOPHAGUS

Esophagoscopy in the patient with a megaesophagus is extremely dangerous and merits particular mention. In advanced achalasia, the esophagus may have a capacity of 1 to 2 liters, and disastrous massive tracheobronchial aspiration may follow attempts to introduce a flexible esophagoscope in the conscious but sedated patient on a casual outpatient basis. The routine pre-endoscopic instructions of "nothing by mouth after midnight" are entirely inadequate in this situation, and "emptying" the esophagus of its retained food particles and debris by use of an intraesophageal nasogastric tube for 24 to 48 hours not only may fail miserably but also may impair effective coughing and preoperative pulmonary hygiene. The patient with a megaesophagus should be placed on a clear liquid diet for 48 hours before endoscopy or the scheduled esophageal operation. Just prior to the endoscopy, an 18 French or larger nasogastric tube is passed orally into the esophagus, and intraesophageal contents are removed as thoroughly as possible by suctioning the tube at various levels and irrigating the esophagus with water as required. When the esophagus is emptied, endoscopy is performed. In patients undergoing an esophagomyotomy for achalasia, the esophagus is emptied as described above, and the endotracheal tube is inserted by means of either an awake endotracheal intubation technique or a "crash" induction, maintaining constant backward pressure on the cricoid cartilage against the cervical spine to prevent regurgitation through UES. When the airway is protected by the inflated endotracheal tube balloon, the rigid esophagoscope is inserted into the esophagus, and evacuation of intraesophageal contents is performed with large suction tubing. The mucosa can then be evaluated prior to operation. Standard flexible esophagoscopy is not ideal in the evaluation of the patient with a megaesophagus. Retained intraesophageal debris in these patients simply cannot be evacuated adequately through the flexible instrument, and a sedated patient with a megaesophagus undergoing a "standard" outpatient fiberoptic esophagoscopy may experience life-threatening pulmonary complications if regurgitation and aspiration occur when his cough reflex is suppressed. Equipment for endotracheal intubation and suctioning must always be available for these patients.

COMPLICATIONS OF ESOPHAGOSCOPY

Esophagoscopy can cause either relatively minor complications (laceration of the lips or tongue, fracture or dislodgment of teeth, pharyngeal lacerations) or catastrophic events (massive tracheobronchial aspiration, esophageal perforation). Fortunately, the complication rate from esophagoscopy is relatively low.[5,17,18] Most minor complications are a result of poor technique and failure to adequately protect the gums, lips, and teeth during the procedure. By far, the leading and most serious complication of esophagoscopy, with or without dilation of a stricture, is perforation, which occurs in 1 to 2 per cent of patients, even in the hands of the most experienced endoscopist. It is a basic surgical principle that *pain or fever after esophageal instrumentation represents an esophageal perforation until proven otherwise* and is an indication for an *immediate* esophagogram.[14] Because the mortality and morbidity of an esophageal perforation are directly related to the time interval between the occurrence of the injury and its diagnosis and repair or drainage, an extremely aggressive position toward diagnosing a perforation after endoscopy must be adopted. A contrast study with *both* a water-soluble agent (Gastrografin) as well as dilute barium, if no perforation is seen, should be obtained, because a perforation may be overlooked on roentgenographic evaluation when only Gastrografin is used (Fig. 3). The treatment of esophageal perforation is discussed elsewhere in this chapter (Part VII).

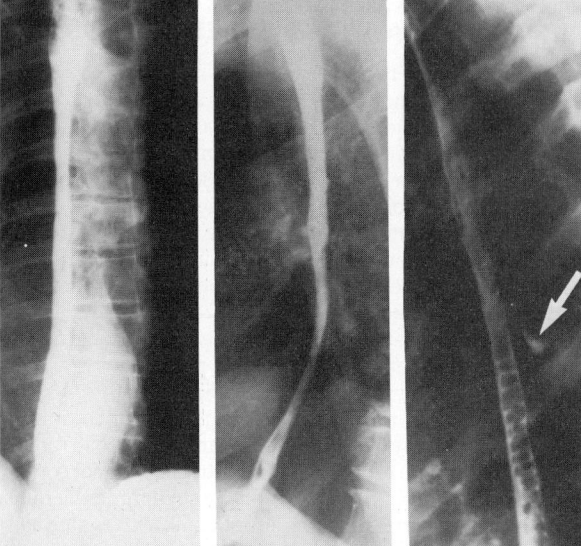

Figure 3. Failure of water-soluble contrast material to demonstrate esophageal perforation. Posteroanterior *(left)* and lateral *(center)* views from a meglumine diatrizoate (Gastrografin) esophagogram of a patient with an acute caustic burn that was dilated prematurely within 10 days of ingestion of Drāno. Despite the developmer' of fever and chest pain, perforation was seen in this study. A barium esophagogram *(right)* demonstrated a perforation (arrow) in the middle third of the thoracic esophagus. (From Orringer, M. B.: Complications of esophageal surgery and trauma. *In* Greenfield, L. J. (Ed.): Complications of Surgery and Trauma, 2nd ed. Philadelphia, J. B. Lippincott Company, 1990, pp. 302–325.)

Perforations proximal to obstructing esophageal lesions are unlikely to heal primarily if repaired and may be treated very effectively by emergent esophagectomy and esophageal substitution using stomach.[15]

RECENT ADVANCES IN ESOPHAGOSCOPY

Several innovations in diagnostic and therapeutic esophagoscopy, although not yet in widespread use throughout the world, warrant mention because they offer significant advances in the esophageal surgeon's armamentarium.

Vital Staining

Squamous cell carcinoma of the esophagus is seldom diagnosed at its earliest stages—carcinoma *in situ* (intraepithelial carcinoma) or microinvasive carcinoma—which may present at esophagoscopy as flat nondescript appearing lesions (leukoplakia or erythroplakia).[4,10,11] Vital staining of the esophageal mucosa with either Lugol's solution or toluidine blue through the esophagoscope offers the ability to diagnose these lesions and hence detect esophageal cancer at an earlier, more readily treatable stage. Three per cent Lugol's solution, a negative tumor marker, stains normal glycogenic esophageal mucosa brown, while pathologic mucosa (early carcinoma, esophagitis, Barrett's mucosa) remains unstained.[7,23] The mucosa is easily evaluated using this technique by means of a swab of the solution applied through a rigid esophagoscope. Biopsy of nonstaining pathologic areas can then be obtained to establish a tissue diagnosis. A 1 per cent aqueous solution of toluidine blue may also be used as a vital stain. It is a metachromatic stain with an affinity for cell nuclei; thus tissues with a high cellular density and nucleus/cytoplasma ratio take up the stain quickly and retain it for approximately 1 hour.[8,12] With this later staining technique, again using rigid esophagoscopy, the esophageal mucosa is first washed with 1 per cent acetic acid to remove excess mucus and food particles, 1 per cent toluidine blue is applied for 1 minute, and the stain is washed away with 1 per cent acetic acid. Those areas of the mucosa that remain stained undergò biopsy and are likely to be neoplastic.[11]

Endoscopic Ultrasonography

Endoscopic ultrasonography is being used with increased frequency as an aid to the standard radiologic (barium esophagogram and computed tomographic scan) and endoscopic assessment of esophageal disease. It provides better definition of benign tumors, specifically leiomyomas[20,21,24]; the potential for more sensitive staging of esophageal carcinoma (detection of depth of invasion and abnormal mediastinal adenopathy)[21,22]; and detection of esophageal varices, which can be monitored before and after sclerotherapy.[1]

Therapeutic Laser Endoscopy

Several types of lasers have proven to be applicable in the treatment of certain esophageal diseases. That in most common use is the Nd-YAG (neodymium:yttrium-aluminum-garnet) laser, which has been used to vaporize unresectable bulky intraluminal carcinomas, thereby providing variable palliation of dysphagia.[3] An even newer generation of contact laser probes have been used to treat some early esophageal carcinomas that have been localized by vital staining.[6,13]

REFERENCES

1. Caletti, G. C., Bolondi, L., Zani, L., Brocchi, E., Guizzardi, G., and Labo, G.: Detection of portal hypertension and esophageal varices by means of endoscopic ultrasonography. Scand. J. Gastroenterol., *21*(Suppl. 123):74, 1986.
2. Castell, D. O., and Johnson, L. F.: Esophageal function in health and disease. *In* Castell, D. O., and Johnson, L. F. (Eds.): Clinical Topics in Gastroenterology. New York, Elsevier, 1983.
3. Fleischer, D., and Sivak, M. U., Jr.: Endoscopic Nd-YAG laser therapy as palliation for esophagogastric cancer: Parameters affecting initial outcome. Gastroenterology, *89*(4):827, 1985.
4. Froelicher, P., and Miller, G.: Esophageal cancer limited to the mucosa and submucosa in Europe. *In* DeMeester, T. R., and Skinner, D. B. (Eds.): Esophageal Disorders: Pathophysiology and Therapy. New York, Raven Press, 1985, pp. 355–357.
5. Gilbert, D. O., Silverstein, F. E., and Tebsco, F. J.: National ASGE survey on upper gastrointestinal bleeding complications. Endosc. Dig. Dis. Sci., *26*:555, 1981.
6. Joffe, S. N.: Contact neodymium-YAG laser surgery in gastroenterology: A preliminary report. Lasers Surg. Med. *6*(2):155, 1986.
7. Mandard, A. M., Tourneux, J., Gignaux, M., Blanc, L., Segol, P., and Mandard, J. C.: In situ carcinoma of the esophagus: Macroscopic study with particular reference to the Lugol test. Endoscopy, *12*:51, 1980.
8. Mashberg, A.: Final evaluation of tolonium chloride rinse for screening of high risk patients with asymptomatic squamous carcinoma. J. Am. Dent. Assoc., *106*:319, 1983.
9. Monnier, P., Hsieh, V., and Savary, M.: Endoscopic treatment of esophageal stenosis using Savary-Gilliard bougies: Technical innovations. Acta Endoscopica *15*(2):119, 1985.
10. Monnier, P., Savary, M., and Anani, P. Endoscopic morphology of "early" esophageal carcinoma. *In* DeMeester, T. R., and Skinner, D. B. (Eds.): Esophageal Disorders: Pathophysiology and Therapy. New York, Raven Press, 1985, pp. 333–345.
11. Monnier, P., Savary, M., and Pasche, R.: Contribution of toluidine blue to bucco-pharyngo-oesophageal cancerology. Acta Endoscopia, *11*(4-5):299, 1981.
12. Monnier, P., Savary, M., Pasche, R., and Anani, P.: Intraepithelial carcinoma of the oesophagus: Endoscopic morphology. Endoscopy, *13*:185, 1981.
13. Ohyama, M.: Treatment of head and neck tumors by contact Nd-YAG laser surgery. Auris Nasus Larynx, *12*(2):138, 1985.
14. Orringer, M. B.: Complications of esophageal surgery and trauma. *In* Greenfield, L. J. (Ed.): Complications in Surgery and Trauma-Second Edition. Philadelphia, J. B. Lippincott Co., 1989, pp. 302–325.
15. Orringer, M. B., and Stirling, M. C.: Esophagectomy for esophageal disruption. Ann. Thorac. Surg., *49*:35, 1990.
16. Savary, M., and Miller, G.: The Esophagus: Handbook and Atlas of Endoscopy. Solothurn, Switzerland, A. G. Gassman, 1978.
17. Shahmir, M., and Schuman, B. M.: Complications of fiberoptic endoscopy: Esophagoscopy and gastroscopy. Gastrointest. Endosc., *26*:86, 1981.
18. Silvis, S. E., Nebel, O., Rogers, G., Sugawa, C., and Mandelstam, P.: Endoscopic complications: Results of the 1974 American Society for Gastrointestinal Endoscopy Survey. J.A.M.A., *235*:928, 1976.
19. Skinner, D. B., and Belsey, R. H. R.: Surgical management of esophageal reflux and hiatus hernia. J. Thorac. Cardiovasc. Surg., *53*:33, 1967.
20. Strohm, W. D., and Classen, M.: Benign lesions of the upper GI tract by means of endoscopic ultrasonography. Scand. J. Gastroenterol., *21* (Suppl. 123):41, 1986.
21. Tio, T. L., and Tytgat, G. N. J. Atlas of Transintestinal Ultrasonography.

Smith, Kline & French. Aalsmeer, The Netherlands, Drukkerij M. Kostuer-loren, B. V., 1986.

22. Tio, T. L., and Tytgat, G. N. J.: Endoscopic ultrasonography in the assessment of intra- and transmural infiltration of tumours in the oesophagus, stomach, and papilla of Vater and in the detection of extra-oesophageal lesions. Endoscopy, 16:203, 1984.

23. Torriie, S., Kohli, Y., Akasaka, Y., and Kawai, K.: New trial for endoscopical observation of esophagus by dye scattering method. Endoscopy, 7:75, 1975.

24. Yasuda, K., Nakajima, M., and Kawai, K.: Endoscopic ultrasonography in the diagnosis of submucosal tumor of the upper digestive tract. Scand. J. Gastroenterol., 21 (Suppl. 123):59, 1986.

VI

TUMORS OF THE ESOPHAGUS

Mark B. Orringer, M.D.

BENIGN ESOPHAGEAL TUMORS AND CYSTS

Benign tumors of the esophagus are rare, constituting 0.5 to 0.8 per cent of esophageal neoplasms.[70,91,133] Benign esophageal tumors are classified into two groups, mucosal and extramucosal (intramural).[49] Leiomyomas are the most common benign intramural tumors of the esophagus. Intramural granular cell myoblastomas, neurofibromas, and mucosal hemangiomas are even rarer benign esophageal tumors.

LEIOMYOMAS. Esophageal leiomyomas are typically found in patients between 20 and 50 years of age, have no clear-cut gender preponderance, are multiple in 3 to 10 per cent of patients, and occur throughout the thoracic esophagus, but rarely in the cervical esophagus.[8,56,94,106] More than 80 per cent occur in the middle and lower thirds of the esophagus. Calcification may occur within a leiomyoma, and this possibility must be considered in the differential diagnosis of a calcified mediastinal mass. Histologically, the tumors consist of interlacing bundles of smooth muscle cells. The tumors vary greatly in size but seldom cause symptoms when they are less than 5 cm. in diameter.[102] When larger than this, patients complain of dysphagia, vague retrosternal pressure, and pain. Most reported leiomyomas have been found incidentally at autopsy and were asymptomatic. Obstruction and regurgitation may occur when these tumors nearly encircle the esophageal lumen, and bleeding is a more common symptom of the malignant form of the tumor, leiomyosarcoma. The potential for malignant degeneration of benign leiomyomas is apparently quite low. In the lower esophagus and cardia of the stomach, large confluent leiomyomas may occur. Another variation is leiomyomatosis, a condition in which multiple leiomyomas occur throughout the esophageal smooth muscle.[56,61]

Esophageal leiomyomas produce a characteristic radiographic appearance on barium swallow examination. They appear in profile as a smooth concave defect with intact mucosa and sharp borders and abrupt sharp angles where the tumor meets the normal esophageal wall. Typically, half the tumor appears to lie within and half outside the esophagus. As with every esophageal tumor, esophagoscopy is indicated to exclude carcinoma, but if a leiomyoma is suspected, a biopsy of the mass should *not* be performed, so that subsequent extramucosal resection is not complicated by scarring at the biopsy site. Endoscopically, these tumors are mobile with intact overlying mucosa; and although they protrude into the esophageal lumen, they can be displaced and passed with the esophagoscope.

Generally, excision of symptomatic leiomyomas or those greater than 5 cm in size is advised. Asymptomatic or smaller tumors discovered incidentally on a barium swallow examination can be observed and followed by periodic barium esophagograms. While excision of the esophageal tumor provides the only absolute proof that it is not malignant, leiomyomas have such a characteristic radiographic appearance, generally slow growth rate, and low risk of malignant degeneration that periodic follow-up of some of these lesions is reasonable. The advent of esophageal ultrasonography has provided yet another means of diagnosing leiomyomas, which appear as hypoechogenic homogenous areas beneath intact mucosa.[128] When resection is indicated, tumors of the middle third of the esophagus are approached through a right thoracotomy; those in the distal third are approached through a left thoracotomy. The tumor is located, and the overlying longitudinal esophageal muscle is split in the direction of its fibers, revealing the mass. The tumor is then gently dissected away from contiguous tissues and underlying submucosa, a relatively simple procedure. When the tumor has been enucleated, the longitudinal muscle may be reapproximated, although large extramucosal defects may be left without complication. Esophageal resection may be required for either giant leiomyomas of the cardia that involve the adjacent stomach (Fig. 1) or for leiomyomatosis, although multiple enucleations may be performed if possible for the latter condition.[61,94,106] The results of resection of leiomyomas are excellent, and recurrence has not been reported.

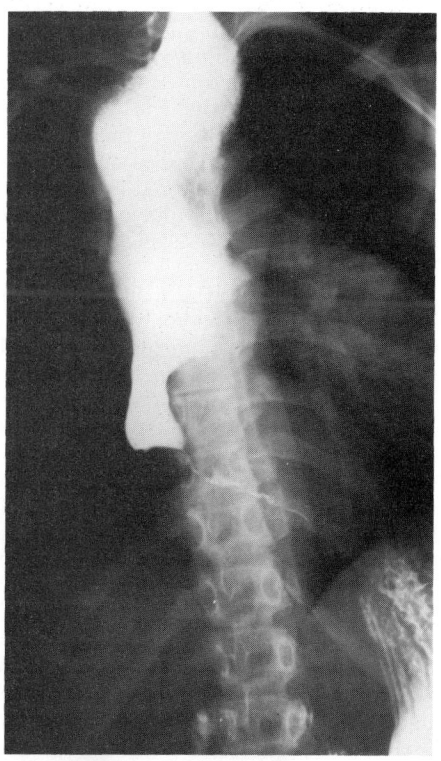

Figure 1. Esophagogram showing a giant leiomyoma involving the distal half of the esophagus and requiring an esophagectomy for resection.

GRANULAR CELL MYOBLASTOMAS. Granular cell myoblastomas are unusual, rare, benign tumors that actually probably arise from Schwann cells, rather than muscle, as their name implies.[38] They are found primarily in the breast, tongue, skin, mouth, upper respiratory tract, and gastrointestinal tract. Approximately one third of gastrointestinal granular cell tumors are located in the esophagus, 50 to 80 per cent in the distal third, and varying in size from 0.5 to 4.0 cm.[54,87] Patients are generally approximately 40 years of age and present with dysphagia, retrosternal or epigastric distress, nausea, and vomiting. The endoscopic diagnosis may be difficult, because these lesions are submucosal and have a gray to yellow appearance. Biopsy specimens may be mistaken for squamous cell carcinoma, because the overlying mucosa typically shows histologic pseudoepitheliomatous hyperplasia.[122] Symptomatic tumors are effectively treated by local excision.

HEMANGIOMAS. Esophageal mucosal hemangiomas constitute 2 to 3 per cent of benign tumors and although usually asymptomatic, may cause intermittent gastrointestinal bleeding, or even less commonly, massive and fatal hematemesis.[84,91,92] Hemangiomas that have bled require treatment, whereas asymptomatic lesions discovered incidentally during esophagoscopy may be followed with periodic endoscopy. Although resection of symptomatic hemangiomas has been the standard approach, newer laser technology offers the potential for effective endoscopic therapy of this mucosal lesion.

PEDUNCULATED INTRALUMINAL TUMORS (POLYPS) OF THE ESOPHAGUS. Benign esophageal polyps are rare but dramatic in their presentation, generally arising in the cervical esophagus, gradually developing progressively longer pedicles, and intermittently extruding into and even out of the mouth.[91] Most of these polyps have occurred in older men, frequently attached to the cricoid cartilage. These tumors cause intermittent dysphagia. Hematemesis or melena may occur if the overlying mucosa becomes ulcerated. The polyps are typically solitary and often long and cylindrical, producing marked esophageal dilation. They are composed of vascular fibroblastic tissue, with varying degrees of associated fat. The barium swallow examination may be nondiagnostic if the polyp is not revealed, or a huge polyp may be misdiagnosed as carcinoma, as a foreign body, or even as achalasia if it has caused marked esophageal dilation. Esophagoscopy similarly may fail to demonstrate the polyp, particularly when the pedicle is not observed and the mucosa overlying the polyp is normal. Although esophageal polyps have been removed endoscopically by electrocoagulation of the pedicle, the preferred approach is resection through a lateral cervical esophagomyotomy, delivering the polyp from the esophagus, and resecting the mucosal origin of the pedicle under direct vision.[88]

MISCELLANEOUS BENIGN TUMORS. Benign esophageal tumors other than leiomyomas and polyps are rare. Papillomas are benign, sessile, lobulated tumors that are covered by squamous mucosa and have a fibrous core. Most occur in the distal esophagus and are associated with some degree of esophageal obstruction. The significance of papillomas has not been established, and they have been postulated to represent localized epithelial hyperplasia or to be premalignant lesions. Occasionally they warrant esophageal exploration to exclude malignancy, and local excision is adequate. Esophageal adenomas, carcinoid tumor, and inflammatory pseudotumors have been reported but are so rare as to be only curiosities.

ESOPHAGEAL CYSTS. Esophageal cysts arise as diverticula of the embryonic foregut. During its embryonic development, the esophagus is initially lined by simple columnar ciliated epithelium, which is eventually replaced by stratified squamous epithelium. Thus, esophageal cysts contain both of these types of epithelium, as well as fat and smooth muscle. A variation of the foregut cyst, the esophageal duplication cyst, extends along the length of the thoracic esophagus, is lined by squamous epi-

thelium, and has submucosal and muscle layers, the latter of which may interdigitate with the outer longitudinal muscle layer of the normal esophagus. Three-quarters of duplication cysts present in childhood. Over 60 per cent are located along the right side of the esophagus.[15,46,136] Esophageal duplication cysts, like other foregut cysts, are often associated with vertebral anomalies (for example, Klippel-Feil deformity or spina bifida) and abnormalities of the spinal cord.[15,124]

More than 60 per cent of congenital esophageal cysts present in the first year of life with either respiratory or esophageal symptoms. The upper third esophageal cysts tend to present in infancy, while the lower third lesions may be asymptomatic initially and present later in childhood. Adults typically remain asymptomatic until bleeding or infection within the cyst causes enlargement,[5,7] which causes dysphagia, choking, or retrosternal pain. Perforation may result from the rare cyst that contains ectopic gastric mucosa. Diagnostically, the cysts may cause displacement of the trachea on a posteroanterior chest roentgenogram or appear as a retrocardiac posterior mediastinal mass on a lateral chest film. The barium esophagogram shows a smooth extramucosal esophageal mass lesion and, very rarely, communication between the esophageal lumen and the cyst. Computed tomography (CT) demonstrates the location of the cyst relative to adjacent mediastinal structures.[135] Spinal films should be obtained prior to resection of a suspected duplication cyst in the event that its origin is the notochord.[127] Because of the potential for bleeding, ulceration, perforation, or infection, excision of these cystic esophageal lesions is recommended. This can generally be achieved with low morbidity by means of an extramucosal resection. If the wall of the cyst cannot be separated from the common esophageal wall, it may be left behind, but the mucosa of the cyst must be stripped away for prevention of recurrence.[69] Marsupialization of the cyst or internal drainage and cauterization of the mucosa are not optimal management. The long-term results of resection are excellent, and recurrence is rare if the initial excision is complete.

MALIGNANT TUMORS OF THE ESOPHAGUS AND CARDIA

INCIDENCE. Esophageal carcinoma remains among the most dismal visceral malignancies, and much energy has been expended by many surgeons attempting to improve the results of resection since Torek performed the first successful esophagectomy in 1913. In the United States, the incidence of this tumor is approximately 4 cases per 100,000 white men per year and 12 cases per 100,000 black men per year,[36] alcohol and tobacco use being strong etiologic factors. Esophageal carcinoma is of epidemic proportion in northeastern Iran, the Transkei of South Africa, the Linxian County in the Hunan province in northern China, certain areas of southern Russia, India, the Middle East, and Singapore.[27] In the Hunan province of China, the prevalence of esophageal carcinoma is 0.9 per cent in the population over 30 years of age, and this extraordinary incidence in humans is matched in the poultry population in the same area. Epidemiologic studies have suggested that the etiology in both instances is the presence of a large amount of carcinogenic nitrosamines in the soil of this region and contamination of foods by fungi, most often Geotrichum candidum, and yeast, which produce mutagens. In northeast Iran the use of opium, which contains pyrrolysates, and ingestion of very hot tea are thought to injure the esophageal mucosa and cause malignant degeneration. In India, Pakistan, and Sri Lanka, the high incidence of esophageal cancer has been linked to chewing tobacco with or without betel nut, betel leaf, slaked lime, or a resin from the acacia. In Singapore, drinking "burning hot" beverages and the use of Chinese tobacco and wine are thought to be etiologic factors in the development of esophageal carcinoma. The South African Bantus and Zulus have a high incidence of esophageal carcinoma that is thought to be related to the high nitrosamine content of their soil as well as contamination of their food by molds, especially the *Fusarium* species, which can produce carcinogens. Alcohol consumption and cigarette smoking appear to be the most consistent risk factors in the populations from Normandy, Brittany, and Europe with the highest incidence of esophageal cancer. Basically, esophageal squamous cell carcinoma is a disease of men (it occurs two to five times more frequently in men than in women) in the sixth and seventh decades of life, but carcinomas of the hypopharynx and cervical esophagus occur almost as often or even more frequently in women than in men. This may be related to the greater incidence of Plummer-Vinson syndrome in women. In Sri Lanka, however, esophageal carcinoma is primarily a disease of women and is the most commonly encountered malignancy of the gastrointestinal tract.[25]

ETIOLOGY. The etiology of esophageal carcinoma is unknown; but as indicated above, certain nutritional factors and potential carcinogens have been incriminated: alcohol, tobacco, zinc, nitrosamines, malnutrition, vitamin deficiencies, anemia, poor oral hygiene and dental caries, previous gastric surgery, and chronic ingestion of hot foods or beverages. There is an increased incidence of esophageal carcinoma in patients with familial keratosis palmaris et plantaris (tylosis), which is inherited as an autosomal dominant trait.[108] A number of esophageal lesions are believed to be premalignant: achalasia,[20,48,90] reflux esophagitis and hiatal hernia, Barrett's (columnar epithelial-lined) esophagus,[72,100,110,114,118] irradiation esophagitis,[43,107] caustic burns,[6] Plummer-Vinson syndrome, leukoplakia, esophageal diverticula, and ectopic gastric mucosa.

PATHOLOGY. Histologically, approximately 95 per cent of esophageal cancers are squamous cell carcinomas. In areas of China where the disease is endemic and mass screening using esophageal brush cytology for detection of early carcinomas is economically and medically justifiable,[109] several macroscopic varieties of early esophageal cancer have been defined. These early forms of esophageal cancer have been variously termed carcinoma *in situ*, superficial spreading carcinoma, and intramucosal carcinoma. They constitute only 2.5 per cent of all resected cases in Japan,[105] are asymptomatic, and may take 3 to 4 years to progress to invasive squamous cell carcinoma.[47] Endoscopically, carcinoma *in situ* most often presents as a slightly raised, granular, reddish plaque-like lesion, although superficial erosions or papillary lesions less than 3 cm. in diameter may also be seen. Microscopically, early esophageal carcinoma is intraepithelial (carcinoma *in situ*), intramucosal (no deeper than the lamina propria), or submucosal, with varying degrees of dysplastic change being observed.[63]

Unfortunately, most esophageal carcinomas are seen in an advanced stage involving the muscular wall and often extending to adjacent tissues. The cervical esophagus is least often (8 per cent) involved by squamous cell carcinoma. Squamous cell esophageal cancer is most frequent in the upper and mid thoracic segments (55 per cent) and the distal third (10 cm.) of the esophagus (37 per cent).[34] The common growth patterns observed are the fungating (60 per cent), ulcerative (25 per cent), and infiltrative (15 per cent) forms.

Esophageal cancer is notorious for its aggressive biologic behavior, with local infiltration, involvement of adjacent lymph nodes, and hematogenous metastatic spread. Lack of a serosal layer tends to favor local tumor extension. Upper and middle third tumors tend to involve the tracheobronchial tree, aorta, and left recurrent laryngeal nerve as it loops around the aortic arch, whereas lower third tumors may invade the diaphragm, pericardium, and stomach. The extensive mediastinal lymphatic drainage, which communicates with cervical and abdominal collaterals, is responsible for the finding of mediastinal, supraclavicular, or celiac lymph node metastases in at least 75 per cent of patients with esophageal carcinoma.[94,120]

Cervical esophageal cancers drain to the deep cervical, paraesophageal, posterior mediastinal, and tracheobronchial lymph nodes. Lower esophageal tumors spread to paraesophageal, celiac, and splenic hilar lymph nodes. Distant spread to liver and lungs is seen in 90 per cent of autopsied cases.[126] The prognosis of invasive squamous cell carcinoma is poor, the overall 5-year survival for treated tumors being 5 to 12 per cent.[34] Extraesophageal tumor extension is present in 70 per cent of cases at the time of diagnosis, and the 5-year survival is only 3 per cent when lymph node metastases are present, compared with 42 per cent when there is no lymph node spread.[63]

Adenocarcinomas constitute 2.5 to 8 per cent of primary esophageal cancers, although this frequency is increasing in the United States. They occur most commonly in the distal third of the esophagus, in the sixth decade of life, and with a male to female ratio of 3 : 1. Esophageal adenocarcinoma may have one of three origins: malignant degeneration of metaplastic columnar epithelium (Barrett's mucosa), heterotopic islands of columnar epithelium, or the esophageal submucosal glands. Gastric cancer may also involve the esophagus secondarily. Patients with a columnar-lined lower esophagus (Barrett's metaplasia) are 40 times more likely to develop adenocarcinoma than the general population.[18,118] While the true incidence of Barrett's esophagus in the general population is unknown, it has been estimated that adenocarcinoma arises in 8 to 15 per cent of patients with a columnar-lined esophagus.[72,100] The finding of dysplasia in Barrett's mucosa is an ominous prognostic sign of impending malignant degeneration,[99] *severe* dysplasia being nearly synonymous with carcinoma *in situ* and being an indication for resectional therapy.

As with squamous cell carcinoma, adenocarcinoma of the esophagus exhibits an aggressive behavior with frequent transmural invasion and lymphatic spread. Since many of these tumors arise in the distal esophagus, spread to paraesophageal, celiac axis, and splenic hilum lymph nodes is common. Metastases to the lung and liver are most frequent. The 5-year survival for esophageal adenocarcinoma is only 0 to 7 per cent,[134] the presence of lymph node metastases exerting a significant negative effect upon survival.[10,50]

Several other rare types of esophageal malignant tumors occur. Anaplastic small-cell (oat cell) carcinoma, apparently arising from the same argyrophillic cells that produce this tumor in the lung,[125] can occur in the esophagus.[123] Like their pulmonary counterparts, they demonstrate neurosecretory granules on electron microscopic examination.[98] They tend to be very aggressive tumors and are commonly associated with distant spread at the time of diagnosis, survival beyond 1 year being unusual. Adenoid cystic carcinoma typically occurs as a middle third esophageal tumor, is discovered late in its course, metastasizes widely, and is associated with a median survival of only 9 months.[35,140] Malignant melanoma may present as a primary esophageal tumor, generally occurring as a large polypoid mass and associated with an average survival of 13.4 months and a 5-year survival of 4.2 per cent.[22,68] Carcinosarcoma of the esophagus is a tumor with histologic elements of both squamous cell carcinoma and malignant spindle cell sarcoma. These typically polypoid tumors most often occur in the distal two thirds of the esophagus, grow to a huge size (10 to 15 cm.), and are associated with only a 2 to 6 per cent 5-year survival.[53,139]

CLINICAL PRESENTATION AND DIAGNOSIS. Symptoms from esophageal carcinoma may be of insidious onset, beginning as nonspecific retrosternal discomfort or indigestion. As the tumor enlarges, the initially intermittent dysphagia becomes progressive and the predominant symptom, with weight loss, odynophagia, chest pain, and occasionally hematemesis following. Any patient who complains of progressive dysphagia warrants *both* a barium esophagogram *and* esophagoscopy to exclude carcinoma. The combination of esophageal biopsy and brushings for cytologic evaluation establishes a diagnosis of carcinoma in 95 per cent of patients with malignant strictures.[58,129,131] The barium esophagogram, particularly using air contrast radiographic technique, has enabled the demonstration of lesions as small as 5 to 15 mm. in early detection programs.[108,115,121] Tumors this small, however, are seldom encountered among Western cultures. The majority of patients present with irregular mucosal filling defects, distortion of the esophageal lumen, or annular constrictions on barium studies (Figs. 2 and 3). Despite these roentgenographic characteristics of esophageal malignancy and, conversely, the smooth, tapered radiographic stricture that generally signifies benign disease, esophagoscopy and biopsy to establish the diagnosis are mandatory in every patient with an esophageal stenosis (see Part V). Unfortunately, programs for early detection of esophageal carcinoma using mass screening of patients with barium esophagograms, flexible fiberoptic esophagoscopy, and exfoliative cytology are not cost-effective in Western cultures, where the incidence of this disease is relatively low.

TREATMENT. When the diagnosis of esophageal carcinoma has been established, therapy must be influenced by the knowledge that *in most of these patients, local tumor invasion or distant metastatic disease precludes cure.* Of the three modalities of treatment available—chemotherapy, radiation therapy, and surgical therapy—none alone has achieved significant and consistent long-term survival. Some chemotherapeutic agents —notably cisplatin, bleomycin, and methotrexate—have demonstrated some effectiveness in the treatment of esophageal squamous cell carcinoma.[23,24,57,59,132] Partial responses of the tumors to these agents occur, but not long-term remission. Despite the fact that squamous cell carcinoma is a radiosensitive and therefore potentially curable tumor, radiation therapy seldom achieves cure in these patients.[30] Radiation therapy is used in the treatment of esophageal carcinoma with one of three theoretic objectives: palliation, cure, or as an adjunct to esophagectomy. Approximately one half of the patients with advanced, metastatic carcinoma and severe dysphagia are able to swallow sufficiently to nourish themselves after receiving a palliative course of radiation to the primary tumor in a dose of 4000 to 5000 rads over a 3- to 4-week period. Supervoltage radiation therapy delivers larger doses (5000 to 7000 rads) over a 5- to 7-week period, utilizing rotational and oblique ports to avoid spinal cord injury as the esophagus is irradiated for cure. Unfortunately, Pearson's report (1966)[89] of a 20 per cent 5-year sur-

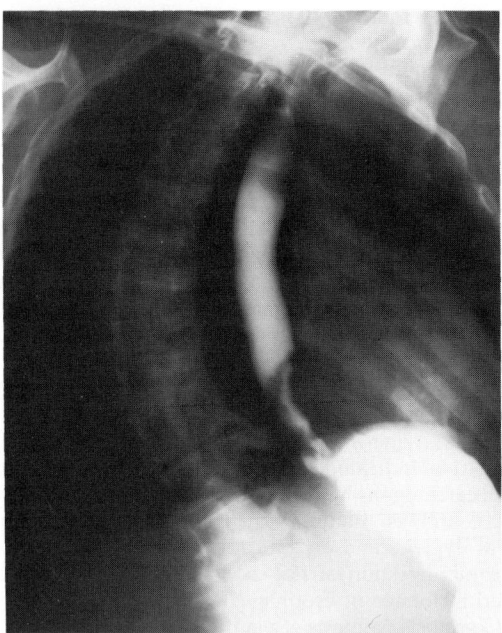

Figure 3. Esophagogram showing a distal esophageal carcinoma presenting as a typical "apple core" constricting lesion.

vival rate in patients with esophageal carcinoma treated by supervoltage radiation has not been duplicated by other investigators, the average 5-year survival rate following this treatment being 6 to 10 per cent.[30] The local tumor is not controlled by radiation; or if it is, it is replaced by stricture or, as is most often the case, continued progression of tumor outside the field of irradiation causes the patient's demise. Similarly, resection, which most effectively relieves the obstruction to swallowing, generally fails to cure the patient with esophageal carcinoma. The explanation is all too apparent: esophageal carcinoma in Western cultures is almost uniformly a *systemic* disease when it is diagnosed; and local therapy, whether with radiation or operation, is simply unable to eradicate this malignancy. This fatalistic attitude toward esophageal carcinoma is borne of the knowledge that the 5-year survival rate from esophageal carcinoma treated by either radiation or operation is less than 10 per cent; more than 80 per cent of the patients die within 1 year of diagnosis.[29,30] In fact, survival is so dismal that some classify a 2-year survival as a "long-term" survival.[85,86] Five-year survival rates of 25 to 37.5 per cent reported by the Japanese using combined preoperative radiation therapy and surgical therapy[1,73] have not been duplicated in Western cultures. Basically, until very recently, the aim of therapy in the patient with esophageal carcinoma has been *palliation,* that is, restoring the patient's ability to swallow comfortably in the most simple and expeditious manner possible.

Palliative transoral intubation of esophageal carcinomas, using any number of tubes that have been described,[21,37,62,71,117] effectively re-establishes a passage for saliva (Fig. 4). These tubes are divided into two types: the *pulsion* tubes, which are pushed through the tumor from above (through the mouth) with the aid of an esophagoscope, and the *traction,* or pull-through, tubes, which are pulled into place by downward traction through a gastrotomy. Unfortunately, although conceptually simple, transoral esophageal intubation has an overall mortality of approximately 14 per cent and a complication rate of at least 25 per cent, largely the result of perforation of the esophagus, migration of the tubes, or obstruction of the tubes by food or tumor overgrowth.[28,41] Although the ability of the patient to handle saliva is improved by intubation of the esophageal tumor, oral intake must be restricted to foods of a consistency compatible with passage through the rigid, indwelling

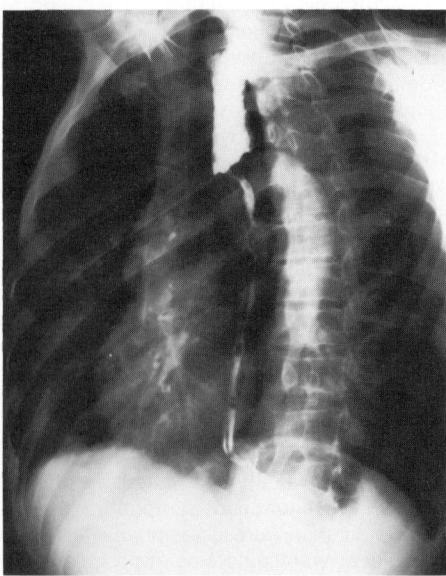

Figure 2. Esophagogram showing an upper esophageal carcinoma at the level of the aortic arch. There is mucosal irregularity and a "shelf" representing the tumor protruding into the esophageal lumen.

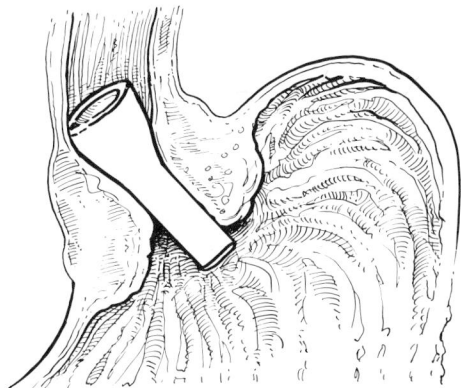

Figure 4. Intubation of unresectable distal esophageal carcinoma with a Celestin tube. (From Payne, W. S., and Olsen, A. M.: The Esophagus. Philadelphia, Lea & Febiger, 1974, p. 250.)

esophageal conduits, and palliation is therefore not optimal. The average survival after palliative intubation for esophageal carcinoma is less than 6 months. This method of therapy appears best suited to patients with malignant tracheoesophageal fistulas, in whom an intraesophageal tube may both occlude the esophageal side of the fistula and permit oral alimentation for the several months of remaining life.[64]

The concept of palliative internal bypass of incurable malignancies of the gastrointestinal tract has been applied to tumors of the stomach, biliary tract, pancreas, and large and small bowel. Bypass of unresectable esophageal carcinomas with a long segment-colonic interposition has been advocated as a method of palliation (Fig. 5). This procedure, however, is of considerable magnitude. Two intra-abdominal gastrointestinal anastomoses are required, and inadequate arterial blood supply

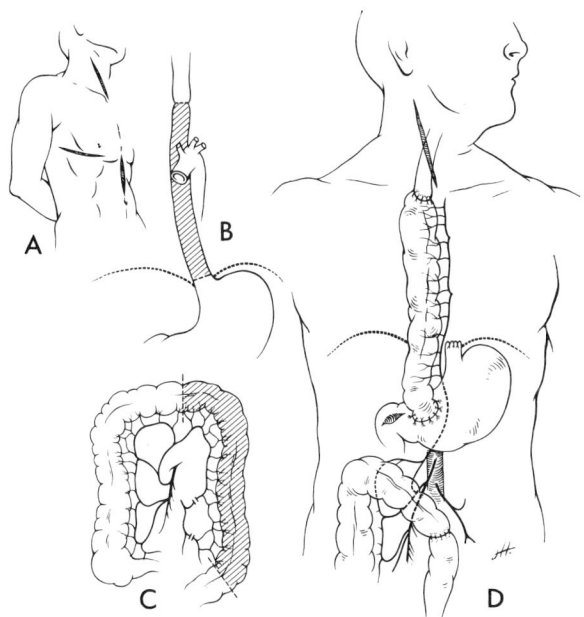

Figure 5. Use of the colon for esophageal replacement or bypass. *A*, Incisions—cervical, right thoracic, and abdominal. *B*, Length of esophagus resected (shaded area). If resection of the tumor is not possible, the cervical esophagus can be divided as shown and the distal end oversewn in preparation for a substernal colonic bypass. *C*, Segment of left colon mobilized for esophageal replacement (shaded area). The ascending, transverse, or descending colon may be used, depending upon the adequacy of the blood supply to the mobilized segment. *D*, Completed operation. The colon may be positioned retrosternally if the esophagus is unresectable or in the posterior mediastinum in the original esophageal bed if resection is possible. A gastric drainage procedure is performed to prevent postvagotomy pylorospasm. (From Payne, W. S., and Ellis, F. H., Jr.: Esophagus and diaphragmatic hernias. *In* Schwartz, S. I. (Ed.): Principles of Surgery. New York, McGraw-Hill Book Company, 1979, pp. 1081–1125.)

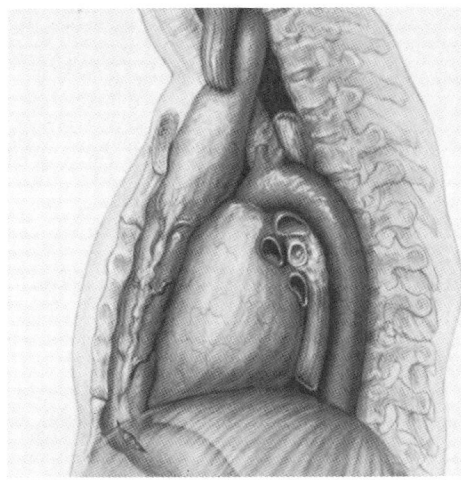

Figure 6. Lateral view showing substernal gastric bypass of the excluded thoracic esophagus. The gastric fundus is suspended from the cervical prevertebral fascia, the anastomosis is on the anterior gastric wall, and the esophagus with its unresectable tumor is excluded in the posterior mediastinum. This technique is now seldom used, because complications from the excluded thoracic esophagus are appreciable and survival after bypassing such an unresectable tumor averages only 6 months. (From Orringer, M. B., and Sloan, H.: Substernal gastric bypass of the excluded thoracic esophagus for palliation of esophageal carcinoma. J. Thorac. Cardiovasc. Surg., 70:836, 1975.)

to or venous drainage from the colonic graft may cause graft necrosis and anastomotic leakage.[13,26,44,74,75,112,137] The mortality for colon bypass of esophageal carcinoma is approximately 15 to 25 per cent.[13,16,26,31,44,96] Gastric tubes to replace or bypass the esophagus have been constructed from the greater curvature of the stomach based on either the left gastroepiploic vessels (the reversed gastric tube)[40,51] or the right gastroepiploic vessels in an isoperistaltic manner.[12,95] These tubes, however, require the construction and healing of a long gastric suture line, and the T formed at the cervical esophagogastric anastomosis frequently causes local ischemia and anastomotic disruption. Retrosternal gastric bypass of the excluded or internally drained unresected esophagus containing a carcinoma has been proposed as a method of achieving palliation in these incurable patients without subjecting them to the morbidity of a thoracotomy to resect the esophagus (Fig. 6).[2,83] Unfortunately, the mortality of retrosternal gastric bypass for esophageal carcinoma is 25 to 40 per cent, the incidence of postoperative anastomotic disruption is high, and survival in these patients again averages less than 6 months.[77]

For most patients with localized esophageal carcinoma, resection, if possible, provides the best palliation. No current data irrefutably demonstrate the superiority of one operative approach for esophageal carcinoma over another. Despite improvements in preoperative evaluation, anesthetic and operative techniques, and postoperative care, esophageal resection and reconstruction remain formidable operations in patients whose nutritional and pulmonary status have been compromised by impaired swallowing. The long-accepted traditional surgical approach to distal esophageal carcinoma has been a left thoracoabdominal incision (Fig. 7). The distal esophagus, proximal stomach, and adjacent lymph node-bearing tissues are resected, and an intrathoracic esophagogastric anastomosis is performed. For higher thoracic esophageal tumors, a thoracoabdominal or separate thoracic and abdominal incisions are used, and a high intrathoracic esophagogastric anastomosis is performed (Fig. 8). In either case, a gastric drainage procedure (pyloromyotomy or pyloroplasty) is recommended to prevent subsequent postvagotomy gastric outlet obstruction due to pylorospasm.

Unfortunately, standard transthoracic esophagectomy has significant disadvantages. A combined thoracic and abdominal

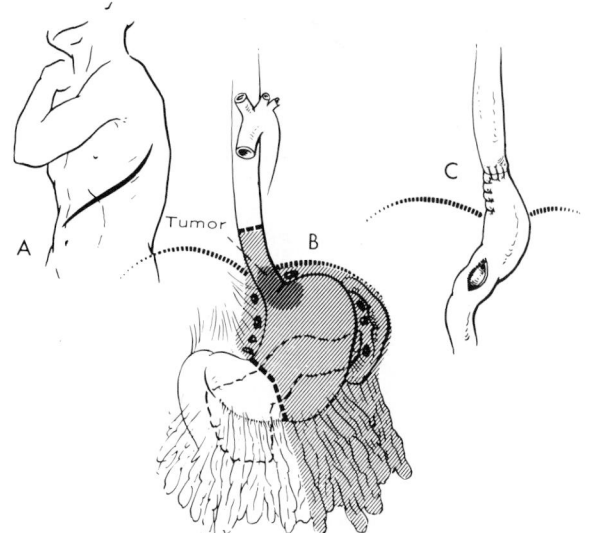

Figure 7. Standard thoracoabdominal esophagogastrectomy for lesions of the distal esophagus and cardia. *A*, Incision. *B*, Tissue to be resected (shaded area). *C*, Completed reconstruction with intrathoracic esophagogastric anastomosis and either pyloromyotomy or pyloroplasty to prevent postvagotomy pylorospasm. (From Ellis, F. H., Jr.: Treatment of carcinoma of the esophagus and cardia. Mayo Clin., Proc., 35:653, 1960.)

operation in a debilitated patient may cause respiratory insufficiency due to postoperative incisional pain and inability to breath deeply, dependence upon mechanical ventilatory assistance, and ultimately death from pneumonia. Disruption of an intrathoracic esophageal anastomosis is the most dreaded complication of this type of operation; mediastinitis and sepsis occur and are fatal in 50 per cent of the patients. The physiologic insult of a combined thoracoabdominal operation and the disastrous results of disruption of an intrathoracic esophageal anastomosis are thus major contributing factors to the morbidity and mortality of this type of esophageal resection and reconstruction and are responsible for reported operative mortality of 15 to 40 per cent, averaging 30 per cent.[32,42,93] Although there are a few reported series of transthoracic esophageal resection and reconstruction for carcinoma with operative mortality less than

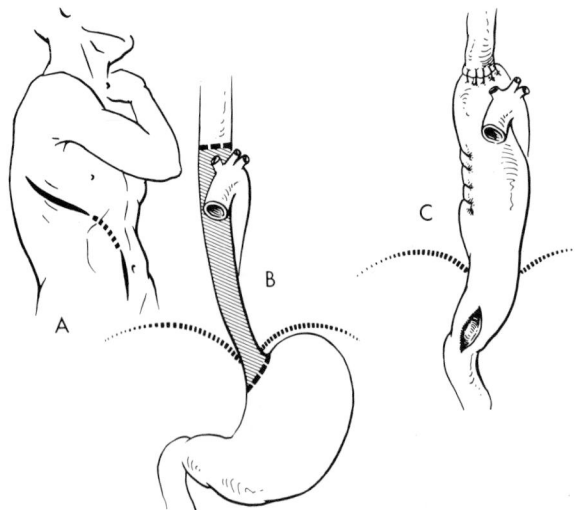

Figure 8. Standard thoracoabdominal Ivor-Lewis esophagogastrectomy for lesions of the lower and middle third of the thoracic esophagus. *A*, The continuous thoracoabdominal incision and the separate thoracic or abdominal incisions which may be used. *B*, Portion of the esophagus to be resected (shaded area). *C*, Completed reconstruction with high intrathoracic esophagogastric anastomosis and gastric drainage procedure. (From Ellis, F. H., Jr.: Treatment of carcinoma of the esophagus and cardia. Mayo Clin., Proc., 35:653, 1960.)

3 per cent,[4,33,65] these are exceptions. An additional disadvantage of this type of esophageal reconstruction is inadequate long-term relief of dysphagia due to either (1) anastomotic suture-line tumor recurrence or (2) the development of reflux esophagitis above the anastomosis. Esophageal carcinoma is notorious for its ability to spread in the submucosal lymphatics well beyond the gross extent of the tumor,[3,17,67,101] and the maximal proximal and distal margins of resection beyond gross tumor are therefore desirable to minimize the possibility of recurrent tumor at the anastomotic suture-line.[66,111] For a patient to undergo a major esophageal resection and reconstruction only to have recurrent dysphagia from tumor within several months is a failure of the operation as a palliative procedure. Finally, intrathoracic esophagogastric anastomoses are almost invariably associated with the development of reflux esophagitis, which follows resection of the LES mechanism.[14,97,116] This not only can produce severe pyrosis and reflux symptoms but also can cause dysphagia from benign stenosis.

In an effort to minimize the aforementioned factors that are responsible for the majority of poor results from esophageal resection and reconstruction in patients with esophageal carcinoma, the technique of transhiatal esophagectomy without thoracotomy was popularized.[78,80,82] In this operation, regardless of the level of the tumor, the entire thoracic esophagus is resected and replaced whenever possible with the stomach, which is anastomosed to the remaining cervical esophagus above the level of the clavicles. This procedure, performed through an upper midline abdominal and a cervical incision, involves resection of the thoracic esophagus through the diaphragmatic hiatus and the neck. The stomach is mobilized by dividing the left gastric and left gastroepiploic vessels, preserving the right gastric and right gastroepiploic arcades, and a Kocher maneuver is performed (Fig. 9). A pyloromyotomy and feeding jejunostomy are performed routinely. The entire thoracic esophagus from the level of the clavicles to the cardia is resected, with careful monitoring at the intra-arterial blood pressure for avoiding prolonged hypotension from cardiac displacement during the transhiatal esophageal dissection (Figs. 10 and 11). The stomach is then transposed to the posterior mediastinum, positioned in the original esophageal bed, and anastomosed to the cervical esophagus (Fig. 12). For distal third esophageal tumors localized to the cardia, the high lesser curvature of the stomach is resected 4 to 6 cm. beyond the gross tumor, preserving that point on the high greater curvature that will reach cephalad to the neck (Figs. 13 and 14). Again, the entire thoracic esophagus is resected, and a cervical esophagogastric anastomosis is performed. Even relatively large intrathoracic esophageal carcinomas have been resectable through the hiatus; if necessary, the tumor can be fractured away from the prevertebral fascia or other adjacent mediastinal structures. For tumors of the upper thoracic esophagus, the addition of a partial upper sternal split facilitates dissection of the esophagus from the trachea under direct vision,[76] and after this the transhiatal esophagectomy can be completed as described previously. In performing a transhiatal esophagectomy, accessible cervical, intrathoracic, and intraabdominal lymph nodes are removed for the purpose of staging, but no attempt is made to perform an *en bloc* resection of the esophagus and its adjacent lymph node–bearing tissue. The advantages of this approach are as follows: (1) A thoracotomy is avoided, thus minimizing the physiologic insult of the operation. (2) An intrathoracic esophageal anastomosis is avoided; and if a cervical leak does occur, it is more easily managed and is not fatal. (3) There are no intra-abdominal or intrathoracic gastrointestinal suture lines, in contrast to the situation with colonic or jejunal interposition, or various gastric tubes. (4) Clinically significant gastroesophageal reflux seldom occurs after a cervical esophagogastric anastomosis. Critics of this operation object to its limited exposure of the intrathoracic esophagus and its blood supply with the accompanying risk of uncontrollable

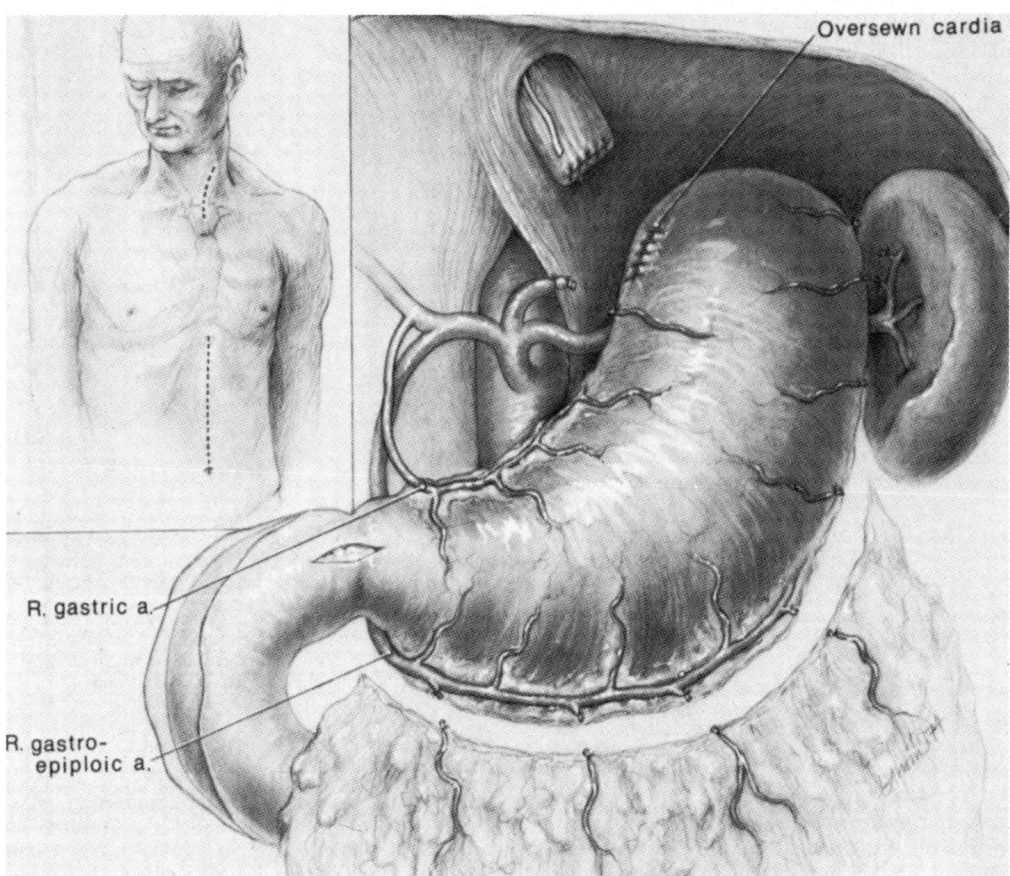

Figure 9. Mobilization of the stomach for either substernal gastric bypass or esophageal replacement after transhiatal esophagectomy. The gastric and right gastroepiploic vessels are preserved, a Kocher maneuver and pyloromyotomy are performed, and the divided cardia is stapled and oversewn. (From Orringer, M. B., and Sloan, H.: Substernal gastric bypass of the excluded thoracic esophagus for palliation of esophageal carcinoma. J. Thorac Cardiovasc. Surg., *70:*836, 1975.)

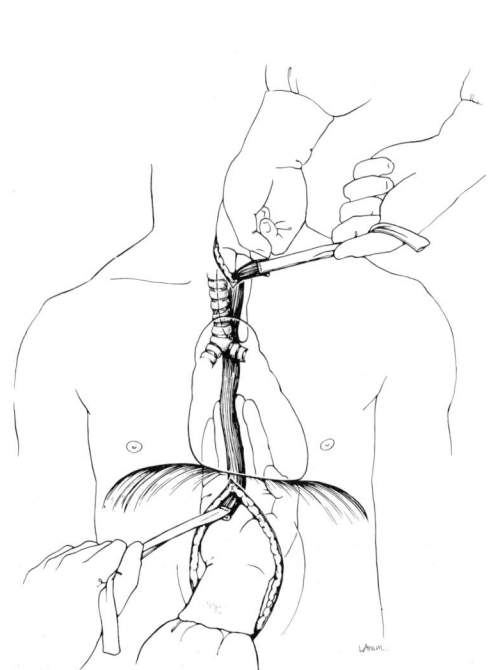

Figure 10. Transhiatal dissection of the lower esophagus through the diaphragmatic hiatus is achieved through an upper midline abdominal incision. Penrose drains around either end of the esophagus are used for traction during the dissection. The upper thoracic esophagus is mobilized through a limited cervical incision. (Modified from Orringer, M. B., and Sloan, H.: Esophagectomy without thoracotomy. J. Thorac. Cardiovasc. Surg., *76:*643, 1978.)

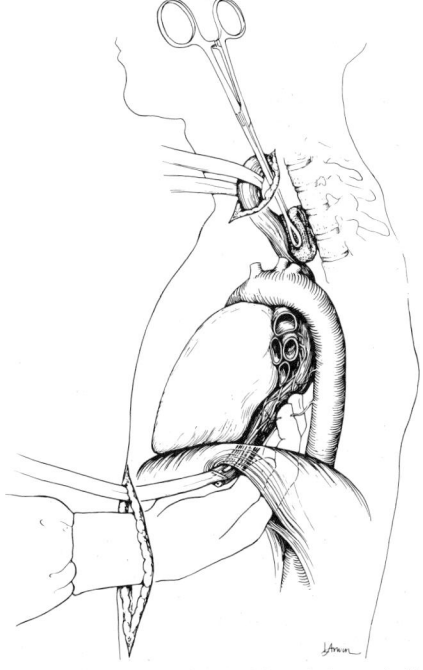

Figure 11. A ''sponge-on-a-stick'' inserted through the cervical incision is used to dissect the upper esophagus away from the trachea and adjacent mediastinal structures in performing a transhiatal esophagectomy without thoracotomy. As the hand inserted through the diaphragmatic hiatus dissects the esophagus free, careful monitoring of the intra-arterial blood pressure is required to prevent prolonged hypotension, which may follow cardiac displacement. (Modified from Orringer, M. B., and Sloan, H.: Esophagectomy without thoracotomy. J. Thorac. Cardiovasc. Surg., *76:*643, 1978.)

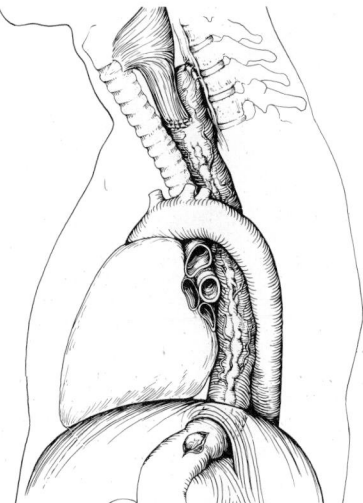

Figure 12. After transhiatal esophagectomy and pyloromyotomy, the stomach is mobilized through the posterior mediastinum, the fundus is sutured to the cervical prevertebral fascia, and an end-to-side esophagogastrostomy is performed. (From Orringer, M. B., and Sloan, H.: Esophagectomy without thoracotomy. J. Thorac. Cardiovasc. Surg., 76:643, 1978.)

hemorrhage, and the inability to perform a complete mediastinal lymph node dissection for purposes of staging and potential cure.

Among the author's last 223 consecutive patients with carcinoma of the thoracic esophagus and cardia, transhiatal esophagectomy without thoracotomy was possible in 215 (96 per cent), local tumor invasion of contiguous structures preventing such resection in 8 patients. The location of the 215 resected tumors

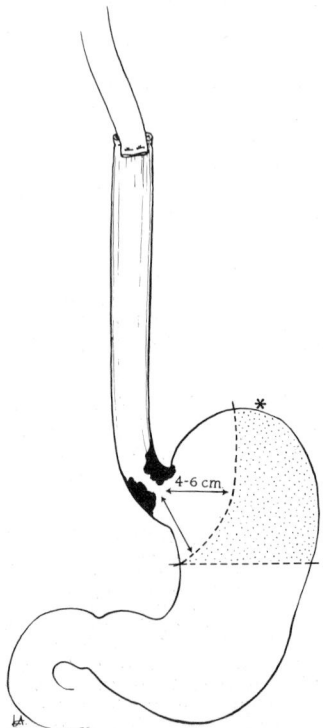

Figure 13. Total thoracic esophagectomy and proximal partial gastrectomy performed for adenocarcinoma limited to the esophagogastric junction and adjacent stomach. Such tumors may be resected with a 4- to 6-cm. gastric margin, and thereby the entire greater curvature aspect of the gastric fundus and that point (*) that reaches most cephalad to the neck are preserved. A proximal hemigastrectomy for such a tumor wastes valuable stomach (stippled area) that can be used for esophageal replacement and contributes little to the operation. (From Orringer, M. B., and Sloan, H.: Esophagectomy without thoracotomy. J. Thorac. Cardiovasc. Surg., 76:643, 1978.)

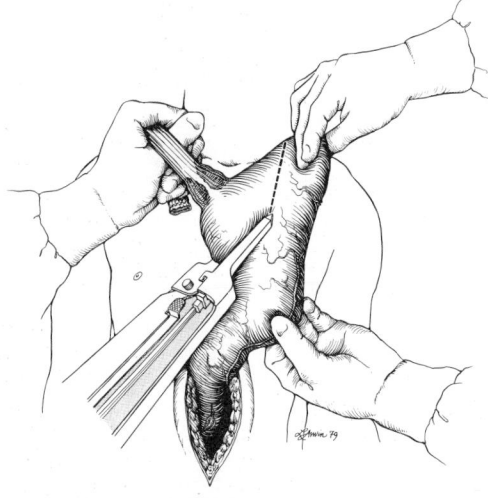

Figure 14. After completing the transhiatal esophagectomy for a localized distal third carcinoma, the surgical stapler is used to fashion a gastric tube from the greater curvature, resecting as much stomach as possible distal to gross tumor. The remaining stomach is then positioned in the posterior mediastinum in the original esophageal bed and is anastomosed to the cervical esophagus. (From Orringer, M. B., and Sloan, H.: Esophageal replacement after blunt esophagectomy. In Nyhus, L. M., and Baker, R. J. (Eds.): Mastery of Surgery. Boston, Little, Brown and Company, 1984, p. 434.)

was the upper third in 12 patients (6 per cent), mid third in 85 patients (39 per cent), and lower third in 118 patients (55 per cent). Ninety-four of the tumors (44 per cent) were squamous cell carcinomas, and 120 (56 per cent) were adenocarcinomas. There was 1 adenosquamous carcinoma. Stomach was used to replace the esophagus in 206 (96 per cent) patients, and colon was used in 9 patients who had undergone prior gastric resections for peptic ulcer disease. *The normal stomach readily reaches to the neck in every patient.* Postsurgical tumor-node-metastasis (TNM) staging (Table 1)[11] of the 215 carcinomas based on histologic evaluation of the resected specimen indicated that in 165 (77 per cent) patients, the carcinomas were either transmurally invasive or metastatic beyond regional lymph nodes (Stage III or IV tumors). In only 15 patients was the tumor confined to the mucosa (Stage I). There were no intraoperative deaths. Intraoperative blood loss averaged less than 1000 ml., hospital mortality was 6 per cent, and 87 per cent of these patients left the hospital able to swallow within 3 weeks of operation. The actuarial survival rates among the 201 operative survivors were 81 per cent at 6 months, 59 per cent at 12 months, 32 per cent at 24 months, 23 per cent at 36 months, and 18 per cent at 48 months. Thirty-nine (19 per cent) of the operative survivors lived 2 years or more, and 16 (8 per cent) are clinically tumor-free. These survival data were neither better nor worse than those achieved by most series of transthoracic resections, but they were accomplished with less postoperative morbidity and mortality.

On the basis of this experience, the author advocates a transhiatal esophagectomy without thoracotomy whenever possible for resectable esophageal carcinomas. If an assessment of the tumor through the diaphragmatic hiatus indicates invasion of contiguous structures that precludes a transhiatal dissection, this approach should be abandoned for the traditional transthoracic esophagectomy. Those who criticize transhiatal esophagectomy without thoracotomy because it denies a formal lymph node dissection to patients with potentially curable tumors have yet to demonstrate that the number of lymph nodes resected has any effect on survival in these patients. When the results of radical transthoracic esophagectomy with *en bloc* dissection of contiguous lymph node–bearing tissues[111] are compared with those of transhiatal esophagectomy without thoracotomy and no formal lymph node dissection, no significant difference in 3-year actuarial survival is apparent (Table 2).

TABLE 1. Tumor-Node-Metastasis (TNM) Staging System for Esophageal Carcinoma

Definition of TNM

Primary tumor (T)

T_X	Primary tumor cannot be assessed
T_0	No evidence of primary tumor
T_{is}	Carcinoma in situ
T_1	Tumor invades lamina propria or submucosa
T_2	Tumor invades muscularis propria
T_3	Tumor invades adventitia
T_4	Tumor invades adjacent structures

Regional lymph nodes (N)

N_X	Regional nodes cannot be assessed
N_0	No regional node metastasis
N_1	Regional node metastasis

Distant metastasis (M)

M_X	Presence of distant metastasis cannot be assessed
M_0	No distant metastasis
M_1	Distant metastasis

Stage Grouping

Stage 0	T_{is}	N_0	M_0
Stage I	T_1	N_0	M_0
Stage IIA	T_2	N_0	M_0
	T_3	N_0	M_0
Stage IIB	T_1	N_1	M_0
	T_2	N_1	M_0
Stage III	T_3	N_1	M_0
	T_4	Any N	M_0
Stage IV	Any T	Any N	M_1

Data from Beahrs, O. H., Henson, D. E., Hutter, R. V. P., and Myers, M. H.: Manual for Staging of Cancer, 3rd ed. American Joint Committee on Cancer. Philadelphia, J. B. Lippincott Company, 1988, pp. 63–67.

It would appear, therefore, that survival after resection of esophageal carcinoma is more a function of individual tumor biology and host resistance than of the extent of the resection performed. Generally, the stomach is preferred over all other organs as a visceral esophageal substitute, being far more resilient than either the colon or jejunum, and easily reaching to the neck to replace the entire thoracic esophagus. Colonic interposition is a tremendous operative undertaking in patients with esophageal carcinoma and should be utilized only when the stomach is not suitable for esophageal replacement.

Recently in an effort to improve survival in patients with local, regional esophageal carcinoma, a trial of two cycles of chemotherapy (cisplatin, vinblastine, and mitoguazone) prior to transhiatal esophagectomy (THE) in 29 patients was undertaken at the University of Michigan.[39] Considerable toxicity from the drugs occurred, and the median survival time of 14 months was not appreciably different from the 12-month median survival time observed in the author's historic controls treated by THE alone.[78] Stimulated by the Wayne State experience with combined preoperative radiation therapy and chemo-

TABLE 2. Effect of Extent of Esophageal Resection for Carcinoma on Survival: Three-Year Actuarial Survival

Esophageal Tumor Site	Radical Esophagectomy with En Bloc Lymph Node Dissection*	Transhiatal Esophagectomy without Formal Lymph Node Dissection†
Middle third	14% (29)	17% (40)
Lower third	33% (37)	31% (47)

* Data from Skinner, D. B.: En bloc resection for neoplasms of the esophagus and cardia. J. Thorac. Cardiovasc. Surg., 85:59, 1983.

†Data from Orringer, M. B.: Transhiatal esophagectomy without thoracotomy for carcinoma of the esophagus. Ann. Surg., 200:282, 1984.

therapy,[60,119] as well as reports of preoperative chemotherapy and postoperative adjuvant radiation therapy,[19] the author and his associates recently conducted a trial of combined preoperative chemotherapy and radiation therapy prior to transhiatal esophagectomy.[79] Forty-three patients, 21 with adenocarcinoma and 22 with squamous cell carcinoma, received 3 weeks of chemotherapy with cisplatin, vinblastine, and 5-FU concurrent with 4500 cGy. radiation therapy. After a 3-week rest, THE was planned. Hematologic toxicity, anorexia, fatigue, and radiation esophagitis were common. There were two preoperative deaths from sepsis due to bone marrow suppression, giving an operability rate in this group of 95 per cent. Two additional patients were found at operation to have unresectable tumors. Thus, the overall resectability rate was 91 per cent (39 of the 43 patients). Transhiatal esophagectomy was performed with no increased morbidity, compared with that of the author's patients, who had no preoperative therapy. Eleven patients had no residual tumor in the resected specimen, giving a pathologic complete response rate of 27 per cent (11 of 41 patients). There was one postoperative death from an unrecognized brain metastasis. At a median follow-up of 27 months, 20 patients (47 per cent) are alive and clinically disease-free and 21 have died, 19 as a result of tumor progression. The median survival time for all 43 patients is 29 months (Kaplan-Meier estimate), a definite improvement over the 12-month median survival time with THE alone.[78] Cumulative survival is 72 per cent at 12 months, 60 per cent at 24 months, and 46 per cent at 36 months, compared with survival in the historic controls treated with THE alone of 59 per cent at 12 months, 32 per cent at 24 months, and 23 per cent at 36 months. All 11 patients with a complete response are alive at a median follow-up time of 36 months, and all are disease-free. Skinner and associates,[113] applying more stringent criteria to their use of radical esophagectomy for carcinoma, have recently reported their results in 31 additional patients, one half with squamous cell and one half with adenocarcinoma. They report an overall 1-year and 2-year survival of 65 per cent and 32 per cent, respectively, which compares with the overall 1- and 2-year survival of 72 per cent and 60 per cent, respectively, in the patients reported above who underwent chemotherapy, radiation therapy and then THE. It would thus appear that multimodality therapy provides better local and regional control of the tumor than can be achieved by radical resection of the esophagus alone. These exciting preliminary results add further support to the growing concept that the natural history of esophageal cancer can be altered and that long-term survival, not just palliation, may be achievable in many patients with this disease. A randomized prospective trial is now in progress to attempt to substantiate the value of such multimodality therapy in the treatment of esophageal carcinoma.

Carcinomas involving the cervicothoracic esophagus (and therefore the larynx) either primarily or secondarily pose the unique problem of esophageal reconstruction after laryngopharyngectomy. Concomitant radical neck dissection is often required because of regional lymph node involvement. Resection of these tumors, which may involve the high retrosternal trachea, is facilitated by removal of the anterior breast plate and construction of a mediastinal tracheostomy.[45,81] Although replacement of the pharynx and cervical esophagus is possible with Wookey skin tubes,[138] Bakamjian flaps,[9] and isolated segments of jejunum anastomosed to a cervical arterial blood supply and venous drainage using microvascular technique,[52,55,104,130] these operations are frequently multistaged, prolonged, and fraught with technical problems. In the author's experience, laryngopharyngectomy for cervicothoracic tumors and concomitant transhiatal esophagectomy without thoracotomy provide the maximal distal esophageal margin beyond the tumor and permit restoration of continuity of the alimentary tract using stomach, which generally reaches cephalad to the remaining pharyngeal margin. A one-stage resection and reconstruction of these carcinomas is as desirable as it is for tumors of the thoracic esophagus, avoiding staged procedures, multiple intestinal anastomoses, and prolonged hospitalization in patients with limited life expectancy.

PREOPERATIVE PREPARATION FOR ESOPHAGECTOMY FOR CANCER. When the diagnosis of esophageal carcinoma has been established, an extensive evaluation for metastatic disease is not customary unless indicated by specific complaints or findings, such as headaches or neurologic signs, bone pain, or abnormal liver chemistries. Bronchoscopic evaluation for evidence of tracheobronchial invasion that contraindicates resection is routine for all upper and middle third intrathoracic carcinomas. The presence of localized intrathoracic or intra-abdominal nodal disease on computed tomographic scan does not preclude a palliative resection; but if hepatic or pulmonary metastases are documented histologically, survival beyond 6 months is unlikely, and no major esophageal resection should be performed.

Patients with esophageal carcinoma are typically cigarette smokers and have had some degree of tracheobronchial aspiration from their esophageal obstruction. Therefore, rigid adherence to a regimen of vigorous pulmonary physiotherapy before operation is consistently rewarded by fewer postoperative complications. Abstinence from cigarette smoking for at least 2 weeks, pulmonary physiotherapy and use of an incentive inspirometer and antibiotics as indicated for associated pneumonitis are routine. In patients in whom severe cachexia has not occurred, relatively little time is spent with preoperative nutritional buildup. However, if the patient is dehydrated or the esophageal obstruction is tight, endoscopic dilation of the malignant stricture and insertion of a nasogastric feeding tube for enteral nutrition is performed so that an intake of 2000 to 3000 calories per day can be ensured. Intravenous hyperalimentation is seldom used in the author's patient population, because this method rarely provides as satisfactory nutrition as do enteral feedings, and the septic and metabolic complications of the intravenous route are avoided. Oral hygiene is often neglected in patients with esophageal carcinoma, and carious teeth should be removed or repaired preoperatively so that the severity of an infection that might follow anastomotic disruption and swallowed oral bacteria is minimized. If there is a history of prior gastric surgery that might preclude the use of the entire stomach as an esophageal substitute, a barium enema examination should be done for assessment of the suitability of the colon for esophageal replacement, and the colon should be prepared in the event that a colonic interposition is required.

SELECTED REFERENCES FOR PARTS I TO VI

Delarue, N. C., Wilkins, E. W., Jr., and Wong, J. (Eds.): Esophageal cancer. *In* International Trends in General Thoracic Surgery. Vol. 4. St. Louis, C. V. Mosby Company, 1988.
With 53 chapters contributed by internationally known authorities in the field, this volume provides a comprehensive overview of the current status of esophageal carcinoma—its epidemiology, the latest diagnostic techniques, staging criteria, pathologic considerations, surgical treatment, postoperative complications, results of multimodality therapy and management of unresectable tumors. The majority of the chapters are followed by brief discussions by authors presenting alternative or additional points of view. This is an up-to-date and all-inclusive reference on the subject of esophageal cancer.

DeMeester, T. R., and Matthews, H. R.: Benign esophageal disease. *In* International Trends in General Thoracic Surgery. Vol. 3. St. Louis, C. V. Mosby Company, 1987.
In the format of International Trends, *this volume on benign esophageal disease contains 26 chapters that span the topics of esophageal physiology, diagnostic techniques, gastroesophageal reflux, reflux strictures and chemical injuries, motility disorders, and upper esophageal diverticula and strictures. Contributing authors are authoritative and present widely varying views that only emphasize that there is no "one right way" to manage many of these complex esophageal problems.*

Henderson, R. D.: The Esophagus: Reflux and Primary Motor Disorders. Baltimore, Williams & Wilkins, 1980.
This monograph provides a modern surgical approach to motor disorders of the esophagus based on detailed manometric and physiologic studies that are well explained and illustrated throughout. Representative case histories, roentgenograms, and illustrations of surgical technique are presented. The clarity and precision of this work are a tribute to the author, whose untimely death occurred in 1989.

Jamieson, G. G. (Ed.): Surgery of the Oesophagus. Edinburgh, Churchill Livingstone, 1988.
This authoritative new textbook achieves its goal: to be an encyclopedic reference on the topic of surgery of the esophagus. The book is a compendium of 105 chapters covering every conceivable aspect of surgical diseases of the esophagus and written by recognized experts in the field. It is perhaps the most comprehensive such text of its kind ever written.

Siewert, J. R., and Holscher, A. H. (Eds.): Diseases of the Esophagus. Berlin, Springer-Verlag, 1988.
This book represents the proceedings of the third triennial congress of the International Society for Diseases of the Esophagus (ISDE), which was held in Munich during International Esophageal Week in September 1986. During this meeting, world leaders in the field of esophageal disease assembled to discuss the most recent advances in their respective areas of expertise. From molecular biology to vital staining, endoscopic ultrasound, multimodality therapy for esophageal cancer, techniques of anastomotic reconstruction—every facet of benign esophageal disease as well as carcinoma—the papers presented here are by necessity brief, but they represent a panorama of the field of esophageal disease as it is being investigated and treated through the world today.

Spechler, S. J., and Goyal, R. K. (Eds.): Barrett's Esophagus: Pathophysiology, Diagnosis, and Management. New York, Elsevier, 1985.
Growing interest in the subject of the columnar cell-lined esophagus on the part of a wide variety of medical and surgical specialists and cell biologists prompted a national symposium on Barrett's esophagus, which was held at the Boston Veterans Administration Medical Center on January 30, 1984. This book is a compilation of the vast amount of material that was presented at this meeting by the 20 speakers and other participants present. It is perhaps one of the most authoritative texts on the subject, with contributions by well-known gastrointestinal pathologists, gastroenterologists, gastrointestinal physiologists, cell biologists, and surgeons. It is an excellent reference text that is clearly written and easily understood by students of surgery at all levels of training.

REFERENCES

1. Akakura, I., Nakamaura, Y., and Kakegaga, T.: Surgery of carcinoma of the esophagus with preoperative radiation. Chest, 57:47, 1970.
2. Akiyama, H., Hiyama, M.: A simple esophageal bypass operation by the high gastric division. Surgery, 75:674, 1974.
3. Akiyama, H., Kogure, T., and Itai, Y.: Role of esophagotomy in the surgical treatment of esophageal cancer. Int. Surg., 59:478, 1974.
4. Akiyama, H., Tsurumaru, M., Kawamura, T., and Ono, Y.: Principles of surgical treatment for carcinoma of the esophagus: analysis of lymph node involvement. Ann. Surg., 194:438, 1981.
5. Akiyama, S., Sakamoto, J., Suyama, M., Imaizumi, M., Ichihashi, H., and Kondo, T.: Esophageal cyst: A case report and a review of the literature. Jpn. J. Surg., 10:338, 1980.
6. Appelquist, P., and Salmo, M.: Lye corrosion carcinoma of the esophagus. Cancer, 45:2655, 1980.
7. Arbona, J. L., Fazzi, J. G. F., and Mayoral, J.: Congenital esophageal cysts: Case report and review of the literature. Am. J. Gastroenterol., 79:177, 1984.
8. Arnorsson, T., Aberg, C., and Torkel, A.: Benign tumors of the oesophagus and oesophageal cysts. Scand. J. Thorac. Cardiovasc. Surg., 18:145, 1984.
9. Bakamijan, V. Y.: A two-stage method of pharyngoesophageal reconstruction with a medially based primary pectoral flap. Plast. Reconstruct. Surg., 36:173, 1965.
10. Balthazar, E. J., Goldfine, S., and Davidian, M. M.: Carcinoma of the esophagogastric junction. Am. J. Gastroenterol., 74:237, 1980.
11. Beahrs, O. H., Henson, D. E., Hutter, R. V. P., and Myers, M. H.: Manual for Staging of Cancer, 3rd ed. American Joint Committee on Cancer. Philadelphia, J. B. Lippincott Company, 1988, pp. 63–67.
12. Beck, C., and Carrell, A.: Demonstration of specimens illustrating a method of formation of a prethoracic esophagus. Ill. Med. J., 7:463, 1905.
13. Bernstein, J. M., and Juler, G. L.: Colon interposition versus esophagogastrostomy for esophageal carcinoma. Am. Surg., 46:216, 1980.
14. Borst, H. G., Dragojevic, D., Stegmann, T., and Hetzer, R.: Anastomotic leakage, stenosis, and reflux after esophageal replacement. World J. Surg., 2:861, 1978.
15. Bower, R. J., Sieber, W. K., and Kiesewetter, W. B.: Alimentary tract duplication in children. Ann. Surg., 188:669, 1978.
16. Burdette, W. J.: Palliative operation for carcinoma of cervical and thoracic esophagus. Ann. Surg., 173:714, 1971.
17. Burgess, H. M., Baggenstoss, A. H., Moersch, H. J., et al.: Carcinoma of the esophagus: Clinicopathologic study. Surg. Clin. North Am., 31:965, 1951.
18. Cameron, A. J., Ott, B. J., and Payne, W. S.: The incidence of adenocarcinoma in columnar-lined (Barrett's) esophagus. N. Engl. J. Med., 313(14):857, 1985.
19. Carey, R. W., Hilgenberg, A. D., Wilkins, E. W., Choi, N. C., Mathisen, D. J.,

and Grillo, H.: Preoperative chemotherapy followed by surgery with possible postoperative radiotherapy in squamous cell carcinoma of the esophagus: Evaluation of the chemotherapy component. J. Clin. Oncol., 4:697, 1986.

20. Carter, R., and Brewer, L. A.: Achalasia and esophageal carcinoma: studies in early diagnosis for improved surgical management. Am. J. Surg., 130:114, 1975.
21. Celestin, L. R.: Improvements in the Celestin tube for endoesophageal intubation in carcinoma and strictures. Armamentarium, 5:10, 1969.
22. Chalkiadakis, G., Wihlm, J. M., Morand, G., Weill-Bousson, M., and Witz, J. P.: Primary malignant melanoma of the esophagus. Ann. Thorac. Surg., 39:472, 1985.
23. Coonley, C. J., Bains, M., Holaris, B., Chapman, K., and Kelsen, D. P.: Cisplatin and bleomycin in the treatment of esophageal carcinoma. Cancer, 54:2351, 1984.
24. DeBesi, P., Salvagno, L., Endrizzi, L., et al.: Cisplatin, bleomycin and methotrexate in the treatment of advanced esophageal cancer. Eur. J. Cancer Clin. Oncol., 20:743, 1984.
25. Doll, R., Payne, P., and Waterhouse, J.: Cancer Incidence in Five Continents: A Technical Report. New York, Springer-Verlag, 1966.
26. Dor, J., Nioclerc, M., Chauvin, G., et al.: Esophagoplasty with the retrosternal transverse colon: Results and comments. Ann. Chir., 32:111, 1978. In International Abstracts in Surgery, 148:131, 1979.
27. Duranceau, A.: Epidemiologic trends and etiologic factors of esophageal carcinoma. In Delarue, N. C., Wilkins, E. W., Jr., and Wong, J. (Eds.): International Trends in General Thoracic Surgery. Vol. 4, Esophageal Cancer. St. Louis, C. V. Mosby Company, 1988, pp. 3–10.
28. Earlam, R., and Cunha-Melo, J. R.: Malignant oesophageal strictures: a review of techniques for palliative intubation. Br. J. Surg., 69:61, 1982.
29. Earlam, R., and Cunha-Melo, J. R.: Oesophageal squamous cell carcinoma. I. A critical review of surgery. Br. J. Surg., 67:381, 1980.
30. Earlam, R., and Cunha-Melo, J. R.: Oesophageal squamous cell carcinoma. II. A critical review of radiotherapy. Br. J. Surg., 67:457, 1980.
31. El-Domeiri, A., Martini, N., and Beattie, E. J., Jr.: Esophageal reconstruction by colon interposition. Arch. Surg., 199:358, 1970.
32. Ellis, F. H., Jr.: Carcinoma of the esophagus. Cancer, 33:264, 1983.
33. Ellis, F. H., Jr., and Gibb, S. P.: Esophagogastrectomy for carcinoma: current hospital mortality and morbidity rates. Ann. Surg., 190:699, 1979.
34. Enterline, H., Thompson, J.: Pathology of the Esophagus. Springer-Verlag, New York, 1984.
35. Epstein, J. I., Sears, D. L., Tucker, R. S., Eagan, J. W.: Carcinoma of the esophagus with adenoid cystic differentiation. Cancer, 53:1131, 1984.
36. Eruster, V. L., Selvin, S., Sacks, S. T., Merrill, D. W., and Holly, E. A.: Major histologic types of cancers of the gum and mouth, esophagus, larynx and lung by sex and by income level. J. Natl. Cancer Inst., 69:773, 1982.
37. Fell, S. C., Yrunwald, R. P., and Hurwitt, E. S.: Palliation of esophageal carcinoma by prosthetic intubation. J. Thorac. Cardiovasc. Surg., 51:272, 1966.
38. Fisher, E. R., and Wechsler, H.: Granular cell myoblastoma-a misnomer: Electron microscopic and histochemical evidence concerning its Schwann cell derivation and nature (granular cell schwannoma). Cancer, 15:936, 1962.
39. Forastiere, A. A., Gennis, M., Orringer, M. B., et al.: Cisplatin, vinblastine, and mitoguazone chemotherapy for epidermoid and adenocarcinoma of the esophagus. J. Clin. Oncol., 5:1143, 1987.
40. Gavriliu, D.: Aspects of esophageal surgery. Curr. Probl. Surg., 12(10), 1975.
41. Giradet, R. E., Ransdell, H. T., Jr., and Wheat, M. W., Jr.: Palliative intubation in the management of esophageal carcinoma (collective review) Ann. Thorac. Surg., 18:417, 1974.
42. Giuli, R., and Gignoux, M.: Treatment of carcinoma of the esophagus: retrospective study of 2400 patients. Ann. Surg., 192:44, 1980.
43. Goffman, T. E., McKeen, E. A., Curtis, R. E., and Schein, P. S.: Esophageal carcinoma following irradiation for breast carcinoma. Cancer, 53:1080, 1983.
44. Griffiths, J. D., and Shaw, H. J.: Cancer of the laryngopharynx and cervical esophagus: Radical resection with repair by colon transplant. Arch. Otolaryngol., 97:340, 1973.
45. Grillo, H. C., Mathisen, D. J.: Cervical exenteration. Ann. Thorac. Surg., 49:401, 1990.
46. Gross, R. E., Holcomb, G. W., Farber, S.: Duplication of the alimentary tract. Pediatrics, 9:444, 1952.
47. Guanrei, Y., He, H., Sungliang, Q., and Yuming, C.: Endoscopic diagnosis of 115 cases of early esophageal carcinoma. Endoscopy, 14:157–61, 1982.
48. Hankins, J. R., and McLaughlin, J. S.: The association of carcinoma of the esophagus with achalasia. J. Thorac. Cardiovasc. Surg., 69:355, 1975.
49. Harrington, S. W.: Surgical treatment of benign and secondarily malignant tumors of the esophagus. Arch. Surg., 58:646, 1949.
50. Heck, H. A., and Rossi, N. P.: Esophageal and gastroesophageal junction carcinoma: an evolved philosophy of management. Cancer, 46:1873, 1980.
51. Heimlich, H. J.: Carcinoma of the cervical esophagus. J. Thorac. Cardiovasc. Surg., 59:309, 1970.
52. Hester, T. R., McConnel, F. M. S., Nahai, F., Jurkiewicz, M. H., and Brown, R. G.: Reconstruction of cervical esophagus, hypopharynx, and oral cavity using free jejunal transfer. Am. J. Surg., 140:487, 1980.
53. Hinderleider, C. D., Aguam, A. S., and Wilder, J. R.: Carcinosarcoma of the esophagus: A case report and review of the literature. Int. Surg., 64:13, 1979.
54. Johnston, J., and Helwig, E. B.: Granular cell tumors of the gastrointestinal tract and perianal region. Dig. Dis. Sci., 26:802, 1981.

55. Jurkiewicz, M. J.: Reconstruction surgery of the cervical esophagus. J. Thorac. Cardiovasc. Surg., 88:893, 1984.
56. Kabuto, T., Taniguchi, K., Iwanaga, T., Terasawa, T., Tateishi, R., and Taniguchi, H.: Diffuse leiomyomatosis of the esophagus. Dig. Dis. Sci., 25:388, 1980.
57. Kelsen, D. P., Bains, M., Hilaris, B., et al.: Combination chemotherapy of esophageal carcinoma using cisplatin, vindesine, and bleomycin. Cancer, 49:1147, 1982.
58. Kobayashi, S., Prolla, J. C., Winans, C. S., et al.: Improved endoscopic diagnosis of gastroesophageal malignancy: Combined use of direct vision brushing cytology and biopsy. J.A.M.A., 212:2086, 1970.
59. Kolaric, K., Maricic, Z., Roth, A., and Dujmovic, I.: Chemotherapy versus chemoradiotherapy in inoperable esophageal cancer. Results of three controlled studies. Oncology, 37: (Suppl. 1):77, 1980.
60. Leichman, L., Steiger, Z., Seydel, H. G., et al.: Preoperative chemotherapy and radiation therapy for patients with cancer of the esophagus: A potentially curative approach. J. Clin. Oncol., 2:75, 1984.
61. Lortat-Jacob, J. L.: Localized myomas and diffuse myomas of the esophagus. [In French.] Arch. Mal. Appl. Dig., 39:519, 1950.
62. Mackler, S. A., and Mayer, R. M.: Palliation of esophageal obstruction due to carcinoma with a permanent intraluminal tube. J. Thorac. Surg., 28:431, 1954.
63. Mandard, A. M., Marnay, J., Gignoux, M., et al.: Cancer of the esophagus and associated lesions: Detailed pathologic study of 100 esophagectomy specimens. Hum. Pathol., 15:660, 1984.
64. Martini, N., Goodner, J. T., D'Angio, G. J., et al.: Tracheoesophageal fistula due to cancer. J. Thorac. Cardiovasc. Surg., 59:319, 1970.
65. Mathisen, D. J., Grillo, H. C., Wilkins, E. W., Moncure, A. C., and Hilgenberg, A. D.: Transthoracic esophagectomy: a safe approach to carcinoma of the esophagus. Ann. Thorac. Surg., 45:137, 1988.
66. McKeown, K. C.: Total three-stage oesophagectomy for cancer of the oesophagus. Br. J. Surg., 63:259, 1976.
67. Miller, C.: Carcinoma of thoracic esophagus and cardia. Br. J. Surg., 49:507, 1962.
68. Mills, S. E., and Cooper, P. H.: Malignant melanoma of the digestive system. Pathol. Ann., 18(2):1, 1983.
69. Milson, J., Unger, S., Alford, B. A., and Rodgers, B. M.: Triplication of the esophagus with gastric duplication. Surgery, 98:121, 1985.
70. Moersch, H. J., and Harrington, S. W.: Benign tumors of the esophagus. Ann. Otol. Rhinol. Laryngol., 52:800, 1944.
71. Mousseau, M., Leforestier, J., Barbin, J., et al.: Place de L'intubation a demeure dans le traitement palliatif du cancer de l'oesophage. Arch. Fr. Mal. App. Dig., 45:208, 1956.
72. Naef, A. P., Savary, M., and Ozzello, L.: Columnar-lined lower esophagus: An acquired lesion with malignant predisposition. J. Thorac. Cardiovasc. Surg., 70:826, 1975.
73. Nakayama, K., and Kinoshita, Y.: Surgical treatment combined with preoperative concentrated irradiation. J.A.M.A., 227:178, 1974.
74. Nicks, R.: Colonic replacement of the oesophagus: Some observations on infarction and wound healing. Br. J. Surg., 54:124, 1967.
75. Ong, G. B.: Resection and reconstruction of the esophagus. Curr. Probl. Surg., 3–56, September 1971.
76. Orringer, M. B.: Partial median sternotomy: Anterior approach to the upper thoracic esophagus. J. Thorac. Cardiovasc. Surg., 87:124, 1984.
77. Orringer, M. B.: Substernal gastric bypass of the excluded esophagus: Results of an ill-advised operation. Surgery, 96:467, 1984.
78. Orringer, M. B.: Transhiatal esophagectomy without thoracotomy for carcinoma of the thoracic esophagus. Ann. Surg., 200:282, 1984.
79. Orringer, M. B., Forastiere, A. A., Perez-Tamayo, C., et al.: Chemotherapy and radiation therapy before transhiatal esophagectomy for esophageal carcinoma. Ann. Thorac. Surg., 49:348, 1990.
80. Orringer, M. B., and Orringer, J. S.: Transhiatal esophagectomy without thoracotomy: A dangerous operation? J. Thorac. Cardiovasc. Surg., 85:72, 1983.
81. Orringer, M. B., and Sloan, H.: Anterior mediastinal tracheostomy: Indications, techniques, and clinical experience. J. Thorac. Cardiovasc. Surg., 78:850, 1979.
82. Orringer, M. B., and Sloan, H.: Esophagectomy without thoracotomy. J. Thorac. Cardiovasc. Surg., 76:643, 1978.
83. Orringer, M. B., and Sloan, H.: Substernal gastric bypass of the excluded thoracic esophagus for palliation of esophageal carcinoma. J. Thorac. Cardiovasc. Surg., 70:836, 1975.
84. Palchick, B. A., Alpert, M. A., Holmes, R. A., Tully, R. J., and Wilson, R. C.: Esophageal hemangioma: Diagnosis with computed tomography and radionuclide angiography. South. Med. J., 76:1582, 1983.
85. Parker, E. F., and Gregorie, H. B., Jr.: Carcinoma of the esophagus: Long-term results. J.A.M.A., 235:1018, 1976.
86. Parker, E. F., Gregorie, H. B., Jr., Arrants, J. E., et al.: Carcinoma of the esophagus. Ann. Surg., 171:746, 1970.
87. Patel, R. M., DeSota-LaPaix, F., Sika, J. V., Mallaiah, L. R., and Purow, E.: Granular cell tumor of the esophagus. Am. J. Gastroenterol., 76:519, 1981.
88. Payne, W. S., and Olsen, A. M.: The Esophagus. Philadelphia, Lea & Febiger, 1974, pp. 229–232.
89. Pearson, J. G.: Radiotherapy of carcinoma of the oesophagus and postcricoid region in southeast Scotland. Clin. Radiol., 17:242, 1966.
90. Pierce, W. S., MacVaughn, H., Johnson, J.: Carcinoma of the esophagus

arising in patients with achalasia of the cardia. J. Thorac. Cardiovasc. Surg., 59:335, 1970.

91. Plachta, A.: Benign tumors of the esophagus: Review of the literature and report of 99 cases. Am. J. Gastroenterol., 38:639, 1962.

92. Postlethwait, R. W.: Benign tumors and cysts of the esophagus. Surg. Clin. North Am., 63:925, 1983.

93. Postlethwait, R. W.: Complications and deaths after operations for esophageal carcinoma. J. Thorac. Cardiovasc. Surg., 85:827, 1983.

94. Postlethwait, R. W.: Surgery of the Esophagus. Norwalk, Conn., Appleton-Century-Crofts, 1979.

95. Postlethwait, R. W.: Technique for isoperistaltic gastric tubes for esophagus bypass. Ann. Surg., 189:673, 1979.

96. Postlethwait, R. W., Sealy, W. C., and Dillon, W. L.: Colon interposition for esophageal substitution. Ann. Thorac. Surg., 12:89, 1971.

97. Raptis, S., and Mearns-Milne, D.: A review of the management of 100 cases of benign strictures of the esophagus. Thorax, 27:599, 1972.

98. Reid, H. A. S., Richardson, W. W., and Corrin, B.: Oat cell carcinoma of the esophagus. Cancer, 45:2342, 1980.

99. Riddel, R. H.: Dysplasia and regression in Barrett's epithelium. In Spechler, S. J., and Goyal, R. K. (Eds.): Barrett's Esophagus—Pathophysiology, Diagnosis, and Management. New York, Elsevier, 1985, pp. 143–153.

100. Sarr, M. G., Hamilton, S. R., Marrone, G. C., and Cameron, J. L.: Barrett's esophagus: Its prevalence and association with adenocarcinoma in patients with symptoms of gastroesophageal reflux. Am. J. Surg., 149:187, 1985.

101. Scanlon, E. F., Morton, D. R., and Walker, J. M.: The case against segmental resection for esophageal carcinoma. Surg. Gynecol. Obstet., 101:290, 1955.

102. Schmidt, H. W., Clagett, O. T., and Harrison, E. G., Jr.: Benign tumors and cysts of the esophagus. J. Thorac. Cardiovasc. Surg., 41:717, 1961.

103. Schwindt, W. D., Bernhardt, L. C., and Johnson, S. A. M.: Tylosis and intra-thoracic neoplasms. Chest, 57:590, 1970.

104. Seidenberg, B., Rosenak, S. S., and Hurwitt, E. S.: Immediate reconstruction of the cervical esophagus by a revascularized isolated jejunal segment. Ann. Surg., 149:162, 1959.

105. Seiffert, E., Borst, H. H., Ostertag, H., Stender, H., Braschke, M., and Misaki, F.: Carcinoma in situ of the esophagus (early esophageal cancer). Endoscopy, 5:147, 1973.

106. Seremetis, M. G., Lyons, W. S., DeGuzman, V. C., and Peabody, J. W.: Leiomyomata of the esophagus. Cancer, 38:2166, 1976.

107. Sherrill, D. J., Grishkin, B. A., Galal, F. S., Zajtchuk, R., and Graeber, G. M.: Radiation associated malignancies of the esophagus. Cancer, 54:726, 1984.

108. Shirakabe, H., Yamaki, G., Maruyama, T., and Nishizawa, M.: Radiologic patterns of early esophageal cancer. In Delarue, N. C., Wilkins, E. W., Jr., and Wong, J., (Eds.): International Trends in General Thoracic Surgery. Vol. 4, Esophageal Cancer. St. Louis, C. V. Mosby Company, 1988, pp. 19–24.

109. Shuy, J.: Cytopathology of the esophagus: An overview of esophageal cytopathology in China. Acta. Cytol. (Baltimore), 27:7, 1983.

110. Sjogren, R. W., Jr., and Johnson, L. F.: Barrett's esophagus: A review. Am. J. Surg., 74:313, 1983.

111. Skinner, D. B.: En bloc resection for neoplasm of the esophagus and cardia. J. Thorac. Cardiovasc. Surg., 85:59, 1983.

112. Skinner, D. B.: Esophageal reconstruction. Am. J. Surg., 139:810, 1980.

113. Skinner, D. B., Ferguson, M. K., Soriano, A., Little, A. G., and Staszak, V. M.: Selection of operation for esophageal cancer based on staging. Ann. Surg., 204:391, 1986.

114. Skinner, D. B., Walther, B. C., Riddell, R. H., Schmidt, H., Iascone, C., and DeMeester, T. R.: Barrett's esophagus: A comparison of benign and malignant cases. Ann. Surg., 198:554, 1983.

115. Skucas, J., and Schrank, W. W.: The routine air-contrast examination of the esophagus. Radiology, 115:482, 1975.

116. Smith, J., and Payne, W. S.: Surgical technique for management of reflux esophagitis after esophagogastrectomy for malignancy: Further application of Roux-en-Y principle. Mayo Clon. Proc., 50:588, 1975.

117. Souttar, H. S.: A method of intubating the oesophagus for in indigent stricture. Br. Med. J., 1:782, 1924.

118. Spechler, J. S., Robbins, A. H., Robbins, H. B., Vincent, M. E., Heeren, T., Doos, W. G., Colton, W. G., and Schimmel, E. M.: Adenocarcinoma and Barrett's esophagus: An overrated risk? Gastroenterol., 87:927, 1984.

119. Steiger, Z., Franklin, R., Wilson, R. F., et al.: Eradication and palliation of squamous cell carcinoma of the esophagus with chemotherapy, radiotherapy, and surgical therapy. J. Thorac. Cardiovasc. Surg., 82:713, 1981.

120. Stout, A. P., and Lattes, R.: Tumors of the Esophagus. In Atlas of Tumor Pathology, Fascicle 29. Washington, D.C., Armed Forces Institute of Pathology, 1957.

121. Suzuki, H., Kobayashi, S., Endo, M., et al.: Diagnosis of early esophageal cancer. Surgery, 71:99, 1972.

122. Swerdlow, M. A., Berry, L. R., and Edwards, A.: Pseudoepitheliomatous hyperplasia associated with myoblastoma: a diagnostic pitfall. U.S. Armed Forces Med. J., 5:831, 1954.

123. Tanoue, S., Shimoda, T., Suzuki, M., Ikegami, M., Ishikawa, E., and Sano, T.: Anaplastic carcinoma of the esophagus. Acta. Pathol. Jpn., 33(4):831, 1983.

124. Tarnay, T. J., Chang, C. H., Nugent, R. G., et al.: Esophageal duplication (foregut cyst) with spinal malfunction. J. Thorac. Cardiovasc. Surg., 59:293, 1970.

125. Tateishi, R., Taniesuchi, H., Wada, A., Horai, T., and Taniguchi, K.: Argyrophil cells and melanocytes in esophageal mucosa. Arch. Pathol., 98:87, 1974.

126. Thompson, W. M.: Esophageal cancer. Int. J. Radiat. Oncol. Biol. Phys., 9:1533, 1983.

127. Thurston, S. E., and Lenn, N. J.: The association of spinal and gastroesophageal anomalies. Clin. Pediatr., 23:652, 1984.

128. Tio, T. L., and Tytgat, G. N. J.: Atlas of Transintestinal Ultrasonography. Smith, Kline and French. Drukkerij Mur-Kostuerloren B. V., Aalsmeer, The Netherlands, 1986.

129. Tytgat, G. N.: Non-radiological investigation of the oesophagus. In Watson, A., and Celestin, L. R. (Eds.): Disorders of the Oesophagus: Advances and Controversies. London, Pitman, 1984, pp. 24–36.

130. Uemichi, A., Invi, K., Onchi, K., et al.: Reconstruction of the cervical esophagus by transplantation and revascularization of a small intestinal segment: 10-year follow-up. Surgery, 81:343, 1977.

131. Vinayeh, R., and Levin, B. Endoscopic diagnosis. In DeMeester, T. R., and Levin, B., (Eds.): Cancer of the Esophagus. New York, Grune & Stratton, 1985, pp. 43–55.

132. Vogl, S. E., Camacho, F., Berenzweig, M., and Ruckdesch, J.: Chemotherapy for oesophageal cancer with mitoguazone, methotrexate, bleomycin and cisplatin. Cancer Treat. Rep., 69:21, 1985.

133. Watson, R. R., O'Connor, T. M., and Weisel, W.: Solid benign tumors of the esophagus (collective review). Ann. Thorac. Surg., 4:80, 1967.

134. Webb, J. N., and Busuttil, A.: Adenocarcinoma of the oesophagogastric junction. Br. J. Surg., 65:475, 1978.

135. Weiss, L. M., Fogelman, D., and Warhit, J. M.: CT demonstration of an esophageal duplication cyst. J. Comput. Assist. Tomogr., 7(4):716, 1983.

136. Whitaker, J. A., Deffenbaugh, L. D., and Cooke, A. R.: Esophageal duplication cyst. Am. J. Gastroenterol., 73:329, 1980.

137. Wilkins, E. W., Jr.: Long-segment colon substitution for the esophagus. Ann. Surg., 192:722, 1980.

138. Wookey, H.: Surgical treatment of carcinoma of the pharynx and upper esophagus. Surg. Gynecol. Obstet., 75:499, 1942.

139. Xu, L., Sun, C., Wu, L., Chang, Z., and Liu, T.: Clinical and pathological characteristics of carcinosarcoma of the esophagus: Report of four cases. Ann. Thorac. Surg., 37:197, 1984.

140. Zardawi, I. M., and Talbot, I. C.: Primary adenoid cystic carcinoma of the oesophagus. Diagn. Histopathol., 6:39, 1983.

VII _____

PERFORATION OF THE ESOPHAGUS: SPONTANEOUS (BOERHAAVE'S SYNDROME), TRAUMATIC, AND FOLLOWING ESOPHAGOSCOPY

David B. Skinner, M.D.

Rupture of the esophagus, an uncommon condition, is a difficult clinical problem. It can be an unexpected cause of rapid death in otherwise healthy individuals, is often difficult to diagnose, and continues to be a challenging surgical problem. Spontaneous rupture of a normal esophagus was first reported under dramatic circumstances by Boerhaave in 1704 in the Netherlands. In Meade's *A History of Thoracic Surgery,*[10] Van Swieten is cited as providing the first English language description of Boerhaave's observation: ". . . the illustrious Baron Wassenaer, Lord High Admiral to the Republick, after intense straining in vomiting, broke asunder the tube of the esophagus, near the diaphragm, so that after the most excruciating pains, the aliments which he swallowed passed, together with the air, into the cavity of the thorax, and he expired in 24 hours."

Pathophysiology

Compared with the incidence of esophageal rupture, spontaneous or instrumental perforation of other portions of the normal alimentary tract is unusual. Consideration of the causes for this difference provides guidance to understanding and management. The esophagus differs from the remainder of the alimentary tract in having no serosal layer. Both serosal and submucosal layers containing collagen and elastic fibers provide strength to the gut wall. The absence of serosa in the esophagus makes it more likely to rupture at lower pressures than the rest of the gut. The distal esophagus lies immediately beneath the left thoracic pleura, and the middle esophagus lies beneath the right pleura. As pressures in the thoracic cavities are less than atmospheric, the gradient across the esophageal wall is greater than intraluminal esophageal pressure. Ruptures of the lower esophagus usually perforate into the left thoracic cavity, and ruptures of the mid esophagus perforate into the right thoracic cavity. There are no surrounding soft tissues to buttress the esophagus in these locations. The esophagus must periodically adjust to rapid forced increases in diameter. During vomiting, the lower esophagus almost momentarily increases in diameter by five times or more.[4] Swallowing of a large bolus requires rapid increase in the esophageal lumen. This combination of factors—the absence of serosa, a pressure gradient across the esophageal wall caused by negative intrathoracic pressures, and the need for rapid dilatation during vomiting and ingestion—provides the setting in which rupture of the esophagus is likely to occur.

Classification and Incidence

Perforations of the esophagus are classified according to etiology and location. The incidence of perforation following a particular cause varies depending on the patient population treated by the reporting hospital or physician. The etiologic classification is listed in Table 1. Commonly recognized categories include spontaneous rupture, instrumental perforation, traumatic perforation, and perforation of intrinsic esophageal disease. Spontaneous or strain-induced rupture occurs less commonly than traumatic or instrumental perforations. Rup-

tures in 22 of 115 patients reported by Nesbitt and Sawyers,[13] in 16 of 68 esophageal perforations described by Rosoff and White,[18] and 8 of 72 from the Massachusetts General Hospital experience[11] occurred spontaneously in a normal esophagus. In these reports, the incidence of spontaneous esophageal rupture was approximately 1 in each 75,000 hospital admissions. Large experiences with strain-induced perforations have been presented by Abbott and co-workers[1] and by Pate and associates.[15] About 90 per cent of ruptures occur in the lower third of the esophagus.

Instrumental perforations of the esophagus may occur during esophagoscopy, esophageal dilatation, the passage of upper alimentary tract tubes, or attempted endotracheal intubation.[5] The risk of perforation during esophagoscopy is approximately 2 per 1000 procedures.[11,19] The incidence is less when the flexible fiberoptic esophagoscope is used routinely, but this does not eliminate the problem of instrumental perforation.[12] Factors that contribute to the frequency of endoscopic perforation include the type and effectiveness of anesthesia, and failure to deflate an endotracheal tube cuff if present. The risk is greater in elderly patients suffering from cervical arthritis.

Instrumental perforation may occur at any level, but it is most common just above the cardia and in the cervical esophagus. Spasm or hypertrophy of the cricopharyngeal sphincter in addition to arthritic vertebral osteophytes explains the frequency of cervical perforations, and the forward and left lateral bend of the distal esophagus contributes to perforation at the lower end. Perforation is also likely to occur at the level of intrinsic esophageal disease. When inflammation or neoplasm has penetrated the submucosa, the strength of the esophageal wall is markedly decreased. Accordingly, patients undergoing esophagoscopy or dilatation are routinely warned of this potential danger, and they must be evaluated shortly following the procedure so that perforation may be detected promptly when it occurs.

Traumatic disruption of the esophagus may be subdivided into five additional categories. Perforations following penetrat-

TABLE 1. Causes of Esophageal Perforation

Spontaneous or strain-induced
Instrumental
    Esophagoscopy
    Dilatation
    Intubation
Traumatic
    Penetrating missile
    Foreign body swallowed
    Blunt chest or abdominal injury
    Surgical dissection
    Ingested caustic agents
Intrinsic esophageal disease
    Carcinoma
    Acid-peptic ulceration
    Anastomotic
    Other

ing wounds of the neck, chest, or abdomen are reported with increasing frequency in recent years, particularly in urban hospitals. In some reports the incidence of these injuries is the highest for all causes.[17,18] The level of the injury depends on the location of the penetrating wound. Rupture of the esophagus from nonpenetrating external trauma is uncommon but must be considered following blows to the chest or upper abdomen. Ingestion of foreign bodies is responsible for a small number of esophageal perforations. These are at the levels at which foreign bodies commonly lodge—the cervical region just below the cricopharyngeal sphincter, the level of the aortic arch, and the distal esophagus just above the cardia. Ingestion of corrosive agents, especially lye, may cause perforation of the esophagus in severe cases. The fifth category of traumatic esophageal perforation follows surgical dissection around the esophagus in the course of other operations. The incidence of esophageal perforation during the performance of abdominal vagotomy is estimated at approximately 0.5 per cent.[24] Esophageal perforation may occur in the course of hiatal hernia repair or other procedures involving esophageal dissection.[20] Perforation of the cervical esophagus during anterior spinal fusion is reported.

Rupture of the esophagus may occur as a complication of primary esophageal disease. Carcinoma of the esophagus may penetrate full thickness through the esophageal wall and cause a mediastinal or pleural cavity perforation. Benign esophageal ulcerations, particularly penetrating gastric ulcers in distal esophagus lined with columnar epithelium, may perforate completely through the esophageal wall. The location of such perforations depends on the level of the intrinsic disease.

Symptoms

Symptoms of esophageal rupture are usually dramatic and signal a catastrophic event. Death may occur within 24 hours in untreated cases. Early collapse of the patient is common. Pain related to the level of perforation is almost a universal complaint. As in the case of Admiral Wassenaer, this is generally severe and of such intensity and distribution that it may mimic the abdominal pain of a perforated gastroduodenal ulcer or severe pancreatitis, and the chest pain of dissection of the aorta or myocardial infarction. Nausea is a common complaint. Vomiting may precede the onset of pain in cases of spontaneous rupture, but disruption of the normal esophagus can occur without prior vomiting.[16] Emesis following the onset of pain often contains blood. Hematemesis and pain also occur following forceful vomiting in the Mallory-Weiss syndrome in which the mucosal laceration is on the stomach side of the cardia, where complete disruption is rare.[9] Evidence of perforation is not part of this syndrome. When a strain-induced tear occurs below the cardia, bleeding rather than perforation is the dominant feature. The reverse is true for tears above the cardia. If perforation occurs into the pleural cavity with resulting pneumohydrothorax, the respiratory symptoms predominate—dyspnea, cyanosis, air hunger, and other symptoms related to a collapsed lung and possible tension pneumothorax.

Physical Findings

Usually fever develops shortly after the onset of pain, and the patient rapidly becomes acutely ill. An early change in vital signs, tachycardia, tachypnea, and hypotension, and clinical evidence of shock are common. When the perforation is limited to the mediastinal tissues, rales in the lung bases are frequently heard. The sound of air in the mediastinum crackling with each heart beat while the patient holds his breath is occasionally present. This is called the *mediastinal crunch sound of Hamman*. More extensive mediastinal emphysema is palpable as crepitus at the base of the neck. In time, this may extend to cause subcutaneous emphysema over the chest wall and neck. If the perforation has penetrated the pleural cavity, findings include those of pneumothorax and pleural effusion. Absence of breath

sounds is observed on the affected side, with dullness to percussion over the lower thoracic cavity and a normal or increased percussion note in the upper chest. Evidence of tension pneumothorax with tracheal shift and limited excursion of the hemithorax occurs in severe cases. In addition to the chest findings, patients with thoracic perforations may have spasm, guarding, and tenderness of the upper abdomen and may complain of abdominal pain. An ileus may develop rapidly along with gastric distention. Perforations limited to the neck cause much less severe abnormalities, often limited to fever, local tenderness and spasm, and crepitus. Abdominal perforations reveal the findings of an acute abdominal emergency but are frequently accompanied by mediastinal emphysema and lower chest abnormalities as well.

Diagnosis

Unfortunate delays in diagnosis occur when rupture of the esophagus is not suspected and the patient is treated promptly for another incorrect diagnosis such as myocardial infarction, dissecting aortic aneurysm, or perforated abdominal viscus, which may cause similar catastrophic symptoms. When the diagnosis of ruptured esophagus is suspected by analysis of symptoms and physical findings, the confirmation is generally easy. Chest radiograph alone may be diagnostic when a hydropneumothorax is seen combined with air dissecting in the mediastinum. When emphysema is limited to the mediastinum, the chest film findings are more subtle. Mediastinal widening may be prominent (Fig. 1). Air in the mediastinum outlined against the left pleural surface and collapsed lung produces a characteristic shadow behind the heart. This may be accentuated by pneumonitis in the partially collapsed basal segments of the left lower lobe.

Esophageal radiographic contrast studies should be performed promptly. A water-soluble medium such as Gastrogra-

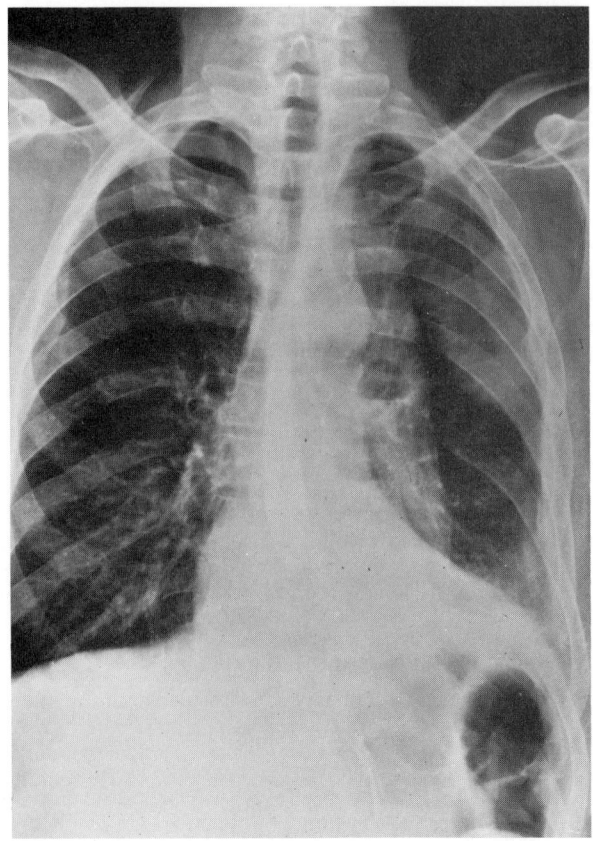

Figure 1. Chest film during a Gastrografin swallow in patient suffering from spontaneous distal esophageal perforation. Notice the mediastinal widening and air-fluid with partial collapse and infiltration of the left lower lobe.

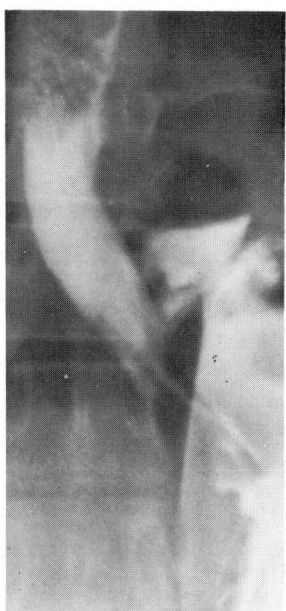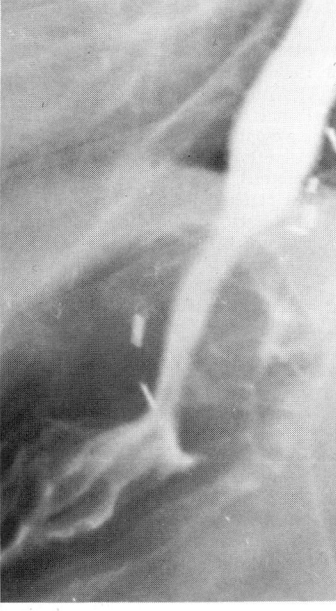

Figure 2. On the left, a Gastrografin swallow demonstrates perforation of the distal esophagus following esophagoscopy. On the right, a postoperative barium swallow demonstrates suture closure of the perforation reinforced by a fundoplication around the distal esophagus.

fin is used initially. If nothing is seen, but the diagnosis is highly suspected, the examination should be repeated with barium (Fig. 2). Even when perforation is obvious by chest radiographs, the esophageal contrast study is essential to document the level and extent of perforation. Generally, an upright abdominal radiograph is taken to exclude the possibility of perforation into the abdomen.

Usual laboratory findings include an elevation in the white blood cell count and hemoconcentration due to fluid loss. Pleural fluid may contain a high amylase level due to swallowed saliva. When the perforation is near the cardia, pleural fluid may be acidic, although neither of these findings is consistent. Serum electrolyte abnormalities and hypoalbuminemia, when present, reflect the duration of the perforation or pre-existing malnutrition, a common problem in alcoholic patients susceptible to esophageal rupture during vomiting. An electrocardiogram is performed to exclude a concomitant myocardial infarction causing a portion of the pain and symptoms. Arterial blood gas determinations provide a useful guide to the severity of pulmonary dysfunction and the progress of resuscitation. The evaluation of the patient with suspected esophageal rupture should require no more than several hours, so that treatment for the correct diagnosis can be undertaken promptly. Only rarely is esophagoscopy necessary to confirm or establish the level of the perforation, but it is useful if underlying esophageal disease such as carcinoma or Barrett's ulcer is suspected.

Treatment

In special circumstances, nonsurgical methods of treating localized esophageal perforations are appropriate and successful.[2] Surgical treatment, however, is usually required for the successful recovery of most patients suffering from this condition. The operative approach depends on the cause and site of the perforation and the time elapsed between the perforation and operation.

CERVICAL PERFORATION. In patients with perforation of the cervical esophagus, limited extravasation, and no thoracic involvement, intensive antibiotic therapy, eliminating oral feeding, and provision of intravenous alimentation are often sufficient treatment. For perforations of the cervical esophagus causing crepitus and dissection of extravasated material in fas-

cial planes, operative drainage coupled with intensive antibiotic therapy is the minimal procedure necessary. If it is possible technically to close the perforation site, this is advantageous. Alternatively, a cervical esophagostomy tube can be inserted through the perforation and led out through a stab wound in the neck to provide drainage and a controlled fistula. With proper treatment, perforations of the cervical esophagus are managed with a low mortality.

THORACIC PERFORATION. Survival following perforation of the thoracic esophagus varies directly with the time interval between perforation and operation. Mortality is 10 to 15 per cent in patients treated in less than 24 hours following injury, whereas the mortality increases up to 50 per cent or more for patients with delayed surgical therapy.[3,11,13]

For the early treatment of spontaneous or instrumental perforation of the esophagus, suture closure of the opening combined with chest drainage is often successful. If adjacent tissue is available to buttress the closure by an onlay patch, this is recommended. The use of adjacent gastric fundus is especially valuable for lower esophageal ruptures. Flaps of diaphragm or adjacent pleura can be placed over the sutured defect.[7]

If perforation is discovered promptly in a patient with an intrinsic esophageal disease and surgical treatment is undertaken early, definitive therapy for the disease is desirable.[20] This may necessitate esophagectomy in patients with carcinoma or stricture, myotomy in patients with achalasia, or an antireflux procedure in patients having reflux esophagitis. Simple closure of a perforation above an obstructing esophageal lesion or in the presence of free acid–peptic reflux cannot be expected to be successful.

When surgical treatment is undertaken late following perforation, operative choices are limited by the dangers of attempting to suture infected and edematous tissues. Nevertheless, aggressive surgical therapy may still salvage an appreciable number of patients.[6] Extensive drainage of infected secretions is essential in all cases and, coupled with intensive nutritional support and antibiotics, may be successful in some patients. It is important to place drainage tubes away from the aorta and major vessels to avoid erosion and serious hemorrhage. Simple suture repair of the neglected perforation is unlikely to be successful. When sepsis and leakage are not readily controlled by drainage alone, other surgical procedures are necessary. In addition to drainage, several approaches to managing the neglected perforation are advocated. Thal and others use a gastric fundus patch sutured over the lower esophageal perforation to achieve closure.[18,21] For early or late perforations, application of a pleural pedicle flap over the defect or suture line is reported to provide good results.[7] For late perforations of the midthoracic esophagus, esophagectomy with closure of the cardia and a cervical esophagostomy may be necessary to control continuing infection in the mediastinum.[8] This approach is especially valuable in patients with extensive destruction of the esophagus or those suffering from esophageal anastomosis breakdown or failure of primary closure.[22] At a later stage, esophageal reconstruction by substernal colon interposition is undertaken. Urschel and colleagues describe a similar approach, but leave the esophagus in place.[23] The cardia is ligated with a large absorbable ligature, and a lateral cervical esophagostomy is performed with tube drainage of the esophagus until the perforation heals. Thereafter, the ligature at the cardia is removed if it has not dissolved. Unfortunately, the ligature at the cardia does not always remain occlusive, as pressure necrosis of the underlying tissue may permit the lumen to reopen. Removal of a permanent large ligature embedded in the esophageal wall may require a limited resection and anastomosis. Results obtained by the several techniques for treating late perforations vary from series to series and appear to be related more to the time interval between perforation and operation and to the underlying disease than to the specific technique used.

Following surgical treatment, continuing infection and its complications are a serious threat. Mediastinitis, empyema, lung or mediastinal abscess, subphrenic abscess, and breakdown of the closure or anastomosis must be diagnosed and drained promptly and thoroughly by the appropriate techniques. Other serious complications include pneumonia, pericarditis, aspiration, and hemorrhage from a major vessel such as the aorta weakened by sepsis and eroded by an adjacent drainage tube. Such infectious complications are the major reason why perforation of the esophagus continues to cause high mortality and morbidity. Adequate restoration of nutrition by parenteral or enteral intubation is essential for ultimate patient survival.

SELECTED REFERENCES

Meade, R. H.: A History of Thoracic Surgery. Springfield, IL, Charles C Thomas, 1961, pp. 649–655.
The history of rupture of the esophagus is presented—from Boerhaave's first described case to the establishment of successful treatment methods in 1958.

Michel, L., Grillo, H. C., and Malt, R. A.: Operative and nonoperative management of esophageal perforation. Ann. Surg., 194:57, 1981.
By analyzing results in 72 patients treated for esophageal perforations, the authors address issues such as criteria for operative versus nonoperative management, the impact of the site and cause of perforation, delays in diagnosis or surgical treatment, and the relative merits of surgical treatment.

Nesbitt, J. C., and Sawyers, J. L.: Surgical management of esophageal perforation. Am. Surg., 53:183, 1987.
This review of 115 patients treated for perforation at Vanderbilt provides an excellent overview of the causes, location, and results of various treatments. The mortality is increased threefold when treatment is delayed more than 24 hours.

Triggiani, E., and Belsey, R.: Oesophageal trauma: Incidence, diagnosis, and management. Thorax, 32:241, 1977.
Experiences in managing 126 patients, including 78 with anastomotic leaks and 16 with chemical perforations, are presented. The value of resection, exteriorization of the cervical esophagus, and gastrostomy for the complicated case is stressed. A good review of the symptoms and diagnostic approach is provided.

REFERENCES

1. Abbott, O. A., Mansour, K. A., Logan, W. D., Jr., Hatcher, C. R., and Symbas, P. N.: Atraumatic so-called spontaneous rupture of the esophagus. A review of 47 personal cases with comments on a new method of surgical therapy. J. Thorac. Cardiovasc. Surg., 59:67, 1970.
2. Cameron, J. L., Kieffer, R. F., Hendrix, T. R., Mehigan, D. G., and Baker, R. R.: Selective nonoperative management of contained intrathoracic esophageal disruption. Ann. Thorac. Surg., 27:404, 1979.
3. Cohn, H. E., Hubbard, A., and Patton, G.: Management of esophageal injuries. Ann. Thorac. Surg., 48:309, 1989.
4. Donner, M. W.: Hemorrhage at the esophagogastric junction (including bleeding esophageal varices). *In* Katz, D., and Hoffman, F. (Eds.): The Esophagogastric Junction. Amsterdam, Excerpta Medica, 1971, pp. 76–77.
5. Dubost, C., Kaswin, D., Duranteau, A., Jehanno, C., and Kaswin, R.: Esophageal perforation during attempted endotracheal intubation. J. Thorac. Cardiovasc. Surg., 78:44, 1979.
6. Finley, R. J., Pearson, F. G., Weisel, R. D., Todd, T. R., Ilves, R., and Cooper, J.: The management of nonmalignant intrathoracic esophageal perforations. Ann. Thorac. Surg., 30:575, 1980.
7. Grillo, H. C., and Wilkins, E. W.: Esophageal repair following later diagnosis of intrathoracic perforation. Ann. Thorac. Surg., 4:387, 1975.
8. Kerr, W. F.: Emergency oesophagectomy. Thorax, 23:204, 1968.
9. Mallory, G. K., and Weiss, S.: Hemorrhage from lacerations of the cardiac orifice of the stomach due to vomiting. Am. J. Med. Sci., 178:506, 1929.
10. Meade, R. H.: A History of Thoracic Surgery. Springfield, IL, Charles C Thomas, 1961, pp. 649–655.
11. Michel, L., Grillo, H. C., and Malt, R. A.: Operative and nonoperative management of esophageal perforations. Ann. Surg., 194:57, 1981.
12. Nashef, S. A. M., and Pagliero, K. M.: Instrumental perforation of the esophagus in benign disease. Ann. Thorac. Surg., 44:360, 1987.
13. Nesbitt, J. C., and Sawyers, J. L.: Surgical management of esophageal perforation. Am. Surg., 53:183, 1987.
14. Pass, L. J., LeNarz, L. A., Schreiber, J. T., and Estrera, A. S.: Management of esophageal gunshot wounds. Ann. Thorac. Surg., 44:253, 1987.
15. Pate, J. W., Walker, W. A., Cole, F. H., Jr., Owen, E. W., and Johnson, W. H.: Spontaneous rupture of the esophagus: A 30-year experience. Ann. Thorac. Surg., 47:689, 1989.
16. Patton, A. S., Lawson, D. W., Shannon, J. M., Risley, T. S., and Bixby, F. E.: Reevaluation of the Boerhaave syndrome. A review of 14 cases. Am. J. Surg., 137:560, 1979.
17. Rea, W. J., Gallivan, G. J., Ecker, R. R., and Sugg, W. L.: Traumatic esophageal perforation. Ann. Thorac. Surg., 14:671, 1972.
18. Rosoff, L., and White, E. J.: Perforation of the esophagus. Am. J. Surg., 128:207, 1974.
19. Sarr, M. G., Pemberton, J. H., and Payne, W. S.: Management of instrumental perforations of the esophagus. J. Thorac. Cardiovasc. Surg., 84:211, 1982.
20. Skinner, D. B., Little, A. G., and DeMeester, T. R.: Management of esophageal perforation. Am. J. Surg., 139:760, 1980.
21. Thal, A. P., and Hatafuku, T.: Improved operation for esophageal rupture. J.A.M.A., 188:826, 1964.
22. Triggiani, E., and Belsey, R.: Oesophageal trauma: Incidence, diagnosis, and management. Thorax, 32:241, 1977.
23. Urschel, H. C., Razzuk, M. A., Wood, R. E., Galbraith, N., Pockey, M., and Paulson, D. L.: Improved management of esophageal perforation: Exclusion and diversion in continuity. Ann. Surg., 179:587, 1974.
24. Wirthlin, L. S., and Malt, R. A.: Accidents of vagotomy. Surg. Gynecol. Obstet., 135:913, 1972.

VIII

HIATAL HERNIA AND GASTROESOPHAGEAL REFLUX

David B. Skinner, M.D.

The subject of hiatal hernia cannot be discussed separately from consideration of gastroesophageal reflux and its complications. Each of these entities has its own history, method of evaluation, indications for treatment, and therapy; however, both conditions involve abnormalities at the gastroesophageal junction and may coexist. Hiatal hernia has been recognized in autopsy studies for several centuries but was not diagnosed in a living human being until early in the twentieth century, following the development of diagnostic radiographic methods. For almost 50 years thereafter, the herniation of the stomach through the esophageal hiatus of the diaphragm was thought to be simply a hernial problem similar to other hernias through the abdominal wall. Early surgical efforts to repair hiatal hernia emphasized anatomic correction by obliteration of the hernia sac and narrowing of the diaphragmatic crura. Large experiences with these types of operation were reported by Harrington, Sweet, and others.

In 1951, Allison clearly described the clinical problem of gastroesophageal reflux with its symptoms and complications.[1] He noted the frequent association of reflux with hiatal hernia and emphasized the importance of phrenoesophageal membrane abnormalities in both conditions. Allison described a method of hiatal hernia repair involving reattachment of the phrenoesophageal membrane, which he hoped would correct the problem of gastroesophageal reflux as well. The Allison repair received wide trials; but before his death, Allison recognized that the incidence of persistence of reflux after repair was too high.[2] It has not been the answer to the problem of gastroesophageal reflux.

Shortly after Allison's report, Belsey and Nissen independently and almost simultaneously developed more effective antireflux operations.[23,32] They recognized the differences in symptoms caused by reflux, compared with those caused by hiatal hernia alone. Although surgical methods for effectively controlling reflux have been known for more than 35 years, the factors that control reflux in normal human beings are only recently being understood and still provoke controversy.

ANATOMY

The anatomy of the esophagus has been described in detail earlier. This discussion concerns the anatomy of the gastroesophageal junction and the passage of the esophagus from the thorax into the abdomen. A precise definition of the gastroesophageal junction is necessary to an understanding of this region, because it is described in several ways that influence clinical thinking. The distal esophagus is perhaps best defined as the narrow-diameter swallowing tube, consisting of two muscle layers, that leads the normal peristaltic contraction to its conclusion. The presence of columnar epithelium within the most distal 2 cm. of the esophagus is a common and normal finding but causes confusion about the location of the gastroesophageal junction. A junction defined as the mucosal border between squamous and columnar epithelium is at a more cephalad level than the junction of the swallowing tube (as defined above) with the digestive pouch or stomach, which is of larger diameter, does not transmit the esophageal peristaltic wave, consists of three muscle layers, and has a serosal covering over a portion of its circumference. For an understanding of the mechanisms that control gastroesophageal reflux, the junction of the muscular swallowing tube with the gastric digestive pouch is a more useful definition of the gastroesophageal junction than the mucosal boundary.

The normal human distal esophagus passes through the diaphragm, and 2 to 4 cm. of distal esophagus lie within the abdomen. The abdomen is defined by its inner boundary, consisting of the endoabdominal fascia. In the region of the esophageal hiatus, this fascia comes off the underside of the diaphragm and bridges the hiatal opening. This fibroelastic fascial tissue inserts through the wall of the esophagus into the submucosa and thereby fixes the entry of the distal esophagus into the abdominal cavity (Fig. 1). The level of entry into the abdomen may be identified by esophageal manometric studies. These demonstrate that intra-abdominal pressure increases with inspiration, whereas intrathoracic pressure decreases. This level of change

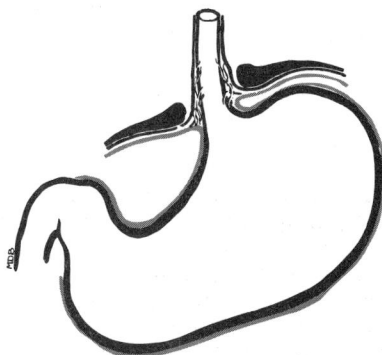

Figure 1. The normal fascial and peritoneal reflections at the diaphragmatic hiatus. The fascia on the deep surface of the diaphragm is reflected onto the esophagus as the phrenoesophageal ligament and fascia propria. Vessels and lymphatics lie between this and the peritoneal reflection. (From Allison, P. R.: Reflux esophagitis, sliding hiatal hernia, and the anatomy of repair. Surg. Gynecol. Obstet., 92:419, 1951.)

in respiratory pressure dynamics occurs over a short distance in normal humans and confirms that 2 to 4 cm. of distal swallowing tube is located within the abdominal positive-pressure environment.[30] Radiographic studies depend upon the air-tissue interface between lung and diaphragm to mark the level of the diaphragm. However, the hiatal opening through the diaphragm is in the posterior mediastinum; so the radiographic identification of the abdominal-thoracic barrier is not accurate for the hiatus. This causes further confusion in identifying a hiatal hernia and the gastroesophageal junction.

The distal esophagus itself differs only slightly from the more proximal esophagus above the phrenoesophageal membrane. There is no anatomically demonstrable circular sphincter muscle in humans and other primates. In cats, Liebermann's dissections demonstrate some specialized muscle fiber arrangements but no distinct sphincter.[18] Some animal species that are frequently used for experimental studies, such as the dog and opossum, have a discrete distal esophageal sphincter. Because this is not present in humans, the results of experimental studies on the lower esophagus in species with this anatomic difference are not readily transferable to humans. Although the muscles of the distal esophagus are similar to those located more proximally, the mucosa demonstrates a change from squamous to columnar epithelium within the lower 2 to 4 cm. of esophagus. Normally, no parietal cells are seen in the mucosa at this level. This zone of simple columnar epithelium resistant to acid digestion is an important protective transitional zone between the neutral pH of esophagus and the acid environment of the stomach.

In addition to the esophagus, the vagus nerve trunks pass through the phrenoesophageal membrane into the abdomen via the esophageal hiatus. No other structures of importance pass through this barrier. The arterial blood supply to the distal esophagus from the ascending branch of the left gastric artery enters the wall of the esophagus below the phrenoesophageal membrane. At the level of the membrane insertion, the vessels in the esophageal wall pass very close to the mucosa, whereas they are normally more deeply situated in the submucosa at higher levels in the esophagus or lower on the stomach.[8] This observation may be responsible for the common location of a ruptured esophageal varix in the lowermost portion of the esophagus, where the veins are most superficial and where the abdominal thoracic pressure difference makes a large change in intraluminal tamponading pressure.

PHYSIOLOGY OF THE ESOPHAGOGASTRIC JUNCTION

The distal esophagus has two important physiologic functions: the transportation of an ingested bolus into the stomach and the prevention of reflux of gastric contents back into the esophagus. Measurements of pressure in the distal esophagus demonstrate a resting pressure between 10 and 20 mm. Hg greater in the distal esophagus than in adjacent stomach. This elevated pressure zone is evidence of the barrier to reflux. When a peristaltic wave occurs, (Fig. 2) the pressure in the distal esophageal segment drops to the level of gastric pressure. This prevents the distal esophageal segment from acting as an obstruction to passage of a bolus of food. The precise mechanism for this decrease in pressure with swallowing is uncertain. Some believe that this is an active muscular relaxation under neural control. Other evidence suggests that shortening of the longitudinal muscle of the esophagus puts tension on the insertion of the phrenoesophageal membrane into the esophageal submucosal layer. Since this membrane enters the esophagus at an angle, the effect of shortening the esophagus is to pull open the lumen of the distal segment and cause a "relaxation" in pressure. In achalasia, in which innervation is disturbed and longitudinal muscle shortening does not occur, the elevated pressure

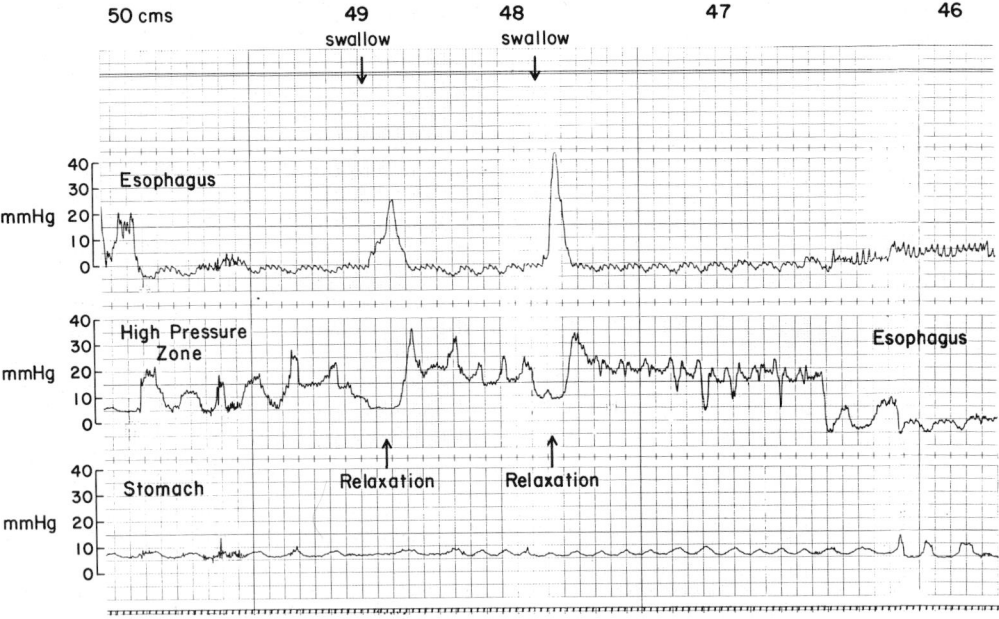

Figure 2. Manometric tracing demonstrating the distal esophageal high-pressure zone. Recordings are made from catheter lumens spaced 5 cm. apart. The catheter train is withdrawn from the stomach into the esophagus so that the proximal, middle, and distal recording channels pass sequentially through the high-pressure zone that measures millimeters of mercury. Notice the relaxation with swallowing.

in the abdominal segment of esophagus does not relax after swallowing. This is thought to be a cause of dysphagia in such patients.

The mechanism for the elevated pressure in the distal esophagus serving as the barrier to reflux is also not completely understood. Some evidence suggests that specialized muscle in the distal esophagus acts as a sphincter under neurohormonal control. This theory of an active intrinsic sphincter is challenged by observations that the laws of physics governing tension in the walls of tubes of different diameter may be responsible for the barrier to reflux.[31] The small-diameter esophageal swallowing tube entering abruptly the large-diameter gastric digestive pouch suggests that the law of Laplace applies and makes it much more difficult to distend the smaller-diameter tube. This may be responsible for a higher resting luminal pressure in the abdominal esophagus. An abnormally low insertion of the phrenoesophageal membrane into the swallowing tube would tend to pull the lumen open, with increases in abdominal pressure, and reduce the difference in diameter at the gastroesophageal junction. The theory that reflux is controlled by physical properties at the gastroesophageal junction depends upon a normal insertion of the phrenoesophageal membrane 3 to 4 cm. above the junction. Hence, pressure in the abdominal cavity does not tend to pull the junction open, and the distal abdominal esophagus is subject to the same external pressure as the larger-diameter gastric tube. As a practical matter, creation of a 3- to 4-cm. segment of intra-abdominal esophagus is a critical part of successful antireflux surgery. Fortunately, the relocation of the distal esophagus into the abdominal environment is much more readily accomplished than an alteration in the neurohormonal control of an intrinsic sphincter if one is present.

HIATAL HERNIA

Hiatal hernia is the herniation of an abdominal organ, usually the stomach, through the esophageal hiatus in the diaphragm. The diagnosis is usually made by radiographic contrast studies demonstrating an abdominal organ higher than the level of the diaphragm. The diagnosis is confirmed by surgical exploration or at autopsy. Because the esophageal hiatus is located in the mediastinum and retroperitoneum, there is no immediately ad-

jacent air-tissue density contrast for radiographic observation. Accordingly, the radiologic diagnosis of hiatal hernia is based on visualization of the lung-diaphragm interface near, but not at, the esophageal hiatus. This is the cause of some error regarding both the frequency and the significance of the radiographic diagnosis of hiatal hernia.

Confusion is increased by failure to recognize that the endoabdominal fascia defines the inner boundary of the abdominal cavity. When the fascia is intact, the significance of a protrusion through the esophageal hiatus is different from a defect in the fascia, allowing a true peritoneal sac to protrude through the endoabdominal lining. To emphasize these important differences in the significance of herniation through the esophageal hiatus, hiatal hernias are classified into two major types (Fig. 3).

Type I Hiatal Hernia

The Type I sliding, or axial, hiatal hernia is the result of an extension of the endoabdominal fascia through the hiatus, which allows a small portion of gastric cardia to slide up into the esophageal hiatus. The phrenoesophageal membrane remains intact. There is no true peritoneal hernia sac. If the phrenoesophageal membrane inserts normally into the esophagus 3 to 4 cm. above the gastroesophageal junction, this type of hernia is generally asymptomatic and is an incidental finding of no consequence. The Type I hiatal hernia is extremely common and can be demonstrated in many adult patients by a radiologist using vigorous compression techniques. This type of hiatal hernia is of no significance unless accompanied by abnormal gastroesophageal reflux. There is no indication for any medical or surgical treatment for a Type I hiatal hernia. If symptoms of reflux are associated with a Type I hiatal hernia, the diagnostic and treatment considerations are directed toward the reflux, rather than the hernia. For this reason, further discussion of this problem focuses upon gastroesophageal reflux.

Type II Paraesophageal Hernia

The Type II hiatal hernia, also termed paraesophageal or rolling hernia, is uncommon and represents a true herniation of the stomach into a peritoneal sac in the mediastinum. The distal esophagus is located in its normal position, anchored by the phrenoesophageal membrane. A defect in the membrane

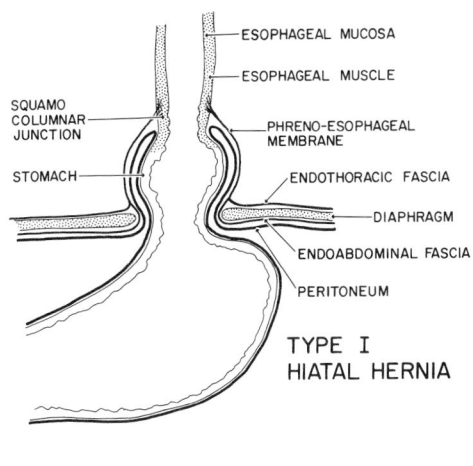

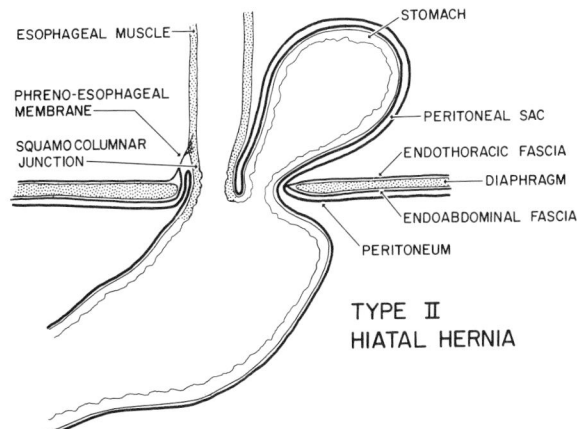

Figure 3. Diagrammatic representation of Type I and Type II hiatal hernias. In the Type I hernia the phrenoesophageal membrane is intact and there is no true peritoneal sac extending into the thorax. In the Type II hiatal hernia there is a defect in the phrenoesophageal membrane, permitting a free peritoneal sac to enter the lower pressure thoracic cavity.

allows a peritoneal sac to protrude alongside the esophagus through the hiatus. This defect usually occurs at the left anterolateral portion of the esophageal hiatus where the greater peritoneal sac reflects off the gastroesophageal junction. A herniation may occur posteriorly as well where the lesser sac peritoneum reflects off the junction. In a large Type II hernia, both greater and lesser peritoneal sacs are commonly present through two defects in the fascia. Because intrathoracic pressure is less than atmospheric and abdominal pressure is positive throughout the respiratory cycle, the natural history of this type of hernia is progressive enlargement. The entire stomach may herniate completely upward into the sacs, so that the pylorus comes to lie near the cardia, which predisposes to gastric volvulus. This causes a giant Type II hernia with an upside-down intrathoracic stomach.

With progressive enlargement of the hernia through the hiatus, the remaining attachments of the phrenoesophageal membrane stretch; so it is common to find a combined, or Type III, hernia in the advanced stages, with components of both sliding and paraesophageal types. With a large defect, other organs, such as the colon, spleen, pancreas, and small intestine, may enter the hernia sac as well and cause a complicated Type IV hiatal hernia with symptoms attributable to the other organs involved.

The Type II hernia may be completely asymptomatic and reach a large size, so that the entire stomach is in an intrathoracic location without the patient's awareness of disabling symptoms. If the distal esophageal segment maintains its intra-abdominal location, there is usually no associated gastroesophageal reflux, and therefore heartburn and regurgitation do not often occur.

When symptoms occur, the patient may complain of fullness after meals, gurgling or splashing noises in the chest, slowness in food passing through the distal esophagus at the level where it is compressed by the adjacent gastric pouch, or early satiety and postprandial vomiting. Acute epigastric or chest pain after meals is an ominous symptom, suggesting intermittent volvulus. Stasis in the incarcerated gastric pouch may cause erosion of gastric mucosa. The result may be an acute or chronic gastric ulcer in the pouch or riding over the diaphragmatic margins ("a riding ulcer"), which may bleed or perforate. Occasionally, bleeding may be quite massive; but more often a chronic unexplained anemia is noted in association with this type of hernia. Gastric volvulus causes gastric obstruction or strangulation, which may cause sudden death.

One prospective study of patients with large asymptomatic Type II hiatal hernias describes 22 such patients without symptoms but with a totally intrathoracic stomach.[32] Within 2 years, 6 had succumbed to one or more complications of the hernia, including gastric strangulation or infarction, bleeding, and acute intrathoracic gastric dilation causing respiratory insufficiency.

Any patient who presents with symptoms of dysphagia should undergo a barium swallow examination or esophagoscopy. This is the most common sequence for the diagnosis of the paraesophageal hernia. Postprandial vomiting, early satiety, and other digestive disturbances may also prompt a barium swallow examination. Radiography is the definitive test for the Type II hiatal hernia, although the diagnosis may be suspected if a chest film shows an air–fluid level in the mediastinum behind the heart (Fig. 4).

When the diagnosis is established, the patient's general condition is evaluated. Unless there is some other life-threatening illness, patients with a large Type II hiatal hernia are generally advised to have surgical correction because of the risk of sudden catastrophic complications. Before operation, esophagogastroscopy is performed because the distortion of the anatomy makes it difficult for the radiologist to exclude other abnormalities of the esophagus or stomach that may require attention or complicate operative management. The presence of the Type II hiatal hernia is an indication for surgical therapy, because there is no effective medical treatment for this condition.

Operative treatment may be performed through an abdominal or thoracic incision. Because of the possibility of intrathoracic adhesions from a long-standing hernia, there is risk of being unable to reduce the hernia through an abdominal approach or of causing injury to the hernia contents within the thoracic sac. For these reasons, many surgeons prefer a thoracic approach for the repair of a giant Type II hiatal hernia.

In principle, all that must be accomplished by the operation is reduction of the hernia, elimination of the sacs, and repair of the large opening in the hiatus. Although this may be achievable in some patients, the dissection necessary to eliminate the hernial sacs often produces the potential for recurrence of a sliding hiatal hernia through the defect or the risk of gastroesophageal reflux. Preoperative esophageal function tests show that approximately two thirds of patients with a Type II hernia also have abnormal reflux as well.[36] For this reason, an antireflux repair is usually performed as part of the operative treatment. The operation consists of full mobilization of the hernia, resection of the redundant anterior and posterior hernia sacs if present, placement of sutures in the diaphragmatic crura posteriorly for narrowing the hiatus, and the creation of an antireflux fundoplication between the stomach and esophagus for eliminating the risk of postoperative gastroesophageal reflux.

Operative treatment for this type of hernia has a mortality risk of approximately 1 per cent. No specific complications from

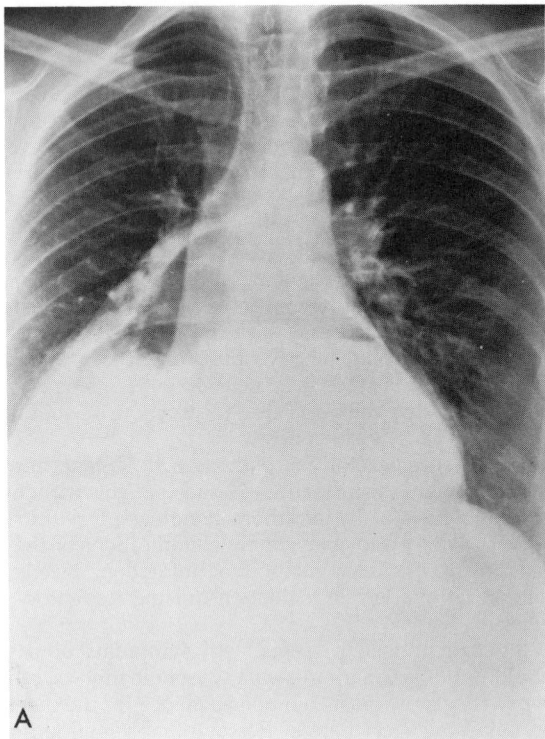

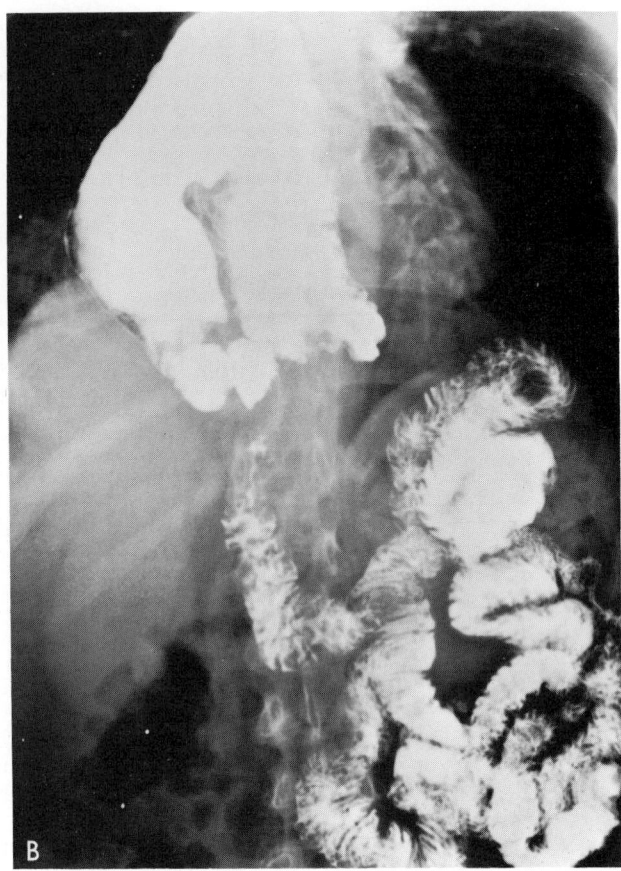

Figure 4. *A* and *B*, Typical radiographic appearance of a large Type II hiatal hernia. As in this case, there is often a loosening of the phreno-esophageal membrane as well, making it a combined sliding and paraesophageal, or Type III, hernia.

the operation are anticipated, although the patient may experience an increased sensation of abdominal fullness and tightness after the repair because of the relocation of the herniated organs back within the abdomen. Long-term recurrence of a hiatal hernia in patients who have previously undergone repair of a paraesophageal hernia occurs in approximately 15 per cent, a rate somewhat higher than that encountered with a repair of a Type I sliding hiatal hernia. The higher recurrence follows the attenuation of tissues caused by the very large hernia. These tissues are less suitable for holding permanent sutures than are the more normal diaphragmatic crura.

GASTROESOPHAGEAL REFLUX

Regurgitation of gastric contents occurs normally in human beings, particularly after a large meal.[9] Distention of the stomach gradually effaces the intra-abdominal segment of esophagus and shortens its length. The gradual conversion of this segment to an inverted-funnel shape permits postprandial reflux to occur normally. Belching, burping, and vomiting are normal experiences. It is only when reflux occurs with increased frequency and at times when the stomach is not distended that pathologic gastroesophageal reflux is observed. An individual who overindulges at mealtimes generally accepts some symptoms of reflux after the meal and does not consider this to be an illness. However, when symptomatic reflux occurs after every meal and between meals, medical advice is often sought.

The precise abnormality causing pathologic gastroesophageal reflux is not completely understood. The study of a population of patients with frequent reflux indicates that the intraluminal tension of the distal esophageal segment is generally reduced and the length of the intra-abdominal esophagus is shorter than normal.[27] The reasons for this loss of intra-abdominal esophageal segment and its high-pressure barrier are not known.

Symptoms

The symptoms of reflux are heartburn and regurgitation aggravated by postural change such as stooping or lying flat and relieved by standing upright. When heartburn is clearly related to postural change and the regurgitation indicates by its sour or bitter taste that it is of stomach origin, the diagnosis of abnormal gastroesophageal reflux can be made on the basis of clinical features alone. Other symptoms can be caused by reflux or the complications of reflux, such as dysphagia, bleeding, substernal chest pain, a sensation of spasm or something sticking in the throat, and respiratory symptoms.

Dysphagia, or difficulty in swallowing, associated with abnormal reflux may occur through three mechanisms. Refluxed gastric contents may serve as an irritant to the esophagus, causing secondary muscle spasm. Direct injury to the esophagus from acid peptic regurgitation may cause edema, inflammation, and spasm—and even fibrosis and a stricture in advanced cases. When a large sliding hiatal hernia is present, the esophageal longitudinal muscle is not fixed at its distal end. As the esophagus contracts, the hernia is pulled up, interfering with efficient progression of peristalsis. The symptom of dysphagia may result.

Bleeding from esophagitis usually presents as chronic anemia and stools positive for occult blood, rather than as frank hematemesis or melena. In a few patients, severe acute esophagitis may cause massive upper gastrointestinal hemorrhage. This is diagnosed by endoscopy. Such bleeding is best managed acutely by intensive medical treatment, including a naso-esophageal antacid drip with the patient in an upright position. Another source of clinically severe bleeding may be an ulcer developing in an esophagus lined with columnar epithelium. The ulcerations on the squamous side of the esophageal mucosal junction are usually superficial. Ulcerations developing in columnar epithelium may become quite deep, similar to gastric ulcers, and may cause rapid gastrointestinal bleeding.

The chest pain caused by reflux is generally described by the patient as heartburn or a burning substernal and epigastric pain. However, another type of pain caused by reflux may mimic the symptoms of angina pectoris, including radiation of the pain to the neck, shoulders, and arms. This type of pain is thought to occur because of esophageal spasm, rather than mucosal irritation. It may be difficult to differentiate from true angina pectoris and ultimately must be diagnosed by objective testing for both reflux and coronary artery disease.

Occasionally, reflux may cause symptoms characterized as "globus hystericus." Such patients have a chronic sensation of a foreign object lodged in the throat, tightness of the throat muscles, and inability to initiate swallowing. The mechanism for this is not completely clear, but it may occur because of reflux into the upper esophagus, causing irritation and spasm in the cricopharyngeal sphincter region. Zenker's diverticulum is now thought to follow cricopharyngeal dysfunction, and about one half of patients with such a diverticulum also have documented reflux.[19]

Respiratory symptoms, including productive cough, frequent respiratory infections, pneumonia, and chronic bronchitis, are common in the general population. Gastroesophageal reflux is also common. Without question, abnormal gastroesophageal reflux may cause chronic aspiration of gastric contents into the lung, with resulting respiratory disease. Recurrent pneumonia, lung abscess, bronchiectasis—with symptoms similar to those of asthma, morning hoarseness, nocturnal cough, and productive morning cough—have all been linked to abnormal reflux as a causative mechanism. However, because respiratory illness and reflux are both common problems, it is an error to assume a cause-and-effect relationship between the two unless that is proved objectively. It is well known that respiratory maneuvers such as a cough, the Müller maneuver, and the Valsalva maneuver may elicit reflux. The attribution of respiratory symptoms to reflux must be based on more than symptomatic evidence.[29]

Diagnostic Studies

RADIOGRAPHY. When symptoms suggestive of reflux cause a patient to consult a physician, several studies are indicated to confirm or eliminate the diagnosis. As for all esophageal disease, a barium swallow and upper gastrointestinal radiography are performed first. It is important to observe the whole esophagus and stomach as a unit, because disorders of the upper esophagus may cause symptoms that may be confused with reflux; and abnormalities of the stomach, including delayed gastric emptying, may aggravate reflux or cause symptoms similar to those of reflux. If the radiologist sees spontaneous free reflux, this alone is clear evidence of pathologic reflux, because it is usually difficult to demonstrate gastroesophageal reflux during the course of a barium swallow examination. Reflux is demonstrated spontaneously during a barium swallow examination in only approximately 40 per cent of patients who ultimately prove to have this disorder. A Type I axial hiatal hernia is a common finding during barium swallow examination. The demonstration of hernia varies directly with the aggressiveness of the radiologic examination. The observation of an axial hiatal hernia without free reflux does not establish the diagnosis of reflux as the cause of the patient's symptoms. Several radiologic reports advocate the use of a "water-sipping" test accompanied by abdominal compression to demonstrate reflux. This is not an accurate test, because swallowing of water is known to cause relaxation or opening of the distal esophagus. If accompanied by compression of the abdomen, this forces reflux to occur in normal subjects. A positive water-sipping test alone should not be considered as conclusive evidence of an incompetent cardia. Because radiographic studies are usually not sufficient for diagnosing symptomatic gastroesophageal reflux, esophageal function tests using pressure and pH measurements in the esophagus are used for more precise diagnosis.

ESOPHAGEAL FUNCTION TESTS. Esophageal function tests have been developed over the past 35 years to investigate various physiologic disorders. No single test is certain to detect all cases of abnormal reflux and avoid false-positive diagnoses. For this reason, the tests are usually performed as a battery to ensure that the results are confirmatory. The techniques for esophageal function testing use manometry for pressure measurements in the stomach and esophagus and the recording of pH in the esophagus using a long gastrointestinal pH electrode. Manometry is frequently performed with fluid-filled catheters bound together with orifices spaced 2 to 5 cm. apart to record pressures at different levels simultaneously. Typically, a manometry study includes three infused catheters with openings at 5-cm. intervals. These are introduced in the same manner that a nasogastric tube is introduced into the stomach, and they are slowly withdrawn across the gastroesophageal junction. The amplitude and length of the abdominal segment of the distal esophagus are recorded. Normal patients have 10 to 20 mm. Hg pressure in the distal esophagus. Approximately 3 cm. of this is located below the respiratory pressure inversion point. Recordings are continued through the length of the esophagus for the purpose of confirming the presence of normal peristalsis and observing whether esophageal spasm or aperistalsis is present. In a large population of patients, those with pathologic reflux have an average distal esophageal pressure and length less than those of normal subjects. Because the range of variability is great, manometry alone is not a satisfactory diagnostic test for an incompetent cardia in an individual patient. Manometry is essential in studying symptomatic esophageal disease for excluding esophageal spasm, achalasia, and scleroderma. Symptoms from these disorders may overlap or mimic those caused by reflux.

A more direct way to measure reflux is pH recording in the esophagus 5 cm. above the distal esophageal high-pressure zone. Declines in pH to less than 4 at this level are clear evidence of reflux. Normal individuals reflux occasionally; so a standardized approach to diagnosing reflux with a pH electrode is used.[33] Following the placement of 300 ml. of 0.1 N HCl into the stomach of an average-sized normal adult, reflux is recorded only once or twice during the performance of a standardized series of respiratory and postural maneuvers. Those with abnormal reflux demonstrate more frequent reflux, or persistence of regurgitated acid in the esophagus. Such a standardized acid reflux test has approximately twice the accuracy of radiographic studies in detecting abnormal reflux but still has an approximate 20 per cent incidence of false-negative or false-positive results.

For esophagitis to develop as a complication of reflux, two events are necessary. The patient must have abnormal frequency of reflux, but there must also be prolonged contact between the irritating gastric contents and the esophageal mucosa to permit penetration of the mucosa and the establishment of esophagitis. For this reason, an acid-clearing test is helpful in identifying patients at risk for esophagitis.[32] This test is performed by instilling 15 ml. of 0.1 N HCl in the midesophagus and instructing the patient to swallow at intervals. Normal individuals clear the acid bolus in 10 swallows or fewer, whereas those with esophagitis frequently are unable to clear the acid and have marked prolongation of acid contact with the mucosa. Salivary neutralization of acid in addition to efficient peristalsis is important for prompt acid clearing.[12]

Symptoms caused by reflux, including epigastric and substernal pain, are similar to those of a variety of other conditions, including gastric and duodenal ulcer, pancreatitis, biliary tract disease, and coronary artery disease. The alternate infusion of 0.1 N HCl and normal saline into the esophagus is a useful test for confirming esophageal origin of symptoms. If the patient's complaints are stimulated by the infusion of hydrochloric acid into the esophagus for 10 minutes or more and are relieved by the infusion of saline, a positive acid perfusion test is recorded. This does not prove that reflux is the cause of the symptoms, but it indicates a likely association.

The battery of esophageal function tests—manometry, the standard acid reflux test, the acid clearing test, and the acid perfusion test—are frequently performed together as an outpatient screening procedure for functional disease of the esophagus.[33] Coupled with analysis of radiographic findings and subsequent endoscopy, these tests enable an accurate diagnosis of esophageal functional disease in nearly all symptomatic patients.

Prolonged monitoring of the pH in the lower esophagus over a 24-hour period is the most precise and useful quantitative method for diagnosing reflux.[17] The pH probe is positioned 5 cm. above the high-pressure zone determined by manometry and left in place while the patient goes through a typical day, with part of the time spent in the upright position and part in the supine position. A neutral pH diet is served. Numerous studies in asymptomatic individuals with normal esophageal function show conclusively that healthy individuals have bouts of postprandial reflux. Patients with abnormal reflux may show distinctive patterns, such as occurrence of reflux only while upright, with a normal neutral pH in the esophagus while reclining; reflux only while in the supine position; or, most frequently, reflux in both positions.[9] There is a clear relationship between the severity of reflux and prolonged gastric emptying.

In patients with atypical symptoms in whom the results of esophageal function tests are equivocal, 24-hour pH monitoring is especially helpful. In atypical syndromes, such as angina-like chest pain, globus hystericus, and respiratory symptoms suspected of being caused by reflux, prolonged monitoring of intraesophageal pH may permit a clear cause-and-effect relationship to be observed between reflux and symptoms.[11] However, the study may demonstrate that reflux and symptoms are unrelated, so that the symptoms are not likely to be caused by reflux. Prolonged pH monitoring is useful in determining reflux as a cause of nonspecific symptoms in young children whose complaints are often minimal and who may present as cases of failure to thrive, chronic anemia, respiratory distress, or difficult feeders. After analyses of radiographic studies of the esophagus and stomach, esophageal function tests, and 24-hour pH monitoring in the esophagus when indicated, sufficient information should be available to establish whether abnormal gastroesophageal reflux is the cause of the illness.

ESOPHAGOSCOPY. When abnormal reflux is diagnosed, esophagoscopy is indicated for assessing the degree of damage to the esophagus and observing other abnormalities that may accompany pathologic reflux. Most important is the determination of whether esophagitis is present. Esophagitis is graded on a scale of 0 to 4, depending on the severity of the changes observed. Grade I esophagitis is recorded when reddening without ulceration is seen. A biopsy of such mucosa may show proximity of the rete pegs to the surface, neovascularization of the squamous epithelium, and hyperplasia of the basal layer. No inflammation is seen in such biopsies; therefore, this is not true esophagitis. Grade II esophagitis is characterized by frank ulcerations just above the gastroesophageal mucosal junction. At more advanced stages, or Grade III esophagitis, some stiffening of the wall is observed. When a frank stricture, which prevents passage of the esophagoscope into the stomach, is encountered, Grade IV esophagitis is diagnosed. The presence of columnar epithelium more than 3 cm. above the junction of the tubular esophagus with the gastric pouch establishes the diagnosis of Barrett's esophagus. Gastric ulceration in the columnar epithelium should be carefully noted. When Barrett's epithelium is seen, multiple biopsies are obtained to exclude dysplasia or neoplasia. This complication, although most likely to be caused by chronic reflux, is a known precursor of adenocarcinoma of the distal esophagus.[34] After endoscopic examination,

sufficient information is available for deciding on treatment for reflux.

Treatment

The indications for surgical treatment of gastroesophageal reflux are primarily the complications of reflux. Patients having ulcerative esophagitis (of Grade II or greater severity) despite medical therapy, stricture, bleeding documented as owing to esophagitis, or aspiration clearly following reflux and causing respiratory illness should be treated by surgical antireflux repair. Patients with less severe reflux are treated medically in an effort to control symptoms. In a few patients whose symptoms cannot be controlled satisfactorily by medical measures, operation may be indicated. Repair should be performed, however, only after the diagnosis is conclusively proved to be abnormal reflux and after a sufficient trial of medical therapy, usually 6 months or more. As stated earlier, patients having a Type II, III, or IV hiatal hernia are treated surgically, and an anti-reflux repair is generally incorporated into the correction of the hiatal hernia.

The medical treatment of gastroesophageal reflux includes methods for reducing the amount of regurgitation by gravity, making the regurgitated gastric contents less damaging to the esophagus, and reducing gastric residual volume. Patients are instructed to sleep with the head of the bed elevated on 6-inch blocks, to take small meals, to avoid eating before bedtime, to avoid lying down after meals, and to avoid stooping whenever possible. Antacids are prescribed to be taken 1 hour after meals, before bedtime, and as necessary to relieve symptoms. If these measures are insufficient, a course of cimetidine or ranitidine is tried in order to reduce the acid content of the regurgitated gastric material. Omeprazole is an alternative and highly effective drug for reducing acid secretion. Drugs such as metoclopramide, which may increase gastric emptying and esophageal peristalsis, may prove valuable. Tranquilizers, muscle relaxants, and anticholinergic drugs are not prescribed, because they interfere with effective esophageal peristalsis, an important safeguard against the development of esophagitis. Weight loss is recommended but is very difficult for patients with chronic symptomatic reflux, because the ingestion of food is an effective neutralizer for the regurgitated acid. With the newer medications for reducing acid, medical therapy generally is successful in controlling symptomatic uncomplicated reflux.

ANTIREFLUX SURGERY. When indications for surgical treatment are clear, the operation performed should be an antireflux repair and not a hiatal hernia repair, as advocated in the past. A number of operations are described to restore the intraabdominal segment of esophagus and to maintain the distal esophagus as a small-diameter tube. All such repairs generally involve mobilization of the cardia and lower esophagus, some type of plication of the stomach around the intraabdominal segment of esophagus, and narrowing of the esophageal hiatus to prevent the reconstituted abdominal esophagus from sliding back into the chest. Three types of antireflux repair have been extensively evaluated. All incorporate similar principles but vary considerably in technical details. Because this type of procedure is of recent origin, the operations carry the names of their developers, the Belsey Mark IV operation, the Nissen fundoplication, and the Hill posterior gastropexy and calibration of the cardia. There is no conclusive evidence yet as to which is the best operation for the long-term control of gastroesophageal reflux.

The Belsey Mark IV operation was first performed by Ronald Belsey in England in 1955. The term *Mark IV* indicates that this was the fourth modification of antireflux surgery from the original operation described by Allison in 1951. The operation is performed only through a thoracic approach.[32] A sixth-interspace incision is preferred. The esophagus is mobilized fully up to the aortic arch to allow restoration of a long segment of

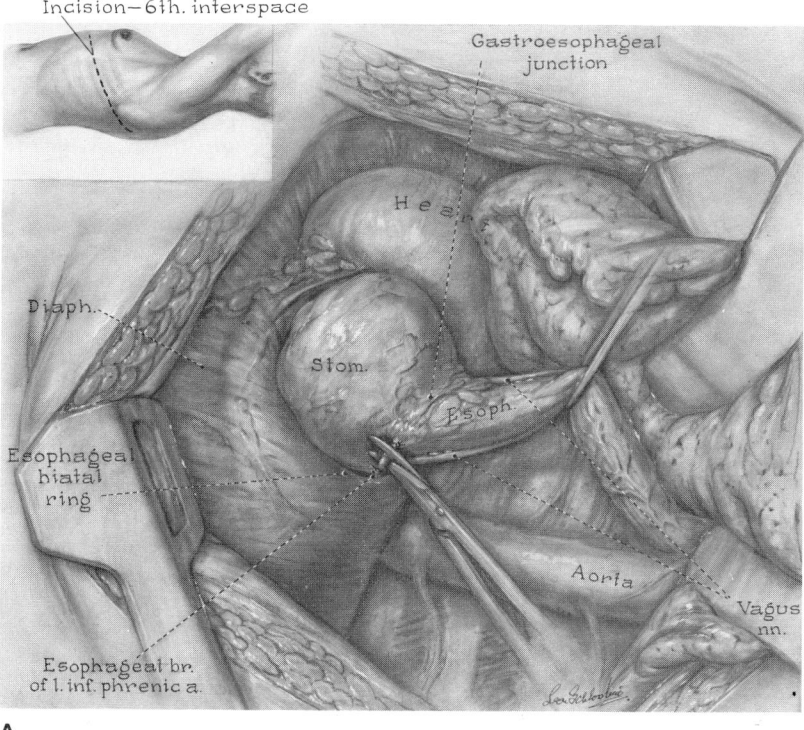

A

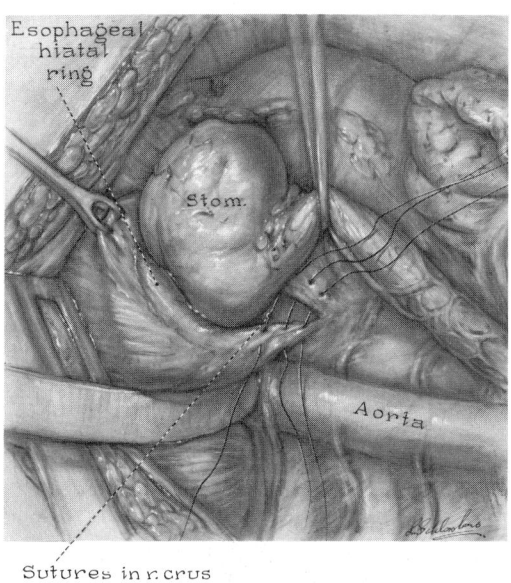

B

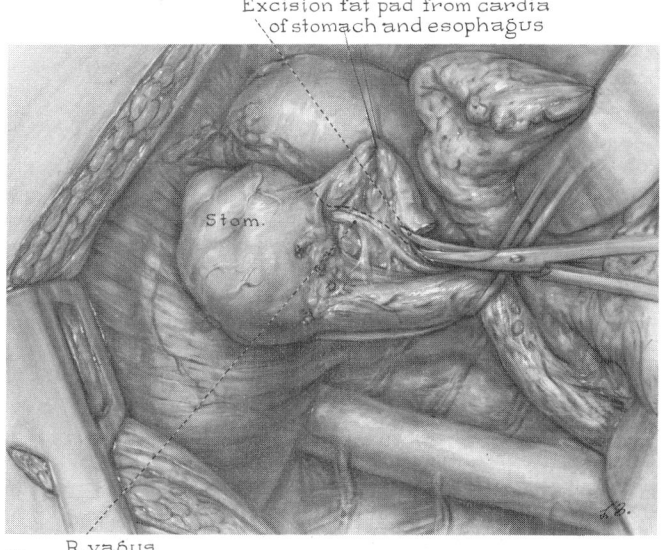

C

Figure 5. The Belsey Mark IV antireflux operation. *A,* Mobilization of the distal esophagus and cardia is done through a left sixth interspace lateral thoracotomy. The esophagus with vagus nerves attached is completely freed up to the lung root. After the hernia sac is entered anteriorly, the entire circumference of the cardia is separated from its attachments. This requires division of branches from the left inferior phrenic artery laterally *(illustrated)* and left gastric artery posteriorly *(not shown). B,* At the start of the repair, sutures are placed in two limbs of the right crus posteriorly, but these are not tied until the completion of the reconstruction. Tension on a clamp applied to the diaphragm anteriorly makes it easier to identify the strong tendinous tissue in the crus where the sutures should be placed. *C,* After complete mobilization of the esophagogastric junction, the pad of fibrofatty tissue at the cardia is excised anteriorly and laterally. The vagus nerves, which tend to be elevated off the esophagus during this dissection, are carefully preserved.

Illustration continued on following page

intra-abdominal esophagus. The cardia is completely freed from its attachments to the diaphragm. The esophageal hiatus is narrowed by the placement of sutures in the crura posteriorly. When eventually tied, these should permit only one finger of the operator to pass through the narrowed hiatus (Fig. 5). The repair is achieved by the plication of the stomach onto approxi-

mately 270 degrees of esophageal circumference, leaving the vagus nerves posteriorly.

The segment of the esophagus not included in the wrap is buttressed against the narrowed hiatus. Two rows of sutures are used, and three mattress sutures are placed in each layer. The first layer imbricates the adjacent gastric fundus onto the lower

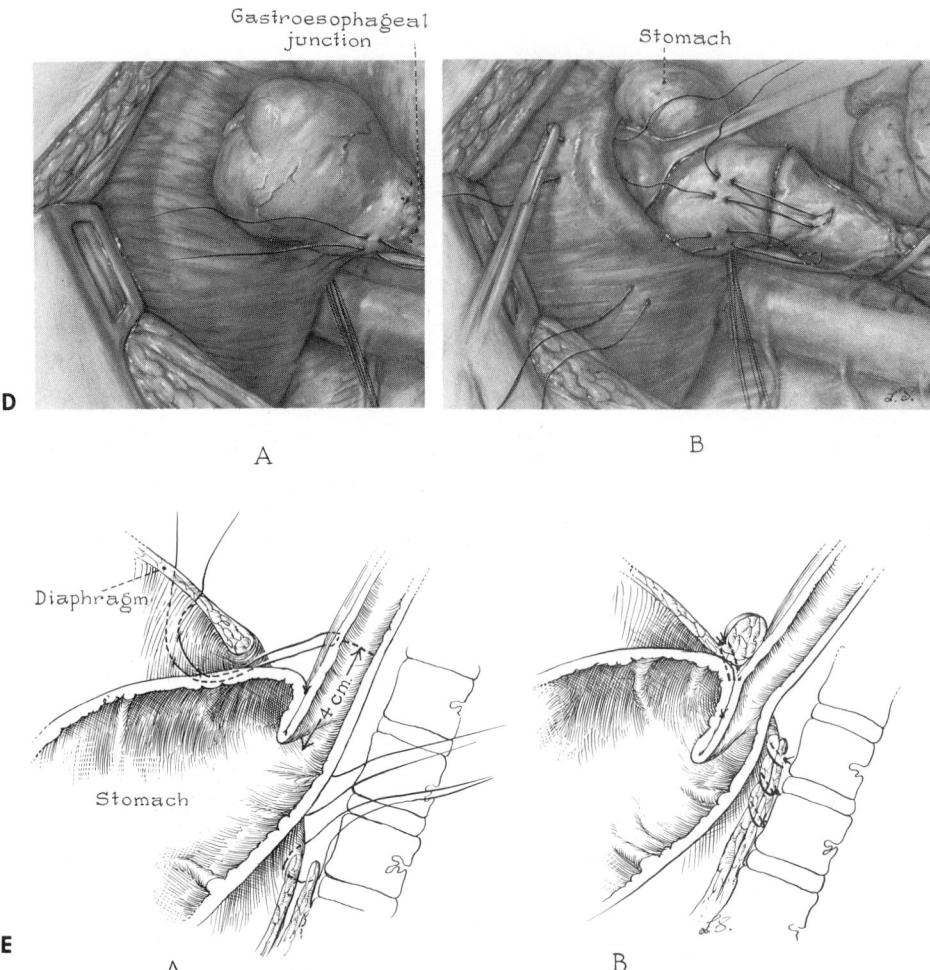

D

A   B

E

A   B

Figure 5 *Continued D*, (A) The reconstruction is started by placing the first of three mattress sutures between the fundus of the stomach and esophagus 2 cm. above the junction. The spacing of these sutures around the circumference of the esophagus is shown in the cross-sectional insert. (B) After completion of the first row of sutures, a second row of three mattress sutures is placed through the diaphragm, fundus, and esophagus. In the illustration, the first suture is in place, and the second is being passed through the diaphragm in the bowl of a spoon retractor, which is used to protect sutures beneath the diaphragm. The posterior sutures in the crus are in place but have not been tied. *E*, Sagittal sections of the repair. (A) The sutures in the crus posteriorly have been placed but not yet tied. The first row of mattress sutures between stomach and esophagus has been tied. One of the mattress sutures in the second row is illustrated. (B) The completed repair. The posterior sutures in the crus and second row of mattress sutures joining diaphragm, stomach, and esophagus are tied after the reconstruction has been placed beneath the diaphragm. (From Belsey, R. H. R., and Skinner, D. B.: Surgical treatment: Thoracic approach. *In* Skinner, D. B., Belsey, R. H. R., Hendrix, T. R., and Zuidema, G. D. (Eds.): Gastroesophageal Reflux and Hiatal Hernia. Boston, Little, Brown & Company, 1972.)

2 cm. of esophagus. A second row of sutures, passing through the edge of the tendinous portion of the diaphragm, the fundus of the stomach, and the esophageal muscle 4 cm. above the gastroesophageal junction is then placed. The esophagus is then reduced manually through the hiatus. It should lie there without tension before the sutures are tied. A postoperative barium swallow should demonstrate a 4-cm. segment of intra-abdominal esophagus. Long-term follow-up studies from Belsey's clinic indicate a recurrence rate of reflux or hiatal hernia after 10 years of approximately 15 per cent.[25] Recurrence rates are higher in patients operated for a large Type II hiatal hernia and lower in those with the more common reflux indications without stricture. Recurrences most commonly are caused by the sutures tearing out of the esophageal muscle or by sutures cutting through the diaphragmatic crura posteriorly.

The fundoplication introduced by Nissen in Switzerland in 1955 is performed through either an abdominal or a thoracic approach.[23,24] In either case, the esophagus is fully detached from the margins of the hiatus. The thoracic approach is selected if more extensive mobilization of the esophagus is required to ensure an adequate intra-abdominal segment of esophagus. For facilitation of a full 360-degree plication of gastric fundus around the abdominal segment of esophagus without tension and without injury to the spleen, several short gastric arteries are ligated and divided. The fundus of the stomach is brought posteriorly around the esophagus. Sutures are placed through the anterior fundus and the wall of the esophagus, and the fundus is brought posteriorly. A 3- to 4-cm. segment of intra-abdominal esophagus is wrapped by the fundus in this manner (Fig. 6). If the fundus is not anchored securely to the

intra-abdominal esophagus, the fundoplication may slip down onto the body of the stomach and cause a double-chamber stomach, with obstruction to the proximal pouch, causing severe reflux. This is a serious complication that can be avoided by adequate mobilization of the esophagus and by placing the wrap around the esophagus above the intact gastrohepatic ligament and hepatic branch of the vagus nerve. The full 360-degree plication of stomach around the esophagus causes a somewhat higher luminal pressure in the abdominal segment of esophagus than does the Mark IV repair.[10] Although this may

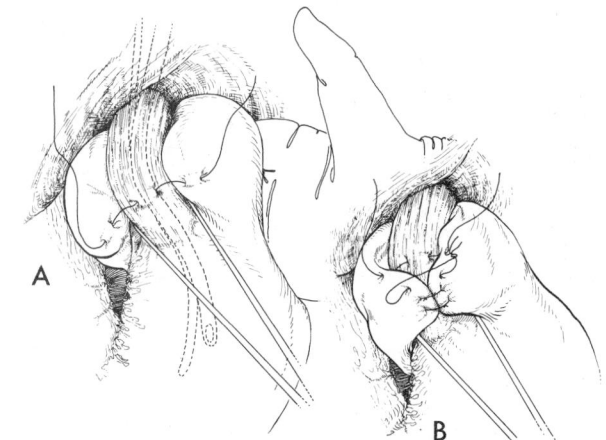

A   B

Figure 6. Nissen's "fundoplication" repair of sliding esophageal hiatal hernia, by the transabdominal approach.

be mechanically a more competent anti-reflux valve, it also introduces a greater risk of postoperative dysphagia as well as inability to belch and vomit. The danger of too tight a repair causing esophageal obstruction is real. Postoperative barium swallow should show the segment of abdominal esophagus and the pseudotumor effect of the fundoplication. Ten-year follow-up results in patients undergoing this repair are comparable to those achieved with the Mark IV repair.[22]

The procedure of posterior gastropexy and calibration of the cardia has undergone several modifications since the operation was first introduced by Hill in 1961.[13] The results achieved with this repair in recent years appear comparable to those achieved with the other two procedures.[14] The operation is done through an abdominal incision. After extensive mobilization of the esophagus through the hiatus, sutures are placed in the diaphragmatic crura to narrow the hiatus. The gastroesophageal junction is anchored to the arcuate ligament just cephalad to the celiac axis. Sutures are placed on both the anterior and the posterior aspects of the gastroesophageal junction for the purpose of causing a partial plication of stomach around the entrance of the esophagus into the stomach. The degree of narrowing of the abdominal esophagus is critical in this operation (Fig. 7); intraoperative manometry is therefore advocated as being essential to the success of this procedure. Postoperative barium swallow examination should demonstrate a narrow segment of abdominal esophagus entering the gastric pouch.

Each of these repairs provides excellent early results in more than 90 per cent of patients. Published follow-up results for each, while not fully comparable, are so similar that it appears unlikely that one repair is clearly superior to the others. Reasons to choose a particular repair include the training and experience of the surgeon, whether an abdominal or thoracic approach is preferred in a particular patient, and the advisability of avoiding a total fundoplication in patients with ineffective peristalsis and a motor disorder.

Side effects of the repair include inability to belch and vomit, symptomatic gaseous distention of the stomach and intestines from aerophagia unrelieved by belching, the risk of dysphagia from too tight a repair, and the risk of injury to the esophagus or stomach owing to the placement of sutures. The incidence of these side effects and the long-term success rates in preventing reflux and recurrent hiatal hernia are factors in judging which is the optimal procedure. A number of modifications of these

basic repairs have been reported. Before any modifications can be generally accepted, they must undergo rigorous assessment of the effect of the operation on controlling reflux, as measured by objective tests such as pH monitoring, and long-term follow-up evaluation.

ESOPHAGUS LINED WITH COLUMNAR EPITHELIUM (BARRETT'S ESOPHAGUS)

In 1950, Barrett described a condition in which columnar epithelium lining the esophagus was associated with either ulceration in the abnormal epithelium or esophagitis at the proximally located squamocolumnar junction.[4,5] The cause of this condition is still undetermined. In some it may be of congenital origin. However, most patients with this condition have severe, chronic, long-standing reflux.[16] It is known that the glandular epithelium may migrate proximally and repopulate the denuded esophageal lining at the junction where the squamous epithelium is eroded by chronic reflux. A stricture or severe esophagitis frequently occurs at the junction of columnar and squamous epithelium. This metaplastic epithelium may undergo dysplasia or neoplastic change. Several types of glandular epithelium may be found in Barrett's esophagus, including cardia type columnar, acid-secreting gastric fundic, and metaplastic intestinal epithelium. A number of patients with adenocarcinoma of the esophagus are seen in whom the cancer appears to arise from the columnar epithelium.[34] When this condition is diagnosed, multiple biopsies must be taken for exclusion of neoplastic change. If high-grade dysplasia or neoplasia is seen, an esophageal resection should be performed.[3] When complications of reflux accompany Barrett's esophagus, an antireflux repair should be performed following dilation of the stricture if necessary. In such patients, long-term observation with repeated endoscopy and biopsy or brush cytology examination is essential to demonstrate that the mucosa is quiescent and not prone to neoplastic degeneration.

REFLUX-INDUCED STRICTURES OF THE ESOPHAGUS

At an advanced stage, reflux may cause sufficient inflammation, ulceration, destruction, and scarring of the esophageal lining to produce a frank stricture. These almost always consist of combinations of edema, inflammation, spasm, and fibrosis. The treatment of the reflux-induced stricture is more difficult and results are less successful than with management of straightforward reflux problems. Therefore, it is important to perform anti-reflux surgery before a stricture develops. For this reason, persistent Grade II ulcerative esophagitis is an indication for antireflux surgery, because this degree of esophagitis is a precursor of the eventual formation of a stricture if reflux persists.

Nearly all patients with reflux-induced strictures, not previously treated surgically, respond to intensive medical therapy and repeated dilatations prior to operation. This has the effect of reducing the inflammation, edema, and spasm and converting the stricture to a lesser degree of esophagitis. Esophageal length is restored. When dilatations to a No. 40 French bougie can be achieved easily prior to operation and the inflammation can be reduced by intensive medical therapy, an antireflux repair alone has a good likelihood of success. If the stricture cannot be easily dilated or if extensive shortening of the esophagus is found at operation, additional operative measures may be necessary. Several approaches are advocated. These include lengthening the esophageal swallowing tube by cutting a tube of stomach from the lesser curvature as a continuation of the esophagus. This procedure is termed a Collis gastroplasty.[7] After the gastroplasty is performed, an antireflux repair (Fig. 8) such as the Mark IV reconstruction or Nissen fundoplication is added to

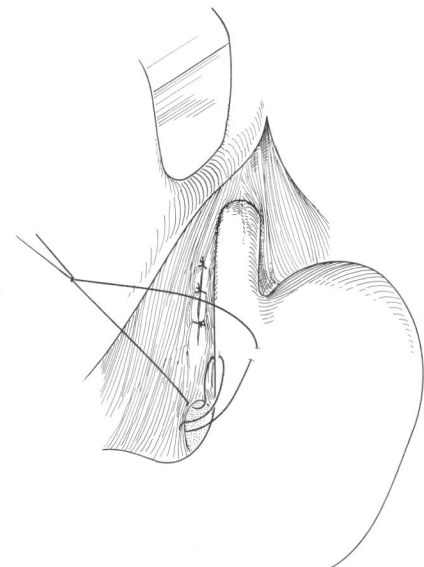

Figure 7. Schematic representation of the Hill posterior gastropexy and calibration of the cardia. This illustration demonstrates the closure of the hiatus and the placement of one of several sutures imbricating the anterior and posterior aspects of the cardia to the arcuate ligament overlying the aorta.

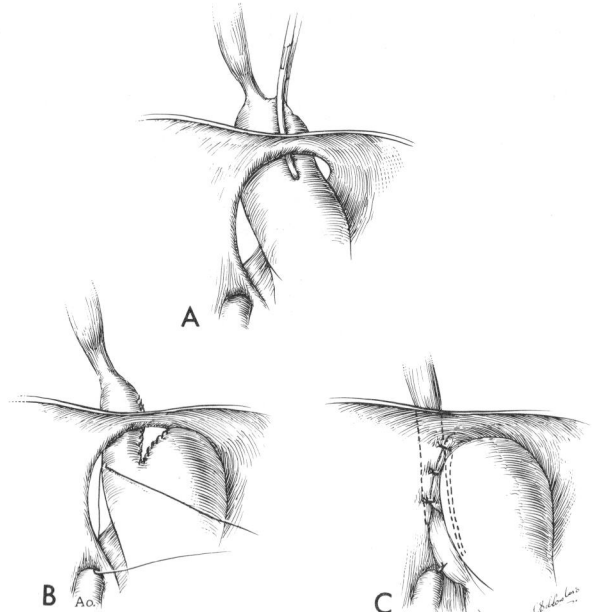

Figure 8. The Collis gastroplasty operation. *A,* A tube is cut from the lesser curvature portion of the stomach. *B,* After suture of the tube and closing of the defect in the fundus, the swallowing conduit is lengthened sufficiently below the stricture to suture the distal end of the tube to preaortic fascia below the diaphragm. *C,* The hiatus is sutured anteriorly around the intra-abdominal portion of the newly created tube. Following this step, a Belsey Mark IV or Nissen fundoplication reconstruction may be performed around the intra-abdominal segment of gastric tube. (From Belsey, R. H. R., and Skinner, D. B.: Management of esophageal strictures. *In* Skinner, D. B., Belsey, R. H. R., Hendrix, T. R., and Zuidema, G. D. (Eds.): Gastroesophageal Reflux and Hiatal Hernia. Boston, Little, Brown & Company, 1972, p. 179.)

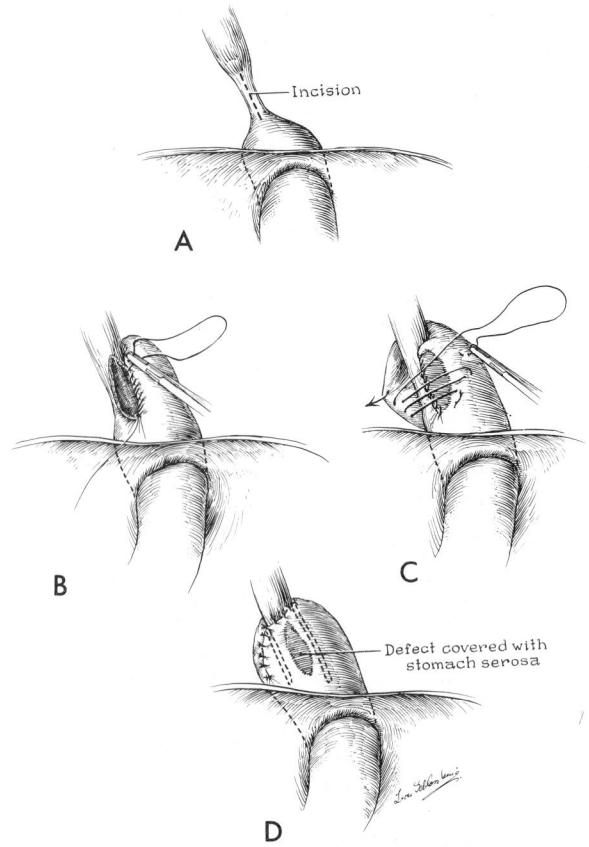

Figure 9. Thal operation for stricture with fundoplication added. *A,* The stricture is incised longitudinally. *B,* The fundus of stomach brought through the hiatus is used to patch the gaping defect in the esophagus. A skin graft may be placed on the serosal surface. *C,* After the gastric patch is completed, the fundus may be wrapped around the distal esophagus as in the Nissen fundoplication procedure. (Interrupted rather than the running sutures illustrated are preferred.) *D,* Completed repair with the opened stricture covered with a gastric patch and surrounded by the fundoplication. The reconstruction remains in the chest. (From Belsey, R. H. R., and Skinner, D. B.: Management of esophageal strictures. *In* Skinner, D. B., Belsey, R. H. R., Hendrix, T. R., and Zuidema, G. D. (Eds.): Gastroesophageal Reflux and Hiatal Hernia. Boston, Little, Brown & Company, 1972, p. 180.)

prevent further reflux into the gastric tube and distal esophagus.[28] Postoperative dilatations of the stricture may be necessary in such cases. It is important that the gastric tube be made around a large-diameter bougie, at least a No. 40 French, to ensure that the tube is not too narrow. It must be cut straight so that the gastroplasty does not cause an inverted funnel at the new gastroesophageal junction.

Another approach to the management of a stricture that cannot readily be dilated preoperatively is the Thal fundic patch operation coupled with a fundoplication. Thal described a technique for cutting longitudinally across the stricture, allowing the opening in the esophagus to gape widely, applying a skin graft across the opening, and then plicating the adjacent fundus of stomach across the opening in the esophagus.[35] This procedure alone does not prevent reflux; but when coupled with a full 360-degree fundoplication of the Nissen type (Fig. 9), satisfactory results are achieved in approximately three quarters of the patients, as reported by Hollenbeck and Woodward.[15]

Another method of treating the esophagus that cannot be reduced into the abdomen is intraoperative dilatation, coupled with a full fundoplication, but with the 360-degree fundoplication left in the chest.[20] When this is done, the hiatus must be opened widely, and the stomach serosa must be carefully anchored to the diaphragm. Despite this, there is a significant risk of progressive enlargement of the iatrogenic hiatal hernia, with further surgical therapy necessary at a later date. An incidence of gastric ulceration in the intrathoracic gastric pouch is seen in these patients as well. None of these approaches, including antireflux surgery for stricture, Collis gastroplasty, Thal fundic patch operation, or intrathoracic Nissen fundoplication, is uniformly satisfactory in patients with stricture. Excellent results, including the relief of dysphagia and long-term control of reflux, are reported in approximately three quarters of the patients after any of these procedures.

When a recurrence develops after previous surgical therapy for a stricture, it is unlikely that further attempts at repair will be successful. In such complicated reoperative cases, a resection of the damaged esophagus with an intestinal interposition using either left colon or jejunum is highly satisfactory.[6,21] The use of stomach to reconstitute the esophagus after resection is not advocated for benign disease, because the incidence of reflux following esophagogastrostomy is too high.[32] The risk of recurrent esophagitis and stricture is minimized by the interposition of an intestinal segment from the esophageal remnant through the diaphragm and into the stomach. Although this operation yields excellent results, it is a procedure of greater magnitude than any of the others and so should be reserved for those patients who have recurrent strictures after failure of previous operative attempts.

SELECTED REFERENCES

Allison, P. R.: Reflux esophagitis, sliding hiatal hernia, and the anatomy of repair. Surg. Gynecol. Obstet. *92*:419, 1951.
In this paper, Allison clearly describes for the first time the symptoms and complications of reflux esophagitis. He identifies the importance of the phrenoesophageal membrane insertion into the esophagus responsible for an intra-abdominal segment of esophagus. He describes a surgical approach that was widely used as the first attempt at an anti-reflux operation. This well-written publication is a landmark paper.

DeMeester, T. R., et al.: Technique, indications, and clinical use of 24-hour esophageal pH monitoring. J. Thorac. Cardiovasc. Surg., *79*:656–670, 1980.
This paper briefly describes the technique for 24-hour intraesophageal pH monitoring. Its main value is in describing the number of atypical syndromes caused by

reflux,, which are difficult to diagnose. In these situations, prolonged intraesophageal pH monitoring has proved to be the most precise diagnostic method and has clarified the pathophysiology of several confusing aspects of reflux-induced symptoms and complications.

Hill, L. D.: An effective operation for hiatal hernia: An eight-year appraisal. Ann. Surg., 166:681, 1967.

In this manuscript, Hill describes the rationale for posterior gastropexy and the technique for exposing the arcuate ligament overlying the aorta. While the subsequent details of the operation have changed somewhat in regard to the fundoplication, the anatomic exposure and basic principles for posterior gastropexy remain unchanged and are well described in this presentation.

Rosetti, M., and Allgower, M.: Fundoplication for treatment of hiatal hernia. Prog. Surg., 12:1, 1973.

The authors describe 1231 patients with hiatal hernia who were operated upon by the Nissen fundoplication technique. Long-term results are reported in 590 patients, of whom 87 per cent have been free of symptoms. Postfundoplication syndromes, recurrence rates, and the use of the operation in patients with a short esophagus are described.

Skinner, D. B., and Belsey, R. H. R.: Surgical management of esophageal reflux and hiatus hernia. J. Thorac. Cardiovasc. Surg., 53:33, 1967.

The paper presents the first description and long-term analysis of the Belsey Mark IV antireflux repair. Results in 832 patients are described. A detailed analysis of symptoms, complications, endoscopic findings, and postoperative results is presented. The detailed operative technique is described.

Skinner, D. B., and Belsey, R. H. R.: *Management of Esophageal Disease.* Philadelphia, W. B. Saunders Company, 1988.

This recently published text describes the authors' lifetime experience in managing patients with gastroesophageal reflux and hiatal hernia. The majority of chapters are devoted to this topic and include extensive illustrations and references.

REFERENCES

1. Allison, P. R.: Reflux esophagitis, sliding hiatal hernia, and the anatomy of repair. Surg. Gynecol. Obstet., 92:419, 1951.
2. Allison, P. R.: Hiatus hernia: A 20-year retrospective survey. Ann. Surg., 178:273, 1973.
3. Altorki, N. K., Sunagawa, M., Little, A. G., and Skinner, D. B. High grade dysplasia in the columnar lined esophagus: To resect or not? Am. J. Surg. In press.
4. Barrett, N. R.: Chronic peptic ulcer of the esophagus and "esophagitis," Br. J. Surg., 38:175, 1950.
5. Barrett, N. R.: The lower esophagus lined by columnar epithelium. Surgery, 41:881, 1957.
6. Belsey, R. H. R.: Reconstruction of esophagus with the left colon. J. Thorac. Cardiovasc. Surg., 49:33, 1965.
7. Collis, J. L.: Gastroplasty. Thoraxchirurgie, 11:57, 1963.
8. DeCarvalho, C. A. F.: Sug L'angio-architecture veineuse de la zone de Transition oesophagogastrique et son interprétation fonctionnelle. Acta Anat., 64:125, 1966.
9. DeMeester, T. R., Johnson, L. F., Joseph G. J., Toscano, M. S., Hall, A. W., and Skinner, D. B.: Patterns of gastroesophageal reflux in health and disease. Ann. Surg., 184:459, 1976.
10. DeMeester, T. R., Johnson, L. F., and Kent, A. H.: Evaluation of current operations for the prevention of gastroesophageal reflux. Ann. Surg., 180:511, 1974.
11. DeMeester, T. R., Wang, C. I., Wernly, J. A., Pellegrini, C. A., Little, A. G., Klementschitsch, P., Bermudz, G., Johnson, L. S., and Skinner, D. B.: Technique, indications, and clinical use of 24-hour esophageal pH monitoring. J. Thorac. Cardiovasc. Surg., 79:656, 1980.
12. Helm, J. F., Dodds, W. J., Pelc, L. R., et al.: Effect of esophageal emptying and saliva on clearance of acid from the esophagus. N. Engl. J. Med., 310:284, 1984.
13. Hill, L. D.: An effective operation for hiatal hernia: An eight-year appraisal. Ann. Surg., 166:681, 1967.
14. Hill, L. D. Intraoperative management of lower esophageal sphincter pressure. J. Thorac. Cardiovasc. Surg., 75:378, 1978.
15. Hollenbeck, J. I., and Woodward, E. R.: The treatment of peptic esophageal stricture with combined fundic patch-fundoplication. Ann. Surg., 182:472, 1975.
16. Iascone, C., DeMeester, T. R., Little, A. G., and Skinner, D. B.: Barrett's esophagus. Arch. Surg. 118:543, 1983.
17. Johnson, L. F., and DeMeester, T. R.: Twenty-four hour pH monitoring of the distal esophagus: A quantitative measure of gastroesophageal reflux. Am. J. Gastroenterol., 62:325, 1974.
18. Liebermann, D., Allgower, M., Schmidt, P., and Blum, A. L: Muscular equivalent of the lower esophageal sphincter. Gastroenterology, 76: 31, 1979.
19. Little, A. G., and Skinner, D. B.: The management of Zenker's diverticulum: cricopharyngeal myotomy and diverticulopexy. *In* Levitsky, S., and Kittle, C. F., (Eds.): Current Controversies in Thoracic Surgery. Philadelphia, W. B. Saunders Company, 1986.
20. Maher, J. W., Hocking, M. P., and Woodward, E. R.: Supradiaphragmatic fundoplication: Long-term follow-up and analysis of complications. Am. J. Surg.,147:181, 1984.
21. Merendino, K. A., and Dillard, D. H.: The concept of sphincter substitution by an interposed jejunal segment for anatomic and physiologic abnormalities at the esophagogastric junction—with special reference to reflux esophagitis, cardio-spasm, and esophageal varices. Ann. Surg., 142:486, 1955.
22. Negre, J. B., Markkula, H. T., Keyrilainen, O., and Matikainen, M.: Nissen fundoplication: Results at 10-year follow-up. Am. J. Surg., 146:635, 1983.
23. Nissen, R.: Eine einfache Operation zur Beeinflussung der Refluxoesophagitis. Schweiz. Med. Wochenschr., 86:590, 1956.
24. Nissen, R.: Gastropexy and "fundoplication" in surgical treatment of hiatal hernia. Am. J. Dig. Dis., 6:954, 1961.
25. Orringer, M. B., Skinner, D. B., and Belsey, R. H. R.: Long-term results of the Mark IV operation for hiatal hernia and analyses of recurrences and their treatment. J. Thorac. Cardiovasc. Surg., 63:25, 1972.
26. Orringer, M. B., and Sloan, H.: Combined Collis-Nissen reconstruction of the esophagogastric junction. Ann. Thorac. Surg., 25:16, 1978.
27. O'Sullivan, G. C., DeMeester, T. R., Joelsson, B. E., Smith, R. B., Blough, R. R., Johnson, L. F., and Skinner, D. B.: Interaction of lower esophageal sphincter pressure and length of sphincter in the abdomen as determinants of gastroesophageal competence. Am. J. Surg., 143:40, 1982.
28. Pearson, F. G., and Henderson, R. D.: Long-term follow-up of peptic strictures managed by dilatation, modified Collis gastroplasty, and Belsey hiatus hernia repair. Surgery, 80:396, 1976.
29. Pellegrini, C. A., DeMeester, T. R., Johnson, L. F., and Skinner, D. B.: Gastroesophageal reflux and pulmonary aspiration: Incidence, functional abnormality, and results of surgical therapy. Surgery, 86:110, 1979.
30. Pellegrini, C. A., DeMeester, T. R., and Skinner, D. B.: Response of the distal esophageal sphincter to respiratory and positional maneuvers in humans. Surg. Forum, XXVII:380, 1976.
31. Skinner, D. B.: Pathophysiology of gastroesophageal reflux. Ann. Surg., 202:546, 1985.
32. Skinner, D. B., and Belsey, R. H. R.: Surgical management of esophageal reflux and hiatus hernia. J. Thorac. Cardiovasc. Surg., 54:33, 1967.
33. Skinner, D. B., and Booth, D. J.: Assessment of distal esophageal function in patients with hiatal hernia and/or gastroesophageal reflux. Ann. Surg., 172:627, 1970.
34. Skinner, D. B., Walther, B. D., Riddell, R. H., Schmidt, H., Iascone, C., and DeMeester, T. R.: Barrett's esophagus: Comparison of benign and malignant cases. Ann. Surg., 198:554, 1983.
35. Thal, A. P., Hatafuku, T., and Kurtzman, R.: New operation for distal esophageal stricture. Arch. Surg., 90:464, 1965.
36. Walther, B., DeMeester, T. R., Lafontaine, E., Courtney, J. V., Little, A. G., and Skinner, D. B.: Effect of paraesophageal hernia on sphincter function and its implication in surgical therapy. Am. J. Surg., 147:111, 1984.

IX

CORROSIVE STRICTURES OF THE ESOPHAGUS

James L. Talbert, M.D.

Despite an enhanced public and legislative awareness, caustic ingestions remain a significant health threat in the United States, affecting between 5000 and 15,000 citizens annually.[21] The incidence is bimodal in age distribution, with over 75 per cent of injuries involving children less than 5 years of age, and a much lower, secondary peak occurring in late adolescence and early adult life.[37] The ingestion is almost always accidental in the young child, who, all too frequently, has been enticed by chemical solutions that have been carelessly placed in familiar soft drink containers or by crystalline caustics that resemble sugar or candy exposed in jars or cans. Instances of caustic ingestion in adolescents and adults usually represent an intentional suicide attempt by an emotionally disturbed or psychotic individual and often involve intake of relatively large volumes of toxic substances with a proportionately greater potential for inflicting serious injury.[7,14,21,33,37,45,46]

Etiology

The most common chemicals implicated in corrosive burns of the esophagus are the alkaline caustics, acid or acidlike corrosives, and household bleaches. Hydrochloric, sulfuric, nitric, and phosphoric acids are contained in automobile battery acids, soldering fluxes, and a variety of commercial cleaners. The alkaline caustics consist of sodium or potassium hydroxide (the active ingredients of household lye and drain cleaners), sodium carbonate (washing soda), sodium metasilicate (dishwashing detergent), and ammonia water (household cleaners). Severe localized esophageal burns can also follow ingestion of Clinitest tablets, which contain significant amounts of anhydrous sodium hydroxide or swallowing the small disc-shaped (button) alkaline batteries commonly used in calculators, cameras, hearing aids, and watches.[4,28,31,39] In the 40 years preceding 1965, most of the caustics ingested in the United States were flakes or solid pellets of sodium hydroxide. However, the introduction at that time of concentrated liquid drain-cleaning products such as Liquid-Plumr, containing 35 per cent sodium hydroxide solution, heralded a relative epidemic of more severe and extensive injuries of the upper gastrointenstinal tract that regressed in the early 1970s only after enforcement of federal legislation limiting the concentration of these agents and requiring the use of child-proof containers.[7,30,45] As one threat subsided, another emerged, when in response to increasing concern for environmental pollution, phosphate dishwashing detergents of relatively mild toxicity were replaced by highly alkaline nonphosphate compounds containing sodium silicate, sodium carbonate, sodium metasilicate, and sodium borate, which presented an increased risk of injury to small children in the home.[23,26] Subsequent modifications in the formulation of the nonphosphate detergents have diminished their potential toxicity, although they may still produce transient, severe respiratory distress when inhaled.[9,45] Moreover, the environment today continues to provide an apparently never-ending array of hazards for young children, as exemplified by recent reports of accidental ingestions of concentrated alkaline solutions used on dairy farms to clean pipelines in milk houses and orofacial burns induced by inquisitive applications of a newly introduced product—oven-cleaning pads.[7,37,44]

Corrosive burns from ingested caustic agents may involve the oropharynx, larynx, esophagus, stomach, and even the small intestine and colon. The site and severity of injury are primarily dependent on the character, quantity, and concentration of the ingested substance. Caustic burns from common household bleaches such as Clorox are encountered with increasing frequency but rarely produce permanent damage unless swallowed in large amounts.[21,34,45,46] Solid lye substances tend to lodge in the oropharynx or upper esophagus, whereas concentrated liquid caustics not only present an increased potential for esophageal injury but may also damage the stomach and distal intestinal tract, especially in young children.[37,46] The ingestion of crystals of lye causes pain, and most children attempt to spit out the caustic material immediately on tasting it.[45] This defense mechanism is absent in the case of liquid caustics, which are often colorless and odorless and may produce serious damage even in concentrations of less than 10 per cent.[2] Because caustic injury induces relaxation of the lower esophageal sphincter, the resultant tendency for gastroesophageal reflux may promote prolonged exposure of the distal lumen to the injurious agent.[37]

In instances of acid ingestion, the esophagus may escape injury because of the relative resistance of the squamous epithelium and the briefness of contact as the liquid rapidly traverses the extent of its lumen. However, upon reaching the stomach, the acid usually induces immediate pylorospasm, which leads to pooling of the destructive chemical in the distal antrum and production of a severe gastritis that may progress within 24 to 48 hours to full-thickness necrosis and perforation.[32] The presence of food in the stomach tends to limit the extent and severity of this process. The immediate pain experienced upon its ingestion makes the consumption of large quantities of acid less common than alkaline poisoning; but an intent, emotionally disturbed person may swallow a significant volume, thereby producing the characteristic clinical pattern.

Like external body burns, caustic injuries of the gatrointestinal tract are categorized as superficial or deep on the basis of histologic appearance and clinical behavior, although at the time of endoscopy differentiation can sometimes prove difficult.[19,33] Characteristically, superficial burns of the mucosa are manifested by erythema, edema, blister formation, or small, isolated ulcers. Deep burns are exemplified by circumferential ulcerations and may extend through the full thickness of the esophageal wall into adjacent mediastinal tissues, penetrating the pleural and peritoneal cavities and even occasionally producing tracheoesophageal or aortoenteric fistulas.[3,23] Sites that appear especially susceptible to injury because of a relative delay in transit include the upper esophagus in the area of the cricopharyngeus; the midesophagus, where the aorta and left mainstem bronchus may partially compress the lumen; and the distal esophagus immediately proximal to the lower sphincter. Following superficial injuries, re-epithelialization of the esophageal mucosa is usually complete by the sixth week; but in instances of full-thickness injury, scarring and contracture may progress for a period of months. Similarly, gastric outlet obstruction may be a later sequela of major acid injury to the stomach as a consequence of progressive antral scarring.[5,33]

Prophylactic Treatment

The most important element in the successful management of a corrosive burn of the esophagus is immediate verification of the etiologic agent and accurate assessment of the depth and extent of injury. Subsequent treatment of the patient must be individualized on the basis of these findings.[19,23,31,45,48] It is essential to seek the container from which the caustic material was obtained in order to confirm the type and to determine the pH. Alkaline solutions with a pH of less than 11.5 are considered relatively safe, whereas those with a pH exceeding this level possess a proportionately increasing potential for injury.[9,21,24,26] First-aid treatment of these patients by antidotal administration is probably ineffective because the corrosive action is largely completed within a time span of seconds, and Ipecac-induced vomiting poses a threat of compounding the original injury by re-exposing tissues to the offending agent.[21] Indeed, previous reports have emphasized an increased incidence of severe laryngeal and esophageal injury following vomiting of ingested caustic substances.[32,45]

The accidental ingestion of a small disc or "button" battery represents a special threat to the small child and demands prompt attention.[28,31,39] Severe local damage to the esophagus may ensue within only 4 to 6 hours as a consequence of the separate or combined effects of generated electrical current, pressure necrosis, and leakage of the highly corrosive contents, either as a result of deterioration of the case or damage sustained during endoscopic retrieval. There is universal agreement that esophageal entrapment of a disc battery is an indication for immediate extraction, although when the object has reached the stomach, spontaneous passage throughout the remainder of the gastrointestinal tract can be anticipated with an extremely low incidence of complications.[21] Although use of a

Foley balloon catheter under fluoroscopic guidance has been advocated for retrieval of these and other esophageal foreign bodies, in this circumstance, endoscopic extraction of disc batteries is preferred because of the importance of identifying any associated injury and, when confirmed, performing a concomitant bronchoscopy to exclude coexistent tracheal damage.[23,39]

Caustic injury is manifested by the symptoms of oral pain, drooling, excessive salivation, and inability or refusal to swallow or drink. When there is a history of ingestion, the mucosa of the lips, tongue, and oropharynx, as well as the skin of the face, hands, and neck must be carefully inspected for evidence of erythema, edema, blistering, or ulceration. Substernal and back discomfort or abdominal pain and rigidity may signify mediastinal or peritoneal perforation. Hoarseness, stridor, and dyspnea suggest laryngeal edema or actual epiglottic and laryngeal destruction through aspiration of the chemical agent. However, the absence of symptoms or visible evidence of oropharyngeal burns does not exclude the possibility of esophageal injury, because in reported series burn damage has been subsequently confirmed by esophagoscopy in 10 to 30 per cent of patients with no external evidence.[1,21,37,45,46] Simultaneously, as many as 70 per cent of patients with evidence of oropharyngeal burns escape associated esophageal injury.[16] It is essential, therefore, that as soon as an appropriate period of time has elapsed to allow gastric emptying and stabilization of the patient esophagoscopy be performed expeditiously, preferably within the first 12 to 24 hours, to confirm the extent and severity of the burn.[12,16] In children, this procedure is best accomplished under general anesthesia in order to avoid undue emotional trauma and minimize the risk of incurring any serious secondary injury that might be induced by the movement of a struggling patient. The only exceptions to proceeding with early endoscopy are those instances in which esophageal or gastric perforation or impending airway obstruction is suspected.

Any evidence of significant pharyngeal or laryngeal damage, identified by direct laryngoscopy or suggested by symptoms of hoarseness, stridor, or dyspnea, demands immediate hospitalization and observation because the period of maximal edema and danger may be delayed for 6 to 24 hours. Esophagoscopy is contraindicated in these situations because of its potential for compounding the original injury, and immediate treatment with steroids and antibiotics should be instituted in all such cases. Blood gases should be monitored serially, and a tracheostomy should be performed if the airway obstruction or respiratory distress appears progressive. Chest films should be studied for evidence of pulmonary infiltrate or free perforation into the mediastinum, pleural, or peritoneal cavities. In the absence of such findings, a barium esophagogram should be obtained for confirmation of the integrity of the upper gastrointestinal tract and assessment of the extent of injury. Although some authors have noted that the initial barium swallow may appear falsely normal in as many as 30 per cent of patients with significant caustic burns, others have found cine-esophagographically visualized abnormalities, especially disordered motility, to be helpful in prognosticating the severity of injury and outcome.[27,41]

The most reliable method for confirming the presence or absence of a caustic burn and estimating its severity is direct visualization. While some authors have suggested that early endoscopy might prove misleading because of insufficient time for the burn wound to mature adequately to permit accurate visual verification, recent clinical experience has refuted this concern, and the importance of instituting early treatment clearly militates against undue delay.[11,14,48] In the past, the endoscopist has also been cautioned against passing a rigid esophagoscope beyond the proximal point of injury because of the potential danger of perforation.[19] However, the advent of the flexible pediatric fiberoptic scope has increased the relative safety of this procedure; and when liquid caustics or acids have been in-

gested, it is especially important to assess the status of the stomach because of the potential of these agents to produce gastric injury, even in the absence of an identifiable esophageal burn.[32]

The depth of burn, as evaluated on the basis of superficial or deep involvement, is an important prognostic guide. In those patients who have sustained only superficial injuries as manifested by erythema, edema, or blistering, the prognosis appears excellent even in the absence of any specific treatment. However, the identification of ulcerations, especially when circumferential, warrants concern because of the inherent high potential for stricture formation.[45,48] In the presence of a validated injury, the status of the esophagus should be serially assessed by contrast studies repeated at intervals of 3 weeks, 3 months, 6 months, and 1 year for excluding the possibility of late stricture formation. In the acute phase of severe injury, the esophagus may appear atonic and dilated, rigid and persistently narrowed, or excessively irritable.[27] Although roentgenographic studies of the stomach during the first 1 to 2 weeks following acid ingestion may demonstrate only prominent mucosal folds, serial examinations frequently demonstrate progressive gastric outlet obstruction or the development of either an hourglass or linitis plastica–like appearance.[14]

In general, two treatment options have been advocated for prevention of stricture: (1) maintenance of an esophageal lumen by mechanical means and (2) pharmacologic modification of wound healing. Unfortunately, because of the continually changing spectrum of ingested caustics over the past 30 years, involving a variety of substances with differing potentials for injury, and the absence of any large, randomized, well-controlled series of patients comparable to that utilized nationally for coordinated evaluations of childhood cancer treatment, management of these injuries has remained controversial, with advocates espousing both forms of treatment, separately or in combination.[14,45] Regardless of the mode of management, clinical reports have increasingly emphasized that in the presence of a full-thickness esophageal injury there is an inherent high potential for stricture formation.[34]

Pharmacologic management of esophageal burns has been predicated on the use of steroids to modify the inflammatory response to the burn injury and antibiotics to control secondary bacterial infection. Experimental studies by Spain and colleagues in 1950 first suggested that early administration of cortisone produced an anti-inflammatory effect that would inhibit fibroplasia in wound healing.[40] These findings were subsequently applied to the treatment of experimental esophageal burns in animals, and the beneficial effects of steroids in reducing the incidence of postinjury stricture appeared to be confirmed when antibiotic coverage was added to control secondary suppurative complications.[17,25] These studies also suggested that steroid therapy should be instituted immediately, and most investigators have discouraged this form of treatment if the patient is seen later than 48 hours after injury.[16,25] In patients treated with steroids and antibiotics, self-bougienage through the ingestion and swallowing of food is probably an important component of treatment; and in a small child who is able to swallow without discomfort, this is the simplest method of achieving esophageal dilation. Moreover, the tendency for early esophageal obstruction to evolve as a consequence of edema and spasm is also minimized by steroid administration, thereby facilitating the early institution of oral feedings.[16] Because the reflux of acidic gastric secretions may potentiate the injury to the esophageal mucosa and further increase the likelihood of stricture formation, prophylactic use of H_2 blockers or administration of therapeutic doses of antacids for 6 to 8 weeks has been recommended.[37]

Steroid treatment is contraindicated in cases of severe caustic burns that are associated with clinical or roentgenographic evidence of perforation of the esophagus or necrosis of the stomach. Concentrated liquid lye preparations are especially likely to produce these complications.[3,23] The use of steroids is also of questionable value in the treatment of acid ingestion, because it may not only mask evidence of peritonitis but also increase the potential for gastric ulceration and bleeding. In contrast, patients with signs of dyspnea, hoarseness, or stridor should be treated immediately with steroids and antibiotics in an effort to relieve the airway obstruction; esophagoscopy is contraindicated. Immediate steroid and antibiotic treatment should also be considered in those patients in whom diagnostic esophagoscopy may be delayed for longer than 12 hours. If no esophageal lesion is subsequently identified by an experienced endoscopist, this treatment can be discontinued.

The steroid and antibiotic regimen that has been used most frequently for treatment of esophageal burns consists of prednisone, administered in divided doses of 2 to 3 mg. per kg. of body weight every 24 hours, and ampicillin, administered in divided doses of 50 to 100 mg. per kg. of body weight every 24 hours for a total of 3 weeks.[16,33] If the patient is initially unable to take oral alimentation, these medications should be administered intravenously with hydrocortisone or methylprednisolone sodium succinate substituted in equivalent doses. Because the act of swallowing food probably contributes to the success of steroid therapy, oral feedings are instituted as soon as they can be tolerated by the patient, beginning with a clear liquid diet and progressing to soft foods over the subsequent 3 to 4 days.

When the initial edema of injury has resolved, usually within 2 to 3 days, the patient's ability to swallow should gradually improve. If dysphagia reappears, stricture formation should be suspected and an immediate barium swallow should be obtained for confirmation. At the end of 3 full weeks of treatment, the steroid dosage should be tapered and finally discontinued. The experience of Middlekamp and associates suggests that prolongation of treatment simply postpones stricture formation and does not alter the eventual outcome.[33] A complete radiographic evaluation of the esophagus is obtained at the termination of steroid therapy and is repeated again at 3 months, 6 months, and 1 year after injury. If stricture formation is evident at any time during this follow-up, dilation should be instituted immediately. Continuation of steroid therapy under these circumstances does not appear to alter the eventual course of stricture formation and may unnecessarily expose the patient to the added hazard of an excessively friable esophagus when esophageal dilation is performed.[33]

The use of bougienage for early treatment of corrosive esophageal burns was introduced by Salzer in 1920 and characteristically has been performed blindly with tapered bougies.[38] A graduated program is established in which esophageal dilation is performed daily for several weeks, then every other day for 2 to 3 weeks, and finally once a week for many months. Previously, it was believed that early bougienage prevented intraluminal adhesions within the injured esophagus, but experimental observations have suggested that this form of treatment may actually enhance cicatrix formation and increase the risk of perforation.[17,25] Certainly in young children, the group most susceptible to caustic burns, esophageal bougienage appears to add psychologic and physical hazards that are unwarranted if other, less traumatic treatment methods can produce equally satisfactory results.

Because of the frequent occurrence of stricture formation in severe esophageal caustic injuries, despite prompt treatment with steroids and antibiotics, an alternative to the bougienage technique, which has been increasingly advocated in such cases, involves mechanical modification of wound healing through placement of intraluminal Silastic stents.[6,10,48] The stent serves to prevent obliteration of the esophageal lumen by either adhesions or scar contracture and to provide a template for epithelial ingrowth. Whether used in concert with or without systemic antibiotics and steroids, several reports have indicated success in decreasing the incidence of stricture formation, even

in the presence of severe, circumferential esophageal mucosal injury, when the stents have been left in place for a minimum of 3 weeks or until the process of re-epithelialization has been completed. However, creation of a gastrostomy may be required for its insertion, and depending on the type and configuration of the stent, a more intense level of monitoring and longer period of hospitalization may be entailed with this form of treatment than with the alternative approach of steroid and antibiotic management.

Management of Corrosive Strictures

The most frequent complication of caustic burns of the esophagus is stricture formation, usually developing within 2 months following the initial injury. In some instances, these lesions are mild and will immediately respond to dilation without subsequent recurrence. All too often, especially when concentrated liquid corrosives have been ingested, lye burns cause extensive full-thickness damage, which eventually produces multiple areas of stricture throughout the extent of the esophagus (Fig. 1). In those cases in which ultimate stenosis can be anticipated on the basis of the severity of the original injury, early passage of a string or small catheter through the patient's nose into the stomach facilitates bougienage.[19] In some instances, a gastrostomy may be necessary in order to maintain satisfactory gastrointestinal alimentation and to facilitate subsequent esophageal dilation. Cases of multiple tight strictures are probably best managed by this approach, retrograde esophageal dilation being performed with rubber tapered-tip Tucker bougies guided by the string or catheter previously passed from above.

The complication of tracheoesophageal fistula may follow an extensive corrosive burn of the esophagus; and it is suggested by progressive pneumonia, choking, coughing with feedings, or aspiration of bile-stained mucus from the airway. These characteristic symptoms usually appear within the first few weeks after injury. The diagnosis can be confirmed by a contrast study utilizing thin barium or Dionosil, avoiding use of water-soluble gastrointestinal contrast media, which are highly irritating when exposed to the bronchi and lungs. Direct operative attack

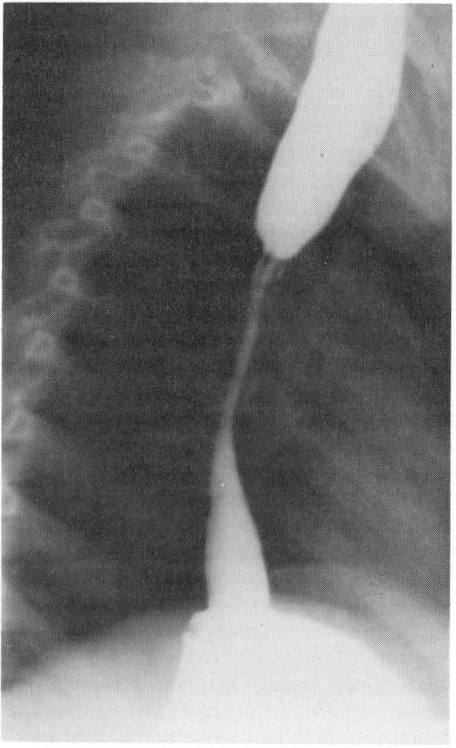

Figure 1. A characteristic extensive esophageal stricture in a child resulting from lye (Liquid-Plumr) ingestion.

on the fistula has frequently been fraught with disaster because the extensive friability and necrosis of the tissues prevent them from holding sutures, patches, or muscle flaps. Instead, successful management entails bipolar exclusion of the esophagus by proximal and distal division and closure in the neck and abdomen in conjunction with a cervical esophagostomy and gastrostomy. A tracheostomy assists in controlling aspiration while the trachea and defunctionalized esophagus heal, usually with complete scarring and obliteration of the latter.[3]

With identification of full-thickness necrosis of the esophagus and stomach as may be incurred by the ingestion of concentrated solutions of alkalis or acids, an emergency gastrectomy and/or transhiatal blunt esophagectomy may be indicated to prevent lethal complications such as overwhelming sepsis or aortoenteric fistula.[10,15] If a gastrostomy is required, it should be positioned on the stomach wall so that a gastric tube can be formed subsequently from the greater curvature, in the event this procedure proves necessary for esophageal reconstruction.[8] It is also important that the antrum and pylorus of the stomach be inspected carefully when a gastrostomy is performed, since a stricture may not be visible from the serosal side and careful intraluminal palpation may be necessary to identify a circumferential thickening. If destruction by the ingested chemical has involved the stomach and pylorus with extensive necrosis and edema, a feeding jejunostomy may be utilized as an alternate route for maintaining enteral alimentation.[49]

Although the safest approach to esophageal dilation is probably retrograde with Tucker bougies passed through a gastrostomy, this method is not necessarily required for all patients. Alternative approaches include antegrade dilation by Sabary-Guillard plastic bougies threaded over a previously positioned guidewire.[43] Another method of dilation that has been found especially helpful in the management of children with isolated or persistent strictures involves use of the Gruntzig inflatable balloon catheter, which was originally devised for transluminal angioplasty. Even in small children with narrow, tortuous strictures, a flexible wire can usually be inserted endoscopically, over which a balloon catheter can be subsequently advanced and optimally positioned under fluoroscopic guidance. As the balloon is inflated with dilute contrast media under radiographic monitoring, the predominant force is focused outward at the site of esophageal scarring and constriction, thereby minimizing the potentially disruptive shearing effect inherently produced by the passage of bougies.[34,42] Chronic cases with minimal or moderate esophageal strictures can also be treated adequately in adults by swallowed mercury-filled Maloney or Hurst bougies when the patient is cooperative.

In cases of localized strictures that extend less than 1.5 cm. in length and fail to respond to bougienage alone, local injection of steroids under direct vision through an esophagoscope into the four quadrants of the circumferential esophageal scar has been reported to be beneficial.[18] This technique was initially suggested by its success in achieving regression of cutaneous hypertrophic scars and burn contractures through local infiltration of triamcinolone diacetate. The steroid injection is followed by bougienage, and the treatment course may be repeated if necessary. Clinitest tablets and disc batteries appear especially prone to produce localized esophageal strictures, and if these lesions fail to respond to dilation, resection and esophageal anastomosis are often feasible.[4]

The need for surgical reconstruction of the esophagus may be indicated by a continuing requirement for frequent dilation of extensive or multiple strictures for longer than 6 months; by failure or refusal of the patient to follow a regimen of regular dilation; by the presence of a fistula between the esophagus and the tracheobronchial tree; or by iatrogenic perforation of the esophagus in the course of an attempted dilation.[11,34] Prolonged unsuccessful attempts at dilation not only expose the patient, frequently a child, to unnecessary physical and psychologic

trauma but also may impede normal growth and development. Use of the right colon with an attached segment of terminal ileum, tunneled through the retrosternal space into the neck, has proved eminently satisfactory in all patients older than 1 year of age with extensive esophageal scarring (Fig. 2).[34,36,47] The inclusion of a short segment of terminal ileum for anastomosis to the proximal esophagus in the neck decreases the bulk of tissue and avoids obstruction at the thoracic inlet, previously a frequent problem in young children undergoing this procedure. Preservation of the ileocecal valve has also appeared to decrease the hazard of aspiration associated with regurgitation from the patulous substernal colonic segment into the proximal esophagus and oropharynx, and incorporation of a pyloroplasty or pyloromyotomy has appeared to diminish the incidence of colitis induced by reflux of acidic secretions from the contiguous stomach.[36,47] An alternate method for colonic interposition is the technique of Waterston, in which transverse and descending colon is brought through the left pleural cavity in an isoperistaltic manner and interposed between the proximal esophagus and the stomach.[13] When the colon proves unsuitable for esophageal substitution because of an aberrant blood supply or an anatomic abnormality such as associated imperforate anus, the gastric tube technique may be utilized.[8] This procedure most frequently employs a reversed, antiperistaltic gastric tube that is based proximally on the greater curvature of the stomach and receives its blood supply from the left gastroepiploic artery. The gastric tube is then passed through a retrosternal tunnel for anastomosis to the cervical esophagus. While the preceding techniques have been demonstrated in children to provide excellent long-term function and allow normal growth and development, the alternative procedure of gastric transposition has gained increasing favor in adults.[35]

Successful management of cases of acid ingestion frequently demands surgical intervention.[5,32] Coexistent esophageal injury is probably much more frequent than previously recognized and esophageal strictures have been reported in 6 to 20 per cent of patients.[49] In a review of 27 patients with gastric injury as a result of acid ingestion, 23 eventually required surgical correction of pyloric stenosis, with gastric resection performed in 17.[32] Gastric outlet obstruction as a result of progressive antral scarring may develop within 3 to 8 weeks or may be delayed for as long as 6 years. Because of the documented incidence of carcinoma occurring in the gastric wall previously subjected to acid injury, subtotal gastrectomy with a Billroth Type I reconstruction is considered the treatment of choice whenever feasible.[32] Prolonged inanition is inevitably encountered in patients sustaining severe gastrointestinal injuries as a result of caustic ingestion, and either total parenteral nutrition or placement of a feeding jejunostomy has proved to be an important adjunct to successful management.[49]

Late Complications

A late complication of corrosive burns of the esophagus that has not been widely recognized is the development of a hiatal hernia 25 to 69 years after injury.[22] Apparently, the fibrotic esophagus contracts and pulls the stomach into the chest. The patient then develops esophagitis and peptic stricture in an already narrowed esophagus secondary to gastroesophageal reflux. Dilation of the esophageal stricture in these patients is not beneficial, because it increases the reflux and the fibrotic stricture becomes tighter. An acquired form of achalasia has also been reported as a consequence of extensive intramural fibrosis.

A final, long-term complication of esophageal scarring and stricture formation is malignant degeneration. It has been estimated that the incidence of esophageal carcinoma in patients who have previously suffered lye stricture is at least 1000-fold greater than in the general population.[29] Any change in symptoms in a patient with a chronic lye stricture, especially one of more than 16 years' duration, should immediately suggest the

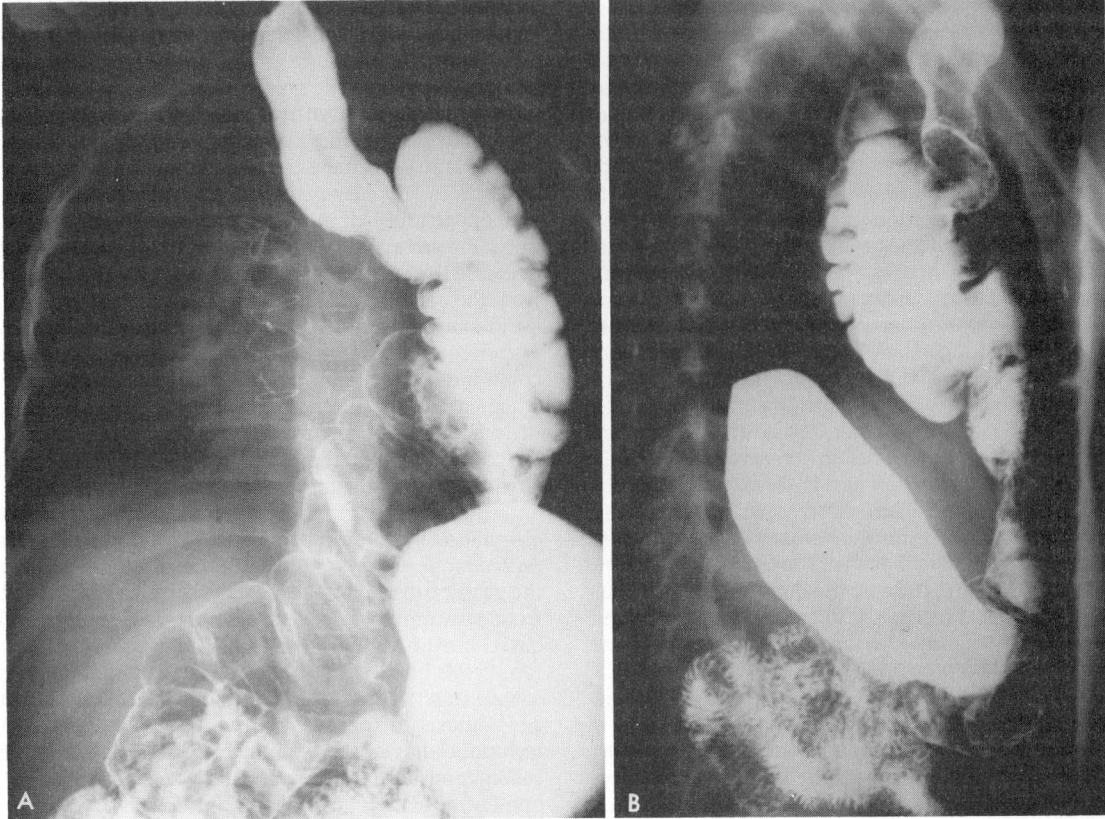

Figure 2. *A*, Anteroposterior, and *B*, lateral views of a retrosternal pull-through of terminal ileum and right colon for bypass of an extensive esophageal lye stricture in a child.

need for radiographic and esophagoscopic examination. Inability to dilate a chronic stricture that has previously responded to treatment or late radiographic evidence of progressive stenosis strongly suggests malignant change. Biopsies performed through the esophagoscope can easily overlook the tumor in such cases, because the carcinoma may be located distal to the area of stenosis and be inaccessible to the biopsy forceps. In these circumstances, therefore, negative biopsies must be considered inconclusive. Fortunately, those carcinomas that develop in scar tissue appear to be less aggressive than the usual esophageal cancer, possibly because the enveloping scar inhibits outward invasion and the resultant intraluminal proliferation produces early obstructive symptoms.[20] Resection of a strictured esophageal segment is indicated in any patient with a chronic lye stricture in whom the aforementioned changes have occurred. Identification of the tumor provides the patient an excellent likelihood of being cured of a lesion that ordinarily has a dismal prognosis.

SELECTED REFERENCES

Haller, J. A., Jr., Andrews, H. G., White, J. J., and Cleveland, W. W.: Pathophysiology and management of acute corrosive burns of the esophagus: Results of treatment in 285 children. J. Pediatr. Surg., 6:579, 1971.
This paper is the classic reference on the physiologic rationale and clinical justification for steroid and antibiotic treatment of esophageal caustic burns.

Kuhns, D. W., and Dire, D. J.: Button battery ingestions. Ann. Emerg. Med., 18:293, 1989.
This comprehensive review focuses on the newest, relatively common source of potentially severe esophageal caustic injury—small disc battery ingestion.

Maull, K. I., Scher, L. A., and Greenfield, L. J.: Surgical implications of acid ingestion. Surg. Gynecol. Obstet., 148:895, 1979.
This paper reviews the treatment of acid ingestion and emphasizes the significant dissimilarities that exist in the early management, late complications, and surgical therapy between cases of acid and alkali ingestion.

Rothstein, F. C.: Caustic injuries to the esophagus in children. Pediatr. Clin. North Am., 33:665, 1986.
This publication presents a comprehensive, current review of the subject of corrosive injuries of the esophagus in children.

Wason, S.: The emergency management of caustic ingestions. J. Emerg. Med., 2:175, 1985.
This review article emphasizes the controversial issues involved in the emergency management of caustic ingestions and attempts to resolve them relative to the formulation of an optimal treatment regimen for the individual patient.

REFERENCES

1. Alford, B. R., and Harris, H. H.: Chemical burns of the mouth, pharynx and esophagus. Ann. Otol. Rhinol. Laryngol., 68:122, 1959.
2. Ashcraft, K. W., and Padula, R. T.: The effect of dilute corrosives on the esophagus. Pediatrics, 53:226, 1974.
3. Burrington, J. D., and Raffensperger, J. G.: Surgical management of tracheoesophageal fistula complicating caustic ingestion. Surgery, 84:329, 1978.
4. Burrington, J. D.: Clinitest burns of the esophagus. Ann. Thorac. Surg., 20:400, 1975.
5. Cochran, S. T., Fonkalsrud, E. W., and Gyepes, M. T.: Complete obstruction of the gastric antrum in children following acid ingestion. Arch. Surg., 113:308, 1978.
6. Coln, D., and Chang, J. H. T.: Experience with esophageal stenting for caustic burns in children. J. Pediatr. Surg., 21:588, 1986.
7. Edmonson, M. B.: Caustic alkali ingestions by farm children. Pediatrics, 79:413, 1987.
8. Ein, S. H., Shandling, B., and Stephens, C. A.: Twenty-one year experience with the pediatric gastric tube. J. Pediatr. Surg., 22:77, 1987.
9. Einhorn, A., Horton, L., Altieri, M., Ochsenschlager, D., and Klein, B.: Serious respiratory consequences of detergent ingestions in children. Pediatrics, 84:472, 1989.
10. Estrera, A., Taylor, W., Mills, L. J., and Platt, M. R.: Corrosive burns of the esophagus and stomach: A recommendation for an aggressive surgical approach. Ann. Thorac. Surg., 41:276, 1986.
11. Ferguson, M. K., Migliore, M., Staszak, V. M., and Little, A. G.: Early evaluation and therapy for caustic esophageal injury. Am. J. Surg., 157:116, 1989.
12. Gaudreault, P., Parent, M., McGuigan, M. A., Chicoine, L., and Lovejoy, F. H.: Predictability of esophageal injury from signs and symptoms: A study of caustic ingestion in 378 children. Pediatrics, 71:767, 1983.

13. German, J. C., and Waterston, D. J.: Colon interposition for the replacement of the esophagus in children. J. Pediatr. Surg., *11*:227, 1976.
14. Goldman, L. P., and Weigert, J. M.: Corrosive substance ingestion: A review. Am. J. Gastroenterol., *79*:85, 1984.
15. Gossott, D., Sarfati, E., and Celerier, M.: Early blunt esophagectomy in severe caustic burns of the upper digestive tract. J. Thorac. Cardiovasc. Surg., *94*:188, 1987.
16. Haller, J. A., Jr., Andrews, H. G., White, J. J., and Cleveland, W. W.: Pathophysiology and management of acute corrosive burns of the esophagus: Results of treatment in 285 children. J. Pediatr. Surg., *6*:579, 1971.
17. Haller, J. A., and Bachman, K.: The comparative effect of current therapy on experimental caustic burns of the esophagus. Pediatrics, *34*:236, 1964.
18. Holder, R. M., Ashcraft, K. W., and Leape, L: The treatment of patients with esophageal strictures by local steroid injection. J. Pediatr. Surg., *4*:646, 1969.
19. Holinger, P. H.: Management of esophageal lesions caused by chemical burns. Ann. Otol. Rhinol. Laryngol., *77*:819, 1968.
20. Hopkins, R. A., and Postlethwait, R. W.: Caustic burns and carcinoma of the esophagus. Ann. Surg., *194*:146, 1981.
21. Howell, J. M.: Alkaline ingestions. Ann. Emerg. Med., *15*:820, 1986.
22. Imre, J., and Kopp, M.: Arguments against long-term conservative treatment of esophageal strictures due to corrosive burns. Thorax, *27*:594, 1972.
23. Kirsh, M. M., Peterson, A., Brown, J. W., Orringer, M. B., Ritter, F., and Sloan, H.: Treatment of caustic injuries of the esophagus: A ten-year experience. Ann. Surg., *188*:675, 1978.
24. Klein, J., Olson, K. R., and McKinney, H. E.: Caustic injury from household ammonia. Am. J. Emerg. Med., *3*:320, 1985.
25. Knox, W. G., Scott, J. R., Zintel, H. A., Guthrie, R., and McCabe, R. E.: Bougienage and steroids used singly or in combination in experimental corrosive esophagitis. Ann. Surg., *166*:930, 1967.
26. Krenzelok, E. P., and Clinton, J. E.: Caustic esophageal and gastric erosion without evidence of oral burns following detergent ingestion. J. Am. Coll. Emerg. Phys., *8*:194, 1979.
27. Kuhn, J. R., and Tunell, W. P.: The role of initial cine-esophagography in caustic esophageal injury. Am. J. Surg., *146*:804, 1983.
28. Kuhns, D. W., and Dire, D. J.: Button battery ingestions. Ann. Emerg. Med., *18*:293, 1989.
29. Lansing, P. B., Ferrante, W. A., and Ochsner, J. L.: Carcinoma of the esophagus at the site of lye stricture. Am. J. Surg., *118*:108, 1969.
30. Leape, L. L., Ashcraft, K. W., Scarpelli, D. G., and Holder, T. M.: Hazard to health: Liquid lye. N. Engl. J. Med., *284*:578, 1971.
31. Litovitz, T. L.: Battery ingestions: Product accessibility and clinical course. Pediatrics, *75*:469, 1985.
32. Maull, K. I., Scher, L. A., and Greenfield, L. J.: Surgical implications of acid ingestion. Surg. Gynecol. Obstet., *148*:895, 1979.
33. Middlekamp, J. N., Ferguson, T. B., Roper, C. L., and Hoffman, F. D.: The management and problems of caustic burns in children. J. Thorac. Cardiovasc. Surg., *57*:341, 1969.
34. Moazam, F., Talbert, J. L., Miller, D., and Mollitt, D. L.: Caustic ingestion and its sequelae in children. South. Med. J., *80*:187, 1987.
35. Orringer, M. B.: Transhiatal esophagectomy for benign disease. J. Thorac. Cardiovasc. Surg., *90*:649, 1985.
36. Rodgers, B. M., Talbert, J. L., Moazam, F., and Felman, A. H.: Functional and metabolic evaluation of colon replacement of the esophagus in children. J. Pediatr. Surg.,*13*:35, 1978.
37. Rothstein, F. C: Caustic injuries to the esophagus in children. Pediatr. Clin. North Am., *33*:665, 1986.
38. Salzer, H.: Early treatment of corrosive esophagitis. Wien. Klin. Wochenschr., *33*:307, 1920.
39. Sigalet, D., and Lees, G.: Tracheoesophageal injuries secondary to disk battery ingestion. J. Pediatr. Surg., *23*:996, 1988.
40. Spain, D. M., Malomert, N., and Haber, A.: The effect of cortisone of the formation of granulation tissue in mice. Am. J. Pathol., *26*:710, 1950.
41. Stannard, M. W.: Corrosive esophagitis in children: Assessment by the esophagogram. Am. J. Dis. Child., *132*:596, 1978.
42. Taub, S., Rodan, B. A., Bean, W. J., Koerner, R. S., Mullin, D. M., and Feng, T. S.: Balloon dilatation of esophageal strictures. Am. J. Gastroenterol. *81*:14, 1986.
43. Tytgat, G. N. J.: Dilation therapy of benign esophageal stenoses. World J. Surg., *13*:142, 1989.
44. Vilogi, J., Whitehead, B., and Marcus, S M.: Oven-cleaner pads: New risk for corrosive injury. Am. J. Emerg. Med., *3*:412, 1985.
45. Wason, S.: The emergency management of caustic ingestions. J. Emerg. Med., *2*:175, 1985.
46. Wasserman, R. L., and Ginsburg, C. M.: Caustic substance injuries. J. Pediatr., *107*:169, 1985.
47. West, K. W., Vane, D. W., and Grosfeld, J. L.: Esophageal replacement in children: Experience with thirty-one cases. Surgery, *100*:751, 1986.
48. Wijburg, F. A., Heymans, H. S. A., and Urbanus, N. A. M.: Caustic esophageal lesions in children: Prevention of stricture formation. J. Pediatr. Surg., *24*:171, 1989.
49. Zargar, S. A., Kochhar, R., Nagi, B., Mehta, S., and Mehta, S. K.: Ingestion of corrosive acids. Gastroenterology, *97*:702, 1989.

27

ABDOMINAL WALL, UMBILICUS, PERITONEUM, MESENTERIES, OMENTUM, AND RETROPERITONEUM

Kevin M. Sittig, M.D., Michael S. Rohr, M.D., Ph.D., and John C. McDonald, M.D.

ABDOMINAL WALL

The abdominal wall is a complex musculoaponeurotic structure that is attached to the vertebral column posteriorly, the ribs superiorly, and the bones of the pelvis inferiorly. It is derived embryonically in a segmental, metameric manner, and this is reflected in its blood supply and innervation.

The abdominal wall protects and restrains the abdominal viscera, and its musculature acts indirectly to flex the vertebral column. The integrity of the abdominal wall is essential to the prevention of hernias, whether congenital, acquired, or iatrogenic. Additionally, the abdominal wall is the repository of the panniculus adiposus, which may reach considerable proportions in some members of the species afflicted with morbid obesity.

EMBRYOLOGY. The abdominal wall begins to develop quite early in the embryo, but it does not achieve its definitive structure until the umbilical cord separates from the fetus at birth. Most of the abdominal wall forms during closure of the midgut and reduction in relative size of the body stalk. The primitive wall is somatopleure (ectoderm and mesoderm without muscle, blood vessels, or nerves). The somatopleure of the abdomen is secondarily invaded by mesoderm from the myotomes that developed on either side of the vertebral column. This mesodermal mass (hypomere) migrates ventrally and laterally as a sheet and the leading edges differentiate, while still widely separated from each other, into the right and left rectus abdominis muscles. The final apposition of these muscles in the anterior midline closes the body wall (Fig. 1).

Before the primordia of the rectus muscles fuse anteriorly, the mesoderm from the hypomere splits into three layers that can be recognized by the seventh week of development. The inner sheet differentiates into the transversus abdominis muscle; the middle sheet becomes the internal oblique muscle; and the superficial sheet becomes the external oblique muscle and aponeurosis. Dorsally, the superior and inferior posterior serratus muscles develop from the superficial layer of the hypomere.

Approximation of the two rectus abdominis muscles in the midline proceeds from both cranial and caudal ends and is complete by the twelfth week, except at the umbilicus. The final closure of the umbilical ring awaits the separation of the cord at birth, but the ring may remain open, in which case an umbilical hernia is present. Most such hernias gradually close spontaneously.

ANATOMY, INNERVATION, AND LYMPHATIC DRAINAGE. The abdominal wall is composed of nine layers. From

without in, they are (1) skin, (2) tela subcutanea (subcutaneous tissue), (3) superficial fascia (Scarpa's fascia), (4) external abdominal oblique muscle, (5) internal abdominal oblique muscle, (6) transversus abdominis muscle, (7) endoabdominal (transversalis) fascia, (8) extraperitoneal adipose and areolar tissue, and (9) peritoneum.

Each layer is discussed individually. The skin of the abdomen is general body skin ordinarily unadorned by heavy hair growth. It may be involved in generalized dermatoses but is otherwise unremarkable. It is rarely the site of cutaneous neoplasia because it usually is protected from exposure to the sun.

The *tela subcutanea* contains a layer of soft adipose tissue that generally increases with age. It contains little fibrous connective tissue and affords little strength in closure of abdominal incisions. The tela subcutanea rests upon the superficial fascia (Scarpa's fascia), which is not to be confused with the investing fascia of the abdominal wall muscles.

Scarpa's fascia is a layer of fibrous connective tissue of modest thickness. The layer contains abundant adipose tissue. A discrete layer of the fascia ordinarily can be demonstrated in the lower abdominal wall, and the layer may be confused with aponeurosis of the external oblique muscle by inexperienced surgeons. The layer affords little strength in wound closure, but its approximation aids considerably in the creation of an aesthetic hairline scar.

The *muscular abdominal wall* is composed of three flat muscles that have broad origins. The muscular wall encloses the largest fraction of the circumference of the torso. Anteriorly, the three flat muscles give way to flat aponeuroses that fuse to form the investing fascia (sheath) of the rectus abdominis muscles.

The *external abdominal oblique muscle* (paired right and left) is the largest and thickest of the flat abdominal muscles. Its broad origin includes the last seven ribs, the thoracolumbar fascia (lumbodorsal aponeurosis), the external lip of the iliac crest, and the inguinal ligament that inserts into the pubic tubercle. The muscle belly gives way to a flat, strong aponeurosis at about the midclavicular line, and it inserts medially into the linea alba (Fig. 2). The aponeurosis of the external oblique passes anterior to the sheath of the rectus abdominis, and, with care, it can be dissected from it. In general, the fascicles of the external oblique muscle pass from superior-lateral to inferior-medial. Thus, the direction of force generated by contraction of muscle is superior-lateral.

The *internal abdominal oblique muscle* originates from the last five ribs, the thoracolumbar fascia, the intermediate lip of the iliac crest, and the lateral half of the inguinal ligament. Its fibers

THE ANTERIOR BODY WALL

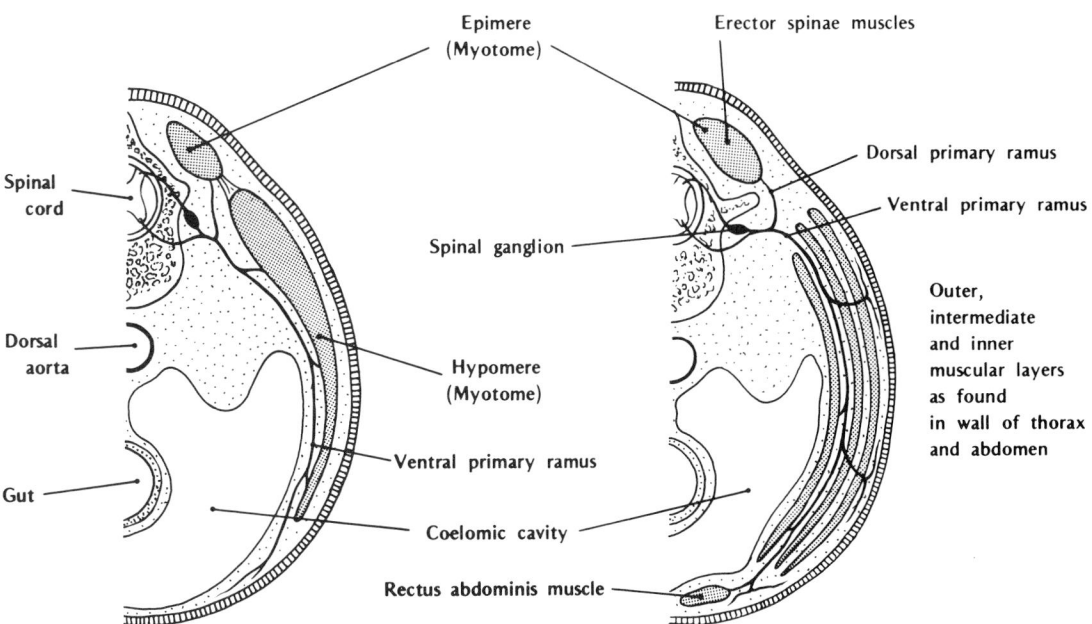

Figure 1. Schematic diagram showing the establishment of the primordia of the abdominal wall muscles. On the left, the relationship of the myotomes to the primitive central nervous system and coelomic cavity is shown. On the right, the differentiation of the hypomere to form the three layers of the abdominal wall musculature is depicted. (Modified from Langman, J.: Medical Embryology. Baltimore, Williams and Wilkins, 1969.)

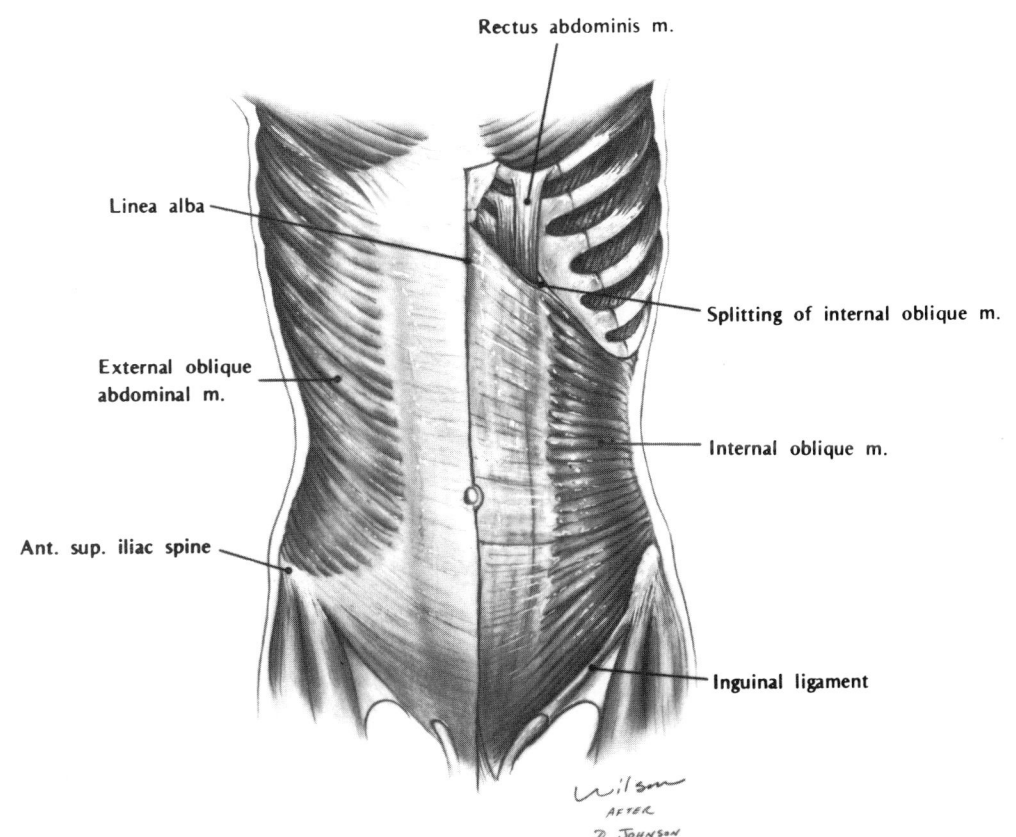

Figure 2. Schematic diagram of abdominal wall muscles showing the external oblique and the internal oblique abdominal muscles. The rectus muscles are seen near the midline. The right rectus muscle is covered by the rectus sheath. (Modified from Healey, J. E., Jr.: A Synopsis of Clinical Anatomy. Philadelphia, W. B. Saunders Company, 1969.)

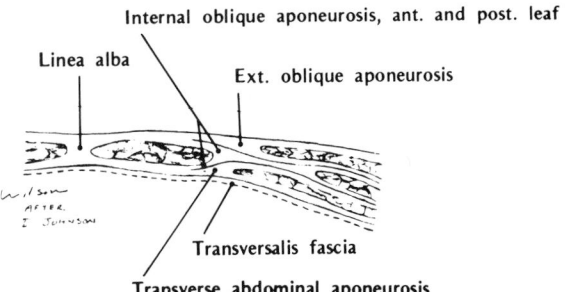

Figure 3. Schematic diagram of transverse section of upper abdominal wall muscles near the umbilicus. The aponeurosis of the internal oblique muscle splits to invest the rectus abdominis muscle. (Modified from Healey, J. E., Jr.: A Synopsis of Clinical Anatomy. Philadelphia, W. B. Saunders Company, 1969.)

course opposite the direction of those of the external oblique. The internal oblique also gives way to a flat aponeurosis medially, which splits to enclose the rectus muscle. The aponeurosis reunites medial to the rectus and inserts into the linea alba (Fig. 3). The fibers that arise from the lateral half of the inguinal ligament pursue a downward course and insert into the os pubis between the symphysis and the tubercle. Some of the lower fibers of the internal oblique muscle are pulled into the scrotum by the testis as it passes through the abdominal wall. These latter fibers are called the cremasteric muscle of the spermatic cord. The cremasteric muscle is responsible for a superficial reflex of the same name in which the testis is retracted from the scrotum in the direction of the inguinal canal.

The *transversus abdominis muscle* is the smallest of the three flat muscles of the abdomen. Its origin is similar to that of the internal oblique muscle. It originates from the lower five ribs, the thoracolumbar fascia, the internal lip of the iliac crest, and the lateral one third of the inguinal ligament. The direction of its fibers is transverse, and they give way to a flat aponeurosis that inserts into the linea alba. The aponeurosis passes behind the rectus sheath in its upper two thirds. The fibers of the trans-

versus abdominis that originate from the inguinal ligament pass downward to insert on the os pubis, as do the fibers of the internal oblique muscle. Occasionally, the lower fibers of both muscles insert by means of a common tendon called the conjoint tendon (Fig. 4). Our experience in the dissecting laboratory and operating room leads us to believe that a true conjoint tendon occurs only infrequently. More often, the muscles insert into the os pubis as a "conjoint muscle."

The plane between the internal oblique and transversus abdominis muscles can properly be considered a neurovascular plane, because it contains the segmental arteries, veins, and nerves that supply the abdominal wall. The anterior primary rami of thoracic spinal nerves T7 to T12 and lumbar nerve L1 supply the abdominal wall in a segmental, sequential manner from above downward. The main trunks of the nerves are found in the neurovascular plane. The anterior cutaneous rami pierce the rectus sheath anteriorly to supply the anterior skin. The anterior cutaneous rami of T10 innervates a dermatome that includes the umbilicus. The lateral cutaneous rami of T7-8-9 supply skin of the thorax and lateral abdominal wall, and the lateral cutaneous rami of T12 and L1 supply the skin of the gluteal region.

The *transversalis fascia* is poorly named and often misunderstood. It more properly should be called the endoabdominal fascia, since it is a continuous lining of the abdominal cavity. Where this fascia lies in direct relation to certain muscles, it is given a special name. Over the psoas muscle, it is called the *psoas fascia*. Where it lies deep to the transversus abdominis muscle, it is properly called the *transversalis fascia*. The integrity of the endoabdominal fascia is absolutely essential for the integrity of the abdominal wall. If this layer is intact, no hernia exists. A hernia may, in fact, be defined as a hole in the endoabdominal fascia or transversalis fascia. This definition applies to esophageal hiatus hernia, umbilical hernia, inguinal hernia, femoral hernia, and incisional hernia.

The transversalis fascia contains a thickened band, the iliopubic tract, which lies deep to the inguinal ligament. Like the

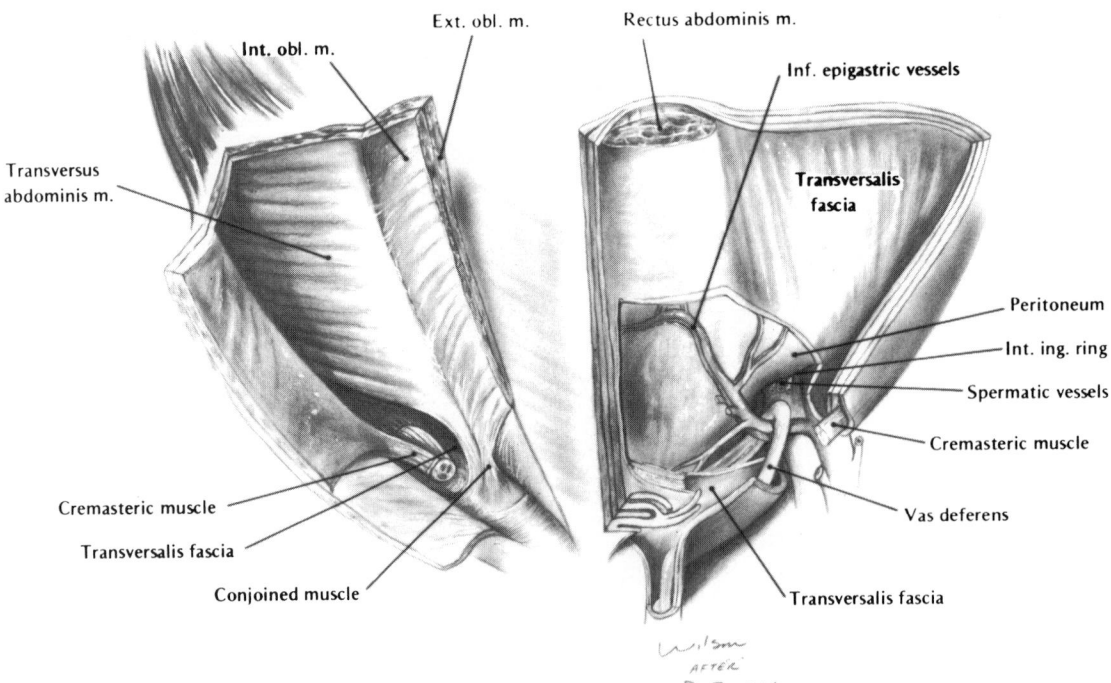

Figure 4. The lower abdominal wall and groin are depicted schematically. On the left, the external abdominal oblique and the internal abdominal oblique muscles are reflected, revealing the transversus abdominis muscle and its origin from the lateral half of the inguinal ligament. The cremaster muscle fibers can be seen originating from the lower part of the internal oblique muscle. The important structures in the inguinal area are depicted. On the right, the transversalis fascia (with a window removed) is shown just superficial to the peritoneum. The inferior epigastric vessels are shown arising from the external iliac vessels. (Modified from Healey, J. E., Jr.: A Synopsis of Clinical Anatomy. Philadelphia, W. B. Saunders Company, 1969.)

inguinal ligament, the iliopubic tract extends from the anterior superior spine of the iliac crest to the pubic tubercle. The iliopubic tract is of considerable importance in the repair of groin hernias.

The *extraperitoneal adipose and connective tissue layer* of the abdominal wall is surgically relatively unimportant. It is found between the endoabdominal fascia and the peritoneum. It contains a greater amount of adipose tissue in obese persons. It also contains the remains of four fetal structures and the inferior epigastric arteries and veins. The latter vessels course from the external iliac vessels upward and medial to the rectus sheath, where they supply the rectus abdominis muscle from below (Fig. 5). The obliterated umbilical arteries arise from the superior vesical arteries and course upward to the umbilicus. They raise a fold of peritoneum (visible from the inside of the peritoneal cavity) called the medial umbilical ligaments, which are paired right and left. In the midline, the obliterated urachus passes from the apex of the bladder to the umbilicus. It is a fibrous cord that represents the remnant of the allantoic stalk. Like the obliterated umbilical arteries, the obliterated urachus also raises a peritoneal fold, the median umbilical ligament.

Above the umbilicus, in the midline, the extraperitoneal adipose tissue projects deep between the two leaves of the falciform ligament of the liver. In the free margin of this sickle-shaped ligament is found the ligamentum teres hepatis, the obliterated umbilical vein, which courses from the umbilicus to the ligamentum venosum. The space between the two leaves of the falciform ligament is filled with extraperitoneal adipose tissue.

The *parietal peritoneum* is the innermost layer of the abdominal wall. It is a thin layer of dense, irregular connective tissue and is covered on the inside by a layer of simple squamous mesothelium. The peritoneal membrane is innervated from above downward in a sequential manner by spinal nerves T7–L1. The peritoneum provides little strength in wound closure but it affords remarkable protection from infection if it remains unviolated.

The rectus muscles and rectus sheath require special description. The muscles are paired right and left, and they extend from the fifth rib superiorly to the pubis inferiorly. They lie in apposition to each other, being separated only by the linea alba. Each muscle is a long, flat ribbon of triangular shape, being wider above than below. Each muscle is composed of long, parallel fascicles interrupted by three tendinous inscriptions (Fig. 6).

The rectus muscles serve to support the abdominal wall and to flex the vertebral column. Each muscle is contained within a fascial sheath, the rectus sheath, which is derived from the aponeuroses of the three flat abdominal muscles. Unfortunately for ease of understanding, the relationship of the aponeuroses of the flat muscles is not constant throughout the course of the rectus muscle. The relationship is different above and below the semicircular line of Douglas, which is about halfway between the umbilicus and pubic symphysis (Fig. 6). Above the semicircular line, the rectus sheath is strong posteriorly. Here the posterior sheath is composed of fascia from the internal oblique muscle, the transversus abdominis muscle, and transversalis fascia. Anteriorly, above the semicircular line, the rectus sheath is composed of the external oblique aponeurosis and the anterior lamella of the internal oblique aponeurosis.

Below the semicircular line, which is the point at which the inferior epigastric artery enters the rectus sheath, the posterior rectus sheath is lacking because the fasciae of the flat muscles pass anterior to the rectus muscle. The muscle, below the semicircular line, is covered posteriorly by a thin layer of transversalis fascia, which is usually transparent when viewed from the inside at operation.

The rectus abdominis muscles are held close together near the anterior midline by the *linea alba*. The linea alba itself has an elongated triangular shape and is based at the xiphoid process of the sternum. The linea alba narrows considerably below the umbilicus so that the medial edge of one rectus muscle may actually overlap the other.

The linea alba is so called because it is a white line. However, it may take on dark pigmentation in women with pregnancy. It is then properly called the *linea nigra*. It never loses its dark pigmentation thereafter.

The lymphatic supply of the abdominal wall follows a simple pattern (Fig. 7). Above the umbilicus, the lymphatic pathways drain into the ipsilateral axillary lymph nodes. Below the umbilicus, they drain into the ipsilateral superficial inguinal lymph nodes. Basically, the superficial lymphatics parallel the superficial veins, which above the umbilicus drain into the axillary vein and below it into the femoral vein.

The arterial supply of the abdominal wall arises from several sources. Above, the superior epigastric arteries enter the rectus sheaths. The superior epigastric artery is a terminal branch of the internal thoracic artery. It has extensive collateral branches within the rectus muscle and the inferior epigastric artery. The

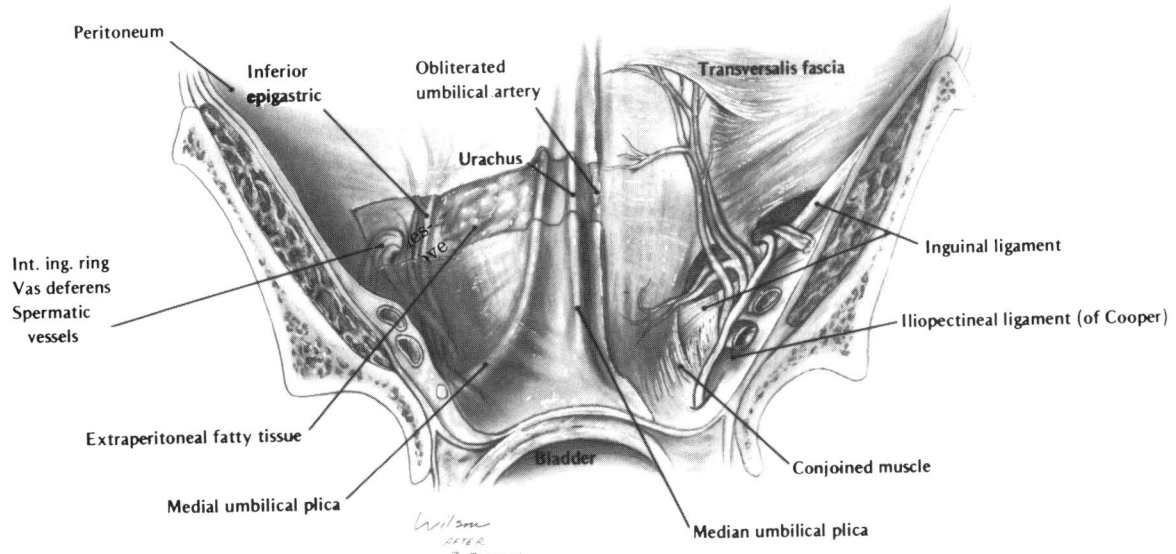

Figure 5. Schematic diagram of the lower abdominal wall as seen from the inside. On the left, the median and medial umbilical folds are apparent. On the right, the peritoneum has been removed, revealing the transversalis fascia. (Modified from Healey, J. E., Jr.: A Synopsis of Clinical Anatomy. Philadelphia, W. B. Saunders Company, 1969.)

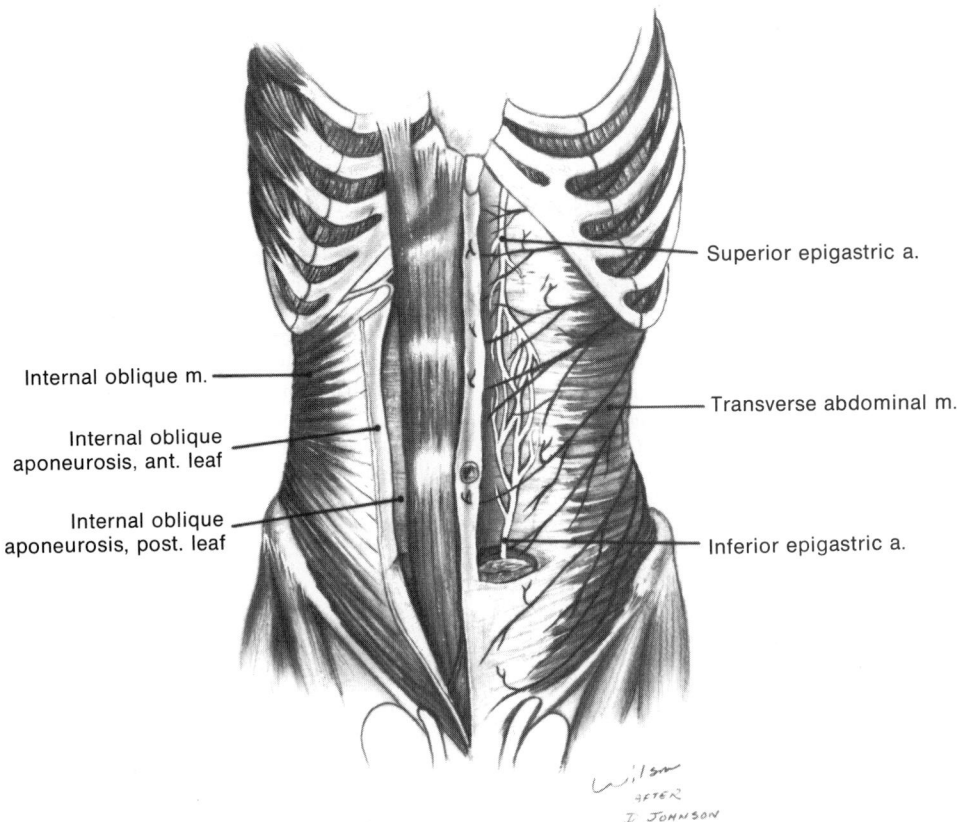

Figure 6. Schematic diagram of abdominal wall, demonstrating the rectus sheath as seen from an anterior dissection. On the right, the blood supply and innervation of the rectus abdominis muscle are depicted. (Modified from Healey, J. E., Jr.: A Synopsis of Clinical Anatomy. Philadelphia, W. B. Saunders Company, 1969.)

inferior epigastric artery arises from the external iliac artery just before the external iliac artery passes into the thigh. The skin and subcutaneous tissues of the lower abdominal wall are supplied bilaterally by several small arteries arising from the femoral artery, which pass upward from the femoral triangle. They are, from medial to lateral, the superficial external pudendal artery, the superficial epigastric artery (misnamed because it really supplies the hypogastrium), and the superficial and deep circumflex iliac arteries.

CONGENITAL ABNORMALITIES

ABDOMINAL WALL. The most common variant of normal anatomy seen in the abdominal wall is diastasis recti. This consists of an upper midline protrusion of the abdominal wall between the right and left rectus abdominis muscles. This abnormality represents a weakness of the linea alba and does not require treatment unless an epigastric hernia occurs in association with the diastasis recti. Frequently, patients or their families need to be counseled about the innocuous nature of the abnormality.

Omphalocele may be seen in the neonate and represents a defect in the closure of the umbilical ring. The herniated viscera are usually covered with a sac composed of amnion. *Gastroschisis* is a defect of the abdominal wall that is located lateral to the umbilicus. It is caused by a failure of closure of the body wall in which abdominal viscera protrude through the defect. No sac is present to cover the herniated intestine. Omphalocele and gastroschisis are discussed in Chapter 38 on pediatric surgery.

OMPHALOMESENTERIC DUCT REMNANTS. Remnants of the omphalomesenteric (vitelline) duct may present as abnormalities related to the abdominal wall. In the fetus, the omphalomesenteric duct connects the fetal midgut to the yolk sac. This normally obliterates and disappears completely. However, any or all of the fetal duct may persist and give rise to symptoms (Fig. 8).

An umbilical *polyp* is a small excrescence of omphalomesenteric duct mucosa that is retained in the umbilicus. Such polyps

resemble umbilical granulomas except that they do not disappear after silver nitrate cauterization. They may be associated with a persistent vitelline duct or umbilical sinus. Appropriate treatment is excision of the mucosal remnant.

Umbilical *sinuses* result from the continued presence of the umbilical end of the omphalomesenteric duct. These resemble umbilical polyps, but close inspection reveals the presence of a sinus tract deep to the umbilicus. The morphology of the sinus tract can be readily delineated with a sinogram. Treatment is excision of the sinus.

Persistence of the entire omphalomesenteric duct is heralded by the passage of enteric contents from the umbilicus. This is seen in the early neonatal period and should be treated promptly with laparotomy and excision of the duct to avoid intussusception or volvulus.

Cystic remnants of the omphalomesenteric duct may persist and be asymptomatic for long periods of time. The cysts may be connected to the ileum with a fibrous band that is a remnant of the obliterated omphalomesenteric duct. Patients may present with acute volvulus and intestinal obstruction or with acute abdomen because of cyst infection. The cysts usually remain undiagnosed until operation, at which time they should be excised.

Meckel's diverticulum results when the intestinal end of the omphalomesenteric duct persists. This is a true diverticulum of the intestine with all layers of the intestinal wall represented. It is discussed in detail in Chapter 38.

URACHAL ANOMALIES. The urachus is a fetal structure that connects the developing bladder to the umbilicus. The urachus normally is obliterated by the time of birth. It may persist *in toto*, resulting in a vesicoumbilical fistula manifested by the drainage of urine from the umbilicus (Fig. 9). Proper treatment is excision of the fistula after distal urinary obstruction has been excluded.

Persistent *urachal sinus* results when the umbilical end of the

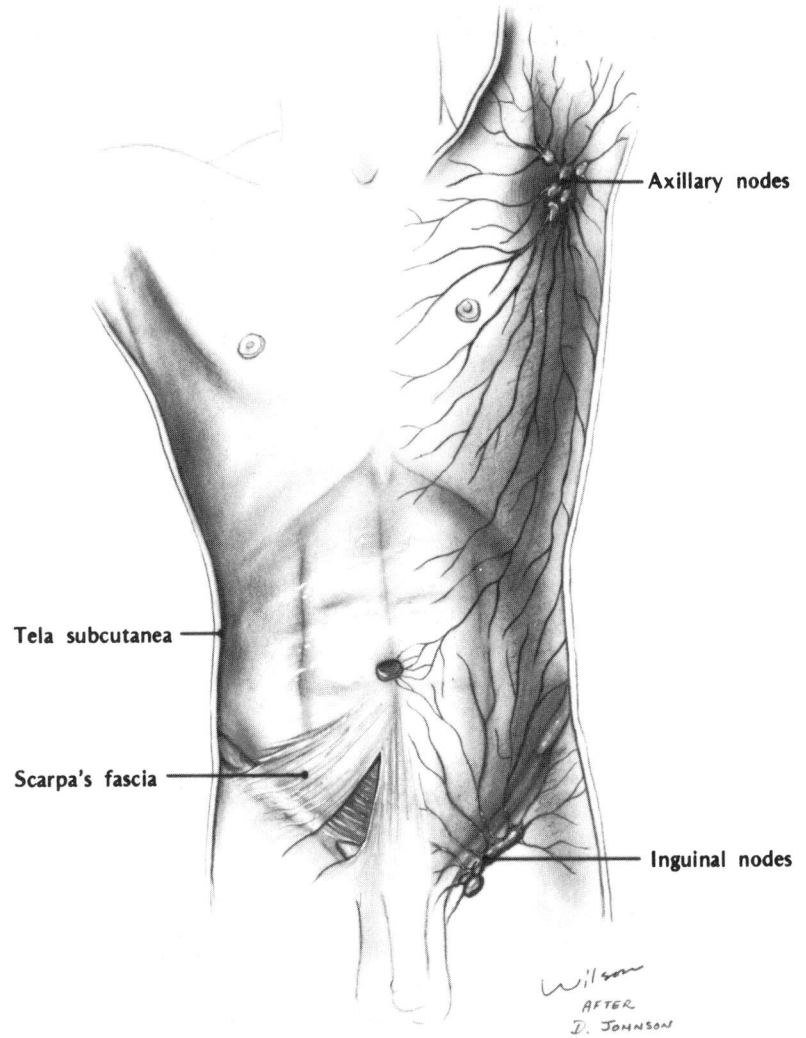

Figure 7. Schematic drawing of the lymphatic drainage of the abdominal wall, revealing drainage of the supraumbilical region to the axillary lymph nodes and drainage of the infraumbilical region to the inguinal lymph nodes. On the left, the tela subcutanea and Scarpa's fascia are depicted. (Modified from Healey, J. E., Jr.: A Synopsis of Clinical Anatomy. Philadelphia, W. B. Saunders Company, 1969.)

urachas does not obliterate normally. Such sinuses present as the chronic drainage of small amounts of material from the umbilicus. They may become infected and should be totally excised. Cystic remnants of the urachus may persist between the bladder and umbilicus when urachal obliteration is incomplete. These cysts may become symptomatic at any time and present as lower abdominal masses or, occasionally, abscesses. They should be excised completely.

True *diverticula* of the urinary bladder result from incomplete obliteration of the distal end of the fetal urachus. They may result in recurrent urinary tract infections and are definitively diagnosed by cystography. Appropriate treatment is excision of the diverticulum and closure of the bladder.

INFECTIONS. The abdominal wall is occasionally the site of dermatoses and subcutaneous infections. Appropriate treatment is directed to the specific cause of the abnormality. The abdominal wall occasionally may be the site of severe bacterial gangrene and necrotizing fasciitis. The most serious form of this infection is seen in elderly patients with necrotizing fasciitis caused by mixed infections of aerobic and anaerobic bacteria. These infections are frequently associated with urinary extravasation or perirectal abscess, but they may present without obvious causes. Necrotizing fasciitis of the abdominal wall is a life-threatening infection that results in necrosis of the skin, subcutaneous tissue, and musculoaponeurotic abdominal wall. The only appropriate treatment is early wide débridement, with exteriorization of all infected planes. Appropriate antibiotic therapy is mandatory. Similar infections occasionally complicate wound healing after intestinal operations.

OMPHALITIS. Infection of the umbilicus may occur in babies and adults. It is generally an innocuous disease that results from poor hygiene and is treated with appropriate cleansing and local care to the umbilicus. However, in the neonatal period, omphalitis may result from bacterial infection and may potentially be associated with serious sequelae, such as portal vein thrombosis. In neonates, treatment includes systemic antibiotics.

RECTUS SHEATH HEMATOMA. Extravasation of blood into the rectus sheath resulting in a hematoma is rarely a life-threatening illness. However, it may mimic other abdominal diseases and must be considered in the differential diagnosis to avoid unnecessary laparotomy. Rectus sheath hematoma is usually the result of trauma, which may be as trivial as a paroxysm of coughing. Patients with rectus sheath hematomas most often give a history of receiving anticoagulant drugs for various conditions. When the hematoma develops, it ordinarily occurs at the level of the semicircular line of Douglas, where the inferior epigastric artery enters the rectus sheath. Patients may complain of an acute illness, with abdominal pain over the hematoma, nausea, and vomiting. Frequently, a tender mass is palpable. Operation is indicated only if more serious conditions cannot otherwise be excluded.

ABDOMINAL WALL TUMORS. *Benign tumors* of the ab-

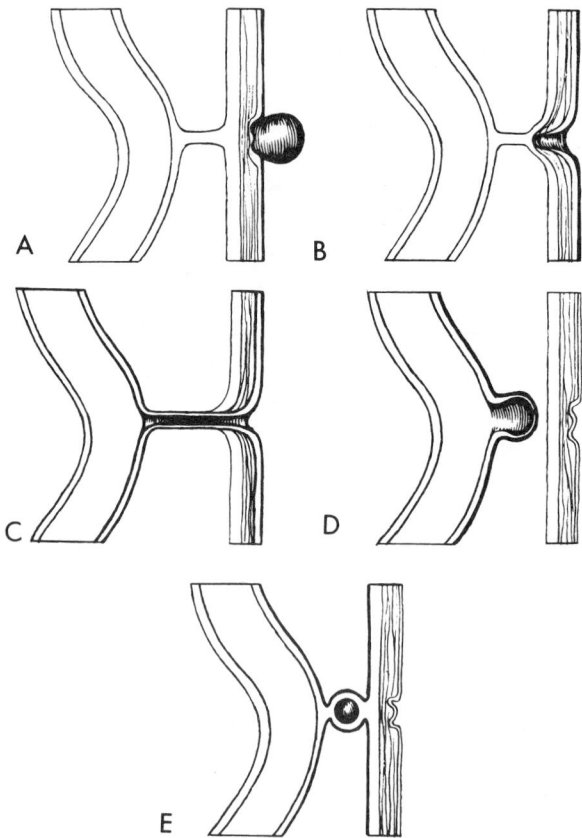

Figure 8. Vestiges of vitelline (omphalomesenteric) duct. *A*, Mucosal polyp (with band from bowel to umbilicus). *B*, Sinus in the umbilicus. *C*, Enteroumbilical fistula (patent omphalomesenteric duct). *D*, Meckel's diverticulum. *E*, Cyst between bowel and abdominal wall, which may communicate with the skin surface. (From Ravitch, M. M., et al.: Pediatric Surgery, 3rd ed. Chicago, Year Book Medical Publishers, 1979.)

dominal wall may arise from any of the elements contained within the abdominal wall itself. Lipomas of the abdominal wall are quite common and are treated by excision. Benign fibromas, hemangiomas, and neurofibromas may be seen. The principles of their treatment are no different from those for similar tumors in other locations.

Desmoid tumors of the abdominal wall are benign fibrous

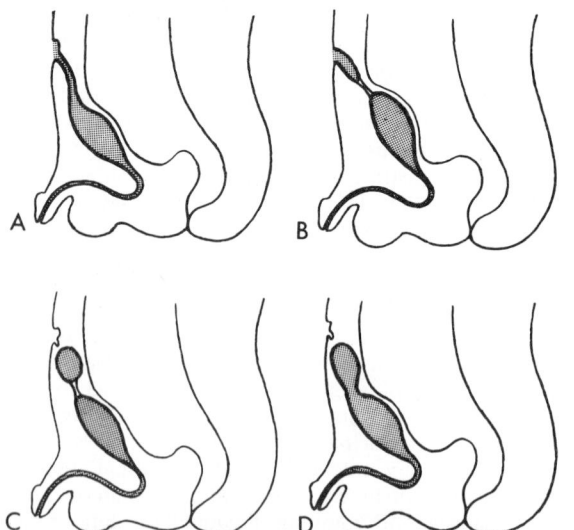

Figure 9. Vestiges of urachus. *A*, Urinary fistula. *B*, Sinus. *C*, Cyst. *D*, Bladder diverticulum. (From Ravitch, M. M., et al.: Pediatric Surgery, 3rd ed. Chicago, Year Book Medical Publishers, 1979.)

tumors that arise from the musculoaponeurotic abdominal wall. These tumors are histologically benign but frequently are locally invasive and are prone to recurrence following local excision. They present as firm, subcutaneous masses that grow slowly. They should be widely excised to prevent local recurrence. They do not have a propensity toward metastasis.

Primary malignancies of the abdominal wall are uncommon. Any of the cutaneous neoplasms may affect the abdominal wall and are treated like skin cancers elsewhere. Sarcomas arising from the abdominal wall are uncommon and are best treated by surgical excision.

The abdominal wall is occasionally the site of metastasis from primary malignancies located elsewhere. In particular, malignancies from the ovary and prostate may metastasize to the lower abdominal wall. The stomach, uterus, lung, kidney, breast, and colon occasionally give rise to metastases located within the abdominal wall.

REFERRED PAIN. A consideration of the innervation of both the abdominal wall and abdominal viscera is appropriate to understand the phenomenon of referred pain. Referred pain is pain of visceral origin (mediated through sympathetic nervous system pathways) that is perceived as somatic or cutaneous pain. None of the abdominal viscera is innervated by somatic afferent fibers, which are traditionally described as pain fibers. However, the abdominal viscera are innervated by afferent sympathetic nervous system fibers. These afferent sympathetic fibers join the central nervous system in a segmental manner, as do the somatic afferent fibers arising from the abdominal wall and skin. When a viscus becomes diseased or distended, the afferent sympathetic nervous system fibers are stimulated. These impulses are transmitted to the central nervous system and are perceived as somatic or cutaneous pain in segments of the body that are innervated from the same central nervous system segment that receives the afferent sympathetic impulses.

An example of referred pain is pain from distention of the vermiform appendix. The vermiform appendix, like all the gastrointestinal tract, has no somatic innervation. However, it has a rich sympathetic innervation. When the appendix becomes distended from obstruction, the resulting pain may be referred to the skin and abdominal wall around the umbilicus. This phenomenon is explained on an anatomic basis by the fact that the region of the umbilicus is innervated by the tenth thoracic spinal cord segment, which is the segment from which the sympathetic innervation of the vermiform appendix is derived. Numerous other examples of referred pain are well documented. These include pain from irritation of the diaphragmatic peritoneum, commonly referred to the shoulder. Referred pain from an obstructed gallbladder is commonly perceived in the region of the scapula. Referred pain from renal colic is frequently perceived in the groin or scrotum.

GENERAL DIAGNOSTIC SIGNS. Many examples exist of diagnostic signs of abdominal and systemic disease that may be manifested in or on the abdominal wall. These include, among others, the Sister Mary Joseph lymph node, which occasionally presents within the substance of the umbilicus. This lymph node, which was first appreciated by an observant operating room nun, is a manifestation of intra-abdominal malignancy. It has the same diagnostic significance as Virchow's node in the neck. Grey Turner's sign of retroperitoneal hemorrhage, which was originally described in hemorrhagic pancreatitis, is well known. Grey Turner's sign also may be visible in patients with ruptured abdominal aortic aneurysm, retroperitoneal hemorrhage from trauma, and retroperitoneal hemorrhage that occurs as a complication of anticoagulation therapy. The caput medusa is a collection of distended veins around the umbilicus that results from portal venous hypertension. The caput medusa sign becomes apparent when there is shunting of blood from the portal venous circulation to the systemic venous system through the abdominal wall. Spider angioma of chronic liver disease may be seen on the abdominal wall. Additionally, petechiae from thrombocytopenia or from fat embolus may present as abdominal wall findings. The striae of Cushing's disease are usually found on the abdominal wall. Distention of the abdomen is most readily appreciated by inspecting the abdominal wall, and the detection of ascitic fluid in the peritoneal cavity is easily appreciated following careful examination.

PERITONEUM

EMBRYOLOGY. The peritoneal cavity is a potential space containing the abdominal viscera. It develops from the primitive coelom, which is formed by a splitting of the lateral mesoderm into somatic and splanchnic layers. Originally there are two bilateral cavities separated by the developing gastrointestinal tract. The somatic mesoderm lines the body wall portion of the coelom, and the splanchnic mesoderm covers the intestine (Fig. 10). As the embryonic body wall closes ventrally, the two coelomic cavities fuse together in the midline. In between, the developing gut is covered on both sides by splanchnic mesoderm. That portion of this double layer of mesoderm from which the gut is suspended is called the mesentery. As the ventral mesentery of the intestine is resorbed, the two coelomic cavities join to become one.

PHYSIOLOGY. The primary functions of the peritoneum have been derived by teleologic reasoning. The peritoneum does provide a frictionless surface over which the abdominal viscera can freely move, and the mesothelial lining secretes fluid that serves to lubricate the peritoneal surfaces. Normally, about 100 ml. of clear, straw-colored fluid is present in the peritoneal cavity of the adult. The quality and quantity of this fluid may change with various pathologic conditions.

When required to do so, the peritoneum serves as a bidirectional dialysis membrane through which water and solutes may move. Such movement is controlled largely by the osmolar gradient. This ability of the peritoneum to absorb substances is the basis for both experimental and clinical administration of fluid, electrolytes, and blood. Isotonic saline administered intraperitoneally is absorbed at a rate of approximately 30 to 35 ml. per hour after an initial equilibration phase. However, if a hypertonic fluid is used, there is a large shift of water (up to 300 to 500 ml. per hour) from the intravascular space into the peritoneal cavity, which can result in hypotension and shock. Studies in humans and animals show that intraperitoneal blood is absorbed at a slower rate, but approximately 70 per cent eventually enters the bloodstream. This absorption occurs primarily through fenestrated lymphatic channels on the undersurface of the diaphragm. Such red blood cells have a normal survival time

in the circulation.[21] Air and gases are also similarly absorbed. Air that enters the peritoneal cavity during laparotomy is present in diminishing amounts for 4 to 5 days.

Peritoneal dialysis is possible because of bidirectional transport across the peritoneal membrane. By adjusting the composition of the dialysate, excess water, sodium, potassium, and products of metabolism can be removed from the bloodstream. In addition, a variety of drugs can be removed with peritoneal dialysis (Table 1). Medications that are not dialyzable are shown in Table 2.

INTRAPERITONEAL FLUID COLLECTION

ASCITES. Normally, there is a balance between fluid secretion and absorption in the peritoneal cavity. Ascites occurs when either the secretion rate increases or the absorption rate decreases disproportionate to the other. This fluid may be a transudate or exudate, and its composition is determined by the etiology of the ascites. A more detailed discussion of ascites is found in Chapter 33 on the liver.

CHYLE. Accumulation of lymph within the peritoneal cavity usually results from trauma or tumor involving lymphatic structures. It differs from other fluid accumulations in the peritoneal cavity in that it has bacteriostatic properties, making infection less likely. In the laboratory, chyle layers out into an upper milky layer, a middle watery layer, and a lower opaque layer. Chylous ascites is further discussed in Chapter 48 on lymphatics.

BILE. Uninfected bile is a mild irritant to the peritoneal cavity. It causes an increased production of peritoneal fluid, resulting in bile ascites or choleperitoneum. Patients with this condition may be relatively well as long as the fluid remains sterile, exhibiting only a mild jaundice from absorption of bile pigments. Infected bile, however, causes a severe peritonitis and necessitates urgent surgical therapy. Most cases of choleperitoneum follow biliary tract operations, but cases of spontaneous perforation of the bile duct have been reported in infants and some adults. This is reported to be the second most common cause of surgical jaundice in infancy.

BLOOD. The most common cause of hemoperitoneum is trauma to the liver or spleen. Less common causes include ruptured ectopic pregnancy, ruptured aortic aneurysm, and other intra-abdominal injuries. As mentioned earlier, approximately two thirds of the red blood cells in the peritoneal cavity are absorbed intact into the bloodstream. However, leaving blood in the peritoneal cavity following operative procedures is not recommended, because it may potentiate infection. It has been shown experimentally that intraperitoneal hemoglobin interferes with the immune response to peritonitis by interfering with clearance of bacteria from the peritoneal cavity.[25]

URINE. Urine collections within the peritoneal cavity are al-

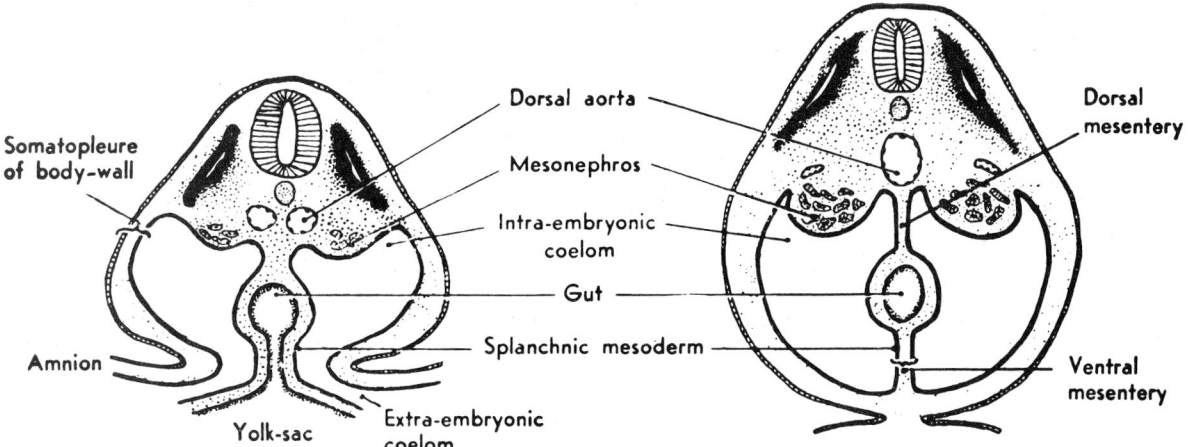

Figure 10. Diagram illustrating early stages in the development of the coelom and mesenteries. (From Patten, B. M.: Human Embryology, 3rd ed. New York, McGraw-Hill Book Company, 1968.)

TABLE 1. Substances That Can Be Removed by Peritoneal Dialysis

Ammonia	Chloral hydrate
Amphetamines	Chlorates
Aniline	Ergotamine
Antibiotics	Ethchlorvynol
Carbenicillin	Fluorides
Gentamicin	Iodides
Isoniazid	Iron (after deferoxamine)
Kanamycin	Lead (after edetate)
Neomycin	Lithium
Nitrofurantoin	Magnesium
Sulfonamides	Meprobamate
Arsenic (after dimercaprol)	Mercury (after dimercaprol)
Aspirin	Methrobenzine
Barbiturates	Mushrooms
Boric acid	Paraldehyde
Bromides	Phenacetin
Calcium	Phenytoin
Carbon tetrachloride	Potassium
	Quinidine

From Schuberth, K. C., and Zitelli, B. J.: The Harriet Lane Handbook, 8th ed. Chicago, Year Book Medical Publishers, Inc., 1979.

most always due to trauma to the urinary tract. These urinomas may present as asymptomatic abdominal enlargement if sterile, but more often they are infected from associated injuries or underlying disease. Such injuries demand operation.

AIR. Pneumoperitoneum is usually secondary to perforation of the gastrointestinal tract or to recent operation. It may result from alveolar rupture in patients on mechanical ventilators. Treatment is directed to the underlying cause of the pneumoperitoneum.

MECONIUM.[6] The neonatal intestine contains sterile meconium. Occasionally, perforation of the intestine occurs *in utero*, and meconium may leak into the peritoneal cavity. This can occur as early as the second trimester of pregnancy, and it results in a sterile inflammatory reaction, fluid accumulation, and eventual calcification of the peritoneal cavity. Depending on the time of the perforation, the newborn infant may present in one of several ways. Remote perforation is shown as fibrous adhesions and calcifications on roentgenograms. The infants may be asymptomatic and may develop problems from obstruction only later. More recent perforation may be walled off, forming a meconium pseudocyst, and infants with this condition present with an abdominal mass. Alternatively, the baby may be born with ascites from recent perforation and require urgent surgical therapy. In many cases, the etiology of the perforation is obstruction of the intestine, with proximal distention and perforation. Some of these infants have meconium ileus and underlying cystic fibrosis.

PERITONITIS. Peritonitis is inflammation of the peritoneum. It can be septic or aseptic, bacterial or viral, primary or secondary, acute or chronic. Most surgical peritonitis is secondary to bacterial contamination from the gastrointestinal tract. Usually

TABLE 2. Substances Not Removed by Peritoneal Dialysis

Amitriptyline	Hallucinogens
Antidepressives	Imipramine
Antihistamines	Methaqualone
Atropine	Methyprylon
Chlordiazepoxide	Nortriptyline
Diazepam	Opiates
Digitalis	Oxazepam
Diphenoxylate	Propoxyphene
Diphenylhydramine	

From Schuberth, K. C., and Zitelli, B. J.: The Harriet Lane Handbook, 8th ed. Chicago, Year Book Medical Publishers, Inc., 1979.

there is underlying pathology or injury to the gut, and this form of peritonitis is discussed elsewhere. Other less common forms of peritonitis are discussed here.

PRIMARY PERITONITIS. Primary peritonitis refers to inflammation of the peritoneal cavity without a documented source of contamination. It occurs more commonly in children than in adults and in women more than in men. This latter distribution is thought to be explained by entry of organisms into the peritoneal cavity through the fallopian tubes. In children, incidence peaks in the neonatal period and again, at age 4 to 5 years. The patients present with an acutely tender abdomen, fever, and leukocytosis. There may be a history of antecedent ear or upper respiratory tract infection. It is often difficult in this situation to differentiate between primary and secondary peritonitis, and the diagnosis ultimately may be made at laparotomy. However, children with nephrotic syndrome and, less commonly, systemic lupus erythematosus are particularly susceptible to primary peritonitis. The bacteria in these cases are usually either hemolytic streptococci or pneumococci. A diagnosis can be made by peritoneal aspiration and Gram's stain after excluding pneumonia and urinary tract infection. Adults with ascites from liver disease have an increased incidence of primary peritonitis.[11] In recent years, the bacterial flora has changed from grampositive to gram-negative organisms. Thus, the distinction between primary and secondary peritonitis is more difficult to make by peritoneal aspirate alone.

TUBERCULOUS PERITONITIS.[26,27,30] Tuberculous peritonitis has decreased in frequency, as have other forms of tuberculosis. In the past, it was seen commonly and carried with it a significant mortality. Presently the mortality rate is less than 5 per cent. The tubercle bacillus presumably gains entry to the peritoneal cavity by one of three mechanisms: transmurally from diseased bowel, from tuberculous salpingitis, or from the bloodstream. The majority of patients do not have radiographic evidence of pulmonary or gastrointestinal tuberculosis, but nearly all have such a focus identified at autopsy. All have positive tuberculin skin tests even if the tuberculosis is confined to the peritoneum.

The clinical manifestations of tuberculous peritonitis are of two types. The moist form consists of fever, ascites, abdominal pain, and weakness. The ascites is progressive and may become massive. The dry form presents in a similar manner but without ascites. Extensive adhesions within the peritoneal cavity result in a "matted" feeling on physical examination. In both forms, tuberculous implants (tubercules) are present on the peritoneal surfaces. Diagnosis may be made most reliably by open or closed peritoneal biopsy and culture. Barium studies are rarely helpful. Recently, laparoscopy has been employed to obtain peritoneal biopsies, which increases the yield over closed biopsy. The ascitic fluid in the moist form is an exudate. On smear examination, lymphocytes are mainly present and rarely acid-fast bacilli are seen. Cultures of the fluid are positive in less than half the cases. Treatment is generally nonoperative and includes appropriate antibiotics. Operation should be reserved for diagnosis if needle biopsy fails or for complications such as fecal fistula.

ASEPTIC PERITONITIS. Aseptic peritonitis is generally due to chemical or foreign body irritants. It may be followed by secondary bacterial peritonitis. Most chemical peritonitis is due to various irritative body fluids (bile, meconium, gastric contents). Foreign bodies may result from external trauma or may be acquired at the time of operation in the form of sutures, sponges, or starch granules. There has been recent interest in starch peritonitis secondary to a reaction to glove powder. It is not clear whether this reaction is allergic or dose related, but the incidence of this complication can be reduced easily by careful glove washing prior to abdominal exploration. Pathologically, there is a granulomatous reaction with giant cell formation. When examined under polarized light, the characteristic birefringent Maltese crosses can be seen in the granulomas.

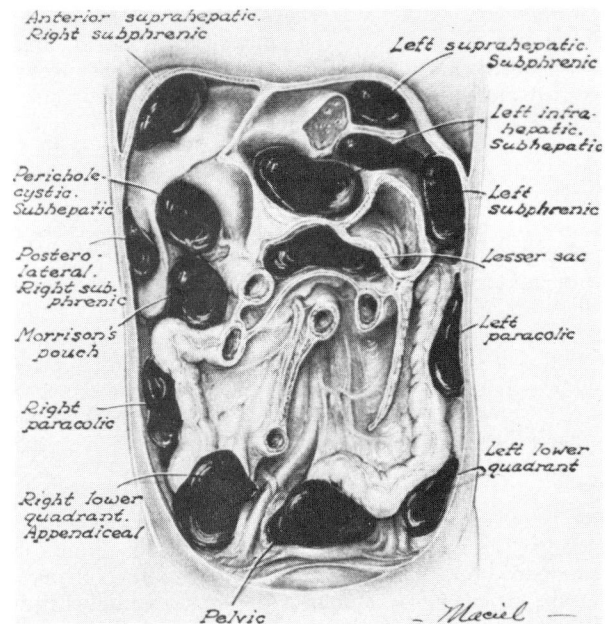

Anterior suprahepatic.
Right subphrenic
Perichole-
cystic.
Subhepatic
Postero-
lateral
Right sub-
phrenic
Morrison's
pouch
Right
paracolic
Right lower
quadrant.
Appendiceal
Left suprahepatic.
Subphrenic
Left infra-
hepatic.
Subhepatic
Left
subphrenic
Lesser sac
Left
paracolic
Left lower
quadrant
Pelvic   *— Maciel —*

Figure 11. Anterior view of abdominal cavity illustrating the types, locations, and anatomic relationship of the various intraperitoneal abscesses. (From Altemeier, W. A., Culbertson, W. R., Fullen, W. D., and Shook, C. D.: Intra-abdominal abscesses. Am. J. Surg., *125*:71, 1973.)

ABSCESSES AND ADHESIONS. Many forms of peritonitis lead to abscess and/or adhesion formation. Intraperitoneal abscess develops two basic patterns. Generalized peritonitis tends to result in abscess formation in anatomically dependent positions, such as the pelvis and paracolic gutters.[3] Localized peritoneal inflammation caused by contiguous disease or injury may result in localized abscesses rather than peritonitis. The common sites of intraperitoneal abscess formation are shown in Figure 11. Adhesions commonly form following peritonitis. Occasionally, adhesions develop to such an extent that the peritoneal cavity is nearly obliterated. This is compatible with life, although intestinal obstruction may occur. Partial obliteration of the peritoneal cavity with bandlike adhesions may also occur. Adhesions form from fibrin produced by the peritoneal surfaces. Most of this fibrin is lysed and absorbed, but some may remain and be invaded with fibroblasts, resulting in dense adhesions. Experimentally, adhesion formation is associated with a reduction in fibrinolysins and may be reduced using steroids, but this has not been validated clinically.[20] Since adhesion formation is a response to peritoneal irritation, meticulous surgical technique is probably the most important factor in prevention.

MESENTERY AND OMENTUM

EMBRYOLOGY. As the peritoneal cavity develops, the splanchnic mesoderm covers the developing gut. Eventually, most of the ventral mesentery is resorbed except for that portion between the liver and the stomach that persists as the gastrohepatic (lesser) omentum. The dorsal mesentery remains intact but changes markedly in size and position as the gastrointestinal tract elongates and rotates. In the gastric region, the cardia of the stomach rotates to the left, and the pylorus moves to the right. The dorsal mesogastrium grows with these changes but does so more than is necessary to accommodate the positional changes in the stomach. The mesogastrium elongates and forms a sac, the omental bursa, which eventually extends caudally over the transverse colon. The omentum fuses with the transverse mesocolon, and the two layers of the omental bursa fuse to become one layer. This apron of dorsal mesogastrium is called the greater omentum.

The intestine begins to elongate during the fifth week of development and forms a loop that extends into the umbilical cord, with the superior mesenteric artery extending from the apex to the loop. This is Stage I of midgut development. Stage II involves return of the duodenum to the abdominal cavity with its 270° counterclockwise rotation around the superior mesenteric artery. In Stage III, the right half of the colon returns to the abdomen and rotates 270° in a counterclockwise direction to lie on the right side anterior to the superior mesenteric artery. This stage is completed with fixation of the intestine and its mesenteries. By the twelfth week of development, rotation is finished but fixation may not be completed until birth. With fusion of the mesentery of the ascending colon to the posterior abdominal wall, the root of the small intestine elongates to extend from the transverse mesocolon to the ileocecal junction. This broad-based mesentery prevents volvulus. Malrotation and volvulus are discussed in Chapter 38.

PHYSIOLOGY. The greater and lesser omenta and the intestinal mesentery are rich in lymphatics and blood vessels. In response to intraperitoneal inflammation, the omentum provides the major source of peritoneal macrophages and aids in removal of foreign material and bacteria. It was previously thought that the omentum, the "policeman of the abdomen," was capable of moving to sites of inflammation, but it has been demonstrated that omental movement is dependent upon intestinal peristalsis and gravity. When in contact with a foreign body or inflamed area, the omentum can adhere quite firmly. In response to intestinal inflammation, the lymph nodes of the mesentery enlarge and may become symptomatic. The etiology of this disorder is presumed to be viral, and it occurs primarily in children.

CONGENITAL INTRAPERITONEAL HERNIAS. Most intraperitoneal hernias result from anatomic variants present at birth. They can be divided into two types, based on etiology and the presence or absence of a hernia sac: hernias that occur through defects in the peritoneum or mesentery do not have sacs, and those that occur secondary to variants in intestinal rotation do have sacs. The first type includes herniation through the epiploic foramen and through congenital defects in the mesentery of the small or large intestine or, less commonly, the broad ligament of the uterus. Some of the mesenteric defects occur secondary to trauma or operation, but most are congenital in origin. Patients with transmesenteric hernia may present with a history of chronic incomplete obstruction or with an acute closed-loop obstruction. In many of these hernias, part of the constricting ring contains major vessels, and care must be taken not to injure these at operation.

The secondary type of intraperitoneal hernia includes the paraduodenal or mesocolic hernias.[29] These occur secondary to abnormal rotation of the intestine. The sac consists of intestinal mesentery, hence the name *mesocolic hernia.* They present more often in adults than in children, in contradistinction to transmesenteric hernias. The right mesocolic hernia occurs secondary to incomplete rotation of the duodenum in Stage II. The duodenum rotates only 90° and remains on the right side of the abdomen, during which time the large intestine rotates normally over it. The proximal small intestine then becomes trapped in the mesentery of the right colon. Operative correction of the right mesocolic hernia is most safely performed by dividing the peritoneal attachments of the right colon, thus moving the colon to the left and leaving the small bowel on the right (Fig. 12). The resulting configuration of intestine is then similar to that of an arrest at Stage I of rotation (nonrotation).

It was formerly thought that left mesocolic hernias occurred as a result of herniation of the small bowel through the paraduodenal fossa near the fourth portion of the duodenum. It is more likely that during Stage II of rotation, the small bowel moves to the left and under the descending colon. With fixation of the colon, the intestine becomes trapped behind the left mes-

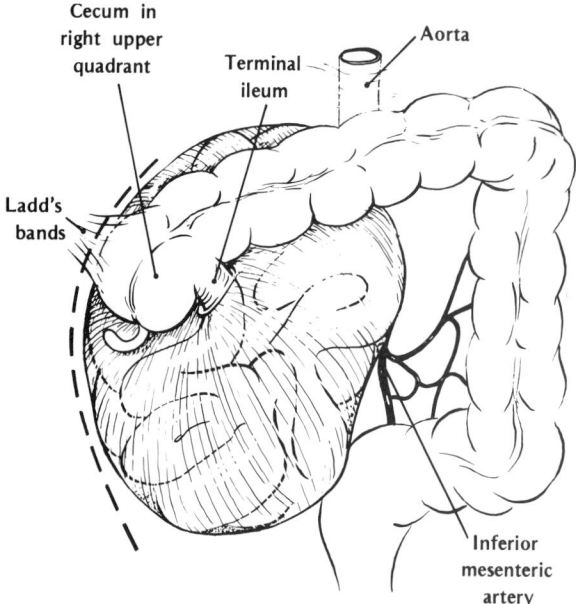

Figure 12. Right mesocolic hernia. The prearterial segment did not rotate during the second stage. The postarterial segment did rotate and has trapped most of the small bowel behind the ascending mesocolon containing the ileocolic, right colic, and middle colic vessels. The dashed line shows the incision for release of the hernia. (From Willwerth, B. M., Zollinger, R. M., Jr., and Izant, R. J., Jr.: Congenital mesocolic (paraduodenal) hernia. Am. J. Surg., 128:358, 1974.)

ocolon. The inferior mesenteric vein often lies along the anterior rim of the neck of the sac. Reduction of this hernia, as with the right side, involves recognizing the anatomic abnormalities and correcting these according to embryogenesis. An incision is made along the border of the inferior mesenteric vein, which is the line of fusion of the left mesocolon, thus releasing the entrapped bowel (Fig. 13).

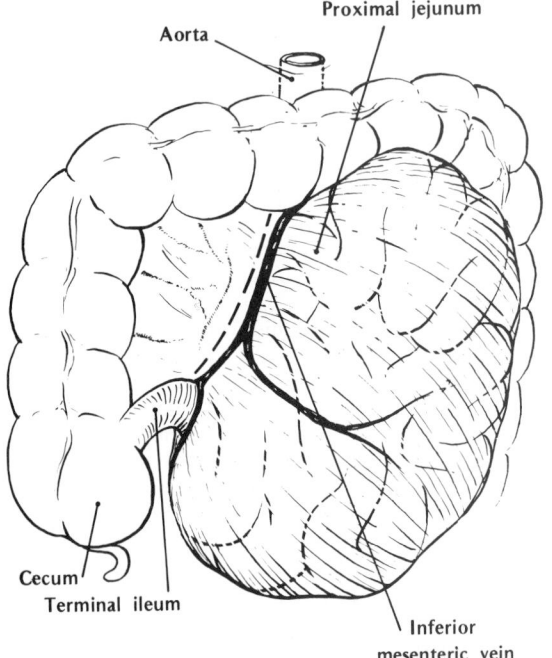

Figure 13. Left mesocolic hernia. A more extensive herniation has occurred, and the sac opening has fused along the dashed line. This line to the right of the inferior mesenteric vein also indicates the area for operative incision. After reduction of the small bowel to the right through this newly created neck, the inferior mesenteric vein, or right lateral margin of the sac, is secured to the retroperitoneum along the left side or root of the small-bowel mesentery. (From Willwerth, B. M., Zollinger, R. M., Jr., and Izant, R. J., Jr.: Congenital mesocolic (paraduodenal) hernia. Am. J. Surg., 128:358, 1974.)

The mesocolic hernias may present with either vague abdominal symptoms or with acute intestinal obstruction. Abdominal films show the small intestine to be confined in one area of the abdomen, but often the diagnosis is not made until laparotomy.

MESENTERIC CYSTS.[17] Mesenteric cysts are most often due to congenital lymphatic spaces that gradually enlarge as they fill with lymph. According to Beahrs[5] and others, they may be divided into four groups based on their etiology: (1) embryonic and developmental cysts, (2) traumatic or acquired cysts, (3) neoplastic cysts, or (4) infective and degenerative cysts.

Mesenteric cysts usually present as abdominal masses accompanied by pain, nausea, and vomiting. These masses usually can be diagnosed on physical examination. They may display a characteristic lateral mobility. They are treated most appropriately by surgical excision. Because of their intimate association with the bowel mesentery, intestinal resection may be required for their complete removal. At operation, they may be confused with duplication cysts of the intestine.[17]

OMENTAL CYSTS. Omental cysts are frequently asymptomatic but may present with vague discomfort or as a mobile abdominal mass that can cause torsion of the omentum. Diagnosis is sometimes difficult, but ultrasound examination may be helpful. On plain films, omental cysts characteristically lie anterior to the intestine. This is best seen in a lateral view. Treatment of omental cysts is by simple excision.

OMENTAL TORSION AND INFARCTION.[2] Torsion of the omentum may be primary or secondary. Primary torsion is rare, and the cause is unknown. Secondary torsion may be due to adhesions, omental cyst, or tumor. The right side of the omentum is involved more than the left, and the torsion generally occurs around two fixed points. Patients often present with signs and symptoms compatible with appendicitis, acute cholecystitis, or a twisted ovarian cyst. Diagnosis is usually not made prior to laparotomy.

Omental infarction may occur secondary to torsion, but it usually is unrelated to torsion. Omental infarction is a rare entity and may follow trauma or may be associated with collagen vascular disease. Treatment for both torsion and infarction entails local resection.

USES OF OMENTUM. The capability of the omentum to wall off infection and its rich vascular and lymphatic supply have led to many uses of omentum in a wide variety of disorders. Free omental grafts generally fibrose and do not function, but with construction of a vascular pedicle, the omentum can reach to the neck or the knee. Omentum has been used as a protective wrapping for intestinal anastomoses to prevent anastomotic leak and promote healing. Enthusiasm for the use of omentum in the treatment of lymphedema of the extremities has waxed and waned. This is discussed in Chapter 48 on lymphatic disorders. However, omental patches have been successfully employed in the closure of perforated duodenal ulcer and for esophageal perforations. Its usefulness has also been demonstrated in operative procedures on the genitourinary tract and in vascular reconstruction. Following hepatic resection or trauma to the liver or spleen, an omental patch aids in hemostasis and in sealing of biliary leaks. In addition, with the advent of microvascular surgery, there are recent reports of the use of omental transplants to improve cerebral vascularity and in chest wall reconstruction.[22]

THE RETROPERITONEUM

ANATOMY (Fig. 14).[15] The retroperitoneum is an actual space located between the peritoneal cavity and the posterior body wall. The diaphragm serves as the superior boundary, whereas the levator muscles of the pelvis delineate the inferior boundary of the retroperitoneal space. Anteriorly, this space is bounded by the posterior parietal peritoneum and the spaces between the leaves of the small and large bowel mesenteries. Posteriorly, it is bounded by the vertebral column and the psoas

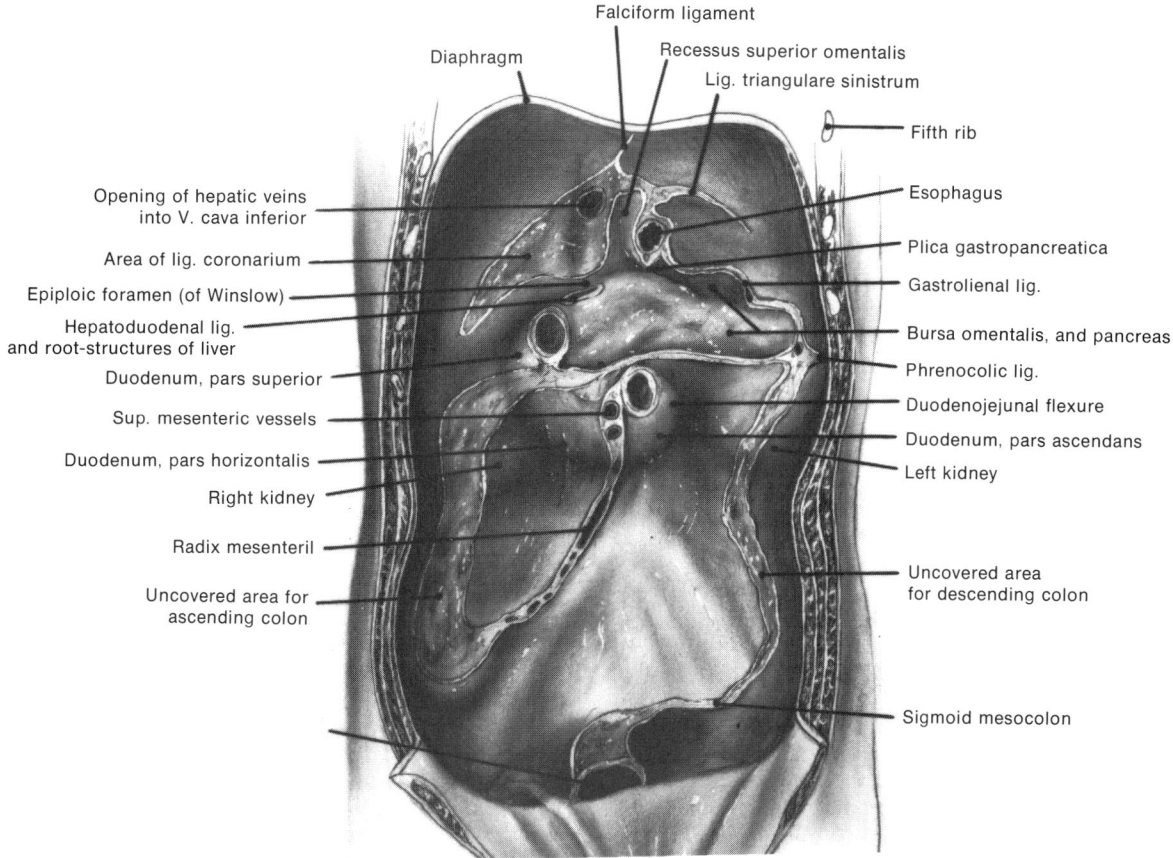

Figure 14. Reflection of the peritoneum on the posterior abdominal wall. (From Schaeffer, J. P. (Ed.): Morris' Human Anatomy, 10th ed. Philadelphia, Blakiston Company, 1951.)

and quadratus lumborum and tendinous portions of the transversus abdominis muscles. Embryologically, ectoderm, mesoderm, and embryonal remnants constitute the contents of the retroperitoneum. It is, therefore, only natural that the majority of abnormalities in the retroperitoneum arise from the aforementioned cell lines. (Table 3 lists the contents of the retroperitoneum.)

Several disorders that lend themselves to surgical treatment can be approached by an extraperitoneal or retroperitoneal exposure. This approach has many advantages over the more commonly used transabdominal approach. By not entering the peritoneal cavity, postoperative ileus is brief, if present at all. This allows the continued use of the alimentary tract to deliver nutritional support to the hypermetabolic postoperative patient. Retroperitoneal exposure avoids manipulation of the intestines and the subsequent development of adhesions. Intra-

TABLE 3. Structures That Can Be Approached Surgically via the Retroperitoneum

Adrenal glands
Kidneys
Ureters
Bladder
Lumbar sympathetic chain
Splenic artery and vein
Renal artery and vein
Distal abdominal aorta
Inferior vena cava
Common iliac artery and vein
Internal iliac artery and vein
External iliac artery and vein
Distal pancreas
Groin hernias

operative fluid and heat loss are markedly lessened, and postoperative atelectasis and pneumonia are seldom seen. If an abscess develops, it will be interstitial and not intraperitoneal. These advantages support the sound judgment to choose retroperitoneal or extraperitoneal exposure over transabdominal exposure when technically feasible.

SURGICAL ANATOMY. The peritoneal "bag" can be dissected easily from the parieties throughout the bulk of its surface area. For practical purposes, dissection is limited in the posterior midline by the major visceral branches of the aorta. Superiorly, dissection is limited by fusion of the peritoneum to the undersurface of the diaphragm, although it can be free from the more caudal aspects of the diaphragm. It becomes progressively more difficult as the ligaments of the liver are approached. It is also easier to dissect the peritoneum from the posterior undersurface of the diaphragm than from the anterior undersurface. Inferiorly, dissection is limited in the depth of the pelvis only by the reflection of peritoneum onto the colon. Anteriorly, the peritoneum is densely fused to the posterior rectus sheath above the semicircular line. Below the semicircular line, dissection can cross the midline readily. Above the semicircular line, it is possible to extend dissection to the midline by dividing the lateral border of the rectus sheath in the semilunar line. This allows the posterior rectus sheath to come away from the rectus muscle while remaining attached to the peritoneum.

The areas where the parietal and visceral peritoneum form a juncture are shown in Figure 14. If the surgeon approaches these areas in the extraperitoneal plane laterally, it is possible to carry the dissection to the midline without entering the peritoneal cavity; however, if operating transperitoneally, it is not possible to reflect the right or left colon without entering the retroperitoneal space.

RETROPERITONEAL INFECTION. Many intra-abdominal

abscesses are localized in such a way that a part of the limiting wall is the parietal peritoneum. Such abscesses, when recognized, are best evacuated through this portion of the abscess, because contamination of the general peritoneal cavity is thereby avoided. The common sites of abscesses, some of which may be drained by the approach, are shown in Figure 11. An abscess can be located by ultrasound studies, computed tomography, or more conventional means such as palpation or fluoroscopy. When operating on a patient with an abscess, the incision should be carefully planned to allow approach of the abscess without transgression of the free peritoneal cavity. Exploratory needle aspiration may be useful. If purulent material is located, the needle may be left in place and the incision extended into the abscess beside the needle.

Some abscesses may present in the retroperitoneal space. This is more common with pancreatic abscesses. Because the pancreas is a retroperitoneal organ, an abscess or a pseudocyst that subsequently becomes infected may dissect behind the pancreas and down either or both sides of the abdomen. It is necessary to recognize the extent of these abscesses in order to obtain adequate drainage. Appendiceal abscesses secondary to perforated retrocecal appendix may also be retroperitoneal.

Reflections of the peritoneum over intra-abdominal organs may influence the localization of intra-abdominal abscesses. From Figure 11, it can be seen that abscesses that arise from sources above the transverse mesocolon usually localize above the mesocolon. If the abscess extends, it will likely extend either up into the subphrenic areas or down lateral to the ascending or descending colon. Abscesses that originate from sources below the mesocolon usually localize within the frame of the colon or extend into the pelvis. Occasionally, giant abscesses encircle the abdomen, going around the colon through the pelvis and into either or both subphrenic spaces (Fig. 15).[4]

RETROPERITONEAL FIBROSIS.[19,29] This unusual disease, which has some similarities to hypersensitivity or autoimmune disease, is relatively rare. The etiology is unknown, although a correlation between the ingestion of methysergide and the disease has been reported.

The most important clinical aspect of retroperitoneal fibrosis

is that the fibrotic process frequently entraps and constricts the ureters, thereby causing obstructive uropathy. Patients' signs and symptoms depend upon the presence or absence of ureteral stenosis, its severity, and the presence or absence of urinary infection. Presentation may vary from mild and nondescript back pain to uremia or sepsis.

The diagnosis of retroperitoneal fibrosis usually can be made accurately by intravenous pyelography if uremia is not present. The characteristic findings are hydronephrosis and hydroureter proximal to the site of extrinsic compression of the ureters. The ureters may be encased over a substantial distance, starting inferiorly and progressing superiorly. The ureters are deviated medially toward the midline. The disease is usually bilateral and symmetric but sometimes may involve only one ureter. When stenosis is severe and/or infection is present, nephrostomy may be urgently required. When the obstruction is minimal, a trial of nonoperative management may be indicated. Such management includes cessation of any drug therapy the patient is receiving, particularly methysergide. Steroid therapy should be instituted. If a response does not occur within a matter of a few weeks, operative treatment should be advised. When renal function has been compromised, nonoperative treatment is not warranted.

Surgical treatment of retroperitoneal fibrosis centers on freeing the encased ureters from their fibrous encapsulation. Once freed, the ureters must be protected from recurrent fibrotic encasement. This has been successfully prevented by converting the ureters into intra-abdominal organs or wrapping them with omentum.[10] Renal autotransplantation also has been used as a means to treat retroperitoneal fibrosis surgically. With vascular and ureteral complications occurring in less than 5 per cent of patients, it is a feasible surgical approach.[12] Nonspecific fibrosis can involve mediastinal structures (nonspecific mediastinal fibrosis), the thyroid gland (Reidel's struma), or the biliary tract (sclerosing cholangitis). These processes are similar and may or may not represent the same disease process involving different anatomic sites.

RETROPERITONEAL TUMORS. At the time of presentation, the majority of retroperitoneal tumors have invaded adjacent organs and have reached considerable size. The relative inaccessibility of the retroperitoneum and the nonspecific symptoms associated with retroperitoneal tumors explain the delay in diagnosis.[9]

Primary retroperitoneal tumors are rare, with a reported incidence of 0.3 to 3 per cent. Ackerman[1] classified these tumors based on their histologic findings: tumors of nerve origin and tumors arising from embryonic origin.[14] The majority of these tumors (60 to 85 per cent) are malignant; 75 per cent are of mesodermal origin and 24 per cent of nerve origin. Included in the mesodermally derived tumors are those arising from adipose tissue, smooth and striated muscles, connective tissues, blood vessels, and lymphatic structures.[9] These tumors are locally aggressive but rarely metastasize.

Computed tomography remains the most effective means of delineating abnormalities of the retroperitoneum. It provides evidence of local extension and resectability.

Successful treatment of these tumors remains primarily surgical. An *en bloc* resection of these malignancies provides the most favorable 5-year survival of 67 per cent.[23] Although partial resection has a 0 per cent 5-year survival, many patients symptomatically improve and may have a better response to radiotherapy and chemotherapy after the tumor has been debulked.

RETROPERITONEAL VASCULAR PROCEDURES. Elective surgical procedures on the aorta and its branches are more commonly being approached from an extraperitoneal route today. Many advantages have already been mentioned, but others warrant discussion. The extraperitoneally exposed visceral aorta and its branches can be easily controlled for bypass, endarterectomy, splenorenal shunting, renal autotransplantation,

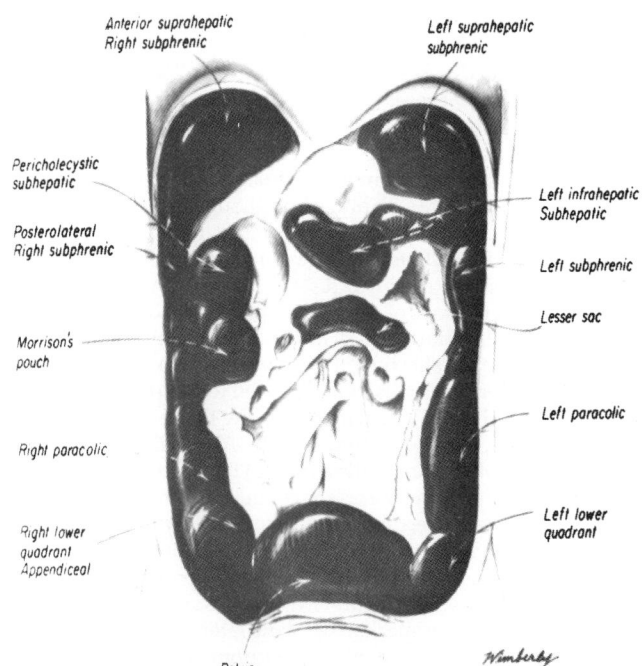

Anterior suprahepatic
Right subphrenic

Left suprahepatic
subphrenic

Pericholecystic
subhepatic

Posterolateral
Right subphrenic

Morrison's
pouch

Right paracolic

Right lower
quadrant
Appendiceal

Left infrahepatic
Subhepatic

Left subphrenic

Lesser sac

Left paracolic

Left lower
quadrant

Pelvic

Figure 15. Anterior view of the abdominal and pelvic cavity illustrating size, component parts, location, and extent of giant horseshoe abscesses. (From Altemeier, W. A., Culbertson, W. R., and Fidler, J. P.: Giant horseshoe intraabdominal abscess. Trans. South Surg. Assoc., *86*:230, 1974.)

and correction of aneurysmal disease. By avoiding the peritoneal cavity, the possibility of iatrogenic intestinal enterotomy and resultant graft contamination is removed. Operative time is also saved by removing the time-consuming and sometimes difficult step of reperitonealizing the aortic graft to prevent graft-enteric fistula formation. The retroperitoneal exposure of an aortic aneurysm does not disturb the periaortic tissue anterior to the proximal anastomosis.[18]

SELECTED REFERENCES

Glenn, J., Sindelar, W. F., Kinsella, T., Glatstein, E., Tepper, J., Costa, J., Baker, A., Sugarbaker, P., Brennan, M. F., Seipp, C., Wesley, R., Young, R. C., and Rosenberg, S. A.: Results of multimodality therapy of resectable soft tissue sarcomas of the retroperitoneum. Surgery, 97:316, 1985.
This article from the National Cancer Institute reviews the use of adjuvant chemotherapy and radiation therapy in patients with resectable retroperitoneal sarcomas. The chemotherapy arm of the study was prospective and randomized and revealed that the chemotherapy regimen administered did not improve survival and was associated with major morbidity.

Hallak, A.: Spontaneous bacterial peritonitis. Am. J. Gastroenterol., 84:345, 1989.
This current article clearly defines the syndrome of spontaneous bacterial peritonitis. It discusses the pathogenesis, clinical presentation, laboratory findings, therapy, and prognosis of this syndrome.

Hau, T., Ahrenholz, D. H., and Simmons, R. L.: Secondary bacterial peritonitis: The biologic basis of treatment. Curr. Probl. Surg., 16:1, 1979.
An up-to-date review of the pathophysiology and treatment of peritonitis. It includes sections on host defenses against peritoneal infection and the role of radical peritoneal débridement.

Healey, J. E., Jr.: A Synopsis of Clinical Anatomy. Philadelphia, W. B. Saunders Company, 1969.
This brief but excellent synopsis of anatomy discusses in depth ten anatomic areas commonly encountered by surgeons. Each section is lucidly illustrated.

McGrath, P. C., Neifeld, J. P., Lawrence, W., Jr., DeMay, R. M., Kay, S., Horsley, J. S., III, and Parker, G. A.: Improved survival following complete excision of retroperitoneal sarcomas. Ann. Surg., 200:200, 1984.
This article concisely discusses the importance of aggressive surgical management of retroperitoneal sarcomas. It clearly illustrates that the improved 5-year survivals achieved were the result of extensive surgical resections with microscopic clear margins.

REFERENCES

1. Ackerman, L. V.: Tumours of the retroperitoneum and peritoneum. In Atlas of Tumor Pathology, Sec II, Fascicle 23–24. Washington, D.C., Armed Forces Institute of Pathology, National Research Council, 1954, p. 136.
2. Adams, J. T.: Primary torsion of the omentum. Am. J. Surg., 126:102, 1973.
3. Altemeier, W. A., Culbertson, W. R., Fullen, W. D., and Shook, C. D.: Intra-abdominal abscesses. Am. J. Surg., 125:70, 1973.
4. Altemeier, W. A., Culbertson, W. R., and Fidler, J. P.: Giant horseshoe intra-abdominal abscess. Am. Surg., 181:716, 1975.
5. Beahrs, O. H., Judd, E. S., Jr., and Dockerty, M. B.: Chylous cysts of the abdomen. Surg. Clin. North Am., 30:1081, 1950.
6. Birtch, A. G., Coran, A. G., and Gross, R. E.: Neonatal peritonitis. Surgery, 61:305, 1967.
7. Blichert-Toft, M., Koch, F., and Neilson, O. V.: Anatomic variants of the urachus relating to clinical appearance and surgical treatment of urachal lesions. Surg. Gynecol. Obstet., 137:51, 1973.
8. Brasfield, R. D., and Das Gupta, T. K.: Desmoid tumors of the anterior abdominal wall. Surgery, 65:241, 1969.
9. Bryant, R. L., Stevenson, D. R., Hunton, D. W., Westbrook, K. C., and Casali, R. E.: Primary malignant retroperitoneal tumors: Current management. Am. J. Surg., 144:646, 1982.
10. Carini, M., Selli, C., Rizzo, M., Durval, A., and Costantini, A.: Surgical treatment of retroperitoneal fibrosis with omentoplasty. Surgery, 91:137, 1982.
11. Conn, H., and Fessel, M.: Spontaneous bacterial peritonitis in cirrhosis: Variations on a theme. Medicine, 50:161, 1971.
12. Deane, A. M., Gingell, J. C., and Pentlow, B. D.: Idiopathic retroperitoneal fibrosis—The role of autotransplantation. Br. J. Urol., 55:254, 1983.
13. Duckett, J. W., Jr.: The prune belly syndrome. In Kelalis, P. P., and King, L. R. (Eds.): Clinical Pediatric Urology. Philadelphia, W. B. Saunders Company, 1976.
14. Kairaluoma, M. I., Krause-Makitalo, B., Pokela, R., Stahlberg, M., Laitinen S., and Mokka, R. E. M.: Primary retroperitoneal tumours in adults. Ann. Chir. Gynaecol., 73:313, 1984.
15. Klein, E. A., Streem, S. B., and Novick, A. C.: Intraoperative consultation for the retroperitoneum and adrenal glands. Urol. Clin. North Am., 12:411, 1985.
16. Kling, S.: Patent omphalomesenteric duct—A surgical emergency. Arch. Surg., 96:545, 1968.
17. Kurzweg, F. T., Daron, P. B., Williamson, J. W., Danna, S. J., and Johnson, J. F.: Mesenteric cysts. Am. J. Surg., 40:462, 1974.
18. Leather, R. P., Shah, D. M., Kaufman, J. L., Fitzgerald, K. M., Chang, B. B., and Feustel, P. J.: Comparative analysis of retroperitoneal and transperitoneal aortic replacement for aneurysm. Surg. Gynecol. Obstet., 168:387, 1989.
19. Ormond, J. K.: Bilateral ureteral obstruction due to envelopment and compression by an inflammatory retroperitoneal process. J. Urol., 59:1072, 1948.
20. Replogle, R. L., Johnson, R., and Gross, R. E.: Prevention of postoperative adhesions with combined promethoxazine and dexamethasone therapy; Experimental and clinical studies. Ann. Surg., 163:580, 1966.
21. Rochlin, D. B., Zill, H., and Blakemore, W. S.: Studies of resorption of chromium-51–tagged erythrocytes from the peritoneal cavity: The absorption of fluids and particulate matter from the peritoneal cavity. Surg. Gynecol. Obstet., 107:1, 1958.
22. Samson, R., and Pasternak, B. M.: Current status of surgery of the omentum. Surg. Gynecol. Obstet., 149:437, 1979.
23. Serio, G., Tenchini, P., Nifosi, F., and Iacono, C.: Surgical strategy in primary retroperitoneal tumours. Br. J. Surg., 76:385, 1989.
24. Shear, L., Swartz, C., Shinaberger, J. A., and Barry, K. G.: Kinetics of peritoneal fluid absorption in adult man. N. Engl. J. Med., 272:123, 1965.
25. Simmons, R. L., Diggs, J. W., and Sleeman, H. K.: Pathogenesis of peritonitis. III. Local adjuvant action of hemoglobin in experimental *E. coli* peritonitis. Surgery, 63:810, 1968.
26. Singh, M. M., Bhargava, A. N., and Jain, K. P.: Tuberculous peritonitis: An evaluation of pathogenic mechanisms, diagnostic procedures, and therapeutic measures. N. Engl. J. Med., 281:1092, 1969.
27. Sochocky, S.: Tuberculous peritonitis: A review of 100 cases. Am. Rev. Respir. Dis., 95:398, 1967.
28. Stiles, Q. R., Raskowski, H. J., and Henry, W.: Rectus sheath hematoma. Surg. Gynecol. Obstet., 12:331, 1965.
29. Suby, H. I., Kerr, W. S., Graham, J. R., and Fraley, E.: Retroperitoneal fibrosis: A missing link in the chain. J. Urol., 93:144, 1965.
30. Viranuvatti, V., Hitanat, S., Boonyapaknavig, V., Plengvanit, V., Kalayasiri, C., and Chearani, O.: Peritoneal biopsy: Experience with blind and direct vision biopsy. Am. J. Proct., 17:489, 1966.
31. Willwert, B. M., Zollinger, R. M., Jr., and Izant, R. J., Jr.: Congenital mesocolic (paraduodenal) hernia. Am. J. Surg., 128:358, 1974.

28

THE ACUTE ABDOMEN

Arnold G. Diethelm, M.D., and Robert J. Stanley, M.D.

Acute abdominal pain continues as a common diagnostic challenge to the surgeon, internist, family practitioner, obstetrician-gynecologist, and pediatrician. Although many patients with sudden or gradual onset of abdominal pain progress to severe abdominal pain requiring operative intervention, others may have the pain resolve over a period of time with eventual recovery without a surgical procedure. The complexity of the entity known as the acute abdomen is such that a careful, methodic diagnostic approach is necessary in order to arrive at a correct diagnosis. Rapid or quick decisions are usually not required and are often incorrect or misleading. If the information from the history, physical examination, laboratory data, and radiographic studies is not conclusive, then periodic re-examination of the patient with appropriate laboratory data and repeat radiologic examination often resolves what earlier appeared to be an uncertain diagnosis. A thorough knowledge of the etiologic basis of abdominal pain and its natural history is essential in the proper management of these patients. In addition, understanding the anatomy and physiology of the peritoneal cavity as well as the pathologic processes that occur within the abdomen is essential for an accurate diagnosis and treatment plan.

HISTORICAL ASPECTS

Acute pathologic conditions of the abdomen have been recognized since Hippocrates and referred to by Paracelsus (1493–1541) and Sydenham (1624–1689) as iliac passion. The reluctance of the surgeon to enter the abdomen by operation prior to the introduction of anesthesia can be appreciated. Moreover, the pathology of many intra-abdominal conditions was not well understood until the late nineteenth century. Appendicitis, recognized by Reginald Fitz in 1886, was previously referred to as typhlitis and recognized only after a careful autopsy study describing the progress of the disease. Similar experiences were true for incarcerated inguinal hernia and intestinal obstruction treated only rarely prior to 1850. The introduction of anesthesia, antiseptic surgical technique, and improved surgical instruments led to exploration of the abdomen with increased frequency at the beginning of the twentieth century. Perhaps no discovery had greater impact on intra-abdominal surgery than the use of antibiotics in combination with operative treatment of intestinal surgery. In the past 15 years the ability to accurately determine intra-abdominal pathologic processes by radiologic imaging has allowed earlier and more accurate diagnosis. Today the combination of improved diagnostic measures, antibiotics, better anesthesia, and pre- and postoperative patient care has decreased morbidity and mortality of patients with acute septic and nonseptic conditions of the abdomen.

ANATOMY AND PHYSIOLOGY OF VISCERAL PAIN

The neurophysiology and anatomy of pain from viscera of the gastrointestinal tract, hepatobiliary tract, pancreas, kidneys,

ureters, bladder, ovaries, fallopian tubes, and uterus are important to the understanding of the patient's complaint during an episode of acute abdominal pain. The lower esophagus receives its sensory innervation through rami from the splanchnic nerves and paravertebral ganglia, whereas pain from the cervical and thoracic esophagus is transmitted by sensory fibers in the vagi (Fig. 1). The sensation of pain from the stomach and duodenum travels via the splanchnic afferent fibers that enter the spinal cord at the seventh and eighth dorsal segments. Distention of the small intestine by a balloon causes discomfort that can be ablated by thoracolumbar ganglionectomy and splanchnicectomy; however, in the presence of colon distention, the sensation of discomfort persists. Thus, colonic afferent axons travel in the sacral nerves. The primary cause of pain from the biliary tract arises from distention of the common duct, cystic duct, gallbladder, and liver capsule. Pain from these structures travels via the major splanchnic nerve to the spinal cord over the seventh through ninth spinal roots. Pancreatic sensory fibers pass in the right and left splanchnic nerves from the celiac plexus. Sensation from the head of the pancreas is via the right splanchnic trunk and from the tail of the pancreas in the left splanchnic trunk. Renal pain and that from the cephalad portion of the ureter pass through fibers in the vascular pedicle to the aorticorenal and celiac ganglia. From here, pain sensory fibers travel to the least splanchnic trunks and to the lowest thoracic ganglion. Thus, the main level of spinal innervation for the kidney and proximal ureter is by the tenth thoracic to the first lumbar segment. The sensory innervation of the bladder, vesical neck, and prostate travels by the second, third, and fourth sacral nerves. Uterine pain travels through the superior hypogastric plexus and the preaortic nerves with afferent fibers passing through the paravertebral ganglia to the twelfth thoracic and first lumbar rami and posterior spinal roots. Sensation of the cervix is transmitted by the sacral parasympathetics to the second, third, and fourth sacral segments. Ovarian pain follows along the sympathetic nerves of the ovarian arteries.

The multiple causes of abdominal pain emphasize the importance of understanding the anatomy and physiology of visceral pain and the patient's subjective interpretation of the pain. Pain can be characterized as sharp, stabbing, or burning or as heavy, diffuse, or dull. The autonomic response to visceral pain, often described as a deep pain, includes sweating and nausea with a decrease in blood pressure and differs from the sharp pricking pain originating from the skin. Visceral pain, that is, pain arising from the abdominal and thoracic cavities, reaches the central nervous system by three routes: (1) the parasympathetic nerves, (2) the sympathetic nerves, or (3) the somatic nerves innervating the body wall and the diaphragm. It has long been recognized that visceral organs can be cut, crushed, or burned with little sensation. However, traction of the mesentery and stimulation of the parietal peritoneum cause pain. Stimulation of the visceral afferent fibers produces pain and includes (1) strong contractions or spasm, (2) sudden distention against resistance, and (3) chemical irritation and mechanical stimulation. Visceral reflexes and organic sensation travel by parasympathetic afferent

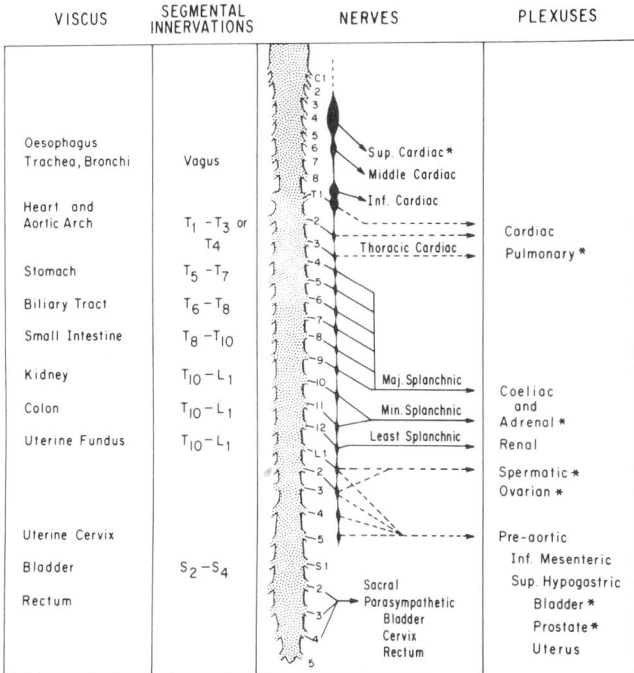

VISCUS	SEGMENTAL INNERVATIONS	NERVES	PLEXUSES
Oesophagus Trachea, Bronchi	Vagus	Sup. Cardiac * Middle Cardiac Inf. Cardiac	
Heart and Aortic Arch	$T_1 - T_3$ or T_4	Thoracic Cardiac	Cardiac Pulmonary *
Stomach	$T_5 - T_7$		
Biliary Tract	$T_6 - T_8$		
Small Intestine	$T_8 - T_{10}$		
Kidney	$T_{10} - L_1$	Maj. Splanchnic	Coeliac and Adrenal *
Colon	$T_{10} - L_1$	Min. Splanchnic	Renal
Uterine Fundus	$T_{10} - L_1$	Least Splanchnic	Spermatic * Ovarian *
Uterine Cervix			Pre-aortic Inf. Mesenteric Sup. Hypogastric
Bladder	$S_2 - S_4$		Bladder *
Rectum		Sacral Parasympathetic Bladder Cervix Rectum	Prostate * Uterus

* No known sensory fibers in sympathetic rami.

Figure 1. Sensory innervations of the viscera. (From White, J. C., and Sweet, W. H.: Pain and the Neurosurgeon. Springfield, IL, Charles C Thomas, 1969, p. 526.)

nerves, whereas the sympathetic nerves conduct visceral pain. The exceptions are the pelvis, the esophagus, and the trachea, where pain can be transmitted by the pelvic and vagus nerves.

Pain from visceral structures may occur at a considerable distance from the organ involved, such as shoulder pain with acute cholecystitis, and is termed referred pain. This important observation has obvious clinical relevance. Visceral pain can be divided into two types: pain caused by stimulation of the parietal peritoneum and pain from the viscera itself. Both types of pain may be referred or nonreferred. The pain caused by inflammation from a perforated duodenal ulcer travels by somatic nerves. Referred parietal pain such as diaphragmatic irritation travels to the shoulder and neck, with the impulse ascending the phrenic nerve and entering the spinal cord via C3 and C4. Pain is then referred to these dermatome segments. The discrepancy between the point of origin of pain and its final point of referral can be explained by the caudal migration of the diaphragm during embryologic development. Referred visceral pain occurs from impulses initiated in the viscera traveling over visceral nerves, usually sympathetic. Unreferred visceral pain (splanchnic pain) such as pain from the gastrointestinal tract is poorly localized and may be interpreted as being elsewhere than the site of stimulation. Visceral pain is usually described as a deep pain or ache. Rigidity and abdominal tenderness are common physical findings representing inflammation of the parietal peritoneum. In this circumstance, pain may be interpreted as regional rather than segmental.

The just abbreviated description of abdominal pain is quite obviously, in clinical situations, dependent on the subjective interpretation by the patient. Careful questioning of the patient by the surgeon may provide additional information, such as whether the attention of the patient can be deflected during the examination and thus lessen the severity of the pain. An inappropriate response may suggest that the subjective expression of pain is less severe than that described by the patient. It is equally important to note the stoic patient who has a high tolerance for pain and may express less discomfort than expected. It should be emphasized that all complaints of abdominal pain

must be considered serious until all reasonable diagnostic efforts prove to the contrary.

The assessment of abdominal pain in the patient who is acutely ill requires a complete knowledge of the anatomic relationship of the intraperitoneal organs, their innervation, and the location of referred pain. Generally, intra-abdominal pain is interpreted by the patient as being localized in various anatomic sites, which may be helpful to the surgeon in analyzing the potential pathologic cause. For example, biliary tract disease is localized more precisely than is disease of the small and large intestines (Fig. 2). Acute cholecystitis presents with right upper quadrant pain and may extend to the epigastric region if pancreatitis or common duct stones are present. Thus, under such circumstances, the location of pain would overlap from the right upper quadrant to the epigastric region. The referral of pain to the right shoulder and scapula is frequently noted in patients with acute cholecystitis and is rarely observed with other causes of abdominal pain. Pain from acute duodenal ulcer disease, nonperforated, is noted in the epigastric region and is often highly circumscribed. If the ulcer is in the posterior wall of the duodenum and erodes into the pancreas, pain is referred directly to the back. This type of pain is often dull and constant and may be impossible to separate from carcinoma of the pancreas. Pain from the small intestine occurs in the periumbilical area and rarely radiates to the back or other intra-abdominal locations. Colon pain is more apparent in the suprapubic location and is ill-defined in terms of character and radiation. Renal pain is not usually abdominal in location and radiates only when the ureter is involved. When a calculus is in the ureter, pain radiates to the testicle and as such is helpful in establishing an accurate diagnosis.

Therefore, localization of pain to the four quadrants of the abdomen has some value to the examiner but may not be relevant to the etiologic origin of the pain. The embryologic development of the gastrointestinal tract is pertinent to the radiation of pain, and the different innervations of the foregut, midgut, and hindgut are important in the assessment of the patient and in understanding that pain from visceral fibers is less well recognized than pain from somatic nerves.

CLINICAL CONSIDERATIONS

An accurate and direct approach to the patient with acute abdominal pain includes a thorough clinical history and physi-

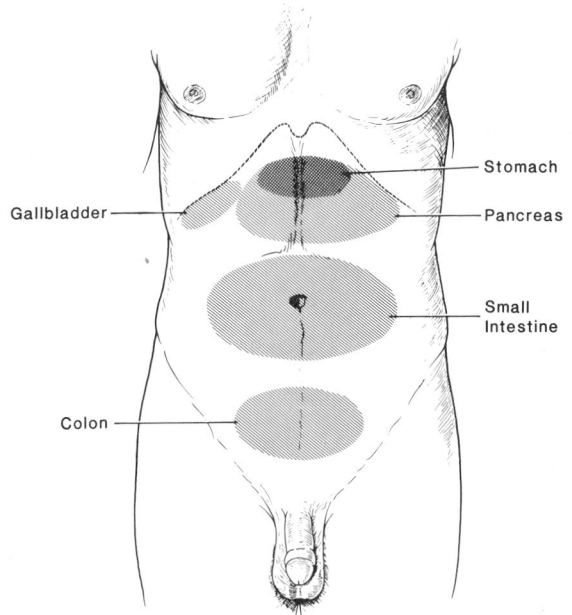

Figure 2. Pain from intra-abdominal viscera.

cal examination by an unhurried physician willing to take the necessary time to establish a correct diagnosis. It is important to assess the clinical situation completely supported by appropriate laboratory work in order to avoid a superficial conclusion. Although most causes of abdominal pain are related to diseases of the gastrointestinal tract and the gynecologic subsystem, all potential causes must be considered in the overall analysis (Fig. 3).

History

PRESENT ILLNESS

PAIN. Abdominal pain, either sudden or gradual in onset, frequently progresses in severity so that it is the paramount feature of the patient's illness. A careful and detailed history defines the time of onset of pain, the location, and change in character and position. Pain that persists for 6 hours or more and is of severe intensity usually requires operative intervention for treatment of the underlying process. The converse is true in those patients with pain of sudden onset who may experience complete resolution in 4 to 6 hours. The exact situation in which the onset of pain occurs may often be important in establishing the diagnosis. Pain that is sharp, severe, and sudden in onset— awakening the patient from sleep, or incapacitating the patient at work—often suggests a perforated viscus. Pain located in the upper abdomen favors peptic ulcer disease, acute cholecystitis, or pancreatitis versus ruptured ovarian cyst, perforated diverticulitis, or ruptured tubo-ovarian abscess when pain is located in the lower abdomen. The character of the pain initially and later is important in the differentiation of small bowel obstruction from strangulation of the intestine. The former pain is a cramping intermittent type of pain, whereas the latter causes a dull constant pain. The original location of the pain and its shifting or changing of position may provide a clue to the diagnosis, as is commonly observed with acute appendicitis. The character of the pain and the patient's description are of major importance. A sudden burning pain in the epigastric region suggests a perforated viscus; severe intermittent cramping pain with short pain-free intervals favors small bowel obstruction. Sudden excruciating tearing pain may be associated with a ruptured aneurysm. Radiation of the pain may be helpful in the diagnosis. Pain of acute cholecystitis frequently radiates around the right costal margin to the right scapula and to the shoulder. Pain in acute pancreatitis is usually epigastric in origin, with subsequent radiation along both costal margins to the back. Ureteral calculi cause pain radiating to the testicle when the stone is in the cephalad portion of the ureter and produce perineal pain when the stone is near the ureterovesical junction. This type of pain is frequently excruciating in severity. A sudden severe

shearing or tearing pain of the chest or intrascapular region extending to the abdomen and occasionally into the upper or lower extremities suggests a dissection of the thoracic aorta.

VOMITING. Vomiting may follow severity of the pain, but in many instances, the cause is related to the gastrointestinal tract. Vomiting occurs uncommonly in the presence of a perforated ulcer but is frequently noted in patients with acute cholecystitis. Vomiting always occurs with obstruction of the small intestine and provides temporary relief from the cramping abdominal pain. The temporal relationship of abdominal pain to vomiting is important and may provide important diagnostic clues to the underlying etiologic factor. Pain almost always precedes vomiting by 3 or 4 hours in patients with appendicitis. The converse is true in gastroenteritis. The frequency of vomiting may be significant in that one or two episodes may occur with gastroenteritis and then subside. Emesis occurs early and repeatedly in patients with small intestinal obstruction, but presents late or not at all in the course of large intestinal obstruction. The character of the emesis, including the color and content, is pertinent in regard to the site of obstruction. Clear vomitus suggests an obstructed pylorus, whereas bile-stained emesis indicates that the obstruction is distal to the entrance of the common bile duct into the duodenum. As the site of obstruction moves distally in the small intestine, the vomitus becomes brown in color and feculent in odor. Cramping abdominal pain that is relieved by vomiting favors small bowel obstruction.

ANOREXIA. It is uncommon for patients with acute abdominal pain to desire food, although true anorexia may not exist. Anorexia is usually associated with acute abdominal pain, and in patients with acute appendicitis, it may precede the onset of pain. This observation becomes especially important in children, in whom anorexia followed by vague periumbilical abdominal pain is suggestive of acute appendicitis.

BOWELS. Constipation, diarrhea, and a recent change in bowel habits are important factors in the diagnosis of patients with abdominal pain. Profuse watery diarrhea for 12 or more hours with cramping abdominal pain is suggestive of gastroenteritis. The failure to pass flatus associated with cramping pain and vomiting strongly supports mechanical obstruction of the gastrointestinal tract. A description of subtle changes in bowel habits, although important, may be difficult to obtain from patients with extreme discomfort during abdominal pain.

MENSTRUATION. An accurate menstrual history is especially valuable in the assessment of abdominal pain in the female. The frequency of the cycle, the duration of the menstrual period, and the exact dates are key factors. Any change in volume of menstrual flow is pertinent, because an ectopic pregnancy may rupture at any time during the cycle as well as simultaneously with the menstrual period. The type of contraception and its duration of use must be considered, because there are specific complications for each method.

PAST ILLNESSES. The patient's history prior to the present illness is of special value, particularly in regard to previous surgical therapy (e.g., appendectomy, cholecystectomy, gastric or intestinal surgery). The previous diagnosis of an abdominal or inguinal hernia may contribute to the diagnosis of the present illness. A history of similar pain is especially valuable, suggesting a recurrent problem. A history of renal calculi or pelvic inflammatory disease may suggest a recurrence of the same illness as contrasted to a new disease. The natural history of a previous attack occasionally predicts the outcome of the current attack.

FAMILY HISTORY. The probability of acute abdominal pain relating to a familial disease is unlikely but may occur in some circumstances. Familial Mediterranean fever (familial recurring polyserositis) occurs in individuals of Armenian or Sephardic Jewish background as an inherited autosomal recessive trait with spontaneous attacks of abdominal pain. Sickle cell anemia in black patients is another example of hereditary influence upon the cause of abdominal pain.

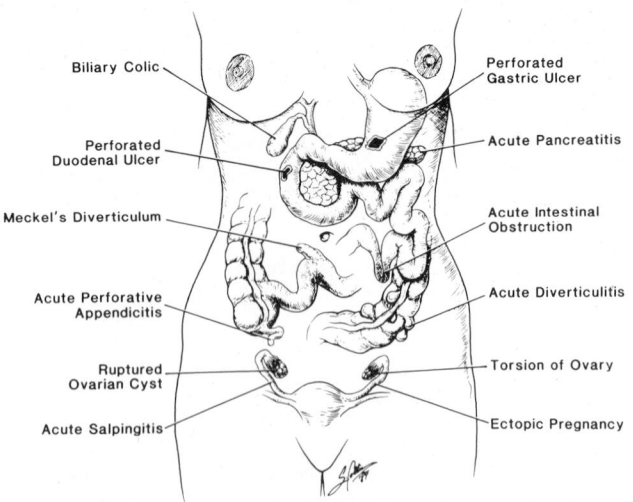

Figure 3. Common causes of abdominal pain.

ORGAN SYSTEM REVIEW. A careful organ system review is essential to the patient's history and should be obtained in detail to avoid overlooking an extra-abdominal cause of pain such as a pulmonary embolus to the lower lobe with diaphragmatic irritation or an acute myocardial infarction. Patients with a systemic illness, such as lupus, nephrotic syndrome, porphyria, and sickle cell crisis, may also develop abdominal pain as a manifestation of their underlying illness and do not require surgical intervention.

Physical Examination

The physical examination coupled with a careful and accurate history, in most instances, provides or at least suggests an accurate diagnosis that may then be confirmed by the appropriately selected laboratory tests and radiologic imaging studies.

The physical examination begins with a brief but complete consideration of the patient's appearance, ability to answer questions, position in bed, and degree of obvious pain or discomfort. The general appearance is noted immediately upon meeting the patient and obtaining the history. An anxious, pale, sweating patient who is either restless or lies quietly in a supine position in bed and complains of abdominal pain has a high probability of intra-abdominal disease or serious extra-abdominal disease referred to the abdomen. The position in bed is important regarding whether the patient lies in a supine position or on the side with the knees and hips flexed. The presence of obvious dehydration with dry mucous membranes, sunken hollow eyes, and rapid shallow respiration all suggest generalized peritonitis. A rapid heart rate with hypotension is noted with hypovolemia and usually is the result of peritonitis and large plasma volume fluid shifts from the intravascular space to the extravascular space within the peritoneum.

Examination of the abdomen always begins with a visual inspection of the chest and abdomen for previous scars, hernia or obvious masses, or abdominal wall defects. The inspection should focus on the size, shape, and contour of the abdomen, with specific consideration focused on the respiration of the patient, including the rate and depth of breathing. Auscultation of the abdomen should include all four quadrants, with special attention given to the frequency and pitch of bowel sounds and rushes of gas audible to the examiner that correlate to the facial expression of pain by the patient. Percussion of the abdomen should begin in the quadrant free of pain and should be performed lightly to avoid eliciting pain at the onset of the examination. This is especially critical in children who have abdominal tenderness, because percussion tenderness may cause the child to lose confidence in the examining physician. The location of maximal tenderness should be confirmed in relation to the area of the abdomen and correlated with the history. Thus, maximal tenderness in the right lower quadrant (RLQ) over McBurney's point is suggestive of appendicitis if there is a history compatible with the disease. The abdomen should be palpated gently, avoiding any undue discomfort to the patient. Palpation should always begin in an area away from that in which pain is described in the history.

A pelvic and rectal examination must always be performed and should preferably be done by the surgeon or physician responsible for the complete assessment of the patient. Umbilical and inguinal hernia should always be sought to document the presence or absence of an incarcerated hernia. The presence of peritoneal irritation can be assessed either by palpation with a quick release of the examining hand (rebound tenderness) or by gently rolling the patient from side to side, with the examiner's hands placed on the patient's pelvis. Rigidity of the rectus muscles may be especially obvious in patients with generalized peritonitis due to a perforated viscus. Examination of the abdomen in such instances may be difficult. Flexion of the lower extremities at the knee and hip helps the patient relax the abdominal wall and allows a more complete examination. The lateral abdominal muscles are less rigid in acute peritonitis than the rectus muscles, and tenderness is less apparent in the older or obese patient with weak abdominal muscles. The abdomen should always be examined for free fluid, liver dullness, and iliopsoas rigidity due to inflammation of the psoas muscle. The pelvic examination reveals the presence of cervical discharge or vaginal bleeding, and bimanual examination confirms or excludes tenderness on uterine or adnexal palpation. A rectal examination should note the existence of a pelvic mass and the presence of a perirectal mass or abscess.

Diagnostic Imaging

The role of the radiologist in the evaluation of the patient with an acute abdomen has evolved greatly in the past decade. Whereas the plain supine and erect radiographs of the abdomen remain the most common first step in the diagnostic imaging evaluation of such a patient, more sensitive and more specific imaging methods, such as computed tomography (CT) and ultrasound, have an increasing role in the evaluation of this complex, emergent clinical problem. Early enthusiasm for more sophisticated imaging technology was tempered by considerations of limited access, high cost, and delay of time required for the imaging procedure. However, CT and ultrasound are now widely available; methods and techniques of examination have been streamlined (e.g., a complete CT examination of the abdomen and pelvis can be accomplished in less than 15 minutes on most current CT units); and although the cost of the more sophisticated examinations remains a factor, recognition is becoming more widespread that CT and sonography often obviate organ-specific imaging studies such as excretory urograms, radionuclide examinations, and diagnostic arteriograms.

As greater experience in the use of CT and ultrasound has been gained, it is recognized that there is a demonstrable morphologic correlate to almost all of the conditions associated with the clinical presentation of an acute abdomen. Although the plain abdominal radiograph may provide specific, diagnostic findings, valuable in making correct therapeutic decisions, more often than not the findings are nonspecific or indeterminate. When approaching acute, severe inflammatory disease affecting the gastrointestinal or genitourinary tract, complications of blunt abdominal trauma, or acute vascular crises (e.g., acute mesenteric venous thrombosis or rupture of a visceral artery aneurysm), the plain film radiographic findings most often are nonrevealing and substantially less informative than is a carefully obtained history and physical examination. In contrast, CT and, to a lesser extent, sonography often provide differential morphologic information not obtainable by any means other than exploratory surgery, allowing the precise diagnosis of most of the entities associated with the acute abdomen.

In this section the appropriate role of the plain film, organ-specific contrast studies of the gastrointestinal and genitourinary tract, radionuclide imaging, CT, sonography, and arteriography, as it applies to the evaluation of the acute abdomen, is presented.

Initial radiologic evaluation of the patient with an acute abdomen most often consists of the plain film of the abdomen obtained in the supine and erect position. The standard erect film of the abdomen, however, is not the most appropriate radiograph for the detection of free intraperitoneal air. This erect radiograph should be obtained with the central ray positioned at the level of the diaphragm in order to optimize the likelihood of detecting small quantities of free air trapped in subdiaphragmatic locations. If the patient is unable to assume the erect position, a lateral decubitus radiograph with the patient's left side down should be requested. In this instance the x-ray beam is in a horizontal cross-table orientation and the central ray should be positioned closer to the right lateral abdominal wall rather than toward the midline of the abdomen. Quantities of free air as small as 5 to 10 cc. can be detected in the space between the lateral aspect of the right lobe of the liver and the lateral abdominal wall.

Free intraperitoneal air, as mentioned, can be the result of many different causes. Those associated with the clinical presentation of an acute abdomen include perforation of a gastric or duodenal peptic ulcer, perforation of the cecum due to obstruction and/or ischemia and necrosis, or perforation associated with colonic diverticulitis. Whereas the quantity of free air associated with a perforated duodenal ulcer is usually relatively small in volume, perforations of the stomach or colon may be associated with much larger quantities of free intraperitoneal air, a distinction of some differential diagnostic value. If the quantity of free air is great enough, its presence can be appreciated on the supine radiograph of the abdomen when the inner and outer surface of the wall of a gas-filled loop of bowel can be clearly defined because of the presence of gas on either side of the soft tissue structure. In a similar manner, the falciform ligament may occasionally be visible as an obliquely oriented soft tissue structure extending from the right upper quadrant toward the umbilicus when sufficiently large quantities of gas are present on either side of it. A sizable hydro- or pyopneumoperitoneum is easily recognized in the erect radiograph of the abdomen by the presence of an air-fluid level that is too great in length for even an obstructed segment of colon (Fig. 4A). This same condition can be recognized on the supine radiograph of the abdomen by the detection of an oval or football-shaped collection of gas beneath the anterior abdominal wall that does not conform to any recognizable loop of bowel (Fig. 4B).

Abnormal calcific densities detectable on a plain radiograph of the abdomen and sometimes associated with the clinical presentation of an acute abdomen include gallstones, renal and ureteral calculi, appendicoliths, intrapancreatic calculi (most often associated with chronic pancreatitis), and curvilinear calcification located in the wall of an abdominal aortic or visceral artery aneurysm. Such plain radiographic information is of value only when correlated with the clinical presentation, since many of these findings are often present in asymptomatic patients.

Plain radiographs of the abdomen have their greatest role in the evaluation of the question of mechanical obstruction of the gastrointestinal tract. Supine and erect radiographs of the abdomen should allow the distinction between gastric outlet obstructions, proximal, mid and distal small bowel obstructions, and colonic obstructive processes. If the plain films suggest a mid to distal small bowel obstruction based on numerous air-fluid levels within loops of dilated small bowel, in association with partial or complete absence of gas within the colon, an immediate full column barium enema clarifies the absence of colonic obstruction. If the ileocecal valve is sufficiently incompetent, the barium permits opacification of collapsed terminal ileum and possibly identifies the point of obstruction. High-grade obstructions of the right colon, such as those caused by a constricting neoplasm, may mimic a distal small bowel obstruction. It is in such cases that an immediate barium enema has its greatest value. Carcinomas of the cecum and ileocecal valve can also produce high-grade obstructions of the small bowel and are readily detected with a barium enema.

In contrast to the high diagnostic yield of a promptly performed barium enema in the presence of mid to distal small bowel obstruction, contrast studies from above, whether with barium or water-soluble contrast medium, frequently have little diagnostic value beyond reinforcing the impression of small bowel mechanical obstruction, and often delay diagnosis and treatment. However, if the clinical presentation as well as the plain radiographs suggest obstruction of the gastric outlet or duodenum, an upper gastrointestinal examination not only is of considerable value in confirming the presence of mechanical obstruction but may suggest the precise cause. Therefore, consultation with the radiologist can be of considerable value when assessing the plain film findings in the patient with an acute abdomen and planning further diagnostic imaging studies.

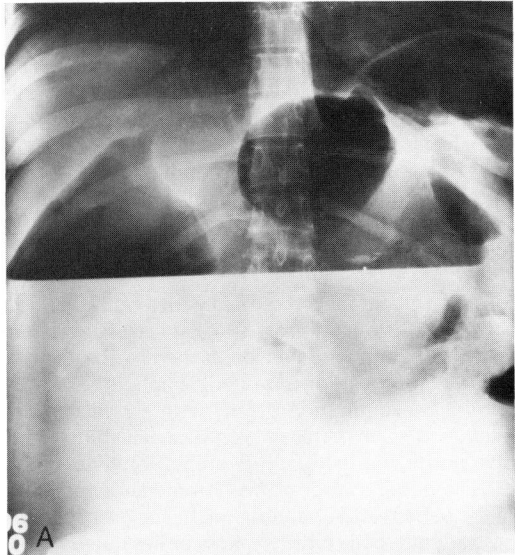

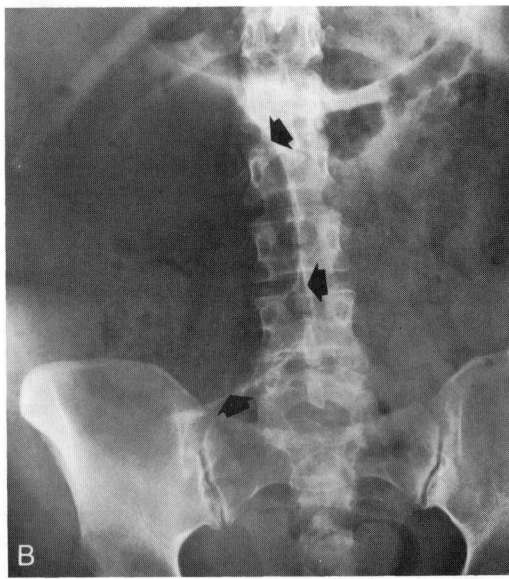

Figure 4. Plain film findings in hydropneumoperitoneum. *A*, Upright view shows fluid level too long to be within a loop of bowel. *B*, In the supine position, the free air is well defined by the interface with the fluid in the peritoneal cavity (arrows).

At times the patient with an acute abdomen presents with a radiographic bowel gas pattern suggestive of mechanical obstruction when, in fact, no mechanically obstructing process is present. Such varied entities as pneumonia, pulmonary infarction, diffuse peritonitis, acute severe pyelonephritis, vascular compromise of the small or large bowel, and a variety of inflammatory processes affecting the gastrointestinal tract as well as metabolic or drug-related effects on the motility of the bowel can all produce an abnormal bowel gas pattern. A decrease in peristalsis or its cessation is referred to as an ileus. This term can be applied to any type of intestinal obstruction, whether mechanical or not. Those conditions that produce diminished or absent bowel motility not due to a mechanical process are attributed to an adynamic or paralytic ileus. It is, of course, crucial in the evaluation of the patient with an acute abdomen to make the important distinction between an adynamic ileus and a mechanical ileus. Plain film findings in a patient with an adynamic ileus include the presence of gas within both the small intestine and colon. There is moderate distention of the caliber of the bowel throughout rather than significant disproportions suggesting a point of transition. Air-fluid levels are at essentially the same level in the same loop of small bowel on the erect radiograph (consistent with complete lack of motility) with an unchanging appearance to the bowel gas pattern over a period of several hours. When it is difficult to differentiate an adynamic ileus pattern from a pattern suggestive of distal colonic obstruction, a carefully performed full column barium enema again provides rapid resolution of this diagnostic problem.

If the patient's clinical presentation suggests a free perforation of the bowel into the peritoneal cavity, and a contrast study of the gastrointestinal tract is still indicated, water-soluble contrast is the appropriate medium to use to avoid the complications of a barium peritonitis.

Other plain film findings of diagnostic value include the detection of gas within the portal and mesenteric venous systems, intramural gas anywhere in the gastrointestinal tract, gas within the biliary tree in the absence of known, surgically created biliary enteric anastomoses, and abnormal gas collections associated with the gallbladder, the urinary tract, or the retroperitoneal spaces in general. In patients with adequate perivisceral and retroperitoneal fat, obscuration of portions or all of the outlines of those organs and structures normally surrounded by fat may be an important clue to an associated or contiguous inflammatory or hemorrhagic process. The inflammation and abscess formation associated with appendicitis, for example, can produce obscuration of the right psoas margin as well as the properitoneal fat flank stripe in the right lower quadrant. Whereas it is important to recognize these findings, they are still nonspecific, and more definitive studies such as computed tomography should be performed.

Experience has shown that when gas is detectable within the portal or mesenteric venous systems on a plain radiograph of the abdomen, the inflammatory or ischemic process that is producing the release of gas into the venous system is generally far advanced and the finding is associated with a high mortality. In contrast, CT can detect minute quantities of gas within the portal and mesenteric venous systems and is often capable of demonstrating the causative condition at a far earlier stage of development. In general, by the time intra-abdominal pathologic processes are detectable on a plain roentgenogram, they are usually far advanced. With the early use of CT, plain films of the abdomen that appear unremarkable or indeterminate have been shown to be insensitive to the readily recognizable morphologic changes on the CT examination associated with the conditions producing an acute abdomen (Fig. 5).

When the signs and symptoms of a patient with an acute abdomen suggest renal colic due to the passage of a renal calculus into the pelvis or ureter, an excretory urogram is often diagnostic. The pain of renal colic can be simulated by other conditions including a renal tumor, acute renal inflammatory disease, or disease processes affecting the renal vascular pedicle, and often the excretory urogram establishes the correct diagnosis.

There are few indications for radionuclide imaging procedures in the evaluation of the acute abdomen. The role of biliary radiopharmaceuticals such as HIDA in the evaluation of patients with suspected acute cholecystitis remains incompletely defined. Strong proponents of their use emphasize the diagnostic importance of the finding of nonfilling of the gallbladder by the radionuclide imaging agent in the presence of good excretion in the remainder of the biliary tree. However, a minimum of 4 hours must elapse before delayed filling of the gallbladder with a patent cystic duct can be excluded. Additionally, chronic cholecystitis has occasionally produced falsely positive studies. It now appears that real-time ultrasonography is the more commonly used imaging study in the assessment of the patient with suspected acute cholecystitis. In a matter of minutes, the caliber of the biliary tree, the presence and location of biliary calculi, the morphologic features of the gallbladder wall, and the presence or absence of tenderness due to the pressure of the transducer directly over the gallbladder can be assessed (Fig. 6).

When acute abdominal pain develops following blunt trauma, radionuclide imaging studies of the liver and spleen are

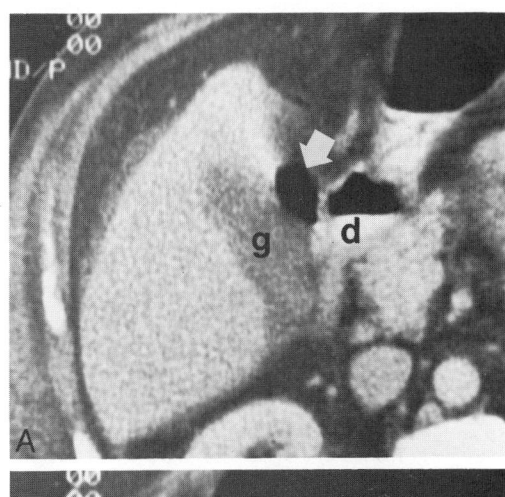

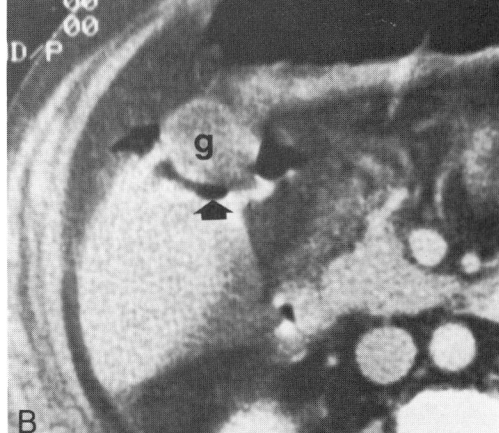

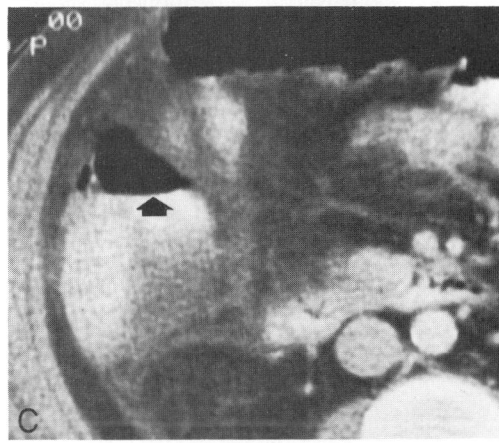

Figure 5. Unsuspected perforated duodenal ulcer. *A,* Small amount of extraluminal gas (arrow) lies lateral to duodenal bulb (d); g, gallbladder. *B,* Three centimeters caudal, gas (arrow) tracks behind the gallbladder laterally. *C,* The air-fluid level (arrow) identifies the loculated extravasated duodenal contents. Inflammatory changes are present in the surrounding mesenteric fat.

generally less informative than is a properly performed CT examination of the abdomen. The radionuclide study is organ-limited, and although it is sensitive to traumatic injuries of the liver and spleen, it is nevertheless insensitive to associated perisplenic or perihepatic processes. A radionuclide study may be indicated in the hemodynamically stable patient in whom the CT findings, for any one of a number of technical problems, are indeterminate.

The indications for the use of CT and ultrasound in the evaluation of the acute abdomen have increased dramatically in the past decade. Ultrasonography can provide rapid morphologic evaluation of liver, spleen, pancreas, and kidney. With the advent of pulsed Doppler ultrasound, the blood vessels of the

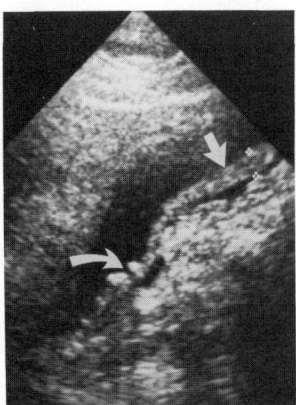

Figure 6. Acute cholecystitis—ultrasound. Two small stones (curved arrow) are present in the neck. The wall of the gallbladder in the fundus (straight arrow) is thickened, and pericholecystic fluid is present.

abdomen can be studied with remarkable precision in a manner not possible as recently as the mid-1980s. Aortic and visceral artery aneurysms, thrombi within veins, arteriovenous fistulas, and vascular anomalies all are amenable to evaluation with modern ultrasound equipment (Fig. 7).

Because of the frequently occurring adynamic ileus in patients with an acute abdomen, large areas of the abdomen are inaccessible for ultrasound evaluation owing to the interposed gas, which transmits a sound wave poorly. Computed tomography is not hampered by overlying gas, bone, or adipose tissue, all of which present relative obstacles to the transmission of a sound wave. Additionally, whereas an experienced sonographer can complete a general survey of the abdomen and pelvis in a relatively short period of time, a complete CT examination of the abdomen and pelvis can be performed in similar time or less with a degree of thoroughness not achievable with ultrasound. Therefore, CT has a more useful role in the early evaluation of the patient with an acute abdomen, unless the signs and symptoms are highly indicative of a disease process in a specific organ system such as acute cholecystitis or renal colic.

Considering one of the more common causes of the acute abdomen, namely, appendicitis, plain films of the abdomen are occasionally helpful and barium enemas have also been shown to clarify some cases with ambiguous findings. However, in the patient with uncomplicated appendicitis, sonography has been found to be more sensitive for the detection of appendicoliths as well as in the demonstration of the abnormally distended and thick-walled appendix itself (Fig. 8). Periappendiceal and pericecal inflammatory changes produce areas of hypoechogenicity, adding support to the diagnosis.

Computed tomography is better in defining the changes associated with complicated appendicitis (Fig. 9). Generally, a periappendiceal phlegmon can be differentiated from an abscess as well as a well-defined, well-localized abscess from a poorly localized, extensive abscess, all of which have therapeutic implications.

The differential diagnosis of appendicitis is extensive and includes acute cholecystitis, perinephric abscess, pyonephrosis, Crohn's disease, cecal or ileocecal carcinoma, psoas abscess, typhlitis (neutropenic enterocolitis), rectus hematoma, intestinal obstruction or infarction, diverticulitis with abscess, and salpingitis, possibly with rupture of the pyosalpinx, as well as other causes of intraperitoneal disease. Computed tomography allows differentiation of many if not all of these entities quickly.

Spontaneous as well as posttraumatic intra-abdominal hemorrhage is readily and accurately diagnosable with CT. Intramural intestinal hemorrhage from whatever cause may also cause acute abdominal pains and produce a characteristic appearance on CT (Fig. 10). Occasionally associated pathologic processes such as pancreatitis, lymphoma, hepatic cirrhosis, and other diseases that produce clotting disorders or vascular fragility are identified. A rare cause of an acute abdomen related to hemorrhage is sudden, spontaneous adrenal hemorrhage, which can also cause an addisonian crisis. The findings on CT are pathognomonic.

The CT findings in bowel ischemia and infarction include wall thickening (a common but nonspecific feature) and, more specific, intramural gas, venous gas, and vascular occlusion (Fig. 11). Pylephlebitis, a septic thrombophlebitis of the portal and mesenteric venous systems usually caused by a suppurative intra-abdominal process, most often appendicitis, is a diagnosis that is rarely, if ever, established on clinical grounds alone and is recognized only late in its course with plain film radiography. However, CT can image the causative inflammatory process, the thrombosed and inflamed vein, and even minute quantities of gas within the mesenteric venous system and the intrahepatic portions of the portal vein (Fig. 12). A similar condition observed in the postpartum patient in which endometritis was a complication is septic thrombosis of the ovarian vein. The CT findings in this entity are characteristic and include an enlarged,

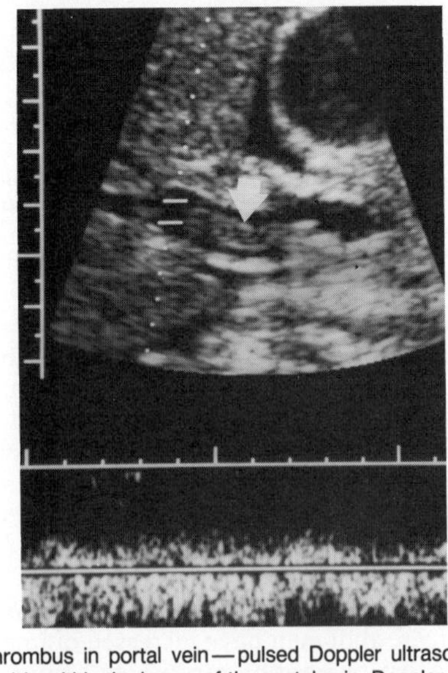

Figure 7. Thrombus in portal vein—pulsed Doppler ultrasound. Echogenic thrombus (arrow) is within the lumen of the portal vein. Doppler tracing indicates flow within the portal vein.

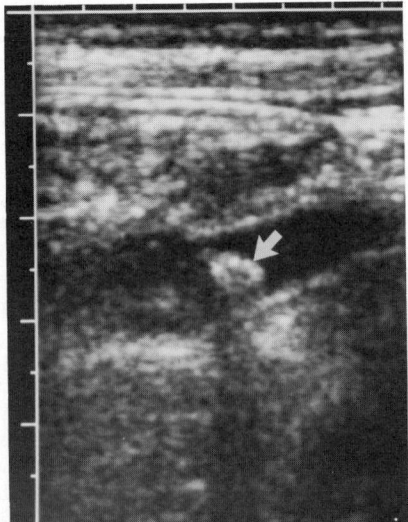

Figure 8. Acute appendicitis—ultrasound. A radiographically nonopaque appendicolith (arrow) is located within a thick-walled distended appendix (longitudinal view).

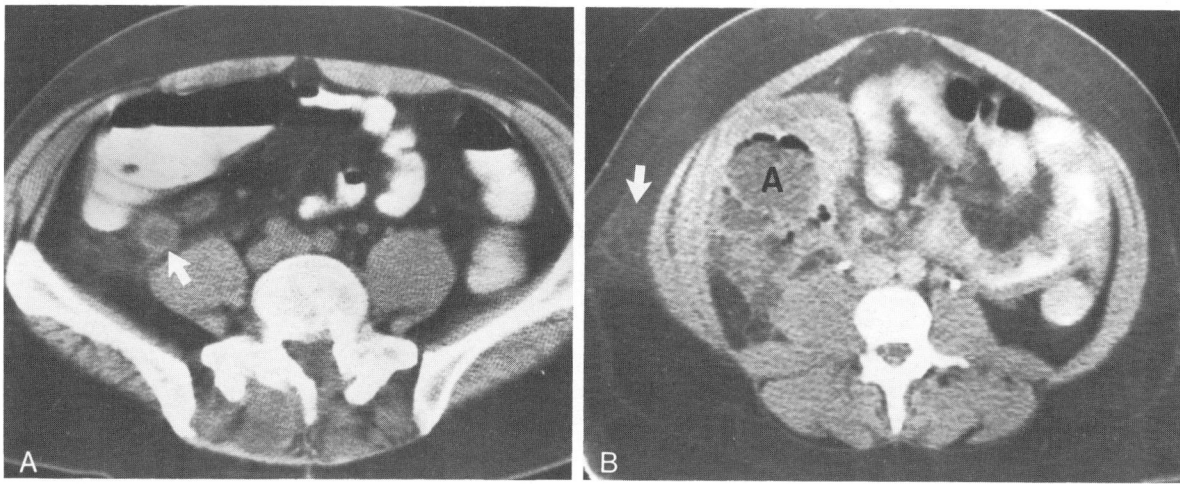

Figure 9. Appendicitis—computed tomography. *A*, Uncomplicated appendicitis. A thick-walled, distended, retrocecal appendix (arrow) with inflammatory change in the surrounding fat. *B*, Complicated appendicitis. Retrocecal appendiceal abscess (A) with associated phlegmon posteriorly in a 3-week postpartum obese female patient. Inflammatory change extends through the flank musculature into the subcutaneous fat (arrow).

thrombosed, thick-walled ovarian vein surrounded by inflammatory changes in the retroperitoneal fat.

Acute pancreatitis frequently presents as an acute abdomen. Since the advent of CT and ultrasound, understanding of the various inflammatory diseases affecting the pancreas has increased by a level of magnitude unsurpassed by that for any of the other disease processes within the abdomen. Prior to the CT-ultrasound era, only the gross changes associated with complicated pancreatitis were recognizable with radiologic techniques. With regard to acute pancreatitis, it is now possible to demonstrate the morphologic changes in this disease of minimal edema of the pancreatic parenchyma in interstitial inflammation to the extensive phlegmon, fluid collections, hemorrhage, and necrosis that develop in fulminant necrotizing hemorrhagic pancreatitis. The diagnosis of uncomplicated acute pancreatitis generally is established by the clinical presentation and biochemical tests without the need for diagnostic imaging. Although CT is not necessary in all cases of acute pancreatitis, it is quite valuable when the diagnosis has not been firmly established clinically or when complications are suspected.

Diagnostic arteriography serves a tertiary role in the evaluation of patients with an acute abdomen and should be considered only when the clinical presentation, supported by highly suggestive findings on CT or ultrasound, indicates a vascular lesion amenable to diagnostic as well as potentially therapeutic angiographic techniques (Fig. 13). For example, spontaneous hemorrhage from an intrahepatic arterial aneurysm, diagnosed

on CT examination, can be confirmed by selective hepatic arteriography and therapeutically managed by selective embolization technique.

In summary, the diagnostic imaging evaluation of the patient with an acute abdomen has undergone significant change in the past decade. Technologically sophisticated imaging methods, primarily involving CT and ultrasound, provide a more rapid and accurate diagnosis. CT and ultrasound should now be considered early in the evaluation of the patient with an acute abdomen, when the diagnosis is not obvious based on the history and physical examination or apparent on the plain radiographs of the abdomen.

Clinical Pathologic Diagnostic Studies

Patients evaluated for acute abdominal pain require certain basic laboratory data that in most instances can be performed rapidly on an emergency basis. The results are important in establishing an early, prompt, and accurate diagnosis. Fortunately those tests requiring a prolonged period for completion are rarely critical for the diagnosis and treatment of patients with abdominal pain. In some instances, the laboratory information may only confirm the clinical diagnosis and in situations of generalized peritonitis have little or no role in the decision for operation. However, patients with abdominal pain and an uncertain diagnosis require frequent periodic examinations of the abdomen before a decision for operation can be achieved. In such circumstances, a repeat complete blood count can be helpful in determining the progress of an acute intra-abdominal inflammatory process.

A complete blood count and urinalysis are essential in all patients evaluated for acute abdominal pain. The results need to be reviewed before a final decision is made regarding surgical intervention unless the urgency is such that immediate operation is required; secured laboratory tests that are especially helpful include serum amylase for patients with acute pancreatitis, aspartate aminotransferase to confirm the presence of acute hepatitis, and human chorionic gonadotropin to confirm the presence of an ectopic pregnancy. Liver function studies may be helpful in those patients with right upper quadrant (RUQ) pain, jaundice, and the possibility of hepatitis. Serum electrolytes obtained on an emergency basis are largely for the therapeutic management of the patient in preparation for admission and observation or in planning for operation.

A peritoneal diagnostic tap may be useful in determining the presence of intraperitoneal blood, fluid, and pus. Peritoneal lavage is more valuable in the presence of blunt abdominal

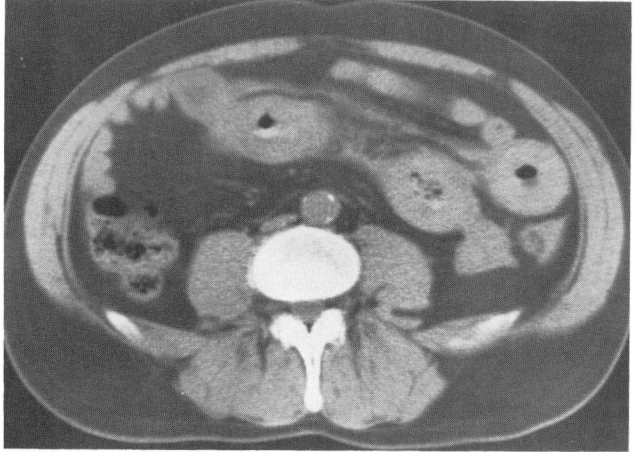

Figure 10. Small bowel intramural hematoma. Uniform, concentric, high-density thickening of the wall of jejunal loops is characteristic.

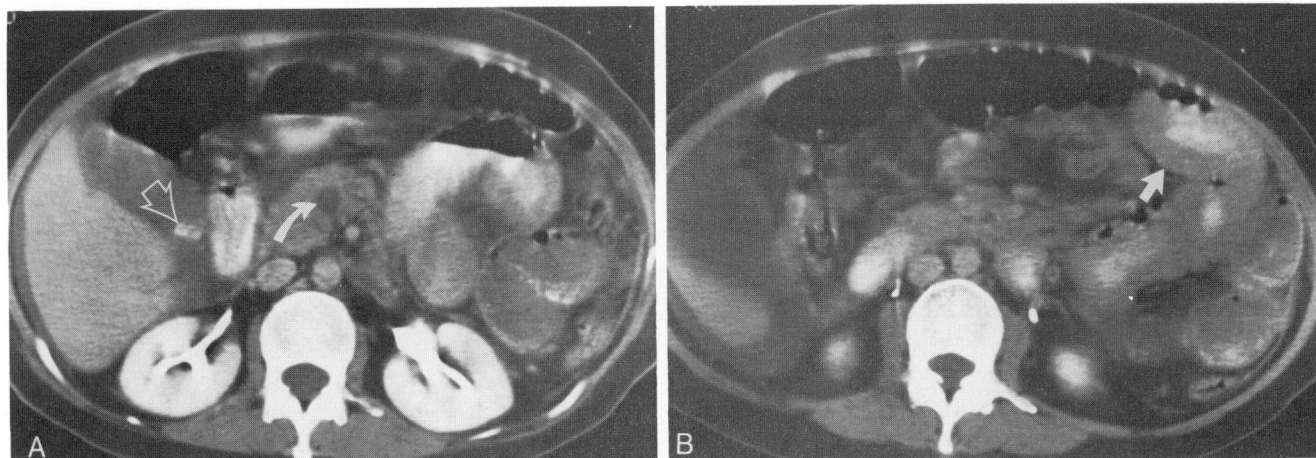

Figure 11. Small bowel infarction associated with mesenteric venous thrombosis. *A*, Low-density thrombosed superior mesenteric vein (arrow); incidental gallstones (open arrow). *B*, Thickening of proximal small bowel wall (arrow) coincided with several feet of infarcting small bowel at time of operation.

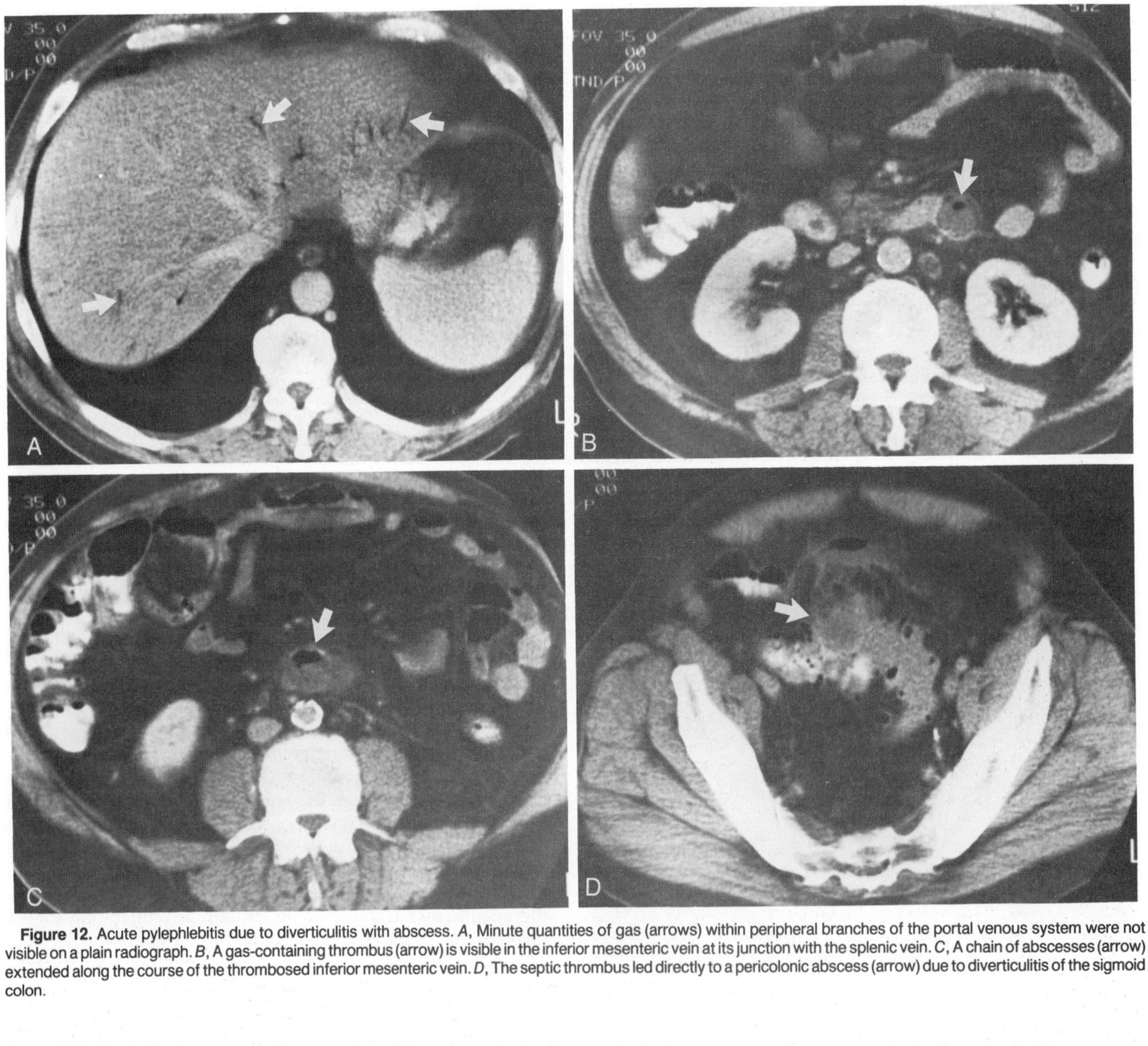

Figure 12. Acute pylephlebitis due to diverticulitis with abscess. *A*, Minute quantities of gas (arrows) within peripheral branches of the portal venous system were not visible on a plain radiograph. *B*, A gas-containing thrombus (arrow) is visible in the inferior mesenteric vein at its junction with the splenic vein. *C*, A chain of abscesses (arrow) extended along the course of the thrombosed inferior mesenteric vein. *D*, The septic thrombus led directly to a pericolonic abscess (arrow) due to diverticulitis of the sigmoid colon.

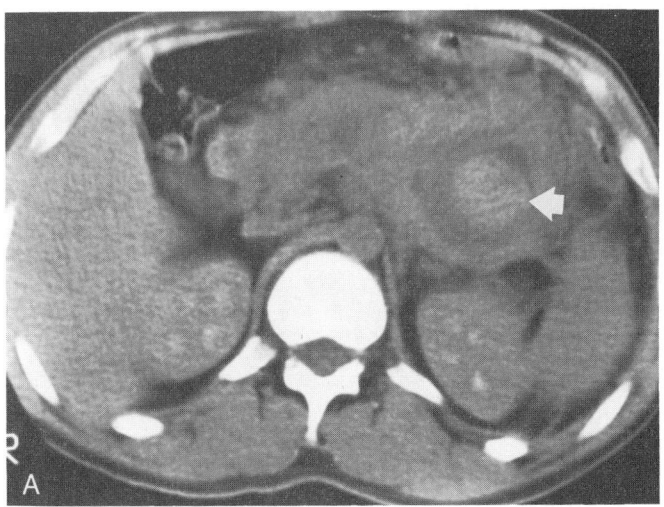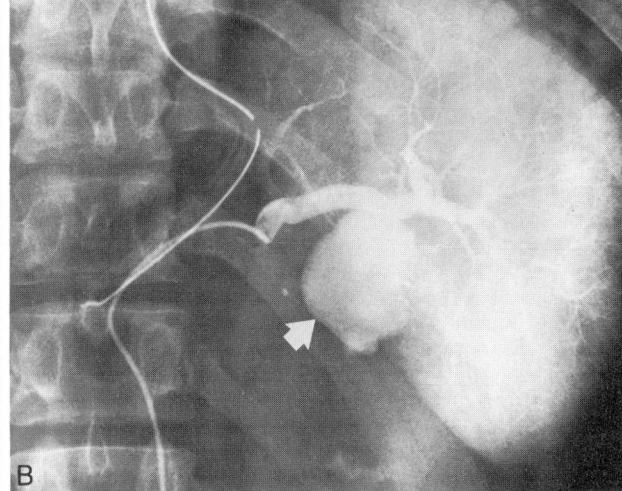

Figure 13. Hemorrhage and false aneurysm complicating pancreatitis. *A,* Intraparenchymal hemorrhage enlarges the body and tail of the pancreas. The lumen of the false aneurysm (arrow) is shown as an area of increased density due to the enhancement of the flowing blood. *B,* Selective splenic arteriogram. False aneurysm (arrow) arises from a branch of the splenic artery. It was successfully treated with transcatheter embolization.

trauma. The presence of blood, purulent material, or bacteria on Gram stain suggests the need for early exploration (Table 1).

PERITONITIS AND THE PERITONEAL CAVITY

The Peritoneal Cavity

The peritoneal cavity is covered by a single layer of mesothelial cells on connective tissue, including collagen, elastic fibers, macrophages, and fat cells. The parietal peritoneum, which covers the abdominal cavity, including the anterior abdominal wall, diaphragm, and pelvis, is immediately adjacent to and reinforced by the transversalis fascia. The visceral peritoneum covers all the intraperitoneal viscera, creating a completely enclosed cavity except for the open ends of the fallopian tubes. The parietal peritoneum is innervated by both somatic and visceral afferent nerves. The peritoneum of the anterior abdominal wall is the area most sensitive to stimuli, and the pelvic peritoneum is the area least sensitive. Patients with abdominal pain may reveal tenderness to palpation of the abdomen, and if peritoneal irritation exists, they have rebound tenderness. Localized inflammation of the anterior parietal peritoneum may cause voluntary muscle guarding. The visceral peritoneum is relatively insensitive and receives afferent innervation only from the autonomic nervous system. Stimuli from the visceral peritoneum are often poorly localized and are perceived as a dull or intermittent cramping type of pain. The visceral afferent nerves have no receptors to mediate pain and temperature but do respond to distention, traction, and pressure. The biliary tract and mesentery of the small bowel have greater innervation than does the small intestine. Thus, pain from the gallbladder and

TABLE 1. Causes of Hemoperitoneum

Gastrointestinal
   Traumatic laceration of liver, spleen, pancreas, mesentery, bowel
Gynecologic
   Ruptured ectopic pregnancy
   Ruptured graafian follicle
   Ruptured uterus
Vascular
   Ruptured aneurysm—aortoiliac, hepatic, renal, and splenic artery
Urologic
   Ruptured bladder
Hematologic
   Ruptured spleen

common duct is more accurately localized than that from the small intestine.

Peritonitis

The inflammatory response of the peritoneum may involve the entire intra-abdominal cavity or only a portion of either the visceral or parietal peritoneum. The peritoneum responds to the trauma of inflammation, and peritonitis occurs with a transudation of fluid, edema formation, and vascular congestion of the tissue layer immediately adjacent to the single layer of mesothelium. The normal volume of 100 ml. of peritoneal fluid increases with the passage of a transudate of fluid from the extracellular compartment. This transudate, rich in protein content, is accompanied by a diapedesis of polymorphonuclear leukocytes, both of which have an important role in conjunction with fibrin in the containment of intraperitoneal infection.

Peritonitis, classified as primary or spontaneous peritonitis, is a diffuse bacterial infection without an apparent intra-abdominal source of infection. The organisms are most commonly those of pneumococcus and hemolytic streptococcus and occur more commonly in children than in adults. Secondary peritonitis implies that it is the result of bacterial contamination from a known source, usually from within the abdomen and often from a perforation of the gastrointestinal tract. Occasionally, the source of infection may follow penetrating trauma or be an extension of a suppurative process from an intra-abdominal organ such as a liver abscess or pyosalpinx. Secondary peritonitis is the most common form of peritoneal infection encountered by the surgeon, and because it is generally of a suppurative type, surgical intervention is required.

Chemical peritonitis refers to the peritoneal inflammation from substances other than bacteria, and although this occurs initially, bacterial contamination soon follows. The substances commonly associated with chemical peritonitis include gastric juice, pancreatic juice, bile, blood, urine, meconium, chyle, and barium. The most severe and common form of chemical peritonitis is that of a perforated peptic ulcer causing a sudden outpouring of gastric juice, which produces an acute inflammatory response in both the visceral and parietal peritoneum.

Bile peritonitis may occur as a result of perforation of the gallbladder, with acute gangrenous cholecystitis. Hemoperitoneum, the result of a ruptured abdominal aneurysm, occurs so quickly that an inflammatory response is minor compared with the catastrophic event itself. However, slow bleeding into the abdomen from a ruptured graafian follicle or splenic injury from trauma produces surprisingly few signs of inflammation. If bacteria are also present, the hemoglobin and ferrous iron act to enhance the inflammatory response to the bacteria in producing suppurative peritonitis. Barium contamination of the peritoneal cavity secondary to spillage during a radiologic contrast examination causes severe peritoneal irritation. The outcome of gastrointestinal perforation is less favorable when both barium and bacteria are combined, producing an increased incidence of sepsis.

The etiologic basis of granulomatous peritonitis includes tuberculosis and iatrogenic causes such as surgical glove powder (talc), which in some circumstances may cause severe inflammation, exudation, and granuloma formation. Tuberculous peritonitis, now much less common than previously, still occurs in the chronically ill or malnourished patient. Although the primary focus of tuberculosis is usually the lung, the source may not be apparent clinically. The disease is, therefore, generally due to the reactivation of pulmonary tuberculosis with hematogenous spread to the peritoneum. The degree of irritation varies from a dull generalized abdominal pain with minimal tenderness to a more severe form of abdominal peritonitis.

SIGNS AND SYMPTOMS. The history of peritonitis is usually associated with the abrupt onset of abdominal pain, often localized at first and then spreading throughout the abdomen. In some circumstances such as perforated diverticulitis, the pain may remain in one quadrant of the abdomen. A careful history often suggests the source of the problem, and this is subsequently confirmed by the physical examination. Perforated peptic ulcer presents suddenly with acute epigastric pain, which then may radiate to the RLQ as the gastric juice drains caudally along the right gutter. The presence of bilateral shoulder pain suggests that peritonitis involves the parietal peritoneum of the diaphragm. Absent or hypoactive bowel sounds indicate generalized peritonitis with an adynamic ileus. Acute appendicitis with sudden perforation occurs rarely and is usually associated with an illness of several or more hours. The pain is eventually localized to the RLQ unless the disease process has progressed to generalized peritonitis. Acute cholecystitis also has a several-hour history of RUQ pain referred to the right scapula or shoulder. Perforation usually occurs after the disease has been in progress for hours or days, and free bile peritonitis develops only after gangrene and perforation of the gallbladder. Peritonitis due to acute ulcerative colitis is usually identified by the history of the primary disease. The peritoneal signs may be severe and generalized if perforation has occurred or diffuse and mild if only colonic inflammation exists without perforation. Crohn's disease may present with acute, severe, localized RLQ pain and may be indistinguishable from acute appendicitis. Free perforation of the distal ileum with generalized peritonitis rarely occurs with Crohn's disease; however, formation of fistula tracts is common. Obstruction and perforation of the small and large intestine are usually not of sudden onset except for cases of acute volvulus. Free perforation of a colonic neoplasm with generalized peritonitis is less common than a walled-off perforation with abscess formation.

The physical findings of patients with peritonitis depend on the etiology and duration and whether the process is diffuse or localized. In the early stages, the patient appears acutely ill and febrile with tachycardia. The blood pressure is normotensive or slightly hypotensive. As the disease progresses and the inflammatory process increases, the patient becomes severely ill, with obvious signs of a decrease in circulating plasma volume. Hypotension and tachycardia are common. The patient may appear anxious and dehydrated with rapid respiration. Fever is always noted in the early hours after onset of peritoneal irritation but may disappear or even become subnormal with progression. The abdomen is distended with hypoactive or absent bowel sounds. Tenderness to percussion and palpation is present in all quadrants of the abdomen. Abdominal masses are

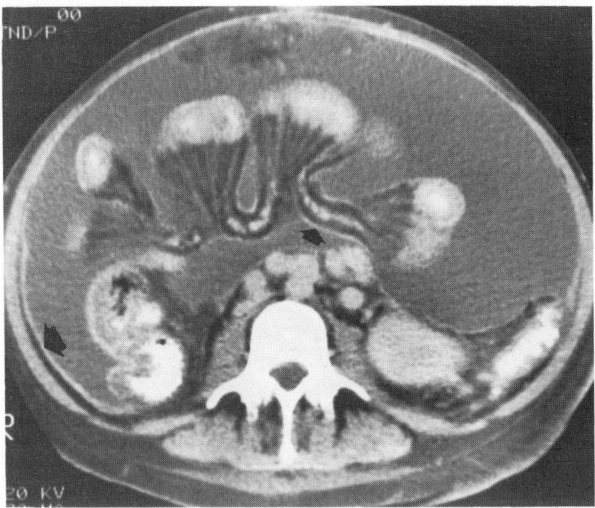

Figure 14. Peritonitis—computed tomography. Inflammatory thickening of the parietal (large arrow) and visceral (small arrow) peritoneum is visible, and the ascitic fluid is of high density characteristic of peritonitis.

rarely palpable in the presence of severe distention and tenderness. Rectal and pelvic examination may or may not identify a pelvic mass but always confirms the peritoneal irritation.

Early recognition of peritoneal irritation is important and proper preoperative management critical if the patient is to survive. This management includes the insertion of a nasogastric tube, restoration of intravascular volume deficit, and improvement in the performance of the cardiovascular and renal subsystem. A Foley catheter should be placed as soon as possible to assess the hourly urinary volume, which provides some indication of intravascular volume replacement. Immediate administration of intravenous antibiotics for broad coverage is essential to control sepsis. Hemodynamic monitoring using a central venous pressure or a Swan-Ganz line may be necessary in patients with hemodynamic instability.

Recent imaging experience has demonstrated that many of the morphologic changes of peritonitis, such as thickening of the parietal and visceral peritoneum, inflammatory changes in the omentum and mesentery, and free or loculated fluid collections, often with higher density than bland ascites, are well demonstrated with CT (Fig. 14). The source of the peritonitis, such as a perforation of bowel, is often apparent as well (Fig. 15).

ORGAN SUBSYSTEM ANALYSIS

The etiology of acute abdominal pain can be separated according to the organ subsystem involved. In considering the body as a whole to be composed of various organ subsystems, the examination of a patient with abdominal pain can be based on the analysis of those subsystems that may cause or contribute to the abdominal pain.

Those body subsystems that contribute to abdominal pain include the gastrointestinal, renal, gynecologic, vascular, cardiac, pulmonary, neurologic, hematologic, metabolic, and musculoskeletal.

Gastrointestinal Subsystem

The most common cause of acute abdominal pain in the gastrointestinal subsystem relates to an inflammatory or mechanical process of the stomach, small and large intestine, gallbladder, common bile duct, liver, or pancreas (Table 2). The symptoms are often nonspecific and affected by the age of the patient, medication taken by the patient, and coexisting disease. For example, older patients, especially those with diabetes, may demonstrate fewer symptoms than do younger patients. Corti-

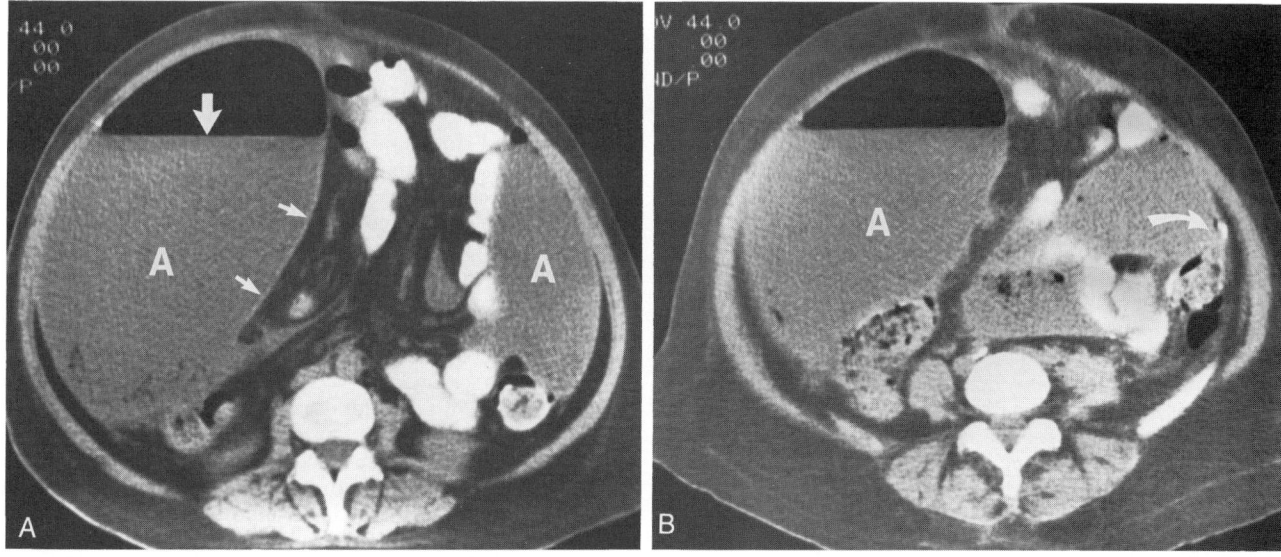

Figure 15. Pyopneumoperitoneum secondary to a perforated descending colon. *A,* Pyo-pneumo interface (large arrow). There is inflammatory thickening of visceral peritoneum (small arrows). Seven liters of grossly infected ascitic fluid (A) were percutaneously drained. *B,* A trail of small gas bubbles in the left flank led to a point of discrete perforation of the descending colon (arrow), confirmed by contrast enema and surgically repaired.

costeroids and other immunosuppressive drugs may mask intraperitoneal inflammatory conditions, and patients receiving such medication are likely to minimize their symptoms. Nausea, vomiting, constipation, and abdominal pain are all common findings and often occur concomitantly.

PERFORATED PEPTIC ULCER. Free perforation of peptic ulcer disease, more often from duodenal ulcer than from gastric ulcer, is usually found in male patients between the third and fourth decades. The perforation may occur in patients in good health without previous symptoms or in patients with a previous history of peptic ulcer disease that worsened several days prior to the episode of pain. Perforation may occur nocturnally and awaken the patient from sleep. The pain is sudden, sharp, and severe and is located first in the epigastrium and later spreads over the entire abdomen. Shoulder pain is common and reflects referred pain from the diaphragmatic irritation. Occasionally, the gastric contents drain to the RLQ, producing pain and tenderness, suggesting acute appendicitis. Nausea is frequent, and although vomiting may occur, it is unusual. Hematemesis is also unusual. The patient with generalized peritonitis from a perforated ulcer usually lies in the supine position, avoiding any undue motion that might increase the abdominal pain.

During the examination, the patient lies quietly, often appearing acutely ill with tachypnea and tachycardia. Hypotension may be present if the process has existed for more than 4 to 6 hours as a result of plasma volume depletion. Respirations are shallow, and deep breathing or coughing produces severe ab-

TABLE 2. Abdominal Pain Secondary to Inflammatory Lesions of the Gastrointestinal Subsystem

Stomach
    Gastric ulcer
    Duodenal ulcer
Biliary tract
    Acute cholecystitis with or without choledocholithiasis
Pancreas
    Acute, recurrent, or chronic pancreatitis
Small intestine
    Crohn's disease
    Meckel's diverticulum
Large intestine
    Appendicitis
    Diverticulitis

dominal pain. The patient may be afebrile soon after perforation but develops fever 6 to 8 hours later. In the first few hours, the abdomen may appear normal or scaphoid but gradually progresses to abdominal distention during the next 12 hours. Percussion reveals the abdomen to be extremely tender, especially in the epigastric region. Palpation of the abdomen reveals a firm "boardlike" appearance with rigidity of the rectus muscles. Rebound tenderness is generally present in all four quadrants, and worse in the epigastric region. Auscultation of the abdomen soon after perforation reveals hypoactive bowel sounds that progress to absent bowel sounds as the process of generalized peritonitis worsens. These findings confirm generalized peritonitis. Rectal examination is unremarkable unless there is pelvic peritonitis, in which case tenderness is present anterior to the examining finger.

Routine laboratory data usually include an elevated white blood cell (WBC) count between 12,000 and 20,000 per cu. mm. with immature forms. The intravascular fluid shifts in the first 6 to 12 hours, confirms the plasma volume loss following peritonitis, and is reflected in the elevated hematocrit. The urinalysis shows a concentrated urine specific gravity, and there is little or no change in liver or renal function if there has been no pre-existing disease.

The plain radiograph of the abdomen or chest usually demonstrates free intraperitoneal air present in approximately 75 per cent of patients with a perforated ulcer. In patients in whom the clinical presentation is atypical and suggests a right mid or lower abdominal inflammatory process such as cholecystitis or appendicitis, a CT examination may demonstrate evidence of localized perforation of the duodenum with leakage in the area of the gallbladder and right flank, without gross free air being apparent (Fig. 5).

ACUTE CHOLECYSTITIS. This disease most commonly occurs in women between the ages of 30 and 60 years who have had a previous history of pregnancy. The younger patients often have a familial history of biliary tract disease. Although the episode of acute cholecystitis may begin several hours after a large meal and often occurs late at night or in the early morning hours, the disease may develop without a prior history of food intake. The attack is characterized by the onset of a constant dull RUQ pain. Some patients move about, attempting to relieve the pain, whereas others lie restlessly in bed. Nausea and vomiting are common, with temporary improvement in the severity of pain after an episode of emesis. The emesis is of moderate quantity and green in color. The pain may subside after several hours; if so, the episode is considered to be biliary colic. The disease process may progress to acute cholecystitis, in which case there is steady severe RUQ pain radiating to the right scapula or shoulder. If there is an associated common duct stone or acute pancreatitis, the pain may also be located in the midline of the epigastrium and may radiate along the right and left costal margins to the back. The temperature is 37° to 39° C. (99° to 101° F.). High fever and chills are not usually common unless the patient has cholangitis. This is rarely noted in the early stages of the disease and becomes apparent after 12 to 24 hours. Blood pressure is usually not altered, and the heart rate is seldom greater than 100 to 110 beats per minute.

Examination of the abdomen reveals mild to moderate distention, and on inspection from the patient's feet, the abdomen may show asymmetry in the RUQ with a mass that distends on deep inspiration. Bowel sounds are hypoactive on auscultation. Tenderness is maximal in the RUQ. In the absence of perforation and generalized peritonitis, tenderness to palpation confirms the RUQ tenderness to be worse with deep inspiration. Frequently, a mass can be palpated along the right costal margin, representing a distended tense gallbladder that descends with deep inspiration. Percussion reveals tenderness over the right rib cage. The rectal examination rarely adds important information to the diagnosis.

Laboratory data reveal the WBC count to be often elevated (10,000 to 13,000); however, a normal WBC count may occur in the presence of severe acute cholecystitis. This is especially true when the patient is over the age of 70 years, with or without diabetes, and in those patients receiving corticosteroid therapy. The urinalysis does not usually contribute to the diagnosis. An electrocardiogram is important to exclude the possibility of an acute myocardial infarction.

An elevated serum bilirubin to 2.0 or 2.5 mg. per 100 ml. may exist with uncomplicated acute cholecystitis. If however, the bilirubin exceeds 3.0 mg. per 100 ml., common duct calculi should be considered. The significance of an increase in serum amylase is difficult to assess because acute cholecystitis may be associated with a mild amylase elevation and may reflect a chemical abnormality with little clinical evidence of pancreatitis.

The radiologic evaluation of acute cholecystitis has changed significantly in the past decade. Studies that formerly had a role, oral cholecystography and intravenous cholangiography, have been essentially abandoned. Ultrasonography, the current most commonly used imaging method, can rapidly assess the caliber of the biliary tree, the presence or absence of biliary calculi, and the appearance of the gallbladder wall and contents, as well as the surrounding structures (Fig. 6). Further support for the diagnosis is provided by demonstrating that pressure from the transducer directly onto the gallbladder elicits the patient's pain pattern.

Radionuclide studies, employing agents such as HIDA, have a supportive role in cases in which the diagnosis is not readily confirmed with ultrasound. If the gallbladder fails to demonstrate uptake of the agent within 4 hours, in the presence of radionuclide activity in the bile duct and small bowel, cystic duct obstruction can be presumed to be present. Computed tomography has a limited role and is usually reserved for evaluating late complications of initially unrecognized acute cholecystitis.

ACUTE PANCREATITIS. Pancreatitis may present with sudden onset characterized by severe epigastric pain radiating directly through to the back and around both costal margins with or without shoulder pain. The similarity of the description of the pain to acute perforation of peptic ulcer is obvious and may also simulate acute cholecystitis. The disease, however, most commonly is associated with biliary tract disease or chronic alcohol intake. Acute pancreatitis usually presents in patients between the ages of 30 and 50 years and has frequently been preceded by a similar episode with a previous diagnosis. The disease is uncommon in children and adolescents and in patients older than 70 years of age. The onset may be rapid with the pain becoming intolerable in 3 to 4 hours. Anorexia, nausea, and vomiting are common, and emesis rarely provides significant relief. Examination reveals an acutely ill patient with obvious severe abdominal pain, tachycardia, and tachypnea. Hypotension, rarely present in the early stages of the disease process, may develop after 4 to 6 hours if retroperitoneal hemorrhage occurs with intravascular volume extravasation. Abdominal tenderness is most evident in the epigastric region and is present with both percussion and palpation. Bowel sounds are usually hypoactive and may be absent. The classic Grey Turner's sign with flank ecchymosis is seldom observed in the early phase of the disease. Cullen's sign, with discoloration of the skin around the umbilicus, is also an uncommon finding in the first few hours.

Routine laboratory tests reveal a leukocytosis of 12,000 to 22,000. The hematocrit is normal in the early phase of the disease but becomes increased if retroperitoneal fluid loss is excessive. The key diagnostic test is the serum amylase, which is elevated within a few hours in most patients who have the acute form of the disease. If the attack is mild, the amylase elevation may be slight and transient, often returning to normal in 24 hours. Urinary amylase levels may be diagnostic in such patients when the serum amylase level has returned to normal. All patients suspected of having acute pancreatitis should have an immediate serum amylase determination; urinary amylase studies should be reserved for those patients with normal serum levels. Serum bilirubin levels may be elevated and, when combined with an increase in serum amylase, present a complex situation in differentiating primary biliary tract disease from pancreatitis. In general, the serum amylase level is not as high in patients with acute cholecystitis, and this elevation seldom persists for more than 2 or 3 days. If the attack of pancreatitis is severe, hypocalcemia may develop from calcium deposition in the pancreas and peripancreatic tissue.

Plain radiographs of the abdomen are often nondiagnostic in patients with acute pancreatitis. Computed tomography and ultrasound are the next studies to confirm the clinical diagnosis or to assess suspected complications. Because of the frequent accompanying adynamic ileus, CT is more reliable to provide images of the entire pancreas and peripancreatic area. Pancreatic edema, intra- or peripancreatic fluid collections, inflammatory or phlegmonous changes in the surrounding anterior pararenal space, changes secondary to pancreatic hemorrhage (Fig. 13) or necrosis, and extension of the inflammatory process into distant intra- and retroperitoneal spaces can all be quickly defined.

ACUTE RELAPSING PANCREATITIS. Acute relapsing pancreatitis differs from acute pancreatitis in that in the former the pain is recurrent with each exacerbation of pancreatitis and is associated with an increase in serum amylase. The patient's previous history of pancreatitis usually confirms the diagnosis. However, the possibility of a pancreatic pseudocyst must always be considered. The physical findings are identical to those noted with acute pancreatitis. The diagnosis can be established by ultrasonography or a CT scan of the pancreas.

CHRONIC PANCREATITIS. Patients with chronic pancreatitis differ from those with recurrent episodes of acute pancreatitis (acute relapsing pancreatitis) in that in the former the pain becomes constant. The history identifies the diagnosis from the patients' previous attacks, and radiographs of the abdomen often reveal calcification in the pancreas. The serum amylase level is elevated if the pancreatic tissue has not been replaced by fibrous tissue.

ACUTE APPENDICITIS. Acute appendicitis is a common cause of abdominal pain and is especially difficult to diagnose in patients younger than 3 years and older than 70 years. Although certain findings by history and physical examination are highly suggestive, establishing the correct diagnosis is often difficult. The symptoms relate to the anatomic position of the appendix and vary according to the age and coexistent disease of the patient. In patients with early acute appendicitis there may be typical findings and an excellent surgical outcome, whereas in those patients with perforation and peritonitis, there may be a different clinical presentation and a less favorable prognosis.

A careful history is essential in making both an accurate and an early diagnosis. Abdominal pain first begins in the epigastrium, then gradually migrates to the periumbilical region and finally to the RLQ. Anorexia, nausea, and vomiting are common. The prodromal symptoms of indigestion, irregularity of the bowels, nausea, and vomiting are all common findings. There is localization of the pain to the RLQ after 6 to 8 hours of onset, with tenderness to palpation and rebound tenderness. Guarding to palpation occurs when the process has progressed to localized peritonitis. Local hyperesthesia of the skin is a common finding. Rigidity is frequently present, although a flaccid abdomen does not preclude acute appendicitis. Abdominal distention is rarely observed in the early stages of the disease but subsequently occurs. It is especially important to remember that a retrocecal appendix may cause only mild abdominal tenderness. Regardless of all the possible findings, the most common complaint is RLQ pain, and the most frequent physical finding is RLQ tenderness to palpation. Rectal examination is especially important, and the findings may vary according to the appendiceal location. Abdominal tenderness is less severe when the appendix is in the retroperitoneum, that is, retrocecal position. However, patients with the appendix lying free in the peritoneal cavity may elicit extreme tenderness on rectal examination, more so on the right side.

Laboratory data are nondiagnostic and often normal. The WBC count may be elevated, but this depends on the duration of the illness. Those patients with symptoms for more than 24 hours with marked abdominal tenderness are more likely to have an elevated WBC count than those patients with symptoms of 6 hours or less. Most patients have a shift to the left in the differential count. The urinalysis is rarely helpful, although occasionally the appendix may lie in contact with the ureter or bladder and cause microscopic hematuria.

The plain film findings are not often helpful, although a fecalith is an exception to this observation. A dilated fluid-filled cecum may be present but is nondiagnostic. A free perforation of the appendix rarely has diagnostic findings, and intraperitoneal air is unusual. Scoliosis of the lumbar spine may occur with psoas spasm and the convex curvature to the right. Recent experience with ultrasound and CT has shown both imaging methods helpful in defining the pathologic changes characteristic of appendicitis as well as its associated complications (Figs. 8 and 9).

Other diagnostic considerations in patients with appendicitis include perforated duodenal ulcer with spillage of gastric contents into the RLQ (Fig. 5). This produces RLQ pain and tenderness. However, the symptoms relating to the peptic ulcer can usually be differentiated from appendicitis. Acute diverticulitis is a common intra-abdominal inflammatory process usually involving the sigmoid colon, especially in patients over the age of 60 years, and when perforated may be difficult to differentiate from appendicitis if the sigmoid colon lies near the midline in the suprapubic area. The occurrence of marked left lower quadrant (LLQ) tenderness in the patient undergoing evaluation for acute appendicitis suggests either perforation with generalized peritonitis or acute diverticulitis. Ruptured graafian follicle is a common cause for RLQ or LLQ pain as a result of bleeding into the peritoneal cavity. The relationship to the menstrual cycle is of obvious importance, and the patient often recollects one or more previous similar episodes. Mittelschmerz pain is usually

sudden in onset, sharp, and often in the pelvis and is not preceded by anorexia, nausea, or vomiting. If the left ovary is involved, the diagnostic considerations are less complicated. The process gradually subsides over a few hours, and most patients are well in a short period of time. Ectopic pregnancy in women of the childbearing years is an important consideration and must be considered in all women with abdominal pain and a history of missed menstrual periods. The pain may be acute, and in the presence of an adnexal mass on pelvic examination, the diagnosis must be considered as a strong possibility.

Pelvic inflammatory disease with acute salpingitis is a frequently encountered process causing acute pelvic pain originating in the RLQ and LLQ. The prime consideration should be to differentiate the disease from acute appendicitis. Acute pelvic inflammatory disease often becomes symptomatic at the completion of or just following a menstrual period. The pain is not related to the gastrointestinal tract and is rarely associated with anorexia, nausea, or vomiting. Pain and tenderness are usually bilateral and are associated with a temperature of 38° to 39° C. (100° to 102° F.). If the patient has had previous symptoms of a similar nature, it is likely that chronic or recurrent pelvic inflammatory disease is the correct diagnosis. Inspection of the abdomen reveals mild to moderate distention in the suprapubic region. Bowel sounds are hypoactive. The abdominal tenderness to palpation usually exists in both lower quadrants, with marked tenderness on palpation of the cervix. Adnexal masses are common findings and often present as thickened areas bilaterally. A vaginal discharge is a frequent sequela. The diagnosis is confirmed by cervical smear and culture with gonococcus being the most frequently found organism. It must be emphasized that salpingitis is primarily a disease of young women and rarely occurs after menopause. Septic thrombosis of the ovarian vein associated with endometritis in the immediate postpartum period can also simulate appendicitis if the right side is involved.

Renal or ureteral calculi may cause abdominal pain; however, when the calculus begins to descend in the ureter, the pain pattern varies with radiation to the groin, testicle, and perineum. The pain is sudden and very severe and may subside in a few minutes. Hydronephrosis on the right side, a right pelvic kidney with pyelonephritis, or a polycystic kidney in a young individual may all cause abdominal pain similar to that of acute appendicitis. Radiographs of the abdomen in patients in a supine position, an intravenous pyelogram, and urinalysis can usually differentiate renal pain from that of nonrenal origin. Acute granulomatous ileocolitis (Crohn's disease) may present in an identical manner to that of acute appendicitis. However, CT demonstration of significant thickening of the wall of the terminal ileum with a surrounding sleeve of inflamed mesenteric fat differentiates the two diseases.

MECKEL'S DIVERTICULITIS. This condition, which involves the persistence of a portion of the vitelline duct on the antimesenteric border of the distal ileum, may produce bleeding, intestinal obstruction, and, less often, acute abdominal pain from diverticulitis. The disease, although uncommon, should always be considered in patients with an acute abdomen and with findings suggestive of acute appendicitis. The signs and symptoms of Meckel's diverticulitis are those of acute appendicitis, and only rarely is the true diagnosis established preoperatively. The usual films of the abdomen in both supine and upright positions are unremarkable, and the WBC count is increased. If surgical exploration is warranted on the basis of the acute abdominal findings, further diagnostic evaluation is not indicated. Whereas a focal inflammatory process in the area of the distal ileum is apparent on CT, the precise diagnosis of Meckel's diverticulitis is usually not possible. Other causes such as perforation by a foreign body (chicken bone) or granulomatous ileitis would also be considered. In the presence of an acute abdomen, barium contrast studies of the intestinal tract would not be indicated. The definitive diagnosis should be confirmed at the time of operation.

ACUTE DIVERTICULITIS. Acute diverticulitis may occur as a result of congenital or acquired diverticula. However, in most instances the diverticulitis is generally a result of the acquired form of the disease, in which the incidence increases with age. Diverticulitis, the result of inflammation of diverticula, is but one of several complications of diverticulosis. The process may involve the entire colon, but more commonly it occurs in the left colon, particularly in the sigmoid colon. The disease presents with LLQ pain, chills, and fever. There is usually a history of constipation. Vomiting and anorexia are uncommon. The patient is febrile with a temperature of 38° to 40° C. (101° to 103° F.).

Abdominal examination reveals the abdomen to be slightly distended, with tenderness in the LLQ. A mass is often palpable just medial to the anterosuperior iliac spine. Bowel sounds are hypoactive, and, if absent, the possibility of peritonitis must be considered. The rectal examination is rarely of diagnostic value unless a pelvic mass can be palpated. Sigmoidoscopy is performed with difficulty because of pain. The lumen is occluded owing to mucosal edema, but no intraluminal masses are noted.

Laboratory data reveal the WBC count to be increased to between 10,000 and 20,000. The urinalysis may contain multiple white cells. Plain radiographs of the abdomen are most often indeterminate unless colonic obstruction or a gas-containing abscess is also present. If the diagnosis of diverticulitis is uncertain or complications are suspected, CT is the most definitive imaging method (Fig. 12). Inflammatory changes in the pericolonic soft tissues and focal abscesses due to diverticulitis are apparent on CT but can be mimicked by a perforated colonic carcinoma. If the patient improves on medical therapy and surgical intervention is not necessary, a barium enema should be performed in 4 to 6 weeks when the patient is asymptomatic to exclude an occult colonic cancer with a focal perforation as the cause of the acute episode.

ACUTE OBSTRUCTION OF THE SMALL INTESTINE. Few conditions are more treacherous and demand a more accurate early diagnosis than obstruction of the small bowel. Small intestinal obstruction from congenital disorders occurs most commonly in children and adolescents and includes intestinal atresia, meconium ileus, and intussusception (Table 3).

The first symptom of acute obstruction of the small intestine is sudden, sharp, colicky abdominal pain, often periumbilical and cramping in nature. Between episodes of colic, the patient is free of pain and may feel quite well. Nausea and vomiting occur soon after the onset of pain, and emesis may relieve the pain. The color of the vomitus is green at first and contains bile. The vomitus then changes to a yellow-brown color, with a feculent odor. Frequent vomiting with epigastric pain is indicative of high small bowel obstruction, whereas cramping lower abdominal pain is noted with more distal abdominal obstruction. Inspection of the abdomen provides important diagnostic clues such as previous incisions, ventral or inguinal hernia, or peristaltic waves. Abdominal distention does not occur with obstruction of the proximal jejunum (high small bowel obstruction) but is common when the site of obstruction occurs in the distal jejunum or ileum. Auscultation of the abdomen reveals hyperactive bowel sounds of increased pitch and intensity, with audible rushes as the intestinal cramps increase in frequency. The increased activity in bowel sounds correlates with the visible peristaltic waves. Tenderness to percussion and palpation is minimal in the early stages but more apparent with the duration of time from the onset of symptoms. Patients with obstruction in the distal jejunum and ileum often have visible peristaltic waves that can be correlated with the patient's symptoms.

Patients with acute obstruction of the small intestine appear acutely ill with anxious facial expressions. Tachycardia is common, and as the disease process continues, hypotension may occur from fluid loss. Temperature is elevated from 37° to 40° C. (99° to 103° F.). During episodes of pain, the patient becomes restless and frequently draws the knees to the chest for relief. Rectal examination is seldom of diagnostic value.

Laboratory data reveal an increase in hematocrit following dehydration and fluid loss from the intravascular space into the intestinal lumen. If the obstruction has existed for several hours or more, the WBC count is increased from 12,000 to 20,000, with an increase in immature forms. The serum amylase level may be normal or slightly elevated and may be misleading regarding an accurate diagnosis concerning acute pancreatitis.

Supine and erect radiographs of the abdomen are most helpful in the evaluation of patients with acute small bowel obstruction. If the level of obstruction is in the mid or distal small bowel, dilated loops of fluid- and gas-filled small bowel are apparent, while the nonobstructed colon appears devoid of gas or feces. A high small bowel obstruction has less impressive plain film findings, especially if the patient has been vomiting. If high obstruction is clinically suspected and the plain film findings are consistent, an oral barium contrast study is valuable in confirming the diagnosis as to the level as well as, in some cases, the cause of obstruction, for example, obstructing carcinoma of the duodenum.

If the initial obstructive series indicates a mid to distal small bowel obstruction, the contrast study of choice to clarify the level and nature of obstruction is a barium enema, not an antegrade small bowel series. This quickly accomplished procedure can confirm that the colon is not involved in the obstructing process. If reflux through an incompetent ileocecal valve can be achieved, the study can also show the collapsed terminal ileum and may define the actual point of obstruction. Further imaging studies are usually not indicated and may only delay needed therapeutic intervention. However, when acute, severe abdominal pain is present and plain radiographs are nonrevealing, CT may show clinically unsuspected small bowel obstruction, such as acute intussusception in an adult due to a small bowel tumor (Fig. 16).

A paralytic ileus can be differentiated from mechanical obstruction of the small intestine by the presence or absence of bowel sounds. However, the progression of cramping abdominal pain and hyperactive bowel sounds to a silent distended abdomen with signs of peritoneal irritation is a most dangerous sign, suggesting intestinal gangrene with necrosis, perforation of the bowel, and generalized peritonitis. Acute venous mesenteric thrombosis is difficult to differentiate from other causes of intestinal obstruction on clinical grounds alone. However, pulsed Doppler ultrasound and CT both are capable of demonstrating thrombosis of the portal and mesenteric venous systems, as well as the associated bowel wall thickening (Figs. 7 and 11). Acute occlusion of the superior mesenteric artery or its branches causes severe acute abdominal pain and is usually

TABLE 3. Abdominal Pain Secondary to Obstructing Lesions of the Gastrointestinal Tract

Jejunum
    Malignancy
    Volvulus
    Adhesions
    Intussusception
Ileum
    Malignancy
    Volvulus
    Adhesions
    Intussusception
Colon
    Malignancy
    Volvulus—cecal or sigmoid
    Diverticulitis

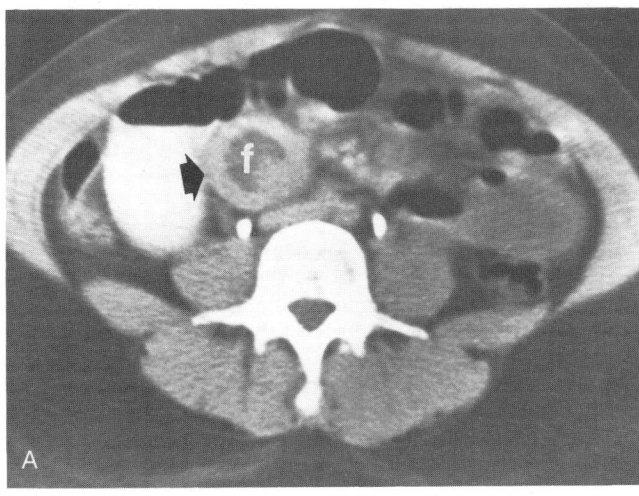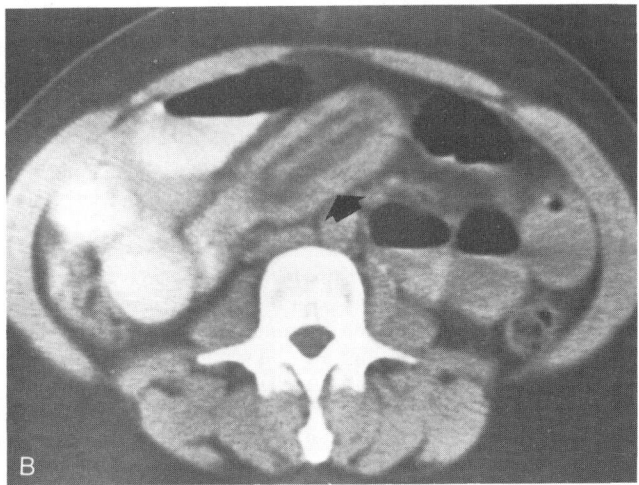

Figure 16. Acute small bowel intussusception — computed tomography. Sudden onset of severe midabdominal pain with nonspecific plain film findings. Cross-sectional (A) and longitudinal (B) images demonstrate a small bowel intussusception (arrows). Mesenteric fat (f) accompanies the intussusception. A benign spindle cell tumor was the cause.

observed in older patients, particularly in those with atrial fibrillation or those with a low cardiac output following surgical procedures. The rapid progression of severe generalized abdominal pain, associated with clinical findings of generalized peritonitis and marked acidosis, suggests mesenteric arterial occlusion and gangrene of the small intestine. In the late stages of this disease, gas may be visible in the portal vein on a plain radiograph of the abdomen. In earlier stages, CT is capable of demonstrating minute quantities of gas in the wall of the affected bowel and in the portal venous system not detectable on a radiograph (Fig. 12).

ACUTE OBSTRUCTION OF THE LARGE INTESTINE. Obstruction of the large intestine occurs more often in patients over the age of 40 years, is gradual in onset, and presents with constipation and abdominal distention. Contrary to obstruction of the small intestine, pain is minimal or absent unless peritonitis occurs. The most common causes of large bowel obstruction include carcinoma of the colon, acute diverticulitis, and volvulus. In many instances, carcinoma of the colon can be diagnosed by a careful history. Progressive constipation over several months with or without thin pencil-sized stools streaked with blood are frequently noted by patients with obstructing carcinoma of the sigmoid or rectosigmoid colon. Nausea and vomiting do not usually occur until the late stage of the disease. The patient may or may not be acutely ill, depending on the duration of the obstruction. The patient's temperature and heart and respiratory rates are often normal. The abdomen appears distended and tympanitic to percussion. Unless peritonitis or peritoneal irritation exists, there is minimal abdominal tenderness to percussion and palpation. The distention may prevent the palpation of abdominal masses, and results of a rectal examination are negative unless the obstructing lesion is within reach of the examining finger.

Laboratory data reveal a normal or near-normal hematocrit and WBC count. The diagnosis can be suggested in most instances by a supine and an upright plain film of the abdomen. The descending and sigmoid colon are dilated to the point of the obstruction and extend cephalad to the cecum if the ileocecal valve is competent. If the ileocecal valve is not competent, the intraluminal air extends retrograde into the ileum. A sigmoidoscopy is necessary to assess the rectum and rectosigmoid with a biopsy of the obstructing tumor if possible. If the obstructing lesion is cephalad to the sigmoidoscope and flexible sigmoidoscopy is not feasible, a barium enema should be obtained to confirm the presence, level, and nature of the obstructing lesion.

Acute diverticulitis with large bowel obstruction occurs most frequently in patients older than 45 years and has often been preceded by other attacks. The location is almost always in the distal descending and sigmoid colon. There is frequently a recent increase in the severity of constipation with pain on defecation. The presenting signs and symptoms include LLQ pain, chills, and fever. The patient usually appears ill, with a distended, tympanitic, tender abdomen, especially marked in the LLQ. A tender mass may be palpable just medial to the left anterior superior iliac spine. Bowel sounds are hypoactive but are rarely absent unless generalized peritonitis has occurred. Rectal examination is usually unrevealing.

Laboratory data reveal a normal hematocrit with a normal or elevated WBC count. Supine and upright film views of the abdomen have similar findings to those observed in patients with carcinoma of the sigmoid colon. Sigmoidoscopy to examine the rectosigmoid colon is essential but usually does not reveal any obvious intrinsic lesions of the lumen. The scope, when passed to the point of inflammation, produces severe pain in contrast to the minimal discomfort observed in patients with carcinoma. When the obstructive diverticulitis is acute, CT is a preferable imaging method to a contrast study of the colon and can demonstrate the presence of an abscess or an inflammatory mass associated with the obstruction (Fig. 12).

Volvulus of the large intestine may cause acute intestinal obstruction and can occur in the cecum or sigmoid portion of the colon. Sigmoid volvulus is more common than cecal volvulus; it occurs more often in patients over the age of 65 years, and frequently in patients residing in nursing homes and psychiatric hospitals where chronic constipation is a serious long-standing problem. Patients with a sigmoid volvulus present with large bowel obstruction of acute onset with little prior history. The patient is usually ill but with normal or near-normal temperature. Examination of the abdomen reveals findings similar to those noted in patients with large bowel obstruction due to carcinoma or diverticulitis. Rectal examination is generally noncontributory to the diagnosis. The diagnosis is established by the supine and upright radiographs of the abdomen, with a contrast enema revealing the characteristic point of torsion and nonfilling of the obstructed loop of sigmoid colon. It should be noted that when a sigmoid or cecal volvulus is strongly suspected, a water-soluble contrast enema is preferable to barium. Sigmoidoscopy can be both diagnostic and therapeutic in that the scope, if passed into the obstructed colon, becomes quickly filled with liquid feces and a release of air. If the scope cannot be passed into the obstructed lumen, a catheter may be passed through the scope into the sigmoid colon and through the obstructed lumen with the same result. Cecal volvulus usually occurs in patients of the middle and older age group, with sudden onset of cramping RLQ and epigastric pain associated with nausea and vomiting. The diagnosis is best established by supine and upright radiographs of the abdomen demonstrating a dilated cecum and ascending colon, often with the gas-distended cecum in the left upper quadrant (LUQ). If the diagnosis is uncertain, a sigmoidoscopy and contrast enema may be required.

An expanding or ruptured abdominal aortic aneurysm generally presents with abdominal pain. If the aneurysm is expanding, a previous history of back pain of several days' duration may be obtained. At physical examination, the aneurysm is palpable, is usually tender, and may be visible if the patient is thin without abdominal obesity. A plain film of the abdomen may demonstrate a calcified border of the aortic aneurysm that is also present in a two-dimensional view obtained with a cross-table lateral film. Ultrasound and CT examinations can confirm the presence and size of the aneurysm as well as provide evidence of active or impending rupture. Operation should be performed as soon as possible in patients with symptomatic aneurysms. If the aneurysm has ruptured, immediate exploration is indicated.

Fecal impaction is a common cause of intestinal obstruction in elderly patients who are bedridden with long-standing constipation. Because of the patient's mental status, an accurate history may be impossible to obtain, and although the abdominal findings do not indicate an acute process, the possibility of the presence of obstructing colon carcinoma or diverticulitis cannot be excluded. Abdominal distention may exist, and although peritoneal signs are uncommon, the colon containing feces is often palpable. Sigmoidoscopy may be limited by the fecal content in the lumen, and multiple enema treatments may be required over a period of several days. After the colon has been emptied of fecal material, colonoscopy and a barium contrast study may be necessary to exclude other causes of intestinal obstruction.

Nonobstructive colonic dilation, also described as pseudo-obstruction of the colon (Ogilvie's syndrome), refers to a clinical entity in which there are signs and symptoms of colonic obstruction without mechanical obstruction. This process, which is poorly understood in regard to causation, may involve the entire colon or a segment of it and creates the risk of bowel rupture. The disease develops more commonly after previous operations and is often associated with other serious medical illnesses. Not infrequently, patients develop pseudo-obstruction while receiving narcotics or psychotropic drugs. Abdominal pain is a frequent complaint and is usually generalized. Vomiting is rare, and the patient may have constipation or frequent watery diarrhea. Abdominal distention is always present, developing over a period of 3 to 4 days, with mild tenderness. Bowel sounds range from normal to hypo- or hyperactive. The WBC count usually exceeds 12,000. Supine radiographs of the abdomen may reveal generalized colon dilation or cecal dilation. When the transverse diameter of the colon exceeds 10 cm., impending rupture of the bowel may exist and surgical or endoscopic intervention is indicated.

Metastatic carcinoma with pelvic implantation may cause extrinsic compression on the sigmoid colon, with obstruction. This rarely presents as a primary illness and usually occurs secondary to other malignant diseases. The patient's history includes progressive constipation over a period of several weeks, and the pelvic and rectal examinations may confirm a pelvic mass. Sigmoidoscopy excludes intrinsic colon lesions involving the mucosa, and a barium enema examination confirms the site of extrinsic compression.

Acute fulminating ulcerative colitis may present with abdominal distention and tenderness to percussion and palpation with hypoactive bowel sounds. The patient's history of chronic ulcerative colitis usually indicates the diagnosis, and the supine and upright abdominal radiographs document dilation of the entire colon, often with pseudopolyps noted as outlined by the intraluminal air. A sigmoidoscopy should confirm the diagnosis by documenting the shaggy, friable bleeding appearance of the mucosa. A barium enema examination should not be performed in these circumstances in order to avoid colon perforation.

Acute Abdominal Pain After Blunt Trauma

Blunt trauma to the abdomen is a major cause of intra-abdominal injury, producing signs and symptoms of the acute abdomen. The injury itself is the inciting event, and the onset of abdominal pain may be immediate or delayed over a period of hours or even days. A careful history is especially important if the patient is alert and able to respond. If the injury is due to a motor vehicle accident in which the patient was a passenger or driver, certain information is particularly important. The speed of the vehicle, whether a seatbelt was used, and the location of the passenger in the car, that is, driver, back seat, or front seat but nondriver, are all important factors in the history.

If the patient is injured in an altercation with another individual, the type of trauma is very pertinent to the diagnosis. Examination of the abdomen often reveals a distended tender abdomen with hypoactive bowel sounds with no visible skin marks or abrasions. The supine and upright plain films of the abdomen may reveal free air with rupture of an intraperitoneal viscus or a ruptured diaphragm with intra-abdominal contents in the pleural cavity. Free blood within the peritoneal cavity may have a "ground-glass" appearance in the abdomen, and if the bleeding is retroperitoneal in location, the radiographic appearance of the psoas margins may be altered. Occasionally, if the duodenum is ruptured, a small amount of air in the retroperitoneal tissues around the duodenum may be visualized. An intravenous pyelogram documents important information regarding the function of both kidneys and the position of the ureters. A cystogram is particularly valuable to exclude rupture of the bladder. Both anteroposterior and oblique views of the bladder during the cystogram are necessary if a small posterior retroperitoneal tear is to be excluded. All patients must have a complete blood count, urinalysis, blood urea nitrogen, creatinine, serum electrolytes, and serum amylase determinations, and a liver profile. Immediate peritoneal lavage is the definitive diagnostic test to confirm the presence of intraperitoneal hemorrhage. Free blood in the peritoneal cavity may follow rupture of the spleen, liver, mesentery, and, occasionally, the pancreas and the bowel. Immediate laparotomy is indicated in these circumstances. A rupture of the pancreas may occur where the body of the organ overlies the vertebral column. This situation is especially common with automobile drivers who have blunt abdominal injury due to compression from the steering wheel. The clinical findings of an acute abdomen after blunt trauma usually prompt surgical intervention. Patients who develop signs and symptoms of an acute abdomen several days after the trauma occurred present a more complex situation and require a careful assessment in which many or all of the original diagnostic procedures are repeated in order to confirm or exclude a perforated viscus, a pancreatic injury, or a delayed rupture of the spleen or liver. For this reason, consideration for admission and careful observation is indicated for individuals who sustain blunt abdominal trauma.

Trauma to the kidney is less common than that to the liver and spleen because of its anatomic location. However, with violent trauma sustained in automobile accidents or in contact sports, the kidney may be ruptured, with severe retroperitoneal bleeding. Because of its location, bleeding may be considerable before it is detected. Ureters are rarely injured in blunt abdominal trauma.

Injury to the large and small intestine and their mesenteric attachments occurs after blunt trauma. Laceration of the mesentery may cause arterial or venous bleeding with hemoperitoneum. Laceration of the bowel wall with a tear in the lumen causing bacterial peritonitis is less common and, when present, suggests generalized peritonitis. The omentum is rarely injured, partly because of its mobility, but it may bleed if the trauma initiates a laceration.

Growing experience with the use of CT in the evaluation of the severely traumatized patient, especially in situations in which the patient has sustained closed head trauma in addition to suspected chest and abdominal trauma, has revealed it to be extremely valuable. In a single CT survey of the abdomen and pelvis, with intravenous contrast medium, complete assessment of the solid viscera, mesentery, retroperitoneum, gastrointestinal tract, abdominal wall, and skeletal structures can be accurately accomplished. The use of CT is advised only if the patient's general medical condition can tolerate the procedure.

Acute Abdominal Pain After Spinal Cord Injury

The progressive improvement in care following spinal cord injuries has allowed a substantial increase in the survival of patients during the past 30 years. However, conditions requiring consideration for abdominal surgery occur in patients with spinal cord injuries and involve the entire gastrointestinal tract. Approximately 10 per cent of all fatalities among patients with spinal cord injuries are the result of a perforated viscus and peritonitis. The ability of a patient to describe the symptoms of acute abdominal pain depends on the location of the spinal cord injury. Conduction of pain to the spinal cord from abdominal viscera may occur by the thoracic, sympathetic, splanchnic, hypogastric, or pelvic nerves and then proceeds to the dorsal root ganglion. Patients with cervical cord injuries are less able to document the site of abdominal discomfort, even though most of these patients experience some type of abdominal pain with a perforated viscus. Patients with lower thoracic and lumbar cord injuries are able to more accurately describe the location and type of pain.

The most frequent signs of such injury are an increase in heart rate and occasionally an increase in blood pressure. Sudden high fever may accompany a perforated viscus. Sweating is frequent, and anorexia or a feeling of "something not right" is a common complaint. Abdominal examination is complicated by the neurologic injury. Distention is a frequent occurrence in patients with spinal cord injury, but tenderness is uncommon. When tenderness does exist, it suggests a perforated viscus or bladder. Palpation of the abdomen may not document rigidity of the rectus muscles because of spasticity or flaccidity. However, a generalized resistance may be present. Shoulder pain is common in patients with a perforated viscus and diaphragmatic irritation. If the spinal cord lesion is at T12 or below and there is normal bowel and bladder function, the sensation to the abdominal viscera is intact.

The incidence rate of gastrointestinal hemorrhage in these patients is 1 to 3 per cent, and the diagnostic evaluation and treatment should be the same as that in patients without neurologic injury. The causes of the acute abdomen are the same in patients with spinal cord injury as in those without neurologic injury. Chronic urinary tract infections, acute pyelonephritis, and fecal impaction are common nonoperative problems that occur in these patients. Complications in the first 30 to 60 days after injury are different from those that occur later. Gastric dilation, ileus, peptic ulcer disease, and pancreatitis may occur in the early period after injury. In a chronic setting, fecal impaction, peptic ulcer disease, hepatitis, diverticulosis, or renal or ureteral calculus may occur. The possibility of appendicitis must be considered at all times, and frequently it has perforated by the time the patient presents. In such circumstances, an RLQ mass is a common finding on examination.

Acute Gynecologic Disease

Acute abdominal pain following disorders of the gynecologic subsystem is one of the most common and serious problems encountered by surgeons. A thorough history and complete

TABLE 4. Abdominal Pain Secondary to Lesions of the Gynecologic Subsystem

Ovary
   Ruptured graafian follicle
   Torsion of ovary
Fallopian tube
   Ectopic pregnancy
   Acute salpingitis
   Pyosalpinx
Uterus
   Uterine rupture
   Endometritis

pelvic and rectal examinations are essential for an accurate diagnosis (Table 4).

ACUTE SALPINGITIS. This disease, most commonly due to gonococcal infection, has an index of highest frequency in patients between the ages of 15 and 35 years and is rarely observed after menopause. The pain begins cephalad to the symphysis in the midline and radiates to the RLQ and LLQ. Occasionally, gonococcal hepatitis may occur and is difficult to differentiate from other forms of hepatitis. The pain of acute salpingitis occurs over a period of hours, and the patient usually has few gastrointestinal complaints. Examination of the abdomen reveals RLQ and LLQ tenderness to percussion and palpation. Bowel sounds are hypoactive. There is severe cervical tenderness to palpation on pelvic examination. A vaginal discharge is frequent, and a positive diagnosis can be established with a cervical smear and culture.

OVARIAN CYSTS. Ovarian cysts may present in an acute manner when torsion occurs. Pain is sudden, is located in the lower abdomen, and is most severe in either the RLQ or LLQ, depending on the ovary involved. Anorexia is rare, but nausea may occur with vomiting in the presence of severe pain. If rupture occurs, generalized peritonitis with free intraperitoneal bleeding results. Pelvic examination is the key diagnostic maneuver, and a palpable mass may confirm the suspicion.

ECTOPIC PREGNANCY. Tubal pregnancy may present as an acute intra-abdominal condition with sudden lower abdominal pain, which is sharp in character and persistent, with or without nausea and vomiting. These symptoms indicate rupture of the fallopian tube and occur in the first trimester of pregnancy. The patient's history is the most important factor in the diagnosis. A missed menstrual period or an abnormally short scanty period precedes the abdominal pain. However, it may be difficult to obtain an accurate history at the time of the acute illness, contributing to the obscurity of the diagnosis.

The patient presents with acute abdominal pain in the lower abdomen that with rupture proceeds to generalized peritonitis, occasional diaphragmatic irritation, and referred pain to the shoulder. The pain worsens with time, and if blood loss is significant, hypotension and tachycardia occur. Examination of the patient reveals moderate distention of the lower abdomen and hypoactive or absent bowel sounds, with marked tenderness to percussion or palpation. Pelvic examination demonstrates blood in the vagina or cervical os. Motion of the cervix is painful, and an adnexal mass is palpable. A hematoma may be present in the cul de sac. The cervix is frequently blue in color, and the uterus is slightly enlarged.

Laboratory data reveal a decrease in hematocrit to 30 per cent or less with a leukocytosis of 15,000. The human chorionic gonadotropin is positive. Peritoneoscopy may be of diagnostic value if the patient's condition is stable. Culdocentesis, paracentesis, or peritoneal lavage may demonstrate bloody peritoneal fluid. Although other conditions that cause acute abdominal pain such as ruptured ovarian cyst, acute appendicitis, or perforated ulcer may be difficult to differentiate from a ruptured ectopic pregnancy, surgical intervention is required for diagnosis and treatment.

Septic thrombosis of the left or right ovarian vein, occurring in the immediate postpartum period, associated with endometritis, is an uncommon and somewhat confusing clinical syndrome that is often misdiagnosed as acute appendicitis, peritonitis, or intra-abdominal abscess. Treatment is nonsurgical and involves measures directed toward the bacterial infection. The role of anticoagulation is uncertain. The appearance of this entity on CT is characteristic.

Acute Abdominal Pain During Pregnancy

The presence of acute abdominal pain during pregnancy is complicated by the duration of the pregnancy, the enlarged uterus, and the difficulty in accurately examining the abdomen. Appendicitis, a common clinical problem of pregnant patients, has many clinical features similar to appendicitis in nonpregnant patients. Acute cholecystitis, another cause of abdominal pain during pregnancy, also presents in a manner similar to that in nonpregnant patients. Acute pancreatitis, perforated ulcer, and acute diverticulitis are observed less frequently, probably because of the age of the patient and her general state of good health. Rupture of a splenic artery aneurysm in pregnant patients has been reported with an increased frequency over that expected in this age group. In this situation, the patient presents with severe epigastric pain, hypotension, and shock. Immediate surgical exploration is indicated for obvious reasons, and the diagnosis is usually established at that time. Rupture of the liver capsule following subcapsular hematoma in the pregnant patient is also an uncommon event presenting as an urgent problem in diagnosis and management. Associated conditions that predispose to this entity include pre-eclamptic toxemia and disseminated intravascular coagulation. This illness most often occurs in women in their late 20s or 30s of whom 80 per cent are multipara. Fifty per cent of women who experience rupture of the liver capsule do so in the third trimester of pregnancy, and 25 per cent do so at term. RUQ and epigastric pain radiating to the back and associated with hypotension, shock, and hemoperitoneum are the usual sequence of events, often followed by death of the fetus. Other causes of abdominal pain during pregnancy include placental abruption, ruptured uterus, torsion of the ovary, pyelonephritis, and pulmonary embolus.

Nonsurgical Causes of the Acute Abdomen

There are a number of nonsurgical causes of acute abdominal pain, which are important for the surgeon to consider in order to avoid operating in those circumstances in which surgical therapy is not indicated (Table 5).

Sickle cell anemia, a hereditary hemolytic disturbance, is observed in patients of the black race. The disease presents early in life and is characterized by attacks of bone and joint pain as well as abdominal pain. The diagnosis can be established by a careful history, because patients usually have had previous episodes of a similar type. Cholelithiasis is common in this group of patients and may present as acute cholecystitis.

Gastroenteritis, if severe, may cause abdominal pain preceded by nausea and vomiting. Diarrhea is common and usually occurs after the onset of abdominal pain. The illness may be related to specific food intake, and other family members may be affected. Fortunately, the process is self-limited and resolves in 6 to 10 hours.

Unrecognized, severe pseudomembranous colitis may present as an acute abdomen, suggesting the need for surgical intervention. Plain abdominal radiographs and sigmoidoscopy often establish the correct diagnosis and obviate operative intervention.

Lead poisoning is associated with colicky abdominal pain, often in the RLQ, and may cause suspicion of acute appendicitis. The history is one of recurrent attacks, and despite the severity of pain, the clinical examination reveals minimal findings of abdominal tenderness.

**TABLE 5. Nonsurgical Causes of
Abdominal Pain**

Cardiac
   Myocardial infarction
   Acute pericarditis
Pulmonary
   Pneumonia
   Pulmonary infarction
Gastrointestinal
   Acute pancreatitis
   Gastroenteritis
   Acute hepatitis
Endocrine
   Diabetic ketoacidosis
   Acute adrenal insufficiency
Metabolic
   Acute porphyria
   Familial Mediterranean fever
   Hyperlipidemia
Musculoskeletal
   Rectus muscle hematoma
Central and peripheral nervous system
   Tabes dorsalis
   Nerve root compression
Genitourinary
   Pyelonephritis
   Acute salpingitis
Hematologic
   Sickle cell crisis

Acute porphyria occurs with recurrent attacks of abdominal pain. The disease is rarely noted prior to puberty, is most common in women, and occurs in the third and fourth decade of life. The abdominal pain is moderate to severe in intensity, may be generalized or localized, and radiates to the back. The abdominal examination reveals minimal tenderness, much less than is expected with the severity of the pain. Fever and leukocytosis may exist, and abdominal radiographs reveal distended loops of bowel. This diagnosis is suggested by a history of previous similar attacks and is confirmed by the excessive porphobilinogen in the urine.

Familial Mediterranean fever, a disorder of individuals of Jewish (Sephardic) or Armenian background, is inherited as an autosomal recessive trait. The paroxysms of abdominal pain are severe, may be associated with chest pain, and precede the fever. Fever may be as high as 40° C. (103° F.), and tachycardia, tachypnea, and abdominal tenderness, especially in the epigastric region, are noted. Because of the recurrent nature of the abdominal findings, a previous surgical exploration has often been performed.

Right or left lower lobe pneumonia with involvement of the diaphragmatic pleura may present as RUQ or LUQ pain, with symptoms of pulmonary infection. The leukocytosis and rapid respiratory rate combined with the radiographic findings of pneumonia suggest a supradiaphragmatic cause for the abdominal pain.

Acute myocardial infarction may produce epigastric pain and may mimic acute pancreatitis or perforated duodenal ulcer. The pain is of sudden onset and is combined with dyspnea and cyanosis. The electrocardiogram provides the correct diagnosis.

Rectus sheath hematoma may cause acute abdominal pain and is frequently preceded by a paroxysm of coughing or straining following heavy exertion. The pain is localized to the rectus sheath, and the abdominal tenderness markedly decreases with tension of the rectus sheath. A tender mass is occasionally palpable. The process is self-limited and is of primary concern only in that it may suggest an acute intra-abdominal condition such as appendicitis. The presence and exact location of an acute hematoma in the abdomen can be rapidly determined with CT.

Acute adrenal insufficiency may occur in the immediate postoperative period, precipitating acute abdominal pain. The diagnosis is straightforward in patients with Addison's disease or in those requiring corticosteroid replacement therapy who are on a subtherapeutic postoperative dosage. However, some patients may develop adrenal hemorrhage after operation, causing adrenal insufficiency characterized by fever, nausea, vomiting, abdominal pain, diarrhea, hypotension, and an apathetic affect. Failure to recognize the entity may cause death. The CT findings in this acute hemorrhagic process are diagnostic.

Hyperlipidemia may occur in patients with acute pancreatitis as well as in those patients with recurrent episodes of abdominal pain occurring in the absence of pancreatitis. The history of hyperlipidemia is the key factor in the diagnosis. The abdominal examination reveals generalized tenderness with occasional hepatomegaly and splenomegaly. The elevated serum amylase may be observed by the high serum lipid level.

All patients with nonsurgical causes of abdominal pain must be evaluated carefully on each recurrence of pain in order to prevent a superficial and erroneous conclusion on the basis that the primary disease is of nonsurgical origin.

SELECTED REFERENCES

Frimann-Dahl, J.: Roentgen Examination in Acute Abdominal Diseases. Springfield, IL, Charles C Thomas, 1974.
This is an outstanding textbook on the radiologic findings of the acute abdomen.

Jeffrey, R. B., Jr.: CT and Sonography of the Acute Abdomen. New York, Raven Press, 1989.
An excellent and comprehensive textbook regarding the use of imaging techniques for the acute abdomen.

Lee, J. K. T., Sagel, S. S., and Stanley, R. J.: Computed Body Tomography with MRI Correlation, 2nd ed. New York, Raven Press, 1989.
A superb textbook with a complete study of CT and MRI of acute and chronic conditions of the abdomen.

Silen, W.: Cope's Early Diagnosis of the Acute Abdomen, 16th ed. New York, Oxford University Press, 1983.
A revised edition of the classic monograph of patients with acute abdominal pain.

REFERENCES

1. Barone, J. E., Gingold, B. S., Arvanitis, M. L., and Nealon, J. F.: Abdominal pain in patients with acquired immune deficiency syndrome. Ann. Surg., 204:619, 1986.
2. Bradley, E. L., Murphy, F., and Ferguson, C.: Prediction of pancreatic necrosis by dynamic pancreatography. Ann. Surg., 210:495, 1989.
3. Brown, C. E. L., Lowe, T. W., Cunningham, F. G., and Weinreb, J. C.: Puerperal pelvic thrombophlebitis: Impact on diagnosis and treatment using x-ray computed tomography and a magnetic resonance imaging. Obstet. Gynecol., 68:789, 1986.
4. Carroll, B. A.: Preferred imaging techniques for the diagnosis of cholecystitis and cholelithiasis. Ann. Surg., 210:1, 1989.
5. Charney, K. J., Juler, G. L., and Comarr, A. E.: General surgery problems in patients with spinal cord injuries. Arch. Surg., 110:1083, 1975.
6. DeBakey, M. E., Crawford, E. S., Cooley, D. A., Morris, G. C., Royster, T. S., and Abbott, W. P.: Aneurysm of the abdominal aorta. Analysis of results of graft replacement therapy 1 to 11 years after operation. Ann. Surg., 160:622, 1964.
7. DeBartolo, H. M., and Van Heerden, J. A.: Meckel's diverticulum. Ann. Surg., 183:30, 1976.
8. Eisenberg, R. L., Heineken, P., Hedgcock, M. W., Federle, M., and Goldberg, H. T.: Evaluation of plain abdominal radiographs in the diagnosis of abdominal pain. Ann. Intern. Med., 97:257, 1982.
9. Feliciano, D.: Management of traumatic retroperitoneal hematoma. Ann. Surg., 211:109, 1990.
10. Glenn, F.: Pain in biliary tract disease. Surg. Gynecol. Obstet., 122:495, 1966.
11. Gore, R. M., Mintzer, R. A., and Calenoff, L.: Gastrointestinal complications of spinal cord injury. Spine, 6:538, 1981.
12. Greenstein, A. J., Sachae, D. B., Mann, D., Lachman, P., Heimann, T., and Aufses, A. H.: Spontaneous free perforation and perforated abscess in 30 patients with Crohn's disease. Ann. Surg., 205:72, 1987.
13. Hattery, R. R., Williamson, B., and Wallace, R. B.: Ultrasonic and computed tomographic imaging of the abdominal aorta. World J. Surg., 4:511, 1980.
14. Lewis, R. F., Holcroft, J. W., Beoy, J., and Dunphy, J. E.: Appendicitis: A critical review of diagnosis and treatment in 1000 cases. Arch. Surg., 110:677, 1975.
15. Ludtke, F. E., Mende, V., Kobles, H., and Lepsien, G.: Incidence and frequency of complications and management of Meckel's diverticulum. Surg. Gynecol. Obstet., 169:537, 1989.
16. Meier, E. E., Imediegwu, O. O., and Tarpley, J. L.: Perforated typhoid enteritis: Operative experience with 108 cases. Am. J. Surg., 157:423, 1989.
17. Ogilvie, H.: Large intestine colic due to sympathetic deprivation. A new clinical syndrome. Br. Med. J., 2:671, 1948.
18. Rodkey, G. V., and Welch, C. E.: Colonic diverticular disease with surgical treatment. A study of 338 cases. Surg. Clin. North Am., 54:655, 1974.
19. Schwartz, M. Z., Tapper, D., and Solenberger, R. I.: Management of perforated appendicitis in children. Ann. Surg., 197:407, 1983.
20. Staniland, J. R., Ditchburn, J., and DeDombal, F. T.: Clinical presentation of acute abdomen: Study of 600 patients. Br. Med. J., 3:393, 1972.
21. Steinheber, F. U.: Medical conditions mimicking the acute surgical abdomen. Med. Clin. North Am., 57:1559, 1973.
22. Strodel, W. E., Nostrant, T. T., Eckhauser, F. E., and Dent, T. L.: Therapeutic and diagnostic colonoscopy in nonobstructive colonic dilatation. Ann. Surg., 197:416, 1983.
23. Svanes, C., Salvesen, H., Espehaug, B., Soreide, O., and Svanes, K.: A multifactorial analysis of factors related to lethality after treatment of perforated duodenal ulcer. Ann. Surg., 209:418, 1989.
24. Tedesco, F. J., Anderson, C. B., and Ballinger, W. F.: Drug induced colitis mimicking an acute surgical condition of the abdomen. Arch. Surg., 110:481, 1975.

29

THE STOMACH AND DUODENUM

James C. Thompson, M.D., M.A.

The stomach and duodenum may be considered logically as a unit, because many physiologic mechanisms and certain diseases are either shared by or interact with these two segments of the gut. They are both affected by peptic ulcer, which is the most common serious inflammatory condition of the gastrointestinal tract. Fortunately, peptic ulceration has a relatively low mortality, but it has a high rate of disability and is responsible for great costs to society in loss of productive time and in medical care. The incidence and prevalence of duodenal ulcer has decreased sharply over the last 3 decades in Western Europe and North America, but not in "developing" countries. Gastric ulcer has remained unchanged.

Carcinoma of the stomach, which has also undergone a dramatic and unexplained diminution in incidence, is discussed in the following chapter, and congenital hypertrophic pyloric stenosis, is covered in Chapter 38. In this section, major attention is directed to the physiology of the stomach and duodenum and peptic ulceration. Other conditions are discussed separately at the end of the chapter.

ANATOMY

The stomach arises as a spindle-shaped dilation of the foregut during the fourth week of embryonic life. With later growth, it undergoes a rotation so that the previous left side of the stomach becomes the anterior wall and the previous right side comes to lie posteriorly (mnemonic—LARP). The duodenum, which was initially suspended between dorsal and ventral mesenteries, also rotates so that the second portion of the duodenum becomes retroperitoneal and encompasses the head of the pancreas in its C loop.

The fully developed stomach is the largest dilation of the gut and lies between the esophagus and the duodenum (Fig. 1). The topographic anatomy of the stomach is quite simple, although it has been confused by the application of overlapping terms by anatomists, surgeons, endoscopists, and radiologists. For gross description, the stomach can be divided into fundus, body, and antrum. The fundus is the dome of the stomach, to the left of and superior to the esophagogastric junction. An angulation approximately 5 to 6 cm. proximal to the pylorus on the lesser curvature, at approximately the midline of the body, is termed the *incisura angularis* (at A on lesser curvature, Fig. 1). The area between the fundus and a line drawn from the incisura angularis to the greater curvature of the stomach (in approximately the position of a line from A to A' in Fig. 1) is the body of the stomach; the area distal to that line and proximal to the pylorus is the gastric antrum. The pylorus may be palpated as a thick ring of muscle and is marked externally by the prominent veins of Mayo.

In terms of *function,* the stomach may be divided into fundus (parietal cell or oxyntic gland area) and antrum (pyloric gland area). The fundus secretes acid-peptic juice, and the antrum, the distal segment, secretes a thick, viscid, relatively alkaline mucus

and the hormones gastrin and somatostatin. The division between the functional area of the fundus and the antrum is a line from A to A'.

The esophagogastric junction, the cardia, is located just to the left of the tenth thoracic vertebra, and the gastroduodenal junction, the pylorus, is located to the right of the midline at approximately the interspace between the first and second lumbar vertebrae. The superior margin of the stomach between the cardia and pylorus (a distance of approximately 12 to 14 cm.) is the lesser curvature of the stomach. It is suspended from the liver by the gastrohepatic ligament, which forms the superior portion of the anterior wall of the lesser omental bursa. The inferior and lateral convex border of the stomach is the greater curvature, which is approximately three times as long as the lesser curvature. From the major portion of the greater curvature is suspended the gastrocolic ligament, which forms the lower portion of the anterior wall of the lesser omental bursa.

The *blood supply of the stomach* is particularly rich. There are innumerable variations in the arrangement of blood vessels, and the schema shown in Figure 1 is only one of many variations. Six vessels provide the main blood supply: the left and right gastric arteries supply the area of the lesser curvature, the right and left gastroepiploic arteries supply the greater curvature, the splenic artery supplies the area of the fundus by way of the short gastric arteries, and the gastroduodenal artery sends branches to the area of the pylorus. The arteries of secondary importance are numbered 7 through 12 in Figure 1. For comparison, the radiologic appearance of the blood supply to the stomach in man, as demonstrated by selective celiac angiography, is shown in Figure 2. A rich anastomotic network is evident, and no area is served by end arteries. Michels[138] studied the blood supply of the stomach in a meticulous manner and called attention to possible surgical hazards (e.g., in more than 20 per cent of patients, the primary or secondary blood supply of the left lobe of the liver would be lost if the left gastric artery were divided at its origin).

The *blood supply of the duodenum* is carried by the supraduodenal and retroduodenal arteries, by the superior pancreaticoduodenal artery, which arises from the gastroduodenal, and by the inferior pancreaticoduodenal artery, which arises from the superior mesenteric artery.

The *parasympathetic nerve supply* to the stomach is from the vagus nerves, which stimulate motility of the stomach and the secretion of acid and pepsin; the vagus appears to have fibers that both stimulate and inhibit release of gastrin. The left and right vagal trunks supply numerous branches and are somewhat inconstant in their relations at the diaphragm (Figs. 1 and 23). The left or anterior vagus nerve supplies a hepatic branch, which also sends fibers to the area of the pylorus. The remaining portion of the left nerve innervates the anterior wall of the stomach. The right or posterior vagus nerve supplies a large branch to the celiac plexus, and the remaining nerve goes to the posterior wall of the stomach.

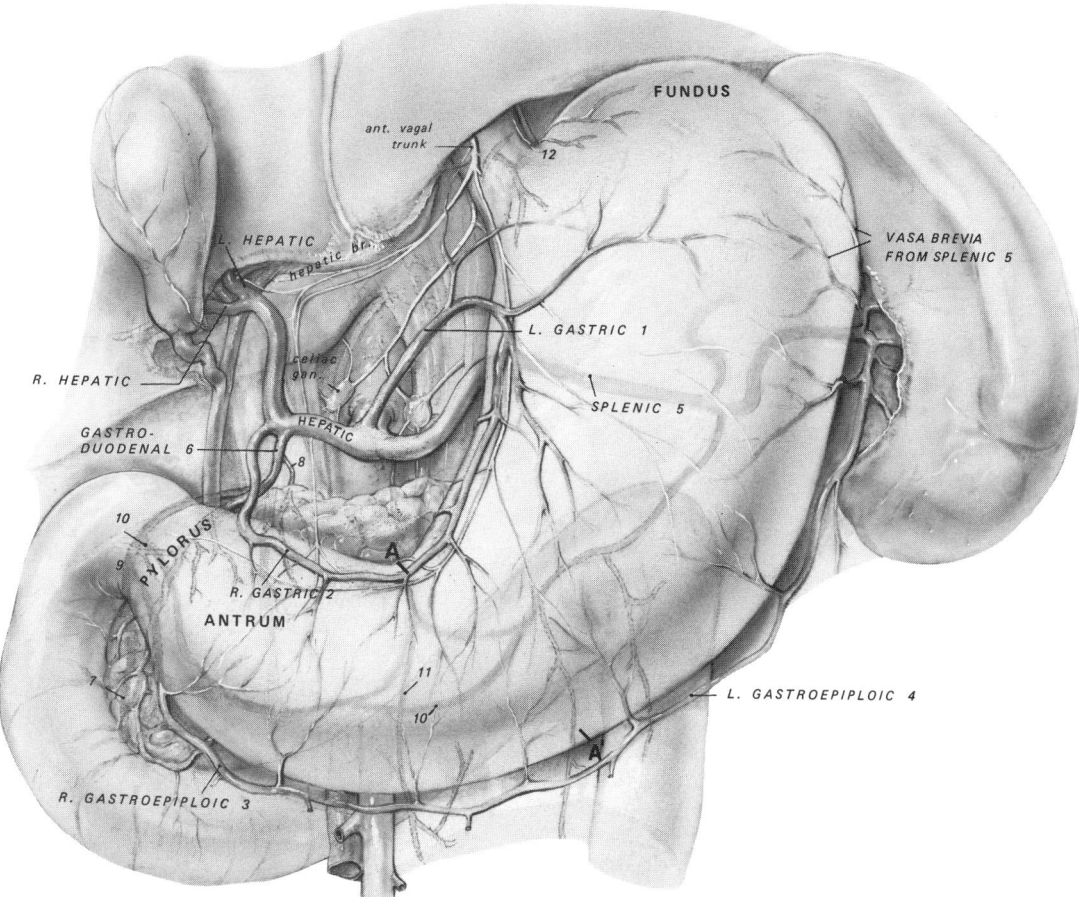

Figure 1. Anatomy of the stomach and duodenum. Grossly, the stomach is divided into fundus (the area superior to the gastroesophageal junction), body, and antrum. The antrum begins proximally at approximately a line drawn from A on the lesser curvature to A' on the greater curvature and extends distally to the pylorus. There are only two important physiologic divisions, the fundic gland (parietal cell) area and the pyloric gland (antral) area. The junction of these two histologic zones is again approximately at a line between A and A'. The blood supply to the stomach is carried by six major vessels and by six other vessels of lesser consequence. The most important vessels are *1*, left gastric artery; *2*, right gastric artery; *3*, right gastroepiploic artery; *4*, left gastroepiploic artery; *5*, splenic artery via the vasa brevia; and *6*, gastroduodenal artery. The remaining vessels are indicated only by a number in the illustration: *7*, superior pancreaticoduodenal artery; *8*, supraduodenal artery of Wilkie; *9*, retroduodenal artery; *10*, transverse pancreatic artery; *11*, dorsal pancreatic artery; and *12*, left inferior phrenic artery. The anterior (left) vagus is shown dividing into a gastric and hepatic branch. Just behind it is also shown the posterior (right) vagus dividing into a gastric and a celiac branch. The duodenal-jejunal flexure is shown here behind the stomach. Its position is variable, and it may often be observed on radiographs protruding above the lesser curvature of the stomach just to the left of the midline.

The wall of the stomach is composed of four layers: mucosa, submucosa, muscle, and serosa. Mucosal architecture varies with the area of the stomach. Several types of cells in the stomach have specific functions: parietal cells manufacture and secrete hydrochloric acid and gastric intrinsic factor; chief cells make and secrete pepsinogen; goblet cells secrete mucus; epithelial cells probably secrete extracellular fluid (nonparietal secretion); and specialized cells (gastrin cells or G cells) within the antral gland synthesize (presumably), store, and secrete gastrin. Somatostatin is presumably synthesized and stored by special cells (delta cells?), located primarily in the antrum. Mast cells (fundus) store heparin, histamine, and other vasoactive substances within granules. The functions of the fundic argentaffin cells are unknown; they probably synthesize or store somatostatin or other peptide hormones. The fundic mucosa contains deep tubular glands (Fig. 3) lined superficially with epithelial cells and containing, in the deeper portions, characteristic parietal cells and chief cells with occasional argentaffin cells. Light and electron micrographs of resting and active fundic glands are shown in Figure 4. The histologic appearance of the mucosa immediately adjacent to the cardia is similar to that of the antrum, except that G cells are lacking. The pyloric glands consist of branching tubules lined predominantly with mucous cells. Some of these epithelial cells, located mainly in the middle third of the glands, react immunochemically with antigastrin anti-

bodies[21] and are the locus of gastrin synthesis and storage. An electron micrograph of a gastrin cell is shown in Figure 5. Each G cell is in direct contact with the lumen, either by actually being on the surface (rarely) or by means of cytoplasmic projections (cell limbs).

The junction between antral and fundic mucosa cannot be differentiated on gross inspection, but application of a pH indicator to the mucosal surface after the stimulation of gastric secretion with pentagastrin quickly and clearly differentiates the proximal acid-secreting mucosa from the distal neutral antrum.

The duodenum begins at the pylorus and ends at the duodenal-jejunal junction just to the left of the second lumbar vertebra (Fig. 6). The duodenum is divided into four portions: superior, descending, transverse, and ascending. The majority of the first portion is occupied by the slightly dilated duodenal bulb, the mucosa of which is characterized by lack of plicae circulares. The common bile duct enters the pancreas immediately posterior to the duodenal bulb and lies within the head of the pancreas. It and the main pancreatic duct open onto the medial wall of the midportion of the second part of the duodenum at the duodenal papilla (ampulla of Vater). The superior mesenteric vessels emerge from behind the pancreas to cross over the third part of the duodenum. The fourth part ascends to the duodenal-jejunal flexure, which is suspended from the posterior body wall by the ligament of Treitz.

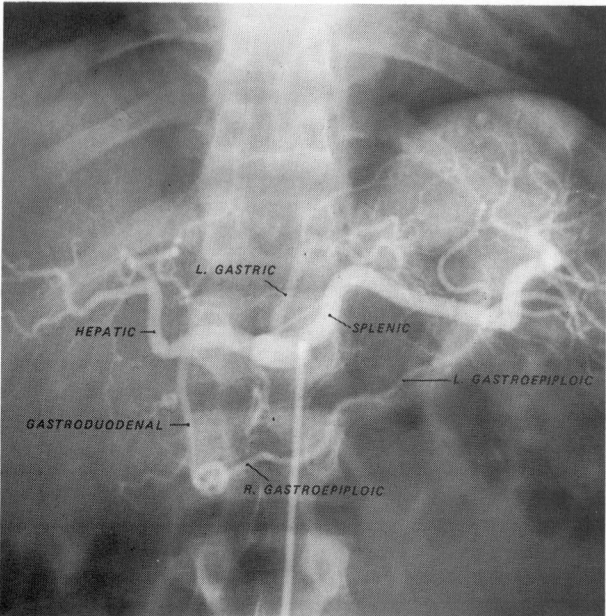

Figure 2. The blood supply of the stomach demonstrated by selective celiac angiography. The angiographic catheter is shown hooked into the orifice of the celiac artery, and injection of radiopaque material outlines the major vessels supplying the stomach (see Fig. 1).

PHYSIOLOGY

The normal flow and ebb of gastric acid secretion in response to a meal provides clear evidence of regulatory mechanisms designed initially to stimulate and later to curtail gastric secretion.[186] Swallowed food enters the stomach where it is mixed with gastric juice and changed to a more liquid form. The viscid, pulpy chyme undergoes only a small amount of digestion in the stomach, mostly proteolysis, before being passed in small boluses into the duodenum, where it is further mixed with bile and pancreatic juice and where major digestion and absorption begin. The function of the mucosa of the small bowel is absorption of food, which is the raison d'être of the gut. The main function of the stomach is to mix and churn the food so that it is delivered slowly, as small particles, into the duodenum. The stomach functions as well as an osmoregulator. Liquids that are highly hyperosmolar are kept in the stomach until they are greatly diluted with secretions from fundic glands. Within the duodenum, the delivered acidic gastric contents are neutralized by bicarbonate from the pancreas, bile, and the duodenal mucosa; the gastric chyme is mixed with pancreatic digestive juices, bile, and enzymes from the duodenal mucosa.

Because *pepsin* is active only in an acid environment (pH less than 5), no peptic ulceration can occur in the absence of acid, so that in one sense, the goal of all ulcer therapy is to maintain the intragastric pH above the level required for activation of pepsin. Because of the important role of acid in digestion and in ulcerogenesis, major attention in gastric physiology has been placed on the study of acid secretion by the stomach. The normal human stomach contains approximately one billion parietal cells, each of which is capable of concentrating hydrogen ions more than one million times. The parietal cell is stimulated by three distinct pathways, each of which delivers chemical messengers capable of eliciting acid secretion from the parietal cell. The first of these, the neurocrine pathway, has nerve transmitters, such as acetylcholine, released from nerves in the stomach wall; the second, the endocrine pathway, delivers hormones such as gastrin; and the third, the paracrine pathway, delivers local factors, such as histamine released from tissue storage sites.[221] There is evidence that the absorbed products of digested

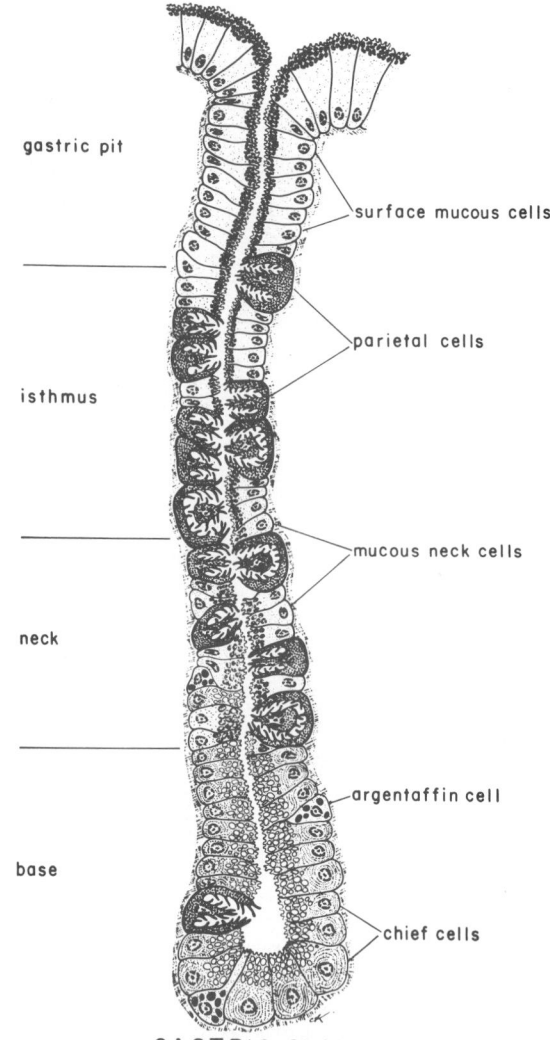

GASTRIC GLAND

Figure 3. Diagram of a simple tubular gastric gland from fundic mucosa. (From Ito, S., and Winchester, R. J.: J. Cell Biol., *16*:541, 1963.)

proteins can stimulate the parietal cell without any chemical intermediary.

STIMULATION OF GASTRIC SECRETION

Gastric juice is composed of parietal and nonparietal components. Pure parietal cell secretion contains between 150 and 170 mEq. H^+ per liter, between 165 and 170 mEq. Cl^- per liter, and 7 mEq. K^+ per liter and is free of sodium.[86,88] In nonparietal secretion, which is nearly identical with extracellular fluid, the chief cation is sodium (about 150 mEq. per liter), and H^+ is nearly absent. Concentration of acid in gastric juice is therefore dependent on the rate of parietal cell secretion and on the degree of admixture with nonparietal secretion.[130] Jacobson and associates[100] have shown that there is a direct relation between the rate of gastric secretion and the blood flow to the mucosa of the stomach. This relationship holds true, except after administration of prostaglandins that suppress acid secretion without affecting the mucosal blood supply.

Gastric secretion has been classified as spontaneous (or interdigestive) and stimulated (or prandial). Spontaneous gastric secretion occurs without intentional stimulation in man and in certain other species and may reflect a background secretion of gastrin and acetylcholine. Pavlov[145] observed that food stimulation of gastric secretion could be effected by a stimulus from the

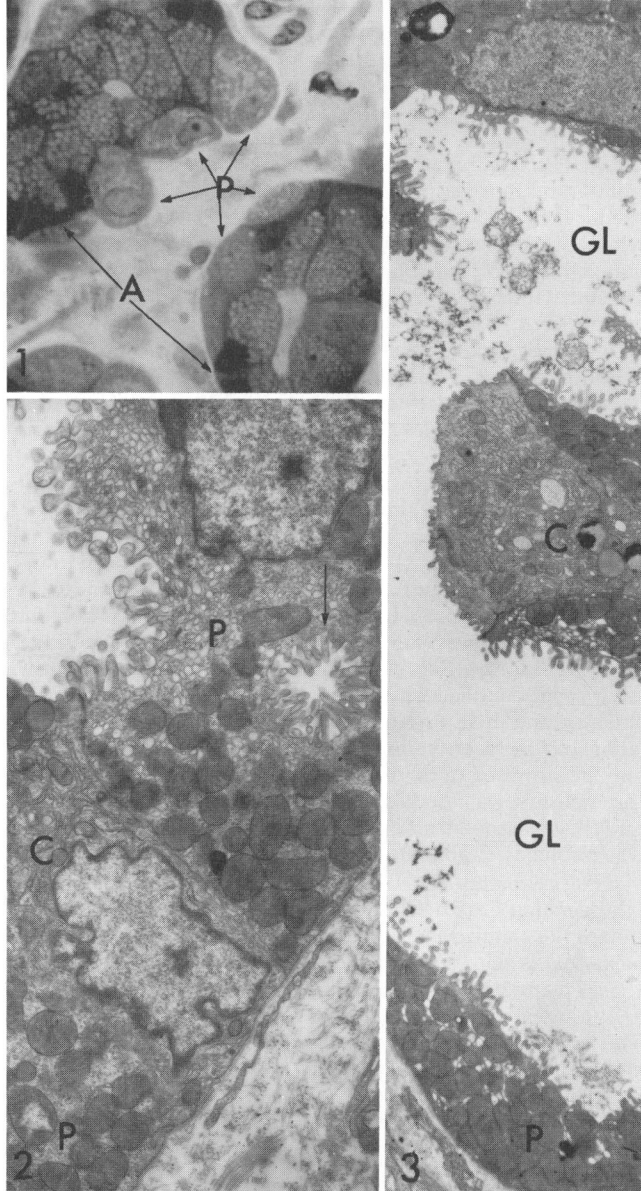

Figure 4. Light and electron micrographs of fundic glands. *1,* Light micrograph (×600, approximate) in which the chief cells are easily recognized by the presence of numerous secretory granules. P, Parietal cells; A, argentaffin cells. *2,* Electron micrograph (×10,800) of resting parietal cells (P) and chief cells (C) of fundic gland. The arrow points to an intracellular canaliculus. *3,* Electron micrograph (×6000) of two parietal cells (P) of a fundic gland. The cells are at their maximal secretory activity and are in the process of discharging the contents of the intracellular canaliculi into the gland lumen (GL). Comparison with the resting parietal cell indicates that the active cell opens out into the gland lumen to expose the entire surface of the intracellular canaliculi into the lumen of the gland. A chief cell (C) is located between the two secreting parietal cells. (Courtesy of Luciano Zamboni, M.D.)

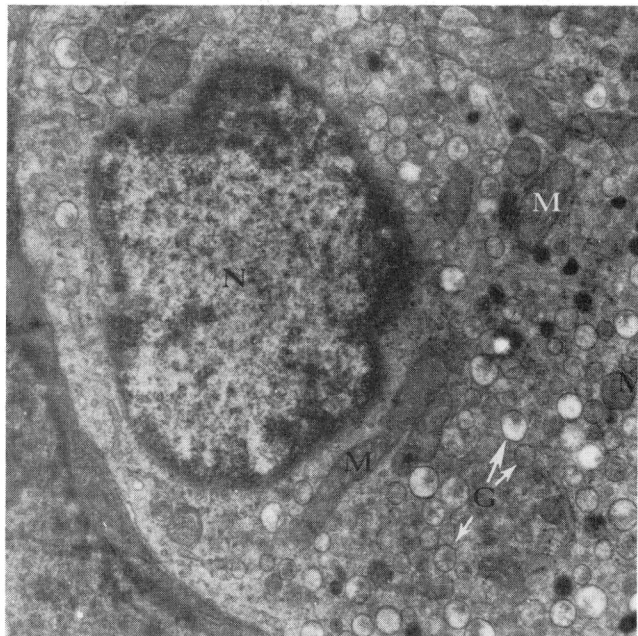

Figure 5. Electron micrograph of a G (gastrin) cell from a pyloric gland. The secretory granules (G), some of which are almost empty, contain gastrin.

are occupied. An adaptation of this suggestion (adding the intestinal phase hormone) is shown schematically in Figure 7. This hypothesis would explain why vagotomy, atropine, and H_2-receptor antagonists inhibit gastric secretion: they each prevent occupation of one of the receptor sites and greatly diminish the response to all stimulants. Local or systemic somatostatin may inhibit parietal acid output. The H_2-receptor appears to be the most important because its blockade causes the greatest suppression of acid release.

When food flows into the intestine, secretin is released in response to acid, cholecystokinin in response to amino acids and fatty acids, glucagon in response to carbohydrates, gastric inhibitory polypeptide in response to carbohydrates and fat, and

head or the stomach, and later it was found that stimuli might arise in the intestine. The *cephalic phase* is stimulated by the sight or smell or chewing of food; the *gastric phase* is stimulated by the presence of food in the stomach; and the *intestinal* phase is stimulated by the presence of food in the small intestine. Although these phases were originally considered distinct, it is now known that various stimuli interact and may potentiate one another, and that they overlap in time.

Grossman and Konturek[75] proposed that the parietal cell has multiple receptor sites on the cell membrane and that maximal stimulation of the cell may be achieved only when all the sites

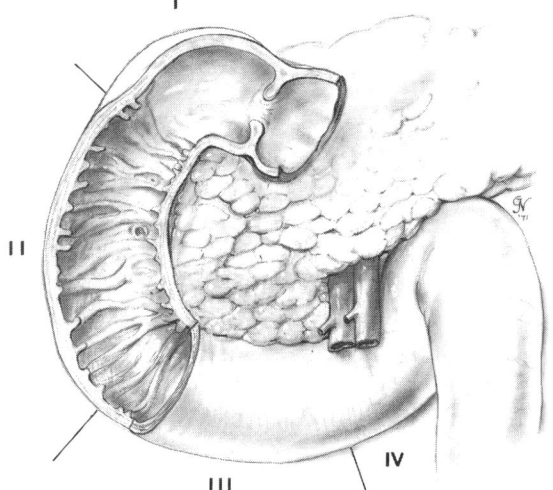

Figure 6. Detailed anatomy of the duodenum. The duodenum is divided into four parts. The first part is occupied almost entirely by the bulb of the duodenum, which has flattened mucosa free of the circular folds (plicae circulares of Kerckring) of mucosa that are characteristic of the rest of the small intestine. The major duodenal papilla is seen in the midpart of the second (descending) portion of the duodenum; the minor duodenal papilla is located about 1 cm. proximally. The third, or transverse, portion of the duodenum extends to the superior mesenteric vessels, and the fourth part extends from the vessels to the duodenal-jejunal flexure.

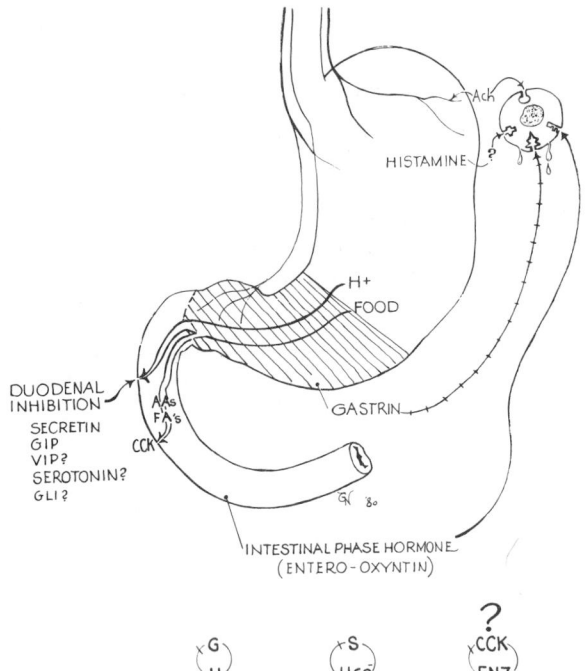

Figure 7. Schematic summary of some of the neurohumoral events that occur when a meal is eaten. Acetylcholine (Ach) is released from vagal nerve endings. Histamine is apparently released from stores within the mucosa. Gastrin is released by food (by a mechanism that is pH-sensitive) from antral mucosa (shaded area). Food in the small bowel stimulates release of the intestinal phase hormone. Each stimulant acts on the parietal cell (perhaps, as shown, each by means of a separate receptor on the cell membrane) to stimulate secretion of H⁺. Delivery of acidified chyme into the duodenum evokes a series of events (some probably reflex, some humoral) that inhibit further gastric secretion. Some of the agents involved are listed. Amino acids and fatty acids (from partially digested food) cause release of cholecystokinin (CCK). Three feedback mechanisms, which act to halt hormone release, are shown diagrammatically across the bottom as typical endocrine closed-loop relationships: acid (H⁺) halts release of gastrin (G) and HCO_3^- halts release of secretin (S). Intraduodenal enzymes (ENZ) may halt release of CCK, but this has not been proved.

pancreatic polypeptide in response to vagal and other humoral stimuli, *inter alia.*

Cephalic Phase

Cephalic phase stimuli (initiated by the sight or smell of food) presumably activate the vagal nuclei in the medulla. Impulses traverse the peripheral vagi and terminate in the gastric mucosa with the release of acetylcholine from vagal nerve endings. Release of acetylcholine in the fundic mucosa directly stimulates acid secretion by the parietal cell and release of pepsinogen by chief cells. Acetylcholine release in the antral mucosa may cause discharge of the antral hormone gastrin. Distention of the stomach excites a vagovagal reflex that also causes release of acetylcholine in the fundic and antral mucosa.

Gastric Phase

The gastric phase of secretion is stimulated by food in the stomach, which by direct contact and by distention causes gastric secretion; it represents almost one half of the postprandial secretion of acid. The humoral mediator of the gastric phase is the hormone gastrin, the activity of which was discovered by Edkins in 1905.[46,47] Gastrin is liberated from the antral mucosa by acetylcholine (released by local reflexes upon antral distention), upon contact with certain substances (for example, two-carbon alcohols, small peptides, and amino acids), and by the vagus itself.

One of the most important aspects of the mechanism for gastrin release is its acid sensitivity. When in the course of gastric secretion the surface pH of the antral mucosa reaches 3.5,

gastrin output is diminished; when it reaches approximately 1.5, further gastrin secretion is halted. As is true with other endocrine organs, there appears to be a closed-loop inverse relation between the concentration of the hormone and the output of the end organ, in this case between gastrin and H⁺ (see Fig. 7).[14]

GASTRIN. Although stimulation of acid secretion by extracts from antral mucosa was reported by Edkins in 1905, the biochemical era in the study of gastrin was not initiated until 1964 when Gregory and Tracy began the experiments that eventuated in the isolation, purification, and synthesis of gastrin.[66,68] The initial form of gastrin (later to be known as *little* gastrin) was composed of 17 linearly arranged L-amino acids with a molecular weight of approximately 2100 (Table 1). The C-terminal four amino acids of the gastrin molecule (Trp-Met-Asp-Phe-NH₂) have been shown to possess the full physiologic range of action of the parent molecule. An analog is available as pentagastrin (Table 1).

Gastrin has been shown to exist in a number of sizes; all the larger sizes apparently contain the smaller forms (Table 1).[152,207] Minigastrin (14 amino acids, G-14) consists of the 14 C-terminal amino acid residues of G-17. G-34 (*big* gastrin) has been found to be the predominant form in circulation; little gastrin can be split enzymatically from big gastrin, which separates it from the apparently inactive N-terminal 17–amino acid tryptic residue. Two larger forms (Rehfeld's Component I and *big-big* gastrin) have been identified by chromatography, but their molecular structure and their physiologic functions are unknown. The relationship between various molecular forms of gastrin could only be surmised until the precise structure of the pre-progastrin molecule was established in 1982.[225] The cDNA to gastrin mRNA was sequenced and the pre-pro-amino acid sequence was resolved[34] (Table 1).

Cholecystokinin, the duodenal hormone that acts to stimulate secretion of pancreatic enzymes and to stimulate contraction of the gallbladder, has a C-terminal group of seven amino acids that is remarkably similar to that of gastrin (Table 1). It shares many physiologic activities with gastrin.[151]

The metabolic functions of gastrin have been reviewed.[152] The most remarkable action of gastrin is its ability to stimulate gastric acid secretion; it is 30 times more potent than histamine by weight and 500 times more potent on a molar basis. In pharmacologic quantities, gastrin appears to have many motor and secretory actions on various target organs in the gut, liver, and pancreas. In addition to its effect on acid secretion, the only other actions of gastrin that have been shown to be physiologic are stimulation of pepsin secretion and stimulation of gastric mucosal blood flow. Gastrin has a pronounced trophic effect on the stomach and pancreas, and it has been shown to stimulate pancreatic enzyme secretion in man. These actions may also prove to be physiologic.

Gastrin appears to be synthesized and is certainly stored by G cells in the pyloric glands of antral mucosa[135] and in the mucosa of the proximal small intestine.[210] Gastrin is present in fundic mucosa in concentrations of 1×10^{-12} by weight, whereas in antral mucosa the concentration is more than 1000 times greater.[98] The duodenum in man contains 10 to 20 per cent as much gastrin as does the antrum[156] and appears to be physiologically active.[121]

Gastrin is released from G cells and is carried by the blood to effector sites in various organs of the gut. Gastrin and cholecystokinin and secretin act on the same target organs, and because of their structural similarity (Table 1), cholecystokinin and gastrin probably act on the same receptor site.[72] Secretin,[197] as well as other members of the secretin family of hormones (glucagon, gastric inhibitory polypeptide [GIP], and vasoactive intestinal polypeptide [VIP])[205] has been shown to block the action of gastrin on the parietal cell and, in addition, to block food-stimulated release of gastrin.[151] Calcium, given intravenously[153] or

TABLE 1. The Gastrin-Cholecystokinin Family

Gastrin[a]	Approximate Molecular Weight		
	I	II	

Little gastrin (G–17)

Position numbers: 1 2 3 4 5 6 7 8 9 10 11 12 13 14 15 16 17

Man — 2098 — 2178

Hog — 2116 — 2196

$$\text{Glp}^b\text{-Gly-Pro-Trp-Leu-Glu-Glu-Glu-Glu-Glu-Ala-Tyr}^c\text{-Gly-Trp-Met-Asp-Phe-NH}_2$$

(SO₂H on position 12: Tyr has SO_2H)

-Met- (Hog, position 5)

Minigastrin (G–14–I, 5–17)

Man — 1833

$$\text{Trp-Leu-Glu-Glu-Glu-Glu-Glu-Ala-Tyr-Gly-Trp-Met-Asp-Phe-NH}_2$$

Big gastrin (G–34–I)

Man — 3839

$$\text{Glp}^b\text{-Leu-Gly-Pro-Gln-Gly-His-Pro-Ser-Leu-Val-Ala-Asp-Pro-Ser-Lys-Lys}^d\text{-}$$
$$\text{Gln-Gly-Pro-Trp-Leu-Glu-Glu-Glu-Glu-Glu-Ala-Tyr-Gly-Trp-Met-Asp-Phe-NH}_2$$

Hog — 3883

$$\text{Glp}^b\text{-Leu-Gly-}Leu\text{-Gln-Gly-His-Pro-}Pro\text{-Leu-Val-Ala-Asp-}Leu\text{-}Ala\text{-Lys-Lys}^d$$
$$\text{Gln-Gly-Pro-Trp-}Met\text{-Glu-Glu-Glu-Glu-Glu-Ala-Tyr-Gly-Trp-Met-Asp Phe-NH}_2$$

Pentagastrin — 768

$$N\text{-t-butyloxycarbonyl-}\beta\text{- Ala-Trp-Met-Asp-Phe-NH}_2$$

Preprogastrin[e]

| Signal Peptide 21 aa | Amino Terminal Extension 37 aa | ArgArg | | LysLys | G17 | GlyArgArg | |

Carboxyl Terminal Extension 9 aa

G34

Cholecystokinin (CCK–33)[f] — 3918

$$\text{Lys-Ala-Pro-Ser-Glu-Arg-Val-}$$
$$\text{Ser-Met-Ile-Lys-Asn-Leu-Gln-Ser-}$$
$$\text{Leu-Asp-Pro-Ser-His-Arg-Ile-Ser-Asp-Arg-Asp-Tyr-Met-Gly-Trp-Met-Asp-Phe-NH}_2$$

(SO₃H attached to Tyr)

CCK-octapeptide (CCK–OP) — 1143

$$\text{-Asp-Tyr-Met-Gly-Trp-Met-Asp-Phe-NH}_2$$

(SO₃H attached to Tyr)

Modified from Thompson, J. C. (Ed.): Gastrointestinal Hormones. Austin, University of Texas Press, 1975, p. 653.

[a] Except where noted, the amino acid sequences for gastrins of different species are identical.

[b] Glp, pyroglutamyl.

[c] Gastrin of each species exists in forms I and II; in form I, there is no SO_3H attached to Tyr in position 12.

[d] Points of cleavage by trypsin.

[e] Modified from Daugherty and Yamada.[34]

[f] Other forms of CCK have been isolated (CCK–58, CCK–39, CCK–20, CCK–12 and CCK–4). All but the smallest possess cholecystokinetic activity.

orally,[154] stimulates gastric secretion by releasing gastrin. Cyclic AMP may be involved as an intraparietal cell second messenger, but the evidence that gastrin works by this pathway is at best inconclusive.[99]

Gastrin has been shown to disappear rapidly from the circulation,[155,196] probably owing to uptake by a widely distributed nonspecific process.[178,193] There is some evidence (especially the hypergastrinemia of patients in chronic renal failure[79]) that the kidneys may have an important role in the uptake of gastrin.

The Zollinger-Ellison syndrome[220,226] of massive gastric hypersecretion and peptic ulceration was shown by Gregory and colleagues[67] to be caused by high levels of circulating gastrin elaborated by gastrinomas of the pancreas or duodenum. Many patients with the Zollinger-Ellison syndrome have serum gastrin levels greater than 1000 pg. per ml., and some have values as high as 100,000 pg. per ml. Hypergastrinemia is also observed in patients with pernicious anemia (due to loss of acid inhibition on antral gastrin release), in patients with the antral exclusion operation (which causes permanent sequestration of antral mucosa in the alkaline environment of the duodenum), in

chronic renal failure (presumably caused by loss of normal renal catabolism),[79] and occasionally in patients with pyloric obstruction.

Because gastrin stimulates secretion of gastric acid and because the duodenal ulcer diathesis is associated with hypersecretion of acid, it might be assumed that patients with duodenal ulcer have high levels of circulating gastrin. Such is not the case. Only in the Zollinger-Ellison syndrome (and in rare patients with antral exclusion) is acid hypersecretion caused by excess gastrin; basal gastrin levels in patients with duodenal ulcer are normal (Fig. 8).

After all vagotomy procedures for duodenal ulcer, there is a *diminished* secretion of gastric acid but *elevated* basal and stimulated levels of gastrin. This postvagotomy hypergastrinemia is caused by a loss of vagal inhibition of gastrin release that appears to arise from the denervated gastric fundus.[194]

Serum gastrin concentrations are higher in patients with gastric ulcer than in patients with duodenal ulcer[203] probably because of lower acid output; in patients with gastric achlorhydria, serum gastrin levels are apt to be very high, and instillation of

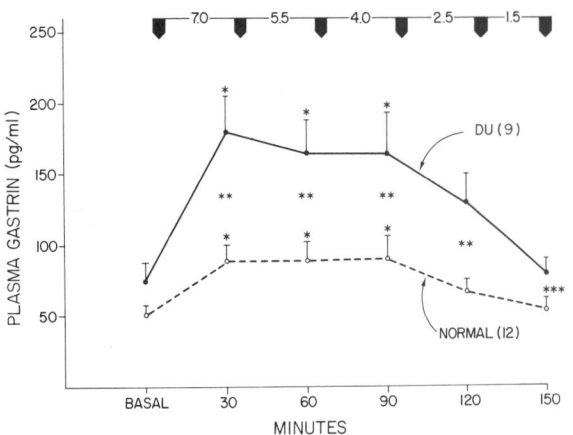

Figure 8. Plasma gastrin levels in response to an amino acid stimulation in duodenal ulcer patients (9) and normal subjects (12). Line at top shows varying pH levels of the 10 per cent amino acid meal (* an increase above basal values; ** significant difference between patients with duodenal ulcer and normal subjects; *** significantly less than peak *and* significant difference between patients with duodenal ulcers and normal subjects). (From Thompson, J. C., and Swierczek, J. S.: Acid and endocrine responses to meals varying in pH in normal and duodenal ulcer subjects. Ann. Surg., *186*:541, 1977.)

acid into the stomach causes an abrupt decrease in serum gastrin.

As a practical consideration, when should a gastrin assay be obtained? Serum gastrin measurements are indicated in any patient in whom the Zollinger-Ellison syndrome is suspected and specifically in patients with the following:

1. Recurrent peptic ulcer or recurrent peptic ulcer symptoms after an acid-reducing operation
2. Duodenal ulcer and massive hypersecretion of acid (greater than 15 mEq. per hour basal)
3. Duodenal ulcer and diarrhea
4. Duodenal ulcer and hypercalcemia
5. Relatives who have the Zollinger-Ellison syndrome or the multiple endocrine neoplasia I syndrome
6. Postbulbar or jejunal ulceration
7. Upper gastrointestinal radiologic studies suggestive of the Zollinger-Ellison syndrome
8. Duodenal ulcer in patients under 20 years of age
9. A previous operation for duodenal ulcer in which antral exclusion is suspected.

Intestinal Phase

There is clear evidence that various stimulants applied to the mid–small bowel can cause secretion of acid from a denervated gastric pouch.[190] The intestinal phase can be stimulated by the instillation of food, particularly proteins, or acids into the proximal jejunum. Distention of the jejunum also stimulates secretion.

The nature of the humoral agent of intestinal stimulation of gastric secretion has not been fully identified; part of the intestinal phase may be the result of absorbed amino acids (which, on parenteral injection, stimulate acid secretion).[95,164]

INHIBITION OF GASTRIC SECRETION

When secretion is stimulated by a meal, what halts the flow of acid? Vagal activity is decreased because cephalic stimulation is removed, but most important, the secretion of acid itself acts to block further release of gastrin and to cause active duodenal suppression of gastric secretion.

Antral acidification has been clearly demonstrated to suppress the release of gastrin.[222] Significant diminution in acid stimulation may occur with an antral pH as high as 5, and at approximately pH 1.5 there is no release of gastrin (Fig. 7).

Antral inhibition is due both to a passive removal of the gastrin stimulus[185] and probably to acid-stimulated release of antral somatostatin, which is probably the long-sought antral chalone.[185] There is clear evidence of active mechanisms of duodenal inhibition.[6,190] Gastric secretion is inhibited by the presence of acid, fat, or hypertonic solutions in the duodenum.

Acidification of the duodenum inhibits gastric secretion; it also releases secretin, and secretin is known to inhibit gastrin-stimulated gastric secretion. The suppressive effect of acidification of the duodenum has been confirmed in man, although the suppression is somewhat less effective in patients with duodenal ulcer than in normal man.[104] Acid-stimulated release of secretin is apparently not altered in patients with duodenal ulcer.[26,198]

Fat in the duodenum in an absorbable form is a highly effective inhibitor of postprandial gastric secretion. Gastric inhibitory polypeptide, secretin, and neurotensin are released by fat and probably have roles in the mediation of this inhibition.

PEPTIC ULCER AND OTHER SYNDROMES OF MUCOSAL INJURY

Peptic ulcer of the stomach and the duodenum afflicts more than 10 million citizens of the United States according to the best statistics, and probably only one half of the cases are recognized.[2] The condition is most common in men between the ages of 20 and 60, and the cost to our society is in excess of $1 billion per year. Evidence indicates that the incidence of duodenal ulcer is decreasing.[136,188] A survey[50] disclosed that hospital admissions for duodenal ulcer in the United States decreased by 43 per cent in the period 1970 to 1978 with no significant change in the number of admissions for gastric ulcer. In that period, deaths from peptic ulcer decreased by 31 per cent; this decrease involved gastric as well as duodenal ulcer. From 1966 to 1979, the number of operations for duodenal ulcer decreased by 40 per cent.[54] This decrease is due primarily to fewer operations for intractability. A comparison of experiences in six British hospitals 5 years before and 4 years after the introduction of cimetidine revealed a 39 per cent decrease in the number of operations for duodenal ulcer.[223] However, for reasons not understood, the incidence of and the number of operations for the life-threatening complications of duodenal ulcer, that is, bleeding and perforation, have not decreased as much.[10,134]

The ratio of men to women with peptic ulcer has decreased steadily; the male : female ratio for hospitalization for ulcer decreased from 2.2 in 1965 to 1.8 in 1981.[119]

Peptic ulcers may occur wherever mucosa is bathed by fundic secretion, and they are found in the esophagus, stomach, and duodenum, adjacent to Meckel's diverticula with ectopic gastric mucosa (rarely), and in any segment of bowel that may be surgically anastomosed to the gastric fundus. Acute ulcers are commonly shallow and multiple, whereas chronic ulcers are apt to be single, deep, and scirrhous.

PATHOGENESIS[71,170]

Abundant information is available from many studies,[76,167] but the pathogenesis of gastroduodenal ulcers is still not fully understood. No single theory explains all types of lesions. Duodenal ulcers tend to be associated with hypersecretion of acid, but only 40 per cent of patients with duodenal ulcers hypersecrete.[74] The increased familial incidence of duodenal ulcer may be explained by evidence that elevated serum pepsinogen I levels may serve as a subclinical marker for duodenal ulcer; 40 per cent of those who have the trait (inherited, apparently, as a mendelian autosomal dominant characteristic) develop an ulcer.[159] Gastric ulcers and stress ulcers associated with acute mucosal injury are not associated with the hypersecretion of acid. Nonetheless, the presence of acid is necessary in order for all peptic ulcers to occur.

It is perhaps worthwhile to use a simplistic model in considering the genesis of ulcers (Table 2). Several factors might be listed that tend to attack the mucosa, and others might properly be thought of as defense mechanisms against mucosal ulceration. Peptic ulcers are caused by acid-peptic digestion, and pepsin is inactive above a pH of 5.4 to 6, having an optimal pH of approximately 1.5. Acid-peptic digestion is the most potent agent attacking the mucosa. Recent studies have shown that nonsteroidal anti-inflammatory drugs (NSAIDs), especially aspirin, may injure the mucosa and allow back-diffusion of acid. The consumption of aspirin has increased enormously in this country (and in Australia), and the incidence of aspirin-induced gastric bleeding has increased concomitantly.

The true pathogenetic role of *Campylobacter pylori* in disrupting mucosal resistance to injury and exercising a causal relationship in ulcerogenesis is still controversial.[170] The organism has been found in the antrum of more than 95 per cent of patients with duodenal ulcer, but it is also present in 20 per cent of healthy volunteers and in 50 per cent of patients with dyspepsia but no ulcer. Some have ascribed the temporary healing of peptic ulcers brought about by the eradication of *Campylobacter*. A suggested model[170] for the pathogenesis of peptic ulcer is shown in Figure 9.

The mechanisms of mucosal defense are not well understood. The greater the fraction of nonparietal cell secretion in gastric juice, the lower is the concentration of H^+, but the mechanisms governing the relative stimulation of the parietal and nonparietal components of gastric secretion are unknown. Emptying of the acid gastric chyme into the crucible of the duodenal bulb where it is neutralized by HCO_3^- from bile and pancreatic juice is one of the most important defenses. The surface epithelium of the stomach and duodenum constitutes a barrier to the back-diffusion of H^+. The integrity of the mucosal barrier is enhanced by the rich blood supply of the mucosa of the stomach and duodenum. Prostaglandins have been shown to enhance mucosal resistance to ulceration; early evidence suggests that patients with duodenal ulcer may have a defect in prostaglandin synthesis.[1]

Classic opinion has held that duodenal ulcer is a condition in which aggressive forces of attack (increased potency of acid-peptic digestion) overcome relatively normal mucosal defenses, whereas in gastric ulcer relatively normal levels of acid-peptic activity overcome impaired gastric mucosal defenses (usually associated with "intestinalization" of stomach mucosa). Recent studies, however, have cast doubt on the normality of mucosal defenses in patients with duodenal ulcer. The secretion of bicarbonate and mucus in the duodenum may well be the main defense mechanism against acid.[57] Mucus adherent to the luminal surface of the mucosa provides a zone of low turbulence (unstirred layer), allowing the development of a gradient for HCO_3^- from the mucosal side and H^+ from the luminal side.[82] Small amounts of bicarbonate protect the mucosa against large

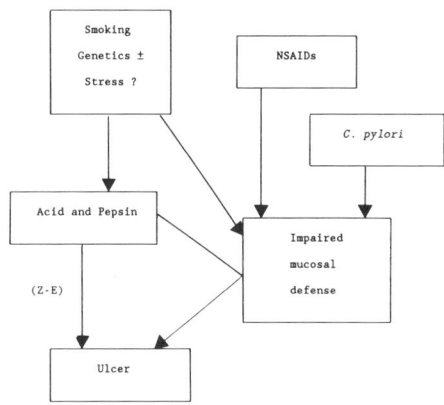

Figure 9. Pathogenesis of peptic ulcer. Mucosal defense mechanisms may be damaged by NSAIDs or *Campylobacter* and facilitate ulceration by acid-peptic juice. Smoking, genetics, and stress may affect both the mucosal defense and acid-pepsin secretion. The massive acid hypersecretion of the Z-E (Zollinger-Ellison syndrome) patient may directly overcome normal mucosa to produce an ulcer. *C. pylori* has been clearly shown to be associated with antral gastritis in children.[43] (Modified from Soll, A. H.: Pathogenesis of peptic ulcer and implications for therapy. N. Engl. J. Med., 322:909, 1990.)

amounts of acid by neutralizing H^+ ions that back-diffuse into the mucus layer. Impaired duodenal bicarbonate secretion is thought to have an important role in the pathogenesis of experimental[22,144,179] and clinical[96] duodenal ulcer disease. Isenberg and colleagues[96] have reported recently that patients with inactive duodenal ulcers have decreased production of bicarbonate, both basal and acid-stimulated, in the mucosa of the proximal duodenum. In this regard, the author has recently studied the problem of the increased incidence of duodenal ulcer that occurs with aging,[18,19,120] despite decreasing acid secretion.[12,74,109,111] Aged rats were found to have a defect in the secretion of duodenal bicarbonate, which suggests that a breakdown in mucosal defenses may be responsible for the age-related increase in duodenal ulcer.[112]

Duodenal Ulcer

The association of duodenal ulcer with acid hypersecretion is firmly established. In most collected series, the mean basal and maximal acid output of patients with duodenal ulcer is one and one half to two times as great as that of control patients, and Cox[33] has shown that the stomachs of patients with duodenal ulcer have almost twice the number of parietal cells as do normal stomachs (normal is about one billion). Samloff and colleagues[161] have shown increased levels of serum Group I pepsinogen in patients with duodenal ulcer and have suggested that the acid secretory potential of the stomach may be reflected by the level of serum Group I pepsinogens. Patients with ulcers show increased acid response to stimulation with protein[198] and with the gastrin analog pentagastrin.[94] In addition, evidence is available that these patients show an increased rate of gastric emptying and an increased acid load delivered to the duodenum[76]; the author[198] was unable to confirm earlier evidence[208] of diminished acid inhibition of gastrin release. There is as yet no evidence that duodenal defense mechanisms are faulty in patients who develop duodenal ulcer.

Strong public opinion holds that emotional factors have an important role in the development of peptic ulcer. Feldman and associates[51] have provided evidence that these patients handle ordinary life-stresses poorly. Diet and alcohol appear to have no role, but smoking appears to predispose to ulcer.

Gastric Ulcer

Whereas duodenal ulcers appear to be caused by increased potency of the acid-peptic forces attacking the mucosa, gastric ulcers may be related primarily to injury of the gastric mucosa, which renders it more susceptible to acid-peptic damage. Most

TABLE 2. Factors Involved in the Pathogenesis of Peptic Ulceration

Enzymatic Digestion of Mucous Membrane

Attack	Defense
Acid-peptic digestion (pH < 4)	Dilution (nonparietal secretion)
Drugs (salicylates, steroids)	Emptying
Trauma	Neutralization (HCO_3^- from bile and pancreas)
Ischemia	Mucosal barrier including mucosal secretion of HCO_3^- (probably most important)
	Rich blood supply
	No acid—no ulcer

studies report that patients with gastric ulcers secrete either low-normal or below-normal amounts of acid, and only 5 per cent of patients with gastric ulcer demonstrate acid hypersecretion.[74] The evidence is now abundant that reflux of bile and pancreatic juice is involved in the pathogenesis of gastric ulcer.[167] Gastric reflux of bile after meals is increased in patients with gastric ulcer,[44,157] which may be caused, at least in part, by dysfunction of the pyloric sphincter.[55] Bile salts apparently damage the mucosa, which is then attacked by acid-peptic digestion.[37,44] Gastric ulcers invariably occur in areas of gastritis.[37,44] Because the gastritis progresses proximally from the pylorus, patients with gastric ulcer have a larger distal area of alkaline mucosa, and gastric ulcers lie in achlorhydric zones of mucosa.[27] The great majority of gastric ulcers (up to 95 per cent) occur on the lesser curvature near the incisura angularis (see Fig. 1).

Acute Mucosal Erosions (Stress Ulcers)[202]

Acute superficial ulcerative lesions of the gastroduodenal area have been variously termed acute mucosal erosions, stress ulcers, acute peptic ulcers, erosive gastritis, hemorrhagic gastritis, and Curling's or Cushing's ulcers. The last two eponymic lesions have specific causes, burns and head injury, respectively; the other terms are approximately synonymous and are often used interchangeably. None of the terms is satisfactory.

The mechanism whereby stress causes mucosal ulceration is poorly understood. If a rat is restrained for 24 hours, it develops multiple superficial gastric erosions.[23] In stress ulceration, the stomach appears to be the target organ for metabolic alterations caused by a number of diseases that in the past progressed rapidly to a fatal outcome. With improved techniques for resuscitation and intensive care, patients now survive these diseases long enough to become susceptible to a sequential series of organ failures: gastrointestinal, pulmonary, renal, hepatic, and cardiac. After long periods of hypotension or sepsis or pulmonary insufficiency, the patients become so debilitated that they may be the victims of whichever organ system fails first. The high concentration of acid and digestive enzymes in the stomach and duodenum renders this area especially vulnerable to autolysis. Much attention has been given to the study of the gastric mucosal barrier, which prevents the back-diffusion of H^+, and to the luminal diffusion of Na^+ ion.[36,84,213] Hollander[87] defined the gastric mucosal barrier as a two-component system consisting of a layer of mucus covering the luminal surface of the stomach and a layer of columnar epithelial cells beneath it. The extent of protection provided by the unstirred layer of mucus is difficult to evaluate. The mucus may facilitate the protective role of duodenal bicarbonate secretion. The row of apical membranes of the epithelial cells is apparently essential. Aspirin has been shown to damage these membranes,[36] and shock and sepsis as well as other metabolic disturbances may also compromise the function of the barrier, but this has never been proved. When acid enters the cell, damage occurs that may allow further back-diffusion of acid with resultant release of histamine, which causes vasodilation and bleeding[35] (Fig. 10). An episode of hemorrhagic or septic shock often precedes acute mucosal bleeding in man. Many critically ill patients have small bowel ileus with consequent bile reflux, which contributes, along with shock, to mucosal injury. A strong correlation between increased gastric mucosal permeability and the incidence of sepsis, hypotension, and respiratory and renal failure has been reported.[63]

There is abundant evidence that many of these desperately ill patients have a great deficit in energy. The deficit is surely enhanced by poor tissue perfusion and poor nutrition. Indeed, the great recent decrease in the number of patients requiring operation for stress bleeding may be a fortuitous dividend of the early application of fluid resuscitation and total parenteral nutrition in severely ill patients who are at risk.

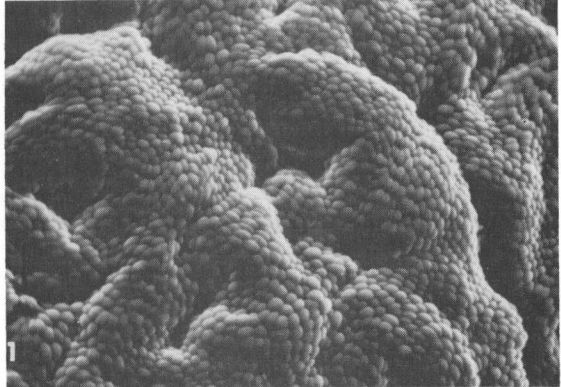
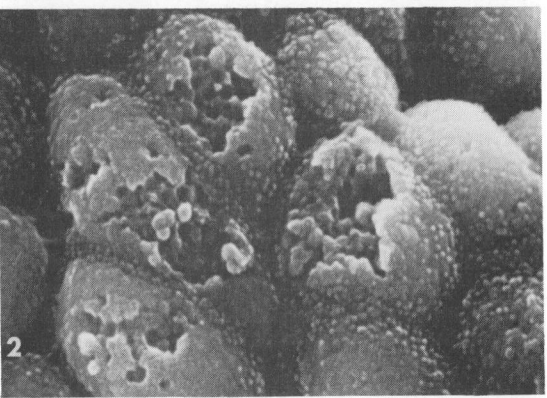
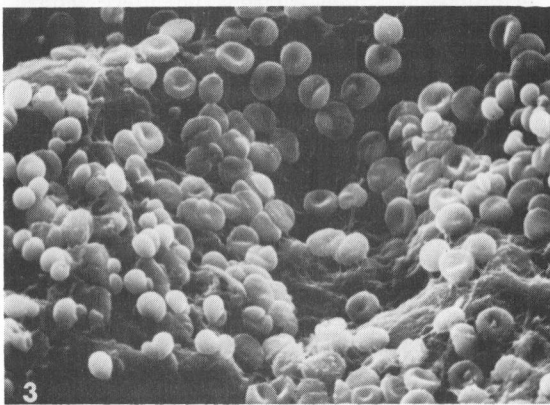

Figure 10. Scanning electron micrographs of gastric mucosa. *1*, Normal surface topography ($\times375$) showing folds, gastric pits, and numerous epithelial cells. *2*, High magnification ($\times8000$) showing damage to four surface epithelial cells demonstrating disruption of apical membrane. *3*, Section taken from area of hemorrhagic gastritis ($\times2000$). Surface of epithelial cells covered with network of fibrin containing many erythrocytes. (From Lucas, C. E., et al.: Natural history and surgical dilemma of "stress" gastric bleeding. Arch. Surg., *102*:266, 1971. Copyright 1971, American Medical Association.)

Sepsis may well be the most important etiologic factor. Undrained pus is responsible for a high proportion of stress ulcers. Upper gastrointestinal bleeding occurring in a critically ill patient is a signal to search for pus.[202]

The pathogenesis of the acute mucosal lesions that occur in neurological or neurosurgical patients (Cushing's ulcer) almost certainly is different from the pathogenesis of other stress-induced lesions. Patients with acute gastric hemorrhage associated with injury to the central nervous system tend to have higher acid secretory levels than do other patients with acute mucosal lesions.[63,177] In a study of 39 United States servicemen injured in Vietnam, Bowen and colleagues[20] found the levels of serum gastrin in patients with central nervous system (CNS) injury to be higher than in patients with injuries not involving the CNS. The higher rate of acid secretion and higher gastrin levels strongly suggest that patients with head injury may have increased vagal activity.

Certain factors appear to be required for the development of acute mucosal erosions: ischemia, the presence of even small amounts of acid, and disruption of the gastric mucosal barrier, which causes increased back-diffusion of H^+.[167]

DUODENAL ULCER

Duodenal ulcer is a chronic disease that was formerly considered to be four times more common in men than in women; Kurata and associates[119] suggest that there may currently be little difference in the sex distribution. Duodenal ulcer may appear at any age but occurs most frequently between the ages of 20 and 60 and has previously been considered to have a peak incidence in the fourth decade of life; recent studies suggest an increasing incidence with increasing age.[18,19,120] The clinical course is characterized by long periods of remission and periods of exacerbation that may last from days to months. The primary symptom is pain, which classically is perceived in the epigastrium in the midline. The pain is often relieved by food or milk or antacid, and the most important differential characteristic of the pain is that it often awakens the patient 2 or 3 hours after going to sleep. After relieving the pain with food or antacid, the patient may go to sleep and awaken in the morning without pain. Heartburn, a burning substernal discomfort, is common in patients with duodenal ulcer and apparently is due to regurgitation of acid into the esophagus (it may be a symptom of hiatal hernia). Early satiety, anorexia, and nausea are often experienced by patients in the early phases of the development of the ulcer. Even during exacerbation, the pain usually lasts for only a few hours at a time. A change in the pattern of pain so that it becomes continuous and no longer is relieved by antacid usually signifies a posterior penetration of the ulcer crater. Atypical pain patterns are often observed in children and in patients with ulcers at the pylorus or distal to the duodenal bulb. Pain is frequently absent in postbulbar ulcers. When present, however, it often has bizarre characteristics and is often unresponsive to antacid therapy.

ASSOCIATED CONDITIONS

It is difficult to prove true statistical relationships between diseases. Increased incidences of duodenal ulcer have been reported in hyperparathyroidism, polycythemia rubra vera, chronic liver disease, uremia, chronic respiratory insufficiency, and certain CNS lesions, as well as after burns and portacaval shunting. One difficulty in establishing statistical relationships is the disparity between the incidence of peptic ulcer in clinical and in autopsy series and the uncertainty as to whether an appropriate control series would consist of chronically ill patients or of patients who are well.[123] The incidence of peptic ulcer in the general population has been variously estimated to be 5 to 15 per cent. In order to be meaningful, any series purporting to demonstrate a slight to moderate increase in the incidence of peptic ulcer must be compared with a local control series.

Evidence for an etiologic relationship with peptic ulcer disease appears to be strongest for hyperparathyroidism, chronic respiratory insufficiency,[58,214] cirrhosis, and nonhypertensive cardiovascular disease.[123] In no instance, however, is the evidence compelling; the purported relationship of cirrhosis and portacaval shunt with peptic ulcer has been reviewed,[183] and the evidence has been found to be insufficient. Healthy skepticism is warranted.

DIAGNOSIS

A presumption of the presence of a duodenal ulcer may be made from a patient's history, but definitive diagnosis depends on either endoscopy or radiology. In the past, radiologic diag-

nosis was given precedence, but fiberoptic endoscopy has now become the standard by which all diagnostic procedures are graded. Even so, if a duodenal ulcer is clearly demonstrated on upper gastrointestinal radiography, there is usually no indication to confirm the finding by endoscopy, unless the patient is bleeding. Radiography costs much less than endoscopy, and this must be considered.

History

Most important in the history is the character of the pain. It may take various forms and be interpreted in various ways. Care should be taken to avoid misunderstanding because of different connotations given to the word "pain." It is often necessary to use several synonyms, "discomfort," "ache," "pressure," or even "hunger pain," in order to be sure that disavowal of pain is valid. The pain is often exacerbated by certain foods, such as tomato sauce, hot spices, fried food, onions, or alcohol. There are many individuals who have frequent episodes of epigastric pain and heartburn for years and who obtain relief with antacids, but in whom a duodenal ulcer is never demonstrated; conversely, after treatment with H_2-antagonists, some patients are found to have persistent ulcer craters, even though their symptoms have long abated. What is important in this disparity between symptoms and pathology is that approximately 15 to 20 per cent of patients who require treatment for perforation or bleeding due to duodenal ulcer have a silent ulcer, that is, they have no antecedent history of ulcer pain.

Radiology

The radiologic diagnosis of duodenal ulcer is 75 to 80 per cent accurate. The patient may show an actual crater deformity indicative of active disease, or may merely demonstrate scarring of the duodenal bulb caused by previous ulceration. Approximately 95 per cent of duodenal ulcers occur in the duodenal bulb (see Fig. 6), and 5 per cent are postbulbar. An indetermin-

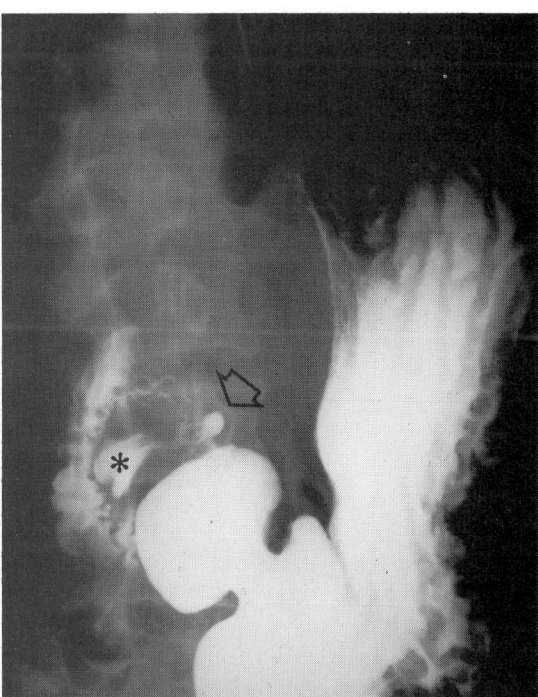

Figure 11. Radiograph of the stomach and duodenum. The arrow points to an ulcer crater of the bulb shown tangentially. The asterisk lies within a pseudodiverticulum produced by scarring. Irritability and scarring prevent filling of the duodenal bulb with barium. (This and subsequent radiographs are from the teaching files of the Department of Radiology, University of Texas Medical Branch, Galveston. They were selected in consultation with Melvyn H. Schreiber, M.D.)

ate number occur in the pyloric canal and are often termed *channel ulcers.*

The normal duodenal bulb is rounded and full. Ulcer disease usually causes irritability, and the bulb becomes difficult to fill with contrast material (Fig. 11).

The most important sign in the diagnosis of duodenal ulcer is the demonstration of the ulcer crater itself. Because ulcer craters are much more commonly located on the anterior or posterior wall of the duodenal bulb, the crater is more likely to be seen *en face* (Fig. 12).

Although postbulbar ulcers (Fig. 13) may occur anywhere in the duodenum distal to the bulb, 75 per cent of postbulbar ulcers occur proximal to the duodenal papilla.[141] They are often small and buried in folds. Because of this and perhaps because of their relative rarity, they are often overlooked. Approximately 15 per cent of patients with postbulbar ulcers also have an ulcer located in the bulb.[31]

With healing, the duodenal ulcer becomes smaller and may finally disappear altogether. At other times, the ulcer may heal as a pitted scar and a tiny excavation may remain, which may erroneously be interpreted as an active ulcer. The cloverleaf deformity of the duodenal bulb seen in healed ulcer disease is the consequence of fibrosis following inflammation. This scarring often makes the incisurae and pseudodiverticula permanent.

Fiberoptic Endoscopy

The development of the flexible fiberoptic panendoscope has greatly facilitated diagnosis of peptic ulcer disease (Fig. 14A to

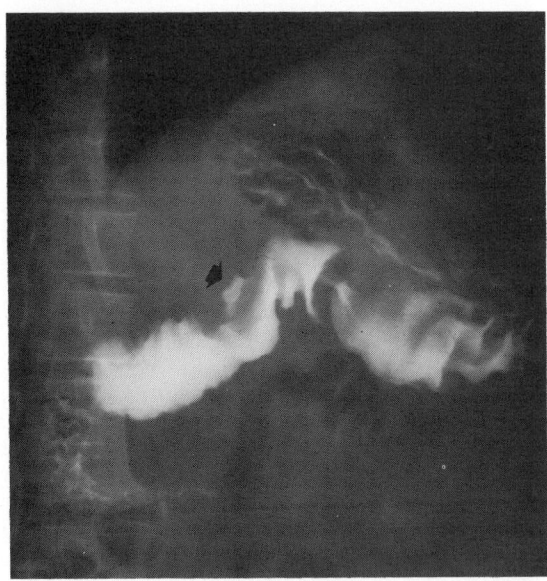

Figure 13. Tangential view of large postbulbar ulcer (arrow) with ring of edematous mucosa around the base of the ulcer.

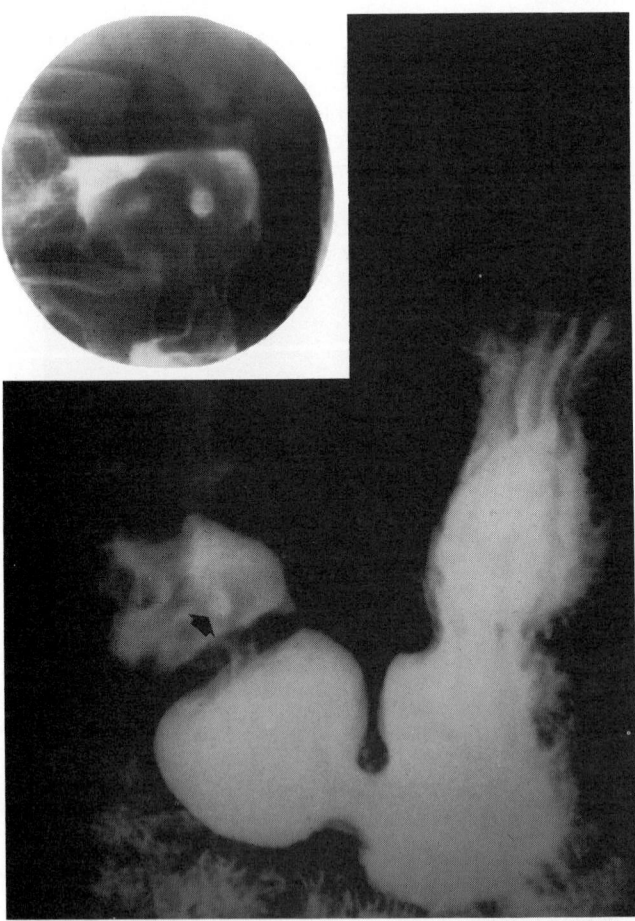

Figure 12. Radiograph of the stomach and duodenum showing a large ulcer crater of the duodenal bulb *en face* (arrow). The mucosal fold just distal to the ulcer crater is thickened and edematous. The compression film (inset) shows displacement of barium by pressure from all areas of the bulb except the ulcer crater, to which the barium remains adherent.

E). A diagnostic accuracy of 95 per cent or even greater may be achieved, and the evidence is clear that endoscopy is superior to radiography in defining the presence of lesions of the esophagus, stomach, and duodenum. In as many as one fourth of patients examined, the side-viewing fiberoptic endoscope is required to correctly visualize the duodenal ulceration. In addition to demonstrating the actual presence of the lesions, endoscopy provides further information: the operator can biopsy the lesion, touch it with the scope to determine its consistency, and most important, detect any bleeding (Fig. 14B). Endoscopy is especially valuable in bleeding patients. Roentgenograms may show an ulcer or esophageal varices, but not the site of bleeding. In addition to providing information on whether varices or ulcers are bleeding, endoscopy has its greatest value in demonstrating Mallory-Weiss tears of the gastroesophageal junction, acute mucosal erosions, gastritis (Fig. 14G), duodenitis, and marginal ulcers (Fig. 14H), none of which is well demonstrated by barium contrast radiologic studies.

Gastric Analysis

The clinical value of gastric secretory tests has been reviewed.[91,122] It is not possible to make a diagnosis of duodenal ulcer by means of gastric analysis (the author recently studied a 70-year-old woman who had a basal acid secretion of 40 mEq. per hour who did not have a peptic ulcer), but very low secretory values (a maximal acid output of less than 12 mEq. per hour, for example) make the diagnosis of duodenal ulcer unlikely.

Is prognosis in a duodenal ulcer patient related to the severity of hypersecretion? The data are not clear, but Krag[116] followed a series of ulcer patients for several years and concluded that those patients with a higher acid output had a significantly more serious clinical course and required operation more often than those with low gastric secretory levels. It should, however, be known that postoperative recurrence cannot be related to the degree of preoperative hypersecretion.[4] In some patients with ulcers, there is a sharp decrease in acid secretory rates when the ulcer heals.[126]

Gastric analysis is currently utilized less because it lacks precise correlation with disease. The test is uncomfortable for the patient, and the physician is often unsure of the role of gastric analysis in planning treatment for the patient. There are three indications for gastric analysis in surgical patients: (1) pre- and postoperative measurement of gastric acid secretion allows the

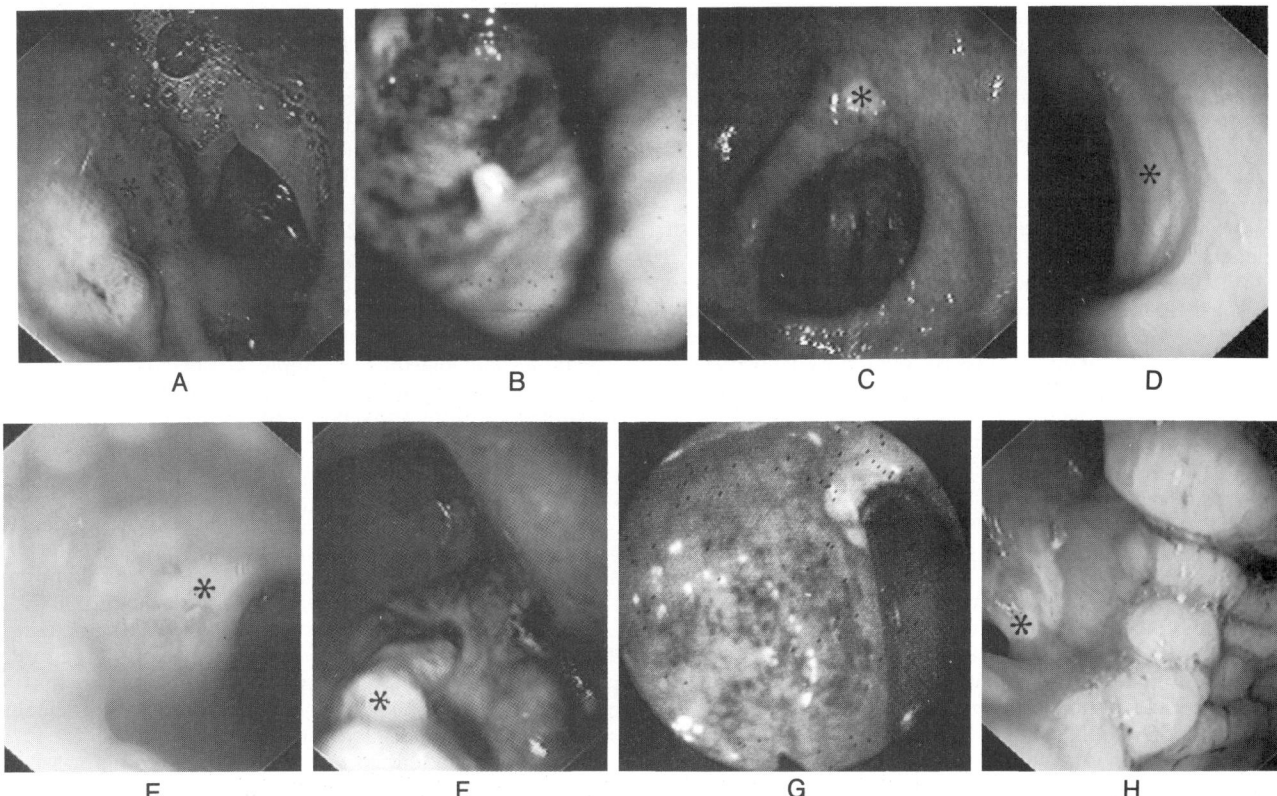

Figure 14. Endoscopic views of gastroduodenal pathology. *A*, Active duodenal ulcer with bile staining of crater. *B*, Bleeding duodenal ulcer with visible vessel. The papillary structure in the center is the vessel. This finding is associated with a 70 per cent likelihood of rebleeding, and many endoscopists believe that it is an indication for either cautery or sclerosis, even when not actively bleeding. *C*, Small benign gastric ulcer at the incisura angularis. *D*, Large gastric ulcer on proximal lesser curvature. Ulcer was benign on biopsy. *E*, Pyloric channel ulcer. *F*, Large fungating gastric cancer with small area of ulceration. *G*, Erosive gastritis. This patient bled massively, but hemorrhage subsided spontaneously. *H*, Bleeding marginal ulcer. Gastric mucosa is to the right, and the folded suture line is in the center. (Endoscopic photographs courtesy of William H. Nealon, M.D.)

best current means for evaluation of the success of any acid-reducing operation; (2) gastric analysis is an important factor in patients in whom the Zollinger-Ellison syndrome is suspected; and (3) in patients with gastric ulcer, the demonstration of achlorhydria would strongly point to carcinoma.

TREATMENT

A large percentage of patients, perhaps most with duodenal ulcer, never have any formal treatment. These patients may manage their difficulties quite well with the occasional administration of a solution of bicarbonate of soda or with proprietary antacid tablets (Tums or Rolaids). Of patients whose ulcer diathesis is sufficiently severe to require medical attention, probably 85 per cent may be managed successfully by medical therapy.

The various H_2-receptor antagonists have proved highly successful in the treatment of uncomplicated duodenal ulcer.[92,181] Approximately 70 per cent of acute ulcers heal,[219] and many do not require chronic treatment. One standard course of therapy is cimetidine 300 mg. four times per day for 4 to 6 weeks. Ranitidine, a related H_2-blocker, is similarly effective in doses of 150 mg. given twice a day; famotidine is even longer acting. There are few side effects (rare gynecomastia and occasional drowsiness). The rate of ulcer recurrence after discontinuing H_2-blockade therapy is high (up to 80 per cent), even after prolonged administration.[93,101]

Medical Treatment

A legitimate aim of all ulcer therapy is to maintain the intraluminal pH above approximately 5.5 so that pepsinogen is not activated. The mainstay of this effort formerly was antacid therapy, but H_2-receptor blockade has proved so effective and

"user-friendly" that it is now the most common and most effective. The choices among different drugs (cimetidine, ranitidine, famotidine, and others) are governed mainly by the cost and duration of action of the drugs. Omeprazole is a relatively new and highly potent suppressor of acid secretion that achieves its effect by blocking the proton-pump in the parietal cell that actually secretes H^+. It is long-lasting and actually renders the stomach achlorhydric for long periods. Because of this, omeprazole treatment may induce sustained hypergastrinemia,[115] which (if prolonged) has the possibility (at least experimentally) of causing carcinoid tumors of the stomach.[49,221]

H_2-receptor blockade treatment was initially designed for a brief intensive period to heal the ulcer. When it became apparent that drug therapy did not alter the basic ulcer diathesis and that recurrence rates after the brief intensive period were approximately 70 to 80 per cent, the concept of maintenance therapy (usually one pill at night) was popularized. The true cost of lifelong maintenance therapy has not been accurately estimated. Costs are a vital consideration today, and governmental agencies are deeply involved in projecting long-term costs. Will surgical therapy, which offers a much higher cure rate and, with selective proximal vagotomy, a low rate of complications, ultimately prove to be more economical than lifelong medical therapy? By current cost estimates, long-term H_2-receptor antagonist treatment appears to be less costly than ulcer surgery for uncomplicated ulcer disease for up to 8 years, but maintenance drug therapy beyond 8 years may be more expensive than elective ulcer surgery.[101] Another study suggests that in Europe (but not in the United States where surgical costs are higher) selective proximal vagotomy proved to be cost-effective in preventing ulcer recurrence after 6 years.[172] Many surgeons have regarded it ironic that the physiologic operation for ulcer disease (selective proximal vagotomy) was devised after there appeared to be a spontaneous diminution in the severity of ulcer disease, and highly effective medical therapy became available. Only time will tell which of the treatments is more cost-effective.

In the past, patients with duodenal ulcers were almost routinely admonished to control their diet in a rigid manner, and the hallmark of having an ulcer was the grueling necessity of adhering to an unpalatable white diet. It is now generally recognized that diet has little role in the treatment of ulcers. If a patient has an exacerbation of pain after eating pizza, onions, or fried foods, he should obviously avoid them. It is probably not wise for the patient to eat just before bedtime. An H_2-receptor blocker or a dose of antacid is recommended. Milk is widely used in the treatment of ulcer disease, but there are few data to support its efficacy; in fact, calcium stimulates gastrin release and acid secretion.[9,153,154]

Many physicians use tranquilizers in managing hyperkinetic, anxious patients who have symptomatic ulcers. Mild sedation may be helpful, rarely, during periods of acute exacerbation, but routine use of sedation should be rigorously avoided.

Indications for Surgical Treatment

Fewer than one in five patients with long-standing duodenal ulcer require operation.[69,200] Surgical techniques in operations on the stomach are discussed in a subsequent section. The complications of duodenal ulcer that require surgical management are hemorrhage, perforation, obstruction, and intractability.

HEMORRHAGE. Bleeding is the most serious complication of peptic ulcer and is responsible for approximately 40 per cent of deaths due to the disease. Bleeding may be chronic and insidious or brisk and life-threatening. Even when large vessels are eroded by enzymatic digestion, bleeding is usually self-limited and it is rare for a patient to bleed continuously to death. Spontaneous remission of the hemorrhage occurs when the blood pressure falls because of hypovolemic shock and a clot then forms on the ulcer crater. Bleeding may be heralded by several days of exacerbation of pain or may arise *de novo* in a patient who has never had ulcer symptoms. Bleeding from duodenal ulcer is usually manifested by passage of black tarry stools (melena), but with rapid bleeding, bright red blood may appear per rectum and blood may also regurgitate into the stomach and be vomited. Hematemesis usually connotes more rapid and serious loss of blood than does melena alone, although some patients with bleeding ulcers may have sufficient pyloric stenosis that they do not regurgitate blood regardless of the briskness of the hemorrhage. Repeated attempts to manage gastrointestinal bleeding by somatostatin have been largely unsuccessful.[30,171]

Mortality for operations on patients during acute bleeding episodes are several times greater than for elective operations. Everything possible must be done to stop the bleeding so that the patient may be resuscitated and evaluated for elective operation. Obviously, however, if the patient continues to bleed, as less than 10 per cent of patients do, emergent operation may be lifesaving.

A patient with signs and symptoms of significant bleeding should receive blood replacement. Blood should be drawn at once for hematocrit measurement and for blood typing and crossmatching. Two large-bore plastic catheters should be inserted into peripheral or central veins; one in the latter position could be used for estimation of central venous blood pressure. If the patient has a history of cardiopulmonary problems, a Swan-Ganz catheter should be placed as well as a nasogastric tube into the stomach and connected to suction. Hematemesis, or the presence of gross blood in the gastric aspirate, indicates that the source of bleeding is proximal to the ligament of Treitz. A urinary catheter should be inserted for measurement of hourly urinary output; a urinary output of more than 30 ml. per hour should be maintained if possible.

The availability of fiberoptic endoscopy has revolutionized the emergency management of patients with massive upper gastrointestinal bleeding. The procedure is safe and accurate and provides critical information quickly (see Fig. 14). In a series of 195 consecutive patients admitted to the author's hospital with massive gastrointestinal hemorrhage (Table 3),[206] 14 were later found to be bleeding from lesions distal to the ligament of Treitz. In three others, no diagnosis was made and the patients stopped bleeding spontaneously. Only five diagnostic errors were made in this series (2.6 per cent). Of the 50 bleeding patients in whom the final diagnosis was duodenal ulcer, a correct endoscopic diagnosis was made in 49 (Fig. 14). Yajko and colleagues[224] reported correct endoscopic diagnosis of the cause of bleeding in 80 per cent of 200 patients with massive upper gastrointestinal bleeding. Multiple prospective studies have provided evidence that early endoscopy in patients with massive upper gastrointestinal hemorrhage does not improve eventual mortality. Nonetheless, endoscopy greatly facilitates therapeutic planning, and most clinicians caring for these patients rely heavily on it.

What are the criteria for deciding which bleeding patients should be operated upon? Any patient who has suffered a massive blood loss, by any of the following criteria, should be considered a *candidate* for operation: (1) loss of 1500 to 2000 ml. of blood; (2) blood loss that causes an acute fall in the hematocrit to 25 or below; (3) acute blood loss causing syncope; (4) after the patient's vital signs have been stabilized, blood loss that requires more than 1000 ml. of blood per 24 hours to maintain a stable hematocrit and stable blood pressure.

If a patient is admitted to the hospital bleeding massively, stops bleeding spontaneously and is completely resuscitated, and then has another massive hemorrhage while hospitalized, operation is indicated. There are other factors that may influence a decision to operate. Usually, the older the patient, the more life-threatening is hemorrhagic shock, and the older patients should be operated upon earlier. When massive hemorrhage intervenes in a patient who is already seriously ill with another disease, the added stress of bleeding may be an intolerable risk and early operation may be indicated. Patients who have had a long history of difficulty with their ulcer, previous hemorrhages, severe pain, or previous perforation should be operated upon earlier than patients in whom hemorrhage is the initial ulcer symptom. Another practical consideration may influence the decision: if the patient has a rare blood type or if there is a shortage of the patient's specific type for any reason, a decision to operate may be precipitated.

When the decision has been made to operate, efforts should be made to empty the stomach. Great care should be taken to

TABLE 3. Final Diagnosis in 195 Consecutive Patients with Gastrointestinal Bleeding

Diagnosis	Number of Patients	Per Cent
Duodenal ulcer	50	25.6
Hemorrhagic gastritis	35	17.9
Bleeding esophageal varices	29	14.9
Mallory-Weiss tears	15	7.7
Gastric ulcer	20	10.3
Esophagitis	7	3.6
Carcinoma	7	3.6
Miscellaneous	15	7.7
Normal (lesions below the ligament of Treitz)	14	7.2
No diagnosis	3	1.5
Total	195	

Modified from Villar, H. V., Fender, H. R., Watson, L. C., and Thompson, J. C.: Emergency diagnosis of upper gastrointestinal bleeding by fiberoptic endoscopy. Ann. Surg., *185*:367, 1977.

prevent vomiting and aspiration of gastric contents during induction of anesthesia by insertion of an endotracheal tube and inflating the balloon cuff around the tube while the patient is still awake. The sequelae of aspiration are often fatal.

At operation, the surgeon should proceed quickly to identify and suture the point of bleeding, following which the procedures of choice are usually vagotomy and a drainage procedure (pyloroplasty or gastroenterostomy) and vagotomy with distal gastric resection. An argument for early operative approach in upper gastrointestinal bleeding is provided in a retrospective study[165] of more than 2100 patients admitted to the emergency hospital at Oxford for a 15-year period, which reported that 81 per cent of the patients had a previous history of gastric symptoms and one third had bled previously. There was a steady decline in surgical mortality during the 15 years, but the overall mortality showed little change. The authors suggested that more patients should be treated by early operation in order to achieve an overall reduction in the mortality.

Hemorrhage occurs when a posterior penetrating ulcer erodes into a blood vessel. Another quite rare complication of posterior penetration of an ulcer is erosion into the common bile duct. Fistulas between the gallbladder and gastrointestinal tract are usually caused by erosion of gallstones, but fistulas between the duodenum and common bile duct are usually caused by peptic ulcers.[40,52]

PERFORATION. Perforation of a duodenal ulcer produces a remarkable series of dramatic changes. Immediately prior to perforation, the patient may feel entirely well, within a few minutes be in great pain, and within an hour be desperately ill. As already noted, hemorrhage is associated with *posterior* erosion of an ulcer; perforation occurs when an anteriorly or laterally placed ulcer erodes through the full thickness of the wall of the duodenum into the free peritoneal cavity, spilling acid-peptic juice, bile, and pancreatic juice into the peritoneal cavity. These chemically active ferments cause havoc; the resultant chemical injury has been aptly compared with a burn of the peritoneum. Within a short time, massive amounts of extracellular fluid may be sequestered in the area of peritoneal injury, and this loss of fluid may cause hypovolemic shock. Perforated ulcers are usually not associated with significant loss of blood.

Diagnosis in most cases is not difficult, but in atypical instances it may be extraordinarily so. Other conditions to be considered are acute pancreatitis, acute appendicitis, acute cholecystitis, and less commonly diverticulitis or acute pyelonephritis.[187]

The patient usually gives a typical history of the sudden development of severe epigastric and later generalized abdominal pain. Movement is painful and the patient lies still. If there is delay in reaching the hospital, shock may ensue.

Examination of the abdomen usually reveals considerable guarding and often boardlike rigidity of the abdominal musculature. With free air in the peritoneal cavity, there is often a loss of the normal dullness on percussion over the liver. If gastric contents have flowed into the right lower quadrant guided by the attachment of the small bowel mesentery, the patient may have signs and symptoms of peritonitis in the right lower quadrant, which may confuse the diagnosis and suggest appendicitis.

Approximately 75 per cent of patients demonstrate free air under the diaphragm on an upright chest film (Fig. 15) or on a lateral decubitus film if the patient is unable to sit. Conversely, this means that approximately one in four patients with perforated duodenal ulcer do not show free air, and that it is perfectly proper, if other evidence warrants, to make the diagnosis of perforation *without* the demonstration of free intraperitoneal air on upright chest films or on lateral abdominal decubitus films.

Although there has been repeated interest in the nonoperative management of perforated duodenal ulcer, the overwhelming consensus of surgeons in the United States is that this cata-

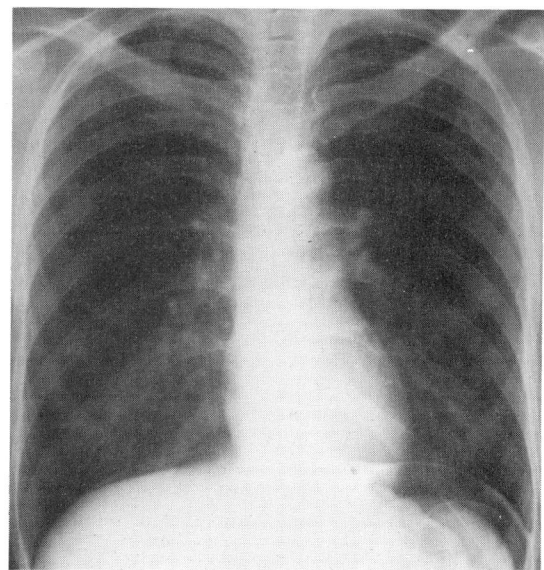

Figure 15. Chest film taken with the patient in the upright position. Free air is clearly visible under both the right and the left leaves of the diaphragm. This patient had a perforated duodenal ulcer.

strophic event should be treated by surgical repair. Mortality for early operation is low, but risk increases with delay. The leak in the duodenum must be closed rapidly in order to reduce the extent of peritoneal contamination.

At operation, the site of perforation should be located and closed with an omental patch (Graham closure) or incorporated into a pyloroplasty, which, when coupled with a vagotomy, not only repairs the perforation by reducing acid secretion but also serves as definitive treatment for the duodenal ulcer. Pyloroplasty of the scarred duodenum is often difficult. For the last 5 years, the author has been pleased with the results of a Graham closure plus truncal vagotomy and gastroenterostomy in patients selected for an acid-reducing operation. Because vagotomy and drainage provide definitive treatment for the ulcer diathesis, and because definitive treatment is required eventually by a large percentage of patients treated initially by simple closure, it is proper to advocate vagotomy and drainage in the treatment of perforated duodenal ulcer in patients with long-standing ulcer disease *except* in instances in which the risk is high. Patients without trouble with an ulcer, or those in whom the ulcer arises from a temporary stressful situation, may be candidates for simple closure of the perforation.[39] There is a close correlation between pre- and postperforation symptoms. A group of patients were studied for the presence of ulcer symptoms after simple closure of perforation; of those who had no symptoms before, 72 per cent were asymptomatic after operation; of those with previous ulcer symptoms, only 23 per cent were asymptomatic.[163]

After management of the perforation, great care should be taken to cleanse the peritoneal cavity with warm Ringer's lactate solution to dilute and remove contamination.

OBSTRUCTION. Patients with chronic duodenal ulcer may develop gastric outlet obstruction caused by chronic cicatrization in which scar contracture gradually narrows the lumen. In this instance, patients with a massively dilated stomach may seek help after months of intermittent obstruction or they may suddenly undergo complete obstruction of the pylorus and vomit perniciously for several days. Because of the massive loss of H^+ and Cl^-, the patient may have a severe hypochloremic alkalosis along with hypokalemia. The potassium deficiency is due to a moderate loss from vomiting (gastric juice has approximately 10 mEq. K^+ per liter) and to an important renal loss caused by substitution of K^+ for H^+. It is necessary to correct the hypokalemia as well as the hypochloremic alkalosis. Administration of sodium chloride and potassium chloride solutions usually suffices; rarely, however (especially in patients with renal failure), it may be necessary to administer hydrochloric acid intravenously to achieve correction of the metabolic alkalosis.[80]

When a patient with gastric outlet obstruction is admitted to the hospital, any significant acid-base and electrolyte abnormalities must be corrected and fluid deficiencies must be restored. In addition, it is important to empty the stomach of retained food. This may require prolonged irrigation and aspiration with a large-bore Ewald tube. Evacuation should be accomplished in order to allow the walls of the stomach to return to their original size and to permit the edema of obstruction to subside. The degree of outlet obstruction can be approximately estimated by means of the saline load test.[59] If the results of the test are abnormal after 3 days of nasogastric suction, operative therapy is indicated. Solids and liquids are emptied by different mechanisms. It is possible for patients to have a normal saline load test and still have great difficulty in emptying solid food. Those patients who have long-standing difficulties usually require operation.

The operative procedure usually recommended is truncal vagotomy either with antrectomy or with gastroenterostomy. The author believes that gastroenterostomy is preferable because it avoids placing an anastomosis or closure in the scarred duodenum. Because the obstructed stomach is edematous and because edematous tissue heals poorly, the stomach should be decompressed for 2 or 3 days before operation. Several days may be required after operation for the stomach to retain its tone and empty normally.

INTRACTABILITY. An ulcer may be intractable because of the extraordinary virulence of the ulcer diathesis or, far more commonly, because the patient is unable to comply with a program of drug treatment. Intractability was formerly the most common indication for operation. Most such patients are now treated with H_2-blockade. Time allows the opportunity to ascertain what percentage of patients can avoid operation. Some fail on H_2-blockade,[93] usually because of poor compliance. In patients with severe ulcer disease, some believe that long-term H_2-blockade may delay, rather than avoid, operative therapy.[5,54] Only surgical therapy can effectively alter the natural history of the majority of patients with duodenal ulcer.[85] Sufficient experience has not been obtained with omeprazole, but the main difficulty is with compliance, not the efficacy of drug treatment; omeprazole is no more effective than cimetidine if not properly used.

Physicians often treat patients who are addicted to alcohol or to aspirin or who have such a disorganized life-style that they cannot adhere to medical treatment of duodenal ulcer. In these instances, the patient may be considered intractable and surgical treatment may be advisable to prevent serious later complications of the ulcer. An acid-reducing operation removes the factor of patient compliance from the therapeutic equation.

On the basis of review of the results of various procedures,[200] it is believed that selective proximal vagotomy is the procedure of choice for elective operations performed for intractability.

GASTRIC ULCER

Gastric ulcers generally become symptomatic later in life than duodenal ulcers and have a peak incidence in the fifth decade. They affect about twice as many males as females, and although variously estimated as only one third to one fifth as common as duodenal ulcers in this country, they are responsible for almost half the deaths due to peptic ulcer disease.[137] The relative incidence of gastric to duodenal ulcer is increasing in the United States.[50]

DIAGNOSIS

History

Although the clinical findings in a patient with gastric ulcer may be quite similar to those in a patient with duodenal ulcer, there are often important differences. The pain pattern is not nearly as clear-cut; pain usually appears just at or slightly to the left of the midline. Although the pain is often relieved by food, many patients with gastric ulcer report an exacerbation on eating, or particularly on drinking warm liquids or alcohol. Early satiety, nausea, and vomiting are often troublesome, and postprandial discomfort may be of such consequence that the patient may decide not to eat in order to relieve the pain. Chronicity is common, and patients often do not seek help from a physician for years. There appears to be some difference in the socioeconomic classes of patients with duodenal and gastric ulcers; gastric ulcer is more common among poor people.

Whereas most patients with duodenal ulcer disease do well on medical management, patients with gastric ulcers have a higher rate of recurrence (62 per cent in 2 years)[73] and of complications, and the complications tend to be more serious than in patients with duodenal ulcer.

Radiology

Although radiographic studies have long been the mainstay of diagnosis of gastric ulcer, gastroscopy is more accurate and affords the additional opportunity for biopsy. An important consideration in the diagnosis of gastric ulcer is the possibility of malignancy. Much has been written about the radiologic criteria for differentiation between benign and malignant ulcers; because of endoscopic biopsy, the matter is less crucial. In most patients with carcinoma of the stomach, there is no confusion with gastric ulcer, but when the patient with carcinoma has an ulceration of the tumor, confusion may arise. The most important differentiating characteristic is whether the ulcer crater penetrates beyond the projected line of the wall of the stomach, which benign ulcers tend to do (Fig. 16), whereas malignant ulcers more often represent an erosion into a filling defect that protrudes into the stomach. Although there are widely respected opinions to the contrary, there appears to be no tendency for malignant ulcers to occur more frequently on the greater curvature of the stomach than elsewhere.[73]

Approximately 95 per cent of benign gastric ulcers are located on or near the lesser curvature, and a majority have been reported in the region of the incisura.[143]

Gastroscopy

Fiberoptic gastroscopy examination allows the endoscopist to directly inspect the gastric ulcer, to obtain a fiberoptic gastrogram, and to obtain with a biopsy forceps small fragments of the edges of the ulcer for histologic examination. Experienced endoscopists can often recognize malignant ulcers (Fig. 14F), but multiple (8 to 12) biopsies provide the answer to the question of possible malignancy. With multiple samples, endoscopic biopsy is remarkably accurate, and surgeons are rarely surprised at operation.

TREATMENT

Most patients with duodenal and gastric ulcers do well on medical (H_2-blockade or antacids) therapy, but there is a higher rate of recurrence in those with gastric ulcers. Because of this and because of the frequency (as high as 63 per cent)[7] and the serious consequences of complications, operation should be considered strongly in patients with recurrent gastric ulcer. Although selective proximal vagotomy has been advocated in patients with gastric ulcer, resection of the distal 50 per cent of the stomach appears to provide the best result. Channel (pyloric)

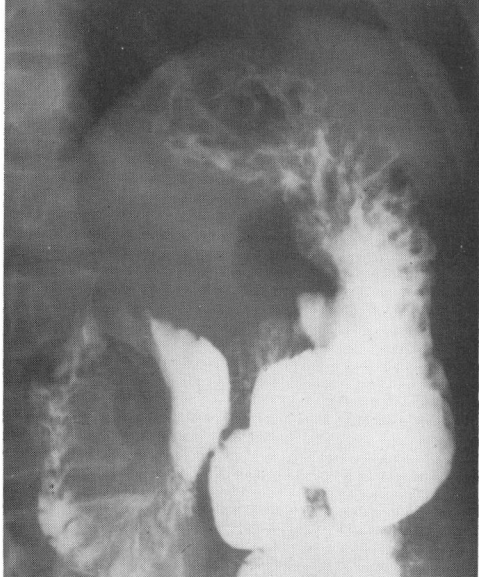

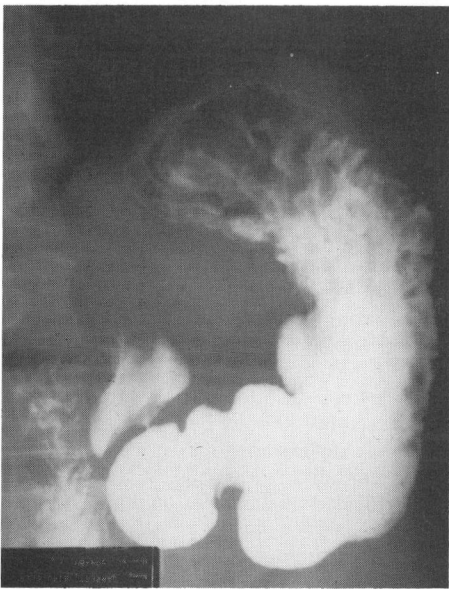

Figure 16. Two views of a benign gastric ulcer located on the lesser curvature of the stomach just proximal to the incisura angularis. After the film on the top was obtained, the patient was placed on a strict antacid regimen for 1 month, after which time the film on the bottom was obtained, which demonstrates enlargement of the crater despite the treatment program. Both films show that the ulcer crater penetrates beyond the projected line of the wall of the stomach, and there is a ring of radiolucent edematous mucosa about the base of the ulcer.

ulcers do not do well with selective proximal vagotomy; they should be resected.

The indications for operation in patients with gastric ulcer are hemorrhage, perforation, obstruction, intractability, and the need to exclude the possibility of carcinoma of the stomach. Since endoscopic biopsy, properly performed, is highly accurate, the last indication is rare. Because malignancy is a possibility in all gastric ulcers, at operation it is important to remove the entire ulcer and obtain pathologic examination by frozen section technique or to obtain biopsy specimens from four quadrants of the ulcer and examine them by frozen section.

The signs and symptoms of bleeding from gastric ulcer are similar to those of bleeding duodenal ulcers. Because patients with gastric ulcers are likely to be older and because bleeding is likely to be more persistent, the outlook is more serious and

operation should be undertaken earlier in patients with gastric ulcers than in patients with duodenal ulcer.

At operation, the ulcer should be excised if possible and included in a distal gastrectomy. If the bleeding ulcer is located high in the stomach, the surgeon may place sutures at the site of bleeding after obtaining a biopsy of the ulcer or (preferably) excise the ulcer locally, repair the defect, and then perform a distal gastrectomy.

Patients with perforation of the stomach due to a gastric ulcer manifest the same signs and symptoms as patients with perforated duodenal ulcer. There is usually free air under the diaphragm, although if the ulcer has perforated into the lesser omental bursa, the air may collect in the bursa and show a characteristic rectangular pattern on radiographs.

Perforated gastric ulcer may be treated either by simple closure of the perforation after biopsy of the ulcer or by gastric resection. Results after resection are clearly superior, so that simple closing should be reserved for poor-risk patients.

Patients with obstructing benign gastric ulcers usually have a large dilated stomach filled with accumulated food. Their preoperative management should be identical to that of patients with obstructing duodenal ulcers. The operative treatment is either a distal gastrectomy or a simple bypass of the obstructed distal stomach, depending on whether the patient is a suitable candidate for a resective procedure. The surgeon must be especially alert for carcinoma.

The main problem in managing patients with gastric ulcer who do not have a complication requiring operation is advocation of surgical intervention. The standard program is to submit the patient to a specified period of intense medical treatment as a test of healing. If the ulcer heals, the patient should be examined at intervals. If the ulcer fails reliably to heal, the patient should have an operation. Although there are advocates of vagotomy for treatment of gastric ulcer, most surgeons are pleased with the good results[65,182] obtained with simple Billroth I distal gastrectomy with excision of the ulcer.[65,182]

In a significant percentage of patients with duodenal ulcer, gastric ulceration develops. In the absence of a specific complication of the gastric ulcer, the patient should be treated as though he had a duodenal ulcer alone.

ZOLLINGER-ELLISON SYNDROME[97,195,220]

Zollinger and Ellison[226] in 1955 described a clinical syndrome that is now recognized to consist of massive gastric hypersecretion, peptic ulceration (often multiple, often jejunal, and frequently fatal), and a non–beta cell islet tumor of the pancreas that produces gastrin. The gastrinoma metastasizes to the liver and regional lymph nodes in more than 50 per cent of cases.[77] Diarrhea and malabsorption are frequently associated with and may precede the development of peptic ulcers.

Patients with Zollinger-Ellison syndrome usually have a basal acid secretion of greater than 15 mEq. per hour; in 12 patients with the Zollinger-Ellison syndrome, a range of basal acid output of between 15 and 76 mEq. per hour was found with a mean of 34.3.[195] Hypergastrinemia measured by radioimmunoassay is the usual finding, although gastrin values (as well as acid secretory output) vary greatly from time to time, and multiple samples may be required for diagnosis (Fig. 17). Release of gastrin by calcium and secretin infusion has proved to be a valuable diagnostic test in patients with gastrinomas. The secretin test is more reliable and is now used almost exclusively.

The diagnosis of Zollinger-Ellison syndrome in full bloom is not difficult. Most patients have severe symptoms of peptic ulcer, although, rarely, patients who have diarrhea without ulcer symptoms seek help. The diarrhea is apparently caused by the massive acid hypersecretion and is not caused by any intrinsic action of gastrin. The diarrhea disappears on institution of

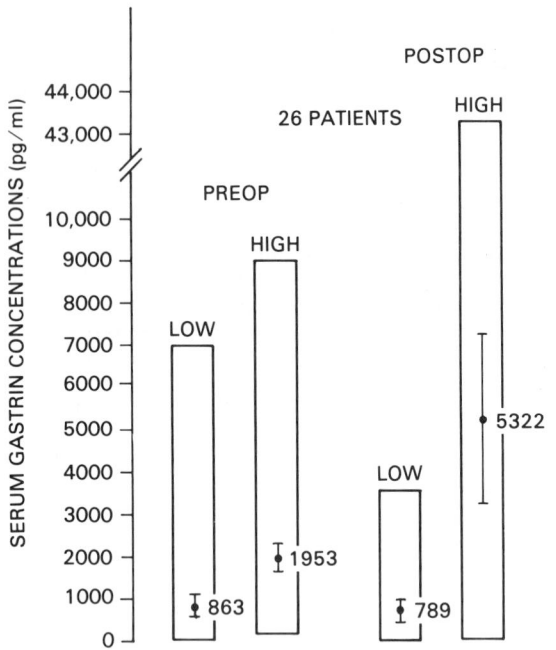

Figure 17. The mean of the lowest and highest basal gastrin concentrations (pg. per ml.) in 26 patients, before and after operation. The range and the means of the high and low values are given. (From Thompson, J. C., et al.: The role of surgery in the Zollinger-Ellison syndrome. Ann. Surg., *197*:594, 1983.)

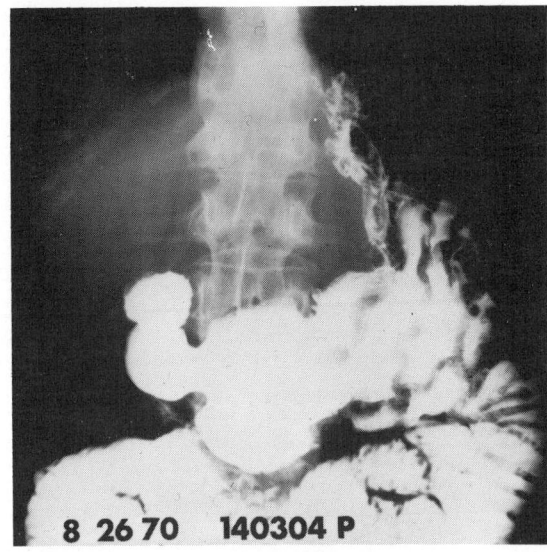

Figure 18. Upper gastrointestinal radiographic study in a patient with the Zollinger-Ellison syndrome. Note the greatly enlarged thickened folds of mucosa in the stomach and in the jejunum, striking representations of mucosal edema.

effective nasogastric suction. Many patients are now seen with milder or atypical manifestations of the syndrome, manifestations that overlap the findings in patients with nonendocrine ulcers. The most important factor in diagnosis is demonstration of elevated levels of serum gastrin (basal or after secretin challenge) along with gastric hypersecretion. A few patients with pyloric obstruction due to chronic duodenal ulcer demonstrate elevation of serum gastrin, but these patients, as well as those with retained antral mucosa, should demonstrate a *decrease* (or, at least, no great rise) in gastrin levels after administration of secretin.

Radiologic studies may be quite helpful. On upper gastrointestinal barium study, the stomach is often observed to be enlarged with thickened edematous mucosa and great folds (Fig. 18). The barium in the stomach is often diluted by the large secretory output, and when the barium column reaches the small intestine, often there are signs of mucosal edema and hypermotility, along with puddling and clumping of the barium. The pancreatic tumor may be demonstrated on selective abdominal angiography in fewer than one third of cases (Fig. 19).

Approximately one of four patients with a gastrinoma is found to have the familial multiple endocrine neoplasia (MEN) syndrome, Type I (that is, multiple endocrine neoplasms involving the parathyroid, pancreas, pituitary, adrenal, and thyroid). Any patient with duodenal ulcer and hypercalcemia should be suspected of having the MEN Type I syndrome with a parathyroid adenoma and a gastrinoma. The gastrinomas are frequently multiple within the pancreas and may arise ectopically in the duodenum or in pancreatic rests in the mesentery or retroperitoneum.

Although the full-blown syndrome is a fulminant one, many patients have been troubled with peptic ulcer symptoms and diarrhea for 5 to 10 years before the syndrome is recognized. The diagnosis is made by demonstrating hypergastrinemia (which is augmented by secretin infusion) in a patient with acid hypersecretion. Demonstration of a gastrin-secreting tumor confirms the diagnosis.

Zollinger and Ellison[226] initially recommended total gastrec-

tomy for patients with gastrinoma. This treatment proved effective and was adopted as standard therapy. Current experience with H_2-blockade treatment appears favorable, however,[102] and many patients are now managed without operation. Omeprazole is effective in patients who are refractory to H_2-blockade.[220] Because of problems in compliance (not deficits in drug potency), the author and others have encountered patients who have failed medical treatment and have required later operation. Because most gastrinomas are malignant, every patient with Zollinger-Ellison syndrome who meets standard criteria for operability should have a laparotomy for possible removal of tumor tissue. The cure rate is not high, but if all tumor tissue can be excised, the patient may be cured. If the patient has intractable symptoms despite repeated attempts on drug therapy, total gastrectomy should be considered. Many patients with gastrinomas do extraordinarily well after total gastrectomy, and the mortality risk is low[192,199]; the author and associates have performed total gastrectomy in 31 patients without mortality.

Patients with gastrinomas may tolerate hepatic metastases for long periods, in a manner similar to patients with the carcinoid syndrome, but the tumors have a clear potential of killing their host, and no spontaneous resolution of the tumor has been observed. An aggressive approach of combined surgical therapy and chemotherapy offers hope of success.[174,192,201,227]

PEPTIC ULCER IN CHILDREN

Although uncommon, peptic ulcer in patients under the age of 15 years often has a complicated and serious clinical course. Ulcers may be primary (true peptic) or secondary to overwhelming disease. True primary ulcers are rare; only 30 patients were seen with primary ulcers during a 30-year period at the Hospital for Sick Children in London.[118] Whenever children develop peptic ulcer, gastrin levels should be measured and patients should be evaluated for the Zollinger-Ellison syndrome. Spontaneous perforations of the gastrointestinal tract in the newborn are apparently due to ischemia induced by remote circulatory disturbances initiated by shock[127] and are often part of the syndrome of necrotizing enterocolitis. Stress ulceration may occasionally be suspected,[29] and medications (aspirin and adrenal steroids) were implicated in 12 of 29 infants and children with acute peptic ulcer.[70]

There appear to be four distinct clinical patterns of peptic

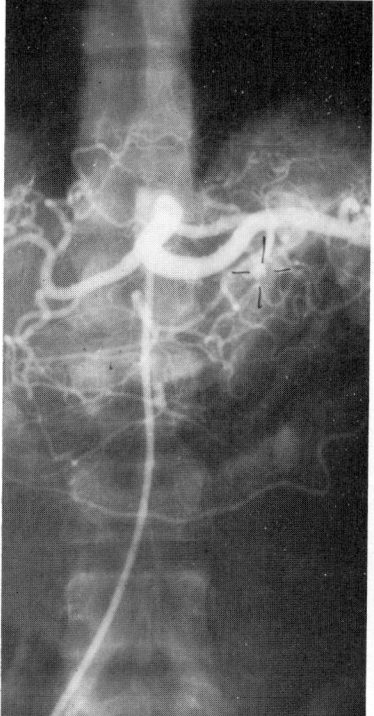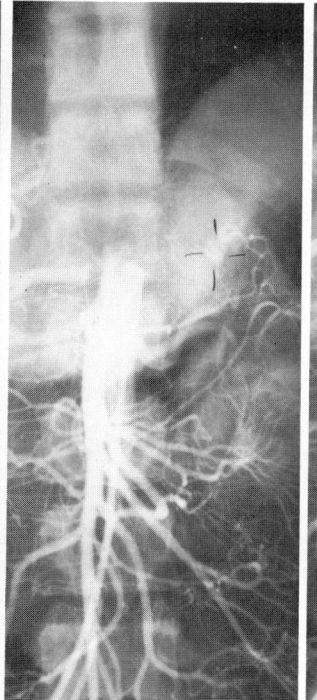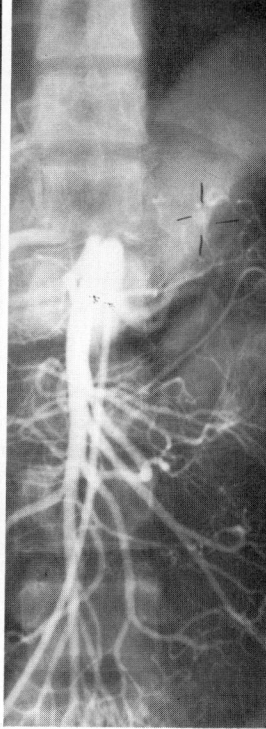

Figure 19. Selective arteriographic demonstration of gastrinoma in a patient with the Zollinger-Ellison syndrome. *Left,* A selective celiac arteriogram. *Center and right,* Superior mesenteric arteriograms. All three views show the small isolated tumor that was found at operation in the midportion of the tail of the pancreas. (From Thompson, J. C., et al: Natural history and experience with diagnosis and treatment of the Zollinger-Ellison syndrome. Surg. Gynecol. Obstet., *140:*721, 1975.)

ulceration in childhood.[105] In the first 2 weeks of life, perforation or hemorrhage may occur without premonitory signs and often with few findings, or none at all, on abdominal examination. If the ulcer has perforated, plain films of the abdomen usually demonstrate free air. Barium studies of the upper gastrointestinal tract in infants who are bleeding may demonstrate a duodenal ulcer.

From the second week of life until the age of 2 years, peptic ulceration may be manifested by bleeding or by poor response to feeding and frequent vomiting. Perforation and massive bleeding are again the principal complications but usually occur with antecedent symptoms of abdominal pain, anorexia, or vomiting, and the radiologist or endoscopist is usually able to demonstrate a distinct ulcer of the duodenum. In the first 2 weeks of life, complications of peptic ulcer have a frightening mortality, and early operation is mandatory. In these infants, it is usually sufficient to close the perforation or to ligate the bleeding point because they do not appear to have an ulcer diathesis and do not later suffer from ulcer disease.[150] After the second week of life, vagotomy and pyloroplasty appear to be the best treatment for complications of peptic ulcer.[105]

From the age of 2 years until 7 years, the incidence of peptic ulceration is the lowest in childhood and, when present, is often associated with lesions of the CNS, sepsis, or other causes of stress ulceration.

After the age of 7 to 8 years, the pathogenesis and clinical course of peptic ulcer disease become more like the typical syndrome observed in adults. Hemorrhage, perforation, obstruction of the gastric outlet, and intractable pain are relatively common. Early in the course of the disease, the radiologic studies are often difficult to interpret, and in the absence of an ulcer crater, the most important findings may be evidence of increased gastric secretion and persistent pylorospasm. The appearance of a duodenal ulcer in a child suggests either a diminished resistance of the mucosa or an especially virulent form of the ulcer diathesis; complications are common and serious. Because of this and because the results with conservative operative approach (vagotomy and drainage) are good and have few detectable later sequelae, early operative treatment of complications of peptic

ulcer in childhood is advisable.[149,150] Measurements of acid secretion in children are rarely reported. A study from Hong Kong reported that both basal and maximal acid secretory rates were elevated in children with duodenal ulcer.[180]

ACUTE MUCOSAL EROSIONS[202]

For reasons that are not clear, the incidence of major bleeding from acute mucosal erosions (stress ulcers or hemorrhagic gastritis) has decreased greatly in the last decade, perhaps because of improvements in the nutrition of severely ill patients. The lesions should, however, still be anticipated in patients who are chronically ill with sepsis and hypotension (see section on pathogenesis). Because the occurrence of these lesions has been clarified, surgeons who manage patients in intensive care units are aware they may find bleeding from acute mucosal erosions in patients who are critically ill for long periods of time, especially those nutritionally depleted patients with sepsis and hypotension.

Production of gastric acid by patients bleeding from acute mucosal lesions has been reported variously to be low, normal, or high. Patients with Cushing's ulcers (associated with lesions of the CNS) appear to have higher levels of acid secretion[63,177] than do patients without CNS trauma, in whom low levels of acid secretion may reflect the severe nature of associated disease or may be due to back-diffusion of acid through the damaged mucosal barrier. Acid output has been found to be low during hypotension caused by hypovolemia or sepsis but often has been found to increase in a striking manner after correction of the fluid losses and hemodynamic abnormalities.[129]

DIAGNOSIS

Acute mucosal lesions should be considered whenever acute upper gastrointestinal bleeding or perforation occurs after a major injury or during the course of an important metabolic insult. Bleeding may begin insidiously, making its initial appearance as coffee-ground flecks in the nasogastric aspirate of postoperative patients, changing during the course of hours or days to brisk bleeding. However, major bleeding may supervene dra-

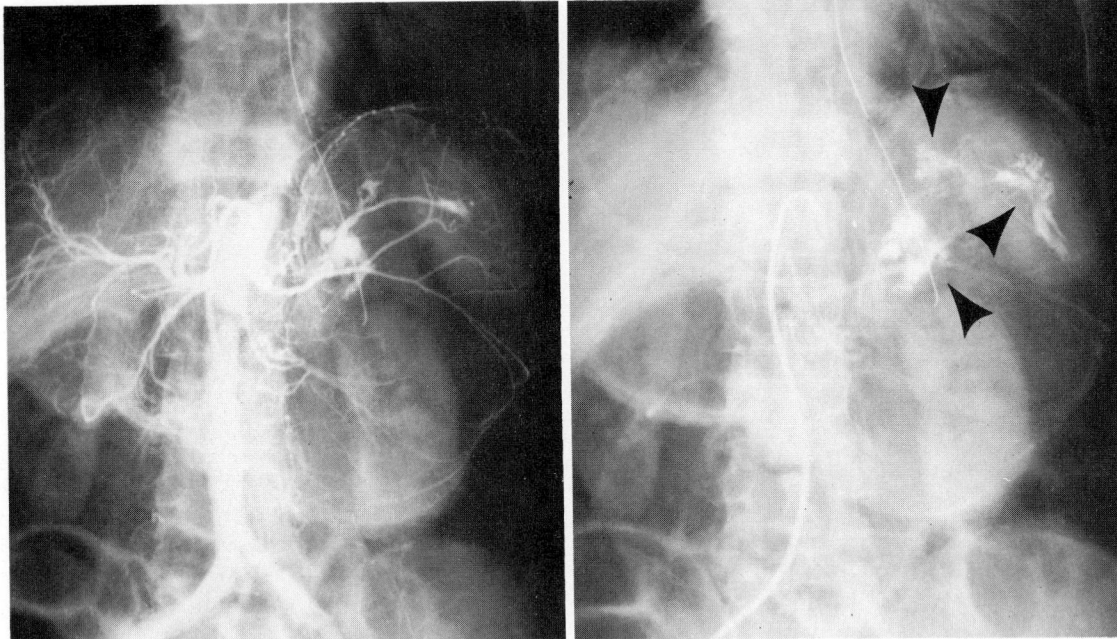

Figure 20. Arteriographic demonstration of acute superficial gastric mucosal lesions. *Left,* Injection of the celiac axis (and aorta) shows extravasation of dye into the lumen of the stomach at the site of acute gastric mucosal erosions. *Right,* After the injection, there is residual dye within the stomach at the point of the superficial gastric erosions (arrowheads).

matically. If the blood initially appears by rectum and if the patient has not vomited, a nasogastric tube should be inserted for diagnosis. Bleeding may be continuous but is usually episodic.

Gastroscopy is the most important diagnostic technique available.[129,206,224] It is usually possible to demonstrate acute, superficial, bleeding gastric lesions when the patients are examined during gastric hemorrhage (Fig. 14G). Upper gastrointestinal radiographs obtained during bleeding episodes are rarely helpful because the erosions are quite superficial. Gastric mucosal changes were observed consistently in all patients in whom gastroscopy was performed within 24 hours of severe trauma by Lucas and associates,[129] and it was possible to follow the progression of the erosions from petechiae to superficial ulceration. The lesions appear first in the proximal stomach on the greater curvature and then spread distally to the antrofundic junction, but rarely beyond. Acute erosions are superficial rather than deep, multiple rather than single, gastric rather than duodenal, and fundic rather than antral, and usually bleed and do not perforate. It is often possible to demonstrate the point of bleeding by selective celiac arteriography (Fig. 20).

TREATMENT

Because bleeding from stress ulceration may vary from minor oozing of blood from a small area of injured mucosa to a brisk, life-threatening hemorrhage, therapeutic programs have varied from iced saline lavage to total gastrectomy.

Regardless of the initial mechanisms of mucosal damage, acid is required for mucosal destruction and bleeding, and *antacid therapy* is, therefore, a logical prophylaxis for all patients who are at risk of stress ulceration.[21,124,169] Intravenous H_2-receptor blockade therapy has been widely used in prophylaxis. Neither antacids nor H_2-blockers can control established bleeding, and in the presence of sepsis, neither is effective in control of acid output.[133] At the first sign of bleeding, antacid therapy may be combined or alternated with iced saline lavage. This regimen is often successful in halting further hemorrhage.[168] Since initiation of antacid treatment in patients at risk for the development of acute mucosal ulceration, operative intervention has rarely

been required. If too much reliance is placed on antacids, however, it is likely that they may be used in excessive quantities, causing severe metabolic alkalosis, small bowel ileus, and diarrhea.[128] Spontaneous cessation of bleeding is common, but hemorrhage may recur. Of more than 300 patients at the Detroit General Hospital who required transfusion for bleeding from acute mucosal erosions, only 38 required operation.[129]

Selective arterial infusion of pitressin into the exact area of bleeding by means of an angiographically placed catheter has been used in the treatment of acute mucosal bleeding. Even in the best of circumstances, however, this is associated with a failure rate of almost 50 per cent,[8] and it may cause ischemic necrosis of the stomach wall.

The percentage of patients requiring operation has continued to decrease. The author avoids operation if possible and has been successful in the majority of cases. Decision to operate is difficult because the patients are often extremely ill. Stress bleeding is usually observed in patients who are experiencing sequential failure of major organs. Surgeons are guided by gastroscopic findings; if the entire gastric mucosa is hemorrhagic and necrotic, total gastrectomy must be considered if operation becomes mandatory.

If the bleeding is found to be caused by a discrete ulcer in the duodenum or proximal stomach, the lesion should be sutured and a vagotomy and drainage procedure performed. If bleeding originates from the distal stomach, a distal gastrectomy, preferably combined with vagotomy, is the best procedure. Because of the high incidence of recurrent bleeding after lesser operations and because the mortality for repeated operations is extraordinary, the author believes that total gastrectomy is warranted if the bleeding sites cannot be completely excised or sutured by means of a lesser operation.[202]

Operative mortality is 35 to 80 per cent and largely reflects the severity of the associated diseases. The survival rate depends largely on control of the process that initiated the stress; most often this requires correction of sepsis. The generally poor results following operation encourage widespread application of prophylactic antacid therapy and H_2-blockade in severely ill patients in whom stress ulcer is likely to develop.

SURGICAL PROCEDURES ON THE STOMACH
HISTORICAL ASPECTS

The initial development of surgical procedures for peptic ulcer was empiric. The subsequent evolution has been guided by demonstration of physiologic mechanisms controlling gastric secretion.[189]

The first operation for peptic ulcer that gained widespread acceptance and one of the most simple operations ever devised for the lesion is gastroenterostomy with anastomosis between the stomach and the jejunum. The procedure was first described in 1881 by Woefler, a colleague of Billroth, who first used it to bypass a carcinomatous obstruction of the pylorus, and then adapted it for peptic ulcer. Because of the simplicity of the procedure and its relative safety, it was quickly adopted by surgeons in Europe and America. By the turn of the century, however, an increasing incidence of marginal ulceration (recurrent peptic ulcer at the margin of the anastomosis) was observed. In 1925, a long-term postoperative study of patients with gastroenterostomy reported a 34 per cent incidence of gastrojejunal ulcer.[125] The operation was gradually abandoned, although it was still in use until the mid-1950s.

The first successful gastric resection was performed by Billroth in Vienna in 1881 when he excised an obstructing carcinoma of the pylorus and performed a gastroduodenostomy. In 1882, von Rydigier performed the first gastric resection for ulcer disease. The first partial gastrectomies were hardly more than pylorectomies, but as operative techniques improved, surgeons became more radical, and by 1940 the term *subtotal gastric resection* was interpreted as denoting removal of the distal 66 to 80 per cent of the stomach. After resection, the continuity of the gut can be restored by anastomosis of the remaining portion of the fundus to the duodenum (gastroduodenostomy or Billroth I anastomosis) or alternatively by closure of the duodenal stump and by anastomosis of the fundic remnant to the first part of the jejunum (gastrojejunostomy or Billroth II anastomosis) (Fig. 21).

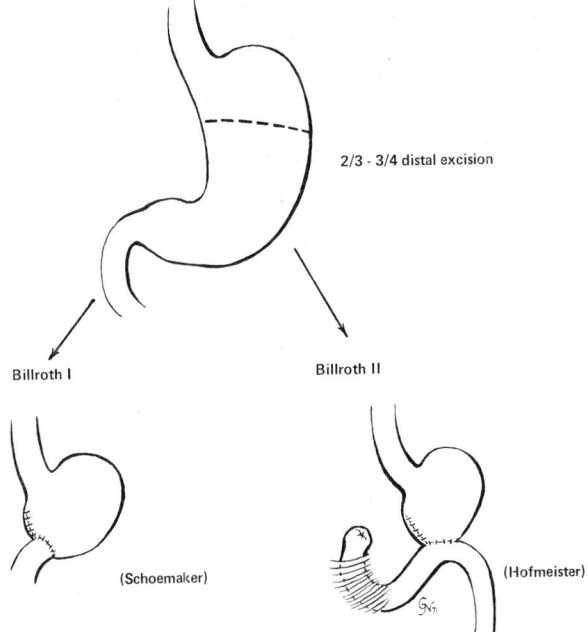

Billroth I

2/3 - 3/4 distal excision

Billroth II

(Schoemaker)

(Hofmeister)

Figure 21. Types of reconstruction after subtotal gastric resection. Resection removes 66 to 75 per cent of the distal stomach, thereby excising the entire antral-gastric mechanism as well as a large portion of the parietal cell mass. Reconstruction of continuity of the gastrointestinal tract may be performed either with a gastroduodenostomy (Billroth I) anastomosis or with a gastrojejunostomy (Billroth II) anastomosis. The Schoemaker modification of the Billroth I anastomosis includes partial closure of the lesser curvature of the stomach, as does the Hofmeister modification of the Billroth II anastomosis.

Subtotal gastrectomy, especially with the Billroth II anastomosis, became very popular in this country by the 1930s, was for 2 decades the standard treatment for peptic ulcer disease, and is still widely used. The objections to the procedure are the relatively high mortality, especially in patients with severe scarring of the duodenum, and the high incidence of postoperative complications.

Dragstedt reasoned that duodenal ulcer disease was usually associated with an increased secretion of acid and that the success of surgical procedures in the stomach was probably related to reduction of the acid-secreting potential. Since the vagus was known to stimulate acid secretion, he concluded that division of the vagus would be beneficial in the treatment of ulcer. His first reports[41,42] of operations in man substantiated this concept.

Gastric emptying is initiated in large part by contraction of the antral musculature; truncal vagotomy denervates the antral pump, causing delayed gastric emptying. Dragstedt later added a drainage procedure (posterior gastroenterostomy) in order to provide emptying of the atonic stomach. Weinberg[212] substituted a modification of the Heineke-Mikulicz pyloroplasty (a procedure in which an incision is made longitudinally through the distal stomach, pylorus, and proximal duodenum and is then closed vertically) as the drainage procedure. There was great initial resistance to the adoption of vagotomy and drainage, but the simplicity of the procedure and low mortality won many converts. Subsequently, the relatively high incidence of recurrence and postoperative diarrhea have demonstrated clearly that the ideal procedure is not yet available.

OPERATIONS CURRENTLY IN USE[189]

All successful current procedures for inflammatory ulcerating lesions of the stomach or duodenum reduce the acid-secreting potential of the stomach. The rationale for this is straightforward in patients with duodenal ulcers whose disease is clearly related to acid hypersecretion. Although peptic ulcers of the stomach and stress ulcers are not associated with acid hypersecretion, acid has at least a permissive role in the pathogenesis of these lesions, and if the stomach is achlorhydric, ulcers do not develop. Although abolition of acid production probably prevents the development of stress ulcers, when they are present abolition of acid production does not, unfortunately, guarantee cessation of bleeding.

The three operations in general use for peptic ulcer are gastric resection without vagotomy, truncal vagotomy and drainage (either gastroenterostomy or pyloroplasty), and truncal vagotomy plus antrectomy. Selective denervation of the acid-secreting portion of the fundus with preservation of innervation to the antrum and to the rest of the abdominal viscera is widely used in Europe and has achieved acceptance in North America. The four procedures are discussed individually.

Subtotal Gastric Resection

Resection of the distal 66 to 75 per cent of the stomach reduces acid production by abolishing the gastrin mechanism and by excision of part of the acid factory, that is, the parietal cell mass. Depending on the extent of parietal cell resection, subtotal gastrectomy diminishes the postoperative maximal gastric secretory response to histamine by 60 to 80 per cent. If a Billroth II reconstruction is planned, it is important that the line of distal resection be distal to the junction of antral and duodenal mucosa. Planned or inadvertent exclusion of antral mucosa with the duodenal stump in a Billroth II anastomosis causes sequestration of antral mucosa in a permanently alkaline environment. Since acid suppression of gastrin release is abolished, a syndrome of hypergastrinemia mimicking the Zollinger-Ellison syndrome results. These patients have a high incidence of recurrent marginal ulceration.[166,204] They can be differentiated from patients with the Zollinger-Ellison syndrome by means of the secretion test. Excision of the retained antral tissue results in cure.

There have been numerous studies in patients with subtotal gastrectomy on the relative superiority of gastroduodenostomy versus gastrojejunostomy. The issue is somewhat confused because gastroduodenostomy appears to be a clearly superior procedure in dogs. In man, however, the incidence of recurrence of peptic ulcer following subtotal gastrectomy without vagotomy is twice as high with a Billroth I anastomosis as it is with a Billroth II.[209]

Reported mortality with subtotal gastrectomy for duodenal ulcer varies between 0.4 and 8.9 per cent[191]; mortality of 3 to 4 per cent is usually quoted.

Truncal Vagotomy and Drainage Procedure

Vagotomy causes a great reduction in gastric secretion, but it also greatly suppresses gastric motility. More than half the patients who have truncal vagotomy alone later require some procedure to enhance emptying of the stomach.

The relatively high incidence of incomplete vagotomy has placed great emphasis on technique. It was initially assumed that with careful attention to detail a complete vagotomy would invariably be possible. Variations in the anatomy of the vagi at the esophageal hiatus and adjacent to the abdominal esophagus and on the stomach make complete interruption of all vagal fibers very difficult indeed in some patients. A common arrangement of the anatomy of the vagi below the diaphragm is shown in Figure 22. Just above the diaphragm, the vagal fibers around the esophagus usually coalesce to form a discrete right and left trunk as they come through the diaphragm; accessory trunks are not uncommon. Many of the fibers that go to the stomach leave the vagal trunks at the hiatus and course inferiorly within the esophageal muscle. The right vagus nerve, usually the larger, lies posteriorly and slightly to the right along the circumference of the esophagus. A few centimeters superior to the esophagogastric junction, the right vagus divides into celiac and gastric branches. The celiac branch usually follows the left gastric artery and joins the celiac plexus, from which it sends branches to the rest of the abdominal viscera; the gastric branch supplies the posterior wall of the stomach. The left vagus lies anteriorly and, again, often to the right of the center of the esophageal circumference. It also divides just above the cardia into a hepatic and a gastric branch. The hepatic division courses within the gastrohepatic omentum to the porta hepatis where it joins the hepatic plexus. There is usually a branch from the hepatic division to the distal stomach and proximal duodenum. The gastric division of the left or anterior vagus supplies the anterior wall of the stomach. The posterior vagus is often located more dorsally and may be found applied to the adventitia covering the anterior surface of the aorta. This is the trunk most often overlooked when vagotomy is incomplete, and, at revagotomy, the surgeon should initially search in the adventitia behind the esophagus for persistent vagal trunks.

At the initial attempt at vagotomy, rarely only one large nerve trunk is present; as many as nine separate trunks have been excised. Demonstration of two (or three or four) nerve trunks by frozen section at operation, therefore, does not guarantee completeness of vagotomy. A transthoracic approach to vagotomy is often used after failure of an earlier abdominal vagotomy. Unfortunately, the results offer little more promise than those with the conventional abdominal approach.[32]

When gastroenterostomy was first added to vagotomy, the anastomosis was usually placed at the most dependent part of the greater curvature of the stomach. Later, in efforts to avoid antral stasis, the anastomosis was performed in the distal antrum, immediately proximal to the pylorus; this placement of the anastomosis is in current use. Pyloroplasty was introduced by Heineke (1886) and Mikulicz (1888) for treatment of peptic ulcer. Weinberg[212] modified the technique to provide a larger

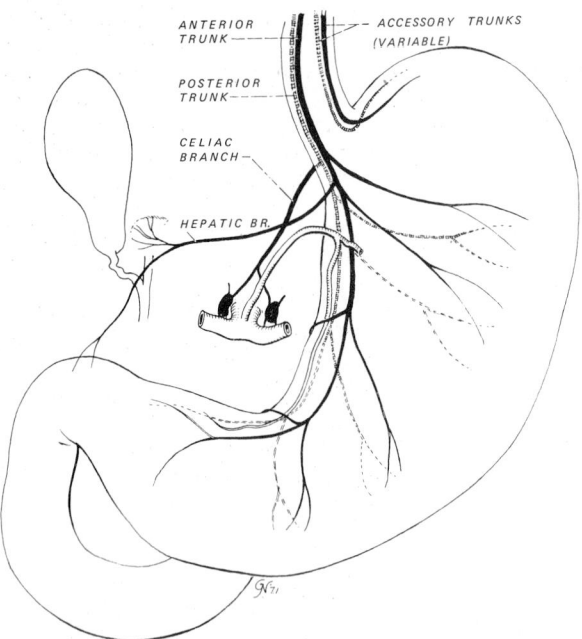

Figure 22. Anatomy of the vagus nerves in relation to the stomach. Both anterior (left) and posterior (right) vagi give off gastric branches. The anterior vagus has a hepatic branch that may send fibers to the region of the pylorus; the posterior vagus has a celiac branch that goes to the celiac ganglia and plexus and from there goes to contribute to the innervation of other abdominal viscera. The remaining fibers descend within the gastrohepatic ligament along the lesser curvature as the anterior and posterior nerves of Latarjet. These give branches to the fundus and cross inferiorly at the incisura angularis onto the antrum, to whose muscle fibers they provide innervation.

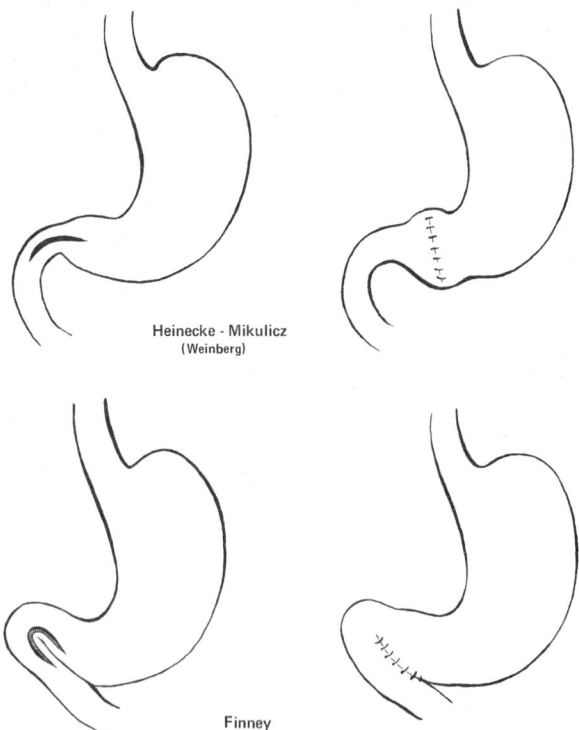

Heinecke - Mikulicz
(Weinberg)

Finney

Figure 23. Two types of pyloroplasties in common use. In the Heinecke-Mikulicz pyloroplasty, a longitudinal incision is made through the distal stomach, pylorus, and proximal duodenum. This incision is then closed in the vertical fashion, which destroys the sphincteric mechanism. The Weinberg modification is a one-layer closure. In the Finney pyloroplasty, a two-layer anastomosis is made between the stomach and duodenum, using a U-shaped incision through the distal stomach, pylorus, and proximal duodenum. It is important that both procedures be performed in such a manner as to ensure a large lumen for gastric drainage.

outlet and advocated its use as superior to gastroenterostomy in that it preserved the normal physiologic pathway of food and that it minimized alkaline regurgitation and possible excitation of the gastrin mechanism. There are multiple techniques for pyloroplasty; of these, the Heineke-Mikulicz and the Finney (Fig. 23) are most commonly used today.

Truncal Vagotomy and Antrectomy

After the introduction of vagotomy and the demonstration that it diminished the capacity of the stomach for acid production, it was inevitable that it should be combined with gastric resection. The resection is limited to the antrum, which usually is a 40 per cent distal gastrectomy. Excision of the antrum and destruction of the vagi remove the major stimulants to acid secretion and leave the entire mass of parietal cells subject to stimulation only by histamine and the intestinal phase secretagogue.

The external landmark for the antrofundic junction on the lesser curvature of the stomach is the incisura angularis. A line drawn inferiorly and 45 degrees to the left down to the greater curvature (see Fig. 1, A–A') approximates the junction of antrum and fundus. It is possible to delineate the junction more precisely by intraoperative demonstration of the differences in surface pH of the two mucosal zones. Experimental studies have shown the neutral pH of the mucosa is well correlated with high gastrin content of the mucosa.[98] The stomach should be divided approximately 2 cm. proximal to the line of pH change. There is no great hazard in leaving a small amount of antral tissue adjacent to acid-producing fundic mucosa.

The addition of vagotomy alters the relative superiority of the Billroth II anastomosis following resection without vagotomy. Experience in patients with vagotomy and antrectomy has indicated that if there is any superiority, the technique of gastroduodenostomy is preferable to that of gastrojejunostomy (presumably, this is a consequence of the preservation of normal duodenal inhibitory mechanisms for the suppression of acid secretion).

Since the aim of all operative procedures for duodenal ulcer is to diminish acid production by the stomach and since vagotomy reliably diminishes acid production at relatively small risk, it has a place in all operations for duodenal ulcer. Simply stated, in the current state of knowledge, if there is no contraindication because of the frailty of the patient, all operations for duodenal ulcer disease should include vagotomy (Fig. 24).

Selective Proximal Vagotomy

Because only the stomach need be denervated for the treatment of peptic ulcer disease and because vagal denervation of the rest of the abdominal viscera has been held responsible for diarrhea and for an increased incidence of gallstones, techniques were developed for selective vagal denervation of the entire stomach with preservation of the hepatic branch of the anterior vagus and the celiac branch of the posterior. Evaluation of results of this operation (selective gastric vagotomy) has shown no superiority over the conventional operation of truncal vagotomy plus an emptying procedure,[184] and the newer operation has not achieved wide acceptance. A further extension of the concept of selective vagotomy[89] suggested that denervation should be limited to only the proximal stomach (approximately to the mass of parietal cells) with preservation of the innervation of the antrum (Fig. 25). In this method (variously termed selective proximal vagotomy, proximal gastric vagotomy, parietal cell vagotomy, supra- or highly selective vagotomy, *inter alia*), the anterior and posterior leaves of the gastrohepatic

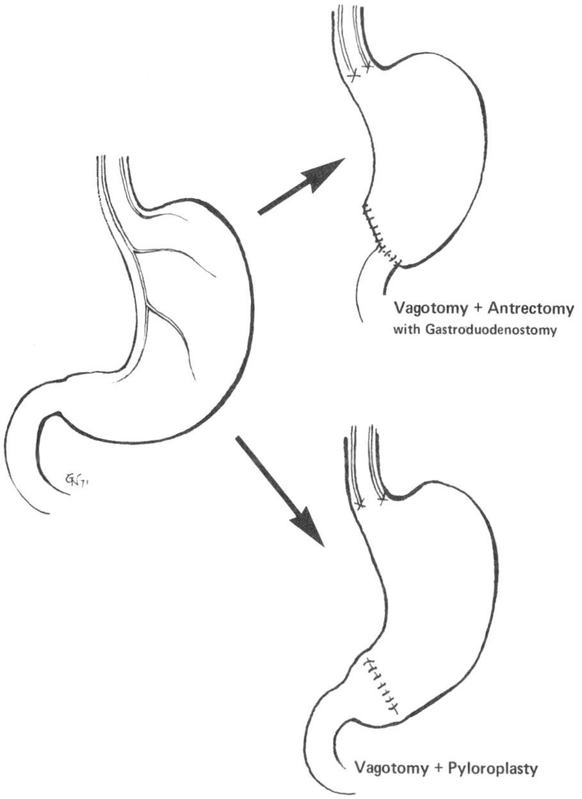

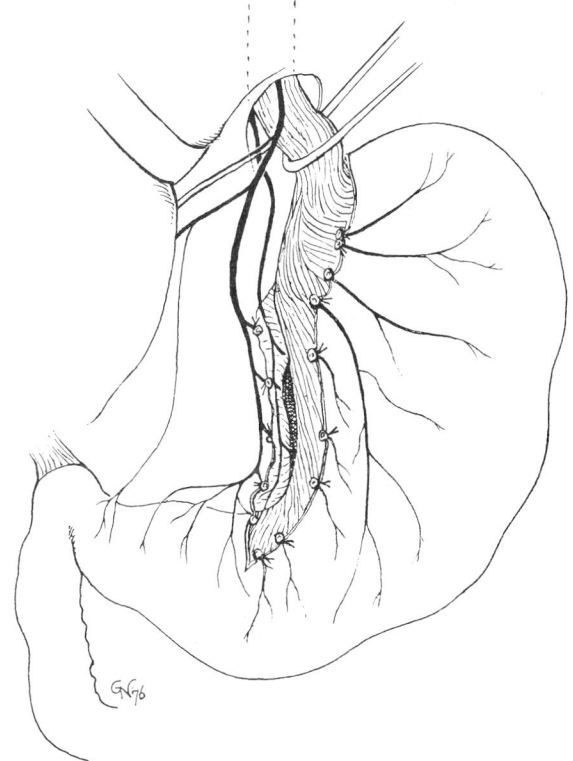

Figure 24. Acceptable operations for duodenal ulcer disease. Because the aim of any surgical procedure for duodenal ulcer is the diminution of acid output, vagotomy should be a part of any such operation if there is no specific contraindication. The choice, therefore, lies between vagotomy plus antrectomy and vagotomy plus drainage. Current information would indicate that gastroenterostomy (with gastric stoma immediately proximal to pylorus) is equally as good a drainage procedure as pyloroplasty.

Vagotomy + Antrectomy
with Gastroduodenostomy

Vagotomy + Pyloroplasty

Figure 25. Technique for selective proximal vagotomy. Fundic branches of the gastric divisions of the anterior and posterior vagi are severed and ligated at the attachment of the gastrohepatic ligament to the lesser curvature of the stomach as well as around the circumference of the fundoesophageal junction. The antral branches of the descending nerves of Latarjet are preserved. As stressed by Goligher[60] and by Hallenbeck and colleagues,[78] it is important that the lower esophagus be completely skeletonized so as to divide any vagal fibers that might reach the fundus by way of the distal esophagus. The hepatic branches of the anterior vagus and the celiac branch of the posterior vagus are preserved.

omentum are divided at their attachment to the stomach, starting at the incisura angularis distally and proceeding proximally to the esophagogastric junction. All the gastric branches of the vagi should be meticulously severed; the antral branches of the nerves of Latarjet should be preserved. Completeness of denervation of the proximal stomach is possible only with meticulous dissection of the distal esophagus to divide all communications between the vagal trunks and the proximal stomach.[60,78] Fear of gastric retention with this procedure led Holle[89] to add an emptying procedure routinely, but analysis of postoperative results suggests that recurrences are a consequence of incomplete denervation of the proximal stomach and not of delayed gastric emptying.

The great appeal of selective proximal vagotomy is that it offers the potential of acid reduction without opening the gastrointestinal tract and without denervating the remainder of the abdominal viscera. Currently, there is great enthusiasm about the procedure; its role in future operative control of duodenal ulcer depends on evaluation of long-term results.

Total Gastrectomy

Total gastrectomy with esophagojejunostomy is used for treatment of the Zollinger-Ellison syndrome or occasionally for hemorrhagic gastritis or for gastric carcinoma. Previous experience with total gastrectomy was associated with a high mortality (10 to 20 per cent) and a high rate of complications. Much of the difficulty was caused by the poor nutritional state of patients with stomach cancer and by postoperative bile reflux esophagitis. Preoperative nutritional therapy with parenteral nutrition and the adoption of the Roux-en-Y esophagojejunal anastomosis, which prevents bile reflux (Fig. 26), have greatly improved the prognosis. Properly performed, total gastrectomy should have a low mortality, even in patients over 70 years of age.[15] The author has performed total gastrectomy in patients with the Zollinger-Ellison syndrome, including over 40 patients with stress ulcers and some with recurring multiple peptic ulcers, both types without mortality. Total gastrectomy has been successful in rare instances of persistent gastric paresis after multiple operative procedures.[45] For reasons that are not well understood but that may be related to the trophic role of gastrin, the mortality and incidence of complications appear to be greatly diminished in patients with the Zollinger-Ellison syndrome.

POSTOPERATIVE COMPLICATIONS

Early Complications

Hemorrhage in the immediate postoperative period may be due to failure to control bleeding from an ulcer or may be due to bleeding at the suture line. The use of gastrostomy tubes for postoperative gastric decompression is attended by a small but definite incidence of complications, including bleeding, leaking of gastric juice into the peritoneal cavity, and, rarely, persistent gastrocutaneous fistulas. Gastrostomy for postoperative gastric decompression has been widely used for more than a decade. The number of complications probably does not justify the purported benefit of gastrostomy tubes in diminishing the incidence of postoperative respiratory complications and aspiration, and many surgeons have abandoned their use.[147] The author employs gastrostomy tubes only in patients in whom anatomic obstruction prohibits placement of a nasogastric tube and in infants and small children.

The scarified duodenum is the bête noire of gastric resection of duodenal ulcer. The most serious common complication following resection is leakage from the duodenal stump (Billroth II) or leakage at the gastroduodenostomy (Billroth I). Both cause peritoneal soilage with gastroduodenal contents and are associated with peritonitis, ileus, sepsis, and significant (10 to 15 per cent) mortality. Resection is associated with a higher incidence

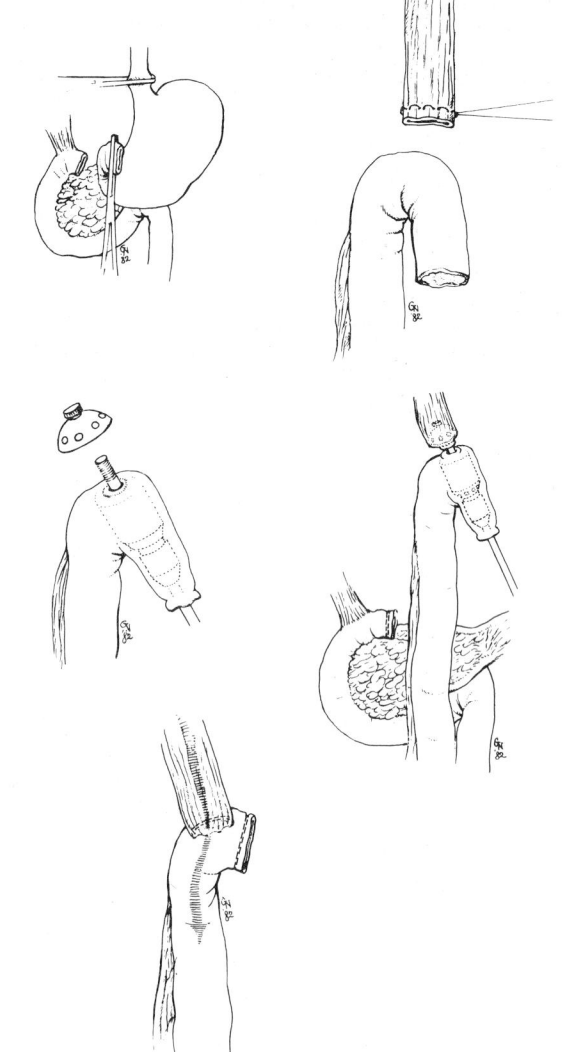

Figure 26. Technique for total gastrectomy. The lesser curvature of the stomach is mobilized by dividing the gastrohepatic omentum and the branches of the left and right gastric vessels. The greater curvature is mobilized by dividing the gastrocolic ligament and the right and left gastroepiploic vessels. The duodenum is divided just distal to the pylorus and is closed. The esophagus is divided proximal to the cardia, and frozen section is obtained to ensure that no gastric mucosa remains with the esophagus. Gastrointestinal continuity is restored with an end-to-side esophagojejunostomy Roux-en-Y, using the EEA stapling device. The isolated jejunal limb should be at least 30 cm. long to prevent bile reflux. (From Thompson, J. C., et al.: The role of surgery in the Zollinger-Ellison syndrome. Ann. Surg., *197*:594, 1983.)

of breakdown of the suture line than are drainage procedures, because dissection is performed in areas of ulcer scarring and the blood supply to the remaining structures is often compromised. Leakage of the suture line is most commonly caused by ischemia. Another factor that may contribute to leakage of a duodenal stump is obstruction of the afferent limb of the gastrojejunostomy. This obstruction, due to a kink in the bowel, causes distention of the obstructed loop with bile and pancreatic juice; the increased pressure may cause perforation of the suture line.

Late Complications

DUMPING SYNDROME. The stomach functions as an osmoregulator by diluting foods and mixing them with gastric juice and by allowing only small amounts of chyme to pass into the duodenum at any one time. Any operative procedure that destroys or bypasses the pylorus may cause sudden emptying of hyperosmolar material into the jejunum, and subsequently a large inflow of extracellular fluid into the jejunum. This rapid fluid shift may clinically produce abdominal colic, nausea, vomiting, diarrhea, faintness, sweating, and pallor. There is a transient but often pronounced decrease in the serum concentration of potassium, which may be associated with alterations in the T and ST segments of the electrocardiogram. There is an early increase in blood sugar, which is often followed by severe hypoglycemia with its characteristic entourage of symptoms.

The early symptoms of abdominal pain and hypermotility of the gut usually occur within 15 to 20 minutes of eating and appear to be most common after a carbohydrate meal; ice cream is a good provocative test. Many patients find they can obtain relief by lying down. Late symptoms associated with hypoglycemia may occur 2 hours after a meal.

The etiology of the dumping syndrome is not well understood. The anatomic requirements for dumping are met in all patients who have had a gastric resection, and at one time or another almost all postgastrectomy patients have minor dumping symptoms. Why is it that only approximately 5 per cent of patients have symptoms severe enough to seek attention and only approximately one in five of these is disabled? Many physicians have observed a correlation of the severity of the dumping syndrome with symptoms of emotional instability. Kellner and Mellinkoff[110] proposed that patients who are chronically unhappy and who complain often of minor problems may lack the motivation necessary to shrug off or adapt to minor symptoms of the dumping syndrome. In such patients, it would be wise to avoid operation (and certainly to avoid extensive resection) if this personality could be recognized prior to operation.

The dumping syndrome is often relieved by eating small dry meals and restricting all intake of fluid during meals. There is no standard operative treatment for the dumping syndrome; good results have been reported following conversion of Billroth I to Billroth II anastomoses (and vice versa) and with the use of a small segment of reversed jejunum to impede gastric emptying. The author believes it wise to delay reoperating on patients with the dumping syndrome and to treat them with alterations of diet together with mild sedation and small doses of anticholinergic drugs in order to avoid operation. Reassurance and supportive therapy often enable patients to cope with their symptoms. Reoperation is often another failure. Fortunately, recent studies have demonstrated that the long-active analog of somatostatin (Sandostatin) is effective in the management of dumping symptoms.[90]

NUTRITIONAL DISTURBANCES. Megaloblastic anemia, iron deficiency anemia, calcium deficiency, and steatorrhea are observed occasionally after gastric resection. Megaloblastic anemia is due to a deficiency of the intrinsic factor, which may follow excision of parietal cells or atrophy of parietal cells as a consequence of postoperative gastritis or of loss of stimuli. Anemia may also be caused by vitamin B_{12} deficiency caused by stasis in the blind loop of the duodenum and proliferation of bacteria. The deficiencies of iron and of calcium after gastric resection are not well understood but occur in 30 to 50 per cent of patients who are studied carefully.

Steatorrhea, which is the loss in the stool of more than 7 per cent of the total amount of fat ingested, is occasionally seen after Billroth II gastrectomy and probably follows bypass of the duodenum, which may interfere with mixing of bile salts and pancreatic lipase with ingested fat. Steatorrhea may be intensified by the development of the blind loop syndrome.

The various nutritional problems are manifested in weight loss by some patients following resection. Except in instances of radical subtotal gastrectomy or total gastrectomy or in a few patients with disabling dumping syndrome, loss of weight is rarely an important consideration, and, in fact, many patients may gain weight postoperatively.[107] Postoperative problems with nutrition appear to be more severe in Great Britain; a survey of 204 patients 15 to 20 years after vagotomy and gastroenterostomy revealed that more than half the patients were ane-

mic and one third had undergone significant loss of weight, which was correlated with diminished food intake and with gastrointestinal symptoms.[216]

DIARRHEA. The foregoing complications are all more common after resection than after vagotomy and drainage procedures. Vagotomy appears to be associated with two complications. One, a suggested increased incidence of gallstones, is difficult to prove statistically and is therefore of questionable importance.

The increased incidence of diarrhea after vagotomy is important. The number of patients with severe diarrhea is small, but symptoms may be disabling. Although approximately 70 per cent of patients report an increase in the frequency of daily bowel movements after vagotomy,[32] this often serves to relieve preoperative constipation and is often considered to be an unexpected benefit of the operation. The incidence of significant postoperative diarrhea varies from approximately 5 to 20 per cent in various series[32,48,107,146]; fortunately, the diarrhea appears to diminish significantly with time.[107]

Diarrhea may occur two or three times every week or may be episodic, once or twice a month and continuing 1 to 3 days at a time. It may be mild or of explosive severity.

The majority of careful studies on postvagotomy diarrhea are from England. The incidence of diarrhea does not appear to be as high in Sweden[24] or in this country.[48,146,217] A study[107] from Houston that reported a 19 per cent incidence of significant diarrhea 1 year after vagotomy and drainage suggests that diarrhea exists if patients are questioned carefully. Most information of value regarding postvagotomy diarrhea is from British studies,[218] one of which reports an incidence of 30 per cent and advocates abandonment of truncal vagotomy in favor of selective proximal vagotomy on this basis.[148]

The etiology of the diarrhea after vagotomy is not understood. It might be predicted that excision of the parasympathetic innervation to the small bowel would mimic the effect of atropine and cause the bowels to be sluggish, but such is not the case. Suggested etiologic factors, such as the loss of the protective action of the hyperacidic stomach with resultant increase in gastroenteritis or an alteration of the growth rate and composition of the small bowel mucosa, are of interest but do not explain the phenomenon.

The treatment of diarrhea should be symptomatic. The patient should be assured that it will usually improve with time. Only in extremely rare instances is an attempt at operative treatment (by interposition of a small segment of reversed jejunum) justified. The author avoids reoperating on these patients.

ALKALINE REFLUX GASTRITIS. A few postoperative patients are troubled with severe continuous burning epigastric pain, usually aggravated by meals. The pain is usually not relieved by vomiting. The condition is diagnosed by gastroscopy, which reveals bile reflux in the stomach and a beefy red, generally inflamed gastric mucosa, often with multiple superficial gastric erosions. Significant blood loss is rare. Although retention and vomiting may occur, there is no organic obstruction of the gastric outlet.

Medical treatment with cholestyramine to bind bile salts has met with scant success. Surgical treatment consists of reoperation to divert bile away from the stomach; if the primary anastomosis had been a gastroduodenostomy, a Henley loop is preferred, whereas after a Billroth II anastomosis, a Roux-en-Y reconstruction is preferable.

Although there is great interest in this condition and although the diagnosis achieved considerable popularity in a very short period, it is believed that great restraint should be exercised in planning reoperation. Ritchie[158] reported a recent critical reappraisal of the syndrome and concluded that it exists but that it has been "overdiagnosed." The author remains somewhat skeptical and advocates caution until the early reported benefits of reoperation are confirmed with time. Patients are now appearing with recurrent ulcer after Roux-en-Y reconstruction. As an expected but unfortunate dividend, many patients now undergo a Roux-en-Y hookup as a primary procedure after gastric resection. The author has reoperated on several patients after this procedure, whose results are predictably bad.

MARGINAL ULCER. Ulcers recur in a small fraction of postoperative patients; 1 to 5 per cent of patients who undergo gastric resection for peptic ulcer may develop recurrent peptic ulceration.[173] Recurrent ulcers after gastric resection and Billroth II anastomosis occur classically on the jejunal side of the margin of the anastomosis. The ulcer may produce periodic episodes of midabdominal pain, it may first appear with massive hemorrhage, or it may erode into the free peritoneal cavity or into the colon, creating a gastrojejunocolic fistula. Any patient in whom ulcer-type pain or occult rectal bleeding develops after a subtotal gastric resection should be suspected of having a marginal ulcer. Diagnosis may be confirmed by radiography or much better by gastroscopy. The diagnostic superiority of endoscopy in patients with marginal ulcer is clearly established. Measurement of serum Group I pepsinogens may be of value in the diagnosis of recurrent ulcer.[162]

In a study of 41 patients in whom stomal ulceration developed over a 15-year period, duodenal ulcer was found to be the original lesion in all but one patient.[17] The average duration of freedom from symptoms after operation was 10 months for gastrectomy and 3 years for gastroenterostomy alone. Pain was the most common symptom (36 of 41 patients had pain as their primary complaint), followed by bleeding (17 of 41 patients). The possibility of the Zollinger-Ellison syndrome should be considered in any patient with a marginal ulcer. Any patient suspected of having a recurrent ulcer should have a determination of serum gastrin. If the level is high, a secretin test should be performed.

Marginal ulcers are often difficult to treat medically. The patient may have a long period of quiescence on a regimen of cimetidine or antacid, only to be suddenly afflicted with a massive hemorrhage. In the absence of a life-threatening bleeding episode, a trial of H_2-blockade therapy is indicated. Of 35 patients with recurrent ulcer after selective proximal vagotomy, only 9 (26 per cent) required reoperation.[16] With the first sign of recurrence of pain or bleeding, however, the patient should be considered for operation.

Whatever the original operation, the best operation for marginal ulcer is truncal vagotomy and distal gastric resection. If the patient has previously had a vagotomy of any type, a truncal vagotomy should be reperformed. If there is a gastroenterostomy, the anastomosis should be taken down, the ulcerated segment of jejunum excised, the jejunum reanastomosed, the distal stomach resected (or re-resected), and another anastomosis between the stomach and jejunum performed. Transthoracic vagotomy does not have a high success rate after initial failure of vagotomy.[32] Reoperation is successful in 70 per cent[173] to 94 per cent[175] of patients.

EVALUATION OF OPERATIONS[200]

Although operations for peptic ulcer disease have been performed regularly for more than 70 years, valid data on the comparative effects of different operations have become available only in the last 20 years. Choice of operative procedures has been dictated by the surgeon's training, experience, or preference. The priority of aims in operative procedures for peptic ulcer should be, first, to preserve the life of the patient; second, to avoid unfavorable side effects; and third, to prevent recurrent ulcer. The best result is an asymptomatic patient. It has been assumed generally that the risk of mortality is less for vagotomy and drainage operations than for resection and that the recurrence rate is lowest with vagotomy and antrectomy, probably intermediate with subtotal gastrectomy alone, and highest with

vagotomy plus a drainage procedure. Study of disparate series clearly reveals that different criteria are used for the selection of patients, that poor-risk patients are often excluded, and that variability exists in the testing of postoperative gastric secretory potential as well as in the vigor with which the study of complications or unfavorable side effects is pursued.

Carefully planned prospective studies with random assignment of surgical procedures to consecutive patients with ulcers are necessary in order to obtain valid data for comparison. The postoperative results of three prospective randomized studies[62,107,146] (as well as those of several nonrandomized series) are summarized in Table 4 (clinical ratings in this table are given on the Visick rating scale; I and II correspond to excellent and good results).

Several points need to be considered in interpreting these studies. As Goligher and Pulvertaft[61] have cautioned, gastric resection is followed by more metabolic ill effects, such as weight loss and anemia, than is vagotomy and drainage. In addition, the fact that there were no deaths in the original series should be interpreted in view of the selection of patients to avoid those with high operative risk. It would appear fair to assume that widespread use of the procedures by the general population of surgeons would be associated with a mortality of approximately 1 per cent in vagotomy plus drainage procedures and of at least 2 per cent in vagotomy and antrectomy.[32] This, then, returns the problem of evaluation to the metaphysical and ultimately unanswerable question: How many ulcer recurrences are equal to one death? Why not tailor the operation to the severity of the ulcer diathesis as estimated by symptoms or acid output? Unfortunately, ulcer recurrence probably cannot be related to the severity of acid secretion before operation.[4]

Although experience is not uniform, there appear to be specific indications for vagotomy and drainage procedures. It appears warranted to advocate this procedure in uncomplicated instances of perforated duodenal ulcer. More important, it is probable that widespread adoption of vagotomy, pyloroplasty, and suture ligation of bleeding duodenal ulcer would cause a diminution in the frightening mortality associated with emergency operations for bleeding. Analysis of mortality following vagotomy, pyloroplasty, and suture ligation for the treatment of bleeding duodenal ulcer reveals some reports as low as 2 and 3 per cent and others as high as 12 per cent, coupled with incidences of rebleeding as high as 25 per cent. Adoption of the U suture-ligation technique[13] for bleeding duodenal ulcers would control bleeding from the transverse pancreatic artery and might well diminish the incidence of rebleeding.

The incidence of recurrent ulceration following vagotomy and drainage appears to be inextricably associated with failure of complete vagus section. Recurrence of ulceration in a patient with great reduction of acid output is extremely rare. Ulcer recurrence is much more closely linked to persistence of vagal innervation than to preoperative secretory activity.

Selective proximal vagotomy is still relatively new, and some believe that it is not yet possible to make any definitive statement about the ultimate role of this operation. Critical comparison with vagotomy and antrectomy led Jordan[108] to conclude that selective proximal vagotomy is superior, even though the recurrence rate of 10 per cent at 10 years was five times greater than with truncal vagotomy and antrectomy; the basis for his judgment is in large part the near-eradication of dumping, diarrhea, and bilious vomiting by selective proximal vagotomy. Inspection of results, as shown in Table 4 and recent summaries,[3,108,117,200] shows that mortality is extremely low and that dumping and diarrhea have been almost eliminated. Recurrences increase with time. An ultimate recurrence rate of 10 to 15 per cent (similar to that with truncal vagotomy) appears likely.[200] There is strong evidence that recurrences are caused by technical failures and that careful attention to the complete denervation of the esophagus will produce substantial improvement.[78]

TABLE 4. Postoperative Results of Operation for Duodenal Ulcer

Procedure	Investigator	Number of Patients	Duration of Study	Per Cent Mortality	Per Cent Recurrence	Per Cent Negative Hollander	Per Cent Dumping	Per Cent Diarrhea	Per Cent Visick I & II
Subtotal gastrectomy	Dinbar et al., 1980	133	5–20 yr.	1.8 elec.	12.7	—	14.2	0	84.2
	Goligher et al., 1968	107	5–8 yr.	0	(5);2	—	—	—	94
	Postlethwait, 1973	346	5 yr.	1.8	3.7	—	12	17.1	89.7
	Walters and Lynn, 1957	549	6–10 yr.	1.7	(1.6);3.7	—	—	—	92
Truncal vagotomy and drainage	Berger et al., 1972	79	9 yr.	0	10	—	1	30	81
	Eisenberg et al., 1969	455	1–10 yr.	1	3.6	—	—	—	—
	Goligher et al., 1969	119	5–8 yr.	0	5.9	—	—	—	89
	Howard et al., 1973	70	2 yr.	0	10	—	8.5	14	—
	Jordan and Condon, 1970	108	2–5 yr.	2	7.4	50(6 mo.)	—	19(1 yr.) 5(5 yr.)	—
	Mulholland et al., 1982	183	0–10 yr.	0	11.6	—	11	16(mild)	62
	O'Leary et al., 1976	348	10 yr.	3	4.9	—	0.3	5(severe)	87
	Pemberton et al., 1980	182	1–17 yr.	3.3 elec.	12.3	—	7.8	6.2	—
	Postlethwait, 1973	337	5 yr.	0.6	6.2	—	12	20.7	83
	Stempien et al., 1971	161	> 10 yr.	—	25.4	46	4.3	1.8	68.3
Truncal vagotomy and antrectomy	Berger et al., 1972	86	9 yr.	0	0	—	7	30(mild)	89
	Goligher et al., 1968	116	5–8 yr.	0	(6);2	—	—	—	92
	Herrington et al., 1973	3584	1–25 yr.	1.6	0.6	—	25(mild)	1	94
	Howard et al., 1973	51	> 2 yr.	0	4	—	27	22	—
	Hubert et al., 1980	412	17.1 yr.	1.1	0.7	—	1	0.7	70.4
	Jordan and Condon, 1970	92	2–5 yr.	0	0	87	—	16	—
	Postlethwait, 1973	331	5 yr.	0.9	0.7	—	17.2	21.5	89.2
Selective vagotomy and drainage	Amdrup and Jensen, 1973	100	5 yr.	0	6	79	34	1	85
	Griffith, 1980	87	12–17 yr.	—	5.7	78	—	—	—
	Humphrey and Wilkinson, 1972	67	1–2 yr.	—	—	—	25	19	64
	Kronborg and Madsen, 1975	50	> 1 yr.	0	8	—	30	32	68
	Siim et al., 1981	105	10–13 yr.	—	15	—	4	3	77
Selective proximal vagotomy	Adami et al., 1980	211	1–6 yr.	0	12.7	—	1.3	2.2	70
	Amdrup, 1974	108	> 2 yr.	0	—	—	5	5	86
	Blackett and Johnston, 1981	233	5–12 yr.	0	10.7	—	—	—	—
	Burge, 1972	130	3 yr.	0	1	—	—	—	—
	Goliger et al., 1978	117	5–8 yr.	0	4.3	—	0.9	5.1	75
	Grassie et al., 1973	79	2–4 yr.	0	1.2	97	0	0	97
	Hedenstedt et al., 1972	131	0.5–3 yr.	0	2.3	94	—	0	—
	Holle et al., 1972	732	1–7 yr.	0.7	0.7	70	—	—	89
	Imperati et al., 1972	62	3–10 mo.	0	—	80	0	—	97
	Johnston, 1974	400	1–5 yr.	0	0.5	60	—	—	88
	Jordan, 1979	35	5 yr.	—	11.4	—	2.5	2.5	95
	Kuzin and Postolov, 1980	210	0–1 yr.	0.5	1.9	—	—	—	—
	Sawyers et al., 1977	86	0.5–4 yr.	1.2	3.5	70	1.2	1.2	95
	Van Heerden et al., 1980	194	6–78 mo.	0	5.1	—	1.5	1.5	—
	Wastell et al., 1977	52	3–7 yr.	0	6	—	6	2	78

Modified from Thompson, J. C., and Wiener, I.: Evaluation of surgical treatment for duodenal ulcer. Acute and long-term effects. Clin. Gastroenterol., 13:569, 1984.

OTHER SURGICAL DISEASES OF THE STOMACH

MALLORY-WEISS SYNDROME

In 1929, Mallory and Weiss[131] described clinical and autopsy findings in four alcoholic patients who had bled from the upper gastrointestinal tract. These patients had longitudinal tears of the esophagogastric mucosa through which the bleeding had occurred. The tears were considered to be due to forceful vomiting. A review of 229 cases[211] revealed an association with alcohol in 60 per cent of cases and with vomiting in 90 per cent. In addition to vomiting, other etiologic conditions were closed-chest massage, or episodes of severe coughing, or other severe increases in intra-abdominal pressure.

Routine application of fiberoptic endoscopy in patients with upper gastrointestinal hemorrhage will almost certainly reveal a much larger incidence of the Mallory-Weiss syndrome than has previously been suspected. The author found an incidence of 7.7 per cent in 195 consecutive patients admitted with massive upper gastrointestinal hemorrhage (see Table 3).[206]

Almost all patients with the Mallory-Weiss syndrome stop bleeding spontaneously. Success may also be achieved with judicious use of the Sengstaken-Blakemore tube. Cautious application of endoscopic cautery techniques offers promise. If bleeding persists, it may rarely be necessary to repair the lesion at operation. A long gastrostomy incision high in the stomach is required for visualization of the tear, which may then best be oversewn from below upward. This laceration should be considered whenever a patient is bleeding vigorously from the upper gastrointestinal tract and there is no obvious diagnosis. There is no indication for performing vagotomy.

ACUTE GASTRIC DILATION

Acute dilation of the stomach is a rare complication observed in patients who are severely ill, who are often comatose, and who have ileus. The condition develops insidiously and may come to medical attention with symptoms of hypovolemia, cardiac failure, or pulmonary edema (after the patient vomits and aspirates massive amounts of gastric juice). Emergency resuscitative measures in patients who have respiratory arrests often introduce massive quantities of air into the stomach.

The vomiting of small amounts of brackish, coffee-ground gastric juice, often associated with hiccups (overflow vomiting), should serve as an immediate indication to the possibility of gastric dilation. The treatment is introduction of a nasogastric tube and aspiration of gastric contents. With accumulation of air and distention of the stomach, there is an outpouring of gastric juice, and as distention increases there may be bleeding. Large amounts of air and 3 to 4 liters of gastric juice may be recovered from the stomach by aspiration. Massive hemorrhage or rupture of the stomach may occur, requiring immediate operative repair.

The most important treatment is prophylaxis. Any patient who has ileus should have a functioning nasogastric tube. If a nasogastric tube is removed from a postoperative debilitated or elderly patient whose bowel function is still questionable, it is wise to assess the gastric residual in 6 to 8 hours to be certain that the stomach has not dilated. Acute gastric dilation may be fatal in a short time if not recognized and corrected.

NONPEPTIC SURGICAL DISEASES OF THE DUODENUM

Those conditions of surgical interest that affect the entire small bowel are discussed in the chapter on the small intestine and are mentioned here only briefly. The duodenum, rarely, and the stomach, even more rarely, are involved with Crohn's disease.[25,53] The symptoms are usually those of upper gastrointestinal obstruction caused by duodenal stenosis. The diagnosis can be made radiographically if the disease involves the rest of the small bowel, but isolated lesions in the duodenum are often difficult to interpret and the diagnosis is commonly made at operation. The symptoms of obstruction are relieved by simple bypass of the stenotic area by gastrojejunostomy or by duodenojejunostomy.

Tumors of the duodenum are classified according to their anatomic relation to the duodenal papilla: 20 per cent are proximal to the papilla, 60 per cent are peripapillary, and 20 per cent are distal.[113] Malignant duodenal tumors may be divided according to the symptoms they produce: obstructing lesions produce vomiting, ulcerating lesions cause bleeding, penetrating lesions may produce refractory pain, and periampullary lesions may produce jaundice and mimic carcinoma of the head of the pancreas. In the last group, the differential diagnosis lies among a primary tumor of the duodenum, a tumor of the head of the pancreas (which may actually erode into the medial wall of the duodenum), and carcinoma of the ampulla.[142] The treatment is the same, but each tumor has a different prognosis (duodenal cancer is intermediate between the other two). The outlook is bleak, but not hopeless.

Villous tumors of the duodenum often appear benign on endoscopy, but multiple biopsies usually reveal malignant changes. Because of their propensity for recurrence after local excision, a strong consideration of primary Whipple resection is worthwhile.[28]

In a study of 24 patients seen at the Mayo Clinic with malignant infrapapillary tumors of the duodenum,[83] the diagnosis was made in 22 cases by radiography, but only half the patients had tumors that were resectable, and of those patients whose tumors were resected, only one third were alive 5 years after operation.

Intramural hematomas of the duodenum may occasionally mimic neoplasms by producing partial obstruction of the duodenum or the common bile duct. There is usually a clear associa-

tion of the lesion with trauma, but occasionally duodenal hematomas may arise spontaneously in patients who have blood dyscrasias or who are on anticoagulant medication. The hematoma usually subsides in time,[103] but because of persistent obstruction or bleeding or an error in diagnosis, the patient may be operated on and, rarely, may require resection of the involved segment.[139]

TRAUMATIC RUPTURE

The duodenum is situated deep in the abdominal cavity and is well protected. Trauma to the duodenum usually involves injury to other organs, and these associated injuries, especially to the pancreas, liver, and inferior vena cava, are a major factor in the prognosis. The injury may be caused by penetrating wounds from knives or gunshot or may be caused by blunt trauma, especially in automobile accidents or falls. Morton and Jordan[140] have reported 131 patients with duodenal injuries, of whom 117 had penetrating wounds and 14 had blunt trauma to the abdomen. Lacerations involved less than half of the circumference of the duodenum in 80 per cent of patients, and 3 per cent had complete transection. Associated injuries to all structures of the upper abdomen were common; the liver was involved in 38 per cent, the pancreas in 28 per cent, and the inferior vena cava in 17 per cent.

Diagnosis prior to operation is unusual, but it may be suspected because of the magnitude of the injury. It is particularly difficult to make the diagnosis of retroperitoneal duodenal rupture after blunt trauma, because symptoms may not occur for 24 to 36 hours. Plain films of the abdomen may reveal free air with penetrating wounds or may show streaks of air in the retroperitoneal tissue around the duodenum and may occasionally outline the kidney. The oral administration of a water-soluble contrast agent may be of help in making the radiologic diagnosis of a duodenal rupture.

Diagnosis of retroperitoneal rupture following blunt trauma may be difficult at laparotomy. Important clues to the diagnosis are bile-staining of the peritoneum of the posterior wall of the abdomen, emphysema of the retroperitoneum or of the mesocolon, and boggy crepitance inferior to the curve of the duodenum.[38] Retroperitoneal hematomas adjacent to the duodenum must be opened and explored; they often conceal duodenal rupture.

If the site of injury is not apparent, the duodenum should be mobilized by dividing the ligament of Treitz, dividing the lateral peritoneal reflection of the second and third part of the duodenum, and freeing the hepatic flexure of the colon. It was possible to treat 85 per cent of patients by débridement and simple closure of the laceration; the serosal patch technique[114] of using an onlay cover of small bowel sutured to the margins of the laceration may be helpful in closing large defects. In severe injuries, defunctionalization of the repaired duodenal laceration has been advocated. This may be accomplished either by pyloric suture and gastrojejunostomy as favored by Graham and colleagues[64] or by gastrostomy and proximal and distal jejunostomy as favored by Stone and Fabian.[176]

In one series, more than one third of 175 patients with duodenal injury were found to have associated pancreatic trauma.[64] Some patients were managed by simple duodenal suture and drainage, but the majority required more extensive procedures, including duodenal diversion and pyloric exclusion and, in the most severe injuries, pancreaticoduodenectomy. The last procedure is rarely justified and clearly should be reserved for the most extreme degree of destructive injury. Reported mortality for duodenal rupture varies between 14 and 50 per cent and depends largely on the severity of the associated injuries and on delay in diagnosis, especially with retroperitoneal rupture after blunt trauma. Death is due to sepsis or to hemorrhage.

The most common postoperative complications are peritonitis, sepsis associated with intraperitoneal abscesses, and fistulas from the duodenum and pancreas.

DIVERTICULITIS

After the colon, the duodenum is the most common site for diverticula. They are fairly rare in patients younger than 40 years of age and are slightly more common in women than in men. Diverticula usually arise in the second or third portion of the duodenum on the concave medial wall but may appear posterior to the pancreas. Inflammation of the diverticula may produce pain, perforation, hemorrhage, pancreatitis, or obstruction of the common bile duct.[106] Gallstones are common in patients with duodenal diverticula, and the biliary tract should be studied in patients who are thought to have symptomatic duodenal diverticulitis. Vague symptoms of upper abdominal discomfort are common, and duodenal diverticula are relatively common, but symptomatic duodenal diverticulitis is rare. The decision to operate on duodenal diverticula should be made with great caution except when there is clear evidence of perforation, bleeding, or obstruction. Rarely, duodenal obstruction is caused by intraluminal protrusion of the duodenal diverticulum.[56]

At operation, the duodenum should be mobilized by dividing the lateral peritoneal attachments and reflecting the duodenum medialward to expose the posterior surface. The diverticulum usually protrudes between the duodenum and pancreas and may be excised and the defect oversewn. If the diverticulum is adjacent to the papilla, care must be exercised to avoid injury to the bile and pancreatic ducts.

The mortality for operations on duodenal diverticula varies between 5 and 10 per cent, and postoperative complications, particularly duodenal fistula, are common.

OBSTRUCTION

The duodenum may be obstructed by scarring caused by peptic ulcer, by duodenal diverticula, by tumors, rarely by diaphragmatic webs,[160] and uncommonly by the pancreas or the superior mesenteric artery.[132]

Annular Pancreas

The envelopment of the second part of the duodenum with a ring of pancreatic tissue is thought to be due to a failure of the ventral anlage of the pancreas to rotate with the duodenum, an event that normally occurs in the sixth and seventh weeks of gestation. The course of the pancreatic duct in patients with annular pancreas suggests that the ventral anlage is fixed anteriorly and in rotating around the duodenum leaves a ring of pancreatic tissue. The age of onset of symptoms depends on the severity of constriction and on whether there is an associated stenosis or atresia of the duodenum. Almost half the children and 15 per cent of the adults with annular pancreas have associated duodenal stenosis. Complications observed with annular pancreas are obstruction of the duodenum, peptic ulcer of the stomach or duodenum observed in one third of patients (probably due to prolonged antral stasis), acute or chronic pancreatitis of the annulus itself (16 per cent), and rare associated biliary obstruction.[215] Infants with neonatal obstruction of the duodenum caused by annular pancreas often are the product of pregnancies that have been complicated by polyhydramnios. Associated anomalies are Down's syndrome, tracheoesophageal fistula, malrotation of the colon, duodenal atresia, and others.[81]

Diagnosis is often made on radiographs, which may show two gas shadows with air-fluid levels (the double-bubble sign) or a dumbbell-shaped shadow. In adults, the diagnosis is often made by the radiologic demonstration of a hugely dilated first portion of the duodenum.

Some patients with annular pancreas may live their entire lives without symptoms. For those patients who have obstruction of the duodenum, the proper treatment is bypass of the area of obstruction by anastomosis of the proximal duodenum with the first part of the jejunum.

SELECTED REFERENCES

Daugherty, D., and Yamada, T.: Posttranslational processing of gastrin. Physiol. Rev., 69:482, 1989.
This is an excellent summary of what is known of the molecular biology of gastrin synthesis, which provides evidence that gastrin cells store and release different molecular forms of gastrin. Purification and techniques of sequencing amino acids of gastrin have allowed determination of the structure of gastrin precursors. These posttranslational-processing events may be crucial in the regulation of gastrin and are thereby related to normal and pathologic acid secretion.

Davenport, H. W.: Salicylate damage to gastric mucosal barrier. N. Engl. J. Med., 276:1307, 1967.
This is the classic article on the effect of salicylates and, by analogy, of all anti-inflammatory drugs, on the gastric mucosal barrier, the protective action of which, as Davenport stresses, is provided primarily by the apical membranes of the gastric epithelial cell. He shows that the apparent diminution in acid secretion, noted after administration of salicylate, is actually due to back-diffusion of secreted acid into the mucosa. This work is the model for all studies on gastric mucosal injury.

DeBakey, M., and Ochsner, A.: Recent advances in surgery. Bezoars and concretions. A comprehensive review of the literature with an analysis of 303 collected cases and a presentation of 8 additional cases. Surgery, 4:934, 1938; 5:132, 1939.
This paper, published in two parts, is included because it provides a near-perfect model of what a review article should be. Having read this article, one believes that there is little further to be known about bezoars.

Dragstedt, L. R.: The physiology of the gastric antrum. Arch. Surg., 75:552, 1957.
This brief article provides a lucid summary of the role of the gastric antrum in gastric secretion. In the process, it provides a concise record of the tremendous contributions that Dragstedt and his colleagues made to the understanding of the role of gastrin and of acid feedback inhibition of gastrin release in gastric physiology.

Goligher, J. C.: A technique for highly selective parietal cell or proximal gastric vagotomy for duodenal ulcer. Br. J. Surg., 61:337, 1974.
This is the classic description of the operative technique for selective vagotomy of the proximal stomach. It could serve as a model for papers on operative technique.

Isenberg, J. I., and Johansson, C. (Eds.): Peptic ulcer disease. Clin. Gastroenterol., 13:287, 1984.
An excellent presentation of the current theories and practices regarding etiology, pathogenesis, natural history, complications, and medical and surgical therapy of peptic ulcer.

Kelly, K. A., and Malagelada, J. R.: Medical and surgical treatment of chronic gastric ulcer. Clin. Gastroenterol., 13:621, 1984.
A clearly arranged integration of medical and surgical approaches to the treatment of gastric ulcer. A summary of recent results of treatment with H$_2$-antagonists is provided. The surgical approaches suggested are interesting. Relatively little discussion is provided for distal 40 to 50 per cent gastrectomy with gastroduodenostomy, which is probably used (with success) by a majority of surgeons over the world to treat gastric ulcer.

Michels, N. A.: Blood supply of the stomach and the esophagus. In Blood Supply and Anatomy of the Upper Abdominal Organs. Philadelphia, J. B. Lippincott Company, 1955, p. 248.
This beautiful description of the anatomic variations of the blood supply to the stomach and esophagus carefully documents the large number of variations and teaches that the standard blood supply that is assumed is actually only a statistical median of huge numbers of possible variants.

Soll, A. H.: Pathogenesis of peptic ulcer and implications for therapy. N. Engl. J. Med., 322:909, 1990.
This up-to-date summary provides information on current concepts of the role of mucosal defense (particularly as impaired by nonsteroidal anti-inflammatory drugs and by Campylobacter pylori) in the pathogenesis of peptic ulcer. Although it was formally considered that duodenal ulcer disease followed increased forces of acid-peptic attack against a relatively normal mucosa, there is now abundant evidence that impaired defense mechanisms, often associated with changes in mucosal bicarbonate secretion, influence ulcer development.

Stabile, B. E., and Passaro, E., Jr.: Duodenal ulcer: A disease in evolution. Curr. Probl. Surg., 21:1, 1984.
A thoughtful and well-organized summary of the entire field of peptic ulcer: etiology, epidemiology, diagnosis, treatment, results, and complications.

Thompson, J. C.: The role of surgery in peptic ulcer. (Editorial.) N. Engl. J. Med., 307:550, 1982.
A review of the diminished incidence of duodenal ulcer and of the reduced need for surgical treatment. The point is made, however, that since complications (bleeding, perforation, and obstruction) continue to occur, and since the recurrence rate after

H₂-blockage treatment is high, and since selective proximal vagotomy offers a cure with little risk, there is likely an important role for surgeons in the future care of patients with peptic ulcer.

Thompson, J. C., Lewis, B. G., Wiener, I., and Townsend, C. M., Jr.: The role of surgery in the Zollinger-Ellison syndrome. Ann. Surg., 197:594, 1983.
A summary of results of 27 patients with the Zollinger-Ellison syndrome, of whom 23 were treated by total gastrectomy without operative mortality. The actuarial survival was 75 per cent at 5 years. The nutritional status after total gastrectomy is excellent (mean postoperative weight loss less than 15 per cent). Authors contend that their results compare well with long-term medical management, the success of which is dependent on serial favorable responses to a lifetime of repeated challenges.

Thompson, J. C., and Marx, M.: Gastrointestinal hormones. Curr. Probl. Surg., 21:1, 1984.
This report summarizes the role of gastrointestinal hormones on the physiology of the gut. The agents covered are gastrin, cholecystokinin, secretin, glucagon, gastric inhibitory polypeptide, vasoactive intestinal polypeptide, pancreatic polypeptide, somatostatin, neurotensin, motilin, substance P, and bombesin, plus discussions of interrelations among gut, brain, and calcium-regulating peptides.

Thompson, J. C., and Wiener, I.: Evaluation of surgical treatment for duodenal ulcer. Acute and long-term effects. Clin. Gastroenterol., 13:569, 1984.
A summary of the current role of operative treatment for peptic ulcer and of the expected results and side effects of various operations. The relative advantages of different procedures are compared, and the specific choices for different operative indications are discussed.

Townsend, C. M., Jr., and Thompson, J. C.: Stress ulceration. In Shires, G. T. (Ed.): Principles of Trauma Care. New York, McGraw-Hill, 1984, p. 548.
A brief summary of the natural history (etiology and pathogenesis) of acute mucosal erosions, along with plans for their prevention and treatment. Attention is directed to causes of stress ulcer (sepsis, hypoxemia, starvation) and the salient need to drain pus. Surgical alternatives are reviewed.

Townsend, C. M., Jr., Lewis, B. G., Grourley, W. K., and Thompson, J. C.: Gastrinoma. Curr. Probl. Cancer, 7:1, 1982.
A brief précis of information regarding the biologic behavior of gastrin-producing tumors. An outline is provided for operative and postoperative management.

Wolfe, M. M., and Jensen, R. T.: Zollinger-Ellison syndrome: Current concepts in diagnosis and management. N. Engl. J. Med., 317:1200, 1987.
These authors have wide experience in the medical management of duodenal ulcer disease and clearly differentiated between the threats of acid hypersecretion versus those of tumor growth. The rationale for various medical regimens are delineated and a logical sequence of management of metastatic gastrinoma is presented, although any enthusiasm for the various chemotherapeutic regimens is hardly justified by the success rate.

Wolfe, M. M., and Soll, A. H.: The physiology of gastric acid secretion. N. Engl. J. Med., 319:1707, 1988.
A clear review of current ideas regarding control mechanisms influencing secretion of acid by the parietal cell. The role of various stimulants and inhibitors of acid secretion on cell membrane receptors and on intracellular cytosolic mechanisms is dissected, and the contributions of various mechanisms are given priority; for example, the gastric phase of acid secretion is said to represent 40 to 50 per cent of the total acid secretory response to a meal. Disorders of acid secretion are discussed in detail, and therapeutic regimens designed to reduce acid secretion are compared and critically examined.

Zollinger, R. M., and Ellison, R. H.: Primary peptic ulcerations of the jejunum associated with islet cell tumor of pancreas. Ann. Surg., 142:709, 1955.
The initial description of the syndrome of gastric hypersecretion, hypergastrinemia, and gastrinoma by Zollinger and Ellison. The authors predicted that the hypersecretory state was caused by a hormone elaborated from a pancreatic islet cell tumor and suggested that total gastrectomy was the treatment of choice. This beautiful description of the case history of two patients clearly demonstrates Pasteur's dictum, "In the field of investigation, chance favors the prepared mind."

REFERENCES

1. Ahlquist, D. A., Dozois, R. R., Zinsmeister, A. R., and Malagelada, J.-R.: Duodenal prostaglandin synthesis and acid load in health and in duodenal ulcer disease. Gastroenterology, 85:522, 1983.
2. Almy, T. P.: Digestive disease as a national problem. II. A white paper by the American Gastroenterological Association, 1967. Gastroenterology, 53:821, 1967.
3. Amdrup, E., Andersen, D., and Jensen, H.-E.: Parietal cell (highly selective or proximal gastric) vagotomy for peptic ulcer disease. World J. Surg., 1:19, 1977.
4. Andersen, D., Amdrup, E., Hostrup, H., and Sorensen, F. H.: The Aarhus County Vagotomy Trial: Trends in the problem of recurrent ulcer after parietal cell vagotomy and selective gastric vagotomy with a drainage. World J. Surg., 6:86, 1982.
5. Andersen, D., Amdrup, E., Sorensen, F. H., and Jensen, K. B.: Surgery or cimetidine? I. Comparison of two plans of treatment: Operation or repeated cimetidine. World J. Surg., 7:372, 1983.
6. Andersson, S.: Gastric and duodenal mechanisms inhibiting gastric secretion of acid. In Code, C. F. (Ed.): American Physiological Society: Handbook of Physiology, Section 6, Alimentary Canal. Vol. 2. Baltimore, Williams & Wilkins, 1967, pp. 865–877.
7. Angel, R. T., Giacobine, J. W., and Jordan, G. L., Jr.: A current evaluation of the problem of gastric ulcers. Am. J. Surg., 114:730, 1967.
8. Athanasoulis, C. A., Baum, S., Waltman, A. C., Ring, E. J., Imbembo, A., and Salm, T. J.: Control of acute gastric mucosal hemorrhage: Intra-arterial infusion of posterior pituitary extracts. N. Engl. J. Med., 209:597, 1974.
9. Barclay, G., Maxwell, V., Grossman, M. I., and Solomon, T. E.: Effects of graded amounts of intragastric calcium on acid secretion, gastrin release, and gastric emptying in normal and duodenal ulcer subjects. Dig. Dis. Sci., 28:385, 1983.
10. Bardhan, K. D., Cust, G., Hinchliffe, R. F. C., Williamson, F. M., Lyon, C., and Bose, K.: Changing pattern of admissions and operations for duodenal ulcer. Br. J. Surg., 76:230, 1989.
11. Barnes, A. D., and Cox, A. G.: Diarrhea. In Williams, J. A., and Cox, A. G. (Eds.): After Vagotomy. London, Butterworth & Company, 1969, p. 211.
12. Baron, J. H.: Studies of basal and peak acid output with an augmented histamine test. Gut, 4:136, 1963.
13. Berne, C. J., and Rosoff, L.: Peptic ulcer perforation of the gastroduodenal artery complex. Ann. Surg., 169:141, 1969.
14. Berson, S. A., and Yalow, R. S.: Gastrin in duodenal ulcers. N. Engl. J. Med., 284:445, 1971.
15. Bittner, R., Schirrow, H., Butters, M., Roscher, R., Wolfgang, K., Wolfgang, O., and Beger, H. G.: Total gastrectomy: A 15-year experience with particular reference to the patient over 70 years of age. Arch. Surg., 120:1120, 1985.
16. Blackett, R. L., and Johnston, D.: Recurrent ulceration after higher selective vagotomy for duodenal ulcer. Br. J. Surg., 68:705, 1981.
17. Bondar, G. F., Yakimets, W. W., Williams, T. G., and MacKenzie, W. C.: Diagnosis and management of stomal ulcer. Can. J. Surg., 7:383, 1964.
18. Bonnevie, O.: The incidence of gastric ulcer in Copenhagen County. Scand. J. Gastroenterol., 10:231, 1975.
19. Bonnevie, O.: The incidence of duodenal ulcer in Copenhagen County. Scand. J. Gastroenterol., 10:385, 1975.
20. Bowen, J. C., Fleming, W. H., and Thompson, J. C.: Increased gastrin release following penetrating central nervous system injury. Surgery, 75:720, 1974.
21. Brechenridge, I. M., Walton, E. W., and Walker, W. F.: Stress ulcers in the stomach. Br. Med. J., 2:1362, 1959.
22. Briden, S., Flemstrom, G., and Kivilaakso, E.: Cysteamine and propionitrile inhibit the rise of duodenal mucosal alkaline secretion in response to luminal acid in rats. Gastroenterology, 88:295, 1985.
23. Brodie, D. A., and Hanson, H. M.: A study of the factors involved in the production of gastric ulcers by the restraint technique. Gastroenterology, 38:353, 1960.
24. Broome, A., and Bergstrom, H.: Selective surgery for duodenal ulcer based on preoperative acid production. Acta Chir. Scand., 132:170, 1966.
25. Burgess, J. N., Legge, D. A., and Judd, E. S.: Surgical treatment of regional enteritis of the stomach and duodenum. Surg. Gynecol. Obstet., 132:628, 1971.
26. Cano, R., Bloom, S. R., and Isenberg, J. I.: Pancreatic bicarbonate secretion in serum secretin in response to graded amounts of duodenal acidification in duodenal ulcer and normal subjects. Gastroenterology, 68:870, 1975.
27. Capper, W. M., Butler, T. J., Buckler, K. G., and Hallett, C. P.: Variation in size of the gastric antrum: Measurement of alkaline area associated with ulceration and pyloric stenosis. Ann. Surg., 163:281, 1966.
28. Chappuis, C. W., Divincenti, F. C., and Cohn, I., Jr.: Villous tumors of the duodenum. Ann. Surg., 209:593, 1988.
29. Chenoweth, A. I., and Dimich, A. R.: Stress ulcer in infants and children. Ann. Surg., 161:977, 1965.
30. Christiansen, J., Ottenjann, R., and Von Arx, F.: Placebo-controlled trial with the somatostatin analogue SMS 201–995 in peptic ulcer bleeding. Gastroenterology, 97:568, 1989.
31. Cook, L., and Hutton, C. F.: Postbulbar duodenal ulceration. Lancet, 1:754, 1958.
32. Cox, A. G.: Vagotomy and drainage procedures. The present position. Prog. Surg., 8:45, 1970.
33. Cox, A. J., Jr.: Stomach size and its relation to chronic peptic ulcer. Arch. Pathol., 54:407, 1952.
34. Daugherty, D., and Yamada, T.: Posttranslational processing of gastrin. Physiol. Rev., 69:482, 1989.
35. Davenport, H. W.: Physiologic structure of the gastric mucosa. In Code, C. F. (Ed.): American Physiologic Society: Handbook of Physiology, Section 6, Alimentary Canal. Vol. 2. Baltimore, Williams & Wilkins, 1967, pp. 759–779.
36. Davenport, H. W.: Salicylate damage to the gastric mucosal barrier. N. Engl. J. Med., 276:1307, 1967.
37. Delaney, J. P., Cheng, J. W. B., Butler, B. A., and Ritchie, W. P., Jr.: Gastric ulcer and regurgitation gastritis. Gut, 11:715, 1970.
38. Deodhar, M. C., Duleep, K. S., Gill, S. S., and Eggleston, F. C.: Retroperitoneal rupture of the duodenum following blunt trauma. Arch. Surg., 96:963, 1968.
39. Donovan, A. J., Venson, T. L., Maulsby, G. O., and Gewin, J. R.: Selective treatment of duodenal ulcer with perforation. Ann. Surg., 189:627, 1979.
40. Dowse, J. L. A.: Spontaneous internal biliary fistulae. Gut, 5:429, 1964.
41. Dragstedt, L. R.: Vagotomy for gastroduodenal ulcer. Ann Surg., 122:973, 1949.

42. Dragstedt, L. R., and Owens, F. M., Jr.: Supradiaphragmatic secretion of vagus nerves in treatment of duodenal ulcer. Proc. Soc. Exp. Biol. Med., 53:152, 1943.

43. Drumm, B., Sherman, P., Cutz, E., and Karmali, M.: Association of *Campylobacter pylori* on the gastric mucosa with antral gastrin in children. N. Engl. J. Med., 316:1557, 1987.

44. Du Plessis, D. J.: Pathogenesis of gastric ulceration. Lancet, 1:974, 1965.

45. Eckhauser, F. E., Knol, J. A., Raper, S. A., and Guice, K. S.: Completion gastrectomy for postsurgical gastroparesis syndrome: Preliminary results with 15 patients. Ann. Surg., 208:345, 1988.

46. Edkins, J. S.: On the chemical mechanism of gastric secretion. Proc. R. Soc. London, 76:376, 1905.

47. Edkins, J. S.: The chemical mechanism of gastric secretion. J. Physiol., 34:133, 1906.

48. Eisenberg, M. D., Woodward, E. R., Carson, T. J., and Dragstedt, L. R.: Vagotomy and drainage procedure for duodenal ulcer: The results of ten years' experience. Ann. Surg., 170:317, 1969.

49. Ekman, L., Hansson, E., Havu, N., Carlsson, E., and Lundberg, C.: Toxicological studies on omeprazole. Scand. J. Gastroenterol. (Suppl.), 108:53, 1985.

50. Elashoff, J. D., and Grossman, M. I.: Trends in hospital admissions and death rates for peptic ulcer in the United States from 1970 to 1978. Gastroenterology, 78:280, 1980.

51. Feldman, M., Walker, P., Green, J. L., and Weingarden, K.: Life events stress and psychosocial factors in men with peptic ulcer disease: A multidimensional case-controlled study. Gastroenterology, 91:1370, 1986.

52. Feller, E. R., Warshaw, A. L., and Schapiro, R. H.: Observations on management of choledochoduodenal fistula due to penetrating peptic ulcer. Gastroenterology, 78:226, 1980.

53. Fielding, J. F., Toye, D. K. M., Beton, D. C., and Cooke, W. T.: Crohn's disease of the stomach and duodenum. Gut, 11:1001, 1970.

54. Finneberg, H. V., and Pearlman, L. A.: Surgical treatment of peptic ulcer in the United States: Trends before and after the introduction of cimetidine. Lancet, 1:1305, 1981.

55. Fisher, R. S., and Cohen, S.: Pyloric-sphincter dysfunction in patients with gastric ulcer. N. Engl. J. Med., 288:273, 1973.

56. Fleming, C. R., Newcomer, A. D., Stephens, D. H., and Carlson, H. C.: Intraluminal duodenal diverticulum. Mayo Clin. Proc., 50:244, 1975.

57. Flemstrom, G., and Turnberg, L. A.: Gastroduodenal defense mechanisms. Clin. Gastroenterol., 13:327, 1984.

58. Glick, D. L., and Kern, F., Jr.: Peptic ulcer and chronic obstructive bronchopulmonary disease. A prospective clinical study of prevalence. Gastroenterology, 47:153, 1964.

59. Goldstein, H., and Boyle, J. D.: The saline load test—a bedside evaluation of gastric retention. Gastroenterology, 49:375, 1965.

60. Goligher, J. C.: A technique for highly selective (parietal cell or proximal gastric) vagotomy for duodenal ulcer. Br. J. Surg., 61:337, 1974.

61. Goligher, J. C., and Pulvertaft, C. N.: Comparison of different operations. In Williams, J. A., and Cox, A. G. (Eds.): After Vagotomy. London, Butterworth & Company, 1969, p. 93.

62. Goligher, J. C., Pulvertaft, C. N., De Dombal, F. T., Conyers, J. H., Duthie, H. L., Feather, D. B., Latchmore, A. J. C., Shoesmith, J. H., Smiddy, F. G., and Willson-Pepper, J.: Five-to-eight-year results of Leeds-York controlled trial of elective surgery for duodenal ulcer. Br. Med. J., 2:781, 1968.

63. Gordon, M. J., Skillman, J. J., Zervas, N. T., and Silen, W.: Divergent nature of gastric mucosal permeability and gastric acid secretion in sick patients with general surgical and neurosurgical disease. Ann. Surg., 178:285, 1973.

64. Graham, J. M., Mattox, K. L., Vaughan, G. D., III, and Jordan, G. L., Jr.: Combined pancreatoduodenal injuries. J. Trauma, 19:340, 1979.

65. Greenall, M. J., and Lehnert, T.: Vagotomy or gastrectomy for elective treatment of benign gastric ulceration? Dig. Dis. Sci., 30:353, 1985.

66. Gregory, R. A.: Memorial lecture: The isolation and chemistry of gastrin. Gastroenterology, 51:953, 1966.

67. Gregory, R. A., Grossman, M. I., Tracy, H. J., and Bentley, P. H.: Nature of the gastric secretagogue in Zollinger-Ellison tumors. Lancet, 2:543, 1967.

68. Gregory, R. A., and Tracy, H. J.: The constitution and properties of two gastrins extracted from hog antral mucosa. Gut, 5:103, 1964.

69. Greibe, J., Bugge, P., Gjorup, T., Lauritzen, T., Bonnevie, O., and Wulff, H. R.: Long-term prognosis of duodenal ulcer: Follow-up study and survey of doctors' estimates. Br. Med. J., 2:1527, 1977.

70. Grosfeld, J. L., Shipley, F., Fitzgerald, J. F., and Ballatine, T. V. N.: Acute peptic ulcer in infancy and childhood. Am. Surg., 44:13, 1978.

71. Grossman, M. I.: Peptic ulcer: Pathogenesis and pathophysiology. In Beeson, P. B., McDermott, W., and Wyngaarden, J. B. (Eds.): Textbook of Medicine. Philadelphia, W. B. Saunders Company, 1979, pp. 1502.

72. Grossman, M. I.: Gastrin and its activities. Nature, 228:1147, 1970.

73. Grossman, M. I.: Résumé and comment. In The Veterans Administration Cooperative Study on Gastric Ulcer. Gastroenterology, 61:635, 1971.

74. Grossman, M. I., Kirsner, J. B., and Gillespie, I. E.: Basal and histalog-stimulated gastric secretion in control subjects and in patients with peptic ulcer or gastric cancer. Gastroenterology, 45:14, 1963.

75. Grossman, M. I., and Konturek, S. J.: Inhibition of acid secretion in dog by metiamide, a histamine antagonist acting on H_2 receptors. Gastroenterology, 66:517, 1974.

76. Grossman, M. I., Guth, P. H., Isenberg, J. I., Passaro, E. P., Jr., Roth, B. E., Sturdevant, R. A. L., and Walsh, J. H.: A new look at peptic ulcer. Ann. Intern. Med., 84:57, 1976.

77. Hallenbeck, G. A.: The Zollinger-Ellison syndrome. Gastroenterology, 54:426, 1968.

78. Hallenbeck, G. A., Gleysteen, J. J., Aldrete, J. S., and Slaughter, R. L.: Proximal gastric vagotomy: Effects of two operative techniques on clinical and gastric secretory results. Ann. Surg., 184:435, 1976.

79. Hansky, J.: Effect of renal failure on gastrointestinal hormones. World J. Surg., 3:463, 1979.

80. Harken, A. H., Gabel, R. A., Fenel, V., and Moore, F. D.: Hydrochloric acid in the correction of metabolic alkalosis. Arch. Surg., 110:819, 1975.

81. Hays, D. M., Greaney, E. M., Jr., and Hill, J. T.: Annular pancreas as a cause of acute neonatal duodenal obstruction. Ann. Surg., 153:103, 1961.

82. Heatley, N. G.: Mucosubstance as a barrier to diffusion. Gastroenterology, 37:313, 1959.

83. Higgins, D. C., Judd, E. S., and Dockerty, M. B.: Surgical aspects of infrapapillary duodenal tumors. Surgery, 49:149, 1961.

84. Hinchey, E. J., Hreno, A., Benoit, P. R., Hewson, J. R., and Gurd, F. N.: The stress ulcer syndrome. Adv. Surg., 4:325, 1970.

85. Hirschowitz, B. I.: Natural history of duodenal ulcer. Gastroenterology, 85:967, 1983.

86. Hollander, F.: Gastric secretion of electrolytes. Fed. Proc., 11:706, 1952.

87. Hollander, F.: Two-component mucous barrier: Its activity in protecting gastroduodenal mucosa against peptic ulceration. Arch. Intern. Med., 93:107, 1954.

88. Hollander, F.: The significance of sodium and potassium in gastric secretion: A review. Gastroenterology, 40:477, 1961.

89. Holle, F.: Surgery of gastroduodenal ulcer based on form and function. Importance, reasoning, technique and results in 580 cases, 300 of them postexamined. Chir. Orthop., 54:1, 1970.

90. Hopman, W. P. M., Wolberink, R. G. J., Lamers, C. B. H. W., and Van Tongeren, J. H. M.: Treatment of the dumping syndrome with the somatostatin analogue SMS 201–995. Ann. Surg., 207:155, 1988.

91. Isenberg, J. I.: Gastric secretory testing. In Sleisenger, M. H., and Fordtran, J. S. (Eds.): Gastrointestinal Disease. Pathophysiology, Diagnosis, Management. Philadelphia, W. B. Saunders Company, 1973, p. 536.

92. Isenberg, J. I.: Peptic ulcer: Medial therapy. In Beeson, P. B., McDermott, W., and Wyngaarden, J. B. (Eds.): Textbook of Medicine. Philadelphia, W. B. Saunders Company, 1979, p. 1513.

93. Isenberg, J. I.: Peptic ulcer. Disease-a-Month, 28:1, 1981.

94. Isenberg, J. I., Grossman, M. I., Maxwell, V., and Walsh, J. H.: Increased sensitivity to stimulation of acid secretion by pentagastrin in duodenal ulcer. J. Clin. Invest., 55:330, 1975.

95. Isenberg, J. I., and Maxwell, V.: Intravenous infusion of amino acids stimulates gastric acid secretion in man. N. Engl. J. Med., 298:27, 1978.

96. Isenberg, J. I., Selling, J. A., Hogan, D. L., and Koss, M. A.: Impaired proximal duodenal mucosal bicarbonate secretion in patients with duodenal ulcer. N. Engl. J. Med., 316:374, 1987.

97. Isenberg, J. I., Walsh, J. H., and Grossman, M. I.: Zollinger-Ellison syndrome. Gastroenterology, 65:140, 1973.

98. Jackson, B. M., Reeder, D. D., Hirose, F., and Thompson, J. C.: Correlation of the surface pH, histology, and gastrin concentration of gastric mucosa. Ann. Surg., 176:727, 1972.

99. Jacobson, E. D., and Thompson, W. J.: Cyclic AMP and gastric secretion: The illusive second messenger. In Greengard, P., and Robison, G. (Eds.): Advances in Cyclic Nucleotide Research. New York, Raven Press, 1976, p. 199.

100. Jacobson, E. D., Linford, R. H., and Grossman, M. I.: Gastric secretion in relation to mucosal blood flow studied by a clearance technique. J. Clin. Invest., 45:1, 1966.

101. Jensen, D. M.: Economic and health aspects of peptic ulcer disease and H_2-receptor antagonists. Am. J. Med., 81(Suppl. 4B):42, 1986.

102. Jensen, R. T., Gardner, J. D., Raufman, J.-P., Pandol, S. J., Doppman, J. L., and Collen, M. J.: Zollinger-Ellison syndrome. Current concepts and management. Ann. Intern. Med., 98:59, 1983.

103. Jewett, T. C., Jr., Caldarola, V., Karp, M. P., Allen, J. E., and Cooney, D. R.: Intramural hematoma of the duodenum. Arch. Surg., 123:54, 1988.

104. Johnston, D., and Duthie, H. L.: Inhibition of gastrin secretion in the human stomach. Effect of acid in the duodenum. Lancet, 2:1032, 1965.

105. Johnston, P. W., and Snyder, W. H.: Vagotomy and pyloroplasty in infancy and childhood. J. Pediatr. Surg., 3:228, 1968.

106. Jones, T. W., and Merendino, K. A.: The perplexing duodenal diverticulum. Surgery, 48:1068, 1960.

107. Jordan, P. H., and Condon, R. E.: A prospective evaluation of vagotomy-pyloroplasty and vagotomy-antrectomy for treatment of duodenal ulcer. Ann. Surg., 172:547, 1970.

108. Jordan, P. H., Jr., and Thornby, J.: Should it be parietal cell vagotomy or selective vagotomy-antrectomy for treatment of duodenal ulcer? Ann. Surg., 205:572, 1987.

109. Kekki, M., Samloff, I. M., Ihamaki, T., Varis, K., and Siurala, M.: Age- and sex-related behaviour of gastric acid secretion at the population level. Scand. J. Gastroenterol., 17:773, 1982.

110. Kellner, H. C., and Mellinkoff, S. M.: The dumping syndrome: An interpretation. Gastroenterology, 44:424, 1963.

111. Khalil, T., Singh, P., Fujimura, M., Townsend, C. M., Jr., Greeley, G. H., Jr., and Thompson, J. C.: Effect of aging on gastric acid secretion, serum gastrin, and antral gastrin content in rats. Dig. Dis. Sci., 33:1544, 1988.

112. Kim, S. W., Parekh, D., Townsend, C. M., Jr., and Thompson, J. C.: Effects of aging on duodenal bicarbonate secretion. Ann. Surg., 211:1990 (in press).

113. Kleinerman, J., Yardumian, K., and Tamaki, H. T.: Primary carcinoma of the duodenum. Ann. Intern. Med., 32:451, 1950.

114. Kobold, E. E., and Thal, A. P.: A simple method for the management of experimental wounds of the duodenum. Surg. Gynecol. Obstet., 118:340, 1963.

115. Koop, H., Willemer, S., Steinbach, F., Eissele, R., Tuch, K., and Arnold, R.: Influence of chronic drug-induced achlorhydria by substituted benzimidazoles on the endocrine stomach in rats. Gastroenterology, 92:406, 1987.

116. Krag, E.: Gastric acid secretion related to prognosis in peptic ulcer. A long-term follow-up study. Acta Med. Scand., 180:461, 1966.

117. Kukral, J. C.: Gastric ulcers: An appraisal. Surgery, 63:1024, 1968.

118. Kumar, D., and Spitz, L.: Peptic ulceration in children. Surg. Gynecol. Obstet., 159:63, 1984.

119. Kurata, J. H., Haile, B. M., and Elashoff, J. D.: Sex differences in peptic ulcer disease. Gastroenterology, 88:96, 1985.

120. Kurata, J. H., Honda, G. D., and Frankl, H.: The incidence of duodenal and gastric ulcers in a large Health Maintenance Organization. Am. J. Public Health, 75:625, 1985.

121. Lamers, C. B., Walsh, J. H., Jansen, J. B., Harrison, A. R., Ippoliti, A. F., and van Tongere, J. H.: Evidence that gastrin 34 is preferentially released from the human duodenum. Gastroenterology, 83:233, 1982.

122. Landor, J. H.: Gastric secretory tests and their relevance to surgeons. Surgery, 65:523, 1969.

123. Langman, M. J. S., and Cooke, A. R.: Gastric and duodenal ulcer and their associated diseases. Lancet, 1:680, 1976.

124. Levine, R. J., and Senay, E. C.: Studies on the role of acid in the pathogenesis of experimental stress ulcers. Psychosom. Med., 32:61, 1970.

125. Lewisohn, R.: The frequency of gastrojejunal ulcers. Surg. Gynecol. Obstet., 40:70, 1925.

126. Littman, A.: Basal gastric secretion in patients with duodenal ulcer. A long-term study of variations in relation to ulcer activity. Gastroenterology, 43:166, 1962.

127. Lloyd, J. R., Bernstein, J., and Espiasse, E.: The etiology of gastrointestinal perforations in the newborn. Harper Hosp. Bull., 22:224, 1960.

128. Lucas, C. E., and Wilson, R. F.: Gastrointestinal complications following trauma. In Walt, A. J., and Wilson, R. F. (Eds.): Management of Trauma. Philadelphia, Lea & Febiger, 1975, p. 545.

129. Lucas, C. E., Sugawa, C., Riddle, J., Rector, F., Rosenberg, B., and Walt, A. J.: Natural history and surgical dilemma of "stress" gastric bleeding. Arch. Surg., 102:266, 1971.

130. Makhlouf, G. M., McManus, J. P. A., and Card, W. I.: A quantitative statement of the two-component hypothesis of gastric secretion. Gastroenterology, 51:149, 1966.

131. Mallory, G. K., and Weiss, S.: Hemorrhages from lacerations of cardiac orifice of the stomach due to vomiting. Am. J. Med. Sci., 178:506, 1929.

132. Mansberger, A. R., Jr., Hearn, J. B., Byers, R. M., Fleisign, N., and Buxton, R. W.: Vascular compression of the duodenum. Emphasis on accurate diagnosis. Am. J. Surg., 115:89, 1986.

133. Martin, L. F., Max, M. H., and Polk, H. C., Jr.: Failure of gastric pH control by antacids or cimetidine in the critically ill: A valid sign of sepsis. Surgery, 88:59, 1980.

134. McConnell, D. B., Baba, G. C., and Deveney, C. W.: Changes in surgical treatment of peptic ulcer disease within a veterans hospital in the 1970s and the 1980s. Arch. Surg., 124:1164, 1989.

135. McGuigan, J. E., and Greider, M. H.: Correlative immunochemical and light microscopic studies of the gastrin cell of the antral mucosa. Gastroenterology, 60:223, 1971.

136. Mendeloff, A. I.: What has been happening to duodenal ulcer? Gastroenterology, 67:1020, 1974.

137. Menguy, R.: Stomach. In Schwartz, S. I. (Ed.): Principles of Surgery. New York, McGraw-Hill, 1969, p. 907.

138. Michels, N. A.: Blood supply of the stomach and the esophagus. In Blood Supply and Anatomy of the Upper Abdominal Organs. Philadelphia, J. B. Lippincott Company, 1955, p. 248.

139. Moore, S. W., and Erlandson, M. E.: Intramural hematoma of the duodenum. Ann. Surg., 157:798, 1963.

140. Morton, J. R., and Jordan, G. L.: Traumatic duodenal injuries. Review of 131 cases. J. Trauma, 8:127, 1968.

141. Mullens, J. E., and Bird, G. S.: Peptic ulceration of the postbulbar portion of the duodenum. Can. J. Surg., 12:27, 1969.

142. Nix, G. A. J. J., Wilson, J. H. P., and Dees, J.: Primary malignant tumours of the duodenum. Fortschr. Geb. Rontgenstr. Nuklearmed. Erganzungsband, 142:385, 1986.

143. Oi, M., Ito, Y., Kumagai, F., Yoshida, K., Tanaka, Y., Yoshikawa, K., Muto, O., and Kijima, M.: A possible dual control mechanism in the origin of peptic ulcer. A study on ulcer location as affected by mucosa and musculature. Gastroenterology, 57:280, 1969.

144. Okabe, S., Ishihare, Y., Inoo, H., and Tanaka H.: Mepirizole-induced duodenal ulcers in rats and their pathogenesis. Dig. Dis. Sci., 27:242, 1982.

145. Pavlov, I. D.: Lectures on the World of the Digestive Glands. London, Charles Griffin & Company, 1902.

146. Price, W. E., Grizzle, J. E., Postlethwait, R. W., Johnson, W. D., and Grabicki, P.: Results of operation for duodenal ulcer. Surg. Gynecol. Obstet., 131:233, 1970.

147. Pricolo, V. E., Vittimberga, G. M., Yellin, S. A., Burchard, K. W., and Slotman, G. J.: Decompression after gastric surgery: Gastrostomy versus nasogastric tube. Am. Surg. 55:413, 1989.

148. Raimes, S. A., Wheldon, E. J., Smirniotis, V., Venables, C. W., and Johnston, I. D. A.: Postvagotomy diarrhea put into perspective. Lancet, 2:851, 1986.

149. Ravitch, M. M.: In discussion of Mander, K. K., Dutta, J., and Mitra, S.: Duodenal ulcer disease in children. World J. Surg., 4:261, 1980.

150. Ravitch, M. D., and Duremdes, G. D.: Operative treatment of chronic duodenal ulcer in childhood. Ann. Surg., 171:641, 1970.

151. Rayford, P. L., Miller, T. A., and Thompson, J. C.: Secretin, cholecystokinin and newer gastrointestinal hormones. N. Engl. J. Med., 294:1093; 1157, 1976.

152. Rayford, P. L., and Thompson, J. C.: Gastrin. Surg. Gynecol. Obstet., 145:257, 1977.

153. Reeder, D. D., Becker, H. D., and Thompson, J. C.: Effect of intravenously administered calcium on serum gastrin and gastric secretion in man. Surg. Gynecol. Obstet., 138:847, 1974.

154. Reeder, D. D., Conlee, J. L., and Thompson J. C.: Effect of calcium carbonate antacid on serum gastrin concentrations in duodenal ulcer patients. Surg. Forum, 22:308, 1971.

155. Reeder, D. D., Jackson, B. M., Brandt, E. N., Jr., and Thompson, J. C.: Rate and pattern of disappearance of exogenous gastrin in dogs. Am. J. Physiol., 222:1571, 1972.

156. Rehfeld, J. F., Stadil, F., Malmstrom, J., and Miyata, M.: Gastrin heterogeneity in serum and tissue: A progress report. In Thompson, J. C. (Ed.): Gastrointestinal Hormones. Austin, University of Texas Press, 1975, p. 43.

157. Rhodes, J., Barnardo, D. E., Phillips, S. F., Rovelstad, R. A., and Hofman, A. F.: Increased reflux of bile into the stomach in patients with gastric ulcer. Gastroenterology, 57:241, 1969.

158. Ritchie, W. P.: Alkaline reflux gastritis: A critical reappraisal. Gut, 25:975, 1984.

159. Rotter, J., Peterson, G., Samloff, I. M., McConnell, R. B., Ellis, A., Spence, M. A., and Rimoin, D. L.: Genetic heterogeneity of hyperpepsinogenemic I and normopepsinogenemic I duodenal ulcer disease. Ann. Intern. Med., 91:372, 1979.

160. Rowe, M. I., Buckner, D., and Clatworthy, H. W., Jr.: Wind sock web of the duodenum. Am. J. Surg., 116:444, 1968.

161. Samloff, I. M., Liebman, W. M., and Panitch, N. M.: Serum group I pepsinogens by radioimmunoassay in control subjects and patients with peptic ulcer. Gastroenterology, 69:83, 1975.

162. Samloff, I. M., Secrist, D. M., and Passaro, E., Jr.: The effect of Betazole on serum group I pepsinogen levels: Studies in symptomatic patients with and without recurrent ulcer after vagotomy and gastric resection or drainage. Gastroenterology, 70:1007, 1976.

163. Sawyers, J. L., Herrington, J. L., Jr., Mulherin, J. O., Whitehead, W. A., Mody, B., and Marsh, J.: Acute perforated duodenal ulcer. An evaluation of surgical management. Arch. Surg., 110:527, 19/5.

164. Schafmayer, A., Teichmann, R. K., Rayford, P. L., and Thompson, J. C.: Effect of parenteral L-amino acids on gastric secretion and serum gastrin in normal dogs and dogs with portacaval transposition. Surgery, 85:191, 1979.

165. Schiller, K., Truelove, S. C., and Williams, D. G.: Haematemesis and melaena with special reference to factors influencing the outcome. Br. Med. J., 2:7, 1970.

166. Scobie, B. A., McGill, D. B., Priestley, J. T., and Rovelstad, R. A.: Excluded gastric antrum stimulating the Zollinger-Ellison syndrome. Gastroenterology, 47:184, 1964.

167. Skillman, J. J.: Pathogenesis of peptic ulcer: A selective review. Surgery, 76:515, 1974.

168. Skillman, J. J., Bushnell, L. S., Goldman, H., and Silen, W.: Respiratory failure, hypotension, sepsis and jaundice: A clinical syndrome associated with lethal hemorrhage from acute ulceration of the stomach. Am. J. Surg., 117:523, 1969.

169. Skillman, J. J., Gould, S. A., Chung, R. S. K., and Silen, W.: The gastric mucosal barrier: Clinical and experimental studies in critically ill and normal man, and in the rabbit. Ann. Surg., 172:564, 1970.

170. Soll, A. H.: Pathogenesis of peptic ulcer and implications for therapy. N. Engl. J. Med., 322:909, 1990.

171. Somerville, K. W., Henry, D. A., Davies, J. G., Hine, K. R., Hawkey, C. J., and Langman, M. J. S.: Somatostatin in treatment of haematemesis and melaena. Lancet, 1:130, 1986.

172. Sonnenberg, A.: Costs of medical and surgical treatment of duodenal ulcer. Gastroenterology, 96:1445, 1989.

173. Stabile, B. E., and Passaro, E., Jr.: Recurrent peptic ulcer. Gastroenterology, 70:124, 1976.

174. Stadil, F., Stage, G., Rehfeld, J. F., Efsen, F., and Fischerman, K.: Treatment of Zollinger-Ellison syndrome with streptozotocin. N. Engl. J. Med., 294:1440, 1976.

175. Steinberg, D. M., Masselink, B. A., and Alexander-Williams, J.: Assessment and treatment of recurrent peptic ulceration. Ann. R. Coll. Surg. Engl., 56:135, 1975.

176. Stone, H. H., and Fabian, T. C.: Management of duodenal wounds. J. Trauma, 19:334, 1979.

177. Stremple, J. F., Molot, M. D., McNamara, J. J., Mori, H., and Jerzy Glass, G. B.: Posttraumatic gastric bleeding. Prospective gastric secretion composition. Arch. Surg., 105:177, 1972.

178. Strunz, U. T., Walsh, J. H., and Grossman, M. I.: Removal of gastrin by various organs. Gastroenterology, 74:32, 1978.
179. Takeuchi, K., Furukawa, O., Tanaka, H., and Okabe, S.: A new model of duodenal ulcers induced in rats by indomethacin plus histamine. Gastroenterology, 90:636, 1986.
180. Tam, P. K. H., and Saing, H.: Gastric acid secretion and emptying rates in children with duodenal ulcer. J. Pediatr. Surg., 21:129, 1986.
181. Thomas, J. M., and Misiewicz, G.: Histamine H$_2$-receptor antagonists in the short- and long-term treatment of duodenal ulcer. Clin. Gastroenterol., 13:501, 1984.
182. Thomas, W. E. G., Thompson, M. H., and Williamson, R. C. M.: The long-term outcome of Billroth I partial gastrectomy for benign gastric ulcer. Ann. Surg., 195:189, 1982.
183. Thompson, J. C.: Alterations in gastric secretion after portacaval shunting. Am. J. Surg., 117:854, 1969.
184. Thompson, J. C.: Standard versus experimental surgical procedures in the treatment of duodenal ulcer. Texas Med., 70:51, 1974.
185. Thompson, J. C.: Antral chalone. In Grossman, J. I., et al.: Candidate hormones of the gut. Gastroenterology, 67:730, 1974.
186. Thompson, J. C.: Hormonal influences on gastric secretion. In Rob, C. (Ed.): Advances in Surgery. Chicago, Year Book Medical Publishers, 1978, p. 53.
187. Thompson, J. C.: Abdominal pain. In Wolf, S. (Ed.): Abdominal Diagnosis. Philadelphia, Lea & Febiger, 1979, p. 1.
188. Thompson, J. C.: The role of surgery in peptic ulcer. N. Engl. J. Med., 307:550, 1982.
189. Thompson, J. C.: Surgical treatment of peptic ulcer disease. Pract. Gastroenterol., 4:9, 1980.
190. Thompson, J. C., and Peskin, G. W.: The intestinal phase of gastric secretion. Am. J. Med. Sci., 241:253, 1961.
191. Thompson, J. C., and Peskin, G. W.: Collective review. The gastric antrum in the operative treatment of duodenal ulcer. Surg. Gynecol. Obstet., 112:205, 1961.
192. Thompson, J. C., Lewis, B. G., Wiener, I., and Townsend, C. M., Jr.: The role of surgery in the Zollinger-Ellison syndrome. Ann. Surg., 197:594, 1983.
193. Thompson, J. C., Llanos, O. L., Teichmann, R. K., Schafmayer, A., and Rayford, P. L.: Catabolism of gastrin and secretin. World J. Surg., 3:469, 1979.
194. Thompson, J. C., Lowder, W. S., Peurifoy, J. T., Swierczek, J. S., and Rayford, P. L.: Effect of selective proximal vagotomy and truncal vagotomy on gastric acid and serum gastrin responses to a meal in duodenal ulcer patients. Ann. Surg., 188:431, 1978.
195. Thompson, J. C., Reeder, D. D., Villar, H. V., and Fender, H. R.: Natural history and experience with diagnosis and treatment of the Zollinger-Ellison syndrome. Surg. Gynecol. Obstet., 140:721, 1975.
196. Thompson, J. C., Rayford, P. L., Ramus, N. I., Fender, H. R., and Villar, H. V.: Patterns of release and uptake of heterogeneous forms of gastrin. In Thompson, J. C. (Ed.): Gastrointestinal Hormones. Austin, University of Texas Press, 1975, p. 125.
197. Thompson, J. C., Reeder, D. D., Bunchman, H. H., Becker, H. D., and Brandt, E. N., Jr.: Effect of secretin on circulating gastrin. Ann. Surg., 176:384, 1972.
198. Thompson, J. C., and Swierczek, J. S.: Acid and endocrine responses to meals varying in pH in normal and duodenal ulcer subjects. Ann. Surg., 186:541, 1977.
199. Thompson, J. C., Way, L. W., Jones, R. S., and Hallenbeck, G. A.: A symposium on the Zollinger-Ellison syndrome. Contemp. Surg., 14:77, 1979.
200. Thompson, J. C., and Wiener, I.: Evaluation of surgical treatment for duodenal ulcer. Acute and long-term effects. Clin. Gastroenterol., 13:569, 1984.
201. Townsend, C. M., Jr., Lewis, B. G., Gourley, W. K., and Thompson, J. C.: Gastrinoma. Curr. Probl. Cancer, 7:1, 1982.
202. Townsend, C. M., Jr., and Thompson, J. C.: Stress ulceration. In Shires, G. T. (Ed.): Principles of Trauma Care. New York, McGraw-Hill, 1984, p. 548.
203. Trudeau, W. L., and McGuigan, J. E.: Relations between serum gastrin levels and rates of gastric hydrochloric acid secretion. N. Engl. J. Med., 284:408, 1971.
204. Van Heerden, J. A., Bernatz, P. E., and Rovelstad, R. A.: The retained gastric antrum: Clinical considerations. Mayo Clin. Proc., 46:25, 1971.
205. Villar, H. V., Fender, H. R., Rayford, P. L., Bloom, S. R., Ramus, N. I., and Thompson, J. C.: Suppression of gastrin release and gastric secretion by gastric inhibitory polypeptide (GIP) and vasoactive intestinal polypeptide (VIP). Ann. Surg., 184:97, 1976.
206. Villar, H. V., Fender, H. R., Watson, L. C., and Thompson, J. C.: Emergency diagnosis of upper gastrointestinal bleeding by fiberoptic endoscopy. Ann. Surg., 185:367, 1977.
207. Walsh, J. H., and Grossman, M. I.: Gastrin. N. Engl. J. Med., 202:1324; 1377, 1975.
208. Walsh, J. H., Richardson, C. T., and Fordtran, J. S.: pH dependence of acid secretion and gastric release in normal and ulcer subjects. J. Clin. Invest., 55:462, 1975.
209. Walters, W., and Lynn, T. E.: Billroth I and Billroth II operations. Arch. Surg., 74:680, 1957.
210. Watson, L. C., Reeder, D. D., Becker, H. D., LaGrone, L., and Thompson, J. C.: Gastrin concentrations in upper gastrointestinal mucosa in dogs. Surgery, 76:419, 1974.
211. Weaver, D. H., Maxwell, J. G., and Castleton, K. B.: Mallory-Weiss syndrome. Am. J. Surg., 118:887, 1969.
212. Weinberg, J. A.: Vagotomy and pyloroplasty in the treatment of duodenal ulcer. Am. J. Surg., 105:347, 1963.
213. Werther, J. L.: The gastric mucosa barrier: Physiological and clinical considerations. Mt. Sinai J. Med. N.Y., 37:482, 1970.
214. West, W. O., Burns, R. O., Daniel, J. M., and Jackson, H. A.: The syndrome of chronic pulmonary disease and gastroduodenal ulceration. Arch. Intern. Med., 103:897, 1959.
215. Whelan, T. J., Jr., and Hamilton, G. B.: Annular pancreas. Ann. Surg., 146:252, 1957.
216. Wheldon, E. J., Venables, C. W., and Johnston, I. D. A.: The nutritional effects of vagotomy and gastroenterostomy 15–20 years after surgery. Br. J. Surg., 56:706, 1969.
217. Whittaker, L. D., Judd, E. S., and Stauffer, M. H.: Analysis of use of vagotomy with drainage procedure in surgical management of duodenal ulcer. Surg. Gynecol. Obstet., 125:1018, 1967.
218. Williams, J. A., and Cox, A. G. (Eds.): After Vagotomy. London, Butterworth & Company, 1969.
219. Winship, D. H.: Cimetidine in the treatment of duodenal ulcer. Review and commentary. Gastroenterology, 74:402, 1978.
220. Wolfe, M. M., and Jensen, R. T.: Zollinger-Ellison syndrome: Current concepts in diagnosis and management. N. Engl. J. Med., 317:1200, 1987.
221. Wolfe, M. M., and Soll, A. H.: The physiology of gastric acid secretion. N. Engl. J. Med., 319:1707, 1988.
222. Woodward, E. R.: The role of the gastric antrum in the regulation of gastric secretion. Gastroenterology, 38:7, 1960.
223. Wyllie, J. H., Alexander-Williams, J., Kennedy, T. L., Clark, C. G., Bell, P. R. F., Kirk, R. M., and MacKay, C.: Effect of cimetidine on surgery for duodenal ulcer. Lancet, 1:1307, 1981.
224. Yajko, R. D., Norton, L. W., and Eiseman, B.: Current management of upper gastrointestinal bleeding. Ann. Surg., 181:474, 1975.
225. Yoo, O. J., Powell, C. T., and Agarwal, K. L.: Molecular cloning and nucleotide sequence of full-length cDNA coding for porcine gastrin. Proc. Natl. Acad. Sci. USA, 79:1049, 1982.
226. Zollinger, R. M., and Ellison, R. H.: Primary peptic ulcerations of the jejunum associated with islet cell tumor of pancreas. Ann. Surg., 142:709, 1955.
227. Zollinger, R. M., Martin, E. W., Jr., and Carey, L. C.: Observation on the postoperative tumor growth behavior of certain islet cell tumors. Ann. Surg., 184:525, 1976.

I ————————————————————

BENIGN TUMORS OF THE STOMACH

Onye E. Akwari, M.D.

Historical Aspects

Amatus Lusitanus[22] described a gastric polyp in 1557, but Morgagni was the first to provide a postmortem description in 1769.[30a] A familial type of multiple colonic adenomatous polyposis was first described by Cripps in 1882.[4] In 1895, Hauser[13] reported an association between familial adenomatous polyposis and multiple gastric polyps. This early association between colonic and gastric polyps may have resulted in the confusing nomenclature of gastric polyps based on the mistaken concept that they are analogous to colorectal polyps in microscopic appearance and natural history. In 1867, Virchow described the pathologic characteristics of leiomyoma.[45] In 1888, Ménétrier described two different gastric diseases under the common term *polyadenomes.*[25,34] He used the term *polyadenoma polypeux* to describe diffuse polyposis and the term *polyadenoma en nappe* to describe giant hyperrugosity of the mucosa of the stomach. Heinz was the first to observe gastric polyps fluoroscopically in 1911, and a gastroscopic diagnosis was first made by Schendler in 1922.[5]

Incidence

Approximately 7 per cent of premortem gastric tumors are benign, including true neoplasms and other lesions that may be confused with neoplastic growths.[27] The reported incidence varies with the method of detection. Benign tumors constitute less than 2 per cent of true gastric neoplasms, approximately 0.5 per cent of neoplasms found at the time of autopsy and approximately 3 per cent of those discovered at the time of endoscopy in symptomatic patients. A classification of benign tumors of the stomach is presented in Table 1. Approximately 40 per cent of these tumors are mucosal epithelial polyps, another 40 per cent are leiomyomas and all the remaining types are rare.[27]

Clinical Presentation

Benign gastric tumors occur predominantly in the middle decades of life and are most commonly located in the gastric antrum or corpus. Tumors of the cardia and pylorus proper are rare.

Because of the propensity of these tumors to ulcerate the associated mucosal epithelium, the resultant occult loss of blood may cause iron deficiency anemia. Deep ulcerations that overlie

TABLE 1. Benign Tumors of the Stomach

Polyps
Hyperplastic polyp (Types I and II in Japanese literature)
Neoplastic or adenomatous polyps (Type III and IV polyps in Japanese literature)
Mixed polyps (hyperplastic and neoplastic)
Fundic gland polyp
Familial polyposis and other polyposis syndromes
Peutz-Jeghers (hamartomatous) polyp
Inflammatory fibroid polyp
Retention (juvenile) polyp

Benign Hyperplastic Gastropathy
Ménétrier's disease (polyadenomes en nappe)
Associated with Zollinger-Ellison syndrome
Glandular type, without hypergastrinemia
Pseudolymphoma

Intramural Tumors
Leiomyoma
Other mesenchymal tumors (lipoma, neurogenic tumors, fibroma, vascular tumors)
Osteoma and osteochondroma
Heterotopic pancreas
Brunner's gland adenoma
Adenomyoma
Xanthoma (xanthelasma)

Inflammatory Tumors
Eosinophilic gastritis
  Diffuse
  Localized (Inflammatory fibroid polyp—see Polyps, above)
Benign histiocytosis X
Granulomatous lesion (sarcoid, Crohn's disease)
Syphilis
Tuberculosis

Cysts
Intramucosal cyst (mucocele)
Submucosal cyst (gastritis cystica profunda)
Duplication cyst

Miscellaneous Conditions
Gastric varices
Aneurysm of gastric vessels (Dieulafoy's disease)
Antral vascular ectasia (watermelon stomach)

intramural tumors are notorious for their association with overt hemorrhage. Ulceration may cause a pain syndrome indistinguishable from that caused by peptic ulcer disease. The patients may therefore have an ill-defined sense of epigastric discomfort and an associated sense of fullness that is often caused by the large size of the tumor or by episodic obstruction of the digestive tract. Leiomyoma and the other mesenchymal tumors may grow to reach a size that is palpable on abdominal examination. Tumors of the cardia and pylorus may cause partial obstruction early, which progresses to complete obstruction as the tumor grows larger. If pedunculated, the tumor, usually pyloric, may create intermittent obstruction as a result of a ball-valve effect. Frank gastroduodenal intussusception secondary to prolapsing gastric tumors may occur.[18]

The current widespread use of upper gastrointestinal endoscopy has undoubtedly greatly increased the rate of detection of benign gastric tumors. Still others are discovered by barium meal radiographs of patients with ill-defined abdominal complaints of pain, indigestion, nausea, weight loss, or unexplained anemia. In many instances, the diagnosis is serendipitous, there being no causal relationship between the lesion discovered on the radiograph and the nonspecific symptoms that prompted the investigation. These lesions cause concern not only because they may simulate their malignant counterparts but also because of their suspected potential for malignant transformation. Neither the radiologist nor the endoscopist can resolve these concerns.

Radiology is fairly sensitive in detecting gastric mucosal polyps, especially with the addition of air contrast techniques to procure good mucosal detail. Small size and the presence of a stalk support the diagnosis of benignancy. Polyps larger than 2 cm. in size (particularly sessile ones with thickening of the gastric wall surrounding them) are more likely to be malignant, although many are benign. Fluoroscopically, benign tumors are more often associated with pliability of the gastric wall. Although an exfoliative cytologic examination that is properly done and expertly interpreted is the most sensitive technique for readily excluding malignancy, it is of no use in diagnosing submucosal lesions. Gastroscopy and biopsy through the fiberoptic gastroscope is usually not diagnostic of a specific type of polyp or hyperplastic gastropathy.[25]

Biopsy material from a patient with intramural tumors is usually inadequate, because the biopsy forceps is unable to penetrate deeply enough for the surgeon to obtain a representative sample of the tumor for histologic examination. This is an especially vexing problem with leiomyomas and other mesenchymal tumors with firm rubbery consistencies.

The indications for extirpation of the tumor are elimination of any clinical malefic effects and the necessity to exclude a diagnosis of malignancy. Ultimately the tumor must be excised and recovered *in toto* either by endoscopic techniques or by surgical excision before a final disposition can be made. Specific aspects of the pathologic features and the management of the more frequently encountered benign tumors are considered individually.

POLYPS

The word *polyp* is derived from the Greek *polypus*, which means "manyfooted" and is generically used to describe any growth that protrudes into the gastric lumen. Almost all gastric polyps arise from the mucosal epithelium.[28] As stated earlier, the nomenclature of gastric polyps is confusing largely because of early attempts to present them as being analogous to colorectal polyps in microscopic appearance and natural history. This is unfortunate because most types of gastric polyps do not have an exact counterpart in the large bowel.[35] Unlike colonic polyps, gastric epithelial polyps are uncommon tumors with an incidence of 0.4 to 0.7 per cent. No distinction appears to exist between the three histologic types of epithelial polyps (hyperplastic, adenomatous, fundic gland) by age, sex, location, symptoms, or endoscopic appearance.[5] The median age for gastric polyps is approximately 65 years, with a gender distribution that is equal or at most includes slightly more females. The histologic appearance of a polyp cannot be predicted on the basis of location within the stomach. However, multiple polyps in the same patient are almost always of the same histologic type.[5,40]

HYPERPLASTIC POLYPS. Hyperplastic polyps (also known as regenerative, inflammatory, hyperplasiogenic, harmartomatous, and Types I and II polyps of Japanese authors) comprise approximately 75 per cent of all gastric epithelial polyps.[5] The polyps may be solitary or multiple and sessile or pedunculated. They are the result of glandular proliferation, since they are regenerative rather than neoplastic. Varying in size from a few millimeters to several centimeters most are less than 2 cm. in diameter. Pedunculation usually occurs in larger polyps. Histologically, they show elongation, tortuosity, and dilatation (often cystic) of the gastric foveolae, with a component of pyloric or, less commonly, fundic type glands in the deeper portion. The stroma is characterized by edema, patchy fibrosis, inflammatory cells, and scattered smooth muscle bundles from the muscularis (Fig. 1).

The gastric lesion termed polyadenomes polypeux by Ménétrier probably corresponds to multiple hyperplastic polyps[25] (see Fig. 1). The polypoid lesion that sometimes develops on the gastric side of gastroenterostomy stomas may also have a microscopic appearance similar to that of a hyperplastic polyp, except for its more diffuse nature and more prominent cystic component referred to as *gastritis polyposis cystica*.[27]

Recent studies[5,38] have demonstrated a modest association between hyperplastic polyps and adenocarcinoma arising in the non-polyp gastric mucosa. A coincident gastric carcinoma was present in 1 of 26 patients with hyperplastic polyps in the series by Deppisch and Rona.[5] The risk, if any, appears to be[28] associated with the atrophic gastritis that frequently accompanies hyperplastic polyps rather than with the polyps themselves. Patients with atrophic gastritis may be predisposed to both polyps and adenocarcinoma. Atrophic gastritis has been reported in 79 per cent of patients with hyperplastic polyps,[44] and Neimarck and Rogers[31] have demonstrated that 5 per cent of patients with atrophic gastritis develop hyperplastic polyps.

NEOPLASTIC POLYPS OR ADENOMAS. Also known as Types III and IV in the Japanese literature, these polyps are usually antral in location, are usually single and large, and may be sessile or pedunculated. Microscopically, they are composed of atypical glands with pseudostratified epithelium that has nuclear abnormalities and a high mitotic count. Like their large bowel counterparts, they can be divided into adenomatous polyps (tubular adenomas), villoglandular polyps (tubulovillous adenomas), and villous adenomas.[26] Scattered endocrine cells that have positive test results for serotonin and a variety of peptide hormones have been identified in them. Carcinoembryonic antigen reactivity is usually found in the cytologically most atypical areas.[35]

Adenomatous polyps have long been associated with gastric adenocarcinoma.[44] This association is directly related to the size of the adenomatous polyp: up to 24 per cent of polyps 2 cm. or greater in diameter were associated with adenocarcinoma. In contrast, only 4 per cent of polyps with a diameter less than 2 cm. were associated with adenocarcinoma.[44] In an analogy to neoplastic polyps of the colorectum, the incidence of dysplasia, carcinoma *in situ*, and invasive adenocarcinoma all appear to increase with gastric polyp size. The exact incidence of malignant transformation of these polyps is not known, but it appears to be relatively low, approximately 3.4 per cent.[38]

FUNDIC GLAND POLYP. Fundic gland polyps (fundic gland hyperplasia, hamartomatous cystic polyps, polyps with fundic glandular cysts) present as multiple small polypoid projections in the gastric fundus or body. Their distinguishing microscopic feature is the presence of microcysts lined by fundic epithelium that includes oxyphilic cells; the overlying foveolae are usually shortened.[35] Fundic gland polyps, although particularly common in those patients with familial polyposis syndromes, are not specific for that disorder, as previously claimed.[46] However, Nishiura and others believe that patients with familial polyposis may be identified by the histochemical findings of their gastric mucus. The presence of O-acylated sialic acid may indicate the necessity of colorectal examination for polyposis in such patients.

INFLAMMATORY FIBROID POLYP. Helwing and Rainer[14] named this lesion, also known as eosinophilic granuloma, granuloblastoma, neurofibroma, and hemangiopericytoma. Frequently associated with hypochlorhydria or achlorhydria, the lesion is probably not a true neoplasm. It is usually located in the antrum and may occur as single or multiple polyps. The gross appearance is similar to that of a pyogenic granuloma.

On microscopic examination, the lesion is shown to be centered in the submucosa and is characterized by fibroblastic proliferation in a whorl-like arrangement that simulates peripheral nerve tumors. There are abundant thin-walled blood vessels and a dense infiltrate of eosinophils, lymphocytes, histiocytes, and plasma cells. Ultrastructurally, many of the proliferating cells have a myofibroblastic appearance, which is in keeping with the presumed reactive nature of the process. An allergic cause has not been established and peripheral eosinophilia is not associated with these polyps. Thus, this condition should be distinguished from diffuse eosinophilic gastritis, in which peripheral eosinophilia is usually present and which probably has an allergic basis.

TREATMENT

SYMPTOMATIC POLYPS. Polyps that cause pain, bleeding, or gastric outlet obstruction should be removed. Total endoscopic excision of pedunculated lesions is advocated so that the nature of the polyp can be firmly established. Open surgical excision is indicated when the benignity of a pedunculated polyp that is greater than 2 cm. in diameter has not been firmly established and/or safe total excision by endoscopic snare and cautery is not feasible; when examination of the tissue removed endoscopically is consistent with invasive malignancy[23]; and when a sessile polyp is present that exceeds 2 cm. in diameter.[4]

The role of individual surgical judgment regarding a specific polypoid lesion cannot be overemphasized. The guiding principle is to perform the least radical operation that allows complete removal.

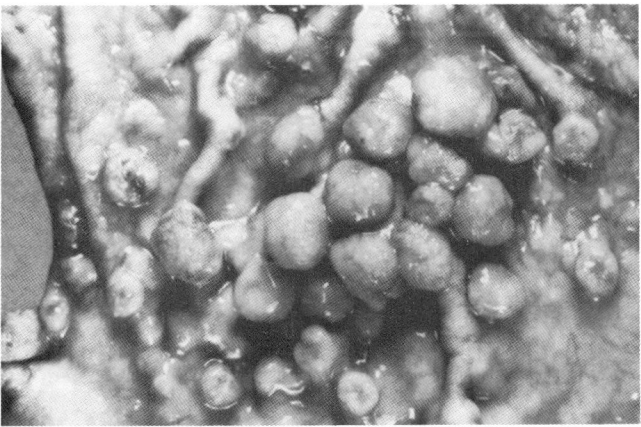

Figure 1. Multiple gastric polyps of the hyperplastic type occurring in a 65-year-old woman. Large sessile polyps of firm consistency occupied a large portion of the gastric mucosa. (From Rosai, J.: Gastrointestinal tract/stomach. *In* Rosai, J.: Ackerman's Surgical Pathology, 7th ed. St. Louis, C. V. Mosby Company, 1989, p. 496.)

A solitary sessile lesion is best excised with a margin of surrounding gastric wall and submitted for frozen section examination. Any further surgical procedure is dictated by the histologic diagnosis. Multiple polyps involving the distal stomach should be treated by subtotal gastrectomy. If a few polyps remain in the proximal pouch, they are removed by endogastric amputation and submitted for frozen section examination. When four to six polyps are randomly located in the stomach, a gastrotomy is indicated; and endogastric excision, frozen section, and further treatment are dictated by the pathologic findings. A group of closely aligned polyps in the gastric corpus can be removed by wide local excision or sleeve resection of the involved segment of gastric corpus. In diffuse polyposis, a large portion of the gastric mucosal surface is involved with innumerable polypoid tumors. Here the decision must also consider the fact that although these polyps are benign, they may be associated with coexisting adenocarcinoma elsewhere in the stomach. An especially difficult circumstance arises when diffuse polyposis involves the fundus of the stomach, where a coexisting adenocarcinoma may be masked and difficult to identify. A total gastrectomy may be indicated in these cases. Local wedge excision is adequate treatment for polyps that appear with focal atypia or carcinoma *in situ*.

ASYMPTOMATIC POLYPS. The availability of endoscopic snare biopsy specimens and the insights provided by recent histologic and statistical studies have helped resolve much of the controversy surrounding these polyps. Biopsy specimens of asymptomatic polyps should be taken by endoscopic snare-cautery excision. Hyperplastic polyps may be safely observed and annual endoscopic follow-up examinations conducted to reexamine the polyps as well as monitor the entire intervening gastric mucosa. If adenomatous epithelium is discovered, total endoscopic or open-wedge excision should be undertaken for lesions greater than 2 cm. in diameter. If reliable histologic diagnosis is unavailable, lesions 2 cm. or greater in diameter, especially if they are broad based and antral in location, should be surgically excised because of their potential risk of malignant transformation.

GASTRIC POLYPS IN POLYPOSIS SYNDROMES

Gastric involvement occurs in over 50 per cent of patients with familial polyposis coli and the related Gardner's syndrome. These patients may also harbor polyps in the duodenum. The gastric polyps can be adenomatous or hyperplastic or of the fundic gland hyperplasia type.[16]

Fundic gland polyps (fundic gland hyperplasia, hamartomatous cystic polyps, polyps with fundic glandular cysts) present as multiple small polypoid projections in the gastric fundus or body. Their distinguishing microscopic feature is the presence of microcysts lined by fundic epithelium, including oxyphilic cells; the overlying foveolae are usually shortened.[35] Fundic gland polyps, although particularly common in patients with polyposis syndromes, are not specific for this disorder, as previously claimed. However, it may well be that the patients with polyposis may be distinguished by histochemical stains characteristic of the mucus. The presence of gastric polyps with O-acylated sialic acid indicates the necessity of examination of the colorectum in such cases.[32]

Other gastric tumors described in association with familial polyposis coli are adenocarcinoma and carcinoid tumors.

All patients confirmed as having familial adenomatous polyposis should have gastroduodenoscopy. Any polyps observed should be recorded, and representative biopsy specimens should be taken. If adenomas are found, they should be eradicated by endoscopic destruction. Since the adenomas are frequently multiple, they often require multiple treatments. Repeat examination should then be undertaken at 6- to 12-week inter-

vals until no polyps remain. The examination is then carried out every 6 months as long as no new polyps are observed. When the initial examination was normal or when only fundic gland polyps are noted, endoscopy is repeated in 3 years.[36]

In Peutz-Jeghers syndrome, hamartomatous gastric polyps have been found in approximately 20 per cent of the patients, with an occasional coexisting adenocarcinoma.[12] These patients require endoscopic surveillance, especially when upper tract symptoms have been reported.

In generalized juvenile polyposis and the related Cronkhite-Canada syndrome, the incidence of gastric retention (juvenile) polyps is very high.[20]

Cowden's syndrome (Cowden is the family name of the index patient) was first described in 1962 by Lloyd and Dennis.[21] The patient presented with multiple orocutaneous hamartomas, a nontoxic goiter, fibrocystic disease of the breasts, and thyroid and breast cancer. This complex can also be accompanied by small sessile gastric polyps, most of which are of the hyperplastic type.[40] The feature of disseminated polyposis in this autosomal dominant disease has recently been emphasized. Gorensek et al.[11] have suggested that the term *disseminated hereditary gastrointestinal polyposis with orocutaneous hamartomatosis* is more descriptive; all four of their patients had hamartomas extending from the oral mucosa to the anus.[11] An increased, evidently genetically determined, incidence of malignant tumors of various organs in patients with Cowden's disease and in their family members has been documented.

INTRAMURAL TUMORS

SMOOTH MUSCLE NEOPLASM. INCIDENCE. Leiomyomas are the most common benign tumor of the stomach reported at autopsy. Meissner[24] found a smooth muscle neoplasm in the gastric wall in 45 per cent of his patients, and most of these neoplasms were less than 1 cm. in diameter. Among benign gastric neoplasms of mesodermal origin, those derived from smooth muscle constitute over 90 per cent and demonstrate no strong sex predilection. Because it is rare for gastric leiomyomas less than 3 cm. in diameter to be symptomatic, considerably less than 2 per cent of gastric neoplasms that are resected surgically are of smooth muscle origin.

PATHOLOGY. Leiomyomas may arise from the muscularis propria, the muscularis mucosae, or the smooth muscle present in the blood vessel wall. They are usually located antrally (25 per cent) or corporally (40 per cent). At an early stage of growth, the leiomyoma is intramural. With expansion, the tumor may protrude into the gastric lumen as a submucosal (endogastric) mass or develop as an exogastric (exophytic) mass. These types of presentation were described by Virchow[45] as "inneren" (submucosal) or "ausseren" (subserosal). Submucosal expansion is by far the more common mode of growth, occurring in about 60 per cent of cases. Rarely, a dumbbell tumor occurs with both submucosal and subserosal components. The tumors may be smooth or lobulated. In time, a central ulceration occurs in the mucosal bulge of the tumor in approximately 50 per cent of submucosal leiomyomas. Ulceration may be present in smaller tumors but absent in very large tumors. Areas of necrosis and cavitation may occur within large tumors. Focal calcifications may develop. The central cavities may communicate with the gastric lumen through one or more sinuses, or they may rupture into the peritoneal cavity. The gross appearance of an ulcerated leiomyoma and the radiologic image of such a lesion are demonstrated in Figure 2.

Gastric leiomyomas are not encapsulated, even though in examination of a tissue section they appear well circumscribed; and in the absence of necrosis, they have a smooth, lobulated, or whorled-silk appearance. Microscopically, the tumor cells at the margin may intermingle with cells of the surrounding gastric

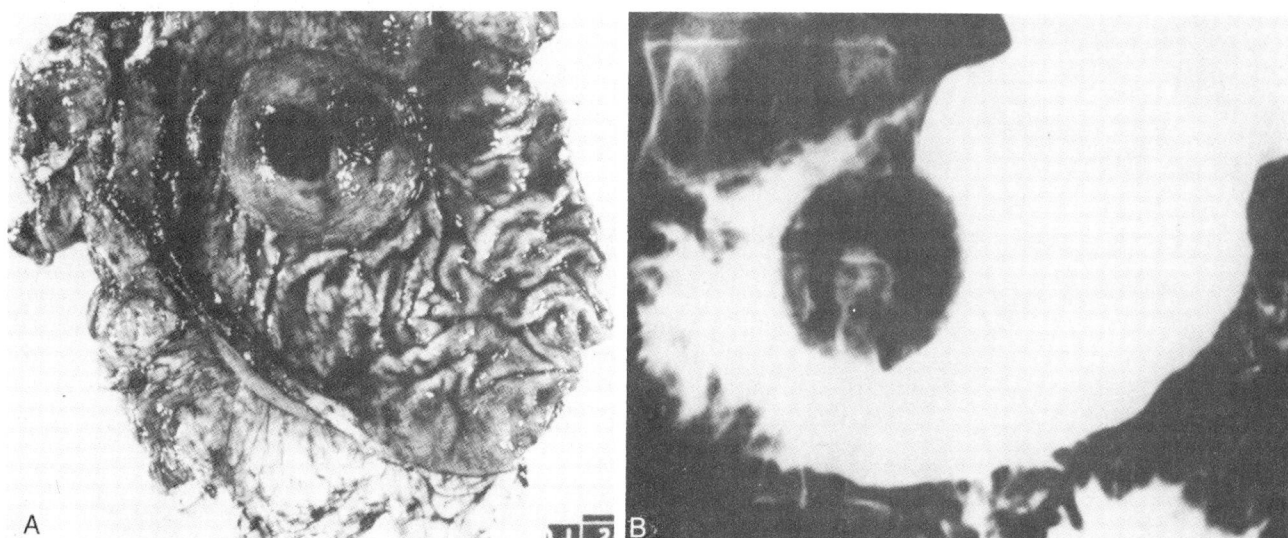

Figure 2. *A,* Leiomyoma of the stomach with two large necrotic ulcers on the surface of the lesion, which produced massive bleeding (specimen of case in *B*). The tumor has been removed by distal antrectomy. *B,* Barium meal examination of the stomach demonstrates a well-circumscribed mass-pedunculated leiomyoma of the proximal gastric antrum. Note the central ulcer with early cavitation of the stomach. (From Stavorovsky M., Mora G. B., Stavorovsky, H., and Papo, J.: Smooth muscle tumors of the alimentary tract. J. Surg. Oncol., 22:109, 1983.)

wall. This is one factor that has led to confusion in distinguishing benign from malignant leiomyoma. Most smooth muscle tumors demonstrate well-differentiated smooth muscle cells with a variable degree of hyalinized connective tissue.[9] However, a relatively large number demonstrate a wide variation from this classic pattern. Peculiar features may include extreme cellularity, presence of occasional large cells with bizarre hyperchromatic nuclei, marked diffuse vascularity, regimentation of nuclei (palisading), and cells with round shape and clear cytoplasm. Palisading leads to confusion between leiomyoma and neurilemmoma. The neurilemmoma is always encapsulated.

Stout[42] described a reasonably distinct variety of gastric smooth muscle tumor, which he called *leiomyoblastoma* (bizarre smooth muscle tumor). The 69 cases he reported were characterized histologically by polyhedral smooth cells with central nuclei and abundant cytoplasm rather than by elongated cells. A clear zone that surrounds the central nucleus is probably an artifact of fixation. The distinguishing histologic features of the leiomyoblastoma type are depicted in Figure 6. Appleman and Helwig[1] more recently suggested the designations *epithelial leiomyoma* or *leiomyosarcoma* for these tumors, depending on whether they have a benign or malignant pattern on histologic examination. Carney[3] described a syndrome characterized by the triad of multiple malignant leiomyoblastoma, pulmonary chondroma, and functioning extra-adrenal paraganglioma.

The criteria for distinguishing benign from malignant smooth muscle tumors are the same for the spindle cell and leiomyoblastoma cell types.[1] There is at present fairly general agreement that the most important criterion for distinguishing a leiomyoma from a leiomyosarcoma is the number of mitotic figures present. Golden and Stout[9] stated that "if two or more mitoses per high power field are present, one can feel fairly secure in predicting malignancy." However, correlation between mitotic activity and the clinical behavior of the tumor is not nearly as good for gastrointestinal smooth muscle tumors as for uterine smooth muscle tumors. Unfortunately, metastasis can occur in a smooth muscle tumor that is by all criteria histologically benign. Thus, the proposal has been made to designate as "smooth muscle tumors of indeterminate malignant potential (STUMP)" those neoplasms that are suspected of being malignant because of high cellularity, atypia, large size, and/or tumor cell necrosis but that have more than five mitoses per ten high-power fields. In the final analysis, the only unchallengeable evidence of ma-

lignancy of a smooth muscle tumor is metastasis or invasive intragastric or extragastric growth that is noted either during a surgical procedure or following surgical resection. All smooth muscle tumors of the stomach should be suspected of being malignant until time and the demonstrable behavior of the tumor provide proof to the contrary. The malignant variant of leiomyoma may invade adjacent organs, may rarely involve lymph nodes except by direct extension, may be seeded in the peritoneal cavity, and may metastasize by hematogenous spread to the liver or lung.[39] In children and adolescents, gastric smooth muscle tumors are very rare; most are malignant.[47]

CLINICAL ASPECTS AND TREATMENT. The propensity of smooth muscle tumors for overlying central mucosal ulceration, which may penetrate deeply into the tumor, results in hematemesis, melena, or anemia caused by occult gastrointestinal blood loss, which draws attention to the tumor. Bleeding from the tumor may be massive and/or intermittent. Although 20 per cent occur near the pylorus, obstruction is rare.[30] An occasional smooth muscle tumor may become pedunculated and may then prolapse through the pylorus, causing gastric outlet obstruction. Huge exogastric tumors are frequently detected by the patient as a palpable mass. Incidental discovery at the time of laparotomy, during the course of a barium meal study, and during gastroscopy for a probably unrelated disease are the most common methods of detection.

The principle of surgical treatment of smooth muscle tumors is local excision with a 2- to 3-cm. margin of surrounding gastric wall. In view of the difficulty in distinguishing between the benign and malignant variants, enucleation is an inappropriate method of treatment. The excised specimen should be submitted for pathologic examination. If a histologic diagnosis of malignancy is made on the basis of frozen section examination, an additional margin of gastric wall may be excised.

In the instance of a very large tumor or a prepyloric tumor, a standard gastric resection may be the most expeditious form of excision. With tumors in the body of the stomach, local excision or sleeve resection is feasible. The more difficult decision is required when the tumor encroaches on the esophagogastric junction. Resection of the esophagogastric junction for a benign leiomyoma would be a surgical misadventure, and a conservative approach is indicated.

Regional lymphadenectomy is not of proven value, and its practice is not consistent with the known biologic behavior of the tumor.

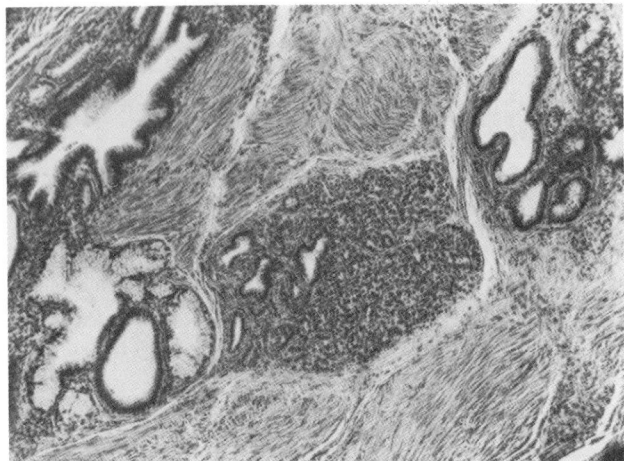

Figure 3. Microscopic appearance of pancreatic rest demonstrating ducts and acini. An islet is present in the middle of the photograph. Magnification, × 90. (From Edis, A. J.: Benign tumors of the stomach. *In* Schwartz, S. I., Ellis, H., and Husser, W. (Eds.): Maingot's Abdominal Operations, 8th ed. New York, Appleton-Century-Crofts, 1985, p. 953.)

HETEROTOPIC PANCREAS

An aberrant rest of pancreatic tissue located in the wall of the stomach presents clinically as a tumor and must be considered in the differential diagnosis of benign gastric neoplasms. Although the tumor may project into the lumen of the stomach and may occasionally cause pyloric obstruction or hemorrhage, it is usually found incidentally at autopsy or laparotomy.[33]

The typical pancreatic rest is a hemispheric mass, a symmetrical cone, or a short cylindrical nipple-like projection measuring 0.5 to 3 cm. in diameter located in the antrum (61 per cent) or the immediate prepyloric area (24 per cent) of the stomach. The most characteristic gross feature is a central ductal orifice that tends to umbilicate the tumor and may be identified by filling during a barium meal or a gastroscopic examination. The orifice usually communicates with a filiform ductal system draining the mass of tightly packed pancreatic acini that form the tumor nodule. Approximately 85 per cent of these lesions are in the submucosa, and most of the others are in the muscular layer.

Technically considered a hamartoma, the mass of heterotopic pancreas is composed of glands and intervening connective tissue. Islets of Langerhans are observed only in one-third of the cases, and if present, their number is generally less than in the normal pancreas (Fig. 3). These lesions may be involved in the same types of pathologic processes that affect the pancreas proper. Debilitating pain may be associated with inflammation occurring in these lesions; ductal dilatation and cyst formation may also occur. Some cases of intramural gastric carcinoma arising in these heterotopic tissues have been reported.[10]

Indeterminate or apparently symptomatic lesions should be excised; but if an accurate radiologic diagnosis can be made and the lesion is asymptomatic, one might be justified in pursuing expectant management. From a practical point of view, however, most patients and physicians prefer surgical excision to avoid the uncertainty and cost of frequent follow-up examinations.

BRUNNER'S GLAND ADENOMA

This lesion may occur in the antrum or juxtapyloric region, representing heterotopic locations of a hamartomatous lesion that is usually found in the duodenum. The Brunner's gland adenoma is composed of intermingled glands and bands of smooth muscle fibers. Islands of pancreatic tissue may be present. Certain of these lesions may be referred to as gastric adenomyomas.[8]

HYPERPLASTIC GASTROPATHY

The general term *hyperplastic gastropathy* refers to a rare condition in which there is enlargement of the rugal folds in the stomach. The etiologic features of the hyperplastic process vary.

Of the two processes that Ménétrier described in 1888 under the common term *polyadenomes*, *polyadenomes polypeux* is probably equivalent to *multiple hyperplastic polyps*, whereas *polyadenomes en nappe* is the form to which the term *Ménétrier's disease* is usually applied at present.

MÉNÉTRIER'S DISEASE. Ménétrier's disease is characterized by gastric mucosal hypertrophy, which may be so extensive that the rugae assume the appearance of convolutions of the brain (Fig. 4). Although this gross appearance is common to all cases of Ménétrier's disease, in an individual case, either the gastric glandular elements or the superficial epithelial elements of the gastric mucosa may predominate. Thus, acid secretion may be high, normal, or low; and hypoproteinemia, formerly considered an essential component of the disease, may not be present. Sundt and associates[43] reported the lack of consensus in the literature regarding which features define the disease. Because the mucosal histologic character, level of acid secretion, and serum albumin levels are semiquantifiable along three graphic axes, Sundt and colleagues suggest describing the three cardinal abnormalities of Ménétrier's disease as *trivalent gastropathy*.

The cardia, fundus, and body of the stomach are usually diffusely thrown into folds and nodular areas that may resemble sessile polyps. The transition between normal and diseased mucosa is always abrupt. A lack of antral involvement is characteristic of the disease.

Microscopically, there is a striking *foveolar hyperplasia* that is accompanied by tortuosity, some degree of cystic dilatation, and extension into the base of the glands. The stroma is edematous

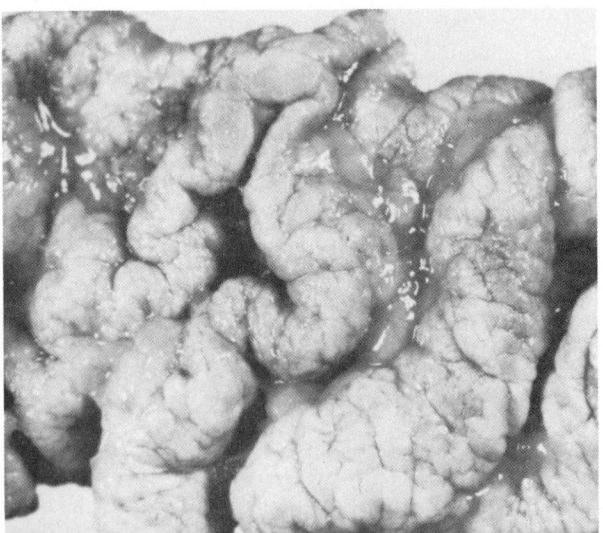

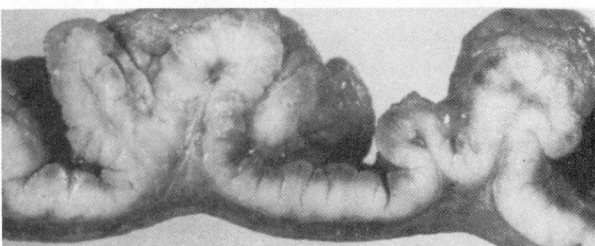

Figure 4. Ménétrier's disease in a 65-year-old woman. The gross pattern of the thickened rugae is reminiscent of convolutions of the brain. (From Rosai, J.: Gastrointestinal tract/stomach. *In* Rosai, J.: Ackerman's Surgical Pathology, 7th ed. St. Louis, C. V. Mosby Company, 1989, p. 499.)

and inflamed. Hyperrugosity may regress, atrophic gastritis may develop, and carcinoma of the stomach may ensue.

Abdominal distress or pain is present in over 80 per cent of patients, blood loss is present in 34 per cent, and symptoms of hypoproteinemia are present in 40 per cent. Weight loss, edema, and malnutrition are common. It should be noted that only one patient described by Ménétrier is suggestive of this entire clinical syndrome.[25]

Ménétrier's disease may be diagnosed at any age.[19] The etiologic factors are unknown.

Treatment is directed to the debilitating effects of the protein-losing gastropathy; and in view of reports of spontaneous resolution, nutritional support and a period of observation are justified when the precise diagnosis has been established.[6] Anticholinergics may be prescribed because they diminish acid secretion and may tighten gastric cell junctions, which limits protein losses by this route. Also, H$_2$ blockers, which have many of the same effects, may be tried if the response to anticholinergics is suboptimal or their side effects become troublesome. Combination therapy with H$_2$ blockers plus anticholinergics or administration of omeprazole may also be useful in conjunction with parenteral nutrition.

If pharmacologic therapy fails, total gastrectomy and reconstruction with a long Roux-en-Y jejunal limb is the best therapy. The operation using a jejunal limb of adequate length obviates reflux esophagitis, eliminates the risk of gastric malignancy, and allows improved nutrition. Also, technical problems posed by the risk of anastomotic leakage and obstruction, which are common when distal gastrectomy is used for Ménétrier's disease, are avoided. The significant incidence of subsequent carcinoma of the stomach in even a small remaining portion of gastric mucosa should discourage the temptation to leave a small rim of stomach below the gastroesophageal junction, a theoretically more secure anastomosis between two serosalized segments of the gastrointestinal tract.

An interesting aspect of the management of patients with Ménétrier's disease is their propensity to be in a hypercoagulable state, sometimes due to an occult gastric malignancy.[43] Hypercoagulability is a well known complication of mucin-producing gastrointestinal adenocarcinomas. Gastric carcinoma occurs in approximately 1 to 15 per cent of all cases of Ménétrier's disease.[37]

Roentgenographically and grossly, Ménétrier's disease can be confused with malignant lymphoma.

PSEUDOLYMPHOMA. Extensive lymphocytic infiltration of a portion of the stomach may occur, predominantly in association with a benign gastric ulcer. A large portion of the stomach may be involved. Submucosal nodules, diffuse thickening, or enlarged rugal folds may be present. The infiltrate has a follicular pattern leading to confusion with "follicular lymphoma." Microscopically, the features favoring the diagnosis of pseudolymphoma are the presence of clearly reactive germinal centers throughout the lesions, a mixed population of inflammatory cells (including mature lymphocytes and plasma cells), and proliferation of blood vessels. Immunohistochemical stains for immunoglobulins usually demonstrate a polyclonal pattern.

The reasonably favorable prognosis reported for gastric lymphoma may reflect inclusion of cases of pseudolymphoma in some series, because the distinctions between the two conditions can be extraordinarily difficult.[2]

OTHER HYPERTROPHIC CONDITIONS

Hyperrugosity may occur in association with gastric cancer and malignant lymphoma. In *chronic hypertrophic gastritis,* described by Schindler in 1963, there is nonneoplastic proliferation of all epithelial elements—mucus-secreting cells as well as parietal cells and chief cells. The lesion is not inflammatory; thus, the term gastropathy is preferred to gastritis.

ZOLLINGER-ELLISON SYNDROME. Zollinger-Ellison (Z-E) syndrome may be associated with gastric changes radiographically and grossly similar to those of Ménétrier's disease. Microscopic examination, however, reveals the hyperplasia of Z-E syndrome to be primarily of the glandular, rather than the foveolar, portion of the fundic gland.

This hyperplasia primarily involves the parietal cells, but there may also be an increased number of enterochromaffin-like cells. Both of these phenomena presumably reflect abnormal gastric stimulation.

The occurrence of cases with features similar to those of Z-E syndrome but without hypergastrinemia, some of them associated with protein loss, suggests the existence of clinicopathologic variations of Z-E syndrome and perhaps as yet unrecognized humoral stimulants.[41]

CYSTIC TUMORS

Cystic tumors constitute a heterogeneous group of developmental anomalies, infections (e.g., hydatid cysts), or truly neoplastic lesions. The mucosal lesions are classified into various types according to their lining and are associated with intestinal metaplasia.[17] The submucosal cysts have also been designated *gastritis cystica profunda.*[7] Both of these cyst conditions are postulated to be more common in patients with gastric carcinoma and are acquired lesions.[15] The most common cystic tumors arise when obstruction of a mucus-secreting gland causes formation of a mucocele in the mucosa or submucosa of the gastric wall. The most important cystic lesion is a reduplication cyst. Usually encountered in the distal stomach, it may but usually does not communicate with the gastric lumen. Distention of the cyst with fluid may cause obstruction and a palpable mass.

SELECTED REFERENCES

Palmer, E. D.: Benign intramural tumors of the stomach: Review with special reference to gross pathology. Medicine, 30:81, 1951.
This exhaustive review of all benign intramural tumors of the stomach is an excellent starting point for students studying both neoplastic and nonneoplastic gastric lesions.

Rosai, J.: Gastrointestinal tract/stomach. *In* Rosai, J.: Ackerman's Surgical Pathology, 7th ed. St. Louis, C. V. Mosby Company, 1989, p. 487.
Both neoplastic and nonneoplastic tumors are reviewed with an exhaustive treatment of polyps. The confusing nomenclature of gastric polyps is clarified, and relevant clinical information is added to the discussion on pathology.

Sivak, M. V.: Symposium. Gastrointestinal endoscopy in clinical practice. Gastrointest. Endosc., 30:101, 1984.
This article reviews the current role of endoscopy—its rationale, technique, and complications—in patients with upper gastrointestinal disorders and complications, including benign gastric tumors.

REFERENCES

1. Appleman, H. D., and Helwig, E. B.: Gastric epithelioid leiomyoma and leimyosarcoma (leiomyoblastoma). Cancer, 38:709, 1976.
2. Brooks, J. J., and Enterline, H. T.: Gastric pseudolymphoma: Its three subtypes and relation to lymphoma. Cancer, 51:476, 1983.
3. Carney, J. A.: The triad of gastric epithelioid leiomyosarcoma, pulmonary chondroma, and functioning extra-adrenal paraganglioma: A five-year review. Medicine [Baltimore], 62:159, 1983.
4. Cripps, H. W.: Two cases of disseminated polyps of the rectum. Trans. Pathol. Soc. Lond. 33:165, 1882.
5. Deppisch, L. M., and Rona, V. T.: Gastric epithelial polyps: A 10-year study. J. Clin. Gastroenterol. 11:110, 1989.
6. Frank, B. W., and Kern, F.: Ménétrier's disease: Spontaneous metamorphosis of giant hypertrophy of the gastric mucosa to atrophic gastritis. Gastroenterology, 53:953, 1967.
7. Franzin, G., and Novelli, P.: Gastritis cystica profunda. Histopathology, 5:535, 1981.
8. Goldberg, H. I., and Margulis, A. R.: Adenomyoma of the stomach: Report of a case. Am. J. Roetgenol. 96:382, 1966.
9. Golden, T., and Stout, A. P.: Smooth muscle tumors of the gastrointestinal tract and retroperitoneal tissues. Surg. Gynecol. Obstet., 73:784, 1941.
10. Golfarb, W. B., Bennett, D., and Monafo, W.: Carcinoma in heterotopic gastric pancreas. Ann. Surg., 158:56, 1963.

11. Gorensek, M., Matko, I., Skralovnik, A., Rode, M., Satler, J., and Jutersek, A.: Disseminated hereditary gastrointestinal polyposis with orocutaneous hamartomatosis (Cowden's disease). Endoscopy, 16:59, 1984.

12. Halbert, R. E.: Peutz-Jeghers syndrome with metastasizing gastric adenocarcinoma: Report of a case. Arch. Pathol. Lab. Med., 106:517, 1982.

13. Hauser, G.: Über polyposis intestinalis adenomatosa und deren Beziehungen zur Krebsentwicklung. Arch. F. Klin. Med., 55:429, 1895.

14. Helwig, E., and Rainer, A.: Inflammatory fibroid polyps of the stomach. Surg. Gynecol. Obstet., 96:355, 1953.

15. Zhu, F. G., Deng, X. J., and Cheng, N. J.: Intramucosal cysts in gastric mucosa adjacent to carcinoma and peptic ulcer: A histochemical study. Histopathology, 11:631, 1987.

16. Iida, M., Yao, T., Itoh, H., Watanabe, H., Matsui, T., Iwashita, A., and Fujishima, M.: Natural history of fundic gland polyposis with familial adenomatous coli/Gardner's syndrome. Cancer, 61:605, 1988.

17. Kato, Y., Sugano, H., and Rubio, C.A.: Classification of intramucosal cysts of the stomach. Histopathology, 7:931, 1983.

18. Kleinhaus, U., Weich, L. Y., and Maoz, S.: Gastroduodenal intussusception secondary to prolapsing gastric tumors. Gastrointest. Radiol., 11:229, 1986.

19. Kraut, J. R., Powell, R., Hruby, M. A., and Lloyd-Still, J. D.: Ménétrier's disease in childhood: Report of two cases and review of the literature. J. Pediatr. Surg., 15:707, 1981.

20. Lipper, S., and Kahn, L. B.: Superficial cystic gastritis with alopecia: A forme fruste of the Cronkhite-Canada Syndrome. Arch. Pathol. Lab. Med., 101:432, 1977.

21. Lloyd, K. N., and Dennis, M.: Cowden's disease: A possible new symptom complex with multiple system involvement. Ann. Intern. Med. 58:136, 1963.

22. Lusitanus, A.: Curatorium medicinalium centuria septima, curatio 23, p. 58:Venet, 1653 [Originally published 1557]. Cited by Marshak.

23. Marshak, R., and Feldman, F.: Gastric polyps. Am. J. Dig. Dis. 10:909, 1965.

24. Meissner, W. A.: Leiomyoma of the stomach. Arch. Pathol., 38:207, 1944.

25. Ménétrier, P.: Des polyadenomes gastriques et de leures rapports avec le cancer de l'estomac. Arch. Physiol. Norm. Pathol. 1:32, 236, PI III, 1888.

26. Miller, J. H., Grisvold, J. J., Weiland, L. H., and McIlrath, D. C.: Upper gastrointestinal tract villous tumors. A. J. R. 134:933, 1980.

27. Ming, S. C.: Tumors of the esophagus and stomach, 2nd series. Washington, D.C., Armed Forces Institute of Pathology, 1973, pp. 82, 101, 125, 127.

28. Ming, S., and Goldman, H.: Gastric polyps: A histogenetic classification and its relation to carcinoma. Cancer, 18:721, 1965.

29. Monaco, A., Roth, S., Castleman, B., and Welch, C.: Adenomatous polyps of the stomach. Cancer, 15:456, 1962.

30. Morgan, B. K., Compton, C., Talbert, M., Gallagher, W. J., and Wood, W. C.: Benign smooth muscle tumors of the gastrointestinal tract. Ann. Surg., 211:63, 1990.

30a. Morgagni, A. B.: Seats and Causes of Disease Investigated by Anatomy (Translated by Alexander, B.). London, England. A. Miller and T. Cadell, 1769. Cited by Spriggs, E. I., and Marxer, O. A.: Polyps of stomach and polypoid gastritis. Quart. J. Med., 12:1, 1943.

31. Neimark, S., and Rogers, A.: Gastric polyps: A review. Am. J. Gastroenterol., 77:585, 1982.

32. Nishiura, M., Hirota, T., Itabashi, M., Ushio, K., Yamada, T., and Oguro, Y.: A clinical and histopathological study of gastric polyps in familial polyposis coli. Am. J. Gastroenterol., 79:98, 1984.

33. Palmer, E. D.: Benign intramural tumors of the stomach: a review with special reference to gross pathology. Medicine, 30:81, 1951.

34. Palmer, E. D.: What Ménétrier really said. Gastrointest. Endosc., 15:83, 1968.

35. Rosai, J.: Ackerman's Surgical Pathology, 7th ed. St. Louis, C. V. Mosby Company, 1989.

36. Sarre, R. G., Frost, A. G. Jagelman, D. G., Petras, R. E., Sivak, M. V., and McGannon, E.: Gastric and duodenal polyps in familial adenomatous polyposis: A prospective study of the nature and prevalence of upper gastrointestinal polyps. Gut, 28:306, 1987.

37. Scharschmidt, B. F.: The natural history of hypertrophic gastropathy (Ménétrier's disease): Report of a case with 16-year follow-up and review of 120 cases from the literature. Am. J. Med. 63:644, 1977.

38. Seifert, E., Gail, K., and Weismuller, J.: Gastric polypectomy. Endoscopy, 15:8, 1985.

39. Shiu, M. H., Farr, G. H., Papachristou, D. N., and Hadju, S. I.: Myosarcomas of the stomach, natural history, prognostic factors and management. Cancer, 49:177, 1982.

40. Snover, D.: Benign epithelial polyps of the stomach. Pathol. Annu., 20(Part 1):303, 1985.

41. Solcia, E., Capella, C., Buffa, R. et al.: Pathology of the Zollinger-Ellison syndrome. In Fenoglio, M., and Wolff, M. (eds.): Progress in Surgical Pathology. New York, Masson Publishing USA, Inc., 1980.

42. Stout, A. P.: Bizarre smooth muscle tumors of the stomach. Cancer, 15:400, 1962.

43. Sundt, T. M., III, Compton, C. C., and Malt, R. A.: Ménétrier's disease. Ann. Surg., 208:695, 1988.

44. Tomasulo, J.: Gastric polyps, histologic types and their relationship to gastric carcinoma. Cancer, 27:346, 1971.

45. Virchow, R. L. K.: Die krankhaften geschwulste. Berlin, A. Hirschwald, 1867.

46. Watanabe, H., Enjoji, M., Yao, T. and Ohsato, K.: Gastric lesions in familial adenomatosis coli: Their incidence and histologic analysis. Hum. Pathol., 9:269, 1978.

47. Wurlitzer, F. P., Mares, A. J., Isaacs, H., Jr., Handling, B. H., and Woolley, M. M.: Smooth muscle tumors of the stomach in childhood and adolescence. J. Pediatr. Surg., 8:421, 1973.

II _____

LYMPHOMA OF THE STOMACH

Theodore N. Pappas, M.D.

The first recorded surgical cure of a lymphoma of the stomach occurred in Cleveland in 1914 when Bunts resected a large antral tumor by means of a subtotal gastrectomy. The patient was reported to have no evidence of disease 19 years later.[25] Since then, major changes have occurred in the treatment of generalized lymphoma, with corresponding changes in the treatment of primary gastric lymphoma.

Non-Hodgkin's lymphoma of the abdomen is a relatively common presentation around the world.[1,4,11,14,28,43] Primary intra-abdominal lymphomas constitute approximately 10 to 20 per cent of all lymphocytic lymphomas, and gastric lymphomas constitute the majority of primary gastrointestinal lymphomas. In contrast, primary gastric lymphomas represent less than 5 per cent of all primary gastric tumors, although the number is increasing. The apparent increase in the incidence of gastric lymphoma is due to an increase in the absolute number of cases or a relative increase compared with gastric cancer.[20,34,37] Controversy continues about the treatment of primary gastric lymphomas, since, unlike the case with other lymphocytic lymphomas, surgical resection is still recommended for localized disease.

Clinical Presentation

The presentation of primary gastric lymphoma is strikingly similar to that of adenocarcinoma of the stomach. These similarities make the clinical distinction between these two disorders very difficult. Patients with primary gastric lymphoma are on average in their mid-50s, with a male to female predominance of 1.7 to 1. The major symptom is abdominal pain, which occurs in over 80 per cent of patients with abdominal lymphoma. This may be associated with anorexia, early satiety, nausea, and vomiting. Vague symptoms such as weakness and malaise are also relatively common. Less than 10 per cent of patients present asymptomatically. Symptoms that occur with diffuse lymphoma can be present in up to 40 per cent of these patients (night sweats, weight loss, and fevers).

In a recent series of patients reported by Green and associates, 42 per cent presented with emergency complications of gastrointestinal lymphoma.[19] These commonly include bleeding, perforation, and obstruction. Gastrocolic fistulas from lymphoma have also been described.[2] In addition, primary gastric lymphoma has been reported to occur following surgical therapy for peptic ulcer disease,[3] following successful treatment of systemic Hodgkin's disease,[15] in conjunction with Crohn's disease of the stomach,[27] or following immunosuppression for renal transplantation.[23,30]

PHYSICAL EXAMINATION. Patients with primary gastric lymphoma may present with abdominal findings suggestive of a mass in the left upper quadrant,[22] but more commonly there are no abnormal findings unless there is a complication of the tumor.[26,34] Splenomegaly is occasionally found in patients with direct extension of the lymphoma to the spleen, but massive splenomegaly may be more indicative of diffuse lymphoma. Other findings that suggest diffuse or abdominal lymphoma include palpable peripheral adenopathy or a large retroperitoneal mass.

Diagnosis

Diagnosis of primary gastric lymphoma can be confirmed by excluding other sites of lymphoma. Spinelli and associates studied 168 consecutive patients with non-Hodgkin's lymphoma; gastroscopy demonstrated a 9 per cent incidence of primary gastric lymphoma and a 20 per cent incidence of a secondary gastric involvement of diffuse lymphoma.[43] Examination should disclose whether the stomach is the primary or secondary site of the lymphoma.

UPPER GASTROINTESTINAL RADIOLOGY. Gastrointestinal series classically have been used to diagnose gastric masses but usually are unable to distinguish adenocarcinoma from lymphoma. Lymphomatous lesions typically involve long segments of the stomach that appear diffuse and infiltrating. Nearly all these lesions have ulcers and enlarged folds. Although very large defects are easily detectable, even small lesions in the range of 3 to 4 cm. can be detected by barium studies with accuracy.[38] Ten to 20 per cent of patients have a completely normal upper GI series in the presence of primary gastric lymphoma.[19,26]

ULTRASOUND. Although seldom used, ultrasound can be helpful in defining the characteristics of an abdominal mass. Derchi and colleagues localized a mass to the stomach wall in 15 of 17 patients studied with ultrasound.[12] The gastric mass in patients with lymphoma may present in a target or a solid homogeneous pattern with a unique hypoechoic appearance, in contrast to patients with adenocarcinoma in whom the stomach wall often has an echo-dense appearance.

ENDOSCOPIC ULTRASOUND. Endoscopic ultrasound has been used in a small number of patients to define the stage of gastric lymphoma. In studies by Caletti and associates, endoscopic ultrasound was useful in defining the layers of the stomach in normal regions and contrasting those with the infiltrative nature of gastric lymphoma.[10] It is also useful in suggesting the presence of local lymph node involvement and contiguous spread of tumor into other organs.

COMPUTED TOMOGRAPHY. Most of the computed tomographic findings in gastric lymphoma are similar to findings in adenocarcinoma of the stomach. Some of the unique characteristics with gastric lymphoma include lesions in more than one region of the stomach or diffuse involvement. In addition, patients with lymphoma are more likely to have widespread adenopathy in the abdomen.[8]

GASTROINTESTINAL ENDOSCOPY. Visual inspection of gastric lesions in patients with primary gastric lymphoma usually suggests gastric malignancy. Unfortunately, the visual diagnosis of gastric lymphoma is correct in only half the patients.[36] The lesions appear as superficial stellate ulcers involving large areas of the stomach. The margin between the normal mucosa and the lesion is often very sharp. This is in contrast to adenocarcinomas, which have a dominant ulceration with an ill-defined margin between normal and abnormal tissue.[17] Biopsies and cytologic examination of these gastric lesions in patients with lymphoma accurately make the diagnosis in 36 to 96 per cent of patients.[14,19,31,32,36,37] Due to insufficient tissue, many patients require exploratory laparotomy for definitive pathologic determination.

Pathology

Although primary gastric lymphoma usually occupies the distal part of the stomach, it can extend through the entire surface of the stomach. The five classifications of the gross morphology of these tumors are (1) infiltrative, (2) ulcerative, (3) nodular, (4) polypoid, and (5) combined (any combination of the other four).

Histological sections of primary lymphoma of the stomach are characterized by mucosally or submucosally based lymphoid tissue. Infiltration of the gastric glands by follicle center cells forming characteristic lymphoid epithelial lesions is pathognomonic.[33] Primary gastric lymphoma is not associated with bone marrow or peripheral node involvement but does metastasize to local nodes by contiguous spread and to the lymphoid tissue in the chest. The prognosis can be determined on the basis of histologic findings, which include size, invasion, and nodal status.[6,35]

Cytologic examination may be an aid in the diagnosis of primary gastric lymphoma. The accuracy of cytologic examination varies from 35 per cent to greater than 80 per cent, depending on the techniques utilized.[9,32,43] Cabre-Fiol and Vilardell state that a combination of direct endoscopic abrasion for cytology plus endoscopic biopsy yielded a correct diagnosis in 14 of 15 patients studied. The experience with cytologic diagnosis for gastric lymphoma from other medical centers has not been as encouraging.[39]

Pseudolymphoma represents 10 per cent of all gastric lymphomas diagnosed. Pseudolymphoma is benign gastric lymphomatosis, which is characterized by lymphoid infiltration of the gastric wall, predominantly in the mucosa, without evidence of nodal disease. Ulceration and extensive fibrosis are present, commonly with chronic peptic ulcer disease.[3,21] The *sine qua non* for the diagnosis is germinal centers present within the gastric lesion.[7] Pseudolymphoma may represent a premalignant lesion that can convert to malignant lymphoma. This has been suggested by the occurrence of both pseudolymphoma and malignant lymphoma in gastrectomy specimens.[26] The current recommended management for pseudolymphoma is conservative surgical resection,[8] and nonoperative observation is reserved for the patient at high risk for surgical therapy. Complete resection offers cure while avoiding the likelihood of malignant conversion. These lesions should not be treated with adjuvant therapy.

Treatment

Many patients with primary gastric lymphoma present with a gastric mass and insufficient tissue to make a definitive diagnosis after endoscopic biopsy. At exploration, half the patients are found to have Stage I or Stage II disease.[31] Current recommendation for treatment of these tumors is attempted cure with surgical resection.[6] All gross tumors should be resected whenever possible. This may include total gastrectomy in patients who are medically suitable. The reported mortality from gastric resection in patients with lymphoma ranges from zero to 10 per cent.[29,32,35,41,42] Intraoperative evaluation to stage the tumor adequately includes adequate sampling of regional lymph nodes and a complete abdominal examination to determine (1) the size of the spleen and (2) the appearance of distant intra-abdominal nodes.

Surgical resection of these tumors affords the greatest likelihood of long-term survival. Although all series in the literature are retrospective and therefore biased, most studies continue to demonstrate that surgically resected patients fare better than those treated with only radiation therapy and chemotherapy. Approximately 75 per cent of patients are resectable on exploration.[14,22,24,41,42] For all stages, curative resection should yield a 5-year survival in the range of 34 to 50 per cent.[13,22,41] Patients who undergo only palliative resections have a 5-year survival ranging from 25 to 35 per cent.[35] The stage of the tumor correlates well with survival. Mentzer and associates report a 4-year survival of 90 per cent in patients with Stage I and Stage II disease, as contrasted with a 4-year survival of 25 per cent in patients with Stage III and Stage IV disease.[31] Shiu reported similar results from the Sloan-Kettering Cancer Center, with a 95 per cent Stage I survival, a 78 per cent Stage II survival, and a 25 per cent Stage IV survival at 5 years.[42]

Surgical resection not only improves survival but also can assist in postoperative palliative care. There are reports of bleeding and perforation in patients receiving adjuvant radiation therapy or chemotherapy prior to resection. Liang and colleagues reviewed 84 patients with primary abdominal lymphomas, 45 of which were primary gastric lymphomas.[28] They found that 38 per cent of the courses of those patients who underwent chemotherapy prior to resection were complicated by bleeding or perforation. Fleming and colleagues reported that preoperative treatment with combination chemotherapy led to upper GI bleeding requiring emergency surgical therapy in 4 of 5 patients.[16] In contrast, Mittal and associates reviewed a series of 37 patients in whom radiation therapy did not lead to perforation or bleeding in any patient prior to resection.[32]

Adjuvant therapy for resected or unresected patients has been recommended for all stages of primary gastric lymphoma. Shimm and colleagues demonstrated that radiation therapy given postoperatively to patients with positive surgical margins improved survival.[40] Shiu and co-workers reviewed a series of 51 patients in whom resection alone yielded a 5-year survival of 33 per cent with a 5-year survival of 67 per cent if radiation was added to surgical resection.[41] Similarly, Hockey and associates showed an improvement of 45 to 73 per cent in 5-year survival if radiation therapy was added to curative surgical resection for patients with Stage I disease.[22] This adjuvant therapy in its aggressive form can include whole abdominal radiation, with a boost to the stomach bed totaling 3700 rads.[41,42] The common chemotherapies include either cyclophosphamide, vincristine, nitrogen mustard, procarbazine, and prednisone (CMOPP) or cyclophosphamide, doxorubicin, vincristine, and prednisone (CHOP).[14,16,31,42]

In summary, all Stage I and Stage II patients (disease confined to stomach and regional nodes) should undergo attempted curative resection followed by adjuvant chemotherapy, radiation therapy, or both. Stage III and Stage IV patients who present with complications of bleeding, obstruction, or perforation should also undergo attempted primary resection followed by adjuvant therapy. Patients without complications who present with preoperative documentation of Stage III or Stage IV disease should be treated with radiation therapy and chemotherapy initially; surgical resection should be reserved for persistent local disease in the stomach or for complications. If preoperative diagnosis and staging are not possible and exploration for diagnosis is made, resection should be attempted unless precluded by the extent of the tumor.

SELECTED REFERENCES

Brooks, J. J., and Enterline, H. T.: Gastric pseudolymphoma: Its three subtypes and relation to lymphoma. Cancer 51:476, 1983.
This represents the most recent complete review of pseudolymphoma of the stomach. The authors characterize the histologic findings in ten cases of pseudolymphoma.

Mentzer, S. J., Osteen, R. T., Pappas, T. N., Rosenthal, D. S., Canellos, G. P., and Wilson, R. E.: Surgical therapy of localized abdominal non-Hodgkin's lymphomas. Surgery 103:609, 1988.
The authors describe a recent series of patients with abdominal lymphoma, with emphasis on presentation and management of these patients. An excellent survival rate with surgical resection for Stage I and Stage II patients is reported.

Rosen, C. B., Van Heerden, J. A., Martin, J. K., Wold, L. E., and Ilstrup, D. M.: Is an aggressive surgical approach to the patient with gastric lymphoma warranted? Ann. Surg. 205:634, 1987.
The authors review 84 patients treated at the Mayo Clinic, all with greater than 5-year follow-up. They emphasize the necessity of attempted surgical cure and also discuss the factors that affect prognosis.

Shiu, M. H., Nisce, L., Pinna, A., Straus, D. J., Tome, M., Filippa, D. A., and Lee, B. J.: Recent results of multimodal therapy of gastric lymphoma. Cancer 58:1389, 1986.
The authors review their experience with multimodal therapy for gastric lymphoma. They show that surgical therapy plus adjuvant chemotherapy yields prolonged survival and represents the best survival data in the literature.

REFERENCES

1. Al-Bahrani, A., Al-Mondhiry, H., Bakir, F., Al-Saleem, T., Al-Eshaiker, M.: Primary gastric lymphoma: Review of 32 cases from Iraq. Ann. R. Coll. Surg. Engl. 64:234, 1982.
2. Allison, J. E.: Gastrocolic fistula as a complication of gastric lymphoma. Am. J. Gastroenterol. 59:499, 1973.
3. Anderson, J. R., Lee, D., Naysmith, A., and Busuttil, A.: Gastric pseudolymphoma. Br. J. Surg. 67:672, 1980.
4. Aozasa, K., Ueda, T., Kurata, A., et al.: Prognostic value of histologic and clinical factors in 56 patients with gastrointestinal lymphoma. Cancer 601:309, 1988.
5. Bonadonna, G., and Valagussa, P.: Should lymphomas of gastrointestinal tract be treated differently from other disease presentations? Eur. J. Cancer Clin. Oncol. 22:1295, 1986.
6. Brooks, J. J., and Enterline, H. T.: Primary gastric lymphoma: A clinicopathologic study of 58 cases with long-term follow-up and literature review. Cancer 51:701, 1983.
7. Brooks, J. J., and Enterline, H. T.: Gastric pseudolymphoma: Its three subtypes and relation to lymphoma. Cancer 51:476, 1983.
8. Buy, J. N., and Moss, A. A.: Computed tomography of gastric lymphoma. AJR 138:859, 1982.
9. Cabre-Fiol, V., and Vilardell, F.: Progress in the cytological diagnosis of gastric lymphoma: A report of 32 cases. Cancer 41:1456, 1978.
10. Caletti, G. C., Zani, L., Bolondi, L., Guizzardi, G., Brocchi, E., and Barbara, L.: Impact of endoscopic ultrasonography on diagnosis and treatment of primary gastric lymphoma. Surgery 103:315, 1988.
11. Dajani, Y. F., and Al-Jitawi, S.: Primary gastrointestinal lymphoma. Trop. Geograph. Med. 35:375, 1983.
12. Derchi, L. E., Banderali, A., Bossi, C., et al.: The sonographic appearance of gastric lymphoma. J. Ultrasound Med. 3:251, 1984.
13. Dworkin, B., Lightdale, C. J., Weingrad, N., et al.: Primary gastric lymphoma: A review of 50 cases. Dig. Dis. Sci. 27:986, 1982.
14. Economopoulos, T., Alexopoulos, C., Stathakis, N., et al.: Primary gastric lymphoma — The experience of a general hospital. Br. J. Cancer 52:391, 1985.
15. Eridani, S., and Singh, A. K.: Gastric non-Hodgkin's lymphoma after successful treatment of Hodgkin's disease. Oncology 43:107, 1986.
16. Fleming, I. D., Mitchell, S., and Dilawari, R. A.: The role of surgery in the management of gastric lymphoma. Cancer 49:1135, 1982.
17. Fork, F. T., Haglund, U., Hogstrom, H., and Wehlin, L.: Primary gastric lymphoma versus gastric cancer. Endoscopy 17:5, 1985.
18. Ghahremani, G. G., and Fisher, M. R.: Lymphoma of the stomach following gastric surgery for benign peptic ulcers. Gastrointest. Radiol. 8:213, 1983.
19. Green, J. A., Dawson, A. A., Jones, P. F., and Brunt, P. W.: The presentation of gastrointestinal lymphoma: Study of a population. Br. J. Surg. 66:798, 1979.
20. Hayes, J., and Dunn, E.: Has the incidence of primary gastric lymphoma increased? Cancer 63:2073, 1989.
21. Highman, L. M., Fantelli, F. J., and Hermann, R. E.: Pseudolymphoma of the stomach. Arch. Surg. 116:227, 1981.
22. Hockey, M. S., Powell, J., Crocker, J., and Fielding, J. W. L.: Primary gastric lymphoma. Br. J. Surg. 74:483, 1987.
23. Jamieson, N. V., Thiru, S., Calne, R. Y., and Evans, D. B.: Gastric lymphomas arising in two patients with renal allografts. Transplantation 31:224, 1981.
24. Jones, R. E., Willis, S., Innes, D. J., and Wanebo, H. J.: Primary gastric lymphoma: Problems in staging and management. Am. J. Surg. 155:118, 1988.
25. Jones, T. E., and Carmody, M. G.: Lymphosarcoma of the stomach. Report of a case with a 19-year surgical cure. Ann. Surg. 101:1136, 1935.
26. Jung, S. S., Wieman, T. J., and Lindberg, R. D.: Primary gastric lymphoma and pseudolymphoma. Am. Surg. 54:594, 1988.
27. Kini, S. U., Pai, P. K., Rao, P. K., and Kini, A. J.: Primary gastric lymphoma associated with Crohn's disease of the stomach. Am. J. Gastroenterol. 81:23, 1986.
28. Liang, R., Todd, D., Chan, T. K., Ng, R. P., and Ho, F. C. S.: Gastrointestinal lymphoma in Chinese: A retrospective analysis. Hematolog. Oncol. 5:115, 1987.
29. Lim, F. E., Hartman, A. S., Tan, E. G. T., Cady, B., and Meissner, W. A.: Factors in the prognosis of gastric lymphoma. Cancer 39:1715, 1977.
30. McTamaney, J. P., Neifeld, J. P., Mendez-Picon, G., and Lee, H. M.: Primary gastric lymphoma following renal transplantation. J. Surg. Oncol. 18:265, 1981.
31. Mentzer, S. J., Osteen, R. T., Pappas, T. N., Rosenthal, D. S., Canellos, G. P.,

and Wilson, R. E.: Surgical therapy of localized abdominal non-Hodgkin's lymphomas. Surgery 103:609, 1988.

32. Mittal, B., Wasserman, T. H., and Griffith, R. C.: Non-Hodgkin's lymphoma of the stomach. Am. J. Gastroenterol. 78:780, 1983.
33. Moore, I., and Wright, D. H.: Primary gastric lymphoma — a tumor of mucosa-associated lymphoid tissue: A histological and immunohistological study of 36 cases. Histopathology 8:1025, 1984.
34. Orlando, R., Pastuszak, W., Preissler, P. L., and Welch, J. P.: Gastric lymphoma: A clinicopathologic reappraisal. Am. J. Surg. 143:450, 1982.
35. Rosen, C. B., Van Heerden, J. A., Martin, J. K., Wold, L. E., and Ilstrup, D. M.: Is an aggressive surgical approach to the patient with gastric lymphoma warranted? Ann. Surg. 205:634, 1987.
36. Russo, A., Grasso, G., Sanfillipo, G., Giannone, G., and Guerrera, G.: Gastroscopy and directed biopsy in the diagnosis of primary gastric lymphomas: Report of 16 personal cases. Tumor, 64:419, 1978.
37. Sandler, R. S.: Has primary gastric lymphoma become more common? J. Clin. Gastroenterol. 6:101, 1984.
38. Sato, T., Sakai, Y., Ishiguro, S., and Furukawa, H.: Radiologic manifestations of early gastric lymphoma. AJR 146:513, 1986.
39. Seybolt, J. F., and Papanicolaou, G. N.: The value of cytology in the diagnosis of gastric cancer. Gastroenterology 33:369, 1957.
40. Shimm, D. S., Dosoretz, D. E., Anderson, T., Linggood, R. M., Harris, N. L., and Wang, C. C.: Primary gastric lymphoma: An analysis with emphasis on prognostic factors and radiation therapy. Cancer 52:2044, 1983.
41. Shiu, M. H., Karas, M., Nisce, L., Lee, B. J., Fillippa, D. A., and Lieberman, P. H.: Management of primary gastric lymphoma. Ann. Surg. 195:196, 1982.
42. Shiu, M. H., Nisce, L., Pinna, A., Straus, D. J., Tome, M., Filippa, D. A., and Lee, B. J.: Recent results of multimodal therapy of gastric lymphoma. Cancer 58:1389, 1986.
43. Spinelli, P., Gullo, C. L., and Pizzetti, P.: Endoscopic diagnosis of gastric lymphomas. Endoscopy 12:211, 1980.

III

THE PATHOGENESIS, PROPHYLAXIS, AND TREATMENT OF STRESS GASTRITIS

Laurence Y. Cheung, M.D.

Erosions of the gastroduodenal mucosa are a common occurrence among patients in surgical, medical, and respiratory intensive care units. Various types of severe physiologic stress are conducive to their development, including major physical or thermal trauma, shock, sepsis, respiratory failure, head injury, or ingestion of a variety of chemical agents such as aspirin and alcohol.[17] For a long time all these lesions have been designated by the term "stress ulcers." Much of the confusion in the past has been the failure to differentiate between these various lesions that occur in different clinical settings.[25] It is now commonly accepted that stress gastritis occurs primarily in patients following severe burn, trauma, hemorrhagic shock, respiratory failure, or sepsis. They are multiple, superficial erosions that occur primarily in the fundus of the stomach. These erosions are clearly different from Cushing's ulcer, ulcers induced by drugs, and reactivation of a preexisting chronic ulcer. A brief description of these other acute lesions should be helpful in distinguishing them from stress gastritis.

Cushing's ulcer, which occurs with intracranial tumors, with head injury, or after cranial surgery, may involve the esophagus, stomach, and duodenum. Morphologically, Cushing's ulcer tends to be a single and deep ulcer. For this reason, perforation is a common complication of Cushing's ulcer but is rarely encountered in the more superficial stress gastritis. Hypersecretion of gastric acid and pepsin is common among patients with Cushing's ulcer but unusual in individuals with stress gastritis. Drug-induced ulcers are often indistinguishable from stress gastritis in their gross and microscopic appearance and distribution. Although both drug-induced and stress-induced ulcers may share the same ultimate pathogenetic events at the cellular level, the initial factors that lead to cellular damage may be different.[11] Occasionally, upper gastrointestinal bleeding in critically ill patients may be caused by a preexisting chronic duodenal or gastric ulcer. It is possible that during the course of another acute illness, activation of a chronic ulcer diathesis could become manifest. Reactivation of a previous chronic ulcer usually occurs at a single site with endoscopic evidence suggesting chronicity, whereas acute stress erosions are usually multiple with no evidence of chronicity. The distinction between these conditions and stress gastritis is important because the prognostic and therapeutic considerations are different.

INCIDENCE

Clinical studies that do not employ endoscopy underestimate the incidence of stress gastritis since most of these erosions do not bleed. It has been shown by gastroscopy that the incidence of such gastric erosions was 100 per cent in 40 severely injured patients.[14] In a similar study at the Brooke Army Surgical Research Institute, gastric erosions were found by sequential endoscopic examinations in 27 of 29 patients with major burns.[9] Acute gastric erosions were also found in a majority of patients in the medical intensive care unit.[18] Most patients developed these lesions within 72 hours of admission to the intensive care unit. Fortunately, only a small number of these patients had significant gastrointestinal hemorrhage.

PATHOGENESIS

Although the precise mechanisms involved in the development of stress gastritis are still unknown, current evidence supports a multifactorial etiology.[25] Most of the factors contribute to the development of stress gastritis by reducing the ability of the stomach to protect itself against acid injury rather than by increasing the amount of acid secretion. This section will focus on some of these factors that have been applied in the clinical approaches to patients at high risk for stress gastritis (Fig. 1).

THE PRESENCE OF LUMINAL ACID

There is no evidence that an increased quantity of acid secretion is the cause of stress gastritis. Although hypersecretion is an unlikely cause, it can be stated with certainty that some hydrogen ions are necessary for the development of stress gastritis. Almost all experimentally induced stress gastritis, under conditions resembling clinical settings, require low gastric luminal pH.

ISCHEMIA

Clinically, most patients who develop stress gastritis have experienced an episode of shock from hemorrhage, sepsis, or cardiac dysfunction. Diminished gastric mucosal blood flow is a

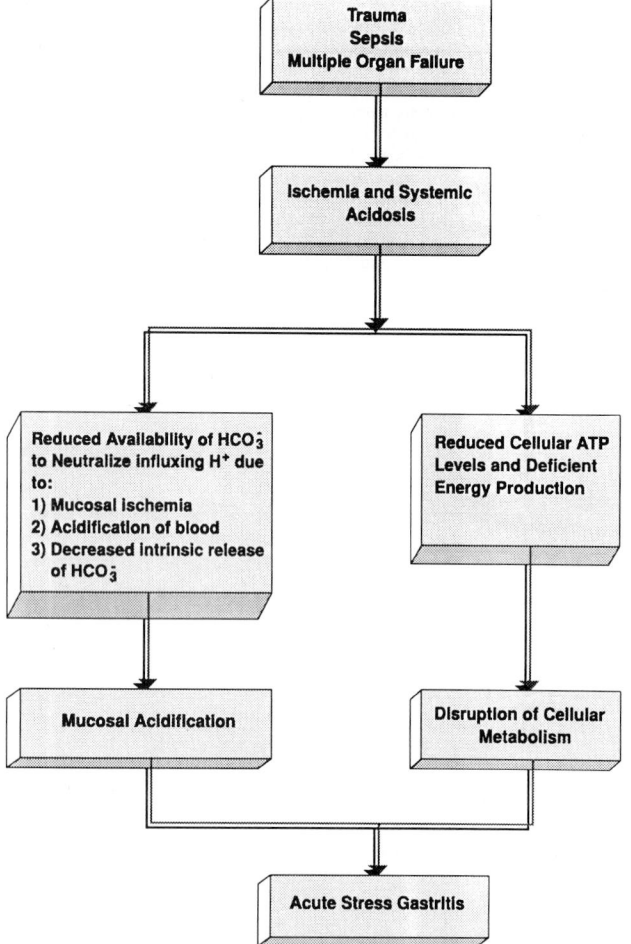

Figure 1. Proposed pathophysiologic mechanism for development of acute stress gastritis.

common denominator in animal experiments that employ restraint, hemorrhage, or endotoxemia for the production of acute ulceration. There is virtual agreement among all investigators that one basic pathogenetic feature of stress gastritis is mucosal ischemia.[6]

The cause-effect relationship between ischemia and stress erosions has been explained by the theory of energy deficit of the gastric mucosa. Ischemia may adversely affect gastric energy metabolism, an important factor in mucosal defense against injury. Menguy and associates have shown in a series of animal experiments that hemorrhagic shock produces a differential energy deficit (decreased levels of ATP and high-energy phosphate) in the gastric mucosa.[15] This deficit is much greater in the fundic mucosa than in the antrum or other tissues such as the liver and muscle. Feeding before hemorrhage has also been shown to result in a lesser degree of injury than fasting, presumably because of greater availability of energy sources. These data support the contention that a differential energy deficit exists between fundus and antrum and provides a possible explanation for the propensity of the fundus rather than the antrum for development of stress ulcers.

The other leading hypothesis is that gastric mucosal blood flow has an important role in the disposal, or buffering, of the H^+ entering the tissue. Under normal conditions, a small amount of H^+ diffuses into the mucosa and may be rapidly cleared or neutralized by adequate mucosal blood flow.[25] Ischemia reduces the capacity of the gastric mucosa to neutralize acid that enters the tissue.[6] This in turn leads to accumulation of H^+ within the tissue, mucosal acidification, and ulceration. Recent studies measuring the mucosal pH with a pH electrode have

supported this hypothesis. Moreover, experimentally induced increases in mucosal blood flow by intra-arterial infusion of isoproterenol prevented ulcerations in dogs subjected to hemorrhagic shock.

SYSTEMIC ACID-BASE BALANCE

Recent studies have suggested that the ability of the gastric mucosa to maintain its neutral pH is dependent not only on the rate of mucosal blood flow, but also on the pH of the arterial blood perfusing the stomach. This concept was first introduced by Cummins, Grossman, and Ivy in 1948.[8] They demonstrated that if systemic acidosis induced by constant intragastric infusion of acid was prevented by intravenous administration of sodium bicarbonate, the gastric and duodenal ulcers that otherwise developed could be prevented. It has also been shown at the University of Kansas that mucosal injury induced by the combination of hemorrhagic shock and topical bile salts can be partially prevented by intravenous infusion of sodium bicarbonate.[7]

SECRETORY STATE OF THE GASTRIC MUCOSA

It is well known that bicarbonate is released intrinsically within the mucosa during active secretion of acid. However, the importance of this intramural release of bicarbonate in mucosal protection against luminal acid has only recently been recognized by Silen and associates.[13] They have clearly shown that an actively secreting stomach is much more resistant to ulceration than a metiamide-inhibited rabbit stomach, supporting the concept that the alkaline tide is of importance in protecting the tissue against ulceration. Acid secretion requires high energy consumption and, therefore, is usually reduced during mucosal ischemia. The reduced acid secretion results in a decrease in the intrinsic release of bicarbonate and, therefore, renders the gastric mucosa more susceptible to acid injury.

REFLUX OF BILE AND DISRUPTION OF GASTRIC MUCOSAL PERMEABILITY BARRIER

Gastric mucosa has a unique ability to contain acid in the lumen and prevent excessive influx of acid into the tissue. This functional capability is defined as the gastric mucosal permeability barrier to acid. A significant amount of research has been done recently to evaluate the relationship between ischemia and the integrity of the gastric mucosal barrier. Most studies have failed to demonstrate disruption of the gastric permeability barrier during hemorrhagic shock.[25] However, it is conceivable that reflux of duodenal contents and bile salts occurs in seriously ill patients, and bile salts are known to disrupt the barrier.[21,25] In addition to the ability of bile salts to increase mucosal permeability to acid, they also produce direct injury to the surface cells of the stomach and render the gastric mucosa more susceptible to acid injury.

PROPOSED MECHANISM OF INJURY TO GASTRIC SURFACE EPITHELIAL CELLS DURING SEVERE PHYSIOLOGIC STRESS

In the last decade, significant progress has been made in understanding the basic mechanism by which surface epithelial cells of the gastric mucosa are protected against luminal acid. Silen and co-workers have proposed a tentative schema by which the surface cells of the gastric mucosa are protected against acidification (Fig. 2).[25] Despite the presence of the gastric mucosal permeability barrier, a small number of hydrogen ions diffuse through the apical cell membrane into the gastric surface epithelial cells. Under normal conditions, influxing hydrogen ions are neutralized by bicarbonate derived from the

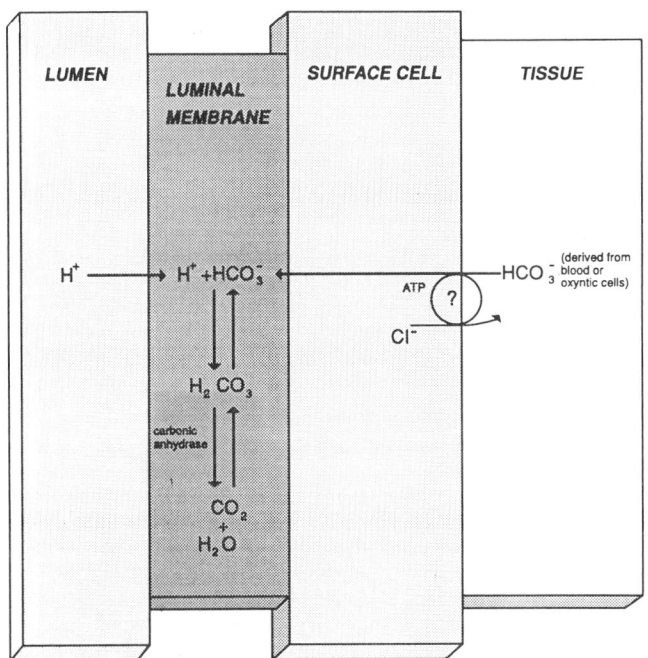

Figure 2. Hypothetical schema of the protective mechanism of surface cells against luminal acid. (Adapted from Silen, W., Merhav, A., and Simson, J. N. L.: The pathophysiology of stress ulcer disease. World J. Surg., 5:165, 1981.)

blood or from actively secreting oxyntic cells in exchange for chloride, possibly as a result of an ATP-dependent step. Dehydration of the resultant H_2CO_3 into harmless CO_2 and H_2O is catalyzed by carbonic anhydrase.

Mucosal ischemia may have several deleterious effects on this protective mechanism of surface epithelial cells in maintaining their intracellular pH. First, less bicarbonate is available to the tissue as a result of ischemia and decreased intrinsic release from oxyntic cells. Systemic acidosis also reduces the availability of bicarbonate to the gastric mucosa. Recently, Ashley and co-workers validated the measurement of intracellular pH of surface epithelial cells of *Necturus* stomach using pH-sensitive intracellular microelectrodes.[2] This technique was used to examine the effect of mucosal or serosal acidification on intracellular pH in gastric surface epithelial cells. It was noted that gastric epithelial cells are much more sensitive to pH changes from the serosal side than from the mucosal side.[3] Such findings are consistent with the concept that systemic acidosis and ischemia render the gastric epithelial cells more susceptible to acid injury. Acidification of intracellular pH may also be explained by the reduced cellular ATP level due to deficient energy metabolism during ischemia, since the exchange of chloride for bicarbonate entering the cell from the serosal side is an ATP-dependent step.

PREVENTION

Based on the various factors identified experimentally as responsible for the pathogenesis of stress gastritis, a variety of prophylactic measures can be instituted in patients at high risk for its development. Since mucosal ischemia may alter a number of mechanisms by which the stomach normally protects itself against injury, vigorous efforts should be made to correct any shocklike state resulting from blood loss and/or sepsis. In addition, efforts should be made to improve ventilatory support, to correct any systemic acid-base abnormality, and to maintain adequate nutrition in these critically ill patients. Despite the lack of documentation, a strong impression exists among clinicians that the incidence and prevalence of stress gastritis have decreased significantly over the past decade, per-

haps as a result of improved general care given to critically ill patients.

The "no acid, no ulcer" dictum has led to the concept that maintaining neutral pH of the gastric contents may prevent development of stress gastritis in critically ill patients. In fact, titration of gastric pH with antacid has been shown to be effective in preventing gastrointestinal bleeding in intensive care unit patients in several controlled prospective trials.[12,19,26]

Several studies have reported that H_2-receptor antagonists are also useful in the prophylaxis of stress ulceration.[18,24,26] In a randomized, double-blinded, placebo-controlled study, Peura and Johnson have shown that cimetidine can alleviate established lesions, prevent bleeding, and diminish the requirement for blood transfusion in patients admitted to a medical intensive care unit.[18] Others have suggested that, when given alone, it does not appear to provide the same degree of protection against mucosal injury as antacids.[19,29] In a recent retrospective analysis of the combined data from 16 prospective trials, Shuman and associates[24] have concluded that acid reduction by either cimetidine or antacid, when compared with placebo, significantly reduces the risk of upper gastrointestinal bleeding in critically ill patients (Fig. 3). When detection of occult blood is used as the minimal criterion for the diagnosis of bleeding, antacids appear to be superior to H_2-receptor antagonists in preventing stress gastritis bleeding. If clinically overt bleeding is used as the minimal criterion, antacids and cimetidine may be equal in their ability to prevent upper gastrointestinal bleeding in critically ill patients. Based on these findings, a strong recommendation can be made for early and aggressive reduction of intragastric acidity by either antacid titration or intravenous

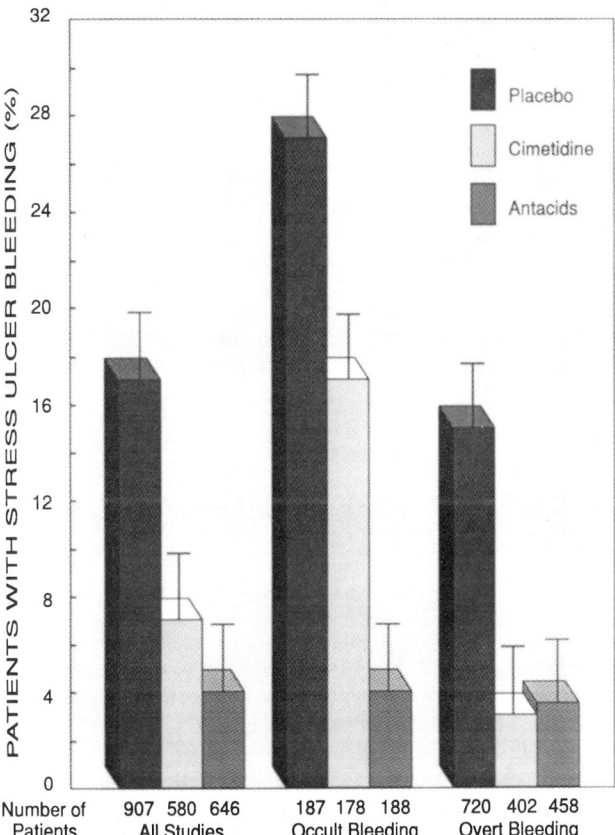

Figure 3. Incidence of stress ulcer bleeding in critically ill patients receiving placebo, cimetidine, or antacids for prophylaxis. Results are shown as percentages (means ± standard deviation). All comparisons between treatment regimens within each group were statistically significant except between antacid and cimetidine treatment in studies requiring overt bleeding. (Adapted from Shuman, R. B., Schuster, D. P., and Zuckerman, G. R.: Prophylactic therapy for stress ulcer bleeding: A reappraisal. Ann. Intern. Med., 106:562, 1987.)

administration of H_2-receptor antagonists in patients at risk for the development of bleeding from stress gastritis.

Most recently, the practice of prophylaxis of stress gastritis in critically ill patients with either antacids or H_2-receptor antagonists has been questioned for the potential serious side effect of neutralization of gastric content. Normal gastric acidity is an important component of the antibacterial defense of the upper gastrointestinal tract. Several recent reports indicate that neutralization of gastric acid or inhibition of acid secretion may increase the risk of nosocomial pneumonia by favoring gastric colonization with gram-negative bacilli.[4,10,28] In a prospective, controlled, randomized study of the prophylaxis of stress bleeding, Tryba compared the effectiveness of sucralfate suspension against antacid in 100 ventilated high-risk patients in a surgical intensive care unit.[28] Sucralfate is a weak buffer that probably acts through pepsin absorption, mucosal protein-binding, and cytoprotection. In this study, sucralfate provided adequate protection against stress bleeding without significantly increasing the intragastric pH. Less nosocomial pneumonia developed in the sucralfate group than in the antacid group, although there was no significant difference in the mortality rate in these two groups.

In a similar prospective study by Driks and associates,[10] gram-negative bacilli were isolated more frequently from tracheal aspirates of patients who were receiving antacid or H_2-blockers than of those receiving sucralfate. The rate of pneumonia was twice as high in the antacid-H_2 group as in the sucralfate group although the difference did not reach statistical significance. Although these results are still preliminary and not yet conclusive, they do suggest that the use of a prophylactic agent such as sucralfate, which preserves the gastric acidity, may be preferable to antacid or H_2-blocker.

TREATMENT

All patients with established stress gastritis with hemorrhage should be given adequate supportive care for shock and sepsis with careful monitoring of the extent of hemorrhage. The patient with bleeding must be assessed for coagulation defects, and any specific clotting abnormalities should be corrected. Initial management to control gastrointestinal hemorrhage should consist of gastric lavage with chilled solutions through a large-bore nasogastric tube. Lavage of the stomach aids in the fragmentation of clots and avoids gastric distention. Another benefit of gastric lavage is removal of duodenal contents that may have refluxed into the stomach as a result of adynamic ileus, since bile salts and pancreatic juice are injurious to gastric mucosa. Fortunately, most patients appear to stop bleeding following this general management. In occasional patients, specific nonoperative or operative treatment is required.[5]

ENDOSCOPIC THERAPY

Techniques for the treatment of stress gastritis via endoscopy include either electrocoagulation or laser photocoagulation.[23] Initial clinical experience with endoscopic therapy reports over 90 per cent permanent hemostasis. However, only a small percentage of the total patients in these studies had bleeding from stress gastritis. Since upper gastrointestinal hemorrhage, whether due to stress gastritis or other causes, ceased spontaneously in a majority of these patients, an evaluation of any new method will require a very large patient population in a controlled study to prove its efficacy. At the present time, this technique provides an opportunity for direct control of bleeding from stress gastritis at institutions where this technique is available.

ANGIOGRAPHIC PHARMACOTHERAPY

The ability to selectively catheterize various branches of the splanchnic arterial circulation using angiographic methods represents an additional therapeutic modality.[5,23] Several initial studies have reported a high success rate with this technique in the treatment of bleeding from stress gastritis. However, control of massive bleeding by selective intra-arterial infusion of vasopressin was not associated with improved survival. Vasopressin therapy is a useful agent in decreasing the amount of blood transfusion required during episodes of hemorrhage, and it provides the interval of time needed for a planned surgical approach to the problem. On the basis of these studies, this technique is recommended if facilities and trained personnel are available before surgical therapy is considered.

SOMATOSTATIN AND PROSTAGLANDINS

Somatostatin is an endogenous gastrointestinal peptide. Exogenous administration of somatostatin has been shown to inhibit acid secretion, reduce mucosal blood flow, and protect the gastric mucosa against stress-induced injury in animal experiments. These data suggest that somatostatin may be a clinically effective peptide in the treatment of stress-induced hemorrhagic gastritis. Recently, several reports indicate that somatostatin is more effective than H_2-receptor antagonists in the control of upper gastrointestinal tract bleeding.[27] Unfortunately, only a small number of the patients in these studies were bleeding from stress gastritis. Therefore, somatostatin has not yet been used in a sufficient number of patients to determine its efficacy and long-term sequelae.

Prostaglandins are a group of long-chain, saturated fatty acids widely distributed throughout the body. The concentrations of various prostaglandins in the stomach are high relative to other tissues, and prostaglandins of the E, F, and I types have been detected in both gastric juice and mucosa. Exogenous prostaglandins have many effects on gastric function, including inhibition of basal and stimulated acid secretion, enhancement of mucosal blood flow, stimulation of mucous secretion, and changes in ion transport.[16] These actions appear to be involved in the ability of prostaglandins to reduce the severity of mucosal injury in a wide variety of experimental ulcer models. The mechanism of this property of prostaglandins is still not completely defined. The antisecretory and other protective effects of some prostaglandins may be useful in the treatment of stress ulceration.[22] Misoprostol, a synthetic prostaglandin E_1 methyl analog, was shown recently to reduce the incidence of gastric lesions in a group of kidney transplant patients.[1] However, the number of patients in this preliminary study was very small, and much more work will be required to determine the effectiveness of prostaglandin therapy for stress-induced mucosal lesions.

SURGICAL THERAPY

Persistent or recurring bleeding that does not respond to all nonsurgical measures is an indication for operative intervention. The operative procedures used for the control of bleeding stress ulcers have ranged from total gastrectomy to procedures of much lesser magnitude, such as pyloroplasty and vagotomy, and oversewing the bleeding lesions. The ideal operation would be one that controls bleeding with the lowest possible mortality and recurrent hemorrhage. In general, it can be said that lesser procedures are associated with lower mortality but with higher incidences of rebleeding. There are no prospective clinical trials to substantiate the superiority of one form of therapy over another.[5,23] Many surgeons advocate general distal gastrectomy combined with bilateral truncal vagotomy. Others have had fairly satisfactory results with vagotomy and pyloroplasty combined with oversewing the bleeding erosions as an initial operation for bleeding stress ulcers. Total gastric resection is reserved for those in whom bleeding continues after the initial operation or for those patients with diffuse bleeding lesions.

An alternative approach, that of gastric devascularization, has been advocated by Richardson and Aust.[20] In this procedure, both the right and left gastric arteries and the right and left gastroepiploic arteries are ligated near their respective origins, with the entire gastric blood supply thereafter derived from the short gastric vessels. The rate of rebleeding following gastric devascularization was low, and no instances of gastric necrosis were reported. Mortality remained high, however. The theoretical advantage of this approach is that serious postgastrectomy sequelae are avoided in those patients who survive the underlying insult.

SELECTED REFERENCES

Cheung, L. Y., and Ashley, S. W.: Gastric blood flow and mucosal defense mechanisms. Clin. Invest. Med., 10:201, 1987.
This review examines the role of mucosal blood flow in the pathogenesis of acute gastric ulceration. Several mechanisms by which ischemia may produce ulceration are presented. The leading hypothesis is that ischemia reduces the capacity of the gastric mucosa to neutralize acid entering the tissue. This, in turn, leads to mucosal acidification and ulceration. Alternatively, ischemia may also render the stomach more susceptible to acute ulceration by causing a severe energy deficit in the mucosa.

Driks, M. R., et al.: Nosocomial pneumonia in intubated patients given sucralfate as compared with antacids or histamine type 2 blockers. N. Engl. J. Med., 317:1376, 1987.
This study compared the rate of nosocomial pneumonia in 130 patients of an intensive care unit given mechanical ventilation. The patients were divided into two groups based on prophylactic treatment for stress ulcer. Patients treated with sucralfate had a higher proportion of gastric aspirates with pH ≤ 4 and lower concentrations of gram-negative bacilli compared with patients in the antacid–histamine type 2 blocker (H₂)group. In addition, the rates of pneumonia and mortality appear higher (although not statistically significant) in the antacid-H₂ group compared with the sucralfate group. These results suggest that antacid-H₂ antagonists that elevate gastric pH favor gastric colonization with gram-negative bacteria, and increase the risk of nosocomial pneumonia in patients receiving mechanical ventilation.

Peura, D. A., and Johnson, L. F.: Cimetidine for prevention and treatment of gastroduodenal mucosal lesions in patients in an intensive care unit. Ann. Intern. Med., 103:173, 1985.
The authors evaluated the efficacy of cimetidine in the prevention and treatment of stress-induced gastroduodenal lesions in a randomized, double-blind study. Patients admitted to a medical intensive care unit without clinical evidence of bleeding were evaluated by serial endoscopy. Endoscopy revealed normal or improved gastroduodenal mucosa in 14 of 21 patients treated with cimetidine, as compared with only 5 of 18 patients given a placebo (p < 0.05). Significantly fewer blood transfusions were given to patients with signs of bleeding in the cimetidine-treated group (0.5 ± 0.3 units) compared with the placebo-treated group (4.5 ± 1.5 units; p < 0.05). The authors concluded that cimetidine reduced both bleeding and the need for transfusions by preventing the progression of established gastroduodenal stress lesions.

Shuman, R. B., Schuster, D. P., and Zuckerman, G. R.: Prophylactic therapy for stress ulcer bleeding: A reappraisal. Ann. Intern. Med., 106:562, 1987.
The authors analyzed published data from 16 prospective trials involving 2133 patients. They suggested that antacids were more effective than cimetidine in preventing stress ulcer bleeding according to the criteria of bleeding by occult blood detection. However, there was no significant difference in the effectiveness of antacids or cimetidine in the prevention of overt bleeding. Both treatments were found to be significantly more effective than placebo in reducing overt bleeding.

Silen, W., Merhav, A., and Simon, J. N. L.: The pathophysiology of stress ulcer disease. World J. Surg., 5:156, 1981.
This is an excellent review of the factors involved in the pathogenesis of stress ulceration. The pathophysiologic differences between stress ulcers and other acute gastroduodenal ulcerations (i.e., Cushing's ulcer, Curling's ulcer, drug-induced gastric lesions) are clearly explained. Although mucosal ischemia appears to be the major inciting event in the development of acute stress ulceration, acid and pepsin must be present for overt ulceration to occur. The significance of other factors, including disturbances in acid-base balance, energy deficit in the fundic mucosa, and steroids and prostaglandins, is discussed in relation to the pathogenesis of stress ulceration.

REFERENCES

1. Alijani, M. R., Benjamin, S. B., Collen, M. J., and Foegh, M. L.: Misoprostol: A prostaglandin E₁ analogue versus antacid in the prevention of stress ulcers in kidney transplant patients. Transplant. Proc., 21:2145, 1989.
2. Ashley, S. W., Soybel, D. I., and Cheung, L. Y.: Measurements of intracellular pH in Necturus antral mucosa by microelectrode technique. Am. J. Physiol., 250:G625, 1986.
3. Ashley, S. W., Soybel, D. I., Moore, C. D., and Cheung, L. Y.: Intracellular pH (pHᵢ) in gastric surface epithelium is more susceptible to serosal than mucosal acidification. Surgery, 102:371, 1987.
4. Bresalier, R. S., Grendell, J. H., Cello, J. P., and Meyer, A. A.: Sucralfate suspension versus titrated antacid for the prevention of acute stress-related gastrointestinal hemorrhage in critically ill patients. Am. J. Med., 83:110, 1987.
5. Cheung, L. Y.: Treatment of established stress ulcer disease. World J. Surg., 5:235, 1981.
6. Cheung, L. Y., and Ashley, S. W.: Gastric blood flow and mucosal defense mechanisms. Clin. Invest. Med., 10:201, 1987.
7. Cheung, L. Y., and Porterfield, G.: Protection of gastric mucosa against acute ulceration by intravenous infusion of sodium bicarbonate. Am. J. Surg., 137:106, 1979.
8. Cummins, G. M., Grossman, M. I., and Ivy, A. C.: An experimental study of the acid factor in ulceration of the gastrointestinal tract in dogs. Gastroenterology, 10:714, 1948.
9. Czaja, A. F., McAlhand, J. C., and Pruitt, B. A. Jr.: Acute gastroduodenal disease after thermal injury. N. Engl. J. Med., 291:925, 1974.
10. Driks, M. R., Craven, D. E., Celli, B. R., Manning, M., Burke, R. A., Garvin, G. M., et al: Nosocomial pneumonia in intubated patients given sucralfate as compared with antacids or histamine type 2 blockers. The role of gastric colonization. N. Engl. J. Med., 317:1376, 1987.
11. Fromm, D.: Drug-induced gastric mucosal injury. World J. Surg., 5:199, 1981.
12. Hastings, P. R., Skillman, J. J., Bushnell L. S., and Silen, W.: Antacid titration in the prevention of acute gastrointestinal bleeding: A controlled, randomized trial in 100 critically ill patients. N. Engl. J. Med., 298:1041, 1978.
13. Kivilaakso, E., Fromm, D., and Silen, W.: Effect of the acid secretory state on intramural pH of rabbit gastric mucosa. Gastroenterology, 75:641, 1978.
14. Lucas, C. E.: Prevention and treatment of acute gastric erosion and stress ulcerations. In Fiddian-Green, R. G., and Turcotte, J. G. (Eds.). Gastrointestinal Hemorrhage. New York, Grune & Stratton, 1980, p. 167.
15. Menguy, R.: Role of gastric mucosal energy metabolism in the etiology of stress ulceration. World J. Surg., 5:175, 1981.
16. Miller, T. A.: Protective effects of prostaglandins against gastric mucosal damage: Current knowledge and proposed mechanisms. Am. J. Physiol., 245:G601, 1983.
17. Miller, T. A.: Stress erosive gastritis. In Moody, F. G., Carey, L. C., Jones, R. S., Kelly, K. A., Nahrwold, D. L., and Skinner, D. B. (Eds.): Surgical Treatment of Digestive Disease. Chicago, Year Book Medical Publishers, 1986, pp. 187–202.
18. Peura, D. A., and Johnson, L. F.: Cimetidine for prevention and treatment of gastroduodenal mucosal lesions in patients in an intensive care unit. Ann. Intern. Med., 103:173, 1985.
19. Priebe, H. J., Skillman, J. J., Bushnell, L. S., Long, P. C., and Silen, W.: Antacid versus cimetidine in preventing acute gastrointestinal bleeding: A randomized trial in 75 critically ill patients. N. Engl. J. Med., 302:426, 1980.
20. Richardson, J. D., and Aust, J. B.: Gastric devascularization: A useful salvage procedure for massive hemorrhagic gastritis. Ann. Surg., 185:649, 1977.
21. Ritchie, W. P. Jr.: Acute gastric mucosal damage induced by bile salts, acid, and ischemia. Gastroenterology, 68:699, 1975.
22. Ritchie, W. P. Jr.: Prostaglandins: A surgeon's perspective. Dig. Dis. Sci., 31:32S, 1986.
23. Robert, R., and Kauffman, G. L. Jr.: Stress ulcers. In: Sleisenger, M. H., and Fordtran, J. S. (Eds.): Gastrointestinal Disease, Pathophysiology, Diagnosis, Management, 3rd ed. Philadelphia, W. B. Saunders Company, 1983, p. 612.
24. Shuman, R. B., Schuster, D. P., and Zuckerman G. R.: Prophylactic therapy for stress ulcer bleeding: A reappraisal. Ann. Intern. Med., 106:562, 1987.
25. Silen, W., Merhav, A., and Simson, J. N. L.: The pathophysiology of stress ulcer disease. World J. Surg., 5:165, 1981.
26. Stothert, J. C., Simonowitz, D. A., Dellinger, E. P., et al.: Randomized prospective evaluation of cimetidine and antacid control of gastric pH in the critically ill. Ann. Surg., 192:169, 1980.
27. Torres, A. J., Landa, I., Hernandez, F., Jover, J. M., Suarez, A., Arias, J., et al.: Somatostatin in the treatment of severe upper gastrointestinal bleeding: A multicentre controlled trial. Br. J. Surg., 73:786, 1986.
28. Tryba, M.: Risk of acute stress bleeding and nosocomial pneumonia in ventilated intensive care unit patients: Sucralfate versus antacids. Am. J. Med., 83:117, 1987.
29. Zinner, M. J., Zuidema, G. S., Smith, P. L., et al.: The prevention of upper gastrointestinal tract bleeding in patients in an intensive care unit. Surg. Gynecol. Obstet., 153:214, 1981.

IV

TUMORS OF THE DUODENUM AND SMALL INTESTINE

G. Robert Mason, M.D., Ph.D.

Current statistics of the American Cancer Society indicate that there are some 2700 new cases of cancer of the small intestine each year, with a distribution of 1400 males and 1300 females and some 900 deaths. This compares with cancer in such organs as the pancreas, which shows an estimated 27,000 new cancers with 25,000 deaths; 10,000 esophageal cancers with 9400 deaths; and 20,000 gastric carcinomas with 13,900 deaths. Benign tumors also may be formed in the small intestine and are found in approximately the same frequency as malignant tumors, except that adenocarcinomas of the small intestine are more common in the proximal portion of the small intestine, whereas other malignancies and benign tumors are found with a slight predominance in the distal portion of the small intestine. Adenocarcinomas of the small intestine represent approximately 1 per cent of all digestive organ cancers, including the liver, pancreas, and esophagus.[74]

The presence of various benign tumors appears to be related to the surface area and general bulk of the intestine. The predilection of adenocarcinoma and of villous tumors of the mucous membrane to the duodenum, and, in particular, to the area of the ampulla of Vater, leads one to suspect that some substance may be excreted in bile or in pancreatic juice that acts as a carcinogen. It has been suggested that secondary bile acids, such as lithocholic acid, may be the agents responsible for these tumors. Conversely, the presence of benzopyrene hydroxylase in small bowel mucosa may serve as a protective mechanism.[83] The use of bile adsorbent substances, such as methylcellulose, in high-fiber diets has been suggested as an anticancer regimen in the prevention of carcinoma of the colon; the use of such agents in the prevention of upper gastrointestinal malignancy is more difficult to ascertain. Relatively speaking, however, the incidence of malignancy in the small intestine is remarkably small, considering its surface area of approximately 4500 sq. m. compared with the relatively high incidence of malignancy in the skin, which has approximately 2 sq. m. of body surface area.[45]

Benign Tumors of the Small Intestine (Table 1)

EPITHELIAL LESIONS. These tumors may be adenomatous or hamartomatous polyps or may derive from the argentaffin (Kulchitsky) or argyrophil cells of the mucosa. Adenomatous polyps may form at the ampulla of Vater and cause obstructive symptoms.[32] These polyps are usually benign. Villous adenomas may also be present in the duodenum or small intestine but are malignant in approximately 50 per cent of patients.[11,25,26,57,61,69,72] These rare tumors (1 per cent of duodenal tumors) may be increasing in incidence or possibly are more evident with increasing endoscopic examinations. Although inflammatory changes may make frozen section diagnosis difficult, permanent sections may be helpful. The intestinal mucosa may be ectopically located and form cysts within the intestinal wall or attached to it. Similarly, there may be a complete duplication of the intestine that may or may not be in continuity with the alimentary tract and may present as a tumor. Polyps are most commonly adenomatous and in the adult may have a relationship to malignancy. In children, however, "juvenile

TABLE 1. Benign Lesions of the Small Intestine

Site	Type of Lesion	Number
Mucosa	Adenoma, adenomatous polyp, Peutz-Jeghers polyp	456
Fibrous tissue	Fibroma, myoma, fibromyoma, myofibroma, fibroadenoma, fibromyxoma, myxoma	484
Fat	Lipoma	219
Vascular	Angioma, hemangiopericytoma, lymphangioma	146
Neurogenic	Neurofibroma, neurinoma, ganglioneuroma	90
Other		4
Total		1399

Adapted from River, L., Silverstein, J., and Tope, J. W.: Benign neoplasms of the small intestine: A critical comprehensive review with reports of 20 new cases. Int. Abstr. Surg., *102*:1, 1956. By permission of Surgery, Gynecology, and Obstetrics.

polyps" may occur, most commonly in association with large intestinal manifestations. These polyps do not have a relationship to malignant change. Hamartomatous polyps are composed of all tissues of the intestinal wall and are usually a manifestation of the Peutz-Jeghers syndrome (see later). Hamartomatous polyps of Brunner's glands are found in the first and second portions of the duodenum; they are similar to Peutz-Jeghers polyps but are not associated with oral pigmentation or familial incidence.[4,7] Adenomatous hyperplasia of Brunner's glands (brunneromas) may also be found.[42] The Cronkhite-Canada syndrome is a variant of polypoid growths, characterized by diffuse mucosal polyposis with edematous lamina propria containing dilated cystic glands.[16] The argentaffin cells contain 5-hydroxytryptamine and may form carcinoid tumors. The argyrophil cells are similar to pancreatic islet cells and the medullary cells of the thyroid that produce calcitonin. These amine precursor uptake and decarboxylation (APUD) cells may give rise to tumors that produce hormones such as gastrin, glucagon, and parathormone.

LYMPHATIC LESIONS. Lymphoid tissue tumors may derive from the intestinal wall and appear to be more common distally than proximally. These tumors may be part of a generalized systemic disease but also may be primary in the intestine. The benign form includes polypoid lymphoid hyperplasia and is more commonly found in the distal ileum. This condition may be an inflammatory response and is not related to malignancy. In some patients, there may be an associated hypogammaglobulinemia. Abnormalities of the lymph channels may also exist and produce lymphatic cysts, lymphangiomas or chylangiomas, and lymphangiectasis.[20,22,44,56]

CONNECTIVE TISSUE TUMORS. Connective tissue may also produce benign tumors. As a collective group, these are the most common tumors of the gastrointestinal tract, and the most common of these are leiomyomas (Table 2). However, lipomas, fibromas, fibromyxomas, ganglioneuromas, neurilemomas,

TABLE 2. Tumors of the Small Intestine: Combined Results of
Fifteen Studies*

	Duodenum	Jejunum	Ileum	Total
Malignant				
Adenocarcinoma	131	119	52	302
Lymphoma	7	69	106	182
Leiomyosarcoma	17	32	28	77
Other sarcoma	0	4	9	13
Islet cell carcinoma	1	0	0	1
Other	2	9	11	22
Total	158	233	206	597
Carcinoid	13	21	233	267
Benign				
Leiomyoma	42	110	82	234
Adenoma	53	55	55	163
Lipoma	32	24	54	110
Hemangioma	6	50	27	83
Neurofibroma	4	7	3	14
Lymphangioma	0	3	5	8
Fibroma/ fibromyoma	2	9	10	21
Pancreatic rest	31	4	1 (Meckel's)	36
Brunner's glands	7	0	1	8
Argentaffin	1	1	5	7
Other	5	17	23	45
Total	183	280	266	729
Grand Total				1593

*See references 17,18,23,24,31,33,35,38,54,58,62,71,80,86,88.

and hemangiomas may also be found. A group of tumors of the duodenum have been described as "chromaffin paragangliomas." Symptomatically, they may resemble peptic ulcer disease, but they are commonly pedunculated tumors that may represent a transition between ganglioneuroma and nonchromaffin paraganglioma.[41] Lipid deposits at the ileocecal valve may be in the form of lipoma or may be diffusely localized as ileocecal lipomatosis. Although lipomas may occur throughout the small intestine, they are most common in the ileum.[51,75]

CONGENITAL ABNORMALITIES. Ectopic tissue, particularly from the pancreas, may be found in the wall of the stomach and small bowel or in Meckel's diverticula. This tissue is not active in an endocrine manner, as are the APUD cells. Diverticula may be found throughout the small intestine. They are usually found on the mesenteric surface of the gut and have been related to muscular weakness at the site of vascular penetration; they may be single but are most often multiple. Traction diverticula may also form secondary to adhesions and are usually single. Diverticula may produce symptoms from bleeding, diverticulitis, or the blind loop syndrome.

INTUSSUSCEPTION. Although often no lesion is found in children, benign and malignant tumors may be present at the leading edge or base of the intussusception, and the intussusception may be palpated as a mass. Meckel's diverticula may also present as intussusception. Symptoms customarily include partial or total bowel obstruction with cramping abdominal pain and, particularly in infants, bloody diarrhea.

INFLAMMATORY DISEASES. Various inflammatory diseases may be considered as small intestinal tumors. These include eosinophilic granulomatous polyps and eosinophilic enteritis.[36] The former are usually single and unassociated with systemic manifestations and cause obstruction, intussusception, or both. The latter is more commonly a thickening of a segment of gut associated with systemic blood eosinophilia and may be associated with malabsorption or protein-losing enteropathy.

Again, the presentation is usually acute obstruction. In both instances, the tissue is edematous with eosinophilic infiltration. Amyloid deposits rarely occur in the intestine, either as primary amyloid or secondary to disease such as ulcerative colitis. Pneumatosis cystoides intestinalis, or gas-filled intestinal cysts, may be associated with scleroderma, instrumentation, ischemic colitis, pulmonary disease, or peptic ulcer disease or may have no known cause. Patients may have rectal bleeding, tenesmus, diarrhea, or no symptoms. Peritoneal signs may follow instrumentation or perforation. Barium contrast studies may show striking indentations of the barium column by gas-filled cysts. Mural thickening, partial obstruction, and malabsorption may be presenting symptoms. Crohn's disease *per se* can also cause similar symptoms and will be discussed elsewhere. Carcinomas of the small intestine may be associated with Crohn's disease and are discussed further under malignant tumors of the small intestine. Connective tissue disorders such as scleroderma are known for their association with esophageal thickening and loss of motility; however, such findings may also be present in the small intestine. Rarely, endometriosis may also present with obstructive symptoms or bleeding. Historically, the relationship may be established with menstrual periods. In the recent past, ulcers and strictures of the small intestine were associated with enteric-coated medications such as potassium chloride. Because these products are no longer commercially available, these lesions appear to be less common; however a careful history of medication ingestion should be elicited in all patients.

RADIATION DAMAGE. Radiation damage to the intestine after therapy for malignancy may cause malabsorption, blood loss, and protein loss, as well as scarring and stenosis that may be mistaken for recurrent malignancy.[50]

Malignant Tumors of the Small Intestine

ADENOCARCINOMA. Adenocarcinoma of the small intestine is said to form less than 1 per cent of all intestinal carcinomas but is the most common small intestinal malignancy. In the Mayo Clinic series, 55 cases of small intestinal cancers were found in contrast to 4597 colon carcinomas and 4315 gastric carcinomas.[62] The duodenum was the most common site for primary carcinoma in Rochlin and Longmire's review, with numbers decreasing distally.[66] Within the duodenum, the most common site appears to be the periampullary region, with otherwise even distribution. Villous tumors of the duodenum are similarly most common in or near the ampulla of Vater, with an approximate 50 per cent incidence of malignancy. This malignancy is not necessarily associated with the size of the lesion, as is described in villous adenomas of the colon. Within the area of the ampulla of Vater, carcinomas may arise from the mucosa of the wall of the duodenum or from the pancreatic ducts or the biliary ducts. Dawson and Connolly emphasize than an analysis of mucin production from these tumors provides better indication of the tissue of origin. Sialomucins arise from true ampullary tumors as a characteristic of biliary ductal epithelium and from duodenal surface mucosa. Brunner's glands secrete neutral mucins, and the pancreatic duct produces predominantly sulfated mucins.[21] This study may be useful prognostically because pancreatic neoplasms have a much lower cure rate than others.

As noted, there is also an apparent increase in incidence of adenocarcinoma of the small intestine associated with Crohn's disease. The presence of cancer in patients with Crohn's disease has been estimated to be from 43 to over 100 times greater than in the population at large. The average age at the time of diagnosis is the late 40s, which is somewhat younger than the average age of all patients with adenocarcinoma of the small bowel in the absence of Crohn's disease. These patients with Crohn's disease and small intestinal cancer have had the disease for approximately 16 years. The mortality is expected to be 80 per cent in 2 years contrasted with a 50 per cent 2-year mortality from cancer associated with ulcerative colitis. As is true with ulcerative colitis, these cancers are multicentric in 20 per cent of patients. A recommendation has been made that screening for dysplasia in patients with Crohn's disease may be helpful in their management.[64]

Adenocarcinomas of the small intestine have been reported to develop in ileostomy stomata and in ileal conduits, as a time-related phenomenon or as a manifestation of recurrence of urethral carcinoma.[5,9,53,68,76,79]

SARCOMA. Lymphomas appear to be the most common small intestinal sarcoma (see Table 2). As noted later, these may be primary or part of a more general disease pattern. Dawson and co-workers have suggested four criteria for the diagnosis of primary bowel lymphoma: (1) no generalized, superficial, or mediastinal lymphadenopathy; (2) normal white blood cell total and differential count; (3) at laparotomy or autopsy, the bowel lesion drainage nodes should be the only ones obviously affected; and (4) the liver and spleen should be free of tumor.[20]

The various manifestations of lymphoma, reticulum cell sarcoma, and Hodgkin's disease may all be primary in the intestine. Patterns of association exist with gluten-sensitive enteropathy and idiopathic steatorrhea. A specific pattern also has been reported of duodenal lymphoma in young individuals in the Middle East.[56] Leiomyomas and other fibrous tumors form approximately 20 per cent of the benign tumors of the small intestine. These lesions have a wide variety of histologic characteristics relating to cellularity, nuclear patterns, and so on. In many cases, metastatic lesions may be found, clearly establishing the malignant nature of the tumor.[77] There is not always a clear diagnosis with solitary lesions. Other sarcomas are relatively rare, that is, fibromyxosarcomas, and liposarcomas. Kaposi's sarcoma has been reported as a primary malignancy in the acquired immune deficiency syndrome.[46]

SECONDARY MALIGNANCIES. Rarely, the small intestine may be a site for metastases from the lung, stomach, colon,

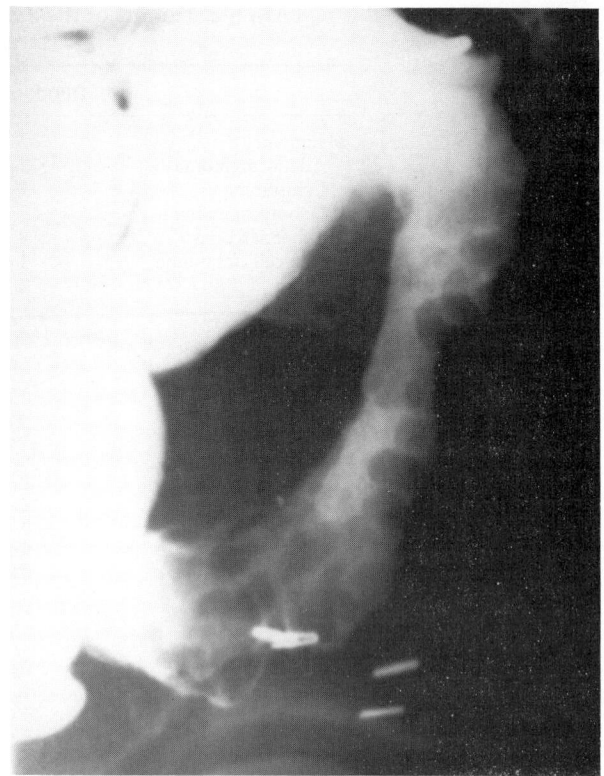

Figure 1. Small intestinal lymphoma showing narrowing of the lumen and edema of the mucosal folds.

adrenal gland, kidney, ovary, uterine corpus, and cervix and from malignant melanoma, plasmacytomas, and leukemia.

CARCINOID AND APUD TUMORS. Carcinoid tumors are most common in the more distal intestine, particularly the appendix, but are found wherever argentaffin cells are located. APUDomas are most common in the stomach and rectum but are also found in the small intestine, most commonly the duodenum. Both of these tumors are well differentiated and slow growing. Criteria of malignancy are invasion of lymph nodes, blood vessels, and nerve sheath or the presence of distant (hepatic) metastasis. Their ill effects are initially primarily endocrine in nature.[87]

RELATIONSHIP TO OTHER NEOPLASTIC GROWTH. Alexander and Altemeir have reported 83 of 112 patients with

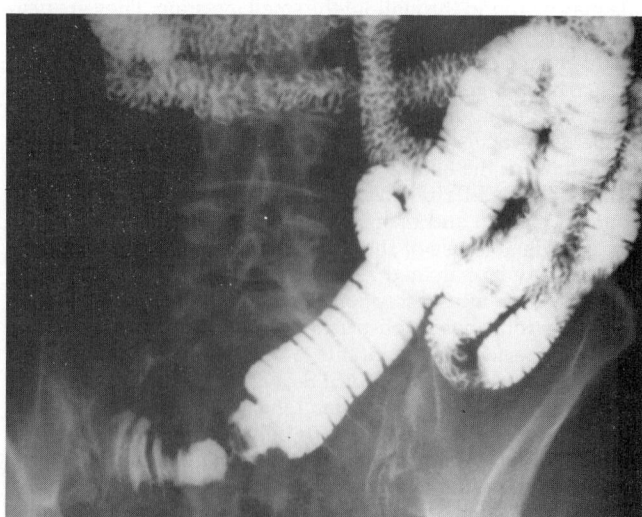

Figure 2. Lymphoma of the small intestine showing narrowing and partial obstruction.

primary neoplasms of the small intestine as having another independent neoplasm at death. Of those with benign intestinal neoplasms, 57 per cent had benign neoplasms elsewhere in the small intestine, and 23 per cent had a second primary malignancy elsewhere.[2]

Syndromes Associated with Small Intestinal Neoplasms

Bessauds-Hillmand-Augier syndrome. Sexual infantilism is associated with intestinal polyposis.[63]

Carter-Horsley-Hughes syndrome. Diffuse polyposis of the small and large intestine was noted in one family.[8]

Cowden disease/multiple hamartoma syndrome. Polyps are present mainly in stomach and colon but are also present in the small intestine.[30]

Cronkhite-Canada syndrome. This is characterized by generalized gastrointestinal polyposis and ectodermal defects, such as alopecia, excessive skin pigmentations, and nail atrophy. In the intestinal polyps, dilated cystic glands are found in an edematous lamina propria. Loss of protein from the gut with calcium, magnesium, and potassium deficiencies may occur.[16,39]

Familial polyposis of the colon. This syndrome is customarily associated with polyps of the colon; however, several cases of generalized polyposis have been recorded with associated malignancy.[67]

Gardner's syndrome. This is generally characterized by rectal and colonic polyposis; however, generalized polyposis has been recorded. These polyps have a relationship to the development of adenocarcinoma. The syndrome also includes cysts of the skin, osteomas, fibrous and fatty tumors of the skin and mesentery, follicular odontomas, and dentigerous cysts and changes in the bony structures of the jaws. This syndrome is familial and is transmitted as an autosomal dominant trait.[27]

Gordon's disease. This is a protein-losing gastroenteropathy, usually manifested as Ménétrier's disease, which involves mucosal hypertrophy, hyperplasia of the superficial epithelium, degeneration in the glandular layer, and hypoproteinemia due to leakage of proteins through the mucous membranes. A diffuse gastrointestinal polyposis associated with protein loss has also been reported.[29]

Juvenile polyposis. This is most commonly found in the colon and rectum; however, isolated examples of generalized gastrointestinal polyposis are reported with and without family history or other congenital abnormalities. The polyps have normal mucosa but have cysts and increased thickness in the lamina propria.[70] No apparent relationship to malignancy is known.

Peutz-Jeghers syndrome. This is characterized by hamartomatous polyps of the gastrointestinal tract (stomach, small bowel, colon), which are associated with mucocutaneous pigmentation (lips, oral mucosa, fingers, forearm, toes, umbilical area). The skin pigmentation may fade after puberty, but that of the mucous membrane is retained.[37,60] Although there is said to be no relation of this syndrome to development of cancer, River and associates reported 10 of 51 cases (19.6 per cent) in which carcinomatous changes were observed in the polyps.[65] The syndrome is probably transmitted as a dominant trait. Peak presentation age in River's series was in the 10- to 29-year-old group.[65] The polyps usually develop later than the pigmentation.

Pseudoxanthoma elasticum. Benign vascular lesions of the intestinal tract have been reported in association with this disease.[49]

Rendu-Osler-Weber disease. This is described as telangiectasia of the nasopharynx or gastrointestinal tract. The disease is characterized by a familial incidence and also by lesions of the palmar surface of the hands and the nail beds.[49]

Torres syndrome. This was described by Muir and co-workers in 1967 and Torres in 1968 to include sebaceous adenomas, epidermoid cysts, fibromas, desmoids, lipomas, fibrosarcomas, and leiomyomas with visceral cancers.[55,81]

Turner's syndrome. Intestinal telangiectasia has been noted in 4 of 55 patients in one series.[34]

von Recklinghausen's disease. Generalized neurofibromatosis with café au lait skin pigmentation may also include neurofibromas of the gastrointestinal tract.[28]

Symptoms and Complications

The numbers and variety of small bowel tumors found at autopsy suggest that many such tumors are asymptomatic. When symptoms do arise, they are usually related to either obstructive phenomena or bleeding. Because the content of the small intestine is largely liquid, the degree of obstruction must be almost complete before symptoms are noted. Epigastric discomfort or cramping pain associated with nausea or with nausea and vomiting slowly increases in severity as the lesion occludes the intestinal lumen. Obstruction is the most common complication (50 per cent) of benign tumors and intussusception is the most common presentation. Bleeding is associated with angiomatous lesions and also with myomas, fibromas, fibromyomas, fibroadenomas, and metastatic tumors. The rate of bleeding may be quite variable, from occult blood loss causing marginal anemia to exsanguinating hemorrhage.

Other complications such as volvulus, necrosis, and peritonitis are less common. Malignant lesions more commonly present with symptoms of pain, anorexia, weight loss, and occult bleeding, whereas benign lesions may bleed more briskly, and the patient may have less anorexia and weight loss. Periampullary duodenal tumors are distinguished by association with painless jaundice, which varies as the tumor undergoes central necrosis and sloughs, with free passage of bile. The presence of a palpable gallbladder further supports the diagnosis of a neoplasm (Courvoisier's law).

Diagnosis

The specific diagnosis of small intestinal neoplasms is possible by direct visualization and biopsy through various fiberoptic endoscopes capable of traversing the entire small bowel from either end. Radiologic contrast studies utilizing various forms of barium are thought to be the best technique for demonstration of lesions in the midrange of the small intestine. Sonography may be useful for large masses, such as leiomyosarcomas.[40] Hypotonic duodenography involves use of drugs such as glucagon, to render the duodenum flaccid and relatively immobile, allowing more accurate delineation of mucosal abnormalities. The radiologic technique of enteroclysis is thought by some to provide better diagnostic results than standard techniques.

The probability is that a routine barium small bowel series is as effective as other radiologic techniques.[73] Lesions bleeding at the time of investigation may be identified by arteriography if blood loss is greater than 1 to 2 ml. per minute. Laparotomy often is the diagnostic technique of choice, particularly for bleeding lesions, and may be combined with intraoperative endoscopy. However, few experiences are more frustrating for the surgeon than the search for a poorly localized bleeding point that ceases to bleed actively with induction of anesthesia.

Management

The majority of small intestinal lesions can be treated successfully by resection and by end-to-end anastomosis of the residual bowel. Villous adenomas have a high incidence of malignancy (50 per cent), but the diagnosis may not be evident on random biopsy or frozen section. Some investigators have recommended local excision, particularly in patients thought at greater risk of death from pancreatoduodenectomy. The degree of differentiation of the tumor is related to the prognosis and bears a strong implication for the recommendation for a procedure; local resections carry less likelihood of cure in undifferentiated tumors. The surgical treatment of duodenal carcinoma is essentially that of carcinoma of the head of the pancreas (Chapter 35).

Results

The results of therapy for carcinoma of the duodenum depend upon the type of tumor, particularly at the ampulla of Vater. Here, duodenal mucosa and the mucosa of the ducts of Wirsung and Santorini and the common bile duct merge in or near the head of the pancreas. Characteristics of pancreatic tumors include perineural invasion, multicentricity, and local nodal metastases. Ampullary and duodenal lesions are more often of a lower grade of malignancy, spread more locally, and do not as frequently invade bile duct perineural lymphatics or local nodes. Small bowel tumors are relatively rare, and malignant tumors are even less common. Therefore, any evaluation of overall success at resection depends upon comparison of small numbers of cases done by various surgeons with varying degrees of skill, as well as on an accurate histologic identification of the tumor source. Because of the liquid content of the small intestine, symptoms are often a late manifestation of adenocarcinoma of the small intestine. The tumor has frequently spread through the wall and into regional lymph nodes and mesentery by the time laparotomy is performed. A 5-year survival rate with *en bloc* resection has been reported by various authors as ranging from 14 to 37 per cent.[3,43,59]

Localized *lymphomas* of the gastrointestinal tract treated by curative resection and 3000 to 4000 rads have shown 5-year survival as high as 85 per cent (11/13).[44] For more advanced disease, combination chemotherapy of doxorubicin, prednisone, cyclophosphamide, and vincristine is said to gain remission in up to 71 per cent of patients.[20,22,52,59]

Leiomyosarcoma and *fibrosarcoma* are said to be the most common lesions in the sarcoma group. Starr and Dockerty report 38 per cent of 26 patients with these lesions, treated by resection, to be well 5 years later.[77] More advanced disease may show some response to a combination of doxorubicin and actinomycin D.[10]

Carcinoid tumors are extremely slow growing, well-differentiated lesions. Some believe that all these lesions are malignant. Macdonald collected 356 gastrointestinal carcinoid tumors and reported an incidence of 31 per cent with nodal metastases and 11 per cent with hepatic metastases at operation.[48] In symptomatic patients, as many as 90 per cent have metastases.[84] Darling and Welch reported a series of 12 patients treated by *en bloc* resection, and of nine operated survivors, eight patients lived 5 or more years.[18] Because of the slow rate of growth of carcinoid tumors, a 5-year span is probably inadequate to predict cures. Carcinoid tumors synthesize 5-hydroxytryptamine (serotonin), as well as kallikrein, bradykinin, and tachykinins.[6,15,48,87] Metastatic carcinoid tumors in the liver may release these and perhaps other substances into the blood to produce episodic symptoms of cutaneous flushing, diarrhea, asthma, and right-sided valvular heart disease ("carcinoid syndrome"). Management of this syndrome may include resection of hepatic masses and oral administration of methysergide and antihistamines. More recently, benefit has been reported with the use of somatostatin analogs.[1,82,85] Strodel and colleagues report a 5-year survival of 35 per cent and 15 per cent at 10 years for patients with hepatic metastases, compared with 72 per cent and 59 per cent, respectively, for patients without hepatic metastases.[78]

SELECTED REFERENCES

Fenoglio-Preiser, C. M., Lantz, P. E., Listrom, M. B., Davis, M., and Rilke, F. O.: Gastrointestinal Pathology. An Atlas and Text. New York, Raven Press, 1989.
A well illustrated text covering a broad variety of clinical entities.

Herlinger, H., and Maglinte, D.: Clinical radiology of the small intestine. Philadelphia, W. B. Saunders, 1989.
Good illustrations of a wide variety of lesions, emphasizing the use of enteroclysis.

River, L., Silverstein, J., and Tope, J. W.: Benign neoplasms of the small intestine: A critical comprehensive review with reports of 20 new cases. Int. Abstr. Surg., 102:1,1956.
This remains the most extensive study available concerning benign small intestinal tumors.

Trimble, I. R., Parsons, J. W., and Sherman, C. P.: A one-stage operation for the cure of carcinomas of the ampulla of Vater and of the head of the pancreas. Surg. Gynecol. Obstet., 73:711, 1941.
The historic development of en bloc resection of the pancreatic head and duodenum is superbly covered in this description of the single-stage "Whipple procedure."

REFERENCES

1. Ahlman, H., and Tisell, L. E.: The use of a long-acting somatostatin analogue in the treatment of advanced endocrine malignancies with gastrointestinal symptoms. Scand. J. Gastroenterol., 22:938, 1987.
2. Alexander, J. W., and Altemeir, W. A.: Association of primary neoplasms of the small intestine with other neoplastic growths. Ann. Surg., 167:958, 1968.
3. Awrich, A. E., Irish, C. E., and Vetto, R. M.: A twenty-five year experience with primary malignant tumors of the small intestine. Surg. Gynecol. Obstet., 151:9, 1980.
4. Bastlein, C., Decking, R., Voeth, C., and Ottenjann, R.: Giant brunneroma of the duodenum. Endoscopy, 20:154, 1988.
5. Baum, R. D.: Re: Adenocarcinoma in an ileal conduit: A late recurrence of urethral adenocarcinoma (letter). J. Urol., 140:382,1988.
6. Bishop, A. E., Hamid, Q. A., Adams, C., Bretherton-Watt, D., Jones, P. M., Denny, P., Stamp, G. W., Hurt, R. L., Grimelius, L., Harmar, A. J., et al.: Expression of tachykinins by ileal and lung carcinoid tumors assessed by combined in situ hybridization, immunocytochemistry, and radioimmunoassay. Cancer, 63:1129, 1989.
7. Boulbourne, I. A., and Busuttil, A.: Brunner's gland hamartoma of the duodenum. J. R. Coll. Surg. Edinb., 32:318,1987.
8. Carter, B. N., Horsley, G. W., Horsley, J. J., and Hughes, R. D.: A new form of diffuse familial polyposis: A probable genetic explanation. Ann. Surg., 167:942, 1968.
9. Carter, D., Choi, H., Otterson, M., and Telford, G. L.: Primary adenocarcinoma of the ileostomy after colectomy for ulcerative colitis. Dig. Dis. Sci., 33:509, 1988.
10. Chang, P., Brenner, C. D., and Wiernik, P. H.: Adriamycin/actinomycin D therapy of advanced sarcomas—increasing response and toxicity. Proc. Am. Soc. Clin. Oncol., 17:422, 1979.
11. Chappuis, C. W., Divincenti, F. C., and Cohn, I., Jr.: Villous tumors of the duodenum. Ann. Surg., 209:593, 1989.
12. Chiotasso, P. J. P., and Fazio, V. W.: Prognostic factors of 28 leiomyosarcomas of the small intestine. Surg. Gynecol. Obstet., 155:197, 1982.
13. Ciccarelli, O., Welch, J. P., and Kent, G. G.: Primary malignant tumors of the small bowel. The Hartford Hospital experience, 1969–1983. Am. J. Surg., 153:350,1987.
14. Cooperman, M., Clausen, K. P., Hecht, C., Lucas, J. G., and Keith, L. M.: Villous adenomas of the duodenum. Gastroenterology, 74:1295, 1978.
15. Creutzfeldt, W., and Stockmann, F.: Carcinoids and carcinoid syndrome. Am. J. Med., 82:4,1987.
16. Cronkhite, L. W., and Canada, W. J.: Generalized gastrointestinal polyposis: An unusual syndrome of polyposis, pigmentation, alopecia, and onychotrophia. N. Engl. J. Med., 252:1011, 1955.
17. Croome, R. D., III, and Newsome, J. F.: Benign and malignant tumors of the small intestine. South. Med. J., 61:271, 1968.
18. Darling, R. C., and Welch, C. E.: Tumors of the small intestine. N. Engl. J. Med., 260:397, 1959.
19. Darman, J. E., Floyd, E., and Cohn, I., Jr.: Malignant neoplasms of the small bowel. Am. J. Surg., 113:131, 1967.
20. Dawson, I. M. P., Coirnes, J., and Morson, B. D.: Primary malignant lymphoid tumors of the intestinal tract. Report of 37 cases with a study of factors influencing prognosis. Br. J. Surg., 49:80, 1961.
21. Dawson, P. J., and Connolly, M. M.: Influence of site of origin and mucin production on survival in ampullary carcinoma. Ann. Surg., 210:173, 1989.
22. Diggs, C. H., and Wiernik, P. H.: The non-Hodgkin lymphomas. In Tice, F. (Ed.): Practice of Medicine. Vol. VI. New York, Harper & Row, 1978.
23. Dundon, C. C.: Primary tumors of the small intestine. Am. J. Roentgenol., 59:492, 1948.
24. Elias, W. S., Lund, C. D., and Yonemoto, R.: Neoplasms of the small intestine. Am. J. Surg., 88:384, 1954.
25. Everett, G. D., Shirazi, S. S., and Mitros, F. A.: Clinical vignette. Villous tumors of the duodenum. Report of two cases. Am. J. Gastroenterol., 75:376, 1981.
26. Galandiuk, S., Hermann, R. E., Jagelman, D. G., Fazio, V. W., and Sivak, M. V.: Villous tumors of the duodenum. Ann. Surg., 207:234, 1988.
27. Gardner, E. J.: Genetic and clinical study of intestinal polyposis. Predisposing factor for carcinoma of colon and rectum. Am. J. Hum. Genet., 3:167, 1951.
28. Ghrist, T. D.: Gastrointestinal involvement in neurofibromatosis. Arch. Intern. Med., 112:357, 1963.
29. Gill, W. J., and Wilken, B. J.: Diffuse gastrointestinal polyposis associated with hypoproteinemia. J. R. Coll. Surg. Edinb., 12:149, 1967.
30. Gold, B. M., Bagla, S., and Zarrabi, M. H.: Radiologic manifestations of Cowden disease. AJR, 135:385, 1980.
31. Good, C. A.: Tumors of the small intestine. Am. J. Roentgenol., 89:685, 1963.

32. Griffen, W. O., Jr., Schaefer, J. W., Schindler, S., Hyde, G., and Bryant, L. R.: Ampullary obstruction by benign duodenal polyps. Arch. Surg., 97:444, 1968.

33. Gupta, S., and Gupta, S.: Primary tumors of the small bowel: A clinicopathological study of 58 cases. J. Surg. Oncol., 20:161, 1982.

34. Haddad, H. M., and Wilkins, L.: Congenital anomalies associated with gonadal aplasia: Review of 55 cases. Pediatrics, 23:885, 1958.

35. Hancock, R. J.: An 11-year review of primary tumors of the small bowel, including the duodenum. Can. Med. Assoc. J., 103:1177, 1970.

36. Higgins, G. A., Lamm, E. W., and Yutzy, C. V.: Eosinophilic gastroenteritis. Arch. Surg., 92:476, 1966.

37. Jegher, H., McKusick, V.A., and Katz, K. H.: Generalized intestinal polyposis and melanin spots of oral mucosa, lips and digits. N. Engl. J. Med., 241:993, 1949.

38. Jenkinson, E. L., Pfisterer, W. H., and Seitz, E. R.: Primary tumors of the small intestine. Radiology, 55:12, 1950.

39. Johnson, M. M., Vosburgh, J. W., Weins, A. T., and Walsh, G. C.: Gastrointestinal polyposis associated with alopecia, pigmentation, and atrophy of the fingernails and toenails. Ann. Intern. Med., 56:935, 1962.

40. Kaftori, J. K., Aharon, M., and Kleinhaus, U.: Sonographic features of gastrointestinal leiomyosarcoma. J. Clin. Ultrasound, 9:11, 1981.

41. Kepes, J. J., and Zacharias, D. L.: Gangliocytic paragangliomas of the duodenum. Cancer, 27:61, 1971.

42. Laarman, G. J., van der Wall, E. E., Muller, J. W., Eggink, H. D., and Hoekstra, J. B.: Extreme adenomatous hyperplasia of Brunner's glands in the proximal jejunum. Netherlands J. Med., 32:20, 1988.

43. Lai, E. C. S., Doty, J. E., Irving, C., and Tompkins, R. K.: Primary adenocarcinoma of the duodenum: Analysis of survival. World J. Surg., 12:695, 1988.

44. Loehr, W. J., Mujahed, Z., Zahn, F. D., Gray, G. F., and Thorbjarnarson, B.:Primary lymphoma of the gastrointestinal tract: A review of 100 cases. Ann. Surg., 170:232, 1969.

45. Lowenfels, B.: Why are small bowel tumors so rare? Lancet, 1:24, 1973.

46. Lustbader, I., and Sherman, A.: Primary gastrointestinal Kaposi's sarcoma in a patient with acquired immune deficiency syndrome. Am. J. Gastroenterol., 82:891, 1987.

47. Macbeth, W. A. A. G., and Gwynne, J. F.: Tumors of the small bowel. Aust. N. Z. J. Surg., 38:206, 1969.

48. Macdonald, R. A.: Study of 356 carcinoids of gastrointestinal tract: Report of four new cases of carcinoid syndrome. Am. J. Med., 21:867, 1956.

49. Manley, K. A., and Skyring, A. P.: Some heritable causes of gastrointestinal disease. Arch. Intern. Med., 107:182, 1961.

50. Mason, G. R., Guernsey, J. M., Hanks, G. E., and Nelson, T. S.: Surgical therapy for radiation enteritis. Oncology, 22:251, 1968.

51. Mayo, C. W., Pagtalunan, R. J. G., and Brown, D. J.: Lipoma of the alimentary tract. Surgery, 53:598, 1963.

52. McKelvey, M. M., Gottlieb, J. A., Wilson, H. E., et al.: Hydroxyldaunomycin (Adriamycin) combination chemotherapy in malignant lymphoma. Cancer, 38:1484, 1976.

53. Meretyk, S., Landau, E. H., Okon, E., Ligumsky, M., and Shapiro, A.: Adenocarcinoma in an ileal conduit: A late recurrence of urethral adenocarcinoma. J. Urol., 138:859, 1987.

54. Miles, R. M., Crawford, D., and Duras, S.: The small bowel tumor problem. Ann. Surg., 189:732, 1979.

55. Muir, E. F., et al.: Multiple primary carcinomata of the colon, duodenum, and larynx associated with keratoacanthosis of the face. Br. J. Surg., 54:191, 1967.

56. Nasr, K., Haghighi, P., Bakhshaden, K., and Haghshenas, M.: Primary lymphoma of the upper small intestine. Gut, 11:673, 1970.

57. Newman, D. H., Doerhoff, C. R., and Bunt, T. J.: Villous adenoma of the duodenum. Am. Surg., 50:26, 1984.

58. Norberg, K., and Emas, S.: Primary tumors of the small intestine. Am. J. Surg., 142:569, 1981.

59. Pagtalunan, R. J. G., Mayo, C. W., and Dockerty, M. B.: Primary malignant tumors of the small intestine. Am. J. Surg., 108:13, 1964.

60. Peutz, J. L. A.: Very remarkable case of familial polyposis of mucous membrane of the intestinal tract and nasal pharynx accompanied by peculiar pigmentation of skin and mucous membrane. Ned. M. Aandschr. Geneeskd., 10:134, 1921.

61. Pollak, E. W., Crow, J., Jacobs, W. H., and Choctaw, W. T.: Villous duodenal adenoma. A less aggressive approach. J. Kansas Med. Soc., 1981, pp. 231–232.

62. Raiford, T. S.: Tumors of small intestine. Arch. Surg., 25:122, 1932.

63. Ravitch, M. M.: Discussion of "A new form of diffuse familial polyposis" by Carter, B. N., Horsley, G. W., Horsley, J. J., and Hughes, R. D. Ann. Surg., 167:942, 1968.

64. Richards, M. E., Rickert, R. R., and Nance, R. C.: Crohn's disease–associated carcinoma: A poorly recognized complication of inflammatory bowel disease. Ann. Surg., 209: 764, 1989.

65. River, L., Silverstein, J., and Tope, J. W.: Benign neoplasms of the small intestine: A critical comprehensive review with reports of 20 new cases. Int. Abstr. Surg., 102:1, 1956.

66. Rochlin, D. B., and Longmire, W. P., Jr.: Primary tumors of the small intestine. Surgery, 50:586, 1961.

67. Ross, J. R. E., and Mara, J. E.: Small bowel polyps and carcinoma in multiple intestinal polyposis. Arch. Surg., 108:736, 1974.

68. Rosvanis, T. K., Rohner, T. J., and Abt, A. B.: Transitional cell carcinoma in an ileal conduit. Cancer, 63:1233, 1989.

69. Ryan, D. P., Schapiro, R. H., and Warshaw, A. L.: Villous tumors of the duodenum. Ann. Surg., 203:301, 1985.

70. Sachatello, C. R., Pickren, J. W., and Grace, J. T., Jr.: Generalized juvenile gastrointestinal polyposis: A hereditary syndrome. Gastroenterology, 58:699, 1970.

71. Schmutzer, K. J., Holleran, W. M., and Regan, J. F.: Tumors of the small bowel. Am. J. Surg., 108:270, 1964.

72. Schulten, M. F., Oyasu, R., and Beal, J. M.: Villous adenoma of the duodenum: A case report and review of the literature. Am. J. Surg., 132:90, 1976.

73. Schwartz S. S.: Book review of "Clinical Radiology of the Small Intestine" by Herlinger, H., and Maglinte, D. Gastroenterology, 97:1347, 1989.

74. Silverberg, E., and Lubera, J. A.: Cancer statistics. Ca, 39:3, 1989.

75. Skaane, P., Eide, T. J., Westgaard, T., and Gauperaa, T.: Lipomatosis and true lipomas of the ileocecal valve. Rontgenstr., 135:663, 1981.

76. Smart, P. J., Sastry, S., and Wells, S.: Primary mucinous adenocarcinoma developing in an ileostomy stoma. Gut, 29:1607, 1988.

77. Starr, G. F., and Dockerty, M. B.: Leiomyomas and leiomyosarcomas of the small intestine. Cancer, 8:101, 1955.

78. Strodel, W. E., Talpos, G., Eckhauser, F., and Thompson, N.: Surgical therapy for small-bowel carinoid tumors. Arch. Surg., 118:39, 1983.

79. Suarez, V., Alexander-Williams, J., O'Connor, H. J., Campos, A., Fuggle, W. J., Thompson, H., Enker, W. E., and Greenstein, A. J.: Carcinoma developing in ileostomies after 25 or more years. Gastroenterology, 95:205, 1988.

80. Thomas, E.: Primary tumors of the small intestine. Aust. N. Z. J. Surg., 37:359, 1968.

81. Torres, D.: Multiple sebaceous tumors. Arch. Dermatol., 98:549, 1968.

82. Vinik, A., and Moattari, A. R.: Use of somatostatin analog in management of carcinoid syndrome. Dig. Dis. Sci., 34:14S, 1989.

83. Wattenberg, L. W.: Studies of polycyclic hydrocarbon hydroxylases of the intestine possibly related to cancer. Cancer, 28:99, 1971.

84. Wiechert, R. F., III, Roth, L. M., Krementz, E. T., et al.: Carcinoid islet cell tumors of the duodenum. Report of 21 cases. Am. J. Surg., 121:195, 1971.

85. Wiedenmann, B., Rath, U., Radsch, R., Becker, F., and Kommerell, B.: Tumor regression of an ileal carcinoid under the treatment with the somatostatin analogue SMS 201-995. Klin. Wochensch., 66:75, 1988.

86. Wig, J. D., Kaushik, S. P., Saleem, M. A., Bhusharmath, S. R., and Talway, B. L.: Primary neoplasms of the small bowel. Ind. J. Cancer, 15:1, 1978.

87. Wilson, J., Cheek, R. C., Sherman, R. T., and Storer, E. H.: Carcinoid tumors. Curr. Probl. Surg., Nov., 1970.

88. Zollinger, R. M., Jr., Sternfeld, W. C., and Schreiber, H.: Primary neoplasms of the small intestine. Am. J. Surg., 151:654, 1986.

V

VASCULAR COMPRESSION OF THE DUODENUM

Bruce Schirmer, M.D.

Historical Aspects

Vascular compression of the duodenum has received varying amounts of attention in medical literature since its initial description by von Rokitansky[43] in 1842. In the late nineteenth century, Kundrat[1,2,31] attributed incomplete duodenal obstruction to compression by the root of the mesentery, and Albrecht[2] described duodenal constriction as arising from mesenteric traction. In the early part of the twentieth century, some reports noted the high frequency of concurrent gastric and duodenal dilatation in patients with the syndrome,[18] whereas others suggested that the duodenal dilatation might be an etiologic factor in gastric disturbances in the postoperative period.[23] In 1907, Bloodgood[12] reported three cases of fatal gastromesenteric ileus and suggested that an operative approach, which involved creating a duodenojejunostomy, might prove helpful in such cases. This operation was first successfully performed 1 year later by Stavely.[45]

Other operative approaches were recommended and, for a brief period, were tried for this condition. These included colon resection[13] and plication[10] to relieve what was perceived as compression of the mesentery from colonic collapse. These operations proved ineffective. In the mid to late 1920s duodenojejunostomy as a surgical treatment for both duodenal obstruction and duodenal stasis was employed relatively frequently in comparison with its application today.[30,31] In 1927, Wilkie[50] reported a series of 64 such operations with a 6 per cent mortality. In the following years indications for the operation were extended to include duodenal stasis from a variety of other causes; operative results were good but less successful.[4,50] Delbert[19] believed some failures were due to a persistence of poor gastric evacuation, and he advocated a gastropyloroduodenojejunostomy.

In 1933, Pool and associates emphasized the consensus that the patient with chronic duodenal stasis could benefit from timely operation under certain circumstances.[40] This report marked the height of the concern regarding this syndrome in the literature of that time. Since the differentiation between duodenal stasis and obstruction was not clearly defined in many of these reports, treatment results were variable, and consequently, surgical treatment of this category of conditions nearly ceased during the next 2 decades. In 1954, Berley and Brown[9] found only seven reported cases from 1944 to that time. Attention to this problem increased during the early 1960s,[29,46] especially because of the comprehensive review by Barner and Sherman.[7] However, with this increased attention, there was also the opinion of some that the syndrome did not truly exist.[16] By the early 1970s there was further interest in the subject and a

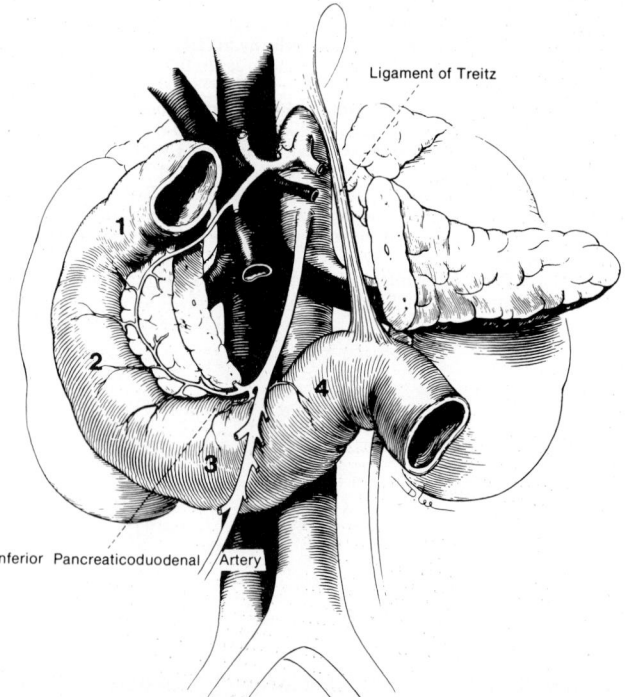

Figure 1. Anatomic structures involved in vascular compression of duodenum. Numerals refer to duodenum's four portions. (From Thompson, N. W., and Stanley, J. C.: Vascular compression of the duodenum and peptic ulcer disease. Arch. Surg., 108:674, 1974. Copyright 1974, American Medical Association.)

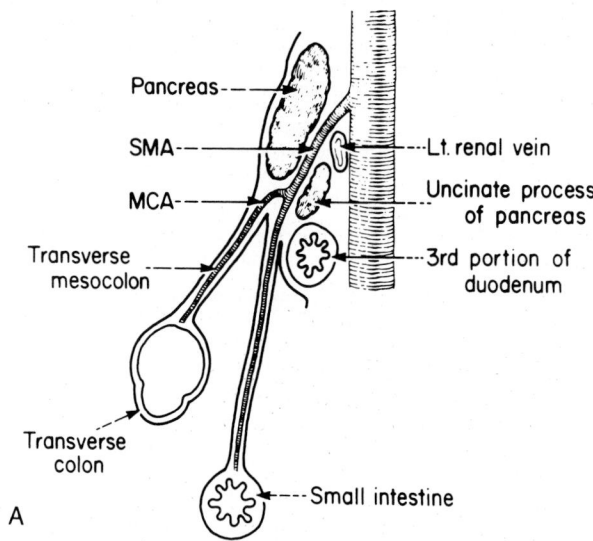

A

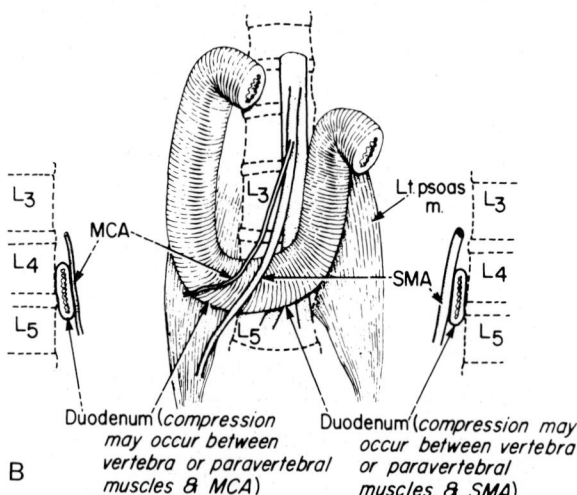

B

Figure 2. *A,* Diagrammatic sagittal section through the neck of the pancreas showing the relation of the third portion of the duodenum to the superior mesenteric artery (SMA), the middle colic artery (MCA), the aorta, and the mesentery. *B,* Anterior view of the duodenum, the superior mesenteric artery (SMA), the middle colic artery (MCA), and the vertebral column. (From Akin, J. T., Jr., Gray, S. W., and Skandalakis, J. E.: Vascular compression of the duodenum: Presentation of ten cases and review of the literature. Surgery, 79:515, 1976.)

growing support for its existence, which were demonstrated by a large number of reports that more clearly defined the anatomic and clinical characteristics of patients with the condition[20,35] as well as by other reports of various clinical settings in which the condition occurred.[8,14,22,26,41,43,48,49]

During the twentieth century this syndrome has been given various names in the literature. *Vascular compression of the duodenum* is the phrase used in our discussion, as it most accurately reflects what is thought to be the true anatomic situation that arises with this collection of symptoms. Another term commonly used to describe this syndrome is *superior mesenteric artery syndrome.*[37] Other names include *Wilkie's syndrome,*[50] *cast syndrome,*[21] *chronic intermittent arteriomesenteric occlusion of the duodenum,*[24] and *arteriomesenteric duodenal obstruction.*[46]

Clinical Presentation

The symptoms that typically are present because of vascular compression of the duodenum arise from obstruction of the third portion of the duodenum as it crosses under the superior mesenteric artery (Fig. 1). These include profound nausea and vomiting, abdominal distention, postprandial epigastric pain,

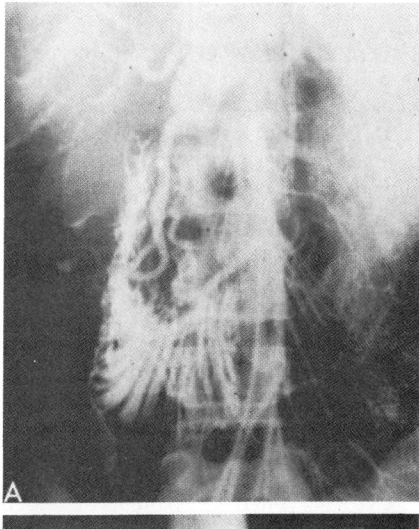

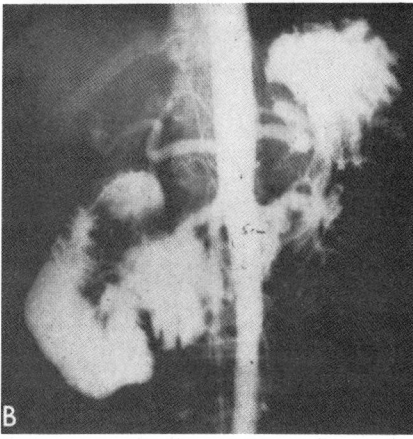

Figure 3. Combined gastrointestinal barium and aortography study revealing the point of compression and abnormal course of the superior mesenteric artery.

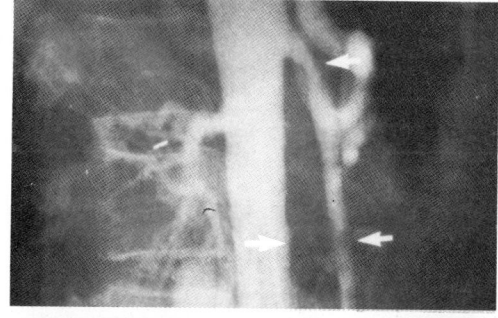

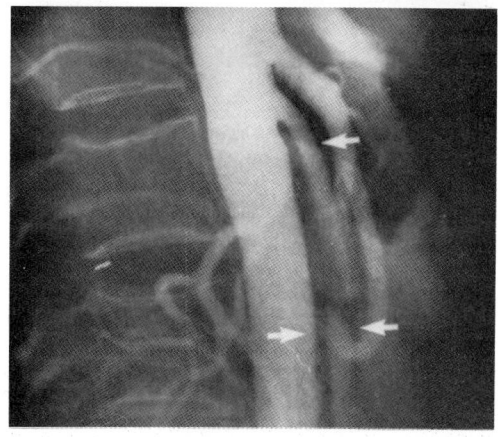

Figure 4. *A*, Abdominal aortography. Lateral projection. Normal case. *B*, Narrowed aortomesenteric angle and decreased aortomesenteric distance. (From Lukes, P. J., Rolny, P., Nilson, A. E., Gamklou, R., Darle, N., and Dotevall, G.: Diagnostic value of hypotonic duodenography in superior mesenteric artery syndrome. Acta Chir. Scand., *144*:39, 1978.)

and weight loss. Acute symptoms are classically relieved when the patient adopts the knee-chest, left lateral, or occasionally prone position. Symptoms have been described as varying from intermittent to constant, depending on the severity of the duodenal obstruction. If nausea and vomiting become protracted, dehydration can follow. Profound dehydration, cachexia, and aspiration as a result of vomiting have all been described as causing death in patients with this problem.

The symptom of weight loss is frequently present prior to the onset of acute gastrointestinal symptoms, and it may in fact precipitate vascular compression of the duodenum. In many case reports where it is noted, weight loss was present in all patients and did in many instances predate the onset of other symptoms. An asthenic body habitus is also frequently described. Most patients with this syndrome are young, and it is slightly more common in females than in males.[1]

Anatomy

The superior mesenteric artery originates behind the neck of the pancreas at the level of the first lumbar vertebra. Its origin is approximately 1.25 centimeters below the celiac axis, and it exits the aorta at an acute angle through which passes the left renal vein and the uncinate process of the pancreas (Fig. 2). The duodenum crosses the lumbar spine from right to left; and there is a distinct ascendancy of the fourth portion of the duodenum relative to the third, which lies more posterior and to the right of the spine (see Fig. 1). It is at this point of passage of the duodenum both upward and over the spine that the bowel is most susceptible to anterior compression leading to obstruction (Fig. 2B). Lumbar lordosis is maximal at approximately the level of

the fourth lumbar vertebra, causing the occasional finding of duodenal compression at this level.

Derrick and Fadhli[20] measured the angle of origin of the superior mesenteric artery from the aorta in 64 specimens and found it to be 41.25 ± 10.65 degrees. Mansberger and associates[35] found the average angle to be only 30 degrees. They also found the average distance from the angle of origin of the vessel to the

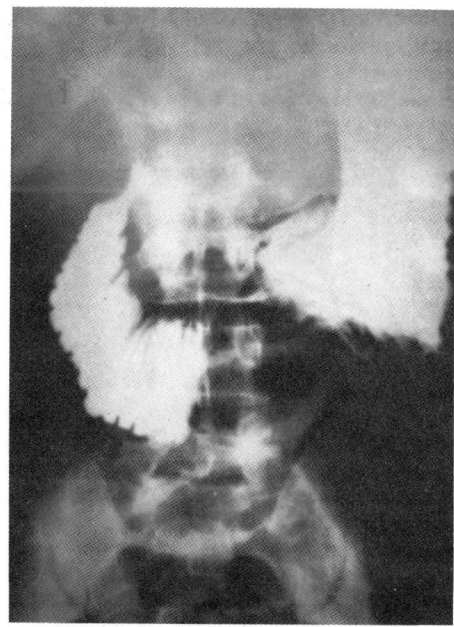

Figure 5. Radiograph from UGI series. Supine position showing complete obstruction of duodenum. (From Reckler, J. M., Bruck, H. M., Munster, A. M., Curreri, P. W., and Pruitt, B. A.: Superior mesenteric artery syndrome as a consequence of burn injury. J. Trauma, *12*:979, 1972. © 1972, Williams & Wilkins.)

TABLE 1. Review of Reported Incidences of Vascular Compression of the Duodenum

Authors*	Number of Cases Reviewed	Number Discovered	Per cent
Goin and Wilk[24]	1,500 (UGI series)	5	0.3300
Goin and Wilk[24]	580 (UGI series)	2	0.4200
Anderson et al.[3]	6,000 (UGI series)	12	0.200
Lee and Mangla[33]	3,108 (chronic care hospital records)	3	0.0965
Lee and Mangla[33]	577,773 (acute care hospital records)	14	0.0024

duodenal midpoint (aortomesenteric distance) to be 10 cm. In studies of *in vivo* subjects by both Mansberger[35] and Hearn[27], measurements were obtained by means of simultaneous barium contrast studies and arteriography to define shortened mesenteric distances and markedly narrowed aortomesenteric angles in patients in whom the syndrome was diagnosed (Fig. 3). Lukes and associates[34] reported an average aortomesenteric angle of only 8 degrees in three patients with vascular compression of the duodenum, compared with 37 degrees in controls, and they reported an average aorta-to-mesentery distance of 3.3 mm. in the three patients versus 18 mm. in controls (Fig. 4 A, B).

Factors that can cause these anatomic differences include weight loss with concomitant loss of fat that is normally located within the aortomesenteric angle, excessive lumbar lordosis, high fixation of the ligament of Treitz, the supine position, and lower origin of the superior mesenteric artery.[35]

Diagnosis

The diagnosis of vascular compression of the duodenum is made radiologically, in association with the appropriate clinical presentation. The most characteristic and reliable diagnostic criteria have been the finding of an abrupt or near-total cessation of flow of barium from the duodenum to the jejunum during an upper gastrointestinal series. Fluoroscopy is necessary to absolutely confirm the diagnosis, since it allows observation of what is usually described as a "to-and-fro peristalsis" of the barium in the proximal duodenum that is associated in most cases with significant disease.[3] This point is usually the distal third portion of the duodenum where the normal anatomic course of the bowel is anterior and travels upward across the spine (Fig. 5). More specific information is obtained if a barium meal can be ingested during an attack of symptoms.[24] A confirmatory finding during fluoroscopy in this setting is the abrupt relief of symptoms correlated with the simultaneous passage of barium past the obstruction point when the patient assumes a position, such as the knee-chest position, which facilitates the relief of the obstruction.

Hypotonic duodenography is most accurate in establishing the diagnosis.[25] It proved accurate, whereas the conventional barium studies were not diagnostic in 3 of 4 patients in one study[34] and in 9 of 11 patients in another.[25] In these patients with duodenal compression there was a significant difference in the aortomesenteric angle and the aortomesenteric distance when compared with those of a matched control group.

The differential diagnosis of symptoms typical for vascular compression of the duodenum includes peptic ulcer disease, biliary lithiasis and its resultant inflammatory conditions, pancreatitis, and duodenitis. Obstruction of the duodenum or proximal jejunum from metastatic or primary tumors or metastatic involvement of the adjacent periaortic lymph nodes represents other considerations.[3] Less common disorders such as visceral neuropathy, collagen vascular diseases such as scleroderma or dermatomyositis, neuromuscular disorders such as vitamin B deficiency, porphyria, or postvagotomy syndrome, or surgical adhesions can also produce symptoms similar to those observed in vascular compression of the duodenum. Traumatic mesen-

teric arteriovenous fistula leading to compression of the duodenum from a false aneurysm has presented as the syndrome.[41]

An association between vascular compression of the duodenum and peptic ulcer disease has been observed. Thompson and Stanley[47] found that 8.4 per cent of the first 281 patients reported with this syndrome had associated peptic ulcer disease, whereas 31.8 per cent of 291 patients described since 1960 had associated peptic ulcer disease. These patients included 44 with duodenal ulcers, 11 with gastric ulcers, and 2 with ulcers in both areas. Peptic ulcer disease was most commonly observed in the chronic form of vascular compression of the duodenum, and the acute form was rare. The reason for this association is unclear. Those patients for whom data are available appear to experience no measured increase in gastric acid secretion. Patients who have both diseases tend not to have the classic asthenic body habitus frequently seen with the syndrome but are typically males of normal body habitus.[47]

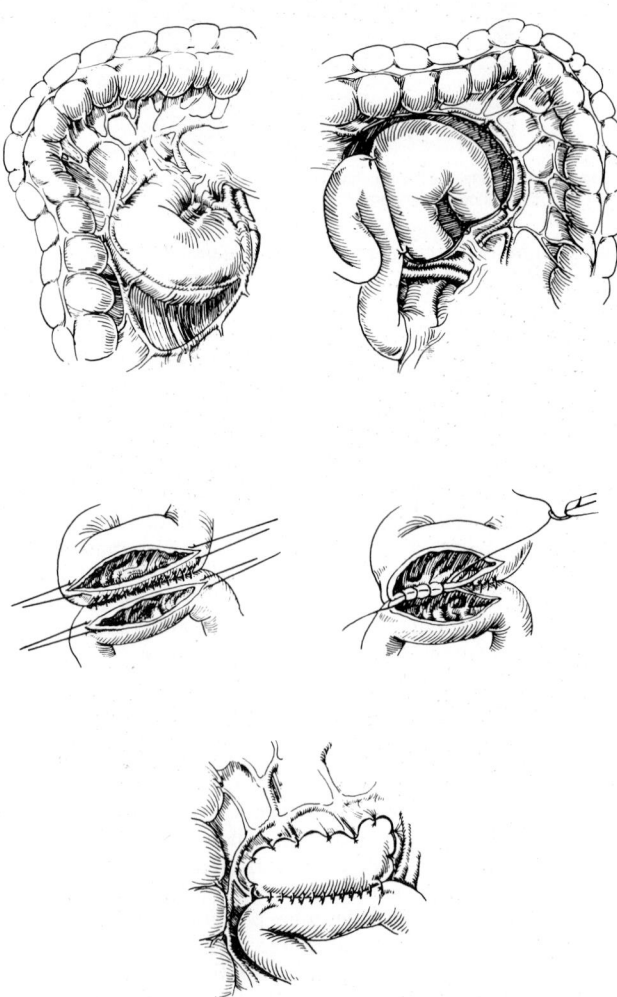

Figure 6. Duodenojejunostomy for vascular compression of the duodenum.

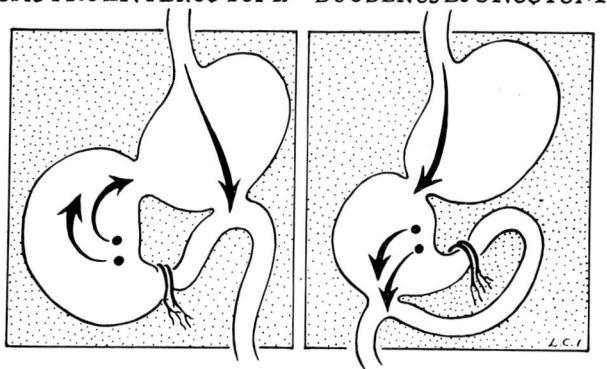

GASTROENTEROSTOMY DUODENOJEJUNOSTOMY

Figure 7. Gastroenterostomy necessitates a regurgitation of bile and pancreatic juice into the stomach, which is eliminated by a duodenojejunostomy. (From Jones, S. A., Carter, R., Smith, L. L., and Joergenson, E. J.: Arteriomesenteric duodenal compression. Am. J. Surg, *100*:262, 1960.)

Incidence

The actual incidence of vascular compression of the duodenum is unknown, but it probably is a rare occurrence in its significantly symptomatic form. The collected incidences of the syndrome as reported by various studies are depicted in Table 1. The majority of these studies involve review of a hospital's experience of upper gastrointestinal series. One report reviewed all hospital records and showed the syndrome to be more common in chronic care hospitals than in acute care hospitals.[33]

Associated Clinical Settings

Associated clinical conditions that are predisposing factors to the precipitation of vascular compression of the duodenum include weight loss, supine immobilization, scoliosis, and the placement of a body cast. Akin and associates[1] found that approximately 25 per cent of patients with vascular compression of the duodenum have one of these etiologic factors, whereas another 25 per cent have weight loss as an aggravating factor, 8 to 10 per cent have possible varied predisposing factors, and 40 per cent have an "idiopathic" form of this condition.

Placement of a body cast with subsequent prolonged nausea and vomiting with gastric and duodenal dilatation was first referred to as the "cast syndrome" by Dorph in 1950.[21] Most cases of the "cast syndrome" have been reported in young patients, many of whom were treated for scoliosis; the number of reported cases is low.[11,21] Windowing of the cast has been shown to be insufficient treatment; but conservative treatment consisting of cast removal, nasogastric decompression, and intravenous fluid replacement is frequently successful.[26] Opera-

tive treatment has been found to be necessary and to be successful.[11,43] A recent report described three cases of cast syndrome successfully treated with total parenteral nutrition.[38]

In 1972, Reckler and associates[41] reported a 1.12 per cent incidence of vascular compression of the duodenum in extensively burned patients treated over a 5-year period. The syndrome occurred exclusively in patients with burns covering more than 30 per cent of their total body surface, and almost all of these patients had experienced significant weight loss (average 25.3 per cent of initial body mass). The syndrome developed in most patients soon after injury; and gastroduodenal ulceration, aspiration, and sepsis were frequent concurrent problems. The authors concluded that nonoperative treatment should be used only in treating the initial onset of the condition, when suitable patient positioning to relieve the obstructive symptoms can be achieved. Otherwise, initial operative treatment produced better survival results.

Two years earlier than Reckler's study Wallace and Howard[48] reported a similar incidence of 0.8 per cent of this syndrome in severely burned patients. These three patients eventually required surgical treatment as well. However, use of the Stryker frame to position patients in the facedown position and successfully relieve the syndrome of duodenal compression was reported by Wayne and associates[49] for four of five bedridden combat casualties in whom this syndrome developed.

Mesenteric compression of the duodenum has been reported in association with anorexia nervosa.[39] It has occurred following total proctocolectomy and J-pouch anal anastomosis,[5,15] where reports implicated the process of pulling the terminal ileum down into the anal canal as possibly placing traction on the mesentery and contributing to duodenal compression. The syndrome has also been reported following resection of an arteriovenous malformation in the cervical cord.[6]

Marchant[36] described the occurrence of the syndrome in 13 pediatric patients observed during the period from 1974 to 1986. Of interest is the fact that 7 of the 13 were within the normal height and weight range for their age group, which indicates that the syndrome need not be preceded by significant weight loss in children. Earlier, Burrington and Wayne[14] reported a large series of pediatric patients with vascular compression of the duodenum but most of these patients had rapid growth or weight loss as part of their clinical pattern. Pediatric patients with this syndrome appear relatively free of the associated peptic ulcer disease observed in adults.

Treatment

Treatment for the syndrome of vascular compression of the duodenum has varied. Generally, conservative measures are initially instituted.[3] Most patients reported in the literature,

TABLE 2. Reported Incidences and Results of Surgical Treatment of Vascular Compression of the Duodenum

Authors*	Type of Operation		
	Duodenojejunostomy*	Lysis of Ligament of Treitz*	Gastrojejunostomy*
Barner and Sherman[7]	161 (95)	6 (?)	31 (71)
Pool et al.[40]	11 (82)		
Marchant et al.[36]		9 (89)	1 (100)
Burrington and Wayne[14]	2 (100)	11 (100)	
Goin and Wilk[24]	2 (100)		
Reckler et al.[41]	5 (80)		2 (100)
Hines et al.[28]	1 (100)		1 (100)
Gustafsson et al.[25]	10 (100)		1 (100)
Jones et al.[29]	12 (100)		5 (40)
Lee & Mangla[33] (own)	8 (87.5)	5 (80)	2 (0)
(reviewed)	50 (92)	24 (87.5)	11 (63.6)
Total	262 (94)	54 (90)	54 (67)

* Data are the number of cases reported and include the percentage of successful operations in parentheses.

TABLE 3. Results of Duodenal Insufflation at Operation

	Amount of Air (cc.)	Preinsufflation Diameter (cm.)	Postinsufflation Diameter (cm.)
Normal patients (n = 10)	230	3.75	4.70
Patients with vascular compression of the duodenum (n = 7)	218	6.7	11.5

Adapted from Jones, A. S., Carter, R., Smith, L. L., and Jorgensen, E. J.: Arteriomesenteric duodenal compression. Am. J. Surg., *100*:262, 1960.

however, have been treated surgically, usually with success. The surgical approach to patients has been generally one of two methods. The first includes detachment of the bowel from the ligament of Treitz, with or without additional derotation and resuspension of segments of the bowel. The other approach, more commonly used in the past, is a diverting bypass, duodenojejunostomy being the most common.

In 1958, Strong[46] was the first to advocate division of the ligament of Treitz with downward displacement of the duodenum as the definitive treatment. The derotation operation, which was developed more recently,[14] involves division not only of the retroperitoneal attachments of the duodenum but also of those of the right colon, followed by placement of the derotated small bowel into the patient's right abdominal gutter. Simultaneously, the colon is placed to the left. This procedure has most commonly been used by pediatric surgeons and probably relates to their experience in treating Ladd's bands in the syndrome of congenital malrotation. The degree of success with this approach in the pediatric patient population has generally been good, reportedly 89 per cent successful.[14,35]

Duodenojejunostomy has been the operative treatment of choice for vascular compression of the duodenum since its early treatment days. The procedure is illustrated in Figure 6. In one early review,[40] the authors dismissed all other operative treatments such as colon plication or gastrojejunostomy as ineffective. The disadvantage of gastroenterostomy is illustrated in Figure 7. The collective major reviews of this subject in the literature and their reported incidence and success of operative treatment are listed in Table 2.

Thompson and Stanley[47] emphasized that patients with peptic ulcer disease and simultaneous vascular compression of the duodenum usually require operative intervention. Intraoperative confirmation of the diagnosis was performed by those authors, as it had been by previous reports,[29] through the use of gastroduodenal insufflation with 150 to 300 ml. of air through a nasogastric tube (Table 3). This maneuver, when followed by duodenal diameter dilatation of greater than 3 to 4 cm, confirms distal duodenal obstruction. The report also emphasized the increased likelihood of marginal ulcer development in patients undergoing duodenojejunostomy after gastric resection or gastrojejunostomy for peptic ulcer disease.

Medical treatment prior to surgical intervention has generally been recommended. Pool and associates[40] emphasized this point, and it has been confirmed in later reviews.[24,29] However, often by the time the diagnosis has been confirmed, patients are in an advanced state of weight loss and deterioration, which leads to a high failure rate of conservative measures.[7] Currently there is only a single report of the use of total parenteral nutrition to treat this syndrome.[38] With this form of nutritional support now widely available, patients whose obstructive symptoms can be relieved with conservative measures are likely to be able to have their weight loss reversed. Also, achieving weight gain is likely to allow more successful conservative treatment of vascular compression of the duodenum in the future.

SELECTED REFERENCES

Akin, J. T., Gray, S. W., and Skandalakis, J. E.: Vascular compression of the duodenum: Presentation of ten cases and review of the literature. Surgery, *79*:515, 1976.

An excellent review of the anatomic considerations important in producing this syndrome, as well as patient demographics and etiologic factors that are involved for patients with this problem.

Anderson, J. R., Earnshaw, P. M., and Fraser, G. M.: Extrinsic compression of the third part of the duodenum. Clin. Radiol., *33*:75, 1982.
An excellent discussion of the diagnostic criteria and the pathognomonic findings in upper gastrointestinal series in patients with this condition.

Burrington, J. D., and Wayne, E. R.: Obstruction of the duodenum by the superior mesenteric artery—does it exist in children? J. Pediatr. Surg., *9*(5):733, 1974.
This article reviews a large series of pediatric patients with the syndrome, with an excellent description of the clinical pattern in children. The authors advocate conservative treatment initially, but this article was the first to propose that if operative intervention is necessary, then division of the ligament of Treitz and duodenal repositioning is the operation of choice.

Gustaffson, L., Falk, A., Lukes, P. J., and Gamklou, R.: Diagnosis and treatment of superior mesenteric artery syndrome. Br. J. Surg., *71*:499, 1984.
A succinct and recent review of the diagnosis and treatment of this condition.

Lee, C. S., and Mangla, J. C.: Superior mesenteric artery compression syndrome. Am J. Gastroenterol., *70*:141, 1978.
This article reviews the incidence of vascular compression of the duodenum as documented in the medical records of several large acute and chronic care facilities. The authors also include an excellent review and comparison of the surgical results in treating this condition as reported in numerous studies.

Mansberger, A. R., Hearn, J. B., Byers, R. M., et al.: Vascular compression of the duodenum. Am. J. Surg., *115*:89, 1968.
This article is the first article to clearly document the anatomic basis for the syndrome with information based on autopsy studies as well as gastrointestinal and arteriographic radiographs in patients.

Marchant, E. A., Alvear, D. T., and Fagelman, K. M.: True clinical entity of vascular compression of the duodenum in adolescence. Surgery, *168*:381, 1989.
An excellent article updating the diagnosis and treatment of this condition in the adolescent population. The authors recommend performance of the derotation operation after division of the ligament of Treitz as the definitive treatment.

Munns, S. W., Morrissy, R. T., Golladay, E. S., and McKenzie, C. N.: Hyperalimentation for superior mesenteric artery (cast) syndrome following correction of spinal deformity. J. Bone Joint Surg., *66A*(8):1175, 1984.
A brief but descriptive article that reviews the cast syndrome and its etiologic factors and diagnosis. The use of total parenteral nutrition to treat this condition is emphasized by these authors.

Jones, A. S., Carter, R., Smith L. L., and Jorgensen, E. J.: Arteriomesenteric duodenal compression. Am. J. Surg., *100*:262, 1960.
This landmark article reviews the clinical experience with this syndrome at that time; it emphasizes the anatomic and diagnostic considerations. The use of intraoperative air insufflation of the duodenum as a diagnostic method is described.

Thompson, N. W., and Stanley, J. C.: Vascular compression of the duodenum and peptic ulcer disease. Arch. Surg., *108*:674, 1974.
This is the only major article that addresses the high association of peptic ulcer disease with vascular compression of the duodenum. The authors review the potential reasons for such an association as well as options for simultaneously treating the conditions.

REFERENCES

1. Akin, J. T., Jr., Gray, S. W., and Skandalakis, J. E.: Vascular compression of the duodenum: Presentation of ten cases and review of the literature. Surgery, *79*:515, 1976.
2. Albrecht, P. A.: Uber arteriomesenterialen Darmverschluss an der Duodenojejunalgrenze, und seine ursachliche Besiehung zur Magenerweiterung. Virchows Arch. Pathol. Anat., *156*:285, 1899.
3. Anderson, J. R., Earnshaw, P. M., and Fraser, G. M.: Extrinsic compression of the third part of the duodenum. Clin. Radiol., *33*:75, 1982.
4. Appelmans, R., Van Goidsenhoven, F., and Boine, J.: Contribution a l'etude des stenoses chroniques du duodenum. Rev. Belge Sci. Med., *2*:1, 1930.
5. Ballantyne, G. H., Graham, S. M., Hammers, L., and Modlin, I. M.: Superior mesenteric artery syndrome following ileal J-pouch anal anastomosis: An iatrogenic cause of early postoperative obstruction. Dis. Colon Rectum, *30*(6):472, 1987.
6. Balmaseda, M. T., Jr., Gordon, C., Cunningham, M. L., and Clairmont, A. C.:

Superior mesenteric artery syndrome after resection of an arteriovenous malformation in the cervical cord. Am. J. Gastroenterol., 82(9):896, 1987.

7. Barner, H. B., and Sherman, C. D.: Vascular compression of the duodenum. Int. Surg., 117:103, 1963.

8. Beck, R. N., and Coulson, D. B.: The body cast syndrome. Radiology, 94:303, 1970.

9. Berley, F. V., and Brown, R. B.: Arteriomesenteric obstruction of the duodenum. U.S. Armed Forces Med. J., 5:1044, 1954.

10. de Beule: Arch. de Mal, d'App. digest et la Nutrit., 21:1103, 1931.

11. Bisla, R.S., and Louis, H. J.: Acute vascular compression of the duodenum following cast application. Surg. Gynecol. Obstet., 140:563, 1975.

12. Bloodgood, J. C.: Acute dilatation of the stomach, gastro-mesenteric ileus. Ann. Surg., 46:736, 1907.

13. Bloodgood, J. C.: Dilatation of the duodenum in relation to surgery of the stomach and colon. J.A.M.A., 59:117, 1912.

14. Burrington, J. D., and Wayne, E. R.: Obstruction of the duodenum by the superior mesenteric artery—does it exist in children? J. Pediatr. Surg., 9(5):733, 1974.

15. Christie, P. M., Schroeder, D., and Hill, G. L.: Persisting superior mesenteric artery syndrome following ileoanal J pouch construction. Br. J. Surg., 75:1036, 1988.

16. Cimmino, C. V.: Arteriomesenteric occlusion of the duodenum: An entity? Radiology, 76:828, 1961.

17. Clairmont, A. C.: Superior mesenteric artery syndrome after resection of an arteriovenous malformation in the cervical cord. Am. J. Gastroenterol., 82(9):896, 1987.

18. Conner, L. A.: Report on acute dilatation of the stomach and its relation to mesenteric obstruction of the duodenum. Trans. Assoc. Am. Physicians, 21:576, 1906.

19. Delbet, P., and deVadder, P.: La gastro-pyloro-duodeno-enterostome. Bull. Acad. Natl. Med. (Paris), 99:274, 1928.

20. Derrick, J. R., and Fadhli, H. A.: Surgical anatomy of the superior mesenteric artery. Ann. Surg., 31(8):545, 1965.

21. Dorph, M. H.: The cast syndrome: Review of the literature and report of a case. New Engl. J. Med., 243:440, 1950.

22. Evarts, C. M., Winter, R. B., and Hall, J. E.: Vascular compression of the duodenum associated with the treatment of scoliosis. J. Bone Joint Surg., 53A(3):431, 1971.

23. Finney, J. M. T.: The relation of the duodenum to gastric disturbances. Bull. Johns Hopkins Hosp., 17:37, 1906.

24. Goin, L. S., and Wilk, S. P.: Intermittent arteriomesenteric occlusion of the duodenum. Radiology, 67:729, 1958.

25. Gustafsson, L., Falk, A., Lukes, P. J., and Gamklou, R.: Diagnosis and treatment of superior mesenteric artery syndrome. Br. J. Surg., 71:499, 1984.

26. Hall, L. W.: The cast syndrome incognito. Am. J. Surg., 127:371, 1974.

27. Hearn, J. B.: Duodenal ileus with special reference to superior mesenteric artery compression. Radiology, 86:305, 1966.

28. Hines, J. R., Gore, R. M., and Ballantyne, G. H.: Superior mesenteric artery syndrome: Diagnostic criteria and therapeutic approaches. Am. J. Surg., 148:630, 1984.

29. Jones, A. S., Carter, R., Smith, L. L., and Jorgensen, E. J.: Arteriomesenteric duodenal compression. Am. J. Surg., 100:262, 1960.

30. Kellog, E. G., and Kellogg, W. A.: Chronic duodenal obstruction with duodenojejunostomy as a method of treatment. Ann. Surg., 73:578, 1921.

31. Kellogg, E. L.: The Duodenum. Hoeber 1933; Radiology, 9:23; 1927.

32. Kundrat: Uber sine siltene Form der inneren Incarceration. Wien. Med. Wochenschr., 41:3512, 1891.

33. Lee, C. S., and Mangla, J. C.: Superior mesenteric artery compression syndrome. Am. J. Gastroenterol., 70:141, 1978.

34. Lukes, P. J., Rolny, P., Nilson, A. E., et al.: Diagnostic value of hypotonic duodenography in superior mesenteric artery syndrome. Acta Chir. Scand., 144:39, 1978.

35. Mansberger, A. R., Hearn, J. B., Byers, R. M., et al.: Vascular compression of the duodenum. Am. J. Surg., 115:89, 1968.

36. Marchant, E. A., Alvear, D. T., and Fagelman, K. M.: True clinical entity of vascular compression of the duodenum in adolescence. Surg. Gynecol. Obstet., 168:381, 1989.

37. McKinnon, D. A., and Spencer, J. R.: Superior mesenteric artery syndrome. Am. J. Surg., 106:552, 1963.

38. Munns, S. W., Morrissy, R. T., Golladay, E. S., and McKenzie, C. N.: Hyperalimentation for superior mesenteric artery (cast) syndrome following correction of spinal deformity. J. Bone Joint Surg., 66A(8):1175, 1984.

39. Pentlow, B. D., and Dent, R. G.: Acute vascular compression of the duodenum in anorexia nervosa. Br. J. Surg., 68:665, 1981.

40. Pool, E. H., Niles, W. L., and Martin, K. A.: Duodenal stasis: duodeno-jejunostomy. Ann. Surg., 98:587, 1933.

41. Reckler, J. M., Bruch, E. M., Munster, A. M., et al.: Superior mesenteric artery syndrome as a consequence of burn injury. J. Trauma, 12(11):979, 1972.

42. Reed, J. K., McGiin, R. F., Gorman, J. F., and Thomford, N. R.: Traumatic mesenteric arteriovenous fistula presenting as the superior mesenteric artery syndrome. Arch. Surg., 121:1209, 1986.

43. Reid, R. L., and Gamon, R. S.: The cast syndrome. Clin. Orthop. Rel. Res., 79:85, 1971.

44. von Rokitansky, C. A.: Handbook der pathologischen anatomic, 1st ed. Wein. Braumuller and Seidel 3:187, 1842.

45. Stavely, A. L.: Acute and chronic gastromesenteric ileus with cure in a chronic case by duodenojejunostomy. Bull. Johns Hopkins Hosp., 19:252, 1908.

46. Strong, E. K.: Mechanics of arteriomesenteric duodenal obstruction and direct surgical attack upon etiology. Ann. Surg., 148:725, 1958.

47. Thompson, N. W., and Stanley, J. C.: Vascular compression of the duodenum and peptic ulcer disease. Arch. Surg., 108:674, 1974.

48. Wallace, R. G., and Howard, W. B.: Acute superior mesenteric artery syndrome in the severely burned patient. Radiology, 94:307, 1970.

49. Wayne, E., Miller, R. E., and Eisenman, B.: Duodenal obstruction by the superior mesenteric artery in bedridden combat casualties. Ann. Surg., 174(3):339, 1971.

50. Wilkie, D. P. D.: Chronic duodenal ileus. Am. J. Med. Sci., 173:643, 1927.

30

CARCINOMA OF THE STOMACH

Aaron S. Fink, M.D., and William P. Longmire, Jr., M.D.

HISTORICAL ASPECTS

Descriptions of gastric cancer specimens probably date to 500 B.C. Cruveilhier,[21] in 1830, attempted to distinguish between benign and malignant gastric ulceration, and in 1856, Bayle[6] published a text describing the symptoms and lesions of gastric malignancy. Despite these early contributions, medicine was largely ignorant of the signs, symptoms, and pathologic anatomy of this disease until techniques of anesthesia and abdominal surgery were improved.

Theodor Billroth, the great nineteenth century Viennese surgeon, reported the first successful gastric resection for malignant disease in 1881.[8] This report, which was one of Billroth's greatest publications, marked the beginning of the "modern" approach to gastric cancer.

The demonstration of the value of gastric analysis by von den Velden in 1879[134] and the development of gastric roentgenography (largely by the German school) around 1910 represented important advances in the diagnosis of gastric cancer. Indeed, roentgenographic visualization of the stomach, as currently refined, has become one of the most useful diagnostic methods currently available. Recent developments have substantially enhanced the accuracy of diagnosing malignant gastric lesions. These include flexible fiberoptic gastroscopy and cytologic studies of gastric washings or endoscopically obtained brushings. The former technique has been adapted to allow photography, biopsy, ultrasound, and laser fulguration of the gastric lining.

As the extent of gastric resection has increased, other methods of gastrointestinal anastomosis have evolved in addition to the Billroth I (end-to-end gastroduodenostomy) and Billroth II (side-to-side gastrojejunostomy) procedures. Of these, the most frequently employed reconstructive procedures after subtotal gastric resection for cancer have been the Hofmeister type of gastrojejunostomy (first performed by von Eiselsberg in 1888[135]), in which the lesser curvature portion of the gastric remnant is closed and only the greater curvature portion anastomosed to the jejunum, and the Polya end-to-side gastrojejunostomy, described in 1911.[103]

Total gastrectomy, first successfully performed by Schlatter in 1897,[113,114] was attended by an almost prohibitive operative mortality until the 1940s, when the introduction of antibiotics and blood replacement, combined with improved anesthetic and surgical techniques, reduced the immediate surgical death rate to about 10 per cent. Two major technical advances of this period included Graham's invaginating esophagojejunostomy,[46] which decreased the risks associated with this treacherous operative step, and Orr's description of the Roux-en-Y esophagojejunostomy,[99] which eliminated reflux esophagitis. During this period, total gastrectomy was proposed as a routine treatment for all resectable cancers of the stomach. After a relatively brief clinical trial, however, the concept was abandoned, since improved survival rates could not be demonstrated and immediate operative mortality and adverse side effects continued to surpass those following subtotal resection. Now, 25 years later, elective or *en principé* total resection is being reconsidered, especially in European and Japanese centers. Recent randomized trials, however, have failed to demonstrate any survival benefit from routine application of total gastrectomy for resectable distal gastric tumors. In North America, total gastrectomy is used infrequently, and extended total gastrectomy is rarely performed.

INCIDENCE

The progressive decrease in the incidence of gastric malignancy throughout the world is one of the most striking features of this neoplasm (Fig. 1). Over the past 50 years, the incidence of gastric carcinoma in the United States has decreased dramatically to about 8 per 100,000.[119] Moreover, as seen in Figure 1, the age-adjusted death rate from stomach cancer has diminished from approximately 30 per 100,000 in 1930 to 6.6 and 3.4 per 100,000 for males and females, respectively.[119] The decline in death rate is independent of sex, race, or age and is believed to be primarily due to the decreasing incidence of the disease, rather than improvements in treatment. It is estimated that there will be 20,000 newly diagnosed cases of gastric cancer in 1990.[119]

In Japan, the mortality from gastric cancer was still increasing in the late 1950s and early 1960s. Currently, although declining, the Japanese mortality from gastric cancer is still second highest in the world (58.8 and 27.5 deaths per 100,000 men and women, respectively).[119] Certainly, the decreasing incidence of gastric cancer in Japan has contributed to the decline in mortality. However, since incidence in Japan now exceeds mortality, and since the percentage change in mortality surpassed that in incidence, it is postulated that the mass screening program has had some impact.[55,66]

Although improvements in nutrition, occupation, and socioeconomic class have been frequently suggested, the reasons for the dramatic decline in the incidence of stomach cancer remain unclear.

ETIOLOGY

The relationships of gastric cancer to a variety of possible etiologic factors have been investigated. These studies have produced several interesting correlations that have identified a series of plausible causal agents. These investigations, however, are limited by their retrospective nature and by the multifactorial pathogeneses of gastric carcinoma. Thus, none of the proposed factors has been conclusively proved to result in the development of gastric cancer. Their association, however, has led to suggestions for further decreasing the incidence of this disease.

ENVIRONMENTAL FACTORS. The incidence of carcinoma varies from country to country as well as regionally within different countries. Migratory studies reveal that the incidence of gastric cancer in the first-generation Japanese (Issei) who migrated to Hawaii was similar to that of the same generation in Japan.[52] In contrast, the second-generation Japanese (Nisei) in Hawaii had a lower incidence than the Issei.[52] In 1980, the

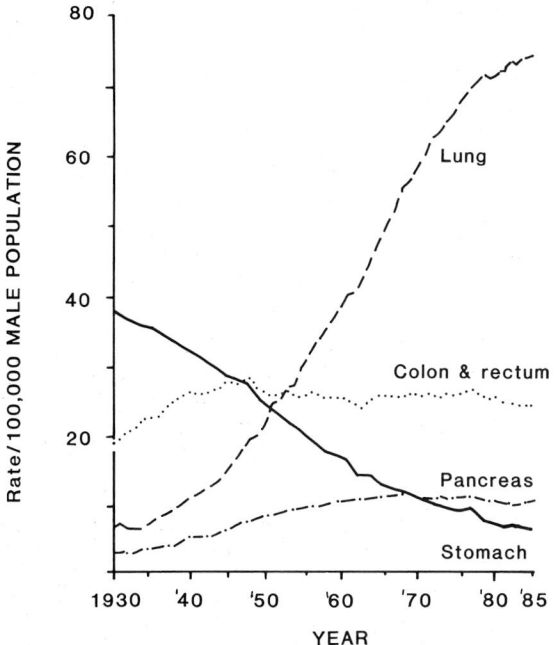

Figure 1. Declining death rate from cancer of the stomach (1930 to 1985) compared with death rates from pulmonary and other gastrointestinal malignancies in the male population. (Redrawn from Silverberg, E.: Cancer statistics, 1989. CA, *39*:3, 1989.)

incidence of gastric cancer in the Hawaiian Japanese approximated that of native Hawaiians. Studies such as these suggest that exposure to environmental agents early in life is a risk factor for developing gastric malignancy. Stocks and Davies[124] proposed a relationship between the amount of zinc and copper in the soil of a particular region and the gastric cancer mortality of that region. More important, however, they also raised the possibility that inhaled or ingested carcinogen(s) might be important etiologic factors.

DIET. Although Hirayama[55] has demonstrated an association between cigarette smoking and gastric carcinoma, much greater attention has been devoted to dietary factors, since the stomach is the first point of prolonged contact with food. In general, gastric cancer appears to be positively correlated with ingestion of starch, pickled vegetables, salted fish, and meat, and negatively correlated with whole milk, fresh vegetables, vitamin C, and refrigeration.[55,62] One of the most consistent observations is an association of increased salt consumption with stomach cancer.[55,62]

Dietary nitrates have also been implicated in the development of gastric cancer; their exact role remains unclear.[35] These agents, which are a common constituent of our diet, can be reduced to nitrites by various enteric bacteria. Nitrite, in turn, can combine with amines and amides, other common dietary compounds, to form nitroso compounds (nitrosamines and nitrosamides); nitrosamides have been shown to be gastric carcinogens in experimental animals.[35] Although nitroso compounds have not been definitely proven to be a cause of gastric cancer in man, a large body of circumstantial evidence supports this hypothesis: some populations at high risk for gastric malignancy ingest large amounts of nitrates.[22,35] Moreover, in hypo- or achlorhydric states, frequently seen in gastric malignancy or premalignant conditions, there is increased intragastric concentration of nitrite-forming bacteria and nitrites.[108,112] Finally, since cold temperatures inhibit the conversion of nitrates to nitrites, the concurrence of the increased refrigeration of food, the decreased use of nitrates as food preservatives, and the progressive fall in the incidence of gastric carcinoma all support an etiologic role for nitrates in the development of gastric malignancy.

RACE AND HEREDITY. In addition to dietary agents, there is evidence to suggest a role for genetic factors. Aird and Bentall, in 1953,[2] observed that blood group A was more frequent in patients with gastric cancer than in controls. In addition, first-degree relatives of individuals with stomach cancer have about a twofold increased risk of subsequently developing the disease.[66] Indeed, in 1958, after analyzing six genetic studies of gastric cancer in humans, Graham and Lilienfeld suggested that cancer of the stomach is more concentrated in certain families.[47] Finally, gastric malignancy has been reported in monozygotic twins.[24]

The increased risk of gastric cancer in certain countries (e.g., Japan, Colombia) as well as in certain ethnic groups (e.g., Hawaiian males and blacks in the United States as compared with Caucasians)[29,52,80] suggests a causal role for racial factors. However, since these groups undoubtedly have similar environmental exposures, it is difficult to distinguish the impact of genetic factors. It is likely that environmental agents are more important as etiologic agents. Their influence, however, may be superimposed on individuals with increased genetic susceptibility.[19]

PRECURSORS OF GASTRIC CANCER

GENERAL RISK FACTORS. Gastric cancer occurs more frequently in males than in females,[29,80,119] the incidence and mortality increasing with age.[29,80,117,119] The incidence is also greater in lower socioeconomic groups,[66] possibly explaining the increased occurrence of the disease in blacks compared with Caucasians.[29,80]

PERNICIOUS ANEMIA. The purported risk of gastric cancer in patients with pernicious anemia was first suggested by Zamcheck and associates in 1955.[140] Based on their autopsy series, they concluded that approximately 10 per cent of these patients develop malignancy. After following a group of 138 patients for an average of 11 years without discovering a single case of gastric cancer, Hoffman[58] questioned the relationship between these two diseases. Regardless of the relationship between these two diseases, it still appears appropriate to screen these patients periodically, since they are also at risk for development of gastric carcinoid.[35]

ADENOMATOUS POLYPS. Although rare, adenomatous gastric polyps may well be the precursor of cancer in a small percentage of gastric tumors. They occur most frequently between the fifth and seventh decades and do not have characteristic symptoms or physical findings; symptoms are more frequent in those with malignant polyps.[86] The diagnosis is usually made on roentgenologic examination, although flexible fiberoptic endoscopy has greatly improved the management of these lesions. The incidence of cancer is increased in polyps larger than 2 cm. in diameter. Huppler and associates[59] reviewed the records of 465 patients with gastric polyps seen at the Mayo Clinic. In approximately 20 per cent of the 300 patients operated upon, the polyp was malignant. Interestingly, 80 per cent of the patients examined were achlorhydric. In 25 per cent of the specimens, zones of adenocarcinoma were discovered at the tip of the polyp without invasion of the stalk, supporting the malignant potential of these lesions. In a more recent review from the Mayo Clinic,[70] the impact of endoscopy is appreciated: only 10 per cent of the 878 patients with gastric polyps underwent operation; the remainder underwent either endoscopic polypectomy or biopsy. In this series, adenocarcinoma was found in 5 per cent of adenomatous polyps; in both cases the polyps were greater than 2 cm. in diameter. Since the possibility of malignancy cannot be completely excluded without removal and pathologic examination of the specimen, endoscopic polypectomy is currently recommended for patients with a single pedunculated polyp less than 2 cm. in diameter and for those who are poor surgical risks. For patients with symptoms (pain or bleeding) or with multiple adenomatous polyps, simple gastrotomy with removal of the polyps and a rim of normal mucosa is recommended. Wedge resection is recommended for patients with sessile polyps larger than 2 cm., as well as for those with carcinoma *in situ*. Finaly, patients with multiple polyposis or a positive family history of polyps associated with carcinoma should undergo subtotal or total gastrectomy. Total gastrectomy is obviously appropriate for patients found to have frank malignancy.

CHRONIC ATROPHIC GASTRITIS. In this condition, normal gastric glands are decreased or absent. Thus, these patients are frequently hypo- or achlorhydric. Several studies[19,20] have suggested that the risk of malignancy is increased when chronic atrophic gastritis coexists with intestinal metaplasia, in which the gastric mucosa is replaced by mucosa closely resembling that of the intestine. The metaplastic mucosa resembles the small intestine in low-risk situations and the large intestine in high-risk situations (elderly, dysplasia, early carcinomatous changes).[19]

The incidence of chronic atrophic gastritis with intestinal metaplasia parallels the increased incidence of gastric cancer in Japan[20] and in high-risk areas of Colombia.[51] In addition, this lesion frequently precedes malignancy in experimental models of gastric carcinoma.[20] Finally, gastric cancer developed in 10 per cent of patients with chronic atrophic gastritis followed for at least 20 years; only 0.6 per cent of patients with normal stomachs or superficial gastritis developed cancer during the same period.[120] The premalignant nature of this entity has been questioned, however, since it is found with increasing frequency in older but normal individuals without stomach cancer.[126] Moreover, it has been found in many patients succumbing to an extragastric malignancy.[50]

PREVIOUS GASTRIC OPERATION. There is considerable evidence that gastric surgery for benign conditions increases the risk of gastric cancer by two- to sixfold.[27,28,41,94,116] Since this increased incidence of malignancy occurred even though the most common site of gastric cancer (antrum) had been resected, the risk may actually be greater. Most cases have occurred after Billroth II anastomosis, 20 years after the original surgical procedure.[94] Burrell and colleagues[14] have recently reviewed the radiologic spectrum of carcinoma of the gastric remnant, suggesting that meticulous technique aided by more careful interpretation might increase the diagnostic yield of barium swallow.

Stump carcinomas were claimed to have an especially poor prognosis.[69,133] This belief has recently been explained by the late presentation of these cases: these lesions tend to present at a more advanced stage in older patients.[69,133] When corrections are made for these patient characteristics, stump cancers are found to have prognoses similar to those of gastric carcinoma arising in the intact stomach.[69,133] These findings support efforts to diagnose stump cancers early. Thus, it has been suggested that radiologic examination and endoscopic assessment with biopsy be done periodically in postgastrectomy patients once they are 15 years beyond their surgical procedure, especially if new symptoms have developed. A recent Danish study,[33] however, questions the degree of cancer risk, as well as the potential benefit of endoscopic screening, for long-term survivors of Billroth II gastrectomy.

HYPERTROPHIC GASTROPATHY (MÉNÉTRIER'S DISEASE). Both the clinical and roentgenologic findings in this condition may closely resemble those of multiple gastric polyps or gastric cancer, and gastric cancer has been reported to occur in such cases.[17] In reviewing the natural history of hypertrophic gastropathy, Scharschmidt[110] suggested that malignant change may be a late complication. He found 120 cases in the literature, which he accepted based on the presence of giant rugal hypertrophic gastropathy. Interestingly, 75 per cent of those tested were hypochlorhydric. Ten cases in which gastric carcinoma and hypertrophic gastropathy are coexistent were excluded

since it was uncertain which entity was primary. Of the remaining cases, 26 had been followed for more than 1 year. Of these, 3 developed carcinoma, suggesting that carcinoma may complicate approximately 10 per cent of cases of Ménétrier's disease.

PATHOLOGY

Gastric adenocarcinoma develops from mucosal cells anywhere within the stomach, although the majority develop in the pyloric and antral regions, particularly along the lesser curvature (Fig. 2). This tumor has been described by a variety of terms depending on various cellular and extracellular characteristics. These features tend to vary not only between different tumors but also within different areas of an individual tumor. Thus, Stout[127] emphasized: "A very small number are exclusively glandular, and another tiny group may consist entirely of undifferentiated cells; but the vast majority show both of these features in different parts of the same tumor. It is this fact which makes the histological classification so hopeless and unrewarding." The majority of pathologists do not accept this view and tend to use one of the several classification schemas described in the following.

The classification proposed by the World Health Organization[98] divides gastric adenocarcinomas into *papillary, tubular, mucinous,* and *signet-ring cell* types, based on the predominant component of the particular tumor. All can be graded as well, moderately, or poorly differentiated. *Papillary* carcinomas are usually polypoid intraluminal masses composed of fingerlike epithelial processes with fibrous cores. *Tubular* neoplasms consist of branching glands embedded in a fibrous stroma; *mucinous* tumors are characterized by large amounts of mucin. Finally, *signet-ring cell* type carcinomas are composed primarily of isolated tumor cells with large amounts of intracellular mucin. In this classification, undifferentiated and unclassified carcinomas are separate groups. According to Day,[25] although there are a fair number of unclassified tumors, this scheme is easy to apply, is reproducible, may aid in the assessment of prognosis, and is a basis for international uniformity.

The Lauren classification, which has been widely used in epidemiologic studies, was introduced in 1965.[73] It crosses the classic descriptions and divides stomach cancers into two main groups, *intestinal* and *diffuse*. The intestinal type tumors have a glandular structure resembling colonic carcinoma with profuse inflammatory cell infiltration and frequent intestinal metaplasia. The intestinal type carcinomas are apparently preceded by a prolonged precancerous process[19] and tend to predominate in regions with high gastric cancer incidence. As regional gastric cancer risk is reduced, the intestinal type tumors represent most of the reduction.[25] Diffuse type tumors are composed of tiny clusters of small, uniform cells. In contrast to intestinal type neoplasms, diffuse type carcinomas are more widely spread

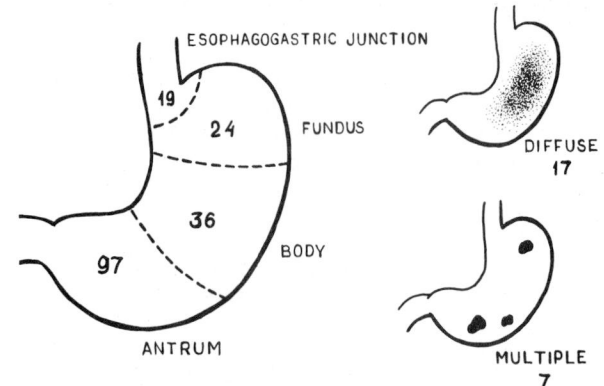

Figure 2. Distribution of the primary site of malignant gastric tumors in 200 surgical specimens studied by Paulino and Roselli.[101] Almost half of the tumors occur in the distal antral region of the stomach.

through the mucosa, have less inflammatory infiltration, and have a poorer prognosis.

Ming's[88] classification separates gastric tumors primarily by their biological behavior as evidenced by their growth patterns, rather than by their architectural structures. Thus, gastric carcinomas are divided into *expanding* type tumors, in which the cells grow by expansion, forming discrete tumor nodules that displace normal structures, and *infiltrative* tumors, in which the cells penetrate individually and widely, eventually causing diffuse involvement of the stomach. Expanding tumors tend to be fungating, whereas the infiltrative tumors tend to be diffuse. Although both types of neoplasms are composed of mucin-producing cells, intestinal metaplasia occurs extensively only in expanding tumors, suggesting that the two types of cancer have a different histogenesis. This scheme is similar to Lauren's, but can be applied to unclassified tumors in Lauren's system.

The histologic appearance and growth patterns of gastric adenocarcinomas may influence prognosis.[25] Thus, for example, tumors with a pronounced lymphocytic and plasma cell infiltrate tend to have a better prognosis.[136] Yet, despite regular recording of the gross and histologic features of stomach cancers, clinicians have become increasingly dissatisfied with the prognostic significance of these descriptive analyses.

Gastric cancers have several methods of extension. These include spread within the gastric wall and into the regional lymphatics as well as direct invasion of adjacent organs, e.g., liver, pancreas, transverse colon, or mesocolon. In addition, hematogenous spread via the portal vein to the liver or via the systemic circulation to the lungs, bones, and elsewhere produces distant metastases. Finally, peritoneal seeding from the involved gastric serosa to the omentum, parietal peritoneum, ovary (Krukenberg's tumor), and other sites, including the pelvic cul-de-sac, also occurs. The last may be palpated as a firm metastatic mass on rectal examination (Blumer's shelf); it is an indication of advanced carcinomatosis.

It is clear that the two major factors influencing survival in resectable tumors are the *extent of spread through the gastric wall* and the presence or absence of *regional lymph node involvement*. In 1970, in hope of providing a more meaningful method of assessing the extent of malignancy, determining prognosis, and aiding selection of treatment, the task force on carcinoma of the stomach of the American Joint Committee for Cancer Staging and End Results Reporting proposed a new staging system,[67] which was revised in 1977.[4] This TNM system emphasized the two prognostic factors; its increased use has facilitated comparing end-results from different sources.

In this staging scheme, the extent of disease is defined in terms of three components (Table 1): The degree of penetration of the primary tumor through the stomach wall is expressed by the letter T; T_1 indicates mucosal and submucosal involvement, T_2 muscularis invasion, and T_3 serosal infiltration. In the revised system, T_4 now implies invasion of contiguous organs. The letter N designates the extent of regional lymph node involvement, from none (subscript 0) to involvement of unremovable intra-abdominal nodes (subscript 3). Distant metastases are described as M_1 if present or M_0 if absent. Finally, in the 1977 revision, the R descriptor was introduced to describe residual tumor: R_0 indicates no residual tumor following surgical therapy, R_1 microscopic residual tumor, and R_2 macroscopic residual tumor. Based on the anatomic extent of disease as determined by all diagnostic methods, findings observed at surgical exploration, and results of pathologic examination of the operative specimens, the tumor is then staged as illustrated in Figure 3. Examination of the survival rates for the various stages under-

TABLE 1. TNM Classification

Primary Tumor (T)

T_1 Tumor limited to mucosa and submucosa regardless of its extent or location

T_2 Tumor involves the mucosa and the submucosa (including the muscularis propria), and extends to or into the serosa, but does not penetrate through the serosa

T_3 Tumor penetrates through the serosa without invading contiguous structures

T_4 Tumor penetrates through the serosa and invades the contiguous structures

Nodal Involvement (N)

N_0 No metastases to regional lymph nodes

N_1 Involvement of perigastric lymph nodes within 3 cm. of the primary tumor along the lesser or greater curvature

N_2 Involvement of the regional lymph nodes, more than 3 cm. from the primary tumor, which are removable at operation, including those located along the left gastric, splenic, celiac, and common hepatic arteries

N_3 Involvement of other intra-abdominal lymph nodes that are not removable at operation, such as the para-aortic, hepatoduodenal, retropancreatic, and mesenteric nodes

Distant Metastasis (M)

M_0 No (known) distant metastasis

M_1 Distant metastasis present

Surgical Results (R)

R_0 No residual tumor

R_1 Microscopic residual tumor

R_2 Macroscopic residual tumor

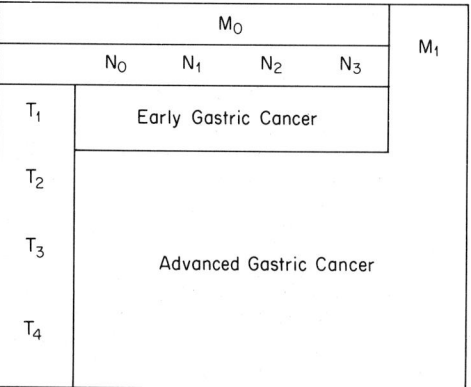

Figure 3. Use of the TNM classification for staging of early and advanced gastric cancer. The vast majority of patients in the United States present with Stage III or IV disease. (Redrawn from Davis, G. R.: Neoplasms of the stomach. *In* Sleisenger, M. H., and Fordtran, J. S. (Eds.): Gastrointestinal Disease. Philadelphia, W. B. Saunders Company, 1983.)

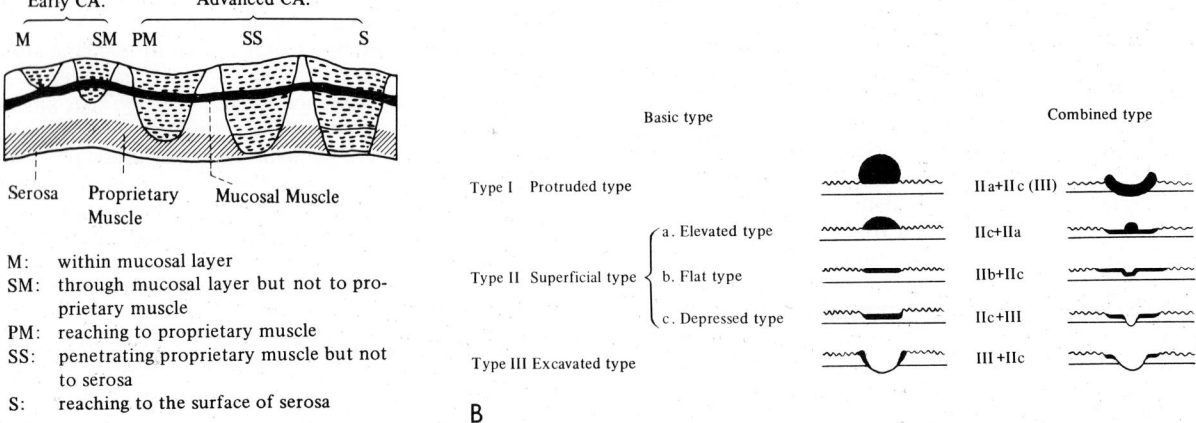

Figure 4. *A,* Schematic drawing of classification of carcinoma of the stomach based on depth of gastric wall penetration. *B,* Further detailed classification of early gastric cancer based on gross and microscopic presentation of the tumor in relation to the surrounding gastric wall. Classification proposed by Japanese Gastroenterological Endoscopic Society. (From Sakita, T., Oguro, Y., Takasu, S., Fukutomi, H., and Miwa, T.: The development of endoscopic diagnosis of early carcinoma of the stomach. Jpn. J. Clin. Oncol., *1:*118, 1971.)

scores the import of extent of mural invasion and regional lymph node involvement: five-year survival is approximately 90 per cent for Stage I, 50 per cent for Stage II, and 10 per cent for Stage III; five-year survival is exceedingly rare for Stage IV disease. Unfortunately, most patients in the United States are Stage III or IV when diagnosed.

EARLY GASTRIC CANCER. With the frequent use of endoscopy in Japan, visualization and recognition of a superficial type of gastric cancer became possible (Figs. 4 and 5). This entity was classified as "early gastric cancer" by the Japanese Gastroenterological Endoscopic Society in 1962[91]; its identification was stressed in hope of decreasing the high Japanese mortality from cancer of the stomach. Although early gastric cancer suggests an early clinical lesion, it is actually defined in pathologic terms (disease involving only the mucosa or submucosa), as illustrated in Figure 4A. Thus, early gastric cancer may be fairly large, may be associated with vague abdominal symptoms, and may have positive lymph nodes (5 to 20 per cent of cases).[48,91]

Early gastric cancer occurs predominantly in the distal stomach. Three types of macroscopic lesions are described (Fig. 4B): *protruded* (Type I), *superficial* (Type II), and *excavated* (Type III); Type II is further divided into three subgroups, of which Type IIc is the most common. Although there have been objections that such a classification offers no special advantage over the TNM classification, and that the TNM system provides greater prognostic significance, the Japanese classification appears to have stimulated recognition of this type of carcinoma by both the endoscopist and the radiologist. For comparison, Figure 3 demonstrates imposition of early gastric cancer into the TNM classification.

Kidokoro[68] reported that the incidence of "early carcinoma" in resectable cases of gastric cancer at the University of Tokyo had increased from 5.7 per cent in 1961 to 34 per cent in 1969. Unfortunately, early gastric cancer represents only 10 to 15 per cent of diagnosed European and North American cases.[31,48] Comparison of early gastric cancer in Japan and Great Britain demonstrated marked similarities, suggesting that the same disease is being described.[31] Five-year survival after resection of early gastric cancer is quite frequent, ranging from approximately 70 to 95 per cent.[32,91,139]

ADVANCED GASTRIC CANCER. If early gastric cancer connotes a potentially curable lesion extending only as far as the submucosa, advanced gastric cancer suggests invasion of the muscularis or beyond. Since these lesions are frequently associated with distant or contiguous spread, they are often not amenable to curative resection.

Grossly, most advanced carcinomas of the stomach may be classified as one of four types proposed by Borrmann in 1926.[12] Listed in order of supposedly increasing degree of malignancy, they are Group I, circumscribed, solitary, polypoid carcinomas without ulceration; Group II, ulcerated carcinomas with wall-like marginal elevation and sharply defined borders; Group III, partially ulcerated carcinomas with marginal elevation and partial diffuse spread; and Group IV, diffuse carcinomas.

DIAGNOSIS

SYMPTOMS. Unfortunately, symptoms are rarely associated with "early" carcinoma of the stomach. When symptoms do occur in early cancer, they are nonspecific.[91] Symptoms are generally not evident until the tumor is advanced and of sufficient size to interfere with either the motor activity of a significant segment of the gastric wall or the normal gastric intraluminal passageway. When these circumstances develop, indigestion, postprandial fullness, eructation, loss of appetite, and heartburn may ensue. Vomiting is a late sign and usually occurs with pronounced dilatation and thickening of the stomach wall. Obstructive symptoms appear earlier with tumors located near the pylorus than with fundic lesions. Weakness may be associated with anorexia and weight loss. Anemia due to chronic blood loss from an ulcerated lesion may also contribute to weakness.

Pain is a common first symptom and has been observed in as many as 96 per cent of patients by the time a diagnosis of gastric carcinoma is made.[72] The type of pain may be similar to that of a benign peptic ulcer and may be relieved by food or antacids. Continuous abdominal pain generally suggests tumor extension beyond the stomach wall. Substernal or precordial pain may be associated with tumors at the cardia. Many patients also note significant weight loss at the time of initial presentation.[72] Infrequently, hematemesis or peritonitis due to free perforation into the peritoneal cavity is the initial manifestation of cancer of the stomach.

The disease may occasionally present with symptoms referable to distant spread. Thus, patients may complain of abdominal swelling from ascites caused by hepatic or peritoneal metastases. Anemia or pleural effusions due to pulmonary metastases may produce dyspnea. Development of a malignant gastrocolic fistula can cause foul-smelling emesis or the finding of recently ingested material in the stool.[84]

Symptoms of fatigue, dyspepsia, weight loss, or anemia in a patient over 40 years of age require diligent examination to exclude gastric cancer. At present, there are no adequate mass screening tests to detect early gastric neoplasms before the onset of such symptoms. Using photofluorography and gastrocamera

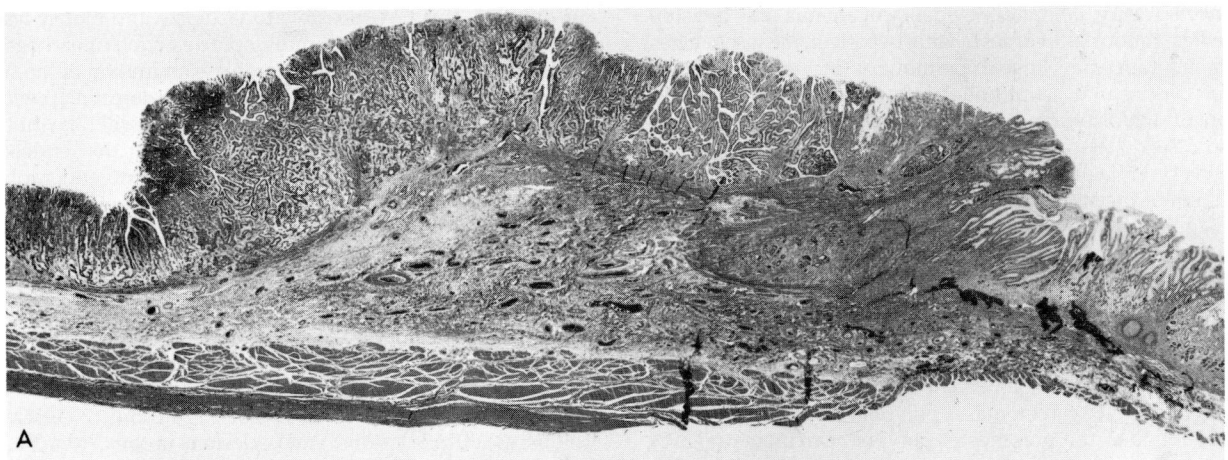

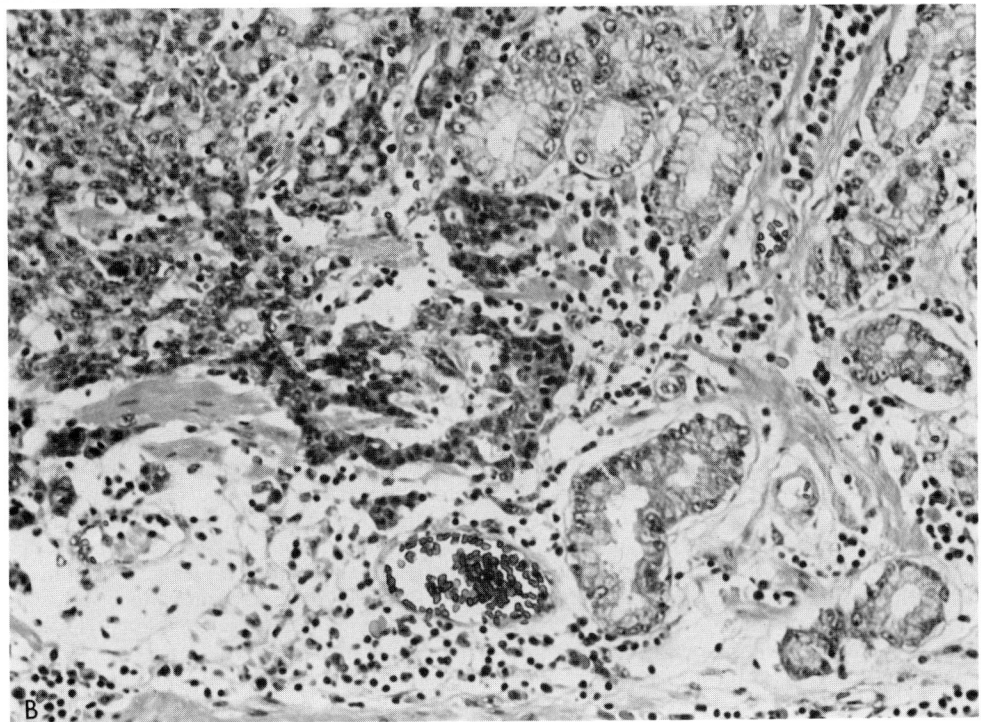

Figure 5. *A*, Photomicrograph of early gastric adenocarcinoma, type IIa (superficial elevated type). *B*, Higher magnification of section from the same lesion, showing the junction of normal and neoplastic mucosa. (Courtesy of Professor Walter F. Coulson, Department of Pathology, UCLA School of Medicine.)

techniques, Japanese mass screening programs diagnosed gastric carcinoma in 0.04 to 0.15 per cent of patients examined; approximately half of these patients had early gastric cancer with excellent 5- and 10-year survivals.[56,65] The increasing percentage of screened individuals in the Japanese population and the decreasing international incidence of gastric carcinoma have contributed to a decrease in the incidence of detection by man screening in Japan.[56] In view of the low incidence of stomach cancer, mass screening would not appear to be cost-effective in the West.[122] It would seem more appropriate to identify and screen high-risk groups, such as those with previous gastrectomy, chronic atrophic gastritis, pernicious anemia, Ménétrier's disease, and adenomatous polyps.

The presence of a low serum pepsinogen I level has been suggested as a specific indicator for intestinal metaplasia,[123] a possible precursor of gastric carcinoma. In another study,[96] serum pepsinogen I was measured in stored sera from 7498 Japanese men living in Hawaii. Fifteen (31 per cent) of the 48 patients subsequently discovered to have gastric cancer had low serum pepsinogen I levels, compared with 6 per cent of age- and sex-matched controls. Markers such as serum pepsinogen I would greatly enhance the ability to identify those at high risk of developing gastric cancer.

PHYSICAL EXAMINATION. There are no specific findings in early cases of gastric cancer. In advanced gastric carcinoma, examination may also be negative or there may be an epigastric mass, hepatomegaly from metastatic disease, or ascites. Although a firm, nontender, movable epigastric mass separate from the liver may suggest cancer of the stomach, the size of the mass alone is not an accurate indicator of operability. Evidence of anemia and weight loss almost certainly appears at some stage in the course of the unattended patient but is rarely present in the early stages of the disease. Signs of distant metastases include Virchow's sentinel node (supraclavicular node, especially on the left), Blumer's shelf, Sister Mary Joseph node (infiltration of the umbilicus), and Krukenberg's tumor.

LABORATORY TESTS. Routine laboratory tests of particular interest are hematocrit, erythrocyte evaluation, liver function tests, and stool examinations for occult blood. These are usually normal in patients with early gastric cancer. In patients with advanced disease, laboratory evidence of anemia may develop, as well as abnormal liver tests with hepatic metastases. Chest roentgenogram may reveal pulmonary or, rarely, osseous spread. Gastric analysis, although infrequently used, allows detection of achlorhydria or hypochlorhydria in the early suspected case.

ROENTGENOGRAPHIC STUDIES. Roentgenographic examination of the stomach after ingestion of barium is often the first diagnostic test obtained in individuals with upper gastrointestinal symptoms. Special compression and double contrast techniques have been added to photofluorography to increase the number of early gastric cancers detected radiographically.[60]

Advanced gastric cancer usually presents as described by Borrmann, i.e., a polypoid mass protruding into the lumen of the stomach, an ulcer crater, or a nondistensible stomach due to diffuse, infiltrating carcinoma. A polypoid mass usually leaves little doubt as to the presence of polypoid carcinoma (Fig. 6). Demonstration of an ulcer crater, however, may present a difficult differential diagnostic problem. As seen radiographically, the characteristic malignant ulcer crater lies in a mass and does not extend outside the boundary of the gastric wall. The mucosal folds do not radiate toward the center of the crater, maintaining their usual contour up to and beyond the ulcer. Malignant ulcers are usually larger than 1 cm. and are surrounded by rigid gastric wall on fluoroscopy. Benign ulcers, usually penetrate beyond the limit of the stomach wall without a surrounding tumor; the rugal folds radiate outward from the center of the crater. Benign ulcers may be of any size.

Several authors have suggested that patients undergo computed axial tomography (CT) scan after identification and verification of a gastric malignancy. This technique has recently been evaluated by Moss and associates.[90] In 22 patients, they demonstrated that the CT scan findings closely correlated with the surgical findings, accurately demonstrating nodal involvement, extragastric extension, and liver metastases. They classified their patients into four categories, based on the CT scan: (1) intraluminal mass without gastric wall thickening, metastases, or tumor extension; (2) gastric wall thickening without extension or metastases; (3) thickening of the gastric wall with direct extension but without metastases; and (4) gastric wall thickening with metastases, with or without direct extension.

GASTROSCOPY. Endoscopy has become an important complementary procedure to the radiologic examination in the diagnosis and management of gastric cancer and other gastrointestinal diseases. It is now possible to visualize and biopsy lesions anywhere in the stomach. Endoscopic detection of early gastric cancers requires thorough and careful examination of the stomach by an endoscopist who is experienced in detecting the subtle changes associated with this lesion and who will take multiple biopsies. Under such conditions, it is evident that endoscopy with biopsy is much more efficient than roentgenography in detecting minute gastric cancers.[97] Endoscopic staining techniques have been developed to facilitate the detection of early gastric malignancy.[128]

Endoscopy with biopsy is currently reported to be over 90 per cent accurate in diagnosing advanced gastric cancer.[7,92] To ensure a high probability of accurate diagnosis, a minimum of eight biopsies has been suggested.[109] Endoscopic as well as radiologic misdiagnosis is most common in four situations: (1) poor local conditions at the site of the lesion; (2) ulcerating lesions; (3) diffuse lesions; and (4) lesions in the cardia.[92] Combining endoscopic biopsy with cytologic specimens obtained by brushing, lavage, or directly irrigating the lesion and collecting the aspirate improves the accuracy of endoscopic diagnosis.[5,7,45,53]

Recently, endoscopic ultrasonography has been developed, allowing direct imaging of the target lesion via the gastrointestinal lumen.[131] This new modality stages gastric tumors quite accurately because of its ability to visualize the degree of tumor infiltration as well as regional lymph node status.[131] Its accuracy may even exceed that of CT scanning.[141]

OTHER DIAGNOSTIC MODALITIES. As mentioned, hypo- or achlorhydria is frequently associated with premalignant and malignant lesions of the stomach. Thus, gastric secretory studies may be of diagnostic value. Other diagnostic modalities that have been proposed include measurement of carcinoembryonic antigen[37,95,130] and fetal sulfoglycoprotein antigens[54] in gastric juice.

PREOPERATIVE STAGING. Determination of the extent of disease may assist in making decisions regarding therapeutic intervention. Any suspicious lesions (lymph nodes or skin nodules) detected on physical examination should be biopsied prior to laparotomy. Liver biopsy should be considered for patients with suspicious CT or liver scans. Moss and associates[90] suggest that the CT scan can be used to avoid unnecessary surgical intervention in appropriate patients. The advisability of deferring surgical therapy based on the CT scan depends on the patient's symptoms as well as the physician's philosophy. This approach is of questionable value if it is believed that most patients should be explored in hope of effecting a cure or at least preventing or treating complications (obstruction, bleeding, or perforation). This attitude was emphasized by McFee and Aust[85] in challenging Moss and associates'[90] conclusion.

TREATMENT

In early gastric cancer, surgical therapy is usually curative. Thus, several Japanese series have reported 5-year survival rates of 95 per cent in patients with malignancy confined to the mucosa.[91,93,139] Although elective total gastrectomy has been proposed for this lesion,[102] most would agree that appropriate subtotal resection combined with adequate lymph node dissection (15 to 20 per cent positive lymph nodes) is the therapy of choice for early gastric cancer. Endoscopic modalities (e.g., laser, ethanol injection) have been proposed for early gastric malignancies found in patients who are not operative candidates.[62]

Unfortunately, the vast majority of patients seen in the West present with advanced gastric cancer. In over 50 per cent of patients, the tumor is no longer localized when first identified, and gastric resection is only moderately beneficial in most of these cases. However, as was true in Billroth's time, surgical resection of the involved portion of the stomach is the only

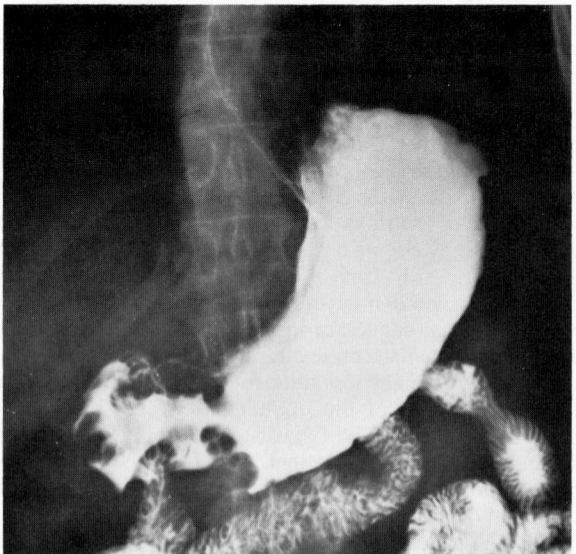

Figure 6. Barium upper gastrointestinal examination revealing classic example of distal polypoid gastric carcinoma. (Courtesy of Drs. Barbara Kadel and Marvin Weiner, Department of Radiology, UCLA School of Medicine.)

method currently capable of curing gastric malignancy. Thus, "denying a patient with gastric cancer the possible benefits of exploratory laparotomy is a great responsibility."[104]

The patient with cancer of the stomach should first be evaluated for profound weight loss or serious cardiovascular, pulmonary, or renal disorders. Although it is unusual that these contraindicate surgical therapy, their identification may reveal the need for special preoperative preparation.

Histologic confirmation of distant spread is currently the most frequent finding that renders surgical intervention inadvisable. Demonstration of metastatic involvement in a Virchow's node, in inguinal lymph nodes, on liver biopsy, in the umbilicus, or in Blumer's shelf indicates that the lesion is incurable. Only definitive, objective evidence of metastatic disease, however, should be accepted as a contraindication to surgical therapy. Thus, if there is any doubt about the presence of distant spread, the patient should be explored.

Exploration should also be recommended if there is an opportunity for palliation, even in the presence of local extension or distant spread. Palliative resection may significantly improve the quality of life remaining for a patient suffering from obstruction or hemorrhage.[30,105] If resection of an obstructing lesion is not possible, gastrojejunostomy can be performed, although results are better following palliative resection.[30,105] In patients with metastatic, obstructing proximal gastric tumors, satisfactory palliation is less frequently achieved. Prosthetic endoesophageal tubes[132] or endoscopic laser therapy[34] may be used in these unfortunate situations. Total gastrectomy, however, should not be performed as a palliative procedure.[78,115]

If laparotomy is selected, it is essential that the initial exploration be thorough, carefully examining and biopsying any suspicious areas in the pelvis, the lower abdomen, the retroperitoneum, and the right upper quadrant, in addition to evaluating fixation and local extension of the primary tumor. If the lesion appears to be confined to the stomach except for possible regional lymphatic spread, a curative resection should be undertaken.

The type and extent of gastric resection must be appropriate for the individual patient and are influenced largely by the location and extent of the gross primary tumor and detectable lymph nodes (Figs. 2 and 7). Zinninger's[142] studies suggested that tumor cells extended proximally in the gastric wall 6 cm. from the primary tumor, mainly within the submucosal lymphatics in the upper stomach and esophagus. Spread toward the

duodenum usually occurred by way of serosal lymphatics and by direct muscular infiltration; the farthest duodenal extension was 3 cm. beyond the pylorus. These observations have been confirmed in a more recent study.[13] In general, then, it would appear that the "standard" resection for the usual distal gastric cancer should include the greater and lesser omenta, division of the duodenum 2 to 3 cm. distal to the pylorus (but with an adequate cuff for a secure closure), ligation of the left gastric artery at the celiac axis, and division of the lesser curvature adjacent to the esophagogastric junction. Division of the greater curvature at the level of the vasa brevia just distal to the spleen completes the resection (Fig. 8). Within such limits, a maximal resection of gastric wall and primary lymphatic drainage areas is performed without making the duodenal stump closure or gastrointestinal anastomosis unduly difficult and thereby potentially hazardous. Minimal trauma occurs to adjacent organs, and widespread secondary lymphatics are not disrupted.[57] More extensive subtotal resection may require removal of the spleen. When the blood supply from the left gastric and splenic arteries is interrupted, the chief blood supply to the gastric remnant is abolished, and the remaining blood supply is precarious. Alimentary continuity following subtotal resection is restored by a gastroduodenostomy (Billroth I) if the ends of the stomach and duodenum can be approximated without tension, or by gastrojejunostomy either anterior or posterior to the transverse colon. In hope of minimizing the risk of obstruction due to tumor recurrence in the gastric bed, many prefer antecolic gastrojejunostomy.

During the late 1940s and early 1950s, several clinics routinely performed total gastrectomy for treatment of gastric cancer. Despite a marked improvement in operative mortality over previous years, the procedure continued to cause more frequent mortality and morbidity than subtotal resection, without improving survival rates.[43,78] Today, total gastrectomy is indicated if it allows removal of all identifiable disease when a large, fungating, or diffusely spreading tumor cannot be removed by subtotal resection. Other indications for total gastrectomy include carcinoma in a gastric remnant following a previous subtotal resection, cancer in a patient with a diffuse mucosal lesion with malignant potential (chronic atrophic gastritis, Ménétrier's disease, pernicious anemia), malignancy in a patient with a strong family history of gastric cancer, and, rarely, cancer developing within diffuse gastric polyposis.[78]

Resectable proximal gastric cancers often pose a difficult therapeutic dilemma. Although Paulino and Roselli[101] recommended an extensive nine-tenths subtotal gastric resection with

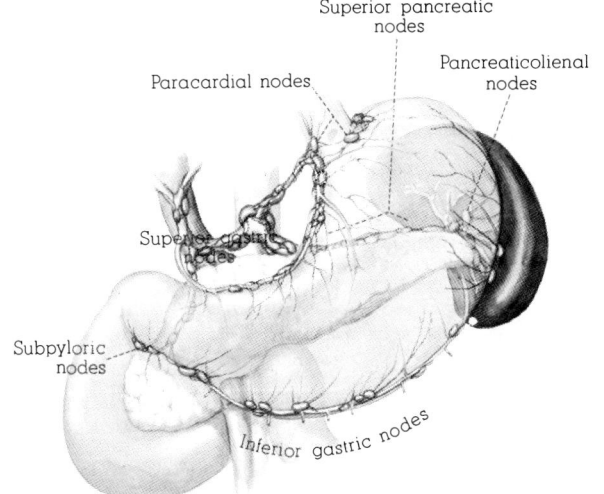

Figure 7. Primary regional lymphatic drainage of the stomach. The frequency of positive lymph nodes depends on the location and depth of invasion of the primary tumor. (From Everson, T. C.: Carcinoma of the stomach. In Everson, T. C., and Cole, W. H. (Eds.): Cancer of the Digestive Tract, Clinical Management. New York, Appleton-Century-Crofts, 1969.)

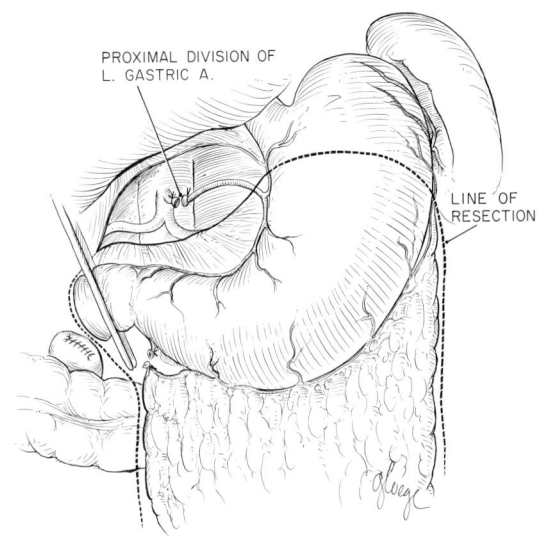

Figure 8. "Standard" subtotal gastric resection for cancer of the distal stomach.

en bloc distal pancreatectomy and splenectomy for carcinoma of the gastric body, the postoperative sequelae of such extensive resections are identical to those of total gastrectomy.[78] Moreover, the potential technical advantage offered by preserving a small gastric remnant is outweighed by the limitations it imposes. The precarious blood supply of the gastric remnant militates against vagotomy (which facilitates the anastomoses) and periesophageal lymph node dissection. Thus, total gastrectomy would also appear to be indicated for cancers of the gastric body.

According to Paulino and Roselli,[101] adenocarcinomas arising in the cardia and esophagogastric junction are best treated by an extensive nine-tenths proximal gastrectomy with distal esophagectomy and interposition of a jejunal segment between the esophagus and the small antral remnant. However, most authors prefer total gastrectomy for resectable tumors in these locations.[78,100,118,125] Regardless of which procedure is chosen, it has been emphasized that any excision of a cancer of the cardia and esophagogastric junction requires a radical operation, most frequently through a thoracoabdominal approach.[3,78] In addition, it is imperative to obtain frozen section control of the proximal and distal resection margins prior to restoring gastrointestinal continuity.[78] These tumors have the poorest prognosis.[87,137]

A recent international review of 15 reports indicated that total gastrectomy was performed in approximately 25 per cent of resections (6.5 to 48.8 per cent).[77] After 20 years of being relegated to a fairly limited role, elective total resection is again being considered. McNeer and associates,[87] Lortat-Jacob and co-workers,[79] and Shiu and colleagues[118] presented data suggesting improved survival following elective total gastrectomy. However, total gastrectomy in each of these small series was frequently associated with an increased operative mortality. Moreover, others[28,43] have not appreciated the improvement in survival rates.

Pichlmayr and Meyer[102] recently reported 299 total resections for both advanced and early gastric cancer. These were performed with an operative mortality of 11 per cent (8 per cent in the last 3 years of the study period). The nutritional status and quality of life were quite acceptable in those patients without recurrent tumor, verifying that total resection is very well tolerated, providing one utilizes reconstructive techniques that avoid bile reflux (Roux-en-Y esophagojejunostomy, jejunal interposition).[71] These authors reported a 41 per cent 5-year survival rate in "curative" elective total gastrectomy. Survival following total resection was no greater than following subtotal resection, although the latter group had a greater number of early, well-differentiated tumors. The authors believe that their data justify continued use of *elective total* gastrectomy for gastric cancer; they admit it does not prove that it will improve survival.

This issue has recently been addressed in a study by Gouzi and associates.[49] They report results of the first randomized prospective trial comparing elective subtotal with total gastrectomy for distal gastric cancers. In this multicenter trial, 169 patients were randomly assigned to either total or subtotal gastrectomy. With the exception of the extent of stomach removed, both groups underwent equally radical resections. On analysis, the two well-matched groups had similar morbidity (33 per cent versus 34 per cent) and mortality (1.3 per cent versus 3.2 per cent). Moreover, there was no difference in 5-year survival between groups (48 per cent), either overall or when patients were matched for nodal and serosal involvement. This critical study indicates that elective total gastrectomy can be performed today without increased postoperative morbidity or mortality. However, subtotal and total gastrectomy appear to offer equal long-term survival following radical resection of distal gastric cancers.

As mentioned previously, early gastric cancer represents approximately one third of all gastric tumors currently diagnosed in Japan.[68,129,139] Since these early tumors spread less exten-

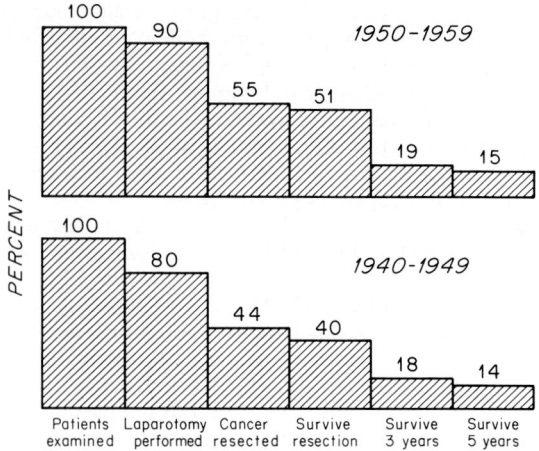

Figure 9. Comparison of ultimate survival rates for gastric cancer patients at the Mayo Clinic diagnosed in 1940 to 1949 and 1950 to 1959. (Redrawn from Remine, W. H., Priestley, J. T., and Berkson, J.: Cancer of the Stomach. Philadelphia, W. B. Saunders Company, 1964.)

sively within the stomach wall with less frequent serosal involvement, several Japanese groups have focused on radical lymph node dissection in lieu of radical resection of the gastric wall.

Majima and colleagues[83] evaluated the effects of an extended lymph node dissection, removing different groups of secondary lymph nodes based on the location of the tumor. They observed no statistically significant improvement in 5-year survival rates following extended as compared with conventional lymph node dissection. In addition, operative mortality was increased by extended lymphadenectomy. In contrast, Soga and co-workers[121] reported improved survival without increased morbidity following radical lymphadenectomy; they emphasized that wide lymphadenectomy is required since lymphatic metastases are frequently quite extensive. The significance of the lymphadenectomy is unclear, however, since different time periods were compared. Preliminary results from an ongoing randomized, prospective trial suggest that radical lymphadenectomy causes significantly greater morbidity (blood transfusion, hospital stay, reoperation) without conferring survival benefit.[26] In addition, results from this randomized trial suggest that most Western patients, in contrast to Japanese, appear to be unsuitable for radical lymphadenectomy.[26]

These results imply a limit beyond which further lymph node resection would yield diminishing returns. At this ill-defined

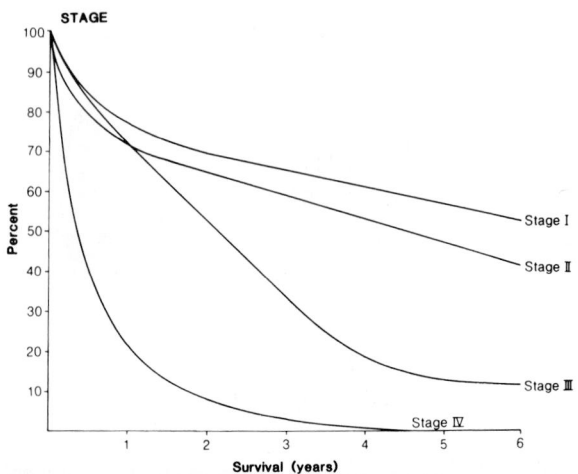

Figure 10. Survival of gastric cancer patients based on stage of their tumor at the time of initial treatment. (From Weed, T. E., Nuessle, W., and Ochsner, A.: Carcinoma of the stomach. Why are we failing to improve survival? Ann. Surg., *193:*407, 1981.)

TABLE 2. Lymph Node Involvement Versus Depth of Invasion of Primary Tumor

Level of Invasion	Number of Patients	Lymph Node Metastases (%)			
		None N_0	Primary N_1	Secondary N_2	Tertiary N_3
Intramucosal	34	88.2	8.8	2.9	—
Submucosal	46	78.3	17.4	4.3	—
Intermediate	94	48.9	30.9	18.1	2.1
Transmural	339	24.8	31.9	33.3	4.7
To neighboring organs	17	23.5	17.6	58.8	—
Total	530	37.7	28.5	30.3	3.4

From Yamada, E., et al.: The surgical treatment of cancer of the stomach. Int. Surg., 65:387, 1980.

limit, involvement of regional lymph nodes must signify systemic spread of the disease. Extensive dissection may in itself be responsible for "opening" lymphatic channels and spreading viable tumor cells. Serosal involvement that reduces 5-year survival by half [67] would appear to be a contraindiction to extensive lymph node dissection. Until further evidence is available, it appears advisable to limit the lymph node dissection to those groups around the pylorus, the hepatoduodenal ligament, and the celiac axis. Excision of additional organs for the removal of lymph nodes is rarely indicated.

CHEMOTHERAPY. Although all gastrointestinal tumors respond poorly, gastric adenocarcinoma may be the least resistant to chemotherapy. Chemotherapy is often used in patients with advanced disease, but the results are generally poor. Only about 15 to 30 per cent of patients respond to single-agent therapy[16,44,75]; responses are usually incomplete and short-lived.[16,44,75] Combinations of cytotoxic drugs appear to be more effective than is single-agent therapy. Response rates may achieve 40 to 50 per cent,[16,36,44,89] but the risks of toxicity are greater. Moreover, the median survival time in responders is increased only to approximately 1 year from 6 months and is no different from single-agent therapy.[23,40,111,138] The fact that responders may live longer than the nonresponders does not prove that the better outcome was entirely due to the chemotherapy. Responders may differ from nonresponders in other ways (perhaps with smaller tumor mass), and chemotherapy may be selecting a subgroup with a better prognosis.[81] Many of the studies do suggest that debulking is important, since removal of as much tumor as possible enhances the response to chemotherapy.[111] This fact supports the concept of resection of the tumor whenever possible.

Another approach involves the use of chemotherapy as an adjuvant to surgical treatment. Several reports have noted prolonged survival and delayed recurrence in patients treated with adjuvant chemotherapy.[38,61,76] The combination of 5-fluorouracil, doxorubicin (Adriamycin), and mitomycin C (FAM) appears particularly efficacious.[82] Unfortunately, studies comparing FAM to control in the adjuvant setting have shown no difference between the treatment arms.[10,18,138]

RESULTS

Reports published 2 decades ago indicated that the overall survival in most gastric cancer series in the United States was dismal. If 100 patients in the United States were randomly selected at the time of diagnosis of their gastric malignancy, approximately 85 would be surgical candidates[29,43,80,106]; 15 per cent would not be explored because of poor surgical risk, distant metastases, or refusal of surgical therapy. At the time of exploration, approximately half of these 85 patients would have disease treatable by "curative" resection (no residual disease), with operative mortality and 5-year survival rates of approximately 10 per cent and 25 per cent, respectively.[29,43,80,106] The other half

of the group would undergo a palliative procedure (resection, bypass) or biopsy only; approximately 75 per cent of these patients would survive surgical therapy but none would survive long term.[29,43,80,106] Thus, only 10 of the original 100 patients would be alive 5 years after diagnosis.

Unfortunately, the literature of the last 25 years is replete with series reporting consistently similar figures for operability, resectability, overall 5-year survival, and 5-year survival following curative resection. Early series published between 1950 and 1970[77,117] reported that 73 to 90 per cent of patients were operable and that 60 to 74 per cent were resectable; overall 5-year survival ranged between 4 and 15 per cent. Five-year survival following curative resection varied from 17 to 29 per cent. Recent series reveal little improvement despite the addition of postoperative radiotherapy and chemotherapy.[9,63,137]

Most,[1,15,107] but not all,[39,121] series comparing sequential results within the same institution fail to reveal any significant improvement, although appreciable progress has been made in decreasing operative mortality.[39] The data from two consecutive time periods at the Mayo Clinic are presented in Figure 9.

Certainly lymph node involvement and distant metastases are the most consistent indicators of the extent of disease and ultimate prognosis in cancer of the stomach (Fig. 10). The absence of lymphatic spread improves the 5-year survival two- to fourfold.[77,117] Since the vast majority of Western patients still

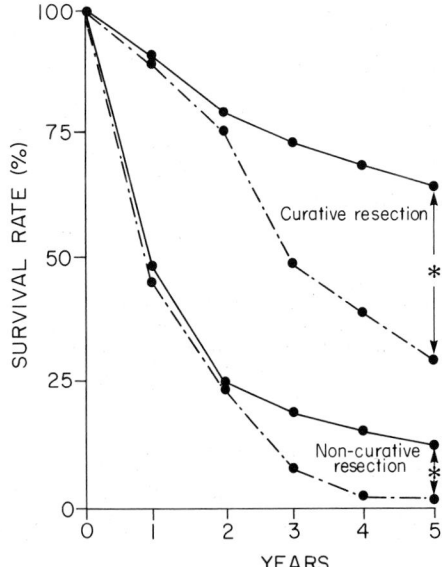

Figure 11. Five-year survival for gastric carcinoma in Japanese patients. The obvious improvement in survival between 1966 and 1975 (solid line) as compared with 1957 to 1963 (dotted line) is primarily due to technical advances allowing increased diagnosis of early gastric cancer. (Redrawn from Yamada, E., et al.: The surgical treatment of cancer of the stomach. Int. Surg., 65:387, 1980.)

present with Stage III or Stage IV disease,[9,119] it is not surprising that there has been little improvement in therapeutic results.

Lymph node involvement is related to the depth of invasion of the primary tumor (Table 2), undoubtedly contributing to the poor prognosis for tumors with serosal penetration.[9,71] Thus, it is apparent that 5-year survival varies with the number of early gastric cancers in the population. In Yamada and associates' series,[139] 31 per cent of their 2421 patients had early gastric cancer. These patients had a 5-year survival of 95 per cent. As would be expected with such a large number of early gastric cancers, the overall 5-year survival for the entire series was 44 per cent. Clearly, the progressive technological advances in the early diagnosis of gastric cancer have enabled the Japanese to significantly improve their therapeutic results with gastric cancer (Fig. 11).

The most promising aspect of this disease is its decreasing incidence worldwide. The excellent results obtainable following treatment of early gastric cancer[42,91,93,139] emphasize the urgent need for the development of a practical mass screening technique that facilitates early diagnosis. The low incidence of the disease in the United States argues against adoption of available mass screening procedures.

SELECTED REFERENCES

Correa, P.: A human model of gastric carcinogenesis. Cancer Res., 48:3554, 1988.
In this fascinating review, gastric carcinoma is discussed as a possible model of human carcinogenesis. A chain of events leading to neoplastic transformation of gastric epithelium is proposed and supported by multiple epidemiologic, pathologic, and clinical observations. In the proposed model, the normal mucosa gradually progresses through inflammatory, atrophic, and dedifferentiated stages and is ultimately transformed into the intestinal type of malignancy. The various phenotypic alterations expressed during this transformation, as well as the forces possibly determining this progression, are thoughtfully reviewed.

Dent, D. M., Madden, M. V., and Price, S. K.: Randomized comparison of R_1 and R_2 gastrectomy for gastric carcinoma. Br. J. Surg., 75:110, 1988.
In Japan, survival rates after surgical therapy for gastric cancer exceed those seen in Western societies. Possible explanations for this finding include the earlier stages of disease generally encountered as well as the more radical surgical approach practiced in Japan. The latter factor is being evaluated in an ongoing South African trial comparing gastrectomy with radical lymphadenectomy (R_2 gastrectomy) to gastrectomy alone (R_1 gastrectomy). The extent of resection was identical in both groups. Over a 5-year period, 608 patients were evaluated as possible trial participants. Of the 403 patients who were surgically explored, only 43 (7 per cent) were found to be eligible (final histologic stage $T_{1-3} N_{0-1} M_0$, age less than 75 years, no previous or coexisting malignancy, distant home). Operative times, blood transfusion requirements, and hospital stay were all significantly greater in patients undergoing R_2 gastrectomy. Reoperation was needed in four R_2 gastrectomy patients and no R_1 gastrectomy patients. Preliminary data (median follow-up of 3.1 years) reveal no significant improvement in survival probability following gastrectomy with radical lymphadenectomy. These findings suggest that in Western societies, surgeons are unlikely to encounter patients suitable for radical lymphadenectomy. Moreover, radical lymphadenectomy appears to have appreciable morbidity without evidence of clear survival benefit.

Fielding, J. W. L., Newman, C. E., Ford, C. H. J., and Jones, B. G. (Eds.): Gastric Cancer. (Advances in the Biosciences, Vol. 32.) Oxford, Pergamon Press, 1981.
This excellent monograph incorporates the papers presented by the participants of an international symposium on gastric cancer held in September 1980 in Birmingham, England. It represents an up-to-date review of cancer of the stomach. Excellent chapters on the incidence, pathogenesis, diagnosis, treatment, and outcome of this disease strongly recommend it as a reference book for anyone interested in gastric carcinoma. Of great interest is Pichlmayr and Meyer's report of 299 elective total gastrectomies performed with 11 per cent operative mortality and 50 per cent 5-year survival following curative resection.

Gouzi, J. L., et al.: Total versus subtotal gastrectomy for adenocarcinoma of the gastric antrum. A French prospective controlled study. Ann. Surg. 209:162, 1989.
This study is the first prospective randomized trial comparing mortality and survival of patients who underwent either total gastrectomy or subtotal gastrectomy for radical resection of adenocarcinoma of the gastric antrum. Two hundred and one patients were entered into this multicenter study and randomly assigned to either subtotal distal gastrectomy (Billroth II reconstruction) or total gastrectomy (Roux-en-Y esophagojejunostomy). Total omentectomy, proximal ligation of the left gastric vessels, duodenal transection at the level of the gastroduodenal artery, and regional lymph node resection were performed in both groups. Thirty-two patients were excluded based on pathologic findings (e.g., early gastric cancer, linitis plastica, lymphoma), leaving 169 patients (76 total and 93 subtotal). On

analysis, the two well-matched groups had similar morbidity (33 per cent versus 34 per cent, total versus subtotal) and mortality (1.3 per cent versus 3.2 per cent, total versus subtotal). Five-year survival was closely related to lymph node status (18 per cent with versus 69 per cent without) and serosal involvement (16 per cent with and 74 per cent without). The extent of resection did not influence survival when patients were matched for nodal and serosal involvement. This critical study indicates that elective total gastrectomy can be performed without increasing postoperative morbidity or mortality, in contrast to conclusions based on earlier retrospective studies. Despite this finding, however, subtotal and total gastrectomy appear to offer equal long-term survival following radical resection of distal gastric cancer.*

Hoerr, S. O.: Carcinoma of the stomach. Am. J. Surg., 101:284, 1961.
From a review of 254 personally treated cases of carcinoma of the stomach, Hoerr presents three cardinal therapeutic principles that are still basically sound today. (1) Every patient with suspected malignant disease of the stomach should have surgical exploration unless there is histologic proof of distant metastases or the patient is physically unable to withstand an operation. (2) At operation, when a careful search for distant metastases proves to be negative, the primary lesion should be excised widely and without biopsy; the adjacent nonessential structures are included in an en bloc resection if they are invaded by the primary tumor. However, neither routine total gastrectomy nor ultraradical lymphadenectomy is advocated. (3) If the lesion is incurable by reason of distant metastases or local extension, one should think carefully before performing a palliative resection. Mortality is high and palliation often fails. Obstruction should be the chief indication for palliation.

Longmire, W. P., Jr.: Gastric carcinoma: Is radical gastrectomy worth while? Ann. R. Coll. Surg. Engl., 62:25, 1980.
This report reviews the results reports by several centers using total gastrectomy as the treatment of choice for gastric carcinoma during the decade 1945 to 1955. The operative mortality was found to be higher, the 5-year survival rate was lower, and the undesirable digestive side effects were greater than those following subtotal resection. The very radical subtotal resections with miniature gastric remnants were also found to cause postgastrectomy symptoms quite similar to those of total gastrectomy. The report reviews 15 reports of gastric cancer treatment from eight countries. Total gastrectomy was utilized in 25 per cent of resections, with an average operative mortality of 22 per cent and a 5-year survival of 12 per cent. Radical resection or total gastrectomy was recommended for certain specific conditions, but for the usual antral gastric cancer, subtotal resection distal to the vasa brevia with preservation of the gastric fundus and spleen was suggested.

Staging System for Carcinoma of the Stomach—1971. Chicago, American Joint Committee for Cancer Staging and End Results Reporting, 1971.
This report describes the purpose, method, and summary of a field trial of the TNM Classification System for carcinoma of the stomach. The system is in keeping with the results of a number of retrospective studies of the life history of gastric cancer. The results of the field trial were reported in Kennedy, B. J.: TNM classification for stomach cancer. Cancer, 26:971, 1970. A uniform system for classification of stomach cancer was developed after a review of 1241 case records from seven participating institutions. Clinical, radiographic, or gastroscopic studies and biopsies of the primary tumor or metastases provided the information necessary to stage a stomach cancer. Survival was dependent on the extent of the penetration of the gastric wall of the tumor. As the depth of penetration increased, the rate of survival decreased. Once the neoplasm involved the regional lymph nodes, a marked reduction in survival was demonstrated. With distant metastases, there was seldom survival beyond 3 years. The system was updated and revised in 1977 as reported in the Manual for Staging of Cancer, American Joint Committee, Chicago, 1977.

Yamada E, et al.: The surgical treatment of cancer of the stomach. Int. Surg., 65:387, 1980.
As an example of the results currently being reported by the Japanese, these authors describe their experience following treatment of 2421 patients with gastric carcinoma between 1965 and 1977. It is important to note that 31 per cent of patients had early gastric cancer. The resectability rate was 80 per cent; 62 per cent of patients underwent curative resection. The 5-year survival rates for early and advanced gastric cancer were 95 and 53 per cent, respectively. Lymph node metastases significantly decreased survival. These impressive survival rates represented a significant improvement from those observed during the previous period (1957 to 1963).

REFERENCES

1. Adashek, K., Sanger, J., and Longmire, W. P., Jr.: Cancer of the stomach. Review of consecutive ten year intervals. Ann. Surg., 189:6, 1979.
2. Aird, I., and Bentall, H. H.: A relationship between cancer of the stomach and the ABO blood groups. Br. Med. J., 1:799, 1953.
3. Akiyama, H., Miyazono, H., Tsurumaru, M., Hashimota, C., and Kawamura, T.: Thoracoabdominal approach for carcinoma of the cardia of the stomach. Am. J. Surg., 137:345, 1979.
4. American Joint Committee for Cancer Staging and End Results Reporting: Manual for Staging of Cancer. Chicago, American Joint Committee, 1977.
5. Au, F. C., Koprowska, I., Berger, A., Maier, W. P., and Ming, S.-C.: The role of cytology in the diagnosis of carcinoma of the stomach. Surg. Gynecol. Obstet., 151:601, 1980.
6. Bayle, A. L. J.: Eléments de pathologie médicale, ou, Précis de médecine

théorique et pratique écrit dans l'esprit due vitalisme hippocratique. Paris, Bailliere, 1956–1957.

7. Bemvenuti, G. A., Hattori, K., Levin, B., Kirschner, J. B., and Reilly, R. W.: Endoscopic sampling for tissue diagnosis in gastrointestinal malignancy. Gastrointest. Endosc., 21:159, 1975.

8. Billroth, T.: Über einen neuen Fall von gelungener Resecktion des Carcinomatosen Pylorus. Wien. Med. Wochenschr., 31:1427, 1881.

9. Bizer, L. S.: Adenocarcinoma of the stomach: Current results of treatment. Cancer, 51:743, 1983.

10. Blake, J. R. S., Hardcastle, J. D., and Wilson, R. G.: Gastric cancer: A controlled trial of adjuvant chemotherapy following gastrectomy. Clin. Oncol., 7:13, 1981.

11. Borch, K., Renvall, H., and Liedberg, G.: Endocrine cell proliferation and carcinoid development: An overview of new aspects of hypergastrinaemic atrophic gastritis. Digestion, 35 (Suppl. 1):106, 1986.

12. Borrmann, R.: Geschwulste des Magens und Duodenums. In Henke, F., and Lubarsch, O.: Handbuch der speziellen pathologischen Anatomie und Histologie. Volume IV, Part 1. Berlin, J. Springer, 1926, pp. 812–1054.

13. Bozzetti, F., Bonfanti, G., Bufalino, R., Menotti, V., Persano, S., Andreola, S., Doci, R., and Gennari, L.: Adequacy of margins of resection in gastrectomy for cancer. Ann. Surg., 196:685, 1982.

14. Burrel, M., Touloukian, J. S., Curtis, A.: Roentgen manifestations of carcinoma in the gastric remnant. Gastrointest. Radiol., 5:331, 1980.

15. Cady, B., Ramsden, D. A., Stein, A., and Haggitt, R. C.: Gastric cancer. Contemporary aspects. Am. J. Surg., 133:423. 1977.

16. Carter, S. K., and Comis, R. L.: Gastric cancer: Current status of treatment. J. Natl. Cancer Inst., 58:567, 1977.

17. Case Records of the Massachusetts General Hospital (Case 38–1980). N. Engl. J. Med., 303:744, 1980.

18. Coombes, R. C., Schein, P. S., Chilvers, C., Palmer, A. J., Wils, J., Rutten, A., Beretta, G., Amadori, D., Cortes-Funes, H., Villar, A., McArdle, C., Boven, E., Vassilopoulos, P., Welvaart, K., Pinto Ferreira, E., Wiig, J., Gisselbrecht, C., and Rougier, P.: A controlled trial of FAM (5-FU, Adriamycin, Mitomycin-C) chemotherapy as adjuvant treatment for resected gastric carcinoma. Cancer Chemother. Pharmacol., 18:A20, 1986.

19. Correa, P.: A human model of gastric carcinogenesis. Cancer Res., 48:3554, 1988.

20. Crespi, M., and Munoz, N.: Gastric precancer states. In Fielding, J. W. L., Newman, C. E., Ford, C. H. J., and Jones, B. G.: Gastric Cancer. Oxford, Pergamon Press, 1981, pp. 65–76.

21. Cruveilhier, J.: Anatomie pathologique du corps humain, ou descriptions, avec figures lithographiées et coloriées, des diverses altérations morbides dont le corps humain est susceptible. Paris, J. B. Bailliere, 1829–1842.

22. Cuello, C., Correa, P., Haenszel, W., Gordillo, G., Brown, C., Archer, M., and Tannenbaum, S.: Gastric cancer in Colombia. I. Cancer risk and suspect environmental agents. J. Natl. Cancer Inst., 57:1015, 1976.

23. Cullinan, S. A., Moertel, C. G., Fleming, T. R., Rubin, J. R., Krook, J. E., Everson, L. K., Windshitl, H. E., Twito, D. L., Marschke, R. F., Foley, J. F., Pfeifle, D. M., and Barlow, J.: A comparison of three chemotherapeutic regimens in the treatment of advanced pancreatic and gastric carcinoma. Fluorouracil vs. fluorouracil and doxorubicin vs. fluorouracil, doxorubicin, and mitomycin. J.A.M.A., 253:2061, 1985.

24. Cwern, M., Garcia, R. L., Davidson, M. I., and Friedman, I. H.: Simultaneous occurrence of gastric carcinoma in identical twins. Am. J. Gastroenterol., 75:41, 1981.

25. Day, D. W.: Histopathology of gastric cancer. In Fielding, J. E., Newman, C. E., Ford, C. H. J., and Jones, B. G.: Gastric Cancer. Oxford, Pergamon Press, 1981, pp. 95–109.

26. Dent, D. M., Madden, M. V., and Price, S. K.: Randomized comparison of R_1 and R_2 gastrectomy for gastric carcinoma. Br. J. Surg., 75:110, 1988.

27. Domellof, L., Eriksson, S., and Janunger, K.-G.: Late precancerous changes and carcinoma of the gastric stump after Billroth I resection. Am. J. Surg., 132:26, 1976.

28. Domellof, L., Eriksson, S., and Janunger, K.-G.: Carcinoma and possible precancerous changes of the gastric stump after Billroth II resection. Gastroenterology, 73:462, 1977.

29. Dupont, J. B., Lee, J. R., Burton, G. R., and Cohn, I., Jr.: Adenocarcinoma of the stomach: Review of 1497 cases. Cancer, 41:941, 1978.

30. Ekbom, G. A., and Gleysteen, J. J.: Gastric malignancy: Resection for palliation. Surgery, 88:476, 1980.

31. Evans, D. M. D., Craven, J. L., Murphy, F., and Cleary, B. K.: Comparison of "early gastric cancer" in Britain and Japan. Gut, 19:1, 1978.

32. Fielding, J. W. L., Ellis, D. J., Jones, B. G., Paterson, J., Powell, D. J., Waterhouse, J. A. H., and Brookes, V. S.: Natural history of "early" gastric cancer: Results of a 10-year survey. Br. Med. J., 281:965, 1980.

33. Fischer, A.: Gastric stump carcinoma. Wien. Klin. Wochenschr., 99:424, 1987.

34. Fleischer, D., and Sivak, M.: Endoscopic Nd-YAG laser therapy as palliative treatment for advanced adenocarcinoma of the gastric cardia. Gastroenterology, 87:815, 1984.

35. Forman, D., Al-Dabbagh, S., Knight, T., and Doll, R.: Nitrate exposure and the carcinogenic process. Ann. N.Y. Acad. Sci., 534:597, 1988.

36. Friedman, M. A., Ogawa, M., Carter, S. K., Sakurai, V., Kimura, K., and Hannigan, J.: Chemotherapy of disseminated gastric cancer. A joint effort of the Northern California Oncology Group and the Japanese Gastric Chemotherapy Group. Cancer, 53:1771, 1983.

37. Fujimoto, S., Kitsukawa, Y., and Itoh, K.: Carcinoembryonic antigen (CEA) in gastric juice as an aid in the diagnosis of gastrointestinal cancer. Ann. Surg., 189:34, 1979.

38. Fujimoto, S., Akao, T., Itoh, B., Koshizuka, I., Koyano, K., Kitsukawa, Y., Takahashi, M., Minami, T., Ishigami, H., Miyazaki, M., Amamiya, K., Ohyama, Y., Ono, K., Kure, M., Itoh, K., and Hikosaka, T.: Protracted oral chemotherapy with fluorinated pyrimidines as an adjunct to surgical treatment for stomach cancer. Ann. Surg., 185:462, 1977.

39. Gal, F. P., and Hermanek, P.: New aspects in the surgical treatment of gastric carcinoma—a comparative study of 1636 patients operated on between 1969 and 1982. Eur. J. Surg. Oncol., 11:219, 1985.

40. Gastrointestinal Tumor Study Group: Randomized study of combination chemotherapy in unresectable gastric cancer. Cancer, 53:13, 1984.

41. Geboes, K., Rutgeerts, P., Broechaert, L., Vantrappen, G., and Desmet, V.: Histologic appearances of endoscopic gastric mucosal biopsies 10–20 years after partial gastrectomy. Ann. Surg., 192:179, 1980.

42. Gentsch, H. H., Groitl, H., and Giedl, J.: Results of surgical treatment of early gastric cancer in 113 patients. World J. Surg., 5:103, 1981.

43. Gilbertsen, V. A.: Results of treatment of stomach cancer. An appraisal of efforts for more extensive surgery and a report of 1983 cases. Cancer, 23:1305, 1969.

44. Giles, G. R., and de Mello, J.: Chemotherapy for gastrointestinal cancer. Br. J. Hosp. Med., 25:15, 1981.

45. Graham, D. V., Spjut, H. J., and Estrada, R. G.: Directed cytology of the esophagus and stomach. A comparison of 3 rapid collection methods. Gastrointest. Endosc., 24:277, 1978.

46. Graham, R.: Total gastrectomy for carcinoma of the stomach: Symposium on gastric cancer. Arch. Surg., 46:907, 1943.

47. Graham, S., and Lilienfeld, A. M.: Genetic studies of gastric cancer in humans: An appraisal. Cancer, 11:945, 1958.

48. Green, P. H. R., O'Toole, K. M., Weinberg, L. M., and Goldfarb, J. P.: Early gastric cancer. Gastroenterology, 81:247, 1981.

49. Gouzi, J. L., Huguier, M., Fagniez, P. L., Launois, B., Flamant, Y., Lacaine, F., Paquet, J. C., and Hay, J. C.: Total versus subtotal gastrectomy for adenocarcinoma of the gastric antrum. A French prospective controlled study. Ann. Surg., 209:162, 1989.

50. Guiss, L. W., and Stewart, F. W.: Chronic atrophic gastritis and cancer of the stomach. Arch. Surg., 46:823, 1943.

51. Haenszel, W., Correa, P., Cuello, C, Guzman, N., Burbano, L. C., Lores, H., and Munoz, J.: Gastric cancer in Colombia. II. Case-control epidemiologic study of precursor lesions. J. Natl. Cancer Inst., 57:1021, 1976.

52. Haenszel, W., Kurihara, M., Segi, M., and Lee, R. K. C.: Stomach cancer among Japanese in Hawaii. J. Natl. Cancer Inst., 49:969, 1972.

53. Hanson, J. T., Thoreson, C., and Morrissey, J. F.: Brush cytology in the diagnosis of upper gastrointestinal malignancy. Gastrointest. Endosc., 26:33, 1980.

54. Heymer, B., and Quentmeier, A.: Biological markers for staging of gastric cancer? In Herfarth, Ch., and Schlag, P.: Gastric Cancer. Berlin, Springer-Verlag, 1979, pp. 157–162.

55. Hirayama, T.: Changing patterns in the incidence of gastric cancer. In Fielding, J. W. L., Newman, C. E., Ford, C. H. J., and Jones, B. G.: Gastric Cancer. Oxford, Pergamon Press, 1981, pp. 1–15.

56. Hirayama, T.: Methods and results (cost-effectiveness) of gastric cancer screening. In Fielding, J. W. L., Newman, C. E., Ford, C. H. J., and Jones, B. G.: Gastric Cancer. Oxford, Pergamon Press, 1981, pp. 77–84.

57. Hoerr, S. O.: Carcinoma of the stomach. Am. J. Surg., 101:284, 1961.

58. Hoffman, N. R.: The relationship between pernicious anemia and cancer of the stomach. Geriatrics, 25:90, 1970.

59. Huppler, E. G., Priestley, J. T., Morlock, C. G., and Gage, R. P.: Diagnosis and results of treatment in gastric polyps. Surg. Gynecol. Obstet., 110:309, 1960.

60. Ichikawa, H., Yamada, T., Horikoshi, H., Doi, H., Tobayashi, K., Sasagawa, M., and Higa, A.: X-ray diagnosis of early gastric cancer. Jpn. J. Clin. Oncol., 1:1, 1970.

61. Imanaga, H., and Nakazato, H.: Results of surgery for gastric cancer and effect of adjuvant mitomycin C on cancer recurrence. World J. Surg., 1:213, 1977.

62. Imaoka, W., Ida, K., Katoh, T., Okuda, J., and Kawai, K.: Is curative endoscopic treatment of early gastric cancer possible? Endoscopy, 19:7, 1987.

63. Irvin, T. T., and Bridger, J. E.: Gastric cancer: An audit of 122 consecutive cases and the results of R_1 gastrectomy. Br. J. Surg., 75:106, 1988.

64. Joossens, J. V., and Geboers, J.: Nutrition and gastric cancer. Proc. Nutr. Soc., 40:37, 1981.

65. Kaneko, E., Nakamura, T., Umeda, N., Fujino, M., and Niwa, H.: Outcome of gastric carcinoma detected by gastric mass survey in Japan. Gut, 18:626, 1977.

66. Kawai, K., Kizu, M., and Miyaoka, T.: Epidemiology and pathogenesis of gastric cancer. Front. Gastrointest. Res., 6:71, 1980.

67. Kennedy, B. J.: TNM classification for stomach cancer. Cancer, 26:971, 1970.

68. Kidokoro, T.: Frequency of resection, metastases and five-year survival rate of early gastric carcinoma in a surgical clinic. In Murakami, T.: Early Gastric Cancer. (Japanese Cancer Association, Gann Monograph on Cancer Research, No. 11, p. 45.). Baltimore, University Park Press, 1972.

69. Kidokoro, T., Hayashida, Y., and Urabe, M.: Long-term surgical results of carcinoma of the gastric remnant: A statistical analysis of 613 patients from 98 institutions. World J. Surg., 9:966, 1985.

70. King, R. M., van Heerden, J. A., and Weiland, L. H.: The management of gastric polyps. Surg. Gynecol. Obstet., 155:846, 1982.

71. Koga, S., Nishimura, O., Iwai, N., Kishi, K., Takeuchi, T., Hinohara, T., and Okamota, T.: Clinical evaluation of long-term survival after total gastrectomy. Am. J. Surg., 138:635, 1979.

72. LaDue, J. S.: The clinical diagnosis of gastric cancer. In McNeer, G., and Pack, G. T.: Neoplasms of the Stomach. Philadelphia, J. B. Lippincott Company, 1967, pp. 102–125.

73. Lauren, P.: The two histological main types of gastric carcinoma: Diffuse and so-called intestinal type carcinoma. An attempt at a histiclinical classification. Acta Pathol. Microbiol. Scand., 64:31, 1965.

74. Lawrence, W., Jr., McNeer, G., Pack, G. T., Paglia, M. A., and Ashley, M. P.: End results and prognosis. In McNeer, G. and Pack, G. T.: Neoplasms of the Stomach. Philadelphia, J. B. Lippincott Company, 1967, pp. 447–491.

75. Lawton, J. O., Giles, G. R., Hall, R., Bird, G. G., and Matheson, T.: Chemotherapy following palliative resection of gastric cancer. Br. J. Surg., 68:397, 1981.

76. Livstone, E.M., and Stablein, D. M.: Adjuvant chemotherapy with 5FU and methyl CCNU prolongs recurrence free interval and survival following curative resection for gastric adenocarcinoma. Gastroenterology 80:1215, 1981.

77. Longmire, W. P., Jr.: Gastric carcinoma: Is radical gastrectomy worth while? Ann. R. Coll. Surg. Engl. 62:25, 1980.

78. Longmire, W. P., Jr.: The place of radical surgery in gastric cancer. In Fielding, J. W. L., Newman, C. E., Ford, C. H. J., and Jones, B. G.: Gastric Cancer. Oxford, Pergamon Press, 1981, pp. 203–217.

79. Lortat-Jacob, J.-L., Giuli, R., Estenne, B., and Clot, Ph.: Intérêt de la gastrectomie totale pour le traitement des cancers de l'estomac. Chirurgie, 101:59, 1975.

80. Lumpkin, W. M., Crow, R. L., Jr., Hernandez, C. M., and Cohn, I.: Carcinoma of the stomach. Review of 1035 cases. Ann. Surg., 159:919, 1964.

81. Macdonald, J. S., and Gohmann, J. J.: Chemotherapy of advanced gastric cancer: Present status, future prospects. Semin. Oncol., 15(Suppl. 4):42, 1988.

82. Macdonald, J. S., Schein, P. S., Woolley, P. V., Smythe, T., Ueno, W., Hoth, D., Smith, F., Boiron, M., Gisselbrecht, C, Brunet, R., and Lagarde, C.: 5-Fluorouracil, doxorubicin, and mitomycin (FAM) combination chemotherapy for advanced gastric cancer. Ann. Intern. Med., 93:533, 1980.

83. Majima, S., Etani, S., Fujita, Y., and Takahashi, T.: Evaluation of extended lymph node dissection for gastric cancer. Jpn. J. Surg., 2:1, 1972.

84. Mallaiah, L., Fructer, G., Brozinsky, S., and Uddin, M. S.: Malignant gastrocolic fistula. Case report and review of the literature. Am. J. Proctol. Gastroenterol. Colon Rectal Surg., 32:12, 1980.

85. McFee, A. S., and Aust, J. B.: Gastric carcinoma and the CAT scan. Gastroenterology, 80:196, 1981.

86. McNeer, G., Joly, D. J., and Berg, J. W.: The significance of adenomatous polyps. In McNeer, G., and Pack, G. T.: Neoplasms of the Stomach. Philadelphia, J. B. Lippincott Company, 1967, pp. 56–68.

87. McNeer, G., Bowden, L., Booker, R. J., and McPeak, C. J.: Elective total gastrectomy for cancer of the stomach. End results. Ann. Surg., 180:252, 1974.

88. Ming, S.-C.: Gastric carcinoma. A pathobiological classification. Cancer, 39:2475, 1977.

89. Moertel, C. G., Mittelman, J. A., Bakemeier, R. F., Engstrom, P., and Hanley, J.: Sequential and combination chemotherapy of advanced gastric cancer. Cancer, 38:678, 1976.

90. Moss, A. A., Schnyder, P., Marks, W., and Margulis, A. R.: Gastric adenocarcinoma: A comparison of the accuracy and economics of staging by computed tomography and surgery. Gastroenterology, 80:45, 1981.

91. Murakami, T.: Early cancer of the stomach. World J. Surg., 3:685, 1979.

92. Nagao, F., and Takahashi, N.: Diagnosis of advanced gastric cancer. World J. Surg., 3:693, 1979.

93. Nagata, T., Ikeda, M., and Nakayama, F.: Changing perspective of gastric cancer in Japan. Histologic perspective of the past 76 years. Am. J. Surg., 145:226, 1983.

94. Nicholls, J. C.: Stump cancer following gastric surgery. World J. Surg., 3:731, 1979.

95. Nitti, D., Farini, R., Grassi, F., Cardin, F., DiMario, F., Piccoli, A., Vianello, R., Farinati, F., Favretti, F., Lise, M., and Naccarato, R.: Carcinoembryonic antigen in gastric juice collected during endoscopy. Cancer, 52:2334, 1983.

96. Nomuro, A. M. Y., Stemmermann, G. N., and Samloff, I. M.: Serum pepsinogen I as a predictor of stomach cancer. Ann. Intern. Med., 93:537, 1980.

97. Oohara, T., Aono, G., Ukawa, S., Takezoe, K., Johjima, Y., Kurosaka, H., Asakura, R., and Tohma, H.: Clinical diagnosis of minute gastric cancer less than 5 mm in diameter. Cancer, 53:162, 1984.

98. Oota, K.: Historical typing of gastric and oesophageal tumours. Geneva, World Health Organization, 1977.

99. Orr, T. G.: A modified technique for total gastrectomy. Arch. Surg., 54:279, 1947.

100. Papachristou, D. N., and Fortner, J. G.: Adenocarcinoma of the gastric cardia. The choice of gastrectomy. Ann. Surg., 192:58, 1980.

101. Paulino, F., and Roselli, A.: Carcinoma of the stomach with special reference to total gastrectomy. In Ravitch, M. (Ed.): Current Problems in Surgery. Chicago, Year Book Medical Publishers, 1973.

102. Pichlmayr, R., and Meyer, H.-J.: Patterns of recurrence in relation to therapeutic strategy. In Fielding, J. W. L., Newman, C. E., Ford, C. H. J., and Jones, B. G.: Gastric Cancer. Oxford, Pergamon Press, 1981, pp. 171–186.

103. Polya, E. A.: Zur stumpfversorgung nach Magenresektion. Zentrabl. Chir., 38:892, 1911.

104. Remine, W. H.: Indications and contraindications for surgery in gastric carcinoma. World J. Surg., 3:709, 1979.

105. Remine, W. H.: Palliative operations for incurable gastric cancer. World J. Surg., 3:721, 1979.

106. Remine, W. H., and Priestley, J. T.: Trends in prognosis and surgical treatment of cancer of the stomach. Ann. Surg., 163:736, 1966.

107. Remine, W. H., Priestley, J. T., and Berkson, J.: Cancer of the Stomach. Philadelphia, W. B. Saunders Company, 1964.

108. Ruddell, W. S. J., Bone, E. S., Hill, M. J., Blendis, L. M., and Walters, C. L.: Gastric-juice nitrite. A risk factor for cancer in the hypochloric stomach? Lancet, 2:1037, 1976.

109. Sancho-Poch, F. J., Balanzo, J., Ocana, J., Presa, E., Sala-Cladera, E., Cusso, X., and Vilardell, F.: An evaluation of gastric biopsy in the diagnosis of gastric cancer. Gastrointest. Endosc., 24:281, 1978.

110. Scharschmidt, B. F.: The natural history of hypertrophic gastropathy (Ménétrier's disease). Report of a case with 16 years follow-up and review of 120 cases from the literature. Am. J. Med., 63:644, 1977.

111. Schein, P. S., Coffey, R., Jr., and Smith, F. P.: Chemotherapy and combined modality treatment of gastric cancer. In Fielding, J. W. L., Newman, C. E., Ford, C. H. J., and Jones, B. G.: Gastric Cancer. Oxford, Pergamon Press, 1981, pp. 139–148.

112. Schlag, P., Ulrich, H., Merkle, P., Bockler, R., Peter, M., and Herfarth, Ch.: Are nitrite and N-nitroso compounds in gastric juice risk factors for carcinoma in the operated stomach. Lancet, 1:727, 1980.

113. Schlatter, C.: A unique case of complete removal of the stomach: Successful esophago-enterostomy. Med. Rec., 52:909, 1897.

114. Schlatter, C.: Further observations on a case of total extirpation of the stomach in the human subject. Lancet, 2:1314, 1898.

115. Schrock, T. R., and Way, L. W.: Total gastrectomy. Am. J. Surg., 135:348, 1978.

116. Schrumpf, E., Stadaas, J., Myren, J., Serck-Hanssen, A., Aune, S., and Osnes, M.: Mucosal changes in the gastric stump 20–25 years after partial gastrectomy. Lancet, 2:467, 1977.

117. Shahon, D. B., Horowitz, S., and Kelly, W. D.: Cancer of the stomach; an analysis of 1152 cases. Surgery, 39:204, 1956.

118. Shiu, M. H., Papacristou, D. N., and Kosloff, C.: Selection of operative procedure for adenocarcinoma of the midstomach. Twenty years experience with implications for future treatment strategy. Ann. Surg., 192:730, 1980.

119. Silverberg, E.: Cancer statistics, 1989. Cancer, 39:3, 1989.

120. Siurala, M.: Gastritis, its fate and sequelae. Ann. Clin. Res., 13:111, 1981.

121. Soga, J., Ohyama, S., Miyashita, K., Suzuki, H., Nashimota, A., Tanaka, O., Sasaki, K., and Muto, T.: A statistical evaluation of advancement in gastric cancer surgery with special reference to the significance of lymphadenectomy for cure. World J. Surg., 12:398, 1988.

122. Sonnenberg, A.: Endoscopic screening for gastric stump cancer—would it be beneficial: A hypothetical cohort study. Gastroenterology, 87:489, 1984.

123. Stemmermann, G. N., Samloff, I. M., Nomura, A., and Walsh, J. H.: Serum pepsinogen I and gastrin in relation to extent and location of intestinal metaplasia in the surgically resected stomach. Dig. Dis. Sci., 25:680, 1980.

124. Stocks, P., and Davies, R. I.: Zinc and copper content of soils associated with the incidence of cancer of the stomach and other organs. Br. J. Cancer, 18:14, 1964.

125. Stone, R., Rangel, D. M., Gordon, H. E., and Wilson, S. E.: Carcinoma of the gastroesophageal junction. A ten year experience with esophagogastrectomy. Am. J. Surg., 134:70, 1977.

126. Stout, A. P.: Gastric mucosal atrophy and carcinoma of the stomach. N.Y. State Med. J., 45:973, 1945.

127. Stout, A. P.: Tumors of the stomach. Atlas of tumor pathology. Section VI, Fascicle 21, Washington, D.C., Armed Forces Institute of Pathology, 1953.

128. Susuki, S., Murakami, H., Suzuki, H., Sakakibara, N., Endo, M., and Nakayama, K.: An endoscopic staining method for detection and operation of early gastric cancer. Int. Adv. Surg. Oncol., 2:223, 1979.

129. Takagi, K.: The incidence of early gastric cancer since the advent of gastroscopy. In Fielding, J. W. L., Newman, C. E., Ford, C. H. J., and Jones, B. G.: Gastric Cancer. Oxford, Pergamon Press, 1981, pp. 159–169.

130. Tatsuta, M., Itoh, T., Okuda, S., Yamamura, H., Baba, M., and Tamura, H.: Carcinoembryonic antigen in gastric juice as an aid in diagnosis of early gastric cancer. Cancer, 46:2686, 1980.

131. Tio, T. L., Schouwink, M. H., Cikot, R. J. L. M., and Tytgat, G. N. J.: Preoperative TNM classification of gastric carcinoma by endosonography in comparison with the pathological TNM system: A prospective study of 72 cases. Hepatogastroenterology, 36:51, 1989.

132. Turnbull, A., Kussin, S., Kurtz, R. C., and Bains, M.: Palliative prosthetic intubation in gastric cancer. J. Surg. Oncol., 15:37, 1980.

133. Viste, A., Eide, G. E., Real, C., Glattre, E., and Soreide, O.: Cancer of the gastric stump: Analyses of 819 patients and comparison with other stomach cancer patients. World J. Surg., 10:454, 1986.

134. von den Velden, R.: Über Vorkommen und Mangel der freien Salzauer in Magensaft bei Gastrektasie. Dtsch. Arch. Klin. Med., 23:396, 1878–79.

135. von Eiselsberg, A.: Über die Magenresectionen und Gastroenterostomieen in Prof. Billroth's Klinik, Marz 1885 bis October 1889. Arch. Klin. Chir., 39:783, 1889.

136. Watanabe, H., Enjoji, M., and Imai, T.: Gastric carcinoma with lymphoid

stroma. Its morphological characteristics and prognostic correlations. Cancer, 38:232, 1976.

137. Weed, T. E., Nuessle, W., and Ochsner, A.: Carcinoma of the stomach. Why are we failing to improve survival? Ann. Surg., 193:407, 1981.

138. Wils, J., and Bleiberg, H.: Current status of chemotherapy for gastric cancer. Eur. J. Clin. Oncol., 25:3, 1989.

139. Yamada, E., Miyaishi, S., Nakazato, H., Kato, K., Kito, T., Takagi, H., Yasue, M., Kato, T., Morimoto, T., and Yamauchi, M.: The surgical treatment of cancer of the stomach. Int. Surg., 65:387, 1980.

140. Zamcheck, N., Grable, E., Ley, A., and Norman, L.: Occurrence of gastric cancer among patients with pernicious anemia at the Boston City Hospital. N. Engl. J. Med., 252:1103, 1955.

141. Ziegler, K., Sanft, C., Zeitz, M., Felsenberg, D., Stein, M., Haring, R., and Riecken, E. O.: Endosonography as a new clinical tool in staging gastric carcinoma. Gastroenterology, 96:A566, 1989.

142. Zinninger, M. M.: Extension of gastric cancer in the intramural lymphatics and its relations to gastrectomy. Am. Surg., 20:920, 1954.

31

THE SMALL INTESTINE

I ———

ANATOMY

R. Scott Jones, M.D.

The small intestine is that portion of the alimentary tract that extends from the pylorus to the cecum. Its major function is absorption, which depends upon the amazingly complex integration of structural, physiologic, and chemical factors. The neurohormonal regulation of gastric, biliary, pancreatic, and intestinal secretion and of motor function provides the appropriate luminal milieu for complete digestion of foodstuffs and presentation of the products of digestion to the specialized intestinal epithelium for absorption.[7] The structure and functions of this segment of the gut are considered in this section.

An essential anatomic characteristic of the small intestine is the large surface area which it provides for absorption. The gross, microscopic, and ultrastructural features of the small intestine in this remarkable arrangement are (1) intestinal length, (2) mucosal folds, (3) villi, and (4) microvilli. The effectiveness of digestion and absorption is also greatly influenced by various types of intestinal movements.

GROSS ANATOMY

GENERAL DESCRIPTION. The length of the alimentary tract in normal individuals is best estimated by means of small polyethylene catheters passed through the intestine via the nose. The average distance from the nose to the anus is 453 cm. The duodenum is approximately 21 cm. long, and the colon is approximately 109 cm. long. The combined length of the jejunum and ileum is 261 cm., or approximately three fifths of the entire canal, or eight fifths of body height.[17] The duodenum is described in Chapter 29. The jejunum begins at the duodenojejunal angle, which is supported by the ligament of Treitz. The proximal two fifths of the small intestine is called the jejunum; the distal three fifths, the ileum. However, this distinction is arbitrary, because there is no clear demarcation between jejunum and ileum. The small intestinal tube, which decreases in luminal diameter as it proceeds distally, is convoluted or folded upon itself and occupies the central and lower part of the abdominal cavity; it is enclosed laterally and superiorly by the colon.[14]

MESENTERY. The small intestine is suspended from the posterior abdominal wall by a large fold of peritoneum, the mesentery, which is attached to the posterior abdominal wall to the left of the second lumbar vertebra, passing obliquely to the right and inferiorly to the right sacroiliac joint. The mesentery contains blood vessels, nerves, lymphatics, and lymph nodes, as well as considerable fat. It is attached to the small intestine along the length of one side, the mesenteric border, leaving the remainder of the surface of the bowel covered by its visceral peritoneum, the serosa. The relationship of the mesentery to the small bowel is important, because the broad-based attachment of the mesenteric root stabilizes the small bowel and prevents it from twisting upon its blood supply. The relationship of the bowel to the mesentery is an important consideration in operative procedures on the intestine.

BLOOD SUPPLY. The small intestine receives its blood supply from the superior mesenteric artery, the second large branch of the abdominal aorta. The superior mesenteric artery courses anterior to the uncinate process of the pancreas and the third portion of the duodenum, where it divides to supply the pancreas, duodenum, and entire small intestine as well as the ascending and transverse colon. The intestinal arteries branch within the mesentery to unite with adjacent arteries to form a series of arterial arcades before sending small, straight arteries to the small intestine. The intestinal arteries contact the small intestine on the mesenteric border, where they pass toward the antimesenteric border, sending small branches into the layers of the intestine. The veins of the small intestine drain into the superior mesentric vein, a major tributary to the portal vein. The unique relationship of the small intestine and its blood supply enables surgical mobilization of long segments of intestine. For example, small intestine may be used to replace the esophagus.

LYMPHATICS. There are aggregated lymphatic nodules, Peyer's patches, in the submucosa of the small intestine. These lymphatic nodules are most abundant in the ileum, but are also present in the jejunum. The lymphatic drainage from the small intestine passes into three sets of mesenteric nodes: the first set is close to the wall of the small intestine, the second set is adjacent to the mesenteric arcades, and the third set is along the trunk of the superior mesenteric artery. The superior mesenteric preaortic group drains into the intestinal trunk, which drains into the cisterna chyli. The lymphatic drainage of the small intestine is the major route by which absorbed lipid is transported into the circulation.

MUCOSA. The mucosal surface of the small intestine contains numerous circular mucosal folds called the plicae circulares (valvulae conniventes, or valves of Kerckring). These folds are 3 to 10 mm. in height, taller and more numerous in the distal duodenum and proximal jejunum, becoming shorter and fewer distally. Rarely visible to the naked eye are the intestinal villi, tiny finger-like processes projecting into the intestinal lumen.

INNERVATION. The efferent nerve supply to the small intestine is from the parasympathetic and sympathetic division of the autonomic nervous system. The parasympathetic innervation is via preganglionic fibers passing through the vagus nerves to synapse with neurons of the intrinsic plexuses of the intestine. The sympathetic innervation of the small intestine is from preganglionic fibers arising from the ninth and tenth thoracic segments of the spinal cord, passing to synapse in the superior mesenteric ganglion. The postganglionic sympathetic fibers pass along the branches of the superior mesenteric artery to the intestine. Pain from the intestine is mediated through thoracic visceral afferents and not vagal afferents, although the vagus does contain large numbers of afferent fibers.[1]

MICROSCOPIC ANATOMY

The small intestine is composed of four layers, which, from the lumen outward, are the mucosa; the submucosa; the muscularis; and the adventitia, or serosa.

Mucosa

The mucosa of the small intestine is composed of (1) the epithelium, (2) the lamina propria, and (3) the muscularis mucosae. The mucosal surface has two important structural features: the villi and the crypts of Lieberkühn (Fig. 1). The villi are finger-like luminal projections having a columnar epithelial surface and a cellular connective tissue core of lamina propria. Each villus contains a central lymphatic vessel called a lacteal, a small artery, vein, and capillary network. Human jejunal villi are approximately 0.5 to 1.0 mm. high, and there are 10 to 40 villi per sq. mm. of mucosal surface. In addition to the vessels, the villi contain smooth muscle fibers extending from the muscularis mucosae, providing contractility to each villus. The crypts of Lieberkühn, or intestinal glands, are adjacent to the bases of the villi and extend down to, but not through, the muscularis mucosae.

The lamina propria is between the intestinal epithelium and the muscularis mucosae and contains blood and lymph vessels, nerve fibers, smooth muscle fibers, fibroblasts, macrophages, plasma cells, lymphocytes, eosinophils, and mast cells, as well as connective tissue elements.[4]

Studies with the scanning electron microscope have provided information on the topography of the mucosal surface. Scanning electron micrographs provide an in-depth perspective of the mucosa with excellent resolution (Fig. 2). The villi vary in shape from circular to flattened or finger-shaped. The finger-shaped villi are 0.1 to 0.25 mm. in diameter. The villi are corrugated by deep horizontal clefts and there are holes 3 to 8 μ across on the surface of the villi representing the openings of the goblet cells.[21] The muscularis mucosae is a thin layer of smooth muscle separating the mucosa from the submucosa.

CELLS OF THE EPITHELIUM

CELLS OF THE VILLI. The columnar epithelial cells are responsible for absorption. These cells are about 22 to 26 μ tall and are characterized by a striated luminal border (brush border) and a basally placed nucleus (Fig. 3). The striated or brush border appearance is due to the microvilli, which are projections 1 μ high and 0.1 μ wide produced by numerous folds in the apical plasma membrane. The microvilli greatly increase the absorptive surface of the epithelial cell. The plasma membranes of the epithelial cells have a three-layer, or trilamellar, appearance and are somewhat thicker over the microvilli than in the lateral and basal portion of the cell. The membrane of the microvillus is continuous, without fenestrations, discernible by electron-microscopic techniques, and separates the lumen of the gut from the interior of the epithelial cell. A coat of fine filaments called the "fuzz" or glycocalyx is closely applied to the luminal surface of the microvillus membrane (Fig. 4). High concentrations of digestive enzymes, particularly disaccharidases, are present in the brush border. The plasma membrane contains 80 to 90 per cent of the disaccharidase activity of the intestinal cell. These findings indicate that the microvilli, in addition to providing increased absorptive surface, perform a very important digestive function.[1]

Three specialized areas of the lateral plasma membrane deserve comment. The "tight junctions" are fusions of the lateral plasma membranes between the terminal web and the intestinal lumen. This tight junction is present about the circumference of the cell. Immediately below the tight junction is an intermediate junction that has an intracellular space of approximately 200 Å. At intervals along the lateral plasma membranes are very close attachments of adjacent membranes called *desmosomes.* The intermediate junction and desmosomes bind adjacent cells together.[1]

The nuclei and mitochondria of absorptive cells are not particularly distinctive. The absorptive cells contain granular and agranular endoplasmic reticulum, which has an important synthetic function in the cell. It is likely that the endoplasmic reticulum synthesizes the protein component of the chylomicron during fat absorption. This organelle has also been shown to be capable of triglyceride synthesis, which is an important step in fat absorption. The endoplasmic reticulum may synthesize the cytoplasmic enzymes of the absorptive cell.

The Golgi material probably stores or modifies substances absorbed or synthesized by the cell. Lysosomes contain lytic enzymes and eliminate waste materials by either lysing them or segregating the noxious substance for extrusion.

GOBLET CELLS. Goblet cells are present in both the villi and the crypts. These cells are characterized by a cytoplasm filled with

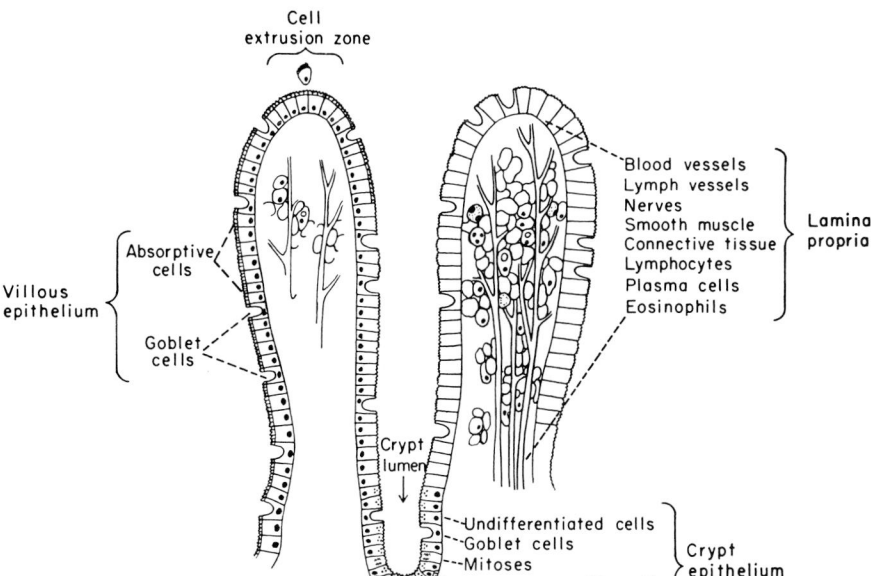

Figure 1. Schematic diagram of two sectioned villi and a crypt to illustrate the histologic organization of the small intestinal mucosa. (From Trier, J. S.: Morphology of epithelium of small intestine. *In* Code, C. F. (Ed.): American Physiological Society Handbook of Physiology, Section 6, Alimentary Canal. Baltimore, Williams & Wilkins, 1968.)

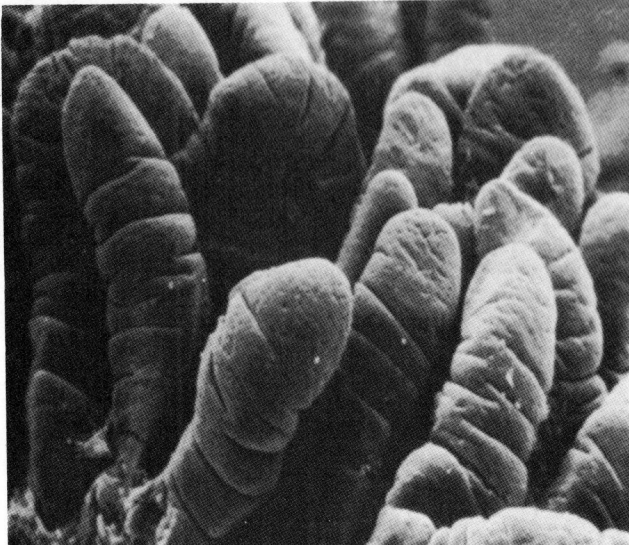

Figure 2. A scanning electron micrograph of human jejunal mucosa. Magnification, ×42. The villi are finger-shaped and are indented with numerous transverse grooves. The pitlike impressions on the villi are the openings of goblet cells. (Courtesy of A. L. Jones, M.D., Associate Professor of Anatomy and Medicine, University of California, San Francisco.)

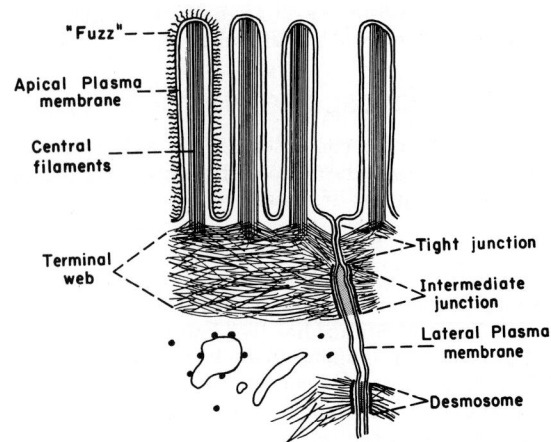

Figure 4. Schematic illustration of the specialization of the apical cytoplasm of the plasma membrane of intestinal absorption cells. (From Trier, J. S., and Rubin, C. E.: Electron microscopy of the small intestine: A review. Gastroenterology, 49:574, 1965.)

mucous granules between the nucleus and the apical brush border. Electron microscopic studies suggest that intestinal goblet cells secrete their mucus by merocrine secretion.[1]

CELLS OF THE CRYPTS

ENTEROCHROMAFFIN CELLS. Enterochromaffin cells are found in the crypts of the small intestine but are in other parts of the gastrointestinal system as well, including the esophagus, stomach, colon, gallbladder, and pancreas. These cells are usually not in contact with the intestinal lumen, and their secretory granules are usually below the nuclei away from the lumen, suggesting secretion into the blood, rather than the lumen. Serotonin has been identified in enterochromaffin cells, but the significance of this observation is unknown. The structure of enterochromaffin cells has suggested an endocrine function. A study using immunocytochemical and radioimmunoassay techniques showed that duodenal acidification caused depletion of

secretin from intestinal endocrine cells associated with increased concentrations of secretin in serum.[28]

PANETH CELLS. Paneth cells occur in the base of the crypts and are structurally similar to cells known to secrete large amounts of protein, such as pancreatic or parotid acinar cells. The function of Paneth cells is unknown.

UNDIFFERENTIATED CELLS. Undifferentiated cells are found only in the crypts, particularly at the bases, where they are the most frequent cell type. These cells exhibit mitosis, because they multiply and differentiate to replace lost absorptive cells.

EPITHELIAL RENEWAL. The epithelium of the small intestine is a dynamic, rapidly proliferating tissue in which old dying cells are constantly replaced by newly formed cells, thus maintaining the structural integrity of the mucosa. Mitotic division of undifferentiated cells occurs in the crypts. An undifferentiated cell may do one of three things: (1) differentiate into an absorptive cell and migrate into the villus, (2) remain in the crypt and continue mitotic activity, or (3) remain in the crypt in a resting stage. The cells entering the villi migrate to the villus tips, where they are shed into the lumen. This process has been studied by observing the fate of injected tritiated thymidine and by means of radioautography on serial biopsies. In the human duodenum and jejunum, cells labeled in this manner are in the crypts for 12 hours after ^{3}H-thymidine injection, appearing at the villus base in 24 hours and at the villus tip in 5 to 7 days. In the ileum, labeled cells reach the villus tips in 3 days. These findings indicate that the population of intestinal epithelial cells is replaced every 3 to 7 days.[1]

Submucosa

The submucosa is a strong fibroelastic and areolar connective tissue layer containing vessels, nerves, and lymph nodules. This layer provides much of the strength for sutures of the intestinal wall, and indeed any method of intestinal suturing should include stitches through the submucosa.

Muscular Layer and Intramural Neural Structures

The muscular portion of the small intestine is formed by two distinct layers of smooth or nonstriated muscle, an outer longitudinal coat and an inner circular coat. Intestinal smooth muscle fibers are spindle-shaped structures about 250 μ long. In the past it was thought that intestinal smooth muscle was a syncytium, but electron microscopic studies show intestinal smooth muscle cells to be discrete structures. However, there are points at which the plasma membrane of adjacent cells is approximated, forming structures called nexuses. It is believed that the

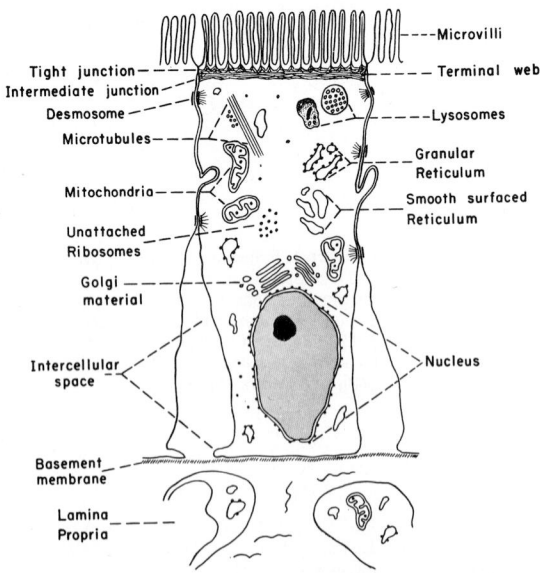

Figure 3. Schematic diagram of an intestinal absorptive cell. (From Trier, J. S., and Rubin, C. E.: Electron microscopy of the small intestine: A review. Gastroenterology, 49:574, 1965.)

nexuses allow electrical continuity between smooth muscle cells and permit conduction through the muscle layer.

There are four identifiable neural plexuses in the small intestine: (1) The subserous plexus is most noticeable on the mesenteric attachment and forms the transition between the mesenteric nerve fibers and the myenteric plexus. Ganglia can be found in the subserous plexus. (2) The myenteric plexus is located between the longitudinal and circular muscle layers and consists of three networks linking varius ganglia and ramifying within the muscle layers. (3) The submucosal plexus is a network of nerve fibers and ganglia in the submucosa. (4) The mucous plexus consists of fibers from the submucosal plexus extending into the mucosa. This plexus does not contain nerve cell bodies.[1]

For references, see page 842.

II

PHYSIOLOGY

R. Scott Jones, M.D.

DIGESTION AND ABSORPTION

Carbohydrate (Fig. 1)

An adult may ingest about 350 gm. of carbohydrate daily, consisting of starch, sucrose, and lactose. Dietary starch contains two glucose polymers, amylopectin and amylose. Amylopectin, the most abundant constituent of starch (80 per cent), is a 1–4 linked straight chain of glucose molecules. In addition, amylopectin possesses a 1–6 branching side chain at approximately every 25 glucose units along the straight chain. Amylose, the other constituent of starch, consists only of 1–4 linkages of glucose molecules in a straight chain.

Pancreas and salivary amylases break the interior 1–4 glucose linkages, and for that reason the end product of amylose digestion by amylase is maltose (glucose-glucose) and maltotriose (glucose-glucose-glucose), which cannot be digested further by amylase because the only linkages present between glucose molecules in this circumstance are terminal bonds.

Because amylopectin contains 1–6 as well as 1–4 glucose linkages, the end products of amylase digestion of amylopectin are maltose, maltotriose, and the residual branched saccharides, the dextrins. The digestion of starch by amylase probably occurs predominantly in the lumen of the alimentary tract. The finding of high concentrations of digestive enzymes in isolated brush border preparations suggests that maltose, maltotriose, and dextrin, as well as the dietary disaccharides, lactose (glucose-galactose) and sucrose (glucose-fructose), are completely broken down to the constituent monosaccharides by the microvilli, probably at the level of the glycocalyx (fuzz coat). It is possible that some disaccharides may be absorbed intact, possibly facilitated by monosaccharide transport, but the significance of that event is not known.

Glucose and galactose are actively transported into the intestinal cells against a concentration gradient. Such transport of these sugars has been demonstrated *in vivo* as well as *in vitro*. Glucose and galactose compete for transport in a manner similar to competitive inhibition in other enzyme substrate systems. The active transport of sugars requires metabolic energy as well as oxygen. Sodium ion has a role in the transport of glucose and galactose; however, only very small concentrations appear to be required. Glucose and galactose are therefore probably absorbed by carrier-mediated active transport. The absorption of glucose and galactose are related to Na^+ movement into the cell produced by the sodium-potassium adenosine triphosphatase (ATPase) located on the basolateral cell membrane. Fructose, the other significant monosaccharide, is not absorbed by active transport, but probably enters the intestinal cells by a process termed facilitated diffusion.[1,8]

Protein

Protein digestion is initiated in the stomach by two factors: (1) the acidic gastric environment favors denaturation of protein, and (2) pepsin hydrolyzes protein to polypeptides. Protein digestion is far from complete when gastric chyme enters the duodenum, where pepsin is inactivated by the higher pH.

Pancreatic proteolytic enzyme precursors are secreted into the duodenum. Trypsinogen is converted to trypsin by the intestinal enzyme enterokinase. The activation of trypsinogen is autocatalytic; i.e., trypsin also activates trypsinogen. Trypsin likewise activates the other pancreatic proteolytic enzyme precursors. Trypsin, chymotrypsin, and elastase are pancreatic endopeptidases that split peptide bonds in the central portion of protein molecules; whereas carboxypeptidases are pancreatic exopeptidases that remove amino acids from the C-terminal position of protein molecules. Aminopeptidases are intestinal exopeptidases that split amino acids from the N-terminal position of protein molecules. Amino acids are the final product of protein digestion and are the molecules that are absorbed. That some dipeptides are absorbed by adult humans is likely, and this is certain in the human neonate for a brief period. The nutritional significance of this phenomenon is undetermined.

Amino acids are absorbed from the intestinal lumen by a process of carrier-mediated active transport.[1] The active transport of amino acids against a concentration gradient has been demonstated *in vitro* by everted intestinal sacs and tissue accumulation methods in animals and man and *in vivo* with intes-

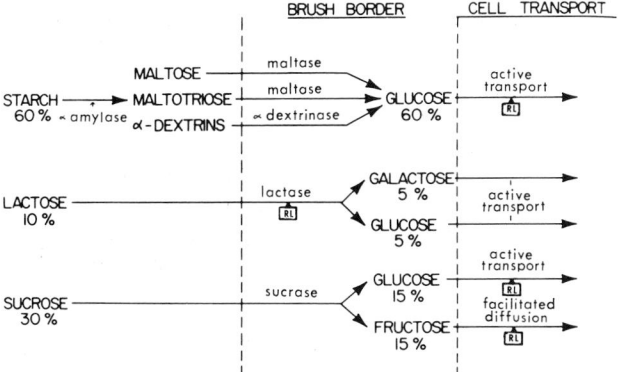

Figure 1. Outline of carbohydrate digestion and absorption in man. Percentages refer to proportion of total carbohydrate in diet; RL locates the rate-limiting step in the overall digestion-absorption process for each carbohydrate ingested. (From Gray, G. M.: Carbohydrate digestion and absorption. Gastroenterology, *58*:96, 1970.)

tinal perfusion methods. The transport of amino acids requires oxygen and sodium. The sodium pump on the basolateral cell membrane of the intestinal epithelial cells maintains an electrical potential across the brush border. Transport of Na$^+$ into the cell is linked to amino acid and oligopeptide movement into the cell.[8] Carrier-mediated active transport is supported by evidence that suggests that certain amino acids exhibit mutual competitive inhibition. Experiments on competitive inhibition of various L-amino acids have suggested several distinct pathways for absorption of amino acids determined by the chemical structure of the amino acids. In normal man, digestion and absorption of protein are usually 80 to 90 per cent completed in the jejunum.

Fat

Although fat emulsification occurs in the stomach, little or no fat digestion occurs except in the small intestine. The entry of gastric chyme into the duodenum is regulated in part by a negative feedback system in which fat in the duodenum inhibits gastric emptying. In the duodenum the dietary fat in the form of triglycerides is mixed with biliary and pancreatic secretions, the important constituents of which are bile salts, pancreatic lipase, and bicarbonate ion.

The naturally occurring bile salts in man are glycine or taurine conjugates of cholic acid, deoxycholic acid, or chenodeoxycholic acid. Bile salts are detergents, being water-soluble at one portion of the molecule and fat-soluble at the other. Such substances tend to produce polymolecular aggregates termed micelles. Bile salt molecules in micelles in biologic solutions are thought to be arranged with the fat-soluble portion of the molecule toward the center of the aggregate and with the water-soluble portion toward the periphery of the aggregate. This phenomenon permits solubilization of lipid in an aqueous environment and causes a micellar solution. Bile salts allow further emulsification to occur, providing an optimal physicochemical environment for the action of pancreatic lipase (Fig. 2). Procolipase is an intraluminal enzyme that is converted to colipase by the action of trypsin. Colipase binds to triglyceride, lipase complexes with colipase, and triglyceride hydrolysis occurs.[5]

Pancreatic lipase catalyzes the hydrolysis of dietary triglyceride into 2-monoglyceride and fatty acids. The 2-monoglyceride and fatty acids then enter the micelles and are held in micellar solution. The bile salt–monoglyceride fatty acid micelle can also solubilize other lipids such as cholesterol, phospholipid, and fat-soluble vitamins. Pancreatic bicarbonate is important in regulating the pH of the intestinal lumen to allow lipase to

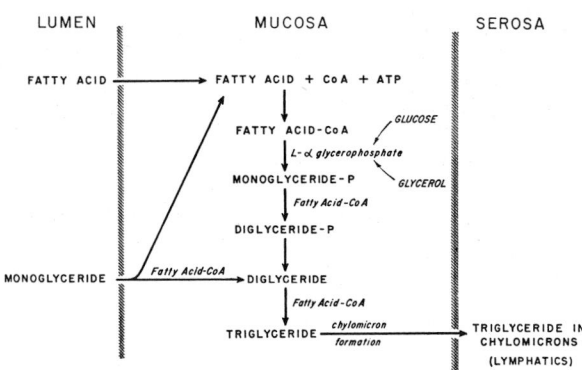

Figure 3. Major biochemical reactions in the transport of long-chain fatty acids and monoglycerides. (From Isselbacher, K J.: Biochemical aspects of lipid malabsorption. Fed. Proc., *26*:1420, 1967.)

function optimally. An alkaline pH favors ionization of fatty acids and bile salts, which increases their solubility in micelles.[18]

An alkaline pH also increases the solubility of bile salts. There are three impediments to the movement of lipids from the intestinal lumen into the absorptive cell: (1) an unstirred water layer, (2) a mucous coat on the brush border, and (3) the lipid bilayer of the brush border membrane. When the micelles encounter the microvilli of the intestinal epithelial cells, the fatty acids and 2-monoglyceride pass into the epithelial cells by a process not requiring energy, probably diffusion.

After entering the epithelial cell, 2-monoglyceride and fatty acids are synthesized into triglyceride in the endoplasmic reticulum. Fatty acid–binding protein participates in the movement of lipid from the brush border to the endoplasmic reticulum. The biosynthesis of triglyceride in the gut may occur by two pathways: (1) the α-glycerophosphate pathway, in which the triglyceride is synthesized from glycerol and fatty acids, and (2) the monoglyceride pathway, in which the triglyceride is formed by the addition of fatty acids to the 1 position of the 2-monoglyceride. The monoglyceride pathway is probably the more important in man (Fig. 3).

After triglyceride synthesis, chylomicrons are formed by triglycerides, phospholipid, cholesterol, cholesterol esters, and protein. Lipoprotein synthesis is necessary for chylomicron formation. Although the lipoprotein content of the chylomicron is relatively small, the various apoproteins are very important in determining subsequent chylomicron metabolism. Chylomicrons pass from the epithelial cells into the lacteals, where they pass through the lymphatics into the venous system (Fig. 4). All

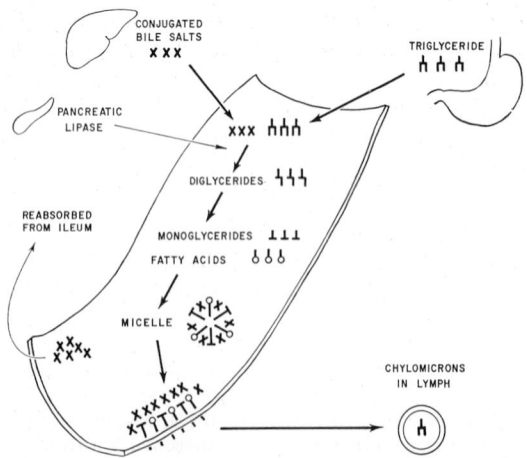

Figure 2. Diagram depicting the intraluminal events in fat absorption. (From Isselbacher, K. J.: Biochemical aspects of lipid malabsorption. Fed. Proc., *26*:1420, 1967.)

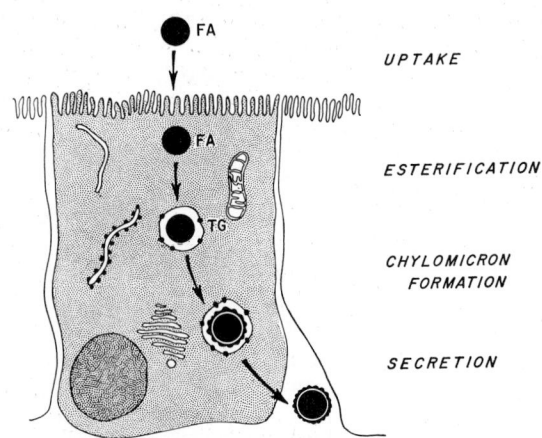

Figure 4. The major steps in the absorption of fat. This diagram depicts the role of the smooth endoplasmic reticulum in esterification and of the rough endoplasmic reticulum in protein synthesis, which is necessary for chylomicron formation. (From Isselbacher, K. J.: Biochemical aspects of lipid malabsorption. Fed. Proc., *26*:1420, 1967.)

long-chain fat is absorbed in the manner just described; however, medium-chain triglyceride (C_8 to C_{10}) may be absorbed without hydrolysis and pass into portal blood, rather than into lymph via chylomicron formation.[1]

Fat is absorbed mainly in the jejunum. Although unconjugated bile acids are absorbed in the jejunum by passive diffusion, the conjugated bile acids that form micelles are absorbed in the ileum by an active transport process. There they are almost completely absorbed and pass via the portal venous blood to the liver, where they are secreted into the bile. Only a small fraction of the total bile salt pool, about 500 to 600 mg., escapes the enterohepatic circulation daily, and this small loss is replaced by hepatic synthesis of bile salts from cholesterol. In a normal adult, the bile acid pool of about 4 to 5 gm. circulates six to eight times daily. Normally, all dietary fat is absorbed and the 5 gm. of fat excreted in the feces daily is derived from desquamated cells and bacteria.

Water and Electrolytes

Large quantities of water are presented to the small intestine. Some water is ingested, but a larger amount is secreted by the digestive glands to provide the appropriate luminal environment for digestion and absorption. It has been estimated that 5 to 10 liters of water enter the small bowel daily, whereas only about 500 ml. or less leave the ileum and enter the colon. The small intestine, therefore, absorbs large quantities of water. Experiments with isotopes reveal that there are simultaneous movements of large quantities of water from intestinal lumen to blood as well as from blood to intestinal lumen. Intestinal absorption is the result of two large oppositely directed fluxes.[37] The net lumen-to-blood flux of water from an isotonic sodium chloride solution containing glucose in the human small intestine is estimated to be 12.7 and 12.1 ml. per hour per cm. in jejunum and ileum, respectively.[10]

The important factors in the movement of water across the intestinal mucosa are diffusion and osmotic filtration caused by osmotic or hydrostatic pressure differences across the membrane. In other words, water absorption follows osmotic gradients established by the active transport of solutes such as sodium ion, glucose, or amino acids into the cells. The intestinal mucosa reacts as if the absorptive cell plasma membrane were penetrated by aqueous channels termed pores.[35,36] These pores allow the transfer of water and water-soluble substances across the lipoidal cell membrane by a process of simple diffusion. The effective pore radii of the jejunum and ileum are estimated to be 7.5 and 3.4 Å, respectively. The small size of the hypothetical pores prevents their identification by electron microscopy. Intestinal absorption cells have on the basolateral cell membrane a sodium pump (Na^+-K^+ATPase) which moves Na^+ out of the cell into the basolateral intercellular space. Movement of K^+ into the cell accompanies the Na^+ movement. The sodium pump produces a concentration gradient that moves Na^+ into the cell from the lumen. This movement by Na^+ by the sodium pump also transports glucose, amino acids, and oligopeptide into the intestinal epithelial cells.[8]

In the human jejunum, sodium ion absorption (net transfer from lumen to blood) (1) occurs against a modest concentration gradient; (2) is dramatically influenced by the rate and direction of water flux; and (3) is stimulated by glucose, galactose, and bicarbonate ions. It appears that in the jejunum a small portion of sodium absorption is mediated by active transport, whereas the major part of jejunal sodium absorption occurs by bulk flow along osmotic gradients. In the jejunum, bicarbonate is effectively absorbed against steep electrochemical gradients. One explanation for this process is that bicarbonate absorption is mediated by H^+ secretion, and the relationship between Na^+ and HCO_3^- transport is explained by an Na^+-H^+ exchange.[36]

The human ileum absorbs Na^+ against steep electrochemical gradients; this absorption is unaffected by water flow and is not stimulated by glucose, galactose, or HCO_3^-. The observations suggest a very efficient Na^+ transport in the ileum. The human ileum also absorbs Cl^- against steep electrochemical gradients. When net ileal Na^+ movement is zero, there is an equimolar exchange of Cl^- and HCO_3^- secretion.[35] It appears that potassium is passively absorbed from the intestine according to its electrochemical gradients.

Calcium is absorbed, particularly in the proximal small intestine (duodenum and jejunum), by a process of active transport. This ion is absorbed better from an acid than from an alkaline environment, which may explain the better absorption in the proximal intestine. Vitamin D and parathyroid hormone enhance calcium absorption.[1]

An important electrolyte absorbed by the small intestine is iron. One of the important functions of the small intestine is the regulation of the body pool of iron. In the individual with normal iron stores, there is only a slight transfer of iron from the intestinal absorptive cell to plasma, and only a small amount of iron enters the mucosal cell from the lumen. In iron deficiency, there is no effective block to the transfer of iron from absorptive cell to plasma and no block to the entry of luminal iron into the mucosal cell.[1]

MOTILITY

There are several types of visible small intestinal muscular activity. The *segmenting contraction* is a localized circumferential contraction of the circular muscle over a length of about 1 cm. of the small intestine. Segmenting contractions divide the luminal content within the area of contraction. Their rhythmic segmenting activity occurs in the proximal small intestine at a rate of approximately 11 contractions per minute and in the distal small intestine at about 9 contractions per minute. Segmenting contractions occurring regularly and rhythmically in adjacent portions of the small intestine divide and subdivide the intestinal content, mixing it and exposing it to larger areas of mucosa, which facilitates digestion and absorption. *Pendular movements* are probably the same or are a minor modification of rhythmic segmentation.

Peristalsis consists of intestinal contractions passing aborally at a rate of 1 to 2 cm. per second through several centimeters of intestine. Peristalsis is somewhat slower in the distal than in the proximal small bowel. The major function of peristalsis is the distal movement of intestinal chyme. Under abnormal circumstances *peristaltic rushes* may occur. Peristaltic rushes usually begin in the proximal small bowel or duodenum and rapidly traverse the entire length of the small intestine. When the peristaltic rush ends, there may be a quiescent period of no motor activity.

The small bowel basal intraluminal pressures are about 8 to 9 cm. H_2O. There are several types of intestinal pressure waves. The Type 1 wave is less than 7½ seconds long, with an amplitude of 15 to 60 cm. H_2O, and is the most common pressure wave observed in man. Type 1 pressure waves generally correlate with segmenting motor activity. The other type of small intestinal pressure wave is the Type 3 wave, which is defined as an elevation of baseline pressures with superimposed Type 1 waves. Type 3 waves last from 10 seconds to 8 minutes and have an amplitude of 5 to 30 cm. H_2O. Type 3 waves have usually been correlated with peristaltic motion.[1]

The Migrating Myoelectrical Complex (MMC)

During the interdigestive period, there are cyclically occurring contractions that move aborally along the intestine. Most of these activity fronts begin in the stomach or duodenum, last about 4½ minutes, and pass along the gut at about 6.8 cm. per min.$^{-1}$. The MMC is thought to sweep or cleanse the intestine during the interdigestive period. Motilin may regulate the MMC.[31]

Regulation of Small Intestinal Motility

MYOGENIC FACTORS. Two types of electrical activity can be recorded from the small intestine. Slow-wave electrical activity begins in the longitudinal muscle layer of the duodenum and is propagated distally. In human adults this activity occurs at 11.7 ± 0.5 (SEM) cycles per minute. This phenomenon, termed the *basic electrical rhythm* (BER), is independent of the intrinsic neural plexuses and is unrelated to motor activity. Intestinal *spike potential* may occur spontaneously during depolarization, or from stretching of the bowel, and is associated with motor activity.

NEUROGENIC FACTORS. Intrinsic neural regulation is initiated by stimulation of the mucosa, or particularly by distention, which causes contraction of longitudinal and circular muscle, propelling luminal content distally. The intrinsic nerve supply regulates, rather than initiates, motor action. In general, sympathetic activity inhibits, whereas parasympathetic activity stimulates, motor function. Epinephrine inhibits small intestinal motor activity, whereas acetylcholine stimulates it. Distention of the small intestine can inhibit small intestinal motility by the intestinointestinal inhibitory reflex. Distention of the ureter, renal pelvis, or biliary system or peritoneal irritation may inhibit intestinal movements.[1]

HORMONAL FACTORS. Gastrointestinal hormones may have an important role in regulating intestinal motility. Gastrin stimulates gastric and intestinal motility and relaxes the ileocecal sphincter. Cholecystokinin-pancreozymin (CCK-PZ) also stimulates intestinal motility and may decrease intestinal transit time. Secretin and chemically similar glucagon inhibit intestinal motility. The role of hormones in regulating intestinal motility is poorly understood.

ENDOCRINE FUNCTION OF THE SMALL INTESTINE

The mucosa of the small intestine is an important source of peptide hormones, the main function of which is the regulation of the gastrointestinal tract.[15]

SECRETIN. Secretin was the first gastrointestinal hormone described. This hormone, a helical polypeptide with 27 amino acid residues, is released from duodenal mucosal S cells in response to intraluminal H^+. Secretin promotes digestion by stimulating copious water and bicarbonate secretion from the pancreas. This action facilitates entry of pancreatic enzymes into the intestinal lumen and provides a pH favoring digestion of fat. Secretin is also a choleretic and in addition inhibits gastric acid secretion and gastrointestinal motility.

CHOLECYSTOKININ-PANCREOZYMIN (CCK-PZ). Cholecystokinin and pancreozymin are the same substance, which is released from intestinal mucosal I cells bathed by amino acids or fatty acids. CCK-PZ facilitates digestion and absorption by stimulating emptying of the gallbladder as well as by increasing bile flow and relaxing the sphincter of Oddi. Another important action of CCK-PZ is stimulation of pancreatic enzyme secretion. CCK-PZ is a linear polypeptide having 33 residues. The C-terminal tetrapeptide of CCK-PZ is identical to that of another gastrointestinal hormone, gastrin, and this fragment possesses the action of both hormones. In general, CCK-PZ and gastrin share actions and differ mainly in potency for a specific action.

NEWER GUT HORMONES. During the past several years, the intestinal mucosa has been recognized as a source of several biologically active peptides. All of these substances do not satisfy rigid physiologic criteria for hormone status but should be described briefly here. *Enteroglucagon* is released from the enteroglucagon (EG) cells occurring predominantly in the distal small intestine. This peptide occurs in two forms: one with a molecular weight of about 3500 and another larger molecule. Enteroglucagon is released by carbohydrate and long-chain fatty acid and inhibits intestinal motility. *Vasoactive intestinal peptide* (VIP) is a member of the secretin-glucagon family of peptides and is found in high concentration in bowel, brain, and peripheral nerve tissue. VIP shares some actions with secretin and glucagon. Blood levels of VIP do not change following meals; so VIP may act as a neurotransmitter or paracrine substance, rather than as a hormone. *Gastric inhibitory polypetide* (GIP) is also a secretin-glucagon–like peptide with 43 amino acids and a molecular weight of about 51000. GIP is released from K cells, predominantly in the jejunum, on stimulation by carbohydrate or fat. Serum GIP concentration increases after meals, and it is believed that its most significant action is to stimulate insulin secretion. *Motilin* is a 22-residue peptide with a molecular weight of about 2700 that is released from the EC cells of the intestine, predominantly the jejunum. Motilin inhibits gastric emptying in man and may also alter the interdigestive myoelectrical complex and cause changes in the lower esophageal sphincter. *Somatostatin*, a tetradecapeptide, was recognized for its growth hormone release–inhibiting characteristics and has subsequently been shown to inhibit release of many hormones. Somatostatin is found in brain, stomach, gut, and pancreas and is probably a paracrine substance. *Bombesin* may be secreted from the small bowel mucosa; and although it possesses several actions, its most important function appears to be stimulation of gastric acid secretion and antral gastrin release.

IMMUNOLOGIC FUNCTION OF THE INTESTINE

The intestine is a source of immunoglobulin, particularly IgA.[34] It is believed that this immunoglobulin arises from plasma cells in the lamina propria and, after linkage with a protein synthesized by epithelial cells, is secreted into the lumen. Secretory IgA contains antibody activities, the exact roles of which are not yet known.

For references, see page 842.

III

INTESTINAL OBSTRUCTION

R. Scott Jones, M.D.

HISTORICAL ASPECTS

Intestinal obstruction was observed and treated by Hippocrates. The earliest recorded operation for intestinal obstruction was probably performed by Praxagoras (350 B.C.), who created an enterocutaneous fistula to relieve the obstruction. However, nonoperative treatment remained the general practice, including reduction of hernias, opium for pain, orally administered mercury or lead shot in an endeavor to open the occluded bowel, electrical stimulation, and gastric lavage.

In the nineteenth century, amid considerable debate, surgical therapy became more frequently employed for intestinal obstruction. Most of the significant advances in the management of this disorder were made after the turn of the twentieth century. Hartwell and Hoguet[16] observed in 1912 that parenteral administration of saline solution prolonged the lives of dogs with intestinal obstruction, and this has become a cardinal principle of the management of intestinal obstruction today. In the second decade of the twentieth century radiographic techniques in the diagnosis of intestinal obstruction were developed. In the 1930s nasogastric or intestinal tubes were employed to prevent or relieve intestinal distention in patients with intestinal obstruction. Antibiotics were added to the therapy of bowel obstruction in the 1940s and 1950s. Fluid replacement, intestinal decompression, antibiotics, and improvements in surgical and anesthetic techniques have reduced mortality in simple intestinal obstruction; however, the recognition and treatment of strangulating intestinal obstruction remain important problems for surgeons today.[39]

ETIOLOGY

When gastrointestinal luminal content is pathologically prevented from passing distally, intestinal obstruction exists. Intestinal obstruction may be caused by mechanical occlusion of the bowel lumen, i.e., *mechanical obstruction,* or by paralysis of the intestinal muscle, i.e., *paralytic ileus.*

MECHANICAL OBSTRUCTION. Three types of abnormalities may produce mechanical obstruction.[24,30]

1. *Obturation of the intestinal lumen* may be caused by several diseases, such as polypoid tumors of the bowel. Intussusception is an invagination of the bowel lumen with the invaginated portion (the intussusceptum) passing distally into the ensheathing outer portion (the intussuscipiens) by peristalsis. This process occludes the blood supply of the intussusceptum. In adults, intussusception is usually caused by an abnormality of the bowel wall, such as a tumor or Meckel's diverticulum; however, in infants and children intussusception may ocur without apparent anatomic cause. Obturation obstruction may be caused by large gallstones, which can enter the intestinal lumen via a cholecystoenteric fistula. This causes a rare condition — gallstone ileus.

Feces, meconium, or bezoars may obstruct the intestine. Bezoars occur more frequently in children, the mentally retarded, and the toothless and in patients after gastrectomy.

2. *Intrinsic bowel lesions* producing intestinal obstruction are often congenital (atresia, stenosis, duplication), are seen most commonly in infants and small children, and are described in the chapter on pediatric surgery. Strictures of the intestine may follow neoplasms, as in carcinoma of the sigmoid colon, or inflammation, as in Crohn's disease. Rarely, one encounters iatrogenic strictures after intestinal anastomosis, after radiation therapy, or after treatment with enteric-coated potassium chloride tablets.

3. *Lesions extrinsic to the bowel* are important causes of intestinal obstruction. Occlusion of the intestine by adhesions from previous surgical procedures or inflammation is the leading cause of small intestinal obstruction. Adhesions may produce obstruction by kinking or angulation or by creating bands of tissue that compress the bowel. External hernias are second only to adhesions as a cause of mechanical small intestinal obstruction. Inguinal, femoral, umbilical, and incisional hernias are important causes of bowel obstruction. The risk of intestinal obstruction is the principal reason for the elective repair of hernias. Internal hernias due to congenital abnormalities of the mesentery or to surgical defects in the mesentery occasionally cause bowel obstruction. Extrinsic masses such as neoplasms and abscesses may cause mechanical bowel obstruction. A volvulus is an extrinsic abnormality in which a portion of the alimentary canal rotates or twists about itself, the twist usually involving the blood supply of the twisted portion of the bowel. This abnormality causes kinking of the gut, producing mechanical obstruction, frequently with occlusion of the blood supply to the bowel. A volvulus is usually associated with some underlying abnormality; for example, midgut volvulus is caused by the mesenteric abnormality of malrotation. Cecal volvulus occurs when the cecum or right colon is on a mesentery, rather than being retroperitoneal. Sigmoid volvulus develops when the sigmoid colon is abnormally long or redundant. Another type of volvulus occurs when adhesions fix the intestine to a point that acts as a pivot for the volvulus. The most common causes of intestinal obstruction in adults are adhesions, usually following previous surgery; hernias; and neoplasms. Neoplasms are the most common cause of colon obstruction.

PARALYTIC ILEUS. Paralytic ileus is a common disorder, occurring to some extent in most patients undergoing abdominal surgery. This abnormality is caused by several neural, humoral, and metabolic factors. There are reflexes that inhibit intestinal motility, such as the intestinointestinal reflex following prolonged intestinal distention. Distention of other organs, such as the ureter, can inhibit intestinal motility. Spinal fracture, retroperitoneal hemorrhage, or trauma may also be associated with paralytic ileus. A humoral factor in paralytic ileus is suggested by experiments in dogs in which motility of transplanted (denervated) intestinal loops was inhibited during experimental peritonitis.[20] The substances responsible for this phenomenon are unknown. Clinically, peritonitis is associated with paralytic ileus. Electrolyte imbalances, particularly hypokalemia, contribute to paralytic ileus by interfering with the normal ionic movements during smooth muscle contraction. Finally, ischemia of the intestine rapidly inhibits motility.

IDIOPATHIC INTESTINAL PSEUDO-OBSTRUCTION. It should be emphasized that most patients with gaseous distention of the intestine have either mechanical intestinal obstruction or paralytic ileus. In the majority of patients with ileus, the disorder can be readily ascribed to peritonitis, metabolic disturbances, or drugs. Idiopathic intestinal pseudo-obstruction is a chronic illness characterized by symptoms of recurrent intestinal obstruction without demonstrable mechanical occlusion of the bowel. Patients with this disease have impaired motor response to intestinal distention, but the duodenal and colonic slow waves may be normal. Some patients have aperistalsis of the esophagus with failure of the lower esophageal sphincter to relax. Although heredity may have a role in this disorder, there is controversy over whether the disease is due primarily to abnormalities of the intramural nerve plexuses or to abnormalities of the intestinal smooth muscle. The symptoms of intestinal pseudo-obstruction are cramping abdominal pain, vomiting, distention, diarrhea, and sometimes steatorrhea. Physical examination reveals abdominal distention. Intestinal pseudo-obstruction is distinguished from mechanical intestinal obstruction by the absence of the radiographic findings of mechanical obstruction. If the diagnosis can be established with certainty, treatment should be conservative and surgical intervention should be avoided. Intravenous hyperalimentation has been reported to be successful in the management of these patients.[11]

PATHOGENESIS

SIMPLE MECHANICAL SMALL INTESTINAL OBSTRUCTION. Mechanical obstruction of the small intestine causes accumulation of fluid and gas proximal to the obstruction, producing *distention* of the intestine. Distention is initiated by ingested fluid, digestive secretions, and intestinal gas. As mentioned earlier, large volumes of saliva, gastric secretion, bile, and pancreatic juice enter the gut daily. The stomach has a very small capacity for fluid absorption; so most alimentary fluid is absorbed by the small intestine.[38]

Intestinal gas normally is propelled aborally by peristalsis and is expelled from the rectum as flatus. Gas accumulating in the intestine proximal to an obstruction originates from (1) swallowed air, (2) carbon dioxide from neutralization of bicarbonate, and (3) organic gases from bacterial fermentation. Swallowed air is the most important source of gas in intestinal obstruction because its nitrogen content is very high and nitrogen is not absorbed by the intestinal mucosa. As a result, the intestinal gas is predominantly (70 per cent) nitrogen. Large quantities of carbon dioxide are produced in the lumen of the gut, but this gas is readily absorbed and therefore contributes little to the distention of intestinal obstruction.

One of the most important events during simple mechanical small bowel obstruction is loss of water and electrolytes from the body, caused mainly by intestinal distention. First, reflex vomiting may follow intestinal distention. In addition, intestinal distention is self-perpetuating in the obstructed small bowel, since distention increases intestinal secretion. Experiments on dogs demonstrate that intestinal distention initially causes decreased absorption (decreased lumen-to-blood flux of water) and may subsequently cause increased secretion (increased blood-to-lumen flux of water) in the obstructed segment, but not in the intestine distal to the obstruction.[32] This phenomenon leads to increased fluid accumulation in the bowel proximal to the obstruction, which may further accentuate dehydration and cause further intestinal distention, which proceeds proximally. Increased secretion in the obstructed bowel has also been demonstrated in man.[40]

The metabolic results of fluid loss in simple mechanical obstruction of the small bowel depend upon the site and the duration of the obstruction. Proximal small bowel obstruction causes relatively greater vomiting and less intestinal distention than distal obstruction. Proximal obstruction causes losses of water, Na^+, Cl^-, H^+, and K^+, producing dehydration with hypochloremia, hypokalemia, and metabolic alkalosis. Distal small bowel obstruction may entail loss of large quantities of fluid into the bowel; however, the abnormalities of serum electrolyte values are usually less dramatic, probably because hydrochloric acid losses are less.[22]

Accompanying dehydration are oliguria, azotemia, and hemoconcentration. If dehydration persists, circulatory changes such as tachycardia, low central venous pressure, and reduced cardiac output may lead to hypotension and hypovolemic shock. Other sequelae of the intestinal distention may be increased intra-abdominal pressure, impeding venous return from the legs and elevation of the diaphragm sufficient to impair ventilation.

Rapid proliferation of intestinal bacteria occurs during intestinal obstruction. Normally the small intestine contains very small quantities of bacteria and may be almost sterile. There may be several causes for the sparse bacterial population of the small intestine, but normal peristalsis with continued aboral progression of luminal content is important in minimizing the small intestinal flora. During small intestinal stasis, whatever the cause, bacteria proliferate rapidly, and this phenomenon is particularly notable in intestinal obstruction. The small intestinal contents thus become "feculent" during obstruction because of large quantities of bacteria. Normally the colon, an organ functioning as a reservoir, contains large numbers of bacteria.

The bacteria in the small intestine probably have no role in the ill effects of simple mechanical small intestinal obstruction, since the bacteria or bacterial toxins do not cross the normal intestinal mucosa.

STRANGULATION OBSTRUCTION. Strangulation develops when the circulation to the obstructed intestine is impaired. The circulation to the bowel may be impaired by sustained increased intraluminal pressure. Closed-loop obstruction occurs when the bowel lumen is occluded at two points along its length. This type of obstruction may proceed more rapidly to strangulation than simple obstruction. Pressure necrosis can develop if the obstructed distending bowel is held by unyielding adhesive bands or hernial rings. The mesenteric vessels can be occluded by deformity or twisting of the mesentery, as in volvulus or intussusception. In strangulation obstruction, the patient may suffer all of the ill effects of simple obstruction in addition to the effects of strangulation. Strangulation causes loss of blood and plasma from the strangulated segment, which may be particularly severe if the vascular obstruction is predominantly venous. This loss of blood and plasma causes shock, particularly if the patient is already dehydrated. If strangulation produces gangrene, peritonitis with its sequelae occurs. Rupture or perforation of a strangulated segment is possible and is a devastating complication.

In addition to the loss of blood and plasma, another important factor in strangulation obstruction is the toxic material from the strangulated loop. The luminal fluid from a strangulated intestinal loop and the bloody, malodorous peritoneal fluid are lethal when administered to normal animals. Bacteria and necrotic tissue appear to be necessary for the development of the toxic fluid. Apparently this lethal fluid is formed in the lumen of the strangulated intestine and passes through the intestinal wall when the gut is injured by distention, vascular compromise, and bacteria. The toxic material is absorbed from the peritoneal cavity, producing systemic effects.[22] Animal experiments show that antibiotics prolong the lives of animals with experimentally introduced strangulation obstruction. The efficacy of antibiotics in humans with intestinal obstruction has not been demonstrated as clearly.

COLON OBSTRUCTION. In general, colon obstruction produces less fluid and electrolyte disturbance than mechanical small bowel obstruction. If the patient has a "competent" ileocecal valve, there may be little or no small bowel distention, but in this instance the colon behaves as a closed loop. When the colon is massively distended by gas, it may perforate, and in this situation, because of its spherical shape and large diameter, the cecum is a likely site for perforation. However, the most common cause of colon obstruction is cancer, and the usual site of perforation is adjacent to the cancer. In patients with "incompetent" ileocecal valves, signs of small bowel distention may accompany colon obstruction. The colon is also subject to strangulation when obstruction compromises the blood supply.

DIAGNOSIS OF INTESTINAL OBSTRUCTION

The questions to ask in evaluating a patient suspected of having intestinal obstruction are as follows: (1) Does the patient have bowel obstruction? (2) If so, where is it? (3) What is the anatomic and pathologic nature of the obstructing lesions? (4) Has strangulation occurred? (5) What is the general condition of the patient (fluid-electrolyte balance, other systemic disease, and so forth)?

The syndrome of intestinal obstruction is characterized by abdominal pain, vomiting, obstipation, abdominal distention, and failure to pass flatus. The pain in intestinal obstruction is typically crampy, with paroxysms occurring at 4- to 5-minute intervals in proximal obstruction and less frequently in distal obstruction. After a longer period of mechanical obstruction, the crampy pain may subside because motility may be inhibited by bowel distention. When crampy abdominal pain is succeeded by continuous severe abdominal pain, strangulation with peritonitis should be suspected.

In patients with proximal intestinal obstruction, vomiting may be profuse and unassociated with abdominal distention. In distal obstruction, the vomiting is less frequent and may be "feculent" because of the large bacterial population of intestinal contents. Obstipation and failure to pass gas from the rectum are characteristic of complete obstruction, but are evident only after the bowel distal to the obstruction has been evacuated. Increase in abdominal girth, due to accumulation of fluid and gas in the intestine, is often noted by patients with distal small bowel obstruction, colon obstruction, or paralytic ileus.

PHYSICAL EXAMINATION. A complete physical examination is indicated, but particular attention should be given to certain points. Tachycardia and hypotension may indicate severe dehydration, peritonitis, or both. Fever suggests the possibility of strangulation. The status of hydration should be estimated by examination of skin turgor and moisture of the mucous membrane. The abdomen is usually distended. Occasionally the examiner must determine whether abdominal distention is due to bowel obstruction or ascites. Ascites is characterized by a fluid wave, shifting dullness, and fullness in the flanks. Peristaltic waves characteristic of small bowel obstruction are sometimes visible through the abdominal wall of thin patients with long-standing obstruction. Surgical scars should be noted because of the etiologic implication of previous surgical procedures; for example, the presence of adhesions or cancer. Incarcerated hernias may be obscure, particularly in obese patients. Abdominal masses (neoplasm, intussusception, abscess) should be sought. Abdominal tenderness is a characteristic finding in patients with intestinal obstruction; however, localized tenderness, rebound tenderness, and guarding suggest peritonitis and the likelihood of strangulation.

Abdominal auscultation in patients with mechanical intestinal obstruction usually reveals periods of increasing or crescendoing bowel sounds separated by relatively quiet periods. The quality of bowel sounds in intestinal obstruction is usually high-pitched, tinkling, or musical in character.

Rectal examination should be done to detect luminal masses. The presence or absence of feces should be noted, and if feces are present, examination for occult blood should be done. Blood in the feces suggests an alimentary mucosal lesion, as may occur with cancer, intussusception, or infarction. Sigmoidoscopic examination should be done if colon obstruction is suspected.

Acute intestinal obstruction can usually be diagnosed on the basis of history and physical examination. Any patient having crampy abdominal pain, vomiting, obstipation, abdominal distention, abdominal tenderness, and peristaltic rushes should be considered to have intestinal obstruction until that diagnosis can be confidently excluded.

RADIOLOGIC EXAMINATION. Radiographs are essential to confirm the clinical diagnosis and to define more accurately the site of obstruction.[12] Abdominal radiographic examination

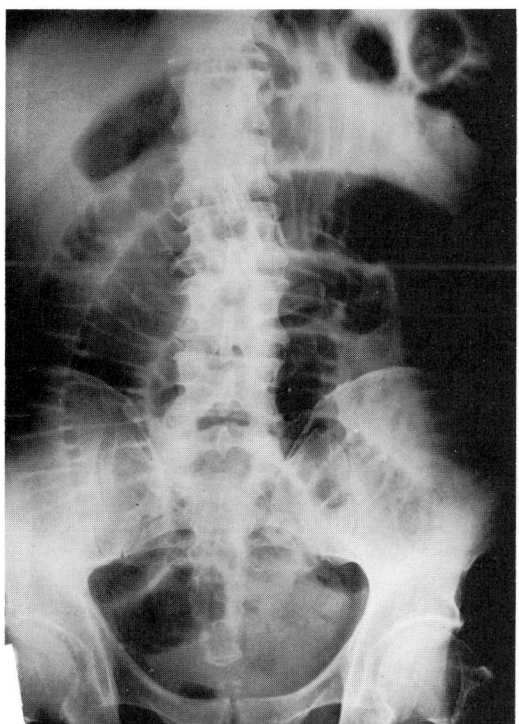
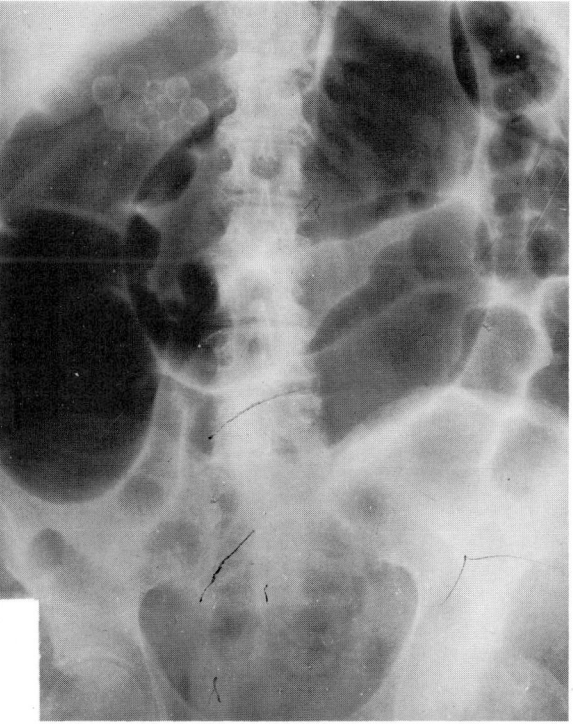

Figure 1. The illustration on the left shows the centrally located loops and clearly depicts the valvulae conniventes, both of which are typical of distended small intestine. On the right the haustral markings and the tendency toward peripheral gas accumulaton typical of colon distention are seen. This patient incidentally had multiple radiopaque gallstones.

of patients with intestinal obstruction usually reveals abnormally large quantities of gas in the bowel. One can usually determine whether small intestine, colon, or both are distended (Fig. 1). Gas in the small bowel outlines the valvulae conniventes, which usually occupy the entire transverse diameter of the bowel image. Colonic haustral markings, however, occupy only a portion of the transverse diameter of the bowel. Typically, the small bowel pattern occupies the more central portions of the abdomen (Fig. 2), whereas the colon shadow is on the periphery of the abdominal film or in the pelvis. Patients with mechanical intestinal obstruction usually have minimal or no colonic gas. Radiographs of patients who have colon obstruction with a competent ileocecal valve show colon distention but little small bowel gas. Patients with colon obstruction and incompetent ileocecal valves usually have radiographic evidence of small bowel and colon distention. Films taken in the upright or lateral decubitus position in patients with mechanical small bowel obstruction usually show multiple gas-fluid levels, with distended bowel resembling an inverted U (Fig. 3). Occasionally, ordinary films fail to distinguish colonic from small intestinal obstruction, and it may be valuable to administer a radiographic contrast agent. Probably the safest and quickest way to distinguish colonic from small bowel obstruction preoperatively is by a carefully performed barium enema study.

It is often difficult radiographically to distinguish paralytic ileus from mechanical obstruction. One radiographic feature of paralytic ileus is that gaseous distention occurs somewhat uniformly in the stomach, small bowel, and colon (Fig. 4). Gas-fluid levels may be seen in paralytic ileus. Examination after a barium meal may assist in distinguishing between paralytic ileus and mechanical obstruction but should be avoided if colon obstruction cannot be excluded. Considerable attention has been directed toward the fact that if the clinical symptoms indicate intestinal obstruction, reliance should not be placed upon abdominal films, because in a number of instances these may appear to be within normal limits at a time when the patient has strangulation obstruction.[13]

LABORATORY TESTS. Any patient with vomiting or evidence of intra-abdominal fluid loss who is suspected of having intestinal obstruction should have laboratory measurements of serum sodium, chloride, potassium, bicarbonate, and creatinine. The hematocrit, white blood cell count, and serum electrolytes should be measured serially to assess adequacy of therapy and to detect the earliest evidence of tissue necrosis.

TREATMENT OF INTESTINAL OBSTRUCTION

In most cases, the appropriate treatment for intestinal obstruction includes surgical relief of the obstruction.[25] Since severe metabolic derangements may accompany bowel obstruction, the decision of when to operate requires careful judgment. The overlapping sequence of events in managing patients with intestinal obstruction should be investigation, resuscitation, and operation. The timing of operation depends upon three factors: (1) duration of obstruction, i.e., severity of fluid, electrolyte, and acid-base abnormalities; (2) improvement of vital organ function — e.g., in the elderly patient with cardiac disease, rapid preoperative digitalization may be helpful; and (3) consideration of the risk of strangulation.[23] Mortality from intestinal obstruction with intestinal gangrene is 4.5 per cent[33] to 31 per cent[25]; whereas in simple mechanical obstruction, when operation is done within 24 hours, mortality is approximately 1 per cent.[30] Because there is no reliable way to detect strangulation preoperatively, operation should be performed as soon as is reasonable. One study suggested that an *absence* of fever, tachycardia, localized tenderness, and leukocytosis indicates a situation in which conservative observation may be safe. However, the presence of *any one or more* of these findings mandates early operative intervention.[33]

A patient with symptoms of short duration, 24 to 30 hours, with minimal metabolic disturbances and no preexisting pulmonary, cardiac, or renal disease, can be operated upon when the diagnosis is made. An elderly patient in whom fluid and electrolyte imbalance develops after several days of illness may profit from 18 to 24 hours of preoperative preparation.

Patients with bowel obstruction are likely to be depleted of

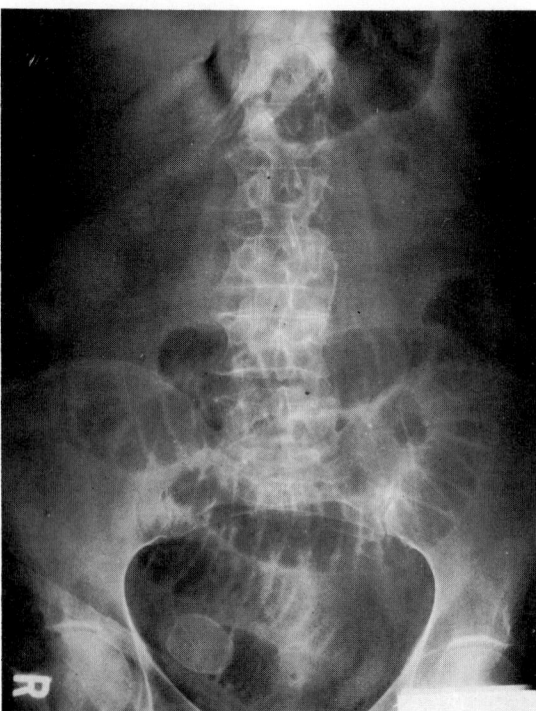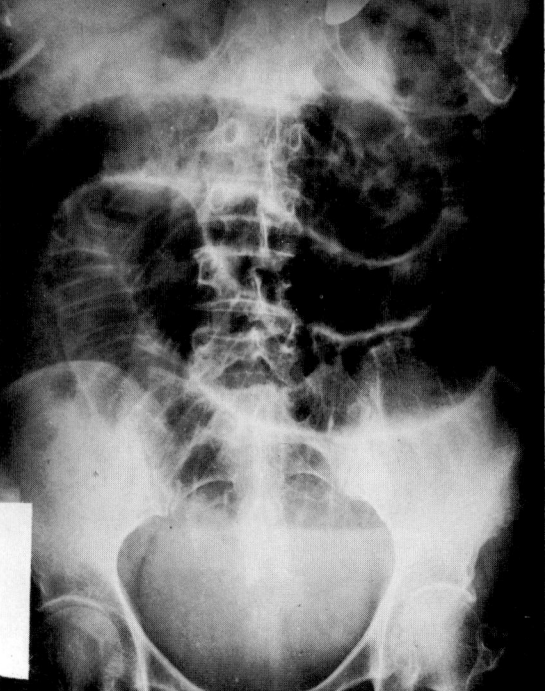

Figure 2. Gallstone ileus is an uncommon cause of intestinal obstruction but often can be diagnosed from plain films when present. The film on the left show complete mechanical smal bowel obstruction caused by a radiopaque gallstone in the right lower abdomen. The film on the right is from another patient with gallstone ileus due to a radiolucent gallstone. The diagnosis was suggested by the presence of gas in the biliary tract.

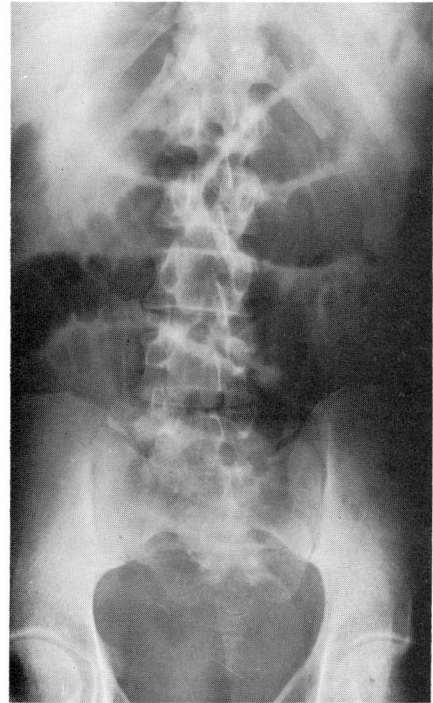
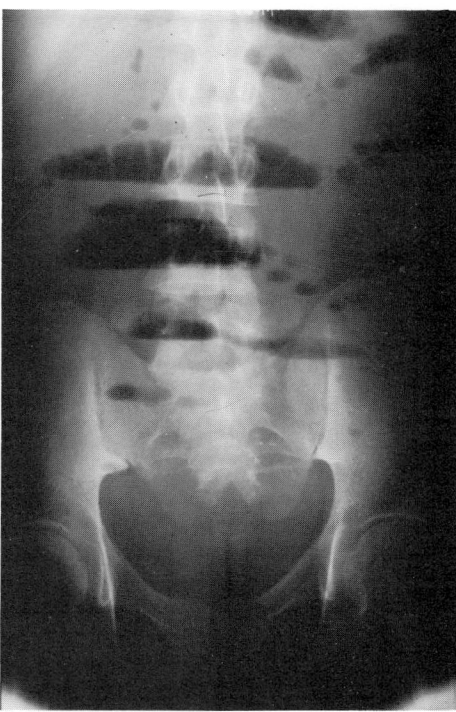

Figure 3. Supine (left upper), upright (right upper), and occasionally lateral decubitus (lower) films usually confirm the diagnosis of acute complete mechanical smal bowel obstruction by revealing distended small bowel loops, gas-fluid levels, inverted U-shaped loops, and the absence of gas in the colon or rectum.

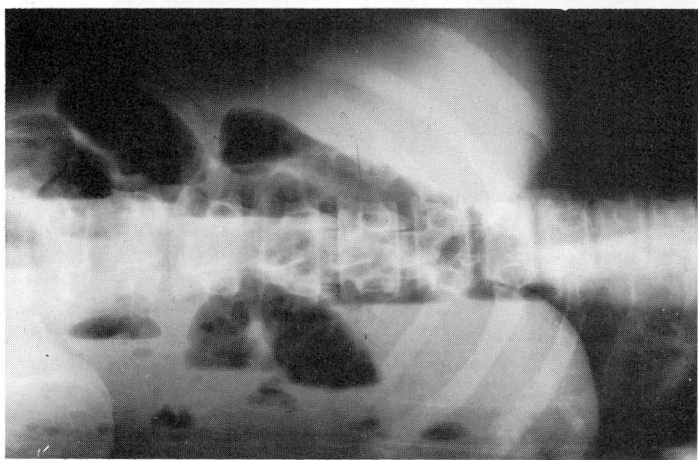

water, sodium, chloride, and potassium, so that intravenous therapy should usually begin with an intravenous isotonic sodium chloride solution. After adequate urine formation is observed, potassium chloride should be added to the infusion. Sufficient fluid should be given to elevate and maintain the central venous pressure to between 5 and 10 cm. of saline. Administration of blood, plasma, or both should be considered if the patient is in shock and if strangulation is suspected. After pulse, blood pressure, central venous pressure, and urinary output are normal, operation may be considered. If marked hemoconcentration and severe electrolyte imbalance were present initially, laboratory studies should be repeated, and if the values are returning to normal, the patient should be operated upon. Antibiotics should be given during the period of resuscitation, particularly if strangulation is suspected.

In addition to fluid therapy, another important adjunct to the supportive care of patients with intestinal obstruction is nasogastric or intestinal suction.[38] Nasogastric suction with a Levin tube empties the stomach, reducing the hazard of pulmonary aspiration of vomitus, as well as minimizing further intestinal distention from swallowed air during the preoperative period. A nasogastric tube is not effective in decompressing distended intestine, and for that reason, long intestinal tubes, such as the Miller-Abbott tube, are often passed through the nostril with the tip of the tube placed in the pyloric antrum. It is usually necessary to position the tube fluoroscopically, and in some patients intubation of the small intestine may be very difficult. When the small bowel is successfully intubated, the tube should be allowed to pass distally, on suction, to deflate the bowel. The principal hazard of the use of long intestinal tubes in small bowel obstruction is that it may delay operative treatment in patients with unsuspected strangulation obstruction. Operation for intestinal obstruction should generally not be delayed if the bowel is not successfully intubated or decompressed preoperatively.

There is controversy concerning the urgency for early operation in patients thought to have partial small bowel obstruction due to adhesions. Some studies reveal that the majority of patients with partial adhesive small bowel obstruction had complete resolution with nasogastric suction, and most patients so treated responded within 24 hours.[3,6,26] Patients with intestinal obstruction due to intra-abdominal cancer usually do not respond well to conservative treatment, but malignant obstruction can frequently be relieved surgically. Judgment is required, however, in managing malignant intestinal obstruction in the terminally ill patient.[3] Certain patients with small bowel ob-

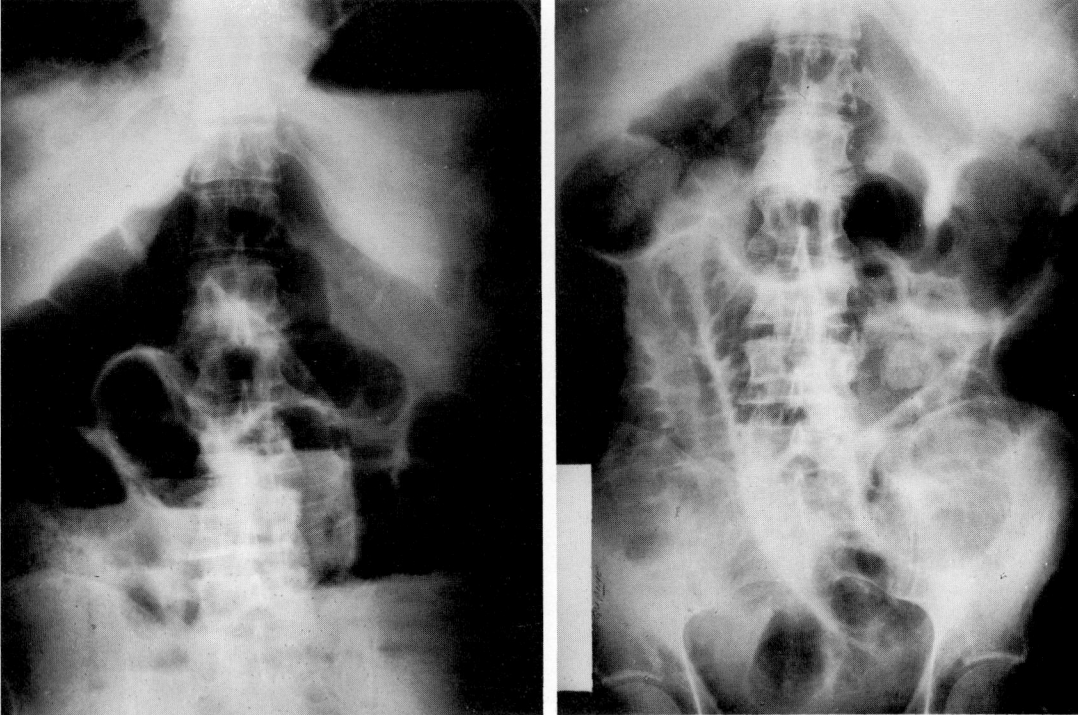

Figure 4. Paralytic ileus is usually difficult to distinguish from mechanical obstruction. The presence of gas in stomach, small bowel, and colon suggests ileus, as shown in these films.

struction should undergo operation within several hours of admission to the hospital. This includes patients with no history of previous abdominal surgery, patients with incarcerated external hernias, patients with signs of peritonitis, and any patient with a suspected strangulated bowel.[2]

Operation may be delayed under the following circumstances: (1) In patients with pyloric obstruction, operation can be postponed safely until the fluid and electrolyte imbalance is completely corrected. (2) The patient in whom intestinal obstruction develops in the period immediately following an abdominal operation initially may be treated conservatively.[27] Overlooked strangulation is, however, a risk in this instance. In one report of 41 patients with early postoperative bowel obstruction, obstruction in 30 patients resolved without operation; however, 2 of those successfully treated patients later required operation for bowel obstruction.[29] (3) Infants with ileocecal intussusception may be managed by hydrostatic reduction of the intussusception, which avoids operation entirely. Adults with intussusception (Fig. 5) should be operated upon because of the high frequency of underlying causes for the intussusception. (4) In patients with sigmoid volvulus, decompression can be performed wth a sigmoidoscope or a colonoscope, but elective operation should be performed later to prevent recurrent volvulus. (5) In patients with intestinal obstruction due to an acute exacerbation of Crohn's disease, a period of conservative treatment may permit resolution of the obstruction. (6) Patients with chronic partial obstruction may be managed by less urgent operative treatment than patients with acute mechanical obstruction.

Operative Treatment for Intestinal Obstruction

In general, the four commonly used approaches to management of intestinal obstruction are determined by the nature of the problem: (1) In simple obstruction, i.e., an incarcerated inguinal hernia, reduction of the hernia suffices, or obstruction caused by peritoneal adhesions can be relieved by division of these structures. (2) A second approach to obstructing lesions is the creation of an intestinal bypass. An example of this therapy

is the treatment of obstructing carcinoma of the cecum by ileo-transverse colon anastomosis. (3) The placement of an entero-cutaneous fistula, such as a colostomy, proximal to the obstruction is a standard form of therapy. (4) Excision of a lesion with restoration of intestinal continuity is used frequently. An example of this therapy is the treatment of obstructing carcinomas of the cecum by right colectomy and ileotransverse colon anastomosis.

With few exceptions, operation for intestinal obstruction should be performed under general anesthesia administered with an endotracheal tube. One of the risks in operating on patients with intestinal obstruction is vomiting and tracheo-bronchial aspiration of the feculent vomitus.

In the absence of external hernia in patients with small bowel obstruction, abdominal exploration should be performed through a midline vertical incision. The obstructed point can be located by following distended bowel distally until collapsed intestine is found. The operative manipulation of obstructed intestine is easier if the intestine has been decompressed preoperatively. It may be desirable to empty the distended bowel during the operation. This can frequently be accomplished by passing an intestinal tube into the intestine at operation.

In operating on patients with multiple intra-abdominal adhesions, the surgeon should be certain that there are no additional sites of obstruction distal to that which is clinically obvious. One may want to express manually the luminal contents into the cecum to exclude other possible distal obstructing points.

It is often difficult to determine whether a segment of bowel is viable. The criteria generally used in determining bowel viability are (1) color, (2) motility, and (3) arterial pulsation. If intestinal viability is questionable, the bowel segment should be completely released and placed in a saline-moistened sponge for 15 to 20 minutes and then re-examined. If normal color has returned and peristalsis is evident, it is safe to retain the bowel. If there is reasonable doubt of the bowel's viability, it should be resected.

The approach to colon obstruction is somewhat different from that to small bowel obstruction. The classic method of

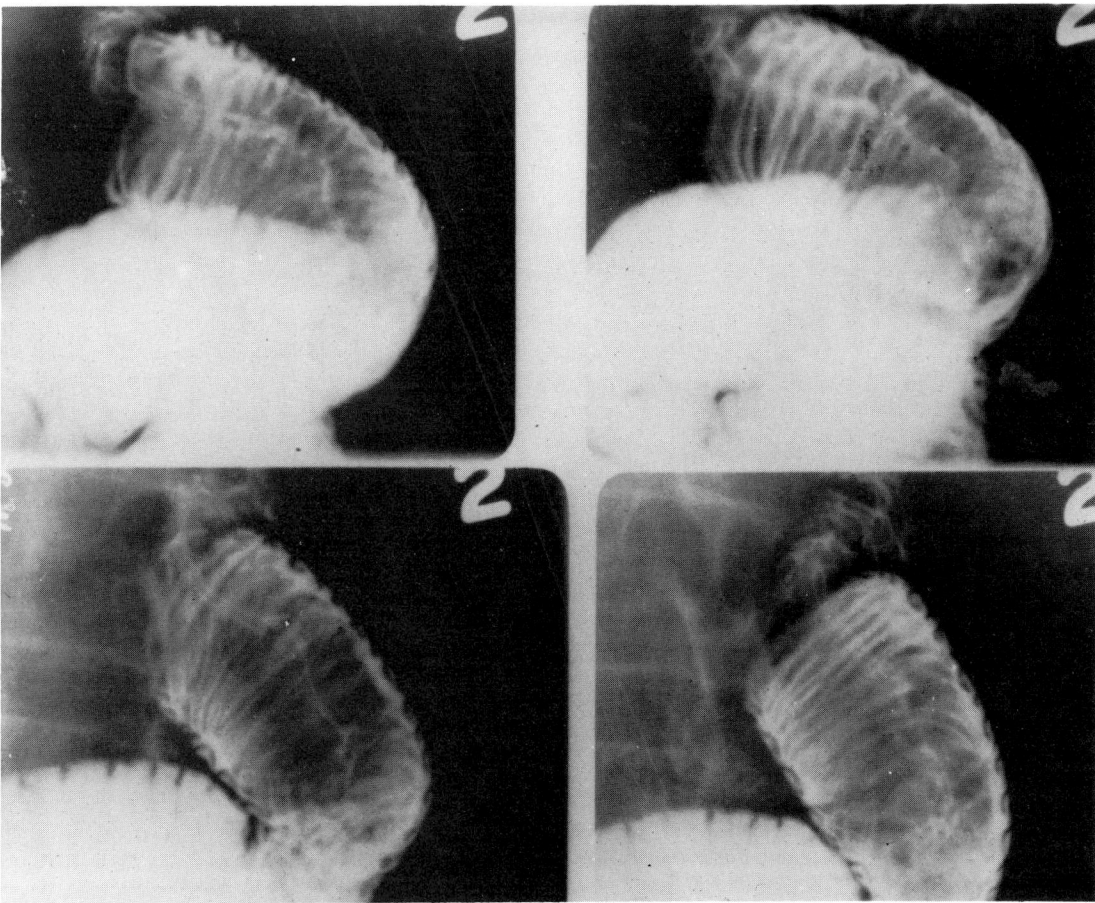

Figure 5. This series of spot films reveals an ileoileal intussusception in an adult.

treating obstruction of the left colon entails three separate operative steps: (1) relief of gaseous distention by colostomy proximal to the obstruction; (2) removal of the diseased segment of colon and anastomosis, leaving the colostomy intact; and (3) closure of the colostomy when healing of the anastomosis is complete. It would also be appropriate to resect the obstructing lesion and to perform a colostomy at one operation and to close the colostomy during a second subsequent operation. The staged procedure is performed for the following reasons: (1) Intestinal obstruction and its sequelae are a significant and immediate threat to life that should be eliminated as simply as possible. Colon resection may be a formidable operation and is more safely performed electively. (2) Surgical anastomosis of distended colon is hazardous. A technically excellent colon anastomosis cannot be made with distended, thin-walled bowel filled with fluid and feces. Colostomies can be performed where the colon is mobile with a mesentery, such as in sigmoid or transverse colon. In most instances, transverse colostomy is the best choice in treating left-sided colon obstruction. In elderly, poor-risk patients with extensive colon distention, a tube cecostomy inserted with local anesthesia may be the procedure of choice.[23]

Obstructive lesions of the cecum and right colon are managed differently. In treating cecal or right colon obstruction due to cancer one must usually choose between right colectomy with ileotransverse colostomy and a bypass operation (ileotransverse colostomy) to relieve the obstruction, with later elective resection of the right colon. The bypass operation should be reserved for poor-risk patients. Right colectomy can be done safely in patients with obstruction because the obstructed colon can be removed and the dilated small bowel can usually be sutured safely to normal colon. The treatment of volvulus of the cecum

depends upon the viability of the cecum. If it is nonviable, right colectomy should be done. If it is viable, detorsion with fixation of the cecum is appropriate.

Recurrent Intestinal Obstruction

Some patients can develop one or more subsequent small bowel obstructions. This appears to be a particular problem for patients with extensive, dense intraperitoneal adhesions. Some recurrent obstructions require reoperation, and most surgeons simply free the intestine as described previously. Plication of the small bowel or its mesentery to reintroduce the small bowel into the peritoneal cavity in an orderly manner without kinks has been suggested for these difficult cases. Another method employed to minimize recurrent small bowel obstruction is the intraoperative passage of a long intestinal tube through the length of the small intestine, leaving it in place for approximately 2 weeks to maintain an adequate intestinal lumen while healing occurs. Available data suggest that the intraluminal tube stent method can be employed with a lower operative mortality and a lower rate of operation.[9]

Treatment of Paralytic Ileus

Paralytic ileus is treated by nasogastric suction and intravenous fluid administration. Correction of electrolyte imbalance, especially hypokalemia, is particularly important in managing this disorder.[23] In some cases of paralytic ileus, particularly with extreme distention, passage of a long tube into the intestine should be tried, since this method of suction provides superior intestinal decompression. If it is clear that mechanical obstruction or intra-abdominal sepsis is not present, parasympathomimetic drugs, such as neostigmine (Prostigmin), may be of value.

Most often, ileus develops after abdominal surgery and is

transient, lasting 2 to 3 days. When ileus persists or occurs without obvious etiology, one should endeavor to exclude mechanical obstruction or intra-abdominal sepsis; a laparotomy may be necessary to exclude those factors confidently.

Some patients with paralytic ileus develop massive distention of the colon and particularly the cecum. Distention secondary to ileus can threaten bowel viability. Patients with this syndrome are frequently elderly or have multisystem disease. Colonoscopy has been reported to be a safe and effective way to decompress massive nonobstructive cecal dilatation in high-risk patients.[19]

SELECTED REFERENCES

American Physiological Society: Handbook of Physiology, Section 6, Alimenatry Canal. Code, C. F. (Ed.). Baltimore, Williams & Wilkins Company, 1967–1968. *The five volumes of this publication sponsored by the American Physiological Society provide an excellent reference source on gastrointestinal function. The authors, all of whom are pre-eminent authorities in their field, provide a comprehensive, detailed, critical description of fact and hypothesis concerning food intake, gastrointestinal secretion, digestion, absorption, and gastrointestinal motility.*

Davenport, H. W.: Physiology of the Digestive Tract, 2nd ed. Chicago, Year Book Medical Publishers, 1966. *This book is an excellent starting point for reading about gastrointestinal physiology. All aspects of intestinal function are discussed clearly, authoritatively, and succinctly.*

Hartwell, J. A., and Hoguet, J. P.: Experimental intestinal obstruction in dogs with especial reference to the cause of death and the treatment by large amounts of normal saline solution. J.A.M.A., 59:82, 1912. *The authors emphasize the importance of fluid loss in the pathogenesis of intestinal obstruction and show that the administration of saline solutions prevented death from high intestinal obstruction in dogs. This paper was presented before the annual session of the American Medical Association in June, 1912, and the authors' observations have stood the test of time.*

Johnson, L. R.: Physiology of the Gastrointestinal Tract, 2nd ed. New York, Raven Press, 1987. *This two-volume textbook provides authoritative and comprehensive descriptions of intestinal function. The material on digestion and absorption is well written and complete.*

Moore, F. D.: Metabolic Care of the Surgical Patient. Philadelphia, W. B. Saunders Company, 1959. *This excellent reference describes the analysis and repair of the metabolic derangements in patients with intestinal obstruction. Small bowel obstruction is classified on the basis of duration or severity of fluid and electrolyte imbalance to assist in planning therapy. This book also provides guides for planning the timing of operation to relieve obstruction. The sections on ileus and postoperative obstruction of the ileus are particularly helpful.*

REFERENCES

1. American Physiological Society: Handbook of Physiology, Section 6, Alimentary Canal. Code, C. F. (Ed.). Baltimore, Williams & Wilkins Company, 1967–1968.
2. Asbun, H. J., Pempinello, C., and Halasz, N. A.: Small bowel obstruction and its management. Int. Surg. 74:23, 1989.
3. Bizer, L. S., Liebling, R. W., Delany, H. M., and Gliedman, M. D.: Small bowel obstruction: The role of nonoperative treatment in simple intestinal obstruction and predictive criteria for strangulation obstruction. Surgery, 89:407, 1981.
4. Bloom, W., and Fawcett, D. W.: A Textbook of Histology, 9th ed. Philadelphia, W. B. Saunders Company, 1968, pp. 560–581.
5. Borgstrom, B., Wieloch, T., and Erlanson-Albertson, C.: Evidence for a pancreatic pro-colipase and its activation by trypsin. F.E.B.S. Lett., 108:407, 1979.
6. Brolin, R. E.: Partial small bowel obstruction. Surgery, 95:145, 1984.
7. Brooks, F. P.: Control of Gastrointestinal Function. New York, Macmillan Company, 1970.
8. Buchan, A. M.: Digestion and Absorption. In Patton, H. D., Fuchs, A. F., Hille, B., Scher, A. M., and Steiner, R. (Eds.): Textbook of Physiology, 21st ed. Philadelphia, W. B. Saunders Company, 1989.
9. Close, W. B. and Christensen, N. M.: Transmesenteric small bowel plication or intraluminal tube stenting. Am. J. Surg., 138:89, 1979.
10. Davenport, H. W.: Physiology of the Digestive Tract, 2nd ed. Chicago, Year Book Medical Publishers, 1966.
11. Faulk, D. L., Anuras, S., and Freeman, M. B.: Idiopathic chronic intestinal pseudo-obstruction. Use of central venous nutrition. J.A.M.A., 240:2075, 1978.
12. Frimann-Dahl, J.: The acute abdomen. In Margulis, A. R., and Burhenne, J. J. (Eds.): Alimentary Tract Roentgenology. Vol. 1. St. Louis, C. V. Mosby Company, 1967, pp. 141–196.
13. Gough, I. R.: Strangulating adhesive small bowel obstruction with normal radiographs. Br. J. Surg. 65:431, 1978.
14. Gross, C. M. (Ed.): Gray's Anatomy of the Human Body, 28th ed. Philadelphia, Lea & Febiger, 1966.
15. Grossman, M. I.: Spectrum of biological actions of gastrointestinal hormones. In Anderson, S. (Ed.): Nobel Symposium XVI: Frontiers in Gastrointestinal Hormone Research. Stockholm, Almqvist & Wiksell/Gebers Forlag, 1973.
16. Hartwell, J. A. and Hoguet, J. P.: Experimental intestinal obstruction in dogs with especial reference to the cause of death and the treatment by large amounts of normal saline solution. J.A.M.A., 59:82, 1912.
17. Hirsch, J. E., Arhens, E. H., Jr., and Blankenhorn, D. H.: Measurement of the human intestinal length in vivo and some causes of variation. Gastroenterology, 31:274, 1956.
18. Hoffman, A. F.: A physiocochemical approach to the intraluminal phase of absorption. Gastroenterology, 50:56, 1966.
19. Kukora, J. S., and Dent, T. L.: The colonoscopic decompression of massive nonobstructive cecal dilatation. Arch. Surg. 112:512, 1977.
20. Landman, M. D., and Longmire, W. P., Jr.: Neural and hormonal influence of peritonitis on paralytic ileus. Am. Surg., 33:756, 1967.
21. Marsh, M. N., and Swift, J. A.: A study of the small intestinal mucosa using the scanning electron microscope. Gut, 10:940, 1969.
22. Miller, L. D., Mackie, J. A., and Rhoads, J. E.: The pathophysiology and management of intestinal obstruction. Surg. Clin. North Am., 42:1285, 1962.
23. Moore, F. D.: Metabolic Care of the Surgical Patient. Philadelphia, W. B. Saunders Company, 1959.
24. Moyer, C. A., Rhoads, J. E., Allen, J. G., and Harkins, H. N.: Surgery, Principles and Practice, 3rd ed. Philadelphia, J. B. Lippincott Company, 1965.
25. Nemir, P., Jr.: Intestinal obstruction: 10-year statistical survey at the Hospital of University of Pennsylvania. Ann. Surg., 135:367, 1952.
26. Peetz, D. J., Gamelli, R. L., and Pilcher, D. B.: Intestinal obstruction in acute mechanical small bowel obstruction. Arch. Surg., 117:334, 1982.
27. Pickleman, J. and Lee R. M.: The management of patients with suspected early postoperative small bowel obstruction. Ann. Sug., 210:216, 1989.
28. Polak, J. M., Pearse, A. G. E., Joffe, S. N., and Bloom, S. R.: Quantification of secretin release by acid using immunocytochemistry and radioimmunoassay. Experientia, 31:462, 1975.
29. Quatramoni, J. C., Rosoff, L., Halls, J. M., and Yellin, A. E.: Early postoperative small bowel obstruction. Ann. Surg., 191:72, 1980.
30. Schwartz, S. I., et al. (Eds.): Principles of Surgery. New York, McGraw-Hill Book Company, 1969, pp. 843–855.
31. Scratcherd, T., and Grundy, D.: The physiology of intestinal motility and secretion. Br. J. Anaesth., 56:3, 1984.
32. Shields, R.: The absorption and secretion of fluid and electrolytes by the obstructed bowel. Br. J. Surg., 52:774, 1965.
33. Stewardson, R. H., Bombeck, C. T., and Nyhus, L. M.: Critical operative management of small bowel obstruction. Ann. Surg., 187:189, 1978.
34. Tomasi, T. B., Jr.: Human immunoglobulin A. N. Engl. J. Med., 279:1327, 1968.
35. Turnberg, L. A. Bieberdorf, F. A., Morawski, S. G., and Fordtran, J. S.: Interrelationships of chloride, bicarbonate, sodium, and hydrogen transport in human ileum. J. Clin. Invest., 49:557, 1970.
36. Turnberg, L. A., Fordtran, J. S., Carter, N. W., and Rector, F. C., Jr.: Mechanism of bicarbonate absorption and its relation to sodium transport in the human jejunum. J. Clin. Invest., 49:548, 1970.
37. Visscher, M. D., Fetcher, E. S., Jr., Carr, C. W., Gregore, H. P., Bushey, M. S., and Barker, D. E.: Isotopic tracer studies on the movement of water and ions between intestinal lumen and blood. Am. J. Physiol., 142:550, 1944.
38. Wangensteen, O. H.: Intestinal Obstructions, 3rd ed. Springfield, Ill., Charles C Thomas, 1955.
39. Wangensteen, O. H.: Historical aspects of the management of acute intestinal obstruction. Surgery, 65:363, 1969.
40. Wright, H. K., O'Brien, J. J., and Tilson, M. D.: Water absorption in experimental closed segment obstruction of the ileum in man. Am. J. Surg., 121:96, 1971.

IV ———————————————————————————————————

CROHN'S DISEASE (REGIONAL ENTERITIS)

Keith A. Kelly, M. D., and Bruce G. Wolff, M. D.

Crohn's disease is a chronic, nonspecific inflammatory disease of the gastrointestinal tract of unknown etiology. It involves mainly the ileum and large intestine, most often producing symptoms of obstruction or localized perforation with fistula. Both medical and surgical treatment are palliative. Nevertheless, operative excision provides effective symptomatic relief and leads to reasonable long-term benefit.

Scattered reports of a chronic inflammatory disease of the small and large intestine appeared in the medical literature during the nineteenth and early twentieth centuries. The report of Crohn and colleagues in 1932, however, crystallized the description of this condition, which subsequently has become known as Crohn's disease.[2] The literature has been abundant since the 1932 report, including the comprehensive review of VanPatter and associates in 1954[15] and the many excellent reports of the National Cooperative Crohn's Disease Study in 1979.[17]

INCIDENCE

The incidence of Crohn's disease in the population is approximately 6 to 7 per 100,000 subjects at risk.[7] The incidence in recent years has been described by some as increasing, whereas others have found it stable. The disease is as common in males as in females at any age, although the peak age of onset is between the second and fourth decades of life. The disease is more common among whites than blacks or Orientals and may be more common among certain ethnic groups. A familial tendency is noted, but the disease is not inherited in an autosomal dominant pattern.

ETIOLOGY

No specific etiology of the disease has been identified. There are two main areas of investigation: the microbiologic and the immunologic. Microbiologists have long sought a specific microorganism that might be the cause of the disease; however, none has yet been identified. Recent reports of the isolation of *Mycobacterium paratuberculosis* from segments of bowel affected with Crohn's disease excited interest, but this organism as a specific cause of the disease has yet to be proven. Also, no virus has been identified as an etiologic agent.

An immunologic origin of the disease has also been sought. Undoubtedly an immunologic response to the condition does exist. Some have postulated that a childhood sensitization to milk impairs mucosal integrity and allows bacteria or bacteriologic products to enter the body. A cellular and humoral immune response to these products then ensues. The ileocolic epithelium, in particular, may be the target of a necrotizing immune response, with ensuing ulceration, tissue destruction, and the clinical appearance of the disease. Although an immunologic response has a role in the pathogenesis of the condition, its role as an etiologic agent is still unclear.

Other data suggest that environmental factors have an etiologic role in the disease. It is more common among individuals living in temperate climates than among those in tropical climates. Smoking may exert a stimulating effect on the disease; many patients with Crohn's disease are heavy smokers.

Spouses of individuals with Crohn's disease have a higher incidence of the disease than those in the general population. Although these data suggest that environmental factors have a role, no specific factor has been identified.

PATHOLOGY

Location of Lesions

Crohn's disease is a generalized inflammatory disorder of the gastrointestinal tract that can involve any area from the mouth to the anus. The disease, however, is discontinous and segmental. The small intestine and the large intestine are the most frequent sites of gross macroscopic involvement. In one large series, 55 per cent of patients had involvement of both small and large intestine, 30 per cent small intestine alone, and 15 per cent large intestine alone.[11] Of those with involvement only of the large intestine, one third (5 per cent of the total) had anorectal involvement only. In contrast, anorectal involvement accompanied more proximal involvement in 48 per cent of patients with Crohn's disease of the large intestine, in 41 per cent of those with small and large intestinal Crohn's disease, and in 23 per cent of those with small intestinal Crohn's disease.

Gross Pathologic Features

APHTHOUS ULCERS. One of the earliest macroscopic signs of Crohn's disease is the appearance of aphthous ulcers in the mucosa of the gastrointestinal tract. These small, flat, soft ulcers have a whitish center and a red border. They are scattered in the mucosa with normal areas of intervening mucosa. As the disease progresses, the aphthous ulcers deepen and coalesce, penetrating through the entire mucosa and forming longer ulcers that may reach 1 cm. in size or larger. The ulcers remain discontinuous and asymmetrical. They often appear first on the mesenteric border of the bowel and have a linear pattern along the wall of the intestine. Because of this, they are sometimes called "rake" ulcers, suggesting that a rake had been pulled across the mucosa in a longitudinal direction to create the pattern. Islands of normal mucosa remain between the ulcers, producing the cobblestone appearance on the surface of the bowel. (Fig. 1).

TRANSMURAL INFLAMMATION. As the ulcers grow and the inflammation spreads, the lesions extend deep into the wall of the bowel through the mucosa and muscularis out to the serosa to form transmural fissures and thornlike defects. The inflammatory response creates a thickening of the bowel wall and a narrowing of its lumen, the so-called "rubber hose" intestine. The inflammatory response on the serosa and adjacent mesentery also thickens these structures, and the fat of the mesentery creeps around the side of the bowel to add to the thickening. The intestinal lymphatic vessels are engorged, and the lymph nodes in the adjacent mesentery are enlarged.

Microscopic Features

FOCAL CHRONIC INFLAMMATION. A chronic inflammatory infiltrate appears in the mucosa and submucosa and extends transmurally through the bowel wall. The areas of inflammation are focal and scattered between areas of uninvolved bowel. Distortion of the normal architecture of the intestinal crypts accompanies the inflammation.

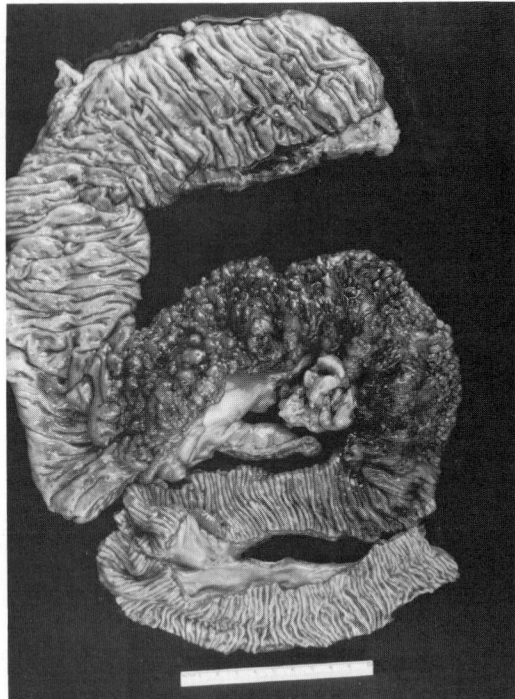

Figure 1. Photograph of ileum, cecum, and ascending colon resected for Crohn's disease of terminal ileum, which demonstrates ulcerated mucosa with a cobblestone appearance, thickened bowel wall, and enlarged adjacent ileal lymph nodes.

GRANULOMAS. The characteristic microscopic lesion of Crohn's disease, however, is the granuloma, which appears in the mucosa, submucosa, or elsewhere in the wall of the bowel or its adjacent lymph nodes, in association with the chronic inflammatory response (Fig. 2). The granulomas are nonspecific and contain chronic inflammatory cells and giant cells. They appear in 50 to 75 per cent of patients.

Intestinal Complications

Two main intestinal complications develop from these lesions: obstruction and perforation. The chronic, fibrosing lesions of Crohn's disease may narrow the lumen of the bowel, producing partial or near-complete *obstruction* with dilatation of the bowel proximal to the lesions and collapse of the bowel distal to the lesions. In contrast, lesions that penetrate into and *perforate* through the bowel wall lead to localized abscesses near the sites of perforation and often fistulas between the sites of

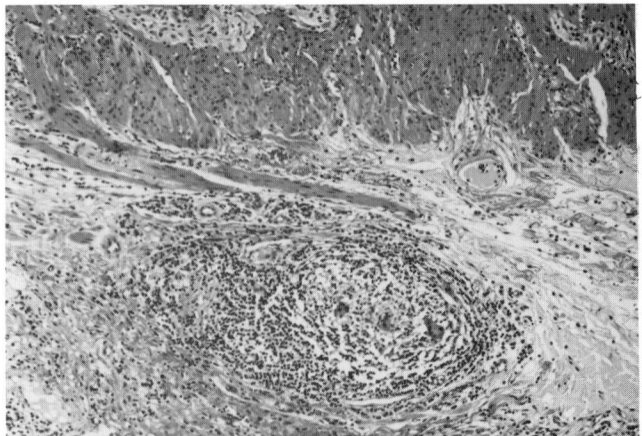

Figure 2. Photomicrograph of ileum with Crohn's disease and a subserosal, noncaseating granuloma.

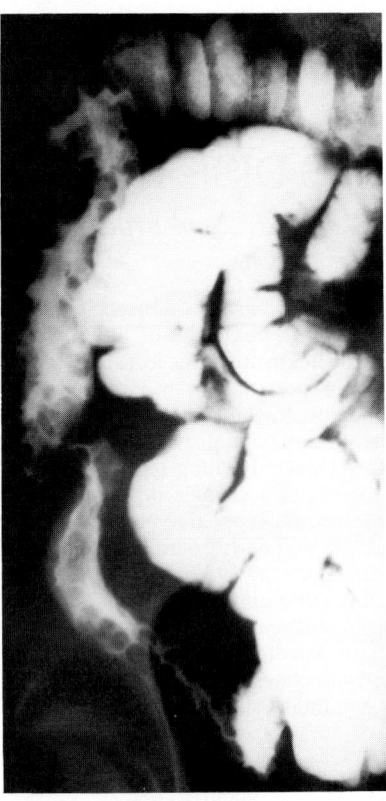

Figure 3. Radiograph of terminal ileum, cecum, and ascending colon involved by Crohn's disease demonstrating mucosal ulceration with a cobblestone appearance, thickened bowel wall, and luminal narrowing.

perforation and adjacent organs, such as loops of small and large intestine, the urinary bladder, the vagina (Fig. 3), the stomach, and sometimes the skin at sites of previous celiotomy. The perienteric fibrous response sometimes causes ureteral destruction. Free perforations can occur directly into the generalized peritoneal cavity, but these are rare. The ulcerating mucosal lesions can also *bleed*, but, again, this is unusual. Patients with Crohn's disease of the large intestine may develop *toxic megacolon*, a condition of marked dilation of the colon, abdominal tenderness, ileus, and systemic signs such as fever, leukocytosis, tachycardia, and severe debility.

Long-standing lesions of the small and large intestine are premalignant. The incidence of *carcinoma* of the small bowel is six times greater in patients with Crohn's disease than in the general population, and the incidence of carcinoma of the large bowel is four to six times greater. The cancers that appear in the small intestine of patients with Crohn's disease have a pattern different from the pattern of those that occur in the small intestine of patients without the disease. These cancers are more likely to occur in males, in young patients, and in the ileum, with a poorer prognosis. Large intestinal cancers associated with Crohn's disease are also usually more advanced when discovered and therefore have a worse prognosis than do cancers arising in a colon without the disease. Cancers usually arise in segments of intestine that have been afflicted with Crohn's disease for 10 years or more. Thus, patients with long-standing Crohn's disease should be examined annually or biannually by means of endoscopy and biopsy for detection of premalignant changes, such as epithelial dysplasia, or cancers.

Extraintestinal Manifestations

Extraintestinal manifestations are present in approximately 30 per cent of patients, reflecting a systemic inflammatory response to the intestinal inflammation. Most common are skin lesions, including erythema nodosum and pyoderma gangreno-

TABLE 1. Extraintestinal Manifestation of Crohn's Disease

Skin
Erythema multiformi
Erythema nodosum
Pyoderma gangrenosum

Eyes
Iritis
Uveitis
Conjunctivitis

Joints
Peripheral arthritis
Ankylosing spondylitis

Blood
Anemia
Thrombocytosis
Phlebothrombosis
Arterial thrombosis

Liver
Nonspecific triaditis
Sclerosing cholangitis

Kidney
Nephrotic syndrome
Amyloidosis

Pancreas
Pancreatitis

General
Amyloidosis

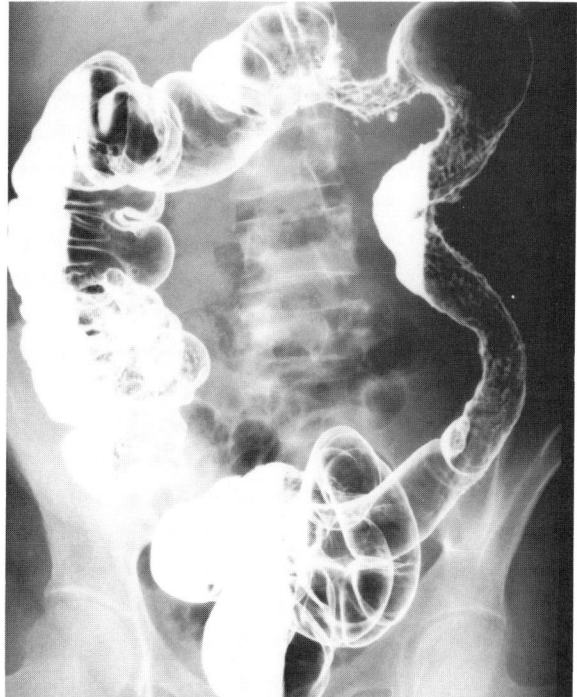

Figure 4. Radiograph of Crohn's disease of the small intestine demonstrating marked narrowing (string sign) of the distal ileum.

sum, and iritis, uveitis, arthritis, spondylitis, pericholangitis/hepatitis, and aphthous stomatitis (Table 1).

SYMPTOMS

The most common symptoms of Crohn's disease are those from the intestinal lesions, with abdominal pain, especially of a cramping nature, heading the list. Diarrhea is frequent; the stools may contain blood, although often do not. The patient experiences abdominal distention or flatulence and sometimes nausea and vomiting. Eating becomes difficult because it induces symptoms. The patient therefore decreases food intake and loses weight. If fistulas develop, the pain and discharge of intestinal contents to the skin or in the perianal area produce localized symptoms. Systemic responses include fever and malaise, while localized pain and discomfort are related to the sites of extraintestinal involvement in the skin, eyes, and joints.

The course of the disease is one of exacerbation and remission; but as the lesions mature and complications develop, the symptoms continue unabated and the disease becomes relentlessly progressive. Approximately 70 per cent of patients eventually undergo operation despite spontaneous remissions and medical or dietary therapy.

DIAGNOSIS

Diagnosis is based on a history, physical findings, and appropriate laboratory tests. The *physical findings* include the palpation of the thickened bowel wall or adjacent inflammatory response or abscesses in the abdomen. Hyperactive bowel tones are detected on auscultation, and peristaltic rushes in the small intestine may be seen through a thin abdominal wall. Abdominal distention occurs. Fistulas are apparent; and when they are present, probes and catheters can be passed through the cutaneous openings and into the lumen of the bowel through the tracts. The perianal skin, on inspection, appears bluish; and perianal fissures, abscesses, and fistulas can be identified.

Proctoscopy often reveals the characteristic rectal aphthous

ulcer with surrounding normal-appearing mucosa. With progressive and extensive involvement, the ulcerations involve more of the wall of the bowel, with isolated segments of normal mucosa remaining. Anoscopy shows perianal abscesses, perianal fistulas, and even rectal-vaginal fistulas. Colonoscopy delineates the extent of the lesions in the large intestine. Sometimes the colonoscope can be passed through the colon and into the ileum for identification of the ileal lesions of the disease. The hallmark of Crohn's disease is the discontinuous and asymmetrical nature of the endoscopic findings. Biopsies taken during endoscopy show chronic inflammation and, sometimes, granulomas.

Roentgenographic examination of the gastrointestinal tract using $BaSO_4$ reveals the ulcerating lesions dispersed in a segmental irregular pattern along the wall of the involved intestine, producing areas of ulceration, narrowing, and thickened bowel wall (Fig. 4). Proximal dilatation of the bowel accompanies obstructing lesions. Long lengths of narowed terminal ileum may reduce the caliber of the lumen to the size of a string (string sign) (Fig. 5). Areas of dilatation may alternate with areas of constriction (Fig. 6). The cobblestone appearance of the mucosa may be apparent, as may the "rake" ulcers. Fissures, fistulas, and perienteric abscesses may be found. Computerized axial tomography may help to delineate thickened bowel, peri-enteric abscesess, and perforations. In toxic megacolon, the transverse colon is greatly dilated and the bowel wall is thickened (Fig. 7). A mass accompanying a narrowed or ulcerated area suggests cancer. Free air in the abdomen is present with free perforation.

The differential diagnosis includes both specific causes of intestinal inflammation and nonspecific causes. Specific microbiologic disease that may be confused with Crohn's disease include bacterial inflammations such as those caused by *Salmonella* and *Shigella*, typhoid fever, intestinal tuberculosis, and protozoan infections such as amebiasis. Appropriate cultures and biopsies reveal the causative organisms in these conditions. With regard to nonspecific intestinal inflammation, chronic ulcerative colitis can usually be differentiated from Crohn's disease (Table 2). Although ulcerative colitis involves the mucosa of the large intestine, it does not extend further into the wall of

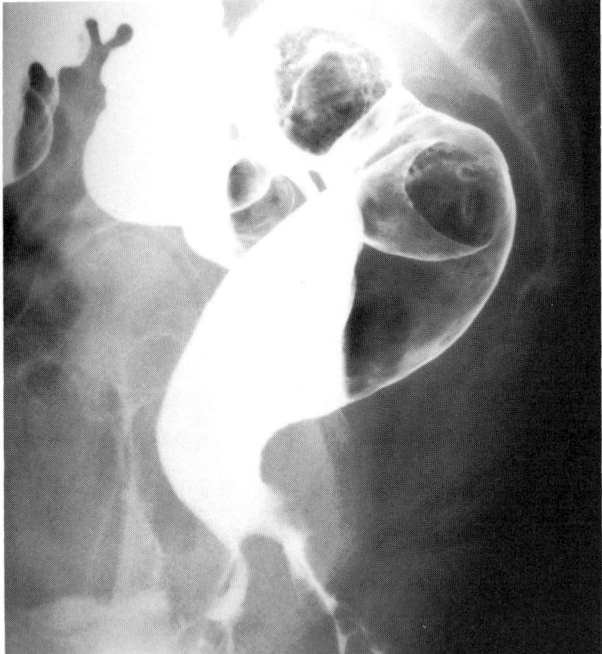

Figure 5. Radiograph of large intestine with Crohn's disease. Areas of narrowing with mucosal ulceration in the transverse colon, descending colon, and sigmoid colon, with spared, healthy-appearing segments of colon and rectum.

the bowel, as does Crohn's disease. Ulcerative colitis generally involves the rectum most severely, with lessening inflammation from the rectum to the ileocolic area. In contrast, Crohn's disease may be worse on the right side of the colon than on the left side, sometimes sparing the rectum. In ulcerative colitis, there is continuous involvement from rectum to proximal segments, whereas segmental lesions are seen in Crohn's disease. Although nonspecific, "backwash" ileitis may be present in ulcerative colitis, ileal and small intestinal involvement suggest Crohn's disease. Bleeding is a common symptom in ulcerative colitis and less common in Crohn's disease. Perianal involvement and rectovaginal fistulas are unusual in ulcerative colitis, but are common with Crohn's disease. In most instances, the two diseases can be clearly separated, but a subgroup of 5 to 10 per cent of all patients with chronic nonspecific inflammatory bowel disease cannot be clearly classified as having ulcerative

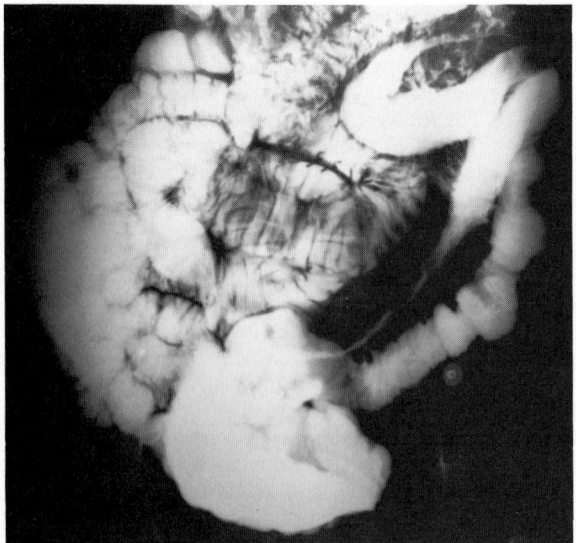

Figure 6. Radiograph demonstrating rectovaginal fistula secondary to Crohn's disease.

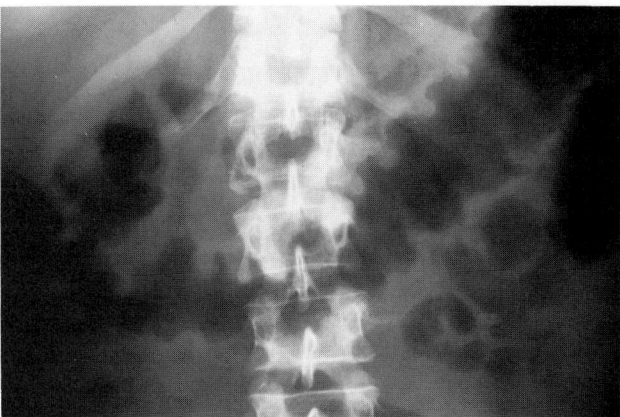

Figure 7. Radiograph of the abdomen in a patient with toxic megacolon secondary to Crohn's disease demonstrating dilatation of the transverse colon with thickening of the bowel wall and edematous haustral folds.

colitis or Crohn's disease. These patients are usually given a diagnosis of "indeterminate" colitis. The true diagnosis often becomes apparent as the patients are followed through the years.

Acute distal ileitis may be a manifestation of early Crohn's disease, but it also may be unrelated, such as when it is caused by a bacteriologic agent such as *Campylobacter* or *Yersinia*. The patient usually presents in a manner similar to that of patients with acute appendicitis, with sudden onset of right lower quadrant pain, nausea, vomiting, fever, and tenderness over the area of involvement. The diagnosis at operation is made by identifying an acutely inflamed segment of terminal ileum. No biopsy or resection should be done. The condition generally subsides spontaneously. If the cecum is not involved, the appendix should be removed for prevention of confusion with appendicitis during subsequent episodes of right lower quadrant inflammation.

THERAPY

Medical and Dietary Therapy

Medical therapy consists of sulfathalazine, 5-aminosalicylic acid, corticosteroids, antibiotics such as metronidazole and ampicillin, and immunosuppressive agents such as azathioprine and cyclosporine. Because no specific etiology has been identified for Crohn's disease, the treatments are also not specific; they suppress inflammation and improve symptoms but are not curative.

Manipulations of the diet ordinarily have little effect on the progress of Crohn's disease. However, complete abstinence from oral intake with total parenteral nutrition may lead to temporary remission of symptoms in some patients with Crohn's disease. Sometimes enteroenteric or enterocutaneous fistulas close. Few long-term benefits of total parenteral nutrition, however, have been achieved. When oral intake is again resumed, the patients usually have recurring difficulty, and the symptoms of the disease return.

Surgical Therapy

INDICATIONS FOR OPERATION. Patients with Crohn's disease are usually operated upon because an intestinal complication of Crohn's disease mandates operation. Approximately 70 per cent of patients with Crohn's disease undergo operation. The most common complications leading to operation are intestinal obstruction, intestinal perforation with fistula formation and abscess, and gastrointestinal bleeding. Obstruction is usually partial and is seldom complete. With nasogastric suction and intravenous nutrition, distended bowel usually decompresses and bowel movements resume. However, failure of

TABLE 2. Diagnosis of Crohn's Colitis Versus Ulcerative Colitis

Observations	Crohn's Colitis	Ulcerative Colitis
Symptoms and Signs		
Diarrhea	70–90%	80–90%
Rectal bleeding	Less common	Prominent
Abdominal pain (cramps)	Moderate to severe	Mild
Palpable mass	At times	No (unless large cancer)
Anal complaints	Frequent (<50%)	Infrequent (<20%)
Radiologic Findings		
Ileal disease	Common	Rare (backwash ileitis)
Nodularity, fuzziness	No	Yes
Distribution	Skip areas	Rectum extending upward and continuously
Ulcer	Linear, cobblestone, fissures	Collar button
Toxic dilatation	Yes	Yes
Proctoscopic Findings		
Anal fissure, fistula, abscess	Common	Rare
Rectal sparing	Common (50%)	Rare (5%)
Granularity	No	Yes
Ulceration	Linear, deep	Superficial erosion

complete resolution or recurrence of obstructive symptoms with resumption of oral feedings usually leads to operation. Perforation with fistula formation and a resultant abdominal mass usually causes continuing pain, fever, malaise, and weight loss until operation can be accomplished. Perianal complications, such as abscess and fistula, commonly lead to operation. Bleeding, a less frequent cause of operation, is usually not massive, but may be persistent and contribute to chronic anemia until the offending lesion or lesions can be resected. Patients with small intestinal Crohn's disease usually require operation for obstruction or perforation, whereas those with large intestinal Crohn's disease are usually operated upon for chronic debility and failure to respond to medical therapy.

Severe systemic symptoms, intractable medical therapy, and weight loss, especially with growth failure in children, also lead to operation. Toxic megacolon and cancer of the small or large intestine are less common intestinal complications requiring operation. Extraintestinal complications (see Table 1) seldom require intestinal operation, but often contribute to the decision for operation. Most of the extraintestinal complications, with the exception of ankylosing spondylitis and the hepatic complications, subside with the excision of intestine grossly involved with Crohn's disease.

PREOPERATIVE PREPARATION. The nutritional status of the patient is optimized before operation. This sometimes, but not often, requires parenteral caloric supplementation. Anemia is treated by blood transfusion. For patients currently on or recently receiving corticosteroid therapy, additional steroids— usually 100 mg. hydrocortisone intravenously every 8 hours— are given to assure adequate supply during the operative stress. The bowels are cleansed with laxatives and enemas for 2 days prior to operation. Alternatively, 4 liters of an electrolyte solution (Go Lytely®) can be given by mouth the night before operation.[18] Diet is restricted to clear liquids the day before operation.

The growth of enteric bacteria is suppressed by administering neomycin, 0.5 gm. every 4 hours, and tetracycline, erythromycin, or metronidazole, 250 mg. every 4 hours, for 36 hours prior to operation. Cefazolin, 0.5 gm., is given intravenously just prior to operation and is continued every 8 hours for two more doses.

GENERAL PRINCIPLES OF OPERATION. Because Crohn's disease involves nearly the entire gastrointestinal tract in most patients, the possibility of totally excising the disease is not reasonable. Thus, surgical treatment is directed to the most severe areas of involvement, including those that represent complications of obstruction, bleeding or perforation.

The two main operative approaches are (1) excision and (2) bypass of the lesions. Currently, most surgeons advise excision rather than bypass. Bypass allows the diseased intestine to remain where it continues to cause symptoms, to require treatment, and perhaps to develop malignancy. The risk of cancer in bypassed small and large intestine with Crohn's disease is greater than the risk in healthy bowel. Excision is done with 5-cm. "disease-free" margins on both sides of the area of involvement. The disease-free margins are established by gross inspection. Most do not use microscopic confirmation of healthy borders. Although the authors have found that a border free of microscopic involvement is followed by fewer recurrences over the long term than when the border is involved,[19] others have not found a higher recurrence when histologic findings of Crohn's disease are present in the margins.[12] Certainly, demanding microscopic borders free of disease may lead to excessively large resections and lead to the "short bowel syndrome." Patients with this syndrome do not have enough remaining intestine to digest and absorb food properly.

After resection of the index segment (or segments) of intestine and anastomosis, fistulas from the index segment to adjacent organs, such as the stomach, the colon, the duodenum, the bladder, or the vagina can usually be closed by suture of the entrance of the fistula into the adjacent segment. Resection of the adjacent segment is seldom required, unless it too is primarily involved with gross Crohn's disease.

SURGICAL TREATMENT OF SPECIFIC SITES

The three most common sites requiring operation for Crohn's disease are the ileum, the colorectum, and the anorectum, with other sites needing surgical treatment less often.

Ileum

A vertical midline abdominal incision is made to the left of the umbilicus. This incision leaves the right lower quadrant of the abdomen unscarred and useful for the site of an ileostomy should one be required at the initial operation or in the future. Careful inspection of the abdominal contents confirms the diagnosis and helps in assessment of the extent of the disease. Ileal Crohn's generally involves the most distal terminal ileum, but "skip areas" can be found more proximally. Mucosal and submucosal lesions may not be apparent unless careful inspection of the small bowel from the stomach to the ileocolic valve is done. Subtle strictures can also be identified by passing a Foley catheter into the lumen of the intestine through an enterotomy, threading the bowel onto the catheter, inflating the balloon of the catheter, and drawing the catheter back along the bowel.

Areas of narrowing impede the withdrawal of the catheter. The diameter of the narrowed lumen can be assessed by noting the diameter of the balloon as it is pulled through the stricture. Strictures detected in this manner may not be apparent on external inspection or palpation of the bowel. The length of healthy intestine from the ligament of Treitz to the first area of involvement should be carefully measured and recorded. The length of intestine grossly involved with Crohn's disease should also be noted.

Crohn's disease of the ileum should be excised with 5-cm. grossly disease-free margins on the proximal and distal end. This usually involves resecting the adjacent ileocolic valve, the cecum, and a small portion of ascending colon (Fig. 8). Obtaining microscopically disease-free margins at each end of the resected specimen appears to prolong the disease-free interval after operation,[19] but controversy exists about this point. Most surgeons do not demand histologic evidence of lack of disease at the margins during operation. No attempt should be made to resect the entire thickened adjacent mesentery; only that amount of mesentery should be resected as needed to facilitate the removal of the diseased bowel and the anastomosis. Intestinal continuity is then restored with an end-to-end ileal-ascending colostomy. The anastomosis can be made with sutures or staples. The authors prefer a two-layer suture technique, using continuous 3-0 absorbable suture on the mucosal-submucosal layer to provide a watertight closure and to control bleeding. Interrupted 4-0 nonabsorbable sutures are used on the seromuscular layer to complete the anastomosis. The defect in the mesentery is closed by approximating the cut mesenteric edges with continuous 3-0 absorbable sutures. Necrotic debris, bowel content, blood, and bacteria are removed by irrigation of the site of excision with isotonic NaCl and aspiration of the irrigant. The abdomen is closed with interrupted No. 1 absorbable sutures.

Crohn's disease of the small bowel may involve segments not only of terminal ileum but of more proximal ileum and even portions of jejunum. Areas of severe involvement (skip lesions) may be interspersed between areas of fairly normal bowel. Skip lesions close to the major area of involvement in the terminal ileum can be resected in continuity with the terminal ileum. However, when the area of small intestine involved in skip lesions or continuous lesions is great, the surgeon is faced with an operative dilemma. Total excision of all gross disease would involve such an extensive resection that the short bowel syndrome would result. Partial excision, however, would leave active, symptom-producing disease. Two options are present cur-

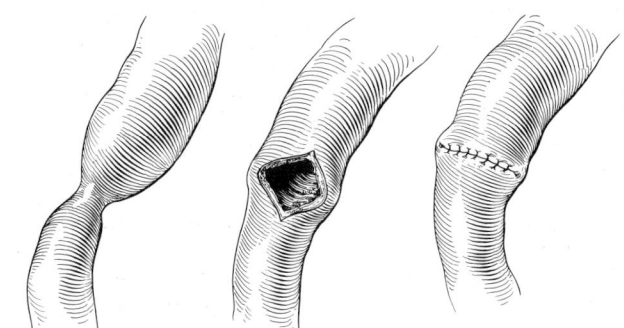

Figure 9. Diagram of "stricturoplasty" for localized segment of Crohn's disease of the small bowel. A longitudinal incision through the strictured segment is made followed by a subsequent transverse closure with sutures. The procedure widens the lumen at the site of stricture and yet resects no bowel.

rently to resolve this dilemma. The first is to bypass the involved segments with a side-to-side anastomosis between the uninvolved proximal small intestine and the adjacent large intestine. This preserves small intestine and bypasses symptom-producing lesions. It does, however, leave diseased and often partially obstructed bowel. A second option is to excise only the most severe areas of involvement and to perform "stricturoplasties" on segments of remaining small bowel to relieve obstruction but to avoid excision.[1,8] The stricturoplasties are performed by making a longitudinal incision through the narrowed areas and closing these incisions in a transverse direction by means of the two-layered technique described above (Fig. 9). This effectively widens the lumen at the sites of the narrowing and yet does not remove any intestine. Stricturoplasty has most application in those patients in whom multiple short areas of narrowing are present over long segments of intestine, in those patients who have already had several previous resections of the small intestine, and when the areas of narrowing are due to fibrous obstruction rather than acute inflammation.

Experience with stricturoplasty has been excellent. In one series, among 24 patients operated upon in whom 86 strictures have undergone stricturoplasty, obstruction has been relieved and healing obtained without fistula formation in all patients.[3] Only one recurrent stricture appeared during a mean follow-up of 40 months.

Ileocolon

Another common distribution of Crohn's disease involves the ileum, cecum, and ascending colon. Under these circumstances, the diseased bowel is removed, again with 5-cm. gross disease-free margins, and an anastomosis made between the ileum and the transverse colon in an end-to-end manner.

Colorectum

The operative approach to Crohn's disease of the colorectum varies, depending on the sites of colorectal involvement and their severity. Patients with severe disease of the colon but mild or minimal rectal disease should have the cecum and colon removed and an ileorectostomy performed. Patients with severe colonic disease and mild rectal disease, but with an anorectal complication, such as an anorectal abscess or fistula, should have a colectomy, an end Brooke ileostomy, and a closure of the proximal rectum, leaving the rectum and anal canal in place but excluded from the fecal stream. The plan is for a subsidence of the anorectal Crohn's disease with the intestinal bypass created by the ileostomy and with further medical and surgical treatment. Subsequent reanastomosis may then be possible at a later date when the rectal disease becomes quiescent or subsides. Patients with toxic megacolon from Crohn's disease should also undergo colectomy, closure of the proximal rectum, and end-ileostomy. This operation can be done expeditiously and leaves no anastomosis in the abdomen. Patients with toxic megacolon

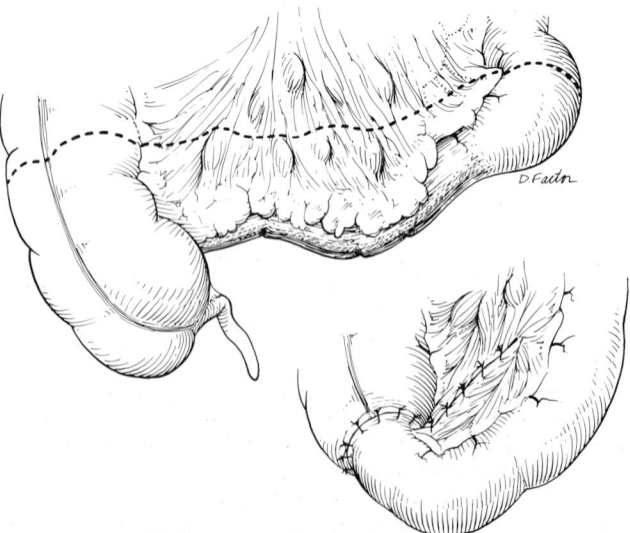

Figure 8. Diagram of resection of the ileum, ileocolic valve, cecum, and ascending colon for Crohn's disease of the ileum. Intestinal continuity is restored by end-to-end ileo-ascending colostomy.

are extremely ill, and anastomoses heal poorly. When both the colon and the rectum are severely involved, protocolectomy with permanent end-ileostomy (Brooke ileostomy) is usually required.

The perineal wound may heal slowly after a complete proctectomy for Crohn's disease. In a past series from the Mayo Clinic, among 32 patients with Crohn's treated by a technique of complete proctectomy and primary closure, only 50 per cent had healed *per primum* by 1 month after operation and only 90 per cent by 1 year.[16] Persistent unhealed perineal wounds require excision of the wound surface and secondary closure, skin grafts, a musculocutaneous flap, or some combination thereof. To avoid the problem of the nonhealing wound, the authors employ endorectal and sphincter-saving excisions rather than wide excisions of the entire anorectum. In these current operations, the diseased mucosa and adjacent underlying and adherent submucosa and muscularis are excised, but most of the muscular complex of the anal sphincter and any associated sinuses or fistulous tracts are left in place. The remaining sphincteric muscle is approximated, and the anal canal is left open. With these techniques, healing is faster, and large, persistent draining wounds are avoided.

Several other options are present for patients with colorectal Crohn's disease but are seldom employed. Localized segments of large intestinal inflammation can sometimes be treated by segmental resection with end-to-end anastomosis of the colon. However, recurrence of Crohn's disease in the remaining colon is so common after segmental resection that most have been reluctant to employ it. Another seldom practiced operation is diverting ileostomy, leaving the entire large intestine in place. The operation may have a role in the patient severely ill with Crohn's colitis. Proponents state that a rapid improvement follows fecal diversion.[6] Continued activity of the colorectal disease producing symptoms and requiring treatment, however, has usually followed this operation. Patients with a diverting ileostomy may eventually have the stoma closed; but after stomal closure, the colonic disease often recurs. Most eventually undergo proctocolectomy and have a permanent ileostomy. Also, stricturoplasty has not been employed in colorectal Crohn's disease; resection of strictured areas is preferred.

Sphincter-saving operations such as the continent ileostomy (Kock pouch) or the ileal pouch-anal anastomosis, both of which are commonly used in ulcerative colitis, are not often used for Crohn's disease. Kock and colleagues have performed the continent ileostomy in a series of patients with Crohn's disease. In this operation, after excision of the large intestine, a pouch is made from 30 cm. of the terminal ileum. A valve that prevents distal outflow from the pouch is created by intussuscepting the terminal ileum retrograde into the pouch and anchoring the intussusceptum in place with stainless steel staples. The end of the terminal ileum is brought to the skin surface as a stoma. When healed, the patient empties the pouch intermittently by passing a catheter through the stoma and valve into the pouch, draining the contents of the pouch directly into the toilet through the tube. Between intubations, the pouch is continent for both gas and stool. Kock and colleagues report that approximately 30 to 50 per cent of the patients have had satisfactory long-term results with the operation. The risk of recurrence of Crohn's disease in the pouch, however, mandates against the use of the continent ileostomy in most patients with Crohn's disease. Also, the ileal pouch–anal anastomosis is not recommended for Crohn's disease of the large intestine. This operation in patients with Crohn's disease has usually led to recurrence of inflammation in the pouch, fistulas at the anastomosis, and peripouch abscesses.

Anorectum

Conservative operations directed to relief of symptoms from anorectal Crohn's disease have been done with increasing frequency in recent years.[5] Abscesses have been drained, fissures

excised, and anal fistulas opened and débrided, sometimes with the aid of a seton, when the fistula extends through the anal sphincter. A seton is a suture of nonabsorbable material passed from the cutaneous opening of the fistula, through the fistula into the lumen of the anal canal, and then back to the skin surface where it is tied to itself. Peritract fibrosis occurs. The fistula can then be opened later without the anal sphincter retracting. Rectovaginal fistulas have been closed by débridement and direct suture of the opening of the fistula, followed by advancement of a rectal mucosal flap from the upper rectum over the opening of the fistula and down to the dentate line.

Emphasis is placed on a conservative approach in anorectal operations for Crohn's disease. Wide excisions of large amounts of tissue should not be performed. Metronidazole, 250 mg. adminstered four times a day, used alone or in combination with operation, aids healing of anorectal Crohn's disease. With conservative medical and surgical therapy, symptoms are often improved, and abscesses, fistulas, and fissures heal.

Some have postulated that anorectal Crohn's disease subsides when more proximal areas of involvement in the small intestine or large intestine are excised. Little evidence exists, however, to support this hypothesis. Removal of a segment of severe ileal Crohn's disease, for example, is unlikely to alter the course of an associated anorectal complication of the disease.

Duodenum

Duodenal Crohn's disease is generally associated with ileal Crohn's disease. It most commonly causes duodenal obstruction, but duodenal perforation with fistulas into the pancreas and peripancreatic areas may also occur. When operation is required, gastrojejunostomy rather than duodenal resection is generally performed, although duodenal stricturoplasty has been employed in selected patients. Vagotomy to prevent marginal ulcer should not be done. The incidence of marginal ulcer is low (<5 per cent) and these ulcers can usually be managed satisfactorily with medical therapy.

Stomach and Esophagus

Gastroesophageal Crohn's disease does not usually require surgical therapy and is almost always managed medically. When localized perforations, bleeding, or fistulas occur, however, local excisions of the grossly diseased areas are required, with closure or anastomosis at sites of excision.

POSTOPERATIVE MANAGEMENT

Postoperatively, the patient takes nothing by mouth, nourishment being administered by intravenous caloric and electrolyte solutions. The stomach and intestines are decompressed by a nasogastric tube. Elastic stockings, sequentially inflating pneumatic cuffs placed on the legs, and early ambulation the day after operation are employed to prevent phlebothrombosis and pulmonary embolism. A urinary bladder catheter is often required for the first 3 to 5 postoperative days.

Instillation of a dilute solution of antibiotics into the wound via a 5-mm. polyethylene catheter placed in the subcutaneous space prior to skin closure and brought to the surface through a puncture site lateral to the wound is initiated the day of operation and continued the following 4 days.[10] The catheter is connected to suction between instillations. This technique has decreased the incidence of wound infection to approximately 1 per cent of patients at risk.

Passage of flatus or bowel contents by the rectum usually begins on or about the third postoperative day, at which time the nasogastric tube can be removed and oral feedings commenced. The authors prescribe a pure liquid diet gradually progressing to solid content, so that patients are taking a soft general diet by the sixth postoperative day. When oral intake is adequate to support caloric, fluid, and electrolyte needs, intravenous feeding can be stopped. The anti-embolism efforts are usually discontinued approximately 5 days postoperatively. Oral prednisone can replace parenteral hydrocortisone when oral intake is resumed. The prednisone is gradually tapered and then discontinued approximately 6 weeks later.

Following discharge from the hospital, continued medical management directed toward prevention of recurrence of Crohn's disease is usually not undertaken. No convincing studies have been published demonstrating that the administration of medical therapy, such as sulfasalazine or prednisone, lessens the incidence of or prolongs the interval to recurrence of Crohn's disease after operation.

COMPLICATIONS OF OPERATION

Early Complications

The main complications of operation in the early postoperative period are intestinal obstruction from adhesions, intra-abdominal abscess, wound infection, anastomotic leaks, bleeding from areas of operation, phlebothrombosis and pulmonary embolism, atelectasis and pulmonary infections, urinary retention, and enterocutaneous fistulas. Most of these complications can be managed nonoperatively; reoperation should be required in less than 10 per cent of patients. Operative mortality is unusual and should be less than 2 per cent of patients at risk.

Late Complications

Resection of the ileum can lead to *malabsorption of vitamin B₁₂*. The ileum is the sole site of absorption of this vitamin. Patients undergoing extensive resections of the ileum should receive 1 mg. vitamin B_{12} parenterally each month on a long-term basis.

The ileum is also the area of intestine where bile salts are actively absorbed. Extensive ileal resections can lead to depletion of the bile salt pool with resulting *steatorrhea* from lack of sufficient bile salts in the enteric lumen for the formation of bile salt micelles. Micelles are necessary for solubilization of fatty acids and their subsequent absorption. Steatorrhea may cause binding of calcium ion by fatty acids, making calcium unavailable in the enteric lumen for binding to oxalates. The unbound oxalate then passes into the large intestine, where it is absorbed. The absorbed oxalate is excreted in the urine, where it may precipitate formation of *oxalate urinary stones*. Uric acid stones may also form in individuals with postresection diarrhea, with resultant sodium, potassium, and water loss. The urinary output decreases, the urine becomes more acidic, and *uric acid urinary stones* can form.

Steatorrhea can be treated by decreasing the intake of fatty food in the diet and ingesting medium-chain triglycerides, and hyperoxaluria can be improved by avoiding food with a high oxalate content, such as spinach, beets, rhubarb, and cocoa. A low-volume acidic urinary output can be combated by vigorous oral fluid intake with increased ingestion of sodium ions.

The loss of bile salts may also lead to the formation of *gallstones*. The bile salt pool becomes depleted, and the concentration of bile salts then becomes insufficient to solubilize the cholesterol in bile. Cholesterol gallstones then develop. Cholecystectomy may be required if symptoms develop from the gallstones.

Failure to absorb bile salts with extensive ileal resection allows unabsorbed bile salts to enter the colon, where they irritate the mucosa and stimulate the outpouring of water and electrolytes into the lumen. Diarrhea results. Cholestyramine, 4 gm. per day orally, binds bile salts and ameliorates diarrhea.

Extensive resections may leave insufficient small intestinal mucosa for digestion and absorption of foodstuffs, vitamins, water, and electrolytes, the *short bowel syndrome* then develops. This condition is characterized by crampy abdominal pain, diarrhea, borborygmi, abdominal distention, and weight loss. The condition often results when less than 100 cm. of jejunoileum remains, although more extensive resections may be tolerated when the ileocolic valve remains. Jejunal losses are tolerated better than ileal losses. The loss of intestine leads to fecal outputs that exceed 1500 ml. per day or more. Malnutrition, dehydration, vitamin deficiencies, and deficiencies of electrolytes can occur. Loss of calcium, for example, may cause osteoporosis.

The short bowel syndrome often requires intravenous administration of nutrients, vitamins, minerals, and water. Elemental diets and liquids are tolerated better by mouth than more complex foods and solids. Gastric hypersecretion of HCl occurs and should be managed with H₂-receptor blockers. Diarrhea can be decreased with antidiarrheal agents such as loperamide hydrochloride. Most patients with the short bowel syndrome improve over time and after 6 months may be able to discontinue intravenous supplementation. Reoperation, other than to drain pus, restore intestinal continuity, close fistulas, and relieve obstruction usually has little benefit.

OUTCOME

Operations for Crohn's disease are palliative; they provide symptomatic relief but not cure. Overall, rates of recurrence are about 6 per cent of patients at risk per year or 30 per cent at 5 years and 60 per cent at 10 years. The 6 per cent rates of recurrence apply to patients after resection and anastomosis for ileal or ileocolic disease. In contrast, the rates of recurrence in the first 10 years after proctocolectomy and permanent ileostomy may be somewhat less. One recent paper reported only 2.5 per cent of patients at risk per year had recurrence over 10 years after proctocolectomy and ileostomy, regardless of whether or not ileal disease was present at the time of operation.[14] Regardless of the type of operation performed, however, rates of recurrence in patients with colonic Crohn's disease usually approach those of patients with ileal or ileocolic Crohn's disease if the patients are followed long enough (25 years) after operation[9] (Fig. 10). The rates of recurrence are not affected or only minimally affected by age, sex, length of intestine involved in disease, interval between onset of disease and operation, and type and duration of medical treatment.[4]

Recurrences usually occur at or just proximal to an anastomosis or stoma. They are diagnosed by symptomatology, physical examination, endoscopy, and radiography and at reoperation with excision. After reoperation for Crohn's disease, recurrence is similar to that following the initial operation. Thus, the results of reoperation, as with initial operation, are usually satisfactory and justify the continued operative approach to the disease. Some patients may require three or more operations. Mortality due to Crohn's disease increases slowly with time and is approximately twofold that of a matched control group of healthy

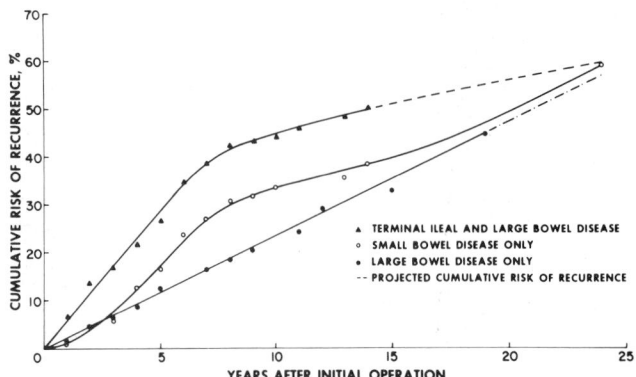

Figure 10. Cumulative rates of recurrence after resection for Crohn's disease of small intestine only, small intestine and large intestine, and large intestine only. (From Lock, M. R., Farmer, R. G., Fazio, V. W., et al.: Recurrence and reoperation for Crohn's disease. N. Engl. J. Med., 304:1586, 1981.)

subjects in the general population.[13] Deaths are due directly to Crohn's disease, its digestive complications, or complications arising from required surgical intervention for the disease.

SELECTED REFERENCES

Lee, E.C.G., and Papaionnou, N.: Minimal surgery for chronic obstruction in patients with extensive or universal Crohn's disease. Ann. R. Coll. Surg. Engl., 64:229, 1982
The authors report that stricturoplasty relieves obstruction in Crohn's disease without resection of bowel, with preservation of intestinal function, and with minimal anastomotic complications.

Lock, M. R., Farmer, R. G., Fazio, V. W., et al: Recurrence and reoperation for Crohn's disease. N Engl. J. Med., 304:1586, 1981.
The authors report that recurrence after operation for Crohn's disease occurs soonest with ileocolic disease, later with ileal disease, and latest with colonic disease, but that, providing the patients are followed long enough (25 years), the eventual rates of recurrence in all three cases are similar.

Mekhjian, H. S., Switz, D. M., Melnyk, C. S., et al: Clinical features and natural history of Crohn's disease. Gastroenterology, 77:898, 1979.
A careful review of the clinical features and natural history of Crohn's disease in a large series of patients.

Van Patter, W. N., Bargen, J. A., Dockerty, M. D., et al: Regional enteritis. Gastroenterology, 26:347, 1954.
An extensive review and description of Crohn's disease, its pathology, its sites of occurrence, and its clinical course.

Wolff, B. G., Beart, R. W., Jr., Frydenberg, H. B., et al: The importance of disease-free margins in resections for Crohn's disease. Dis. Colon Rectum, 26:239, 1983.
An analysis of the continuing controversy regarding the extent of resection in Crohn's disease, favoring the position that achieving a disease-free margin at the time of resection lessens the likelihood of subsequent recurrence of the disease.

REFERENCES

1. Alexander-Williams, J., and Haynes, I. G.: Conservative operations for Crohn's disease of the small bowel. World J. Surg., 9:945, 1985.
2. Crohn, B. B., Ginzburg, L., and Oppenheimer, G. D.: Regional enteritis: A pathologic and clinical study. J.A.M.A., 99:1323, 1932.
3. Dehn, T. C. B., Kettlewell, M. G. W., Mortensen, N. J. McC., et al.: Ten-year experience of stricturoplasty for obstructive Crohn's disease. Br. J. Surg., 76:339, 1989.
4. Farmer, R. G., Whelan, G., and Fazio, V. W.: Long-term follow-up of patients with Crohn's disease. Gastroenterology, 88:1818, 1985.
5. Fry, R. D., Shemesh, E. I., and Kodner, I. J.: The management of anal and perineal Crohn's disease: Techniques and results. Surg. Gynecol. Obstet., 168:42, 1989.
6. Harper, P. H., Truelove, S. C., Lee, E. C. G., et al.: Split ileostomy and ileocolostomy for Crohn's disease of the colon and ulcerative colitis: A 20-year survey. Gut, 24:106, 1983.
7. Hellers, G.: Crohn's disease in Stockholm County, 1955–1974: A study of epidemiology, results of surgical treatment and long-term prognosis. Acta Chir. Scand. Suppl., 490:1, 1979.
8. Lee, E. C. G., and Papaionnou, N.: Minimal surgery for chronic obstruction in patients with extensive or universal Crohn's disease. Ann. R. Coll. Surg. Engl., 64:229, 1982.
9. Lock, M. R., Farmer, R. G., Fazio, V. W., et al.: Recurrence and reoperation for Crohn's disease. N. Engl. J. Med., 304:1586, 1981.
10. McIlrath, D. C., vanHeerden, J. A., Edis, A. J., et al.: Closure of abdominal incisions with subcutaneous catheters. Surgery, 80:411, 1976.
11. Mekhjian, H. S., Switz, D. M., Melnyk, C. S., et al.: Clinical features and natural history of Crohn's disease. Gastroenterology, 77:898, 1979.
12. Pennington, L., Hamilton, S. R., Bayless, T. M., et al.: Surgical management of Crohn's disease: influence of disease at margin of resection. Ann. Surg., 192:311, 1980.
13. Prior, P., Gyde, S., Cooke, W. T., et al.: Mortality in Crohn's disease. Gastroenterology, 80:307, 1981.
14. Scammell, B. E., Andrews, H., Allan, R. N., et al.: Results of proctocolectomy for Crohn's disease. Br. J. Surg., 74:671, 1987.
15. Van Patter, W. N., Bargen, J. A, Dockerty, M. B., et al.: Reginal enteritis. Gastroenterology, 26:347, 1954.
16. Waits, J. O., Dozois, R. R., and Kelly, K. A.: Primary closure and continuous irrigation of the perineal wound after proctectomy. Mayo Clin. Proc., 57:185, 1982.
17. Winship, D. H., Summers, R. W., Best, W. R., et al.: National Cooperative Crohn's Disease Study: Study design and conduct of the study. Gastroenterology, 77:829, 1979.
18. Wolff, B. G., Beart, R. W., Jr., Dozois, R. R., et al.: A new bowel preparation for elective colon and rectal surgery. Arch. Surg., 123:895, 1988.
19. Wolff, B. G., Beart, R. W., Jr., Frydenberg, H. B., et al.: The importance of disease-free margins in resections for Crohn's disease. Dis. Colon Rectum, 26:239, 1983.

V

THE SURGICAL APPROACH TO MORBID OBESITY

Walter J. Pories, M.D.

Morbid obesity is a serious disease associated with a high incidence of medical complications and a significantly shortened life span. Obesity is "morbid" when the patient is 100 pounds or more over ideal body weight. The problem, unfortunately, is common. People in the United States tend toward obesity, with an estimated 12 million persons being seriously overweight. Of these, at least 3 million are morbidly obese; some have estimated the number to be closer to 7 million.

COMPLICATIONS

There is a direct relationship between the amount of excess weight and the incidence of arthritis, coronary heart disease, cerebrovascular disease, congestive heart failure, hypertension, diabetes mellitus, cancer of the stomach, and cholecystitis (Figs. 1 and 2).[33,55] *Mortality* accelerates steeply when an individual becomes 50 per cent overweight; morbidly obese young men have a 12-fold increase in mortality.[76,77,85] In women of this age group, the prognosis is equally bleak. Sudden, unexplained deaths are common.

Hypertension is the most common complication associated with morbid obesity, occurring in 59 per cent of patients. As might be expected, the principal cause of death in the morbidly obese is directly related to cardiovascular disease in the form of stroke, acute coronary thrombosis, or arryhthmias. The role of the obesity is underscored by the observation that weight reduction alone lowers blood pressure in over one half of hypertensive obese patients.

Adult-onset diabetes (noninsulin-dependent diabetes mellitus, or NIDDM) or impaired glucose tolerance occurs in one third of the morbidly obese, with the frequency and severity of glucose intolerance being directly related to the degree of excess weight.[84] NIDDM is not due to a lack of insulin; in fact, patients generally exhibit significant hyperinsulinemia. The insulin resistance in these obese individuals, according to the studies of Caro and his associates[12] in the laboratories at East Carolina, is not due to alterations in the structure of the insulin receptors but to complex defects in the metabolism of the cell membrane, the cytoplasm, and the nucleus. So far, these data[16,74] and those of others[24,34,36,46] suggest (1) a decreased availability of the recep-

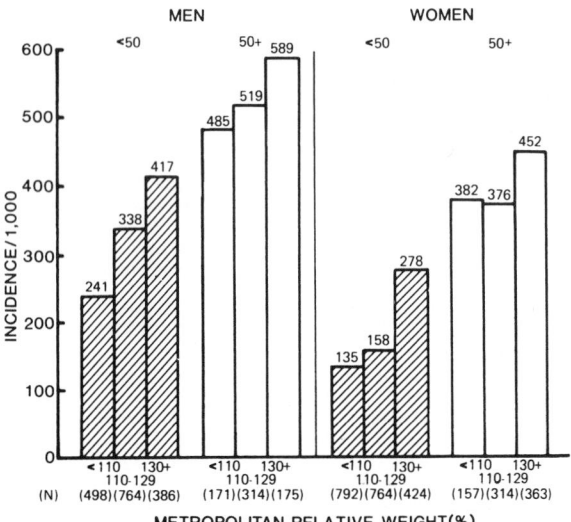

Figure 1. The 26-year incidence of cardiovascular disease by Metropolitan Relative Weight at entry among Framingham Study men and women younger than age 50 years and age 50 years or older. N, the number at risk for an event. Numbers above the bars give the actual incidence rates per 1000. (From Hubert, H. B., Feinleib, M., McNamara, P. M., et al.: Obesity as an independent risk factor for cardiovascular disease: A 26-year follow-up of participants in the Framingham Heart Study. Circulation, 67:968, 1983. By permission of the American Heart Association, Inc.)

tors on the cell membrane, (2) decreased insulin receptor kinase activity, (3) inadequate generation of second messengers, and (4) diminished activity of specific glucose transport proteins. When diabetes complicates morbid obesity, mortality increases 40 per cent.[18]

Pulmonary insufficiency develops in almost all morbidly obese individuals to some degree as the expiratory reserve volume declines with the continuing gain in weight. In those who develop the full-blown pickwickian hypoventilation syndrome, the mortality exceeds 30 per cent.[17] *Cholelithiasis* is increased threefold, and some maintain that all morbidly obese people either have or will develop chronic cholecystitis.[82] Morbidly obese individuals often have difficulty conceiving; their *infertility* and the frequently seen *amenorrhea* generally reverse after surgically induced weight loss. Pregnancy, when it does occur, is associated with an increased risk of *preeclampsia*, hypertension, poor fetal weight gain, diabetes mellitus, and *wound infec-*

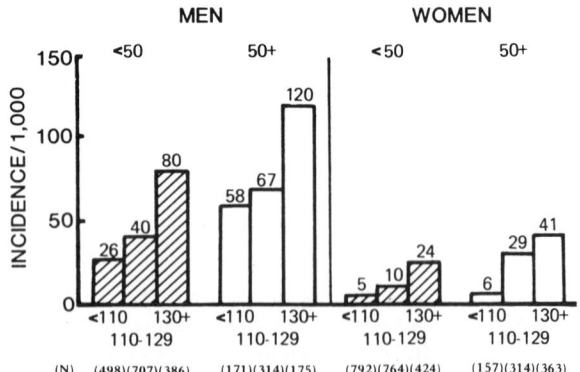

Figure 2. The 26-year incidence of sudden death by Metropolitan Relative Weight at entry among Framingham Study men and women younger than age 50 years and age 50 years or older. N, the number at risk for an event. Numbers above the bars give the actual incidence rates per 1000. (From Hubert, H. B., Feinleib, M., McNamara, P. M., et al.: Obesity as an independent risk factor for cardiovascular disease: A 26-year follow-up of participants in the Framingham Heart Study. Circulation, 67:968, 1983. By permission of the American Heart Association, Inc.)

tions.[60] The debilitating symptoms of *degenerative arthritis* are compounded by the severe stress placed on articulating joint surfaces by the patient's excessive weight. Other complications of obesity include *gout, skin diseases, proteinuria, increased hemoglobin concentration, and immunologic impairment.*

In fact, morbid obesity probably affects every organ system, and particularly the heart. Obese patients have an increased cardiac output, stroke volume, central blood volume, plasma volume, and total blood volume; they also have decreased peripheral resistance. If they are also hypertensive, the peripheral resistance is elevated as well. As the left ventricular volume is augmented in response to the high stroke volume, afterload is correspondingly increased. It is not surprising that left ventricular function becomes impaired early in morbidly overweight patients, regardless of arterial pressure.[51] The skeleton, stressed by the massive and poorly distributed weight, undergoes early joint and bone deterioration. The lungs expand poorly because the weight of the chest wall, breasts, and abdominal organs limits the function of the intercostal and diaphragmatic muscles. Accordingly, morbidly obese individuals show significant decreases in vital capacity, expired respiratory volume, and ventilatory ventilation and sharp increases in carbon monoxide diffusing capacity.[64]

Morbid obesity also exerts profound *hormonal effects* as a result of the excessive production of estrogen by the large volume of fat cells. In morbidly obese women, this hormonal change results in dysfunctional uterine bleeding, amenorrhea, and an inadequate luteal phase.[67] In men, the high estrogen blood concentrations are associated with low serum testosterone and low testosterone-estradiol-binding globulin levels, although in both sexes the hypothalamic-pituitary-gonadal axis remains normal. The increased incidence of breast cancer in obese women may well be due to these high levels of estrogen.

Of greater immediate concern to the patients, however, and the major reason for seeking surgical therapy, are the *psychologic and socioeconomic consequences* of morbid obesity. Fat people are frequently objects of public scorn and malicious ridicule. They are viewed as lacking self-esteem and slovenly by nature, with insufficient will power to curtail excessive eating.[48] Their obese physiques are the antithesis of the lean, trim, and muscular body habitus so highly prized in today's exercise-conscious Western society. Obese patients are often unable to fit into armchairs, find suitable clothing, obtain access to public toilets, and enter public conveyances. If they can enter an automobile, they may be unable to get out.

Employers usually consider the morbidly obese poor candidates because of their unfavorable appearance, their inability to fit into office furniture or into factory environments, and their high absenteeism due to illness. In relationships with their peers, the severely obese make few friendships and seldom find satisfactory marital or sexual partners, although the libidos of these obese individuals are often as great as their size. Obese women, particularly, tend to marry inadequate spouses who are afraid to accept the challenge of more desirable women. Frequently the object of jokes, morbidly obese people assume the role of the jolly fat person, hiding their misery in public and soothing it by eating even more. Obesity limits the availability of educational opportunities[11] and the opportunities for finding a mate.

Finally, patients frequently mention their inabilities to meet their parental and other social roles: their children and other family members are ashamed to be seen with them at school, at athletic events, and in social situations. In short, the environment of the morbidly obese is neither happy nor filled with opportunities. Kral[41] summarized it well when he concluded that the morbidly obese are severely handicapped by every measure: physically, emotionally, economically, and socially. Morbid obesity is indeed a serious disease.

THE ETIOLOGY OF HUMAN OBESITY: GENETIC OR ENVIRONMENTAL?

Although there is wide acceptance of the observation that "obesity runs in families," the cause of that obesity, whether genetic or environmental, continues to be disputed. In a superb summary of the various studies to be discussed, Stunkard, in his Salmon Lecture,[79] concludes that both etiologies have a role. The genetic argument rests on several findings: (1) the demonstration that most of the offspring of thin parents are thin and most of the children of fat parents are fat; (2) the strong inverse relationship between the current socioeconomic status and obesity in women holds just as strongly when analyzed for socioeconomic status of origin; (3) analysis of the Twin Register of the National Academy of Sciences/National Research Council shows that the concordance rates for obesity in monozygotic twins were approximately twice those at lesser degrees of overweight and even higher at greater degrees of overweight; and (4) body mass index (BMI) of adoptees is strongly related to the BMI of the biologic parents and not to that of the adoptive parents.

Similarly, there is evidence that environmental factors are also strong: (1) adoptees who are raised in a rural environment are more overweight than those who have been raised in an urban setting; (2) studies of Danish draftees showed no change in the average weight of these men from 1943 to 1960, but in the following 12 years there was an eightfold increase in the number with severe obesity, certainly too short a time for a change in the gene pool; and (3) the higher attendance at "smorgasbord restaurants" by obese people on the nights that buffets were featured. Currently, most authorities concur that both genetic and environmental factors have a role and that the genetic influences appear to be stronger.

Considerable interest exists in the area of energy requirements by the obese. It is clear that obesity, and especially morbid obesity, is not simply a matter of excessive food intake; it also may be caused by decreased energy expenditure from lessened activity or by altered metabolism, such as a reduced thermogenic response to food or attenuated loss of heat through the thickened subcutaneous fat.[5,35] The current examinations by Ravussin and colleagues[63] of the energy expenditure in Pima Indians suggest that some persons with similar physical characteristics are more "energy efficient" and thus more capable of weight gain than others. Some have suggested that an increased rate of gastric emptying in the obese may be the cause of abnormal energy utilization.[89]

Others[38] continue to explore the "set point" theory, which is based on the observation that the body weight of animals is remarkably constant, and concludes that the body weight is "set at a point," perhaps controlled at the hypothalamic level, which is defended at that level even when circumstances change in the environment. DuBois[19] suggests that the set point is based on a gene that allows storage of energy in the form of fat during periods of plenty and that favors the survival of such fat individuals during times of famine. For such a gene to be fully expressed, one has to be in a situation in which unlimited amounts of food are continuously available. The best example is the desert rat, which gorges after each rain and starves during dry spells. If placed in a cage with food available at all times, the rat will become so fat that it eventually will be unable to move. The Pima Indians, with their high prevalence of obesity, may have developed such a thrifty genotype through centuries of desert existence.

In the Minnesota starvation study,[39] volunteers lost 25 per cent of their body weight, whereas in the Vermont prison study,[72] men gained 50 or more pounds. In each study, body weight rapidly returned to normal when subjects were allowed to control their own food intake. The pursuit of an appetite

control center, perhaps in the ventromedial hypothalamus,[32] is another fertile area for investigation of obesity. Studies of parabiotic rats,[31] i.e., surgically produced Siamese twins, showed that when hypothalamic lesions cause obesity in one twin, the other twin decreases its food intake and may even die of starvation. The body weight of the artificial twins appears to be regulated as a unit. Studies of lipectomy[21] support theories of the regulation of body weight; removing fat from one adipose depot is followed by compensatory increase in fat in other depots.

The controversy about the etiology of obesity is not merely academic. Obesity is the most common form of malnutrition in the United States today. Billions of dollars are spent each year in the United States in the pursuit of diets, slimming programs, and the management of obesity. Additional billions are spent by pharmaceutical companies pursuing research to formulate various dietary supplements and to find the compounds that could safely alter metabolic rate, to introduce dietary fats that cannot be digested, or to change the appetite control center. Even the smallest towns in the United States have stores that specialize in clothing for the "stout or larger woman." Control of obesity, if achieved, would probably have an effect at least equal to that of control of smoking in terms of the nation's health.

The largest price, however, is paid by the morbidly obese: not only do they have high health care costs, they also cannot meet their costs of daily living because they are often unemployed and indigent. It is time to recognize, as the National Institutes of Health Consensus Conference on Obesity[55] concluded, that morbid obesity is a serious, disabling, and common disease, and that morbid obesity, like other diseases, deserves treatment and insurance coverage for therapy.

THE DEFINITION OF OBESITY

A number of indices have been developed for the quantification of obesity. The most useful is the list of 1983 Height and Weight Standards of the Metropolitan Life Insurance Company, shown in Table 1. The midpoint of the medium weights listed on that table has been arbitrarily accepted, for bariatric studies, to be the ideal body weight (IBW) for an individual of given sex and size.

The term *morbid obesity* was coined to reflect the life-threatening consequences of being more than 100 pounds (45 kg.) over ideal body weight. Recently, some researchers have adopted the term *malignant obesity* to identify those who exceed their ideal weight by 200 per cent, or 200 pounds.

Height and weight also can be manipulated in various mathematical formulas. Of these ratios, the most useful is the body mass index (weight/height^2), which provides a convenient estimate of excess fat and can be related to health risks with Bray's nomogram shown in Figure 3.[8] His data, organized in Figure 4 to compare BMI versus all-cause mortality, show a J-shaped curve, with the minimal mortality for both men and women occurring among individuals somewhat below the average BMI. Deviations in BMI above and below this are associated with an increase in mortality. Note that above 40 kg./m.^{2} the curve becomes steep. The digestive and respiratory diseases comprise the low-weight mortalities, whereas cardiovascular diseases, diabetes, and gallbladder disease represent the high-weight causes of mortality.

The most accurate and clinically useful measure of obesity is probably provided by hydrodensitometry. Israel and colleagues[20] have developed a head-above-water approach that measures body composition in a clinically acceptable manner. They showed a significant inverse correlation (r = −0.21) between per cent fat and relative fat-free weight (rel FFW = actual FFW/ideal FFW). As individuals increase body fat, they also add FFW to support the increased load during ambulation;

TABLE 1. Height and Weight Standards of the Metropolitan Life Insurance Company

Men				Women			
Height	Small	Medium	Large	Height	Small	Medium	Large
5'2"	128–134	131–141	138–150	4'10"	102–111	109–121	118–131
5'3"	130–136	133–143	140–153	4'11"	103–113	111–123	120–134
5'4"	132–138	135–145	142–156	5'0"	104–115	113–126	122–137
5'5"	134–140	137–148	144–160	5'1"	106–118	115–129	125–140
5'6"	136–142	139–151	146–164	5'2"	108–121	118–132	128–143
5'7"	138–145	142–154	149–168	5'3"	111–124	121–135	131–147
5'8"	140–148	145–157	152–172	5'4"	114–127	124–138	134–151
5'9"	142–151	148–160	155–176	5'5"	117–130	127–141	137–155
5'10"	144–154	151–163	158–180	5'6"	120–133	130–144	140–159
5'11"	146–157	154–166	161–184	5'7"	123–136	133–147	143–163
6'0"	149–160	157–170	164–188	5'8"	126–139	136–150	146–167
6'1"	152–164	160–174	168–192	5'9"	129–142	139–153	149–170
6'2"	155–168	164–178	172–197	5'10"	132–145	142–156	152–173
6'3"	158–172	167–182	176–202	5'11"	135–148	145–159	155–176
6'4"	162–176	171–187	181–207	6'0"	138–151	148–162	158–179

Courtesy of Metropolitan Life Insurance Company.

however, at some critical point (fatness, total weight, cardiorespiratory impairment, orthopedic complications, and so on), mobility of morbidly obese patients becomes restricted, so that they "lose" or "atrophy" in the fat-free compartment. The initial data suggest that this pathologic threshold for adiposity is 45 per cent fat. Israel's work may soon lead to a badly needed redefinition of morbid obesity: instead of the traditional measures related to height and weight, the disease also should be described in degree of adiposity and loss of function.

Other indices of relative adiposity include skinfold thickness, total body potassium, total body water, uptake of fat-soluble inert gases, energy balance, nitrogen balance, and various combinations of height versus weight calculations. Except for special research protocols, no clinical advantage is evident for any of these approaches.[13]

WHO LIVES LONGER, APPLES OR PEARS?

Fat is not symmetrically distributed throughout the body but is more likely to be concentrated in the abdomen in men and on the hips in women. One of the most important developments in understanding the health risks associated with obesity has been the recognition of the importance of body fat distribution. Bray[7] notes that five prospective studies have examined the relation of fat distribution to morbidity and mortality. Whether the abdominal-to-gluteal circumference ratio or waist-to-hip ratio (WHR) or the subscapular skinfold or a combination of skin folds was used as the indicator of abdominal fat, all five studies found a clear-cut and highly significant increase in the risk of death and/or an increased risk of diabetes, hypertension, or stroke in those individuals with large bellies and narrow hips (apples) versus those with a more gynecoid distribution (pears). Fat distribution was a more important risk factor for morbidity and mortality than overweight or obesity per se and had a relative risk ratio of 2 or more. The data for the WHR divided into

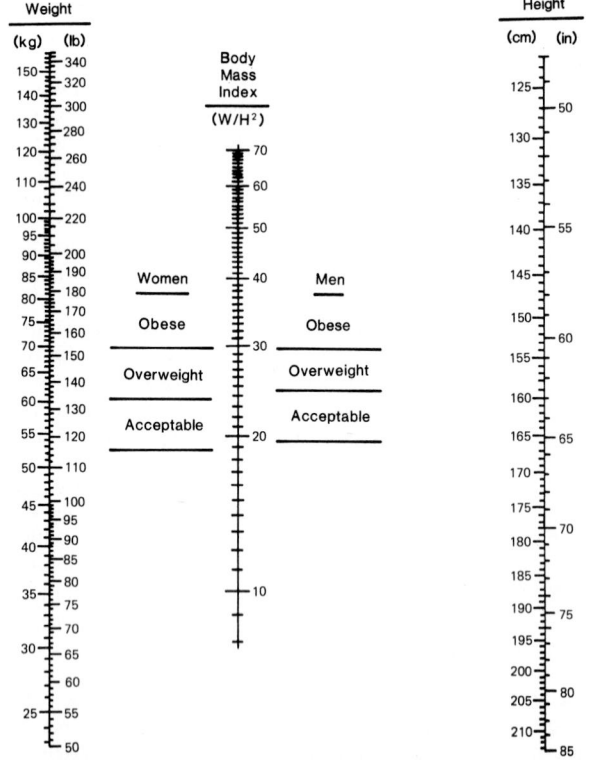

Figure 3. Excess body fat is conveniently estimated by the Body Mass Index Scale, which can be calculated by dividing nude weight in kg. by the square of barefoot height in meters. Alternatively, this nomogram can be used. When a ruler is aligned at the weight and height values, the point where it intersects the scale in the middle gives the body mass index. Obese patients of either sex have index values greater than 30. (From Bray, G. A.: Management options in obesity. Hosp. Pract. *4*:104a, 1982. As redrawn by Albert Miller from original by George A. Bray.)

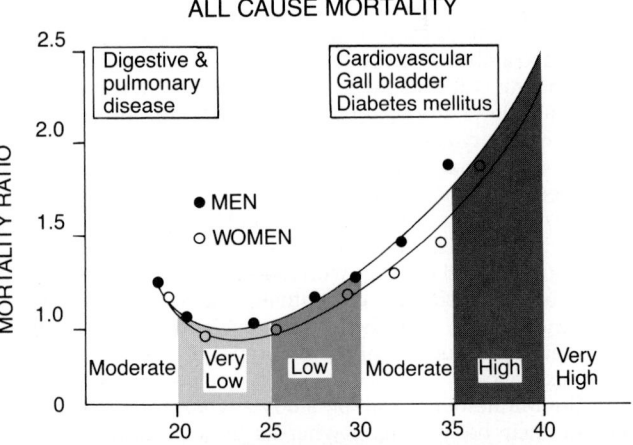

Figure 4. Deviations in body mass index (BMI) are associated with an increase in mortality. Above 40 kg. per m², the curve becomes steep. (Redrawn from Bray, G. A.: Obesity. West. J. Med. *149*:429, 1988.)

fifths for a cohort of residents of Gothenburg, Sweden[45] showed a much greater chance of remaining free of myocardial infarction and of long-term survival in the quintile with the lowest WHR compared with the quintile with the highest WHR. This effect was independent of total fatness. Before fully accepting the concept that "pears outlive apples," however, it is necessary to heed Kuczmarski's[43] warning that the definitions of waist and hip measures are inexact and vary throughout the literature. Future studies with computed tomographic scans, ultrasound, and magnetic resonance imaging and more accurately defined circumference measurements are badly needed to clarify this important question.

NONOPERATIVE TREATMENT OF MORBID OBESITY

THE FAILURE OF DIETING. Although dieting remains the most useful method of weight control for most individuals, it is generally ineffective for morbidly obese individuals.[8,26] In most cases, even when massively obese patients are aided by groups such as Weight Watchers, by psychotherapy, by diuretics, by thyroid preparations, or by anorectic agents such as amphetamines, the lost pounds are usually regained together with additional ones as soon as the intense weight-reducing regimen has ceased. In fact, weight loss is usually disappointingly low. In a study of 100 patients subjected to an intensive weight-reducing regimen by four dietitians, 77 per cent lost less than 10 pounds and only one patient lost more than 20 pounds.[68]

Stunkard and McLaren-Hume[80] have reported similarly disappointing results. In a review of the literature on the failure rate of nonsurgical management of the grossly obese, they found that only 25 per cent of the patients lost as much as 20 pounds, and only 5 per cent lost 40 pounds or more. In their series of 100 consecutive patients, only 12 per cent lost 20 pounds, 1 per cent (one patient) lost 40 pounds, and 28 per cent failed to return after the first visit. Even when compared with the least effective of the gastric operations, the horizontal gastroplasty, diets were not as effective as the operation in a randomized trial conducted by Andersen and associates.[3] Initial weight losses were similar, but the group treated by diet alone regained significantly more weight by the end of the 2-year trial.

After pooling the data from several studies, Bray[7] found that the overall success rate over 1 year with diet alone is about 25 per cent, with diet and medication about 40 per cent, and with behavior modification nearly 50 per cent. For individuals losing 40 pounds but still weighing 250 or 300 pounds, such losses are not adequate. Bray concluded that the long-term success rate by any of the conservative (i.e., nonoperative) methods is not much more than 10 to 15 per cent.

WIRING THE TEETH. Wiring the teeth deserves mention as another generally unsuccessful approach to morbid obesity. Anyone who has cared for a patient with a fractured jaw is aware that with the jaws wired shut such individuals are limited to liquids. They almost always lose weight, even though such loss could be prevented by the use of appropriate liquid nutrient formulas. Similarly, morbidly obese individuals lose weight if the jaws are wired shut. However, the approach has been abandoned for three reasons: (1) many morbidly obese patients are edentulous and therefore are not suitable candidates, (2) they tolerate the wiring poorly because of their personality patterns and generally demand removal of the wires within a few days, and (3) most important, as soon as the wires are removed, even if a major change in appearance is apparent, they resume previous eating habits and quickly return to their original weight.[37] There may still be limited indications for wiring teeth in poor-risk obese patients who are in cardiac or pulmonary failure and who are being prepared for operation. However, if this is done, it must be remembered that many morbidly obese patients are severely malnourished despite their size and that their liquid diets may require considerable nutritional enrichment in order to minimize postoperative complications.

SURGICAL THERAPY FOR MORBID OBESITY

Because diets are ineffective in the management of morbid and malignant obesity, most authorities now agree with Stunkard and Wadden's[81] recommendation: "During the past 10 or so years, surgery has become the treatment of choice of that small percentage of persons who suffer from severe obesity."

The cost of surgical therapy is not insignificant. Approximately 150,000 bariatric operations are performed each year in the United States alone, at a cost of $250 million. These estimates do *not* include the additional charges incurred by the intensive follow-up or the care of the complications seen after bariatric surgery, such as malnutrition, anastomotic stenoses, incisional hernias, staple line breakdowns, psychiatric problems, bowel obstructions, and so on.

Surgical therapy may now be accepted as the therapy of choice, but the evidence for that supremacy has accumulated slowly. The history of bariatric surgery is a story of procedures that are developed, enthusiastically adopted, and rapidly dropped without further follow-up as soon as the next operation or modification is described. Recently, however, excellent rigorous studies are under way that indicate that the two commonly performed operations, the Greenville gastric bypass (GGB) and the vertical banded gastroplasty (VBG), provide effective weight control with acceptable mortality and morbidity rates.

HISTORICAL ASPECTS

The progress of surgical therapy for obesity is interesting not only because of its historical value but also because it represents a remarkable and useful record of physiologic and metabolic studies of the human gut.

THE INTESTINAL BYPASS. Although it had long been known that loss of major portions of the small bowel led to weight loss, Kremen and associates first conceived the idea of therapeutically reducing the length of functional intestine.[42] In 1954, after careful study in dogs, they reported a patient in whom an end-to-end jejunoileostomy was performed for weight reduction. In the discussion of that paper, Sandblom mentioned that Henrikson of Gothenburg, Sweden, had resected "an appropriate amount of small intestine" in a patient because of obesity and had induced weight loss but had encountered difficulty in achieving nutritional balance. In 1956, Payne and associates initiated the first clinical program of surgical therapy for obesity.[58] As illustrated in Figure 5A, their initial procedure was designed to bypass most of the small intestine and half of the colon by an end-to-side anastomosis of the proximal 36 cm. of jejunum to the mid-transverse colon. When Payne and associates reported their series of patients in 1963, it was evident that the procedure produced dramatic weight loss, but that liver failure was prohibitive. One patient died, and each of the remaining nine required reoperation. In six of these individuals, the original intestinal continuity was restored. However, in three patients, in recognition of the essentiality of the terminal ileum, end-to-side jejunoileostomy was performed with good results, except that these patients regained weight. Encouraged by the success of the jejunoileostomies, Payne and DeWind,[59] Sherman and associates,[71] and others initiated a series of trials and adopted the "14 + 4" procedure because of its reasonably predictable weight loss. The procedure, illustrated in Figure 5B, was named "14 + 4" because 14 inches (36 cm.) of proximal jejunum was anastomosed to 4 inches (10 cm.) of distal ileum.

Because the end-to-side jejunoileostomy permits considerable reflux up the bypassed ileum and thus extends the absorptive surface area in an unpredictable fashion, other groups, no-

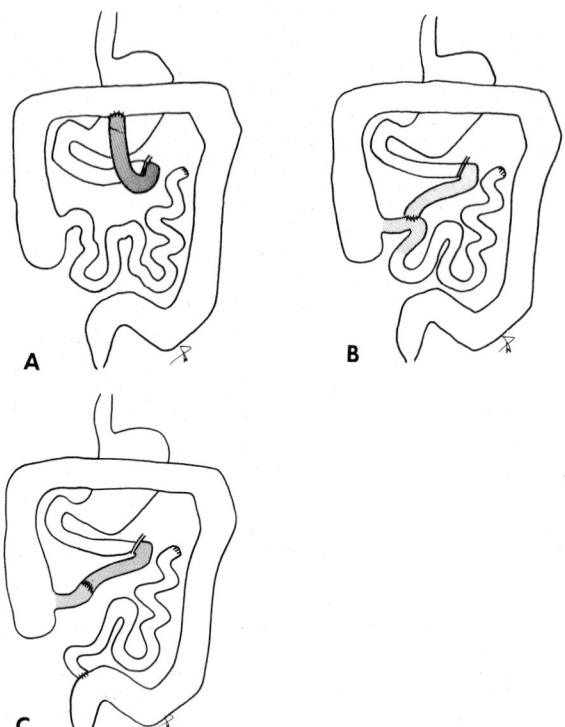

Figure 5. Various types of intestinal bypass. The absorptive surfaces are shaded. The early Payne jejunotransverse colostomy (A) bypassed the terminal ileum with prohibitive metabolic consequences. The end-to-side jejunoileostomy (B) has a somewhat larger absorptive surface than the end-to-end jejunoileostomy (C) because of backwash into the bypassed segment. A, Payne's first operation.[58] Jejunotransverse colostomy with a 60-cm. jejunal segment. B, Payne's second operation.[59] End-to-side jejunoileostomy. C, Scott's end-to-end jejunoileostomy with drainage of remaining small bowel into sigmoid colon.[30]

tably those of Scott[70] and Buchwald,[10] came to prefer the end-to-end jejunoileostomy. Scott joined 30 cm. of proximal jejunum to 20 cm. of terminal ileum, whereas Buchwald utilized corresponding 40-cm. and 4-cm. segments (Fig. 5C). (In massively obese patients who weigh over 158.9 kg. or 350 pounds, Scott employed 30-cm. and 15-cm. segments.) Note that the end-to-end anastomosis required a second anastomosis to drain the totally bypassed ileojejunal loop into the cecum, the transverse colon, or the sigmoid colon.

The direct relationship between intestinal length and weight loss was demonstrated by Weismann.[86] As shown in Figure 6, operations with more than 64 cm. (25 inches) of intestine in continuity produced unsatisfactory weight loss.

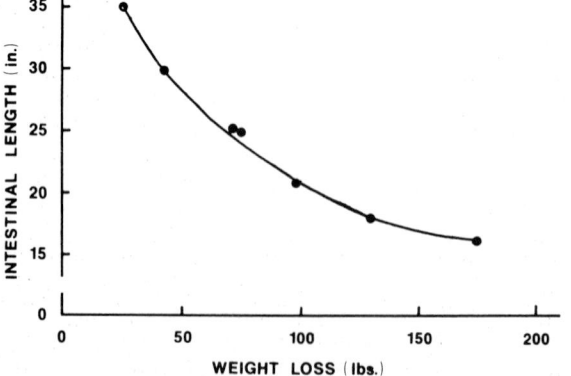

Figure 6. The relationship of intestinal bypass length to weight loss. Operations with more than 64 cm. (25 inches) in continuity produce unsatisfactory weight loss. (From Bray, G. A., Barry, R. E., Benfield, J. R., et al.: Intestinal bypass as a treatment for obesity. Ann. Intern. Med., 85:97, 1976. Modified from Weismann, R. E.: Surgical palliation of massive and severe obesity. Am. J. Surg., 125:437, 1973.)

RESULTS OF INTESTINAL BYPASS. Most groups performing intestinal bypass procedures preferred an end-to-end jejunoileostomy, which excluded all but about 50 cm. of small intestine from the digestive stream; good results, in terms of weight loss, were reported in about 80 per cent of their patients, with an average weight loss of 45 kg., or 100 pounds. Massively obese individuals lost more than those less obese; younger patients lost more than those in middle age. Most weight loss occurred during the first year after operation, with the jejunocolic bypass resulting in an average total weight loss of 41 per cent and the jejunoileal bypass, an average weight loss of 35 per cent.[10] By the second or third year, almost all patients reached a plateau, and many regained their weight as adaptations for better absorption occurred in their intestines.

COMPLICATIONS OF INTESTINAL BYPASS PROCEDURES. Jejunoileal bypass was associated with a high complication rate. The early in-hospital mortality and complications in six series of intestinal bypass operations are shown in Table 2. The mortality rate varied from 1 to 8 per cent, and the major complications included wound problems (10 to 20 per cent), pulmonary emboli (1 to 4 per cent), and hepatic failure (1 to 2 per cent). Bray and co-workers[6] reviewed 989 patients collected in the literature and reported the following causes for the 29 deaths (3 per cent) during the first postoperative month: liver failure (five deaths), pulmonary embolism (eight deaths), cardiac failure (two deaths), surgical technique including anastomotic leaks and sepsis (seven deaths), and other complications (seven deaths). They also reported a long-term follow-up of 1500 patients and found the complications shown in Table 2. Of particular concern were the metabolic problems. Some resulted from the severe loss of minerals associated with diarrhea, including hypocalcemia, hypokalemia, hypomagnesemia, and iron and zinc deficiency. Hypoproteinemia and anemia were common. The diarrhea usually began about the fifth postoperative day and soon reached 12 to 20 liquid movements per day, gradually subsiding to 6 to 10 semi-formed movements per day. Serum electrolyte, mineral, and vitamin levels had to be carefully monitored and corrected to avoid serious and occasionally uncontrollable symptoms. Vitamin B_{12} and folic acid deficiencies were common.

TABLE 2. Complications of Jejunoileostomy Used for Treatment of Obesity

Complications	Per Cent
Major Complications	
Early	
Operative mortality	0–6.5
Pulmonary emboli	1–6
Wound infection	2–10
Gastrointestinal hemorrhage	0–6
Renal failure	0–9
Later	
Urinary calculi	3–30
Liver disease	0–14
Anemia	0–3
Acute cholecystitis	0–7
Intestinal obstruction	0–3.5
Minor Complications	
Diarrhea	100
Minor electrolyte abnormalities	40–80
Hypoproteinemia	40–100
Vomiting	10–80
Polyarthritis	0–6
Hair loss	0–100

From Bray, G. A., Barry, R. E., Benfield, J. R., et al.: Intestinal bypass operation as a treatment for obesity. Ann. Intern. Med., 85:97, 1976.

Gastrointestinal complications included intractable diarrhea with associated rectal problems, hemorrhage, and "bypass enteritis." The last is a syndrome that is probably due to pathologic bacterial colonization of the bypassed bowel from the colon and is characterized by diarrhea, abdominal pain, fever of up to 39° C., and occasionally even pneumatosis cystoides.

Even more worrisome were the long-term problems associated with intestinal bypass. First, as noted earlier, 20 per cent of the patients failed to lose weight satisfactorily, and some lost no weight at all. A significant number regained some of the lost weight during the second and third year after operation, and some of these patients required another procedure in which an additional segment of the now-adapted small bowel was removed.

The long-term side effects of jejunoileal bypass consisted of diarrhea, electrolyte imbalance, and impaired absorption of a variety of nutrients. Wise and Stein[88] reported that biliary or urinary calculi developed in 8 per cent of their patients following intestinal bypass, possibly as a result of increased bile salt and glycine synthesis and hyperoxaluria. Gregory and associates[28] also found urologic stone disease in 6 per cent of 435 ileal bypass patients and suggested that excessive glycine reabsorption with hepatic conversion to oxalate, increased exogenous oxalate absorption, hepatic failure, and dehydration all contributed to the problem.

There appears to be a significant inverse correlation between oxalate absorption and fecal fat excretion. Oxalate (soluble) has a high affinity for calcium, resulting in formation of the insoluble precipitate, calcium oxalate. When dietary fat combines with calcium, oxalate remains available for adsorption. After intestinal bypass, fatty acids are present in large amounts; these combine with calcium even more readily than they combine with oxalate, effectively increasing the amount of soluble oxalate for absorption.[6] In addition, renal failure severe enough to require surgical restoration of bowel continuity was also reported, with recovery after operation.[14]

Liver disease was the most feared complication of intestinal bypass, and a number of fatalities were reported. Many morbidly obese patients were particularly vulnerable because fatty metamorphosis is common among the morbidly obese even prior to operation — that is, their fatty livers resemble those of force-fed geese. Payne and DeWind[58] reported that 95 per cent of their patients weighing over 113 kg. (250 pounds) had fatty infiltration of the liver preoperatively, and during the period of initial rapid weight loss this fatty infiltration was clearly increased. Salmon[66] found that two thirds of his patients had fatty metamorphosis at the time of operation, and in one tenth of the group the change was severe. Following bypass, 95 per cent developed moderate-to-great infiltration that gradually cleared, according to serial needle biopsies, within 4 years. In the first series of 43 patients reported by O'Leary and associates,[56] 42 per cent developed significant postoperative abnormalities of liver function. One patient died as a result of liver failure, and another required reversal of the intestinal bypass because of progressive liver dysfunction.

Abnormalities in liver function occurred in about 40 per cent of patients with an intestinal bypass. These changes were unpredictable and dangerous, appearing as early as 3 weeks or as late as 2 years after operation. Nausea, vomiting, jaundice, and enlargement of the liver were reported frequently; ascites and anasarca were rare. Hepatic coma and death occurred in 1 per cent of all bypass patients. Although many patients showed improvement 6 to 12 months after operation, in 3 to 5 per cent the changes were progressive and associated with marked fibrosis. In severe cases, the terminal changes were histologically indistinguishable from alcoholic cirrhoses. Hepatic deterioration progressed in some patients despite restoration of good nutrition by hyperalimentation.[9]

O'Leary and associates[56] postulated that liver failure following intestinal bypass is caused by the excluded intestinal limb, inasmuch as liver dysfunction is not seen in either humans or experimental animals with subtotal enterectomy. Cultures from the excluded intestinal limb of the patient who was subjected to a second operation revealed disappearance of aerobic organisms and marked overgrowth of *Bacteroides*. Prompted by this observation, O'Leary's group performed jejunoileal shunts in dogs and found that animals protected with antibiotics specific for *Bacteroides* survived without liver dysfunction. All the control animals died of liver failure within 4 months, however, and in all these experiments *Bacteroides* was cultured from the excluded loop. These investigators suggested, therefore, that *Bacteroides* may be a contributing agent in the development of liver failure, because it produces a hepatotoxic endotoxin.

In addition to hepatic dysfunction and urinary and biliary calculi, a large number of reports cited a variety of problems, including unmanageable diarrhea, polyarthrosis, fatigue, lethargy, muscle cramps, uncontrollable nausea and bloating,[2] tuberculosis,[4] and nontuberculous granulomas.[6] In addition to the various metabolic problems, patients developed mechanical complications, including obstruction of the bypassed small intestine and intussusception of the blind loop into the colon. These two problems can be particularly puzzling and dangerous, because roentgenographic findings may not be helpful, since the characteristic small bowel loops with air-fluid levels may not be present. Scott and associates[70] reviewed late results of bypass in a series of 200 patients and found that the procedure is followed by a 2.5 per cent operative mortality rate and a 25 per cent complication rate, with only 66 per cent of the survivors obtaining good results. Moreover, Halverson's group[30] reported that 58 per cent had life-endangering complications and that 23 per cent required reversal of the intestinal bypass because of complications such as liver dysfunction, severe malnutrition or weakness, and late electrolyte imbalance.

In summary, after intestinal bypass most patients lost one third of their total body weight with some improvement of insulin resistance, hypertension, cardiac failure, pulmonary function, and hyperlipidemia. Unfortunately, the long-term complications were serious, with persistent diarrhea, hypokalemia, profound hypomagnesemia and hypocalcemia, arthalgias, neurologic signs, enteropathies, intussusceptions, avitaminoses, trace element deficits, cholelithiasis, renal disease, and liver failure. Thousands of operations were done, however, before it became evident that 50 per cent of these patients required rehospitalization and many had to have the bypasses reversed to prevent death from hepatic failure. Equally sad, most patients' intestinal function adapted, and they began to regain their weight in the second year. Griffen and associates[29] finally abandoned the procedure after a review of the results: "Jejunoileal bypass is not an appropriate operation for morbidly obese patients and should be abandoned."

CONVERSION FROM INTESTINAL TO GASTRIC BYPASS

Because the intestinal bypass is associated with so many long-term complications and because these complications are unpredictable, most bariatric surgeons agree that patients with these intestinal configurations should be converted to either a gastric bypass or a vertical banded gastroplasty. Simple reversal is, of course, another option, but in almost all cases the patients will quickly revert to morbid obesity, merely trading one set of complications for another. Since many of these patients are severely malnourished, 2 to 3 weeks of parenteral nutrition may be needed to prepare them for operation.

THE BILIOPANCREATIC BYPASS

Despite the frightening experience with the intestinal bypass, the malabsorption operation has not been abandoned completely. Scopinaro[1,25,78] of Italy has stimulated some interest

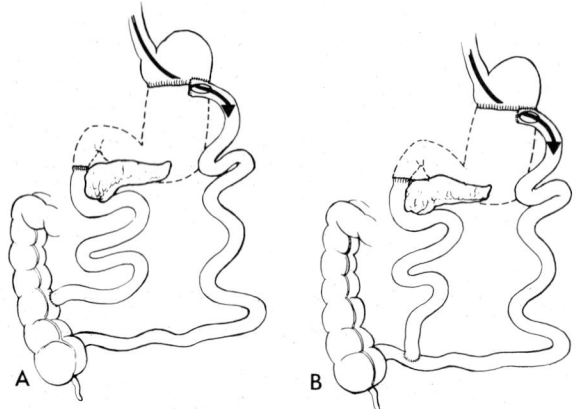

Figure 7. Two versions of Scopinaro's intestinal bypass, (*A*, total; *B*, partial). The operation not only shortens the intestine but also includes a 25 to 75 per cent gastric resection. This irreversible operation has not yet been tested adequately.

with his biliopancreatic bypass, a procedure, shown in Figure 7, that diverts pancreatobiliary secretions via the duodenum and the jejunum into the ileum or colon, with the remaining small intestine being anastomosed to the stomach after antrectomy. It thus combines some of the characteristics of the intestinal bypass with a gastric resection; in contrast with the other common bariatric procedures, it is not reversible. The operation produces significant weight loss but, as might be expected, is associated with serious malnutrition and other complications. Further studies of the procedure under carefully controlled conditions are indicated before the operation can be recommended for wide use.

GASTRIC OPERATIONS FOR MORBID OBESITY

In 1969, Mason and Ito,[49] concerned by the frequency and seriousness of the complications from intestinal bypass, devised the gastric bypass (Fig. 8), which was designed to interfere with food intake rather than with digestion and absorption. In their original approach, the stomach was transected proximally to form a small gastric pouch that was anastomosed to a loop of proximal jejunum, thus bypassing the distal stomach and duodenum. The procedure and various modifications were rapidly adopted when others, such as Alden,[2] Griffen,[29] Hermreck,[60] and their associates confirmed that the gastric bypass was not only safer but was as effective as the intestinal bypass in producing weight loss in morbidly obese patients.

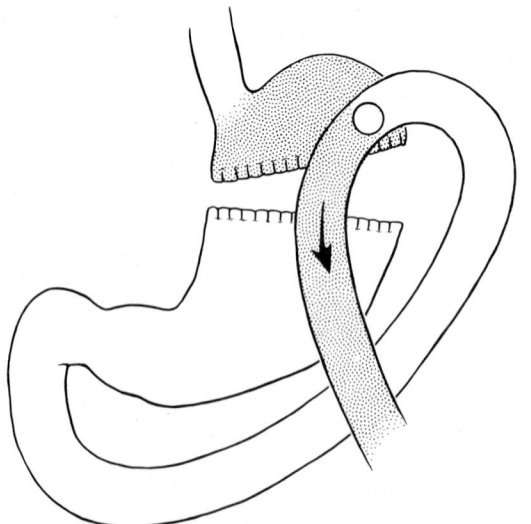

Figure 8. Mason's first gastric bypass.[49] The stomach is transected to form a small pouch, and a loop of jejunum restores gastrointestinal continuity.

The subsequent two decades have seen a host of new procedures, which can be divided into four types: (1) gastroplasties, (2) gastric bypasses, (3) external constricting prostheses, and (4) artificial bezoars or gastric balloons. All reduce the gastric reservoir; the gastroplasties, gastric bypasses, and banding procedures also delay gastric emptying with a small gastric outlet; and the gastric bypass, in addition, bypasses the antrum, duodenum, and about a foot of proximal jejunum. These four types are shown in Figure 9.

THE VERTICAL BANDED GASTROPLASTY. Since Mason's first gastric bypass was a major technical challenge, especially in morbidly obese patients, other alternatives, called gastroplasties, were developed that also could provide a small gastric pouch and a limited outlet without requiring gastric division or an intestinal anastomosis. A large variety of gastroplasties evolved around the same principle: the partition of the stomach with a stapler leaving a small passage, about 1 cm. in diameter, (1) in the center of the staple line or (2) at the greater or (3) lesser curvature. Others solved the problem with a gastrogastroplasty, forming a small anastomosis between the two separated gastric pouches. All these eventually failed, either because of stretching of the opening or the breakdown of the staple line.

Mason, the real pioneer in bariatric surgery, persevered through a number of model procedures and, in 1980, developed the VBG, which, today, is the most commonly performed bariatric operation in the United States. The operation requires close attention to detail; for more information the reader is directed to Mason's recent and detailed description in the *Surgical Clinics of North America.*

THE PROCEDURE. The abdomen is entered through a midline incision and carefully explored. If no contraindications are found, a 32-French Ewald tube is passed into the stomach and positioned against the lesser curvature. A Penrose drain is then passed around the esophagus just above the cardia and the thin gastrohepatic ligament is entered. The fingers of the left hand are inserted into the lesser sac to open the passage between the gastric neurovascular bundle and the gastric wall. The Penrose

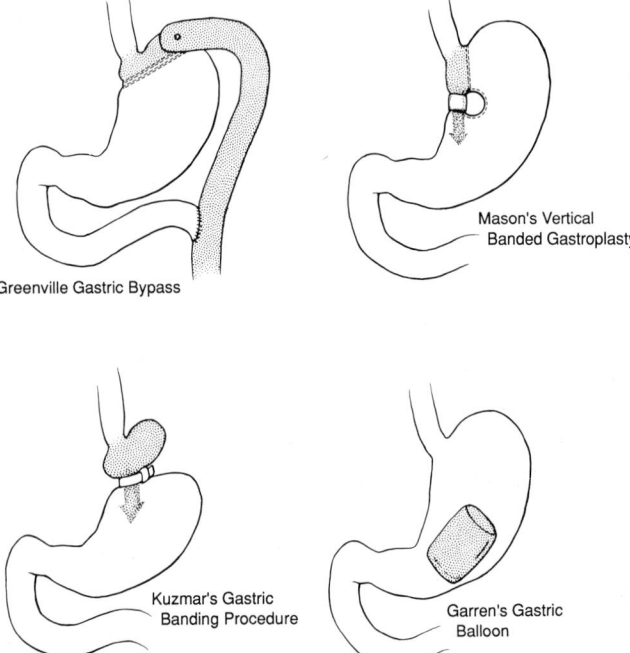

Greenville Gastric Bypass

Mason's Vertical Banded Gastroplasty

Kuzmar's Gastric Banding Procedure

Garren's Gastric Balloon

Figure 9. Four gastric interventions to induce weight control. The gastric bypass produces the greatest weight loss; the vertical banded gastroplasty is a somewhat less effective bariatric procedure but produces fewer nutritional deficits; the gastric banding is a promising new idea; the Garren balloon proved to be dangerous and ineffective and was removed from the market by the Food and Drug Administration.

drain is brought through, closely encompassing only esophageal and gastric tissue, i.e., excluding the vessels and branches of the vagus nerves. A 25-mm. diameter end-to-end (EEA) stapler is used to create a window adjacent to the Ewald tube, which is positioned against the lesser curvature. The window may require reinforcement with absorbable sutures, especially if there is any doubt about the "doughnut" specimens excised by the stapler. The linear 4-row stapler is then applied through the gastric window parallel to the Ewald tube to produce the pouch. The final pouch volume is adjusted to values of 9 to 25 ml., with an average of 15 ml. as measured through the tube. The collar is created with a 1.5- by 7.0-cm. strip of Marlex mesh marked and sewn so that a 5.0-cm. opening will be used for morbidly obese patients and a 4.5-cm. opening for malignantly obese patients.

At the end of the procedure, the integrity of the pouch is tested with the insufflation of air with the abdomen filled with saline. The mesh is then covered with omentum. If other conditions are found during the exploration that require additional procedures, such as cholelithiasis, these generally can be treated during the same procedure. The abdomen is closed with an absorbable suture and the skin reapproximated with staples.

RESULTS. Mason recently reported a combined series of 900 patients from the University of Iowa Hospitals and Clinics in Iowa City and the St. Francis Memorial Hospital in San Francisco. The operative mortality was 0.33 per cent. Three-year results show sustained weight control with a loss of 35 kg. (54 per cent excess weight loss) in 45 patients whose initial weight was greater than 225 per cent of ideal. During the study, the size of the collar, i.e., the gastric pouch outlet, was changed. No data were provided regarding the intensity of the follow-up. Similarly, Deitel and associates reported a series of 233 patients and confirmed Mason's excellent results, but after 12 months 16 patients were not available for follow-up; after 18 months, only 146 patients were included in the evaluation; and at 24 months, only 87 were available for study.[15] In summary, the vertical banded gastroplasty is an effective procedure that can be performed with an acceptable morbidity and mortality. The operation deserves rigorous study to determine its long-term effectiveness and late complications.

THE GREENVILLE GASTRIC BYPASS. Of the Roux-en-Y gastric exclusion procedures, the GGB appears to be the most effective operation. That procedure, shown in Figure 10,[61] produces the following anatomic changes: (1) a small proximal gastric pouch, measuring 20 to 30 ml.; (2) a Roux-en-Y anastomosis with a limb measuring about 40 cm.; (3) an 8-mm. gastrojejunostomy, sewn with a continuous double-layered suture to limit dilatation; and (4) application of four staple lines in parallel manner to prevent staple line failure.

THE OPERATION. The abdomen is entered through a midline incision and exposure is provided by the Gomez retractor. If the exploration demonstrates no contraindications, the upper stomach is isolated by inserting the index finger gently into the angle at the cardia to the left of the esophagus. At this point, there is a weak, thin area of the posterior peritoneum that is easily entered by the dissecting finger. The dissection is gently continued behind the esophagus and cardia and the finger brought out, not at the right side of the esophagus but between the ascending branches of the left gastric artery, 2.5 to 3.0 cm. below the esophagogastric junction. A large Malecot catheter, from which the bulbous end has been cut, is used to pull a doubleheaded TA 90 Auto Suture stapling instrument through the passage. A proximal pouch measuring 4 cm. in width and 1.5 cm. in height is then prepared by firing the staples. A figure-eight suture is placed at each end of the staple line to close the ends securely and to serve as guy sutures. The jejunum is divided at its apex, about 30 to 40 cm. from the ligament of Treitz, with the GIA stapling instrument and the distal end is then sutured to the gastric pouch. The anastomosis is sewn to fit snugly around a

0.8-cm. Salem Sump tube in two layers with continuous Prolene. The Roux-en-Y enteroenterostomy is then completed by joining the proximal jejunum end-to-side to the distal jejunum with GIA and TA 55 stapling instruments. It is important to fasten the Roux loop to the mesocolon to prevent an internal hernia and to oversew any bleeders in the enteroenterostomy before closing it. The abdomen is closed with a running double-stranded 0 PDS absorbable suture. The skin is stapled. The operation can usually be performed in 60 to 75 minutes; blood loss rarely exceeds 300 ml.

RESULTS. From February 1980 to April 1990, the identical GGB was performed in 475 morbidly obese patients, a group composed of 337 white and 72 black women as well as 56 white and 10 black men. Within this group, 331 were married, 42 were divorced, 74 were single, 18 were separated, and 8 were widowed. Also within this group, 296 were employed, 176 were not employed, and 3 were between jobs.

Follow-up has been and continues to be rigorous: over the 9 years of the study, personal contact was maintained with all but 9 patients for a follow-up rate of 98 per cent.

The operation produced significant *weight loss* and, during the 9 years of observation, patients maintained that loss well (Table 3). If morbid obesity is defined as 100 pounds over ideal weight, 94 per cent of the patients were no longer morbidly obese within 2 years. There was, however, some weight gain between 24 and 108 months (179 to 206 pounds, or 15.1 per cent), reflecting the individuals who learn to "outeat their pouch" with high-calorie liquids and continue snacking, as well as those individuals who had a staple line breakdown.

The GGB effectively reduced the proportion of *body fat*. Measurements of body composition by Israel[20] with hydrodensitometry (underwater immersion weighing) in 220 of the patients demonstrated that the women fell from a preoperative mean of 50.92 per cent to 38.46 per cent fat and men from 46.70 per cent to 31.93 per cent fat.

The GGB produced remarkable improvement in the abnormal glucose metabolism of those morbidly obese individuals who were either glucose impaired or had frank adult-onset *diabetes mellitus* (Table 4). NIDDM was present in 100 (21 per cent), and impaired glucose tolerance was present in another 62 (13 per cent) of these 475 patients. All but three of these (98 per cent) became euglycemic after operation. This normalization of glucose metabolism occurs with surprising speed, even before there is significant weight loss. After 10 days, there is no further evidence of NIDDM in most patients, even in patients who had required over 100 units of insulin preoperatively. Forty-two recent patients with diabetes, therefore, were studied intensively. Of these, 12 had been maintained on insulin, another 9 were on sulfonylureas, and another 2 were on both medications prior to the gastric bypass. None now receive any antidiabetic medication or special diets (however, the gastric bypass with its small pouch reduces the daily intake to approximately 1300 calories per day). As shown in Table 5, fasting blood glucose, fasting insulin, and glycosylated hemoglobin were restored to normal levels in all the patients while insulin release, insulin resistance, and utilization of glucose sharply improved. The remarkable reversal of NIDDM is probably not only due to weight loss or decreased caloric intake, but also may be due to the bypass of the neuroendocrine axis of the antrum and duodenum. There is increasing evidence that (1) the gut hormones affect insulin action; (2) insulin can be recovered from the exocrine secretions of the human pancreas; and (3) the mucosa of the duodenum and proximal jejunum contains insulin receptors. These findings suggest the existence of a foregut hormonal regulatory mechanism for glucose metabolism with the following sequence: (1) carbohydrate absorbed from the stomach stimulates the islets to secrete insulin; (2) the insulin is not only released into the blood as an endocrine secretion but is also secreted into the duodenum through the pancreatic duct; (3)

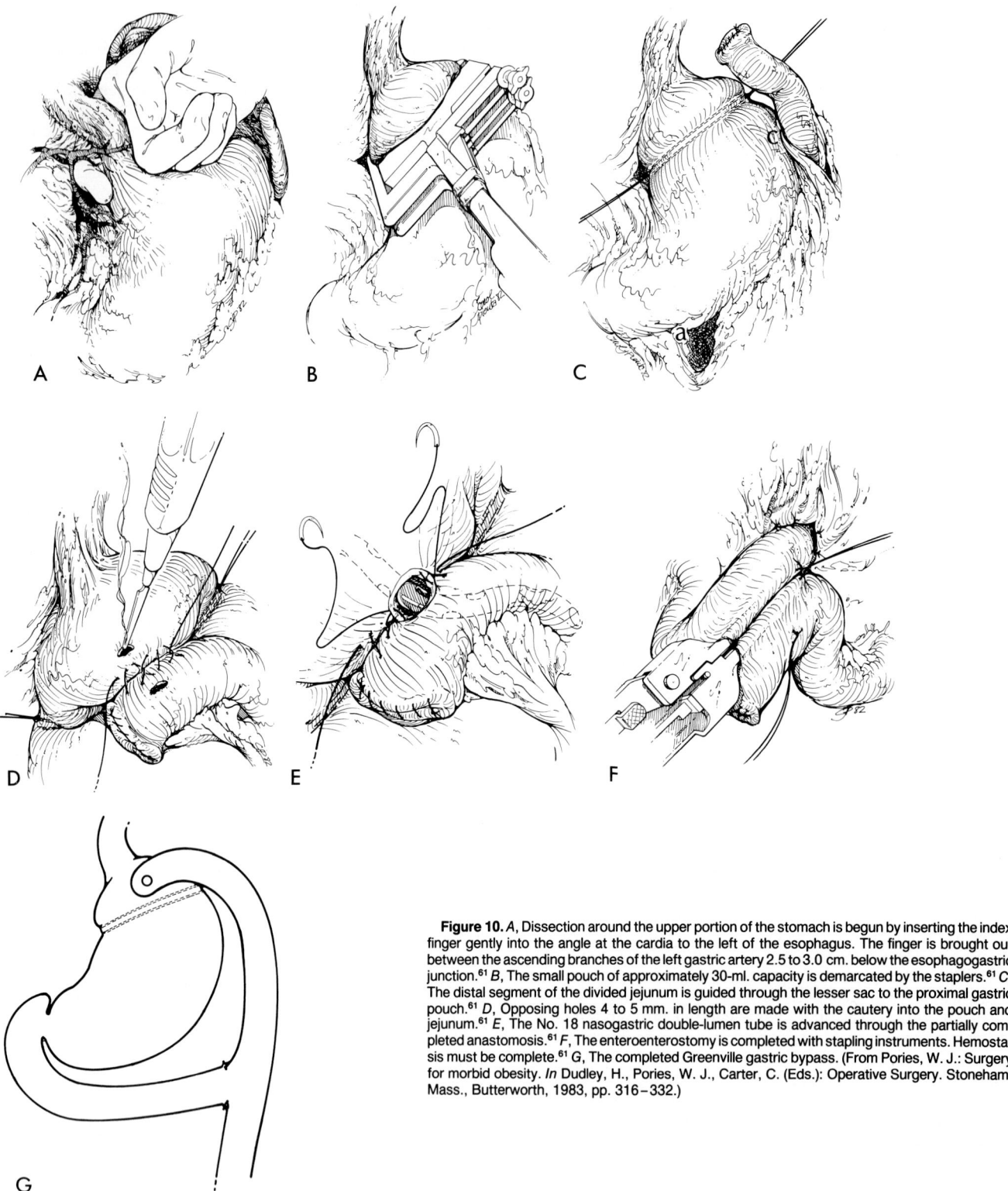

Figure 10. *A*, Dissection around the upper portion of the stomach is begun by inserting the index finger gently into the angle at the cardia to the left of the esophagus. The finger is brought out between the ascending branches of the left gastric artery 2.5 to 3.0 cm. below the esophagogastric junction.[61] *B*, The small pouch of approximately 30-ml. capacity is demarcated by the staplers.[61] *C*, The distal segment of the divided jejunum is guided through the lesser sac to the proximal gastric pouch.[61] *D*, Opposing holes 4 to 5 mm. in length are made with the cautery into the pouch and jejunum.[61] *E*, The No. 18 nasogastric double-lumen tube is advanced through the partially completed anastomosis.[61] *F*, The enteroenterostomy is completed with stapling instruments. Hemostasis must be complete.[61] *G*, The completed Greenville gastric bypass. (From Pories, W. J.: Surgery for morbid obesity. *In* Dudley, H., Pories, W. J., Carter, C. (Eds.): Operative Surgery. Stoneham, Mass., Butterworth, 1983, pp. 316–332.)

when the blood glucose and the consequent insulin levels become high enough, the exocrine insulin stimulates the insulin receptors in the foregut and (4) stimulates the mucosa to secrete an anti-insulin that produces insulin resistance by blocking the insulin receptor. Such a mechanism, still unproved, could be one of the ways, in addition to the weight loss, that the gastric bypass restores the morbidly obese patient with diabetes to euglycemia. It is still too early to predict whether the correction of the glucose metabolism also leads to prevention of diabetic lesions.

The GGB also favorably affected *hypertension.* Of the 475 patients, 280 (59 per cent) were hypertensive before the operation, and of these, 155 (33 per cent) were on antihypertensive medication. After the GGB, 95 (20 per cent) remained hypertensive and 77 (16 per cent) were kept on medication by their physicians.

Concern about the *fate of the bypassed stomach* led to retrograde endoscopic and histologic studies of the distal pouch.[22,50,57,73] Initial studies demonstrated gastritis in the bypassed pouches, but further studies of patients prior to opera-

TABLE 3. Weight Loss after Gastric Bypass for the GGB Cohort

Time	N	Mean Weight (lb.)	Mean Percentage of Excess Original Weight	Mean Percentage of Ideal Body Weight
Preoperative	475	293 (196–565)	0	214 (140–377)
3 mo.	439	238 (124–490)	37 (6–103)	174 (97–307)
6 mo.	391	210 (124–441)	55 (14–95)	154 (104–282)
12 mo.	370	185 (104–397)	72 (23–124)	135 (85–268)
24 mo.	275	179 (105–367)	74 (9–116)	131 (88–248)
36 mo.	230	193 (118–407)	66 (6–108)	140 (91–256)
48 mo.	197	193 (114–413)	64 (21–112)	141 (87–253)
60 mo.	181	199 (107–428)	63 (2–116)	144 (86–263)
72 mo.	140	198 (121–399)	60 (9–104)	146 (96–270)
84 mo.	114	201 (113–378)	60 (−5–109)	148 (94–273)
96 mo.	65	193 (130–300)	58 (11–91)	144 (107–214)
108 months	30	206 (155–320)	56 (16–86)	148 (112–196)

tion and up to 2 years after operation indicate that gastritis is common in morbidly obese patients; that it is equally common after operation; that bile washes back into the excluded antrum; and that no metaplastic or dysplastic changes of the gastric mucosa were noted on the late postoperative endoscopic biopsies. Longer-term observations are needed and are under way.

Although the GGB produced long-term improvement in the health and physical functioning of morbidly obese patients, the emotional and social changes for the better proved to be temporary. There is significant improvement in both physical and role functioning throughout the first 24 months after operation; but by the end of 36 months, the previously significant improvement erodes to a nonsignificant difference (Table 6). Similarly, the *RAND mental health measures* (Table 7) show marked improvement 6 months after operation, but self-control erodes first to a nonsignificant difference even at 12 months. By 3 years, all the emotional improvement has returned to preoperative levels. The patients feel better and look better, but one would presume from these early findings that those with inadequate preoperative personalities return to that state despite how well they look and feel. Whether counseling or other psychiatric intervention can alter this regression bears investigation. Relevant to these findings is the report by Ryden and associates,[65] who found depression to be more common in those patients who had an excellent result after bariatric surgery and concluded that "the marked weight loss leads to problems of adaptation, which in turn may trigger depressive reactions."

The *complications* associated with the GGB are summarized in Table 8. The perioperative mortality of 1.3 per cent (6 of 475) is low for this group of high-risk patients with such complicating preoperative factors as pickwickian syndrome, inadequately managed diabetes, cardiopulmonary failure, asthma, chronic skin infections, and disabling arthritis. The average length of stay was 8.6 days (range, 5 to 34 days). Of the 475 patients, 11 per cent had a complication serious enough to prolong their hospital stay. The most common perioperative complications included wound problems (minor infections, 10.1 per cent; seromas and liquefied fat, 10.1 per cent; major infections, 3.8 per cent; dehiscence, 1.0 per cent) and anastomotic leak or subphrenic abscess in 2.5 per cent. Infectious complications

were most common in patients with NIDDM or glucose impairment. Reoperation was required in 2.3 per cent; 7.9 per cent were readmitted during the first 30 days after operation.

There were 16 late deaths among the 475 operated patients (3.4 per cent) during the 9 years of follow-up. The high rate of depression seen among morbidly obese individuals may be responsible for the three deaths from suicide, the death from malnutrition bulimia, and the two deaths caused by progressive cirrhosis from extensive alcohol abuse. Initially, it was suspected that the two auto accidents also might be due to emotional stress, but both proved to be bona-fide accidents on eastern North Carolina's dangerous rural highways. The five deaths from sepsis and the two deaths from cancer (liver and larynx) raise questions about the 18 to 24 months of immunocompromise that probably occurs with the malnutrition induced by the procedure.

Patients with bariatric surgery require rigorous follow-up because late complications are common. The most common was dumping (70.6 per cent), an initially bothersome but desirable outcome because it alters behavior and, probably, affects the long-term effectiveness of the procedure.[75] The other complications are not as desirable: nutritional deficits, primarily during the period of major weight loss, manifested by hair loss, 49.0 per cent; constipation, 43.4 per cent; anemia, 43.6 per cent; vitamin B_{12} deficiency, 37.3 per cent; psychiatric problems, 41.4 per cent; nausea and vomiting usually due to initial overeating, 35.3 per cent; incisional hernias, 16.2 per cent; neuropathies usually due to vitamin B complex deficits, 12.4 per cent; cholelithiasis, 9.2 per cent; bile reflux and esophagitis, 5.8 per cent; small bowel obstruction due to adhesions, 4.3 per cent (usually self-limited); marginal ulcer (all but one healed with H_2 blockers), 3.8 per cent; pouch dilatation, 2.9 per cent; staple line failures, 2.6 per cent; anastomotic dilatation, 2.7 per cent; and anastomotic stenosis requiring dilatation, 1.3 per cent. Over the 9-year follow-up, 31.3 per cent of the patients re-entered the hospital, primarily for cholecystectomies, incisional hernia repairs, abdominal pain, psychiatric problems, and nutritional deficits.

The most serious complications are the neuropathies that may occur when these patients fail to take their vitamin B com-

TABLE 4. Effect of the Gastric Bypass on Diabetes and Hypertension (N = 475)

	Before Operation		After Operation	
	N	%	N	%
Diabetes				
No. of diabetic patients	100	21.1	3	0.6
No. of glucose-impaired patients	62	13.1	0	0

TABLE 5. Effect of the Gastric Bypass on Measures of Glucose Metabolism

	Before Operation (N = 42)	Year After Operation (N = 32)
Fasting blood glucose (mg%)	213 ± 15	117 ± 8
Fasting insulin (μU./ml.)	53 ± 7	14 ± 1
Glycosylated hemoglobin (%)	12.3 ± 1.1	6.6 ± 0.6
Maximum insulin release (μU./ml.)	76 ± 11	62 ± 15
Kg. rate (%/min. glucose disappearance)	0.65 ± 0.08	0.88 ± 0.07

TABLE 6. Effect of the Gastric Bypass on Physical Functioning and Role Functioning

| | Preoperative | | | | | | | |
| | 6 Months (N = 78) | | 12 Months (N = 65) | | 24 Months (N = 36) | | 36 Months (N = 15) | |
Scale	Mean Diff.	p	Mean Diff.	p	Mean Diff.	p	Mean Diff.	p
Physical functioning	1.94	0.001	3.11	0.001	2.64	0.001	1.07	NS
Role functioning	1.00	0.001	1.26	0.001	1.28	0.001	0.53	NS

plex or vitamin B_{12} supplements. These syndromes, which are manifested by weakness, peripheral tingling, dizziness, anorexia, and confusion, should be treated promptly because they can progress rapidly. Hospitalization with total parenteral nutrition may be needed.

Despite these problems, only one patient has requested and undergone reversal of the gastric bypass; and in patients in whom the operation failed because of pouch dilatation, anastomotic widening, and staple failure, all but one requested that the defect be corrected as quickly as possible before they regained their previous weight. Few operations are performed that have that high a level of patient satisfaction.

EXTERNAL CONSTRICTING PROSTHESES. The application of external prostheses to the stomach offers another way to limit the size of the reservoir. The concept of using gastric banding for the treatment of obesity originated in 1976, when Wilkinson and Peloso[87] performed the first operation, using a strip of Marlex mesh to pull the stomach into an hourglass configuration. When this approach failed to produce adequate weight loss, Wilkinson wrapped the entire stomach, but this operation failed as well. Molina[53] of the United States and Kolle[40] of Norway continued to explore banding with nylon and later with Dacron bands. Molina's surgical technique differs significantly from all other operations for obesity because it involves only a very small skin incision and is done mainly by palpation. The most successful approach appears to be that of Kuzmak,[44] who uses a 1-cm. wide soft, radiopaque, partly inflatable silicone band with a subcutaneous reservoir to develop a pouch that is measured with an inflatable balloon. The stoma is precisely sized to a diameter of 12 to 13 cm. with a banding instrument equipped with an electronic sensor. His experience with the inflatable band remains small, but he reported 152 patients with a noninflatable band operated since 1983, with a 92.1 per cent follow-up. With patients' average preoperative weight of 293 pounds, the average per cent of excess weight lost at 1 year postoperatively was 42.1 ± 25.5 per cent; at 2 years, 60.1 ±

27.3 per cent; at 3 years, 72.0 ± 26.5 per cent; and at 4 years, 76.0 ± 22.8 per cent. Slightly more than 28 per cent of the patients reached a weight that is less than 30 per cent above their estimated ideal weight. There was one mortality (from a pulmonary embolus); one embolism of the femoral artery; three stomal obstructions; and one migration of the band. There were no wound infections, intra-abdominal infections, or dehiscences. Others, however, report less satisfactory results. Granstrom and Backman,[27] in 72 patients followed for 12 to 54 months after gastric banding, had two operative deaths, and 22 of their patients required 33 reoperations. Even so, according to Kuzmak, gastric banding has become the prevailing procedure for controlling severe obesity in the Scandinavian countries and Australia. The operation is also being performed in the United States, Poland, and Czechoslovakia. With Kuzmak's introduction of precise calibration, the operation appears to be a promising and far less traumatic approach.

THE GASTRIC BALLOON. The *gastric balloon* was introduced by Garren,[23] on the premise that this artificial bezoar would produce early satiety and thus diminish food intake. The device enjoyed rapid acceptance and widespread application through massive publicity and the scheduling of multiple, well-attended national courses. Within several years, thousands of balloons had been implanted. The Food and Drug Administration recently took the device off the market because of its lack of long-term effectiveness, the unjustifiable cost ($7000 per year), and the high complication rates (obstruction, ulceration, perforation, and so on).

Comparison Between the Gastric Bypass, the Gastroplasties, and Gastric Banding

Several prospective studies compared the old gastroplasties, i.e., those prior to the vertical banded gastroplasty, with gastric bypasses. In each of these, the gastric bypass proved to be the better procedure. In each of the versions, whether the stoma was on the lesser or the greater curvature or whether it was in

TABLE 7. Effect of the Gastric Bypass on the RAND Measures of Mental Health

| | Preoperative | | | | | | | |
| | 6 Months (N = 78) | | 12 Months (N = 65) | | 24 Months (N = 36) | | 36 Months (N = 15) | |
Scale	Mean Diff.	p	Mean Diff.	p	Mean Diff.	p	Mean Diff.	p
Anxiety	3.09	0.001	3.25	0.001	1.31	NS	0.27	NS
Depression	2.15	0.001	1.82	0.001	1.00	NS	1.20	NS
General health	2.86	0.001	3.65	0.001	3.47	0.001	2.60	NS
Positive well-being	3.97	0.001	4.26	0.001	2.81	0.003	0.27	NS
Self-control	0.96	0.03	0.51	NS	0.06	NS	0.13	NS
Vitality	4.90	0.001	5.36	0.001	4.33	0.001	1.27	NS
Mental Health Index*	10.18	0.001	9.63	0.001	5.17	NS	1.07	NS

* Anxiety + depression + positive well-being + self-control.
NS, not significant.

TABLE 8. Deaths and Perioperative Complications after the GGB with an Incidence over 1 Per Cent (February 1, 1980 to April 31, 1990; N = 475)

Complication	N	%
Perioperative Deaths	6	1.3
Sepsis	2	
Pulmonary embolus	1	
Late deaths (over ten years)	16	3.4
Sepsis	1	
Myocardial infarction	1	
Cancer		
Liver	1	
Larynx	1	
Suicide	3	
Cirrhosis	2	
Auto accident	3	
Malnutrition	1	
AIDS	1	
Unknown	1	
Wound complications		
Severe wound infection	17	3.8
Minor wound infection	48	10.1
Seroma or liquefied fat	48	10.1
Dehiscence	5	1.1
Technical complications		
Subphrenic abscess	12	2.5
Splenic tear	13	2.7
Other postoperative complications		
Pneumonia	9	1.9
Arrhythmias	7	1.5
Required Perioperative Reoperation	11	2.3

the middle of the staple line, the gastric pouches enlarged and the stomas stretched so that, within 1 or 2 years, the 20 per cent mean weight loss was soon regained. Naslund and co-workers,[62] in a series of 57 patients followed for 2 years, found that weight loss at 1 year was significantly greater and failures significantly fewer in the 29 who underwent the gastric by-pass.[54] Our own prospective and randomized series of 87 patients, comparing the GGB with gastric partition (gastric pouch stapling with a gastrogastrostomy), demonstrated that the GGB patients lost 15 per cent more of their original weight at 12 months and 21 per cent at 18 months, with fewer failures and a similar complication rate.

Only one well-controlled series comparing the gastric bypass with the true Mason's vertical banded gastroplasty has been published. Sugerman and associates[83] stopped the randomization at 9 months after 20 patients had undergone each procedure because greater weight loss (p<0.05) was noted after the gastric bypass. The difference increased (p<0.01) with each 3-month interval during 3 years. In a later study, the same investigators obtained their best results by assigning patients addicted to sweets to the gastric bypass and recommended that vertical banded gastroplasty should not be performed in patients who are so addicted.[83]

In summary, all three procedures — the Greenville gastric bypass, Mason's vertical banded gastroplasty, and the gastric banding procedures — have been shown to be effective therapies for morbid obesity. Each has been reported to produce effective weight loss, to reverse hyperglycemia and hypertension, and to provide significant rehabilitation. All can be done with surprisingly low operative mortalities (less than 1 per cent) and acceptable morbidity.

At present, the VBG is still the most commonly performed bariatric operation.[15] Even though the data remain incomplete, it would appear that the gastric bypass produces the greatest weight loss but is also associated with the highest rate of complications and nutritional deficiencies. The vertical banded gastroplasty is less effective in terms of weight reduction but is technically easier and has fewer long-term nutritional problems. Finally, gastric banding is technically the easiest procedure and may have few complications, but the data are still inadequate to assess the long-term effectiveness of the operation.

PREOPERATIVE MANAGEMENT OF THE MORBIDLY OBESE PATIENT

PATIENT SELECTION. Most groups operating for morbid obesity use similar criteria for the selection of their patients and, in general, manage their patients in the same way. Patients are considered to be candidates if they exceed their ideal weight, as defined by the 1983 Height and Weight Standards of the Metropolitan Life Insurance Company, by at least 100 pounds. Another good measure is whether their body composition by hydrodensitometry exceeds 45 per cent fat. Patients tend to be better candidates and their families appear to be more supportive of surgical therapy if they have been morbidly obese for 5 or more years and if there have been one or two documented attempts to lose weight, either under a doctor's supervision or with one of the bariatric commercial programs such as TOPS, Weight Watchers, or Nutri-System. Moreover, surgical therapy is considered especially indicated if the patients have developed one or more of the complications of morbid obesity, including hypertension, diabetes mellitus, cardiac failure, pulmonary failure, pickwickian syndrome, sleep apnea, or arthritis, or have become too disabled to find employment or to function daily. Contraindications include a recent history of alcohol or substance abuse, inadequate intelligence to understand the procedure and its consequences, a previous pattern of severe depression or suicidal attempts, and, occasionally, a hostile and unsupportive family.

PREOPERATIVE EVALUATION. The authors' preoperative evaluation process is designed to move slowly to ensure that the patient is well educated about the procedure and to emphasize that the operation is a serious undertaking. The protocol begins with initial interviews, which, if possible, include the family. Usually two visits suffice for determining whether the patient is an appropriate candidate; if so, the preoperative workup is begun. That evaluation includes a complete medical and dietary history; physical examination; a complete blood count; urinalysis; 12-test serum profile (SMA-12); electrolyte testing; skin tests to common antigens to determine whether the patient is anergic; a glucose tolerance test; serum levels of T_3, T_4, thyroid-stimulating hormone, and vitamin B_{12}; an electrocardiogram; posteroanterior and lateral chest roentgenograms; and a pulmonary function test with arterial blood gases. All patients are screened for psychopathology by the project psychologist or psychiatrist. Additional members of the family, if available, are counseled regarding the operation. For ongoing studies, the authors also do a series of psychometric tests, special tests for glucose metabolism, and immersion hydrostatic weighing. If indicated by the results of the workup, patients may need to undergo more sophisticated studies, such as upper gastrointestinal series, fiberoptic endoscopy, echocardiography, stress testing, and cardiac angiography. Bariatric surgery is a major undertaking; it is important that the patients be well prepared.

PREOPERATIVE PREPARATION. In general, patients are admitted either the night before or on the morning of operation, depending on their level of surgical risk. Complicated cases, however, such as those of patients with cardiorespiratory failure, may require several days of preparation in the hospital to bring the patient to an optimal preoperative status. A cephalosporin is given intravenously for prophylaxis the morning of operation and for 2 days thereafter. Serious health problems need to be stabilized before operation. Skin lesions need to clear as much as possible, and chronic problems such as asthma, chronic pulmonary infections, diabetes, and hypertension need to be stabilized; if the patient is taking medications, these need to be reviewed and adjusted to appropriate levels.

POSTOPERATIVE CARE. In general, the postoperative care of bariatric patients resembles that following standard abdominal surgery and will, therefore, not be described in detail, except to emphasize the need for prophylactic antibiotics; careful monitoring of vital signs, fluid balance, and glucose metabolism; and the need for appropriate furniture and equipment to manage these massive individuals.

The first 24 hours are particularly critical because of the great seriousness of a leak or intra-abdominal infection. If the pulse remains over 120, if there is a rise in temperature to over 38.8° C. (102° F.), or if the patient appears ill despite normal vital signs, emergency exploration and the addition of other antibiotics may be required. Barium swallows may be helpful but are not always reliable; several patients have been observed with anastomotic leaks who demonstrated normal passage of barium without extravasation. Neglect of a perforation or intra-abdominal infection is associated with a high mortality rate. If there is doubt, it is best to proceed with operation; an unnecessary exploration is safer than an overlooked perforation.

Patients usually spend the first night in the critical care unit for close monitoring and intensive nursing care. Most spend the rest of their hospital stay (usually a total of 5 to 6 days) on the surgical wards. Patients are maintained NPO until they pass flatus, usually the third day, are begun on half-strength Ensure (30 ml. t.i.d.) with water (30 ml. q.h.) on the fourth day, and full-strength Ensure with water, in the same doses, on the fifth and usually last day. After discharge, the patients are maintained on full fluids for 2 weeks and then cautiously progress to a full diet by the end of 6 weeks. Most patients gradually return to their previous diet in terms of variety but with a marked reduction in quantity because of satiety and because the gastric pouch empties slowly. Most patients do not tolerate carbohydrates well because of the induced dumping; meats may present difficulties: the East Carolina program begins slowly with fish, then progresses to chicken, and finally to red meat. By the end of 3 months most patients eat a small but well-balanced diet.

The most common early complications seen in the clinic are wound abscesses, and these, as might be expected, occur most commonly in the diabetic patients. The wound infections generally present as red bulges that drain spontaneously or that can be drained through a small, 1- to 2-cm. opening of the incision. It is not necessary to open the entire wound or significant lengths of the incision; such interventions may lead to long-term wound care and delays in healing. Late subphrenic abscesses usually can be drained percutaneously with interventional radiologic techniques.[52]

LONG-TERM FOLLOW-UP. Patients generally do remarkably well and are a delight to follow with their new body image, their freedom from diabetes, and their new lifestyle. Even so, they need to be cautioned before operation that long-term follow-up is essential. Of particular importance is the maintenance of vitamin intake; omission of vitamins may lead to severe anemias, Korsakoff-Wernicke syndrome, or other neuropathies. Glucose tolerance, blood pressure, and emotional status need to be followed closely. Weight gain exceeding 12 per cent above the minimal postoperative weight is generally the result of staple line breakdown, pouch or anastomotic dilatation, or compulsive snacking. Abdominal pain is most commonly due to cholecystitis, although some patients may develop marginal ulcers that, fortunately, clear quickly with H₂ blockers. Recurrent vomiting usually signals overeating but may be due to stenosis of the gastrojejunostomy. Such strictures almost always can be relieved with one or two dilatations of the anasto-

mosis.[47] Finally, these patients require considerable emotional support from their referring physician, the surgical staff, and their own families. The encouragement is especially needed during the period of adjustment to their new body image and, perhaps more important, to the new expectations of performance by the patient and the family. Some workers have found support groups for patients useful; for selected patients, consultation with a psychiatrist may be necessary.

REVISION OF FAILED BARIATRIC PROCEDURES. All bariatric procedures have a failure rate, ranging from 80 per cent or more for horizontal gastroplasties to about 5 to 10 per cent for the vertical banded gastroplasties and gastric bypasses. Most of the failures are due to failed staple lines, stenosis of the gastric outlets, distended gastric pouches, or dilated gastrojejunostomies. Revision of these failures is difficult and associated with a high complication and second failure rate.[69] A variety of approaches have been explored, but the best results have been obtained with the creation of a new gastric pouch and anastomosis and full division of the stomach below the new staple line, as shown in Figure 11.

CONCLUSION. Morbid obesity is a serious and increasingly common disease that represents a severe handicap and that is associated with major health problems, including diabetes, hypertension, biliary disease, arthritis, and a number of other disorders. Because diets rarely produce sustained weight loss in these patients, surgical therapy has become the treatment of choice. Two operations, the Greenville gastric bypass and Mason's vertical banded gastroplasty, have produced the best results to date; both are no longer experimental and can be considered effective procedures that can sharply ameliorate or

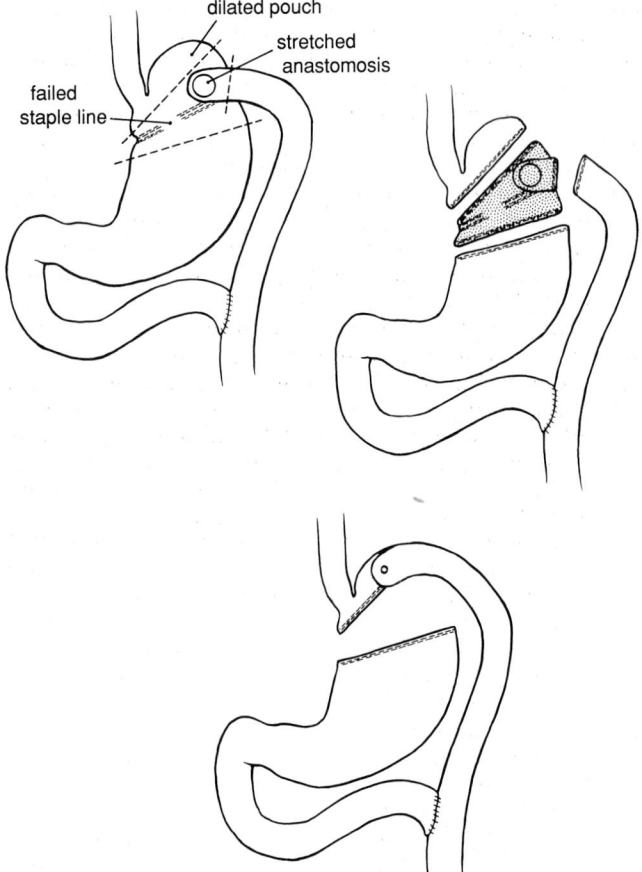

Figure 11. Our most successful revision for failed gastric bypass procedures, whether due to staple line breakdown, pouch distension, or anastomotic dilatation. The previous anastomosis and the staple line are removed with GIA stapling devices to avoid spillage. A new 8-mm. anastomosis is then sewn with a double layer of polypropylene suture between the new gastric pouch and the Roux-en-Y loop.

reverse not only the excessive weight but also the complications of the disorder. The operations are difficult, and the management of these patients is challenging but rewarding. Long-term follow-up is essential for the proper management of such late complications as nutritional deficiencies and psychologic problems. Failures due to pouch distention, anastomotic dilatation, and staple line breakdown are unusual, but revisions, though technically challenging, can be done with acceptable results.

SELECTED REFERENCES

Bray, A. G.: Obesity; basic aspects and clinical application. Med. Clin. North Am., 73:1, 1989.
This is an excellent and updated review of the basic aspects of obesity and the clinical applications of current knowledge by a distinguished authority in the field. The bibliography is comprehensive and current.

Deitel, M. (Ed.): Surgery for the Morbidly Obese Patient. Philadelphia, Lea & Febiger, 1989, p. 400.
This text provides the most complete review of bariatric surgery to date. The authors are distinguished workers in the field, and the bibliography is excellent.

Stunkard, A. J.: The Salmon Lecture. Some perspectives on human obesity: Its causes. Some perspectives on human obesity: Treatment. Bull. N.Y. Acad. Med., 64:901, 1988.
This brief monograph is divided into two sections: the first provides a thoughtful and complete examination of the various controversies regarding the genetic vs. the environmental etiologies of obesity. The second examines the success and lack of success of the various forms of therapy in individuals with mild, moderate, and severe types of obesity.

Workshop on Basic and Clinical Aspects of Regional Fat Distribution. Bethesda, Md., National Institutes of Health, September, 1989.
A comprehensive collection of abstracts reviewing the relationship of fat distribution to human morbidity and mortality by the leaders in that area of study.

REFERENCES

1. Adami, G., Gianetta, E., Barreca, A., et al: Body composition after "very-little-stomach" biliopancreatic bypass. Eur, Surg. Res., 19:91, 1987.
2. Alden, J. F.: Comparison of gastric bypass and jejunoileal bypass. *In* Najarian, J. S., and Delaney, J. P. (Eds.): Gastrointestinal Surgery. Chicago, Year Book Medical Publishers, 1979.
3. Andersen, T., Backer, O. G., Stokholm, K. H., et al.: Randomized trial of diet and gastroplasty compared with diet alone in morbid obesity. N. Engl. J. Med., 310:352, 1984.
4. Battershill, J. H.: Tuberculosis after intestinal bypass surgery for obesity. Chest, 70:318, 1976.
5. Bessard, T., Schutz, Y., and Jequier, E.: Energy expenditure and postprandial thermogenesis in obese women before and after weight loss. Am. J. Clin. Nutr., 38:680, 1983.
6. Bray, G. A., Barry, R. E., Benfield, J. R. et al.: Intestinal bypass operation as a treatment for obesity. Ann. Intern. Med. 85:97, 1976.
7. Bray, G. A.: Surgical treatment of morbid obesity. Trans. Assoc. Life Insur. Med. Directors 62:107, 1979.
8. Bray, G. A.: Management options in obesity. Hosp. Pract., April, 1982.
9. Brown, R. G., O'Leary, J. P., and Woodward, E. R.: Hepatic effects of jejuno-ileal bypass for morbid obesity. Am. J. Surg. 127:53, 1974.
10. Buchwald, H., Varco, R. L., Moore, R. B., et al.: Intestinal bypass procedures. Curr Problems in Surgery. Chicago, Year Book Medical Publishers, 1975, pp. 1–51.
11. Canning, H., and Mayer, J.: Obesity—its possible effect on college acceptance. N. Engl. J. Med., 275:1172, 1966.
12. Caro, J. F., Dohm, L. G., Pories, W. J., Sinha, M. K.: Cellular alterations in liver, skeletal muscle, and adipose tissue responsible for insulin resistance in obesity and type II diabetes. Diabetes Metab Rev. 5(8):665, 1989.
13. Colliver, J. A., Frank, S., and Frank, A.: Similarity of obesity indices in clinical studies of obese adults. A factor analytic study. Am. J. Clin. Nutr., 38:640, 1983.
14. Cryer, P. E., Garber, A. J., Hoffsten, P., et al.: Renal failure after small intestinal bypass for obesity. Arch. Intern. Med., 135:1610, 1975.
15. Deitel, M., Jones, B. A., Petrov, I., et al.: Vertical banded gastroplasty: Results in 233 patients. Can. J. Surg., 29:322, 1986.
16. Dohm, G. L., Tapscott, E. B., Pories, W. J., Dabbs, D. J., Flickinger, E. G., Meelheim, D., Fushiki, T. J., Atkinson, S. M., and Caro, J. F.: An in vitro human muscle preparation suitable for metabolic studies. Decreased glucose transport in muscle from morbidly obese subjects. J. Clin. Invest., 82:486, 1988.
17. Drenick, E. J.: Risk of obesity and surgical indications. Int. J. Obesity, 5,385, 1980.
18. Dublin, L. I., and Marks, H. H.: Mortality Among Insured Overweights in Recent Years. New York, Recording and Statistical Recording Press, 1952.
19. Dubois, A.: Obesity and gastric emptying. Gastroenterology, 84:875, 1983.
20. Evans, P. E., Israel, R. G., Flickinger, E. G., O'Brien, K. F., and Donnely,
J. E.: Hydrostatic weighing without head submersion in morbidly obese females. Am. J. Clin. Nutr., 50:400, 1989.
21. Faust, I. M., Johnson, P. R., and Hirsch, J.: Surgical removal of adipose tissue alters feeding behavior and the development of obesity in rats. Science, 197:393, 1977.
22. Flickinger, E. G., Sinar, D. R., and Pories, W. J.: The bypassed stomach. Am. J. Surg., 149:151, 1985.
23. Garren, L. R.: Intragastric balloon in the treatment of morbid obesity. Presented at the Symposium on Surgical Treatment of Morbid Obesity, Los Angeles, Calif., 1984.
24. Gerich, J. E.: Role of insulin resistance in the pathogenesis of type II (non-insulin–dependent) diabetes mellitus. Bailliere's Clin. Endocrinol. Metab., 3:307, 1988.
25. Gianetta, E., Friedman, D., Adami, G. F., et al.: Etiological factors of protein malnutrition after biliopancreatic diversion. Gastroenterol. Clin. North Am., 16:503, 1987.
26. Gotto, A. M., Foreyt, J. P., and Goodrick, G. K.: Evaluating commercial weight loss clinics. Arch. Intern. Med., 142:682, 1982.
27. Granstrom, L., and Backman, L.: Technical complications and related reoperations after gastric banding. Acta Chir. Scand. 153:215, 1987.
28. Gregory, J. G., Starkloff, E. B., Miyai, K., et al.: Urologic complications of ileal bypass operation for morbid obesity. J. Urol., 113:521, 1975.
29. Griffen, W. O., Jr., Bivins, F. A., and Bell, R. M.: The decline and fall of the jejunoileal bypass. Surg. Gynecol. Obstet.157:301, 1983.
30. Halverson, J. D., and Koehler, R. E.: Assessment of patients with failed gastric operations for morbid obesity. Am. J. Surg., 145:357, 1983.
31. Hervey, G. R.: The effects of lesions in the hypothalamus in parabiotic rats. J. Physiol., 154:336, 1959.
32. Hoebel, B. G., and Teitelbaum, P.: Weight regulation in normal and hypothalamic rats. J. Comp. Physiol. Psychol., 61:189, 1966.
33. Hubert, H. B., Feinleib, M., McNamara, P. M. et al.: Obesity as an independent risk factor for cardiovascular disease: A 26-year follow-up of participants in the Framingham Heart Study. Circulation, 67:986, 1983.
34. James, D. E., Brown, R., Navarro, J., and Pilch, P. F.: Insulin regulatable tissues express a unique insulin-sensitive glucose transport protein. Nature, 333:183, 1988.
35. James, W. P. T.: Energy requirements and obesity. Lancet, 2:386, 1983.
36. Kahn, C. F., and White, M. F.: The insulin receptor and the molecular mechanism of insulin action. J. Clin. Invest., 82:1151, 1988.
37. Kark, A. E.: Jaw wiring. Am. J. Clin. Nutr., 33:420, 1980.
38. Keesey, R. E., and Corbett, S. W.: Metabolic defense of the body weight set point. *In* Stunkard, A. J., and Stellar, E. (Eds.): Eating and Its Disorders. New York, Raven Press, 1983, pp. 87–96.
39. Keys, A., Borzek, J., Henschel, A., et al.: The Biology of Human Starvation. Minneapolis, University of Minnesota Press, 1950.
40. Kolle, K.: Gastric banding. OMGI, 17th Congress, Stockholm, 1982, Abstract No. 145, p. 37.
41. Kral, J. G., Strauss, R. J., and Wise, L.: Perioperative risk management in obese patients. *In* Deitel, M. (Ed.): Surgery for the Morbidly Obese Patient. Philadelphia, Lea & Febiger, 1989.
42. Kremen, A. J., Linner, J. H., and Nelson, C. H.: An experimental evaluation of the nutritional importance of the proximal and distal small intestine. Ann. Surg., 140:439, 1954.
43. Kuczmarski, R. J.: The assessment of body fat distribution in population based surveys. *In* Workshop on Basic and Clinical Aspects of Regional Fat Distribution. Washington, D.C., National Institutes of Health, Sept., 1989, pp. 47–51.
44. Kuzmak, L. I.: Gastric banding. *In* Deitel, M. (Ed.): Surgery for the Morbidly Obese Patient. Philadelphia, Lea & Febiger, 1989, pp. 225–259.
45. Lapidus, L., Bengtsson, C., Larsson, B., et al.: Distribution of adipose tissue and risk of cardiovascular disease and death. Twelve-year followup of participants in the population study of women in Gothenburg, Sweden. Br. Med. J., 289:1257, 1984.
46. Larner, J.: Banting Lecture, 1987: Insulin signaling mechanism(s); Lessons from the Old Testament of glycogen metabolism and a New Testament of molecular biology. Diabetes, 37:1597, 1988.
47. Lineaweaver, W., Ryckman, F., and Hawkins, I.: Endoscopic balloon dilation of outlet stenosis after gastric bypass. Am. Surg., 51:194, 1985.
48. Linner, J.: Surgery for Morbid Obesity. New York, Springer-Verlag, 1984.
49. Mason, E. E., and Ito, C.: Gastric bypass. Ann. Surg., 170,329, 1969.
50. McCarthy, H. B., Rucker, R. D., Jr., and Chan, E. K.: Gastritis after gastric bypass surgery. Surgery, 98:68, 1985.
51. Messerli, F. T., Sundgaard-riise, K., Resising, E., et al.: Disparate cardiovascular effects of obesity and arterial hypertension. Am. J. Med., 74:808, 1983.
52. Mishkin, J. D., Meranze, S. G., Burke, D. R., et al.: Interventional radiologic treatment of complications following gastric bypass surgery for morbid obesity. Gastrointest. Radiol. 13:9, 1988.
53. Molina, M.: Gastric banding, an experience with more than 500 cases. Presented at Symposium on Surgical Treatment of Obesity, Los Angeles, Calif., 1984.
54. Naslund, I., Wickbom, G., Christoffersson, E., et al.: A prospective randomized comparison of gastric bypass and gastroplasty. Acta Chir. Scand., 152:681, 1986.
55. National Institutes of Health: Consensus development statement. Health implications of obesity. Washington, D.C., 11–13, 1985.
56. O'Leary, J. P., Maher, J. W., Hollenbeck, J. I., et al.: Pathogenesis of hepatic failure after obesity bypass. Surg. Forum 25:356, 1974.

57. Park, H. K., Sinar, D. R., and Sloss, R. R.: Histologic and endoscopic studies before and after gastric bypass surgery. Arch. Pathol. Lab. Med., 110:1164, 1986.
58. Payne, J. H., and DeWind, L. T.: Surgical treatment of obesity. Am. J. Surg., 118:141, 1969.
59. Payne, J. H., DeWind, L. T., and Commons, R. R.: Metabolic observations in patients with jejunocolic shunts. Am. J. Surg., 106:273, 1963.
60. Peltier, G., Hermreck, A. S., Moffat, R. E., et al.: Complications following gastric bypass procedures for morbid obesity. Surgery, 86:648, 1979.
61. Pories, W. J.: Surgery for morbid obesity. In Dudley, H., Pories, W. J., Carter, C. (Eds.): Operative Surgery. Stoneham, Mass., Butterworth, 1983, pp. 316–322.
62. Pories, W. J., Flickinger, E. G., Meelheim, H. D., et al.: The effectiveness of gastric bypass over gastric partition in morbid obesity. Ann. Surg., 196:389, 1982.
63. Ravussin, E., Lillioja, S., Knowler, W. C., et al.: Reduced rate of energy expenditure as a risk factor for body-weight gain. N. Engl. J. Med. 318:467, 1988.
64. Ray, C. S., Sue, D. Y., Bray, G., et al.: Effects of obesity on respiratory function. Am. Rev. Respir. Dis., 128:501, 1983.
65. Ryden, O., Olsson, S. A., and Danielsson, B. A.: Weight loss after gastroplasty: Psychological sequelae in relation to clinical and metabolic observations. J. Am. Coll. Nutr., 8:15, 1989.
66. Salmon, P. A.: The results of small intestinal bypass operations for the treatment of obesity. Surg. Gynecol. Obstet., 132:965, 1971.
67. Schneider, G., Kirschner, M. A., Berkowitz, R., et al.: Increased estrogen production in obese men. J. Clin. Endocrinol. Metab., 48:633, 1979.
68. Schumacher, N., Groth, B., Kleinsek, J., et al.: Successful weight control for employees. J. Am. Diet. Assoc. 74:466, 1979.
69. Schwartz, R. W., Strodel, W. E., Simpson, W. S., et al.: Gastric bypass revision: Lessons learned from 920 cases. Surgery, 104:806, 1988.
70. Scott, H. W., Jr., Dean, R. H., Shull, H. J., et al.: Results of jejunoileal bypass in two hundred patients with morbid obesity. Surg. Gynecol. Obstet., 145:661, 1977.
71. Sherman, C. D., Jr., May, A. G., Nue, W., et al.: Clinical and metabolic studies following bowel bypassing for obesity. Ann. N.Y. Acad. Sci., 131:614, 1965.
72. Sims, E. A. H., and Horton, E. S.: Endocrine and metabolic adaptation to obesity and starvation. Am. J. Clin. Nutr., 21:1455, 1986.
73. Sinar, D. R., Flickinger, E. G., Park, H. K., et al.: Retrograde endoscopy of the bypassed stomach segment after gastric bypass surgery. South. Med. J., 78:255, 1985.
74. Sinha, M. K., Pories, W. J., Flickinger, E. G., Meelheim, D., and Caro, J. F.: Insulin receptor kinase activity of adipose tissue from morbidly obese humans with or without noninsulin-dependent diabetes. Diabetes, 36:620, 1987.
75. Sirinek, K. R., O'Dorisio, T. M., Howe, B., et al.: Neurotensin, vasoactive intestinal peptide, and Roux-en-Y gastrojejunostomy. Arch. Surg., 120:605, 1985.
76. Society of Actuaries: Build and Blood Pressure Study, 1959.
77. Sonne-Holm, S., Sorensen, T. I. A., and Christensen, U.: Risk of early death in extremely overweight young men. Br. Med. J., 287:795, 1983.
78. Stock-Damge, C., Aprahamian, M., Raul, F., et al.: Small-intestinal and colonic changes after biliopancreatic bypass for morbid obesity. Scand. J. Gastroenterol., 21:1115, 1986.
79. Stunkard, A. J.: The Salmon Lecture. Some perspectives on human obesity: Its causes. Some perspectives on human obesity: Treatment. Bull. N.Y. Acad. Med., 64:902, 1988.
80. Stunkard, A., and McLaren, H.: The results of treatment for obesity. Arch. Intern. Med., 103:79, 1979.
81. Stunkard, A. J., and Wadden, T. A.: Obesity. In Rakel R. E.: Conn's Current Therapy. Philadelphia, W. B. Saunders Company, 1987, pp. 459–463.
82. Sturdevant, R. A. L., Pearce, J. L., and Dayton, S.: Increased prevalence of cholelithiasis in men ingesting a serum cholesterol-lowering diet. N. Engl. J. Med., 288:24, 1973.
83. Sugerman, H. J., Starkey, J. V., and Birkenhauer, R.: A randomized prospective trial of gastric bypass versus banded gastroplasty for morbid obesity and their effects on sweets versus non-sweets eaters. Ann. Surg., 205:613, 1987.
84. Toeller, M., Gries, F. A., Dannehl, X.: Natural history of glucose intolerance in obesity: A ten-year observation. Int. J. Obesity, 6:145, 1982.
85. VanItallie, T. B.: Morbid obesity: A hazardous disorder that resists conservative treatment. Am. J. Clin. Nutr. (Suppl.), 33:358, 1982.
86. Weismann, R. E.: Surgical palliation of massive and severe obesity. Am. J. Surg., 125:437, 1973.
87. Wilkinson, L. H., and Peloso, O. A.: Gastric (reservoir) reduction for morbid obesity. Arch. Surg., 116:602, 1981.
88. Wise, L., and Stein, T.: Biliary and urinary calculi. Pathogenesis following small bowel bypass for obesity. Arch. Surg., 110:1043, 1975.
89. Wright, R. A., Krinsky, S., Fleeman, J., et al.: Gastric emptying and obesity. Gastroenterology, 84:747, 1983.

VI

MECKEL'S DIVERTICULUM

Ward O. Griffen, Jr., M.D., Ph.D.

The most frequently encountered diverticulum of the small intestine, first noted in 1730 by Ruysch, was described completely by Johann Meckel in 1808. Meckel's diverticulum occurs in the terminal ileum 45 to 90 cm. proximal to the ileocecal valve. Almost invariably the diverticulum arises from the antimesenteric border of the ileum and is a true diverticulum, since it contains all layers of the intestinal wall (Fig. 1). It varies in length and diameter from 1 to 10 or 12 cm. In autopsy studies, the incidence of Meckel's diverticulum is 0.3 per cent but may be placed as high as 2 per cent when surgical cases are reviewed.

The embryologic origin and usual location of Meckel's diverticulum are explained by the development of the midgut. During the first few weeks of fetal life, the primitive yolk sac divides into two portions, the larger becoming the primitive gut, the smaller continuing as a yolk sac near the placenta. These two portions remain connected by a tube contained within the umbilical cord. This tube, the omphalomesenteric or vitelline duct, ordinarily is obliterated by the seventh week. Persistence of this duct may lead to (1) a fistula between the umbilicus and the ileum when the entire duct remains patent, (2) Meckel's diverticulum due to failure of closure of the intestinal end of the duct, (3) an umbilical sinus when the umbilical side of the duct is not obliterated, (4) a fibrous cord between the umbilicus and the ileum representing the obliterated duct and its vessels, or (5) any combination of these four entities, the most frequent being

Meckel's diverticulum connected to the umbilicus by a fibrous strand.

Charles W. Mayo is credited with having stated, "Meckel's diverticulum is frequently suspected, often looked for, and seldom found." The clinical manifestations are most common in the pediatric age group, but the diverticulum can produce symptoms at all ages. The average mortality from Meckel's diverticulum as reported in several surgical series is 6 per cent, with a large proportion of the deaths occurring in the elderly. As with many other less common intra-abdominal conditions, death frequently occurs because of delay in diagnosis and proper therapy. For this reason, techniques in detection of Meckel's diverticulum have been evaluated recently. The use of technetium scanning appears to hold the greatest promise as a diagnostic aid (Fig. 2). ^{99m}Tc-pertechnetate (^{99m}Tc) is taken up by gastric mucosa, and, therefore, in patients who have ectopic gastric mucosa in a Meckel's diverticulum (about 50 per cent), this may be a helpful diagnostic maneuver. In a recent report, 90 per cent of patients presenting with bleeding from a Meckel's diverticulum were correctly diagnosed preoperatively. There was one false-negative, but pentagastrin stimulation prior to the scan may increase its sensitivity. An important controversy is whether a diverticulum should be removed if found incidentally. Diverticulectomy under these circumstances has an extremely low morbidity and mortality. However, many individ-

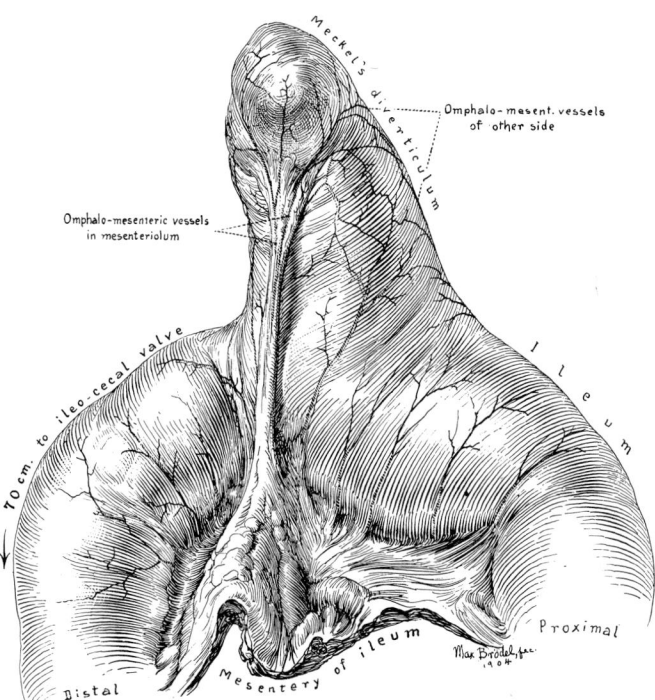

Figure 1. Typical anatomic example of a Meckel's diverticulum. Note the separate blood supply and gross appearance. (From Kelly, H. A., and Hurdon, E.: The Vermiform Appendix and Its Diseases. Philadelphia, W. B. Saunders Company, 1905.)

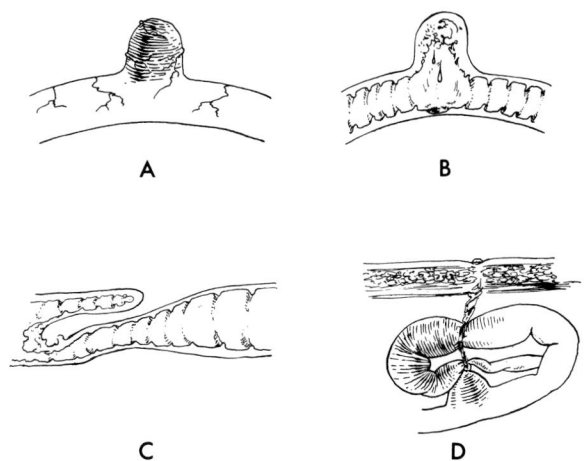

Figure 3. Presenting clinical manifestations of Meckel's diverticulum. *A*, Diverticulitis. *B*, Peptic ulcer secondary to heterotopic gastric mucosa within the diverticulum. *C*, Intussusception with the diverticulum acting as the leading portion of the intussusceptum. *D*, Volvulus of a segment of small bowel about a fibrous strand connecting the diverticulum to the umbilicus.

uals have a Meckel's diverticulum without developing any symptoms from it. Therefore, the current recommendations are (1) leave the diverticulum alone if there is no evidence of ectopic tissue (e.g., localized thickening of the diverticulum) and if the orifice is wide, and (2) remove the diverticulum if there is evidence of ectopic mucosa, if the orifice draining the diverticulum is narrow, or if there is any concern that the patient's symptoms are secondary to an abnormality of the diverticulum.

The important mechanisms of the clinical presentation of a Meckel's diverticulum are depicted in Figure 3. The most common clinical problem associated with Meckel's diverticulum is bleeding, which usually presents as melena or bright red blood per rectum. The usual source of the bleeding is a chronic ileal ulcer associated with heterotopic gastric tissue within the diverticulum. Owing to a high index of suspicion, bleeding from this source is usually treated during childhood. However, it is not

unusual to encounter an adult with a history of three or more isolated episodes of intestinal bleeding before a celiotomy was advised. This complication of Meckel's diverticulum occurs in about 50 per cent of patients with symptoms associated with the diverticulum.

The second most common symptom associated with a Meckel's diverticulum is intestinal obstruction. The cause of this obstruction may be volvulus of the small bowel around a diverticulum that is attached to the anterior abdominal wall, intussusception, or, rarely, incarceration of the diverticulum in a hernia (Littre). In the first instance, acute mechanical obstruction is usually present and, if allowed to progress, may result in strangulation of the involved bowel. The intussusception may be ileoileal or ileocolic and presents as acute obstruction associated with an urge to defecate and the passage of the classic "currant jelly" stool. This complication occurs in about 25 per cent of patients reported in surgical series. Barium enema reduction of an intussusception secondary to a Meckel's diverticulum can be performed. However, if the diverticulum is identified at the time of the barium enema, the patient should undergo resection of the diverticulum.

The next most common complication, occurring in about 20 per cent of patients, is diverticulitis. It often presents as acute appendicitis except for the location of the pain and may or may not be associated with enteroliths within the diverticulum. Failure to establish a prompt diagnosis may lead to perforation of the diverticulum, peritonitis, and death. As a corollary to prompt intervention in patients with Meckel's diverticulitis, when a patient is operated upon for acute appendicitis and the appendix is found to be normal, it is imperative that the distal 90 cm. of terminal ileum be inspected for the presence of a Meckel's diverticulum, which, if present, should be resected.

Occasionally a Meckel's diverticulum may be detected on small bowel follow-through roentgenograms or barium enema (Fig. 4). In an entirely asymptomatic patient, it should be left alone. However, if the patient has any abdominal complaints that may be related to the presence of the diverticulum, its removal should be advised. The mortality and morbidity for resection of an uncomplicated Meckel's diverticulum should be and are negligible. Usually the diverticulum can be excised by stapling its base so that the staple line is diagonal or transverse. The transected area may be left alone or inverted in accordance with the surgeon's preference.

Surgical treatment of a complicated Meckel's diverticulum does not have such favorable results. Mortality is reported to be between 5 and 10 per cent; morbidity as high as 25 per cent has

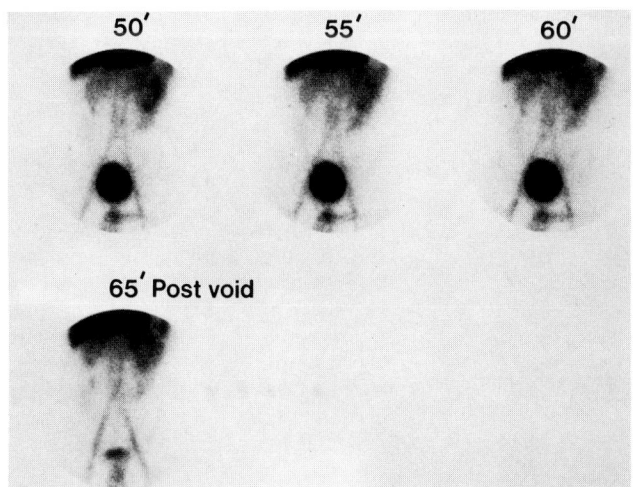

Figure 2. Positive 99mTc-pertechnetate scan in a 28-year-old patient presenting with rectal bleeding. Note dark area above and lateral to the vessel bifurcation on the patient's right.

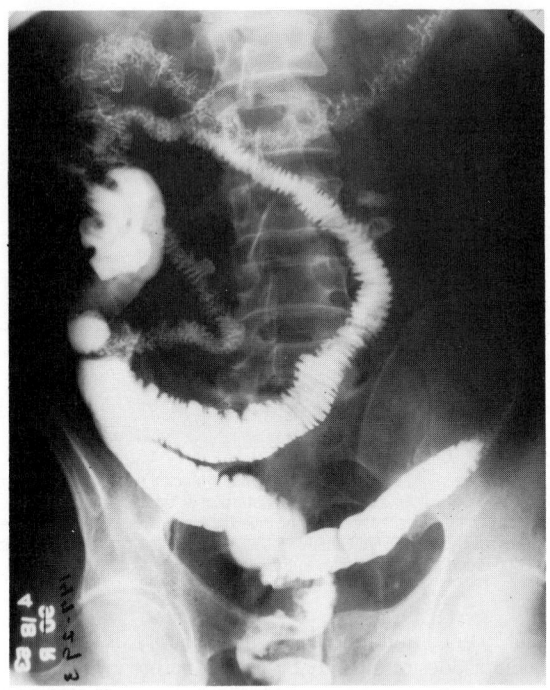

Figure 4. Meckel's diverticulum noted on a small bowel follow-through x-ray examination.

SELECTED REFERENCES

DeBartolo, H. M., Jr., and van Heerden, J. A.: Meckel's diverticulum. Ann. Surg., 183:30, 1976.
This is an updated review of the wide experience of the Mayo Clinic with Meckel's diverticulum. One hundred and ninety patients are presented in this important and detailed review.

Mackey, W. C., and Dineen, P.: A fifty year experience with Meckel's diverticulum. Surg. Gynecol. Obstet., 156:56, 1983.
The authors report a 50-year experience with Meckel's diverticulum at the New York–Cornell Medical Center. There were 402 patients. Emphasis was placed upon the fact that symptoms referable to the diverticulum occurred in 68 patients (17 per cent), and intestinal obstruction, inflammation, and lower gastrointestinal bleeding represented 90 per cent of the presenting symptoms.

Moses, W. R.: Meckel's diverticulum, a report of 2 unusual cases. N. Engl. J. Med., 237:118, 1947.
The largest collected series of Meckel's diverticulum, 1605 cases. One of the two cases reported is a leiomyosarcoma in a Meckel's diverticulum, a rare occurrence, seen in only 24 cases of the 1605 reviewed.

Soderlund, S.: Meckel's diverticulum. A clinical and histologic study. Acta Chir. Scand. [Suppl. 248], 1959.
A detailed report including a histologic review, a clinical review of 413 cases of Meckel's diverticulum, and a complete histologic survey. Included in the discussion is the embryologic explanation for heterotopic tissue in a Meckel's diverticulum and the physiologic reason for the occurrence of peptic ulceration when there is gastric mucosa in the diverticulum.

Vane, D. W., West, K. W., and Grosfeld, J. L.: Vitelline duct anomalies. Experience with 217 childhood cases. Arch. Surg., 122:542, 1987.
A large experience in Meckel's diverticulum in the pediatric age group; 85 patients (40 per cent) had symptoms, the majority of them with rectal bleeding. Diverticulectomy was the procedure of choice.

been cited. The only technical controversy concerns the choice between diverticulectomy and segmental resection. Since bleeding associated with a Meckel's diverticulum is from a peptic ulcer of the adjacent ileal mucosa, simple diverticulectomy usually will not remove the ulcer. Postoperative bleeding may occur, and for this reason most surgeons prefer wider excision of the diverticulum or segmental resection of the portion of ileum containing the lesion.

Recent articles about a Meckel's diverticulum have reported the unusual occurrence of a neoplasm in the diverticulum. The most common benign neoplasms of a Meckel's diverticulum are lipoma, leiomyoma, neurofibroma, and angioma. Malignant lesions of this diverticulum are leiomyosarcoma and carcinoid, which represent 80 per cent of such lesions, and adenocarcinoma and metastatic lesions, which constitute the remainder.

SUMMARY

Meckel's diverticulum is an uncommon clinical disorder. Only a high index of suspicion leads to proper diagnosis by use of further radiologic studies. Bleeding and obstruction are the most common manifestation of this lesion. Earlier diagnosis will enhance the surgical statistics.

REFERENCES

1. Berman, E. J., Schneider, A., and Potts, W. J.: Importance of gastric mucosa in Meckel's diverticulum. J.A.M.A., 156:6, 1954.
2. Cooney, D. R., Duszynski, D. O., Camboa, E., Karp, M. P., and Jewett, T. C., Jr.: The abdominal technetium scan (a decade of experience). J. Pediatr. Surg., 17:611, 1982.
3. Enge, I., and Frimann-Dahl, J.: Radiology in acute abdominal disorders due to Meckel's diverticulum. Br. J. Radiol., 37:775, 1964.
4. Jewett, T. C. Jr., and Butsch, W. L.: Meckel's diverticulum. The abdominal masquerader. Surgery, 46:440, 1959.
5. Kiesewetter, W. B.: Meckel's diverticulum in children. Arch. Surg., 75:914, 1957.
6. Passaro, E. Jr., Richmond, D., and Gordon, H. E.: Surgery for Meckel's diverticulum in the adult: Factors in morbidity and mortality. Arch. Surg., 93:315, 1966.
7. Rutherford, R. B., and Akers, D. R.: Meckel's diverticulum: A review of 148 pediatric patients with special reference to the pattern of bleeding and to mesodiverticular bands. Surgery, 59:618, 1966.
8. Sharma, G., and Benson, C. K.: Enteroliths in Meckel's diverticulum: Report of a case and review of the literature. Can. J. Surg., 13:54, 1970.
9. Silk, Y. N., Douglass, H. O. Jr., and Penetrante R.: Carcinoid tumor in Meckel's diverticulum. Am. Surg., 54:664, 1988.
10. Weinstein, E. C.: Meckel's diverticulum. J. Am. Geriatr. Soc., 13:903, 1965.
11. Wine, C. R., Nahrwold, D. L., and Waldhausen, J. A.: Role of the technetium scan in the diagnosis of Meckel's diverticulum. J. Pediatr. Surg., 9:885, 1974.

VII

CARCINOID TUMORS AND THE CARCINOID SYNDROME

Haile T. Debas, M.D.,
and Susan L. Orloff, M.D.

Although Merling described the gross pathology of a carcinoid tumor of the appendix in 1838, it was Oberndorfer in 1907 who coined the phrase "Karzinoide."[16,27] In 1930, Kramer described similar tumors that arose from the Kultschitzsky cells of the bronchial mucosa.[13] That these tumors secreted humoral substance(s) was suspected for a long time, but it was only in 1952 that Erspamer and Asero showed that carcinoid tumors secreted serotonin.[8,33] Secretion of large quantities of 5-hydroxyindoleacetic acid (5-HIAA), the metabolite of serotonin, in the urine of patients with carcinoid tumors was recognized by Page and associates[30] in 1955. The carcinoid syndrome consisting of watery diarrhea, facial flushing, and right-sided cardiac valvular lesions was described by Pernow and Waldenstrom in 1954.[32]

CARCINOID TUMORS

INCIDENCE

Carcinoid tumors are the most common gut endocrine tumors. They constitute 55 per cent of all the gut endocrine tumors and 13 to 34 per cent of all tumors of the small bowel. The incidence is 1.5 cases per 100,000 of the general population.[6,26]

THE APUD CONCEPT

In 1968, Pearse reported that certain cells in the gut and elsewhere share common histochemical characteristics: they (1) have high *a*mine content in their cytoplasm; (2) are capable of amine *p*recursor *u*ptake; and (3) are able to *d*ecarboxylate these to produce amines and/or peptides. From this description, he coined the acronym APUD, and suggested that all APUD cells derive from the embryonic neural crest.[31] In addition, these cells commonly produce neuron-specific enolase and chromogranins, both of which may be used as tumor markers. In this section, the authors are concerned with carcinoid tumors that arise from the different portions of the gut itself: the foregut, the midgut, and the hindgut. Foregut carcinoid tumors arise mainly in the stomach[42] and other embryologic derivatives of the foregut of which the pancreas and lungs are important sites. Midgut carcinoids arise from the distal duodenum, jejunum, ileum and appendix, and ascending and right transverse colon. Of these, the appendix and terminal ileum are the most frequent sites. Hindgut carcinoids develop mainly in the rectum. The differential characteristics of carcinoid tumors from the different portions of the gut are cited in Figure 1.

SECRETORY PRODUCTS

Carcinoid tumors secrete a wide variety of products, including amines, tachykinins (substance P, neurokinin A, neuropeptide K), and other peptides. The secretory products vary from tumor to tumor. The most common secretory products are listed in Table 1.

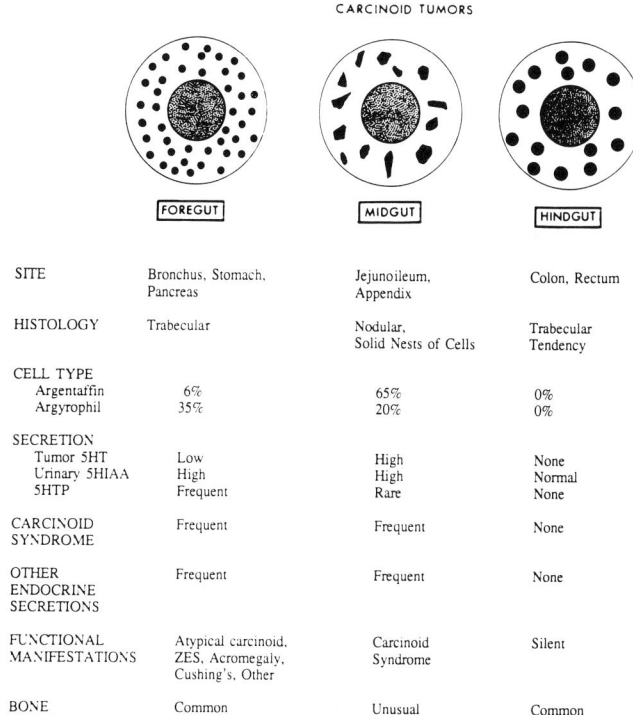

CARCINOID TUMORS

	FOREGUT	MIDGUT	HINDGUT
SITE	Bronchus, Stomach, Pancreas	Jejunoileum, Appendix	Colon, Rectum
HISTOLOGY	Trabecular	Nodular, Solid Nests of Cells	Trabecular Tendency
CELL TYPE			
Argentaffin	6%	65%	0%
Argyrophil	35%	20%	0%
SECRETION			
Tumor 5HT	Low	High	None
Urinary 5HIAA	High	High	Normal
5HTP	Frequent	Rare	None
CARCINOID SYNDROME	Frequent	Frequent	None
OTHER ENDOCRINE SECRETIONS	Frequent	Frequent	None
FUNCTIONAL MANIFESTATIONS	Atypical carcinoid, ZES, Acromegaly, Cushing's, Other	Carcinoid Syndrome	Silent
BONE METASTASES	Common	Unusual	Common

Figure 1. Cytologic, histochemical, biochemical, and clinical characteristics of carcinoid tumors arising in structures derived from the foregut, midgut, and hindgut. (Modified from Orloff, M. J.: Carcinoid tumors of the rectum. Cancer, *28*:175, 1971.)

PATHOLOGY

Classically, carcinoid tumors are formed by solid nests of small monotonous cells with exceedingly rare mitoses and occasional acinar or rosette formation. However, there is variability in histology and five histologic types may be identified:[34]

A type: tumors with nodular solid nests and peripheral invading cords.

B type: tumors with a trabecular or ribbon-like structure forming a frequent anastomosing pattern.

C type: tumors with a tubular, acinar, or rosette-like structure.

D type: tumors with structures of lower or atypical differentiations.

Mixed type: tumors with mixed structures of any combination of the above four types.

The mixed tumors that show an acinar and a glandular pattern have the best median survival time (4.4 years), whereas the undifferentiated pattern is associated with the poorest median survival (0.5 year).[12]

Determination of the benign or malignant nature of carcinoid tumors cannot be made histologically; only the presence of metastases or invasion of adjacent structures is a true indicator of

TABLE 1. Secretory Products of Carcinoid Tumors

Amines	Tachykinins	Peptides	Other
5-HT	Kallikrein	Pancreatic polypeptide (40%)	Prostaglandins
5-HIAA (88%)	Substance P (32%)	Chromogranins (100%)	
5-HTP	Neuropeptide K (67%)	Neurotensin (19%)	
Histamine		HCG$_a$ (28%)	
Dopamine		HCG$_b$	
		Motilin (14%)	

5-HT, 5-hydroxytryptamine; 5-HIAA, 5-hydroxyindoleacetic acid; 5-HTP, 5-hydroxytryptophan. Figures in parentheses represent percentage frequency. Data obtained from reference 37.

malignancy. Even when carcinoid tumors are malignant, however, they may be compatible with long survival. The overall 5-year survival has been quoted as high as 62 per cent for ileal carcinoid[42] with the 5-year survival for malignant carcinoids being 20 to 40 per cent.[39] The average duration from the onset of symptoms to death from the disease is 8 years.[44]

SITE OF ORIGIN

Carcinoid tumors may originate from neuroendocrine cells all along the gastrointestinal (GI) tract. About 85 per cent of the tumors are located in the intestine, but they may also occur in the lungs or occasionally in the pancreas, biliary tract, or thymus.[11] The most common location of carcinoid tumors in the GI tract is in the appendix. Appendiceal carcinoids rarely metastasize. Ileal carcinoids have the highest propensity to metastasize. The site of origin and rate of metastases from data on carcinoid tumors distilled from two large clinical series are listed in Table 2.[13,42]

The age distribution of carcinoid tumors includes patients as young as 10 years and those in their ninth decade, with a peak incidence in the sixth and seventh decades.

CLINICAL MANIFESTATIONS

Carcinoid tumors differ in their presentation depending on their location. The most common carcinoid tumors of the foregut are those that occur in the stomach and bronchus. Gastric carcinoid tumors may be silent. When symptomatic, however, they may cause either upper abdominal pain or bleeding. Bronchial carcinoid tumors present with hemoptysis, with pneumonitis occurring behind the bronchus occluded by the tumor, or with localized wheezing. Midgut carcinoid tumors frequently occur in the appendix and small intestine. The tumors may be silent at both locations and found incidentally at operation for another condition. Appendiceal carcinoid tumors, however, may cause acute obstructive appendicitis. Carcinoid tumors of

TABLE 2. Site of Origin of Carcinoid Tumors and Metastases

Tumor Site	Cases (%)	Metastases (Average %)
Stomach	2.8	23
Duodenum	2.9	20
Jejunoileum	25.5	34
Appendix	36.2	2
Colon	6.0	60
Rectum	16.4	18
Bronchus	9.9	—
Ovary	0.5	6
Miscellaneous	0.2	—
Unknown Primary	3.3	—

Data distilled from a study of 3718 cases[44] and 6965 cases.[42]

the small intestine are slow-growing and may be present for years without overt symptoms, and thus escape attention. One third of the patients with carcinoid tumors present with years of intermittent abdominal pain often ascribed to the irritable bowel syndrome. Malignant carcinoid tumors generally induce advanced fibrosis, which, by kinking of the intestine and by fibrous adhesions, may cause mechanical obstruction even when the primary tumor is small. Other symptoms include diarrhea, upper intestinal bleeding, weight loss, intussusception, and a palpable abdominal mass. The most frequent site of hindgut carcinoid tumors is the rectum. These rectal tumors may cause bleeding and are frequently detected by digital or endoscopic examination. When hindgut carcinoid tumors occur in the colon, they may cause abdominal pain, a palpable mass, and rectal bleeding.

DIAGNOSIS
BIOCHEMICAL

1. Tryptophan $\xrightarrow{\text{Tryptophan 5-hydroxylase}}$ 5-hydroxytryptophan (5-HTP)

2. 5-hydroxytryptophan $\xrightarrow{\text{Dopa-decarboxylase}}$ 5-hydroxytryptamine (5-HT)

3. 5-hydroxytryptamine $\xrightarrow{\text{Monoamine oxidase}}$ 5-hydroxyindoleacetaldehyde

4. 5-hydroxyindoleacetaldehyde $\xrightarrow{\text{Aldehyde dehydrogenase}}$ 5-hydroxyindoleacetic acid (5-HIAA)

The biochemical steps in the production of 5-HT and 5-HIAA are given. In patients with *typical* carcinoid tumors, the rate-limiting step in the synthesis of serotonin is the conversion of tryptophan into 5-HTP by the enzyme tryptophan 5-hydroxylase. Once formed, 5-HTP is rapidly converted to 5-HT in the tumor. Most of the secreted 5-HT is taken up by platelets and stored in their secretory granules. The rest remains free in the plasma and is then largely converted into the urinary metabolite 5-HIAA by the ubiquitous enzyme monoamine oxidase (MAO) and by aldehyde dehydrogenase (AD). These enzymes are abundant in the kidney, and the urine typically contains large amounts of 5-HIAA. The normal range for 5-HIAA secretion is 2 to 8 mg. per 24 hours. Typical tumors are usually both argentaffin- and argyrophil-positive.

In patients with foregut tumors (*atypical* carcinoid tumors), the urine contains relatively little (but above-normal) 5-HIAA but large amounts of 5-HTP and 5-HT. It is thought that these tumors are deficient in dopa-decarboxylase and have impaired conversion of 5-HTP into 5-HT, leading to 5-HTP secretion into the vascular compartment. Some 5-HTP is converted into 5-HT and 5-HIAA in extrarenal sites. Some of the 5-HTP is decarboxylated in the kidney and excreted into the urine as 5-HT, but some of the 5-HTP is excreted directly into the urine. Atypical carcinoid tumors are usually argentaffin-negative and argyrophil-positive. Serotonin-rich items of food, such as bananas, plantains, pineapples, kiwi fruits, walnuts, hickory nuts, pecans, and avocados, and the analgesic acetaminophen, may artificially increase 5-HIAA. False-negative results may be obtained in patients taking salicylates or L-dopa. Approximately 50 per cent of patients with carcinoid tumors of GI origin have evidence of serotonin production (manifested by elevated urinary 5-HIAA) whether or not an associated carcinoid syndrome is present.[9] Therefore, urinary 5-HIAA should be determined in patients with a carcinoid tumor even in the absence of the carcinoid syndrome. In carcinoid tumors, neurotensin is elevated in 43 per cent, substance P in 32 per cent, motilin in 14 per cent, somatostatin in 5 per cent of cases, and VIP rarely.[42]

LOCALIZATION

A number of techniques have been used to identify the primary site of the tumor and to evaluate the extent of the disease and the presence of metastases. A chest radiogram or CT is sufficient to detect a bronchial carcinoid tumor. Carcinoid tumors of the colon and rectum are usually demonstrable by barium enema examination or by colonoscopy. Routine barium studies often fail to demonstrate carcinoid tumors of the small intestine. Enteroclysis is more likely to give positive results. Ultrasound, abdominal CT, and magnetic resonance scanning are usually not helpful because the tumors are too small for detection. Advanced intestinal carcinoid tumors may be visualized on barium examination when mesenteric fibrosis produces foreshortening, rigidity, fixation, and kinking of the bowel loops.[23,36] CT is of value for demonstration of the mesenteric fibrosis and can be used to evaluate tumor extension in the mesentery, the retroperitoneal space, and the liver.[19] Superior mesenteric angiography in advanced tumors may show segmental caliber changes or occlusions of branches of the superior mesenteric artery, which together with the mesenteric veins may be trapped by tumor or fibrosis. Angiography is the superior method for demonstration of hepatic metastases from carcinoid tumors. Recently, midgut tumors have been identified by ^{131}I-metaiodobenzylguanidine (^{131}-MIBG) scintigraphy.[10]

The presence of a carcinoid tumor should be established by biopsy whenever this is clinically feasible. Positive argentaffin and argyrophil stains suggest the carcinoid nature of the tumor. However, electron microscopic demonstration of neurosecretory granules is probably the most specific test available. Endoscopy and biopsy have a valuable role in the diagnosis of primary gastric and rectal carcinoid tumors.[38]

Patients with ileal carcinoid tumors have a propensity to develop a second neoplasm elsewhere, especially in the colon. The incidence of a second tumor has been reported as 36 per cent in one series and 40 per cent in another.[23,38] Thus, a search for synchronous, metachronous, and metastatic neoplasms should be undertaken.

TREATMENT

Early resection, while the tumor is small, offers the patient the best chance for cure. Carcinoid tumors should be treated by resection regardless of the presence of metastases, since growth of the primary neoplasm is slow and local complications, such as obstruction and intussusception, are frequent. The incidence of metastases is dependent on the size and location of the primary tumor.[3] Appendiceal carcinoid tumors are rarely malignant, and lesions smaller than 1.5 cm. may be safely treated by routine appendectomy. If the tumor is at the base of the appendix, a cecectomy may be necessary. For the rare appendiceal tumor larger than 1.5 cm., ileocolectomy is recommended. This procedure is also justified when local invasion or lymph gland metastases are present. Gastroduodenal carcinoid tumors smaller than 1 cm. may be excised endoscopically.[3] For larger, invasive tumors, appropriate wide resection that may include

subtotal gastrectomy and omentectomy is recommended.[43] Rectal carcinoid tumors less than 1 cm. in size may be treated by endoscopic excision. Tumors measuring 1 to 2 cm. should be excised operatively with margins, and those larger than 2 cm. may require anterior resection. When local excision has been performed, the depth of invasion should be investigated histologically. If there is invasion of the muscularis propria, wider excision or anterior resection is necessary.[38] The resection of midgut carcinoid tumors, originating from the ileum and jejunum, may sometimes present a technical problem because of the fibrosis and foreshortening of the mesentery. Appreciation of this difficulty obviates more extensive resection than is necessary, and thus avoids creation of short gut syndrome. At clinical discovery, a large percentage (up to 70 per cent) of the small intestinal tumors are metastatic to lymph nodes and/or liver.[36] Those tumors with distant metastases should be managed by wide *en bloc* resection regardless of the size of the primary. This may include ileocolectomy for lesions located in the distal ileum.[4,36]

OUTCOME

The published survival rates vary. In general, the larger the primary tumor (> 2 cm.), the worse the prognosis. Patients with noninvasive appendiceal and rectal tumors of less than 2 cm. have 5-year survival rates that approach 100 per cent.[38] The survival rate declines to 40 per cent when the tumor diameter is greater than 2 cm. Invasion of the muscle wall or the presence of lymph node metastases is a poor prognostic sign. In the presence of liver metastases, 5-year survival rates of 21 to 42 per cent have been quoted.[4,23,36]

THE CARCINOID SYNDROME

CAUSES

The carcinoid syndrome occurs in less than 10 per cent of patients with carcinoid tumors. The carcinoid syndrome is encountered when venous drainage from the tumor gains access to the systemic circulation so that vasoactive secretory substances escape hepatic degradation. This situation obtains in three circumstances: (1) when hepatic metastases are present; (2) when venous blood from extensive retroperitoneal metastases drains into paravertebral veins; and (3) when the primary carcinoid tumor is outside the gastrointestinal tract, e.g., bronchial, ovarian, or testicular.

CLINICAL MANIFESTATIONS

The principal features of carcinoid syndrome include flushing, sweating, wheezing, diarrhea, abdominal pain, cardiac valvular fibrosis, and pellagra dermatosis. Diarrhea is found in 83 per cent of patients, flushing in 49 per cent, dyspnea in 20 per cent, and bronchospasm in 6 per cent.[41] Two types of carcinoid flush are described.[42] With midgut carcinoid tumors, the flush is usually transient, is faint pink to red, and involves the face and the upper trunk. It may be provoked by alcohol, blue cheese, chocolate, and red wines. In contrast, the flush in foregut tumors is often more intense, is more protracted, is purplish in hue, involves the upper trunk and limbs, and leads to telangiectasias.

A substantial number of patients develop right-sided cardiac valvular disease with congestive heart failure. Serotonin and possibly other neurohumors produced by the tumor cause fibrosis, and eventual incompetence of the tricuspid and pulmonic valves. The lungs metabolize serotonin and the other mediators and serve to protect the left side of the heart from fibrosis. If one can establish that the tumor is slow-growing, patients with carcinoid-induced cardiac lesions are candidates for valve replacement.

BIOCHEMICAL MEDIATORS

The specific etiologic agent(s) for each of the protean manifestations of the carcinoid tumors is not known. Serotonin, prostaglandins, 5-hydroxytryptophan, substance P, kallikrein, histamine, dopamine, and neuropeptide K are thought to be involved in the clinical manifestations of carcinoid tumors (Table 1). Pancreatic polypeptide and motilin levels are often raised,[41] and may serve as markers of tumor activity and provide a means of monitoring tumor growth and response to therapy.

Serotonin is thought to be largely responsible for both the diarrhea and fibrosis. The cardiac lesions, tricuspid and pulmonic insufficiency, are considered to be a component of this fibrosing phenomenon. The vasomotor changes, however, are considered to be mediated by kinins and such vasoactive peptides as substance P, neuropeptide K (NPK), neurokinin A (NKA), and neurotensin. Other substances, such as histamine vasoactive intestinal peptides (VIP), and prostaglandins, may also contribute to the systemic manifestations in the carcinoid syndrome.

DIAGNOSIS

Urinary 5-HIAA or whole blood and platelet-poor plasma 5-HT is the most reliable test to confirm the diagnosis of carcinoid syndrome. Occasionally, the measurement by radioimmunoassay of plasma levels of substance P and neurotensin may also be helpful. Measurements of neuron-specific enolase and chromogranins, when available, provide nonspecific evidence for the presence of a neuroendocrine tumor.

A useful diagnostic aid is the pentagastrin provocative test, which induces facial flushing, gastrointestinal symptoms, elevation in circulating 5-HT, and release of the peptides substance P, NKA, and NPK.[1,25,35]

TREATMENT

SURGICAL

Surgical cure of patients with the carcinoid syndrome is almost impossible in the presence of intra-abdominal and hepatic metastases. In rare instances in which the syndrome is secondary to bulky carcinoid tumors originating in teratomas or in the lung, total excision of all neoplastic tissue can be accomplished with cure of both the malignant neoplasm and the clinical syndrome.[3] Surgical attempts at palliation should be considered because the slow progression of this neoplasm will often allow the patient many months or years of comfortable life if immediately life-threatening complications can be controlled.[7] Thus, metastatic tumors in the abdomen should be treated with *en bloc* resection, regardless of the size of the primary lesion.[36] Hepatic metastases can be treated with lobectomy, local resection, or enucleation.[2] Debulking procedures have resulted in significant relief of flushing and diarrhea with decreased levels of urinary 5-HIAA.[2,7] Another palliative approach involves ischemic treatment of the liver, which can be achieved by temporary surgical liver dearterialization[5,24] or by hepatic artery embolization.[2,24]

LIVER TRANSPLANTATION

Orthotopic liver transplantation has been used for the treatment of patients with unresectable hepatic metastases from carcinoid tumors.[17,28] Two patients with malignant carcinoid syndrome who received orthotopic liver transplants by O'Grady and associates were free of associated symptoms at 6 and 10 months after operation. Hepatic transplantation may be considered as a potential therapeutic approach for some highly selected patients with unresectable hepatic metastases from carcinoid tumors. The usual fear that immunosuppressive therapy may induce growth of occult metastases pertains to this form of therapy.

PHARMACOLOGIC

Four types of pharmacologic agents are available for symptomatic control: (1) serotonin antagonists (cyproheptadine, methotrimeprazine, and methysergide maleate); (2) interferon (IFN); (3) chemotherapeutic agents; and (4) somatostatin and its analogs. The response to serotonin antagonists has been largely poor. Interferon, which acts by stimulating macrophages and T lymphocytes, has shown promising results in the control of flushing and stabilization of disease.[21,22] Moertel and associates have reported objective responses with chemotherapeutic agents in more than 200 patients at the Mayo Clinic. These drugs include 5-fluorouracil (5-FU) (26 per cent response), doxorubicin (21 per cent), streptozotocin (17 per cent), dacarbazine (DTIC) (13 per cent), and cis-platinum (10 per cent).[20] In a randomized multi-institutional trial performed by ECOG, the combination of 5-FU and streptozotocin had a response rate of 33 per cent compared with that of cyclophosphamide plus streptozotocin. A Mayo Clinic trial of hepatic arterial occlusion followed by combination chemotherapy with DTIC and doxorubicin, alternating with 5-FU and streptozotocin, resulted in complete relief of the carcinoid syndrome and 63 to 100 per cent decrease in urinary 5-HIAA in 9 out of 10 patients. The early results of this program appear to show more frequent, more complete, and more lasting responses than either hepatic artery occlusion or chemotherapy alone.[14]

Most recently, somatostatin-14 and its long-acting analog, Octreotide, have been used successfully to control symptoms of diarrhea and flushing.[14,26,40,42] The single largest series is from the Mayo Clinic where 66 patients with hepatic metastases and carcinoid syndrome have been treated with Octreotide. Flushing was abolished or significantly reduced in 87 per cent and diarrhea in over 75 per cent. A fall of 50 per cent or more in urinary 5-HIAA was observed. More important, the median survival of patients was increased by 3 years.[15] No major clinical side effects have been observed. Another trial by Vinik and associates has indicated that tumor growth is retarded in two thirds of patients treated with Octreotide up to 4 years. Octreotide has also been used to rapidly reverse life-threatening hypotension during induction of anesthesia[18] and has been used successfully to treat and prevent life-threatening carcinoid crisis.

REFERENCES

1. Ahlman, H., Dahlstrom, A., Gronstad, K., Tisell, L. E., Oberg, K., Zinner, M. J., and Jaffe, B. M.: The pentagastrin test in the diagnosis of the carcinoid syndrome: Blockade of gastrointestinal symptoms by Ketanserin. Ann. Surg., 201:81, 1985.
2. Ahlman, H., Schersten, T., and Tisell, L. E.: Surgical treatment of patients with the carcinoid syndrome. Acta Oncol., 28[Fasc. 3]:403, 1989.
3. Akerstrom, G.: Surgical treatment of carcinoids and endocrine pancreatic tumours. Acta Oncol., 28[Fasc. 3]:409, 1989.
4. Aranha, G. V., and Greenlee, H. B.: Surgical management of carcinoid tumors of the gastrointestinal tract. Am. Surg., August:429, 1980.
5. Bengmark, S., Ericsson, M., Lunderquist, A., Martensson, H., Nobin, A., and Sako, M.: Temporary liver dearterialization in patients. World J. Surg., 6:46, 1982.
6. Buchanan, K. D., Johnston, C. F., O'Hare, M. M. T., et al.: Neuroendocrine tumors. A European view. Am. J. Med., 81[Suppl. 66]:14, 1986.
7. Davis, Z., Moertel, C. G., and McIlrath, D. C.: The malignant carcinoid syndrome. Surg. Gynecol. Obstet., 137:637, 1973.
8. Erspamer, V., and Asero, B.: Identification of enteramine, the specific hormone of the enterochromaffin cell system, as 5-hydroxytryptamine. Nature, 169:800, 1952.
9. Feldman, J. M., and Jones, R. S.: Carcinoid syndrome from gastrointestinal carcinoids without liver metastasis. Ann. Surg., 196:33, 1982.
10. Feldman, J. M., Russel, A. B., Lucas, K. J., and Coleman, R. E.: Iodine-131 metaiodobenzylquanidine scintigraphy of carcinoid tumors. J. Nucl. Med., 27:1691, 1986.
11. Godwin, J. D. II: Carcinoid tumors: An analysis of 2837 cases. Cancer, 36:560, 1975.

12. Johnson, L. A., Lavin, P., Moertel, C. G., et al.: Carcinoids: The association of histologic growth pattern and survival. Cancer, *51*:882, 1983.
13. Kramer, R.: Adenoma of bronchus. Ann. Otol. Rhinol. Laryngol., *39*:689, 1930.
14. Kvols, L. K.: Therapeutic considerations for the malignant carcinoid syndrome. Acta Oncol., *28*[Fasc. 3]:433, 1989.
15. Kvols, L. K., et al.: Treatment of malignant carcinoid syndrome with long acting somatostatin analogue. Metabolism *39*(9):Suppl. 2, Sept. 1990.
16. Lubarsch, O.: Über den primaren Krebs des Ileum nebst Bemerkungen über das gleichzeitige vorkommen von Krebs und Tuberculos. Virchows Arch. Pathol., *111*:281, 1888.
17. Makowka, L., Tzakis, A. G., Mazzaferro, V., Teperman, L., Demetris, A. J., Iwatsuki, S., and Starzl, T.: Transplantation of the liver for metastatic endocrine tumors of the intestine and pancreas. Surg. Gynecol. Obstet., *168*:107, 1989.
18. Marsh, H. M., Martin, J. K. Jr., Kvols, L. K., et al.: Carcinoid crisis during anesthesia: Successful treatment with a somatostatin analogue. Anesthesiology, *66*:89, 1987.
19. McCarthy, S. M., et al.: Computed tomography of malignant carcinoid disease. J. Comput. Assist. Tomogr., *8*:846, 1984.
20. Moertel, C. G.: Treatment of the carcinoid tumor and the malignant carcinoid syndrome. J. Clin. Oncol., *1*:727, 1983.
21. Moertel, C. G., and Hanley, J. A.: Combination chemotherapy trials in metastatic carcinoid tumors and the malignant carcinoid syndrome. Cancer Clin. Trials, *2*:327, 1979.
22. Moertel, C. G., Rubin, J., and Kvols, L. K.: Therapy of metastatic carcinoid tumor and the malignant carcinoid syndrome with recombinant leukocyte and interferon. J. Clin. Oncol., *7*:865, 1989.
23. Moertel, C. G., Sauer, W. G., Dockerty, M. B., and Baggenstoss, A. H.: Life history of the carcinoid tumor of the small intestine. Cancer, *14:5*:901, 1961.
24. Nobin, A., Mansson, B., and Lunderquist, A.: Evaluation of temporary liver dearterialization and embolization in patients with metastatic carcinoid tumor. Acta Oncol., *28*[Fasc. 3]:419, 1989.
25. Norheim, I., Theodorsson-Norheim, E., Brodein, E., and Oberg, K.: Tachykinins in carcinoid tumors; their use as a tumor marker and possible role in the carcinoid flush. J. Clin. Endocrinol. Metab., *63*:605, 1988.
26. Oberg, K., and Eriksson, B.: Medical treatment of neuroendocrine gut and pancreatic tumors. Acta Oncol., *28*[Fasc. 3]:425, 1989.
27. Oberndorfer, S.: Karzinoide Tumoren des Dunndarms. Z. Pathol., *1*:426, 1907.
28. O'Grady, J. G., Polson, R. J., Rolles, K., Calne, R. Y., and Williams, R.: Liver transplantation for malignant disease: Results in 93 consecutive patients. Liver Transplant. Malignant Dis., *207*:373, 1988.
29. Orloff, M. J.: Carcinoid tumors of the rectum. Cancer, *28*:175, 1971.
30. Page, I. H., Corcoran, A. C., Udenfriend, S., Sjoersma, A., and Wiessbach, H.: Argentaffinoma as an endocrine tumor. Lancet, *1*:198, 1955.
31. Pearse, A. G. E., and Takor, T. T.: Neuroendocrine embryology and the APUD concept. Clin. Endocrinol., *5*[Suppl.]:229s, 1976.
32. Pernow, B., and Waldenstrom, J.: Paroxysmal flushing and other symptoms caused by 5-hydroxytryptamine and histamine in patients with malignant tumors. Lancet, *2*:951, 1954.
33. Rappaport, M. M., Green, A. A., and Page, I. H.: Serum vasoconstrictor (serotonin) IV isolation and characterization. J. Biol. Chem., *176*:1243, 1948.
34. Soga, J., and Tazawa, K.: Pathologic analysis of carcinoids: Histologic reevaluation of 62 cases. Cancer, *28*:990, 1971.
35. Strodel, W. E., Vinik, A. I., Jaffe, B. M., Eckhauzir, F., and Thompson, N. W.: Sus P in the totalization of a carcinoid tumor. J. Surg. Oncol., *27*:106, 1984.
36. Strodel, W. E., Vinik, A. I., Thompson, N. W., Eckhauser, F. E., and Talpas, G. B.: Small bowel carcinoid tumors and the carcinoid syndrome. *In* Thompson, N. W., and Vinik, A. I. (Eds.): Endocrine Surgery Update. New York, Grune & Stratton, 1983, pp. 277–291.
37. Theodorsson, E.: Regulatory peptides as tumour markers. Acta Oncol., *28*[Fasc. 3]:319, 1989.
38. Thompson, G. B., van Heerden, J. A., Martin, J. K. Jr., Schutt, A. J., Ilstrup, D. M., and Carney, J. A.: Carcinoid tumors of the gastrointestinal tract: Presentation, management, and prognosis. Surgery, *98*:1054, 1985.
39. Tilson, M. D.: Carcinoid syndrome. Surg. Clin. North Am., *54*:409, 1974.
40. Vinik, A., and Moattari, A. R.: Use of somatostatin analog in management of carcinoid syndrome. Dig. Dis. Sci., *34*[Suppl.]:14s, 1989.
41. Vinik, A. I., Strodel, W. E., Lloyd, R. V., and Thompson, N. W.: Unusual gastroenteropancreatic (GEP) tumors and their hormones. *In* Thompson, N. W., and Vinik, A. I. (Eds.): Endocrine Surgery Update. New York, Grune & Stratton, 1983, pp. 293–320.
42. Vinik, A. I., Thompson, N., Eckhauser, F., and Moattari, A. R.: Clinical features of carcinoid syndrome and the use of somatostatin analogue in its management. Acta Oncol., *28*[Fasc. 3]:389, 1989.
43. Welch, J. P., and Malt, R. A.: Management of carcinoid tumors of the gastrointestinal tract. Surg. Gynecol. Obstet., *145*:223, 1977.
44. Wilson, H., Cheek, R. C., Sherman, R. T., and Storer, E. H.: Carcinoid tumors. Curr. Prob. Surg., November: 1, 1970.

VIII

MALABSORPTION SYNDROMES

John P. Grant, M.D.

Malabsorption may be defined as any disorder with impaired absorption of fat, carbohydrate, protein, vitamin, electrolytes, minerals, and/or water. This abnormal physiologic state is observed in a wide variety of diseases involving the gastrointestinal tract. Knowledge of malabsorption dates to antiquity, being mentioned in the Ebers Papyrus, originating before the time of Christ. Aretaeus of Cappadocia (A.D. 120–220) may be credited with the earliest description of sprue. William Hillary (1722–1762) published the first report of sprue in the English language. The term *steatorrhea* apparently was first used in 1824 by Kunzmann. Modern understanding of absorption and malabsorption is a result of advances in knowledge concerning physiochemical and biochemical processes involved in intestinal absorption and transport, the advent of the electron microscope, and the use of radioisotopes and intestinal biopsy procedures.

DETECTION OF MALABSORPTION

The major clinical manifestations of malabsorption are unexplained weight loss, steatorrhea and diarrhea, anemia, tetany, bone pain and pathologic fractures, bleeding, dermatitis, neuropathy, glossitis, and edema. Although there may be malabsorption of both carbohydrate and protein, there is generally a selectively greater defect in fat absorption.

TESTS FOR MALABSORPTION. Tests for malabsorption may be grouped as follows:

1. *Screening tests.* Screening tests detect the more clinically significant degrees of malabsorption.
    a. *Gross inspection of the stool.* With steatorrhea, the stool is bulky, sticky, and tends to float. It is often very malodorous.
    b. *Microscopic examination of the stool for fat.* Increased fat by Sudan III staining suggests impaired fat absorption. Increased numbers of striated muscle fibers suggests impaired protein digestion.
    c. *Determination of random stool fat content.* Normal stool fat content is 5 to 6 gm. per day when dietary fat intake is 50 to 150 gm. per day. With steatorrhea, fat content may increase to 25 gm. per day or more.
    d. *Determination of random stool protein content.* Normally 2.5 gm. protein or less per day is lost in the stool with a dietary protein intake of 100 to 120 gm. per day. More than 3 gm. per day is definitely abnormal.
    e. *Serum carotene determination.* Carotene, a fat-soluble vitamin, is poorly absorbed in the presence of even moderate steatorrhea. If dietary intake is adequate, low serum concentrations strongly suggest fat malabsorption.
    f. *D-Xylose–carbohydrate malabsorption.* Normally, 5 gm. D-

xylose is excreted in the urine over 5 hours after oral administration of 25 gm. Improved sensitivity and reliability have been reported when only 5 gm. of D-xylose is given orally and blood xylose concentrations at 1 hour are corrected to a constant body surface area.[29] D-xylose absorption is also abnormal in the majority of patients with steatorrhea of intestinal origin.

   g. *Radiologic evaluation.* Radiologic examination is used in evaluating intestinal transit time, fistulas, motility, and strictures, and in identifying certain mucosal diseases such as Crohn's disease, diverticula, and cancer.

2. *Intake-output balance tests.* Balance tests are more sensitive than screening tests and identify even mild degrees of malabsorption.

   a. *Fat balance tests.* Measurement of fecal fat in 3- to 5-day stool collections while the patient is ingesting a relatively constant mixed-fat diet (usually 100 gm. fat per day) should normally result in less than 6 gm. over 24 hours, or less than 5 per cent of ingested fat.

   b. *Radioactive tracer tests.* A ^{14}C-triolein breath test is used in evaluating intestinal absorption of neutral fat.[9] ^{13}C-Trioctanion, a stable nonradioactive isotope, is also used in detecting and quantitating fat malabsorption through measurement of 2-hour [13]CO_2 respiratory excretion in a breath test.[67] Measurement of stool content of intravenously administered radioactive macromolecules (^{131}I-albumin, ^{51}Cr-albumin, and [67]Cu-ceruloplasmin) identifies patients with protein-losing enteropathy.

3. *Tests for specific compounds.*

   a. *Lactose tolerance test.* Abnormal absorption occurs with deficiency of brush-border lactase and in many disorders of the small intestine.

   b. *Schilling test—vitamin B_{12} absorption.*

   c. *Other radioactive compounds.* Procedures are available to test specifically for malabsorption of iron, calcium, amino acids, folic acid, pyridoxine, vitamin D, and nearly all compounds that are easily labeled with radioisotopes. These tests are clinically rarely useful. Recently, bile salt malabsorption has been found to be estimated quite accurately by [75]SeHCAT, a taurine conjugate of selenahomocholic acid.[47]

4. *Small bowel biopsy.* Peroral small bowel biopsy has been helpful in diagnosing celiac disease, tropical sprue, Whipple's disease, parasitic enteritis, intestinal lymphangiectasia, diffuse primary intestinal lymphoma, amyloidosis, abetalipoproteinemia, and hypogammaglobulinemia.

SURGICAL CONDITIONS ASSOCIATED WITH MALABSORPTION

Many classifications of malabsorption syndromes have been suggested. A useful classification is that of Johnson[35] shown in Table 1. A review of the list indicates that a significant number of conditions occur in the surgeon's domain, some being cured by operation, others being the sequel to operative removal or rearrangement of parts of the gastrointestinal tract. In the dis-

TABLE 1. Classification of Malabsorption Syndromes

Intraluminal factors	Tropical sprue
Decrease in effective length	Disaccharidase deficiency
Resection of stomach or small bowel	Radiation enteritis
Intestinal fistulization	Drug-induced (neomycin, etc.)
Hypermotility (hyperthyroidism)	Triglyceride enzyme deficiency
Decreased digestive activity	Ground substance
Pancreatic juice	Lymphoma, leukemia
Pancreatitis	Whipple's disease
Carcinoma of pancreas	Regional enteritis
Pancreatectomy	Systemic mast cell disease
Cystic fibrosis	Amyloidosis
Pancreatic duct lithiasis with	Tuberculosis
obstruction	Carcinoma, sarcoma
Pancreaticocutaneous fistula	
Bile	Abnormalities in blood or lymphatic channels
Hepatitis	Blood
Cirrhosis	Arterial or venous insufficiency
T-tube drainage	Congestive heart failure
Biliary obstruction	Vasculitis
Inadequate resorption of bile salts	Lymphatics
Congenital absence of bile salts	Intestinal lymphangiectasis
Changes in microorganism population	Lymphatic obstruction
Blind loop	
Small intestinal diverticula	Indeterminate
Intestinal stasis	Zollinger-Ellison syndrome
Visceral neuropathy (diabetes mellitus)	Malignant carcinoid
Primary neurologic diseases	Abetalipoproteinemia
Scleroderma	Protein-losing enteropathy
Partial obstruction	Pernicious anemia
Oral antibiotics (neomycin)	Hyperthyroidism
Giardiasis (also hookworm, whipworm)	Hypoparathyroidism
Acute infectious diarrhea	Pneumatosis cystoides intestinalis
Gastric achlorhydria	Hemochromatosis
	Kwashiorkor
Changes in intestinal wall	Hypogammaglobulinemia
Mucosal epithelial cell	Adrenal-pituitary insufficiency
Celiac disease of childhood	Tabes mesenterica
Gluten-induced enteropathy	

From Johnson, C.F.: Malabsorption syndromes: Clinical and theorectical consideration. Postgrad. Med. J., 37:667, 1965.

cussion that follows, emphasis is placed on the disorders seen in surgical patients.

Following Esophagectomy and Esophagogastrectomy

Absorption studies on patients undergoing esophagectomy or esophagogastrectomy for either benign or malignant disease are few. Two independent studies, involving 30 patients, in which absorption studies were done after esophagogastrectomy, revealed the presence of fat malabsorption of moderate degree.[52,59] The amount of nitrogen excreted in the stool was only slightly abnormal. Both D-xylose and vitamin B_{12} absorption and a small bowel biopsy were normal. The malabsorption of fat observed in patients after esophagectomy or esophagogastrectomy is most likely related to the vagotomy performed as a part of the esophageal resection.

Following Total Gastrectomy

Total gastrectomy commonly leads to rather severe nutritional abnormalities. The etiology of weight loss, steatorrhea, and anemia is complex. There is loss of gastric storage capacity, inadequate mixing of food with digestive enzymes, loss of intrinsic factor, and anorexia. Reduced nutrient intake in patients following total gastrectomy has been related to the pain asso-

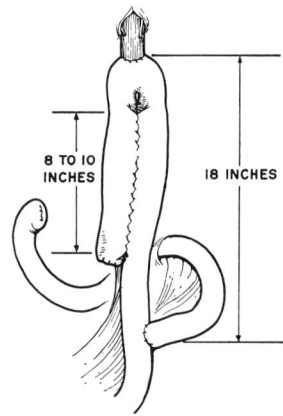

Figure 2. Alimentary reconstruction after total gastrectomy by Hunt-Lawrence jejunal pouch and Roux-en-Y esophagojejunostomy. (From Scott, H. W., Jr., Law, D. H., IV, Gobbel, W. G., Jr., and Sawyers, J. L.: Clinical and metabolic studies after total gastrectomy with a Hunt-Lawrence jejunal food pouch. Am. J. Surg., *115*:148, 1968.)

ciated with peptic esophagitis and to an inadequate food reservoir. Scott and Weidner[57] suggested that a 16- to 18-inch Roux-en-Y esophagojejunostomy would eliminate esophagitis. Longmire and Beal[4,43] found that interposition of an isoperistaltic segment of jejunum between the esophagus and the duodenum accomplished the same result. The end-to-side esophagojejunostomy with an enteroenterostomy between the ascending and descending limbs does not protect as well against development of esophagitis.

Various techniques for construction of reservoir pouches as gastric substitutes have been described (Fig. 1).[33,46,49,62] Scott and associates[56] studied the nutritional status of eight patients in whom a pouch was created from a double loop of jejunum that was anastomosed side to side just below the esophagojejunostomy anastomosis (Fig. 2). All eight patients were in a good state of nutrition 10 months to 3 years postoperatively. However, none underwent fat or protein absorption studies. Everson[18] collected results of all reported metabolic studies on patients who had undergone total gastric resection from 1897 to 1952 and found strong evidence for defective fat and protein absorption. Bradley and co-workers[7] evaluated 10 patients who had undergone total gastrectomy, 6 for Zollinger-Ellison syndrome and 4 for giant gastric ulcers or complicated marginal ulcers, and combined their data with the data of 12 similar patients reported in the medical literature. Sixty-nine per cent of 22 patients showed fat malabsorption (more than 10 per cent of ingested fat), and 42 per cent demonstrated protein malabsorption. There was no significant difference between patients who had undergone creation of a jejunal pouch and those patients who had not. A major factor contributing to weight loss and failure to gain weight was inadequate caloric intake. Lygidakis, using a surgical reconstruction procedure in 32 patients after total gastrectomy (Fig. 3), reported, after 10 to 15 years, weight gain in 30 patients, normal serum albumin in 26, normal D-xylose absorption in 29, and normal 72-hour stool fat in 30.[45] Armbrecht and associates[1] studied intestinal absorption in 11 patients after Roux-en-Y reconstruction. Loss of 0 to 8 kg. was observed over an average of 19 months. D-xylose and lactose absorption were normal. All 11 had signs of steatorrhea, and the median transit time to the cecum was only 110 minutes. They attributed weight loss to a combination of rapid transit, bacterial overgrowth of the small intestine, and pancreatic understimulation.

The incidence of pernicious anemia in patients subjected to total gastrectomy is considerably less than the theoretic 100 per cent. One explanation is the normally large hepatic reserve of intrinsic factor and the relatively poor survival record (perhaps

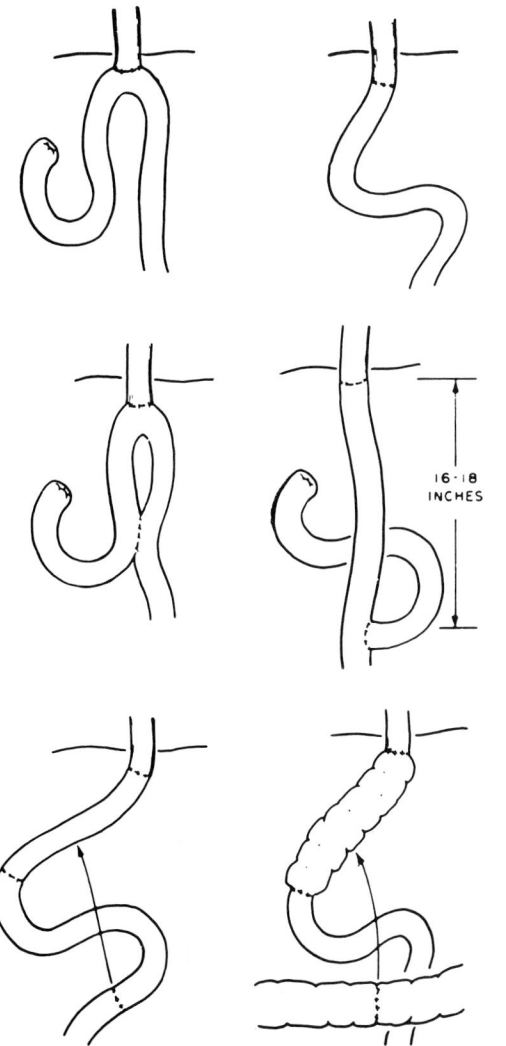

Figure 1. Methods of alimentary tract reconstruction most frequently used after total gastrectomy. (From Scott, H. W., Jr., Gobbel, W. G., Jr., and Law, D. H., IV: Malabsorption syndromes. Surg. Gynecol. Obstet., *121*:1231, 1965. By permission of Surgery, Gynecology and Obstetrics.)

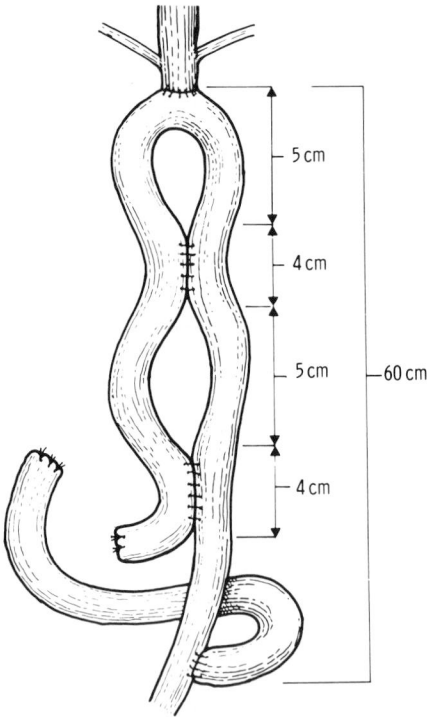

Figure 3. Alimentary reconstruction after total gastrectomy described by Lygidakis. (From Lygidakis, N. J.: Long term results of a new method of reconstruction for continuity of the alimentary tract after total gastrectomy. Surg. Gynecol. Obstet., *158*:335, 1984. By permission of Surgery, Gynecology and Obstetrics.)

3 or 4 years) of those patients undergoing the operative procedure for gastric cancer. Another explanation is the unknowing retention of as little as 1 to 2 cm. of normal fundic mucosa, which can provide sufficient intrinsic factor to prevent development of pernicious anemia. Hypochromic anemia has been observed in both humans and dogs after total gastrectomy. Such anemia usually responds favorably to oral iron therapy.

Following Partial Gastrectomy

Partial gastrectomy is also associated with nutritional problems in some patients. Intestinal continuity after subtotal gastrectomy can be restored by anastomosis of the stomach to the duodenum (Billroth I) or to a loop of jejunum (Billroth II). Opinions are divided as to which operative procedure best preserves the nutritional state of patients. All studies agree that the most common nutritional impairment following either type of anastomosis is loss of weight. In 1954, Zollinger and Ellison[72] reported that 127 of 203 patients were underweight after partial gastrectomy. Two thirds of the Billroth II patients were underweight, compared with one third of the Billroth I patients. Harkins and Nyhus[27] reported that 74 per cent of their patients with Billroth II anastomosis lost significant weight, compared with 42 per cent of patients with Billroth I anastomosis. However, Fischer[20] reported minimal nutritional problems following Billroth II anastomoses in a 25-year follow-up study. Weight loss of 1 to 10 kg. was found in 37 per cent of patients and over 10 kg. in only 11 per cent of patients.

There is further debate concerning the relative importance of inadequate caloric intake versus impaired digestion and/or absorption of ingested food after partial gastrectomy. Clinical evidence substantiates both points of view. Certainly partial gastrectomy reduces the gastric reservoir and smaller meals are taken. If frequency of intake is not increased, inadequate nutrition follows. The fact that a variable number of patients remain or become poorly nourished despite an adequate diet suggests the possibility of nutrient malabsorption. Metabolic balance studies in patients following partial gastrectomy have shown

variable degrees of fat and protein malabsorption.[6,70] Malabsorption of fat is generally greater in patients who have had a Billroth II procedure, approximately 50 per cent demonstrating steatorrhea greater than 8 gm. in 24 hours. Nonetheless, less than 20 per cent of patients develop clinically significant malabsorption. In contrast, only 25 per cent of patients who have undergone a Billroth I procedure demonstrate steatorrhea, and less than 10 per cent show clinically significant malabsorption.[17,35,71]

Several factors appear significant in the development of malabsorption after gastric procedures. With either Billroth I or II anastomosis, there is decreased gastric digestion, more rapid and less regulated gastric emptying, and decreased intestinal transit time. Additional factors leading to malabsorption following a Billroth II anastomosis include (1) defective stimulation of biliary and pancreatic secretions due to bypass of the duodenum (this has recently been challenged as a mechanism by the findings of increased cholecystokinin release in patients with a Billroth I or II procedure, compared with normal individuals, after ingestion of a fatty meal)[32]; (2) possible inadequate mixing of pancreatic enzymes and bile salts with the gastric contents; (3) possible stasis in the afferent loop leading to bacterial overgrowth and abnormalities of bile salt metabolism; and (4) loss of the duodenum as the principal surface for iron, calcium, fat, and carotene absorption. Small bowel biopsy studies have shown inconsistent and nonspecific histologic changes in the mucosa that are not adequate to explain the changes in function.

The most common metabolic complication of subtotal gastrectomy is anemia, which occurs in up to 30 per cent of patients within 15 years.[58] Causes include malabsorption of iron, folate, and, rarely, vitamin B[12]. Oral administration of iron is usually helpful, although refractory cases may require intramuscular or intravenous iron administration or blood transfusions. A metabolic bone disease similar to osteomalacia occurs in up to 33 per cent of patients after 10 to 20 years owing to malabsorption of vitamin D and calcium.[42]

The treatment of patients with malnutrition secondary to a subtotal gastrectomy consists of the administration of a diet high in calories, fat, and protein. The administration of pancreatic enzymes may be of use in some patients. Occasionally, for patients in whom severe malnutrition with hypoalbuminemia develops after partial gastrectomy, optimal treatment must include intravenous nutrition during clinical investigation and dietary manipulations. There has been variable interest in the use of further surgical procedures for improvement of the nutritional status. Conversion of a Billroth II to a Billroth I anastomosis or interposition of a jejunal segment (reversed or isoperistaltic) between the stomach and the duodenum (Fig. 4) has been employed. Except on rare occasions, surgical intervention for postgastrectomy malnutrition should be undertaken only as a last resort.

Following Vagotomy

When vagotomy is combined with a drainage procedure or with partial resection of the stomach, it becomes very difficult to determine which aspect of the operation contributes most to the nutritional problems that may follow. Experimental studies have indicated that vagal denervation alters to some degree the normal physiology of the stomach, pancreas, biliary system, and small bowel.[3,29] Weight loss following vagotomy with gastroenterostomy is generally thought to be less severe than that following partial gastrectomy. Yet Scott and associates[56] reported that 604 of 715 patients who had undergone antrectomy with truncal vagotomy maintained their ideal weight.

Malabsorption following vagotomy may be due in part to diarrhea, poor mixing of pancreatic secretions and bile salts with food, and, with truncal vagotomy, diminished release of cholecystokinin and secretin. The reported incidence of diar-

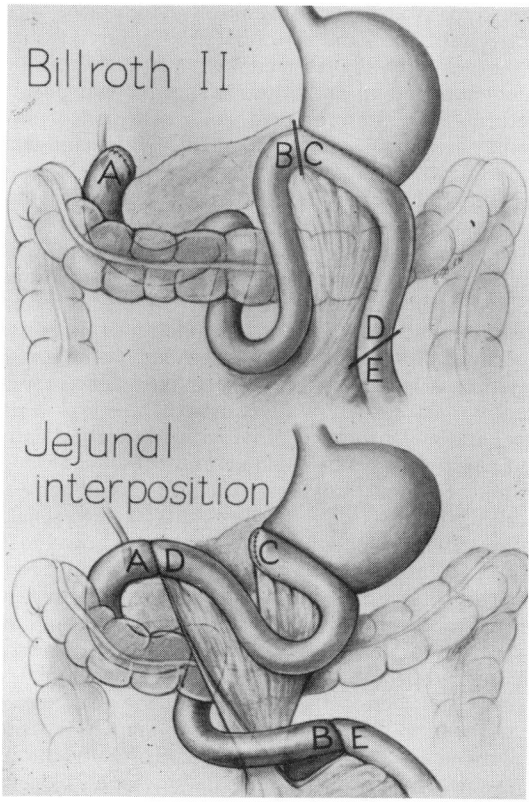

Figure 4. Diagram illustrating conversion of Billroth II anastomosis to the jejunal interposition of Henley. (From Wirts, C. W. Templeton, J.Y., Fineberg, C., and Goldstein, F.: The correction of postgastrectomy malabsorption following a jejunal interposition operation. Gastroenterology, 49:141, 1965.)

rhea following truncal vagotomy varies from 28 to 68 per cent, but it is troublesome in only approximately 5 per cent.[19,28,39] The diarrhea is often intermittent, appearing suddenly with explosive, loose stools. The incidence of diarrhea following selective vagotomy is less than 10 per cent.[38] The diarrhea may be due to stasis of food in the stomach and small bowel, causing bacterial overgrowth; uncontrolled gastric emptying with dumping, supported by the lower incidence following selective vagotomy; and/or rapid small bowel transit due to vagal denervation.[12,31] Aggravation of diarrhea following cholestyramine suggests a role of bile acids.[16]

Steatorrhea is common after vagal denervation. Fox and Grimson[23] reported that after truncal vagotomy without a drainage procedure, eight of nine patients showed excess excretion of fat. Doty and Meyer[15] demonstrated in a dog model that vagotomy and antrectomy interfered with absorption of solid fat but not liquid dietary fat. Abnormalities of gastric grinding and sieving of food particles were implicated with larger fat particles being malabsorbed. Shingleton and associates[60] reported that the amount of excess fat excreted in the stool was less after vagotomy and drainage than after partial gastrectomy with Billroth II anastomosis. Because the ileocecal valve is under vagal control, truncal vagotomy may alter valvular competence, causing the sulcus entericus to spend less time in the terminal ileum. Malabsorption of bile salts may therefore be a contributing factor in postvagotomy steatorrhea. There appears to be no difference between fecal fat levels after truncal vagotomy and after selective vagotomy.[44]

Alterations in glucose absorption and metabolism following vagotomy and pyloroplasty have been well documented. Using tracer methods, Radzuik and Bondy[53] demonstrated a reduction in glucose absorption from 92 to 60 per cent in five patients following vagotomy and pyloroplasty. The malabsorption was attributed to rapid gastric emptying and decreased small bowel

transit time leading to overloading of the limited glucose absorbing capacity of the gut. Plasma glucose and insulin peaks, however, were two to four times higher than in normal subjects, reflecting rapid gastric emptying and initial gut glucose absorption. Clearance of glucose from the blood was unaltered, compared with that of normal patients. The relatively short absorption period with normal glucose clearance leads to the typically observed "reactive" hypoglycemia. The overall response to glucose intake is an early postprandial hyperglycemia accompanied by hyperinsulinemia followed by reactive hypoglycemia.

Following Gastrointestinal Fistula

GASTROCOLIC FISTULAS. Gastrocolic fistulas can occur as a result of a penetrating marginal ulcer at a gastrojejunostomy, direct erosion of a large gastric ulcer or gastric or colonic carcinoma, or Crohn's disease. Malabsorption can be due either to bypass of ingested food into the colon or to severe enteritis due to reflux of colonic bacteria into the stomach with bacterial overgrowth of the stomach and small intestine.

ENTEROCUTANEOUS FISTULAS. Enterocutaneous fistulas can occur following gastrointestinal surgery, trauma, or Crohn's disease. If the fistula is located distally, little malabsorption occurs and nutritional depletion is uncommon. If the fistula is proximal, however, significant loss of ingested food may occur. Low-output fistulas (less than 200 ml. per day) seldom cause significant malnutrition. High output fistulas (especially more than 1000 ml. per day) can be associated with marked malnutrition and formidable skin care problems. Biliary and pancreatic fistulas may lead to malabsorption of fat, protein, and starch, depending on the amount of daily loss.

Pancreatic Insufficiency

In various types of pancreatic disease, malabsorption may not be present due to the organ's large functional reserve. However, when advanced, pancreatic disease is a well-established cause of malabsorption. Chronic pancreatic insufficiency may be the end result of relapsing pancreatitis; cystic fibrosis of the pancreas; or tumors, either primary or metastatic. Resection of a major portion of the pancreas, ligation of its duct, or loss of enzyme-rich fluid through pancreatic fistulas can also lead to pancreatic insufficiency.

The diagnosis of exocrine pancreatic insufficiency is suggested by pancreatic calcification with a normal D-xylose absorption test in the presence of steatorrhea and/or increased loss of protein in the stool. The secretin test has been used for evaluation of pancreatic function. Secretin is injected intravenously with timed samples of duodenal juice obtained through an indwelling gastroduodenal tube. Depression of secretin stimulation in patients with pancreatic tumors depends upon the degree and site of pancreatic duct obstruction. The greatest depression of secretin stimulation is observed in advanced pancreatic destruction due to pancreatitis and in large tumors involving the head of the pancreas.

Treatment of patients with disorders of the pancreas leading to malabsorption and malnutrition depends upon the nature of the underlying disease. Patients with chronic relapsing pancreatitis and severe malabsorption are benefited by the administration of a pancreatic enzyme preparation. Patients with chronic relapsing pancreatitis with a dilated partially or completely obstructed pancreatic duct can be benefited by anastomosis of the dilated duct to a portion of the gastrointestinal tract, restoring intestinal flow of pancreatic enzymes. Patients with an external pancreatic fistula can benefit from replacement of the fistula drainage via intestinal feeding tubes or by implantation of the fistula tract into a segment of the intestine. Patients with a tumor in the head of the pancreas occluding the major pancreatic duct should undergo resection of the tumor with reimplantation of the tail of the pancreas into the upper small bowel.

Total pancreatectomy produces both diabetes and malabsorption. Although insulin requirements are not as high as might be expected, control of the diabetes may be difficult. Studies by Braga and associates[8] in patients after subtotal pancreatectomy and acinar destruction with polychloroprene injection of the pancreatic duct confirm that enterocyte function is normal in the absence of exocrine function with no evidence for bacterial overgrowth or rapid transit. The lack of lipase and protease production represented all observed malabsorption. They reported complete reversal of malnutrition with oral pancreatic enzymes.

NON–BETA ISLET CELL TUMORS. Gastrin-secreting tumors of the pancreas cause marked gastric hypersecretion and hyperacidity. Because of increased volume of gastric secretions, increased secretory response of the duodenal mucosa due to irritation from excess acid, and inactivation of pancreatic exocrine enzymes by the duodenal acidity, malabsorption and diarrhea are severe. Total gastrectomy as treatment of the gastric hypersecretion can lead to severe malabsorption as previously described. Chronic administration of H_2 receptor antagonists has fewer side effects than total gastrectomy and is finding increasing application. Recently, subcutaneous somatostatin, which suppresses gastrin production, has been found quite effective. The long-term metabolic effects of global hormonal suppression by somatostatin are unknown.

Vasoactive intestinal peptide, when released in large amounts from pancreatic tumors, leads to a massive secretory response of the small intestine and severe diarrhea with at times dramatic wasting of electrolytes.

Biliary Tract Disease

Hepatobiliary diseases may cause malabsorptive states through two mechanisms: (1) the absence of adequate amounts of bile in the intestinal tract and (2) the hepatic disease itself. Thus, steatorrhea has been described in patients suffering from acute viral hepatitis, chronic intrahepatic cholestasis, chronic extrahepatic obstructive jaundice, and cirrhosis of the liver.[2,58,63] The frequency of bone disease in patients with chronic intrahepatic cholestasis indicates a disturbance of calcium metabolism as well.[63] Bony changes may be those of both osteoporosis and osteomalacia.[2] It is presumed that the clinical abnormalities follow both malabsorption of vitamin D and calcium loss in the stools.

Treatment of patients with chronic cholestasis or obstructive jaundice, whether caused by bile duct obstruction or acute cholestasis, must include administration of fat-soluble vitamins A, D, E, and K, and calcium salts.[58] Diarrhea may be partially reduced by limiting fat intake, which may also reduce losses of fat-soluble vitamins and calcium in the stool. If obstructive jaundice is present, surgical intervention is indicated to re-establish bile flow into the intestinal tract. In patients with biliary fistulas, bile collected from the fistula should be returned to the gastrointestinal tract through a stomach tube as a temporary measure until the fistula closes spontaneously or is closed surgically.

Following Small Bowel Resection

Generally, resection of a short segment of small bowel is well tolerated, with few, if any, signs of malabsorption. Yet even with removal of only short segments of bowel, chronic vitamin D and calcium malabsorption leading to osteomalacia has been observed.[11] Malabsorption increases as more small bowel is removed. When more than 50 per cent of the small bowel is removed, malabsorption becomes a significant clinical problem. Although there have been reports of patients surviving extensive resection of the small bowel,[48,64] resections of all but 40 cm. or less usually lead to progressive weight loss, sepsis, and death. The use of total intravenous nutrition, preventing complications of starvation, has improved survival significantly. Given time and adequate nutrition, the remaining small bowel undergoes

adaptive hyperplasia, increasing absorptive surface, enhancing absorptive processes, and assuming absorptive functions normally performed by the resected segment.[69] Patients in whom the duodenum and 40 cm. or more of small bowel distal to the ligament of Treitz are preserved along with part of the large bowel may eventually tolerate an oral diet with maintenance of body weight to within 70 to 80 per cent of usual. Long-term home parenteral nutrition is probably necessary if less intestine can be preserved.[34]

Malabsorption following small bowel resection is due to several factors: (1) Resection of the distal small bowel, more so than of proximal segments, especially with loss of the ileocecal valve, induces a marked reduction in intestinal transit time, affecting absorption of all foodstuffs.[61] (2) Resection of as little as 15 cm. of the terminal ileum may lead to vitamin B_{12} deficiency as well as bile salt malabsorption with diarrhea. Depletion of the bile salt pool and malabsorption of fat with steatorrhea lead to increased calcium losses in the stool and subsequent increased absorption of soluble oxalate salts (instead of excretion as insoluble calcium oxalate salts). Oxaluria may lead to renal stone formation. (3) Resection of the proximal small bowel may lead to calcium and iron malabsorption. (4) Intestinal resection leads to gastric hypersecretion and hyperacidity in direct proportion to the amount of small bowel removed.[24] The high solute load may exceed the absorptive capacity of the remaining small bowel; injury of the small bowel mucosa by acid may impair absorption and increase secretions; and the acidic secretions may inactivate the digestive enzymes lipase and trypsin—all leading to malabsorption and diarrhea. (5) Finally, intolerance to some sugars, especially lactose, may become clinically evident.

The treatment of patients with extensive resection of the small bowel requires careful observation and management. After moderate resections, frequent feedings of low-fat, low-oxalate, and high-protein dry diets are usually well tolerated. With more extensive resections, total parenteral nutrition should be initiated within the first week and continued until intestinal adaptation permits an adequate oral diet. Chronic home intravenous nutrition may be necessary. Addition of bile salts to treat steatorrhea or cholestyramine to treat bile salt diarrhea has been advocated but is rarely beneficial. Calcium carbonate administered orally may reduce steatorrhea and does decrease oxalate absorption. Gastric hypersecretion should be treated aggressively with frequent antacids (calcium carbonate or aluminum hydroxide) and an H_2-receptor antagonist for up to 6 months to prevent peptic ulcer disease as well as diarrhea and malabsorption.[50] Interestingly, the hypergastrinemia and need for H_2-receptor antagonists diminish over time. Finally, multi-vitamin supplements, including vitamin B_{12}, folic acid, and vita-min K, essential fatty acids as an intravenous fat emulsion, and various minerals, including copper, zinc, iron, iodide, magnesium, manganese, and selenium, should be provided to prevent deficiencies.

Blind Loop Syndrome

Although the term blind loop syndrome was originally used to describe complications of blind loops of the small intestine following surgical therapy, there are many other conditions that give rise to this syndrome, such as stricture of the intestine, Crohn's disease, small bowel stasis as in intestinal pseudo-obstruction, postvagotomy syndromes, scleroderma, and small bowel diverticula.[14,55] All have in common stasis and subsequent infection. The syndrome is characterized by diarrhea, steatorrhea, anemia, loss of weight, abdominal pain, and multiple vitamin deficiencies.

The hematologic aspect of the intestinal stagnation syndrome revolves mainly around the features of vitamin B_{12} deficiency, although it is possible that folic acid deficiency may be a complicating factor. The diagnosis of blind loop syndrome can be confirmed by the Schilling test demonstrating intrinsic factor resistant vitamin B$_{12}$ malabsorption.[54] There are two main hypotheses for the development of vitamin B$_{12}$ deficiency: (1) bacteria in the stagnant area utilize vitamin B$_{12}$ leaving an inadequate amount for absorption, (2) the bacteria produce a toxin that inhibits the absorption of vitamin B$_{12}$ across the small bowel mucosa.

The importance of steatorrhea in patients with blind loop syndrome has been emphasized. Evidence has been presented to suggest that the bacteria present in the blind loop cause structural alterations of bile salts that interfere with absorption of fat.[36]

Treatment of the blind loop syndrome should include surgical correction of the underlying cause of intestinal stasis if feasible. If operation cannot be undertaken, use of antibiotics can improve symptoms. The recommended antibiotic is tetracycline given in a dosage of 1 gm. daily. Other useful drugs include chlortetracycline, clindamycin, and Flagyl. Neomycin is ineffective against anaerobes. With effective antibiotic therapy, the Schilling test should return to normal or near normal and the diarrhea and steatorrhea should subside within a week. After treatment for 2 to 3 weeks, the antibiotics can be given intermittently (1 to 2 weeks out of each month) to continue suppression of clinical symptoms.

Miscellaneous Small Bowel Lesions of Surgical Interest

Regional enteritis (Crohn's disease) and granulomatous ileocolitis often cause a multiplicity of absorptive defects, including malabsorption of protein, fat, vitamin B$_{12}$, and iron.[5]

Radiation enteritis and tuberculosis may cause malabsorption as a result of intrinsic involvement of the bowel wall or lymphatics or stasis due to partial obstruction. Resection of involved segments may be required. Vascular occlusive lesions involving two or more major intestinal vessels commonly lead to altered intestinal motility and malabsorption, causing slow but progressive malnutrition. If possible to perform, percutaneous dilatation of the involved vessels or surgical revascularization can be curative if the intestine has not become fibrotic, with complete loss of the mucosal surface. Intravenous or oral hyperalimentation in the pre- and postoperative periods in these patients is most helpful. Intestinal lymphangiectasis and intestinal lymphatic obstruction due to tumor or infection are rare causes of malabsorption.

SELECTED REFERENCES

Baron, J. H., Alexander-Williams, J., Allgower, M., Muller, C., and Spencer, J. (Eds.): Vagotomy in Modern Surgical Practice. London, Butterworths, 1982.
This is a comprehensive review of normal vagal function with special attention to consequences of vagotomy in surgical practice. It consists of a series of articles presented at an international symposium in Basel in 1981.

Booth, C. C., and Neale, G. (Eds.): Disorders of the Small Intestine. Oxford, Blackwell Scientific Publications, 1985.
This is an excellent review of current understanding of diseases of the small intestine. Although devoted mainly to medical diseases, there are separate chapters on the effects of surgical procedures on malabsorption.

Koo, J., Lam, S. K., Chan, P., Lee, N. W., Lam, P., Wong, J., and Ong, G. B.: Proximal gastric vagotomy, truncal vagotomy with drainage, and truncal vagotomy with antrectomy for chronic duodenal ulcer: A prospective, randomized controlled trial. Ann. Surg., 197:265, 1983.
The metabolic side effects of three current operative procedures for peptic ulcer disease were compared in 152 patients—the largest of recent studies. Proximal gastric vagotomy had the fewest side effects of dumping, epigastric fullness, and diarrhea.

REFERENCES

1. Armbrecht, U., Lundell, L., Lindstedt, G., and Stockbruegger, R. W.: Causes of malabsorption after total gastrectomy with Roux-en-Y reconstruction. Acta. Chir. Scand., 154:37, 1988.
2. Atkinson, M., Nordin, B. E. C., and Sherlock, S.: Malabsorption and bone disease in prolonged obstructive jaundice. Q. J. Med., 25:299, 1956.
3. Baldwin, J. N., Albo, R., Jaffe, B., and Silen, W.: Metabolic effects of selective and total vagotomy. Surg. Gynecol. Obstet., 120:777, 1965.
4. Beal, J. M., Briggs, J. D., and Longmire, W. P., Jr.: Use of a jejunal segment to replace the stomach following total gastrectomy. Am. J. Surg., 88:194, 1954.
5. Beeken, W. L.: Remedial defects in Crohn's disease. Arch. Intern. Med., 135:686, 1975.
6. Bohmansson, G.: Studien über die chiurgische Behandlung von Gastroduodenalgeschwüren mit besonderer Berücksichtigung der Operationsanatomie und der postoperativen Digestionsphysiologie nebst einem Beitrag zur Frage der chirurgischen Behandling akuter Ulkusblutungen. Acta Chir. Scand., Suppl. 7, 1926.
7. Bradley, E. L., Isaacs, J., Hersh, T., Davidson, E. D., and Millikan, W.: Nutritional consequences of total gastrectomy. Ann. Surg., 182:415, 1975.
8. Braga, M., Cristallo, M., DeFranchis, R., Mangiagalli, A., Agape, D., Primignani, M., and DiCarlo, V.: Correction of malnutrition and maldigestion in patients with surgical suppression of exocrine pancreatic function. Surg. Gynecol. Obstet., 167:485, 1988.
9. Butler, R. N., Gehling, N. J., Lawson, M. J., and Grant, A. K.: Clinical evaluation of the 14C triolein breath test: A critical analysis. Aust. N.Z. J. Med., 14:111, 1984.
10. Cattel, R. B.: Massive resection of the small intestine. Lahey Clin. Bull., 4:167, 1945.
11. Compston, J. E., Ayers, A. B., Horton, L. W. L., Tighe, J. R., and Creamer, B: Osteomalacia after small-intestine resection. Lancet, 1:9, 1978.
12. Condon, J. R., Robinson, V., Suleman, M. I., Fan, V. S., and McKeown, M. D.: The cause and treatment of post-vagotomy diarrhoea. Br. J. Surg., 62:309, 1975.
13. Doig, A., and Girdwood, R. H.: The absorption of folic acid and labeled cyanocobalamin in intestinal malabsorption. Q.J. Med., 29:333, 1960.
14. Donaldson, R. M., Jr.: Small bowel bacterial overgrowth. Adv. Intern. Med., 16:191, 1970.
15. Doty, J. E., and Meyer, J. H.: Vagotomy and antrectomy impairs canine fat absorption from solid but not liquid dietary sources. Gastroenterology, 94:50, 1988.
16. Duncombe, V. M., Bolin, T. D., and Davis, A. E.: Double-blind trial of cholestyramine in post-vagotomy diarrhoea. Gut, 18:531, 1977.
17. Ellison, E. H.: Nutritional problems following gastric resection. Surg. Clin. North Am., 35:1683, 1955.
18. Everson, T. C.: Nutrition following total gastrectomy, with particular reference to fat and protein assimilation. Collective review. Surg. Gynecol. Obstet., 95:209, 1952.
19. Farris, J. M., and Smith, G. K.: Vagotomy and pyloroplasty for bleeding duodenal ulcer. Am. J. Surg., 105:388, 1963.
20. Fischer, A. B.: The long-term results following Billroth II resection for duodenal ulcer. Dan. Med. Bull., 33:319, 1986.
21. Fletcher, R. F., Henly, A. A., Sammons, H. G., and Squire, J. R.: Case of magnesium deficiency following massive intestinal resection. Lancet, 1:522, 1960.
22. Floch, M. H.: Recent contributions in intestinal absorption and malabsorption. Am. J. Clin. Nutr., 22:327, 1969.
23. Fox, H. J., and Grimson, K. S.: Defective fat absorption following vagotomy. J. Lab. Clin. Med., 35:362, 1950.
24. Frederick, P. L., Sizer, J. S., and Osborne, M. P.: Relation of massive bowel resection to gastric secretion. N. Engl. J. Med., 272:509, 1965.
25. Goulston, K., Bhanthumnavin, K., and Harrison, D.: Investigation of steatorrhea. Med. J. Aust., 2:462, 1968.
26. Grant, J. P.: Handbook of Total Parenteral Nutrition. Philadelphia, W. B. Saunders Company, 1980.
27. Harkins, H. N., and Nyhus, L. M.: A comparison of the Billroth I and Billroth II procedures: Clinical and experimental studies. Bull. Soc. Int. Chir., 15:111, 1956.
28. Harkins, H. N., Stavney, L. S., Griffith, C. A., Savage, L. E., Kato, T., and Nyhus, L. M.: Selective gastric vagotomy. Ann. Surg., 158:448, 1963.
29. Hayama, T., Magee, D. F., and White, T. T.: Influence of autonomic nerves on the daily secretion of pancreatic juice in dogs. Ann. Surg., 158:290, 1963.
30. Haymond, H. E.: Massive resection of the small intestine: An analysis of 257 collected cases. Surg. Gynecol. Obstet., 61:693, 1935.
31. Hobsley, M: Dumping and diarrhoea. Br. J. Surg., 68:681, 1981.
32. Hopman, W. P. M., Jansen, J. B. M. J., and Lamers, C. B. H. W.: Plasma cholecystokinin response to oral fat in patients with Billroth I and Billroth II gastrectomy. Ann. Surg., 199:276, 1984.
33. Hunnicutt, A. J.: Total gastrectomy for Ca; a new procedure. Bull. Alameida County Med. Assoc., 5:16, 1949.
34. Jeejeebhoy, K. N., Zohrab, W. J., Langer, B., Phillips, M. J., Kuksis, A., and Anderson, G. H.: Total parenteral nutrition at home for 23 months without complication, and with good rehabilitation. Gastroenterology, 65:811, 1973.
35. Johnson, C. F.: Malabsorption syndromes: Clinical and theoretical consideration. Postgrad. Med. J., 37:667, 1961.
36. Kim, Y. S., Spritz, N., Blum, M., Terz, J., and Sherlock, P.: The role of altered bile acid metabolism in the steatorrhea of experimental blind loop. J. Clin. Invest., 45:956, 1966.
37. Kirsner, J. B.: Clinical observations on malabsorption. Med. Clin. North Am., 53:1169, 1969.
38. Knight, C. D., Van Heerden, J. A., and Kelly, K. A.: Proximal gastric vagotomy. Ann. Surg., 197:22, 1983.
39. Koo, J., Lam, S. K., Chan, P., Lee, N. W., Lam, P., Wong, J., and Ong, G. B.:

Proximal gastric vagotomy, truncal vagotomy with drainage, and truncal vagotomy with antrectomy for chronic duodenal ulcer: A prospective, randomized controlled trial. Ann. Surg., *197*:265, 1983.

40. Law, D. H.: Medium chain triglyceride therapy of malabsorption. Clin. Res., *14*:48, 1966.

41. Laws, J. W., Shawdon, H., Booth, C. C., and Stewart, J. S.: Correlation of radiological and histological findings in idiopathic steatorrhea. Br. Med. J., *1*:1311, 1963.

42. Leading Article. Osteomalacia after gastrectomy. Lancet, *1*:77, 1986.

43. Longmire, W. P., Jr., and Beal, J. M.: Construction of a substitute gastric reservoir following total gastrectomy. Ann. Surg., *135*:637, 1952.

44. Losowsky, M. S., Walker, B. E., and Kelleher, J.: Malabsorption in Clinical Practice. London, Churchill-Livingstone, 1974, p. 191.

45. Lygidakis, N. J.: Long term results of a new method of reconstruction for continuity of the alimentary tract after total gastrectomy. Surg. Gynecol. Obstet., *158*:335, 1984.

46. McCorkle, H. J., and Harper, H. A.: The problem of nutrition following complete gastrectomy. Ann. Surg., *140*:467, 1954.

47. Merrick, M. V., Eastwood, M. A., Anderson, J. R., and Ross, H. McL.: Enterohepatic circulation in man of a gamma-emitting bile-acid conjugate, 23-selena-25-homotaurocholic acid (SeHCAT). J. Nucl. Med., *23*:126, 1982.

48. Meyer, H. W.: Acute superior mesenteric artery thrombosis. Recovery following extensive resection of the small and large intestine. Arch. Surg., *53*:298, 1946.

49. Moroney, J.: Colonic replacement and restoration of the human stomach. Ann. R. Coll. Surg. Engl., *12*:328, 1953.

50. Murphy, J. P., Jr., King, D. R., and Dubois, A.: Treatment of gastric hypersecretion with cimetidine in the short-bowel syndrome. N. Engl. J. Med., *300*:80, 1979.

51. Newcomer, A. D., Hofmann, A. F., DiMagno, E. P., Thomas, P. J., and Carlson, G. L.: Triolein breath test: A sensitive and specific test for fat malabsorption. Gastroenterology, *76*:6, 1979.

52. Phillips, D. F., Wollaeger, E. E., Ellis, F. H., Jr., and Power, M. H.: Fecal excretion of fat and nitrogen after esophagogastrectomy in man. Surgery, *49*:433, 1961.

53. Radziuk, J., and Bondy, D. C.: Abnormal oral glucose tolerance and glucose malabsorption after vagotomy and pyloroplasty. Gastroenterology, *83*:1017, 1982.

54. Reilly, R. W., and Kirsner, J. B.: The blind loop syndrome. Gastroenterology, *37*:491, 1959.

55. Rutgeerts, P., Ghoos, Y., Vantrappen, G., and Eyssen, H.: Ileal dysfunction and bacterial overgrowth in patients with Crohn's disease. Eur. J. Clin. Invest., *11*:199, 1981.

56. Scott, H. W., Jr., Herrington, J. L., Jr., Edwards, L. W., Shull, H. J., Stephenson, S. E., Jr., Sawyers, J. L., and Classen, K. L.: Results of vagotomy and antral resection in surgical treatment of duodenal ulcer. Gastroenterology, *39*:590, 1960.

57. Scott, H. W., Jr., and Weidner, M. G.: Total gastrectomy with Roux-en-Y esophagojejunostomy in treatment of gastric cancer. Ann. Surg., *143*:682, 1956.

58. Sherlock, S.: Primary biliary cirrhosis (chronic intrahepatic obstructive jaundice). Gastroenterology, *37*:574, 1959.

59. Shils, M. E., and Gilat, T.: The effect of esophagectomy on absorption in man: Clinical and metabolic observations. Gastroenterology, *50*:347, 1966.

60. Shingleton, W. W., Baylin, G. J., Isley, J. K., Sanders, A. P. and Ruffin, J. M.: A study of fat absorption after gastric surgery using I-131 labeled fat. Ann. Surg., *144*:433, 1956.

61. Singleton, A. O., Redmond, D. C., and McMurray, J. E.: Ileocecal resection and small bowel transit and absorption. Ann. surg., *159*:690, 1964.

62. State, D., Barclay, T., and Kelly, W. D.: Total gastrectomy with utilization of a segment of transverse colon to replace the excised stomach. Ann. Surg., *134*:1035, 1951.

63. Summerskill, W. H. J., and Moertel, C. G.: Malabsorption syndrome associated with anicteric liver disease. Gastroenterology, *42*:380, 1962.

64. Todd, W. R., Ditterbrandt, M., Montague, J. R., and West, E. S.: Digestion and absorption in a man with all but three feet of the small intestine removed surgically. Am. J. Dig. Dis., *7*:295, 1940.

65. Tovey, F. I., and Clark, C. G.: Anaemia after partial gastrectomy: A neglected curable condition. Lancet, *1*:956, 1980.

66. Tuna, N., Mangold, H. K., and Mosser, D. G.: Re-evaluation of the I-131-triolein absorption test. J. Lab. Clin. Med., *61*:620, 1963.

67. Watkins, J. B., Schoeller, D. A., Klein, P. D., Ott, D. G., Newcomer, A. D., and Hofmann, A. F.: ^{13}C-trioctanoin: A non radioactive breath test to detect fat malabsorption. J. Lab. Clin. Med., *90*:422, 1977.

68. Wilkins, R., Garvey, C., and DeLacey, G.: Radiological examination. *In* Booth, C. C., and Neale, G. (Eds.): Disorders of the Small Intestine. Oxford, Blackwell Scientific Publications, 1985, pp. 5–11.

69. Williamson, R. C. N., and Chir, M.: Intestinal adaptation. N. Engl. J. Med., *298*:1393, 1444, 1978.

70. Wilson, T. H.: Intestinal Absorption. Philadelphia, W. B. Saunders Company, 1962.

71. Wollaeger, E. E., Waugh, J. M., and Power, M. H.: Fat-assimilating capacity of the gastrointestinal tract after partial gastrectomy (Billroth I anastomosis). Gastroenterology, *44*:25, 1963.

72. Zollinger, R. M., and Ellison, E. H.: Nutrition after gastric operations. J.A.M.A., *154*:811, 1954.

IX

RADIATION INJURY TO THE INTESTINE

Jerome J. DeCosse, M.D., Ph.D.

Radiation therapy is the primary method of management in some forms of curable cancer, such as squamous cell carcinoma of the cervix, carcinoma of the intrinsic larynx, and seminoma of the testis. Radiation therapy complements surgical therapy or is an alternative form of therapy for curable tumors at other sites, such as squamous cell carcinoma of the oral cavity, adenocarcinoma of the endometrium, and carcinoma of the breast. Both radiation therapy and chemotherapy may be used in the curative treatment of lymphoma and pediatric tumors, such as Ewing's sarcoma and Wilms' tumor, and in bone marrow transplantation. Radiation therapy also is used frequently in the palliative management of incurable cancer. Today more than half of all patients with cancer receive curative or palliative radiation therapy.[5] However, because the number of long-term survivors of cancer who have received radiation therapy has greatly increased in recent years, the number of those who have persistent radiation damage to normal tissue also has increased.[1,11]

Roentgen, a physicist, discovered x-rays in 1895. The diagnostic potential of this discovery became apparent in January 1896 when he radiographed a colleague's hand for demonstration purposes. The next decade revealed both the therapeutic possibilities and the hazards of radiation, but radiation therapy for cancer did not become routine in the United States until after World War II.

The goal of radiation therapy is local control of tumor with minimal damage to normal tissue. To achieve this goal, the therapist must consider the total duration of a course of radiation therapy, the total dose, the number and size of fractions (small daily doses), the extent of the portal (area of the body to be exposed to radiation), and the organ system or systems being irradiated. It is nearly impossible to expose a tumor to radiation without also exposing normal tissue. Both tumors and normal tissue vary in sensitivity to radiation. The amount of radiation that tissues can receive and still remain functional is their radiation tolerance. Intestinal tolerance is a major constraint on radiation therapy of the abdomen and pelvis.

The energy absorbed in a biologic system is measured by the rad, which is defined as 100 ergs or 10^{12} primary ionizations per gram of tissue. One rad equals 0.01 Gy. The curative dose for cervical cancer is 7000 to 7500 rads, whereas the maximal tolerance dose for intestine is 5500 to 6500 rads. About 5 per cent of patients who receive radiation therapy for abdominal or pelvic tumors experience late radiation injury requiring surgical intervention.[22]

THE BIOLOGIC BASIS OF RADIATION INJURY

Therapeutic radiation may be administered by a variety of external sources; by direct application to the tumor, as with radium; and by intravenous, intracavitary, or interstitial insertion with radioisotopes. Different forms of radiation vary in their linear energy transfer (LET)—the amount of energy they lose—as they traverse a given tissue. Gamma rays have high penetration and a relatively low LET; that is, they dissipate energy evenly over a long distance. Alpha particles have low penetration and higher LET; they travel a shorter distance, and the energy concentration is higher at the end of their path. The penetration and LET of x-rays fall between these extremes (Table 1). Differences in LET, among other variables, cause similar doses of different types of ionizing radiation to differ in their biologic effects on a specific organ or site.

Within irradiated tissue, energy transferred by ionizing radiation generates a series of biochemical events. The molecules initially ionized by radiation transfer energy to other molecules. Radiation interacts with intracellular water. These events produce free radicals and cause synthesis of abnormal macromolecules. Within the cell, DNA appears to be the critical target associated with radiation-induced cell death. The cell membrane also may have a role in longer-term damage.

Radiation may cause rapid cell death from mitotic arrest, but sometimes death is preceded by a nonmitotic period of cell growth, hence the clinical experience that a tumor may not appear to respond to radiation therapy until several weeks after initiation of treatment.

In addition to causing cell death, any type of ionizing radiation can induce, as Muller demonstrated in his Nobel Prize–winning studies, true point mutations with breakage and rearrangement of chromosomes (Fig. 1).[24] These effects of radiation, a linear function of dose, are persistent and cumulative over long periods of time.

Different types of cells vary considerably in their sensitivity to ionizing radiation. In general, the more frequently cells divide routinely, the greater their sensitivity to radiation. Hematopoietic cells, reproductive cells, and the stem cells in the intestinal crypts proliferate very rapidly and are at the greatest risk of radiation injury.[26] Static cell populations, such as nerve cells, are relatively resistant to radiation injury.

Tissue and whole organ effects depend on age, sex, temperature, oxygenation, metabolic activity, weight, stress, species variation, and other variables. In addition to causing cellular injury, radiation causes progressive changes in fine vasculature and interstitial connective tissue. Subendothelial proliferation and medial thickening may progressively deplete blood supply to the irradiated tissue (Fig. 2). Interstitial collagen deposition also may cause severe scarring and further obliterate blood flow, causing tissue hypoxia and eventual necrosis, while fibrotic barriers may inhibit revascularization and repair.

ACUTE INTESTINAL INJURY

The acute effects of a given dose of ionizing radiation are inversely proportional to field size; that is, with small portals, other physical factors being equal, large amounts of radiation may be given safely, whereas with total-body radiation, approximately 400 rads constitute the median lethal dose (LD_{50}) in man. Such injuries have followed nuclear disasters and accidental radiation exposures, such as the nuclear accident at Chernobyl in 1986. Radiation at this level affects the proliferating cells in the crypts of Lieberkühn, which are no longer able to supply replacements for the cells on the intestinal villi. The villi become flattened, and intestinal barrier function fails. Leakage of fluids into the intestinal lumen causes the patient to become dehydrated, while bacteria that normally live within the gastrointestinal tract enter the bloodstream, causing systemic toxemia. In a context of total-body radiation, damage to the bone marrow compounds the effect; pancytopenia due to hematopoietic depression may lead inexorably to the patient's death. At lower levels of total-body irradiation, prolonged and vigorous water and electrolyte replacement, antibiotic protection, and in some cases, bone marrow transplantation (used with some success among Chernobyl victims with total body doses less than 7 Gy) may enable patients to survive acute injury.[7]

The intestinal alterations that follow therapeutic irradiation are less devastating. The basic pathophysiologic mechanisms are more transient, self-limited, and localized. Epithelial changes may include decreased mitoses in the intestinal crypts, necrosis of crypt epithelial cells, and decreased height of crypts and villi. Patients with mucosal lesions and steatorrhea may have few or no gastrointestinal symptoms.

Intensive radiation therapy is often administered to the pelvis for carcinoma of the cervix, endometrium, ovary, bladder, or prostate (placing the patient at risk for acute radiation-induced or factitial proctitis) or to the para-aortic area for lymphosarcoma or testicular tumors (placing the patient at risk for transient injury to the intestine). Complications of radiation therapy to extensive visceral cancer, such as small bowel perforation in intestinal lymphosarcoma, should be distinguished from complications of radiation directed to other organs or tissues.

Patients with proctitis usually present with diarrhea, tenesmus, and rectal bleeding. Diarrhea also may follow impaired bile salt reabsorption in the injured terminal ileum. Nausea is common, and crampy abdominal pain may be present. Ordinar-

TABLE 1. Some Types of Ionizing Radiation and Their LET Values

Particle	Charge	Energy (MeV)	Description	LET (keV/μ)
Alpha	+2	5	Helium nucleus	100.0
Proton	+1	2	Hydrogen nucleus	16.0
		5		8.0
		10		4.0
Neutron	0	2.5	Neutron	20.0
		14.1		7.0
Electron	−1	0.001	Electron	12.3
		0.010		2.3
		0.100		0.42
		1.000		0.25
X-ray		3.000	Electromagnetic radiation	0.3
Gamma ray			Cobalt 60	0.3

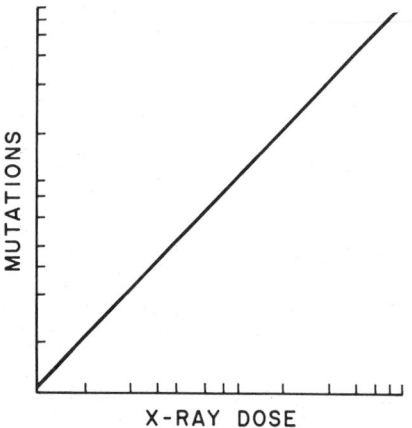

Figure 1. The frequency of mutations in *Drosophila* spermatozoa relates directly to the intensity of radiation administered.

ily, these symptoms subside shortly after completion of radiation therapy, and patients require only supportive therapy with antidiarrheal, anticholinergic, and antispasmodic medication. An elemental diet, cholestyramine, and perhaps glutamine[17,18] may be beneficial.

LATE INTESTINAL INJURY

In some patients, gastrointestinal symptoms persist after radiation therapy. Overt radiation injury to the intestine may take weeks, months, or even years to become evident clinically. Late radiation injury is caused by progressive vasculitis and diffuse collagen deposition and fibrosis rather than altered epithelial proliferative kinetics. The vasculitis causes tissue hypoxia, which may progress to necrosis, ulceration, and perforation. Collagen deposition may lead to obstruction of the intestine.[4]

Some patients with acute injury progress to chronic injury with a continuous display of intestinal symptoms; others experience a long symptom-free period before their chronic radiation injury becomes evident. Subclinical injury may become overt when low-flow states, such as congestive heart failure or vascular narrowing from hypertension and arteriosclerosis, in-

crease the hypoxia from radiation vasculitis until, finally, cellular oxygenation and nutrition are reduced below critical levels (Fig. 3).[9]

Prior surgical therapy or prior intra-abdominal infection may increase the risk of injury because following operation or infection loops of small or large intestine may adhere to tissue being irradiated.[8] Surgeons performing procedures that are to be followed by radiation therapy may reduce the risk of intestinal injury by accurately outlining the area to be treated with radiopaque markers, by reperitonealization, by excluding small bowel from the pelvis through omental transposition or other measures,[3,15,23] and by scrupulous cleansing of the peritoneal cavity before closure.

Some chemotherapeutic drugs, such as dactinomycin, doxorubicin, and 5-fluorouracil, enhance the effect of radiation. Both treatments need not be administered at the same time; if they are applied sequentially, the subsequent effect is labeled a recall phenomenon. Although linked, the specific cellular damage caused by chemotherapy is probably different from that caused by radiation; in the gut, chemotherapy accelerates the depletion of crypt stem cells in zones of focal radiation ischemia.[27]

Chronic radiation injury of the intestine is frequently associated with injury to cutaneous, bony, and other visceral structures encompassed by the radiation portals. The radiation portal may be demarcated by a chronic dermatitis with capillary telangiectasia, epidermal atrophy, hyperkeratosis, and indolent ulceration. Sterility in men and amenorrhea in women may be evident. Gastrointestinal injury may be associated with genitourinary injury.[29,30] Since genitourinary injury may be more life-threatening, investigation of intestinal injury should include assessment by intravenous pyelography, cystoscopy, and computed axial tomography (CT scanning) for cystitis or urethral injury, as well as for radiation nephritis.

Radiation injury of the small or large intestine may cause malabsorption, acute or chronic obstruction, ulceration, perforation, abscess formation, and fistulization.[28] Radiation-induced enteritis should be regarded as a possible cause for abdominal pain after abdominal or pelvic irradiation.

Short of biopsy, there are no specific tests to distinguish radiation damage from recurrent tumor or ischemic or inflammatory bowel disease, although CT scanning and magnetic resonance imaging may help to identify recurrent tumor. However, a patient who appears well and maintains body weight but continues to have crampy abdominal pain often has a radiation injury rather than residual or recurrent cancer. Conditions associated with malabsorption, such as steatorrhea and hypocalcemia, also point to a diagnosis of radiation injury to the small intestine.

Symptoms of partial obstruction may be insidious: limited nausea, no vomiting, only slight crampy pain, and modest distention. In the presence of such symptoms, a small intestinal

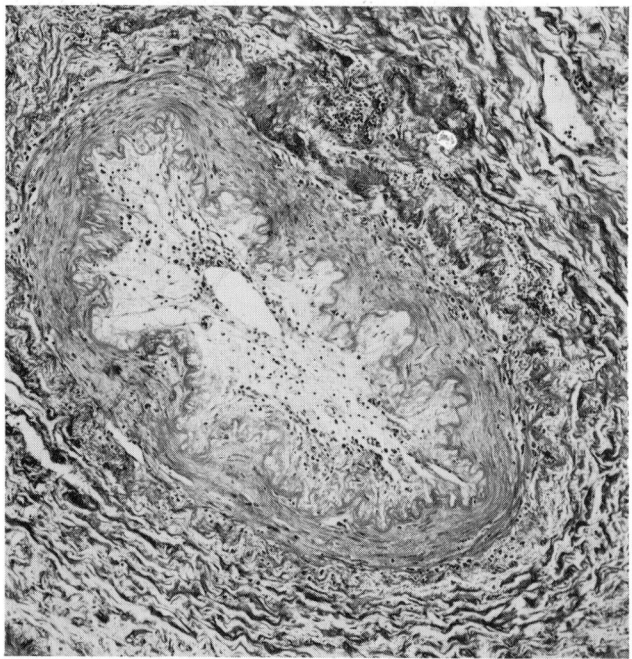

Figure 2. Photomicrograph (×80) of an ileal arteriole demonstrating occlusive radiation vasculitis and surrounding perivascular fibrosis, findings characteristic of chronic radiation injury.

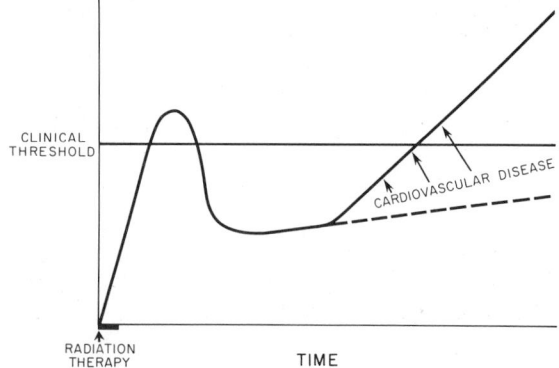

Figure 3. A model suggesting a pattern for radiation injury: early transient symptoms, a latent period of subclinical activity, and precipitation of clinical symptoms, often by onset of cardiovascular disease. (After Rubin, P., and Casarett, G. W.: Clinical Radiation Pathology. Philadelphia, W. B. Saunders Company, 1968.)

barium examination should be conducted. However, the results may be difficult to interpret; the film may appear negative even when considerable pathologic change has occurred.[31]

Constricted, narrow loops of intestine or puddling of barium are indicative of partial obstruction (Fig. 4).[21] It is important not only to determine whether the obstruction is complete or partial but also to establish whether it involves vascular compromise. Patients with vascular compromise may have continuous abdominal pain between cramps, back pain suggesting torsion in the mesentery, involuntary guarding, localized and persistent tenderness to percussion or palpation, reduced or absent peristaltic sounds, a rectal temperature above 38° C., and a white blood count in excess of 12,000 cells per cu. mm.

Both vascular compromise and complete obstruction require surgical exploration: in the former case, exploration is urgent; in the latter, it should be preceded by nasogastric intubation and drainage, as well as volume repletion. At laparotomy, radiation-injured bowel is stenotic and thick-walled. The serosal surface is gray and opaque from serositis. Loose fibrinous adhesions congeal loops of small intestine to one another and to adjacent surfaces. Wide resection of the diseased bowel is the treatment of choice. Occasionally a bypass is necessary.[10,20] Normal, unirradiated intestine should be used for the enteroenterostomy.

Partial obstruction from radiation-induced stenosis of the small intestine may not require resection and should be managed initially by conservative intestinal decompression and fluid replacement. Oral steroids, sulfasalazine, and a low-residue diet may reduce symptoms to a tolerable level.[14]

Obstruction and vascular occlusion can lead to hypoxia, necrosis, and perforation of the intestine. Perforation can cause (1) a diffuse peritonitis if the perforated loop has free access to the peritoneal cavity; (2) a localized abscess if matted loops of intestine and adjacent structures obstruct access to the peritoneal cavity; or (3) fistulization if the perforation occurs into the bladder, ureter, vagina, intestine, or an operative wound agglutinated to the injured intestine. Operative management requires exteriorization of the perforated bowel, drainage, and proximal defunctionalization.[11]

Patients who have had both an operation and radiation therapy for carcinoma of the cervix or endometrium are at risk for fistulization into the posterior vaginal fornix. Following a prodromal period of pelvic inflammation that may last hours, days, or weeks, the bowel contents emerge in the vagina. Fistulization between loops of bowel may exclude a segment of intestine and cause diarrhea or a blind loop syndrome with vitamin B_{12} deficiency. Urinary tract infections and pneumaturia (passage of air in the urine) may herald fistulization into the bladder. It is important to localize the site of the injury as accurately as possible by endoscopy, oral and rectal contrast studies, CT scanning, and fistulograms (by instillation of iodinated water-soluble dyes) and to exclude recurrent cancer.

Patients with intestinal fistulas are usually severely ill— wasted, dehydrated, and toxic from chronic infection. Radiation-induced intestinal fistulas rarely heal spontaneously; excision is almost always necessary.[2] However, a preliminary program of gastrointestinal decompression, resolution of pelvic sepsis, and nutritional replacement or total parenteral nutrition reduces operative risk and improves the likelihood of healing.

Because the rectum is apposed to the uterine cervix and body, most patients receiving radiation therapy for cancer at these sites have transient and self-limited diarrhea that can be managed effectively by simple supportive measures. Some patients have persistent proctitis with severe pelvic pain, pain on defecation, and rectal bleeding. Persistence of these symptoms after radiation therapy merits assessment by endoscopy and barium enema examination. Generally, radiation-induced proctitis can be managed successfully with a low-residue diet, stool softeners, sedation, antispasmodics, and general supportive measures. Oral steroids, sulfasalazine, and steroid enemas are beneficial in more severe injuries. Some patients with severe rectal bleeding or intractable pain may require a proximal defunctionalizing colostomy, but this procedure is not always successful in relieving pain.

Proctitis may progress to ulceration. At proctoscopy, the ulcer is located anteriorly at the level of the cervix or uterus and has a gray, shaggy, friable base without the elevated perimeter suggestive of carcinoma. Rectal ulcers that do not heal may progress to perforation or the formation of a rectovaginal fistula. Rectovaginal fistulas often are associated with recurrent carcinoma and therefore require biopsy.

Rectovaginal fistulas from radiation injury are rarely self-healing; they usually require defunctionalization of the rectum by colostomy.[16] If pelvic fibrosis is extensive and the fistula involves a strictured distal rectum, the colostomy may be permanent. However, in recent years, some patients have had gut continuity restored successfully by coloanal "sleeve" anastomosis[13,25] (sometimes with some associated incontinence[32]) or by interposition of a rotated flap of sigmoid colon.[6]

Radiation injury may cause both genitourinary and rectal obstruction. Radiation fibrosis in the pelvis simulates recurrent cancer and requires biopsy. Another sequela of continued proctitis is rectal stenosis, which usually can be managed by conservative measures including instrumental or digital dilations but sometimes requires a sigmoid or descending colon colostomy to defunctionalize the rectum.

Another long-term risk from radiation therapy is the development of neoplasia. The initial point of action of ionizing radiation in the induction of cancer is not known but may involve chromosomal damage. Low to moderate doses of radiation may be more carcinogenic than intensive therapeutic doses, in which fibrosis and vasculitis may impair subsequent cellular proliferation.[19]

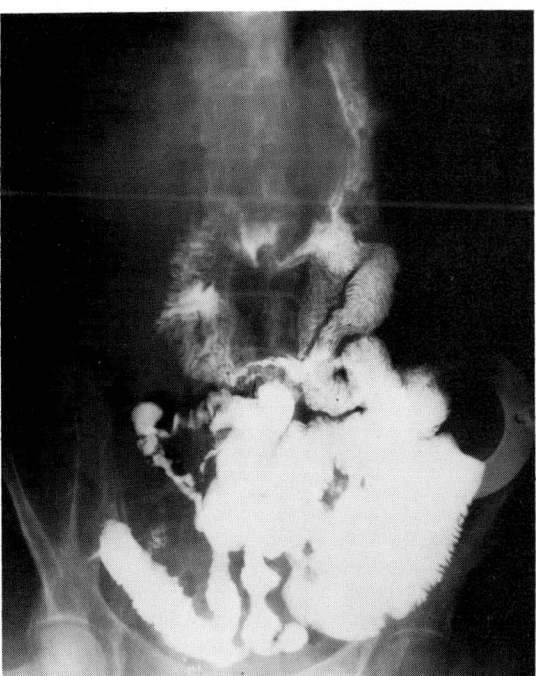

Figure 4. The relatively normal feathery appearance of the upper jejunum can be contrasted with stenosis, loss of valvular markings, and puddling evident in the distal radiation-injured small intestine.

SELECTED REFERENCES

Kohn, H. I., and Fry, R. J. M.: Radiation carcinogenesis. N. Engl. J. Med., 310:304, 1984.
    A review of the epidemiology of radiation carcinogenesis and the relation of epidemiologic observation to experimental radiation biology.

Muller, H. J.: Radiation damage to genetic material. Am. Sci., 38:33, 1950.
   The author reviews his Nobel Prize–winning work on mutation frequency. His publications about this subject began in 1927, and the cited report summarizes his many important contributions.

Quastler, H.: The nature of intestinal radiation death. Radiat. Res., 4:303, 1956.
   The cell kinetic evidence for radiation injury to the proliferative epithelium of the intestine is developed by an outstanding contributor to the field of cell cycle studies.

Rubin, P.: The Franz Bushke Lecture: Late effects of chemotherapy and radiation therapy: A new hypothesis. Int. J. Radiat. Oncol. Biol. Phys., 10:5, 1984.
   The author reviews previously published work about the pathophysiology of radiation effects and draws on documented histopathologic changes in clinical situations and in vivo *and* in vitro *laboratory modeling to suggest a basis for differences between the late effects of chemotherapy and those of radiation therapy.*

Rubin P, and Casarett, G. W.: Clinical Radiation Pathology. Vols. I and II. Philadelphia, W. B. Saunders Company, 1968.
   A classic text on the cytologic and histologic findings in radiation injury, setting forth the radiation effect time course paradigm that characterizes the clinical events based on histopathologic alterations in irradiated tissue.

Warren, S. L., and Whipple, G. H.: Roentgen ray intoxication. I. Unit dose over thorax negative—over abdomen lethal. Epithelium of small intestine—sensitive to x-rays. J. Exp. Med., 35:187, 1922.
   Two distinguished investigators and leaders of American medicine describe intestinal epithelial necrosis after radiation. This pioneering work is the first of a series by these authors on the pathology of acute and chronic radiation injury.

REFERENCES

1. Allan-Mersh, T. G., Wilson, E. J., Hope-Stone, H. F., and Mann, C. F.: Has the incidence of radiation-induced bowel damage following treatment of uterine carcinoma changed in the last 20 years? J. R. Soc. Med., 79:387, 1986.
2. Allen-Mersh, T. G., Wilson, E. J., Hope-Stone, H. F., and Mann, C. V.: The management of late radiation-induced rectal injury after treatment of carcinoma of the uterus. Surg. Gynecol. Obstet., 164:521, 1987.
3. Bakare, S. C., Shafir, M., and McElhinney, A. J.: Exclusion of small bowel from pelvis for postoperative radiotherapy for rectal cancer. J. Surg. Oncol., 35:55, 1987.
4. Berthrong, M.: Pathologic changes secondary to radiation. World J. Surg., 10:155, 1986.
5. Brady, L. W., Markoe, A. M., Sheline, G. E., Suntharalingam, N., and Sutherland, R. M.: Radiation oncology: Programs for the present and future. Cancer, 55:2037, 1985.
6. Bricker, E. M., Kraybill, W. G., and Lopez, M. J.: Functional results after postirradiation rectal reconstruction. World J. Surg., 10:249, 1986.
7. Champlin, R.: The role of bone marrow transplantation for nuclear accidents. Implications of the Chernobyl disaster. Semin. Hematol., 24:1, 1987.
8. Cox, J. D., Byhardt, R. W., Wilson, J. F., Haas, J. S., Komaki, R., and Olson, L. E.: Complications of radiation therapy and factors in their prevention. World J. Surg., 10:171, 1986.
9. DeCosse, J. J., Rhodes, R. S., Wentz, W. B., Regan, J. W., Dworken, H. J., and Holden, W. D.: The natural history and management of radiation-induced injury of the gastrointestinal tract. Ann. Surg., 170:369, 1970.

10. Fenner, M. N., Sheehan, P., Nanavanati, P. J., and Ross, D. S.: Chronic radiation enteritis: A community hospital experience. J. Surg. Oncol., 41:246, 1989.
11. Galland, R. B., and Spencer, J.: Surgical management of radiation enteritis. Surgery, 99:133, 1986.
12. Galland, R. B., and Spencer, J.: Surgical aspects of radiation injury to the intestine. Br. J. Surg., 66:135, 1979.
13. Gazet, J.-C.: Parks' coloanal pull-through anastomosis for severe, complicated radiation proctitis. Dis. Colon Rectum, 28:110, 1985.
14. Goldstein, F., Khoury, J., and Thornton, J. J.: Treatment of chronic radiation enteritis and colitis with salicylazosulfapyridine and systemic corticosteroids: A pilot study. Am. J. Gastroenterol., 65:201, 1976.
15. Kavanah, M. T., Feldman, M. I., Devereux, D. F., and Kondi, E. S.: New surgical approach to minimize radiation-associated small bowel injury in patients with pelvic malignancies requiring surgery and high-dose irradiation. Cancer, 56:1300, 1985.
16. Kimose, H.-H., Fischer, L., Spjelldnaes, N., and Wara, P.: Late radiation injury of the colon and rectum: Surgical management and outcome. Dis. Colon Rectum, 32:684, 1989.
17. Klimberg, V. S., Souba, W. W., Dolson, D. J., Salloum, R. M., Hautamaki, R. D., Plumley, D. A., Mendenhall, W. R., Bova, F. C., Bland, K. I., and Copeland, E. M.: Prophylactic glutamine protects the intestinal mucosa from radiation injury. Cancer, 66:62, 1990.
18. Klimberg, V. S., Souba, W. W., Kasper, M., Salloum, R. M., Plumley, D. A., Dolson, D. J., Hautamaki, R. D., Mendenhall, W. R., Bova, F. C., Bland, K. I., and Copeland, E. M.: Oral glutamine supports gut metabolism and structure, promotes "bowel rescue," improves survival, and decreases morbidity following abdominal radiation. Arch. Surg., 125:1040, 1990.
19. Kohn, H. I., and Fry, R. J. M.: Radiation carcinogenesis. N. Engl. J. Med., 310:304, 1984.
20. Makela, J., Nevasaari, K., and Kairaluomo, M. I.: Surgical treatment of intestinal radiation injury. J. Surg. Oncol., 36:93, 1987.
21. Mason, G. R., Dietrich, P., Friedland, G. W., and Hanks, G. E.: The radiological findings in radiation-induced enteritis and colitis. Clin. Radiol., 21:232, 1970.
22. Miholic, J., Schwarz, C., and Moeschl, P.: Surgical therapy of radiation-induced lesions of the colon and rectum. Am. J. Surg., 155:761, 1988.
23. Morgenstern, L., Hart, M., Lugo, D., and Friedman, N.: Changing aspects of radiation enteropathy. Arch. Surg., 120:1225, 1985.
24. Muller, H. J.: Radiation damage to genetic material. Am. Sci., 38:33, 1950.
25. Parks, A. G., Allen, C. L. O., Frank, J. D., and McPartlin, J. F.: A method of treating post-irradiation rectovaginal fistulas. Br. J. Surg., 65:417, 1978.
26. Quastler, H.: The nature of intestinal radiation death. Radiat. Res., 4:303, 1956.
27. Rubin, P.: The Franz Bushke Lecture: Late effects of chemotherapy and radiation therapy: A new hypothesis. Int. J. Radiat. Oncol. Biol. Phys., 10:5, 1984.
28. Russell, J. C., and Welch, J. P.: Operative management of radiation injuries to the intestinal tract. Am. J. Surg., 137:433, 1979.
29. Schellhammer, P. F., Jordan, G. H., and El-Mahdi, A. M.: Pelvic complications after interstitial and external beam irradiation of urologic and gynecologic malignancy. World J. Surg., 10:259, 1986.
30. Schofield, P. F., Carr, N. D., and Holden, D.: Pathogenesis and treatment of radiation bowel disease: Discussion paper. J. R. Soc. Med., 79:3030, 1986.
31. Smith, D. H., and DeCosse, J. J.: Radiation damage to the small intestine. World J. Surg., 10:189, 1986.
32. Varma, J. S., and Smith, A. N.: Anorectal function following coloanal sleeve anastomosis for chronic radiation injury to the rectum. Br. J. Surg., 73:285, 1986.

X

APPENDICITIS

Robert E. Condon, M.D., and Gordon L. Telford, M.D.

Acute appendicitis must be considered in any patient who complains of abdominal pain or who presents with symptoms suggestive of peritoneal irritation. Acute appendicitis is the most frequent cause of persisting, progressive abdominal pain in teenagers. It is a common, sometimes confusing, and often treacherous cause of an acute abdomen at all ages. There is no way to prevent the development of appendicitis. The only way to reduce morbidity and to prevent mortality is to perform appendectomy before perforation or gangrene occurs.[4]

INCIDENCE

The incidence of acute appendicitis decreased markedly between 1940 and 1960, possibly as a result of the widespread use of antibiotics. At present, appendectomy represents about 1 per cent of all surgical operations.[30,37] Appendicitis is rare in infants, becomes increasingly common throughout childhood, and reaches its maximal incidence in the teens and twenties. Thereafter the incidence declines, although appendicitis occurs

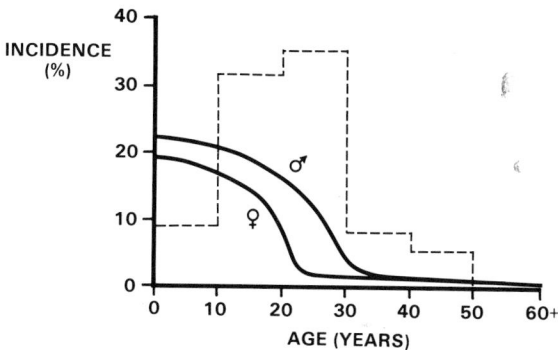

Figure 1. The age distribution of the incidence of appendicitis, in 1000 cases reported by Lewis et al.,[30] is indicated for each decade by the histogram (broken line). The future risk of appendicitis developing, as derived from the data of Ludbrook and Spears,[31] is indicated by the solid curved lines for men (♂) and women (♀).

throughout adulthood and into old age (Fig. 1). Among teenagers and young adults, the male-female ratio is about 3:2. After age 25, the excess male incidence gradually declines until the sex ratio is equal.

HISTORICAL ASPECTS

Curiously, a condition as common as appendicitis was not recorded in medical literature until about 500 years ago.[34]

When first recognized as a distinct disease entity in the sixteenth century, appendicitis was called "perityphlitis" because the inflammatory process that brought about the death of the patient was thought to have originated in the cecum. It now appears obvious that what was so described was perforative appendicitis.

Although Melier, in 1827, had correctly ascribed the origin of purulent "iliac tumor" to inflammation of the appendix, it was not until 1886 that Fitz clearly defined appendicitis as the initial process in cases previously diagnosed as "perityphlitis." Fitz suggested that appendectomy would be essential to cure.

The first surgeon to correctly diagnose acute appendicitis prior to rupture, perform appendectomy, have the patient recover, and report his experience was Senn, in 1889.[43] Groves,

practicing in rural Canada, apparently had done a successful appendectomy 6 years earlier, but his case was not reported until 1961. In 1889, McBurney described the clinical findings of acute appendicitis prior to rupture, including a description of the point of maximal abdominal tenderness that now bears his name. The gridiron incision commonly attributed to McBurney actually was devised by McArthur.

Over the relatively short span of somewhat less than a century, acceptance of prompt appendectomy as the treatment of appendicitis has improved the prognosis from that of a usually fatal disease to one in which death is uncommon, even in very complicated cases.[4]

ANATOMY

Embryologically, the appendix is a continuation of the cecum, arising from its inferior tip. Suppression of the development of the apical segment of the cecum is followed by appendicular hypoplasia or agenesis. During infancy, more rapid growth of the right and anterior portions of the cecum causes rotation of the appendix posteriorly and medially to its adult position, about 2.5 cm. below the ileocecal valve (Fig. 2).

The appendix averages 10 cm. in length in adults, although it is not uncommon to find an appendix more than twice that long. The narrow lumen of the appendix is lined by colonic epithelium. There are a few submucosal lymphoid follicles present at birth; these gradually increase in number to a peak of approximately 200 follicles between the ages of 12 and 20. After age 30, there is an abrupt reduction to less than half that number, and, subsequently, to a trace or a total absence of lymphoid tissue after age 60.

The walls of the appendix are muscular; the inner circular layer is a continuation of the same muscle in the cecum. The outer longitudinal muscle coat is formed by coalescence of the three taeniae coli at the junction of the cecum and appendix. Thus the taeniae, particularly the anterior taenia, may be used as a landmark to locate an elusive appendix. The mesentery of the appendix passes behind the terminal ileum to join the mesentery of the small intestine. The appendicular artery courses in the free border of the mesoappendix and is a branch of the

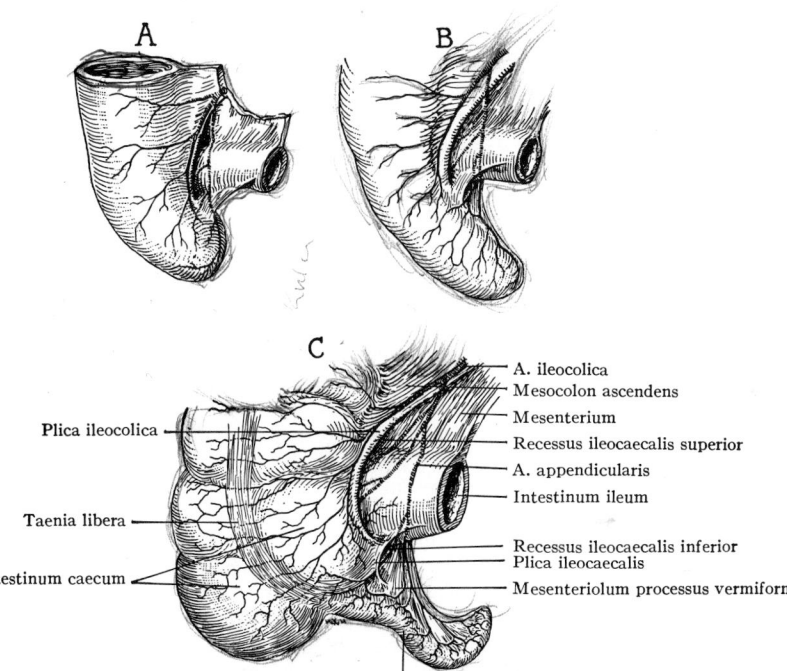

Figure 2. Development of the appendix. Lagging growth of the inferior tip of the cecum during early intrauterine development *(A)* produces the infantile appendix *(B)*. Continued differential growth of the lateral cecal wall leads to the posteromedial position *(C)* of the appendix in older children and adults. (From Anson, B., and McVay, C. B.: Surgical Anatomy, 5th ed. Philadelphia, W. B. Saunders Company, 1971.)

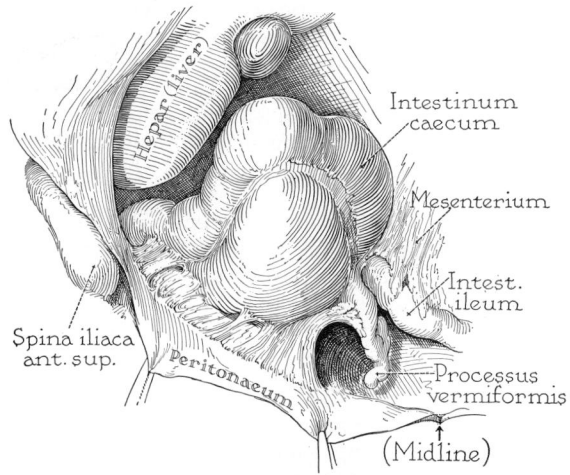

Figure 3. The most common position of the appendix is behind the cecum. (From Anson, B., and McVay, C. B.: Surgical Anatomy, 5th ed. Philadelphia, W. B. Saunders Company, 1971.)

ileocolic artery. In many patients, in addition, an accessory appendicular branch from the posterior cecal artery supplies the base of the appendix at its junction with the cecum.

The relation of the base of the appendix to the cecum is constant, but the tip of the appendix may be found in a variety of locations. Most commonly, the appendix lies behind the cecum, although still in an intraperitoneal location.[52] This low retrocecal position is found in 65 per cent of patients (Fig. 3) and is due to the fact that several inches of the cecum usually remain in an intraperitoneal position, since the reflection of the peritoneum to the parietes from the cecum occurs opposite the ileocecal junction. The second most common position of the tip of the appendix, found in about 30 per cent of patients, is at the brim of, or in, the pelvis. In about 5 per cent of patients, the tip of the appendix lies extraperitoneally, either behind the cecum and ascending colon or passing behind the distal ileum along the right margin of the ascending colon.

Malrotation or maldescent of the cecum is associated with abnormal locations of the appendix, which may be found anywhere between the right iliac fossa and the left infrasplenic area. In cases of situs inversus the appendix is in the left lower quadrant. Such abnormal positions of the cecum introduce difficulties in diagnosis if appendicitis supervenes.

PATHOPHYSIOLOGY

Appendicitis is caused by obstruction followed by infection. Approximately 60 per cent of cases are related to hyperplasia of submucosal lymphoid follicles, 35 per cent to the presence of fecal stasis or a fecalith, 4 per cent to the presence of other foreign bodies, and 1 per cent to strictures or tumors of the wall of the appendix or the cecum. Lymphatic hyperplasia leading to obstruction is most frequent in children; the lymphoid follicles in the appendix respond to a variety of infections. Obstruction due to a fecalith is more frequent in older adults. Fecalith formation may be promoted by the relatively tenacious feces of urbanized Westerners who consume a low-fiber, high-carbohydrate diet.

The amount of lymphoid tissue in the appendix parallels the incidence of acute appendicitis, the peak for both occurring in the early teens. Hyperplastic follicles may partially obstruct the lumen, setting the stage for development of appendicitis. Hyperplasia of lymphoid tissue may be a response to an acute respiratory infection, measles, mononucleosis, or other diseases producing a generalized reaction of lymphatic tissue. The follicles of the appendix also respond to infections in the gut; ap-

pendicitis has been reported, for example, in association with *Salmonella* and *Shigella* enterocolitis.

Formation of an appendiceal fecalith begins with entrapment of a bit of vegetable fiber in the lumen of the appendix, stimulating the secretion and deposition of calcium-rich mucus. The mucus subsequently becomes inspissated around the bit of fiber; this causes a second round of irritation and deposition of mucus. Eventually, concretions reach a diameter of approximately 1 cm., at which point, if not expelled, they may obstruct the lumen; appendicitis ensues.

Among other intraluminal objects that may obstruct to precipitate an attack of appendicitis, pinworms (*Enterobius vermicularis*) are the commonest parasites reported in the United States, but *Taenia* and *Ascaris* also have caused appendicitis. Other foreign bodies include vegetable seeds, cherry stones, and inspissated barium. In older patients, obstruction by a cecal carcinoma, and in younger adults, a carcinoid tumor, are occasional causes of appendicitis. Metastases to the appendix, particularly from carcinoma of the breast, also may cause appendicitis.

The events that follow obstruction of the appendix depend upon interactions among four factors: the content in the lumen, the degree of obstruction, the continued secretion by the mucosa, and the inelastic character of the appendiceal serosa. The sequence following obstruction of the appendix probably is as follows: mucus accumulates in the lumen, and pressure within the organ begins to increase; virulent bacteria convert the accumulating mucus into pus; continued secretion combined with the relative inelasticity of the serosa leads to a further rise in pressure within the lumen; obstruction of lymphatic drainage ensues, leading to edema of the appendix, beginning diapedesis of bacteria, and the appearance of mucosal ulcers. This is the stage of *acute focal appendicitis*.

The inflammation and increased pressure in the lumen present at this stage are perceived by the patient as poorly localized visceral pain tending to be periumbilical or epigastric in location, accompanied by anorexia, nausea, and occasional vomiting. It is because the appendix and the small bowel have the same nerve supply that visceral pain is first perceived in the epigastrium or periumbilical area.

Continued secretion causes a further rise in intraluminal pressure, which produces venous obstruction and further edema and ischemia in the appendix. Bacterial invasion spreads through the wall of the appendix. This stage is called *acute suppurative appendicitis*. The inflamed serosa of the appendix contacts the parietal peritoneum. Somatic pain, arising from the peritoneum as a result of contact with the inflamed appendix, is perceived as the classic shift and localization of pain in the right lower quadrant.

Continuation of this pathologic process eventually leads to venous thrombosis and then to compromise of the arterial blood supply. The area of the appendix with the poorest blood supply, the midportion of the antimesenteric border, undergoes gangrene with the appearance of ellipsoidal infarcts. The development of *gangrenous appendicitis* is the first stage of complicated appendicitis; morbidity increases, since these infarcts functionally act as perforations, permitting escape of bacteria from the lumen of the appendix and contamination of the peritoneal cavity.

Continued secretion from viable portions of the appendiceal mucosa and continued high intraluminal pressure finally lead to perforation through a gangrenous infarct, spilling accumulated pus. *Perforative appendicitis* is now present; morbidity and mortality increase. Fortunately, in most cases, the obstruction that initially led to appendicitis blocks continued spillage of feces from the cecum through the perforated appendix. If appendicitis has not progressed too rapidly, inflammatory adhesions have formed between loops of bowel, peritoneum, and omentum to hem in the appendix. Perforation then leads to localized peritonitis; a periappendiceal abscess forms eventually if untreated. In 1 to 2 per cent of patients, particularly the very young and the very old, rapidity of progression of the disease or disabled or otherwise ineffective defense mechanisms permit development of generalized peritonitis.

PROGNOSIS

Seventy-five years ago, 15 of every 100,000 persons in the United States could expect to die each year of appendicitis. Today, mortality has decreased to less than 1 in 100,000 persons annually. The mortality risk of an individual patient with acute but not gangrenous appendicitis is less than 0.1 per cent. In gangrenous appendicitis mortality rises to about 0.6 per cent. The mortality of perforated appendicitis today is approximately 5 per cent, down from over 50 per cent just over a half century ago. Although the mortality of appendicitis has declined progressively, morbidity from appendicitis continues to be high. Overall, morbidity currently occurs in 10 per cent of all patients with appendicitis. Wound infections represent one third of all morbidity. The presence of gangrene or perforation increases the morbidity risk four- or fivefold, with wound infection rates of 15 to 20 per cent.[30]

The role that delay in diagnosis and treatment has in mortality and serious morbidity cannot be overemphasized. Delay in performing appendectomy often is due to uncertainty of diagnosis or to a trial of antibiotic therapy. The use of antibiotics in an attempt to avoid or postpone appendectomy ignores the fact that acute appendicitis begins as an obstruction. Observation until typical or definite symptoms appear is ill-advised. Exploration to discover the cause of minimal but unexplained symptoms, even in poor-risk patients, is safer than waiting.[16,18]

CLINICAL DIAGNOSIS

The diagnosis of acute appendicitis is the classic example of the application of clinical skills. Ancillary laboratory and radiologic tests are not essential in making the diagnosis. Recently, algorithms[10,49] and symptom ranking systems[47] have been reported, but these aids have not really improved the overall accuracy of preoperative diagnosis. Although symptoms and signs in many cases are atypical, it is a tribute to the acumen of medical students and physicians that the findings at operation usually confirm the clinical diagnosis.

SYMPTOMATIC HISTORY. The sequence of symptoms in acute appendicitis usually begins with diffuse abdominal pain, felt most prominently in the epigastrium or around the umbilicus, followed by anorexia and some nausea. Vomiting, if it occurs, appears next. After a variable time, pain shifts toward the right side and then into the right lower quadrant and becomes localized. Anorexia of some degree generally accompanies appendicitis in adults, although it is a less frequent complaint in children.

Abdominal pain is present in all patients with appendicitis except those with transverse myelitis or similar disabilities. Pain may be characterized as either typical or atypical. Typical pain consists of initial diffuse, central, not very severe visceral pain, followed by somatic pain that is more severe and well localized in the right lower quadrant. This classic pain sequence is found in 55 per cent of patients with appendicitis but also may occur in one fourth of patients with other intra-abdominal conditions.

Atypical abdominal pain is common in acute appendicitis, occurring in 45 per cent of patients who prove to have appendicitis and 75 per cent of patients in whom appendicitis initially is suspected but who prove to have some other disease. Atypical pain is defined as pain that fails to follow the classic visceral-somatic sequence. Atypical appendicitis pain may be entirely so-matic, often well localized in the right lower quadrant, from the beginning. Conversely, atypical pain may never become localized and may remain diffuse throughout the preoperative course of acute appendicitis. Atypical pain is found more frequently in older patients, in whom pain is always less intense and characteristically localizes much later, and in patients receiving chronic antibiotic therapy for some unrelated condition, such as acne.

Nausea, at least of some degree, is present in 9 of 10 patients with appendicitis. Vomiting is more variable; children and teenagers frequently vomit; vomiting may be entirely absent in older adults. Vomiting in appendicitis is not persistent or prolonged; most patients vomit only once or twice. Vomiting appears after the onset of pain. If vomiting precedes pain, the diagnosis should be questioned. The character of bowel function is of little diagnostic value. Many patients admit to constipation; a few voluntarily state that defecation may relieve their pain. Diarrhea occurs in some patients, especially young children.

The pain of appendicitis in the past was said to be relieved immediately after perforation, remaining diminished in severity for a short time, until pain due to diffuse peritonitis supervened. Relief of pain was attributed to decreased pressure in the appendix. In fact, relief of pain following perforation occurs rarely. In most patients, pain continues or increases in severity. The characteristic feature of pain following perforation is that it is no longer so discretely localized. In addition, the patient is more ill and abdominal distention begins to develop.

Any patient with an abnormally located appendix is likely to have an atypical history, particularly of pain. A high retrocecal appendicitis commonly causes nothing more than diffuse pain in the right flank and loin. An inflamed appendix entirely within the true pelvis may never produce somatic pain involving the anterior abdominal wall but may instead cause tenesmus and only vague discomfort in the suprapubic area. It should be emphasized that the precise anatomic location of the appendix varies, and its position has a definite relationship to the specific signs and symptoms (Fig. 4).

PHYSICAL EXAMINATION. The traditional physical signs of appendicitis are local tenderness, rebound tenderness, and muscle guarding. Cutaneous hyperesthesia, pelvic tenderness on the right side on rectal examination, and the presence of the

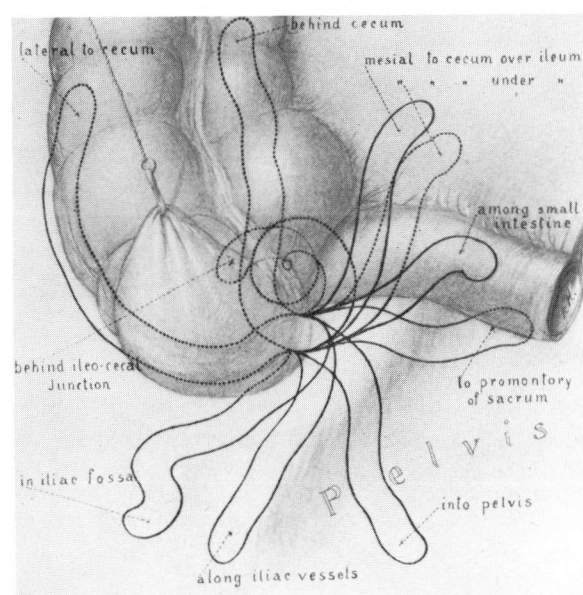

Figure 4. Diagram showing the various directions in which an appendix may point. (From Kelly, H. A., and Hurdon, E.: The Vermiform Appendix and Its Diseases. Philadelphia, W. B. Saunders Company, 1905.)

psoas and obturator signs are frequently listed in textbooks but are rarely seen in patients. Appendicitis may cause a rise in temperature up to 38° C., but higher fever is unusual with uncomplicated appendicitis. A normal temperature often is present even with advanced appendicitis. The pulse rate usually remains normal. In fact, all physical diagnostic signs are fallible.

If symptoms have been present for more than a few hours, inspection may disclose some limitation of respiratory movement in the lower half of the abdomen. Systematic gentle palpation detects an area of maximal tenderness that corresponds to the position of the appendix and usually is located in the right lower quadrant at or near McBurney's point (Fig. 5).

The presence of peritoneal inflammation can be suspected if a cough or percussion of the abdominal wall elicits pain. The classic method of demonstrating peritoneal inflammation is rebound tenderness following release of abdominal palpation pressure. The finding of rebound tenderness may be of occasional help in doubtful cases, but it is unnecessary to distress a patient with clear signs of appendicitis by eliciting rebound tenderness as a routine maneuver. Rovsing's sign, pain in the right lower quadrant when palpation pressure is exerted in the left lower quadrant, is a manifestation of referred rebound tenderness and is sometimes helpful in supporting a diagnosis of appendicitis.

Muscle guarding, or resistance to palpation, approximately parallels the severity of the inflammatory process, particularly in younger patients. As peritoneal irritation progresses, voluntary muscle guarding increases and eventually is replaced by reflex involuntary rigidity. True rigidity does not diminish during expiration, a finding that allows it to be differentiated by palpation from voluntary guarding.

Cutaneous hyperesthesia is reported by an occasional patient able to distinguish the difference in sensation elicited by light stroking of the skin on the right and left sides of the abdomen. This sign, although classic, is unreliable, since the degree of discrimination required is beyond the capacities of most patients with appendicitis.

On occasion, especially in patients who seek care relatively late in the course of their appendicitis, a periappendiceal mass may be palpated in the right lower quadrant. The mass may be due to an abscess or due only to omentum and coils of bowel adherent about the inflamed appendix.

When appendicitis is sufficiently advanced so that inflamma-

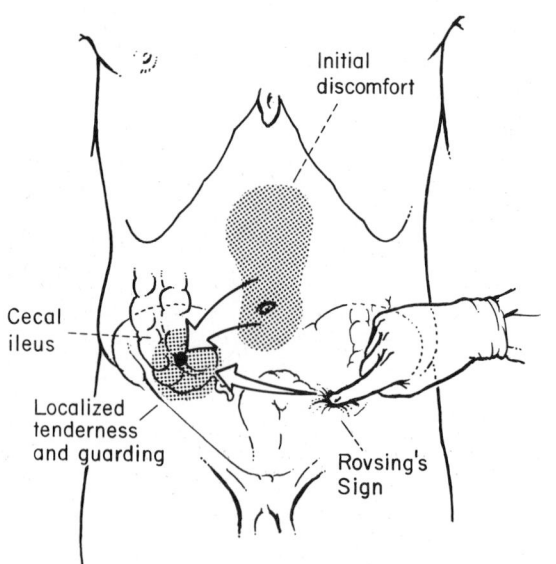

Figure 5. Some physical signs of appendicitis prior to rupture. McBurney's point is indicated by the black dot in the right lower quadrant. (From Gelin, L. E., Nyhus, L. M., and Condon, R. E.: Abdominal Pain: A Guide to Rapid Diagnosis. Philadelphia, J. B. Lippincott Company, 1969.)

tion involves the anterior abdominal wall, the posture of the patient becomes a useful corroborative sign. Movement is avoided. If asked to turn or sit up, the patient does so gingerly to avoid pain caused by sudden movement of the abdominal wall. The right hip often is slightly flexed. Further active flexion against resistance or passive extension of the hip stretches the iliopsoas muscle; the patient may complain of increased pain. This is a positive psoas sign, said to indicate irritation of the psoas muscle by the inflamed appendix. A psoas sign rarely is present early in appendicitis; whenever it can be elicited, other clinical signs of appendicitis usually are clear. The obturator sign, hypogastric or adductor pain elicited by passive internal rotation of the flexed thigh, is said to indicate an inflamed appendix lying against the internal obturator muscle. This sign is positive less often than is the psoas sign.

Rectal examination is essential in every patient suspected of having appendicitis. In addition, all women must have a pelvic examination. The primary purpose is to exclude pelvic lesions such as ovarian cyst or tubal abscess in females. A secondary purpose is to elicit tenderness in cases of pelvic appendicitis. Tenderness of the pelvic peritoneum must be distinguished from the general discomfort commonly felt during rectal examination. There rarely is any acute disorder posterior to the rectum, so that a useful baseline of discomfort due only to insertion of the examining digit through the anal canal can be established by first palpating the sacrum and coccyx. The rectal examination occasionally identifies the presence of a mass or tenderness specifically localized to the right side. In those few patients in whom the inflamed appendix lies wholly within the pelvis, tenderness on rectal examination may be the only positive physical sign.

Following rupture, physical signs usually become much more definite. If the rupture is contained in the right lower quadrant, a boggy, tender mass usually can be palpated. Tenderness, which classically is fingerpoint with simple acute appendicitis, now encompasses the whole right lower quadrant. Rebound tenderness and muscular rigidity are more marked. The temperature may rise to 39° C., and there is a corresponding rise in the pulse rate.

If the rupture fails to localize, signs of spreading peritonitis ensue. Tenderness becomes diffuse and there is more generalized rigidity of the abdominal muscles. The temperature usually is above 38° C., with spikes to 40° C.; the pulse rate rises to over 100 per minute.

Complicated appendicitis mimicking or associated with mechanical small bowel obstruction is particularly prevalent in elderly patients. Inflammatory adhesive bands secondary to appendicitis cause the obstruction. The clinical history typically is of 2 to 5 days of diffuse abdominal pain; there are signs of peritoneal irritation on physical examination in addition to signs of mechanical small bowel obstruction.

LABORATORY EXAMINATIONS. Far too much emphasis has been placed upon the alleged value of laboratory work in the diagnosis of acute appendicitis. The differential white cell count and the total leukocyte count usually are abnormal in appendicitis, but the degree of abnormality does not correlate with the degree of abnormality in the appendix.[5,30] Up to one third of patients, particularly older adults[20] and blacks,[21] have a normal total leukocyte count in the presence of acute appendicitis. Most patients, however, have a shift to the left in the differential white cell count, even when the total count is normal.[5,41] Less than 4 per cent of patients with acute appendicitis have both a normal differential count and a normal total white cell count. In cases of suspected appendicitis, whenever the clinical findings are at variance with the white cell count, clinical findings should take precedence. The hematocrit is normal in appendicitis. If an older patient presents with symptoms suggesting appendicitis and has a significant anemia, carcinoma of the cecum should be suspected.

Minimal albuminuria and some white blood cells in the urine are present in 20 per cent of male patients with appendicitis. The presence of some white blood cells in the urine is so common in women that urinary findings are of no diagnostic value. Identification of significant numbers of microorganisms in the urinary sediment confirms the presence of a urinary tract infection but does not exclude the diagnosis of appendicitis. The finding of a few red blood cells in the urine of a patient with appendicitis also is not unusual. It is not necessary for the appendix to be in contact with the ureter or bladder for an occasional red cell to be found. However, patients with more than 30 red cells in a centrifuged specimen of voided urine should be suspected of having primary urinary tract disease.[27]

RADIOGRAPHIC EXAMINATION. Radiographic examination of the abdomen does not show any pathognomonic signs in early acute appendicitis with the exception of occasional demonstration of an appendiceal fecalith. Plain films may show a distended cecum with a fluid level (cecal ileus) early in appendicitis. If radiographs demonstrate a mass extrinsic to the cecum, the appendix nearly always is gangrenous and often perforated. In late complicated acute appendicitis, radiographs may reveal scoliosis to the right, absence of the right psoas shadow, absence of small bowel gas in the right lower quadrant although abundantly present elsewhere, edema of the abdominal wall, or interruption of the properitoneal fat line in the flank.

Barium enema examination, formerly believed to be contraindicated because of the risk of spill if the appendix were perforated, has been shown to be a safe procedure in patients with appendicitis.[25,40] This procedure obviously is unnecessary in most cases of acute appendicitis in which the diagnosis is reasonably clear on clinical grounds. A barium enema can, however, be of diagnostic aid in two clinical situations in which avoidance of a negative laparotomy is desirable: first, in those patients, typically children, with a pre-existing debilitating systemic disease, such as leukemia, which markedly increases operative risk; second, in those patients, typically young women with abdominal pain, in whom the diagnosis continues to be obscure after 6 to 12 hours of observation and in whom the negative laparotomy rate is high. The positive findings to be sought during the barium enema are nonfilling or partial filling of the appendix, often associated with extrinsic pressure defects ("reverse 3") on the cecum. The false-negative rate of barium enema in selected patients with appendicitis is about 10 per cent.[11,40]

The possible utility of laparoscopy for women with indefinite abdominal findings and of ultrasonography, magnetic resonance imaging, or computed tomography for patients in whom the diagnosis is obscure remains to be established.

DISTINCTIVE CLINICAL SETTINGS OF APPENDICITIS

APPENDICITIS IN INFANTS AND YOUNG CHILDREN. Accurate diagnosis of appendicitis in infants and young children is very difficult. First, the patient is, for obvious reasons, unable to provide a history of the illness; second, acute nonspecific abdominal pain is common in infants and young children; and third, appendicitis is infrequent in infants. These features serve to decrease the level of diagnostic suspicion. Because the diagnosis frequently is difficult to establish, treatment is delayed, complications develop, and subsequent management becomes more involved.

Appendicitis is uncommon in infants, probably because the conical configuration of the appendix makes obstruction of the lumen unlikely. Before differential growth of the cecum occurs, the lumen of the appendix is larger at its junction with the cecum than at the tip (see Fig. 2). Perforative appendicitis in the first month of life often is associated with Hirschsprung's disease.[33]

Despite the fact that every child with appendicitis has abdominal pain, it can be so similar to nonspecific gastroenteritis that suspicion of appendicitis may not be aroused. Not until after rupture has occurred and the child is obviously ill is a diagnosis of appendicitis seriously entertained. Two thirds of young children with appendicitis have had symptoms for more than 3 days preceding appendectomy.[45]

The unavoidable fact that a young child cannot provide a history means that other clinical aspects of appendicitis become the diagnostic features. The diagnosis can be missed easily if the classic pattern of appendicitis is expected. Vomiting, fever, irritability, flexing of the thighs, and diarrhea are likely to be early complaints. "Beware of diarrhea in a child whose illness begins with abdominal pain" is good advice. The most consistent finding on physical examination is abdominal distention. Leukocyte counts are not reliable. The presence of a fecalith noted on a plain abdominal film in a child with suspicious symptoms is sufficient evidence to consider the diagnosis of appendicitis as established.[12]

The incidence of perforation in acute appendicitis approaches 100 per cent in infants less than a year of age, is between 70 and 80 per cent in infants under 2 years of age, and remains above 50 per cent up to the age of 5 years. Because of the high incidence of perforation, the mortality of acute appendicitis in this age group remains high overall (about 5 per cent) but is much lower in specialized pediatric centers.[23] The improving results in this age group are illustrated by a series of 89 consecutive children with perforated appendicitis treated surgically with no mortality.[32]

The higher mortality in young patients often has been attributed to the absence of a fully developed omentum, with consequent widespread peritonitis following rupture of the appendix. While the omentum is undoubtedly a factor, a most important element is failure of the physician to consider the diagnosis. In one reported series, nearly 40 per cent of children with gangrenous or perforative appendicitis previously had been seen by a physician who failed to appreciate the nature of the disease process.[45]

APPENDICITIS IN YOUNG WOMEN. The diagnosis of acute appendicitis in women 20 to 30 years of age is fraught with a higher rate of error than is true in women of other ages or in men. While the overall incidence of negative laparotomy in patients with suspected appendicitis is about 15 to 20 per cent, the incidence in young women is 30 to 45 per cent. The diagnostic dilemma is compounded by the fact that the incidence of true appendicitis is almost twice as high during the latter half of the menstrual cycle as during the first half.[2] Pain or discomfort associated with ovulation (mittelschmerz), diseases involving the ovary, tube, or uterus, and infections or other disorders of the urinary system represent some, but not all, of the misdiagnoses.

When faced with the problem of possible appendicitis in a young woman, careful observation may be in order if the pain is atypical, there is no muscular spasm in the right lower quadrant on physical examination, and fever and leukocytosis are absent. The possible role of laparoscopy in clarifying this diagnostic dilemma remains to be established. If symptoms and signs do not progress over several hours, a careful barium enema examination that visualizes the appendix may be helpful in excluding appendicitis as the cause of the symptoms. However, it must be remembered that a negative exploration is to be preferred, in most circumstances, to permitting evolution of an acute appendicitis to the stage of perforation.

APPENDICITIS DURING PREGNANCY. The incidence of appendicitis during pregnancy parallels that in nonpregnant women of the same age. Appendicitis occurs once in every 2000 pregnancies and is the most common extrauterine condition requiring an abdominal operation during pregnancy. Appendicitis occurs more frequently during the first two trimesters,

compared with the third. During the first 6 months of pregnancy, symptoms of appendicitis do not differ much from those
in the nonpregnant woman.[13] This fact needs emphasis, since
the manifestations of appendicitis often are assumed to be
markedly different even during early pregnancy.

Appendectomy should be performed upon suspicion of the
presence of appendicitis, just as if the pregnancy were not
present. If performed before the appendix ruptures, appendectomy often does not disturb the pregnancy. Moreover, the effects of a negative laparotomy are sufficiently minor that early
operation for acute appendicitis should be performed whenever
the diagnosis is entertained.[9]

During the third trimester, the clinical situation is slightly
altered; displacement and lateral rotation of the cecum and appendix by the enlarged uterus lead to localization of pain higher
in the abdomen or in the right flank. In addition, appendicitis
during the final trimester tends to be more serious, if less frequent, since delay in diagnosis leads to an increased incidence of
perforation, and the normal responses within the peritoneal
cavity are impaired. The displaced omentum often is unable to
reach the area of the inflamed appendix to help contain the
infection. In addition, contractions of the nearby uterus serve to
impair localization. Rupture is often followed by diffuse peritonitis.

Premature labor occurs in about half of women who develop
appendicitis during the third trimester; the prognosis for the
infant in cases of uncomplicated appendicitis is directly related
to the infant's birth weight. In cases of appendicitis with peritonitis and other septic complications, fetal loss is much higher
and is due not only to prematurity but also to the effects of
sepsis on the fetus.

Acute pyelitis of pregnancy and torsion of an ovarian cyst,
when they occur during pregnancy, can be difficult to distinguish from appendicitis. However confusing differential diagnosis may be, one fact must be kept in mind: the mortality of
appendicitis in pregnancy is due to delayed diagnosis and operation. Early appendectomy is the treatment of choice for appendicitis at all stages of a pregnancy.

APPENDICITIS IN THE ELDERLY. The incidence of appendicitis in older patients is rising, in contrast to the incidence in
the population generally. The increase is due almost entirely to
improved longevity among the aged. As is true of infants, acute
appendicitis among older patients has a mortality much greater
than that in young adults.[38,48] The higher mortality is due both
to delay by the patient in seeking medical care and to delay by
physicians in removing the appendix. The concomitant presence in elderly patients of other diseases that lower physiologic
reserve has a role, but the major reason for increased mortality is
delay in treatment.

The classic symptoms of pain, anorexia, and nausea are
present in most older patients but are less pronounced than in
younger adults. Pain in the right lower quadrant is the most
frequent complaint but often is mild and causes little initial
concern. Localization occurs later than in younger patients.

Physical examination in elderly patients with appendicitis
differs mainly by the paucity of findings in the presence of
severe disease. The initial examination may reveal nothing abnormal, although tenderness in the right lower quadrant is elicited eventually in most patients. Distention of the abdomen, as
is also true of infants, is prominent in elderly patients, even in
the absence of perforation. Symptoms and signs mimicking mechanical small bowel obstruction are not uncommon. Subnormal temperatures are more frequently encountered in the aged,
especially with an abscess or generalized peritonitis. An occasional older patient enters the hospital with a painless right
lower quadrant mass, denying any previous history suggestive
of appendicitis. Conversely, some elderly patients present with
generalized peritonitis of obscure etiology; they, too, deny previous acute symptoms.

More than 30 per cent of elderly patients have a ruptured

appendix at the time of operation. Impaired blood supply and
structural weakness of the appendix are said to produce earlier
perforation in older patients. Although such factors may have a
role, it is delay in getting the patient to the operating room that is
responsible for the high incidence of perforation. If it is probable that an aged patient has acute appendicitis, an urgent operation should be advised. More elderly patients die because surgeons do not operate in doubtful cases than die from
misdiagnosis and operative removal of a normal appendix.[18]

Whenever appendicitis develops in a patient in the sixth decade of life or later, a concomitant carcinoma of the right colon
may be present and should be specifically sought during exploration.

DIFFERENTIAL DIAGNOSIS

Differential diagnosis of abdominal pain is one of the fascinating exercises of clinical surgery. This is particularly true in a
patient with suspected appendicitis. However, before too much
time and effort are expended in diagnostic investigation, it must
be remembered that most of the entities that enter into the
differential diagnosis of appendicitis require operative therapy
in any case. If they do not, at least they usually are not made
worse by an exploratory operation. The essential differential
diagnostic maneuver then is to eliminate those entities that do
not need operative therapy, for example, myocardial infarction,
basilar pneumonia, and acute pancreatitis.

In young children, the diseases most frequently mistaken for
appendicitis are acute gastroenteritis, mesenteric lymphadenitis, pyelitis, Meckel's diverticulitis, intussusception, enteric duplication, Henoch-Schönlein purpura, and primary peritonitis.
In this age group, basilar pneumonia (even on the left side) may
mimic appendicitis and should be particularly sought.[24] Acute
gastroenteritis is usually associated with cramping abdominal
pain and watery diarrhea. In mesenteric adenitis, an upper respiratory tract infection often is present or has recently subsided.
Mesenteric lymphadenitis due to *Yersinia* infection leading to
pseudoappendicitis has been reported recently with increasing
frequency.

It is important to differentiate intussusception from acute appendicitis. Appendicitis is uncommon under 2 years of age,
whereas most attacks of idiopathic intussusception occur in that
age group. A sausage-shaped mass may be palpable in the right
lower quadrant. The preferred treatment of intussusception is
reduction by gentle barium enema.

Children with acute lymphocytic leukemia may have inflammation progressing to necrosis and perforation of the appendix
or the adjacent ileum or cecum.[44] This entity, "typhlitis" or the
"leukemic ileocecal syndrome," is of importance not only because of its clinical similarity to acute appendicitis but also because controversy exists concerning surgical intervention. Reports indicate that aggressive surgical therapy may improve
survival.[42,50]

In teenagers and young adults, differential diagnosis is directed by the patient's sex. In some young women, obstipation
needs to be considered. Diseases of the ovary and tube commonly mimic appendicitis; ruptured ectopic pregnancy, mittelschmerz, endometriosis, and salpingitis (pelvic inflammatory
disease) must be differentiated.

Ruptured ectopic pregnancy may produce right lower quadrant pain, but in most patients there is a palpable tubal mass on
pelvic examination, and culdocentesis yields nonclotting blood.
Mittelschmerz is distinguished by its characteristic onset in
midmenstrual cycle; symptoms spontaneously subside in a few
hours. Endometriosis can be differentiated by the repetitive recurrence of pain with each menses. Salpingitis may cause the
greatest diagnostic difficulty, but usually the pain is bilateral,
low in the abdomen, and symptoms occur at the end of a menstrual period. Women taking birth control pills sometimes report right lower abdominal discomfort at the end of the second

week of each pill cycle; pain is diffuse, and leukocytosis and fever are absent. Regional enteritis (Crohn's disease) can be confusing; cramps and diarrhea are more frequent with this disorder than with appendicitis.

In a young man, the list of alternative diagnoses is quite small: acute regional enteritis, right renal or ureteral calculus, torsion of a testis, and acute epididymitis. The frequent presence of cramps and diarrhea and the infrequency of anorexia are hints that the process is regional enteritis. Renal or ureteral calculi characteristically cause severe pain, more severe than that of acute appendicitis, but the pain does not persist or progress, since it is related to movement of the calculus; there will be associated microscopic hematuria. Torsion of a testis and acute epididymitis are easily diagnosed by examination of the external genitalia.

In adults, diseases that must be considered in the differential diagnosis of acute appendicitis are diverticulitis, perforated duodenal or gastric ulcer, acute cholecystitis, pancreatitis, intestinal obstruction, perforating cecal carcinoma, torsion of an ovarian cyst, perforated ileal diverticulum, mesenteric vascular occlusion, rupturing aortic aneurysm, and idiopathic infarction of an epiploic appendage or the omentum.

TREATMENT

PREOPERATIVE PREPARATION. No patient with acute appendicitis needs to be rushed directly to the operating room upon admission to the hospital. All patients, but especially those in whom perforation and peritonitis are suspected, should receive aggressive preoperative preparation. This rarely re-

TABLE 1. Placebo-Controlled Clinical Trials of Parenteral Antibiotics

Study	Year	Antibiotic(s) Studied	Placebo		Treated		Significance ($p < 0.05$)
			No. Infected/ Total	Per cent Infected	No. Infected/ Total	Per cent Infected	
1	1956	Tetra	5/82	6	1/83	1	NS
2	1971	Amp or Tetra	29/86	34	19/82	23	NS
3	1973	Cephaloridine	5/22	23	4/25	16	NS
4	1976	Tobra-Linco	4/14	29	0/14	0	NS
5*	1976	Linco	17/100	17	6/100	6	Yes
6	1976	Metro	11/46	24	5/49	10	NS
7	1977	Cephaloridine	18/63	29	7/70	1	Yes
8	1978	Genta-Clinda	5/49	10	3/57	5	NS
9	1978	Metro	16/47	34	4/241	2	Yes
10	1979	Clindamycin	24/72	33	14/81	17	Yes
					30/85	35	NS
11*	1979	Metro	12/51	24	1/49	2	Yes
12	1979	Metro	7/48	15	2/42	5	NS
13	1980	Metro	21/83	25	17/87	20	NS
14	1980	Metro-Perf	13/173	8	1/200	1	Yes
		Metro-Noperf	15/33	45	0/35	0	Yes
15	1980	Metro	7/91	8	5/96	5	NS
16	1980	Metro	11/50	22	1/54	2	Yes
17	1980	Cefaz	20/66	30	14/71	20	NS
		Metro			14/67	21	NS
		Cefaz + Metro			2/67	3	Yes
18	1981	Cefamandole	6/45	13	1/46	2	Yes
		Cefamandole-Carben			0/45	0	Yes
19	1981	Metro	27/115	23	32/260	12	Yes
20	1981	Metro	15/33	45	2/62	3	Yes
21	1981	Metro	16/97	16	3/87	3	Yes
22	1982	Metro	17/154	11	1/124	1	Yes
23	1982	Metro	19/103	19	8/71	11	NS
24	1982	Metro	5/63	8	2/58	3	NS
25	1982	Metro	12/55	22	5/58	9	Yes
26	1982	Amp-Genta	75/168	45	14/46	30	NS
		Amp-Genta-Clinda			5/86	6	Yes
27	1983	Cefoxitin	5/52	10	0/51	0	Yes
28	1983	Metro	4/42	10	2/30	7	NS
29	1983	Metro					
30*	1983	Cefamandole	12/60	20	10/42	24	NS
31	1983	Metro	11/66	17	11/67	16	NS
32	1983	Pen-Genta	4/37	11	8/62	13	NS
		Pen-Genta-Clinda			5/64	8	NS
		Ceforanide-Clinda			3/34	4	Yes
33	1983	Metro	16/136	12	6/151	4	Yes
34†	1983	Metro	15/42	36	10/48	21	NS
35*	1984	Genta-Clinda	9/36	25	0/40	0	Yes
36	1984	Trinidazole	21/177	12	18/288	6	Yes
37	1985	Metro	5/61	8	0/67	0	Yes
38	1989	Cefoxitin	74/890	8	21/845	3	Yes

* Topical povidone-iodine.

† Ampicillin.

Amp, ampicillin; Carben, carbenicillin; Cefaz, cefazolin; Clinda, clindamycin; Genta, gentamicin; Metro, metronidazole; Pen, penicillin; Tetra, tetracycline; Perf, perforating; Noperf, nonperforating.

quires more than 2 to 3 hours and often can be accomplished in an hour or less. Patients with a palpable periappendiceal mass may, in selected cases, be managed initially without an operation.

Fluid replacement should be initiated as rapidly as possible, with the objective of establishing a good urinary output. Nasogastric suction is helpful in all patients with appendicitis but particularly in those with peritonitis. Hyperpyrexia often is a problem in children and should be treated with salicylates in addition to hydration and antibiotics. If fever does not subside, a cooling mattress may be required. Anesthesia should not be induced in patients whose temperature is over 39° C. until appropriate measures have been initiated to reduce the fever.

Antibiotics are administered preoperatively to help control any local or generalized sepsis that may be present and to reduce the incidence of postoperative wound infection. Although prophylactic administration of antibiotics continues to be a matter of controversy, the evidence that has accumulated over approximately the past decade is clearly in favor of antibiotic administration.[28]

Controlled trials comparing antibiotics to placebo have consistently shown that antibiotics effective against anaerobes, either alone or in combination, are effective in reducing the risk of wound infection (Tables 1 and 2). Antibiotics primarily active only against aerobes were not consistently effective. This is a curious finding, because the most frequently isolated organism associated with wound infection complicating appendectomy is *Escherichia coli,* an aerobe. Nonetheless, anti-anaerobe activity appears to be essential for antibiotic efficacy in acute appendicitis.

Antibiotics probably are of minor benefit unless the appendix

is gangrenous or has perforated, but that fact cannot be determined until after the appendix is exposed during operation. It has been clearly established that if antibiotics are to have any favorable effect at all in reducing the incidence of wound infection, they must be started preoperatively. Therefore, the authors administer antibiotics to all patients with suspected appendicitis but continue administration intraoperatively only in those patients in whom acute appendicitis has been demonstrated. Antibiotic therapy is not continued beyond 24 hours postoperatively unless the appendix is gangrenous or perforated. The authors' current choice of antibiotic is cefoxitin.

EXAMINATION UNDER ANESTHESIA. After the patient has been anesthetized, the abdomen should be carefully and systemically palpated once more. On occasion, such examination shows the gallbladder to be the real cause of the patient's symptoms. If an appendiceal mass is detected, it may be due to a periappendiceal phlegmon without perforation, to a collection of fluid and pus associated with gangrene or localized perforation of the appendix, or to a frank periappendiceal abscess.

MANAGEMENT OF THE PATIENT WITHOUT A PALPABLE MASS (PRESUMED UNCOMPLICATED APPENDICITIS). In this case, there is no question about what operation needs to be done: the patient needs appendectomy. The questions to be considered concern the choice of incision, the handling of the appendiceal stump, whether or not to employ drains, and the method of wound closure.

TRANSVERSE INCISION. This incision (Fowler-Weir; Davis-Rockey) is made at a level 1 to 3 cm. below the umbilicus and is centered on the midclavicular-midinguinal line. The length of the incision needs to be 1 cm. or so longer than the breadth of the surgeon's hand. The aponeurosis and muscles of the ab-

TABLE 2. Clinical Trials Comparing Parenteral Antibiotic Regimens

		Group 1			Group 2			
Study	Year	Drug(s)	No. Infected/ Total	Per cent Infected	Drug(s)	No. Infected/ Total	Per cent Infected	Significance (p < 0.05)
1	1979	Clinda	14/81	17	Cefazolin	30/85	35	Yes
2	1980	Amp	15/32	47	Metro	5/31	16	Yes
3	1982	Genta-Clind	1/40	3	Cefaman	11/48	23	Yes
					Cefoper	6/42	14	Yes
4	1982	Metro	7/52	13	Cefoxitin	7/55	13	NS
5	1983	Moxalact	1/27	4	Cephalor	10/32	31	Yes
6	1983	Amp-Metro	19/42	13	Metro	33/141	23	Yes
7	1983	Metro	31/102	30	Metro-Cefotax	14/103	14	Yes
					Cefotax	13/103	13	Yes
8	1983	Genta-Metro	8/28	29	Metro	11/31	35	NS
9	1983	Metro	50/219	23	Metro-Cefotax	15/162	9	Yes
10	1983	Metro	9/98	9	Ticar	8/92	9	NS
11	1983	Genta-Clind	1/52	2	Cefaman	11/48	23	Yes
					Cefoper	7/47	15	Yes
12	1983	Cefoxitin	20/46	43	Metro	22/48	46	NS
13	1983	Genta-Amp	7/31	23	Genta-Amp-Clinda	1/33	3	Yes
14	1984	Amp-Metro	22/106	21	Cefoxitin	13/103	13	NS
15	1984	Genta-Amp-Metro	7/81	9	Metro	9/73	12	NS
16	1985	Metro	21/116	18	Amoxicillin-Clavulanate	13/115	11	NS
17	1985	Moxalactam	13/290	5	Cefotax	24/289	8	Yes
					Cefoper	20/285	7	NS
18	1985	Genta-Clind	0/38	0	Amp-Sulbactam	8/67	12	Yes
19	1985	Doxycycline	9/36	25	Nalidix-Metro	1/22	5	Yes
20	1986	Pen-Strep-Metro	8/34	24	Amp-Metro	7/33	21	NS
21	1986	Genta-Clind	0/66	0	Imipenem	1/33	3	NS
22	1986	Genta-Metro	5/151	3	Cefoxitin	6/156	4	NS
23	1986	Amp-Sulbact	3/35	9	Cefotax-Metro	5/38	13	NS
24	1987	Genta-Clind	2/51	4	Cefoxitin	4/54	7	NS
25	1988	Cefoxitin	6/82	7	Ceftriax	8/85	9	NS
26	1989	Genta-Amp-Metro	5/100	5	Ceftriax	3/100	3	NS

Amp, ampicillin; Cephalor, cephaloridine; Cefaman, cefamandole; Cefoper, cefoperazone; Cefotax, cefotaximine; Ceftriax, ceftriaxone; Clind(a), clindamycin; Genta, gentamicin; Metro, metronidazole; Moxalact, moxalactam; Nalidix, nalidixic acid; Pen, penicillin; Strep, streptomycin; Sulbact, sulbactam; Ticar, ticarcillin.

dominal wall are split or incised in the direction of the skin wound (Fig. 6). The incision lies in the direction of skin wrinkle lines and yields a cosmetically superior scar even if of necessity it is not sutured.

Exposure of the appendix through this approach is better than through the gridiron (McBurney) incision, particularly in patients with a retrocecal appendix and in those who are obese. There is no substitute for good exposure in any operation, and for this reason the transverse incision is preferred.

After the peritoneum is opened, the appendix is identified by following the anterior cecal taenia, and the inflamed appendix is coaxed into the wound, cupped in the palm of the hand. If the appendix is retrocecal (common) or retroperitoneal (uncommon) or if local inflammation and edema are intense, exposure is improved by dividing the lateral peritoneal reflection of the cecum. If the mobilization is done properly, the cecum lies within the wound at the level of the abdominal musculature and the appendix is at the level of the anterior abdominal wall. It is unnecessary for vigorous retraction to be maintained throughout the operation.

GRIDIRON INCISION. The muscle-splitting incision (McArthur-McBurney) is the time-honored approach and one widely used today (Fig. 7). Its advantage is that separation of muscles in the line of their fibers produces a wound that does not depend entirely upon sutures for restoration of tissue continuity. The skin incision is made obliquely in the right lower quadrant. As in all incisions across skin wrinkle lines, the scar widens with time and the cosmetic result is less than optimal. Exposure of the

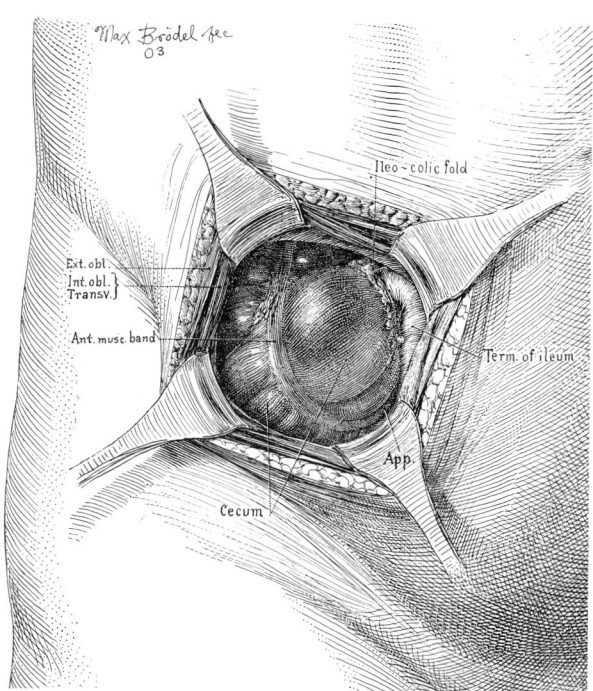

Figure 7. Gridiron incision. All musculoaponeurotic layers have been split, the peritoneum opened transversely, and the wound margins retracted. (From Kelly, H. A., and Hurdon, E.: The Vermiform Appendix and Its Diseases. Philadelphia, W. B. Saunders Company, 1905.)

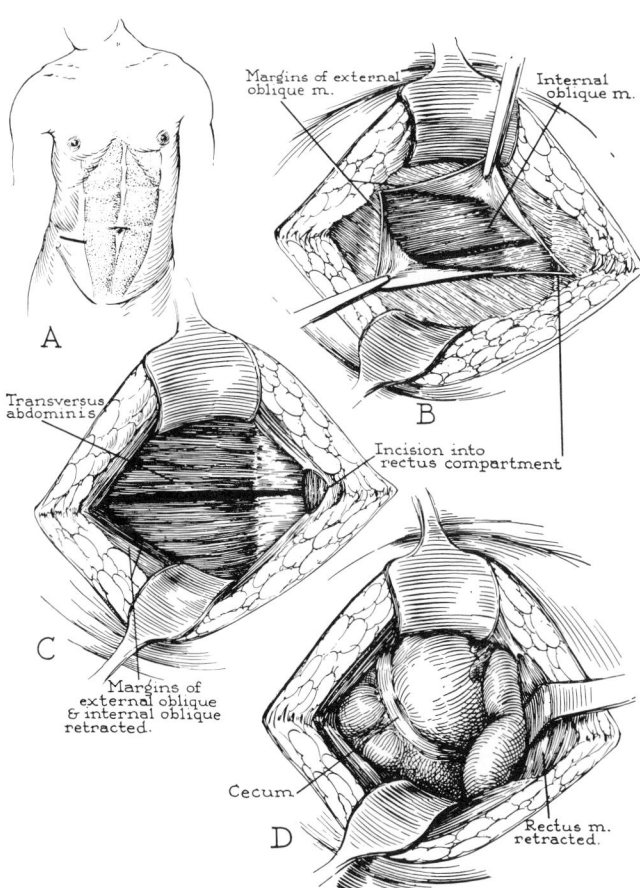

Figure 6. Transverse incisions for appendectomy. *A*, Placement of skin incision. *B*, External oblique muscle may be split, as illustrated, or incised transversely. The internal oblique and transversus abdominis muscles are split, and the rectus sheath, but not the rectus muscle, is incised (*B* and *C*). Retraction exposes the cecum *(D)*, which is rotated into the wound. (From Shackelford, R. T.: Surgery of the Alimentary Tract. Philadelphia, W. B. Saunders Company, 1977.)

appendix, especially a retrocecal appendix, through a gridiron incision can be awkward unless the appendix lies immediately below the incision. The gridiron incision can be extended medially, partially transecting the rectus sheath, which usually provides the additional exposure required to approach a pelvic appendix but often does not improve exposure of a retrocecal appendix. Under desperate circumstances, a gridiron incision can be extended vertically; this maneuver destroys the rationale of this incision but is occasionally necessary to expose a retrocecal appendix.

OTHER INCISIONS. Some surgeons use a vertical right paramedian incision or a pararectus (Battle) incision. Neither provides access to the appendix that is as good as that achieved through a transverse or gridiron incision. In addition, the Battle incision is particularly prone to disruption or development of a ventral hernia should wound infection occur.

If there is doubt about the diagnosis, so that general exploration of the abdomen is indicated, a vertical midline incision centered on the umbilicus is preferred. Appendectomy usually can be done through such an incision, although exposure is not ideal. If gangrenous or perforated appendicitis is encountered, the midline incision can be closed and a more direct approach made to the appendix.

THE APPENDICEAL STUMP. The mesoappendix is transected beginning at its free border by taking small bits of tissue between pairs of hemostats placed approximately 1 cm. from and parallel to the appendix. A suture should be passed through the mesoappendix and into the wall of the cecum close to the base of the appendix in order to secure the intramural accessory branch of the posterior cecal artery. If exposure of a long appendix is difficult, the mesoappendix can be transected in a retrograde manner beginning at the base of the appendix.

In most cases of appendicitis, inversion of the unligated stump with a Z stitch, rather than the more conventional purse-string suture, is preferred (Fig. 8). This maneuver accomplishes inversion of the appendiceal stump without spillage of cecal content. The appendix that is to be inverted should not be ligated, because ligation plus inversion does not reduce the risk of

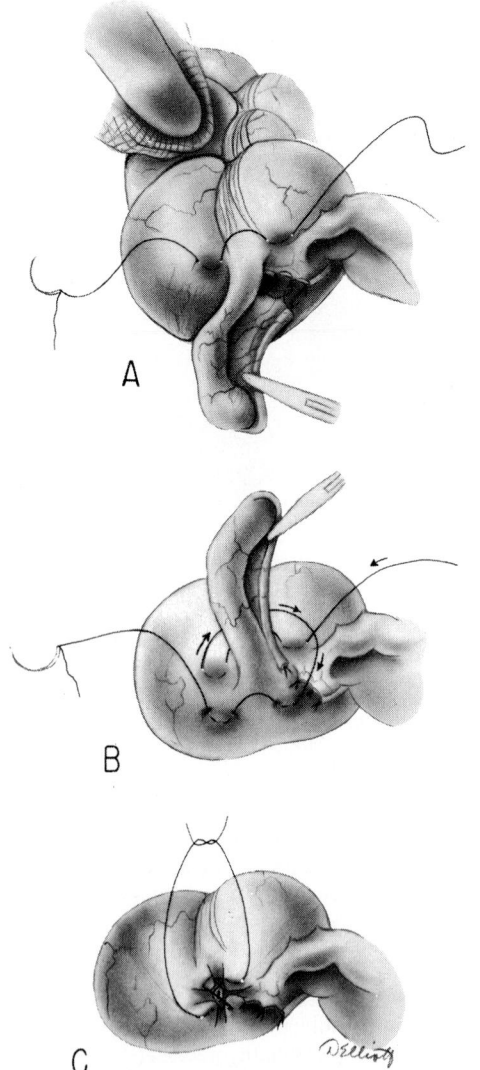

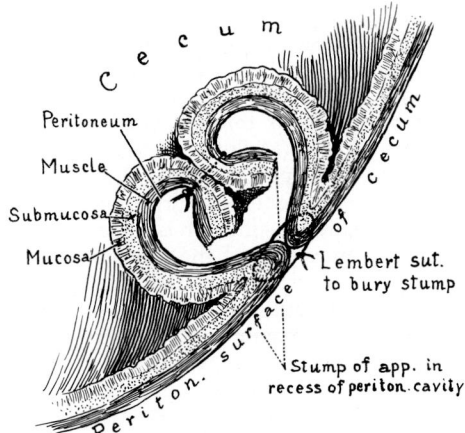

Figure 9. Ligation plus inversion of an appendix stump leads to a closed space and sets the stage for future trouble. (From Kelly, H. A., and Hurdon, E.: The Vermiform Appendix and Its Diseases. Philadelphia, W. B. Saunders Company, 1905.)

Figure 8. The upper level of the Z stitch is placed as a Lembert suture in the cecum near the base of the appendix (A). The suture is brought back behind the appendix and continued as a second Lembert suture at the lower margin of the appendix (B). After the appendix is transected between clamps, the stump is inverted into the cecum and the proximal clamp removed. The ends of the Z stitch are drawn up and tied over the stump of the appendix (C). (From Adams, J. T.: Z-stitch suture for inversion of the appendiceal stump. Surg. Gynecol. Obstet., 127:1321, 1968. By permission of Surgery, Gynecology & Obstetrics.)

septic complications,[26] but does create conditions conducive to development of an intramural abscess or mucocele (Fig. 9). In addition, the ligated plus inverted appendiceal stump may later appear as a cecal tumor and be a vexing source of diagnostic difficulties.[36]

If the appendix is edematous, turgid, or otherwise unsuitable for inversion, it should be doubly ligated at its base, the distal ligature being placed as a suture ligature. It is unnecessary to paint the appendiceal stump with alcohol or iodophor or to suture the mesoappendix or omentum over the base of the cecum.

Unexpected Findings (Appendix Abnormal). Although clinical symptoms may have led to a preoperative diagnosis of acute appendicitis, on occasion the operative findings in the appendix are those of another entity. The presence of a yellow-gray bulbous mass in the appendix should suggest the presence of a carcinoid tumor or a mucocele.[35] In the absence of metastases, simple appendectomy is sufficient therapy for these lesions.[22,53] Carcinoma of the appendix[1] or the cecum,[17] or an appendiceal metastasis,[6] can be associated with appendicitis. Patients with a

large periappendiceal mass or abscess are particularly likely to harbor a hidden cancer. Right hemicolectomy usually is required to manage carcinoma of the appendix or cecum. The discovery of a markedly enlarged, diffusely thickened, and indurated appendix should lead to a suspicion of appendiceal Crohn's disease,[54] especially when the duration of preoperative symptoms has exceeded 5 days. Simple appendectomy usually is sufficient therapy.

Erroneous Diagnoses (Appendix Normal). Although every surgeon feels somewhat chagrined at removing a "lily-white" appendix, the diagnosis of appendicitis is not always clear and a finite number of normal appendices always are going to be excised in appropriate clinical circumstances. As Ravitch has said, "there is only one way to have a 100 per cent accurate diagnostic record for acute appendicitis, and that is to wait until they all rupture." Intensive in-hospital observation of selected patients may reduce, but not eliminate, the incidence of removal of a normal appendix.

In the context of removal of a normal appendix, the unfortunate term "unnecessary appendectomy" has been used, a pejorative phrase that only serves to confuse the real issues. A judgment that appendectomy was "unnecessary" can be made only in retrospect. The removal of a normal appendix in appropriate clinical circumstances never constitutes an unnecessary appendectomy. A policy of active surgical intervention on the basis of minimal clinical suspicion has been demonstrated to reduce both the morbidity and the mortality of appendicitis.[17,19] Watchful waiting, however careful it may be, risks increasing both morbidity and mortality. In addition, cost-benefit analysis supports a policy of a low threshold of suspicion leading to early appendectomy.[39]

If exploration reveals a normal appendix, orderly investigation for the cause of the patient's symptoms must be done. The first maneuver is to obtain a specimen of any peritoneal fluid or exudate for Gram's stain to determine whether bacteria are present; this specimen also should be cultured for aerobes and anaerobes. Next, the cecum should be inspected; in 3 per cent of patients older than age 40, the symptoms mimicking appendicitis are secondary to malignant disease of the colon. The cecum and adjacent ileum also are examined for evidence of a perforated diverticulum. The small intestine is examined in retrograde manner for regional enteritis or a Meckel's diverticulum; the pelvic organs are palpated and inspected, seeking disease in that area. The intra-abdominal colon should be palpated next, after which the gallbladder and the duodenum in the right upper quadrant and the stomach in the midepigastrium should be sought. If enlarged lymph nodes are present in the small bowel mesentery, a representative node should be excised and sent for culture. The presence of infection by *Yersinia* organisms has been recognized in several cases that clinically appeared to be mesenteric adenitis; the diagnosis can be confirmed both by culture of involved nodes and by measurement of serum antibody titers. Exploration should not cease until the cause of the acute abdominal symptoms has been identified or the surgeon is certain that no remediable lesion is present within the abdominal cavity.

WOUND CLOSURE. The area of the cecum, the right iliac fossa, and the margins of the wound are irrigated prior to closure with dilute antibiotic solution: 500 mg. kanamycin and 50,000 units bacitracin dissolved in 500 ml. sterile normal saline. Irrigation should be repeated after the muscles and aponeuroses have been sutured.

Closure of the peritoneum is not necessary and may promote formation of adhesions. Each fascial layer is closed with nonabsorbable or slowly absorbable (polyglycolic acid) sutures. It is preferable not to place sutures in subcutaneous fat.

Drainage of either the muscular or the subcutaneous portions of the wound is unnecessary, and possibly harmful, when an unperforated appendix has been removed intact. If there has been contamination of the subcutaneous tissue by periappendiceal pus, it is preferable to pack the subcutaneous portion of the wound loosely open for 24 to 48 hours; the pack is then removed, but the skin is not reapproximated with paper tape until the wound is clean and granulations can be seen, usually about the fifth postoperative day.

Antibiotic therapy should not be continued postoperatively unless the appendix is gangrenous or perforated. The patient may be discharged as early as the third postoperative day provided there is no undue wound tenderness or fever and antibiotics have not been administered for 48 hours prior to discharge.

MANAGEMENT OF THE PATIENT WITH A PERIAPPENDICEAL MASS (PRESUMED GANGRENOUS OR LOCALLY PERFORATED APPENDICITIS) DETECTED AFTER INDUCTION OF ANESTHESIA. Appendectomy is the treatment of choice for patients with a mass detected by examination under anesthesia. The incision should be made transversely over the most prominent portion of the mass and the muscles and aponeuroses split by the gridiron principle. The medial aspect of the wound should be packed for prevention of contamination of the peritoneal cavity by spillage from the periappendiceal phlegmon.

Fluid and pus, if present, are aspirated after a specimen has been obtained for culture and sensitivity tests. The tissues are dissected sufficiently to expose the appendix. Care should be taken not to disturb adherent coils of intestine or omentum on the medial side of the mass when accomplishing appendectomy. More often than not, the base of the appendix is quite turgid and the surgeon has to settle for double ligation of the stump, inversion being impossible.

The question of whether to drain in these cases has been debated for years. In most patients with a gangrenous but unperforated appendix and without a collection of periappendiceal pus, closure without subfascial drainage is preferred. If a periappendiceal abscess is present or the tissues are so turgid as to create a rigid cavity, then the cavity should be drained with soft rubber drains brought out through a separate stab incision to avoid wound infection and incisional hernia.

The right iliac fossa and the wound should be liberally irrigated with dilute antibiotic solution prior to layer closure of the muscles with interrupted nonabsorbable sutures. Although some surgeons close the skin incision in these cases, leaving a drain in the subcutaneous tissues, it is preferable to leave the skin and subcutaneous tissues unsutured. Gauze soaked in the antibiotic irrigating solution is placed within the wound, and a dressing is applied. After 24 hours, the dressing and gauze pack are removed and the wound is covered with a dry dressing. If needed, the skin may be loosely approximated on the fifth or sixth postoperative day with paper tape. If the wound does not appear clean and healthy at this time, it should not be closed; granulation occurs rapidly, and the wound heals spontaneously in 3 to 6 weeks.

Systemic antibiotics should be continued for 4 to 5 days after operation. A rectal examination is conducted daily to detect development of pelvic abscess. Discharge from the hospital is delayed until the patient has been afebrile for 2 days, has not had antibiotics for 72 hours, and has no evidence of wound infection or intraperitoneal or pelvic abscess.

MANAGEMENT OF THE PATIENT WITH A FIXED PERIAPPENDICEAL MASS (PRESUMED APPENDICEAL ABSCESS). If a patient is first seen when symptoms are subsiding and a well-localized periappendiceal mass is found by physical examination, it is reasonable in most adults to start systemic antibiotics and to continue expectant treatment. However, children, pregnant women, and most elderly patients should not be managed by expectant treatment of the appendiceal mass; drainage of the appendiceal abscess should be done as soon as the patient can be prepared for operation. In two of three adults in whom expectant treatment of the appendiceal mass is indicated, symptoms continue to subside and a subsequent interval appendectomy can be accomplished. In one of three such patients, however, symptoms do not continue to subside, and prompt appendectomy or drainage of the appendiceal abscess should be performed.

The location of an appendiceal abscess corresponds with the anatomic location of the tip of the appendix: about 66 per cent are situated behind the cecum, 30 per cent form in the pelvis, and 4 per cent are found behind the terminal ileum or extraperitoneally behind the ascending colon.

The incision for drainage is made just medial to the crest of the ilium at the level of the most prominent portion of the periappendiceal mass. The muscles are split, and the lateral edge of the peritoneum is exposed and pushed medially so that the mass surrounding the appendix is approached from its lateral retroperitoneal aspect. If pus is present under pressure, the abscess may rupture spontaneously. If not, a finger should be slowly introduced into the abscess and its loculations broken down by blunt dissection. Care is taken not to break down adhesions walling off the medial aspect of the abscess mass. If the appendix is readily accessible, appendectomy can be performed.

In infants, appendectomy should be accomplished in addition to drainage of the abscess. The reason is that the conical shape and broad lumen of the infant appendix promote continued drainage of feces from the cecum through the perforation. Accomplishment of appendectomy at the time of drainage of the abscess is less important in adults, since the narrow obstructed lumen of the adult appendix usually prevents retrograde drainage of feces. If the appendix is not removed when the abscess is drained, interval appendectomy should be done 6 to 8 weeks after drainage from the abscess has ceased and the wound has healed.

A sump drainage tube should be inserted into the abscess cavity and extracted through a stab wound in the flank. The wound is irrigated with dilute antibiotic solution, the muscular layers are closed, and the subcutaneous tissues and skin incision are packed open as described previously for patients with a mobile periappendiceal mass. The sump tube should be left undisturbed until it is draining less than 2 ounces each day. The tube then should be rotated but not advanced. If drainage does not resume, a sinogram should be obtained. Only when the abscess cavity has been obliterated should the drain be progressively advanced and removed.

Systemic antibiotics should be continued for at least 5 days postoperatively, and longer if clinically indicated. A daily rectal examination is made to detect a developing pelvic abscess. The head of the bed should be elevated 15 to 30 degrees (semi-Fowler position); while this position does not prevent the development of a subphrenic abscess, it promotes drainage toward the pelvis and is more comfortable for the patient.

If, after a week or so, the patient is afebrile and shows no signs of complications secondary to the drained appendiceal abscess, continued treatment in a hospital is not strictly necessary, although it often is found more convenient. Criteria for discharge are the same as those noted previously for patients with a mobile periappendiceal mass.

MANAGEMENT OF PATIENTS WITH DIFFUSE PERITONITIS DUE TO APPENDICITIS. Spreading peritonitis is the principal cause of continuing mortality from appendicitis and requires careful and energetic treatment. It is generally agreed that appendectomy must be performed in children whether peritonitis is diffuse or not, since any other course is associated with a higher mortality.

There is continuing controversy about the management of adults. The patient with perforative appendicitis in whom diffuse peritonitis develops, and who has failed to wall off the process so that the perforated appendix is a continuing source of peritoneal contamination, benefits from appendectomy. However, a patient whose perforation initially leads to diffuse peritonitis, but in whom the perforated appendix is subsequently walled off as an appendiceal abscess, is best managed by operation limited to drainage of the abscess. In both types of patients, general principles governing the management of bacterial peritonitis apply.

The question of if and what to drain in patients with diffuse appendiceal peritonitis also has been an issue of controversy for years. Although drainage of each localized collection of pus is certainly indicated, prophylactic placement of multiple drains within the abdominal cavity is an unwarranted practice.[14,55] Such prophylactic intra-abdominal drains are rapidly walled off and do not succeed in draining the peritoneal cavity except for a few hours. They may be detrimental rather than helpful, because they perpetuate inflammation by the presence of an unnecessary foreign body and lead to formation of adhesions that may later cause intestinal obstruction.

The principles of wound management in these cases are irrigation of the wound with dilute antibiotic solution, subfascial drains only to localized collections of pus, closure of musculoaponeurotic layers, skin and subcutaneous tissues packed open rather than sutured and drained, daily rectal examination to detect development of a pelvic abscess, and nursing the patient in a semiupright position for the initial postoperative week. Systemic administration of antibiotics should be continued for as long as clinically indicated.

RECURRENT, SUBACUTE, AND CHRONIC APPENDICITIS. There are a few patients in whom an initial attack of acute appendicitis subsides spontaneously. If the initial diagnosis is clear, the risk of a recurrent episode of appendicitis is high; following nonoperative treatment or simple abscess drainage without appendectomy, the incidence of recurrent appendicitis is approximately 28 per cent.[3] Elective appendectomy within 6 to 8 weeks therefore should be advised.

Even if a full-blown appendicitis does not ensue, the appendix thereafter may become, in Maingot's phrase, a "grumbler," precipitating recurrent attacks, usually milder than the initial attack, of right lower quadrant pain. Characteristically, patients are symptom-free between attacks; physical examination is normal unless the patient is examined while symptoms are present. If abdominal films demonstrate the presence of a fecalith, a barium enema shows nonfilling of the obstructed appendix, or observation of repeated attacks provides evidence that the patient is suffering from recurrent subacute appendicitis, elective appendectomy should be undertaken.

The presence of retained barium in the appendix or of an asymptomatic fecalith, noted on investigation of the patient for

other symptoms, is an indication for elective interval appendectomy, because appendicitis is likely to develop in such patients within 2 to 3 years.[8,51]

In order to sustain a diagnosis of chronic appendicitis as justification for appendectomy in patients with persistent right lower abdominal complaints, the resected appendix must show fibrosis in the appendiceal wall, partial to complete obstruction of the lumen, evidence of old mucosal ulceration and scarring, and infiltration by chronic inflammatory cells. It is not sufficient to diagnose chronic appendicitis on the basis of a few polymorphonuclear leukocytes found within the wall of an excised appendix. This latter degree of "inflammatory response" can be elicited by the manipulations required for excision of a normal appendix.

INCIDENTAL APPENDECTOMY. Opinion regarding the advisability of incidental appendectomy routinely during other intra-abdominal operations is not unanimous.[15] Some studies have shown that the removal of the appendix en passant does not increase total operative time, length of hospital stay, or the incidence of infectious postoperative complications. The most recent studies, however, indicate that incidental appendectomy in most clinical contexts does increase the risk of wound infection by 2 or 3 per cent.

The rationale for performing incidental appendectomy is that it obviates the future development of appendicitis and thereby reduces the overall morbidity due to appendicitis. In most cases, however, the operation is done after the period of maximal risk for development of appendicitis has passed. Analysis of the risk-benefit balance indicates that incidental appendectomy is appropriately done only in infants and children.[7] Incidental appendectomy requires that the patient needs an abdominal operation for another reason, and such opportunities are relatively uncommon in children. Most patients undergoing incidental appendectomy are women undergoing a hysterectomy or cholecystectomy who are more than 30 years of age,[46] whose future risk of developing appendicitis is minimal, and who therefore do not receive a measurable benefit greater than the risk undertaken.

COMPLICATIONS OF APPENDECTOMY

Postoperative complications occur in only 5 per cent of patients if an unperforated appendix is removed intact, but in over 30 per cent of patients with gangrenous or perforated appendicitis. The incidence of perforation is less than 20 per cent in the first 24 hours of symptoms but rapidly climbs to over 70 per cent after 48 hours. There is considerable urgency in making a correct diagnosis and accomplishing appendectomy within 24 hours after the onset of symptoms in order to reduce the incidence of complications. The more frequent complications of appendectomy include wound infection, pelvic, subphrenic, and intraperitoneal abscesses, fecal fistula, pylephlebitis, and intestinal obstruction.

Infection of the subcutaneous tissues is the most common complication following appendectomy. The organisms recovered from the appendiceal fossa in cases of acute appendicitis are most frequently anaerobic Bacteroides species, followed by the aerobes Klebsiella, Enterobacter, and E. coli.[29] However, E. coli are the most frequent bacteria recovered from an infected wound. Because wound infections in cases of appendicitis are caused by fecal organisms, the classic signs of infection (calor, dolor, rubor, tumor) often are not present. The early signs of a fecal wound infection are undue pain and modest edema around the wound. If such signs are present, the skin and subcutaneous tissue should be opened. A rush of pus should not be expected. Fecal infections induce necrosis of subcutaneous fat, often of considerable extent, but only as damaged fat liquifies does much pus form.

Pelvic, subphrenic, or intra-abdominal abscess occurs in up to

20 per cent of patients with gangrenous or perforative appendicitis. Abscesses usually are due to preoperative contamination of the peritoneal cavity by organisms leaking from a gangrenous or perforated appendix. Less often contamination ensues from intraoperative spillage. Occasionally, an abscess forms around a retained fecalith or other foreign body. The presence of an abscess is manifested by recurrent fever, malaise, and anorexia, usually beginning about 1 week after appendectomy. A pelvic abscess may cause diarrhea and may be palpated on vaginal or rectal examination. Subphrenic abscess can be diagnosed by the classic signs of effusion in the overlying thorax and immobility of the involved diaphragm. Computed tomography is of great help in diagnosing the presence of an intra-abdominal abscess. Confirmation of the presence of an intra-abdominal abscess may require an exploratory laparotomy. All abscesses must be drained, either percutaneously or surgically.

Fecal fistula usually is not a dangerous complication of appendectomy. Fistulas may be due to a retained foreign body, such as a sponge, a pursestring suture tied too tightly, a ligature slipping from a tied but noninverted appendiceal stump, necrosis from a periappendiceal abscess encroaching on the cecum, erosion of the wall of the cecum by a drain, regional enteritis, colon obstruction by an undetected neoplasm, or retention of a mucus-producing tip of the appendix.

Some fecal fistulas close spontaneously; all that is required is to ensure that the tract remains open until drainage ceases. Fecal fistulas do not close spontaneously if the tip of the appendix or a foreign body is present, if the bowel beyond the fistula is obstructed, or if the mucous membrane of the gut is continuous with the skin. In such cases, closure of the fistula requires an operation.

Pylephlebitis, or portal pyemia, is a serious illness characterized by jaundice, chills, and high fever. It is due to septicemia of the portal venous system, leading to development of multiple liver abscesses. Pylephlebitis is associated with gangrenous or perforated appendicitis and may appear either preoperatively or postoperatively. The infecting organism is usually *E. coli*. Fortunately, now that antibiotics are utilized both before and after appendectomy, this complication has become rare.

Intestinal obstruction, initially paralytic but occasionally progressing to true mechanical obstruction, may occur with slowly resolving peritonitis in complicated appendicitis. Late mechanical obstruction following appendicitis is uncommon. The development of a mechanical bowel obstruction usually requires operative relief.

SELECTED REFERENCES

Fitz, R. H.: Perforating inflammation of the vermiform appendix, with special reference to its early diagnosis and treatment. Trans. Assoc. Am. Phys., 1:107, 1886.
In this paper Reginald Fitz describes 25 patients, correlating pathologic findings with clinical symptoms to demonstrate conclusively that "perityphlitis" begins with inflammation of the appendix. Fitz was the first physician to use the term "appendicitis." This classic study marks the beginning of modern operative treatment of acute appendicitis.

McBurney, C.: Experience with early operative interference in cases of disease of the vermiform appendix. N.Y. Med. J., 50:676, 1889.
The purpose of this paper was to report successful treatment by appendectomy of appendicitis prior to perforation. In describing the early clinical symptoms of his patients, McBurney said, "The seat of greatest pain, determined by the pressure of one finger, has been very exactly between an inch and a half and two inches from the anterior spinous process of the ilium on a straight line drawn from the process to the umbilicus." This is now known as McBurney's point. He also recommended the gridiron incision which had been described earlier by McArthur. Despite McArthur's priority, this incision is universally known today as the McBurney incision.

Melier, F.: Memoire sur des tumeurs phlegmoneuses occupant la fosse de l'appendice cecal. J. Gen. Med., 100:317, 1827.
Melier was a young medical graduate working in Paris. He correctly deduced from his observations of a series of autopsies that what was then called iliac tumor was, in reality, an appendiceal abscess. Melier suggested that this then fatal disease began with inflammation of the appendix rather than of the cecum. His hypothesis

was brutally publicly rejected by Dupuytren, the dominant surgeon of the day. Melier's correct deduction about appendicitis lapsed into obscurity, another victim of authoritarianism.

van Zwalenburg, C.: The relation of mechanical distention to the etiology of appendicitis. Ann. Surg., 41:437, 1905.
This is a remarkably prescient paper by a turn-of-the-century surgeon practicing in California. In this paper, van Zwalenburg first proposed, based on his clinical observations of cases of appendicitis, that obstruction was the basic pathophysiologic process in this disease. His hypothesis was later supported by the work of Wangensteen and Dennis, cited below.

Wangensteen, O. H., and Dennis, C.: Experimental proof of obstructive origin of appendicitis in man. Ann. Surg., 110:629, 1939.
In a group of patients with carcinoma of the colon, but with a normal appendix, who were undergoing decompressive colostomy, the appendix was exteriorized and ligated at its base for the purpose of producing obstruction, and the tip was cannulated and connected to a recording manometer. Intraluminal pressures up to 126 cm. H_2O (93 mm. Hg) developed in less than 24 hours. Despite the very high pressure in the lumen, the appendiceal mucosa continued to secrete mucus. This paper clearly established obstruction-secretion as the fundamental process in acute appendicitis.

Worcester, A.: Early operations for appendicitis. N. Engl. J. Med., 218:651, 1938.
A delightfully candid account of some of the first patients in the United States to have an appendectomy. The year was 1886. Dr. Worcester himself was one of the patients.

REFERENCES

1. Andersson, Å., Bergdahl, L., and Boquist, L.: Primary carcinoma of the appendix. Ann. Surg., 183:53, 1976.
2. Arnbjörnsson, E.: Varying frequency of acute appendicitis in different phases of the menstrual cycle. Surg. Gynecol. Obstet., 155:709, 1982. Also published as: Acute appendicitis risk in various phases of the menstrual cycle. Acta Chir. Scand., 149:603, 1983.
3. Arnbjörnsson, E.: Management of appendiceal abscess. Curr. Surg., 41:4, 1984.
4. Berry, J., Jr., and Malt, R. A.: Appendicitis near its centenary. Ann. Surg., 200:567, 1984.
5. Bolton, J. P., Craven, E. R., Croft, R. J., and Menzies-Gow, N.: An assessment of the value of the white count in the management of suspected acute appendicitis. Br. J. Surg., 62:906, 1975.
6. Burney, R. E., Koss, N., and Goldenberg, I. S.: Acute appendicitis secondary to metastatic carcinoma of the breast. Arch. Surg., 108:872, 1974.
7. Condon, R. E.: Incidental appendectomy is rarely indicated. *In* Simmons, R. L., and Udekwu, A. O. (Eds.): Debates in Clinical Surgery. Chicago, Year Book Medical Publishers, 1990, pp. 91–98.
8. Copeland, E. M., and Long, J. M., III: Elective appendectomy for appendiceal calculus. Surg. Gynecol. Obstet., 130:439, 1970.
9. Cunningham, F. G., and McCubbin, J. H.: Appendicitis complicating pregnancy. Obstet. Gynecol., 45:415, 1975.
10. DeDombal, F. T., Leaper, D. J., Horrocks, J. C., Staniland, J. R., and McCann, A. P.: Human and computer-aided diagnosis of abdominal pain: Further report with emphasis on performance of clinicians. Br. Med. J., 1:376, 1974.
11. Fee, H. J., Jones, P. C., Kadell, B., and O'Connell, T. X.: Radiologic diagnosis of appendicitis. Arch. Surg., 112:742, 1977.
12. Gill, B., and Cudmore, R. E.: Significance of faecoliths in the diagnosis of acute appendicitis. Br. J. Surg., 62:535, 1975.
13. Gomez, A., and Wood, M.: Acute appendicitis during pregnancy. Am. J. Surg., 137:180, 1979.
14. Haller, J. A., Jr., Shaker, I. J., Donahoo, J. S., Schnaufer, L., and White, J. J.: Peritoneal drainage versus non-drainage for generalized peritonitis from ruptured appendicitis in children. Ann. Surg., 177:595, 1973.
15. Hays, R. J.: Incidental appendectomies. Current teaching. J.A.M.A., 238:31, 1977.
16. Hobson, T., and Rosenman, L. D.: Acute appendicitis—when is it right to be wrong? Am. J. Surg., 108:306, 1964.
17. Hossain, M. A.: Unrecognized carcinoma of caecum presenting as acute appendicitis or appendix abscess. Br. Med. J., 2:709, 1962.
18. Howie, J. G. R.: Death from appendicitis and appendicectomy. Lancet, 2:1334, 1966.
19. Howie, J. G. R.: The place of appendicectomy in the treatment of young adult patients with possible appendicitis. Lancet, 1:1365, 1968.
20. Hubbell, D. S., Barton, W. K., and Solomon, O. D.: Leukocytosis in appendicitis in older persons. J.A.M.A., 175:139, 1961.
21. Hyman, P., and Westring, D. W.: Leukocytosis in acute appendicitis: Observed racial difference. J.A.M.A., 229:1630, 1974.
22. Hughes, J.: Mucocele of the appendix with pseudomyxoma peritonei: A benign or malignant disease? Ann. Surg., 165:73, 1967.
23. Janik, J. S., and Firor, H. V.: Pediatric appendicitis: A 20-year study of 1,640 children at Cook County (Illinois) Hospital. Arch. Surg., 114:717, 1979.
24. Jona, J. Z., and Belin, R. P.: Basilar pneumonia simulating acute appendicitis in children. Arch. Surg., 111:552, 1976.
25. Jona, J., Belin, R., and Selke, A.: Barium enema as a diagnostic aid in children with abdominal pain. Surg. Gynecol. Obstet., 144:351, 1977.

26. Kingsley, D. P. E.: Some observations on appendicectomy with particular reference to technique. Br. J. Surg., *56*:491, 1969.

27. Kretchmar, L. H., and McDonald, D. F.: The urine sediment in acute appendicitis. Arch. Surg., *87*:209, 1963.

28. Krukowski, Z. H., Irwin, S. T., Denhohn, S., and Matheson, N. A.: Preventing wound infection after appendectomy: A review. Br. J. Surg., *75*:1023, 1988.

29. Leigh, D. A., Simmons, K., and Norman, E.: Bacterial flora of the appendix fossa in appendicitis and postoperative wound infection. J. Clin. Pathol., *27*:997, 1974.

30. Lewis, F. R., Holcroft, J. W., Boey, J., and Dunphy, J. E.: Appendicitis: A critical review of diagnosis and treatment in 1,000 cases. Arch. Surg., *110*:677, 1975.

31. Ludbrook, J., and Spears, G. F. S.: The risk of developing appendicitis. Br. J. Surg., *52*:856, 1965.

32. Marchildon, M. B., and Dudgeon, D. L.: Perforated appendicitis: Current experience in a children's hospital. Ann. Surg., *185*:84, 1977.

33. Martin, L. W., and Perrin, E. V.: Neonatal perforation of the appendix in association with Hirschsprung's disease. Ann. Surg., *166*:799, 1967.

34. Meade, R. H.: The evolution of surgery for appendicitis. Surgery, *55*:741, 1964.

35. Moertel, C. G., Weiland, L. H., Nagorney, D. M., and Dockerty, M. B.: Carcinoid tumor of the appendix: Treatment and prognosis. N. Engl. J. Med., *317*:1699, 1987.

36. Myllarniemi, H., Perttala, Y., and Peltokallio, P.: Tumor-like lesions of the cecum following inversion of the appendix. Am. J. Dig. Dis., *19*:547, 1974.

37. Noer, T.: Decreasing incidence of acute appendicitis. Acta Chir. Scand., *141*:431, 1975.

38. Owens, B. J., III, and Hamit, H. F.: Appendicitis in the elderly. Ann. Surg., *187*:392, 1978.

39. Parker, S. G., and Kassirer, J. P.: Therapeutic decision making: A cost-benefit analysis. N. Engl. J. Med., *293*:229, 1975.

40. Rajagopalan, A. E., Mason, J. H., Kennedy, M., and Pawlikowski, J.: The value of the barium enema in the diagnosis of acute appendicitis. Arch. Surg., *112*:531, 1977.

41. Sasso, R. D., Hanna, E. A., and Moore, D. L.: Leukocytic and neutrophilic counts in acute appendicitis. Am. J. Surg., *120*:563, 1970.

42. Schaller, R. T., and Schaller, J. F.: The acute abdomen in the immunologically compromised child. J. Pediatr. Surg., *1*:937, 1983.

43. Senn, N.: A plea in favor of early laparotomy for catarrhal and ulcerative appendicitis, with the report of two cases. J.A.M.A., *12*:630, 1889.

44. Sherman, N. J., and Woolley, M. M.: The ileocecal syndrome in acute childhood leukemia. Arch. Surg., *107*:39, 1973.

45. Stone, H. H., Sanders, S. L., and Martin, J. D., Jr.: Perforated appendicitis in children. Surgery, *69*:673, 1971.

46. Sugimoto, T., and Edwards, D.: Incidence and costs of incidental appendectomy as a preventive measure. Am. J. Public Health, *77*:471, 1987.

47. Teicher, I., Landa, B., Cohen, M., Kabnick, L. S., and Wise, L.: Scoring system to aid in diagnosis of appendicitis. Ann. Surg., *198*:753, 1983.

48. Thorbjarnarson, B., and Loehr, W. J.: Acute appendicitis in patients over the age of sixty. Surg. Gynecol. Obstet., *125*:1277, 1967.

49. VanWay, C., Murphy, J., Dunn, E., and Elerding, S. C.: A feasibility study of computer-aided diagnosis in appendicitis. Surg. Gynecol. Obstet., *155*:685, 1982.

50. Ver Steeg, K., LaSalle, A., and Ratner, I.: Appendicitis in acute leukemia. Arch. Surg., *114*:632, 1979.

51. Vukmer, G. J., and Trummer, M. J.: Barium appendicitis—report of a case. Arch. Surg., *91*:630, 1965.

52. Wakeley, C. P. G.: Position of vermiform appendix as ascertained by analysis of 10,000 cases. J. Anat., *67*:277, 1933.

53. Wesser, D. R., and Edelman, S.: Experiences with mucoceles of the appendix. Ann. Surg., *153*:272, 1961.

54. Yang, S. S., Gibson, P., McCaughey, R. S., Arcari, F. A., and Bernstein, J.: Primary Crohn's disease of the appendix—report of 14 cases and review of the literature. Ann. Surg., *189*:334, 1979.

55. Yates, J. L.: An experimental study of the local effects of peritoneal drainage. Surg. Gynecol. Obstet., *1*:473, 1905.

32

THE COLON AND RECTUM

I

SURGICAL ANATOMY AND OPERATIVE PROCEDURES

Joel J. Roslyn, M. D., and Michael J. Zinner, M. D.

The colon and rectum are the site of numerous pathologic processes, which often require surgical intervention. These problems are generally of congenital, traumatic, inflammatory, mechanical, vascular, or neoplastic etiology. The large intestine or colon extends from the ileocecal valve to the anus and is somewhat arbitrarily divided into the cecum, ascending and transverse colon, splenic flexure, descending and sigmoid colon, rectosigmoid, rectum, and anus. Although the average length of the large intestine is approximately 135 to 150 cm., the location of the various anatomic divisions varies from patient to patient. The function of the colon, i.e., water absorption and evacuation of fecal waste, has been well known for many years, but the mechanisms by which these specific activities are accomplished continue to be the focus of investigation. Surgical procedures are frequently required in the management of patients with colonic diseases. A successful outcome is dependent largely on the physicians' understanding and appreciation of anatomy, physiology, pathology, and microbiology of the colon.

SURGICAL ANATOMY

The large intestine, or colon, extends from the ileocecal valve, generally in the right lower quadrant, and courses in a horseshoe manner around the upper abdomen and down the left side of the abdominal cavity and into the pelvis. Its anatomic relationships to both peritoneal and retroperitoneal organs, when coupled with its unique histologic and gross anatomic features, are important for the surgeon to comprehend when managing patients with diseases of the colon. There are several distinct anatomic differences between the large and small intestine. The vermiform appendix has the characteristic muscular coating of the small intestine. The remainder of the colon contains the same inner circular muscular layer below the serosa as does the small bowel, but its outer longitudinal muscle layer is quite distinct. This outer longitudinal muscular coat is concentrated into three separate longitudinal strips, "taeniae coli," which give the colon a characteristic appearance. These are found throughout the length of the colon down into the sigmoid area. At the level of the rectosigmoid junction, the taeniae generally coalesce and provide a complete longitudinal muscular coat for the rectum. The configuration of the taeniae coli and their state of contraction are responsible for the formation of "haustra." This term refers to the sacculations or protrusions of the bowel wall between the taeniae. Unlike the valvulae conniventes, which are characteristic of the small intestine, the haustra of the colon only partially encircle the large intestine. Their appearance on simple radiographs of the abdomen is quite characteristic and often allows distinction of the colon from the small intestine. The third gross characteristic unique to the colon is the "appendices epiploicae," which are extensions of peritoneal fat. These appendages have no demonstrable function and are occasionally involved with inflammatory processes of the colon.

Although the colon is generally considered to be an intraperitoneal organ, the ascending and descending segments are frequently fixed by retroperitoneal attachments that give a portion of the circumference of the lumen a certain retroperitoneal location. Developmental anomalies may affect the anatomic location of the ascending or sigmoid colon. The transverse colon is usually supported by a mesentery and may be found in a horizontal position or in a more dependent position traversing freely into the lower abdomen. The propensity to develop a cecal or sigmoid volvulus, i.e., a twist of the colon around its mesentery is due in large measure to the extent to which these organs are fixed retroperitoneally. The variability in the location of the transverse colon may, in addition, cause differing symptoms in patients with disorders in this segment.

THE ILEOCECAL VALVE AND CECUM. The ileocecal valve refers to a functional anatomic sphincter located at the junction of the terminal segment of the ileum as it enters the posterior medial aspect of the proximal segment of the colon, the cecum. The fusion of an upper and lower lip, the muscular nature of which is not unlike the cecum itself, serves to function as a sphincter that prevents the reflux of material from the cecal lumen back into the terminal ileum. The internal diameter of the colon is largest at the cecum and frequently measures 7 to 9 cm. The cecum is therefore the most proximal and widest segment of the colon and is typically situated in the right iliac fossa. The cecum is generally enveloped by peritoneum in the majority of patients and is fixed posteriorly in only a small percentage of individuals. Therefore, the cecum usually has a certain degree of mobility. Depending on the degree to which embryologic intestinal rotation occurs, the cecum may be found in a variety of positions, including the right upper or left upper quadrants. This abnormality, in which the cecum and ascending colon may be completely mobile and not fixed to the retroperitoneal or paracolic gutter, makes possible the development of cecal volvulus. As a result of the large diameter of the cecum, lesions such as tumors in this area rarely cause obstructive symptoms. Carcinomas arising within the cecum are typically associated with a more indolent course, and patients frequently present with anemia and generalized fatigue or other constitutional symptoms. Distal colonic obstruction secondary to carcinoma, or diverticulitis, may be complicated by the development of cecal perforation. This occurrence can be explained by the physical characteristics of the cecum and by an understanding of

Laplace's law. This physical principle states that the tension in the wall of a viscus is proportionally related to the internal pressure and the radius of the tube, (tension = pressure × radius). Therefore, it is not surprising that the segment of the colon with the largest radius is the site where tension is the greatest and the most likely site for perforation in the presence of distal obstruction.

The vermiform appendix generally projects from the inferior aspect of the medial portion of the cecum. Its length is quite variable, and it may ultimately come to lie in a pelvic or retrocecal position.

ASCENDING COLON AND HEPATIC FLEXURE. Coursing upward from the cecum to the transverse colon is the ascending colon and the hepatic flexure, which specifically is the portion of the colon that turns medially and joins the transverse colon. The ascending colon has great importance in colonic function as well as in its anatomic relationships to the retroperitoneal organs, including the right kidney and ureter and the duodenum. During mobilization of the ascending colon and hepatic flexure, care must be exercised by the surgeon not to injure the right ureter or the duodenum. Occasionally tumors involving the hepatic flexure can erode into the duodenum, and this possibility should be considered in appropriate clinical settings.

THE TRANSVERSE COLON. The transverse colon generally measures 35 to 50 cm. in length and lies between the hepatic flexure in the right upper quadrant and the splenic flexure in the left upper quadrant. It is the most mobile portion of the colon and may be found in the upper abdomen or as far down as the pelvis. With the exception of its most proximal and distal connections with the hepatic and splenic flexures, respectively, the transverse colon is generally considered to be completely intraperitoneal. It is suspended by the transverse mesocolon and is frequently enveloped anteriorly by the junction of the greater omentum and mesocolon. This area is frequently the site of either primary colonic tumors or neoplastic involvement from contiguous spread from gastric or pancreatic malignancies.

SPLENIC FLEXURE. The angle between the distal transverse colon and the descending colon is designated the splenic flexure and is frequently angulated and in a more cephalad position than is the hepatic flexure. The anatomic importance of this segment of the colon is considerable, in large measure because of its attachment and intimate relationship to the spleen. The phrenocolic and splenocolic attachments should be carefully considered during mobilization of the splenic flexure.

DESCENDING COLON. The descending colon courses from the splenic flexure down into the sigmoid colon at the level of the pelvic brim and generally measures 20 to 25 cm. It is only partially peritonealized, is frequently in intimate association with the left ureter, and rarely has a free mesentery.

SIGMOID COLON. The sigmoid colon is the S-shaped segment of the colon that extends from the pelvic brim to the peritoneal reflection, where the next segment of bowel is designated as the rectum. This segment of the bowel is frequently redundant to a varying degree and may be 10 to 30 cm. in length. In most individuals, it has a short mesentery. However, this may become quite elongated, as is the bowel itself in patients with sigmoid volvulus. Regardless of the extent and length of sigmoid colon, a rather constant finding is that it is situated approximately 15 to 18 cm. from the anus. Therefore, the sigmoid colon, which is frequently the site of malignancy and/or diverticulitis, can be easily visualized with a rigid sigmoidoscope.

RECTUM. The rectum is quite distinct from the more proximal colon in many important respects. The junction of the rectosigmoid is frequently marked by a distinct flexure in the bowel, this segment being directed posteriorly and downward to conform to the curve of the sacrum. As it proceeds distally, the lumen becomes quite enlarged, and the most distal fusiform segment is frequently known as the rectal ampulla. There is considerable mobility in the rectum, and it is generally not fixed to the sacrum. Perhaps most important to the surgeon is the relationship of the pelvic peritoneum to the rectum. As the rectum descends into the pelvis, the complete peritoneal investment which is found more proximally becomes less apparent, such that the distal portion of the rectum has essentially no peritoneal covering. Therefore, much of the rectum can be considered extraperitoneal. The mobility of the rectum is responsible for the variability and apparent change in location of rectal tumors as assessed preoperatively, compared with during surgical procedures, when the patient is in a different position. The relationship of the rectum to the surrounding sphincteric mechanism has provided the rationale for sphincter-saving operations, which are being performed with increasing frequency for patients with ulcerative colitis and familial polyposis.[6]

BLOOD SUPPLY OF THE COLON. A comprehensive understanding of the vascular supply to the colon (Fig. 1) is essential for all surgeons performing primary colonic procedures as well as procedures in which the colon is used as a conduit, such as in esophageal replacements and urologic reconstructions. The cecum, ascending colon, hepatic flexure, and proximal portion of the transverse colon derive arterial blood supply from the ileocolic, right colic, and middle colic branches of the superior mesenteric artery. The inferior mesenteric artery supplies blood to the distal transverse colon, splenic flexure, descending colon, and sigmoid via the left colic artery and branches of the sigmoid and superior hemorrhoidal vessels. The rectum is supplied by a rich network of vessels from the middle hemorrhoidal and inferior hemorrhoidal arteries. As the main vessels course through the mesentery toward the bowel wall, they frequently bifurcate, and the arcades are formed 1 to 2 cm. from the mesenteric border of the bowel. In this manner, a continuous chain of communicating vessels is formed, and this has been referred to as the marginal artery of Drummond. The anastomosis or linking of arcades between the superior and inferior mesenteric vessels has been referred to as the long anastomosis of Riolan.

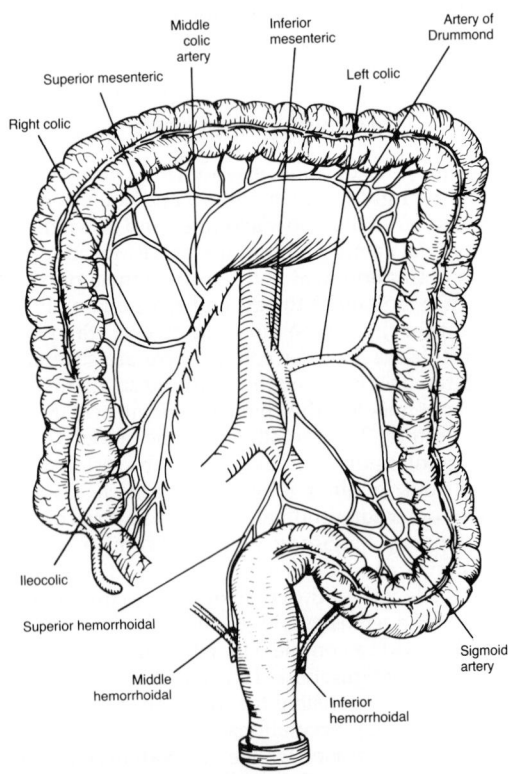

Figure 1. Anatomy and blood supply of the large intestine. (From Beart, R. W., Jr., Nivatvong, S., and Wolff, B.: The colon, rectum, and anus. *In* Nora, P. F. (ed.): Operative Surgery, 3rd ed., Philadelphia, W. B. Saunders Co., 1990.)

The colon is drained by a rich and vast network of lymphatics which frequently follow the course of the major vessels. The nodes may be involved with inflammatory or neoplastic diseases, and knowledge of their location is critical to curative cancer resections.

SURGICAL PROCEDURES

Surgical procedures for diseases of the colon continue to be among the most common operative procedures performed by surgeons. Although most of these procedures are standardized and are surrounded by a rich heritage and tradition (Fig. 2), nonetheless an evolution in management of selected patients with differing colonic diseases is occurring. Although other chapters concern specific disease entities and details of specific procedures, it appears quite appropriate to review the more general operations and principles involved with each.

In planning resection of the colon, certain specific factors should be carefully considered by the surgeon. It is essential to ensure adequate vascularity to all colonic anastomoses. The blood supply to the colon can be variable, specifically in segments that depend on good collateral vessels or marginal arcades. Ideally, one should be able to palpate pulsating vessels in the colonic mesentery; and, at the very least, active bleeding from the cut edges of the colon should be documented. Adequate mobilization of the colon is necessary to minimize tension on an anastomosis. The bacterial flora of the colon is significantly different both qualitatively and quantitatively from that of the small bowel, and efforts should be made to achieve adequate bowel preparation prior to colonic anastomoses. Atten-

tion to these general details increases the likelihood of a successful colon resection and reanastomosis, whether by means of the traditional hand-sewn technique or with the use of stapling devices.

The basic principles of surgical oncology apply to tumors involving the colon. Curative operations of the colon should be performed whenever possible. The surgeon should attempt to remove all of the malignant tissue from both the primary organ and any other structures locally involved as well as the lymphatic channels and tissue through which the primary tumor is likely to spread. In the context of tumors involving the large intestine, adherence to these principles requires ligation of the appropriate vessels at their origin. The exact distance of proximal and distal bowel that should be removed with a tumor has been the subject of considerable debate in recent years. Nonetheless, certain standard principles still apply. These include (1) obtaining tumor-free margins and (2) removing all lymphatic drainage. The goals and concepts concerning benign lesions of the colon are different from those for neoplastic disease. As such, the nature of the recommended operations also differs. In general, in benign conditions of the colon, it is not necessary to remove the mesentery, and one can stay closer to the bowel wall. This is usually a safer surgical approach.

Tumors of the cecum and ascending colon are generally managed by a right hemicolectomy with resection of the ileocecal valve, entire ascending colon, and proximal transverse colon to the level of, but not including, the middle colic vessels. If one follows the concepts that have previously been stated, malignant lesions in this area necessitate ligation of the ileocolic and right colic vessels at their origin from the superior mesenteric artery. Reconstruction is generally by an ileotransverse colos-

Figure 2. Extent of resection recommended for malignant lesions of colon. (From Beart, R. W., Jr., Nivatvongs, S., and Wolff, B.: The colon, rectum and anus. *In* Nora, P. F. (Ed.): Operative Surgery Principles and Techniques. Philadelphia, W. B. Saunders Company, 1990.

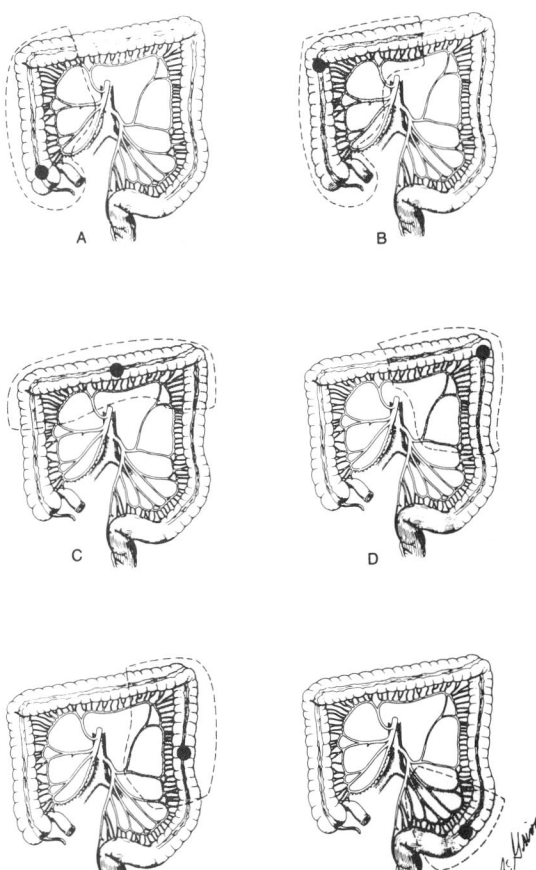

tomy. Lesions involving the hepatic flexure are managed by a similar operative approach with resection of the transverse colon beyond the middle colic vessels. Lesions involving the mid transverse colon are managed by transverse colectomy. For lesions involving the descending colon, the splenic flexure and descending colon are generally removed, with an end-to-end anastomosis. Sigmoid resections are frequently performed for malignant disease as well as benign conditions secondary to complications arising from diverticulosis. The length of bowel resected as well as mesentery varies in accordance with the indication for operation. For a malignant process, the inferior mesenteric artery should be ligated at its origin from the aorta. Reanastomosis following resection of lesions from the rectosigmoid can be safely performed either with a hand-sewn technique or with stapling devices. In fact, the advent of stapling

devices and the continuing refinement in their development have allowed surgeons to perform low anastomoses (low anterior resection) that previously would not have been technically possible (Fig. 3). Tumors involving the rectum that preclude low anterior resection and restoration of gastrointestinal continuity are best managed by a combined excision of the distal rectum and anus with anterior resection and abdominoperineal resection.

The operations described above are frequently modified where benign disease is concerned. Total proctocolectomy—complete resection of the colon, rectum, and anus—has been the standard of care for patients with severe ulcerative colitis. In recent years, newer procedures that preserve sphincteric and anal function have been introduced, and considerable experience has been gained by a number of surgeons.[6,7,25,46,60] Al-

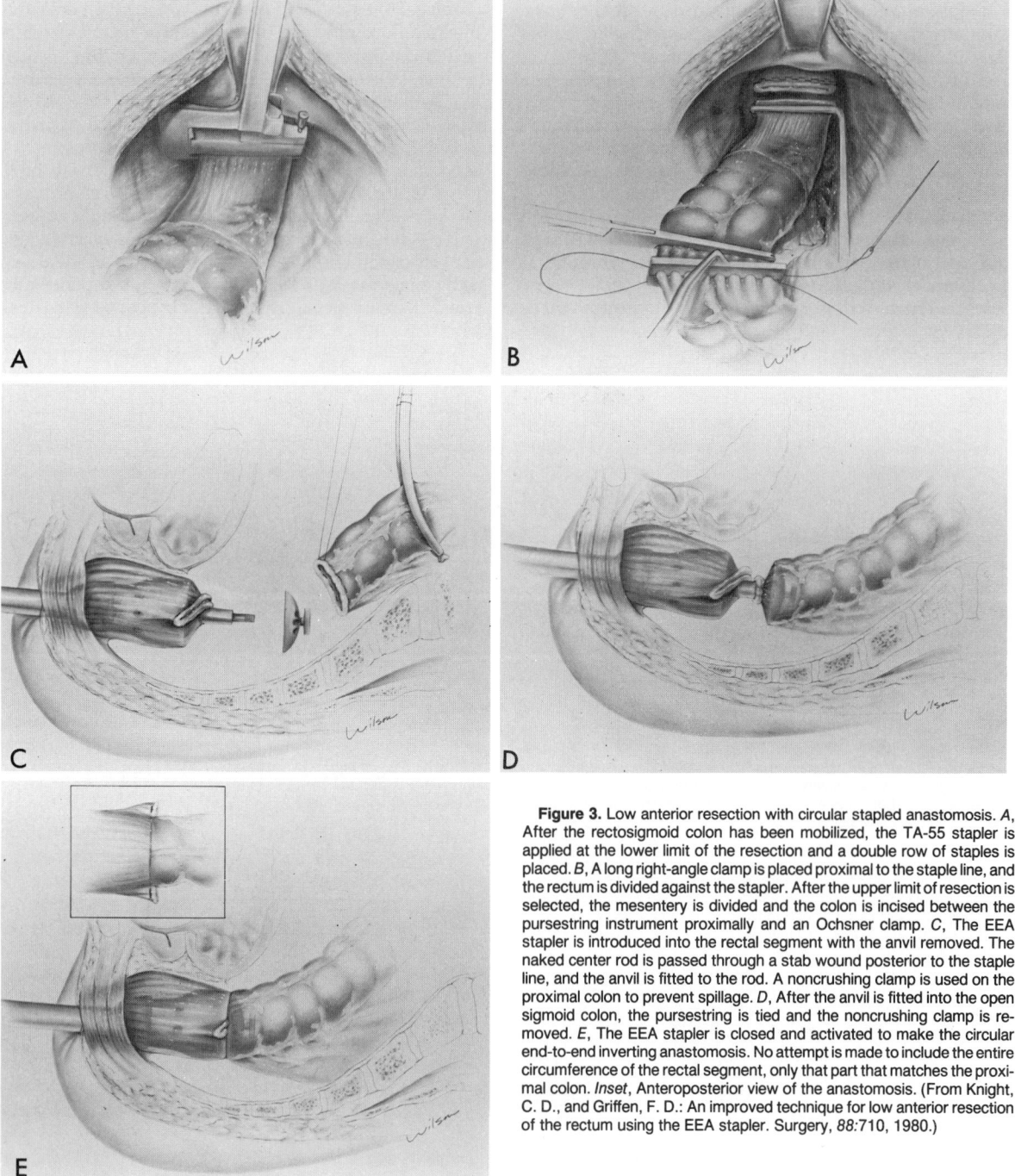

Figure 3. Low anterior resection with circular stapled anastomosis. *A*, After the rectosigmoid colon has been mobilized, the TA-55 stapler is applied at the lower limit of the resection and a double row of staples is placed. *B*, A long right-angle clamp is placed proximal to the staple line, and the rectum is divided against the stapler. After the upper limit of resection is selected, the mesentery is divided and the colon is incised between the pursestring instrument proximally and an Ochsner clamp. *C*, The EEA stapler is introduced into the rectal segment with the anvil removed. The naked center rod is passed through a stab wound posterior to the staple line, and the anvil is fitted to the rod. A noncrushing clamp is used on the proximal colon to prevent spillage. *D*, After the anvil is fitted into the open sigmoid colon, the pursestring is tied and the noncrushing clamp is removed. *E*, The EEA stapler is closed and activated to make the circular end-to-end inverting anastomosis. No attempt is made to include the entire circumference of the rectal segment, only that part that matches the proximal colon. *Inset*, Anteroposterior view of the anastomosis. (From Knight, C. D., and Griffen, F. D.: An improved technique for low anterior resection of the rectum using the EEA stapler. Surgery, *88:*710, 1980.)

though the specific details of these procedures may vary, the concepts are similar. These procedures are described in greater detail in another chapter.

Colostomy

The term *colostomy* refers to the creation of a stoma, which in effect is an opening of the bowel onto the surface of the abdomen. Colostomies, whether temporary or permanent, are performed for a number of indications in patients with colonic and gastrointestinal disorders. Several techniques for performing a colostomy have been described, and each has specific advantages and disadvantages applicable in different settings. It is essential that surgeons caring for patients with colonic disorders be well informed concerning the surgical options in the creation of a large bowel stoma.[1]

Colostomy may be necessary (1) to function as the site of elimination of feces when the distal colon or rectum has been removed; (2) to divert the fecal stream to protect a distal anastomosis; (3) to decompress a more distal colonic obstruction and serve as a "vent"; and (4) to temporarily divert the fecal stream from a pathologic process to be managed at a later date. Depending on the specific indication and individual setting, the surgeon may choose to perform either a temporary or a permanent colostomy. The ideal temporary colostomy should provide adequate fecal diversion, be safe to construct, and be easy to reanastomose when one is restoring gastrointestinal continuity. A loop, or "double-barreled" colostomy, is typically performed when diversion is temporary. This is generally achieved by exteriorizing a segment of the colon and then making an opening in the loop of bowel through the taeniae. This procedure is relatively straightforward and can be performed expeditiously without significant manipulation or dissection. Question has arisen whether or not this procedure is completely *diverting* in nature.[62] To address this concern, many surgeons have developed the practice of stapling the distal segment and thereby creating, in essence, an end-colostomy. Although a transverse colostomy is a satisfactory temporary stoma, in general, it should not be performed in clinical settings where permanent diversion is anticipated. Several problems can occur with this type of stoma, which, although not life-threatening, can cause considerable nuisance and discomfort for the patient. The material discharged from a transverse colostomy is frequently semi-liquid, and achieving a satisfactory seal with an appliance may therefore be difficult. In addition, the size of the stoma is frequently bulky, and this adds to the difficulty of appliance management. Moreover, there appears to be a predisposition for prolapse and peristomal hernias with this type of colostomy. In general, permanent fecal diversion from this portion of the gastrointestinal tract can best be achieved by creation of an ileostomy rather than a proximal transverse loop colostomy.

When distal resection of the colon is indicated but primary anastomosis ill-advised because of associated inflammation and/or intra-abdominal sepsis, a Hartmann procedure is often performed. This involves sigmoid resection with oversewing or closure of the distal rectal pouch and creation of an end descending colostomy. This type of stoma although generally temporary should be created with the use of the same principles and techniques of a more permanent stoma. A permanent colostomy is generally performed following abdominoperineal resection in patients with rectal tumors. Because of the position of the stoma in the distal colon, many of these patients are able to eliminate feces on a schedule and may not require a bag or appliance. Creation of sigmoid colostomies should be performed meticulously, and great attention paid to the location of the stoma. The ideal stoma should be situated in the left iliac fossa and pierce the abdominal wall through the rectus muscles. Positioning of the stoma in this location reduces the likelihood of peristomal herniation. Internal hernias around the colostomy can be avoided by securing the mesentery to the left paracolic gutter and closing this defect with a series of interrupted sutures. The key to providing an adequate cutaneous stoma for application of an appliance is having the mesentery elevated through the stomal site and on minimal tension. Ideally, one should strive to have a stoma that although not as high as an ileostomy is nevertheless a quarter to a half an inch above the skin to permit application and good fitting of an appliance. The frequency with which patients eliminate feces through a colostomy is individual, although it can be regulated to some extent in most patients by diet. Attention to the details described above for creation of colostomies should reduce the associated complications, which include stomal stenosis and necrosis secondary to ischemia, prolapse and peristomal hernias, internal hernias, and more life-threatening complications such as bleeding and perforation.[57]

Colostomy takedown and restoration of gastrointestinal continuity is not an innocuous procedure and has been associated with significant morbidity.[40,42,54] Experience suggests that takedown of an end-colostomy has significantly more morbidity than takedown of a simple loop colostomy. These data should be considered at the time of initial laparotomy when the decision is made as to which type of stoma to use. Before colostomy closure, patients should undergo radiographic or endoscopic evaluation and bowel preparation. These procedures should be approached and managed with the same concern and principles that apply to primary colonic resections.

For references, see page 908.

II

PHYSIOLOGY

Joel J. Roslyn, M.D., and Michael J. Zinner, M.D.

Unlike the small intestine, which has been the subject of countless *in vivo* and *in vitro* physiologic investigations, the physiologic mechanisms that govern function of the colon have remained poorly defined until recent years. Although it has been known that the primary functions of the colon are to serve as an organ for storage and elimination of intestinal contents, only now are the complicated interaction and interdependence between the physiochemical factors, central and enteric nervous system, and gut peptides that serve to coordinate and facilitate the absorptive activity of the colon and colonic motility appreciated. Simply stated, the four primary functions of the human colon are (1) to absorb sodium and water and thereby concentrate fecal contents; (2) to secrete potassium and bicarbonate; (3) to serve as a storage reservoir for fecal contents; and (4) to facilitate elimination of intestinal waste. The mechanisms that govern this latter function and maintenance of continence are quite elaborate and are focused in the rectum.[15] Interested readers should see the references on page 908 for several excellent reviews on this subject.

ABSORPTION

Although the small intestine is largely responsible for the absorption of essentially all nutrients that enter the gastrointestinal tract, the colon is responsible for absorption of large amounts of water from the feces, so in essence drying the fecal mass. Although the entire length of the colon (approximately 135 cm.) has the capacity to absorb water and specific electrolytes, the majority of this absorptive activity actually occurs in the ascending colon. The total absorptive area of the large bowel is estimated to be approximately 900 sq. cm. Its capacity to absorb water and electrolytes is reflected by the 10-fold reduction in water volume that occurs there regularly. Numerous studies have suggested that approximately 1000 to 1500 ml. of water is delivered from the ileum into the cecum during a 24-hour period. This effluent has a sodium concentration of approximately 200 mEq. per liter. The total volume of stool water is estimated to be only 100 to 150 ml. per day, with a sodium concentration of 25 to 50 mEq. per liter.[56] Therefore, despite the significant concentration effect and absorption of water, which is continuing, the sodium concentration is paradoxically quite low in the stool effluent. Numerous *in vivo* and *in vitro* electrophysiologic studies have demonstrated that the mechanism (Fig. 1) by which this occurs is an active transport process directed against a combined transepithelial chemical concentration and electropotential difference.[12,64,66] Numerous factors have been identified that influence water and electrolyte movement by the colon. These include the mucosal cyclic adenosine monophosphate (cAMP) level,[11] pH, osmolarity, and ions such as fatty acids[13] and bile acids.[48] More recent information suggests that water and electrolyte movement is also controlled to some extent by the hormonal milieu.[10,26,32] The net effect of active sodium transport is that this process influences the return of water from the lumen, and therefore absorption of water is a passive process.

In addition to being the site of sodium and water absorption, the colon also has an important role in the enterohepatic circulation of bile acids insofar as there is some absorption of these solutes (less than ileum) from the colon by nonionic or passive fusion.[49] This activity assumes even greater significance in patients in whom the terminal ileum is either diseased or surgically absent. In addition, the colon is the site of bile acid dehydroxylation, the process by which primary bile acids are converted to secondary bile acids. Bile acids affect colon transport of water and electrolytes. In the setting of ileal disease or following resection, conjugated bile acids that are normally absorbed in the distal small bowel are hydrolyzed by colonic bacteria and may induce a form of secretory diarrhea.

SECRETION

Studies in both animals[24] and humans[34] would suggest that potassium is actively secreted by colonic epithelium. This activity is stimulated by exogenous or endogenous mineralocorticoids. There is also evidence that bicarbonate is secreted by the human colon as an active process directed against both a chemical concentration difference and an electrical potential difference.[23] Alterations in net fluid and electrolyte movement in the colon have been documented after administration of a number of laxatives[9,61] as well as in disease states, such as ulcerative colitis, granulomatous colitis, congenital chloridorrhea and watery diarrhea syndrome.[59]

During the past 15 years, considerable attention and investigative efforts have focused on the hormonal regulation of ion transport in the small and large intestine in both health and disease. Although there is considerable evidence that several peptides and bioactive amines modulate small intestinal ion transport, several studies suggest that cAMP,[11] prostaglandins,[58] and gut peptides, including vasoactive intestinal polypeptide[10,59] influence colonic ion transport. The true physiologic role of these substances on colonic absorptive and secretory function remains to be defined.

COLONIC MOTILITY

As mentioned previously, the storage and excretory functions of the colon are closely intertwined and are dependent on a series of neural-mediated reflexes and smooth muscle contractions that are probably regulated to some extent by the autonomic nervous system. The advent of new manometric methodology and studies of electrical activity have facilitated the characterization of colonic motor activity. It is thought that ingestion of food stimulates the production of mass movements, strong, propulsive contractions moving in a caudad direction, which serve to move fecal material down into the descending and distal colon. These propulsive contractions may be altered in patients with irritable bowel syndrome and may actually be modified by laxatives or antidiarrheal drugs. Increased understanding of colonic motor activity has improved management of patients with gastrointestinal disease in the preoperative and postoperative state. The importance of understanding colonic motor activity is underscored by the recent recognition of a number of "dysmotility" syndromes that can mimic mechanical bowel obstruction.[18,19,39,47]

Evacuation of stool and rectal continence are key activities of the normal human colon. The sphincteric mechanism surrounding the anorectum is composed of an internal and external anal sphincter. The internal sphincter consists of circular smooth muscle, and its tonically contracted state prevents passage of stool. As the rectum becomes distended, the internal sphincter relaxes and the striated muscle of the external sphincter is stimulated, and its activity in conjunction with the levator muscle groups serves to facilitate defecation and passage of stool.[15,29,43] The anorectum is richly innervated, and the sensory and motor pathways that regulate and control continence and defecation have been well defined.[70] The interested reader is referred to the references on page 908 for more detailed descriptions of this most important process. Increased understanding of the processes and anatomic structures responsible for defecation and continence have greatly facilitated the development of new and innovative procedures for sphincter preservation in patients with such diseases as ulcerative colitis and familial polyposis.

For references, see page 908.

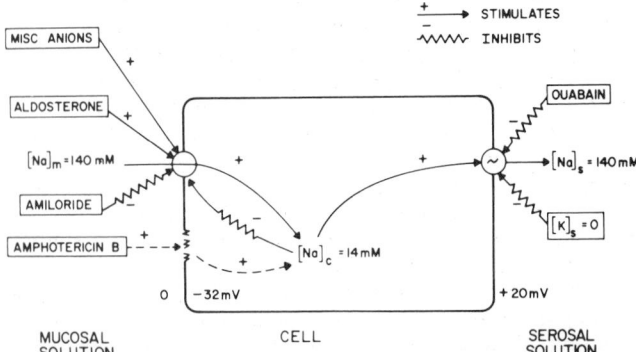

Figure 1. A cellular model for active sodium transport by mammalian colon. (From Schultz, E. G.: Ion transport by mammalian large intestine. *In* Johnson, L. R. (Ed.): Physiology of the Gastrointestinal Tract. New York, Raven Press, 1981.)

III ————————————————————————————————————

DIAGNOSTIC STUDIES

Joel J. Roslyn, M.D., and Michael J. Zinner, M.D.

The astute physician is directed toward the colon as the site of pathology on the basis of the patient's complaints and history. Given the critical nature that the colon has in storage and evacuation of feces, diseases of the colon, whether inflammatory or neoplastic in etiology, frequently lead to alteration of gastrointestinal function. This is frequently reflected by change in the caliber of the stool, diarrhea (contrasted with steatorrhea), constipation or obstipation, hematochezia, melena, or rectal tenesmus or urgency. Insofar as many systemic diseases and/or medications can affect colonic activity, it is essential that a complete history be obtained from all patients presenting for evaluation of a gastrointestinal disorder that may involve the colon or rectum. It is not uncommon for patients with carcinomas of the ascending colon or cecum to be asymptomatic in terms of gastrointestinal function but present with general fatigue, evidence of hypochromic, microcytic anemia, or heme-positive stools. In contrast, those individuals with malignant processes involving the sigmoid colon frequently present with obstructive symptoms and may have marked alterations in their bowel habits. All patients in whom a diagnosis of colonic disease is being considered should undergo a complete physical examination including pelvic and rectal examinations. Considerable information can often be gained from visualization and palpation, with specific attention given to systemic disease processes that may affect the colon, and the presence of stigmata of portal hypertension, malnutrition, or the palpation of masses that may be inflammatory or neoplastic in origin. Examination of the stool for blood either directly or by guaiac testing is an essential part of all physical examinations, especially in the setting where carcinoma of the colon is being considered.[2] The efficacy of mass screening, however, remains to be defined.[65,69]

Other diagnostic studies should be considered based on the individual clinical setting. Ordering tests for the sake of completeness should be avoided; and attention is focused on the specific problem with diagnostic tests ordered only as necessary. While no serum study is specific for any colonic disease, many laboratory evaluations can be helpful. Varying degrees of malnutrition may be present in individuals with either long-standing inflammatory bowel disease, whether ulcerative colitis or granulomatous colitis, or in individuals with malignancies involving the colon. Baseline biochemical assessment of the patient's nutritional status provides important information concerning the problem and may assist in planning the timing of definitive therapy. Liver function tests are particularly helpful in the clinical evaluation of systemic processes or when liver metastases may be present. The utility of carcinoembryonic antigen (CEA) continues to be a source of considerable controversy.[14,51] Most agree that a CEA level is appropriate for monitoring patients after resection for colon carcinomas. One must be cognizant of the fact that this assay, while perhaps sensitive, is not specific for carcinoma of the colon and may be elevated with other malignant processes as well as a number of benign causes. Perhaps the most controversial issue regarding the utility of monitoring CEA levels concerns the appropriate clinical course that should be followed in patients with rising CEA levels after colon resection who have no symptoms or other evidence of recurrent disease. Interested readers should refer to appropriate references.

In addition to the history, physical examination, and labora-

tory evaluation, a number of other diagnostic modalities should be considered in specific clinical settings. For many years, radiographic evaluation with contrast studies was the standard in evaluating colonic problems. While this technique remains invaluable, particularly for identifying anatomic location, it is now apparent that endoscopy with direct visualization of the colonic mucosa has become the single most important diagnostic (and occasionally therapeutic) modality available. Nuclear medicine studies and angiography continue to have important roles in the evaluation and management of patients with hemorrhage from the large intestine.

RADIOGRAPHIC EVALUATION

Plain abdominal radiographs and contrast studies of the large intestine continue to be invaluable diagnostic methods in the evaluation of patients with suspected colonic disease. These tests are quick, easy to perform, noninvasive, and associated with essentially no morbidity. They are frequently quite helpful in directing the endoscopist and/or surgeon to the site of pathology and in general provide important information. Today, contrast studies of the colon, and colonoscopy should be viewed as complementary procedures. While barium studies fail to detect small polyps and/or carcinomas, they continue to be an important screening test in patients with colon lesions. It is essential when ordering a barium enema that the clinician inform the radiologist of the presumptive diagnosis and in addition provide as much clinical information as possible. This dialogue facilitates the interpretation of the radiograph and enhances the ability to make an accurate diagnosis. The communication between clinician and radiologist is particularly important when the concern is colonic obstruction and/or perforation. In these settings, consideration should be given to the use of a water-soluble agent such as Gastrografin.

ENDOSCOPY

Although the importance of visualization of the gastrointestinal tract was recognized by Hippocrates, the discipline of fiberoptics became a reality in the 1960s and 1970s, and the endoscopic era began. With an ever expanding technology, ability to visually inspect the colon from the rectum to the cecum is such that this can now be performed safely in outpatient endoscopic units routinely. With improving optics in a higher quality instrument, diagnostic and therapeutic colonoscopy has become routine and has, in effect, revolutionized diagnostic capabilities in the management of patients with colonic disorders. Although colonoscopy should be performed only by trained surgical and gastrointestinal endoscopists, the recent introduction of a 60-cm. flexible sigmoidoscope has allowed the nonspecialist to participate in diagnostic evaluation of the colon. Nevertheless, expertise is required to manipulate the flexible sigmoidoscope, and all individuals practicing this technique should have basic training. Currently, endoscopic evaluation of the colon remains the most important technique in the accurate diagnosis of colonic disease, especially carcinoma.[52] A variety of endoscopic instruments are available, depending on the expertise of the endoscopist and the presumed site of the lesion. The anoscope or proctoscope is invaluable for the assessment of internal hemorrhoids and rectal tumors that are within 8 to 10 cm. of the anal verge. Generally no premedication or anesthetic is required for introduction, but care must be taken in passing the instrument through the anus and allowance made for relaxation of the sphincteric mechanism prior to complete insertion. Rigid sigmoidoscopy allows visualization of the distal 20 to 25 cm. of the colon. This technique should be mastered by all general surgeons and internists. Physicians performing rigid sigmoidoscopy should be aware of the anatomic features of the rectum and sigmoid, including the posterior orientation and angulation, which generally occurs at the junction of the rectosigmoid and sigmoid colon. This examination can be performed with the patient in the knee-chest, jackknife, or lateral position. In some cases, flexible sigmoidoscopy has advantages over the rigid instrument. In essence, this 60-cm. colonoscope, which is state of the art in terms of fiberoptics, allows the same flexibility as does full colonoscopy regarding cauterization, polypectomy, and biopsy. With training, individuals should be able to master this technique and thereby perform a more meticulous examination of the colon.

Colonoscopy is the most accurate method of assessing colonic disease. A skilled endoscopist can maneuver the scope to visualize the entire colon from the anus to the cecum. There are several general indications for flexible sigmoidoscopy or for colonoscopy, including (1) diagnosis, (2) biopsy to confirm or establish the nature of a disease process or malignant lesion, (3) therapeutic removal of polyps,[30] (4) management of bleeding lesions,[63] (5) surveillance and follow-up of lesions previously removed endoscopically or surgically, (6) detection and removal of foreign bodies, and (7) early cancer detection or another screening process. In addition, colonoscopy has also been used to facilitate endoscopic dilatation of anastomotic strictures.[8] Although vast experience throughout the world has suggested that colonoscopy is a safe procedure that can be performed with minimal morbidity and essentially no mortality,[33,44] a number of potential contraindications should be considered. These include (1) suspected colonic perforation, (2) acute fulminating inflammatory bowel disease, (3) peritonitis with secondary paralytic ileus, and (4) acute inflammatory disease of the anus. Unlike rigid or flexible sigmoidoscopy, satisfactory performance of colonoscopy generally requires varying degrees of intravenous sedation. Therefore, the general medical condition of the patient and specifically cardiopulmonary status should be carefully considered before proceeding with a colonoscopic procedure. A number of medications are employed by endoscopists; some of the more popular ones are meperidine and the benzodiazepines, alone or in combination. In addition, glucagon administered intravenously is frequently used as an adjunct to facilitate smooth muscle relaxation. General anesthesia is generally not required for colonoscopy.

The efficacy and safety of diagnostic and/or therapeutic colonoscopy are dependent on the presence of a well-cleansed bowel. A satisfactory bowel preparation can be achieved by means of a number of techniques, including mechanical preparation with enemas and simple irrigation of the gastrointestinal tract with saline, mannitol preparation, or commercially available physiologic preparations.[20,28,31,50] The commercially available preparations, including solutions containing polyethylene glycol (PEG), are easy and safe and can be completed in a matter of hours. In the authors' experience, these latter preparations have largely replaced the more traditional regimens, which required the patient's being maintained on clear liquids for 24 to 48 hours prior to the procedure as well as the administration of citrate of magnesia, castor oil, and tap water enemas. The specific regimen to be employed for bowel preparation should be carefully considered in patients with advanced diverticular disease, inflammatory bowel disease, or severe constipation. In those individuals in whom partial or total colonic obstruction is suspected, the use of tap water enemas is recommended, rather than irrigating solutions. Individuals performing colonoscopy should be aware of their limitations and be well trained in maneuvers that may be required to manipulate the scope through a tortuous or redundant sigmoid colon and should become familiar with the endoscopic appearance of colonic mucosal and malignant diseases.

OTHER DIAGNOSTIC TESTS

The use of intravenous pyelography and ureteral stents in the management of patients undergoing laparotomy for colonic disease continues to be controversial. The ureters, either right or left, may be primarily or secondarily involved with inflammatory or malignant processes of the colon. Moreover, in patients who have already undergone previous laparotomy for gastrointestinal or vascular disease, the normal anatomic position of the ureters may be altered. Although it has not been the authors' practice routinely to obtain these studies or place stents preoperatively in all patients undergoing colonic or pelvic surgery, these measures are helpful in individuals with large malignant lesions, those with complex inflammatory processes, those undergoing reoperation, or those having had prior pelvic radiation. Computed tomographic (CT) scans and more recently magnetic resonance imaging (MRI) have been particularly helpful in the assessment of patients with rectal tumors with regard to resectability. The evolving management of these patients including the neoadjuvant use of radiation therapy has heightened awareness of the utility of these studies. In addition, these scans may be helpful in the assessment of other malignant processes that may involve the gastrointestinal tract, contiguous organs, or the liver. The decision to proceed with one of these studies again should be individualized on the basis of the clinical setting. Other serum and radiologic examinations may be indicated, depending on the specific colonic disorder. A precise anatomic and pathologic diagnosis is now feasible in most patients with colonic disorders. The recognition of a number of motor disturbances involving primarily the anorectum has provided impetus for the development of several new diagnostic modalities that attempt to quantify motor activity in this region.[41,45,71] The ultimate role of these tests remains to be defined.

For references, see page 908.

IV

INTESTINAL ANTISEPSIS

Joel J. Roslyn, M.D., and Michael J. Zinner, M.D.

The microflora and microbiology of the colon are important to the activity of this organ in both health and disease. Maintenance of the normal ecologic relationships is responsible for the physiologic role that the colon has in the enterohepatic circulation of bile acids. Alterations in the microflora may be observed in clinically significant syndromes. Perhaps more important to the surgeon, however, is the effect that the qualitative and quantitative characteristics of the microbiologic environment in the colon have on the outcome of colonic surgery. Through the years, investigative efforts have focused on understanding this interaction, and attempts have been directed to control the environment to facilitate safe surgical therapy. The methods employed in preparing the bowel for both endoscopic and surgical procedures have evolved over the past 30 to 40 years. Understanding the scientific basis for this evolution is critical for the surgeon involved in planning and management of patients with colonic disease.

MICROBIOLOGY OF THE COLON

The human colon is site of more than 400 bacterial species. Unlike the stomach and proximal small bowel, both of which have a bacterial count generally considered no greater than 10^5 organisms, the colon has a bacterial concentration that approaches 10^{12} CFU ml. The organisms found in the colon vary widely, depending on the clinical situation, but, in general, include large numbers of both aerobic and anaerobic bacteria (Table 1). Nearly one third of the fecal dry weight consists of bacteria. The predominant bacteria are anaerobic and include *Bacteroides, Bifidobacterium,* and *Eubacterium.* There are a number of host and microbial factors that interact to maintain a relatively stable microfloral population within the colon. When these factors are altered, groups of bacteria may proliferate and normal physiologic function may be impaired, or the patient may be at increased risk for development of subsequent infection. A series of epidemiologic studies have attempted to demonstrate a link between colon cancer and intestinal microflora.[3,16] The exact mechanism responsible for this link remains to be identified. Perhaps the most important clinical manifestation of colonic microflora concerns the risk of infection following colonic surgical procedures. Analysis of the available litera-

TABLE 1. Concentration of Bacteria Present in Normal Human Small and Large Intestine

Bacteria	Ileum	Colon
Total bacterial count	10^3-10^9	10^8-10^{12}
Anaerobes		
Bacteroides sp.	10^3-10^7	10^9-10^{12}
Lactobacillus	10^2-10^5	10^6-10^{12}
Clostridia sp.	10^2-10^4	10^3-10^{10}
Aerobes		
Coliforms	10^2-10^7	10^5-10^8
Streptococcus sp.	10^2-10^6	10^4-10^7
Lactobacillus	10^2-10^5	10^3-10^7
Staphylococcus sp.	10^2-10^4	10^2-10^4

ture suggests that the rate of wound infection in patients undergoing colonic procedures who have not received prophylactic antibiotics may be as high as 75 per cent.[17,37,68] This concept has been largely responsible for the development of approaches for intestinal antisepsis.

HISTORICAL ASPECTS

Much of the progress observed during the past 50 years in the development of colonic surgery as a discipline has followed increased understanding of the factors responsible for postoperative septic complications and the mechanisms by which these can be controlled. The earliest attempts to control postoperative infection in colonic surgery focused on surgical manipulations that reduced the amount of intraoperative soilage. These included innovative colostomy techniques, extraperitoneal techniques for bowel anastomosis, and the development of special clamps and closed suture techniques. Despite these measures, the postoperative infection rate continued to be unacceptably high. Improved microbiologic and culture techniques demonstrating the high bacterial count in the colon ultimately prompted the introduction of bowel preparation as a preoperative adjunctive measure. The goals of bowel preparation include a mechanical cleansing of the bowel and an antibiotic reduction of micro-organisms. Through the years, these goals and concepts have remained crucial, although the mechanisms by which they are achieved have varied widely and continue to be the source of considerable controversy and investigation. A large number of controlled, prospective, randomized studies have clearly demonstrated that mechanical preparation (by whatever technique) and antibiotic protection (by a number of routes and agents) are most appropriate for intestinal antisepsis in preparation for colonic surgery.[4] The affirmation of these findings has prompted several investigators to emphasize that future studies of colon antisepsis should not include a true placebo arm in which mechanical preparation or antibiotic protection is omitted.[5] Nevertheless, methods employed for mechanical cleansing of the bowel and antibiotic protection continue to be investigated and are varied.

MECHANICAL PREPARATION

As previously stated, much of the dry weight of feces is bacteria. To reduce the bulk of feces and bacteria within the colon, mechanical cleansing of the colon has long been an integral feature of intestinal antisepsis and colon preparation. However, it appears that mechanical cleansing alone does not produce a significant reduction in the colony count of bacteria within the colon. For many years, mechanical preparation of the bowel consisted of a 3-day period during which the patient was maintained on clear liquids and received a variety of purgatives and laxatives. While the details of the specific regimens may have varied from institution to institution, they all shared certain potential problems. They were time-consuming, frequently requiring several days of hospitalization preoperatively, and were associated with varying degrees of physical exhaustion, patient compliance, and dissatisfaction. During the past 10 years, colonic lavage with a variety of solutions has been introduced as a viable alternative to the 3-day mechanical preparation component of the intestinal antisepsis program. The earliest attempts at colonic lavage with saline were associated with problems and potential risks, especially in elderly patients, due to sodium and water retention.[20] This system was modified to include the use of oral mannitol.[50] During the past several years, a commercially available electrolyte-polyethylene glycol solution has been introduced and widely tested.[28] Clinical trials have examined the efficacy of this solution as compared with more conventional mechanical preparations for colonoscopy and have clearly determined the newer solution to be safe, well tolerated, and cost-effective. This type of solution administered orally in 4 liters the day before operation generally provides excellent mechanical preparation of the bowel. Use of this solution has become the standard regimen for mechanical bowel preparation for elective colonic surgery.

ORAL VERSUS PARENTERAL ANTIBIOTICS FOR COLONIC SURGERY

The rationale for the use of antibiotics preoperatively for patients undergoing colonic surgery is to reduce the number of bacteria within the colon. This concept is well accepted. However, there continues to be controversy concerning the most efficacious way of achieving this goal. The role of oral antibiotics rather than parenteral agents, together with the selection of specific agents, continues to be debated and studied. In 1973, Nichols and associates[53] demonstrated the benefit of orally administered, nonabsorbable antibiotics in combination with mechanical cleansing, contrasted with only the latter. The findings of this rather limited study were confirmed several years later in a prospective, randomized, multi-institutional trial. This study of over 1000 patients undergoing colonic surgery suggested that there was no significant benefit from the addition of parenteral antibiotic prophylaxis to an appropriate mechanical preparation with oral nonabsorbed antimicrobial agents.[4] A large number of studies have subsequently attempted to identify the ideal agents for either oral antimicrobial therapy or parenteral administration.[21,22,27,35-38,67] There are certain characteristics that any ideal prophylactic antibiotic regimen, whether oral or parenteral, should include. The regimen selected should provide broad suppression of fecal flora with high activity against aerobic and anaerobic organisms. Toxicity should be minimal, and there should be no emergence of resistant organisms. Additionally, a single agent is preferable to multiple drugs, there should be a short term of administration, and the drugs should be cost-effective. Orally administered neomycin and erythromycin base or metronidazole have become the most common agents used for oral antibiotic preparation (Table 2). These agents are generally administered at 1:00 P.M., 2:00 P.M., and 11:00 P.M. the day before operation. It was initially thought that absorption of these drugs was not desirable. It is now thought that increased tissue levels of the drug at sites distant from the colon aid the normal host resistance mechanisms when contamination of the wound occurs.

Appropriate regimens for parenteral antibiotics should include agents that have considerable activity against aerobes and anaerobes. Several investigators have reviewed multiple-drug regimens, including aminoglycosides and metronidazole or clindamycin, rather than single-agent regimens. In recent years, the second-generation cephalosporins have gained considerable popularity as useful agents for antimicrobial prophylaxis. However, these combinations or single agents are not effective against group D streptococci (enterococci). More recent studies have compared the third-generation cephalosporins used as a single dose compared to multiple dose administration of the second-generation cephalosporins.[35,55] These types of studies may ultimately help define the nuances of antibiotic utilization in patients undergoing colonic surgery. In the future, continuation of the evolution in management of patients undergoing elective and emergent colonic surgery will ensue. Undoubtedly, new antibiotics will be described, and perhaps understanding of the host factors that dictate the response to clinical infection will be such that whole new techniques will be described for colon and intestinal antisepsis.

SELECTED REFERENCES

Corman, M. D.: Colon and Rectal Surgery. Philadelphia, J. B. Lippincott Company, 1989.
  A very thorough and up-to-date discussion of all facets of colon and rectal surgery, this text contains excellent reviews of technical considerations.

DeCosse, J. J., and Todd, I. P.: Anorectal Surgery. Edinburgh, Churchill Livingstone, 1988.
  In addition to an excellent overview of surgical principles pertinent to anus and rectum, this volume contains an outstanding discussion and review of anorectal physiology.

Goligher, J., Duthrie, H., and Nixon, H.: Surgery of the Anus, Rectum, and Colon, 5th ed. London, Bailliere-Tindall, 1983.
  This work continues to be the classic text and provides an authoritative and thorough review of all clinical problems involving the large intestine, rectum, and anus.

Kelvin, F. M., and Gardiner, R.: Clinical Imaging of the Colon and Rectum. New York, Raven Press, 1987.
  This is a radiology text that is beautifully written and provides an excellent reference book for all clinicians involved in the care of patients with colorectal disease.

Shinya, H.: Colonoscopy: Diagnosis and Treatment of Colonic Diseases. New York, Igaku-Shoin, 1982.
  This work is a simple, well-written text covering the fundamentals of colonoscopy. The book is written by a surgical endoscopist and provides basic information.

REFERENCES

1. Abrams, J. S.: Abdominal Stomas: Indications, Operative Techniques, and Patient Care. Boston, John Wright. PSG, Inc., 1984.
2. American Cancer Society. Guidelines for the cancer-related checkup. CA, 30:208, 1980.
3. Aries, V., Crowther, J. S., Drassar, B. S., Hill, M. J., and Williams, R. E. O.: Bacteria and the aetiology of cancer of the large bowel. Gut, 10:334, 1969.
4. Bartlett, J. G., Condon, R. E., Gorbach, S. L., et al.: Veterans Administration's cooperative study on bowel preparation for elective colorectal operations. Ann. Surg., 188:249, 1978.
5. Baum, M. L., Anish, D. S., Chalmers, T. C., et al.: A survey of trials of antibiotic prophylaxis in colon surgery: Evidence against further use of no-treatment controls. N. Engl. J. Med., 305:795, 1981.
6. Becker, J. M.: Anal sphincter function after colectomy, mucosal proctectomy, and endorectal ileoanal pull-through. Arch. Surg., 119:526, 1984.
7. Becker, J. M., and Raymond, J. L.: Ileal pouch-anal anastomosis: A single surgeon's experience with 100 consecutive cases. Ann. Surg., 204:375, 1986.
8. Bedogni, G., Ricci, E., Pedrazzoli, C., et al.: Endoscopic dilatation of anastomotic colonic stenosis by different techniques: an alternative to surgery? Gastrointest. Endosc., 33:21, 1987.
9. Binder, H. J.: Pharmacology of laxatives. Annu. Rev. Pharmacol. Toxicol., 17:355, 1977.
10. Binder, H. J.: New modes for regulating intestinal ion transport. Gastroenterology, 78:642, 1980.
11. Binder, H. J., Felburn, C., and Volpe, B. T.: Bile salt alteration of colonic electrolyte transport: Role of cyclic adenosine monophosphate. Gastroenterology, 68:503, 1975.
12. Binder, H. J., Foster, E. S., Budinger, M. E., and Hayslett, J. P.: Mechanism of electroneutral sodium chloride absorption in distal colon of the rat. Gastroenterology, 93:449, 1987.
13. Binder, H. J., and Mehtan, P.: Short-chain fatty acids stimulate active sodium

TABLE 2. Common Regimens for Oral Antibiotic Bowel Preparation

Drugs	Regimen
I. Neomycin	1 gm. orally at 1 P.M., 2 P.M., and 11 P.M. the day before surgery
Erythromycin base	1 gm. orally at 1 P.M., 2 P.M., and 11 P.M. the day before surgery
II. Metronidazole	750 mg. every 8 hours for 72 hours

and chloride absorption in vitro in the rat distal colon. Gastroenterology, 96:989, 1989.

14. Bland, K. I., and Polk, H. C., Jr.: Therapeutic measures applied for the curative and palliative control of colorectal carcinoma. Surg. Annu., 15:123, 1983.

15. Burleigh, D. E., and D'Mello, A.: Physiology and pharmacology of the internal anal sphincter. In Henry, M. M., and Swash, M. (Eds.): Coloproctology and the Pelvic Floor: Pathophysiology and Management. London, Butterworths, 1985.

16. Burkitt, D. P.: Epidemiology of cancer of the colon and rectum. Cancer, 28:3, 1971.

17. Burton, R. C.: Postoperative wound infection in colonic and rectal surgery. Br. J. Surg., 60:363, 1973.

18. Christensen, J.: Motility of the colon. In Johnson, L. R. (Ed.): Physiology of the Gastrointestinal Tract. New York, Raven Press, 1990.

19. Christensen, J.: Intestinal pseudo-obstruction and paralytic ileus. In Moody, F. G., et al. (Eds.): Surgical Treatment of Digestive Disease. Chicago, Year Book Medical Publishers, 1990.

20. Chung, R. S., Gurll, N. J., and Berglund, E. M.: A controlled clinical trial of whole gut lavage as a method of bowel preparation for colonic operations. Am. J. Surg., 137:75, 1979.

21. Clarke, J. S., Condon, R. E., Bartlett, J. G., et al.: Preoperative oral antibiotics reduce septic complications of colon operations: Results of a randomized double-blind clinical trial. Ann. Surg., 186:251, 1977.

22. Condon, R. E., et al.: Efficacy of oral and systemic antibiotic prophylaxis in colorectal operations. Arch. Surg., 118:496, 1983.

23. Donowitz, M., Asarkof, N., and Pike, G.: Calcium dependence of serotonin induced changes in rabbit ileal electrolyte transport. J. Clin. Invest., 66:341, 1980.

24. Donowitz, M., and Binder, H. J.: Mechanism of fluid and electrolyte secretion in the germ free rat cecum. Dig. Dis. Sci., 24:551, 1979.

25. Dozois, R. R., Kelly, K. A., Welling, D. R., et al.: Ileal pouch-anal anastomosis: Comparison of results in familial adenomatous polyposis and chronic ulcerative colitis. Ann. Surg., 210:268, 1989.

26. Edmonds, C. J., and Marriott, J.: Electrical potential and short-circuit current in rat colon in vivo and the effect of aldosterone. J. Physiol., 210:1021, 1970.

27. Edmondson, H. T., and Rissing, J. P.: Prophylactic antibiotics in colon surgery: Cephaloridine vs. erythromycin and neomycin. Arch. Surg., 118:227, 1983.

28. Ernstoff, J. J., Howard, D. A., Marshall, J. B., Jumshyd, A., and McCullough, A. J.: A randomized blinded clinical trial of a rapid colonic lavage solution (Golytely) compared with standard preparation for colonoscopy and barium enema. Gastroenterology, 84:1512, 1983.

29. Felt-Bersma, R. J. F., Strijars, R. L. M., Janssen, J. J. W. M., et al.: The external anal sphincter: Relationship between anal manometry and anal electromyography and its clinical relevance. Dis. Colon Rectum, 32:112, 1989.

30. Forde, K. A.: Colonoscopic management of polypoid lesions. Surg. Clin. North Am., 69:1287, 1989.

31. Fordtran J. S., Santa Ana, C. A., vB. Cleveland, M.: A low-sodium solution for gastrointestinal lavage. Gastroenterology, 98:11, 1990.

32. Foster, E. S., Zimmerman, T. W., Hayslett, J. P., and Binder, H. J.: Corticosteroid alteration of active electrolyte transport in rat distal colon. Am. J. Physiol., 245:G668, 1983.

33. Ghazi, A., and Grossman, M.: Complications of colonoscopy and polypectomy. Surg. Clin. North Am., 62:889, 1982.

34. Gingell, J. C., Davies, M. W., and Shields, R.: Effect of a synthetic gastrin-like pentapeptide upon the intestinal transport of sodium, potassium, and water. Gut, 9:111, 1968.

35. Goransson, G., Nilsson-Ehle, I., Olsson, S., et al.: Single versus multiple dose doxycycline prophylaxis in elective colorectal surgery. Acta Chir. Scand., 150:245, 1984.

36. Groner, J. I., Edmiston, C. E. Jr., Krepel, C. J., et al.: The efficacy of oral antimicrobials in reducing aerobic and anaerobic colonic mucosal flora. Arch. Surg., 124:281, 1989.

37. Guglielmo, B. J., Hohn, D. C., Koo, P. J., et al.: Antibiotic prophylaxis in surgical procedures: A critical analysis of the literature. Arch. Surg., 118:943, 1983.

38. Khubchandani, I. T., Karamchandani, M. D., Sheets, J. A., et al.: Metronidazole vs. erythromycin, neomycin, and cefazolin in prophylaxis for colonic surgery. Dis. Colon Rectum, 32:17, 1989.

39. Klatt, G. R.: Role of subtotal colectomy in the treatment of incapacitating constipation. Am. J. Surg., 145:623, 1983.

40. Knox, A. J. S., Birkett, F. D. H., and Collins, C. D.: Closure of colostomy. Br. J. Surg., 58:669, 1971.

41. Lestar, B., Penninckx, F. M. and Kerremaus, R. P.: Defecometry: A new method for determining the parameters of rectal evacuation. Dis. Colon Rectum, 32:197, 1989.

42. Livingston, D. H., Miller, F. B., and Richardson, J. D.: Are the risks after colostomy closure exaggerated? Am. J. Surg., 158:17, 1989.

43. Lubowski, D. Z., Nicholls, R. J., Swash, M., and Jordan, M. J.: Neural control of internal anal sphincter function. Br. J. Surg., 74:668, 1987.

44. Macrae, F. A., Tank, G., and Williams, C. B.: Toward safer polypectomy: A report on the complications of 5000 diagnostic or therapeutic colonoscopies. Gut, 24:376, 1983.

45. Mahieu, P., Pringot, J., and Bodart, P.: Defaecography: description of a new procedure and results in normal patients. Gastrointest. Radiol., 9:247, 1984.

46. Martin, L. W., Lecoultre, C., and Schubert, W. K.: Total colectomy and mucosal proctectomy with preservation of continence in ulcerative colitis. Ann. Surg., 186:477, 1977.

47. McCready, R. A., and Beart, R. W.: The surgical treatment of incapacitating constipation with idiopathic megacolon. Mayo Clin. Proc., 54:779, 1979.

48. Mekhjian, H. S., and Phillips, S. F.: Perfusion of the canine colon with unconjugated bile acids: Effect of water and electrolyte transport, morphology, and bile acid absorption. Gastroenterology, 59:120, 1970.

49. Mekhjian, H. S., Phillips, S. F., and Hofmann, A. F.: Colonic absorption of unconjugated bile acids: Perfusion studies in man. Dig. Dis. Sci., 24:545, 1979.

50. Minervini, S., Alexander-Williams, J., I. A., Bentley, S., and Keighley, M. R. B.: Comparison of three methods of whole bowel irrigation. Am. J. Surg., 140:400, 1980.

51. Moertel, C. G., Schutt, A. J., and Go, V. L. W.: Carcinoembryonic antigen test for recurrent colorectal carcinoma: Inadequacy for early detection. J.A.M.A., 239:1065, 1978.

52. Neugut, A. I., and Pita, S.: Role of sigmoidoscopy in screening for colorectal cancer: A critical review. Gastroenterology, 95:492, 1988.

53. Nichols, R. L., Broido, P., Condon, R. E., et al.: Effect of preoperative neomycin-erythromycin intestinal preparation on the incidence of infectious complications following colon surgery. Ann. Surg., 178:453, 1973.

54. Parks, S. E., and Hastings, P. R.: Complications of colostomy closure. Am. J. Surg., 149:672, 1985.

55. Periti, P., Mazzei, T., and Tonelli, F.: Single-dose cefotetan vs. multiple-dose cefoxitin-antimicrobial prophylaxis in colorectal surgery: Results of a prospective, multicenter, randomized study. Dis. Colon Rectum, 32:121, 1989.

56. Phillips, S. F., and Giller, J.: The contribution of colon to water and electrolyte conservation in man. J. Lab. Clin. Med., 81:733, 1973.

57. Porter, J. A., Salvati, E. P., Rubin, R. J., and Eisenstat, T. E.: Complications of colostomies. Dis. Colon Rectum, 32:299, 1989.

58. Racusen, L. D., and Binder, H. J.: Effect of prostaglandin on ion transport across isolated colonic mucosa. Dig. Dis. Sci., 25:900, 1980.

59. Rambaud, J. C., Modigliani, R., Matuchansky, C., et al.: Pancreatic cholera studies on tumoral secretions and pathophysiology of diarrhea. Gastroenterology, 69:110, 1975.

60. Ravitch, M. M., and Sabiston, D. L., Jr.: Anal ileostomy with preservation of the sphincter: A proposed operation in patients requiring total colectomy for benign lesions. Surg. Gynecol. Obstet., 84:1095, 1947.

61. Saunders, D. R., Sillery, J., and Rachmilewitz, D.: Effect of dioctyl sodium sulfosuccinate on structure and function of rodent and human intestine. Gastroenterology, 69:380, 1975.

62. Schofield, P. F., Cade, D., and Lambert, M.: Dependent proximal loop colostomy: Does it defunction the distal colon? Br. J. Surg., 67:201, 1980.

63. Schrock, T. R.: Colonoscopic diagnosis and treatment of lower gastrointestinal bleeding. Surg. Clin. North Am., 69:1309, 1989.

64. Schultz, S. G.: Ion transport by mammalian large intestine. In Johnson, L. R. (Ed.): Physiology of the Gastrointestinal Tract. Vol. 2. New York, Raven Press, 1983.

65. Simon, J. B.: Occult blood screening for colorectal carcinoma: A critical review. Gastroenterology, 88:820, 1985.

66. Smith, F. W., and Sleisenger, M. H.: Physiology of the colon. In Sleisenger, M. H., and Fordtran, J. S. (Eds.): Gastrointestinal Disease: Pathophysiology, Diagnosis, Management. Philadelphia, W. B. Saunders Company, 1989.

67. Tonelli, F., Ficari, F., DeFarra, F., et al.: Short or long term prophylaxis with cefoxitin in elective colonic surgery. Coloproctology, 7:84, 1985.

68. Washington, J. A., Dearing, W. H., Judd, E. S., and Elveback, L. R.: Effect of postoperative antibiotic regimen on development of infection after intestinal surgery: A prospective, double-blind study. Ann. Surg., 180:567, 1974.

69. Winawer, S. J.: Detection and diagnosis of colorectal cancer. Cancer, 51:2519, 1983.

70. Womack, N. R., Morrison, J. F. B., and Williams, N. S.: The role of pelvic floor denervation in the aetiology of idiopathic faecal incontinence. Br. J. Surg., 73:404, 1986.

71. Womack, N. R., Williams, N. S., Holmfield, J. H., Morrison, J. F., and Simpkins, K. C.: New method for the dynamic assessment of anorectal function in constipation. Br. J. Surg., 72:994, 1985.

V _____

DIVERTICULAR DISEASE OF THE COLON

Anthony L. Imbembo, M.D., and Robert W. Bailey, M.D.

HISTORICAL ASPECTS

Diverticular disease of the colon has often been termed a disease of the twentieth century.[41] Until the early 1900s, the condition was only of occasional pathologic interest, being described in sporadic case reports. In 1904, its anatomic basis was defined, and it was suggested that diverticular inflammation was due to impaction of a fecalith.[4] The latter observation also was correlated with the pathologic findings of perforation, abscess formation, and fistulization. In 1907, the first report advocating surgical resection for complicated diverticulitis was presented by Mayo at the American Surgical Association.[29] Even in this early report, the advantages of creating a diverting colostomy ("temporary anus") or of performing a primary resection, when technically feasible, were expressed. In 1917, Telling and Gruner published an extensive report providing one of the most thorough reviews of diverticular disease to that time.[55] Since these initial accounts, the incidence of diverticular disease in Western countries has apparently increased from an estimated 5 per cent in 1910 to more than 40 per cent in 1970.[22] This dramatic increase has been attributed both to increased recognition of diverticular disease and to changing environmental conditions. The rapid evolution of an industrialized society corresponds with the observed increase in prevalence of the disease in the United States, Great Britain, and Western Europe.

DEFINITION

Diverticula are saclike protrusions of the colonic wall, varying in size from a few millimeters to several centimeters. They can be classified as either "true" or "false" diverticula. True diverticula contain all layers of the bowel wall present in normal colon. True diverticula are believed to be congenital in origin, whereas the much more common false diverticula are thought to be acquired. False diverticula, or "pseudodiverticula," represent herniations of the mucosa and submucosa through the muscular layer of the bowel wall. Unless otherwise stated in the text, the term *diverticula* refers to the predominant lesion, namely, colonic pseudodiverticula. The term *diverticulosis* simply indicates the presence of multiple diverticula of the colon. The mere existence of diverticula does not connote significant morbidity or mortality. The morbidity associated with this disease relates primarily to the development of diverticular inflammation or of hemorrhage.

INCIDENCE AND ETIOLOGY

The current prevalence of diverticular disease in the general population is between 35 and 50 per cent, as estimated by several large autopsy and radiographic series.[22] The incidence appears, therefore, to have strikingly increased over the last 50 years since earlier studies reported an overall incidence of only 5 to 10 per cent. The incidence is also clearly related to patient age. Prevalence is estimated to be less than 5 per cent at age 40, increasing to 30 per cent by age 60, and as high as 65 per cent by age 85.[41] Males and females appear to be affected equally. Geographically, diverticular disease is much more common in the United States and Western Europe than in other, less industrialized regions such as Africa, South America, and Asia. Although dietary factors are thought to contribute significantly to the

development of diverticular disease, the complete etiology is likely to involve other as yet unrecognized influences. For example, diverticular disease in Oriental populations is localized predominantly to the right colon, in distinct contrast to the left-sided predilection observed in Western populations.[53] Such variations in the anatomic distribution of diverticula among populations might suggest that factors other than diet alone exert a substantial influence on the character of this disease worldwide.

MECHANICAL FACTORS. Clinical and experimental studies within the last 30 years have implicated low-fiber diets as a prominent etiologic factor in the development of diverticular disease.[39,41] Diets lacking vegetable fiber are presumed to predispose to the development of diverticula by altering colonic motility. Colonic motility is a complex process serving to transport feces distally, while also permitting storage, thereby facilitating fluid and electrolyte absorption. Colonic motility is modulated by myogenic, hormonal, and neural influences.[23] There is evidence that patients with diverticular disease manifest exaggerated contractile responses to feeding and hormonal stimuli.[23,43] These abnormal muscular contractions are believed to cause colonic smooth muscle hypertrophy, a characteristic of diverticular disease. Some patients with diverticulosis also exhibit various types of colonic dysmotility thought to contribute to formation of diverticula. Normal fecal transport is modulated by coordinated, segmental muscular contractions that serve to separate the colonic lumen into a series of chambers[39,42] (Fig. 1). Contraction of any one chamber tends to increase intraluminal pressure within that segment. Under normal circumstances, the chamber is open at one end, thereby allowing passage of feces, which causes lowering of intraluminal pressure. Patients with diverticulosis exhibit such segmentation, but individual chambers tend to become occluded at both ends during muscular contraction. When outflow from a particular segment is obstructed both proximally and distally, massive increases in intraluminal pressures, as high as 90 mm Hg, have been noted.[42] Such isolated increases of intraluminal pressure are thought to predispose to herniation of mucosa through the bowel wall and thus to the development of diverticula (see Fig. 1).

The possible role of dietary fiber in the development of diverticula is best explained by effects on colonic diameter and stool consistency. It has been postulated that colonic segments with bulky fecal contents and large luminal diameters are less likely to exhibit exaggerated segmentation. Low-fiber diets are associated with a narrowed colon filled with small, hardened feces. Segmentation is enhanced, and high luminal pressures tend to develop. Although this concept has been widely disseminated, definitive evidence for a causal relationship between low dietary fiber and the development of diverticular disease does not exist.[47,54] Nonetheless, high-residue diets are in widespread use in the management of diverticular disease. Whether or not such therapy has a significant influence on the natural history of diverticular disease is unclear. Most clinical studies, however, tend to suggest favorable results when patients are treated with supplementary dietary fiber.[40,54]

ANATOMIC FEATURES. Diverticula tend to develop at specific points in the circumference of the colon. This localization is determined in part by the anatomic relationship between the colonic musculature and its nutrient blood supply (Fig. 2). Diverticula form at so-called weak points, where the nutrient

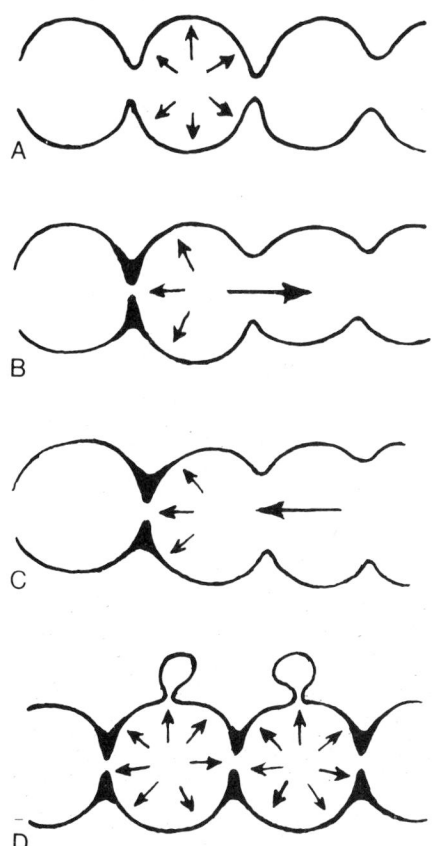

Figure 1. Schema demonstrating the process of segmentation. *A*, Contraction of a single chamber results in increased intraluminal pressure. Under normal circumstances the chamber is not completely isolated, thereby preventing dramatic increases in pressure. *B*, Relaxation at one end of a chamber during contraction allows fecal matter to be transported distally along the lumen. *C*, Failure to relax at one end of a chamber can reduce or even halt transit of intestinal contents along the lumen. *D*, Complete isolation of one or more chambers during contraction causes dramatic increases in intraluminal pressure, thereby predisposing to diverticular formation. (From Painter, N. S.: The aetiology of diverticulosis of the colon with special reference to the action of certain drugs on the behavior of the colon. Ann. R. Coll. Surg., 34:111, 1964.)

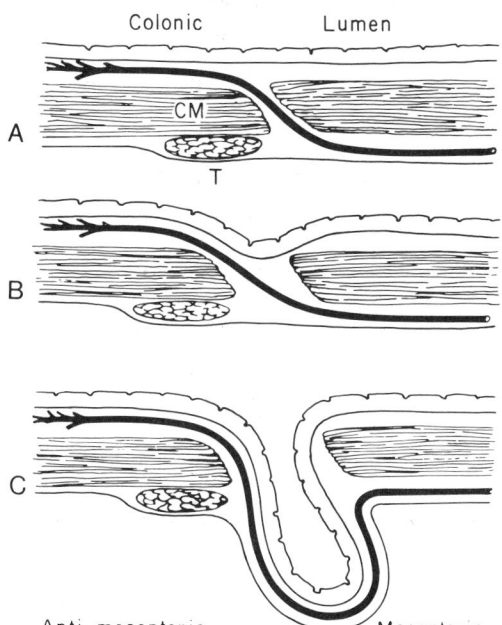

Figure 2. Schematic demonstration of the relation of a diverticulum to mural vasculature. *A*, The vasa recta penetrate the colonic wall obliquely at specific sites in the circular muscle (CM), usually along the mesenteric side of the taeniae (T). *B*, As a diverticulum begins to herniate through the colonic wall, the blood vessels are drawn along. *C*, The vasa recta eventually become draped over the dome of the diverticulum and are prone to rupture after injury arising from within the lumen of the colon. (From Meyers, M. A., et al.: Pathogenesis of bleeding colonic diverticulosis. Gastroenterology, 71:577, 1976.)

blood vessels (vasa recta) penetrate the circular muscle layer en route to the mucosa. These "perforating" vessels tend to penetrate the colonic wall along the mesenteric border of the two antimesenteric taeniae. The gaps in the circular muscle layer where the vasa recta penetrate constitute points of potential weakness through which the mucosa and submucosa can herniate, forming diverticula. Diverticula, therefore, are usually located between the single mesenteric taenia and one of the two antimesenteric taeniae (Fig. 3). They rarely occur along the antimesenteric border of the colon, i.e., between the two antimesenteric taeniae.

The distribution of diverticula throughout the colon also tends to follow a distinct pattern (Fig. 4). The majority of diverticula occur in the descending and sigmoid colon. It is estimated that 90 to 95 per cent of patients with diverticulosis have involvement of the sigmoid colon.[22,47,48] Approximately 65 per cent of patients have disease limited to the sigmoid colon alone.[44,47] Conversely, only a small number of patients (2 to 10 per cent) have disease confined to the ascending or transverse colon.[47]

NATURAL HISTORY

Most patients with diverticulosis remain asymptomatic throughout their lifetime. It is estimated that between 10 and 25 per cent of patients eventually develop signs and symptoms of diverticulitis.[1,44] Another 15 per cent present with diverticular

hemorrhage. As with most conditions, the prognosis of any one episode of bleeding or diverticulitis varies according to the patient's general health and the severity of the underlying disease process. Patients with mild diverticulitis can be treated conservatively with excellent results, whereas patients with free intra-abdominal perforation of a diverticulum require emergent surgical therapy and can be expected to incur a 20 per cent mortality.[48] An overall mortality of less than 5 per cent can be expected in association with an initial attack of diverticulitis.[44]

Following the first episode of diverticulitis, approximately one third of patients sustain a second attack, usually within 3 to 5 years.[44] Another 30 to 40 per cent suffer from intermittent symptoms of discomfort and crampy abdominal pain, without

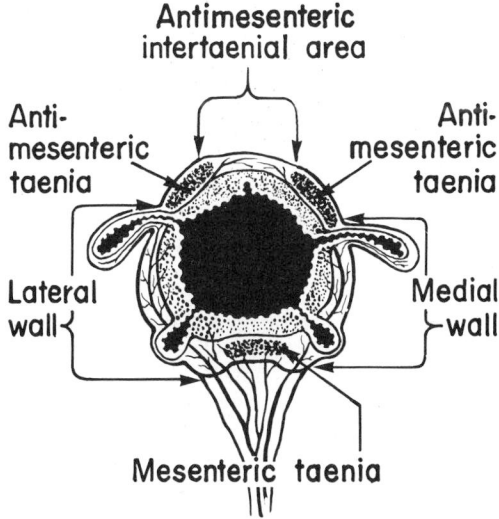

Figure 3. Transverse section of the colon demonstrating the relationship of diverticula to colonic taeniae and vasculature. (From Goligher, J.: Diverticulosis and diverticulitis of the colon. *In* Duthie, H., and Nixon, H.: Surgery of the Anus, Rectum, and Colon. London, Bailliere, 1984, p. 1083.)

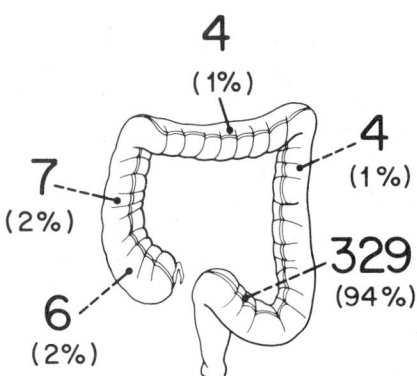

Figure 4. Diagram illustrating the prevalence of diverticular disease by location within the colon. (From Rodkey, G. V., and Welch, C. E.: Changing patterns in the surgical treatment of diverticular disease. Ann. Surg., 200:466, 1984.)

requiring hospitalization. The remainder can be expected to remain symptom-free. The prognosis is worse following a second attack, with only 10 per cent of patients remaining symptom-free. The morbidity and mortality from recurrent attacks also are higher than those associated with an initial episode. Complications such as abscess formation or fistulization develop in approximately 20 per cent of patients following a single attack of diverticulitis, and the complication rate approaches 60 per cent in patients who have had previous episodes.[44]

Since diverticulosis is an acquired disease, the incidence of which clearly increases with age, it would appear logical that the number and size of diverticula would also increase with time. Not all patients, however, are destined to an inevitable course of worsening disease. In fact, only 30 per cent of patients demonstrate radiologic evidence of progression of their disease, either in the form of an increased number of diverticula or involvement of other segments of the colon. Progression of disease following resection of involved colon is also unusual, occurring in less than 10 to 15 per cent of patients.[6]

COMPLICATIONS OF DIVERTICULOSIS

Hemorrhage

Diverticular disease is the most common cause of massive lower gastrointestinal bleeding. Although, overall, colon carcinoma is the most common source of gastrointestinal blood loss, such bleeding is usually sparse, often being detected only as occult blood on chemical testing.

INCIDENCE AND ETIOLOGY. Bleeding can be expected to develop in 15 per cent of patients with diverticulosis, and until the recent introduction of angiography and emergent colonoscopy, diverticula were thought to represent up to 90 per cent of significant lower intestinal hemorrhage.[31] Actual localization of bleeding to a diverticulum was uncommon, however, as the diagnosis often was established primarily by excluding other potential sources of hemorrhage, such as carcinoma.[5] With the advent of improved localization techniques, angiodysplastic lesions, also known as *arteriovenous malformations*, have been implicated with increasing frequency as a cause of colonic bleeding. Currently, it is estimated that 30 to 50 per cent of massive colonic bleeding is due to diverticulosis, while angiodysplasia is responsible for another 20 to 30 per cent.[8,27,56] Remaining causes include colonic neoplasms, inflammatory bowel disease, ischemic colitis, and rare congenital lesions. Since as many as 30 to 40 per cent of patients with lower intestinal hemorrhage never have the site of bleeding accurately determined, there is significant variation in the reported incidence of diverticular bleeding.[8,56]

Diverticular hemorrhage arises from the right colon in 70 to 90 per cent of patients.[11] The explanation for this right-sided predilection is not entirely clear, but may be related to the thinner wall of the right colon. Approximately 70 per cent of patients with diverticular hemorrhage cease bleeding spontaneously, often prior to presentation at the hospital. The risk of rebleeding is only 30 per cent but increases to 50 per cent in patients who have suffered a second episode of hemorrhage.[5,31]

Diverticular hemorrhage is thought to follow injury and subsequent rupture of blood vessels lying adjacent to a diverticulum. Anatomic studies have identified several dynamic relationships that may be responsible for the development of diverticular hemorrhage (Fig. 5). Diverticula develop at potential weak points in the colonic wall where the nutrient blood vessels penetrate the circular muscle layer en route to the mucosa. As a diverticulum begins to herniate, it tends to carry one of the penetrating vessels with it. Eventually, the vessel becomes draped over the dome of the diverticulum, separated from the colonic lumen only by the thin mucosal layer. This anatomic relationship predisposes to injury with subsequent rupture. Characteristic pathologic changes in the vasa recta of bleeding diverticula have been observed. These consist of eccentric thickening of the intima and thinning of the underlying media.[33] In all cases, rupture occurs eccentrically into the lumen of the diverticulum.

CLINICAL FEATURES. Most patients with diverticular hemorrhage present with only minor or occult bleeding. Patients often describe intermittent, sporadic passage of bright red or maroon blood from the rectum. Fifty percent of patients give a history of a previous episode or colonic hemorrhage.[11] Abdominal pain or discomfort is usually absent. Diverticular hemorrhage does not normally occur in the presence of acute inflammation; in fact, active diverticulitis is extremely uncommon during a bleeding episode.[33] Physical examination is usually unremarkable.

One third of patients with diverticular hemorrhage (or approximately 5 per cent of all patients with diverticulosis) present with massive, exsanguinating hemorrhage. Such patients demand immediate resuscitation and therapeutic intervention. The overwhelming majority of these patients are elderly, usually in their seventh or eighth decade. Consequently, 70 per cent of these patients have serious associated diseases, with the more common co-morbid conditions being atherosclerosis, hypertension, diabetes mellitus, congestive heart failure, renal insufficiency, and peripheral vascular disease. These associations undoubtedly contribute to the high morbidity and mortality (10 to 20 per cent) associated with diverticular hemorrhage.[8,31,56]

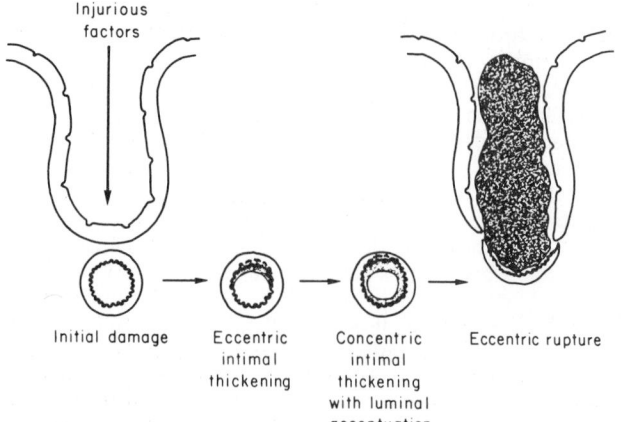

Figure 5. Schematic demonstrating proposed mechanism of diverticular hemorrhage. Arterial branches of the vasa recta lie in proximity to the dome of the diverticulum. Over time, the artery is subjected to injury, but only along the side of the vessel facing the diverticular lumen. Eccentric (toward the colonic lumen) intimal thickening develops, with eventual rupture into the colon. (From Meyers, M. A., et al.: Pathogenesis of bleeding colonic diverticulosis. Gastroenterology, 71:577, 1976.)

DIAGNOSIS. The first step in the management of any patient with massive gastrointestinal hemorrhage is immediate resuscitation. Monitoring should be instituted rapidly, as for any patient with the potential for hypovolemic shock. The passage of a nasogastric tube helps to exclude an upper gastrointestinal source of bleeding. Resuscitative measures should commence before any further diagnostic maneuvers are undertaken.

All patients with massive lower gastrointestinal hemorrhage should undergo proctoscopy as soon as possible. The main purpose of this examination is to exclude the rectum as the bleeding source. Although difficult in the face of active hemorrhage, identification of bleeding from hemorrhoids or other rectal lesions is extremely important. Emergency subtotal colectomy for exsanguinating colonic hemorrhage should not be performed until every effort has been made to exclude the rectum as the site of bleeding. Failure to do so results occasionally in a patient who continues to bleed postoperatively from a previously unidentified rectal source.

Seventy to 80 per cent of patients stop bleeding spontaneously; such patients should undergo elective evaluation. Continued massive bleeding in a hemodynamically unstable patient is an indication for emergent surgical intervention.[14] However, in actively bleeding patients who maintain relative hemodynamic stability, attempts at localization of the bleeding site should be made, either by selective mesenteric arteriography, radioisotope scanning, or colonoscopy. Emergent selective mesenteric arteriography successfully identifies the site of hemorrhage in 40 to 60 per cent of patients[11,56] (Fig. 6). The high rate of spontaneous cessation of bleeding following initial resuscitative management probably contributes to the relatively high incidence of nondiagnostic arteriograms.[5,31,56] In order for arteriography to be diagnostic, bleeding must be active at a minimal rate of 0.5 ml. per minute. Therefore, performing selective mesenteric arteriography in all patients with lower gastrointestinal hemorrhage, regardless of the rate of bleeding, produces lower diagnostic yields. Limiting arteriography to those patients with ongoing hemorrhage produces a diagnostic yield of 70 to 100 per cent.[8]

Another alternative, even in the actively bleeding patient, is to perform diagnostic colonoscopy. Jensen and Machicado recently have demonstrated that combined colonoscopy/esophagogastroduodenoscopy is extremely effective in localizing the site of bleeding, provided the colon has been rapidly and adequately purged with large amounts of nonabsorbable, polyethylene-glycol solution (GoLytely).[24] In a group of 80 patients with lower gastrointestinal hemorrhage, they reported an 86 per cent diagnostic accuracy rate. They either detected lesions in the colon (in 74 per cent of patients) or noted the absence of such lesions in patients with bleeding emanating above the ileocecal valve (20 per cent of patients). Emergent colonoscopy was not associated with an increased technically related complication rate. However, congestive heart failure, secondary to the voluminous (3 to 7 liters) purge of the gastrointestinal tract, occurred in 4 per cent of patients.

Radioisotope scans are of two basic types, ^{99m}Tc-labeled sulfur colloid or red blood cells. ^{99m}Tc-sulfur colloid, once injected intravenously, is cleared from the circulation by the liver, spleen, and bone marrow within several minutes. However, any labeled colloid that extravasates into the intestinal lumen is not cleared and remains, it is hoped, near the site of bleeding. Any abnormal radioactive pooling can be detected on scanning. The study is completed within a short time, and bleeding rates as low as 0.1 ml. per min. can be detected reliably (Fig. 7). Labeled erythrocytes, however, have a relatively long half-life within the circulation. Scanning can be repeated at 24 or 36 hours after injection. Therefore, the tagged red blood cell scan may be useful in detection of chronic or intermittent bleeding.[20]

Although extremely accurate in detection of active bleeding, radioisotope scans have had variable success in accurately localizing the site of hemorrhage. In one series of 59 patients, the site of bleeding was suggested in 36 (61 per cent) but in only 25 patients (42 per cent) did the activity on scintigraphy correlate with an actual pathologic lesion demonstrated by other means (endoscopy, angiography, or surgical therapy).[20] Others have reported localization accuracy rates of 24 to 91 per cent.[57]

One reason for the relatively poor localization rates is that blood within the intestinal lumen does not remain stationary. For example, blood originally extravasated into the cecum may pass rapidly into the distal colon after only a few peristaltic waves. Similarly, with an incompetent ileocecal valve, blood may reflux proximally into the small intestine. In either case, subsequent scanning might not determine accurate localization. Normal anatomic relationships also may be responsible for diagnostic errors. Bleeding lesions in the upper gastrointestinal tract may superimpose on adjacent colon, thereby causing an incorrect diagnosis of colonic hemorrhage. Similarly, lesions in the transverse colon, although an unusual site for hemorrhage, may be interpreted as an upper intestinal bleeding source. Bleeding from a redundant loop of sigmoid colon, which drapes toward the patient's right lower quadrant, may be falsely identified as bleeding from the right colon. For all these reasons, segmental colon resection based solely upon the results of a positive bleeding scan should be undertaken with extreme caution.

Despite the wide variations noted, such scans are frequently obtained as the initial diagnostic study in patients with intestinal hemorrhage. Currently, several centers utilize nuclear scanning as a screening test to determine the need for subsequent arteriography.[2,52] Patients with positive bleeding scans proceed to selective arteriography, whereas those with no evidence of active bleeding are observed for signs of further hemorrhage. Bleeding scans are extremely sensitive in detecting active bleeding, with acceptable false-negative and false-positive rates of less than 10 per cent.[57] By reserving arteriography for the patient with a positive scan, the diagnostic accuracy of this study can be substantially improved, often to greater than 90 per cent.

In patients who have ceased bleeding, diagnostic studies can

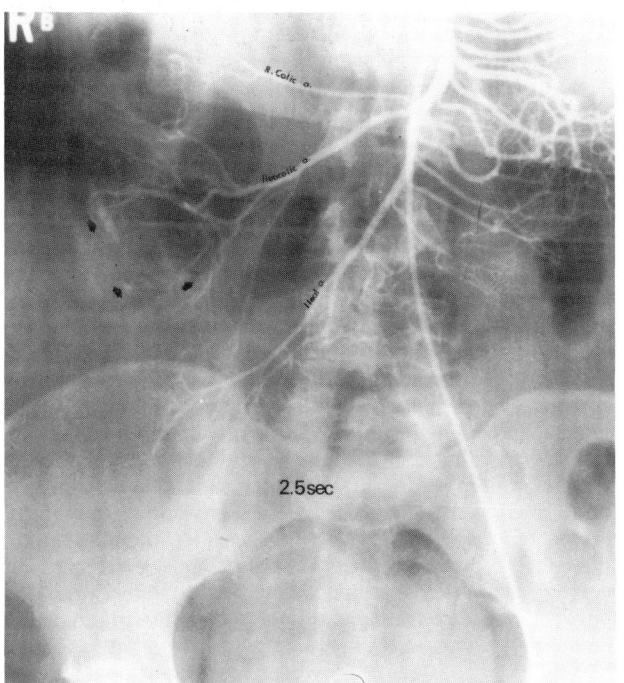

Figure 6. Selective mesenteric radiograph demonstrating extravasation of contrast (arrows) from diverticular hemorrhage. The specific case represents an unusual situation in which multiple, simultaneous bleeding sites were detected.

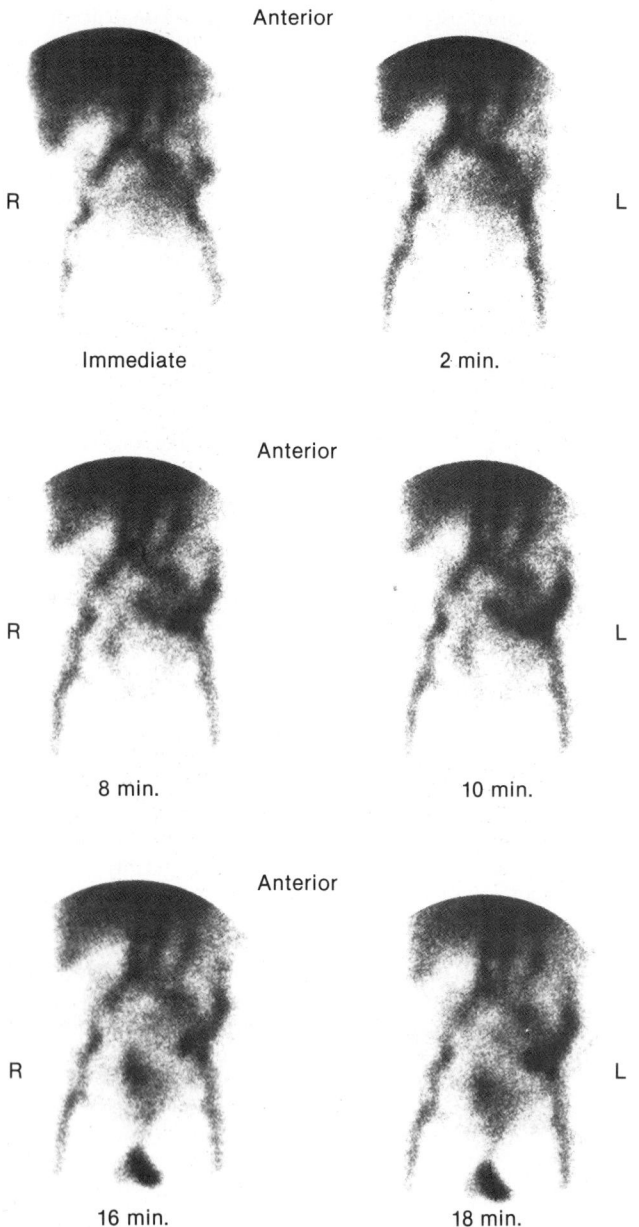

Anterior

R   L

Immediate   2 min.

Anterior

R   L

8 min.   10 min.

Anterior

R   L

16 min.   18 min.

Figure 7. Radionuclide scan with technetium-99m demonstrating rapid extravasation of tracer into the left colon of a patient with bleeding diverticular disease. The tracer can be almost observed immediately in the left colon. At 8 to 10 minutes tracer is clearly present within the sigmoid colon, and by 16 to 18 minutes tracer has already passed distally into the rectum.

be performed on a more elective basis. The colon can be adequately prepared and colonoscopy performed with excellent results. Elective colonoscopy should have a diagnostic sensitivity of 90 per cent in detecting nonbleeding lesions of the colon. The double-contrast barium enema is still a useful test but may have a sensitivity of only 70 per cent in this situation. A barium enema should rarely, if ever, be obtained in the early diagnostic period. When barium contrast has been introduced into the colon, it obscures any subsequent attempts to visualize by arteriography or colonoscopy. The contrast enema, therefore, is not routinely recommended as the initial diagnostic test in the elective or emergent evaluation of patients with colonic hemorrhage.[52,56]

TREATMENT. Initial resuscitative measures, as for any patient with gastrointestinal hemorrhage and hypovolemia, should be instituted promptly. With adequate fluid resuscitation, blood transfusion, and correction of coagulation abnor-

malities, 70 to 80 per cent of patients cease bleeding spontaneously. However, approximately 15 per cent of all patients presenting with massive diverticular hemorrhage require emergency surgical intervention before further diagnostic information can be obtained. The mortality in this group is high, often approaching 30 to 50 per cent.[56]

If a bleeding source can be localized at arteriography, selective intra-arterial infusion of vasopressin (0.1 to 0.4 unit per minute) or embolization with thrombotic agents, such as absorbable gelatin (Gelfoam) or autologous clot, has been used with success. In patients with an identifiable site of bleeding, selective intra-arterial infusion of vasopressin (a potent vasoconstrictor) can be expected to control hemorrhage in over 90 per cent of patients.[8] The infusion should be initiated at a rate of 0.2 unit per minute. If the bleeding is not controlled promptly, the rate can be increased to a maximum of 0.4 unit per minute. Continued bleeding despite vasopressin infusion is an indication for other therapeutic measures, which may include embolization, colonoscopy, or, more likely, surgical intervention. If, however, bleeding ceases with the administration of vasopressin, the infusion should be maintained for another 24 hours. If bleeding does not recur, the infusion should be tapered gradually and discontinued over the subsequent 12 hours. The catheter should be left in place for an additional 8 to 12 hours for use if bleeding recurs. Selective vasopressin infusion, however, is not without problems. Its vasoconstrictive effects often are only temporary, with up to 50 per cent of patients rebleeding after the infusion has been discontinued.[8] Vasopressin is also associated with infrequent but potentially serious side effects. Major complications can include myocardial, mesenteric, and cerebral ischemia, arrhythmias, hypertension, hyponatremia, and fluid overload.[51] Embolic, thrombotic, and septic complications due to the indwelling arterial catheter also contribute to an overall complication rate of 4 to 6 per cent.[2] Still, selective arterial infusion of vasopressin may convert an emergent situation to an elective or semi-elective one, thereby decreasing the operative mortality in this elderly, high-risk patient population.

Transcatheter embolization might be an alternative to vasopressin, especially in situations where vasopressin has not been effective or is contraindicated. However, use of embolization for the treatment of lower intestinal hemorrhage is controversial.[3] Because of a postembolic colon infarction rate of 13 per cent, transcatheter embolization has been used more often for control of upper intestinal hemorrhage.[49] On rare occasions, colonoscopy may reveal an actively bleeding lesion at the base of a diverticulum, thereby permitting attempts at electrocoagulation or laser photoablation. Diverticular hemorrhage, however, is usually not amenable to endoscopic therapy.[24] Although the barium enema has been used in the past in an attempt to tamponade diverticular hemorrhage, the validity of this approach is questionable.[52]

Emergent surgical intervention is recommended in any patient who continues to bleed despite all resuscitative and therapeutic maneuvers. Indications for emergent operation include persistent hemodynamic instability, a transfusion requirement of greater than 6 units over a 24-hour period, and recurrent hemorrhage. Emergent surgical therapy can be either "directed" or "nondirected," depending on the success or failure of preoperative localization. If a bleeding site has been identified by colonoscopy, arteriography, or nuclear scanning, a segmental resection can be performed with the expectation that bleeding is controlled in over 90 per cent of patients. If the source of bleeding has not been identified, subtotal colectomy is the treatment of choice.[14] Emergency subtotal colectomy without preoperative localization of the bleeding site has an operative mortality of 30 to 50 per cent.[8] However, even with angiographic localization and a more limited resection, an operative mortality of 20 to 30 per cent can be expected with emergency intervention. This can be reduced to less than 10 per cent when surgical therapy is performed on an elective basis.[8] Segmental resection or hemicolectomy should not be performed when the site of colonic hemorrhage has not been identified. Such procedures are associated with an extremely high rate of rebleeding (35 to 50 per cent) and an increased operative mortality (30 per cent), as compared with the rates of rebleeding (10 per cent) and mortality (10 per cent) after subtotal colectomy.[14] Attempts to intraoperatively localize previously unidentified bleeding sites, either by multiple enterotomies or divided colostomies, are usually unsuccessful. Other maneuvers that have been used sporadically to localize bleeding intraoperatively include Doppler scanning, transillumination of the bowel lumen, and intra-arterial injection of methylene blue dye, also with very limited success. Several centers have reported intraoperative endoscopic localization to be helpful.[7,52]

Elective colon resection is recommended in any patient with a history of previous diverticular bleeding who presents with a second episode of hemorrhage. As previously mentioned, the mortality associated with elective colon resection in this setting should be 10 to 20 per cent. The incidence of rebleeding following elective operation should be less than 10 per cent.[8] This is dependent, however, upon the accuracy of preoperative localization.

Diverticulitis

The term *diverticulitis* simply refers to inflammation of one or more diverticula. It constitutes a spectrum from mild, well-localized inflammation to a fulminant process causing free perforation and generalized peritonitis. It is thought that diverticulitis represents, at an anatomic level, perforation of a diverticulum into the pericolic, or so-called "peridiverticular," space. However, as many as one third of patients undergoing colon resection for symptomatic diverticulitis do not have pathologic evidence of inflammation on subsequent histologic inspection.[37] Since many patients may have abdominal symptoms in the absence of active inflammation, a clear distinction between diverticulitis and painful colonic spasm is often difficult.[37,40] Moreover, patients with diverticulosis may also suffer from other, coexistent conditions that cause abdominal pain such as irritable bowel syndrome. Thus, a patient's symptoms may be totally unrelated to the diverticular disease.

The inflammatory process may be classified as either simple or complicated. Simple diverticulitis can be expected to resolve, in most cases, with standard medical therapy. Patients with complicated diverticulitis manifest one or more of the serious sequelae of the disease, such as abscess formation, obstruction, free perforation, or fistulization. Such patients generally require surgical intervention.

INCIDENCE AND ETIOLOGY. Diverticulitis develops in 15 to 20 per cent of patients with diverticulosis sometime during their lifetime. Although 65 per cent of diverticula are confined solely to the sigmoid colon, inflammation is limited to this segment in over 90 per cent of patients.[48] Right-sided diverticular inflammation occurs in only 5 per cent of patients with diverticulitis.[18,19,50]

The pathogenesis of diverticulitis generally is believed to be secondary to perforation, either microscopic or macroscopic, of a diverticulum. The perforation is preceded by chronic effacement and erosion of the diverticular wall by increased intraluminal pressure or inspissated food particles trapped within the diverticular lumen. Eventually, sufficient inflammation and focal necrosis ensues, leading to perforation. In most settings, the inflammatory process is relatively mild and of sufficient duration so that the entire perforation is walled off by the pericolic fat and surrounding mesentery. Involvement of other abdominal organs in this walling-off process occasionally leads to intestinal obstruction or fistulization. Following contained perforation, the inflammatory process may cause intra-abdominal abscess formation. If the perforation is not well contained, gen-

eralized peritonitis may supervene. The pathogenesis of diverticulitis previously was thought to be quite similar to that of appendicitis. However, luminal obstruction of a diverticular neck by a fecalith or inspissated food particles is believed to be an extremely rare event.[47]

CLINICAL FEATURES. The presenting clinical features of diverticulitis vary according to the location and severity of the underlying inflammatory process. Patients with painful colonic spasm or irritable bowel syndrome may present with abdominal complaints similar to those associated with mild, acute diverticulitis. Patients with diverticulitis, however, usually manifest signs and symptoms of ongoing inflammation, such as progressive localized pain, anorexia, fever, leukocytosis, and the presence of peritoneal findings on abdominal examination.

Left lower quadrant pain is the most common complaint of patients with diverticulitis. It is present in over 70 per cent of patients and is the most common reason for hospitalization.[45,47] The pain is usually present for several days prior to hospitalization, thus helping to differentiate the condition from other acute surgical conditions, such as appendicitis or perforated peptic ulcer. Only 17 per cent of patients present with symptoms of less than 24 hours' duration.[48] A history of previous episodes of pain is elicited by one half of patients.[28] Other symptoms often are present in association with an acute attack. Nausea and vomiting are found in only 20 per cent of patients.[45] Diarrhea is present in one third and constipation in almost one half of patients. Urinary tract symptoms such as dysuria, urgency, and increased frequency are present in only 10 to 15 per cent of patients.[28,45] Although most of these symptoms are nonspecific, their presence is associated with an overall worsened prognosis.[44,45]

Physical examination usually reveals abdominal tenderness, characteristically localized to the left lower quadrant. A tender abdominal mass is found in 20 per cent of cases, and its presence portends a worse prognosis.[45] Occasionally, tenderness may be manifest in the right lower quadrant. This may be due to either right-sided diverticulitis or inflammation of a redundant loop of sigmoid colon. Overall, abdominal distention is reported in up to two thirds of patients. Low-grade fever and mild leukocytosis are commonly present.[28] Patients with white blood cell counts greater than 15,000 per cu. mm. are more likely suffering from an intra-abdominal abscess or generalized peritonitis. Urinalysis may demonstrate an increased number of white blood cells if the inflammatory process is adjacent to the ureter or bladder. The presence of bacteria, especially colonic flora, in the urine is a strong indication that a fistula exists between the inflamed colon and the urinary tract.

DIAGNOSIS. Most patients can be diagnosed on the basis of their clinical presentation. However, since other acute surgical conditions such as appendicitis, perforated colon cancer, or perforated duodenal ulcer can present with a similar clinical pattern, confirmation of the diagnosis by radiographic or endoscopic means is of utmost importance.

Routine abdominal and chest radiographs are usually unremarkable. Only one third of such films demonstrate any abnormality.[36] Despite this, they are helpful in excluding other acute surgical problems such as intestinal obstruction or a perforated viscus. Free air beneath the diaphragm is an unusual finding with diverticulitis. Occasionally, plain films may demonstrate retroperitoneal air or a mass effect secondary to a large paracolic abscess.

Contrast radiography or colonoscopy should be undertaken with caution in patients with suspected acute diverticulitis. The increased luminal pressure from the injected contrast material or from insufflation of air may lead to free rupture of a previously well-localized peridiverticular abscess or phlegmon.[47] The fear of extravasation of barium and/or feces into the peritoneal cavity causes most clinicians to delay contrast studies until signs of active inflammation have subsided. Although studies

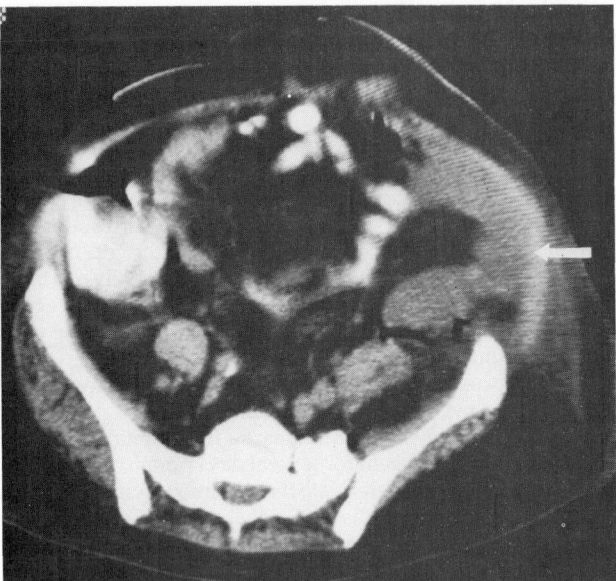

Figure 8. CT scan of the abdomen demonstrating severe diverticulitis. A pericolic abscess (arrow) is present in the left lower quadrant, and significant signs of inflammation (bowel wall edema, "dirty fat" appearance to the mesentery) are present through the lower abdomen.

have suggested that both contrast enemas and colonoscopy, when performed by experienced personnel, can be done safely with a high diagnostic yield, the introduction of computed tomography (CT) has substantially reduced their use. CT scanning has been shown to be as accurate as barium enema in diagnosing diverticulitis (Fig. 8). Evidence of pericolic inflammation, bowel wall edema, abscess formation, and even fistulization is present in 63 to 95 per cent of patients.[36] CT scanning has the advantages of being noninvasive, avoiding increased intraluminal pressure, and being able to detect extraluminal disease, i.e., the presence of ureteral obstruction or distant ab-

scess formation. CT scanning is especially useful in identifying and localizing abscess or phlegmon formation. It is also an objective way to follow resolution of the inflammatory process.

In contrast, elective evaluation of a patient following complete resolution of an episode of diverticulitis should include colonoscopy, barium enema, or both. Contrast studies of the colon may reveal co-existent lesions such as polyps or colon cancer. It is imperative that the entire colon be evaluated in any patient with suspected diverticulitis in order to establish the extent of the underlying disease (Fig. 9). Even if a patient has an otherwise normal-appearing colon by barium study, colonoscopy can add important information. For example, diverticular inflammation can lead to severe stricture formation, which mimics colon cancer (Fig. 10). Colonoscopy with multiple biopsies should be undertaken in such a situation. Even with multiple negative biopsies, the gross appearance of the lesion may resemble carcinoma so closely that urgent resection is recommended.

TREATMENT. Some patients with minor episodes of diverticulitis can be treated as outpatients with oral antibiotics and a clear liquid diet. Patients who do not improve on such treatment require hospitalization. Except for the most minor of attacks, however, a patient with acute diverticulitis should be hospitalized for treatment and close observation. Standard inpatient therapy consists of bowel rest (including the use of nasogastric suction if nausea, vomiting, or abdominal distention is present), intravenous antibiotics, and fluid restoration. Antispasmodics and analgesia often are added in order to improve patient comfort. The antibiotic regimen should provide coverage of normal colonic flora. Common programs include an aminoglycoside in combination with either clindamycin or metronidazole. With resolution of clinical evidence of inflammation, oral intake can be instituted. Prior to discharge the patient should be taught the elements of a high-fiber diet. Psyllium seed preparations may be prescribed to add bulk to the stool with the aim of minimizing segmentation. Barium enema or colonoscopy should be scheduled within several weeks of the acute episode.

Patients who fail to respond or deteriorate within the first 24 to 48 hours usually require urgent surgical treatment. Occasionally, patients who are known to have a diverticular abscess can be stabilized temporarily by percutaneous CT-guided drainage.

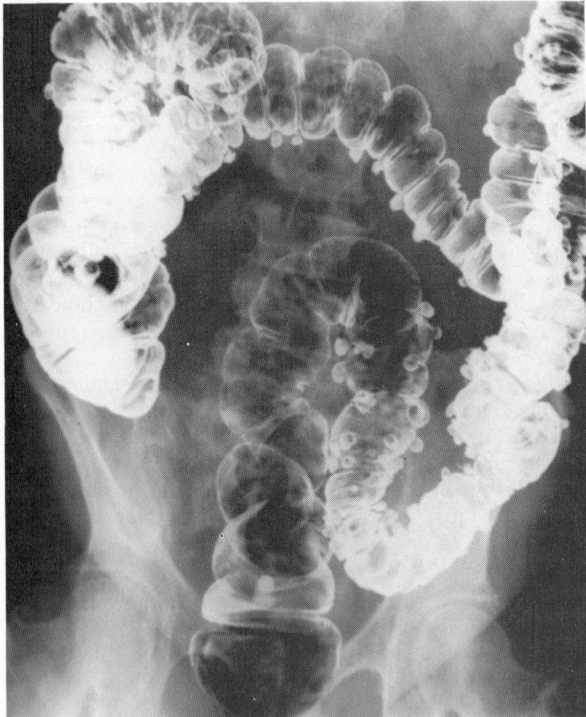

Figure 9. Barium enema demonstrating a typical case of severe diverticulosis. This patient has pancolonic disease, but the highest concentration is in the left and sigmoid colon.

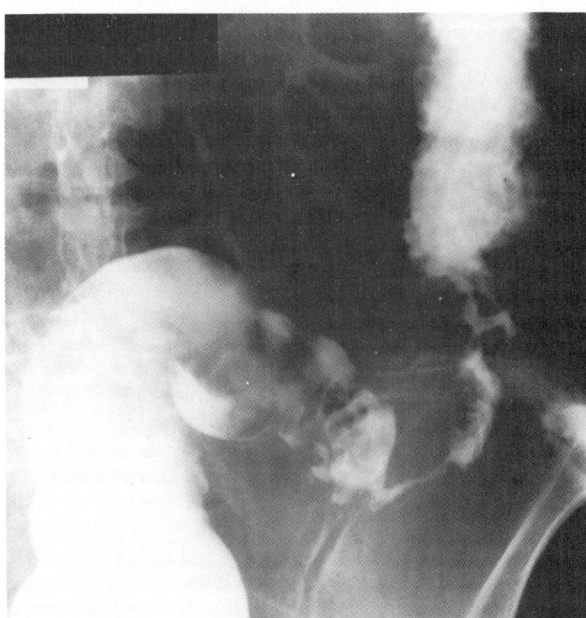

Figure 10. Barium enema demonstrating a severe stricture in the sigmoid colon secondary to diverticular disease. Severe disease such as demonstrated is often difficult to differentiate from colon carcinoma; therefore, colonoscopy is often necessary to exclude malignancy.

Recent studies have suggested that this maneuver may provide valuable time for adequate resuscitation of a critically ill patient prior to further management.[38] However, such drainage should never be construed as definitive treatment.

Approximately 20 per cent of patients who develop acute diverticulitis eventually require surgical therapy.[21,48] After a second attack, the incidence of complications approaches 50 to 60 per cent, with a mortality that is twice that associated with an initial attack.[44] Most agree that recurrence of acute diverticulitis warrants surgical resection when active inflammation has subsided.[47] Indications for surgical therapy are listed in Table 1. Septic complications such as abscess formation and free perforation are the most common indications for operation. Other less common indications include intestinal obstruction, fistulization, intractable abdominal pain, the presence of a persistent abdominal mass, and the inability to exclude the presence of colonic carcinoma. In several additional distinct subgroups, surgical treatment also is recommended; patients under the age of 40, those with suspected right-sided diverticulitis, and those who are immunocompromised usually do not respond to standard medical therapy.

SURGICAL OPTIONS. The form of surgical treatment depends largely on the severity and extent of the underlying inflammatory process. Patients undergoing elective operation for recurrent attacks, the presence of a persistent abdominal mass, or intractable symptoms usually are best served by resection of the involved segment and primary anastomosis. Adequate bowel preparation usually is possible, and both oral and systemic antibiotics can be administered safely and easily. The mortality for elective colon resection after the resolution of inflammatory diverticular disease should be less than 2 per cent.[48]

Patients presenting with progressive or fulminant disease usually require emergent intervention. Because bowel preparation is not usually possible, two- and three-stage procedures have been advocated (Fig. 11). The two-stage procedure initially entails resection of the involved colon with creation of an end-colostomy. The colostomy then is closed at a subsequent procedure, often deferred for 8 to 12 weeks. An alternative, less commonly employed two-stage approach is to resect the involved segment and perform a primary anastomosis, protected by a proximal, diverting colostomy. The proximal colostomy is then closed at a later date. The three-stage procedure consists of drainage of the involved segment along with creation of a proximal diverting colostomy. This is followed by resection of the diseased segment with primary anastomosis as a second procedure. The third operation consists of closure of the proximal colostomy. If the inflammatory process is well localized and if the colon can be safely mobilized, resection is preferred, usually with creation of an end-colostomy and mucous fistula or Hartmann's pouch. The traditional three-stage approach is now largely of historical interest. Numerous studies have docu-

TABLE 1. Indications for Operation

Absolute
    Complications of the disease
        Hemorrhage
        Sepsis (abscess, peritonitis)
        Fistula
        Obstruction
    Recurrent episodes of inflammation
    Intractable symptoms or signs (persistent pain or mass)
    Clinical deterioration
    Inability to exclude carcinoma

Relative
    Chronic stricture
    Young patient
    Steroid use
    Right-sided diverticulitis

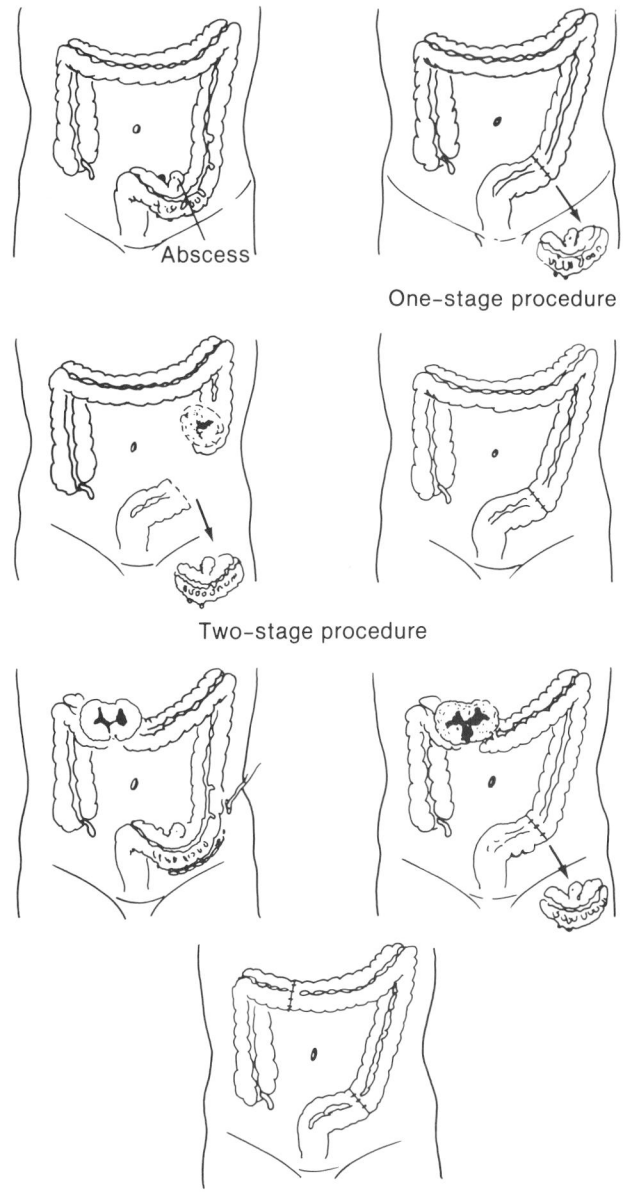

Figure 11. Schematic illustration of the options in the surgical treatment of diverticular disease. One-stage procedure: (1) Resection of the diseased segment of colon with primary anastomosis. Two-stage procedure: (1) Resection of the diseased segment with formation of a temporary end colostomy. (2) Closure of colostomy. Three-stage procedure: (1) Simple drainage of the diseased region with formation of a proximal, diverting colostomy. (2) Resection of the diseased segment with primary anastomosis. The colostomy is left intact. (3) Closure of colostomy. (Redrawn from Rege, R. V., and Nahrwold, D. L.: Diverticular disease. Curr. Probl. Surg., 26:136, 1989.)

mented that primary resection is associated with a significantly lower mortality (0 to 10 per cent) and morbidity (25 to 30 per cent), compared with simple drainage of the abscess with proximal colostomy. The mortality and morbidity following the latter approaches 30 per cent and 50 per cent, respectively.[15,28,48] Only in the extremely rare circumstance where the diseased segment is densely adherent to adjacent structures, such as the ureter or iliac vessels, should resection be abandoned in favor of drainage and proximal colostomy.

SEQUELAE OF DIVERTICULITIS. Common sequelae of diverticulitis include abscess formation, free intraperitoneal perforation, intestinal obstruction, and fistulization (Fig. 12). Each of these conditions may coexist in any patient. Complications develop in up to 25 per cent of patients with active diverticulitis,

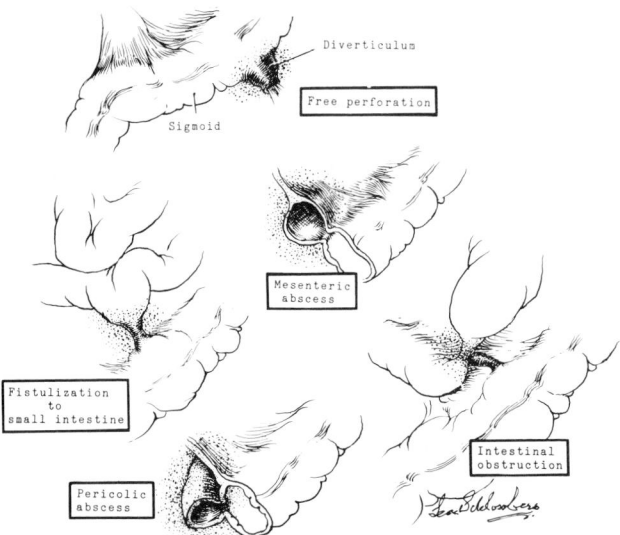

Figure 12. Complications of diverticulitis.

and surgical intervention is necessary in nearly all such instances.[21,48] Of patients requiring surgical intervention, the distribution of the various complications is abscess formation, 40 to 50 per cent; intestinal obstruction, 10 to 30 per cent; free perforation, 10 to 15 per cent; and fistulization, 4 to 10 per cent.[28,45,48]

OBSTRUCTION. Diverticulitis may progress to large bowel obstruction. Such obstruction is rarely complete. Occasionally, a loop of small intestine may become densely adherent to the inflammatory process in the colon, causing partial or complete small bowel obstruction. Primary resection of the involved segment with either primary anastomosis or colostomy is the treatment of choice, depending upon the adequacy of bowel preparation proximal to the diseased segment.

FREE PERFORATION. Although most episodes of perforated diverticulitis are confined to the peridiverticular region or pelvis, an occasional patient presents with signs of generalized peritonitis. Free intraperitoneal contamination may develop secondary to rupture of an inflamed diverticulum or of an established diverticular abscess. These patients require emergent surgical intervention. The overall mortality is high (20 to 40 per cent), largely because of complications such as septic shock and multiple organ failure.[21] Resection of the perforated segment with end-colostomy followed by copious irrigation of the peritoneal cavity is the appropriate treatment.

ABSCESS FORMATION. Diverticular abscesses are extremely common and are characterized, according to their location, as peridiverticular, retroperitoneal, mesenteric, or pelvic. Occasionally, such collections spread to adjacent structures and present as hip, thigh, or anterior abdominal wall abscesses. Occasionally, a hepatic abscess may develop as a secondary complication. Primary resection of the involved segment with colostomy and adequate local drainage is the most appropriate treatment. Recently, interventional radiologists have reported success with percutaneous drainage of diverticular abscesses; such measures may help to stabilize critically ill patients. Many of these patients are then able to undergo elective, one-stage resection of the diseased colon at a later date. However, since the underlying focus of infection is not removed, overall success and acceptance of this procedure have not been clearly established.

FISTULIZATION. Although less common than abscess formation or intestinal obstruction, colonic fistulas may develop secondary to diverticulitis. Over 90 per cent of cases of acute diverticulitis are localized to the sigmoid colon; therefore, fistulization most commonly involves this segment. The most common type is the colovesical fistula, representing up to two thirds of all internal diverticular fistulas.[58] Colocutaneous fistulas are the second most common type of diverticular fistula, followed by colovaginal and coloenteric fistulas, in decreasing order of frequency.[17] Other fistulas, such as colouterine, coloureteric, and colosalpingian, are extremely rare.

The most common diverticular fistula, the colovesical fistula, serves as an excellent example of the clinical features, diagnostic evaluation, and therapeutic options in management of this complication. Colovesical fistula is 3 to 5 times more common in men than in women. This discrepancy has been attributed to the presence of an intervening uterus in females, which serves as a protective anatomic barrier between the inflamed colon and the bladder. This is supported by the fact that 61 per cent of women who develop a colovesical fistula have had a previous hysterectomy.[35] Patients with colovesical fistulas present with dysuria (94 per cent), fecaluria (75 per cent), and pneumaturia (75 per cent) as the most frequent complaints.[34] Only 25 to 30 per cent of patients present with abdominal pain or evidence of systemic infection. Recurrent urinary tract infections are a common presentation.

The diagnosis of a colovesical fistula can often be made on the basis of a history of pneumaturia and the finding of fecaluria on urinanalysis. These findings do not, however, identify the underlying etiology of the fistulization. Colovesical fistulas may develop secondary to diverticulitis, granulomatous colitis, or carcinoma. Therefore, further diagnostic evaluation is necessary. Cystoscopy and barium enema are the studies most likely to confirm the presence of a colovesical fistula and to define its cause. Cystoscopy is usually more helpful, with a diagnostic accuracy of 80 to 95 per cent. The most common finding on cystoscopy is localized inflammation and bullous edema of the bladder mucosa, with actual demonstration of the fistula occurring in only 20 per cent of patients. Barium enema demonstrates nonspecific colonic abnormalities in nearly all cases; however, actual visualization of the fistula tract can be expected in only 30 per cent.[34] Other diagnostic options include cystography, colonoscopy, and CT scanning. Of these, CT scanning is probably the most helpful.[26] CT scanning has the advantage of making it possible to evaluate the extent of disease outside the colon or bladder. The low diagnostic yield (20 per cent) of cystography and colonoscopy in detecting colovesical fistula has limited their use.

Surgical therapy should be performed in all patients with a well-established diagnosis of colovesical fistula. Most patients with a colovesical fistula present with long-standing disease and usually, therefore, can be prepared for operation on an elective basis. After antibiotic administration (oral and systemic) and mechanical preparation, segmental colon resection, primary bladder repair, and primary colon anastomosis can usually be performed. A one-stage repair can be performed safely in 90 per cent of patients with colovesical fistula of diverticular origin.[30] The mortality associated with a colovesical fistula is 4 to 5 per cent.[58] The surgical treatment of diverticular fistula involving organs other than the bladder usually consists of segmental colon resection and primary anastomosis with repair and resection of the involved organ.

SPECIAL CONSIDERATIONS

DIVERTICULAR DISEASE IN THE IMMUNOCOMPROMISED PATIENT. Immunosuppression is associated with an increased incidence of colon perforation in patients with diverticular disease.[9] The most common form of immunosuppression is long-term corticosteroid therapy. Immunocompromised patients with diverticulitis tend to present with minimal or no symptoms or suggestive physical findings. The masking of the clinical features of colon perforation is an important reason for delayed diagnosis in this group. While medical treatment of acute diverticulosis is successful in 75 per cent of nonimmunocompromised patients, surgical intervention is required in nearly all patients who are immunocompromised.[46] Patients with impaired immune response are more likely to present with a free intraperitoneal perforation due to the inability of the immunocompromised patient to adequately wall off an inflammatory process. Early operative intervention should be considered in any immunocompromised patient with acute diverticulitis. Some advocate elective colon resection in patients with diverticular disease who are scheduled for kidney transplantation.[10]

DIVERTICULAR DISEASE IN YOUNG PATIENTS. Symptomatic diverticular disease in patients under the age of 40 comprises only 2 to 4 per cent of all patients with diverticulosis.[16] Although diverticular disease is unusual in younger patients, several important distinctions exist. Of patients less than 40 years of age with diverticulitis, 90 per cent are men.[12] The reason for this predominance is unclear. The correct admitting diagnosis of acute diverticulitis is made in only 15 to 35 per cent of these patients.[12,16] Because of the uncommon occurrence of diverticula in this age group, the diagnosis of acute diverticulitis often is not considered in the evaluation of abdominal pain. Despite the fact that the inflammatory process originates in sigmoid colon in 70 to 85 per cent of patients, a preoperative diagnosis of acute appendicitis is made in one third of patients.[12,16] The disease also tends to follow a more fulminant course and is associated, therefore, with a higher incidence of complications. Up to 70 per cent of patients with diverticulitis in this age group eventually require operative intervention.[12,16] Therefore, symptomatic diverticular disease in patients under 40 is a strong indication for surgical resection.

RIGHT-SIDED DIVERTICULITIS. Isolated diverticula of the right colon occur in 1 to 3 per cent of all patients with diverticular disease; however, right-sided diverticulitis represents 4 to 9 per cent of all operations for inflammatory complications.[18]

Two types of diverticula are generally recognized. Acquired right-sided diverticula are false diverticula, their walls consisting only of mucosa, submucosa, and serosa. They develop secondary to the same pathologic process that causes formation of diverticula concentrated in the sigmoid colon. The incidence of these acquired lesions also increases with age. Congenital diverticula usually are solitary lesions and are most commonly found in the right colon, with 88 per cent located in the cecum. Their incidence does not increase with age. Congenital diverticula often contain fecaliths that may cause inflammation and perforation.

The average age of patients with right-sided diverticula (44 years) is less than that of patients with sigmoid diverticula. Patients usually present with right lower quadrant pain, thereby leading to a diagnosis of acute appendicitis. Appendicitis is the preoperative diagnosis in 60 per cent of patients with right-sided diverticulitis.[18,50] Several clinical features, however, may help to differentiate diverticulitis from appendicitis. Patients with diverticulitis are usually older. Symptoms are often of longer duration (average, 3.3 days) as opposed to less than 24 hours in patients with appendicitis.[18,19] The pain begins in the right lower quadrant and remains there, unlike the migrating history typical of appendicitis. Episodes of nausea and vomiting are less common (~ 20 per cent of patients) than with appendicitis (~ 80 per cent of patients).[19] Right-sided diverticulitis is diagnosed correctly in only 5 to 7 per cent of cases, the diagnosis frequently being made at laparotomy.[18,50] Physical examination is usually not helpful in making the correct diagnosis. Barium enema and, more recently, CT scanning occasionally provide diagnostic assistance.[13] In patients with an atypical clinical presentation for acute appendicitis, consideration should be given to obtaining one of these studies. At exploration, two thirds of patients have an isolated, inflamed diverticulum that can be treated by local resection. One third of patients have developed a large, inflammatory mass that is extremely difficult to distin-

guish from a neoplasm. Right partial or hemicolectomy is then indicated.

GIANT DIVERTICULA. Giant colonic diverticula are extremely uncommon.[25,32] Giant diverticula, otherwise known as *giant air cysts*, most commonly present with vague abdominal pain and an enlarging abdominal mass that is mobile and tympanitic on physical examination. Plain abdominal radiographs reveal a large, usually solitary, air-filled cystic cavity. Although, on rare occasions, the gallbladder, urinary bladder, small intestinal diverticula, and intra-abdominal abscesses can present as large, air-filled cavities, volvulus of the colon is the major differential diagnosis. Three distinct pathologic forms of giant colonic diverticula have been identified.[32] One variant represents an unusual enlargement of the commonly recognized *false* colonic diverticula and occurs in the absence of perforation or active inflammation. The second variant develops after perforation of a diverticulum with subsequent formation of an abscess cavity. The abscess cavity remains in communication with the colonic lumen, with enlargement of the cavity occurring secondary to either a continued air leak or the presence of gasforming organisms. The third variant contains all three layers of the colonic wall, representing, therefore, a true congenital lesion. Giant diverticula usually arise from the sigmoid colon and are treated by resection of the involved bowel segment.

SELECTED REFERENCES

Meyers, M. A., Alonso, D. R., Gray, G. F., and Baer, J. W.: Pathogenesis of bleeding colonic diverticulosis. Gastroenterology, 71:577, 1976.
The authors describe the presumed pathogenesis of diverticular hemorrhage. Precise anatomic localization of the sites of diverticular hemorrhage was obtained by arteriographic and microangiographic techniques. Consistent changes in the microvasculature of the colon were identified on histologic section. Excellent diagrams are provided describing the development of bleeding colonic diverticula.

Painter, N. S.: The cause of diverticular disease of the colon, its symptoms and its complications: Review and hypothesis. J. R. Coll. Surg. Edinb. 30:118, 1985.
The author provides an in-depth summary of the roles of segmentation and dietary factors in the development of diverticular disease. The discussion also concerns the development of symptoms and the proposed etiology of complications secondary to diverticulitis.

Parks, T. G.: Natural history of diverticular disease of the colon. Clin. Gastroenterol., 4:53, 1975.
The author provides an excellent and detailed review of the natural history of diverticular disease. The discussion is divided into clear, concise subgroups that relate prognosis to factors such as age, sex, the number of diverticula, the extent of the disease, the nature of the symptomatology, and numerous other aspects that are not readily discussed in most texts.

Rege, R. V., and Nahrwold, D. L.: Diverticular Disease. Curr. Probl. Surg., 26:136, 1989.
An in-depth and clear discussion of the pathogenesis, clinical manifestations, complications, and management of diverticular disease is provided. An extensive review and discussion of the currently available data on important and controversial aspects of diverticular disease is superbly provided. Readers interested in a more detailed analysis of diverticular disease are referred to this monograph.

Rodkey, G. V., and Welch, C. E.: Changing patterns in the surgical treatment of diverticular disease. Ann. Surg. 200:466, 1984.
This well-recognized work summarizes a 70-year surgical experience with diverticular disease at the Massachusetts General Hospital. Clinical features, complications, and management are expertly reviewed.

Steer, M. L., and Silen, W.: Diagnostic procedures in gastrointestinal hemorrhage. N. Engl. J. Med., 309:646, 1983.
This is an excellent review of the important considerations involved in evaluation of gastrointestinal hemorrhage. Although not specifically directed toward diverticular bleeding, the key advantages and disadvantages of various diagnostic modalities are discussed. The reader is provided with a good understanding of available techniques and, therefore, a basis for making appropriate therapeutic decisions in the management of gastrointestinal hemorrhage.

REFERENCES

1. Almy, T. P., and Howell, D. A.: Diverticular disease of the colon. N. Engl. J. Med., 302:324, 1980.
2. Athanasoulis, C. A.: Angiography in the management of patients with gastrointestinal bleeding. Adv. Surg., 16:1, 1983.
3. Athanasoulis, C. A.: Therapeutic applications of angiography [first of two parts]. N. Engl. J. Med., 302:1117, 1980.

4. Beer, E.: Some pathological and clinical aspects of acquired (false) diverticula of the intestine. Am. J. Med. Sci., 128:135, 1904.

5. Behringer, G. E., and Albright, N. L.: Diverticular disease of the colon: A frequent cause of massive rectal bleeding. Am. J. Surg., 125:419, 1973.

6. Benn, P. L., Wolff, B. G., and Ilstrup, D. M.: Level of anastomosis and recurrent colonic diverticulitis. Am. J. Surg., 151:269, 1986.

7. Bowden, T. A., Jr., Hooks, V. H., III, and Mansberger, A. R.: Intraoperative gastrointestinal endoscopy in the management of occult gastrointestinal bleeding. S. Med. J., 72:1532, 1979.

8. Browder, W., Cerise, E. J., and Litwin, M. S.: Impact of emergency angiography in massive lower gastrointestinal bleeding. Ann. Surg., 204:530, 1986.

9. Canter, J. W., and Shorb, P. E., Jr.: Acute perforation of colonic diverticula associated with prolonged adrenocorticosteroid therapy. Am. J. Surg., 121:46, 1971.

10. Carson, S. D., Krom, R. A. F., Uchida, K., Yokota, K., West, J. C., and Weil, R., III: Colon perforation after kidney transplantation. Ann. Surg., 188:109, 1978.

11. Casarella, W. J., Kanter, I. E., and Seaman, W. B.: Right-sided colonic diverticula as a cause of acute rectal hemorrhage. N. Engl. J. Med., 286:450, 1972.

12. Chodak, G. W., Rangel, D. M., and Passaro, E., Jr.: Colonic diverticulitis in patients under age 40: Need for earlier diagnosis. Am. J. Surg., 141:699, 1981.

13. Crist, D. W., Fishman, E. K., Scatarige, J. C., and Cameron, J. L.: Acute diverticulitis of the cecum and ascending colon diagnosed by computed tomography. Surg. Gynecol. Obstet., 166:99, 1988.

14. Drapanas, T., Pennington, D. G., Kappelman, M., and Lindsey, E. S.: Emergency subtotal colectomy: Preferred approach to management of massively bleeding diverticular disease. Ann. Surg., 177:519, 1973.

15. Eng, K., Ranson, J. H. C., and Localio, S. A.: Resection of the perforated segment: A significant advance in treatment of diverticulitis with free perforation or abscess. Am. J. Surg., 133:67, 1977.

16. Eusebio, E. B., and Eisenberg, M. M.: Natural history of diverticular disease of the colon in young patients. Am. J. Surg., 125:308, 1973.

17. Fazio, V. W., Church, J. M., Jagelman, D. G., Weakley, F. L., Lavery, I. C., Tarazi, R., and VanHillo, M.: Colocutaneous fistulas complicating diverticulitis. Dis. Colon Rectum, 30:89, 1987.

18. Gouge, T. H., Coppa, G. F., Eng, K., Ranson, J. H. C., and Localio, S. R.: Management of diverticulitis of the ascending colon: 10 years' experience. Am. J. Surg., 145:387, 1983.

19. Graham, S. M., and Ballantyne, G. H.: Cecal diverticulitis: A review of the American experience. Dis. Colon Rectum, 30:821, 1987.

20. Gupta, S., Luna, E., Kingsley, S., Prince, M., and Herrera, N.: Detection of gastrointestinal bleeding by radionuclide scintigraphy. Am. J. Gastroenterol. 79:26, 1984.

21. Haglund, U., Hellberg, R., Johnsen, C., and Hulten, L.: Complicated diverticular disease of the sigmoid colon: An analysis of short and long term outcome in 392 patients. Ann. Chir. Gynecol., 68:41, 1979.

22. Hughes, L. E.: Postmortem survey of diverticular disease of the colon. I. Diverticulosis and diverticulitis. Gut, 10:336, 1969.

23. Huizinga, J. D.: Electrophysiology of human colon motility in health and disease. Clin. Gastroenterol., 15:879, 1986.

24. Jensen, D. M., and Machicado, G. A.: Diagnosis and treatment of severe hematochezia: The role of urgent colonoscopy after purge. Gastroenterology, 95:1569, 1988.

25. Kempczinski, R. F., and Ferrucci, J. T., Jr.: Giant sigmoid diverticula: A review. Ann. Surg., 180:864, 1974.

26. Labs, J. D., Sarr, M. G., Fishman, E. K., Siegelman, S. S., and Cameron, J. L.: Complications of acute diverticulitis of the colon: Improved early diagnosis with computerized tomography. Am. J. Surg., 155:331, 1988.

27. Leitman, I. M., Paull, D. E., and Shires, G. T., III.: Evaluation and management of massive lower gastrointestinal hemorrhage. Ann. Surg., 209:175, 1989.

28. Letwin, E. R.: Diverticulitis of the colon: Clinical review of acute presentations and management. Am. J. Surg., 143:579, 1982.

29. Mayo, W. J., Wilson, L. B., and Giffin, H. Z.: Acquired diverticulitis of the large intestine. Surg. Gynecol. Obstet., 5:8, 1907.

30. McConnell, D. B., Sasaki, T. M., and Vetto, R. M.: Experience with colovesical fistula. Am. J. Surg., 140:80, 1980.

31. McGuire, H. H., Jr., and Haynes, B. W., Jr.: Massive hemorrhage from diver-

32. McNutt, R., Schmitt, D., and Schulte, W.: Giant colonic diverticula — Three distinct entities: Report of a Case. Dis. Colon Rectum, 31:624, 1988.

33. Meyers, M. A., Alonso, D. R., Gray, G. F., and Baer, J. W.: Pathogenesis of bleeding colonic diverticulosis. Gastroenterology, 71:577, 1976.

34. Mileski, W. J., Joehl, R. J., Rege, R. V., and Nahrwold, D. L.: One-stage resection and anastomosis in the management of colovesical fistula. Am. J. Surg., 153:75, 1987.

35. Miller, R. E.: Role of hysterectomy in predisposing the patient to sigmoidovesical fistula complicating diverticulitis. Am. J. Surg., 147:660, 1984.

36. Morris, J., Stellato, T. A., Haaga, J. R., and Lieberman, J.: The utility of computed tomography in colonic diverticulitis. Ann. Surg., 204:128, 1986.

37. Morson, B. C.: The muscle abnormality in diverticular disease of the sigmoid colon. Br. J. Radiol. 36:385, 1963.

38. Neff, C. C., VanSonnenberg, E., Casola, G., Wittich, G. R., Hoyt, D. B., Halasz, N. A., and Martini, D. J.: Diverticular abscesses: Percutaneous drainage. Radiology, 163:15, 1987.

39. Painter, N. S.: The cause of diverticular disease of the colon, its symptoms and its complications: Review and hypothesis. J. R. Coll. Surg. Edinb., 30:118, 1985.

40. Painter, N. S., Almeida, A. Z., and Colebourne, K. W.: Unprocessed bran in treatment of diverticular disease of the colon. Br. Med. J., 2:137, 1972.

41. Painter, N. S., and Burkitt, D. P.: Diverticular disease of the colon: A 20th century problem. Clin. Gastroenterol., 4:3, 1975.

42. Painter, N. S., Truelove, S. C., Ardran, G. M., and Tuckey, M.: Segmentation and the localization of intraluminal pressures in the human colon, with special reference to the pathogenesis of colonic diverticula. Gastroenterology, 49:169, 1965.

43. Parks, T. G., and Connell, A. M.: Motility studies in diverticular disease of the colon. I. Basal activity and response to food assessed by open-ended tube and miniature balloon techniques. Gut, 10:534, 1969.

44. Parks, T. G.: Natural history of diverticular disease of the colon. Clin. Gastroenterol., 4:53, 1975.

45. Parks, T. G.: Reappraisal of clinical features of diverticular disease of the colon. Br. Med. J., 4:642, 1969.

46. Perkins, J. D., Shield, C. F., III., Chang, F. C., and Farha, G. J.: Acute diverticulitis: Comparison of treatment in immunocompromised and nonimmunocompromised patients. Am. J. Surg., 148:745, 1984.

47. Rege, R. V., and Nahrwold, D. L.: Diverticular disease. Curr. Probl. Surg., 26:136, 1989.

48. Rodkey, G. V., and Welch, C. E.: Changing patterns in the surgical treatment of diverticular disease. Ann. Surg., 200:466, 1984.

49. Rosenkrantz, H., Bookstein, J. J., Rosen, R. J., Goff, W. B., II, and Healy, J. F.: Postembolic colonic infarction. Radiology, 142:47, 1982.

50. Sardi, A., Gokli, A., and Singer, J. A.: Diverticular disease of the cecum and ascending colon: A review of 881 cases. Am. Surg., 53:41, 1987.

51. Sherman, L. M., Shenoy, S. S., and Cerra, F. B.: Selective intra-arterial vasopressin: Clinical efficacy and complications. Ann. Surg., 189:298, 1979.

52. Steer, M. L., and Silen, W.: Diagnostic procedures in gastrointestinal hemorrhage. N. Engl. J. Med., 309:646, 1983.

53. Sugihara, K., Muto, T., Morioka, Y., Asano, A., and Yamamoto, T.: Diverticular disease of the colon in Japan: A review of 615 cases. Dis. Colon Rectum, 27:531, 1984.

54. Talbot, J. M.: Role of dietary fiber in diverticular disease and colon cancer. Fed. Proc., 40:2337, 1981.

55. Telling, W. H. M., and Gruner, O. C.: Acquired diverticula, diverticulitis, and peridiverticulitis of the large intestine. Br. J. Surg., 4:468, 1917.

56. Uden, P., Jiborn, H., and Jonsson, K.: Influence of selective mesenteric arteriography on the outcome of emergency surgery for massive lower gastrointestinal hemorrhage: A 15-year experience. Dis. Colon. Rectum, 29:561, 1986.

57. Winzelberg, G. G., Froelich, J. W., McKusick, K. A., Waltman, A. C., Greenfield, A. J., Athanasoulis, C. A., and Strauss, H. W.: Radionuclide localization of lower gastrointestinal hemorrhage. Radiology, 139:465, 1981.

58. Woods, R. J., Lavery, I. C., Fazio, V. W., Jagelman, D. G., and Weakley, F. L.: Internal fistulas in diverticular disease. Dis. Colon Rectum, 31:591, 1988.

VI

BENIGN NEOPLASMS OF THE COLON, INCLUDING VASCULAR MALFORMATIONS

Anthony L. Imbembo, M.D., and J. Lawrence Fitzpatrick, M.D.

Benign lesions of the colon are being identified with increasing frequency largely because of the use of colonoscopy in the evaluation and follow-up of patients with a variety of disorders. Many benign lesions remain asymptomatic. The most frequent clinical presentation is occult bleeding. Occasionally, vague abdominal pain or a change in the character or frequency of stools may develop. Most discussions of benign neoplasms and polyps of the colon have been hampered by variable terminology. The framework outlined in Table 1 may be helpful.[2]

SUBMUCOSAL LESIONS

Submucosal lesions either cause a mass effect or assume a polypoid appearance. Frequently, biopsy of submucosal lesions is nondiagnostic, revealing only colonic mucosa, often with some degree of inflammation or ulceration. Hypertrophied lymph follicles may mimic a mass or polyp or occasionally form the lead point for an intussusception. Malignant lymphoma arising in the colon is quite rare. Fibromas and lipomas may arise throughout the colorectum but also are uncommon.

Carcinoid tumors arise from remnants of the neural crest. Thirty-five to 40 per cent of gastrointestinal carcinoids arise in the appendix, 15 per cent in the rectum, and 10 per cent in the remainder of the colon.[17] Rectal carcinoids appear to exhibit a more benign course than do those arising in the small bowel. Therefore, lesions less than 2 cm. in diameter are excised safely via the transanal route. However, the risk of malignancy is estimated to be approximately 20 per cent for tumors greater than 2 cm. in size. A more aggressive approach, such as abdominoperineal resection, may be warranted for large rectal carcinoids. Carcinoids of the intraperitoneal colon tend to be malignant. Segmental resection encompassing the lymphatic drainage constitutes standard treatment.

Air-filled cysts in the submucosa of the colon may assume the appearance of polyps. Full-thickness biopsy establishes the diagnosis of pneumatosis cystoides intestinalis. The condition may develop secondary to a fulminant colitis with invasion of the bowel wall by gas-forming bacteria. Pneumatosis also may occur in association with conditions such as chronic obstructive pulmonary disease or scleroderma. The pathophysiology of these associations is not understood, but an infectious etiology is doubtful, and resection is not required.

NONNEOPLASTIC MUCOSAL LESIONS

HYPERPLASTIC (METAPLASTIC) POLYPS. Hyperplastic polyps are smooth, rounded lesions that are typically sessile and less than 1 cm. in size. They are usually multiple, probably constituting the most common colonic polyp. Hyperplastic polyps are found most frequently in the distal colon or rectum. Their incidence increases with age, occurring in as many as 75 per cent of individuals over age 60.[8] At endoscopy, they may be indistinguishable from adenomatous polyps and, therefore, usually require removal.

Although hyperplastic polyps are not neoplastic, there is no certainty as to their genesis. Microscopically, the mucosa has an orderly papillary configuration with elongated crypts. There is no atypia. Although mitotic activity at the base of the crypts is normal, maturation and migration of cells appear to be delayed. Failure to slough cells may be responsible for polyp formation.[26]

As a consequence of their prevalence, multiplicity, and increasing frequency with age, hyperplastic polyps are encountered in up to 90 per cent of patients with colonic carcinoma. However, there does not appear to be an increased incidence of carcinoma in patients with hyperplastic polyps. Hyperplastic polyps are not considered premalignant.[26] Because their natural history is to remain small or regress, no specific therapy is required. Follow-up colonoscopy is not mandated merely by the presence of hyperplastic polyps.

INFLAMMATORY POLYPS (PSEUDOPOLYPS). Inflammatory polyps arise in response to colonic injury. They may develop secondary to any severe inflammatory process of the colon, including amebic colitis and other infectious processes but most often are associated with idiopathic ulcerative colitis. They consist either of residual intact mucosa or of regenerating epithelium. Inflammatory polyps themselves have no malignant potential. In the setting of ulcerative colitis, however, premalignant changes can coexist in adjacent areas of denudation.

Benign lymphoid polyps can arise in response to inflammation. They are found most frequently in the rectum and terminal ileum. When lymphoid aggregates undergo diffuse hypertrophy, nodular lymphoid hyperplasia, a condition observed more often in children, is said to exist.

TABLE 1. Classification of Colorectal Polyps

I. Neoplastic mucosal lesions
   A. Benign (adenoma)
      1. Tubular adenoma
      2. Tubulovillous adenoma
      3. Villous adenoma
   B. Malignant (carcinoma)
      1. Carcinoma *in situ* (intramucosal)
      2. Invasive carcinoma (through muscularis mucosae)
II. Nonneoplastic mucosal lesions
   A. Normal epithelium (in a polypoid configuration)
   B. Hyperplastic polyp (metaplastic polyp)
   C. Juvenile polyp (retention polyp)
   D. Inflammatory polyps (pseudopolyps)
      1. Inflammatory bowel disease
      2. Bacterial infections or amebiasis
      3. Schistosomiasis
III. Submucosal lesions
   A. Pneumatosis cystoides intestinalis
   B. Lymphoid polyps (benign and malignant)
   C. Lipomas
   D. Carcinomas
   E. Metastatic neoplasms
   F. Other rare lesions

Modified from Boland, C. R., and Kim, Y. S.: Colonic polyps and the gastrointestinal polyposis syndrome. *In* Sleisenger, M. H., and Fordtran, J.: Gastrointestinal Disease, W. B. Saunders Company, 1983.

JUVENILE POLYPS. Although juvenile or retention polyps are nearly always found in children under the age of 10, with the average age at discovery being 4.1 years, they can be observed at any age. They are found in approximately 4 per cent of individuals under age 21. There is a slight male predominance (3:2).

Juvenile polyps are thought to be hamartomas, up to 25 per cent of patients having multiple lesions. They are cherry-red and pedunculated, with a smooth surface contour. Size varies from a few millimeters to 2 cm. The distal colon is involved most frequently, with over three quarters occurring in the rectum. Microscopically, the abundant glands are elongated and dilated, with areas of mucous-filled, cystic dilatation; hence the term *retention polyp*. An intense inflammatory infiltrate and excessive lamina propria are usually present. Both the columnar and numerous goblet cells demonstrate little atypia. The stroma is usually edematous and markedly vascular. Abundant lymphoid tissue and hamartomatous elements such as bone also may be present. Areas of necrosis and ulceration are often observed.

Owing to the rich blood supply of juvenile polyps, along with their tendency to ulcerate, bleeding per rectum is the most common presentation. Nearly all patients with juvenile polyps have hematochezia, although massive hemorrhage is rare. Because most of these polyps are pedunculated, torsion can cause infarction and resultant sloughing. Prolapse occurs in approximately one third of patients, the child presenting with a cherry-red or "beefy" protrusion from the anus. Propulsion of the polyp and its stalk by peristalsis creates traction, which may cause crampy abdominal pain. Intussusception is rare. Because screening endoscopy is not done in children, juvenile polyps rarely are detected incidentally. Thus, their prevalence in the general pediatric population is not known.

Juvenile polyps have no malignant potential. They should be removed for histologic confirmation and relief of symptoms. Most can be removed endoscopically with care being taken to control completely the highly vascular pedicle. Lesions low in the rectum or those that have prolapsed can be removed transanally. Recurrence is very rare after excision.[20]

NEOPLASTIC MUCOSAL LESIONS

Adenomatous polyps are benign epithelial neoplasms with an estimated incidence in the general population of 5 to 10 per cent. Adenomas are classified according to their histologic glandular pattern. Tubular adenomas, which are the most common, have a complex, branching glandular arrangement, whereas villous tumors have glands arranged in long fingerlike projections. There is also an intermediate polyp demonstrating features of each. The degree of dysplasia varies considerably, villous lesions usually demonstrating the most severe changes; each neoplastic polyp can be either pedunculated or sessile.

In adenomatous polyps cellular proliferation is no longer limited to the base of a crypt and apical cells no longer slough into the bowel lumen. New glands form by folding or branching. The type of polyp formed is determined by the interrelationship between the abnormal mucosa and the underlying connective tissue and capillaries. With a pedunculated polyp, the connective tissue stalk contains normal mucosa and is not neoplastic, since it is formed by traction on the polyp exerted by peristalsis.

TUBULAR ADENOMAS. Tubular adenomas constitute 60 to 80 per cent of neoplastic polyps.[36] They are extremely rare in patients younger than 20 years of age; thereafter, the incidence increases steadily with age. There is no sexual predilection. Tubular adenomas tend to remain small, less than 2 cm. in diameter. They are dome-shaped and more intensely colored than the surrounding mucosa. Ulceration is usually a sign of malignancy. An increased predilection for the right colon has become apparent in recent years. In a series of 5786 polyps, the distribution was: rectum, 5.7 per cent; sigmoid, 46.3 per cent; left colon, 24.3

per cent; transverse, 10.7 per cent; right colon, 13 per cent.[36] Tubular polyps are usually pedunculated.

Most tubular adenomas demonstrate only mild dysplasia (Fig. 1). However, in 20 per cent severe atypia, carcinoma *in situ*, or invasive carcinoma is present.[36] Typically, these changes are confined to larger lesions. Because lymphatic channels arise in the muscularis mucosa, extension of malignancy to this level defines invasion. The overall incidence of carcinoma arising in a tubular adenoma is approximately 15 per cent. A polyp of over 1 cm. diameter has approximately a 10 per cent likelihood of being malignant, whereas with one over 2 cm. the risk increases to nearly 35 per cent.[31]

VILLOUS ADENOMAS. Villous tumors comprise at most 10 per cent of colonic polyps. They occur slightly more often in men (3:2). Although tubular adenomas are found throughout the colon, villous adenomas tend to occur distally. In a report typical of many, of 219 villous tumors, 144 were in the rectum and 54 in the sigmoid.[32] Villous adenomas are usually sessile. Unlike tubular adenomas, they may become quite large, over 60 per cent being greater than 2 cm. Diameters of nearly 12 cm. have been reported.[5] Grossly, villous adenomas have a cauliflower appearance and a very soft consistency. They are compressed easily and, therefore, may not be recognized on rectal examination. Areas of firmness or ulceration usually indicate malignancy. Microscopically, they are characterized by fingerlike epithelial projections resembling villi (Fig. 2).

Intermediate lesions exhibiting characteristics of tubular and villous lesions are termed variously tubulovillous adenomas, villoglandular adenomas, or mixed polyps. Generally, tubular adenomas with a villous component of 10 to 30 per cent are termed tubulovillous, whereas those in which it is greater are classified as villous adenomas. The greater the villous component, the greater the possibility of malignant change.

Although some villous adenomas are asymptomatic, particularly if small, two thirds of patients develop rectal bleeding, and one half complain of mucous or watery rectal discharge. Prolapse is rare because of their sessile base. Large villous adenomas can encompass the entire circumference of the bowel. A large rectal lesion may cause tenesmus or a sense of incomplete evacuation after defecation. Because of their soft texture and compressibility, colonic obstruction rarely occurs.

Rarely, a villous adenoma secretes a profuse discharge of water and/or mucus. Several liters per day can be lost, with resultant hypovolemia and/or dehydration. There also may be marked loss of potassium from the surface of the tumor. As much as several hundred milliequivalents of potassium replacement per day may be required. Because the potassium losses greatly exceed serum concentration, the existence of an active electrolyte pump at the mucosal surface has been suggested.[37]

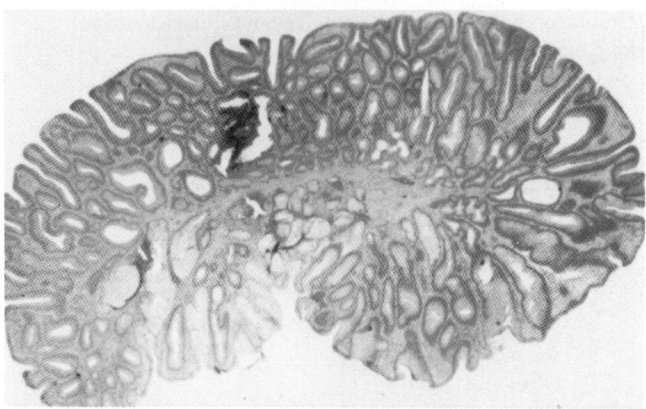

Figure 1. Tubular adenoma. Overgrowth of columnar epithelium shows tubules lined by adenomatous cells, decreased goblet cells, and decreased mucosa. (Modified from Watne, A. L.: The syndromes of intestinal polyposis. Curr. Probl. Surg., 24(4):282, 1987. Courtesy of W. Chang, M.D.)

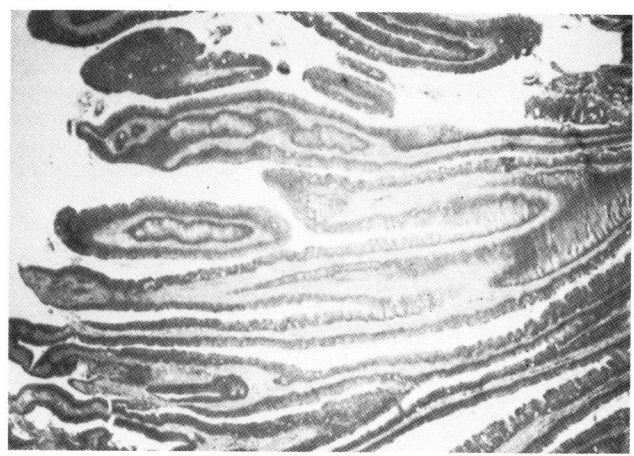

Figure 2. Villous adenoma. Deep, interlacing crypts with hyperchromatic cells and atypia. (Modified from Watne, A. L.: The syndromes of intestinal polyposis. Curr. Probl. Surg., 24(4):282, 1987.)

Treatment of Adenomatous Polyps

Most adenocarcinomas of the colon originate in areas of adenomatous change. Several lines of evidence support this concept. Adenoma prevalence within a population group, as well as the number of adenomas per individual, parallels the prevalence of cancer.[10] The prevalence of both adenomatous polyps and cancers increases with age, with the development of adenomas preceding that of carcinomas by approximately 5 to 10 years. The anatomic distribution of adenomatous polyps and cancer generally is similar.[42] In addition, adenomatous elements, particularly villous tumors, frequently are found adjacent to colonic carcinoma.[16] Overall, it is estimated that approximately 70 per cent of adenomas remain static, 8 per cent regress, and another 8 per cent disappear.[29] Approximately 5 per cent increase in size, and 1 per cent develop into invasive carcinoma.

The risk of malignant degeneration depends, in large measure, on the characteristics of the adenoma. Nearly 5 per cent of the tubular adenomas, 22.5 per cent of tubulovillous polyps, and 40 per cent of villous adenomas contain carcinoma.[9] When adenomas are less than 1 cm. in diameter, only 1 per cent of tubular polyps contain carcinoma, as compared with 3.5 per cent of tubulovillous and 10 per cent of villous adenomas. In tumors over 2 cm. in size, carcinoma is present in 35 per cent of tubular adenomas and over 50 per cent of villous lesions.

In a study reported by Gilbertson and the Minnesota Cancer Detection Center Program, an 85 per cent decrease in the expected cancer rate among study participants was attributed to removal of detected adenomas.[16] Generally, all polypoid lesions greater than 1 cm. in diameter should be removed completely. Lesions less than 1 cm. must be followed or removed, with the decision often depending on technical considerations. Enlarging polyps must always be removed.

Tubular or tubulovillous polyps containing carcinoma *in situ* (neoplastic cells not involving the muscularis mucosa) are treated adequately by simple total excision, including the stalk if present. A more extensive resection is indicated if *in situ* changes are present at the excision margin or if the carcinoma actually proves to be invasive. Since tubular polyps containing invasive carcinoma are rarely associated with lymph node metastases, segmental resection is usually adequate.[9]

All villous adenomas should be considered premalignant. Characteristics such as firmness or ulceration should strongly suggest malignant degeneration. A negative biopsy in larger villous tumors does not exclude cancer, because sampling errors are common. Villous tumors above the peritoneal reflection should be removed by segmental resection. If there is any suggestion of malignancy, resection with adequate margins including the regional lymphatics must be performed.

The management of villous tumors of the rectum is less clearly defined. If biopsy reveals invasive cancer, either low anterior or abdominoperineal resection of the rectum is indicated. If malignancy has not been established, the entire tumor must be excised, if possible. The transanal approach is used for distal lesions. Lesions higher in the rectum may be resected via the posterior transsacral approach[41] (Fig. 3). *En bloc* resection is preferred to allow complete pathologic examination. Morcellation of the tumor does not permit this. If complete excision is not possible, repeat excision and fulguration with electrocautery or laser may be an option.

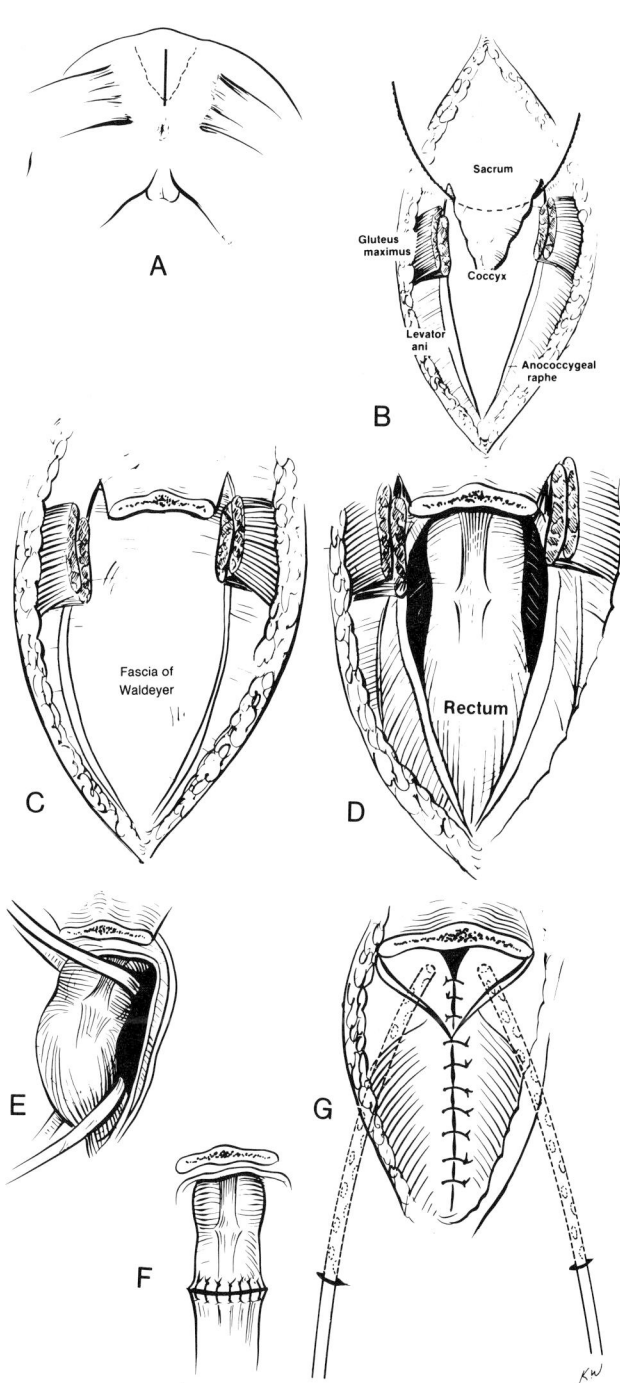

Figure 3. Posterior sacral approach to rectum. *A,* Patient in prone position. *B,* Division of anococcygeal raphe and freeing of sacrum. *C,* After division of the sacrum, fascia of Waldeyer is evident. *D,* Exposure of rectum. *E,* Mobilization of rectum. *F,* Resection and anastomosis. *G,* Closure in layers. (Modified from Westbrook, K., Lang, N., Broadwater, J. R., and Thompson, B. W.: Posterior surgical approaches to the rectum. Ann. Surg., 195:677, 1982. Courtesy of W. Chang, M.D.)

GASTROINTESTINAL POLYPOSIS SYNDROMES

FAMILIAL POLYPOSIS COLI. Familial polyposis coli is the most common of the hereditary polyposis syndromes.[19] Diagnosis requires the demonstration of at least 100 adenomatous polyps, although the number may be 5000. The average number in total colectomy specimens has been approximately 1000.[5] Adenomatous polyps usually form after puberty. Initially, the polyps appear in the rectum and distal colon and progress until the entire colon is carpeted. The diagnosis usually is made between ages 20 and 40, the average age being 36 years. Ninety per cent of all cases are identified by age 50.[5,6]

It has been difficult to determine the number of patients with familial polyposis coli. The reported incidence is 1:6800 to 1:24,000, with an average of 1 per 12,000 births.[6] Although reported most frequently in well-studied, industrialized areas, familial polyposis coli has been identified worldwide in all racial and ethnic groups.

The polyps are small initially, less than 5 mm., and tend to remain so. They exhibit the full spectrum of adenomatous changes, from tubular to villous. Even with the presence of hundreds of polyps, patients may be asymptomatic. Many are diagnosed only on screening evaluation. Others develop problems such as crampy abdominal pain, diarrhea, hematochezia, and iron deficiency anemia. Late cases may present with symptoms of colonic carcinoma. The diagnosis is made by endoscopy and/or contrast barium enema. Biopsy is essential to verify that the lesions are adenomatous. Although the colon usually is involved uniformly, skip areas may occur, and occasionally polyps greater than 2 cm. may be observed.

Familial polyposis coli is associated with extracolonic manifestations.[4] For example, mandibular osteomas, often multiple, and other sclerotic bony lesions are found on occasion. Adenomatous polyps develop elsewhere in the gastrointestinal tract, including particularly the gastric antrum, duodenum, periampullary region, and ileum. Gastric and periampullary malignancy have been reported. Therefore, endoscopic surveillance of the upper gastrointestinal tract is indicated. Although there is an increased risk of malignancy throughout the gastrointestinal tract, prophylactic resection is not indicated for any segment other than the colon.

Colorectal cancer must be considered an inevitable consequence of familial polyposis coli. Since the exact age of onset of polyps is not always known, the usual interval between polyp formation and malignant degeneration has not been established, although a latency period of 10 to 15 years has been suggested.[6] In approximately 12 per cent of patients cancer develops within the first 5 years after diagnosis; after 15 years cancer develops in over 50 per cent. The average age for detection of cancer is approximately 40. Multiple synchronous carcinomas occur in over 40 per cent of patients.[19]

Because of the almost inexorable progression to malignancy, resection of the colon is indicated. Controversy exists only regarding the timing and extent of the procedure. Surveillance colonoscopy is not sufficiently reliable for detection of malignancy at an early stage. Generally, colonic resection is advised at the time of diagnosis. In asymptomatic children and teenagers, the procedure may be deferred to allow physical and psychosocial maturation, so long as regular endoscopic examination is performed. However, colonic malignancies have been reported in individuals less than 20 years old. Total proctocolectomy and ileostomy definitively eliminate the possibility of colorectal carcinoma. However, the consequence of a permanent abdominal stoma is unacceptable to many patients. Total abdominal colectomy with ileoproctostomy has been an alternative approach used by many. This procedure preserves reservoir function and continence, and the patient usually has about three bowel movements per day. Unfortunately, retention of

the rectum does not eliminate the risk of malignancy. Following total abdominal colectomy and ileoproctostomy, spontaneous regression of rectal polyps is not infrequent, regression rates of over 60 per cent having been reported.[13] Despite regression, all patients require close endoscopic follow-up for removal of any polyps that reappear. The reasons for regression have not been defined. Unfortunately, in most patients new polyps develop at some time.

The risk of developing cancer despite close observation in the retained rectum is 20 per cent at 20 years to as high as 60 per cent after 25 years.[28] The time course between ileoproctostomy and the development of rectal cancer is from months to as much as 25 years. Thus, abdominal colectomy with ileoproctostomy is an acceptable choice only in the elderly, who presumably have a shortened follow-up period, or for patients in whom the rectum is not heavily invaded by polyps.

The current alternative to ileostomy after total abdominal colectomy is rectal mucosectomy and ileoanal pull-through. The unstable mucosa is removed, leaving a short sleeve of rectal musculature through which the ileum is brought for anastomosis to the anus. Continence is preserved in the majority of patients and there is nearly no risk of resultant sexual dysfunction since dissection external to the rectum is eliminated. With a straight ileoanal anastomosis, the patient tends to experience about eight to ten bowel movements per day. In an attempt to improve reservoir function, a variety of ileal pouches have been proposed for use in conjunction with the procedure (Fig. 4). Overall, the more frequent complications include pouch inflammation due to fecal stasis, dehydration, and nocturnal incontinence to some degree. Acceptance of these procedures is increasing steadily as techniques become refined.

GARDNER'S SYNDROME. Gardner's syndrome is a familial disease consisting of gastrointestinal polyposis, osteomas of the mandible, skull and long bones, and a number of soft tissue tumors including sebaceous cysts, fibromas, lipomas, and desmoid tumors.[14] The colon is the most common site for polyposis, but the stomach, duodenum, small bowel, and periampullary areas also may be involved. The diagnostic evaluation, malignant potential, and management are identical to those for familial polyposis coli.

The extracolonic manifestations of Gardner's syndrome are frequent and varied. The small intestine, particularly the duodenum and periampullary area, is subject to neoplastic development, with an overall incidence of malignant degeneration as high as 12 per cent in these locations. In the stomach multiple

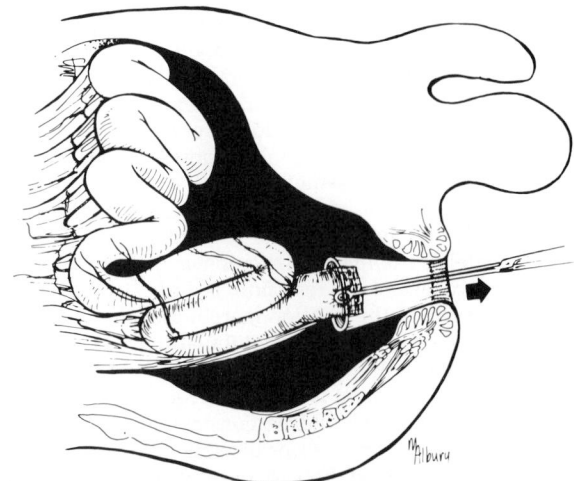

Figure 4. After abdominal colectomy and removal of mucosa from the rectum, the distal ileum is pulled through the rectal muscle sleeve before anastomosis to the anus. Note that an S-pouch ileal reservoir has been created. (Modified from Wong, W. D., Rothenberger, D. A., and Goldberg, S. M.: Ileoanal pouch procedures. Curr. Probl. Surg. 22(3):9, 1985.)

adenomas, microcarcinoids, hyperplastic polyps, and/or lymphoid polyps can develop. Frequent endoscopy, biopsy, and/or polypectomy are essential. Generally, the gastric lesions can be followed by surveillance. In the West, gastric carcinoma is rare in association with Gardner's syndrome. Bony abnormalities, consisting of osteomas, exostoses, and cortical thickening, can occur in the skull, mandible, facial bones, and long bones. Associated dental anomalies include odontomas, dentigenous cysts, supernumerary teeth, and unerupted teeth. The bony changes may predate the colonic manifestations of the disease.

It is the presence of cutaneous and subcutaneous lesions that most often serves to differentiate Gardner's syndrome from familial polyposis coli. Epidermal cysts, fibromas, and lipomas can occur on the face, neck, trunk, and scalp. Desmoid tumors are quite rare in the general population (0.03 per cent) but are observed in up to 4 per cent of patients with neoplastic polyposis.[24] These locally aggressive tumors in the abdominal wall usually arise from a surgical scar or are secondary to trauma; however, spontaneous occurrence also is observed. Histologically, desmoid tumors vary from well-differentiated fibromas to borderline fibrosarcomas. Cultured fibroblasts from patients with polyposis have exhibited an enhanced tritiated thymidine incorporation and increased tetraploidy. These findings suggest that impaired control of fibroblast proliferation constitutes a significant defect. An enlarging desmoid tumor may extend intra-abdominally, usually when the tumor has arisen in a preexistent scar. Diffuse mesenteric or retroperitoneal fibrosis may ensue, causing gastrointestinal, vascular, or ureteral obstruction. Desmoid tumors occur in up to 20 per cent of patients with Gardner's syndrome and are the second leading cause of death. Because of encasement of vital structures, they usually are not completely resectable. Occasional responses to radiation have been reported.[25]

Familial polyposis coli and Gardner's syndrome are inherited as autosomal dominant traits. Growing evidence suggests that all forms of neoplastic polyposis constitute a single inherited defect, individual manifestations being due to variations in genetic expression.[15]

HAMARTOMATOUS POLYPOSIS SYNDROMES. CRONKHITE-CANADA SYNDROME. This entity is characterized by (1) diffuse gastrointestinal polyposis extending from stomach to rectum; (2) skin and nail changes consisting of alopecia, hyperpigmentation, and finger and toenail atrophy; and (3) weight loss, diarrhea, and malnutrition. It does not follow a familial pattern and is usually identified in adults, most cases being diagnosed at over 50 years of age.[11] Hamartomatous polyps similar to juvenile (retention) polyps are found in 52 to 96 per cent of patients.[12] Although these nonneoplastic polyps are not considered premalignant, reports have documented the occasional development of carcinoma, which emphasizes the need for surveillance.

The etiology of Cronkhite-Canada syndrome is not certain, but it may be related to malabsorption, malnutrition, or vitamin deficiencies. Gastrointestinal manifestations may include diarrhea, bulky stools due to steatorrhea, hematochezia, intussusception, and rectal prolapse. Fluid, electrolyte, vitamin, and mineral deficiencies are coupled typically with large protein losses. Surgical intervention is reserved for complications such as bleeding, gastric outlet obstruction, rectal prolapse, intussusception, and resection of short segments of massively involved intestine.

Treatment is directed to vigorous nutritional and metabolic support. Both partial and complete remissions have been reported to follow weeks or months of treatment.[12] Anecdotal benefit has been ascribed to corticosteroids, anabolic steroids, and oral antibiotics.[12]

FAMILIAL HAMARTOMATOUS POLYPOSIS SYNDROME. NEUROFIBROMATOSIS. Neurofibromatosis (von Recklinghausen's disease) is a neuroectodermal disease manifested by cutaneous pigmentation (café au lait spots) along with visceral and cutaneous neurofibromas. It is inherited as an autosomal dominant trait. Gastrointestinal involvement occurs in up to 25 per cent of patients.[21] Neurofibromas occur most frequently in the stomach and jejunum, but the colon also may be involved. The lesions consist of an overgrowth of neural tissue together with other mesenchymal elements. Any layer of the bowel wall may be affected. Gastrointestinal neurofibromas may cause occult bleeding, luminal obstruction, or intussusception. Therapy is directed to symptomatic lesions only.

PEUTZ-JEGHERS SYNDROME. This syndrome is characterized by mucocutaneous pigmentation and gastrointestinal polyposis. It appears to be inherited as an autosomal dominant trait. Melanin deposits may appear in infancy or early childhood and tend to occur on or around the lips, buccal linings, nostrils, hands, feet, or perianal area. The gastrointestinal polyps are hamartomas with a very prominent smooth muscle component deriving from the muscularis mucosa. They are usually multiple; and although they may occur anywhere within the gastrointestinal tract, they are most frequently found in the small bowel.[22] The most common complications are intussusception, obstruction, and bleeding. Although carcinoma of the colon and duodenum have been reported in patients with Peutz-Jeghers syndrome, the incidence is only 2 to 3 per cent. There does appear to be a significantly increased risk of the development of small-bowel carcinoma. Ovarian and testicular tumors also may develop with greater frequency in these patients.[43]

MULTIPLE HAMARTOMA SYNDROME. The multiple hamartoma syndrome (Cowden's syndrome) is an autosomal dominant trait characterized by multisystem hamartomas. The manifestations may include orocutaneous lesions, severe fibrocystic disease of the breast, multiple cancers of the breast, goiter, thyroid adenomas, and carcinoma, as well as gastrointestinal polyps.

JUVENILE POLYPOSIS SYNDROMES. Juvenile polyps are distinct hamartomas of the retention variety. There are at least three distinct syndromes, depending on whether the polyps are located in the stomach or the colon or diffusely involve the entire gastrointestinal tract.[34] Unlike the multiple adenomatous polyposis syndromes, which rarely present before adulthood, juvenile polyposis produces symptoms in childhood. Typical manifestations include obstruction, bleeding, and intussusception. Although the juvenile polyps are hamartomas, and as such do not have malignant potential, it now appears that the risk of the development of colon cancer is increased.[38] The findings of associated adenomatous polyps and changes in the stability of colonic epithelium appear to be responsible. Therefore, patients with juvenile polyposis must be followed closely and associated adenomas removed. The syndrome now must be regarded as premalignant.

VASCULAR MALFORMATIONS

ANGIODYSPLASIA. The terms *angiodysplasia* and *arteriovenous malformation* are now used interchangeably. There are two broad groups. Those occurring in younger individuals are thought to be congenital and are distributed throughout the gastrointestinal tract. Those lesions identified in older patients, usually over 50, are found most frequently in the cecum and right colon. The latter lesions are considered to be acquired and are far more frequent. It has been suggested that acquired angiodysplasia arises from chronic, progressive dilatation of venules within the bowel wall secondary either to partial obstruction of draining veins or to increased intraluminal pressure. As these veins become more distended and tortuous, there is disruption of the capillary network with its associated system of sphincters. A minute arteriovenous shunt forms in the submucosa.[3] The predilection for the right colon has not been explained.

Angiodysplasia is estimated to occur in approximately 2 per cent of individuals over 50 years old and may cause chronic blood loss with anemia or acute episodes of gross lower gastrointestinal hemorrhage. In some studies, 15 to 25 per cent of the patients with angiodysplasia have had aortic stenosis[27]; however, in only approximately 1 per cent of patients with acquired aortic stenosis does gastrointestinal hemorrhage develop.[66] Patients with chronic renal failure may also have an increased likelihood of bleeding from angiodysplasias. In renal failure, however, the lesions tend to be diffuse.

The diagnosis of angiodysplasia may be difficult. Despite multiple investigations, many patients have a long history of occult blood loss. Selective mesenteric angiography probably is the most effective diagnostic approach.[35] Diagnostic findings include an early filling vein, a localized vascular tuft, blush or stain, and a slowly draining tortuous vein which is usually visualized late in the sequence (Fig. 5). Angiodysplastic lesions are usually located on the antimesenteric border. Since angiodysplasia is nearly impossible to identify at laparotomy, preoperative localization is imperative.

Recently, colonoscopy has been advocated as the primary diagnostic modality. Successful visualization has been reported in up to 80 per cent of patients, in the absence of significant hemorrhage. Diagnostic findings include visible telangiectasias, distinct cherry-red areas, and tortuous dilated vessels with erosions. Colonoscopic electrocoagulation and/or laser photoablation have been effective in over 60 per cent of patients, with a complication rate of less than 10 per cent. Surgical resection is definitive treatment, provided the bleeding sites have been localized. Many now reserve resection for those cases in which endoscopic coagulation fails or for ongoing gross hemorrhage.[39]

HEMANGIOMAS. Hemangiomas of the gastrointestinal tract are much less frequent than angiodysplasia. They occur in both the colon and the small intestine. Histologically, hemangiomas are composed of large blood-filled sinuses within a connective tissue framework. Gastrointestinal hemangiomas are classified as capillary, cavernous, or mixed and probably arise from the rich submucosal vascular plexus. Most often they are solitary and of the cavernous type.[1]

Kaposi's sarcoma is a neoplastic vascular malformation and a common manifestation of the acquired immune deficiency syndrome. It has been considered a variety of hemangioma.[40] Fifty per cent of Kaposi's sarcomas are found in the gastrointestinal tract, the duodenum being the most common location. The colon and rectum may also be involved.

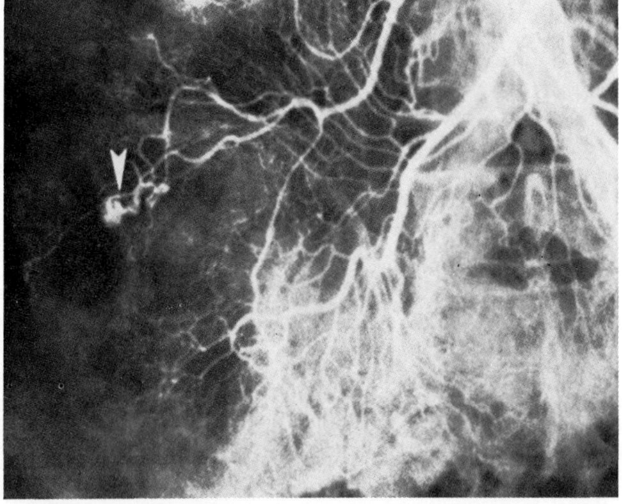

Hemangiomas may cause occult blood loss or gross hemorrhage, even in childhood. Overall, the rectum is the most common location. Endoscopy is often an effective diagnostic modality. On angiography, hemangiomas demonstrate a characteristic tumor blush and abnormal vessels. On barium contrast study, a mass effect may be observed, but this is nonspecific. Thirty per cent of hemangiomas contain phleboliths visible on plain films.

Hemangiomas are treated either by local excision or segmental resection of the involved segment of bowel. Because of their vascularity and the potential for serious hemorrhage, endoscopic coagulation should not be attempted. Kaposi's sarcoma is considered for resection only in the presence of obstruction or bleeding.

MESENTERIC VARICES. Colonic varices develop secondary to portal hypertension or from localized mesenteric venous outflow obstruction due to tumor, lymphadenopathy, or adhesions. Both endoscopy and mesenteric angiography with attention to the late venous phase are effective diagnostic studies. Asymptomatic varices require no treatment. Bleeding varices are addressed according to etiology. Diffuse intestinal varices may require portal decompression therapy. Isolated varices are best treated by segmental resection, if possible. Varices involving a colostomy can be a very significant problem, because repeated local trauma usually causes chronic bleeding.

TELANGIECTASIAS. Telangiectasias of the colon usually occur as part of the hereditary hemorrhagic telangiectasias syndrome (also known as Osler-Weber-Rendu syndrome). Telangiectasias also are present in the skin, nose, liver, or central nervous system. Epistaxis is the most frequent form of hemorrhage, but gastrointestinal bleeding occurs in up to 40 per cent of patients, often not until middle age. There is often a family history for the disease. The lesions usually are multiple, and new ones can develop over time. Telangiectasias are usually small and do not produce a mass effect. The diagnosis is best made by endoscopy or angiography.

The tendency to multiplicity makes management of telangiectasias difficult. Endoscopic photoablation or electrocoagulation has been used. Unfortunately, other lesions may subsequently become symptomatic.[33] Extensive surgical resection is not indicated for episodic bleeding, but may be required, on occasion, for massive hemorrhage. Some have suggested that oral estrogens may decrease the tendency of these lesions to bleed.

SELECTED REFERENCES

Feinberg, S. M., Jagelman, D. G., et al.: Spontaneous resolution of rectal polyps in patients with familial polyposis following abdominal colectomy and ileorectal anastomosis. Dis. Colon Rectum, 31:169, 1988.
An extensive experience with this procedure is reviewed. The natural history of the residual rectal segment is defined.

Haggitt, R. C., et al.: Hereditary gastrointestinal polyposis syndromes. Am. J. Surg. Pathol., 10:871, 1986.
This is an in-depth review article summarizing recent pathologic and clinical literature concerning polyposis syndromes. It compares and contrasts the different syndromes and pathologic details. There is an extensive bibliography.

Muto, T., Bussey, H. J. R., and Morson, B. C.: The evolution of cancer of the colon and rectum. Cancer, 36:2251, 1975.
The authors provide data supporting the polyp-cancer sequence, with an in-depth discussion of polyps. This remains the classic reference on neoplastic polyps.

Trudey, J. L., Fazio, V. W., and Sivak, M. V.: Colonoscopic diagnosis and treatment of arteriovenous malformations in chronic lower gastrointestinal bleeding. Dis. Colon Rectum, 31:107, 1988.
The authors present an experience with endoscopy for diagnosis and treatment and recommend colonoscopy as the initial diagnostic procedure.

REFERENCES

1. Abrahamson, J., and Shandling, B.: Intestinal hemangiomata in childhood and a syndrome for diagnosis: A collective review. J. Pediatr. Surg., 8:487, 1973.
2. Boland, C. R., Itzkowitz, J. A., and Kim, Y. S.: Colonic polyps and the gastroin-

Figure 5. Angiodysplasia. Selective superior mesenteric arteriogram in the arterial phase. The arrow points to a small vascular tuft in the cecum. (From Marx, F. W., et al.: Angiodysplasia as a source of intestinal bleeding. Am. J. Surg., *134:*126, 1977.)

testinal polyposis syndromes. *In* Sleisenger, M. H., and Fordtran, J. S. (Eds.): Gastrointestinal Diseases, 4th ed. Philadelphia, W. B. Saunders Company, 1989, p. 1483.

3. Boley, S. J., Sammartano, R., Adams, A., DiBiase, A., Kleinhaus, S., and Sprayregen, S.: On the nature and etiology of vascular ectasias of the colon: Degenerative lesions of aging. Gastroenterology, 72:650, 1977.

4. Bussey, H. J. R.: Extracolonic lesions associated with polyposis coli. Proc. R. Soc. Med., 65:294, 1972.

5. Bussey, H. J. R.: Familial polyposis coli. Baltimore, Johns Hopkins University Press, 1975.

6. Bussey, H. J. R., Veale, A. M. O., and Morson, B. C.: Genetics of gastrointestinal polyposis. Gastroenterology, 74:1325, 1978.

7. Cello, J. P., and Grendell, J. H.: Endoscopic laser treatment for gastrointestinal vascular ectasias. Ann. Intern. Med., 104:352, 1986.

8. Clark, J. C., Collan, Y., Eide, T. J., Esteve, J., Ewen, S., Gibbs, N. M., Jensen, O. M., Koskela, E., MacLennan, R., Simpson, J. G., Stalsberg, H., and Zaridze, D. G.: Prevalence of polyps in an autopsy series from areas with varying incidence of large-bowel cancer. Int. J. Cancer, 36:179, 1985.

9. Cooper, H. S.: Surgical pathology of endoscopically removed malignant polyps of the colon and rectum. Am. J. Surg. Pathol., 7:613, 1983.

10. Correa, P.: Epidemiology of polyps and cancer. *In* Morson, B. C. (Ed.): The Pathogenesis of Colorectal Cancer. Philadelphia, W. B. Saunders Company, 1978, p. 126.

11. Cronkhite, L. W., and Canada, W. J.: Generalized gastrointestinal polyposis: An unusual syndrome of polyposis, pigmentation, alopecia and onychotrophia. N. Engl. J. Med., 252:1011, 1955.

12. Daniel, E. S., Ludwig, S. L., Lewin, K. J., Ruprecht, R. M., Rajacich, G. M., and Schwabe, A. D.: The Cronkhite-Canada syndrome: An analysis of the pathologic features and therapy in 55 patients. Medicine, 61:293, 1982.

13. Feinberg, S. M., et al.: Spontaneous resolution of rectal polyps in patients with familial polyposis following abdominal colectomy and ileorectal anastomosis. Dis. Colon Rectum, 31:169, 1988.

14. Gardner, E. J.: A genetic and clinical study of intestinal polyposis, a predisposing factor for carcinoma of the colon and rectum. Am. J. Hum. Genet., 3:167, 1951.

15. Gardner, E. J.: Familial polyposis coli and Gardner's syndrome—Is there a difference? *In* Ingall, J. R. F., and Mastromarino, A. J. (Eds.): Prevention of Hereditary Large Bowel Cancer. New York, Alan R. Liss, Inc., 1983, p. 39.

16. Gilbertson, V. A., and Nelms, J. M.: The prevention of invasive cancer of the rectum. Cancer, 41:1137, 1978.

17. Godwin, J. D.: Carcinoid tumors: An analysis of 2837 cases. Lancet, 36:560, 1975.

18. Greenstein, R. J., McElhinney, A. J., Reuben, D., and Greenstein, A. J.: Colonic vascular ectasias and aortic stenosis: Coincidence or causal relationship? Am. J. Surg., 151:347, 1986.

19. Haggitt, R. C., et al.: Hereditary gastrointestinal polyposis syndromes. Am. J. Surg. Pathol., 10:871, 1986.

20. Hill, J. J., Morson, B. C., and Bussey, H. J. R.: Aetiology of adenomacarcinoma sequence in large bowel. Lancet, 1:245, 1978.

21. Hochberg, F. H., Dasilva, A. B., Galdabini, J., and Richardson, Jr., E. P.: Gastrointestinal involvement in von Recklinghausen's neurofibromatosis. Neurology, 24:1144, 1974.

22. Jeghers, H., McKusick, V. A., and Katz, K. H.: Generalized intestinal polyposis and melanin spots of the oral mucosa, lips and digits. N. Engl. J. Med., 241:993, 1031, 1949.

23. Jensen, D., and Bown, S.: Gastrointestinal angiomata: Diagnosis and treatment with laser therapy and other endoscopic modalities. *In* Fleisher, D., Jensen, D., and Bright-Asare, P. (Eds.): Therapeutic Laser Endoscopy in Gastrointestinal Disease. The Hague, Martinus Nijhoff Publishers, 1983, p. 151.

24. Jones, I. T., Jagelman, D. G., Fazio, V. W., Lavery, I. C., Weakley, F. L., and McGannon, E.: Desmoid tumors in familial polyposis coli. Ann. Surg., 204:94, 1986.

25. Kiel, K. D., and Suit, H. D.: Radiation therapy in the treatment of aggressive fibromatoses (desmoid tumors). Cancer, 54:2051, 1984.

26. Lane, N., Kaplan, H., and Pascal, R. R.: Minute adenomatous and hyperplastic polyps of the colon: Divergent patterns of epithelial growth with specific associated mesenchymal changes. Gastroenterology, 60:537, 1971.

27. Meyer, C. T., Troncale, F. J. Galloway, S., and Sheahan, D. G.: Arteriovenous malformations of the bowel: An analysis of 22 cases and a review of the literature. Medicine, 60:36, 1981.

28. Moertel, C. G., Hill, J. R., and Adson, M. A.: Management of multiple polyposis of the large intestine. Cancer, 28:160, 1971.

29. Morson, B. C.: Genesis of colorectal cancer. Clin. Gastroenterol., 5:505, 1976.

30. Morson, B. C., and Bussey, H. J. R.: Predisposing causes of intestinal cancer. Curr. Probl. Surg., February 1970, p. 8.

31. Muto, T., Bussey, H. J. R., and Morson, B. C.: The evolution of cancer of the colon and rectum. Cancer, 36:2251, 1975.

32. Quan, S. H. Q., Castro, E. B.: Papillary adenomas (villous tumors): A review of 215 cases. Dis. Colon Rectum, 14:267, 1971.

33. Reilly, P. J., and Nostrant, T. T.: Clinical manifestations of hereditary hemorrhagic telangiectasia. Am. J. Gastroenterol., 79:363, 1984.

34. Sachatello, C. R., Pickren, J. W., and Grace, J. T.: Generalized juvenile gastrointestinal polyposis: A hereditary syndrome. Gastroenterology, 58:699, 1970.

35. Salem, R. R., Wood, C. B., Rees, H. C., Kheshavarzian, A., Hemingway, A. P., and Allison, D. J.: A comparison of colonoscopy and selective visceral angiography in the diagnosis of colonic angiodysplasia. Ann. R. Coll. Surg. Engl., 67:225, 1985.

36. Shinya, H., and Wolff, W. I.: Morphology, anatomic distribution and cancer potential of colonic polyps. Ann. Surg., 190:679, 1979.

37. Solomon, S. S., et al.: Villous adenoma of the rectosigmoid accompanied by electrolyte depletion. J.A.M.A., 194:5, 1965.

38. Stemper, T. J., Kent, T. H., and Summers, R. W.: Juvenile polyposis and gastrointestinal carcinoma: A study of a kindred. Ann. Intern. Med., 83:639, 1975.

39. Trudey, J. L., Fazio, V. W., and Sivak, M. V.: Colonoscopic diagnosis and treatment of arteriovenous malformations in chronic lower gastrointestinal bleeding. Dis. Colon Rectum, 31:107, 1988.

40. Wall, S. D., Friedman, S. L., and Margulis, A. R.: Gastrointestinal Kaposi's sarcoma in AIDS: Radiographic manifestations. J. Clin. Gastroenterol., 6:165, 1984.

41. Westbrook, K. C., Lang, N. P., Broadwater, J. R., and Thompson, B. W.: Posterior surgical approaches to the rectum. Ann. Surg., 195:677, 1982.

42. Williams, A. R., Balasooriya, B. A. W., and Day, D. W.: Polyps and cancer of the large bowel: A necropsy study in Liverpool. Gut, 23:835, 1982.

43. Wilson, D. M., Pitts, W. C., Hintz, R. L., and Rosenfeld, R. G.: Testicular tumors with Peutz-Jeghers syndrome. Cancer, 57:2238, 1986.

VII ————————————————

ULCERATIVE COLITIS

James M. Becker, M.D., and Frank G. Moody, M.D.

Ulcerative colitis, a diffuse inflammatory disease of the mucosal lining of the colon and rectum, is characterized by bloody diarrhea that exacerbates and abates without apparent cause. It is difficult to realize that a disease so devastating remains without an identified etiology or specific medical therapy. Total removal of the affected organs—the colon and rectum—provides a complete cure, but at a sacrifice, since patients so treated must learn to live with an external abdominal stoma (an ileostomy) for the remainder of their lives. Since the disease has its peak onset in early and middle adulthood, living with an ileostomy represents a long time span for most patients. Fortunately, new surgical alternatives have eliminated the need for a permanent ileostomy without sacrificing definitive treatment of the disease.

HISTORICAL ASPECTS

Although diarrheal illnesses have been described since the early medical writings of Hippocrates (ca. 400 B.C.),[1] there is little evidence that they were distinguished from the all too common infectious enteritides until the court testimony concerning the appearance of the colon of a Mrs. Banks by Wilkes in 1859. This case was documented more formally in 1875, but by that time the pathologic anatomy of the disease had been described in a study of over 200 cases that occurred in the Union Army during the Civil War (Fig. 1).[16] By the turn of the century, the disease was fully characterized as to its nonspecific nature and was distinguishable by clinical as well as pathologic criteria.

Goligher and colleagues have traced the evolution of surgical approaches to ulcerative colitis in an authoritative manner.[35] Sigmoid colostomy, curiously enough, was the first well-documented surgical pro-

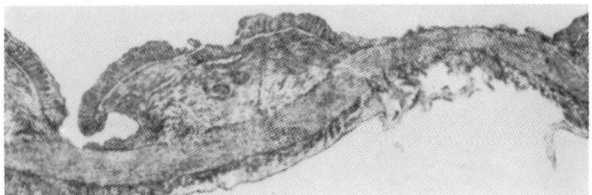

Figure 1. This classic photomicrograph of ulcerative colitis taken during the Civil War reveals the mucosal ulceration so characteristic of the disease. (From Crohn, B. B.: Letters to the Editor. Gastroenterology, 42:366, 1962. © by Williams & Wilkins, 1962.)

cedure for inflammatory bowel disease (Pennel, 1850). During the remainder of the nineteenth century, a variety of diverting procedures were performed, but without success. Appendicostomy, first performed in 1902 for ulcerative colitis, represented a major advance. This procedure soon was displaced by a completely diverting ileostomy (1913), which was accompanied by piecemeal resection of the diseased colon. Not until approximately 1940 did it become clear that definitive treatment required either total proctocolectomy or at least subtotal or total colectomy with ileostomy. Ileostomy itself was associated with a high complication rate until Brooke proposed immediate maturation of the stoma in 1952. Proctocolectomy with Brooke ileostomy thus emerged as the procedure of choice for ulcerative colitis. This has recently been challenged by anal sphincter–sparing operations, as originally proposed by Ravitch and Sabiston in 1947.[79]

ETIOLOGY

The etiology of ulcerative colitis remains unknown despite intensive work by many investigators. The examination of bacterial and viral agents continues to be an area of great activity. Despite scattered reports suggesting that *Chlamydia*, cytomegalovirus, or *Yersinia* is involved in the pathogenesis of ulcerative colitis, these reports have not been substantiated by further work. *Clostridium difficile* toxin activity has been associated with relapses of ulcerative colitis but appears to be better correlated with prior antibiotic administration than with disease activity. Ljungh and Wadstrom[57] have isolated *Escherichia* with unique binding characteristics from patients with ulcerative colitis. The immune response to this strain is being investigated, in an effort to examine factors that might lead to chronic infections with a resultant chronic autoimmune inflammatory disease of the colon. A viral cause also appears unlikely, since the disease cannot be transmitted and viral particles have not been identified. Specifically, rotavirus and Norwalk agents cannot be identified serologically as important factors in recurrences. A cytopathic agent with physical and chemical characteristics suggestive of a 16-nm. RNA virus has been identified in patients with ulcerative colitis, but this finding has not been duplicated. Although serum lysozymes are elevated in patients with Crohn's disease, they are normal in those with ulcerative colitis.[26,101]

Genetic factors may have a role, since most studies have suggested that ulcerative colitis is two to four times more common in Jewish than in non-Jewish white populations and is probably about 50 per cent less frequent in nonwhite than in white populations.[2,52] Gilat and colleagues,[32] however, in a study of Jews in Tel Aviv, reported a remarkably decreased incidence of ulcerative colitis in that city (3.7 per 100,000 population) compared with the incidences reported from Copenhagen (7.3 per 100,000), Oxford, England (7.3 per 100,000), and Rochester, Minnesota (7.2 per 100,000). In addition, the female to male ratio was only 0.8, as compared with 1.3 for the other studies. A greater frequency (10 to 15 per cent) of ulcerative colitis has been identified in family members of patients with confirmed ulcerative colitis. Some families have reportedly had up to six members affected. The disease occurs with greater frequency in monozygotic twins. Finally, HLA phenotypes AW24 and BW35 are associated with ulcerative colitis in those Israeli Jews of

European origin mentioned previously. The AW24 phenotype is also increased in frequency in patients with early onset of chronic ulcerative colitis and moderate to severe disease. Obviously, geographic as well as racial differences influence the occurrence of the disease.

Psychological factors have long been thought to have a critical role in exacerbations of the disease.[25] It is now clear that patients with ulcerative colitis have no unusual predisposing factors when compared with matched controls.[65] Moreover, colectomy is usually followed by a marked improvement in preexisting morbid psychologic states such as depression or social estrangement. Psychosomatic factors most likely only facilitate the colonic mucosal reaction to another as yet unidentified causative agent.

There has been considerable speculation that ulcerative colitis is an autoimmune disease.[54] For example, many patients have circulating antibodies to normal colonic epithelium that cross react with specific enterobacterial lipopolysaccharide antigens.[66] In addition, lymphocytes may be rendered cytotoxic to colonic epithelium by incubation with serum from patients with ulcerative colitis. These patients have also been found to have alterations of their T- and B-cell lymphocyte activation and homing properties. Whereas total lymphocyte and T-cell lymphocyte counts are normal in patients with ulcerative colitis, thymosine-dependent T-lymphocyte response may be abnormal, suggesting an immune-deficient state.[11] These interesting aberrations have been reviewed by members of Work Group Eight on Progress in Digestive Disease, who point out that these changes may not necessarily contribute to the pathogenesis of the disease, but may indeed be a consequence of its activity.[15] In fact, Brandtzaeg and colleagues[8] have demonstrated quite clearly that rather than a defect occurring in immunoglobulin activity at the tissue level in the remaining glands of patients with ulcerative colitis, IgA transport is normal, whereas IgG immunocyte response is five times that of control patients. It is possible, therefore, that IgG antibodies have a role in the chronicity of the disease but may not be involved in its onset.

Another area of great interest has been that of cytokines and immunoregulatory molecules involved in the control of the immune response.[58] The production of interferon during inflammation could have a significant role in the differentiation of mature memory and effector cells within the intestine. The inflammatory mediators interleukin-4 and interleukin-5 have been shown to greatly affect IgA production. Lower levels of interleukin-2 have been identified in both ulcerative colitis and Crohn's disease patients. Abnormalities in complement function or metabolism have also been reported. The finding of deficient activity of interleukin-2 in patients with ulcerative colitis suggests abnormal T-cell proliferation and clonal expansion at the gut mucosal level, thereby inducing a defective immune response leading to a chronic inflammatory reaction. Low levels of interleukin-2, however, have not correlated with duration, activity, or anatomic location of disease or response to corticosteroid therapy.[29,89,93] Other investigators have explored the role of helper T cells, suppressor-inducer T cells, and contrasuppressor T cells in controlling intestinal immune responses. In conclusion, although abnormalities in immune regulation have been implicated in ulcerative colitis, definitive proof of basic immunologic defects or autoimmune phenomena in this disorder is still lacking.

Several exciting alternative approaches to the pathogenesis of ulcerative colitis have been taken. Roediger[80] has suggested that ulcerative colitis represents an energy-deficient disease of the colonic epithelium. Colonocytes from patients with ulcerative colitis demonstrated lower oxidation of butyrate to carbon dioxide and decreased free coenzyme A (CoA). In pigs, it was found that the induction of low colonic mucosal CoA content produced a colitis that resembled human ulcerative colitis. In this model, resolution of the colitis occurred when CoA deficiency was corrected with pantothenic acid. The precise cause of the decreased fatty acid oxidation was not speculated on, but this failure of fatty acid oxidation was thought to represent a state of energy deficiency of the colonic mucosal cells.

A further clue comes from the work of Soergel and associates.[41] Five patients with diversion colitis were found to have reduced short-chain fatty acid (SCFA) levels within the bypassed segments. Treatment with intraluminal instillation of an isotonic SCFA solution caused complete endoscopic healing in all 5 patients and recurrence when saline was substituted for the SCFA solution. Luminal SCFAs have also been shown to accelerate healing of surgical anastomoses,[81] increased regional blood flow, and oxygen intake[55] and have contrasting effects on epithelial proliferation *in vitro* as compared with *in vivo*.[86,100] Thus, whereas short-chain fatty acids may have a role in the pathogenesis and treatment of inflammatory bowel disease, this requires further study in patients with ulcerative colitis.

Podolsky and Isselbacher[74] have suggested that there might be alterations in colonic mucosal glycoprotein composition in patients with ulcerative colitis. Mucin profiles were performed on mucosa from patients with ulcerative colitis, and a selective decrease in mucin species IV was identified. Normal mucin profiles were found in patients with Crohn's disease, ischemic colitis, infectious colitis, and radiation colitis. Patients with ulcerative colitis were found to have this abnormality even in the absence of active disease. It was thought, therefore, that this alteration might be "permissive" for injury by an additional factor or factors. It is unclear, however, whether this defect is a cause or an effect of the disease.

A relationship between cigarette smoking and ulcerative colitis has been suggested. Several studies have found that current and former smoking has opposite effects on the risks of this disease. Boyko[7] critically reviewed the available literature on this topic and found that current smokers had a 60 per cent reduction in risk of ulcerative colitis compared with those who never smoked, whereas former smokers had a two-fold increase in risk compared with those who never smoked. Plausible biological mechanisms for these relationships have yet to be defined.

A decided disadvantage to accumulation of knowledge in regard to etiology is the lack of an appropriate animal model. The ingestion of amylopectin, a substance found in high concentrations in seaweed and a potent antipepsin agent, leads to pathologic change in the colon of several species, similar to that observed in ulcerative colitis in man.[16] The gibbon also acquires a pathologic entity analogous to human ulcerative colitis.[96] Possibly, further detailed study of this model may yield important clues to the etiology of this curious, almost mysterious, condition.

PATHOLOGY

Ulcerative colitis, for the most part, is a disease confined to the mucosal and submucosal layers of the colonic wall. It is a continuous colonic disease with the rectum essentially always involved. In 10 per cent of patients, the terminal ileum may show mild inflammation and dilation, a process that has been called "backwash ileitis." On gross inspection, the colonic mucosa demonstrates healed granular superficial ulcers superimposed on a friable and thickened mucosa with increased vascularity. Patients may also demonstrate superficial fissures and small and regular pseudopolyps. This is in contradistinction to the transmural inflammatory changes found in Crohn's disease of the colon, in which all layers may be involved in a granulomatous inflammatory process. The pathologic changes observed in ulcerative colitis, however, are nonspecific and can be seen in shigellosis, amebiasis, and gonorrheal colitis.

In its earliest stage, the typical lesion consists of infiltration of round cells and polymorphonuclear leukocytes into the crypts of Lieberkühn at the base of the mucosa, forming crypt abscesses. Light microscopy reveals poor staining and vacuolization of overlying epithelial cells. There is swelling of mitochondria, widening of intercellular spaces, and broadening of the endoplasmic reticulum observed by transmission electron microscopy. As the lesions progress, there is a coalescence of crypt abscesses and desquamation of overlying cells to form an ulcer. This is associated with undermining of adjacent, relatively normal mucosa, which becomes edematous and assumes a polypoid configuration as it becomes isolated between adjacent ulcers. Collagen and a luxurious growth of granulation tissue occupy the areas of ulceration, which extend down to, but rarely through, the muscularis. The histologic features of a typical ulcer and pseudopolyp are shown in Figure 2. In fulminating ulcerative colitis and toxic megacolon, such lesions may penetrate through the full thickness of the bowel wall and lead to perforation into the peritoneal cavity. Fortunately, these forms of the disease are infrequent (15 and 3 per cent, respectively). The pathologic changes described, therefore, offer a very clear

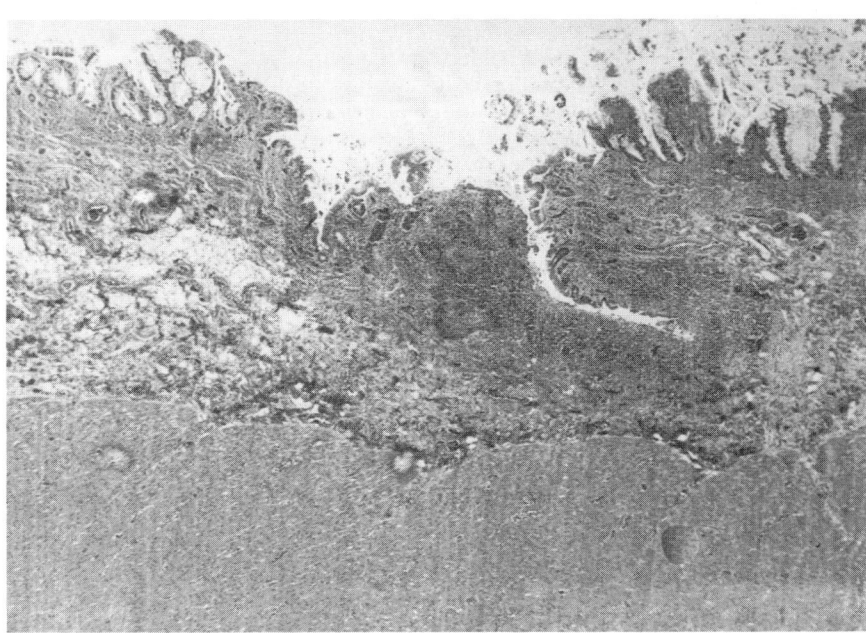

Figure 2. This low-power photomicrograph reveals the details of a chronic mucosal ulceration of the colon in ulcerative colitis. Note the round cell infiltration and granulation tissue at its base. The mucosa at its margins is edematous and hypertrophic, providing a pseudopolypoid appearance. The poor staining of the mucosal cells is a characteristic finding. (From Goligher, J. C., de Dombal, F. T., Watts, J. M., and Watkinson, G.: Ulcerative Colitis. Baltimore, Williams & Wilkins, 1968.)

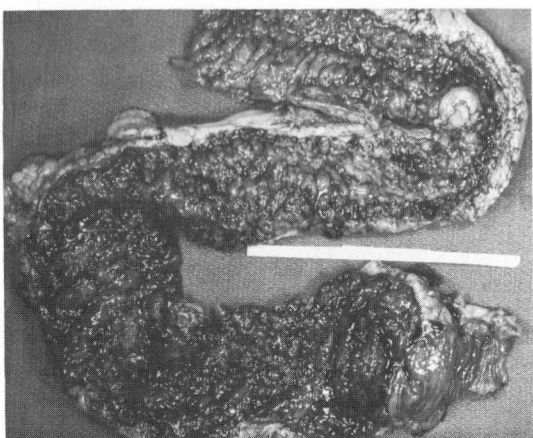

Figure 3. As shown in this photograph, the mucosal lining of the colon in ulcerative colitis is remarkably disturbed. Islands of edematous mucosa are isolated by ulcerations that are contiguous throughout the entire colon in this case. Note that the process stops abruptly at the ileocecal valve.

explanation of the clinical manifestations of the disease. It is little wonder that a colon as shown in Figure 3 allows almost constant passage of 20 or more bloody bowel movements per day. The denuded, remarkably distorted mucosal lining provides little opportunity for absorption of sodium or water. Each bowel action milks large volumes of blood from the exposed hillocks of granulation tissue. Loss of haustral markings, an early roentgenographic finding, is thought to be due to paralysis of the muscularis mucosa. The foreshortening of the colon, and its rigid "stovepipe" appearance on barium roentgenograms, is a consequence of repeated injury and the scar that forms with repair of these injuries (Fig. 4).

Little is known as to why some patients have involvement only of the rectum, whereas others may develop changes throughout the colon. Moreover, the factors determining the severity and time course of the disease are poorly understood. Possibly these factors relate to the extent of immunologic disturbance engendered by the initial attack. There is also some

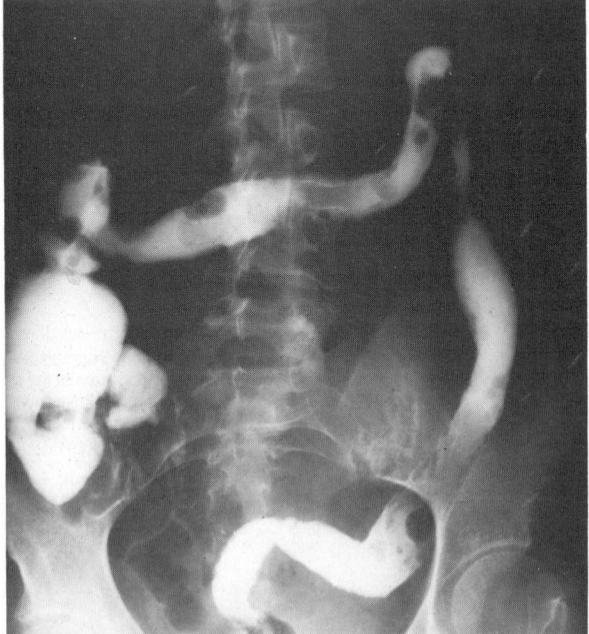

Figure 4. The contracted, "stovepipe" appearance of this colon, as viewed by barium roentgenogram, is typical of advanced ulcerative colitis in its chronic phase. The large lucent areas in the barium column probably represent fecal matter, whereas the smaller, more subtle shadows along the left colon are most likely pseudopolyps.

evidence that prostaglandins may have a role in acute episodes of the disease.[90] Unfortunately, a positive response to prostaglandin synthetase inhibitors, such as indomethacin, has not yet been reported. More recent evidence suggests that acute episodes of colitis may in fact be associated with prostaglandin deficiencies.[77]

CLINICAL MANIFESTATIONS

The initial presentation of ulcerative colitis may take many forms. Bloody diarrhea is the most common early symptom. Occasionally, arthritis, iritis, hepatic dysfunction, and skin lesions may be paramount. The most common clinical manifestations are enumerated in Table 1. The disease presents as a chronic, relatively low-grade illness in most patients. In a small number of patients (15 per cent), it has an acute and catastrophic fulminating course. Such patients present with frequent bloody bowel movements (up to 30 per day), high fever, and abdominal pain. The disease, therefore, offers a wide spectrum of clinical manifestations ranging from a mild diarrheal illness to an overwhelming life-threatening event of short duration that demands immediate medical attention.

Onset of the disease occurs in patients less than 15 years of age in approximately 15 per cent of cases, and presentation in patients over 40 years of age is not uncommon. The incidence of ulcerative colitis is 3.5 to 6.5 per 10^5 population and the prevalence 60 per 10^5. A slight female predominance has been reported.[11]

Physical findings are directly related to the duration and presentation of the disease. Weight loss and pallor are usually present. In the active phase, the abdomen, in the region of the colon, is usually tender to palpation. There may be signs of an acute abdomen accompanied by fever and decreased bowel sounds. This is especially true during acute attacks or in the fulminating form of the disease. Abdominal distention is unusual, except in patients who have toxic megacolon, in which instance the patient is usually febrile and has signs of an acute abdomen. The perianal area may be excoriated from the numerous wipings associated with bowel movements. There may be evidence of perianal inflammation in the form of a fissure, abscess, or fistula-in-ano, although the last is more common in Crohn's disease. Rectal examination is almost always painful and in the presence of perianal inflammation should be done with gentle care. Examination of the integument, tongue, joints, and eyes is important, since the presence of disease in these areas may suggest ulcerative colitis as a likely cause of the diarrheal illness.

Proctosigmoidoscopy is a helpful and specific diagnostic aid, since ulcerative colitis involves the distal colon and rectum in 90 to 95 per cent of the cases. In fact, the mucosa of both the rectum and the sigmoid colon is usually erythematous and granular and bleeds easily when touched by the endoscope or rubbed with a cotton swab. Normal colonic vascular markings may be absent

TABLE 1. Principal Symptoms of Ulcerative Colitis (525 Cases)

Diarrhea	79%
Abdominal pain	71%
Rectal bleeding	55%
Weight loss	18%
Tenesmus	16%
Vomiting	14%
Fever	11%
Constipation	5%
Arthralgia	2%

From Peete, W. P. J., and Sabiston, D. C., Jr.: Ulcerative colitis. *In* Sabiston, D. C., Jr. (Ed.): Davis-Christopher Textbook of Surgery, 10th ed. Philadelphia, W. B. Saunders Company, 1972.

or the mucosa may be hyperemic. In the disease-bearing mucosa, superficial (less than 2 mm.) mucosal alterations are seen. The intercolonic haustra are thick and blunted. Cobblestoning and deep linear ulceration, which are common endoscopic findings in Crohn's disease, are unusual in ulcerative colitis. In advanced disease, ulcers may be present, surrounded by hyperplastic areas of granulation tissue and edematous mucosa, which may assume a polypoid appearance (pseudopolyps). Mucosal bridging is also commonly found. In chronic advanced disease, the lumen of the rectosigmoid may be remarkably contracted. The use of flexible sigmoidoscopy has improved diagnostic accuracy and patient acceptance. Colonoscopic examination is of value in determining the extent and activity of the disease. Unless a distinct granuloma is identified, endoscopic biopsies are of little value in differentiating ulcerative colitis from Crohn's colitis.

Although recent studies have suggested that previous reports may have overestimated the risk of cancer in the adult population with ulcerative colitis, patients with this disease still appear to be confronted with at least a 10 to 20 per cent likelihood of developing carcinoma within 20 years of the diagnosis of ulcerative colitis.[91] Adenocarcinoma in association with ulcerative colitis is multicentric in 15 per cent of patients. In addition, the cancers tend to be flatter and perhaps more infiltrating. These tumors are more evenly distributed throughout the colon, with approximately 50 per cent being found proximal to the splenic flexure. Carcinoma in association with ulcerative colitis is more difficult to diagnose by history and physical examination, stool guaiac testing, and radiographic studies. The likelihood of carcinoma in patients with ulcerative colitis appears to relate both to the extent of colonic involvement and the duration of disease. Although it is generally accepted that patients with extensive total ulcerative colitis are at increased risk of developing carcinoma, the question of what constitutes extensive colitis is still not fully resolved. In addition, the assessment is variable if judged radiographically or colonoscopically. The evidence that patients with left-sided ulcerative colitis, by any criteria, are at increased risk when compared with the general population, which carries a 4 to 6 per cent likelihood of developing colorectal carcinoma with three fourths of these cancers occurring on the left side, is far from overwhelming. The likelihood of cancer may be related to duration of activity and age of onset, although this has not been clearly established. Although it was held for some time that the carcinoma associated with ulcerative colitis was more aggressive than that in the general population, recent studies have demonstrated that the natural evolution of the cancer is likely the same in both groups.[40]

Rectal biopsies have also been advocated to assess the presence or absence of dysplasia. Morson and Pang[67] have advocated a surveillance program of rectal biopsy in order to assess the point at which a patient becomes at high risk for colonic cancer. When dysplasia of the rectal mucosa is identified, colectomy has been advocated. Other investigators in this field have found the test less useful, with false-negative results of 20 to 40 per cent and false-positive results of 30 to 40 per cent.[85] Colonoscopy may improve the accuracy of surveillance; however, random biopsies have a very low yield because of the immense sampling problem. Between 20 and 25 equally spaced biopsies are required on a 10-cm. length of colon to reasonably detect a patch of dysplasia 2 cm. in diameter. Moreover, the endoscopic appearances of both dysplasia and carcinoma in ulcerative colitis remain nearly undocumented. The biopsy of target lesions, that is, any lesion that cannot be reasonably accepted as part of the chronic disease state, is recommended. In addition, the end point of surveillance remains controversial. Many gastroenterologists recommend colectomy only in the presence of high-grade dysplasia, a dysplasia-associated mass lesion, or a frank carcinoma. Unfortunately, the presence of dysplasia, whether low-grade or high-grade, can give rise directly to an invasive

carcinoma, and all large centers have had patients under surveillance who developed and died of colorectal carcinoma. To date, no study has demonstrated that surveillance lowers the mortality from colorectal cancer in association with ulcerative colitis.[14]

A plain abdominal film may reveal a variant of the disease called *toxic megacolon*, in which there may be free air within the peritoneal cavity from perforation of the colon. A more common sign is a remarkable dilation of the transverse colon (Fig. 5).

Barium enema examination, usually with air contrast, can be performed safely in most patients and is extremely helpful in identifying the extent and the severity of the disease. Barium roentgenographic signs include loss of haustral markings and irregularities of the colon wall, which represent small ulcerations. These are well demonstrated in Figure 6, which contrasts the appearance of the left side of the splenic flexure and that of the right. As the disease progresses, pseudopolyps become a prominent roentgenographic sign (Fig. 7). In advanced disease, the colon assumes the appearance of a rigid contracted tube (see Fig. 4). The barium roentgenogram, although useful, should be used with discretion. Preparation of the colon should be avoided, since it may exacerbate the colitis. When diarrhea is not present, a liquid diet for 3 days prior to examination is recommended. Barium roentgenogram should be omitted when the clinical signs of toxic megacolon are present. With these admonitions in mind, a barium view of the colon should be obtained in all patients with ulcerative colitis at a convenient time in the disease process, in order to exclude the presence of cancer. How often repeat examination is necessary remains an open question. However, because the incidence of malignancy is strikingly high, after 10 years of the disease it is appropriate to obtain a yearly barium examination alternating at 6-month intervals wth colonoscopy. Upper gastrointestinal contrast studies are also indicated in most patients to exclude Crohn's disease.

The aforementioned clinical manifestations and simple diag-

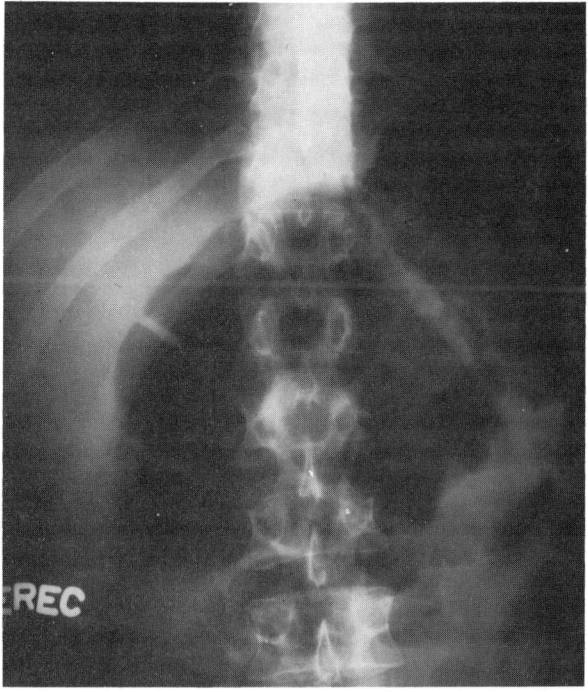

Figure 5. Toxic megacolon is characterized by massive distention of the right colon by air as shown in this upright roentgenogram of the abdomen. Distention of the cecum in excess of 12 to 14 cm. is felt to represent a sign of impending perforation. The irregularities in the air column represent pseudopolyps within the lumen of the colon.

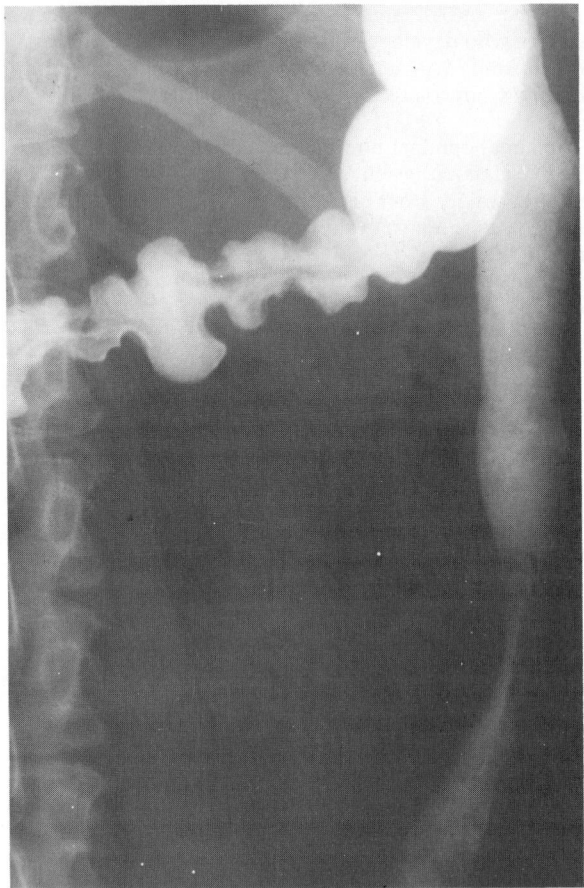

Figure 6. This barium roentgenogram of the splenic flexure of the colon reveals loss of haustral markings in the descendng colon, in contrast to their presence in the transverse colon. The irregular appearance of the barium column in the descending colon is indicative of the inflammation and ulceration of its mucosal lining.

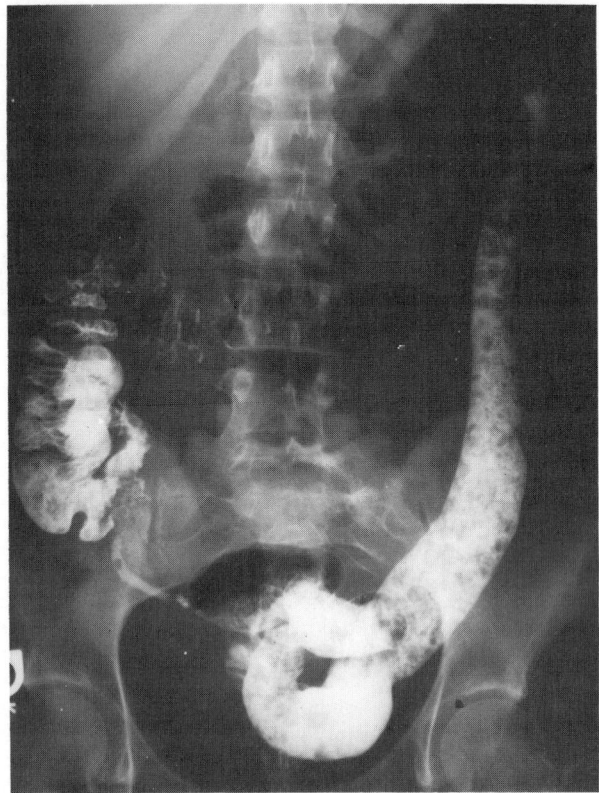

Figure 7. Mucosal pseudopolyp formation is well demonstrated in the descending colon in this barium roentgenogram. The right colon appears relatively spared.

nostic tests usually help identify the presence of ulcerative colitis. It is necessary, however, to obtain stool smears and cultures to exclude colitis due to viruses, *Chlamydia*, bacterial pathogens, and parasites. Particularly important and difficult to exclude are pseudomembranous colitis, the proctocolitis seen increasingly in homosexual males, and traveler's diarrhea. Cello and Meyer[12] have provided a useful schema for distinguishing ulcerative colitis from granulomatous colitis (Table 2). Note, however, the low frequency of discriminating clinical characteristics except for associated small bowel disease or skip areas within the colon when the etiology is Crohn's disease.

The strong association of cancer of the colon with ulcerative colitis bears further emphasis.[101] For example, 2 of 5 patients with total colonic involvement may die of cancer if they survive their disease and the colon is left in place.[59] Three per cent of children with ulcerative colitis have cancer of the colon at 10 years; 20 per cent develop cancer during each ensuing decade.[18] With the availability of far more acceptable surgical alternatives to proctocolectomy and ileostomy, it is hoped that patients will obtain definitive treatment for the disease well before they enter the phase of accelerating cancer risk. These data support close medical management for such patients and surgical intervention, on this basis alone, when chronicity is well established.

The extracolonic manifestations of ulcerative colitis can be categorized as the colitic group, the pathophysiologic group, and the miscellaneous group of disorders. The colitic group of extracolonic manifestations in general parallels the activity of the underlying bowel disease, being present and most active when the colitis is active and usually subsiding when the colitis goes into remission induced by medical therapy or by surgical

intervention or spontaneously. It appears most likely that these extracolonic disorders may represent antigen-antibody immune complex disorders. Ocular manifestations are common in ulcerative colitis and include conjunctivitis, iritis, and choroiditis. These are closely related to disease activity and respond to steroid therapy. More severe and rare eye diseases, including ulcerative panophthalmitis, are more difficult to treat even with

TABLE 2. Pathologic Features Distinguishing Crohn's Colitis from Ulcerative Colitis

	Percentage of Cases with Finding	
Pathologic Finding	**Crohn's Colitis**	**Ulcerative Colitis**
Macroscopic		
Bowel wall thickened	74	17
Superficial discrete ulcers	53	13
Confluent linear ulcers	37	0
Deep fissures	37	0
Skip lesions	21	0
Bowel lumen narrowing	68	35
Cobblestoning of mucosa	21	0
Microscopic		
Transmural inflammation	95	17
Submucosal thickening	79	4
Fissures	95	35
Increased submucosal cellularity	100	30
Granulomas	100	0
Submucosal fibrosis	63	4
Full mucosal thickness ulceration	79	43

From Cello, J. P., and Meyer, J. H.: Crohn's disease of the colon. *In* Sleisenger, M. H., and Fordtran, J. S. (Eds.): Gastrointestinal Disease. Philadelphia, W. B. Saunders Company, 1978, p. 1660.

high-dose steroid suppression. Articular disorders, including peripheral joint disease, arthralgias, swelling, pain, and redness with migratory involvement, usually parallel the intensity of the colitis and respond to medical or surgical treatment. The joints of the lower extremities are most frequently involved. Fortunately, permanent deformity of these joints is very uncommon. A certain percentage of patients go on to develop clear evidence of rheumatoid arthritis even after colectomy. Ankylosing spondylitis and sacroiliitis, in contrast, can cause permanent fixation of the spine and need to be treated aggressively. Bone involvement specific to the axial skeleton is less closely related to severity of the inflammatory state of the colon and, in fact, may precede frank evidence of ulcerative colitis. Patients with ulcerative colitis frequently experience dermatologic disorders, including erythema nodosum and pyoderma gangrenosum. Although in most patients these difficult problems resolve after colectomy, in others they may precede the colonic disease or may not become manifest until after proctocolectomy has been performed.

Pathophysiologic disorders are more often seen in Crohn's disease than in ulcerative colitis, since in ulcerative colitis the normal physiology of the terminal ileum is not disturbed. Liver disease is common in patients with both ulcerative colitis and Crohn's disease. Nonspecific inflammation and fatty metamorphosis manifested by mild increases in the serum transaminase values are common in ulcerative colitis. Pruritus and elevation of the alkaline phosphatase are seen commonly in association with the pericholangitis that occasionally accompanies ulcerative colitis. The most dreaded complication, sclerosing cholangitis, presents with pruritus, alkaline phosphatase elevation, right upper quadrant pain and tenderness, and jaundice. The diagnosis is most often made by endoscopic retrograde cholangiopancreatography or transhepatic cholangiography. It has been estimated that 50 per cent of patients who present with sclerosing cholangitis already have or will develop frank ulcerative colitis. Controversy surrounds the treatment of this disorder. Whereas some patients respond to colectomy, many others show progression of their disease even after colon resection. Surgical drainage, internal stent placement, antibiotics, and ultimately liver transplantation have all been reported to be of value in the treatment of symptomatic sclerosing cholangitis. Cholangiocarcinomas have also been reported in patients with ulcerative colitis, usually after many years of sclerosing cholangitis.[38,50]

MEDICAL MANAGEMENT

The outcome of an acute episode of ulcerative colitis relates to the severity of the disease as manifested by systemic symptoms. Duration of the disease or extent of involvement of the colon does not appear to be a determinant of survival if ulcerative proctitis is excluded from consideration. Those who present with advanced signs of acute illness require hospitalization and supportive, as well as specific, therapy for associated metabolic and hematologic derangements. Because of the massive fluid and electrolyte loss per rectum, such patients usually present with metabolic acidosis, contracted extravascular volume, and prerenal azotemia. The serum potassium level is usually low because of excessive loss in stool and urine. Intravenous administration of balanced salt solutions in amounts sufficient to replace these losses is an initial step in management. Patients with long-standing disease may have lost considerable protein and probably are in a depleted nutritional state. The precise role of specialized nutritional support in ulcerative colitis, and, in particular, of total parenteral nutrition, is unclear. Despite early enthusiasm, total parenteral nutrition does not appear to have a specialized therapeutic role in this disease. Total parenteral nutrition does improve the overall nutritional state of patients with ulcerative colitis and may reverse growth retardation in chil-dren, but it certainly does not replace conventional medical treatment or prevent or delay colectomy in patients with ulcerative colitis. In fact, in patients with severe acute colitis, it may be impossible to attain positive nitrogen balance while the colon is still in place.[20,24,62,79]

Corticosteroids and immunosuppressive agents have both been demonstrated to be effective in the management of ulcerative colitis. Both agents, however, are capable of producing significant side effects. In general, corticosteroids have been more readily accepted by the medical community as therapeutic agents and remain the mainstay of therapy in acute attacks. Between 40 and 60 mg. of prednisone in a single daily dose is effective in inducing remission.[98] Rectal steroids have been shown to be effective in left colon disease or proctitis and may have therapeutic efficacy in universal colitis as well, perhaps because approximately 30 per cent of the steroid given rectally is absorbed into the systemic circulation. The controversy of intravenous steroids versus intravenous adrenocorticotropic hormone (ACTH) has now been resolved by a randomized trial that revealed a similar response to equipotent doses of either hormone.[48] A recent study suggests that ACTH may be more effective in patients not previously treated with corticosteroids, whereas corticosteroids appear preferable for patients already receiving steroid therapy.[64] A steroid-induced remission is not more likely to exacerbate than a spontaneous remission, and an ACTH-induced remission is not more likely to exacerbate than a corticosteroid-induced remission. The usual doses recommended are in the range of 300 mg. of hydrocortisone or 40 units of ACTH per day. Occasionally, massive doses of steroids (over 1 gm. pr day) are required. The usual response is rapid, and acute signs of inflammation subside within a few days. The optimal duration of intravenous steroid therapy is 5 to 7 days, although this may be extended in patients supported nutritionally with total parenteral nutrition. Proctoscopic examination is useful in following response to therapy. There is still controversy as to whether maintenance steroid therapy reduces recurrence of the disease. Although maintenance steroids may be useful in controlling symptoms of patients with continuing activity, maintenance therapy with low-dose corticosteroids for patients with inactive disease has not been demonstrated to prevent relapse.[56]

Sulfasalazine has enjoyed widespread use in the chronic phases of ulcerative colitis. Its mode of action is unknown. Sulfasalazine may exert its prophylactic effect by inhibiting mucosal prostaglandin synthesis,[46] although not all studies have supported this mechanism.[76] Whatever the mechanism of action, sulfasalazine appears to be associated with fewer exacerbations as assessed by controlled randomized trials.[19,97] The drug appears to be of lesser value in severe ulcerative colitis. Sulfasalazine is metabolized by bacteria to 5-aminosalicylic acid (5-ASA) and sulfapyridine. Dose-related side effects of sulfasalazine include nausea, vomiting, headache, and abdominal discomfort. Hypersensitivity effects include fever, skin rash, agranulocytosis, and hemolytic anemia. Studies have indicated that the sulfapyridine produced by bacterial degradation of sulfasalazine is responsible for the majority of the side effects, whereas the 5-ASA component appears to be the effective moiety of the drug. Five-aminosalicylic acid is now available in this country for clinical use. Studies have shown that 5-ASA enemas are superior to a placebo for the healing of proctitis.

A third approach has been through the use of immunosuppressive agents. Rosenberg and colleagues[83] have concluded, based on a well-controlled study, that azathioprine allows reduction of the use of steroids in chronic cases but does not, in itself, control exacerbation of the disease. In a more recent controlled trial, however, Kirk and Lennard-Jones[51] demonstrated that clinical improvement may occur in about 25 per cent of patients treated with a dose of azathioprine at 2 to 2.5 mg. per kg. Uncontrolled trials have demonstrated a favorable response to 6-mercaptopurine (6-MP) in 64 to 70 per cent of patients with refractory ulcerative colitis.[76] Unpublished studies have similarly suggested that cyclosporine may be of value in controlling patients who have failed conventional medical management. A trial of 6-MP or cyclosporine may be warranted when steroids and sulfasalazine have failed, when the disease is confined to the left side of the colon or rectum, when the patient is compliant, and when there is no absolute indication for immediate surgical therapy.[75] However, before prescribing these immunosuppressive agents, one must be fully familiar with the dosing, monitoring, toxicity, and possible induction of lymphoma or other malignancies associated with these drugs.

Although widely prescribed for both ulcerative colitis and Crohn's disease, metronidazole and other antibiotics are of no proven value in the treatment of inflammatory bowel disease.

The major therapeutic problem between acute episodes is control of diarrhea and maintenance of nutrition. Diet therapy is no longer recommended, and patients are encouraged to eat a substantial diet of their choice. Milk products are to be avoided only if they cause problems such as increasing diarrhea or cramps (as they may in about half the patients with ulcerative colitis). The reason for this is not clear but relates to something specific in cow's milk rather than to the lactase deficiency that exists in many patients with ulcerative colitis. Opiates such as codeine or paregoric should be avoided. Nocturnal diarrhea can be controlled by anticholinergics or diphenoxylate with atropine. The synthetic peripheral-acting opioid loperamide may be more effective than diphenoxylate in this situation and avoids the atropine side effects associated with this drug.[70] Stool bulk formers, such as psyllium, are also helpful. Finally, the importance of rest and peace of mind cannot be overemphasized. Patients are advised to remain at rest during episodes of exacerbation.

INDICATIONS FOR SURGICAL TREATMENT

Since total removal of the colon and rectum (proctocolectomy) cures ulcerative colitis, one might reasonably ask why all patients with established chronicity are not so treated. The incidence of surgical intervention appears to be related to the availability of skilled and knowledgeable gastrointestinal surgeons and enlightened physicians. For example, the clinic at Leeds offers surgical care to approximately half of their patient population,[35] whereas in other series the operative rate is below 10 per cent.[32] There are several well-identified complications that require urgent operation for survival.[33] These include (1) massive, unrelenting hemorrhage; (2) toxic megacolon with impending or frank perforation; (3) fulminating acute ulcerative colitis that is unresponsive to steroid therapy; (4) obstruction from stricture; and (5) suspicion or demonstration of colonic cancer. Surgical therapy is also recommended in children who fail to mature at an acceptable rate. The largest number of colectomies for ulcerative colitis are performed for less dramatic indications, as the disease enters an intractable chronic phase and becomes both a physical and a social burden to the patient.

Acute perforation occurs infrequently, with the incidence directly related to both the severity of the initial episode and extent of the disease in the bowel. Specifically, although the overall incidence of perforation during a first attack is less than 4 per cent, if it is severe the incidence rises to 9.7 per cent. If the total colon is involved, the perforation rate is 14.6 per cent, and if the attack is both severe and involves the total colon, it increases to 19.2 per cent.[34]

Obstruction caused by benign stricture formation occurs in 11 per cent of patients, 34 per cent of these occurring in the rectum.[17] They usually follow submucosal fibrosis and occasionally mucosal hyperplasia. Although they do not usually cause acute obstruction, the lesions must be differentiated from carcinoma by biopsy or excision, and particular attention should be given to excluding Crohn's disease. Strictures caused by carcinoma are less common than those caused by benign disease and are more prone to perforate.

Massive hemorrhage secondary to ulcerative colitis is rare, occurring in fewer than 1 per cent of patients.[34] Prompt surgical intervention is indicated after hemodynamic stabilization. More than 50 per cent of patients with acute colonic bleeding have toxic megacolon, so one should be suspicious of the coexistence of the two complications. Uncontrollable hemorrhage from the entire colorectal mucosa may be the one clear indication for emergency proctocolectomy. If possible, the rectum should be spared for later mucosal proctectomy with ileoanal anastomosis.

Acute toxic megacolon can occur in both ulcerative colitis and Crohn's disease. Its incidence ranges between 6 and 13 per cent in patients with ulcerative colitis.[28] Patients usually present clinically with the onset of abdominal pain and severe diarrhea (greater than 10 stools per day), followed by abdominal distention and generalized tenderness. Once megacolon and toxicity develop, fever, leukocytosis, tachycardia, pallor, lethargy, and shock ensue. It is important to note that any of these manifestations can be masked by chronic steroid use and the generally poor nutritional condition of the patient. An abdominal radiograph usually shows dilation of the transverse and occasionally sigmoid colon, which is greater than 5 cm. and averages 9.2 cm. (Fig. 5).[28] Thickening and nodularity of the bowel wall due to mucosal inflammation are also noted. Caprilli[10] recently noted abnormal gaseous distention of the small bowel in association with toxic megacolon; thus, this finding may be a useful predictor of its development in patients with severe colitis.

The morbidity and mortality for acute toxic megacolon remain high. Soyer and Aldrete[94] reported, in 12 patients, an incidence of postoperative sepsis of 50 per cent, wound infection of 58 per cent, abscess or fistula of 33 per cent, and delayed wound healing of 25 per cent. Postoperative mortality ranges from 11 to 16 per cent, and for the subset of patients with perforation, 27 to 44 per cent.[39,44] These data support the use of combined aggressive medical and surgical treatment of this disease.

Initial treatment for toxic megacolon includes intravenous fluid and electrolyte resuscitation, nasogastric suction, broadspectrum antibiotics to include anaerobic and aerobic gramnegative coverage, and total parenteral nutrition to improve nutritional status. Proctoscopy may be helpful in determining the etiology of the attack, as may culture of the stool. Although the efficacy of steroids is still in question,[63] most patients presenting with toxic megacolon are already on steroid therapy and thus need stress doses of corticosteroids to prevent adrenal crisis. Most clinicians think that steroids help reduce the inflammation and may "cool down" an acute toxic episode in up to 50 per cent of patients, although long-term remissions are not achieved.[37] Moreover, the short-term use of corticosteroids does not appear to increase surgical morbidity. Long-term use of larger doses, however, does increase the incidence of wound and septic complications. The authors agree with Fazio[28] that provided the patient is stable, an initial medical trial is warranted in order to make the operation elective rather than urgent. If no clear response is obtained within 24 to 48 hours, surgical therapy is warranted. It is likely that larger doses of steroids after initial medical failure will not benefit the patient and, as noted, may be deleterious. During the time of medical therapy, serial blood counts, serum electrolyte levels, and abdominal roentgenograms should be closely monitored.

In the presence of acute toxic megacolon caused by ulcerative colitis, surgical therapy can be associated with a high operative morbidity and mortality. Block and colleagues[6] noted an overall mortality following emergency operation of 8.7 per cent; 6.1 per cent after total abdominal colectomy, and 14.7 per cent after proctocolectomy. This suggests that more conservative surgical intervention is appropriate in the acute setting. Also, with the recent popularity of anal sphincter–sparing procedures, when operating for acute ulcerative colitis one should weigh the possibility of subsequent surgical correction for continence. Specifically, leaving the rectum intact allows its use for subsequent mucosal proctectomy and ileoanal anastomosis. When urgent colectomy is required, total abdominal colectomy, Brooke ileostomy, and Hartmann's pouch are appropriate.[36,88] Although ileostomy alone for acute complications has been abandoned, it has been used in the recent past with good success by Turnbull and co-workers,[99] in combination with skin level transverse and sigmoid colostomies for toxic megacolon. This is a relatively simple procedure that spares such desperately ill patients a major operative intervention until their acute illness has subsided. Because the procedure involves only decompression of the colon and does not remove the acutely inflamed tissue, most surgeons have instead preferred colon resection.

SURGICAL MANAGEMENT

Total proctocolectomy with permanent Brooke ileostomy, by eliminating diseased mucosa and the risk of malignant transformation, offers definitive treatment for ulcerative colitis but, nevertheless, remains controversial and poorly accepted by patients and their physicians. Patients with a permanent ileostomy are incontinent of gas and stool and must wear a collecting bag day and night. As high as 40 to 50 per cent of patients with a Brooke ileostomy have appliance-related problems, and the psychological and social implications, particularly for young patients, are tremendous.[73,84] Therefore, the search has continued for adequate alternatives to proctocolectomy and ileostomy.

Until recently, single-stage total proctocolectomy was the procedure of choice when complications of the disease were treated electively. This procedure is performed through a midline incision. The rectum may be excised from the abdomen by division at the level at the anal verge or by circumferential incision from the perineum. When cancer is not suspected, excision is performed rapidly with division of the mesentery close to the bowel wall. This principle is especially important in the pelvic colon and rectum, where injury to the sacral parasympathetic nerves may lead to bladder and sexual dysfunction. Endorectal mucosal resection, as described later, appears to offer the surest way to avoid such serious complications.[31] After standard proctocolectomy, management of the perineal wound is a problem, since chronic infection and poor healing may cause a lingering sinus tract between the buttocks. The authors' preference is to apply active closed drainage to this area for 3 to 5 days following operation. Gauze packing of the perineum should be reserved for pelvic hemorrhage that cannot otherwise be controlled.

The importance of providing the patients with a well-functioning, trouble-free ileostomy cannot be overemphasized. Most surgeons have accepted the technique of Brooke (Fig. 8). The principles include passing the end of the ileum through an opening in the mid-aspect of the right rectus muscle at a point below the umbilicus that allows convenient placement of the forepiece of an ileostomy bag. Placement that is too low or too lateral may lead to serious problems in ileostomy care and function. The length of the stoma is important. Approximately 5 cm. should be withdrawn above the skin so that when the tip is folded back upon itself, 2 to 3 cm. protrude from the surface. The folding back or "maturing" prevents the development of an inflammatory response in the serosa and provides more substance to the protruding ileal nipple. Simple and easily applied receptacles are now available. In the final analysis, it is the need for an external stoma that limits the more general use of colectomy for patients with established ulcerative colitis.

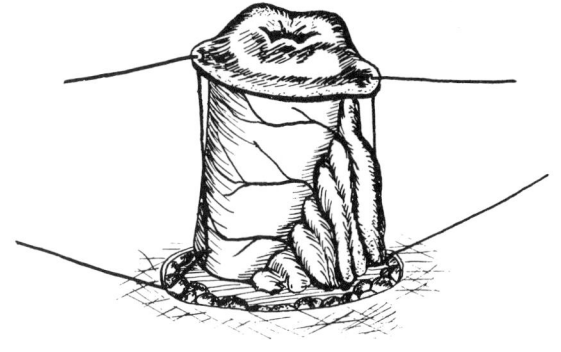

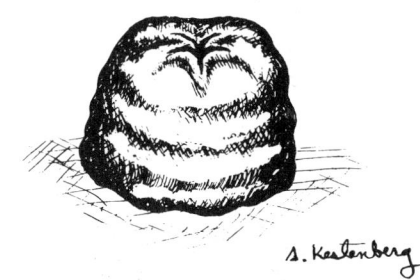

Figure 8. Technique of construction of an end-ileostomy as described by Brooke. The ileum is brought 5 cm. through an abdominal defect and then everted and sutured to the dermis to "mature" the ileostomy.

At present, there are several alternatives to proctocolectomy and Brooke ileostomy (Table 3). Subtotal colectomy with ileorectal anastomosis has been employed as a compromise operation for ulcerative colitis for decades (Fig. 9). One advantage of the operation is that it eliminates an abdominal ileostomy and can be offered to patients who adamantly refuse ileostomy. In addition, since the pelvic autonomic nerves are not disturbed, impotence or bladder dysfunction is not encountered. The disadvantages of ileorectal anastomosis, however, are considerable, and with the availability of newer alternatives, these disadvantages may outweigh any advantages. The operation does not eliminate the proctitis. At least 10 per cent of patients require proctectomy for control of the inflammatory disease alone. Patients with ileorectal anastomosis have a considerable risk of developing carcinoma in the rectal remnant, from 15 per cent at 30 years in Baker and associates' series[3] to 17 per cent after 20 years in the series of Johnson and colleagues.[47] Functional results also vary, with a high stool frequency necessitating subsequent proctectomy in another 10 per cent of patients.[27] The authors believe, therefore, that subtotal colectomy with ileorectal anastomosis should be considered only in patients who are not candidates for ileoanal pull-through and who refuse proctectomy.

In 1969, Kock described a new type of ileostomy, a continent ileostomy, made entirely of terminal ileum and consisting of a pouch that would hold intestinal contents and an ileal conduit that led from the pouch to a cutaneous stoma. This was modified in 1973 to include an intestinal valve between the pouch and stoma, the valve being constructed by intussuscepting the terminal ileum in a retrograde manner into the pouch for 3 to 4 cm. (Fig. 10). Patients would then empty the pouch by passing a tube through the valve into the pouch via the stoma. This technique offered the patient a new life-style by making the ileostomy continent, thereby avoiding the need for an external appliance.[53] Although results with the Kock pouch have improved, technical and anatomic complications remain that necessitate reoperation in up to 40 to 50 per cent of patients. The majority of

TABLE 3. Outcome of Operations for Ulcerative Colitis

Procedure	Fecal Continence Preserved	Stoma Present	Intubations Required	Disadvantages
Brooke ileostomy	No	Yes	No	Ileostomy bag required
Ileal pouch–anal anastomosis	Yes	No	No	Frequent stooling, occasional fecal leakage, pouchitis may appear
Kock pouch	Yes	Yes	Yes	Valve malfunction, pouchitis may appear
Ileorectostomy	Yes	No	No	Rectal mucosa may cause symptoms, develop cancer

From Kelly, K. A.: Ileoanal anastomosis. *In* Bayless, T. M. (Ed.): Current Management of Inflammatory Bowel Disease. Philadelphia, B. C. Decker, 1989, pp. 129–133.

the problems revolve around the nipple valve, including valve disintussusception and stenosis.[22]

In 1947, Ravitch and Sabiston proposed an anal sphincter-sparing operation that consisted of abdominal colectomy, mucosal proctectomy, and endorectal ileoanal pull-through and anastomosis[71,79] (Fig. 11). As initially proposed, the operation was performed by first resecting the colon in the standard manner. Rather than removing the entire rectum and anus, the disease-bearing mucosa of the rectum was dissected free and resected, preserving an intact rectal muscular cuff and anal sphincter mechanism. Continuity of the intestinal tract was reestablished by extending the terminal ileum into the pelvis within the muscular tube and circumferentially suturing it to the anus. The potential advantages of this approach are elimination of all diseased mucosa, preservation of parasympathetic innervation to the bladder and genitalia, and thus avoidance of impotence, avoidance of a permanent abdominal ileostomy, and preservation of the anorectal sphincter apparatus, which is responsible for fecal continence. Despite these theoretic advantages, the operation was initially associated with a high complication rate and an unpredictable functional result, and, therefore, enthusiasm for ileoanal anastomosis among surgeons declined. During the late 1970s, there was a resurgence of interest in the ileoanal pull-through operation, in part because of disillusionment with the Kock pouch, but mainly because of the improved success of the operation. This improvement was in part a result of the generalized advancement in perioperative and intraoperative surgical care, but specifically it was the result of several technical alterations in the operation.

Perhaps the most important modification of the operation was the creation of an ileal pouch or reservoir proximal to the ileoanal anastomosis. This addition was partially prompted by the physiologic studies of Heppel and co-workers,[45] which showed an inverse correlation between ileal compliance or capacity and stool frequencies in patients following straight ileoanal pull-through. Several pouch configurations exist: J, S, and W (in increasing size) (Fig. 12). Studies comparing the functional result following ileoanal anastomosis with and without an ileal reservoir have found that 24-hour stool frequency was significantly reduced in patients with ileal pouches, particularly in the early postoperative period.[42,60,69]

Technically the operation involves abdominal colectomy, mucosal proctectomy, endorectal ileal pouch–anal anastomosis, and diverting loop ileostomy. Eight weeks later the ileostomy is closed. If a previous colectomy with ileostomy has been performed for severe colitis or frank toxic megacolon, a second major operation is required for mucosal proctectomy and ileoanal anastomosis.

The functional results in the authors' series of 230 patients after ileoanal anastomosis (78 per cent for ulcerative colitis and 22 per cent for familial polyposis coli) have been encouraging.[5] A two-loop J pouch has been employed (Fig. 13), and it has been found that by providing an adequate intestinal reservoir and preserving nearly normal anal sphincter function, the operation provides anal continence and acceptable stool frequency. The

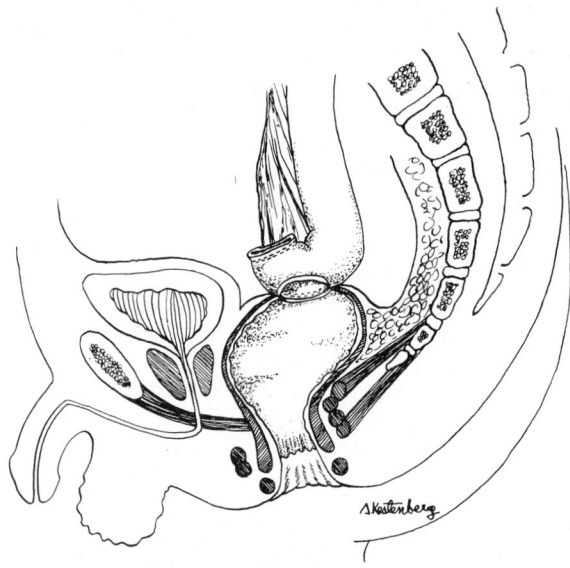

Figure 9. Ileorectal anastomosis following subtotal colectomy. This operation eliminates proctectomy with its attendant complications but does not provide definitive treatment for ulcerative colitis.

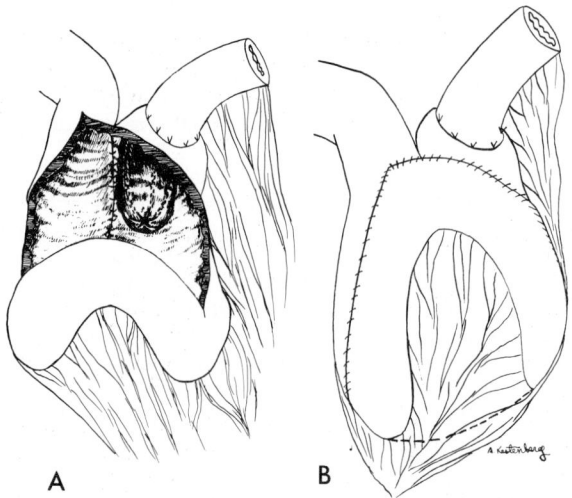

Figure 10. *A* and *B*, The Kock continent ileostomy consists of an intestinal reservoir and nipple valve constructed by intussuscepting the efferent limb of ileum and tacking it in place with sutures or staples. This provides a continent internal reservoir that the patient can drain by intubating the pouch several times throughout the day.

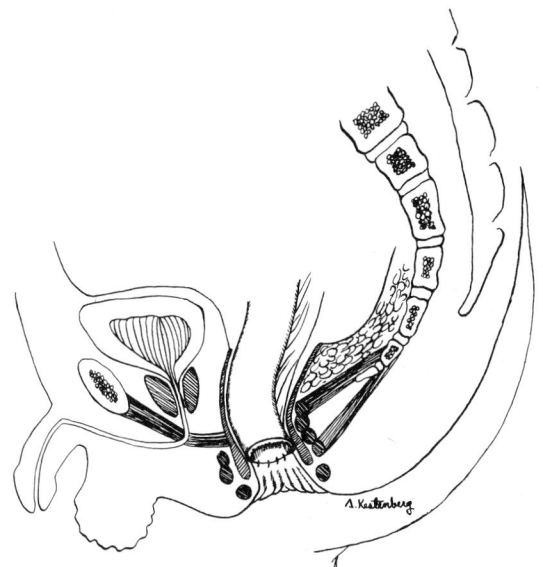

Figure 11. End-to-end ileoanal anastomosis following colectomy, mucosal proctectomy, and endorectal ileoanal pull-through. After abdominal colectomy, the rectal mucosa is circumferentially dissected from the rectal muscle and anal sphincter. The ileum is then extended down into the pelvis endorectally and anastomosed to the dentate line of the anus.

functional results of ileoanal anastomosis in the largest series with adequate late follow-up data are summarized in Table 4. These studies demonstrated that the number of bowel movements is in the range of four to nine daily, with an average of six. Nocturnal bowel movements occur one to two times nightly, with a mean of slightly more than one. Of greater importance were control and urgency of bowel movements, which were variable depending on the time after the operation. Daytime incontinence was extremely uncommon, although nocturnal seepage occurred in 10 to 50 per cent of patients. Improvement in these functions continued for more than 2 years postoperatively.

When urgent or emergency surgical therapy is required for the more devastating complications of ulcerative colitis, less than total proctocolectomy may be a wise decision.[88] For example, subtotal colectomy with ileostomy and Hartmann closure of the rectum avoids rectal excision in an acutely ill patient and yet does not eliminate the possibility of mucosal proctectomy with

ileoanal anastomosis at a later date. This procedure is known to be effective when acute fulminating disease or toxic megacolon is the indication for surgical intervention.[36] Perhaps the only indication for emergency total proctocolectomy is life-threatening hemorrhage from the entire colorectal mucosa.

Mortality for elective surgical therapy is in the range of 0 to 2 per cent; for emergency operation it is about 4 to 5 per cent; and for toxic megacolon it rises to 17 per cent.[36] These are remarkable statistics when one considers the debilitating nature of the disease and the fact that many patients have had long-term steroid therapy. The major complication in all reported series is sepsis, either in the wound or in the intra-abdominal cavity. There is little evidence that the development of more potent and specific antibiotics has significantly reduced the incidence of this complication; attention to details of operative management continues to be the most secure way to ensure a smooth postoperative course. The most common late complication of resectional therapy with ileostomy or ileoanal anastomosis is intestinal obstruction, which occurs in about 10 per cent of patients. Other bothersome but nonlethal complications following proctocolectomy include delay in perineal closure (25 per cent), sexual dysfunction (5 to 10 per cent), and renal stones (10 per cent). Ileostomy dysfunction as a consequence of stenosis has been reduced to 2 per cent by the Brooke-Turnbull ileostomy. Additional uncommon complications include prolapse, herniation, and ulceration of the stoma, which is usually a sign of the development of Crohn's disease within the ileal stoma. Whether, in fact, the outcome following surgical therapy for Crohn's disease of the colon is as favorable as for ulcerative colitis continues to be a source of controversy.[95]

Stomal complications are, of course, not found in patients after ileoanal anastomosis. The most frequent late complication in this group of patients is the poorly defined problem of ileal pouch dysfunction or pouchitis, which has been reported to occur in 10 to 20 per cent of patients undergoing ileoanal anastomosis for ulcerative colitis. Pouchitis is an incompletely defined and poorly understood clinical syndrome consisting of increased stool frequency, watery stools, cramping, urgency, malaise, and fever. Fortunately, treatment with a short course of metronidazole is successful in most patients.

Results with ileoanal anastomosis in patients with ulcerative

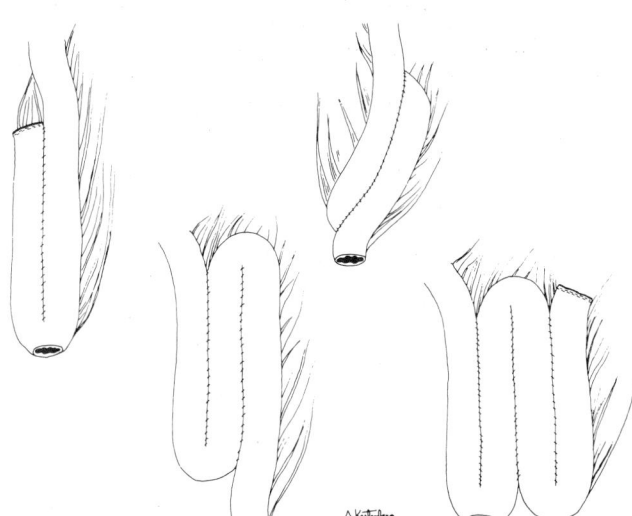

Figure 12. Ileal pouch configurations in patients undergoing endorectal ileoanal anastomosis. (From Becker, J. M., and Parodi, J. E.: Total colectomy with preservation of the anal sphincter. Surg. Annu., 21:263, 1989. Used with permission.)

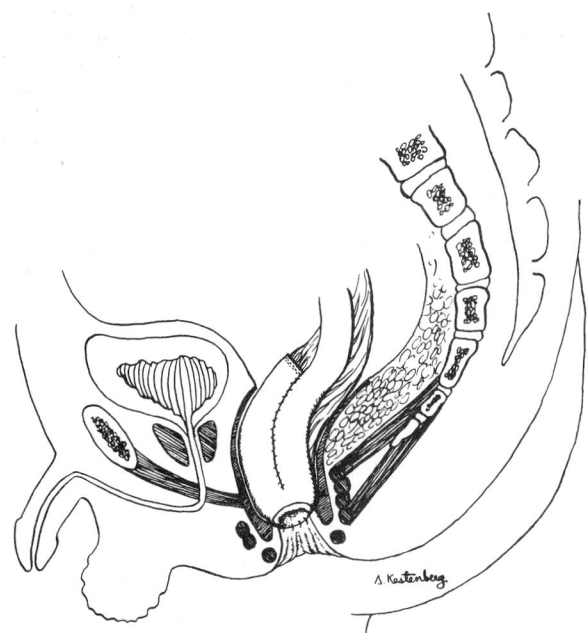

Figure 13. Ileal "J" pouch–anal anastomosis. The two-loop ileal pouch is simple to construct, provides adequate storage capacity, and is evacuated spontaneously and fully.

TABLE 4. Stooling Pattern in Patients After Ileoanal Anastomosis

Author	Number of Patients Evaluated	Type of Reservoir	24-hour Stool Frequency in the Postoperative Period	
			Early	Late
Becker and Parodi[4]	183	J pouch	7.8	5.8
Pemberton et al.[73]	390	J pouch	5.0	6.0
Martin et al.[60]	93	S pouch	6–8	2–4
	7	S pouch	8–12	6–8
Nasmyth et al.[68]	12	S pouch	6.0	5.0
	4	L pouch	7.0	7.0
	7	J pouch	6.2	7.0
	8	J pouch (modified)	6.7	6.2
Keighley[49]	12	J pouch (endoanal)	—	6.4
	10	J pouch (abdominal)	6.1	—
Schoetz et al.[87]	69	J pouch	7.0	5.1
	22	S pouch	—	—
Smith[92]	19	J pouch	—	6.0
Bubrick et al.[9]	21	S pouch	9.8	6.2
Cohen et al.[13]	50	J pouch	6.5	5.0
	6	S pouch	—	—
Fonkalsrud[30]	77	Side-to-side	8–12	7.0
Nicholls and Pezim[69]	58	S pouch	3.7	—
	12	J pouch	5.5	—
	18	W pouch	4.1	—
Heimann et al.[43]	17	Straight	10–12	6.0

From Becker, JM, Parodi, JE: Total colectomy with preservation of the anal sphincter. Surg. Annu., 21:263, 1989.

colitis are such that this operation is preferable in most patients. The authors[4] and others[21,61] have found that more than 90 per cent of patients are satisfied with their results, would not consider another alternative, and have fewer restrictions in their daily activities than do patients with Brooke ileostomies or Kock pouches (Table 5).

The formation of social groups (ileostomy clubs) has provided an important mechanism for the education of patients with abdominal stomas. The preparation of an individual for surgical therapy should include one or more visits with a patient who has mastered the techniques of ileostomy management. Some hospitals have enterostomal therapists. These professionals are individuals who are highly skilled in dealing with the physical and emotional problems of stomal management. In institutions that perform a large number of ileal pouch operations, specialized patient-oriented support groups are essential.[23]

These are extraordinary advances for patients who suffer from this poorly understood disease. New advances in surgical therapy have made the operative approach even more attractive to patients with ulcerative colitis. The cumulative mortality, as reported by Goligher and associates in their excellent monograph on the subject,[35] suggests that operative therapy should

be administered quite liberally in the chronic or acutely fatal forms of the disease. In most patients, fortunately, ulcerative colitis is episodic and mild. Unfortunately, the high incidence of cancer in the presence of persistent disease (especially after 10 years' duration) does not allow even these patients a life free of concern.

SELECTED REFERENCES

Bayless, T. M.: Current Management of Inflammatory Bowel Disease. Philadelphia, B. C. Decker, 1989.
    A recent, concise review of current diagnosis and treatment of inflammatory bowel disease.

Becker, J. M., and Parodi, J. E.: Total colectomy with preservation of the anal sphincter. Surg. Annu., 263:302, 1989.
    This article represents a more recent analysis of results in patients following ileoanal anastomosis.

Cello, J. P., and Schneiderman, D. J.: Ulcerative colitis. *In* Sleisenger, M. H., and Fordtran, J. S. (Eds.): Gastrointestinal Disease. Philadelphia, W. B. Saunders Company, 1989.
    The authors provide a very readable, authoritative text on the various facets of ulcerative colitis that relate to diagnosis, medical management, and natural history of the disease. The discussion of newer concepts of etiology places the numerous variables in a contemporary perspective.

TABLE 5. Performance Status After Proctocolectomy

Type of Operation	Number of Patients		Activities					
	Total	Wanting Change	Sex		Social		Sports	
			Improved	Restricted	Improved	Restricted	Improved	Restricted
Brooke	675	40%	15%	29%	28%	21%	15%	43%
Kock pouch	330	11%	31%*	29%	38%*	17%	26%*	21%*
Ileoanal	50	6%	34%†	8%‡	52%†	12%†	40%†	8%‡

* Differs from Brooke, $p < 0.05$.
† Ileoanal > Brooke, $p < 0.02$.
‡ Ileoanal < Brooke, $p < 0.002$.

Modified with permission from Dozois, R. R., and Kelly, K. A.: Newer operations for ulcerative colitis and Crohn's disease. *In* Kirsner, J. B., and Shorter, R. G. (Eds.): Inflammatory Bowel Disease, 3rd ed. Philadelphia, Lea & Febiger, 1988, p. 661.

Dozois, R. R.: Alternatives to conventional ileostomy. Chicago, Year Book Medical Publishers, 1985.
A comprehensive review of the current surgical alternatives for patients requiring colectomy for chronic ulcerative colitis.

Lukash, W. M., and Johnston, R. B. (Eds.): The Systemic Manifestations of Inflammatory Bowel Disease. Springfield, IL, Charles C Thomas, 1975.
This monograph describes in detail the various colonic as well as extracolonic manifestations of ulcerative colitis. It is recommended because of the discussion of extracolonic manifestations, in which associated liver, eye, skin, joint, blood, metabolic, and endocrine problems are covered in detail.

Pemberton, J. H., Heppell, J., Beart, R. W., et al.: Endorectal ileoanal anastomosis. Surg. Gynecol. Obstet, 155:417, 1982.
This article reviews in detail the history, the physiologic and anatomic rationale, and the early results with this exciting alternative to proctocolectomy and Brooke ileostomy.

Turnbull, R. B., Jr., and Weakley, F. L.: Atlas of Intestinal Stomas. St. Louis, C. V. Mosby, 1967.
The authors provide a stepwise, reliable method of constructing an ileostomy. The technical features offered cannot be overemphasized and, if adhered to, minimize ileostomy problems.

REFERENCES

1. Adams, F.: The genuine works of Hippocrates. Baltimore, Williams & Wilkins, 1939.
2. Almy, T. P., and Sherlock, P.: Genetic aspects of ulcerative colitis and regional enteritis. Gastroenterology, 51:757, 1966.
3. Baker, W. N. W., Glass, R. E., Ritchie, J. K., and Aylett, J. S. O.: Cancer of the rectum following colectomy and ileorectal anastomosis for ulcerative colitis. Br. J. Surg., 5:862, 1978.
4. Becker, J. M., and Parodi, J. E.: Total colectomy with preservation of the anal sphincter. Surg. Annu., 21:263, 1989.
5. Becker, J. M., and Raymond, J. L.: Ileal pouch–anal anastomosis: A single surgeon's experience with 100 consecutive cases. Ann. Surg., 204:375, 1986.
6. Block, G. E., Moosa, A. R., Siminowitz, D., et al.: Emergency colectomy for inflammatory bowel disease. Surgery, 82:531, 1977.
7. Boyko, E. J.: A critical review of the association between cigarette smoking and risk of ulcerative colitis. In MacDermott, R. P. (Ed.): Inflammatory Bowel Disease: Current Status and Future Approach. Amsterdam, Excerpta Medica, 1988, pp. 671–676.
8. Brandtzaeg, P., Baklien, K., Fausa, O., and Hoel, P. S.: Immuno-histochemical characterization of local immunoglobulin formation in ulcerative colitis. Gastroenterology, 66:1123, 1974.
9. Bubrick, M. P., Jacobs, D. M., and Levy, M.: Experience with the endorectal pullthrough and S pouch for ulcerative colitis and familial polyposis in adults. Surgery, 98:689, 1985.
10. Caprilli, R., Vernia, P., Catella, G., et al.: Early recognition of toxic megacolon. J. Clin. Gastroenterol., 9:160, 1987.
11. Cello, J. P.: Ulcerative colitis. In Sleisenger, M. H., and Fordtran, J. S. (Eds.). Gastrointestinal Disease. Philadelphia, W. B. Saunders Company, 1983, pp. 1122–1168.
12. Cello, J. P., and Meyer, J. H.: Crohn's disease of the colon. In Sleisenger, M. H., and Fordtran, J. S. (Eds.): Gastrointestinal Disease. Philadelphia, W. B. Saunders Company, 1978, p. 1660.
13. Cohen, Z., McLeod, R. S., Stern, H., et al.: The pelvic pouch results. Am. J. Surg., 105:601, 1985.
14. Collins, R. H., Feldman, M., and Fordtran, J. S.: Colonic cancer, dysplasia, and surveillance in patients with ulcerative colitis. A critical review. N. Engl. J. Med., 316:1654, 1987.
15. Colonic and inflammatory bowel disease. Work Group VIII. Gastroenterology, 69:1140, 1975.
16. Crohn, B. B.: An historic note on ulcerative colitis. (Letter.) Gastroenterology, 42:366, 1962.
17. deDombal, F. T., Watts, J., Watkinson, G., and Goligher, J. C.: Local complications of ulcerative colitis: Stricture, pseudopolyposis and carcinoma of the colon and rectum. Br. Med. J., 1:1142, 1966.
18. Devroede, G. H., Taylor, W. F., Sauer, W. G., et al.: Cancer risk and life expectance of children with ulcerative colitis. N. Engl. J. Med., 285:17, 1971.
19. Dick, A. P., Grayson, M. J., Carpenter, R. G., and Petrie, A.: Controlled trial of sulphasalazine in the treatment of ulcerative colitis. Gut, 5:437, 1964.
20. Dickinson, R. J., Ashton, M. G., Axon, A. T. R., et al.: Controlled trial of intravenous hyperalimentation and total bowel rest as an adjunct to the routine therapy of acute colitis. Gastroenterology, 79:1199, 1980.
21. Dozois, R. R.: Ileal pouch–anal anastomosis. Surg. Rounds, 10:34, 1987.
22. Dozois, R. R., Kelly, K. A., Bert, R. W., and Beahrs, O. H.: Improved results with continent ileostomy. Ann. Surg., 192:319, 1980.
23. Dunnegan, D., and Becker, J. M.: Support groups for ileal pouch patients. In Bayless, T. M. (Ed.): Current Management of Inflammatory Bowel Disease. Philadelphia, B. C. Decker, 1989.
24. Elson, C. O., Layden, T. J., Nemchausky, B. A., et al.: An evaluation of total parenteral nutrition in the management of inflammatory bowel disease. Dig. Dis. Sci., 25:41, 1980.
25. Engle, G. L.: Studies of ulcerative colitis. III. The nature of the physiological process. Am. J. Med., 19:231, 1955.
26. Falchuk, K. R., Perotto, J. L., and Isselbacher, K. J.: Serum lysozyme in Crohn's disease and ulcerative colitis. N. Engl. J. Med., 292:395, 1975.
27. Farnell, M. B., Van Heerden, J. A., Bert, R. W., Jr., et al.: Rectal preservation in non-specific inflammatory diseases of the colon. Ann. Surg., 192:249, 1980.
28. Fazio, V. W.: Toxic megacolon: Natural history and management. In D. G. Jagelman (Ed.): Mucosal Ulcerative Colitis. New York, Futura Publishing, 1986, pp. 159–175.
29. Fiocchi, C., Hilfiker, M. L., Youngman, K. R., Doerder, N. C., and Finke, J. H.: Interleukin-2 activity of human intestinal mucosa mononuclear cells. Decreased levels in inflammatory bowel disease. Gastroenterology, 86:734, 1984.
30. Fonkalsrud, E. W.: Endorectal ileal pullthrough with isoperistaltic ileal reservoir for ulcerative colitis and polyposis. Ann. Surg., 202:145, 1985.
31. Fonkalsrud, E. W., and Ament, M. E.: Endorectal mucosal resection without proctectomy as an adjunct to abdominoperineal resection for nonmalignant conditions. Ann. Surg., 188:245, 1978.
32. Gilat, T., Ribak, J., Benaroya, Y., Zemishlany, Z., and Weissman, I.: Ulcerative colitis in the Jewish population of Tel-Aviv Yafo, Gastroenterology, 66:335, 1974.
33. Golligher, J. C.: Surgical aspects of ulcerative colitis and Crohn's disease of the large bowel. Adv. Surg., 11:71, 1977.
34. Goligher, J. C.: Ulcerative colitis. In J. C. Goligher (Ed.): Surgery of the Anus, Rectum and Colon. New York, Macmillan, 1980, pp. 689–826.
35. Goligher, J. C., deDombal, F. T., Watts, J. M., and Watkinson, G.: Ulcerative Colitis. Baltimore, Williams & Wilkins, 1968.
36. Goligher, J. C., Hoffman, D. C., and deDombal, F. T.: Surgical treatment of severe attacks of ulcerative colitis with special reference to the advantages of early operation. Br. Med. J., 4:703, 1970.
37. Grant, C., and Dozois, R. R.: Toxic megacolon and ultimate fate of patients after successful medical management. Am. J. Surg., 147:106, 1984.
38. Greenstein, A. J., Janowitz, H. D., and Sachar, D. B.: The extra-intestinal complications of Crohn's disease and ulcerative colitis: A study of 700 patients. Medicine, 55:401, 1976.
39. Greensten, A. J., Sachar, D. B., Gibas, A., et al.: Outcome of toxic dilatation in ulcerative and Crohn's colitis. J. Clin. Gastroenterol., 7:137, 1985.
40. Gyde, S. N., Prior, P., Thompson, H., et al.: Survival of patients with colorectal cancer complicating ulcerative colitis. Gut, 25:228, 1984.
41. Harig, H. M., Soergel, K. H., Komorowski, R. A., and Wood, C. M.: Treatment of diversion colitis with short-chain–fatty acid irrigation. N. Engl. J. Med., 230:23, 1989.
42. Harms, B. A., Pellet, J. R., and Starling, J. R.: Modified quadruple-loop (W) ileal reservoir for restorative proctocolectomy. Surgery, 101:234, 1987.
43. Heimann, T., Gelernt, I., Bauer, J., et al.: Mucosal proctectomy without reservoir. Am. J. Surg., 145:674, 1983.
44. Heppel, J., Farkouh, E., Dube, S., et al.: Toxic megacolon, an analysis of 70 cases. Dis. Colon Rectum, 29:789, 1986.
45. Heppel, J., Kelly, K. A., Phillips, S. F., et al.: Physiologic aspects of continence after colectomy, mucosal proctectomy and endorectal ileoanal anastomosis. Ann. Surg., 195:435, 1982.
46. Hoult, J. R. S., and Moore, P. K.: Sulphasalazine is a potent inhibitor of prostaglandin 15-hydroxydehydrogenase: Possible basis for therapeutic action in ulcerative colitis. Br. J. Pharmacol., 64:6, 1978.
47. Johnson, W. R., McDermott, F. T., Pihl, E., and Hughes, E. S. R.: Mucosal dysplasia, a major predictor of cancer following ileorectal anastomosis. Dis. Colon Rectum, 26:697, 1983.
48. Kaplan, H. P., Portnoy, B., Binder, H. J., et al.: A controlled evaluation of intravenous adrenocorticotropic hormone and hydrocortisone in the treatment of acute colitis. Gastroenterology, 69:91, 1975.
49. Keighley, M. R. B.: Abdominal mucosectomy reduces the incidence of soiling and sphincter damage after restorative proctocolectomy and J pouch. Dis. Colon Rectum, 30:386, 1987.
50. Kern, F.: Extra-intestinal complications of chronic ulcerative colitis and Crohn's disease of the colon. In Kirsner, J. B., and Shorter, R. G. (Eds.): Inflammatory Bowel Disease. Philadelphia, Lea & Febiger, 1980, pp. 217–240.
51. Kirk, A. P., and Lennard-Jones, J. E.: Controlled trial of azathioprine in chronic ulcerative colitis. Br. Med. J., 284:1291, 1982.
52. Kirsner, J. B.: Genetic aspects of inflammatory bowel disease. Clin. Gastroenterol, 2:557, 1973.
53. Kock, N. G.: Continent ileostomy. Prog. Surg., 12:180, 1973.
54. Kraft, S. C., and Kirsner, J. B.: Present status of immunological mechanisms in ulcerative colitis. Gastroenterology, 51:788, 1966.
55. Kvietys, P. R., and Granter, D. N.: The effect of volatile fatty acids on blood flow and oxygen uptake by the dog colon. Gastroenterology, 80:962, 1981.
56. Lennard-Jones, J. E., Misiewica, J. J., Connell, A. M., et al.: Prednisone as maintenance treatment for ulcerative colitis in remission. Lancet, 1:188, 1965.
57. Ljungh, A., and Wadstrom, T.: Subepithelial connective tissue protein binding of Escherichia coli isolated from patients with ulcerative colitis. In MacDermott, R. P. (Ed.): Inflammatory Bowel Disease: Current Status and Future Approach. Amsterdam, Excerpta Medica, 1988, pp. 571–575.
58. MacDermott, R. P.: Overview of current and future approaches to research in the inflammatory bowel diseases. In MacDermott, R. P. (Ed.): Inflammatory Bowel Disease Current Status and Future Approach. Amsterdam, Excerpta Medica, 1988, pp. v–ix.
59. MacDougall, I. P. M.: The cancer risk in ulcerative colitis. Lancet, 2:655, 1964.

60. Martin, L. W., Sayers, H. S., Alexander, F., et al.: Anal continence following Soave procedure. Ann. Surg., 203:525, 1986.

61. McHugh, S. M., Diamont, N. E., McLeod, R., and Cohen, Z.: S-pouches versus "J" pouches colon: A comparison of functional outcomes. Dis. Colon Rectum, 30:671, 1987.

62. McIntyre, P. B., Powell-Tuck, J., Wood, S. R., Lennard-Jones, J. E., Lerebours, E., Hecketsweiler, P., Galamiche, J-P., and Colin, R.: Controlled trial of bowel rest in the treatment of severe acute colitis. Gut, 276:481, 1986.

63. Meyers, S., and Janowitz, H. D.: The place of steroids in the therapy of toxic megacolon. Gastroenterology, 75:729, 1978.

64. Meyers, S., Sachar, D. B., Goldberg, J. D., and Janowitz, H. D.: Corticotrophin versus hydrocortisone in the intravenous treatment of ulcerative colitis. A prospective, randomized, double-blind clinical trial. Gastroenterology, 85:351, 1983.

65. Monk, M., Mendeloff, A. I., Siegel, C. I., and Lilienfeld, A.: An epidemiological study of ulcerative colitis and regional enteritis among adults in Baltimore. III. J. Chron. Dis., 22:565, 1970.

66. Montiero, E., Fossey, J., Shiner, J. M., Drasser, B., and Allison, A.: Antibacterial antibodies in rectal and colonic mucosa in ulcerative colitis. Lancet, 1:249, 1971.

67. Morson, B. C., and Pang, L. S.: Rectal biopsy as an aid to cancer control in ulcerative colitis. Gut, 8:423, 1967.

68. Nasmyth, D. G., Williams, N. S., and Johnston, D.: Comparison of the function of triplicated and duplicated pelvic ileal reservoir after mucosal proctectomy and ileoanal anastomosis for ulcerative colitis and adenomatous polyposis. Br. J. Surg., 73:361, 1986.

69. Nicholls, R. J., and Pezim, M. E.: Restorative proctocolectomy with ileal reservoir for ulcerative colitis and familial adenomatous polyposis: A comparison of three reservoir designs. Br. J. Surg., 72:470, 1985.

70. Palmer, K. R., Corbett, C. L., and Holdsworth, C. D.: Double-blind crossover study comparing loperamide, codeine, and diphenoxylate in the treatment of chronic diarrhea. Gastroenterology, 79:1272, 1980.

71. Pemberton, J. H., Heppel, J., Bert, R. W., et al.: Endorectal ileoanal anastomosis. Surg. Gynecol. Obstet., 155:417, 1982.

72. Pemberton, J. H., Kelly, K. A., Beart, R. W., Jr., et al.: Ileal pouch–anal anastomosis for chronic ulcerative colitis. Ann. Surg., 206:504, 1987.

73. Pemberton, J. H., Phillips, S. F., Dozois, R. R., et al.: Current clinical results of conventional ileostomy. In Dozois, R. R. (Ed.): Alternatives to Conventional Ileostomy. Chicago, Year Book Medical Publishers, 1985, pp. 40–50.

74. Podolsky, D. K., and Isselbacher, K. J.: Glycoprotein composition of colonic mucosa. Specific alterations in ulcerative colitis. Gastroenteroloy, 87:991, 1984.

75. Present, D. H.: Mercaptopurine and other immunosuppressive agents in the treatment of Crohn's disease and ulcerative colitis. Gastroenterol. Clin. North Am., 18:57, 1989.

76. Present, D. H., Chapman, M. G., and Rubin, P. H.: Efficacy of 6-mercaptopurine in refractory ulcerative colitis (abstract). Gastroenterology, 94:A359, 1988.

77. Rampton, D. S., McNeil, N. I., and Sarner, M.: Analgesic ingestion and other factors preceding relapse in ulcerative colitis. Gut, 24:187, 1983.

78. Rampton, D. S., Sladen, G. E., and Youlten, L. J. F.: Rectal mucosal prostaglandin E$_2$ release and its relation to disease activity, electrical potential difference, and treatment in ulcerative colitis. Gut, 21:591, 1980.

79. Ravitch, M. M., and Sabiston, D. L., Jr.: Anal ileostomy with preservation of the sphincter: A proposed operation in patients requiring total colectomy for benign lesions. Surg. Gynecol. Obstet., 84:1095, 1947.

80. Roediger, W. E. W.: The colonic epithelium in ulcerative colitis. An energy deficiency disease? Lancet, 2:712, 1980.

81. Rolandelli, R. H., Koruda, M. J., Settle, R. G., et al.: The effect of enteral feedings supplemented with pectin on the healing of colonic anastomoses in the rat. Surgery, 99:703, 1986.

82. Rombeau, J. L., Barot, L. R., Williamson, C. E., et al.: Preoperative total parenteral nutrition and surgical outcome in patients with inflammatory bowel disease. Am. J. Surg., 143:139, 1982.

83. Rosenberg, J. L., Wall, A. J., et al.: A controlled trial of azathioprine in the management of chronic ulcerative colitis. Gastroenterology, 69:96, 1975.

84. Roy, P. H., Sauer, W. G., Beahrs, O. H., et al.: Experiences with ileostomies: Evaluation of long-term rehabilitation in 497 patients. Am. J. Surg., 119:77, 1970.

85. Rubio, C. A., Johansson, C., Slezak, P., Ohman, V., and Hammarberg, C.: Villous dysplasia: An ominous histologic sign in colitic patients. Dis. Colon Rectum, 27:283, 1984.

86. Sakata, T.: Stimulatory effect of short-chain fatty acids on epithelial cell proliferation in rat intestine: A possible explanation for trophic effects of fermentable fibre, gut microbes and luminal trophic factors. Br. J. Nutr., 58:95, 1987.

87. Schoetz, D. J., Jr., Coller, J. A., and Veidenheimer, M. C.: Ileoanal reservoir for ulcerative colitis and familial polyposis. Arch. Surg., 121:404, 1986.

88. Scott, H. W., Jr., Sawyers, J. L., Gobbel, W. G., Jr., et al.: Surgical management of toxic dilatation of the colon in ulcerative colitis. Ann. Surg., 179:647, 1974.

89. Sharon, P., and Stenson, W. F.: Enhanced synthesis of leukotriene B$_4$ by colonic mucosa in inflammatory bowel disease. Gastroenterology, 86:453, 1984.

90. Sharon, P., Ligumsky, M., Rachmilewitz, D., and Zor, V.: Role of prostaglandins in ulcerative colitis. Gastroenterology, 75:638, 1978.

91. Sinclair, T. S., Brunt, P. W., and Mowat, N. A. G.: Nonspecific proctocolitis in northeastern Scotland: A community study. Gastroenterology, 85:1, 1983.

92. Smith, L. E.: A review of twenty-one rectal mucosectomy and ileal pouch pull-through procedures. Am. Surg., 52:182, 1986.

93. Smolen, J. S., Gangl, A., Polterauer, P., Menzel, E. J., and Mayr, W. R.: HLA antigens in inflammatory bowel disease. Gastroentrology, 82:34, 1982.

94. Soyer, M. T., and Aldrete, J. S.: Surgical treatment of toxic megacolon and proposal for a program of therapy. Am. J. Surg., 140:421, 1980.

95. Steinberg, D. M., Allan, R. D., Brooke, B. N., et al.: Sequelae of colectomy and ileostomy: Comparison between Crohn's colitis and ulcerative colitis. Gastroenterology, 68:33, 1975.

96. Stout, C., and Snyder, R. L.: Ulcerative colitis–like lesion in saimang gibbons. Gastroenteroloy, 57:256, 1969.

97. Taffet, S. L., and Das, K. M.: Sulfasalazine. Adverse effects and desensitization. Dig. Dis. Sci., 28:833, 1983.

98. Truelove, S. C., et al.: Cortisone in ulcerative colitis. Final report on a therapeutic trial. Br. Med. J., 2:1041, 1955.

99. Turnbull, R. B., Jr., Hawk, W. A., and Weakley, F. L.: Surgical treatment of toxic megacolon, ileostomy and colostomy to prepare patient for colectomy. Am. J. Surg., 122:325, 1971.

100. Whitehead, R. H., Young, G. P., and Bhathal, P. S.: Effects of short-chain fatty acids on a new human colon carcinoma cell line (LIM1215). Gut, 27:1457, 1986.

101. Yardley, J. H., Bayless, T. H., and Diamond, M. P.: Cancer in ulcerative colitis. Gastroenterology, 76:221, 1979.

102. Yoshimura, H. H., Estes, M. K., and Graham, D. Y.: Search for evidence of a viral etiology for inflammatory bowel disease. Gut, 25:347, 1984.

VIII

VOLVULUS OF THE COLON

Anthony L. Imbembo, M.D., and Karl A. Zucker, M.D.

Volvulus is the abnormal twisting or rotation of a portion of the bowel around its mesentery. This may cause occlusion of the lumen at each end of the segment with resultant obstruction and/or vascular compromise. Colonic volvulus has plagued mankind since antiquity. Descriptions of this disorder and its natural history were detailed in the Egyptian Papyrus Ebers.[1] Colonic volvulus was also described in the writings of ancient Greek and Roman physicians, who administered purgatives as the preferred treatment. Hippocrates is credited with the use of a 12-inch-long suppository and of anal insufflation with air to untwist the bowel, a method very similar to that used currently in treating sigmoid volvulus.[2] Today volvulus is an uncommon cause of obstruction in English-speaking countries, representing approximately 1 to 3 per cent of all admissions for bowel obstruction.[3] It remains, however, a major health problem in parts of Russia, Iran, and Africa, where volvulus may constitute the most common cause of intestinal obstruction. In Ethiopia, for example, sigmoid volvulus represented 54 per cent of all intestinal obstructions.[4]

The various forms of colonic volvulus were described by Rokitansky in the mid nineteenth century. The sigmoid colon, cecum or right colon, transverse colon, or splenic flexure may be involved.[5] Colonic volvulus generally occurs in the setting of a large redundant colonic segment that has a narrow mesenteric base. The redundant segment is freely mobile within the peritoneal cavity, and the points of fixation are quite close, serving as foci for development of volvulus. These features may be acquired, as in sigmoid volvulus, or congenital in origin, as is likely with cecal volvulus. Left untreated, volvulus generally progresses rapidly from colonic obstruction to strangulation and gangrene.

SIGMOID VOLVULUS

The sigmoid colon is the most common site for colonic volvulus, comprising overall about three quarters of the cases of large bowel volvulus. In Olmstead County, Minnesota, where comprehensive medical records are available for all residents, there was an incidence of 1.47 episodes of sigmoid volvulus per 100,000 population per year. Sigmoid volvulus was also found to be twenty times more common in individuals above age 60 than in those who were younger.[3]

Much of the international literature has ascribed the pathogenesis of sigmoid volvulus to an acquired redundancy of sigmoid colon secondary to the ingestion of high-residue diets.[6,7] In the United States, the most prominent association appears to be chronic constipation. Almost all patients have a long-standing history of disordered bowel habits, with excessive reliance on laxatives or enemas. Other contributing factors may include underlying neuropsychiatric disorders such as Parkinson's disease, Alzheimer's disease, multiple sclerosis, traumatic paralysis, chronic schizophrenia, pseudobulbar palsy, and senility. These associations have generally been attributed to the usual bedridden state of these patients and/or the use of various neuropsychotropic drugs, which are both known to alter bowel motility. Thus, in the United States up to 50 per cent of patients admitted with sigmoid volvulus are referred from chronic care facilities.[6,7] Adhesions from prior abdominal procedures have also been implicated as a causative factor in some patients, with the scar tissue serving as a pivot point around which the bowel can twist. In one study, 53 per cent of 59 patients with sigmoid volvulus gave a history of prior abdominal surgery.[3] Although an uncommon complication in pregnant women, sigmoid volvulus appears to be the most frequently encountered cause of intestinal obstruction during pregnancy.[6,7]

The age and sex distributions of patients with sigmoid volvulus have been detailed in a number of international reports, with two distinct patterns emerging. Patients in Iran, Africa, India, and Eastern Europe are predominantly middle-aged males (mean age, 40 to 50 years); whereas in the United States, Australia, the United Kingdom, and Canada volvulus occurs in elderly patients (mean age, 60 to 70 years) of both sexes. In a large collected series from the United States, approximately two thirds of the patients were black; racial differences, however, have not been noted in reports from other countries.[6,7]

The diagnosis of sigmoid volvulus usually is easy to make based on the patient's history, physical examination, and plain abdominal radiographs. The acute sigmoid volvulus generally presents with the sudden onset of severe, colicky abdominal pain, obstipation, and abdominal distention. Distention is usually rapidly progressive as the twisted sigmoid continues to fill with gas and feces without the possibility of egress. The development of generalized abdominal pain, tenderness, fever, and hypovolemia should suggest that strangulation has occurred. Occasionally, patients present with a history of intermittent abdominal pain and distention consistent with chronic intermittent volvulus.

Plain abdominal radiographs often reveal a dilated colon forming the "bent inner tube" or "omega loop" sign. The convexity of the loop points toward the right upper quadrant, or

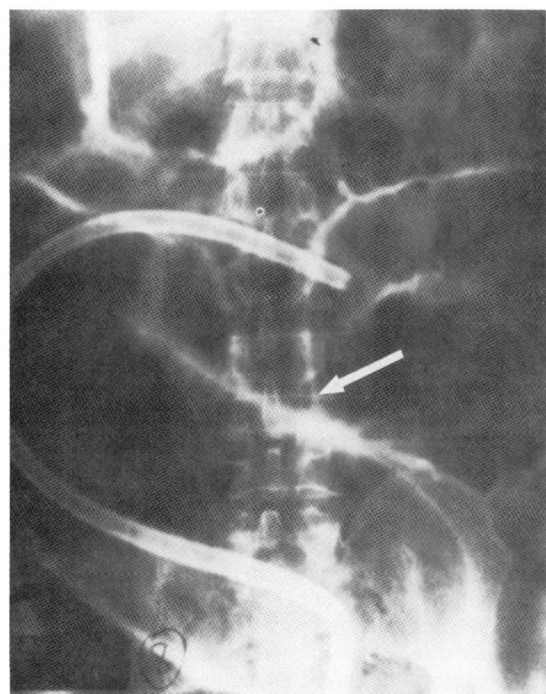

Figure 1. Sigmoid volvulus with rectal tube placement for decompression. The convexity of the loops (arrow) points toward the right upper quadrant. (Courtesy of G. H. Ballantyne, M.D.)

away from the point of obstruction (Fig. 1). Also visible on plain abdominal films is the narrowed segment of colon, the "bird's beak," which points towards the site of obstruction. Two air-fluid levels are frequently observed within the sigmoid loop. Barium enema is usually not required for diagnosis and is contraindicated whenever strangulation is suspected.

The treatment for acute sigmoid volvulus has evolved from attempts to untwist the bowel nonoperatively, as advocated by Hippocrates and his successors, to primary operative detorsion, to a combination of early nonoperative reduction followed by definitive surgical therapy. Operative detorsion of sigmoid volvulus was popularized in the late nineteenth century with Atherton reporting the first successful experience in the United States in 1883.[8] However, operative mortality was found to be high, especially since surgical intervention generally occurred very late in the course of the disease. Nonoperative reduction of sigmoid volvulus was rapidly adopted after the report of Bruusgard in 1947,[9] who found that 82 per cent of 148 patients with sigmoid volvulus were successfully reduced by a combination of rigid proctoscopy and rectal tube insertion. With this approach, the overall mortality was only 14.2 per cent.

The initial treatment of sigmoid volvulus consists of attempted nonoperative reduction, which can be expected to be successful in approximately 70 to 80 per cent of patients.[6,7] Successful detorsion of a sigmoid volvulus permits deferral of surgical intervention in an acutely ill patient with an unprepared bowel. Techniques that have been successfully employed to reduce the sigmoid colon volvulus include proctoscopy alone, enemas alone, proctoscopy and placement of a rectal tube, and barium/water-soluble contrast enemas. The latter modality is occasionally employed as part of the radiologic evaluation if there is question as to the diagnosis after plain films and may itself untwist the volvulus. Recently, fiberoptic colonoscopy has been advocated in those patients who fail rigid proctoscopy. In a report from Nigeria, colonoscopic decompression was successful in 83 of 92 patients (90.2 per cent) with sigmoid volvulus.[10] The fiberoptic colonoscope is especially useful when the sigmoidoscope fails to reach the point of volvulus. Some have now advocated its use as the primary modality for detorsion. However, the safety and overall efficacy of this approach is still unclear.

The most widely used nonoperative procedure for reduction of sigmoid volvulus is the combination of proctoscopy and rectal tube placement. With the patient in the lateral knee-chest position, a rigid proctoscope is carefully advanced through the rectum into the distal sigmoid colon. The advancing proctoscope along with the gentle insufflation of air to distend the bowel often will untwist the colon. A well-lubricated rectal tube is then passed through the proctoscope and eased past the point of torsion. With reduction of the volvulus, there is usually explosive decompression with passage of gas and liquid feces. At the time of proctoscopy, careful attention is paid to the appearance of the colonic mucosa. Evidence of vascular compromise on proctoscopy necessitates immediate surgical intervention.

If there is no evidence of bowel wall ischemia and nonoperative reduction is successful, delayed sigmoid colon resection is recommended for most patients. This procedure should be performed when the patient has been adequately resuscitated, nutritionally repleted, and has undergone appropriate bowel preparation. With a delayed, elective resection, primary anastomosis may be performed safely in most patients. However, in those patients who fail nonoperative reduction, the appropriate surgical approach can be much less clear. Colostomy alone, proximal to the site of volvulus, is contraindicated, because this procedure does not prevent strangulation of the segment or recurrent volvulus. Operative detorsion alone has a high rate of recurrence of up to 40 per cent and is not an acceptable procedure in most cases.[11] Other procedures that have been used in conjunction with operative detorsion include tube sigmoidostomy, extraperitonealization of the sigmoid colon, sigmoidopexy to the transverse colon, sigmoidopexy to the peritoneum, fixation of the sigmoid mesentery, and resection with end colostomy (with or without mucus fistula).[6,7] Unfortunately, there is insufficient experience reported to evaluate the efficacy of each of these procedures. Most currently recommend initial operative reduction followed by delayed resection and primary anastomosis. If gangrene is present at the time of laparotomy, immediate resection is indicated, usually with end-colostomy and mucus fistula or Hartmann's pouch.

The main determinant of patient mortality from acute sigmoid volvulus is viability of the sigmoid colon. In the United States, patients undergoing successful nonoperative reduction followed by elective resection have an expected mortality of 6 to 10 per cent. Patients with gangrenous colons have a mortality of 50 to 70 per cent.[6,7] Prompt nonoperative or operative intervention in hope of preventing strangulation of sigmoid volvulus appears to be the most important principle of treatment. Recurrence of volvulus after nonoperative reduction is 55 to 90 per cent. The mortality relative to recurrent volvulus or its treatment can be as high as 20 to 30 per cent.[6,7] Therefore, maximal survival is achieved by early elective resection, even in an elderly population.

CECAL VOLVULUS

Cecal volvulus represents 20 to 40 per cent of all cases of colonic volvulus. In 502 patients with volvulus of the colon collected from 16 series, 34 per cent were found to be cecal.[3] Approximately 90 per cent of patients with cecal volvulus have an axial twist of a segment of the proximal colon (Figs. 2, 4B) or even of the entire right colon, while in the remainder there is a cephalad fold of the cecum across the ascending colon (cecal bascule) (Figs. 3, 4A). A mobile cecum is a prerequisite for development of a cecal volvulus. Various anomalous patterns of cecal attachment allow such mobility. A detailed study of 125 cadavers revealed that over one third of cecums examined were mobile enough to allow a volvulus to occur.[12] Poor fixation usually follows malrotation of the colon, setting the stage for torsion, often around the pedicle of the ileocolic artery.

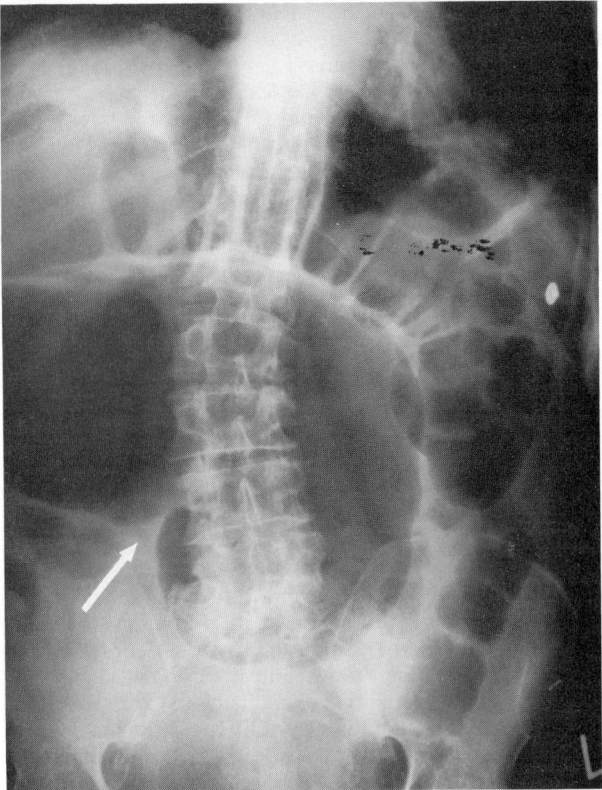

Figure 2. Cecal volvulus with an axial twist at the level of the mid-ascending colon. In contrast to sigmoid volvulus, the convexity of the loops (arrow) points toward the left upper quadrant. (Courtesy of G. H. Ballantyne, M.D.)

Various risk factors have been implicated in the development of cecal volvulus. As with sigmoid volvulus, high-fiber diets among Eastern European and African inhabitants and the use of various neuropsychotropic drugs in Western populations have

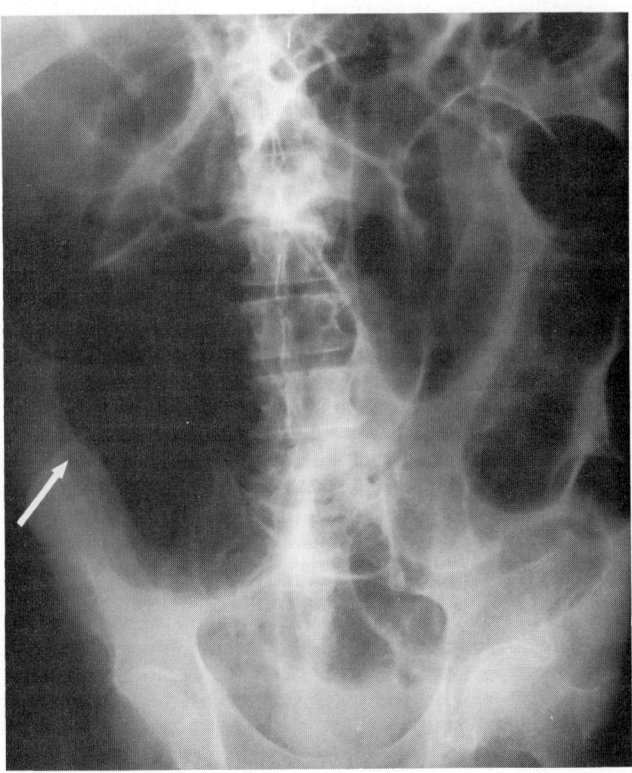

Figure 3. Cecal bascule with a cephalad fold of the cecum across the ascending colon (arrow). The ileocecal valve and terminal ileum are visible over the L2–3 interspace. (Courtesy of G. H. Ballantyne, M.D.)

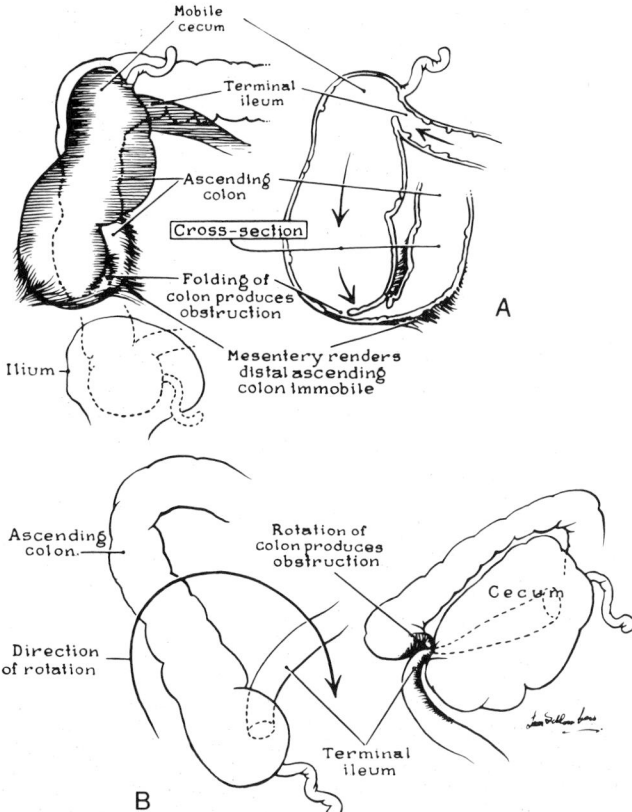

Figure 4. *A*, Diagrammatic representation of cecal volvulus caused by an anterior cephalad displacement of the cecum, resulting in obstruction at the site of transverse folding. Dotted lines show usual position of the cecum in relation to the ilium. *B*, Demonstration of cecal volvulus produced by a clockwise rotation of the terminal ileum, cecum, and ascending colon. (From O'Mara, C. S., Wilson, T. M., Jr., Stonesifer, G. L., and Cameron, J. L.: Cecal volvulus. Ann. Surg., *189:*724, 1979.)

been implicated. In the United States, as many as one half to two thirds of these patients have undergone previous abdominal surgical procedures; in one series, 68 per cent of these operations were appendectomies.[13] Colonic distention following distal obstruction has also been implicated in the development of cecal volvulus and should be excluded in all such patients.

Cecal volvulus generally presents with the acute onset of severe, colicky pain, nausea, vomiting, and obstipation. Often, abdominal distention develops along with a compressible mass extending from the right lower quadrant to the midabdominal region. Chronic abdominal symptoms occur in many patients because of the tendency for cecal volvulus to resolve spontaneously, only to recur subsequently. These patients often obtain relief by the self-administration of enemas or by assumption of the knee-chest position. Plain abdominal roentgenograms reveal marked distention of the cecum as well as small bowel dilatation. Barium enema classically reveals the narrowing accompanying the twisting of the colon ("bird's neck" deformity); however, such studies may be misinterpreted as demonstrating obstruction secondary to neoplasm. The filling of the entire left colon on barium enema can serve to differentiate cecal from sigmoid volvulus.

Nonoperative techniques for the reduction of cecal volvulus have been much less successful than for sigmoid volvulus. Reduction of the volvulus by barium enema is accomplished in a small number of patients; however, early recurrence is the general course.[14] Colonoscopic reduction has been reported in a small number of patients but is accompanied by a high failure rate, often delays necessary operative reduction, and may be unwise in the setting of ischemic bowel.[15]

The physical examination as well as the presence of fever and leukocytosis correlate poorly with the presence or absence of

gangrenous bowel in patients with cecal volvulus.[13] Approximately 25 per cent of patients are found to have gangrenous changes at the time of laparotomy. Mortality in the setting of gangrenous bowel approaches 40 per cent, while in patients with viable bowel it is generally less than 10 per cent.[16] Therefore, when the diagnosis of cecal volvulus has been made, prompt surgical intervention is advised. When the cecum is gangrenous, resection is mandatory, usually with ileotransverse colostomy. However, in the setting of viable bowel the procedure of choice is less clear. Several options are available, including detorsion alone, cecopexy, cecostomy, and colonic resection. Operative detorsion alone without fixation is associated with a high recurrence rate and consequent mortality.[3,16] Cecopexy performed by suturing the colon to the parietal peritoneum eliminates hypermobility, with quite satisfactory overall results. Cecostomy accomplishes both fixation and venting of the obstructed colon; however, this procedure inevitably causes spillage of colonic contents, increasing the risk of intra-abdominal sepsis or prolonged wound complications. Right hemicolectomy for nongangrenous cecal volvulus was first recommended by Melchior in 1948 and is the procedure of choice in a number of institutions.[16,17] In this way, the possibility of recurrent volvulus is eliminated. However, results from 15 recent reports of patients with cecal volvulus comparing these procedures have revealed no significant difference in overall mortality.[16] Controlled trials are necessary to determine whether there is an optimal procedure.

VOLVULUS OF THE TRANSVERSE COLON

Less than 100 cases of transverse colon volvulus have been reported. In a collected series of international reports, these patients were found to be middle-aged, women outnumbering men two to one.[3] Patients present with the typical signs and symptoms of colonic obstruction. Diagnosis of transverse colon volvulus is difficult on plain abdominal films and in most series was not suspected preoperatively. Contrast radiologic studies may be more specific. Reported attempts at nonoperative reduction of transverse colon volvulus have been few and generally unsuccessful. Urgent surgical intervention is recommended in all patients, and the principles of treatment are similar to those for cecal volvulus. If gangrenous bowel is encountered, resection is mandatory. In patients with viable colon, detorsion alone appears to be associated with a high rate of recurrence and mortality.[3] Transverse colectomy, colopexy, and transverse tube colostomy have each been successfully utilized. The procedure of choice is unknown at this time.

VOLVULUS OF THE SPLENIC FLEXURE

The splenic flexure is the least common site for colonic volvulus, and less than 50 cases have been reported. The splenic flexure is fixed in position by the gastrocolic, splenocolic, and phrenocolic ligaments. Congenital absence or iatrogenic division of one or more of these attachments may predispose to splenic flexure volvulus. Approximately two thirds of reported patients with splenic flexure volvulus have undergone previous abdominal surgery.[3] Urgent surgical intervention is recommended. Resection is mandated in cases of ischemic bowel. Most patients with nongangrenous bowel have also been treated by resection, although there have been successful reports of patients treated by colopexy or splenic flexure colostomy.

SELECTED REFERENCES

Ballantyne, G. H.: Review of sigmoid volvulus: History and results of treatment. Dis. Colon Rectum, 25:494, 1982.
A lucid summary of the history of sigmoid volvulus along with a summary of various forms of therapy from the international literature. Results of the various surgical options in the treatment of nongangrenous sigmoid volvulus are presented.

Ballantyne, G. H., Brandner, M. D., Beart, R. W., and Ilstrup, D. M.: Volvulus of the colon: Incidence and mortality. Ann. Surg., 202:83, 1985.

This is an excellent and up-to-date review of colonic volvulus. One hundred thirty-seven patients with sigmoid, cecal, transverse, and splenic volvulus from 1960 to 1980 are described in detail. Methods of diagnosis, treatment, and outcome are discussed in these patients and compared with the current experience in the literature.

O'Mara, C. S., Wilson, T. H., Stonesifer, G. L., and Cameron, J. L.: Cecal volvulus: Analysis of 50 patients with long-term follow-up. Ann. Surg., 189:724, 1979.

The authors report the diagnosis, management, and outcome of 50 patients with cecal volvulus. The diagnosis of cecal volvulus was made preoperatively in less than half of the patients. Thirty-eight per cent of the patients had undergone one or more previous abdominal operations, the majority being appendectomies. When gangrene of the cecum was present, resection was performed. Otherwise the authors recommend cecopexy because of the low mortality and recurrence rate.

Tejler, G., and Jiborn, H.: Volvulus of the cecum: Report of 26 cases and review of the literature. Dis. Colon Rectum, 31:445, 1988.

The management of 26 patients with cecal volvulus is described along with a review of 350 patients in the literature. The pathogenesis of cecal volvulus as a result of colonic malrotation with a common ileocolic mesentery is discussed. The authors recommend resection as the treatment of choice when there is no gangrene present.

REFERENCES

1. Brothwell, D., and Sandison, A. T. (Eds.): Diseases in Antiquity: A Survey of the Diseases, Injuries, and Surgery of Early Populations. Springfield, Charles C Thomas, 1967.
2. Adams, F. (Trans. and Ed.): The Genuine Works of Hippocrates. London, Sydenham Society, 1849.
3. Ballantyne, G. H. Brandner, M. D., Beart, R. W., and Ilstrup, D. M.: Volvulus of the colon. Ann. Surg., 202:83, 1985.
4. Johnson, L. P.: Recent experience with sigmoid volvulus in Ethiopia. Ethiopia Med. J., 4:197, 1965.
5. Von Rokitansky: A Manual of Pathologic Anatomy. London, Sydenham Society, 1849.
6. Ballantyne, G. H.: Review of sigmoid volvulus: Clinical patterns and pathogenesis. Dis. Colon Rectum, 25:823, 1982.
7. Ballantyne, G. H.: Review of sigmoid volvulus: History and results of treatment. Dis. Colon Rectum, 25:494, 1982.
8. Atherton, A. B.: Cases of internal strangulation of the bowels: Laparotomy. Boston Med. Surg. J., 108:531, 1883.
9. Bruusgaard, C.: Volvulus of the sigmoid colon and its treatment. Surgery, 22:466, 1947.
10. Arigbabu, A. O., Badejo, O. A., and Akinola, D. O.: Colonoscopy in the emergency treatment of colonic volvulus in Nigeria. Dis. Colon Rectum, 28:795, 1985.
11. String, S. T., and DeCosse, J. J.: Sigmoid volvulus: An examination of the mortality. Am. J. Surg., 121:293, 1971.
12. Wolfer, J. A., Beaton, L. E., and Anson, B. J.: Volvulus of the cecum: Anatomical factors in its etiology. Surg. Gynecol. Obstet., 74:882, 1942.
13. O'Mara, C. S., Wilson, T. H., Stonesifer, G. L., and Cameron, J. L.: Cecal volvulus. Ann. Surg., 189:724, 1979.
14. Hjelmstedt, A.: Volvulus of the right colon. Acta. Chir. Scand., 118:455, 1960.
15. Anderson, M. J., Okike, N., and Spencer, R. J.: The colonoscope in cecal volvulus: Report of three cases. Dis. Colon Rectum,, 21:71, 1978.
16. Tejler, G., and Jiborn, H.: Volvulus of the cecum: Report of 26 cases and review of the literature. Dis. Colon Rectum, 31:445, 1988.
17. Melchior, E.: Volvulus of the cecum: An appeal for primary resection with report of six cases. Surgery, 25:251, 1949.

IX

CARCINOMA OF THE COLON, RECTUM, AND ANUS

Anthony L. Imbembo, M.D., and Alan T. Lefor, M.D.

Carcinoma of the colon and rectum is the second most common malignancy occurring in the United States, exceeded in frequency only by lung cancer. It is also the second leading cause of cancer death. In 1989, the American Cancer Society estimated that there would be 151,000 new cases of colorectal cancer (constituting approximately 15 per cent of all new cases of cancer) and 61,300 deaths from colorectal cancer in the United States.[2] The probability of developing colorectal cancer is 1 in 25 adults in the United States. It is obviously a major public health problem with which all physicians must be familiar and one in which surgical resection remains the primary form of therapy for most patients. Unfortunately, the overall survival after treatment has not improved in the past 40 years. There has been, however, a decrease in surgical mortality largely due to improvements in critical care. Aggressive approaches directed to identification of patients with early lesions and development of new therapeutic modalities are needed to improve survival.

EPIDEMIOLOGY AND ETIOLOGY

Carcinoma of the colon and rectum is generally a disease of older individuals with an approximately equal incidence in men and women. In a report of 862 patients from a single institution, only 31 (3.6 per cent) were under the age of 41.[30] The incidence is increasing gradually, as it is for most other malignancies, in the Western hemisphere.

The etiology of carcinoma of the colon and rectum remains unclear. However, many studies have suggested a correlation between colorectal cancer, economic status, geographic location, and dietary exposure. In industrialized countries, including the United States and those of Western Europe, a great deal of animal fat, protein, and refined carbohydrates are consumed; in these geographic areas the incidence of colorectal cancer is much higher than in the developing countries of Africa, South America (excluding Argentina and Uruguay, where meat consumption is high), and Japan, where considerably less meat is consumed and the diet is significantly higher in vegetable fiber. Specifically, the death rate from carcinoma of the colon in the United States is approximately 17 per 100,000 population; however, it is as high as 24 per 100,000 in New Zealand to a low of 3 per 100,000 in Mexico. These variations are not thought to be due to genetic differences, primarily because certain immigrant groups tend to assume the colon cancer incidence rates of their adopted countries. For example, in a study comparing Japanese immigrants to Hawaii, with second-generation Japanese immigrants already resident, a higher incidence of large bowel cancer was found in individuals who discontinued the practice of eating at least one Japanese-style meal daily. The increased consumption of meat is the major dietary difference between residents of Japan and Hawaii, and such an increase in beef consumption paralleled the higher risk of bowel cancer among Japanese immigrants. A correlation between the daily consumption of meat and the incidence of large bowel cancer also has been noted in individuals from many countries, suggesting an etiologic role.[15] In most international studies, colorectal cancer risk linked to economic development has been attributed to similar dietary variation among study groups. Some investigators believe that metabolic products of biliary metabolism, low dietary fiber content, and/or bacterial enzymes may be important factors in increasing colon cancer risk. Despite data from many population and experimental studies, definitive proof that any specific dietary or environmental factor is causally related to variations in the incidence of colon cancer has not been established.

There are also a number of diseases with hereditary predisposition to colorectal cancer. Familial polyposis is an autosomal dominant genetic defect that is expressed phenotypically in approximately 80 per cent of patients. In this condition, adenomatous polyps are not present at birth but usually tend to develop in the second decade of life. The majority of adenomas in familial polyposis are tubular, with the number of polyps observed varying from over 100 to well over 5000 in an individual patient. If untreated, nearly all patients develop colorectal carcinoma by age 40. Gardner's syndrome is a variant of familial polyposis that is also an autosomal dominant disorder demonstrating a high degree of penetrance. In conjunction with the adenomatosis, multiple osteomas of the skull and mandible, multiple epidermoid cysts of the skin, and desmoid tumors of the abdominal wall or small bowel mesentery are characteristic features. Turcot's syndrome has been described as polyposis coli associated with malignant tumors of the central nervous system.

Peutz-Jeghers syndrome is an autosomal dominant inherited disease with variable expression. Typically, pigmented spots develop on the lips and buccal mucosa, and occasionally on the dorsal aspects of the hands and feet. Tumors consisting of normal intestinal epithelium and abnormal amounts and arrangements of smooth muscle occur throughout the gastrointestinal tract; these lesions are considered hamartomas. The condition can occur with polyps and without pigmentation or vice versa. The tumors were originally considered to have a low malignant potential. However, a number of cases of cancer have been reported involving stomach, duodenum, and colon. Adenomas have been found to coexist with the hamartomatous lesions, with carcinoma believed to arise from the adenomas. Thus, the true malignant potential of Peutz-Jeghers syndrome remains to be established.

Other than the definition of familial polyposis and its variants, it has been difficult to identify or analyze the role of hereditary disposition in the development of colorectal cancer. Overall, inheritance presently is thought to have a minor role in the genesis of colorectal cancer. However, even when dominant inherited syndromes are excluded, familial association in colon cancer is somewhat higher than in control groups. It has been recognized that a significant percentage of patients with colorectal cancer have family members who also have had colorectal cancer and that relatives of colorectal cancer patients are at a somewhat increased risk, compared with the general population.[24] Patients under the age of 40 in whom colorectal cancer develops have been noted to be more likely to have a family history of colorectal cancer. The probability of developing a new colorectal cancer is increased in patients who have had prior colorectal cancer, adenomatous polyps, female genital cancers, breast cancer, or bladder cancer.

In patients with a previous colorectal cancer, the probability of developing a second or metachronous lesion is approximately three times higher than that in the general population. When colonic polyps are found in a specimen resected for primary colorectal cancer, the risk may be as high as six times the expected development. If the initial tumor was in the cecum, the likelihood of developing a second primary colon cancer is greatest. Metachronous lesions vary in incidence from 1.9 per cent in patients with colonic cancer to a high of 5 per cent after 25 years. The average elapsed time for development of a metachronous lesion is approximately 13.5 years.[26]

The risk of developing colorectal carcinoma is increased in patients with chronic ulcerative colitis. The lifetime cancer risk is nearly 60 per cent, with increased risk beginning after the first 10 years of disease. The number of colorectal carcinomas arising from ulcerative colitis currently is thought to be comparable with that arising from familial polyposis. The risk of developing carcinoma in association with ulcerative colitis is highest in patients having continuous disease, total colonic involvement, and onset before age 25. During the past decade, there has been increasing recognition that adenocarcinoma also can develop in association with Crohn's disease.

POPULATION SCREENING

As with many malignancies, patients with carcinoma of the colon and rectum who are diagnosed and treated at an earlier stage tend to have improved survival. If overall cost were not a consideration and the risk of screening tests nonexistent, an aggressive search for malignancies could be advocated in all. However, since this is not the case, it is necessary to determine who should be screened for occult carcinoma of the colon and what screening tests should be performed.

The screening of stool specimens for occult blood remains the simplest and least expensive screening test for carcinoma of the lower gastrointestinal tract. However, its value as a method of reducing mortality has yet to be demonstrated.[46] In a study from Kansas, 41,519 stool guaiac test kits were sent out, and only 18,198 kits returned. At least one test was positive for each 448 patients, and information could be obtained on 336 of these. Of these, 20 patients had malignancies, for a total incidence of 0.11 per cent and a 6 per cent incidence of those with positive stool guaiac test results.[8] These data are similar to those reported in other community screening projects. In this study, the total cost for each cancer detected was $12,300. If only the diagnostic tests were considered, the cost was still $5,000 per cancer. Such studies demonstrate that mass population screening in this manner may not be cost effective.

In a physician-based program in Virginia, 33,318 patients were screened over 26 months. Positive fecal occult blood tests were found in 3.3 per cent of asymptomatic patients and 14.8 per cent of symptomatic patients. Malignancies were found in 94 patients, of whom 33 per cent were asymptomatic. Eighty per cent of the asymptomatic patients were found to have relatively early lesions (Dukes A or B), and only 8 per cent had distant metastases. The screening of patients by primary care physicians in this study was concluded to be effective in detecting malignancies at an early stage, and yet the overall yield was quite low.[45]

Although the value of population screening for occult fecal blood remains to be established, there are a number of groups with a consistently increased risk of the development of carcinoma of the colon and rectum. These include patients with long-standing ulcerative colitis, Crohn's disease, previous history of cancer of the large intestine, previously resected polyps, Peutz-Jeghers syndrome, familial colon cancer, Gardner's syndrome, and familial polyposis. Such patients must be aggressively evaluated and re-evaluated for the development of malignancy. However, most patients with newly diagnosed large intestinal malignancy are not classified in these high-risk groups.

Sigmoidoscopy is an important technique for evaluation of the lower intestinal tract; and with use of the flexible instrument, nearly 50 per cent of all colonic malignancies should be reached (Fig. 1). The value of flexible sigmoidoscopy as a screening method in patients with inguinal hernia was demonstrated in a study of 110 patients (99 per cent male) in which colorectal cancers were identified in 3.6 per cent of patients. In this select group, with a mean age of 63, the yield of neoplasms was relatively high.[32]

Current recommendations of the American Gastroentero-

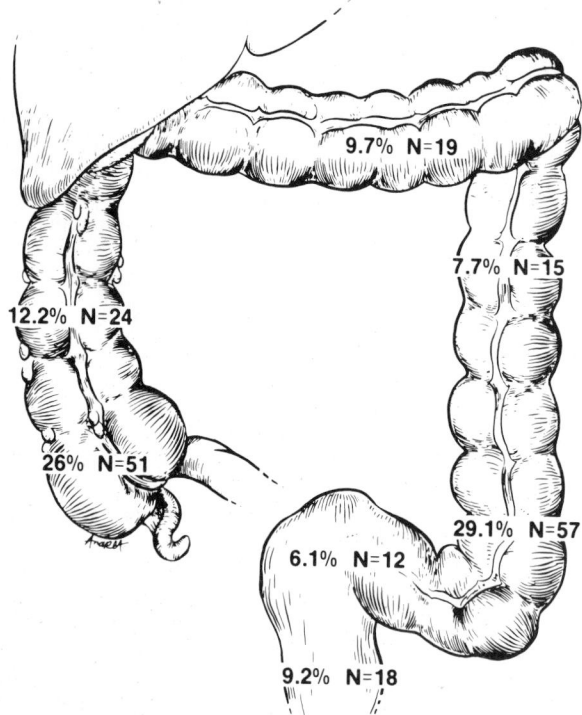

Figure 1. Incidence of malignant lesions and various locations in the colon. (Modified from Oren, J., Folse, R., Kraudel, K., and Lewis, D.: The preoperative liver scan and surgical decision-making in patients with colorectal cancer. Am. J. Surg., *151:*452, 1986.)

logic Association include digital rectal examination and fecal occult blood tests annually beginning at age 40, and flexible sigmoidoscopy at age 50 for the individual with average risk.[11] A negative endoscopy in 2 consecutive years is followed by endoscopy every 3 years thereafter. High-risk individuals should undergo earlier and more frequent endoscopic studies. Even a single positive fecal occult blood test requires evaluation by colonoscopy or flexible sigmoidoscopy coupled with double-contrast barium enema. Positive fecal occult blood tests are often ascribed to coexistent hemorrhoids. This can be a fatal error; the possibility of a proximal malignancy must never be excluded without evaluation.

In screening patients, age alone must not unduly lower the index of suspicion for colorectal malignancy. The 5-year survival rate in patients under age 40 is considerably lower than that for older patients. In a series of 31 patients under age 40 with colorectal carcinoma, 5-year survival was only 22 per cent.[30] Delay in diagnosis in the younger age group has also been documented. In a group of 9 patients under age 20 with colon cancer, the diagnosis was made 3 to 36 months after the onset of symptoms, with a mean delay of 11.6 months. Clearly, an increased awareness of this disease in the younger patient is necessary for improved survival.

SYMPTOMS AND SIGNS

Unfortunately, many of the signs and symptoms of colorectal cancer are nonspecific. Ideally, patients would be identified as having this disease while asymptomatic. In fact, when symptoms appear, the prognosis is significantly worsened; early diagnosis within the symptomatic period does not necessarily improve survival.

Malignant lesions of the right colon typically grow as bulky, fungating, ulcerated masses that project into the lumen of the bowel. These lesions are commonly a cause of significant anemia, because the rather large surface area tends to bleed rather freely. Generally, blood loss is not noted by the patient because

it is fully mixed with the stool. Right-sided carcinomas tend to be associated with vague, dull abdominal pain which is quite difficult to localize. One third of patients present with a palpable abdominal mass, reflecting the paucity of early symptoms with these lesions.

Carcinoma of the left colon tends to grow in an annular manner and gradually encircles the bowel lumen, often leading to progressive obstruction. Obstructive symptoms are more apt to develop with left-sided lesions because of this pattern of growth, coupled with luminal contents that are more solid. Typical symptoms include constipation, diarrhea, or alternating periods of each. Red blood of the surface of the stool may be noted. Other obstructive symptoms may include crampy abdominal pain with or without change in stool caliber. Although a much less frequent presentation overall, complete large bowel obstruction is due to colonic cancer in more than one half of patients. Basically, any change in bowel habits in an adult over 35 years of age warrants investigation.

Rectal carcinoma tends to cause hematochezia and, with larger lesions, tenesmus or a sense of incomplete evacuation. Anal lesions can also cause hematochezia. The appearance of bright red blood per rectum should not be ascribed to hemorrhoids without complete evaluation for carcinoma of the large intestine.

DIAGNOSIS

After obtaining a thorough history, with particular emphasis on bowel habits and family history, a complete physical examination is the first step in establishing a diagnosis. Visual and manual examination of the perianal area is essential. Unusual lesions may be sites of anal carcinoma. Digital examination of the rectum is mandatory. The anal mucosa must be examined completely in a circumferential manner in a search for mucosal irregularities. By having the patient perform a Valsalva maneuver, a high rectal lesion may be pushed within reach of the examining finger.

Endoscopy of the large bowel provides an opportunity to identify and biopsy suspicious areas. Anoscopy is simple and useful in examining and biopsying any lesions palpated by the examining finger. It is of no value in screening asymptomatic patients, however. Proctosigmoidoscopy with a rigid endoscope can be performed with relative ease to 25 cm., and thus as many as 40 per cent of the cases of carcinoma of the colon and rectum can be identified (see Fig. 1). The flexible sigmoidoscope allows visualization of the colon to approximately 40 to 60 cm. from the anal verge, thus increasing the diagnostic yield, and generally is better tolerated by the patient. Colonoscopy is the most complete modality, enabling the experienced endoscopist to visualize the entire colon. Biopsies can be taken from any suspicious area. However, even the most able endoscopist cannot always reach the cecum. Colonoscopy should probably be performed in all patients with colorectal cancer to exclude coexistent polyps or a synchronous carcinoma. Synchronous lesions were reported to occur in 3.6 per cent of patients with colorectal cancer in the precolonoscopy era; the frequency is now thought to be considerably higher.

Barium enema usually identifies lesions as small as 1 cm., especially when air contrast is used. A typical carcinoma appears as a constricting segmental lesion (Fig. 2). If barium enema has been used as the primary diagnostic method, the distal rectum and anus should be evaluated endoscopically, since imaging of these areas on barium enema is much less satisfactory.

Various additional studies may be helpful in staging the disease. Abnormal renal function mandates further evaluation to exclude secondary obstruction; however, the routine use of preoperative intravenous pyelograms has not been demonstrated to reduce the incidence of postoperative urologic complications. Chest films may demonstrate pulmonary metastases. Hema-

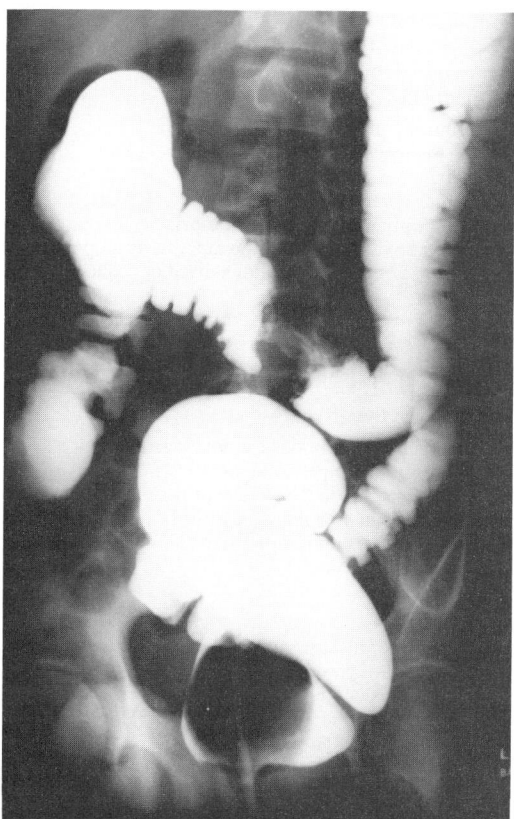

Figure 2. Barium enema showing a typical carcinoma of the transverse colon.

turia or pyuria should suggest the need for cystoscopic evaluation to exclude bladder invasion.

Liver function tests and carcinoembryonic antigen (CEA) level should be obtained. Elevation of both alkaline phosphatase and CEA has been shown to be associated with a high incidence of liver metastases in patients with colorectal cancer.[43] It is important to determine the preoperative CEA level, because if it is elevated before excision of the primary lesion and returns to normal postoperatively, it can be of value in following patients for metastasis or recurrence. The CEA level is of little value as a screening test for carcinoma of the colon and rectum. However, it is elevated in association with a number of unrelated benign conditions as well as other malignancies, including cancers of the breast and lung. The CEA level is normal in as many as 20 per cent of patients with colorectal cancer, including some with widespread metastases.

Preoperative computed tomographic (CT) scanning of the abdomen and pelvis is an important step in the evaluation of all patients with colorectal cancer, especially those with rectal lesions. CT scans can identify retroperitoneal adenopathy, assess the degree of lateral spread of pelvic malignancy, determine whether transperitoneal seeding, including ovarian involvement, has occurred, occasionally identify hepatic metastases, identify ureteral obstruction (when performed with water-soluble contrast), and provide a baseline for long-term follow-up. The latter is an especially important consideration for those patients who do not have an elevated CEA level preoperatively. By obtaining the scan preoperatively, it can be correlated with intraoperative findings, thereby increasing its utility as a baseline study in long-term follow-up.

Hematogenous spread to liver, bone, lungs, and brain is quite common. A bone scan is indicated in any patient with complaints referable to the skeletal system. Chest films are appropriate in all patients, whereas CT scanning of the brain is reserved for those with neurologic abnormalities or mental status changes.

PATHOLOGY

Grossly, colonic malignancies are described as fungating, ulcerating, or stenosing. In one review of 1376 tumors, 25 per cent were fungating, 61 per cent ulcerating, 7 per cent stenosing, and 7 per cent described as "other."[39] Classically, tumors of the right colon are bulky polypoid lesions with friable surfaces, and lesions of the left colon are infiltrative constricting lesions that grossly appear as a "napkin ring."

The distribution of primary carcinomas of the colon apparently has been changing over time, with an increase in the number of right-sided lesions being reported. Slater and co-workers reported cancers from a single institution over a 40-year period and found an increase in right-sided lesions from 16.8 per cent in 1946/47 to 28.6 per cent in 1976/77.[38] The explanation for this is unclear by may relate to the increased use of colonoscopy.

Histologically, most colonic malignancies are adenocarcinomas with varying degrees of differentiation. The histopathology was used, as early as 1915, by Broders to predict the outcome of cancer treatment.[5] Broders' method of grading was based on cytologic study evaluating the degree of cellular differentiation and the number of mitotic figures. In a Grade I tumor, at least three fourths of the lesion was differentiated epithelium, whereas in a Grade IV tumor, 75 to nearly 100 per cent was undifferentiated. Rankin and Broders studied 598 specimens of rectal cancer graded by this system and correlated tumor grades with the incidence of lymph node metastases and survival.[31] The incidence of lymph node metastases increased directly with the grade of malignancy: 27 per cent with Grade I, 44 per cent with Grade II, 56 per cent with Grade III, and 65 per cent with Grade IV. Survival decreased as the grade of malignancy increased: with Grade I, survival was 68 per cent; Grade II, 43 per cent; Grade III, 27 per cent; and Grade IV, 20 per cent. They also recognized that the prognostic value of grading is more marked in patients with positive lymph nodes: of patients with Grade I tumors and positive lymph nodes, 55 per cent survived; but none of the patients with Grade IV tumors and positive lymph nodes did so.

A variety of other grading systems have been proposed. These have been based on such factors as tumor architecture alone, tumor architecture in addition to cellular differentiation, and complex histologic grading systems including consideration of glandular arrangement, invasiveness, loss of nuclear polarity, number of mitoses, papillary character, mucin secretion, and both size and variation in size of nuclei.[14] Of the latter, only gradation of glandular arrangement, invasiveness, loss of nuclear polarity, and number of mitoses correlated with outcome. The advantages of more complex systems over Broders' system have not been established. All grading systems are limited by the inhomogeneity of the primary tumor and relative lack of discriminatory power except at extremes of the grade.

There are several histologic subtypes that may affect prognosis. Mucoid adenocarcinomas secrete large amounts of mucus and are thought to be associated with a 5-year survival of 34 per cent as compared with 53 per cent in control tumors. These tumors may have a particularly poor prognosis when occurring in the rectum (18 per cent 5-year survival as compared with 49 per cent survival with control nonmucous tumors). This poor prognosis appears to hold even if the tumor is well-differentiated and nodes are not involved.[41]

When the accumulation of large amounts of mucoid material is primarily intracellular, individual cells have a "signet ring" appearance. Survival with signet ring adenocarcinomas is unusual. Scirrhous adenocarcinomas contain extensive fibrous tissue, and their histologic grade tends to be more poorly differentiated than usual. In a group of 93 patients with scirrhous carcinoma of the terminal 25 cm. of the large bowel, only 18 per cent survived 5 years.[48] Symptoms appear to occur late in the course with these tumors, which usually are obstructive in nature; bleeding is very unusual, a fact that may contribute to a relative delay in diagnosis.

Lymphoma of the colon occurs, but is quite rare and, like other lymphomas, is a systemic disease. Leiomyosarcomas of the large bowel are extremely uncommon.

STAGING OF DISEASE

When the diagnosis of carcinoma has been made, it is important to determine the stage of the disease in order to assess prognosis. Clinical staging is based only on preoperative examination and laboratory and radiologic tests, whereas pathologic staging is based on gross and histologic study of the resected specimen. The true stage of the disease is accurately determined only after surgical exploration and histologic examination of the lesion and regional lymph nodes. New technologies such as flow cytometry and labeled monoclonal antibodies are being evaluated for use in staging.

Since clinical staging attempts to delineate extent of disease, an understanding of the biology of the tumor and modes of spread is essential. Carcinoma of the colon and rectum extends beyond the primary tumor in the following ways: intramural extension, direct invasion of adjacent structures, lymphatic spread, hematogenous spread, intraperitoneal seeding, and implantation at an anastomotic site. With use of the studies outlined previously, clinical staging prior to laparotomy can be assessed with moderate accuracy.

During the past 60 years, a variety of pathologic staging systems have been employed. These systems have included consideration of factors such as depth of bowel wall invasion, involvement of regional lymph nodes, and the presence of distant metastases in an attempt to provide prognostic information.

The original staging system for carcinoma of the rectum was proposed in 1932 by Dukes, a pathologist.[10] He proposed three categories: A lesions involved the rectal wall only, B lesions had spread to perirectal tissues without nodal involvement, and C lesions had regional nodal metastases. Kirklin modified the original Dukes system by specifying B_1 and B_2 lesions, and Astler and Coller in 1954 included C_1 and C_2 lesions (Table 1). The Astler-Coller modification of the Dukes system is used quite frequently today, although a D stage has been added for those patients with distant metastases.[21]

In any report, it is essential that the staging system be specified, because similar designations can have quite disparate significance. Many advocate the adoption of a standard descriptive system, such as the TNM system recently recommended by the American Joint Committee on Cancer (Table 2).[3] The TNM system includes more variables than the modification of the Dukes

TABLE 1. Astler Coller Modification of Dukes Classification of Colon Carcinoma

Stage A	Lesion limited to mucosa
Stage B_1	Lesion extending into muscularis propria but not through it Negative lymph nodes
Stage B_2	Lesion penetrating muscularis and extending into the serosa Negative lymph nodes
Stage C_1	Lesion involves any layer of bowel wall except serosa Positive lymph nodes
Stage C_2	Lesion involves all layers of the bowel wall including serosa Positive lymph nodes

From Lineweaver, W.: Staging Colon Cancer. Contemp. Surg., 25: 19, 1984.

TABLE 2. American Joint Committee on Cancer TNM Classification Scheme

Primary Tumor (T)

T_x	Primary tumor cannot be assessed
T_0	No evidence of primary tumor
T_{is}	Carcinoma *in situ*
T_1	Tumor invades submucosa
T_2	Tumor invades muscularis propria
T_3	Tumor invades through the muscularis propria into the subserosa or into nonperitonealized pericolic or perirectal tissues
T_4	Tumor perforates the visceral peritoneum or directly invades other organs or structures (including invasion of other segments of the colon across serosa)

Regional Lymph Nodes (N)

N_x	Regional lymph nodes cannot be assessed
N_0	No regional lymph node metastasis
N_1	Metastasis in 1 to 3 pericolic or perirectal lymph nodes
N_2	Metastasis in 4 or more pericolic or perirectal lymph nodes
N_3	Metastasis in any lymph node along the course of a named vascular trunk

Distant Metastasis (M)

M_x	Presence of distant metastasis cannot be assessed
M_0	No distant metastasis
M_1	Distant metastasis

Stage Grouping				Dukes Stage
Stage 0	T_{is}	N_0	M_0	
Stage I	T_1	N_0	M_0	A
	T_2	N_0	M_0	A
Stage II	T_3	N_0	M_0	B
	T_4	N_0	M_0	B
Stage III	Any T	N_1	M_0	C
	Any T	N_2, N_3	M_0	C
Stage IV	Any T	Any N	M_1	

From American Joint Committee on Cancer: Manual for Staging of Cancer: Colon and Rectum. Philadelphia, J. B. Lippincott Company, 1988, pp. 75–80.

system, specifies more accurate staging of the primary lesion, and includes clinical data reflecting the local extent of tumor. This system also permits comparison with cases previously staged by the Dukes system.

The incidence and survival of patients in two series staged by the Astler-Coller modification of the Dukes system are provided in Table 3. These data are representative of numerous other studies that have been reported.

New technologies are being evaluated in an effort to improve prognostic accuracy. It has been suggested that the proton mag-

TABLE 3. Incidence and Survival by Stage of Disease

	Incidence		5-Year Survival	
Stage	Series 1[21] (N = 352) (%)	Series 2[36] (N = 264) (%)	Series 1[21] (N = 352) (%)	Series 2[36] (N = 264) (%)
A	0.3	5.3	100	93
B_1	13.6	17.4	67	85
B_2	46.6	37.1	54	63
C_1	4	19.3	43	55
C_2	35.5	9.1	23	28
D		11.7		0

netic resonance spectral patterns of colon tumors may be used to predict the likelihood of metastasis. The level of natural killer cytotoxicity against a standard target has been shown to be predictive of tumor recurrence, with patients having low activity at increased risk.[42] Recently, it was shown that for primary tumors, abnormal DNA content (i.e., aneuploidy) was an independent prognostic factor in predicting both relapse-free and overall survival. However, in patients with hepatic metastases, DNA content of the metastatic lesions had no influence on survival.[18,36]

TREATMENT

Excision of the primary tumor with adequate margins of bowel and inclusion of the lymphatic drainage remains the cornerstone of therapy. The options are dependent on the location of the primary tumor. Extensive lymphatic dissection beyond the regional drainage is probably unnecessary.

PREOPERATIVE PREPARATION. Preoperative preparation should include mechanical cleansing of the bowel, because it has been shown that reduction of colonic microflora decreases the risk of postoperative infectious complications. The traditional approach has consisted of a 3-day program of clear liquids, oral cathartics, and enemas. More recently, whole gut lavage with polyethylene glycol-electrolyte solution has become quite standard. Four liters of this solution is administered orally or through a nasogastric tube on the day prior to the procedure. Oral antibiotics frequently are prescribed on the preoperative day to further reduce the bacterial count. Erythromycin base and neomycin are commonly used. Intravenous antibiotics usually are administered for wound infection prophylaxis just prior to the procedure and continued for a few doses postoperatively.

Psychologic preparation of the patient must be considered. Male patients should be counseled regarding incidence of sexual dysfunction, primarily impotence, following pelvic surgery, especially if abdominoperineal resection is contemplated (25 to 75 per cent). Patients with low-lying lesions should be advised of the possible necessity of either a permanent or temporary colostomy. All patients in whom colostomy is contemplated

should have preoperative consultation with an enterostomal therapist.

EXTENT OF OPERATION. The type of resection depends on the location and extent of the tumor. As the lymphatic drainage parallels the regional circulation, the major vessels must be resected near their origin. Invasion into adjacent structures, such as small bowel, ovaries, uterus, or abdominal wall mandates *en bloc* resection. Assessment of the presence and extent of metastatic disease is mandatory. A distal margin of 5 cm. of normal bowel beyond the tumor, measured in the unstretched state before resection, is generally recommended. However, some reports state that a 2-cm. margin is adequate, especially for rectal lesions, where the extent of the distal margin could jeopardize retention of the anal sphincter. For rectal lesions, the lateral extent of resection is of paramount importance in the prevention of local recurrence.

Lesions of the right colon require right hemicolectomy (Fig. 3). This procedure includes approximately 10 to 15 cm. of terminal ileum, the cecum, and the ascending and right transverse colon. The ileocolic vessels, the right colic and right branch of the middle colic artery, along with the mesentery, which includes the regional lymphatics, are resected. For lesions at the hepatic flexure, resection is extended to include the middle colic artery at its origin.

Lesions in the transverse colon are treated by transverse colectomy (Fig. 4) or by extension of the right hemicolectomy to include the entire transverse colon (Fig. 3). The middle colic artery is resected to the base of its mesentery. Carcinomas of the splenic flexure and proximal descending colon require resection of the left transverse colon and the descending colon to the first branch of the inferior mesenteric artery, including the left colic vessels but preserving the sigmoid branch of the inferior mesenteric vessels (Fig. 5).

Sigmoid carcinomas require an extended resection that includes the inferior mesenteric artery close to its origin (Fig. 6). Lesions in the upper third of the rectum are treated similarly, with resection and primary anastomosis (low anterior resection). A variety of methods are available to accomplish the anastomosis with low anterior resection, including intraluminal

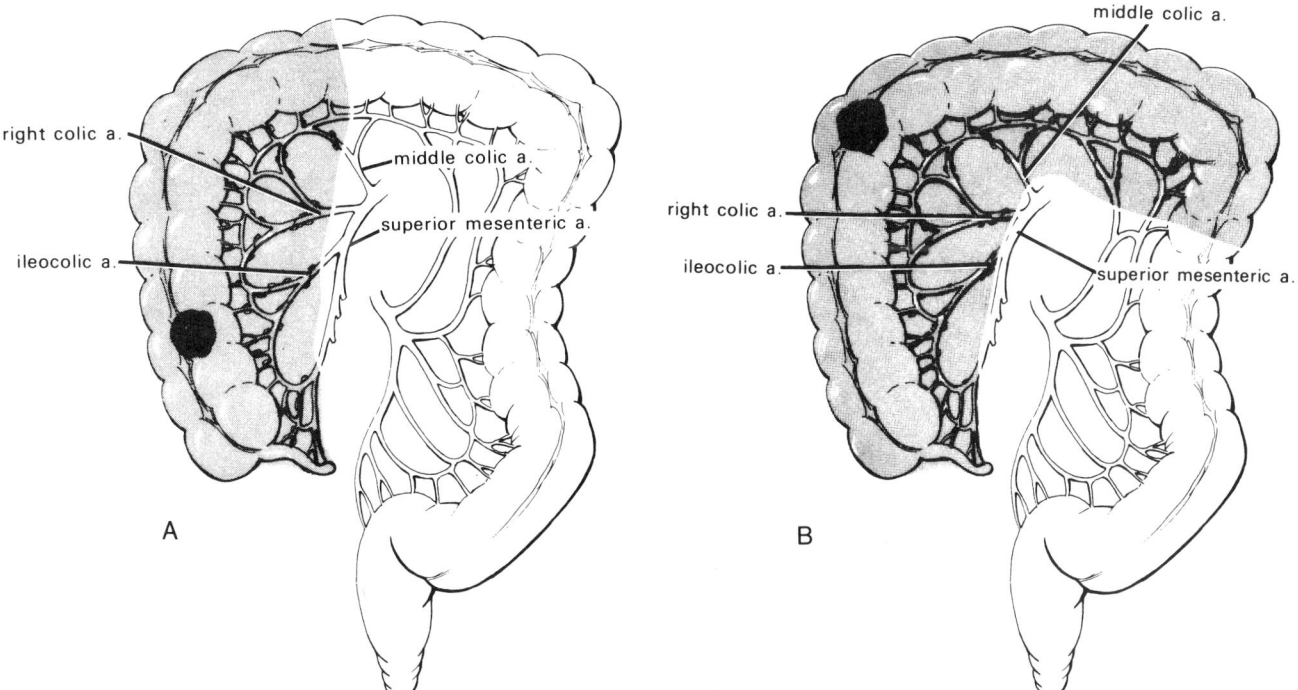

Figure 3. Diagrammatic outline of right hemicolectomy (A) and extended right hemicolectomy (B). (Modified from Grage, T. B., Ferguson, R. M., and Simmons, R. L.: *In* Horton, J., and Hill, G. J. II (Eds.): Clinical Oncology. Philadelphia, W. B. Saunders Company, 1977.)

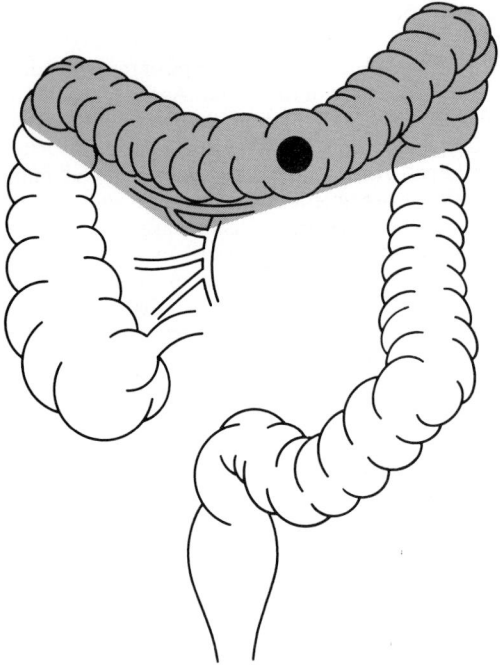

Figure 4. Transverse colectomy with resection of mesentery and ligation of middle colic artery at its origin. (Modified from Elias, E. G.: Handbook of Surgical Oncology. Boca Raton, Fla., C.R.C. Press, 1989.)

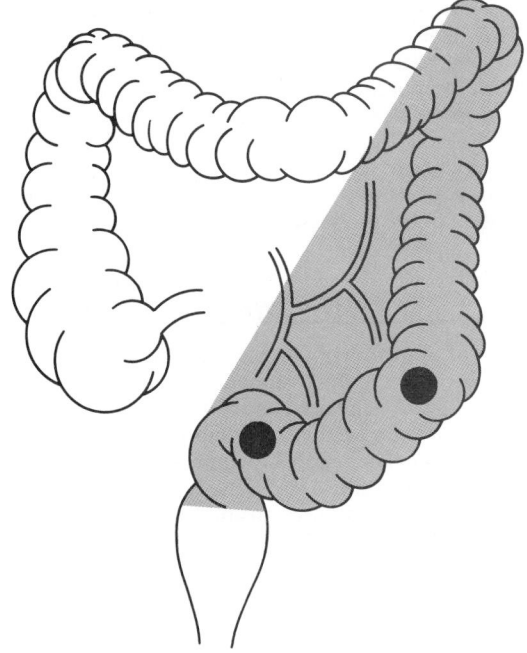

Figure 6. Sigmoid lesions require extended sigmoid resection with sacrifice of the inferior mesenteric artery at its origin. (Modified from Elias, E. G.: Handbook of Surgical Oncology. Boca Raton, Fla., C.R.C. Press, 1989.)

staplers, single layer sutures, and the end-to-side technique if significant luminal disparity exists. Some have advocated a proximal diverting colostomy to "protect" a less than perfect anastomosis after low anterior resection; the best approach is to correct any problem that might exist.

Treatment of carcinomas located in the middle and lower thirds of the rectum remains somewhat controversial. Local excision is an option to be considered in less than 5 per cent of all patients with carcinoma of the rectum. Such therapy is limited to patients with small, mobile, well-differentiated lesions, con-

fined to the mucosa (Dukes A), in a patient with a normal CT scan and normal CEA level. It is, perhaps, most applicable to older patients with a significantly compromised cardiopulmonary status. When restricted to these highly selected patients, results are comparable to those obtained with radical resection.[33] Electrocoagulation also has been applied selectively as primary therapy of rectal cancer. In a report of 81 patients treated with curative intent by electrocoagulation, Salvati and associates reported an overall 5-year survival of 47 per cent.[34] The best results were achieved in patients with tumors 4 cm. or less in diameter. Further evaluation of these modalities is necessary to define more completely their possible role in the primary treatment of rectal cancer.

For most patients, complete operative extirpation is recommended. The standard approach for rectal cancer has been the abdominoperineal resection first introduced by Miles in 1908. Lesions of the lower third of the rectum are usually treated in this manner, because after resection of the tumor there is insufficient bowel remaining for re-establishment of intestinal continuity. In abdominoperineal resection a combined abdominal and perineal approach is employed, often with two operative teams working simultaneously. The sigmoid and rectum are mobilized via the abdominal approach down to the levator ani muscles and coccyx, while the anal canal below the levators is excised from the perineal approach. It is essential that wide resection of the perirectal fat be included. Regional lymphatics are encompassed through resection of the sigmoid mesentery to include ligation of the inferior mesenteric artery near its origin, and all perirectal tissue in the pelvis. The proximal sigmoid colon is brought out as a permanent colostomy (Figs. 7 to 9).

The procedure chosen for midrectal carcinoma depends on a number of variables, the decision often not being made until well into the procedure. If the lesion can be palpated easily on rectal examination, abdominoperineal resection is indicated. If at the time of resection, the tumor can be mobilized to the level of the abdominal incision, low anterior resection can be safely performed. Generally, abdominoperineal resection is required for lesions distal to 8 cm. from the anal verge. For lesions above 12 cm., anterior resection can nearly always be done. For lesions located between 8 and 12 cm., the procedure chosen may de-

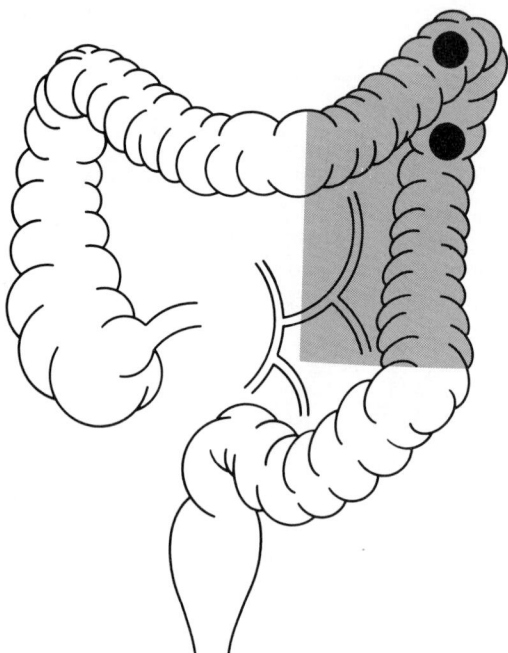

Figure 5. Splenic flexure lesions require left colectomy with resection of left colic vessels and preservation of the sigmoid branch of the inferior mesenteric artery. (Modified from Elias, E. G.: Handbook of Surgical Oncology. Boca Raton, Fla., C.R.C. Press, 1989.)

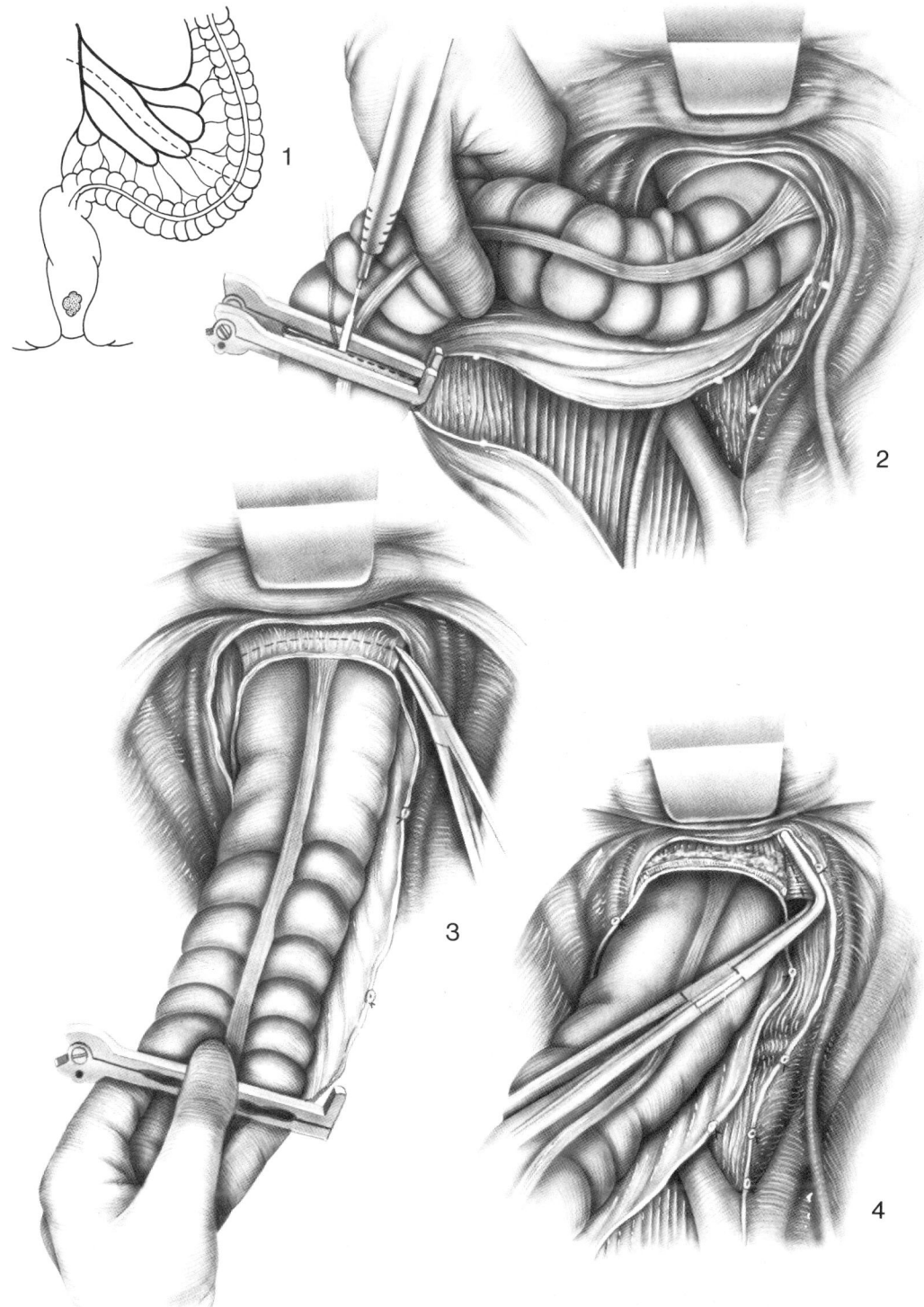

Figure 7. The patient is placed in the lithotomy position with both the abdomen and perineum draped. This permits two surgical teams to proceed with the abdominal and perineal procedures simultaneously. Alternatively, the abdominal procedure is performed first (as depicted). The patient is then repositioned for the perineal procedure. (1) The abdomen is approached through a midline incision extending above the umbilicus. The proximal boundary is the midportion of the sigmoid colon, with all distal bowel, mesentery, and surrounding soft tissues resected. (2) The lateral peritoneal attachments of the sigmoid colon are incised. Both ureters are identified and protected throughout. The sigmoid mesentery has been divided and the distal segment dissected from the retroperitoneum. The colon itself is best divided with staplers. (3) With the ureters carefully avoided and well-visualized, Denonvillier's fascia between the rectum and the bladder is divided. (4) The rectum is bluntly dissected posteriorly to the level of the coccyx, staying anterior to the prevertebral fascia. The lateral stalks which include the middle hemorrhoidal arteries are dissected close to the pelvic wall. (Modified from Gliedman, M. L.: Atlas of Surgical Techniques. New York, McGraw-Hill, 1990.)

pend on factors such as the extent of tumor and exposure that can be achieved in the pelvis.

The dissection for a low anterior resection is similar to that used for abdominoperineal resection, including removal of is-chiorectal fat and sigmoid mesentery, and rectal mobilization to the level of the levator ani muscles. The important issues are adequacy of exposure and margin distal to the tumor. If both are acceptable, the low anterior resection with anastomosis below the level of the peritoneal reflection is completed. However, if the surgeon believes that anastomosis cannot be completed safely, abdominoperineal resection is performed. The extent of resection should not be affected by an understandable desire to preserve the anal sphincter.

SPECIAL OPERATIVE TECHNIQUES. A variety of special techniques have been proposed for use with resection of carcinoma of the colon and rectum. While many of these concepts have intuitive or potential theoretic advantages, few have been subjected to prospective study. One is the "no-touch technique" as advocated by Turnbull. This procedure involves ligation of the venous and arterial trunks prior to manipulation of the primary tumor and was designed to prevent the intraoperative embolization of tumor into the portal circulation. In a careful review of reported data, Sugarbaker and Corlew have found no evidence supporting the superiority of this approach.[40]

Luminal ligation, originally described as part of the no-touch technique, might be of benefit. The authors recommend the use of umbilical tapes secured proximal and distal to the tumor to prevent intraluminal tumor cell dissemination. Recently, it has been suggested that a reduced incidence of anastomotic recurrence can be achieved by intraoperative cell fixation employing dilute formalin solution introduced into the lumen of such an occluded segment.[22]

Stapling devices have become very popular in the United States. Their use permits construction of anastomoses at lower levels in the rectum than has been possible with the standard sewn techniques. The use of an end-to-end intraluminal stapler has increased the number of patients who are candidates for low anterior resection, reducing the need for abdominoperineal resection and permanent colostomy. After the specimen has been removed, the intraluminal stapler in inserted through the anus and passed through a purse-string suture that has been placed in the cut end of the rectum. The head of the stapler is passed into the proximal sigmoid colon, which is then tied down about it. With the bowel ends closely approximated, the stapler is fired to complete the anastomosis (Fig. 10).[49] Several reports have documented the safety of stapled anastomoses as compared with the conventional handsewn method. A randomized prospective trial of patients with Dukes B and C rectal carcinoma has now provided evidence that the sphincter-saving resection is not associated with attenuated survival or an increased incidence of treatment failure as compared with abdominoperineal resection.[47]

UNEXPECTED FINDINGS AT LAPAROTOMY. One of the most common findings is the presence of synchronous hepatic metastases. Despite this ominous discovery, palliation is still necessary. In the presence of multiple bilobar hepatic metastases, simple resection of the primary, without significant attention to margins, is indicated to prevent bowel obstruction. Hepatic metastases in a patient with a low rectal primary carcinoma can present a therapeutic dilemma. The authors recommend an aggressive approach, including resection and anastomosis, when feasible. Patients in whom resection is not performed nearly always develop severe pain, tenesmus, incontinence, or hemorrhage before death. Since the quality of remaining life is significantly improved for such patients, an abdominoperineal resection may be indicated for palliation. If resection proves not to be feasible, the bowel should be diverted with the proximal end brought out as a colostomy and the distal end as a mucous fistula. Oversewing the distal end proximal to the tumor is contraindicated since further tumor growth may cause complete obstruction and formation of a mucocele.

If a single isolated metastatic lesion is identified in an accessible location on the surface of the liver, wedge resection of the metastasis can be performed simultaneously with resection of the primary lesion. However, if there is question about other deeper hepatic lesions, it is best to confine treatment to resection of the primary lesion and fully evaluate the liver after recovery.

The incidence of development of complete large bowel ob-

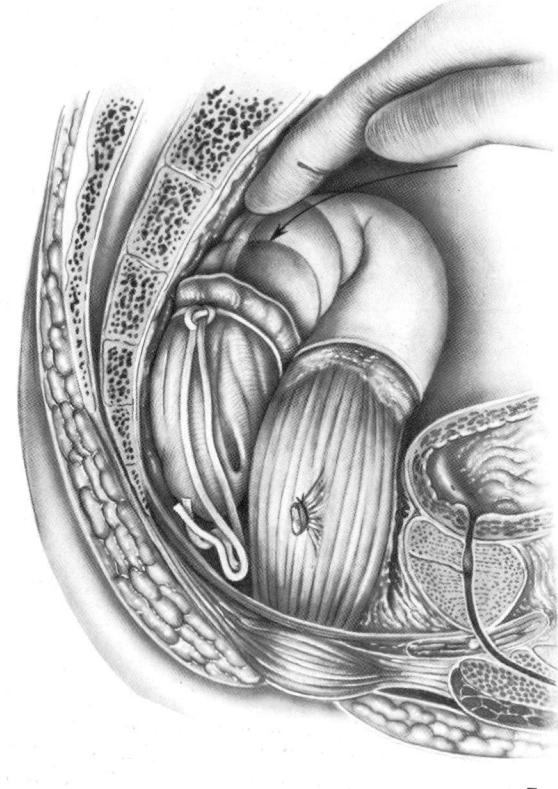

5

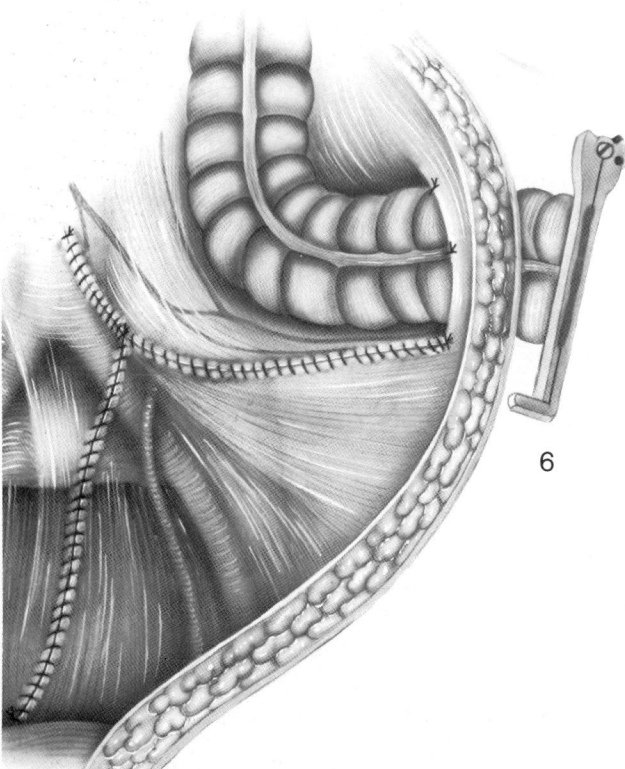

6

Figure 8. (5) The colon is mobilized completely to the level of the levator ani muscles. It is then placed in the prevertebral space and the pelvic floor closed with absorbable sutures. (6) The proximal sigmoid is brought out through a separate incision to create a permanent colostomy. The colostomy is usually matured after the abdomen has been closed. (Modified from Gliedman, M. L.: Atlas of Surgical Techniques. New York, McGraw-Hill, 1990.)

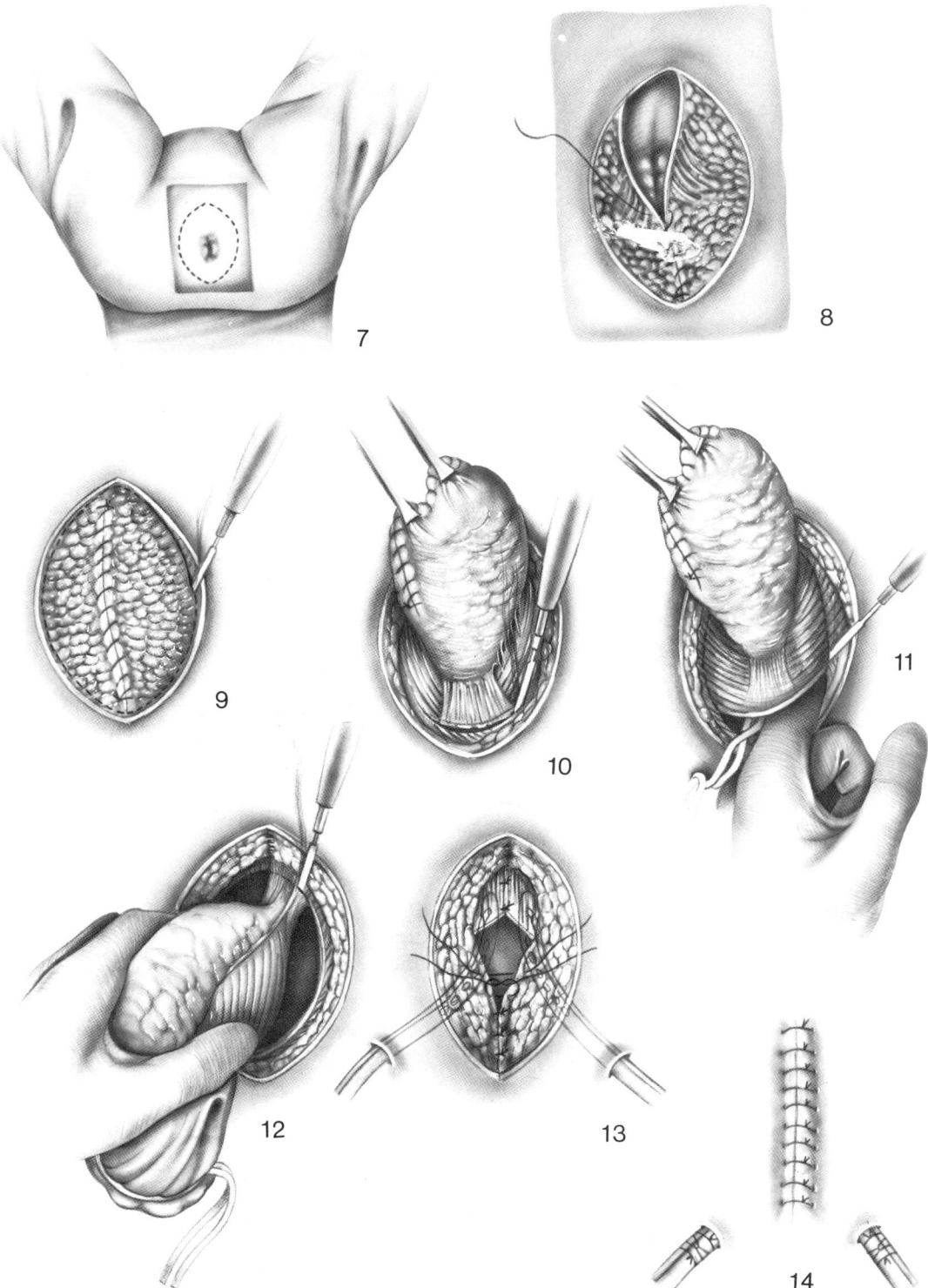

Figure 9. (7) and (8) With the patient in lithotomy position and the anus sewn closed, an incision is made in the skin surrounding the anus. (9) The subcutaneous tissues are divided laterally and posteriorly until the levator ani muscles are reached. (10) The anococcygeal membrane is opened just anterior to the coccyx, thereby permitting entry into the pelvis above. (11) The dissection continues laterally. (12) When the opening is sufficiently large, the distal sigmoid is retracted into the perineal wound. This retraction facilitates anterior dissection when the rectum must be carefully separated from the prostate or vagina. (13) and (14) Sump drains (as illustrated) or a large Foley catheter are placed into the pelvis. The levators are reapproximated to the extent possible. The subcutaneous tissues and skin are closed. (Modified from Gliedman, M. L.: Atlas of Surgical Techniques. New York, McGraw-Hill, 1990.)

struction in patients with colonic carcinoma is 8 to 21 per cent. For most patients with left-sided obstructing lesions in whom bowel preparation is not possible, primary resection with temporary colostomy and mucous fistula is usually necessary. With right-sided obstructing lesions, resection followed by primary anastomosis often can be performed safely. For any perforated colonic carcinoma, resection with temporary diversion is most prudent. As a group, patients with obstructing or perforating colonic carcinomas have a higher operative mortality and considerably shorter overall survival.[17] However, when curative *en bloc* resection proves to be possible for a colonic carcinoma extending directly into adjacent organs, 5-year survival may be

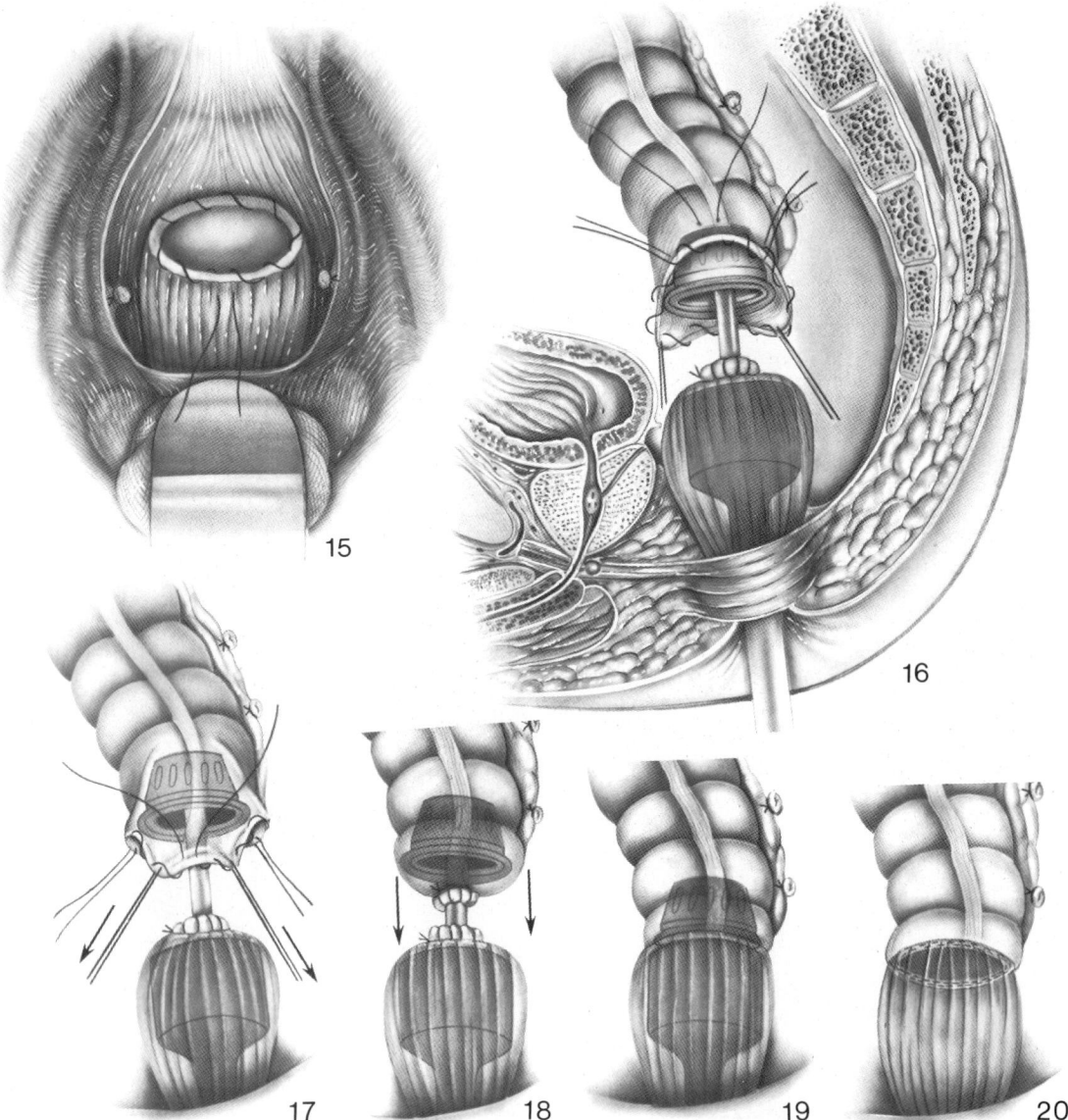

Figure 10. With this technique the stapler is introduced through the anus. (15) A purse-string suture is placed around the circumference of the rectal stump. (16) A similar purse-string is placed around the cut end of the sigmoid colon. Stay sutures are placed to facilitate introduction of the anvil into the sigmoid. The rectal purse-string has been tied to the body of the stapler. (17) and (18) The sigmoid pursestring is tied around the stalk of the stapler. The body and anvil of the stapler are brought together. (19) The stapler is fired to complete the anastomosis. (20) The stapler is withdrawn. Two complete tissue rings should be present. (Modified from Gliedman, M. L.: Atlas of Surgical Techniques. New York, McGraw-Hill, 1990.)

identical to that achieved for all patients undergoing curative resection. However, simple lysis between the tumor and an adjacent involved organ is doomed to failure due to dissemination of tumor cells and inevitable local recurrence.[40]

While unusual, the combination of an abdominal aortic aneurysm and a colon carcinoma presents a difficult problem. Generally, any symptomatic lesion should be treated initially. If both lesions are asymptomatic, the aneurysm is initially resected. Elective aneurysm repair generally can be accomplished with low mortality and minimal long-term sequelae. Conversely, colon resection may cause local septic problems which may delay aneurysm repair unduly.[28]

ROLE OF OOPHORECTOMY. Oophorectomy is recommended by some for all postmenopausal women at the time of resection of the primary tumor. A 6 per cent incidence of ovarian metastases has been reported in women with carcinoma of the colon and rectum.[4] Bilateral oophorectomy also may be advised in the presence of disseminated disease to prevent development of symptomatic ovarian masses.[25] Oophorectomy should be considered for premenopausal women in the presence of gross abnormalities on the surface of the ovary. Al-

though oophorectomy may not improve survival, it tends to decrease morbidity.

ADJUVANT THERAPY. The use of adjuvant modalities such as irradiation, chemotherapy, or immunotherapy in the treatment of colorectal cancer remains controversial. Adjuvant therapy is generally limited to patients at highest risk for recurrence, those with Dukes B_2 or C lesions. This lack of enthusiasm for adjuvant therapy derives from numerous controlled studies which demonstrate that the overall survival benefit is probably small. However, a recent study suggests an improvement in overall survival of patients with Dukes C colon carcinoma who receive adjuvant 5-fluorouracil (5-FU) and levamisole.[24a]Adjuvant radiation therapy may be appropriate for a few patients, such as those in whom complete *en bloc* resection is not possible.

Most studies of adjuvant therapy have focused on patients with rectal cancer. Although several trials of adjuvant 5-FU alone in patients with colorectal cancer have not demonstrated consistent benefit, a few have reported a small improvement in survival when rectal cancers were considered separately. A few studies of adjuvant radiation therapy for patients with rectal cancers have demonstrated improved local recurrence rates. For example, in a randomized clinical trial studying the effect of preoperative radiation therapy in conjunction with radical excision, the local recurrence rate was 15 per cent in the adjuvant group as opposed to 30 per cent in the control group. However, in this and other studies, no statistically significant benefit in overall survival has been demonstrated.[13] However, in a study from the Gastrointestinal Tumor Study Group (GITSG), 227 patients with Dukes B_2 or C rectal lesions were randomized to receive no adjuvant therapy, postoperative radiation therapy alone, postoperative chemotherapy alone, or a combination of chemotherapy and radiation therapy (5-FU and methyl CCNU). In the patients receiving combined therapy, there was an approximately 20 per cent increased survival rate at 6 years, and the recurrence rate was lowest.[12]

A number of issues await resolution concerning the use of adjuvant radiation therapy for rectal cancer. One of the most significant complications of postoperative treatment is radiation injury to the small bowel following its descent into the pelvis after resection. A recent approach to prevent this problem is insertion of an absorbable polyglycolic acid mesh sling at the pelvic brim. A variety of radiation schedules, including pre- or postoperative treatment, or both, with intervening surgical therapy ("sandwich" technique) have been employed. However, the single best approach has not been defined.

A number of trials involving adjuvant immunotherapy also are under way, including the use of BCG, autologous tumor cell vaccines, and biologic response modifiers such as interleukin-2. Currently, there is no definitive information regarding their efficacy.

POSTOPERATIVE FOLLOW-UP. Most tumors recur in the first 2 years following curative resection. Careful follow-up is necessary to identify these recurrences early, so that therapy might provide a reasonable likelihood of increased survival. The authors recommend both colonoscopy and barium enema in the postoperative period, usually within 2 to 3 months, to establish a baseline. Colonoscopy should be repeated annually for at least the first 4 years following resection[19] and then every 2 to 3 years. Barium enema is reserved for evaluation of colonoscopic findings or to permit complete visualization if this is not possible by colonoscopy. Routine physical examination, as well as complete blood count and liver function tests, should be obtained every 3 months for 2 years, then every 6 months for 2 years, and then annually. A chest film should be obtained every 6 months for 3 years, then annually. CEA levels should be obtained every 2 months for 2 years, every 4 months for 2 years, then annually. While the absolute level is important, trends must also be noted. A gradual increase in CEA level is usually a sign of recurrence. However, a number of benign conditions, as well as other malignancies, can cause elevation of the CEA. An aggressive approach appears to be warranted when the CEA level increases during follow-up.[23] If an elevated level is confirmed on repeat assay, the patient should undergo thorough imaging evaluation. A second-look operation should be considered if extra-abdominal spread is not identified on these studies. Of 146 patients with increasing CEA levels evaluated at Ohio State University, 139 were found to have recurrences, and 81 of these were resectable for potential cure.[23]

THERAPY OF RECURRENT DISEASE. Recurrent disease most often appears in the form of hepatic metastases or local recurrence. A third major site of treatment failure is the peritoneal surface. Most patients have combined recurrences involving more than one of these locations. Pulmonary and cerebral metastases also occur but are much less common.

Approximately 35 per cent of all patients with colorectal carcinoma develop hepatic metastases during the course of their disease. It is estimated that 10 to 20 per cent of these patients may benefit from hepatic resection. While the presence of extrahepatic metastases negates any survival benefit from hepatic resection, it has been demonstrated that resection of isolated liver metastases can provide improved survival. Before undertaking hepatic resection, a staging evaluation including CT scanning of both the chest and abdomen should be performed in an effort to identify any extrahepatic disease prior to laparotomy. Bone scans are indicated only for those patients with skeletal symptoms.

In the absence of demonstrable extrahepatic disease, laparotomy for hepatic resection is indicated in the patient with reasonable operative risk. Extrahepatic disease may be encountered at laparotomy. In a study of 107 patients, extrahepatic metastases were found in 26 per cent, despite negative staging work-up.[20] In the absence of extrahepatic metastases at laparotomy, resection may be performed for cure if the distribution of lesions in the liver permits. In a multi-institutional retrospective study of 607 patients who underwent hepatic resection for metastatic disease, 21 per cent of patients remained disease-free at 5 years. Of those who subsequently developed recurrent disease, most occurred in the liver or lungs.[16] The factors that best correlated with hepatic recurrence after resection were positive margins and the presence of bilobar disease. On the basis of this study, relative contraindications to hepatic resection are the presence of positive hepatic nodes, extrahepatic metastases, or four or more hepatic metastases. The best candidates for hepatic resection remain those with a solitary metastasis in one lobe of the liver. While this is a rare situation, resection has achieved a 5-year survival as high as 25 per cent with a median survival of 29 months.[6] For small metastases, the type of resection, whether wedge or lobectomy, does not appear to affect survival. However, for large solitary metastases (greater than 4 cm.), lobectomy appears to offer an advantage.

Treatment of those patients with unresectable hepatic metastases remains a complex issue. Although response rates using 5-FU infusions are in only the 20 per cent range, no other agent has demonstrated superiority. Thus, most trials have involved 5-FU or its active metabolite, 5-fluorodeoxyuridine (5-FUDR). The optimal route for administration of the drug has been investigated in various centers. Hepatic metastases have been shown to receive most of their blood supply from the hepatic arterial circulation. Most clinical trials have relied on hepatic artery infusion; and in a recent trial, such administration was demonstrated to be superior to portal vein infusion in terms of objective response.[9] Much of the initial experience with regional infusion chemotherapy of hepatic metastases was obtained with percutaneously placed hepatic artery catheters connected to extracorporeal pumps. These systems were associated with significant mechanical and infectious complications. Most centers now employ an implantable pump that allows continuous infusion. The pump has proven to be very reliable, being nearly without mechanical complications. At laparotomy, the pump catheter is usually inserted into the gastroduodenal artery and positioned at its junction with the common hepatic artery. The distal gastroduodenal artery is ligated, as are any branches supplying the stomach or duodenum distal to the gastroduodenal takeoff. A cholecystectomy is performed to avoid chemical cholecystitis.

In a carefully controlled, prospectively randomized study, Chang and co-workers examined the efficacy of continuous hepatic artery infusion of 5-FUDR as compared with systemic infusion in patients with unresectable hepatic metastases from colorectal carcinoma.[7] They found considerable toxicity associated with intra-arterial administration and overall no survival benefit. However, they did find a significantly increased response rate with the hepatic artery infusion (62 per cent versus 17 per cent). Subgroup analysis demonstrated a small survival benefit for those with negative hepatic lymph nodes. However, they thought that this small benefit was offset by the toxicity, which included chemical hepatitis (79 per cent), biliary sclerosis (21 per cent), and gastritis/duodenitis (21 per cent).

For patients who develop a second, separate primary lesion in the colon after curative resection, subtotal colectomy with ileosigmoid colostomy or ileoproctostomy, if possible, is recommended. Future evaluation of the remaining colon then becomes an easily performed outpatient procedure. Close follow-up is essential for such patients.

Anastomotic recurrences develop in 2 to 15 per cent after curative resection and represent approximately 10 per cent of all local failures. The risk is highest after resection of sigmoid or rectal carcinomas. The resectability of a recurrent lesion can be determined only by re-exploration. Local recurrence after low anterior resection usually requires abdominoperineal resection for complete extirpation of the tumor. Pelvic recurrence after abdominoperineal resection is usually unresectable, leaving patients eligible only for palliative radiotherapy. Wanebo has suggested the selective use of abdominal sacral resection for posterior recurrences and perineal recurrences involving bone or ligamentous structures; long-term survival has been achieved in a few instances.[44]

Recurrent disease is predicted most accurately by elevation in CEA levels. Metastases can be difficult to identify at operation, and new technologies are being developed to approach this problem. For example, administration of monoclonal radioisotope labeled antibodies preoperatively permits use of a detection probe (radioimmunoguided surgery, RIGS) to identify metastatic disease.[35] With the development of superior antibodies, this system could greatly improve the detection of occult disease.

The treatment of peritoneal surface implants remains difficult. Some success has been reported with use of intraperitoneal 5-FU delivered by peritoneal dialysis catheter. New approaches, however, are needed.

MALIGNANCIES OF THE ANUS

Neoplasms of the anus are relatively uncommon. Anal canal tumors occur at or just above the dentate line, whereas anal margin tumors are those found below the dentate line. Tumors in this region drain into inguinal, hypogastric, and pelvic lymphatics, the inguinal nodes being the most frequent metastatic site. Anal cancers represent approximately 2 per cent of all malignancies of the large bowel.[1] There are a number of pathologic types, squamous cell carcinoma comprising about 70 per cent. Other less common types include cloacogenic carcinoma, mucoepidermoid carcinoma, adenocarcinoma, basal cell carcinoma, and melanoma. The incidence is increased in association with chronic anal fistulas and chronic Crohn's disease. Epidemiologic studies have suggested a higher risk of anal cancer in male homosexuals, as well as in single versus married men. A possible correlation between anal cancer and habitual anal intercourse has been suggested. Conjecture has also been made as to the possible role of a transmissible agent, such as the papillomavirus which causes condylomata acuminata, in development of anal malignancy.

Anal cancers often remain asymptomatic for long periods, the disease being discovered late in its course in a majority of patients. It is fairly common for anal tumors to be discovered incidentally during routine examinations. Pain and bleeding are the most common symptoms; the symptoms are often indistinguishable from those associated with lesions such as hemorrhoids, fissures, or pruritus ani.

Squamous cell carcinoma, cloacogenic carcinoma, and mucoepidermoid carcinoma are grouped together as epidermoid carcinomas. They occur in the anal canal and are biologically aggressive. Local excision is most appropriate for small lesions (2.0 cm. or less) of the anal margin. If this approach is selected, all involved skin must be excised while preserving anal function. The resultant denuded surface frequently requires a split thickness skin graft for coverage. A fairly high 5-year survival, averaging approximately 70 per cent, can be expected, so long as local excision is restricted to well-differentiated, superficial tumors of the perianal area. Local excision is occasionally se-

lected for high-risk individuals who might not tolerate a more aggressive approach.

Abdominoperineal resection has been the standard approach for more advanced squamous cell cancers of the anal margin and for nearly all such tumors of the anal canal. The resection must include a particularly wide margin of perianal skin. The reported 5-year survival rates are 47 to 65 per cent.

The addition of either routine prophylactic pelvic lymphadenectomy or of radical inguinal lymphadenectomy to resection has proved to provide no survival benefit. However, therapeutic groin dissection for histologically positive synchronous inguinal lymph node metastases is thought to be advisable, although the patient continues to have a guarded prognosis. In contrast, groin dissection for metachronous inguinal lymph node metastases may provide better survival, at least in some centers, 5-year survival of 0 to 83 per cent having been reported.

Radiation therapy has also been advocated. Using a combination of interstitial radiation and external beam therapy, a 5-year disease-free survival of 68 per cent has been achieved.[29] Nigro has advocated a combined program of chemotherapy and external beam radiation followed by definitive surgical therapy. The patient receives 30 cGY. of radiation to the primary tumor and regional nodes from day 1 to day 21. Systemic 5-FU is administered on days 1 to 4 and 28 to 31, and mitomycin-C is given on day 1. Approximately 4 to 6 weeks after completion of the radiation, the patient undergoes local excision of the primary site. If no tumor is found, the patient is followed closely. If there is residual tumor, abdominoperineal resection is performed. A 78 per cent survival rate, with follow-up of 2 to 11 years has resulted.[27] Similar survivals now have been confirmed by others suggesting that this approach is as effective as radical surgical intervention applied uniformly.

Adenocarcinoma of the anus is rare, usually occurring in conjunction with chronic anal fistulas. If no fistula is present and a primary rectal cancer with distal extension has been excluded, the lesion may arise from sweat glands, apocrine glands, or anal intramuscular glands. Treatment of adenocarcinoma of the anal canal is identical to that for adenocarcinoma of the rectum.

Anorectal melanoma comprises 1.6 per cent of all melanomas and 1 per cent of all anal cancers. It has a very poor prognosis. No patient with a lesion of greater than 1.6 mm. in thickness has survived 5 years. The optimal extent of surgical resection has not been established. Local excision removing the entire lesion is imperative. If this is not possible, abdominoperineal resection probably is indicated. Routine inguinal lymph node dissection is of no benefit; the procedure is reserved for those with clinically positive nodes.

SELECTED REFERENCES

Adam, Y., and Efron, G.: Current concepts and controversies concerning the etiology, pathogenesis, diagnosis, and treatment of malignant tumors of the anus. Surgery, 101:253, 1987.
This is a thorough review of factors that influence the biologic behavior of anal carcinoma, as well as a review of treatment options for this uncommon disease. There is a complete discussion of the anatomy, pathology, pathogenesis, and staging of anal malignancies. The therapeutic options are also discussed, including the use of multimodality approaches. In addition to discussing squamous cell carcinoma, some of the rare lesions of the anus, including adenocarcinoma, melanoma, basal cell carcinoma, and mesenchymal tumors, are also discussed. This review has a large, current list of references in this area.

Chang, A. E., Schneider, P. D., Sugarbaker, P. H., Simpson, C., Culnane, M., and Steinberg, S. M.: A prospective randomized trial of regional versus systemic continuous 5-fluorodeoxyuridine chemotherapy in the treatment of colorectal liver metastases. Ann. Surg., 206:685, 1987.
This article reports a prospective randomized study of adjuvant 5-fluorouracil (5-FU) for patients with colorectal liver metastases. The study directly compares the results with intravenous (IV) and intraarterial (IA) therapy. Although patients treated with IA 5-FU had a significantly higher rate of response to therapy (tumor shrinkage on CT scan), compared with the IV treated group, there was no improvement in overall survival. The 2-year survival for the IA and IV groups was 22 per cent and 15 per cent respectively. The presence of metastatic disease in hepatic lymph nodes was associated with a poorer prognosis. Although a subgroup of

patients with negative nodes treated with IA 5-FU had a slightly improved survival, the small gain in survival appeared to be offset by the toxicity of IA 5-FU, including chemical hepatitis, biliary sclerosis, peptic ulcers, and gastritis/duodenitis.

Fleischer, D. E., Goldberg, S. B., Browning, T. H., and Cooper, J. N.: Detection and surveillance of colorectal cancer. J.A.M.A., 261:580, 1989.
This article presents guidelines for improving early detection and management of colorectal cancer and the lesions that precede the development of malignancy. Included is a discussion of risk factors and symptoms and signs. There is a good discussion of the diagnostic tests available, including fecal occult blood testing, proctosigmoidoscopy, barium enema, and colonoscopy. There is a concise summary of current recommendations for screening, surveillance in high-risk groups, and postoperative follow-up. This article is followed in J.A.M.A. (in the same issue) by detailed discussions on fecal occult blood testing and sigmoidoscopy as screening tests, from the U.S. Preventive Services Task Force. These articles represent detailed analyses of each method of screening and, together with the first article, represent a complete discussion of screening for colorectal carcinoma.

Galloway, D. J., Cohen, A. M., Shank, B., and Friedman, M. A.: Adjuvant multimodality treatment of rectal cancer. Br. J. Surg., 76: 440, 1989.
The authors of this review article discuss the limitations of surgical intervention alone in the therapy of rectal malignancies and include a critical evaluation of adjuvant therapies currently in use. They discuss some of the major issues concerning the use of adjuvant radiation, such as dose, sequencing, and field size. The major trials in the literature are reviewed, and their results, nicely tabulated. Combined adjuvant modalities are also discussed. The article concludes with a discussion of major issues in the use of adjuvant therapy.

Hughes, K. S., Simon, B., Songhorabodi, S., Adson, M. A., et al.: Resection of the liver for colorectal carcinoma metastases: A multi-institutional study of patterns of recurrence. Surgery, 100:278, 1986.
The authors have collected data on patients undergoing resection for metastatic carcinoma of the colon and rectum to the liver from a total of 24 institutions from 1948 through 1985, including a total of 899 patients. This paper analyzes a subgroup of 607 patients who underwent curative resection of hepatic metastases for recurrence. A 5-year survival rate of 33 per cent was noted, with a 5-year disease free survival rate of 25 per cent. Recurrences were noted in 424 patients. Recurrences were initially limited to a single organ in 59 per cent. The liver was a site of initial recurrence in 35 per cent of patients and the lung in 18 per cent. Only 12 per cent had an initial recurrence that did not involve liver, lung, or the initial site of disease. Hepatic recurrence was increased in patients with bilobar disease or positive margins. The authors conclude that adjuvant therapy must approach the lung and liver to effectively control recurrent disease.

Pilipshen, S. J., Heilweil, M., Quan, S. H. Q., Sternberg, S. S., and Enker, W. E.: Patterns of pelvic recurrence following definitive resections of rectal cancer. Cancer, 53:1354, 1984.
This is a review of patterns of local and distal recurrence after curative surgical therapy for rectal cancer of 412 patients treated at Memorial Sloan-Kettering Cancer Center. The pelvis was the predominant site of recurrence, either alone or with other sites concomitantly. There were significantly fewer recurrences in patients with Stage B_2 and C_1, compared with C_2 lesions. There were more pelvic recurrences in patients with low and midrectal lesions, compared with those with lesions above 12 cm. The procedure used (low anterior resection versus abdominoperineal resection) was not associated with a difference in the rate of pelvic recurrence, except in those patients with low rectal cancers treated with low anterior resection.

Sugarbaker, P. H., and Corlew, S.: Influence of surgical technique on survival in patients with colorectal cancer: A review. Dis. Colon Rectum, 25:545, 1982.
The authors have reviewed a large number of studies that suggest special techniques alter the survival of patients after surgical intervention for colorectal malignancies. Particularly, they evaluated distal resection margin, en bloc removal of adjacent involved organs, radical resections, "no-touch" techniques, and the control of intraluminal spread of tumor cells. They found the en bloc removal of adjacent organs to be important, but found no data to support the use of "no-touch" techniques or radical resections. Data regarding distal margin of resection were inconsistent, and they recommend the application of methods to reduce intraluminal spread of tumor cells. They note a great deal of variability in the treatment of what many believe is a standard approach.

REFERENCES

1. Adam, Y. G., and Efron, G.: Current concepts and controversies concerning the etiology, pathogenesis, diagnosis, and treatment of malignant tumors of the anus. Surgery, 101:253, 1987.
2. American Cancer Society: Cancer statistics. CA, 39:12, 1989.
3. American Joint Committee on Cancer: Manual for Staging of Cancer: Colon and Rectum. Philadelphia, J.B. Lippincott Company, 1988, pp. 75–80.
4. Birnkrant, A., Sampson, J., and Sugarbaker, P. H.: Ovarian metastasis from colorectal cancer. Dis. Colon Rectum, 29:767, 1986.
5. Broders, A. C.: Carcinoma grading and practical application. Arch. Pathol., 2:376, 1926.
6. Butler, J., Attiyeh, F. F., and Daly, J. M.: Hepatic resection for metastases of the colon and rectum. Surg. Gynecol. Obstet., 162:109, 1986.
7. Chang, A. E., Schneider, P. D., Sugarbaker, P. H., Simpson, C., Culnane, M.,

and Steinberg, S. M.: A prospective randomized trial of regional versus systemic continuous 5-fluorodeoxyuridine chemotherapy in the treatment of colorectal liver metastases. Ann. Surg., 206:685, 1987.
8. Chang, F. C., Jackson, T. M., and Jackson, C. R.: Hemoccult screening for colorectal cancer. Am. J. Surg., 156:457, 1988.
9. Daly, J. M., Kemeny, N., Sigurdson, E., Oderman, P., and Thom, A.: Regional infusion for colorectal hepatic metastases. Arch. Surg., 122:1273, 1987.
10. Dukes, C. E.: The classification of cancer of the rectum. J. Pathol. Bacteriol., 50:527, 1940.
11. Fleischer, D. E., Goldberg, S. B., Browning, T. H., Cooper, J. N., Friedman, E., Goldner, F. H., Keefe, E. B., and Smith, L. E.: Detection and surveillance of colorectal carcinoma. J.A.M.A., 261:580, 1989.
12. Gastrointestinal Tumor Study Group: Prolongation of the disease-free interval in surgically treated rectal carcinoma. N. Engl. J. Med., 312:1465, 1985.
13. Gerard, A., Buyse, M., Nordlinger, B., Loygue, J., Pene, F., Kempf, P., Bosset, J., Gignoux, M., Arnaud, J., Desaive, C., and Duez, N.: Preoperative radiotherapy as adjuvant treatment in rectal cancer: Final results of a randomized study of the European Organization for Research and Treatment of Cancer (EORTC). Ann. Surg., 208:606, 1988.
14. Grinnell, R. S.: The grading and prognosis of carcinoma of the colon and rectum. Ann. Surg., 109:500, 1939.
15. Haenszel, W., and Kurihara, M.: Studies of Japanese migrants. I. Mortality from cancer and other diseases among Japanese in the United States. J. Natl. Cancer Inst., 40:43, 1968.
16. Hughes, K. S., Simon, R., Songhorabodi, S., Adson, M. A., et al.: Resection of the liver for colorectal carcinoma metastases: A multi-institutional study of patterns of recurrence. Surgery, 100:278, 1986.
17. Kelley, W. E., Brown, P. W., Lawrence, W., and Terz, J. J.: Penetrating, obstructing, and perforating carcinomas of the colon and rectum. Arch. Surg., 116:381, 1981.
18. Kokal, W. A., Duda, R. B., Azumi, N., Sheibani, K., Kemeny, M. M., Terz, J. J., and Harada, J. R.: Tumor DNA content in primary and metastatic colorectal carcinoma. Arch. Surg., 121:1434, 1986.
19. Larson, G. M., Bond, S. J., Shallcross, C., Mullins, R., and Polk, H. C.: Colonoscopy after curative resection of colorectal cancer. Arch. Surg., 121:535, 1986.
20. Lefor, A. T., Hughes, K. S., Shiloni, E., Steinberg, S. M., Vetto, J. T., Papa, M. Z., Sugarbaker, P. H., and Chang, A. E.: Intra-abdominal extrahepatic disease in patients with colorectal hepatic metastases. Dis. Colon Rectum, 31:100, 1988.
21. Lineweaver, W.: Staging colon cancer. Contemp. Surg., 25:19, 1984.
22. Long, R. T. L., and Edwards, R. H.: Implantation metastasis as a cause of local recurrence of colorectal carcinoma. Am. J. Surg., 157:194, 1989.
23. Martin, E. W., Minton, J. P., and Carey, L. C.: CEA directed second-look surgery in the asymptomatic patient after primary resection of colorectal carcinoma. Ann. Surg., 202:310, 1985.
24. Moertel, C. G., Bargan, J. A., and Dockerty, M. B.: Multiple carcinomas of the large intestine: Review of the literature and study of 261 cases. Gastroenterology, 34:385, 1958.
24a. Moertel, C. G., Fleming, T. R., Macdonald, J. S., Haller, D. G., Laurie, J. A., Goodman, P. J., Ungerleider, J. S., Emerson, W. A., Tormey, D. C., Glick, J. H., et al.: Levamisole and fluorouracil for adjuvant therapy of resected colon carcinoma. N. Engl. J. Med. 322:352, 1990.
25. Morrow, M., and Enker, W. E.: Late ovarian metastases in carcinoma of the colon and rectum. Arch. Surg., 119:1385, 1984.
26. Morson, B. C.: Genesis of colorectal cancer. Clin. Gastroenterol., 5:505, 1977.
27. Nigro, N. D., Seydel, H. G. Facr, M. S., et al.: Combined preoperative radiation and chemotherapy for squamous cell carcinoma of the anal canal. Cancer, 51:1826, 1983.
28. Nora, J. D., Pairolero, P. C., Nivatvongs, S., Cherry, K. J., Hallett, J. W., and Gloviczki, P.: Concomitant abdominal aortic aneurysm and colorectal carcinoma: Priority of resection. J. Vasc. Surg., 9:630, 1989.
29. Papillon, J.: Radiation therapy in the management of epidermoid carcinoma of the anal region. Dis. Colon Rectum, 17:181, 1974.
30. Pitluk, H., and Poticha, S. M.: Carcinoma of the colon and rectum in patients less than 40 years of age. Surg. Gynecol. Obstet., 157:335, 1983.
31. Rankin, F. W., and Broders, A. C.: Factors influencing prognosis in carcinoma of the rectum. Surg. Gynecol. Obstet., 46:660, 1928.
32. Rubin, B. G., Ballantyne, G. H., Zdon, M. J., Zucker, K. A., and Modlin, I. M.: The role of flexible sigmoidoscopy in the preoperative screening of patients with inguinal hernia. Arch. Surg., 122:296, 1987.
33. Saadia, R., and Schein, M.: Local treatment of carcinoma of the rectum. Surg. Gynecol. Obstet., 166:481, 1988.
34. Salvati, E. P., Rubin, R. J., Eisenstat, T. E. Siemons, G. O., and Mangione, J. S.: Electrocoagulation of selected carcinoma of the rectum. Surg. Gynecol. Obstet., 166:393, 1988.
35. Sardi, A., Workman, M., Mojzisik, C., Hinkle, G., Nieroda, C., and Martin, E. W.: Intra-abdominal recurrence of colorectal cancer detected by radioimmunoguided surgery (RIGS system). Arch. Surg., 124:55, 1989.
36. Scott, N. A., and Beart, R. W. Jr.: Colorectal cancer: Flow cytometric DNA analysis. Aust. N.Z. J. Surg., 58:189, 1988.
37. Scott, N. A., Wieand, H. S., Moertel, C. G., Cha, S. S., Beart, R. W., and Lieber, M. M.: Colorectal cancer: Dukes' stage, tumor site, preoperative plasma CEA level, and patient prognosis related to tumor DNA ploidy pattern. Arch. Surg., 122:1375, 1987.
38. Slater, G. I., Haber, R. H., and Aufses, A. H.: Changing distribution of carcinoma of the colon and rectum. Surg. Gynecol. Obstet., 158:216, 1984.

39. Sugarbaker, P. H., Gunderson, L. L., and Wittes, R. E.: Colorectal cancer. *In* Devita, V. T., Hellman, S., and Rosenberg, S. A. (eds): Cancer: Principles and Practice of Oncology. Philadelphia, J. B. Lippincott, 1985, pp. 795–884.

40. Sugarbaker, P. H., and Corlew, S.: Influence of surgical technique on survival in patients with colorectal cancer. Dis. Colon Rectum, 25:545, 1982.

41. Symonds, D. A., and Vickery, A. L.: Mucinous carcinoma of the colon and rectum. Cancer, 37:1891, 1976.

42. Tartter, P. I., Steinberg, B., Barron, D. M. and Martinelli, G.: The prognostic significance of natural killer cytotoxicity in patients with colorectal cancer. Arch. Surg., 122:1264, 1987.

43. Tartter, P. I., Slater, G., Gelernt, I., Aufses, A. H.: Screening for liver metastases from colorectal cancer with carcinoembryonic antigen and alkaline phosphatase. Ann. Surg., 193:357, 1981.

44. Wanebo, H. J., and Marcove, R. C.: Abdominal sacral resection of locally recurrent rectal cancer. Ann. Surg., 194:458, 1981.

45. Wanebo, H. J., Fang, W. L., Mills, A. S., and Zfass, A. M.: Colorectal cancer: A blueprint for disease control through screening by primary care physicians. Arch. Surg., 121:1347, 1986.

46. Winchester, D. P., Sylvester, J., and Maher, M. L.: Risks and benefits of mass screening for colorectal neoplasia with the stool guaiac test. CA, 33:333, 1983.

47. Wolmark, N., and Fisher, B.: An analysis of survival and treatment failure following abdominoperineal and sphincter-saving resection in Dukes B and C rectal carcinoma: A report of the NSABP clinical trials. Ann. Surg., 204:480, 1986.

48. Woolam, G. L., Jackman, R. J., Ramirez, R. F., Beahrs, O. H., and Dockerty, M. B.: Scirrhous carcinoma of the lower intestine. Surg. Gynecol. Obstet., 121:753, 1965.

49. Yeatman, T., and Bland, K.: Sphincter-saving procedures for distal carcinoma of the rectum. Ann. Surg., 209:11, 1989.

X

DISORDERS OF THE ANAL CANAL

James P. S. Thomson, M.S.
and Onye E. Akwari, M.D.

ANATOMY

The anal canal is the terminal muscular membranous channel of the gastrointestinal tract. Ranging in length from 4 to 4.5 cm., it extends from just below the level of the puborectalis muscle to the anal opening. At the level of the puborectalis the alimentary tract changes its direction acutely, so that the anal canal courses posteriorly and downward. Together with the rectosigmoid above, the anorectum has a double-7 configuration, which is probably important in the maintenance of continence in resistance to positive intra-abdominal pressure.

Embryologically, the upper part of the canal is formed from the cloanal expansion of the hindgut, in which a longitudinal septum eventually separates the alimentary tract posteriorly from the genitourinary tract anteriorly. The lower part of the canal is derived from the proctodeal dimple of the ectoderm. The two parts are initially separated by a cloanal membrane, which then normally disappears, leaving the anal valves as a vestigial remnant.

The structure of the anal canal and its junction with the distal rectum may be conceptualized as two tubular parts, one of which forms a sheath over the other for the length of the anal canal (Fig. 1). The inner component is the termination of the gut tube, the inner circular layer of smooth muscle expanding to form the internal sphincter; the outer component is the striated muscle of the pelvic floor, which consists of the levator ani muscle, the puborectalis muscle, and the external anal sphincter. In effect, these form one continuous sheet of striated muscle. The intersphincteric space represents the plane of fusion between these components (Fig. 2). Modern concepts of the functional anatomy of the anorectum are owed in large measure to the work of Parks.[36,51]

The columnar epithelium of the rectum is replaced by a mixture of columnar and squamous epithelium in the upper anal canal, corresponding to the zone of fusion between the embryonic hindgut and the proctodeum. This mucocutaneous junction at the level of the anal valves is designated as the dentate or pectinate line. Distal to this line the anal canal is lined by stratified squamous epithelium (the pecten), which is tightly bound onto the internal sphincter; at the anus this changes to normal skin with hair follicles and a number of apocrine sweat glands. It is fortunate that the pecten that extends into the canal for about 2 cm. is devoid of hair, sweat glands, and sebaceous glands. This epithelium does not secrete mucus; therefore, the perineum is not continuously soiled by mucous discharge.

The canal above the dentate line is longitudinally corrugated by the anal columns of Morgagni, the distal ends of which fuse into the crescentic anal valves. In the zone that extends cephalad from the anal valves for a distance of about 3 to 11 mm., the epithelial type has been described as transitional, resembling that of the lower urinary tract, stratified squamous, stratified columnar, simple columnar, or cuboidal. The surfaces of the columns of Morgagni tend to retain the rectal character, although heterotopic stratified squamous epithelium may also be found within the columnar type. This array of epithelial cell types is of great importance in the origin of lesions of this area.[22,36,51]

The perineum is supplied with many sensory nerve endings

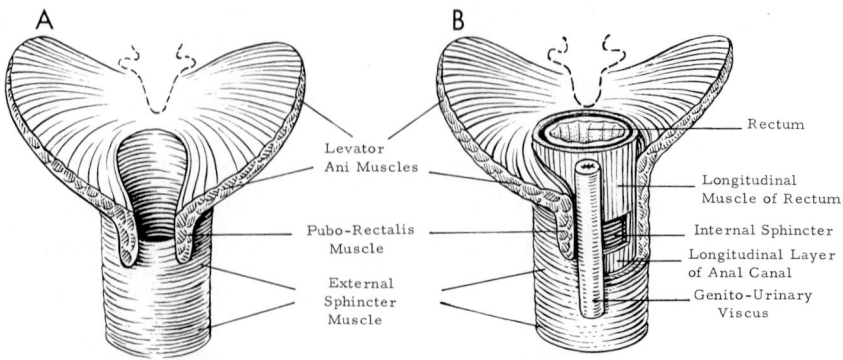

A

B

Levator
Ani Muscles

Pubo-Rectalis
Muscle

External
Sphincter
Muscle

Rectum

Longitudinal
Muscle of Rectum

Internal Sphincter

Longitudinal Layer
of Anal Canal

Genito-Urinary
Viscus

Figure 1. The anal mechanism comprises two components, visceral and somatic, each of which is tubular. The visceral tube is enclosed by a skeletal muscle tube by means of which continence is maintained. *A,* Diagrammatic representation of the skeletal muscle component. *B,* Composite arrangement after insertion of the simple visceral component. (From Parks, A. G.: Hemorrhoidectomy. *In* Welch, C. E. (Ed.): Advances in Surgery. Copyright © 1971, Year Book Medical Publishers. Used by permission.)

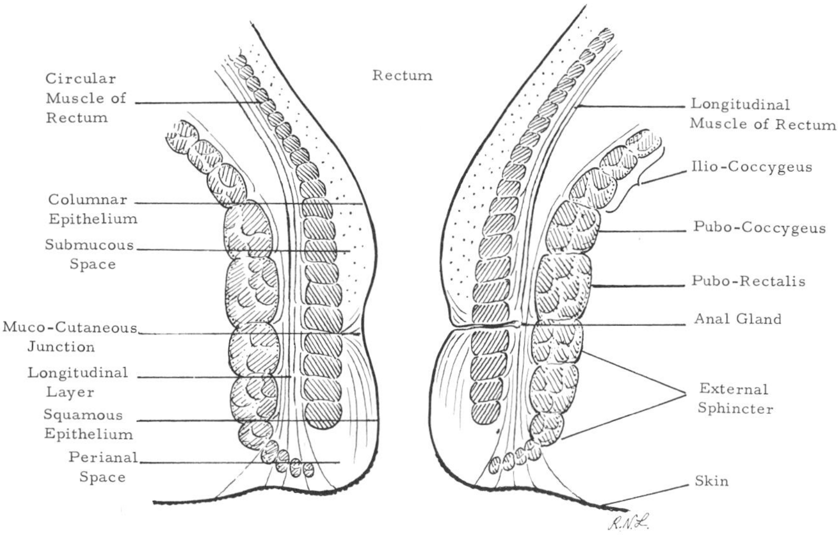

Figure 2. Diagrammatic section through the pelvic floor. The visceral and skeletal muscle components are apparent, separated by the intersphincteric space. Squamous mucosa lines the lower half of the anal canal, up to the level of the anal crypts. (From Parks, A. G.: Hemorrhoidectomy. *In* Welch, C. E. (Ed.): Advances in Surgery. Copyright © 1971, Year Book Medical Publishers. Used by permission.)

of a specialized type, especially at the level of the valves. These nerve endings supply information to the spinal centers, which regulate the mechanisms of continence.

The *internal sphincter* is the lowermost part of the circular muscle of the rectum. Its distal border is denoted by the intersphincteric groove. The internal sphincter is surrounded by the deep and superficial parts of the external sphincter.

The internal sphincter derives innervation from the autonomic nervous system and is not subject to voluntary control. It is most important in maintaining closure of the anal canal. Internal sphincter tone is normally maximal, relaxation being activated in response to rectal distention. This reflex (rectosphincteric) is mediated by neural pathways of the myenteric and submucosal nerve plexuses.

PHYSIOLOGY

Contrary to the previously held belief that sympathetic nerve is stimulatory and parasympathetic nerve inhibitory to the internal sphincter, it has been found that both the sympathetic and parasympathetic nerves are inhibitory to the anal sphincter. The external sphincter and puborectalis are supplied by the inferior rectal branch of the internal pudendal and the perineal branch of the fourth sacral nerve. The levator ani is supplied not only by the pudendal but also by the direct branch of the third, fourth, and frequently fifth sacral nerves, which lie above the pelvic floor.

The sensory nerve supply of the anal canal is the interior rectal nerve, a branch of the pudendal nerve. The epithelium of the anal canal is profusely innervated with sensory nerve endings, especially in the vicinity of the dentate line. Pain sensation in the anal canal can be felt up to 1.5 cm. proximal to the dentate line.

THE INTERSPHINCTERIC SPACE. The intersphincteric space lies between the internal and external sphincters (see Fig. 2). It contains a variable amount of smooth muscle, representing the terminal fibers of the longitudinal muscle of the alimentary tract. It also contains areolar tissue and the anal glands or ducts. These glands and ducts are branching tubes that extend from the anal crypts mainly posteriorly and penetrate to the internal sphincter to varying depths.[20] They are important in the genesis of anal and perianal suppuration, and the space is one in which infection spreads rapidly.[37] The anal glandular ducts are lined by transitional or stratified columnar epithelium and contain mucin-producing cells. They may undergo cystic dilatation. Because there are very few blood vessels in the intersphincteric space, it may be developed surgically in various operations because the areolar tissues are easily separated. These operations

include lateral sphincterotomy for fissure *in ano*, excision of the rectum and the anal canal in patients with inflammatory bowel disease, posterior anal sphincter repair, and exploration of the posterior pelvic cavity as may be required for removal of dermoid cysts.

THE EXTERNAL SPHINCTER AND PELVIC FLOOR. The external sphincter is located inferior to the pelvic floor. It is formed by a series of three muscular rings that act as one functional unit. The three parts are described as subcutaneous, superficial, and deep. The somatic musculature of the pelvic floor consisting of the levator ani and puborectalis muscles is continuous with the external sphincter. Their nerve supplies derive from S2, S3, and S4 and consist of direct branches to the levator ani and the puborectalis muscles and internal pudendal nerve to the external sphincter. These muscles have an unusual physiologic tone maintained even at rest and during sleep by a spinal reflex centered in the cauda equina.[10] The reflex is maintained by stretch receptors in the muscles. Several factors influence this basal resting tone, some of them increasing it and others inhibiting it altogether. For example, a rise in intra-abdominal pressure during coughing causes an immediate reflex rise in the tone of the pelvic floor muscles (Fig. 3). This tends to counteract stress incontinence liable to occur at such a time and also prevents a tendency for prolapse on the part of the pelvic viscera.[39] Several factors decrease the resting tone of the external sphincters, defecation straining being one of the most potent. This is probably part of the normal physiologic mechanism, but excessive straining produces abnormalities, most notably transanal prolapse of the rectum.[57] Micturition also induces total cessation of external sphincter activity. Extreme distention of the rectum as occurs in impaction of feces totally abolishes sphincter tone and is responsible for the incontinence that such patients suffer. The direct effect of sphincter activity is not the only factor nor is it the most important one in establishing anorectal control. The structural arrangements of the anorectal region are certainly of equal importance, although these are indeed maintained by muscle action. The lower rectum makes a right angle with the axis of the anal canal; as a result, the mucosa of the anterior wall of the lower rectum is firmly apposed to the top of the closed anal canal. The force of abdominal pressure is transmitted directly through the anterior rectal wall, thus pressing it firmly into the anal canal and effectively closing it (Fig. 3). The greater the force of abdominal pressure, the more secure the closure, and thus the tendency for stress incontinence is counteracted. This valvelike action is similar to the one present at the esophagogastric junction and indeed is found at most sites where a viscus passes from a cavity of high pressure to one of low pressure. The rise in pressure in the high-pressure system

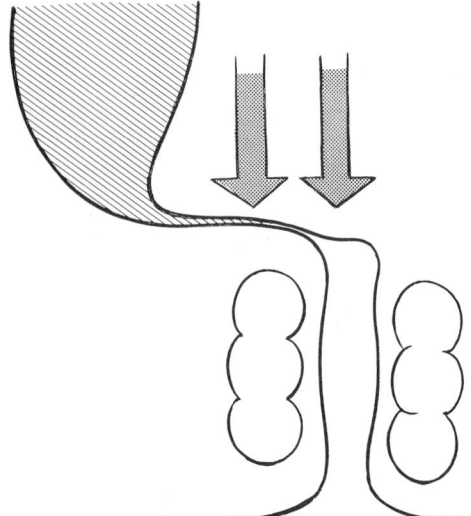

Figure 3. The gut makes two right angles in its course through the anorectal region. This arrangement is mostly maintained by the contraction of the puborectalis muscle. The lowermost part of the anterior rectal wall is opposed to the closed anal canal, thereby forming a valve. Increase in abdominal pressure will automatically increase the firmness of closure of the valve. (From Parks, A. G.: Hemorrhoidectomy. *In* Welch, C. E. (Ed.): Advances in Surgery. Copyright © 1971. Year Book Medical Publishers. Used by permission.)

makes the valve more secure; the most potent force unlocking the valve is a rise in pressure in the viscus itself. The measurement of the anorectal angle alone has been used in assessing the effectiveness of the flap valve mechanism, although whether this is a valid functional assessment is debatable.[43]

The upper parts of the external sphincter are continuous with the levator ani muscles; they form a unified muscle mass and contract as one. The lowest muscle of the levator group is the puborectalis, which has a strong sphincter action as it passes as a sling behind the upper anal canal. The upper parts of the levator ani muscle, the pubococcygeus and iliococcygeus, close off the pelvic hiatus on either side of the visceral outlet. They divide the pelvic cavity from the perineum. Below them on either side of the anal canal is the ischiorectal fossa, containing mainly fat; above is the fat of the supralevator space. These structures are especially important in relation to the anatomy of fistula *in ano*.[35]

PRINCIPLES OF DIAGNOSIS

Systematic evaluation of anorectal diseases includes a careful history and physical examination prior to the use of special investigations.

History

Two symptoms that may occur with reference to the region are of special importance because they suggest the presence of neoplastic or inflammatory disease. These symptoms are anorectal bleeding and alteration of bowel habit. Anorectal bleeding is a very common sign of disease in this area, but only approximately 12 per cent of patients with this sign have serious bowel disease above the level of the anorectum. The majority of the other patients have hemorrhoids or a fistula *in ano*. Further inquiry provides more information as to the time of bleeding (for instance, with defecation or on other occasions), the quantity of blood, its site (that is, whether it is merely on toilet paper or mixed together with the stool), and its character (whether the blood is clotted, dark, or bright red). It is important to recognize that in order to ascertain an alteration in bowel habit, it is necessary to establish the previous pattern. This can be accomplished

only by careful inquiry, allowing the surgeon to understand exactly what the patient means when he complains of diarrhea or constipation. Moreover, the use of or any change in the use of laxatives must be noted, because this may indicate a change in bowel habit and function. Other signs and symptoms of disease of this region may include anal discharge (purulent or mucoid), perianal swelling, prolapse, pain, or pruritus (itching, irritation, or soreness).

Examination

A general assessment of the condition of the *whole* patient should be made, but the main areas of the examination are the abdomen and lower alimentary tract. The abdomen is carefully examined for the presence of tenderness, a mass, or enlargement of an intra-abdominal organ and ascites. The opportunity should be taken to examine the inguinal regions for lymphadenopathy, because these may occur with diseases of the perianal skin or lower anal canal such as a primary chancre or carcinoma.

Prior to the examination of the lower part of the alimentary tract, the patient must be suitably positioned. The knee-elbow position is perhaps the best for the physician, but it may be an ordeal for the patient. The left lateral position is widely used because it is more comfortable for the patient although somewhat less convenient for the doctor. Other positions used include the jackknife and lithotomy positions. Preparation for this examination is again the subject of dispute. Any interference causes some abnormality in the appearance of the epithelium, and some reddening of the mucosa with loss of vascular pattern is not uncommon after administration of enemas and evacuant suppositories. Mucus is also produced, which may raise unnecessary suspicion of a lesion higher up in the colon. Systematic examination begins with visual study of the anus and perineum, followed by a careful digital and rectal examination, including stool inspection and simple assessment of perianal sensation. A digital examination of the anus should be performed with a well-lubricated finger. The anal sphincter is relaxed by having the patient strain down against the examining finger. This maneuver avoids traumatic pain during the examination. The presacral and perineal area can be examined by thumb and index finger to exclude areas of inflammation or tumor. Loss of perianal skin sensation should be carefully noted, because this may be associated with various neurologic diseases of the spinal cord and lumbosacral nerve root lesions.

When this preliminary evaluation of the patient has been completed, a disposable enema enables satisfactory visualization of the anorectum by means of the proctoscope. The scope should be passed, if possible, to 25 cm.; however, if it is not possible to pass this instrument further than the rectosigmoid junction at 15 cm., undue force should not be used; it is necessary to have the patient's full cooperation. The procedure should be discontinued if the patient is unduly uncomfortable or unable to tolerate a higher examination.

Gross lesions such as carcinomas or polyps are identified with ease, and the presence of mucosal inflammation should be noted. The earliest sign of inflammation is the loss of the typical pattern of the submucosal vessels; this is followed by reddening of the mucosa, granular change, and occasional frank ulceration. If the mucosa is normal, care is taken to notice the presence of blood, mucus, or pus in the lumen of the bowel, which may indicate the presence of a lesion above the reach of the instrument. The surgeon should always be prepared to have a biopsy performed when there are suspicious lesions so that a precise histopathologic diagnosis can be made. Finally the anoscope is passed and used for examining the anal canal. It enables anterior mucosal prolapse, hemorrhoids, anal polyps, and internal openings of fistulas to be visualized. It is important to emphasize the necessity of performing anorectal assessment in *all* patients and particularly those with signs and symptoms of anorectal disease.

SPECIAL INVESTIGATIONS

RADIOLOGY. A plain film of the abdomen is useful for determining the fecal distribution and detecting grossly abnormal dilatation of the large intestines. However, if a plain film of the abdomen is made immediately after proctoscopy, defining excessive gaseous distention should be interpreted with caution, because air may have been insufflated at the time of instrumentation. The most commonly performed investigation, however, is a barium enema. This requires careful preparation of the patient to empty the large bowel of fecal matter and along with proctoscopy allows an opinion on the state of the whole large intestine to be made. Only after gross abnormalities of the rest of the large intestine have been excluded can signs and symptoms, especially bleeding, be attributed to anal disease alone.

ENDOSCOPY. The advent of flexible fiberoptic sigmoidoscopy has made it possible for the entire left colon to be evaluated at the time of the initial examination. This is a valuable diagnostic aid, permitting mucosal biopsies to be taken. It also has a therapeutic role, because with it, polyps can be removed and vascular malformations coagulated.

MICROBIOLOGY. Microbiologic examination of the feces for pathogenic bacteria and parasites is an important part of the assessment of patients with diarrhea. In patients with pruritus, a fungal infection may be present, and perianal skin scrapings should be examined in the mycology laboratory. In patients with a possible sexually transmitted disease, a rectal swab may be examined for gonorrhea, and darkfield microscopic examination of a smear taken from a perianal ulcer may show spirochetes pathognomonic of syphilis.

The advent of AIDS poses a unique diagnostic challenge for the surgeon, because a wide number of infectious and neoplastic processes can involve the anorectum in these patients.[25] Any patient with cramping abdominal pain presenting with unexplained diarrhea, especially if there is evidence of perineal trauma, should alert the surgeon to the possibility of "gay bowel syndrome". The term refers to proctocolitis due to trauma or a wide number of enteric organisms, including *Herpesvirus hominis, Salmonella, Shigella* or *Campylobacter* species; *Entamoeba histolytica; Cryptosporidium; Giardia lamblia; Chlamydia trachomatis; Neisseria gonorrhoeae*, and *Treponema pallidum.* In some of these patients cytomegalovirus may cause diffuse gastrointestinal tract disease responsible for bleeding, diarrhea, and inflammation of the digestive tract. The diagnosis may be made by tissue biopsies and careful microbiologic studies. Attention is paid to the identification of the specific infecting organism and therapy directed to the organism.

HISTOPATHOLOGY. The histopathologic examination of a biopsy specimen is a most valuable method in determining the different types of inflammatory bowel disease and is essential in the assessment of patients with neoplastic disease. All mucosal biopsy specimens should be oriented on a piece of filter paper before fixation so that sections taken subsequently will be right angles to the surface. This provides the histopathologist the best likelihood of providing a useful report.

MANOMETRY, SPHINCTER ELECTROMYOGRAPHY, AND DEFECOGRAPHY. Anorectal manometry measures anorectal intraluminal pressure by the use of a balloon probe attached to a catheter that is connected to a pressure transducer and to a polygraph. A continuously perfused open-tip catheter may be used. Electromyography of the anal sphincters can be performed with either needle or surface electrodes able to detect the contractual activity of striated muscle and to obtain separate recordings from the external sphincter and from the puborectalis muscle. Sphincter electromyography is used for exploring functionally the perineal surface and for detecting the size and site of the anal sphincter. This technique finds greatest application in the assessment of sphincter injuries or congenital abnormalities, allowing identification of good active sphincter muscle in the right anatomic positions, and thus helping in the performance of effective transposition operations during anal reconstruction. The combination of anorectal manometry and electromyography can help not only in studies for assessing anorectal and pelvic floor neuromuscular disorders but also in the diagnosis and management of incontinence, prolapse, megarectum, and other functional anorectal disorders. With these studies one can assess preoperative and postoperative anorectal function and not only diagnose anorectal disorders but also make an objective assessment of the results of therapy.[29,41]

PELVIC FLOOR PROBLEMS

Complete Rectal Prolapse (Procidentia)

This uncommon condition is caused mainly by a disorder of anorectal physiology. The rectal wall, including its muscle layer, literally turns inside out like a glove. The rectum may prolapse 3 or more inches, its outer surface now being mucus-secreting epithelium. Not only is the presence of the prolapse unpleasant, but the mucosa secretes quantities of mucus (traumatic proctitis), which causes soiling and perineal excoriation. Initially the prolapse occurs only with defecation and is relatively easily replaced. Later it occurs with any rise of intra-abdominal pressure such as coughing, lifting, and even when walking.

This condition occurs most commonly at the extremes of life, in children under the age of 5 and in elderly women. It is occasionally seen from the third decade onward, but again, almost always in women. In children it usually disappears spontaneously by the age of 5. Why it occurs in this age group, apart from those with cystic fibrosis, is unknown; defecation straining in children can be excessive, and this is possibly the cause. Seldom is operative treatment indicated in children; simple bowel training advice is usually sufficient.

In adults the most obvious abnormality to be found, apart from the prolapse, is laxity of the anal sphincters. Usually, the anal canal gapes because of the lack of sphincter tone; but even if this is not apparent on inspection, it can be readily induced by asking the patient to strain. Sphincter response to voluntary contraction is also poor and may be absent. Seldom, however, is there any frank neurologic defect, and the preponderance of cases in women indicates some anatomic cause for the functional abnormality. However, oddly enough, the condition is more common in women who have not borne children; it is not possible, therefore, to ascribe it to birth trauma. The deficient sphincter function causes the most distressing symptom. About two thirds of patients with rectal prolapse are frankly incontinent of feces. They regard themselves as social outcasts and are usually unwilling to leave their homes. This symptom is usually elicited only on direct questioning, because the patient may be too ashamed to mention it spontaneously.

Complications of rectal prolapse, although rare, have been described and include incarceration, strangulation, and gangrene. Ulceration of the exposed mucosa may cause minor or rarely severe hemorrhage. Rupture of the prolapse is an exceedingly rare complication. Complicated prolapse may require emergency rectosigmoidectomy.

Treatment otherwise depends on the severity of the symptoms and the age and general condition of the patient. There has been a trend in recent years to perform major surgical procedures at an earlier stage than was previously considered desirable. This is partly because lesser procedures are so often ineffective and also because patients tolerate the abdominal repairs very well, no matter how old they are. The operation performed is one of the several types of abdominal rectopexy currently practiced. Through a lower abdominal incision the rectum is mobilized and a procedure is performed that causes adherence of the rectum to the sacrum, thus preventing it from prolapsing.[57] One effective approach is to surround the rectum partially with polyvinyl alcohol sponge. The success rate from the point of view of correction of the prolapse is high, and the incidence of incontinence is reduced. However, one third of the patients are still incontinent to some degree.[27]

If the patient is such a poor operative risk that an abdominal procedure is considered unjustified, a local anal operation may be helpful. This usually takes the form of some modification of the Theiersch wire operation initially introduced in 1891. A ring of silver (or nylon) wire is inserted into the tissues around the canal through two small puncture wounds in the perineum, one in front and one behind the anus. The ring is about 3 cm. in diameter, just large enough to allow the passage of stool but not large enough to allow the prolapse to appear. This is effective provided the patient clears the rectum adequately; if not, fecal impaction rapidly develops. It has no beneficial effect whatsoever on incontinence.

It should be remembered that there are other causes of anorectal prolapse. These include hemorrhoids, mucosal prolapse, anal fibroepithelial polyps, and adenomas, especially large sessile adenomas of the rectum.

Fecal Incontinence

The distressing nature of fecal incontinence has already been emphasized. It is usually found accompanying quite severe degrees of rectal prolapse. However, it occasionally occurs without any obvious degree of prolapse. It has the same female preponderance. In most cases no obvious cause can be found, but some interesting work[40] suggests there may be a myopathy due to damage to the pudendal nerves either by entrapment in the pudendal canal or by stretching (excessive defecatory straining efforts over a prolonged period or even during childbirth). In those under 65 years of age it can be treated by a muscle-tightening procedure performed behind the anal canal (postanal sphincter repair).[6] The levator ani muscles, the puborectalis muscle, and the external sphincter muscles are apposed behind the anorectal junction. The effect of this is to thrust the anal canal forward and upward to restore the anorectal angle and to shorten the muscles, which makes their action more efficient. A more physiologic approach has been suggested. Electrodes can be implanted into the muscles and activated by a buried induction coil, or stimulation can be achieved by two electrodes inserted into the anal canal in the form of a plug. Unfortunately, the results of this method in the treatment of idiopathic incontinence have been uniformly disappointing, probably owing to the myopathy described by Parks and co-workers.[40]

Incontinence may be secondary to organic disease or abnormality in the colon or anal canal. An individual with a normal pelvic sphincter mechanism may nevertheless lose control if there is severe diarrhea, and this is the state in which many patients with colitis find themselves. If there is a mild sphincter weakness, diarrhea may cause frank incontinence. This is commonly found in the elderly patient whose pelvic floor muscles have lost their tone and who has diverticulitis. Elimination of the factor causing diarrhea restores normal continence.

Trauma or abnormality of the sphincters may cause incontinence. In anorectal agenesis the external sphincter muscle is often grossly deficient and may be inadequate to restore the rectal lumen. Childbirth may cause total severance of the muscle ring anteriorly, causing varying degrees of incontinence. Total section of the sphincters may occur as the result of fistula surgery or direct trauma. Fortunately, this situation can be remedied by sphincteroplasty; but a temporary colostomy is required.[6] The key factors that regulate normal continence are summarized in Table 1. Alterations of these physiologic mechanisms are generally associated with fecal incontinence.

Impaction of Feces

This is a condition caused by disordered anorectal physiology. The rectum becomes overloaded and filled with a hard mass of feces that cannot be spontaneously evacuated. It may be secondary to idiopathic megacolon ("lazy colon"), which is found in children and young adults. Fecal impaction occurs spontaneously in the aged and may complicate convalescence after orthopedic, pelvic, or abdominal operations. If a patient has a painful anal fissure, this sometimes causes such an inhibition to defecation that rectal overloading occurs. This tendency is increased if codeine-containing tablets for pain relief are ingested. The large fecal mass causes reflex relaxation of the anal sphincters. Liquid stool passes around the impaction and then leaks out in a totally uncontrolled manner. The patient complains of diarrhea and incontinence. Manual disimpaction under anesthesia is often necessary, followed by a brief enema regimen to allow the rectal wall to recover its tone.

HEMORRHOIDS

The condition generally termed hemorrhoids is divided into three components: (1) abnormal prolapse of upper anal and lower rectal mucosa; (2) venous engorgement in the submucosa of the upper anal canal; and (3) protuberances at the anal margin, commonly termed skin tags or external hemorrhoids. These can exist independently of one another, but all three are usually found together. Some degree of physiologic prolapse of the anal mucosa occurs during normal defecation, and there is partial eversion of the anal canal. Abnormal mucosal prolapse is merely an exaggeration of the normal; the reason is unknown. Perhaps it is due to the constipating habits induced by the dietary and physical limitations of the current culture. The first symptom is bleeding; the veins in the submucosa of the prolapsing tissue contain blood at high pressure, because they communicate directly with the abdominal cavity. During prolapse this region is exposed to atmospheric pressure, and the pressure gradient causes bleeding that is characteristically arterial in type. The arterial nature of the venous blood may be due to the presence of arteriovenous fistulas.[52]

With time there is further downward descent of the anal mucosa. Rectal mucosa passes into the anal canal, forcing the squamous mucosa of the lower anal canal downward and outward so that it comes to lie at the anal margin. The columnar, goblet cell mucosa of the upper anal canal is intermittently exteriorized and, owing to the minor trauma it receives, secretes mucus. The mucus is produced below the level of effective sphincter action, so that leakage occurs. Mucous soiling of the perineum causes excoriation of the perianal skin, soreness, and pruritus. Later, production of mucus may be somewhat diminished by squamous metaplasia, which occurs in the columnar mucosa of the upper anal canal as a result of repeated prolapse.

The squamous mucosa of the lower anal canal is forced out, and it forms bulging excrescences termed either external hemorrhoids or anal skin tags. This is particularly likely to occur in women after delivery and may cause discomfort or quite marked pain. The squamous mucosa is highly sensitive and, when exposed, can cause considerable soreness and pruritic symptoms. An understanding of the nature of the descent of the anal mucosa in hemorrhoidal change is essential for proper treatment.

The veins in the submucosa of the upper anal canal may

TABLE 1. Factors Important in the Control of Anal Continence

Anorectal high-pressure zone
Anorectal angle/flap valve
Rectal compliance and capacity
Anal and rectal sensory mechanisms
Colonic transit time
Stool volume and consistency
Rectal motility
Anal canal motility

become greatly dilated and varicose. In this event, considerable bleeding is particularly likely to occur. The protrusion of the hemorrhoidal tissue into the anal canal exaggerates any tendency to mucosal prolapse, because the tissue is forcibly exteriorized during defecation. The prolapsed mass may return spontaneously after defecation, or it may require manual replacement. In the prolapsed state, the presence of the hemorrhoidal mass through the anal sphincter mechanism may cause such irritation that the sphincter experiences paroxysms of severe spasm. The pain of sphincter spasm is further compounded by the pain from the relative ischemia of the hemorrhoidal mass so trapped by the sphincter. Manual replacement of the acutely prolapsing hemorrhoidal mass, if successful, provides the patient a great deal of immediate and often dramatic relief. Some patients have an associated laxity of the external sphincters; in this event large internal hemorrhoids tend to prolapse with any transitory rise in intra-abdominal pressure such as occurs during coughing or even walking. When this stage, which is sometimes termed third-degree hemorrhoidal change (Fig. 4), is reached, the patient is likely to have acute anal discomfort at any time. The prolapsed hemorrhoidal mass causes perineal aching and soilage from persistent mucus discharge. When this state has been reached, conservative treatment is usually of little help.

Complications

There are two main complications of hemorrhoids, (1) anemia due to continued and excessive bleeding and (2) acute thrombosis. So uncommon is anemia as a result of hemorrhoidal bleeding that other causes of this condition should be sought, such as carcinoma of the stomach or cecum, before a firm diagnosis is made. Thrombosis is common and can occur in the external anal plexus under the squamous mucosa, in the main hemorrhoidal plexus of the submucosa of the upper anal canal, or in both. External anal thrombosis is common and is often seen in patients who have no other stigmata of hemorrhoids. The cause is unknown, but it is possibly due to the high venous pressures that develop during excessive straining efforts that cause distention and stasis in the veins. The patient notices an acute swelling situated at the anal verge that may be intensely painful. Pain may continue for several days and then gradually subside spontaneously. The swelling may disappear in 3 to 4 weeks. Occasionally the clot wears through the overlying skin and is extruded, causing soiling of the clothing with dark clotted blood (Fig. 5). Treatment is usually symptomatic only, because the condition subsides in a relatively short time. However, if pain is severe, it may be justified to incise the hemorrhoid and enucleate the clot under local anesthesia.

Acute thrombosis of the internal hemorrhoidal plexus is a much more unpleasant situation (see Fig. 5). The patient experiences sudden severe anal pain followed by protrusion of the thrombosed area. The pain can be extremely severe and may

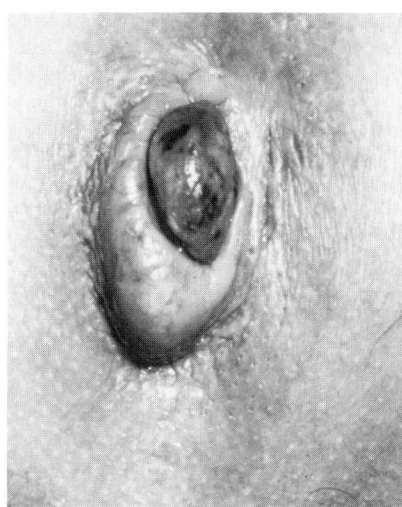

Figure 5. Prolapsed, thrombosed right posterior hemorrhoid.

continue for as long as a week. Gradually the edema subsides, and the thrombus is absorbed. Treatment is conservative in the first instance, consisting of analgesics to relieve the pain and a mild laxative to prevent constipation. Various local applications are used, such as lead and spirit lotion or ice packs, but it is doubtful whether they have any specific effects. If symptoms continue to be severe for several days, surgical treatment may be considered, but this is not a light undertaking. The surgical technique is not particularly difficult despite the presence of the thrombosis, but the postoperative course is more subject to pain and complication than that of an ordinary hemorrhoidectomy.

Management

Some patients with hemorrhoids do not require treatment, only reassurance that they do not have a serious cause for their symptoms. However, if there is a history of bowel irregularity, this requires attention. If the hemorrhoids are very troublesome, many treatments are available (Table 2).

BOWEL REGULATION. In many patients hemorrhoidal symptoms can be relieved by attention to hygiene and by avoiding excessive defecation straining. Such is the artificiality of our dietary and other habits that constipation with consequent defecation straining is often the rule, rather than the exception. Straining causes descent of the pelvic floor, weakening of the sphincter muscles, and both rectal and gynecologic prolapse. It would appear sensible, therefore, that individuals with these tendencies compensate by taking sufficient fruit and bran in their diet; failing this, a hydrophilic laxative taken as often as necessary is usually effective and quite harmless.

Recently, the hypothesis that hemorrhoids follow chronic constipation was investigated by studying bowel habit, anal pressure profiles, and anal compliance in 13 men and 10 women with prolapsing hemorrhoid, 12 women with severe constipation and 14 male and 11 female control subjects. Hemorrhoids were not necessarily associated with constipation, but these pa-

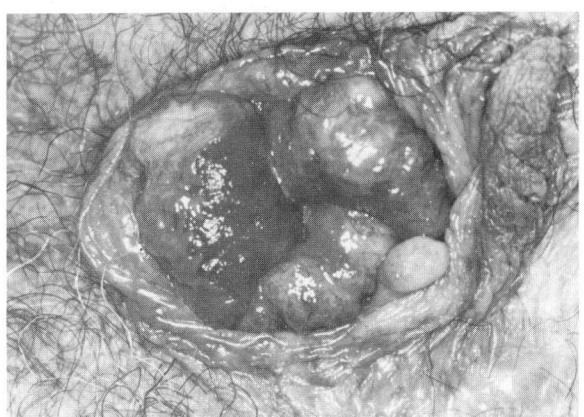

Figure 4. Third-degree hemorrhoids. Note the squamous epithelial change and the darkened mucosa.

TABLE 2. Techniques for Treating Hemorrhoids

Mode of Action	Technique
Fixation of mucosa	Injection therapy
	Infrared coagulation
	Direct current from galvanic generator and probe
Fixation of mucosa and removal of redundant mucosa	Elastic band ligation
	Cryotherapy
Relaxation of internal sphincter	Maximal anal dilatation
	Internal sphincterotomy
Radical excision of hemorrhoids	Hemorrhoidectomy

tients had abnormal anal pressure profiles (significantly longer high-pressure zones) and poorer anal compliance.[11] The hypothesis that hemorrhoids are caused by constipation may need reconsideration. Shafik[49] has proposed that patients with hemorrhoids have "high rectal neck pressure and straining at defecation, even with soft and bulky stools." He attributes hemorrhoids to a "persisting anorectal band and concomitant failure of rectal neck remodeling which results in mucosal prolapse and venous congestion." Also the long-held classic view that they are analogous to varicose veins, subject to thrombosis and hematoma formation, is being replaced by the concept that they are normal submucosal or dermal pads in which the supporting and anchoring connective tissue deteriorates with age, excessive straining, trauma, overuse of laxatives, and so on. This allows the vascular pad or cushion to slide downward, with distention of veins as they lose their support.[13] Whatever the underlying cause may be, a physiologic abnormality present in these patients, in both sexes, is elevation of anal sphincter pressure.[11]

INJECTION THERAPY. Injection therapy has been practiced for about 100 years and gives considerable relief for varying periods of time. Many different substances have been used, such as sterilized arachis oil containing a small percentage (5 per cent) of phenol or a mixture of quinine and urea. The injection is placed in the submucosa of the upper anal canal well above the sensitive squamous epithelium. It is quite simply performed through an anoscope and if properly done produces very little pain. There is no direct effect on the veins themselves, as is commonly thought, but a fibrous tissue reaction is induced in the submucosa of the upper anal canal and lower rectum, thereby drawing the dropped mucosa upward toward the normal site. Injection therapy is particularly valuable in early cases when it prevents the excessive mucosal prolapse from occurring at defecation and so stops bleeding. It is less successful for the more advanced type of hemorrhoid but even so can sometimes be most helpful in the elderly or others in whom there is a contraindication to operative treatment.

INFRARED COAGULATION. Infrared coagulation is a recent innovation. A small controlled burn is created at the anorectal junction, which causes mucosal fixation. This treatment has been found to be as effective as injection therapy and has the advantage of being less invasive. However, there is a risk of secondary hemorrhage, greater than with injection therapy, and the equipment required is more expensive.

ELASTIC BAND LIGATION. Each hemorrhoid is visualized through an anoscope; the upper part above the mucocutaneous line is grasped by an instrument, and a small elastic band is slipped over it. A special instrument has been designed to perform this maneuver.[3] The tissue distal to the elastic band undergoes necrosis, and excess mucosa in the upper anal canal is removed. The lower anal mucosa is drawn up by the ensuing fibrosis, which also causes adherence of the mucosa to the underlying muscle. This method accomplishes its tasks satisfactorily, but it is associated with pain, which may be very severe in some cases associated with perianal and systemic sepsis. Secondary hemorrhage has been reported.

CRYOTHERAPY. Another new form of therapy involves freezing the tissues of the hemorrhoid for a time sufficient to cause necrosis.[23] If carefully used and applied only to the upper part of the hemorrhoidal area at the anorectal junction, it achieves a result similar to that of elastic banding, but there is no pain associated with it. The effectiveness of this form of cryosurgery is at present being evaluated. Both these methods may well come to occupy a midposition between injection therapy and surgical excision. In the advanced case they do little to correct the anal mucosal descent, nor do they remove the external anal tags that are the result of this descent. They are, therefore, unlikely to replace surgical therapy for this disorder but may nevertheless be a valuable addition to conservative therapy.

DIRECT CURRENT FROM GALVANIC GENERATOR AND PROBE. This new modality delivers direct current in relatively low amperage of 8 to 16 mA. for a period of 8 to 10 minutes to the root of the hemorrhoid. A popping sound is often heard during treatment, and an eschar develops, with subsequent contraction and shrinking of the hemorrhoidal complex.

In a study comparing infrared photocoagulation, heater probe coagulation, and direct current therapy, Ultroid was found to be associated with the least discomfort and complications. The best results were in small hemorrhoids.[59]

MAXIMAL ANAL DILATATION. It has been debated that the tightness of the internal sphincter is responsible for many of the symptoms of hemorrhoids. Maximal anal dilatation was introduced in an attempt to disrupt this tight band. There is no doubt that this procedure reduces many of the symptoms, especially in young patients. However, it does not eliminate redundant tissue; and if maximal anal dilatation is used, it must be remembered that there is a significant incidence of incontinence (not only for flatus but also for solid feces) in a few patients, especially the elderly and those with pelvic floor problems.

INTERNAL SPHINCTEROTOMY. Surgical division of the

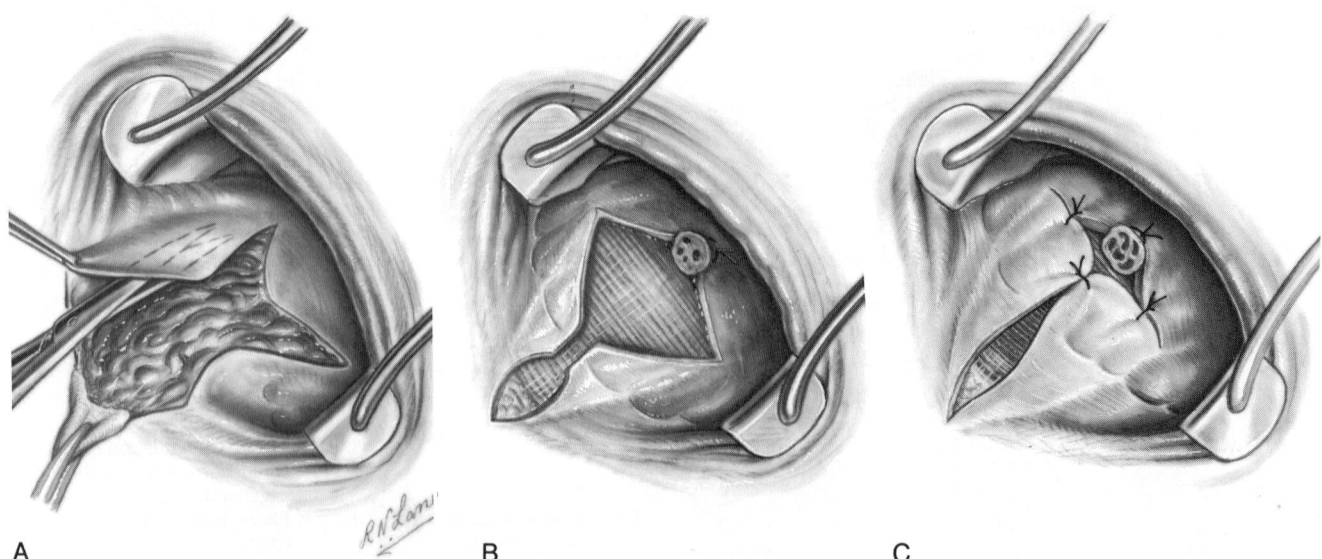

A   B   C

Figure 6. Submucosal hemorrhoidectomy. *A,* The mucosa of the anal canal is dissected off the vascular submucosa. The submucosa is then itself stripped off the internal sphincter. *B,* The vascular hemorrhoidal tissue has been removed, leaving the floor of the wound formed by the internal sphincter. The two mucosal flaps are demonstrated. *C,* Mucosal anatomy is reconstituted. Squamous mucosa is fixed at the correct level in the anal canal.

tight unyielding distal internal sphincter is the alternative to maximal dilatation. This simple, safe procedure has been widely adopted in the treatment of fissure, but its role in the treatment of hemorrhoids is unclear.

HEMORRHOIDECTOMY. There is no doubt that a correctly performed hemorrhoidectomy is the best treatment for curing a patient of hemorrhoids. Often, though, it is not well done, and there may be persistence or an early return of symptoms. In most series, only 5 to 10 per cent of patients require operative treatment: those who have large prolapsing hemorrhoids with squamous epithelial change, those with a significant external component, those whose symptoms have not responded to other treatments, and those who have recurrent episodes of external thrombosis. There are three currently used operative techniques for hemorrhoids: (1) ligation and excision technique,[31] (2) submucosal hemorrhoidectomy[35] (Fig. 6), and (3) closed hemorrhoidectomy.[12]

The most significant shift in the operative treatment of hemorrhoids is that it is now often performed in an ambulatory setting. Although open hemorrhoidectomy is performed in some centers, the closed technique has gained rapidly in popularity.[17,18] In a series of 2274 patients, only 14 patients had secondary hemorrhage requiring packing and five postoperative abscesses, only one of whom required hospitalization. However, the postoperative period may be marked by pain (especially during the first bowel movement) and, in addition to bleeding, a small incidence of urinary or fecal retention. Thus, patients must be closely observed in the early postoperative period. Hemorrhoidectomy, however, is an operation that benefits the patient considerably and should not be withheld if the patient has troublesome symptoms.

ANORECTAL SUPPURATION

There are many possible types of anorectal suppuration (Table 3). Of these, the most common is an abscess or a fistula, or both, due to nonspecific anal gland infection. The pathogenesis of these two apparently separate conditions is often the same: the abscess is the acute phase and the fistula the chronic phase.[35]

Abscess

Infection starts in the intersphincteric space, probably in one of the anal glands. A small abscess may be formed at this site (an intersphincteric abscess). The infection may spread from there vertically (Fig. 7), horizontally (Fig. 8), or circumferentially (Fig. 9), producing a number of different clinical situations.

An *intersphincteric abscess* is limited to the primary site. It may be symptomless, but it can cause throbbing pain that resembles the pain of a fissure, in that it is initiated by defecation and goes on for many hours. The pain may be so severe as to prevent sleep. A fissure may sometimes be present, and so the diagnosis

TABLE 3. Causes of Anorectal Suppuration

Abscess and fistula
    Nonspecific anal gland infection
    Crohn's disease
    Tuberculosis
    Perforation by foreign body
    External trauma
    Carcinoma
Pilonidal infection
Hidradenitis suppurativa
Infected epidermoid cyst
Skin sepsis (staphylococcal)
Intrapelvic suppuration
    Acute appendicitis
    Diverticular disease
    Crohn's disease

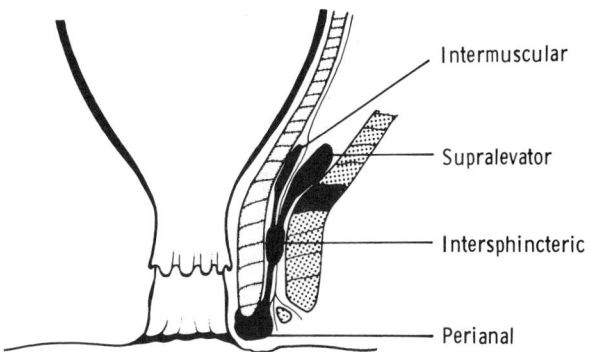

Figure 7. Upward and downward vertical spread of infection from an intersphincteric abscess. (From Parks, A. G., and Thomson, J. P. S.: Abscess and fistula. *In* Thomson, J. P. S., Nicholls, R. J., and Williams, C. R. (Eds.): Colorectal Disease. Copyright © 1981, William Heinemann Medical Books, London, and Appleton-Century-Crofts, New York. Used by permission.)

may be overlooked. Chronic infection may persist at this site, causing intermittent anal pain.

A *perianal abscess* is the result of distal vertical spread of the infection to the anal margin. It presents as a tender, red swelling, which occasionally is misdiagnosed as an external anal thrombosis.

Proximal vertical spread of infection produces an *intermuscular abscess* within the rectal wall or a *supralevator abscess*, depending upon which side of the longitudinal muscle the sepsis has tracked. These abscesses are often difficult to diagnose, because there are no external manifestations. Patients usually complain of vague pelvic discomfort, but rectal examination should reveal indurated swelling. Often an examination under anesthesia is required to established the diagnosis.

Horizontal spread of infection may cause a track across the internal sphincter into the anal canal or across the external sphincter into the ischiorectal fossa, where an *ischiorectal abscess* results. At this site, a quite large abscess may be formed, extending upward to the top of the fossa and sometimes into the supralevator space by passing across the levator ani muscle as well as downward to the perineal skin. The patient may complain of pain and fever before a swelling is visible. Induration then occurs under the skin over the ischiorectal fossa, and finally a typical red fluctuant abscess is seen.

Circumferential spread may occur from one side to the other in the intersphincteric space, the supralevator space, or the ischiorectal fossa, producing a *horseshoe abscess*. It is evident that a very complicated septic process can develop.

MANAGEMENT. The management of abscess in this area is relatively straightforward. They should be drained as soon as diagnosed. An intersphincteric abscess is drained by dividing

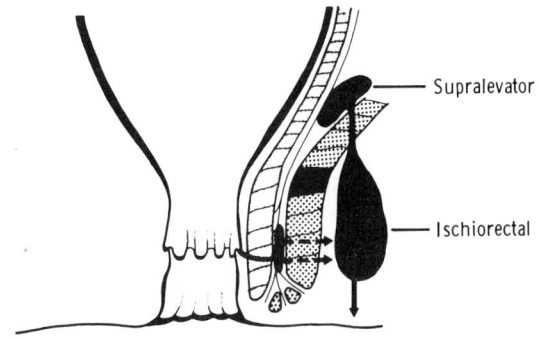

Figure 8. Horizontal spread of infection medially into the anal canal and laterally into the ischiorectal fossa. The level at which the primary tract crosses the external sphincter may not be the same as the level of the internal opening. Vertical spread of infection may then occur across the levator ani muscle. (From Parks, A. G., Thomson, J. P. S.: Abscess and fistula. *In* Thomson, J. P. S., Nicholls, R. J., and Williams, C. R. (Eds.): Colorectal Disease. Copyright © 1981, William Heinemann Medical Books, London, and Appleton-Century-Crofts, New York. Used by permission.)

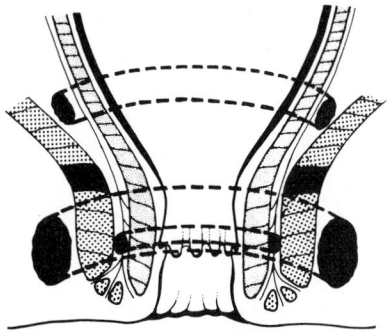

Figure 9. Circumferential spread of infection may occur in the intersphincteric and supralevator spaces and the ischiorectal fossa. (From Parks, A. G., and Thomson, J. P. S.: Abscess and fistula. *In* Thomson, J. P. S., Nicholls, R. J., and Williams, C. R. (Eds.): Colorectal Disease. Copyright © 1981, William Heinemann Medical Books, London, and Appleton-Century-Crofts, New York. Used by permission.)

the internal sphincter up to the level of the abscess. A perianal abscess requires only a simple skin incision. Both an intermuscular abscess and a supralevator abscess (providing it does not rise from an extension of an ischiorectal abscess), being inside the striated muscle of the pelvic floor, need to be drained into the lower rectum and upper anal canal. An ischiorectal abscess often requires removal of a circle of skin over the ischiorectal fossa to provide adequate drainage. Because this abscess may extend quite high in the fat of the fossa and spread circumferentially, it is wise to explore the cavity digitally and gently break down any loculations that may be present, but great care must be exercised. It should be remembered that drainage is always the primary treatment. The pus should be sent for culture, and antibiotics should be used only if the infection does not respond to drainage and perhaps in immunocompromised patients.

Treatment of the presenting abscess is often only the initial stage of management, because there may be other associated infection, especially in the intersphincteric space. This is suggested when there is a history of recurrent abscess, when gut organisms are detected on pus culture, when induration is detected, or when there is a known fistula. Under these circumstances, after 7 days or so, a further examination under anesthesia should be undertaken and the residual sepsis drained. A preliminary computed tomographic (CT) scan of the perineum and pelvis may identify unsuspected collections of pus.

The importance of urgent drainage of perianal abscesses cannot be overemphasized. In a recent unpublished review of institutional and reported experience, neglected abscesses were the single most important cause of devastating necrotizing infections of the perineum. Infection in this area can spread with amazing rapidity.

Fistula in Ano

A fistula is by definition an abnormal communication between any two epithelial surfaces. Fistula *in ano* is indeed such a communication, but the situation is not quite a straightforward one. The external opening of the fistula onto the perineal skin (whether spontaneous or created after incision and drainage of an abscess) is a sinus leading down to a small chronic abscess in the intersphincteric space. However, this abscess is usually due to infection in the anal gland or the surrounding lymphoid tissue, and only a minute duct communicates between it and the anal canal at the level of the mucocutaneous junction. In about half the cases the intersphincteric abscess also discharges into the anal canal, so that there is now a larger sinus entering the canal. What is the incidence of fistula *in ano* complicating anorectal sepsis? Henrichsen and Christiansen[14] studied 50 consecutive patients and noted a 26 per cent incidence of fistula either in the acute phase or during follow-up within 6 months. Half of the fistulas diagnosed at follow-up were unrecognized by the

patients and no fistulas developed in patients where culture from the abscess only revealed skin-derived bacteria. Fistulas occurred when intestinal microorganisms were cultured from the anorectal abscess.

CLINICAL PRESENTATION. A fistula may present as an acute abscess or in a number of less dramatic ways. The patient may notice a small discharging sinus, and the discharge from the sinus may cause skin excoriation and pruritus.

On examination, subcutaneous induration can often be traced from the external opening to the anal margin, and this is indicative of an underlying track. On digital examination, there may be a nodule palpable in the wall of the anal canal that indicates the site of the primary abscess. A probe is classically used in the diagnosis of the fistula, but it can be a dangerous instrument in inexperienced hands. It is possible to create false openings into the anal canal or into the rectum by injudicious probing. A probe passed into the external sinus usually demonstrates the site of the fistula in the anal canal. If there is an opening of reasonable size, the probe passes into the canal. Under no circumstances should force be used in this maneuver, because a false track may result.

ANATOMY. The path that fistulas follow is largely determined by the anatomy of the region. They tend to course in fascial or fatty planes, the most usual being the intersphincteric space between the two groups of sphincters and the fat of the ischiorectal fossa. In most cases, the track passes directly to the perineal skin. However, much more complex situations occasionally occur. In particular, circumferential spread is not uncommon; this usually occurs in the ischiorectal fossa, and the track may pass from one fossa to the other behind the rectum, constituting what is known as a horseshoe fistula.

Fistulas are usually found to conform to one of four main anatomic types, which are now briefly considered (Table 4).[28]

INTERSPHINCTERIC FISTULA. This is the most common type, constituting about 70 per cent of all cases. The infection passes directly downward to the anal margin. There are some less common and more complicated variants of this fistula; for instance, a track may pass upward into the rectal wall and discharge into the rectal ampulla. This high intersphincteric fistula, frequently and erroneously termed a submucous fistula, may cause intermittent rectal wall abscesses but is still quite easy to treat.

TRANSSPHINCTERIC FISTULA. In this type, the track crosses the external sphincter and enters the ischiorectal fossa en route to the skin. If it passes through muscle at a low level, it is easy to treat. However, it may pass through the upper part of the sphincter mass and constitute a more difficult therapeutic problem. A further complication of this type of fistula is the presence of a high extension that causes induration and can be palpated on digital examination through the rectal wall. A probe passes directly into the high extension and thus may mislead the surgeon into thinking that the fistula has a much higher connection with the rectum itself. Overenthusiastic probing may produce an artificial connection between the high part of the fistula and the rectum, with disastrous results for the patient. Transsphincteric fistulas constitute about 25 per cent of all fistulas and are

---

TABLE 4. Classification of Anorectal Fistulas

Type 1:	Intersphincteric, the most common, in which the fistulous track is confined to the intersphincteric plane.
Type 2:	Transsphincteric, in which the fistula connects the intersphincteric plane with the ischiorectal fossa by perforating the external sphincter.
Type 3:	Suprasphincteric, similar to Type 2, but the track loops over the external sphincter and perforates the levator ani.
Type 4:	Extrasphincteric, in which the track passes from rectum to perineal skin completely external to the sphincteric complex.

generally not difficult to treat. A horseshoe pattern of sepsis in the ischiorectal fossae from one side to the other is, in fact, less difficult to treat than might appear, although quite a large wound may be necessary to drain it.

SUPRASPHINCTERIC FISTULA. The remaining 5 per cent of fistulas are made up of two rare types in which treatment is difficult as well as hazardous when done by the inexperienced. The first of these is a suprasphincteric fistula, in which the track passes first upward in the intersphincteric space, then laterally over the top of the puborectalis muscle, and finally downward into the ischiorectal fossa to the skin. It passes above all the muscles of continence before pursuing a downward course to the perineal skin. Clearly, division of all the external sphincter muscle will make the patient incontinent, so that this fistula constitutes a therapeutic challenge. This fistula may also have a high extension in the pelvis that runs pararectally. It produces high induration that can be palpated in the rectum.

EXTRASPHINCTERIC FISTULA. The final type is fortunately rarest and constitutes perhaps 1 per cent of all fistulas. It passes from the skin of the perineum up through the ischiorectal fat, through the levator ani muscles, and then communicates with the rectum. The track of this fistula passes outside all the muscles of continence. It is therefore termed extrasphincteric. If treated in the classic manner, incontinence would be inevitable. There are a variety of causes, some of them gross disease such as Crohn's disease or carcinoma. Trauma, either direct external or internal, as, for example, a swallowed fish bone penetrating the rectal wall, is another cause. There is the type previously mentioned, a transsphincteric fistula with a high extension passing upward that may burst spontaneously into the rectum or a communication forcibly produced by probing. Whatever the cause, this type of fistula has an additional cause for its persistence, because high rectal pressures allow mucus and feces to enter into the internal opening. Treatment entails abolishing these pressure changes by means of a temporary colostomy. Whatever the cause of extrasphincteric fistula, treatment is difficult and usually lasts several months.

MANAGEMENT. The management of a fistula needs to be considered in three parts:

1. *Accurate definition of the pathoanatomy.* This may be determined (a) by palpation for induration—a most important physical sign that is difficult for the inexperienced to detect; (b) by gentle probing; (c) by partially laying open the wound and using a curette to detect granulation tissue; and (d) only very occasionally by radiology (probably of value only in extrasphincteric fistulas). Goodsall's rule, although generally helpful, cannot be a guide for the definition of anatomy in complex cases (Fig. 10).

2. *Drainage of the sepsis.* This consists of draining the primary intersphincteric infection in all types of fistulas and the primary track across the external sphincter and secondary tracks within the ischiorectal fossae in transsphincteric fistulas. Suprasphincteric and extrasphincteric fistulas are very unusual and complicated to manage. They should be referred to specialists in this field of management.

3. *Careful nursing care of the wound.* There should be a twice daily routine of baths, irrigation of the wound, and placement of a dressing to ensure healing from the depths of the wound to the surface. It is essential for the surgeon to instruct and assist the nurses in this most important aspect of management. Because these perineal wounds are closed body cavities and may communicate with the peritoneum, hydrogen peroxide irrigation should not be used. The oxygen released has no egress, and the hydrogen peroxide is readily absorbed from the peritoneal surfaces. Oxygen bubbles entering the bloodstream in this manner have caused physiologic derangement and nearly fatal cases of gas embolism.[30,54]

A seton[45] of monofilament nylon or fine silicone tubing may be used to drain the primary track across the external sphincter,

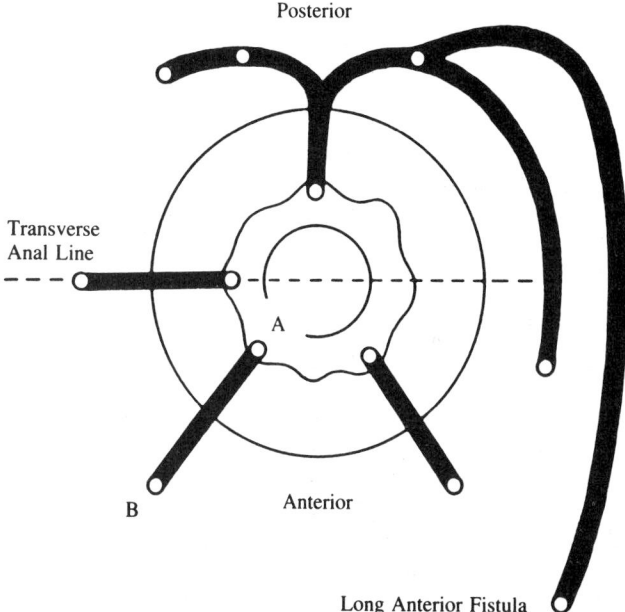

Figure 10. Goodsall's rule. The usual relationship of primary and secondary fistula orifices is diagrammed. The internal (primary orifice) is marked A. The rule predicts that if a line is drawn transversely across the anus, an external opening (B) anterior to this line will lead to a straight radial tract, whereas an external opening that lies posterior to the line will lead to a curved tract and an internal opening in the posterior commissure. The long anterior fistula is an exception to the rule. (From Schrock, T. R.: Benign and malignant disease of the anorectum. *In* Fromm, D. (Ed.): Gastrointestinal Surgery. New York, Churchill Livingstone, 1985, p. 612.)

especially if the track is above the level of the anal valves. It should not be tied tightly, so that the wound is allowed to heal around it. When it is removed, usually after 2 to 3 months, the remaining track may close spontaneously. If this does not occur, the track may need to be divided, as the muscle is fixed by fibrosis, which causes minimal separation of the cut ends.

If a fistula wound fails to heal, a number of factors should be considered. There may have been failure to drain the sepsis completely. The postoperative care may have been inadequate, causing (1) pockets of sepsis in the depths of the wound (it may be necessary to evaluate these wounds once or twice postoperatively under anesthesia in the operating room), (2) overgrowth of granulation tissue (readily cauterized with silver nitrate), or (3) ingrowth of hairs due to lack of shaving. In addition, there may be a specific cause for the fistula, such as Crohn's disease[53] or tuberculosis,[50] that had not been previously recognized. It must be remembered that congenital fistula *in ano* may occur in the first few months of life.[44] Congenital anovulvar fistula has been reported in a 30-year-old woman.[42] An innovative and attractive technique is sliding flap advancement for the treatment of difficult and persisting chronic high anal fistulas. A rectal flap consisting of mucosa, submucosa, and circular muscle fibers is outlined around the internal opening and extended 5 cm. cephalad. The flap is mobilized and drawn down to cover the internal orifice of the fistula. Wedell and others[58] had satisfactory results in 29 of 30 patients with this approach. A new nonoperative approach using a multistrand stainless steel wire to accomplish progressive fistulotomy in the office setting has been described.[32]

ANAL FISSURE

The squamous mucosa of the lower half of the anal canal is prone to superficial ulceration, which presents clinically as an anal fissure. It is a linear ulcer, usually situated in the posterior commissure of the canal (Fig. 11). Because it involves the highly sensitive squamous epithelium, it is often a painful condition. With each act of defecation the ulcer is stretched, causing pain,

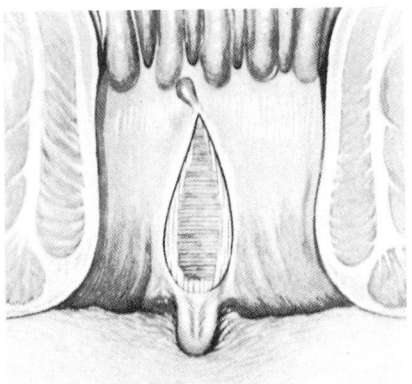

Figure 11. The typical appearance of a posterior anal fissure showing the sentinel tag and the circular muscle fibers in the floor of the ulcer. (From Morgan, C. N., and Thompson, H. R.: Surgical anatomy of the anal canal with special reference to the surgical importance of the internal sphincter and conjoint longitudinal muscle. Ann. R. Coll. Surg. Engl., *19*:88, 1956.)

which may continue for several hours, and also bleeding, which is characteristically anal in type. The natural sequel of anal pain is that the patient avoids defecation, with the resultant formation of a hard, constipated stool. When the event can be delayed no longer, pain may be excruciating. The condition tends to be cyclic, pain continuing for 1 to 2 months followed by a remission. Should the patient become constipated, the healed fissure splits open and another episode is initiated. Although the cause of fissure is unknown, when it occurs it is readily reactivated by constipation. It is very common in women just before and after childbirth and is frequently misdiagnosed as hemorrhoids at this time. Oddly enough, over one third of all patients with Crohn's disease have an anal fissure, although the latter is far too common for this disease to be responsible in more than a small fraction of cases.[53]

Patients learn to keep the stool soft by the use of laxatives; but this, coupled with the fibrous tissue response to the ulceration, causes a contracted anal canal. The internal sphincter ring becomes narrower than normal and the submucosa infiltrated with scar tissue. Return to an even normally formed stool may cause immediate recurrence of the condition. It is not uncommon for patients to take laxatives regularly for 20 or more years before seeking advice; yet the disorder is remediable with rapid and complete cure.

The history of pain during and after defecation is typical. On examination the fissure can usually be seen situated posteriorly (see Fig. 11). There may be a skin tag protruding from the anal margin, the sentinel pile, and an anal polyp or hypertrophied anal papilla at the dentate line. The fissure is usually situated just within the anus and may be overlooked; it can readily be revealed by traction on the anal skin that partially everts the canal. Pain may cause an exaggerated anal reflex so that any attempt at digital examination is impossible because of intense external sphincter spasm. Rectal examination is usually possible, however, and the fissure can again be detected by local tenderness.

There are several important conditions to bear in mind in the differential diagnosis. Crohn's disease causes a fissure of the nonspecific type; other symptoms alert the physician to this possibility. Primary syphilis may cause a fissure-like lesion, but this lesion does not have the same predilection for the commissures and is often laterally situated. The inguinal lymph nodes are usually enlarged. Carcinoma of the anal canal occasionally causes symptoms entirely compatible with fissure and indeed in the early stages may have the same appearance on examination. It is a useful axiom to be suspicious of any fissure-like lesion that is not in the posterior or anterior commissure or that does not rapidly respond to therapy.

Treatment is usually entirely satisfactory. In about one third of the patients the fissure heals with conservative measures, the

remainder requiring a minor surgical procedure for cure. There are many types of local treatment. A local anesthetic application diminishes pain and abolishes the exaggerated anal reflex. Healing is more rapid if the local anesthetic is applied to an anal dilator and passed twice a day for 5 minutes. Avoidance of constipation by the use of a bland laxative is essential. If these measures fail, the division of the lower half of the internal sphincter is generally curative.[19,29] This operation, usually done laterally in the anal canal, enlarges the lower anal canal and eliminates defecation trauma.

CROHN'S DISEASE IN THE ANORECTUM

This form of anorectal inflammation is becoming increasingly common, or perhaps it is more frequently being recognized as a distinct entity separate from granular proctitis. It can resemble the latter in every way (except histologically) but usually causes a more patchy inflammation with intervening areas of normal epithelium. Granulomatous infiltration of the submucosa can cause nodular areas readily detectable with the examining finger. Frank ulceration, rather than the diffuse granular change of granular proctitis, is not uncommon. The diagnosis is again established by the proctoscopic appearance and the histologic changes seen on biopsy. Dense lymphocytic infiltration of the submucosa occurs, with occasional giant cell–containing granulomas.

There may be associated anal manifestations in up to 75 per cent of patients. These include a bluish discoloration, edematous tags, ulceration (both perianal and anal), and sepsis (Fig. 12).[53] The course of this disease is not as benign as that of granular proctitis. Simultaneous occurrence in the ileum and colon is common. The fibrotic changes, so characteristic of granulomatous enteritis, cause narrowing and stenosis of the rectum.

Treatment is conservative in the first instance and a regimen similar to that in granular proctitis is employed. If severe stenosis or fistulization occurs, administration of oral prednisone in adequate doses may be justified. Some good reports have appeared on the use of immunosuppressive drugs, but as yet there is conflicting evidence and opinion on the desirability of this mode of therapy. Occasionally the disease can progress to such a degree that excision of the rectum is the only possible course. In any case in which excision of the rectum has to be performed for benign disease such as this, it is essential that it be accom-

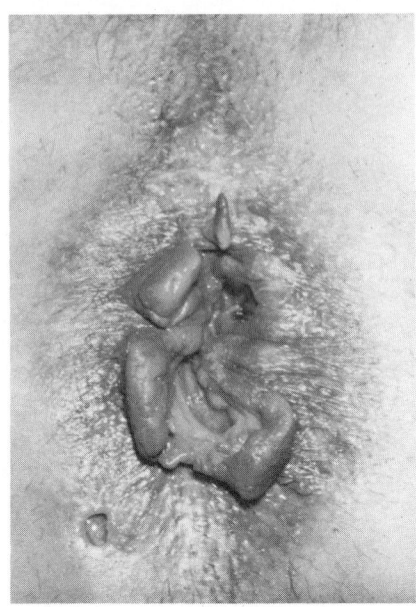

Figure 12. The anal manifestations of Crohn's disease.

plished in a manner quite different from that of excision for carcinoma. The dissection is performed as close to the rectal muscle as possible so that damage to other pelvic structures and, in particular, the nervi erigentes is avoided. Failure to observe this precaution in young individuals (and this disease affects the young predominantly) may cause severe bladder or sexual dysfunction.

PERIANAL DISORDERS

There are a number of conditions that affect the perianal skin which should be borne in mind in the assessment of patients with anorectal symptoms. The most common symptoms are itching (pruritus) or soreness in the region, but other symptoms outlined previously may occur.

Infections

BACTERIAL. Although most septic conditions occurring in this region are in association with fistula *in ano* or pilonidal infection, occasionally a simple staphyloccal boil may occur. There is another infection that affects the perianal skin caused by *Corynebacterium minutissimum*: erythrasma. This can be readily diagnosed by the salmon-pink fluorescence in ultraviolet light and is treated with erythromycin.

The apocrine sweat glands of the area may be involved in an inflammatory process which is probably bacterial, known as *Hidradenitis suppurativa*. This produces a purulent discharge, and the treatment is essentially operative. The infected areas are opened and allowed to heal by secondary intention. If there is extensive involvement, the skin may have to be excised and the defect covered with a split-thickness skin graft.

Infection with *Treponema pallidum* (syphilis) may produce a chancre or condylomata lata. The former should always be considered when a fissure *in ano* is diagnosed and the latter when viral condylomata acuminata are being considered. It is diagnosed by direct examination of a smear of perianal skin scrapings or by culture. Treatment is directed to some predisposing condition, such as hemorrhoids if present, and appropriate antibiotic therapy.

PARASITIC. Patients with a threadworm infestation of the gastrointestinal tract may complain of pruritus; it can be treated with piperazine. Other infestations include scabies and pediculosis.

TUMORS OF THE ANUS

Benign Tumors

Condyloma acuminatum (perianal warts)[4] is the perineal homologue of the common viral wart. It is caused by a papovavirus and presents as multiple papillary acanthotic and parakeratotic growths, covering the perianal skin, sometimes extensively. They may also be present on the male external genitalia and on the vulva, vagina, and cervix in the female. In addition, warts may be present in the anal canal and in the lower rectum. While a proportion of patients may practice anal intercourse, this is by no means the rule.

Histologically, the lesions may show conspicuous vacuolation (poikilocytosis) of superficial cells. As in other sites, koilocytotic cell nuclei may show irregular outlines, but dysplasia is not usually a feature. However, transformation to invasive squamous carcinoma is recognized; and in these cases varying degrees of dysplasia, away from obvious cancer, may be encountered. The giant variety of condyloma acuminatum may also occur in the anorectum but less commonly than in the genital area. The clinical and histologic resemblance to *verrucous carcinoma* is such that currently most observers regard these lesions as essentially identical, and fortunately their treatments are the same. If there is a subtle transition from giant

condyloma to verrucous carcinoma, it should be remembered that the former can also evolve into conventional invasive squamous carcinoma. When a few perianal warts are present, the local application of podophyllin is usually effective; but when the condition is extensive, both in the perianal area and in the anal canal, excisional treatment under general anesthesia is required. These warts are probably sexually transmitted, and so other forms of sexually transmitted disease should be excluded.

Polyps (papillae) of the anal canal, a condition in which the stroma is hyperplastic and occasionally atypical, have been described. There is a structural resemblance to vaginal polyps. The polypoid expression of the *solitary rectal ulcer* syndrome may also present in the anal transitional zone, where it has been termed *inflammatory cloacogenic polyp*. Benign adnexal tumors of apocrine origin have been described as rare lesions of the anal area.[47]

MALIGNANT TUMORS

Malignant tumors of the anus histologically reflect the composite derivation of the anus from both the embryologic hindgut and the proctodeal dimple of ectoderm. Thus, tumors of the proximal anus are adenocarcinomas, derived from the colorectal type of glandular epithelium. The lymphatic spread of these tumors is largely along the superior hemorrhoidals to the pelvic organs.

A more distal transitional zone of stratified epithelium with interspersed glandular cells includes the valves and sinuses. It is distinguished by its gray-blue surface and may have nonkeratinizing squamous epithelium. The uniqueness of this zone is reflected by the fact that mucus secreted by this epithelium appears to be distinct from that found in rectal mucosa. Tumors arising in this zone of "unstable transitional epithelium"[9] may be histologically squamous, pseudoadenoid, pseudosarcomatous, cloacogenic, mucoepidermoid, or neuroendocrine or have the characteristics of melanoma, carcinoid, perianal mucinous carcinoma, lymphoma, or small cell carcinoma. The lymphatic drainage from this zone is either directly along the inferior and middle hemorrhoidal chain of lymph nodes to the hypogastric and obturator nodes or indirectly via the submucosal plexus of nodes to the rectal nodes, superior hemorrhoidal nodes and plexuses of nodes associated with the pelvic organs.

The most distal anus is a zone of nonkeratinized squamous epithelium, devoid of hair, sweat glands, and sebaceous glands. This zone then merges into the keratinized perianal skin with glands and follicles. Well-differentiated keratinizing carcinoma arising in this distal zone may spread to the superficial inguinal nodes.

For the appropriate diagnosis to be established, a biopsy is required. The histologic types of tumor encountered in the anus, and some of their characteristics are summarized in Table 5. Anal carcinoma presents clinically with bleeding (50 per cent), pain (40 per cent; much higher than in colonic carcinoma), a mass (25 per cent), and pruritus (15 per cent). About 25 per cent of the patients are asymptomatic! Women are more frequently afflicted (2:1 to 4:1). Development of the tumor has been associated with Crohn's disease, lymphogranuloma venereum, condyloma acuminatum, and independent lower genital tract carcinomas (especially cervical) in women. An evolving strong association found between anal carcinoma and receptive anal intercourse related to homosexual behavior may be independent of human immunodeficiency virus (HIV) infection in the homosexual male population.[5,26,47]

It is important to distinguish between squamous carcinoma of the anal canal[8] and squamous carcinoma of the anal margin, which, although it has a similar age of incidence as the former, is more common in men (4:1) and has a more favorable prognosis despite the fact that most anal margin tumors are treated by local excision. Grossly, anal canal cancers may present as local-

TABLE 5. Histologic Classification of Malignant Neoplasms of the Anus

	Comments
Epithelial tumors	
Intraepithelial carcinoma (Bowen's disease)	Rare. Slow growing. Total excision of involved skin with split-thickness grafting curative.[48]
Paget's disease	Arises in intraepithelial segments of apocrine gland ducts. Contains mucin.[24]
Primary invasive carcinoma	3% of anorectal carcinomas.[26]
Keratinizing and nonkeratinizing carcinoma	
Basaloid, cloacogenic, or transitional carcinoma	
Adenocystic carcinoma	
Mucoepidermoid carcinoma	Distinguished by presence of mucin.
Basal cell carcinoma	Rodent ulcer. Presents as "piles" or sore spot with raised edges. Local excision 70+% survival.
Adenocarcinoma	Arise from anal glands or ducts[21] in congenital duplications; associated with chronic fistula *in ano*.[15]
Spindle cell (pseudosarcomatous) carcinoma	
Small cell carcinoma	Resemble oat cell carcinoma of the lung.[47]
Nonepithelial tumors	
Malignant melanoma	Anus is the most common site of primary gastrointestinal melanoma. Electron microscopy and identification of S-100 protein may be needed to differentiate anaplastic carcinoma from melanoma.
Mesenchymal neoplasms	Very rare. Treated by abdominoperineal resection after unequivocal histologic diagnosis is established.
Leiomyosarcoma[52]	
Granular cell tumors[46]	
Rhabdomyosarcoma	

ized ulcers or raised ulcerated warty growths, frequently on the anterior wall. They may extend to surround the anus completely or become distinctly polypoid. Others present as indurated poorly defined intramural masses without ulceration.

Careful clinicopathologic staging is important in management and prognosis. The different protocols recognize the basic levels of carcinoma *in situ*, submucosal versus sphincteric muscle involvement, and metastases to nodes or distant sites. Epidermoid, cloacogenic, and transitional cell carcinomas of this region have for years been treated by abdominoperineal resection, which has a 5-year survival of 24 to 70 per cent, with an average of about 55 per cent for the larger series.[26]

Recent reports show that external irradiation in combination with 5-fluorouracil and mitomycin has a 5-year survival of 78 per cent (Table 6).[34] This rate is superior to that of abdominoperineal resection combined with chemotherapy, or abdominoperineal resection combined with radiation. Residual tumor after combined therapy and unresponsive bulky tumors are treated by local excision[38] or abdominoperineal resection.[47] Combined chemotherapy and radiation therapy (chemoradiation therapy) may thus negate a permanent colostomy, making it very attractive to patient and physician alike.

TABLE 6. Chemoradiation Therapy for Cancer of the Anus

External irradiation
    3000 rads (30 Gy) to the primary tumor and pelvic and inguinal nodes. Start: day 1 (200 rad/day).

Systemic chemotherapy
    1. 5-FU: 1000 mg./sq. m. per 24 hr as a continuous infusion for 4 days. Start: day 1.
    2. Mitomycin C: 15 mg./sq. m. intravenous bolus. Start: day 1 *only*.
    3. 5-FU: Repeat 4-day infusion. Start: day 28.

Data from Nigro, N. D.: Multidisciplinary management of cancer of the anus. World J. Surg. 11:446, 1987.

MALIGNANT MELANOMA OF THE ANAL CANAL

Anorectal melanoma is seen about once for every eight squamous cell carcinomas of the anal region. They constitute 0.4 to 0.8 per cent of colorectal malignancies and less than 2 per cent of all melanomas. Since the initial report by Moore in 1857,[33] approximately 500 cases of malignant melanoma have been reported in the literature. Commonly presenting with intermittent rectal bleeding and pain, these lesions may be ignored because they are thought to be hemorrhoids. Histologic examination reveals pigment in hematoxylin and eosin–stained sections in about half of the cases. The tumor may be positively identified on electron microscopy and S-100 protein analysis.[1]

Malignant melanoma spreads rapidly, involving the superior hemorrhoidal group of lymph nodes early. Spread to the nodes of the lateral wall of the pelvis and the para-aortic and inguinal nodes then occurs. Death follows widespread blood-borne deposits, predominantly in the liver and lungs. Survival after surgical excision of the anorectum is measured in months, although 5-year survival has been reported in a few patients undergoing abdominoperineal resection. These lesions were less than 3 mm. in thickness.[56]

OTHER NONEPITHELIAL TUMORS

Connective tissue sarcomas are rarely seen, but leiomyosarcoma arising from the internal sphincter[2] and perianal rhabdomyosarcomas and myoblastomas arising from the external sphincter have been reported. Malignant lymphoma involving the anus is rare. Endocrine tumors (carcinoids) have been classified as arising in the rectum, but they may originate from the endocrine cell population of the anal canal. Abdominoperineal resection is advocated for those carcinoids exceeding 2 cm. in diameter, although lymph nodal spread may be associated with smaller lesions.

OTHER ANAL DISORDERS: PRURITUS ANI

There are a variety of other disorders that may occur, and these include psoriasis, contact dermatitis, lichen sclerosis, and multiple sebaceous cysts.

Pruritus is a symptom that may be caused by any of the disorders previously mentioned, by poor hygiene, or as the result of certain anorectal conditions such as hemorrhoids, fissure, anal polyps, proctitis, rectal prolapse, and neoplasms. The investigation of the patient with pruritus should follow the usual pattern, with a thorough examination of the perianal skin, anal canal, and rectum with a proctoscope. The special investigations performed may include (1) urine testing for glycosuria; (2) perianal skin scrapings for mycologic examination, which should be taken before lubricant is placed on the skin; (3) examination of the perianal skin under ultraviolet light; and (4) biopsy.

Treatment consists of managing any underlying or aggravating cause. However, in a large proportion of patients, the situation can be relieved by simple attention to anal hygiene. This involves not only cleanliness but the avoidance of rubbing and scratching. Cure is nearly impossible in a patient who persists in the latter habits.

Shafik[49] has proposed that idiopathic pruritus is initiated by the antigenic action of either "epithelial debris," which he identified in remnants of the anorectal sinuses in the lower rectal neck, or the secretions from these sinuses. He has proposed that scleropathy (5 per cent solution of phenol in almond oil in the subcutaneous tissue of the rectal neck) destroys the epithelial debris or entraps them in a fibrous tissue mass, alleviating pruritus. This hypothesis of an anatomic basis for pruritus is as yet unproven, and the complications of anal sclerotherapy can be severe, including sloughing, cellulitis, and abscess formation.[49]

SELECTED REFERENCES

Beahrs, O. H., Ravo, B., and Khubchandani, I. T. (Eds.): Techniques of Colorectal Surgery. Surg. Clin. North Am., *68*(6), 1988.
This excellent issue of Surgical Clinics *brought together an international field of surgeons, surgical anatomists, and physiologists. The result was a comprehensive update of colorectal surgery.*

Sir Alan Parks, 1920–1982—Surgeon and Scientist. Symposium Proceedings, November 1983, Royal College of Surgeons of England, London.
This collection of the contributions of the late Sir Alan Parks to colorectal surgery highlights his role in the molding of modern concepts of the anatomy and physiology of the anorectal region.

REFERENCES

1. Ackerman, D. M., Polk, H. C., Jr., and Schrodt, G. R.: Desmoplastic melanoma of the anus. Hum. Pathol., *16*:1277, 1985.
2. Akwari, O. E., Dozois, R. R., Weiland, L. H., and Beahrs, O. H.: Leiomyosarcoma of the small and large bowel. Cancer, *42*:1375, 1978.
3. Barron, J.: Office ligation of internal hemorrhoids. Am. J. Surg., *105*:563, 1963.
4. Bogomoletz, W. V., Potet, F., and Molas, G.: Condylomata acuminata, giant condyloma acuminatum (Buschke-Lowenstine tumour) and verrucous squamous carcinoma of the perianal and anorectal region: A continuous precancerous spectrum? Histopathology, *9*:1155, 1985.
5. Boman, B. M., Moertel, C. G., O'Connell, M. J., Scott, M., Weiland, L. H., Beart, R. W., Gunderson, L. L., and Spencer, R. J.: Carcinoma of the anal canal: A clinical and pathologic study of 188 cases. Cancer, *54*:114, 1984.
6. Browning, G. G. P., and Motson, R. W.: Results of Parks operation for faecal incontinence after anal sphincter injury. Br. Med. J., *286*:1873, 1983.
7. Browning, G. G. P., and Parks, A. G.: Post anal repair for neuropathic faecal incontinence: Correlation of clinical results and anal canal pressures. Br. J. Surg., *70*:101, 1983.
8. Dougherty, B. G., and Evans, H. L.: Carcinoma of the anal canal: A study of 79 cases. Am. J. Clin. Pathol., *83*:159, 1985.
9. Fenger, C.: The anal transitional zone. Acta Pathol. Microbiol. Scand. [A], *86*:225, 1978.
10. Floyd, W. F., and Wells, E. W.: Electromyography of the sphincteri ani externus in man. J. Physiol., *122*:599, 1953.
11. Gibbons, C. P., Bannister, J. J., and Read, N. W.: Role of constipation and anal hypertonia in the pathogenesis of haemorrhoids. Br. J. Surg., *75*:656, 1988.
12. Goldberg, S. M.: Closed haemorrhoidectomy. *In* Todd, I. P., and Fielding, L. P. (Eds.): Rob and Smith's Operative Surgery, 4th ed. Colon, Rectum and Anus. London, Butterworths, 1983.
13. Haas, P. A., Fox, T. A., and Hass, G. P.: The pathogenesis of hemorrhoids. Dis. Colon Rectum, *27*:442, 1984.
14. Henrichsen, S., and Christiansen, J.: Incidence of fistula-in-ano complicating anorectal sepsis: A prospective body. Br. J. Surg., *73*:371, 1986.
15. Jones, E. A., Morson, B. C.: Mucinous adenocarcinoma in anorectal fistulae. Histopathology, *8*:279, 1984.
16. Kalogeropoulos, N. K., Antonakopoulos, G. N., Agapitos, M. B., and Papacharalampous, N. X.: Spindle cell carcinoma (pseudosarcoma) of the anus: A light, electron microscopic and immunocytochemical study of a case. Histopathology, *9*:987, 1985.
17. Khubchandani, I., Trimpi, H., and Sheets, J. A.: Closed hemorrhoidectomy with local anesthesia. Surg. Gynecol. Obstet., *135*:955, 1972.
18. Khubchandani, I. T.: Operative hemorrhoidectomy. Surg. Clin. North Am., *68*:1411, 1988.
19. Khubchandani, I. T., and Reed, J. F.: Sequelae of internal sphincterotomy for chronic fissure in ano. Br. J. Surg., *76*:431, 1989.
20. Kratzer, G. L., and Dockerty, M. B.: Histopathology of the anal ducts. Surg. Gynecol., *84*:333, 1947.
21. Lee, S. H., Zucker, M., and Sato, T.: Primary adenocarcinoma of an anal gland with secondary perianal fistulas. Hum. Pathol., *12*:1034, 1981.
22. Levin, S. E., et al.: Transitional cloacogenic carcinoma of the anus. Dis. Colon Rectum, *20*:17, 1977.
23. Lewis, M. D.: Cryosurgical hemorrhoidectomy. Dis. Colon Rectum, *15*:128, 1972.
24. Linder, J. H., and Myers, R. T.: Perianal Paget's disease. Am. J. Surg., *36*:342, 1970.
25. Lipsett, P., and Allo, M. D.: AIDS and the surgeon. Surg. Clin. North Am., *68*:73, 1988.
26. Lopez, M. J., Bliss, D. P., Kraybill, W. G., and Soybel, D. I.: Carcinoma of the anal region. Curr. Probl. Surg. *26*(8):525, 1989.
27. Mann, C. V.: Rectal prolapse. *In* Morson, B. C.: Diseases of the Colon, Rectum and Anus. New York, Appleton-Century-Crofts, 1969.
28. Marks, C. G., and Ritchie, J. K.: Anal fistulas at St. Mark's Hospital. Br. J. Surg., *64*:84, 1977.
29. McNamara, M. J., Percy, J. P., and Fielding, I. R.: A manometric study of anal fissure treated by subcutaneous lateral internal sphincterotomy. Ann. Surg., *211*:235, 1990.
30. Miller, R. D.: Gas embolism produced by hydrogen peroxide irrigation. Anesthesiology, *63*:316, 1985.
31. Milligan, E. T. C., Morgan, C. N., Jones, L. E., and Officer, R.: Surgical anatomy of the anal canal, the operative treatment of hemorrhoids. Lancet, *11*:1119, 1937.
32. Misra, M. C., and Kapur, B. M. L.: A new non-operative approach to fistula in ano. Br. J. Surg., *75*:1093, 1988.
33. Moore, W.: Recurrent melanoma of the rectum after previous removal from the verge of the anus in a man aged 65. Lancet, *11*:290, 1857.
34. Nigro, N. D.: Multidisciplinary management of cancer of the anus. World J. Surg., *11*:446, 1987.
35. Parks, A. G.: The surgical treatment of hemorrhoids. Br. J. Surg., *43*:337, 1956.
36. Parks, A. G.: Modern concepts of the anatomy of the anorectal region. Postgrad. Med., *34*:360, 1958.
37. Parks, A. G.: Pathogenesis and treatment of fistula-in-ano. Br. Med. J., *1*:463, 1961.
38. Parks, A. G.: Squamous carcinoma of the anal canal. Ann. Gastroenterol. Hepatol., *17*:103, 1981.
39. Parks, A. G., Porter, N. H., and Melzak, J.: Experimental study of the reflex mechanism controlling the muscles of the pelvic floor. Dis. Colon Rectum, *5*:407, 1962.
40. Parks, A. G., Swash, M., and Urich, H.: Sphincter denervation in anorectal incontinence and rectal prolapse. Gut, *18*:656, 1977.
41. Pescatori, M., and Ravo, B.: Diagnostic anorectal functional studies. Manometry, sphincter electromyography and defecography. Surg. Clin. North Am., *68*:1231, 1988.
42. Pescatori, M., Vulpio, C., and Castiglioni, G. C.: Congenital anovulvar fistula in a 30-year-old woman. Br. J. Surg., *73*:161, 1986.
43. Phillips, S. F., and Edwards, D. A.: Some aspects of anal continence and defecation. Gut, *6*:396, 1965.
44. Pople, I. K., and Ralphs, D. N. L.: An etiology for fistula in ano. Br. J. Surg., *75*:904, 1988.
45. Ramanujam, P. S., and Prasad, M. L.: The role of seton in fistulotomy of the anus. Surg. Gynecol. Obstet., *157*:419, 1983.
46. Rickert, R. R., Larkey, I. G., Kantor, E. B.: Granular-cell tumors (myoblastomas) of the anal region. Dis. Colon Rectum, *21*:413, 1978.
47. Rosai, J.: Anus. *In* Rosai, J. (Ed.): Ackerman's Surgical Pathology, 7th ed. St. Louis, C. V. Mosby Company, 1989.
48. Scoma, J. A., and Levy, E. L.: Bowen's disease of the anus: Report of two cases. Dis. Colon Rectum, *18*:137, 1975.
49. Shafik, A.: A new concept of the anatomy of the anal sphincter mechanism and physiology of defecation. Treatment of hemorrhoids: Report of a technique. Am. J. Surg., *148*:393, 1984.
50. Shukla, H. S., Gupta, S. C., Singh, G., and Singh, P. A.: Tubercular fistula in ano. Br. J. Surg., *75*:38, 1988.

51. Sir Alan Parks, 1920–1982—Surgeon and Scientist. Symposium Proceedings, November 1983, Royal College of Surgeons of England, London.

52. Stelzer, F., Staubesand, J., and Machleidt, H.: Das Corpus cavernosum recti—Die Grundlage der inneren Hamorrhoiden. Langenbecks Arch. Klin. Chir., 299:302, 1962.

53. Thomson, J. P. S.: The surgical management of perianal manifestations of Crohn's disease. In Allan, R. N., Keighley, M. R. B., Alexander-Williams, J., and Hawkins, C. (Eds.): Inflammatory Bowel Diseases. New York, Churchill Livingstone, 1983.

54. Tsai, S.-K., Lee, T.-Y., and Mok, M. S.: Gas embolism produced by hydrogen peroxide irrigation of an anal fistula during anesthesia. Anesthesiology, 63:316, 1985.

55. Walls, E. W.: Observations on the microscope anatomy of the human anal canal. Br. J. Surg., 45:504, 1958.

56. Wanebo, H. J., Woodruff, J. M., Farr, G. H., and Wuan, S. H.: Anorectal melanoma. Cancer, 47:1891, 1981.

57. Wassef, R., Rothenberger, D. A., and Goldberg, S. M.: Rectal prolapse. Curr. Probl. Surg., 23(6):397, 1986.

58. Wedell, J., Meier zu Eissen, P., Banzhaf, G., and Kleine, L.: Sliding flap advancement for the treatment of high level fistulae. Br. J. Surg., 74:390, 1987.

59. Zinberg, S. S., Stern, D. H., Furman, D. S., and Wittles, J. M.: A personal experience in comparing three non-operative techniques for treating internal hemorrhoids. Am. J. Gastroenterol., 84:488, 1989.

33

THE LIVER

William C. Meyers, M.D.

DEVELOPMENT OF HEPATOBILIARY SURGERY

For centuries the liver has been a mysterious organ with complex anatomy, an overwhelming number of functions, and an extraordinary capability to regenerate. The organ's large size and abundant blood supply contributed to the respect paid to this organ in most civilizations and operating theaters. Improved understanding of anatomy and physiology, combined with a number of recently developed surgical techniques, has led from myth and mystery to the emergence of the specialty of hepatobiliary surgery.

The Liver in Early History

For the Babylonians (3000–2000 B.C.) the liver was the primary instrument used in the art of divination in astronomy and occasionally in settling major disputes. In this practice, pegs were inserted into clay liver models. A record was kept of the variations from normal anatomy encountered in livers of sacrificed animals and the overall prognosis determined by the similarity of the sacrificed liver to the model. This mystical practice, which still goes on today in sections of Burma, Borneo, and Uganda, formed the basis for the understanding of the anatomy of the liver in early civilizations.

The liver was also considered by the Babylonians to be the seat of the soul. The soul's seat changed to the heart for the Egyptians, but early Greeks restored the importance of the liver in the beginning of the humoral theory of medicine. Hippocrates (ca. 460–377 B.C.) incorporated the four basic substances (fire, water, air, and earth) into man, and these four elements were transformed from food by the heat of digestion into the four body humors: blood, phlegm, black bile, and yellow bile. The soul had three parts, the nutritive part residing in the liver. Galen viewed the liver as a focus for formation of heat, blood, and blood vessels. The humoral theory of medicine, with the liver as a central focus, prevailed until the seventeenth century. Undoubtedly, the Greeks' respect for the liver stemmed in part from their knowledge of the prodigious regenerative power of the liver, indicated by the myth of Prometheus.

Development of Anatomy

Knowledge of the liver's gross anatomy developed slowly until the latter half of the present century. Considerable appreciation of the topographic anatomy was evident to the Babylonians (Fig. 1), including the locations of the gallbladder, falciform ligament, and caudate and quadrate lobes, and the portal venous and vena caval anatomy. The Egyptians contributed to the understanding of topographic anatomy through their permissive attitude in the practice of human necropsy. The Greeks provided more detailed description as well as an understanding of some variability of the topographic lobes. Galen (A.D. 130–201) believed that the hepatic, arterial, and portal systems terminated in minute connections where blood gradually passed to hepatic veins and ultimately the vena cava.

Knowledge of anatomy was in general rudimentary until the sixteenth and seventeenth centuries. Da Vinci masterfully sketched the liver. Vesalius produced his masterpiece, *De Humani Corporis Fabrica,* and Fabricius accurately described the umbilical, portal, and hepatic veins and also the gross anatomy of the biliary tract. In 1654, Glisson published his *Anatomia Hepatis* in which he redefined hepatic function as well as described the liver capsule, which followed the branching pattern of the portal vein and bile duct.

In the latter part of the nineteenth century, the liver's anatomy was suspected to be not quite so simple as its topographic features (principally the falciform ligament) suggested. In 1888, Rex provided an accurate gross anatomic description of the mammalian liver and this was followed by a similar description of man by Cantlie in 1897. The principal basis of this description is that the liver is divided into two relatively equal masses, the right and left lobes, by an interlobar plane passing obliquely through the bed of the gallbladder to the sulcus of the inferior vena cava. This gross anatomy was later confirmed by McIndoe and Counseller and others. A more recent second classification of the gross anatomy was initially described by Couinaud in 1954; in this classification (now known as the "French" system), the liver is divided into eight segments.

An understanding of the microscopic anatomy of the liver originated in the later seventeenth century with Malpighi. Using a primitive scope, he recognized a lobular arrangement of the liver although he did not identify hepatocytes. Two centuries later, Kiernan (1833) described a basic hepatic unit of lobules centered on hepatic venules. He accurately described portal triads, which became known as "Kiernan's spaces." Important observations concerning the hepatocytes and cell plates occurred later in the nineteenth century. Kupffer described his cells in 1876 and Disse his periendothelial space in 1890. The concepts of canaliculi and sinusoids developed at the turn of the nineteenth century. In 1954, Rappaport developed the concept of liver acini consisting of cylindrical masses of hepatic tissue surrounding portal triads, with various functions served by hepatocytes depending on proximity to the portal inflow.

Biliary anatomic variability has been the cause of confusion for years. Galen described a dual system with separate insertions into the stomach and duodenum, which now, of course, is known to be unusual. As late as the nineteenth century the gallbladder was commonly described as usually connecting to the right ductal system. Rex and Cantlie's descriptions recognized that the biliary system consisted of two main divisions with the gallbladder usually connecting to a common duct. Only in the past century have there been accurate estimates of biliary variability.

Physiology

Although understanding of hepatic function has been expanded greatly in this century, knowledge concerning hepatic physiology developed slowly until the mid-nineteenth century with the work of Bernard. The Hippocratic-Galenic theory that the liver was the center of nutrition is realized to be partly correct, although the strict dogmatic principles espoused by the promoters of this concept took many centuries to correct. Galen

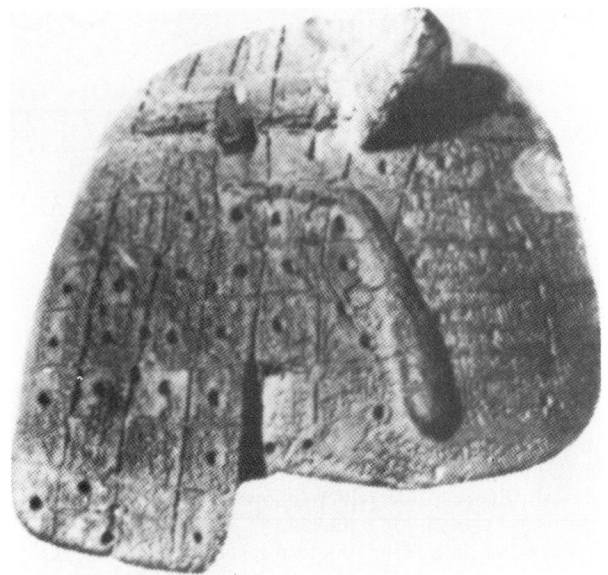

Figure 1. Clay model of sheep's liver from the Assyro-Babylonian era, ca. 2000 B.C. (Reproduced from the British Museum of Art.)

believed strongly that a natural spirit resided in the liver which directed the overall process of nutrition and blood flow. His strict principles included that all functions of the liver were related to a filtering action into hepatic venous blood, lymph, or bile. A central observation that contributed to the erosion of some of these strict principles was the finding by Bartholin in 1652 that some mesenteric lacteals reached the liver and the realization by Rudbeck a year later that lymph flowed from the liver rather than to it, which challenged the Galenic concept of the liver as the source of "sanguification." The concept of the liver as a center of metabolism was developed in the nineteenth century from an appreciation of the microscopic anatomy; development of inorganic and organic chemistry, biochemistry, and physiology; discoveries such as synthesis of urea; analysis of the composition of food; and the identification of nutritional deficiencies, such as for vitamin A and protein. In 1843, Bernard reported a number of physiologic discoveries of importance to the liver. His work included recognition of the importance of liver in glucose production and storage, as well as integrative functions with gastric and pancreatic juice. A number of bile acids became recognized in the mid-nineteenth century, although their structure was not elucidated until the twentieth century. Most of what is known about other important hepatic functions such as protein and vitamin synthesis and the liver's role in coagulation also developed since the latter half of the nineteenth century.

Origins of Hepatobiliary Surgery

Although there were some origins in earlier centuries, hepatobiliary surgery is primarily a twentieth century art with many of the refinements occurring in the past two to three decades. Therapy of liver disease began in the ancient civilizations with numerous empiric formulas for the treatment of various abdominal ailments. Hippocrates attached great importance to the diet and hygiene as a basis for medical therapy. Hepatic abscess drainage was advocated by Hippocrates (ca. 500 B.C.), Erasistratus (ca. 300 B.C.), Celsus (ca. A.D. 200), and Aretaeus (ca. A.D. 200). Hippocrates probably encountered cases of hydatid cysts.

New treatments of hepatobiliary disorders emerged in the eighteenth and nineteenth centuries, including prophylactic therapy. In 1793, Baillie suggested the avoidance of alcohol in the dietary treatment of cirrhosis. In the mid-1800s, Frerichs, considered by many to be the father of hepatology, recommended alkaline mineral waters and herb juices for dissolution of fat. Salt and water restriction became standard for the treatment of ascites in the 1800s. Of note also in that century was that some physicians confused the practice of phlebotomy with drainage of hepatic abscesses and advocated direct hepatic puncture with a trochar, with a mortality rate of 80 to 90 per cent. Various medical problems were attributed to a "wandering liver" or "hepatoptosis." Surgical therapy included "ventrofixation" of a lobe of the liver, performed by Billroth in 1882. The first elective resection was performed in 1888 by Langenbuch for that syndrome. The "corset tumor" removed in that resection probably represented an adenoma.

Surgical therapy for portal hypertension began at the turn of the nineteenth-twentieth century. Eck performed his famous fistula operation consisting of a side-to-side mesocaval shunt with portal vein ligation in 1877 and had one long-term surviving dog. Of great importance was the development of Carrel's vascular surgery techniques. Carrel was said to be greatly stimulated by the death of French President Sadi Carnot, who died from a stab wound of the portal vein in 1884. Although there were some isolated reports of portosystemic shunts performed in the later nineteenth and early twentieth centuries, extensive experience with shunts is considered to have been initiated in 1945 with the report of Whipple, Blakemore, and Lord.

Biliary operations have a longer history than those on the liver. The first procedure was done for gallstones. The first successful procedure was probably performed by Ibn Sina, who drained an abdominal abscess leading to a biliary fistula, probably a complication of gallstone disease. Trendelenburg reported that Fabricius performed a cholecystolithotomy in 1618. Bobbs of Indiana performed the first well-documented cholecystolithotomy in 1867. One interesting early biliary operation was a cholecystolithotomy performed in 1881 by Halsted on his mother in the middle of the night. Langenbuch performed the first successful cholecystectomy in 1882. Significant advances in biliary surgery include the development of the technique of oral cholecystography in 1922 by Graham and Cole, choledochoscopy in 1923 by Bakes, the discovery of vitamin K by Dam in 1929, and intraoperative cholangiography introduced in 1932 by Mirizzi. The first successful resection of cholangiocarcinoma was reported in 1903. Cholecystectomy became established as a safe surgical procedure in the 1940s and 1950s. Endoscopic and retrograde cholangiography are products of the 1970s. Developing refinements of the 1980s and 1990s include intraoperative ultrasonography and laparoscopic cholecystectomy.

The development of hepatobiliary surgery culminates in the rise and increased safety of hepatic resections and liver transplantation. A number of series of hepatic resections are now reported in excess of 100 patients. The mortality has steadily decreased from 20 per cent 2 decades ago to consistently less than 5 per cent and, in several centers, to less than 1 per cent in elective operations. The increased safety has followed improved technology and understanding of the anatomy and physiology of the liver. With improved safety has come an increased confidence and a wide expansion of the indications for resection. The most common indication for partial liver resection in most centers remains tumor.

A spectacular advance in hepatic surgery and hepatic therapy in general has been the success of liver transplantation. Welch performed the first experimental liver transplant in 1955 using a heterotopic technique in dogs, but the procedure was abandoned because of difficulties in maintaining vascular inflow and adequate biliary drainage. In 1959, Moore and Starzl (Fig. 2) independently achieved successful orthotopic liver transplantation in dogs, the same year that Kasai and Suzuki reported their first hepatoportoenterostomy for biliary atresia. The first human liver transplant was performed by Starzl in Colorado in 1963. Subsequently, Starzl and Calne developed large series of liver transplant patients. Other important advances in transplantation include identification of the immunosuppression characteristics of cyclosporine by Borel in 1972 and

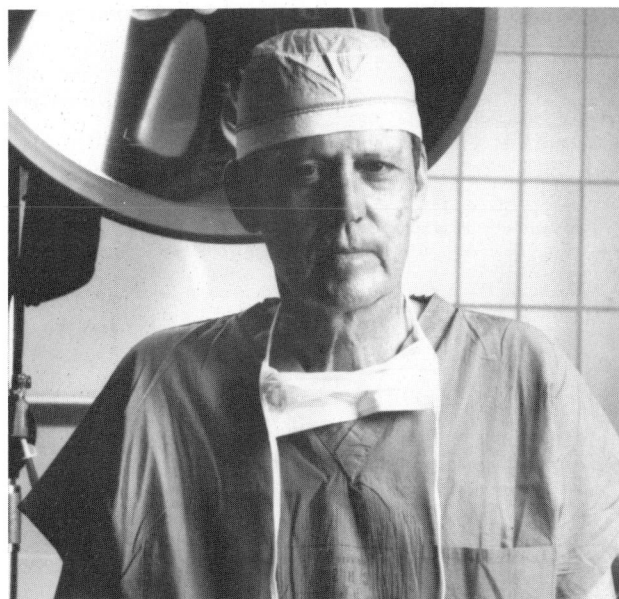

Figure 2. Recent photograph of Thomas Starzl (born 1926), who performed the first liver transplant.

the first clinical trials of cyclosporine in 1978. Early reports now indicate that there may be even more effective agents than cyclosporine. A recent important achievement, which combines the advances made in hepatic resection and transplantation, is the successful transplantation of the left lateral segment from a live parent to a child, performed in 1989 at the University of Chicago.

It is interesting to note the exchange of roles surgery and medicine have had in the treatment of hepatobiliary disorders over the past 2 decades. The development of endoscopic, percutaneous, and other lithotriptic approaches may be radically changing the treatment of gallstones. However, many of the medical disorders such as cirrhosis and metabolic deficiencies are being treated by liver transplantation. With refinements in techniques and the emergence of a specialty, changes in the structure of the field of hepatobiliary surgery are likely to continue. Two international organizations now exist, the International Biliary Association (IBA) and the Hepato-Biliary-Pancreatic Society (HPB), and efforts are being made to consolidate the two with formation of national chapters, from which it is hoped that much needed cooperative studies will be conducted. Drastic changes are likely to occur in the next few years in both the surgical techniques and training of hepatobiliary surgeons to include comprehensive use of endoscopy, radiology, and more invasive procedures.

SELECTED REFERENCES

Beal, J. M.: Historical perspective of gallstone disease. Surg. Gynecol. Obstet., *158*:181, 1984.
Detailed article on surgical aspects of gallstone disease.

Chen, T. S., and Chen, P. S.: Understanding the Liver, a History. Westport, CT, Greenwood Press, 1984.
Remarkable book on the development of hepatology. Examines in detail the historical aspects of the understanding of anatomy, physiology, and diseases pertinent to hepatobiliary surgery.

Meyers, W. C., and Jones, R. S.: Development of liver and biliary surgery. *In* Meyers, W. C., and Jones, R. S. (Eds.): Textbook of Liver and Biliary Surgery. Philadelphia, J. B. Lippincott Company, 1990.
Includes details on many of the historical aspects of hepatobiliary surgery.

Starzl, T. E., Iwatsuki, S., Van Thiel, D. H., et al.: Evolution of liver transplantation. Hepatology, 2:614, 1982.
Historical review of liver transplantation by the individual who has contributed the most.

REFERENCES

General

1. Beal, J. M.: Historical perspective of gallstone disease. Surg. Gynecol. Obstet., *158*:181, 1984.
2. Beck, J.: Surgery of the liver. J.A.M.A., *78*:1063, 1902.
3. Budd, G.: Diseases of the Liver. Philadelphia, Blanchard and Lea, 1853.
4. Chakravorty, R. C., and Wanebo, H. J.: Historic preamble: Liver and biliary cancer. In Wanebo, H. J. (Ed.): Hepatic and Biliary Cancer. New York, Marcel Dekker, 1987.
5. Chen, T. S., and Chen, P. S.: Understanding the Liver, a History. Westport, CT, Greenwood Press, 1984.
6. Frerichs, F. T.: A Clinical Treatise on Diseases of the Liver. Vols. I and II. C. Murchinson, trans. London, New Sydenham Society, 1860–1861.

Early History

7. Cahill, K. M.: Platonic concepts of hepatology. Arch. Intern. Med., *111*:819, 1963.
8. Celsus: De medicina. Books I, II, IV, and VII. W. G. Spencer, trans. Cambridge, MA, Loeb Classical Library, Harvard University Press, 1935.
9. Glenn, F.: Biliary tract disease since antiquity. Acad. Med. Bull. N.Y., *47*:329, 1971.
10. Jastrow, M.: The Liver in Antiquity and the Beginnings of Anatomy. Philadelphia, Trans. Coll. Physicians, 1907.
11. Lloyd, G. E. R.: Hippocrates, the Sacred Disease: Hippocratic Writings. Harmondsworth, Penguin Books, 1978.
12. Siegel, R. E.: Galen's System of Physiology and Medicine. Basel, S Karger, 1968, p. 241.
13. Singer, C.: A Short History of Anatomy and Physiology from the Greeks to Harvey. New York, Dover, 1975.

Anatomy and Physiology

14. Admirand, W. H., and Small, D. M.: The physiochemical basis of cholesterol gallstone formation in man. J. Clin. Invest., *47*:1043, 1968.
15. Bernard, C.: Du suc gastrique et de son role dans la nutrition. These Paris, Rignoux 38, 1843.
16. Bernard, C.: Sur le mecanisme de la formation du sucre dans le foie. Compt. Rend., *41*:461, 1855.
17. Bernard, C.: Lecon sur les proprietes physiologiques et les alterations pathologiques des liquides de l'organisme. Vol. 2. Paris, Balliere, 1859, p. 192.
18. Cantlie, J.: On a new arrangement of the right and left lobes of the liver. J. Anat. Physiol. (London) (Section Proc. Anat. Soc. Great Britain and Ireland), *32*:iv, 1877.
19. Charcot, J. M.: Leçons sur les Maladies du Foie, des Voies Biliaries, et des Reins. Paris, Progress Medical, 1877.
20. Couinaud, C.: Bases anatomiques des hepatectomies gauche et droite réglées, techniques que en deroulent. J. Chir. Paris, *70*:933, 1954.
21. Disse, J.: Über die Lymphbahnen der Saugetierleber. Arch. Mikr. Anat., *36*:203, 1890.
22. Glisson, F.: Anatomia Hepatis. Amsterdam, Ravesteyn, 1659. Cited in Heaton, K. W. (Ed.): Bile Salts in Health and Disease. Edinburgh, Churchill Livingstone, 1972.
23. Healey, J. E., Jr., and Schroy, P. C.: Anatomy of the biliary ducts within the human liver. Arch. Surg., *66*:599, 1953.
24. Hjortsjo, C. H.: The topography of the intrahepatic duct systems. Acta Anat. (Basel), *11*:599, 1951.
25. Kiernan, F.: The Anatomy and Physiology of the Liver. Phil. Trans., 1833.
26. Kupffer, C. von: Über Sternzellen der Leber. Arch. Mikr. Anat., *12*:353, 1876.
27. Lipman, T. O.: Wohler's preparation of urea and the fate of vitalism. J. Chem. Educ., *41*:452, 1964.
28. Mall, F. P.: A study of the structural unit of the liver. Am. J. Anat., *5*:2270, 1906.
29. Morgagni, J. B.: The Seats and Causes of Disease. Vol. 2. B. Alexander, trans. New York, Hafner, 1960 (reprint of 1769 London edition).
30. Rappaport, A. M.: The structural and functional units in the human liver (liver acinus). Anat. Rec., *130*:673, 1958.
31. Rex, H.: Beitrage zur Morphologie der Saugerleber. Morphol. Jahrb. (Leipzig), *14*:517, 1888.
32. Young, F. G.: Claude Bernard and the discovery of glycogen: A century of retrospect. Br. Med. J., *1*:1431, 1957.
33. Young, J.: Malpighi. N. Z. Med. J., *20*:1, 1921.

Hepatobiliary Surgery

34. Beal, J. M.: The surgeon's library; historical perspective of gallstone disease. Surg. Gynecol. Obstet., *158*:181, 1984.
35. Berman, C.: Primary Carcinoma of the Liver. London, HK Lewis, 1951.
36. Calne, R. Y., and Williams, R.: Survival after orthotopic liver transplantation: A followup report of two patients. Br. Med. J., *3*:436, 1970.
37. Charcot, J. M.: Lecons sur les Maladies du Foie, des Voies Biliaires, et des Reins. Paris, Progress Medical, 1877.
38. Courvoisier, L. G.: Casuistish-statistiche Beitrage zur Pathologie und Chirurgie der Gallenwege. Leipzig, Vogel FCW, 1890.
39. Donovan, A. J., and Covey, P. C.: Early history of the portacaval shunt in humans. Surg. Gynecol. Obstet., *147*:423, 1978.

40. Eck, N. V.: The question of ligature of the portal vein. Voen. Med. J. (St. Petersburg), *130*:1877. Transl. into English in Child, C. G.: Eck's fistula. Surg. Gynecol. Obstet., *96*:375, 1953.

41. Frerichs, F. T.: Diseases of the Liver. Vols. I and II. London, The New Sydenham Society, 1860–1861.

42. Glenn, F., and Grafe, W. R., Jr.: Historical events in biliary tract surgery. Arch. Surg., *93*:848, 1966.

43. Goldsmith, N. A., and Woodburne, R. T.: The surgical anatomy pertaining to liver resections. Surg. Gynecol. Obstet. *105*:310, 1957.

44. Keen, W. W.: On resection of the liver. Boston Med. Surg. J., *126*:405, 1892.

45. Langenbuch, C.: Ein Fall von Extirpation der Gallenblase wegen chronischer Cholelithiasis. Berlin Klin. Wochenschr., *48*:725, 1882.

46. Langenbuch, D.: Ein Fall von Resektion eines linksseitigen Schnurlappens der Leber. Heilung Berl. Klin. Wochenschr., 1888.

47. Moore, F. D. et al: One-stage homotransplantation of the liver following total hepatectomy in dogs. Transplant. Bull., *6*:103, 1959.

48. Rokitansky, C.: A Manual of Pathological Anatomy. Transl. by E. Sieveking. Philadelphia, Blanchard and Lea, 1855.

49. Starzl, T. E., et al.: Homotransplantation of the liver in humans. Surg. Gynecol. Obstet., *117*:659, 1963.

50. Starzl, T. E., Iwatsuki, S., Van Thiel, D. H., et al.: Evolution of liver transplantation. Hepatology, 2:614, 1982.

51. Tiffany, L. M.: Surgery of the liver. Boston Med. Surg. J., *122*, 1890.

52. Trendelenburg, F.: Die ersten 25 Jahre der deutschen Gesellschaft für Chirurgie. Berlin, V. Springer, 1923.

53. Warren, W. D., et al.: Selective trans-splenic decompression of gastroesophageal varices by distal splenorenal shunt. Ann. Surg., *166*:437, 1967.

54. Welch, C. S.: A note on transplantation of the whole liver in dogs. Transplant. Bull., 2:54, 1955.

55. Whipple, A. O.: Problem of portal hypertension in relation to hepatosplenopathies. Ann. Surg., *122*:449, 1945.

I

ANATOMY AND PHYSIOLOGY

William C. Meyers, M.D.

ANATOMY

The liver lies in the right upper quadrant of the abdomen, beneath the diaphragm and connected to the digestive tract via the portal vein and the biliary drainage system. Its large size and central location suggest a broad importance for the function of other organs. Anatomic features that enable the liver to function as an important integrator between the digestive system and the remainder of the body include (1) a dual blood supply with portal blood from the splanchnic system and the hepatic artery, (2) a specific architectural arrangement of single cells and cell masses that facilitates exchange between blood and hepatocytes, (3) a specific orientation of the hepatocytes that compartmentalizes biliary versus blood pathways, and (4) an organized biliary excretory system that regulates the enterohepatic circulation. This section considers aspects of the anatomic organization of the liver that are important for understanding both hepatic physiology and surgery.

NORMAL DEVELOPMENT. The liver begins as a diverticulum (Fig. 1) at the superior intestinal portal, below the heart, on day 22 after ovulation. Within several days the diverticulum grows into the transverse septum, which contains the vitelline and umbilical veins. Although undoubtedly differentiation occurs before the primordium becomes visible, the exact processes involved in the differentiation remain unclear. At least two separate inductive endodermal processes are likely to be involved.[6] In the first, lateral splanchnic mesoderm migrates anteriorly to fuse across the midline with the embryonic pharynx. The hepatic bud appears as hepatic and cardiac mesenchyme segregates. In the second, hepatic mesenchyme stimulates endodermal cord cells to differentiate into hepatocytes, and conversely the endoderm stimulates the mesenchyme to form sinusoids. Individual endodermal cells migrate freely with mesenchymal cells of the transverse septum. An alternative suggestive source of hepatocytes is from mesodermal coelomic lining.

The right umbilical vein regresses in the sixth week, leaving the left to carry placental blood to the fetus. The intrahepatic veins attain their arrangement by the next week. Inflow vasculature, bile ducts, and reduction of the thickness of hepatic cords from 3 to 5 cells to a single cell occurs later. Blood cells are produced in the liver between the ninth and twenty-fourth week. The liver protrudes from the transverse septum into the abdomen with the bare area a reminder of its origin. Bile ducts

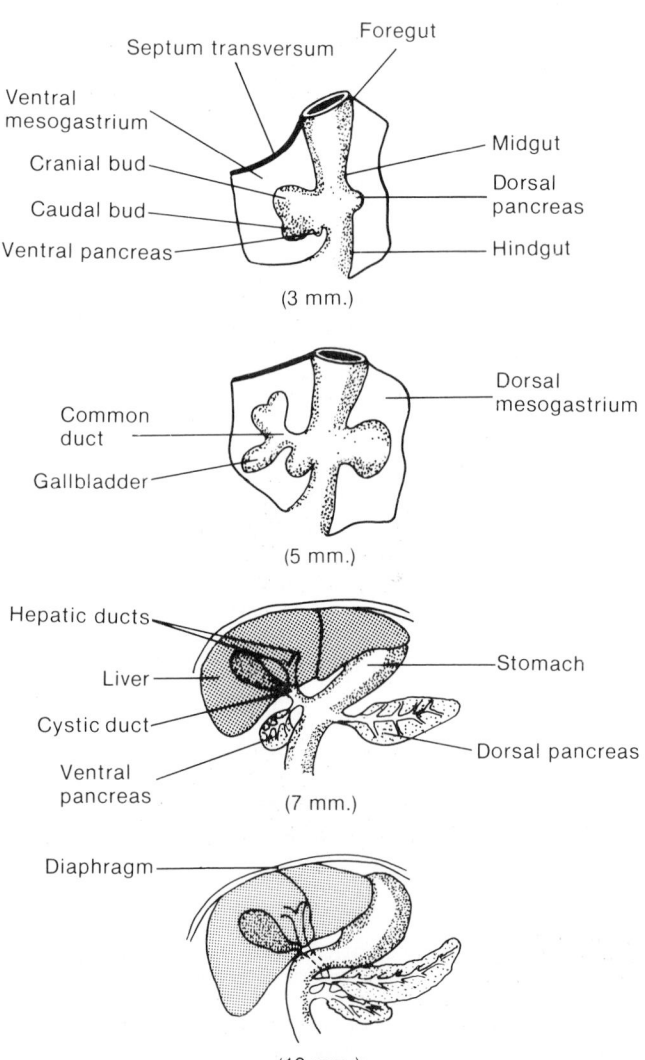

Figure 1. Embryologic development of the liver through the 3-mm., 5-mm., 7-mm., and 12-mm. somite stages. (From Theler, M. M., and Law, L. W.: Anatomy and embryology. *In* Sleisenger, M. M., and Fordtran, J. S., Gastrointestinal disease, 2nd ed. Philadelphia, W. B. Saunders Company, 1978, p. 1245.)

differentiate from hepatic cells and join an extrahepatic biliary system, appearing first in the hilum and then spreading peripherally. Bile formation may be evident as early as the third month.

The relative size of the liver decreases to approximately 5 per cent of body volume from 10 per cent in the ninth week of gestation. The right lobe increases in size with the left lobe decreasing and a left to right orientation of the hepatic artery occurs that reduces in relative caliber.

GENERAL DESCRIPTION. The topographic anatomy of the liver has been recognized for centuries.[1] It was not until this century, however, that corrosion casts and stereoscopic x-ray films[11,14,16] confirmed previous anatomic dissections and the true lobar anatomy of the liver was appreciated.[7,8,18] Studies by Rappaport and others, beginning in the 1950s, have provided a clearer concept of the hepatic functional unit, based on the organization of hepatocytes around portal triads.[17]

The liver is the largest gland in the body, weighing approximately 1500 gm. in the adult (Fig. 2). It represents about one fiftieth of the body weight of the adult and about one twentieth of the body weight of the newborn owing to its blood-forming activity during fetal life. The liver is covered by a fibrous capsule (Glisson's capsule) that extends into the parenchyma along the blood vessels and bile ducts. The superior surface conforms to the undersurface of the diaphragm, and the inferior surface is in contact with the duodenum, colon, kidney, adrenal gland, esophagus, and stomach. In the adult, the normal liver extends in the midclavicular line from approximately the right fifth intercostal space down to slightly below the costal margin. Therefore, it is essentially under the protection of the ribs. The gallbladder lies in a transpyloric plane on the undersurface of the liver. The entire liver is invested by peritoneum except for a "bare" area on the posterior superior surface adjacent to the inferior vena cava where Glisson's capsule is in direct contact with the diaphragm.

TOPOGRAPHIC ANATOMY. Reflections of peritoneum attach the liver to the abdominal wall, diaphragm, and abdominal viscera. These "ligaments" are as follows:

1. The falciform ligament, which attaches the liver to the anterior abdominal wall from the diaphragm to the umbilicus and incorporates in its deep border the ligamentum teres hepatis with the obliterated left umbilical vein. This venous system is usually atrophied in the adult but may remain patent, connecting the periumbilical superficial venous system to the portal system, particularly in patients with cirrhosis.

2. The anterior and posterior right and left coronary ligaments, which are continuous with the falciform ligament connecting the diaphragm to the liver. The lateral aspects of the anterior and posterior coronary ligaments form the right and left triangular ligaments. The area encompassed by the falciform, coronary, and triangular ligaments and the inferior vena cava and diaphragm defines the "bare" area of the liver.

3. The anterior layer of the lesser omentum, or gastrohepatic and hepatoduodenal ligaments, which is continuous with the left triangular ligament and contains the hepatic artery, portal vein, and common bile duct. The hepatoduodenal ligament is the anterior boundary of the epiploic foramen of Winslow. The two major hepatic veins that return blood to the systemic circulation drain directly into the inferior vena cava posterior to the liver.

There are four lobes of the liver: right, left, quadrate, and caudate. The topographic right lobe includes a portion of the liver to the right of the falciform ligament, and the left lobe a portion to the left. The quadrate lobe represents a rectangular junction on the inferior surface bounded by the umbilical fissure on the left, the gallbladder fossa on the right, and the portal triad posteriorly. The posterior (transverse) extension of the falciform ligament (ligamentum venosum) on the left and the impression of the inferior vena cava on the right delineate the caudate ("spigelian") lobe. The liver resembles the lung[17] because of its bilobar anatomy, a dual blood supply with both a venous and arterial source, and an important system of exchange with the outside environments (biliary and bronchial system). However, the liver's parenchymal mass exhibits many vascular and biliary intercommunications between the right and left systems. An example of the importance of these intercommunications is that biliary drainage of one lobe sometimes decompresses effectively the entire liver despite persistent obstruction of the other lobe.

LOBAR ANATOMY. The distribution of the major branches of the veins, arteries, or bile ducts of the liver do not conform precisely with the topographic anatomy. The relationships between the hepatic veins and portal vein branches determine the lobar anatomy of the liver. The lobar anatomy of the liver is best demonstrated by direct injection of its blood supply with substances such as methylene blue or colored celloidin (Fig. 3). A plane called the *portal fissure* ("Cantlie's line") passes from the left side of the gallbladder fossa to the left side of the inferior vena cava to divide the liver into *right* and *left lobes*. The left lobe

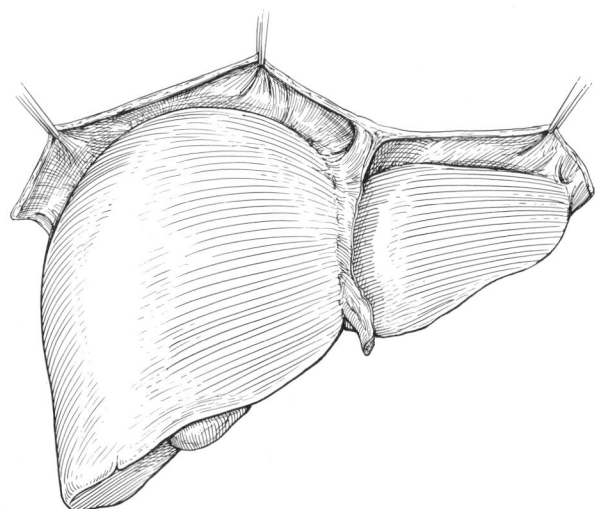

Figure 2. The anterior surface of the liver is viewed with the falciform ligament separating the lateral from the medial segments of the left lobe of the liver. Whereas the falciform ligament is the primary topographic landmark, this does not divide the two lobes of the liver. The vasculature and biliary systems divide into two lobes approximately determined by an anterior-posterior plane through the gallbladder and vena cava. On the right is the upper layer of the right coronary ligament and on the left is the left coronary ligament, which ends as the left triangular ligament.

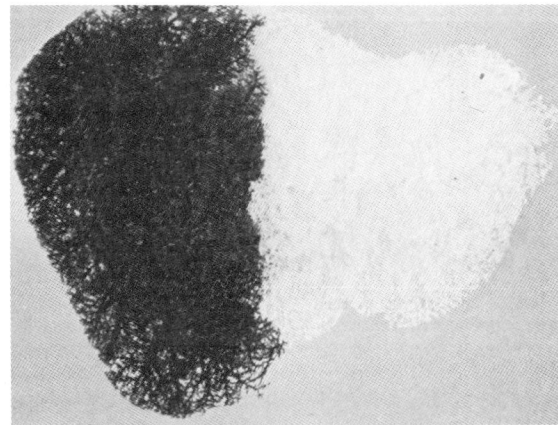

Figure 3. A corrosion case with the right and left portal veins injected with vinyl acetate of different colors demonstrates the true lobar anatomy of the liver, which is quite different from the topographic anatomy demonstrated in Figure 2. (From Mays, E. T.: In Calne, R. Y., and Della Rovere, G. Q. (Eds.): Liver Surgery. Philadelphia, W. B. Saunders Company, 1982.)

consists of a *medial segment* lying to the right of the falciform ligament and umbilical fissure plus a *lateral segment* to the left of the falciform ligament. The right lobe consists of an *anterior* and *posterior* segment. No visible surface marking designates this segmental separation. Conventionally most of the caudate "lobe" is in the medial segment of the left lobe, but it extends over the plane between the gallbladder and the inferior vena cava into the anatomic right lobe. This concept of lobar and segmental anatomy of the liver forms the basis for the classic types of major hepatic resection that correspond to "segments" described in the French system, as follows.

FRENCH "SEGMENTAL" SYSTEM. Another nomenclature system for hepatic anatomy was developed by Soupalt, Couinaud, and Bismuth (Fig. 4). This system considers not only the

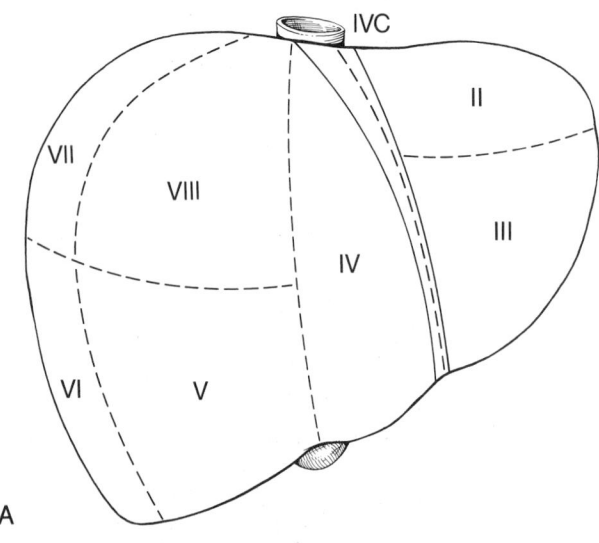

A

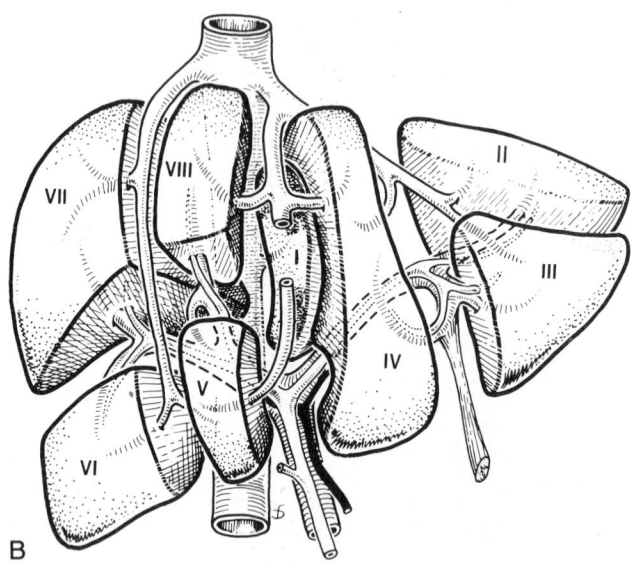

B

Figure 4. Segmental anatomy as defined by Couinaud. *A*, Intact liver. *B*, Schematic representation to emphasize segmental divisions according to the hepatic veins. Except for the falciform ligament, there are few topographic landmarks, and the subsegmental anatomy is generally not helpful surgically, using present techniques. The caudate lobe according to this scheme is subsegment 1 and is not shown. The line of demarcation between the right and left lobes is marked. The left lobe is divided into two segments, medial and lateral, by the falciform ligament in this illustration. Segment IV corresponds to the medial segment, and segments II and III correspond to the lateral segment. The right lobe has an anterior and a posterior segment. (*B* from Bismuth, H.: Surgical anatomy and anatomical surgery of the liver. *In* Blumgart, L. H. (Ed.): Surgery of the Liver and Biliary Tract. Edinburgh, Churchill Livingstone, 1988.)

hepatic venous drainage but also the portal, biliary, and arterial anatomy. Instead of four, there are eight segments: four on the right, three on the left, and one corresponding to the caudate lobe. Segment I corresponds to the caudate lobe. Segments II to IV compose the left lobe, and segments V to VIII the right. The three main hepatic veins divide the liver into four *sectors.* The planes containing the right, middle, and left hepatic veins are termed *portal* scissurae; the planes containing portal pedicles are termed *hepatic* scissurae. The caudate lobe is its own autonomous segment in the French system. "Segments," according to French, correspond generally to the "subsegments" described in the lobar anatomic classification.

PORTAL VEIN. The portal vein carries approximately 75 per cent of the blood supply to the liver. It is formed by the junction of the superior mesenteric and splenic veins behind the head of the pancreas and passes posterior to the first part of the duodenum at the level of the second lumbar vertebra. It usually measures between 1 and 3 cm. in diameter and 5 and 8 cm. in length before it divides into a right and left branch in the porta hepatis. In approximately 10 per cent of the population, the portal vein has three branches, with two going to the right lobe and one to the left lobe. It consistently courses behind the bile duct and hepatic artery and the hepatoduodenal ligament. Variants from the normal branching system are extremely rare. Other anatomic features of particular surgical importance include the following:

1. The portal vein has no valves, so that its pressure is easily estimated via all its branches. For example, during surgical procedures for portal hypertension, portal pressure may conveniently be measured in a small mesenteric or omental vein.

2. The intrahepatic portal venous channels must offer an extremely low resistance to blood flow in order to provide the large amount of flow to the liver, since much kinetic energy has already been lost passing through the capillary network of the digestive system. In addition, the intrahepatic architecture must be highly specialized to accommodate both the high-pressure hepatic arterial stream and the portal flow.

3. A long segment of portal vein proximal (in terms of flow) to its hepatic division usually exists, and the major branching usually occurs outside the liver.

4. Numerous tributaries of the portal vein outside the liver connect with the systemic venous system. Whereas these communications are of little importance in normal individuals, they often develop into large channels with a great deal of collateral flow in patients with portal hypertension.

The most important natural portal-systemic anastomoses include (1) the left gastric or coronary vein, which joins the splenic or portal vein near its confluence and connects with the esophageal venous plexus and also with tributaries of the superior vena cava; this is often the most important anastomotic system in the development of esophageal varices; (2) the short gastric and left gastroepiploic veins, which connect to the splenic vein and contribute to the formation of gastric and esophageal varices; (3) umbilical and periumbilical veins, which communicate with the left portal vein and may cause spectacular physical findings such as caput medusae or the loud Cruveilhier-Baumgarten bruit; (4) tributaries of the inferior mesenteric vein, which include superior hemorrhoidal veins that communicate with the middle and inferior hemorrhoidal veins of the systemic circulation and may cause large hemorrhoids; (5) other retroperitoneal communications, such as connections to the renal and adrenal veins.

The portal trunk divides into the left and right hepatic branches in the portal fissure (Fig. 5). The left branch is longer than the right and consists of two sections, the pars transversa and the pars umbilicus. Two branches to the lateral segment of the left lobe usually arise from the pars umbilicus near the plane of the falciform ligament. Branches from both sections supply

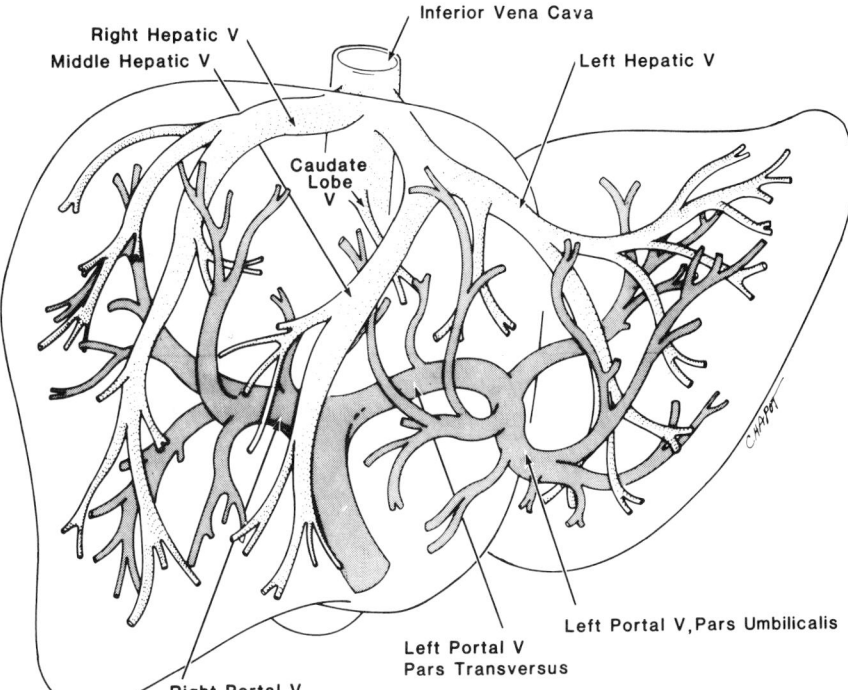

Figure 5. Hepatic veins and portal vein. There are three major hepatic veins: right, middle, and left. The portal vein divides into a right and left trunk with the left curving in the falciform ligament as the pars umbilicus, where the umbilical vein usually joins it. (From Campra, J. L., and Reynolds, T. B.: The hepatic circulation. *In* Arias, I., et al. (Eds.): The Liver: Biology and Pathobiology. New York, Raven Press, 1982, pp. 627–645.)

the medial segment of the left lobe. The right main branch of the portal vein divides into anterior and posterior segments. Both systems branch into small veins and venules and finally into hepatic sinusoids. Abundant intercommunication exists at the sinusoidal level.

HEPATIC ARTERY. The extrahepatic arterial system does not parallel the portal channels, although the intrahepatic system does (Fig. 6). A usual pattern is present in slightly over 50 per cent of individuals.[25] The proper hepatic artery arises from the celiac axis and passes along the upper border of the pancreas toward the liver. Posterior or superior to the duodenum it gives off the gastroduodenal artery and is then termed the common hepatic artery. Within the porta hepatis it divides into right and left branches and subsequently into smaller branches corresponding to the portal venous system and subsegmental anatomy. Because of abundant collaterals, ligation of the hepatic artery proximal to the gastroduodenal artery can be performed without injury to the liver. In fact, ligation of even the proper hepatic artery can often be performed without serious consequence because of development of a rich collateral extrinsic blood supply from the celiac axis and superior mesenteric and inferior phrenic arteries. Ligation of the right or left hepatic artery usually leads to enzyme elevation, although often there are no clinical manifestations. The proper hepatic artery contributes to a diffuse subcapsular plexus that may also contribute significantly to the collateral circulation.

The most important variations of the hepatic arterial system are the right or common hepatic artery arising from the superior mesenteric trunk, the left lateral segmental artery arising from the left gastric artery, the right hepatic artery traversing anterior rather than posterior to the bile duct, and the right hepatic artery traveling posterior to the portal vein (Fig. 7). In addition, the right hepatic artery often has a curved extrahepatic course, which may lead to inadvertent ligation during cholecystectomy. The cystic artery usually arises from the right hepatic artery, although there is some variability. The most common variant is origination of the cystic artery from the gastroduodenal artery; the next most common variations are origination from the left or common hepatic artery. There may also be double cystic arteries.

HEPATIC VEINS. Three major hepatic veins (right, middle,

and left) are of surgical importance. Short segments of these veins emerge posteriorly from the liver and drain into the inferior vena cava. The right hepatic vein is the largest of the three, follows along the intersegmental plane between the anterior and posterior segments, and provides the principal drainage for the right lobe of the liver. The middle hepatic vein lies in the lobar fissure and drains principally the medial segment of the left lobe as well as a variable portion of the anterior segment of the right lobe. It joins the left hepatic vein in 80 per cent of dissections. The left hepatic vein drains principally the left lateral segment. In addition, there are multiple small veins that drain the posterior aspect of the liver directly into the vena cava. In general, the short extrahepatic segments of the major hepatic veins may make accessibility difficult, particularly for control of traumatic bleeding. The course and drainage area of the middle hepatic vein may be variable, which may be of importance during hepatic resection. With thrombosis of the major hepatic veins (Budd-Chiari syndrome), the small posterior veins as well as the portal collateral circulation become more important.

BILIARY SYSTEM. The biliary drainage system begins at the hepatocyte level where portions of the hepatocyte membrane form small channels termed canaliculi. Bile drains from the canaliculi into intrahepatic ducts that follow the segmental anatomy determined primarily by the vascular supply. The convergence of canaliculi and proximal ductal systems is termed the canal of Hering. The ductal pattern becomes more variable distally. The left lobar duct forms in the umbilical fissure from the union of ducts from segments II, III, and IV, and then passes to the right across the base of segment IV (medial segment of the left lobe, "quadrate lobe"), and unites with the right lobar duct to form the common hepatic duct. The right hepatic duct drains segments V to VIII and arises from the junction of the right anterior and posterior segmental ducts. The right posterior duct has almost a horizontal course prior to its junction with the anterior duct when it descends more vertically. The junction of the two main right biliary channels usually occurs above the right branch of the portal vein.

The shorter extrahepatic right lobar duct joins the longer left duct at the base of the right lobe. The extrahepatic portion of the left lobar duct characteristically measures above 2 cm. in length. The right and left lobar ducts join outside the liver to become the

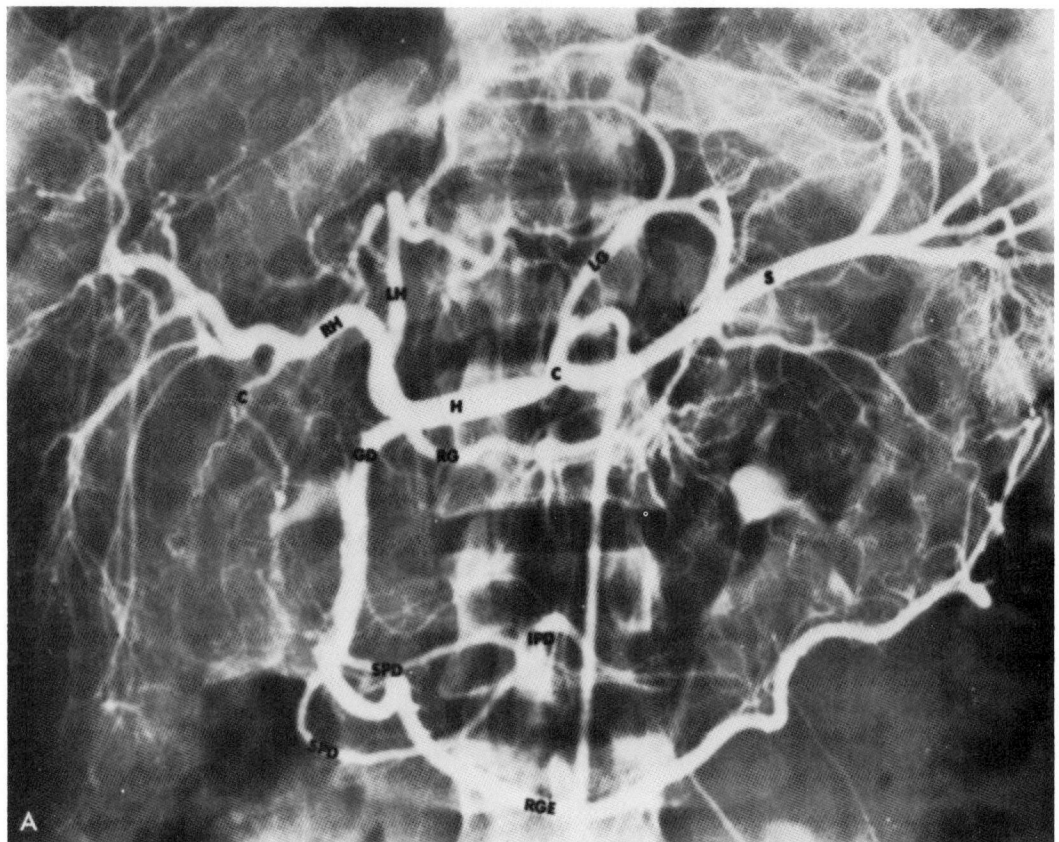

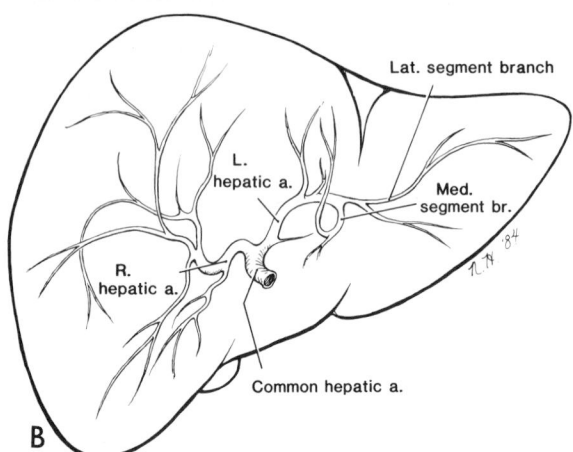

Figure 6. A, Celiac axis with a usual branching pattern is demonstrated. The angiographic catheter is located at the origin of the celiac axis (C) and shown are the following arteries: splenic (S), left gastric (LG), hepatic (H), cystic (C), gastroduodenal (GD), right gastric (RG), superior and inferior pancreaticoduodenal (SPD and IPD), and right gastroepiploic (RGE). The hepatic artery proximal to the gastroduodenal artery (H) is usually called the "proper" hepatic artery, whereas the artery distal to the gastroduodenal artery and before its next major division is the common hepatic artery (B). (From Campra, J. L., and Reynolds, T. B.: The hepatic circulation. In Arias, I. M., Jakoby, W. B., Popper, H., Schacter, D., and Shafritz, D. A. (Eds.): The Liver: Biology and Pathobiology, 2nd ed. New York, Raven Press, 1988.) B, Diagram of the branches of the common hepatic artery.

common hepatic duct, which, of course, passes anterior to the portal vein in most individuals. The left hepatic duct joins the right at a much more anterior and acute angle, an anatomic consistency that becomes important during common duct exploration or cholangiography. The length of the common hepatic duct varies according to the location of its junction with the cystic duct, where it becomes the common bile duct. The hepatic duct confluence varies considerably with respect to the union of the right anterior, right posterior, and left main hepatic ducts. The biliary drainage of the caudate "lobe" (segment I) varies considerably but enters both the right and left hepatic duct systems in approximately 80 per cent of patients. In approximately 15 per cent of patients, the caudate lobe drains only into the left hepatic duct system, and in 5 per cent, it drains only into the right hepatic duct.

The upper limit of normal for the diameter of the common bile duct is controversial. Most references list the upper limit as 6 to 8 mm. except after cholecystectomy when it may dilate to 10 to 12 mm. Intra- and extrahepatic ducts usually lie anterior to the corresponding portal branches. The extrahepatic bile ducts lie within the hepatoduodenal ligament. The common hepatic artery ascending to the left of the common bile duct gives off the right hepatic artery, which usually courses dorsal to the bile duct. Like the common hepatic duct, the common bile duct varies in length. It passes posterior to the first part of the duodenum and then courses through the pancreas and the wall of the duodenum to form the papilla of Vater on the medial duodenal wall. The major pancreatic duct (duct of Wirsung) joins the common duct in approximately 90 per cent of patients, forming the ampulla of Vater.

SPHINCTER OF ODDI. The circular smooth muscle fibers in the ampulla of Vater area comprise the sphincter of Oddi, which regulates the flow of bile from the liver into the duodenum. The three principal parts of the sphincter of Oddi are (1) the sphincter of the choledochus, that is, the circular muscle fibers surrounding the intramural and submucosal bile duct, (2) the pancreatic sphincter, which consists of the amuscular septum between the bile and pancreatic ducts, and (3) an ampullary

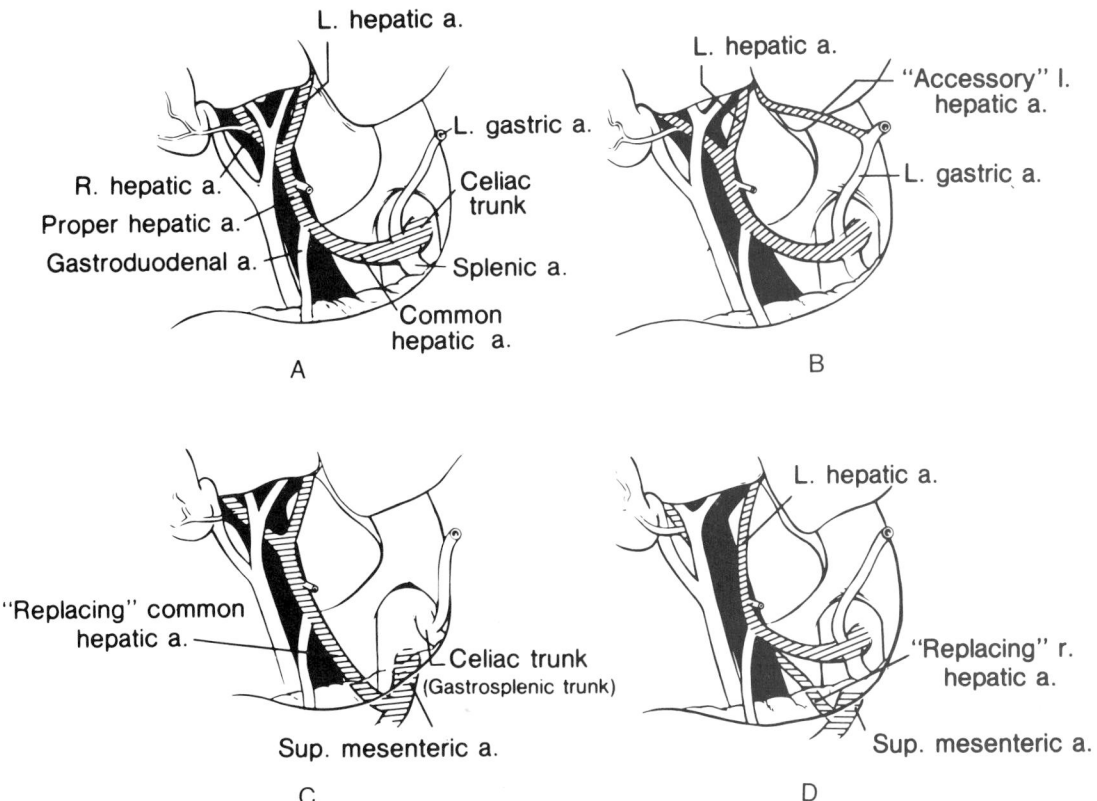

Figure 7. Four most common variations of the hepatic arterial system. (From Skandalakis, L. J., Gray, S. W., Colburn, G. L., and Skandalakis, J. E.: Surgical anatomy of the liver and associated extrahepatic structures. *In* Contemporary Surgery, 1987. Glenview, Ill., Bobit Publishing Company.)

sphincter. The ampullary sphincter, the most important component of the sphincter of Oddi, includes a layer of longitudinal muscle fibers that help prevent reflux of intestinal contents into the ampulla. Relaxation of the ampullary sphincter may promote reflux into the pancreatic duct. In approximately 10 per cent of patients, papillae have clearly distinct, separate openings of the common bile duct and pancreatic duct. The blood supply of the common bile duct arises from the gastroduodenal, common hepatic, and right hepatic arteries. A plexus formed on the duct provides two axial vessels: the "three o'clock" and "nine o'clock" arteries, named for the positions related to a cross section of the duct.

GALLBLADDER. The gallbladder, a pear-shaped, distensible appendage of the extrahepatic biliary system, usually contains 30 to 50 ml. of bile. It has a fundus, body, and neck. The gallbladder fills and empties through the cystic duct, which varies in length and usually contains the spiral valves of Heister that regulate bile flow. The valves may be extremely tortuous, making intraoperative cannulation difficult for cholangiography. Englargement of the neck of the gallbladder, such as from a stone, may form a pouch (Hartmann's pouch). The triangle bounded by the cystic duct, common hepatic duct, and inferior border of the liver forms the triangle of Calot. The gallbladder obtains its blood supply from the cystic artery that originates from the right hepatic artery, usually after the latter passes beneath the common hepatic duct. Venous drainage of the gallbladder enters principally into the portal vein. The lymphatics drain into cystic duct nodes near the superior aspect of the cystic duct. Venous and lymphatic channels also enter into the liver parenchyma.

BILIARY SYSTEMS VARIANTS. Variations in the gallbladder and related anatomy assume importance in surgical therapy, particularly because failure to recognize variants allows iatrogenic injury. Small accessory ducts between the liver and gallbladder easily escape detection. Occasionally, liver parenchyma partially embeds the gallbladder, and rarely one may encounter a completely intrahepatic gallbladder. The length of the cystic duct varies and occasionally passes for several centimeters ensheathed with the common hepatic duct (Fig. 8). Passage of the cystic duct posterior and around the common hepatic duct to form a left-sided junction (spiral union) occurs in less than 5 per cent of patients. The cystic duct may also join the right or left hepatic duct, receive an accessory or right hepatic duct, or be absent. Rarely, major hepatic ducts drain separately into the gallbladder. Common variations in the anatomy of the hepatic artery that have relevance to this biliary anatomy include a bend in the course of the hepatic artery that can mimic the cystic artery origin, a short cystic artery takeoff from the right hepatic artery, dual cystic arteries, or an artery that courses anterior to the hepatic ductal system.

NERVES. A complex system of nerves is located in the portal and pericapsular regions. The clinical importance of these nerves generally is not known. An anterior neural plexus consists primarily of sympathetic fibers derived bilaterally from ganglia T7 to T10 and synapsing in the celiac plexus and fibers from the right and left vagus nerves and right phrenic nerve. The anterior plexus surrounds the hepatic arteries. A posterior plexus, which intercommunicates with the anterior plexus, is located around the portal vein and bile ducts. The hepatic arteries are innervated by the sympathetic system. A branch of the posterior vagal trunk provides the principal source of parasympathetic fibers to the biliary passages. Pain in the liver capsule and gallbladder is referred to the right shoulder and scapula via the third and fourth cervical nerves. Interruption of the anterior neural plexus may have various physiologic effects, such as on the composition of secreted bile[40] and the accumulation of fat in the liver. The significance of these findings is not known.

LYMPHATICS. Hepatic lymphatic fluid from the perisinusoidal spaces of Disse and clefts of Mall drains into large lymphatics in the porta hepatis, then into the cisterna chyli, and subsequently into the thoracic duct. Lymphatic vessels are also found around hepatic veins, in Glisson's capsule, and around

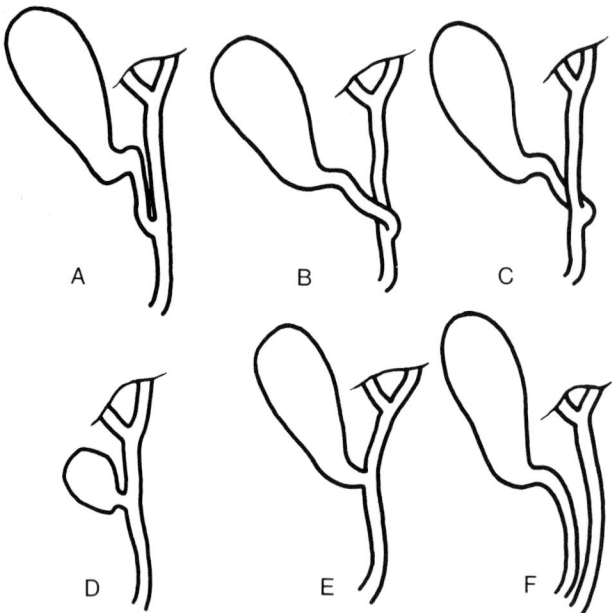

Figure 8. Most common variations of the cystic duct. (From Skandalakis, L. J., Gray, S. W., Colburn, G. L., and Skandalakis, J. E.: Surgical anatomy of the liver and associated extrahepatic structures. *In* Contemporary Surgery, 1987. Glenview, Ill., Bobit Publishing Company.)

bile ducts. They may pass through the diaphragm into the thoracic duct. Draining lymph nodes are located in the porta hepatis, in the celiac region, and near the inferior vena cava. Lymph vessel dilation occurs in cirrhosis, veno-occlusive disease, and glycogenosis. Change in the permeability of the endothelial cells of the hepatic sinusoids (e.g., with cirrhosis or histamine injection) may alter lymph flow and protein content. This mechanism may be important in the pathogenesis of ascites. In addition, numerous lymph vessels are located around the extrahepatic biliary system. Injection of dye into the bile duct with superphysiologic pressure demonstrates communication with the hepatic lymph vessels, but the importance of these communications under physiologic conditions is not known. The term *cystic node* commonly refers to lymphatics superior to the cystic duct, and *hiatal node* those inferior to the cystic duct along the anterior border of the epiploic foramen.

MICROSCOPIC ANATOMY. Descriptions of the histologic character of the liver have classically focused on a generalized scheme of small lobules with a tributary of the hepatic vein at the "center" and branches of the portal vein, artery, and bile duct (portal triad) at the "periphery."[48] The functional anatomy is different from this description in that the portal triad forms the axis about which parenchymal cells and peripherally the hepatic venule are situated. This orientation led to the concept of the liver acinar unit described later. The "classic" liver lobule measures about 0.7 by 2 mm. in size and is approximately hexagonal in shape with interlobular portal canals at the periphery containing connective tissue stroma and triads (portal venule, hepatic arteriole, and bile ductule). In the center of the lobule is the central vein or terminal hepatic venule. The hepatic parenchymal cells are arranged in single layers (cell plates) between minute vascular channels termed sinusoids. The hepatocytes radiate from the central vein to the portal canals. Spaces that interconnect these cell plates are sometimes referred to as lacunae. Terminal branches of the triads penetrate the periphery of the lobule where lacunae are less numerous. Lobulation in the human liver is less well defined than in other species.

MICROCIRCULATION. The major inflow system, that is, the portal vein, and the outflow system of hepatic veins have been likened to large branching trees with their main trunks at a 90-degree angle.[46] The terminal branches of the two systems do not meet but are regularly interspersed, with the space between the "twigs" from each system filled with hepatic cell plates and sinusoids. The portal veins and their branches become progressively smaller as they penetrate the liver substance. Terminal veins connect with the sinusoidal bed, piercing through closely applied cell plates. Flow of the portal blood into the sinusoids is regulated in part via the periphery of the cell plates.

The branches of the hepatic artery similarly decrease in caliber as they penetrate the parenchyma, although their size and wall structure vary considerably. They form a general plexus that eventually terminates in the sinusoids. A special capillary plexus encompasses the bile ducts and also empties terminally into the sinusoids. The peribiliary plexus may have an important role in bile secretion and absorption. Cuffs of smooth muscle surrounding the terminal arterioles may also help regulate flow into the sinusoids.[26]

The hepatic sinusoids are approximately 7 to 15 μ wide, but the width may increase up to 180 μ under physiologic conditions (Fig. 9). Pressure within the sinusoids is only 2 to 3 mm. Hg, making this an extremely low resistance system. The low pressure and remarkably functional system can in part be explained by three anatomic features: (1) The sinusoids are lined by Kupffer and endothelial cells, which overlap loosely and are not attached to each other. (2) The endothelial cells are flat and markedly fenestrated, with openings varying from 0.1 to 2 μ in diameter. (3) Hepatocyte and membrane microvilli project through the fenestrae of the endothelial cells and are readily exposed to sinusoidal contents. Sinusoids are freely permeable to low- and high-molecular-weight substances in solution. The sinusoids empty into terminal hepatic venules, which empty into hepatic veins of increasing caliber.

SPACE OF DISSE. The space between the thin endothelial lining of the sinusoid and the hepatocytes is the perisinusoidal space of Disse (Fig. 10). This is thought to be the primary site for formation of hepatic lymph. Because of the marked porosity of the sinusoids, high- and low-molecular-weight substances may enter this space, which communicates with large spaces apposed to the portal connective tissue. Albumin and very-low-density lipoprotein, about 500 Å in diameter, easily pass from the sinusoid to the space of Disse. The stellate Kupffer cells often cannot be differentiated from endothelial cells by light microscopy. However, the former are much larger and have irregular surfaces with folds and microvilli. The Kupffer cells take up ^{99}Tc-labeled sulfur colloid, useful in liver scans, and endogenous peroxidase is also a cytochemical marker. These active phagocytes may have an important antitumor role. Other important activities of these cells, which are a topic of intensive research, include secretion of lysosomal enzymes and endogenous production of pyrogens. The most important cells within the perisinusoidal space are the lipocytes, fibroblasts, and neurons.

HEPATOCYTES AND SITES OF BILE FORMATION. Hepatocytes represent approximately 60 per cent of the cells of the liver and comprise approximately 80 per cent of the cytoplasmic mass. Their diameter varies between 13 and 30 μ and they have eight or more surfaces. Although their structure, shape, and function vary considerably, particularly in relation to the distance from the portal venule, each hepatocyte is probably capable of performing all hepatocytic functions. The cell has both a microvillar and a straight surface. Microvilli face the perisinusoidal space and extend into the pericellular space. Even the straight surface of the membrane is capable of forming microvilli, particularly during regeneration or cholestasis. The microvilli of the hepatocyte are not as extensive as those of the intestinal absorptive cells. The microvilli of the intestine increase the surface area of the apical membrane by 24-fold, whereas the hepatocyte surface area is increased by a factor of only 1.6.[47] Approximately 15 per cent of the plasma membrane encompasses bile canaliculi that remain separated from the pericellular space by junc-

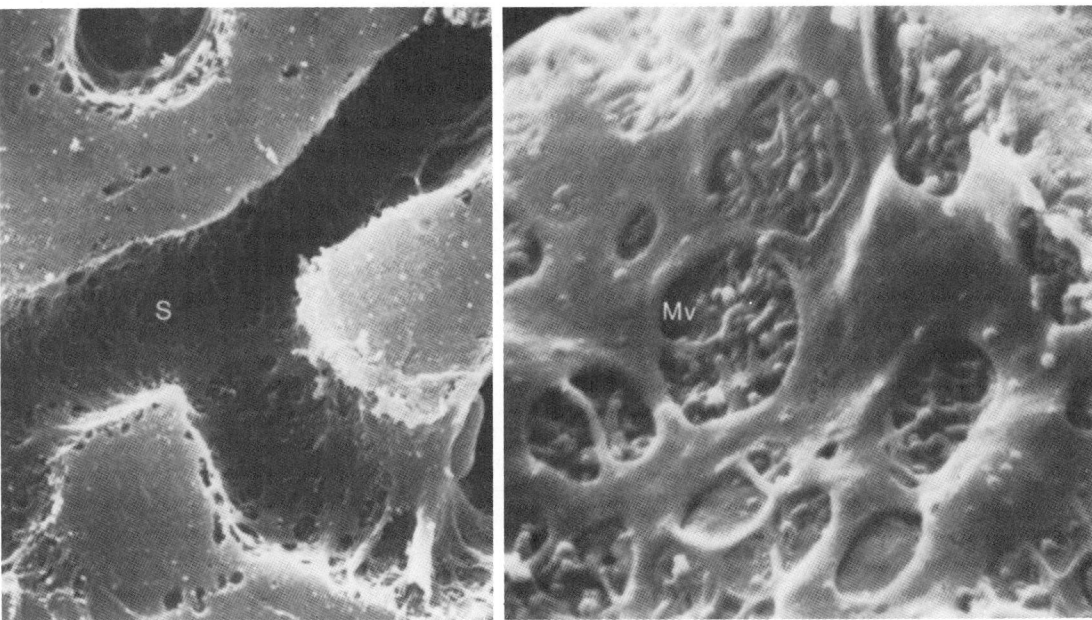

Figure 9. On the left, this scanning electron micrograph demonstrates hepatic sinusoids with varying-sized fenestrations in the endothelial lining cells. On the right, an enlargement demonstrates the microvilli of underlying hepatocytes protruding through fenestrations. (From Tissues and Organs: A Text-Atlas of Scanning Electron Microscopy. By Richard G. Kessel and Randy H. Kardon. Copyright © 1979 by W. H. Freeman and Company. Reprinted with permission.)

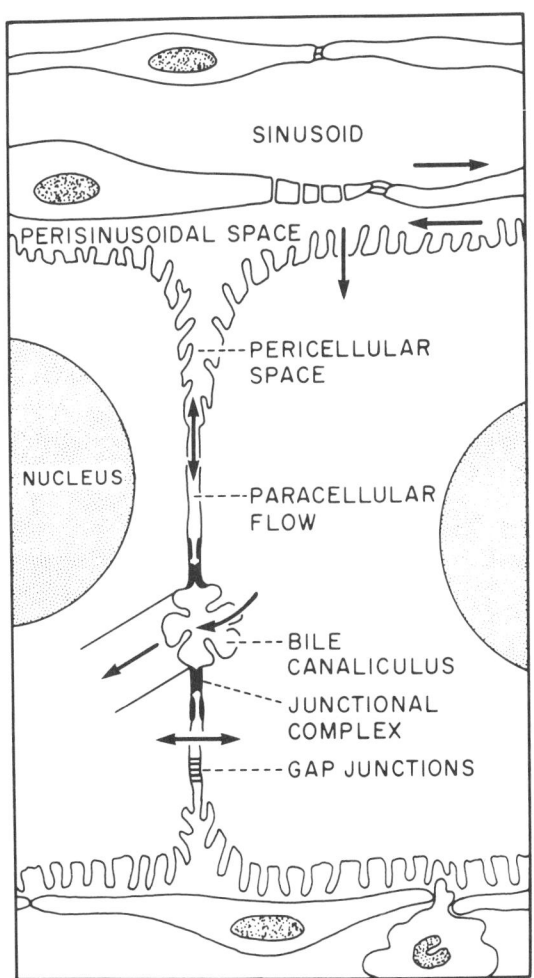

Figure 10. Diagram of sinusoids, perisinusoidal space of Disse, and principal hepatocyte surfaces. Arrows show direction of fluid flow. (From Arias, I., et al. (Eds.): The Liver: Biology and Pathobiology. New York, Raven Press, 1982.)

tional complexes of tight junctions and desmosomes (Fig. 10). Gap junctions provide some direct communication between the cells. The main source of canalicular bile is across the canalicular membrane, although some paracellular flow of small solutes also occurs. The canaliculi measure approximately 1 μ in diameter. The epithelial ductular or ductal lining cells measure 10 μ in diameter and have distinct basement membranes, in contrast to the hepatocytes.

ULTRASTRUCTURE. The average volume of the hepatocyte is 11,000 μl. The organization and structure of the organelles of the hepatocyte stimulate much current research, and information about their function is accumulating. For example, an area with a diameter 1 μ wide adjacent to the bile canalicular membrane of the adult hepatocyte contains a large number of junctional complexes, microfilaments, vesicles, and multivesicular bodies, as well as some microtubules, smooth endoplasmic reticulum, lysosome-like structures, and frequently a Golgi complex.[47]

This busy area contributes actively to the secretion of canalicular bile. Mitochondria occupy approximately 18 per cent of the liver cell volume and participate in oxidative phosphorylation and the oxidation of fatty acids. Lysosomes catabolize endogenous substances as well as some endogenous wastes. Multivesicular bodies contain large quantities of proteins derived from plasma. Microtubules and associated mechanotransducers may regulate the direction of vesicular transport in the cell. Smooth endoplasmic reticulum is associated with glycogen deposits, and microsomes derived from both smooth and rough endoplasmic reticulum conduct many of the synthetic and other metabolic functions of the liver. As many as 50 Golgi complexes occupy a hepatocyte.[52] These organelles perform multiple functions, including synthesis of lipoprotein, glycoprotein, and albumin as well as bile secretion and bile acid transport. Transcytoplasmic transport is facilitated by the hepatocyte's cytoskeleton, which has been the focus of much recent research.

Recent research has revealed some other features of the hepatic ultrastructure. Mitochondria are more numerous, larger, and longer around portal tracts. The sinusoidal surface has both phagocytic and endocytic properties that are reflected in the formation of a trimer lattice-forming protein called clathrin. New techniques, such as high-voltage electron microscopy and elimination of embedding material, are rapidly increasing knowledge of the cytoarchitecture.

THE LIVER ACINAR UNIT (Fig. 11). The anatomy of the microcirculation led to the concept that the liver is divided into microscopic masses of cells functionally situated around terminal portal venules.[49-51] In an acinar unit, the portal venule is accompanied by a hepatic arteriole, a bile ductule, lymphatics, and nerves. Blood flows from the terminal portal venules into the sinusoids and comes into contact with hepatocytes within the unit until it drains into the terminal hepatic venules. The solutes are removed by the hepatocytes, and their concentration in sinusoidal blood decreases as blood flows toward the terminal hepatic venule. The hepatocytes around the portal venule axis have been arbitrarily divided into three zones. In Zone 1, the area immediately adjacent to the portal venule, the sinusoids are smaller in diameter and more anastomotic than in Zone 2 and Zone 3, which are farther away from the portal venule. This concept explains the "centrilobular" necrosis seen with hypotension. Zone 1 cells are the first to receive blood and oxygen and are therefore the last to undergo necrosis. Reciprocally, Zone 3 cells are more susceptible to oxygen deprivation. Zone 3 hepatocytes may also be less resistant to hepatotoxins since they receive blood of less nutritional value. Liver cell heterogeneity appears to be explained to a large degree by the liver acinus. For example, Golgi apparatus are much more numerous in the hepatocytes of Zone 1 and are more likely to be involved in bile salt transport, based on the decreasing sinusoidal bile salt concentration gradient from Zone 1 to Zone 3.

ANOMALOUS DEVELOPMENT OF THE LIVER. Incomplete or maldevelopment of the hepatobiliary system can cause a number of anomalies that can be encountered clinically. Complete absence of the liver is rare and not seen after birth. Absence of the left lobe has been reported. Hepatic transposition is associated with situs inversus. Occasionally, a tongue of liver tissue extends inferiorly from the right lobe, usually in female patients. The ascending (Riedel's lobe) is nearly always asymptomatic but has caused colonic or pyloric obstruction. The principal clinical concern is an undiagnosed mass. Heterotopic liver has also been seen from the left lobe, on or in the gallbladder, pancreas, adrenal, spleen, and omphalocele sac. Four cases of supradiaphragmatic liver lobes have been reported in the absence of a hernia sac. Small amounts of portal tissue are commonly seen microscopically in the hepatic ligaments.[6]

Although biliary variants are extremely common, true anomalies are not. Biliary atresia and choledochocele are the most common serious biliary problems seen shortly after birth. Other abnormalities include congenital absence of the gallbladder, intrahepatic or left-sided gallbladder, multiple gallbladders, and

abnormalities in shape of the gallbladder. There appears to be a familial predisposition for absence of the gallbladder. Both this anomaly and intrahepatic gallbladder have a higher than expected association with common duct stones. No more than three gallbladders have been reported in a single patient except in Siamese twins. Other gallbladder abnormalities include septation, bilobulation, and duplication of the cystic duct. The definition of multiple gallbladders is determined by the presence of more than one cystic duct. Occasionally, the gallbladder has a long mesentery predisposing it to torsion. Portal vascular abnormalities include portal agenesis, congenital portacaval shunt, a preduodenal portal vein, and anomalous pulmonary veins that traverse the diaphragm and enter the portal system.

PHYSIOLOGY

The liver is an amazingly dynamic organ, active in the uptake, storage, distribution, and disposition of various nutrients from the intestine or blood, and responsible for the synthesis, transformation, and metabolism of many endogenous and exogenous substrates. Although being rather uniform in appearance, as outlined in the previous section, the liver performs a remarkable variety of important functions. Some of these functions, by inference from the correctability of certain disease processes with transplantation, are now being recognized. For example, certain metabolic defects have been found to reside in the liver, such as familial hypercholesterolemia in which the liver appears functionally and histologically normal but the afflicted patient dies with severe arteriosclerotic coronary disease. A second example is the recent success of liver transplantation for hemophilia (factor XII deficiency).

General Considerations

The liver receives blood from the arterial and portal circulations, takes up various nutrients, pollutants, and other substrates, and stores, transforms, or distributes them at vascular, biliary, and lymphatic systems. To accomplish this, the liver expends approximately 20 per cent of the body's energy[64] and consumes 20 to 25 per cent of the total oxygen utilized despite constituting only 4 to 5 per cent of the total body weight. Most of the body's metabolic needs are regulated in some way by the liver. Much recent research has focused on the conductants of cellular and paracellular traffic and appears to be leading to the development of some important new concepts; however, many of the specific molecular events remain elusive.

Blood Flow

Mean total hepatic blood flow has been estimated by the sulfobromophthalein (Bromsulphalein or BSP) technique to be approximately 1500 ml. per minute per 1.73 m².[72,73] Approximately, 70 to 75 per cent of total hepatic blood flow comes from the portal vein and the remaining 25 to 30 per cent from the hepatic artery.[75,85] There is a reciprocal increase in hepatic arterial flow in response to reduction in portal venous flow, but the converse does not occur. Portal flow does not increase with occlusion of the hepatic artery. Portacaval shunt or ligation of the superior mesenteric artery leads to a nearly 100 per cent increase in hepatic arterial flow.[80,85] The compensation is not complete, however, so that total hepatic blood flow does not return to normal. Reflex neural control appears to be an important regulator of the hepatic artery but not the portal vein. These reflexes are mediated by the periarterial neural plexus. Autoregulation, a method by which organs preserve local blood flow during alterations in their major vascular system, is also apparent in the hepatic arterial system but not in the portal venous system.

Hepatic inflow increases with expiration and decreases with inspiration, which is opposite that of phasic flow into the inferior vena cava from the lower portion of the body. Hepatic

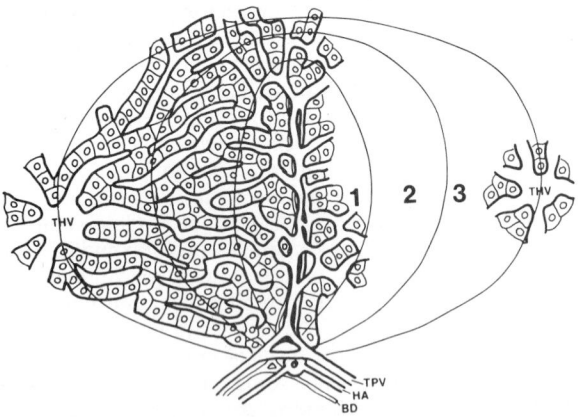

Figure 11. Diagram of a liver acinar unit as described by Rappaport. Terminal extensions of a portal venule (TPV), hepatic arteriole (HA), and bile ductule (BD) are labeled. Zone 1 represents the area nearest the sinusoidal axis, and blood flows sequentially through Zone 2 and Zone 3 into terminal hepatic venules (THV). (From Gumucio, J. J., and Miller, D. L.: Liver cell heterogeneity. In Arias, I., et al. (Eds.): The Liver: Biology and Pathobiology. New York, Raven Press, 1982, pp. 647-661.)

blood flow is also increased during mild exercise. During vigorous exercise, total hepatic blood flow is decreased as a result of shunting to the muscles and brain. Approximately 1000 ml. of blood can be made available to the rest of the body by the liver in periods of stress. Elevation of hepatic venous pressure causes hepatic arterial constriction and decreased blood flow regulated by myogenic properties within the arterial wall. Portal pressure may be estimated using radiologic techniques by wedging a catheter in a small hepatic venule. this occludes the sinusoidal outflow system so that sinusoidal pressure becomes a reflection of portal pressure. Portal pressure is determined by constriction or dilation of the mesenteric and splenic vasculature and intrahepatic resistance. Portal flow is increased by food, bile salts, secretin, cholecystokinin, pentagastrin, epinephrine, vasoactive intestinal polypeptide, glucagon, and isoproterenol. Portal flow is inhibited by serotonin, angiotensin, and vasopressin. Effects on the hepatic arterial system of many of these substances are more variable. Hepatic arterial pressure reflects the systemic arterial pressure. Portal vein pressure ranges from 7 to 10 mm. Hg (10 to 14 cm. of saline). Sinusoidal pressure is 2 to 4 mm. Hg above inferior vena caval pressure, and hepatic vein pressure is only slightly higher than that of the inferior vena cava.

The portal and arterial systems converge in the sinusoidal bed where the pressure remains remarkably constant and low. The reduction in arterial pressure occurs as the branches penetrate thick cell plates of hepatic parenchyma. Small inlet venules to the sinusoids regulate portal flow into the bed. Commonly employed methods of measuring hepatic blood flow include (1) electromagnetic flow probes; (2) hepatic clearance of substances such as indocyanine green or colloidal particles; (3) indicator dilution with markers such as ^{131}I-labeled albumin; and (4) various other physical measurements, such as injection of ^{133}Xe gas and measurement of the speed of its removal using an external probe. Arteriographic estimates are in general unreliable. It is usually easier to obtain hepatic arterial measurements than it is to document portal venous inflow by indirect methods.

Deprivation of portal blood flow causes deterioration in hepatic structure and function, marked pathologically by Zone 3 ("centrilobular") hepatocyte atrophy and fatty infiltration.[76,87] In addition, ultrastructural changes in the rough endoplasmic reticulum, polyribosomes, and number of glycogen granules may be prominent.[84] In 1877, Eck performed the first portacaval shunts and erroneously concluded that his fistula, an anastomosis between the portal or superior mesenteric vein and the vena cava with hilar portal ligation (Fig. 12), did not cause "any danger to the body."[77] This conclusion was based on almost no data. Eight dogs underwent portacaval shunts for Eck fistulas, and seven of the eight died perioperatively. The eighth recovered fully but escaped from the laboratory 2½ months postoperatively. Sixteen years later, Pavlov correctly recognized that the portal diversion was not harmless. His dogs developed a neurologic disorder that included ataxia and convulsions and died. This encephalopathic syndrome was termed "meat intoxication."[78]

Over the ensuing years, there was great debate over whether these adverse effects were caused by reduction in blood flow or by diversion of nutrient or hormonal factors from the portal circulation. The former hypothesis was supported by the observation that portacaval transposition avoided many of the adverse effects of the Eck fistula.[81] However, further work demonstrated that many of the histologic abnormalities persisted after transposition. More recently, complicated double liver preparations demonstrated that the portal blood contains factors that maintain the anatomic and functional integrity of the liver.[82,83,86]

Bile Formation

Bile secretion is an active process, relatively independent of total hepatic blood flow except during conditions simulating

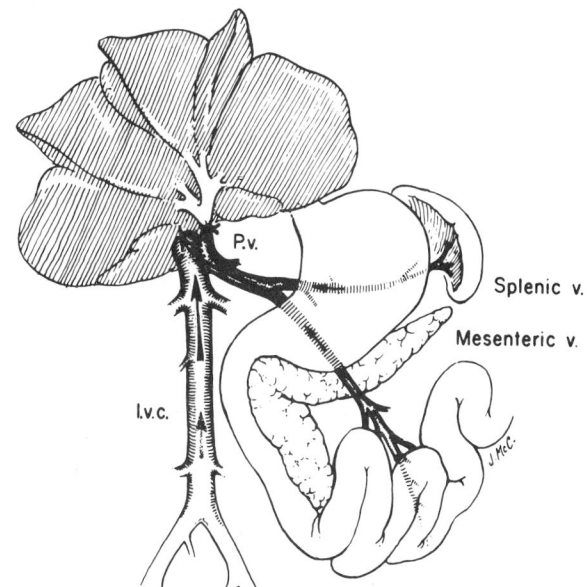

Figure 12. Eck fistula as diagrammed by Starzl and associates. A side-to-side anastomosis between the portal or superior mesenteric vein and inferior vena cava has been constructed with hilar ligation of the portal vein distal (in terms of flow) to the anastomosis, essentially creating an end-to-side portacaval shunt. (From Starzl, T. E., et al.: The influence of portal blood upon lipid metabolism in normal and diabetic dogs and baboons. Surg. Gynecol. Obstet., *140:*381, 1975.)

shock.[92] Bile is formed at two sites (Fig. 13): (1) the canalicular membrane of the hepatocyte and (2) the bile ductules or ducts. The bile canaliculus is a long, narrow channel that begins as a space of approximately 1 μ in diameter bounded by two or three hepatocyte canalicular membranes. It has no wall of its own, but the membrane has numerous microvilli. Until recently micropuncture of these channels has been generally unsuccessful, so that knowledge of hepatocyte bile production was obtained by indirect methods. The best method of determining canalicular flow is by the clearance of metabolically inert, freely permeable neutral solutes such as erythritol or mannitol, although there is some question whether the bile duct epithelial cells are also slightly permeable to these sugars.[89] There appears to be both a transcellular and a paracellular route for canalicular and probably ductular bile formation.

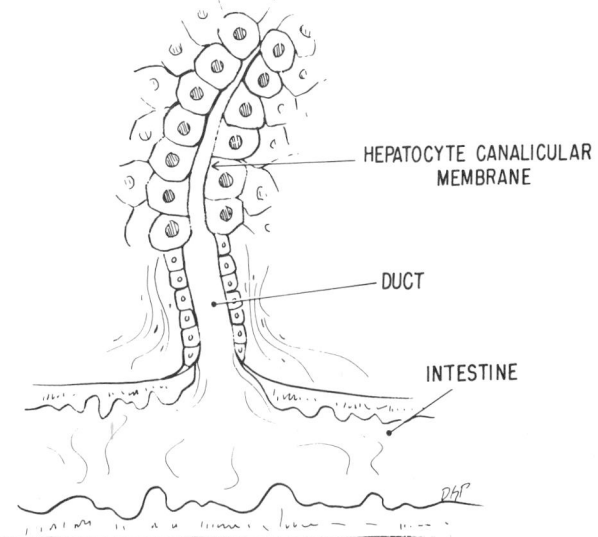

Figure 13. Schematic diagram demonstrating the two principal cellular sites of bile production: (1) the canalicular membrane of the hepatocytes, and (2) epithelial cells of the bile ductules or ducts distally. In addition to these sites, a paracellular route is also operative (see Fig. 10).

Key regulatory factors in bile formation include organic anion uptake and intracellular pH regulation. Studies using isolated hepatocyte completion such as via direct measurement of intracellular pH and membrane potential have provided some insight into the mechanism involved. Organic anions appear to be taken up by specific proteins on the sinusoidal membrane. Na^+-K^+-ATPase provides the driving force for bile acid uptake, which is sodium linked. A canalicular membrane carrier facilitates movement across that membrane. A Na^+-H^+ antiprotein is also located on the sinusoidal membrane, which coupled with a cytosolic carbonic anhydrase acts as a driving force for canalicular secretion of bicarbonate via a canalicular $Cl^-HCO_3^+$ exchanger.

The principal organic compounds in bile are the conjugated bile acids, cholesterol, phospholipid, bile pigments, and protein (Table 1). Because of the excellent correlation between bile acid output and bile flow, the term bile acid–dependent flow describes this fraction of bile formation. In addition, canalicular flow may be generated in near absence of bile acids or during stabilized bile acid–dependent flow, and this fraction is termed the bile acid–independent canalicular fraction. Abundant evidence now exists that this bile salt–independent fraction may not be as "independent" as previously thought; however, this term is still useful. Secretion of cholesterol and phospholipid is closely linked to the output of bile acids, which are powerful detergents and form micelles. Stimulation of bile salt–independent canalicular flow, for example, by the hormone glucagon, may paradoxically decrease cholesterol output.[102]

As bile passes through the biliary ductules or ducts, it is modified by secretion or absorption of water and electrolytes by the epithelial cells. The only known function of the gallbladder is to concentrate and store hepatic bile during fasting. Approximately 90 per cent of the water in gallbladder bile is absorbed within 4 hours, which causes a highly concentrated solution.[75] Bile acids in the gallbladder may reach 50 times their concentration in hepatic bile. Cholecystokinin appears to be the principal physiologic stimulator of gallbladder contraction and is released from the mucosa of the proximal small intestine in response to food. Cholecystokinin also simultaneously relaxes the sphincter of Oddi. Other peptides, such as vasoactive intestinal polypeptide, neuropeptide Y, motilin, pancreatic polypeptide, and somatostatin, may be involved in control of gallbladder storage and emptying. Histamine and prostaglandins may also be involved. Intestinal mucosa contains a similar substance ("pancreatone") that inhibits gallbladder contraction after a meal. However, pancreatone has not been identified definitively. Cholinergic stimulation causes contraction of the gallbladder and relaxation of the sphincter of Oddi. Bile acids in the intestine appear to have a negative feedback effect on release of cholecystokinin from the intestine. The importance of gallbladder function is debatable, as humans have no apparent nutritional consequences after cholecystectomy.

Total unstimulated bile flow in a 70-kg. man has been estimated to be 0.41 to 0.43 ml. per minute.[91,103] Of this, 0.15 to 0.16 ml. per minute is bile acid–dependent flow, another 0.16 to 0.17 ml. per minute is bile acid–independent canalicular flow, and approximately 0.11 ml. per minute is from ductular secretion. Under physiologic conditions, total bile flow in 1 day is estimated to be 600 to 1000 ml. The total amount can vary considerably, depending on the presence or absence of various physiologic stimulants or inhibitors. There are also diurnal variations and changes in flow with the rhythmic motility of the gastrointestinal tract during fasting.

Substances that have a bile acid–like choleretic effect include BSP, fluorescein, indocyanine green, various radiologic agents, and phloridzin. Bilirubin is incorporated into micelles and does not cause choleresis, even with an infusion of quantities close to its T_m. Feeding stimulates both the bile salt–dependent and the bile salt–independent canalicular fractions of bile secretion. Bile acid–independent canalicular flow may be stimulated by barbiturates, thyroid hormone, insulin, glucagon, vasoactive intestinal polypeptide, theophylline, dibutyryl cyclic adenosine monophosphate (dibutyryl cyclic AMP), prostaglandins A_1, E_1, and E_2, and salicylates. It is inhibited by ouabain, ethacrynic acid, amiloride, chlorpromazine, and somatostatin. Ductal secretion is stimulated by secretin, cholecystokinin, bombesin, cerulein, and gastrin. Somatostatin inhibits both canalicular and ductal flow, and serotonin inhibits ductular flow. Of all the stimulants of independent flow, secretin, glucagon, and cholecystokinin are most likely to be physiologic regulators of bile formation. The vagus nerve appears to have little physiologic effect on bile formation or composition.

Bile is a mixed micellar solution. Normal ranges of the concentrations of major inorganic and organic solutes in hepatic bile are listed in Table 1. Sodium is the most important cation involved in canalicular secretion, and bicarbonate is secreted in large quantities at the ductular level. Osmolality is approximately 300 mOsm. per kg., which is isosmotic with plasma. The low osmolality reflects in part the aggregation of bile acids in micelles and the consequent loss of osmotic activity. Note in Table 1 that the concentrations of the major electrolytes approximate those of Ringer's lactate. This solution may be administered for water and electrolyte replacement in a patient with a bile fistula. A prolonged bile fistula with adequate water and electrolyte replacement causes some impairment in lipid and vitamin absorption, anorexia, and malaise. These effects are reversed by replacement of bile into the upper gastrointestinal tract. Surprisingly, many patients with bile fistulas tolerate drinking their own bile disguised in orange juice or other ways. Bile secretory pressure is usually 10 to 20 cm. of saline. Maximal secretory pressure is 30 to 35 cm. even in the presence of complete biliary obstruction. Numerous proteins are present physiologically in bile. The most abundant are albumin and IgA. The presence of IgA depends on an active secretory process, whereas albumin does not. It is likely that IgA is important to the immunocompetence of the gastrointestinal tract.

Lymphatics

The lymph collects and transports large and small molecules, plasma protein, debris, bacteria, other foreign substances, and fluid. Lymph is 3 to 5 per cent protein, mainly albumin, and its electrolyte composition approximates that of plasma. Movement is mainly passive, depending on tissue turgor, blood flow, and body position. Thoracic duct or inferior vena caval obstruction decreases lymph flow. In cirrhosis, there is widening, increased permeability, and increased number of lymph channels. Few studies have been performed on the physiologic or pathophysiologic significance of hepatic lymph.

Enterohepatic Circulation

Bile salts secreted into the biliary system empty into the intestine where they are efficiently reabsorbed into the portal circulation. The liver extracts the bile acids and transports them to the canalicular membrane where they are resecreted back into the biliary system. This process is referred to as the enterohepatic circulation (Fig. 14). Total bile salt pool size in humans is

TABLE 1. Composition of Hepatic Bile

Inorganic Ions (mEq./L.)	Organic Solutes
Na^+ (140–165)	Bile acid (5–50 mmol./L.)
K^+ (3.8–5.8)	Cholesterol (100–340 mg./100 ml.)
Cl^- (93–123)	Phospholipid (150–800 mg./100 ml.)
HCO_3^- (15–55)	Protein (25–500 mg./100 ml.)
Ca^{++} (1.4–5.0)	
Mg^{++} (1.5–3.0)	

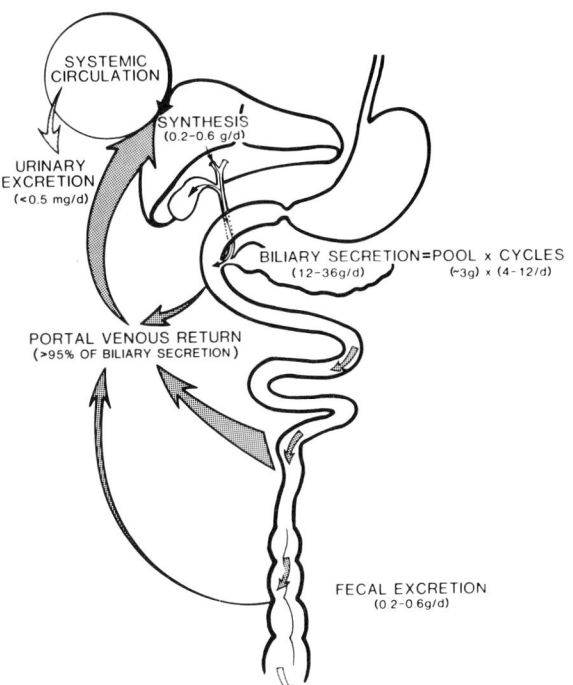

Figure 14. The enterohepatic circulation of bile salts with some general kinetic values for man. (From Carey, M. C.: The enterohepatic circulation. *In* Arias, I., et al. (Eds.): The Liver: Biology and Pathobiology. New York, Raven Press, 1982, pp. 429–465.)

2 to 5 gm. and undergoes this circulation two to three times per meal and six to ten times daily, depending on dietary habits. In addition, 0.2 to 0.6 gm. is lost per day in the stool, and this quantity is replaced by newly synthesized bile acids. Therefore, 20 to 40 times more bile acid than is normally synthesized is delivered into the intestine, underscoring the remarkable efficiency of this system. Under normal circumstances, serum bile acid levels are low because of the 95 per cent or greater efficiency of extraction by the liver from the portal circulation. The liver can remove more than 80 per cent of bile salts carried to it in a single pass. Serum bile acid levels are frequently increased in patients with liver disease. The pruritus associated with obstructive jaundice may be related to elevated serum bile acid levels, although it has been difficult to demonstrate much deposition of bile acids in skin.

The active secretion of bile acids across the canalicular membranes into bile is the primary metabolic pump of the enterohepatic circulation. Bile acids are conjugated by the liver with glycine or taurine prior to secretion in bile. The principal primary bile acids in humans are cholic acid and chenodeoxycholic acid. Secondary bile acids formed in the intestine by bacterial alteration include deoxycholic acid and lithocholic acid. Lithocholic acid induces cirrhosis in experimental animals. In the intestine, bile acids aid in fat and vitamin absorption. Various gastrointestinal problems such as regional enteritis, ileal resection, Zollinger-Ellison syndrome, radiation enteritis, and blind loop syndrome may be associated with deficient primary bile acid absorption, which leads to diarrhea, steatorrhea, or vitamin B_{12} deficiency. A decreased bile salt pool size may also predispose to the formation of gallstones. In blood, bile salts are tightly bound by both serum albumin and lipoproteins, particularly high-density lipoprotein. Hepatic uptake is carrier mediated and follows Michaelis-Menten kinetics.

Bilirubin Metabolism

Bilirubin, a breakdown product of heme, is excreted almost entirely in the bile. With hepatocellular disease or extrahepatic biliary obstruction, free bilirubin may accumulate in blood and

tissues and may cause toxic effects. Kernicterus in children is an extreme example of this toxicity. The liver retains a remarkable ability to clear bilirubin in the presence of partial ductal obstruction. With ligation of the right or left hepatic duct in dogs or humans, marked liver enzyme abnormalities usually occur, particularly elevation of the canalicular markers alkaline phosphatase and 5'-nucleotidase; yet, serum bilirubin levels often remain normal for a long period of time. Approximately 75 per cent of bilirubin is derived from senescent erythrocytes. Bilirubin circulates bound to albumin, which protects tissues from its toxicity. It is rapidly removed from plasma by the liver via a carrier-mediated transport system. In the hepatocyte, bilirubin is bound to other proteins (Y and Z), which probably have a role in transport. It is conjugated with glucuronide, a sugar group, before being secreted in bile. Conjugated bilirubin may then form a permanent covalent bond with albumin. The resultant structure is known as delta bilirubin. The implications of delta bilirubin in disease are still being investigated.

Disorders of bilirubin metabolism leading to predominantly unconjugated hyperbilirubinemia include neonatal hyperbilirubinemia, Crigler-Najjar Type 1, which usually leads to kernicterus and death; the more benign Crigler-Najjar syndrome Type 2; and Gilbert's syndrome. Disorders characterized by predominantly conjugated hyperbilirubinemia include Dubin-Johnson syndrome, Roter's syndrome, and "recurrent intrahepatic cholestasis"; patients with these disorders usually have a benign course.

In the intestine, bilirubin is reduced by bacteria to mesobilirubinogen and stercobilinogen, collectively termed urobilinogen, both of which are excreted in the stool. A fraction of urobilinogen is oxidized to urobilin, which is a brown pigment and gives stool its normal color. Part of urobilinogen is reabsorbed from the intestine and is excreted in the urine. With complete biliary obstruction, urobilinogen is not formed and therefore cannot be reabsorbed, so it does not appear in the urine.

Bilirubin is only one of many pigments in bile. Another class of pigments is the porphyrins, which are involved in the formation of heme. The liver participates in their synthesis. Defects in heme synthesis may cause overproduction of these precursors. A clinical feature of the porphyrias is abdominal pain, which sometimes may be considered in the differential diagnosis of the acute abdomen.

Other Hepatocyte Functions

PROTEIN METABOLISM. Hepatic protein synthesis and catabolism are vitally important, and measurement of these functions often provides a useful indication of the degree of liver impairment. At least 17 of the major human plasma proteins are synthesized and secreted by the liver.[125] The liver is the only organ that produces serum albumin and alpha globulin, and it synthesizes most of the urea in the body. Hepatic regulation of protein metabolism profoundly affects the coagulation system. Production of various serum proteins is an important index of liver function; for example, the marker enzymes aspartate aminotransferase and alanine aminotransferase are useful clinical indicators of hepatocellular necrosis, and alkaline phosphatase, 5'-nucleotidase, leucine aminopeptidase, and gamma glutamyl transpeptidase are markers of cholestasis. Reduced serum fibrinogen may indicate severe liver dysfunction, because synthesis of this protein is remarkably preserved until late in the course of severe liver disease. Measurement of the maximal rate of urea synthesis has provided important research information about hepatic function, although this test is not practical for routine clinical use.

Albumin, the major protein in human serum, has been the most studied of the various proteins synthesized by the liver. Hepatic synthesis of this large protein (584 amino acids, molecular weight 66,000) is influenced by nutrition, various hormones, and oncotic pressure. Fasting decreases the synthesis of a number of proteins, including albumin, which is reduced by 40 to 50 per cent within 24 hours.[126] Refeeding rapidly reverses this, and the essential amino acid tryptophan may be crucially involved. Serum albumin levels are often decreased in cirrhotic patients. Conflicting studies exist as to whether ethanol has a direct toxic effect on protein synthesis. Androgens, thyroxine, glucocorticoids, and growth hormone increase albumin synthesis, whereas glucagon decreases albumin production in isolated hepatocytes. Insulin appears to have no effect. Interestingly, albumin synthesis is not controlled by the serum albumin concentration itself, but is regulated indirectly by plasma oncotic pressure, which is largely determined by albumin. Protein synthesis occurs mainly in the membrane-bound ribosomes of the rough endoplasmic reticulum.

The liver expresses a number of genes that are not expressed in other organs, for example, albumin and tyrosine aminotransferase. Transferrin and alpha$_1$-antitrypsin are examples of proteins expressed mainly in the liver but to a lesser extent in other organs. In addition, other genes such as the housekeeping genes for actin, myosin, tubulin, and cytokeratins are expressed in liver and many other tissues. Ongoing studies of liver-specific gene regulation fall into the categories of (1) response of liver-specific genes to exogenous stimuli, (2) liver-specific gene expression in hepatomas, (3) extinction of expression in somatic cell hybrids, (4) introduction of identified regulatory sequences into homologous or heterologous cell lines, and (5) transgenic mice.

GLUCOSE AND LIPID METABOLISM. The liver has a central role in energy metabolism. It helps provide a continuous supply of glucose for the central nervous system and red blood cells, which rely on this substrate for energy. It integrates the supply and demand of fuels required for tissues, such as muscle and adipose tissue, during changing nutritional balance. During the fed stage, approximately 50 per cent of glucose reaching the liver is converted to glycogen. The liver has a maximal storage capacity of 65 gm. per kg. of liver tissue. Fatty acids may also be synthesized from glucose, which may be esterified and secreted as very-low-density lipoprotein. Fructose is generally a better substrate for lipogenesis than is glucose. Galactose appears to be more important in infancy and childhood. Approximately half the energy made available to the liver is used in various types of transport, particularly sodium transport, and secretory function. In the postabsorptive state, the liver adds glucose to the blood rather than removing it. Glycogen stored during feeding is broken down to glucose, which supplies the central nervous system, red blood cells, and other tissues such as muscle.

During fasting, fatty acids begin to supplant ingested glucose as the principal fuel for most tissues. Hepatic glycogen stores are depleted within 48 hours of fasting. Gluconeogenesis then begins, using carbons from amino acids of muscle protein. Energy is also supplied by ketone bodies produced in the liver using fatty acids stored in adipose tissue. Two important signals for these adaptive responses of the liver are the concentration of glucose in sinusoidal blood and levels of insulin, catecholamines, and glucagon. Much is known about the biochemical and physiologic events of metabolism of glucose and fatty acids by the normal liver. In contrast, relatively little is known about changes in metabolism in the diseased liver. For example, clinically significant hypoglycemia is unusual with chronic liver disease, although it may be pronounced following major hepatic resection. Another example of this lack of knowledge is the poor understanding of the significance of fatty liver. The finding of fatty liver on liver biopsy may represent an appropriate response of the liver or may indicate an intrinsic hepatic derangement.

The liver also has a central role in lipoprotein and cholesterol metabolism. Many of the protein constituents of lipoproteins, termed apoproteins, are synthesized in the liver. Apoprotein E may be responsible for determining when the lipoproteins are removed by the liver.[131] The liver is the most active site of cholesterol and bile salt synthesis. Hydroxymethylglutaryl coenzyme A (HMG CoA) reductase is the rate-limiting enzyme of cholesterol synthesis. Bile salt synthesis is the major catabolic pathway of cholesterol in the liver, and 7α-hydroxylase is the rate-limiting enzyme for conversion of cholesterol to bile salts. The other important route of cholesterol elimination is direct secretion into bile. Cholesterol can enter the liver cell with four different species of lipoproteins: chylomicrons, very-low-density lipoprotein, low-density lipoprotein, and high-density lipoprotein. The chylomicron remnant, formed after degradation of the chylomicrons in the capillary beds, is probably the single most important source of hepatic cholesterol. Very-low-density lipoprotein remnants are removed inefficiently by the human liver, except in patients with hypertriglyceridemia. The amount of low-density lipoprotein, the major plasma carrier of cholesterol, removed by the human liver is unknown. High-density lipoprotein may be the most important lipoprotein involved in transport of cholesterol from peripheral tissues to the liver for excretion, a process known as reverse cholesterol transport. The amount of hepatic cholesterol produced by the liver itself is unknown, although approximately 20 per cent of biliary cholesterol appears to come from a newly synthesized pool.

VITAMIN METABOLISM. The liver has many important roles in uptake, storage, and mobilization of vitamins. The initial step in vitamin D activation occurs in the liver, where vitamin D$_3$ is converted to 25-hydroxycholecalciferol [25(OH)D$_3$]. The transport protein for vitamin D, called DBP, is manufactured in the liver. Vitamin A nutritional status can be estimated by vitamin A stores in the liver. The water-soluble B vitamins pass into the portal vein, and riboflavin, nicotinic acid, vitamin B$_{12}$, folic acid, and pantothenic acid are preferentially retained in the liver. These may be needed as cofactors in numerous enzyme-catalyzed reactions or may be metabolized for storage or synthesis of active forms. Vitamin B$_{12}$ is metabolically altered and then recycled in the enterohepatic circulation. Examples of active forms of B vitamins processed by the liver are thiamine, pyrophosphate, and pyridoxine phosphate. Some vitamins are transported by plasma proteins that are synthesized in the liver. An important example is transcobalamin II for vitamin B$_{12}$ transport. The metals iron, copper, zinc, manganese, selenium, and cobalt are essential for normal liver function. Vitamins E and C participate with some of the metals to perform several important hepatic functions.

Of particular surgical significance was the discovery of fat-soluble vitamin K. This vitamin is vital for carboxylation of coagulation factor precursors. Henrik Dam in 1929 observed that chicks developed hemorrhages when fed fat-free diets.[134] He designated the active ingredient in normal feed as vitamin K, for the German word "koagulation." The veterinary hematologic disorder "sweet clover disease," first reported in 1922 in cattle that developed fatal hemorrhages,[137] was found later to be caused by bis-hydroxycoumarin, a vitamin K antagonist.[133] It was not until the 1960s and early 1970s that vitamin K was shown to be required for the formation of blood factors II, VII, IX, and X. The minimal daily requirement of vitamin K is extremely small, approximately less than 0.1 μg. per kg. of body weight. Vitamin K is usually administered in pharmacologic doses, however, to counteract anticoagulation effects. Vitamin K coagulation disorders may be caused by chronic obstructive liver disease when intestinal bile salt deficiency causes insufficient absorption of the vitamin or by malabsorptive syndromes or administration of oral anticoagulants. In contrast, hepatocellular disease severe enough to prolong clotting times does not respond well to parenteral vitamin K. In fact, correction of the prothrombin time by vitamin K can be used as an index of severity of the hepatocellular disease.

BLOOD COAGULATION. The liver synthesizes 11 proteins critical for hemostasis: fibrinogen (factor I), prothrombin (factor

II), factors V, VII, VIII, IX, X, XI, and XII, prekallikrein, and high-molecular-weight kininogen.[138] In addition, the reticuloendothelial system of the liver is the major mechanism of clearance of the coagulation proteins. The liver may also affect coagulation in many other ways. For example, cirrhosis may cause portal hypertension, which may cause hypersplenism and a low platelet count. The most valuable tests to assess liver-induced coagulation dysfunction remain the prothrombin and partial thromboplastin times. Fresh frozen plasma is theoretically attractive to administer to patients with coagulation problems from hepatocellular disease. It contains the labile proteins V and VIII as well as many of the prothrombin complex proteins. The limiting factor, however, is the volume of administration, in that 1 or 2 liters are required for 50 per cent clotting activity.[139] Factor VII is one of the proteins with a short half-life, and frequent therapy may be required to maintain adequate levels of this factor.

METABOLISM OF DRUGS AND TOXINS. Drug and toxin metabolism is primarily a hepatic function. The range of metabolic transformations that foreign compounds undergo is conveniently categorized into two types: the Phase I reactions of oxidation, reduction, and hydrolysis; and the Phase II reactions, in which a compound is combined with an endogenous molecule to form a conjugate. The enzymes of biotransformation are localized primarily in the membranes of the endoplasmic reticulum. When liver cells are homogenized and centrifuged, the tubular reticulum fragments, and bits of the membranes form tiny vesicles called microsomes. Oxidative reactions represent most of the hepatic Phase I transformation in what has become known as the cytochrome P-450 system. This system may be separated chromatographically into three components: cytochrome P-450, NADPH–cytochrome P-450 reductase, and phospholipid.[141] Both the newborn and the elderly are particularly sensitive to many drugs, probably as a result of a lack of development or decreased activity of this system. The dietary protein:carbohydrate ratio, malnutrition, and other nutritional factors alter the rate of metabolism of pentobarbital, strychnine, aminopyrine, theophylline, and other drugs oxidized in the system. There appears to be much individual variability in the rates of drug metabolism.[142] For example, eating cabbage or Brussels sprouts considerably alters antipyrine metabolism. Other environmental factors such as alcohol intake, smoking habits, and occupational exposures definitely have a role in the marked individual variations.

Immunology

Only recently have various immunologic functions of the liver become appreciated. The liver has a major role in the development of the immune system from the time of early embryonic life. The lymphocytes begin to develop during the first 5 weeks of gestation, initially from mesenchymal cells of the yolk sac and later within the massive hematopoietic tissue of liver and spleen. Primitive lymphocytes, known as stem cells, then divide and form T and B lymphocytes. Certain stem cells also give rise to Kupffer cells, which are observed within the developing liver before bone marrow formation. Kupffer cells probably have an extensive role in the immune system. For example, these cells secrete cytokines, such as interleukin-1 and tumor necrosis factor, and contain surface receptors for immunoglobulin Fc fragment and complement. Liver parenchymal cells have an important role in the transport of immunoglobulin A into bile and intestine. The exact role of IgA in the liver or bile is not known. Up to half of biliary IgA may be produced in the liver, and a small number of immunoglobulin-containing cells are found in the portal tracts. In addition to the above-mentioned functions, the cells of the liver likely have important roles in the pathogenesis of many hepatic and extrahepatic immunologic diseases. For example, transplantation is likely to provide considerable knowledge in the next few years on the role the liver and other organs have in harboring of viruses such as hepatitis B and C and the retroviruses.

Liver Regeneration

It has been known for centuries that the liver has a remarkable capacity to regenerate. The liver can regain its normal size after 75 to 90 per cent hepatectomy provided the liver remnant is normal. After a suitable growth stimulus, rat hepatocytes proliferate at least once within 24 to 36 hours.[147] Nonparenchymal cells proliferate later. Regeneration occurs first in the hepatocyte zones that are more seriously damaged. For example, carbon tetrachloride injury occurs mainly in Zone 3 and subsequent regeneration occurs initially in this zone.[146] Little is known about the time reference of regeneration in humans, except that liver size approaches normal within weeks to months after resection. Despite much research, a clear concept of the mechanism of regeneration has not emerged, although insulin, glucagon, and epidermal growth factor may be involved. Recent speculation has focused on the possibility that there may be two types of cells capable of proliferation, parenchymal cells and "stem" cells, which may produce normal or neoplastic tissue.

SELECTED REFERENCES

Anatomy

Bismuth, H.: Surgical anatomy and anatomical surgery of the liver. *In* Blumgart, L. H.: Surgery of the Liver and Biliary Tract. Edinburgh, Churchill Livingstone, 1988.
This is an excellent review of the French segmental system of liver anatomy.

Jones, A. L.: Anatomy of the normal liver. *In* Zakim, D., and Boyer, T. D. (Eds.): Hepatology. Philadelphia, W. B. Saunders Company, 1982.
This chapter describes some basic concepts concerning anatomy and function.

Rappaport, A. M.: The microcirculatory hepatic unit. Microvasc. Res., 6:212, 1973.
The work of this investigator permits the understanding of the functional unit of the liver and the heterogeneity of hepatocyte function.

Skandalakis, L. J., Gray, S. W., Colborn, G. L., and Skandalakis, J. E.: Surgical anatomy of the liver and associated extrahepatic structures. Contemporary Surgery, 1987.
This article provides many details of anatomy including observations on vascular and biliary variability.

Physiology

Arias, I. M., Jakoby, W. B., Popper, H., Schachter, D., and Shafritz, D. A.: The Liver: Biology and Pathobiology. New York, Raven Press, 1988.
This is an excellent detailed analysis of a number of important topics in hepatobiliary physiology and pathobiology.

Scharschmidt, B. F., and Schmid, R.: Bile secretion, intestinal lipid absorption and the enterohepatic circulation of bile salts. *In* Way, L. W., and Pellegrini, C. A. (Eds.): Surgery of the Gallbladder and Bile Ducts. Philadelphia, W. B. Saunders Company, 1987, p. 23.
This is a review of the basic concepts of bile formation.

Sherman, M.: Molecular biology of the liver and liver disease. *In* Gitnick, G. (Ed.): Current Hepatology. Vol. 9. Chicago, Year Book Medical Publishers, 1989, p. 55.
This is a recent review of an area of intense ongoing research likely to have important implications in future concepts and treatment.

Zakim, D., and Boyer, T. D.: Hepatology, 2nd ed. Philadelphia, W. B. Saunders Company, 1990.
This recent edition includes basic physiologic principles concerning many disease processes.

REFERENCES

Anatomy

General

1. Bender, G. A.: Great Moments in Medicine. Detroit, Northwood Institute Press, 1966, pp. 50–55.
2. Campra, J. L., and Reynolds, T. B.: The hepatic circulation. *In* Arias, I. M., Popper, H., Schacter, D., and Shafritz, D. A. (Eds.): The Liver: Biology and Pathobiology. New York, Raven Press, 1982, pp. 627–645.
3. Jones, A. L.: Anatomy of the normal liver. *In* Zakim, D., and Boyer, T. D. (Eds.): Hepatology. Philadelphia, W. B. Saunders Company, 1982, pp. 3–31.

4. Longmire, W. P., Jr., and Tompkins, R. K.: Anatomy. *In* Longmire, W. P., Jr., and Tompkins, R. K. (Eds.): Manual of Liver Surgery. New York, Springer-Verlag, 1981, pp. 13–25.
5. Rappaport A. M.: Physioanatomic considerations. *In* Schiff, L., and Schiff, E. R. (Eds.): Diseases of the Liver, 5th ed. Philadelphia, J. B. Lippincott Company, 1982, pp. 1–57.
6. Skandalakis, L. J., Gray, S. W., Colborn, G. L., and Skandalakis, J. E.: Surgical anatomy of the liver and associated extrahepatic structures. *In* Contemporary Surgery, 1987.

Lobar Anatomy

7. Cantlie, J.: On a new arrangement of the right and left lobes of the liver. J. Anat. 32:4, 1897.
8. Cantlie, J.: On a new arrangement of the right and left lobes of the liver. J. Anat. Physiol. (London) (Section Proc. Anat. Soc. Great Britain and Ireland) 32:iv, 1898.
9. Couinaud, C.: Les enveloppes vasculobiliaires de foie ou capsule de Glisson. Leur interet dans la chirurgie vesiculaire, les resections hepatiques et l'abord du hile du foie. Lyon Chir., 49:589, 1954.
10. Couinaud, C.: Controlled hepatectomies and exposure of the intrahepatic bile ducts. Paris, C. Couinaud, 1981.
11. Elias, H., and Petty, D.: Gross anatomy of the blood vessels and ducts within the human liver. Am. J. Anat., 90:59, 1952.
12. Goldsmith, N. A., and Woodburne, R. T.: The surgical anatomy pertaining to liver resections. Surg. Gynecol. Obstet., 105:310, 1957.
13. Hahn, P. F., et al.: Physiological bilaterality of portal circulation; streamline flow of blood into liver as shown by radioactive phosphorus. Am. J. Physiol., 143:105, 1945.
14. Hjortsjo, C.-H.: The topography of the intrahepatic duct systems. Acta Anat. (Basel), 11:599, 1951.
15. Junes, M. P.: Les arborisations biliovasculaires intrahepatiques: (etude anatomo-chirurgicale en vue des hepatectomies) d'apres 50 moulages hepatiques en matieres plastiques. Bordeaux Chir., 1:5, 1954.
16. McIndoe, H. A., and Counseller, V. S.: A report on the bilaterality of the liver. Arch. Surg., 15:589, 1927.
17. Rappaport, A. M.: Physioanatomic considerations. *In* Schiff, L., and Schiff, E. R. (Eds.): Diseases of the Liver, 5th ed. Philadelphia, J. B. Lippincott Company, 1982, pp. 1–57.
18. Rex, H.: Beitrage zur Morphologie der Saugerleber. Morphol. Jahrb., 14:517, 1888.

Portal Vein

19. Gilfillan, R. S.: Anatomic study of the portal vein and its main branches. Arch. Surg., 61:449, 1950.
20. Gupta, S. C., Gupta, C. D., and Arora, A. K.: Intrahepatic branching patterns of portal vein. A study by corrosion cast. Gastroenterology, 72:621, 1977.
21. Lam, K. C., Juttner, H. U., and Reynolds, T. B.: Spontaneous portosystemic shunt: Relationship to spontaneous encephalopathy and gastrointestinal hemorrhage. Dig. Dis. Sci., 26:346, 1981.
22. Toni, G., Testoni, P. P., Trombetta, N., and Favero, A.: Lexone epatiche. Institutio di Anatomia Umana Trieste. Cited by Sedgwick, C. E., and Poulantzas, J. K.: Portal Hypertension. Boston, Little, Brown and Company, 1959.

Hepatic Artery

23. Healey, J. E., Jr.: Clinical anatomic aspects of radical hepatic surgery. J. Int. Coll. Surgeons, 22:542, 1954.
24. Healey, J. E., Jr., Schroy, P. C., and Sorensen, R. J.: The intrahepatic distribution of the hepatic artery in man. J. Int. Coll. Surgeons, 20:133, 1953.
25. Michels, N. A.: Newer anatomy of the liver and its variant blood supply and collateral circulation. Am. J. Surg., 112:337, 1966.
26. Rappaport, A. M., and Schneiderman, J. H.: The function of the hepatic artery. Rev. Physiol. Biochem. Pharmacol., 76:129, 1976.
27. Rhodin, J. A.: The ultrastructure of mammalian arterioles and precapillary sphincters. J. Ultrastruct. Res., 18:181, 1967.

Hepatic Veins

28. Elias, H., and Sherrick, J. C.: Morphology of the Liver. New York, Academic Press, 1969.
29. Nakamura, S., and Tsuzuki, T.: Surgical anatomy of the hepatic veins and the inferior vena cava. Surg. Gynecol. Obstet., 152:43, 1981.
30. Rappaport, A. M.: Anatomic considerations. *In* Schiff, L. (Ed.): Diseases of the Liver, 4th ed. Philadelphia, J. B. Lippincott Company, 1975, pp. 1–50.

Biliary System

31. Boyden, E. A.: The sphincter of Oddi. Surgery, 1:25, 1937.
32. Chenderovitch, J.: Les conceptions actuelles de la secretion biliaire. Presse Med., 71:2645, 1963.
33. Elias, H., and Petty, D.: Gross anatomy of blood vessels and ducts within the human liver. Am J. Anat., 90:59, 1952.

34. Higgins, G. M.: The biliary tract of certain rodents with and those without a gallbladder. Anat. Rec., 232:89, 1926.
35. Job, T. T.: The anatomy of the duodenal portion of the bile and pancreatic ducts. Anat. Rec., 32:212, 1926.
36. Johnston, E. V., and Anson, B. J.: Variations in the formation and vascular relationships of the bile ducts. Surg. Gynecol. Obstet., 94:669, 1952.

Nerves

37. Amenta, F., Cavallotti, C., Ferrante, F., and Tonelli, F.: Cholinergic nerves in the human liver. Histochem. J., 13:419, 1981.
38. Gray, H.: Anatomy of the Human Body, 29th ed. Philadelphia, Lea and Febiger, 1973.
39. Jayle, G. E.: Les nerfs du foie, etude anatomique et histologique. Nutrition, 7:57, 1937.
40. Mallet-Guy, P., et al.: Etude experimentale de la neurectomie periartere hepatique. I. Effets de la resection du "pedicule nerveux anterieure" sur le foie normal. Lyon Chir., 51:45, 1956.

Lymphatics

41. Disse, J.: Über die Lymphbahnen der Saugetierleber. Arch Mikr. Anat., 36:203, 1890.
42. Jdanov, D. A.: Anatomy and function of the lymphatic capillaries. Lancet, 2:895, 1969.
43. Mall, F. P.: A study of the structural unit of the liver. Am. J. Anat., 5:227, 1906.
44. Mallet-Guy, P., et al.: Recherches experimentales sur la circulation lymphatique du foie. I. Donnes immediates sur la permeabilite biliolymphatique. Lyon Chir., 58:847, 1962.
45. Szabo, G., et al.: The effect of occlusion of liver lymphatics on hepatic blood flow. Res. Exp. Med. (Berlin), 169:1, 1976.

Microscopic Anatomy

46. Campra, J. L., and Reynolds, T. B.: The hepatic circulation. *In* Arias, I. M., Popper, H., Schachter, D., and Shafritz, D. A. (Eds.): The Liver: Biology and Pathobiology. New York, Raven Press, 1982, pp. 627–645.
47. Jones, A. L., and Schmucker, D. L.: Current concept of liver structure as related to function. Gastroenterology, 73:833, 1977.
48. Kiernan, F.: The anatomy and physiology of the liver. Philos. Trans. R. Soc. Lond. 123:711, 1833.
49. Rappaport, A. M.: The microcirculatory hepatic unit. Microvasc. Res., 6:212, 1973.
50. Rappaport, A. M.: Hepatic blood flow: Morphologic aspects and physiologic regulation. *In* Javitt, N. B. (Ed.): Liver and Biliary Tract Physiology. International Review of Physiology. Vol. 21. Baltimore, University Park Press, 1980.
51. Rappaport, A. M., Borowy, Z. J., Lougheed, W. M., and Lotto, W. N.: Subdivision of hexagonal liver lobules into a structural and functional unit. Role in hepatic physiology and pathology. Anat. Rec., 119:11, 1954.

Ultrastructure

52. Claude, A.: Growth and differentiation of cytoplasmic membranes in the course of lipoprotein granule synthesis in the hepatic cell. J. Cell. Biol., 47:745, 1970.
53. Jones, A. L., Schmucker, D. L., Mooney, J. S., et al.: Alterations in hepatic pericanalicular cytoplasm during enhanced bile secretory activity. Lab. Invest., 40:512, 1979.
54. Jones, A. L., Schmucker, D. L., Renston, R. H., et al.: The architecture of bile secretion: A morphological perspective of physiology. Dig. Dis. Sci., 25:609, 1980.
55. Jones, A. L.: Anatomy of the normal liver. *In* Zakim, D., and Boyer, T. D. (Eds.): Hepatology. Philadelphia, W. B. Saunders Company, 1982, pp. 17–21.
56. Zakim, D., and Boyer, T. D.: Hepatology. Philadelphia, W. B. Saunders Company, 1982, Chapters 1–12.

Liver Development

57. Baum, S., Locko, R. C., and d'Avignon, M. B.: Functional anatomy and radionuclide imaging: Riedel's lobe of the liver. Anat. Clin., 4:121, 1982.
58. Braasch, J. W.: Congenital anomalies of the gallbladder and bile ducts. Surg. Clin. North. Am., 38:627, 1958.
59. Ekberg, H., Tranberg, K. G., Anderson, R., Jeppsson, B., and Bengmark, S.: Major liver resection: Perioperative course and management. Surgery, 100:1, 1986.
60. Elias, H.: Appositional growth of the embryonic liver. Rev. Int. Hepatic, 14:317, 1964.
61. Feigl, W., Firbas, W., Sinzinger, H., and Wicke, L.: Truncus coeliacus und seiner Anastomosen mit der Arteria mesenterica superior. Acta Anat., 92:272, 1975.
62. Gray, S. W., and Skandalakis, J. E.: Embryology for Surgeons. Philadelphia, W. B. Saunders Company, 1972.

Physiology

General

63. Arias, I. M., Jakoby, W. B., Popper, H., Schachter, D., and Shafritz, D. A.: The Liver: Biology and Pathobiology. New York, Raven Press, 1988.
64. Baldwin, R. L., and Smith, N. E.: Molecular control of energy metabolism. In Sink, J. D. (Ed.): The Control of Metabolism. University Park, PA, The Pennsylvania State University Press, 1974, p. 17.
65. Bujanover, Y., Amarri, S., Lebenthal, E., and Petell, J. K.: The effect of dexamethasone and glucagon on the expression of hepatocyte plasma membrane proteins during development. Hepatology, 8:722, 1988.
66. Corless, J. K., and Middleton, H. M.: Normal liver function—a basis for understanding hepatic disease. Arch. Intern. Med., 143:2291, 1983.
67. Gitnick, G.: Current Hepatology. Vol. 9. Chicago, Year Book Medical Publishers, 1989.
68. Heyworth, M. F., and Jones, A. L.: Immunology of the Gastrointestinal Tract and Liver. New York, Raven Press, 1988.
69. Meyers, J. D.: The hepatic blood flow and splanchnic oxygen consumption of man—their estimation from urea production or bromsulfalein excretion during catheterization of the hepatic veins. J. Clin. Invest., 26:1130, 1947.
70. Schiff, L., and Schiff, E. R.: Diseases of the Liver, 6th ed. Philadelphia, J. B. Lippincott Company, 1987.
71. Zakim, D., and Boyer, T. D.: Hepatology. Philadelphia, W. B. Saunders Company, 1990.

Blood Flow

72. Bradley, E. L., III: Measurement of hepatic blood flow in man. Surgery, 75:783, 1974.
73. Bradley, S. E., Inglefinger, F. J., Bradley, G. P., and Curry, J. J.: The estimation of hepatic blood flow in man. J. Clin. Invest., 24:890, 1945.
74. Campra, J., and Reynolds, T.: The hepatic circulation. In Arias, I. M., Jakoby, W. B., Popper, H., Schachter, D., and Shafritz, D. A. (Eds.): The Liver: Biology and Pathobiology. New York, Raven Press, 1988, p. 911.
75. Chiandussi, L., Greco, F., Stardi, G., Vaccarino, A., Ferraris, C. M., and Curti, B.: Estimation of hepatic arterial and portal venous blood flow by direct catheterization of the vena porta through the umbilical cord in man. Preliminary results. Acta Hepatosplenol. (Stuttg.), 15:166, 1968.
76. Child, C. G., Barr, D., Holswade, G. R., and Harrison, C. S.: Liver regeneration following portacaval transposition in dogs. Ann. Surg., 138:600, 1953.
77. Eck, N. V., and Voprosu, K.: O perevyazkie vorotnois veni. Predvaritelnoye soobshtshjenye (Ligature of the portal vein). Voen. Med. J. (St. Petersburg), 130:1, 1877. (English translation provided by Child, C. G., III: Surg. Gynecol. Obstet., 960:375, 1953.)
78. Hahn, M., Massen, O., Nencki, M., and Pavlov, J.: Die Eck'sche fistel zwischen der unteren Hohlvene und der Pfortader und ihre Folgen für den Organismus. Arch Exp. Pathol. Pharmakol., 32:161, 1893.
79. Jones, A. L.: Anatomy of the normal liver. In Zakim, D., and Boyer, T. D.: Hepatology. Philadelphia, W. B. Saunders Company, 1990, pp. 3–29.
80. Kock, N. G., Hahnloser, P., Roding, B., and Schenk, W. G., Jr.: Interaction between portal venous and hepatic arterial blood flow: An experimental study in the dog. Surgery, 72:414, 1972.
81. Mann, F. C.: The portal circulation and restoration of the liver after partial removal. Surgery, 8:225, 1940.
82. Marchioro, T. L., Porter, K. A., Dickinson, T. C., Faris, T. D., and Starzl, T. E.: Physiologic requirements for auxiliary liver homotransplantation. Surg. Gynecol. Obstet., 121:17, 1965.
83. Pouyet, M., Berard, P., Ruckebusch, Y., Grivel, M. L., Bousquet, G., and Vauzelle, J. L.: Derivations portohepatiques: Selectives origine pancreatique due facteur hepatotrophique portal. Ann. Chir., 23:393, 1969.
84. Putnam, C. W., Porter, K. A., and Starzl, T. E.: Hepatic encephalopathy and light and electron micrographic changes of the baboon liver after portal diversion. Ann. Surg., 184:155, 1976.
85. Schenk, W. G., Jr., McDonald, J. C., McDonald, K., and Drapanas, T.: Direct measurement of hepatic blood flow in surgical patients: With related observations on hepatic flow dynamics in experimental animals. Ann. Surg., 156:463, 1962.
86. Sexton, A. W., Marchioro, T. L., Waddell, W. R., and Starzl, T. E.: Liver deglycogenation after portacaval transposition. Surg. Forum, 15:120, 1964.
87. Starzl, T. E., Francavilla, A., Halgrimson, C. G., Francavilla, F. R., Porter, K. A., Brown, T. H., and Putnam, C. W.: The origin, hormonal nature, and action of hepatotrophic substances in portal venous blood. Surg. Gynecol. Obstet., 137:179, 1973.
88. Starzl, T. E., Porter, K. A., and Francavilla, T.: The Eck fistula in animals and humans. Curr. Probl. Surg., 20:687, 1983.

Bile Formation

89. Barnhart, J. L., and Combes, B.: Erythritol and mannitol clearances with taurocholate and secretin-induced cholereses. Am. J. Physiol., 234:E146, 1978.
90. Behar, J., and Biancani, P.: Effects and mechanisms of action of motilin on the cat sphincter of Oddi. Gastroenterology, 95:1099, 1988.
91. Boyer, J. L., and Bloomer, J. R.: Canalicular bile secretion in man. Studies utilizing the biliary clearance of ^{14}C mannitol. J. Clin. Invest., 54:773, 1974.
92. Brauer, R. W.: Hepatic blood supply and the secretion of bile. In Taylor, R. W. (Ed.): The Biliary System. Oxford, Blackwell Scientific Publishers, 1965, p. 41.
93. Buanes, T., Grotmol, T., Landsverk, T., and Raeder, M. G.: Secretin empties bile duct cell cytoplasm of vesicles when it initiates ductular HCO_3^- secretion in the pig. Gastroenterology, 95:417, 1988.
94. Coehlo, J. C. U., Runkel, N., Herfarth, C., Senninger, N., and Messmer, K.: Effect of analgesic drugs on the electromyographic activity of the gastrointestinal tract and sphincter of Oddi and on biliary pressure. Ann. Surg., 204:53, 1986.
95. Erlinger, S.: Secretion of bile. In Schiff, L., and Schiff, E. R. (Eds.): Diseases of the Liver. Philadelphia, J. B. Lippincott Company, 1987, p. 77.
96. Forker, E. L.: Mechanisms of hepatic bile formation. Ann. Rev. Physiol., 39:323, 1977.
97. Graf, J.: Canalicular bile salt–independent bile formation: Concepts and clues from electrolyte transport in rat liver. Am. J. Physiol., 244:G233, 1983.
98. Hoover, E. L., Jaffe, B. M., Webb, H., and England, D. W.: Effects of female sex hormones and pregnancy on gallbladder prostaglandin synthesis. Arch. Surg., 123:705, 1988.
99. Jones, R. S., and Meyers, W. C.: Regulation of hepatic biliary secretion. Ann. Rev. Physiol., 141:67, 1979.
100. Kaminski, D. L., Deshpande, Y. G., and Beinfeld, M. C.: Role of glucagon in cholecystokinin-stimulated bile flow in dogs. Am. J. Physiol., 254:G864, 1988.
101. Lillemoe, K. D., Webb, T. H., and Pitt, H. A.: Neuropeptide Y: A candidate neurotransmitter for biliary motility. J. Surg. Res., 45:254, 1988.
102. Meyers, W. C., and Jones, R. S.: Glucagon or insulin suppressed biliary lipid excretion in dog and man. Ann. Surg., 190:709, 1979.
103. Prandi, D., Erlinger, S., Glasinovic, J. C., and Dumont, M.: Canalicular bile production in man. Eur. J. Clin. Invest., 5:1, 1975.
104. Scharschmidt, B. F., and Van Dyke, R. W.: Mechanisms of hepatic electrolyte transport. Gastroenterology, 85:1199, 1983.
105. Scharschmidt, B. F., and Schmid, R.: Bile secretion, intestinal lipid absorption and the enterohepatic circulation of bile salts. In Way, L. W., and Pellegrini, C. A. (Eds.): Surgery of the Gallbladder and Bile Ducts. Philadelphia, W. B. Saunders Company, 1987, p. 23.
106. Takeshige, K., Kuroda, H., Fukaya, Y., Suzuki, H., Hasegawa, M., and Yamamoto, S.: The role of portal blood factors in regeneration of the liver. World J. Surg., 6:603, 1982.
107. Wheeler, H. O.: Water and electrolytes in bile. In Code, C. F. (Ed.): Handbook of Physiology. Section 6, Alimentary Canal, Vol. 5. Washington, D.C., Am. Physiology Society, 1968, pp. 2409–2431.
108. Wolfe, B. M., Walker, B. K., Shaul, D. B., Wong, L., and Ruebner, B. H.: Effect of total parenteral nutrition on hepatic histology. Arch. Surg., 123:1084, 1988.

Lymphatics

109. Disse, J.: Über die Lymphbahnen der Saugetierleber. Arch. Mikr. Anat., 36:203, 1890.
110. Jdanov, D. A.: Anatomy and function of the lymphatic capillaries. Lancet, 2:895, 1969.
111. Mall, F. P.: A study of the structural unit of the liver. Am. J. Anat., 5:227, 1906.
112. Mallet-Guy, P., et al.: Recherches experimentales sur la circulation lymphatique du foie. I. Donnes immediates sur la permeabilite biliolymphatique. Lyon Chir., 58:847, 1962.
113. Szabo, G., et al.: The effect of occlusion of liver lymphatics on hepatic blood flow. Res. Exp. Med. (Berlin), 169:1, 1976.

Enterohepatic Circulation

114. Carey, M. C., and Cahalane, M. J.: The enterohepatic circulation. In Arias, I. M., Jakoby, W. B., Popper, H., Schachter, D., and Shafritz, D. A. (Eds.): The Liver: Biology and Pathobiology. New York, Raven Press, 1988, p. 573.
115. Heaton, K. W.: The importance of keeping bile salts in their place. Gut, 10:857, 1969.
116. Hofmann, A. F.: The enterohepatic circulation of bile acids in man. Clin. Gastroenterol., 6:3, 1977.
117. Small, D. M., Dowling, R. H., and Redinger, R. N.: The enterohepatic circulation of bile salts. Arch. Intern. Med., 130:552, 1972.

Bilirubin Metabolism

118. Berk, P. D., Howe, R. B., Bloomer, J. R., and Berlin, N. I.: Studies of bilirubin kinetics in normal adults. J. Clin. Invest., 48:2176, 1969.
119. Chowdhury, J. R., Wolkoff, A. W., and Arias, I. M.: Heme and bile pigment metabolism. In Arias, I. M., Jakoby, W. B., Popper, H., Schachter, D., and Shafritz, D. A. (Eds.): The Liver: Biology and Pathobiology. New York, Raven Press, 1988, p. 419.
120. Cramer, G. L., Greenberg, B. D., Sack, E. M., and Layden, T. J.: Intrahepatic cholestasis, bile excretory function, and hyperbilirubinemia. In Gitnick, G. (Ed.): Current Hepatology. Chicago, Year Book Medical Publishers, 1989, p. 285.
121. Robinson, S. H.: Origins of the early-labeled peak. In Berk, P. D., and Berlin, N. I. (Eds.): The Chemistry and Physiology of Bile Pigments. Washington, D.C., U.S. Government Printing Office, 1977, p. 175.

Protein Metabolism

122. Becker, W., Konstantinides, B. S., Eyer, S., et al.: Plasma amino acid clearance as an indicator of hepatic function and high energy phosphate in hepatic ischemia. Surgery, *102*:777, 1987.
123. Donohue, T. M., Jennet, R. B., Tuma D. J., and Sorrell, M. F.: Synthesis and secretion of plasma proteins by the liver. *In* Zakim, D., and Boyer, T. D. (Eds.): Hepatology. Philadelphia, W. B. Saunders Company, 1990, p. 124.
124. Farrell, G., and Koltai, A.: Hepatic testosterone metabolism in male rats with portal bypass. Gastroenterology, *95*:425, 1988.
125. Knowles, B. B., et al.: Human hepatocellular carcinoma cell lines secrete the major plasma proteins and hepatitis B surface antigen. Science, *209*:497, 1980.
126. Rothschild, M. A., et al.: Effects of a short-term fast on albumin synthesis studied in vivo, in the perfused liver, and on amino acid incorporations by hepatic microsomes. J. Clin. Invest., *47*:2591, 1968.
127. Sherman, M.: Molecular biology of the liver and liver disease. *In* Gitnick, G. (Ed.): Current Hepatology. Chicago, Year Book Medical Publishers, 1989, p. 55.
128. Zern, M. A., Shafritz, D. A., and Shields, D.: Hepatic protein synthesis and its regulation. *In* Arias, I. M., Jakoby, W. B., Popper, H., Schachter, D., and Shafritz, D. A. (Eds.): The Liver: Biology and Pathobiology. New York, Raven Press, 1982, p. 103.

Glucose and Lipid Metabolism

129. Cooper, A. D.: Role of the liver in the degradation of lipoproteins. Gastroenterology, *88*:192, 1985.
130. Cooper, A. D.: Hepatic lipoprotein and cholesterol metabolism. *In* Zakim, D., and Boyer, T. D. (Eds.): Hepatology. Philadelphia, W. B. Saunders Company, 1990.
131. Shelbourne, F., Hanks, J. B., Meyers, W. C., et al.: Effect of apoproteins in hepatic uptake of triglyceride emulsions in the rat. J. Clin. Invest., *65*:652, 1980.
132. Zakim, D.: Metabolism of glucose and fatty acids by the liver. *In* Zakim, D., and Boyer, T. D. (Eds.): Hepatology. Philadelphia, W. B. Saunders Company, 1990.

Vitamin Metabolism

133. Bikle, D. D.: Metabolism and functions of vitamins A, D, and K. *In* Zakim, D., and Boyer, T. D. (Eds.): Hepatology. Philadelphia, W. B. Saunders Company, 1990.
134. Campbell, H. A., and Link, K. P.: Studies on the hemorrhagic sweet clover disease. IV. The isolation and crystallization of the hemorrhagic agent. J. Biol. Chem., *138*:21, 1941.
135. Dam, H.: Cholesterinstoffwechsel in Huhnereiern und Huhnchen. Biochem. Z., *215*:475, 1929.
136. Friedman, P. A.: Vitamin K. *In* Arias, I. M., Jakoby, W. B., Popper, H., Schachter, D., and Shafritz, D. A. (Eds.): The Liver: Biology and Pathobiology. New York, Raven Press, 1982, p. 359.
137. Schofield, F. W.: Damaged sweet clover: Cause of a new disease in cattle simulating hemorrhagic septicemia and blackleg. J. Am. Vet. Med. Assoc., *64*:553, 1924.

Blood Coagulation

138. Colman, R. W., and Rubin, R. N.: Blood coagulation. *In* Arias, I. M., Jakoby, W. B., Popper, H., Schachter, D., and Shafritz, D. A. (Eds.): The Liver: Biology and Pathobiology. New York, Raven Press, 1988, p. 1033.
139. Penny, R., Rosenberg, M. C., and Firkin, B. G.: The splenic platelet pool. Blood, *27*:1, 1966.

Metabolism of Drugs and Toxins

140. Alvares, A. P.: Oxidative biotransformation of drugs. *In* Arias, I. M., Jakoby, W. B., Popper, H., Schachter, D., and Shafritz, D. A. (Eds.): The Liver: Biology and Pathobiology. New York, Raven Press, 1982, p. 265.
141. Lu, A. Y. H., and Coon, M. J.: Role of hemoprotein P-450 in fatty acid δ-hydroxylation in a soluble enzyme system from liver microsomes. J. Biol. Chem., *243*:1331, 1968.
142. Pantuck, E. J., Hsaio, K.-C., Loub, W. D., Wattenberg, L. W., Kuntzman, R., and Conney, A. M.: Stimulatory effect of vegetables on intestinal drug metabolism in the rat. J. Pharmacol. Exp. Ther., *198*:278, 1976.
143. Vessey, D. A.: Hepatic metabolism of drugs and toxins. *In* Zakim, D., and Boyer, T. D. (Eds.): Hepatology. Philadelphia, W. B. Saunders Company, 1990.

Liver Regeneration

144. Gumucio, J. J., Katz, M. E., Miller, D. L., Balabaub, C. P., Greenfield, J. M., and Wagner, R. M.: Bile salt transport after selective damage to acinar zone 3 hepatocytes by bromobenzene in the rat. Toxicol. Appl. Pharmacol., *50*:77, 1979.
145. Kahn, D., Hickman, R., Terblanche, J., and von Sommoggy, S.: Partial hepatectomy and liver regeneration in pigs — the response to different resection sites. J. Surg. Res., *45*:176, 1988.
146. Leffert, H. L., Koch, K. S., Lad, P. J., Shapiro, I. P., Skelly, H., and deHemptinne, B.: Hepatocyte regeneration, replication and differentiation. *In* Arias, I. M., Jakoby, W. B., Popper, H., Schachter, D., and Shafritz, D. A. (Eds.): The Liver: Biology and Pathobiology. New York, Raven Press, 1988, p. 833.
147. Rabes, H. M.: Kinetics of hepatocellular proliferation as a function of the microvascular structure and functional state of the liver. *In* Hepatotrophic Factors. CIBA Foundation Symposium, No. 55. Amsterdam, Elsevier, 1978, p. 31.
148. St. Hilaire, R. J., and Jones, A. L.: Epidermal growth factor: Its biologic and metabolic effects with emphasis on the hepatocyte. Hepatology, *2*:601, 1982.

Immunologic Function

149. Heyworth, M. F., and Jones, A. L.: Immunology of the Gastrointestinal Tract and Liver. New York, Raven Press, 1988.
150. Shiratori, Y., Kawase, T., Shina, S., Okano, K., Sugimoto, T., Teraoka, H., Matano, S., Matsumoto, K., and Kamii, K.: Modulation of hepatotoxicity by macrophages in the liver. Hepatology, *8*:815, 1988.
151. Lim, G. M., Sheldon, G. F., and Alverdy, J.: Biliary secretory IgA levels in rats with protein-calorie malnutrition. Ann. Surg., *207*:635, 1988.

II

PYOGENIC AND AMEBIC LIVER ABSCESS

Gene D. Branum, M.D., and William C. Meyers, M.D.

Liver abscess remains a formidable diagnostic and therapeutic problem. Changing etiologies of liver abscess reflect both improvements in health care and increased recognition of the condition in sicker, often immunocompromised patients. Pyogenic (bacterial) and amebic abscesses share many clinical features and are classically discussed together. The pyogenic type is much more common in most sections of the United States, yet amebic abscess is endemic in most areas and requires clinical suspicion for correct diagnosis. Fungi, cytomegalovirus, and other organisms also cause liver abscess, predominantly in the immunocompromised host but are less common and usually cause more diffuse hepatic disease. Echinococcosis generally has a different clinical presentation from pyogenic or amebic abscess unless there is secondary bacterial involvement and is discussed in a later chapter.

Liver abscess has been recognized since Hippocrates (circa 400 B.C.), who speculated that prognosis is related to the type of fluid within the lesion.[30] In the early nineteenth century, Bright[11] suggested that amebae might contribute to formation of hepatic abscess, and Koch in 1883 described amebae in the wall of a hepatic abscess. Fitz[19] and Dieulafoy[18] emphasized the importance of intra-abdominal (bacterial) sources of infection in the pathogenesis of the disease. Dieulafoy coined the term *la foie appendiculaire* in describing multiple hepatic abscesses subsequent to perforated appendicitis with pyelophlebitis (Fig. 1). Ochsner and DeBakey provided classic treatises on pyogenic and amebic hepatic abscess in 1938[49] and 1943.[47,48] The latter authors reviewed a large personal experience and the world literature and emphasized the similarity in clinical presentation between the two types of abscesses. Major advances in both

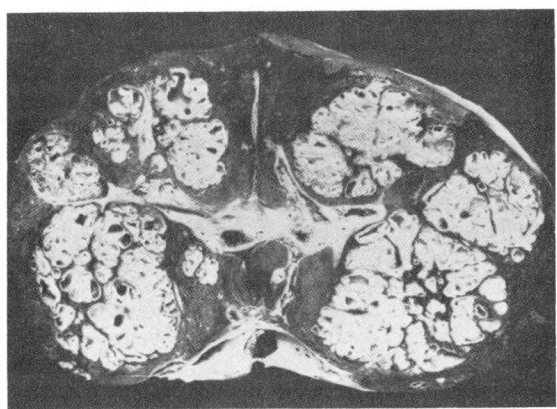

Figure 1. "Foie appendiculaire." Liver with multiple pyogenic abscesses. Patient died 3 weeks after operation for suppurative appendicitis. (From Bras, G., and Brandt, K. H.: Vascular disorders. In MacSween, R. N. M., Anthony, P. P., and Scheuer, P. J. (Eds.): Pathology of the Liver. Edinburgh, Churchill Livingstone, 1987, p. 481.)

diagnosis and treatment of liver abscess have occurred during the past 15 years. Although clinical signs have remained the same, radiologic methods of diagnosis have greatly improved, and it is rare to overlook a lesion with ultrasonography or computerized tomography. Antibiotic therapy has also improved, but the principal advance in the management of hepatic abscess has been the application of percutaneous aspiration techniques for diagnosis or treatment.

INCIDENCE

The overall incidence of liver abscess remains relatively stable, although the distribution of causes is changing. Pyogenic abscess represents approximately 80 per cent of the cases in the United States, and superinfection, another 10 per cent. Amebae are the primary cause of about 10 per cent, and fungi and other organisms cause the remainder. The overall rate of pyogenic abscess in the United States is estimated between 8 and 15 per 100,000 population. The incidence of both pyogenic and amebic abscess is higher in nations where medical care is not immediately available. For example, in Malaysia pyogenic abscess constitutes 0.85 per cent of total hospital admissions.[4]

Amebic infestation is higher in (1) countries in tropical or subtropical zones, (2) locations with poor sanitation, and (3) mental institutions. In 1975, the Centers for Disease Control (CDC) (Atlanta, Georgia) noted 1.3 cases of amebiasis reported per 100,000 population. The CDC recorded 3500 cases of amebiasis per year, data that probably underestimate the actual number of cases. Immigrants and tourists from developing countries have a higher incidence, and American tourists to tropical areas are more likely to develop invasive amebiasis than permanent residents. Amebae are estimated to infest 15 to 30 per cent of the population of Mexico, Africa, Southeast Asia, and South America. Local inhabitants are less likely than visitors to manifest symptoms, presumably due to partial immunity.[4]

Hepatic abscess is the most common extraintestinal manifestation of amebiasis.[1] Hepatic amebiasis is reported in 3 to 10 per cent of afflicted patients.[4] DeBakey and Ochsner found an average incidence of hepatic involvement associated with intestinal disease to be 13.2 per cent.[16] Certain severely infested locations report up to a 40 per cent incidence of hepatic involvement. Liver abscess of both types affects both sexes and all age groups. In recent years, pyogenic abscess affected slightly more males than females, which is consistent with earlier series. The 40- to 60-year-old age group is the most commonly afflicted, and children represent a distinct group because of a higher rate of immunosuppression in hospitalized youth. In a recent series from Duke University,[10] all six patients with pyogenic abscess less

than 15 years of age were male. Over the past several years in Los Angeles, the male-to-female ratio has been nearly 2:1 in young patients.[22] This changing sex distribution in younger patients probably reflects the impact of the acquired immunodeficiency syndrome (AIDS). Amebic abscess affects males more than females in as much as a 9 to 10:1 ratio. In general, the patients are younger, with the highest incidence in the 20- to 50-year-old age group. Several recent reports indicate a marked increase in the incidence of amebic liver abscess in children under the age of 3. There does not appear to be any particular racial susceptibility except for that related to living conditions. Examples include Mexican-Americans in the American Southwest and the predisposition of South African blacks, compared with South African whites.[2,6]

PATHOGENESIS

Pyogenic Abscess

The pathophysiology of liver abscess in general or pyogenic abscess in particular involves two basic elements: (1) the presence of the organism and (2) the vulnerability of the liver. The spread of bacterial or other organisms to the hepatic parenchyma may occur via (1) the portal system, (2) ascension from the biliary tree, (3) the hepatic artery during generalized septicemia, (4) direct extension from subhepatic or subdiaphragmatic infection, or (5) a direct route following trauma (Fig. 2).

Most organisms enter the liver through the portal route. Hepatic clearance of portal bacteria is probably a very common event in healthy individuals. The human liver remains sterile in most circumstances because of an efficient clearance mechanism that prevents colonization of hepatic sinusoids or parenchyma. Multiplication, tissue invasion, and abscess formation occur secondary to the introduction of other factors such as necrotic tissue, hepatic injury, malignant tumors, microemboli, poor perfusion, or congenital or acquired biliary or vascular obstruction. Pyogenic hepatic abscess usually represents an infective process in another organ. The process is usually, but not always, within the abdomen. Appendicitis was by far the common source in most earlier series, representing 35 per cent of the total group in Ochsner's patients.[49] Appendicitis is involved in only approximately 10 per cent of cases in more recent series (Table 1).[10,28,29]

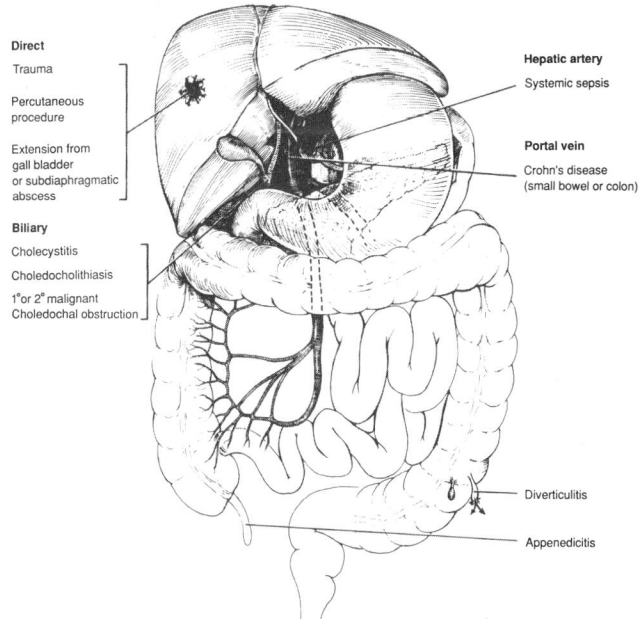

Figure 2. Sources of organisms invading the liver in pyogenic hepatic abscesses.

TABLE 1. Source of Pyogenic Abscess in Four Series of Patients Since 1985 (n = 171)

	No.	%
Cryptogenic	32	18.7
Biliary		
Benign	41	23.9
Malignant	17	9.9
Colonic		
Benign	29	16.9
Malignant	2	1.2
Hematogenous (arterial)	14	8.2
Other portal	12	7.0
Trauma	10	5.8
Other (chronic granulomatous disease, local extention, abdominal surgery)	9	5.3

The other most common sources are cholecystitis, biliary or pancreatic cancer with obstruction, diverticulitis, regional enteritis, trauma, generalized sepsis, and pelvic inflammatory disease.[13,56,59] Patients receiving chemotherapy for hematologic or solid malignancies are at increased risk. Other important associations with hepatic abscess in adults include colon cancer, diabetes, and cardiopulmonary disease. Associated conditions in children are malignancy, non-AIDS immunodeficiency states, AIDS, polycystic disease, cholecystitis, necrotizing enterocolitis, and congenital hepatic fibrosis. The most common non-AIDS immunodeficiency states occur after transplantation, as a result of liver failure, following treatment of malignancy, or with chronic granulomatous disease.[22]

Despite advances in diagnostic techniques and an aggressive search for a source, no probable cause of hepatic abscess has been identified in 13 to 35 per cent of cases since 1984.[6,9,10,23,26,34] Cryptogenic abscesses constituted 22 per cent of Ochsner's collected series in 1938.[49] This incidence may increase further with more use of percutaneous drainage techniques because of fewer opportunities for abdominal exploration. In most previous series, cryptogenic abscesses were usually solitary, and the associated mortality, low. It is also possible that mortality associated with cryptogenic abscess could increase because of more undetected problems such as underlying malignancy.

Portal pyelophlebitis is an infection of the portal vein, usually manifested radiographically by air in the portal vein. Although portal venous infection undoubtedly occurs more frequently than the demonstration of portal venous air, the latter complication is usually lethal. Pyelophlebitis is a likely cause of hepatic abscess. In this condition, mesenteric veins at the site of an inflammatory process thrombose and subsequently extend into the portal system and embolize to the liver. The septic emboli block venous radicles, giving rise to polymorphonuclear leukocyte, lymphocyte, and macrophage migration to the region and an intense inflammatory reaction. Foci are usually multiple, but multiple sites may coalesce into a "solitary" abscess, with or without septations. Multiple microscopic hepatic abscesses are often found at autopsy in patients dying of sepsis with portal pyelophlebitis. More abscesses occur in the right than in the left lobe. This is probably secondary to preferential laminar drainage of the superior mesenteric vein to the right lobe, although some controversy exists concerning this explanation.[41]

Abscess formation secondary to biliary obstruction follows a slightly different pattern, with similar results. After obstruction of bile ducts, bacteria multiply and ascend into intrahepatic biliary radicles and canaliculosinusoidal channels, producing cholangitis. Bacterial proliferation causes further biliary distention with lymphatic and portal invasion and formation of a pyelophlebitic abscess. Further coalescence allows escape of pus into surrounding hepatic tissue with formation of multiple pockets and subsequent septations of a predominant cavity.

Biliary tract disease has supplanted appendicitis as the most common gastrointestinal problem associated with liver abscess.[4,10,41,44,50,51] Bile ducts, biliary lymphatics, and periductal vascular channels are the primary routes by which abscesses develop in association with biliary infection. Liver abscess occurs most commonly with cholecystitis, choledocholithiasis, and malignant or benign biliary stricture. Malignant obstruction of the bile duct by pancreatic carcinoma, cholangiocarcinoma, or metastatic adenocarcinoma causes more cases of liver abscess than observed previously because of improved palliative treatments, such as percutaneous or endoscopic biliary drainage techniques. Patients undergoing biliary-enteric bypass are at increased risk of abscess formation, even when there is no demonstrable stricture. Several studies suggest that choledochoduodenal anastomoses are associated with a higher incidence of bacteremia or abscess than Roux-en-Y hepatico- or choledochojejunostomy. A greater potential for reflux of foodstuffs in the former drainage procedure supports the latter observation. The incidence of a potential biliary source in association with liver abscess is currently estimated at 30 to 50 per cent.[6,9,10,26,34]

Trauma predisposes hepatic parenchyma to abscess formation by several mechanisms: bile leakage, decreased perfusion, foci of hepatic necrosis, direct introduction of bacteria via penetrating high- or low-velocity missiles, and hematoma formation. The combination of bile leakage, hematoma, and necrotic tissue provides a rich culture medium for bacteria introduced by the trauma itself or entrapment of blood or bile-borne bacteria.

Pathology and Microbiology

Pyogenic hepatic abscesses have some characteristic gross and microscopic pathologic features. In most series, right hepatic abscesses predominate by a nearly 3:1 ratio. The presumed explanation for this is streaming of the superior mesenteric vein fraction of portal flow to the right lobe of the liver as well as its relatively greater volume.[4] Bilobar metastases occur in 10 per cent of patients. Most series indicate a nearly equal distribution between solitary and multiple liver abscesses. Abscesses vary in size from less than a millimeter to several centimeters. They may appear honeycombed with multiple lesions, although this appearance is unusual except with fungal organisms. Interestingly, the size of solitary abscesses nearly tripled in one study between 1945 to 1957 and 1971 to 1983.[44] Grossly, hepatic abscesses appear yellow, compared with the normal deep maroon hepatic parenchyma which surrounds them. The organ is usually subtly enlarged, and palpation may reveal fluctuant areas corresponding to the pus-filled cavity. The liver is often adherent to surrounding organs or the diaphragm because of associated capsular inflammation. Small abscesses deep within the parenchyma rarely exhibit these findings. Most traumatic abscesses are solitary and localized near the site of injury. Microscopically, acute inflammatory reaction is observed with necrosis and hepatocyte cords in the portal triad regions. Cholestasis may be evident in adjacent tissue.

Organisms recovered from liver abscesses vary greatly but generally reflect bile or enteric flora (Table 2). Reasons for the variability include differences in antibiotics prior to culture, cul-

TABLE 2. Most Common Organisms Isolated in Five Series of Pyogenic Abscess Reported Since 1985 (n = 219)[6,9,10,26,34]

	No.	%
Escherichia coli	72	33
Klebsiella pneumoniae	39	18
Bacteroides species	53	24
Streptococcal species	80	37
Microaerophilic streptococci	26	12

ture techniques, or patient populations.[17,35,39,42] In most recent series, most patients have a positive culture, and over half grow more than one organism. Solitary abscesses are more likely than multiple ones to grow multiple organisms.[39,42,46,53] The high frequency of "sterile" abscesses found in earlier studies was probably due primarily to an inability to isolate anaerobic or microaerophilic organisms. At present, the most likely reason for a sterile culture is effective antibiotic therapy. The most common aerobic organisms in most series are *Escherichia coli, Klebsiella*, and enterococci. The most common anaerobes are *Bacteroides*, anaerobic streptococci, and *Fusobacterium* species. Streptococcal species (aerobic, anaerobic, or microaerophilic) are found in 25 to 30 per cent of cultured abscesses and are believed to be of increasing importance in the pathogenesis of pyogenic abscess.[46,52] The presence of isolated colonies of *E. coli* or *Klebsiella* should raise the suspicion of a biliary source, while the presence of anaerobes suggests a colonic source. One interesting observation is the more common appearance of staphylococcal abscesses in young males, compared with other patient groups.[10] More than half of patients not receiving antibiotics may have microorganisms cultured from the peripheral blood.

AMEBIC ABSCESS

Amebic liver abscess follows intestinal infestation by *Entamoeba histolytica*. The most common mode of transmission of *E. histolytica* is by individual contact rather than contaminated drinking water or food. Venereal transmission usually causes genital, gut, or visceral disease. Two forms of the protozoan may be found in stool specimens: trophozoites and cysts. Trophozoites are the invasive form and are derived from cysts. The factors that determine clinically significant disease are poorly understood. The simple finding of trophozoites or cysts in the stool is so common that this alone is not evidence of active disease.[4]

The incidence of liver disease in patients with intestinal amebiasis is reported to be between 3 and 25 per cent.[2,4,16] There is a latency period of several weeks between intestinal infection and observable hepatic involvement. The amebae reach the liver through the portal vein. The trophozoites either degenerate in the portal venous radicles or migrate to an adjacent area, causing necrosis and liquefaction. The areas of destruction coalesce to form most commonly a single large cavity in the right lobe. The abscess may vary in size from less than a centimeter to 25 cm. in diameter. The contents are a mixture of necrotic hepatic parenchyma and blood that yields a classic "anchovy paste" appearance. This is usually sterile and odorless. Secondary bacterial infection occurs in approximately 10 per cent of cases and may change the color and odor of the contents.[5,6] Protozoa are usually found only in a rim of necrotic tissue and are therefore unlikely to be aspirated.

Seventy-five to 90 per cent of abscesses are found in the right lobe.[4,5,6] Left lobe or bilobar involvement usually indicates more advanced disease. Right lobe lesions are more likely to rupture intraperitoneally, and left lobe lesions, into the pericardium or pleural space[4,31] (Fig. 3). As with pyogenic abscess, the liver is usually enlarged. Capsular adhesions to the diaphragm or adjacent tissue are generally not as numerous. Early or acute lesions have thin walls with little fibrosis, whereas older abscesses have a more well-formed fibrous capsule, sharply demarcating them from normal liver parenchyma. There is usually marked necrosis of hepatic parenchyma within the lesions, with little polymorphonuclear cell infiltration. As the abscess matures, it becomes spherical, and more eosinophilic staining debris develops. Calcification is unusual except in chronic abscesses.

Like pyogenic hepatic abscess, the amebic variety may be associated with depressed immunologic states. Experimental infection is easier to induce after splenectomy, probably because of decreased macrophage clearance of the parasite. Antimacrophage serum exacerbates and BCG improves host defenses against amebae. Cell-mediated immunity is impaired during the first 2 weeks of infection in normal patients without

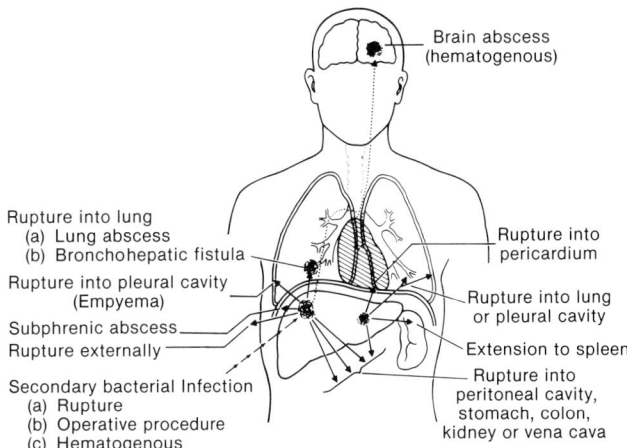

Figure 3. Sites of rupture or extension of amebic abscess. A slight but real possibility of hematogenous spread exists, as illustrated by the development of a brain abscess.

treatment. Therefore, suppression of immune response during systemic infection may have a role in amebic liver abscess.

DIAGNOSIS

The diagnosis of hepatic abscess is challenging because clinical signs are usually not specific. Early differentiation between pyogenic and amebic liver abscess may be even more difficult because of the similarity in signs, symptoms, and radiologic features. Both pyogenic and amebic abscess should be considered lethal unless detected early. For pyogenic abscess, two diagnoses are necessary for optimal management: (1) the abscess condition itself and (2) the underlying source. Neither diagnosis may be apparent initially, but both can usually be discovered with appropriate evaluation. The diagnosis of hepatic abscess is apparent at the time of admission in a minority of patients but if suspected is readily diagnosed by ultrasonography or computed tomography (CT) in over 95 per cent of patients.

The majority of patients with hepatic abscess have symptoms of less than 2 weeks' duration, although one third have been affected a month or longer. The primary symptoms are fever, malaise, chills, anorexia, weight loss, abdominal pain, and nausea. With amebic abscess, a recent diarrheal syndrome can be documented in only a minority of patients. An occasional historical feature is a long-standing respiratory infection prior to the development of abdominal symptoms. Fever of unknown origin is the presentation in a significant number of patients. Rarely, patients with either amebic or pyogenic abscess are admitted with diffuse peritonitis, shock, or hepatic failure. Possible physical findings include right upper quadrant tenderness, pleural dullness to percussion, fever, hepatomegaly, and jaundice. Tenderness may be elicited by either direct palpation or percussion of the right rib cage. Most patients have a leukocytosis and some liver enzyme abnormality. The most common findings on plain abdominal or chest radiographs are right-sided atelectasis, an elevated hemidiaphragm, pleural effusion, and pneumonia. Occasionally, a subdiaphragmatic air-fluid collection is observed with pyogenic abscess or a superinfected amebic abscess (Fig. 4). In addition to ultrasonography or liver CT, a liver scan usually accurately localizes the abscess. CT should routinely be performed with intravenous contrast in order to demonstrate the relative hypovascularity of the abscess.[27]

Specific Imaging Tests

ULTRASONOGRAPHY (Fig. 5*A* and *B*). Ultrasonography is the most useful screening test when the suspicion of hepatic abscess arises.[12,45] The test is highly sensitive (85 to 95 per cent),

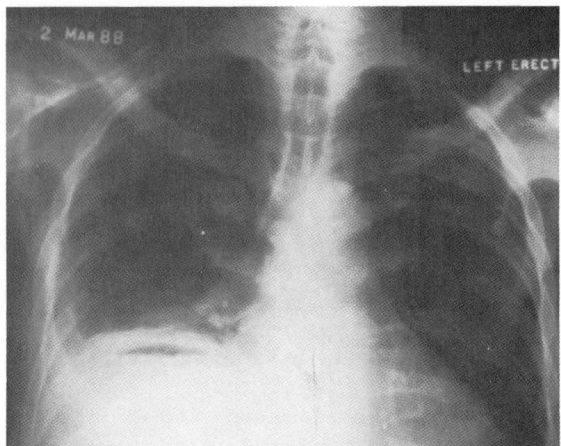

Figure 4. Typical appearance of a pyogenic abscess on a plain chest roentgenogram. Note the elevated right hemidiaphragm, blunted right costophrenic angle, and intrahepatic air-fluid level. (From Meyers, W. C., and Jones, R. S.: Textbook of Liver and Biliary Surgery. Philadelphia, J. B. Lippincott Co., 1990, p. 133.)

is more accurate than CT in imaging the biliary tree, and allows diagnostic or therapeutic drainage or biopsy at the time of performance. Limitations of ultrasonography arise in nonhomogeneous livers, in those situated high beneath the thoracic cage, and in extremely obese or uncooperative patients.[26]

COMPUTED TOMOGRAPHY (Fig. 5C). CT scanning is the most sensitive of the imaging procedures (95 to 100 per cent) and allows diagnostic or therapeutic intervention to be performed.[12,27] The appearance of an abscess on a CT scan is variable, and lesions may appear cystic or isodense, with solid meta-

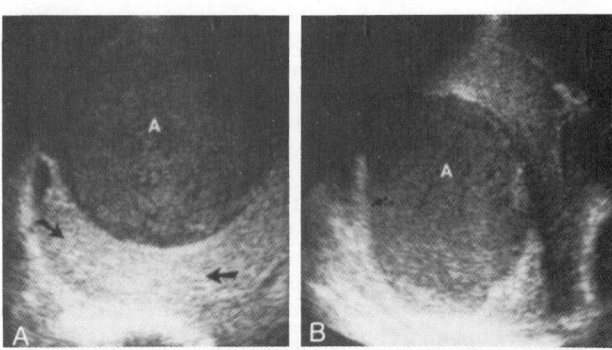

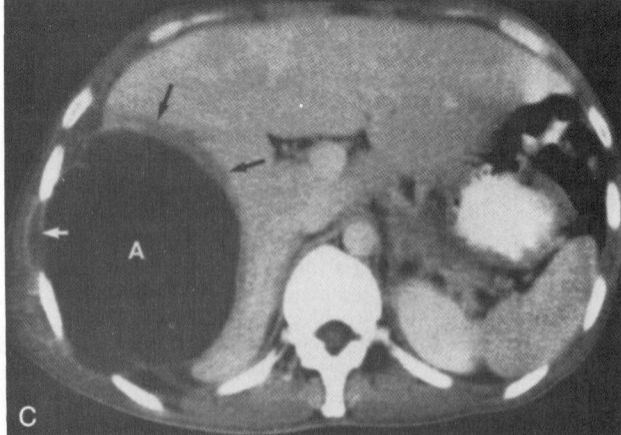

Figure 5. Sonographic and computed tomographic (CT) appearance of an amebic abscess. *A*, Large, rounded abscess (A) in the right lobe with slight distal acoustic enhancement (arrows). *B*, Location of the abscess immediately adjacent to the diaphragm (arrow). *C*, CT scan revealing abscess (A) with surrounding low-density peripheral zone of edema (black arrows) and extrahepatic extension of abscess into intercostal space (white arrow). (From Jeffrey, R. B., Jr.: CT and Sonography of the Acute Abdomen. New York, Raven Press, 1989, p. 25.)

static lesions. A minority of hepatic lesions contain gas, making this criterion generally of little use, but diagnostic if present. The phenomenon of an enhancing rim surrounding an abscess is apparent in a small percentage of cases.[27]

RADIONUCLIDE SCANS. Technetium 99m sulfur colloid scanning has been useful in the diagnosis of abscesses for 4 decades. The labeled colloid is engulfed by hepatic Kupffer cells where the Tc is reduced to a lower energy state, and the radiation emitted is measured by a photon-sensitive crystal. The ability of the test to demonstrate an abscess lies in the difference of Kupffer cell activity within and surrounding the abscess. The test is very sensitive but has the significant limitations of (1) being unable to detect lesions smaller than 2 cm. and (2) being unable to discriminate between solid and cystic structures. The liver scan is an adequate screening test but is not useful in planning treatment strategies. Newer radionuclide scans utilizing gallium and indium have been reported but add nothing to the standard technetium scan and are not as useful as ultrasonography or CT scanning.

OTHER TECHNIQUES. Hepatic arteriography has been used in the past in diagnosing pyogenic abscesses, but this invasive technique offers no benefit over CT scan with percutaneous aspiration for diagnosis.[3,55,57] At present, magnetic resonance imaging offers no advantage over CT scanning and cannot be used for percutaneous procedures. The diagnosis of the underlying source may be apparent from the history, physical examination, or initial laboratory tests. If ultrasonography and CT do not reveal the underlying source, barium studies, colonoscopy, ERCP, or other tests may be indicated.

Differential Diagnosis

Correct and expedient diagnosis of pyogenic versus amebic abscess is important because the treatments are radically different. The standard treatment of pyogenic abscess remains external drainage with an appropriate course of antibiotics. Management also includes consideration of the underlying cause of the abscess. Treatment of uncomplicated amebic abscess is primarily nonsurgical.

When an abscess has been demonstrated, the distinction must be made between pyogenic and more unusual types (Table 3). *Echinococcus* can usually be excluded by history. Serum antibody titer for *E. histolytica* or counterimmunoelectrophoresis are highly specific and of great benefit when positive.[5,6,33] Major centers should have results available in 24 to 36 hours. Percutaneous aspiration may help in the identification of a bacterial organism. However, such aspiration is not usually helpful in the diagnosis of amebae, and in only 10 to 20 per cent of cases can amebae be found on microscopic analysis of rectal mucosa secretions. If the latter results are positive, the finding still may be

TABLE 3. A Comparison of Characteristics in Amebic Versus Pyogenic Abscess in the United States

	Amebic	Pyogenic
Demographics		
Age	Mean under 40	Mean over 50
Sex	Males 9–10:1	Approximately equal
Race	>90% Latin origin	No predisposition
Symptoms		
Right upper quadrant pain	60–65%	30–40%
Fever	95–100%	95–100%
Chills	<30%	75–80%
Laboratory		
Serologic tests positive for *Entamoeba histolytica*	98–100%	<5%
Mortality	<5%	10–15%

and Nyhus, L. M.: Ultrasonic examination during surgery for abdominal abscess. World J. Surg., 7:409, 1983.

37. Mandel, S. R., Boyd, D., Jaques, P. F., Mandell, V., and Staab, E. V.: Drainage of hepatic, intraabdominal, and mediastinal abscesses guided by computerized axial tomography. Am. J. Surg., 145:120, 1983.

38. Martin, E. C., Karlson, K. B., Fankuchen, E., Cooperman, A., and Casarella, W. J.: Percutaneous drainage in the management of hepatic abscesses. Surg. Clin. North Am., 61:157, 1981.

39. Maza, L. M. de la, Naeim, F., and Berman, L. D.: The changing etiology of liver abscess, further observations. J.A.M.A., 227:161, 1974.

40. McCorkell, S. J., and Niles, N. L.: Pyogenic liver abscesses: another look at medical management. Lancet, 1:803, 1985.

41. McDonald, A. P., and Howard, R. J.: Pyogenic liver abscess. World J. Surg., 4:369, 1980.

42. McDonald, M. I., Corey, G. R., Gallis, H. A., and Durack, D. R.: Single and multiple pyogenic liver abscesses: Natural history, diagnosis and treatment, with emphasis on percutaneous drainage. Medicine, 63:291, 1984.

43. McFadzean, A. J. S., Chang, K. P. S., and Wong, C. C.: Solitary pyogenic abscess of the liver treated by closed aspiration and antibiotics: A report of 14 consecutive cases with recovery. Br. J. Surg., 41:141, 1953.

44. Miedema, B. W., and Dineen, P.: The diagnosis and treatment of pyogenic liver abscesses. Ann. Surg., 200:328, 1984.

45. Monroe, L. S., Leopold, G. R., Brown, J. W., and Smith, J. L.: The ultrasonic scan in the management of amebic hepatic abscess. Am. J. Dig. Dis., 16:523, 1971.

46. Moore-Gillon, J. C., Eykyn, S. J., and Phillips, I.: Microbiology of pyogenic liver abscesses. Br. Med. J., 283:819, 1981.

47. Ochsner, A., and DeBakey, M.: Amebic hepatitis and hepatic abscess, an analysis of 181 cases with review of the literature. Part 1. Surgery, 13:460, 1943.

48. Ochsner, A., and DeBakey, M.: Amebic hepatitis and hepatic abscess, an analysis of 181 cases with review of the literature. Part 2. Surgery, 13:612, 1943.

49. Ochsner, A., DeBakey, M., and Murray, S.: Pyogenic abscess of the liver. II. An analysis of forty-seven cases with review of the literature. Am. J. Surg., 40:292, 1938.

50. Pitt, H. A., and Zuidema, G. D.: Factors influencing mortality in the treatment of pyogenic hepatic abscess. Surg. Gynecol. Obstet., 140:228, 1975.

51. Ranson, J. H. C., Madayag, M. A., Localio, S. A., and Spencer, F. C.: New diagnostic and therapeutic techniques in the management of pyogenic liver abscesses. Ann. Surg., 181:508, 1975.

52. Rubin, R. H., Swartz, M. N., and Malt, D.: Hepatic abscess: changes in clinical, bacteriologic and therapeutic aspects. Am. J. Med., 57:601, 1974.

53. Sabbaj, J., Sutter, V. L., and Finegold, S. M.: Anaerobic pyogenic liver abscess. Ann. Intern. Med., 77:629, 1972.

54. Satiani, B., and Davidson, E. D.: Hepatic abscesses: Improvement in mortality with early diagnosis and treatment. Am. J. Surg., 135:647, 1978.

55. Sheinfeld, A. M., Steiner, A. E., Rivkin, L. B., Dermer, R. H., Shemesh, O. N., and Dolberg, M. S.: Transcutaneous drainage of abscesses of the liver guided by computed tomography scan. Surg. Gynecol. Obstet., 155:662, 1982.

56. Silver, S., Weinstein, A., and Cooperman, A.: Changes in the pathogenesis and detection of intrahepatic abscess. Am. J. Surg., 137:608, 1979.

57. vanSonnenberg, E., Ferrucci J. T. Jr., Mueller, P. R., Wittenberg, J., and Simeone, J. F.: Percutaneous drainage of abscesses and fluid collections: Technique, results, and applications. Radiology, 142:1, 1982.

58. Wallace, R. J., Jr., Greenberg, S. B., Lau, J. M., Kalchoff, W. P., Mangold, D. E., and Martin, R. R.: Amebic peritonitis following rupture of an amebic liver abscess. Arch. Surg., 113:322, 1978.

59. Wallack, M. K., Brown, A. S., Austrian, R., and Fitts, W. T., Jr.: Pyogenic liver abscess secondary to asymptomatic sigmoid diverticulitis. Ann. Surg., 184:241, 1976.

60. Yiengpruksawan, A., Ganepola, G. P., and Freeman, H. P.: Extended applications of ultrasonography by the surgeon: A preliminary report. Am. J. Surg., 153:221, 1987.

III

NEOPLASMS OF THE LIVER

William C. Meyers, M. D.

Surgeons encounter more liver tumors today, and techniques for diagnosing and treating these lesions are rapidly evolving. Therefore, it has become particularly important to be knowledgeable of the advances in this field in order to manage these patients most efficiently. The increase in number of tumors being found is due to four principal factors: an apparent increased incidence, improved detection, enthusiasm generated by the greater success of surgical treatment, and development of combined, aggressive approaches to reduce tumor volume in apparently incurable situations. Over the past 25 years several new categories of tumors have been recognized. New etiologic factors have been identified, such as the hepatitis B virus, exposure to vinyl chloride, use of oral contraceptives, and injection of Thorotrast. Progress includes improved radiologic diagnosis, such as with ultrasonography, computed tomography (CT), magnetic resonance imaging, and, most recently, CT-angiography. There have also been advances in the correlation of pathologic features with the clinical courses of both benign and malignant neoplasms. This section reviews some of the clinical features of these tumors, with emphasis on recent advances in their causes and treatment.

The earliest hepatic surgery was performed almost exclusively for trauma. The earliest resection for tumor was by Langenbuch in 1888. In 1899, Keen reviewed the liver resections performed to that time. In 1911, Wendel performed the first successful major hepatic resection using selective hilar ligation of the vessels. With improved understanding of the anatomy and physiology of the liver has come an increased confidence in surgical treatment, a significant increase in the number of resections performed, a wide expansion of the indications for resection, and a reduction in the mortality from major hepatic resection to 1 to 5 per cent.

PRIMARY MALIGNANT TUMORS

Hepatocellular Carcinoma

Hepatocellular carcinoma may be the most prevalent malignant disease worldwide today. Hepatoma is much more common in sub-Saharan Africa, Southeast Asia, Japan, the Pacific Islands, Greece, and Italy than it is in North and Central America, Britain, most parts of Europe, the Middle East, the Soviet Union, and Australia. The incidence in Africa is 16 per 100,000 inhabitants of Nigeria to 164.6 per 100,000 individuals in Mozambique. The standardized incidence in the United States is estimated to be 1 to 7 per 100,000 individuals annually. Three autopsy series demonstrate that hepatocellular carcinoma has nearly doubled in the United States over the past 20 years. Hepatocellular carcinoma occurs four to nine times more frequently in males than in females, except in the group without pre-existent liver disease in whom the ratio is 1:1. Orientals in the United States are approximately eight times at risk of developing the tumor compared with white populations.

ETIOLOGY. Epidemiologic and laboratory studies have now firmly established a strong and specific association between hepatitis B virus and hepatocellular carcinoma. Several other risk factors have also become well documented. These include alcoholic cirrhosis, blood group B, and hepatic adenoma. Implicated risk factors for hepatocellular carcinoma include aflatoxin, other mycotoxins, plant alkaloids, oral contraceptives, androgen, vinyl chloride, Thorotrast, smoking, parasites, porphyria cutanea tarda, and organochloride pesticides. Hepatitis B virus is the most important etiologic agent identified worldwide. The association of this virus is restricted to the "chronically persistent" form, that is, characterized by a positive hepatitis B surface antigen (HBsAG) in serum. Correlation, case control, and cohort studies have established a relationship epidemiologically.

Studies from Asia and Africa suggest that hepatitis B virus is present in as many as 70 to 80 per cent of patients with hepatocellular carcinoma. In 97 consecutive autopsy studies of patients with hepatocellular carcinoma in Los Angeles, 21 per cent had hepatitis B. In addition, 40 per cent of 55 patients dying of hepatitis B viral cirrhosis had hepatocellular carcinoma at autopsy. One third of the patients with hepatocellular carcinoma studied by autopsy had cryptogenic cirrhosis. Whether hepatocellular carcinoma occurs as a consequence of chronic hepatitis B infection or as a result of chronic liver disease is not certain. Since hepatitis B vaccine has been available for only a short time, it is not known if this will have a significant impact on the incidence of the disease in endemic areas. Alcoholic cirrhosis is the major predisposing factor for hepatocellular carcinoma in the United States; 8 to 10 per cent of patients dying of alcoholic cirrhosis have hepatocellular carcinoma. In one study, 55 per cent of alcoholic cirrhotics who had stopped drinking had hepatocellular carcinoma at autopsy, leading to the suggestion that abstinence from alcohol allows the alcoholic patient to live long enough to develop the tumor.

Aflatoxins are potent carcinogens in experimental animals. They are products of the fungus *Aspergillus flavus*, which is found in wheat, soybeans, corn, rice, oats, bread, milk, cheese, and peanuts. The United States Food and Drug Administration limits the amount of aflatoxins allowed in peanut butter to 20 parts per billion.

The exact risk of hepatocellular carcinoma that develops with use of oral contraceptives is not clear, although a number of such tumors have been reported to arise within benign adenomas in oral contraceptive users. A type of carcinoma termed fibrolamellar carcinoma characteristically develops under the age of 35, and it is possible that some of these tumors are linked etiologically to oral contraceptives. A number of cases of hepatoma have been reported in males following administration of androgens or other anabolic steroids for the treatment of aplastic anemia, although it is possible that multiple transfusions contributed to the anemia in these patients. There does appear to be a degree of hormone responsiveness in these androgen-related hepatocellular carcinomas.

Interestingly, primary biliary cirrhosis does not appear to be associated with hepatocellular carcinoma. The reported association of hepatocellular carcinoma with hemochromatosis is approximately 10 per cent.

In populations with low incidences of hepatocellular carcinoma, the elderly are the predominant group affected. In the Far East, hepatocellular carcinoma develops predominantly in the fifth and sixth decades. In sub-Saharan Africa, the tumor develops at a younger age, with the peak incidence in the third through fifth decades. In high-incidence locations, the tumor more often occurs in patients treated for cirrhosis for a long time.

SYMPTOMS AND SIGNS. The most common symptoms are weakness, malaise, upper abdominal or shoulder pain, and weight loss. In one series from the United States, an abdominal mass was a main complaint in 19 of 144 patients (14 per cent) with primary hepatic malignant tumors, and jaundice was present in 34 patients (24 per cent). Approximately two thirds of the patients are hospitalized with an obvious cancer in the liver and symptoms or signs including abdominal pain and tenderness, dyspnea, asthenia, weight loss, hepatomegaly, jaundice, ascites, peripheral edema, or evidence of portal hypertension. A

minority of patients initially experience an acute abdominal event such as rupture of the tumor or hemorrhage, fever of unknown origin, or an occult process. Approximately 5 per cent of patients are initially found to have metastatic lesions, of which pulmonary metastases are the most common. In endemic areas, hepatocellular carcinoma is the most common cause of nontraumatic acute hemoperitoneum in males. The duration of symptoms is often surprisingly short. In one series, over 75 per cent of patients had symptoms of less than 6 weeks' duration. Physical findings depend on the stage of the disease. Hepatomegaly is the most common sign in the patients. Interestingly, an arterial bruit can be heard in approximately 15 to 20 per cent of patients, which may be diagnostically valuable. It is important to note that many of the signs, including jaundice, ascites, splenomegaly, protein wasting, and spider angiomas, may be a manifestation of the underlying chronic liver disease rather than of the tumor.

A large number of paraneoplastic manifestations are associated with hepatocellular carcinoma. These include serum protein abnormalities of alpha-fetoprotein, globulins, haptoglobin, ceruloplasmin, alpha-antitrypsin, choriogonadotropins and choriosomatotropins, alkaline phosphatase, and isoferritins. Associated hematologic abnormalities include erythrocytosis, hemolysis, plasmacytosis, antifibrinolysis, and dysfibrinogenemias. Other abnormalities include hypercholesterolemia, hypertriglyceridemia, porphyria, cystathioninuria, ethanolaminuria, hypoglycemia, pseudohyperparathyroidism, sexual changes, hypertrophic pulmonary osteoarthropathy, increased thyroxine-binding globulin, and carcinoid syndrome. Increased carcinoembryonic antigen may also occur.

DIAGNOSIS. The oncofetoprotein alpha-fetoprotein (AFP) deserves special mention because of its diagnostic value. This protein has a molecular weight of 64,000 to 74,000 daltons. It is present in large quantities during fetal development but decreases rapidly after birth and thereafter remains at the normal adult level of 10 ng. per ml. or less. Using a relatively insensitive immunodiffusion method, 28 to 87 per cent of patients with hepatocellular carcinoma have significant elevations of AFP in serum. Radioimmunoassay for AFP increased positivity for tumor detection in Chinese patients 69 to 93 per cent. In the United States, 75 per cent of patients with hepatocellular carcinoma arising in association with hepatitis B cirrhosis had AFP levels above 400 ng. per ml. Sixty-five per cent of patients with hepatocellular carcinoma secondary to alcoholic cirrhosis had positive results, whereas only 33 per cent of patients with carcinoma arising in a noncirrhotic liver had positive assays. In one study, 14 of 16 patients who underwent laparotomy for a positive AFP level found on screening tests had resectable cancers. AFP may return to normal after successful surgical resection and is a useful level to follow. Mild elevations of AFP may be found in acute viral hepatitis, chronic liver disease, and some cases of metastatic cancer. Higher levels may be found in adult patients with fulminant type B hepatitis. Markedly elevated levels may also be found in patients with teratocarcinomas, yolk sac tumors, and, rarely, hepatic metastatic carcinomas from the stomach or pancreas.

Over the past several years, the value of real-time ultrasonography has been realized in both Japan and Taiwan as a screening test for hepatocellular carcinoma in high-risk populations. One study in Japan disclosed that ultrasonography detected 72.5 per cent of tumors that developed in a group of patients with chronic liver disease undergoing routine follow-up evaluation. In another study, ultrasonography detected 92 per cent of hepatocellular carcinomas less than 5 cm. in diameter, compared with scintigraphy, which demonstrated only 50 per cent. Arteriography confirmed the majority of lesions. It was also learned that ultrasonography performed at 4- to 5-month intervals theoretically detects all tumors less than 3 cm. in diameter. The time interval was determined by calculation of estimated tumor growth rate. In one study, 4.6 months ensued for a rapidly growing 1 cm. hepatocellular carcinoma to reach the size of 3 cm. In one prospective study of 115 patients with cirrhosis in Japan, hepatocellular carcinoma developed in 12 (10.4 per cent). Seven of 30 (23 per cent) hepatitis B serum antigen positive and 5 of 85 (6 per cent) seronegative patients developed hepatocellular carcinoma. A recent development is the use of intraoperative ultrasonography for the detection of occult tumors. Several reports now document the utility of this technique in combination with preoperative AFP determinations.

Alkaline phosphatase is elevated in over 50 per cent of patients with hepatocellular carcinoma. Transaminase elevations are less predictable, and serum bilirubin is usually elevated late in the disease process.

A number of radiologic investigations may be helpful in the diagnosis of hepatocellular carcinoma. Plain radiographs are nonspecific and may show an enlarged liver, elevated hemidiaphragm, and, rarely, calcification of the tumor. Ultrasonography is a noninvasive and inexpensive method to visualize a suspected mass in the liver. Radionuclide scans are extremely sensitive but have more false-positive results than does ultrasonography or CT (Fig. 1A). Lesions less than 2 to 3 cm. in diameter are often not detected by ultrasonography or radionuclide

scans. CT scanning, with or without intravenous contrast material, appears to be increasing in accuracy and may detect lesions as small as 1 cm. in diameter. It may also differentiate fatty, cystic, and solid lesions.

Hepatic arteriography (Fig. 1B) may be helpful in identifying the number and location of multiple lesions. It occasionally provides an accurate preoperative diagnosis of a lesion such as a hemangioma. Hepatocellular carcinoma may be either hyper- or hypovascular. The preoperative arteriogram also outlines the vasculature to the liver, which may be helpful, particularly if there is anatomic variability. A disadvantage of arteriography is the possibility of causing thrombosis in an artery of the remaining lobe when major hepatic resection is anticipated. Splenoportography may demonstrate the intrahepatic spread of tumor or invasion of the portal vein, but this procedure is not widely used because invasion may also be seen during the venous phase of arteriography. Percutaneous cholangiography or retrograde cholangiography may be helpful in selected patients. Laparoscopy to obtain an accurate needle biopsy of a lesion has not gained wide acceptance.

Percutaneous needle biopsy or fine-needle aspiration for cytodiagnosis generally adds little to the evaluation of potentially resectable, indeterminant liver masses, although needle biopsy

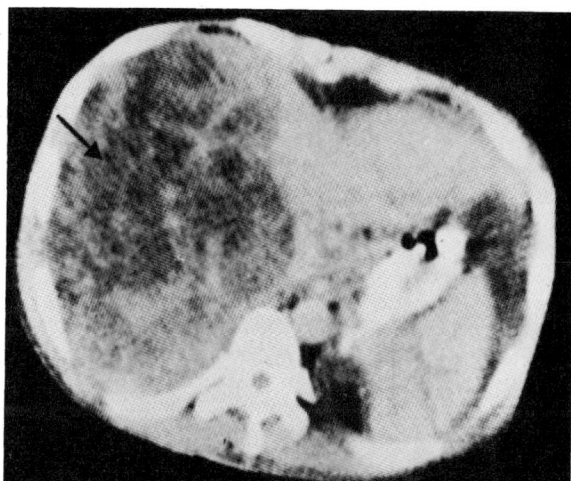

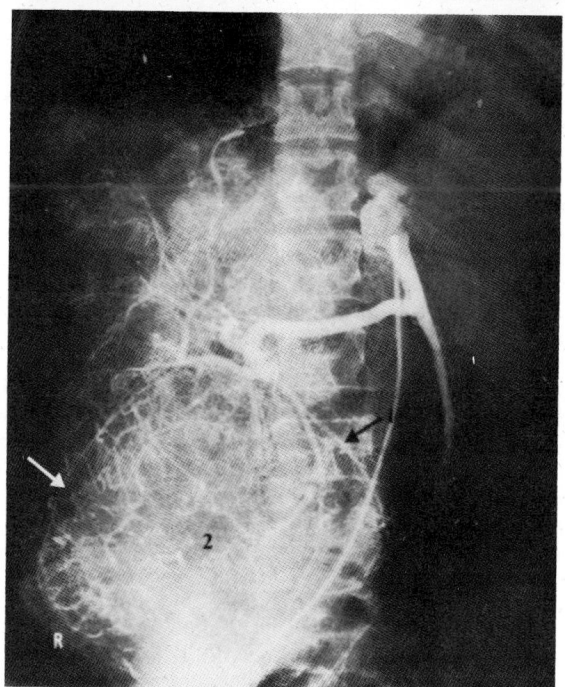

Figure 1. Computed tomogram (A) and arteriogram (B) of a moderately vascular hepatoma of right lobe of liver. Note displacement of vessels (1) and neovascularity (2) in B. (From Sherlock, S., and Summerfield, J. A. (Eds.):Color Atlas of Liver Disease. Chicago, Year Book Medical Publishers, 1979.)

or aspiration has some hazard for hypervascular masses. These techniques are reported to diagnose two thirds of hepatocellular carcinomas, and an indeterminant or negative biopsy aspirate adds little to the decision-making process, except perhaps to establish cirrhosis. Magnetic resonance imaging may have a developing role in the diagnosis of equivocal masses demonstrated by other tests, but at present this examination is generally considered too costly for routine use.

TREATMENT AND PATHOLOGY. The overall survival of patients with untreated hepatocellular carcinoma is approximately 3 to 4 months after symptoms appear, although in the United States the course may be more benign. If the lesion is resected, average survival is reported to be approximately 3 years. Five-year survival rates after resection in large series are 11 to 46 per cent. Liver resection at present is the only therapy that substantially prolongs survival. Exploration is indicated unless there is obvious unresectable tumor, distant metastases, or end-stage cirrhosis. Operative mortality from major hepatic resection has decreased from nearly 20 per cent before 1950 to approximately 5 per cent currently. Much of the mortality is due to postoperative liver failure from accompanying cirrhosis.

Prognostic indices have been developed to calculate risk of hepatectomy and hepatocellular carcinoma. Most are based on modifications of the Child's classification, percentage of uninvolved liver tissue, indocyanine green dye retention rate, and patient age. Hepatic resection is accomplished in approximately half of patients undergoing laparotomy. Wedge resection is as effective as more radical procedures in many patients and is the procedure of choice for patients with cirrhosis. In addition to detection of occult lesions, intraoperative ultrasonography may help determine the extent of resection by identifying the precise segment of liver involved, sometimes with injection of stain into the involved vasculature.

The impact of discovery and treatment of subclinical hepatocellular carcinoma is best depicted in studies from Shanghai. The overall 5-year survival increased dramatically from 1.7 per cent in the period from 1958 to 1966 to 7.1 per cent in the period from 1967 to 1975 and 19.5 per cent in the period from 1976 to 1984. This dramatic increase was clearly the result of improved detection and resective treatment of subclinical hepatocellular carcinoma. No 5-year survival was reported in the absence of resection. Most patients underwent a limited resection, which usually consisted of a 1- to 3-cm. margin around the tumor.

Liver transplantation has been performed for otherwise unresectable tumors, but with only approximately 20 per cent 1-year survival. A higher prolonged survival with transplantation is observed in selected groups, such as the 80 to 90 per cent cure rate with cancers found coincidentally with cirrhosis on pathologic examinations. Fibrolamellar hepatocellular carcinoma is one group with a generally better prognosis with transplantation, 30 to 40 per cent 1-year tumor-free survival compared with only 10 per cent for nonfibrolamellar tumors. Most deaths after transplantation for tumor are directly attributable to tumor recurrence.

Nonsurgical treatment of hepatocellular carcinoma includes hepatic artery ligation, arterial embolization, intra-arterial chemotherapy, targeting radiation or chemotherapy, direct tumor injection, or a combination of methods. [131]I antiferritin therapy combined with external radiation and/or chemotherapy has not achieved satisfactory results. Mean survivals were 5 and 10 months, respectively, to AFP-negative and AFP-positive patients in one carefully designed study. Interestingly, arterial embolization has yielded the best results in unresected patients. However the improvement in survival is still less than 6 months. Some recent studies have suggested improved survival with the combination of an external beam linear accelerator and direct percutaneous ultrasound-guided alcohol injection. Because hepatitis B infection is now unequivocally linked to development of hepatocellular carcinoma, it would appear that hepati-

tis B vaccine would reduce the incidence of this disease in endemic populations. However, economic factors have thus far prohibited wide distribution of this vaccine in endemic parts of the world. Recently, a significant response rate has been reported with doxorubicin (adriamycin) in the treatment of black South African patients, indicating that further studies of this drug and trials of various drug combinations are still reasonable.

There is some indication that survival differs according to the histologic pattern of hepatocellular carcinoma. For example, fibrolamellar carcinoma occurs more frequently in young adults and may have a better prognosis than other types. However, a recent paper suggested that although these tumors may be resectable more often, the cure rate after resection is no different from that with non-fibrolamellar hepatocellular carcinomas. The gross appearance of hepatocellular carcinoma varies according to the presence or absence of pre-existent cirrhosis (Fig. 2). It is usually a single mass when it develops in the noncirrhotic liver but is multinodular in the cirrhotic organ. Carcinoma in a normal liver begins as a fairly homogeneous mass and may develop small satellite nodules. Some carcinomas in cirrhotic livers have a pseudocapsule and appear nodular, which resembles micro- or macronodular cirrhosis. Grossly, the tumor nodules may be difficult to distinguish from the neoplastic nodules. Histologic patterns of hepatocellular carcinoma have been classified into trabecular, pseudoglandular, solid, scirrhous, pleomorphic, and clear cell. The trabecular pattern is by far the most common. The fibrolamellar variant is an unusual cell type arising in the normal liver and characterized microscopically by parallel bundles of collagen that separate clusters of acidophilic hepatocytes. This tumor appears to have a better prognosis. Even when the tumor is unresectable, the patient may survive 1 or 2 years. Long-term survival has been reported after resection even when there is lymph node metastasis.

Bile Duct Cancer (Cholangiocarcinoma)

Bile duct cancers represent 5 to 30 per cent of primary carcinomas of the liver. They may occur within the liver parenchyma and small ducts or ductules or arise from major hepatic ducts outside the liver substance. The intrahepatic type of cholangiocarcinoma is associated with chronic cholestasis, cirrhosis, hemochromatosis, and congenital cystic disease of the liver. *Clon-*

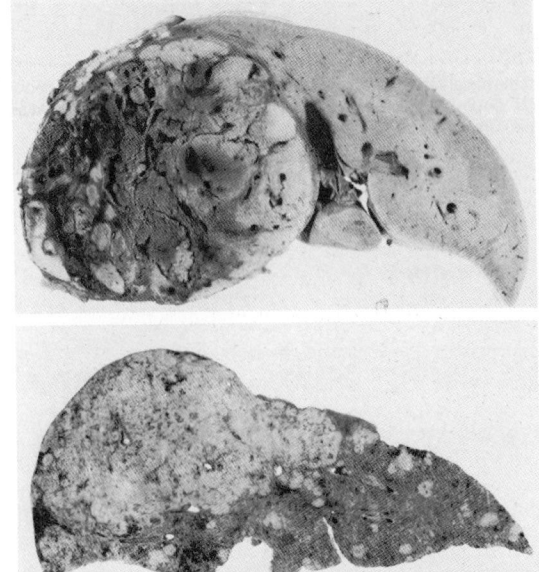

Figure 2. Solitary *(A)* and multiple *(B)* hepatocellular carcinomas in fixed specimens. Tumor in *A* occurred in a noncirrhotic liver. (From Okuda, K., and Ishak, K. G. (Eds.): Neoplasms of the Liver. New York, Springer-Verlag, 1987, pp. 82–83.)

orchis sinensis infestation is associated with more than 90 per cent of cholangiocarcinomas in Hong Kong. However, one third of patients without bile duct carcinoma also have infestation with this fluke. Extrahepatic bile duct cancers arise anywhere along the hepatic ducts or common bile duct and represent 10 per cent of primary hepatic malignancies. There is a 3:2 predominance of males to females. Pruritus, vague abdominal pain, mild cholangitis, and jaundice are the usual initial symptoms. Physical examination may reveal slight hepatomegaly and jaundice but usually no other findings except an enlarged gallbladder when the lesion is distal. Both intra- and extrahepatic bile duct cancers have been associated with ulcerative colitis and may also be confused with sclerosing cholangitis. There is no association of these tumors with cirrhosis, hemochromatosis, or Thorotrast injection, although there is an association with cystic disease of the liver and biliary tree as well as with gallstones.

On pathologic examination, the lesion is often a markedly sclerosing adenocarcinoma. The tumor may extend into the parenchyma along the biliary ducts. Approximately 20 to 25 per cent of the tumors are found to be resectable even when the lesion involves the bifurcation of the hepatic ducts (Klatskin tumors) (Fig. 3). The treatment of choice probably remains surgical resection, which provides longest survival. The average survival in one series after surgical resection was approximately 2 years. There is an approximately 15 to 30 per cent 5-year survival rate after resection. Most cures occur after resection of distal third lesions; cure is unusual for proximal bile duct cancers. If the tumor cannot be resected, a bypass or intubation procedure may provide excellent palliation. Prior to these palliative procedures, survival was usually only several months. With more aggressive palliation, average survival has been extended to 1 or 2 years. Adjunctive iridium seed implantation through a biliary drainage tube is immediately employed, with or without external beam iridium, but whether this leads to significant improvement in survival remains unclear. Percutaneous or endoscopic biliary drainage is offered as a primary treatment for poor-risk surgical patients or those with obviously unresectable tumors. The long-term results of percutaneous or endoscopic drainage compared with open dilation and intubation have not been fully evaluated. Intrahepatic ductal enteric anastomoses such as the Longmire or falciform ligament approaches have had mixed success in the treatment of unresectable cholangiocarcinoma.

One might expect that patients with bile duct cancer would be a particularly favorable group for hepatic transplantation because of the slow-growing and localized nature of the tumor. However, results of transplantation have generally been disappointing, primarily because of tumor recurrence. This has, in part, been the stimulus for "cluster" operations recently being performed by several transplant groups in which most of the upper abdominal viscera are transplanted *en bloc*. No firm data on results of this aggressive surgical procedure are yet available. Nonsurgical treatment has consisted primarily of the placement of a permanent indwelling tube, either by percutaneous or endoscopic methods. At present chemotherapy is considered an ineffective primary treatment modality.

Other Primary Malignant Tumors

A variety of other malignant hepatic tumors may occur that are treated similarly to the tumors just discussed. Hepatoblastoma is an epithelial malignant tumor occurring primarily in childhood. Sixty per cent occur in individuals younger than 2 years of age. This tumor has a notoriously poor prognosis, although there have been reports of up to a 60 per cent 5-year cure rate with surgical resection. Increased cure rates are now being reported with combination approaches, using chemotherapy and radiation therapy followed by surgical therapy. Other tumors include combined hepatocellular and cholangiocarcinoma, bile duct cystadenocarcinoma, and squamous cell carcinoma. Carcinoid, adrenal cancers, teratomas, and other mixed malignant tumors have also been reported in the liver. Primary hepatic sarcomas have received much attention because of their association with vinyl chloride and Thorotrast. Angiosarcoma is the principal tumor associated with these agents. These tumors usually occur as multiple nodules of variable size, and no cure is yet reported. Solid sarcomas such as leiomyosarcoma, fibrosarcoma, rhabdomyosarcoma, and mesenchymal sarcoma also rarely appear in the liver.

Epitheloid hemangioendotheliomas are considered malignant neoplasms because of their characteristic diffuse involvement within the liver and ability to metastasize. The clinical

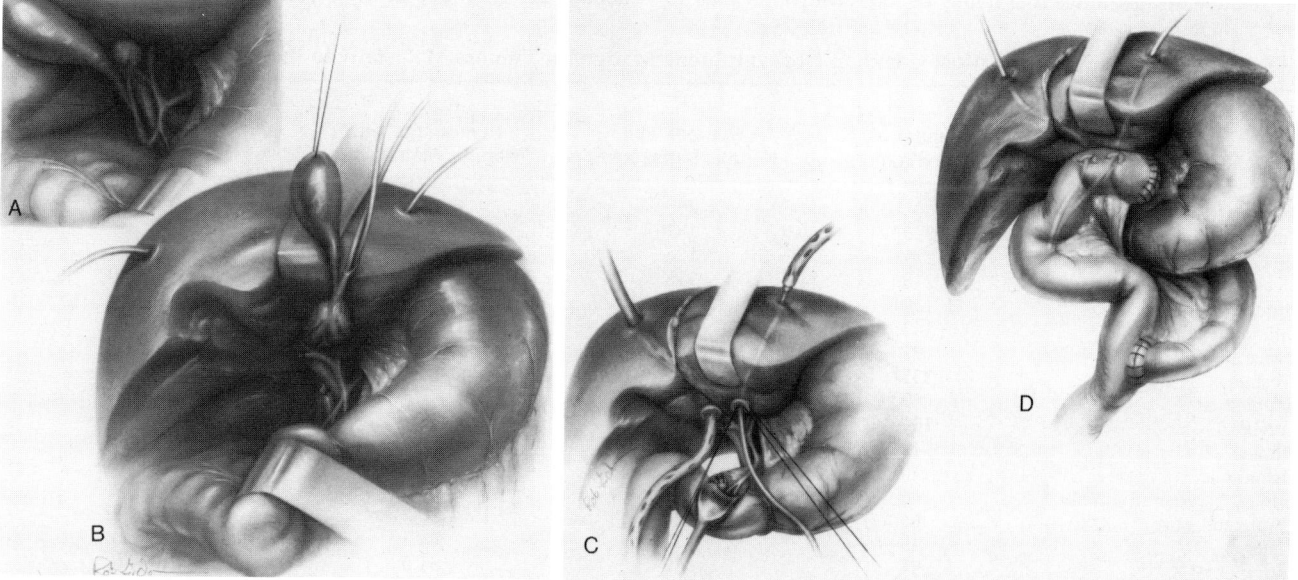

Figure 3. Illustration of proximal bile duct tumor resection. *A*, Intact anatomy with tumor. *B*, The distal common duct has been divided, and the proximal system with gallbladder, radiologic tubes, and tumor has been lifted up to complete the dissection. *C*, The tumor has been resected, and percutaneous tubes are being replaced with larger ones. The left tube is in the process of being exchanged. The multiple side holes in the tubes permit internal biliary drainage. The proximal ends of the tubes exit percutaneously. The biliary reconstruction depicted in *D* is with a Roux-en-Y jejunal limb. The posterior biliary-jejunal anastomosis can be seen ghosted near the closed end of the jejunum. (From Meyers, W. C., and Jones, R. S., (Eds.): Textbook of Liver and Biliary Surgery. Philadelphia, J. B. Lippincott Company, 1990.)

presentation and course are extremely variable with most patients dying eventually of liver failure 1 to 10 years after diagnosis. Other malignant tumors reported rarely as primary lesions in the liver include malignant fibrocystiosarcoma, familial erythrophagocytic cytosis, lymphohistiocytosis, and lymphoma.

Metastatic Tumors

Metastatic cancer comprises the largest group of malignant tumors in the liver. Most arise in the liver probably as a result of primary tumor cell shedding into the vascular system. According to one autopsy study, bronchogenic carcinoma was the most common primary lesion causing hepatic metastases (Table 1). Next in frequency were colon, pancreas, breast, and stomach tumors. The most common symptoms of hepatic metastatic disease are pain, ascites, jaundice, palpable mass, weight loss, anorexia, fever, and vague gastrointestinal complaints. Most of these symptoms generally indicate advanced disease.

Most lesions favorable for resection have been found by early laboratory detection before the development of symptoms or signs. For this reason, liver enzymes and carcinoembryonic antigen assays have been recommended for routine follow-up of patients with resected colorectal cancer. If an elevated carcinoembryonic antigen level returns to normal after removal of the primary colorectal cancer, an elevation at a later time appears to be an extremely sensitive test for evaluation of recurrence. Imaging studies such as radionuclide or CT have usually been performed when a serum abnormality is detected, but a recent prospective study at the National Institutes of Health concluded that serum laboratory tests alone detected liver metastases inadequately. The consensus group recommended using a single liver imaging study plus selected blood tests for patients being screened for colorectal metastases. The most commonly used imaging studies (Fig. 4) for this purpose are ultrasonography, CT, and radionuclide imaging. Magnetic resonance imaging is rapidly becoming a useful test in some medical centers but is likely to have little screening role in the next several years because of time and expense. In some centers, the most sensitive imaging test for detection of colorectal metastases has been dynamic CT performed during the portal venous phase of selective hepatic or mesenteric arteriography. Depicted tumors are radiolucent because of their primary arterial inflow. Angio-CT has the relative disadvantage that it may be too sensitive, in that it

also demonstrates many benign lesions of no pathologic significance.

The liver is the most common site of metastatic colorectal cancer. Approximately one fourth of metastatic colorectal cancers to the liver are resectable. Several studies have documented the unfavorable prognosis of untreated hepatic metastases from colorectal cancer, as 60 to 75 per cent of patients are dead at 1 year and nearly 100 per cent at 3 years. Whereas earlier reports indicated that patients who had untreated solitary liver metastases did not live much longer than the group as a whole, a recent critical analysis demonstrated small but significant differences in survival among patients with solitary, multiple unilateral, or widespread metastases (Fig. 5). A review of 345 patients who underwent surgical therapy for hepatic metastases revealed that 70 per cent had primary colorectal lesions. Wilms' tumors, melanomas, and leiomyosarcomas represented another 10 per cent, and a variety of other tumors the remaining 20 per cent. Cumulative 5-year survival after hepatic resection of colorectal metastases was 22 per cent. Patients with tumors greater than 5 cm. in diameter had a poorer outcome. There is no correlation of survival with the time interval between resection of the primary tumor and the hepatic metastases. Wedge resection with a generous margin of normal tissue was as effective as lobectomy. There was no difference in survival between synchronous versus metachronous lesions or solitary versus multiple lesions in the same lobe or based on the status of colonic lymph node involvement in the resected primary tumor. Recent information indicates a survival advantage for resection of two, or even three, lesions in separate sections of the liver.

Three-year survival in recent reports of resection for metastatic colorectal cancer is approximately 35 to 40 per cent. Five-year survival appears to be about 20 to 30 per cent. This compares favorably with a 5-year survival approaching zero for patients with metastases who did not undergo resection. Favorable results have also been reported with resection for Wilms' tumor. Nine of 15 patients in one series were free of disease 18 months to 7 years after surgical therapy. En bloc wedge resections of the liver along with the primary tumor have been advocated for stomach, gallbladder, kidney, and adrenal cancers. Cancers reported not to respond favorably after resection of metastatic hepatic lesions include carcinoma of the stomach, pancreas, gallbladder, ovary, breast, and head and neck. Major hepatic resection has been performed for palliation of symp-

TABLE 1. Most Common Nonlymphoma Malignant Tumors Metastatic to the Liver

Tumor	Number of Primary Tumors	Number with Hepatic Metastases	Percentage with Hepatic Metastases	Percentage of Patients with Hepatic Metastases Who Were Icteric
Bronchogenic	682	285	41.8	9
Colon	323	181	56.0	34
Pancreas	179	126	70.4	51
Breast	218	116	53.2	30
Stomach	159	70	44.0	60
Unknown primary	102	59	57.0	35
Ovary	97	47	48.0	0
Prostate	333	42	12.6	0
Gallbladder	49	38	77.6	60
Cervix	107	34	31.7	10
Kidney	142	34	23.9	15
Melanoma	50	25	50.0	13
Urinary bladder and ureter	66	25	37.9	11
Esophagus	66	20	30.3	29
Testis	45	20	44.4	14
Endometrial	54	17	31.5	<20
Thyroid	70	12	17.1	14

Data obtained at Los Angeles County University of Southern California Medical Center and John Wesley County Hospital. From Edmondson, H. A., and Peters, R. L.: Neoplasms of the liver. In Schiff, L., and Schiff, E. R. (Eds.): Diseases of the Liver, 5th ed. Philadelphia, J. B. Lippincott Company, 1982, pp. 1101–1157.

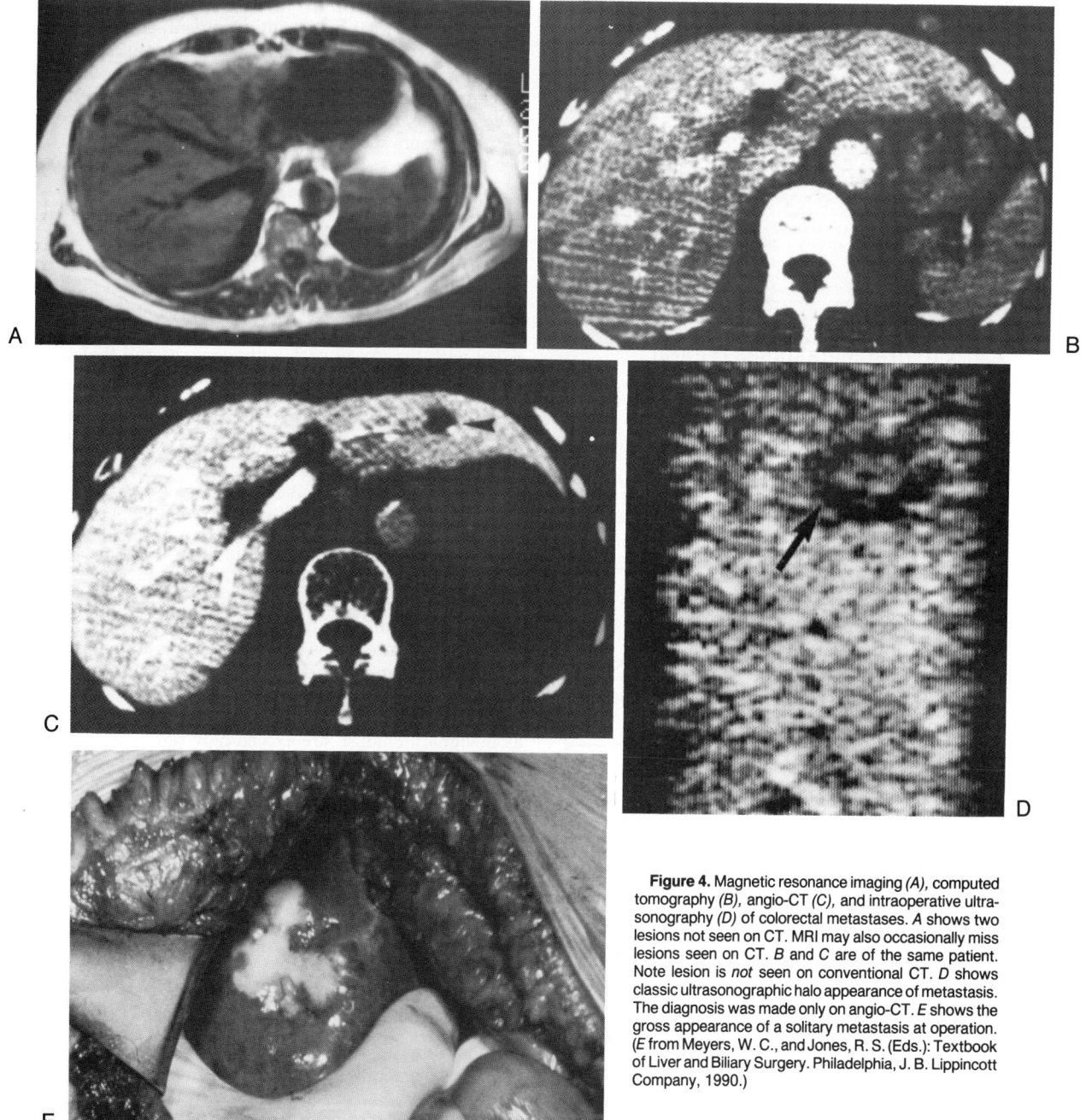

Figure 4. Magnetic resonance imaging (A), computed tomography (B), angio-CT (C), and intraoperative ultrasonography (D) of colorectal metastases. A shows two lesions not seen on CT. MRI may also occasionally miss lesions seen on CT. B and C are of the same patient. Note lesion is *not* seen on conventional CT. D shows classic ultrasonographic halo appearance of metastasis. The diagnosis was made only on angio-CT. E shows the gross appearance of a solitary metastasis at operation. (E from Meyers, W. C., and Jones, R. S. (Eds.): Textbook of Liver and Biliary Surgery. Philadelphia, J. B. Lippincott Company, 1990.)

toms for carcinoid tumors or insulinomas. This procedure has also been performed for gastrinoma with good results. When synchronous hepatic metastasis is found during operation for the primary colorectal malignancy, the hepatic lesion may be removed simultaneously or at a second procedure. This decision is based on the adequacy of the colon preparation, magnitude of the principal procedure, extent of hepatic resection involved, and general status of the patient. Because no randomized prospective studies have been performed, it has not been proved whether the prolongation of survival after resection of hepatic metastases is a function of the resection or the natural biology of the tumor.

With improved safety of hepatic resection, indications for hepatic resection of metastases have expanded. Examples include resection of large symptomatic lesions in the presence of extrahepatic disease, resection of residual hepatic disease in combination with aggressive chemotherapy, and/or resection of multiple lesions. There is little question that such aggressive

surgical therapy benefits selected patients, but how many remains unclear. Data are beginning to indicate that a number of factors are predictors of survival following resection of colorectal hepatic metastases. These include size, number of metastatic lesions, and presence of residual local disease. Logically, relatively few data suggest that the colonic lymph node status should be another predictor. Interestingly, some information suggests that females have better survival after hepatic resection of colorectal hepatic metastases.

A variety of other treatment modalities have been advocated for treatment of metastatic colorectal cancer to the liver. The chemotherapeutic agent 5-fluorouracil (5-FU) has a 20 per cent reported response rate in treatment of tumors of the gastrointestinal tract, but the response appears to be less in the presence of hepatic metastases. Leucovorin or levamisole appears to add to this rate. A hepatic artery infusion pump is used in some centers. An increase in 1-year survival in a prospective Phase II trial was reported in patients receiving continuous floxuridine (FUDR)

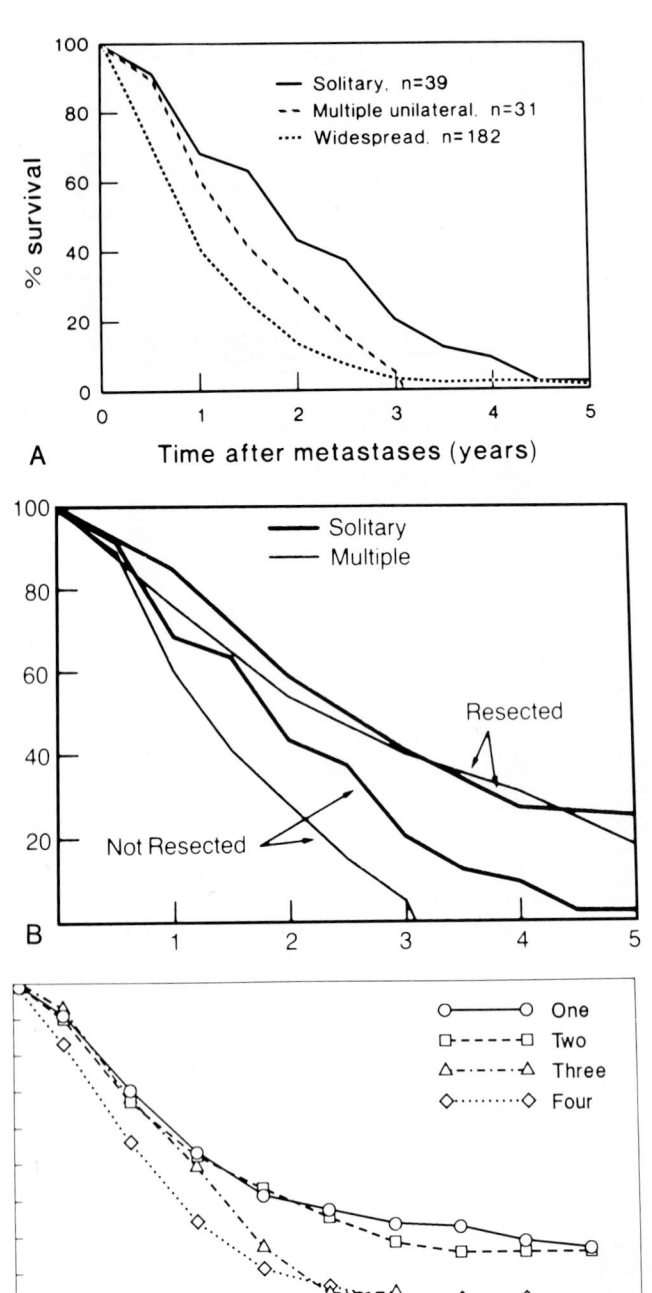

Figure 5. Survival graphs for colorectal cancer patients with *A*, unresected hepatic metastases; *B*, unresected versus resected hepatic metastases; and *C*, 1 to 4 resected hepatic metastases. (*A* from Wagner, J. S., et al.: Ann. Surg., *199*:502, 1984. By permission of the Mayo Foundation.)

with this pump compared with controls. The best results are presently being reported with a combination of 5-FU and FUDR. Intra-arterial chemotherapy was associated with a 62 per cent response rate, although 2-year survival was not greatly changed. FUDR is also associated with a 10 to 20 per cent evidence of biliary sclerosis. However, definitive results of this mode of treatment are still not available, and these patients may represent a subgroup with metastatic cancer with a more favorable natural history. Hyperthermia is being investigated in several centers, and temporary or permanent hepatic artery occlusion is still being tested. Radiation therapy has had no real success.

Contraindications to major hepatic resection for metastatic disease include total hepatic involvement, advanced cirrhosis, jaundice except when caused by extrinsic or hepatic ductal obstruction, vena caval or main portal vein invasion, and extrahepatic tumor involvement. Transplantation of the liver for metastatic disease has generally been unsuccessful except with selected tumors such as carcinoid.

BENIGN HEPATIC NEOPLASMS

Adenomas and Focal Nodular Hyperplasia

Liver cell adenoma and focal nodular hyperplasia are frequently difficult to differentiate although each has its own distinct pathologic and clinical features. The striking similarities are that both occur primarily in young women and are associated with the use of oral contraceptives and that pathologically both are composed of hepatocytes. Hepatic adenomas are usually solitary and may vary in size up to 38 cm. in diameter. Occasionally they may be multiple but cluster in families. They are prone to hemorrhage and necrosis, and tumor rupture or dramatic bleeding occurs in approximately one third of patients. Malignant change is possible. The remaining patients present because of pain or a palpable mass. The patient with an unresected adenoma who discontinues oral contraceptives and becomes pregnant is at considerable risk for tumor rupture and hemorrhage. Microscopically, the adenomas are closely approximated cords of hepatocytes that have vacuolated sinusoidal borders. Centers of the adenomas may undergo degenerative changes. Adenomas have an abundant blood supply; the benign tumor appears separate from adjacent normal hepatic tissue. In contrast, focal nodular hyperplasia does not produce symptoms, and hemorrhage, rupture, or other problems, such as malignant change, are exceedingly rare. Histologically this lesion has a central stellate scar and no true encapsulation, and the cells, which are slightly different in color, usually blend with the normal hepatic parenchyma. The ultrastructure of the hepatocytes in nodular hyperplasia is similar to that of normal hepatocytes. The blood supply to areas of focal nodular hyperplasia is quite different from that to hepatic adenomas, with most of the supply arising centrally rather than peripherally.

Nodular Regenerative Hyperplasia

Nodular regenerative hyperplasia is, by definition, a noncirrhotic diffuse hepatocellular process characterized by multiple nodules in intervening areas of hepatic atrophy. It is similar to focal nodular hyperplasia in that both are not true neoplasms. Nodular regenerative hyperplasia is more frequently confused with cirrhosis. Both are frequently associated with portal hypertension, but the former is distinguished by the absence of severe fibrosis. Although this condition is considered generally rare, because of the understandable confusion between this entity and cirrhosis the incidence is reported quite variably.

Cavernous Hemangiomas

Cavernous hemangiomas occur in all age groups, often grow during pregnancy, and are usually successfully diagnosed by ultrasonography, CT, magnetic resonance imaging, radionuclide scan, or arteriography. Approximately 2 per cent of livers at autopsy contain cavernous hemangiomas, making this the most common liver tumor encountered coincidentally at laparotomy. Most hemangiomas are small and do not cause symptoms. However, they may be large and when associated with diffuse hemangiomatosis can nearly replace the liver. Spontaneous rupture is unusual but can be dramatic. Rare complications include congestive heart failure due to arteriovenous shunts and consumptive coagulopathy. Biopsy of a cavernous hemangioma may lead to severe, uncontrollable hemorrhage. Indications for resection are usually determined by the presence of symptoms, the danger of rupture, and the amount of liver tissue involved.

Hemangioendotheliomas

These rare, vasoformative, cellular tumors usually appear during the first 2 years of life and may be accompanied by similar tumors in the skin and other parts of the body. They may have significant degrees of arteriovenous shunting causing congestive heart failure. Malignant change rarely occurs. Prednisone may be successful in treatment, and resection may be indicated when there is no response to prednisone.

Other Benign Solid Tumors

Other benign solid tumors that may appear in the liver include lipomas, fibromas, leiomyomas, myxomas, teratomas, carcinoid tumor, and mesenchymal hamartomas. Carcinoid is an exceedingly rare primary liver tumor and is associated with the carcinoid syndrome. Mesenchymal hamartomas are rare but are important to recognize because they grow to an extremely large size in an infant or young child and require surgical resection. Biliary cystadenomas and bile duct adenomas are exceedingly rare and may cause pain or extrahepatic biliary obstruction. Other even rarer benign biliary tumors include meningioma, fibroma, granular cell myoblastoma, and carcinoid. Small biliary hamartomas, or tufts of biliary hyperplasia, appear to be extremely common. Another lesion usually of little pathologic significance, but relatively common, is focal fatty change.

Some benign conditions that can be confused with hepatic neoplasms include hereditary hemorrhagic telangiectasia, peliosis hepatis, and hepatic pseudotumor. Hereditary hemorrhagic telangiectasia is a diffuse telangiectatic process in the liver with numerous arteriovenous fistulas, it is rare, associated with fibrosis, and considered by some authorities to be a form of cirrhosis. Peliosis hepatis is also a rare lesion characterized by variably sized blood lakes and the most common association is with anabolic steroid therapy. Rarely is the condition clinically important. Eighteen cases of inflammatory "pseudotumor" have been reported, most probably resulting from healed abscesses.

NONPARASITIC CYSTS

Cysts of the liver are generally benign. They may be solitary or multiple and may or may not communicate with the hepatic ductal system. Large solitary parenchymal cysts appear to be exceedingly rare; only 19 have been observed by investigators at a major medical center in the past 20 years. Most cysts are lined by biliary epithelium but may also have a mesothelial cell lining or rarely other types. They are more common in the right lobe of the liver. It has been presumed that most of these cysts are congenital. They occur four times as frequently in females as in males. Although most cysts are small and asymptomatic, they may be quite large; in fact, one reported cyst contained 17,000 ml. of fluid. The most common presenting symptoms of large cysts are increased abdominal girth, vague pain, occasional bleeding or infection, and rarely evidence of significant hepatocyte compromise such as obstructive jaundice. Small cysts require no treatment, although if discovered incidentally at the time of operation, they may simply be aspirated. For large cysts from which clear fluid is aspirated, the preferred treatment is excision. However, major vascular and ductal structures may be proximal to the wall, in which case unroofing and external drainage is the treatment of choice. An infected cyst should be treated like an abscess, that is, with open drainage. If the cyst contains biliary contents, a communication to the bile duct system should be presumed and excision or Roux-en-Y cystojejunostomy is the treatment of choice.

Polycystic liver disease often accompanies polycystic kidneys. The number of cysts varies, but most do not cause liver function compromise, and rupture, hemorrhage, and infection are rare. When indicated, they may be treated in a manner similar to solitary cysts. Injection of formalin and other sclerotic solutions has been suggested but has never gained significant acceptance. The surgical procedure of choice for a symptomatic dominant cyst in polycystic disease is the fenestration operation, in which the symptomatic cyst is made to communicate with the peritoneal cavity.

Cysts may also form as a consequence of trauma or inflammation; however, these are not true cysts, since they have a fibrous rather than an epithelial lining. There are no special aspects of treatment of these cysts. Cystadenomas, cystadenocarcinomas, and other neoplasms with necrotic centers obviously may present as cysts and should be treated by excision. Cystadenoma is thought to be a precursor of cystadenocarcinoma. Other unusual cysts include teratomas, necrotic cysts secondary to infarction, intrahepatic duodenal duplications, and cysts associated with congenital hepatic fibrosis. Peliosis hepatis is a dilation of the hepatic sinusoids often associated with tuberculosis and steroids.

Choledochal or other solitary ductal cysts are more common in the Orient than in the United States. They occur more commonly in females than in males, but the pathogenesis is unknown. Sixty per cent are diagnosed before the age of 10. Associated intrahepatic ductal dilation is frequent. The most common type of choledochal cyst is one that involves the common bile duct and cystic duct but does not involve the junction of the common hepatic duct. A number of other types may occur, including a diverticulum, diffuse biliary ductal involvement, and segmental dilation. Treatment of choledochal or hepatic ductal cysts or dilation is surgical and is supplemented by antibiotics to control infection. Because of the significant likelihood of biliary obstruction, cholangitis, calculi, and carcinoma, the procedure of choice is excision whenever possible. However, this may not be practical anatomically. In addition, the pancreatic duct may on occasion drain into the cyst, and then drainage procedures such as hepaticoenterostomy or cystoenterostomy are preferred. The incidence of carcinoma in congenital biliary duct cysts appears to be approximately 5 to 8 per cent. Occasionally this occurs after cyst excision. The incidence of stricture after cystoenterostomy has been reported to be as high as 40 to 50 per cent.

Multiple cystic dilations of the intrahepatic ducts (Caroli's disease) is a congenital malformation often associated with congenital hepatic fibrosis. It may be confined to one segment or lobe but is usually diffuse. This problem also appears to be more common in the Orient. Symptoms of biliary tract disease such as colic or cholangitis may be associated with Caroli's disease. Treatment depends on the location and extent of the intrahepatic ductal dilation. Both drainage and resection in selected patients have been reported to provide good results.

ECHINOCOCCAL CYSTS

Echinococcosis, or hydatidosis, is the most frequent cause of liver cysts in the world. The problem is endemic in Greece, other parts of Eastern Europe, South America, Australia, and South Africa. Echinococcosis is rare in the United States, although it is prevalent enough to be seen by most general surgeons during their careers. The most common form is due to *Echinococcus granulosus*, although occasionally *Echinococcus multilocularis* is the infective agent. The adult *E. granulosus* is a tapeworm that resides in the jejunum of dogs. Eggs are passed in the stool and ingested by cows, sheep, moose, caribou, or humans. Embryos pass through the intestinal mucosa into the portal circulation and are filtered by the liver and occasionally by the lungs. They then develop into cysts that have two layers, an outer fibrous layer and an inner parasite-derived layer. The inner layer is the

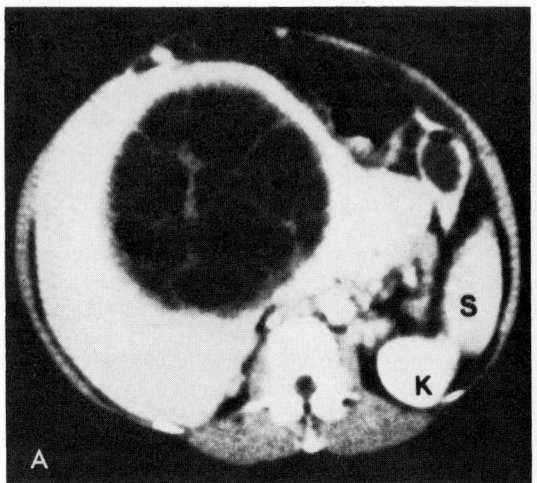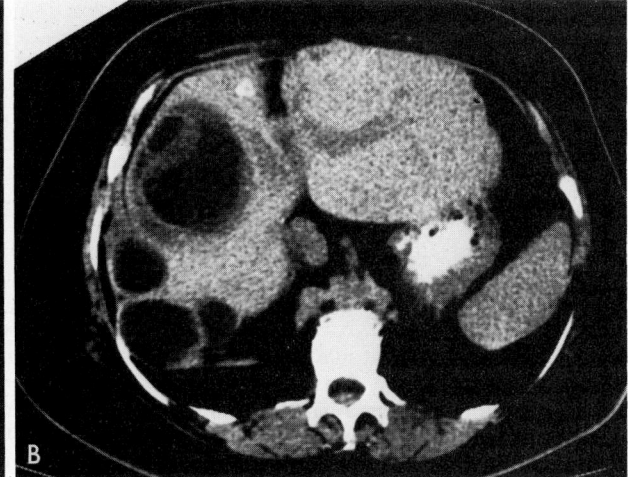

Figure 6. Solitary (A) and multiple (B) recurrent echinococcal cysts with septa seen on computed tomography (K, kidney; S, spleen). (A from Gutierrez, O. H., and Schwartz, S. I. (Eds.): Atlas of Hepatic Tumors and Focal Lesions. New York, McGraw-Hill Book Company, 1984.)

germinal membrane that contains the scolices and daughter cysts and may float freely in the clear cyst fluid.

Approximately 80 per cent of hydatid cysts are initially single and in the right lobe. The most common presenting symptoms or signs are abdominal pain and palpation of a mass in the right upper quandrant. The cysts are usually greater than 5 cm. in diameter when they cause symptoms. The complications of echinococcal cysts include infection, rupture, anaphylaxis, biliary obstruction, and liver replacement. The patient may have mildly elevated liver function tests and eosinophilia. Of the serologic tests, the indirect hemagglutination test and the Casoni skin test have approximately an 85 per cent sensitivity. Problems with the Casoni skin test are that the test itself may sensitize the host, which may cause false-positive serologic tests or even anaphylaxis, and there is a high frequency of false-positive tests due to poor standardization of the nitrogen content in the antigen. The complement fixation test has approximately a 70 per cent sensitivity. Calcification of the cystic wall is present in over half the patients. Liver scan, ultrasonography, CT (Fig. 6), and arteriography all have nearly 100 per cent sensitivity. Endoscopic retrograde cholangiopancreatography and cholangiography have been reported to be helpful occasionally. The finding of daughter cysts or hydatid "sand" on ultrasonography and CT scan helps differentiate this cyst from pyogenic or amebic liver abscess. This entity must be suspected in order to avoid percutaneous needle aspiration, which may cause spillage and spread of the cysts. Communication of the cyst with the biliary tract may be seen on the preoperative cholangiogram or intraoperatively in approximately one fourth of patients. Treatment is primarily surgical.

At exploration, the abdomen is carefully packed with pads around the cysts to reduce the risk of peritoneal soilage. The cyst may then be apirated as completely as possible with a closed system. If the fluid color suggests biliary communication, a sclerosing solution should not be used. Hypertonic saline, chlorhexidine, 80 per cent alcohol, and 0.5 per cent cetrimide are all useful as scolecidal agents and may be instilled into the cyst cavity. Formalin is no longer used because of the risk of systemic toxicity. After 5 minutes the procedure is repeated and then the cyst cavity is unroofed. The fluid in the echinococcal cyst cavity is highly antigenic, and therefore anaphylaxis as well as spread is a risk of cyst rupture. Instillation of scolecidal agents is effective in destroying 80 to 90 per cent of scoleces. There are two alternatives in the management of the cyst cavity: drainage and obliteration without drainage. Except in cases with biliary communication, drainage is accompanied by greater postopera-

tive morbidity and prolonged hospitalization. Therefore, most surgeons prefer not to drain the cyst cavities. Small intra- or extrahepatic cysts may be excised. Recently, mebendazole has been found to be an effective agent in some cases of echinococcal cysts, and this drug may be used for cases not amenable to surgical therapy.

The treatment of the more aggressive *E. multilocularis*, or alveolar hydatid disease, is excision whenever possible. However, this is rarely possible. This disease is limited geographically to the Northern Hemisphere, being endemic in Alaska and Canada. Natural hosts include the fox, coyote, and small rodents.

MAJOR HEPATIC RESECTION

With reduction of operative mortality to less than 5 per cent, elective major hepatic resection has gained acceptance as the primary mode of therapy for many primary and metastatic tumors of the liver and other selected benign conditions. Those conditions include segmental Caroli's disease or hepatolithiasis, echinococcosis, or solitary hepatic abscesses in chronic granulomatous disease of childhood. Classically, four types of major resection have been employed, based on the lobar and segmental anatomy of the liver (Fig. 7): (1) right hepatic lobectomy (Fig. 8), (2) left hepatic lobectomy, (3) right trisegmentectomy (resec-

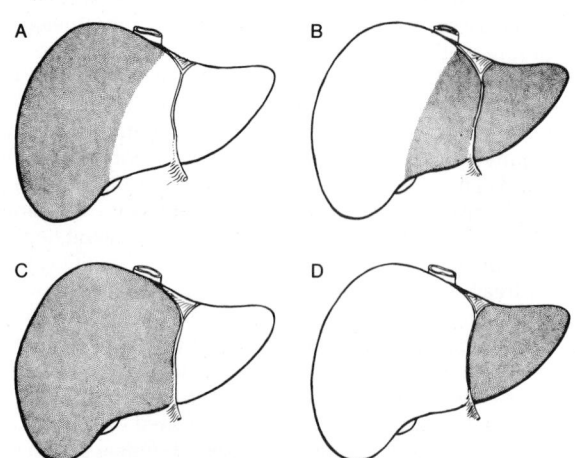

Figure 7. Four classic major hepatic resections: A, right hepatic lobectomy; B, left hepatic lobectomy; C, right trisegmentectomy; and D, left lateral segmentectomy.

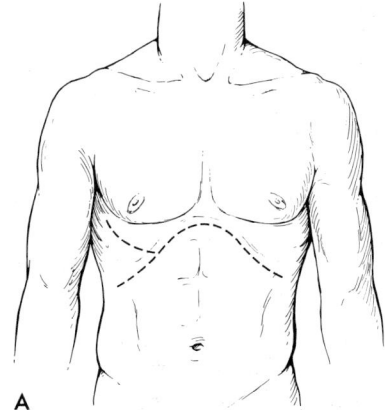

Figure 8. One technique of hepatic lobectomy. *A,* Subcostal incision with possible extension into right thorax or left side. *B,* Mobilization of right lobe of liver is performed with division of peritoneum overlying the inferior vena cava from the diaphragm to the foramen of Winslow. *C,* Cholecystectomy after ligation of the cystic artery and duct or right hepatic artery and duct. *D,* Clamping and ligation of the right hepatic vein after ligation and division of the right branch of the portal vein and hepatic artery. Ligation of the hepatic veins may be more safely performed during parenchymal dissection. *E,* Parenchymal dissection with ligation of multiple vascular and biliary branches after ligation and division of portal vein, hepatic artery, and bile duct to the right lobe.

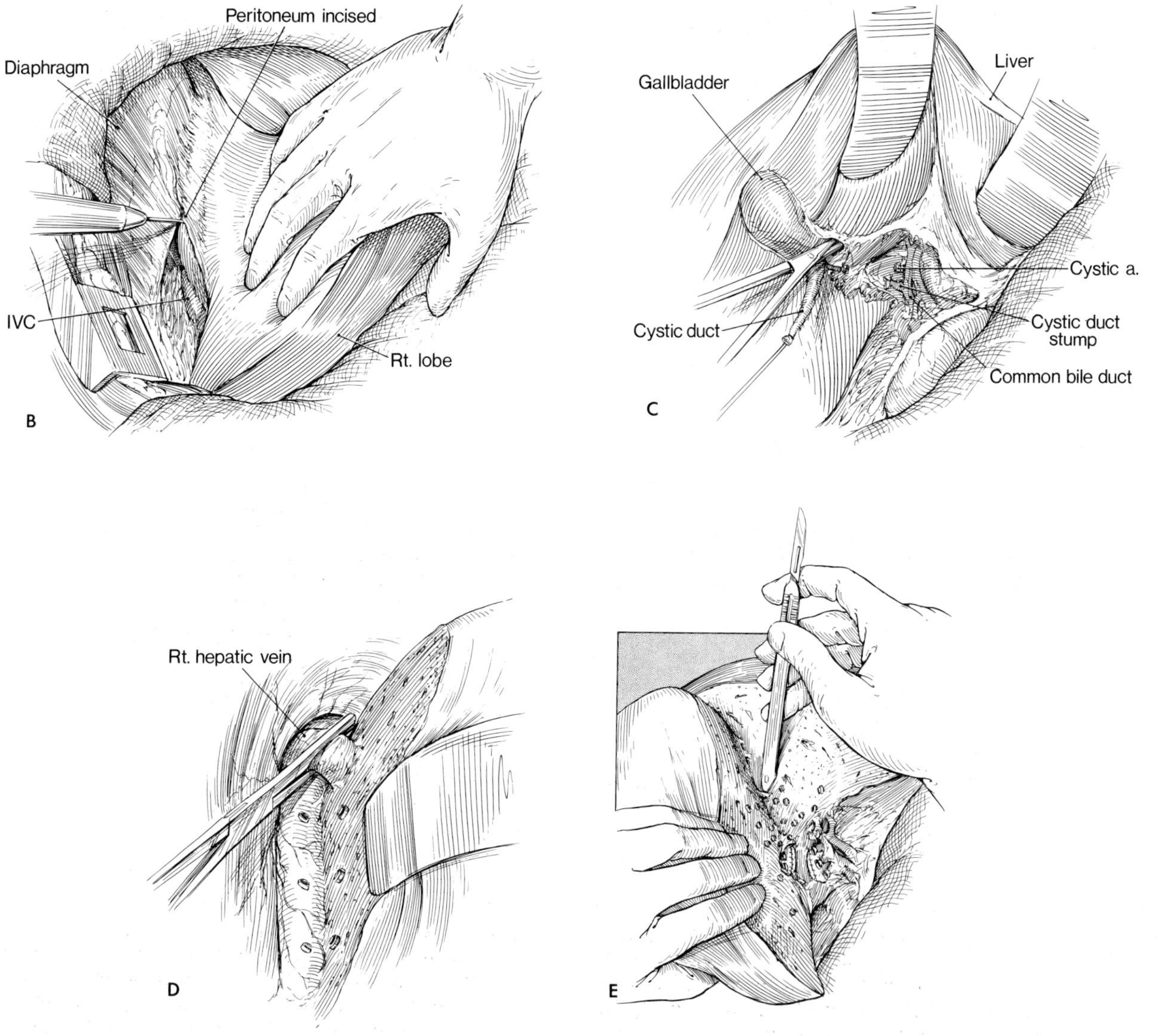

Peritoneum incised

Diaphragm

IVC

Rt. lobe

B

Gallbladder

Liver

Cystic a.

Cystic duct

Cystic duct stump

Common bile duct

C

Rt. hepatic vein

D

E

tion of the right lobe with the medial segment of the left lobe), and (4) left lateral segmentectomy. With improvement in techniques, several new categories of resection have become much more common (Fig. 9). Two types of resection that are occasionally performed in several centers are the left trisegmentectomy (resection of the left lobe plus the anterior segment of the right lobe) and left medial segmentectomy (left middle lobectomy).

Bismuth has popularized resection according to the French segmental anatomic nomenclature.

Major hepatic resections for abdominal trauma are usually nonanatomic and do not usually require hilar dissection. In addition, development of a new surgical instrument, the CUSA, has permitted large, nonanatomic wedge resections in a relatively bloodless field (Fig. 10). This instrument has a metal tip

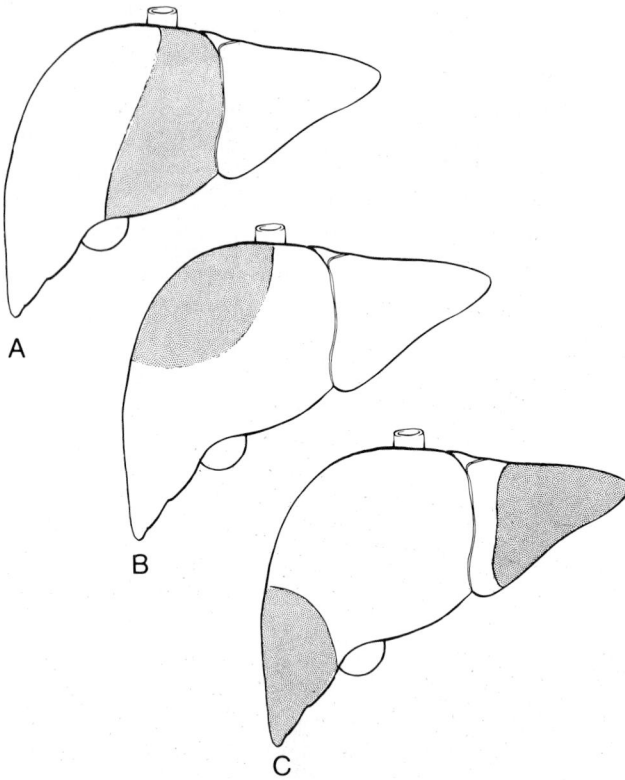

Figure 9. Examples of three "newer" types of hepatic resection. *A*, Example of segmental resection, in this case segment 4 (medial segment of left lobe). *B*, Nonanatomic resection, in this case resection of dome of liver (portions of anterior segment of right lobe and medial segment of left). *C*, Multiple resections. (From Meyers, W. C., and Jones, R. S. (Eds.): Textbook of Liver and Biliary Surgery. Philadelphia, J. B. Lippincott Company, 1990.)

thoractomy and a midline or paramedian incision. Lobectomy and trisegmentectomy require hilar dissection, whereas the left lateral segmentectomy generally does not. Branches of the portal vein, hepatic artery, and bile duct of the lobe to be removed are ligated and divided. Then the hepatic vein system may be occluded or ligated and divided, or in many cases the hepatic venous system may be ligated during parenchymal dissection. The parenchymal dissection is performed with the handle of the knife or finger fracture, and the biliary vascular bundles are ligated. A variety of noncrushing liver clamps may be applied to control parenchymal bleeding during this stage of the operation. Some surgeons advocate routine use of temporary occlusion of the portal triad (the Pringle maneuver) during major resections.

Hypoglycemia and hypoproteinemia frequently occur in the postoperative period following major hepatic resection. These should be treated supportively and usually resolve within 1 week after the operation. Alkaline phosphatase and transaminase elevations frequently occur, and transient hyperbilirubinemia is not uncommon. Up to 80 to 90 per cent of the liver may be removed without serious consequence if the remaining liver is normal. Patients with pre-existent diffuse liver disease are at greatly increased risk of liver failure following resection. There is no good liver function test to predict the adequacy of function of the remaining liver.

SELECTED REFERENCES

Blumgart, L. H.: Surgery of the Liver and Biliary Tract. Vol. 2, Secs. 9, 12, 14. New York, Churchill Livingstone, 1988.
  This is a collection of work from a number of authoritative figures in the field. A number of topics are discussed from widely opposing viewpoints.

Blumgart, L. H., and Benjamin, I. S.: Liver resection for bile duct cancer. Surg. Clin. North Am., 69:323, 1989.
  This is an excellent update of common indications for liver resection.

Foster, J. H., and Berman, M. M.: Solid Liver Tumors. Philadelphia, W. B. Saunders Company, 1977.
  This is landmark monograph on the subject.

Hanks, J., and Jones, R. S.: The pathogenesis, detection, and surgical treatment of hepatic metastases. Curr. Probl. Cancer, 10:217, 1986.
  This is an excellent review of surgical aspects of metastatic tumors.

Kew, M. C.: Hepatic tumors. Semin. Liver Dis., 4:89, 1984.
  This issue provides an excellent overview of understanding of the etiology and pathogenesis of several of the more common and important hepatic tumors.

Meyers, W. C., and Jones, R. S.: Textbook of Liver and Biliary Surgery. Philadelphia, J. B. Lippincott Company, 1990.
  This recent, comprehensive textbook covers hepatobiliary surgery with emphasis on the pathobiology and historical perspectives that guide current therapy.

that vibrates at an ultrasonic frequency that fragments parenchymal cells easily. An irrigation port lifts the cells up and a suction port removes them. The advantage of this instrument is that major biliary and vascular structures remain intact during parenchymal dissection, which permits isolation and ligation of these structures without hilar dissection. Using this or similar techniques, many more lesions can be safely resected and even partial hepatic transplantation is now possible.

A variety of incisions may be used, including subcostal incisions with possible extension as a median sternotomy or right

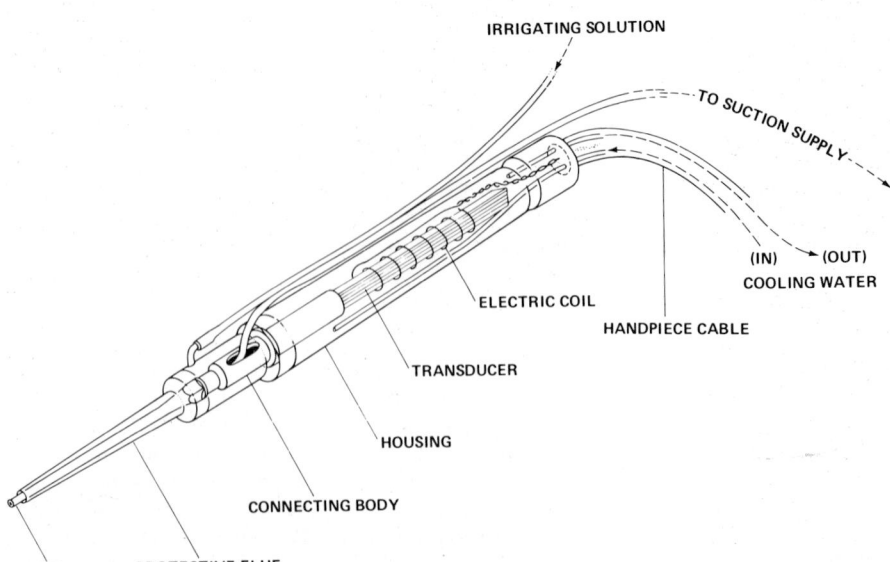

IRRIGATING SOLUTION

TO SUCTION SUPPLY

(IN) → (OUT)
COOLING WATER

ELECTRIC COIL

HANDPIECE CABLE

TRANSDUCER

HOUSING

CONNECTING BODY

TIP   PROTECTIVE FLUE

Figure 10. Instrument, the CUSA, used for hepatic parenchymal dissection. Other new instruments such as a waterjet and new clamps are also being commonly employed. This instrument has a metal tip that vibrates at an ultrasonic frequency and may aspirate fragmented parenchymal cells and leave vascular and biliary structures intact for ligation, which may permit the surgeon to perform segmental and nonanatomic resections more safely. (Reproduced from CUSA brochure by permission from Cooper LaserSonics, Santa Clara, CA.)

Nakayama, F.: Progress in the treatment of bile duct cancer: Multidisciplinary approach—introduction. World J. Surg., 12:1, 1988.

Okuda, K., and Ishak, K. G.: Neoplasms of the Liver. New York, Springer-Verlag, 1987.
These are the most authoritative pathology texts in the field.

REFERENCES

General

1. Blumgart, L. H.: Surgery of the Liver and Biliary Tract. Vol. 2, Secs. 9, 12, 14. New York, Churchill Livingstone, 1988.
2. Calne, R. Y., and Della Rovere, G. Q.: Liver Surgery. Philadelphia, W. B. Saunders Company, 1982.
3. Edmondson, H. A., and Peters, R. L.: Neoplasms of the Liver. *In* Schiff, L., and Schiff, E. R. (Eds.): Diseases of the Liver. Philadelphia, J. B. Lippincott Company, 1982, pp. 1101–1157.
4. Fortner, J. G., et al.: Surgery in liver tumors. Curr. Probl. Surg., June, 1972.
5. Foster, J. H., and Berman, M. M.: Solid Liver Tumors. Philadelphia, W. B. Saunders Company, 1977.
6. Kew, M. C.: Tumors of the liver. *In* Zakim, D., and Boyer, T. D. (Eds.): Hepatology. Philadelphia, W. B. Saunders Company, 1982, pp. 1048–1083.
7. Longmire, W. P., Jr., and Tompkins, R. K.: Manual of Liver Surgery. New York, Springer-Verlag, 1981.
8. Meyers, W. C., and Jones, R. S.: Textbook of Liver and Biliary Surgery. Chapters 6 and 7. Philadelphia, J. B. Lippincott Company, 1990.
9. Okuda, K., and Ishak, K. G.: Neoplasms of the Liver. New York, Springer-Verlag, 1987.

Hepatocellular Carcinoma

10. Alpert, E.: Human alpha-1 fetoprotein. *In* Okuda, K., and Peters, R. L. (Eds.): Hepatocellular Carcinoma. New York, John Wiley & Sons, 1976, p. 353.
11. Anthony, P. P.: Primary carcinoma of the liver: A study of 282 cases in Ugandan Africans. J. Pathol., 101:37, 1973.
12. Aoki, K.: Cancer of the liver—international mortality trends. World Health Stat. Rep., 31:28, 1978.
13. Berman, C.: Primary carcinoma of the liver. London, HK Lewis and Company, 1951.
14. Bismuth, H., Castaing, D., and Garden, O. J.: The use of operative ultrasound in surgery of primary liver tumors. World J. Surg., 11:610, 1987.
15. Blumberg, B. S., and London, W. T.: Primary hepatocellular carcinoma and hepatitis B virus. Curr. Probl. Cancer, 6:1, 1982.
16. Doll, R., Muir, C., and Waterhouse J.: Cancer incidence in five continents. Acta Un Int. Contra Cancrum, 2:1, 1970.
17. Dunham, L. J., and Bailar, J. C.: World maps of cancer mortality rates and frequency rates. J. Natl. Cancer Inst., 41:155, 1968.
18. Edmondson, H. A., and Peters, R. L.: Neoplasms of the liver. *In* Schiff, L., and Schiff, E. R. (Eds.): Diseases of the Liver. Philadelphia, J. B. Lippincott Company, 1982, pp. 1101–1157.
19. Exelby, P. R., Filler, R. M., and Grosfeld, J. L.: Liver tumors in children in the particular reference to hepatoblastomas and hepatocellular carcinoma: American Academy of Pediatrics Surgical Section Survey—1974. J. Pediatr. Surg., 10:329, 1975.
20. Forbes, A., Portmann, B., Johnson, P., and Williams, R.: Hepatic sarcomas in adults: A review of 25 cases. Gut, 28:668, 1987.
21. Heyward, W. L., Lanier, A. P., McMahon, B. J., Fitzgerald, M. A., Kilkenny, S., and Paproxki, T. R.: Early detection of primary hepatocellular carcinoma. J. A. M. A., 254:3052, 1985.
22. Higginson, J.: The geographical pathology of primary liver cancer. Cancer Res., 23:1624, 1963.
23. Iwatsuki, S., Gordon, R. D., Shaw, B. W., and Starzl, T. E.: Role of liver transplantation in cancer therapy. Ann. Surg., 202:401, 1985.
24. Kew, M. C.: Alpha-fetoprotein. *In* Read, A. E. (Ed.): Modern Trends in Gastroenterology. Vol. 5. London, Butterworth, 1975, p. 91.
25. Liaw, Y.-F., Tai, D.-I., Chu, C.-M., Lind, D.-Y., Sheen, I.-S., Chen, T.-J., and Pao, C. C.: Early detection of hepatocellular carcinoma in patients with chronic type B hepatitis. A prospective study. Gastroenterology, 90:236, 1986.
26. Longmire, W. P., Jr., Passaro, E. P., and Joseph, W. L.: The surgical treatment of hepatic lesions. Br. J. Surg., 53:852, 1966.
27. Mallory, F. B.: Cirrhosis of liver. N. Engl. J. Med., 205:1231, 1932.
28. Nagorney, D., Adson, M., Weiland, L., Knight, C., Jr., Smalley, S., and Zinsmeister, A.: Fibrolamellar hepatoma. Abstract presented at 1984 meeting of the Society for Surgery of the Alimentary Tract, New Orleans, La.
29. Okuda, K., Kubo, Y., Okazaki, N., et al.: Clinical aspects of intrahepatic bile duct carcinoma including hilar carcinoma. Cancer, 39:232, 1977.
30. Okuda, K., Obata, H., Nakajima, Y., et al.: Prognosis of primary hepatocellular carcinoma. Hepatology, 4:35, 1984.
31. Peters, R. L.: Pathology of hepatocellular carcinoma. *In* Okuda, K., and Peters, R. L. (Eds.): Hepatocellular Carcinoma. New York, John Wiley & Sons, 1976.
32. Purtilo, D. R., and Gottlieg, L. S.: Cirrhosis and hepatoma occurring at Boston City Hospital (1917–1968). Cancer, 32:458, 1973.
33. Ramming, K. P., Haskell, C. M., and Tesler, A. S.: Gastrointestinal tract neoplasms. *In* Haskell, C. M. (Ed.): Cancer Treatment. Philadelphia, W. B. Saunders Company, 1980, pp. 231–357.
34. Shikata, T.: Studies on the relationship between hepatic cancer and liver cirrhosis. Acta Pathol. Jpn., 9:267, 1959.
35. Waterhouse, J., Muir, C., Correa, P., et al.: Cancer incidence in five continents. Lyon World Health Organization, 1977.
36. Wu, M.-C., Chen, H., Chang, H.-H., Yuo, H.-P., and Yang, C.-M.: Resection of primary hepatic carcinoma during a period of eighteen years. Shanghai, First Affiliated Hospital of the 2nd Military Medical College (private publication), 1979.

Cholangiocarcinoma

37. Belmaric, J.: Malignant tumors in Chinese. Int. J. Cancer, 4:560, 1979.
38. Blumgart, L. H., Benjamin, I. S., Hadis, N. S., and Beazley, R.: Surgical approaches to cholangiocarcinoma at confluence of hepatic ducts. Lancet, 1:66, 1984.
39. Chitwood, W. R., Meyers, W. C., Heaston, D. K., Herskovic, A. M., McLeod, M. E., and Jones, R. S.: Diagnosis and treatment of primary extrahepatic bile duct tumors. Am. J. Surg., 143:99, 1982.
40. Klatskin, G.: Adenocarcinoma of the hepatic duct at its bifurcation within the porta hepatis. Am. J. Med., 38:241, 1965.
41. Terblanche, J.: Carcinoma of the proximal extrahepatic biliary tree. *In* Nyhus, L. M. (Ed.): Surgery Annual. New York, Appleton-Century-Crofts, 1979, pp. 249–265.

Metastatic Tumors

42. Adson, M. A.: Resection of liver metastases—when is it worthwhile? World J. Surg., 11:511, 1987.
43. Adson, M. A.: The resection of hepatic metastases. Another view. Arch. Surg., 124:1023, 1989.
44. Adson, M. A., and Van Heerfen, J. A.: Major hepatic resection for metastatic colorectal cancer. Ann. Surg., 191:576, 1980.
45. Balch, C. M., Urist, M. M., Soong, S.-J., and McGregor, M. A.: A prospective phase II clinical trial of continuous FUDR regional chemotherapy for colorectal metastases to the liver using a totally implantable drug infusion pump. Ann. Surg., 198:567, 1983.
46. Bengmark, S., and Hafstrom, L.: The natural history of primary and secondary malignant tumors of the liver. I. The prognosis for patients with hepatic metastases from colonic and rectal carcinoma by laparotomy. Cancer, 23:198, 1968.
47. Bismuth, H., and Castaing, D.: Echographie per-operatoire du foie et des voies biliares. Paris, Flammarion Medecine-Sciences, 1985.
48. Flanagan, L., and Foster, J. H.: Hepatic resection for metastatic cancer. Am. J. Surg., 113:551, 1967.
49. Folkman, J.: Proceedings: Tumor angiogenesis factor. Cancer Res., 34:2109, 1974.
50. Fortner, J. G., Silva, J. S., Golbey, R. B., Cox, E. B., and Maclean, B. J.: Multivariate analysis of a personal series of 247 consecutive patients with liver metastases from colorectal cancer. I. Treatment by hepatic resection. Ann. Surg., 199:306, 1984.
51. Foster, J. H.: Survival after liver resection for secondary tumors. Am. J. Surg., 135:389, 1978.
52. Hanks, J. B., Meyers, W. C., Filston, H. C., Killenberg, P. G., and Jones, R. S.: Surgical resection for benign and malignant disease. Ann. Surg., 191:584, 1980.
53. Hughes, K., Scheele, J., and Sugarbaker, P. H.: Surgery for colorectal cancer metastatic to the liver. Optimizing the results of treatment. Surg. Clin. North Am., 69:339, 1989.
54. Jaffe, B. M., Donegan, W. L., Watson, F., and Spratt, J. S., Jr.: Factors influencing survival in patients with untreated hepatic metastases. Surg. Gynecol. Obstet., 127:1, 1968.
55. Kortz, W. J., Meyers, W. C., Hanks, J. B., Schirmer, B. D., and Jones, R. S.: Hepatic resection for metastatic cancer. Ann. Surg., 199:182, 1984.
56. Lundstedt, C., Ekberg, H., Hederstrom, E., Stridbeck, H., Torfason, B., and Transverg, K. G.: Radiologic diagnosis of liver metastases in colo-rectal carcinoma. Prospective evaluation of the accuracy of angiography, ultrasonography, computed tomography and computed tomographic angiography. Acta Radiol., 28:431, 1987.
57. Lundstedt, C., Ekberg, H., Lunderquist, A., and Tranberg, K. G.: Site and number of liver tumors recorded at angiography and computed tomography compared with the findings at laparotomy and of resected liver specimens. Acta Radiol., 28:153, 1987.
58. Parker, G. A., Lawrence, W., Jr., Horsley, J. S., Neifeld, J. P., Cook, D., Walse, J., Brewer, W., and Koretz, M. J.: Intraoperative ultrasound of the liver affects operative decision making. Ann. Surg., 209:569, 1989.
59. Pestana, C., Reitemeier, R. J., Moertel, C. G., Judd, E. S., and Dockerty, M. B.: The natural history of carcinoma of the colon and rectum. Am. J. Surg., 108:826, 1964.
60. Silen, W.: Hepatic resection for metastases from colorectal carcinoma is of dubious value. Arch. Surg., 124:1021, 1989.
61. Taylor, K. J.: Intraoperative ultrasound in detecting hepatic metastases. Hepatology, 8:426, 1988.

62. Wagner, J. S., Adson, M. A., Van Heerden, J. A., Adson, M. H., and Ilstrup, D. M.: The natural history of hepatic metastases from colorectal cancer. Ann. Surg., *199*:502, 1984.
63. Wanebo, H. J., Semoglou, C., Attiyeh, F., et al.: Surgical management of patients with primary operable colorectal cancer and synchronous liver metastases. Am. J. Surg., *135*:81, 1978.
64. Wilson, S., and Adson, M. A.: Surgical treatment of hepatic metastases from colorectal cancer. Arch. Surg., *3*:330, 1976.

Other Solid Neoplasms

65. Blumgart, L. H. and Benjamin, I. S.: Liver resection for bile duct cancer. Surg. Clin. North Am., *69*:323, 1989.
66. Edmondson, H. A.: Tumors of the liver and intrahepatic bile ducts. *In* Atlas of Tumor Pathology, Section 7, Fascicle 25. Washington, D.C., Armed Forces Institute of Pathology, 1958, pp. 32–112.
67. Ehren, H., Mahour, G. H., and Isaacs, H.: Benign tumors in infancy and childhood. Am. J. Surg., *145*:325, 1983.
68. El-Domeiri, A. A., Huvos, A. G., Goldsmith, H. S., and Foote, F. W., Jr.: Primary malignant tumors of the liver. Cancer, *27*:7, 1971.
69. Fechner, R. E.: Benign hepatic lesions and orally administered contraceptives. Hum. Pathol., *8*:255, 1977.
70. Goodman, Z. D.: Benign tumors of the liver. *In* Okuda, K., and Ishak, K. G. (Eds.): Neoplasms of the Liver. New York, Springer-Verlag, 1987, pp. 105–125.
71. Kerlin, P., Davis, G. L., McGill, D. B., Weiland, L. H., Adson, M. A., and Sheedy, P. F.: Hepatic adenoma and focal nodular hyperplasia: Clinical, pathologic, and radiological features. Gastroenterology, *84*:994, 1983.
72. Okuda, K., and Ishak, K. G.: Neoplasms of the Liver. New York, Springer-Verlag, 1987.
73. Walt, A. J.: Cysts and benign tumors of the liver. Surg. Clin. North Am., *57*:449, 1977.

Benign Cysts

74. Bristowe, J. S.: Cystic disease of the liver associated with similar disease of the kidneys. Trans. Pathol. Soc. Lond. *7*:229, 1856.
75. Caroli, J., and Couinaud, C.: Une affection nouvelle, sans doute congenitale, des voies biliaires: La dilatation kystique unilobaire des canaux hepatiques. Sem. Hop. Paris, *34*:496, 1958.
76. Glenn, F., and Moody, F. G.: Intrahepatic calculi. Ann. Surg., *153*:711, 1961.
77. Hadad, A. R., Westbrook, K. C., Graham, G. G., Morris, W. D., and Campbell, G. S.: Symptomatic nonparasitic liver cysts. Am. J. Surg., *134*:739, 1977.
78. Jones, R. S.: Liver cysts. *In* Comeron, J. L. (Ed.): Current Surgical Treatment, 2nd ed. St. Louis, C. V. Mosby, 1986, pp. 157–160.
79. Longmire, W. P., Jr., and Tompkins, R. K.: Cystic disease. *In* Longmire, W. P., Jr., and Tompkins, R. K. (Eds.): Manual of Liver Surgery. New York, Springer-Verlag, 1981, pp. 118–156.
80. Sanfilippo, P. M., Behars, O. H., and Weiland, L. H.: Cystic disease of the liver. Ann. Surg., *179*:922, 1974.

81. Sherlock, S.: Cysts and congenital biliary abnormalities. *In* Diseases of the Liver and Biliary System, 7th ed. Oxford, Blackwell Scientific Publications, 1985, pp. 429–441.
82. Todani, T., Tabuchi, K., Watanabe, Y., and Kobayashi, T.: Carcinoma arising in the wall of congenital bile duct cysts. Cancer, *44*:1134, 1979.

Echinococcal Cysts

83. Barros, J. L.: Hydatid disease of the liver. Am. J. Surg., *135*:597, 1978.
84. Brown, H. W.: Basic Clinical Parasitology, 3rd ed. Chapters 10–13. New York, Appleton-Century-Crofts, 1969,
85. Kasai, Y., Koshino, I., Kawanishi, N., Sakamoto, H., Sasaki, E., and Kumagai, M.: Alveolar echinococcosis of the liver: Studies on 60 operated cases. Ann. Surg., *191*:145, 1980.
86. Langer, J. C., Rose, D. B., Keystone, J. S., Taylor, B. R., and Langer, B.: Diagnosis and management of hydatid disease of the liver: A 15 year North American experience. Ann. Surg., *199*:412, 1984.
87. Longmire, W. P., and Tompkins, R. K.: Infections. *In* Longmire W. P., and Tompkins, R. K. (Eds.): Manual of Liver Surgery. New York, Springer-Verlag, 1981, pp. 62–76.
88. Wilson, J. F., and Rausch, R. L.: Alveolar hydatid disease: A review of clinical features of 33 indigenous cases of *Echinococcus multilocularis* infection in Alaskan Eskimos. Am. J. Trop. Med. Hyg., *29*:1340, 1980.

Major Hepatic Resections

89. Bismuth, H.: Surgical anatomy and anatomical surgery of the liver. World J. Surg., *6*:3, 1982.
90. Bismuth, H., Castaing, D., and Garden, D. J.: Major hepatic resection under total vascular exclusion. Ann. Surg., *210*:13, 1989.
91. Bismuth, H., Houssin, D., and Castaing, D.: Major and minor segmentectomies "reglees" in liver surgery. World J. Surg., *6*:10, 1982.
92. Castaing, D., Garden, O. J., and Bismuth, H.: Segmental liver resection using ultrasound-guided selective portal venous occlusion. Ann. Surg., *210*:20, 1989.
93. Couinaud, C.: Bases anatomiques des hepatectomies gauche et droite reglees, techniques qui en deroulent. J. Chir. (Paris), *70*:933, 1954.
94. Jones, R. S.: The Liver: Malignant and benign tumors, nonparasitic cysts, parasitic cysts, abscess, liver anatomy, technique of liver resection. *In* Moody, F. G., et al. (Eds): Surgical Treatment of Digestive Disease. Chicago, Year Book Medical Publishers, 1986, p. 377.
95. Keen, W. W.: Report of a case of resection of the liver for the removal of a neoplasm, with a table of 76 cases of resection of the liver for hepatic tumors. Ann. Surg., *30*:267, 1899.
96. Langenbuch, C.: Ein Fall von Resektion eines linksseitigen Schnurlappens der Leber, Heilung. Berl. Klin. Wochenschr., *25*:37, 1888.
97. Longmire, W. P., Jr., and Tompkins, R. K.: Manual of Liver Surgery. New York, Springer-Verlag, 1981.
98. Wendel, W.: Beitrage zur Chirurgie der Leber. Arch. Klin. Chir., *95*:887, 1911.
99. Wendel, W.: Über Leberlappenresektion. Arch. Klin. Chir., *114*:982, 1920.

IV

HEMOBILIA

Francis S. Rotolo, M.D., Gene D. Branum, M.D., and William C. Meyers, M.D.

Bleeding into the biliary tract is common, usually inconsequential, but occasionally may be life-threatening, particularly if unrecognized. Glisson provided the first modern description of bleeding into the biliary tract in 1654 and recognized that it was probably an extremely common event:

I believe that if the liver is injured by a contusion, it may lead to blood leaving the body by way of vomit or the stool; for there is no doubt that the biliary duct takes unto itself (to the great good of the patient) some of the blood issuing into the liver and leads it down to the intestines; from there it is either impelled upwards through reverse peristalsis or downwards through normal peristalsis.

In 1948 Sandblom combined Greek and Latin derivations to apply the term "hemobilia" to the syndrome of gastrointestinal bleeding caused by hemorrhage into the biliary tract. Rupture of a hepatic artery aneurysm into the biliary tract was first reported by Jackson in 1921. The most common cause of hemobilia has been trauma. More recently, the most common causes of identified hemobilia reflect advances in hepatobiliary diagnostic and therapeutic techniques. These have included percutaneous liver biopsy, transhepatic and endoscopic cholangiography, and, most recently, direct or extracorporeal lithotripsy.

Causes

Bleeding may arise anywhere within the biliary system, i.e., liver parenchyma, intra- or extrahepatic bile ducts, gallbladder, pancreas, or the ampullary region. The communication between the vascular and biliary systems may be caused by laceration, pressure necrosis, tumor, or infection. In addition, thrombolysis in bile may contribute to continued bleeding. Because of its higher pressure, the arterial system is more often involved than the venous system.

In a 1972 review of 545 patients, trauma was the most important causative factor in 48 per cent of cases, infection in 28 per cent, gallstones in 10 per cent, aneurysms in 7 per cent, and tumor in 5 per cent. Trauma included both blunt and penetrating injuries, automobile accidents leading the list. Blunt trauma may cause deep liver injury with or without disruption of Glisson's capsule. Probably the most frequent reason for hemobilia following liver injury is bleeding deep within the substance of the liver when the capsule remains intact, is sutured closed, or heals superficially. If the resultant hematoma expands, it may rupture into the biliary system, or a false aneurysm may occur and in a more delayed manner lead to the same problem. These are the principal reasons that suture closure of a liver laceration is generally not recommended. Penetration may cause hemobilia by a similar mechanism or by creating a direct communication of a vascular structure with the biliary system.

In earlier reviews, operative trauma represented approximately 15 per cent of cases of hemobilia. Major procedures on or near the liver that may cause minor or major bleeding include liver, stomach, or colon resections; cholecystectomy; or extraction of intrahepatic calculi (Fig. 1). The procedure most likely to cause some degree of bleeding within the biliary system is common bile duct exploration. The peribiliary arterial plexus is often involved in the bleeding. Hepatic artery false aneurysms may follow unsuspected injury and later erode into the bile duct. Postoperative dislodgment of a T-tube may produce the problem. Diagnosis of thrombus within the biliary tree is easily made by cholangiogram if there is a catheter such as a T-tube within the common bile duct. Thus, thrombus may occasionally be confused with a retained stone. Recently, percutaneous cholangiography has become an important cause of bleeding into the biliary system. Hemobilia follows 4 per cent of percutaneous transhepatic cholangiograms and 9 per cent of percutaneously placed biliary drainage catheters. Some degree of hemobilia occurs in 5 to 10 per cent of therapeutic endoscopic procedures. In these patients, thrombus in the biliary tree usually evolves from the sphincterotomy site. Some degree of hemobilia occurs in 8 to 14 per cent of extracorporeal hepatic biliary lithotripsy and 4 to 8 per cent of extracorporeal gallstone lithotripsy. In nearly all of the latter cases reported bleeding has been minor and inconsequential.

Infection may be an important factor in the development of hemobilia. In the Far East the parasites *Clonorchis sinensis* and *Ascaris* may cause cholangitis or pericholangiticar abscesses, which may cause hemobilia. Less commonly, amebic abscess, tuberculosis, and *Echinococcus* infestation are implicated. Biliary tract infection in North America is more often caused by calculi, which may also cause hemobilia by direct trauma to the ampulla or other sites within the duodenal ductal system. Prior to the development of oral cholecystography, the coexistence of biliary colic with blood in the stool was considered a reliable sign of gallstones. The term *hemocholecyst* refers to bleeding within the gallbladder, which rarely may be the cause of biliary colic. Pyogenic liver abscess may lead to hemobilia by direct erosion into a vessel, by formation of a pseudoaneurysm, or as a complication of treatment. Hemobilia may also follow a mycotic aneurysm complicating subacute bacterial endocarditis or another disease process. Pancreatitis may cause hemobilia by erosion of a large vessel such as the splenic or gastroduodenal artery and communication with the pancreatic duct; the outcome is usually fatal. Hemobilia due to pancreatic disease is unusual except when cancer has by erosion entered the biliary system.

Various aneurysms may cause hemobilia by pressure necrosis. Arteriosclerotic, false, or mycotic aneurysms of the hepatic or gastroduodenal artery have all been reported to cause this problem. In one series, 43 of 103 ruptured hepatic artery aneurysms (42 per cent) led to hemobilia. Hepatoma secondary to cirrhosis is the most common tumor causing hemobilia. Other tumors that have been reported to induce hemobilia include gallbladder cancer, cholangiocarcinoma, hemangioma, angiosarcoma, adenomas, cystadenomas, cystadenocarcinomas, and metastatic lesions of the liver parenchyma, gallbladder, and bile ducts. Hemobilia may also occur in association with choledochal cyst or may appear spontaneously in association with vasculitis, heterotopic gastric mucosa, or hemolytic disease such as sickle cell anemia.

Symptoms and Signs

The classic triad of gastrointestinal bleeding, right upper quadrant pain, and jaundice suggests the possibility of hemobilia. Of course, these symptoms may suggest other diseases, such as terminal cancer; but in the setting of trauma, general good

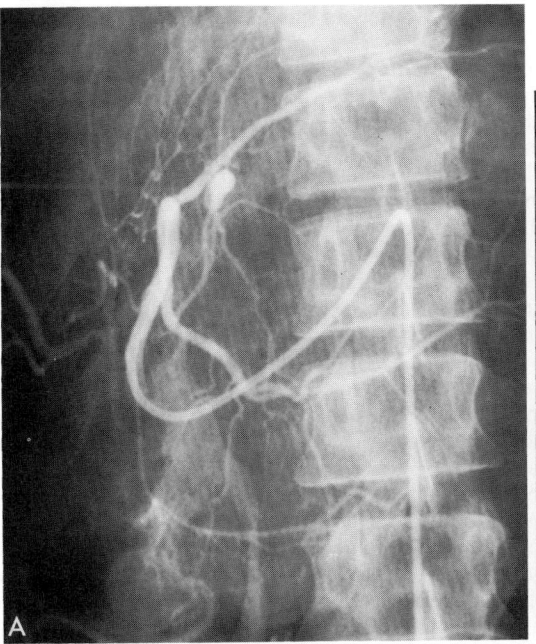
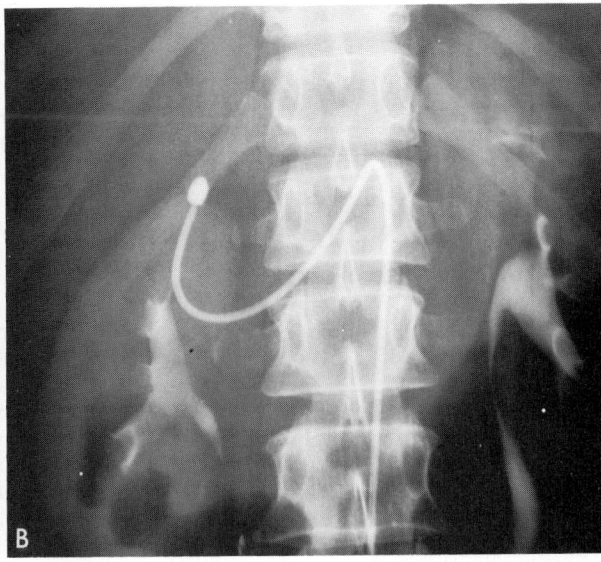

Figure 1. *A,* Intraparenchymal hepatic artery aneurysm causing hemobilia following percutaneous liver biopsy. *B,* Arteriographic balloon used to occlude and thrombose artery and aneurysm. (X-ray films selected with the assistance of N. Reed Dunnick, M.D., from a case reported in Dunnick, N. R., Doppman, I. L., and Brereton, H. D.: Balloon occlusion of segmental hepatic arteries: Control of biopsy induced hemobilia. J.A.M.A., *238:*2524, 1977.)

health, or biliary tract manipulation, this triad should suggest the possibility of hemobilia. All three symptoms are not necessarily present. Acute bleeding usually first causes pain, followed by hematemesis or melena. Hemobilia may occur days, weeks, or months following trauma. A palpable mass representing the liver or gallbladder may accompany these symptoms. When a right upper quadrant bruit is heard with the classic triad, a visceral artery aneurysm causing hemobilia should be considered.

Aids in Diagnosis

Early diagnosis may be lifesaving with severe hemobilia. Arteriography remains the single most accurate and helpful diagnostic test in evaluation of patients in whom bleeding into the biliary ducts is suspected. Liver or biliary scans, ultrasonography, computed tomography, or magnetic resonance imaging may provide helpful information such as evidence of anatomic defects or abnormalities in the liver or bile ducts. Endoscopic retrograde cholangiopancreatography (ERCP) or percutaneous transhepatic cholangiography (PTC) may be helpful, but these procedures, particularly PTC, may confuse the diagnosis because this manipulation may also create a new source of bleeding. Ultrasonography may yield an erroneous impression of normal duct size in the presence of fresh blood or clot because of its variable echogenicity. Technetium-labeled or another red blood cell scan may occasionally be an efficient way of establishing a diagnosis, particularly in stable patients but may also delay definitive diagnosis and treatment in severely bleeding patients. An external biliary drainage catheter may demonstrate the bleeding, or injection of the catheter with contrast material may document thrombus within the biliary system (Fig. 2). Immediate surgical therapy is rarely required to establish the diagnosis of severe hemobilia, although it may occasionally be indicated for treatment purposes. If the operation is performed prior to diagnosis, a cause such as hepatic artery aneurysm, calculi, or tumor may be evident, or the biliary system may be found to be distended with blood.

Management

The conditions associated with hemobilia can cause severe blood loss and in some cases hemorrhagic shock. Initial management of the patient should be general evaluation and resuscitation, with blood transfusions as needed (Fig. 3). Careful

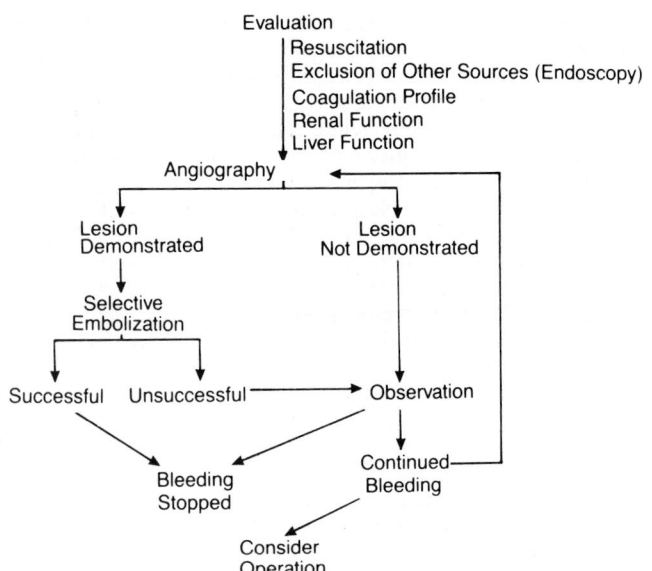

Figure 3. Management scheme for patients with suspected hemobilia. (From Czerniak, A., et al.: Hemobilia—A disease in evolution. Arch. Surg., *123*:718, 1988. Copyright 1988, American Medical Association.)

monitoring of blood replacement is important in the care of these patients. If anticipated, coagulopathy may be prevented or managed by administration of blood components such as fresh frozen plasma or platelets. After the diagnosis of hemobilia is established, several options for treatment exist. The majority of cases of hemobilia, particularly those involving intrahepatic false aneurysms, may be effectively treated with arteriographic techniques such as embolization with clot, steel coils, or other suitable material.

Selection of operative versus nonoperative treatment should be based upon the severity of bleeding, the underlying cause, and the age and general state of the patient. If the bleeding appears to be minor and easily monitored, e.g., in a postoperative situation, it is best managed expectantly. With acute trauma and hemoperitoneum, management of the acute bleeding is a primary concern. Hepatic parenchymal bleeding may be controlled by a variety of methods, including direct ligation of the bleeding vessel, resection, packing, or ligation of the proper, common, right, or left hepatic artery. Ligation of the proper hepatic artery rarely causes any clinical problem because of abundant collaterals. Ligation of the common, right, or left hepatic artery more often causes enzyme abnormalities but is usually tolerated by the patient, particularly when this is a lifesaving maneuver. Cholecystectomy is curative with bleeding into the gallbladder. A false aneurysm within the parenchyma of the liver is best treated nonoperatively by embolization of the involved arterial branch or balloon tamponade with arteriographic control (see Fig. 1B). Underlying processes such as biliary calculi or infection are usually best managed simultaneously with control of hemobilia. If a common bile duct exploration is performed, selective occlusion of the right or left hepatic artery may indicate which system is involved in the bleeding. In addition, selective occlusion of the right and left hepatic ducts may determine which duct is bleeding after extraction of multiple intrahepatic calculi. In selected cases, moderate to severe bleeding in children has been treated by vigorous supportive therapy, including blood replacement and serial angiography to monitor progressive healing. Visceral artery aneurysms may be treated operatively by ligation, usually with arterial repair.

Hemobilia after percutaneous transhepatic cholangiography (PTC) is usually minor and ceases spontaneously. However, it may cause several problems including ineffective biliary drainage (see Fig. 2), difficulty in determining the diagnosis of the

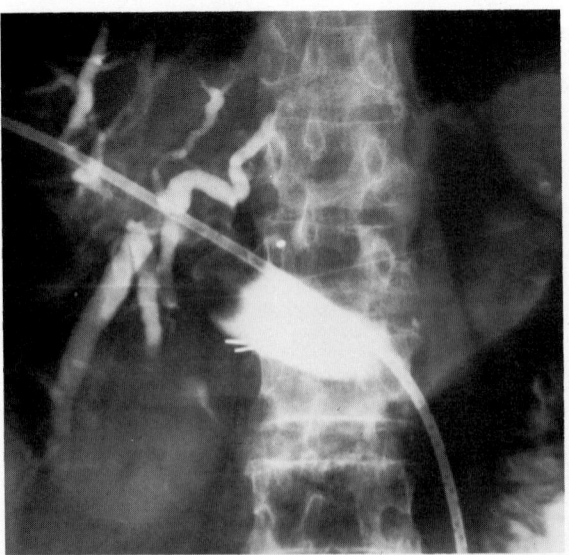

Figure 2. Large amount of thrombus within a markedly dilated common duct in a patient with obstructing carcinoma of the head of the pancreas. Thrombus prevented effective drainage of the catheter, and significant intraperitoneal hemorrhage at the hepatic entrance site occurred.

primary problem, or continued bleeding from the catheter into the biliary system or into the peritoneal cavity. If these problems do not resolve, operation may be indicated. All reported cases after gallstone lithotripsy have been minor; but with increased use of this technique, severe bleeding is likely to occur occasionally. The overall mortality from severe hemobilia is estimated to be between 10 and 20 per cent, depending on the age of the patient and the underlying etiology, but mortality decreases with increased awareness of the condition and prompt, appropriate therapy.

SELECTED REFERENCES

Czerniak, A., Thompson, J. N., Hemingway, A. P., et al.; Hemobilia — A disease in evolution. Arch. Surg., 123:718, 1988.
This is a review that provides a sound approach to diagnosis and management.

Fagan, E. A., Allison, D. J., Chadwick, V. S., et al.: Treatment of haemobilia by selective arterial embolization. Gut, 21:541, 1980.
Arterial embolization comprises a very important therapy for hemobilia.

Goodnight, J. E., Jr, and Blaisdell, F. W.: Hemobilia. Surg. Clin. North. Am. 61:973, 1981.
This is a short, excellent review of hemobilia. Current diagnostic techniques and both surgical and nonsurgical treatment are discussed.

Sandblom, P.: Hemobilia. (Biliary Tract Hemorrhage). Springfield, Ill., Charles C Thomas, 1972.
This is a classic monograph on the subject. Sandblom reviews the cases of hemobilia in the world literature up to 1972.

V

SURGICAL COMPLICATIONS OF CIRRHOSIS AND PORTAL HYPERTENSION

Layton F. Rikkers, M.D.

Cirrhosis was first described in a fourth century B.C. Hippocratic aphorism: "In cases of jaundice it is a bad sign when the liver becomes hard." [6] Although the deleterious effect of alcohol on the liver was appreciated by Galen and his contemporaries in the second century A.D., alcoholic liver disease as an entity was first recognized by Baillie and other English writers following the "gin plague" in the eighteenth century. Shortly thereafter, Laennec introduced the term *cirrhosis,* which was derived from the Greek word *kirrhos,* meaning "orange-yellow." Nineteenth century European and English pathologists, including Carswell and Rokitansky, described the gross and histopathologic characteristics of the disease. Although alcoholic cirrhosis was thought to be due to toxins other than alcohol or to malnutrition during much of the twentieth century, recent investigations have established alcohol itself as a hepatotoxin.

Cirrhosis is the end result of mechanisms causing hepatocellular injury, including toxins (alcohol), viruses (hepatitis B and hepatitis C), prolonged cholestasis (extrahepatic and intrahepatic), autoimmunity (lupoid hepatitis), and metabolic disorders (hemochromatosis, Wilson's disease, alpha$_1$-antitrypsin deficiency). Although the mechanisms are diverse, the pathologic response is quite uniform: hepatocellular necrosis followed by fibrosis and nodular regeneration. Each of these elements may exist alone (necrosis, uncomplicated hepatitis; fibrosis, congenital hepatic fibrosis; nodular regeneration, partial nodular transformation), but all three are required for the development of cirrhosis. Cirrhosis is always a diffuse process and may be classified either morphologically or by etiology. Alcoholic cirrhosis, which is usually micronodular, and posthepatitic cirrhosis, which is generally macronodular, are most common in the United States. Because the pathologic responses to various mechanisms of hepatocellular injury are so similar, occasionally the cause cannot be ascertained (cryptogenic cirrhosis).

Cirrhosis causes two major phenomena, hepatocellular failure and portal hypertension. Even after the noxious agent is removed (e.g., abstinence from alcohol), the disease may progress. Although the mechanism is not clear, both ischemia, secondary to extensive fibrosis and intra- and extrahepatic shunts, and autoimmune factors may have roles. The altered hepatic architecture and perisinusoidal fibrosis cause increased hepatic vascular resistance, leading to portal hypertension and its associated complications of variceal hemorrhage, encephalopathy, ascites, and hypersplenism.

Autopsy studies suggest an incidence of cirrhosis of between 3.5 and 5.0 per cent. In only 15 per cent of heavy drinkers does alcoholic cirrhosis develop. However, because of the large number of alcoholics in the United States as well as a significant percentage of patients with nonalcoholic causes of chronic liver disease, cirrhosis presently ranks as the fifth leading cause of death between the ages of 35 and 54. Hepatic failure and variceal hemorrhage are the first and second most common causes of death, respectively, in patients with cirrhosis.

Historically the treatment of cirrhosis has been the treatment of the complications of portal hypertension. Currently, medical treatment of cirrhosis with antifibrogenesis drugs such as colchicine and penicillamine is experimental. In contrast, since 1980 the surgical management of chronic liver disease with hepatic transplantation has been highly successful, with long-term survival generally above 70 per cent. A major challenge to the physician or surgeon managing patients with cirrhosis is to determine when definitive treatment (transplantation), rather than palliative treatment (e.g., operations to prevent recurrent variceal hemorrhage), should be applied.

ANATOMY, PHYSIOLOGY, AND PATHOPHYSIOLOGY OF PORTAL HYPERTENSION

The liver is a unique organ in that it has a dual blood supply, portal venous and hepatic arterial. The portal vein is formed from the confluence of the superior mesenteric and splenic veins (Fig. 1). The left gastric, or coronary, vein drains the distal esophagus and lesser curvature of the stomach, generally entering the portal vein near its origin. The splenic vein lies beneath the pancreas and is usually joined by the inferior mesenteric vein just before its confluence with the superior mesenteric vein.

The hepatic artery, one of three major branches of the celiac axis, lies medial to the common bile duct and portal vein in the hepatoduodenal ligament. Common variations include origins

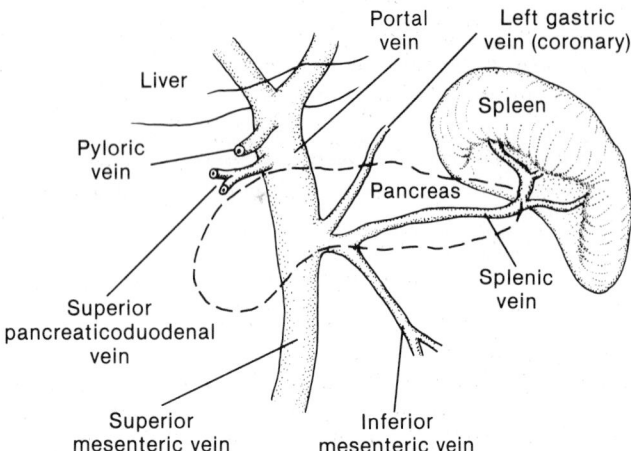

Figure 1. The extrahepatic portal venous circulation.

of the right and left hepatic arteries from the superior mesenteric artery and left gastric artery, respectively, both of which occur in approximately 20 per cent of the population.

Hepatic blood flow averages 1500 ml. per min., which represents approximately 25 per cent of the cardiac output. The portal vein contributes two thirds of the total hepatic blood flow, whereas hepatic arterial perfusion represents over half of the liver's oxygen supply. The volume of portal venous flow is indirectly regulated by vasoconstriction and vasodilation of the splanchnic arterial bed. In contrast, hepatic arterioles respond to circulating catecholamines and sympathetic nervous stimulation; thus, hepatic arterial flow is directly regulated. However, even intense vasoconstrictive influences can be overcome by a hepatic arterial autoregulatory, or "buffer," response, which maintains total hepatic blood flow as near to normal as possible when portal perfusion is decreased in patients with shock or in those with either disease-induced or surgically created portal systemic shunts.[19]

Many splanchnic hormones are important regulators of hepatic metabolism. Insulin is particularly important because it is a hepatotrophic hormone and is essential for maintenance of liver structure and function. Thus, even if the quantity of hepatic blood flow is maintained in the normal range by hepatic arterial compensation for decreased portal flow, hepatic physiology may be impaired.

Because increased portal venous resistance is usually the initiator of portal hypertension, classifications of this disorder are generally based on the site of elevated resistance. However, increased portal venous inflow secondary to a hyperdynamic systemic circulation and splanchnic hyperemia is often a major contributor to the maintenance of portal hypertension. The cause of the elevated cardiac output and splanchnic hyperemia is not known; but splanchnic hormones, such as glucagon, and decreased sensitivity of the splanchnic vasculature to catecholamines probably have a role.[2]

The most common cause of prehepatic portal hypertension is portal vein thrombosis, which represents approximately 50 per cent of cases of portal hypertension in the pediatric age group. When the portal vein is thrombosed in the absence of liver disease, hepatopetal (to the liver) portal collaterals develop to restore portal perfusion. This combination is termed *cavernomatous transformation* of the portal vein. Isolated splenic vein thrombosis (left-sided portal hypertension) is usually secondary to pancreatic inflammation or neoplasm. The result is gastrosplenic venous hypertension; superior mesenteric and portal venous pressures remain normal. The left gastroepiploic vein becomes a major collateral, and gastric varices are generally more prominent than esophageal varices. This variant of portal hypertension is important to recognize because it is easily reversed by splenectomy alone.

The site of increased resistance in intrahepatic portal hyper-

tension may be at the presinusoidal, sinusoidal, or postsinusoidal level. Frequently, more than one level is involved. The most common cause of intrahepatic, presinusoidal hypertension is schistosomiasis. In addition, many causes of nonalcoholic cirrhosis also cause presinusoidal portal hypertension, especially early in their course. Alcoholic cirrhosis, the most common cause of portal hypertension in the United States, usually causes increased resistance to portal flow at the sinusoidal (secondary to deposition of collagen in Disse's space) and postsinusoidal levels (secondary to regenerating nodules distorting small hepatic veins). Postsinusoidal causes of portal hypertension are rare and include the Budd-Chiari syndrome (hepatic vein thrombosis), constrictive pericarditis, and heart failure. Rarely, increased portal venous flow alone, secondary either to massive splenomegaly (idiopathic portal hypertension) or to a splanchnic arteriovenous fistula, causes portal hypertension.

A portal pressure above the normal level of 5 to 10 mm. Hg stimulates portal-systemic collateralization. Collaterals usually develop where the portal and systemic venous circulations are in proximity (Fig. 2). Although the collateral network through the coronary and short gastric veins to the azygos vein is the most important one clinically, because it leads to formation of esophagogastric varices, other sites include a recanalized umbilical vein from the left portal vein to the epigastric venous system, retroperitoneal collaterals, and the hemorrhoidal venous plexus. In addition to extrahepatic collaterals, a significant fraction of portal venous flow passes through both anatomic and physiologic (capillarization of hepatic sinusoids) intrahepatic shunts. As hepatic portal perfusion decreases, hepatic arterial flow generally increases ("buffer" response).[19]

EVALUATION OF THE PATIENT WITH CIRRHOSIS

Key aspects of the assessment of an individual with suspected chronic liver disease or one of the complications of portal hypertension are the following: (1) diagnosis of the underlying liver disease, (2) estimation of functional hepatic reserve, (3) definition of portal venous anatomy and hepatic hemodynamic evaluation, and (4) identification of the site of upper gastrointestinal hemorrhage if present. These diagnostic categories assume varying levels of importance, depending on the clinical situation. For example, estimation of functional hepatic reserve is useful in determining the risk of therapeutic intervention and whether definitive (hepatic transplantation) or palliative treat-

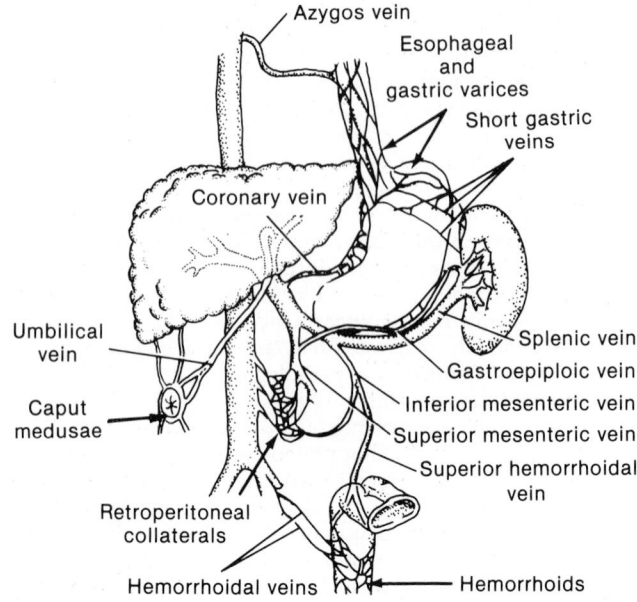

Figure 2. Portal systemic collateral pathways develop where the portal venous and systemic venous systems are in apposition (large arrows).

ment (e.g., endoscopic sclerotherapy or shunt surgery) is indicated. Knowledge of portal anatomy and physiology guides selection of an appropriate operation for control of variceal bleeding. Precise identification of the site of bleeding is essential, because hemorrhage secondary to portal hypertension may be from esophageal varices, gastric varices, or portal hypertensive gastropathy and because a significant fraction of patients with portal hypertension bleed from other lesions.

HISTORY AND PHYSICAL EXAMINATION

In a patient with nonspecific constitutional complaints such as weight loss, malaise, and weakness, a past history of chronic alcoholism, hepatitis, complicated biliary disease, or exposure to hepatotoxins should prompt inclusion of cirrhosis in the differential diagnosis. Subtle clues of the presence of underlying chronic liver disease on physical examination are spider angiomata, palmar erythema, testicular atrophy, and gynecomastia. A palpable spleen in association with these signs suggests portal hypertension. Confirmatory evidence of cirrhosis is provided by signs of hepatic functional decompensation or advanced portal hypertension such as jaundice, ascites, palpation of a firm irregular liver edge, dilated abdominal wall veins, and impairment of mental status or the presence of asterixis (liver flap).

LABORATORY TESTS

Cirrhosis is often accompanied by anemia, leukopenia, and thrombocytopenia. Anemia may be secondary to bleeding, nutritional deficiencies, hemolysis, or bone marrow depression secondary to alcoholism. Although many patients with portal hypertension have some degree of hypersplenism, it is unusual to find a platelet count of less than 50,000 per cu. mm. or a white blood cell count less than 2,000 per cu. mm. In addition to thrombocytopenia, coagulation may be impaired by a prolonged prothrombin time, because many of the coagulation factors are synthesized by the liver and by primary fibrinolysis, which is present in many patients with chronic liver disease.

A chemistry profile is helpful in both the diagnosis and assessment of severity of cirrhosis. Hypoalbuminemia is usually a reliable index of chronic, rather than acute, liver disease. Elevation of the hepatocellular enzymes, aspartate aminotransferase and alanine aminotransferase, to more than three times their normal level is indicative of significant, ongoing hepatocellular necrosis, which is often present in patients with alcoholic hepatitis and chronic active hepatitis due to a variety of causes. Increased disease activity may be an important risk factor in patients who undergo surgical therapy. A ratio of alanine aminotransferase to aspartate aminotransferase of greater than 2 is highly suggestive of alcohol as the cause of liver disease. Although mild elevations of the enzymes alkaline phosphatase and gamma glutamyl transpeptidase are nonspecific, marked increases in these enzymes are indicative of either intrahepatic or extrahepatic cholestasis (primary or secondary biliary cirrhosis). In the absence of prior blood transfusions, a total bilirubin

level of greater than 3 mg. per 100 ml. is indicative of severe hepatic decompensation and a high operative risk status.

Hepatitis serology should be obtained in most patients with cirrhosis. A significant fraction of patients with hepatitis B and hepatitis C develop cirrhosis, whereas hepatitis A generally causes only acute liver disease. The most common internal malignancy worldwide is hepatocellular carcinoma, which is frequently secondary to hepatitis B. However, this malignancy frequently develops in patients with other causes of cirrhosis and occasionally in patients without chronic liver disease. Unexpected hepatic functional deterioration is sometimes caused by development of hepatocellular carcinoma, which can be diagnosed in approximately 60 per cent of patients by an elevated alpha-fetoprotein level.

Common serum electrolyte abnormalities in cirrhosis are hyponatremia, hypokalemia, and metabolic alkalosis. These metabolic disorders are secondary to hyperaldosteronism, diarrhea, and recurrent emesis, which frequently accompany cirrhosis. Deleterious consequences of metabolic alkalosis are shifting of the oxyhemoglobin disassociation curve to the left, impairment of tissue oxygen delivery, and conversion of ammonium chloride to ammonia, which facilitates transport of this purported cerebral toxin across the blood-brain barrier.

LIVER BIOPSY

Percutaneous liver biopsy is a useful technique for establishing the cause of cirrhosis and for assessing activity of the liver disease. When the diagnosis is known and the chemistry profile suggests quiescent disease, liver biopsy is probably not necessary prior to surgical intervention for variceal hemorrhage. Percutaneous liver biopsy should not be done when either coagulopathy or moderate ascites is present.

MEASUREMENT OF HEPATIC FUNCTIONAL RESERVE

The time-honored method of assessing hepatic functional reserve is Child's classification (Table 1). Although this classification scheme includes three clinical variables in addition to two biochemical indices and, therefore, is not a direct measure of hepatic functional reserve, no other test has surpassed it with respect to predicting operative outcome or assessing long-term prognosis in the patient who does not undergo surgical therapy. In most clinical series, operative mortality for Child's A, B, and C class patients is 0 to 5 per cent, 10 to 15 per cent, and greater than 25 per cent, respectively. Because many patients with acute variceal hemorrhage present with decompensated hepatic function as reflected by Child's class, an interval of medical management to improve the patient from a Child's class C to class A or B is worthwhile prior to surgical intervention.[14]

True quantitative measures of hepatocellular function, such as galactose elimination capacity, aminopyrine breath test, and hepatic clearance of amino acids, are not available in most institutions. However, these tests may be valuable indicators of limited hepatic reserve in some patients with nearly normal con-

TABLE 1. Child's Criteria for Hepatic Functional Reserve

	A Minimal	B Moderate	C Advanced
Serum bilirubin (mg./dl.)	< 2.0	2.0–3.0	> 3.0
Serum albumin (gm./dl.)	> 3.5	3.0–3.5	< 3.0
Ascites	None	Easily controlled	Poorly controlled
Neurologic disorder	None	Minimal	Advanced, "coma"
Nutrition	Excellent	Good	Poor, "wasting"

From Boyer, T. D.: Portal hypertension and its complications: Bleeding esophageal varices, ascites, and spontaneous bacterial peritonitis. *In* Zakim, D., and Boyer, T. D. (Eds.): Hepatology: A Textbook of Liver Disease. Philadelphia, W. B. Saunders Company, 1982, pp. 464–499.

ventional measures of liver function. Now that hepatic transplantation has become a realistic option for many patients with cirrhosis, accurate quantitation of hepatocellular function to determine which patients are transplant candidates has become even more important.

HEPATIC HEMODYNAMIC ASSESSMENT

In patients with alcoholic cirrhosis and many types of nonalcoholic cirrhosis, portal pressure can be indirectly estimated by measurement of hepatic venous wedge pressure. Because hepatic venous wedge pressure is normal in patients with presinusoidal portal hypertension, portal pressure in these individuals can be measured only directly by transhepatic or umbilical venous cannulation of the portal venous system or by percutaneous puncture of the spleen. However, because the magnitude of portal venous pressure predicts neither likelihood of bleeding nor ultimate prognosis, the only useful application of these techniques is in differentiating between presinusoidal and sinusoidal/postsinusoidal causes of portal hypertension.

Because splanchnic venous thrombosis may be the cause of portal hypertension or develop secondary to cirrhosis, portal venous anatomy should be defined prior to performing a portal-systemic shunt operation. Selective visceral angiography has been the most frequently used method for visualization of the portal venous system and for qualitative estimation of hepatic portal perfusion.[22] A complete angiographic study generally consists of selective injections of radiographic contrast into the superior mesenteric and splenic arteries, followed by late venous phase films to define splenic, superior mesenteric, and portal veins. If the renal vein is to be used in shunt construction, this vessel should also be cannulated and opacified. Hepatic portal perfusion can be estimated from the venous phase of the superior mesenteric angiogram and graded as follows: Grade 1, normal perfusion; Grade 2, visualization of intrahepatic portal venous radicles; Grade 3, opacification of portal vein only; Grade 4, nonvisualization of the portal vein (Fig. 3).[22] This grading system is particularly valuable for assessment of portal blood flow before and after a selective shunt, because one of the objectives of such a procedure is preservation of hepatic portal perfusion. Postoperative venography, either indirectly after arterial injection or directly via venous shunt cannulation, is the most accurate method of determining shunt patency.

Duplex ultrasonography is a noninvasive alternative to angiography for assessment of portal venous patency, direction of portal flow, and shunt patency status.[24] This technique is less accurate in assessing superior mesenteric and splenic vein anatomy and flow characteristics. Duplex ultrasonography usually accurately assesses patency status of central shunts (e.g., portacaval), but is of less value in evaluation of more peripheral shunts (e.g., distal splenorenal).

DIAGNOSIS OF BLEEDING

In the absence of hematemesis, a nasogastric tube should be inserted to determine whether bleeding is from the upper gastrointestinal tract. The key procedure for diagnosing the site of upper gastrointestinal hemorrhage in a patient with portal hypertension is endoscopy. Prior to endoscopy, the patient should be hemodynamically stabilized and the stomach evacuated of blood clots with a large-bore lavage tube. Iced lavage solutions have no advantages over those at room temperature.

Upper gastrointestinal bleeding in patients with portal hypertension is secondary to portal hypertension in approximately 90 per cent of instances. The remaining 10 per cent of patients bleed from Mallory-Weiss tears, gastric ulcers, and duodenal ulcers, all of which are more common in patients with alcoholic cirrhosis than in the general population. Portal hypertensive bleeding is most commonly from esophagogastric varices (esophageal varices, 90 per cent; gastric varices, 10 per cent). The endoscopic diagnosis of variceal hemorrhage can be established by observation of a bleeding varix (25 per cent of patients) or by observation of moderate to large-sized varices and no other lesions in a patient who has recently experienced a major upper gastrointestinal hemorrhage (more than 2 units of blood).

The only nonvariceal cause of portal hypertensive bleeding is portal hypertensive gastropathy.[21] The frequency of this recently defined lesion is unknown, but it is probably more common after eradication of varices by endoscopic sclerotherapy. Portal hypertensive gastropathy mainly involves the fundus and body of the stomach and has an endoscopic appearance of a white reticular network with enclosed erythematous areas. Because varices and portal hypertensive gastropathy often coexist, it may be difficult to determine which lesion is responsible for any specific episode of bleeding. Occasionally, massive bleeding in a patient with cirrhosis makes an endoscopic diagnosis initially impossible, in which case endoscopy should be repeated after bleeding is controlled.

Although a barium esophagram is also a sensitive means of detecting varices, the disadvantage of this technique is that it does not determine whether the varices are the source of hemor-

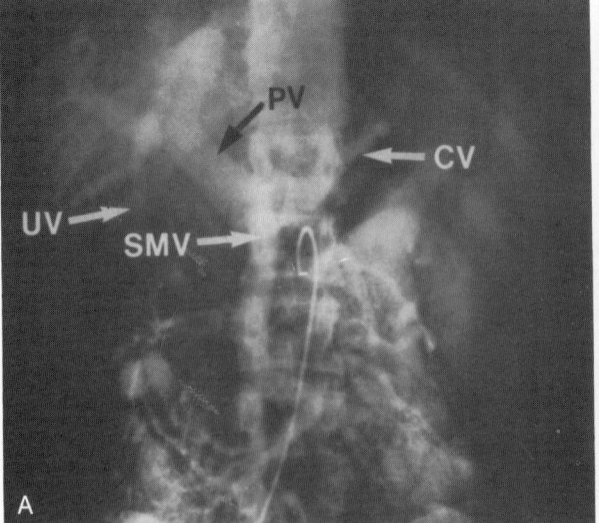
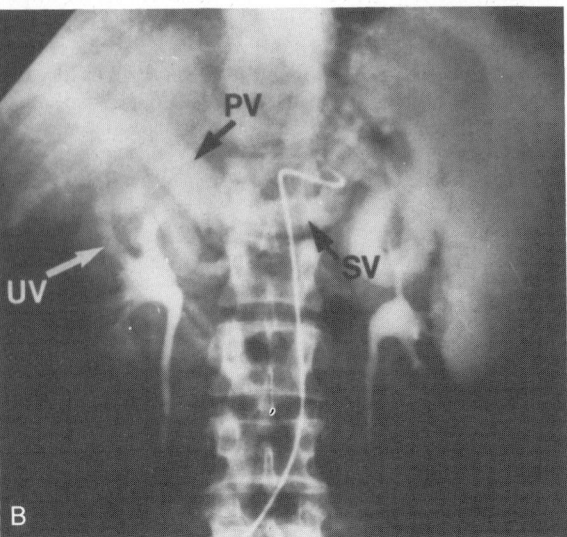

Figure 3. Venous phase films following superior mesenteric (A) and splenic (B) angiograms in a patient with portal hypertension secondary to alcoholic cirrhosis. The portal perfusion grade is 2. PV, portal vein; SMV, superior mesenteric vein; UV, umbilical vein; CV, coronary vein; SV, splenic vein. (From Rikkers, L. F.: Portal hypertension. In Goldsmith, H. (Ed.): Practice of Surgery. Philadelphia, Harper & Row, 1981, pp. 1–37.)

rhage. Thus, barium studies are never indicated in the acute setting. Rarely, a radioisotope-labeled red blood cell scan may be helpful in evaluating upper gastrointestinal bleeding in patients with portal hypertension.

VARICEAL HEMORRHAGE

Bleeding from esophagogastric varices is the single most life-threatening complication of portal hypertension, responsible for approximately one third of all deaths in patients with cirrhosis. The risk of death from bleeding in any individual patient is mainly related to the underlying hepatic functional reserve. Patients with extrahepatic portal venous obstruction and normal hepatic function rarely die of bleeding varices, whereas individuals with decompensated cirrhosis (Child's class C) have a mortality in excess of 50 per cent. The greatest risk of death due to variceal bleeding is within the first few days after the onset of hemorrhage and declines rapidly after 6 weeks, when it returns to the prebleeding risk level.[32] The relationship between the risk of mortality and the time from onset of bleeding is important to consider when one is interpreting the results of clinical studies (Fig. 4). Investigations of elective treatment often omit the patients with the highest risk, many of whom die soon after the onset of acute variceal hemorrhage.

PATHOGENESIS OF VARICEAL HEMORRHAGE

Varices in the distal esophagus and proximal stomach are a component of the collateral network, which diverts high-pressure portal venous flow through the left and right gastric veins and the short gastric veins to the azygos system. Less commonly, varices develop at other sites in the gastrointestinal tract but are less prone to rupture in those locations. Esophagogastric varices do not develop until portal pressure exceeds 12 mm. Hg and, once present, bleed in only 30 to 50 per cent of patients.

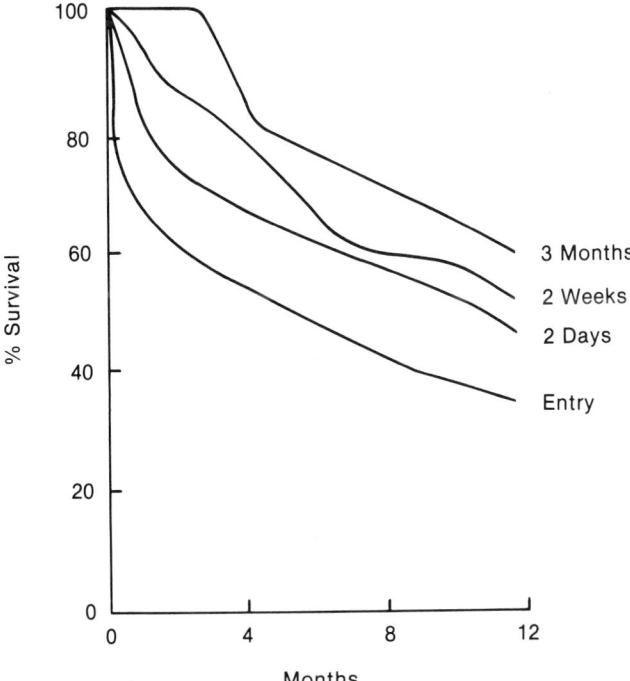

Figure 4. Effect on survival curves (life-table analysis) by zero-time selection. Survival is lowest when the time from hospital admission is used, but considerably higher when the initial 2 weeks after the onset of variceal hemorrhage are not considered (e.g., many of the elective surgical therapy and chronic sclerotherapy series). These data represent subsets of the same patients. (From Smith, J. L., and Graham, D. Y.: Variceal hemorrhage: A critical evaluation of survival analysis. Gastroenterology, 82:968, 1982.)

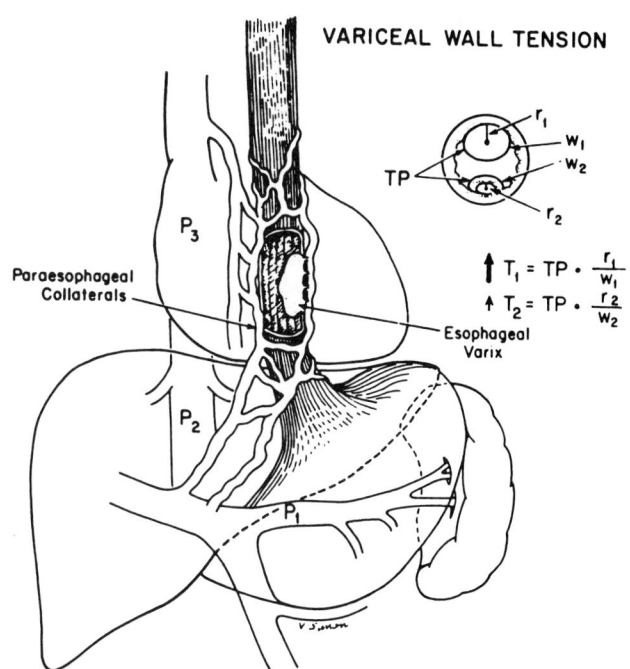

Figure 5. Variceal wall tension (likelihood of rupture) can be derived from Laplace's law. In varices with the same transmural pressure (TP) but different radii ($r_1 > r_2$) and wall thickness ($w_1 < w_2$), wall tension (T) is greatest in the varix with the largest radius (r_1) and thinner (w_1) wall. P_1, portal pressure; P_2, inferior vena cava pressure; P_3, right atrial pressure. (From Polio, J., and Groszmann, R. J.: Hemodynamic factors involved in the development and rupture of esophageal varices: A pathophysiologic approach to treatment. Semin. Liv. Dis., 6:318, 1986.)

The pathogenesis of variceal rupture is incompletely understood but is most likely multifactorial. Polio and Groszmann[25] presented a unifying hypothesis of variceal rupture based on Laplace's law (Fig. 5). Although it has been observed that variceal size, magnitude of portal pressure, and thickness of the epithelium overlying the varix all significantly separate bleeders from nonbleeders, the overlap between groups is large when any one of these variables is considered independently. Laplace's law states that variceal wall tension is directly related to transmural pressure and varix radius and inversely related to variceal wall thickness, thus combining all three of these variables (see Fig. 5). Because all of these parameters cannot be measured clinically, there are inherent inaccuracies in predicting which patients with varices will bleed. However, endoscopic classification schemes that consider size of varices and characteristics such as cherry red spots and red wale markings, which are related to the thickness of the overlying epithelium, have improved the predictability of variceal hemorrhage. These prognostic indices are especially important when one is considering prophylactic therapy (treatment for varices that have not previously bled).

TREATMENT OF VARICEAL HEMORRHAGE

Therapy for portal hypertension and variceal bleeding has evolved over the past 100 years. The many treatment modalities available suggest that no single therapy is entirely satisfactory for all patients or for all clinical situations. Nonoperative treatments are generally preferred for acutely bleeding patients because they are often high operative risks because of decompensated hepatic function. Therapies that are effective (result in a low rebleeding rate) and minimally alter hepatic physiology are optimal for long-term prevention of recurrent bleeding. Only treatments associated with minimal morbidity and mortality can be considered for prophylaxis, since many patients would be treated unnecessarily (only a third to half of patients with varices eventually bleed).

HISTORY OF TREATMENT FOR PORTAL HYPERTEN-

SION.[6] A chronology of the treatment of portal hypertension, which began with the description of the Eck fistula (end-to-side portacaval shunt) in 1877, is presented in Table 2. Eck's main concerns were to determine whether survival was possible after complete portal flow diversion and to develop a treatment for ascites. Probably the most important contribution to this field was made by Pavlov's group in 1893. These investigators perfected the technique of portacaval shunting and, after carefully observing 20 surviving dogs, described in detail the syndrome of "meat intoxication" or portasystemic encephalopathy, which they believed was due to intestinally absorbed cerebral toxins bypassing the site of metabolism in the liver. They also found from autopsy studies that dogs with encephalopathy had patent portacaval shunts and atrophic livers, whereas animals with normal cerebral function and preserved hepatic structure had thrombosed shunts and maintenance of hepatic portal perfusion via collaterals.

The modern era of treatment for variceal hemorrhage can be dated from 1945, when Blakemore, Lord, and Whipple introduced the portacaval and conventional splenorenal shunts into clinical practice. Although balloon tamponade and endoscopic sclerosis of varices were initially described in the 1930s, these were found to be only temporizing measures. During the ensuing 20 years, several varieties of nonselective shunts (complete portal decompression and portal flow diversion) were described and the portacaval shunt was evaluated in randomized, controlled trials. Motivated by the discouraging results of these trials, Warren, Zeppa, and Fomon introduced the concept of selective variceal decompression (distal splenorenal shunt) in 1967.[42] An initial wave of enthusiasm for the distal splenorenal shunt (partial portal flow diversion) was followed by several randomized trials, which produced inconsistent results. A report from Johnston and Rodgers in 1973 of a large series of patients successfully treated by endoscopic sclerotherapy led to a resurgence of interest in this treatment, which has now become the most widely applied therapy for bleeding varices.[17] Although pharmacotherapy was first used for acute hemorrhage in 1956, pharmacologic treatment for long-term prevention of initial or recurrent hemorrhage was a phenomenon of the 1980s. Improved immunosuppression (cyclosporine) and surgical techniques led to the widespread application of hepatic transplantation during that decade.

TREATMENT OF THE ACUTE BLEEDING EPISODE.[3] Since many patients with acute variceal bleeding have decompen-

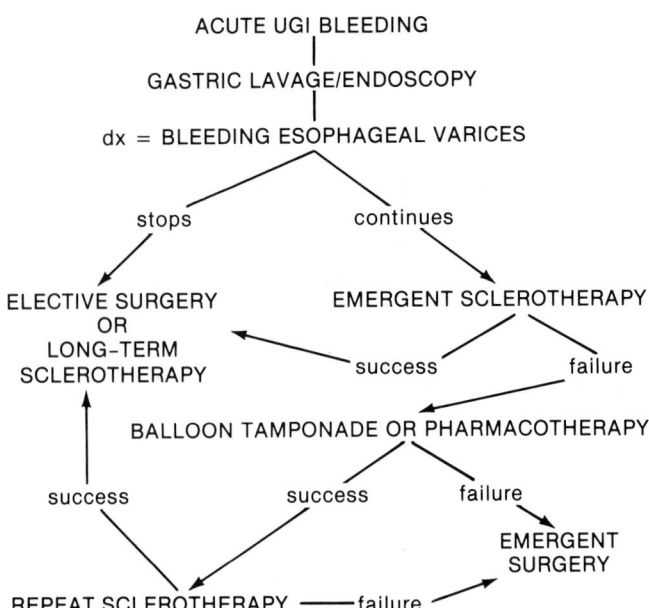

Figure 6. Algorithm for management of acute variceal hemorrhage (see text). (Redrawn from Burnett, D. A., and Rikkers, L. F.: Nonoperative emergency treatment of variceal hemorrhage. Surg. Clin. North. Am., 70:291, 1990.)

sated hepatic function secondary to either recent alcoholism or hypotension, they are high risks for emergency surgical intervention. In addition, these individuals often have other complications of chronic liver disease such as encephalopathy, ascites, coagulopathy, and malnutrition. Therefore, emergency treatment should be nonoperative whenever possible. Endoscopic sclerotherapy, which has become the mainstay of nonoperative treatment of acute hemorrhage in most centers, controls bleeding in over 85 per cent of patients, allowing an interval of medical management for improvement of hepatic function, resolution of ascites and encephalopathy, and enhancement of nutrition prior to definitive treatment for prevention of recurrent bleeding. Although pharmacotherapy and balloon tamponade still have an important role in emergency management in some patients—e.g., those with sclerotherapy failure and those bleeding from gastric varices—these modalities are used less frequently than in the past. A management scheme for acute variceal hemorrhage is outlined in Figure 6.

RESUSCITATION AND DIAGNOSIS. The highest priority in emergency management is restoration of circulating blood volume, which should be accomplished prior to upper gastrointestinal endoscopy. Although initial resuscitation is usually with isotonic crystalloid solutions, a minimum of 6 units of blood should be typed and cross-matched for most patients with variceal bleeding. Volume status is assessed by central venous pressure measurements, urinary output via a Foley catheter, and a Swan-Ganz pulmonary artery catheter if necessary. If the prothrombin time is prolonged more than 3 seconds, fresh frozen plasma should be a component of the resuscitation volume. Although moderate hypersplenism is a common accompaniment of portal hypertension, platelet transfusions are necessary only when the platelet count is less than 50,000 per cu. mm.

Endoscopy to determine the cause of bleeding should be performed as soon as the patient is stabilized. If a bleeding esophageal varix is observed or suspected because of an overlying clot, sclerotherapy should be performed during the initial endoscopy if the expertise is available. Bleeding from gastric varices or from portal hypertensive gastropathy should be initially treated with pharmacotherapy. Because these lesions are often incompletely controlled by nonsurgical means, such patients frequently require early surgical intervention.

PHARMACOTHERAPY. Vasopressin, which is a potent splanchnic

TABLE 2. History of Treatment for Portal Hypertension

Year	Author	Contribution
1877	Eck	Portacaval shunt (dog)
1893	Pavlov et al.	Encephalopathy (dog)
1903	Vidal	Clinical portacaval shunt (ascites)
1930	Westphal	Balloon tamponade
1939	Crafoord, Frenckner	Endoscopic sclerotherapy
1945	Blakemore, Lord, Whipple	Clinical portacaval and splenorenal shunts (bleeding)
1950	Sengstaken, Blakemore	Balloon tamponade
1956	Kehne	Vasopressin
1967	Warren, Zeppa, Fomon	Distal splenorenal shunt
1967	Starzl	First successful liver transplant
1968	Inokuchi	Left gastric–vena caval shunt
1973	Johnston, Rodgers	Reintroduction of endoscopic sclerotherapy
1973	Sugiura, Futagawa	Extensive esophagogastric devascularization
1980	Calne	Cyclosporine for transplantation
1981	Lebrec et al.	Propranolol for bleeding

vasoconstrictor, has been the most commonly used drug in the acute setting and controls hemorrhage in approximately 50 per cent of patients. Vasopressin is usually administered intravenously as a bolus dose of 20 units over 20 minutes and then as a continuous infusion of 0.4 unit per minute. Because vasopressin also constricts systemic arterioles, it frequently causes hypertension, bradycardia, decreased cardiac output, and coronary vasoconstriction. Therefore, the use of this drug should be confined to the intensive care unit, where the patient can be appropriately monitored. The adverse systemic effects of vasopressin can be effectively counteracted by simultaneous infusion of nitroglycerin or nitroprusside. The combination of vasopressin and nitroglycerin may also be more effective in controlling variceal hemorrhage than vasopressin alone.[9]

Glypressin, an analog of vasopressin with a longer duration of action, and somatostatin have more recently been used for control of acute variceal bleeding. Preliminary trials suggest that both of these agents may be more effective than vasopressin and have fewer adverse side effects. However, further controlled trials are needed.

Because acute variceal hemorrhage can be controlled by sclerotherapy in the majority of patients, pharmacotherapy is used less frequently than in the past. However, it remains an important component of treatment for patients awaiting endoscopy, for sclerotherapy failures, and for those individuals bleeding from portal hypertensive gastropathy or gastric varices, neither of which can be effectively treated by sclerotherapy.

BALLOON TAMPONADE. The major advantages of variceal tamponade with the Sengstaken-Blakemore tube (Fig. 7) are immediate cessation of bleeding in more than 85 per cent of patients and the widespread availability of this device, even in small community hospitals. Significant disadvantages of balloon tamponade are frequent recurrent hemorrhage after balloon de-

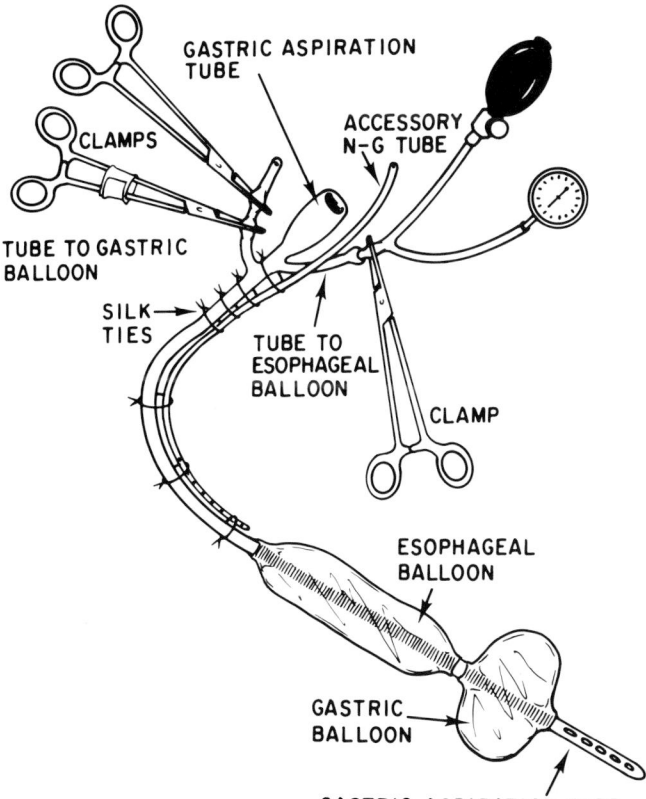

Figure 7. The modified Sengstaken-Blakemore tube. Note the accessory nasogastric tube for suctioning of secretions above the esophageal balloon and the two clamps, one secured with tape, to prevent inadvertent decompression of the gastric balloon. (From Rikkers, L. F.: Portal hypertension. In Goldsmith, H. (Ed.): Practice of Surgery. Philadelphia, Harper & Row, 1981, pp. 1–37.)

TABLE 3. Protocol for the Use of the Sengstaken-Blakemore Tube

A. Before insertion
1. Consider nasotracheal intubation.
2. Use new tube and inspect balloons for leaks.
3. Attach No. 18 Salem sump tube above esophageal balloon.
4. Evacuate blood from stomach with large tube.
5. Insert through nose using ring forceps if necessary
B. After insertion
1. Apply low, intermittent suction to stomach tube.
2. Apply constant suction to Salem sump.
3. Inflate gastric balloon with 25-ml. increments of air to 100 ml., observing the patient for pain.
4. Snug gastric balloon to gastroesophageal junction and affix to nose, under slight tension, with soft rubber pad.
5. Add 150 ml. of air to gastric balloon.
6. Place two clamps (one taped closed) on tube to gastric balloon.
7. Inflate esophageal balloon to 24–45 mm. Hg, clamp, and assess every hour.
8. Perform heavily penetrated upper abdomen–lower chest film (portable) to confirm balloon positions.
9. Determine serial hematocrits every 4–6 hours (gastric tube may occlude and fail to detect recurrent hemorrhage).
10. Tape scissors to head of bed so tube can be transected and rapidly removed if respiratory arrest develops.
11. Deflate esophageal and gastric balloons after 24 hours.
2. Remove tube in additional 24 hours if there is no recurrent hemorrhage.

Modified from Rikkers, L. F., and Edney, J. A.: Portal hypertension. In Goldsmith, H. (Ed.): Practice of Surgery. Woodbury, Conn., Woodbury Press, 1988, pp. 1–37.

flation, considerable discomfort for the patient, and a high incidence of serious complications when the device is used by inexperienced personnel. The potentially lethal complications of esophageal perforation secondary to intraesophageal inflation of the gastric balloon, ischemic necrosis of the esophagus secondary to overinflation of the esophageal balloon, and aspiration can be avoided by using balloon tamponade only in an intensive care unit and adhering to a strict protocol (Table 3).

Because of the effectiveness of sclerotherapy for acute variceal bleeding in most patients, balloon tamponade is infrequently required. However, it may be lifesaving when exsanguinating hemorrhage prevents acute sclerotherapy and in patients with sclerotherapy failure who do not respond to pharmacotherapy. Because balloon deflation is followed by a high rebleeding rate, definitive treatment such as endoscopic variceal sclerosis or surgical therapy should be planned for most patients in whom the Sengstaken-Blakemore tube is used.

ENDOSCOPIC SCLEROTHERAPY. Although first described in 1939, endoscopic variceal sclerosis was abandoned after the introduction of portal systemic shunt surgery. Currently, endoscopic sclerotherapy is the most commonly utilized treatment for both management of the acute bleeding episode and prevention of recurrent hemorrhage. In early trials, variceal sclerosis was performed through a rigid esophagoscope under general anesthesia. However, most sclerotherapists now prefer a flexible endoscope because complications are fewer and general anesthesia can be avoided. Both intravariceal and paravariceal techniques of injection are used, and often these two techniques are purposefully or inadvertently combined. The most commonly used sclerosants in the United States are morrhuate sodium and sodium tetradecyl sulfate.

When experienced personnel are available, the initial sclerotherapy injections often can be done during the endoscopy at which diagnosis of variceal bleeding is made. Each varix is usually injected with 1 to 2 ml. of sclerosant just above the esophagogastric junction and 5 cm. proximal to it. A subsequent sclerotherapy session is planned for 4 to 6 days later. Additional endoscopies and sclerosis treatments depend on the effectiveness of the initial efforts in controlling bleeding and whether sclerotherapy has been selected as definitive treatment for that patient.

Emergency sclerotherapy of esophageal varices has been highly effective with control of hemorrhage in over 85 per cent of patients.[34] However, this technique has been generally unsuccessful for bleeding gastric varices. Few controlled trials comparing endoscopic sclerotherapy with other treatments have been conducted in the acute setting. One study found sclerotherapy to be superior to balloon tamponade, and another demonstrated that this technique was equivalent to the emergency portacaval shunt in Child's class C patients.[34]

Minor complications of sclerotherapy, including retrosternal chest pain, esophageal ulceration, and fever, occur commonly. More serious complications, which represent the 1 to 3 per cent mortality of this procedure, are esophageal perforation, worsening of variceal hemorrhage, and aspiration pneumonitis. Sclerotherapy failure should be declared when two sessions fail to control hemorrhage. Unless urgent surgical therapy is performed in these patients, mortality exceeds 60 per cent.

EMERGENCY SURGICAL THERAPY. Although nonoperative therapies are both preferable and effective for the majority of patients with acute variceal bleeding, emergency surgery should be promptly done when less invasive measures fail to control hemorrhage or are not indicated. The most common situations requiring urgent or emergency surgery are (1) failure of acute sclerotherapy, (2) failure of long-term sclerotherapy, and (3) hemorrhage from gastric varices or portal hypertensive gastropathy. Selection of the appropriate emergency operation should mainly be guided by the experience of the surgeon. Esophageal transection with a stapling device is rapid and relatively simple, but rebleeding after this procedure is quite high, and there is little evidence that operative mortality is less than that after surgical portal decompression. The most commonly performed shunt operation in the emergency setting is the portacaval shunt because it rapidly and effectively decompresses the portal venous circulation.[23] However, when the patient is not actively bleeding at the time of operation and in those individuals in whom bleeding is temporarily stayed by vasopressin infusion or balloon tamponade, a more complex operation such as the distal splenorenal shunt may be appropriate. Although some have advocated early emergency shunt operation for all patients with variceal hemorrhage, there is no evidence that this approach is superior to acute sclerotherapy followed by elective operative intervention or by chronic variceal sclerosis.[23] The major disadvantage of emergency surgical therapy is that operative mortality exceeds 25 per cent in most reported series.

PREVENTION OF RECURRENT HEMORRHAGE. When a patient has bled from varices, the likelihood of a repeat episode exceeds 70 per cent. Since most patients with variceal bleeding have chronic liver disease, the challenge of long-term management is both prevention of recurrent bleeding and maintenance of satisfactory hepatic function. Options available for definitive treatment include pharmacotherapy, chronic sclerotherapy, three hemodynamic types of shunt operation (nonselective, selective, and partial), a variety of nonshunt procedures, and hepatic transplantation.

PHARMACOTHERAPY. Pharmacotherapy for the prevention of recurrent variceal bleeding was introduced in 1981 by Lebrec and co-workers, who reported that a dose of propranolol sufficient to decrease heart rate by 25 per cent led to a decreased frequency of recurrent hemorrhage and prolongation of survival in good-risk patients with alcoholic cirrhosis.[20] Stimulated by this initial positive investigation, pharmacotherapy has become the most intense area of clinical investigation in portal hypertension. Unfortunately, two subsequent controlled trials comparing propranolol with a placebo in patients with all Child's classes failed to demonstrate a beneficial influence of this drug on either frequency of rebleeding or survival.[5,39] Mul-

tiple subsequent investigations have shown inconsistent results.[4] Invasive hemodynamic monitoring of patients on propranolol has demonstrated minimal or no reduction of portal pressure in many individuals and no correlation between decrease in portal pressure and reduction in pulse rate, which has been the index used in most studies for assessing therapeutic effect. Thus, two obstacles to effective treatment with propranolol are variability of response to the drug and the lack of an easily measured hemodynamic index for monitoring therapy.

Although beta blockade may be effective for some patients with portal hypertension, until more convincing evidence is presented that recurrent hemorrhage is consistently prevented, the use of this drug as well as other agents should be confined to controlled trials. Multiple studies assessing other drugs, including long-acting nitrates, calcium channel blockers, and serotonin antagonists, are in progress, with preliminary results in some cases. If a reliable drug or combination of drugs can be found, the major advantage of pharmacotherapy is its noninvasiveness. However, drug treatment for prevention of recurrent bleeding requires strict patient compliance, which may be a considerable problem for active alcoholics.

ENDOSCOPIC SCLEROTHERAPY. During the past decade, chronic sclerotherapy has become the most common treatment for prevention of recurrent variceal hemorrhage. The increasing popularity of endoscopic variceal sclerosis can be attributed to several factors: (1) There is disenchantment with shunt surgery among several gastroenterologists and surgeons. (2) Sclerotherapy is less invasive than surgical therapy. (3) Sclerotherapy has no adverse hemodynamic effects. (4) It can be performed by gastroenterologists to whom most patients are initially referred. (5) Several controlled trials have confirmed the therapeutic efficacy of variceal sclerosis.[34]

The objective of chronic sclerotherapy is to eradicate esophageal varices. Although the timing of repeat sclerotherapy sessions varies from series to series, variceal eradication is usually successful in approximately two thirds of patients. After eradication is achieved, diagnostic endoscopy should be performed at 6-month to 1-year intervals, because varices do recur and recurrent varices can bleed. Some investigators have noted an increased frequency of bleeding from gastric varices and portal hypertensive gastropathy after eradication of esophageal varices.

Several controlled trials comparing chronic sclerotherapy with conventional medical management have been completed.[34] Survival was significantly prolonged in the sclerotherapy group of only one of these studies.[43] Although fewer sclerotherapy patients than medically treated patients rebled in all of the investigations, recurrent bleeding still occurred in approximately 50 per cent of sclerotherapy patients. Rebleeding is most frequent during the initial year, and the rate decreases to approximately 15 per cent per year thereafter. Although a single episode of recurrent hemorrhage does not signify sclerotherapy failure, uncontrolled hemorrhage, multiple major episodes of rebleeding, and hemorrhage from gastric varices and portal hypertensive gastropathy all require that sclerotherapy be abandoned and another treatment modality be substituted. Data from randomized, controlled trials of shunt operations versus sclerotherapy indicate that sclerotherapy failure secondary to rebleeding occurs in approximately one third of patients.[29,40] Thus, chronic sclerotherapy is a rational initial treatment for many patients who bleed from esophageal varices; but subsequent treatment with a shunt procedure, nonshunt operation, or hepatic transplantation should be anticipated for a significant percentage of patients.

PORTAL SYSTEMIC SHUNTS. Portal systemic shunts are clearly the most effective means of preventing recurrent hemorrhage in patients with portal hypertension. These procedures are effective because they decompress to some degree the portal venous system by shunting portal flow into the low-pressure systemic venous system. However, diversion of portal blood, which contains hepatotrophic hormones, nutrients, and cerebral toxins, is also responsible for the adverse consequences of shunt operations, namely, portal systemic encephalopathy and accelerated hepatic failure. Depending on whether they completely decompress, compartmentalize, or partially decompress the portal venous circulation, portal systemic shunts can be classified as nonselective, selective, or partial. In addition to variceal decompression, the goal of selective and partial portal systemic shunts is preservation of hepatic portal perfusion, thereby preventing or minimizing the adverse consequences of these procedures.

Nonselective Shunts. Commonly used types of nonselective shunts, all of which completely divert portal flow, include the end-to-side portacaval shunt (Eck fistula), the side-to-side portacaval shunt, large-diameter interposition shunts, and the conventional splenorenal shunt (Fig. 8). The end-to-side portacaval shunt is the prototype of nonselective shunts and is the only shunt procedure that has been compared with conventional medical management in randomized, controlled trials.[28] Survival data from the four controlled investigations of the therapeutic portacaval shunt (performed in patients with prior variceal hemorrhage) are depicted in Figure 9. The most common causes of death in medically treated and shunted patients were rebleeding and accelerated hepatic failure, respectively. Although no survival advantage could be demonstrated for shunt patients, all of these studies had a crossover bias in favor of medically treated patients, several of whom received a shunt when intractable recurrent variceal hemorrhage developed. In addition, nearly all of the trial patients had alcoholic cirrhosis; so these results do not necessarily apply to other causes of portal hypertension. Other important findings of these randomized trials included (1) reliable control of bleeding in shunted patients; (2) variceal rebleeding in over 70 per cent of medically treated patients; and (3) spontaneous, often severe, encephalopathy in 20 to 40 per cent of shunted patients.

All of the other nonselective shunts in Figure 8 maintain continuity of the portal vein, thereby connecting the portal and systemic venous systems in a side-to-side manner. Therefore, these procedures decompress both the splanchnic venous circulation and the intrahepatic sinusoidal network. Because the liver

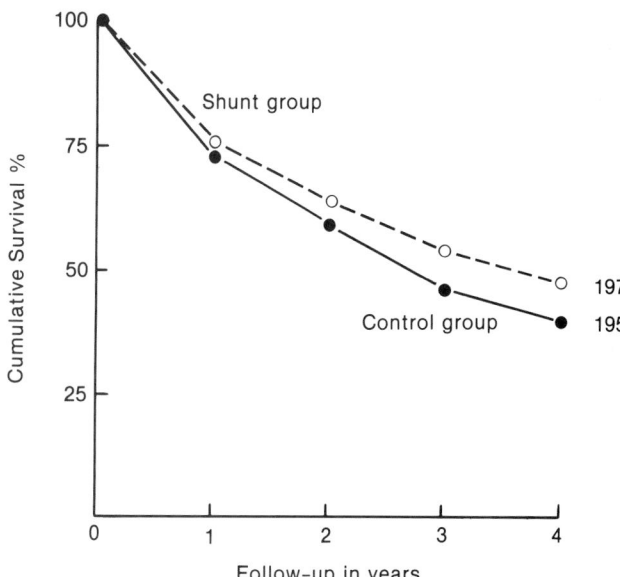

Figure 9. Cumulative survival data from four controlled trials of the portacaval shunt versus conventional medical management. (From Boyer, T. D.: Portal hypertension and its complications: Bleeding esophageal varices, ascites, and spontaneous bacterial peritonitis. *In* Zakim, D., and Boyer, T. D. (Eds.): Hepatology: A Textbook of Liver Disease. Philadelphia, W. B. Saunders Company, 1982, pp. 464–499.)

and intestines are both important contributors to ascites formation, side-to-side portal systemic shunts are the most effective in relieving ascites as well as preventing recurrent variceal bleeding. However, because they completely divert portal flow like the end-to-side portacaval shunt, side-to-side shunts also accelerate hepatic failure and lead to frequent post-shunt encephalopathy. One controlled investigation of the end-to-side versus the side-to-side portacaval shunt showed no significant clinical differences between these procedures.[26]

Synthetic grafts or autogenous vein may be interposed between the portal and systemic venous circulations at a variety of locations (see Fig. 8). The interposition mesocaval shunt in particular became popular during the 1970s after an initial report showed a lower frequency of encephalopathy following this procedure than after other nonselective shunts. However, subsequent data, including a randomized trial of the interposition mesocaval shunt versus the direct side-to-side portacaval shunt, have documented that there are no clinical or hemodynamic differences between these two operations.[36] A major disadvantage of prosthetic interposition shunts is a high graft thrombosis rate which approaches 35 per cent during the late postoperative interval.[33] However, advantages of these procedures are that they are technically relatively easy; the hepatic hilum is avoided, thereby making subsequent liver transplantation less complicated; and they can be easily occluded if intractable post-shunt encephalopathy develops.

The conventional splenorenal shunt consists of anastomosis of the proximal splenic vein to the renal vein. Splenectomy is also done. Because the smaller proximal, rather than the larger distal, end of the splenic vein is used, shunt thrombosis is more frequent after this procedure than after the distal splenorenal shunt. Although early series noted that postshunt encephalopathy was less common after the conventional splenorenal than it was after the portacaval shunt, subsequent analyses have suggested that this low frequency of encephalopathy was probably due to restoration of hepatic portal perfusion after the development of shunt thrombosis in many patients. A conventional splenorenal shunt that is of sufficient caliber to remain patent gradually dilates and eventually causes complete portal decompression and portal flow diversion. A purported advantage of the procedure is that hypersplenism is eliminated by splenec-

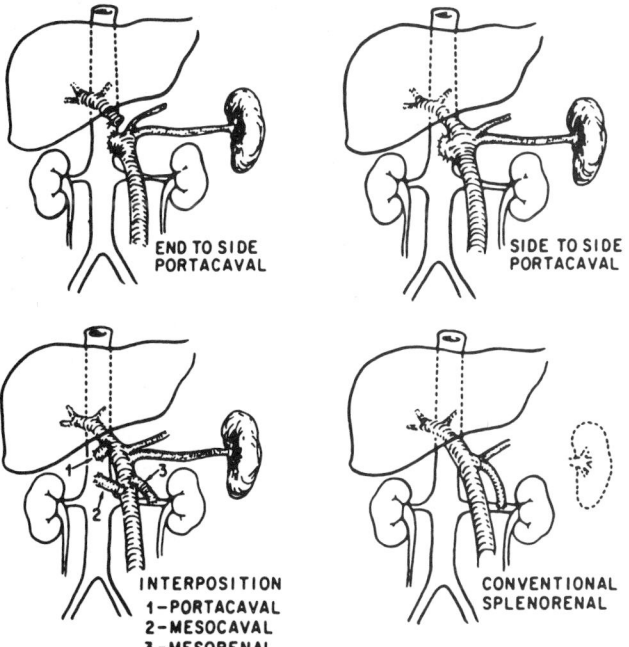

Figure 8. Nonselective shunts completely divert portal blood flow away from the liver. (From Rikkers, L. F.: Portal hypertension. *In* Moody, F. G., et al. (Eds.): Surgical Treatment of Digestive Disease. Chicago, Year Book Medical Publishers, 1986, pp. 409–424.)

tomy. However, the thrombocytopenia and leukopenia that accompany portal hypertension are rarely of clinical significance, making splenectomy an unnecessary procedure in most patients.

In summary, nonselective shunts effectively decompress varices. However, because of complete portal flow diversion, they are complicated by frequent postoperative encephalopathy and accelerated hepatic failure. Side-to-side nonselective shunts effectively relieve ascites as well as prevent variceal hemorrhage. Presently, the only indications for nonselective shunts are in the emergency setting, in patients with both variceal hemorrhage and medically intractable ascites, and as a bridge to hepatic transplantation in patients in whom bleeding is not controlled by sclerotherapy.

Selective Shunts. The hemodynamic and clinical disadvantages of nonselective shunts stimulated development of the concept of selective variceal decompression. In 1967, Warren, Zeppa, and Fomon[42] introduced the distal splenorenal shunt, and in the following year Inokuchi reported his initial results with the left gastric vena caval shunt.[15] The latter procedure consists of interposition of a vein graft between the left gastric (coronary) vein and the inferior vena cava, and thus directly and selectively decompresses esophagogastric varices. However, only a minority of patients with portal hypertension have appropriate anatomy for this operation, experience with it has been limited to Japan, and no controlled trials have been conducted.

The distal splenorenal shunt consists of anastomosis of the distal end of the splenic vein to the left renal vein and interruption of all collaterals, such as the coronary and gastroepiploic veins, connecting the superior mesenteric and gastrosplenic

components of the splanchnic venous circulation (Fig. 10). This causes separation of the portal venous circulation into a decompressed gastrosplenic venous circuit and a high-pressure superior mesenteric venous system that continues to perfuse the liver. Although the procedure is technically demanding, it can be mastered by most well-trained surgeons who are knowledgeable in the principles of vascular surgery.

Not all patients are candidates for the distal splenorenal shunt. Because sinusoidal and mesenteric hypertension is maintained and important lymphatic pathways are transected during dissection of the left renal vein, the distal splenorenal shunt tends to aggravate, rather than relieve, ascites. Thus, patients with medically intractable ascites should not undergo this procedure. However, the larger population of patients in whom transient ascites develops after resuscitation from a variceal hemorrhage are candidates for a selective shunt. Other contraindications to a distal splenorenal shunt are prior splenectomy and a splenic vein diameter of less than 7 mm.

Although selective variceal decompression is a sound physiologic concept, the distal splenorenal shunt remains controversial after an extensive clinical experience spanning more than 20 years.[11] The key questions regarding this procedure are (1) How effective is it in preserving hepatic portal perfusion? and (2) Is it superior to nonselective shunts with respect to duration or quality of survival?

Although the distal splenorenal shunt leads to portal flow preservation in over 85 per cent of patients during the early postoperative interval (Fig. 11), the high-pressure mesenteric venous system gradually collateralizes to the low-pressure shunt, causing loss of portal flow in approximately 50 per cent of patients by 1 year. The degree and duration of portal flow

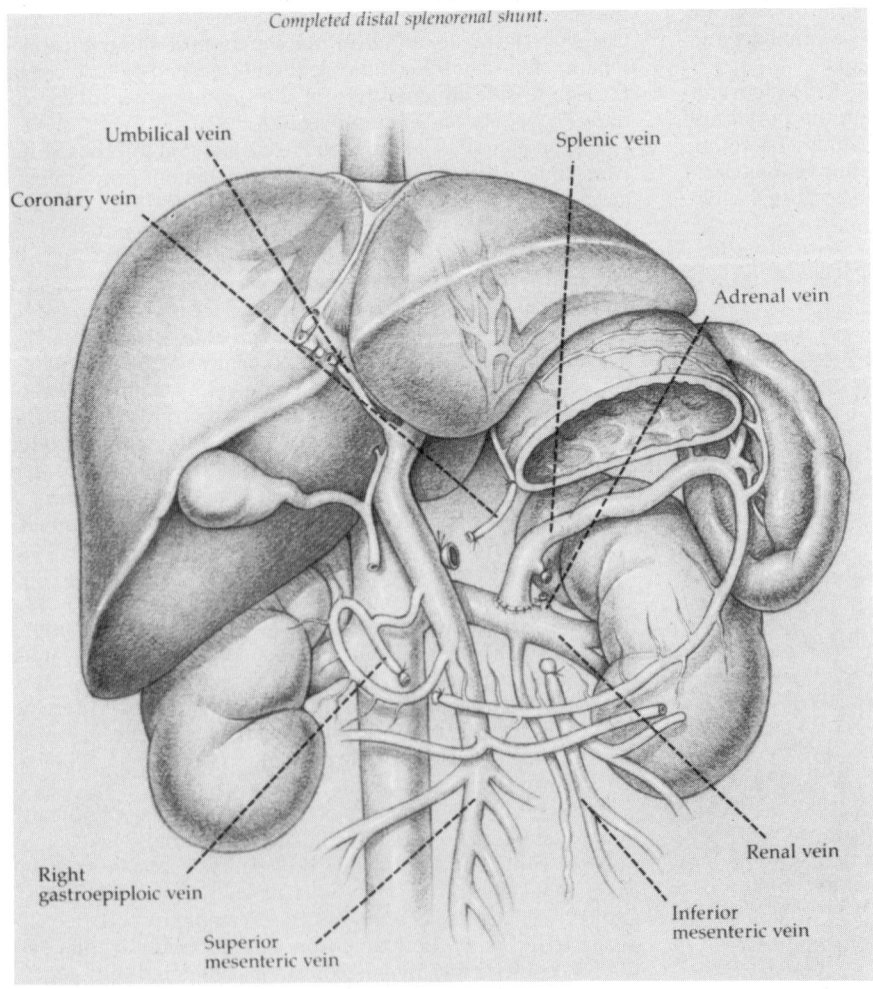

Completed distal splenorenal shunt.

Umbilical vein

Splenic vein

Coronary vein

Adrenal vein

Right gastroepiploic vein

Renal vein

Superior mesenteric vein

Inferior mesenteric vein

Figure 10. The distal splenorenal shunt provides selective variceal decompression through the short gastric veins, spleen, and splenic vein to the left renal vein. Hepatic portal perfusion is maintained by interrupting the umbilical, coronary, gastroepiploic veins, and any other prominent collaterals. (From Rikkers, L. F.: Distal splenorenal shunt for portal hypertension. Surgery Illustrated, 1988. Drawing by William B. Westwood. Courtesy of LTI Medica and The Upjohn Company. Copyright 1988 by Learning Technology Incorporated.)

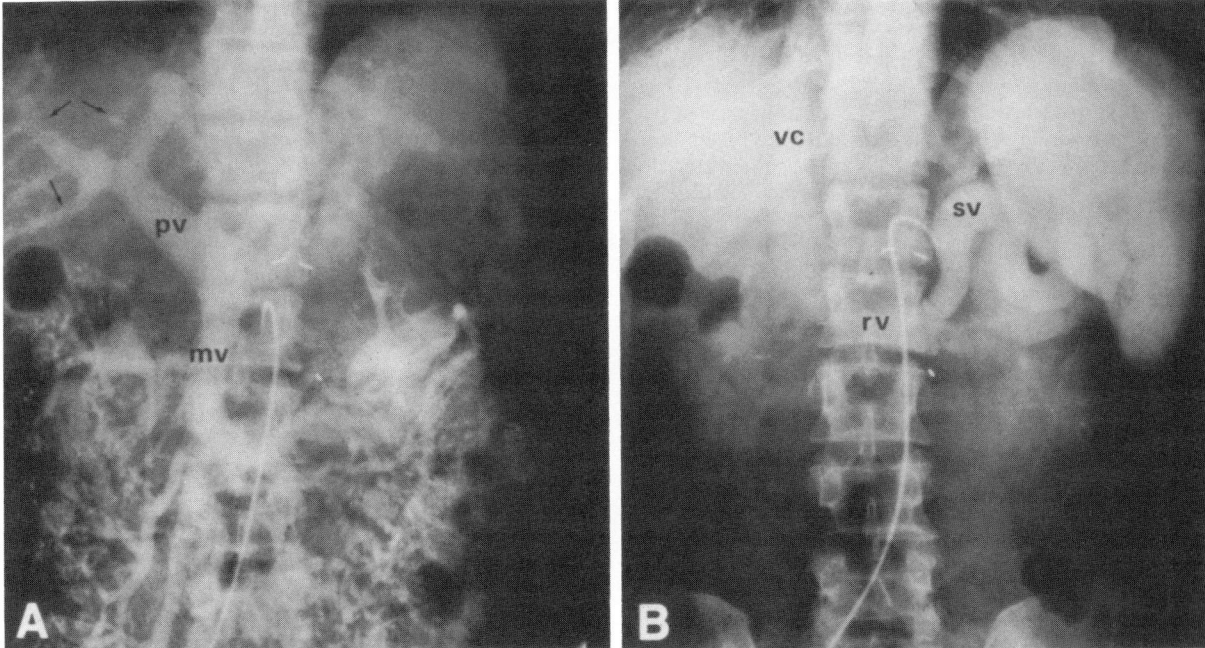

Figure 11. Selective superior mesenteric *(A)* and splenic *(B)* angiograms after a distal splenorenal shunt. The venous phase of the superior mesenteric angiogram visualizes the superior mesenteric vein (MV), portal vein (PV), and intrahepatic portal vein branches (arrows). The venous phase of the splenic angiogram opacifies the splenic vein (SV), left renal vein (RV), and inferior vena cava (VC). (From Rikkers, L. F., Rudman, D., Galambos, J. T., et al.: A randomized, controlled trial of the distal splenorenal shunt. Ann. Surg., *188:*271, 1978.)

preservation depend both on the cause of portal hypertension and on technical details of the operation (the extent to which the mesenteric circulation and the gastrosplenic venous circulation are separated). Henderson and co-workers[12] have shown that portal flow is maintained in the majority of patients with nonalcoholic cirrhosis and noncirrhotic portal hypertension (e.g., portal vein thrombosis). In contrast, portal flow rapidly collateralizes to the shunt in individuals with alcoholic cirrhosis.

Modification of the distal splenorenal shunt by purposeful or inadvertent omission of coronary vein ligation leads to early loss of portal flow. Even when all major collaterals are interrupted, portal flow may be gradually diverted through a pancreatic collateral network (pancreatic siphon). This pathway can be discouraged by dissecting the full length of the splenic vein from the pancreas (splenopancreatic disconnection). In an uncontrolled series, the Emory group has shown that portal flow can be preserved into the late postoperative interval in most patients with alcoholic cirrhosis when splenopancreatic disconnection is done.[13] However, this extension of the procedure makes it technically more challenging, which may be a significant disadvantage in an era when fewer shunts are being done because of increasing utilization of endoscopic sclerotherapy and hepatic transplantation.

Six of the seven controlled comparisons of the distal splenorenal shunt with nonselective shunts have included predominantly alcoholic cirrhotic patients.[27,28] None of these trials have demonstrated an advantage with either procedure with regard to long-term survival. Three of the studies demonstrated a lower frequency of encephalopathy after the distal splenorenal shunt, whereas the other trials have shown no difference in the incidence of this postoperative complication. In contrast to survival, encephalopathy is a subjective end point that was assessed with a variety of methods in the different trials. One of the more objective investigations quantified encephalopathy by the number of postoperative hospital admissions required for the treatment of this complication.[18] This trial demonstrated significantly fewer admissions for encephalopathy in the selective than it did in the nonselective shunt group (Fig. 12). Another important end point in comparing treatments for variceal

hemorrhage is the effectiveness with which recurrent bleeding is prevented. In nearly all uncontrolled and controlled series of the distal splenorenal shunt, this procedure has been equivalent to nonselective shunts.[11] A single exception is one of the controlled trials that was complicated by a high rebleeding rate in the distal splenorenal shunt group (30 per cent).[10] Mainly because of these inconsistent results of the controlled trials, there is no consensus as to which shunting procedure is superior in patients with alcoholic cirrhosis. However, because the quality of life (encephalopathy rate) was significantly better in the distal splenorenal shunt group in three of the trials, there would appear to be an advantage to selective variceal decompression even in this population.[27]

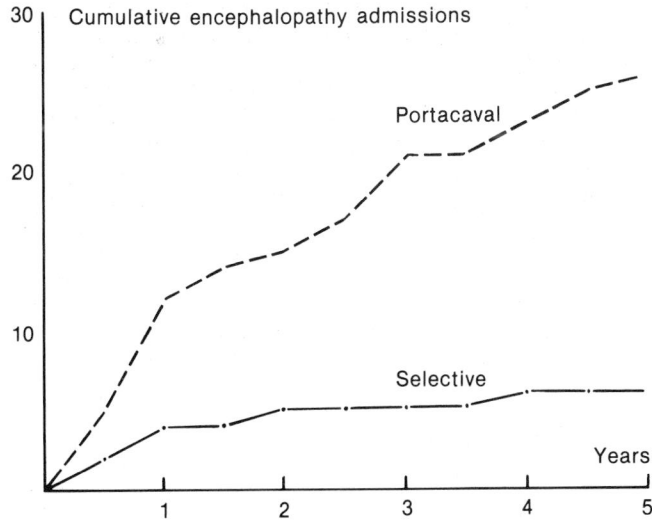

Figure 12. In the Toronto controlled trial of the distal splenorenal shunt versus the portacaval shunt, there were significantly fewer cumulative hospital admissions for encephalopathy in the selective shunt group. (From Langer, B., Taylor, B. R., Mackenzie, D. R., et al.: Further report of a prospective randomized trial comparing distal splenorenal shunt with end-to-side portacaval shunt: An analysis of encephalopathy, survival, and quality of life. Gastroenterology, *88:*424, 1985.)

There are considerably fewer data regarding selective shunting in nonalcoholic cirrhosis and in noncirrhotic portal hypertension. Because hepatic portal perfusion after the distal splenorenal shunt is better preserved in these disease categories, one might expect improved results. A single controlled trial in patients with schistosomiasis (presinusoidal portal hypertension) demonstrated a lower frequency of encephalopathy after the distal splenorenal shunt than after a conventional splenorenal shunt (nonselective).[7] There were few deaths in either limb of this trial. Two large uncontrolled series of the distal splenorenal shunt have demonstrated better survival in patients with nonalcoholic than in those with alcoholic cirrhosis.[41,44] However, this has not been a consistent finding in all centers in which the distal splenorenal shunt is performed.

Recently completed controlled trials have also compared the distal splenorenal shunt with chronic endoscopic sclerotherapy.[29,40] In these investigations, recurrent hemorrhage was much more effectively prevented by selective shunting than by sclerotherapy, but hepatic portal perfusion was maintained in a significantly higher fraction of sclerotherapy patients. Despite this hemodynamic advantage, encephalopathy rates have been similar after both therapies. The two North American trials were dissimilar with respect to the effect of these treatments on long-term survival (Fig. 13). Sclerotherapy with surgical rescue for the one third of sclerotherapy failures led to significantly better survival than selective shunt alone in the Atlanta study.[40] In this investigation, 85 per cent of sclerotherapy failures could be salvaged by surgical therapy. In contrast, a similar investigation conducted in a sparsely populated area (Intermountain West and Plains) showed no significant difference in survival between groups.[29] Only 25 per cent of sclerotherapy failures could be salvaged by surgical therapy in this trial. The survival results of these two studies suggest that sclerotherapy is a rational initial treatment for patients who bleed from varices if sclerotherapy failure is recognized and such patients promptly undergo surgical therapy. However, patients living in remote areas are less likely to be salvaged by shunt operations when sclerotherapy fails, and a selective shunt may be preferable initial treatment for these patients.

Partial Shunts. Because the small-diameter portacaval H-graft shunt incompletely decompresses, rather than compartmentalizes, the portal circulation, it is a partial, rather than a selective, shunt. Sarfeh and associates have demonstrated that when an 8- to 10-mm. polytetrafluoroethylene graft is interposed between the portal vein and inferior vena cava, hepatic portal perfusion can be maintained in most patients.[30] In their initial uncontrolled series, encephalopathy was less frequent and survival longer in patients with continuing portal flow than in those with complete portal diversion. An advantage of the small diameter interposition shunt is its relative technical simplicity. A potential disadvantage may be a high shunt thrombosis rate, which has been observed in the late postoperative interval after large-diameter interposition shunts. Therefore, the results of a recently initiated controlled trial between small and large diameter interposition shunts are anxiously anticipated.

NONSHUNT OPERATIONS. The objectives of these procedures are either ablation of varices or, more commonly, extensive interruption of collaterals connecting the high-pressure portal venous system with the varices. One exception is splenectomy, which is effective in left-sided portal hypertension caused by splenic vein thrombosis.

The simplest nonshunt operation is transection and reanastomosis of the distal esophagus with a stapling device. This operation, which has generally been applied to the emergency setting, is frequently followed by recurrent hemorrhage. The most effective nonshunt operation is extensive esophagogastric devascularization, combined with esophageal transection and splenectomy. The Sugiura procedure preserves the coronary and paraesophageal veins to maintain a portal systemic collateral

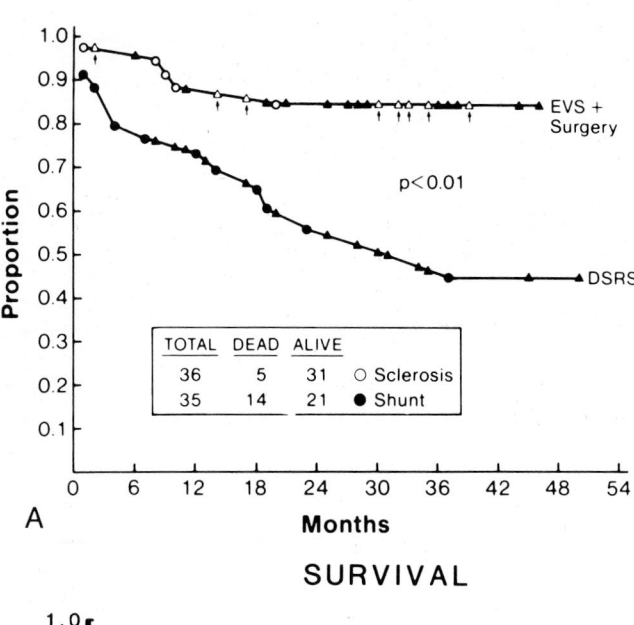

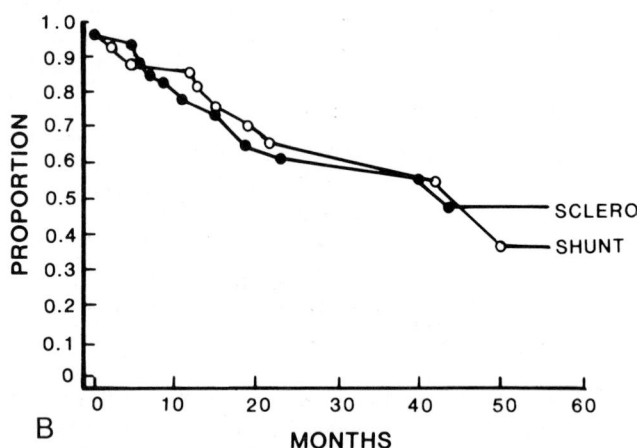

Figure 13. Kaplan-Meier survival analyses for sclerotherapy and distal splenorenal shunt groups in the Atlanta *(A)* and Omaha *(B)* controlled trials. Sclerotherapy plus surgical therapy for the one third of patients who failed sclerotherapy led to significantly longer survival than the distal splenorenal shunt in the Atlanta trial *(A)* but not in the Omaha *(B)* trial. Surgical therapy for sclerotherapy failures was less frequent in the Omaha trial because many patients lived in geographically remote areas. (*A*, From Warren, W. D., Henderson, J. M., Millikan, W. J., et al.: Distal splenorenal shunt versus endoscopic sclerotherapy for long-term management of variceal bleeding: A preliminary report of a prospective, randomized trial. Ann. Surg., *203:*454, 1986. *B*, from Rikkers, L. F., Burnett, D. A., Volentine, G. D., et al.: Shunt surgery versus endoscopic sclerotherapy for long-term treatment of variceal bleeding: Early results of a randomized trial. Ann. Surg., *206:*261, 1987.)

pathway and thus discourage reformation of varices.[37] The results with this operation in Japan have been excellent, with rebleeding less than 5 per cent and 10-year survival of 72 per cent after elective procedures. However, extensive devascularization procedures have generally been less successful in North American patients with alcoholic cirrhosis. Long-term followup in American series has revealed rebleeding in 35 to 55 per cent, which is similar to the endoscopic sclerotherapy experience. In many centers, esophagogastric devascularization procedures are used mainly for unshuntable patients with diffuse splanchnic venous thrombosis and for individuals with distal splenorenal shunt thrombosis.

HEPATIC TRANSPLANTATION. Of the numerous therapeutic options for prevention of recurrent variceal hemorrhage, hepatic transplantation is the only one that addresses the underlying liver disease in addition to providing reliable portal decompression.[16] However, because of economic factors and a limited supply of donor organs, hepatic transplantation is not available to all patients. In addition, transplantation is not indicated for some of the more common causes of variceal bleeding, such as schistosomiasis (normal liver function) and active alcoholism (noncompliant).

Patients with variceal bleeding who are transplant candidates include nonalcoholic cirrhotics and abstinent alcoholic cirrhotics with either limited hepatic functional reserve (Child's class C) or a poor quality of life secondary to disease (e.g., encephalopathy, fatigue, or bone pain). In such individuals, the acute hemorrhage should be treated with sclerotherapy and the patient's transplant candidacy immediately activated. If sclerotherapy is ineffective, an interposition shunt that avoids the hepatic hilum is a reasonable temporizing procedure until a donor organ becomes available.

There are few data available concerning the best therapy for eventual transplant candidates who have well-compensated liver disease (Child's classes A and B) when they bleed from varices. Although most of these individuals should initially be treated with chronic sclerotherapy, it is unclear whether hepatic transplantation or a nontransplant operation is preferable for patients in whom sclerotherapy has failed and for patients who bleed from gastric varices or from portal hypertensive gastropathy. The issue is not whether these patients should undergo transplantation, but when this formidable procedure should be undertaken. If a nontransplant operation (e.g., selective shunt or devascularization procedure) is performed initially, these patients should be carefully assessed at 6-month to 1-year intervals and hepatic transplantation considered when other complications of cirrhosis develop or hepatic functional decompensation is evident either clinically or by careful assessment with quantitative tests of liver function.

OVERALL TREATMENT PLAN. An algorithm for definitive management of variceal hemorrhage is shown in Figure 14. Patients are first grouped according to their transplant candidacy. This decision is based on multiple factors: etiology of portal hypertension, abstinence for alcoholic cirrhotics, the presence or absence of other diseases, and physiologic, rather than chronologic, age. Transplant candidates with decompensated hepatic function or a poor quality of life secondary to liver disease should undergo transplantation as soon as possible. Most future transplantation and nontransplantation candidates should undergo initial sclerotherapy unless they bleed from gastric varices or portal hypertensive gastropathy or live in remote geographic locations and have limited access to emergency tertiary care. These latter individuals and those who fail sclerotherapy should undergo a selective shunt procedure if they meet the criteria for this operation. Patients with medically intractable ascites and those with diffuse splanchnic venous thrombosis are best treated with a side-to-side portal systemic shunt and a devascularization procedure, respectively. Future transplantation candidates should be carefully monitored so that they undergo transplantation at the appropriate time, before their operative risk is poor. Finally, pharmacotherapy for prevention of recurrent variceal bleeding is experimental at the present time.

PREVENTION OF INITIAL VARICEAL HEMORRHAGE (PROPHYLACTIC THERAPY). The rationale for treating a patient with varices before he bleeds is the high mortality (approximately 50 per cent) associated with the initial hemorrhage. However, because only a third of patients with varices eventually bleed, unless potential bleeders are more reliably identified, approximately two thirds of patients undergoing prophylactic therapy would be treated unnecessarily.

The first trials of prophylaxis for variceal hemorrhage compared the portacaval shunt with conventional medical therapy.[28] In these investigations, survival of shunted patients was actually less than that of medically treated patients because of accelerated hepatic failure secondary to complete portal diversion. In addition, in a significant fraction of patients with shunts postshunt encephalopathy developed.

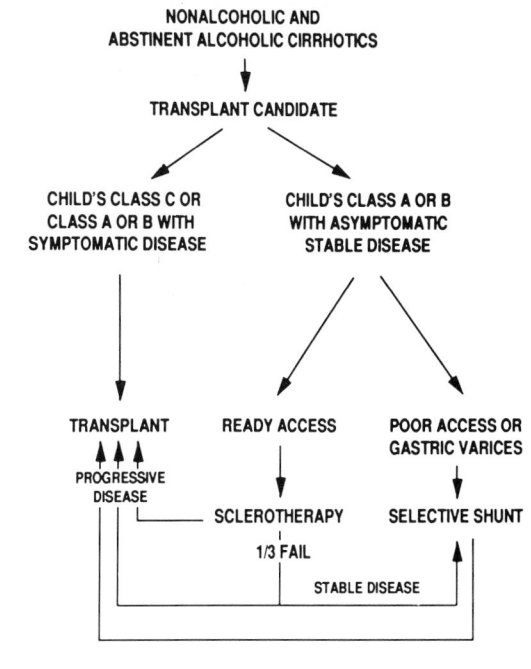

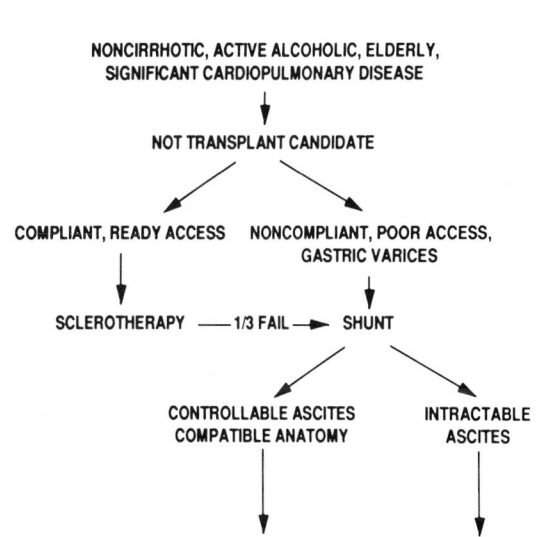

Figure 14. Algorithm for definitive therapy of variceal hemorrhage (see text). (Redrawn from Rikkers, L. F.: Definitive therapy for variceal bleeding: A personal view. Am. J. Surg., *162*(1):8085, 1990.)

The major impetus to reconsideration of prophylactic therapy was the development of relatively noninvasive treatments (endoscopic sclerotherapy and pharmacotherapy), which should be associated with less morbidity than major operative procedures. However, currently sclerotherapy cannot be advocated for prophylaxis because controlled trials have demonstrated no consistent benefit and some have demonstrated a high rebleeding rate and a lower survival in the sclerotherapy group than in medically treated controls.[38] In contrast, all trials of beta blockade as prophylactic therapy have found a reduced incidence of initial variceal hemorrhage in treated patients.[4] In several of these studies, the decreased bleeding rate in the treatment group was statistically significant; and in one study, survival was prolonged in patients receiving beta blockade. Because beta blockade has been associated with few adverse side effects, it can be recommended for reliable patients with varices who have never bled.

PORTAL SYSTEMIC ENCEPHALOPATHY

Portal systemic encephalopathy[8,31] is a psychoneurologic syndrome that may have a number of manifestations, including alterations in the level of consciousness, intellectual deterioration, personality changes, and neurologic findings such as the flapping tremor, asterixis. Although encephalopathy may sometimes develop spontaneously in patients with chronic liver disease, it more often occurs after portal systemic shunt procedures. It is particularly common (20 to 40 per cent of patients) in individuals who undergo nonselective shunts.

Although the pathogenesis of encephalopathy is uncertain, most theories are based on circulating cerebral toxins which are intestinally absorbed and bypass the liver via shunts or fail to be inactivated by the liver's decreased metabolic capacity. Purported cerebral toxins include ammonia, mercaptans, and gamma amino butyric acid. The false neurotransmitter hypothesis, based on the high ratio of aromatic to branched-chain amino acids present in the blood of patients with chronic liver disease, has also been proposed to explain the neuropsychologic disturbances observed.

Encephalopathy develops spontaneously in less than 10 per cent of patients. More commonly, one or more of the following precipitating factors induce the syndrome: gastrointestinal hemorrhage, excessive diuresis, azotemia, constipation, sedatives, infection, and excess dietary protein.

Most episodes of encephalopathy can be successfully treated by identifying and then eliminating the precipitating factors responsible. Dietary protein should be restricted, infections should be treated, all sedatives should be discontinued, and intestinal catharsis to remove blood within the gastrointestinal tract should be accomplished. Stool softeners and dietary protein restriction should be prescribed for patients who have chronic encephalopathy.

Pharmacologic treatment of encephalopathy is indicated for individuals with chronic, intermittent symptoms and for those with persistent, acute psychoneurologic disturbances despite elimination of precipitating factors. The only drugs with proven effectiveness are neomycin, a poorly absorbed antibiotic that suppresses urease-containing bacteria, and lactulose, a nonabsorbable disaccharide that acidifies colonic contents and also has a cathartic effect. Acute episodes of encephalopathy can be treated equally effectively by neomycin and lactulose. Neomycin is orally administered in a dose of 1.5 gm. every 6 hours, whereas in the acute setting lactulose should be given in a dose of 30 gm. every hour or 2 until a cathartic effect is noted. The patient should then be maintained with 20 to 30 gm. of lactulose 2 to 4 times daily or as needed to produce two soft bowel movements daily. Neomycin should not be used for treatment of chronic encephalopathy because nephrotoxicity or ototoxicity may develop. Lactulose combined with mild protein restriction (60 to 80 gm. daily) is the preferred treatment for chronic intermittent encephalopathy.

Enteral or parenteral administration of nutritional formulas enriched in branched-chain amino acids has been suggested as a treatment for both acute and chronic encephalopathy. These solutions have improved mental status in some, but not all, controlled trials. Further research is necessary before these expensive formulations can be routinely recommended.

Surgical therapy has a minor role in the management of encephalopathy. Cerebral function has been improved in some patients with chronic encephalopathy after interruption of a completely diverting portal systemic shunt (nonselective shunt). Also, in isolated cases occlusion of a major portosystemic collateral such as the coronary vein has reversed encephalopathy after the distal splenorenal shunt. Although both total colectomy and colonic exclusion have resolved encephalopathy in some patients, the significant morbidity and mortality following these operations in patients with decompensated hepatic disease have prevented their widespread use.

ASCITES

Ascites[31] is another complication of portal hypertension that rarely requires surgical treatment. Portal hypertensive ascites is initiated by altered hepatic and splanchnic hemodynamics that cause transudation of fluid into the interstitial space. When the rate of interstitial fluid formation exceeds lymph drainage capacity, ascites accumulates. This pathophysiologic process leads to an intravascular volume deficit, which initiates compensatory mechanisms such as aldosterone secretion to restore plasma volume. Both the liver and intestines are important sites of ascites formation, and clinically detectable ascites is rare in patients with extrahepatic portal hypertension.

Medical management resolves ascites in approximately 95 per cent of patients. Dietary salt restriction and diuretic therapy are the mainstays of medical treatment. A rational first-line diuretic is spironolactone, because secondary hyperaldosteronism is present in most patients. A combination of salt restriction (20 to 30 mEq. per day) and spironolactone in a dose of 100 to 400 mg. per day leads to effective diuresis in approximately two thirds of patients. If this regimen fails to mobilize ascites, a more potent diuretic such as hydrochlorothiazide or furosemide should be added. Recent studies have demonstrated that intermittent, large-volume paracentesis either with or without intravenous infusion of colloid is also effective.[1] Contrary to earlier beliefs, large-volume paracentesis in a stable patient does not markedly alter systemic hemodynamics or renal function.

Surgical therapy should be reserved for the unusual patient with medically intractable ascites. The safest and most effective surgical procedure is the peritoneovenous shunt. However, recent controlled trials have demonstrated that this relatively simple operation is followed by significant morbidity and that survival is not prolonged when compared with that associated with medical management.[35] Although side-to-side portal systemic shunts are also effective in relieving ascites, these operations should not be used for ascitic patients unless they have bled from esophagogastric varices.

SELECTED REFERENCES

Groszmann, R. J. (Ed.): Portal Hypertension: Circulatory and Renal Abnormalities. Semin. Liver Dis., 6 (4), 1986.
This is a compendium of eight chapters by authorities in the areas of pathophysiology of portal hypertension, variceal rupture, and ascites. Excellent chapters on hemodynamic evaluation of the patient with portal hypertension and treatment of ascites are also presented. Each chapter contains a comprehensive and up-to-date bibliography.

Langer, B., Taylor, B. R., Mackenzie, D. R., et al.: Further report of a prospective randomized trial comparing distal splenorenal shunt with end-to-side portacaval shunt: An analysis of encephalopathy, survival, and quality of life. Gastroenterology, 88:424, 1985.
This is probably the "purest" of the several controlled trials comparing nonselective and distal splenorenal shunts. Eighty patients with cirrhosis and at least one proven episode of variceal hemorrhage were prospectively randomized. Although survival and rebleeding were similar after portacaval and distal splenorenal shunts, encephalopathy, quantified by the number of required hospital admissions, was significantly more frequent in the portacaval shunt group.

Rikkers, L. F., (Ed.): Management of variceal hemorrhage. Surg. Clin. North Am., 70(2), 1990.
This series of 14 chapters by recognized authorities concerns all aspects of acute and definitive treatment of variceal hemorrhage. Individual chapters are devoted to pharmacotherapy, endoscopic sclerotherapy, each of the major types of portal systemic shunt, nonshunting operations, and hepatic transplantation. Additional chapters consider pathophysiology of portal hypertension, nonoperative emergency treatment, emergency surgery, diagnosis and hemodynamic evaluation, prophylactic therapy, and management of children with variceal bleeding.

Sherlock, S.: Diseases of the liver and biliary system, 8th ed. London, Blackwell Scientific Publications, 1989.
This is one of the few as well as one of the finest textbooks on this subject by a single

author. The chapters on ascites, the portal venous system and portal hypertension, hepatic encephalopathy, and hepatic cirrhosis are concise but comprehensive and well illustrated. They present excellent background information for this chapter.

Terblanche, J., Burroughs, A. K., Hobbs, K. E. F.: Controversies in the management of bleeding esophageal varices. N. Engl. J. Med., *320:*1393, 1469, 1989.
This excellent and up-to-date review consists of three parts: emergency management, long-term management, and prophylactic management of esophageal varices. The many controlled trials of pharmacotherapy, endoscopic sclerotherapy, and surgical therapy are summarized. The several remaining controversies concerning the treatment of variceal hemorrhage are discussed; and, where appropriate, the authors' conclusions are presented. The bibliography is comprehensive and current.

Warren, W. D., Henderson, J. M., Millikan, W. J., et al.: Distal splenorenal shunt versus endoscopic sclerotherapy for long-term management of variceal bleeding: Preliminary report of a prospective, randomized trial. Ann. Surg., *203:*454, 1986.
This is the first of three published controlled trials comparing chronic sclerotherapy and the distal splenorenal shunt. Seventy-one patients with cirrhosis (44 per cent Child's C) and prior variceal hemorrhage were randomized. Rebleeding was more frequent after sclerosis (53 per cent) than after the distal splenorenal shunt (3 per cent). Approximately one third of sclerotherapy patients failed, but nearly all were salvaged by surgical therapy, leading to significantly better survival in the sclerotherapy group. A survival advantage for sclerotherapy has not been found in any of the subsequent trials. Although hepatic portal perfusion and quantitative hepatic function were better maintained in the sclerotherapy group, frequencies of posttreatment encephalopathy were similar in the two groups. The authors concluded that sclerotherapy should be the initial definitive treatment for most patients with variceal bleeding as long as surgical rescue is readily available.

REFERENCES

1. Arroyo, V., Gines, P., Planas, R., et al.: Paracentesis in the management of cirrhotics with ascites. *In* Epstein M. (Ed.): The Kidney in Liver Disease, 3rd ed. Baltimore, Williams & Wilkins Company, 1988, pp. 578–592.
2. Benoit, J. N., and Granger, D. N.: Splanchnic hemodynamics in chronic portal hypertension. Semin. Liver Dis., *6:*287, 1986.
3. Burnett, D. A., and Rikkers, L. F.: Nonoperative emergency treatment of variceal hemorrhage. Surg. Clin. North Am., *70:*291, 1990.
4. Burroughs, A.: The management of bleeding due to portal hypertension. 2. Prevention of variceal rebleeding and prevention of the first bleeding episode in patients with portal hypertension. Q. J. Med., *68:*507, 1988.
5. Burroughs, A. K., Jenkins, W. J., Sherlock, S., et al.: Controlled trial of propranolol for the prevention of recurrent variceal hemorrhage in patients with cirrhosis. N. Engl. J. Med., *309:*1539, 1983.
6. Chen, T. S., and Chen, P. S.: Understanding the Liver. Westport, Greenwood Press, 1984.
7. da Silva, L. C., Strauss, E., Gayotto, L. C. C., et al.: A randomized trial for the study of the elective surgical treatment of portal hypertension in Mansonic schistosomiasis. Ann. Surg., *204:*148, 1986.
8. Fraser, C. L., and Arieff, A. I.: Hepatic encephalopathy. N. Engl. J. Med., *313:*865, 1985.
9. Gimson, A. E., Westaby, D., Hegarty, J., et al.: A randomized trial of vasopressin and vasopressin plus nitroglycerin in the control of acute variceal hemorrhage. Hepatology, *6:*410, 1986.
10. Harley, H. A., Morgan, T., Redeker, A. G., et al.: Results of a randomized trial of end-to-side portacaval shunt and distal splenorenal shunt in alcoholic liver disease and variceal bleeding. Gastroenterology, *91:*802, 1986.
11. Henderson, J. M.: The distal splenorenal shunt. Surg. Clin. North Am., *70:*405, 1990.
12. Henderson, J. M., Millikan, W. J., Jr., Wright-Bacon, L., et al.: Hemodynamic differences between alcoholic and nonalcoholic cirrhotics following distal splenorenal shunt: Effect on survival? Ann. Surg., *198:*325, 1983.
13. Henderson, J. M., Warren, W. D., Millikan, W. J., et al.: Distal splenorenal shunt with splenopancreatic disconnection: A 4-year assessment. Ann. Surg., *210:*332, 1989.
14. Holman, J. M., and Rikkers, L. F.: Success of medical and surgical management of acute variceal hemorrhage. Am. J. Surg., *140:*816, 1980.
15. Inokuchi, K., Beppu, K., Koyanagi, N., et al.: Fifteen years' experience with left gastric venous caval shunt for esophageal varices. World J. Surg., *8:*716, 1984.
16. Iwatsuki, S., Starzl, T. E., Todo, S., et al.: Liver transplantation in the treatment of bleeding esophageal varices. Surgery, *104:*697, 1988.
17. Johnston, G. W., and Rodgers, H. W.: A review of 15 years' experience in the use of sclerotherapy in the control of acute haemorrhage from oesophageal varices. Br. J. Surg., *60:*797, 1973.
18. Langer, B., Taylor, B. R., Mackenzie, D. R., et al.: Further report of a prospective randomized trial comparing distal splenorenal shunt with end-to-side portacaval shunt. Gastroenterology, *88:*424, 1985.
19. Lautt, W. W., and Greenway, C. V.: Conceptual review of the hepatic vascular bed. Hepatology, *7:*952, 1987.
20. Lebrec, D., Poynard, T., Bernau, J., et al.: A randomized controlled study of propranolol for prevention of recurrent gastrointestinal bleeding in patients with cirrhosis: A final report. Hepatology, *4:*355, 1984.
21. McCormack, T. T., Sims, J., Eyre-Brook, I., et al.: Gastric lesions in portal hypertension: inflammatory gastritis or congestive gastropathy? Gut, *26:*1226, 1985.
22. Nordlinger, B. M., Nordlinger, D. F., Fulenwider, J. T., et al.: Angiography in portal hypertension: Clinical significance in surgery. Am. J. Surg., *139:*132, 1980.
23. Orloff, M. J., Bell, R. H., Jr., Hyde, P. V., et al.: Long-term results of emergency portacaval shunt for bleeding esophageal varices in unselected patients with alcoholic cirrhosis. Ann. Surg., *192:*325, 1980.
24. Ozaki, C. F., Anderson, J. C., Lieberman, R. P., and Rikkers, L. F.: Duplex ultrasound as a noninvasive technique of assessing portal hemodynamics. Am. J. Surg., *155:*70, 1988.
25. Polio, J., and Groszmann, R. J.: Hemodynamic factors involved in the development and rupture of esophageal varices: A pathophysiologic approach to treatment. Semin. Liver Dis., *6:*218, 1986.
26. Resnick, R. H., Iber, F. L., Ishihara, A. M., et al.: A controlled study of the therapeutic portacaval shunt. Gastroenterology, *67:*843, 1974.
27. Rikkers, L. F.: Is the distal splenorenal shunt better? Hepatology, *8:*1705, 1988.
28. Rikkers, L. F.: Portal hypertension. *In* Moody, F. G. (Ed.): Surgical Treatment of Digestive Disease, 2nd ed. Chicago, Year Book Medical Publishers, 1990, pp. 363–380.
29. Rikkers, L. F., Burnett, D. A., Volentine, G. D., et al.: Shunt surgery versus endoscopic sclerotherapy for long-term treatment of variceal bleeding. Ann. Surg., *206:*261, 1987.
30. Sarfeh, I. J., Rypins, E. B., and Mason, G. R.: A systemic appraisal of portacaval H-graft diameters: Clinical and hemodynamic perspectives. Ann. Surg., *204:*356, 1986.
31. Sherlock, S.: Diseases of the Liver and Biliary System. Oxford, Blackwell Scientific Publications, 1989.
32. Smith, J. L., and Graham, D. Y.: Variceal hemorrhage: A critical evaluation of survival analysis. Gastroenterology, *82:*968, 1982.
33. Smith, R. B., III, Warren, W. D., Salam, A. A., et al.: Dacron interposition shunts for portal hypertension: An analysis of morbidity correlates. Ann. Surg., *192.*9, 1980.
34. Snady, H.: The role of sclerotherapy in the treatment of esophageal varices: Personal experience and a review of randomized trials. Am. J. Gastroenterol., *82:*813, 1987.
35. Stanley, M. M., Ochi, S., Lee, K. K., et al.: Peritoneovenous shunting as compared with medical treatment in patients with alcoholic cirrhosis and massive ascites. N. Engl. J. Med., *321:*1632, 1989.
36. Stipa, S., Ziparo, V., Anza, M., et al.: A randomized controlled trial of mesentericocaval shunt with autologous jugular vein. Surg. Gynecol. Obstet., *153:*533, 1981.
37. Sugiura, M., and Futugawa, S.: Esophageal transection with paraesophagogastric devascularization (the Sugiura procedure) in the treatment of esophageal varices. World J. Surg., *8:*673, 1984.
38. Terblanche, J., Burroughs, A. K., and Hobbs, K. E. F.: Controversies in the management of bleeding esophageal varices. N. Engl. J. Med., *320:*1469, 1989.
39. Villeneuve, J. P., Pomier-Layrargues, G., Infante-Riwand, C., et al.: Propranolol for the prevention of recurrent variceal hemorrhage: A controlled trial. Hepatology, *6:*1239, 1986.
40. Warren, W. D., Henderson, J. M., Millikan, W. J., et al.: Distal splenorenal shunt versus endoscopic sclerotherapy for long-term management of variceal bleeding: Preliminary report of a prospective, randomized trial. Ann. Surg., *203:*454, 1986.
41. Warren, W. D., Millikan, W. J., Jr., Henderson, J. M., et al.: Ten years' portal hypertensive surgery at Emory. Ann. Surg., *195:*530, 1982.
42. Warren, W. D., Zeppa, R., and Fomon, J. J.: Selective transsplenic decompression of gastroesophageal varices by distal splenorenal shunt. Ann. Surg., *166:*437, 1967.
43. Westaby, D., MacDougall, B. R. D., and Williams, R.: Improved survival following injection sclerotherapy for esophageal varices: Final analysis of a controlled trial. Hepatology, *5:*827, 1985.
44. Zeppa, R., Hutson, D. G., Levi, J. U., and Livingstone, A. S.: Factors influencing survival after distal splenorenal shunt. World J. Surg., *8:*733, 1984.

VI ———————————————————————————

PERITONEOVENOUS SHUNTS FOR INTRACTABLE ASCITES

Paul D. Greig, M.D.
and Bernard Langer, M.D.

Ascites is the pathologic accumulation of fluid in the peritoneal cavity. It may be part of a generalized third-space fluid loss in conditions such as chronic renal disease, congestive heart failure, or massive fluid overload, but is more often related to intra-abdominal factors that lead to formation of peritoneal fluid at a more rapid rate than that at which it can be absorbed (Table 1). Of these conditions, chronic liver disease is by far the most common.

PATHOPHYSIOLOGY OF ASCITES FORMATION IN CIRRHOSIS

The formation of ascites in the cirrhotic patient follows the interaction of three factors: intrahepatic and portal hypertension, hypoalbuminemia, and alterations of sodium and water excretion by the kidneys.[1]

PORTAL HYPERTENSION. The fibrosis and nodular regeneration that occur in the cirrhotic liver increase the resistance to blood flow. With postsinusoidal obstruction, there are increases in both the sinusoidal and intrahepatic pressure and the pressure in the portal and splanchnic veins. This increased hydrostatic pressure promotes the movement of fluid from the intravascular to the extravascular compartment and then into the peritoneal cavity from the surfaces of the liver, bowel, and mesentery. In conditions of presinusoidal portal hypertension, including schistosomiasis and portal vein thrombosis, ascites is uncommon, whereas in postsinusoidal obstruction, including acute right-sided heart failure and the Budd-Chiari syndrome, ascites is characteristic. Postsinusoidal obstruction also increases hepatic lymph production and both pressure and flow in intrahepatic and intestinal lymphatics, which may contribute to the generation of ascites.

HYPOALBUMINEMIA. A decrease in plasma oncotic pressure as a result of hypoalbuminemia also contributes to the formation of ascites. Ordinarily, the fluid that passes out of the

TABLE 1. Causes of Ascites

General extravascular fluid accumulation
  Chronic renal failure
    Nephrotic syndrome
  Chronic right heart failure
    Constrictive pericarditis, cardiac tamponade, tricuspid stenosis or insufficiency
  Malnutrition
  Marked fluid overload
Intra-abdominal causes
  Acute liver disease
    Viral hepatitis
    Acute hepatic necrosis
  Chronic liver disease
    Cirrhosis
    Budd-Chiari syndrome
  Pancreatic ascites
  Chylous ascites
  Malignancy, especially ovary, colon, metastatic breast
  Tuberculosis

capillary wall is low in protein and the higher plasma protein concentration in the post-capillary venule exerts an osmotic pressure that draws extravascular fluid back into the intravascular space. In cirrhotic patients with low plasma albumin levels, this osmotic gradient is lower and fluid recovery from the extravascular compartment by this mechanism is impaired.

SODIUM AND WATER RETENTION. Changes in renal function are commonly observed in the cirrhotic patient and are manifested by sodium and water retention. In "well-compensated" cirrhosis, the renal changes may be characterized only by an impairment in the ability to excrete a sodium load without formation of ascites. More severe renal dysfunction occurs in uncompensated cirrhotic patients with ascites. These patients have a reduction in total renal blood flow with a decreased glomerular filtration rate (GFR) from intrarenal shunting of blood to medullary nephrons despite normal or increased circulating blood volume and cardiac output. Associated with these renal and hemodynamic changes are increases in plasma renin, angiotensin, and aldosterone levels. These factors contribute to sodium retention with low urinary volumes and sodium concentrations.[13]

Progression of salt and water retention may lead to marked oliguria, with rising urea and creatinine levels and persistently low urine sodium concentration. This form of functional renal failure has been termed *hepatorenal syndrome* and represents the end stage of the spectrum of renal dysfunction observed in advanced liver disease.[32] In this condition, the kidney is histologically normal and the renal abnormality is potentially reversible, as has been demonstrated by the return of normal function following transplantation of such kidneys, by liver transplantation, and, in some cases, following peritoneovenous shunting.

These alterations in renal salt and water handling in the cirrhotic patient with ascites have been attributed to two different mechanisms, neither of which has been satisfactorily proven. The "classic theory" postulates that portal hypertension and hypoalbuminemia produce an imbalance of Starling forces across the splanchnic bed with the loss of intravascular volume as ascites. Despite a normal or increased total blood volume, there is a marked increase in splanchnic blood volume (as a result of portal hypertension with venous vasodilation and the development of portosystemic collateral vessels), which, with the third-space loss of ascitic fluid, leads to a decrease in the "effective circulating volume." This is responsible for the decreases in renal blood flow and glomerular filtration rate and stimulation of the renin-angiotensin-aldosterone system, which produce sodium and water retention. This retention of sodium and water further aggravates the ascites. Alternatively, the "overflow theory" postulates that there is a primary abnormality of renal function with progressive sodium and water retention in patients who have intrahepatic and portal hypertension. The cause of this abnormality has yet to be defined; however, a reduction in the responsiveness of the systemic vasculature to catecholamines may be responsible for the vasodilation and low peripheral vascular resistance in cirrhotic patients. This is thought to lead to the redistribution of renal blood flow, reduction in glomerular filtration rate (GFR), increase in renin secretion and aldosterone formation, and sodium and water retention. These changes lead to increased plasma volume and, in the presence of portal hypertension and hypoalbuminemia, produce ascites through overflow of fluid into the hepatic and splanchnic extravascular compartments.[13]

The peritoneovenous shunt has been useful in studying the pathogenesis of ascites in patients with cirrhosis.[4] Acutely, it produces the physiologic maneuver of decompressing the peritoneal cavity and establishing a sustained volume expansion. Studies of shunted patients have been valuable in identifying the role of systemic and renal hemodynamics,[5,20] the renin-angiotensin-aldosterone axis,[5,20] vasopressin,[37] prostaglandins,[40] catecholamines,[7] and atrial natriuretic factor[26] in the etiology of the sodium and water retention observed in these patients.

CLINICAL MANIFESTATIONS OF ASCITES IN CHRONIC LIVER DISEASE

Although the development of ascites usually is chronic, ascitic fluid may accumulate rapidly in the presence of a hepatoma, hepatic vein thrombosis, or acute hepatitis superimposed on chronic cirrhosis. Transient ascites may develop after a laparotomy or from aggressive resuscitation of patients with variceal bleeding with large volumes of fluid. The presence of ascites in the patient with chronic liver disease usually indicates an advanced degree of liver dysfunction and is associated with a poor prognosis. One-year survival statistics of less than 50 per cent have been reported for patients with resistant ascites,[9] a prognosis that is similar to that of patients who have bled from esophageal varices.

In well-compensated cirrhotic patients, a small amount of ascites may go unnoticed, other than for a slight increase in abdominal girth, and requires no treatment. Severe ascites, however, may become grossly disabling with significant interference with activities of daily living. There may be associated pleural effusions and atelectasis with shortness of breath, swelling of the legs, and the development of umbilical and inguinal hernias. Patients with significant ascites are at risk of developing spontaneous bacterial peritonitis. Abdominal distention may produce anorexia and, when combined with therapeutic dietary restrictions, may lead to protein-calorie malnutrition.

MEDICAL TREATMENT OF ASCITES

When ascites becomes symptomatic, treatment is directed toward reduction of, but not necessarily the complete elimination of, ascites. Many patients can be managed with dietary restriction to 400 mg. of sodium and 1 liter of fluid per day. If the ascites is more resistant, diuretics may be added, beginning with an aldosterone antagonist such as spironolactone or amiloride. If this is insufficient, a thiazide or a loop diuretic such as furosemide should be added. In general, loop diuretics should not be used alone because of their tendency to produce potassium depletion. The addition of diuretics to dietary restriction should be done cautiously and, in the patient with massive ascites, should aim to mobilize no more than 1 liter of fluid or 1 kg. of body weight per day.

Serious complications can follow chronic and overly-aggressive use of diuretics in cirrhotic patients, particularly when combined with intermittent therapeutic paracentesis. These include hypokalemia and metabolic alkalosis, hyponatremia, hypocalcemia, and hypomagnesemia. Excessive diuresis can aggravate hypovolemia and produce prerenal failure with oliguria and acute tubular necrosis or may precipitate the hepatorenal syndrome. There is also a problem of compliance in the cirrhotic patient in whom, although controlled in the hospital, ascites redevelops at home.

SURGICAL TREATMENT OF ASCITES

Over 90 per cent of patients with ascites respond to diet and diuretic therapy. In those with persistent ascites and reasonable hepatic function, surgical intervention may be indicated. Surgical procedures for intractable ascites have been directed toward either decreasing production of ascites or increasing its resorption (Table 2).

Paracentesis can be immediately effective in removing all ascites, but rapid reaccumulation occurs, accompanied by a decrease in plasma volume and its attendant risks. Paracentesis alone has been rarely employed for chronic hepatic ascites. Therapeutic paracentesis may be necessary in patients with tense ascites, particularly if the patient is short of breath from the increased intra-abdominal pressure and elevated diaphragm. Paracentesis, combined with reinfusion of filtered ascitic fluid[34] or an equivalent amount of plasma or 5 per cent albumin,[19] provides the same type of palliation as paracentesis alone, but without the risk of hypovolemia. The volume replacement must be carefully titrated so that rapid reaccumulation of the ascites is avoided. More liberal use of repeated paracentesis (4 to 6 liters per day) combined with albumin infusions has been recently reported as being as successful as diuretic therapy in bringing chronic ascites under control;[19] however, these patients must be carefully monitored for complications. Often the effect is only transient, because ascites reaccumulates in most patients. This is, however, a useful temporizing measure in the patient with acute ascites that may occur after portosystemic shunt, particularly a distal splenorenal shunt, to avoid an ascitic leak through the wound.

Physiologic side-to-side portosystemic shunts (side-to-side portacaval, mesocaval, or proximal splenorenal anastomoses) lower pressure in both the splanchnic system and the intrahepatic portal system, which theoretically should decrease the rate of ascites formation. There is substantial evidence from animal models and in patients with the Budd-Chiari syndrome to support the use of side-to-side shunting when both bleeding and uncontrolled ascites require surgical treatment.[33] Side-to-side shunting has been employed for intractable ascites alone; but because of the risk of the procedure plus the risk of postshunt encephalopathy, peritoneovenous shunting has become preferred. More recent experience with portosystemic shunting for ascites in selected patients has confirmed the effectiveness of the operation in controlling ascites, but the 50 per cent incidence of encephalopathy is a strong argument against its general acceptance.[16]

Lymphovenous anastomosis consists of reimplantation of the thoracic duct into the subclavian vein to increase lymph flow and decrease ascites formation. The effectiveness of this therapy is unproved.

Peritoneovenous Shunting

Peritoneovenous shunting is based on an extension of the principles of paracentesis with reinfusion studies and involves the implantation of a prosthetic conduit with a one-way valve between the peritoneal cavity and the intrathoracic vascular compartment. The shunt that has received the most extensive

TABLE 2. Surgical Management of Intractable Ascites

To decrease production of ascites:
 Lymphovenous anastomosis
 Side-to-side portosystemic shunting
 Omentopexy
To increase removal or resorption of ascites:
 Paracentesis
 Paracentesis with reinfusion
 Peritoneovenous anastomosis
 Peritoneovenous shunting

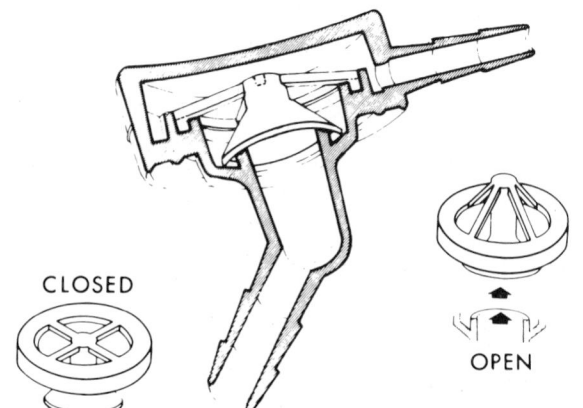

Figure 1. A cross section of the LeVeen valve. Note that the silicone rubber struts are attached to a ring that attaches to the valve casing. The valve is in the normally closed position and opens with 3 cm. of water pressure. (From LeVeen, H. H., et al.: Further experience with peritoneovenous shunt for ascites. Ann. Surg., *184*:574, 1976.)

use and most careful study is that devised by LeVeen and first reported in 1974 (Fig. 1).[30,31] It consists of a pressure-activated one-way valve to which peritoneal and venous Silastic catheters are connected. The pressure gradient between positive intraperitoneal and negative intrathoracic pressures promotes fluid flow from the abdomen to the intravascular space.

Other valves, such as the Denver shunt (Fig. 2),[43] have been developed as alternatives to the LeVeen valve and incorporate features that allow active pumping of fluid from the peritoneal cavity to the venous compartment. Other shunts have incorporated a multimicroorifice filter to remove proteinaceous debris from the ascites fluid.[23] One randomized trial in 21 cirrhotic patients has suggested that the LeVeen valve has a superior patency rate of 40 per cent at 2 years, compared with the Denver shunt; however, survival was similar in the two groups.[17]

INDICATIONS. The most common indication for a peritoneovenous shunt is chronic intractable ascites due to cirrhosis. As many as 10 per cent of patients with significant ascites become refractory to conservative management by diet and diuretic therapy. These patients often require repeated hospital admissions for treatment of ascites and under strict medical supervision on a diet of 20 mEq. of sodium and 1 liter of fluid excrete less than 10 mEq. of sodium per day despite large doses

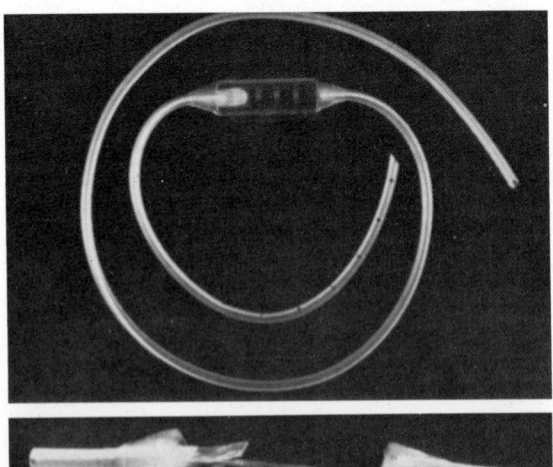

Figure 2. Denver peritoneovenous shunt. The shunt is made of silicone rubber and consists of a fenestrated peritoneal catheter, a pump chamber with a one-way valve, and a venous catheter. The valve is shown magnified with the pump chamber partly removed. (From Turner, W. W., Jr., and Pate, R. M.: The Denver peritoneovenous shunt: Relationship between hepatic reserve and successful treatment of ascites. Am. J. Surg., *144*:619, 1982.)

of diuretics. The results of peritoneovenous shunting vary, depending on the severity of the renal dysfunction and the degree of hepatocellular dysfunction of the patient being shunted. The shunt should not be employed in patients who can be managed with diet and diuretics but should be reserved only for those who fail closely supervised medical management.

The peritoneovenous shunt may also be effective in the treatment of the hepatorenal syndrome. This form of "functional renal failure" must be distinguished from the form of "prerenal" failure that follows central blood volume constriction or acute tubular necrosis. In many of these patients, the peritoneovenous shunt may reverse the hepatorenal syndrome; but because of their advanced liver disease, these patients are at particularly high risk for the procedure and postoperative complications.[12]

Postoperative ascites may develop in the cirrhotic patient following any abdominal operation, but especially following portosystemic shunting procedures. This may be secondary to aggressive intravenous therapy in the perioperative period combined with the division of periportal or retroperitoneal lymphatics at the time of the procedure. Therapeutic paracentesis with maintenance of urinary output by colloid infusion is successful in most patients. If the postoperative ascites is severe and reaccumulates rapidly, an early peritoneovenous shunt is usually effective.

CONTRAINDICATIONS. In general, peritoneovenous shunting is contraindicated in any patient with infected peritoneal fluid or another source of sepsis, acute viral or alcoholic hepatitis, end-stage liver disease, or uncorrectable coagulopathy. A serum bilirubin of more than three times the upper limit of normal has generally been considered a contraindication.[18,41] In addition, the presence of any one of the following risk factors has been reported to be associated with a 50 per cent mortality within the first postoperative month and should be considered a relative contraindication[42]: an episode of gastrointestinal bleeding or peritonitis within the previous month; hepatic encephalopathy greater than Grade 1; complications of alcoholism such as pancreatitis, cardiomyopathy, or neuropathy; an uncomplicated hernia; severe malnutrition; a prothrombin time more than 4 seconds prolonged; and a serum creatinine more than 2.3 times the upper limit of normal (Table 3). Patients who have had a previous significant variceal bleeding remain at risk of rebleeding after peritoneovenous shunting as a result of the transient increase in portal pressure and the coagulopathy that accompany the reinfusion of the ascitic fluid. If the esophageal varices have not been obliterated by repeated injection sclerotherapy, or there has been recent bleeding, patients are better treated by a side-to-side portosystemic shunt.

PROCEDURE

PREOPERATIVE ASSESSMENT. A diagnostic paracentesis is performed to exclude infection (negative culture and a cell count less than 250×10^6 per liter) or malignancy. Liver biopsy (transjugular) and detailed liver tests including coagulation studies are performed. Perioperatively, prophylactic antibiotics, such as a cephalosporin and an aminoglycoside, should be administered to cover both skin and gastrointestinal tract organisms.

OPERATIVE PROCEDURE. The shunt may be inserted under local or general anesthetic (Fig. 3). The LeVeen valve is placed in the abdominal wall deep to the rectus muscle. A pumpable valve (e.g., Denver shunt) is placed over the chest wall or lower end of the sternum. The peritoneal end lies freely in the ascites in the peritoneal cavity. The venous limb is tunneled subcutaneously and may be inserted into the superior vena cava (SVC) via either the internal jugular or the subclavian vein. During the operation, the tip is directed under radiologic control to lie just below the junction of the superior vena cava and the right atrium. A tip that is left too high in the SVC or innominate vein predisposes to catheter blockage and venous thrombosis. Meticulous hemostasis is important in preventing the occurrence of hematoma and

TABLE 3. Risk Factors for Peritoneovenous Shunting

	Group 1	Group 2	Group 3	Group 4
Gastrointestinal bleeding	None or 1 > 1 year ago	At least 1 > 1 month ago	At least 1 > 1 month ago	One within past month
Peritonitis or sepsis	None	At least 1 > 1 month ago	At least 1 > 1 month ago	One within past month
Encephalopathy (grade)	0–1	0–2	0–2	3–5
Complications of alcoholism	None	One mild to moderate	One mild to moderate	Multiple or severe
Other serious illness	None	Uncomplicated hernia	Uncomplicated hernia	Complicated hernia or heart failure
Nutritional index (% of standard)	>80	40–80	40–80	<40
Total bilirubin (mg./100 ml.)	≤3.0	3.1–6.0	≤6.0	>6.0
Prothrombin time (sec. above control)	≤2.0	2.1–4.0	≤6.0	≥6.0
Creatinine (mg./100 ml.)	<1.4	1.4–2.3	≥2.4	>2.4 (with acute or chronic lesion)

Adapted from Stanley, M. M., et al.: Peritoneovenous shunting as compared with medical treatment in patients with alcoholic cirrhosis and massive ascites. N. Engl. J. Med., 321:1632, 1989.

ecchymosis. The incidence of postoperative coagulopathy may be reduced by draining all of the ascitic fluid and replacing it with body-temperature Ringer's lactate.[3,24] The ascitic fluid can be discarded at the time of operation so that the incidence of pulmonary edema is also reduced.[41]

POSTOPERATIVE MANAGEMENT. Postoperatively, prophylactic antibiotics are continued for 48 hours. An abdominal binder is used to increase intra-abdominal pressure, and intrathoracic pressure is intermittently reduced by inspiratory exercises to increase the gradient across the valve and promote ascites flow. Small doses of intravenous furosemide may be necessary for maintaining the urinary output at greater than 60 ml. per minute. Body weight, abdominal girth, and the hematocrit, serum electrolytes, and coagulation status are monitored closely in the postoperative period.

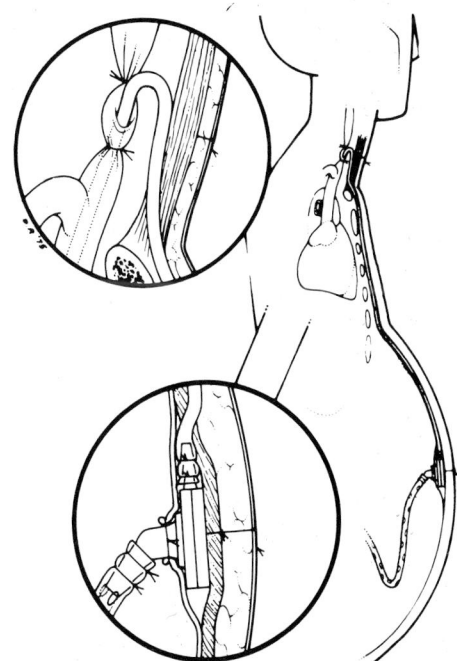

Figure 3. The valve lies outside the peritoneum and deep to the abdominal muscles. The venous collecting tube traverses the subcutaneous tissue of the chest wall into the neck, where it enters the internal jugular vein. The top of the tubing is pushed into the superior vena cava (7.5 cm.). (From LeVeen, H. H., et al.: Further experience with peritoneovenous shunt for ascites. Ann. Surg., 184:574, 1976.)

RESULTS

EARLY (DAYS 1 TO 14). With reinfusion of the ascitic fluid, there is an increase in the total circulating blood volume, a hemodilutional fall in hematocrit, an increase in the cardiac output, and a decrease in the systemic vascular resistance. There is an early rise in renal blood flow and glomerular filtration rate and a resultant decrease in renin and aldosterone levels. In some patients, spontaneous natriuresis and diuresis occur; however, in most, small doses of furosemide are required to produce and maintain the significant diuresis and natriuresis that are characteristic of a functioning shunt and that lead to progressive loss of ascitic fluid documented by abdominal girth and weight changes.[5]

Early postoperative complications occur in up to 80 per cent of patients[2,8,22,24,27] and include infection, leaking of ascitic fluid, variceal hemorrhage, pulmonary edema, coagulation disorders, shunt migration or blockage, and cardiac arrhythmias. In all patients a degree of coagulopathy with prolongation of the prothrombin and partial thromboplastin times and a fall in platelet count develops, and in up to 20 per cent clinical manifestations of disseminated intravascular coagulation (DIC) may develop.[39] The degree of coagulopathy and the incidence of DIC have been reduced by discarding most of the ascites intraoperatively, with or without replacement with saline or Ringer's lactate.[3,24,41] The DIC is treated by temporarily ligating the shunt and providing fresh frozen plasma, cryoprecipitate, and platelets. ε-Aminocaproic acid may also be useful in this setting.[29] The coagulation defect is usually self-limited, resolving after a few days.

Patients undergoing peritoneovenous shunting are a high-risk group for infectious complications as a result of a pre-existing protein-calorie malnutrition and reduced cell-mediated immunity.[14] Previous episodes of spontaneous bacterial peritonitis increase the risk of postoperative shunt infection; and in patients with a prolonged hospitalization immediately prior to operation, the colonizing nosocomial organisms tend to be more virulent. When it occurs, shunt infection is a serious complication that always requires removal of the shunt as well as systemic antibiotics.

Blockage of the shunt may occur by kinking or the formation of a fibrin sheath with the development of a thrombus at the tip of the venous limb or by the collection of fibrin and other peritoneal debris within the valve. The diagnosis of shunt occlusion can be made with either an intraperitoneal injection of technetium-99m sulfur colloid and scanning of the chest[25] or a direct percutaneous injection of radiopaque contrast into the venous limb and imaging of the shunt tip.[38] With the latter technique, a more precise identification of point of occlusion (valve, venous tubing, or intravascular thrombin sheath) can be made. In the event of a blocked valve with a patent venous limb, it is not necessary to revise the complete shunt, but only replace the valve and peritoneal limb.

The operative mortality ranges up to 30 per cent.[22,24,27] The major causes of early death are infection and complications of the underlying liver disease, including hepatic failure and variceal hemorrhage. Variations in operative mortality and survival reported in the literature reflect the severity of the liver disease and renal dysfunction in the groups of patients being selected for shunting procedures.

LATE (1 TO 12 MONTHS). The renal and hemodynamic changes persist in the late postoperative period. Most patients have normal levels of renin and aldosterone and persistent improvement in creatinine clearance and sodium and water excretion. However, many continue to retain sodium when challenged with a diet of 100 mEq. of sodium, and most patients require small doses of diuretics even though the shunt is patent and functioning.[21] Others become ascites-free without diet or diuretic therapy.[14] In some patients, ascites remains under control with diuretics, even if the shunts become blocked.[15]

With the control of ascites, many patients demonstrate an improvement in nutritional status with an increase in serum albumin and transferrin,[14] an improvement in cell-mediated immunity,[14] and an increase in lean body mass[6,14] with an obvious gain in muscle bulk. These improvements probably are a result of improvement and increase in appetite and dietary intake.[6]

Late complications occur in a significant number of surviving patients and include shunt blockage, infection, SVC thrombosis, and small bowel obstruction. The shunt patency rate of 5-year survivors has been reported to be as low as 40 per cent, and the incidence of SVC thrombosis has been over 25 per cent.[15] Most of the late postoperative deaths are due to bleeding esophageal varices and hepatic failure.

Peritoneovenous shunting does not appear to prolong life. One randomized study comparing the peritoneovenous shunt with diuretic therapy in 28 patients refractory to sodium restriction alone suggested improved survival with the shunt.[44] However, two subsequent multicenter, randomized studies of 57 patients in France[8] and 299 males in the United States[24] demonstrated no difference between diet and diuretic therapy and peritoneovenous shunting. The early mortality (30 days) was 20 to 50 per cent, depending on the severity of the liver disease, and the 1-year survival was 25 to 79 per cent. These authors did identify a modest benefit in favor of the shunt, which was limited to control of ascites and was predominantly in the first month. In other uncontrolled series, life survival curves following insertion of the peritoneovenous shunt have been similar to older studies of patients who developed ascites prior to the introduction of the LeVeen valve, with a 50 to 75 per cent 1-year survival and 30 to 40 per cent survival at 2 years.[2,17,18,41]

In cirrhotic patients with intractable ascites, peritoneovenous shunting should be considered as only a palliative procedure. Although the operation is appealing because of its apparent technical simplicity and the dramatic early postoperative diuresis, the postoperative complication rate is significant, particularly in patients with advanced hepatocellular failure. Long-term survival is determined primarily by the natural history of the liver disease.

Patients must be selected carefully. In a patient who is a candidate for liver transplantation, peritoneovenous shunting should be avoided—it is unlikely to alter the course of the underlying liver disease, and the occurrence of SVC thrombosis poses a significant relative contraindication to the transplant operation. Two groups of patients appear to be the best candidates for peritoneovenous shunting: (1) those in whom uncontrollable ascites develops immediately after portosystemic de-

compression or other abdominal surgery and (2) those whose chronic, intractable ascites is disproportionate to the other complications of portal hypertension and end-stage liver disease, particularly hepatocellular dysfunction.

PERITONEOVENOUS SHUNT FOR MALIGNANT ASCITES. Malignant ascites occurs most frequently with intraperitoneal spread of ovarian, colonic, or breast cancer as a result of lymphatic obstruction, peritoneal surface inflammation, or secretion of fluid from a tumor. Approximately half of these patients obtain useful palliation from a combination of paracentesis and chemotherapy and/or radiotherapy. In selected patients who are unresponsive to this treatment and who do not have loculated fluid, peritoneovenous shunting may be indicated.[28]

Complications are similar to those in the cirrhotic population,[11,24] and the operative mortality is similar.[6] Shunt occlusion is more frequent, especially in patients with bloody or viscid ascitic fluid, high protein content (greater than 4.5 gm. per liter), or positive cytology.[10,35] These factors are therefore relative contraindications to its use. Tumor embolism occurs in approximately 5 per cent of patients and occasionally leads to acute respiratory failure and death.[10] Despite these complications, 60 to 75 per cent of patients obtain useful palliation, with the best results occurring in patients with carcinoma of the ovary or breast.[11,36] Median reported survival, however, is only 3 months.[10,11,24,27]

SELECTED REFERENCES

Blendis, L. M., Greig, P. D., Langer, B., Baigrie, R. S., Ruse, J., and Taylor, B. R.: The renal and hemodynamic effects of the peritoneovenous shunt for intractable hepatic ascites. Gastroenterology, 77:250, 1979.
This is a report of the clinical, hemodynamic, and metabolic changes in 15 patients with chronic liver disease having peritoneovenous shunts. The initial rapid movement of fluid into the intravascular compartment is demonstrated by changes in hematocrit and cardiac output. The resultant increases in renal blood flow and creatinine clearance are accompanied by decreases in renin and aldosterone levels. Despite these changes, small doses of furosemide are usually required to produce diuresis and natriuresis. This study also documents the significant complication rate associated with this procedure in poor-risk patients with advanced liver disease.

Bories, P., Compean, D. G., Michel, H., Bourel, M., Capron, J. P., Gauthier, A., Lafon, J., Levy, V. G., Pascal, J. P., Quinton, A., Tournieux, B., and Weill, J. P.: The treatment of refractory ascites by the LeVeen shunt: A multi-centre controlled trial (57 patients). Journal of Hepatology, 3:212, 1986.
This multicenter prospective trial randomized 57 patients with alcoholic cirrhosis and refractory ascites to either LeVeen shunt or conventional medical therapy. Although the LeVeen shunt was more effective in controlling ascites within the first month, there was no difference between medical and surgical groups at 1 year. Moreover, the complication rate was higher in the shunted group (86 per cent), compared with the medical group (29 per cent); and the 1-month mortality was higher in the surgical group (41 per cent versus 18 per cent). At 1 year the mortality of one group was similar to that of the other (79 per cent and 75 per cent). The authors suggest that the poor prognosis for refractory ascites in alcoholics makes the LeVeen shunt inadvisable. The similar survival rates in the medical and surgical groups indicate that the LeVeen shunt does not alter the natural history of alcoholic cirrhosis complicated by ascites. The benefit of improved control of ascites in the first month in the surgical group was negated by the higher mortality in this group. The risk of the operation is dependent upon the degree of preoperative hepatocellular and renal dysfunction. This study suggests that there is a group of patients in whom the risk of LeVeen shunting is prohibitive. The poor overall survival in both medical and surgical groups is similar to that reported historically.

Franco, D., Meakins, J. L., Wu, A., Smadja, C., Bonnet, P., Gouffier, E., and Campillo, B.: Long term results (> 5 years) in patients with peritoneovenous shunting for intractable ascites: liver function and cancer mortality. H.P.B. Surg., 1:185, 1989.
Of the 107 patients receiving a LeVeen shunt from 1976 through 1981, 28 patients survived at least 5 years. Thirty-nine per cent had a patent shunt, and there was SVC thrombosis in 26 per cent. If one combines the 26 per cent 5-year survival with the 39 per cent patency in the survivors, there was a 5-year patency rate of only 12 per cent of the 107 shunts.
This is one of the first reports of the long-term survival and outcome following peritoneovenous shunting. The 26 per cent actual 5-year survival is very low and probably reflects the natural history of the underlying liver disease. The high incidence of SVC thrombosis is significant and represents a significant contraindication for the patient who might be considered for liver transplantation. Of particular interest is the lack of ascites in the patients with blocked shunts. This suggests

that the "sodium-retaining lesion" that these patients had preoperatively is reversible in the long term.

LeVeen, H. H., Christoudias, G., Ip, M., Luft, R., Falk, G., and Grosberg, S.: Peritoneovenous shunting for ascites. Ann. Surg., 180:580, 1974.
This is the first report of the clinical use of the LeVeen valve. It outlines the principle of the pressure-activated valve and the experimental data behind the first clinical application of the device. The dramatic decreases in abdominal girth and weight in conjunction with the increase in urinary output are documented in their first 34 patients. This publication and its follow-up (see LeVeen et al.[31]) are responsible for the popularization of peritoneovenous shunting for intractable hepatic ascites.

Stanley, M. M., Ochi, S., Lee, K. K., Nemchausky, B. A., Greenlee, H. B., Allen J. I., et al.: Peritoneovenous shunting as compared with medical treatment in patients with alcoholic cirrhosis and massive ascites. N. Engl. J. Med., 321:1632, 1989.
This prospective study randomized 299 men with alcoholic cirrhosis and ascites resistant to a standard medical regimen to receive a LeVeen shunt or intensive diet and diuretic therapy. Patients were grouped into four risk categories on the basis of the severity of liver dysfunction, previous complications, and renal dysfunction. The time to resolution of ascites was less for surgical patients; however, within in each risk group both in-hospital mortality and median long-term survival were similar between surgical and medical therapies. The duration of hospitalization was longer in the medical patients, and there was a more rapid recurrence of ascites in the medical group. The authors conclude that peritoneovenous shunting alleviates disabling ascites more rapidly than medical management and delays its recurrence; however, the duration of survival was more closely related to the severity of the illness and was not altered by shunting.
This is an important study that has identified a number of risk factors that constitute contraindications to LeVeen shunting (see Table 3). It is evident that peritoneovenous shunting does not alter the natural history of alcoholic cirrhosis complicated by massive ascites.

REFERENCES

1. Arroyo, V., Bernardi, M., Epstein, M., Henriksen, J. H., Schrier, R. W., and Rodes, J.: Pathophysiology of ascites and functional renal failure in cirrhosis. J. Hepatol., 6:239, 1988.
2. Bernhoft, A., Pellegrini, A., and Way, L. W.: Peritoneovenous shunt for refractory ascites: Operative complications and long-term results. Arch. Surg., 117:631, 1982.
3. Biagini, J. R., Belghiti, J., Fekete, F.: Prevention of coagulopathy after placement of peritoneovenous shunt with replacement of ascitic fluid by normal saline solution. Surg. Gynecol. Obstet., 163:315, 1986.
4. Blendis, L. M.: The use of peritoneovenous shunting in unravelling the pathogenesis of ascites in cirrhosis. Isr. J. Med. Sci., 22:78, 1986.
5. Blendis, L. M., Greig, P. D., Langer, B., Baigrie, R. S., Ruse, J., and Taylor, B. R.: The renal and hemodynamic effects of the peritoneovenous shunt for intractable hepatic ascites. Gastroenterology, 77:250, 1979.
6. Blendis, L. M., Harrison, J. E., Russell, D. M., Miller, C., Taylor, B. R., Greig, P. D., and Langer, B.: Effects of peritoneovenous shunting on body composition. Gastroenterology, 90:127, 1986.
7. Blendis, L. M., Sole, M. J., Campbell, P., Lossing, A. G., Greig, P. D., Taylor, B. R., and Langer, B.: The effect of peritoneovenous shunting on catecholamine metabolism in patients with hepatic ascites. Hepatology, 7:143, 1987.
8. Bories, P., Compean, D. G., Michel, H., Bourel, M., Capron, J. P., Gauthier, A., Lafon, J., Levy, V. G., Pascal, J. P., Quinton, A., Toumieux, B., and Weill, J. P.: The treatment of refractory ascites by the LeVeen shunt: A multi-centre controlled trial (57 patients). J. Hepatol., 3:212, 1986.
9. Capone, R. R., Buhac, I., Kohberger, R. C., et al.: Resistant ascites in alcoholic liver disease: course and prognosis. Dig. Dis. Sci., 23:867, 1979.
10. Cheung, D. K., and Raaf, J. H.: Selection of patients with malignant ascites for a peritoneovenous shunt. Cancer, 50:1204, 1982.
11. Edney, J. A., Hill, A., and Armstrong, D.: Peritoneovenous shunts palliate malignant ascites. Am. J. Surg., 158:598, 1989.
12. Epstein, M.: Peritoneovenous shunt in the management of ascites and the hepatorenal syndrome. Gastroenterology, 82:790, 1982.
13. Epstein, M. (Ed.): The Kidney in Liver Disease, 3rd ed. Baltimore, Williams & Wilkins, 1988.
14. Franco, D., Charra, M., Jeambrun, P., Belghiti, J., Cortesse, A., Sossler, C., and Bismuth, H.: Nutrition and immunity after peritoneovenous drainage of intractable ascites in cirrhotic patients. Am. J. Surg., 146:652, 1983.
15. Franco, D., Meakins, J. L., Wu, A., Smadja, C., Bonnet, P., Gouffier, E., and Campillo, B.: Long term results (> 5 years) in patients with peritoneovenous shunting for intractable ascites: Liver function and cancer mortality. H.P.B. Surg., 1:185, 1989.
16. Franco, D., Vons, C., Traynor, O., and de Smadja, C.: Should portosystemic shunt be reconsidered in the treatment of intractable ascites in cirrhosis? Arch. Surg., 123:987, 1988.
17. Fulenwider, J. T., Galambos, J. D., Smith, R. B., III, Henderson, J. M., and Warren, W. D.: LeVeen vs Denver peritoneovenous shunts for intractable ascites of cirrhosis: A randomized, prospective trial. Arch. Surg., 121:351, 1986.
18. Fulenwider, J. T., Smith, R. B., III, Redd, S. C., Ansley, J. D., Henderson, J. M., Millikan, W. F., Galambos, J. T., and Warren, W. D.: Peritoneovenous shunts: Lessons learned from an eight-year experience with 70 patients. Arch. Surg., 119:1133, 1984.
19. Gines, P., Arroyo, V., Quintero, E., Planas, R., Bory, F., Cabrera, J., Rimola, A., Viver, J., Camps, J., Jimenez, W., Mastai, R., Gaya, J., and Rodes, J.: Comparison of paracentesis and diuretics in the treatment of cirrhotics with tense ascites. Gastroenterology, 93:234, 1987.
20. Greig, P. D., Blendis, L. M., Langer, B., Ruse, J., and Taylor, B. R.: The acute effects of sustained volume expansion on the renin-aldosterone system and renal function in human hepatic ascites. J. Lab. Clin. Med., 98:127, 1981.
21. Greig, P. D., Blendis, L. M., Langer, B., Taylor, B. R., and Cola-pinto, R. F.: Renal and hemodynamic effects of the peritoneovenous shunt. II. Long term effects. Gastroenterology, 80:119, 1981.
22. Greig, P. D., Langer, B., Blendis, L. M., Taylor, B. R., Glynn, M. F. X.: Complications after peritoneovenous shunting for ascites. Am J. Surg., 139:125, 1980.
23. Guzman, E., Wigness, B. D., Dorman, F. D., Rohde, T. D., and Buchwald, H.: A new peritoneovenous shunt. Surgery, 100:691, 1986.
24. Holm, A., Halpern, N. B., and Aldrete, J. S.: Peritoneovenous shunt for intractable ascites of hepatic, nephrogenic, and malignant causes. Am. J. Surg., 158:162, 1989.
25. Kirchmer, N., and Hart, U.: Radionuclide assessment of LeVeen shunt patency. Ann. Surg., 185:145, 1977.
26. Klepetko, W., Muller, C., Hartter, E., Miholics, J., Schwarz, C., Woloszczuk, W., and Moeschl, P.: Plasma atrial natriuretic factor in cirrhotic patients with ascites: Effect of peritoneovenous shunt implantation. Gastroenterology, 95:764, 1988.
27. Kostroff, K. M., Ross, D. W., and Davis, J. M.: Peritoneovenous shunting for cirrhotic versus malignant ascites. Surg. Gynecol. Obstet., 161:204, 1985.
28. Lacy, J. H., Wieman, T. J., and Shively, E. H.: Management of malignant ascites. Surg. Gynecol. Obstet., 159:397, 1984.
29. LeVeen, H. H., Ahmed, N., Hutto, R. B., Ip, M., and LeVeen, E. G.: Coagulopathy post peritoneovenous shunt. Ann. Surg., 205:305, 1987.
30. LeVeen, H. H., Christoudias, G., Ip, M., Luft, R., Falk, G., and Grosberg, S.: Peritoneo-venous shunting for ascites. Ann. Surg., 180:580, 1974.
31. LeVeen, H. H., Wapnick, S., Grosberg, S., and Kinney, M. J.: Further experience with peritoneo-venous shunt for ascites. Ann. Surg., 184:574, 1976.
32. Levy M.: Pathophysiology of the hepatorenal syndrome and potential for therapy. Am. J. Cardiol., 60:661, 1987.
33. Orloff, M. J.: Pathogenesis and surgical treatment of intractable ascites associated with alcoholic cirrhosis. Ann. N.Y. Acad. Sci., 170:202, 1970.
34. Parboo, S.P., Ajdukiewicz, A., and Sherlock, S.: Treatment of ascites by continuous ultrafiltration of plasma and reinfusion of protein concentrate. Lancet, 1:949, 1974.
35. Qazi, R., and Savlov, E. D.: Peritoneovenous shunt for palliation of malignant ascites. Cancer, 49:600, 1982.
36. Reinhold, R. B., Lokich, J. J., Tomashefski, J. and Costello, P.: Management of malignant ascites with peritoneovenous shunting. Am. J. Surg., 145:455, 1983.
37. Reznick, R. K., Langer, B., Taylor, B. R., Seif, S., and Blendis, L. M.: Hyponatraemia and arginine vasopressin secretion in patients with refractory hepatic ascites undergoing peritoneovenous shunting. Gastroenterology, 84:713, 1983.
38. Schwartz, M. L., and Miller, R. P.: Angiographic assessment of peritoneovenous shunt malfunction. Arch. Surg., 116:435, 1981.
39. Schwartz, M. L., Swaim, W. R., and Vogel, S. B.: Coagulopathy following peritoneovenous shunting. Surgery, 85:671, 1979.
40. Shaw-Stiffel, T., Campbell, P. J., Sole, M. J., Greig, P. D., Wong, P. Y., and Blendis, L. M.: Renal prostaglandin E_2 and other vasoactive modulators in refractory hepatic ascites: response to peritoneovenous shunting. Gastroenterology, 95:1332, 1988.
41. Smadja, C., Franco, D.: The LeVeen shunt in the elective treatment of intractable ascites in cirrhosis. Ann. Surg., 201:488, 1985.
42. Stanley, M. M., Ochi, S., Lee, K. K., Nemchausky, B. A., Greenlee, H. B., Allen, J. I., et al.: Peritoneovenous shunting as compared with medical treatment in patients with alcoholic cirrhosis and massive ascites. N. Engl. J. Med., 321:1632, 1989.
43. Turner, W. W., and Pate, R. M.: The Denver peritoneovenous shunt: Relationship between hepatic reserve and successful treatment of ascites. Am. J. Surg., 144:619, 1982.
44. Wapnick, S., Grosberg, S. J., and Evans, M. I.: Randomized prospective matched pair study comparing peritoneovenous shunt and conventional therapy in massive ascites. Br. J. Surg., 66:667, 1979.

VII

VIRAL HEPATITIS AND THE SURGEON

John D. Hamilton, M.D.

Much has been learned about viral hepatitis in the past two decades, and although this entity is not strictly a surgical disease, it is of considerable importance to both the surgical patient and the surgeon. This section summarizes some current concepts about hepatitis. Excellent texts, monographs, symposia, and papers should be consulted for more detailed consideration of specific points.[6,12,38,52,57]

DEFINITION

Viral hepatitis is an infection of the liver caused by one of five groups of viruses: hepatitis A (HAV), formerly infectious hepatitis; hepatitis B (HBV), formerly serum hepatitis; hepatitis C (HCV), the recently recognized virus that is associated with parenterally transmitted non-A, non-B hepatitis (PT-NANB); hepatitis D (HDV), known also as delta-associated hepatitis; and hepatitis E (HEV), the virus responsible for enterically transmitted non-A, non-B hepatitis (ET-NANB).

ETIOLOGY

VIRUS CHARACTERIZATION. Selected features of each viral agent are listed in Table 1. Until fairly recently, the causes of viral hepatitis were not distinguished other than by certain epidemiologic criteria. It is evident from Table 1, however, that the viral causes are very different. Other viral agents such as cytomegalovirus (CMV), Epstein-Barr virus (EBV), and rubella affect the liver as well, but usually only as a part of a more general systemic disease.

NOMENCLATURE. New terminology has been developed to describe the hepatitis virus antigens and antibodies, and familiarity with the terms and their meanings is essential to the understanding of this group of diseases. The currently recommended terms and their interpretation are shown in Table 2.

To date, no antigens common to two or more viral agents have been identified. Within each class of virus, no differences in the virulence or the nature of the ultimate disease have been found between subtypes or strains. Whereas all of these agents are infectious for animals, have been visualized by electron microscopy, and, in one case, HAV, have been cultured *in vitro*, the standard diagnostic tests are serologic, specific for viral antigens and IgG and IgM antibodies.

PATHOGENESIS

The pathogenesis of viral hepatitis is incompletely understood, but two alternative theories have been proposed as mechanisms for the viral-induced diseases. One hypothesis suggests direct cytopathogenicity of liver cells by virus, and the other proposes humoral and cell-mediated immunopathogenetic mechanisms for all types of viral hepatitis. It is possible that both mechanisms occur sequentially. The extrahepatic manifestations of HBV, HCV, and HDV are thought to be due to the localization of antigen-antibody complexes in the affected tissue (synovium, arteries, kidneys, and skin).[23,24]

EPIDEMIOLOGY

A consideration of the trends in occurrence, risk factors, and modes of transmission is extremely important to the understanding of viral hepatitis. In 1988, 26,000 cases of HAV, 22,000 cases of HBV, and 2500 cases of NANB were reported to the Centers for Disease Control. From these figures, they project that there are 300,000 cases of HBV and 5000 deaths due to viral-induced cirrhosis and hepatocellular carcinoma per year in the U.S. Generally, hepatitis A has been decreasing but represents about 50 per cent of all reported cases of hepatitis. Hepatitis B and PT-NANB hepatitis (HCV) have been increasing and comprise 40 and 10 per cent, respectively, of the reported cases.

TABLE 1. Characteristics of the Hepatitis Viruses

Virus	Virus Family/ Genus	Size	Nucleic Acid	Sequenced and/or Cloned	Grown in Tissue Culture	Identified by Electron Microscopy	Specific Serologic Tests	Infectious for Animals	Special Characteristics
HAV	Picornaviridae/ Enterovirus 72	27 nm.	Single-stranded RNA	Yes	Yes	Yes	Yes	Yes	—
HBV	Hepadnaviridae* Hepadnavirus type 1	42 nm. Dane particle	Primarily circular, double-stranded DNA	Yes	Yes†	Yes	Yes	Yes	
		22 nm. surface antigen							
HCV	Togavirus-like	36–62 nm.	Positive strand RNA	Yes	No	Yes	Yes	Yes	—
HDV	Defective virus	35–37 nm.	Negative strand RNA	Yes	No	Yes	Yes	Yes	Requires HBV for replication
HEV	Calicivirus-like	27–32 nm.	Unknown	No	No	Yes	Yes	Yes	Recognized only in developing countries

* Proposed.
† Reported but unconfirmed.

TABLE 2. Nomenclature of the Hepatitis Virus Antigens and Antibodies and their General Interpretation

Virus	Antigens		Antibodies	
	Name	Interpretation	Name	Interpretation
Hepatitis A virus (HAV)	HA Ag (major antigen of HAV)*	Acute infection	Anti-HA IgG IgM	Immune to HAV Recurrent or current acute infection
Hepatitis B virus (HBV)	HBsAg (surface antigen of HBV) Subtypes adr, adw, ayw, ayr HBcAg (core antigen of HBV)* HBeAg (core-related antigen)	Prior exposure to HBV Distinctive strains of HBV Infectivity—acute or chronic Infectivity—acute or chronic	Anti-HBs Anti-HBc Anti-HBe	Immune to HBV Early or late convalescence or chronic hepatitis Late convalescence
Post-transfusion non-A, non-B hepatitis virus (HCV)	Not available	Not available	Anti-HBc*	Immune to HCV
Delta-associated agent (HDV)	Delta antigen*	Acute delta-associated hepatitis	Anti-delta	Immune to delta-associated hepatitis (low titer) or chronic HDV
Enterically transmitted non-A, non-B hepatitis virus (HEV)	Virus-like particles by immune electron microscopy*	Acute infection	Anti-HEV*	Immune to HEV

* Research methods only.

A mortality of 0.8 per cent has been associated with these cases.[33]

Some of the epidemiologic characteristics relative to disease transmission are summarized in Table 3. HAV and HEV are transmitted, by the fecal-oral route, as might occur with close personal contact or the ingestion of contaminated food or water. Both HAV and HEV are present in the feces of infected patients during the 1 to 2 weeks preceding and the 1 to 2 weeks following the onset of clinical disease, but there is no known chronic fecal carrier. Theoretically, both viral infections have a brief viremic period and could therefore be transmitted parenterally, but this is considered to be most unlikely. Moreover, HEV has not been recovered yet in the U.S. Hepatitis A and HEV, therefore, do not appear to constitute any special risk for the surgeon.

HBV, HCV, and HDV are typically, but not exclusively, transmitted by parenteral routes.[1,6,36,37,52] HBV is present in high concentrations in the blood and in nearly all other body fluids but may not be present in an infectious form in feces owing to enzymatic inactivation. It is worthwhile to emphasize that HBsAg is not infectious itself but rather serves as a marker for the possible presence of the infectious virus, which is most accurately measured by the core (HBcAg) and core-related antigens (HBeAg). No viral markers currently exist to identify HCV antigen/virus.

The classic route of transmission of HBV and HCV is by transfused blood.[6,7] This mechanism is facilitated by the capability of HBV and HCV to exist as asymptomatic but infectious viruses in the serum of otherwise normal blood donors or patients with other conditions, making the period of infectivity potentially very long. HDV, a defective virus that requires HBV for replication, is not known to exist as a chronic, asymptomatic viremia. It is of particular importance to recognize that blood and blood products from different sources have a greater or lesser risk of possessing infectious virus. Most whole blood and its derivatives, which are not prepared by pooling of units, have a relatively smaller risk of inducing infection with HBV. This is largely due to the infrequency of HBV presence in the normal adult population, the exclusion of potentially infected donors, and, perhaps most important, the routine testing of donor blood for HBsAg. Preparations generally considered to be safe include serum albumin, thrombin, profibrinolysin, fibrinolysin, immune serum globulin (ISG), and all hyperimmune globulins. Higher-risk blood and blood products are those derived from commercial as opposed to volunteer donors and from pools of plasma and clotting factors, including I, II, VII, IX, and X.[13,21,32,42,45,54] Washed and frozen human blood cells are not reliably virus-free.[2] Moreover, since no tests are available to exclude HCV and HDV viruses from blood or blood products, none of the aforementioned measures are known to eliminate this virus. As might be expected, then, post-transfusion hepatitis is most often due to HCV.[3] Recently, however, donated blood is subjected to testing for elevation of alanine aminotransferase (ALT) and HBcAg as surrogate markers to identify blood more likely to be infected with HCV. Hepatitis due to HBV, HCV, or HDV may be acquired by other parenteral routes more commonly in the individual who uses intravenous drugs. The prevalence of hepatitis in this group approaches 100 per cent. Other predictable means of exposure include accidental needlestick or accidental injury such as might occur during a surgical procedure. It is this occupational risk that represents a

TABLE 3. Epidemiology of Viral Hepatitis Transmission

Virus	Major Infectious Body Fluid	Route*				
		Transfusion/ IV Drug Use	Fecal/Oral	Sexual	Vertical	Occupational
HAV	Feces	−	4+	1+	−	+/−
HBV	Blood and other body fluids	−/4+	+/−	3+	3+	3+
HCV	Blood	2+/4+	+/−	1+	+/−	2+
HDV	Blood	−/4+	1+	3+	3+	−
HEV	Feces	−	4+	Unknown	Unknown	Unknown

* Estimates of the relative frequency and/or efficiency.

continuous threat during the period of a surgical career and that constitutes the basis for individual protection through careful surgical procedures, appropriate surveillance when necessary, and HBV vaccine for all surgical personnel.

There is strong evidence that HAV and HEV certainly, but also HBV and HCV viruses, may be transmitted by close, personal contact. Sexual transmission is a route for HAV, HBV, and probably HCV.[4,5,20,51] It is not possible at present to quantitate the frequency of nonparenteral transmission in nonepidemic circumstances, but episodes of hepatitis B and HCV occur without a prior known opportunity for parenteral inoculation. It appears likely that the efficiency of disease transmission is much lower in these cases.

Vertical transmission *in utero* and perinatal transmission occur with HBV, HCV, and HDV. Occupational exposure is a realistic possibility for HBV and HCV particularly and a much lower possibility for HAV and HDV.

Previous experience with one of the hepatitis viruses does not protect against a subsequent infection with any of the others. Apparent second cases of the same viral disease are more likely to result from a chronic infection, a relapse, or, most likely, a new infection with an unrelated virus.[41]

CLASSIFICATION AND CLINICAL DISEASE

All five hepatitis viruses cause a wide spectrum of clinical disease, and in the majority of instances the resultant syndromes are indistinguishable. Some of the characteristic clinical events are summarized in Table 4. Typically, there are three more frequent types of infection: (1) inapparent and asymptomatic, (2) anicteric but symptomatic, and (3) icteric and symptomatic. The precise incidence of these alternatives is unknown, but inapparent disease appears to occur several to many times more frequently than symptomatic clinical disease, especially in children. The clinical illness typically found in about 90 per cent of symptomatic patients may include lassitude, anorexia, weakness, nausea, dark urine, fever, vomiting, headache, chills, and abdominal discomfort, other miscellaneous symptoms occurring somewhat less commonly.[40] Laboratory abnormalities reflect liver cell necrosis including primarily an elevation of aminotransferase and, less commonly, elevations of alkaline phosphatase and bilirubin.[14,29,39,44] Tests for viral antigens and antibodies are helpful to make specific diagnoses.[22] The usual sequence of events is illustrated in Figure 1; additional information regarding the interpretation of these tests is provided in Table 2.

In most typical cases of viral hepatitis, the pathologic findings in the liver consist of combinations of portal, periportal, and lobular hepatitis. There is an accumulation of inflammatory cells and parenchymal cell necrosis throughout the liver.[34] Differences in histopathology generally correlate with the clinical severity and resolve completely with recovery from the illness.

The management of hepatitis is supportive, without need or demonstrated value of any known intervention. This includes attention to normal nutrition, avoidance of hepatotoxins, and activity as tolerated. Antibiotics and immune serum globulin are of no known benefit. Recovery is complete in about 85 to 90 per cent of patients in 2 to 6 weeks following the onset of illness.[43] Apart from the occasional patient ($<$ 1 to 2 per cent) with HAV who develops fulminant hepatitis or relapsing clinical illness over a period of several weeks, there are no further complications of this viral infection. HEV appears to act similarly, although a particular predilection for pregnant women has been noted.

HBV and HCV, however, have variants of typical disease. In sum, they represent the course of 10 and 30 per cent of the clinically detectable cases of HBV and HCV, respectively. With respect to hepatitis B, atypical manifestations include those that are atypical by virtue of the type of abnormality and those that are atypical by virtue of the severity or duration of the abnormality. Regarding the first possibility, extrahepatic manifestations of hepatitis B most frequently occur in the form of arthralgias, predominantly involving the small joints.[46] Other reported "immune phenomena" include arteritis, nephritis, and dermatitis.[23] Extrahepatic manifestations occur with HCV and HDV as well. Viral hepatitis may atypically present with a primarily cholestatic profile of liver function abnormalities, particularly HCV.[49] Such patients may have profound jaundice and itching but no anatomic obstruction of the biliary system.

Atypical viral hepatitis manifestations differing in duration or severity may be classified as follows, as defined by the expert panel contributing to the Hepatitis Knowledge Base.[11]

Benign Sequelae
1. Prolonged viral hepatitis
2. Relapsing viral hepatitis
3. Posthepatitis hyperbilirubinemia
4. Chronic persistent hepatitis
5. Carrier

Serious Sequelae
1. Fulminant hepatitis
2. Chronic aggressive hepatitis
3. Viral hepatitis with confluent hepatitis necrosis
4. Cirrhosis
5. Hepatoma

A brief consideration will be given to each of these atypical presentations. *Prolonged viral hepatitis* is defined simply as typical acute disease lasting 4 to 12 months. It differs from *relapsing viral hepatitis* in that the latter resolves within several months but only after an unsettling relapse or two of typical disease. *Prolonged viral hepatitis* is not easily distinguished from *chronic persistent hepatitis*, which appears to share most of its features.[11,19] All three entities share the features of an ultimately self-limited disease, no demonstrated effective therapy, and no sequelae. *Posthepatitis hyperbilirubinemia* may persist as the sole

TABLE 4. Clinical Characteristics and Consequences of Viral Hepatitis

Virus	Asymptomatic (%)	Incubation Period	Acute	Extrahepatic Manifest.	Fulminant/ Mortality	Chronic Hepatitis			Associated with Cirrhosis/Hepatocellular Carcinoma
						Persistent	Aggressive	Carrier	
HAV	Children $>$80% Adults $<$20%	25 days	+	−	+/1–4%	−	−	−	−/−
HBV	$>$50%	75 days	+	+	+/1–4%	2–4%	2–4%	5%	+/+
HCV	75%	14–28 days	+	+	+/0.1– 0.2%	15%	30%	+(?%)	+/−
HDV	Unknown	28–90 days	+	+	+/+	2–4%	2–4%	5%	+/−
HEV	Unknown*	22–60 days	+	−	+/+ pregnant women	−	−	−	−

* Usually recognized as part of epidemic.

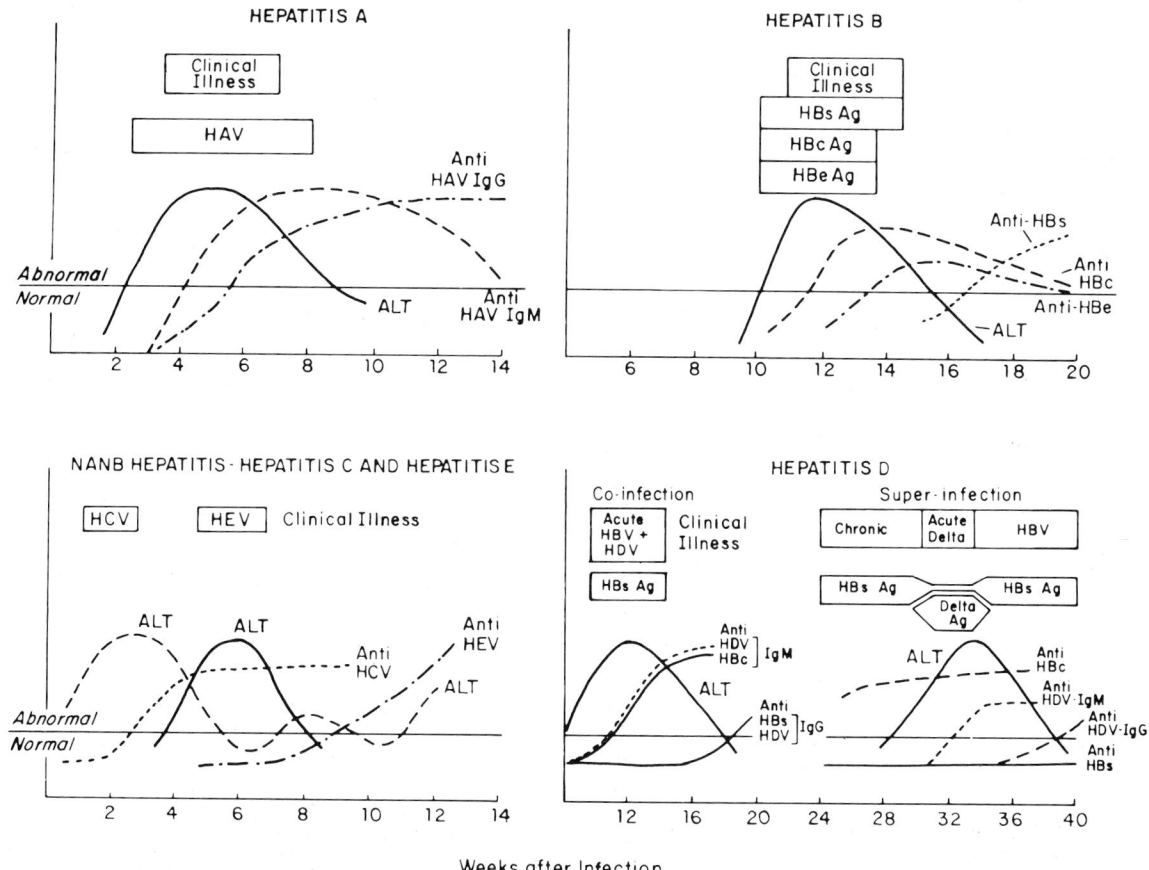

Figure 1. Laboratory findings in hepatitis A and hepatitis B.

abnormality, in the presence of normal liver histology, following typical acute viral hepatitis, only to resolve spontaneously.

Carriers of HBsAg about whom most is known are asymptomatic and represent less than 1 per cent of normal populations in this country, although worldwide there are estimated to be about 216 million carriers.[33] Acute HBV infections result in long-term carriage of HBsAg and sometimes other markers of HBV in approximately 5 per cent of clinically identified cases. It is not unusual to lack a history of prior infection. The carrier may or may not be infectious. Currently there are no available tests which make that distinction, but several guidelines may be useful: (1) the closer the HBsAg-positive individual is to his acute infection, (2) the higher the titer of anti-HBc, (3) the higher the titer of HBeAg, and (4) the more immunocompromised the carrier, the more likely the carrier is to be infectious. In contrast, the presence of antibodies to HBsAg or HBeAg makes the individual less likely to be infectious. From a practical point of view, all carriers should be considered potentially infectious, particularly when an invasive procedure is contemplated. Judgments as to the timing for a surgical procedure are, of course, dictated primarily by the indications for operation. In elective procedures, however, when it is not possible to distinguish the true chronic carrier from an individual with incubating acute viral hepatitis, a period of observation is a worthwhile precaution to allow the circumstances to clarify. HCV carriers are of less certain importance. That they occur appears certain in view of the frequency of post-transfusion hepatitis.

Of some concern to the surgeon is the possibility that he may be or will become a carrier of HBV or HCV.[25] Although the risk to patients has not been conclusively defined, most agree that disease transmission from physician to patients is a very unusual event and that common hygienic measures, not to mention scrupulous surgical technique, reduce that risk perhaps to

the vanishing point.[30,35] Therefore, no authorities on this subject wish or are prepared to institute control measures that might preclude further practice of their profession. Routine determination of HBsAg or HCV markers in asymptomatic physicians is not currently recommended.

Of the serious sequelae, *acute fulminant viral hepatitis* occurs unpredictably, and hepatic encephalopathy, coagulation defects, renal failure, and death may supervene within 4 weeks. No specific intervention, including exchange transfusion, steroids, or hyperimmune globulin, has been found useful. *Chronic aggressive hepatitis* (CAH) and *viral hepatitis with confluent hepatic necrosis* (subacute hepatic necrosis, or SHN) appear to represent points on a spectrum from more to less advanced and chronic disease.[11,56] A prior episode of typical hepatitis may or may not have occurred. Pathologically, SHN shows necrosis of hepatocytes with bridging, cholestasis, and early scar formation. CAH shows piecemeal necrosis and lymphocyte infiltration of portal tracts and lobules. Corticosteroids have been used for both conditions, but beneficial results have not been proved. Either entity may progress to *cirrhosis* with its complications. Finally, there is an association between *hepatoma* (hepatocellular carcinoma) and HBV, suggesting the oncogenic potential of this virus.[8,9] No association with carcinoma has been identified with other classes of hepatitis virus.

HCV appears to cause chronic hepatitis even more frequently than HBV. Initially, chronic hepatitis due to HCV was considered to be more benign than that associated with HBV.[10] Subsequently, however, in follow-up biopsy studies, as many as 30 per cent of the originally detected CAH had become cirrhosis.[55]

Since HDV does not cause disease in the absence of HBV, the contribution to chronicity is somewhat complicated. Available evidence suggests that chronic HDV infection worsens the microscopic presentation and accelerates the liver disease.[15,16,52,55]

TABLE 5. Recommendations for Use of Immune Globulins

Virus Exposure	Time of Evaluation	Nature of Exposure	Immune Globulin Recommended	
			ISG*	HBIG†
HAV	Pre-exposure	Travel to endemic area	+	NA
	Postexposure	Household	+	NA
		School or work	−	NA
		Institution	+	NA
		Primate handler	+	NA
		Medical and paramedical personnel	+	NA
		Common-source epidemic	+	NA
HBV	Pre-exposure	Personnel or family members attending an infected patient	+	−
	Postexposure	Parenteral		
		Transfusion of HBsAg-positive blood	−	+
		Accidental		
		Needle-stick or surgical injury or blood on open wound or mucous membrane	−	+
		Nonparenteral		
		Intimate contact	+	−
		Postnatal	−	+
HCV	Postexposure	Parenteral		
		Transfusion	+	−
		Accidental	+	−
HDV	−	−	−	−
HEV	−	−	−	−

* ISG dose 0.01 to 0.02 ml. per kg. body weight within 14 days of exposure if possible
† HBIG dose 0.05 to 0.07 ml. per kg. within 7 days of exposure and repeated 1 month later

PREVENTION

General measures, including case finding and attention to standard principles of cleanliness and hygiene and specific measures directed toward the interdiction of recognized modes of transmission, are the mainstays of disease prevention for all hepatitis viruses.[27] Unfortunately, these methods are only partially successful, and the need for consideration of passive immunity or active immunization is common. The current recommendations for the use of immune serum globulin or hyperimmune hepatitis B immune globulin are summarized in Table 5. There is general, but not complete, agreement on these recommendations among authorities.[33,47,48]

Active immunization is now commercially available for HBV. The recommended indications are summarized in Table 6. One vaccine (Heptavax B, Merck, Sharp and Dohme) has been widely tested in randomized, controlled, double-blind trials. Normal recipients of vaccine develop high titers of antibody to HBsAg and are protected against naturally acquired disease, and the vaccine has been conclusively shown to be safe. Other vaccine preparations are now available that have been prepared by recombinant DNA technology (Recombivax, Merck, Sharp

TABLE 6. Hepatitis Vaccine Recommendations

	HBIG	Vaccine
HBV pre-exposure		
Health care workers	−	+
Institutions for mentally retarded		
Staff	−	+
Clients	−	+
Hemodialysis patients	−	+
Homosexually active males	−	+
Illicit injectable drug users	−	+
Recipients of certain blood products	−	+
Household and sexual contacts of HBV carriers	−	+
HBV postexposure		
Perinatal	+	+
Percutaneous	+	+
Sexual	+	+

and Dohme; and Energix, Smith, Kline and French). These preparations have been demonstrated to be immunogenic and safe.[18,28,33,50,53] This method of disease prevention should be very important in the prevention of disease in selected high-risk populations.[25,31,33] Booster immunization has not yet been recommended by the CDC. Although several vaccines for HAV are being tested, none are commercially available.

TREATMENT

There are no currently accepted, effective modes of specific therapy for any of the types of viral hepatitis. Trials have been reported, however, of a variety of agents including alpha interferon. Critical analysis of these trials, however, does not reveal compelling evidence of efficacy.[17,33]

SELECTED REFERENCES

Arankalle, V. A., Ticehurst, J., Sreenivasan, M. A., et al.: Aetiological association of a virus-like particle with enterically transmitted non-A, non-B hepatitis. Lancet, 1:550, 1988.
Although hepatitis E has not been recognized in the U.S., its description in this paper is among the very first to confirm a second cause of non-A, non-B hepatitis. The epidemiologic distinctions from HCV are nicely outlined, as are some of the basic virologic features.

Beasley, R. P.: Hepatitis B virus: The major etiology of hepatocellular carcinoma. Cancer, 61:1942, 1988.
This paper details the evidence that implicates HBV as the cause of hepatocellular carcinoma from an epidemiologic point of view. It summarizes the author's own seminal work done in government workers in Taiwan.

Choo, Q. L., Kuo, G., Weiner, A. J., et al.: Isolation of a cDNA clone derived from a blood-borne non-A, non-B viral hepatitis genome. Science, 244:359, 1989.
This is the first description of a portion of the molecular composition of one of the causes of non-A, non-B hepatitis, now called hepatitis C. Identified by a novel molecular method, this discovery is of major importance in the study of the various causes of viral hepatitis.

Proceedings of an International Symposium on Hepatitis Delta Virus. Rizzetto, M., Gerin, J. L., and Purcell, R. H. (Eds.). Saint Vincent, Italy, Alan R. Liss, Inc., 1987.
For the reader interested in the latest information on HDV or delta hepatitis, this book is essential. This viral infection is discussed from nearly every perspective — basic science, epidemiology, clinical features, prevention, and treatment.

Viral Hepatitis and Liver Disease. Proceedings of the International Symposium on Viral Hepatitis and Liver Disease. Zuckerman, A. J. (Ed.). London, Alan R. Liss, Inc., 1988.
This volume is a compendium of the most recent information available from international authorities on viral hepatitis. It is an especially useful reference for accurate, up-to-date information on a wide range of subjects.

REFERENCES

1. Aach, R. D., Szmuness, W., Mosley, J. W., Hollinger, F. B., Kahn, R. A., Stevens, C. E., Edwards, V. M. and Werch, J.: Serum alanine aminotransferase of donor in relation to the risk of non-A, non-B hepatitis in recipients. N. Engl. J. Med., *304*:989, 1981.
2. Alter, H. J., Tabor, E., Meryman, H. T., Hoofnagle, J. H., Kahn, R. A., Holland, P. V., Gerety, R. J., and Barker, L. F.: Transmission of hepatitis B virus infection by transfusion of frozen deglycerolized red blood cells. N. Engl. J. Med., *298*:637, 1978.
3. Alter, M. J.: Non-A, non-B hepatitis: Sorting through a diagnosis of exclusion. Ann. Intern. Med., *110*:583, 1989.
4. Alter, M. J., Ahtone, J., Weisfuse, I., Starko, K., Vacalis, T. D., and Maynard, J. E.: Hepatitis B virus transmission between heterosexuals. J.A.M.A., *256*:1307, 1986.
5. Alter, M. J., Coleman, P. J., Alexander, W. J., Kramer, E., Miller, J. K., Mandel, E., Hadler, S. C., and Margolis, H. S.: Importance of heterosexual activity in the transmission of hepatitis B and non-A, non-B hepatitis. J.A.M.A., *262*:1201, 1989.
6. Alter, M. J., Hadler, S. C., Francis, D. P., and Maynard, J. E.: The epidemiology of non-A, non-B hepatitis in the U.S. *In* Dodd, R. Y., and Barker, L. F. (Eds.): Infection, Immunity and Blood Transfusion. New York, Alan R. Liss, Inc., 1985, p. 71.
7. Barker, L. F., and Murray, R.: Relationship of virus dose of incubation time of clinical hepatitis and time of appearance of hepatitis-associated antigen. Am. J. Med. Sci., *263*:27, 1972.
8. Beasley, R. P.: Hepatitis B virus. The major etiology of hepatocellular carcinoma. Cancer, *61*:1942, 1988.
9. Beasley, R., Hwang, L-Y., Lin, C-C., and Chien, C-S.: Hepatocellular carcinoma and hepatitis B virus: A prospective study of 22,707 men in Taiwan. Lancet, *2*:1129, 1981.
10. Berman, M., Alter, H. J., Ishak, K. G., Purcell, R. H., and Jones, E. A.: The chronic sequelae of non-A, non-B hepatitis. Ann. Intern. Med., *91*:1, 1979.
11. Bernstein, L. H., Koff, R. S., Siegel, E. R., Merritt, A. D., Goldstein, C. M., and Panel, E.: The hepatitis knowledge base—a prototype information transfer system. Ann. Intern. Med., *93*:169, 1980.
12. Blumberg, B. S.: Polymorphisms of the serum proteins and the development of iso-precipitin in transfused patients. Bull. N.Y. Acad. Med., *40*:377, 1964.
13. Boeve, N. R., Winterscheid, L. C., and Merendino, K. A.: Fibrinogen-transmitted hepatitis in the surgical patient. Ann. Surg., *170*:833, 1969.
14. Boggs, J. D., Melnick, J. L., Conrad, M. E., and Felsher, B. F.: Viral hepatitis: Clinical and tissue culture studies. J.A.M.A., *214*:1041, 1970.
15. Bonino, A., Negro, F., Baldi, M., Brunetto, M. R., Chiaberge, E., Capalbo, M., Maran, E., Lavarini, C., Rocca, N., and Rocca, G.: The natural history of chronic delta hepatitis. Prog. Clin. Biol. Res., *234*:145, 1987.
16. Bonino, F., Smedile, A., and Verme, G.: Hepatitis delta virus infection. Adv. Intern. Med., *32*:345, 1987.
17. Burke, C. A.: A statistical view of clinical trials in chronic hepatitis B. J. Hepatol., *3*:S261, 1986.
18. Centers for Disease Control: Hepatitis B virus vaccine safety: Report of an inter-agency group. M.M.W.R., *31*:465, 1982.
19. Chadwick, R. G., Galizzi, J. Jr., Heathcote, J., Lyssiotis, T., Cohen, B. J., Scheuer, P. J., and Sherlock, S.: Chronic persistent hepatitis: Hepatitis B virus markers and histologic follow-up. Gut, *20*:372, 1979.
20. Corey, L., and Holmes, K. K.: Sexual transmission of hepatitis A in homosexual men: Incidence and mechanism. N. Engl. J. Med., *302*:435, 1980.
21. Craske, J., Dilling, N., and Stern, D.: An outbreak of hepatitis associated with intravenous injection of factor VIII concentration. Lancet, *2*:221, 1975.
22. Czaja, A. J.: Serologic markers of hepatitis A and B in acute and chronic liver disease. Mayo Clin. Proc., *54*:721, 1979.
23. Dienstag, J. L.: Immunopathogenesis of the extrahepatic manifestations of hepatitis B virus infection. Springer Semin. Immunopathol., *3*:461, 1981.
24. Dienstag, J., Bhan, A., Klingenstein, R., and Savarese, A.: Immunopathogenesis of liver disease associated with hepatitis B. *In* Szmuness, W., Alter, H., and Maynard, J. E. (Eds.): Viral Hepatitis. Philadelphia, Franklin Institute Press, 1982, p. 221.
25. Dienstag, J. L., and Ryan, D. M.: Occupational exposure to hepatitis B virus in hospital personnel: Infection or immunization. Am. J. Epidemiol., *115*:26, 1982.
26. Dienstag, J. L., Szmuness, W., Stevens, C. E., et al.: Hepatitis A virus infection: New insights from sero-epidemiological studies. J. Infect. Dis., *137*:328, 1978.
27. Favero, M. S., Maynard, J. E., Leger, R. T., Graham, D. R., and Dixon, R. E.:

Guidelines for the care of patients hospitalized with viral hepatitis. Ann. Intern. Med., *91*:872, 1979.
28. Francis, D., Hadler, S., Thompson, S., Maynard, J., Ostrow, D., Altman, N., Braff, E., O'Malley, P., Hawkins, D., Judson, F., Denley, K., Nylund, T., Christie, G., Meyers, F., Moore, Y., Gardner, A., Doto, I., Miller, J., Reynolds, G., Murphy, B., Schable, C., Clark, B., Curran, J., and Redeker, A.: The prevention of hepatitis B with vaccine: Report of the Centers for Disease Control multicenter efficacy trial among homosexual men. Ann. Intern. Med., *97*:362, 1982.
29. Goldberg, D. M., and Campbell, D. R.: Biochemical investigation of outbreak of infectious hepatitis in a closed community. Br. Med. J., *2*:1435, 1962.
30. Grady, G. F.: Hepatitis B from the medical professions—how rare? How preventable? N. Engl. J. Med., *296*:995, 1977.
31. Hamilton, J. D.: Hepatitis B virus vaccine. An analysis of its potential use in medical workers. J.A.M.A., *250*:2145, 1983.
32. Holland, P. V., Alter, H. J., Purcell, R. H., Lander, J. J., Sgouris, J. T., and Schmidt, P. J.: Hepatitis B antigen and antibody in cold ethanol fractions of human plasma. Transfusions, *12*:363, 1972.
33. Immunization Practices Advisory Committee: Update on hepatitis B prevention. M.M.W.R., *36*:353, 1987.
34. Ishak, K.: Light microscopic morphology of viral hepatitis. Am. J. Clin. Pathol., *65*:787, 1976.
35. Kiernan, T. W., and Powers, R. J.: Hepatitis B virus. Inappropriate reactions to transmission risks. J.A.M.A., *241*:585, 1979.
36. Krugman, S., Giles, J.: Viral hepatitis, type B (MS-2 strain): Further observations on natural history and prevention. N. Engl. J. Med., *288*:755, 1973.
37. Krugman, S., Giles, J. P., and Hammond, J.: Infectious hepatitis: Evidence for two distinctive clinical epidemiological and immunological types of infection. J.A.M.A., *200*:365, 1967.
38. Lemon, S. M.: Type A viral hepatitis—new developments in an old disease. N. Engl. J. Med., *313*:1059, 1985.
39. Madsen, S., Bang, N. U., and Iversen, K.: Serum glutamic oxalacetic transaminase in disease of the liver and biliary tract. Br. Med. J., *1*:543, 1958.
40. Mosley, J. W., and Galambos, J.: Viral hepatitis. *In* Schiff, L. (Ed.): Diseases of the Liver. Philadelphia, J. B. Lippincott Company, 1975.
41. Mosley, J. W., Redeker, A. G., Feinstone, S. M., and Purcell, R. H.: Multiple hepatitis viruses in multiple attacks of acute viral hepatitis. N. Engl. J. Med., *296*:75, 1977.
42. Oken, M. M., Hootkin, L., and DeJager, R. L.: Hepatitis after Konyne administration. Am. J. Dig. Dis., *17*:271, 1972.
43. Redeker, A. G.: Viral hepatitis: Clinical aspects. Am. J. Med. Sci., *270*:9, 1975.
44. Schneider, A. J., and Mosley, J. W.: Studies of variations of glutamic-oxalacetic transaminase in serum in infectious hepatitis. Pediatrics, *24*:367, 1959.
45. Schroeder, D. D., and Mozen, M. M.: Australia antigen: Distribution during Cohn cold ethanol fractionation of human plasma. Science, *168*:1462, 1970.
46. Schumacher, H. R., and Gall, E. P.: Arthritis in acute hepatitis and chronic active hepatitis. Am. J. Med., *57*:655, 1974.
47. Seeff, L. B., and Koff, R. S.: Passive and active immunoprophylaxis of hepatitis B. Gastroenterology, *86*:958, 1984.
48. Seeff, L. B., Wright, E. C., Zimmerman, H. J., Alter, H. J., Dietz, A. A., Felsher, B. F., Finkelstein, J. D., Garcia-Pont, P., Gerin, J. L., Greenlee, H. B., Hamilton, J., Holland, P. V., Kaplan, P. M., Kiernan, T., Koff, R. S., Leevy, C. M., McAuliffe, V. J., Nath, N., Purcell, R. H., Schiff, E. R., Schwartz, C. C., Tamburro, C. H., Vlahcevic, Z., Zemel, R., and Zimmon, D. S.: Type B hepatitis after needle-stick exposure: Prevention with hepatitis B immune globulin. Ann. Intern. Med., *88*:285, 1978.
49. Shouval, D., Levij, I. S., and Eliakim, M.: Chronic active hepatitis with cholestatic features. I. A clinical and immunologic study. II. A histopathological study. Am. J. Gastroenterol., *72*:542, 1979.
50. Stevens, C. E., Alter, H. J., Taylor, P. E., Zang, E. A., Harley, E. J., Szmuness, W., and Dialysis Vaccine Study Group: Hepatitis B vaccine in patients receiving hemodialysis. N. Engl. J. Med., *311*:496, 1984.
51. Szmuness, W., Much, M. I., Prince, A. M., Hoofnagle, J. H., Cherubin, C. E., Harley, E. J., and Black, G. H.: On the role of sexual behavior in the spread of hepatitis B infection. Ann. Intern. Med., *83*:489, 1975.
52. Szmuness, W., Prince, A. M., Grady, G. F., Mann, M. K., Levine, R. W., Friedman, E. A., Jacobs, M. J., Josephson, A., Ribot, S., Shapiro, F. L., Stenzel, K. H., Suki, W. N., and Vyas, G.: Hepatitis B infection. A point-prevalence study in 15 U.S. hemodialysis centers. J.A.M.A., *227*:901, 1974.
53. Szmuness, W., Stevens, C. E., Harley, E. J., Zang, E. A., Olesko, W. R., William, D. C., Sadovsky, R., Morrison, J. M., and Kellner, A.: Hepatitis B vaccine: Demonstration of efficacy in a controlled clinical trial in a high-risk population in the United States. N. Engl. J. Med., *303*:833, 1980.
54. Trepo, C., Hantz, D., Jacquier, M. F., Nemoz, G., Cappel, R., and Trepo, D.: Different fates of hepatitis B markers during plasma fractionation: A clue to the infectivity of blood derivatives. Vox Sang., *35*:143, 1978.
55. Vyas, G. H.: Viral Hepatitis—1984. Proceedings of the 4th International Symposium on Viral Hepatitis. San Francisco, CA, 1984.
56. Whitcomb, F. F., Jr.: Chronic active liver disease. Definition, diagnosis, and management. Med. Clin. North Am., 1979.
57. Zuckerman, A. J.: Viral Hepatitis and Liver Disease. Proceedings of the International Symposium on Viral Hepatitis and Liver Disease. New York, Alan R. Liss, Inc., 1988.

34

THE BILIARY SYSTEM

David L. Nahrwold, M.D.

HISTORICAL ASPECTS

Most of the progress in the diagnosis and treatment of biliary tract disease has been made in the last century, but gallstones and their sequelae, which cause most of the clinical problems, are not a malady of modern times. The earliest known gallstone dates back to the twenty-first Egyptian Dynasty (1085–945 B.C.), having been discovered in the mummy of a priestess of Amen. Ironically, this ancient specimen was destroyed in the bombing of England during World War II. Much later, during the time of the Roman Empire, Pliny described the rare anomaly of double gallbladder,[28] and the well-known physician Soranus of Ephesus described jaundice and the associated signs of extrahepatic obstruction, including acholic stools, dark urine, and itching.[4] Gallstones were first described in the fifth century by a Greek physician, Alexander Trallianus, who wrote about calculi within the bile ducts.

The surgical relevance of biliary tract disease was first made obvious by the Islamic physician Ibn Sina (980–1037), who stated that a biliary-cutaneous fistula could follow drainage of an abdominal wall abscess. Perforation of an acutely inflamed gallbladder into the abdominal wall with abscess formation may have been the underlying problem. Joenisius first extracted gallstones through a biliary fistula that had formed from spontaneous drainage of an abdominal wall abscess. According to Power,[30] Jean Louis Petit (1674–1760) noted that a gallbladder could become adherent to the abdominal wall and proposed that it be punctured through the wall of the abdomen by a trocar. He believed the wound should be enlarged with a knife if stones could be palpated with a sound passed through the trocar. It is not clear that he actually performed the procedure, however.

The first cholecystostomy is credited to John Stough Bobbs, in Indianapolis on June 15, 1867.[9] His patient, a 32-year-old woman, had a large abdominal mass, which proved to be the gallbladder filled with clear serous fluid and gallstones. Obviously, she had hydrops of the gallbladder. He opened the gallbladder, removed the stones, and closed it by suture. His operation actually was a cholecystotomy; an opening to the outside was not established. His patient survived until the age of 77, when she died of arteriosclerosis.

Carl Langenbuch of Berlin performed the first cholecystectomy in June of 1882, using the aseptic technique that Joseph Lister had initiated in 1868, the year in which Bobbs had reported the first cholecystostomy. The patient was a 43-year-old man who had suffered from biliary colic for 16 years. He was released from the hospital 8 weeks after operation. Four years later, in 1886, the first cholecystectomy in the United States was performed by Justus Ohage, of St. Paul, Minnesota. Ludwig Courvoisier of Basel performed the first successful choledocholithotomy in 1890 and made several contributions to the understanding of bile duct obstruction at the turn of the century.

Important discoveries in the area of diagnostic testing have been made in the twentieth century. This field was opened by the development of cholecystography by Graham and Cole, culminating in the first cholecystogram in man in 1924.[13] Cholescintigraphy was first reported in 1953.[44] Improved imaging techniques and better dyes and nuclides led to the present high-resolution oral cholecystography and cholescintigraphy. Operative cholangiography was described in 1932; cholangiography by the percutaneous transhepatic and the endoscopic retrograde routes has been developed since 1950. The applications of ultrasonography, computed tomography, choledochoscopy, and interventional radiologic techniques to the diagnosis and management of biliary tract disease have occurred in the past 2 decades.

Alternatives to traditional cholecystectomy were developed during the 1980s and are currently under evaluation. They include oral chemolysis, extracorporeal shock wave lithotripsy, percutaneous dissolution and extraction, and laparoscopic cholecystectomy.

ANATOMY

The gallbladder and extrahepatic bile ducts are derived from the primitive foregut and are formed in conjunction with the liver. The shape of the gallbladder is approximately that of a pear, with a bulbous fundus at the distal end, a middle corpus that tapers to a neck, and a proximal cystic duct that enters the common bile duct (Fig. 1). The organ is about 7 cm. long and holds 30 to 50 ml. of bile. The corpus nestles into the substance of the liver for a variable distance and the entire organ is held to the liver by a peritoneal covering, which is a reflection of the visceral peritoneum covering the liver. The fundus may protrude slightly beyond the edge of the liver and lies anteriorly in the region of the costal arch at the lateral border of the rectus muscle. The cystic duct lies posteriorly on a plane with the duodenum, but superiorly to it at the level of the first lumbar vertebra. The infundibulum of the gallbladder is lax, because it is not bound to the liver by peritoneum. When distended by a stone, it has the appearance of a diverticulum, which is called Hartmann's pouch. The cystic duct is 2 to 4 cm. long and contains the spiral valves of Heister, which allow easy entry of bile into the gallbladder but offer resistance to its outflow.

The extrahepatic bile ducts lie within the hepatoduodenal ligament. Normally, the right anterior and posterior segmental bile ducts join to form the right hepatic duct, a confluence that usually is just within the substance of the liver. The left lateral and left medial segmental ducts form the left hepatic duct, which joins the right hepatic duct to form the common hepatic duct. The right and left hepatic ducts are 1 to 4 cm. long, with the left more accessible because it has a more transverse course prior to entering the liver. The length of the common hepatic duct is extremely variable because it is determined by the point at which the cystic duct joins it. The common bile duct courses through the pancreas and the wall of the duodenum to form the papilla of Vater on the medial wall of the duodenum (Fig. 2). Its distal end is enveloped by the sphincter of Oddi, which regulates the flow of bile from the liver into the duodenum. The pancreatic duct may share a common orifice on the papilla of Vater with the common bile duct or may join the common duct

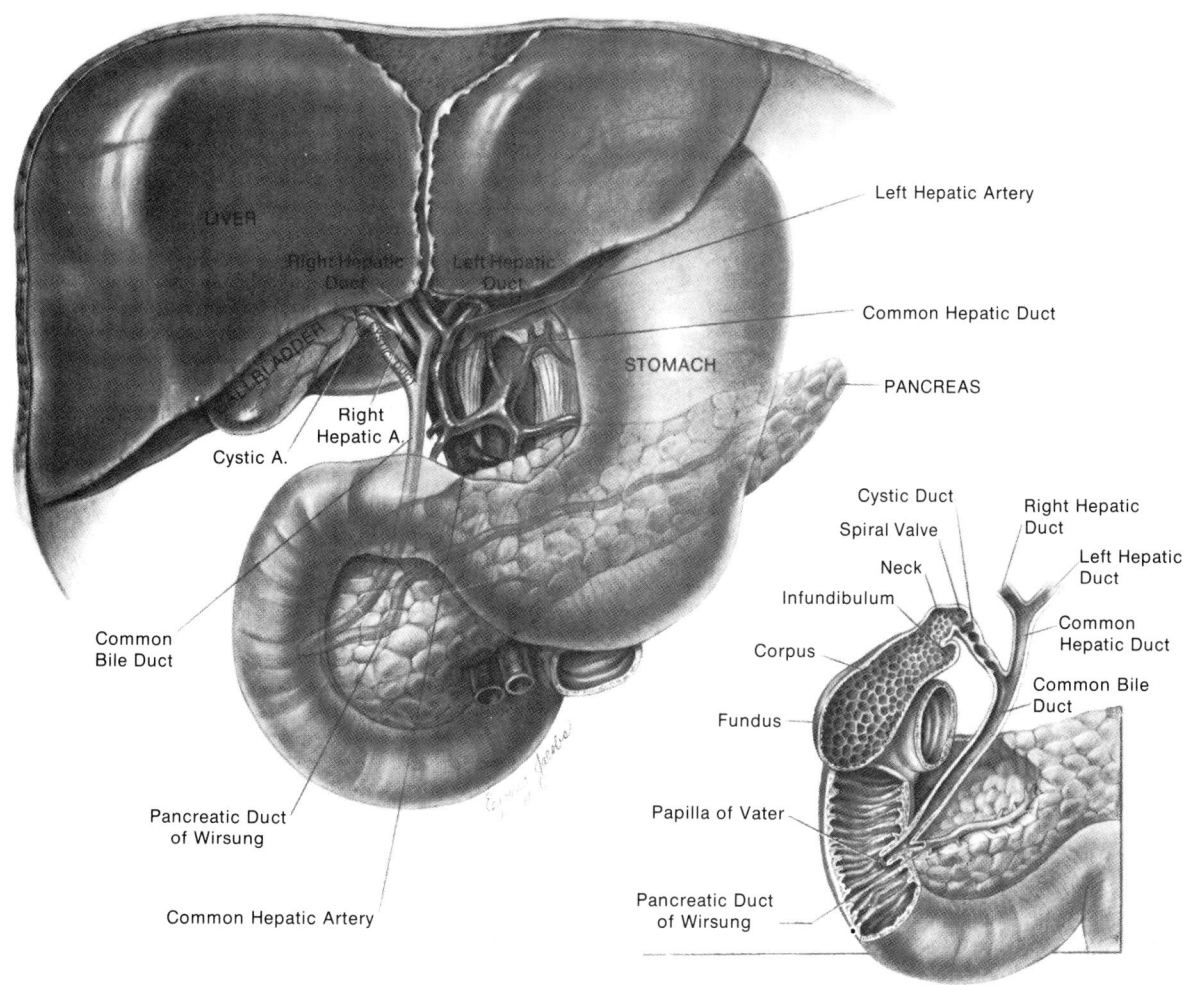

Figure 1. Anatomy of the biliary system.

proximal to its entrance into the duodenum; or the two ducts may open separately on the papilla (Fig. 2). A common channel, 1 mm. to several centimeters in length, is present in approximately 75 per cent of individuals, and in about 25 per cent the common bile duct and pancreatic duct open separately on the papilla.

The common bile duct receives its blood supply from the retroduodenal, the common hepatic, and the right hepatic arteries. Their branches form a plexus on the duct that is joined together by two axial vessels, the three o'clock and nine o'clock arteries, named for their positions in reference to a cross section of the duct. The gallbladder is supplied by branches of the cystic artery, which originates from the right hepatic artery after the latter passes beneath the common hepatic duct. The venous drainage of the gallbladder and extrahepatic ducts is into the portal vein. Lymphatics from the gallbladder drain into the cystic duct lymph node, located near the superior aspect of the junction of the infundibulum of the gallbladder and the cystic duct. Lymph nodes along the posterior aspect of the common bile duct and the common hepatic duct drain these structures.

The triangle of Calot is bounded by the cystic duct, the common hepatic duct, and the inferior border of the liver. The right hepatic and cystic arteries are located within it, and anomalous structures often pass through it, so that care must be taken to identify them during cholecystectomy.

SIGNIFICANCE OF VARIATIONS IN ANATOMY. Variations in the anatomy of the gallbladder, the bile ducts, and the arteries that supply them and the liver are important to the surgeon because failure to recognize them causes iatrogenic in-

jury to the biliary tract. The significant variations in ductal anatomy are shown in Figure 3. The cystic duct may be long, illustrating the need for its complete dissection. The duct may pass behind the common hepatic duct to enter on its posterior wall or on its left lateral aspect. In chronic cholecystitis, the gallbladder may be small and shrunken, and the cystic duct may be absent or extremely short; in this circumstance, the common bile duct may easily be mistaken for the cystic duct as dissection proceeds from the gallbladder fundus toward the cystic duct. A very long cystic duct may enter the common bile duct a variable distance from the sphincter of Oddi and may be fused with the common duct, in which case the two ducts should not be separated because they share a common wall. In addition, an "accessory" duct from the liver may enter the cystic duct or the common hepatic duct. Actually, this is not an accessory duct, but rather an anomalous course and entry of either the right anterior or right posterior segmental duct from the liver.

Variations in the anatomy of the hepatic and cystic arteries that are of surgical significance are shown in Figure 4. A bend in the course of the hepatic artery, curving into the configuration of a "caterpillar hump," invites injury unless carefully dissected free. A very short cystic artery also places the hepatic artery at risk.

CONGENITAL ANOMALIES OF THE GALLBLADDER

Absence of the gallbladder is a very rare condition that appears to have a genetic predisposition because several family

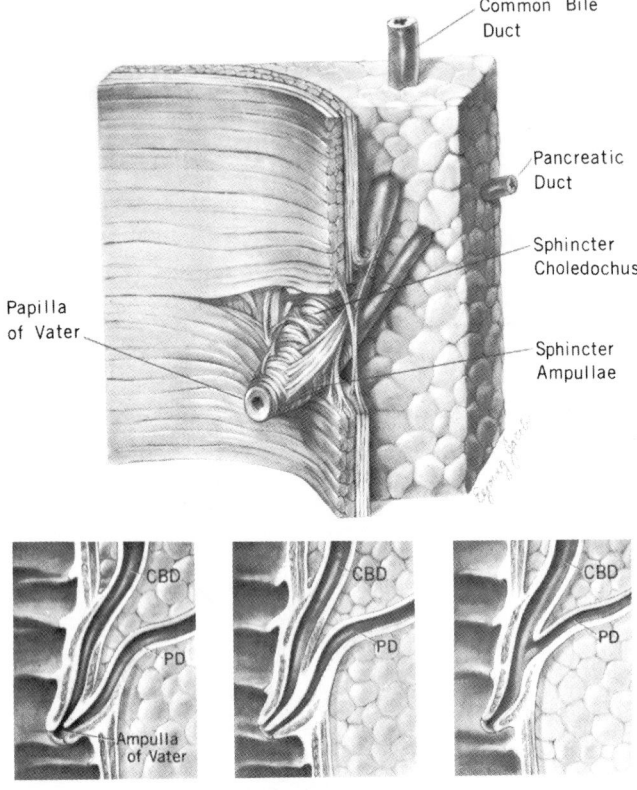

Figure 2. The choledochoduodenal junction.

members may be affected.[43] The condition is associated with an increased incidence of primary sclerosing cholangitis and carcinoma of the bile ducts.[31]

The nearly 400 cases of gallbladder agenesis were reviewed recently.[5] They formed three categories. Approximately one third were asymptomatic, and absence of the gallbladder was discovered incidentally at autopsy or operation for another condition. Slightly more than half had symptoms suggestive of biliary tract disease and underwent operation. In addition to

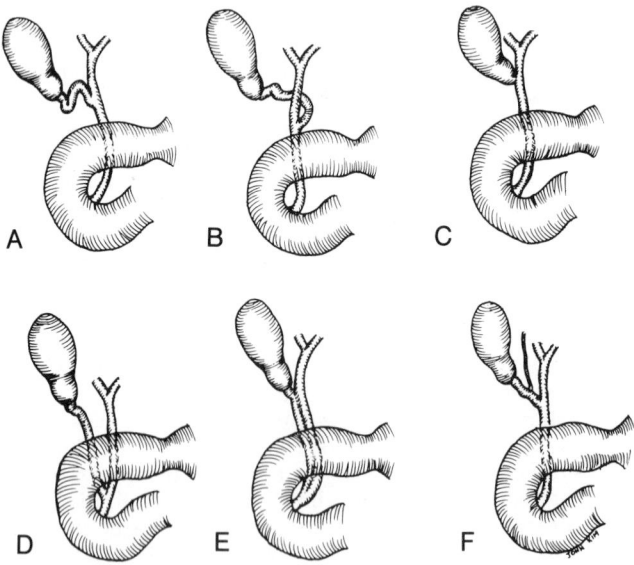

Figure 3. Surgically significant variations in ductal anatomy. A, Long, tortuous cystic duct. B, Cystic duct crosses common hepatic duct posteriorly and joins common duct on left side. This junction is seen posteriorly in some patients. C, Very short or absent cystic duct, usually observed in severe, chronic inflammation. D, Long cystic duct with low insertion into common duct. E, Long cystic duct fused to common hepatic duct. F, Anomalous entry of right anterior or posterior segmental duct into cystic duct; may also enter common hepatic duct.

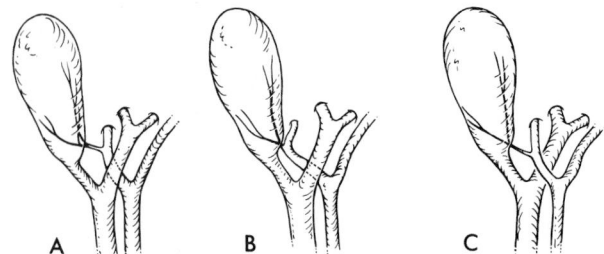

Figure 4. Important variations in the anatomy of the cystic and right hepatic arteries. A, Normal. B, "Caterpillar hump" right hepatic artery, which could cause injury to it. C, Right hepatic artery passing anterior to common hepatic duct where it could be mistaken for cystic duct or cystic artery.

absence of the gallbladder, one third of these had dilation of the common bile duct and 27 per cent had a stone or stones in the bile duct. The remaining 13 per cent of patients were children who died of multiple congenital anomalies.

Agenesis of the gallbladder is rarely diagnosed preoperatively because in symptomatic patients the sonogram is interpreted as demonstrating a small, contracted gallbladder, and on oral cholecystography and scintigraphy the gallbladder is not visualized, all of which suggest the presence of disease. A thorough search for the gallbladder should be made at operation. If none is found, operative cholangiography is indicated.

Double and triple gallbladders have been reported, the latter being extremely rare. Double gallbladders may share a common cystic duct and be completely separated, or they may be divided by a septum. When they do not share a common outlet, the cystic ducts of double or triple gallbladders open separately into the common bile duct or, less commonly, into the right hepatic duct.[17]

An ectopic location of the gallbladder is also very rare. Intrahepatic location on the right side makes cholecystectomy hazardous, and a cholecystostomy with removal of the stones is the preferred treatment of cholelithiasis in this anomaly. A left-sided gallbladder is located to the left of the falciform ligament and usually is partially embedded in the substance of the left lobe of the liver. The cystic duct may drain into the left hepatic duct or the common hepatic duct. In retrodisplacement of the gallbladder the organ is located beneath the posterior and inferior surfaces of the liver. Torsion may occur in a "floating" gallbladder, in which the organ is completely peritonealized and free from the liver, or attached to the liver by a long mesentery.

Choledochal Cysts

Cysts of the biliary duct system are very uncommon, and understanding of them is incomplete. Approximately 80 per cent are diagnosed during childhood, but the remainder become apparent in adulthood. Originally, they were described as cystic dilations of the extrahepatic duct system, which Alonso-Lej classified with regard to their location and their fusiform or diverticular configuration.[2] During the past decade, attention has been brought to their frequent association with cystic dilation of the duct system within the liver, a condition described in 1958, now known as Caroli's disease.[12] The more common variants are shown in Figure 5. The solitary fusiform extrahepatic cyst (Fig. 5A) is the most common, and the supraduodenal diverticulum the most rare. The etiology is uncertain; one speculation is that the supraduodenal diverticulum follows a confined, localized perforation of the bile duct. Some evidence suggests that fusiform dilation follows distal obstruction and destruction of the proximal duct epithelium by pancreatic juice, because the pancreatic duct enters proximal to the ampulla in most of these patients; distal obstruction and damage to the epithelium cause cysts in puppies.[24,28]

The classic symptoms are abdominal pain, jaundice, and an

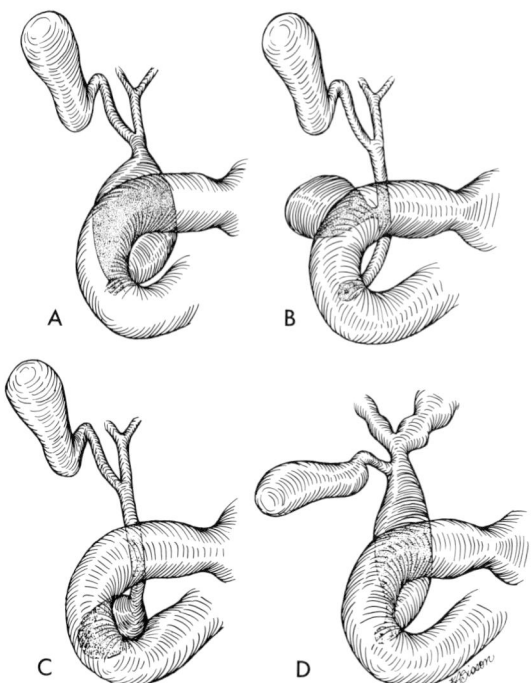

Figure 5. Cysts of the extrahepatic bile ducts. *A*, Classic, fusiform choledochal cyst. *B*, Extrahepatic supraduodenal diverticulum. *C*, Choledochocele. *D*, Fusiform extrahepatic and intrahepatic cysts. (After Alonso-Lej, F., Rever, W. B., Jr., and Pessagno, D. J.: Congenital choledochal cyst, with a report of 2, and an analysis of 94 cases. Surg. Gynecol. Obstet., *108*:1, 1959.)

abdominal mass, but not all children have a mass. In both children and adults, cholangitis is frequent, probably because of bile stasis and colonization with bacteria. Most cysts can be detected by ultrasonography or by radionuclide scanning, but the definitive diagnosis requires cholangiography.

Until recently, drainage of the cyst into the duodenum or a Roux-en-Y limb of jejunum has been recommended. However, the long-term results of procedures in which the cyst remains *in situ* are not good because of recurrent pancreatitis in approximately a third of patients and the development of carcinoma in the cyst in about one fourth of them.[21] Therefore, choledochal cysts should be treated by excision and Roux-en-Y hepaticojejunostomy whenever possible.[26]

CHOLEDOCHOLITHIASIS

Common duct stones are found in 8 to 16 per cent of patients who have cholelithiasis. The incidence increases with age and reaches approximately 25 per cent in patients over 60 years. In most cases, bile duct stones migrate from the gallbladder; the fact that they often are larger than the cystic duct suggests that they are able to grow within the bile duct system. Most are cholesterol stones, in keeping with their high incidence in the gallbladder.

Stones may form *de novo* within the bile ducts. These calculi, termed primary common duct stones, are usually composed of calcium bilirubinate and always are associated with bile duct obstruction. Frequently, infection or bacterbilia is present. Arbitrarily, those stones discovered more than 2 years after cholecystectomy are designated primary common duct stones. The causation of calcium bilirubinate stones is thought to be precipitation of unconjugated bilirubin as the calcium salt. Normally, bilirubin is conjugated as the glucuronide. Stone formation begins when the soluble bilirubin diglucuronide is deconjugated by beta-glucuronidase, an enzyme produced by bacteria such as *Escherichia coli* and by the epithelium of the biliary tract, leaving insoluble, unconjugated bilirubin to precipitate with

calcium.[27] The clinical settings in which this occurs include posttraumatic biliary stricture, a narrowed biliary-enteric anastomosis, stenosis of the sphincter of Oddi, sclerosing cholangitis, and Oriental cholangiohepatitis. A suspected but unproved cause of primary common duct stones is malfunction of the choledochal sphincter mechanism, with bile stasis and marked dilation of the bile duct system. Calcium bilirubinate stones are also termed "earthy" stones, because they are brown and tend to crumble easily. They are ovoid, in contrast to the faceted appearance of cholesterol stones.

CLINICAL MANIFESTATIONS AND DIAGNOSIS. Common duct calculi may be asymptomatic or cause biliary colic, bile duct obstruction, cholangitis, or pancreatitis. The pain may be mild or severe and cannot be differentiated from pain arising in the gallbladder. Jaundice is intermittent if the obstruction is partial and intermittent, or it may be progressive if a stone becomes impacted in the distal duct. Chills and fever are usually associated with slight abdominal discomfort and a mild elevation of serum bilirubin, but any of these signs of cholangitis may be absent. Occasionally symptoms of cholangitis are accompanied by shock and confusion, coma, or other central nervous system symptoms, which signal the presence of acute toxic cholangitis, a condition in which infected bile or pus is under pressure within the duct system. Immediate resuscitation and emergency decompression of the duct system are necessary to prevent death. In routine cases of choledocholithiasis, the physical examination may be normal. Jaundice and mild tenderness in the epigastrium and right upper quadrant may be present.

The white blood cell count usually is elevated when cholangitis is present, but in the absence of active infection it is normal. Elevations of the serum bilirubin and alkaline phosphatase are characteristic. The mean serum bilirubin in choledocholithiasis is approximately 9 mg. per 100 ml., and values above 15 are rare.[42] Serum amylase measurement always should be done; when this is elevated, gallstone pancreatitis must be considered.

The early symptoms of choledocholithiasis cannot be distinguished easily from gallbladder colic or acute cholecystitis. Ultrasonography should be done to detect the presence or absence of gallstones and dilation of the bile ducts. Ultrasonography is not reliable in detection of common duct stones. Endoscopic retrograde cholangiography is indicated for most patients who have bile duct obstruction, as manifest by persistent jaundice or bile duct dilation on ultrasonography. Percutaneous transhepatic cholangiography is an alternative, but endoscopic retrograde cholangiography permits visualization of other portions of the gastrointestinal tract and allows the performance of pancreatography and endoscopic sphincterotomy, when indicated. Patients who have transient bilirubin or amylase elevation and cholelithiasis may be expected to have choledocholithiasis. If cholecystectomy is planned, preoperative cholangiography is not necessary, but the surgeon should be alert to the need for operative cholangiography and possible common duct exploration.

TREATMENT. When present, cholangitis should be treated with antibiotics. Defervescence usually occurs rapidly. If it does not, acute toxic cholangitis may be present, and decompression of the duct system must be performed immediately. This can be done by establishing percutaneous transhepatic biliary drainage or by endoscopic sphincterotomy, but immediate laparotomy and insertion of a T-tube should be done if these simpler procedures fail or are not available.

Most common duct stones are found and removed at the time of cholecystectomy. Operative cholangiography should be done routinely to detect choledocholithiasis. If it is not, common duct exploration is necessary when choledocholithiasis is suspected, a practice that frequently causes an unnecessary, negative common duct exploration. This is potentially harmful because the addition of common duct exploration increases the mortality, morbidity, and expense of cholecystectomy.[3] Common duct stones are found in well over 90 per cent of patients in whom they are palpated at operation and in patients with a recent history of cholangitis with jaundice.[42] These findings should serve as indications for common duct exploration. Patients with findings that may have served as indications in the past, such as a history of pancreatitis, a dilated duct, small stones in the gallbladder, and an enlarged cystic duct, should have common duct exploration only when the operative cholangiogram is positive or suggestive. Routine operative cholangiography at cholecystectomy detects calculi in approximately 5 per cent of patients in whom the history and clinical findings are not suggestive of choledocholithiasis. The common duct should be opened longitudinally and explored carefully with stone forceps, scoops, and balloon catheters. The author uses choledochoscopy routinely. The flexible scope is more maneuverable, but visualization is better with the rigid type. Choledochoscopy is especially valuable to exclude intraductal papillary tumors and occult cancers. Stones impacted in the distal duct may be impossible to remove from above, and a duodenotomy and sphincterotomy may be necessary. After the stones have been removed, the duct should be closed around a Moss-Whelan T-tube, which has a large side arm, allowing percutaneous stone removal later, if necessary. T-tube cholangiography should be done before the abdomen is closed to assess the position of the tube and to be certain no stones remain.

Consideration must be given to a common duct drainage procedure in certain circumstances. The author's preference is a large side-to-side choledochoduodenostomy, but division of the common duct and an end-to-side anastomosis are preferred by some. One of these procedures should be done when there are more than five stones, when there is marked dilation of the duct, when not all stones can be removed, and when a previous choledocholithotomy has been done.

In some situations, sphincteroplasty is more efficacious than choledochoduodenostomy, especially when a stone is impacted in the distal duct, ampullary stenosis is present, or the duct is small in diameter.

Following choledocholithotomy, the T-tube should not be removed prior to a postoperative cholangiogram, nor should it be removed earlier than 10 days postoperatively. When stones are present, the tube should be left in place for approximately 6 weeks, at which time percutaneous extraction of the calculi can be performed through the mature, fibrous tract created by the tube (Fig. 6).

Dissolution of common duct stones by continuous perfusion of cholic acid or mono-octanoin (glycerol-1-mono-octanoate) through the T-tube is possible, but is not always effective, and requires 1 to 2 weeks.[34,42] Only cholesterol stones respond to these agents. When percutaneous extraction and attempts at dissolution fail, endoscopic sphincterotomy should be attempted. If this is not possible or an attempt is unsuccessful, extracorporeal shock wave lithotripsy should be tried. Finally, reoperation may be necessary.

Choledocholithiasis in a patient who previously underwent cholecystectomy is best treated by endoscopic sphincterotomy. The success rate for endoscopic sphincterotomy and extraction of stones is approximately 90 per cent,[14,32] and the mortality is 1.0 to 1.5 per cent,[15] which compares favorably with the mortality for surgical choledocholithotomy. Extraction of stones larger than 1.5 cm. in diameter is seldom possible, and the success rate for clearance of the duct when numerous stones are present is low. In such instances, surgical choledocholithotomy may be necessary. The endoscopic approach cannot be used in patients who have had a Billroth II reconstruction, and it should also be avoided when a distal common duct stricture is present. Other contraindications include the presence of duodenal diverticula in certain locations, coagulation disorders, and recent pancreatitis.

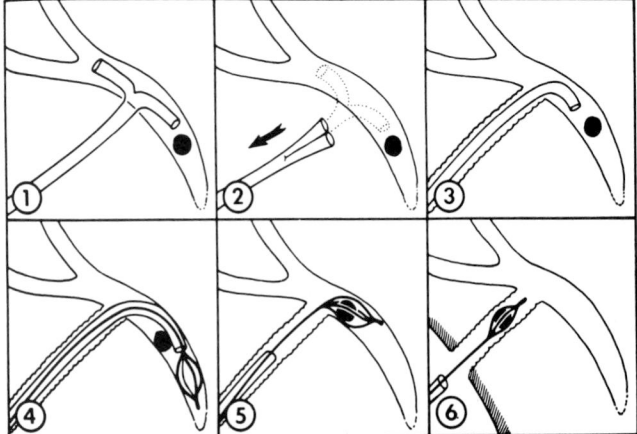

Figure 6. Steps in instrument extraction of retained common duct stone. 1. Repeat T-tube cholangiogram is obtained on the day of stone extraction 4 to 5 weeks after choledochotomy. 2. After the location of the retained stone has been ascertained, the T-tube is withdrawn. 3. Using the sinus tract of the T-tube, the steerable catheter is guided into the bile duct, and its movable tip is advanced beyond the retained stone. 4. The basket is inserted through the steerable catheter, the catheter is withdrawn, and the basket is opened. 5. The open basket is withdrawn in order to engage the stone. The basket is only retracted, never advanced, outside the enclosure of the steerable catheter. 6. The stone is extracted through the drain tract. (From Burhenne, H. J.: Nonoperative retained biliary tract stone extraction. A new roentgenologic technique. Am. J. Roentgenol., *117*:388, 1973.)

Extracorporeal shock wave lithotripsy is used when stones are too large to extract via the endoscopic approach. Endoscopic sphincterotomy is done, and a nasobiliary catheter is placed for injection of contrast material. Lithotripsy fragments the stones so that they pass spontaneously or can be extracted. Early results suggest that complete clearance of stones can be achieved in 70 to 85 per cent of these complicated cases.[6,33]

The best method for management of patients who present with cholelithiasis and choledocholithiasis is not clear. If their symptoms are clearly due to cholelithiasis, cholecystectomy and choledocholithotomy would appear to be the best approach, but preliminary endoscopic sphincterotomy and clearance of stones from the duct, followed by cholecystectomy, may be more cost-effective.[22,26]

Elderly and high-risk patients who present with cholangitis or other manifestations of choledocholithiasis should have early endoscopic sphincterotomy and extraction of stones. Most of them also have cholelithiasis, but cholecystectomy is not without risk in this group of patients. Experience to date suggests that fewer than 20 per cent eventually require cholecystectomy, although the length of follow-up is relatively short.[25,36]

BILE DUCT STRICTURES

More than 90 per cent of bile duct strictures are due to iatrogenic injury during cholecystectomy or bile duct surgery. The remainder follow abdominal trauma, chronic pancreatitis, impaction of a calculus within the duct system, or chemical injury. Over 80 per cent follow cholecystectomy and are due to inadvertent injury to the common hepatic or common bile duct. A knowledge of anatomic variants, routine operative cholangiography, and meticulous care in dissection are required in prevention of injuries. Iatrogenic strictures of the distal common bile duct usually follow injuries by probes, forceps, or dilators during common duct exploration. The healing of bile duct injuries is characterized by extensive scarring and fibrosis, probably because of damage to the blood supply of the duct system and the fibrosing effect of bile on injured tissue.[23] More than 70 per cent of iatrogenic strictures involve the common hepatic duct or the confluence of the right and left hepatic ducts.[41]

CLINICAL MANIFESTATIONS AND DIAGNOSIS. Strictures due to bile duct injury present in the immediate postoperative period or many years later. In the early postoperative period, jaundice, drainage of bile from a drain or through the wound, or sepsis may herald the presence of an injury and development of a stricture. Recurrent cholangitis is the most common manifestation of a stricture that develops months or years after operation. Stricture is a rare cause of acute suppurative cholangitis, in which the biliary duct system contains pus under pressure. In long-standing strictures, jaundice may be the only manifestation; sometimes this is due to the formation of stones proximal to the site of narrowing. The threat to life that is posed by a stricture includes sepsis from cholangitis and the development of cirrhosis, portal hypertension, and hemorrhage from esophageal varices. Therefore, symptoms of biliary tract obstruction following cholecystectomy or other biliary tract operations always should be investigated. The development of jaundice or symptoms of cholangitis is an indication for liver function tests. Elevated serum bilirubin and alkaline phosphatase are indicative of obstruction. In postoperative patients, leakage of bile may be detected by paracentesis and confirmed by a ^{99m}technetium-IDA scan. The most important study is cholangiography, which demonstrates the exact location and extent of the stricture. Percutaneous transhepatic cholangiography is more useful because it provides better information about the proximal extent of the lesion, which determines the type of repair and its degree of difficulty. Simultaneous insertion of a Ring catheter aids in the subsequent repair. The differential diagnosis of cholangitis and jaundice that occur months or years after cholecystectomy includes stricture, stones, and cancer. The diagnostic tests and the order in which they are utilized must be individualized for the patient, depending on the history and physical findings.

TREATMENT. The goal of treatment is to construct a wide, tension-free anastomosis, with mucosa-to-mucosa apposition, between normal bile duct and the intestine. This is best accomplished by an end-to-side choledochoduodenostomy or a Roux-en-Y hepaticojejunostomy (Fig. 7). The former is applicable to distal bile duct strictures such as those caused by chronic pancreatitis. Most iatrogenic strictures are in the proximal portion of the extrahepatic duct system and cannot be treated by choledochoduodenostomy because a tension-free anastomosis is not possible. The Roux-en-Y limb permits a tension-free anastomosis that can be sized according to the diameter of the bile duct. A stent is left in place for approximately 3 months, although this length of time is arbitrary. The only solid data on the length of time a stent should be kept in place indicate that patients stented for longer than 1 month have better results than those stented for less than a month.[29]

Excellent results are obtained in over 70 per cent of patients. The percentage of excellent results is inversely related to the

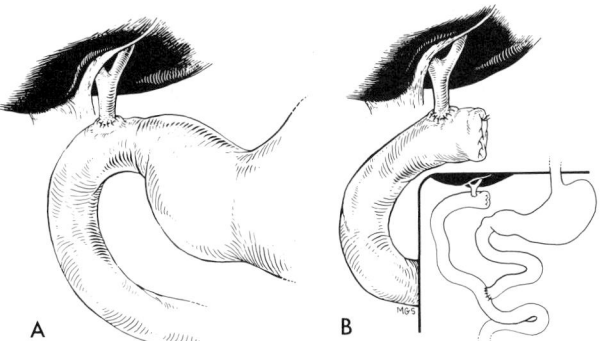

Figure 7. Choledochoduodenostomy (A) and anastomosis to a Roux-en-Y limb (B). Note that the end of the jejunum is closed so that a precise, appropriately sized mucosa-to-mucosa anastomosis can be done to the jejunum.

number of previous repairs. Serum bilirubin and alkaline phosphatase should be monitored, and if either is elevated persistently, cholangiography is indicated. A stricture may recur as long as 20 years after repair.

The role of percutaneous transhepatic balloon dilation of benign strictures is not yet clear. Immediate success can be achieved in most patients, but recurrence is frequent, and long-term results favor surgical therapy. Some have suggested initial balloon dilation and stenting, and operation later if nonsurgical management fails.[16] Clearly, balloon dilation and stenting have a role in poor-risk patients.[37]

BILE DUCT CANCER

Carcinomas of the extrahepatic bile ducts are rare and are usually recognized late in their course. Because of their location in proximity to the liver, hepatic artery, and portal vein, they may not be resectable. Nevertheless, these tumors do not have a high propensity to metastasize, so that palliation for significant periods of time may be possible.

The average age of onset is approximately 60 years; males and females are equally affected. Bile duct cancer has been categorized according to anatomic location[20]; the upper third includes cancers between the undersurface of the liver and the cystic duct. Half to three fourths are located in this area. Mid-third lesions are between the cystic duct and the superior border of the pancreas; 10 to 25 per cent are found there. Lower-third lesions are located between the superior border of the pancreas and the ampulla, representing 10 to 20 per cent of lesions, but carcinomas of the ampulla itself are not included in this category.

ASSOCIATED DISORDERS. The etiology is unknown, but several associations have been found. The most frequent is with chronic ulcerative colitis, in which those patients who develop cancer are younger than those without ulcerative colitis. Colectomy does not affect the potential for the development of bile duct cancer. Patients with sclerosing cholangitis also have an increased incidence of bile duct cancer. Sclerosing cholangitis appears to progress to carcinoma in some patients. A common etiologic factor between these diseases has not been identified. Other conditions in which the incidence of bile duct cancer is increased include infestation with *Clonorchis sinensis*, the chronic typhoid carrier state, choledochal cyst, and Caroli's disease.[7] These associations offer no clue to the etiology. Aflatoxins cause bile duct cancers in animals.

CLINICAL MANIFESTATIONS AND DIAGNOSIS. Approximately 90 per cent of patients present with jaundice.[1,39] Weight loss and pain occur in approximately half, but the pain is not severe; pruritus is frequent. Sometimes the disease presents with cholangitis—chills and fever, abdominal pain, and jaundice. Physical examination reveals an enlarged, tender liver. The gallbladder may be palpable in lesions distal to the entrance of the cystic duct when obstruction is complete. The presence of ascites and splenomegaly signifies portal vein invasion and implies a grave prognosis. Laboratory tests demonstrate elevation of the bilirubin and the alkaline phosphatase.

As in all cases of extrahepatic bile duct obstruction, cholangiography is necessary to determine the location of the tumor and its resectability. The author prefers percutaneous transhepatic cholangiography because the proximal extent of the lesion can be visualized. Computed tomography may be helpful in determining the extent of the lesion in the radial direction, and angiography may delineate growth into a major vessel, usually the portal vein.[8] In distal lesions, endoscopy may be helpful to exclude carcinoma of the ampulla of Vater. Cytologic diagnosis is possible by percutaneous directed fine-needle aspiration of the tumor or by brushings obtained via the endoscope. The value of these procedures depends on the skill of the cytologist.

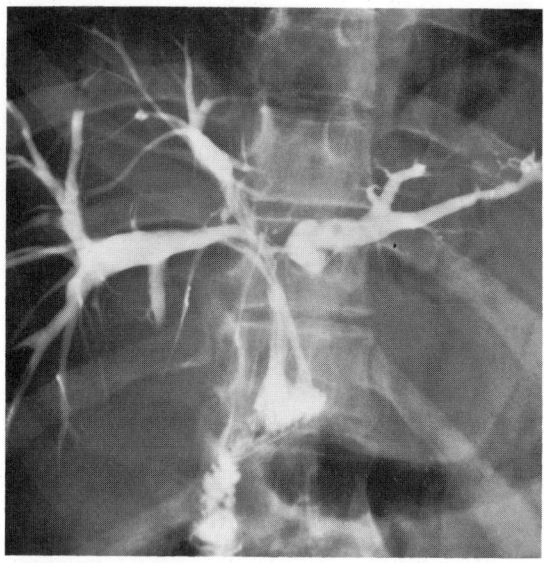

Figure 8. Carcinoma involving the common hepatic duct and both hepatic ducts through which a tube has been passed for palliation.

TREATMENT. Surgical resection of the tumor is the only likelihood for cure. Proximal-third lesions may require resection of both the right and left hepatic ducts, if the tumor is at their confluence.[10] Reconstruction should be by Roux-en-Y hepaticojejunostomy, splinted by Silastic tubes that are brought out through the liver and the skin proximally. The ability to change these tubes under fluoroscopic guidance has obviated the need to bring the distal end out through the Roux-en-Y limb and the skin. Growth of the cancer into the liver and the branches of the portal vein and hepatic artery makes resection inadvisable. Usually the tumor can be dilated sufficiently to pass a tube through it for relief of jaundice, although episodes of cholangitis are frequent (Fig. 8). Radiation therapy may be helpful in prolonging life.

Middle-third lesions should also be resected, with reconstruction by Roux-en-Y hepaticojejunostomy. Although an indwelling splint may not be necessary to protect the anastomosis, especially if it is large, one should be used if radiation therapy is contemplated because bile duct epithelium is easily damaged by radiation.[35]

Carcinomas in the distal third of the bile duct are by definition in the intrapancreatic portion of the duct and must be treated by the Whipple procedure. Often, it is not possible to differentiate them from pancreatic cancers preoperatively.

The prognosis is poor. Approximately 10 per cent of patients who have bile duct cancer are cured. Cure is rare for proximal-third lesions, approximately 10 per cent for middle-third cancers, and about 25 per cent for those in the lower third. The role of radiation therapy and chemotherapy in enhancing survival is not clear.

SCLEROSING CHOLANGITIS

Sclerosing cholangitis is an inflammatory disease of the bile ducts that causes fibrosis and thickening of their walls and multiple short, concentric strictures. Both the intrahepatic and extrahepatic portions of the duct system as well as the gallbladder may be involved. The outer diameter of the ducts may be normal. Segments of the ducts between the strictures are slightly dilated or of normal size. The disease is progressive and gradually causes cirrhosis, portal hypertension, and death from hepatic failure. Sclerosing cholangitis may predispose to the development of cholangiocarcinoma, which may have a similar cholangiographic appearance.

Many cases occur primarily, but some are associated with inflammatory bowel disease, most notably ulcerative colitis, with which about 70 per cent of cases are associated.[18] Retroperitoneal and mediastinal fibrosis, pancreatitis, pancreatic fibrosis, orbital pseudotumors, and Peyronie's disease have also been reported in association with sclerosing cholangitis. The etiology has been linked to altered immunity, toxins, and infectious agents, and there is indirect evidence to support each of these theories.

Approximately two thirds of cases occur in individuals under the age of 45, and the male to female ratio is 3:2. Fatigue, anorexia, weight loss, and the insidious development of jaundice and pruritus are the usual findings. Vague upper abdominal pain is sometimes present. Cholangitis may develop and may become a vexing problem after surgical intervention or the placement of indwelling tubes or stents percutaneously. The diagnosis is made by the typical cholangiographic appearance, usually obtained by endoscopic retrograde cholangiography, the clinical findings, and liver biopsy.

Medical therapy consists of corticosteroids and long-term antibiotic administration when cholangitis is a recurrent problem. Immunosuppressants, bile acid–binding agents, colchicine, and penicillamine have been used. There is no solid evidence that these agents alter the slow, progressive course of the disease. Ursodeoxycholic acid, which improves primary biliary cirrhosis, is now being evaluated.[19]

Surgical intervention in the form of a biopsy of an extrahepatic bile duct and liver biopsy may be necessary, especially when cholangiocarcinoma cannot be excluded. More often, consideration of surgical therapy or percutaneous balloon dilation arises when the patient is jaundiced and clearly has one or more points of obstruction within the biliary tree. The treatment of each patient must be individualized; in the rare patient who has an isolated obstruction within the extrahepatic duct system, a Roux-en-Y choledochojejunostomy proximal to the obstruction is indicated. Intraoperative or percutaneous dilation of strictures may be a useful adjunct. Some have advocated Roux-en-Y choledochjejunostomy and placement of a large Silastic tube through the biliary-enteric anastomosis and the duct system, bringing the proximal end out through the substance of the liver and the abdominal wall, and the distal end out through the Roux-en-Y jejunal limb and the abdominal wall as well. Usually, the tube is brought through the right hepatic duct and the right lobe of the liver. Holes are cut in those portions of the tube that are placed within the liver, bile ducts, and jejunum to allow free drainage of bile from liver to jejunum. The tube, known as a transhepatic U-tube stent, should be flushed daily with a small amount of sterile saline and can be changed if it becomes occluded. No study has shown that this procedure is beneficial, and many believe that it should not be done.

When the extrahepatic duct system is severely involved, the most severe constriction may be at or near the bifurcation of the common hepatic duct. In this situation, Cameron and associates[11] have recommended excision of the extrahepatic duct system distal to the bifurcation and individual anastomoses of the right and left hepatic ducts to a Roux-en-Y limb of jejunum. Each of the anastomoses is then splinted with a transhepatic U-tube stent as described previously. The short-term results have been good.

Stones and sludge may form within the bile ducts of patients with multiple strictures, and surgical intervention to remove the stones and to dilate strictures and permanently stent them may be helpful in individual cases. The decision for surgical intervention must be based on the circumstances in the individual case. A limiting factor in the surgical approach is that significant dilation proximal to a stricture does not occur in sclerosing cholangitis. This obviates a large, freely draining biliary-enteric anastomosis and invites recurrent stricture at the anastomosis. When the biliary tract has been violated, recurrent episodes of cholangitis are frequent, and this problem must be balanced against the potential benefits of relieving partial biliary obstruction. Ultimately, the success of surgical procedures is limited by recurrent cholangitis and the progressive nature of the disease. Therefore, although surgical therapy may be lifesaving in some circumstances, it must be regarded as palliative in the overall context of the disease.

Insertion of a T-tube, popular in the past, should not be done. Transhepatic U-tube stents are more effective. Cholecystectomy should not be done unless there is definite evidence of cholecystitis or cholelithiasis. Ideally, patients should have surgical therapy, when indicated, prior to the development of significant biliary cirrhosis and portal hypertension. Operation is hazardous and probably contraindicated in most of these far-advanced cases. Removal of the colon has no effect on the course of sclerosing cholangitis in those patients who have chronic ulcerative colitis.

The definitive management of patients with sclerosing cholangitis is hepatic transplantation. At present, the 5-year survival rates are approximately 60 per cent, generally the same as those for other types of chronic liver disease.

SELECTED REFERENCES

Cotton, P. B., and Vallon, A.: British experience with duodenoscopic sphincter-otomy for removal of bile duct stones. Br. J. Surg., 68:373, 1981.
A large experience by an expert is recorded and the complications, pitfalls, and nuances are described.

Glenn, F., and Grafe, W. R., Jr.: Historical events in biliary tract surgery. Arch. Surg., 93:848, 1966.
The authors review the significant events in biliary tract surgery and provide excellent references for those who wish to study this interesting subject.

Jordan, G. L., Jr.: Choledocholithiasis. Curr. Probl. Surg., 19:723, 1982.
This is an extensive review of the subject and provides the author's views on diagnostic testing and technical details. The pathophysiology of choledocholithiasis is discussed.

LaRusso, N. F., Wiesner, R. H., Ludwig, J., and MacCarty, R. L.: Primary sclerosing cholangitis. N. Engl. J. Med., 310:899, 1984.
This is a concise review of the medical aspects of the disease, in which the causes and pathogenesis are discussed. Criteria for diagnosis in questionable cases are given, and medical management is outlined and emphasized.

Nagorney, D. M., McIlrath, D. C., and Adson, M. A.: Choledochal cysts in adults: Clinical management. Surgery, 96:656, 1984.
The large Mayo Clinic experience with problems in management of choledochal cysts is presented. The complications of carcinoma and pancreatitis are emphasized.

Pitt, H. A., Miyamoto, T., Parapatis, S. K., Tompkins, R. K., and Longmire, W. P., Jr.: Factors influencing outcome in patients with postoperative biliary strictures. Am. J. Surg., 144:14, 1982.
This review of a large series of patients treated by the UCLA group provides follow-up data on recurrence. The outcomes of various surgical approaches and procedures are given.

Tompkins, R. K., Thomas, D., Wile, A., and Longmire, W. P., Jr.: Prognostic factors in bile duct carcinoma: Analysis of 96 cases. Ann. Surg., 194:447, 1981.
Bile duct tumors were classified according to location and the results of surgical treatment are analyzed. This is a scholarly review of the subject.

REFERENCES

1. Alexander, F., Rossi, R. L., O'Bryan, M., Khettry, U., Braasch, J. W., and Walkins, E., Jr.: Biliary carcinoma. A review of 109 cases. Am. J. Surg., 147:503, 1984.
2. Alonso-Lej, F., Rever, W. B., Jr., and Pessagno, D. J.: Congenital choledochal cyst, with a report of 2, and an analysis of 94 cases. Surg. Gynecol. Obstet., 108:1, 1959.
3. Bartlett, M. K., and Waddell, W. R.: Indications for common duct exploration; evaluation in 1000 cases. N. Engl. J. Med., 258:164, 1958.
4. Beal, J. M.: Historical perspective of gallstone disease. Surg. Gynecol. Obstet., 158:181, 1984.
5. Bennion, R. S., Thompson, J. E., Jr., and Tompkins, R. K.: Agenesis of the gallbladder without extrahepatic biliary atresia. Arch. Surg., 123:1257, 1988.
6. Bland, K. I., Jones, R. S., Maher, J. W., et al.: Extracorporeal shock-wave lithotripsy of bile duct calculi. Ann. Surg., 209:743, 1989.
7. Bloustein, P. A.: Association of carcinoma with congenital cystic conditions of the liver and bile ducts. Am. J. Gastroenterol., 67:40, 1977.
8. Blumgart, L. H., Hadjis, N. S., Benjamin, I. S., and Beazley, R.: Surgical ap-

9. Bobbs, J. S.: Case of lithotomy of the gallbladder. Trans. Ind. State Med. Soc., 18:68, 1868.
10. Cameron, J. L., Broe, P., and Zuidema, G. D.: Proximal bile duct tumors. Ann. Surg., 196:412, 1983.
11. Cameron, J. L., Pitt, H. A., Zimmer, M. J., Herlong, H. F., Kaufman, S. L., Boitnott, J. K., and Coleman, J.: Resection of hepatic duct bifurcation and transhepatic stenting for sclerosing cholangitis. Ann. Surg., 207:614, 1988.
12. Caroli, J., Soupalt, R., Kossakowski, J., Plocker, L., and Paradowska, M.: La dilatation polikistique congenitale des voies biliares intrahepatiques. Essai de classification. Sem. Hop. Paris, 34:488, 1958.
13. Cole, W. H.: The development of cholecystography; the first fifty years. Am. J. Surg., 136:541, 1978.
14. Cotton, P. B.: Endoscopic management of bile duct stones (apples and oranges). Gut, 25:587, 1984.
15. Frost, R. A.: Prospective multi-center study of British sphincterotomy: Initial results and complications. Gut, 25:549, 1984.
16. Gallcher, D. J., Kadir, S., Kaufman, S. L., Mitchell, S. E., Kinnison, M. L., Chang, R., Adams, P., White, R. I., Jr., and Cameron, J. L.: Nonoperative management of benign postoperative strictures. Radiology, 156:625, 1985.
17. Harlaftis, N., Gray, S. W., and Skandalakis, J. E.: Multiple gallbladders. Surg. Gynecol. Obstet., 145:928, 1977.
18. LaRusso, N. F., Wiesner, R. H., Ludwig, J., and MacCarty, R. L.: Primary sclerosing cholangitis. N. Engl. J. Med., 310:899, 1984.
19. Leuschner, U., Fischer, H., Kurtz, W., Guldutuna, S., Hubner, K., Hellstern, A., Gatzen, M., and Leuschner, M.: Ursodeoxycholic acid in primary biliary cirrhosis: Results of a controlled double-blind trial. Gastroenterology, 97:1268, 1989.
20. Longmire, W. P., Jr.: Tumors of the extrahepatic biliary radicles. Curr. Probl. Cancer, 1:1, 1976.
21. Nagorney, D. M., McIlrath, D. C., and Adson, M. A.: Choledochal cysts in adults: Clinical management. Surgery, 96:656, 1984.
22. Neoptolemos, J. P., Carr-Locke, D. L., and Fossand, D. P.: Prospective randomized study of preoperative endoscopic sphincterotomy versus surgery alone for common bile duct stones. Br. J. Surg., 294:470, 1987.
23. Northover, J. M. A., and Terblanche, J.: A new look at the arterial supply of the bile duct in man and its surgical implications. Br. J. Surg., 66:379, 1979.
24. Okada, A., Oguchi, Y., Kamata, S., Ikeda, Y., Kawashima, Y., and Saito, R.: Common channel syndrome: Diagnosis with endoscopic retrograde cholangiopancreatectography and surgical management. Surgery, 93:634, 1984.
25. Olaison, G., Kald, B., Karlqvist, P., Lindstrom, E., and Anderberg, B.: Endoscopic removal of common bile duct stones without subsequent cholecystectomy. Acta Chir. Scand., 153:541, 1987.
26. O'Neill, J. A., Templeton, J. M., Schnaufer, L., Bishop, H. C., Ziegler, M. M., and Ross, A. J., III: Recent experience with choledochal cyst. Ann. Surg., 205:533, 1987.
27. Ostrow, J. D.: The etiology of pigment gallstones. Hepatology, 4:2155, 1984.
28. Palmisano, D. J.: Double gallbladder. Am. J. Surg., 118:463, 1969.
29. Pitt, H. A., Miyamoto, T., Parapatis, S. K., Tompkins, R. K., and Longmire, W. P., Jr.: Factors influencing outcome in patients with postoperative biliary strictures. Am. J. Surg., 144:14, 1982.
30. Power, D.: Gallstones; a plea for earlier operation. Br. J. Surg., 1:12, 1913.
31. Richards, R. N.: Congenital absence of the gallbladder and cystic duct associated with primary carcinoma of the common bile duct. Can. Med. Assoc. J., 94:859, 1966.
32. Safrany, L.: Endoscopic treatment of biliary tract disease. Lancet, 2:983, 1978.
33. Sauerbruch, T., and Stern, M.: Fragmentation of bile duct stones by extracorporeal shock waves. Gastroenterology, 96:146, 1989.
34. Sharp, K. W., and Gadacaz, T. R.: Selection of patients for dissolution of retained common duct stones with mono-octanoin. Ann. Surg., 196:137, 1982.
35. Sindelar, W. F., Tepper, J., and Travis, E. L.: Tolerance of bile duct to intraoperative radiation. Surgery, 92:533, 1982.
36. Tanaka, M., Ikeda, S., Yoshimoto, H., and Matsumoto, S.: The long-term fate of the gallbladder after endoscopic sphincterotomy: Complete follow-up study of 122 patients. Am. J. Surg., 154:505, 1987.
37. Teplick, S. K., Walferth, C. C., Hayes, M. F., and Amron, G. I.: Balloon dilation of benign post-surgical biliary-enteric anastomotic strictures. Gastrointest. Radiol., 7:307, 1982.
38. Todani, T., Watanabe, Y., Fujii, T., and Uemura, S.: Anomalous arrangement of the pancreatobiliary ductal system in patients with choledochal cyst. Am. J. Surg., 147:672, 1984.
39. Tompkins, R. K., Thomas, D., Wile, A., and Longmire, W. P., Jr.: Prognostic factors in bile duct carcinoma: Analysis of 96 cases. Ann. Surg., 194:447, 1981.
40. Van Stiegmann, G., Pearlman, N. W., Goff, J. S., Sun, J. H., and Norton, L. W.: Endoscopic cholangiography and stone removal prior to cholecystectomy. Arch. Surg., 124:787, 1989.
41. Warren, K. W., Mountain, J. C., and Midell, A. I.: Management of strictures of the biliary tract. Surg. Clin. North Am., 51:711, 1971.
42. Way, L. W., Admirand, W. H., and Dunphy, J. E.: Management of choledocholithiasis. Ann. Surg., 176:347, 1972.
43. Wilson, J. E., and Dietrick, J. E.: Agenesis of the gallbladder: Case report and familial investigation. Surgery, 99:106, 1986.
44. Yuhl, E. T., Stirrett, L., Hill, M. R., Jr., and Beal, J. M.: The cholescintigram: A preliminary report. Surgery, 34:724, 1953.

I

ACUTE CHOLECYSTITIS

David L. Nahrwold, M.D.

Acute cholecystitis is a chemical or bacterial inflammation of the gallbladder that may cause severe peritonitis and death unless proper treatment is instituted. In approximately 95 per cent of patients, gallstones are present in the gallbladder (calculous cholecystitis), and in about 5 per cent they are not (acalculous cholecystitis).

ACUTE CALCULOUS CHOLECYSTITIS

The incidence of acute calculous cholecystitis is higher in females, with a 3:1 ratio of females to males to approximately the age of 50 years and a ratio of approximately 1.5:1 thereafter.

The exact incidence of acute cholecystitis among patients with gallstones is not known, but approximately 20 per cent of patients who enter a hospital for biliary tract disease have acute cholecystitis. The percentage of cholecystectomies done for acute cholecystitis has increased recently, especially in the elderly.[8] Patients who have symptoms from gallstones should be advised to have elective cholecystectomy to avoid the mortality and morbidity of acute cholecystitis and its complications.

Acute calculous cholecystitis appears to be caused by obstruction of the cystic duct or the junction of the gallbladder with the cystic duct by a stone, or by edema formed as the result of local mucosal erosion and inflammation caused by the stone. The obstruction causes gallbladder distention, followed by subserosal edema, venous and lymphatic obstruction, cellular infiltration, and localized areas of ischemia. Perforation at the site of ischemic gangrene may cause bile peritonitis or, if surrounded by omentum, a localized pericholecystic abscess. Rarely, a gangrenous area may perforate into the wall of the duodenum or small intestine, causing a cholecystoenteric fistula. Gallstones then may enter the small intestine, and if one is sufficiently large, the rare syndrome of mechanical obstruction of the distal ileum, gallstone ileus, may ensue. Fortunately, early treatment has reduced the incidence of these complications of acute cholecystitis.

The role of bacteria in the pathogenesis of acute cholecystitis is not clear; positive cultures of bile or gallbladder wall are found in 50 to 75 per cent of patients.[3,17,27,28] Nevertheless, deaths and complications from untreated cholecystitis are usually associated with septic complications of the disease, and the organisms involved are those that most often colonize the stone-containing gallbladder. A very important feature of the pathogenesis may be erosion of the mucosa by a stone, allowing highly concentrated bile salts access to tissue planes. Bile salts are toxic to cells because they have detergent properties that allow them to solubilize the lipids in cell membranes. This causes destruction of cells, necrosis, and, eventually, perforation of the gallbladder.

Although obstruction by a stone is essential for the development of acute calculous cholecystitis, other factors appear to be involved, because acute cholecystitis is not the inevitable consequence of obstruction. Hydrops of the gallbladder, in which the outlet is obstructed by a stone, produces marked distention, but acute inflammation does not follow. In animals, ligation of the cystic duct alone does not produce acute cholecystitis. Thus, it appears that outlet obstruction plus another factor is essential for the development of acute cholecystitis. The other factor

could be erosion of the mucosa by a stone, permitting bile salts or bacteria access to the tissues of the gallbladder wall. In animal experiments, the presence of pancreatic juice, gastric juice, or concentrated bile in the lumen of the obstructed gallbladder causes acute cholecystitis.[36,41]

PATHOLOGY. The inflamed gallbladder is enlarged and the serosal surface is congested and may have areas of gangrene or necrosis; the wall is edematous and thickened. The obstructing stone is usually impacted in the infundibulum or the cystic duct; bloody bile or pus may be found within the lumen. Mucosal sloughing is usually present, although this may be apparent only on microscopic examination. Neutrophils are found within 24 hours and become more prominent as time progresses; the neutrophilic response is more prominent in gangrene, perforation, and empyema. *Empyema* is the term used to denote the acutely inflamed gallbladder that contains pus. Empyema of the gallbladder is the equivalent of an intra-abdominal abscess and may be associated with severe sepsis. Cystic duct obstruction is the *sine qua non* for its development. In neglected cases, spontaneous drainage of the gallbladder through the abdominal wall may occur, a circumstance termed empyema necessitans.

Approximately 65 per cent of gallbladders involved with acute cholecystitis also have the manifestations of chronic cholecystitis: fibrosis of the wall, chronic inflammatory cell infiltrate, Rokitansky-Aschoff sinuses, and mucosal flattening.[19] This is evidence that recurrent attacks of acute cholecystitis are frequent. As the acute process resolves, fibrosis of the wall and a chronic inflammatory infiltrate become prominent features.

SYMPTOMS. A majority of patients have symptoms referable to the gallbladder prior to the development of acute cholecystitis, but 20 to 40 per cent are asymptomatic. Persistent pain in the area of the gallbladder is present in almost every case. In fact, the absence of pain essentially excludes the diagnosis. Frequently, the pain develops after ingestion of a meal and probably follows forceful contraction of the gallbladder against a fixed obstruction, usually a stone impacted in the infundibulum or the cystic duct. As the development of acute cholecystitis progresses through the sequence of distention, edema, venous and lymphatic obstruction, and ischemia, the pain probably is caused by gallbladder distention and, later, by inflammation of the gallbladder and adjacent peritoneal surfaces. Depending on the habitus of the patient and the precise location of the organ, the pain may be in the right upper quadrant, in the epigastrium, or in both areas. Radiation of the pain is around the right side toward the tip of the scapula. Pain in the right shoulder is present when the diaphragm is irritated by the inflammatory process. The persistence and severity of pain serve to distinguish the development of acute cholecystitis from an attack of gallbladder colic. The former may last for several days, but the latter rarely lasts for more than a few hours.

Nausea and vomiting, which occur in 60 to 70 per cent of patients, are the only other significant symptoms. This appears to be a reflex phenomenon, associated with a rapid rise in gallbladder pressure. Frequently, patients attempt to induce vomiting, having the sensation that this will relieve their symptoms.

PHYSICAL FINDINGS. The inflammatory nature of acute cholecystitis causes an elevated temperature in approximately 80 per cent of patients. Fever may be absent in elderly or immunocompromised patients and in those who take steroids or nonsteroidal anti-inflammatory drugs. Just as pain is present in almost all patients, the most common and reliable finding on physical examination is tenderness in the right upper quadrant, the epigastrium, or both areas. Subjective tenderness is so common that its absence should raise serious question about the diagnosis. Approximately half of all patients have muscle rigidity in the right upper quadrant, and about one fourth have rebound tenderness. The frequency of these findings, which are indicative of peritonitis, increases as the disease progresses. Murphy's sign, consisting of inspiratory arrest during deep palpation of the right upper quadrant, is not a consistent finding but is almost pathognomonic when present. Unless generalized peritonitis has developed, acute cholecystitis usually does not cause paralytic ileus distal to the duodenum; therefore, bowel sounds are absent in only approximately 10 per cent of patients. A mass in the region of the gallbladder is palpable in nearly 40 per cent. Because gallbladder distention is inherent in the pathogenesis of the disease, the organ itself is palpable in some patients, but in many a mass is palpable because the omentum becomes attached to the gallbladder in response to the inflammation. The presence of a mass late in the course of the disease may signify the development of a pericholecystic abscess. A palpable, tender gallbladder is almost pathognomonic of acute cholecystitis.

Jaundice, usually mild, occurs in approximately 10 per cent of patients and has been attributed to an accompanying cholangitis. Although the extrahepatic bile ducts are obviously involved in the inflammatory process, they are not obstructed. The jaundice is more likely due to entry of bile pigments into the circulation through the damaged gallbladder mucosa or to physiologic obstruction of the bile duct system from choledochal sphincter spasm induced by the adjacent inflammatory process.[31] The presence of jaundice should suggest the possibility of concomitant choledocholithiasis, which occurs in 10 to 15 per cent of patients; otherwise, it is an insignificant finding.

LABORATORY FINDINGS. The white blood cell count is elevated in 85 per cent of patients, but it may not be increased in those who take anti-inflammatory drugs or in the elderly. One half have elevation of the serum bilirubin, and the serum amylase is increased in one third. In general, the blood tests are nonspecific and not especially helpful, except for the white blood cell count.

RADIOLOGIC STUDIES. Roentgenograms of the abdomen in the supine and erect positions and an upright chest film are frequently obtained in patients with acute abdominal conditions. When acute cholecystitis presents with a classic history and physical findings, the usefulness of these radiologic studies must be questioned because the only information potentially available is documentation of the presence of gallstones or air in the gallbladder and biliary tract. Only approximately 15 per cent of gallstones are opaque, and both emphysematous cholecystitis and cholecystoenteric fistulas are very rare; therefore, the yield of useful information is minimal. Plain roentgenograms may be helpful in complicated cases, or when the specific diagnosis in the patient with an acute abdominal condition is not clear.

The specific test for acute cholecystitis is cholescintigraphy with a derivative of [99m]technetium-iminodiacetic acid (technetium-IDA scan). Normally, the scan outlines the liver and the extrahepatic biliary tract, including the gallbladder, and demonstrates the nuclide flowing into the upper small intestine as well (Fig. 1). In acute cholecystitis, the gallbladder is not observed on the scan, presumably because the gallbladder outlet or the cystic duct is obstructed (Fig. 2). In acute calculous cholecystitis, cholescintigraphy has a sensitivity of nearly 100 per cent, meaning that the test is positive in almost all patients who have acute cholecystitis, and a specificity of 95 per cent, meaning that the scan is negative in 95 per cent of individuals who do not have the disease.[39] Complete obstruction of the common

bile duct or the common hepatic duct is detectable on the technetium-IDA scan, but the degree of resolution is not sufficient to diagnose stones or other lesions.

Calculi within the gallbladder can be accurately detected by ultrasonography, but this test is not specific for acute calculous cholecystitis. A thickened gallbladder wall and pericholecystic fluid are sometimes present. Ultrasonography can detect right upper quadrant masses and enlargement of the bile ducts and pancreas, so it may be useful in complicated cases or when the diagnosis is obscure.[6] Although some have advocated routine ultrasonography in suspected acute cholecystitis to confirm the presence of gallstones, the technetium-IDA scan is more specific and is the indicated test in patients with the classic clinical manifestations.

DIFFERENTIAL DIAGNOSIS. Acute cholecystitis must be differentiated from other acute abdominal conditions, including acute appendicitis, perforated or penetrating duodenal ulcer, acute or perforated gastric ulcer, and acute pancreatitis. Most cases of acute appendicitis can be differentiated easily, but those in which the tip of a long, retrocecal appendix lies near the gallbladder can be vexing. Cholescintigraphy is helpful in this situation.

In approximately 15 per cent of cases of acute cholecystitis, the serum amylase is elevated, causing concern over the possibility of acute pancreatitis. The cause of hyperamylasemia in uncomplicated acute cholecystitis is unknown; hyperamylasemia does not necessarily indicate that clinically significant pancreatitis is present.

Gallstone-associated pancreatitis is a self-limiting process associated with the passage of a stone through the distal common bile duct and into the duodenum.[1] Elevation of the serum amylase is common in this situation, and acute cholecystitis is estimated to be present in as many as a third of patients with gallstone pancreatitis. The pathophysiologic mechanisms and sequence of events that lead to the simultaneous presence of acute cholecystitis and gallstone pancreatitis are not clear, but both processes appear to resolve when the stone has passed into the duodenum. The importance of the association is that acute cholecystitis should be considered in patients known to have acute pancreatitis, and the possibility of gallstone pancreatitis should be considered in patients who have acute cholecystitis and elevation of serum amylase.

The differential diagnosis must also include conditions that cause pain due to rapid liver enlargement or hepatic inflammation, including viral hepatitis, acute alcoholic hepatitis, right-sided heart failure, and gonococcal perihepatitis. These usually can be distinguished from acute cholecystitis without difficulty. Gallbladder colic rarely lasts longer than 3 hours and does not have the clinical manifestations of an inflammatory process. Other acute abdominal conditions such as small bowel obstruction and acute regional enteritis can be differentiated easily by a carefully elicited history and a thorough physical examination.

COMPLICATIONS. Complications of acute cholecystitis are perforation, pericholecystic abscess, and fistula. All are consequences of gallbladder wall ischemia and gangrene. Free perforation, which represents approximately one third of these complications, occurs when a gangrenous area becomes necrotic and bile leaks into the peritoneal cavity. Diffusion of bile throughout the peritoneal cavity frequently causes generalized peritonitis with systemic sepsis and death unless treated promptly. The mortality from perforation is approximately 20 per cent.[21,28]

Pericholecystic abscess follows perforation of the gallbladder that is walled off by omentum or adjacent organs such as the colon, stomach, or duodenum. The abscess forms between the gallbladder and the surrounding structures. An abscess may also form between the gallbladder and the bare area of the liver behind the gallbladder. Pericholecystic abscess is the most common complication, representing approximately 50 per cent, but

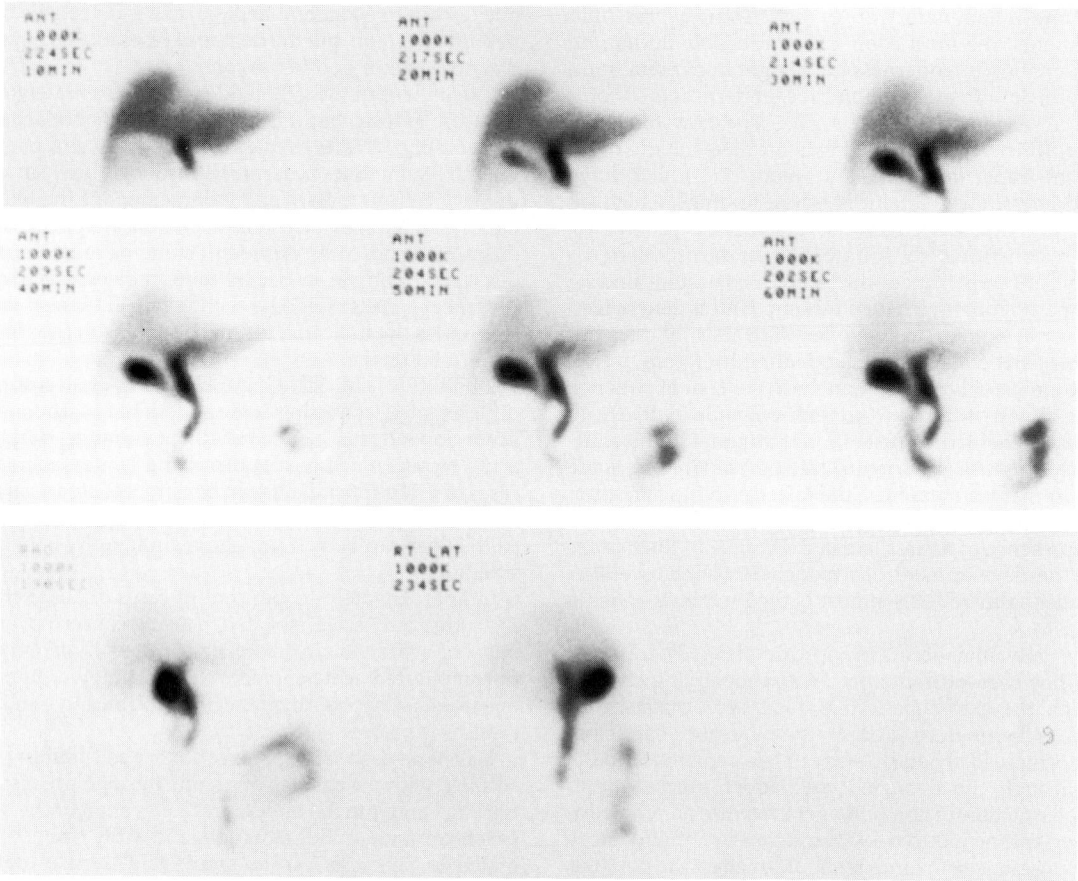

Figure 1. Normal cholescintigram showing liver, bile duct, gallbladder, and small intestine. From left to right, scans were done every 10 minutes in the anterior view. The bottom scans are the right anterior oblique view (left) and the right lateral view (right).

is the least virulent with a mortality of approximately 15 per cent.

Fistulization occurs when the gallbladder becomes attached to a portion of the gastrointestinal tract and perforates it. The duodenum is the most common site followed by the colon. Cholecystojejunal and cholecystogastric fistulas are rare. Fistulization represents approximately 15 per cent of the complications of acute cholecystitis, but fistulas into the gallbladder may follow other diseases such as penetrating peptic ulcer, Crohn's disease, trauma, tuberculosis, and intra-abdominal abscess. When a stone is discharged from the gallbladder into the small intestine and is sufficiently large to obstruct the narrow terminal ileum, the resulting "gallstone ileus" creates an additional hazard for the patient with a cholecystoenteric fistula.

The symptoms of these complications are generally indistinguishable from those of acute cholecystitis. In one series, only 59 per cent of patients had signs of peritoneal irritation, and fewer than half had diffuse abdominal tenderness or absent bowel sounds.[21] In addition, none of the three types of complications is consistently manifested by a specific symptom complex. The findings then are similar to those of acute cholecystitis.

Complications may develop as early as 2 days following the onset of the symptoms of acute cholecystitis and as late as several weeks. The average onset is approximately a week, but this information is not helpful in managing the individual case. The overall mortality from complications is approximately 20 per cent.[9,13,21,38] Because the mortality of complications is more than four times that of surgically treated uncomplicated acute cholecystitis, early cholecystectomy should be done as soon as the diagnosis of acute cholecystitis is made and the patient is in optimal condition.

TREATMENT. Patients suspected of having acute cholecystitis should be hospitalized. Initial management should include administration of an antibiotic that is effective against the enteric organisms found in the bile of approximately 80 per cent of patients with gallstones and acute cholecystitis. These organisms include both gram-positive and gram-negative aerobes and anaerobes. Those present most frequently are *Escherichia coli, Klebsiella aerogenes, Streptococcus faecalis, Clostridium welchii, Proteus* species, *Enterobacter* species, and anaerobic streptococci. A single organism is found in approximately 40 per cent of cases, two species in about 30 per cent, three in 20 per cent, and four or more in the remainder.[23] Obviously, no single antibiotic is effective against all these organisms. The broadest coverage would be achieved by the combination of ampicillin, clindamycin, and an aminoglycoside, but the toxicity of the last is of concern. Therefore, the author favors administration of a second-generation cephalosporin for most cases of acute cholecystitis and reserves the triple-drug combination for patients who are seriously ill with sepsis. The incidence of postoperative septic complications is markedly reduced by antibiotic administration.[3,37] The incidence of wound infection, for example, is reduced to the extent that it is difficult to demonstrate that prophylactic administration of one antibiotic protects against wound infection more efficaciously than another. Antibiotic therapy should be initiated as soon as the diagnosis is made and should be continued for 24 hours postoperatively, unless the degree of peritonitis in surrounding tissues is severe, in which case it should continue for 7 days. Changes in the regimen may be indicated by the course of the patient and the result of the cultures of bile and gallbladder wall taken at operation.

The definitive treatment of acute cholecystitis is cholecystectomy. The timing of operation was debated until recently when

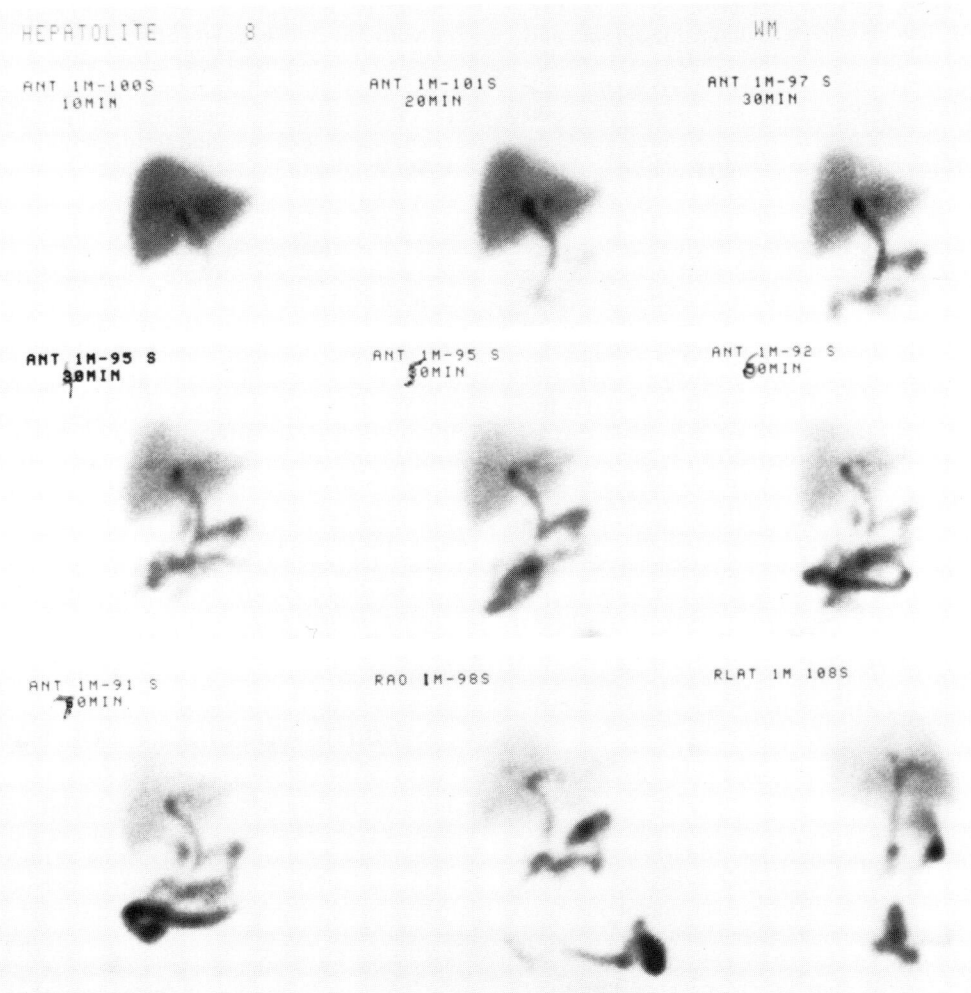

Figure 2. Abnormal cholescintigram in a patient with acute calculous cholecystitis. The gallbladder is not visualized. From left to right, scans were done every 10 minutes in the anterior view. Last two scans are the right anterior oblique view and the right lateral view, respectively.

data from several studies became available. Some thought that patients should be treated nonoperatively, allowing resolution of the acute inflammation, followed by elective cholecystectomy approximately 6 weeks later. Others maintained that operation should be done as soon as the diagnosis was made. Several prospective trials demonstrate that the mortality for early and delayed surgical therapy is equal, and that there are no significant differences in the frequency or severity of postoperative complications.[22,30] These and other studies have also demonstrated that length of hospital stay is shorter and return to productivity is sooner when early cholecystectomy is performed. In addition, some patients for whom delayed cholecystectomy is planned require emergency operation because they become worse or do not improve, and this group has higher mortality and morbidity.[42] Approximately 25 per cent of patients for whom delayed operation is contemplated have a recurrence of acute cholecystitis prior to the planned operation and may require cholecystectomy sooner than intended.[24] The data clearly favor early cholecystectomy.

PREOPERATIVE MANAGEMENT. In all patients with the tentative diagnosis of acute cholecystitis, the author initiates antibiotic therapy, nasogastric suction, intravenous fluid administration, and monitoring of hemodynamic parameters and urinary output while diagnostic studies are in progress. High priority is placed on obtaining cholescintigraphy. Serum amylase, bilirubin, alkaline phosphatase, electrolytes, blood sugar, and creatinine are measured, and a complete blood count is done. The

electrocardiogram is correlated with the clinical history for evidence of a recent myocardial infarction, ischemia, or unstable angina pectoris. Chest and abdominal roentgenograms are obtained to assist in the assessment of cardiopulmonary disease and evidence of emphysematous cholecystitis or pericholecystic abscess. Other clinical investigation, such as ultrasonography or noninvasive carotid blood flow measurement, is done as warranted by the history and physical examination. During the evaluation period, which usually takes less than 12 hours, frequent examinations are done. When the diagnosis is reasonably certain, a decision is made for early or delayed cholecystectomy. Early operation is performed in all patients who do not have significant risk factors and is done as soon as the patient is in optimal condition as determined by hemodynamic monitoring and urinary output, generally within 12 to 24 hours of admission. Delayed operation is elected in the few patients who have significant risk factors, including unstable angina, clinically significant carotid artery disease, congestive heart failure, cirrhosis, and other conditions that significantly increase the risk of operation.

TECHNICAL ASPECTS. Cholecystectomy for acute cholecystitis is more difficult than elective cholecystectomy for chronic symptoms, and the risk of injury to the extrahepatic bile ducts is higher. The first problem is the tense, distended gallbladder, which cannot be displaced to visualize the triangle of Calot adequately. Usually, the gallbladder must be decompressed by aspiration of its contents through a trocar placed in the fundus.

Care must be taken not to spill infected bile during this maneuver, and samples of bile should be cultured for aerobic and anaerobic organisms. No attempt should be made to remove the stones. After decompression, the junction of the cystic duct with the common duct can be identified, and the cystic duct dissected free. When accurate identification of these structures is difficult because of inflammation and edema, the dissection should proceed from the fundus toward the cystic duct. Because common duct stones are present in 10 to 15 per cent of cases of acute cholecystitis, the same incidence seen in elective cholecystectomy, an operative cholangiogram should be obtained through the cystic duct when it is safe to do so. Occasionally, the cystic duct and the common duct are very friable, in which case the risk of duct injury is high, and cholangiography should not be done. Mild hyperbilirubinemia and hyperamylasemia are not absolute indications for choledochotomy and exploration of the common duct in acute cholecystitis because these tests are frequently elevated. However, when operative cholangiography demonstrates common duct stones or there is clinical evidence of them, choledocholithotomy should be done. If the condition of the patient is too precarious, a large Moss-Whelan T-tube can be inserted for decompression, and the stones can be extracted percutaneously through the T-tube tract at a later date.

Cholecystostomy should be done only when cholecystectomy is too dangerous. Although the procedure relieves the obstruction that is requisite for the development of acute cholecystitis, the inflamed organ is not removed, and cure is dependent on the ability of the patient's defenses to resolve the inflammatory process.

Ideally, if cholecystostomy is planned, it should be done under local anesthesia to minimize risk. Unplanned cholecystostomy is performed in lieu of cholecystectomy where the degree of inflammation in the area of Calot's triangle is so severe that dissection is too dangerous to proceed. When this occurs, care must be taken to be certain that any collection of pus near the neck of the gallbladder is drained, because cholecystostomy does not ameliorate the sepsis associated with a pericholecystic abscess. Cholecystostomy is done by placing pursestring sutures in the fundus of the gallbladder, aspirating and culturing its contents through a stab wound, removing the calculi with

stone forceps, inserting a large catheter, and securing the catheter with the pursestring sutures. The catheter is brought through a stab wound in the abdominal wall, and the gallbladder fundus is sewn to the peritoneum (Fig. 3). The importance of removal of the stones cannot be overemphasized because subsequent removal of the cholecystostomy tube may cause gallbladder symptoms if a stone is impacted within the infundibulum or the cystic duct. Cholangiography through the tube prior to its removal identifies retained stones, which usually can be extracted percutaneously under fluoroscopic guidance.

TREATMENT OF COMPLICATIONS. The basic treatment of complications of acute cholecystitis is cholecystectomy. The peritoneal cavity should be evacuated of bile and irrigated copiously in cases of free perforation. Pericholecystic abscesses should be drained; they are usually completely evacuated in the process of cholecystectomy. Fistulization is managed by cholecystectomy and closure of the involved segment of small intestine or colon. Medical treatment of these complications is dangerous because of the accompanying sepsis and, in the case of free perforation and pericholecystic abscess, the need to establish drainage. The results with prompt cholecystectomy and drainage and closure of fistula, when present, are superior to nonoperative therapy.[21] Cholecystostomy should be avoided unless cholecystectomy is absolutely contraindicated because insertion of a tube into the gallbladder does not prevent leakage from a perforation or control an abscess.

ACUTE ACALCULOUS CHOLECYSTITIS

Acute acalculous cholecystitis is acute inflammation of the gallbladder in the absence of gallstones and represents approximately 4 to 8 per cent of all cases of acute cholecystitis. The condition is estimated to be increasing in frequency,[18] but this has not been proved. In contrast to calculous cholecystitis, which is more common in females, the male to female ratio is approximately 1.5 : 1.[20]

The disease has a tendency to occur after, or in association with, other conditions, especially major trauma, burns, or operations. Other conditions known to be precedents include multiple transfusions, childbirth, bacterial sepsis, and debilitating diseases such as sarcoidosis, polyarteritis nodosa, and lupus erythematosus. These patients are often critically ill, requiring extensive monitoring and life support procedures. Acute acalculous cholecystitis associated with administration of total parenteral nutrition has been reported.[33] No apparent precipitating factor is present in as many as 50 per cent of patients.

Acute postoperative cholecystitis and *acute posttraumatic cholecystitis* are used to describe the most frequently associated conditions. Not all such cases are of the acalculous variety, however. Approximately two thirds of those that occur postoperatively and 15 per cent of posttraumatic cases are associated with gallstones.[20,32]

The pathologic process of acute acalculous cholecystitis does not differ from that of the calculous type, except that the incidence of gangrene and perforation is higher. Whether this is an inherent feature of the disease or the result of delayed diagnosis and treatment is conjectural. The obscured symptoms and findings by the effect of recent trauma, operative procedures, or other illness frequently lead to a delay in recognition of the condition. This could be partially responsible for the higher mortality observed in acalculous cholecystitis, although coexisting disease may also add to the usual risk factors.[1] Thus, the association with other conditions does not denote the presence or absence of gallstones.[18,20,32]

ETIOLOGY. The etiology of acute acalculous cholecystitis is uncertain and may be multifactorial. The theories can be grouped into three categories: stasis, sepsis, and ischemia. Stasis of gallbladder bile occurs in the absence of regular contraction, stimulated by cholecystokinin, which is released by the pres-

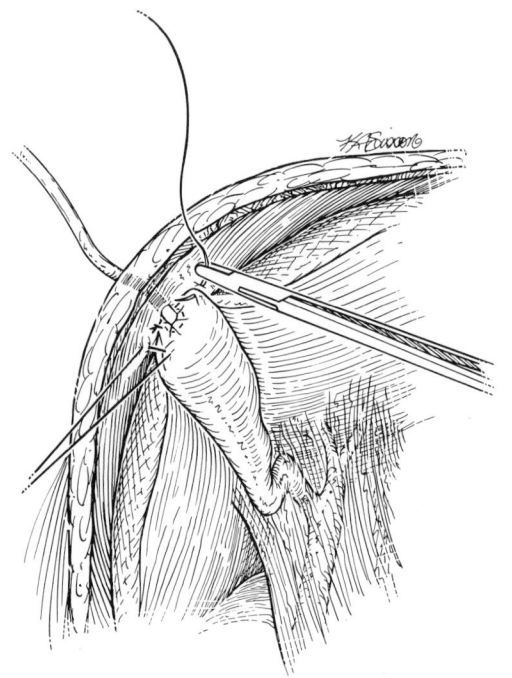

Figure 3. Technique of cholecystostomy. Gallbladder is sutured to the peritoneum to create a seal that prevents leakage of bile into the peritoneal cavity.

ence of certain products of digestion in the upper small intestine. Maximal concentration and extraction of water from gallbladder bile reduce it to a viscid material known as sludge, which may even contain soft concretions. Presumably, viscid bile and sludge may produce a functional obstruction of the gallbladder outlet, with the ensuing sequence of edema, venous and lymphatic obstruction, ischemia, and necrosis. Stasis of gallbladder bile may also render it more susceptible to colonization with bacteria and the possibility of bacterial invasion of the gallbladder wall during functional outlet obstruction. Lack of oral intake frequently accompanies several of the conditions with which acalculous cholecystitis occurs, including trauma, major operative procedures, and serious debilitating disease. Administration of narcotics may be a contributing factor. Thus, stasis may be an important mechanism in some patients with these conditions, as well as in long-term total parenteral nutrition patients. However, acute acalculous cholecystitis occurs in patients who have eaten normally, and other factors must be involved.

Ischemia has been implicated because of the high incidence of gangrene and necrosis. Brief or prolonged periods of hypotension or low flow are not uncommon during operations, following trauma and burns, or in association with sepsis. Decreased blood flow to the gallbladder epithelium could cause it to slough, and concentrated bile acids, which are toxic to tissues, would then have access to the gallbladder wall. Although this theory is plausible, acute acalculous cholecystitis is a very rare consequence of hypotension, so that its validity remains questionable.[20]

Interest in factor XII as an etiologic agent has been strong because it is activated by transfusion of blood products and by bacterial endotoxin. Injection of *E. coli* endotoxin into dogs causes ischemia and other findings compatible with early acute cholecystitis[2]; therefore, sepsis may be important in the development of acalculous cholecystitis in some patients.

DIAGNOSIS. Recognition of the disease may be delayed when the patient cannot communicate well because of concomitant disease or the postoperative or posttraumatic state. The symptoms are identical to those of acute calculous cholecystitis, except that they may be absent or masked by symptoms of an underlying or precedent condition. Pain in the right upper quadrant or the epigastrium, or both, occurs in approximately 70 per cent and vomiting in 35 per cent. Whereas pain is almost always present in acute calculous cholecystitis, it may be absent or obscured in the acalculous variant because of narcotic administration, decreased level of consciousness, or abdominal pain from an incision or other disease process.

The most significant physical findings include tenderness in the right upper quadrant and fever, which occur in approximately 75 per cent. Abdominal distention and absent or hypoactive bowel sounds are present in approximately 25 per cent, and a right upper quadrant mass and jaundice are present less frequently.[33] Usually, the diagnosis can be made from the physical examination, but only approximately half the cases are correctly diagnosed preoperatively when abdominal surgery or trauma have been antecedent.

The inflammation is reflected in an elevated white blood cell count in 70 per cent, and the alkaline phosphatase or aspartate aminotransferase is elevated in over 50 per cent.

Cholescintigraphy should be done when acute acalculous cholecystitis is suspected,[14] but the accuracy, approximately 88 per cent, is not as high as in calculous cholecystitis.[16] The problem is a higher incidence of false-positive scans.[12] Patients at risk for acute acalculous cholecystitis may have inadequate oral intake, and their gallbladders may contain viscid bile from lack of contraction. Therefore, the radionuclide may not be able to enter the otherwise normal gallbladder. Ultrasonography may be helpful by demonstrating distention and thickening of the wall. However, these signs are not always present, and when

they are, they may be nonspecific. For example, thickening of the gallbladder wall occurs in ascites, congestive heart failure, and hypoalbuminemia. Percutaneous aspiration of bile from the gallbladder and establishment of a percutaneous tube cholecystostomy is being employed more often as a combined diagnostic and therapeutic maneuver. The bile is examined for the presence of bacteria and leukocytes.

TREATMENT. The standard treatment has been emergency cholecystectomy. In contrast to the calculous form, for which some have advocated delayed operation, the high risk of gangrene and perforation mandate early treatment. Unless the inflammation is so severe as to make it dangerous, operative cholangiography should be done to exclude the possibility of passage of a single gallstone into the common bile duct. Mortality from acute acalculous cholecystitis is higher than that from acute calculous cholecystitis because the antecedent or concomitant condition usually increases the risk and because the diagnosis is often delayed. Some have advocated either periodic ingestion of fat or cholecystokinin administration in total parenteral nutrition patients to empty the gallbladder and prevent stasis and, presumably, the development of acute cholecystitis.[26,33]

A small experience with percutaneous cholecystostomy in the treatment of acute cholecystitis in the high-risk patient has accumulated. A summary of reported cases revealed a success rate of 99 per cent, and morbidity and mortality of 25 and 10 per cent, respectively.[40]

UNUSUAL TYPES OF ACUTE CHOLECYSTITIS

ACUTE EMPHYSEMATOUS CHOLECYSTITIS. This form of acute cholecystitis represents only approximately 1 per cent of all cases and is characterized by the presence of gas in the wall and the lumen of the gallbladder.

Emphysematous cholecystitis is more common in diabetics; approximately 40 per cent of the reported cases have this association.[29] Approximately 75 per cent have occurred in males, and the average age of afflicted patients is approximately 60 years. The onset of emphysematous cholecystitis is abrupt, and in addition to right upper quadrant pain, nausea, and vomiting, patients rapidly become toxic.

The pathognomonic diagnostic sign is the presence of gas within the lumen and the wall of the gallbladder on a plain roentgenogram of the abdomen (Fig. 4). The gas is produced by bacteria; *Clostridium perfringens*, *E. coli*, *Klebsiella*, or a mixture of organisms is usually found. *C. perfringens* has been cultured in approximately half the reported cases.[29] Gangrene of the gallbladder is usually present; stones are absent in approximately 30 per cent of cases. Emergency cholecystectomy is the

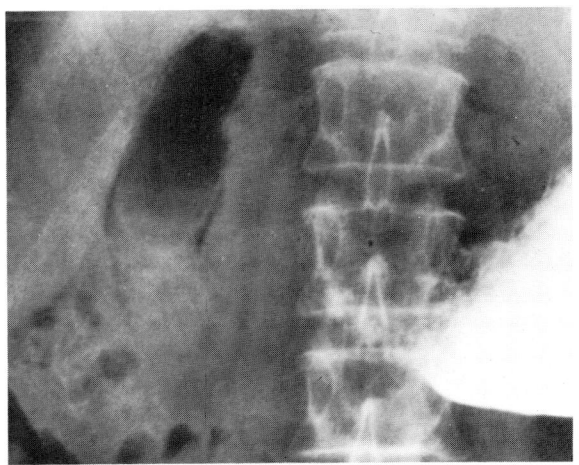

Figure 4. Radiograph showing air in the wall and lumen of the gallbladder in acute emphysematous cholecystitis.

appropriate treatment. The high incidence of gangrene invites perforation and sepsis unless the gallbladder is removed.

TYPHOID CHOLECYSTITIS. Acute cholecystitis occurs rarely in patients who have typhoid fever, usually during the third week of the illness or later. Gallstones are not present, and the offending organism, *Salmonella typhi*, is found in the bile. Perforation of the gallbladder is very common.

A more common problem is the colonization of the gallbladder bile with *S. typhi* in patients who have had typhoid fever, which may or may not have been clinically apparent. These individuals become typhoid carriers and excrete the organism in their feces. Gallstones and chronic cholecystitis may develop. Ampicillin in large doses has been effective in eradicating the carrier state in a majority of patients,[34] but when gallstones are present, they serve as a continuing nidus for infection and cholecystectomy may be necessary.[10,15]

TORSION OF THE GALLBLADDER. Hemorrhagic infarction of the gallbladder occurs when the organ twists 180 degrees or more. Two anatomic anomalies permit torsion. In the most rare type, the gallbladder has no mesentery or attachment to the liver and is completely peritonealized. It lies free in the peritoneal cavity, suspended only by the cystic duct and cystic artery, both of which may have a short mesentery. The propensity for infarction is obvious, and it usually occurs in childhood.[5] More commonly, the gallbladder is suspended from its usual position on the liver by a mesentery that is sufficiently long to allow torsion in either direction. Gallstones are present in a significant number of cases,[25] and it has been suggested that the weight of the stones contributes to the torsion. However, the weight of gallstones is not much different from the weight of the bile they displace.

Acute torsion causes abdominal pain on the right side, and the twisted, infarcted gallbladder may be palpable as a mass in the right lower quadrant. The correct diagnosis often is not made preoperatively, the symptoms frequently being mistaken for acute appendicitis. Some patients have periodic episodes of abdominal pain that are presumed to be caused by incomplete volvulus and spontaneous reduction. The treatment of torsion of the gallbladder is cholecystectomy.

TUMORS. Carcinoma of the gallbladder occasionally presents as acute cholecystitis. This is not surprising, because of the frequent association with gallstones and the possibility that the cancer itself may obstruct the gallbladder outlet.

Granular cell myoblastomas, firm yellow nodules that are thought to be of neuroectodermal origin, are found in the wall of the cystic duct, the common bile duct, or the gallbladder.[7] They are benign tumors that tend to occur in young black females. Gallstones may be present. Those obstructing the cystic duct may cause acute cholecystitis, empyema, or hydrops of the gallbladder.[35] The treatment is cholecystectomy with excision of the portion of the cystic duct that bears the tumor.

Tumors of the gallbladder often are incidental findings, even though they may cause acute cholecystitis. This serves to reinforce the dictum that the excised gallbladder should always be opened in the operating room and inspected for a neoplasm, so that gallbladder cancer can be treated appropriately.

SELECTED REFERENCES

Glenn, F.: Acute acalculous cholecystitis. Ann. Surg. 189:458, 1979.
  A large experience with 139 cases is described and the associated illnesses are emphasized. The author's management led to a mortality of 6.5 per cent, one of the lowest reported in the literature.

Glenn, F.: Acute cholecystitis. Surg. Gynecol. Obstet., 143:56, 1976.
  This is a classic review of over 2000 cases by the late master biliary tract surgeon, Frank Glenn. He emphasized the serious risk factors and the increased mortality in elderly patients. An aggressive approach to the patient with acute cholecystitis is described.

Norrby, S., Herlin, P., Holmin, T., Sjodahl, R., and Tagesson, C.: Early or delayed

cholecystectomy in acute cholecystitis? A clinical trial. Br. J. Surg., 70:163, 1983.
  This is the report of a trial to determine the best method of management of the patient with acute cholecystitis. The results demonstrate that mortality and morbidity are the same with early and delayed operation, but that length of hospital stay is reduced and patients return to productivity sooner with early surgical therapy.

Weedon, D.: Pathology of the gallbladder. New York, Masson Publishing USA, Inc., 1984.
  This book describes the pathogenesis, clinical findings, and pathology for all known conditions that affect the gallbladder, as well as their complications. The illustrations are excellent and the references are very complete. The individual who wishes to have a comprehensive knowledge of acute cholecystitis or to study the nuances of individual cases will find this monograph very helpful.

Werbel, G. B., Nahrwold, D. L., Joehl, R. J., Vogelzang, R. L., and Rege, R. V.: Percutaneous cholecystostomy in the diagnosis and treatment of acute cholecystitis in the high-risk patient. Arch. Surg., 124:782, 1989.
  An experience with percutaneous cholecystostomy in critically ill patients who have acute acalculous or calculous cholecystitis is presented. The role of this technique in diagnosis is emphasized. The results of other reports are summarized.

REFERENCES

1. Acosta, J. M., Pellegrini, C. A., and Skinner, D. B.: Etiology and pathogenesis of acute biliary pancreatitis. Surgery, 88:118, 1980.
2. Becker, C. G., Dubin, T., and Glenn, F.: Induction of acute cholecystitis by activation of Factor XII. J. Exp. Med., 151:81, 1980.
3. Chetlin, S. H., and Elliott, D. W.: Biliary bacteremia. Arch. Surg., 102:303, 1971.
4. Chetlin, S. H., and Elliott, D. W.: Preoperative antibiotics in biliary surgery. Arch. Surg., 107:319, 1973.
5. Chilton, C. P., and Mann, C. V.: Torsion of the gallbladder in a 9-year-old boy. J. R. Soc. Med., 73:141, 1980.
6. Deitch, E. A., and Engle, J. M.: Acute acalculous cholecystitis. Ultrasonic diagnosis. Am. J. Surg., 142:290, 1981.
7. Dewar, J., Dooley, J. S., Lindsay, I., George, P., and Sherlock, S.: Granular cell myoblastoma of the common bile duct treated by biliary drainage and surgery. Gut, 22:70, 1981.
8. Diettrick, N. A., Cacioppo, J. C., and Davis, R. P.: The vanishing elective cholecystectomy. Arch. Surg., 123:810, 1988.
9. Diffenbaugh, W. G., Sarver, F. E., and Strohl, E. L.: Gangrenous perforation of the gallbladder. Analysis of 19 cases. Arch. Surg., 59:742, 1949.
10. Dinbar, A., Altmann, G., and Tulcinsky, D. B.: The treatment of chronic biliary salmonella carriers. Am. J. Med., 47:236, 1969.
11. DuPriest, R. W., Jr., Khaneja, S. C., and Cowley, R. A.: Acute cholecystitis complicating trauma. Ann. Surg., 189:84, 1979.
12. Echevarria, R. A., and Gleason, J. L.: False-negative gallbladder scintigram in acute cholecystitis. J. Nucl. Med., 21:841, 1980.
13. Essenhigh, D. M.: Perforation of the gallbladder. Br. J. Surg., 55:175, 1968.
14. Fox, M. S., Wilk, D. J., Weissmann, H. S., Freeman, L. M., and Gliedman, M. L.: Acute acalculous cholecystitis. Surg. Gynecol. Obstet., 159:13, 1984.
15. Freitag, J. L.: Treatment of chronic typhoid carriers by cholecystectomy. Public Health Rep., 79:567, 1964.
16. Freitas, J. E.: Cholescintigraphy in acute and chronic cholecystitis. Semin. Nucl. Med., 12:18, 1982.
17. Fukunaga, F. H.: Gallbladder bacteriology, histology and gallstones. Study of unselected cholecystectomy specimens in Honolulu. Arch. Surg., 106:169, 1973.
18. Glenn, F., and Becker, C. G.: Acute acalculous cholecystitis: An increasing entity. Ann. Surg., 195:131, 1982.
19. Gunn, A. A.: A surgeon's appraisal of cholecystitis. J. R. Coll. Surg. Edinb., 20:180, 1975.
20. Howard, R. J.: Acute acalculous cholecystitis. Am. J. Surg., 141:194, 1981.
21. Isch, J. H., Finneran, J. C., and Nahrwold, D. L.: Perforation of the gallbladder. Am. J. Gastroenterol., 55:451, 1971.
22. Jarvinen, H. J., and Hastabacka, J.: Early cholecystectomy for acute cholecystitis, a prospective randomized study. Ann. Surg., 191:501, 1980.
23. Keighley, M. R. B.: Microorganisms in the bile. Ann. R. Coll. Surg. Engl., 59:329, 1977.
24. Lahtinen, J., Alhava, E. M., and Aukee, S.: Acute cholecystitis treated by early and delayed surgery. A controlled clinical trial. Scand. J. Gastroenterol., 13:673, 1978.
25. Levene, A.: Acute torsion of the gallbladder. Postmortem finding in two cases. Br. J. Surg., 45:338, 1958.
26. Long, T. N., Heimbach, D. M., and Carrico, C. J.: Acalculous cholecystitis in critically ill patients. Am. J. Surg., 136:31, 1978.
27. Lou, M. A., Mandal, A. K., Alexander, J. L., and Thadepalli, H.: Bacteriology of the human biliary tract and the duodenum. Arch. Surg., 112:965, 1977.
28. Mason, G. R.: Bacteriology and antibiotic selection in biliary surgery. Arch. Surg., 97:533, 1968.
29. Mentzer, R. M., Jr., Golden, G. T., Chandler, J. G., and Horsley, J. S., III: A comparative appraisal of emphysematous cholecystitis. Am. J. Surg., 129:10, 1975.
30. Norrby, S., Herlin, P., Holmin, T., Sjodahl, R., and Tagesson, C.: Early or

delayed cholecystectomy in acute cholecystitis? A clinical trial. Br. J. Surg., 70:163, 1983.

31. Ostrow, J. D.: Absorption of bile pigments by the gallbladder. J. Clin. Invest., 46:2035, 1967.
32. Ottinger, L. W.: Acute cholecystitis as a postoperative complication. Ann. Surg., 184:162, 1976.
33. Petersen, S. R., and Sheldon, G. F.: Acute acalculous cholecystitis: A complication of hyperalimentation. Am. J. Surg., 138:814, 1979.
34. Scioli, C., Fiorentino, F., and Sasso, G.: Treatment of *Salmonella typhi* carriers with intravenous ampicillin. J. Infect. Dis., 125:170, 1972.
35. Serpe, S. J., Todd, D., and Baruch, H.: Cholecystitis due to granular cell myoblastoma of the cystic duct. Am. J. Dig. Dis., 5:824, 1960.
36. Stephenson, S. E., Jr., and Nagel, C. B.: Acute cholecystitis: An experimental study. Ann. Surg., 157:687, 1963.
37. Stone, H. H., Hooper, C. A., Kolb, L. D., Geheber, C. E., and Dawkins, E. J.:

Antibiotic prophylaxis in gastric, biliary and colonic surgery. Ann. Surg., 184:443, 1976.

38. Strohl, E. L., Diffenbaugh, W. G., Baker, J. H., and Cheema, M. H.: Gangrene and perforation of the gallbladder. (Int. Abstr. Surg.) Surg. Gynecol. Obstet., 114:1, 1962.
39. Weissmann, H. S., Badia, J., Sugarman, L. A., Kluger, L., Rosenblatt, R., and Freeman, L. M.: Spectrum of ^{99}m-Tc-IDA cholescintigraphic patterns in acute cholecystitis. Radiology, 138:167, 1981.
40. Werbel, G. B., Nahrwold, D. L., Joehl, R. J., Vogelzang, R. L., and Rege, R. V.: Percutaneous cholecystostomy in the diagnosis and treatment of acute cholecystitis in the high-risk patient. Arch. Surg., 124:782, 1989.
41. Womack, N. A., and Bricker, E. M.: Pathogenesis of acute cholecystitis. Arch. Surg., 44:658, 1942.
42. Wright, H. K., and Holden, W. D.: The risks of emergency surgery for acute cholecystitis. Arch. Surg., 81:341, 1960.

II

CHRONIC CHOLECYSTITIS AND CHOLELITHIASIS

David L. Nahrwold, M.D.

The term *chronic cholecystitis with cholelithiasis* often is used to connote symptomatic gallbladder disease. Chronic inflammatory changes are found in the gallbladders of many symptomatic patients with gallstones, but gallstones may also be present in an otherwise normal gallbladder, and gallbladder symptoms may occur in the absence of inflammation.[23] Approximately 98 per cent of patients with symptomatic gallbladder disease have gallstones. Understanding of the pathogenesis of gallstones and their relationship to gallbladder disease is central to the management of patients with chronic cholecystitis.

PATHOGENESIS OF GALLSTONES

An estimated 20 million people in the United States harbor gallstones. Approximately 475,000 cholecystectomies are done annually. The prevalence increases with increasing age. Women of childbearing age have an incidence higher than that of men of the same age; in an autopsy series, gallstones were found in approximately 17 per cent of women and 8 per cent of men over age 20.[18] Much of the present knowledge of cholesterol gallstones is derived from the study of Pima Indian women in the Southwestern United States, who have an incidence of approximately 75 per cent between the ages of 25 and 34 years.[31] In the Far East, pigment gallstones predominate, and their incidence in American blacks is higher than in Caucasians. Gallstones are classified into cholesterol, pigment, and mixed types, but the majority of stones cannot be classified in this rigid system. Pure cholesterol stones, having the appearance of white pearls, are rare. Most cholesterol stones contain significant amounts of pigment and are more aptly termed predominantly cholesterol stones. Pigment calculi are classified into black pigment stones, which are associated with hemolysis and cirrhosis, and the earthy calcium bilirubinate type, which is associated with infection in the biliary system.

Predominantly Cholesterol Stones

The primary constituents of bile are water, electrolytes, pigments, cholesterol, lecithin, and bile salts. Cholesterol and lecithin, insoluble in water, are soluble in bile because, at their concentration in bile, bile salts form micelles, groups of molecules arranged with their hydrophilic polar group on the outside and the hydrophobic group on the inside. Lecithin is incorporated into the bile salt micelle. Mixed bile salt–lecithin micelles become swollen following water penetration, allowing cholesterol to be "packaged" within them and, therefore, solubilized in bile. Because cholesterol, lecithin, and bile salts form micelles and make it possible for lecithin and cholesterol to dissolve in bile, the total amount of any one of these substances relative to the total amounts of the other two determines the maximal amount of cholesterol, for example, that can be solubilized. When the relative amounts of the three substances are insufficient to "package" all the cholesterol in micelles, and therefore solubilize it, cholesterol crystals appear in bile, making possible the formation of a cholesterol gallstone. Bile is said to be lithogenic when the solubility of cholesterol is exceeded. The relationships between the three substances were first expressed by Admirand and Small[1] by a triangular coordinate graph and were later modified by Holzbach and associates[14] (Fig. 1). The solubility of cholesterol also can be expressed through a mathematical formula that provides the ratio of the solubility of cholesterol in specific bile to the maximal solubility of cholesterol in that bile.[21] Bile with a lithogenic index greater than 1.0 is supersaturated.

Bile salts are secreted by the liver, concentrated and stored in the gallbladder, and released into the intestine during a meal. Approximately 95 per cent are reabsorbed in the intestine, mainly in the ileum; approximately 5 per cent are excreted in the feces, and this amount is replaced by hepatic synthesis. In health, the size of the bile salt pool remains fairly constant, and the pool circulates six to ten times each day. The primary bile acids, cholic and chenodeoxycholic acids, are conjugated with taurine or glycine in the liver. Bacteria in the distal ileum and colon may deconjugate and dehydroxylate them, forming the secondary bile acids deoxycholic and lithocholic acid that are absorbed by passive diffusion in the colon. The constant recycling of bile acids is known as the enterohepatic circulation, and the size of the pool and its frequency of cycling may be important in the formation of predominantly cholesterol stones. Bile acids are synthesized in the liver from cholesterol, a process influenced by a negative feedback system. Sequestration of bile acids in the gallbladder during fasting contracts the pool and initially causes a decrease in bile acid secretion relative to cholesterol secretion, with formation of lithogenic bile. However, after 24 hours, bile acid secretion increases, and the bile is no longer saturated. Cholecystectomy causes redistribution of the

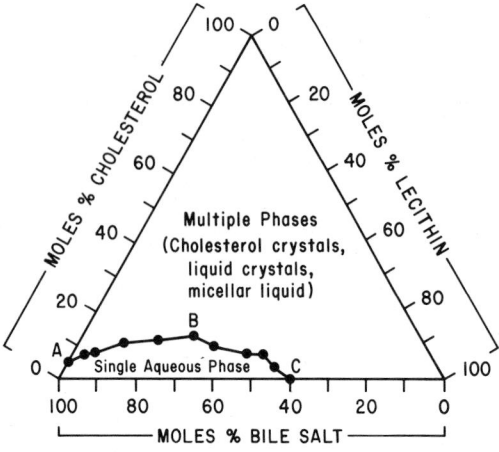

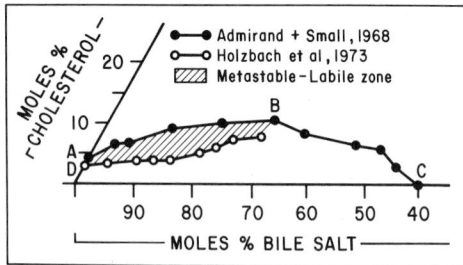

Figure 1. Triangular diagram in which the amounts of lecithin, bile salt, and cholesterol can be used to express the lithogenicity of bile. Lines are drawn into the triangle perpendicular from the appropriate point on each side of the triangle. If the point at which they intersect is above line ABC, cholesterol is completely soluble; if beneath, the bile is supersaturated. Between lines ABC and DBC is a metastable-labile zone in which stone formation could occur if specific nucleating factors are present.

bile acid pool in the enterohepatic circulation and increases the frequency of cycling. This exerts negative feedback on bile acid synthesis and causes a reduction in the pool size. These changes favor formation of a nonlithogenic bile in many patients after cholecystectomy.

Stone formation is initiated by nucleation, a complex process that requires more than saturation with cholesterol alone. Bacteria, cellular debris, gallbladder mucus, bile pigments, calcium salts, and other substances have been implicated as nucleating agents. Saturation of bile with cholesterol is known to be associated with stasis of bile in the prairie dog model of gallstone formation, and gallbladder emptying is also compromised.[22] In addition, cholesterol saturation of bile within the gallbladder causes increased secretion of gallbladder mucus, which enhances nucleation of cholesterol crystals. Growth of a stone is also a complicated process that is not clearly understood. The mixed nature of predominantly cholesterol stones gives rise to many unanswered questions regarding incorporation of pigment and other bile constituents in a stone as it enlarges.

The precise cause of predominantly cholesterol gallstones is not yet known, and current evidence suggests that it is multifactorial. Cholesterol saturation of bile, stasis of bile within the gallbladder, and nucleating factors appear to be important. The incidence of predominantly cholesterol gallstones is increased with age and in females. Obesity, exogenous estrogen administration, truncal vagotomy, and pregnancy are other predisposing factors. Recently, gallstones have been found to be a consequence of caloric restriction in individuals on certain diets.[4] Genetic factors, as exemplified by the high incidence in the Pima and Chippewa Indians, may also have a role.

Pigment Stones

Approximately 30 per cent of patients with cholelithiasis in the United States have pigment stones. They are of two types:

black pigment stones and earthy calcium bilirubinate stones. Pigment stones are much more common in Asian than in Western countries, but the extent to which they are found in the United States has not been recognized until recently. Stones associated with ileal resection or disease and total parenteral nutrition are the pigment type.[8, 26]

Black pigment stones (black or dark brown in color) are found almost exclusively in the gallbladder. They are associated with cirrhosis and conditions that cause hemolysis, including sickle cell disease, thalassemia, hereditary spherocytosis, and artificial cardiac valves. They consist of an insoluble black pigment polymer, some calcium bilirubinate, calcium carbonate, and calcium phosphate; 10 to 60 per cent of the weight is residue, probably a mucin glycoprotein. Typically, the bile of patients with black stones is sterile. The black pigment is a polyvinyl network polymer of bilirubinate.

Earthy calcium bilirubinate stones (earthy brown to orange in color) are soft in consistency and are found almost exclusively in the bile ducts. They form in circumstances that predispose to bacterbilia and infection, such as in the bile ducts of patients who have had a previous biliary-enteric anastomosis, and in patients with strictures or Caroli's disease. Earthy calcium bilirubinate stones are found within the ducts of the liver and extrahepatic ducts in recurrent pyogenic cholangitis, or Oriental cholangiohepatitis, a common disease in Southeast Asia in which the bile duct system is infected with parasites and/or enteric organisms, usually *Escherichia coli*. These stones consist mainly of calcium bilirubinate, the calcium soaps of fatty acids derived from lecithin, and cholesterol. The mucin glycoprotein residue found in black pigment stones is also present in calcium bilirubinate stones.

The etiology of the two types of pigment stones is not completely clear, but the bile of patients with pigment stones contains an excess of unconjugated bilirubin, compared with individuals with cholesterol stones or no stones. Many also have abnormally high activity of beta-glucuronidase, an enzyme produced by bacteria, especially *E. coli*, which is also found in the epithelium of the biliary tract. Presumably, beta-glucuronidase hydrolyzes soluble bilirubin glucuronide to insoluble unconjugated bilirubin and glucuronic acid. The unconjugated bilirubin may then form insoluble calcium bilirubinate.[19] There is some evidence that unconjugated bilirubin may be secreted into bile and at least partially solubilized by bile salts in the presence of calcium. Theoretically, a decrease in the amount of bile salts present could cause precipitation of calcium bilirubinate. The mechanisms by which calcium bilirubinate precipitates and forms a calcium bilirubinate stone or polymerizes and forms a black pigment stone are not known. The presence of ova or other foreign bodies at the center of calcium bilirubinate stones suggests that a nucleating factor may be necessary. Precipitates of calcium phosphate or carbonate could serve this function in formation of black pigment stones. Stasis of bile in the gallbladder may be a factor, as it appears to be in cholesterol stone formation. Sludge, a soft, black, amorphous substance, is found in gallbladders that have not contracted normally and has been identified as calcium bilirubinate. Sludge is often present in the gallbladders of patients on long-term total parenteral nutrition therapy. These patients have an increased incidence of pigment gallstones.[29]

PATHOLOGY

The pathologic findings in chronic cholecystitis are best interpreted from the clinical manifestations of the disease. Two types of chronic cholecystitis emerge: that which follows an episode of acute cholecystitis, and that which occurs primarily without antecedent acute cholecystitis. The former is termed secondary chronic cholecystitis, and the latter primary chronic cholecystitis.[10]

Acute cholecystitis is caused by gallbladder outlet obstruction, almost always by a stone. Marked thickening of the gallbladder wall from edema is characteristic and there is subserosal hemorrhage, a marked inflammatory infiltrate, and mucosal necrosis. In cases that do not progress to perforation, these abnormalities gradually resolve over 3 to 4 weeks. Simultaneously, granuloma formation begins at the end of the first week, and after 2 or 3 weeks, fibroblast proliferation and collagen formation ensue. These features, typical of chronic cholecystitis, become the dominant findings by 5 weeks. The granulomas frequently contain cholesterol clefts, and Rokitansky-Aschoff sinuses, outpouchings of the mucosa, are present. The mucosa itself becomes thin and loses its villous appearance; fibrosis occurs in the muscular coat.

In contrast, primary chronic cholecystitis is characterized by a thin-walled gallbladder, with an intact mucosa that retains its villous configuration. Sometimes the muscular coat is hypertrophic, and in these cases, crypt formation is frequent. The inflammatory cell infiltrate is primarily lymphocytic. Stones are almost always present in both forms of chronic cholecystitis. Primary chronic cholecystitis lacks an initial, acute inflammatory phase, and the exact pathophysiologic events leading to its development are not known.

DIAGNOSIS

Chronic cholecystitis is characterized by recurrent attacks of right upper quadrant or epigastric pain or discomfort, which usually follow meals. Nausea and vomiting may occur during the attack, and self-induced vomiting frequently makes the patient feel better. The discomfort may persist for several days or only a few hours. Intervals between attacks are variable; they may be almost continuous or separated by several years. Patients often complain of the sensation of right upper quadrant fullness or of bloating between attacks. These symptoms may follow an episode of acute cholecystitis or they may begin insidiously. No fever or other signs of inflammation are present.

It is unlikely that the pain in primary chronic cholecystitis, and in most cases of secondary chronic cholecystitis, is related to inflammation of the gallbladder. Rather, the pain is gallbladder colic, which follows the temporary obstruction of the gallbladder outlet by a stone in the cystic duct or the infundibulum. The frequent occurrence after a large meal is explained by gallbladder contraction, induced by cholecystokinin, against the fixed obstruction. The pain persists for the duration of the contraction and is relieved as the gallbladder relaxes, a process that may be hastened by opiates. Gallbladder pain characteristically radiates around the side toward the tip of the right scapula. However, some patients complain of radiation straight through to the back, or radiation into the substernal area. Approximately 10 per cent of patients with cholelithiasis have choledocholithiasis, and their gallstones sometimes first become manifest by the symptoms of cholangitis.

Patients with gallstones may complain of intolerance to fatty foods, flatulence, bloating, belching, pyrosis, and vague upper abdominal sensations; reliable evidence suggests that these symptoms alone probably are not due to chronic cholecystitis or cholelithiasis.[28] The cardinal symptom of chronic cholecystitis and cholelithiasis is pain.

Physical findings are present only during an attack of pain. They include right upper quadrant or epigastric tenderness to palpation and voluntary muscle guarding, but signs of peritonitis are absent. The gallbladder is not palpable and the temperature is normal. Jaundice is not a feature of cholelithiasis or chronic cholecystitis unless common duct obstruction is present. Blood tests are unremarkable; specifically, the white blood cell count and the differential counts are normal.

The diagnosis is confirmed by ultrasonography of the gallbladder, which is a highly sensitive and accurate test for the diagnosis of gallstones. Experts using real-time gray-scale scanning have achieved a sensitivity and specificity of 98 per cent.[7]

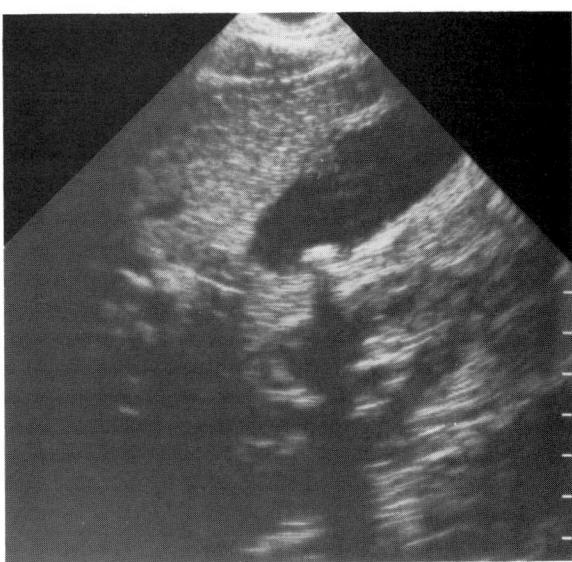

Figure 2. Ultrasound of the gallbladder demonstrating a stone with acoustic shadowing.

The important criteria include demonstration that the stones move to the dependent portion of the gallbladder when the position of the patient is changed and that the stone produces acoustic shadowing (Fig. 2). Reverberation at the edges of small stones is also a helpful sign. The advantages of ultrasonography are that it is accurate, is safe, does not use radiation, and can be performed rapidly without preparation. For these reasons, it has replaced oral cholecystography, in which oral administration of iopanoic acid is followed by radiographic examination of the right upper quadrant 12 to 24 hours later. The dye enters the gallbladder and outlines the stones (Fig. 3). Nonvisualization of the gallbladder indicates obstruction of the cystic duct, presumably by a stone, and, therefore, also confirms the diagnosis of cholelithiasis. However, this finding may be falsely positive if the patient did not ingest the dye tablets, if the tablets were not absorbed, or if liver function is compromised as indicated by a serum bilirubin value above approximately 3.0 mg. per 100 ml. Although ultrasonography should be the initial diagnostic test, oral cholecystography should be done when the symptoms are suggestive and ultrasonography is negative or nondiagnostic. The combination of these tests is very accurate and helpful in questionable cases, but both are unnecessary when ultrasonography is clearly positive.

Acute cholecystitis is best diagnosed by cholescintigraphy, but this test also is based on the presence or absence of cystic duct obstruction and is not useful in the detection of gallstones. Cholangiography, by the percutaneous or endoscopic routes, has no place in the diagnosis of chronic cholecystitis or cholelithiasis, unless jaundice or other evidence of disease of the biliary duct system is present.

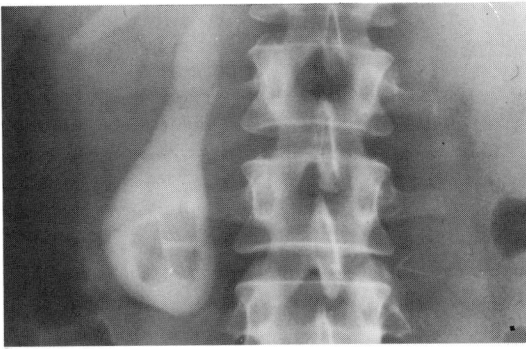

Figure 3. Oral cholecystogram demonstrating faceted gallstones outlined by the contrast material.

The differential diagnosis includes acute cholecystitis. The characteristics of pain and the physical examination are most helpful. The pain of acute cholecystitis is relentless and becomes progressively more severe, whereas biliary colic persists no longer than a few hours. Involuntary guarding, muscle rigidity, and rebound and percussion tenderness, all indicative of peritoneal irritation, become evident as acute cholecystitis progresses. In biliary colic associated with chronic cholecystitis, voluntary muscle guarding is characteristic, but the signs of peritonitis are not. Pancreatitis, duodenal and gastric ulcer, right pyelonephritis, and gastroesophageal reflux can produce upper abdominal symptoms that may be confused with those of chronic cholecystitis and cholelithiasis. Occasionally, arthritic changes in the thoracic spine cause radicular pain that radiates around the side to the right upper quadrant. This can easily be mistaken for pain originating in the right upper quadrant and radiating around to the back, as occurs in gallbladder disease. Conditions causing rapid expansion of the liver, such as congestive heart failure or hepatitis, also can be suggestive of gallbladder disease.

In addition, the symptoms of coronary artery disease may be confused with biliary colic. Nitroglycerin relieves the pain of biliary colic and angina pectoris. The prevalence of both diseases makes this a serious problem. Some evidence suggests that gallbladder disease may cause electrocardiographic changes and arrhythmias in patients with coronary artery disease, but there is no evidence that cholecystectomy has a favorable effect on coronary artery disease. The problem goes beyond diagnostic considerations, because cholecystectomy in the presence of coronary artery disease, and especially after a recent myocardial infarction, has a very significant risk of death. The only certain way to exclude coronary artery disease is by coronary angiography.

The importance of a complete history cannot be overemphasized. A complex of symptoms not including pain probably is not due to cholelithiasis or chronic cholecystitis, even if gallstones are demonstrated on ultrasonography. In addition, cholecystectomy is not likely to eliminate the symptoms. With the techniques available to diagnose upper abdominal problems, including endoscopy, ultrasonography, computed tomography, and angiography, almost every condition can be detected and adequately evaluated.

TREATMENT

Cholecystectomy

The initial treatment of biliary colic, after the diagnosis has been made, is parenteral administration of a narcotic to relieve pain. This may help to induce relaxation of the gallbladder as well. Nasogastric suction probably is of no benefit. Hospitalization is not necessary, unless the diagnosis is obscure. Many patients believe that a low-fat diet is helpful, but this has not been proved scientifically.

Cholecystectomy is the definitive treatment for patients with symptomatic gallstones. During the past 2 decades, the mortality for elective cholecystectomy in several large series of patients has been zero to 0.5 per cent[11,12,25] The risk of death for elective cholecystectomy done for chronic cholecystitis was 0.5 per cent in a large series of over 7000 patients.[20] In patients under age 50, the mortality was approximately 0.1 per cent. The most frequent cause of death after elective cholecystectomy is cardiovascular disease. This emphasizes the importance of obtaining a good history to detect angina pectoris and careful examination of the electrocardiogram for ischemia or evidence of previous myocardial infarction. Symptoms of cerebrovascular disease, especially transient ischemic attacks, also should be sought, and a noninvasive carotid artery flow study should be done if the history is positive or questionable. Elective cholecystectomy should be delayed until after coronary artery bypass or carotid artery revascularization, if either is indicated. Diseases of the liver and biliary tract, principally cirrhosis, are second to cardiovascular disease as a cause of death after elective cholecystectomy. Intraoperative hemorrhage is the primary problem, but hepatic failure and sepsis also occur.[33]

Septic complications after elective cholecystectomy have been reduced markedly since the introduction of prophylaxis in selected patients. The biles of 10 to 15 per cent of patients with chronic cholecystitis are colonized with bacteria; this rises to approximately 50 per cent in patients with resolving acute cholecystitis, and 80 per cent in patients with florid acute cholecystitis. The organisms are enteric, most commonly *E. coli*, *Klebsiella aerogenes*, and *Streptococcus faecalis*. *Clostridium*, *Bacteroides*, and *Proteus* also are found frequently. The incidence of bacterbilia increases significantly with age. With cholelithiasis and chronic cholecystitis, antibiotic prophylaxis should be given to patients over age 60, those recovering from an episode of acute cholecystitis, and those known to have concomitant common duct stones. The author prefers a second-generation cephalosporin administered 1 hour before operation.

TECHNICAL CONSIDERATIONS. The gallbladder can be exposed adequately through a midline or paramedian incision, but a generous subcostal incision provides the best exposure for routine gallbladder and bile duct surgery. There is controversy over whether dissection of the gallbladder should proceed from the fundus to the cystic duct or in the opposite direction. The two most important facets of the procedure are that the gallbladder not be removed prior to operative cholangiography and that the junction of the cystic duct, common hepatic duct, and common bile duct be dissected completely prior to division of any structure. After these procedures are accomplished and the cystic artery has been ligated at its entrance into the gallbladder, the organ can be removed in whichever direction the surgeon deems most efficacious (Fig. 4). Approximately 10 per cent of patients have concomitant choledocholithiasis. The author does operative cholangiography in all cases to detect stones and anomalous anatomy, for which the benefit of cholangiography often is overlooked. Intraoperative manometry and intraoperative ultrasonography have also been used to detect common duct stones. Drains should not be used after elective cholecystectomy unless a bile leak is present.

Gallstone Dissolution

Two oral agents have been developed for dissolution of cholesterol gallstones. Chenodeoxycholic acid (chenodiol) was approved in 1983, but the side effect of dose-related diarrhea has precluded its widespread acceptance. Ursodeoxycholic acid (ursodiol), approved in 1988, has become the drug of choice because it is at least as effective as chenodiol and has no known side effects. Both drugs act by reducing the amount of cholesterol in bile, thereby permitting solubilization of the cholesterol in stones and gradual dissolution. They reduce bile cholesterol saturation by different mechanisms. Chenodiol decreases the amount of hepatic hydroxymethylglutaryl-CoA reductase the rate-limiting enzyme for the synthesis of cholesterol by hepatocytes, whereas ursodiol reduces the absorption of cholesterol from the intestine.[2,17] The two mechanisms provided a rationale for administering them together; interestingly, diarrhea does not occur with the combination, and there is some evidence that the results are slightly better than with single-drug therapy.[27]

Using ideal criteria, ursodiol or a combination of ursodiol and chenodiol effectively dissolves cholesterol gallstones in approximately 50 per cent of patients. Patients should have radiolucent stones less than 2 cm. in diameter in a gallbladder that functions on oral cholecystography. Criteria favoring dissolution include ideal body weight, small stones, floating stones, and a small number of stones.[32] Dissolution therapy is more likely to be successful in young patients, because the gallstones of older patients are more likely to contain larger amounts of pigment and calcium.

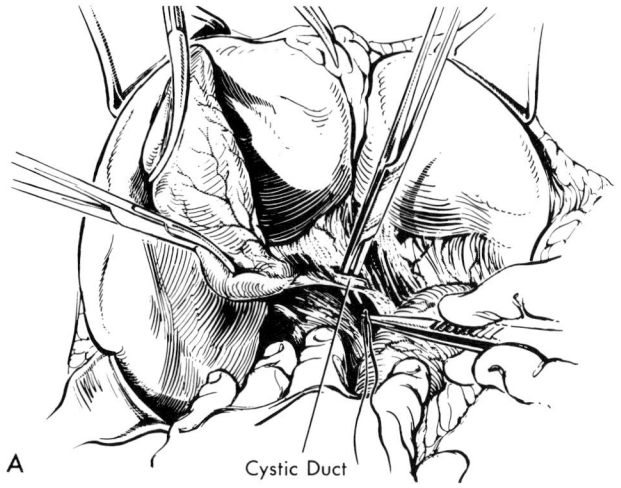

A — Cystic Duct

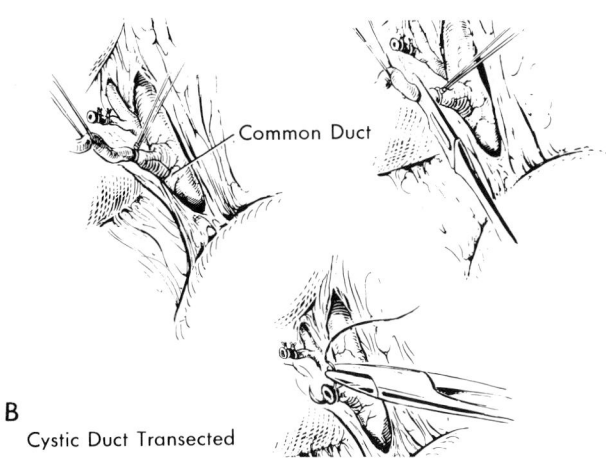

Common Duct

B — Cystic Duct Transected

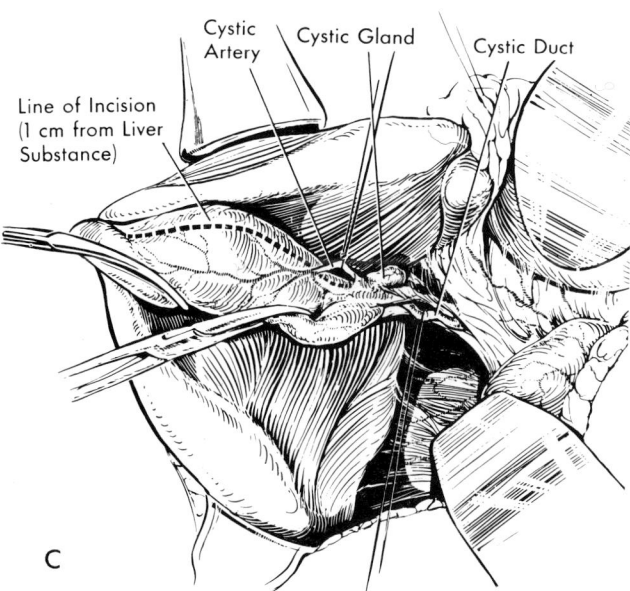

Cystic Artery Cystic Gland Cystic Duct

Line of Incision (1 cm from Liver Substance)

C

Figure 4. Gallbladder removed from cystic duct toward fundus after complete dissection of the junction of the cystic duct with the common hepatic and common bile ducts. Cystic duct has been dissected free throughout its length, and cystic artery has been ligated at its entrance into the gallbladder. (From Glenn, F.: Atlas of Biliary Tract Surgery. New York, The Macmillan Company, 1963. Illustrations by Caspar Henselmann.)

Extracorporeal Shock Wave Lithotripsy

Lithotripsy is used in the treatment of highly selected patients with gallstones. Lithotripters generate longitudinal, large-amplitude acoustic waves within a water medium, which is coupled to the skin of the patient by direct contact or a membrane that allows passage of the waves into the body. The machines differ according to the energy source used to generate the shock wave and the mechanism by which the shock wave is focused on the gallstones. One device uses an electrical current passed across a spark gap located within a metal ellipse. Shock waves are reflected off the sides of the ellipse, causing them to be focused at the fixed point (F_2) within about 10 cm. of the spark gap. In another machine, shock waves are generated by piezoelectric crystals, which are arrayed so that their ouput is focused on the gallstone. Other devices use electromagnetic energy focused by an acoustic lens or even microexplosions of lead azide pellets.

Acoustic waves pass unimpeded through water as well as through human tissue, which is composed primarily of water. Gallstones fragment when acoustic energy is focused on them. Typically, 1500 to 2000 shock waves are utilized during a treatment, but this varies according to the strength of each shock wave, the acoustic impedance of the tissue through which the waves must pass, and the characteristics of the stones. The goal is to fragment stones into pieces small enough to pass out the cystic duct and the sphincter of Oddi; the maximal size is thought to be about 5 mm. The effectiveness of lithotripsy is primarily related to the volume and the characteristics of the stones.

The selection of patients for lithotripsy was specified in the clinical trials for safety and efficacy. Patients should have symptoms attributable to gallstones, but common duct stones, recent acute cholecystitis, cholangitis, and pancreatitis are contraindications. Patients should have fewer than four stones, each less than 3 cm. in diameter. Lithotripsy should not be done in patients with pigment or calcified stones. The gallbladder must be visualized on oral cholecystography, and the stones should be easily observed on ultrasound. No cysts or aneurysms may be in the shock wave path. The presence of a pacemaker or an arrhythmia is a contraindication because the shock wave discharges are gated to the electrocardiogram.

Ursodiol or a combination of ursodiol and chenodiol should be given as adjuvant therapy after the procedure; this regimen should be continued until the gallbladder is free of fragments. Presumably, adjuvant bile acid therapy is effective because the surface areas of the original calculi are expanded by the fragmentation.

Repeat lithotripsy is necessary after 4 to 6 weeks if fragments larger than 5 mm. are present. Fragments larger than this are unlikely to pass through the cystic duct. Retreatment rates are approximately 10 to 40 per cent depending on the experience of the operator, the size of the original stone burden, the power of the machine, the body habitus of the patient, and the criteria for retreatment.

In these highly selected patients, and using the criteria outlined, the stone-free rates are approximately 35 per cent at 6 months, 65 per cent at 12 months, and over 90 per cent at 2 years.[5,30]

Complications of lithotripsy include minor bruising over the area of entry of the shock waves. Gross hematuria at the first urination occurs occasionally, and microscopic hematuria is frequent, because of the proximity of the right kidney. Approximately one third of patients have pain on passage of the fragments. The pain is typical of biliary pain and is usually located in the right upper quadrant or the epigastrium. Common duct obstruction requiring endoscopic sphincterotomy, gallstone pancreatitis, and the need for cholecystectomy have occurred in less than 5 per cent of patients.

Although lithotripsy does not require general or regional anesthesia, most patients require intravenous analgesia. Patients can be treated as outpatients and may return to normal activity immediately after the procedure.

Contact Dissolution

Percutaneous catheterization of the gallbladder under local anesthesia and systemic analgesia, using fluoroscopic guidance, has become a routine procedure in advanced interventional radiology units. Thistle and colleagues at the Mayo Clinic have pioneered use of the percutaneously placed catheter to infuse methyl tert-butyl ether (MTBE) into the gallbladder to dissolve cholesterol gallstones.[34] Although still an investigational agent in the United States, MTBE is an alkyl ether that remains liquid at body temperature and rapidly dissolves cholesterol. When small aliquots of 3 to 6 ml. are infused and withdrawn four to six times per minute, stones dissolve in 1 to 3 days, leaving little or no residue in the gallbladder. Care must be taken to avoid introduction of MTBE into the common bile duct and the duodenum because duodenitis as well as anesthesia has been reported. Infusion and withdrawal has been done by hand using syringes, but automated systems designed to avoid overfilling and loss of MTBE outside of the gallbladder are being tested.

The early results have been excellent. In carefully selected patients, 95 per cent of the stone mass was dissolved in almost all patients within an average of 12.5 hours. Bile leaks have been prevented by the introduction of a Gelfoam plug within the transhepatic tract of the catheter.

Experience with the combination of lithotripsy followed by contact dissolution with MTBE is also accumulating, but the indications for this combined therapy are not clear.[24]

Percutaneous Cholecystolithotomy

Surgeons have extracted stones from the gallbladder weeks or months after surgical tube cholecystostomy using cystoscopes, stone baskets, and instruments designed for nephrolithotomy. With the advent of percutaneous cholecystostomy, for which general anesthesia is not necessary, a variety of techniques for stone removal have been used. The tract can be dilated and the stones removed with a Dormia basket, using a choledochoscope or nephroscope for visualization.[3,16] Kellett and associates catheterized the gallbladder under general anesthesia, removed the calculi under endoscopic visualization, and inserted a Foley catheter, which was removed when the tract was mature.[15] Stones too large to extract manually have been fragmented with the rigid ultrasonic lithotripter, an electrohydraulic lithotripter, or a laser fiber, all of which can be passed through an Amplatz sheath placed within the gallbladder through the percutaneous tract.

Gallstone Recurrence

Because the gallbladder is left in place in all the alternatives to cholecystectomy, recurrence of stones is likely. Recurrent stones have been reported after lithotripsy, but the long-term recurrence rate is unknown because the follow-up period is too short. However, data on patients who have had oral dissolution suggest that the recurrence rate is approximately 10 per cent per year for about the first 5 years, following which it remains relatively stable. Prevention of recurrence and management of patients after recurrence are being investigated.

Laparoscopic Cholecystectomy

Cholecystectomy can be performed with the use of instruments designed for laparoscopic gynecologic procedures, and this method is currently being evaluated. Using general anesthesia, a needle is introduced through the umbilicus, and a pneumoperitoneum with carbon dioxide is created. An endoscope is inserted through a small incision adjacent to the umbilicus, and the gallbladder is examined to determine the feasibility of laparoscopic cholecystectomy. Three other access sites are established, one for grasping the gallbladder, another for suction and irrigation, and the third for introducing instruments for dissection and applying clips.[9]

The risks include uncontrolled bleeding, bile duct injury, and injury to other organs. The absence of a large scar and the short hospital stay are obviously advantageous. Additional experience and follow-up will provide data for comparison with open cholecystectomy.

Asymptomatic Stones

The indications for treatment of patients with cholelithiasis include the symptoms that can reasonably be attributed to the presence of gallstones. Asymptomatic stones may be discovered at surgical therapy for other illnesses or on routine testing for unrelated abdominal complaints. The question is whether cholecystectomy should be done in healthy asymptomatic patients to prevent the development of acute cholecystitis and its complications. The best evidence suggests that the rate of development of symptoms is approximately 2 per cent per year in patients with truly asymptomatic stones, and that mortality and morbidity in this group are approximately equal to that of cholecystectomy.[13] The author does not believe that truly asymptomatic patients should have cholecystectomy, unless it can be done safely at operation for another condition. Cholecystectomy is recommended by some in asymptomatic patients who are candidates for heart or renal transplantation, for patients who must receive total parenteral nutrition indefinitely, and during bariatric surgical procedures for morbid obesity.

SPECIAL CONSIDERATIONS

CHRONIC ACALCULOUS CHOLECYSTITIS. Acute inflammation of the gallbladder without stones is a recognized entity that requires cholecystectomy. Occasionally, patients have signs and symptoms of gallbladder disease, but stones cannot be demonstrated by repeated ultrasound or oral cholecystography. The criteria for cholecystectomy in this situation are not clearly defined, but a significant number of patients are found to have gallbladder disease and subsequently are free of symptoms. How many patients have relief because of the "placebo effect" of surgical therapy is unknown, however. The presence of cholesterol crystals in bile has been considered an indication that small gallstones may be forming and causing symptoms as they pass through the biliary tract. Recently, duodenal drainage during administration of cholecystokinin has been used to obtain samples of bile from the gallbladder for examination for crystals. Prior to the test, iopanoic acid is administered to opacify the gallbladder and to monitor its contraction fluoroscopically. Criteria for a positive test include the presence of crystals, reproduction of pain, and either hypocontraction or hypercontraction of the gallbladder. Positive responders have a high incidence of chronic acalculous cholecystitis, cholelithiasis, cholesterolosis, and adenomyomatosis, and about three fourths of the cholecystectomized patients become asymptomatic.[6] More experience is needed with this diagnostic test.

HYDROPS OF THE GALLBLADDER. Hydrops of the gallbladder is caused by obstruction of the outlet, usually by an impacted stone, but occasionally by a tumor or fibrosis. The organ becomes filled with mucoid material and distends to an extremely large size (Fig. 5). There is little evidence of inflammation. The mucoid material undoubtedly comes from the gallbladder epithelium, but the pathophysiologic mechanism is not known. Although most cases occur in adults, children develop hydrops in association with a wide range of infectious diseases and as the result of congenital narrowing of the cystic duct. The average age is approximately 5 years.

Hydrops causes pain in the area of the gallbladder, which may be located as far inferiorly as the pelvis, depending on its size. The gallbladder usually is palpable and may be tender.

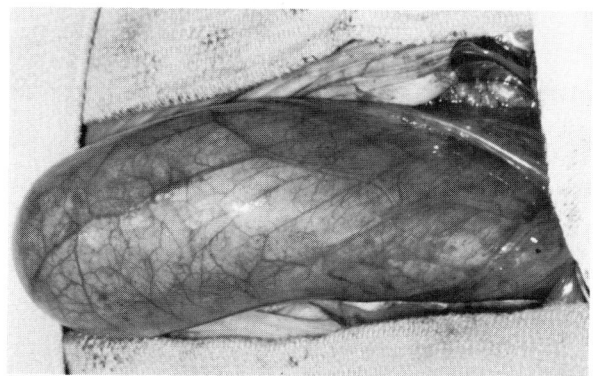

Figure 5. Hydrops of the gallbladder. Elongated, tense gallbladder filled with clear, mucoid material protrudes through wound.

Some patients are asymptomatic. The gallbladder does not visualize on oral cholecystography because of the cystic duct obstruction but may be identified easily by ultrasonography. In children, the process usually resolves without treatment; in adults, cholecystectomy is indicated.

SELECTED REFERENCES

Carey, M. C., and Cahalane, M. J.: Whither biliary sludge? Gastroenterology, 95:508, 1988.
This is a comprehensive discussion of the mechanisms involved in the formation of gallstones. The relevant literature is explained in a simple, coherent manner.

Dubois, F., Icard, P., Berthelot, G., and Levard, H.: Coelioscopic cholecystectomy: Preliminary report of 36 cases. Ann. Surg., 211:60, 1990.
The technique of laparoscopic cholecystectomy is outlined in a series of 36 patients together with the indications and complications encountered in the early part of the series. By the time the article went to press the series had been expanded to 220 patients with no complications for the last 180 patients.

Fromm, H.: Gallstone dissolution therapy. Current status and future prospects. Gastroenterology, 91:1560, 1986.
The epidemiology and natural history of gallstones, together with a comprehensive discussion of the mechanisms by which bile acids and solvents dissolve gallstones are presented. The indications, treatment regimens, and complications of bile acid therapy are described.

McSherry, C. K., and Glenn, F.: The incidence and causes of death following surgery for nonmalignant biliary tract disease. Ann. Surg., 191:271, 1980.
The causes of death following 11,808 biliary tract operations are reported. Detailed information about mortality for subgroups is presented. This experience provides a standard with which the results in other hospitals or individual practices can be compared. High-risk groups are identified.

Ostrow, J. D.: The etiology of pigment gallstones. Hepatology, 4:2155, 1984.
The types of pigment stones and the latest concepts about mechanisms by which they are formed are presented in a scholarly, comprehensible manner. The problems that currently obviate pigment gallstone dissolution are described.

Peters, J. H., Ellison, E. C., Innes, J. T., Liss, J. L., Nichols, K. E., Lomano, J. M., Roby, S. R., Front, M. E., and Carey, L. C.: Safety and efficacy of laparoscopic cholecystectomy: A prospective analysis of 100 patients. Ann. Surg. 213:3, 1991.
This is a detailed, well-illustrated description of operative technique, coupled with extensive statistical analysis of patient profile, laboratory data, operative data, complications, postoperative course, hospital cost, and follow-up.

Sackmann, M., Delius, M., Sauerbruch, T., Holl, J., Weber, W., Ippisch, E., Hagelauer, U., Wess, O., Hepp, W., Brendel, W., and Paumgartner, G.: Shock-wave lithotripsy of gallbladder stones: The first 175 patients. N. Engl. J. Med., 318:393, 1988.
This is the first report of a large number of patients treated by lithotripsy. Most other studies of this therapy have used a similar protocol, and the results are comparable.

REFERENCES

1. Admirand, W. H., and Small, D. M.: The physicochemical basis of cholesterol gallstone formation in man. J. Clin. Invest., 47:1043, 1968.
2. Ahlberg, J., Angelin, B., and Einarsson, K.: Hepatic 3-hydroxy-3-methylglutaryl coenzyme A reductase activity and biliary lipid composition in man: Relation to cholesterol gallstone disease and effect of cholic acid and chenodeoxycholic acid treatment. J. Lipid Res., 22:410, 1981.
3. Akiyama, H., Nagusa, Y., Fujita, T., Shirane, N., Sasao, T., Iwamori, S., Hidaka, T., and Okuhara, T.: A new method for nonsurgical cholecystolithotomy. Surg. Gynecol. Obstet., 161:73, 1985.
4. Broomfield, P. H., Chopra, R., Sheinbaum, R. C., Bonorris, G. G., Silverman, A., Schoenfield, L. J., and Marks, J. W.: Effects of ursodeoxycholic acid and aspirin on the formation of lithogenic bile and gallstones during loss of weight. N. Engl. J. Med., 319:1567, 1988.
5. Burnett, D., Ertan, A., Jones, R., O'Leary, J. P., Mackie, R., Robinson, J. E., Jr., Salen, G., Stahgren, L., Van Thiel, D. H., Vassy, L., Greenberger, N., and Hoffman, A. F.: Use of external shock-wave lithotripsy and adjuvant ursodiol for treatment of radiolucent gallstones. Dig. Dis. Sci., 34:1011, 1989.
6. Burnstein, M. J., Vassal, K. P., and Strasberg, S. M.: Results of combined biliary drainage and cholecystokinin cholecystography in 81 patients with normal oral cholecystograms. Ann. Surg., 196:627, 1982.
7. Cooperberg, P. L., and Burhenne, H. J.: Real-time ultrasonography. Diagnostic treatment of choice in calculous gallbladder disease. N. Engl. J. Med., 302:1277, 1980.
8. Coyle, J. J., Hoyt, D. B., and Sedaghat, A.: Relationship of intestinal bypass operations and cholelithiasis. Gastroenterol. Forum, 31:139, 1980.
9. Dubois, F., Icard, P., Berthelot, G., and Levand, H.: Celioscopic cholecystectomy. Preliminary report of 36 cases. Ann. Surg., 211:60, 1990.
10. Edlung, Y., and Zettergren, L.: Histopathology of the gallbladder in gallstone disease related to clinical data. Acta Chir. Scand., 116:460, 1958.
11. Ganey, J. B., Johnson, P. A., Prillaman, P. E., and McSwain, G. R.: Cholecystectomy: Clinical experience with a large series. Am. J. Surg., 151:352, 1986.
12. Gillaland, T. M., and Traverso, L. W.: Modern standards for comparison of cholecystectomy with alternative treatments for symptomatic cholelithiasis with emphasis on long-term relief of symptoms. Surg. Gynecol. Obstet., 170:39, 1990.
13. Gracie, W. A., and Ransohoff, D. F.: The natural history of silent gallstones. Gastroenterology, 80:1161, 1981.
14. Holzbach, R. T., Marsh, M., Olszewski, M., and Holan, K.: Cholesterol solubility in bile with evidence that supersaturated bile is frequent in healthy man. J. Clin. Invest., 52:1467, 1973.
15. Kellet, M. J., Wickham, J. E. A., and Russell, R. C. G.: Percutaneous cholecystolithotomy. Br. J. Med., 296:453, 1988.
16. Kerlan, R. K., Jr., LaBerge, J. M., and Ring, E. J.: Percutaneous cholecystolithotomy: Preliminary experience. Radiology, 157:653, 1985.
17. LaRusso, N. F., and Thistle, J. L.: Effect of litholytic bile acids on cholesterol absorption in gallstone patients. Gastroenterology 84:265, 1983.
18. Lieber, M. M.: The incidence of gallstones and their correlation with other diseases. Ann. Surg., 135:394, 1952.
19. Maki, T.: Pathogenesis of calcium bilirubinate gallstones: Role of E. coli, β-glucuronidase, and coagulation by inorganic ions, polyelectrolytes, and agitation. Ann. Surg., 165:90, 1966.
20. McSherry, C. K., and Glenn, F.: The incidence and causes of death following surgery for nonmalignant biliary tract disease. Ann. Surg., 191:271, 1980.
21. Metzger, A. L., Heymsfield, S., and Grundy, S. M.: Lithogenic index—a numerical expression for the relative lithogenicity of bile. Gastroenterology, 62:499, 1972.
22. Meyer, P. D., DenBesten, L., and Gurll, N. J.: Effects of cholesterol gallstone induction on gallbladder function and bile salt pool size in the prairie dog model. Surgery, 83:599, 1978.
23. Nahrwold, D. L., Rose, R. C., and Ward, S. P.: Abnormalities in gallbladder morphology and function in patients with cholelithiasis. Ann. Surg., 184:415, 1976.
24. Peine, C. J., Petersen, B. T., Williams, H. J., Bender, C. E., Patterson, D. E., Segura, J. W., Nagorney, D. M., Warner, M. A., and Thistle, J. L.: Extracorporeal shock-wave lithotripsy and methyl tert-butyl ether for partially calcified gallstones. Gastroenterology, 97:1229, 1989.
25. Pickleman, J., and Gonzalez, R.: Improving results of cholecystectomy. Arch. Surg., 121:930, 1986.
26. Pitt, H. A., Berquist, W. E., Mann, L. L., Porter-Fink, V., Fonkalsrud, E. W., and Ament, M. E.: Parenteral nutrition induces calcium bilirubinate gallstones. Gastroenterology, 84:1274, 1983.
27. Podda, M., Zuin, M., Battezzati, P. M., Ghezzi, C., deFazio, C., and Dioguandi, M. L.: Efficacy and safety of a combination of chenodeoxycholic acid and ursodeoxycholic acid for gallstone dissolution: A comparison with ursodeoxycholic acid alone. Gastroenterology, 96:222, 1989.
28. Price, W. H.: Gallbladder dyspepsia, Br. Med. J., 2:138, 1963.
29. Rosyln, J. J., Berquist, W. E., Pitt, H. A., Mann, L. L., Kangarloo, H., DenBesten, L., and Ament, M. E.: Increased risk of gallstones in children receiving total parenteral nutrition. Pediatrics, 71:784, 1983.
30. Sackmann, M., Delius, M., Sauerbruch, T., Holl, J., Weber, W., Ippisch, E., Hagelauer, U., Wess, O., Hepp, W., Brendel, W., and Paumgartner, G.: Shock-wave lithotripsy of gallbladder stones: The first 175 patients. N. Engl. J. Med., 318:393, 1988.
31. Sampliner, R. E., Bennett, P. H., Comess, L. J., Rose, F. A., and Burch, T. A.: Gallbladder disease in Pima Indians: Demonstration of high prevalence and early onset by cholecystography. N. Engl. J. Med., 283:1358, 1970.
32. Schoenfield, L. J., Lachin, J. M., et al.: Chenodiol (chenodeoxycholic acid) for dissolution of gallstones: The National Cooperative Gallstone Study. Ann. Intern. Med., 95:257, 1981.
33. Schwartz, S. I.: Biliary tract surgery and cirrhosis: A critical combination. Surgery, 90:577, 1981.
34. Thistle, J. L., May, G. R., Bender, C. E., Williams, H. J., LeRoy, A. J., Nelson, P. E., Peine, C. J., Petersen, B. T., and McCullough, J. E.: Dissolution of cholesterol gallbladder stones by methyl tert-butyl ether administered by percutaneous transhepatic catheter. N. Engl. J. Med., 320:633, 1989.

III

CHOLANGITIS

David L. Nahrwold, M.D.

Cholangitis, originally described by Charcot in 1877,[3] is a bacterial or parasitic inflammation of the bile duct system that is invariably associated with partial or complete biliary tract obstruction. Bacteria can be present within the biliary tract (bacterbilia) without clinical symptoms, but whether asymptomatic bacterbilia causes pathologic changes in the bile ducts, the liver, or the gallbladder is not known. In clinical practice, the term *cholangitis* is used to connote the signs and symptoms produced by bacterial inflammation of the biliary duct system, without regard to the presence or absence of inflammatory changes within the walls of the bile ducts or the parenchyma of the liver. Thus, today the term is used in a clinical context, just as it was used by Charcot in his original description over a century ago. During those 100 years, and especially during the past 2 decades, degrees of severity of inflammation of the biliary tract have become apparent, from clinically inapparent bacterbilia to an episode of cholangitis manifested by mild, short-lived fever and abdominal pain, to a lethal form of the disease, acute suppurative cholangitis, in which complete bile duct obstruction converts the biliary duct system into an abscess cavity that contains pus under pressure. The concept of this spectrum of cholangitis is important because the severity of clinical signs and symptoms determines the appropriate therapy and its timing. Because cholangitis does not occur in the absence of other biliary tract disease, the treatment varies according to the type of obstructing lesion present. When the diagnosis of cholangitis is made, appropriate tests must be done to locate the associated lesion.

PATHOGENESIS

The development of cholangitis is predicated upon the presence of bacteria and partial or complete obstruction of the biliary tract. The origin of bacteria in bile is unclear, but normally small numbers of bacteria pass into the portal venous system from the intestine, enter the liver, and are phagocytosed by the reticuloendothelial system. The best evidence suggests that bacteria do not colonize bile in healthy individuals, but that they frequently do so when a foreign body such as a stone or other lesion is present within the biliary duct system. Presumably, stasis of bile, produced by the obstructing lesion or foreign body, facilitates bacterial colonization and growth, but this has been inferred from clinical data and has not been proved by scientific investigation. Clinical cholangitis occurs when bacteria enter the circulation from the biliary duct system. This occurs only when pressure within the system is sufficiently high. Either complete or partial obstruction of the biliary tract may cause increased intraductal pressure.

The relationships between intraductal pressure and entry of bacteria into the circulation have been investigated in animals and man. Early observations that T-tube cholangiography caused cholangitis led to the demonstration that small particles appeared in the bloodstream after cholangiography, and that pressures of about 20 cm. of water are necessary for cholangiovenous reflux to occur.[12] Bile canaliculi, the terminal tributaries of the biliary duct system that are lined by hepatocytes, communicate directly with hepatic sinusoids at their terminal ends, so that the anatomic arrangement within the liver permits reflux of bacteria from canaliculi directly into the venous circulation.[4,6]

Small particles approximately the size of a virus can pass into the circulation at pressures less than the secretory pressure of the liver,[7] and radioactively labeled bacteria enter the circulation at pressures slightly higher than the secretory pressure of the liver.[8]

Cholangitis often occurs in patients who have only partial biliary duct obstruction, and it is logical to assume that intraductal pressure could be normal in the absence of complete obstruction. This question has been approached experimentally, and higher than normal pressures have been found in patients and animals with partial obstruction, although they are not as high as when complete obstruction is present.[20] The exact circumstances under which cholangiovenous reflux occurs in patients with partial obstruction are not known, but high intraductal pressure for varying lengths of time could be caused by temporary impaction of an otherwise freely movable stone. Short-lived increases in intra-abdominal pressure caused by movement, coughing, or other maneuvers also could produce cholangiovenous reflux when the choledochal sphincter mechanism is closed.

ASSOCIATED PATHOLOGY

The conditions that affect the biliary tract and are associated with cholangitis are listed in Table 1. The most common cause of acute cholangitis is choledocholithiasis, which represents approximately 60 per cent of the cases.[18] Common duct stones usually occur in association with cholelithiasis but may also be found in patients who have had cholecystectomy. Common duct stones associated with cholelithiasis probably migrate from the gallbladder. It is clear that stones may form *de novo* within the bile ducts, or they may have been present, but overlooked, at the time of cholecystectomy. Stones that form *de novo* are termed primary or recurrent common duct stones, and those that are not discovered at cholecystectomy are called retained or secondary stones. The distinction between the two types is not always possible, so that, arbitrarily, common duct stones discovered more than 2 years after cholecystectomy are assumed to have formed *de novo* (Fig. 1). Although primary common duct stones are encountered less frequently than retained stones, the relative frequency of cholangitis is higher in patients with the primary type.

Calcium bilirubinate is the predominant constituent of primary common duct stones, whereas retained stones are composed primarily of cholesterol. The most plausible theory for the formation of calcium bilirubinate stones is that bilirubin diglucuronide, the soluble conjugate of bilirubin excreted in bile, is

TABLE 1. Biliary Tract Conditions Associated with Cholangitis

Choledocholithiasis
Malignant tumors
Benign strictures
Biliary-enteric anastomoses
Invasive procedures
Foreign bodies
Parasitic infestations

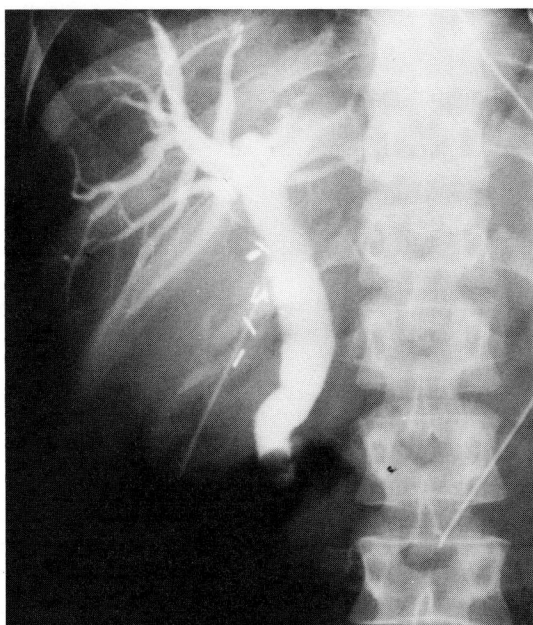

Figure 1. Cholangiogram in a patient who had cholecystectomy 3 years previously and presented with cholangitis. A stone was impacted in the distal common bile duct.

deconjugated by beta-glucuronidase, an enzyme produced by some bacteria that may be present in bile, especially *Escherichia coli.* The unconjugated bilirubin, insoluble in bile, combines with calcium and forms a calculus. This theory is supported by the fact that common duct stones made of calcium bilirubinate are found in association with bacterbilia and in conditions lending themselves to bacterbilia, such as biliary-enteric anastomoses, benign strictures, and the presence of foreign bodies. The signs and symptoms of acute cholangitis are the most frequent manifestations of both primary and secondary common duct stones, and the diagnosis of acute cholangitis usually prompts the studies leading to their discovery.

Malignant tumors that cause bile duct obstruction are carcinoma of the head of the pancreas, carcinoma of the bile ducts, and carcinoma of the ampulla of Vater. Strictures associated with these tumors are an infrequent cause of cholangitis[2,18] so that studies leading to their detection usually are prompted by the occurrence of jaundice, rather than signs and symptoms of infection. Malignant strictures are associated with bacterbilia in one fourth to one third of cases, less frequently than other lesions that predispose to cholangitis. However, cases of cholangitis associated with malignancies are much more likely to be severe and life-threatening than are those associated with other obstructive lesions. Approximately half the cases reported by Boey and Way[2] had acute suppurative cholangitis, the most severe form of the disease. This high incidence probably is due to the completeness of obstruction in malignant disease.

Benign strictures of the duct system are often heralded by an episode of cholangitis. Most of them are due to primary sclerosing cholangitis, but a few follow operative trauma during cholecystectomy.

Almost all patients with stricture have bacterbilia. As mentioned previously, calcium bilirubinate stones are prone to form proximal to a stricture, so the development of cholangitis may be the result of both stricture and stone. Another cause of bile duct stricture, observed with increasing frequency, is chronic pancreatitis. This stricture, located in the intrapancreatic portion of the common bile duct, may first become manifest through the development of acute cholangitis.

Patients who have biliary-enteric anastomoses are prone to bacterbilia because of reflux of chyme into the biliary tract, even

though some protection may be afforded by a Roux-en-Y anatomic arrangement. There is no solid evidence that bacterbilia in such patients is harmful, or that such patients are predisposed to cholangitis. However, when the anastomosis is too narrow, cholangitis does occur (Fig. 2). Acute suppurative cholangitis is rare in patients with a biliary stricture or a biliary-enteric anastomosis in the absence of an accompanying stone that produces complete obstruction, but benign strictures are second only to choledocholithiasis as a cause of acute cholangitis.

Invasive procedures frequently precipitate acute cholangitis. The frequency of chills and fever after T-tube cholangiography has led to various regimens to prevent it, including drainage of bile for 24 hours after the procedure and antibiotic coverage. This complication, which follows cholangiovenous reflux and bacteremia, can be avoided by careful attention to sterile technique and slow injection of the contrast material. The T-tube should not be removed or clamped for approximately 24 hours after cholangiography, but antibiotic coverage is unnecessary. Acute cholangitis may follow percutaneous transhepatic cholangiography, endoscopic retrograde cholangiopancreatography, or cholangiography done by injection of contrast through other indwelling biliary drainage tubes, such as the U-tubes sometimes used to splint biliary-enteric anastomoses. Other biliary tract procedures that may be complicated by cholangitis include percutaneous transhepatic biliary drainage, endoscopic sphincterotomy, percutaneous extraction of calculi, and insertion of an endoprosthesis. Obviously, contamination of bile may occur during these procedures, and they are almost always performed for conditions that are associated with bacterbilia. Temporary increases in biliary tract pressure are frequent during these procedures, and concomitant cholangiography is frequently necessary, so the high incidence of cholangitis is not surprising.

The presence of a T-tube or stent within the biliary duct system causes bacterial colonization of the bile within a week in over 90 per cent of cases.[16] This is responsible for the high frequency of cholangitis in these patients, especially when obstruction and increased pressure occur after indwelling tubes are clamped or become occluded with the "sludge" that typically forms on foreign bodies in the biliary tract. This problem has led to the recommendation that tubes and catheters expected to be indwelling on a long-term basis be irrigated daily, when possible.

Parasites are a cause of cholangitis and biliary strictures in the Orient. They include *Clonorchis sinensis, Trichuris trichiura,* and *Ascaris lumbricoides,* which obstruct the biliary duct system and

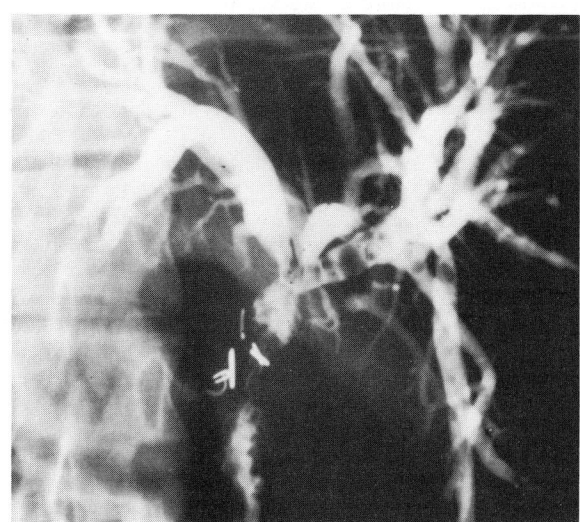

Figure 2. Cholangiogram in a patient who had a bile duct injury at cholecystectomy, followed by a Roux-en-Y choledochojejunostomy, which is now strictured. Note the many calculi within the intrahepatic ducts.

are associated with bacterbilia. This problem is rare in the United States.

The high incidence of cholangitis in patients with obstruction and a foreign body in the biliary tract, such as a stone, an indwelling tube, or a parasite, suggests that bacterbilia is favored by the presence of a foreign body. This also appears to be true in the gallbladder, in which the presence of a stone may be associated with bacterbilia even though the organ is histologically normal, whereas in the absence of a stone the normal gallbladder never contains bacteria.

CLINICAL MANIFESTATIONS

The original description of cholangitis by Charcot consisted of intermittent chills and fever, jaundice, and abdominal pain. Charcot's triad, as this combination is now known, remains the hallmark of acute cholangitis, by definition. His original description referred to the presence of pus or purulent mucus mixed in stagnant bile, a circumstance that has more recently been termed *acute suppurative cholangitis*. Reynolds and Dargan described patients who had shock and central nervous system (CNS) depression in addition to Charcot's triad, and noted that this lethal combination of symptoms, now known as Reynolds' pentad, occurred in the presence of complete obstruction of the biliary duct system that contained pus under pressure.[17] They termed this syndrome *acute obstructive cholangitis*. It is now known that pus may be present in partially obstructed as well as completely obstructed ducts, and that some patients with cholangitis may develop shock and coma without having frank pus within the duct system. The significance of Reynolds' pentad (intermittent chills and fever, abdominal pain, jaundice, shock, and CNS depression) is that this condition is rapidly lethal without emergency intervention, whereas Charcot's triad is an acute but less toxic condition for which immediate intervention usually is not necessary. Therefore, it has been suggested that the latter condition be termed *acute cholangitis,* and the former *acute toxic cholangitis*. These designations imply the requisite therapy, which of necessity must be chosen without knowledge of whether the biliary duct system contains pus and whether the biliary tract is completely obstructed. Acute suppurative cholangitis and acute obstructive cholangitis are final diagnoses that can be applied only after the appropriate therapy has been accomplished, or at autopsy. Therefore, the terms *acute cholangitis* and *acute toxic cholangitis* are used in discussing clinical manifestations and treatment, even though the differences in symptoms between the two conditions may be subtle in many cases, and the correlation between clinical findings and pathologic findings may be weak in others.

Acute Cholangitis

The average ages of patients reported in several large series are approximately 55 to 70 years, which reflect the ages at which diseases associated with cholangitis occur, as well as the increased incidence of bacterbilia that occurs with age. Patients who have choledocholithiasis without cholangitis are, on the average, younger than those who develop cholangitis. The incidence in men and women is approximately equal.

An accurate history is essential in making the diagnosis. The details of previous biliary tract problems or operations should be obtained, bearing in mind the possibilities of retained or primary common duct stones, operative injury to the bile ducts, or a previous biliary-enteric anastomosis, all of which may predispose to cholangitis. Recurrent episodes of pancreatitis may suggest a distal common duct stricture. Similarly, the possibility of malignant stricture should be explored by questioning the patient about anorexia, pain, and weight loss.

The complete symptom triad of chills and fever, abdominal pain, and jaundice occurs in only 50 to 70 per cent of patients who have cholangitis.[2,13] The most frequent symptom is fever,

which is present in over 90 per cent, but a history of chills is not as frequent. Abdominal pain, usually in the right upper quadrant, occurs in about 80 per cent and is characteristically mild. Severe abdominal pain is very unusual. Clinically apparent jaundice is present is approximately 80 per cent. Nausea and vomiting, not part of Charcot's triad, are the only other frequent symptoms.

Other than elevated temperature and jaundice, the positive physical findings are limited to the abdomen. Sixty to 80 per cent of patients have abdominal tenderness, which is generally in the right upper quadrant or epigastrium. Signs of peritoneal irritation are not commonly found. In general, the abdominal tenderness is mild to moderate. Bowel sounds are usually normal. Occasionally, a mass may be present in the right upper quadrant due to an enlarged gallbladder, a tumor, or an abscess. In patients with biliary stricture and biliary cirrhosis, the liver may be enlarged. They may have other stigmata of biliary cirrhosis as well.

The laboratory findings in acute cholangitis reflect the infectious nature of the disease and the fact that biliary tract obstruction is a prerequisite for its development. The white blood cell count is elevated in approximately 75 per cent of cases. In some instances, a shift to the left is the only abnormality. The presence or absence of an abnormal white blood cell count depends on the interval between symptoms and the time of measurement. Obviously, the patient who had an episode of chills and fever a week prior to examination is unlikely to have an abnormal count, whereas the opposite is true for the patient who has bacteremia at the time of testing. More than 90 per cent of patients with acute cholangitis have hyperbilirubinemia. The degree of hyperbilirubinemia varies according to the underlying biliary tract problem, but 20 per cent of patients have a serum value of 2.0 mg. per 100 ml. or less.[2,11] As mentioned previously, 70 to 80 per cent have jaundice detectable on physical examination, so measurement of serum bilirubin is essential to detect the remaining 20 to 30 per cent of patients. Serum alkaline phosphatase values are elevated in over 90 per cent, and the same is true of aspartate aminotransferase and alanine aminotransferase levels. Serum amylase is frequently increased, but this is probably a nonspecific finding, except in patients with concomitant pancreatitis, in whom the values are elevated to at least twice normal. The importance of measuring serum bilirubin, alkaline phosphatase, and aminotransferases in patients who are not jaundiced cannot be overemphasized, because they direct attention to the biliary tract in the setting of combinations of nonspecific symptoms such as nausea and vomiting, chills, fever, and abdominal pain. The possibility of cholangitis must be raised in any patient who has intermittent fever without other symptoms. This aspect of the diagnostic process in patients with fever of undetermined origin often is overlooked.

In many cases, the clinical pattern of cholangitis suggests bacteremia, especially when chills and fever are present. Patients suspected of having acute cholangitis should have cultures of their blood drawn during a chill, when possible, because of the importance of determining the sensitivity of the organism to specific antibiotics in the event the initial antibiotic treatment fails. Slightly less than half of patients with acute cholangitis have positive blood cultures.[2,11,18] Most patients who have chills and fever probably would have positive cultures if it were possible to obtain blood samples more frequently and at the most appropriate times. Not surprisingly, the type of organisms cultured and the frequency with which each is found in the blood correlates very well with the types found later at operation in the bile of the patient. The organisms most frequently cultured from the blood of patients with acute cholangitis are, in decreasing order, *E. coli, Klebsiella pneumoniae,* and *Streptococcus faecalis.* These organisms are those most commonly found in bile, in the same order of frequency, although approximately two thirds of patients have multiple organisms present in the bile. Anaerobic organisms, usually *Bacteroides fragilis,* are found rarely in both bile and blood, but anaerobic cultures of blood should be made.

Acute Toxic Cholangitis

This form of cholangitis is the most severe, causing death if prompt therapy is not administered. The presumption is that such cases are associated with continuing sepsis, usually due to pus under pressure within the bile duct system, but the correlation between severity of symptoms and the presence or absence of pus in the duct system is not perfect. Approximately 15 per cent of all patients with cholangitis have the acute toxic form, the symptoms of which are more likely to include shock and CNS depression. The CNS depression may assume the form of coma, disorientation, drowsiness, confusion, or inappropriate behavior and is not different from the CNS symptoms observed in patients with severe, persistent sepsis from other causes. In general, the symptoms of acute toxic cholangitis are more severe, but the characteristic features are the persistent and progressive nature of the symptoms and the failure of the patient to respond rapidly to conventional therapy for sepsis. This, of course, is characteristic of the course of patients who have an untreated source of sepsis, and it is the signal for emergency measures to locate the septic focus and to drain it immediately. In acute toxic cholangitis, this means emergency decompression of the biliary duct system.

The laboratory findings in acute toxic cholangitis are apt to reveal a higher white blood cell count and bilirubin, but the differences are not sufficient to distinguish between the acute and acute toxic forms. In fact, there is no reason to categorize cholangitis other than to emphasize the high mortality and the need for emergency surgical treatment in the most severe cases.

DIFFERENTIAL DIAGNOSIS

The condition most commonly confused with acute cholangitis is acute cholecystitis because right upper quadrant pain, fever, jaundice, and elevated bilirubin and white blood cell count are clinical manifestations common to both conditions. The only clinical features that tend to distinguish the two conditions are the frequency and severity of right upper quadrant pain and the degree of tenderness on physical examination. In acute cholecystitis, persistent pain is present in almost every patient, whereas pain is absent in approximately 20 per cent of patients with acute cholangitis and tends to be less severe. Similarly, abdominal tenderness is absent in approximately 20 per cent of patients with acute cholangitis but is invariably present in acute cholecystitis. Peritoneal signs, frequent in acute cholecystitis, are absent in acute cholangitis. Nevertheless, these differences are not always sufficient to distinguish between the two conditions, and some believe that cholangitis frequently occurs in association with acute cholecystitis. Cholescintigraphy, specific for the diagnosis of acute cholecystitis, should be done when uncertainty exists.

Pyogenic liver abscess should be considered in the differential diagnosis. The symptoms may be identical, and liver abscess is a complication of acute cholangitis. Liver abscesses may be detected by ultrasonography, radionuclide scanning, and computed axial tomography. Hepatitis may present with right upper quadrant pain and tenderness, fever, and jaundice, but the differentiation from acute cholangitis usually can be made from the tests of hepatic function. Aminotransferase values are much higher in hepatitis than in cholangitis. Acute pancreatitis may present with fever and an increased serum bilirubin, but the pain and tenderness associated with pancreatitis are usually more striking than in cholangitis. Although serum amylase values may be increased in both conditions, the degree of elevation is much higher in pancreatitis.

Perforated or penetrating duodenal ulcer presents with upper abdominal pain and may be accompanied by fever and slight elevation of serum bilirubin. A carefully elicited history usually differentiates these conditions from acute cholangitis. The clinical pattern in some cases of right pyelonephritis, acute appendicitis, right lower lobe pneumonia, and pulmonary infarct may be suggestive of acute cholangitis, but the correct diagnosis usually becomes apparent with frequent serial examinations and careful correlation of the history and physical examination with the laboratory data. Fever, chills, and jaundice or elevated serum bilirubin may occur in bacterial sepsis from any cause. Although it is important not to ascribe all such cases to acute cholangitis, it is equally important to consider acute cholangitis when the source of sepsis is not readily apparent.

DIAGNOSIS OF THE UNDERLYING CONDITION

The underlying biliary tract disease must be delineated when the diagnosis of acute cholangitis is made. Cholangiography is the definitive test and is necessary for planning the definitive therapy, but it should not be done until the acute process is under control. Injection of contrast material under pressure into the biliary tract may produce cholangiovenous reflux and exacerbate the sepsis unless appropriate antibiotic therapy has controlled the infection. Patients with acute cholangitis should have an ultrasound examination, with special emphasis on the presence or absence of cholelithiasis, bile duct dilation, masses in the head of the pancreas or within the porta hepatis, and choledocholithiasis. Ultrasonography is highly accurate in the detection of gallbladder calculi and bile duct enlargement, but less so in the delineation of common duct calculi.

When the cholangitis is under control, further testing may proceed, using the ultrasound examination as a guide. If a mass in the pancreas or the porta hepatis is suspected, computed axial tomography should be done to delineate its extent as well as to assess the liver for hepatic metastases. Cholescintigraphy is helpful in differentiating between acute cholecystitis and acute cholangitis, but its role in the diagnosis of conditions that underlie cholangitis is limited. Complete bile duct obstruction can be diagnosed by cholescintigraphy, but delineation of lesions causing incomplete obstruction is not possible (Fig. 3).

The essential procedure is cholangiography, which can be performed by the percutaneous transhepatic or endoscopic retrograde techniques. Percutaneous transhepatic cholangiography should be done when ultrasonography demonstrates a dilated proximal duct system, and endoscopic retrograde cholangiography is indicated when the duct system is normal. The endoscopic technique should be considered when concomitant upper gastrointestinal endoscopy is indicated such as in a suspected carcinoma of the ampulla of Vater, or when pancreatography is necessary such as in chronic pancreatitis. Certain aspects of percutaneous transhepatic cholangiography and endoscopic retrograde cholangiopancreatography that influence the therapy of acute cholangitis and acute toxic cholangitis are discussed in the following.

TREATMENT

The principles of therapy for acute cholangitis are first to achieve complete control of the septic process, and second to correct the underlying cause. All patients with significant symptoms of acute cholangitis or acute toxic cholangitis should receive antibiotic therapy. An occasional patient may have a history of mild, short-lived symptoms suggestive of acute cholangitis but is asymptomatic at the time of examination. Under these circumstances clinical investigation for the underlying cause may proceed without antibiotic coverage, except when indicated for invasive procedures. To date, there is no ideal antibiotic regimen. The choice should be based on the organisms most often cultured from the blood, which are *E. coli, K.*

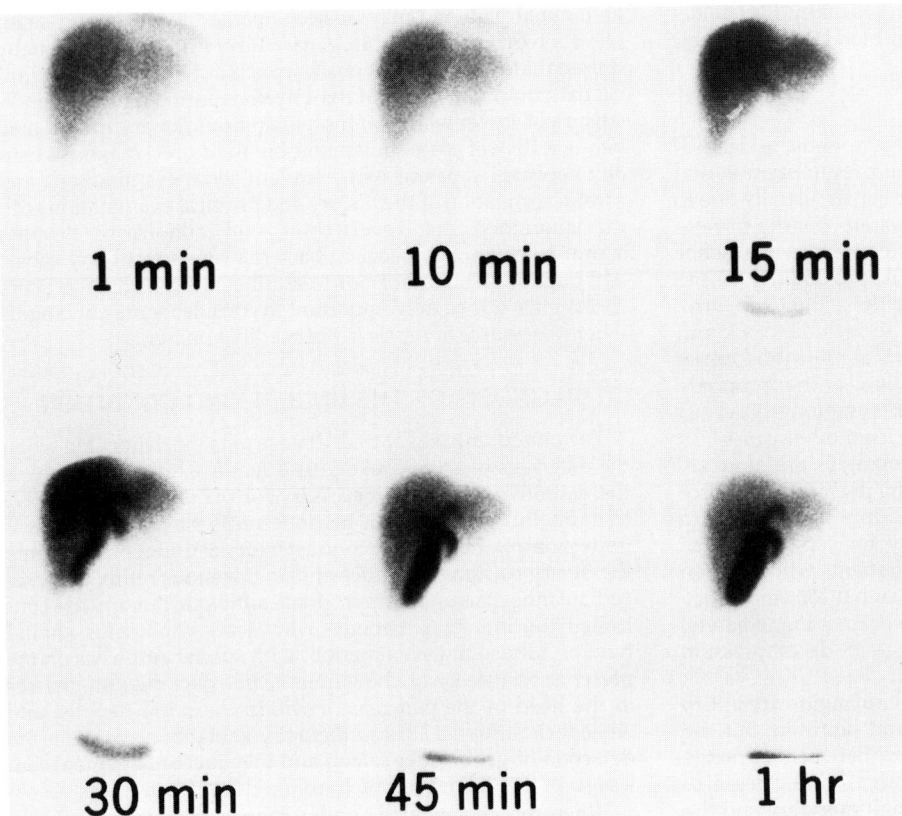

Figure 3. Hepatobiliary scan demonstrating complete obstruction of the distal common bile duct.

pneumoniae, and *S. faecalis.* The first two organisms are best treated by an aminoglycoside such as gentamicin or tobramycin, but these agents are not effective against *S. faecalis* or other enterococci. Enterococci are best managed by a combination of a penicillin and an aminoglycoside. To further complicate the situation, anaerobes, most commonly *B. fragilis,* are cultured from bile in one fourth to one third of patients. This organism is best treated by clindamycin or metronidazole. Therefore, the author treats patients with severe acute cholangitis, and all patients with acute toxic cholangitis, by a combination that includes a penicillin such as ampicillin, an aminoglycoside, and either clindamycin or metronidazole. Some might dispute the need for gram-negative anaerobe coverage because of the relatively low frequency in which these organisms are actually cultured from the blood in patients with cholangitis. The major disadvantage of this regimen is the nephrotoxicity of the aminoglycosides, which is made even more likely because of the septic shock and hyperbilirubinemia observed in some patients with cholangitis. Serum levels of aminoglycosides and creatinine should be monitored to minimize this problem.

In patients with mild cholangitis, and no evidence of continuing, severe sepsis, antibiotic therapy with a second- or third-generation cephalosporin is adequate. These agents are effective against *E. coli, K. pneumoniae,* and other gram-negative aerobic organisms, but not against the more rarely cultured *S. faecalis* and other enterococci. The newer penicillins, such as piperacillin, mezlocillin, and imipenem, appear to be effective against gram-negative aerobes and enterococci and may prove to be the safest and most effective agents for acute cholangitis. The results of blood cultures and sensitivities should be used to adjust antibiotic therapy and to discontinue nephrotoxic agents when less toxic agents can be substituted. The emphasis on the concentration of antibiotics in bile may be less important than originally thought. Although there are theoretic advantages to high bile concentrations, such as the elimination of organisms from bile, tissue and serum concentrations may be more important. In acute toxic cholangitis with complete bile duct obstruc-

tion, for example, high concentrations might not be achieved because of failure of the liver to secrete the antibiotic into bile.

Elderly and debilitated patients who have acute cholangitis and all patients with acute toxic cholangitis require careful monitoring of hemodynamic parameters, urinary output, and blood gases. Direct arterial blood pressure monitoring should be instituted if the blood pressure is unstable or urinary output is abnormal. In such cases, measurements of central venous and pulmonary wedge pressures are necessary, and frequent determinations of cardiac output and systemic vascular resistance should be made so that decisions concerning volume replacement, inotropic agents, and vasoactive drugs can be made on the basis of the available data. Coagulation parameters should also be monitored, especially in patients who have chronic liver disease.

Most patients with cholangitis respond rapidly to therapy. After they have been afebrile for approximately 48 hours, cholangiography and other indicated studies should be done under continuing antibiotic coverage, and when the underlying condition is delineated, appropriate therapy should be instituted. Accurate diagnosis is essential, because in at least one series,[18] recurrent cholangitis postoperatively caused some deaths. When carefully analyzed, these deaths were due to inadequate or incomplete surgical treatment because of inadequate preoperative information. Some patients with very mild episodes of cholangitis who have special problems, such as a mild biliary stricture and other reasons militating against surgical correction, have been managed by chronic antibiotic therapy with ampicillin, a cephalosporin, or a trimethoprim and sulfamethoxazole combination. However, the decision not to correct a benign, underlying condition surgically must be made very judiciously because, although convenient, it may cause the development of biliary cirrhosis, portal hypertension, and death (Fig. 4). Conservative definitive management with percutaneous biliary drainage or internal stenting is appropriate in malignant conditions known to be incurable.

Patients with acute cholangitis or acute toxic cholangitis who

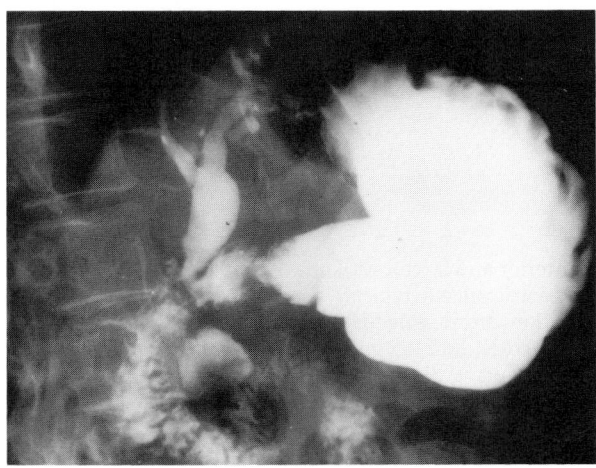

Figure 4. Barium examination of the upper gastrointestinal tract in a patient who had choledochoduodenostomy many years previously. Note the narrowed anastomosis and dilated bile ducts. Biliary cirrhosis was present.

do not respond to antibiotic therapy and supportive care as described previously should have emergency decompression of the biliary duct system. The time-honored, successful method is insertion of a T-tube into the common bile duct and gentle irrigation of the duct to remove the pus, with no further manipulation or procedure directed toward treatment of the underlying condition. The principle of emergency decompression of the duct system still pertains, but less traumatic and simpler means of accomplishing this should be used when possible. The most efficacious is percutaneous transhepatic biliary drainage, in which the dilated duct is located by a needle, a guidewire is passed into the duct, and a catheter is introduced over the guidewire.[5] This procedure does not require general anesthesia and is simple and safe. The disadvantage is that the catheter is small and requires frequent, careful irrigation to maintain adequate decompression. Another approach is endoscopic sphincterotomy and extraction of obstructing stones from the duct.[10] This approach combines emergency decompression with definitive therapy in the approximately 60 per cent of patients with cholangitis whose obstruction is due to choledocholithiasis. The author favors percutaneous drainage, but the endoscopic approach is equally effective. The availability of facilities and personnel with expertise in these techniques influences management of the individual patient. When they are unavailable, laparotomy and common duct decompression should be done without delay. Cholecystostomy does not decompress the biliary duct system adequately and should not be done.

RESULTS AND COMPLICATIONS

The results of treatment of mild acute cholangitis are excellent. Deaths are almost always related to complications of the operation performed for the underlying condition and are unrelated to the original episode of cholangitis. However, the mortality of severe acute cholangitis and acute toxic cholangitis is high, especially when shock and CNS symptoms are present. In one review of 86 patients, the mortality was 100 per cent in untreated patients and 50 per cent in those who had bile duct decompression.[1] The high mortality of nonoperative therapy has been confirmed in other reviews.[13,14] More recent data suggest that the mortality of properly-treated acute toxic cholangitis is 20 to 25 per cent.[9,13]

The most serious complication of acute cholangitis and acute toxic cholangitis is hepatic abscess. Biliary tract disease, including cholangitis, represents approximately half of all cases of hepatic abscess.[15] Because they occur in association with cholangitis, hepatic abscesses are often overlooked. They should be suspected in all patients who fail to respond to treatment of cholangitis. Antibiotic treatment should include coverage for anaerobic organisms because they are frequently cultured from hepatic abscesses. Hepatic abscesses are successfully treated by surgical or percutaneous drainage, but the mortality approaches 100 per cent when multiple abscesses are present. The best approach to this problem is to prevent them by prompt attention to biliary tract obstruction and cholangitis.

SELECTED REFERENCES

Boey, J. H. and Way, L. W.: Acute cholangitis. Ann. Surg., *191*:264, 1980.
A large series of 99 patients with cholangitis was analyzed for associated conditions, symptoms, laboratory findings, and outcome after treatment. They found that the correlation between clinical manifestations and biliary suppuration was inexact. They emphasize that cholangitis has a wide spectrum of severity.

Pitt, H. A., and Longmire, W. P., Jr.: Suppurative cholangitis. *In* Hardy, J. M. (Ed.): Critical Surgical Illness, 2nd ed. Philadelphia, W. B. Saunders Company, 1980, pp. 380–408.
This is a comprehensive review of the literature on cholangitis with emphasis on the more lethal forms. Treatment, both supportive and definitive, is explained in detail. Excellent case descriptions are used to supplement the material presented.

REFERENCES

1. Andrew, D. J., and Johnson, S. E.: Acute suppurative cholangitis, a medical and surgical emergency. Am. J. Gastroenterol., *54*:141, 1970.
2. Boey, J. H., and Way, L. W.: Acute cholangitis. Ann. Surg., *191*:264, 1980.
3. Charcot, J. M.: Lecons sur les maladies du foie des voies filiares et des reins. Paris, Faculté de Medecine de Paris, 1877.
4. Edlund, Y., and Hanzon, V.: Demonstration of the close relationship between bile capillaries and sinusoid walls. Acta Anat., *17*:105, 1953.
5. Gould, R. J., Vogelzang, R. L., Neeman, H. L., Pearl, G. L., and Poticha, S. M.: Percutaneous biliary drainage as an initial therapy in sepsis of the biliary tract. Surg. Gynecol. Obstet., *160*:523, 1985.
6. Hampton, J. C.: An electron microscope study of the hepatic uptake and excretion of microscopic particles injected into the blood stream and into the bile duct. Acta Anat., *32*:262, 1958.
7. Hultborn, A., Jacobsson, B., and Rosengren, B.: Cholangiovenous reflux during cholangiography. Acta Chir. Scand., *123*:111, 1962.
8. Jacobsson, B., Kjellander, J., and Rosengren, B.: Cholangiovenous reflux. Acta Chir. Scand., *123*:316, 1962.
9. Lai, E. C. S., Tam, P. C., Paterson, I. A., Ng, M. M. T., Fan, S., Choi, T., and Wong, J.: Emergency surgery for severe acute cholangitis. Ann. Surg., *211*:55, 1990.
10. Leese, T., Neoptolemos, J. P., Baker, A. R., and Carr-Locke, D. L.: Management of acute cholangitis and the impact of endoscopic sphincterotomy. Br. J. Surg., *73*:988, 1986.
11. Longmire, W. P., Jr.: Suppurative cholangitis. *In* Hardy, J. M. (Ed.): Critical Surgical Illness. Philadelphia, W. B. Saunders Company, 1971, p. 397.
12. Mixer, H. W., Rigler, L. G., and Gonzales-Oddone, M. V.: Experimental studies on biliary regurgitation during cholangiography. Gastroenterology, *9*:64, 1947.
13. O'Connor, M. J., Schwartz, M. L., McQuarrie, D. G., and Sumner, H. W.: Acute bacterial cholangitis. Arch. Surg., *117*:437, 1982.
14. Pitt, H. A., and Longmire, W. P., Jr.: Suppurative cholangitis. *In* Hardy, J. M. (Ed.): Critical Surgical Illness, 2nd ed. Philadelphia, W. B. Saunders Company, 1980, p. 380.
15. Pitt, H. A., and Zuidema, G. D.: Factors influencing mortality in the treatment of pyogenic hepatic abscess. Surg. Gynecol. Obstet., *140*:228, 1975.
16. Pitt, H. A., Postier, R. G., and Cameron, J. L.: Bacteremia after tube cholangiography. Ann. Surg., *191*:30, 1980.
17. Reynolds, B. M., and Dargan, E. L.: Acute obstructive cholangitis. A distinct clinical syndrome. Ann. Surg., *150*:299, 1959.
18. Saharia, P. C., and Cameron, J. L.: Clinical management of cholangitis. Surg. Gynecol. Obstet., *142*:369, 1976.
19. Saik, R. P., Greenburg, A. G., Farris, J. M., and Peskin, G. W.: Spectrum of cholangitis. Am. J. Surg., *130*:143, 1975.
20. Williams, R. D., Fish, J. C., and Williams, D. D.: The significance of biliary pressure. Arch. Surg., *95*:374, 1974.

IV

GALLSTONE ILEUS AND FISTULA

Francis E. Rosato, M.D.

BILIARY FISTULAS

A biliary fistula is an established and abnormal connection between any portion of the biliary tree and some other area. If this abnormal connection is between the biliary tree and the exterior, it is termed an *external fistula*, whereas connections between the biliary tree and an internal structure constitute an *internal fistula*. Gallstones, peptic ulcer, trauma, and neoplasia are common causes of such fistulas. In general, external fistulas are most likely due to trauma, particularly operative trauma; internal fistulas most often follow peptic ulcer, gallstone disease, and cancer.

The mode of presentation varies, depending on the cause and the type of fistula. Most external fistulas occur in a postoperative setting and usually after the formation of an extrabiliary accumulation of bile. Internal biliary fistulas are more insidious in their presentation, since the antecedent neoplastic or inflammatory adherence to another body structure occurs over a protracted period of time. The most common biliary fistulas and their symptom complex are listed in Table 1. Cholangitis is a likely associated problem with any biliary fistula. In addition, there have been reported biliary tract connections made into the kidney, urinary bladder, uterus, vagina, portal vein, inferior vena cava, and pericardial sac.

External Biliary Fistula

The common setting for external biliary fistula is after operation on the biliary tree, particularly when exploration or reconstruction of the common bile duct is included. If bile leakage occurs, a walled-off collection of bile results, producing a chemical peritonitis. This is usually accompanied by a characteristic rise in conjugated serum bilirubin due to absorption from the peritoneal cavity and several days later by an elevation of serum alkaline phosphatase, probably due to pericholangitis.[11] Rarely, bile peritonitis may pursue a more indolent course, producing a mild jaundice and abdominal distention termed bile ascites.[17] Usually, however, a walled-off bile collection occurs, typically productive of fever and abdominal tenderness that are persistent until such time as the bile is removed, either operatively by the placement of drains (or reopening of drain tracts) or spontaneously.[8] Occasionally, in the absence of any bile duct obstruction, such external fistulas may rapidly close. With sonographic or computed tomographic scan imaging, percutaneous catheter placement successfully resolves 80 per cent of fistulas.[15] Even with distal common duct obstruction, endoscopic papillotomy allows improved bile flow and passage of common duct stones, permitting nonoperative closure.[6,14]

Internal Biliary Fistula

Ninety per cent of internal biliary fistulas are from gallstone disease, whereas 5 per cent are secondary to peptic ulcer. Ulcers on the posterior duodenum invade the common duct; those on

TABLE 1. Symptoms of Biliary Fistulas

Fistula Type	Symptom Complex
Biliary-cutaneous	Bile peritonitis and/or external bile leakage
Biliary-intestinal	Gallstone ileus
Biliary-pleurobronchial	Bile-tinged sputum (biloptysis)

the anterior and lateral wall attach and erode into the gallbladder. Gastric ulcers typically erode into the gallbladder also where they produce fistulas.[12] Tumors of the stomach, gallbladder, pancreas, and common duct erode into contiguous structures, producing different types of fistulas.[10] After the connection between the biliary tree and adjacent structure has been established, the symptom complex of cholangitis ensues. At times an internal biliary fistula in the same manner as an external biliary fistula may first be a localized bile collection; for example, a choledochobronchial fistula usually follows a bile collection that leads to an inflammatory process producing connection between these two physically disparate structures.[9]

Complications of Fistula

There are three important complications of biliary fistula, regardless of the type of fistula or the particular structures involved[13] (Fig. 1).

1. *Hyponatremia.* The sodium content of bile is approximately 150 mEq. per liter, and the loss of such bile externally or even internally into the bronchial tree or bladder can produce a severe hyponatremia.

2. *Inanition and weight loss.* The critical role of bile as an emulsifying agent facilitating the absorption of fats and fat-soluble vitamins is well established. The external loss of bile produces a malabsorption problem, and the resultant diarrhea may additionally jeopardize protein and carbohydrate absorption. When internal biliary fistulas have been formed, particularly between the biliary system and the upper reaches of the intestinal tract, this complication is minimized.

3. *Infection.* There are two principal modes by which infection ensues in the biliary fistula setting. The first is from a transient

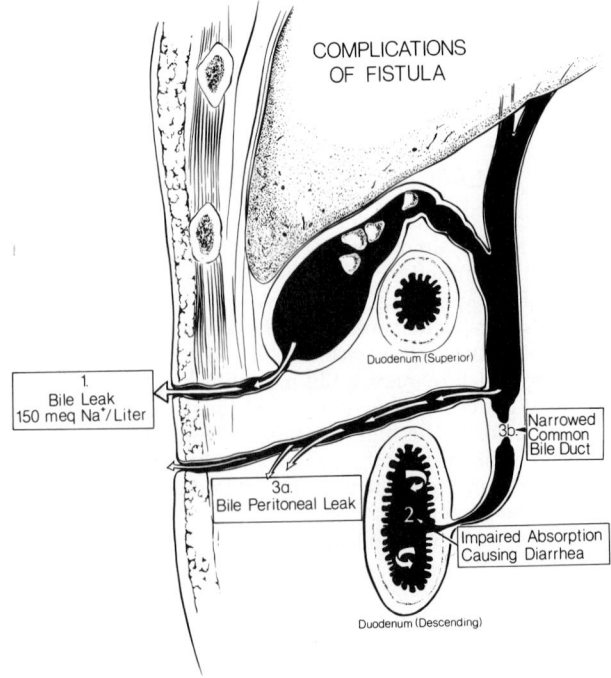

Figure 1. Diagrammatic representation of major biliary fistula complications.

leakage of bile from the tract, with resultant contamination of the peritoneal space. Bile is not sterile and especially in fistulas contains coliform organisms and occasionally anaerobic clostridia. Bile leakage into body cavities produces, therefore, transient episodes of bacterial infection, in addition to the anticipated chemical inflammation. The second factor in infection is cholangitis, which occurs in about 10 to 15 per cent of cholecystoduodenal fistulas. It is an unusual occurrence in choledochoduodenal fistula. The exact mechanism is not clearly understood, since in general the pressure gradients favor the distal flow of bile; in addition, cholangitis does not ensue even when reflux has been demonstrated in surgically created biliary-enteric fistulas. Some degree of bile stasis and obstruction appears essential, therefore, in the production of cholangitis. Cholangitis is ushered in with the classic Charcot's triad of jaundice (either appearing for the first time or aggravated), fever, and shaking chills.

Gallstone ileus, the last complication, is considered separately in this section.

Therapy

The management of a biliary fistula should be considered in sequential steps.

1. ESTABLISH THE ANATOMY OF THE FISTULA. When the fistula is established to the outside, a No. 8 or 10 French red rubber tube can be inserted in the external orifice and snugged in place with a pursestring suture of 2–0 silk. Injection of contrast material serves to delineate the site of origin and the fistula tract as well (Fig. 2). Where internal fistula is present, attempts are made through upper gastrointestinal series, barium enema, cholangiography, bronchoscopy, or cystography to delineate the anatomic extent of the fistula[1] (Fig. 3). Endoscopic retrograde cholangiopancreatography allows visualization of the distal biliary tree; transhepatic cholangiography demonstrates the intrahepatic biliary system and the extrahepatic ductal system as well, often pinpointing the biliary origins of the fistula.

2. ATTEMPT TO ESTABLISH THE CAUSE OF THE FISTULA. In attempting to localize the fistula, one can often obtain additional information on the underlying cause. Studies such as gastroduodenoscopy, radioactive scanning of the liver, sonography (particularly to detect nonopacified gallstones), and cytologic evaluation of a number of aspirated specimens may be required. The value of surgical exploration for final determination of the cause cannot be overemphasized; very often initial studies localize the fistula, and surgical therapy delineates its cause. Historically, those 10 per cent of fistulas due to peptic ulcer disease can be suspected when there is a lessening of ulcer

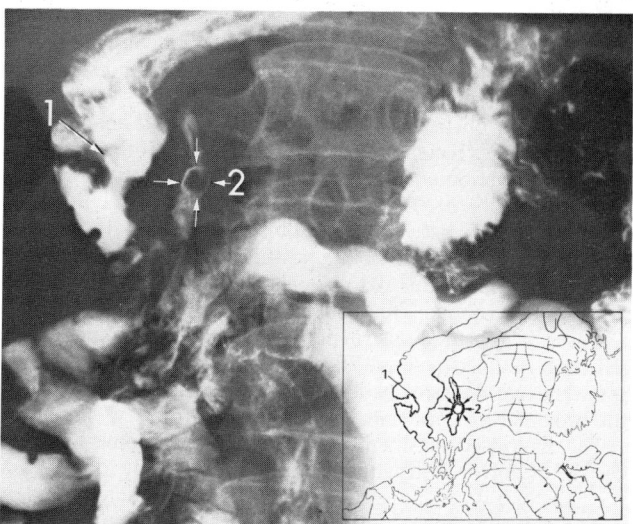

Figure 3. Upper gastrointestinal series showing duodenum (1) and shortly thereafter opacification of common bile duct. This sequence is pathognomonic of choledochoduodenal fistula. Note stone in common bile duct (2).

symptoms consonant with the appearance of the fistula, presumably due to alkaline bathing of the ulcer through the choledochoduodenal fistula.

3. CONTROL INFECTION. Since infection is one of the major complications of fistula, appropriate antibiotics must be chosen to combat infection. Cultured bile, in the case of external fistula, is often helpful in making the correct choice of antibiotics. In general, drugs with a high degree of enterohepatic recirculation effective against gram-negative bacilli, at times including those with a spectrum against anaerobes, would be ideal for the preparation of such patients. Ampicillin or cefoxitin (Mefoxin) is an ideal initial agent.

4. CORRECT ELECTROLYTE ABNORMALITIES. Particular attention should be paid to possible sodium depletion. With the advent of intravenous hyperalimentation, nutritional problems can be corrected during the preparative period while studying the type and cause of the fistulas.

5. SURGICAL THERAPY. As mentioned, the initial approach to both internal and external biliary fistulas is to establish drainage (usually by computed tomographic or ultrasound guidance) and to relieve obstruction, where it exists, by endoscopic papillotomy. Thus, most fistulas can "dry out" without surgical intervention.[4] However, continuing jaundice, sepsis, or electrolyte disturbances may force a surgical approach.

When inflammation is the cause of the fistula, the surgical separation of the adjacent structures is usually done with surgical closure of each. When neoplasia is the underlying problem, separation may not be possible, although, wherever possible, it is obviously urged. Often the relief of distal obstruction to bile flow may be sufficient to cause complete resolution of the fistula without direct operative intervention. In general, operative cholangiography may be of help in deciding appropriate surgical therapy. Inflammatory fistulas are usually "taken down" and attention given to relief of any attendant biliary obstruction.

Neoplastic fistulas often cannot be closed, and in this situation relief of obstruction to bile flow is recommended. For example, cholangitis in cholecystogastric fistulas due to prepyloric tumors often can be controlled by gastrojejunostomy alone.

GALLSTONE ILEUS

This particular complication follows internal fistulas in which a gallbladder or common duct stone, through an internal biliary fistula, gains entrance into the intestinal tract. One would anticipate the usual potential complications attendant on any internal biliary fistula, particularly ascending cholangitis. In addi-

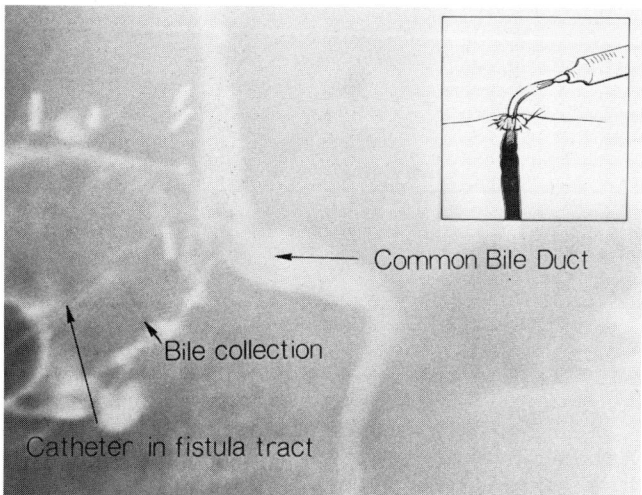

→ Common Bile Duct

Bile collection

Catheter in fistula tract

Figure 2. Catheter (inset) introduced into fistula tract, and resultant fistulogram demonstrating a choledochocutaneous fistula. The tortuosity of the common bile duct resulted from bile-induced inflammation.

tion, in this condition, the presence of a large stone in the intestinal tract produces obstruction at the point where its diameter exceeds that of the intestinal lumen. A typical presentation for gallstone ileus would include frequent previous episodes of partial bowel obstruction, which exacerbate and abate as the stone negotiates its way into a narrower region of the intestinal tract. This phenomenon is called "tumbling" obstruction.

Three fourths of the spontaneous fistulas underlying gallstone ileus occur between the gallbladder and the duodenum. Most gallstones that enter the gastrointestinal tract are either passed or vomited, but 10 to 15 per cent may lead to the condition described above. This disorder represents only 1 per cent of all cases of intestinal obstruction but 25 per cent of simple obstruction in those over age 70. The common site of obstruction, found in two thirds of patients, is the terminal ileum, whereas the proximal jejunum is the least likely.[7]

The diagnosis is easily made if a large mass lesion is found at the site of bowel obstruction; this "mass" is readily identified if the gallstone is opaque, and sometimes, even if nonopaque, it can be observed because of surrounding intestinal air. In addition, the finding of air in the biliary tree makes the diagnosis almost certain. Ultrasound, more recently, has been helpful.

Treatment

The proper treatment of gallstone ileus is relief of the intestinal obstruction, usually by the performance of an enterotomy and removal of stones. Concomitant definitive correction of the internal fistula is advocated if the patient is in good condition and has sustained no prolonged preoperative losses or intraoperative complications and there is not significant inflammatory reaction at the fistula site.[5] Since spontaneous closure of the underlying biliary fistula only rarely occurs, there is a 10 per cent recurrence of gallstone ileus after enterotomy alone. In addition, recurrent cholecystitis, recurrent cholangitis, and a reportedly higher incidence of gallbladder carcinoma in association with biliary enteric fistula all reinforce the recommendation favoring complete corrections after enterotomy. This may be delayed as a separate procedure when the patient is judged too ill to withstand the prolonged single operation.[3]

SELECTED REFERENCES

Deitz, D. M.: Improving the outcome in gallstone ileus. Am. J. Surg., 151:572, 1986.
The authors present a retrospective 32-year experience covering 24 patients with gallstone ileus. They emphasize the preponderance of females over 70 years of age who have this condition, the small percentage with correct preoperative diagnosis, and the significant mortality of 13 per cent. A very thorough and recent review.

Fox, P. F.: Planning the operation for cholecystoenteric fistula with gallstone ileus. Surg. Clin. North Am., 50:93, 1970.

This reference reviews 13 patients with gallstone ileus but includes considerable effort in detailing surgical operative aspects. This is a fine reference in planning operative intervention and provides some technical detail.

Papanicolaou, N.: Abscess-fistula association: Radiologic recognition and percutaneous management. A.J.R., 143:811, 1984.
This is one of the larger earlier series detailing the new and critically important contribution of percutaneous catheter drainage to successful resolution of biliary fistulas, even when such fistulas are associated with abscesses.

Safaie-Shirazi, S.: Spontaneous enterobiliary fistulas. Surg. Gynecol. Obstet., 137:769, 1973.
This is one of the larger case review series presenting data on 92 patients with spontaneous enterobiliary fistula. It emphasizes clinical presentation, diagnosis, and long-term results of management.

REFERENCES

1. Calonje, M. A., Ozenstark, J. L., and Nice, C. M., Jr.: Internal biliary fistula. J.A.M.A., 179:112, 1962.
2. Constant, E., and Turcotte, J. G.: Choledochoduodenal fistula: The natural history and management of an unusual complication of peptic ulcer disease. Ann. Surg., 167:220, 1968.
3. Cooperman, A. M., Dickson, E. R., and ReMine, W. H.: Changing concepts in the surgical treatment of gallstone ileus: A review of 15 cases with emphasis on diagnosis and treatment. Ann. Surg., 167:377, 1968.
4. Czerniak, A., Thompson, J. N., Soreido, O., et al.: The management of fistulas of the biliary tract after injury to the bile duct during cholecystectomy. Surg. Gynecol. Obstet., 167:33, 1988.
5. Day, E. A., and Marks, C.: Gallstone ileus. Review of the literature and presentation of thirty-four new cases. Am. J. Surg., 129:552, 1975.
6. Del Olmo, L., Mero-no, E., Moreira, V. F., et al.: Successful treatment of postoperative external biliary fistulas by endoscopic sphincterotomy. Gastrointest. Endosc., 34:307, 1988.
7. Dietz, D. M., Standage, B. A., Pinson, C. W., et al.: Improving the outcome in gallstone ileus. Am. J. Surg., 151:572, 1986.
8. Fitchett, C. W.: Spontaneous external biliary fistula. Trans. South. Surg. Assoc., 80:214, 1969.
9. Gugenheim, J., Ciardullo, M., Traynor, O., and Bismuth, H.: Bronchobiliary fistulas in adults. Ann. Surg., 207:90, 1988.
10. Hicken, N. F., and Coray, Q. B.: Spontaneous gastrointestinal biliary fistulas. Surg. Gynecol. Obstet., 82:723, 1946.
11. McCarthy, J. D., and Picazo, J. G.: Bile peritonitis—diagnosis and course. Am. J. Surg., 116:664, 1968.
12. Misra, M. C., Grewal, H., and Kapur, B. M.: Spontaneous choledochoduodenal fistula complicating peptic ulcer disease—a case report. Jpn. J. Surg., 19:367, 1989.
13. Norcross, J. W., and Dadey, J. L.: Medical complications of operative bile-duct injuries. N. Engl. J. Med., 257:1216, 1957.
14. O'Rahilly, S., Duignan, J. P., Lennon, J. R., and O'Malley, E.: Successful treatment of a postoperative external biliary fistula by endoscopic papillotomy. Endocrinology, 15:68, 1983.
15. Papanicolaou, N., Mueller, P. R., Ferrucci, J. R., Jr., et al.: Abscess-fistula association: Radiologic recognition and percutaneous management. A.J.R., 143:811, 1984.
16. Renner, W., Went, J., McLean, J., and Plattner, G.: Ultrasound demonstration of a non-calcified gallstone in the distal ileum causing small bowel obstruction. Radiology, 144:884, 1982.
17. Rosato, E. F., Berkowitz, H. D., and Roberts, B.: Bile ascites. Surg. Gynecol. Obstet., 130:494, 1970.
18. Safaie-Shirazi, S., Zike, W. L., and Printen, K. J.: Spontaneous enterobiliary fistulas. Surg. Gynecol. Obstet., 137:769, 1973.

V

CARCINOMA OF THE GALLBLADDER

David Fromm, M.D.

Although carcinoma of the gallbladder is the most common malignant lesion of the biliary tract, it represents only 5 per cent of all cancers found at autopsy.[1] Ninety-one per cent of patients who develop this malignancy are at least 50 years of age or older[15] (Fig. 1). The incidence of the cancer in women is three to four times that for men, and this is in contrast to the predominance of cancer of the bile ducts in men.

INCIDENCE AND ASSOCIATIONS

The highest incidence of cancer of the gallbladder occurs in American Indians, Americans of Mexican origin, Alaskan natives, northeastern Europeans, Israelis, and Japanese immigrants to the United States. The frequency of this cancer in Alaskan natives is about the same as that for the Indians of New

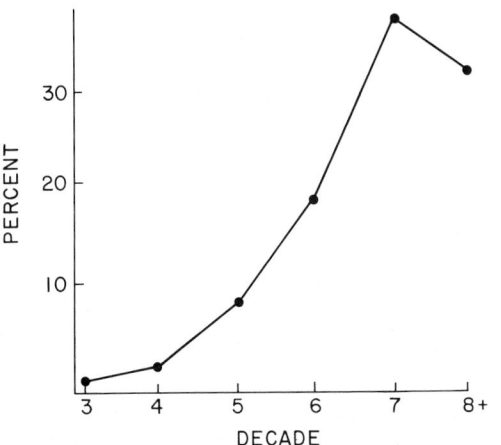

Figure 1. Frequency of carcinoma of the gallbladder relative to age. Note the increase with each decade. Data compiled from 1728 patients from 29 reports. (From Piehler, J. M., and Crichlow, R. W.: Primary carcinoma of the gallbladder. Surg. Gynecol. Obstet., *147*:929, 1978.)

Mexico,[3] which has been estimated to be more than six times that of the non-Indian population. American Indian women are twice as likely to develop the cancer than are Spanish American women, who are almost ten times as likely to develop the cancer than are non–Spanish American whites.[4] The lowest rates are reported for black Americans, black Rhodesians, Indians in India, and Spaniards in Spain.

There is a well-established association between cancer of the gallbladder and gallstones, which are present in at least 70 per cent of patients, a figure far greater than that found in the age-matched general population. A parallel exists between the epidemiology of cancer of the gallbladder and gallstones. In both conditions there is a higher incidence in females, an increasing incidence with age, and variation among ethnic groups. Cancer of the gallbladder associated with cholelithiasis is found in about 0.5 per cent of autopsies, whereas this figure ranges from about 1 to 2 per cent in patients undergoing cholecystectomy. There is no predilection for development of carcinoma in a gallbladder containing single or multiple stones. However, there may be some relationship to the size of a stone, as it has been suggested that the risk for developing carcinoma in a patient with a 3-cm. gallstone is ten times that for one with a stone less than 1 cm.[5]

In addition to gallstones, there are at least three other pathologic conditions of the gallbladder presumably associated with the development of carcinoma: cholecystoenteric fistula, porcelain gallbladder, and adenoma. There is believed to be a 15 per cent incidence of development of carcinoma of the gallbladder in patients who have or have had a cholecystoenteric fistula,[2] and the tumor may develop as much as 16 years later. The incidence of carcinoma in a calcified, or porcelain, gallbladder is reported to range from 12.5 to 61 per cent. However, it is difficult to assess the isolated roles of these two complications of biliary tract disease in neoplastic degeneration of the gallbladder, since the majority of cholecystoenteric fistulas are due to stones and porcelain gallbladders contain stones. The relationship of relatively rare, usually asymptomatic, adenoma of the gallbladder to carcinoma is controversial, but adenomatous residue has been found in 19 per cent of cases of invasive carcinoma.[13]

There are also other related conditions. Cancer of the gallbladder is more frequent in the presence of congenital biliary dilation, in which case there appears to be a lower incidence of associated gallstone.[12] However, congenital biliary ductal dilation is frequently related to a long common channel, distal to the entry of the pancreatic duct. This circumstance alone is believed to be associated with a higher incidence of gallbladder carci-

noma.[11] Ulcerative colitis has a well-known association with biliary tract malignancy. Although the majority involve the bile ducts, as many as 13 per cent originate in the gallbladder.

PATHOGENESIS

The etiology of carcinoma of the gallbladder is unknown. A few experimental studies suggest that malignant transformation may be caused by foreign bodies. Not only are these data controversial, but they also do not account for the instances in which gallstones are not found. Other experimental data suggest that stones alone do not cause carcinoma, but in the presence of a carcinogen, stones facilitate the development of the tumor. It is possible that bacteria associated with gallstones produce a carcinogen, but such has not yet been identified in man.

TYPE

Adenocarcinoma comprises 82 per cent of cases and may be scirrhous, papillary, or mucin-producing. Undifferentiated carcinoma occurs in 7 per cent and squamous cell occurs in 3 per cent. The latter is believed to arise from pluripotential cells in the basal layers of the epithelium. Mixed carcinoma, or adeno-acanthoma, comprises 1 per cent. Unusual tumors include lymphosarcoma, rhabdomyosarcoma, reticulum cell sarcoma, fibrosarcoma, melanoma, carcinoid,[18] and carcinosarcoma.

ROUTES OF METASTASIS

Carcinoma of the gallbladder spreads by several routes: lymphatic, vascular, intraperitoneal seeding, neural, intraductal, and direct extension.[7] All four major types of tumor (adenocarcinoma, undifferentiated, squamous, and mixed) appear to spread in a similar manner. Although metastases to practically every organ can occur, this is a late phenomenon that probably occurs through venous routes. Spread to adjacent organs occurs with some frequency and usually involves liver, stomach, duodenum, hepatic flexure of the colon, abdominal wall at the site of a previous cholecystectomy, omentum, or a combination of these. Lymphatic metastases involve the pericholedochal nodes in the lesser omentum and those behind the first portion of the duodenum (Fig. 2). Most of the lymphatic trunks that drain the left side of the gallbladder terminate in the cystic lymph node. The lymphatic trunks on the right side pass into the pericholedochal nodes lying to the right of the common duct. There are extensive connections between the various sets of lymph vessels, but the lymphatics along the hepatic artery do not connect with those from the gallbladder.

Liver, like lymphatic, involvement generally occurs early. The various forms of liver involvement include spread along the bile ductules, veins, and lymphatics and by direct extension. However, the usual mode of spread to the liver is by direct extension and through lymphatic vessels. The disseminated multinodular form of liver involvement is probably due to retrograde lymphatic spread or is the first manifestation of widespread vascular metastases. The lymphatic drainage of the liver on the right side empties for the most part into the pericholedochal nodes (Fig. 2). Involvement of the liver can occur in the absence of lymph node metastases.

Venous metastases most often involve cholecystic veins draining into the gallbladder bed, terminating in the quadrate lobe (segment IV). The venous system along the peritoneal side of the gallbladder also drains into the quadrate lobe (Fig. 3). The tumor may also extend along the cystic duct into the common duct. This is more typical for papillary adenocarcinoma but does not occur in all cases of this tumor. Cases of intraductal spread may represent instances of multifocal cancer.

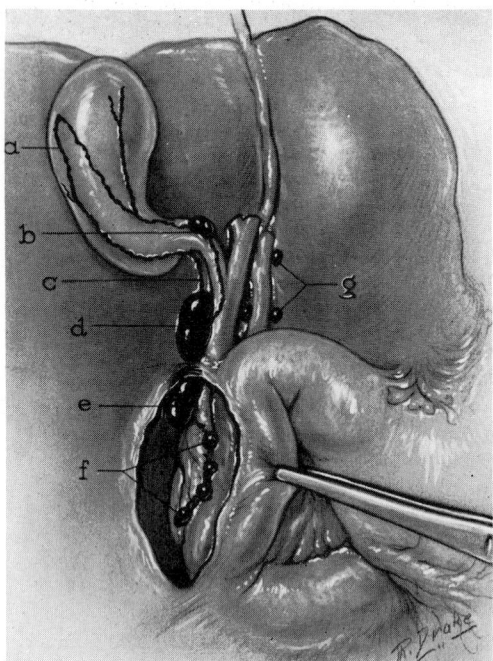

Figure 2. Lymphatic drainage of the gallbladder: a, subserosal lymphatics; b, cystic node; c, lymph vessels ending in lower lymph nodes; d, node of hiatus; e, superior pancreatoduodenal node; f, posterior pancreatoduodenal nodes; g, nodes along the hepatic artery do not connect with those draining the gallbladder. (From Fahim, R. B., McDonald, J. R., Richards, J. C., and Ferris, D. O.: Carcinoma of the gallbladder: A study of its modes of spread. Ann. Surg., *156:*114, 1962.)

DIAGNOSIS

The symptoms of carcinoma of the gallbladder are not specific. Pain occurs in 66 per cent, weight loss in 59 per cent, jaundice in 51 per cent, anorexia in 40 per cent, and right upper quadrant mass in 40 per cent of patients.[17,19] The clinical presentation differs depending on stage of the disease, but there is no distinct pattern because the presenting symptoms and their duration are dependent on the site of the lesion, its extent, and the presence or absence of pre-existing biliary symptoms. Malig-

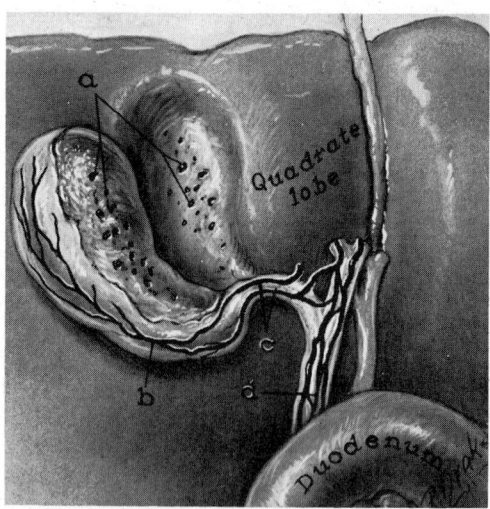

Figure 3. Venous drainage of the gallbladder: a, cholecystic veins entering the gallbladder bed and draining into the quadrate lobe; b, subserosal cholecystic veins communicating with veins of the gallbladder neck; c, veins of the neck drain into the quadrate lobe or venous plexus around the bile ducts; d, the latter also drain into the quadrate lobe. The venous drainage from the gallbladder emptying into the quadrate lobe ultimately communicates with the hepatic veins. (From Fahim, R. B., McDonald, J. R., Richards, J. C., and Ferris, D. O.: Carcinoma of the gallbladder: A study of its modes of spread. Ann. Surg., *156:*114, 1962.)

nancy in patients with pre-existing biliary symptoms generally produces a noticeable change in symptoms.

Neither the physical findings nor the laboratory features are specific. A right upper quadrant mass may be apparent and is usually tender. The presence of a palpable gallbladder represents advanced disease. Jaundice most often is due to invasion of the common duct or compression from involved pericholedochal lymph nodes and, less frequently, involvement of the liver; rarely, it is due to concurrent stones in the biliary tract.[19] The jaundice is accompanied by pain in the majority of patients, which may be of use in distinguishing this disease from a periampullary carcinoma. A gallbladder involved with malignant disease can perforate into adjacent organs or into the free peritoneal cavity. The latter has been reported in as many as 5 per cent of patients.[1]

Fistulization or symptomatic invasion of an adjacent organ frequently leads to the diagnosis of carcinoma originating in the symptomatic organ. Invasion of the upper gastrointestinal tract can cause obstruction or bleeding, mimicking peptic ulcer disease. Hemorrhage follows invasion of adjacent organs, hematobilia, or liver failure as a terminal manifestation of the disease. Patients presenting with acute cholecystitis tend to have less advanced disease, most likely due to the incidental presence of tumor.

Because of the deceptive nature of presentation of the disease and its relative rarity, the correct preoperative diagnosis is made infrequently. However, certain combinations of signs and symptoms should arouse suspicion. These include an elderly female with biliary complaints presenting with a change in frequency or severity of pain, right upper quadrant mass or hepatomegaly, and constitutional symptoms of malignant disease. By the time these factors are noted, however, the disease is rarely (if at all) at a curable stage. Those with early, resectable lesions tend to have symptoms of benign biliary disease.

The diagnosis is infrequently made by radiographic studies. A nonfunctioning gallbladder is apparent on the majority of oral cholecystograms. The rare occurrence of visualization (1 to 2 per cent) is usually of poor quality and the diagnosis is not evident. Upper gastrointestinal barium study may show compression of the antroduodenal area, but this can also be found in benign, acute inflammatory gallbladder disease. Patients with an abnormal upper gastrointestinal series from carcinoma of the gallbladder have been found to have extensive disease. Nearly two thirds of patients may be correctly diagnosed by computed tomographic scans.[10] A few cases have been diagnosed by sonography. Angiography is reported to give the highest degree of diagnostic accuracy, but the majority of tumors diagnosed in this manner are unresectable.

PROGNOSIS

Malignancy of the gallbladder usually is associated with a dismal prognosis. About 88 per cent died within a year of diagnosis and only about 4 per cent were alive after 5 years in a review of nearly 6000 patients.[15] Most of the long-term survivors are those in whom the surgeon was unaware of the presence of the tumor at the time of cholecystectomy (approximately 12 per cent of cases of carcinoma), the diagnosis being made by the pathologist. It is a rare patient who is symptomatic from the tumor and who enjoys prolonged survival following operative treatment.

Localized tumors are generally associated with a longer survival. However, regional lymph nodes are involved and invasion of the liver occurs in the majority of patients by the time they undergo operation. Papillary adenocarcinoma, which tends to be localized, has a median survival of almost 6 months after diagnosis with 24 per cent of patients alive at the end of 1 year.[8] In contrast, other types of adenocarcinoma have a median survival of 2 months after diagnosis with 10 per cent of patients alive after 1 year, whereas anaplastic carcinoma has a median survival of less than 1 month with only 4 per cent of patients alive after 1 year. Squamous cell tumors of the gallbladder tend to behave as anaplastic carcinomas. For those with localized disease, knowledge of the depth of invasion is important prognostically. Nearly all patients with invasion confined to the mucosa and muscularis and who survive operation are alive at 5 years, whereas only about 7 per cent with serosal (or adventitial) involvement are alive at 5 years.[14]

TREATMENT

Knowledge of the routes of spread suggests that the extent of the tumor can be excised in some patients with invasion beyond the confines of the gallbladder wall. However, there continues to be debate over the utility of radical resection of the tumor. Proponents of a radical approach optimistically maintain that up to 30 per cent of patients present with tumors that could be encompassed by radical cholecystectomy, which includes in-continuity resection of the hepatic bed or right hepatic lobectomy (or even trisegmentectomy) and regional lymph node dissection. Yet, only a few long-term survivors have been reported following radical resection. Moreover, the operative morbidity and mortality of radical resection remain high for a disease associated with an extremely poor prognosis. Radical excision may be followed by death from disseminated metastases as soon as 2 months later,[17] despite what appeared to be adequate resection at operation. There are insufficient data to support the proposition that the patient with unexpected carcinoma found histologically should undergo reoperation with intent for radical excision. Nevertheless, it is generally held that radical procedures do not significantly influence prognosis.

Moderate palliation can occasionally be achieved by operation, even though its benefits are usually of short duration. Palliation is chiefly employed for relief of common duct obstruction or for bypassing an obstructed portion of the gastrointestinal tract. Some palliation may also be achieved by removing the gallbladder, when feasible, in the hope of delaying obstruction of surrounding structures. There are few reports dealing with chemotherapy and/or radiation therapy, which thus far have questionable benefit.

Obstructive jaundice occurring sometime after cholecystectomy can be difficult to treat by operation because of tumor encroachment in the porta hepatis. Endoscopic sphincterotomy followed by placement of a prosthesis retrogradely through a malignant stricture in the common duct or at the hepatic bifurcation can successfully reduce symptoms relating to biliary obstruction. However, long-term palliation appears more related to tumor extent than to resolution of jaundice.[9] Percutaneous insertion of a biliary prosthesis can also be used to decompress the biliary tree, but such catheters tend to be painful and occasionally are complicated by the appearance of painful malignant deposits along the catheter site.[16]

The bleak outlook for carcinoma of the gallbladder has led some to maintain that practically all patients with asymptomatic gallstones should undergo cholecystectomy. One less death from cancer of the gallbladder probably occurs for every 100 cholecystectomies done during the preceding year.[6] However, given the incidence of gallstones, this proposition would place an inordinate drain on surgical resources in order to prevent a generally fatal condition of relatively low incidence in the general population. In fact, the chances of other complications from cholelithiasis are much greater than the eventual development of malignancy. Yet, there appears to be an association between the increasing rate of cholecystectomy and what appears to be a decreasing mortality from cancer of the gallbladder. This may be fortuitous, since the incidence of carcinoma of the stomach has also been declining but not as a result of prophylactic gastrectomy.[4]

SELECTED REFERENCES

Arminski, T. C.: Primary carcinoma of the gallbladder. A collective review with the addition of twenty-five cases from The Grace Hospital, Detroit, Michigan. Cancer, 2:379, 1949.
This is an excellent review of the literature prior to 1948.

Diehl, A. K.: Epidemiology of gallbladder cancer: A synthesis of recent data. J.N.C.I., 65:1209, 1980.
This is a particularly good summary of the epidemiology of gallbladder cancer.

Fahim, R. B., McDonald, J. R., Richards, J. C., and Ferris, D. O.: Carcinoma of the gallbladder: A study of its modes of spread. Ann. Surg., 156:114, 1962.
This is a classic study of the routes of metastases and provides the anatomic basis for radical excision.

Piehler, J. M., and Crichlow, R. W.: Primary carcinoma of the gallbladder. Surg. Gynecol. Obstet., 147:929, 1978.
This is a thorough review of the literature extending that of Arminski to 1976.

Strauch, G. O.: Primary carcinoma of the gallbladder. Presentation of seventy cases from the Rhode Island Hospital and a cumulative review of the last ten years of the American literature. Surgery, 47:368, 1960.
This is another excellent review.

REFERENCES

1. Arminski, T. C.: Primary carcinoma of the gallbladder. A collective review with the addition of twenty-five cases from The Grace Hospital, Detroit, Michigan. Cancer, 2:379, 1949.
2. Berliner, S. D., and Burson, L. C.: One-stage repair of cholecyst-duodenal fistula and gallstone ileus. Arch. Surg., 90:313, 1965.
3. Boss, L. P., Lanier, A. P., Dohan, P. H., and Bender, T. R.: Cancers of the gallbladder and biliary tract in Alaskan natives: 1970–79. J.N.C.I., 69:1005, 1982.
4. Diehl, A. K.: Epidemiology of gallbladder cancer: A synthesis of recent data. J.N.C.I., 65:1209, 1980.
5. Diehl, A. K.: Gallstone size and the risk of gallbladder cancer. J.A.M.A., 250:2323, 1983.
6. Diehl, A. K., and Beral, V.: Cholecystectomy and changing mortality from gallbladder cancer. Lancet, 1:187, 1981.
7. Fahim, R. B., McDonald, J. R., Richards, J. C., and Ferris, D. O.: Carcinoma of the gallbladder: A study of its modes of spread. Ann. Surg., 156:114, 1962.
8. Hart, J., and Modan, B.: Factors affecting survival of patients with gallbladder neoplasms. Arch. Intern. Med., 129:931, 1972.
9. Huibregtse, K., Schneider, B., Coene, P. P., and Tytgat, G. N. J.: Endoscopic palliation of jaundice in gallbladder cancer. Surg. Endosc., 1:143, 1987.
10. Itai, Y., Araki, T., Yoshikawa, K., Furui, Sh., Yashiro, N., and Tasaka, A.: Computed tomography of gallbladder carcinoma. Radiology, 137:713, 1980.
11. Kimura, K., Ohto, M., Saisho, H., Unozawa, T., Tsuchiya, Y., Morita, M., Ebara, M., Matsutani, S., and Okuda, K.: Association of gallbladder carcinoma and anomalous pancreaticobiliary ductal union. Gastroenterology, 89:1258, 1985.
12. Kinoshita, H., Nagata, E., Hirohashi, K., Skai, K., and Kobayashi, Y.: Carcinoma of the gallbladder with an anomalous connection between the choledochus and the pancreatic duct. Cancer, 54:762, 1984.
13. Kozuka, S., Tsubone, M., Yasui, A., and Hachisuka, K.: Relation of adenoma to carcinoma in the gallbladder. Cancer, 50:2226, 1982.
14. Nevin, J. E., Moran, T. J., Kay, S., and King, R.: Carcinoma of the gallbladder. Staging, treatment, and prognosis. Cancer, 37:141, 1976.
15. Piehler, J. M., and Crichlow, R. W.: Primary carcinoma of the gallbladder. Surg. Gynecol. Obstet., 147:929, 1978.
16. Shorvon, P. J., Leung, J. W. C., Corcoran, M., Mason, R. R., and Cotton, P. B.: Cutaneous seeding of malignant tumours after insertion of percutaneous prosthesis for obstructive jaundice. Br. J. Surg., 71:694, 1984.
17. Solan, M. J., and Jackson, B. T.: Carcinoma of the gall-bladder. A clinical appraisal and review of 57 cases. Br. J. Surg., 58:593, 1971.
18. Strauch, G. O.: Primary carcinoma of the gallbladder. Presentation of seventy cases from the Rhode Island Hospital and a cumulative review of the last ten years of the American literature. Surgery, 47:368, 1960.
19. Tanga, M. B., and Ewing, J. B.: Primary malignant tumors of the gallbladder: Report of 43 cases. Surgery, 67:418, 1970.

35

THE PANCREAS

Charles J. Yeo, M.D., and John L. Cameron, M.D.

Historically, the first description of the pancreas is credited to Herophilus of Chalkaidon around the year 300 B.C. Four centuries later, in approximately 100 A.D., this abdominal organ was named the pancreas by Rufus of Ephesus.[20] The first operative intervention on the pancreas has been attributed to LeDentu in the year 1862, involving percutaneous aspiration of a pancreatic mass with an unfavorable outcome.[33] Much evidence has accumulated during the years, adding to knowledge of the basic anatomy and physiology of the pancreas and to the pathophysiology of pancreatic disease.

EMBRYOLOGY

The pancreas begins development during the fourth week of gestation, when the embryo is 3 to 4 mm. in size. Pancreatic tissue originates from the endodermal lining of the duodenum, from which form two pouches that develop into a large dorsal and a smaller ventral pancreas (Fig. 1). The dorsal pouch arises first, directly from the duodenal endoderm, and normally forms the bulk of adult pancreatic tissue. The ventral pouch forms from the endoderm of the hepatic diverticulum, and it maintains a close association with the common bile duct throughout development. As the duodenum rotates to assume a C configuration, the ventral pancreatic pouch migrates dorsally in a clockwise direction to assume a position adjacent to the posterior inferior surface of the more rapidly expanding dorsal pancreatic primordium (Fig. 2). At approximately the eighth week of gestation, the parenchyma of the dorsal and ventral primordia fuse, as do their respective ductal systems. The ventral primordium forms the uncinate process and the inferior aspect of the head of the adult gland. The dorsal primordium becomes the superior aspect of the head as well as the entirety of the neck, body, and tail of the gland.

The fusion of the pancreatic ductal systems during fetal development produces the most typical anatomic arrangement of the pancreatic ductular structures. More than 85 per cent of the time the ventral pancreatic duct fuses with the more distal dorsal pancreatic duct to create the duct of Wirsung, also known as the main pancreatic duct. This duct joins with the common bile duct in an intrapancreatic location and empties pancreatic exocrine secretions through the ampulla of Vater at the major duodenal papilla. The proximal aspect of the dorsal pancreatic duct (duct of Santorini) often remains in communication with the duct of Wirsung and may empty small amounts of exocrine pancreatic secretions through a separate minor duodenal papilla located on the medial aspect of the duodenum proximal to the major papilla.

Clinically recognized malformations of pancreatic embryology include heterotopic pancreas, pancreas divisum, and annular pancreas. The development of pancreatic tissue outside the confines of the main gland is a congenital abnormality referred to as heterotopic pancreas. Most commonly, heterotopic pancreatic tissue is found in the stomach, duodenum, small bowel, or Meckel's diverticulum. In most locations heterotopic pancreatic tissue resides in a submucosal location, presenting as firm, yellow, irregular nodules that vary in size from millimeters to several centimeters. The mucosa overlying typical heterotopic pancreatic tissue commonly has a central umbilication. There may be a duct draining exocrine pancreatic secretions from the aberrant tissue into the intestinal lumen. Histologically, heterotopic pancreatic tissue can vary from entirely normal architecture, including ductular structures, acini, and islets of Langerhans, to rudimentary pancreatic structures with markedly aberrant histology. The clinical significance of heterotopic pancreas is dependent upon resultant complications. Intestinal obstruction may ensue as a result of the heterotopic tissue, rarely being due to the size of the mass, and more commonly following intussusception, with the ectopic pancreatic tissue serving as the intussusceptum. Other complications of heterotopic pancreas include ulceration and hemorrhage. Appropriate treatment is indicated for the complications of heterotopic pancreas, usually involving local excision of the heterotopic tissue, with histologic examination to exclude the presence of malignancy.

Pancreas divisum is an anatomic variant that follows failure of fusion of the two primordial ductal systems. This anomaly has been recognized in up to 10 per cent of patients undergoing endoscopic retrograde pancreatography for presumed pancreatic disease. In this entity, the major portion of the pancreas is drained via the duct of Santorini into the minor duodenal papilla. The major duodenal papilla usually communicates with a small duct of Wirsung, which drains the ventral pancreas, consisting of the inferior head and uncinate process. The significance of pancreas divisum remains controversial. In selected patients undergoing endoscopic pancreatography for "idiopathic pancreatitis," the incidence of pancreas divisum approaches 25 per cent. In these cases, it is unknown whether the ductal anomaly has any causal relationship to the pancreatitis. Some have speculated that pancreas divisum, when associated with relative stenosis of the minor duodenal papilla, can cause pancreatitis. Patients with this suspected abnormality have been treated with transduodenal sphincteroplasty of the minor papilla, with mixed surgical results. Pancreas divisum associated with extensive dorsal pancreatic parenchymal injury or multiple ductular stenoses is not optimally treated with transduodenal minor papillary sphincteroplasty alone and instead may require pancreatic resection or pancreatic ductular drainage via longitudinal pancreaticojejunostomy.

Annular pancreas is a rare condition that results when histologically normal pancreatic tissue completely or partially encircles the second portion of the duodenum. Annular pancreas is thought to arise from failure of normal clockwise rotation of the ventral pancreatic primordia, possibly related to abnormal fixation at the free end. With annular pancreas, the tissue originating from the ventral primordium lies anterior to the duodenum, where it can fuse with the dorsal pancreas to form a complete ring, or may remain as an incomplete ring. Varying degrees of duodenal obstructive symptomatology may be observed in this condition. In children, there is a common association with other serious congenital anomalies such as intracardiac defects, mongolism, and intestinal malrotation. For an unexplained reason,

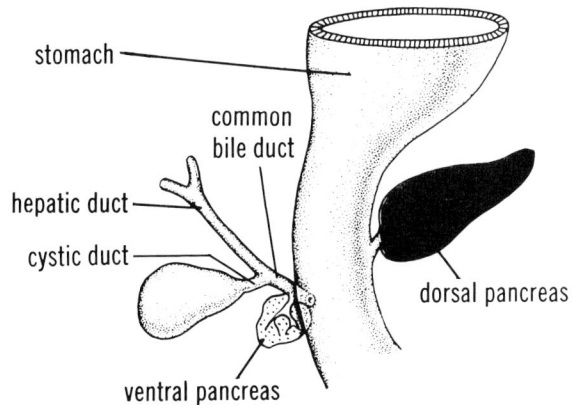

Figure 1. The smaller ventral pancreas initially develops as an outpouching from the hepatic diverticulum. The larger dorsal pancreas originates directly from the endodermal epithelium of the duodenum. (From Langman, J.: Medical Embryology, 3rd ed. Baltimore, Williams & Wilkins, 1975, p. 287.)

some children have no symptoms from this anomaly, and instead they may present as adults, commonly in the fourth decade of life. In adults, symptoms may appear to be those of upper gastrointestinal obstruction, chronic pancreatitis, or peptic ulcer. Obstructive symptoms are an indication for operation. Resection or division of the normal pancreatic tissue comprising the annulus is not recommended, because of the high incidence of duodenal or pancreatic fistula. Instead, bypass surgery in the form of duodenojejunostomy is indicated.

ANATOMY

The pancreas occupies a retroperitoneal position in the abdomen, lying posterior to the stomach and lesser omentum. It extends obliquely from the duodenal C loop to a more cephalad position in the hilum of the spleen (Fig. 3). The normal adult pancreas varies in weight from 75 to 125 gm., in length from 10 to 20 cm., and in cephalad to caudad width from 3 to 5 cm. In the anteroposterior axis, the pancreas is thickest at the head, varying from 1.5 to 3.5 cm., and thinnest at the tail, 0.8 to 2.5 cm. The gland has a distinctive yellow/tan/pink color, and is multilobulated. The pancreas is covered by peritoneum anteriorly, and posteriorly it lies in proximity to the inferior vena cava, right renal vein, aorta at the level of the first lumbar vertebra, superior mesenteric vessels, and splenic vein.

The gland is divided into four portions: the head (which includes the uncinate process), the neck, the body, and the tail. That portion of the pancreas anterior to the superior mesenteric vein is designated the neck of the gland. The head of the gland extends to the right of the neck, lying within the confines of the duodenal C loop; and it includes the posteroinferior extension arising from the ventral primordium, designated the uncinate process. The uncinate process extends posterior to the superior

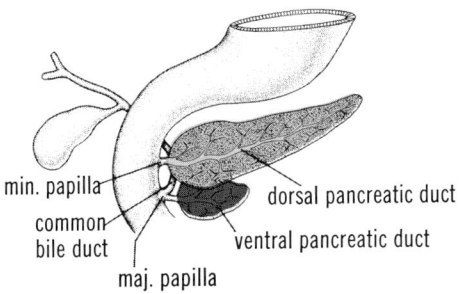

Figure 2. After clockwise rotation in a dorsal direction, the ventral pancreas comes to lie adjacent to the dorsal pancreas, as shown here. The dorsal pancreatic duct enters the duodenum at the minor papilla and the ventral pancreatic duct at the major papilla. (From Langman, J.: Medical Embryology, 3rd ed. Baltimore, Williams & Wilkins, 1975, p. 288.)

mesenteric vein ending at the right margin of the superior mesenteric artery. The body of the pancreas lies immediately to the left of the neck; the tail of the pancreas extends to the left of the body into the splenic hilum.

An extensive arterial system originating from multiple sources supplies the pancreas. The head of the pancreas is intimately associated with the second portion of the duodenum, and these two structures are jointly supplied by two arterial arcades known as the anterior and posterior pancreaticoduodenal arteries. These arteries originate from the superior and inferior pancreaticoduodenal vessels as branches of the celiac axis and superior mesenteric artery, respectively. The blood supply to the body and tail of the pancreas is via a more variable complex of arteries. The distal body and tail of the pancreas are supplied by short branches of the splenic and left gastroepiploic arteries. Within the posterosuperior and posteroinferior aspects of the body of the pancreas lie the superior and inferior pancreatic arteries, respectively.

The venous drainage of the pancreas corresponds with the arterial anatomy. Veins draining the pancreatic parenchyma eventually terminate in the portal vein, which arises posterior to the neck of the pancreas at the junction of the splenic and superior mesenteric veins.

Multiple lymph node groups drain the pancreas. From the head of the gland, nodes in the pancreaticoduodenal groove communicate with subpyloric, portal, mesocolic, mesenteric, and aortocaval nodes. Lymphatics in the body and tail of the pancreas drain to retroperitoneal nodes in the splenic hilum, or to celiac, aortocaval, mesocolic, or mesenteric nodes.

A dual sympathetic and parasympathetic innervation subserves the pancreas. Preganglionic sympathetic axons arise from cell bodies within the thoracic sympathetic ganglia and travel as the greater, lesser, and lowest splanchnic nerves to terminate within the celiac ganglia. From these, postganglionic sympathetic fibers traverse retroperitoneal tissue to innervate the pancreas, serving as the principal pathways for pain of pancreatic origin. This sympathetic pathway is the target during splanchnicectomy for the relief of pain of pancreatic origin. The parasympathetic innervation of the pancreas commences with preganglionic fiber cell bodies that reside within the vagal nuclei, the axons of which terminate in parasympathetic ganglia within the pancreatic parenchyma. Postganglionic parasympathetic fibers then traverse a short course to innervate the pancreatic islets, acini, and ducts, serving an exclusively efferent function.

HISTOLOGY

Two distinct organ systems share residence within the human pancreas. The endocrine portion of pancreatic function is served by the structures termed the islets of Langerhans. The islets are nearly spherical collections of cells scattered throughout the pancreatic parenchyma. Up to a million islets per gland exist. Each islet has an extensive blood supply, marked by a network of intercommunicating sinusoids, and is composed of several distinctive cell types. The insulin-producing beta cells compose the majority of the islet population. The alpha cells produce glucagon and constitute approximately 20 to 25 per cent of the total islet cell number. Scattered about the periphery of the islets, constituting approximately 5 per cent of the islet cells, are the somatostatin-producing delta cells, which appear to function as paracrine modulators of islet cell function. Small minorities of islet cells have been shown by immunohistochemical techniques to contain pancreatic polypeptide (PP), gastrin, and vasoactive intestinal polypeptide (VIP).

The acini and ductal systems constitute the exocrine portion of the pancreas (Fig. 4). On a macroscopic level, the exocrine pancreas is analogous to clusters of grapes (representing individual acini) on a vine (representing minor ducts) and terminat-

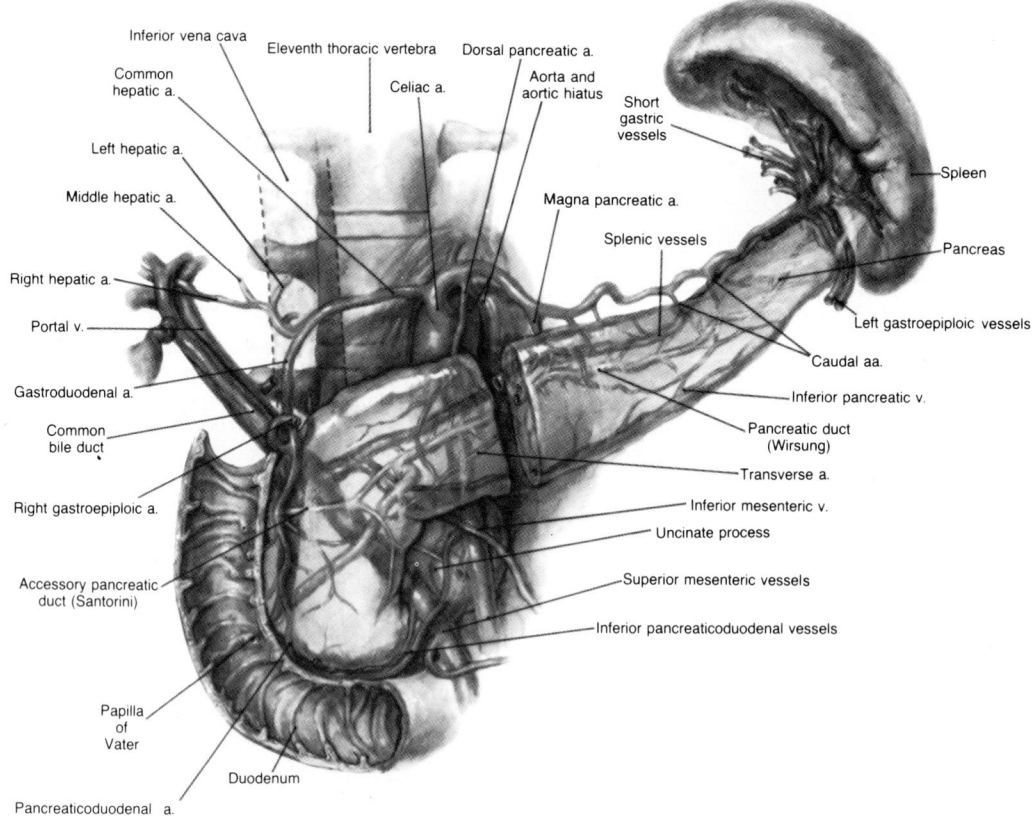

Figure 3. Anatomic relationships of the pancreas, including the adjacent viscera, arterial and venous systems, and pancreatic ducts. (From Schlossberg, L., and Zuidema, G. D.: The Johns Hopkins Atlas of Human Functional Anatomy, 3rd ed. Baltimore, The Johns Hopkins University Press, 1986, Plate 48.)

ing in a major trunk (representing the major pancreatic duct). Each acinus has an approximately spheroid configuration and is composed of a single layer of acinar cells. Acinar cells contain zymogen granules (Fig. 5) in their narrow, centrally located apical portion and rest on a distinct basal lamina supported by delicate reticular fibers at the periphery. The pancreatic ductal system originates in the centroacinar cells of each individual acinus, includes intercalated duct cells along the ductal pathway, and terminates in the main excretory duct of the pancreas.

PHYSIOLOGY

EXOCRINE. Investigation of the physiology of exocrine pancreatic secretion has attracted much attention for more than a

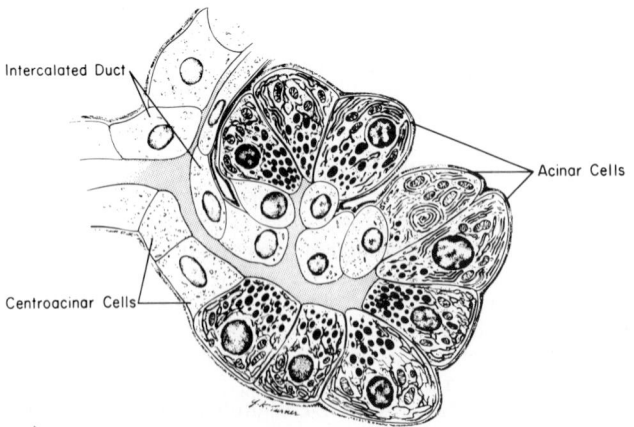

Figure 4. Illustration demonstrating the relationships of a terminal branch of the pancreatic ductal system to the centroacinar cells and acinar cells. (From Bloom, W., and Fawcett, D. W.: A Textbook of Histology, 10th ed. Philadelphia, W. B. Saunders Company, 1975, p. 738.)

century. Heidenhain in 1875 first demonstrated the effect of vagal stimulation on pancreatic secretion.[25] This work was extended by Pavlov and later by Babkin,[2] who reported the cholinergic nature of the stimulus to pancreatic exocrine secretion. Bayliss and Starling[5] first demonstrated the presence of a substance in duodenal mucosa, secretin, which stimulated pancreatic secretion.

The final products of pancreatic exocrine secretion derive from the interplay of an intricate system of acinar and ductal cell functions. The final secretory product of the human exocrine pancreas is a clear isotonic solution with a pH in the range of 8 and a specific gravity that varies between 1.007 and 1.035. There are two distinct components of pancreatic exocrine secretion: enzyme secretion originates from acinar cells, and water and electrolyte secretion originates from the centroacinar and intercalated duct cells. From endoscopic pancreatic cannulation studies, basal secretory rates of pancreatic exocrine products average 0.2 to 0.3 ml. per minute, with rates approaching 5.0 ml. per minute with maximal secretin stimulation.

The secretion of water and electrolytes is under both vagal and humoral control. The electrolyte composition of exocrine pancreatic juice varies with the rate of pancreatic secretion (Fig. 6). Over the entire spectrum of secretory rates, the composition of sodium and potassium in the pancreatic exocrine effluent remains constant with the concentrations of these cations being approximately equivalent to plasma. In contrast, the anion concentration of pancreatic exocrine secretion is dependent upon the secretory rate. At low secretory rates, the concentrations of chloride and bicarbonate ions are nearly equivalent to those of plasma, whereas with neurohumoral stimulation the bicarbonate component increases in concentration and the chloride anion concentration decreases. Secretin is the most potent endogenous stimulant of pancreatic bicarbonate secretion. The term *hormone* was first used in reference to secretin, a 27−amino acid peptide. Secretin is synthesized in the mucosal S cells of the

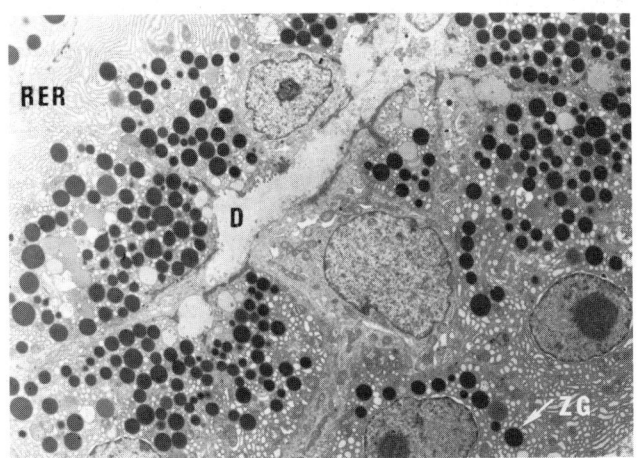

Figure 5. Electron micrograph of multiple acinar cells and a portion of a terminal duct (D). The acinar cells contain extensive rough endoplasmic reticulum (RER) and electron-dense zymogen granules (ZG). Uranyl acetate and lead citrate, ×2000.

crypts of Lieberkühn of the proximal small intestine and is released in the presence of luminal acid and bile. Secretin circulates in the blood, binds to secretin receptors on pancreatic ductal cells, effecting signal transduction via the intracellular adenylate cyclase system, to yield an increase in intracellular cyclic adenosine monophosphate (cAMP).

An entirely distinct sequence of intracellular events mediates the synthesis and excretion of the digestive enzyme exocrine products from pancreatic acinar cells. Experiments using radioactive labeling techniques have delineated a sophisticated and stepwise sequence of intracellular events that produce the final exocrine digestive enzyme products. Messenger RNA is translated into proenzymes on the microsomes of the rough endoplasmic reticulum. These proenzymes subsequently pass to the Golgi apparatus, where they are packaged within a glycoprotein vesicular membrane. These zymogen granules formed at the level of the Golgi apparatus contain a full complement of digestive enzymes. Zymogen granules then migrate to the acinar cell apex, where zymogen granule membranes fuse with the acinar cell plasma membrane (exocytosis), yielding extrusion of the zymogen granule contents into the centroacinar luminal space. Specific enzymes synthesized and released include endopeptidases such as trypsin, chymotrypsin, elastase, and kallikrein, as well as exopeptidases such as carboxypeptidase A and B. Other synthesized enzymes include phospholipase, lipase, colipase, nonspecific carboxylesterase, amylase, ribonuclease, and deox-

yribonuclease. The peptidases synthesized by acinar cells are released into the pancreatic ductal system in inactive forms. Peptide activation commences after the peptidase enters the duodenum, where mucosal enterokinase cleaves trypsinogen to trypsin, leaving trypsin to further activate the other peptidases. In contrast to the peptidases, ribonuclease, deoxyribonuclease, amylase, and lipase are released into the pancreatic ductal system in their active forms. The control of pancreatic acinar cell secretion is mediated by specific secretogogues acting upon acinar cell receptors. Secretagogues such as cholecystokinin (CCK) and acetylcholine stimulate acinar cell enzyme secretion via a membrane transduction process involving the accumulation of intracellular cyclic guanosine monophosphate (cGMP) and the mobilization of intracellular calcium. CCK is the most potent endogenous hormone known to stimulate pancreatic enzyme secretion.

Three classical phases of digestion describe the response of the pancreas to a meal. During the cephalic phase of digestion, stimuli such as the smell, sight, and taste of food activate vagal efferent signals, which follow parasympathetic pathways to stimulate pancreatic enzyme release. In addition, cephalic phase stimulation of gastric acid secretion causes duodenal acidification, which stimulates secretin release and subsequent pancreatic bicarbonate secretion. In all, the net effect of cephalic phase stimulation is the secretion of an enzyme-rich bicarbonate-poor fluid. During the gastric phase of digestion, the gastric G cell product, gastrin, serves a major function. Antral distention and antral protein stimulate the release of gastrin, which promotes gastric acid secretion and also serves as a weak stimulator of pancreatic enzyme secretion. The ability of gastrin to serve as a weak stimulator of pancreatic enzyme secretion can be explained by the sequence homology between gastrin and the C terminal pentapeptide-amide sequence of CCK, yielding an affinity for the CCK receptor on pancreatic acinar cells that is 1/1000 times as strong as CCK. Gastrin-stimulated gastric acid secretion contributes to pancreatic bicarbonate secretion via duodenal acidification and subsequent secretin release. Stimulation of vagal afferents by antral distention also has a role in the gastric phase of pancreatic exocrine secretion, as is proven by the reduction in antral distention-induced pancreatic exocrine secretion following truncal vagotomy. During the intestinal phase of digestion, the hormones secretin and CCK serve a major function in mediating pancreatic exocrine secretion. Duodenal acid and bile stimulate secretin release, with resultant pancreatic bicarbonate secretion from duct cells. Duodenal fat and protein releases CCK, with subsequent stimulation of pancreatic enzymes from acinar cells. In addition to these humorally mediated events, bile salts, fatty acids, and amino acids in the duodenum can stimulate pancreatic exocrine secretion via neural pathways.

ENDOCRINE. The best known endocrine function of the pancreas involves glucose homeostasis. The association between diabetes mellitus and the pancreas was established more than a century ago, in 1889, in a canine experiment where glucose intolerance developed after removal of the pancreas.[53] In the 1920s Banting and Best isolated pancreatic extracts that were highly active against hyperglycemia.[3] Later insulin was crystallized and found to contain two polypeptide chains linked by a disulfide bridge. Insulin is the secretory product of the beta cell within the islets of Langerhans. The secretory granules of beta cells contain the storage form of insulin (Fig. 7). The release of insulin from the beta cell into the portal blood is controlled by multiple factors including the level of glycemia, vagal interactions, and local concentrations of somatostatin, among other factors.

Glucagon is a single-chain 29–amino acid peptide synthesized and released from islet alpha cells. A major stimulus for glucagon release is a substantial drop in serum glucose. Glucagon causes hyperglycemia by promoting hepatic glycogenolysis and gluconeogenesis from proteins. Although the primary ef-

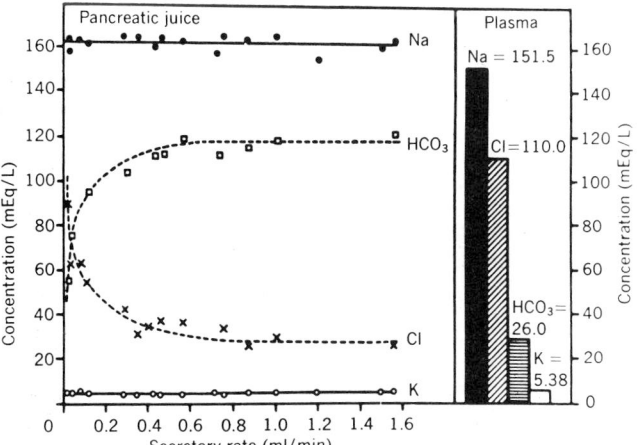

Figure 6. Relationship between the rate of secretion and the concentration of electrolytes in pancreatic juice, compared with the electrolyte composition of plasma. (From Bro-Rasmussen, F., Killmann, S. A., and Thaysen, J. H.: The composition of pancreatic juice as compared to sweat, parotid saliva and tears. Acta Physiol. Scand., 37:97, 1956.)

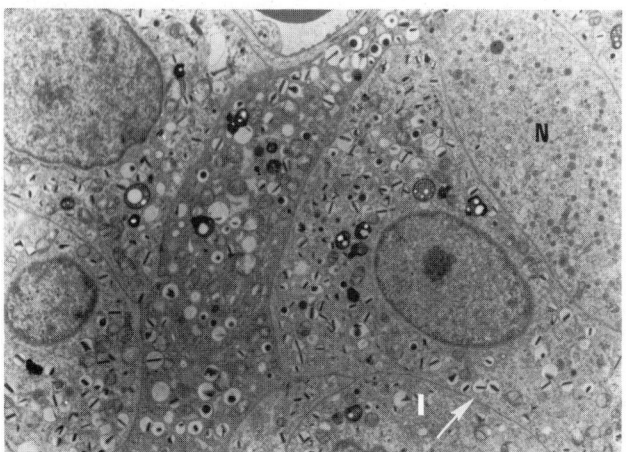

Figure 7. Electron micrograph of a portion of an islet of Langerhans. Most of the cells are beta cells, with characteristic insulin-containing granules (I) seen as tubular densities within clear vacuoles. A non-beta cell (N) is seen near the top right. Uranyl acetate and lead citrate, ×3000.

fect of glucagon appears to be on glucose homeostasis, other effects of glucagon have been described, including inhibition of gastric acid secretion, inhibition of gastrointestinal motility, and stimulation of choleresis and triglyceride lipolysis.

Pancreatic polypeptide (PP) is a 36–straight-chain amino acid peptide localized predominantly to non–beta islet cells of the head and uncinate process of the pancreas. PP is released into the blood in a biphasic manner following a meal, with both cholinergic and adrenergic modulation. At physiologic levels, PP has been reported to decrease pancreatic exocrine secretion and to alter biliary tract motility. It has also been implicated as a glucoregulatory hormone. In PP-deficient states such as postpancreatectomy or chronic pancreatitis, there has been demonstrable hepatic resistance to insulin, reversed by chronic,[47] but not acute, administration of PP.[4]

Somatostatin is a cyclic tetradecapeptide synthesized and released from islet delta cells as well as other brain-gut sources. The gastrointestinal tract contains 70 per cent of the body's somatostatin. Stimulants of somatostatin release into the blood include a meal, vagal stimulation, bombesin, CCK, gastrin, and secretin. Somatostatin has a broad spectrum of gastrointestinal activity including inhibition of hormone release (gastrin, secretin, VIP, PP, insulin, and glucagon), inhibition of gastric acid and pepsin secretion, inhibition of pancreatic exocrine secretion, and inhibition of gastrointestinal motor activity, as well as reduction of gastrointestinal blood flow.

ACUTE PANCREATITIS

Although the disease now classified as acute pancreatitis has been recognized since antiquity, it was not until the mid nineteenth century that appreciation of the importance of the pancreas and the severity of its inflammatory disorders became evident. Operative intervention for acute pancreatitis associated with pancreatic gangrene or abscess formation was suggested by Senn in 1886.[46] In 1889, Fitz presented a succinct clinical and pathologic description of acute pancreatitis.[19] In 1901, Opie, at the Johns Hopkins Hospital, documented a gallstone impacted in the ampulla of Vater during the postmortem examination of a patient, operated upon by Halsted, who died of gallstone pancreatitis, thereby first describing the pathogenetic mechanism of gallstone pancreatitis.[38] Moynihan in 1925 described acute pancreatitis as "the most terrible of all the calamities that occur in connection with the abdominal viscera."[36] This statement still underscores the importance of acute pancreatitis as a major cause of morbidity and mortality today.

Acute pancreatitis includes a broad spectrum of pancreatic

disease, which varies from mild parenchymal edema to severe hemorrhagic pancreatitis associated with loss of parenchymal viability, with subsequent gangrene and necrosis. The clinical presentation of acute pancreatitis is quite variable, from episodes of mild abdominal discomfort alone to a severe illness associated with hypotension, metabolic derangements, sepsis, fluid sequestration, multiple organ failure, and death. Nine out of 10 patients experience the disease with mild to moderate symptoms and a self-limited course, and improve with supportive care. In contrast, in 1 of 10 patients a severe life-threatening form of acute pancreatitis evolves. Two recent autopsy studies have reviewed the causes of death in acute pancreatitis. In 126 patients with fatal acute pancreatitis, the late complications of multisystem organ failure and pancreatic abscess contributed to most of the deaths.[57] In a review of 405 postmortem examinations, the dominant pathologic finding in 95 per cent of patients dying within 7 days of admission was pulmonary edema and congestion. In contrast, the dominant finding in 77 per cent of patients expiring after day 7 was infection.[43]

Etiology

Many causes of acute pancreatitis exist (Table 1). In 90 per cent of the cases the cause is related to excessive alcohol intake or biliary tract disease. The relative frequency of these two principal causes of acute pancreatitis varies according to patient population. In urban settings in the United States, alcohol abuse is the principal cause of acute pancreatitis. In other areas of the United States, and in many regions of Asia and Europe, gallstone-associated pancreatitis predominates.

Alcohol is implicated as the etiologic agent in many patients with acute pancreatitis. Although the exact mechanism of alcohol-related injury is unknown, the association between alcohol abuse and acute pancreatitis is undeniable. Several theories exist to explain alcohol-related acute pancreatitis. First, alcohol-related pancreatitis may be the result of pancreatic exocrine hypersecretion in the presence of partial ampullary obstruction. Alcohol is a known stimulant of gastric acid secretion, and the resultant duodenal acidification is a stimulus for the release of secretin, which increases the exocrine secretion of pancreatic water and bicarbonate. Alcohol is also known to increase the resistance of the sphincter of Oddi at the ampulla of Vater, thereby at least theoretically causing partial obstruction to the flow of pancreatic exocrine secretion. In a feline model, enterally administered alcohol has been shown to increase pancreatic

TABLE 1. Causes of Acute Pancreatitis

Alcohol
Biliary tract disease
Hyperlipidemia
Hypercalcemia
Familial
Trauma
External
Operative
Retrograde pancreatography
Ischemia
Hypotension
Cardiopulmonary bypass
Atheroembolism
Vasculitis
Pancreas duct obstruction
Tumor
Pancreatic divisum
Ampullary stenosis
Ascaris infestation
Duodenal obstruction
Viral infection
Scorpion venom
Drugs
Idiopathic

duct pressure and permeability to macromolecules. Thus, this first theory implicating alcohol in the etiology of acute pancreatitis suggests that the pancreatic parenchyma is injured by pancreatic enzyme extravasation, facilitated by an increase in pancreatic ductal permeability, and occurs in the presence of exocrine hypersecretion and partial ampullary obstruction. A second mechanism to explain the etiologic role of alcohol suggests that alcohol may initiate enzyme extravasation and cause pancreatic injury as a result of protein obstruction of the pancreatic duct. A third postulated mechanism to explain alcohol-induced pancreatitis involves the intermediate state of hypertriglyceridemia. Transient hypertriglyceridemia is known to occur after alcohol ingestion in some individuals. Clinical and laboratory studies have suggested that toxic levels of free fatty acids, produced from the lipolysis of triglycerides, may induce pancreatic injury by causing acinar cell or capillary endothelial cell injury.

The etiologic role of gallstones in the pathogenesis of acute pancreatitis first suggested by Opie now involves gallstone migration through the ampulla of Vater, causing diversion of bile into the pancreatic duct and subsequent bile-induced pancreatic parenchymal injury.[38] Evidence supporting this mechanism is derived from clinical studies documenting the retrieval of gallstones in the stool of approximately 90 per cent of patients with acute gallstone pancreatitis. These data suggest that it is the migration of a gallstone, and not necessarily the impaction of a gallstone, that initiates the pancreatic injury. Further evidence to support the gallstone migration theory evolves from cholangiographic studies that demonstrate a common channel between the common bile duct and the pancreatic duct in up to 90 per cent of patients with a history of gallstone pancreatitis, compared with only a 20 to 30 per cent incidence of a common channel in patients with calculous biliary tract disease and no history of pancreatitis. Additional evidence is demonstrated on intraoperative cholangiograms performed at cholecystectomy, which show that pancreatic duct reflux is demonstrable in more than 60 per cent of patients with a history of pancreatitis, a nearly fourfold increase, compared with those patients lacking a history of pancreatitis. Thus, gallstone-associated pancreatitis is associated with the anatomic existence of a common channel between the pancreatic and bile ducts, and it occurs in the setting of gallstone migration through the ampullary region.

Many other causes of acute pancreatitis exist. Hyperlipidemia alone, without excessive alcohol intake, is an etiologic agent. Hyperlipidemia may occur secondary to nephritis, castration, or exogenous estrogen administration, or it may occur as hereditary hyperlipidemia (Fredrickson Types 1 and 5) notable for hypertriglyceridemia and chylomicronemia.

Hypercalcemia is associated with acute pancreatitis, generally arising as a result of hyperparathyroidism. The mechanism of hypercalcemia-related pancreatitis may involve calcium-induced trypsinogen activation with subsequent parenchymal autodestruction, calcium-associated stone precipitation in the pancreatic duct causing ductal obstruction, or calcium-stimulated pancreatic exocrine hypersecretion.

Familial cases of acute pancreatitis have been reported with no definite mechanism defined. Acute pancreatitis may also occur after pancreatic trauma, i.e., penetrating or blunt external trauma, intraoperative manipulation, or ampullary manipulation and pancreatic ductal overdistention during retrograde pancreatography.

Pancreatic ischemia is also implicated in the etiology of acute pancreatitis. Ischemic episodes may occur during systemic hypotension or cardiopulmonary bypass or may be associated with visceral atheroembolism or vasculitis. Ischemic pancreatitis has been produced with the use of an *ex vivo* isolated canine pancreatic preparation.[45] In this model pancreatic ischemia has caused parenchymal edema, hyperamylasemia, and pathologic findings mimicking acute pancreatitis.

Numerous drugs (Table 2) have been linked to the initiation of acute pancreatitis. The most substantive evidence supports estrogens and azathioprine in the direct causation of pancreatitis. Direct causation has not been definitively proven for other substances.

The actual events on a cellular and molecular level responsible for initiation of pancreatic parenchymal injury causing acute pancreatitis remain largely unknown. To assist in delineating the cellular and subcellular events that incite acute pancreatitis, a number of animal models have been developed. In 1975, Lombardi and co-workers reported that in young female mice fed a choline-deficient diet supplemented by 0.5 per cent ethionine (the CDE diet) acute hemorrhagic pancreatitis developed with a reproducible mortality.[34] Lampel and Kern, in 1978, showed that the intravenous infusion of supramaximal doses of the cholecystokinin analog cerulein caused reproducible acute edematous pancreatitis in rats.[32] Results of CDE diet and cerulein infusion experiments involving pulse labeling techniques and tritiated amino acid incorporation into zymogen granules, as well as cytochemical and immunohistochemical analyses, suggest that some pancreatitis-inducing stimuli prevent the extrusion of zymogen granules from individual acinar cells. This prevention of zymogen granule exocytosis causes fusion of the zymogen granules with intracellular lysosomes, activation of the zymogen proenzyme trypsinogen (Fig. 8), and generation of active intracellular trypsin, which is capable of cellular autodigestion.[48] Pathologic examination of human tissue examined by electron microscopy during acute pancreatitis confirms the findings of zymogen granule enlargement and formation of large autophagosomes. Although this mechanism is supported by several models of acute pancreatitis, it appears not to be applicable to all.

Clinical Presentation

In acute pancreatitis, a diverse spectrum of illness is seen, varying from a mild, short-lived, self-limited disease to a severe toxic condition associated with shock, hypovolemia, multiple metabolic derangements, and ultimate death. The clinical presentation alone may be quite suggestive of the diagnosis. The predominant clinical feature of acute pancreatitis is abdominal pain. Pain normally begins in the mid epigastrium, achieving maximal intensity several hours into the illness. Paroxysmal pain is uncommon. In most patients, the pain has a penetrating quality, radiating to the back. Although the pain is most commonly located in the mid epigastrium, it may predominate in the right or left upper quadrants. Generalized nonlocalized abdominal pain may also be observed. In patients with alcohol-associated pancreatitis, pain often commences between 12 and 48 hours after an episode of inebriation. In contrast, patients with gallstone-associated pancreatitis typically experience the onset

Table 2. Drugs Implicated in the Initiation of Acute Pancreatitis

Definite Association	Probable Association
Azathioprine	Thiazide diuretics
Estrogens	Furosemide
	Ethacrynic acid
	Sulfonamides
	Tetracycline
	L-asparaginase
	Corticosteroids
	Phenformin
	Procainamide
	Valproic acid
	Clonidine
	Pentamidine
	Dideoxyinosine

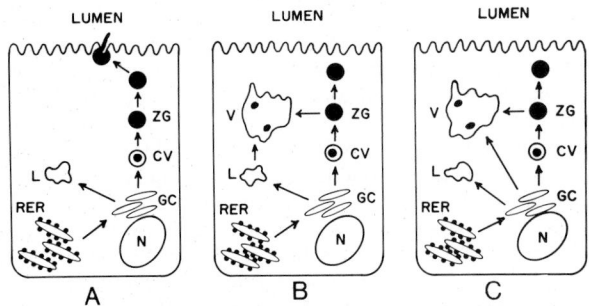

Figure 8. Intracellular transport of digestive enzymes and lysosomal hydrolases. *A*, Normal pattern, with synthesis of digestive enzymes and lysosomal hydrolases in the rough endoplasmic reticulum (RER), with subsequent transport to the Golgi complex (GC) adjacent to the nucleus (N). Lysosomal hydrolases are then transported to lysosomes (L), while digestive enzymes are concentrated in condensing vacuoles (CV) and zymogen granules (ZG). Zymogen granules fuse with the luminal plasma membrane and release their contents by exocytosis. *B*, Changes in mice fed the CDE diet, which blocks exocytosis and causes digestive enzymes and zymogen granules to accumulate. The zymogen granules fuse with lysosomes in a process termed crinophagy, causing the formation of large vacuoles (V). *C*, Changes in rats given supramaximal doses of cerulein. Here, transport to the Golgi complex is unaffected, but impaired separation of lysosomal hydrolases and digestive enzymes results in the formation of abnormal large vacuoles that contain both types of enzymes. Mature zymogen granules also fuse with these vacuoles, and exocytosis at the luminal plasma membrane is prevented. (From Steer, M. L., and Meldolesi, J.: The cell biology of experimental pancreatitis. N. Engl. J. Med., *316*:144, 1987.)

of pain after a large meal. Nausea and vomiting frequently accompany the abdominal pain. The vomiting may be severe and protracted. Rare patients with acute pancreatitis may present without abdominal pain, but with a severe systemic illness marked by hypotension, hypoperfusion, and depression of mental status. In these patients, the diagnosis of acute pancreatitis may be particularly difficult to establish.

Typical findings on physical examination in patients with acute pancreatitis include fever, tachycardia, epigastric tenderness, and abdominal distention. Abdominal distention may be the result of a paralytic ileus arising from retroperitoneal irritation or may occur secondary to a retroperitoneal phlegmon. Severe pancreatitis associated with hemorrhage into the retroperitoneum may produce two distinctive physical signs: Turner's sign (bluish discoloration in the left flank) and Cullen's sign (bluish discoloration of the periumbilical region). These physical signs, which occur in less than 3 per cent of patients with pancreatitis, are the result of the tracking of blood-stained retroperitoneal fluid through the tissue planes of the abdominal wall to the flank or along the falciform ligament to the umbilical area. These signs signal the presence of a severe episode of acute hemorrhagic pancreatitis, with an overall mortality exceeding 30 per cent.

Jaundice is an uncommon finding at the initial presentation with acute pancreatitis. Jaundice may occasionally be seen in patients with gallstone-associated pancreatitis, where it represents distal common bile duct obstruction by gallstones. Jaundice may also follow compression of the distal common bile duct by edema of the pancreatic head.

Patients with severe pancreatitis may manifest major circulatory derangements such as hypotension, hypovolemia, hypoperfusion, and obtundation. Formerly, the etiology of this shock state was attributed to a putative circulating myocardial depressant factor thought to be elaborated during severe hemorrhagic pancreatitis. Recent investigations have shown instead that the detrimental effects of acute pancreatitis on cardiovascular function are related primarily to hypovolemia and decreased preload to the heart and are not related to a depressant factor released in response to the disease.

Extra-abdominal manifestations of acute pancreatitis may be found on careful physical examination in many patients. Up to one third of patients have evidence of a left pleural effusion or left hemidiaphragm elevation. Less frequently, patients mani-

fest signs of acute pulmonary failure, marked by tachypnea, dyspnea, and cyanosis. The etiology of this respiratory dysfunction remains unclear, although it has been linked to abnormalities of circulating phospholipase A, circulating free fatty acids generated from triglyceride lipolysis, pulmonary surfactant, and volume overload in the setting of pulmonary capillary leakage. Nonpulmonary findings associated with acute pancreatitis include subcutaneous fat necrosis and cerebral abnormalities of a nonlateralizing nature, including belligerence, confusion, psychosis, and coma. It has been speculated that these cerebral abnormalities follow hyperosmolarity, hypoperfusion and hypoxia, cerebral fat embolism, or disseminated intravascular coagulopathy.

Diagnosis

Acute pancreatitis is often suspected on the basis of clinical presentation, with the diagnosis supported by appropriate laboratory determinations and radiographic findings (Table 3).

LABORATORY DETERMINATIONS. The determination of serum amylase is the most widely used laboratory test in the diagnosis of acute pancreatitis. In most cases hyperamylasemia is observed within 24 hours of the onset of symptoms, with gradual return to normal values during the subsequent 7 days. Persistent hyperamylasemia beyond the initial week of the illness may indicate the development of complications such as pancreatic pseudocyst, phlegmon, or abscess or may indicate ongoing acute pancreatic inflammation. The degree of initial hyperamylasemia is not a reliable predictor of the severity of pancreatitis. However, the magnitude of hyperamylasemia is an independent predictor that differentiates gallstone-associated pancreatitis from alcohol-induced pancreatitis when examined by regression analysis in patient populations with diverse causes of pancreatitis.

Despite its widespread use, serum amylase is not an ideal marker for the diagnosis of acute pancreatitis. Serum amylase alone is limited as a predictor of acute pancreatitis because of high false-positive and high false-negative rates. In an acute hospital setting, nearly one third of the detected elevations of serum amylase are unrelated to acute pancreatitis (false-positive). A multitude of other causes of hyperamylasemia exists (Table 4). In addition, there is a false-negative rate of approximately 10 per cent, indicating that hyperamylasemia is observed in only 90 per cent of patients subsequently proven to have acute pancreatitis. Thus, the absence of hyperamylasemia does not exclude the diagnosis of acute pancreatitis. There are several possible explanations for the absence of hyperamylasemia in cases of acute pancreatitis. In some only brief hyperamylasemia may occur prior to medical evaluation, normoamylasemia being observed at the initial presentation. The lack of hyperamylasemia may also reflect extensive pancreatic necrosis or failure of a chronically diseased gland to elaborate sufficient circulating amylase at the time of acute inflammation. Moreover, most patients with hyperlipidemia-induced acute pancreatitis present with normoamylasemia, possibly related to a circulating inhibitor of amylase activity in these hyperlipidemic patients.

The measurement of pancreatic isoenzyme components im-

TABLE 3. Diagnosis of Acute Pancreatitis

Laboratory Tests	Radiographic Procedures
Serum amylase	Plain chest roentgenogram
Serum amylase isoenzymes	Plain abdominal roentgenogram
Urinary amylase	Upper gastrointestinal contrast series
Amylase-creatinine clearance ratio	Ultrasonography
Serum lipase	Computed tomography
Serum methemalbumin	Magnetic resonance imaging
Peritoneal fluid analysis	

TABLE 4. Disorders Associated with Hyperamylasemia

Intra-abdominal	Extra-abdominal
Pancreatic disorders	Salivary gland disorders
Acute pancreatitis	Mumps
Chronic pancreatitis	Parotitis
Trauma	Trauma
Carcinoma	Calculi
Pseudocyst	Irradiation sialadenitis
Pancreatic ascites	
Abscess	Impaired amylase excretion
	Renal failure
Nonpancreatic disorders	Macroamylasemia
Biliary tract disease	
Intestinal obstruction	Miscellaneous
Mesenteric infarction	Pneumonia
Perforated peptic ulcer	Pancreatic pleural effusion
Peritonitis	Mediastinal pseudocyst
Afferent loop syndrome	Cerebral trauma
Acute appendicitis	Severe burns
Ruptured ectopic pregnancy	Diabetic ketoacidosis
Salpingitis	Pregnancy
Ruptured aortic aneurysm	Drugs
	Bisalbuminemia

proves the accuracy of the diagnosis in acute pancreatitis. Normally P type amylase isoenzyme arises from the pancreas, representing 40 per cent of circulating amylase. The remaining 60 per cent of total circulating amylase, designated S type isoamylase, derives from salivary glands, fallopian tubes, ovaries, endometrium, prostate, breast, lung, and possibly liver. Isoenzyme analyses have been shown to be of some benefit in excluding the diagnosis of acute pancreatitis, particularly in patients with hyperamylasemia and an absence of P type isoenzyme elevation.

The measurement of urinary amylase excretion has also been proposed as a sensitive index of the disease. Urinary amylase elevations persist for a longer period of time than serum elevations, with the magnitude of urinary elevations frequently surpassing the magnitude of serum elevations. However, hyperamylasuria alone is not diagnostic of pancreatitis and may be observed in most other disorders associated with hyperamylasemia. In addition, a normal urinary amylase value does not preclude the diagnosis of acute pancreatitis.

The measurement of the renal clearance of amylase has been suggested as a means of improving the accuracy of the diagnosis of acute pancreatitis. The equation for the calculation is

$$\frac{\text{urine amylase}}{\text{serum amylase}} \times \frac{\text{serum creatinine}}{\text{urine creatinine}} \times 100$$

= the amylase-creatinine clearance ratio

Many authors have supported the use of the amylase-creatinine clearance ratio in the diagnosis of acute pancreatitis, noting that the renal glomerular permeability to amylase appears to be increased in the disease. Normally this ratio varies from 1 to 4 per cent. A ratio of greater than 6 per cent is consistent with the diagnosis of acute pancreatitis, ratios up to three times this level frequently being observed in severe pancreatitis. Unfortunately, acute pancreatitis may occur with a normal amylase-creatinine clearance ratio. Additionally, false-positive elevated ratios may be seen in disease states such as renal insufficiency, perforated peptic ulcer, pancreatic carcinoma, burns, and diabetic ketoacidosis. Thus, the amylase-creatinine clearance ratio is not a totally specific or totally sensitive indicator of acute pancreatitis.

The elevation of serum lipase is a more accurate indicator of acute pancreatitis than is the elevation of serum amylase because lipase is solely of pancreatic origin. In addition, the duration of hyperlipasemia often exceeds that of hyperamylasemia, making this test beneficial in patients with late clinical presenta-

tion. However, hyperlipasemia is not entirely specific for acute pancreatitis, being observed in other disease states such as perforated peptic ulcer, acute cholecystitis, and intestinal ischemia.

The finding of serum lactescence is one of the most specific indicators of acute pancreatitis. Lactescent serum occurs when circulating triglyceride values exceed 500 mg. per 100 ml. Serum lactescence may be seen in patients with hereditary hyperlipidemia-associated pancreatitis or in alcohol-associated pancreatitis. Patients with lactescent serum usually have falsely normal serum amylase levels, making the demonstration of serum lactescence a valuable diagnostic indicator supporting the diagnosis of acute pancreatitis.

Additional support for the diagnosis of acute pancreatitis can be derived from a number of standard laboratory tests. Although these tests are not specific for the diagnosis of acute pancreatitis, they may provide important information substantiating the diagnosis. Hematologic evaluation may reveal hemoconcentration from third-space fluid sequestration. An elevated white blood cell count above 10,000 cells per cu. mm. is typical. Serum chemistries often reveal hyperglycemia, mild azotemia, abnormalities of liver function tests, and hypocalcemia. Hyperglycemia appears to be the result of relative hypoinsulinemia, and relative hyperglucagonemia, and it is associated with the degranulation of beta cells by electron microscopy.[60] Mild azotemia is related to fluid sequestration, resultant hypovolemia, and diminished cardiac output. Hypocalcemia is the consequence of dilutional hypoalbuminemia, calcium deposition in areas of fat necrosis, and resistance of skeletal bone to parathyroid hormone stimulation. Derangements of calcitonin and vitamin D do not appear to be acutely implicated in pancreatitis-induced hypocalcemia. Abnormalities of liver function tests are more commonly found in gallstone-associated pancreatitis, in which they reflect some obstruction to the free flow of bile through the ampulla of Vater. Using stepwise logistic regression analyses, a number of investigators have confirmed that elevated bilirubin, alkaline phosphatase, γ-glutamyl transferase, alanine aminotransferase, and aspartate amino transferase serve as independent predictors favoring a common bile duct stone as the initiator of the attack of pancreatitis.

In a minority of patients with pancreatitis, arterial blood gas abnormalities occur. However, in up to 10 per cent of patients, generally those with severe attacks, severe progressive pulmonary dysfunction marked by dramatic hypoxemia and hyperventilation may occur. Severe pancreatitis may also cause dramatic coagulation abnormalities marked by hypercoagulability, disseminated intravascular coagulation, and hypofibrinogenemia.

Diagnostic paracentesis is occasionally utilized to confirm the diagnosis of acute pancreatitis. Elevations in peritoneal fluid amylase and lipase may be found in settings where their respective serum levels are normal. However, diagnostic paracentesis is not an ideal test for the confirmation of the diagnosis of acute pancreatitis due to its invasive nature, potential for complications, and the lack of complete specificity of peritoneal fluid enzyme elevations for acute pancreatitis.

RADIOGRAPHIC PROCEDURES. Clinical and laboratory evidence of acute pancreatitis can be supported by radiographic procedures such as plain chest and abdominal radiographs, gastrointestinal contrast studies, sonography, computed tomography (CT), and magnetic resonance imaging (MRI) studies.

Chest film findings supportive of the diagnosis of acute pancreatitis, but not specific for the disease, include left basalar atelectasis, elevation of the left hemidiaphragm, and left pleural effusion. These findings reflect the presence of a significant peridiaphragmatic, retroperitoneal inflammatory process occurring in the region of the pancreas. Chest films are also useful in eliminating other diagnoses from the differential diagnosis in a patient with abdominal pain. For example, the findings of pneumoperitoneum or lobar pneumonia on an upright chest film would lead the clinician away from the diagnosis of acute pancreatitis.

There are no specific indicators of acute pancreatitis on abdominal radiographs. However, they reveal nonspecific abnormalities in the majority of patients. Most frequently seen on the abdominal plain film is the presence of air in the duodenal loop, representing a local duodenal ileus secondary to the adjacent inflammatory reaction in the head of the gland. Also common is the abnormality referred to as the "sentinal loop sign," representing a dilated proximal jejunal loop localized to the upper abdomen, adjacent to the pancreatic bed. The "colon cutoff sign" may also be observed, indicative of distention of the colon to the level of the transverse colon with little to no air being present in the splenic flexure and more distal colon. Other possible findings on abdominal films include gallstones in the gallbladder, obliteration of the psoas margin secondary to retroperitoneal edema, or a nonspecific ileus pattern. One specific marker of pancreatic disease is the presence of pancreatic calcifications, although this is not an indicator of acute pancreatitis.

Upper gastrointestinal contrast studies were used formerly to assist in the diagnosis of acute pancreatitis. Typical findings on upper GI series included widening of the duodenal C loop, anterior displacement of the stomach by an inflamed retroperitoneal process, and subtle duodenal mucosal abnormalities reflecting duodenal wall inflammation. However, no findings on upper GI series are specific for acute pancreatitis, and more sensitive and specific radiographic evaluations are now available.

Abdominal sonography may be used to assist in the diagnosis of acute pancreatitis. Unfortunately, the value of ultrasonography is often limited by the presence of air and fluid-filled loops of bowel overlying and obscuring the pancreas. In the absence of this limitation, ultrasound can be used to detect pancreatic edema and acute peripancreatic fluid collections. In addition, in patients with suspected gallstone-associated pancreatitis, the gallbladder can be assessed for gallstones, and the common bile duct can be evaluated for size and the presence of stones.

Currently the most widely accepted and sensitive method used to confirm the diagnosis of acute pancreatitis is CT. The accuracy of CT scanning is improved with both oral and intravenous contrast enhancement. Nearly all patients with acute pancreatitis have some abnormalities on CT scan. Specific CT findings in acute pancreatitis can be categorized into pancreatic and peripancreatic changes (Table 5). Pancreatic changes include diffuse or focal parenchymal enlargement, edema, or necrosis with liquefaction. Peripancreatic changes include blurring or thickening of the surrounding tissue planes and the presence of fluid collections. An approximate correlation exists between the degree of CT abnormality and the clinical course and severity of the acute pancreatitis. CT is additionally useful

for the demonstration of structural complications that develop during the course of acute pancreatitis such as pancreatic abscess, phlegmon, or pseudocyst.

MRI holds promise for more sophisticated imaging and more accurate diagnosis of acute pancreatitis. Currently, MRI and CT appear to provide equivalent information regarding the presence and extent of fluid collections and parenchymal irregularity. High-resolution ^{31}P spectral analysis has been used in longitudinally evaluating the severity of acute pancreatitis in several experimental settings. The stepwise depletion of the high-energy compounds adenosine triphosphate and phosphocreatine was found to parallel the progression of the acute pancreatitis in one study[29] and to be associated with the presence of ischemic pancreatitis in another.[14] Active investigation is currently under way to elucidate the role of magnetic resonance imaging and spectroscopy in the clinical assessment of pancreatitis.

Endoscopic retrograde pancreatography is an invasive procedure that has proven utility in occasional patients with recurrent attacks of acute pancreatitis without obvious etiology. In these settings, endoscopic pancreatography has been useful in identifying potentially correctable abnormalities in up to 50 per cent of patients. In such patients, the findings of pancreas divisum, stenosis of the ampulla of Vater, and focal pancreatic duct abnormalities may be demonstrated. Significantly, endoscopic retrograde pancreatography has no role in the standard diagnostic evaluation of the majority of patients with acute pancreatitis.

Clinical Course

The clinical course of up to 90 per cent of patients with acute pancreatitis follows a mild self-limited pattern. However, in 10 to 15 per cent of patients with acute pancreatitis a severe form of illness develops that may be attended by lengthy hospitalization and specific complications, with significant associated morbidity and mortality. Patients with severe pancreatitis provide a major management challenge, often requiring intensive care settings, invasive hemodynamic monitoring, frequent laboratory and radiographic evaluation, and experienced management.

It is possible to predict the severity of an attack of pancreatitis and the overall prognosis using routinely available clinical and laboratory determinations. The most widely used predictive criteria involve 11 prognostic signs identified by Ranson in 1974[41] (Table 6). These prognostic signs are clinically valuable in guiding the therapy of each individual patient with acute pancreatitis. Patients that present with two or fewer prognostic signs have essentially no mortality, and generally simple supportive care suffices in their management. Patients with three or four prognostic signs have a mortality that approximates 15 per cent, with nearly half the patients requiring intensive care unit support. If five or six prognostic signs are present, intensive care unit support is usually required, and mortality approaches 50

TABLE 5. Computed Tomographic Findings in Acute Pancreatitis

Pancreatic changes
  Parenchymal enlargement
    Diffuse
    Focal
  Parenchymal edema
  Necrosis

Peripancreatic changes
  Blurring of fat planes
  Thickening of fascial planes
  Presence of fluid collections

Nonspecific findings
  Bowel distention
  Pleural effusion
  Mesenteric edema

TABLE 6. Ranson's Early Prognostic Signs of Acute Pancreatitis

At Admission	During Initial 48 Hours
Age over 55 years	Hematocrit fall > 10 percentage
WBC > 16,000 cells/cu. mm.	points
Blood glucose > 200 mg./dl.	BUN elevation > 5 mg./dl.
Serum lactate dehydrogenase >	Serum calcium fall to < 8
350 I.U./L.	mg./dl.
SGOT > 250 U./dl.	Arterial Po$_2$ < 60 torr
	Base deficit > 4 mEq./L.
	Estimated fluid sequestration >
	6 L.

Data from Ranson, J. H. C., Rifkind, K. M., Roses, D. F., et al.: Prognostic signs and the role of operative management in acute pancreatitis. Surg. Gynecol. Obstet., 139:69, 1974.

per cent. Patients with seven or more prognostic signs have an even higher predicted mortality and represent a group of patients that test the limits of modern medicine. The application of this prognostic scoring system allows early stratification of patients based on predicted outcome and allows the triaging of patients to appropriate treatment modalities. Patients assessed to have severe pancreatitis are at risk for the development of life-threatening complications, and they are optimally managed in the intensive care setting with hemodynamic monitoring, aggressive fluid resuscitation, and consideration of antibiotic administration as prophylaxis against infectious complications.

While the Ranson prognostic scoring system has gained widespread use, many other predictive indicators have been proposed. Methemalbuminemia loosely correlates with the presence of severe hemorrhagic pancreatitis. Diagnostic peritoneal lavage can assess the severity of illness and serves as a predictor of prognosis. Serum ribonuclease activity has been suggested as a marker of severe parenchymal necrosis. Other scoring systems based on laboratory and radiographic evidence have also been proposed. However, currently the 11 prognostic indicators first delineated by Ranson stand as the most widely used method for the assessment of patients with acute pancreatitis.

Nonoperative Management

Following initial clinical assessment, confirmation of diagnosis by laboratory and radiographic study, and prediction of prognosis, the initial management of patients with acute pancreatitis is nonoperative (Table 7). Standard therapy in all patients includes intravenous fluid resuscitation, electrolyte replacement, and analgesics. Nasogastric decompression is reserved for patients with significant ileus, in which it is used to prevent emesis and aspiration. Patients with severe pancreatitis often require nutritional support via parenteral alimentation, antibiotic administration for prevention or treatment of septic complications, or respiratory support for pulmonary dysfunc-

TABLE 7. Proposed Nonoperative Therapies for Acute Pancreatitis

Supportive measures
    Intravenous fluid therapy
    Electrolyte replacement
    Analgesia
    Nutritional support
    Antibiotics
    Respiratory support

Pancreatic exocrine secretion suppression
    Nasogastric suction
    Histamine receptor antagonists
    Antacids
    Anticholinergics
    Glucagon
    Calcitonin
    Somatostatin
    Cholecystokinin receptor antagonists

Pancreatic enzyme inhibition
    Protease inhibitors
        Aprotinin
        Gabexate
        Fresh frozen plasma
    Antifibrinolytics
    Phospholipase A inhibitors

Pancreatic protection from oxygen-derived free radicals
    Free radical scavengers
    Xanthine oxidase inhibitors

Elimination of toxic intraperitoneal compounds
    Peritoneal dialysis

tion. In addition to these standard supportive measures, a number of specific therapies have undergone trial under experimental or clinical conditions as a test of efficacy in reducing the degree of pancreatic parenchymal injury, subsequent complications, and overall mortality.

STANDARD SUPPORTIVE MEASURES. Acute pancreatitis is commonly associated with massive fluid sequestration. Fluid can accumulate within the bowel lumen secondary to paralytic ileus, or there can be marked edema in the peripancreatic region. External fluid losses may also occur in the form of emesis. An essential initial step in the management of acute pancreatitis involves generous fluid resuscitation directed to correction of hypovolemia and restoration of circulating blood volume. The adequacy of volume replacement is assessed by the response of the heart rate, blood pressure and urinary output. In patients with preexisting cardiac, pulmonary, or renal disease, or in patients with severe pancreatitis, invasive monitoring including urethral catheterization, central venous pressure measurement, or measurement of cardiac output and cardiac filling pressures via a Swan-Ganz catheter is often indicated. In rare cases, shock may be intractable to fluid resuscitation alone, requiring the use of potent vasopressor agents during initial resuscitation. Crystalloid solutions are generally used for fluid resuscitation in acute pancreatitis. Severe hemorrhagic pancreatitis may require blood transfusion or the transfusion of clotting factors to correct a markedly abnormal coagulation status. However, clinical trials of colloid therapy have failed to delineate benefit from routinely administering fresh frozen plasma as a specific therapy in acute pancreatitis.

During the initial phase of resuscitation, a variety of electrolyte abnormalities may be encountered. A hypochloremic contraction alkalosis may follow persistent emesis and is treated with vigorous volume replacement with normal saline, supplemented with exogenous potassium chloride. Intravascular volume contraction may cause hypernatremia correctable by isotonic volume replacement. Serum calcium is often depressed secondary to hypoalbuminemia; however, if the ionized calcium level is normal, the patient does not require exogenous calcium replacement. Patients with depressed ionized calcium levels should receive supplementation. Hypomagnesemia may also be observed and should be corrected, because this may hasten the normalization of serum ionized calcium. Mild hyperglycemia is a frequent finding that improves with volume resuscitation. Marked hyperglycemia or glycosuria mandates cautious insulin administration.

Abdominal pain is treated with careful administration of narcotic analgesics. Meperidine is the preferred drug. Morphine is avoided because of its potential for causing sphincter of Oddi spasm, an entity that could theoretically potentiate ongoing pancreatic parenchymal injury. Infrequently used techniques to manage the abdominal pain of acute pancreatitis include percutaneous splanchnic nerve blocks and epidural anesthesia.

In patients with acute pancreatitis oral intake is initially prohibited. Oral intake can generally be resumed during the first week of treatment when abdominal pain and tenderness have improved, ileus has resolved, and hyperamylasemia is normalizing. Premature return to oral intake has been associated with the formation of pancreatic abscess and reactivation of pancreatic inflammation. In a subgroup of patients, the return to eating is necessarily delayed as a result of persistent pain, ileus, or the occurrence of a complication such as pseudocyst, phlegmon, or abscess. Under these circumstances, standard parenteral nutrition using carbohydrate and amino acid–based solutions is indicated. Intravenous lipids can also be used as a calorie source in most patients. Lipid administration should be restricted in patients with underlying hyperlipidemia and in those rare patients who demonstrate hypertriglyceridemia with exogenous intravenous lipid administration.

Antibiotics are not indicated in the routine treatment of mild to moderate pancreatitis. In severe pancreatitis, there has as yet been no prospective study of the use of prophylactic antibiotics to reduce infectious complications. However, it appears appropriate to advise the use of prophylactic antibiotics in patients with severe pancreatitis, defined as the presence of three or more Ranson prognostic signs. Respiratory complications of acute pancreatitis such as atelectasis, effusion, pneumonia, and mild respiratory insufficiency generally require supportive care with supplemental oxygen administration, physical therapy, and treatment of infection. Progressive respiratory failure unresponsive to lesser supportive modalities may require endotracheal intubation and positive pressure ventilation.

PANCREATIC EXOCRINE SECRETION SUPPRESSION. Therapeutic attempts to suppress pancreatic enzyme secretion have included nasogastric suction, histamine H_2-receptor antagonists, antacids, anticholinergics, glucagon, calcitonin, somatostatin, and cholecystokinin-receptor antagonists such as proglumide. All these therapies have some theoretic potential to improve the outcome in patients with acute pancreatitis based on the hypothesis that pancreatic exocrine hypersecretion in the presence of partial ampullary obstruction is important in the pathogenesis of the disease. In fact, currently, none of these therapies has proved effective in shortening the duration of the disease, reducing complications, or reducing mortality.

Treatment directed to reduction of gastric acid delivery to the duodenum (such as nasogastric suction, histamine H_2-receptor antagonists, antacids, and anticholinergics) is designed to reduce duodenal acidification-induced secretin release from the duodenum, thereby reducing the volume of pancreatic exocrine secretion. However, no beneficial effect of any of these has been demonstrated. Nasogastric suction is, however, indicated in a subset of patients who present with gastric distention, persistent emesis, or altered mental status at risk for aspiration. Histamine H_2-receptor antagonists or antacids are indicated as prophylaxis against upper gastrointestinal tract hemorrhage in patients with severe pancreatitis. The adverse side effects of anticholinergics, such as urinary retention, tachycardia, and prolongation of ileus, make them unattractive for use in the treatment of acute pancreatitis.

Both glucagon and calcitonin, the hormonal product of the thyroid parafollicular C cell, suppress pancreatic exocrine and gastric acid secretion. Neither has documented efficacy in altering the outcome of acute pancreatitis.

Somatostatin is also a potent inhibitor of pancreatic exocrine secretion and gastric acid output. Native somatostatin has a circulating half-life in the blood of less than 3 minutes and thus must be delivered by continuous intravenous infusion. Octreotide is a long-acting octapeptide analog of the native tetradecapeptide which is now available for clinical use. In animal models of established experimental pancreatitis, somatostatin has been effective in reducing mortality from bile-induced pancreatitis and in hastening the return to normoamylasemia. However, multicenter clinical trials have failed to document statistically significant reduction in overall mortality in patients with acute pancreatitis. Evaluation of octreotide therapy in acute pancreatitis is continuing.

The cholecystokinin receptor antagonist proglumide has proved efficacious in models of experimental pancreatitis. In animal models using both cerulein-induced and CDE diet–induced pancreatitis, proglumide treatment has reduced mortality. Further investigations are needed to clarify the role of cholecystokinin receptor antagonists in the management of clinical pancreatitis.

PANCREATIC ENZYME INHIBITION. The treatment of acute pancreatitis by inhibition of pancreatic enzyme activation has a sound theoretic basis. Protease inhibitors such as aprotinin, gabexate, and fresh frozen plasma have been studied. However, in clinical trials none was of value in the treatment of acute pancreatitis.

Clinical studies have also failed to demonstrate a beneficial effect of antifibrinolitics such as ϵ-aminocaproic or p-aminomethylbenzoic acid. Phospholipase A inhibitors such as calcium disodium-EDTA also have not decreased morbidity or mortality in human pancreatitis.

PANCREATIC PROTECTION FROM OXYGEN-DERIVED FREE RADICALS. Systemic hypotension, low flow states associated with cardiopulmonary bypass, emboli to mesenteric vessels, or obstruction to visceral flow from vasculitis can cause relative pancreatic ischemia with resultant acute pancreatitis. Experimental models of acute pancreatitis have been used to demonstrate that free radical scavengers such as superoxide dismutase and catalase or xanthine oxidase inhibitors such as allopurinol can prevent acute experimental pancreatitis when administered before initiation of the parenchymal injury.[45] However, these treatments are not effective in arresting the progression of established experimental pancreatitis, and thus these therapies are unlikely to be clinically beneficial in the treatment of established acute pancreatitis.

ELIMINATION OF TOXIC INTRAPERITONEAL CONTENTS. Potentially toxic intraperitoneal compounds such as histamine, vasoactive kinins, elastase, prostaglandins, phospholipase A, trypsin, and chymotrypsin have been identified in the peritoneal exudate from acute pancreatitis. These compounds may mediate many adverse systemic effects such as hypotension, pulmonary failure, hepatic failure, and altered vascular permeability. Peritoneal dialysis appears theoretically attractive as a means of accelerating the removal of these activated toxic compounds. Studies in experimental pancreatitis have yielded favorable responses to peritoneal dialysis with improvement in outcome. Two prospective randomized trials using nonlavaged control groups compared with lavage treatment groups have failed to reveal any beneficial effect of peritoneal lavage on overall outcome.[27,35] One prospective study[49] and two noncontrolled trials[9,42] have suggested that peritoneal lavage may be of benefit in reducing the early systemic complications of severe pancreatitis. Currently, peritoneal dialysis appears best considered as a possible benefit in patients with severe pancreatitis associated with early clinical deterioration despite maximal intensive care support.

Operative Management

Operative intervention in patients with acute pancreatitis is indicated in four specific circumstances: (1) uncertainty of diagnosis, (2) treatment of pancreatic sepsis, (3) correction of associated biliary tract disease, and (4) progressive clinical deterioration despite optimal supportive care.

UNCERTAINTY OF CLINICAL DIAGNOSIS. Since there is no single test or combination of studies which is capable of diagnosing acute pancreatitis with 100 per cent accuracy, it may occasionally be difficult to exclude other diagnoses that mimic acute pancreatitis and require operative intervention. Examples of such conditions include perforated viscus or acute mesenteric ischemia. In these situations, when the clinical diagnosis is not firm, exploratory laparotomy may be indicated to exclude a surgically correctable disease with potentially fatal outcome in the unoperated state. With the widespread availability of abdominal CT scanning, these situations are becoming even less frequent. At the time of exploration any ascitic fluid present is sampled for amylase, lipase, aerobic and anaerobic culture, and cell counts. If no extrapancreatic disease is discovered, the gastrocolic omentum is opened to fully expose the body and tail of the pancreas. If uncomplicated acute pancreatitis is present, no manipulation is indicated, and the operation is terminated. In patients with systemic toxicity and gross evidence of severe pancreatitis associated with large amounts of peritoneal fluid exudate, the placement of a peritoneal dialysis catheter for postoperative lavage should be considered. In patients with cholelithiasis and presumed gallstone-associated pancreatitis, definitive biliary surgery including cholecystectomy and intra-operative cholangiography is favored if the clinical circumstances permit. In patients with severe hemorrhagic pancreatitis with necrosis but without frank infection, formal pancreatic resection is no longer favored. Instead, cautious débridement of necrotic tissue is performed, and wide retroperitoneal drainage is established.

TREATMENT OF PANCREATIC SEPSIS. Pancreatic abscess is a serious and life-threatening complication of acute pancreatitis, occurring in up to 5 per cent of all patients. It occurs with increasing frequency in direct proportion to the severity of acute pancreatitis. In patients with six or more Ranson's prognostic signs, over 50 per cent of patients develop a pancreatic abscess. Pancreatic abscess formation follows secondary infection of necrotic pancreatic and peripancreatic tissue. The organisms may arise from transmural migration of bacteria from adjacent inflamed bowel or from hematogenous seeding. Enteric organisms predominate. Polymicrobial infection is common, occurring in the majority of cases. Fungal infection is being recognized with increased frequency. The abscesses may be unilocular but are usually multilocular, and they may be located in any region adjacent to the pancreas. It is not uncommon to find large abscesses that extensively dissect retroperitoneal planes, residing behind the ascending or descending colon laterally or extending in the midline inferior to the base of the small bowel mesentery.

Typically, pancreatic abscesses are diagnosed after the first week of illness. Abscess development should be suspected in patients with severe pancreatitis, in patients with documented bacteremia, in patients with clinical deterioration after the first week, and in patients in whom pancreatitis fails to resolve within the first week to 10 days. Clinical manifestations of pancreatic abscess include fever, abdominal pain, abdominal distention, and a palpable abdominal mass. Associated laboratory abnormalities include persistent hyperamylasemia, nonspecific elevations of liver function tests, and leukocytosis. The diagnosis of pancreatic abscess is assisted by radiographic studies. Plain abdominal films may show extraluminal retroperitoneal air, described as the "soap bubble sign," present in 15 per cent of patients. Abdominal ultrasonography and nuclear medicine scans using gallium and indium-labeled leukocytes may suggest a diagnosis of pancreatic abscess but cannot accurately differentiate abscess from phlegmon. Currently CT scanning is the most widely used and accurate procedure for evaluating potential pancreatic abscess. Findings on a CT scan such as air bubbles in the retroperitoneum are diagnostic of a pancreatic abscess, but unfortunately are absent in many cases. The combination of abdominal CT scan with guided percutaneous needle aspiration has been demonstrated to be highly reliable in differentiating pancreatic abscess from sterile peripancreatic phlegmon. Fluid sampled at percutaneous needle aspiration is immediately Gram-stained and cultured. The aspiration is considered positive for pancreatic abscess if either Gram's stain or the culture reveals organisms.

Treatment of pancreatic abscess combines antibiotic therapy with prompt surgical drainage. Operative débridement is necessary to remove the thick, debris-filled, pastelike collections of infected necrotic material. The two accepted alternatives for management of pancreatic abscess are (1) laparotomy with débridement and wide sump drainage and (2) laparotomy with débridement and open packing. In either case the anterior transperitoneal approach to the abdomen is used to facilitate exposure. The gastrocolic omentum is divided, and the retroperitoneum is débrided of devitalized tissues. Anatomic resection is usually avoided. The abscess is copiously irrigated with saline and topical antibiotic solutions. Subsequently, wide sump drainage of the retroperitoneum or open packing is instituted. The wide sump drainage technique allows fascial closure of the abdomen and places multiple large-bore drains in dependent

positions to drain the abscess cavities. Using this technique, 16 to 40 per cent of patients require reoperation for persistent peripancreatic sepsis, and mortality varies from 5 to 50 per cent, averaging 30 per cent. The alternative to wide sump drainage involves open packing (marsupialization) of the pancreatic abscess cavity. With this technique, the abdominal fascia is not closed; and multiple packing changes, initially in the operating room and subsequently in the intensive care unit, allow repetitive access to the abscess cavity. Retrospective studies have observed an improvement in outcome for the open drainage technique, compared with the wide sump drainage technique. However, no randomized prospective trials have been reported.

CORRECTION OF ASSOCIATED BILIARY TRACT DISEASE. Formerly, definitive biliary tract surgery for gallstone-associated pancreatitis was often deferred up to 8 weeks after the acute episode of pancreatitis. This approach has gradually lost favor, primarily because the natural history of gallstone-associated pancreatitis without early surgical intervention is that of frequent recurrences. Up to 50 per cent of patients awaiting deferred elective operation have experienced a recurrence of gallstone-associated pancreatitis. Since typical episodes of gallstone-associated pancreatitis follow a mild short-lived clinical course and since definitive biliary tract surgery within 5 to 7 days of the index admission has proved safe and cost-effective, early biliary tract surgery is now favored. This approach eliminates the need for a second hospitalization and reduces the overall hospital length of stay. At this time, most surgeons proceed with biliary tract surgery during the index admission, after clinical resolution of pancreatitis. The one exception to this treatment plan involves patients with severe gallstone pancreatitis who have a prolonged clinical course marked by ileus, abdominal distention, a CT scan showing multiple peripancreatic fluid collections, and slow resolution of hyperamylasemia. These patients appear to benefit from a delay in elective operation. In these cases a nonoperative management course is followed as long as clinical improvement persists, thereby allowing resolution of pancreatic and peripancreatic inflammation. Two to 4 weeks are allowed to elapse between hospitalization for acute pancreatitis and readmission for definitive biliary tract surgery.

Another option for operative intervention in patients with gallstone-associated pancreatitis involves early surgical intervention within the first 72 hours of the onset of the disease. The rationale for such early intervention is that early elimination of ampullary obstruction by a common duct calculus can theoretically reduce the severity of the episode of pancreatitis. In studies comparing historical controls managed by delayed operative intervention with a group undergoing immediate cholecystectomy and common bile duct exploration for calculus retrieval, mortality was 16 per cent versus 2 per cent, respectively. However, the mortality in this historical control group is inappropriately high by today's standards, and the conclusion that immediate surgery is indicated in all patients with gallstone pancreatitis is unsupported. In a randomized study of patients with gallstone-associated pancreatitis, it has been demonstrated that early operation within 72 hours of admission can be performed safely, with equivalent morbidity and mortality when compared with patients undergoing delayed procedures 3 months after the acute illness.[50] However, patients undergoing early operation required more complicated surgical procedures because the incidence of choledocholithiasis was 64 per cent, versus 18 per cent in the delayed operative group. Further data have failed to reveal any advantage to early operation in patients with gallstone pancreatitis. Early surgical therapy appears to offer no advantage in the majority of patients, often requires more complicated operative intervention, and appears to be overly aggressive, since most patients improve with standard supportive measures, passing their common bile duct calculi without further incident. Thus, the current recommendation for management of patients with gallstone-associated pancreatitis favors initial supportive care, followed by delayed biliary surgery during the index admission.

In those patients with a prolonged deteriorating clinical course, the use of endoscopic retrograde cholangiopancreatography (ERCP) or percutaneous transhepatic cholangiography can document the presence of choledocholithiasis and impacted ampullary stones may be retrieved nonoperatively by endoscopic sphincterotomy (ES) or percutaneous transhepatic techniques.[37] For those patients with severe gallstone-associated pancreatitis, recent data support the use of early ERCP and ES in management.[37] In this study, 121 patients with acute gallstone pancreatitis were randomized to treatment with ERCP and ES versus conventional therapy. ERCP was performed within 72 hours of admission; and if common bile duct stones were identified, ES and stone extraction were performed. In the subgroup of 46 patients with severe pancreatitis, significantly fewer complications occurred with ERCP and ES (such as pseudocyst, pulmonary insufficiency, and death) and a shorter mean hospital stay, as compared with the group managed with supportive care alone. Therefore, in patients with severe attacks of gallstone pancreatitis, the use of early ERCP, combined with ES in the presence of common bile duct stones, appears appropriate.

DETERIORATION OF CLINICAL STATUS. In patients with acute pancreatitis and a deteriorating clinical condition who fail to respond to nonoperative supportive care, operative intervention has been advocated.[7] This issue remains the most controversial indication for surgical therapy in patients with acute pancreatitis. Among proponents of early operative intervention, recommended operative procedures range from local débridement of obviously necrotic tissue (necrosectomy) to formal total pancreatectomy. Beger and associates have recently generated renewed interest in early necrosectomy in patients judged to have necrotizing pancreatitis by clinical and CT criteria.[7] However, to date, no controlled randomized clinical trials allow realistic evaluation of the efficacy of such early resectional therapies. In a canine model, in a comparison with a nonoperated control group, resectional therapy increased mortality.[26] Overall, there are few objective clinical or experimental data to support the use of routine early pancreatic resection in patients with severe pancreatitis. Nonetheless, operative intervention may still be indicated in selected patients with clinical deterioration and the presumed diagnosis of pancreatitis for exclusion of another surgically correctable lesion or detection and treatment of early pancreatic abscess formation.

CHRONIC PANCREATITIS

Chronic pancreatitis defines a clinical entity that includes recurrent or persistent abdominal pain and evidence of exocrine and endocrine pancreatic insufficiency. It is marked pathologically by irreversible parenchymal destruction of pancreatic tissue. Pathologic findings in chronic pancreatitis in both humans and animal models[60] include evidence of acinar loss, glandular shrinkage, proliferative fibrosis, calcification, and ductal stricturing. Electron microscopic findings in chronic pancreatitis reveal evidence of dense collagen and fibroblastic proliferation in the parenchyma, this fibroproliferative response separating large clusters of islet cells with normal or nearly normal ultrastructural features.

Etiology

Chronic pancreatitis is associated with alcohol abuse, hyperparathyroidism, congenital anomalies of the pancreatic duct such as pancreas divisum, and pancreatic trauma. The most common cause of chronic pancreatitis in industrialized countries is alcohol abuse. The exact mechanism whereby alcohol induces the disease is unknown. Dietary factors may have a permissive role in alcohol-related chronic pancreatitis, since the risk of chronic pancreatitis associated with alcohol intake in-

creases in proportion to the protein intake and is maximized by ingestion of a high-fat diet. In underdeveloped or developing countries, chronic pancreatitis appears to be related to nutritional factors. In patients with hyperparathyroidism, the associated hypercalcemia is believed to be responsible for the chronic pancreatitis, possibly by overstimulation of the exocrine secretions of the gland and by predisposing to precipitation of protein aggregates within the main pancreatic ductal system. In some patients with idiopathic chronic pancreatitis, the etiology of the disease is unknown.

Clinical Presentation

The incidence of chronic pancreatitis in the United States approximates 4 per 100,000 population. Typically, patients present with a history of alcohol abuse in the fourth or fifth decades of life. Abdominal pain is the feature that prompts consultation. The pain is commonly epigastric in location but may be localized to the right or the left side of the midline. Radiation of the pain to the back is common. Some patients have continuous and unremitting pain, whereas others have recurrent episodes of pain that entirely resolve between attacks. Anorexia and weight loss may be present. Insulin-dependent diabetes mellitus occurs in up to one third of patients. Up to one quarter have steatorrhea, indicative of a major reduction in pancreatic exocrine function. Thus, the clinical tetrad of abdominal pain, weight loss, diabetes, and steatorrhea serves as a classic presentation in patients with chronic pancreatitis. Additionally, many patients present with a history of narcotic analgesic abuse in an effort to control their abdominal pain.

Diagnosis

Chronic pancreatitis is usually suspected on clinical findings. Routine laboratory tests are rarely helpful. Radiographic evaluation may reveal pancreatic calcifications on plain abdominal films, a finding at least 95 per cent specific for chronic pancreatitis.

A CT scan of the abdomen is useful in the evaluation of both parenchymal and ductal disease. The size and texture of the gland are evaluated and inspected for pancreatic parenchymal calcifications, nodularity, inhomogeneous densities, as well as pseudocyst formation or dilatation of the pancreatic ductal system. Important information is gained by the use of endoscopic retrograde pancreatography. Pancreatography can document ductal abnormalities not convincingly demonstrated by CT scan. Also, pancreatography has an essential role in guiding surgical therapy, by providing anatomic information that directs therapy to specific pathology (Fig. 9). Characteristic early changes in chronic pancreatitis observed via pancreatography include ductal dilatation and filling of secondary and tertiary branches, which ordinarily are not visualized. Patients with well-established chronic pancreatitis demonstrate ductal strictures and calculi and often show pseudocyst formation. The characteristic "chain of lakes" pancreatogram, representing ductal dilatation in concert with ductal stricturing, is a classic finding in chronic pancreatitis, but it is not observed as frequently as uniform ductal dilatation. An entirely normal pancreatogram in a patient with abdominal pain safely eliminates the diagnosis of chronic pancreatitis.

Pancreatic function tests are occasionally used in the workup of chronic pancreatitis. These tests are generally reserved for difficult diagnostic problems and clinical research and are not essential for preoperative evaluation. The purpose of these tests is to document exocrine pancreatic insufficiency as a marker for parenchymal pathology. Tests such as the Lundh test meal, duodenal essential amino acid perfusion, and the intravenous secretin and cholecystokinin stimulation tests require gastroduodenal intubation with collection of the pancreatic effluent for assessment. A simpler approach is to examine the stool for increased fat with a 72-hour fecal fat measurement and the Sudan stain.

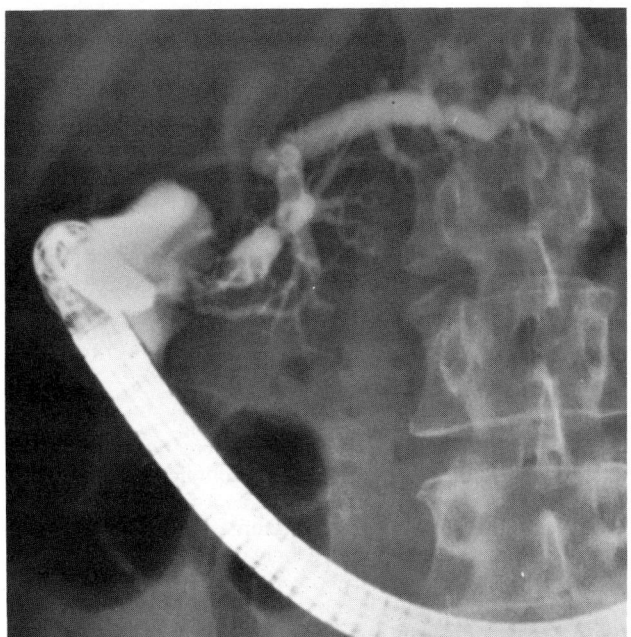

Figure 9. Endoscopic retrograde pancreatogram in a patient with chronic pancreatitis, showing a dilated pancreatic duct with areas of ductal stricturing and calculi.

Pancreatic endocrine function is normally assessed by glucose tolerance testing. More than two thirds of all patients with chronic pancreatitis have abnormal studies. Fortunately, less than one third of patients are insulin-dependent. Chronic pancreatitis-associated diabetes is generally mild and is rarely associated with ketoacidosis or vascular complications. Peripheral neuropathy is a common finding and appears to be related to both the diabetes and the effects of alcohol. Experimental data in a canine model suggest that pancreatic parenchymal fibrosis associated with chronic pancreatitis is associated with abnormal islet responsiveness causing a circulating insulin deficiency and glucose intolerance, in the presence of histologic and ultrastructural evidence of intact islets of Langerhans.[60] Endocrine function is generally unaffected by ductal drainage procedures but is reduced by resectional therapies.

Nonoperative Management

Three areas are encompassed in the nonoperative management of chronic pancreatitis: control of abdominal pain, treatment of endocrine insufficiency, and treatment of exocrine insufficiency.

The control of abdominal pain can be a major problem, and it is generally the sole indication for operative intervention. In the typical setting of alcohol-related chronic pancreatitis, total abstinence from alcohol is mandatory for nonoperative pain relief and is successful in some patients. In addition to abstinence, dietary manipulation, including small-volume, frequent, low-fat meals, is recommended, although controlled data proving efficacy are lacking. High-dosage regimens of exogenous pancreatic enzyme supplements, which theoretically decrease pancreatic secretion and thereby reduce pain, have had limited efficacy. Attempts to control pain often require early use of nonnarcotic analgesics, followed later by narcotic analgesics.

Exogenous insulin therapy in patients with chronic pancreatitis-associated diabetes must be used cautiously: one must attempt to control glycosuria and avoid hypoglycemia. In this group of patients, hypoglycemia following insulin administration can arise as the result of poor nutrient absorption secondary to malabsorption or the irregular caloric intake typical of alcoholics.

Digestive enzyme insufficiency with associated steatorrhea or malabsorption occurs in a minority of patients with chronic

pancreatitis. When present, exocrine insufficiency is treated with exogenous pancreatic enzyme supplementation. During a typical 4-hour postprandial period, adequate digestion requires the administration of approximately 30,000 I.U. of lipase and 10,000 I.U. of trypsin. Should malabsorption persist even with adequate exogenous pancreatic enzyme supplementation, the addition of histamine H_2-receptor antagonists may prove efficacious by diminishing the gastric acid-induced degradation of the exogenous enzyme preparations.

Operative Management

Surgical treatment of chronic pancreatitis can be broadly categorized into three groups: ampullary procedures, ductal drainage procedures, and ablative procedures. Ablative procedures are usually considered as the last step in surgical treatment for patients with chronic pancreatitis because of the fear of producing insulin-dependent diabetes mellitus. The primary goal of operative management is relief of pain, the secondary consideration being to preserve maximal endocrine and exocrine function. Prior to consideration of surgical intervention, mandatory evaluation of pancreatic disease involves parenchymal imaging by CT scan as well as assessment of pancreatic ductal anatomy by endoscopic retrograde pancreatography. Should preoperative pancreatography be unobtainable, intraoperative pancreatography can be performed.

AMPULLARY PROCEDURES. Favorable results following sphincteroplasty of the ampulla of Vater for chronic pancreatitis were reported by Doubilet and Mulholland in 1956.[17] At that time, the procedure was designed to eliminate pancreatitis by preventing bile reflux into the pancreatic duct in the setting of a common channel between the distal common bile duct and the pancreatic duct. Results in the intervening years in patients treated by sphincteroplasty have not been favorable, and therefore enthusiasm for the procedure has diminished. Ampullary procedures currently have limited application. In patients with the rare finding of a focal obstruction at the ampullary orifice, transduodenal sphincteroplasty of the major pancreatic duct orifice may be helpful. Also, for patients with recurrent pancreatitis associated with pancreas divisum and relative stenosis of the minor pancreatic duct papilla, transduodenal sphincteroplasty of the minor papilla may be successful in up to 85 per cent of patients. However, the results are less favorable in patients with pancreas divisum and established chronic pancreatitis.

DUCTAL DRAINAGE PROCEDURES. A ductal drainage procedure intended to decompress the pancreatic duct in a retrograde manner was described by Duval in 1954.[18] This procedure involved a limited distal pancreatectomy and an end-to-end pancreaticojejunostomy. It was used as treatment to relieve proximal pancreatic duct obstruction. While this procedure was successful in selected patients, the enthusiasm for caudal pancreaticojejunostomy diminished as failures of the operation were reported and as knowledge of pancreatic ductal pathology revealed more widespread ductal disease. Currently, caudal pancreaticojejunostomy is perhaps best applied to the uncommon cases of isolated proximal pancreatic ductal stenosis not involving the ampulla.

In 1958 Peustow and Gillesby described the side-to-side pancreaticojejunostomy,[40] a procedure subsequently modified by Partington and Rochelle.[39] This procedure is now more widely used than the caudal pancreaticojejunostomy, and it has been evaluated in many large clinical series with success rates of 60 to 90 per cent. It is theoretically more appealing than the caudal pancreaticojejunostomy because it decompresses nearly the entire pancreatic duct. Determinants of success for the side-to-side pancreatocojejunostomy include a pancreatic duct greater than 1 cm. in diameter, the presence of pancreatic calcifications, and a pancreatic-jejunal anastomosis longer than 6 cm. Currently side-to-side pancreaticojejunostomy is the most commonly applied pancreatic ductal drainage procedure, and it is recommended in patients with a dilated pancreatic duct in need of operative therapy for chronic pancreatitis. Ductal drainage does not improve established pancreatic exocrine or endocrine dysfunction, although it may delay the rate of progressive functional impairment in patients with early disease.

ABLATIVE PROCEDURES. The operative treatment of chronic pancreatitis by surgical resection of the pancreas is associated with variable success and the potential for significant postoperative complications. In carefully selected patients with isolated parenchymal disease in the body and tail of the pancreas, often secondary to trauma, limited distal pancreatectomy (40 to 80 per cent pancreatectomy) has documented success. Such a resection extends no further than to the neck of the pancreas, to the level of the superior mesenteric vein. Subtotal distal pancreatectomy (95 per cent pancreatectomy) involves distal pancreatic resection extending beyond the pancreatic neck to the level of the intrapancreatic portion of the common bile duct (Fig. 10). It has been applied to patients with severe diffuse parenchymal disease. Subtotal distal pancreatectomy has a nearly universal risk of postoperative insulin-dependent diabetes mellitus. Sixty to 80 per cent of patients treated by subtotal distal pancreatectomy obtain adequate pain relief. This operation should be reserved for patients who have diffuse parenchymal destruction without duct dilatation or in whom prior lesser procedures have failed.

Pylorus-preserving pancreaticoduodenectomy (modified Whipple operation) should be considered in cases of chronic pancreatitis without ductal dilatation where parenchymal disease primarily affects the head of the gland. In these circumstances, resection of the head of the pancreas and duodenum by pancreaticoduodenectomy provides relief of associated biliary or duodenal obstruction and preserves a substantial mass of islet cell tissue in the body and tail of the gland. Up to 80 per cent of properly selected patients obtain satisfactory results after pancreaticoduodenectomy. Finally, total pancreatectomy for chronic pancreatitis, combined with the necessary duodenal resection, is usually utilized as a completion pancreatectomy in patients with refractory pain after lesser procedures. In such circumstances, over 60 per cent of patients have been rendered pain-free. However, the significant problems associated with labile insulin sensitivity, steatorrhea, and weight loss dictate that total pancreatectomy be best applied as a last resort in carefully selected patients.

Several newer surgical treatments have been reported for the management of patients with chronic pancreatitis. Warren and associates proposed a duodenum-preserving resection of the pancreatic head combined with denervation of the body and tail.[54] Beger and associates reported a similar duodenum-preserving resection of the pancreatic head combined with Roux-

en-Y drainage of the retained pancreatic duct.[6] A modified side-to-side pancreaticojejunostomy with an anterior central resection or "coring out" of the pancreatic head has been utilized by Frey and Smith.[21] None of these newer procedures has had sufficiently widespread use to allow adequate evaluation.

Pancreatic autotransplantation remains an uncommonly used procedure in patients with chronic pancreatitis. Autotransplantation following resectional therapy, using either islet cell suspensions or segmental grafts, has theoretical value in preserving endocrine function but has had only limited success. Currently, pancreatic autotransplantation for chronic pancreatitis, intended to avert surgically induced diabetes mellitus, has limited indication and utility.

DISRUPTIONS OF THE PANCREATIC DUCT

In adults, disruptions of the main pancreatic duct are most commonly found in the setting of alcoholic pancreatitis, although they may occasionally occur as a result of pancreatic trauma or neoplasms. In children, trauma is the leading cause of pancreatic duct disruption. In pancreatic duct disruption pancreatic exocrine secretions exit the duct at the site of the disruption. Disruptions of the main pancreatic duct cause external or internal pancreatic fistulas. If the pancreatic exocrine secretions drain externally through a drain site or a wound, an external pancreaticocutaneous fistula results. If the exocrine secretions extravasate into the peritoneal cavity but are walled off by adjacent tissues, a pancreatic pseudocyst may occur. Pancreatic ascites occurs when the exocrine secretions extravasate anteriorly from the pancreatic duct, are not walled off, but drain freely into the peritoneal cavity. Pancreatic pleural effusion can result if the secretions extravasate into the retroperitoneum and track cephalad through the diaphragm to enter the thorax, draining into one or both pleural spaces. Rarely, pancreatic secretions may extravasate into a hollow viscus, forming a pancreatic-enteric fistula.

External Pancreatic Fistula

Drainage of pancreatic fluid through an abdominal wound or drain tract that persists for greater than 7 days is, by definition, an external pancreatic fistula. Pancreaticocutaneous fistulas follow pancreatic surgery in as many as 25 per cent of patients. Fistulas that drain less than 200 ml. per day are classified as low-output fistulas, whereas those in excess of 200 ml. per day are high-output fistulas. Complications of pancreaticocutaneous fistulas include sepsis, fluid and electrolyte abnormalities, and skin excoriation. Sinography and CT are used to delineate the anatomy of the fistulous tract and to exclude the presence of undrained cavities. The skin surrounding the fistulous tract is protected by means of appropriate skin care products. Attention is paid to fluid and electrolyte status, with appropriate replacement. Total parenteral nutrition is often utilized to avoid pancreatic stimulation by oral intake and to maximize tissue anabolism. The long-acting somatostatin analog octreotide has been reported to be of benefit in expediting closure of external pancreatic fistulas that fail to close by standard treatment. The majority of external pancreatic fistulas close with nonoperative management. Refractory fistulas may require surgical management. Prior to operation, endoscopic retrograde pancreatography is essential in delineating the anatomy of the pancreatic duct. Fistulas originating from the tail of the pancreas in association with a normal proximal pancreatic duct may best be managed by distal pancreatectomy. Distal pancreatic fistulas associated with abnormalities of the proximal pancreatic duct may be managed by distal pancreatectomy and pancreaticojejunostomy or by pancreaticojejunostomy to the fistula site itself. Fistulas localized in the head, neck, or body of the gland are best managed by Roux-en-Y pancreaticojejunostomy to the fistula tract.

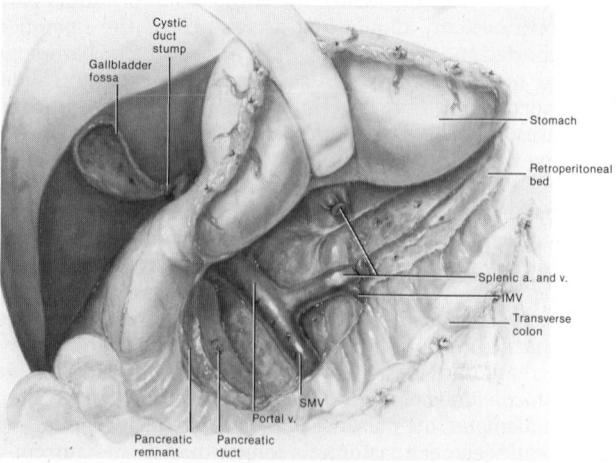

Figure 10. Illustration of a 95 per cent pancreatectomy, performed for chronic pancreatitis. (From Cameron, J. L.: Atlas of Surgery. Vol. 1. Toronto, B. C. Decker, 1990, p. 365. Illustration by Corinne Sandone.)

Internal Pancreatic Fistula

PANCREATIC PSEUDOCYST. Pancreatic pseudocysts are localized collections of pancreatic secretions in a cystic structure that lack an epithelial lining and occur as a result of surrounding tissues walling off and containing a pancreatic duct disruption. Pancreatic pseudocysts may be located within the pancreatic parenchyma but more often are adjacent to or near the pancreas in one of the potential spaces that separate the pancreas from adjacent abdominal viscera. Pancreatic pseudocysts represent well over 75 per cent of cystic lesions of the pancreas. Electrolyte concentrations in pseudocyst fluid are equivalent to those in plasma. Pseudocysts contain high concentrations of pancreatic enzymes, including amylase, lipase, and trypsin. Pseudocysts persist for as long as the cyst remains in continuity with the disrupted pancreatic duct. Should the communication between the pancreatic duct and the pseudocyst close secondary to cicatrization, the fluid contents of the cyst are absorbed and the pseudocyst disappears. Pancreatic pseudocysts develop in up to 10 per cent of patients after an attack of acute alcoholic pancreatitis. Pseudocysts are also associated with acute pancreatitis with other causes, as well as with chronic pancreatitis, pancreatic trauma, and pancreatic neoplasm.

Clinically, patients with pancreatic pseudocysts most often present with upper abdominal pain, which may be found in up to 90 per cent of patients. Nonspecific symptoms at presentation include nausea and vomiting as well as weight loss. Physical examination reveals abdominal tenderness in the majority of patients, and an abdominal mass is present in less than half. The most common clinical scenario of a patient with a pancreatic pseudocyst involves abdominal pain as well as early satiety, nausea, and vomiting secondary to gastroduodenal obstruction from the mass effect of the pseudocyst. More uncommon modes of clinical presentation include pruritis and jaundice secondary to common bile duct obstruction, variceal bleeding secondary to either splenic vein or portal vein obstruction, evidence of sepsis secondary to pseudocyst infection, and evidence of intra-abdominal hemorrhage secondary to bleeding from a pseudoaneurysm in adjacent visceral vessels.

Laboratory findings in patients with pancreatic pseudocysts are nonspecific. Many have elevations of serum amylase, and a small percentage of patients have evidence of liver function test abnormalities. Although a pancreatic pseudocyst may be suspected by clinical and laboratory findings, radiographic studies are necessary for definitive diagnosis. A CT scan of the abdomen is the favored study in an initial assessment for determining the presence of a pancreatic pseudocyst (Fig. 11). Ultrasound evaluation is nearly as accurate as CT scanning and can be recommended in the follow-up of patients with known pseudocysts for assessment of interval size changes.

The management of patients with pseudocysts is guided by the natural history. Previous reports have suggested that spontaneous resolution of pseudocysts occurred in less than 25 per cent of patients. The natural history of pseudocysts followed by ultrasound has been reported by Bradley and associates.[10] These data indicated that pseudocysts documented to be present for less than 6 weeks had a 40 per cent spontaneous resolution rate with a 20 per cent complication rate, whereas pseudocysts present for greater than 12 weeks never resolved and were associated with a complication rate of 67 per cent. Pseudocyst size has also been considered to be a factor determining the need for surgical therapy, most authors suggesting operative therapy for pseudocysts greater than 5 to 6 cm. With these criteria for operation, the operative treatment of pancreatic pseudocysts has a mortality varying from 5 to 12 per cent and morbidity of 21 to 53 per cent. The advent of CT scanning for patients suspected of having pancreatic pseudocysts has allowed more precise documentation of the natural history. In a recent report of 75 patients followed at the Johns Hopkins Hospital, patients with asymptomatic pseudocysts were preferen-

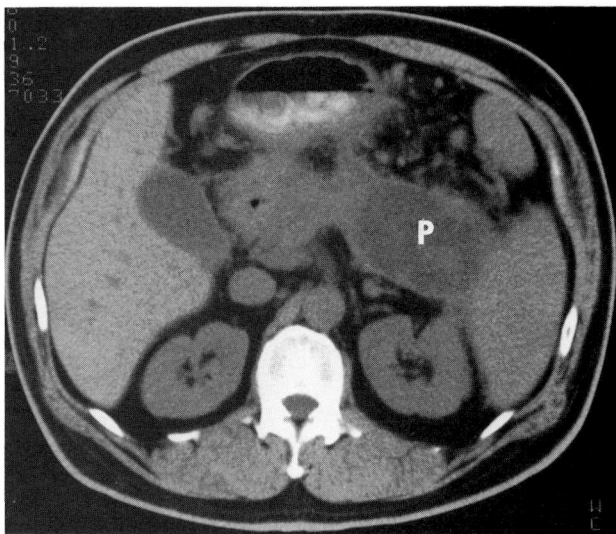

Figure 11. CT scan of a patient with a pseudocyst (P) in the body and tail of the pancreas that developed after an episode of acute pancreatitis.

tially managed nonoperatively, independent of pseudocyst size.[58] Operative management was performed only for persistent abdominal pain, pseudocyst enlargement, or pseudocyst complications. Forty-eight per cent of the entire group were successfully managed nonoperatively, whereas 52 per cent required surgical therapy. In the group managed without operation, with a mean follow-up of 1 year, 60 per cent had complete pseudocyst resolution documented radiographically and 40 per cent had pseudocysts that remained stable or decreased in size. No pseudocyst-related mortality occurred in either group. CT data, including the number of pseudocysts per patient, location, and wall thickness, were identical in the two groups. The only CT criterion that was significantly different between the two groups was pseudocyst size, with pseudocysts in the group operated upon averaging 7.4 ± 0.6 cm. in diameter, and pseudocysts in the group not operated upon average 5.8 ± 0.8 cm. in diameter. Pseudocyst size correlated with eventual need for operation; 67 per cent of patients with pseudocysts larger than 6 cm. required surgical therapy, and those with pseudocysts 6 cm. or less required surgery significantly less frequently. Twenty-seven per cent of pseudocysts greater than 10 cm. in size were successfully managed nonoperatively. These data suggest that strict size criteria alone are not sufficient to determine the need for operative versus nonoperative management.

Currently, treatment of patients with pancreatic pseudocysts is based upon the clinical setting, the presence or absence of symptoms, the age and size of the pseudocyst, and the presence or absence of complications. In the most common clinical settings a pseudocyst is discovered after an episode of acute alcoholic pancreatitis. With the resolution of pancreatitis, free of complications and able to tolerate oral intake, the patient is discharged from the hospital, with follow-up CT or ultrasound studies obtained at monthly intervals in assessment for pseudocyst enlargement, stability, or resolution. In contrast, if after an episode of acute pancreatitis a pseudocyst is associated with pain or early satiety precluding oral intake and hospital discharge, the patient remains hospitalized, supported with total parenteral nutrition, while pseudocyst size and clinical symptoms are assessed. Persistent symptoms, failure to tolerate oral intake, or pseudocyst-related complications require operative intervention. A 6-week period is generally allowed between the episode of pancreatitis and elective operative intervention, to allow satisfactory internal drainage.

Occasional patients are encountered without an obvious history of pancreatitis or trauma and with a pseudocyst of indeterminate age. If asymptomatic, these patients are followed with outpatient CT or ultrasound studies for several months, with observation of pseudocyst resolution or size diminution. However, if at the time of presentation significant symptoms exist, operative intervention is indicated, if one assumes that pseudocyst wall maturation has already occurred.

For pseudocysts that fail to resolve and require operative intervention, specialized preoperative studies other than abdominal ultrasound or CT scan are not mandatory. Endoscopic retrograde pancreatography is not essential prior to surgical therapy, although it may be useful in recurrent pseudocysts, multiple pseudocysts, or to help better define pancreatic duct anatomy prior to operative intervention. If endoscopic pancreatography is employed prior to surgical intervention, it is recommended that it be performed within 24 hours of operation to reduce the risk of pseudocyst infection. Options for the management of pseudocysts include internal drainage, pseudocyst excision, external drainage, and percutaneous or endoscopic techniques. When possible, treatment of pancreatic pseudocysts includes biopsy of the pseudocyst wall to exclude the possibility of a cystic neoplasm.

The preferred therapy in uncomplicated pseudocysts requiring operation is internal drainage. Three options for operative internal drainage of pseudocysts include drainage to a defunctionalized Roux-en-Y jejunal limb (cystojejunostomy), drainage into the stomach (cystogastrostomy), and drainage into the duodenum (cystoduodenostomy). Cystojejunostomy is the most versatile and useful method of cyst drainage (Fig. 12), being particularly appropriate when the pseudocyst presents at the base of the transverse mesocolon or is not adherent to the posterior gastric wall. Cystogastrostomy can be used when the pseudocyst is adherent to the posterior wall of the stomach. When feasible, cystogastrostomy is a faster and less technically demanding procedure than Roux-en-Y cystojejunostomy. The final option for internal drainage involves cystoduodenostomy. This procedure has limited utility, being applicable to pseudocysts in the head of the pancreas within 1 cm. of the duodenal lumen. Cystoduodenostomy has the potential for the formation of a duodenal fistula. It is best performed in a way similar to the way in which cystogastrostomy is performed, by opening the lateral duodenal wall and creating a connection between the pancreatic pseudocyst and the duodenum through a medial duodenotomy. The majority of pancreatic pseudocysts are drained internally by means of cystojejunostomy or cystogastrostomy.

Excisional therapy of pancreatic pseudocysts is utilized in a minority of cases, usually limited to distal pancreatic resections for pseudocysts in the tail of the gland. Distal pancreatectomy with or without splenectomy in this setting may be a technically challenging procedure because of peripancreatic and pericystic inflammation. Following distal pancreatectomy, if an obstructed proximal pancreatic duct is present, drainage of the pancreatic remnant by means of a Roux-en-Y pancreaticojejunostomy is indicated.

External drainage of pancreatic pseudocysts is indicated with gross infection, in the intraoperative patient with instability precluding more complex surgical intervention, and with immature pseudocysts with thin nonfibrous walls that do not allow safe internal drainage. A pancreaticocutaneous fistula occurs after external drainage, which often closes spontaneously. Persistent pancreaticocutaneous fistulas may require operative closure.

Percutaneous or endoscopic drainage of pancreatic pseudocysts has been reported but is only infrequently indicated. Percutaneous drainage is associated with high recurrence rates and a small but real potential for visceral injury. Also, adequate biopsy of the pseudocyst wall is not possible. However, diagnostic percutaneous aspiration of pancreatic pseudocyst fluid is a safe and accurate method of detecting pseudocyst infection. Endoscopic techniques to drain pseudocysts, using either the transgastric or transampullary route, have been reported. These techniques, while successful in small numbers of selected patients, have yet to be sufficiently assessed for one to recommend their use. Percutaneous or endoscopic drainage of pseudocysts appears best indicated in patients who are not operative candidates and who require decompression of large pseudocysts for management of symptoms. Asymptomatic patients with stable pseudocysts are not well served by percutaneous or endoscopic management techniques.

PANCREATIC ASCITES AND PANCREATIC PLEURAL EFFUSION. Similar pathophysiology and etiology apply to the entities of pancreatic ascites and pancreatic pleural effusion.[12] Both entities occur as a result of a pancreatic duct disruption secondary in most cases to alcohol abuse. Often these entities occur in the absence of a history of clinical pancreatitis. In pancreatic ascites, pancreatic exocrine secretions exiting a pancreatic duct disruption drain anteriorly into the peritoneal cavity. In pancreatic pleural effusion, the exocrine secretions drain from a duct disruption posteriorly into the retroperitoneum and then in a cephalad direction into the mediastinum and pleural space.

Patients with pancreatic ascites usually present with painless massive ascites and are often thought to have alcoholic cirrhosis with ascites. The diagnosis of pancreatic ascites is best made by paracentesis, in which analysis of the ascitic fluid reveals it to be high in amylase (greater than 1000 units per liter) and high in albumin (greater than 3 gm. per 100 ml.). Patients with pancreatic pleural effusion generally present with primary pulmonary symptoms such as dyspnea, chest pain, and cough. Abdominal symptoms may be absent. Findings on physical examination are

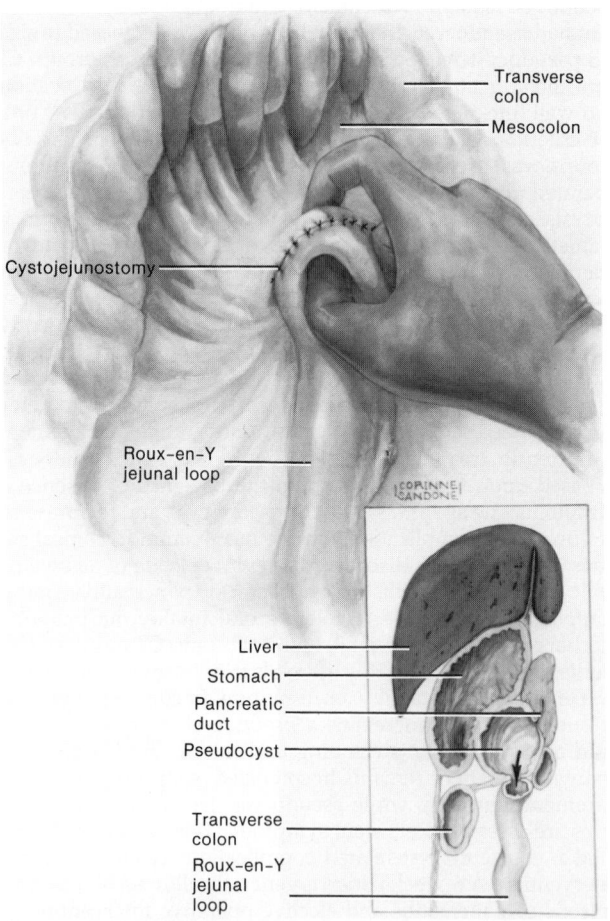

Figure 12. Illustration of internal drainage of a pancreatic pseudocyst by Roux-en-Y cystojejunostomy through the base of the transverse mesocolon. (From Cameron, J. L.: Atlas of Surgery. Vol. 1. Toronto, B. C. Decker, 1990, p. 379.)

TABLE 8. Management of Patients with Internal Pancreatic Fistula

Nonoperative treatment
  Prohibition of oral intake
  Nasogastric tube suction
  Paracentesis (for pancreatic ascites)
  Thoracentesis or chest tube (for pancreatic pleural effusion)
  Hyperalimentation
  ? Somatostatin (octreotide)

Operative treatment
  Direct duct leak
    Roux-en-Y drainage of duct leak
    Pancreatic resection for distal duct leak, with Roux-en-Y drainage of proximal pancreatic remnant if proximal duct disease present

  Leaking pseudocyst
    Roux-en-Y drainage of pseudocyst to jejunum
    Small, distal pseudocyst—possible resection, with Roux-en-Y drainage of proximal pancreatic remnant if proximal duct disease present
    External drainage

consistent with pleural effusion. The diagnosis of pancreatic pleural effusion is made by thoracentesis, again revealing a greatly elevated pleural fluid amylase and a high albumin content. Up to one quarter of patients may present with both pancreatic ascites and pancreatic pleural effusion. In both conditions the serum amylase is usually but not invariably elevated.

Nonoperative treatment is initially indicated in patients with pancreatic ascites and pancreatic pleural effusion (Table 8). The rationale of treatment is to decrease pancreatic exocrine secretion, thereby encouraging the pancreatic duct disruption to seal. Management includes the prohibition of oral feeding, nasogastric suction, total parenteral nutrition, and the use of paracentesis or thoracentesis, as appropriate, to eliminate the ascites or pleural fluid and thereby encourage the apposition of serosal surfaces. The long-acting somatostatin analog octreotide may be of some benefit in selected cases. Nonoperative management is recommended for a 2- to 3-week period and may resolve the

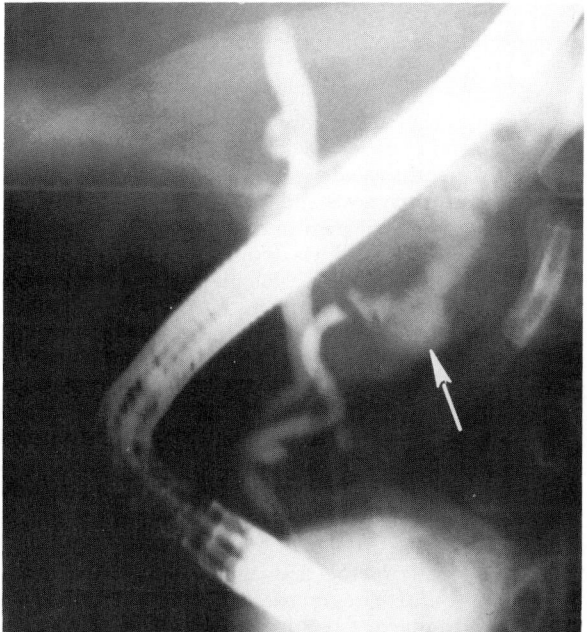

Figure 13. Endoscopic retrograde cholangiopancreatogram in a patient with pancreatic ascites. The pancreatic duct disruption is well visualized, demonstrating an abrupt cutoff with contrast extravasating into the lesser sac (arrow).

clinical entity in 50 per cent of patients. In patients not cured by nonoperative management, surgical therapy is indicated after delineation of pancreatic duct anatomy using endoscopic retrograde pancreatography (Fig. 13). Most patients with pancreatic ascites or pancreatic pleural effusion are leaking from an incompletely formed or ruptured pseudocyst, and a minority have direct duct leaks. Surgical therapy is based upon the findings of pancreatography. Distal pancreatic duct disruption or a leaking pseudocyst in the body or tail of the pancreas may be treated with distal pancreatectomy or with Roux-en-Y pancreaticojejunostomy. Pancreatic duct leaks in the more proximal aspects of the gland are treated with Roux-en-Y pancreaticojejunostomy to the site of pancreatic duct or pseudocyst disruption.

PANCREATIC ENTERIC FISTULA. Spontaneous decompression of a pancreatic pseudocyst or abscess into an adjacent hollow viscus can produce the unusual finding of a pancreatic enteric fistula. Most commonly, these fistulas occur between the pancreas and the splenic flexure or transverse colon. Less frequently involved organs include the stomach, duodenum, small bowel, and extrahepatic biliary tree. Symptomatic pancreatic pseudocysts have rarely been reported to be cured by spontaneous decompression into an enteric structure. In most cases, however, spontaneous rupture of a pseudocyst or abscess into a hollow viscus causes bleeding or sepsis, and appropriate operative intervention becomes necessary for correction of the disorder.

NEOPLASMS OF THE PANCREAS

EXOCRINE TUMORS

CANCER OF THE EXOCRINE PANCREAS

In the United States there are approximately 28,000 cases of cancer of the exocrine pancreas diagnosed each year. Cancer of the pancreas is the fifth most common cause of cancer death, exceeded only by lung, colorectal, breast, and prostate cancer. Ninety per cent of patients die within the first year after diagnosis. In both men and women pancreatic cancer represents 3 per cent of all cancers and 5 per cent of all cancer deaths. Since 1960 the relative 5-year survival rate for all cases of pancreatic cancer has increased from 1 per cent to 3 per cent. Considering only cancers of the digestive tract, cancer of the pancreas ranks second, behind colorectal cancer, in incidence and cancer death rates. Cancer of the pancreas is more common in blacks than in whites, more common in smokers than in nonsmokers, and more common in males than in females and appears to be linked to the presence of diabetes mellitus and the use of alcohol. Cancer of the pancreas is possibly linked to both a history of previous pancreatitis and the ingestion of a high-fat diet.

Pathologically, over 90 per cent of malignant pancreatic exocrine tumors are classified as duct cell adenocarcinomas. The most common site of origin of duct cell adenocarcinomas is the pancreatic head, where two thirds of the cases are localized. Subtypes of duct cell adenocarcinoma include mucinous and adenosquamous varieties. Less common types of pancreatic exocrine cancer include cystadenocarcinoma and acinar cell carcinoma.

Periampullary Adenocarcinoma

DIAGNOSIS. Neoplasms originating in the region of the ampulla of Vater are categorized as periampullary tumors. Clinically, radiographically, intraoperatively, and pathologically, it is often difficult to accurately differentiate cancer of the head of the pancreas from three other malignant periampullary neoplasms: ampullary carcinoma, duodenal carcinoma, and carcinoma of the distal common bile duct. Approximately 85 per cent of these tumors arise from the head of the pancreas, less than 10 per cent represent ampullary carcinomas, and duodenal carcinomas and carcinomas of the distal common bile duct represent less than 5 per cent each. The most common clinical features in patients with periampullary carcinoma are jaundice, weight loss, and abdominal pain. Approximately three quarters of the patients present with jaundice, and it is this symptom that normally causes the patient to seek medical attention. Weight loss occurs in over 75 per cent of patients. Abdominal pain is found in 70 per cent of patients, generally reflected as a dull aching pain in the midepigastrium or the right upper quadrant, with possible radiation to the back. Anorexia, weakness, pruritis, and alteration of bowel habits may also be present. The most common physical finding at initial presentation is jaundice. Hepatomegaly and a palpable gallbladder may also be noted.

The majority of patients with periampullary carcinoma have laboratory abnormalities marked by elevated serum bilirubin and alkaline phosphatase with mild elevations of hepatic transaminases. Serologic markers for pancreatic carcinoma have been evaluated, including carcinoembryonic antigen (CEA), CA 19-9, DU-PAN-2, alpha-fetoprotein (AFP), and pancreatic oncofetal antigen (POA). No currently available serologic test is completely accurate for diagnosis, the tests being limited by cross-reactivity with other tumors and low sensitivity for small, potentially resectable lesions.

In patients with suspected periampullary carcinoma, radiologic intervention is extremely important for diagnosis, staging, and management. Older techniques such as barium upper GI series may be positive in patients with large tumors, showing widening of the duodenal sweep or the "inverted 3" sign. Sonography is a useful screening examination, particularly in patients less than 40 years old, who are more likely to have cholestatic jaundice. In older patients, CT scanning is an essential procedure for the evaluation of periampullary neoplasms. CT scanning is superior to sonography in that it allows visualization of the entire pancreas, without distortion from overlying bowel gas, and it provides better accuracy in detecting hepatic metastases and in determining the size of the periampullary neoplasm.

After CT scanning, the site of biliary obstruction is defined by cholangiography. Cholangiography can suggest the site of tumor origin and is essential in planning successful resection and reconstruction (Fig. 14). In patients with high-grade biliary obstruction, percutaneous transhepatic cholangiography (PTHC) is favored because it allows delineation of the proximal biliary anatomy to be used for reconstruction. PTHC has nearly a 100 per cent success rate in visualizing the biliary tree in the

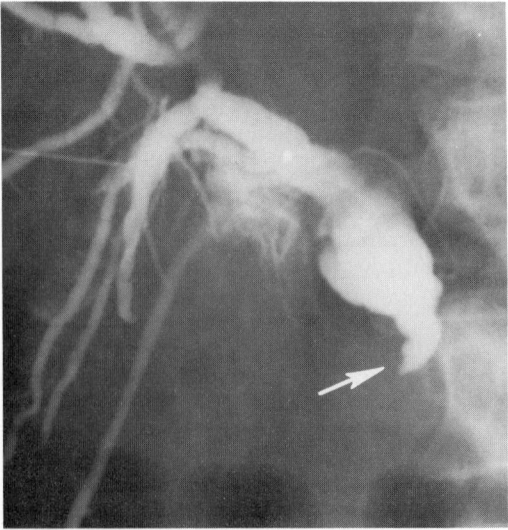

Figure 14. Percutaneous transhepatic cholangiogram of a patient with periampullary adenocarcinoma, showing a dilated intrahepatic and extrahepatic biliary tree with a typical "bird's beak" obstruction (arrow) at the level of the common bile duct.

setting of dilated intrahepatic ducts, with a 75 per cent success rate in visualizing the biliary tree in settings of nondilated ducts. PTHC in the setting of an obstructing periampullary neoplasm is generally combined with catheter drainage of the biliary tree via the percutaneous transhepatic route. Endoscopic retrograde cholangiopancreatography (ERCP) has a role in patients with periampullary neoplasms. ERCP is particularly valuable in the diagnosis of duodenal or ampullary carcinoma, where diagnostic tissue can be obtained by endoscopic biopsy. ERCP may also be useful in cases of partial biliary obstruction, where the endoscopically injected contrast can fill the proximal biliary tree above the tumor, thus defining the proximal biliary anatomy for subsequent biliary-enteric reconstruction. Biliary endoprostheses may be placed at the time of ERCP in carefully selected patients who are not candidates for exploration and resection, as a means of palliating the obstruction.

Selective celiac and mesenteric angiography combined with the evaluation of portal venous anatomy is generally used for delineation of major arterial and venous anatomy and for staging for resectability. Angiography has no role in tumor localization in patients with periampullary carcinoma. In a recent review of the use of staging angiography for 90 patients with periampullary neoplasms at the Johns Hopkins Hospital, the resectability rate was 77 per cent in patients with normal studies, 35 per cent in patients with encasement of the portal or superior mesenteric veins or the superior mesenteric or hepatic arteries, and 0 per cent in patients with visceral vessel occlusion.[16] Currently the combined use of CT (for assessment of both the primary tumor and the liver for metastases) and visceral angiography (to identify local tumor extension causing vessel occlusion or widespread encasement) is recommended for preoperative staging of periampullary neoplasms. Laparoscopy has been advocated by some as a means of improving staging, particularly addressing the issue of small unsuspected liver metastases or peritoneal implants. MRI has also shown promise in the evaluation of periampullary carcinomas, yielding information regarding tumor size and location, presence of hepatic metastases, and patency of portal venous and hepatic arterial structures. Prospective comparison of CT, MRI, laparoscopy, and visceral angiography for staging of periampullary neoplasms awaits study.

MANAGEMENT. The majority of patients presenting with periampullary neoplasms are operative candidates and are treated surgically. In a minority of patients, nonoperative therapy may be appropriate.

NONOPERATIVE THERAPY. Nonoperative therapy is an option in patients with documented distant metastases, unresectable local disease, and in patients with acute or chronic debilitating illnesses. In patients treated nonoperatively, attempts are made to acquire a tissue diagnosis and to palliate features of the disease such as abdominal pain and biliary obstruction. Tissue diagnosis can be obtained via biopsy of distant metastases, biopsy of hepatic metastases, cytologic specimens acquired by ERCP or PTHC, or by percutaneous needle biopsy of the primary pancreatic neoplasm. Percutaneous needle biopsy of the primary tumor is generally reserved for those patients who are to be treated nonoperatively and is not used preoperatively in patients with localized, apparently resectable tumors. Following tissue diagnosis, palliation of tumor-associated pain commences with oral analgesics. Poorly controlled pain may require percutaneous celiac ganglion blocks. Palliation of biliary obstruction can be achieved nonoperatively via a percutaneous transhepatic drainage catheter or by an endoprosthesis. Percutaneous transhepatic internal drainage allows constant access to the biliary tree but requires an external catheter. Endoprostheses have the advantage of avoiding external catheters, but their use is limited by prosthesis migration and side hole obstruction by biliary sludge, which mandate repeat endoscopy for manipulation or replacement. Nonoperative palliation of duodenal obstruction, which occurs in up to one third of patients, can be difficult, with very limited possibilities for success with the use of systemic chemotherapy or external beam radiotherapy. High-grade duodenal obstruction generally requires operative intervention for gastroenterostomy.

OPERATIVE THERAPY. The majority of patients with periampullary carcinoma are managed operatively. Preoperative preparation includes (1) assessment and supplementation of nutritional status, (2) standard mechanical and oral antibiotic bowel preparation, (3) assessment of coagulation status with correction of prolonged prothrombin time by exogenous vitamin K, (4) intravenous antibiotic prophylaxis administered perioperatively to reduce the possibility of a wound infection, and (5) consideration of placement of a percutaneous transhepatic catheter for preoperative decompression of the biliary tree, intraoperative use during the dissection, and postoperative decompression of the biliary-enteric anastomosis. Catheter drainage of the biliary tree appears best applied in patients with biliary sepsis secondary to cholangitis or in patients with major nutritional deficiency states and high-grade biliary obstruction. Randomized, prospective studies have shown that routine percutaneous transhepatic biliary drainage does not reduce operative mortality and may prolong hospital stay.

Resectional Therapy. At exploration, care is taken to assess distant intra-abdominal metastases. Hepatic metastases, serosal implants, and lymph node metastases outside of the resection area indicate unresectable disease. The duodenum and head of the pancreas are elevated from the retroperitoneum, lifting these structures off the inferior vena cava and the aorta (Kocher maneuver). The superior mesenteric artery is palpated for the purpose of ensuring that the vessel is not encased by tumor extending from the uncinate process. The common bile duct is isolated in the porta hepatis, as is the anterior surface of the portal vein, and the hepatic artery. At the inferior aspect of the neck of the pancreas the anterior surface of the superior mesenteric vein is identified. The plane between the neck of the pancreas and the anterior surface of the superior mesenteric vein is developed, fully elevating the pancreatic neck from the vein. If no tumor is encountered outside of the resection margin during these maneuvers, resection is performed. The role of intraoperative biopsy to obtain a tissue diagnosis prior to resection remains controversial. Benign periampullary lesions presenting as solid periampullary masses in patients in their sixth and seventh decades causing pain, weight loss, and jaundice are unusual; therefore, few resections are performed for benign disease in this setting. If resection is performed and the permanent pathology reveals chronic pancreatitis, the resection remains appropriate and effective therapy. Currently, for all patients explored with curative intent for a preoperative diagnosis of periampullary carcinoma, the resectability rate approaches 35 to 40 per cent. The resectability rate is lowest for adenocarcinoma of the head of the pancreas (15 to 20 per cent), is approximately 80 per cent for ampullary carcinoma, and averages 60 per cent for duodenal and distal common bile duct tumors. Preoperative staging using MRI, visceral angiography, and/or preoperative laparoscopy can significantly improve these resectability rates.[16]

The first successful resection of a periampullary carcinoma was performed by Halsted at the Johns Hopkins Hospital in 1898.[24] He performed a local resection of an ampullary tumor. Presently, standard resection for periampullary carcinoma involves a pancreaticoduodenectomy, first described by Whipple in 1935.[55] The gallbladder, common bile duct, entire duodenum, head of the pancreas to the level of the superior mesenteric vein, pylorus, and distal stomach are resected (Fig. 15). Restoration of gastrointestinal tract continuity utilizes the proximal jejunum brought through the transverse mesocolon for pancreaticojejunostomy, hepaticojejunostomy, and gastrojejunostomy. The standard Whipple resection remains the classic therapy for periampullary carcinoma and can be successfully

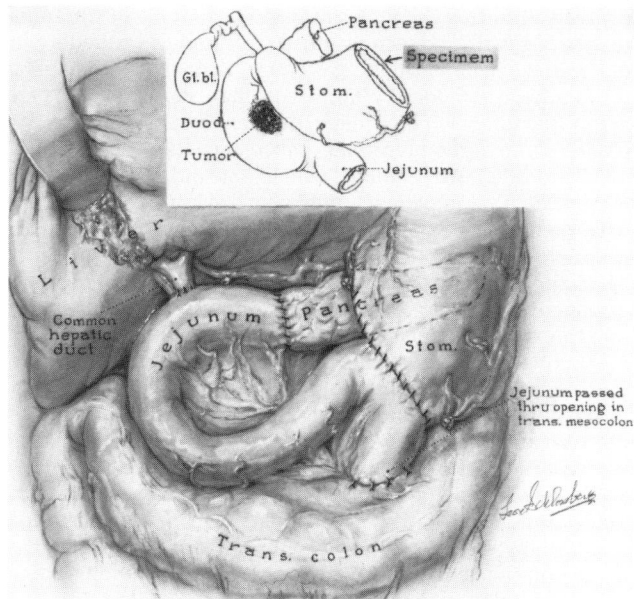

Figure 15. Illustration of a standard pancreaticoduodenectomy (Whipple procedure) and the subsequent reconstruction. The inset at the top depicts the resected specimen. (From Cameron, J. L.: Current status of the Whipple operation for periampullary carcinoma. Surg. Rounds, September: 77, 1988.)

performed in experienced hands with a perioperative mortality of less than 5 per cent. A modification of the standard Whipple resection, the pylorus-preserving pancreaticoduodenectomy (Fig. 16), has gained popularity in recent years. This modification eliminates gastric resection and leaves a 2-cm. cuff of duodenum for enteric reconstruction as a duodenojejunostomy. Operative time is shortened somewhat, and the incidence of postgastrectomy complications such as dumping and marginal ulceration associated with the standard Whipple procedure are

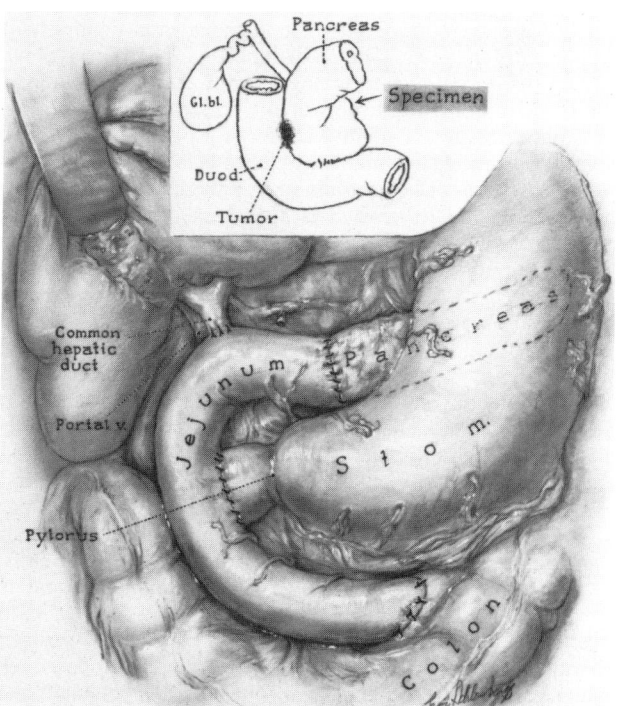

Figure 16. Illustration of a pylorus-preserving pancreaticoduodenectomy and the subsequent reconstruction. The inset at the top depicts the resected specimen. (From Cameron, J. L.: Current status of the Whipple operation for periampullary carcinoma. Surg. Rounds, September: 77, 1988.)

reduced. A further theoretic advantage is that the postprandial release of gastrin and secretin are nearly normal in patients who undergo the pylorus-saving procedure, compared with patients who undergo a standard Whipple resection. Particularly in periampullary tumors of ampullary, duodenal, and distal bile duct origin, the pylorus-preserving pancreaticoduodenectomy appears indicated. Accumulated data to date indicate no compromise in survival in patients undergoing pylorus preservation.

Formerly, total pancreatectomy was proposed as a more appropriate operation for pancreatic carcinoma. Support was based on a reported 30 to 40 per cent incidence of multifocality of pancreatic cancer, a concern about tumor cell implantation into the remnant pancreatic duct at Whipple resection, and the high mortality and morbidity associated with the pancreaticojejunostomy required in the Whipple reconstruction. It now appears that concerns about tumor seeding and multicentricity are not relevant, because the 5-year survival rate in patients who undergo the classic total pancreatectomy is equivalent to that in patients who undergo Whipple resection. Also, improved techniques and postoperative management have made pancreaticojejunostomy safer. Total pancreatectomy necessarily removes all exocrine and endocrine pancreatic function, requiring exogenous pancreatic enzyme and insulin administration.

At present the overall 5-year survival rate for all patients with resected periampullary carcinoma approximates 15 to 25 per cent. A major determinant of survival is the site of origin of the tumor. Resectable cancers of the duodenum, distal bile duct, and ampulla are associated with 5-year survival rates of 40 to 60 per cent, whereas resectable carcinoma of the head of the pancreas is associated with a 5-year survival rate of 5 to 20 per cent. Other determinants of survival in patients with adenocarcinoma of the head of the pancreas following resection include lymph node status and intraoperative blood transfusion requirements. In a recent review from the Johns Hopkins Hospital of patients with adenocarcinoma of the head of the pancreas undergoing Whipple resection, the actuarial 5-year survival rate approached 50 per cent for patients with negative lymph nodes, compared with less than 5 per cent for patients with one or more positive lymph nodes.[15] In addition, an inverse relationship was found between intraoperative blood transfusion requirements and the survival rate.[13] The median postoperative survival was 36 months for patients receiving 2 or fewer units of blood, as compared with 10 months for patients receiving 3 or more units.

Palliative Surgery. Palliative surgery for periampullary carcinoma is performed in patients with unresectable disease discovered at the time of laparotomy or in patients with prohibitive risk for resectional therapy (advanced age, limited cardiopulmonary reserve, and so forth) whose symptoms are poorly alleviated nonoperatively. Palliative surgery seeks to alleviate biliary obstruction, duodenal obstruction, and tumor-associated pain. Multiple authors have extensively reviewed the results of palliative operations for unresectable periampullary cancer. Biliary obstruction is treated with biliary-enteric bypass, by means of the gallbladder or the common hepatic duct. Although symptomatic gastroduodenal obstruction is uncommon at initial diagnosis of periampullary cancer, up to one third of patients with unresectable tumors develop obstructive symptoms prior to death. For this reason, gastrojejunostomy is usually performed at the time of biliary bypass. Prophylactic gastrojejunostomy does not add to the morbidity or mortality of palliative surgery for unresectable disease. Abdominal and back pain associated with unresectable periampullary tumors can be a major problem. Chemical splanchnicectomy using either 6 per cent phenol or 50 per cent alcohol can be performed intraoperatively in an effort to achieve pain control with reported benefit in over 80 per cent of patients, although controlled studies of this technique are absent.

ADJUVANT THERAPY. Chemotherapy alone currently has no role after curative resection or palliative therapy of periampullary carcinoma. Single-agent therapy with 5-fluorouracil, mitomycin C, streptozotocin, or high-dose methotrexate yields partial response rates of 10 to 20 per cent, but it does not prolong survival. While combination drug therapy appears to improve response rates in carefully selected patients, there has been no significant improvement in survival demonstrated for any chemotherapeutic regimens.

The combination of radiation and chemotherapy has been shown to prolong survival following curative Whipple resection. In a controlled prospective trial reported by the Gastrointestinal Tumor Study Group (GITSG), patients receiving 40 Gy external beam radiation therapy (EBRT) and weekly intravenous 5-fluorouracil following curative resection demonstrated a significantly longer median survival (20 months), compared with the resected group receiving no adjuvant therapy (11 months).[28] In this study, the 2-year actuarial survival was 42 per cent in the treated group versus 15 per cent for the control group. A follow-up study by the GITSG confirmed improved survival with combination radiation and chemotherapy.[23]

Results of adjuvant treatment of unresectable periampullary cancer are not as promising as for resectable tumors. The median survival in patients with unresectable tumors is approximately 6 to 9 months. EBRT alone does not prolong survival. The combination of EBRT with chemotherapy, usually 5-fluorouracil, has yielded mixed results on overall survival, with several reports suggesting improved outcome, compared to EBRT alone and others showing no advantage. In an effort to boost the irradiation dose delivered directly to unresectable tumors, several studies of intraoperative radiation therapy (IORT) have been undertaken. IORT alone does not improve survival. IORT in combination with EBRT with or without chemotherapy has had conflicting results, with most studies showing improved local control of the tumor but little improvement in long-term survival.

Carcinoma of the Body and Tail of the Pancreas

Adenocarcinomas of the body and tail of the pancreas represent up to 30 per cent of all cases of pancreatic carcinoma. Tumors in this location generally grow to large size prior to the development of symptoms. This silent course occurs as a result of the retroperitoneal location of the body and tail of the pancreas away from the common bile duct and duodenum. Thus, these tumors do not cause early obstructive jaundice or gastrointestinal obstructive symptoms.

The clinical presentation of patients with carcinoma of the body and tail of the pancreas generally involves weight loss and pain, which are present in up to 90 per cent of patients. Weight loss may be significant, often involving up to 20 per cent of the patient's body weight. Because of the distance between the primary tumor and the intrapancreatic portion of the common bile duct, less than 10 per cent of patients present with jaundice. On physical examination, the findings are often nonspecific. Vague abdominal tenderness may be present, or an abdominal mass may be palpated. Evidence of metastatic dissemination may be found and can include hepatomegaly, ascites, a Blumer's shelf, or lymph node metastases to Virchow's nodes.

The diagnosis of carcinoma of the body and tail of the pancreas depends upon radiographic assessment. Serum tests for tumor-associated antigens such as CEA and CA 19–9 are usually positive with large tumors, but they may be negative. The abdominal CT scan is the best initial radiographic study (Fig. 17). The CT scan can demonstrate the primary tumor in the pancreas, be used for assessment for liver metastases, and may give information regarding involvement of adjacent visceral and vascular structures or lymph node metastases. Endoscopic retrograde pancreatography usually documents a pancreatic duct abnormality. The most common abnormality on ERCP is a pancreatic duct cutoff, representing obstruction to the flow of

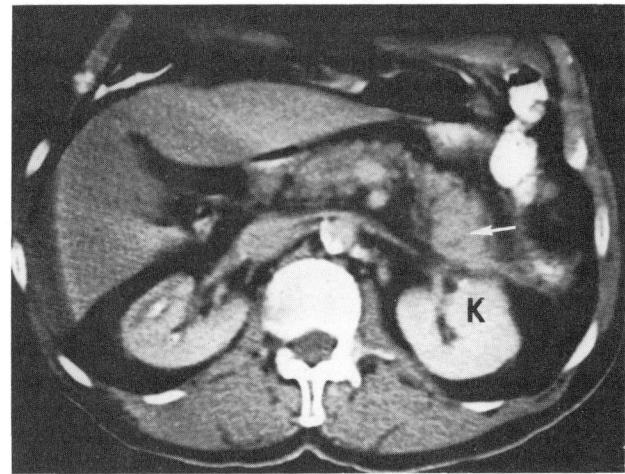

Figure 17. CT scan of a patient with adenocarcinoma of the body and tail of the pancreas. The tumor (arrow) is seen anterior and adjacent to the left kidney (K). At operation the tumor was invading Gerota's fascia.

contrast material by the neoplasm. The proximal pancreatic duct is generally normal. In the absence of prior abdominal trauma and an otherwise normal pancreatogram, a finding such as stenosis or obstruction of the pancreatic duct in the region of the body or tail of the pancreas is highly suggestive of a pancreatic neoplasm.

Following the radiographic identification of an abnormality in the body or tail of the pancreas, accurate tissue diagnosis is indicated. The necessity for tissue diagnosis arises from the need to differentiate pancreatic adenocarcinoma, which is rarely resectable in this region, from more favorable neoplasms such as pancreatic islet cell tumors or benign pancreatic neoplasms, which are often resectable. Tissue diagnosis may be obtained at laparotomy or via percutaneous needle aspiration of the primary mass. Prior to laparotomy, visceral arteriography may be helpful. Evaluation of the celiac axis, splenic artery and vein, and superior mesenteric artery and vein is performed. Splenic artery or vein involvement by tumor does not preclude curative resection. However, tumor involvement of the main trunk of the celiac axis, superior mesenteric artery, or superior mesenteric vein usually indicates unresectability. Good risk patients without evidence of metastatic disease and with favorable arteriographic findings are best served by abdominal exploration with the intent of tumor resection. In the unusual patient with a resectable adenocarcinoma, distal pancreatectomy and *en bloc* splenectomy provide an opportunity for cure and serve as good palliation of tumor-associated pain. In patients with unresectable disease diagnosed at laparotomy, intraoperative chemical splanchnicectomy can be used to palliate pain. In the majority of patients with carcinoma of the body and tail of the pancreas, biliary bypass and duodenal bypass are not indicated. However, a proportion of patients with carcinoma of the body and tail of the pancreas have tumor encroachment at the level of the duodenojejunal junction, and this small group of patients may be well served by a palliative gastroenterostomy. Poor-risk patients or those with evidence of metastatic or clearly unresectable tumors by CT scan or arteriography are not explored and instead undergo percutaneous biopsy for tissue diagnosis.

The resectability rate for carcinoma of the body and tail of the pancreas is low (less than 7 per cent), and the prognosis is generally dismal (mean survival, 5 to 6 months). The few reported 5-year survivors following resection have had their tumors discovered as incidental findings during evaluation of other intra-abdominal pathology. Patients undergoing resection of adenocarcinoma of the body and tail of the pancreas with curative intent may be benefited by adjuvant chemotherapy and postoperative external beam radiation therapy, al-

though confirmatory data are lacking. Unresectable tumors respond poorly to radiation or chemotherapy.

Cystadenocarcinoma of the Pancreas

Cystadenocarcinoma generally arises in females between the ages of 40 and 60, and it represents less than 2 per cent of all pancreatic exocrine neoplasms. Cystadenocarcinomas often present as cystic masses in the body and tail of the pancreas, associated with abdominal and back pain. CT scan of the abdomen typically reveals a tumor mass with associated cysts, which may be misinterpreted as representing a pancreatic pseudocyst. Histologically, these cystic tumors are lined with an epithelium with disordered columnar cells associated with mucin production and papillary features. When this diagnosis is suspected by CT scan, and in the absence of distant metastases, resectability is assessed by arteriography. Tissue diagnosis in patients with metastatic or unresectable disease may be obtained by percutaneous biopsy. Patients without evidence of metastatic or unresectable disease are candidates for exploration. At the time of laparotomy it may be impossible to distinguish between a malignant cystadenocarcinoma and a benign cystadenoma. Resectable lesions in the body and tail of the pancreas are treated by distal pancreatectomy and *en bloc* splenectomy. Resectable lesions in the head of the pancreas, which are less common, are treated by pancreaticoduodenectomy. The long-term survival rate for resected cystadenocarcinomas approaches 50 per cent, greatly in excess of the rate for the more common pancreatic ductal adenocarcinoma.

Acinar Cell Carcinoma of the Pancreas

This is a rare malignancy of the pancreas that has no sexual predominance. These tumors are usually discovered when large in size and are associated with weight loss and pain. Histologically, they consist of epithelium with tall cylindric cells, containing an eosinophilic cytoplasm with periodic acid–Schiff (PAS) positivity in their apical regions. Electron microscopy reveals classic features of intracellular zymogen granules. These tumors are diagnosed, assessed for resectability, and managed as pancreatic ductal adenocarcinomas in the same fashion.

BENIGN NEOPLASMS OF THE EXOCRINE PANCREAS

Cystadenoma

The majority of cystic lesions of the pancreas are pancreatic pseudocysts. Cystadenomas comprise less than 10 per cent of cystic pancreatic lesions, with a predilection for middle-aged and older women. It is frequently difficult to differentiate between benign and malignant cystic neoplasms of the pancreas based upon clinical, radiographic, or gross pathologic findings. Symptoms are often vague and may include abdominal pain, gastrointestinal obstructive symptoms, or, rarely, obstructive jaundice. Grossly, these tumors appear as large multilobulated cystic masses. Histologically, they have a characteristic lining epithelium incorporating papillary projections with branching villous processes. These tumors have no malignant potential, and patients are therefore cured by appropriate resection. Because it may be difficult to distinguish this benign neoplasm from the more common pancreatic pseudocyst both radiographically or intraoperatively, biopsy of all pancreatic cystic structures is indicated at the time of definitive therapy.

Solid and Papillary Neoplasms of the Pancreas

These unusual tumors have a notable female predominance and usually are found in patients between 10 and 35 years of age. Most occur in the body or tail of the gland. These tumors tend to grow to a large size, evidence of local invasion being observed frequently. On gross examination these neoplasms are large, rounded masses often containing hemorrhagic areas. Histologic findings reveal a mixture of solid, papillary, and micro-

TABLE 9. Classification of Functional Pancreatic Endocrine Tumors

Tumor Name	Major Hormone(s)	Cell Type	Syndrome	Malignancy Rate	Extrapancreatic Location
Insulinoma	Insulin	Beta-cell	Hypoglycemia	<15%	Rare
Gastrinoma (Zollinger-Ellison syndrome)	Gastrin	Non-beta-cell	Peptic ulcer Diarrhea	50%	Frequent
VIPoma (Verner-Morrison syndrome)	VIP Prostaglandins	Non-beta-cell	Watery diarrhea Hypokalemia Achlorhydria	Majority	Occasional
Glucagonoma	Glucagon	Alpha-cell	Hyperglycemia Dermatitis	Majority	Rare
Somatostatinoma	Somatostatin	Delta-cell	Hyperglycemia Steatorrhea	Majority	Rare

cystic changes with cystic degeneration. These tumors are potentially curable by resection, and most patients have long-term survival. Appropriate pancreatic resection involves distal pancreatectomy for lesions of the body and tail of the pancreas and pancreaticoduodenectomy for lesions of the head.

ENDOCRINE TUMORS

Endocrine tumors of the pancreas are rare, with an annual clinically recognized incidence of 5 per 1 million population. In contrast, the prevalence of these tumors in unselected autopsy material approximates 1 per 100 where they are usually noted as incidental findings. Pancreatic endocrine cells are presumed to originate from neural crest cells. Cells of this origin are termed APUD cells, indicating that they have a high content of *a*mine, have capacity for amine *p*recursor *u*ptake, and contain an amino acid *d*ecarboxylase. A generalized derangement of the APUD system may cause abnormalities of multiple endocrine cells, as is observed in the multiple endocrine neoplasia (MEN) syndromes.

Functional endocrine tumors of the pancreas are conventionally named according to the major hormone produced by the tumor (Table 9). The majority (more than 75 per cent) of tumors discovered *pre mortem* are functional and elaborate one or more hormonal products into the bloodstream. Patients with normal serum levels of hormones and no recognized clinical manifestations who have pancreatic endocrine tumors are considered to have nonfunctional islet cell tumors.

All endocrine tumors of the pancreas have a similar light microscopic appearance. Routine histologic examination does not predict the biologic behavior or endocrine manifestations of these neoplasms. Immunofluorescence techniques and the peroxidase-antiperoxidase procedure allow demonstration of specific hormones within tumor cells. Malignancy is determined by the presence of local invasion, spread to regional lymph nodes, or the existence of hepatic or distant metastases.

The general principles applicable to the management of patients with suspected functional pancreatic endocrine tumors involve first, the recognition of the abnormal physiology or characteristic syndrome; second, the detection of hormone elevations in serum by radioimmunoassay; and third, the localization and staging of the tumor in preparation for operative therapy. Characteristic clinical syndromes have been well described for insulinoma, gastrinoma, VIPoma and glucagonoma. Radioimmunoassay is widely available for measurement of serum insulin, gastrin, VIP, and glucagon. Less widely available are the assays for somatostatin, PP, prostaglandins, and other hormonal markers. The standard radiographic techniques used for pancreatic endocrine tumor localization include CT scanning

with intravenous and oral contrast, visceral angiography, transhepatic portal venous sampling, and intraoperative ultrasonography. The place of MRI in the evaluation of pancreatic islet cell tumors remains to be defined. The accuracy of the CT scan in detecting the primary tumor within the pancreas varies from 35 to 85 per cent and is largely based on the size of the tumor. Larger lesions are more easily detectable (Fig. 18). The CT scan is also used in evaluation for hepatic metastases. In a patient with biochemical documentation of hormone excess, particularly for insulinoma and gastrinoma, it is not uncommon for the CT scan to be normal. The next step in radiographic assessment involves visceral angiography. The angiogram is particularly useful in identifying an enhancing tumor blush in lesions less than 1 cm. in size not demonstrated by CT scan (Fig. 19). Tumors not visualized by CT scan or angiography may be localized by means of transhepatic portal venous sampling. In experienced hands, this technique appears safe and useful, based on the ability to demonstrate a step-up in hormone concentration at the portal venous drainage site of the primary tumor. With the use of the combination of CT scan, angiography, and portal venous sampling, over 80 per cent of pancreatic endocrine tumors can be localized preoperatively. If the primary tumor cannot be localized and there is no biochemical question about the diagnosis, exploratory surgery is indicated.

At exploration, a thorough evaluation of the pancreas and

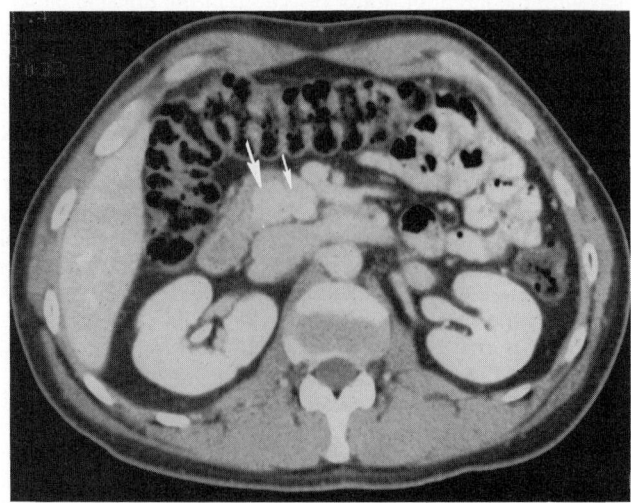

Figure 18. Contrast-enhanced CT scan of a patient with a malignant insulinoma of the head and uncinate process of the pancreas. The 3-cm. tumor (large arrow) lies adjacent to the superior mesenteric vein (small arrow). The tumor was resected by pylorus-preserving pancreaticoduodenectomy, and the hyperinsulinism was cured.

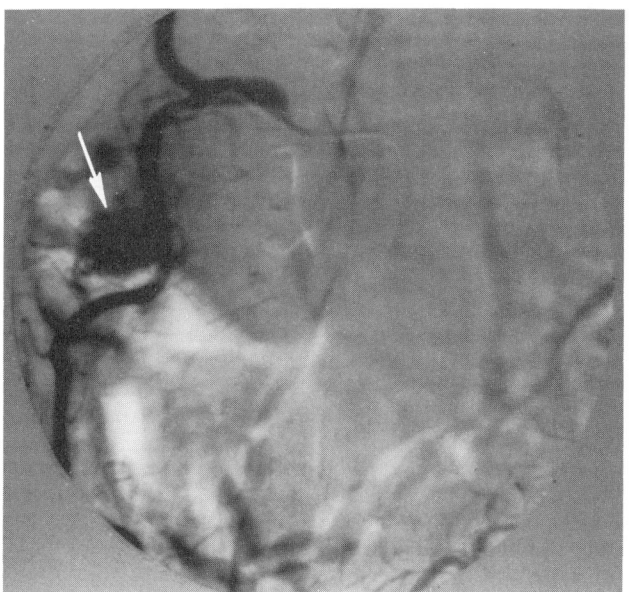

Figure 19. Selective celiac arteriogram in a patient with the Zollinger-Ellison syndrome. The hepatic artery injection fills the gastroduodenal artery, which reveals a tumor blush (arrow) in the region of the duodenum or head of the pancreas. At exploration a 2-cm. benign duodenal gastrinoma was identified and locally resected.

peripancreatic region is undertaken. The pancreatic head is assessed bimanually by means of the Kocher maneuver, and the body and tail are explored by dividing the gastrocolic ligament and the peritoneum at the inferior pancreatic margin. The liver is carefully assessed for evidence of hepatic metastases. Tumors are sought at common extrapancreatic sites, such as the duodenum, small bowel mesentery, and lymph nodes. Small pancreatic lesions may be difficult to detect by bimanual palpitation alone, and intraoperative real-time ultrasound may assist in their identification. The distribution of pancreatic endocrine tumors varies, gastrinomas, somatostatinomas, and PPomas most commonly found in the head of the gland and insulinomas and glucagonomas tending to be evenly distributed throughout the pancreas. The goals of surgical therapy for pancreatic islet cell tumors include control of symptoms due to hormone excess, excision of maximal neoplastic tissue, and prevention of tumor recurrence. Operative strategies vary for the different tumors.

Insulinoma

The most common endocrine tumor of the pancreas is the insulinoma. The first recognition of the insulinoma syndrome is attributed to Whipple and associates.[56] Insulinoma is associated with Whipple's triad, which consists of (1) symptoms of hypoglycemia at fasting, (2) documentation of blood glucose levels of less than 50 mg. per 100 ml., and (3) relief of symptoms following administration of glucose. Insulinomas synthesize and secrete insulin autonomously in the presence of low blood glucose levels, causing spontaneous hypoglycemia and characteristic clinical symptoms. These symptoms can be categorized into two groups: hypoglycemia-induced catecholamine-surge symptoms (tremor, irritability, weakness, diaphoresis, tachycardia, and hunger) and neuroglycopenic symptoms (personality change, confusion, obtundation, seizure, and coma). Typically, the relief of symptoms is achieved by the consumption of carbohydrate-rich foods.

In an adult population, the differential diagnosis of hypoglycemia includes functional hypoglycemia associated with gastrectomy or gastroenterostomy, chronic adrenal insufficiency, hypopituitarism, extensive hepatic insufficiency, surreptitious administration of insulin or ingestion of sulfonylureas, and reactive hypoglycemia. Of these diagnoses, reactive hypoglyce-

mia is the most common, normally causing symptoms 3 to 5 hours after meals and not associated with fasting hypoglycemia.

The most reliable method for diagnosing insulinomas involves a monitored 72-hour fast. Blood for glucose and insulin determinations is sampled every 4 to 6 hours during the fast and particularly when symptoms develop. Symptomatic hypoglycemia with fasting is usually associated with concurrent serum insulin levels greater than 25 μU. per ml. Additional support for the diagnosis of insulinoma is derived from the calculation of the insulin-to-glucose ratio. Normal values are less than 0.3, whereas nearly all patients with insulinomas demonstrate insulin to glucose ratios greater than 0.4 after an overnight fast. C peptide and proinsulin are synthesized in excess along with insulin by insulinoma cells. C peptide and proinsulin levels are usually elevated in the presence of insulinoma, while they are low in patients self-administering insulin. Further support for the diagnosis of insulinoma is obtained by screening for the possibility of surreptitious insulin or sulfonylurea administration. Sulfonylureas are a group of oral hypoglycemic agents that stimulate insulin secretion and are used for the treatment of non–insulin-dependent adult-onset diabetes. The presence of sulfonylureas can be assessed by serum screening.

Following biochemical diagnosis and appropriate localization studies, the treatment of insulinoma is surgical. Up to 90 per cent of patients have benign solitary pancreatic adenomas amenable to surgical cure. Malignant insulinoma is present in 10 to 15 per cent of cases.

At the time of exploration, insulinomas are found evenly distributed throughout the pancreas, with one third located in the head, one third in the body, and one third in the tail. Small benign adenomas not in proximity to the pancreatic duct, located anywhere in the gland may be enucleated (Fig. 20). In the body and tail of the gland, larger benign lesions or those in proximity to the pancreatic duct are usually excised by distal pancreatectomy. Large benign lesions in the head of the pancreas, not amenable to local excision, may be resected by pancreaticoduodenectomy. If at the time of exploration no tumor is identified, a blind distal pancreatic resection to the level of the superior mesenteric vein is recommended, in the hope of excising a previously unidentified adenoma.

In cases of malignant insulinoma, resection of the primary tumor and accessible metastases should be considered. Such resections may include distal pancreatectomy for lesions of the body and tail of the gland or pancreaticoduodenectomy for resectable lesions of the head of the gland. Tumor debulking may be helpful in reducing hypoglycemic symptoms in patients not well controlled by medical therapy preoperatively. Pharmacologic therapy may be useful in patients with residual tumor following resection where symptomatic hypoglycemia is not avoided by frequent feedings. Diazoxide, in doses of 600 and 1000 mg. per day, can improve hypoglycemic symptoms because of its ability to directly inhibit the release of insulin from beta cells. Salt and water retention following diazoxide therapy can be improved by the use of a thiazide diuretic, which also has a synergistic effect in improving hypoglycemia via inhibition of insulin secretion. As with other pancreatic islet cell tumors, there is evidence to support the use of adjuvant chemotherapy or hormonal therapy in patients with unresectable disease (e.g., streptozotocin, octreotide).

Gastrinoma (Zollinger-Ellison Syndrome)

Following the first report of an islet cell tumor of the pancreas associated with peptic ulcer disease in 1946,[44] Zollinger and Ellison in 1955 described 2 patients with florid peptic ulcer disease and pancreatic islet cell tumors.[61] The diagnostic triad proposed for this syndrome at that time included (1) the presence of primary peptic ulcerations in unusual locations, (2) gastric hypersecretion of gigantic proportion persisting despite ad-

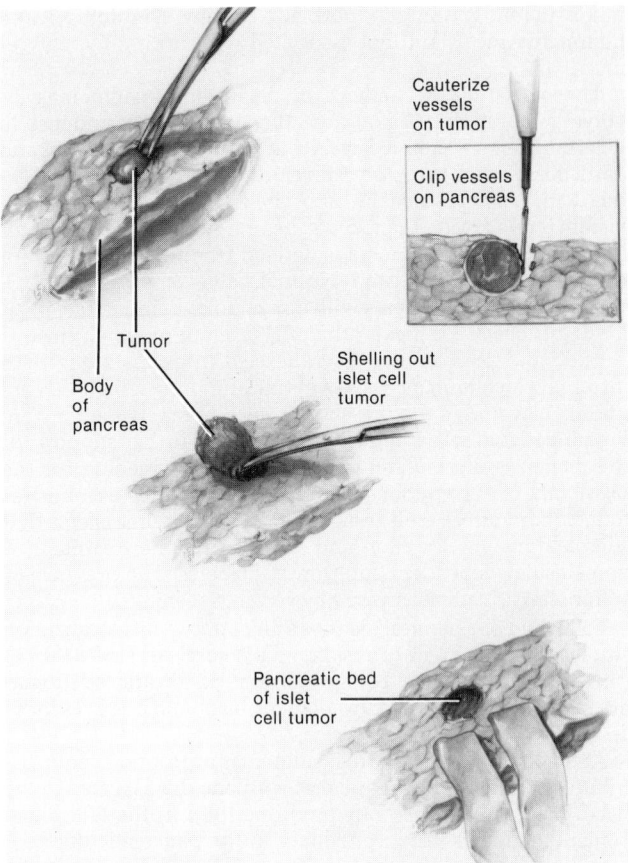

Figure 20. Technique used for enucleation of a benign insulinoma, using the scissors (top left and center) or the electrocautery (top right). After enucleation, the site of tumor excision is drained (bottom right). (From Cameron, J. L.: Atlas of Surgery. Vol. 1. Toronto, B. C. Decker, 1990, p. 441.)

equate therapy, and (3) the identification of an islet cell tumor of the pancreas. In the intervening decades, much information has accumulated regarding these gastrin-secreting tumors and the associated Zollinger-Ellison syndrome.[1,59] It is estimated that 0.1 per cent of patients with primary duodenal ulcer disease and up to 2 per cent of patients with recurrent ulcers following standard ulcer therapy may harbor a gastrinoma. Seventy-five per cent of gastrinomas occur sporadically, in the absence of other endocrinopathies, whereas 25 per cent are associated with the MEN-I syndrome (hyperparathyroidism and pituitary tumors). Formerly, over 60 per cent of gastrinomas were regarded as malignant on the basis of the findings of metastatic disease at the time of laparotomy. More recent information suggests that as screening for hypergastrinemia becomes more widespread, the diagnosis of gastrinoma is being made earlier, with discovery of a higher percentage of solitary, benign curable tumors.

Clinical manifestations of gastrinoma are nearly exclusively related to hypergastrinema. Peptic ulceration of the upper gastrointestinal tract and abdominal pain are the most common findings, occurring in 90 per cent of patients. While the finding of postbulbar duodenal ulcers is suggestive of the Zollinger-Ellison syndrome, the most frequently found ulcer is in the duodenal bulb. Diarrhea occurs in up to 50 per cent of patients, and 10 per cent of patients present with diarrhea as the sole manifestation of the syndrome. The diarrhea observed in patients with gastrinoma arises as a result of gastric hypersecretion, and it can be eliminated by nasogastric suction. A history compatible with peptic esophageal injury can be obtained in up to 10 per cent of patients, representing acid injury to the esophagus as a result of gastroesophageal reflux.

The diagnosis of gastrinoma requires a proper level of suspicion in several clinical settings (Table 10). When suspected, fasting serum gastrin levels should be obtained. In patients with gastrinoma, the fasting serum gastrin level is usually elevated above the normal range of 100 to 200 pg. per ml. A fasting gastrin over 1000 pg. per ml. is generally diagnostic of gastrinoma when accompanied by well-established acid peptic disease or hyperchlorhydria. Many patients with gastrinomas have fasting gastrin values in an intermediate range of 200 to 1000 pg. per ml. The documentation of fasting hypergastrinemia alone is not sufficient for diagnosis. Gastrin is the normal secretory product of antral G cells, and hypergastrinemia may exist in other pathophysiologic states, both ulcerogenic and nonulcerogenic (Table 11). Identification of the correct cause of hypergastrinemia utilizes knowledge of the clinical setting as well as two additional diagnostic modalities: gastric acid analysis and provocative testing.

Gastric acid analysis differentiates ulcerogenic from nonulcerogenic states. The analysis is performed after stopping antisecretory medications and allows the measurement of the basal acid output (BAO) and the maximal acid output (MAO). A BAO in excess of 15 mEq. per hour in nonoperated patients or in excess of 5 mEq. per hour in patients with previous acid-reducing operations supports the diagnosis of gastrinoma. A BAO/MAO ratio in excess of 0.6 provides additional support for the diagnosis.

Provocative testing should be employed when the diagnosis is considered, particularly in patients with fasting gastrin levels in the range of 200 to 1000 pg. per ml. Provocative testing can be helpful in differentiating between gastrinoma, antral G-cell hyperplasia/hyperfunction, and other causes of ulcerogenic hypergastrinemia. Secretin has supplanted calcium as the provocative agent of choice. The test is performed after an overnight fast, by administering 2 units of Kabi secretin per kilogram of body weight as an intravenous bolus and obtaining serum samples for gastrin for up to 30 minutes. An absolute increase in the gastrin level of 200 pg. per ml. over the baseline level is diagnostic of gastrinoma. Patients with antral G-cell hyperplasia/hyperfunction have a flat gastrin response to secretin. The gastrin response to a test meal is additionally helpful in distinguishing the causes of ulcerogenic hypergastrinemia. In the fasting state, serum gastrin levels are measured before and at 15-minute intervals for 1 hour after a test meal. Patients with gastrinoma have little to no postprandial change in serum gastrin (a less than 50 per cent increase over basal), whereas patients with antral G-cell hyperfunction have a greater than 100 per cent increase in serum gastrin.

After the diagnosis of gastrinoma, patient management follows two distinct, yet interrelated, pathways: (1) control of gastrin acid hypersecretion and (2) alteration of the natural history of the gastrinoma (i.e., tumor localization, assessment of metastatic disease, and resection of localized tumor for cure). Formerly, patients with gastrinoma died of complications from overwhelming gastric acid hypersecretion. At that time, total gastrectomy provided the most reliable means of controlling the ulcer diathesis without effect on the natural history of the gas-

TABLE 10. Diagnosis: Suspect and Screen for Gastrin

Initial diagnosis of peptic ulcer disease
Recurrent peptic ulcer
Failure of medical therapy for peptic ulcer
Postoperative peptic ulcer
Postbulbar peptic ulcer
Family history of peptic ulcer
Peptic ulcer and diarrhea
Prolonged undiagnosed diarrhea
MEN-I kindred
Known nongastrinoma pancreatic endocrine tumor
Prominent gastric rugal folds on upper gastrointestinal series

TABLE 11. Disease States Associated with Hypergastrinemia

Ulcerogenic (Hyperchlorhydric)	Nonulcerogenic (Nonhyperchlorhydric)
Zollinger-Ellison syndrome	Postvagotomy
Retained excluded antrum	Pernicious anemia
Gastric outlet obstruction	Atrophic gastritis
Antral G-cell hyperplasia/hyperfunction	Short-gut syndrome
	Renal failure

trinoma. Since the advent of powerful antisecretory medications such as histamine H_2-receptor antagonists and substituted benzimidazoles, the pharmacologic control of gastric acid hypersecretion has improved and total gastrectomy is rarely indicated. However, it is now recognized that tumor progression continues in the presence of antisecretory medications, and the majority of patients with unresected gastrinoma succumb to their neoplastic process. The current strategy for patients with gastrinoma, particularly those with "sporadic" gastrinomas not associated with the MEN-I syndrome, involves careful evaluation at initial diagnosis for potential curative resection.

Histamine H_2-receptor antagonists have been used successfully in the long-term management of acid hypersecretion in patients with gastrinoma. Failure rates for medical therapy range up to 60 per cent, with the major cause of failure being inadequate drug dosage. The appropriate dose of antisecretory medication should be determined for each patient by gastric acid analysis, since symptoms alone are not adequate for judging treatment efficacy. Patients not operated upon or patients with vagotomy alone are treated with sufficient antisecretory medications to lower gastric acid output to less than 10 mEq. per hour during the last hour before the next dose of the drug. In contrast, patients with previous distal gastrectomy require sufficient antisecretory medication to lower their gastric acid output to less than 5 mEq. per hour during the last hour before the next dose. The median doses of oral histamine H_2-receptor antagonists needed to achieve the proper reduction of gastric acid hypersecretion approximate 4 to 5 gm. per day for cimetidine, 1.5 to 3 gm. per day for ranitidine, and 0.3 gm. per day for famotidine. The pharmacologic approach to reduction of gastric acid hypersecretion has been recently improved by the introduction of a new class of antisecretory agents: the substituted benzimidazoles, of which omeprazole is currently available. Omeprazole acts to selectively inhibit the H^+-K^+-adenosine triphosphatase (proton pump) on the luminal surface of the gastric parietal cell. Omeprazole is effective in patients with gastrinoma either as primary treatment or in patients who are not well-controlled on high-dose histamine H_2-receptor antagonist therapy. Effective omeprazole doses have ranged from 40 mg. per day in a single dose to 160 mg. per day in two divided doses. The safety and efficacy of long-term omeprazole therapy remains to be established.

Prior to the advent of effective pharmacologic control of gastric acid hypersecretion, total gastrectomy was the therapy of choice in patients with gastrinoma, because it served as the best solution to the pathophysiologic state of hyperchlorhydria. Although total gastrectomy markedly diminished the mortality and morbidity from acid peptic disease, it was attended by an operative mortality of up to 15 per cent, caused partially by the need to operate on an emergent basis in patients with life-threatening complications of peptic ulcer. Although early reports suggested that total gastrectomy had a favorable impact on tumor progression in patients with unresected disease, this contention is no longer accepted. Total gastrectomy is now best reserved for patients with unresectable tumors who cannot or will not take adequate doses of antisecretory medications or whose gastric hypersecretion cannot be pharmacologically controlled. The operative mortality for total gastrectomy in elective settings is currently less than 2 per cent.

A lesser surgical procedure useful as an adjunct in the management of selected patients with Zollinger-Ellison syndrome is parietal cell vagotomy. Parietal cell vagotomy can reduce antisecretory drug requirements, and it is a safer, less morbid operation than total gastrectomy. At present, the role of parietal cell vagotomy in the management of gastrinoma patients remains controversial. Its use should be considered in three situations: (1) in the setting of a negative exploration for gastrinoma in a patient without past ulcer complications but whose gastric hypersecretion is inadequately controlled with antisecretory medications; (2) in the setting of a resectable gastrinoma in the pancreas or peripancreatic lymph nodes, where there is a moderately high "no cure" rate, in an effort to reduce antisecretory drug requirements if there is persistent postoperative hypergastrinemia; and (3) in the setting of unresectable disease in a patient adequately medically managed but on very high doses of antisecretory medication (i.e., cimetidine greater than 5 gm. per day or its equivalent).

After the institution of appropriate pharmacologic therapy to control gastric hypersecretion, all patients undergo radiographic studies in an effort to localize the primary tumor and to assess metastatic disease. Localization and staging by abdominal CT scanning, selective angiography, and selective venous sampling for gastrin have previously been discussed. Patients with radiographically suspected unresectable metastatic disease to the liver should undergo percutaneous biopsy for histologic verification. If unresectable metastatic tumor is documented, the patient is not explored and is maintained on antisecretory medication. In the absence of documented unresectable disease, all patients should undergo exploration with curative intent.

At the time of exploration the entire abdomen is carefully assessed, paying particular attention to the pancreas and to the known locations of extrapancreatic gastrinomas. Abnormal masses and peripancreatic lymph nodes are excised and submitted for frozen section. Intraoperative ultrasound may be valuable in identifying nonpalpable intrapancreatic disease. If no tumor is encountered, a longitudinal duodenotomy is performed at the second portion of the duodenum (Fig. 21), and the duodenum is bimanually palpated and carefully everted in a search for duodenal gastrinomas. Duodenal gastrinomas are typically submucosal in location, and they are resected with a small margin of normal duodenal tissue. Tumors within the pancreas are resected by enucleation or partial pancreatectomy. Tumors easily accessible to the pancreatic surface, small (less than 2 cm.), and well-encapsulated may be carefully enucleated. Larger tumors without defined capsules or situated deep in the pancreatic parenchyma usually require pancreatic resection. Tumors of the neck, body, and tail are treated by distal pancreatectomy; whereas tumors in the pancreatic head or uncinate process are resected by pancreaticoduodenectomy.

Despite extensive preoperative localization studies and meticulous surgical exploration, some patients with gastrinoma have no tumor demonstrable at laparotomy. The percentage of such patients varies from 5 to 40, depending on such factors as the security of the diagnosis, the availability and experience with localization techniques, the experience of the surgeon, and the use of blind resection based solely upon transhepatic portal venous sampling results. If exploration is negative, several alternatives are available to the operating surgeon, including clo-

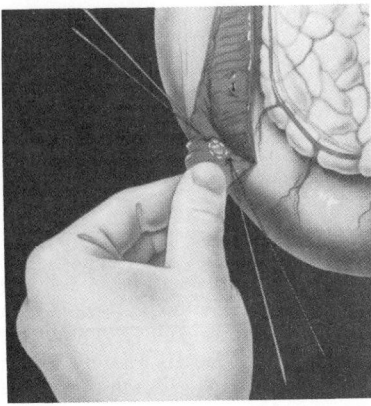

Figure 21. Illustration depicting a longitudinal duodenotomy used to identify a duodenal gastrinoma (indicated by dashed white circle) that is to be locally resected. (From Thompson, N. W., Vinik, A. I., and Eckhauser, F. E.: Microgastrinomas of the duodenum: A cause of failed operations for the Zollinger-Ellison syndrome. Ann. Surg., *209:*396, 1989.)

sure without intervention, parietal cell vagotomy, and total gastrectomy. Closure without intervention would appear appropriate in patients with controlled acid hypersecretion. Parietal cell vagotomy may be considered a means of reducing antisecretory drug requirements in patients on high-dose therapy but without previous life-threatening complications while taking appropriate pharmacologic treatment. Total gastrectomy appears best reserved for patients with past life-threatening complications of ulcer disease while under appropriate medical management.

Results of selected recent series of patients with gastrinoma treated surgically have been recently reviewed.[59] Of the 130 patients who underwent exploration, 81 per cent had tumor located at the time of operation, 19 per cent had a negative exploration, and 13 per cent had liver metastases unsuspected by various preoperative localization studies. Primary tumors were identified in 64 per cent of the patients explored and were distributed in the ratio of 4:2:3 (pancreatic, duodenal, and other). Thirty-five per cent of the patients who underwent exploration and resection were considered to have had surgical cures, as defined by fasting postoperative eugastrinemia, negative postoperative secretin stimulation testing, and negative imaging studies on follow-up. Considering only those patients who underwent exploration and who were thought to have had successful resection, the cure rate was 60 per cent. These results represent a major change in the management of these patients during the past several decades and support the practice of initial short-term pharmacologic control of gastric hypersecretion, followed by aggressive tumor localization and staging in anticipation of curative resection.

At present, the cause of death in the majority of gastrinoma patients is tumor growth and dissemination. Chemotherapy, hormonal therapy with octreotide, hepatic transplantation, hepatic embolization, and interferon have all been used in treating patients with unresectable or metastatic gastrinoma. The overall response to chemotherapy is poor. A recent prospective study of monthly cycles of streptozotocin, 3 gm. per cu. m., 5-fluorouracil, 1.2 gm. per cu. m., and doxorubicin, 40 mg. per cu. m., in patients with metastatic gastrinoma showed that 60 per cent of the patients failed to respond and that in the 40 per cent of patients with a response, no complete responses occurred. Survival rates have not been significantly altered by the use of chemotherapy. Hormonal therapy with the long-acting somatostatin analog octreotide has been reported to ameliorate symptoms, reduce hypergastrinemia, and diminish hyperchlorhydria in patients with metastatic gastrinoma. However, the role of octreotide, which must be parenterally administered, will probably remain limited, because adequate doses of oral

antisecretory medications can control hyperchlorhydria and acid peptic symptoms in most patients. Neither hepatic transplantation nor embolization therapy have proven benefit in the management of gastrinoma metastatic to the liver. Human leukocyte interferon has been used in small numbers of patients and has been reported to cause a 50 per cent reduction in tumor size or serum gastrin levels. Overall, further trials are awaited in an effort to define the proper role of these adjuvant therapies either alone or in combination in the management of patients with unresectable metastatic gastrinoma.

VIPoma (Verner-Morrison syndrome)

Verner and Morrison described two cases of islet cell tumor and diarrhea in 1958[52] and have been credited with the definition of the syndrome. Pancreatic islet cell tumors associated with watery diarrhea, hypokalemia, and either achlorhydria or hypochlorhydria (WDHA) can produce a variety of biologically active substances. The primary candidates for the active agent in this syndrome include vasoactive intestinal polypeptide (VIP) and prostaglandins. This syndrome has many names, including *Verner-Morrison syndrome*, *WDHA syndrome*, and *pancreatic cholera*.

Patients typically present with intermittent severe diarrhea, often of a watery nature. Unlike the diarrhea associated with the Zollinger-Ellison syndrome, the diarrhea in the WDHA syndrome is not relieved by nasogastric suction, since it represents a secretory diarrhea caused by elevated circulating hormones. Cutaneous flushing may be observed in some patients. Gastric analysis usually reveals hypochlorhydria, although patients usually respond to pentagastrin with an increase in acid production. The diagnosis is generally suspected on the basis of the clinical syndrome, and elevations in serum VIP or pancreatic polypeptide (a marker for islet cell tumors) may provide further support for the diagnosis.

Tumor localization and staging is performed by the standard tests used for endocrine tumors of the pancreas, as previously discussed. Preoperative preparation must include correction of fluid and electrolyte losses by volume and electrolyte replacement. The long-acting somatostatin analog, octreotide, has proven efficacious in reducing circulating VIP levels and controlling diarrhea in selected cases.

The definitive treatment of the WDHA syndrome is surgical excision of the tumor. Half of the reported cases have had evidence of malignancy, with documented tumor metastases outside of the confines of the pancreas. The majority of the tumors have been found in the body or tail of the pancreas. In less than 20 per cent of the cases, diffuse islet cell hyperplasia has been found as the etiology of the syndrome. If no tumor is found in the pancreas, a careful exploration of the retroperitoneum, including both adrenals, is performed. If no tumor is identified, subtotal pancreatectomy to the level of the superior mesenteric vein is considered. When the tumor is identified as incurable because of metastatic spread, palliative debulking of safely resectable tumor is indicated. In patients with symptomatic unresectable or recurrent tumor, indomethacin or octreotide therapy may be beneficial.

Glucagonoma

The hallmarks of the glucagonoma syndrome are mild diabetes and severe dermatitis. In addition, patients may demonstrate malnutrition, anemia, glossitis, hypocholesterolemia, hypoproteinemia, and venous thrombosis. The diabetes characteristic of this disorder is mild and only rarely associated with ketoacidosis. The characteristic skin rash (necrolytic migratory erythema) usually exhibits cyclic migrations, with spreading margins and a healing point of resolution within its center. It is typically located on the lower abdomen, perineum, perioral area, or feet. In patients with the syndrome, glucagon determinations usually show values in excess of 500 pg. per ml., with normal levels being less than 120 pg. per ml. Elevated basal insulin levels are also characteristic.

Preoperative management consists of treatment of the dermatitis and stabilization of the diabetes, with concurrent tumor localization and staging by means of standard tests. The dermatitis has been reported to improve with steroid and zinc therapy as well as with the institution of total parenteral nutrition.

Exploration is recommended in essentially all patients suspected of having glucagonoma. The majority of glucagonomas have been found in the body and tail of the pancreas and have tended to be large at the time of exploration. Metastases have been found in up to 80 per cent of patients, and complete resection has been possible in only 30 per cent. Tumor debulking is performed when feasible and safe and has been associated with a return to euglycemia and complete resolution of the dermatitis. Patients with incurable or recurrent disease have been treated with the chemotherapeutic agents streptozotocin and dacarbazine (DTIC) with some success. Hormonal therapy with octreotide has also been reported to control the hyperglycemia and dermatitis.

Somatostatinoma

The somatostatinoma syndrome, encompassing the presence of gallstones, diabetes, and steatorrhea, was first described by Ganda and associates in 1977[22] and shortly thereafter by Kregs and co-workers.[31] Much of the symptomatology observed in this syndrome is related to the ability of somatostatin to inhibit the function of most of the digestive organs. Somatostatin has also been shown to reduce the circulating levels of a number of hormones. Somatostatinoma is a rare pancreatic endocrine tumor. The syndrome is difficult to diagnose because the early findings are nonspecific. From the small number of cases reported in the English literature, the primary tumor was located in the head of the pancreas in the majority of the patients, often with liver metastases present at exploration. Management of patients with somatostatinoma encompasses preoperative treatment of hyperglycemia and malnutrition combined with standard radiographic localization and staging studies. Gallbladder ultrasonography should be performed to determine the presence of gallstones. At exploration, resection for cure has been uncommon, although safe resection and debulking are indicated. Cholecystectomy appears indicated because of the known increased incidence of cholelithiasis with persistent hypersomatostatinemia.

Nonfunctional Islet Cell Tumors

The majority of clinically detected islet cell tumors of the pancreas are associated with characteristic clinical syndromes caused by hypersecretion of hormonal products. Fifteen to 25 per cent of pancreatic endocrine tumors are found to be nonfunctional, on the basis of the absence of a defined clinical syndrome and the lack of elevated serum hormone levels. Nonfunctioning or clinically silent tumors are morphologically indistinguishable from their functional counterparts. These nonfunctioning islet cell tumors frequently have clinical manifestations similar to the more common exocrine malignancies. Thus, these patients frequently present with abdominal pain, weight loss, and jaundice, all related to the mass effect of the tumor. Nonfunctioning islet cell tumors are associated with a higher malignancy rate (90 per cent) than their functioning counterparts, and they are most commonly located in the head of the pancreas. However, in contrast to the poor prognosis associated with ductal adenocarcinoma of the exocrine pancreas, these nonfunctional islet cell tumors are often indolent and slow-growing. Surgical exploration follows routine radiographic studies and staging efforts. At operation localized tumors are resected by pancreaticoduodenectomy when lesions are located in the head and distal pancreatectomy when they are in the distal gland. Patients with surgically incurable disease

may benefit from primary tumor debulking or surgical palliation of jaundice and gastric outlet obstruction by biliary-enteric or gastroenteric bypass, respectively. Five-year survival for all patients averages 25 to 45 per cent. Five-year survival without curative resection has been documented in several cases. Chemotherapy with 5-fluorouracil and streptozotocin may be associated with a favorable objective response.

PANCREATIC LYMPHOMA

Primary involvement of the pancreas with non-Hodgkin's lymphoma occurs and represents an unusual neoplasm of the pancreas. Equal numbers of males and females have been reported. The clinical presentation commonly includes weight loss and abdominal pain and may include jaundice and symptoms of gastric outlet obstruction. The most common physical finding is a palpable abdominal mass. The abdominal CT scan may suggest the diagnosis by revealing a large soft tissue mass in the vicinity of the pancreas with peripancreatic lymphadenopathy (Fig. 22). In suspected cases of pancreatic lymphoma, radiographically guided needle biopsy can establish the diagnosis. After the pathologic diagnosis of non-Hodgkin's lymphoma, further staging is performed via bone marrow biopsy and accurate review of the chest and abdominal CT scan. Staging laparotomy is generally not necessary. There is no role for extensive resection in the management of patients with pancreatic lymphoma. Nonjaundiced patients appear to be best treated by doxorubicin-based combination chemotherapy regimens. In patients with obstructive jaundice, temporary biliary decompression is performed with a percutaneous transhepatic catheter. Chemotherapy begins with nonhepatotoxic agents such as cyclophosphamide and prednisone until resolution of jaundice, and then doxorubicin-containing regimens are initiated. Long-term remission can be obtained with chemotherapy alone. Surgical exploration appears best reserved for patients with the suspected diagnosis of pancreatic lymphoma and nondiagnostic percutaneous needle biopsy results.

PANCREATIC TRAUMA

The pancreas is injured in less than 2 per cent of patients with abdominal trauma. Two thirds of pancreatic injuries are associated with penetrating abdominal trauma, and one third are associated with blunt abdominal trauma. As a consequence of the retroperitoneal location of the pancreas, a significant pro-

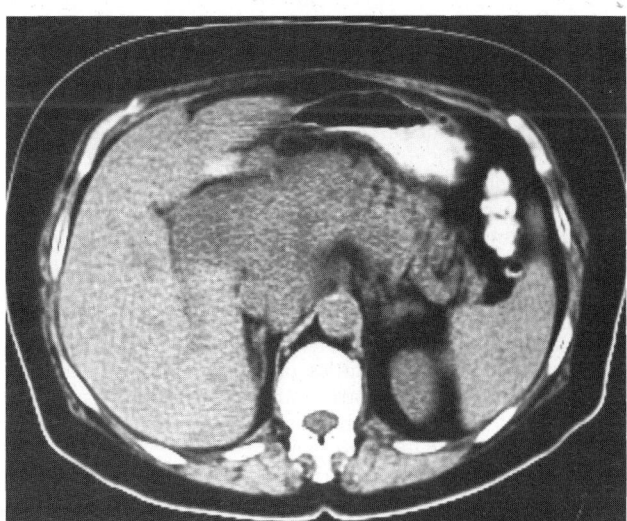

Figure 22. CT scan of a patient with pancreatic lymphoma demonstrating a large soft tissue mass in the region of the pancreas. (From Webb, T. H., Lillemoe, K. D., Pitt, H. A., et al.: Pancreatic lymphoma: Is surgery mandatory for diagnosis or treatment? Ann. Surg., 209:25, 1989.)

portion of patients with pancreatic trauma have injuries to adjacent organs and major vascular structures. Penetrating pancreatic injuries have the lowest mortality for stab wounds (approximately 5 to 10 per cent), with intermediate mortality associated with gunshot wounds, and the highest mortality (50 per cent) observed with close-range shotgun wounds. Blunt pancreatic trauma is associated with mortality of 15 to 50 per cent. In the majority of fatal cases, death is the result of hemorrhage from nearby vascular structures. The second most common cause of death involves delayed mortality from intra-abdominal sepsis.

In blunt abdominal trauma, the extent and location of pancreatic injury are determined by the mechanism of injury and the location of impact. Injuries occurring secondary to midline forces, such as classic steering wheel injuries, are associated with pancreatic neck transections, which occur when the vertebral column acts as a fulcrum over which the pancreas is sheared. Forces to the left of the vertebral column in the left upper quadrant are associated with distal pancreatic contusions or injuries of the spleen or left kidney. Forces confined to the right of the vertebral column may cause contusions to the pancreatic head, liver laceration, gallbladder injury, duodenal injury, avulsion of the common bile duct, or right renal injury.

Clinical Presentation

Pancreatic injury is associated with many clinical presentations. Patients with penetrating abdominal trauma generally present with obvious external injury and frequently show signs of ongoing hemorrhage, progressive peritonitis, and hypovolemia. The presentation of blunt abdominal trauma with pancreatic injury may be varied. Patients with pancreatic injury and solid organ injury to the liver or spleen may present with signs of obvious hypovolemia and peritonitis requiring exploration. In contrast, blunt abdominal trauma without other solid organ injury may produce subtle pancreatic injury difficult to diagnose. Such patients can present with mild epigastric pain and abdominal tenderness with otherwise unimpressive physical findings. In these patients, progressive clinical deterioration may herald the diagnosis of a pancreatic injury.

Diagnosis

No laboratory test is sufficiently accurate for the specific diagnosis of pancreatic injury. Hyperamylasemia is present in up to 90 per cent of patients with blunt pancreatic injury but is only present in a minority of patients with penetrating pancreatic injury. Moreover, hyperamylasemia may occur in up to 50 per cent of patients with blunt abdominal trauma without pancreatic injury. Thus, hyperamylasemia is an insensitive and nonspecific indicator of pancreatic injury. Nonspecific laboratory tests such as the hematocrit and the white blood cell count provide little assistance in the initial assessment of patients with suspected pancreatic injury, although they may be useful during serial observation of such patients. Peritoneal lavage, which has proven useful in the assessment of patients with blunt abdominal trauma, is inaccurate and unreliable for the diagnosis of pancreatic trauma. This is due to the retroperitoneal location of the pancreas and the existence of other sources for intraperitoneal amylase other than the pancreas, such as the bile duct, intestine, and fallopian tubes.

Chest and abdominal films are often not helpful in diagnosing pancreatic injury. Unusual and often late findings on abdominal films associated with pancreatic injury include obliteration of the psoas shadow, the presence of retroperitoneal air, and displacement of the stomach secondary to a retroperitoneal mass. Injury to the head of the pancreas with associated duodenal injury can be evaluated by means of an upper gastrointestinal series with water-soluble contrast. Extraluminal contrast extravasation indicates disruption of duodenal integrity and a major injury. A duodenal hematoma may be diagnosed by the typical "coiled spring" appearance of duodenal luminal narrowing.

In the setting of blunt abdominal trauma, the CT scan has gained importance in the serial evaluation of pancreatic injury. An abdominal CT scan obtained within hours of pancreatic trauma may reveal subtle abnormalities suggestive of pancreatic injury such as hemorrhagic infiltration of the peripancreatic fat or peripancreatic thickening due to fluid sequestration. In the appropriate clinical setting, serial assessment by CT scan may be of benefit in following subtle peripancreatic abnormalities and documenting early pancreatic pseudocyst, phlegmon, or abscess formation.

Endoscopic retrograde pancreatography (ERP) is occasionally useful in the acute setting following abdominal trauma. In general, however, abnormalities found at the time of acute injury, such as minor pancreatic ductal extravasation or small pseudocyst formation, require only expectant observation. Thus, the information gained by acute ERP is of little benefit in the management of such patients. In contrast, the use of ERP in a delayed setting following blunt abdominal trauma is important in defining pancreatic ductal abnormalities associated with pancreatic pseudocysts or other pancreatic ductal disruptions. In this setting, the definition of duct anatomy and pathology is of great importance in planning definitive operative management.

Management

Patients with pancreatic injury suggested by clinical and radiographic examination who have stable vital signs and lack a specific indication for exploration may initially be managed nonoperatively. In this setting, patients are serially observed clinically, with laboratory evaluation of the hematocrit, white blood cell count, and serum amylase, and with abdominal CT scan. Such patients are followed for the development of complications such as pancreatic abscess, acute pseudocyst formation, or retroperitoneal phlegmon.

Patients who undergo laparotomy for abdominal trauma require complete assessment of the pancreas at the time of surgical exploration. Assessment involves performance of the Kocher maneuver for evaluation of the duodenum and the head of the pancreas and division of the gastrocolic ligament for entrance into the lesser sac for visualization of the neck, body, and tail of the pancreas. Bimanual palpation of the body and tail may be accomplished by opening the peritoneum inferior to the pancreas and by reflecting the spleen and distal pancreas from the retroperitoneum toward the midline. In the setting of blunt or penetrating trauma, all peripancreatic hematomas should be explored to exclude and repair any major vascular injury.

The goals of operative therapy for pancreatic injury include control of hemorrhage, débridement of nonviable tissue with maximal preservation of viable pancreatic tissue, and adequate drainage of exocrine secretions. Operative therapy is dependent upon the degree of pancreatic injury. Pancreatic injury can be categorized into four classes. In order of increasing severity, they are (1) pancreatic contusion without capsular rupture, (2) pancreatic capsular and parenchymal rupture without injury to the main pancreatic duct, (3) severe pancreatic parenchymal injury with rupture of the main pancreatic duct, and (4) combined severe pancreatic and duodenal injuries.

CLASS I INJURY. Pancreatic contusion without capsular rupture is treated by external drainage alone. External drainage for Class I injuries is recommended because of the difficulty in assessing pancreatic capsular injury intraoperatively. By draining Class I injuries, occult capsular disruptions that could potentially cause accumulation of pancreatic secretions and subsequent pancreatic pseudocyst, abscess, or pancreatic ascites are prevented. Drains are usually left in place until oral intake is re-established.

CLASS II INJURY. More severe pancreatic injuries that involve pancreatic capsular or parenchymal rupture but are not associated with injury to the main pancreatic duct constitute Class II injuries. These injuries are treated by cautious débridement of devitalized tissue, achievement of adequate hemostasis, careful suture closure of major capsular disruption, and external drainage of the injury site.

CLASS III INJURY. Pancreatic parenchymal injuries associated with rupture or destruction of a major pancreatic duct constitute Class III injuries. These injuries require individualization of treatment, based on injury location and associated injuries to adjacent structures. Class III injuries may be diagnosed preoperatively by endoscopic retrograde pancreatography, or they may be discovered at the time of laparotomy via intraoperative pancreatography or operative findings. Class III injuries to the body and tail of the pancreas are best treated by distal pancreatectomy encompassing the site of the injury, with or without splenectomy. Following distal pancreatectomy, the transected surface of the pancreatic remnant is closed, and the closure is externally drained. Distal resection up to the level of the superior mesenteric vein can be performed with reasonable rapidity, rarely causes pancreatic endocrine insufficiency, and has a low incidence of persistent external pancreatic fistula. As an alternative to distal pancreatectomy, Class III injuries to the body of the pancreas may be treated with Roux-en-Y pancreaticojejunostomy to the distal pancreatic remnant with oversewing of the proximal pancreas. This procedure requires the creation of a Roux-en-Y jejunal limb, but no distal pancreatic resection is performed. This procedure requires more time than distal pancreatic resection, requires two gastrointestinal anastomoses, and may be complicated by postoperative leak from the pancreatic-enteric anastomosis. Thus, it is not commonly chosen for Class III injuries to the body of the pancreas.

Class III injuries to the head of the pancreas not associated with duodenal injury are uncommon and usually follow penetrating trauma. Isolated injuries of the inferior head or uncinate process may be débrided and externally drained or drained via Roux-en-Y pancreaticojejunostomy. Injuries in the proximity of the pancreatic neck may be treated by distal pancreatectomy to the level of the injury. Injuries adjacent to the duodenal C loop in the central aspect of the pancreatic head are treated as Class IV injuries.

CLASS IV INJURY. Combined severe injuries to the pancreas and duodenum represent a minority of cases of pancreatic trauma. These Class IV injuries are frequently associated with injuries to adjacent visceral or major vascular structures, and they are attended by mortality of up to 45 per cent. There are several different surgical options for the treatment of Class IV injuries. First, the serosal patch technique employs healthy small bowel serosa to patch defects in the duodenal wall that cannot be safely closed primarily. This technique has utility when discrete duodenal injuries occur in combination with injury to the head of the pancreas not requiring pancreatic resection. In such instances, a serosal patch may provide secure duodenal closure, whereas the pancreatic injury is managed with hemostasis, débridement, and external drainage.

More extensive injuries to the duodenum and head of the pancreas can be treated by a second approach: duodenal decompression with triple ostomy. This technique uses tube gastrostomy, retrograde tube jejunostomy for duodenal drainage, and antegrade tube jejunostomy for enteral feeding. These triple ostomies are combined with secure duodenorrhaphy and wide drainage of the duodenum and head of the pancreas.

Patients with more severe injuries to the duodenum and head of the pancreas may be managed by a third technique: the duodenal diverticularization procedure.[8] This procedure, as initially described, involved closure of the duodenal defect, placement of a proximal tube duodenostomy, pyloroantrectomy with gastrojejunostomy, truncal vagotomy, T-tube placement, and wide drainage of the retroperitoneum. The goal of this therapy is to achieve widespread drainage of the retroperitoneum and a re-

duction in the flow of luminal contents through the duodenum. The pyloric exclusion procedure is a more recent modification of the duodenal diverticularization technique. In the exclusion procedure, the pylorus is closed from within the gastric lumen with an absorbable suture. A gastrojejunostomy is performed, and the injury to the duodenum is primarily repaired. Vagotomy and antrectomy are not performed, thus avoiding their late complications and saving operative time. Marginal ulceration at the gastrojejunal anastomosis is prevented by histamine H_2-receptor antagonist therapy. Both the diverticularization and exclusion procedures are applicable to intermediate severity pancreaticoduodenal injuries.

Devitalizing injuries of the duodenum and head of the pancreas not amenable to lesser procedures are treated by pancreaticoduodenectomy. Indications for pancreaticoduodenectomy in the setting of abdominal trauma include massive destruction of the duodenum and pancreatic head, avulsion of the bile duct and pancreatic duct at the ampulla of Vater, and, rarely, jeopardized vascularity of the pancreaticoduodenal region. Pylorus-preserving pancreaticoduodenectomy may be accomplished if the most proximal duodenum is free of injury. Mortality following pancreaticoduodenectomy in the setting of abdominal trauma varies from 0 to 60 per cent. Mortality is related to many factors, including the magnitude of the injury to associated structures, the condition of the patient prior to operation, the length of operation, the overall blood loss, and the experience of the surgeon.

PANCREATIC TRANSPLANTATION

In the United States there are approximately 1 million Type I diabetics. Half of these diabetics develop significant long-term metabolic complications such as nephropathy, neuropathy, vasculopathy, and retinopathy within 20 years of the onset of their disease. Well-controlled glucoregulation in these patients prevents not only ketoacidosis, hypercholesterolemia, and hyperlipidemia, but also appears to reduce the long-term metabolic complications. Until recently, the primary therapy for insulin-dependent diabetes involved intermittent administration of subcutaneous insulin. Now, newer methods of treatment include (1) fine regulation of serum glucose by sophisticated insulin delivery systems, (2) pancreatic islet cell transplantation, and (3) vascularized pancreas (segmental or whole) transplantation.

A number of insulin delivery systems are currently available; others are undergoing testing. Delivery systems can involve external or internal (implantable) devices with an open-loop format or a closed-loop format using a glucose sensor. Results with delivery systems indicate that insulin-dependent diabetes can be successfully treated without daily parenteral injections, with doses of insulin that mimic physiologic secretion, and with satisfactory glycemic control as assessed by glycosylated hemoglobin. For the future, the most attractive system appears to be an implantable pump with a peritoneal insulin delivery arm combined with a glucose-sensing closed-loop system.

Pancreatic transplantation serves as an alternative method of treating insulin-dependent diabetes. The first human pancreas transplant was performed by Kelly and associates in 1966.[30] In the ensuing years, multiple different techniques have evolved and varied experiences have been gained in the field of experimental and human pancreatic transplantation.[11,51]

Pancreas transplantation remains confined to a select group of patients with insulin-dependent diabetes mellitus. Pancreas transplantation can be performed (1) in a nonuremic patient, (2) simultaneously with a kidney transplant in a uremic patient with end-stage diabetic nephropathy, or (3) at an interval after successful kidney grafting in a patient with renal failure. Contraindications for pancreas transplantation vary but generally include the presence of malignancy, active infection, advanced cardiovascular disease, and major amputations or blindness.

Enthusiasm for pancreatic islet transplantation has exacerbated and abated over the past 3 decades. Theoretically, islet cell grafting is attractive because it avoids transplantation of the antigenic exocrine tissue and because it has the potential to allow harvesting of islets for multiple recipients from a single donor. The isolation, processing, and purification of islet tissues have been topics of renewed inquiry. Prevention of islet rejection has been recently studied with standard immunosuppressive regimens as well as immunoalteration and immunoisolation techniques. In animal models the kidney capsule or a peritoneal omental pouch appears ideal as a recipient site for islet transplantation. To date, there have been no consistently successful human islet transplants reported.

Enthusiasm for segmental or whole pancreas transplantation has increased greatly since the late 1970s. Worldwide a number of techniques for vascularized pancreatic allotransplantation are utilized. In the United States, whole organ grafts are generally performed, providing exocrine drainage via a duodenal segment to the urinary bladder. In Europe, segmental pancreatic grafts are preferred, with exocrine secretion managed by drainage into a Roux-en-Y jejunal limb or prevented by ductal polymer injection. A recent report by Sutherland and associates indicates that bladder-drained grafts achieve significantly better 1-year function than enterically drained or duct-injected grafts.[51] The improvement in function observed with bladder-drained grafts has been attributed largely to the ability to serially follow urinary amylase excretion as a measure of graft function. Immunosuppressive regimens for segmental or whole pancreas transplantation usually involve quadruple drug therapy with prednisone, azathioprine, cyclosporine, and polyclonal anti-T-lymphocyte antibody. Initial therapy for rejection episodes usually involves monoclonal antibody therapy with OKT-3.

Specific surgical complications are well recognized after vascularized pancreatic transplantation. These include posttransplant pancreatitis, transplant vascular thrombosis, peritransplant hemorrhage, and sepsis. Posttransplant pancreatitis may have several causes, including injury to the pancreas during the procurement procedure, preservation injury, rejection, and ductal obstruction. No specific treatment is available for the management of posttransplant pancreatitis. The incidence of graft thrombosis following transplantation has been reported to be as high as 20 per cent. Graft thrombosis is more frequent after segmental pancreatic transplantation, partially because of the low flow through the graft and the large caliber of the draining splenic vein. Attempts to prevent graft thrombosis have included the creation of a distal arteriovenous fistula at the time of segmental grafting, as well as the use of posttransplant anticoagulation therapy with dextran, heparin, and warfarin. Local sepsis after pancreatic transplantation is not uncommon, particularly after enteric drainage of the pancreatic graft. Infection may be the result of an anastomotic leak or may arise from small areas of necrotic transplanted pancreatic tissue.

The results of pancreatic allotransplantation using vascularized grafts have been steadily improving. The most recent data available[11] indicate a 60 to 80 per cent 1-year graft survival for synchronous pancreas and kidney transplants. The graft survival rates are lower for pancreas transplants performed alone or after renal transplantation. Although there appears to be no distinct advantage in pancreatic graft survival between segmental or whole organ grafts, bladder-drained grafts appear to be favored over enterically drained or polymer-injected grafts.

After successful pancreatic transplantation, carbohydrate metabolism reliably improves. Posttransplant patients with functioning grafts demonstrate nearly normal glucose tolerance testing, fasting euglycemia, and improved functional status. Although graft function eliminates the need for exogenous insulin

therapy, standard immunosuppressive therapy is substituted. The ultimate purpose of pancreatic transplantation is to reverse or halt the secondary complications of diabetes. Patients receiving successful combined pancreatic and renal transplants have been noted to have an absence of electron microscopic evidence of diabetic nephropathy in the transplanted kidney, supporting a protective effect of pancreatic transplantation against diabetic nephropathy. Successful pancreatic transplantation has also been associated with a subjective improvement in peripheral neuropathy, as well as an objective improvement in motor nerve conduction velocities in the upper and lower extremities. The effects on diabetic retinopathy have not been as universally favorable, although subjective visual improvement or stabilization has been observed after successful grafting. Overall, accumulating evidence supports a beneficial effect of pancreas transplantation on the various end organs commonly injured by diabetes mellitus.[51]

SELECTED REFERENCES

Banting, F. G., and Best, C. H. L.: The internal secretion of the pancreas. J. Lab. Clin. Med., 7:251, 1922.
The authors describe their classic work with potent hypoglycemic extracts from a duct-ligated pancreas, which led to the isolation of insulin.

Bayliss, W. M., and Starling, E. H.: The mechanism of pancreatic secretion. J. Physiol., 28:325, 1902.
This article describes the experiments that led to the discovery of the first hormone — secretin.

Brooks, J. R.: Where are we with pancreas transplantation? Surgery, 106:935, 1989.
A review of the current status of pancreas transplantation that addresses many of the current controversies.

Cameron, J. L.: Chronic pancreatic ascites and pancreatic pleural effusions. Gastroenterology, 74:134, 1978.
An article that reviews the entities of pancreatic ascites and pancreatic pleural effusion.

Crist, D. W., Sitzmann, J. V., and Cameron, J. L.: Improved hospital morbidity, mortality and survival after the Whipple procedure. Ann. Surg., 206:358, 1987.
This paper reviews the recent Johns Hopkins Hospital experience with Whipple resections for periampullary neoplasms. The authors document improvements in mortality and morbidity rates, as well as reductions in operative time, blood loss, and blood transfusion requirements.

Halsted, W. S.: Contributions to the surgery of the bile passages, especially the common bile duct. Boston Med. Surg. J., 141:645, 1899.
This paper includes a description of the first successful resection of a periampullary tumor.

Halsted, W. S.: Retrojection of bile into the pancreas: A cause of acute hemorrhagic pancreatitis. Bull. Johns Hopkins Hosp., 12:179, 1901.

Opie, E. L.: The etiology of acute hemorrhagic pancreatitis. Bull. Johns Hopkins Hosp., 12:182, 1901.
These two papers, published together, laid the groundwork for the "common channel theory" of the etiology of gallstone pancreatitis.

Neoptolemos, J. P., Carr-Locke, D. L., London, N. J., et al.: Controlled trial of urgent endoscopic retrograde cholangiopancreatography and endoscopic sphincterotomy versus conservative treatment for acute pancreatitis due to gallstones. Lancet, 2:979, 1988.
The authors describe the results of ERCP plus sphincterotomy to retrieve stones versus supportive care alone in patients with gallstone pancreatitis. In patients with severe pancreatitis the endoscopic intervention reduced the complication rate and the length of hospital stay.

Ranson, J. H. C., Rifkind, K. M., Roses, D. F., et al.: Prognostic signs and the role of operative management in acute pancreatitis. Surg. Gynecol. Obstet., 139:69, 1974.
In this paper the authors show that the severity of an attack of acute pancreatitis can be predicted, at or soon after hospital admission, by the presence or absence of easily obtainable clinical criteria.

Sarr, M. G., and Cameron, J. L.: Surgical management of unresectable carcinoma of the pancreas. Surgery, 91:123, 1982.
An extensive review of over 8000 patients who underwent palliative surgery for unresectable pancreatic cancer.

Steer, M. L., and Meldolesi, J.: The cell biology of experimental pancreatitis. N. Engl. J. Med., 316:144, 1987.
A recent review of the pathophysiology and cellular mechanisms involved in the pathogenesis of acute pancreatitis.

Whipple, A. O., Parsons, W. B., and Mullins, C. R.: Treatment of carcinoma of the ampulla of Vater. Ann. Surg., 102:763, 1935.

This paper describes the first successful pancreaticoduodenectomy, which was performed in two stages.

Yeo, C. J., Bastidas, J. A., Lynch-Nyhan, A., et al.: The natural history of pancreatic pseudocysts documented by computed tomography. Surg. Gynecol. Obstet., 170:411, 1990.
The authors present data pertaining to the natural history of pancreatic pseudocysts, as documented by computerized tomography at the Johns Hopkins Hospital. In this review 48 per cent of the patients were managed nonoperatively, and 52 per cent were treated operatively. Algorithms for patient management are depicted.

Yeo, C. J., Bastidas, J. A., Schmieg, R. E., Jr., et al.: Pancreatic structure and glucose tolerance in a longitudinal study of experimental pancreatitis-induced diabetes. Ann. Surg., 210:150, 1989.
Using the canine pancreatic duct ligation model of pancreatitis the authors serially evaluated pancreatic histology and electron microscopy, as well as glucose tolerance and insulin response to glucose loading. The data support the conclusion that chronic pancreatitis is associated with abnormal islet responsiveness, leading to circulating insulin deficiency and glucose intolerance.

Zollinger, R. M., and Ellison, E. H.: Primary peptic ulcerations of the jejunum associated with islet cell tumors of the pancreas. Ann. Surg., 142:709, 1955.
This paper proposed the association between islet cell tumors of the pancreas and peptic ulcer disease, now known to be the result of a gastrinoma.

REFERENCES

1. Andersen, D. K.: Current diagnosis and management of Zollinger-Ellison syndrome. Ann. Surg., 210:685, 1989.
2. Babkin, B. P.: Secretory Mechanisms of the Digestive Glands, 2nd ed. New York, Hoeber Medical Division, Harper and Row, 1950.
3. Banting, F. G., and Best, C. H. L.: The internal secretion of the pancreas. J. Lab. Clin. Med., 7:251, 1922.
4. Bastidas, J. A., Couse, N. F., Yeo, C. J., et al.: The effect of pancreatic polypeptide infusion on glucose tolerance and insulin response in longitudinally studied pancreatitis-induced diabetes. Surgery. 107:661, 1990.
5. Bayliss, W. M., and Starling, E. H.: The mechanism of pancreatic secretion. J. Physiol., 28:325, 1902.
6. Beger, H. G., Buchler, M., Bittner, R. R., et al.: Duodenum-preserving resection of the head of the pancreas in severe chronic pancreatitis: Early and late results. Ann. Surg., 209:273, 1989.
7. Beger, H. C., Buchler, M., Bittner, R., et al.: Necrosectomy and postoperative local lavage in patients with necrotizing pancreatitis: Results of a prospective clinical trial. World J. Surg., 12:255, 1988.
8. Berne, C. J., Donovan, A. J., White, H. J., et al.: Duodenal "diverticularization" for duodenal and pancreatic injury. Am. J. Surg., 127:503, 1974.
9. Bolooki, H., and Gliedman, M. L.: Peritonal dialysis in the treatment of acute pancreatitis. Surgery, 64:466, 1968.
10. Bradley, E. L. III, Clements, J. L., Jr., Gonzalez, A. C.: The natural history of pancreatic pseudocysts: A unified concept of management. Am. J. Surg., 137:135, 1979.
11. Brooks, J. R.: Where are we with pancreas transplantation? Surgery, 106:935, 1989.
12. Cameron, J. L.: Chronic pancreatic ascites and pancreatic pleural effusions. Gastroenterology, 74:134, 1978.
13. Cameron, J. L., Crist, D. W., Sitzmann, J. V., et al.: Factors influencing survival following pancreaticoduodenectomy for pancreatic cancer. Am. J. Surg. In press.
14. Clemens, J. A., Chacko, V. P., Olson, J. L., et al.: Correlation of high-energy phosphate metabolism and electron microscopic morphology changes in acute experimental pancreatitis. Surg. Forum, 40:152, 1989.
15. Crist, D. W., Sitzmann, J. V., and Cameron, J. L.: Improved hospital morbidity, mortality and survival after the Whipple procedure. Ann. Surg., 206:358, 1987.
16. Dooley, W. C., Cameron, J. L., Pitt, H. A., et al.: Is preoperative angiography useful in patients with periampullary tumors? Ann. Surg., 211:649, 1990.
17. Doubilet, H., and Mulholland, J. H.: Eight-year study of pancreatitis and sphincterotomy. J.A.M.A., 160:521, 1956.
18. Duval, M. K., Jr.: Caudal pancreatico-jejunostomy for chronic relapsing pancreatitis. Ann. Surg., 140:775, 1954.
19. Fitz, R. H.: Acute pancreatitis. Boston Med. Surg. J., 120:181, 1889.
20. Fitzgerald, P. S.: Medical anecdotes concerning some diseases of the pancreas. In Fitzgerald, P. J. (Ed.): The Pancreas. Baltimore, Williams & Wilkins, 1980, pp. 1–29.
21. Frey, C. F., and Smith, G. J.: Description and rationale of a new operation for chronic pancreatitis. Pancreas, 2:701, 1987.
22. Ganda, O. P., Weis, G. C., and Soeldner, A.: Somatostatinoma: A somatostatin-containing tumor of the endocrine pancreas. N. Engl. J. Med., 296:963, 1977.
23. Gastrointestinal Tumor Study Group: Further evidence of effective adjuvant combined radiation and chemotherapy following curative resection of pancreatic cancer. Cancer, 59:2006, 1987.
24. Halsted, W. S.: Contributions to the surgery of the bile passages, especially the common bile duct. Boston Med. Surg. J., 141:645, 1899.
25. Heidenhain, R.: Beitrage sur Kenntnis des Pancreas. Arch. Ges. Physiol., 10:557, 1875.
26. Henry, L. G., and Condon, L. E.: Ablative surgery for necrotizing pancreatitis. Am. J. Surg., 131:125, 1976.
27. Ihse, I., Evander, A., Holmberg, J. T., et al.: Influence of peritoneal lavage on objective prognostic signs in acute pancreatitis. Ann. Surg., 204:122, 1986.
28. Kalser, M. H., and Ellenberg, S. S.: Pancreatic cancer: Adjuvant combined radiation and chemotherapy following curative resection. Arch. Surg., 120:899, 1985.
29. Kaplan, O., Kushnir, T., Sandbank, V., et al.: Acute pancreatitis in rats: A ^{31}P nuclear magnetic resonance study. J. Surg. Res., 43:172, 1987.
30. Kelly, W. D., Lillehei, R. C., Merkel, F. K., et al.: Allotransplantation of the pancreas and duodenum along with the kidney in diabetic nephropathy. Surgery, 61:827, 1967.
31. Kregs, G. J., Orei, L., Conlon, M., et al.: Somatostatinoma syndrome. N. Engl. J. Med., 301:285, 1979.
32. Lampel, M., and Kern, H. F.: Acute interstitial pancreatitis in the rat induced by excessive doses of a pancreatic secretagogue. Virchows Arch. (Pathol. Anat.), 373:97, 1977.
33. LeDentu, M.: Rapport sur l'observation precedente. Bull. Soc. Anat. Paris, 10:197, 1865.
34. Lombardi, B., Estes, L. W., and Longnecker, D. S.: Acute hemorrhagic pancreatitis (massive necrosis) with fat necrosis induced in mice by DL-ethionine fed with a choline-1 deficient diet. Am. J. Pathol., 79:465, 1975.
35. Mayer, A. D., McMahon, M. J., Corfield, A. P., et al.: Controlled clinical trial of peritoneal lavage for the treatment of severe acute pancreatitis. N. Engl. J. Med., 312:399, 1985.
36. Moynihan, B.: Acute pancreatitis. Ann. Surg., 81:132, 1925.
37. Neoptolemos, J. P., Carr-Locke, D. L., London, N. J., et al.: Controlled trial of urgent endoscopic retrograde cholangiopancreatography and endoscopic sphincterotomy versus conservative treatment for acute pancreatitis due to gallstones. Lancet, 2:979, 1988.
38. Opie, E. L.: The etiology of acute hemorrhagic pancreatitis. Bull. Johns Hopkins Hosp., 12:182, 1901.
39. Partington, P. F., and Rochelle, R. E. L.: Modified Peustow procedure for retrograde drainage of the pancreatic duct. Ann. Surg., 152:1037, 1960.
40. Peustow, C. B., and Gillesby, W. J.: Retrograde surgical drainage of the pancreas for chronic relapsing pancreatitis. Arch. Surg., 76:898, 1958.
41. Ranson, J. H. C., Rifkind, K. M., Roses, D. F., et al.: Prognostic signs and the role of operative management in acute pancreatitis. Surg. Gynecol. Obstet., 139:69, 1974.
42. Ranson, J. H. C., and Spencer, F. C.: The role of peritoneal lavage in severe acute pancreatitis. Ann. Surg., 187:565, 1978.
43. Renner, I. G., Savage, W. T., III, Pantoja, J. L., et al.: Death due to acute pancreatitis: A retrospective analysis of 405 autopsy cases. Dig. Dis. Sci., 30:1005, 1985.
44. Sailer, S., and Zinninger, M. M.: Massive islet cell tumor of pancreas without hypoglycemia. Surg. Gynecol. Obstet., 82:301, 1946.
45. Sanfey, H., Bulkley, G. B., and Cameron, J. L.: The role of oxygen-derived free radicals in the pathogenesis of acute pancreatitis. Ann. Surg., 200:405, 1984.
46. Senn, N.: The Surgery of the Pancreas. Philadelphia, W. J. Dorman, 1886, pp. 71–107.
47. Seymour, N. E., Brunicardi, F. C., Chaiken, R. L., et al.: Reversal of abnormal glucose production after pancreatic resection by pancreatic polypeptide administration in man. Surgery, 104:119, 1988.
48. Steer, M. L., and Meldolesi, J.: The cell biology of experimental pancreatitis. N. Engl. J. Med., 316:144, 1987.
49. Stone, H. H., and Fabian, T. C.: Peritoneal dialysis in the treatment of acute alcoholic pancreatitis. Surg. Gynecol. Obstet., 150:878, 1980.
50. Stone, H. H., Fabian, T. C., and Dunlop, W. E.: Gallstone pancreatitis: Biliary tract pathology in relation to time of operation. Ann. Surg., 194:305, 1981.
51. Sutherland, D. E. R., Dunn, D. L., Goetz, F. C., et al.: A 10-year experience with 290 pancreas transplants at a single institution. Ann. Surg., 210:274, 1989.
52. Verner, J. V., and Morrison, A. B.: Islet cell tumor and a syndrome of refractory diarrhea and hypokalemia. Am. J. Med., 25:374, 1958.
53. Von Mering, J., and Minkowski, O.: Diabetes mellitus nach Pancreasextirpation. Arch. Exp. Pathol. Pharmakol., 26:371, 1890.
54. Warren, W. D., Millikan, W. J., Jr., Henderson, J. M., et al.: A denervated pancreatic flap for control of pain in pancreatitis. Surg. Gynecol. Obstet., 159:581, 1984.
55. Whipple, A. O., Parsons, W. B., Mullins, C. R.: Treatment of carcinoma of the ampulla of Vater. Ann. Surg., 102:763, 1935.
56. Whipple, A. O., and Frantz, V. K.: Adenoma of islet cells with hyperinsulinism: A review. Ann. Surg., 101:1299, 1935.
57. Wilson, C., Imrie, C. W., Carter, D. C.: Fatal acute pancreatitis. Gut, 29:782, 1988.
58. Yeo, C. J., Bastidas, J. A., Lynch-Nyhan, A., et al.: The natural history of pancreatic pseudocysts documented by computed tomography. Surg. Gynecol. Obstet., 170:411, 1990.
59. Yeo, C. J.: ZES: Current approaches. Contemp. Gastroenterol. 3:17, 1990.
60. Yeo, C. J., Bastidas, J. A., Schmieg, R. E., Jr., et al.: Pancreatic structure and glucose tolerance in a longitudinal study of experimental pancreatitis-induced diabetes. Ann. Surg., 210:150, 1989.
61. Zollinger, R. M., and Ellison, E. H.: Primary peptic ulcerations of the jejunum associated with islet cell tumors of the pancreas. Ann. Surg., 142:709, 1955.

36

THE SPLEEN

George F. Sheldon, M.D., Robert D. Croom III, M.D.,
and Anthony A. Meyer, Ph.D., M.D.

HISTORICAL ASPECTS

For over 2500 years, knowledge of the biologic functions of the spleen has been elusive. Removal of the spleen, however, has long been known to be compatible with life. Galen (131–201) described the spleen as an "organ of mystery." Aristotle (384–322 B.C.) assumed that the spleen was not necessary for life. Pliny in the first century thought the spleen's weight might hinder the speed of runners and could be "taken out of the body by way of incision," but with the complication of the loss of the ability to laugh. In both the Babylonian Talmud (second to sixth centuries) and the ancient Jewish writings of Judah Halevi (1086–1145), the concept of the spleen's role in laughter was developed. As laughter was believed to be a "cleansing process," it was postulated that the spleen "cleanses the blood and spirit from unclear and obscuring matter." Maimonides, in his *Aphorisms of Moses* (mid-twelfth century), re-emphasized the concept of the blood-purifying function of the spleen.[42] Between the eighteenth and early twentieth centuries, experiments in numerous species of animals supported the concept of the nonessential nature of the spleen, although postsplenectomy peripheral blood changes were described.[33,42]

In 1919, Morris and Bullock performed the first experimental studies in animals that suggested an essential role of the spleen in host defense. Their conclusion, based on experiments in splenectomized rats infected with bacillus of rat plague, was that "the spleen aids . . . tremendously in resisting infectious processes . . . and . . . removal temporarily robs the body of its resistance."[42] The concept of an essential role of the spleen in immune function was disputed by the noted English surgeon Hamilton Bailey (1927). Pfeiffer (1924), however, expressed concern that inadequate follow-up of splenectomized patients precluded a scientific conclusion regarding the effects of splenectomy. The first major challenge to the concept of the dispensable nature of the spleen was King and Shumacker's (1952) report on the increased susceptibility to infection in infants following splenectomy.[29,42]

The proper surgical procedure for diseases or injury of the spleen has undergone frequent revision. Galen and other ancient anatomist-physiologists probably performed splenectomy in experimental animals such as monkeys, and may have done so in humans. The first recorded splenectomy was performed for a "stopped-up" (perhaps malarial) spleen in 1549 by Adrian Zaccarelli.[42] Malpighi (1666) proved that ligation of the splenic artery of dogs was not fatal. Clark (1676) performed splenectomy in dogs with survival. In 1673, Clark removed a portion of a spleen that extruded from an abdominal knife wound 3 days after an attempted suicide. The first total splenectomy for trauma (Matthias) was in another case of attempted suicide (1678) associated with evisceration.[42] The first splenectomy for trauma in the United States was performed by a Navy surgeon, O'Brien, in San Francisco in 1816.[42] The patient was a Mexican sailor who had been eviscerated by a knife wielded by a woman he had assaulted. Splenectomy was accomplished by ligation of the splenic pedicle. In both cases, the patients recovered and returned to their usual pursuits without ill effects, lending credence to the concept of the nonessential nature of the spleen.

Numerous partial and total splenectomies were performed as surgery became established as a specialty in the nineteenth and twentieth centuries. A high mortality from elective splenectomy for hypersplenism, however, resulted in controversy in Germany, with temporary cessation of splenectomy for hematologic diseases. Billroth (1881) postulated that the spleen was capable of repair after injury, a conclusion based on an autopsy performed on a trauma victim who died of head injury with a contained splenic injury.[42] Spencer Wells (1887) performed a splenectomy for hypersplenism in a patient who subsequently was shown to have hereditary spherocytosis.[40] William Mayo (1910) performed splenorraphy for a gunshot wound of the spleen.[42]

By the early twentieth century, total splenectomy was considered the only proper operation for diseases or injury of the spleen, a conclusion based on three premises: the belief that the spleen could be removed without early or late complications; the almost universal mortality of splenic injury treated without operation; and, perhaps the most widely cited reason for advocating splenectomy for splenic injury, the popularity of the concept of "delayed rupture" of the spleen.

Modern imaging techniques have improved understanding of splenic injury, with the concept of "delayed rupture" now discarded in favor of "delayed diagnosis." New diagnostic methods and operative techniques have made possible a variety of operations and therapeutic approaches to splenic disease and injury.

ANATOMY

Embryonic development of the spleen begins in the fifth week of gestation as a small cluster of mesenchymal cells in the dorsal mesogastrium between the stomach and pancreas. Mesenchymal remnants that do not fuse with the main splenic mass account for the high incidence (15 to 30 per cent) of accessory spleens in adjacent tissues.

The spleen is the second largest organ of the reticuloendothelial system. It is located in the posterior left upper quadrant of the abdomen, where its relationships to the diaphragm, stomach, pancreas, left kidney, and splenic flexure of the colon are maintained by suspensory ligaments. The splenophrenic, splenorenal, and splenocolic ligaments are usually relatively avascular, except in patients with portal hypertension, and their transection allows the spleen to be displaced medially and anteriorly. The gastrosplenic ligament, which extends from the greater curvature of the body and fundus of the stomach to the spleen, contains the short gastric arteries and veins. Located in the most medial aspect of the splenorenal ligament and attached to the spleen at the hilum, the splenic pedicle contains the splenic artery and vein, lymphatic structures, and often the tail of the pancreas (Fig. 1).

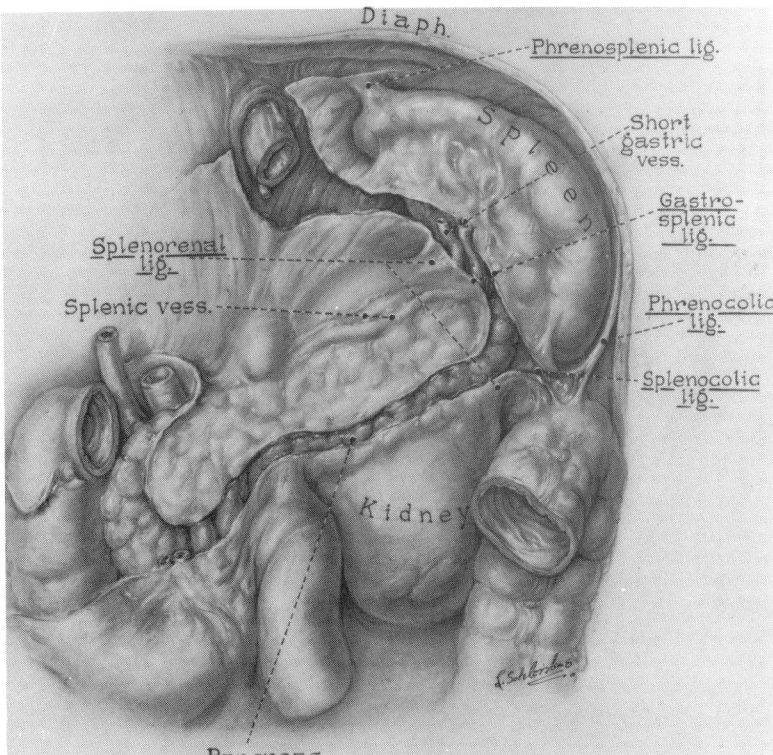

Figure 1. Suspensory ligaments of the spleen. (From Ballinger, W. F., and Erslev, A. J.: Splenectomy: Indications, technic and complications. Curr. Probl. Surg., 1–51, February 1965.)

The arterial supply to the spleen is derived from the celiac artery via both the splenic artery and the short gastric arteries, which usually arise as branches of the gastroepiploic or the splenic arteries (Fig. 2). The splenic vein is formed by a coalescence of polar veins in the splenic hilum and courses with the splenic artery along the dorsal surface of the pancreas to enter the portal system.

The normal adult spleen is a slightly concave, solid, dark red organ, which measures approximately 3 by 8 by 14 cm., weighs between 100 and 175 gm., and frequently has fetal lobulations on its anterior edge. A thin peritoneal capsule encloses the deeper organ pulp and easily strips from it. In elderly individuals or in those with prior splenic injury, irradiation, or recurrent infarction, the splenic capsule may become firm and thickly scarred ("sugar-coated") and adherent to the diaphragm.

A trabecular connective tissue framework extends into the splenic pulp from the internal capsular surface to subdivide the

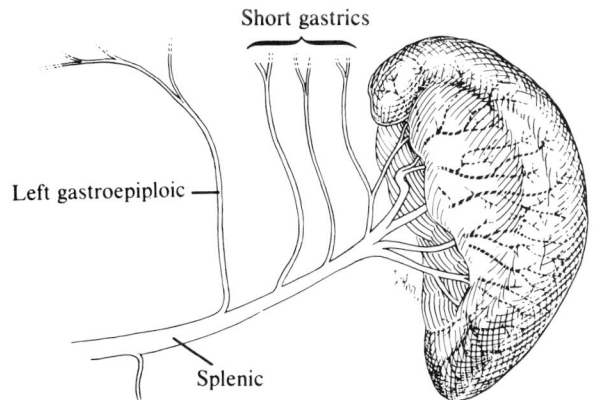

Figure 2. The arterial supply of the spleen is derived from the splenic artery through five or six branches that arise in or proximal to the hilus. The most proximal branch of the splenic artery is the left gastroepiploic artery. Four to six short gastric arteries are present in the gastrosplenic ligament between the proximal greater curvature of the stomach and the spleen. (From Blaisdell, F. W., and Trunkey, D. D.: Trauma Management. New York, Thieme-Stratton, 1982, p. 186.)

organ into small communicating compartments. After entering the spleen at the hilum, arterial vessels branch into the trabeculae to enter the pulp. Veins and lymphatics draining the pulp also pass in the trabeculae to leave the spleen at the hilum. The splenic pulp is conventionally divided into three areas: red pulp, white pulp, and an interfacing marginal zone. The red pulp, so designated because of its gross appearance from the presence of blood, is composed almost entirely of large, branching, thin-walled blood vessels called splenic sinuses or sinusoids and thin plates or cords of cellular tissue lying between the sinuses to form splenic cords. Within this cordal meshwork, erythrocytes, platelets, and some granulocytes are crowded with macrophages and plasma cells, macrophages often being the predominant cells. Lying within and surrounded by the red pulp are small gray-white zones of lymphatic tissue, consisting of lymphocytes, plasma cells, and macrophages, that constitute the white pulp. The white pulp forms periarterial lymphatic sheaths and lymphatic nodules, which, like those of lymph nodes, may contain germinal centers. The marginal zone constitutes the interface between the red and white pulp and is an ill-defined vascular space where many arterial vessels terminate.[48]

Controversy has surrounded the exact nature of the splenic microcirculation for 300 years. Theodor Billroth receives credit for the "open circulation" theory, in which either arterioles empty blood directly into tissue spaces or arterial capillaries open into pulp cords, with blood cells then passing through pores in the walls of splenic sinusoids to enter the venous circulation. In the "closed circulation" theory, splenic blood follows an endothelialized pathway throughout to flow directly into sinusoids (Fig. 3). Studies in rabbits, using plastic microspheres too large to pass through pores of the venous sinuses, confirm the unique "open" splenic microcirculation. Ninety per cent of splenic arterial flow enters the "open circulation" of the red pulp, with only 10 per cent of the blood in arterial capillaries emptying directly into venous sinuses. Blood cells and particles, such as particulate antigens, must circulate through the meshwork of splenic cords before squeezing through 0.5- to 2.5-μm. pores between endothelial cells of the sinuses to center the venous circulation.[8]

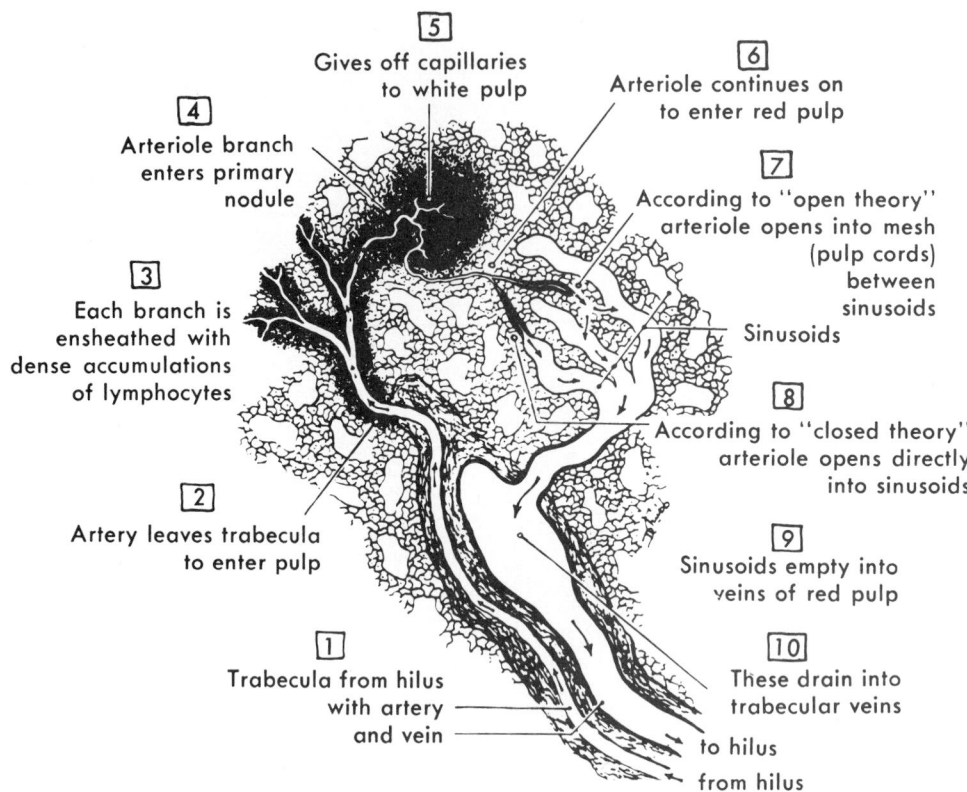

Figure 3. Diagram of the blood circulation through the spleen, illustrating the "open" and "closed" theories of blood flow. (From Blaustein, A.: The Spleen. New York, McGraw-Hill Book Company, 1963, p. 15.)

FUNCTION

During early fetal development, the spleen produces red and white blood cells. By the fifth month of gestation, the spleen and other extramedullary sites of blood cell production no longer have hematopoietic function but retain the capability throughout life. As a result of a singular microcirculation, the spleen is a sophisticated filter with both blood cell monitoring and management functions and important immune functions. When the spleen is removed, these functions are lost.

Normal red cells usually traverse the splenic circulation but may undergo "repair" by having surface abnormalities such as pits or spurs removed. Reticulocytes pass through the spleen more slowly than do mature red cells and lose nuclear remnants and excess membrane before entering the circulation as mature cells. In reducing the membrane surface area, the spleen converts the red cell from a target appearance to a biconcave disc. The spleen also removes high molecular weight surface protein, Howell-Jolly bodies (nuclear remnant), Heinz bodies (denatured hemoglobin), Pappenheimer bodies (iron granules), and spur cells. These "cleaned" red cells, if they have the deformability to pass through the splenic circulation, re-enter the bloodstream. Aged red cells (120 days) that have lost enzymatic activity and membrane plasticity are trapped and destroyed in the spleen[8] (Table 1).

The normal filtering function of the spleen also enables it to remove abnormal blood cells. Morphologically abnormal erythrocytes, such as the spherocytes of hereditary spherocytosis, fixed sickled cells, and rigid hemoglobin C cells, are trapped by the splenic filter. Blood cells coated with immunoglobulin G (IgG) are destroyed by the splenic monocytes, which have surface receptors for the Fc fragment of the IgG coating the cells.[8] Because the spleen removes cells coated with IgG or IgM, it is the site of destruction in diseases such as autoimmune hemolytic anemia, immune thrombocytopenic purpura, and probably Felty's syndrome. Parasites with intraerythrocytic habita-

tion, such as malaria, can be "pitted" from the red cell by the spleen.[8] Red cells that are unable to deform in order to pass into the splenic sinuses are eventually destroyed by the histiocytes/ macrophages of the red pulp.

In addition to blood cell morphology and surface characteristics, the rate of blood flow through the splenic microcirculation and alterations of splenic pulp pressure affect the filtering function of the spleen. For example, patients with splenic vein thrombosis have slow red cell passage through the splenic microcirculation owing to elevated portal-splenic pulp pressure with resulting increased red cell sequestration and destruction.[8,40]

The spleen is involved in specific and nonspecific immune responses. Properdin and tuftsin, which are synthesized in the spleen, are opsonins. Tuftsin binds to granulocytes to promote phagocytosis, whereas properdin can initiate the alternative

TABLE 1. Biologic Substances Removed by the Spleen

In Normal Subjects
Red blood cell membrane
Red blood cell surface pits and craters
Howell-Jolly bodies
Heinz bodies
Pappenheimer bodies
Acanthocytes
Senescent red blood cells
Particulate antigen

In Patients with Disease
Spherocytes (hereditary spherocytosis)
Sickled cells, Hb C cells
Antibody-coated RBC
Antibody-coated platelets
Antibody-coated WBC

Modified from Eichner, E. R.: Splenic function: Normal, too much and too little. Am. J. Med., 66:311, 1979.

pathway of complement activation to produce destruction of bacteria as well as foreign and abnormal cells. Because these opsonic proteins also are produced in other organs, the loss of the splenic contribution to their synthesis is probably small. However, serum levels of both tuftsin and properdin are below normal after splenectomy and in some diseases associated with hyposplenism.[8]

The macrophages and histiocytes of the spleen remove bacteria and abnormal or foreign cells and are especially effective in removing bacteria coated with antibody or opsonic proteins. If bacteria for which the host lacks pre-existing antibody are present in the bloodstream, the spleen's unique circulation makes it the major site for clearance of these bacteria as well as the initial site for synthesis of immunoglobulin M (IgM).[8] When radioactively labeled bacteria are administered to animals, the liver clears most of the well-opsonized microorganisms while the spleen removes those that are poorly opsonized.[8] When specific antibody is lacking to facilitate bacterial removal by the liver, the spleen becomes the primary site for clearance. Encapsulated bacteria, which resist antibody binding, are less effectively removed in an asplenic individual than in a normal host.[8]

The role of the spleen in removing malignant tumor cells is probably underestimated. Although large metastases to the spleen are uncommon, micrometastases occur frequently, with one study reporting 50 per cent of spleens from patients with solid tumors containing neoplastic cells. Experimental evidence suggests that intense destruction of malignant cells in the spleen limits the incidence of clinically apparent metastases.[8]

A third important immune function of the spleen is the production of specific antibody, especially IgM. Particulate antigens, such as salmonella flagella, lodge in the splenic red pulp and are transported by macrophages into the germinal centers where the IgM response is thought to occur.[8] In asplenic individuals, IgM levels fall, and the antibody response to a blood-borne antigen diminishes.[8] Because of the anatomy of the splenic microcirculation, humoral and cellular antigens remain in contact with macrophages and lymphocytes for longer periods than in other areas of the reticuloendothelial system. The importance of an adequate time period for interaction of these cells after antigen exposure is becoming apparent as lymphocyte and macrophage subpopulations responsible for humoral and cellular immunity are identified.

INDICATIONS FOR SPLENECTOMY

Two large series illustrate the changing indications for splenectomy that have accompanied improved diagnosis and therapy of hematologic diseases.[45,49] In one report of a 30-year experience, splenectomy was performed for primary and secondary hypersplenism (41 per cent), incidental to other operations (30 per cent), trauma (10.5 per cent), diagnosis (9 per cent). Hodgkin's staging (8 per cent), and non-Hodgkin's lymphoma (1.5 per cent). The most recent 5-year experience in this institution showed the indications for splenectomy in 473 cases to be Hodgkin's staging (27 per cent), incidental to other operations (20 per cent), hypersplenism (16 per cent), trauma (14 per cent), non-Hodgkin's lymphoma (7 per cent), and diagnosis (7 per cent).[45]

In a comparison between two series of splenectomies performed for hematologic disorders between 1946 and 1962 and 1963 and 1982, 400 splenectomies (20 per year) were performed between 1963 and 1982, compared with 94 (5.5 per year) during the earlier interval.[49] A sharp decline occurred in the number of splenectomies performed each year between 1974 and 1982. The evolution of the staging laparotomy for lymphomas, particularly Hodgkin's disease, with the decline in the average annual incidence of staging laparotomies since 1974 was the major factor responsible. Contributing to the differences was an increase in the total number of splenectomies for hereditary

spherocytosis, idiopathic hypersplenism, and myeloproliferative disorders. The average number of splenectomies for immune thrombocytopenic purpura increased significantly between the two time periods. Hairy cell leukemia and Felty's syndrome emerged as indications for splenectomy during the second time period. Of the 400 splenectomies performed for hematologic disorders at this institution between 1963 and 1982, the indications were therapeutic splenectomy (57 per cent), Hodgkin's staging (40 per cent), and diagnosis (3 per cent).[49]

An improved understanding of immune anemia, thrombocytopenia, and neutrocytopenia has clarified the role of splenectomy in many hematologic diseases. Some diseases, such as immune thrombocytopenic purpura, appear to be increasing in incidence. Splenectomy as a means of staging Hodgkin's disease is no longer such an important diagnostic test in the overall approach to that disease, which now can be controlled in most patients using radiotherapy and chemotherapy. Splenectomy for splenomegaly associated with selected leukemias and non-Hodgkin's lymphomas is less commonly indicated as chemotherapy and radiation therapy have become more effective. Hypersplenism, both primary and secondary, is now diagnosed less commonly owing to better definition and classification of diseases that previously were labeled as hypersplenic syndromes. The most frequent indications for splenectomy now are traumatic injury, immune thrombocytopenic purpura, and hypersplenism (Table 2).

In another report of splenectomy for hematologic disease, 81 per cent of the patients underwent splenectomy to control anemia, thrombocytopenia, neutropenia, or discomfort from splenomegaly.[35] In 19 per cent, splenectomy was performed for diagnostic purposes, most commonly Hodgkin's disease staging. The morbidity of 25 per cent accurately reflects the frequency of complications, which are related primarily to bleeding and infection. Sepsis is the usual cause of death following splenectomy for hematologic disease, and the mortality ranges from 5 to 27 per cent[35] (Table 3).

Splenic Trauma

The spleen is the most common intra-abdominal organ injured in blunt trauma and is a frequently injured organ in penetrating abdominal injury. Selected older reports reveal mortality for splenic injury as high as 20 per cent. Although some recent series report no deaths from splenic trauma, others still show a

TABLE 2. Indications for Splenectomy

To Control or Stage Basic Disease
Hereditary spherocytosis
Autoimmune anemia
Hodgkin's disease
Ruptured spleen
Immune thrombocytopenic purpura (ITP)
Thrombotic thrombocytopenic purpura (TTP)
Primary cysts or tumors

For Chronic and Severe Hypersplenism
Hairy cell leukemia
Lymphoproliferative disorders (NHL, CLL)
Felty's syndrome
Agnogenic myeloid metaplasia
Thalassemia major
Gaucher's disease
Hemodialysis splenomegaly
Splenic vein thrombosis
Sickle cell disease, HbS/C disease
Acquired immune deficiency syndrome (AIDS)
Thrombocytopenia associated with drug abuse

Modified from Eichner, E. R.: Splenic function: Normal, too much and too little. Am. J. Med., 66:311–320, 1979.

TABLE 3. Characteristics of 306 Patients Who Underwent Splenectomy for Hematologic Disease

Diagnosis	Number of Patients	Mean Age (Range)	Sex (M:F)	Number with Complications (%)	Deaths (%)	Mean Spleen Weight (gm) (Range)
Idiopathic thrombocytopenic purpura (ITP)	65	35 (0.5–73)	0.3	14 (22)	1 (2)	171 (26–660)
Hodgkin's disease	40	26 (5–57)	1.5	4 (10)	2 (5)	349 (50–1698)
Hereditary spherocytosis	39	15 (4–44)	0.8	2 (5)	0	430 (57–1500)
Non-Hodgkin's lymphoma	25	49 (7–76)	0.9	9 (36)	1 (4)	573 (60–2050)
Idiopathic hypersplenism	21	48 (5–74)	2.0	9 (43)	5 (24)	798 (357–2050)
Myelofibrosis	17	55 (30–72)	2.4	8 (47)	3 (18)	1776 (205–5180)
Felty's syndrome	16	56 (20–80)	0.6	3 (19)	0	766 (225–1250)
Hairy cell leukemia	16	52 (32–68)	15.0	3 (19)	1 (6)	1904 (319–5400)
Autoimmune hemolytic anemia	14	44 (16–67)	0.6	3 (21)	0	762 (175–2800)
Chronic myelogenous leukemia	9	49 (21–87)	3.5	5 (56)	3 (33)	2981 (1102–6040)
Splenomegaly with portal hypertension	9	44 (21–62)	0.1	4 (44)	0	862 (500–1830)
Chronic lymphocytic leukemia	7	62 (49–71)	2.4	5 (71)	0	2113 (685–5500)
Other*	28	35 (1–77)	0.6	7 (25)	0	773 (120–3060)
Total	306			76 (25)	16 (5)	

* This category includes ill-defined myeloproliferative disorders (4), pure red cell aplasia (3), pyruvate kinase deficiency (2), thalassemia (2), aplastic anemia (2), splenomegaly without cytopenia (2), infectious mononucleosis (2), congenital nonspherocytic hemolytic anemia (1), systemic lupus erythematosus (1), amyloidosis (1), sickle cell anemia (1), Letterer-Siwe disease (1), Gaucher's disease (2), polycythemia vera (1), mast cell leukemia (1), and subacute monocytic leukemia (1).

From Musser, G., Lazar, G., Hocking, W., Busuttil, R. W.: Splenectomy for hematologic disease: The UCLA experience with 306 patients. Ann. Surg., 200:41, 1984.

mortality approaching 10 per cent because of the frequent association of other major organ injuries.

DIAGNOSIS. Injury to the spleen should be suspected in blunt upper abdominal injuries that commonly occur in motor vehicle or bicycle accidents. Splenic injuries are commonly associated with fractured ribs of the left chest. The diagnosis and clinical course of an isolated splenic injury are variable. The spleen receives approximately 5 per cent of the cardiac output, and a large laceration through the body of the spleen can extend into the splenic pedicle, causing extensive and continued hemorrhage, abdominal distention with hemoperitoneum, and shock. More commonly, a laceration deep into the pulp occurs, or an adhesion between the spleen and its ligaments or diaphragm results in capsular avulsion with cessation of hemorrhage after an initial blood loss of 500 to 750 ml. If the injury does not involve the major splenic vasculature and is limited to the pulp or capsule, the patient may remain hemodynamically stable. However, subcapsular hematomas can form that have the potential to rupture at a time remote from the injury, representing the phenomenon of "delayed" rupture of the spleen. Alternatively, some subcapsular hematomas evolve into splenic cysts, whereas others resolve with fibrosis and scarring (Fig. 4). Unfortunately, in the acute setting of evaluating the stable patient with splenic injury, it is difficult to identify which splenic injuries will resolve without operative management.

If a splenic injury is suspected, admission to the hospital for monitoring is mandatory. Although many useful measures are available to aid in the diagnosis of splenic injury, their application requires a high index of clinical suspicion. A careful history should be obtained to include delineation of pain and a mechanism of injury consistent with splenic trauma. Usually injury to the left upper abdomen associated with fractured ribs of the left anterior chest will alert the clinician to proceed with evaluation by specific diagnostic tests. If the patient is in shock with hemoperitoneum, the diagnosis of splenic injury is established at laparotomy.

The signs and symptoms of splenic trauma are those of hemoperitoneum. Generalized and nonspecific abdominal pain in the left upper quadrant occurs in approximately one third of patients with splenic injury. Pain referred to the tip of the left shoulder (Kehr's sign) is inconstant, varying in incidence from

15 to 75 per cent, and is unreliable for excluding splenic injury but is useful for enhancing the diagnostic probability, if present. Kehr's sign is elicited by bimanual compression of the left upper quadrant after the patient has been in Trendelenburg's position for several minutes preceding the maneuver. On rare occasions, patients with splenic injury have a palpable tender mass in the left upper quadrant (Ballance's sign), resulting from an extracapsular or subcapsular hematoma with omentum adherent to the injured spleen.

Patients with splenic trauma usually have hemoglobin/hematocrit values that are 10 to 30 per cent below normal and a moderate leukocytosis. Diagnostic peritoneal lavage is a useful and inexpensive maneuver that may reveal gross blood or an elevated red blood cell count diagnostic of intraperitoneal hemorrhage. When intraperitoneal hemorrhage is diagnosed by peritoneal lavage, laparotomy is performed to diagnose and treat all bleeding viscera, including the spleen.

A variety of imaging techniques are useful in the diagnosis of

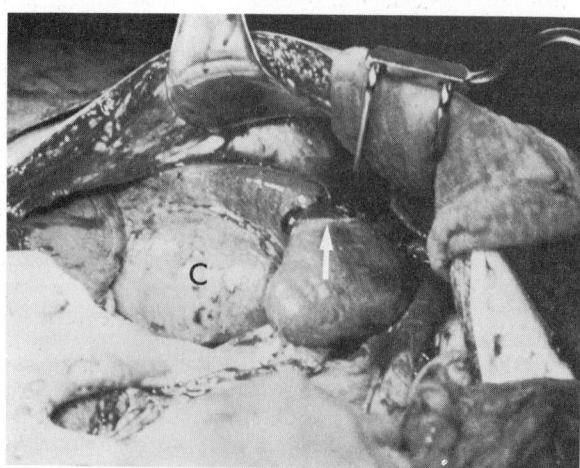

Figure 4. Operative photograph showing a traumatic laceration (arrow) producing avulsion of the lower pole of the spleen and a splenic cyst (C), an incidental finding produced by an untreated injury 8 years previously. Splenic salvage was precluded by dense inflammatory adhesions between the spleen and the diaphragm.

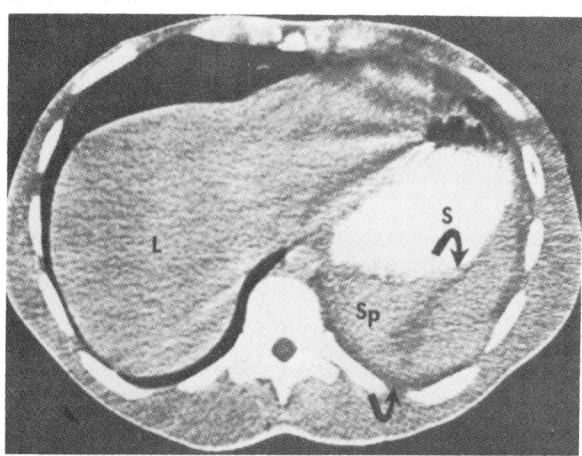

Figure 5. Computed tomogram (CT scan) revealing a laceration of the spleen (Sp) (arrows). The liver (L) and stomach (S) were uninjured. (From Federle, M. P., Crass, R. A., Jeffrey, R. B., and Trunkey, D. D.: Computed tomography in blunt abdominal trauma. Arch. Surg. *117*:645, 1982. Copyright 1982, American Medical Association.)

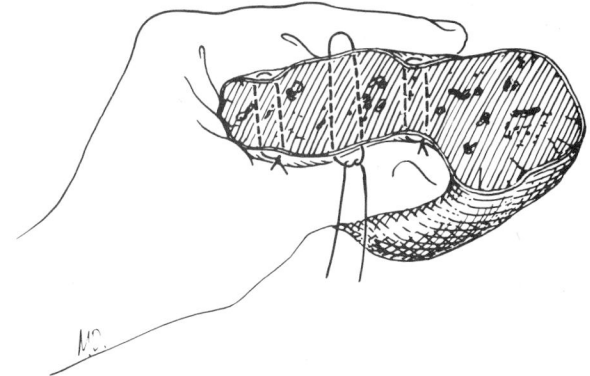

Figure 6. Technique of hemostasis following partial splenectomy. The spleen should be adequately mobilized to identify and control the injury. Compression facilitates identification of bleeding vessels, which are occluded by sutures or small metal clips, and placement of absorbable mattress sutures to control bleeding from the raw surface. (From Blaisdell, F. W., and Trunkey, D. D.: Trauma Management. New York, Thieme-Stratton, 1982, p. 194.)

splenic injury. Standard abdominal or contrast radiography may reveal depression of the splenic flexure of the colon and medial displacement of the stomach in patients with an injured spleen but is less reliable in establishing the diagnosis of splenic trauma than isotope or scanning techniques. Splenic angiography can demonstrate a variety of splenic injuries but is used infrequently because of the equal or greater accuracy of diagnostic peritoneal lavage and less invasive imaging techniques. Ultrasonography of the spleen can provide evidence of free blood and hematoma surrounding the splenic capsule with reasonable accuracy. Isotope scans (^{99m}Tc sulfur colloid) are popular in many centers for the acute diagnosis of splenic injury with a diagnostic accuracy rate exceeding 90 per cent. However, computed tomography (CT) is probably the most accurate method available for diagnosing splenic injury (Fig. 5).

Reports of imaging techniques reveal a high sensitivity and specificity (more than 90 per cent) for the diagnosis of splenic injury; however, considerable variation exists in the skill and enthusiasm of different radiologic units performing the tests for suspected splenic injury. Although CT scanning and isotope imaging techniques are accurate methods for establishing the diagnosis of an injured spleen, the accuracy in individual instances is in large part dependent on the skill of the radiologist.

CHANGING CONCEPTS IN TREATMENT OF RUPTURED SPLEEN. In recent years, the spleen's important role in cellular and humoral immunity has been clarified, and the danger of overwhelming bacterial infection in asplenic patients has been established.[8,29,39,42] Consequently, operative techniques for splenic preservation have been developed, and a concept for nonoperative management of selected splenic injuries is evolving.[32,34,36,39,42] Although periodic reports of repairing injured spleens by use of suture or cauterization have been available for many years, interest in partial splenectomy has been rekindled since 1960. In animal and human studies, it has been shown that segmental resection of the spleen is practical and safe.[39,42] In addition to partial splenectomy, splenorrhaphy, ligation of segmental vessels, and capsular repair are useful techniques for splenic salvage (Figs. 6 and 7). Splenic salvage operations have been greatly aided by the development and use of topical hemostatic agents such as microfibrillar collagen (Avitene) and a variety of absorbable "envelopes" to aid in hemostasis from splenic injuries.[27] Although technically more difficult than splenectomy, splenic repair can be performed with comparable transfusion requirements, reoperation rates, and morbidity.

Conservatism in the management of splenic injury has extended beyond repairing and preserving an injured spleen when possible. Because bleeding from splenic trauma appears to be more self-limited in children than in adults, nonoperative therapy may prove to be safe in selected pediatric patients. Nonoperative therapy requires a stable patient who is found by diagnostic tests to have an isolated splenic injury. At The Hospital for Sick Children (Toronto), where nonoperative management of splenic injury has been pioneered, 75 children with splenic injury were treated between 1981 and 1986. Ten (13 per cent) required splenectomy or splenorrhaphy, but the remaining 65 patients (87 per cent) were successfully managed nonoperatively. Of those patients treated nonoperatively, only 23 per cent required blood transfusions. In contrast with an earlier report, current guidelines for management have resulted in an increased number of patients managed nonoperatively, a reduction in the number of patients receiving blood transfusions, and a decrease in the length of both hospital stay and time spent in the intensive care unit.[36]

A large series of injuries associated with splenic trauma suggests an appropriate note of caution before nonoperative management of splenic trauma is adopted.[47] In 258 patients with splenic injury, concomitant injuries requiring operative therapy were present in 36.5 per cent of those with blunt trauma and 94 per cent of patients with penetrating injury. Children under the age of 16 years had an incidence of intra-abdominal injuries in addition to the spleen of 32.6 per cent for blunt trauma and 100 per cent for penetrating trauma.[47]

One pitfall of nonoperative management of splenic trauma

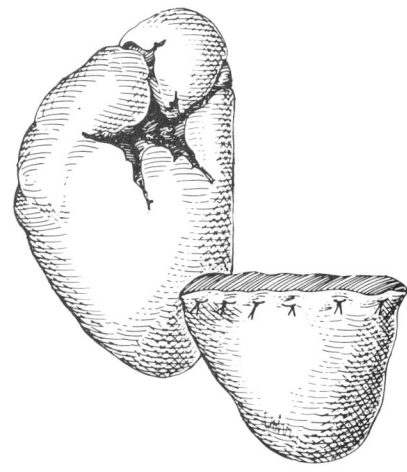

Figure 7. Technique of splenorrhaphy. Stellate lacerations that are deep or involve the hilus are best treated by resection of the injured segment. (From Blaisdell, F. W., and Trunkey, D. D.: Trauma Management. New York, Thieme-Stratton, 1982, p. 194.)

lies in the significant possibility of failing to diagnose and treat concomitant intra-abdominal injuries. An additional concern is that most reported series of nonoperative management of splenic injuries include patients with blood transfusion requirements substantial enough to expect an incidence of transfusion-related hepatitis greater than the statistical probability of postsplenectomy sepsis. In addition, hospital time is usually longer for nonoperative management (13 to 16 days) compared with operative management (7 days), with a longer period for convalescence.[47]

The recommended management in adults with hemoperitoneum and demonstrated splenic injury is laparotomy, with the expectation that 30 to 50 per cent of spleens may be salvaged with sufficient (over 50 per cent) splenic pulp retained to preserve immune function. In both children and adults with splenic injury secondary to penetrating wounds, laparotomy should be performed because of the risk of significant injury to other intra-abdominal organs. All patients in shock or with significant transfusion requirement should have exploratory laparotomy for control of hemorrhage from the spleen and management of any other injured structures.

Nonoperative treatment of splenic trauma in children is prudent only for the stable patient who is being followed in an appropriate hospital area by surgeons experienced in nonoperative management. There should be no hesitation to proceed with laparotomy and splenic repair. Operation is well tolerated, and splenic salvage techniques are probably more feasible in children than adults because of the higher ratio of splenic capsule to pulp. Any mortality from nonoperative management of splenic injury in children is unacceptable.

DELAYED RUPTURE OF THE SPLEEN. As early as 1866, Evans suggested that the spleen might bleed catastrophically at a time remote from injury.[42] It was postulated that injury to the pulp of the spleen could not be contained indefinitely by the thin splenic capsule under continuous arterial pressure. The usual interval between injury and the onset of clinically apparent intra-abdominal hemorrhage (*period de latence*, Baudet, 1907) is within 2 weeks, although longer intervals have been reported.[42] Although the incidence of delayed rupture of the spleen has been reported to be 15 to 30 per cent, the criteria for diagnosis are variable and unconvincing.[42] It is apparent from splenic injuries managed nonoperatively that many heal by fibrosis and without sequelae. The entity of delayed rupture of the spleen is more properly termed *delayed diagnosis* of splenic injury. As imaging techniques for follow-up of suspected or proved splenic trauma become commonplace, it is likely that delayed rupture of the spleen will cease to be an entity with clinical meaning or application.

SPLENOSIS AND SPLENIC IMPLANTS. Splenosis is the autotransplantation of splenic tissue following splenic trauma. Although less than 200 cases have been reported, the true incidence of splenosis undoubtedly is more common because of the high incidence of traumatic injury to the spleen. Appearing as sessile or pedunculated dark red nodules, splenic implants vary in size from a few millimeters to several centimeters in diameter. Splenic implants depend upon a blood supply from small arteries penetrating the capsule and usually remain small or outgrow their blood supply and undergo infarction. Splenosis may occur anywhere in the peritoneal cavity and has been reported on the pericardium and the pleura as well as in the subcutaneous tissue of abdominal incisions.[10] Splenosis seldom causes symptoms and usually is discovered as an incidental finding at reoperation years after splenic trauma. Isolated reports have described splenosis producing intestinal obstruction from adhesions, stomach masses simulating carcinoma, and pain, presumably from torsion.[10]

Interest in the postsplenectomy sepsis syndrome has heightened interest in splenosis as potentially valuable for preservation of immune function by providing splenic implants at the time of removal of an injured spleen. Splenosis can be produced in a variety of animals by transplantation of splenic pulp.[10] Von Stubenrauch seeded crushed splenic pulp throughout the peritoneal cavity in dogs and thought that "splenoids" arose *de novo* from the peritoneum. Perla described the histologic sequence of splenic transplants in rats. After transplantation, splenic implants underwent degeneration, with only the reticulum cells at the periphery remaining viable after 24 hours. Regeneration of splenic tissue appeared to originate from the reticulum cell precursor.[10] Investigators interested in preserving the immune function of the spleen have injected splenic pulp into the liver in order to avoid mechanical problems from adhesions that sometimes develop in association with splenosis.

Splenosis, "the born-again spleen," may provide the blood management functions of the spleen.[37] The absence of Howell-Jolly bodies, siderocytes, and other postsplenectomy blood changes, as well as the recurrence of the hematologic disease for which splenectomy was performed, should raise suspicion of splenosis or the presence of accessory splenic tissue.[22,37,40,41,50] Splenosis has been reported in conjunction with the expected postsplenectomy blood changes, suggesting that a critical mass of splenic tissue is needed for recovery of splenic function. Residual splenic tissue can be detected by isotope scanning using ^{99m}Tc sulfur colloid (Fig. 8).

Splenic reticuloendothelial function has been investigated in a series of patients who previously had total splenectomy, partial splenectomy and splenic repair, and splenic autotransplantation.[46] Partial splenectomy and splenorrhaphy resulted in normal splenic reticuloendothelial function that was indistinguishable from a control group of patients sustaining trauma but who had intact spleens. Extraperitoneal splenic autotransplantation resulted in the preservation of a small amount of reticuloendothelial function. The subnormal reticuloendothelial function achieved by splenic autotransplantation was clearly superior to that resulting from total splenectomy without deliberate splenic autotransplantation. Splenic autotransplantation, which in this study involved placing thin slices of spleen weighing a total of 25 to 30 gm. into an anterolateral extraperitoneal pocket, appeared to be safe and was not associated with increased postoperative complications.[46]

Although autotransplanted splenic tissue, accessory splenic tissue, and splenosis can restore some of the spleen's blood management functions and antibody synthesis, it is unclear how much splenic tissue is needed for protection against overwhelming postsplenectomy sepsis. Studies have failed to identify re-establishment of resistance to postsplenectomy sepsis after autotransplantation of splenic tissue. Death from postsple-

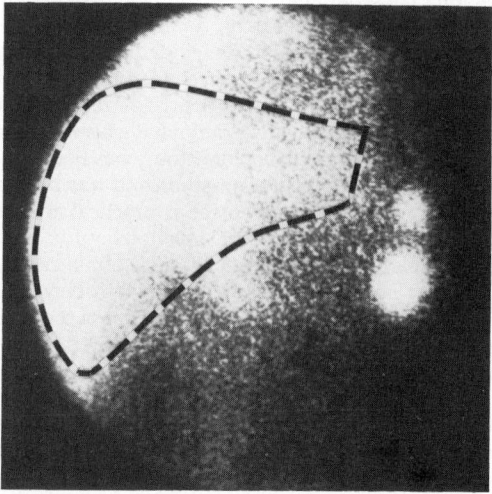

Figure 8. Technetium-99m sulfur colloid scan reveals two accessory spleens in the left upper quadrant. The liver is outlined.

nectomy sepsis has occurred in children and adults having a total mass of residual splenic tissue weighing 3 to 92 gm.[46] Although residual splenic tissue can restore some of the spleen's functions, a critical amount of splenic tissue is required for full protection against postsplenectomy sepsis.[8,29,39]

Immune Thrombocytopenic Purpura

Immune thrombocytopenic purpura (ITP) (previously idiopathic thrombocytopenic purpura) is a syndrome characterized by a persistently low platelet count. The thrombocytopenia is caused by a circulating antiplatelet factor that results in platelet destruction by the reticuloendothelial system. In most patients, the antiplatelet factor is an immunoglobulin (IgG) antibody directed toward a platelet-associated antigen. Circulating immune complexes may have a causal role in some cases, but their precise role is unclear. Proof of autoimmunity is lacking.[30]

The majority of patients with ITP are young women. In the series of Schwartz and colleagues, the average age was 36 years, and the duration of clinical symptoms before splenectomy was 24 weeks, with an average preoperative platelet count of 33,000 per cu. mm.[41] ITP is increasing in frequency, and the disease is being diagnosed more often now in men. This increase results in part from the association of immune thrombocytopenia with the acquired immunodeficiency syndrome (AIDS) and an increasing occurrence of ITP in three groups of patients at risk for developing AIDS—homosexual men positive for human immunodeficiency virus (HIV), parenteral drug abusers, and hemophiliacs receiving multiple transfusions.[20] The diagnosis of ITP is suggested by spontaneous and easy bruising, petechiae, and mucosal bleeding. Menorrhagia is common, and prolonged bleeding after shaving trauma may be an initial complaint in men. Intracranial hemorrhage is a rare and usually fatal complication.

The propensity for hemorrhage is reflected by the level of thrombocytopenia. A bleeding diathesis is unlikely with thrombocytopenia in the range of 50,000 to 100,000 per cu. mm. Bleeding with minor trauma or surgical therapy can be expected with platelet counts in the range of 20,000 to 100,000 per cu. mm. Spontaneous bleeding with purpura and petechiae, epistaxis, menorrhagia, and gingival bleeding occurs commonly with platelet counts below 20,000 per cu. mm. and especially below 5000 per cu. mm.[25]

Crosby has suggested classifying patients with thrombocytopenia into those with "dry purpura" (petechiae and ecchymoses) and those with "wet purpura" (active bleeding from mucosal surfaces). This distinction postulates that patients with wet purpura are at increased risk for central nervous system bleeding and thus require aggressive treatment.[30]

Patients with easy bruisability or hemorrhage require a careful history, with special emphasis on recent exposure to quinine, quinidine, sulfonamides, and thiazides that may produce drug-dependent antibodies and immune thrombocytopenia. Isoantibodies against transfusion products also can cause thrombocytopenia. Collagen vascular disease such as systemic lupus erythematosus may be indistinguishable in initial presentation from ITP.[25,30] Pseudothrombocytopenia, a phenomenon in which the platelet count is spuriously low, results when antibodies in the patient's serum react with platelets in blood anticoagulated with EDTA causing agglutination. Platelet clumping results in a falsely low platelet count that will be at variance with the estimated number of platelets present on a peripheral blood smear obtained by fingertip puncture. EDTA-dependent platelet antibodies have been detected in several patients erroneously diagnosed as having ITP.[22,50] Diagnosis of ITP requires the exclusion of drug-dependent antibodies, isoantibodies, collagen vascular disease, lymphoproliferative disorders, thyroid disease, recent viral illness, and spurious thrombocytopenia.[22,25,30,50] Patients with "classic" ITP rarely have a palpable spleen (less than 2 per cent), whereas a palpable spleen that

reflects mild-to-moderate enlargement and an associated high incidence of generalized lymphadenopathy have been found in ITP associated with AIDS.[22,50]

ITP is diagnosed definitively only after exclusion of other illnesses or conditions that cause or are associated with thrombocytopenia. Except for thrombocytopenia, patients with ITP usually have normal blood counts. Antinuclear antibodies are rarely present, but autoantibodies have been noted in some patients. A peripheral blood smear shows thrombocytopenia, occasionally with an increased number of large platelets. A bone marrow aspirate reveals normal granulocytic and erythrocytic elements with an increased megakaryocyte count.[22,30,50]

PLATELET KINETICS AND THE IMMUNE SYSTEM. Platelet kinetics in patients with ITP are markedly altered, with an increased platelet production (four to five times normal) and an increased megakaryocyte mass being present in association with a greatly shortened platelet survival.[30] In patients with ITP, body surface counts show primarily splenic sequestration of platelets, with significant liver sequestration occurring only in patients with severe disease. The amount of platelet-associated antibody reflects the severity of the clinical disease and is inversely correlated with the patient's platelet count and intravascular platelet life span. The antiplatelet factor probably is an IgG antibody directed against a platelet-associated antigen. In some patients, the IgG antibody functions in combination with IgM, IgA, or both.[30] Antiplatelet antibody assays are now routinely available, and the value for platelet-associated IgG normally is less than 1200 gamma globulin molecules per platelet.

The spleen is an important site of antibody production, and splenic cells from patients with chronic ITP produce five to six times more IgG in culture than control splenic cells.[30] The initial immune response to the platelet antigen probably occurs in the spleen, or in the bone marrow where intramedullary platelets and megakaryocytes share antigenic determinants and may trigger a response. In its function as a monitor of the intravascular space, the spleen probably is more important in the early response. Less involved initially, the marrow assumes an important role as the immune response becomes generalized. With development and recirculation of memory cells (both B and T lymphocytes), the marrow becomes a major site of antibody production. The liver produces little or no antiplatelet antibody, and the lymph nodes are not deeply involved in the response to intravascular antigens.[30]

Platelet destruction in ITP requires sufficient quantities of antigen (platelets), antibody, and phagocytic cells in an environment that provides time for antibody binding and subsequent platelet phagocytosis.[30] The spleen is ideally suited for this function, and once platelet sensitization has occurred, phagocytosis is triggered by the Fc portion of the IgG molecule or by complement activation with C3b fixation to the platelet surface. The macrophage Fc-receptor mechanism clearly is important, as increased platelet-bound IgG is present in essentially all patients with ITP. Macrophage Fc and C3b receptors may act synergistically, resulting in a greatly enhanced phagocytic efficiency.[30]

Because 30 per cent of the total circulating platelet mass is within the spleen at all times as an exchangeable platelet pool, the spleen is the most active site of platelet destruction.[30] The stagnant blood flow in the splenic microcirculation allows sensitized platelets to be readily removed by phagocytic cells lining the reticular network of the red pulp. Having no resident platelet pool and possessing a rapid microcirculation by contrast, the liver assumes a major role in platelet destruction when severe disease and high antibody titers result in heavily sensitized platelets. The bone marrow is the most likely source of antibody in patients who have undergone splenectomy.[30] Intramedullary platelet destruction and inhibition of thrombopoiesis may occur as a result of antiplatelet antibody binding to both platelets and megakaryocytes, although the efficiency of the marrow reticuloendothelial system is below that of the liver and the spleen.[30]

A recent study investigating the mechanisms of increase in the platelet count following treatment of immune thrombocytopenic purpura determined the survival time and localization of radiolabeled autologous platelets and measured platelet-associated immunoglobulin levels before and after prednisone therapy or splenectomy.[11] Prednisone therapy resulted in an increased platelet count from increased platelet production. The increased platelet count following splenectomy correlated with increased platelet survival. The degree of radiolabeled platelet localization in the liver was normal in patients in whom splenectomy was effective and was increased to above normal in patients in whom splenectomy was ineffective. The conclusion that prednisone improves platelet counts primarily by increasing platelet production requires modification of the pathophysiologic concept of immune thrombocytopenia to incorporate the hypothesis that in some patients the predominant cause of thrombocytopenia is ineffective marrow production of platelets rather than accelerated platelet removal.[11]

In summary, thrombocytopenia in patients with immune thrombocytopenic purpura usually occurs because of a combination of intramedullary platelet removal by reticuloendothelial cells resulting in ineffective platelet production and decreased survival of circulating platelets due to peripheral sequestration and destruction in the spleen and liver. Successful therapy may produce an increase in the platelet count either by increasing the effective production of platelets or by decreasing peripheral platelet sequestration and destruction. Splenectomy appears to increase platelet survival by removing a major organ of peripheral destruction. If the liver is the major site of platelet destruction, splenectomy may not result in improvement in the platelet count.[11]

TREATMENT. The goal of therapy in chronic ITP is to obtain a complete and sustained remission of the disease and to remove the patient from the risks of hemorrhage.[30] This can be achieved in 80 to 90 per cent of patients (Table 4).

When ITP is initially diagnosed, the patient should be hospitalized. A patient with active bleeding should remain at bed rest, and specific therapy should be instituted. Platelet transfusions provide immediate benefit and should be administered as needed to control bleeding. Although transfused platelets rapidly become coated with antibody and are destroyed, providing only transient benefit, they afford protection against life-threatening bleeding.[25,30] High-dose intravenous gamma globulin also is useful but requires several days for a beneficial platelet increase to occur.

Corticosteroid therapy (prednisone, 1 mg. per kg. per day or the therapeutic equivalent) is instituted at the time of diagnosis. Most patients with ITP are improved with steroids, an increase in the platelet count occurring within 3 to 7 days and reaching a maximum in several weeks.[30] Complete and sustained remission with steroids is rare, although rates as high as 25 per cent have been reported.[30] In most cases, even if the platelet count becomes normal with steroids, the response is transient and thrombocytopenia recurs as the steroid dose is tapered.

Splenectomy should be performed in patients with ITP that is refractory to corticosteroid therapy. In the majority of patients, splenectomy is performed electively. Emergency splenectomy is necessary in patients with ITP who have evidence of central nervous system bleeding.

Complete remission following splenectomy is more likely in patients who have shown a response to steroids. Additional clinical features indicating the likelihood of a favorable response to splenectomy include patients who are less than 60 years old, who have disease of relatively short duration, and who exhibit a prompt thrombocytosis with platelet counts reaching 500,000 per cu. mm. or more following splenectomy.[25,30] Most patients, however, are improved following splenectomy even if their platelet counts were not significantly increased by steroid therapy.

Eighty-eight per cent of Schwartz and associates' patients responded to splenectomy and developed normal platelet counts. Of those responding to splenectomy, 20 per cent had platelet counts exceeding 100,000 per cu. mm. by the third postoperative day, and 90 per cent of them had normal platelet counts after 1 week. The remaining responders developed normal platelet counts within 1 to 6 months postoperatively. In 3 patients, thrombocytopenia recurred after a long interval and was attributed in 1 patient to an accessory spleen.[41]

The level of platelet-associated IgG falls to normal following a response to splenectomy, because of the removal of a large site of antiplatelet antibody production.[30] A steroid response also is accompanied by a decrease in platelet-associated IgG. An increase in the platelet count often occurs before platelet-associated IgG falls because of the steroid influence on the reticuloendothelial system. A response to immunosuppressants such as cyclophosphamide and vincristine also is associated with a decrease in platelet-associated IgG.[30]

ITP DURING CHILDHOOD. In children, particularly those under the age of 6 years, ITP often appears following a viral upper respiratory infection. In contrast to the adult form of the disease, childhood ITP usually undergoes spontaneous remission without specific therapy. A short course of prednisone therapy usually is prescribed; however, a clear benefit has not been demonstrated.[25]

Intracranial hemorrhage is a life-threatening complication of childhood ITP and occurs in 1 to 2 per cent of cases. It is responsible for the majority of deaths from the disease in this age group. The risk of intracranial hemorrhage is greatest during the first month of the illness. Most reported cases appear to be spontaneous, but minor head trauma may result in intracranial hemorrhage in patients with platelet counts below 10,000 to

TABLE 4. Results of Therapy in Immune Thrombocytopenic Purpura

Therapy	Number of Cases	Average Dose	Response Time (Days)	Response* Excellent	Good (%)	Fair	Poor
Splenectomy	756	—	1–14	80	← 20 →		
Steroids	253	60–100 mg./day	14	19	← 34 →		47
Cyclophosphamide	61	50–200 mg./day	14–56	42	14	12	32
Vinblastine	20	10 mg./wk.	10	5	← 56 →		39
Vincristine	21	2 mg./wk.	10	← 28 →		48	24
Azathioprine	92	100–250 mg./day	60–120	8	18	26	48

* Response definitions: excellent, normal platelet count after therapy; good, normal platelet count during therapy; fair, improved platelet count during therapy; poor, no response. In some cases, details of the reports did not permit accurate placement, and in those cases percentages may apply to more than one response category (arrows).

Modified from McMillan, R.: Chronic idiopathic thrombocytopenic purpura. N. Engl. J. Med., 304:1135, 1981.

20,000 per cu. mm.[51] Development of intracranial hemorrhage in ITP is an indication for emergency splenectomy.

Spontaneous and complete remission occurs in approximately 85 per cent of children with ITP. Those in whom spontaneous remission does not occur within 1 year are considered to have chronic ITP and usually undergo elective splenectomy to avoid the risks of chronic thrombocytopenia.

SPLENECTOMY AND PERIOPERATIVE THERAPY FOR ITP. Most patients are referred for splenectomy after steroid therapy has failed to achieve a complete and sustained remission. In a small group of patients, ITP is diagnosed as a result of abnormal bleeding during surgical therapy or after injury. A third group of patients requires emergency splenectomy for intracranial hemorrhage.

High-dose intravenous gamma globulin is very effective in achieving an increase in the platelet count preoperatively in patients who do not respond to steroids or are not candidates for steroid therapy. It is postulated that intravenous gamma globulin therapy promotes a rise in the platelet count because it temporarily reduces platelet destruction by saturating macrophage Fc receptors, thus producing a transient blockade of the reticuloendothelial system. A significantly improved platelet count (100,000 to 250,000 per cu. mm.) occurs within 4 to 6 days and provides a "therapeutic window" for performance of splenectomy.[22,50] In addition to effecting an increase in the platelet counts of patients who fail to respond to steroids or who are not candidates for steroid therapy, high-dose gamma globulin therapy is appropriate for the patient with ITP needing urgent splenectomy in whom a trial of steroids is not warranted, and in the pregnant patient with ITP late in the third trimester of pregnancy.

Immunizations with polyvalent pneumococcal vaccine (Pnu-Imune 23 or Pneumovax 23), *Haemophilus influenzae* vaccine, and *Neisseria meningitidis* vaccine should be administered as soon as it becomes likely that splenectomy will be performed. Ideally, these immunizations should be administered 10 to 14 days preoperatively. It is probable that patients receiving steroids will have a suboptimal early response to these vaccines but ultimately will develop protective antibody titers. The availability of blood and platelets for transfusion should be ensured, although the need for blood transfusion is rare. Intraoperative thrombocytopenic bleeding usually ceases after the splenic artery is ligated. In Schwartz's series, platelets were not used preoperatively and were administered intraoperatively or postoperatively in only 9 of 120 patients who had splenectomy for ITP.[41] Although a nasogastric tube is advisable for postoperative gastric decompression in most patients undergoing splenectomy, one of the authors (G.F.S.) avoids use of a nasogastric tube in patients with ITP because of the potential risk of precipitating hemorrhage from the nose or nasopharynx.

Splenectomy can be performed through a variety of abdominal incisions. The midline incision is preferred in ITP as it allows entry into the peritoneal cavity without transection of abdominal muscles and thus reduces the potential for postoperative muscle hematoma. The spleen, usually of normal size, is assessed for adhesions and the nature of its ligamentous attachments. Splenic ligaments vary considerably in composition; some are thin membranes affording easy dissection, and others are thick and tendinous. The technique for splenectomy is a matter of personal preference. The authors prefer the sequence of initially incising the posterior splenic ligaments, followed by mobilizing the spleen and tail of the pancreas toward the midline for subsequent dissection of the splenic vessels in the hilus. Caution is taken to avoid excessive traction or trauma to the tail of the pancreas. Division of the gastrosplenic ligament is performed with suture ligation of the gastric ends of the short gastric arteries. Following removal of the spleen, laparotomy pads are placed in the left upper quadrant while a search is made for accessory splenic tissue. Approximately 20 per cent of

patients have an accessory spleen; common sites are the splenic hilus, adjacent to the splenic vessels and tail of the pancreas, the greater omentum, and the gastrosplenic and gastrocolic ligaments. Rarely has an accessory spleen been found in the intestinal mesentery or presacral and gonadal regions.[9,40] The left upper quadrant is not drained routinely. Indications for closed suction drainage are injury to the pancreas during hilar dissection and incomplete hemostasis.

During the immediate postoperative period, steroid therapy is continued intravenously and the platelet count is monitored. It usually is possible to begin tapering the steroid dose immediately. In patients demonstrating a satisfactory thrombocytosis, steroids are gradually reduced over 4 to 6 weeks and discontinued.

The mortality rate for splenectomy in ITP is under 2 per cent and occurs primarily in patients with intracranial hemorrhage. In approximately 80 per cent of adult patients who have splenectomy for ITP, the platelet count returns to normal or above normal levels within the first 6 weeks following operation.[30] In approximately 15 per cent, there is substantial improvement in the platelet count from preoperative levels, but it will not reach a normal level. Only about 5 per cent of patients remain severely thrombocytopenic after splenectomy and require some form of chronic therapy. In these patients with refractory ITP, therapy with the least severe side effects is chosen to maintain the platelet count at a safe level (30,000 to 50,000 per cu. mm.). Ingestion of antiplatelet drugs, trauma, azotemia, fever, and infection increase the bleeding tendency in thrombocytopenic patients.[30] Immunosuppressants such as cyclophosphamide, vinca alkaloids (vincristine and vinblastine), and azathioprine and danazol, a modified androgen, have been used to treat patients with refractory ITP with variable results (see Table 4).

Thrombotic Thrombocytopenic Purpura

Thrombotic thrombocytopenic purpura (TTP) (Moschcowitz's syndrome) is a syndrome characterized by thrombocytopenia, microangiopathic hemolytic anemia, fluctuating neurologic abnormalities, progressive renal failure, and fever. TTP is produced by widespread deposition of platelet microthrombi, and the pentad of clinical manifestations results from occlusion of arterioles and capillaries by subendothelial and intraluminal deposits of "hyaline" material composed of aggregated platelets and fibrin. The etiology of TTP is unknown, and approximately 90 per cent of the cases of TTP are idiopathic. The pathologic response in TTP may be initiated by various stimuli, including viral and bacterial infection, pregnancy, drugs (oral contraceptives, mitomycin, and cyclosporine), and nonspecified toxins. The syndrome has been associated with systemic lupus erythematosus and other connective tissue disorders, malignancies, and more recently with AIDS. TTP has a peak incidence in the third decade of life and occurs more frequently in women than in men.[22,50]

The differential diagnosis includes hemolytic-uremic syndrome, disseminated intravascular coagulation (DIC), drug reaction, eclampsia, aplastic anemia, idiopathic autoimmune hemolytic anemia, ITP, leukemia, paroxysmal nocturnal hemoglobinuria, periarteritis nodosa, infection, systemic lupus erythematosus, and exposure to toxins. The exact role of the spleen in TTP is unclear, but approximately 20 per cent of patients have splenomegaly.[22,50]

The prognosis for untreated patients with TTP is very poor, with less than 10 per cent surviving beyond 1 year.[22] The current therapeutic regimen of infusions of fresh-frozen plasma results in dramatic improvement for the majority of patients with TTP. A combined therapeutic approach using plasma therapy, antiplatelet agents (aspirin and dipyridamole), and high-dose corticosteroid therapy is instituted immediately after the diagnosis is established. Plasma infusion or plasma exchange using plasmapheresis and replacement with fresh-frozen plasma achieves response rates of between 70 and 90 per cent.[22] It is speculated that plasma infusion or plasma exchange replaces a deficient plasma component or removes some toxic substance.[22,50] Immunosuppressive drugs (vincristine and azathioprine) also are beneficial adjunctive agents in the present combined therapeutic approach for TTP. If combined modality therapy fails, splenectomy should be performed. Splenectomy occasionally results in spectacular improvement, particularly when combined with high-dose corticosteroid therapy and antiplatelet drugs.[22] Although a clear physiologic explanation is lacking for this occasional response to splenectomy, prior experience has documented that 70 per cent of the long-term survivors with TTP were patients who had undergone splenectomy.[41]

Hypersplenism

Hypersplenism is a concept, probably first used by Chauffard in 1907, that refers to a variety of ill effects resulting from increased splenic function which may be improved by splenectomy.[22,50] Criteria for diagnosis include (1) anemia, leukopenia, thrombocytopenia, or combinations thereof, (2) compensatory bone marrow hyperplasia, (3) splenomegaly, and (4) improvement following splenectomy.[8,22,50] Hypersplenism is classified as *primary* when an underlying disease cannot be identified to account for the exaggerated splenic function. *Secondary hypersplenism* refers to those cases in which a specific or more or less well-defined disorder has been diagnosed. Because it now is possible to obtain more specific diagnoses for many patients who previously would have been thought to have primary hypersplenism, primary hypersplenism is now diagnosed much less frequently than secondary hypersplenism.

Primary hypersplenism was initially described in 1939 by Doan and Wiseman as an illness consisting of neutropenia and splenomegaly for which splenectomy was curative.[40] The definition of the syndrome subsequently was broadened to include patients with variable degrees of anemia, thrombocytopenia, or pancytopenia. Subclassification of primary hypersplenism is used to describe splenic hyperfunction resulting in depression of one or more of the formed elements of the blood (red cells, white cells, and platelets). Primary splenic panhematopenia (pancytopenia) refers to depression of all formed elements, whereas in primary splenic neutropenia, depression of the white blood cells is the prominent feature.

Most patients with primary hypersplenism are women. Clinical manifestations depend upon the specific formed elements that are depressed and include pallor and other signs of anemia, fever, recurrent infections, oral ulcerations, ecchymoses, and petechiae. Splenomegaly is common. The peripheral blood smear shows leukopenia or varying degrees of pancytopenia without evidence of leukemia or myeloproliferative disorders. Pancellular hyperplasia is present in the bone marrow.

Primary hypersplenism is a diagnosis of exclusion and should be accepted only after an exhaustive search for a specific etiology of hypersplenism has been unrewarding. Corticosteroids are seldom of benefit in primary hypersplenism. Splenectomy is indicated when the diagnosis is established and usually results in marked hematologic improvement for nearly all patients. Occasional patients have subsequently developed reticulum cell sarcoma or histiocytic lymphoma.[40,50]

Lymphoma with primary presentation in the spleen may present as asymptomatic splenomegaly with or without hypersplenism. Radionuclide, CT, and magnetic resonance imaging usually reveal nonspecific, featureless organ enlargement. If parenchymal expansion secondary to tumor infiltration and congestion becomes massive, splenic pooling and increased regional blood flow may result in hypersplenism. Lymphoma with primary presentation in the spleen may result in the diagnosis of "idiopathic splenomegaly" until splenectomy permits accurate histopathologic diagnosis.

TABLE 5. Etiology of Splenomegaly

Mechanism	Example
Work hypertrophy: immune response	Subacute bacterial endocarditis Infectious mononucleosis Felty's syndrome
Work hypertrophy: red cell destruction	Spherocytosis Thalassemia major Pyruvate kinase deficiency
Congestive	Cirrhosis Splenic vein thrombosis
Myeloproliferative	Chronic myelocytic leukemia Myeloid metaplasia
Infiltrative	Sarcoidosis Amyloidosis Gaucher's disease
Neoplastic	Lymphoma Hairy cell leukemia Chronic lymphocytic leukemia Metastatic cancer

Modified from Eichner, E. R.: Splenic function: Normal, too much and too little. Am. J. Med., 66:311, 1979.

Secondary hypersplenism classically refers to a syndrome of pancytopenia (anemia, thrombocytopenia, and leukopenia) associated with portal hypertension from intrahepatic or extrahepatic portal or splenic vein obstruction. Hypersplenism associated with portal hypertension secondary to cirrhosis seldom requires splenectomy. Cytopenias commonly are improved after a shunt between the portal and systemic circulations, presumably resulting from relief of congestive splenomegaly.[40] Splenic vein thrombosis with bleeding from gastric varices should be treated by splenectomy, which usually cures the gastric variceal bleeding and any existing hypersplenism.[6,39]

Secondary hypersplenism includes a number of diseases sharing the common feature of splenomegaly. Rather than listing these, it is more appropriate to consider the mechanisms producing splenic enlargement[8] (Table 5). Work hypertrophy from immune response and/or red blood cell destruction, venous congestion, myeloproliferation, infiltration, and neoplastic proliferation within the spleen produce variable degrees of splenomegaly. Diverse pathophysiologic mechanisms are involved in the resulting hypersplenism[8] (Table 6). In both pri-

TABLE 6. Etiology of Hypersplenism in Selected Diseases

Disease	Probable Mechanism
Hairy cell leukemia	Retention of hairy cells in splenic pulp
Portal hypertension (cirrhosis, splenic vein thrombosis)	Increased pooling of blood cells
Felty's syndrome	Immune system work hypertrophy
Thalassemia major	Reticuloendothelial system work hypertrophy
Hemodialysis splenomegaly	Immune and reticuloendothelial system work hypertrophy
Gaucher's disease	Increased pooling and flow-induced dilutional anemia
Agnogenic myeloid metaplasia	Extramedullary hematopoiesis

Modified from Eichner, E. R.: Splenic function: Normal, too much and too little. Am. J. Med., 66:311, 1979.

mary and secondary hypersplenism, the degree of splenomegaly does not correlate closely with the severity of clinical symptoms or the degree of depression of formed elements of the blood.

Hyposplenism

Hyposplenism is a potentially lethal syndrome characterized by diminished splenic function. Hyposplenism was first described by Dameshek in 1955 in a patient with sprue who had an asplenic peripheral blood pattern with Howell-Jolly bodies and target cells.[8] As in the asplenic patient, other peripheral blood findings that suggest hyposplenism are the presence of acanthocytes and siderocytes, a long-term lymphocytosis and monocytosis, and a mild thrombocytosis.[8] Diagnosis of hyposplenism is confirmed by an isotope scan (^{99m}Tc sulfur colloid) revealing an atrophic spleen. Hyposplenism can occur in the presence of a normal-sized or an enlarged spleen (Table 7).

The danger of hyposplenism is the risk of developing potentially lethal sepsis (see section on Overwhelming Postsplenectomy Sepsis). Sickle cell anemia is the most common disease associated with hyposplenism. Children with sickle cell anemia are vulnerable to overwhelming pneumococcal infection similar to that seen in asplenic children. The child with sickle cell anemia is most vulnerable when the spleen is enlarged. By the time the spleen becomes atrophic from recurrent infarctions ("autosplenectomy"), the patient has developed some immunity from exposure to different pneumococcal strains.[8]

The most common surgical disease associated with hyposplenism is chronic ulcerative colitis, in which 40 per cent or more of patients develop hyposplenism as the pancolitis progresses. Other conditions associated with hyposplenism in which the surgeon is commonly involved include thyrotoxicosis, corticosteroid administration, and when patients have received Thorotrast (thorium dioxide) as a radiocontrast agent.[8] If a patient is suspected of having or proved to have hyposplenism, the same precautions against sepsis recommended for asplenic patients should be instituted.

Hodgkin's Disease

Described by Thomas Hodgkin in 1832, Hodgkin's disease is a malignant lymphoma characterized by the presence of typical, multinucleate giant cells. The unique cell, described by Sternberg and later Reed around the turn of the century, is essential for diagnosis. Hodgkin's disease is relatively rare, with a bimodal age-incidence curve that peaks in the late twenties and declines to the mid-forties. After age 45 years, the incidence of Hodgkin's disease increases with age. The disease is slightly more common in men than in women.[3,22,50]

Most patients with Hodgkin's disease have asymptomatic lymphadenopathy at the time of diagnosis. The site of initial nodal involvement is the cervical area in most patients (65 to 80 per cent), followed by the axillary (10 to 15 per cent) and inguinal (6 to 12 per cent) regions. Retroperitoneal lymph nodes may be involved, but lymphangiography or computed tomography (CT scan) is required for diagnosis. Mediastinal involvement occurs in 6 to 11 per cent of patients at the time of diagnosis.[3,22,50]

Constitutional symptoms (B symptoms), such as fever, night sweats, weight loss, and pruritus, usually indicate widespread involvement and are unfavorable prognostic signs. They may appear simultaneously with lymph node enlargement or may precede development of lymphadenopathy. A typical fever pattern is a high temperature alternating for a few days with an afebrile period (Pel-Ebstein fever). Less specific constitutional symptoms include localized acute discomfort in areas of adenopathy following ingestion of alcoholic beverages, malaise, lethargy, easy fatigability, generalized weakness, and anorexia.[3,22,50]

Many patients have a mild normochromic normocytic anemia. One third have a leukocytosis due to a neutrophil increase, and eosinophilia is present frequently. Lymphopenia is common in the later stages of the disease. The platelet count is normal initially but is frequently depressed in advanced disease. There is a progressive loss of T-lymphocyte function with reduced cell-mediated immunity.

A classification of Hodgkin's disease was developed by the International Symposium held in Rye, New York, in 1965, at which time the earlier classifications were simplified. In the "Rye classification," there are four histopathologic subtypes of Hodgkin's disease: lymphocyte predominance, nodular sclerosis, mixed cellularity, and lymphocyte depletion. Lymphocyte predominance and nodular sclerosis subtypes have a more favorable prognosis than mixed cellularity and lymphocyte depletion subtypes. However, the prognostic implications of subtyping are becoming less useful because of the excellent results of current aggressive treatment.[3,22,50]

Hodgkin's disease metastasizes initially in a predictable, nonrandom pattern via lymphatic channels to contiguous lymph node groups and organs with a prominent lymphatic tissue component. The predictable mode of spread of Hodgkin's disease provides the basis for irradiation of adjacent lymph node areas in patients with apparently localized disease.[3] Treatment and ultimate survival of the patients with Hodgkin's disease depend on the anatomic distribution of the disease and the presence or absence of specific symptoms, the stage of the disease, and the histopathologic subtype.[3,22,50]

Histopathologic diagnosis is made by examining specimens from lymph node biopsy, in which the largest and most centrally placed node should be selected for excision. In a matted group or cluster of nodes, a central node from the group should be excised or a generous incisional biopsy obtained. Nodes from the lower cervical or axillary areas provide the most satisfactory tissue for histopathologic evaluation, because nodes from the parotid, submandibular, and inguinal regions often show changes due to previous inflammatory processes in their regions of drainage. When only mediastinal adenopathy is present, biopsy is performed through mediastinoscopy or thoracotomy, as indicated. Laparotomy is seldom required to obtain the initial diagnosis in Hodgkin's disease.[3]

Since the concept of staging was introduced approximately 25 years ago, the staging process has undergone continued modification with the intent of accurately defining the anatomic sites of involvement and thus improving patient selection for the most appropriate type and amount of therapy. Stage I disease indicates nodal involvement in only one lymph node region. Stage II disease is limited to two or more lymph node regions on the same side of the diaphragm. Stage III refers to disease involving lymph node regions on both sides of the diaphragm (the spleen is considered a lymph node). Stage IV disease encompasses diffuse or disseminated involvement of one

TABLE 7. Diseases Associated with Hyposplenism

Atrophic spleen
    Ulcerative colitis
    Celiac disease
    Dermatitis herpetiformis
    Thyrotoxicosis (Graves' disease)
    Hemorrhagic thrombocythemia
    Thorotrast administration
    Sickle cell anemia (chronic)

Normal-sized or enlarged spleen
    Sickle cell anemia, HbS/C disease
    Sarcoidosis
    Amyloidosis
    Corticosteroid administration (?)

Modified from Eichner, E. R.: Splenic function: Normal, too much and too little. Am. J. Med., 66:311, 1979.

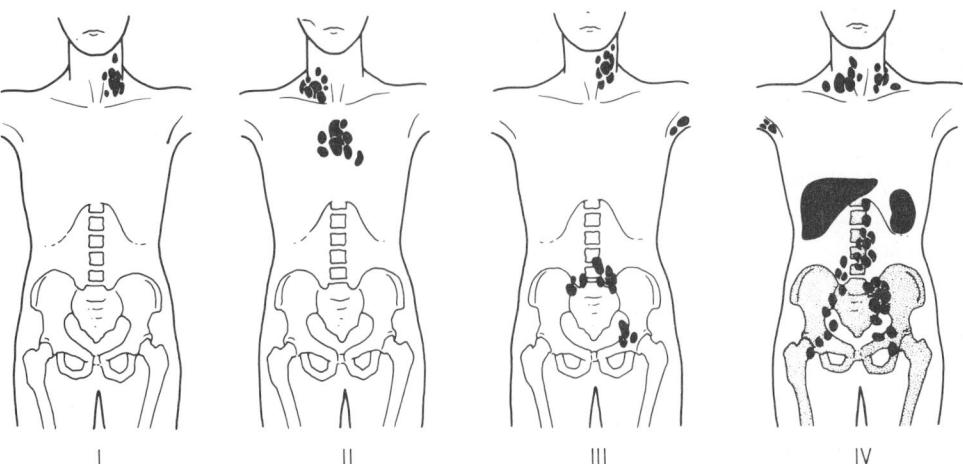

Figure 9. Ann Arbor Staging Classification for Hodgkin's disease. (From Hoffbrand, A. V., and Pettit, J. E.: Essential Haematology. Oxford, Blackwell Scientific Publications, 1980, p. 141.)

or more distant extranodal organs with or without associated lymph node involvement. Stage is further classified as A (absence) or B (presence) with regard to fever, night sweats, weight loss, and pruritus. The subscript E is used to classify selected patients having localized extranodal disease in Stages I, II, and III (e.g., lung, muscle, bone, skin) contiguous to involved nodes. In general, the E designation is reserved for patients having extralymphatic disease so limited in extent and/or location that it is amenable to definitive treatment by radiotherapy. The S subscript indicates splenic involvement.[3,21,22,39,50] Anatomic substages of Stage IIIA disease have been designated to differentiate between upper abdominal disease (III_1) and lower abdominal disease (III_2). A biologic difference or prognostic significance has not been clearly shown with respect to 5-year survival or disease-free survival between upper and lower abdominal involvement.[39] Both a clinical stage designation and a pathologic stage designation are implied by the Ann Arbor staging classification (Fig. 9).

Clinical stage is dependent on history and physical examination, the initial diagnostic biopsy, laboratory tests, and the results of radiographic and imaging studies. *Pathologic stage* is more accurate than the clinical stage because histopathologic data from the bone marrow, liver, spleen, intra-abdominal lymph nodes, and other involved tissues (e.g., bone, skin, lung) provide precise knowledge of the extent of the disease.[3,22,23,50]

Lymphangiography and abdominal CT scanning are reliable and complementary tests to evaluate retroperitoneal and abdominal nodal involvement. Lymphangiography has an overall accuracy of 80 to 90 per cent, with high sensitivity and specificity, and can detect disease in nodes that are not significantly enlarged. Shortcomings include the need for bipedal incisions and a failure to adequately visualize the celiac, splenic hilar, and portal nodes. These and other enlarged lymph nodes can be detected by CT scanning, which has lower overall accuracy, sensitivity, and specificity than lymphangiography.[39] CT is not helpful in detecting splenic involvement unless extensive splenic disease exists.[23,24] When the lymphangiogram is positive, the involvement of retroperitoneal nodes by Hodgkin's disease is confirmed by staging laparotomy in 80 to 90 per cent of cases.[23,39] Additionally, approximately 40 per cent of patients with abnormal lymphangiograms have another site of Hodgkin's disease within the abdomen, most commonly the spleen.[23] A normal lymphangiogram usually indicates that the retroperitoneal lymph nodes are uninvolved (10 to 15 per cent incidence of false-negatives) but does not exclude other abdominal sites of occult disease. Approximately 20 per cent of patients with negative lymphangiograms have intra-abdominal disease, usually in the spleen.[23]

Subdiaphragmatic Hodgkin's disease frequently is confined to the spleen and splenic hilar lymph nodes. The probability of subdiaphragmatic Hodgkin's disease is related closely to histopathologic subtype, with mixed cellularity and lymphocyte depletion subtypes having greater likelihood of subdiaphragmatic extension than lymphocyte predominance and nodular sclerosis subtypes. The probability of splenic involvement increases with increasing spleen size and is almost always present in spleens weighing more than 400 gm.[22,23,50] The absence of splenomegaly does not exclude splenic involvement. Hodgkin's disease involving the spleen commonly is apparent on gross examination as grayish white nodules ranging from several millimeters to several centimeters in size (Fig. 10). Liver involvement with Hodgkin's disease rarely, if ever, occurs in the absence of splenic disease.[22-24,39,50] Hepatic disease, in contrast to splenic disease, may not be apparent from inspection and palpation.

In a report of the Stanford experience, the spleen was found to be involved with Hodgkin's disease in 39 per cent of patients undergoing staging laparotomy.[39] In 50 per cent of these, the spleen was the only site of intra-abdominal disease detected by staging laparotomy. Splenic involvement consisted of fewer than five nodules in 27 per cent, with all the nodules being too small to have been detected by CT or found on random biopsy. All positive liver and accessory spleen specimens were associated with positive splenic involvement, suggesting that the spleen is the trigger for visceral dissemination.[39]

Staging laparotomy, which in the past was frequently em-

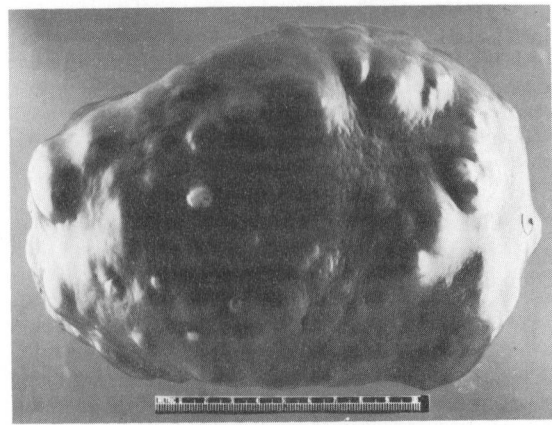

Figure 10. Spleen weighing 960 gm. exhibits typical gross nodules of Hodgkin's disease. The spleen, which was palpable preoperatively, was removed during staging laparotomy.

ployed for pathologic staging of Hodgkin's disease, now is being used less frequently. Its use as a diagnostic test has been based upon the following: (1) Hodgkin's disease generally begins in a single area and spreads initially in a predictable and nonrandom manner via lymphatic channels to contiguous lymph node areas and organs having a prominent lymphatic tissue component. (2) Selection of therapy is dependent upon pathologic stage. (3) Assignment of stage using clinical criteria alone frequently is inaccurate. Approximately 25 to 30 per cent of clinically staged patients have their stage of disease increased (upstaged), and approximately 10 to 15 per cent are downstaged following laparotomy, for a total alteration in stage of approximately 40 per cent.[23,24,39] (Patients with AIDS who develop Hodgkin's disease have great likelihood of being upstaged by laparotomy.) (4) Prognosis is related primarily to the pathologic stage of the disease.

The role of staging laparotomy continues to be re-evaluated as a routine staging procedure for Hodgkin's disease. Diagnostic advantages and contributions of staging laparotomy have helped significantly to change the understanding and therapeutic management of patients with Hodgkin's disease, and the current success and widespread use of combination chemotherapy have challenged the need to know the precise anatomic extent of the disease required for treatment by radiation therapy.[38] Staging laparotomy is not applicable to all patients with Hodgkin's disease and should be performed only in patients in whom the results may change management decisions and plans for therapy. Patients with advanced disease, clinical Stage IIIB or Stage IV, do not benefit from staging laparotomy because treatment is with combination chemotherapy. (If splenomegaly is present or develops in these advanced stages of Hodgkin's disease, splenectomy may be of value to control cytopenias and reduce tumor burden.) Staging laparotomy has been restricted by the recent recognition of the limitations of radiation therapy for patients with extensive mediastinal presentation or with multiple extranodal sites. The success of combination chemotherapy in treating minimal or occult disease and for controlling recurrent disease after radiation therapy is a major consideration in further restricting the use of staging laparotomy.[38] Recently, splenectomy in Hodgkin's staging has been shown to be a predisposing risk factor for acute leukemia in patients over the age of 40 years who have received combination chemotherapy (MOPP—mustard, vincristine, procarbazine, and prednisone). This surprising association suggests that staging laparotomy with splenectomy should not be done in patients of this age group who may eventually require MOPP-like chemotherapy.[38]

Controversy continues regarding the role of staging laparotomy, and improved noninvasive diagnostic tests and the introduction of more effective and less toxic chemotherapy will continue to reduce the indications for this procedure.[38] Currently, staging laparotomy is appropriate for selected patients with Hodgkin's disease of low clinical stage (Stages IA, IIA, and IIIA) in whom the results have major influence on therapeutic management.

Staging laparotomy is based upon a systematic abdominal exploration with an organized approach to tissue sampling and consists of splenectomy, liver biopsy, and selective excision of abdominal and retroperitoneal lymph nodes based upon CT, lymphangiographic, and operative findings. The operation is performed through a midline incision. The liver is examined initially and, if no gross evidence of disease is identified, a 2-cm. wedge of tissue is excised from the left hepatic lobe. Deep biopsies are obtained from the right and left lobes with a Trucut needle. Splenectomy is then performed, with biopsy of splenic hilar lymph nodes and placement of identifying metal clips on the splenic pedicle. (Partial splenectomy does not provide an adequate degree of accuracy in staging to justify its use as an alternative to splenectomy.[24,39,43]) The lesser omentum is in-

cised, and a lymph node is removed from the celiac axis region. The hilum of the liver, the cystic duct, and distal common duct areas are inspected, and representative lymph nodes are removed. Representative nodes are excised from the small intestinal mesentery and mesocolon. Exposure of the para-aortic, paracaval, and iliac lymph nodes is necessary to examine these areas adequately. If any abnormal or suspicious retroperitoneal nodes were demonstrated on lymphangiogram, the nodes are excised and the sites marked with metal clips. Confirmation that the specific node(s) has been excised can be obtained by comparing an intraoperative abdominal radiograph with the lymphangiogram. (Ten to 15 per cent of patients with normal lymphangiograms have involvement of the retroperitoneal lymph nodes by Hodgkin's disease (false-negative), and representative nodes should be excised even if the lymphangiogram is normal.) A bone marrow biopsy should be obtained from the iliac crest to conclude the staging aspects of the operation. Preoperative bone marrow biopsy has a false-negative rate of 2 to 3 per cent and would constitute a significant treatment error if not corrected by staging laparotomy findings.[39]

Oophoropexy (ovarian translocation) is advisable in the premenopausal woman in whom radiation therapy using an inverted Y port is likely. Both ovaries should be moved from the potential field of radiation and identified with metal clips. Lead shielding is an important adjunct to the protective effects offered by oophoropexy, and menstrual function is retained in approximately 55 per cent of women receiving pelvic irradiation for Hodgkin's disease after oophoropexy and lead shielding.[44] Ancillary procedures, such as appendectomy or cholecystectomy, add an unnecessary risk to the staging laparotomy and are not recommended.

Staging laparotomy has minimal morbidity, and the mortality rate is less than 0.5 per cent. The risk of developing postsplenectomy sepsis in patients with Hodgkin's disease is 10 per cent or higher.

Current treatment of Hodgkin's disease integrates radiation therapy and combination chemotherapy to achieve the maximal potential for cure. The success of combination chemotherapy in controlling and even curing Hodgkin's disease in patients demonstrating recurrence after radiation therapy has been a major therapeutic advance. In the Stanford experience from 1974 to 1980 for patients at all stages of Hodgkin's disease, survival was 86 per cent, and freedom from progression (FFP) was 77 per cent in surgically staged patients.[39] For Stages IA and IIA patients being treated by irradiation only, survival and FFP were 91 per cent and 82 per cent, respectively, with no advantage being shown by adding chemotherapy (usually MOPP). Adding chemotherapy to radiation improved survival from 65 to 92 per cent and FFP from 70 to 82 per cent in Stage IIIA patients. Stage IIIB patients had a generally poorer prognosis even with combination therapy, but alternating chemotherapy and radiation therapy has significantly improved survival. Extensive extranodal disease (Stages IIE, IIIE, and IV) has a poor survival rate (approximately 60 per cent at 5 years), whether radiation or combined therapy is used.[39]

Non-Hodgkin's Lymphomas

Non-Hodgkin's lymphomas (NHLs) constitute a diverse group of primary malignancies of lymphoreticular tissue. The clinical course and natural history of NHL are more variable than those of Hodgkin's disease, the pattern of spread is irregular, and more patients have leukemic features.[3,21,22,50] Current histologic classifications incorporate the nomenclature based on light and electron microscopic morphology, histochemical studies, and selected cell-surface antigens.[3,21,22,50] For prognostic and therapeutic purposes, NHL is classified according to nodular (favorable) and diffuse (unfavorable) types.

In contrast to Hodgkin's disease, only about two thirds of patients with NHL initially have asymptomatic lymphadenopathy. In 20 to 35 per cent of patients, the onset of NHL occurs in an extranodal site.[3] In addition to peripheral and mediastinal lymphadenopathy, NHL commonly is found initially as an abdominal mass (retroperitoneal or mesenteric) or as hepatic and/or splenic enlargement. Constitutional symptoms such as fever, weight loss, and night sweats are frequently present. Occasionally the first manifestation of NHL is an oncologic emergency, such as superior vena caval syndrome, spinal cord compression, or ureteral obstruction.

In NHL, the mode of spread generally is unpredictable, and most patients have disseminated disease at the time of presentation.[3,22,50] In patients with initial nodal involvement, early spread may be limited to contiguous lymphatic sites or adjacent extranodal sites. More often, NHL spreads rapidly to distant nodal and extranodal sites through the bloodstream. Progression of NHL arising in extranodal areas may be through (1) local invasion of adjacent structures, (2) extension to regional lymph nodes, and/or (3) dissemination to noncontiguous lymph nodes and/or distant extranodal sites. The extranodal spread of NHL is comparable to the pattern of metastasis observed in carcinoma.[3]

The median age at the time of diagnosis is 50 years, without sex preference. Patients under age 35 years and over age 65 years are more apt to have diffuse histology. The majority of non-Hodgkin's lymphomas are monoclonal B-cell tumors that are sometimes associated with an IgM or IgG protein. In some patients, particularly children with a mediastinal mass, the disease is thymic in origin.[21,22,50]

As with Hodgkin's disease, chemotherapy, radiation therapy, or both are the primary forms of treatment. Therapeutic considerations are based on the histopathologic type of lymphoma and the stage (extent) of disease. Because the majority of patients with NHL have disseminated disease at the time of presentation, staging laparotomy seldom is required and is indicated only for the patient with limited disease in whom laparotomy findings may influence selection of therapy.

NHL that has primary presentation in the spleen may present as asymptomatic splenomegaly with or without hypersplenism. Radionuclide, CT, and magnetic resonance imaging usually reveal nonspecific, featureless organ enlargement. If parenchymal expansion secondary to tumor infiltration and congestion becomes massive, splenic pooling and increased regional blood flow may result in hypersplenism. NHL with primary presentation in the spleen may result in the diagnosis of "idiopathic splenomegaly" until splenectomy permits accurate histopathologic diagnosis.

Splenectomy in NHL also is performed for hematologic depression secondary to hypersplenism or to relieve symptomatic splenomegaly or discomfort from recurrent splenic infarctions. Hypersplenism may produce symptomatic anemia requiring red blood cell transfusions, dangerous levels of thrombocytopenia, and leukopenia with recurrent infections. The severity of the cytopenia may require withholding of chemotherapy and radiotherapy.[1,12,22,50] Immunohemolysis or autoimmune hemolytic anemia (AIHA) occasionally contributes to the anemia in NHL and is diagnosed by a positive Coombs' test.

The bone marrow typically has significant infiltration by neoplastic cells and additionally shows erythroid hypoplasia and decreased megakaryocytes. Because most patients with NHL have received chemotherapy or radiation therapy prior to becoming candidates for splenectomy, the splenic contribution to the pancytopenia can be determined only by the response to splenectomy.[12] Almost all patients with NHL undergoing splenectomy for hypersplenism require red cell and platelet transfusions preoperatively.

Significant therapeutic benefit can be achieved by splenectomy in 80 to 90 per cent of patients with advanced lymphomas (including Hodgkin's disease).[1,12] Although patients with both non-Hodgkin's lymphomas and Hodgkin's disease may develop remission with reinstituted chemotherapy following correction of cytopenias, the eventual outcome of the underlying disease is unchanged. Most patients with well-differentiated lymphocytic lymphoma survive for 5 years, and many live 10 years after the diagnosis is made. The prognosis is more favorable for the nodular than for the diffuse forms of NHL.[12,22,50]

Chronic Lymphocytic Leukemia

Chronic lymphocytic leukemia (CLL) is a lymphoproliferative abnormality that occurs primarily in the elderly (sixth decade of life or older) with a male predominance (2 : 1). Proliferation and accumulation of abnormal lymphocytes in lymphatic tissues result in the major signs of lymphadenopathy, splenomegaly, and lymphocytosis in the peripheral blood. The most constant abnormality on physical examination is lymph node enlargement, which frequently is found either by the patient or on routine physical examination. Splenomegaly is present in most patients and is progressive during the course of the disease. Hepatomegaly is a frequent finding, and lymphocytic infiltration of the skin and gastrointestinal and respiratory tracts occurs as the disease progresses. The diagnosis is based on the increase in the total leukocyte count due to a large number of abnormal, small, immature lymphocytes. Bone marrow examination demonstrates a variable and progressive degree of infiltration by abnormal lymphocytes.[22,50]

Current therapy for CLL incorporates the judicious use of chemotherapeutic agents, corticosteroids, irradiation, and splenectomy.[21,22,50] Although chronic lymphocytic leukemia is not cured by available therapeutic modalities, effective palliation is achieved in most patients, and many lead relatively normal lives. The disease progresses over 5 to 10 years, with gradual increases in lymphadenopathy, splenomegaly, and hepatomegaly and development of weakness, weight loss, anemia, and thrombocytopenia. CLL frequently is complicated by development of immune hemolysis (autoimmune hemolytic anemia, AIHA) in which the hemolytic anemia is nearly always Coombs-positive. If hemolysis becomes severe and cannot be controlled by medical therapy, splenectomy is useful to ameliorate the hemolytic process. As with non-Hodgkin's lymphoma, splenectomy in chronic lymphocytic leukemia is performed primarily for hematologic depression secondary to hypersplenism and for palliation of symptomatic splenomegaly (Fig. 11). Significant hematologic improvement follows splenectomy in 80 to 90 per cent of patients, but the natural course of chronic lymphocytic leukemia is unchanged.[1,12,22,50] Unless another illness supervenes, death usually occurs from hemorrhage or infection.

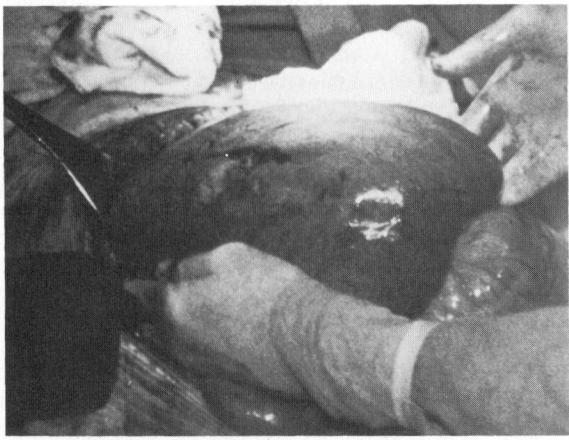

Figure 11. Operative photograph showing removal of a 5660-gm. spleen in a patient with chronic lymphocytic leukemia and hypersplenism.

Chronic Myeloid Leukemia

Chronic myeloid (granulocytic, myelocytic) leukemia (CML, CGL) is a myeloproliferative abnormality characterized by marked elevation of the leukocyte count from myeloid cells in all stages of maturation and by neoplastic overgrowth of granulocytes in the bone marrow. The incidence of CML increases with age and is more frequent in men than in women (ratio, 3 : 2). Splenomegaly is the most common physical finding, and sternal tenderness, lymphadenopathy, and hepatomegaly are frequently present.[22,50] A unique chromosomal abnormality, designated the Philadelphia chromosome (Ph[1]), occurs in 90 per cent of patients with CML. Patients who are Ph[1]-negative have an atypical course and a poorer prognosis than patients with CML who have the Ph[1] chromosome.[22,50] Chemotherapy (busulfan, hydroxyurea), irradiation, radioactive phosphorus, and extracorporeal irradiation of the blood can control symptoms and most physical and laboratory abnormalities of CML during the chronic or "treatable" phase, which lasts from 1 to 4 years.[22,50] Development of "myeloblastic crisis" appears to be an intrinsic feature of CML and indicates an accelerated or acute stage of the disease, which results in death from infection or hemorrhage within 3 to 6 months.[22,50]

Splenectomy may be of benefit in selected patients during the chronic stage of CML to palliate severe thrombocytopenia and/or anemia and to relieve pain from splenic infarctions or massive splenomegaly. Splenectomy offers no benefit in delaying the onset of blastic transformation, improving the quality of life after the development of blastic crisis, or prolonging survival.[31]

Hairy Cell Leukemia

Hairy cell leukemia (HCL, leukemic reticuloendotheliosis) is an uncommon form of leukemia characterized by pancytopenia, splenomegaly without significant lymphadenopathy, and characteristic mononuclear cells in the blood and bone marrow. The disease is more common in men (ratio, 4 : 1). The typical patient is a middle-aged man with moderate splenomegaly, absence of significant peripheral adenopathy, and variable hepatomegaly.[15]

Initial complaints among symptomatic patients are abdominal fullness or discomfort due to splenomegaly; nonspecific symptoms of fatigue, weakness, and weight loss; and easy bruising from thrombocytopenia or recurrent infections associated with leukopenia. In approximately 25 per cent of patients, splenomegaly and cytopenias are detected during a routine examination or during evaluation for an unrelated illness.

HCL is characterized by the presence of malignant cells that have irregular, filamentous cytoplasmic projections on light microscopy that give the cells a hairy appearance. The surface projections are demonstrable by electron microscopy as broadbased, undulating ruffles and patches of short, blunt microvilli.

A pancytopenia of moderate severity is present in approximately two thirds of patients at the time of diagnosis. Hairy cells frequently are present in the peripheral blood and often account for a large proportion of the total white cell count. Demonstration in the hairy cells of *tartrate-resistant acid phosphatase* (TRAP) isoenzyme activity as a red reaction product is helpful supporting evidence for diagnosis. Although not required for diagnosis, the TRAP-positive reaction product occurs in 90 to 95 per cent of patients with hairy cell leukemia. Bone marrow biopsy permits definitive diagnosis of HCL from characteristic morphology.[15]

Approximately 10 to 15 per cent of HCL patients have an indolent course with a nearly normal life expectancy and require no specific therapy. These are usually elderly men who have minimal splenomegaly, relatively few hairy cells in the blood, and asymptomatic neutropenia. The remaining 85 to 90 per cent of patients require treatment because of one or more cytopenias resulting in symptomatic anemia requiring transfusions, thrombocytopenic bleeding, and repeated infections attributable to neutropenia. Pancytopenia develops from concurrent splenic pooling secondary to infiltrative splenomegaly and bone marrow replacement with hairy cells. Symptomatic splenomegaly and recurring splenic infarctions are other indications for therapy. For the majority of patients who require some form of therapy shortly after diagnosis, splenectomy continues to be an early consideration. Splenectomy is most appropriate for those patients with severe cytopenias, a large spleen, and patchy bone marrow infiltration. Splenectomy results in rapid palliation, and almost all patients have hematologic improvement. Blood counts return to normal in approximately 40 to 50 per cent of patients. The response lasts for many years, and almost half the patients require no further therapy.[16,17]

Patients with hairy cell leukemia who have diffuse infiltration of the bone marrow, minimal splenomegaly, and severe cytopenias gain only minor or short-term benefit from splenectomy and require additional therapy. In the past 5 years, interferon-α (IFN-α) and pentostatin (deoxycoformycin) have been found to be highly effective systemic therapy for hairy cell leukemia. Randomized trials of IFN-α versus pentostatin currently are in progress, both for newly diagnosed HCL patients and those patients who previously had splenectomy. Presently IFN-α remains the systemic therapy of choice, with pentostatin being indicated for patients with hairy cell leukemia refractory to IFN-α. Splenectomy likely will continue to have a place in the sequential treatment of those patients with hairy cell leukemia requiring therapy.[16,17]

SPLENECTOMY FOR ANEMIA

Hemolytic anemia results from an increase in the rate of red cell destruction. The adult bone marrow can produce red cells at six to eight times the normal rate, and hemolysis must be reasonably severe before laboratory or clinical evidence of anemia occurs.[21,22,50] Diagnostic evaluation should include a detailed family history, because many hemolytic anemias benefited by splenectomy have a hereditary basis. Congenital hemolytic anemias have a defect intrinsic to the red cell that may involve the cell membrane (hereditary spherocytosis), cellular metabolism (pyruvate kinase deficiency, glucose-6-phosphate dehydrogenase (G-6-PD) deficiency), hemoglobin structure (sickle cell anemia), or hemoglobin chain synthesis rates (thalassemia). Acquired hemolytic anemias have an extracorpuscular factor that affects normal red cells. ^{51}Cr-labeled red cell survival studies are sometimes useful to confirm hemolysis and a shortened red cell life span and to determine sites of red cell destruction.[21,22,50]

Clinical features include variable pallor related to the degree of anemia; mild, fluctuating jaundice; and splenomegaly. Pigment gallstones are common after childhood and may produce biliary tract symptoms. Valuable laboratory studies include serum direct and total bilirubin and haptoglobin levels. Jaundice associated with hyperbilirubinemia resulting from hemolysis is caused by an excess of unconjugated (free) bilirubin and is measured by an increase in the indirect-reacting fraction of bilirubin. The unconjugated bilirubin that is bound to albumin does not enter the urine, and indirect hyperbilirubinemia thus is not associated with biliuria. Reticulocytosis and bone marrow erythroid hyperplasia reflect increased red cell production. Red cell morphology is often abnormal, as is osmotic fragility. ^{51}Cr-tagged red cell studies demonstrate a shortened red cell survival.[21,22,50]

Hereditary Spherocytosis

Hereditary spherocytosis is a relatively common, genetically determined red blood cell membrane disorder that causes hemolytic anemia. The erythrocyte membrane defect results from a deficiency in spectrin, a major component of the membrane skeleton that is thought to be responsible for the shape, strength, and reversible deformability of the red blood cell.[2,22,50] The membrane abnormality leads to a gradual loss of red cell surface area, so that instead of remaining a flexible biconcave disc, the red cell becomes small and spherical. Lacking adequate deformability to traverse the splenic microcirculation, spherocytes are trapped in the splenic red pulp and are eventually destroyed by reticuloendothelial cells.

Hereditary spherocytosis occurs primarily by autosomal dominant inheritance with variable expression. Twenty to twenty-five per cent of the cases appear sporadically.[2,22,50] The severity of the anemia and other clinical manifestations are variable. The disease may be so severe that repeated blood transfusions are required to maintain a functional hemoglobin level, or it may be so mild as to go unnoticed in childhood, becoming manifest in adult life with development of symptomatic cholelithiasis. Aplastic crisis, which usually is precipitated by a viral illness such as that caused by human parvovirus (HPV), may produce a rapidly worsening anemia that may be life-threatening. Fluctuating jaundice due to hemolysis is common, and pigment gallstones are frequent, the incidence being directly related to the severity of the hemolysis and patient age. Cholelithiasis develops in 20 to 55 per cent of patients with hereditary spherocytosis but is uncommon before age 10 years. Moderate splenomegaly is a characteristic physical finding.[7] Diagnosis is established by the presence of spherocytes in the peripheral blood, reticulocytosis (usually 5 to 20 per cent), an increased osmotic fragility, and a negative Coombs test.[21,22,50]

Splenectomy is indicated in nearly all patients. In children, splenectomy usually is performed after age 6 years but can be done at a younger age if warranted by the severity of the anemia and the need for frequent transfusions. Following splenectomy, hemolysis is alleviated, and clinical cure of the anemia is achieved in most patients. The intrinsic red cell membrane defect is unaltered by splenectomy, but red cell survival becomes normal. With resolution of hemolysis, jaundice disappears, and the increased risk of calculous biliary tract disease is removed. Gallbladder ultrasonography is advisable prior to splenectomy in anticipation of combining cholecystectomy with splenectomy if gallstones are demonstrated.[7]

Hereditary Elliptocytosis

Hereditary elliptocytosis is a relatively common heterogeneous red blood cell membrane disorder characterized by an abundance of elliptical red cells. The abnormality usually results in a mild anemia of which most patients have no symptoms throughout their lifetimes.[5,22,50] Like hereditary spherocytosis, hereditary elliptocytosis results from an abnormal erythrocyte membrane skeleton. Several defects in the red cell membrane skeleton have been identified in hereditary elliptocytosis and include impaired association of spectrin chains and a quantitative deficiency of protein 4.1.[2,22,50] Symptomatic individuals have a mild hemolytic anemia, with clinical and laboratory features similar to those of hereditary spherocytosis except for the elliptical appearance of the erythrocytes. Splenectomy is indicated in symptomatic patients and results are uniformly good, although the abnormal erythrocyte morphology persists.[5,22,50]

Hereditary Pyropoikilocytosis

Hereditary pyropoikilocytosis (HPP) is a rare congenital hemolytic anemia that is catalogued along with hereditary elliptocytosis because of certain molecular and morphologic similarities. Distinguished from hereditary elliptocytosis (and hereditary spherocytosis) by marked alterations in red cell morphology and by the pattern of inheritance, this severe hemolytic disorder occurs most commonly in blacks. Erythrocytes in HPP are severely deformed, and nearly all red cells are poikilocytic,

fragmented, spherocytic, or elliptocytic. Osmotic fragility is increased, and red cells in HPP exhibit increased susceptibility to thermal injury. The decision for splenectomy in HPP is deferred until the natural course of the disease has been established. In some newborn infants, HPP gradually evolves into morphologic features characteristic of hereditary elliptocytosis. "True" HPP persists as a severe hemolytic anemia that usually requires early splenectomy, which greatly reduces hemolysis.[22,50]

Hereditary Nonspherocytic Hemolytic Anemia

A number of erythrocyte enzyme deficiencies associated with hemolytic syndromes constitute this group of hemolytic anemias. Pyruvate kinase (PK) deficiency is the prototype of the enzymopathies involving the Embden-Meyerhof pathway of anaerobic glycolysis in the red cell. PK deficiency is inherited as an autosomal recessive trait and affects both sexes equally. An unusually high incidence exists among the Pennsylvania Amish.[22,50] A discrepancy between red cell energy needs and ATP-generating capacity results in irreversible membrane injury, with cellular distortion, rigidity, dehydration, and premature destruction of the red cells by the spleen.[22,50] The severity of the anemia is variable. Splenectomy results in improvement, but hemolysis is not abolished and mild anemia persists. After splenectomy, transfusion requirements are reduced, young children experience a period of rapid "catch-up" growth, and the danger from aplastic crises is reduced.[22,50]

It is important to differentiate between pyruvate kinase deficiency and other erythrocyte enzymopathies resulting in hemolytic anemia, such as G-6-PD deficiency and its variants. Specific enzyme assays are employed for this purpose. In G-6-PD deficiency, hemolysis is precipitated by infection and other acute illness, certain drugs, and fava beans. Splenic enlargement is rare, in contrast to frequent splenomegaly with PK deficiency, and splenectomy is not indicated for patients with G-6-PD deficiency.[5,22,50] A role for splenectomy in other erythrocyte enzyme deficiency states has not been established.

Sickle Cell Anemia

Sickle cell anemia is a hereditary hemolytic anemia occurring in blacks who are homozygous for the sickle hemoglobin gene. Sickle hemoglobin (HbS) differs from normal adult hemoglobin (HbA) only in the substitution of valine for glutamic acid in the sixth position of the beta chain. HbS, which results from this single amino acid substitution, imparts the sickle shape to deoxygenated red cells and is responsible for the wide spectrum of clinical features that characterize sickle cell anemia. The highest incidence of HbS occurs among black Africans and descendants of emigrants from equatorial Africa. Sickle cell anemia (homozygous state for HbS) occurs in approximately 0.5 per cent of the black population, and sickle cell trait (heterozygous state for HbS) is present in approximately 8 per cent of African-Americans. In the homozygous state, HbA is totally lacking and the red cells contain predominantly HbS. The red cells of individuals with sickle cell trait contain both HbA and HbS, with the relative amount of HbS ranging between 35 and 45 per cent. A combination of two variant hemoglobin genes or a combination of a variant hemoglobin and an interacting thalassemia gene results in doubly heterozygous states designated by both aberrant gene products, e.g., HbS/C, HbS/beta-thalassemia.[22,50]

Under conditions of reduced oxygen availability, red cells containing HbS acquire the sickle-shaped deformity due to the intracellular polymerization of the HbS molecules. Sickling of erythrocytes containing HbS occurs more readily with a reduced pH, higher intracellular concentration of HbS, low intracellular concentration of HbF (fetal hemoglobin), and conditions favoring hemoglobin deoxygenation. Increased blood viscosity due to the sickled cells and an increased adhesion of sickled cells to vascular endothelium result in circulatory stasis and stagnation that lead to further reduction in oxygen tension, further sickling, and a "vicious cycle" of erythrostasis. The consequent thrombosis, ischemia, necrosis, and organ fibrosis result in the clinical features of sickle cell anemia.[22,50]

Patients with sickle cell anemia characteristically are without symptoms until the second half of the first year of life because of an initial sufficiency of HbF that limits clinically significant sickling. Clinical features of sickle cell anemia, which are both acute and episodic ("crises") and chronic and progressive, are more a consequence of the rheologic properties of the sickle cells than of the anemia itself. Patients with sickle cell crisis often have severe abdominal pain and signs of peritoneal irritation similar to those of acute surgical illnesses, such as acute cholecystitis and appendicitis. Clinical features of abdominal crises in patients with sickle cell anemia tend to be similar for a given individual, and deviation from previous patterns may be an important differentiating feature of an acute surgical illness in patients with sickle cell anemia.[26] Chronic features of sickle cell anemia include retarded growth and development after the first decade; bone and joint disease; cardiovascular, pulmonary, hepatobiliary, genitourinary, and neurologic manifestations; hematuria; priapism; and ulcerations over the malleoli and distal portions of the legs. The incidence of pigment gallstones in patients with sickle cell anemia increases with age. Calculi appear first in childhood (2 to 4 years of age) and are present in approximately 70 per cent of adult patients.[22,50]

Diagnosis is established by the presence of characteristic sickle cells on blood smear, hemoglobin electrophoresis demonstrating predominantly HbS, variable amounts of HbF (5 to 15 per cent) and no HbA, and the presence of the sickle cell trait in both parents. Treatment is palliative and is directed toward minimizing complications of the disease. Many patients die during childhood from infections, renal failure, and heart failure. Rarely will a patient with sickle cell anemia have a relatively normal life span.[22,50]

The role of the spleen in sickle cell anemia is unclear. Sequestration crisis characterized by sudden trapping of blood in the spleen is a complication that occurs almost exclusively in infants and young children whose spleens are chronically enlarged. Further enlargement of the spleen occurs rapidly at the expense of the blood volume, and hypovolemic shock and death may occur within hours.[22,50] Splenomegaly first becomes apparent after 6 months of age and characteristically persists throughout childhood. Despite splenomegaly, splenic hypofunction may be documented as early as 5 months of age, and the risk of overwhelming infection exists in a child with sickle cell anemia by age 1 year.[22,50] By adolescence or early adult life, recurrent infarctions have resulted in splenic atrophy and functional asplenia (hyposplenism). (See sections on hyposplenism and overwhelming postsplenectomy sepsis.) Splenectomy may be beneficial to the occasional child with sickle cell anemia in whom excessive red cell sequestration occurs in an enlarged spleen.[22,50]

Sickle cell trait is rarely associated with significant clinical or hematologic manifestations, although splenic infarction has occurred in patients flying at high altitudes in unpressurized aircraft.[22,50]

Thalassemia (Thalassemia Syndromes)

These hereditary hemolytic anemias result from a defect in hemoglobin synthesis in which one of the hemoglobin polypeptide chains is synthesized at a markedly reduced rate. Specific pairs of genes are responsible for synthesis of the alpha, beta, gamma, and delta chains of the hemoglobin molecule, and a deficiency in synthesis of one of these subunits may lead to one of the thalassemia syndromes. Thalassemia is classified by the deficient peptide chain.[22,50] Beta-thalassemia, in which there is a quantitative reduction in the rate of beta chain synthesis, is the most common type of thalassemia. When the abnormal gene is inherited from both parents (homozygous), severe anemia termed *thalassemia major* results. Heterozygous patients have a mild anemia termed *thalassemia minor*. The term *thalassemia intermedia* is used to describe some homozygous patients who have a milder than usual course and some heterozygous patients who have a more severe course than usual. In thalassemia major, the reduction in the rate of beta chain synthesis produces a marked decrease in the amount of normal adult hemoglobin (HbA) with a compensatory increase in fetal hemoglobin (HbF). Homozygous alpha-thalassemia is incompatible with life, and these infants are stillborn or die shortly after birth. Patients with heterozygous alpha-thalassemia have a mild form of anemia similar to that in heterozygous beta-thalassemia.[22,50]

The pathogenesis of hemolysis in thalassemia lies in the unbalanced synthesis of the polypeptide chains. Due to the absence of the complementary polypeptide chain with which to bind, the overproduced normal chains form aggregates that precipitate within the red cell cytoplasm and lead to premature cell destruction. In homozygous beta-thalassemia (thalassemia major), the deficiency of beta chain synthesis results in a relative overproduction of alpha chains, which undergo aggregation to form insoluble inclusions in bone marrow erythroid precursors. Ineffective erythropoiesis occurs as a result of the death of many of these cells. Additionally, the inclusion-bearing red cells are detained in the spleen, where they sustain mechanical and metabolic injury that facilitates their ultimate destruction.[22,50]

Thalassemia major results in a severe anemia and clinical manifestations, usually within the first year of life. Pallor, retarded growth, and enlargement of the head with "thalassemic facies" are present, along with splenomegaly and hepatomegaly. The intense erythroid hyperplasia in the bone marrow results in expansion of the medullary cavities and attenuation of the cortex, producing bony abnormalities and a predisposition to fractures. Due to defective iron utilization, coupled with increased iron absorption and frequent blood transfusions, iron overload is a common complication.

The peripheral blood smear in thalassemia major shows a microcytic hypochromic anemia with a severe degree of poikilocytosis, anisocytosis, and polychromatophilia. Nucleated red cells invariably are present and may outnumber the leukocytes. Reticulocytosis and leukocytosis are characteristic, but the platelet count generally is normal. Hemoglobin electrophoresis in thalassemia major reveals absence or almost complete absence of HbA with the presence of large amounts of HbF.

Treatment consists of transfusion therapy and iron chelation, and splenectomy is effective in selected patients. Although the basic hematologic disease is not influenced, splenectomy decreases blood transfusion requirements and relieves discomfort from splenomegaly. Most patients with thalassemia major die during the second decade of life from complications of iron excess with myocardial hemosiderosis. Patients with alpha-thalassemia minor and beta-thalassemia minor rarely need treatment, and an important therapeutic consideration for patients with thalassemia minor is avoidance of therapeutic iron to minimize the risk of iron overload.[22,50]

Autoimmune Hemolytic Anemia

Autoimmune hemolytic anemia (AIHA) is an acquired hemolytic anemia resulting from antibody that is produced by the body against its own red cells. Patients with AIHA have the usual manifestations of hemolysis, with anemia, reticulocytosis, a shortened erythrocyte survival time, fluctuating jaundice, and splenomegaly. The blood smear in AIHA shows spherocytes and microspherocytes in numbers exceeded only in hereditary spherocytosis. The distinguishing feature of AIHA is a positive direct Coombs test, which identifies antibody on the red cell surface. The type of antibody attached to the red cell determines the mechanism of hemolysis as well as the site for primary destruction of the sensitized cells. Anti–red cell antibodies are classified as warm-reactive or cold-reactive, depending upon whether they bind to red cells most avidly at 37° C. or have progressively greater affinity for erythrocytes as the temperature approaches 0° C.[22,50]

Warm-reactive antibodies usually are IgG (less commonly IgM, IgA, or a combination) and facilitate sequestration and destruction of sensitized erythrocytes in the spleen. When IgG-coated red cells become attached to splenic macrophages, which have receptors for the Fc portion of the IgG molecule, portions of the red cell membrane are removed, rendering the erythrocyte more spherical and more susceptible to sequestration and premature destruction. Red cells coated by both IgG and complement are destroyed by the reticuloendothelial system generally and not primarily by the spleen.[21,22,50] Cold-reactive antibodies usually are IgM (rarely IgG or IgA) and bind to red cells mainly in the peripheral circulation where the blood temperature is cooled. Cold-reactive antibodies may cause either immediate intravascular hemolysis by complement-mediated mechanisms or sequestration and destruction of sensitized red cells by the liver. These patients usually have chronic hemolysis that is acutely worsened by cold exposure and often demonstrate acrocyanosis (Raynaud's phenomenon) due to intracapillary red cell agglutination.[22,50]

The designation *autoimmune* in AIHA must not obscure the fact that in many cases the hemolytic process is associated with or related to a drug or a reversible disease that can be eliminated. Drugs associated with AIHA include penicillin, cephalothin, streptomycin, methyldopa (Aldomet), quinidine, quinine, phenacetin, PAS, and several sulfonamides.[22,50]

Autoimmune hemolytic anemia may occur in association with another disease, such as mycoplasmal pneumonia, viral infections, chronic lymphocytic leukemia, lymphoma, Hodgkin's disease, systemic lupus erythematosus, infectious mononucleosis, and AIDS. When a drug exposure or an underlying disease is identified, AIHA is termed *secondary.* When no other etiologic association is demonstrable, AIHA is classified as *primary,* or idiopathic. AIHA occurs at any age and in both sexes but is more common in women over age 50 years. Pallor and splenomegaly are the main physical findings in idiopathic AIHA, whereas in secondary AIHA additional clinical features of the underlying disease are present. The severity and duration of the hemolytic anemia may vary, and in some patients the course is rapid and fulminating. Severe hemolysis may produce hemoglobinuria and acute tubular necrosis. When AIHA follows mycoplasmal pneumonia, the disease may be acute and self-limited over several weeks and require no therapy. More often the disease is chronic, with varying degrees of severity over months or years.[21,22,50]

Treatment is directed toward the hemolytic anemia and any underlying disease. Blood transfusions, corticosteroid therapy, and splenectomy are important aspects of treatment for the anemia. Splenectomy usually is performed in patients with AIHA in whom steroids are ineffective or an excessive steroid dose is required, or when complications preclude steroid use. ^{51}Cr-labeled red cell studies are useful to measure the degree of splenic sequestration and to serve as a guide for selecting patients who are most likely to respond to splenectomy.[22,40,50] Splenectomy results in a favorable response with complete hematologic remission in approximately 80 per cent of patients demonstrating significant splenic sequestration. Lack of significant red cell sequestration by the spleen does not preclude a good response to splenectomy. Splenectomy is more likely to induce a complete and sustained remission in primary (idiopathic) AIHA in which only IgG (warm-reactive) antibodies coat the red cells. In addition to removing the primary site for destruction of the sensitized red cells, splenectomy can be expected to significantly reduce production of anti-red cell antibody, because the spleen is a major site for IgG antibody production.

The prognosis for patients with secondary AIHA depends mainly on the underlying disease and is generally favorable when the hemolytic anemia follows a viral illness or is related to a drug exposure. Prognosis is poor when AIHA is associated with an underlying malignancy or one of the collagen diseases. The presence of complement indicates a greater likelihood of association with an underlying disease than the presence of IgG alone coating the red cells.

AIHA caused by cold-reactive antibodies usually is not benefited by splenectomy, and treatment for these patients consists of avoiding cold temperatures, treating any underlying disease, suppression of antibody production, and plasmapheresis in acutely ill patients.[21,22,50]

Hereditary Hydrocytosis and Xerocytosis

Hereditary hydrocytosis and xerocytosis are rare forms of hemolytic anemia that result from a primary alteration in red cell membrane monovalent cation permeability.[5,22,50] If the major effect involves membrane permeability to sodium, sodium gain exceeds potassium loss with an increase in total intracellular cation content and water movement into the red cell. The water-distended red cells (hydrocytes) have increased fragility, a low mean corpuscular hemoglobin concentration (MCHC) and an elevated mean corpuscular volume (MCV), and a characteristic fish-mouth (stomatocyte) appearance on peripheral blood smear. When the permeability disorder allows potassium loss to exceed sodium gain, total intracellular cation content decreases, with resulting loss of water and cell dehydration. The dehydrated red cells (xerocytes) have a low MCV, an elevated MCHC, and a dense appearance on blood smear. Xerocytosis is differentiated from hereditary spherocytosis, elliptocytosis, or other conditions in which the MCHC is elevated by red cell morphology and resistance of the cells to osmotic lysis.[5,22,50]

Splenectomy is effective in hydrocytosis by reducing hemolysis and eliminating the need for transfusion and the potential risk for life-threatening aplastic crises. In contrast to hereditary spherocytosis, mild hemolysis persists after splenectomy, and the risk of pigment gallstone formation continues. Splenectomy seldom is required for xerocytosis because the hemolysis usually is not severe.[5,22,50]

Miscellaneous Anemias Sometimes Benefited by Splenectomy

Splenectomy occasionally is performed for rare disorders such as acquired idiopathic sideroblastic anemia, congenital dyserythropoietic anemia, and porphyria erythropoietica. In these syndromes, splenectomy may offer significant benefits by improving the hemolytic anemia and reducing transfusion requirements.[5,22,50]

MISCELLANEOUS DISEASES SOMETIMES BENEFITED BY SPLENECTOMY

Myeloid Metaplasia (Agnogenic Myeloid Metaplasia, Myelofibrosis, Myelosclerosis)

Myeloid metaplasia is an unusual illness with numerous names but no known cause. There is gradual and progressive impairment of normal hematopoiesis due to continued fibroblastic proliferation, which ultimately produces sclerosis of the bone marrow and myelofibrosis.[5,22,50] The panproliferative process results in increased connective tissue proliferation also in the liver, spleen, and lymph nodes and concomitant proliferation of hematopoietic elements in the spleen, liver, and long bones.[22,40,50] Myeloid metaplasia is closely related to polycythemia vera, myelocytic (myelogenous) leukemia, and essential (idiopathic) thrombocytosis, and together these conditions constitute a disease spectrum termed *myeloproliferative disorders.*

Characteristic features of myeloid metaplasia are (1) progressive fibrosis of the bone marrow, (2) extramedullary hematopoiesis, (3) presence in the peripheral blood of immature erythroid and granulocyte precursors (leukoerythroid response), and (4) massive splenomegaly. In some patients the enlarged spleen provides an expanded vascular space with an associated increase in plasma volume. By serving as a "shunt," the enlarged spleen may result in a decreased peripheral vascular resistance and an increased cardiac work load. Portal hypertension with varices and ascites may develop in some patients from hepatic fibrosis, increased forward blood flow through the splenoportal system, or a combination of these factors.[22,40,50]

Most patients are middle-aged or older and have symptoms related to anemia and splenomegaly. Malaise, dyspnea, and weight loss are common, and symptoms due to splenomegaly include abdominal fullness and discomfort, early satiety, and intermittent pain from splenic infarction. Less common symptoms include episodes of spontaneous bleeding, recurrent infections, bone pain, pruritus, and complications of hyperuricemia. Splenomegaly due primarily to extramedullary hematopoiesis is invariably present, and myeloid metaplasia (myelofibrosis) has been responsible for some of the largest spleens encountered (Fig. 12). Hepatomegaly is present in 50 to 75 per cent of the patients.[22,40,50]

The peripheral blood smear characteristically shows immature red cells, anisocytosis, poikilocytosis, and numerous teardrop and elongated shapes. Most patients have a mild normochromic anemia that worsens as myelofibrosis progresses. The white blood cell count usually is depressed but may reach levels of 50,000 per cu. mm. or higher. Immature granulocyte forms are present, and these, along with the red cell abnormalities, constitute a leukoerythroblastic anemia. A normal platelet count is present in 25 per cent of patients, and thrombocytopenia occurs in approximately a third. Thrombocytosis of over 1,000,000 per cu. mm. occurs in 25 per cent of the patients. The leukocyte alkaline phosphatase (LAP) score is usually normal or high. Hyperuricemia is present frequently and should be anticipated, to avoid episodes of gouty arthritis and renal calculi. Bone marrow biopsy reveals varying degrees of fibrosis with scattered foci of hematopoietic elements.[22,40,50]

Treatment of patients with myeloid metaplasia is directed toward the anemia, thrombocytosis, and splenomegaly and includes blood transfusions, corticosteroid and androgen therapy, chemotherapy (busulfan, hydroxyurea), and splenic irradiation. Hydroxyurea is of great value in rapidly reducing and controlling the marked thrombocytosis associated with this disease. In addition, hydroxyurea may be beneficial in slowing development of splenomegaly.

Splenectomy is effective in controlling anemia and thrombocytopenia and relieving symptoms due to painful or massive splenomegaly.[22,39,40,50] Splenectomy should be performed early rather than late in the course of the illness, since the risk of complications following splenectomy increases with progression of the disease. Indications for splenectomy are (1) an increasing transfusion requirement, (2) thrombocytopenic bleeding episodes, (3) symptomatic splenomegaly, (4) high-output cardiac failure, and (5) portal hypertension with bleeding varices.[22,39,50] Although the course of myeloid metaplasia is not altered by splenectomy, certain prognostic factors are associated with favorable long-term survival. These include a hemoglobin level greater than 10 gm. per dl., a platelet count greater than 100,000 per cu. mm., a normal LAP score, and a spleen weighing less than 3000 gm.

Loss of the spleen as a major site of extramedullary hematopoiesis rarely has an adverse influence on the hematologic status of patients with myeloid metaplasia.[22,40,50] Morbidity and mortality rates after splenectomy, however, are significantly higher for patients with myeloid metaplasia than for patients with other hematologic disorders.[22,39,40,50] In advanced disease, the patients are in poor general condition, and the risk of postoperative hemorrhage and infection is great. Additionally, following splenectomy many of these patients have a marked thrombocytosis that is associated with an increased risk of thromboembolic complications, which include thrombosis of the portal vein and major mesenteric veins.[18,22,50] Specific antiplatelet therapy may be needed in the preoperative preparation and postoperative care of patients undergoing splenectomy for myeloid metaplasia.[18,22,50] The spectrum of antiplatelet therapy includes administration of aspirin, dipyridamole, heparin, dextran, hydroxyurea, and busulfan. Hydroxyurea is especially valuable in reducing and controlling the marked thrombocytosis that can occur following splenectomy. A rapid reduction in the platelet count can be achieved by plateletpheresis (thrombocytopheresis) in patients who have thrombohemorrhagic manifestations and severe thrombocythemia.[18,22,50]

In some patients with myeloid metaplasia, there is transition to another form of myeloproliferative disorder, and in approximately 10 per cent of patients, acute myeloid leukemic transformation occurs. The median survival after diagnosis of myeloid metaplasia is 5 years, but many patients live longer. Death usually results from hemorrhage, infection, or cardiac or renal failure.[22,39,50]

Felty's Syndrome

Felty's syndrome consists of the triad of severe rheumatoid arthritis, granulocytopenia, and splenomegaly. It usually occurs in patients with a long history of rheumatoid arthritis. Patients with Felty's syndrome fail to show a substantial granulocytosis in response to infection, and severe, persistent, and recurrent infections are characteristic. Antibody directed against granulocytes is demonstrable in most patients. Mild anemia and thrombocytopenia are present in some cases. Moderate splenomegaly is common and results from expansion of the red pulp.[22,28,50]

Splenectomy is effective in most patients with Felty's syndrome and should be performed in those having significant recurrent infections and chronic leg ulcers. The granulocyte response is immediate, and most patients show resolution or significant improvement of granulocytopenia within 48 to 72 hours after splenectomy. Long-term correction of the granulocytopenia is achieved in the majority of patients, with a marked reduction in the incidence of infections and healing of leg ulcerations. Controversy exists regarding the advisability of splenectomy for patients with Felty's syndrome who have severe granulocytopenia (less than 500 granulocytes per cu. mm.) but have not yet developed severe or recurrent infections.[22,28,50]

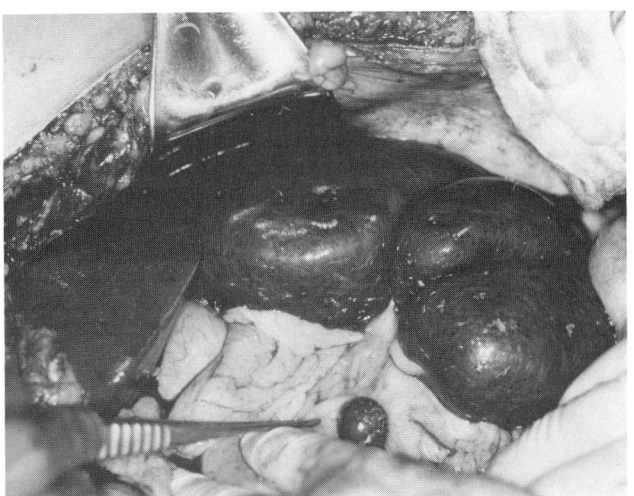

Figure 12. A massively enlarged spleen (2400 gm.) along with an accessory spleen in a patient with myelofibrosis undergoing splenectomy for anemia and thrombocytopenia.

Gaucher's Disease

Gaucher's disease is a disorder of lipid metabolism that may result in massive splenomegaly and hypersplenism. Genetically transmitted as an autosomal recessive trait, the disease is most commonly found in Ashkenazic Jews. Caused by a deficiency of β-glucocerebrosidase, an enzyme responsible for breaking down certain lipid complexes, Gaucher's disease ultimately leads to retention of glucocerebroside in macrophages, especially those of the spleen, liver, bone marrow, and lungs.[22,50]

Diagnosis is made by finding the typical Gaucher cells in biopsied tissues. These large-diameter (20 to 80 μm.) cells, which contain dense fibrillar deposits of glucocerebroside in the cytoplasm, may be found in any tissue having a fixed macrophage population (e.g., bone marrow, spleen, and liver).[22,50]

The appearance of clinical manifestations is earliest and progression of disease is most rapid in patients having the least glucocerebrosidase activity.[22,50] Of the three clinical forms of the disease, the adult form is most common. Splenomegaly, which may be massive, is usually the presenting feature and may be discovered accidentally or as a result of symptoms of early satiety, abdominal fullness, or painful infarctions. Bone pain is common due to bone destruction, which may result in collapse of vertebral bodies, pathologic fractures, and crippling. Central nervous system abnormalities are absent in the adult form of Gaucher's disease. Thrombocytopenia results in recurrent bleeding from the nose and gums, purpura, and petechiae.[5,22,50]

The infantile form, in which the central nervous system is the major site of involvement, is a much less common form of Gaucher's disease. Retarded development, early appearance of neurologic signs, seizures, hepatosplenomegaly, and cachexia are followed by death, usually before 3 years of age. The juvenile form appears during childhood and usually becomes apparent due to splenomegaly. In contrast to the adult form of Gaucher's disease, there is progressive neuronal damage and development of central nervous system abnormalities.[22,50]

Moderate-to-severe thrombocytopenia is present in most patients and is the most troublesome hematologic manifestation. Moderate normocytic anemia and leukopenia are common. Splenectomy is almost uniformly effective in correcting the cytopenias and relieves symptoms due to splenomegaly and recurring splenic infarction, although there is no evidence that splenectomy influences other aspects of the disease.[22,50]

Subtotal splenectomy has been performed for patients with the adult form of Gaucher's disease who have developed massive splenomegaly and hypersplenism.[19] Hypersplenism was controlled, and dramatic improvement occurred in appetite and general feeling of well-being after resection of approximately 85 per cent of the spleen. Functioning residual splenic tissue was demonstrable postoperatively. In addition to controlling cytopenias and eliminating symptoms related to splenomegaly, subtotal splenectomy in Gaucher's disease may provide a splenic remnant large enough to afford protection against overwhelming sepsis.[19]

Cysts and Tumors of the Spleen

The differential diagnosis of splenomegaly and isolated splenic masses includes cysts and primary tumors of the spleen other than systemic neoplasms of lymphoid tissue and the reticuloendothelial system. Splenic cysts and primary tumors are rare but must be considered in the differential diagnosis of a left upper quadrant mass.

Cystic lesions of the spleen comprise parasitic and nonparasitic cysts. Parasitic cysts are due almost exclusively to echinococcal disease and comprise 60 to 70 per cent of splenic cysts in countries where hydatid disease is endemic (South America, Australia, and Greece). Because echinococcal disease is rare in the United States, nonparasitic cysts are encountered much more frequently. Nonparasitic cysts are classified as primary or true cysts, which have an epithelial lining, and pseudocysts. Pseudocysts are much more common and probably result from liquefaction of old hematomas or areas of infarction and inflammation. True cysts of the spleen are very rare and include epidermoid and dermoid cysts, cystic hemangiomas, and cystic lymphangiomas.

Symptoms of splenic cysts are vague and result primarily from mass effect, compression of adjacent viscera, and diaphragmatic irritation. Although selected nonparasitic cysts may be effectively managed by aspiration, splenectomy should be performed for all large cysts and those with uncertain diagnosis. In some patients a splenic cyst may be suitably located for excision by partial splenectomy. Intraoperative drainage may facilitate dissection and splenectomy for very large cysts. External drainage and marsupialization have an unacceptable incidence of infection, bleeding, and cyst reaccumulation and are inappropriate techniques for management of splenic cysts.

Malignant and benign primary tumors of the spleen are rare. Most primary malignant tumors are angiosarcomas, although primary splenic lymphoma may occur. Before primary parenchymal lymphoma is diagnosed in the spleen, the bone marrow, nodal regions, liver, and other areas must be evaluated and found to be free of disease. Benign splenic tumors include hamartomas, lymphangiomas, hemangiomas, and lipomas.[39]

Except for involvement with Hodgkin's disease and non-Hodgkin's lymphomas, metastatic disease to the spleen is diagnosed infrequently (Fig. 13). The spleen's effective filtering mechanism and high blood flow suggest that the spleen would develop metastatic lesions more often. Although spleens from patients dying of metastatic tumors frequently reveal malignant cells, metastatic deposits are rare. Studies in rodents have confirmed that metastatic tumors rarely develop in the spleen fol-

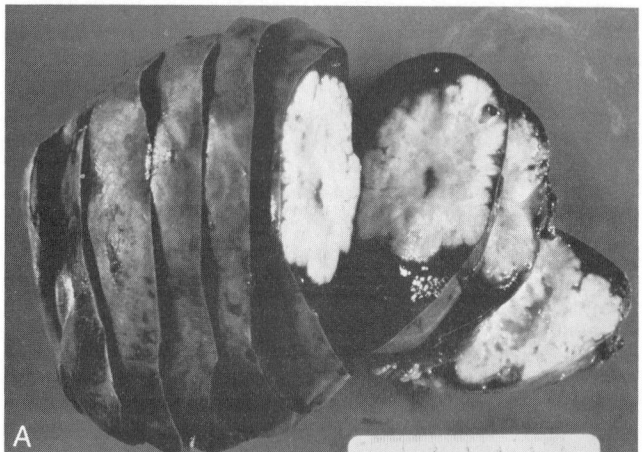

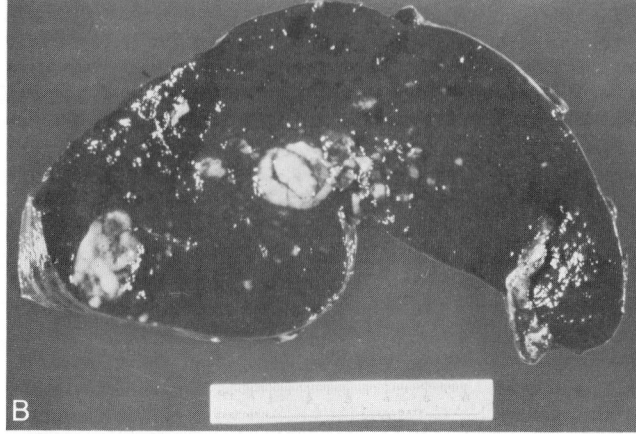

Figure 13. A, Large metastatic deposit in the spleen (480 gm.) from gastric adenocarcinoma. B, Metastatic plasmacytomas in the spleen (1000 gm.) of a patient with multiple myeloma who developed hypersplenism.

lowing injection of tumor cells into the splenic artery. It is probable that the splenic immune mechanisms that so efficiently destroy abnormal red cells also eliminate the majority of metastatic tumor cells that are trapped in the red pulp.[8]

Splenic Vein Thrombosis

Since the pathophysiology of splenic vein thrombosis was first elucidated 50 years ago, this uncommon cause of upper gastrointestinal variceal hemorrhage has been found to be eminently curable by splenectomy.[6] Pancreatitis is the cause of splenic vein thrombosis in more than half the reported cases. Other causes include pancreatic carcinoma, pancreatic pseudocyst, penetrating gastric ulcer, retroperitoneal fibrosis, and myeloproliferative disorders.[6] The underlying disease produces thrombosis of the splenic vein, with subsequent development of venous collateral channels. Because the collateral pathways are usually the short gastric veins to the submucosal venous plexus of the gastric cardia and fundus, gastric varices develop.

Splenic vein thrombosis should be suspected in a patient with upper gastrointestinal hemorrhage, isolated gastric varices on endoscopy, and a history of pancreatitis or pancreatic cancer. Splenomegaly is variable, and if present it is not associated with other stigmata of cirrhosis. Anemia usually is present, but tests of liver function are normal. Definitive diagnosis is made by celiac angiography, which demonstrates absence of the splenic vein. Splenomegaly may be noted along with venous collaterals in the splenic hilus.[6,39]

Splenectomy is curative and eliminates the increased blood flow through collaterals to the gastric venous plexuses. Although no studies have followed the course of asymptomatic patients with splenic vein thrombosis, it appears prudent to consider splenectomy if this diagnosis is made.

Infectious Mononucleosis

Infectious mononucleosis is a disease characterized by fever, sore throat, lymphadenopathy, and atypical lymphocytes in the blood smear. The atypical lymphocytes are believed to be T cells reacting against B lymphocytes infected with Epstein-Barr virus. Most patients are young adults, but the disease also occurs in middle-aged individuals.[21,22,50] The diagnosis is made by finding a pleomorphic atypical lymphocytosis and heterophile antibodies in the serum as demonstrated by a "mono" spot test.

Clinical symptomatology is akin to that of a severe upper respiratory infection. The spleen is enlarged and palpable in over 50 per cent of young patients, in contrast to the 3 per cent incidence of a palpable spleen found normally in this age group.[8,22,50] Hepatomegaly is present in 15 per cent of patients.

Splenic rupture may occur, probably resulting from minor trauma to an enlarged and diseased spleen rather than from spontaneous rupture. There has been minimal experience with splenic preservation for rupture associated with infectious mononucleosis. Most series of splenectomy for bleeding in patients with infectious mononucleosis report a higher mortality than with splenectomy for trauma.

Incidental Splenectomy

The spleen is vulnerable to injury during operative procedures in the upper abdomen. Operations on the stomach, esophageal hiatus, vagus nerves, pancreas, left kidney and adrenal gland, and transverse and descending colon carry risk of splenic injury. When the splenic capsule is torn, splenectomy frequently is performed (Table 8).

In most series, morbidity and mortality are higher with iatrogenic injury requiring incidental splenectomy than with splenectomy for a specific disease. One large series reported an earlier (before 1974) morbidity rate of 44 per cent and a mortality rate of 14 per cent.[45] The recent experience from the same institution revealed a pronounced decrease in the incidence of incidental splenectomy but a continued significant morbidity (26 per cent)

TABLE 8. Morbidity and Mortality in Splenectomy, 1948 to 1978

Indication	Number of Patients	Per Cent	Morbidity (%)	Mortality (%)
Hypersplenism	999	41	15	7
Primary	557	23	10	2
Secondary	442	18	22	13
Incidental	659	27	36	13
Trauma	257	10.5	30	16
Hodgkin's staging	203	8	4	0
Other	299	12	—	—
Total	2417	100	34	9.25

Modified from Traetow, W. D., Fabri, P. J., and Carey, L. C.: Changing indications for splenectomy: 30 years' experience. Arch. Surg., *115*:447, 1980. Copyright 1980, American Medical Association.

and mortality (12 per cent). Awareness of the risk for overwhelming postsplenectomy sepsis and the high complication and death rates from incidental splenectomy indicate and emphasize the need for avoiding intraoperative splenic injury. Most iatrogenic injuries occur to the capsule, and techniques for splenic repair and preservation should be employed instead of splenectomy.

SPLENECTOMY

Operations for splenic injury or disease should be preceded by specific preoperative preparations. All patients should receive polyvalent pneumococcal vaccine (Pnu-Imune 23 or Pneumovax 23), polyvalent meningococcal vaccine, and *Haemophilus influenzae* type b conjugate vaccine as early as possible before operation. Blood and blood products should be sought sufficiently in advance to allow crossmatching, which may be difficult in patients with acquired hemolytic anemia, thalassemia, or isoantibodies from previous transfusions. Platelet availability is advisable in severely thrombocytopenic patients for use after removal of the spleen if thrombocytopenic bleeding occurs. The operating room and blood and blood products should be warmed prior to use. This is especially important in patients with chronic lymphocytic leukemia or lymphoma who may have developed cold hemagglutinin disease and thus have an increased risk for hemolysis.

Splenectomy can be performed through several standard abdominal incisions. It is rarely, if ever, necessary to use a thoracoabdominal incision, even to remove massively enlarged spleens. The midline incision is preferred, although a left subcostal incision is favored by some surgeons, especially in children. Palpation is done to detect any inflammatory adhesions to the spleen that might result in a capsular tear and troublesome bleeding if not carefully divided. The spleen is mobilized by dividing its posterior ligamentous attachments, which may contain blood vessels requiring control by electrocauterization or ligation. The short gastric vessels are divided and suture-ligated, avoiding injury or ischemia to focal areas of the greater gastric curvature that might result in necrosis and gastric fistula formation. Some instances of postsplenectomy bleeding are due to inadequately secured short gastric vessels in patients who develop gastric distention postoperatively. A nasogastric tube is advisable for most patients undergoing splenectomy, although one of the authors (G. F. S.) does not use a nasogastric tube in ITP patients because of the potential risk of causing bleeding from the nose or nasopharynx.

The spleen may be removed by either of two techniques. Splenic ligaments may be divided and the spleen mobilized toward the midline prior to securing the hilar vessels, a technique applicable for normal-sized, slightly enlarged, and ruptured spleens (Fig. 14). Initial ligation of the splenic artery and

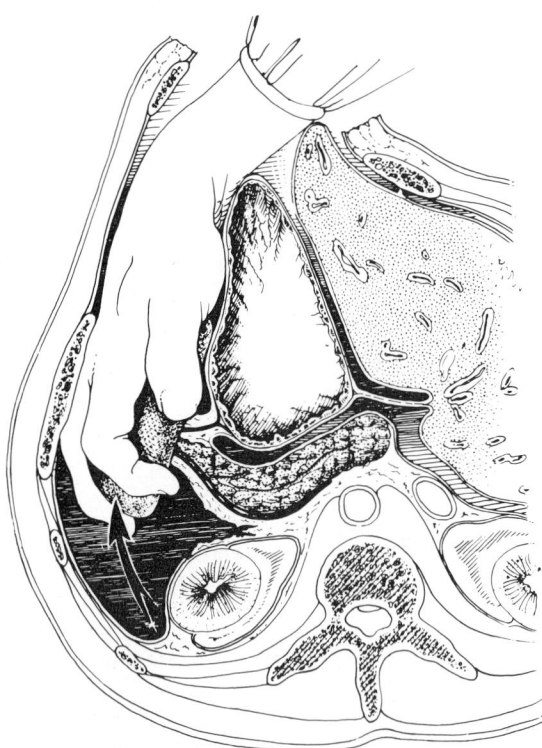

Figure 14. Technique of splenic mobilization for splenectomy or splenorrhaphy. The spleen is easily mobilized to the midline after dividing its posterior ligaments. The plane of dissection lies posterior to the body and tail of the pancreas and can be developed rapidly by blunt dissection. (From Blaisdell, F. W., and Trunkey, D. D.: Trauma Management. New York, Thieme-Stratton, 1982, p. 190.)

vein along the upper edge of the pancreas before splenic mobilization is a very useful technique with massive splenomegaly, as it controls the major portion of the vascular supply and allows safer mobilization of the spleen and dissection of its hilar branches[14] (Fig. 15). Isolation and ligation of blood vessels in the hilus should be performed carefully to avoid injuring the tail of the pancreas. Accessory splenic tissue occurs in approximately 20 per cent of patients, and a thorough search for an accessory spleen should be made in all patients undergoing splenectomy

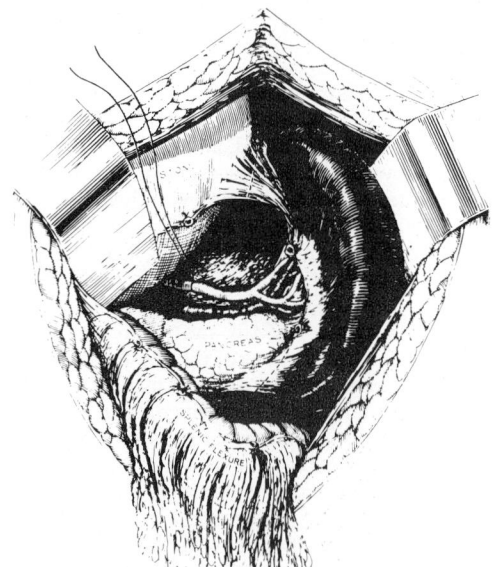

Figure 15. Technique of splenectomy showing in continuity ligation of the splenic artery and vein prior to mobilizing the spleen. The gastrosplenic ligament has been partially divided. Initial control of the splenic artery and vein in this manner minimizes the danger of major bleeding in performing splenectomy for very large spleens. (From Cooper, P.: The Craft of Surgery, 2nd ed. Boston, Little, Brown, & Company, 1971, p. 1314.)

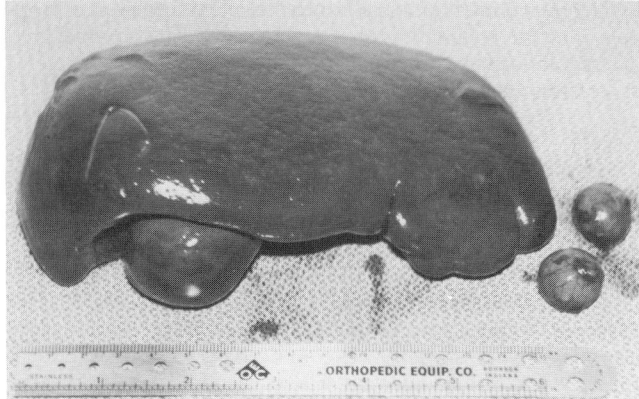

Figure 16. A spleen (440 gm.) demonstrating prominent fetal lobulations and two accessory spleens, from a patient with hereditary elliptocytosis.

for hematologic disease (Fig. 16). The left upper quadrant should not be drained routinely. When injury to the tail of the pancreas or incomplete hemostasis indicates the advisability for left upper quadrant drainage, a system of closed suction drainage should be employed. Depending upon the indication for splenectomy, most patients tolerate the operation well. The most common postoperative complication is left lower lobe atelectasis. Other more serious complications include postoperative hemorrhage, subphrenic abscess, pancreatitis, pneumonia, wound infection, and portal vein and mesenteric venous thrombosis.

BLOOD COMPOSITIONAL CHANGES IN THE ASPLENIC OR HYPOSPLENIC PATIENT

The absence of functional splenic tissue results in characteristic compositional changes in the circulating blood. Some of these are predictable and desirable results of splenectomy and are a measure of its success when splenectomy is performed for a hematologic disease.

In its normal filtering function, the spleen removes excess red cell membrane, surface abnormalities such as pits and spurs, and a variety of intracellular inclusions. Red cells that cannot be adequately molded and pitted are culled.[8] In the absence of the spleen, this function is lost and several characteristic red cell changes can be identified in the peripheral blood. Howell-Jolly bodies (nuclear remnants) typically are present in asplenic patients, and absence of Howell-Jolly bodies after splenectomy suggests the presence of functional residual splenic tissue (accessory spleen or splenosis).[8,37] Target cells, red cells with fine inclusions (stippled red cells), acanthocytes (spur cells), Heinz bodies (denatured hemoglobin), and Pappenheimer bodies (iron granules) also are predictable findings in asplenic patients. Granulocytosis, lymphocytosis, and monocytosis commonly occur after splenectomy but are variable in occurrence, magnitude, and duration.[8,22,50]

Thrombocytosis occurs immediately after splenectomy in most patients and is often the desired therapeutic result. Up to 75 per cent of patients who have had splenectomy develop thrombocytosis (platelet count of greater than 400,000 per cu. mm.), and platelet counts in excess of 1,000,000 per cu. mm. develop in some patients. Generally this has not been associated with an increased risk of thromboembolism.[4] An exception to this is seen in patients with myeloproliferative disorders who clearly have an increased risk of thromboembolic complications following splenectomy.[18,22,50] In these patients, and especially in those with thrombocytosis preoperatively, specific antiplatelet therapy should be utilized. The spectrum of antiplatelet therapy includes administration of aspirin, dipyridamole, heparin, dextran, hydroxyurea, and busulfan. Hydroxyurea is especially useful in controlling thrombocytosis. A rapid reduction of the thrombocytosis can be achieved by plateletpheresis (thrombocytopheresis) in patients with thrombohemorrhagic manifestations.[18,22,50]

After splenectomy, depression of serum levels of at least two important opsonins occurs. Diminution in these two opsonic proteins, tuftsin and properdin, is partially responsible for the increased susceptibility of asplenic patients to infection from encapsulated bacteria. The exact role of these opsonins is unclear. Children with sickle cell anemia have low levels of properdin and an impaired alternate pathway of complement activation, which decrease their ability to opsonize pneumococci. However, children who have undergone splenectomy for trauma have normal pneumococcal opsonizing activity despite subnormal levels of properdin and tuftsin.[8]

THE PROBLEM OF OVERWHELMING POSTSPLENECTOMY SEPSIS

Asplenic patients and those with deficient splenic function have an increased susceptibility to the development of overwhelming infection characterized by fulminant bacteremia, meningitis, or pneumonia. Although it was suggested as early as 1919 that removal of the spleen would increase susceptibility to infection (Morris and Bullock), the increased risk of fatal sepsis was first documented by King and Shumacker in 1952.[29,39,42] Singer's review of 2796 patients with splenectomy described a 4.2 per cent incidence of sepsis and a 2.5 per cent mortality rate (Table 9). The risk of overwhelming sepsis is approximately 60 times greater than normal following splenectomy and may be as high as 0.5 to 1.0 per cent per year. Although a lifetime risk of fulminant sepsis is incurred with splenectomy, the risk is greatest in children under 4 years of age and within 2 years of splenectomy (80 per cent of cases).[8] In one series of adults, the average time period between splenectomy and fulminant sepsis was 5.8 years, with a range of 7 months to 25 years.[29] A follow-up of 740 servicemen who had undergone splenectomy for trauma demonstrated an increased mortality rate from pneumonia and ischemic heart disease.[29,39]

The risk for overwhelming postsplenectomy sepsis is highest in patients requiring splenectomy for thalassemia and reticuloendothelial system diseases, such as Hodgkin's disease, histiocytosis X, or the Wiskott-Aldrich syndrome.[8,29] It is lowest for patients with splenectomy for trauma, ITP, and hereditary spherocytosis[8] (Table 9).

The postsplenectomy sepsis syndrome typically occurs in a previously healthy individual following a mild upper respiratory infection associated with fever. Within hours, nausea, vomiting, headache, confusion, shock, and coma occur, and death follows within 24 hours. Laboratory studies reveal hypoglycemia, acidosis, electrolyte abnormalities, and disseminated intravascular coagulation.[8,29] Blood cultures reveal *Streptococcus pneumoniae*, *Neisseria meningitidis*, *Escherichia coli*, or *Haemo-*

philus influenzae in 75 per cent of the cases, with *S. pneumoniae* comprising 50 per cent.[29] Patients with pneumococcal sepsis have no obvious site of primary infection, and the bacteremia, which may reach extraordinary proportions (more than 10^6 bacteria/per ml.), is of cryptic origin. The peripheral blood smear shows vacuolated polymorphonuclear leukocytes, thrombocytopenia, and occasionally pneumococci.[8,29] The fulminant nature of the syndrome makes it difficult to diagnose early enough for therapy to be effective. Adrenal hemorrhage is a common autopsy finding.[29]

The spleen has both mechanical and humoral roles in protecting against bacterial infection, and the exact mechanism by which postsplenectomy sepsis develops is unclear. Among the immunologic defects that occur after splenectomy are decreased serum properdin and tuftsin levels, decreased serum IgM, impaired alternate pathway of complement activation, and a reduced response to particulate antigens.[8,29,39] Opsonization is critically important in the phagocytosis of *S. pneumoniae*, but animal studies indicate that an adequate splenic mass also is important in pneumococcal clearance.[29,39] Evidence suggests that approximately 50 per cent of the normal mass of splenic tissue is necessary to preserve protection against encapsulated bacteria.[29,39] Because postsplenectomy sepsis and death have occurred in patients who had a total mass of residual splenic tissue weighing 3 to 92 gm., preservation of a sufficient "critical" splenic mass appears necessary for the maintenance of normal host defenses.[8,39]

Antibiotic prophylaxis or early antibiotic therapy may be effective in reducing the incidence of postsplenectomy sepsis. Because half the patients develop sepsis from *S. pneumoniae*, penicillin can be administered prophylactically or immediately with the onset of a febrile upper respiratory illness. In patients who have had splenectomy for Hodgkin's disease staging, the incidence of overwhelming sepsis has been reduced by penicillin prophylaxis.[29] The authors' practice is to administer penicillin prophylactically for an indefinite period after splenectomy in young children. If allergy to penicillin exists, erythromycin or trimethoprim/sulfamethoxazole is substituted. Each adult patient is instructed to obtain and wear a Medic Alert medal indicating their asplenic state and increased risk for infection. In addition, the danger of overwhelming postsplenectomy sepsis and the importance of seeking immediate medical attention with the onset of a febrile upper respiratory illness are stressed to adult patients and to the parents of children who have had splenectomy.

Considerable hope exists for preventing postsplenectomy sepsis by immunization with specific vaccines. Ideally, patients should be immunized well in advance of splenectomy (2 to 3 weeks preoperatively) to allow development of protective antibodies. Polyvalent vaccines against capsular polysaccharides from pneumococcal strains responsible for the majority of seri-

TABLE 9. Incidence of Postsplenectomy Sepsis

Reason for Splenectomy	Number of Patients	Number of Patients with Sepsis (%)	Number of Fatalities from Sepsis (%)	Increased Risk of Death from Sepsis (X)
Trauma	688	10 (1.4)	4 (0.58)	58
Incidental to operation	233	5 (2.1)	2 (0.86)	86
ITP	489	10 (2.0)	7 (1.43)	140
Hereditary spherocytosis	850	30 (3.5)	19 (2.23)	220
Acquired hemolytic anemia	67	5 (7.5)	2 (2.90)	290
Portal hypertension	221	18 (8.2)	13 (5.90)	590
Primary anemia	70	6 (8.5)	5 (7.01)	700
Reticuloendothelial disease	69	8 (11.5)	7 (10.10)	1000
Thalassemia	109	27 (24.8)	12 (11.00)	1100
Total	2796	119 (4.2)	71 (2.50)	

Modified from Singer, R.: Postsplenectomy sepsis. Perspect. Pediatr. Pathol., 1:285, 1973.

ous pneumococcal disease [Pnu-Imune 23 (23 strains) and Pneumovax 23 (23 strains)] are available. Polyvalent meningococcal vaccines also are available, and *Haemophilus influenzae* type b conjugate vaccines provide immunization against type b *Haemophilus,* a leading cause of serious systemic bacterial disease. Although the efficacy of vaccination to reduce the incidence of overwhelming infection is difficult to assess due to the infrequent occurrence of postsplenectomy sepsis, polyvalent pneumococcal vaccine has provided significant protection from pneumococcemia in children with sickle cell anemia.[8,29]

Not all splenectomized patients are capable of developing protective antibody titers following vaccination. Children less than 2 years of age and patients with Hodgkin's disease who are receiving chemotherapy and/or radiation therapy do not respond consistently to polyvalent pneumococcal vaccine. An additional shortcoming of immunization is that current vaccines do not immunize against all bacteria capable of producing overwhelming postsplenectomy sepsis. It is unclear whether and how often patients should be reimmunized after splenectomy. As new vaccines become available and further studies are completed, a more definitive immunization program may become standard. Presently, repeat immunization every 5 years appears reasonable.

Rare Splenic Disorders

WANDERING (ECTOPIC) SPLEEN. Congenital deficiency or acquired laxity of the suspensory ligaments of the spleen may result in extreme splenic mobility. This rare condition, which is termed *wandering* or *ectopic spleen*, permits a normal-sized spleen to be palpable in the lower abdomen or in the pelvis. The majority of cases of wandering spleen have occurred in young and middle-aged women in whom multiparity and laxity of the abdominal wall and splenic ligaments due to the hormonal effects of pregnancy have been cited as predisposing causes. A wandering spleen may be an incidental finding on physical or radiographic examination. An enlongated splenic pedicle predisposes a wandering spleen to torsion, leading either to development of acute symptoms due to splenic volvulus and infarction or chronic and intermittent abdominal discomfort due to spontaneous torsion and detorsion. Useful diagnostic tests in the patient who is asymptomatic or has chronic and recurring symptoms include abdominal CT or ultrasonography, a splenic radionuclide scan, and visceral arteriography. Splenic volvulus with infarction requires emergency splenectomy. Selected asymptomatic patients and those with chronic and recurring symptoms may sometimes be managed successfully by splenopexy, which preserves splenic function and avoids the potential danger of postsplenectomy sepsis.

SPLENIC ARTERY ANEURYSM. Aneurysms of the splenic artery are rare and occur more frequently in women, in whom the most common etiology is medial dysplasia of the arterial wall. Atherosclerosis accounts for the majority of splenic artery aneurysms in men. Additional causes include focal arterial injury from pancreatitis, trauma or arteritis from septic emboli, portal hypertension with splenomegaly, and an ill-defined pathogenesis associated with multiparity.[39] Most splenic artery aneurysms are asymptomatic, and characteristic eggshell calcification of an arteriosclerotic aneurysm may be an incidental finding on an abdominal radiograph (Fig. 17). When symptoms are present, they are variable and consist primarily of vague left upper quadrant discomfort. Aneurysmal rupture may occur, and the rupture initially may be contained within the lesser sac. Initial aneurysmal rupture into the peritoneal cavity or delayed rupture from the lesser sac are associated with findings of hemoperitoneum and exsanguinating hemorrhage. Rarely, a splenic artery aneurysm ruptures into the gastrointestinal tract, pancreatic duct, or splenic vein. The mortality with a ruptured splenic artery aneurysm remains high. Excision of the aneurysm is advisable for symptomatic aneurysms and for asymptomatic aneurysms in patients who are acceptable operative risks. This is especially important for women of childbearing age who have an increased propensity for aneurysmal rupture during pregnancy. Elective surgery has a low risk of mortality and minimal morbidity. In the treatment of splenic artery aneurysm, the spleen should be preserved if possible.[39]

SPLENIC ABSCESS. Splenic abscess occurs rarely and usually results from (1) bacteremia associated with a primary septic focus such as bacterial endocarditis or lung abscess, or (2) secondary infection in an area of the spleen damaged by infarction (sickle cell anemia or leukemia), trauma, or parasitic infestation. Clinical features of splenic abscess are those of left subphrenic suppuration and include fever, chills, left upper quadrant tenderness, and often splenomegaly. Imaging techniques (sonography and radionuclide and CT scans) are useful in differentiating splenic abscess from left subphrenic abscess and in determining whether there is a single abscess or multiple abscesses within the spleen. CT scan is probably the most direct way of evaluating the spleen and establishing an early diagnosis.[39]

Splenectomy has been the preferred treatment for most patients in the past and remains a standard means of safe and rapid management. Splenotomy and abscess drainage may be advisable for selected patients with a single abscess and extensive adhesions between the spleen and adjacent structures. Image-guided percutaneous drainage may be appropriate in the management of some patients with splenic abscess. Percutaneous drainage is most likely to be successful if the abscess is

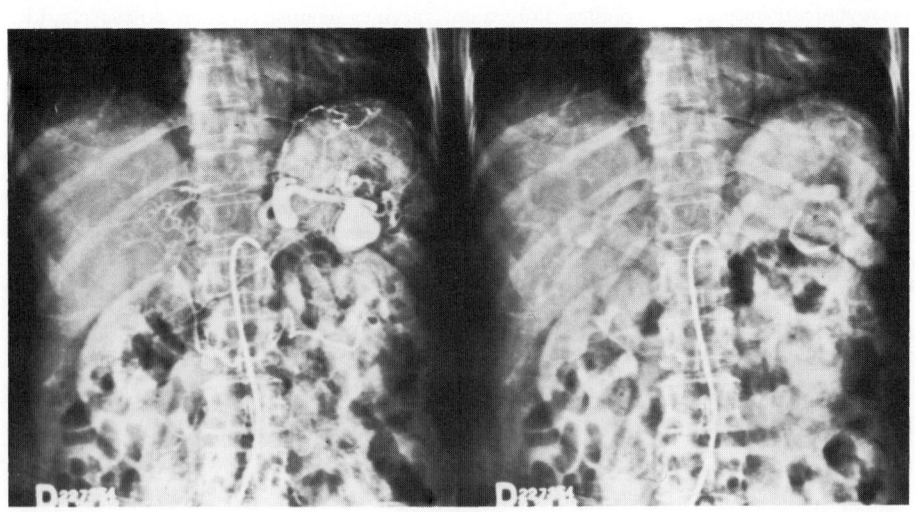

Figure 17. A splenic arteriogram disclosing an aneurysm of the distal splenic artery. *A,* The aneurysm is filled with contrast material. In a later radiograph, *B,* the eggshell calcification characteristic of an arteriosclerotic aneurysm is evident. Excision of the aneurysm was performed and required splenectomy.

A   B

unilocular and if the abscess contents are amenable to complete evacuation by an indwelling suction catheter.[13]

SELECTED REFERENCES

Croom, R. D., McMillan, C. W., Sheldon, G. F., and Orringer, E. P.: Hereditary spherocytosis: Recent experience and current concepts of pathophysiology. Ann. Surg., 203:34, 1986.

A thorough review of this important hemolytic anemia is presented along with case reports that illustrate the recently identified, recessively inherited form of hereditary spherocytosis. This article contains a concise description of the hypothesized erythrocyte membrane skeleton and the relationship to current concepts of pathophysiology of this disease.

Eichner, E. R.: Splenic function: Normal, too much and too little. Am. J. Med., 66:311, 1979.

This exceptionally thoughtful and complete review article discusses splenic function in normal and pathologic conditions. The indications for splenectomy are presented from the viewpoint of a hematologist.

Leonard, A. S., Giebink, G. S., Baesl, T. J., and Krivit, W.: The overwhelming postsplenectomy sepsis problem. World J. Surg., 4:423, 1980.

This article contains a complete discussion of the postsplenectomy sepsis syndrome and the postulated immune defects. Invited commentary by Filler, Grosfeld, Lynn, and Singer is included, along with their experiences with this problem and therapeutic recommendations.

McMillan, R.: Chronic idiopathic thrombocytopenic purpura. N. Engl. J. Med., 304:1135, 1981.

This article provides a complete discussion of this complex immune syndrome and reviews the mechanisms of pathogenesis and results of therapy.

Schwartz, S. I.: Progress symposium — Diseases affecting the spleen. World J. Surg., 9:377, 1985.

This symposium focuses on traumatic, infectious, vascular, neoplastic, and selected hematologic indications for operations on the spleen and its blood vessels. Indications, results, and complications of operation are reviewed, and a thorough overview of postsplenectomy sepsis is presented.

Schwartz, S. I., Adams, J. T., and Bauman, A. W.: Splenectomy for Hematologic Disorders. Chicago, Year Book Medical Publishers, 1971.

Although published 20 years ago, this monograph by a premier surgical hematologist is a classic. The immunologic mechanisms have undergone some revision since publication, but the presentation of surgical concepts and the clear writing style are noteworthy.

Sherman, R.: Perspectives in management of trauma to the spleen: 1979 Presidential Address, American Association for the Surgery of Trauma. J. Trauma, 20:1, 1980.

This article provides a comprehensive and scholarly review of the evolution of concepts and techniques for management of splenic trauma.

REFERENCES

1. Adler, S., Stutzman, L., Sokal, J. E., and Mittelman, A.: Splenectomy for hematologic depression in lymphocytic lymphoma and leukemia. Cancer, 35:521, 1975.
2. Agre, P., Orringer, E. P., and Bennett, V.: Deficient red-cell spectrin in severe, recessively inherited spherocytosis. N. Engl. J. Med., 306:1155, 1982.
3. Bonadonna, G., and Santoro, A.: Current Diagnosis and Treatment of Malignant Lymphomas. Evansville, Ind., Mead Johnson & Company, 1983.
4. Boxer, M. A., Braun, J., and Ellman, L.: Thromboembolic risk of postsplenectomy thrombocytosis. Arch. Surg., 113:808, 1978.
5. Brain, M. C., and McCulloch, P. B.: Current Therapy in Hematology – Oncology 1983 – 1984. Ontario, B. C. Decker, 1983.
6. Bunt, T. J., Hackler, M. T., and Greene, F. L.: Isolated splenic vein thrombosis: The curable variceal hemorrhage. South. Med. J., 76:936, 1983.
7. Croom, R. D., McMillan, C. W., Sheldon, G. F., and Orringer, E. P.: Hereditary spherocytosis: Recent experience and current concepts of pathophysiology. Ann. Surg., 203:34, 1986.
8. Eichner, E. R.: Splenic function: Normal, too much and too little. Am. J. Med., 66:311, 1979.
9. Eraklis, A. J., and Filler, R. M.: Splenectomy in childhood; A review of 1413 cases. J. Pediatr. Surg., 7:382, 1972.
10. Fleming, C. R., Dickson, E. R., and Harrison, E. G., Jr.: Splenosis: Autotransplantation of splenic tissue. Am. J. Med., 61:414, 1976.
11. Gernsheimer, T., Stratton, J., Ballem, P. J., and Slichter, S. J.: Mechanisms of response to treatment in autoimmune thrombocytopenic purpura. N. Engl. J. Med., 320:974, 1989.
12. Gill, P. G., Souter, R. G., and Morris, P. J.: Splenectomy for hypersplenism in malignant lymphomas. Br. J. Surg., 68:29, 1981.
13. Gleich, S., Wolin, D. A., and Herbsman, H.: A review of percutaneous drainage in splenic abscess. Surg. Gynecol. Obstet., 167:211, 1988.
14. Goldstone, J.: Splenectomy for massive splenomegaly. Am. J. Surg., 135:385, 1978.
15. Golomb, H. M.: Hairy cell leukemia: Lessons learned in twenty-five years. J. Clin. Oncol., 1:652, 1983.
16. Golomb, H. M., and Ratain, M. J.: Recent advances in the treatment of hairy cell leukemia. N. Engl. J. Med., 316:870, 1987.
17. Golomb, H. M., and Ratain, M. J.: What is the choice of treatment for hairy cell leukemia? J. Clin. Oncol., 7:156, 1989.
18. Gordon, D. H., Schaffner, D., Bennett, J. M., and Schwartz, S. I.: Postsplenectomy thrombocytosis: Its association with mesenteric, portal, and/or renal vein thrombosis in patients with myeloproliferative disorders. Arch. Surg., 113:713, 1978.
19. Guzzetta, P. C., Connors, R. H., Fink, J., and Barranger, J. A.: Operative technique and results of subtotal splenectomy for Gaucher disease. Surg. Gynecol. Obstet., 164:359, 1987.
20. Hoballah, J. J., Kim, E. H., and Dumont, A. E.: Thrombocytopenic purpura in parenteral drug abusers. Surg. Gynecol. Obstet., 168:497, 1989.
21. Hoffbrand, A. V., and Pettit, J. E.: Essential Haematology. London, Blackwell Scientific Publications, 1980.
22. Jandl, J. H.: Blood: Textbook of Hematology. Boston, Little, Brown & Company, 1987.
23. Jones, S. E.: Importance of staging Hodgkin's disease. Semin. Oncol., 7:126, 1980.
24. Kinsella, T. J., and Glatstein, E.: Staging laparotomy and splenectomy for Hodgkin's disease: Current status. Cancer Invest., 1:87, 1983.
25. Koller, C. A.: Immune thrombocytopenic purpura. Med. Clin. North Am., 64:761, 1980.
26. Kudsk, K. A., Tranbaugh, R. F., and Sheldon, G. F.: Acute surgical illness in patients with sickle cell anemia. Am. J. Surg., 142:113, 1981.
27. Lange, D. A., Zaret, P., Merlotti, G. J., Robin, A. P., Sheaff, C., and Barrett, J. A.: The use of absorbable mesh in splenic trauma. J. Trauma, 28:269, 1988.
28. Laszlo, J., Jones, R., Silberman, H. R., and Banks, P. M.: Splenectomy for Felty's syndrome: Clinicopathological study of 27 patients. Arch. Intern. Med., 138:597, 1978.
29. Leonard, A. S., Giebink, G. S., Baesl, T. J., and Krivit, W.: The overwhelming postsplenectomy sepsis problem. World J. Surg., 4:423, 1980.
30. McMillan, R.: Chronic idiopathic thrombocytopenic purpura. N. Engl. J. Med., 304:1135, 1981.
31. Medical Research Council's Working Party for Therapeutic Trials in Leukaemia: Randomized trial of splenectomy in Ph¹-positive chronic granulocytic leukaemia, including an analysis of prognostic features. Br. J. Haematol., 54:415, 1983.
32. Morgenstern, L.: Salvaging the spleen. Contemp. Surg., 23:27, 1983.
33. Morgenstern, L.: The Surgical Inviolability of the Spleen: Historical Evolution of a Concept. London, Wellcome Institute of the History of Medicine, 1974, pp. 62 – 68.
34. Morgenstern, L., and Uyeda, R. Y.: Nonoperative management of injuries of the spleen in adults. Surg. Gynecol. Obstet., 157:513, 1983.
35. Musser, G., Lazar, G., Hocking, W., and Busuttil, R. W.: Splenectomy for hematologic disease: The UCLA experience with 306 patients. Ann. Surg., 200:40, 1984.
36. Pearl, R. H., Wesson, D. E., Spence, L. J., Filler, R. M., Ein, S. H., Shandling, B., and Superina, R. A.: Splenic injury: A 5-year update with improved results and changing criteria for conservative management. J. Pediatr. Surg., 24:428, 1989.
37. Pearson, H. A., Johnston, D., Smith, K. A., and Touloukian, R. J.: The bornagain spleen: Return of splenic function after splenectomy for trauma. N. Engl. J. Med., 298:1389, 1978.
38. Rosenberg, S. A.: Exploratory laparotomy and splenectomy for Hodgkin's disease: A commentary. J. Clin. Oncol., 6:574, 1988.
39. Schwartz, S. I.: Progress Symposium — Diseases affecting the spleen. World J. Surg., 9:377, 1985.
40. Schwartz, S. I., Adams, J. T., and Bauman, A. W.: Splenectomy for Hematologic Disorders. Chicago, Year Book Medical Publishers, 1971.
41. Schwartz, S. I., Hoepp, L. M., and Sachs, S.: Splenectomy for thrombocytopenia. Surgery, 88:497, 1980.
42. Sherman, R.: Perspectives in management of trauma to the spleen: 1979 Presidential Address, American Association for the Surgery of Trauma. J. Trauma, 20:1, 1980.
43. Sterchi, J. M., Buss, D. H., and Beyer, F. C.: The risk of improperly staging Hodgkin's disease with partial splenectomy. Am. Surg., 50:20, 1984.
44. Stillman, R. J., Schiff, I., and Schinfeld, J.: Reproductive and gonadal function in the female after therapy for childhood malignancy. Obstet. Gynecol. Surv., 37:385, 1982.
45. Traetow, W. D., Fabri, P. J., and Carey, L. C.: Changing indications for splenectomy. Arch. Surg., 115:447, 1980.
46. Traub, A., Giebink, G. S., Smith, C., Kuni, C. C., Brekke, M. L., Edlund, D., and Perry, J. F.: Splenic reticuloendothelial function after splenectomy, spleen repair, and spleen autotransplantation. N. Engl. J. Med., 317:1559, 1987.
47. Traub, A. C., Perry, J. F., Jr.: Injuries associated with splenic trauma. J. Trauma, 21:840, 1981.
48. Weiss, L.: Cell and Tissue Biology: A Textbook of Histology, 6th ed. Baltimore, Urban & Schwarzenberg, 1988.
49. Wilhelm, M. C., Jones, R. E., McGehee, R., Mitchener, J. S., Sandusky, W. R., and Hess, C. E.: Splenectomy in hematologic disorders: The everchanging indications. Ann. Surg., 207:581, 1988.
50. Wintrobe, M. M.: Clinical Hematology, 9th ed. Philadelphia, Lea & Febiger, 1990.
51. Woerner, S. J., Abildgaard, C. F., and French, B. N.: Intracranial hemorrhage in children with idiopathic thrombocytopenic purpura. Pediatrics, 67:453, 1981.

37

HERNIAS

Lloyd M. Nyhus, M.D., C. Thomas Bombeck, M.D., and
Michael S. Klein, M.D.

HISTORICAL ASPECTS

The early history of interest in hernia is that of the discipline of surgery. The names associated so intimately with the subject of hernia are familiar because of the pioneering thrust these men gave to surgery in general, e. g., Celsus, Henri de Mondeville, Guy de Chauliac, and Ambroise Paré.[88]

The Egyptian papyri do not contain reference to the operative treatment of hernia, but the Papyrus Ebers (1552 B.C.) recommended diet and externally applied pressure (truss?) for its treatment. The word *barbaric* is frequently used for surgery during the Middle Ages, and no less so for the treatment of hernia. Major developments in the knowledge of hernial anatomy and treatment occurred during the eighteenth century. Percival Pott of London refuted many of the old theories.[66] He was probably the first to suggest the congenital origin of hernias.

Early in the nineteenth century, four men contributed important descriptions of inguinal anatomy: Camper,[13] Cooper,[19] Hesselbach,[38,39] and Scarpa.[73] In 1801, Camper published the description of the fascia that bears his name. The skilled anatomist Sir Astley Cooper (1768–1841) published his two-volume work, *The Anatomy and Surgical Treatment of Abdominal Hernia,* in 1804 and 1807. First descriptions credited to Cooper include transversalis fascia, internal ring, inguinal canal, correct formation of femoral sheath by the transversalis fascia, and the complete description of Camper's fascia. He paid little attention to the "ligament of the pubis," now called Cooper's ligament, and he certainly had no idea how important this structure would become in the modern treatment of hernia. Hesselbach described the triangle that bears his name in 1814 while he was prosector in the anatomic theater of Würzburg. Finally, in this quartet of anatomists must be included Scarpa, for whom a superficial layer of fascia is named. He is also credited with being the first to describe a sliding hernia (1821).

The nineteenth century brought anesthesia, hemostasis, and antisepsis, which made modern surgery possible. As in every area of surgery, these advances allowed rapid development of the science of hernial surgery. Wide acceptance soon was attained in Europe and America for the operation consisting of ligature and excision of the sac at the external ring and suturing of the pillars around the cord to reduce the size of the ring. This procedure was described in 1877 by Czerny.[20] It is to Marcy of Boston that the modern era of hernial surgery is credited.[53,54] His understanding of the importance of the transversalis fascia and of the anatomic contribution of fascial repair of the internal ring was reported in 1871. Parenthetically, this was 12 years before Bassini did his first operation for hernia and 16 years before Bassini published his first paper on the subject.

Marcy's writings, however, did not stimulate the imagination of his contemporary surgeons, and further refinements in technique were suggested by Macewen (1886),[52] Lucas-Championniére (1892),[50] and Ferguson (1899).[25]

It remained for Bassini to develop a technique for reconstruction of the inguinal floor with transposition of the cord.[85] His operation (1884) included high ligation of the sac and reinforcement of the floor of the canal by suturing the transversus abdominis aponeurosis to the inguinal ligament beneath the cord, thus placing the cord under the external oblique aponeurosis. Bassini at this time held the chair of clinical surgery at the University of Padua. Independently and almost simultaneously, Halsted (1852–1922) developed an operation similar to that of Bassini. The Halsted operation (Halsted I) transposed the cord above the external oblique aponeurosis.[34,68] This procedure was first mentioned in 1889. The Halsted II operation (1893) did not transpose the cord but added imbrication of the aponeurosis of the external oblique muscle in performing the closure. The first mention of imbrication is credited to Andrews. The ludicrous overuse of eponyms in this field can be appreciated when it is learned that the Halsted II procedure is also known as the Ferguson-Andrews operation, since Ferguson left the cord in its normal anatomic position and Andrews stressed the imbrication of the external oblique aponeurosis. The technique of imbrication today is popular and used regularly by devotees of the Canadian, or Shouldice, repair.[86]

The use of the iliopectineal ligament (Cooper's ligament), or ligamentum pubicum superius, B.N.A., to anchor the medial parietal wall in the repair is credited to Lotheissen of Innsbruck.[48] The use of this structure is an integral part of the hernial repair made popular by McVay,[56] and the operation is known throughout the United States as the McVay repair.

The importance of the posterior inguinal wall in the etiology as well as in the repair of hernias was recognized relatively late. One of the strongest advocates of the transversalis fascia layer repair was Harrison (1883–1962).[37] A thickening in the transversalis fascia layer, the iliopubic tract, has received minimal attention from anatomists and surgeons alike. Depicted by Hesselbach (1814), it was described in detail in 1836 by Thomson.[78] In the past several decades, use of this structure has been recommended by a small number of surgeons interested in the anatomy of the groin (Clark and Hashimoto, 1946[14]; Donald, 1948[21]; Griffith, 1959[32]; Condon, 1964[16]; Nyhus, 1964[59]; and Howard, 1974[40]).

After such a long period of interest in this anatomic area, controversy still abounds. The last chapter in the history of groin anatomy and operative repair of hernia defects has not been written.

GROIN HERNIA

Anatomy of the Inguinal and Femoral Canals

As in all areas of the abdomen, the abdominal wall in the groin is composed of multilaminar arrangements of muscle, their aponeuroses, fascia, fat, and either skin or peritoneum. The abdominal wall at the level of the groin may be divided into two groups of laminae, an outer and an inner. These two groups are mirror images of each other and are divided by the inguinal canal and spermatic cord (Table 1; Fig. 1).

By definition, a hernia is a protrusion of normal cavity con-

TABLE 1. Layers of the Abdominal Wall

Skin	
Fat (abdominal panniculus)	
Fascia (Scarpa's)	
Aponeurosis and muscle (external oblique)	Superficial stratum
Inguinal canal, muscle (internal oblique) and spermatic cord	
Aponeurosis and muscle (transversus abdominis)	
Fascia (transversalis)	Deep stratum
Fat (preperitoneal fat)	
Peritoneum	

tents through the fascial and muscular layers designed to contain them. Thus, groin hernias are due to failure of the laminae of the abdominal wall to contain the enclosed viscera.

EXTERNAL OBLIQUE APONEUROSIS. The external oblique muscle arises from the lower eight ribs posteriorly and sweeps downward and around the trunk as a broad, flat muscle. The muscle fibers give way to its flat tendon of insertion, the external oblique aponeurosis, at the linea semilunaris, located in approximately the midclavicular line. The aponeurosis is attached to the iliac crest and the anterior superior iliac spine laterally (Fig. 2) and inserts rather broadly into the linea alba medially. It comprises a portion of the rectus sheath only very medially and does not attach to the lateral edge of the sheath, that structure being composed of deeper layers. Inferiorly, the aponeurosis is slightly thickened and folded back upon itself to form the inguinal ligament. As such, this structure is not a true ligament, since its function is not to stabilize bone. The lower edge of the inguinal ligament is loosely bound to the fascia lata by the innominate fascia. This fascia also serves to bind together the collagenous fibers of both the aponeurosis and the inguinal ligament. Medially, the inguinal ligament inserts on the pubic tubercle and fans downward onto the superior pubic ramus as the lacunar ligament. The medial attachment of the inguinal ligament is continuous with the insertion of the aponeurosis into the linea alba.

EXTERNAL INGUINAL RING. Just above the inguinal liga-

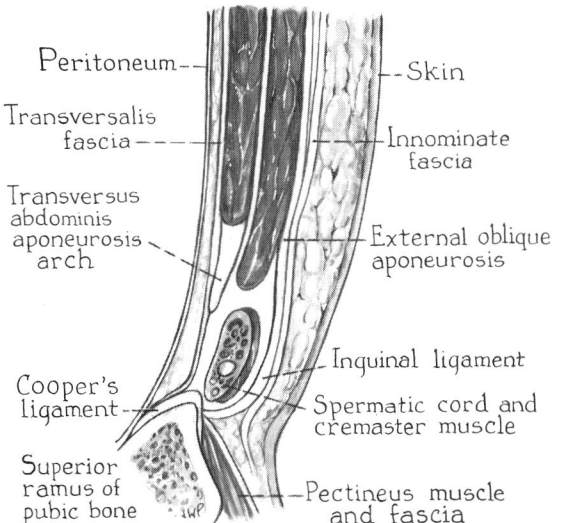

Figure 1. A parasagittal schematic representation of the musculoaponeurotic relationships in the middle of the right inguinal canal, viewed from the lateral aspect of the section. The closer approximation, via their common insertion into the pectineal line of the pubis, of the superficial (external oblique, inguinal ligament) layer to the deep (transversus abdominis, transversalis fascia) musculoaponeurotic layer in the medial portion of the groin is demonstrated. (From Condon, R. E.: The anatomy of the inguinal region and its relation to groin hernia. In Nyhus, L. M., and Condon, R. E.: Hernia, 3rd ed. Philadelphia, J. B. Lippincott Company, 1989.)

ment and lateral to its insertion onto the pubic tubercle, the fibers of the external oblique aponeurosis split to form a triangular opening, the external or superficial inguinal ring (Fig. 3). The ring serves as the point of egress for the spermatic cord in the male and the round ligament in the female. It has no role in diagnosis, prevention, or treatment of inguinal hernia.

INTERNAL OBLIQUE MUSCLE. The internal oblique muscle is the central and most muscular layer of the abdominal wall. It originates from the lateral half of the inguinal ligament and the iliac fascia, from the anterior two thirds of the middle lip of the iliac crest, and from the lower portion of the lumbar aponeurosis near the crest. The aponeurosis of this muscle proceeds medially to fuse with the aponeurosis of the transversus abdominis muscle to form the anterior and, in the upper abdomen, posterior rectus sheaths. The fused aponeuroses then proceed medially to insert into the linea alba as the rectus sheath. The lowermost portion of the internal oblique, below the semilunar line of Douglas, contributes only to the anterior rectus sheath. In that area, it fuses with the transversus abdominis aponeurosis to form the sheath, but in only 5 per cent of individuals does it fuse laterally to the sheath to form a "conjoined tendon." That anatomic structure is more a rarity than a constant finding, and its description should be deleted from the hernia literature.

Inferiorly and laterally, the internal oblique originates from the inguinal ligament and the iliac crest and from deeper structures derived from the transversalis fascia. The medial margin of this insertion forms an arch over the internal inguinal ring. From this point, fibers of the muscle arch downward and envelop the spermatic cord as it issues from the internal ring (Fig. 4). These fibers form the cremaster muscle. This muscle is important in hernia repair only in that it should be completely removed to expose the internal ring.

TRANSVERSUS ABDOMINIS. This is the most internal of the three flat muscles of the abdominal wall. It rises by fleshy fibers from the lateral portion of the iliopubic tract, from the inner lip of the iliac crest, the lumbodorsal fascia, and from the inner surfaces of the cartilages of the lower six ribs. It passes medially in a transverse manner around the lateral aspect of the abdomen onto the anterior abdominal wall. At a point lateral to the rectus sheath, its muscular fibers are replaced by a tendinous aponeurosis, which fuses with the internal oblique aponeurosis to form the rectus sheath. The lower free margin of this muscle arches with the internal oblique from the lateral origin of that muscle over the internal inguinal ring to form a free edge over the ring and above the floor of the inguinal canal medial to the ring (Fig. 5). This arch, termed the *transversus abdominis aponeurotic arch*, occasionally fuses with the arch of the internal oblique aponeurosis to form a "conjoined tendon" or falx inguinalis, but only in 5 per cent of cases. The common finding is that the transversus aponeurosis joins the internal oblique at the rectus sheath. The arch forms the upper margin of the area through which inguinal hernias of all types protrude. The arch itself forms a basic component of the anatomic repair of all inguinal hernias.

ENDOABDOMINAL FASCIA. The endoabdominal or transversalis fascia is an important layer in the prevention of groin and other abdominal wall hernias. This fascial layer forms a bag that holds the abdominal viscera within, and separates them from, the muscular and bony layers of the abdomen without. Various portions of the bag are known by different names, depending on the external structure at that point. Thus, the endoabdominal fascia underlying the transversus abdominis muscle and its aponeurosis is known as the transversalis fascia.

HESSELBACH'S TRIANGLE. This classic anatomic designation is given to the area bounded superiorly by the falx inguinalis, laterally by the inferior epigastric vessels, and inferiorly by the inguinal ligament. As is already clear, the designation is confusing, because none of the three borders of the triangle is in the same layer of the abdominal wall. The inguinal ligament is

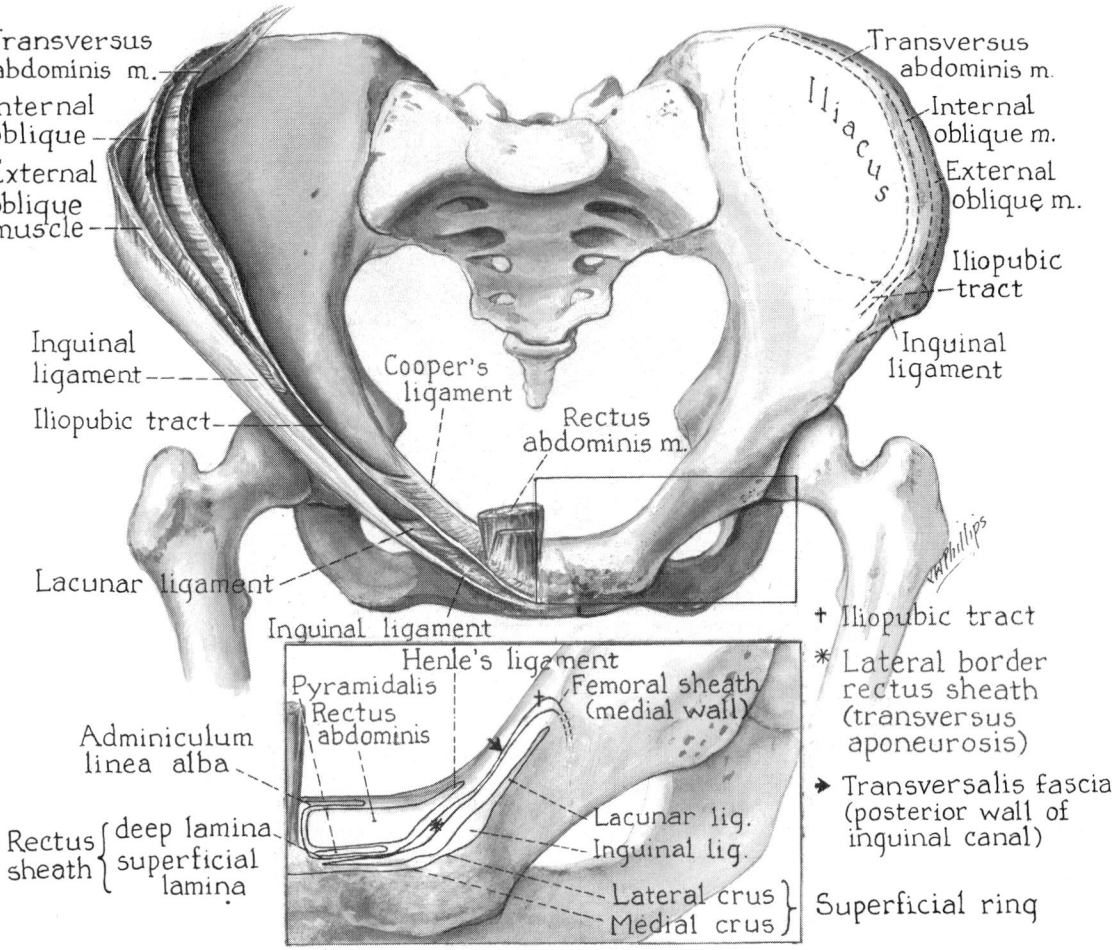

Figure 2. The skeletal origins of the three flat muscles are indicated in the main illustration. The origins of the internal oblique and transversus abdominis muscles are not only from the crest of the ilium but also partly from iliacus fascia and the iliopectinal arch (not shown). The complex insertions of the muscle layers of the groin into the body and superior ramus of the pubis are depicted in the inset (left side). The inferior portions of each of the three muscles of the groin have been preserved in this dissection to illustrate the relationships between these layers. The drawing shows well the relationship between the femoral sheath and canal (removed) and the insertions of the iliopubic tract and lacunar ligament. The internal oblique muscle arches above the spermatic cord and across the groin to insert into the deep lamina of the rectus sheath, usually somewhat superior to the line of transection depicted here. (From Condon, R. E.: The anatomy of the inguinal region and its relation to groin hernia. *In* Nyhus, L. M., and Condon, R. E.: Hernia, 3rd ed. Philadelphia, J. B. Lippincott Company, 1989.)

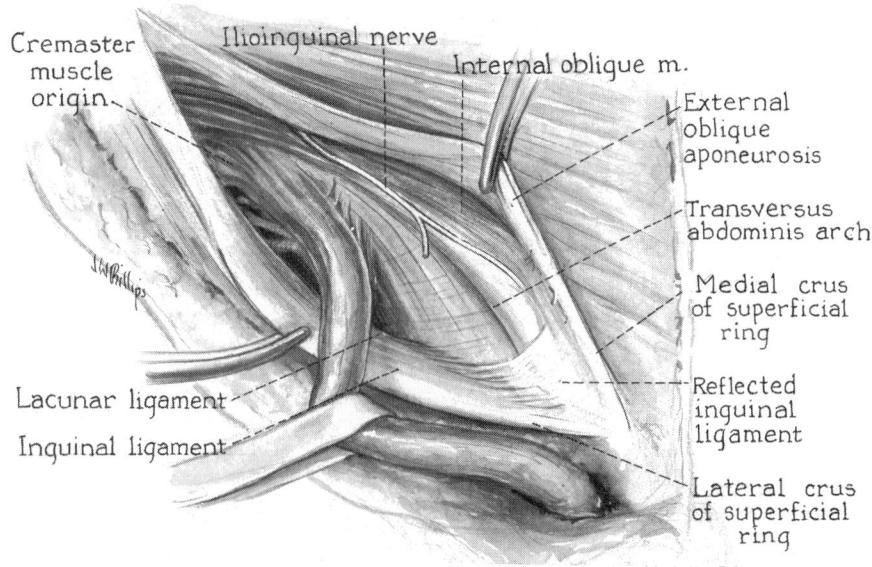

Figure 3. Dissection of the inguinal canal. The external oblique aponeurosis has been opened widely and the spermatic cord mobilized by transection of many of its areolar (cremasteric fascia) attachments to the walls of the inguinal canal. (From Condon, R. E.: The anatomy of the inguinal region. *In* Nyhus, L.M., and Harkins, H. N. (Eds.): Hernia. Philadelphia, J. B. Lippincott Company, 1964.)

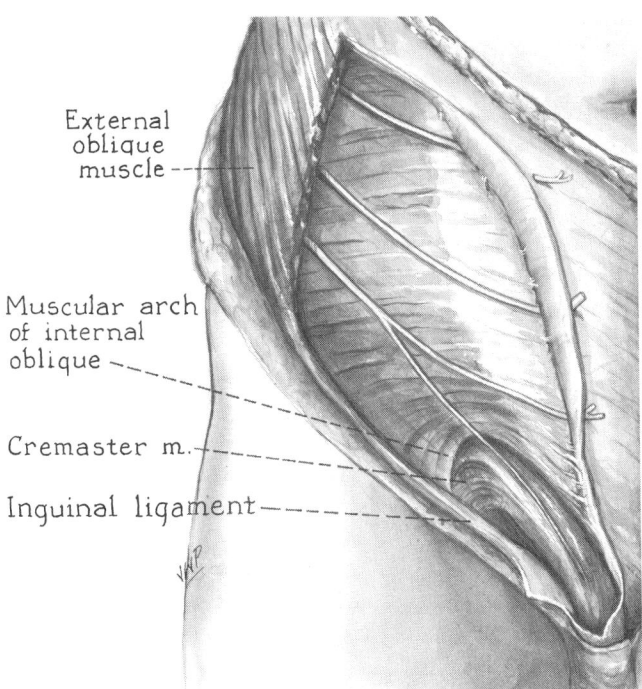

External
oblique
muscle ---

Muscular arch
of internal
oblique ~~

Cremaster m.-

Inguinal ligament ------

Figure 4. Deeper dissection of the groin (right side) to show the internal oblique muscle layer. The spermatic cord has been left *in situ*. (From Condon, R. E.: The anatomy of the inguinal region. *In* Nyhus, L. M., and Harkins, H. N. (Eds.): Hernia. Philadelphia, J. B. Lippincott Company, 1964.)

superficial to the falx inguinalis (when one exists), and both layers are superficial to the inferior epigastric vessels. Use of this term in the description of hernia repair should be abandoned. More correctly, the boundaries of the floor of the inguinal canal, which is what Hesselbach intended to describe, should be limited to structures within that floor. These comprise the transver-

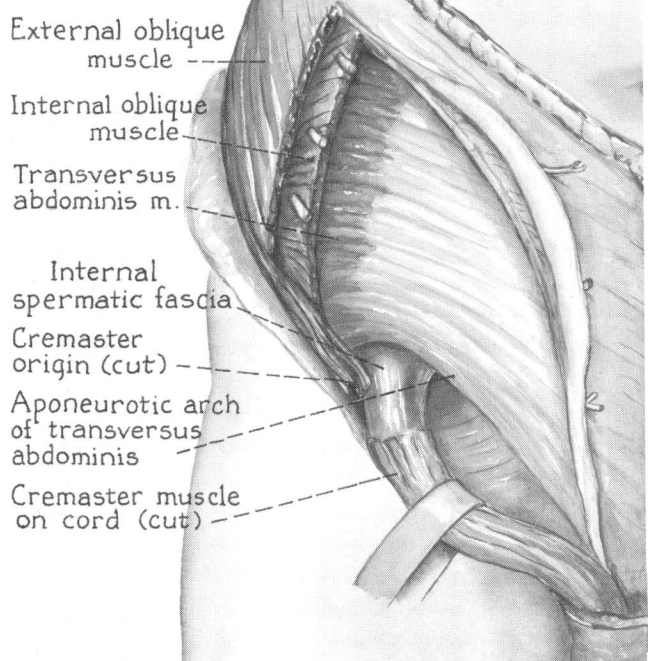

External oblique
muscle ---

Internal oblique
muscle --

Transversus
abdominis m. --

Internal
spermatic fascia

Cremaster
origin (cut) ---

Aponeurotic arch
of transversus
abdominis ---

Cremaster muscle
on cord (cut) ---

Figure 5. Dissection to show the deepest of the three muscle layers of the groin. The spermatic cord has been mobilized to show the arching muscular and aponeurotic lower margin of the transversus abdominis (the transversus abdominis arch). Inferior to this arch, the posterior wall of the inguinal canal is formed by transversalis fascia. (From Condon, R. E.: The anatomy of the inguinal region. *In* Nyhus, L. M., and Harkins, H. N. (Eds.): Hernia, Philadelphia, J. B. Lippincott Company, 1964.)

salis fascia and its analogs. For a complete understanding of these structures, the most important of the groin structures in hernia surgery, the reader is referred to classic works by Condon[16] and by Anson, Morgan, and McVay.[7] A full understanding of the anatomy and physiology of this layer is basic to a successful treatment of groin hernia.

TRANSVERSALIS FASCIA ANALOGS. In several locations in the endoabdominal fascial sac there exist thickenings or condensations of the fascia, which are continuous with and integral to the sac itself. These condensations, termed *transversalis fascial analogs*, are usually formed at points of insertion of various muscle groups, or at points of attachment at other fascial or aponeurotic structures into the fascial sac itself. Four important fascial analogs are the transversalis fascial sling, the transversus abdominis aponeurotic arch, the iliopubic tract, and the iliopectineal ligament (Cooper's ligament).

TRANSVERSALIS FASCIAL SLING. The transversalis fascial sling reinforces the medial margin of the internal inguinal ring. The internal ring itself is the site of exit of the spermatic cord from the abdominal cavity. It is located midway between the anterior superior iliac spine and the pubic tubercle and is 2 cm. above the inguinal ligament. As the cord exits through the ring, it turns medially and inferiorly to traverse the inguinal canal. As it perforates the transversalis fascia at the internal ring, it carries a prolongation of the transversalis fascia, the internal spermatic fascia. Because of the abrupt inferomedial turn the cord structures take, this tubular projection of fascia is bent inferomedially, forming a fold at its lower medial margin. This fold forms a slinglike thickened condensation in the transversalis fascia at the medial and inferior margin of the ring.

TRANSVERSUS ABDOMINIS APONEUROTIC ARCH. The transversus abdominis aponeurotic arch has already been mentioned. It forms the superior border of the floor of the inguinal canal and consists of the fused aponeurosis of the transversus abdominis with the transversalis fascia.

ILIOPUBIC TRACT. The iliopubic tract is another fascial condensation wholly intergral to the endoabdominal fascial sac. It arises from the iliopectineal arch, which is a fibrous condensation of endoabdominal fascia, spanning the iliopsoas muscle as it exits from the pelvis. Via this arch, the tract gains insertion on the anterior superior iliac spine and inner lip of the wing of the ilium. From its insertion, it extends inferomedially above and slightly behind the inguinal ligament. Immediately after its origin, it arches over the femoral vessels, forming the anterior portion of the femoral sheath. It then fans out to insert along the superior border of the pubic ramus and the pubic tubercle and into the body of the pubis. Its lateral recurved portion, that is, the portion that curves down to the pubic ramus immediately after the ligament passes over the femoral vessels, forms the medial boundary of the femoral canal. It is this fanlike recurved portion and not the lacunar ligament, which is external to it, that ordinarily closes the femoral canal.

COOPER'S LIGAMENT. On the posterior aspect of the superior ramus of the pubis and extending posterolaterly from it along the rim of the true pelvis is the iliopectineal line. Periosteum of the pelvis along the line is intimately fused with another condensation of the transversalis fascia and iliopubic tract to form Cooper's ligament. It is anatomically constant and always strong in character.

PREPERITONEAL SPACE AND PREPERITONEAL FAT. Between the transversalis fascia and peritoneum is the preperitoneal space, which is loosely filled with fat and fibrous tissue and is the internal analog of the abdominal panniculus without. It varies in thickness and density with the body habitus of the individual and may in the extremely thin person represent only a potential space.

PERITONEUM. Deep to the preperitoneal space and forming its innermost boundary is the peritoneum. In the groin, as elsewhere, the peritoneum is a thin elastic membrane that serves only to provide a lubricating surface for its contained viscera. Because of the elastic character of the peritoneum, it does not act in the prevention of hernia.

SPERMATIC CORD. The spermatic cord is formed at the internal ring by the confluence of the vas deferens from the testis and the spermatic artery and veins, which descend into the ring to the testis. In men and boys with normal anatomy, these structures are also joined by a slip of fibrous tissue, the ligamentum vaginale, which is the remnant of the processus vaginalis of the peritoneum. At the ring the testicular vein is formed by the confluence of the pampiniform plexus of veins, which provides venous drainage of the spermatic cord and testis. As these structures exit through the deeper layers of the abdominal wall, they pursue an oblique downward course for 5 to 7 cm. into the scrotum, through the inguinal canal.

As the cord structures pass through the internal ring, transversalis fascia is reflected onto the cord as the internal spermatic fascia. The internal oblique muscle then contributes muscular fibers, which invest the cord as the cremaster muscle. The cremaster-covered cord then proceeds downward toward the pubic tubercle and the external inguinal ring. As it passes through the external ring, the investing fascia of the external oblique aponeurosis, Gallaudet's fascia,[26] is reflected onto the cord, covering the remaining slips of the cremaster muscle as the external spermatic fascia. The cord then enters the scrotum.

FEMORAL CANAL. This space, the femoral canal, is ordinarily closed by the reflected fibers of the iliopubic tract as they swing around the external iliac vein to attach to Cooper's ligament. It is a common misconception that the medial boundary of this canal is formed by the recurved fibers of the inguinal ligament. Those fibers, and indeed that entire fascial layer, are within the superficial stratum of the abdominal wall. The next most superficial layer is the inguinal ligament and its recurrent portion, the lacunar ligament. Thus, a femoral hernia sac protrudes through the internal femoral ring lateral to the recurved portion of the iliopubic tract, across Cooper's ligament, which is posterior to the sac, and beneath the inguinal ligament. It protrudes through the fossa ovalis, which is the defect in the fascia lata left for entrance of the greater saphenous vein. The fossa ovalis is loosely closed with the cribriform fascia, which is a prolongation of the innominate fascia from the abdominal wall.

Physiology of Inguinal Canal Structures

In the normal individual, two mechanisms act to preserve the integrity of the inguinal canal and to prevent protrusion of abdominal contents through the internal ring. The first of these is the sphincter action of the transversus abdominis and internal oblique muscles at the internal ring. The ring is attached to the transversus abdominis muscle via the transversalis fascial sling, which reinforces the medial and inferior margin of the ring. When the transversus abdominis contracts, it pulls the transversalis fascial sling superiorly and laterally. This serves both to close the internal ring around the cord structures and to pull the internal ring superiorly and laterally, under the buttress formed by the internal oblique. For this action to be effected, the transversalis fascia and its structures must be movable beneath the internal and external obliques. Any operative procedure that fixes the transversalis fascia or internal ring to a more superficial fixed structure, such as the inguinal ligament, destroys the sphincter action of the transversus abdominis.

The second mechanism closing the inguinal canal is the shutter action of the transversus abdominis aponeurotic arch, which normally is upwardly convex at rest and is straightened and flattened when the transversus abdominis and internal oblique muscles are tensed. Any tensing action brings the arch in apposition to the inguinal ligament, thereby covering the cord and buttressing the floor of the inguinal canal. It has been postulated that the occurrence of direct inguinal hernia is due primarily to a higher than normal position of this transversus aponeurotic arch, so that when the abdominal musculature is stimulated and the arch brought down, it does not reach the inguinal ligament and iliopubic tract, thereby leaving a weakened area in the floor of the inguinal canal, which is defended only by the transversalis fascia. The incidence of recurrent hernia following various repairs and, indeed, of all direct hernias has been attributed to this "congenital" malformation.

The Biology of Inguinal Herniation

Both indirect and direct inguinal hernias are considered to originate from congenital variants, such as the presence of a preformed sac or processus vaginalis in the former and the failure of the shutter action of the transversus abdominis aponeurotic arch in the latter. The search for other explanations had to await the arrival of sophisticated investigators knowledgeable in the biochemistry of connective tissues. Studies now have been undertaken in these areas.[63,64,84]

The rectus sheath near inguinal hernias in adults was found to be thinner than normal. Indeed, on careful analysis, specimens obtained from patients without hernia weighed more than similar specimens in patients with hernia. This decrease in actual weight of the specimens from patients with hernia was found to correlate with a decrease in hydroxyproline and thus collagen content. Fibroblasts were cultured from the anterior rectus sheath of patients with and without hernia. The rate of cell proliferation was less by a factor of 50 per cent in patients with herniation. Other studies were performed, and all results appeared to indicate a reduced collagen synthesis as part of the etiologic process in development of herniation in the adult. Peacock[61] has made a strong plea for further studies to elucidate both sides of the collagen equation, i.e., synthesis versus degradation. These are important and refreshing approaches to the study of inguinal hernia.

DIAGNOSIS, INCIDENCE, AND PROGNOSIS

DIAGNOSIS. Diagnosis of hernia is made usually on the basis of physical examination, rather than history. In children, however, the mother's insistence on having observed a lump in the groin should alert the examiner to the presence of a groin hernia even if the first examination is negative. Similarly, chronic use of a truss may cause such a degree of scarring that the hernial sac does not readily fill with bowel. A negative examination in this setting should be followed after several days by success if the truss is not used in the interim. A dragging sensation or pain in the groin suggest the presence of a hernia. Minor pain is common at the outset; but in time, sensations in the area become those of only vague discomfort.

Examination of the groin is best accomplished with the examiner seated on a low chair before the standing patient. The examination consists of the following: (1) observation of the groin area for evidence of a bulge or swelling while the patient coughs or tenses the abdominal musculature, preferably while holding a deep breath; (2) repetition of the preceding step with the index finger invaginated into the external ring for palpation of bulges or significant pressure impulses against the examining finger (note that an enlarged external ring without a palpable mass or impulse does not connote the presence of a hernia); and (3) repetition of steps 1 and 2 while the patient is lying down. Formerly it was considered important to differentiate preoperatively between direct and indirect hernias during examination, but this appears less important now when surgeons are able to make an accurate diagnosis and perform an appropriate technical procedure at operation. Femoral hernias must be differentiated from inguinal hernias during the examination because a different operative approach is indicated. The common error is to overlook a femoral hernia. If, on accurate palpation, the swelling protrudes below the inguinal ligament, it is femoral; if above, it is inguinal. A number of other "lumps and bumps" appear in the groin which must be differentiated from hernial expansion. These include (1) inguinal adenitis, (2) ectopic testis, (3) hydrocele of the cord, (4) psoas abscess, (5) femoral adenitis, and (6) saphenous varix.

INCIDENCE. The accurate incidence of hernias is difficult to obtain. Statistics available are those from the 1960 survey of the United States Department of Health, Education and Welfare,[80] which found that hernia occurred in approximately 15 per 1000 of the population interviewed, i.e., 3 million Americans. The same government agency found that 40 million days of restricted activity per year could be attributed to this problem. Each individual with a hernia averaged almost 16 days of restricted activity as a result of the condition. More important, the total amount of work loss by the populace with hernias was 10 million days, a figure that reflects the prevalence of hernias in the male population. The economic aspects of the hernial problem are further revealed by the National Center for Health Statistics study of 1980.[81] In one year, 537,000 hernial repairs were performed. Most of those operations were performed on inpatients. In 1990, more than half of these hernial operations are predicted to be performed on outpatients. Simple excisions and biopsies were the only nongynecologic operative procedures performed with greater frequency.

Approximately 50 per cent of all hernias are indirect inguinal and 25 per cent are direct inguinal. Incisional and ventral abdominal hernias represent approximately 10 per cent, followed by femoral, 6 per cent; umbilical, 3 per cent; esophageal hiatal, 1 per cent; and miscellaneous rarer types, 2 per cent. The total balance favors groin hernias, approximately 75 per cent. Parenthetically, it should be noted that 86 per cent of all groin hernias occur in males; yet, 84 per cent of all femoral hernias occur in females. It must be emphasized, however, that the most common groin hernia found in females is the indirect inguinal, and the proportion of femoral hernias in females is high only because of the relatively rare incidence of femoral hernia in males.

PROGNOSIS AFTER TREATMENT. Today, recurrence of a hernia after operative treatment remains a difficult problem. The poorer results are related to many factors, including (1) failure to understand the fine nuances of the surgical anatomy within the groin; (2) failure to use meticulous operative technique for a common hernial repair; and (3) failure to follow all patients operated on so that there is awareness of technical shortcomings.[33] Until this subject is judiciously approached, 100,000 patients annually are at risk for recurrence of what was thought to be a simple problem.

The Danger of Hernia

MORTALITY. Morbidity and economic factors have been discussed. Unfortunately, death rates from this potentially curable entity remain high. A 1964 survey of the Department of Health, Education and Welfare showed that 2030 individuals died from intestinal obstruction due to hernia. A similar report in 1967 listed hernia associated with intestinal obstruction as one of the 10 leading causes of death in the United States.[27] Constantly improving surgical techniques have been shown to decrease this prohibitive rate of mortality.[77]

INCARCERATION, STRANGULATION, AND INTESTINAL OBSTRUCTION. The *sine qua non* of danger is protrusion of a hollow viscus outside its normal environment through a ring of variable size. If the viscus becomes caught by the ring and cannot be replaced, it becomes incarcerated. If, in addition, blood flow to or from the protruding viscus is compromised, the process of strangulation begins, with ultimate necrosis of the bowel if left unattended. Incarcerated hernias are difficult to differentiate from those in which the strangulating process has begun and therefore are considered to be surgical emergencies. Incarcerated hernias may or may not cause intestinal obstruction, but essentially all hernias involving bowel that reach the stage of vascular compromise do cause the signs and symptoms

of intestinal obstruction. There are two exceptions, namely, Richter's hernia — i.e., one side of the bowel wall is involved — and Littre's hernia — i.e., the incarceration and strangulation of a Meckel's diverticulum. In all patients with signs and symptoms of intestinal obstruction, all potential hernia sites must be visualized and palpated, and contrariwise, all patients with incarcerated or strangulated hernia should be carefully reviewed for the presence of intestinal obstruction. Femoral, indirect inguinal, and umbilical hernias are more likely to cause strangulation of bowel because these sacs have smaller necks that tend to be surrounded by rings of rigid tissue. Direct inguinal hernias usually have a broad neck.

Recognition of impending or actual strangulation is extremely important, since emergency measures (operation) are indicated. Pain in the region of the hernial swelling and, particularly, tenderness to palpation are ominous signs. Sudden change from a state of hernial reducibility to irreducibility and discoloration of the tissues over the swelling are additional signs of strangulation.

Without signs of strangulation, an incarcerated hernia of short duration may be carefully reduced by gentle but firm pressure upon the swelling. It is possible to reduce the bowel content from its extracavitary position but not release the bowel from the peritoneal sac, i.e., reduction en masse. Thus, one must observe the patient for a period following reduction to ensure restoration of normal bowel activity.

INGUINAL HERNIAS IN ADULTS

Hernias may be classfied as either funicular or diffuse. The former type protrudes through a tight fibrous ring of some type, almost always at the site of exitus of some structure from the endoabdominal fascial sac. Indirect inguinal hernias, femoral hernias, and umbilical hernias are all funicular. These hernias tend to incarceration, obstruction, and even strangulation because of the tight ring through which the herniating viscera protrudes. In addition to causing the usual symptoms of dragging discomfort at the site of herniation, these hernias are always potentialy disastrous and must be repaired whenever found.

Diffuse hernias, however, lack the tight constricting ring at the site of exitus from the endoabdominal fascial sac. Most ventral hernias, direct inguinal hernias, and lumbar hernias meet this classification.

In the indirect inguinal hernia, the protruding viscus exits from the endoabdominal fascial sac through the internal inguinal ring. The herniating viscus, therefore, always has the same covering as the investments of the spermatic cord and does not actually protrude through any layer of the abdominal wall. By its nature, it always requires a preformed or at least a potential sac, which, in this instance, is the patent processus vaginalis. It is therefore a true congential defect. Depending on the length of the patent processus vaginalis, the indirect inguinal hernia may protrude into the inguinal canal or through the external ring or extend into the scrotum.

INDIRECT HERNIA. The processus vaginalis is the peritoneal tube along which the fetal testis moves from its retroperitoneal origin into the scrotum. This occurs in the seventh to eighth month of gestation. Normally, the processus vaginalis obliterates completely to form a fibrous cord, the ligamentum vaginale, which extends from a dimple on the parietal peritoneum deep to the internal ring down through the inguinal canal into the scrotum to the tunica vaginalis and testis. It may only partially obliterate anywhere along the course of its descent. The various anomalies of obliteration of the processus are frequently associated. An undecended testicle or a testicle in the inguinal canal is always associated with an indirect inguinal hernia. The high association of either testicular or cord hydroceles with inguinal hernias is well known.

Indirect inguinal hernias may be further subdivided with regard to the extent of dilatation of the internal inguinal ring. An infantile or childhood hernia may have a normal or only slightly enlarged internal inguinal ring, with the major defect being only protrusion of bowel into a patent processus vaginalis. It should be emphasized that a simple patent processus vaginalis is not a hernia, but that it possesses a high potential of becoming one.

If the hernia has been present for some time, the internal ring may be enlarged. Such a hernia is frequently found in the young adult. If the ring enlarges sufficiently to begin to push the inferior epigastric vessels medially, a simple adult hernia is present. If the enlargement impinges on the floor of the inguinal canal, a combined indirect-direct hernia is present. Occasionally the ring is dilated sufficiently without displacement of the inferior epigastric vessels to impinge on the floor of the inguinal canal. This condition leads to an outpouching of peritoneum around the inferior epigastric vessels, so that both direct and indirect hernial sacs exist, straddling those vessels. This is the pantaloon hernia.

DIRECT HERNIA. In a direct hernia, the protruding viscus does not herniate through a preformed ring. The transversalis fascia weakens and bulges outward in front of the hernial mass. In the case of the direct inguinal hernia, the weakness in the wall of the sac is in the floor of the inguinal canal medial to the internal inguinal ring and medial to the inferior epigastric vessels. In the past, the location of the inferior epigastric vessels lateral to the hernia has been considered important. In the author's experience, these vessels may be anywhere with regard to the location of the direct hernia and may even be a part of the wall of the hernial sac.

Most recurrent hernias are direct, resulting after the repair of indirect inguinal hernia. A few recurrent hernias are indirect. In every instance, a recurrent indirect hernia is due to failure of the initial operation to remove the patent processus vaginalis (hernial sac) from the cord at the internal ring. As long as a peritoneal outpouching is left through the internal ring, hernia is a threat. The sac may be left in the cord if the sac is divided at the internal ring.

Inguinal Hernia Repair

Currently, controversy exists regarding the proper layers of the abdominal wall to be used for repair of inguinal hernia. On this basis, the types of repair have been divided into the posterior (transversalis fascia lamina) and anterior (external-internal oblique lamina). Proponents of the posterior repair insist that the reconstruction of the inguinal canal and of the internal inguinal ring should be accomplished with preservation of deep groin anatomy. Transversalis fascial structures should be sutured to transversalis fascial structures. Layers normally found superficial to the inguinal canal and its contents should not be used to reinforce the posterior wall of the inguinal canal. This approach is based on the concept that the basic hernial defect lies within the deep structures of the abdominal wall, that is, those deep to the internal oblique, and therefore the repair should reside within those layers.

However, proponents of the anterior type of repair do not make the distinction between superficial and deep layers of the abdominal wall and consequently use superficial structures such as the external oblique aponeurosis and inguinal ligament as either anchoring points or artificial buttresses for repair of the internal ring and floor of the inguinal canal. Surgeons who use the anterior lamina ignore the fact that the superficial stratum of the abdominal wall musculature is movable upon the deep stratum and vice versa. Artificial attachment of the deep layer to the superficial layer leads to strain at the suture line or attachment, and this may be the reason for the high incidence of recurrence with this type of hernia repair. Nonetheless, a large fund of experience has been reported with repairs described by Halsted, Bassini, Andrews, and Ferguson. Rarely, the anatomic layers of

the deep stratum of the abdominal wall may be insufficient to permit repair strictly within that layer, and the more superficial procedures may be required.

A single operative technique is not appropriate in all patients. The approach must be designed at the operating table to properly manage the following variations: (1) small indirect inguinal, (2) medium indirect inguinal, (3) large indirect and direct inguinal, and (4) femoral hernias.

SMALL INDIRECT INGUINAL HERNIA. The basic pathologic feature here is a patent processus vaginalis with minimal dilatation of the internal abdominal ring. After removal of the hernial sac and high ligation of the neck of the sac, restoration of the transversalis fascia surrounding the spermatic cord at the internal ring suffices. Since the hernial sac tends to enlarge the ring medially, the sutures are placed medial to the cord structures. Although this is the simplest of all hernial defects to correct, it is also the most common, and a meticulous anatomic dissection and repair give great satisfaction. Griffith[32] in 1959 described a technique for this repair, an anterior approach to the posterior inguinal wall. Condon[17] also has given a lucid presentation of the anterior approach and use of the transversalis fascia analogs for repair of the internal ring.

MEDIUM INDIRECT INGUINAL HERNIA AND ATTENUATED POSTERIOR INGUINAL FLOOR. Occasionally, the internal ring has expanded (enlarged) further medially, and the posterior inguinal wall appears attenuated. In this instance, the sutures are "walked" from the internal ring closure medially between the aponeurotic arch of transversus abdominis and iliopubic tract until the pecten of the pubis is reached. Thus, in addition to the plastic closure of the internal ring, the posterior inguinal floor has been strengthened. Small direct hernias are managed in the same manner except that dissection of the internal ring is unnecessary.

STANDARD ANTERIOR INGUINAL WALL REPAIRS. It is to the small or medium indirect inguinal hernia that the classic Bassini operation consisting of sutures between the transversus abdominis aponeurotic arch and the lacunar-inguinal ligaments is best suited. The various modifications of Halsted,[34,50] Lucas-Championniére,[50] Andrews,[5] and Ferguson[25] are well known (Figs. 6 and 7). Literally millions of pateints with hernias have been cured by these techniques. Yet an increased risk of recurrence persists (5 to 20 per cent) after the anterior wall repair of all (small and large, direct and indirect) inguinal hernias. If selected for use in repair of small or medium indirect inguinal hernias, this technique should provide satisfactory overall results.

LARGE INDIRECT AND DIRECT INGUINAL HERNIA. These are the most difficult problems. As the indirect hernia enlarges, it breaks down the posterior inguinal wall medial to the internal ring, so that in essence the surgeon must reconstruct the entire posterior inguinal wall and form a new internal inguinal ring. McVay has popularized Cooper's ligament repair for this problem and has reported a 3.6 per cent overall recurrence rate (see Fig. 8).[57]

THE SHOULDICE REPAIR. Shouldice founded a hospital in Toronto, Canada, that treats only patients with hernial defects. He and his colleagues have reported excellent results: a 0.6 per cent recurrence rate after 13,108 primary repairs of inguinal hernias.[29,75] Multiple layers of fascia, including both the posterior and the anterior strata of the inguinal wall, are used in the repair. Good results have been reported by others.[9,86]

FEMORAL HERNIA

By popular usage, femoral hernia has been separated from indirect and direct inguinal hernias because of its exit beneath the inguinal ligament. The authors believe, as do others,[35] that femoral hernia should be considered a third variety of inguinal hernia. Its anatomic boundaries are familiar after study of the posterior inguinal wall: (1) superior—iliopubic tract (anterior

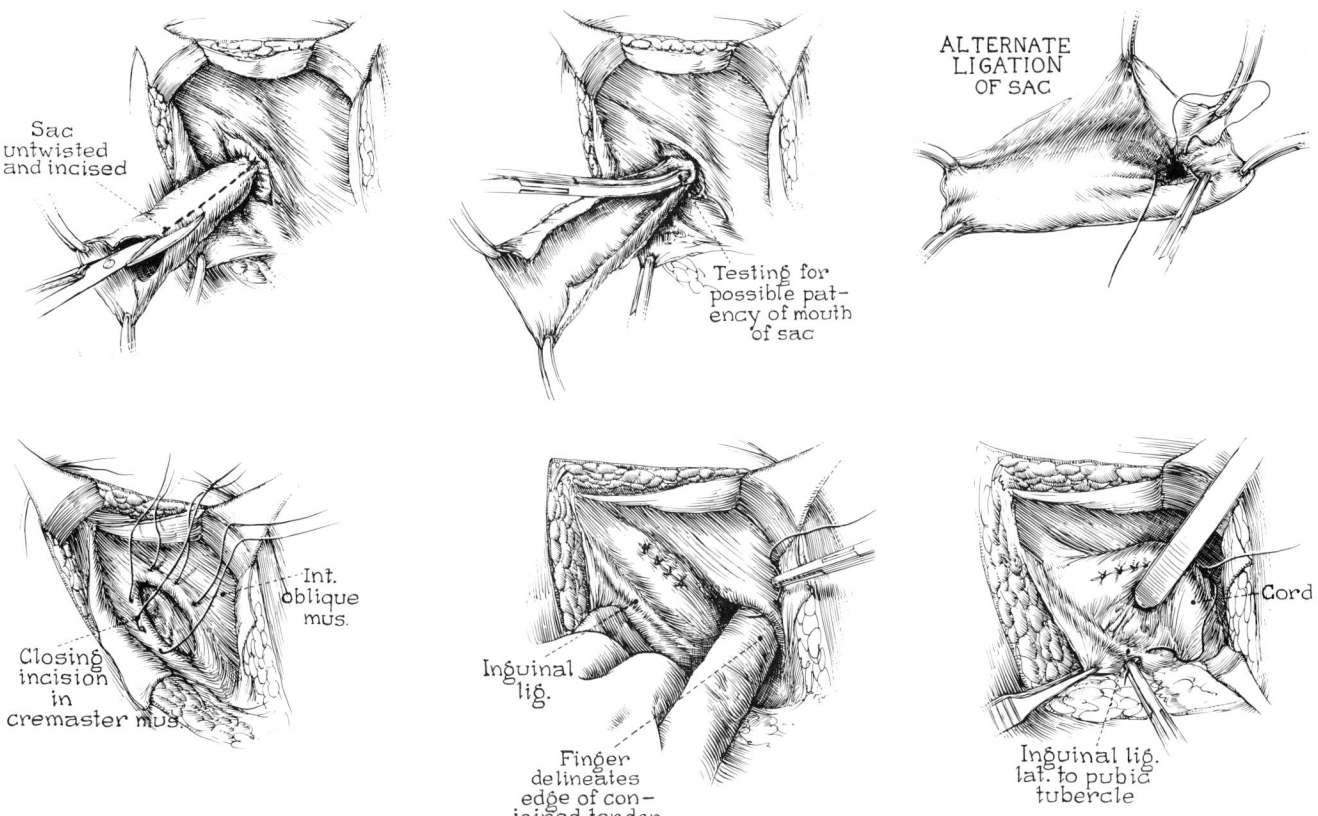

Figure 6. The classic Halsted-Ferguson operation. The anterior approach has reached the stage of high ligation of the periotoneal sac. The arch of the transversus abdominis aponeurosis (frequently called conjoined tendon) is delineated as well as the inguinal ligament. (From Ravitch, M. M.: Repair of Hernias. Copyright © 1969 by Year Book Medical publishers, Inc., Chicago. Used by permission.)

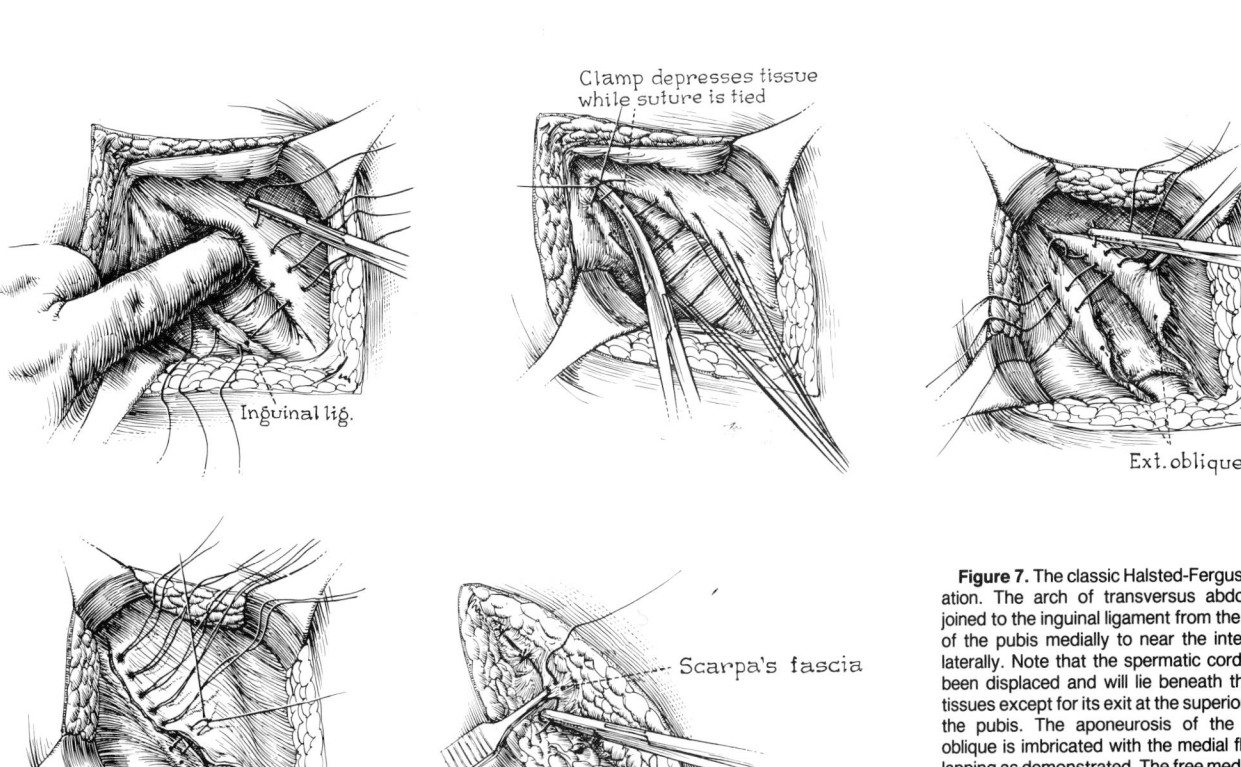

Figure 7. The classic Halsted-Ferguson operation. The arch of transversus abdominis is joined to the inguinal ligament from the tubercle of the pubis medially to near the internal ring laterally. Note that the spermatic cord has not been displaced and will lie beneath the joined tissues except for its exit at the superior edge of the pubis. The aponeurosis of the external oblique is imbricated with the medial flap overlapping as demonstrated. The free medial flap of aponeurotic fascia is then sutured to the lateral flap. (From Ravitch, M. M.: Repair of Hernias. Copyright © 1969 by Year Book Medical Publishers, Inc., Chicago. Used by permission.)

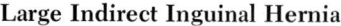

Large Indirect Inguinal Hernia   Direct Inguinal Hernia

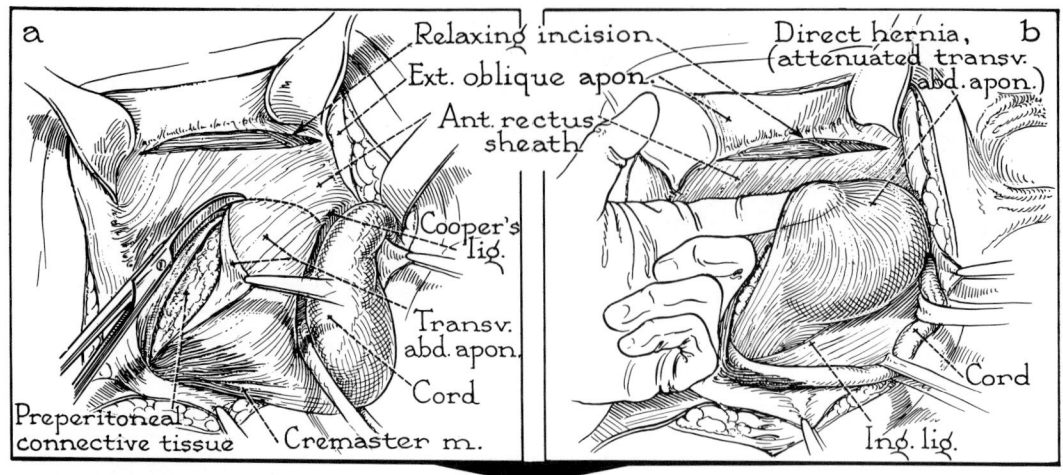

RECONSTRUCTION OF THE POSTERIOR INGUINAL WALL

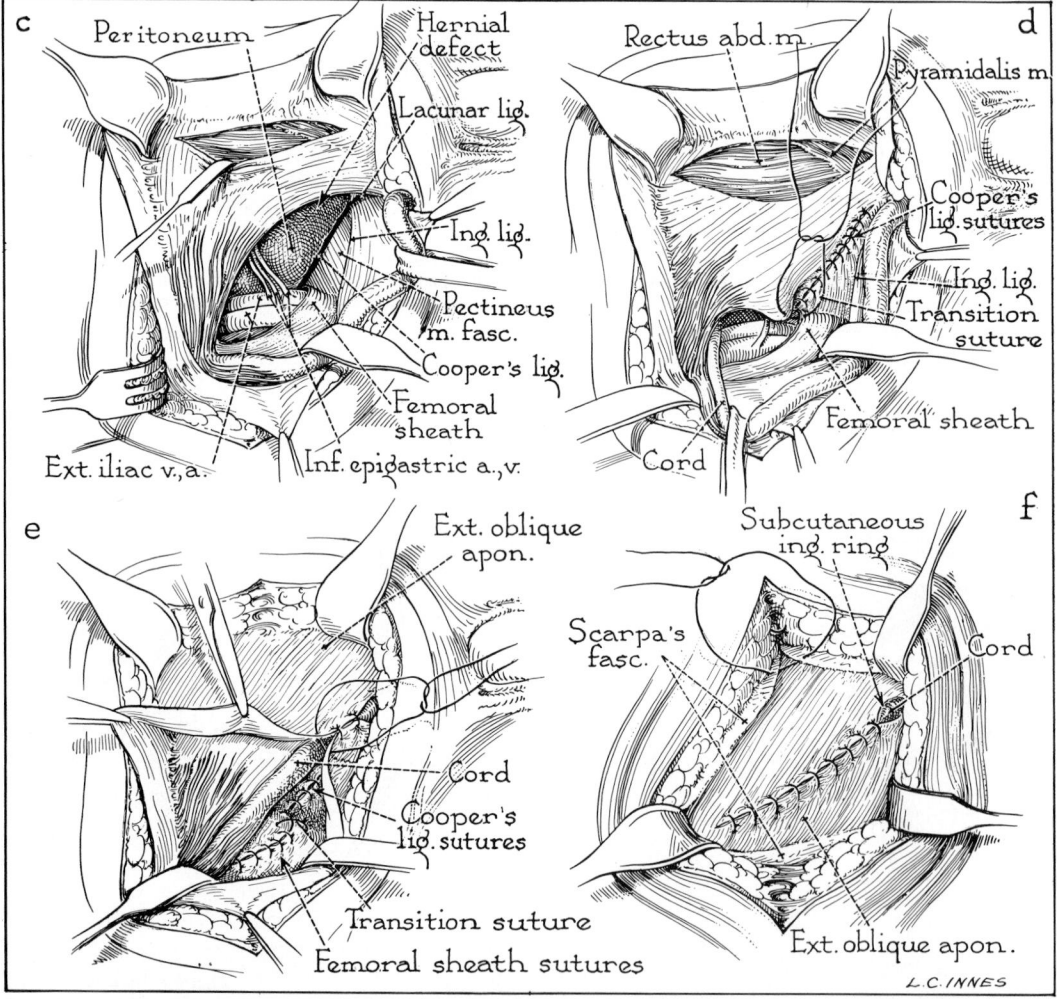

L.C.INNES

Figure 8. Hernioplasty for large indirect inguinal and direct inguinal hernias (reconstruction of the posterior inguinal wall). *a,* Trimming out the attenuated transversus abdominis layer. Not shown is the excision of the hypertrophied fascia and cremaster muscle from the spermatic cord and the excision of the hernial sac. *b,* Trimming out the attenuated posterior inguinal wall in a direct inguinal hernia that consists only of a thin transversalis fascia. The relaxing incision has been made in both *a* and *b. c,* The defect after incision of all attenuated layers as shown in *a* and *b. d,* The reconstruction of the posterior inguinal wall by suturing the strong edge of the transversus abdominis aponeurosis and fused transversalis fascia to Cooper's ligament. Note the "slide" and the widening of the defect in the rectus sheath where the relaxing incision was made. The transition suture has not been tied. *e,* The transversalis fascia has been sutured to the anterior femoral sheath, and the closure of the external oblique aponeurosis over the cord has begun medially. *f,* The completed closure of the external oblique aponeurosis. (From McVay, C. B.: The hernias. *In* Davis, L.: Christopher's Textbook of Surgery, 9th ed. Philadelphia, W. B. Saunders Company, 1968.)

femoral sheath); (2) inferior—Cooper's ligament; (3) lateral—femoral vein; and (4) medial—insertion of iliopubic tract into Cooper's ligament (previously said to be the lacunar ligament).

The McVay Cooper's ligament repair is satisfactory for repair of femoral hernias. Other techniques include the "low approach"[51,85] and the inguinal approach.[6,58,71] There has been a resurgence of interest in the preperitoneal approach, particularly for femoral hernias, during the past decade.[59] For safety, for visualization of anatomic structures, and for ease of performance of ancillary procedures, the posterior or preperitoneal approach to the repair of a femoral hernia is recommended. This approach is unquestionably superior to the direct anterior and subinguinal approaches.

POSTERIOR (PREPERITONEAL) APPROACH TO FEMORAL HERNIA. The skin incision for the preperitoneal approach is different from that used for the anterior approach (Fig. 9). It is oriented horizontally and is placed approximately three fingerbreadths above the pubic tubercle. One third of the incision extends over the rectus muscle and two thirds lateral to it. The edges of the skin incision are retracted, and dissection is carried to the preperitoneal space. With blunt dissection the preperitoneal fat is dissected away from the lower abdominal wall.

The hernial sac can readily be seen protruding into the femoral canal medial to the external iliac vein and just lateral to the reflected fibers of the iliopubic tract and anterior to Cooper's ligament (Fig. 10). The femoral canal is closed by apposition of the iliopubic tract to Cooper's ligament[62] (Fig. 11).

A direct hernia may also be repaired through this approach with excellent results.[61,69] Cooper's ligament repair may be done from the same approach. Cooper's ligament is readily identifiable at the inferomedial aspect of the wound as it proceeds posteriorly from the pubic tubercle along the iliopectineal line. As with the anterior approach, sutures are placed through the transversus abdominis aponeurotic arch and Cooper's ligament in the medial aspect of the repair; a transition suture is placed between the transversus arch, iliopubic tract, and Cooper's ligament; and finally the lateral portion of the repair is completed with sutures through the transversus arch and the iliopubic tract.

When Cooper's ligament repair is performed through the posterior approach, the transversus abdominis aponeurosis is observed to be apposed to Cooper's ligament with a deceptive

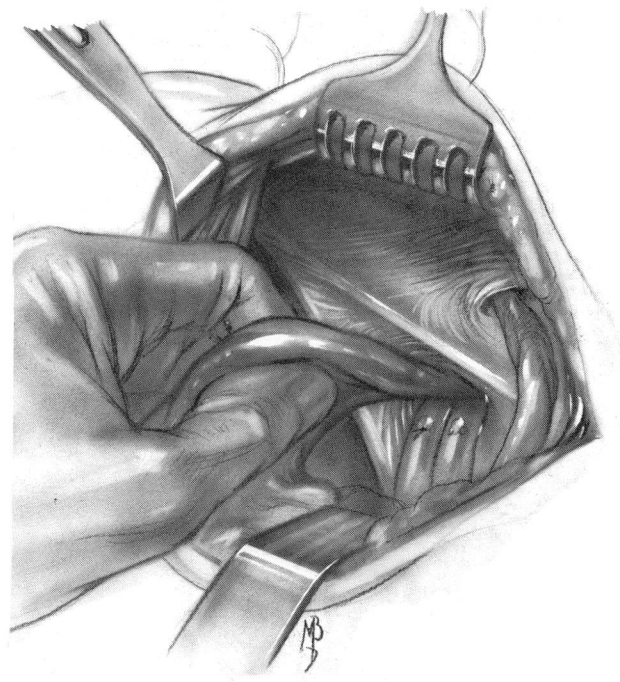

Figure 10. Femoral hernia. The peritoneal sac of the femoral hernia is reduced by traction and blunt dissection. (From Nyhus, L. M.: The preperitoneal approach and iliopubic tract repair of all groin hernias. In Nyhus, L. M., and Harkins, H. N. (Eds.): Hernia. Philadelphia, J. B. Lippincott Company, 1964.)

lack of tension. This lack of tension is due to the incision in the transversus abdominis, which was used for entering the preperitoneal space. When the operative wound in the transversus abdominis is closed at the end of the procedure, tension again is placed on this aponeurosis and therefore upon the suture line. Consequently, a relaxing incision is used to relieve tension on the line of repair.

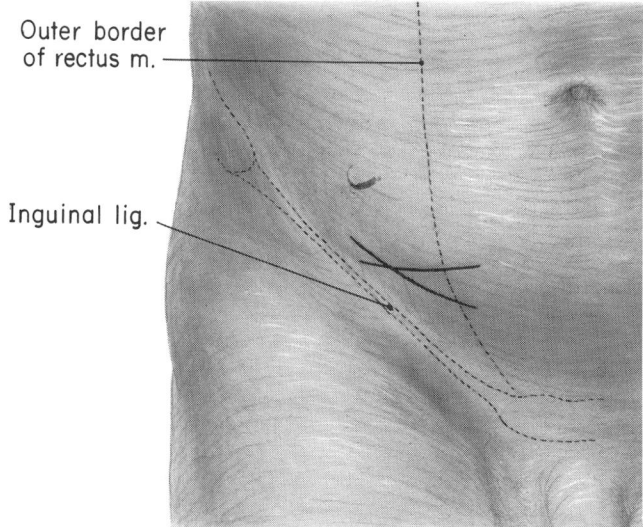

Figure 9. Incisions used in the anterior and preperitoneal approaches. the preperitoneal area is approached through the short, horizontal incision. The direct anterior approach is achieved through the longer incision in the lines of skin tension. (From Nyhus, L. M., and Bombeck, C. T.: The anatomic and physiologic repair of groin hernia. GP, 33:115, 1966.)

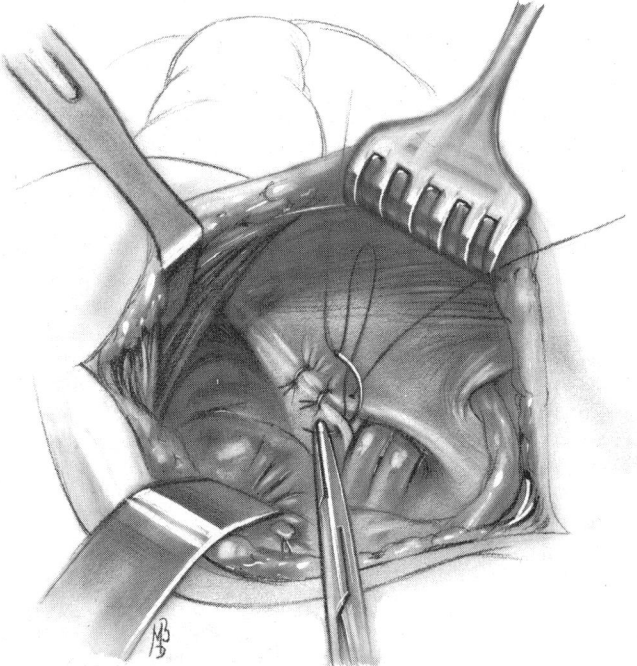

Figure 11. Femoral hernia. The femoral canal is narrowed by sutures placed between the iliopubic tract above and Cooper's ligament below. (From Nyhus, L. M.: The preperitoneal approach and iliopubic tract repair of all groin hernias. In Nyhus, L. M., and Harkins, H. N. (Eds.): Hernia. Philadelphia, J. B. Lippincott Company, 1964.)

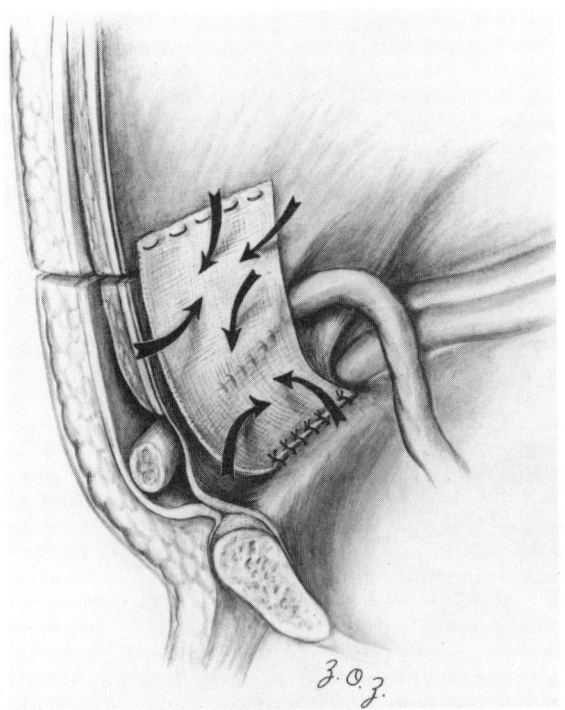

Figure 12. Marlex mesh positioned to buttress repair of a recurrent direct groin hernia as seen from the posterior approach. Arrows depict uniform pressures applied to mesh leading to complete protection of adjacent abdominal wall. (From Nyhus, L. M.: Recurrent groin hernia: Therapeutic solutions. World J. Surg., 13:541, 1989.)

POSTERIOR (PREPERITONEAL) APPROACH FOR RECURRENT GROIN HERNIA. Whereas use of prosthetic materials for primary repair of groin hernias usually is not recommended, the authors hold the opposite position about difficult recurrences. Prosthetic materials used to buttress the hernial repair from the posterior approach have been very effective in preventing further recurrence (Fig. 12).[60]

SPECIAL PROBLEMS, UNUSUAL HERNIAS, AND MISCELLANEA

APPENDECTOMY. In the past it was debatable whether the appendix should be removed during the repair of a right inguinal hernia. A good rule for the experienced surgeon is to do so if the appendix is adequately exposed and the patient can tolerate the procedure. It is unlikely that any harm results from removal of the appendix in an otherwise uncomplicated hernia repair,[23] although most surgeons generally do not perform the procedures simultaneously.

DIVISION OF THE SPERMATIC CORD. Surgical castration, with removal of the testicle on the involved side, division of the spermatic cord at the internal ring, and complete closure of the ring, has been used as a method of treatment of inguinal hernia, particularly in aged men and after multiple recurrent hernias. Prior written permission must be obtained if this is contemplated.

If cord division is planned without removal of the testicle, great care must be exercised in dissection of the cord to prevent embarrassment of the collateral blood supply of the testicle (Fig. 13).

PROSTHETIC MATERIALS. Many artificial aids to hernial repair have been used in past years. These include fascial sutures, fascia lata grafts taken from the thigh, ox fascia, dermal grafts, and all of the various prosthetic meshes such as stainless steel, nylon, tantalum, and Marlex or polypropylene.[28,45] With available methods of repair, these ancillary measures should seldom be required. There is currently more use of prosthetic

materials in repairs of primary hernias; however, because most hernial defects can be repaired satisfactorily without these foreign materials, they should not be used routinely. Nonetheless, should the autogenous tissues be so deficient as to make it impossible to close the defect of a direct inguinal hernia, the newer plastic meshes such as polypropylene can be used. To improve results when the posterior approach to repair recurrent hernias is employed, the authors do add a synthetic mesh buttress[60] (see Fig. 12).

COOPER'S HERNIA. The sac follows the femoral canal, but additional tracts pass into the scrotum, toward the labium majus, and toward the obturator foramen.[2]

HESSELBACH'S HERNIA (EXTERNAL FEMORAL HERNIA). This hernial sac passes into the pelvis lateral to the femoral vessels but below the inguinal ligament and iliopubic tract. It is usually associated with an indirect hernia on the same side.

INCARCERATED AND STRANGULATED HERNIAS. An incarcerated hernia is, by definition, simply an irreducible one. Incarceration of itself would not be a particularly emergent condition were it not for the possible supervention of strangulation of the incarcerated viscus. Strangulation of a hernia is a true surgical emergency and must be treated as soon as the diagnosis is made. The most commonly strangulated groin hernia is the femoral, but because it is an uncommon hernia compared with the inguinal hernia, there are fewer strangulated femoral hernias than there are strangulated inguinal hernias.

The usual vigorous efforts of the surgeon to reduce an incarcerated hernia must be tempered with the awareness of two possible complications. The first of these is "reduction en masse," wherein the hernia, with sac, is reduced within the endoabdominal fascia, so that even though the external bulge is reduced, the hernia remains incarcerated within the sac. Therefore, following reduction of any incarcerated hernia the patient must be carefully observed for signs of continuing intestinal obstruction.

The second possibility is the potentially catastrophic event of reduction of a strangulated, nonviable piece of bowel within the abdominal cavity. At the first sign of strangulation of a hernia, all attempts at reduction must be abandoned and the patient operated upon immediately.

INGUINAL HERNIA IN THE FEMALE. Indirect inguinal hernia does occur in the female, in which case the sac is adher-

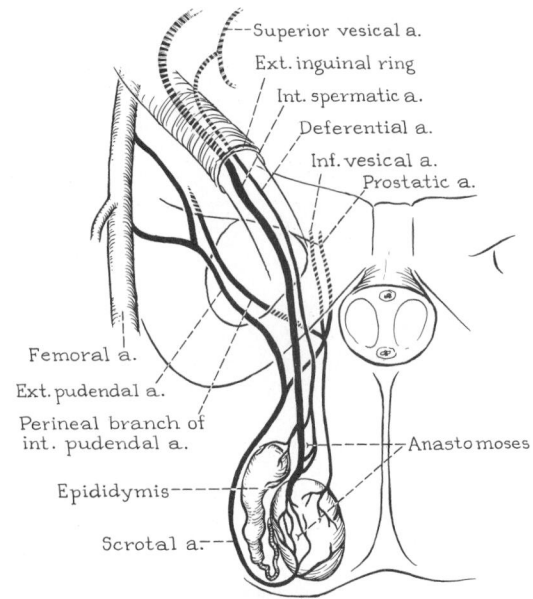

Figure 13. Schematic drawing of both primary and collateral circulation of the testis. (From Nyhus, L. M.: Complications of hernia repair. In Artz, C. P., and Hardy, J. D. (Eds.): Complications in Surgery and Their Management, 2nd ed. Philadelphia, W. B. Saunders Company, 1967.)

ent to the round ligament, since there is no spermatic cord. Because the round ligament serves no useful function, it can be divided at its exit from the internal ring and, following excision of the sac, the entire internal ring can be closed tightly. Inasmuch as no compromise is required to preserve a spermatic cord, recurrent hernia is almost unknown in the female.

INTERPARIETAL AND INTERSTITIAL HERNIAS. These hernias represent a subgroup of inguinal hernia. The sac or sacs, in addition to the normal course, burrow within the abdominal wall, i.e., preperitoneally, where the sac lies between the peritoneum and the transversalis fascia; in the abdominal wall, where the sac lies between the transversalis fascia and the transversus abdominis, internal oblique, and external oblique muscles; or superficially, where the sac lies between the external oblique aponeurosis and the skin.[47,49]

LACUNAR LIGAMENT HERNIA (LAUGIER'S HERNIA OR VELPEAU'S HERNIA). These hernias pass through Gimbernat's ligament. Incision of the ligament may be necessary for reduction of the incarcerated mass.[67]

LIPOMA OF THE CORD. Lobulated preperitoneal fat may project down the cord at the internal ring. Since this fat pad presents as a mass, it may be mistaken for an indirect inguinal hernia. Whenever a lipoma of the cord is identified (usually found at the lateral margin of the cord), it should be excised to prevent confusion as to diagnosis at a later date.

OBTURATOR HERNIA. This hernia passes through the obturator foramen or canal in the os innominatum. It is a "hidden" hernia, and diagnosis is difficult. The diagnosis is suggested by a pain that passes down the inner side of the thigh to the knee (Howship-Romberg sign). The thigh adductor reflex may be absent as well. If the hernial sac content is incarcerated or strangulated, a mass may be palpated on rectal examination. These hernias are five times more commonly seen in females than in males. Most of the patients who have this type of hernia are elderly, weak, and often emaciated. Because of the rigid walls of the orifice, strangulation frequently occurs.

The defect may be approached by the abdominal, preperitoneal, inguinal, or obturator route.[83] Tissue surrounding the defect is of poor quality, and it is often necessary to patch the defect with prosthetic material such as Marlex.[70]

PECTINEAL HERNIA (CLOQUET'S HERNIA). This hernia enters the femoral canal and then perforates the aponeurosis of the pectineus muscle. Thus it does not present at the fossa ovalis. This hernia was first described by Callisen[12] and later in more detail by Cloquet.[15]

PERINEAL HERNIA. Defects occur in the muscle floor of the pelvis through which peritoneal sacs project. Fortunately these hernias are usually reducible, and strangulation seldom occurs. There are three types: (1) The anterior type, which protrudes anterior to the transverse perinei muscles and begins as a defect in the levator ani, usually contains bladder and is found most often in females. (2) The posterior type, which is similar to the anterior type but protrudes posteriorly in the levator ani or between this muscle and the coccyx, contains ileum and is also most commonly found in females. (3) Complete rectal prolapse may be approached by the abdominal and perineal routes or by both routes synchronously.[30,46]

PREVASCULAR HERNIA. Prevascular hernias are found within the femoral sheath but anterior to the femoral vessels. They are rare and may be treated by either Cooper's ligament or the iliopubic tract repair.[11,79]

RETROVASCULAR HERNIA (SERAFINI'S HERNIA). Retrovascular hernias pass within the femoral sheath but exit posterior to the femoral vessels.[74]

SCIATIC HERNIA. The rarest of all hernias, a sciatic hernia makes its exit through the greater or lesser sacrosciatic foramen. The mass presents below the fold in the buttock. It may be approached by the abdominal or sciatic route, but occasionally a synchronous technique is favorable.

SLIDING INGUINAL HERNIAS. Occasionally the cecum on the right or the sigmoid colon on the left makes up a portion of the sac wall in an indirect inguinal hernia. In that instance, special care must be exercised to avoid opening the intestine or devascularizing it when managing the sac. For this reason, since it is difficult to determine whether a sliding hernia is present until the hernial sac is opened, the sac of an indirect hernia is always opened at its anterior medial aspect. The hernia itself is caused by failure of fusion of the two leaves of peritoneum as they cover the colon; these leaves are allowed to evert around the colon as it protrudes into a hernial sac. When the sac has been inverted, the repair is done as for any other indirect inguinal hernia. In women, especially girls and infants, the sliding hernia may also contain portions of the female genital tract, but these are managed in the same manner as the colon, by imbrication of the peritoneal sac behind the protruding structure.

SUPRAVESICAL HERNIA. This is another rare hernia, first described by Sir Astley Cooper. Keynes[42] has cataloged the types and treatment extensively.

ABDOMINAL WALL HERNIA

Abdominal wall hernia may be defined as any protrusion of the abdominal viscera through the endoabdominal fascial sac. Examples are umbilical, epigastric, lumbar (both superior and inferior), spigelian, and ventral incisional hernia.

UMBILICAL HERNIA. Umbilical hernia is a true congential defect, occurring through the patent umbilical ring following obliteration of the umbilical vessels after delivery. It is considerably more common in black infants than in white, but the reason for this difference is not clear. True umbilical hernia is to be distinguished from omphalocele, which is due to failure of abdominal wall closure in the midline around the umbilicus in early intrauterine life.

The hernia is present in 10 per cent of white infants and in 40 to 90 per cent of black infants. In almost all of these, the patent umbilical ring closes spontaneously by the age of 2 years. Opinion is currently divided as to whether any umbilical hernia in a child ever requires operation except for urgent indication. Some surgeons advise only observation of the hernia until the child is 2 years old, and then surgical correction should a defect greater than 1 cm. persist. Other authors, on the basis of a large series of patients observed for many years, recommend no operation at all on the assumption that all umbilical hernias eventually close.[43]

Incarceration and strangulation of umbilical hernias, although rare, do occur. Rupture of an umbilical hernia may also occur, especially in cases of blunt abdominal trauma. In these instances, the hernia is managed in the same way as any strangulated hernia or any external rupture of the abdominal viscera.

In contrast to infantile umbilical hernia, umbilical hernia in the adult must always be treated with the same dispatch used for the treatment of an inguinal hernia because it is known to be liable to incarceration or strangulation, or both. Spontaneous or traumatic rupture of umbilical hernia in pregnancy or in cirrhosis with ascites is not uncommon. The concept that surgical repair of an umbilical hernia in the cirrhotic patient may precipitate variceal hemorrhage is disputed.[65]

THE REPAIR. The classic repair for umbilical hernia is that proposed by Mayo[55] in 1907, the "pants-over-vest" method. Farris[24] has proposed that the Mayo repair for umbilical hernia may not be necessary. On the basis of both experimental and human operative experience, he has advocated a simple transverse closure of the defect with good result.

The poor results with umbilical hernia repair prior to the use of the Mayo operation were probably due to the poor surgical technique and unsuitable suture material that characterized the period. With advances in surgical technique, better suture material, and better anesthesia, simple closure of the defect, whether in the transverse or vertical plane, has become the treatment of choice.

Recurrence of an umbilical hernia is rare, and only isolated reports have appeared in the literature. Should hernia recurrence become a problem in any individual patient, owing to the size of the umbilical hernia, a prosthetic mesh repair may be required.

EPIGASTRIC HERNIA. All hernias occurring in the midline of the abdomen, with the exception of those of the umbilicus, are collectively referred to as hernias of the linea alba. These hernias are far more common above the umbilicus than below and are termed epigastric hernias. They are much more common than is generally realized, occurring in approximately 5 per cent of the general population at autopsy. Most are small and asymptomatic and therefore undiagnosed.

It may be difficult to diagnose a small epigastric hernia consisting only of a tag of omentum herniated through the linea alba. The presence of unexplained upper abdominal symptoms, especially in the obese patient, which are aggravated when the patient reclines on his back, should lead one to suspect this diagnosis. This latter finding, pain on reclining, is thought to be due to traction on the incarcerated tissue.

Pain in the linea alba is also a common presenting finding in other upper abdominal disease. Therefore, a thorough survey for intra-abdominal disease must be done before epigastric hernia is incriminated. The diagnosis is easily made by palpation of a small subcutaneous mass in the linea alba.

Current accepted treatment of epigastric hernia is simple closure of the defect. These hernias are frequently multiple, and a wide exposure of the linea alba through a vertical midline skin incision is indicated.

VENTRAL (INCISIONAL) HERNIA. Incisional hernia is the one true iatrogenic hernia. Principles of treatment of incisional hernia should therefore begin with principles of proper wound closure. The most common cause of incisional hernia is wound infection, and this should be borne in mind during closure of possibly contaminated wounds. Proper principles of wound closure are considered elsewhere in this volume.

Transverse incisions are associated with a significantly lower incidence of wound disruption and incisional hernia than are vertical incisions. Nonetheless, vertical incisions continue to be used for operations on the alimentary tract when transverse incisions would suffice. The anatomic reason for the superiority of transverse incisions is simple. All strata of the abdominal wall, except the rectus abdominis muscle, are collections of fibers, either muscular or fascial, that are oriented in a horizontal direction. The tension exerted by the muscular layers of the abdominal wall is directed horizontally. Vertical incisions are therefore always placed across the lines of force exerted by the abdominal musculature and are always closed under tension. In transverse incisions, tension exerted by the abdominal musculature tends more to appose the edges of the incision than to disrupt them.

More than with any other hernia of the abdominal wall, obesity has a role in recurrence after ventral hernia repair. Extreme obesity may be regarded as a contraindication to the repair of any incisional hernia, except in the emergent situation.

Incisional hernias, if small, are subject to the same complications as funicular hernias in any other area of the body. They are usually large and diffuse, however. Because of the trauma that has occurred at the operative site, incarceration is relatively common in these hernias, but since they are diffuse, strangulation is rare. One dreaded complication is spontaneous rupture of an incisional hernia with evisceration. Because of the relative fragility of the overlying scar in the superficial layer covering the hernia, this complication is relatively more common with this type of hernia than it is with others.

The treatment of incisional hernia is simple closure of the defect, but this may require a complicated procedure. An incisional hernia is always due to separation of the suture line origi-

nally used to close the operative wound. Frequently, the same factors that caused the suture line separation and herniation originally are still operable when a second suture line is placed at the same site. Moreover, each time a wound disrupts the defect, it grows larger and more difficult to close. This is especially true of hernias that have occurred through vertical incisions. The surgeon is frequently faced with an ovoid, ever-widening defect that is oriented vertically and must be closed under tension.

As might be expected because of the difficult nature of the defect, the absence of suitable contiguous tissues to be used in the repair, and the consequent high recurrence rate, the number of operative procedures proposed for the correction of incisional hernia is high. Prosthetic meshes, autogenous or heterologous fascia, and special suture techniques were first devised for repair of these hernias.[82]

Preoperative treatment of the patient includes correction of any nutritional or metabolic deficits that may be present to contribute to recurrence of the hernia, reduction of weight if the patient is obese, and finally treatment of ancillary systemic conditions that, through augmentation of intra-abdominal pressure, may contribute to recurrence. Some measures to increase intra-abdominal volume may also be necessary in patients with chronic pulmonary dysfunction. Progressive pneumoperitoneum has proved to be very effective.[31] Reinsertion of abdominal content that has been within the hernial sac for an indeterminate length of time may severely limit diaphragmatic excursion in these patients, and possibly lead to severe embarrassment of pulmonary function. Very large incisional hernias may contribute to pulmonary dysfunction by compromise of the efficiency of the cough mechanism in patients with chronic bronchitis and emphysema. Under these circumstances, repair of the hernia is indicated because of respiratory disease, not despite it.

Incisional hernias are treated by three types of operation, varying as to their complexity. In the first, simple closure, nothing is necessary except simple reapproximation of the edges of the fascial defect at the transversalis fascial level and above. This repair is probably sufficient for hernias occurring through transverse incisions and for other small incisional hernias. Special attention must be paid to the ends of the wound created, for it is here that recurrent herniation is most likely to occur.

For larger incisional hernias and those with gaping fascial defects, two relatively complicated types of operation are used, those using autogenous tissues and those using prosthetic devices.

SPIGELIAN HERNIA. Spigelian hernia, or spontaneous lateral ventral hernia, as it is sometimes termed, may be defined as a protrusion through the spigelian fascia. The spigelian fascia is that area of the transversus abdominis aponeurosis lateral to the edge of the rectus sheath but medial to the spigelian line. The spigelian line is the point of transition of the transversus abdominis muscle to its aponeurotic tendon. The fascia begins at approximately the level of the eighth or ninth costal cartilage and extends downward to the pubic tubercle. It is widest at a point just below the umbilicus in the region of the semilunar line of Douglas. Most spigelian hernias occur at the widest and therefore weakest area of the spigelian fascia, but they have been reported at the lowermost extent of this fascia, wherein they are easily confused with direct inguinal hernia. The distinction is easily made, since a lower spigelian hernia always protrudes through the transversus abdominis aponeurotic arch, whereas a direct hernia protrudes below it. Spigelian hernias, being small, are of the funicular type and have a high incidence of incarceration and strangulation. The diagnosis may be difficult because of the frequent absence of a palpable mass. Spangen has found ultrasonic scanning of the abdominal wall to be of major diagnostic assistance in patients in whom this unusual hernia is suspected.[76]

The treatment is straightforward. A transverse skin incision is made over the defect and carried down through the external oblique aponeurosis, which is opened in the direction of its fibers. The hernial sac is identified, isolated, opened, ligated, and closed in the usual manner. The transversus abdominis aponeurotic defect can usually be closed with a few interrupted nonabsorbable sutures. Wound closure is performed in the usual manner. Cases reported in the literature are too few for assessment of recurrences.

LUMBAR HERNIA (PETIT'S TRIANGLE HERNIA AND GRYNFELTT'S HERNIA). These are also relatively rare hernias, only 250 to 300 cases having been reported in the literature. The more common of the two is superior lumbar hernia, or Grynfeltt's. Probably superseding both of these, however, are incisional hernias following nephrectomy or traumatic hernias of the lumbar region.

The inferior lumbar triangle, or triangle of Petit, is an anatomic area of weakness, bounded posteriorly by the latissimus dorsi, anteriorly by the external oblique, and inferiorly by the iliac crest. The floor is formed by the internal oblique and transversus abdominis muscles. The superior triangle, or triangle of Grynfeltt-Lesshaft, is situated above and anterior to Petit's triangle and is normally covered by the latissimus dorsi and serratus posterior inferior muscle. The boundaries of the triangle are the twelfth rib above, which forms the base, and the anterior border of the internal oblique anteriorly. The floor is ordinarily the quadratus lumborum muscle mass. It is more constant and larger than Petit's triangle, which represents the higher incidence of hernia. Etiologically, hernias through these triangles are either spontaneous or traumatic. Congenital hernias have also been described in this region. The incidence of strangulation is approximately 10 per cent.

Because of the anatomy of these hernias, treatment is difficult. Until the advent of satisfactory mesh repairs, the basic principle of treatment of Petit's triangle hernia was that advocated by Dowd[22] in 1907, which involved closure of the defect by a pedicle flap of tensor fascia lata and gluteus maximus from below the iliac crest, with side-to-side apposition of the external oblique and latissimus dorsi. Repair of the upper triangle is essentially the same, depending on the development of flaps from adjacent structures. The basic principle of repair of all lumbar hernias is initial closure of the transversalis fascial defect.

With the increasing use of mesh prostheses, it appears likely that the treatment of choice is the employment of one of these aids. If the hernia is small, operative repair by suture of the external oblique to the latissimus dorsi, with or without fascia lata reinforcement, has been successful.

In addition to the aforementioned two varieties of lumbar hernia, there have been isolated reports of hernias occurring through congenital defects or eventrations of other portions of the posterior abdominal wall. Most of these are treated by simple closure of the defect, or by pedicle flap or prosthetic closure should the defect be large. The most common posterior hernia is the postnephrectomy incisional hernia. Repair is essentially the same as that for incisional hernia in any location.

SELECTED REFERENCES

Condon, R. E.: Surgical anatomy of the transversus abdominis and transversalis fascia. Ann. Surg., 173:1, 1971.
By reproducing in color a photograph of the posterior inguinal wall, Condon has helped overcome many anatomic misconceptions of groin anatomy. This report provides a succinct but exceptionally clear description of the posterior inguinal wall.

Devlin, H. B.: Management of Abdominal Hernias. London, Butterworths, 1988.
As stated by the author—a neat, practical book on hernia.

Fruchaud, H.: Traitement chirurgical des hernias de l'aine chez l'adulte. Paris, G. Doin et Cie, 1956.

Fruchaud, H.: Anatomie chirurgical des hernies de l'aine. Paris, G. Doin et Cie, 1956.
These two monographs are beautifully illustrated. All interested in this subject should review these fine works.

Glassow, F.: Short-stay surgery (Shouldice technique) for repair of inguinal hernia. Ann. R. Coll. Surg. Engl. 58:133, 1976.
The Shouldice Hospital in Thornhill, Ontario, is unique because the only operations performed there are related to the problem of hernia. Glassow reports his personal 21-year experience with 14,982 consecutive inguinal hernial repairs, with an overall recurrence of 0.6 per cent using the Shouldice method, which includes a multiple-layer closure of continuous stainless steel wire sutures.

Griffith, C. A: Inguinal hernia: An anatomic-surgical correlation. Surg. Clin. North Am., 39:531, 1959.
Crediting Marcy for original work relating to plastic closure of the internal ring, Griffith provides a fine technique for repair of the small indirect hernia in the adult.

Lytle, W. J.: The deep inguinal ring: Development, function, and repair. Br. J. Surg., 57:531, 1970.
The closing mechanism of the internal ring is well described in this short paper. The student of hernial repair should read carefully all the works of Lytle.

Madden, J. L.: Abdominal Wall Hernias: An Atlas of Anatomy and Repair. Philadelphia, W. B. Saunders Company, 1989.
The genius of the late Frank Robinson, illustrator of renown, is highlighted by his illustrations of the works of McVay, Nyhus, Lytle, Usher, and Ponka.

McVay, C. B.: Anson and McVay's Surgical Anatomy, 6th ed. Philadelphia, W. B. Saunders Company, 1984.
This two-volume monograph includes the finest review of hernial anatomy available today. The section on the abdominal wall represents a distillate of over 43 years of active study, both in the anatomy laboratory and at the operating room table.

McVay, C. B., Read, R. C., and Ravitch, M. M.: Inguinal hernia. Curr. Probl. Surg., October 1967.
This monograph provides a tripartite summary of hernial repair today. McVay presents the complete repair of the posterior inguinal wall that he has popularized so successfully. Read reviews the preperitoneal approach, and Ravitch presents the classic Halsted-Ferguson procedure.

Nyhus, L. M. (Ed.): Hernias. Surg. Clin. North Am., 64:183, 1984.
A report of new developments in the field of herniology during the 1970s.

Nyhus, L. M. (Ed.): Progress symposium. Selected topics in hernia. World J. Surg. 13:489, 1989.
Fourteen presentations updating current hernial concepts.

Nyhus, L. M., and Condon, R. E. (Eds.): Hernia, 3rd ed. Philadelphia, J. B. Lippincott Company, 1989.
Details of all facets of hernial problems are presented. A multiauthor text, it contains diverse views as to the appropriate approach to groin hernias. It also includes sections on diaphragmatic hernia and medicolegal problems related to hernia surgery.

Skandalakis, J. E., Gray, S. W., Mansberger, A. R., Jr., Colborn, G. L., and Skandalakis, L. J.: Hernia: Surgical anatomy and technique. New York, McGraw-Hill, 1989.
Anatomic truths are stressed.

Pollak, R., and Nyhus, L. M.: Complications of groin hernia repair. Surg. Clin. North Am., 63:1363, 1983.
A comprehensive review of the pre- and postoperative sequelae of inguinal and other groin hernias.

Ponka, J. L.: Hernias of the Abdominal Wall. Philadelphia, W. B. Saunders Company, 1980.
A personal approach to the subject of hernia.

Usher, F. C.: The repair of incisional and inguinal hernia. Surg. Gynecol. Obstet., 131:525, 1970.
The use of prosthetic material in hernial repair has been largely a result of the work of Usher.

REFERENCES

1. Abel, A. L., and Hunt, A. H.: Stainless steel wire for closing abdominal incisions and for the repair of herniae. Br. Med. J., 2:379, 1948.
2. Aird, I.: A Companion in Surgical Studies, 2nd ed. Baltimore, Williams & Wilkins Company, 1957.
3. Ali, M.: Cutis strip and patch repair of large inguinal hernias. N. Engl. J. Med., 251:932, 1954.
4. Allgower, M.: Sphincter-splitting approach to rectum. Am. J. Surg., 145:5, 1983.
5. Andrews, E. W.: Imbrications or lap joint method: A plastic operation for hernia. Chicago Med. Rec., 9:67, 1895.
6. Annandale, T.: Case in which a reducible oblique and direct inguinal and femoral hernia existed on the same side and were treated by operation. Edinburgh Med. J., 21:1087, 1876.
7. Anson, B. J., Morgan, E. H., and McVay, C. B.: Surgical anatomy of the inguinal region based upon a study of 500 body-halves. Surg. Gynecol. Obstet., 111:707, 1960.
8. Bassini, E.: Nuovo metodo per la cura radicale dell'ernia. Atti Cong. Ass. Med. Ital. (1887), 2:179, 1889.
9. Berliner, S. D.: Adult inguinal hernia: Pathophysiology and repair. Surg. Annual, 15:307, 1983.

10. Black, S.: Sciatic hernia. *In* Nyhus, L. M., and Condon, R. E. (Eds.): Hernia, 3rd ed. Philadelphia, J. B. Lippincott Company, 1989.
11. Burton, C. C.: Inguinopectineal hernias—a classification and correlation. Int. Abstr. Surg., 97:419, 1953.
12. Callisen, H.: Herniorum rariorum biga acta societatis medicae hafniae. Hanniae, 2:321, 1777.
13. Camper, P.: Icones herniarum. Francofurti ad Moenum, Varrentrapp and Wenner, 1801.
14. Clark, J. H., and Hashimoto, E. I.: Utilization of Henle's ligament, iliopubic tract, aponeurosis transversus abdominis and Cooper's ligament in inguinal herniorrhaphy. Surg. Gynecol. Obstet., 82:480, 1946.
15. Cloquet, J.: Recherches anatomiques sur les hernies de l'abdomen. Thèse. Paris, 1817.
16. Condon, R. E.: The anatomy of the inguinal region. *In* Nyhus, L. M., and Harkins, H. N. (Eds.): Hernia. Philadelphia, J. B. Lippincott Company, 1964.
17. Condon, R. E.: Anterior iliopubic tract repair. *In* Nyhus, L. M., and Condon, R. E. (Eds.): Hernia, 3rd ed. Philadelphia, J. B. Lippincott Company, 1989.
18. Condon, R. E.: Inside looking in—posterior repair of groin hernias. J. Surg. Pract., 8:34, 1979.
19. Cooper, A. P.: The Anatomy and Surgical Treatment of Abdominal Hernia. 2 volumes.London, Longman & Co., 1804–1807.
20. Czerny, V.: Studien zur Radikalbehandlung der Hernien. Wien. Med. Wochenschr., 27:497, 1877.
21. Donald, D. C.: The value derived from utilizing the component parts of the transversalis fascia and Cooper's ligament in the repair of large indirect and direct inguinal hernias. Surgery, 24:622, 1948.
22. Dowd, C. N.: Congenital lumbar hernia at the triangle of Petit. Ann. Surg., 45:245, 1907.
23. Eiseman, B., Robinson, R. M., and Brown, J. H.: Simultaneous appendectomy and herniorrhaphy without prophylactic antibiotic therapy. Surgery, 53:578, 1962.
24. Farris, J. M.: Umbilical hernia. *In* Nyhus, L. M., and Harkins, H. N.: Hernia, Philadelphia, J. B. Lippincott Company, 1964.
25. Ferguson, A. H.: The Technique of Modern Operations for Hernia. Chicago, Cleveland Press, 1907.
26. Gallaudet, B. B.: A Description of the Planes of Fascia of the Human Body. New York, Columbia University Press, 1931.
27. Gaster, J.: Hernia—One Day Repair. Darien, Conn., Hafner Publishing Company, 1970.
28. Gilsdorf, R. B., and Shea, M. M.: Repair of massive septic abdominal wall defects with Marlex mesh. Am. J. Surg., 130:634, 1975.
29. Glassow, F.: The Shouldice repair for inguinal hernia. *In* Nyhus, L. M., and Condon, R. E. (Eds.): Hernia, 2nd ed. Philadelphia, J. B. Lippincott Company, 1978.
30. Goligher, J. C.: Prolapse of the rectum. *In* Nyhus, L. M., and Harkins, H. N.: Hernia. Philadelphia, J. B. Lippincott Company, 1964.
31. Goni Moreno, I.: Chronic eventrations and large hernias—preoperative treatment by progressive pneumoperitoneum—original procedure. Surgery, 22:945, 1947.
32. Griffith, C. A.: Inguinal hernia: An anatomic-surgical correlation. Surg. Clin. North Am., 39:531, 1959.
33. Guy, C. C., Werelius, C. Y., and Bell, L. B., Jr.: Five years' experience with tantalum mesh in hernia repair. Surg. Clin. North Am., 35:175, 1955.
34. Halsted, W. S.: The radical cure of hernia. Bull. Johns Hopkins Hosp., 1:12, 1889.
35. Halverson, K., and McVay, C. B.: Inguinal and femoral hernioplasty. Arch. Surg., 101:127, 1970.
36. Hannington-Kiff, J. G.: Absent thigh adductor reflex in obturator hernia. Lancet, 1:180, 1980.
37. Harrison, P. W.: Inguinal hernia: A study of the principles involved in the surgical treatment. Arch. Surg., 4:680, 1922.
38. Hesselbach, F. K.: Anatomisch-chirurgische Abhandlung über den Ursprung der Leistenbrüke. Würzburg, Baumgärten, 1806.
39. Hesselbach, F. K.: Neueste anatomisch-pathologische Untersuchungen über den Ursprung und das Forschreiten der Leistenund Schenkel-brüche. Würzburg, Baumgärten, 1814.
40. Howard, P. M.: Let's simplify and clarify the anatomy and surgery of groin hernias. Am. J. Surg., 128:65, 1974.
41. Jones, T. I.: An experience with the Shouldice repair. *In* Nyhus, L. M., and Condon, R. E. (Eds.): Hernia, 2nd ed. Philadelphia, J. B. Lippincott Company, 1978.
42. Keynes, W. M.: Supravesical hernia. *In* Nyhus, L.M., and Harkins, H. N.: Hernia. Philadelphia, J. B. Lippincott Company, 1964.
43. Kiesewetter, W. B.: Hernias—inguinal and umbilical. Am. J. Surg., 101:656, 1961.
44. Kiesewetter, W. B., and Oh, K. S.: Unilateral inguinal hernias in children: What about the opposite side? Arch. Surg., 115:1443, 1980.
45. Koontz, A. R.: The use of tantalum mesh in inguinal hernia repair. Surg. Gynecol. Obstet., 92:101, 1951.
46. Koontz, A. R.: Perineal hernia. *In* Nyhus, L. M., and Harkins, H. N.: Gynecol. Obstet., 92:101, 1951.
47. Koontz, A. R., and Stafford, E. S.: Unusual types of interparietal hernia. Arch. Surg., 71:723, 1955.
48. Lotheissen, G.: Zur Radikaloperation der Schenkelhernien. Zentralbl. Chir., 25:548, 1898.

49. Lower, W. E., and Hicken, N. F.: Interparietal hernias. Ann. Surg., 94:1070, 1931.
50. Lucas-Championnière, J.: Cure radicale des hernies; avec une étude statistique de deux cents soizante-quinze opérations et cinquante figures intercalées dans le texte. Paris, Rueff et Cie, 1892.
51. Lytle, W. J.: Femoral hernia. Ann. R. Coll. Surg. Engl., 21:244, 1957.
52. Macewen, W.: On the radical cure of oblique inguinal hernia by internal abdominal peritoneal pad, and the restoration of the valved form of the inguinal canal. Ann. Surg., 4:89, 1886.
53. Marcy, H. O.: A new use of carbolized catgut ligatures. Boston Med. Surg. J., 85:315, 1871.
54. Marcy, H. O.: The radical cure of hernia by the antiseptic use of the carbolized catgut ligature. Trans. A.M.A., 29:295, 1878.
55. Mayo, W. J.: Radical cure of umbilical hernia. J.A.M.A., 48:1842, 1907.
56. McVay, C. B.: Inguinal and femoral hernioplasty: Anatomic repair. Arch. Surg., 57:524, 1948.
57. McVay, C. B.: The hernias. *In* Davis, L. (Ed.): Christopher's Textbook of Surgery, 9th ed. Philadelphia, W. B. Saunders Company, 1968.
58. Moschcowitz, A. V.: Femoral hernia: A new operation for the radical cure. N.Y. J. Med., 7:396, 1907.
59. Nyhus, L. M.: An anatomic reappraisal of the posterior inguinal wall: Special consideration of the iliopubic tract and its relation to groin hernias. Surg. Clin. North Am., 44:1305, 1964.
60. Nyhus, L. M.: The recurrent groin hernia: Therapeautic solutions. World J. Surg., 13:541, 1989.
61. Nyhus, L. M.: The preperitoneal approach and iliopubic tract repair of inguinal hernia. *In* Nyhus, L. M., and Condon, R. E. (Eds.): Hernia, 3rd ed. Philadelphia, J. B. Lippincott Company, 1989.
62. Nyhus, L. M.: The preperitoneal approach and iliopubic tract repair of femoral hernia. *In* Nyhus, L. M. and Condon, R. E. (Eds.): Hernia, 3rd ed. Philadelphia, J. B. Lippincott Company, 1989.
63. Peacock, E. E., Jr.: Biology of hernia. *In* Nyhus, L. M., and Condon, R. E. (Eds.): Hernia, 2nd ed. Philadelphia, J. B. Lippincott Company, 1978.
64. Peacock, E. E., Jr., and Madden, J. W.: Studies on the biology and treatment of recurrent inguinal hernia. II. Morphological changes. Ann. Surg., 179:567, 1974.
65. Rescovitz, M. D.: Umbilical hernia repair in patients with cirrhosis: No evidence for increased incidence of variceal bleeding. Ann. Surg., 199:325, 1984.
66. Pott, P. A.: A Treatis on Ruptures. London, C. Hitch and L. Hawes, 1756.
67. Priesching, A: Laugerische Hernia. Arch. Klin. Chir., 281:411, 1956.
68. Ravitch, M. M.: Repair of Hernias. Chicago, Year Book Medical Publishers, 1969.
69. Read, R. C.: Preperitoneal exposure of inguinal herniation. Am. J. Surg., 116:653, 1968.
70. Rogers, F. A: Strangulated obturator hernia. *In* Nyhus, L. M., and Harkins, H. N. (Eds.): Hernia. Philadelphia, J. B. Lippincott Company, 1964.
71. Ruggi, G.: Metodo operative nuova per la cura radicale dell'ernia crurale. Bull. Sci. Med. Bologna Sev., 7:223, 1892.
72. Santulli, T. V., and Shaw, A.: Inguinal hernia: Infancy and childhood. J.A.M.A., 176:110, 1961.
73. Scarpa, A.: Sull'ernia del revineo. Pavia, P. Bizzoni, 1821.
74. Serafini, G.: Sulle varieta dell'ernia crurale e particolarmente sull'ernia crurale retrovascolare intravaginale e sull'ernia pettina. Policlinico (Chir.), 24:230, 1917.
75. Shearburn, E. W., and Myers, R. N.: Shouldice repair of inguinal hernia. Surgery, 66:450, 1969.
76. Spangen, L.: Spigelian hernia. Surg. Clin. North Am., 64:351, 1984.
77. Stewardson, R. H., Bombeck, C. T., and Nyhus, L. M.: Critical oprative management of small bowel obstruction. Ann. Surg., 187:189, 1978.
78. Thomson, A: Cause anatomique de la hernie inguinale externe. J. Conn. Méd. Prat. 4:137, 1836.
79. Turner, D. P. B.: Prevascular femoral hernia. Br. J. Surg., 41:77, 1953.
80. U.S. Department of Health, Education and Welfare: National Health Survey on Hernias. Series B, No. 25, Washington, D.C., U.S. Government Printing Office, Dec. 1960.
81. U.S. Department of Health and Human Services, Public Health Service, National Center for Health Statistics: National Health Survey: Utilization of Short-Stay Hospitals, Annual Summary for the United States, 1980. Series 13, No. 64. Washington, D.C., U.S. Government Printing Office, March 1982.
82. Usher, F. C.: The repair of incisional and inguinal hernias. Surg. Gynecol. Obstet., 131:525, 1970.
83. Wakely, C. P. G.: Obturator hernia. Br. J. Surg., 26:515, 1939.
84. Wagh, P. V., and Read, R. C.: Defective collagen synthesis in inguinal herniation. Am. J. Surg., 124:819, 1972.
85. Wantz, G. E.: The operation of Bassini as described by Attilio Catterina. Surg. Gynecol. Obstet. 168:67, 1989.
86. Wantz, G. E.: The Canadian repair of inguinal hernia. *In* Nyhus, L. M., and Condon, R. E. (Eds.): Hernia, 3rd ed. Philadelphia, J. B. Lippincott Company, 1989.
87. Wheeler, M. H.: Femoral hernia: Analysis of the results of surgical treatment. Proc. R. Soc. Med., 68:177, 1975.
88. Zimmerman, L. M., and Anson, B. J.: Anatomy and Surgery of Hernia, 2nd ed. Baltimore, Williams & Wilkins, 1967.

38

PEDIATRIC SURGERY

Jay L. Grosfeld, M.D.

HISTORICAL ASPECTS

The first text in pediatric surgery is credited to the Swiss surgeon Felix Wurtz in the year 1563.[141] Further development of the specialty followed the publication of a pediatric surgical text by Forster (England)[37] and published lectures on childhood surgical conditions by Guersant (France) in 1864.[54] In the late 1870s, the Hospital for Sick Children, Great Ormond Street in London, and the Hopital des Enfants Malades in Paris developed separate surgical programs within each institution. The first textbook of pediatric surgery in the United States was published by Kelley in 1909.[70] By 1920 a number of surgeons began to devote much of their energies to the care of children. Herbert Coe of Seattle was one of these individuals and was a founder of the Surgery Section of the American Academy of Pediatrics. Following World War II, the growth of pediatric surgery flourished under the direction of William E. Ladd and Robert E. Gross at the Boston Children's Hospital, Willis Potts of Chicago, and Sir Denis Browne in London.[53,75,106] Their special clinical and educational contributions to the field are well recognized. Their trainees extended these concepts to other regions of the country and abroad, leading to significant improvement in the surgical care of infants and children. Other pioneers included Swenson, Koop, Clatworthy, Bill, Benson, Randolph, Martin, Holder, and Hendren, who developed new techniques and established postgraduate training programs in the field. The first journal dedicated to pediatric surgery *(The Journal of Pediatric Surgery)* was published in 1966 with Koop as editor-in-chief. The American Pediatric Surgical Association was founded in 1970 with Gross elected the first president. In 1975, the American Board of Surgery developed a special certificate in pediatric surgery, formally recognizing the specialty. The number of training programs in pediatric surgery has increased significantly over the past few years with more than 26 training centers now in America and Canada. The approval of training programs is determined by criteria established by the Residency Review Committee for Surgery. The evolution of sophisticated neonatal intensive care, parallel development of other pediatric subspecialties, early detection of numerous anomalies by prenatal ultrasonography, the development of high-risk obstetric centers, combined programs of cancer care, and the emergence of other pediatric surgical subspecialties (neurosurgery, orthopedics, urology, cardiology, pathology, anesthesia, and radiology) have further enhanced the growth, importance, and popularity of pediatric surgery. In 1988, the specialty established its first independent Surgical Forum session at the annual meeting of the American College of Surgeons, indicative of expansion of efforts in the field to promote clinical excellence, quality education, and innovative scientific research.

SPECIAL CONSIDERATIONS

Newborn Physiology

The newborn infant is a unique surgical patient who is physically and physiologically different from the adult. The neonate presents a significant challenge in patient care management involving both congenital and acquired conditions. Due to small size, limited volume capacities, and functional immaturity of organ systems, the infant's response and ability to cope with stress of serious illness and major operative procedures may be marginal.

Cardiovascular System

The cardiovascular system of the newborn must convert from a fetal circulation that bypasses the lung to a postnatal state with both systemic and pulmonary circulations. In the absence of intracardiac defects or anomalies of the aortic arch, the newborn heart functions quite well. The elevated pulmonary artery pressure in the neonate in association with a patent foramen ovale and ductus arteriosus may cause right-to-left shunting. The neonate's cardiac output is rate-dependent, and the heart has limitations in increasing the stroke volume and develops decreased cardiac output with episodes of bradycardia. The pathophysiology of congenital heart defects is covered elsewhere in this text.

Thermoregulation

The newborn infant must be kept in a neutral thermal environment (22.7° C. [73° F.]) to minimize caloric expenditure, reduce oxygen consumption, and diminish metabolic demands. The baby's temperature must be closely monitored by skin probes or axillary probes, because the rectal temperature does not reflect an accurate measure of body temperature in the neonate, and insertion of a rectal thermometer may also cause rectal perforation. The normal skin temperature is 36 to 36.5° C. The infant's relatively large body surface area, lack of hair and subcutaneous tissue, and increased insensible losses make the patient vulnerable to hypothermia. The neonate cannot shiver but responds to cold stress by increasing metabolic rate and oxygen consumption by mobilizing brown fat deposits in the neck, axilla, mediastinum, and perirenal area (nonshivering thermogenesis).[76] Continued exposure to cold ultimately leads to decreased perfusion and metabolic acidosis. Heat loss can occur as a result of radiant and evaporative heat loss and by conduction and/or convection.[23] Overhead radiant heaters, warming lights, tinfoil caps, heat shields, extremity wraps, and warmed preparation solutions are measures frequently used to reduce skin exposure and heat loss.

Pulmonary Function

The lung is not fully mature at birth. There are 17 subdivisions of the tracheobronchial tree *in utero,* and the lung continues to add new respiratory units (terminal bronchioles and alveoli) until 8 years of age. The more immature the patient, the fewer number of pulmonary units present. The premature baby has fewer Type II pneumocytes and lower surfactant levels, making the patient susceptible to alveolar collapse, atelectasis, hyaline membrane formation, and barotrauma. The neonate is also at risk for the development of persistent pulmonary hypertension (formerly designated persistent fetal circulation), a con-

TABLE 1. Tracheal Tube Size in Infants and Children

Age of Patient	Internal Tracheal Tube Diameter
Premature	2.5 mm.
0–3 months	3.0 mm.
3–7 months	3.5 mm.
7–15 months	4.0 mm.
15–24 months	4.5 mm.
2–10 years	$\dfrac{16 + \text{age (yr.)}}{4} = \text{mm.}$
10–19 years	6.0–8.0 mm. (cuffed)

From Coran, A. G.: Perioperative care of the pediatric surgery patient. *In* Wilmore, D. W., Brennan, M. F., Harken, A. H., Holcroft, J. W., and Meakins, J. L. (Eds.): Care of the Surgical Patient. Vol. 1. New York, Scientific American, Inc., 1989, p. 9.

dition in which the pulmonary vascular resistance is equal to or greater than systemic vascular resistance causing hypoxemia due to extrapulmonary right-to-left shunting. This may occur in a variety of conditions including hyperviscosity, decreased lung mass (diaphragmatic hernia), or with a decreased vessel radius (reactive vasoconstriction, pulmonary venous obstruction, total anomalous venous drainage, or hypoplastic left heart). The tidal volume in the neonate is 6 to 10 ml. per kg. The airway diameter is quite small (trachea 2.5 to 4 mm.) and is easily obstructed with secretions (Table 1). The respiratory rate may be as high as 60 per minute and still be normal. Respiratory distress is heralded by tachypnea, grunting, nasal flaring, intercostal and substernal retraction, and cyanosis. Infants are nasal and diaphragmatic breathers; the newborn infant does not breath by mouth. If a newborn baby needs gastric drainage, the tube should be inserted through the mouth rather than the nose. Any condition that obstructs the nasal passages (e.g., choanal atresia) or interferes with diaphragmatic function (e.g., eventration, diaphragmatic hernia) may lead to severe respiratory distress.

Normal blood gas tensions in the newborn are different from the adult's because of shunting (foramen ovale, patent ductus) and a more rapid respiratory rate. The Pao_2 is usually 75 to 80 mm. Hg in a blood sample obtained from the right radial artery (above the ductus) and may be only 60 mm. Hg from a sample taken from the umbilical artery (below the ductus). The $Paco_2$ is usually 30 to 35 mm. Hg because of the relatively rapid respiratory rate. The lower the $Paco_2$, the less the risk of pulmonary vasoconstriction. The apH is usually normal, 7.3 to 7.4. Pulse oximetry is a very useful method of monitoring oxygen saturation.

Renal Function

Although the newborn kidney may not concentrate urine normally, it functions quite well otherwise and responds very well to a fluid load. This occurs despite a reduced glomerular filtration rate and immature tubular function. A urine osmolality of less than 150 mOsm. may indicate overhydration, whereas greater than 400 mOsm. may reflect dehydration. A urinary output of 1 to 2 ml. per kg. per hour is considered normal in infants.

Immunologic Function

The neonate is relatively immunodeficient since decreased levels of opsonins, IgG and IgM, and the C3b component of complement are present. The more immature the infant, the less capable is the ability of the polymorphonuclear leukocytes to phagocytize bacteria. The premature infant is, therefore, at an increased risk for severe infection.[23] Prolonged rupture of fetal membranes, perinatal asphyxia, and maternal peripartum infection increase the risk of neonatal infection. The evaluation of

sepsis in the newborn requires an extensive work-up including cerebrospinal fluid cultures, chest films, urinalysis, complete blood count and differential smear, platelet count, culture of any eye drainage, ear examination (otitis), evaluation of intravenous or arterial catheter sites including the umbilicus, careful evaluation of the wound in a postoperative patient, and in premature infants evaluation for possible necrotizing enterocolitis. Combination antibiotic therapy is administered empirically after acquisition of cultures. Group B beta-streptococcus (gram-positive) and *Escherichia coli* (gram-negative) are the two most common serious infections.

Metabolic and Endocrine Function

Liver function in the newborn is immature. Most infants have some deficiency in hepatic enzyme function, particularly those involved in the conjugation of indirect to direct bilirubin (glucuronyl transferase, Y and Z protein) and detoxification of certain drugs (sulfonamides) and anesthetic agents. The premature infant is prone to hyperbilirubinemia and the risk of kernicterus owing to passage of indirect bilirubin across the blood-brain barrier. Most endocrine activity in the full-term neonate functions at a near-normal level. Hypoglycemia is the major cause of seizures in the newborn and is defined as a concentration of less than 20 mg. per 100 ml. in the premature infant and 30 mg. per 100 ml. in the full-term infant.[12] Hypoglycemia is most commonly noted in babies who are small for gestational age. These infants have intrauterine growth retardation and inadequate glycogen stores in the liver. Progeny of diabetic mothers may also have hypoglycemia from a temporary excess insulin production stimulated during intrauterine life by the mother's elevated glucose levels. Infants with nesidioblastosis have severe hypoglycemia that may be resistant to treatment with steroids and diazoxide and require a somatostatin analog or total parenteral nutrition to maintain the blood sugar level until a 95 per cent pancreatectomy can be performed.

Hypocalcemia (less than 7 mg. per 100 ml.) may also present with jitteriness, hypotonicity, or seizures and is most frequently observed in premature infants, infants of diabetic mothers, and asphyxiated infants. Hypomagnesemia and pyridoxine deficiency are more rare causes of seizures in the newborn.

Fluid and Electrolyte Balance

In the newborn, the total body water space is 80 per cent of body weight in the term infant.[23] The extracellular water space composes more than two thirds of the total body water space. The neonate has increased insensible water losses (30 to 35 ml. per kg. per day) when compared with the adult (15 ml. per kg. per day). In premature infants weighing less than 1500 gm., insensible losses are significantly higher (45 to 60 ml. per kg.). Radiant heat warmers, phototherapy for hyperbilirubinemia, fever, and respiratory distress increase the insensible losses. Water requirements for maintenance in the normal newborn varies from 100 to 125 ml. per kg. per day in the full-term infant and up to 140 ml. per kg. per day in the premature (Table 2). Ten per cent dextrose in 0.25 per cent saline is used as a maintenance solution. Potassium and sodium requirements are 2 to 3 mEq. per kg. per day. Fluid losses related to gastric drainage are replaced in equal volumes with lactated Ringer's solution if bilious and 5 per cent dextrose in 0.45 per cent normal saline if clear. The postoperative patient may need somewhat less fluid because of antidiuretic hormone secretion and cortisol release. Body weight, skin turgor, urine and serum osmolality, and urine specific gravity are reasonable parameters to assess fluid requirements. Normal serum osmolarity is 280 mOsm. Poor urinary output and high urine specific gravity may reflect third space interstitial fluid shifts requiring an additional intravenous bolus (10 ml. per kg. of lactated Ringer's solution over ½ hour). Large volume losses from an enterostomy can be replaced with 0.5 ml. of lactated Ringer's solution per 1 ml. of stomal effluent.

TABLE 2. Daily Fluid Requirements for Neonates and Infants

Weight	Volume
Premature < 2.0 kg.	140–150 ml./kg./day
Neonates and infants (2–10 kg.)	100 ml./kg./day (for first 10 kg.)
Infants and children (10–20 kg.)	1000 ml + 50 ml./kg./day > 10 kg.
Children > 20 kg.	1500 ml. + 20 ml./kg./day > 20 kg.

From Coran, A. G.: Perioperative care of the pediatric surgery patient. *In* Wilmore, D. W., Brennan, M. F., Harken, A. H., Holcroft, J. W., and Meakins, J. L. (Eds.): Care of the Surgical Patient. Vol. 1. New York, Scientific American, Inc., 1989, p. 6.

The total blood volume in the newborn is approximately 8 per cent of body weight and decreases to approximately 5 per cent in older infants. This can be calculated as 80 ml. per kg. A safe transfusion for the infant is 10 ml. per kg. (packed red blood cells). In instances of thrombocytopenia, 10 ml. per kg. of platelets is an adequate transfusion volume. If an infant has hypotension, a rapid infusion of 20 ml. per kg. of lactated Ringer's solution reduces the pulse rate, increases the blood pressure, and often restores hemodynamic stability.

Nutrition

The neonate has a metabolic rate that is higher than the older child's and 2.5 times that of the adult. The neonate requires 120 calories per kg. per day for growth. Most infant formulas contain 20 calories per ounce; the caloric need can be determined by weight (kg.) $\times$ 6 oz. = volume of formula necessary to deliver 120 calories per kg. Major illness (sepsis), trauma, or fever may increase the caloric requirements. Half of the calories provided are carbohydrates, 35 per cent fat, and 15 per cent protein. Infants require more protein, vitamins, and minerals than the adult patient does. Linoleic acid is an essential fatty acid and histidine, tyrosine, and cystine are essential amino acids in the infant and are added to eight other essential amino acids required by adult patients. Breast milk (296 mOsm.) is the advisable formula for most infants when possible. In some instances modification of the diet is necessary. Following gastrointestinal surgery, lactose-containing formulas (Enfamil, Similac) should be avoided because flattening of the intestinal villi occurs in the unfed neonate associated with decreased lactase levels, leading to poor absorption and diarrhea. Lactose also produces a large curd, which may obstruct a small anastomosis. Low osmolar nonlactose formulas such as Isomil or Prosobee (260 mOsm.) (soybean formulas) are useful in the postoperative patient. Feedings are initiated when the gastric returns are clear and of low volume (2 ml. per hour). Initial feedings should be diluted (e.g., quarter strength; half strength; and so on) and gradually increased in volume and then density as tolerated. The swallowing mechanism in premature infants is immature, indicating that these babies should be fed by small, frequent gavage feedings. In patients with the short bowel syndrome, a more defined formula (elemental diet) given by a continuous drip technique may be necessary. Infants with obstructive jaundice thrive on Vital, a non-long-chain fat–containing diet that delivers 30 calories per ounce. If the infant cannot tolerate an enteral diet, intravenous nutrition may be required.

Total Parenteral Nutrition

Parenteral nutrition is one of the most important developments in pediatric surgical care. This technique permits the delivery of adequate amounts of carbohydrates, fat, and amino acids to ensure appropriate caloric intake leading to growth of an infant even in the absence of enteral intake. The most common cases managed with total parenteral nutrition therapy include short bowel syndrome, necrotizing enterocolitis, severe gastroenteritis due to nonspecific diarrhea syndromes, Crohn's disease with internal fistulas, gastroschisis, extensive thermal burns, pediatric oncology patients, following correction of intestinal atresia, and in many nonsurgical pediatric patients with inadequate enteral intake.[23] The nonprotein calorie:gm. of nitrogen ratio is maintained at greater than 150:1. A continuous drip of a solution containing 25 per cent carbohydrate concentration, 2.5 gm. per kg. of amino acids in the newborn and 3.5 gm. per kg. per day in older children, and no more than 4 gm. per kg. of fat emulsion administered as either a 10 per cent or 20 per cent solution of intralipid usually delivers 120 to 130 calories per kg. per day. Venous access for total parenteral nutrition is most readily achieved by inserting a Silastic catheter (Broviac or Hickman) into the external jugular vein and under fluoroscopic control placing the end of the catheter in a central high-flow location in the superior vena cava at the entrance of the right atrium. The cephalic vein, facial vein, internal jugular vein, and saphenofemoral entry can be used as alternative venotomy sites. The amount of fat must be reduced (0.5 gm. per kg. per day) if the patient is jaundiced or the triglyceride level is greater than 200 mg. per 100 ml. Appropriate sodium (3 to 4 mEq. per kg. per day) and potassium (2 to 3 mEq per kg. per day) are added to the infusate. Multivitamins, calcium, phosphorus, magnesium, zinc, copper, and folate are also added to the solution. A weight gain of 15 to 30 gm. per day is anticipated barring the presence of untoward events (e.g., sepsis, or other complications) that increase metabolic demand and require additional calories. Technical complications may be encountered at the time of central venous catheter insertion and include bleeding, pneumothorax, and vein perforation. Late complications include catheter-related sepsis, vena caval thrombosis, and, rarely, a pulmonary embolus. A myriad of metabolic complications have been observed including hyperglycemia, hyperosmolality, hypoglycemia, hypocalcemia, hypophosphatemia, fluid overload characterized by pulmonary and peripheral edema, fatty acid and mineral deficiencies, and cholestatic jaundice.[23] Most of the metabolic problems can be avoided by careful monitoring, the addition of fat infusions, and trace element solutions. Cholestatic jaundice remains a problem and is most often observed in premature infants with sepsis including peritonitis. Inability of the premature infant to tolerate the high amino acid load due to immature enzyme function is suspected. The amount of amino acids infused may need to be reduced to 1 gm. per kg. per day. Cholestasis is often improved by initiating enteral feedings or with administration of cholecystokinin. Chronic liver disease (cirrhosis) and a few instances of hepatoblastoma or hepatoma have been observed as late complications of prolonged total parenteral nutrition administration in the neonatal period.

ALIMENTARY TRACT OBSTRUCTION

Neonatal alimentary tract obstruction is often heralded by a number of cardinal signs. These include maternal polyhydramnios, bilious vomiting, abdominal distention, and failure to pass normal amounts of meconium in the first 24 hours of life. Although none of these observations is pathognomonic of obstruction, all are consistent with an obstructive phenomenon and should be carefully evaluated.

1. *Polyhydramnios* refers to the presence of excess fluid in the amniotic sac (greater than 2000 ml.). Twenty-five to 40 per cent of amniotic fluid is swallowed by the fetus (usually in the fourth to fifth fetal month) and is reabsorbed in the first 25 to 35 cm. of jejunum. Instances of high alimentary tract obstruction are associated with maternal polyhydramnios including esophageal atresia without tracheoesophageal fistula, pyloric atresia, duodenal atresia, and high jejunal atresia. Other fetal causes include swallowing problems due to central nervous system dis-

orders such as anencephaly, diaphragmatic hernia, and cystic adenomatoid malformations that compress the esophagus and interfere with swallowing.[1] There are also maternal causes related to cardiac, renal, and hepatic disease and toxemia; some cases are idiopathic in nature. Any pregnant female with abnormalities of amniotic fluid should be studied by a prenatal ultrasound examination. Many of the above-noted lesions are detected on the sonogram and can be anticipated at the time of delivery, allowing early treatment and, it is hoped, improved results.

2. *Bilious vomiting* is always pathologic whether noted in the neonate or an octogenarian. The presence of bile in the stomach at birth should be carefully investigated. The newborn infant's stomach usually contains less than 15 ml. of clear gastric juice at birth. Greater than 20 to 25 ml. of clear gastric juice or any bile may signify the presence of alimentary tract obstruction.[47,101] Bilious vomiting may also be seen in instances of neonatal sepsis with adynamic ileus. The presence of bile indicates the level of obstruction is distal to the ampulla of Vater.

3. *Abdominal distention* is a sign of distal intestinal obstruction. The normal contour of the newborn abdomen is round, unlike the usual scaphoid appearance of the adult abdomen. Physical findings associated with distention include visible veins on the abdominal wall due to attenuation, visible loops of intestine ("intestinal patterning") with or without noticeable peristalsis, and occasionally respiratory distress caused by elevation of the diaphragm. A recumbent and an erect abdominal radiograph are obtained to evaluate the nature of the distention. Distention may be due to free air (perforated viscus), fluid (hemoperitoneum from birth injury, chyloperitoneum), or distended bowel (intestinal obstruction or adynamic ileus).

4. *Failure to pass normal amounts of meconium in the first 24 hours of life* is another cardinal sign of potential bowel obstruction. Normal meconium is composed of amniotic fluid and debris (squames, lanugo hairs), succus entericus, and intestinal mucus. Meconium is dark green or black in color and sticky in consistency, and up to 250 gm. may be passed per rectum. Failure to pass this material in the first day of life may be pathologic. Infants with Hirschsprung's disease, meconium plug syndrome, small left colon syndrome, and colonic neuronal dysplasia may present with failure to pass meconium. There are other causes, however, including sepsis with adynamic ileus, hypothyroidism, and infants born to narcotics addicts.

Esophageal Atresia and Tracheoesophageal Fistula

Infants with esophageal atresia frequently present with severe respiratory distress and excessive salivation. Choking, coughing, and cyanosis are often encountered on the first attempted feeding. Infants with an associated tracheoesophageal fistula may also develop acute gastric dilation due to air entering the distal esophagus and stomach with each inspired breath. As most neonates have an incompetent lower esophageal sphincter, this ultimately leads to reflux of gastric acid through the fistula into the tracheobronchial tree leading to aspiration and chemical pneumonitis. There are five recognized anatomic variants of esophageal atresia (Fig. 1).[63,99] These include proximal esophageal atresia with a distal tracheoesophageal (TE) fistula (Gross Type C, which is the most common variant occurring in 85 per cent), proximal esophageal atresia without a TE fistula (Type A, 8 per cent), "H-type" TE fistula without esophageal atresia (Type E, 4 per cent), proximal esophageal atresia with a proximal TE fistula (Type B, 1 per cent), and proximal esophageal atresia with a double TE fistula (proximal and distal; Type D, 2 per cent). The incidence of this anomaly is 1 in 1500 to 3000 live births with both sexes equally affected. Esophageal atresia without a TE fistula is associated with maternal polyhydramios. Approximately 33 per cent of infants have low birth weight and 60 to 70 per cent have associated anomalies (gastrointestinal, cardiac, genitourinary, musculoskeletal, and central nervous system). Esophageal atresia has been noted in infants with Down's and trisomy-18 syndromes. In addition, many of the patients (10 per cent) have the VATER association, an acronym for a nonhereditary concurrence of anomalies including V, vertebral or vascular defects; A, anal anomalies; T, TE fistula; E, esophageal atresia; and R, radial limb or renal anomalies.

The diagnosis of esophageal atresia is not difficult to confirm. Attempted passage of a firm red rubber catheter through each nares (to exclude choanal atresia) demonstrates the level of atresia by encountering an obstruction. Frontal and lateral chest films confirm the location of the tube in the blind proximal pouch. If gas is present in the gastrointestinal tract below the diaphragm, an associated TE fistula must also be present.[63,99,121] If no gas is seen below the diaphragm, a distal fistula is highly unlikely. These simple observations yield a diagnosis in 95 per cent of patients. Bronchoscopy demonstrates the fistula in Type B, Type D, and Type E ("H-type"). Contrast study with isosmolar and sterile Omnipaque is an alternative but entails the risk of aspiration.

Emergency care of the infant includes insertion of a sump suction catheter in the proximal pouch that is placed on constant suction to control oral secretions. The infant is evaluated for other associated anomalies by physical examination and ultrasound studies of the heart and kidneys. The ultrasound studies should also note the location of the aortic arch (left or right). Parenteral antibiotics are administered using ampicillin (100 to 200 mg. per kg. per day) and gentamicin (5 to 7 mg. per kg. per day). Although the Waterston risk classification[136] was used for many years to determine the timing of operative therapy (immediate versus staged), more recent assessment of the physiologic status of the neonate has refined these criteria and ex-

ESOPHAGEAL ATRESIA
TE FISTULA

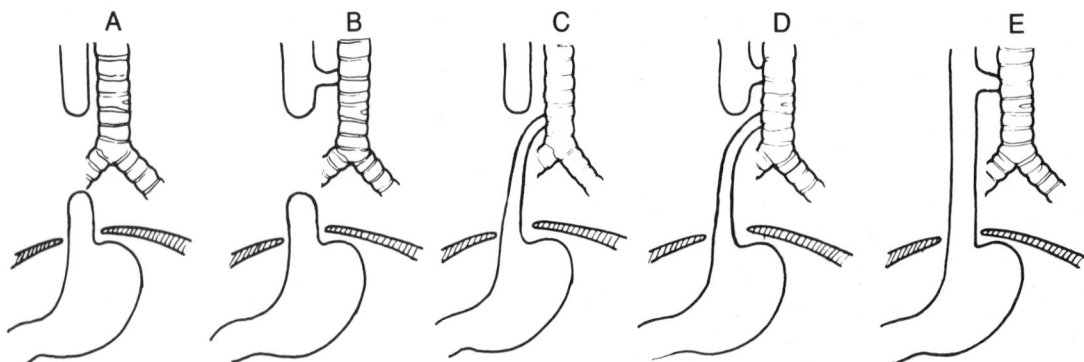

Figure 1. The five variants of esophageal atresia and transesophageal (TE) fistula. Proximal atresia with a distal TE fistula (Type C) is the most common type observed.

cludes birth weight, gestational age, and the pulmonary status previously considered essential determinants.[99,117] Currently, infants with stable cardiac and respiratory status undergo immediate thoracotomy and repair.[99] Anomalies that are not life-threatening or a physiologic derangement that is easily correctable is included in the determination of stability. Intercostal retractions, oxygen requirements, endotracheal intubation, and minor pulmonary infiltrates are not considered contraindications for immediate repair as long as the infant is stable.[99] The operation is performed through a right extrapleural thoracotomy in the fourth intercostal space. The procedure can be done through the left side of the chest if there is a right aortic arch. The TE fistula is usually identified at the site where the azygous vein passes over the trachea to enter the superior vena cava. The azygous vein is divided between 4-0 silk ties and the fistula is identified. The tracheal end is sutured with interrupted 5-0 silk or polypropylene suture. The tracheal suture line is covered with mediastinal pleura to reduce the risk of a recurrent TE fistula should an anastomotic leak occur. The proximal blind atretic esophageal pouch is identified and dissected superiorly into the neck (if possible) to attain adequate length. The dissection along the esophagotracheal plane must be done very cautiously to avoid weakening the tracheal wall in an attempt to reduce the incidence of postoperative tracheomalacia. If there is an excessive gap between the two ends of the esophagus, a proximal circular myotomy (Livaditis technique) is performed 1 to 2 cm. above the blind end of the atresia, producing a tension-free end-to-end anastomosis accomplished with one layer of interrupted 4-0 silk or absorbable Maxon suture with the knots on the outside[81,114] (Fig. 2). In stable patients, a gastrostomy (formerly used in almost every patient with esophageal atresia and TE fistula) is avoided.[99,117] A high incidence of gastroesophageal reflux is noted in patients with esophageal atresia and is enhanced by a Stamm gastrostomy.[15,93] A small orogastric tube is passed through the anastomosis to drain the stomach postoperatively. A barium swallow is obtained on the sixth to seventh postoperative day to evaluate the anastomosis for a leak; if none is observed, oral feedings are initiated. The patient can usually be discharged in 10 days barring complications.

Infants considered unstable are candidates for either delayed primary repair or staged repair. Instability is determined by the presence of significant cardiac defects with heart failure, hyaline membrane disease, and pulmonary insufficiency due to aspiration pneumonia.[99] In these infants, the proximal atretic pouch remains on suction and a temporary Stamm gastrostomy is inserted, often under local anesthesia using 0.25 per cent xylocaine without epinephrine. When the underlying problems subside and the patient becomes stable, primary repair is performed as previously noted. Some babies with severe cardiac anomalies and/or severe pulmonary compromise who require ventilator support may require staging and lifesaving division of the TE fistula because of inability to ventilate the infant due to air loss through the fistula. If they survive, eventually they may become candidates for thoracotomy and an attempted anastomosis.

Another group of patients who benefit from staging are those infants with Type A atresia without a TE fistula. These babies undergo a Stamm gastrostomy as a newborn and daily dilations of the atretic proximal pouch for a 6- to 8-week period. Some investigators suggest that the proximal segment grows and extends farther into the mediastinum without dilations. The proximal pouch is also maintained on long-term suction. At thoracotomy, most of these infants require a single or double circular esophageal myotomy (or spiral myotomy) to achieve an end-to-end esophageal anastomosis.[81,114,117] This technique has led to esophageal salvage and has obviated the need for esophageal replacement procedures (gastric tube, colon interposition, or gastric pull-up) in most patients. A few infants have an extra long gap separation between the two ends of the esophagus that

HAIGHT-TELESCOPIC ANASTOMOSIS

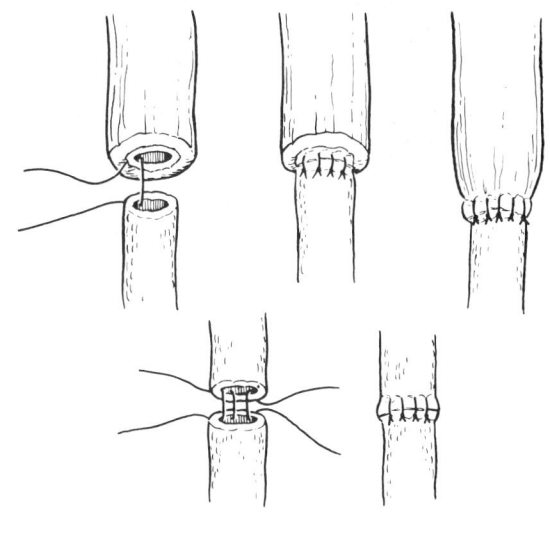

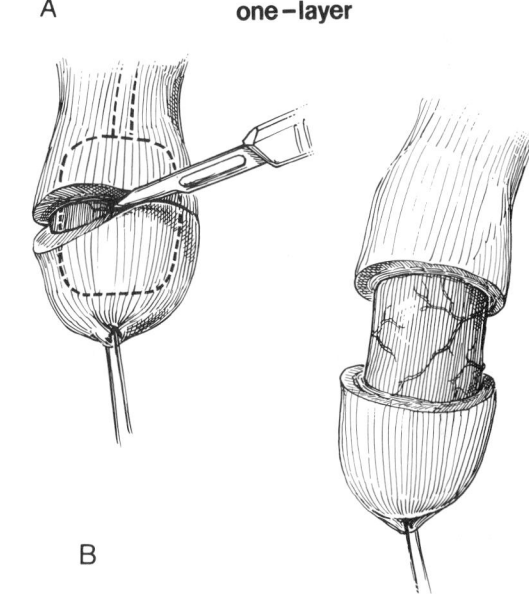

Figure 2. A, Primary anastomosis is accomplished using the telescopic technique described by Haight or a single-layer end-to-end anastomosis, which is favored by most surgeons currently. B, In instances of long gap atresia, a proximal esophagomyotomy may permit the safe performance of a primary anastomosis and avoid the need for esophageal replacement. (B from Ballantine, T. V. N.: Surgery of the esophagus. In Waldhausen, J. A., and Pierce, W. E. (Eds): Johnson's Surgery of the Chest, 4th ed. Chicago, Year Book Medical Publishers, 1985, p. 199.)

cannot be successfully brought together. Under these circumstances, the distal esophagus is at the level of the diaphragm. A proximal cervical esophagostomy is constructed between the heads of the sternocleidomastoid muscle on either the left side (if a gastric tube is contemplated) or the right side of the neck if a substernal colon interposition is considered.

In infants with an "H-type" TE fistula without atresia, the repair can often be performed through a cervical approach.[63] Division of the TE fistula is facilitated by endoscopic passage of a small catheter through the fistula to aid in its intraoperative identification. Rotation of a strap muscle between the esophageal and tracheal suture lines promotes healing and avoids recurrence of the fistula.

Postoperative complications are common and include atelectasis, pneumonia, esophageal motility disorders, gastroesophageal reflux (25 to 50 per cent), anastomotic stricture (15 to 30 per cent), and leak (10 to 20 per cent).[99] Owing to the use of the extrapleural approach, a leak does not lead to empyema, and spontaneous closure occurs. Most strictures respond to esophageal dilation except those in which the anastomotic suture line is continually bathed with gastric acid due to significant gastroesophageal reflux. If the stricture is resistant to dilation, an antireflux procedure should be performed. The most popular antireflux procedure is the Nissen fundoplication. Owing to poor esophageal motility in instances of esophageal atresia, an antireflux operation occasionally causes a physiologic obstruction. In addition, the success rate of antireflux procedures is lower in infants with esophageal atresia. Survival is achieved in all good-risk patients who are considered stable at initial evaluation and most patients with staged procedures (more than 90 per cent). Deaths are attributed to severe cardiac defects, pulmonary insufficiency with end-stage bronchopulmonary dysplasia, and chromosomal disorders.

Pyloric Atresia

Pyloric atresia represents 1 per cent of all cases of alimentary tract obstruction. There may be a familial history with cases observed in siblings and occasionally associated with epidermolysis bullosum. Maternal polyhydramnios is observed in more than 60 per cent of patients.

These infants present with vomitus of clear gastric juice or any attempted feedings. Plain films of the abdomen show a single upper abdominal gas bubble consistent with swallowed air in the stomach or a gastric air-fluid level. The infant may develop hypochloremic alkalosis from vomiting and loss of hydrochloric acid. An orogastric tube should be inserted to aspirate the stomach, prevent vomiting, and avoid the risk of aspiration. Intravenous fluids are administered to replenish electrolytes and fluid losses from previous vomiting. At operation, the atretic lesion is most often a mucosal web. Excision of the prepyloric atretic web with pyloroplasty is an efficacious procedure. Occasionally, the distal stomach and duodenum are separated, requiring a gastroduodenostomy. Postoperatively, an orogastric tube is left in place for gastric drainage until normal motility and appropriate gastric emptying are demonstrated.

Duodenal Obstruction

Duodenal atresia probably occurs during early intrauterine life. The most frequently encountered anomaly is an in-continuity mucosal atresia. Occasionally the two ends are separated by a small distance. In some cases, an intrinsic obstructive web has a "windsock" deformity. Obstruction may be complete (atresia) or incomplete (stenosis). In 85 per cent of patients, the obstruction occurs just distal to the ampulla of Vater and presents with bilious vomiting.[101] In 15 per cent, however, the obstruction occurs proximal to the ampulla and the infant may vomit clear gastric juice. Polyhydramnios is noted in 33 to 50 per cent, and the anomaly can be detected by prenatal ultrasound examination. Infants with duodenal obstruction are often premature (40 to 50 per cent), 33 per cent have Down's syndrome, and 50 to 70 per cent have associated anomalies including cardiac, renal, and other gastrointestinal defects (esophageal atresia with TE fistula and imperforate anus). At birth, the infant usually fails to tolerate attempted feeding. Bilious vomiting is observed and prompts diagnostic evaluation. Plain films of the abdomen demonstrate a "double-bubble" with one air bubble in the stomach and the second in the duodenum proximal to the obstruction (Fig. 3). If atresia is present, no air is seen distal to the duodenum. However, if stenosis is present, air is seen in the intestine beyond the duodenum. Contrast studies are usually unnecessary to confirm the diagnosis. An orogastric tube is passed into the stomach to decompress the area of obstruction and avoid aspiration. Fluid and electrolyte disturbances are cor-

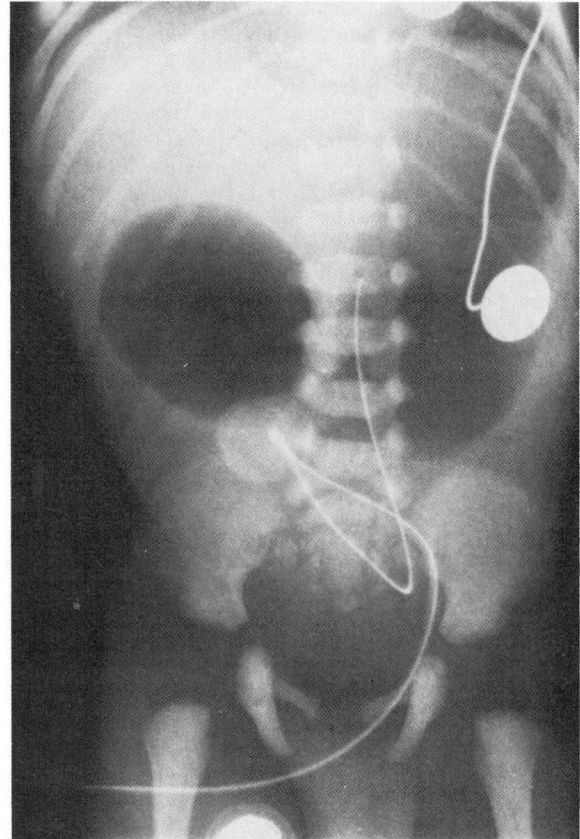

Figure 3. Plain roentgenogram of the abdomen demonstrates a "double-bubble" sign consistent with a diagnosis of duodenal obstruction. Air outlines the stomach and the first part of the duodenum. (From Rescorla, F. J., and Grosfeld, J. L.: Intestinal atresia and stenosis: Analysis of survival in 120 cases. Surgery, 98:668, 1985.)

rected to replenish any losses related to prior vomiting and dehydration. Antibiotics are administered, especially if the infant also has a cardiac anomaly. Ampicillin (100 mg. per kg. per day) and gentamicin (5 to 7 mg. per kg. per day) are given parenterally in divided doses. Peak and trough levels are obtained for gentamicin. During the preoperative preparation, a cardiac echogram and electrocardiogram are obtained and reviewed by the pediatric cardiologist.

When stable (usually within 24 to 48 hours), the infant undergoes laparotomy under general endotracheal anesthesia through a right upper quadrant transverse incision. The operation of choice is a duodenoduodenostomy to bypass the obstruction. In instances of windsock web, a duodenotomy and excision of the web at its origin is preferred. The ampulla should be identified by gently compressing the gallbladder, which produces a jet of bile from the ampulla. The anastomosis is accomplished in either one or two layers of interrupted 5-0 silk sutures. An end-to-end or diamond-shaped anastomosis is an effective procedure. At the time of the procedure, a small (No. 8 to 10 French) red rubber catheter should be passed distally to exclude a second mucosal web. An annular pancreas and/or malrotation are observed in 25 to 30 per cent of patients. Although side-to-side duodenojejunostomy was a popular procedure formerly, this anastomosis is rarely indicated currently. When the proximal atretic duodenal pouch is grossly dilated, an antimesenteric tapering is a useful adjunct. Although gastrostomy was previously recommended, the author rarely uses a gastrostomy tube because of the potential risk of gastroesophageal reflux and aspiration. An orogastric tube effectively decompresses the stomach until the anastomosis functions.

Postoperatively, the infant receives intravenous maintenance support with 100 ml. per kg. per day of 0.25 per cent saline in 10 per cent dextrose in water with 2 to 3 mg. per kg. per day of KCl added. Antibiotics are continued for 72 hours and then discontinued. Feedings are started when bowel movements are observed and the volume of gastric drainage is minimal. Half-strength, low osmolar, small-curd formula such as a soybean-based formula or quarter-strength Pregestimil is a useful diet. When tolerated, the density and volume can be increased to full-strength 20 calories per ounce in amounts adequate to deliver 120 calories per kg. per day. The current survival is 88 to 90 per cent with most deaths related to associated anomalies, particularly those affecting the cardiovascular system. There are some late complications including gastroesophageal reflux and delayed gastric emptying. Duodenal stenosis presents with a partial obstruction and may not be detected until beyond the newborn period. Poor eating habits, bilious vomiting, and failure to thrive are often observed. Plain abdominal films often show dilation of the stomach and proximal duodenum with air noted distally. Duodenal stenosis may be due to annular pancreas, malrotation with Ladd's bands (incomplete rotation and fixation), an anterior portal vein, or a mucosal web with a small diaphragm. Preparation and operative treatment are similar to that noted for duodenal atresia.

Jejunoileal Atresia and Stenosis

Small bowel atresia is due to a late mesenteric vascular accident as a result of intrauterine volvulus, malrotation, internal hernia, intussusception, or strangulation in a tight abdominal wall defect (e.g., gastroschisis and omphalocele). Atresias occur slightly more commonly in the jejunum than in the ileum. Most are single; however, in 10 to 15 per cent of patients, multiple atresias are observed. Ten to 12 per cent occur in infants with cystic fibrosis, which suggests that a sweat chloride determination should be obtained in each instance prior to hospital discharge. The pathologic findings are classified as Type I, a mucosal web or diaphragm (that may be due to epithelial obstruction), or Type II, in which an atretic cord exists between two blind ends of the bowel with an intact mesentery. In Type IIIa, there is a complete separation of the blind ends of the bowel by a V-shaped mesenteric "gap" defect. Type IIIb represents instances of atresia with an apple-peel or Christmas tree deformity in which the distal bowel receives a retrograde blood supply from the ileocolic or right colic artery. Type IV represents instances of multiple atresias often characterized by a "string of sausage" appearance (Fig. 4).

Jejunal Atresia

High jejunal atresia usually presents with bilious vomiting and three to four air-fluid bubbles on plain abdominal films. A history of polyhydramnios may be elicited in 35 per cent of patients. These patients are more often full-term infants and have fewer associated anomalies than do babies with duodenal atresia. Jaundice is noted in as many as 40 per cent. An orogastric tube is inserted into the stomach and fluid and electrolyte replenishment is accomplished with administration of parenteral electrolyte solution. Fluid resuscitation is accomplished within a short time, and exploratory laparotomy should be performed expeditiously through a right upper quadrant transverse incision. The proximal dilated atretic segment is often atonic and should be resected back to the ligament of Treitz (in instances with near-normal bowel length) where an end-to-end anastomosis is performed. The distal bowel should be evaluated for additional atresias or stenosis by passage of a soft red rubber catheter or by injection of saline. In cases with the short bowel syndrome due to a volvulus, the proximal atretic segment can be preserved by performing an antimesenteric tapering enteroplasty. Disparity in the size of the dilated proximal bowel and the smaller distal end may be corrected by an end-to-oblique interrupted anastomosis with 5-0 silk (Fig. 5). Anastomotic

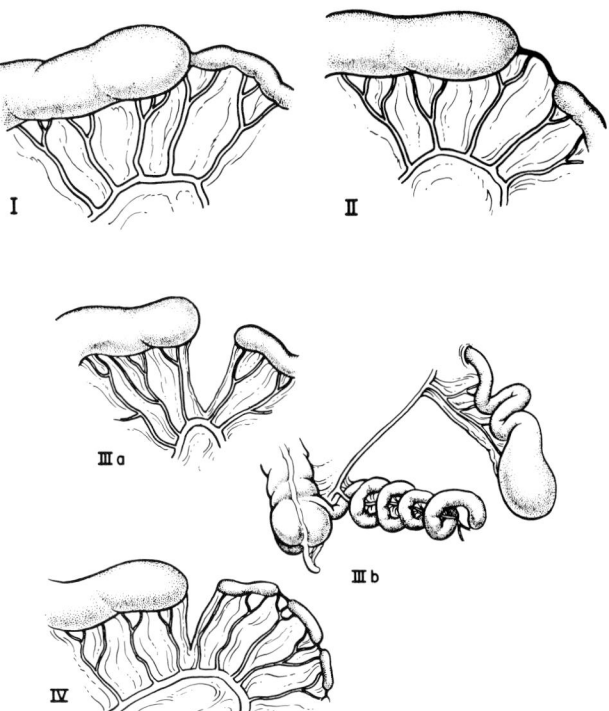

Figure 4. Classification of jejunoileal atresia. The most common type of atresia noted was Type IIIa gap defect. (From Grosfeld, J. L., et al.: Operative management of intestinal atresia based on pathologic findings. J. Pediatr. Surg., *14*:368, 1979.)

function may be delayed for 7 to 10 days. The stomach is decompressed by an orogastric tube; nutritional support is accomplished with parenteral nutrition using glucose (25 per cent), amino acids (2.5 per cent), and intralipid (4 gm. per kg. per day) until bowel function is restored. When bowel motions are observed and the gastric volume decreases, the orogastric tube can be removed and diet instituted. A low osmolar, small-curd, easily absorbed formula such as Pregestimil, or a soybean-based formula can be used. Feedings are increased in both density and volume as tolerated. Most infant formulas contain adequate vitamin and iron supplements. However, with some formulas that do not contain supplements, iron must be administered on

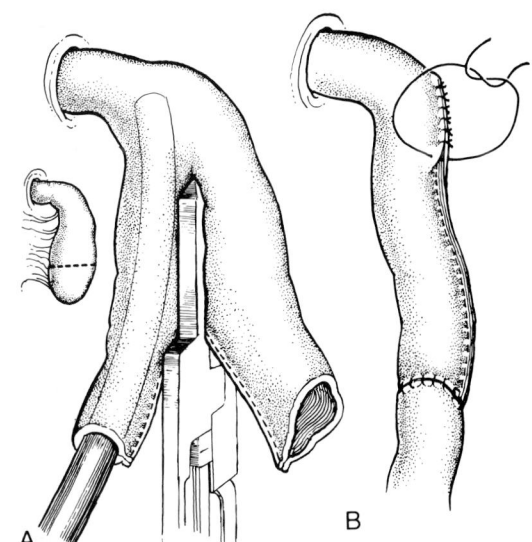

Figure 5. Illustration demonstrates the technique employed in the performance of a tapering jejunostomy in cases of proximal jejunal atresia. (From Grosfeld, J. L., et al.: Operative management of intestinal atresia based on pathologic findings. J. Pediatr. Surg., *14*:368, 1979.)

a daily basis for the first year of life (0.6 ml. Fer-in-sol per day). In instances of short bowel syndrome, special formulas may be required in addition to long-term total parenteral nutrition to ensure adequate caloric intake for growth.

Ileal Atresia

Infants with ileal atresia frequently present with abdominal distention, bilious vomiting, and failure to pass meconium. Erect and recumbent abdominal radiographs demonstrate many dilated intestinal loops often with air-fluid levels. The atretic loop may be much larger than the other loops of bowel. Since haustral markings are not present on the abdominal films of a neonate, a barium enema must be performed in each case of low intestinal obstruction. The first enema the newborn baby receives is a barium enema. Preparation of the colon for this study is unnecessary. The barium enema provides information regarding small intestinal or colonic distention, determines whether the colon is used or unused ("microcolon"), and, therefore, identifies the level of obstruction (e.g., small bowel or colon) and the position of the cecum in regard to possible anomalies of intestinal rotation and fixation.[101] Occasionally, areas of calcification are observed on abdominal radiographs signifying the presence of "meconium peritonitis." This is a sign of intrauterine bowel perforation (12 per cent of cases). The sterile fetal meconium leads to an intense local inflammatory reaction and eventually becomes calcified. The two most common causes of low small bowel obstruction in the newborn are ileal atresia and meconium ileus.

Barium enema usually demonstrates a microcolon (unused) limiting the obstruction to the small bowel (Fig. 6A and B). The majority of patients have Type IIIa pathology, and when reasonably normal bowel length is preserved, operative management includes resection of the dilated atretic loop and an interrupted 5-0 silk end-to-oblique anastomosis (Fig. 6C). At the time of the procedure, the distal bowel should be inspected for additional areas of atresia or stenosis. This can be demonstrated by injecting saline into the distal bowel. In cases associated with short bowel syndrome, a tapering ileostomy is performed to preserve an intestinal length compatible with survival. In the presence of severe peritonitis or when bowel viability is in question, a temporary enterostomy may be required. Infants with ileal atresia who have an intact ileocecal valve have better absorptive capability and survival than do those infants in whom the ileocecal valve is resected. This is probably associated with improved fat and vitamin B$_{12}$ absorption and an improved enterohepatic circulation of bile from the distal ileum rather than the valve itself.

Meconium Ileus

Meconium ileus is a unique form of congenital obstruction that occurs in 10 to 15 per cent of infants born with cystic fibrosis.[85,86,90] A deficiency of pancreatic enzymes and abnormality in the composition of the meconium are the factors responsible for presence of the solid meconium concretions that lead to an obturator form of obstruction. A careful family history should be obtained at the time of birth. The occurrence of low small bowel obstruction in identical twins is generally due to meconium ileus. Infants present with abdominal distention, bilious vomiting, and failure to pass meconium. Certain abdominal radiographic findings may help distinguish between ileal atresia and meconium ileus. Babies with meconium ileus often demonstrate significant dilation of similar sized bowel loops with few if any air-fluid levels. A ground-glass appearance in the right lower quadrant (Neuhauser's sign or "soap-bubble" sign) may be observed and represents viscid meconium mixed with air.[85,104] Although this is not pathognomonic of meconium ileus (e.g., seen in some cases of colon atresia), it is a frequent finding. Barium enema commonly demonstrates an unused "microcolon" similar to ileal atresia; however, reflux of contrast material into the distal ileum may identify the small obstructive concretions characteristic of this hereditary disorder. The treatment of meconium ileus depends on whether it is uncomplicated (simple obturator obstruction) or complicated by atresia, volvulus, perforation, or giant cystic meconium peritonitis.[16,56,104] The treatment of choice in uncomplicated meconium ileus is nonoperative clearance of the obstructive intraluminal meconium pellets using a Gastrografin enema.[86,104] This radiopaque substance allows direct visualization under fluoroscopic control while its hypertonicity draws fluid into the bowel lumen, which separates the abnormal meconium pellets from the bowel wall leading to relief of obstruction (Fig. 7). This form of therapy causes significant fluid shifts and requires infusion of crystalloid and/or colloid during the procedure to prevent hypovolemia. Careful attention to fluid balance, blood pressure, pulse rate, and urinary output is essential. Occasionally the Gastrografin enema must be repeated to relieve the obstruction. This technique is successful in 50 per cent of uncomplicated cases. Unsuccessful nonoperative attempts in uncomplicated cases and all cases of meconium ileus with complications require operative intervention. The procedure currently favored by the author in uncomplicated cases is intraoperative irrigation of the viscid meconium and clearing of the obstructive pellets through an enterotomy.[56,104] The bowel is irrigated with saline and dilute Hypaque or Gastrografin, which lowers the viscosity of the meconium, flushes the debris, and relieves the obstruc-

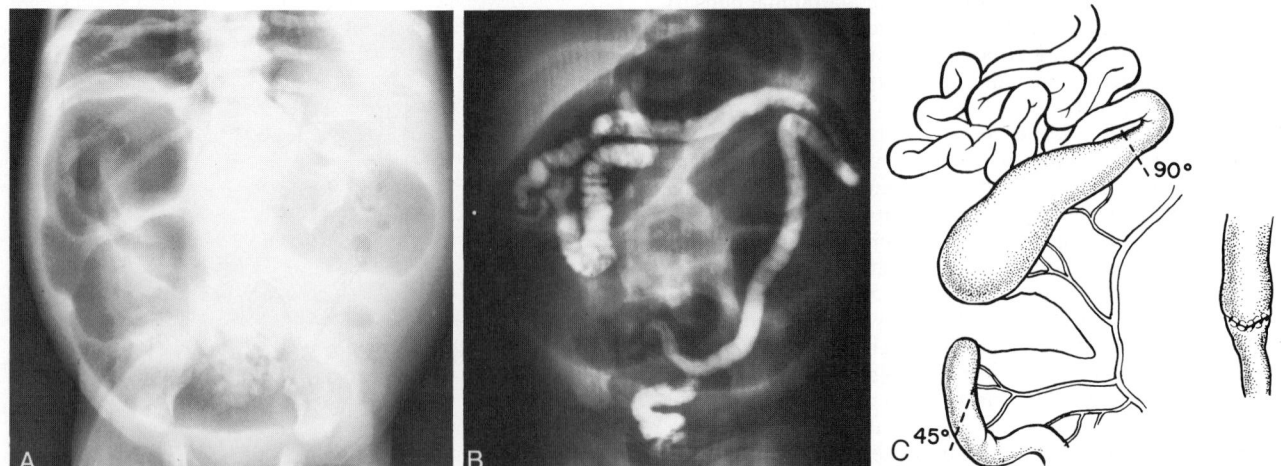

Figure 6. Flate plate of abdomen demonstrates distended intestine *(A)* and barium enema demonstrates a microcolon *(B)* in an infant with ileal atresia. *C,* The technique for an end-to-oblique anastomosis of the ileum. (*C* from Grosfeld, J. L., et al.: Operative management of intestinal atresia based on pathologic findings. J. Pediatr. Surg., *14*:368, 1979.)

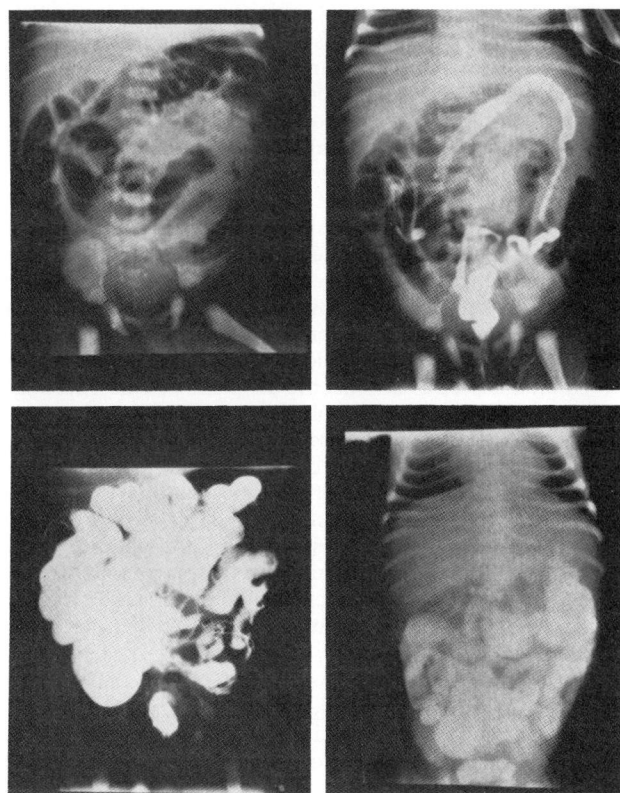

Figure 7. Composite of abdominal roentgenograms demonstrating the diagnosis and successful treatment of uncomplicated meconium ileus using a hypertonic Gastrografin enema. (From Rescorla, F. J., et al.: Changing patterns of treatment and survival in neonates with meconium ileus. Arch. Surg., *142*:837, 1989. Copyright 1989, American Medical Association.)

tion by washing the pellets into the colon, from which evacuation follows (Fig. 8). This procedure avoids the need for enterostomy in most uncomplicated cases and a second operation (e.g., enterostomy closure). The Bishop-Koop enterostomy or double-barrel enterostomy, which were popular methods of treatment formerly, are rarely necessary at present.[10] Avoidance of an enterostomy facilitates early discharge from the hospital and reduces the risk of hospital-acquired cross-infection. In in-

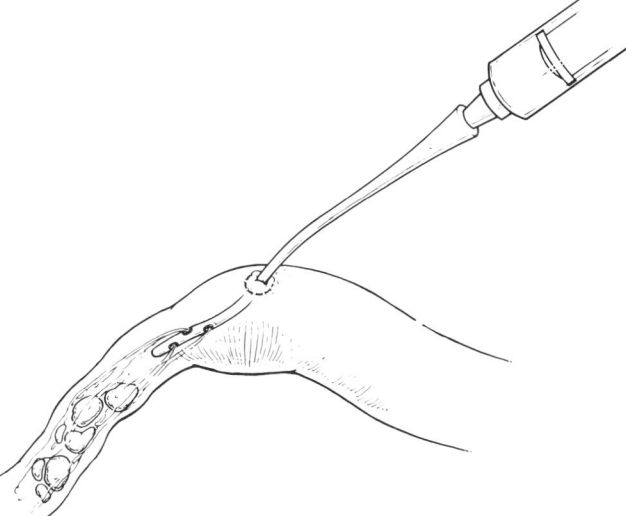

Figure 8. Illustration demonstrates the technique of intraoperative enterotomy and catheter irrigation of the obstructing meconium pellets. (From Rescorla, F. J., et al.: Changing patterns of treatment and survival in neonates with meconium ileus. Arch. Surg., *124*:837, 1989. Copyright 1989, American Medical Association.)

stances of meconium ileus complicated by atresia, volvulus, perforation, or gangrenous bowel, bowel resection and anastomosis or temporary enterostomy are required. Gastrografin enema is contraindicated in these cases.

After correction of the obstruction, careful family counseling and parental instruction regarding diet, enzyme replacement, and pulmonary toilet using percussion and postural drainage are important components in the overall care of these patients. Survival of this condition has improved dramatically in recent years with more than 90 per cent of patients currently surviving the neonatal period.

Long-term follow-up is essential. In addition to the occurrence of severe chronic pulmonary disease, these children are at risk of developing meconium ileus equivalent as a result of poor enzyme compliance and decreased fluid intake during episodes of infection. This leads to severe intraluminal obstruction with inspissated fecal material that mimics the findings of meconium ileus in the neonate. Recognition of this late complication of cystic fibrosis allows nonoperative intervention with either a Gastrografin swallow or enema; operation can be avoided in most cases.

COLONIC OBSTRUCTION

Causes of colon obstruction in the neonate include meconium plug syndrome, aganglionic megacolon (Hirschsprung's disease), colon atresia, small left colon syndrome, neuronal colonic dysplasia, and the various presentations of imperforate anus.

Colon Atresia

Colon atresia as an isolated entity (unassociated with imperforate anus or cloacal exstrophy) is relatively uncommon. Failure to pass meconium in the first 24 hours of life, abdominal distention, and bilious vomiting are the usual clinical manifestations.[101] Infants with colon atresia are usually full-term and rarely have associated anomalies. Erect and recumbent abdominal radiographs demonstrate dilated intestine with air-fluid levels. The atretic loop often has a soap-bubble appearance due to the admixture of meconium and air. Diagnosis is confirmed by barium enema, which demonstrates a blind-ending distal end of a microcolon and dilated air-filled loops of proximal intestine. Most cases occur in the right colon and are Type IIIa atresias with a V-shaped gap between the atretic ends probably following a vascular injury (volvulus) to the mesentery. The sigmoid colon is the second most common site of colon atresia. Type I mucosal atresia has also been noted in the colon. Colon atresia has been treated with a preliminary colostomy in the newborn period and subsequent closure with anastomosis at age 3 to 6 months. All 12 infants with isolated colon atresia treated at the author's institution in this manner have survived. Other reports concerning colon atresia recommend primary anastomosis for right-sided lesions and a temporary colostomy for atresia affecting the sigmoid colon.

Meconium Plug Syndrome

The meconium plug syndrome was first described in 1956. The exact etiology is unknown and is thought to be due to some factor or factors that dehydrate the meconium. Meconium plug syndrome is unrelated to meconium ileus and in the vast majority is not a sequela of cystic fibrosis. Although an occasional infant with meconium plug syndrome has a positive sweat chloride determination consistent with cystic fibrosis, most do not.[90,107] Infants typically present with significant abdominal distention and failure to pass meconium in the first 24 hours of life. Plain abdominal radiographs demonstrate many loops of distended bowel with air-fluid levels. Barium enema demonstrates a microcolon extending up to the descending or transverse colon, at which point the colon becomes dilated and copious intraluminal material (thick meconium plug) is observed.

The barium enema is often both diagnostic and therapeutic. Following instillation of the contrast material, large pieces of inspissated meconium plugs are passed and the obstruction is completely relieved. Occasionally, a second enema (usually using Gastrografin) is required to effect a complete evacuation of the thickened meconium. If any signs of obstruction recur, aganglionic megacolon must be considered as the cause of these symptoms. Five per cent of cases of Hirschsprung's disease present with a clinical pattern of meconium plug syndrome in the neonatal period. Under these circumstances, a screening submucosal suction biopsy should be performed and the tissues examined for the presence or absence of ganglion cells.

Aganglionic Megacolon (Hirschsprung's Disease)

Aganglionic megacolon is a neurogenic form of intestinal obstruction in which there is an absence of ganglion cells in the myenteric (Auerbach's) and submucosal (Meissner's) plexuses. Hypertrophic nerve fibers are often observed. The absence of parasympathetic innervation causes failure of relaxation of the internal anal sphincter. Aganglionosis begins at the anorectal line and in 80 per cent of patients involves the rectosigmoid area; aganglionosis extends proximal to the splenic flexure in 10 per cent, and in 10 per cent the entire colon and distal ileum or more proximal small bowel may be involved. Relatively rare cases of total aganglionosis of the entire gastrointestinal tract have also been reported. Three to 5 per cent of patients have Down's syndrome. Hirschsprung's disease has a definite family history. The risk of a second child being born with Hirschsprung's disease in a family in whom the first infant had rectosigmoid involvement is approximately 6 per cent. The incidence of a second child's having Hirschsprung's disease in cases in which the first infant had total colonic aganglionosis is 12 per cent. Eighty per cent of the cases occur in males; in instances of total colonic aganglionosis, 35 per cent are females. Occasionally this condition occurs with other neurocristopathies including Klippel-Feil syndrome, Ondine's curse (sleep apnea), von Waardenburg's syndrome, and neuroblastoma.[108]

Most infants with Hirschsprung's disease are symptomatic at birth. More than 95 per cent present with delayed passage of meconium in the first 24 hours of life. Almost all the infants with aganglionosis are full-term infants with an average birth weight of more than 3 kg. Abdominal distention and bilious vomiting are other presenting findings. Abdominal distention is often severe with obvious dilated loops of bowel visible on the abdominal wall (intestinal patterning). In some instances (10 to 15 per cent of cases), the distended infants may have severe diarrhea alternating with constipation. This diarrhea is known as the enterocolitis of Hirschsprung's disease and is associated with an increased morbidity and mortality. Erect and recumbent abdominal radiographs demonstrate many dilated loops of bowel. A barium enema is performed in each suspected case of aganglionic megacolon. This contrast study usually demonstrates that the colon is slightly dilated; however, in most newborns there is no definitive "cut-off" point indicating the transition zone where the narrow distal aganglionic rectum or rectosigmoid meets the obstructed dilated normal proximal colon containing ganglion cells. In some patients, the transition zone may not become apparent until 3 to 6 weeks. Unlike the normal newborn infant who evacuates the contrast from a barium enema in 10 to 18 hours, infants with Hirschsprung's disease retain the barium for 24 to 48 hours. This observation emphasizes the importance of obtaining a delayed (later than 24 hours) follow-up abdominal radiograph. In older infants, the transition zone is usually appreciated on the barium study. The barium enema may appear entirely normal in infants with short segment disease affecting the rectum only and demonstrates a comma-shaped rectosigmoid, flattened flexures, and occasionally a microcolon in instances of total colonic aganglionosis.

The differential diagnosis of Hirschsprung's disease includes hypothyroidism, meconium plug syndrome, colonic neuronal dysplasia, adynamic ileus associated with sepsis, intestinal pseudo-obstruction, and infants born to narcotics addicts. These conditions are also associated with delayed passage of meconium at birth. The diagnosis of Hirschsprung's disease is confirmed by obtaining a rectal biopsy. A submucosal suction biopsy is adequate in 90 per cent of patients. Ganglion cells are either identified or are absent in the Meissner's submucosal plexus. This determination must be done with permanent stains and is not amenable to frozen section techniques. In more emergent circumstances, a definitive diagnosis requires a full-thickness operative rectal biopsy, which can be evaluated for the presence or absence of ganglion cells in Auerbach's myenteric plexus by frozen section technique. If no ganglion cells are observed on at least 10 sections, the diagnosis of Hirschsprung's disease is confirmed. Acetylcholinesterase staining is also a useful diagnostic method. Increased acetylcholinesterase staining of neurofibrils is characteristic of Hirschsprung's disease. Anorectal manometry may be a useful diagnostic adjunct. This technique measures the anorectal intraluminal pressure with a balloon probe connected to a pressure transducer and polygraph recorder. In infants with Hirschsprung's disease, this study usually demonstrates an absent rectoanal inhibitory reflex, indicating a lack of relaxation of the internal sphincter characteristic of aganglionosis.

The treatment of choice in the neonatal period is a temporary decompressing colostomy at least 10 cm. proximal to the transition zone. This site is evaluated at the time of operation for the presence of ganglion cells on frozen section to avoid placing the stoma in obstructed aganglionic bowel. If there are no ganglion cells present in the sigmoid colon, a biopsy is obtained in the transverse colon. If no ganglion cells are noted, the appendix should be removed. If no ganglion cells are noted in the appendix, the disease process extends into the small bowel and the biopsy process continues until ganglion cells are identified. At 9 months to 1 year of age, a definitive pull-through procedure using the Soave (endorectal), modified Duhamel (retrorectal), or Swenson (rectosigmoidectomy) procedure is performed in infants with rectosigmoid disease. The choice of the procedure employed is made by the pediatric surgeon. All of these operations are acceptable procedures with the Soave and Duhamel being the most often employed at present. In cases of total colonic aganglionosis, the pull-through procedure may be delayed until 18 months of age. Most pediatric surgeons favor the modified Duhamel operation for total colonic aganglionosis. When the aganglionic process extends proximal to the mid-small bowel, a vascularized antimesenteric aganglionic patch of right colon has been a useful adjunct to aid fluid absorption and slow transit time.[71,74] The extended side-to-side Martin modification of the "long" Duhamel procedure, which employed the entire aganglionic colon in an anastomosis with the distal small bowel, has been abandoned because of significant complications associated with this technique, particularly recurring enterocolitis. In rare cases of aganglionosis affecting the entire small bowel, an extensive enteromyotomy and myectomy as advocated by Ziegler and associates may lead to relief of obstruction.[142] Infants with extensive aganglionosis extending into the proximal small intestine generally require total parenteral nutrition to achieve adequate caloric intake. In addition, special care of the perineal and perianal skin is necessary to prevent skin breakdown from diarrhea. The survival of babies with Hirschsprung's disease has improved significantly in the past decade. Rare deaths occur in infancy owing to delays in diagnosis complicated by enterocolitis and sepsis and in instances of total colonic aganglionosis with significant proximal extension into the small intestine. Many of the deaths have been observed in babies with Down's syndrome. Infants who presented with enterocolitis preoperatively are more likely to have this unusual complication in the postoperative course following both colostomy and pull-through procedures. Overall, survival is achieved in more than 90 per cent of patients. Long-term follow-up is important. Most infants (greater than 96 per cent) are continent; however, soiling is a problem (2 to 3 per cent), and rarely (1 per cent) incontinence is observed. Some patients (10 per cent) may have constipation; however, this can usually be improved with a high-fiber diet and stool softeners. Most children with postoperative symptoms improve with age.

ANORECTAL ANOMALIES

There is a wide spectrum of anorectal anomalies within the general category of anal atresia, imperforate anus, and rectal atresia. A recent symposium leading to a unified international classification of these anomalies was held in 1984 and is termed the Wingspread Classification[119] (Table 3). Anal atresia refers to an inappropriate ascent of the proctodeum leading to a thin veil-like membrane covering the normal anal canal and residing within the normal sphincter. This is treated simply by puncturing the skin membrane that is often seen protruding with meconium. Anal dilations avoid the need for any extensive surgical procedures. These lesions can be categorized as low, intermediate, or high according to whether the rectal atresia has descended below the puborectalis sling, is at the level of the puborectalis, or remains above that level.[28,119,130]

Eighty-five to 90 per cent of infants with imperforate anus and rectal atresia have an associated fistulous tract originating from the rectal segment. In males, the fistulous tract is usually to the perineum (low lesion) or to the verumontanum of the urethra (intermediate or high). Anal atresia with a perineal fistula can be treated definitively in the neonatal period with a "cutback" perineal Y-V anoplasty. Infants with rectal atresia and a fistula to the urethra are best managed with a diverting sigmoid colostomy in the neonatal period with a subsequent posterior sagittal anoplasty (as advocated by Peña) performed between 9 and 12 months of age[28,29,96] (Figs. 9 and 10). In females, a variety of anomalies are observed. Anal atresia with a rectoperineal fistula can be repaired in a neonate by performing a perineal Y-V anoplasty. Rectal atresia with a rectoforchette fistula (to the forchette of the vagina), an intermediate level lesion, can be treated by transplantation of the fistula to a site within the circular fibers of the external sphincter.[83,130] The timing of the procedure varies. This could be accomplished in the neonatal period; however, the author usually prefers to gently dilate the

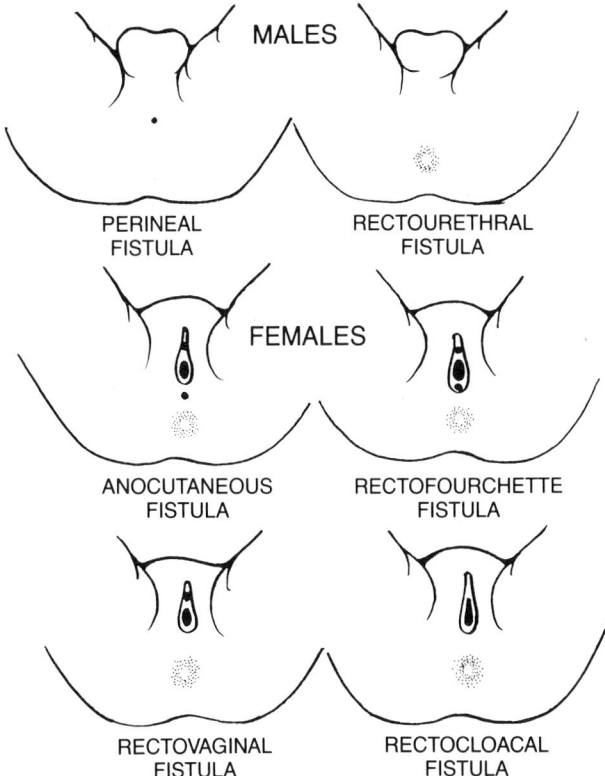

Figure 9. Perineal appearance of anorectal anomalies in males and females. (From Grosfeld, J. L.: Anorectal malformations. *In* Zuidema, G., and Condon, R. E. (Eds.): Surgery of the Alimentary Tract, 3rd ed. Vol. 4. Philadelphia, W. B. Saunders Company, 1990.)

fistula on a daily basis to maintain evacuation of feces and then performs a transplant anoplasty at age 3 to 6 months when the tissues are more firm. Transplantation of the fistula allows preservation of the perineal body and an improved perineal appearance. Separation of the rectal and vaginal openings by the perineal body reduces the risk of urinary tract infection and vaginal soiling. If the tissues appear fragile at the time of the repair, a backup colostomy to divert the fecal stream may facilitate healing and avoid breakdown of the repair. Females with intermediate or high rectal atresia and rectovaginal fistula require a colostomy in the neonatal period. Subsequent division of the fistula and posterior sagittal anoplasty is performed at 9 to 12 months of age. The colostomy is left in place postoperatively in both sexes until adequate healing of the anoplasty has occurred and the anoplasty site is dilated to a No. 13–14 Hegar dilator size.[130] This is usually accomplished in 3 to 6 months.

The operations for children with imperforate anus should be performed by pediatric surgeons with considerable expertise in the management of these cases. The first operation is the most important and there is no room for error. Infants undergoing perineal anoplasty in the newborn period develop good external sphincter tone with increased potential for developing continence. The higher the rectal atresia, the poorer the potential outcome of the operation in regard to obtaining fecal continence. Long-term care and follow-up are required in these patients, and their families must be carefully counseled not to expect the normal progression of bowel training in these children. If the puborectalis sling and deep and superficial fibers of the external sphincter are preserved at the time of the pull-through procedure, many of these children have a reasonable likelihood of obtaining socially acceptable continence. This may not be achieved, however, until a stage of maturity is reached (6 to 9 years) so that the child voluntarily participates in attempts to remain clean to avoid fecal odor. Perfect continence may never be achieved owing to the absence of a true internal

TABLE 3. Wingspread Classification of Anorectal Anomalies (1984)

Level	Female	Male
High	Anorectal agenesis with rectovaginal fistula	Anorectal agenesis with rectoprostatitis, urethral fistula
	Rectal atresia	Rectal atresia
Intermediate	Rectovestibular fistula	Rectobulbar urethral fistula
	Rectovaginal fistula	
	Anal agenesis without fistula	Anal agenesis without a fistula
Low	Anovestibular fistula	Anocutaneous fistula
	Anocutaneous fistula	Anal stenosis*
	Anal Stenosis*	Rare Malformations
	Cloacal malformations	
	Rare malformations	

* Previously called "covered anus."
From Smith, E. D.: The bath water needs changing but don't throw out the baby: An overview of anorectal anomalies. J. Pediatr. Surg., 22:335, 1988.

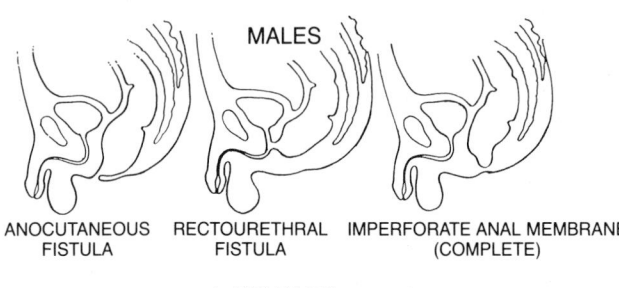

MALES

ANOCUTANEOUS   RECTOURETHRAL   IMPERFORATE ANAL MEMBRANE
FISTULA   FISTULA   (COMPLETE)

FEMALES

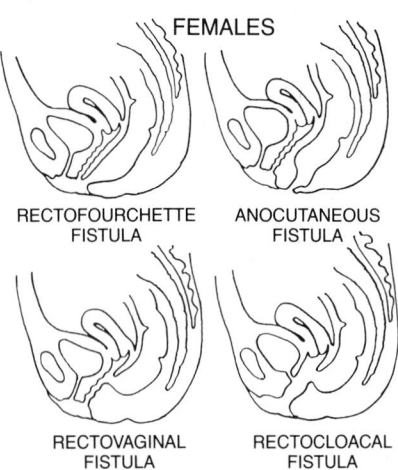

RECTOFOURCHETTE   ANOCUTANEOUS
FISTULA   FISTULA

RECTOVAGINAL   RECTOCLOACAL
FISTULA   FISTULA

Figure 10. Lateral view of pelvis demonstrating the anorectal anomalies of males and females. (From Grosfeld, J. L.: Anorectal malformations. *In* Zuidema, G., and Condon, R. E. (Eds.): Surgery of the Alimentary Tract, 3rd ed. Vol. 4. Philadelphia, W. B. Saunders Company, 1990.)

sphincter component in many of these patients. Many of the children with imperforate anus have an associated spinal dysraphic syndrome that may not be detected until they are older.[68,131] These anomalies are best detected by magnetic resonance imaging of the spinal canal and pelvic musculature. Neural contribution to continence is also quite important and must be thoroughly evaluated in problematic cases. Infants with imperforate anus have a high rate of associated anomalies in other systems. A careful system review involving other areas of the gastrointestinal tract (esophageal atresia; duodenal atresia), cardiovascular system, musculoskeletal system, genitourinary tract, and central nervous system (as noted before) should be done in early infancy to delineate these problems and initiate treatment before they become catastrophic and lead to the unnecessary demise of the patient.

NECROTIZING ENTEROCOLITIS

Necrotizing enterocolitis is a life-threatening intra-abdominal condition affecting 1 to 2 per cent of patients in most neonatal intensive care facilities. The majority of cases occur in premature and low-birth-weight infants. The exact etiology is unknown; however, a number of conditions appear to predispose to the onset of this potentially catastrophic illness. These include shock, hypoxia, the respiratory distress syndrome, apneic episodes, sepsis, polycythemia, hyperviscosity, exchange transfusions, patent ductus arteriosus, hyperosmolar feedings, and cyanotic heart disease.[20] The common underlying pathophysiologic insult involves splanchnic vasoconstriction, diminished splanchnic perfusion, mucosal ischemic injury, and probable bacterial invasion. Symptoms and signs include increased gastric residuals with gavage feedings, abdominal distention, vomiting (often bilious), lethargy, occult or gross rectal bleeding, fever or hypothermia (below 36° C. [96.5° F.]), abdominal mass, abdominal wall erythema, oliguria, jaundice, and apnea-bradycardia. Any evidence of these signs or symptoms should prompt cessation of attempted feedings and immediate evaluation.

These observations may be accompanied by a variety of abdominal radiographic findings that include fixed dilated intestinal loops, pneumatosis intestinalis, portal vein air, free fluid (ascites), and free air (Fig. 11). Laboratory data frequently show a leukocytosis with a shift to the left on the differential smear, anemia, hypoalbuminemia, electrolyte disturbances, metabolic acidosis, hyper- or hypoglycemia, and a progressive decrease of the platelet count. In some instances, disseminated intravascu-

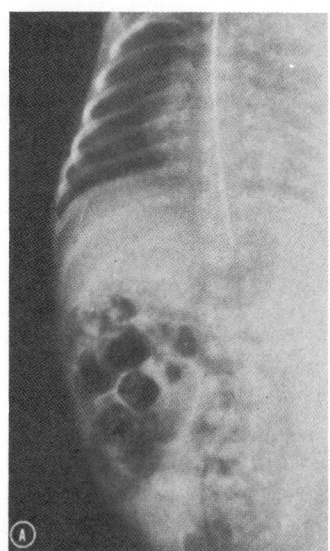

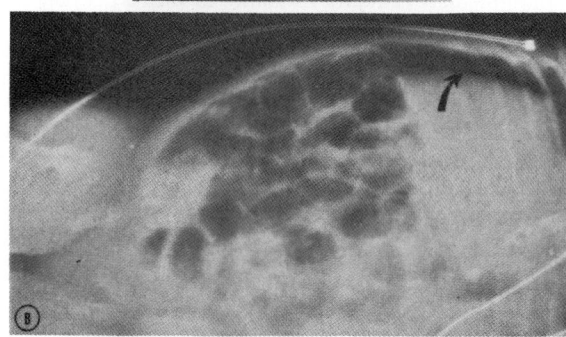

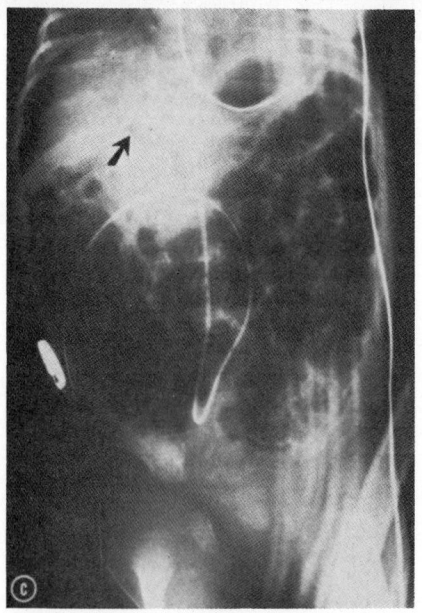

Figure 11. *A* to *C*, Abdominal roentgenographs demonstrating the presence of pneumatosis intestinalis consistent with the diagnosis of necrotizing enterocolitis. (From Cikrit, D., et al.: Necrotizing enterocolitis: Factors affecting mortality in 101 surgical cases. Surgery, 96:648, 1984.)

lar coagulation may also be present. Resuscitation of the patient involves cessation of feedings, insertion of an orogastric tube, repletion of intravascular volume with crystalloid and colloid infusions, ventilator support as indicated, acquisition of blood cultures, parenteral administration of systemic antibiotics (ampicillin, gentamicin, and clindamycin), blood transfusion, and platelet transfusion as necessary.

Some infants demonstrate a prompt response to supportive therapy with improvement of their general status. They are maintained without enteral intake and on gastric drainage, antibiotics, and parenteral nutrition support for 7 to 10 days. If serial abdominal radiographs demonstrate improvement of the pneumatosis and decreased distinction, nonoperative therapy can often be successful. Infants with evidence of free air on abdominal radiographs, abdominal wall erythema (consistent with perforation and abscess), and/or the presence of an abdominal mass require operative intervention. In addition, infants on nonoperative therapy who demonstrate progressive clinical deterioration characterized by shock, unstable vital signs, decreasing serial platelet counts, continued gross rectal bleeding, persistent acidosis, rising serum phosphorus levels, increasing abdominal distention, or the presence of turbid brown fluid containing bacteria on paracentesis (in instances with ascites) require operation. When an operation is necessary, these high-risk premature infants require expert pediatric anesthesia support and the availability of blood, platelets, and fresh frozen plasma in the operating theater.

At laparotomy, the surgical treatment of the patient is individualized according to the pathologic findings noted in each case. Patients with ischemic necrosis and perforation require bowel resection. The author has usually elected to create a temporary stoma to facilitate the procedure and control peritonitis. Extensive involvement from the duodenum to mid-transverse colon is observed in 15 per cent of patients. Under these dire circumstances, no resection is performed, the abdomen is closed, and supportive care is continued for 24 to 48 hours. If the infant improves, a second-look laparotomy is performed to observe any viable bowel. This procedure has been successful in a few patients. The majority of infants with extensive necrotizing enterocolitis succumb. Under very unusual circumstances when the ischemic involvement is limited to a short segment of bowel, a primary anastomosis may be considered.

Postoperative complications are common. These include further bowel necrosis, gram-negative sepsis, disseminated intravascular coagulation, wound infection and breakdown, cholestasis, short bowel syndrome, and severe malabsorption with dietary intolerance.[20,56] Intestinal stenosis may occur in the distal bowel following surgical management and may also be a complication of nonoperative management. Intestinal stricture following treatment of necrotizing enterocolitis is most likely due to mucosal destruction and healing by the formation of a circumferential cicatrix. Stenotic lesions are more commonly observed in the colon than in the small bowel. Recognition of this complication is very important, especially when a proximal stoma is in place and closure of the enterostomy is being considered. These patients should be evaluated preoperatively by a barium enema examination. Mortality varies according to treatment, severity and extent of disease, the presence of multiorgan failure, gestational age, birth weight, and the development of postoperative complications. Patients who respond to medical therapy are often less ill and have less disease. Surgically treated patients have already failed attempted medical therapy, which constitutes a more severe form of the disease. Survival after medical therapy is approximately 75 per cent but is only 50 to 60 per cent following surgical treatment. An increased mortality is observed in infants with birth weight less than 1000 gm., gestational age less than 29 weeks, an umbilical artery catheter, acidosis and/or poor urinary output, and abdominal wall erythema, or following treatment with aminophylline or caffeine

for apneic episodes and vitamin E for retrolental fibroplasia.[20] The presence of portal vein air is a sign of advanced disease and frequently is associated with rapid clinical deterioration.[20] Late complications are frequently noted and an additional 20 per cent of survivors of early therapy subsequently succumb to these problems. Long-term survivors continue to have problems with both motor and intellectual developmental delays, cerebral palsy, failure to thrive, below-level school performance, and attention deficits.

MALROTATION AND MIDGUT VOLVULUS

Anomalies of intestinal rotation follow failure of normal bowel rotation from the fifth to twelfth week of fetal development. The small bowel lacks appropriate fixation to the posterior wall, the cecum fails to migrate to the right lower quadrant, and the colon fails to attach to the lateral abdominal wall. This leads to a right upper abdominal position for the cecum, which may extend fixation bands across the duodenum and cause obstruction. The bowel hangs from a narrow pedicle based on the superior mesenteric artery and vein. Due to the presence of abnormal bands, the small bowel can twist in a clockwise direction, leading to volvulus of the midgut. Congenital diaphragmatic hernia, abdominal wall defects, duodenal atresia, and prune belly syndrome are conditions associated with anomalies of rotation and fixation.

Approximately a third of all cases of midgut volvulus occur in the first week of life, and 85 per cent of cases are recognized by 1 year of age. Infants usually present with the sudden onset of bilious vomiting and become seriously ill. If the condition is not recognized promptly, midgut infarction may ensue, leading to either death or the need for massive enterectomy. On physical examination, the abdomen may be tender and distended. Bilious material is usually observed when an orogastric tube is passed into the stomach. In some patients, bloody tissue can be passed per rectum. The plain abdominal radiograph may demonstrate an airless abdominal cavity beyond the level of the duodenum or many air-fluid levels. Both barium enema and upper gastrointestinal barium studies may prove useful in achieving a diagnosis. The barium enema documents the fact that the cecum is in an abnormal position in the upper abdomen. The upper gastrointestinal contrast study demonstrates obstruction at the level of the second to third portion of the duodenum at the point of volvulus around the superior mesenteric vessels ("corkscrew effect"). The infant is given intravenous antibiotics and fluid resuscitation with crystalloid solutions (lactated Ringer's solution). The patient is taken to the operating room on an emergent basis.

At the time of laparotomy, the volvulus is identified and reduced counterclockwise. Although the bowel may appear dusky, it often returns to a normal appearance. The use of a sterile intraoperative Doppler probe or fluorescein with a Wood's light may be useful in documenting the viability of the intestine. Obviously infarcted intestine is resected. Any fixation bands (Ladd's bands) from the abnormally located cecum across the duodenum or jejunum are divided, and the colon is moved to the left side of the abdomen with the cecum placed next to the sigmoid colon. The small bowel then falls straight down from the duodenum on the right side of the abdomen. An appendectomy is also performed because the cecum is located in an atypical position, making the diagnosis of possible appendiceal disease in the future difficult. If the viability of most of the bowel remains in question at the time of detorsion, the abdomen is closed and the patient given supportive therapy. A second-look procedure is performed at 24 to 36 hours to determine if the bowel is viable. The mortality for midgut volvulus remains high (18 to 25 per cent). Even those infants who can be salvaged may have significant morbidity since the short bowel syndrome may be a consequence of extensive bowel resection.[50] Because of the fact that midgut volvulus can occur at any time, when malrotation is identified either *de novo* or at the time of a laparotomy for another condition, a Ladd procedure and appendectomy should be performed.

ABDOMINAL WALL DEFECTS

Defects of the anterior abdominal wall (gastroschisis and omphalocele) represent a relatively common cause of admission to most major children's centers.

Omphalocele

An omphalocele is a covered defect of the umbilical ring into which abdominal contents herniate. The sac is composed of an outer layer of amnion and an inner layer of peritoneum. Omphalocele occurs in approximately 1 in 5000 births. There is a high incidence of associated anomalies. More than 50 per cent of the patients have other serious defects involving the alimentary tract and the cardiovascular, genitourinary, musculoskeletal, and central nervous systems. Many infants with omphalocele are premature. Others may be affected by a number of syndromes including the Beckwith-Wiedemann syndrome (gigantism, macroglossia, and an umbilical defect–umbilical hernia or omphalocele), chromosomal abnormalities (trisomy 13–15, 16–18), exstrophy of the bladder or cloaca, and the pentalogy of Cantrell (omphalocele, anterior diaphragmatic hernia, sternal cleft, ectopia cordis, and intracardiac defects, most commonly a ventricular septal defect and occasionally a diverticulum of the left ventricle). The size of the omphalocele defect varies from 2 to 10 cm. (Fig. 12). The smaller the defect, the better the prognosis. The contents of the sac may include only bowel; however, frequently the liver as well as the entire gastrointestinal tract is within the sac. The extra-abdominal location of the viscera *in utero* leads to a small abdominal cavity that may make attempts at primary repair difficult. In addition, malrotation is almost always present as a coexisting anomaly.

The emergency care of patients with omphalocele includes the insertion of an orogastric tube to decompress the stomach and prevent swallowed air from causing bowel distention, which may interfere with attempted reduction of the viscera at the time of repair. If the infant requires transfer to a tertiary high-risk pediatric center, the intact omphalocele sac should be kept covered with a sterile dressing and protected from injury and the patient transported in a thermally neutral environment. Excessively wet dressings may macerate the sac and also cause temperature loss by cooling and evaporative loss. Intravenous fluids (10 per cent dextrose in water with 0.25 per cent normal saline) and parenteral antibiotics are administered (ampicillin 100 mg. per kg. per day and gentamicin 5 mg. per kg. per day).

The patient's general condition should be carefully assessed in regard to cardiorespiratory status and the occurrence of additional anomalies. Since the viscera are covered by a physiologic sac, there are a number of options available regarding treatment. Operative management depends on the circumstances and the anatomy in each patient. Small defects (2 cm.) can be managed by direct primary closure of the abdominal wall. Medium to large defects may require a staged closure using a Dacron-reinforced Silastic silo as temporary housing for the bowel. The prosthesis is sutured to the edge of the defect with continuous 3-0 Prolene suture. The silo can gradually be reduced over 3 to 7 days and the baby returned to the operating room for closure of the abdominal wall. On rare occasions, when the defect is very large (greater than 10 cm.) or in cases of suspected chromosomal syndromes (trisomy 13, 18), conservative management using topical application of an escharotic agent is reasonable therapy. Topical therapy is also useful as a temporizing measure in a premature infant with an omphalocele and hyaline membrane disease or in heart failure. The definitive repair can be delayed until the infant's cardiopulmonary status is improved. Escharotic agents include 0.25 per cent mercurochrome and 0.5 per cent silver nitrate solution. Twice-daily application allows the sac to thicken and epithelialize. The overall survival for infants with omphalocele depends on the size of the defect, whether the infant is premature, if the sac ruptures, and how many associated anomalies coexist and of what severity they are. Infants with chromosomal syndromes and those with the pentalogy of Cantrell have a significant mortality. The overall mortality at the author's institution is 37 per cent.

Gastroschisis

Gastroschisis (Greek for belly cleft) is a defect of the anterior abdominal wall just lateral to the umbilicus. The defect is generally to the right of an intact umbilical cord. This anomaly is probably the result of a defect that occurs at the site where the second umbilical vein involutes. Unlike omphaloceles, there is no peritoneal sac so that antenatal evisceration of the bowel occurs through the defect during intrauterine life. The irritating effects of amniotic fluid (pH 7) on the exposed bowel wall leads to a chemical form of peritonitis characterized by a thick edematous membrane that is occasionally exudative. The exposed viscera may be congested and the bowel appears foreshortened (Fig. 13). Nonrotation always accompanies this condition. In contrast to omphalocele, the incidence of associated anomalies in patients with gastroschisis is relatively infrequent. The exception to this general observation is the occurrence of intestinal atresia, which may complicate gastroschisis in 10 to 15 per cent of patients. Atresia of the bowel is often due to intrauterine volvulus or an interruption of the blood supply to a segment of exposed intestine by compression in a very tight defect in the abdominal wall. The liver is almost never eviscerated; however, in young females occasionally the ovaries and fallopian tubes are found outside the defect. The sexes are equally affected, and 40 per cent of the patients are either premature or small for gestational age. Of interest is the fact that 20 to 25 per cent of the patients are born to unwed teenaged mothers.

Gastroschisis can frequently be detected on a prenatal ultrasound study. If possible, the pregnant woman should be referred to a high-risk obstetric unit with available neonatal intensive care facilities and pediatric surgical expertise. There is no evidence to suggest that early cesarean section improves the outcome. Spontaneous vaginal delivery is reasonable for these infants. When delivered, the infant with gastroschisis is subject to a variety of problems due to an increase in insensible losses related to exposure of the eviscerated bowel. Hypothermia, hypovolemia, and sepsis are the major problems to avoid. Significant "third space" fluid deficits occur as the result of sequestra-

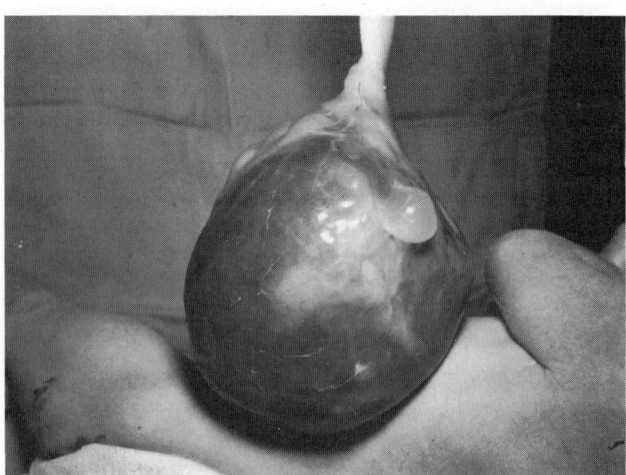

Figure 12. A large omphalocele containing the liver. (From Grosfeld, J. L., et al.: Contemporary management of abdominal wall defects. Surg. Clin. North Am., *61*:1037, 1981.)

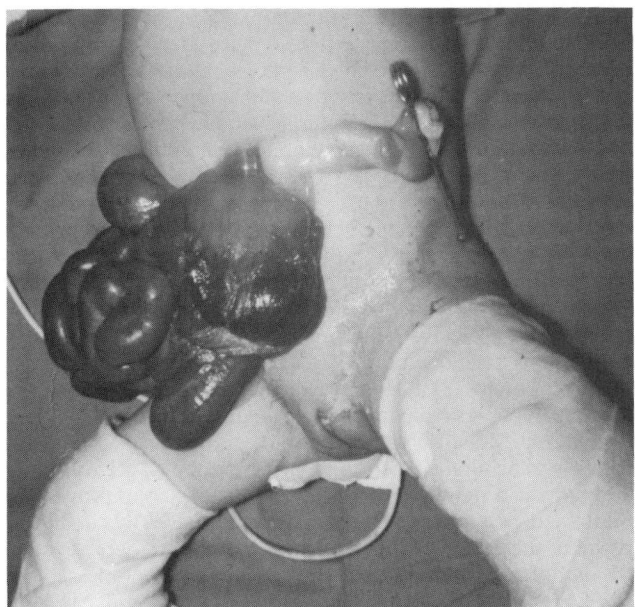

Figure 13. The typical appearance of an infant with gastroschisis. The viscera herniated *in utero* through a small defect in the abdominal wall just to the right of the umbilicus. (From Grosfeld, J. L., et al.: Contemporary management of abdominal wall defects. Surg. Clin. North Am., *61*:1037, 1981.)

tion of interstitial fluid. The lower half of the infant (including the eviscerated bowel) is placed into a sterile bowel bag. Fluid requirements are two and a half times that of a normal newborn in the first 24 hours of life. The infant is resuscitated with a bolus of 20 ml. per kg. of 10 per cent dextrose in lactated Ringer's solution given over 30 minutes. Additional fluid is administered until urinary output is established. Acid-base balance is closely monitored since metabolic acidosis is commonly observed owing to poor perfusion related to hypovolemia. An orogastric tube is placed in the stomach to prevent air swallowing and aspirate intestinal contents because the infant with gastroschisis has an associated adynamic ileus. The infant is given parenteral antibiotics (ampicillin and gentamicin). At operation, the abdominal wall and exposed viscera are prepared with an iodophor solution. The defect is enlarged 1 to 2 cm. in both a cephalad and caudad direction. The stomach contents are aspirated by the anesthesiologist, and meconium in the left colon is evacuated through the rectum by external compression of the viscera. The abdominal wall is manually stretched in order to enlarge the relatively small peritoneal cavity. Primary reduction of the viscera is attempted using a maximal ventilatory pressure of 35 cm. H_2O and Pao_2 as a guide and is successful in 70 per cent of patients. Abdominal closure is accomplished using one layer of through and through interrupted 3-0 polypropylene sutures. The umbilicus can be preserved for cosmetic purposes. Some infants, however, require a staged closure using a Dacron-reinforced Silastic silo as a temporary extra-abdominal housing. The viscera can be gradually reduced by gentle pressure starting on the second to third postoperative day. The silo can usually be removed and closure of the abdominal wall completed within a week in most patients. Antibiotics are discontinued when the silo is removed.

Owing to a prolonged adynamic ileus, most infants with gastroschisis require total parenteral nutrition for adequate caloric support. Total parenteral nutrition may be required for 3 to 4 weeks. Most infants tolerate oral intake by 3 weeks of age and can usually take all of their calories enterally by 1 month. In infants with an associated intestinal atresia, a temporary enterostomy is constructed at the time of the initial abdominal wall repair. Closure can be accomplished at a later date. Although a primary anastomosis can be performed, due to inflammatory changes in the bowel wall at birth, these are complicated by

stricture in a significant number of patients. Patients with atresia often have longer delays in gastrointestinal recovery and prolonged hospitalization. With appropriate neonatal resuscitation, surgical treatment, and nutritional support, the current survival in infants with gastroschisis is greater than 90 per cent.

SURGICALLY CORRECTABLE CAUSES OF RESPIRATORY DISTRESS

Congenital Diaphragmatic Hernia

Congenital posterolateral diaphragmatic hernia (foramen of Bochdalek) is a defect in the developing pleuroperitoneal fold through which the viscera ascend and enter the chest usually in the eighth to tenth week of fetal life. The herniated bowel acts as a space-occupying lesion and prevents normal lung development. The risk of occurrence is 1 in 2200 live births; males are more commonly affected. The infants are often full-term and weigh more than 3 kg. The defect is on the left side in 88 per cent of patients, on the right side in 10 per cent, and rarely bilateral (1 to 2 per cent).[27] The defect can be detected *in utero* by prenatal ultrasonography. Polyhydramnios may be noted and is a poor prognostic sign.[1] High-risk mothers are brought to a tertiary care obstetric center with the immediate availability of neonatal intensive care, pediatric surgical expertise, and resources for extracorporeal membrane oxygenation (ECMO). At birth, infants with diaphragmatic hernia develop symptoms of respiratory distress either in the delivery room or shortly thereafter as the bowel in the chest becomes distended with swallowed air. This further compresses the ipsilateral lung (which is often hypoplastic), and in addition causes a mediastinal shift interfering with ventilation of the contralateral lung. The infant appears dyspneic, tachypneic, and cyanotic and has severe retractions with an increased chest diameter and a relatively scaphoid abdomen. Bowel sounds may be heard on auscultation of the affected chest. Anteroposterior and lateral chest films demonstrate air-filled viscera in the chest, confirming the diagnosis (Fig. 14). The infant may have severe hypoxia and respiratory acidosis. A combined metabolic acidosis may also be present when insufficient tissue perfusion coexists with pulmonary embarrassment.

Treatment can be conveniently divided into three main areas: (1) stabilization and preoperative preparation, (2) operative treatment, and (3) postoperative respiratory, circulatory, metabolic, and nutritional support. Infants with diaphragmatic hernia should have direct endotracheal intubation and ventilatory support with high oxygen flow (Fio_2 of 1). The respiratory rate is set intentionally rapid to induce a respiratory alkalosis. Excessive ventilatory pressure should be avoided to reduce the risk of contralateral pneumothorax. An arterial catheter should be inserted in the right wrist to serially monitor preductal Pao_2, pH, and $Paco_2$. An umbilical artery catheter is a viable alternative and monitors postductal blood gas tensions. An orogastric tube is inserted to decompress the stomach and prevent further air from entering the gastrointestinal tract. If the infant becomes stabilized and demonstrates a Pao_2 greater than 100 mm. Hg and an arterial-alveolar gradient of less than 600 mm. Hg, operative correction of the defect is attempted. This is best accomplished by a transabdominal approach using a subcostal incision on the affected side.[27] The bowel is carefully reduced from the chest, avoiding injury to the spleen on the left side and the liver on the right side. Infants with diaphragmatic hernia have malrotation, and if coloduodenal or duodenojejunal bands are noted, a Ladd procedure should be performed. The hernia defect is evaluated, and the distal rim can usually be identified above the renal fossa. A chest tube is inserted under direct vision. Primary repair is accomplished when feasible using horizontal 3-0 or 2-0 nonabsorbable mattress sutures. If there is inadequate diaphragmatic tissue or an absent diaphragm, a syn-

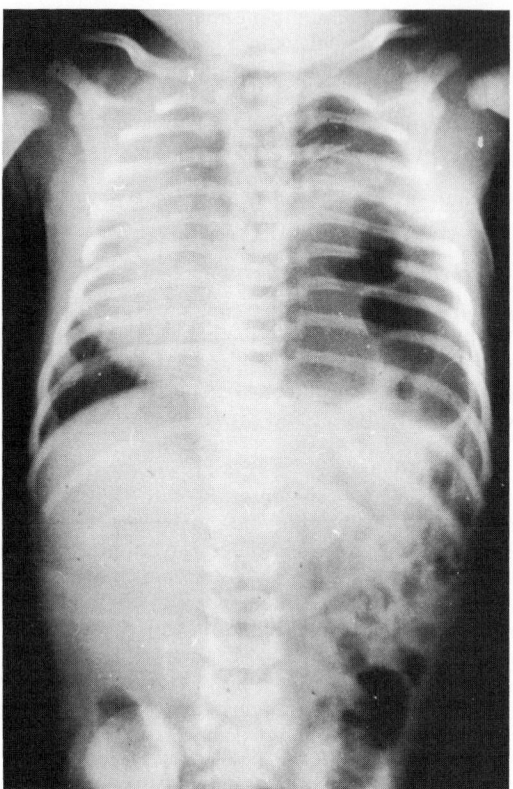

Figure 14. Chest film demonstrates bowel gas in the left chest consistent with the diagnosis of congenital diaphragmatic hernia.

thetic patch is necessary to reconstruct the barrier between the abdominal and thoracic cavities. The author prefers the use of a Gore-Tex patch. The abdomen is closed in layers if not excessively tight. In some instances, the abdominal cavity is extremely small and either an intentional ventral hernia with skin closure or application of a temporary Dacron-reinforced silastic housing may be necessary.

Postoperatively, the infant is monitored in the neonatal intensive care unit in a thermal neutral environment with the endotracheal tube in place and ventilation supported using an Fio_2 of 1, and maintaining the Pao_2 above 150 mm. Hg for a period of time. The infant is slowly weaned from high inspired oxygen requirements over a 48- to 72-hour period to avoid the "honeymoon" phenomenon with sudden pulmonary vasoconstriction and potentially lethal persistent pulmonary hypertension.

Unfortunately, few of the neonates with diaphragmatic hernia who present shortly after birth have this benign course. More often the babies have severe hypoxemia and some degree of hypercarbia that may not respond to mechanical ventilation or administration of pharmacologic agents such as prostaglandins, tolazoline, acetylcholine, and thorazine used to induce pulmonary vasodilation. The response to these agents has generally been disappointing. The survival has been less than 30 per cent and is even lower if polyhydramnios is observed (15 per cent).[1,27,57] Mortality is directly related to the degree of pulmonary hypoplasia (especially if the contralateral lung is also hypoplastic) and the presence of associated congenital anomalies including cardiac defects or chromosomal abnormalities. The advent of prenatal ultrasound and early recognition of the defect *in utero* allowing optimal prenatal and perinatal care has not improved the overall survival of these patients with conventional therapy.[1] In fact, the mortality appears to be increasing in many centers. This observation is probably related to early recognition (prenatal ultrasound), better neonatal transport services, and improved techniques of resuscitation allowing arrival

of patients with diaphragmatic hernia to a tertiary neonatal intensive care center prior to their demise. In Canada and certain centers in Europe, infants with diaphragmatic hernia are stabilized and observed on ventilator support (often using a high-frequency jet ventilator) for a 24-hour period. Only those infants who demonstrate adequate oxygenation (Pao_2 greater than 100 mm. Hg on Fio_2 of 1) and the ability to ventilate at the alveolar level of Pco_2 less than 60 mm. Hg are subjected to operative repair (approximately 50 per cent of the patients survive). In the United States, the rapid development of ECMO has led to a number of innovative clinical programs.[7,8] The infant who develops persistent pulmonary hypertension following an apparently successful repair of a diaphragmatic hernia ("the honeymoon phenomenon") can almost always be salvaged by the use of ECMO (Fig. 15). However, infants with severe pulmonary hypoplasia have not had the same postoperative benefits from ECMO and continue to have a high mortality.[1] More recently, placing the infant on ECMO preoperatively has been attempted.[7] When the infant's general condition improves, the infant can be successfully weaned from the ECMO circuit and repair of the defect can be performed. In other centers, repair of the diaphragmatic hernia is performed while the infant is still on the ECMO circuit. There have been some survivors in each clinical setting; however, not enough data are available for definitive recommendations at this time.

There is no doubt that ECMO has a significant role in the management of certain patients with diaphragmatic hernia but is not a panacea for all patients.[7,8] An oxygenation index (O.I.) greater than 40 has a mortality risk of 80 per cent and is an indication for ECMO (O.I. = MAP [mean airway pressure] × Fio_2 × 100/Pao_2) based on three of five postductal arterial blood gas determinations.[7] Gestational age under 34 weeks, intracranial hemorrhage, neurologic impairment, anomalies incompatible with a meaningful life expectancy, and irreversible lung disease are contraindications for ECMO. Although some patients with diaphragmatic hernia and presumed bilateral pulmonary hypoplasia, (e.g., Pao_2 less than 50 mm. Hg without adequate oxygenation during a honeymoon period) do not improve on ECMO, others surprisingly have survived, indicating that the criteria are not absolute. Recent reports indicate survival of 70 to 90 per cent using ECMO for all diaphragmatic hernia candidates who fail conventional treatment and have no

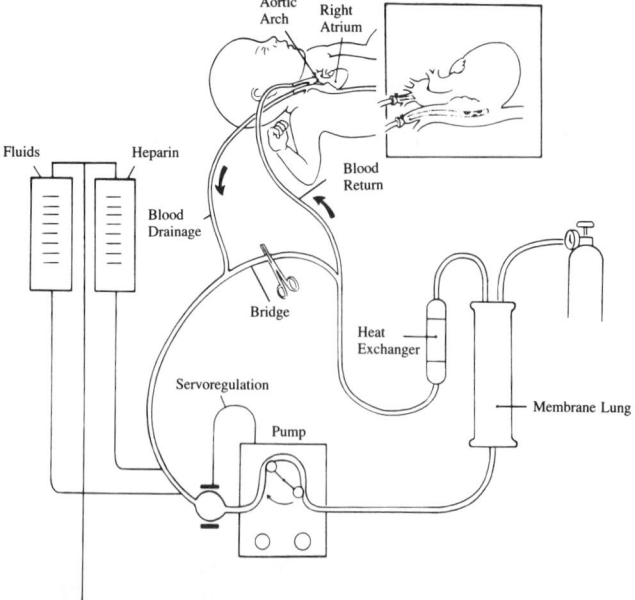

Figure 15. The ECMO circuit used for extracorporeal support in the neonatal unit. (From Bartlett, R. H.: Extracorporeal life support in neonatal respiratory failure. Surg. Rounds, *12*:41, 1989.)

other contraindications for life support therapy. The decision to employ ECMO must be individualized until more definitive and absolute criteria become available.

Prenatal intrauterine surgical repair of congenital diaphragmatic hernia with a live birth has been successfully accomplished by Harrison and co-workers.[57] However, this must be considered a courageous undertaking and remains an experimental program that has significant ethical overtones and cannot be routinely recommended.[57] In a smaller percentage of patients, the diagnosis of diaphragmatic hernia is not achieved until after the infant is 24 hours old. All of these patients should survive following successful repair without the need for ventilator support. Rare instances of delayed presentation of right diaphragmatic hernia are noted in association with beta-hemolytic streptococcal infection.[4,103] Some cases are not detected until later in infancy, presenting with failure to thrive, obstructive jaundice, and chronic recurring pulmonary symptoms.

There are other congenital abnormalities of the diaphragm that may also lead to respiratory compromise. These include anterior parasternal diaphragmatic hernia into the space of Larrey, commonly referred to as a *Morgagni hernia,* and *eventration of the diaphragm.* The Morgagni hernia is relatively uncommon in infants and children and usually presents with respiratory distress or abdominal or substernal pain due to entrapment of the transverse colon in the defect. In rare instances, there may be bilateral defects on either side of the sternum. Diagnosis can be suspected on the lateral chest film demonstrating an air-filled structure in the anterior mediastinum. This can be confirmed by ultrasound examination or a barium enema study demonstrating the colon in the chest. Repair is best accomplished through an abdominal approach. Eventration refers to a thin, floppy attenuation of the central portion of the diaphragm allowing the intra-abdominal viscera to push the diaphragm upward and encroach on the lung. This condition may occur *de novo,* but is more often a complication of phrenic nerve injury from a difficult breech delivery or is due to inadvertent trauma during the performance of congenital heart surgery. Atelectasis, tachypnea, dyspnea, and cyanosis may be noted. The elevated diaphragm alters the esophagogastric angle and may cause gastroesophageal reflux, vomiting, and aspiration pneumonia. Severe hypoxia may require intubation and ventilator support. When the infant is stable, plication of the eventrated diaphragm can be more safely accomplished on an elective basis with a thoracotomy. The infant can generally be extubated in the first 24 hours postoperatively.

Congenital Cystic Lung Disease

The lung is derived as an outpouching of the primitive foregut. A number of foregut malformations may present with severe respiratory distress. These include instances of congenital and acquired lobar emphysema, pulmonary sequestration, congenital cystic adenomatoid malformation, bronchogenic cyst, and enteric duplication.[27] *Lobar emphysema* presents in young infants in the first 4 to 5 months of life with an overdistended, hyperaerated lobe (usually upper or middle lobe) that compresses the ipsilateral lung causing atelectasis and leads to a shift of the mediastinum to the contralateral side. The treatment of choice is thoracotomy and lobectomy. *Sequestrations* may be *intralobar* (in older children) or *extralobar* (infants) and both have a systemic blood supply with direct arterial inflow from the aorta. Extralobar lesions drain into the azygous venous system and do not communicate with the lung, whereas intralobar lesions are within the lung tissue (lower lobes), drain through the pulmonary veins, and are associated with pulmonary infection. The arterial supply can be detected by ultrasonography and may arise from the subdiaphragmatic aorta. The treatment of choice is resection, which includes a lobectomy for intralobar lesions. *Congenital cystic adenomatoid malformations* have a "swiss cheese" appearance on chest films and a disproportion

of cartilaginous elements in relation to alveoli. Air is trapped in the lesion, causing overdistention and compression of normal tissues. One third of the patients are stillborn. Maternal polyhydramnios is often observed. Many of these lesions can be detected by prenatal ultrasonography. The infants can develop severe respiratory compromise shortly after birth with persistent pulmonary hypertension, and, in some instances, pulmonary hypoplasia may coexist. A few have been salvaged with ECMO after lobectomy failed to alleviate the respiratory distress. These observations indicate that these patients should be managed at high-risk obstetric and neonatal intensive care centers with immediate pediatric surgical expertise and ECMO resources available. *Bronchogenic cysts* are usually located near the bifurcation of the trachea and cause compression of the bronchus (most commonly on the left side). Diagnosis is achieved by chest radiography and ultrasonography. The treatment of choice is excision of the cyst. *Enteric cysts* of the esophagus can compress the trachea and in some instances may communicate with the tracheobronchial tree, the lung, or the spinal canal (neurenteric cyst). Rarely, hemorrhage into the tracheobronchial tree as a result of peptic ulceration from ectopic gastric mucosa in the cyst has been observed. Diagnosis is achieved with barium esophagram and ultrasonography. Extramucosal resection of the esophageal cyst is the operation of choice.

Other Causes

Congenital abnormalities of the oropharynx, nasopharynx, jaw, tongue, and trachea may also be the cause of respiratory distress, including micrognathia with Pierre Robin's and Stickler's syndromes; choanal atresia or stenosis; and hemangiomas, lymphangiomas, and teratomas of the pharynx or tongue that can cause obstruction of the airway. Tracheomalacia, subglottic stenosis, laryngotracheal clefts, and congenital tracheal stenosis are often important conditions to consider. The appropriate diagnosis can usually be made with a careful physical examination, laryngoscopy, and bronchoscopy.[27]

PYLORIC STENOSIS

Pyloric stenosis is a common condition in infancy of unknown etiology. This condition is hereditary and occurs in 1 in 750 births. It is far more common in males and often noted in the first-born son. Pyloric obstruction is the result of hypertrophy of the circular smooth muscle of the pylorus. The condition presents with progressive, often projectile, nonbilious vomiting following attempted feeding. The onset of vomiting usually begins between the second and third weeks of life and increases in frequency and force. The infant fails to gain weight and may actually lose weight. The number of bowel motions and times of voiding diminish. Eight per cent of patients have bloody gastric vomitus related to gastritis or esophagitis. Five to 8 per cent of patients are jaundiced owing to an elevation of indirect bilirubin as a result of decreased glucuronyl transferase levels caused by a lack of substrate delivered to the liver from limited caloric intake. On physical examination, visible gastric waves may be observed progressing across the upper abdomen from left to right during feedings. Diagnosis can be established by palpation of a pyloric mass (olive-shaped) in the midline, one third to one half the distance from the umbilicus to the xiphoid when the stomach is empty. This is best accomplished while offering the infant an oral feeding of dextrose and water. If the "olive" cannot be palpated, an ultrasound examination may demonstrate an elongated pyloric channel (greater than 15 mm.) and thickened muscle wall (greater than 3.5 mm.). If the ultrasound study is not diagnostic, a barium contrast study is obtained to evaluate the pylorus as well as other possible causes of nonbilious vomiting. The gastrointestinal series may demonstrate an elongated pylorus with an antral shoulder and either a single string sign or a double railroad tract sign consistent with pyloric stenosis. The differential diagnosis includes pylorospasm, milk allergy, hiatal hernia, pyloric duplication, prepyloric antral web, gastroesophageal reflux, adrenogenital syndrome (salt-losing type), and certain aminoacidurias associated with electrolyte derangements and gastric waves. If the diagnosis is made early in the course of the illness (prior to the onset of dehydration), operative correction can be accomplished without excessive preparation. Infants with prolonged vomiting, however, may present with dehydration associated with hypochloremic alkalosis. Hypokalemia may coexist as a result of excessive urinary losses of K^+. Serum pH, electrolytes, blood urea nitrogen, urinary output and specific gravity, and the infant's weight should be carefully evaluated.

Pyloric stenosis is never a surgical emergency, but may be a medical emergency requiring aggressive intravenous resuscitation in the dehydrated infant and the occasional patient with peripheral collapse and shock due to severe hypovolemia. Dehydration and metabolic derangements must be corrected prior to operation. Percutaneous insertion of a scalp vein (23-gauge) or a short Silastic (22-gauge) intravenous catheter is used to administer parenteral fluid therapy. Cutdown by venesection is almost never required. The infant receives no oral intake and the stomach is emptied of old formula and retained secretions using a No. 10 French orogastric tube. In the infant with severe dehydration, an initial fluid infusion of 20 ml. per kg. of 5 per cent dextrose in 0.9 per cent (normal) saline or 5 per cent plasmanate (colloid) is rapidly administered over a 30-minute period. This volume load usually stabilizes the infant and improves renal plasma flow. The infusion is then continued with 5 per cent dextrose in 0.45 per cent saline at a rate of 200 ml. per kg. per day for an 8-hour period. Potassium (3 to 4 mEq. per kg. per day) is added when urinary output is established. A safe rate of K^+ infusion is 4 mEq. per 100 ml. of infusate (40 mEq. per liter). After the first 8 hours, the intravenous infusion rate is reduced slightly to 125 to 150 ml. per kg. per day for the next 16 hours. Patients with mild isotonic dehydration can be safely prepared with an infusion of 5 per cent dextrose in 0.25 per cent saline at a rate of 125 ml. per kg. per day. All but the most severely depleted infants are usually ready for operation after 24 hours of fluid therapy. In the past decade, it has not been found necessary to use ammonium chloride to correct the alkalosis. Operation may be safely performed when the pH is less than 7.5, serum chloride is greater than 88 mEq. per liter, serum CO_2-combining power is less than 30 mEq. per liter, serum potassium is greater than 3.2 mEq. per liter, urinary output is satisfactory (1 to 2 ml. per kg. per hour), and specific gravity is less than 1.020.

A No. 10 or No. 12 French orogastric catheter or sump drainage tube is inserted just prior to the anticipated operation to empty the stomach and diminish the risk of aspiration. The infant is similarly intubated awake to prevent possible aspiration because of gastric outlet obstruction. General endotracheal anesthesia is employed. Operation is performed through a small transverse right upper abdominal incision made over the oblique muscles and the lateral border of the rectus muscle, which is retracted medially. The stomach is mobilized and the pylorus is brought into the wound. Pyloromyotomy (Ramstedt-Fredet procedure) is accomplished by an incision on the relatively avascular anterior surface of the white glistening "pyloric tumor," starting at the pyloric vein (pyloroduodenal line) distally and extending proximally onto the normal prepyloric antrum. Downward pressure over the incision site using the back of the scalpel handle will split the muscle. Gentle spreading of the thick, hypertrophic circular muscle with a hemostat or pyloric spreader allows the submucosa and mucosa to protrude and relieve the obstruction. Independent motion of the two sides of the divided pyloric muscle indicates an adequate pyloromyotomy. If the distal extent of the incision is at the pyloroduodenal line, entry into the duodenum is avoided. If entry does occur, the opening is sutured with 4-0 Vicryl and then covered with omentum. Closure of the abdomen is accomplished in layers of continuous 4-0 Vicryl. A 4-0 white Vicryl subcuticular suture is used to appose the skin edges, which may be sealed and supported with either collodion or Steri-Strips.

Postoperatively, the patient is placed in a crib with the head elevated at a 30-degree angle. The orogastric tube is maintained on suction for 6 hours and then removed and feeding is initiated. In cases in which intraoperative duodenal entry occurred, feedings are withheld for 24 hours. Feedings are started by offering 15 ml. (½ ounce) of Pedialyte every 2 hours for two feedings. If tolerated, feedings are advanced to 15 ml. of half-strength (10 calories per ounce) formula every 2 hours for two feedings. The volume of intake is increased to 30 ml. (1 ounce) of half-strength formula every 3 hours. On the following day the concentration of the formula is increased to full strength (20 calories per ounce), which is offered every 3 hours. An intravenous infusion is kept in place, using 5 per cent dextrose in 0.25 per cent saline at a rate of 100 ml. per kg. per day for the first 24 to 36 hours to prevent hypoglycemia and dehydration if the early feedings are not well tolerated. Early postoperative vomiting is not uncommon but is usually self-limited. If repeated vomiting occurs, an orogastric tube is reinserted and the stomach gently lavaged with normal saline or 5 per cent sodium bicarbonate. Feedings are then resumed. If the infant was breast-fed prior to operation, nursing may be resumed on the second day. If feedings are well tolerated, the volume of full-strength formula is advanced and the infant is usually discharged on the second postoperative day. Pyloromyotomy is one of the most gratifying of all surgical procedures. The infant rapidly resumes an adequate caloric intake and gains weight to the delight of both parents and physician. The expected morbidity is quite low (occasional wound infection), and mortality should be zero.

GASTROESOPHAGEAL REFLUX

In the past decade, gastroesophageal reflux (GER) has become one of the most common clinical conditions managed by pediatric surgeons. The largest group of patients with clinically symptomatic GER are infants and children with neurologic impairment; more than 70 per cent of GER cases are reported in this impaired patient population. Infants with apnea and bradycardia and children with chronic pulmonary conditions due to asthma, bronchopulmonary dysplasia, and cystic fibrosis represent an additional group of patients with significant GER. Many of these children receive bronchodilator medications (e.g., aminophylline) that reduce the lower esophageal sphincter pressure and may lead to active GER. Choking, asthmalike symptoms, coughing at night, and recurring episodes of pneumonia related to aspiration of gastric contents are being recognized with an increasing frequency as symptoms of GER. Dysfunction of the lower esophageal sphincter may also be observed in children with scleroderma, familial dysautonomia, Cornelia de Lange's syndrome, dystrophia myotonia, and nemaline myopathy of infancy. GER has also been implicated as an etiologic factor in the sudden infant death syndrome.[6,17,94] High risk for GER is found in those infants with congenital anomalies including esophageal atresia with or without tracheoesophageal fistula and following repair of omphalocele and gastroschisis where the tight closure of the abdominal wall is associated with increased abdominal pressure. GER is also common in disorders associated with diaphragmatic distortion such as eventration, diaphragmatic hernia, and severe elevation due to a large upper abdominal mass that may alter the esophagogastric angle. Dysfunction of the lower esophageal sphincter, reduced length of the sphincter, disordered esophageal motility, poor esophageal clearance, and delayed gastric emptying all have a role in the severity of the symptoms.[11,25,94]

The common presenting findings of symptomatic GER include failure to thrive, vomiting, and repeated episodes of respiratory infection due to aspiration of gastric contents. Diagnosis can be achieved by a number of tests including barium esophagram with fluoroscopic control, lower esophageal sphincter manometrics, gastric scintigraphy, 24-hour pH-probe measurements, and esophagoscopy. Delayed gastric emptying is observed in 25 to 50 per cent of patients.[35,64,65,94] This is documented with a quantitative gastric scintiscan using radiolabeled scrambled eggs in older children and labeled thickened formula in infants. Medical therapy includes the administration of antacids, H_2-blockers, and parasympathomimetic agents (bethanechol, metoclopramide). Keeping infants in a head-up position on an incline board reduces the risk of reflux. In infants, small frequent feedings and occasionally nasojejunal feedings are useful. Prospective randomized double-blind studies evaluating the effects of parasympathomimetic medications unfortunately demonstrate little benefit.[36,92] Indications for operative intervention include continued failure to thrive, persistent vomiting, repeated episodes of respiratory infection, and the presence of Barrett's esophagus, esophagitis (with blood-tinged or coffee-ground vomitus), and stricture. Simultaneous demonstration of decreased esophageal pH (less than 4) associated with apnea and bradycardic episodes is also an indication for fundoplication in these patients.

A number of antireflux operations are used to treat GER. These include the Nissen fundoplication procedure (360-degree wrap), Thal procedure, Dor modification of the Nissen procedure (270 degrees), Hill repair, and anterior plication of Boix-Ochoa.[5,11,35] The most popular antireflux operation is the Nissen fundoplication procedure. This is constructed using a short-floppy gastric wrap (no longer than 3 cm. in length) performed over the largest size esophageal dilator that safely fits within the lumen of the intra-abdominal portion of the esophagus at the time the sutures are inserted. Suture placement is important and requires a healthy seromuscular bite of stomach (using 3-0 silk in neonates and 2-0 silk in older infants, children, and teenagers), a bite of the anterior wall of the esophageal smooth muscle (avoiding esophageal lumen entry), and then another healthy bite on the wrapped portion of the gastric fundus. Heavy sutures are necessary to prevent wrap breakdown. In some cases, one or two short gastric vessels must be divided to acquire a tension-free wrap. The vagus nerves are carefully preserved to avoid postoperative gastric atony. If the crura of the hiatus were dissected to free the distal intra-abdominal esophagus, these should be carefully reapproximated with interrupted 2-0 silk suture in infants and 0-silk in older children to prevent herniation of the fundic wrap into the mediastinum.[26] If delayed gastric emptying is identified preoperatively, a concomitant pyloroplasty is performed.[35,94] The author prefers a one-layer technique using a Gambee stitch of 4-0 interrupted silk in infants and 3-0 silk in older children. The sutures are left long, and a portion of omentum is placed over the pyloroplasty site and tied. In patients with severe neurologic impairment and swallowing disorders, a gastrostomy tube is inserted for feeding purposes. In otherwise normal children the gastrostomy is omitted. Both clinical and laboratory evidence is available that indicates that a Stamm gastrostomy placed along the anterior gastric wall near the greater curvature results in GER.[15,93,94] This has been documented in many patients in whom a gastrostomy was initially performed for feeding purposes only to be followed by severe postoperative vomiting due to GER. The incidence of postgastrostomy GER is similar after percutaneous endoscopically placed gastrostomy tubes as well, indicating that fixation of the stomach to the anterior abdominal wall is responsible for this event.[93] These observations strongly suggest that a complete work-up to evaluate both the esophagus and stomach should be done prior to the performance of feeding gastrostomy. Recent information suggests that a gastrostomy placed along the lesser curvature avoids the complication of GER postoperatively.

The success rate of antireflux procedures is in the 90th per-

centile. Significant complications are observed in 16 per cent of patients.[26] The complication rate is significantly higher in infants and children with neurologic impairment and in patients with esophageal atresia. The most frequent complications involve the wrap (8 per cent) itself, with wrap breakdown or herniation into the mediastinum being most common. Postoperative small bowel obstruction occurs in 4 per cent of patients. Of interest is that some of these events are related to postoperative small bowel intussusception rather than adhesions.[26] Wound infection, dehiscence, inadvertent splenectomy, and pancreatitis have also been documented as complications of fundoplication. Gagging, gas-bloat syndrome, and early satiety are postprandial problems that may be related to disordered gastric motility.[35,64,94] In some instances, significant delays in gastric emptying can be documented by gastric scintigraphy, and these postoperative symptoms have been ameliorated by performance of an emptying procedure (pyloroplasty). These observations further indicate the importance of a complete preoperative work-up of patients with feeding disorders and GER. In children with recurrent symptoms of GER due to wrap breakdown, a second Nissen fundoplication procedure has the same success rate as a primary procedure (greater than 90 per cent).[26] It is, therefore, reasonable to recommend reoperation in these cases. Multiple failures of a Nissen fundoplication procedure (more than three) usually require resection of the lower esophagus and jejunal interposition.

INTUSSUSCEPTION

Intussusception is a relatively frequent cause of intestinal obstruction in infancy and early childhood. More than 50 per cent of cases are observed between the ages of 3 months and 1 year and 80 per cent by 2 years. Intussusception is more common in males and most are well nourished and otherwise healthy infants.[139] The exception is the child with cystic fibrosis who may fail to thrive or as a sequela of Henoch-Schönlein purpura. Approximately 30 per cent of cases follow an episode of viral gastroenteritis or an upper respiratory infection. The clinical presentation of intussusception typically includes the sudden onset of abdominal pain (85 per cent) characterized by episodic screaming and drawing the legs up. This may be followed by vomiting (60 per cent), which initially may be clear but eventually becomes bilious in nature as obstruction progresses. The appearance of blood in the stool is a common finding and may vary from occult blood to bright red bleeding with the classic description of currant-jelly stool consisting of blood mixed with mucus being the most common observation. On physical examination, the abdomen is often distended, the right lower quadrant may feel empty, and a sausage-shaped mass may be palpable in the upper right to midabdomen (65 per cent). The intussusceptum may occasionally be palpated on rectal examination. The child may appear gravely ill if symptoms are present for more than 24 to 48 hours, sometimes mimicking the symptoms of meningitis. The child is often febrile and has a leukocytosis. Plain erect and recumbent radiographs of the abdomen may demonstrate dilated loops of small intestine, air-fluid levels, or a soft tissue mass effect in the right upper quadrant. A diagnostic barium enema may demonstrate the intussusceptum with a coil-spring sign at the point of bowel invagination (Fig. 16).

The infant with intussusception is managed by insertion of a nasogastric tube, intravenous fluid resuscitation, and antibiotics. After rehydration, the child is taken to the radiology suite for an attempted hydrostatic reduction of the intussusception. A sedative should be administered prior to the examination when hypovolemia has been corrected. The surgical staff should be in attendance for the attempted reduction with the anesthesiologist and operating room staff alerted and standing by should reduction by unsuccessful. A hydrostatic barium enema has been the mainstay of nonoperative treatment. The enema is

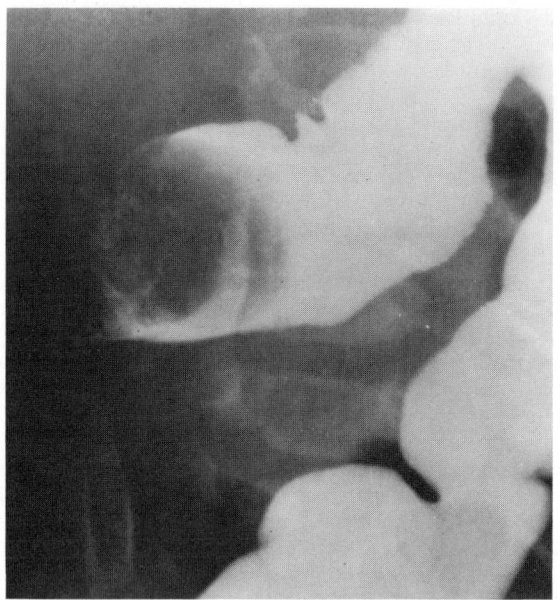

Figure 16. Barium enema in an infant with idiopathic ileocolic intussusception demonstrates the intussusceptum in the right upper quadrant.

performed with a 3-foot column and limitation of continuous hydrostatic pressure to 5-minute time frames.[139] Reduction is considered satisfactory when the intussusceptum is reduced through the ileocecal valve and the contrast material refluxes into multiple small bowel loops. Recently, air reduction of intussusception has been performed successfully in a large number of patients in China.[55] This technique is now being performed in the United States and Canada, and early reports suggest this technique is as effective as barium enema reduction. The air pressure must be monitored with a maximum of 110 mm. Hg in children and 80 mm. Hg in infants. The procedure is also monitored under fluoroscopic control, and two to three attempts at reduction can be safely performed. The perforation rate is similar to that observed with hydrostatic barium enema. This generally occurs in the uninvolved intussuscipiens. Perforation occurs more commonly in infants less than 6 months of age with symptoms present for more than 3 days.[30]

The rate of successful reduction varies from center to center but is 50 to 75 per cent.[31,139] Some centers do not attempt reduction if the infant has symptoms for greater than 72 hours and has a severe obstructive bowel pattern on plain abdominal films. Unsuccessful reduction is followed by laparotomy through a right lower quadrant transverse abdominal incision. The intussusception is identified, and manual reduction is attempted using a milking technique to squeeze the mass retrograde through the ileocecal valve. Following reduction, an appendectomy is performed and, when present, a Jackson's veil is divided. This band of tissue tends to draw the terminal ileum toward the cecum. Recurrence of intussusception after barium or air reduction is between 8 and 12 per cent, whereas recurrence following surgical reduction is extremely rare. Failure of manual reduction often is a sign of bowel necrosis. Reduction attempts should cease when bowel wall muscle splitting is noted to avoid intraoperative perforation and soiling. Bowel resection is required in 37 to 41 per cent of patients. Although performance of a primary anastomosis in obstructed unprepared bowel is controversial, many cases have been performed successfully. In the presence of bowel obstruction with severe distention or in those cases complicated by perforation and barium peritonitis, resection should be followed by formation of a temporary enterostomy. Intussusception in older children may be due to a pathologic lead point. These cases include instances of B cell lymphoma, Peutz-Jeghers polyps, inversion of a

Meckel's diverticulum, submucosal hemangioma, carcinoid tumor, juvenile polyposis coli, and *Ascaris lumbricoides* worm infestation.

Postoperative complications include prolonged adynamic ileus, fever, wound infection, pneumonitis, urinary tract infection, enterostomy stenosis, wound dehiscence, and subhepatic abscess. Despite considerable morbidity, in recent studies mortality has been zero.[139] A high index of suspicion, early recognition, and diagnostic barium enema often allow a prompt diagnosis and nonoperative reduction. When symptoms have been present for more than 72 hours and a severe obstructive pattern is noted on the plain abdominal radiograph, a low success rate with hydrostatic reduction might be anticipated. In these cases, confirmation of the diagnosis is suggested with a gentle barium enema and prompt operation without attempted hydrostatic reduction.

MECKEL'S DIVERTICULUM

Meckel's diverticulum is the most common form of persistent vitelline duct remnant. The diverticulum occurs on the antimesenteric border of the ileum usually within 60 cm. of the ileocecal valve and contains all layers of the intestinal wall. Other vitelline duct anomalies include a persistent vitelline duct (which presents at the umbilicus as a draining fistula), a fibrous band connecting the ileum to the undersurface of the umbilicus, a patent vitelline sinus beneath the umbilicus and an obliterated bowel portion, and a vitelline duct cyst (Fig. 17). Ectopic tissue is

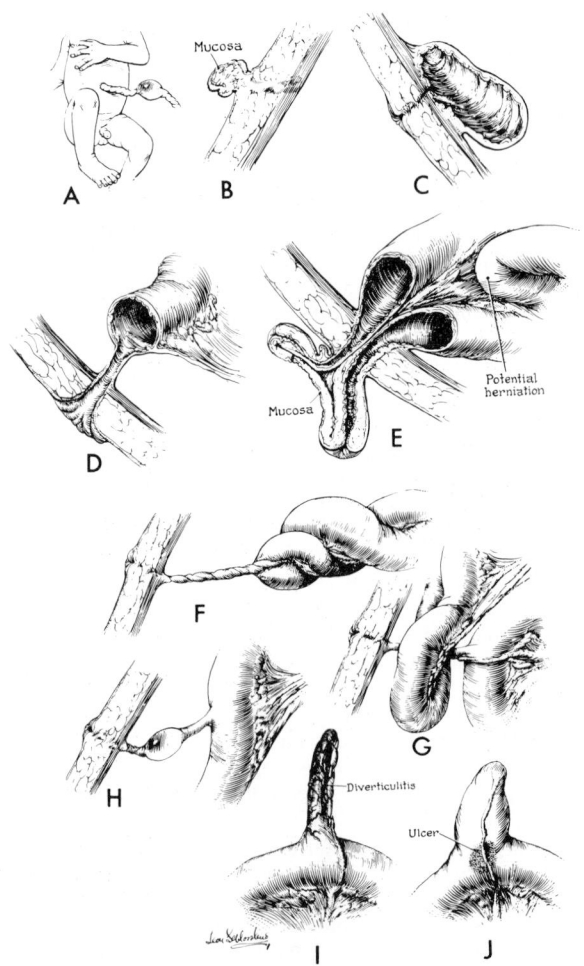

Figure 17. Variants of a persistent vitelline duct. The most common variant is a Meckel's diverticulum. (From Ravitch, M. M.: In Rhoads, J. E., et al.: Surgery: Principles and Practice. 4th ed. Philadelphia, J. B. Lippincott Co., 1970.)

frequently noted in these lesions (gastric, pancreatic). Ectopic gastric mucosa is most common and is responsible for the most frequent complication of this anomaly — peptic ulceration with hemorrhage (22 per cent).[132] Other complications include inflammation (2 per cent), bowel obstruction due to internal hernia around a vitelline duct band (13 per cent), intussusception (with Meckel's diverticulum acting as a lead point; less than 1 per cent), and a T-shaped prolapse of both efferent and afferent intestine through a persistent vitelline duct fistula at the umbilicus in the neonate (less than 1 per cent). Hemorrhage is related to peptic ulceration occurring at the margin of ectopic gastric mucosa with ileal mucosa. Hemorrhage from a Meckel's diverticulum presents as painless rectal bleeding that is often significant. The hemoglobin is often less than 8 gm. per 100 ml., and frequently blood transfusion is required. Spontaneous cessation of bleeding is customary; however, life-threatening hemorrhage may occur.

Diagnostic evaluation of a patient with a suspected bleeding Meckel's diverticulum should begin with a ^{99m}technetium-pertechnetate scan (Fig. 18). This isotope is picked up by gastric mucosa and may be enhanced by giving the infant cimetidine and pentagastrin prior to the test. Ectopic mucosa is also present in intestinal duplications, a lesion that must be included in the differential diagnosis. Barium studies are usually unrewarding. A visceral angiogram may occasionally be useful when the rate of bleeding is greater than 1 ml. per minute. The treatment of choice is resection of the Meckel's diverticulum. This can be accomplished by a wedge excision, bowel resection, and anastomosis or by use of a stapling device.[132] In some patients, a primitive persistent right vitelline artery originating from the mesentery supplies the diverticulum and must be identified and ligated. Instances of bowel obstruction may be related to a volvulus around a persistent vitelline band or under a persistent vitelline artery leading to bowel infarction. These patients often present with fever, leukocytosis, and sepsis. In addition to this type of occurrence, cases of inflammation and perforation are also treated with antibiotics (ampicillin, gentamicin, and clinda-

mycin). All of these complications of vitelline duct anomalies usually require resection and bowel anastomosis.

MESENTERIC AND OMENTAL CYSTS

Both mesenteric and omental cysts are probably the result of an abnormality of the lymphatic system. These cysts have a fibrous wall that is lined by a single layer of endothelial cells and have small lymphatic spaces. In most patients, omental cysts are detected in the first few years of life and present with an asymptomatic large abdominal mass. Omental cysts are often located anteriorly and displace the stomach posteriorly. Almost all omental cysts are serous and contain clear straw-colored fluid of low specific gravity. Mesenteric cysts may be single or multiple and can occur anywhere in the abdominal cavity. Patients with mesenteric cysts frequently present with abdominal pain, vomiting, abdominal distention, and evidence of intestinal obstruction due to volvulus around the cysts. Sudden enlargement has been observed after relatively minor episodes of blunt abdominal trauma leading to hemorrhage into the mesenteric cyst. The most common sites include the ileal mesentery, lesser sac, and jejunal mesentery. Those cysts affecting the small bowel may be chylous, whereas most mesenteric cysts involving the colon are serous. Diagnosis is easily achieved with an abdominal ultrasound examination, which demonstrates a large unilocular or septated nonspecific sonolucent cystic mass with a smooth wall. The treatment of choice is resection of the cyst. In some instances, this requires resection of the cyst with a segment of intestine because of adherence of the cyst wall and the adjacent bowel.

ENTERIC DUPLICATIONS

Enteric duplications are relatively rare anomalies that can occur anywhere in the alimentary tract from the mouth to the anus. The most common site is the small intestine. Enteric duplications share a common mesenteric blood supply and bowel wall with the normal intestine. These lesions may be cystic or tubular and in 20 per cent of cases communicate with the normal intestine. The duplication cyst may contain ectopic gastric mucosa and in some instances pancreatic tissue as well. Clinical presentation includes a shifting abdominal mass (due to its mesenteric attachment) that may be palpated in different areas of the abdomen at separate examinations. Symptoms include cramping abdominal pain or vomiting due to compression of the normal bowel by the duplication cyst. In some instances, the presenting finding is melena related to hemorrhage from peptic ulceration due to ectopic gastric mucosa in the duplication that communicates with the normal bowel. An ultrasound examination of the abdomen detects a cystic mass and a ^{99m}technetium-pertechnetate scintiscan demonstrates the presence of ectopic gastric tissue. The therapy of choice is resection of the duplication cyst. This may require resection of the involved segment of normal intestine. In long tubular duplications, the mucosal lining may be stripped to remove potential sites of ectopic mucosa and the duplication joined side-to-side with the normal bowel to obviate the need for extensive bowel resection. A similar technique can be used for duodenal duplications to avoid the necessity of a pancreatoduodenectomy. A blind loop syndrome due to bacterial overgrowth in a tubular duplication that communicates proximally but not distally may also occur. This unusual occurrence may be detected with the use of a diagnostic small bowel barium enteroclysis.

INTESTINAL POLYPS

A number of polypoid conditions may affect the alimentary tract of children. These include juvenile polyps of the colon, Peutz-Jehgers syndrome with hamartomatous polyps, Cronk-

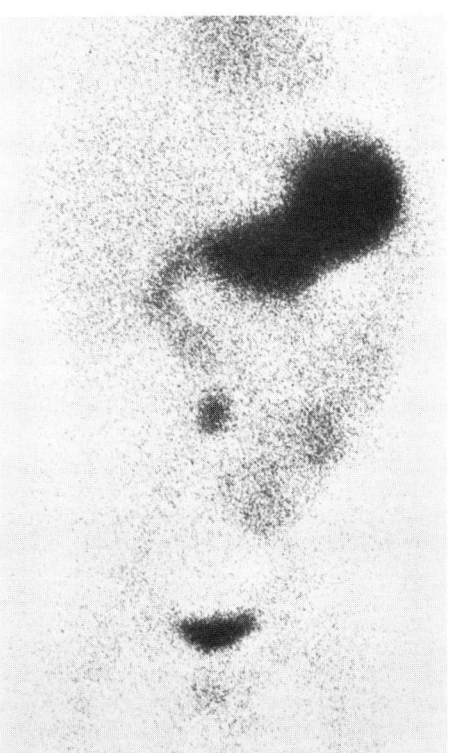

Figure 18. ^{99m}Technetium scintiscan identifies an area of lower abdominal isotope pickup consistent with ectopic gastric mucosa in a Meckel's diverticulum.

hite-Canada syndrome, familial polyposis, Gardner's syndrome, Turcot's syndrome, and generalized juvenile polyposis coli.

Juvenile polyps are the most frequent polyps noted in children. These present between the ages of 4 and 14 years. These polyps are inflammatory in nature and have a cystic component. The polyp may contain eosinophils, which may implicate an allergenic cause. The most common symptom is rectal bleeding. In some patients, a polyp with a long stalk can prolapse out the rectum with a bowel motion. The most accurate method of diagnosis is by proctosigmoidoscopy, which detects 85 per cent of cases. In more than 80 per cent, the polyp is solitary. Multiple polyps may occur, and an air contrast barium enema and colonoscopy should be performed to determine the exact site of the polyps. The natural history of most juvenile polyps is autoamputation and spontaneous involution. Very few require treatment except for those associated with significant bleeding, cramping abdominal pain from intussusception, and recurring prolapse. In most, polypectomy can be accomplished with the use of the sigmoidoscope or colonoscope without the need for laparotomy. Children with familial generalized juvenile polyposis coli have a myriad of polyps throughout the entire colon and present with failure to thrive, anemia, hypoproteinemia, and hypokalemia from rectal bleeding and loss of mucus rich in protein and potassium. These children require abdominal colectomy and ileorectal anastomosis. Proctoscopy is performed every 6 months to evaluate the rectal segment for polyps. Although juvenile polyposis is not a premalignant condition, recurring rectal polyps may require resection of the rectal mucosa and an ileoanal pull-through procedure in the future. Unlike solitary juvenile polyps, in children with generalized polyposis the polyps persist into adult life and may involve the small intestine. The other polypoid conditions noted are covered extensively elsewhere in this text.

BILIARY TRACT DISORDERS

Cholestasis in Infancy

Neonatal jaundice is a common occurrence and is considered a physiologic event following immaturity of the enzyme glucuronyl transferase. Appropriate delivery of substrate (caloric intake) to drive the enzyme system usually resolves the jaundice in a week to 10 days. The elevation in serum bilirubin is almost entirely due to increase in the indirect unconjugated fraction. Jaundice persisting more than 2 weeks following birth must be considered pathologic and is accompanied by an elevation of the direct fraction (conjugated) of bilirubin (greater than 2 mg. per 100 ml.), indicating some form of cholestatic syndrome or obstruction. Infants with hepatic dysfunction are at risk for developing sequelae from cholestasis regardless of its etiology. A prompt evaluation of the cause of jaundice is required.

The differential diagnosis of persistent jaundice includes a wide spectrum of disorders including breast milk jaundice, Rh and ABO incompatibilities, hemolytic disease (hereditary spherocytosis), Gilbert's disease, and Crigler-Najjar syndrome where the indirect unconjugated bilirubin fraction is elevated (greater than 80 per cent). Those patients in whom more than 20 per cent of the total bilirubin is direct have either cholestasis or obstruction; and these cases include metabolic conditions (tyrosinemia, Gaucher's disease, galactosemia, cystic fibrosis, hypothyroidism, iron storage disease, infantile copper overload, fructosemia, and alpha$_1$-antitrypsin deficiency), infectious agents (cytomegalovirus, herpesvirus, rubella virus, hepatitis B virus, varicella, coxsackievirus, echovirus, toxoplasmosis, and syphilis), sepsis, total parenteral nutrition, intrahepatic disorders (idiopathic neonatal hepatitis, intrahepatic cholestasis due to arteriohepatic dysplasia [Alagille's syndrome], Byler's disease, Zellweger's syndrome, and absence of bile ductules),

and those conditions that affect the extrahepatic biliary tree leading to obstruction (biliary atresia, biliary hypoplasia, bile duct stenosis, spontaneous perforation of the bile duct, inspissated bile syndrome).

A number of tests are available to separate some of the causes of cholestasis from obstructive jaundice. The presence of bile in the duodenal aspirate, green- or brown-colored stool, sweat chloride determination, thyroxine and thyroid-stimulating hormone levels, cultures, TORCH screen and VDRL titers, metabolic screen for aminoacidurias, evaluation of urine-reducing substances, and normal alpha$_1$-antitrypsin level eliminate most causes of cholestasis that do not require surgical intervention. Most infants with biliary atresia have persistent and progressive jaundice associated with elevation of the serum alkaline phosphatase levels. Hepatomegaly is the most common finding on physical examination. The liver is often quite firm on palpation. Splenomegaly is also noted but in slightly older infants (more than 6 weeks). Ascites and the presence of prominent venous patterning on the abdominal wall above the level of the umbilicus is usually a sign of more advanced liver disease (with portal hypertension) and is less common in infants evaluated in the first 6 weeks to 2 months of life. The stools are acholic and the urine may appear dark and contains bile but no urobilinogen.

None of the clinical findings and tests currently available for evaluation of infants with biliary atresia are pathognomonic. The tests simply indicate instances of obstruction. Ultrasound examination of the biliary tree may demonstrate the presence of a gallbladder or rarely a choledochal cyst; neither of these findings, however, excludes biliary atresia. The intrahepatic bile ducts are never enlarged in cases of biliary atresia. In a jaundiced infant with elevated direct bilirubin fraction, acholic stools, and a negative duodenal aspirate, a ^{99m}Tc-DISIDA (^{99m}technetium–diisopropyl iminodiacetic acid) scintiscan should be obtained. If the radioisotope appears in the intestine, obstruction can be excluded; failure of hepatic clearance indicates obstruction. Although many centers pretreat the infant with a 5-day course of phenobarbital prior to the DISIDA scan, recent reports indicate that babies with obstructive jaundice who receive phenobarbital have a higher incidence of liver failure when given a halogenated general anesthetic at the time of definitive surgical correction of biliary atresia. These observations suggest avoidance of phenobarbital administration or, if it is deemed vital for diagnosis, indicate a slight delay in proceeding with surgical therapy if required. In addition, a nonhalogenated anesthetic agent can be employed. Seventy-five to 80 per cent of infants with an obstructive DISIDA scan have biliary atresia. Although percutaneous needle biopsy may be helpful in differentiating between biliary atresia (proliferating bile ducts) and idiopathic neonatal hepatitis (giant cells and focal areas of necrosis), there is a significant overlap, with patients with atresia often demonstrating the presence of giant cells. A minilaparotomy with operative cholangiography (when possible) should be performed. This differentiates neonatal hepatitis, biliary hypoplasia, and Alagille's syndrome by demonstrating an intact but small patent biliary tree with tiny intrahepatic branches and passage of contrast into the duodenum. A confirmatory open liver biopsy should be obtained and the abdomen closed. If biliary atresia is documented, however, the incision can be enlarged and an exploration of the porta hepatis performed.

Biliary Atresia

The etiology of biliary atresia is probably related to a dynamic intrauterine inflammatory process leading to fibrosis of both the intrahepatic and extrahepatic biliary tree. Although biliary atresia was considered a postnatal condition, a number of cases with associated cystic dilation of the atretic duct have been identified *in utero* by prenatal ultrasound examination or at laparotomy in the newborn for other congenital anomalies such as duodenal and jejunal atresia.[52] Some reports suggest the inflammatory process responsible for fibrosis of the bile ducts may be the result of an REO-3 viral infection; however, solid scientific evidence is needed to confirm this relationship.[52,79] The incidence of biliary atresia is 1 in 15,000 live births; this condition is slightly more common in females. Infants with biliary atresia have associated anomalies in 25 to 30 per cent, including duodenal atresia or stenosis, annular pancreas, malrotation, polysplenia syndome, situs inversus, and anterior (preduodenal) portal vein. In addition, 15 per cent of patients may have a congenital heart defect.

An important consideration in the management of infants with biliary atresia is to recognize the disadvantages of delayed diagnosis and treatment; early laparotomy should be performed by 2 months of age.[52,69,79,88,134] A number of recent reports clearly indicate that the success of surgical correction of biliary atresia is much improved when done in the first 2 months of life and that the operation is probably a useless technical exercise after 3 months of age because of progressive ductular fibrosis (extra- and intrahepatic). At operation, the pathologic variants of biliary atresia include fibrous obliteration of the gallbladder with a fibrous bile duct up to the level of the porta hepatis in the majority of patients (80 per cent), a "correctable" form of atresia with a blind-ending cystic dilation of the common hepatic duct in 5 to 6 per cent, and a patent gallbladder (containing white bile) and distal common bile duct with no evidence of proximal ducts in 15 per cent of patients.[52] The procedure of choice is a modification of the Kasai hepatoportoenterostomy.[52,69,79] The fibrous cord representing the bile duct is followed to the porta hepatis and a frozen section of the thick fibrous structure above the bifurcation of the portal vein is obtained. If microscopic bile ductules are observed by the pathologist, a Roux-en-Y hepatoportoenterostomy is performed using one layer of 5-0 interrupted absorbable suture (Maxon). The bifurcation of the portal vein must be mobilized and retracted inferiorly to allow incorporation of the entire porta hepatis in the anastomosis (Fig. 19). The Roux limb is brought out as a temporary biliostomy to evaluate bile flow and perhaps reduce the incidence and severity of postoperative cholangitis. Some pediatric surgeons do not use a cutaneous stoma but prefer to establish an antireflux intussuscepted valve between the distal end of the limb and the duodenum.[79,105] Others have used a vascularized pedicle of appendix in a hepatoporto-appendicoduodenostomy with the distal appendix tunneled in the muscular wall of the duodenum to prevent reflux.[24] When the gallbladder and distal common duct are patent, a hepatoportocholecystostomy has been a useful technique to restore bile flow.[79,88]

Postoperatively, the infant is placed on trimethoprim-sulfamethoxazole as a prophylactic biliary antibiotic and also given phenobarbital to stimulate bile flow. Ursodeoxycholic acid and prostaglandins have been used in some centers as choleretics. Fat-soluble vitamins (including A, D, E, and K) are administered daily. Postoperative complications include cholangitis, progressive cirrhosis manifested by portal hypertension with bleeding esophageal varices, ascites, hypoalbuminemia, hypoprothrombinemia, fat-soluble vitamin deficiencies (vitamins D, E, A, and K), micronutrient deficiency (calcium, phosphorus, and zinc), and malabsorption of long-chain triglycerides. Cholangitis is characterized by a decrease in bile secretion, recurrence of jaundice, fever, and leukocytosis. This event should be documented by a positive blood culture that identifies the offending organism. However, this is not always the case, and the infant should be started on a third-generation cephalosporin or imipenem and choleretics (phenobarbital, glucagon, and steroids)[68,79] even in the absence of a positive blood culture. Intravenous aminoglycoside can be added if there is no response to treatment. Reoperation should be limited to patients with recurring episodes of cholangitis and to re-establish bile flow in those infants who drain adequate bile after the initial hepatoportoenterostomy and are anicteric who then suddenly

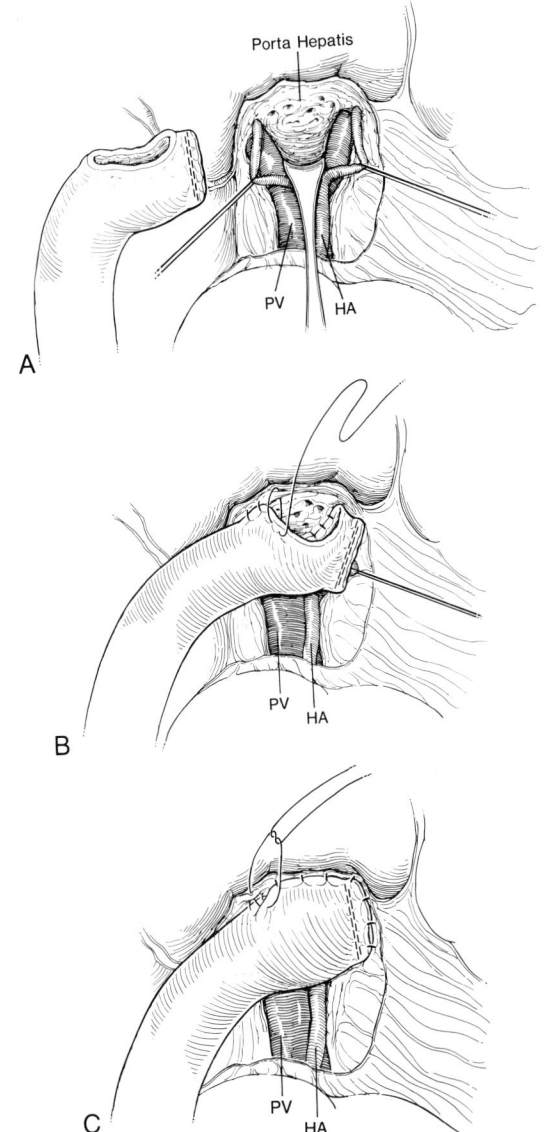

Figure 19. *A* to *C*, The bifurcation of the portal vein is the landmark for the dissection of the porta hepatis in infants with biliary atresia. The bifurcation is freed and retracted inferiorly so that the entire fibrous porta can be included in the hepatoportoenterostomy anastomosis. (*B* and *C*). PV, portal vein; HA, hepatic artery. (From Grosfeld, J. L., et al.: The efficacy of hepatoportoenterostomy in biliary atresia. Surgery, *106*:692, 1989.)

develop jaundice.[38,52] In these cases, a mechanical cause for obstruction of the Roux loop may be the underlying cause.

Successful outcome following hepatoportoenterostomy is related to proper performance of the procedure, the age of the patient (less than 2 months) and severity of the liver disease at the time of the operation, the presence of microscopic ductules at the porta hepatis, and whether adequate bile flow is achieved. Patients can be staged postoperatively and placed in prognostic groups by 4 to 6 weeks after the procedure. Infants who produce adequate amounts of bile (greater than 6 mg. per 100 ml. per day) from the biliostomy and are completely relieved of their jaundice indicate success of the procedure with long-term survival and maintenance of normal or near-normal liver function, and liver transplantation is rarely required.[52,79,134] If the bile flow is moderate but the infant remains jaundiced and the liver disease is stabilized, extended survival can be expected; however, the infant requires a liver transplantation at a future time (in years).[52] In instances in which no bile flow is achieved and the infant's liver disease is progressive, the procedure must be considered a failure and the patient becomes a candidate for early liver transplantation (in months).[52,79] Infants in whom the diagnosis is delayed, and referral for surgical evaluation occurs after 3 months of age when the diagnosis is confirmed, are candidates for liver transplantation as the primary procedure of choice.[52,79,134] Most infants with biliary atresia should undergo hepatoportoenterostomy; approximately 30 per cent of those patients operated upon early have a successful outcome and may never require liver transplantation. An additional group of patients are improved, have an extended survival, and can delay the timing of the liver transplant when the donor organ pool size is larger. In the remaining infants who either fail to improve following hepatoportoenterostomy or are referred late, liver transplantation is a vital and lifesaving procedure. In these more urgent cases, the use of reduced-size orthotopic grafts has decreased the waiting period for a donor organ and improved the overall survival of candidates for liver transplantation, particularly those who previously died awaiting a donor organ.

Choledochal Cyst

Cystic enlargement of the common bile duct is referred to as a choledochal cyst. The etiology of choledochal cyst is controversial and includes a common channel theory with destructive effects of pancreatic enzymes causing damage in the wall of the common duct. These lesions are more common in females (4 : 1), and approximately half the patients present with jaundice, a right upper quadrant mass, and abdominal pain. Both the pain and jaundice may be intermittent. In some instances, the initial presentation is acute pancreatitis due to an abnormal insertion of the pancreatic duct. Cholelithiasis and cirrhosis may complicate choledochal cysts that are not recognized early.

There are five main variants of choledochal cyst (Fig. 20); I, fusiform dilation of the common hepatic and common bile duct with the cystic duct entering the cyst (the distal common bile duct may be stenotic); II, a lateral saccular cystic dilation; III, a choledochocele represented by an intraduodenal cyst; IV, multiple extra- or intrahepatic cysts or both; and V, single or multiple intrahepatic cysts. Type I is the most common form observed; diagnosis is achieved by ultrasound examination, which usually demonstrates the choledochal cyst and dilated intrahepatic ducts. Although preoperative percutaneous transhepatic cholangiography and endoscopic retrograde cholangiopancreatography have demonstrated the cyst and biliary system, these studies are probably unnecessary in most cases. Definitive operation is performed through a transverse or subcostal right

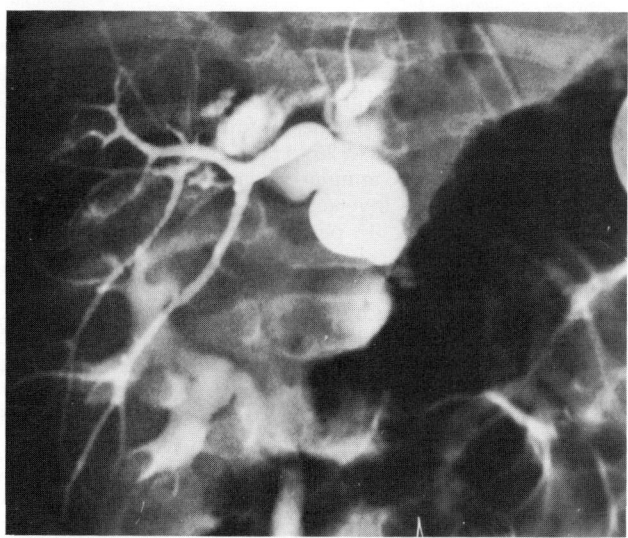

Figure 21. Intraoperative cholangiogram demonstrates a Type I choledochal cyst.

upper quadrant incision. An operative cholangiogram is performed through the gallbladder or the cyst wall and clarifies the pathologic process, including the site of an abnormally inserted pancreatic duct (Fig. 21). Internal drainage procedures such as cystduodenotomy and cystjejunostomy, which were popular procedures in the past, are no longer recommended.[19,91] The choledochal cyst is devoid of epithelium and the wall is fibrous and fails to contract, leading to poor emptying and significant bile stasis. These diversionary procedures were complicated by cholangitis, cholelithiasis, cirrhosis, and malignant degeneration in the cyst wall. At the present time, the operation of choice is complete resection of the cyst and a Roux-en-Y hepatojejunostomy performed with interrupted 5-0 absorbable suture (Maxon).[19,91] The cyst wall must be carefully dissected from the anterior surface of the portal vein, and an abnormally high insertion of the pancreatic duct must be identified to prevent injury. The distal end of the bile duct is oversewn at the duodenum. When significant inflammation is present, the cyst can be resected leaving the outer posterior layer of the cyst wall in place on the portal vein to decrease the risk of excessive hemorrhage.[19] Postoperative complications are few, and the operative mortality has been negligible. The risks of cholangitis, anastomotic stricture, progressive liver disease, and carcinoma are significantly reduced by resection of the choledochal cyst. Long-term follow-up, however, is important.

Cholelithiasis

The etiology of gallstones in infants and children differs somewhat from that in adults. The most common cause of cholelithiasis in pediatric patients is pigment stones due to congenital hemolytic disorders including hereditary spherocytosis, thalassemia, pyruvic-kinase deficiency, and sickle cell disease. Other causes include cholestasis as a result of long-term treatment with total parenteral nutrition and cystic fibrosis. Children with extensive bowel resection due to malrotation with midgut volvulus, necrotizing enterocolitis, or intestinal atresias who have distal ileum resection have an abnormal enterohepatic circulation of bile and secrete a more concentrated cholesterol in the bile that increases the rate of gallstone formation. In adolescent females, use of birth control pills, a positive family history of gallstones, and teenage pregnancy are associated with an increased risk of gallstone formation. Diagnosis is achieved in a manner similar to adult patients, relying heavily on the results of ultrasonographic studies and the occasional use of endoscopic retrograde cholangiopancreatography when indicated. The treatment of choice is cholecystectomy.

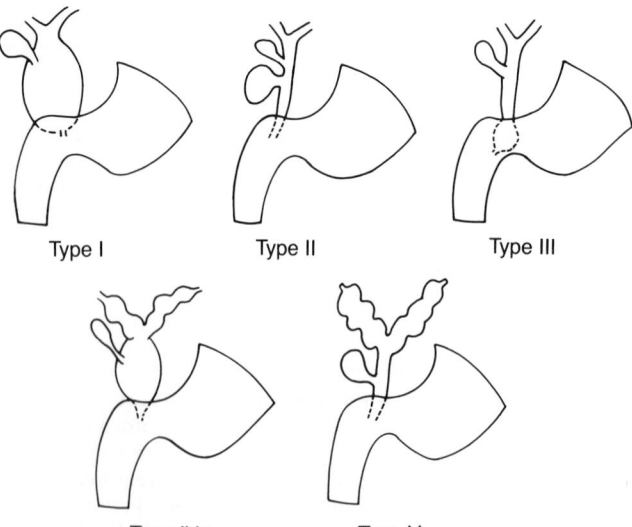

Figure 20. There are five types of choledochal cyst. Type I is the most common form. (From O'Neill, J. A., et al.: Recent experience with choledochal cyst. Ann. Surg., 205:533, 1985.)

ACUTE APPENDICITIS

Acute appendicitis is one of the most common causes of acute abdomen in the childhood group. A careful clinical history and thorough physical examination are the hallmarks of making an early, accurate diagnosis of appendicitis. The pathophysiologic mechanism of appendicitis involves obstruction of the appendix by a fecalith producing a "close-loop" obstruction. The classic presentation of appendicitis includes the onset of epigastric or periumbilical pain followed by anorexia, nausea, and vomiting. The pain then radiates to the right lower quadrant, becoming more localized and intense than the early periumbilical pain.[58]

The appendix is a fingerlike projection that may be in a variety of locations including in the pelvis, in the right upper quadrant under the gallbladder, across the top of the bladder, or in a retrocecal site. Other unusual locations of the appendix are the left lower quadrant in cases of situs inversus and the upper midabdomen in instances of malrotation. Under these circumstances, the site of localized pain may occur at locations other than the classic presentation of this disease process in the right lower quadrant. When the appendix lies behind the cecum, irritation of the parietal peritoneum often does not occur, and the classic shift of pain to the right lower quadrant may be absent. Localized right lower quadrant pain indicates the patient may have appendicitis, and in the absence of other findings, prompt operation should be performed to prevent perforation. In young children, perforation may occasionally occur after 12 to 15 hours of documented pain[46]; perforation is present in 25 per cent at 24 hours from the onset of symptoms, 50 per cent by 36 hours (half will be gangrenous or perforated), and 80 per cent at 48 hours.[58] Gangrenous or perforated appendicitis occurs in one third to one half of patients admitted to most children's hospitals.[46,58,111] At least half of these patients have been seen in a physician's office or an emergency room and sent home with an incorrect diagnosis. This is especially true for infants less than 2 years of age, in whom appendicitis is relatively unusual.[40] The young child with ruptured appendix commonly has free perforation and peritonitis because of the inability of the short, flimsy omentum to wall off the process. Appendiceal perforation in the newborn period may be related to distal obstruction from Hirschsprung's disease, meconium plug syndrome, or a localized process due to necrotizing enterocolitis.[46]

A careful, detailed history is important to establish the exact time of the onset of pain and the sequence of events.[58] Vomiting follows periumbilical pain in appendicitis, but often precedes abdominal pain in gastroenteritis. Documenting the character and frequency of diarrhea may prove useful. Mucoid, infrequent, small-volume episodes of diarrhea may be associated with pelvic irritation due to appendicitis and follow the onset of abdominal pain. High-volume, frequent, watery diarrhea that may or may not precede the onset of crampy abdominal pain may be indicative of gastroenteritis or other conditions of inflammatory bowel disease. Careful documentation of symptoms in other systems is important, such as recent urinary tract infection; in adolescent females, information regarding the menstrual cycle, previous episodes of pelvic inflammatory disease, mittelschmerz, and an accurate sexual history is important. The physical examination is the most important single determinant in the child with an acute abdomen and forms the basis for decisions regarding surgical intervention. In some patients, observation and periodic re-examination by the same physician may be necessary to confirm or exclude the diagnosis of appendicitis. Physical examination must include a careful and meaningful abdominal and rectal examination with the patient cooperative to make the evaluation valid. The examination should document guarding, muscle spasm, and possible rebound tenderness consistent with peritoneal irritation. Evaluation of the obturator and psoas signs may be helpful. The rectal examination may reveal a mass in the pelvis consistent with a pelvic abscess or elicit tenderness due to irritation of the pelvic peritoneum from exudate or fluid from pelvic appendicitis. In some patients, the rectal examination may reveal a fecal impaction due to severe constipation, which may cause significant abdominal pain. If the child is not cooperative, a short-acting nonanalgesic medication (secobarbital, 2 mg. per pound intramuscularly) is administered to relieve anxiety but not reduce the pain response. Most patients with appendicitis have a low-grade temperature (37 to 39° C. [98.6 to 102° F.]). Patients with pyelonephritis, pelvic inflammatory disease, and gastroenteritis from a variety of organisms (Salmonella, Shigella, Campylobacter, Yersinia) often have a higher temperature.

The laboratory evaluation includes a complete blood count with differential smear and urinalysis. Although the white blood cell count is greater than 10,000 per cu. mm. in more than 90 per cent of patients, a normal count should not delay surgical exploration in a child with localized right lower quadrant tenderness or peritonitis. The urinalysis is important in differentiating between pyelonephritis or a renal calculus and acute appendicitis. The urine may contain a few red blood cells and white blood cells if an inflamed appendix lies near the ureter or bladder. An elevated urine specific gravity is consistent with hypovolemia and dehydration and is more common in cases with perforation. In teenaged girls, an erythrocyte sedimentation rate should be obtained. This test is normal in appendicitis, but if elevated it may reflect the presence of pelvic inflammatory disease. Other laboratory tests are unnecessary unless the patient is severely dehydrated and hypovolemic and blood urea nitrogen and serum electrolytes are obtained. Radiologic evaluation should include a chest film to exclude right middle or lower lobe pneumonia and flat and erect abdominal radiographs. Although the abdominal radiographs may be nonspecific, a calcified appendicolith may be observed in 15 per cent of patients and is consistent with a diagnosis of appendicitis. Although there has been recent enthusiasm for use of a diagnostic barium enema to exclude acute appendicitis, the author has not found this useful. Both false-negative and false-positive studies have been reported.[59] Ultrasound imaging may demonstrate an appendiceal abscess but is not useful in detecting early appendicitis.[58]

In addition to the conditions previously mentioned, the differential diagnosis includes idiopathic intussusception, intestinal obstruction and volvulus, Meckel's diverticulum, Crohn's disease, ovarian torsion (cyst or tumor), perforated ulcer, pancreatitis, mittelschmerz, Henoch-Schönlein purpura, pelvic inflammatory disease, ruptured ectopic pregnancy, hemorrhage from a tumor (Wilms' tumor, neuroblastoma), and other pathologic processes.

In instances of early acute appendicitis, the child is promptly prepared for operation with an intravenous infusion in the left upper extremity and a preoperative dose of cefoxitin or triple antibiotics (ampicillin, gentamicin, and clindamycin) given at least 30 minutes before operation, since one cannot always exclude gangrenous changes or perforation. In ruptured appendicitis, the child may be severely dehydrated and have a high temperature, a rapid pulse, and adynamic ileus related to peritonitis. The patient must be carefully resuscitated with a rapid intravenous infusion of lactated Ringer's solution 20 ml. per kg. over ½ hour and then at a rate of 200 ml. per kg. per day until the pulse rate decreases and urinary output is established. Triple antibiotics (as noted) and pain medication are administered, and a nasogastric tube is inserted and placed on intermittent suction. Two to 4 hours may be required to adequately prepare the patient with perforation for operation. Appendectomy is accomplished through a right lower quadrant (Rockey-Davis) incision. Nonperforated cases are managed by appendectomy (with inversion of the stump) and closure of the wound in layers. Antibiotics are discontinued after two doses. Patients can usually resume oral intake after 24 hours, and in most cases the child is discharged in 72 hours. In instances of perforation, however, all pus is drained, cultures are obtained, an appendectomy is performed, and the pelvis and right gutter are irrigated with saline (or an antibiotic solution) and aspirated dry. If there is a localized abscess, this may be drained through a separate stab wound below the main wound. In instances of generalized peritonitis, the peritoneal cavity is irrigated and aspirated dry but drainage is not performed.[46,58,115] The muscular layers of the wound are closed in layers, but the skin is packed open. Antibiotics are continued for 5 to 7 days at least until the temperature returns to normal and the white blood cell count diminishes. In some centers, the use of triple antibiotics has reduced the incidence of intra-abdominal abscess and postoperative wound infection even when the wound is primarily closed and no intra-abdominal drains are employed.[115] The nasogastric tube remains in place until alimentary tract function returns. Diet is advanced, and the patient is discharged when afebrile and a postoperative rectal examination confirms no evidence of pelvic abscess. The morbidity and mortality of appendicitis in children have gradually decreased over the past 2 decades despite the fact that the incidence of ruptured appendix at diagnosis remains high. Most deaths are noted in the very young when the diagnosis is not considered and long delays in treatment occur and in those patients with ruptured appendix who are poorly prepared for operation and develop renal failure, hyperpyrexic events (including seizures), and gram-negative sepsis.

INFLAMMATORY BOWEL DISEASE

Crohn's disease may occur in childhood and adolescence and often presents with growth failure, cramping abdominal pain, diarrhea, perianal disease, and stricture leading to bowel obstruction. This transmural condition most commonly affects the distal ileum and right colon. Multiple areas of small intestine may be involved and in some patients the only area of involvement is the colon. Rare cases of duodenal involvement have also been documented in children.[77] Diagnosis is usually achieved by barium enteroclysis of the small bowel, barium enema, and proctosigmoidoscopy and biopsy. Conservative therapy includes the use of sulfadine and steroids.[78] In resistant cases, both cyclophosphamide (Cytoxan) and cyclosporine have been used to produce a remission.[2,14] Indications for surgical intervention in children include growth failure, intestinal obstruction, perforation with internal fistulas, and the presence of a mass indicating perforation into the mesentery. The patients are often anemic, hypoalbuminemic, and malnourished. Leukocytosis, an elevated erythrocyte sedimentation rate, and an elevated platelet count are frequently noted. A course of total parenteral nutrition and administration of metronidazole often leads to significant improvement of the patient's nutrition and general status in preparation for surgical therapy.[23] Limited resection of obstructive segments or sites of fistulas with preservation of bowel length when possible is recommended. Occasionally a total colectomy is required for granulomatous colitis. In cases of duodenal involvement, gastroenterostomy with vagotomy is a useful procedure. Recurrence following surgical intervention occurs in as many as 50 per cent of patients and symptoms extend into adult life. Long-term follow-up is essential. This condition is presented in great detail elsewhere in this text.

TRAUMA

Accidents are the leading cause of death in children between the ages of 1 and 15 years. Each year approximately 15,000 deaths occur in children as a result of traumatic events, which represent approximately 50 per cent of all deaths reported in the pediatric age group.[98] Motor vehicle accidents are responsible

for the greatest number of deaths followed by falls, bicycle injuries, drowning, burns, and the unique aspects of pediatric trauma such as child abuse and birth trauma.[23] In recent years, an increasing number of deaths have been related to violence including the use of firearms. In addition, more than 20 million children sustain some type of injury each year requiring treatment, causing more than 100,000 cases of permanent disability.[102]

Although there are many similarities in the management of the adult and childhood trauma patient, there are several differences worthy of mention. These include response to stress, psychological trauma and communication difficulties, thermoregulation, a relatively small total blood volume, increased metabolic requirements related to growth and an increased metabolic rate, aerophagia with acute gastric dilation and an increased risk of aspiration, smaller airway diameter that can be more easily obstructed by secretions and difficult to intubate, greater risk for postsplenectomy sepsis, and a different physiologic response to severe head injury (with incomplete sutures, and so on) than in the adult.[23,98,139] In addition, the accident pattern is quite different since most pediatric injuries are the result of blunt trauma, whereas injuries in adults are relatively evenly divided between blunt and penetrating trauma. Moreover, the trauma scores utilized to evaluate injury severity in adult patients are inadequate for the pediatric patient and this has led to the development of the pediatric trauma score (Table 4).[23] A pediatric trauma score of less than 8 to 9 indicates an

TABLE 4. Pediatric Trauma Score

Parameter	Coded Value
Size	
> 20 kg.	+2
10–20 kg.	+1
< 10 kg.	−1
Airway	
Normal	+2
Maintainable	+1
Not maintainable	−1
Systolic Blood Pressure	
> 90 mm. Hg	+2
50–90 mm. Hg	+1
< 50 mm. Hg	−1
In the absence of a proper size BP cuff, assess BP by assigning these values:	
Pulse palpable at wrist	+2
Pulse palpable at groin	+1
Pulse not palpable	−1
Central Nervous System Status	
Awake	+2
Partially conscious or unconscious	+1
Comatose or decerebrate	−1
Open Wounds	
None	+2
Minor	+1
Major	−1
Skeletal Injury	
None	+2
Closed Fracture	+1
Open/multiple fractures	−1
Total score	Range −6 to +12

Scoring triage criterion for direct transport of the child to a Level 1 trauma center is <9.

From Coran, A. G.: Perioperative care of the pediatric surgical patient. In Wilmore, D. W., Brennan, M. F., Harken, A. H., Holcroft, J. W., and Meakins, J. L. (Eds.): Care of the Surgical Patient. Vol. 1. New York, Scientific American, Inc., 1989, p. 20.

injury that places the child at risk for dying and suggests that the patient be transported to a pediatric trauma facility. Although adult trauma centers have reduced the mortality for adult patients, this has not been the case for the severely injured child. Pediatric trauma patients should have access to appropriate transport and receive care at a regional pediatric trauma center that is experienced in managing the complex requirements for the treatment of the seriously injured child. This represents between 5 and 10 per cent of the total number of children injured because the majority of the cases (more than 90 per cent) can be managed at most local medical facilities, emphasizing the importance of adequate trauma outreach programs designed to educate ambulance transport and emergency room personnel at the community level.

The pediatric trauma center includes a multidisciplined group of pediatric surgical, anesthetic, and medical specialists in an integrated system of care. Multiple injury patients are ideally admitted to the pediatric surgical trauma service for initial resuscitation and complete evaluation of the patient's status. Other surgical specialists are available as necessary for evaluation of injuries in their area of expertise (e.g., neurosurgery, orthopedics) and have a vital role in the overall care of the patient. Head injuries are more common in children and represent the most frequent cause of death in the pediatric age group.[23] Early identification of severe head injury and aggressive management of increased intracranial pressure elevation has significantly reduced the mortality of pediatric head injury in the last decade to less than 10 per cent.

The resuscitation of the pediatric trauma victim follows the basic guideline of adult trauma care by initiating the traditional ABCs including establishing an airway, controlling external sources of bleeding, and restoring the circulating volume. The cervical spine should be stabilized and the oropharynx cleared of blood and debris (food, broken teeth). If necessary, intubation is accomplished with a noncuffed pediatric endotracheal tube using the fifth fingernail as a guide for sizing. A large-bone intravenous catheter is inserted in either the upper or lower extremity, and if the blood pressure is low (less than 90 mm. Hg), crystalloid (lactated Ringer's solution) is rapidly infused at a rate of 20 ml. per kg. to restore the circulating volume, reduce the rapid pulse rate, and increase blood pressure to above 90 mm. Hg. A nasogastric tube is inserted to decompress the distended stomach and prevent aspiration. A Foley catheter is inserted to monitor urinary output. If the blood pressure drops again, an additional bolus of crystalloid is administered. Continued low blood pressure and rapid pulse rate are indicative of ongoing blood loss and O-negative uncrossmatched blood is adminstered. The possibility of intrathoracic trauma and pneumothorax should be considered. If this is excluded, the unstable patient who does not respond to fluid resuscitation most likely has a significant intra-abdominal injury with bleeding and requires immediate operation.[98] However, when the patient becomes hemodynamically stable if an abdominal injury is considered, a more definitive evaluation can be accomplished by obtaining a computed tomography (CT) scan.[66,89,102] If the patient has an associated head injury, the CT scan of the head is followed by a study of the abdomen. The CT scan with both intravenous and oral contrast documents injury to the liver and spleen, evaluates possible duodenal laceration or hematoma, images the pancreas, localizes abnormal fluid collections, identifies free air from bowel perforation, and adequately evaluates both kidneys with one examination. Although most adult trauma centers commonly use diagnostic peritoneal lavage as an important clinical maneuver to establish the presence of an intra-abdominal injury, bloody lavage fluid return in children does not necessarily indicate the need for laparotomy. Nonoperative management of the injured spleen and liver is an accepted method of therapy in the childhood group.[66,72,89,95,102] As long as the child's vital signs remain stable and blood loss is minimal (less than 40 ml. per kg.), operation is unnecessary.[95] The child with a stable spleen or liver injury is transferred to the pediatric intensive care facility on the pediatric surgical service. The facility must have in-house surgical staff available on a 7-days-a-week, 24-hours-a-day basis. The patient may resume oral intake after 48 hours and is transferred from the intensive care unit to a regular pediatric floor. One-week hospitalization is usually all that is necessary for children with an isolated splenic injury. This child must refrain from any physical activity for a few weeks and avoid contact sports for 3 months.

Continued bleeding (more than half the blood volume), multiple injuries, or the presence of free air are indications for operative intervention. Following complete mobilization, the injured spleen can be salvaged by a number of techniques including topical hemostatic agents, splenorrhaphy, partial splenectomy, and splenic artery ligation.[72,95,102] The fact that infants and children are more susceptible to overwhelming postsplenectomy infection due to encapsulated bacteria with a cell wall (pneumococcus, *Haemophilus influenzae*) makes conservative management and splenic salvage important considerations.[139] Complete splenectomy is rarely indicated. When the spleen is removed, the child should be immunized with Pneumovax vaccine (which contains 23 serotypes of pneumococcus) and placed on oral prophylactic penicillin. For children under 8 years of age, immunization with a vaccine against *H. influenzae* should be considered. In children with liver injury, the major indication for surgical intervention is significant intra-abdominal bleeding (greater than 40 ml. per kg.). These cases are usually identified early with the patient's course unstable from the onset of care.[89,102] Careful control of hemostasis (with the aid of the Pringle maneuver) and adequate débridement of devitalized liver tissue and drainage are the essential aspects of surgical care. The cell saver and rapid autotransfuser are helpful intraoperative adjuncts. Hepatic resection is rarely indicated. In some instances with coagulation defects due to excessive bleeding and multiple transfusions, the only method to control hemorrhage is by placing packs in the right upper quadrant.[102] The packs are removed in the operating room at a second-look procedure 24 to 48 hours later when levels of coagulation factors return to normal.

Injuries to the small intestine are less common than those of the spleen and liver.[51] These injuries are related to blunt trauma that compresses the second and third portion of the duodenum against the spine.[140] Duodenal hematomas can be identified by contrast studies and can be treated conservatively in most patients with nasogastric suction and total parenteral nutrition.[140] Although a duodenal laceration can be detected by the presence of free air or air bubbles in the retroperitoneum, the best method of diagnosis is administration of oral contrast material at the time of a CT scan of the abdomen. Surgical management includes primary suture of the duodenal laceration and drainage, jejunal serosal patch, and, occasionally in severe injuries, pyloric exclusion with temporary gastroenterostomy or duodenal diverticulization.[113,135] The last procedures are more commonly required with an associated injury to the head of the pancreas. Pancreatic injuries are also related to direct compression of the midportion of the gland against the vertebral column.[133] The CT scan is the most accurate diagnostic method in pancreatic injury.[125,133] Most patients can be treated conservatively; however, if the pancreatic duct is transected, a distal pancreatectomy with splenic salvage (when possible) is advised. Serial ultrasound studies are employed to follow the course of the injury and determine if a pseudocyst or abscess develops. Some pseudocysts resolve spontaneously; others that persist can be treated with ultrasound-guided percutaneous drainage. Failure of these techniques usually indicates an overlooked ductal injury that can be confirmed by endoscopic retrograde cholangiopancreatography and often requires either an internal drainage procedure or a distal pancreatectomy. Pancreatic abscesses are usually associated with a febrile course often complicated by sepsis and require operative débridement and drainage.[133]

Renal injuries require surgical intervention in less than 20 per cent of patients. Leakage of pyelogram contrast material from the kidney and failure to visualize the kidney suggestive of a hilar vascular injury (confirmed by angiogram) are the two major indications for operation. Bleeding from the urethra is a common finding in pelvic fractures. A urethrogram should be performed to detect a urethral rupture prior to attempted passage of an indwelling urinary catheter. A suprapubic cystostomy is necessary to establish urinary drainage.

Although the survival following severe blunt polytrauma has improved in recent years, the key to improvement rests with innovative prevention programs to reduce the number of victims. The topic of trauma is also covered elsewhere in this text and the reader is encouraged to peruse this section for further information about other aspects of injury management.

NECK MASSES

The appearance of a neck mass is a common occurrence in infancy and childhood and is a source of parental alarm. The etiology of the neck mass may be infectious, congenital, or neoplastic.

Lymphadenitis

Lymphadenitis is characterized by the presence of enlarged, often tender lymph nodes. Most are the result of a local infection that is controlled by the natural barrier established in the lymphoid tissue. Most cases revolve with treatment of the primary source of infection (e.g., otitis media, tonsillitis). Cervical lymph gland enlargement is often the result of a suppurative bacterial infection due to *Staphylococcus* or *Streptococcus* infection. Acutely infected lymph nodes often enlarge rapidly and are painful, and erythema (cellulitis) may be observed in the skin overlying the mass. Fever and leukocytosis are often present. Antibiotics are started using a third-generation cephalosporin. The therapy of choice for suppurative lymphadenitis is incision and drainage of the infected lymph node when it becomes fluctuant. Appropriate cultures are obtained. Antibiotics are discontinued after 48 hours if the temperature returns to normal. Daily dressing changes of the packing inserted at the time of drainage are made by the parents at home. Recurring suppurative lymphadenitis may be caused by an immunodeficiency syndrome (e.g., chronic granulomatous disease, acquired immune deficiency syndrome, Bruton's syndrome).

Lymphadenitis may also be caused by a more indolent chronic inflammatory process such as atypical mycobacterial infection, cat-scratch disease, or fungal infection (histoplasmosis).[3] Lymph node enlargement is of longer duration than in the acute infectious cases, and multiple lymph nodes may be affected. The lymph nodes are also less tender and may be complicated by a draining sinus with enlarged lymph nodes in the mediastinum as well. A chest film should always be obtained when a chronic inflammatory process is suspected. The chest film is usually normal in instances of atypical mycobacterial infection but may demonstrate enlarged mediastinal lymph nodes in histoplasmosis. Skin tests should be planted using intermediate PPD (which is usually positive for atypical mycobacterium), and complement fixation titers for histoplasmosis should also be obtained. The therapy of choice for chronic lymphadenitis due to mycobacteria and occasionally fungi is complete excision of the involved lymph nodes in order to eradicate the infection, which may be resistant to drug therapy. In some instances, a modified radical neck dissection is necessary to accomplish this goal. Cultures of the lymph node should be sent for evaluation of mycobacterium and fungi in addition to bacterial cultures.

Cervical Anomalies

The most common benign cervical anomalies include branchial cleft cysts and sinuses, thyroglossal duct cysts, cystic hygroma, dermoid cysts, hemangiomas, and torticollis.[34,128]

Branchial cleft anomalies are remnants of the four paired embryonic branchial arches, clefts, and pouches. These lesions may present as sinuses, fistulas, or cartilaginous rests in infants and more commonly present as cysts in older children, adolescents, and adults. The first branchial cleft sinus presents anterior to the ear and connects with the eustachian tube. The most frequently observed anomaly involves the second branchial cleft remnant, which may present clinically anywhere along the anterior border of the sternocleidomastoid muscle from the angle of the jaw (as a cystic mass) to the lower third of the neck (as a sinus tract). The sinus tract passes cephalad in a deeper path under the digastric muscle, between the branches of the carotid artery and under the hypoglossal nerve to end in the tonsillar fossa. The tract is excised using a stepladder technique (two incisions) with high ligation at the tonsillar fossa. The third and fourth branchial clefts develop into the lower and upper parathyroid glands, respectively. These may be deficient in their development as part of a pharyngeal pouch deficiency syndrome characterized by absent parathyroids, absent or depleted thymus (DiGeorge's syndrome) leading to an immunosuppressive syndrome (T cell depletion), hypocalcemia, and seizures. Aortic arch vascular anomalies may also coexist. Therapy includes administration of vitamin D and calcium and transplant of fetal thymic tissues or bone marrow transplantation. The fifth embryonic branchial cleft involutes.

Thyroglossal duct anomalies are midline lesions that originate at the base of the tongue at the foramen caecum and pass through the central portion of the hyoid bone. The thyroglossal duct usually obliterates in the sixth intrauterine week. Persistence of this fetal structure postnatally causes a midline swelling over the hyoid bone that moves with deglutition. Infection is the most common complication. A sinus tract may develop as a result of infection. The differential diagnosis of upper midline neck masses includes inflamed submental lymph node, pretracheal dermoid cyst, or ectopic thyroid tissue. The lymph node usually responds to antibiotics, is movable, and is separate from the hyoid bone. Ectopic thyroid is rare, does not get infected, and always appears solid on ultrasonography. Dermoid cysts are usually small and spherical and contain keratin-like material. They do not go through the hyoid bone and separate easily from the pretracheal fascia at operation. In older individuals, the thyroglossal duct may contain thyroid remnants that occasionally become malignant. This is extremely rare in children. The treatment of choice is complete excision of the mass with the central portion of the hyoid bone and high suture ligation of the duct at the foramen caecum (Sistrunk procedure). The recurrence rate is 6 to 9 per cent and is more common following infection. Inadequate resection of the hyoid centrum and recurrence of duct patency at the base of the tongue are the most frequent findings at reoperation.

Cystic hygroma is another neck mass frequently encountered in children. The most common site of cystic hygroma is the neck. This developmental lymphangioma is derived from the primitive embryonic jugular venolymphatic sacs. In some instances the mass may be detected by prenatal ultrasound. More commonly, however, the mass either is noted at birth or presents when sudden enlargement of a neck hygroma occurs during an upper respiratory infection and may lead to severe tracheal compression and air hunger. Ten per cent of cystic hygromas extend into the axilla or mediastinum. A chest film or neck and chest ultrasonography usually identify these masses. Complete excision is the therapy of choice; however, this is not always possible since the mass may be more solid in nature and infiltrate structures such as the tongue or pharynx, and the cystic form is frequently intimately adherent to vital structures (e.g., vagus nerve, phrenic nerve), which should not be sacrificed since this lesion is benign. The use of sclerosing agents, steroid injection, and irradiation have been attempted but have not been effective measures. Recent reports indicate that injection of a bleomycin-fat emulsion may eradicate the lesion.

Torticollis refers to a hard, spindle-shaped, fibrous tumor within the sternocleidomastoid muscle. The mass is usually detected in the first 2 to 4 weeks of life. The incidence of this occurrence is 0.4 per cent of live births. The most likely cause of this lesion is a birth injury. Torticollis occurs more commonly following breech delivery and may be associated with eventration of the diaphragm and Erb's palsy on the same side. Clinical presentation includes a hard mass within the sternocleidomastoid muscle, ipsilateral facial hemihypoplasia, plagiocephaly, head turned away from the side of the mass, and, occasionally, ipsilateral trapezius atrophy. An underlying cervical vertebral abnormality should be excluded by obtaining a radiograph of the cervical spine. In older children, a spinal cord tumor at the cervical level should be suspected. In 80 per cent of patients, the mass responds to conservative therapy that includes ipsilateral stimulation to feeding, light, and sound and range-of-motion exercises twice daily. Approximately 20 per cent of patients require division of the affected sternocleidomastoid muscle below the level of the exit of the spinal accessory nerve. The two ends should be separated and any adhesions to the cervical fascia divided.

Neck masses in children may also be caused by a benign or malignant tumor.[34] Primary tumors that arise in the neck in the pediatric age group include teratomas, neurofibromas, salivary gland tumors (submandibular and parotid), thyroid and parathyroid tumors, Hodgkin's disease, non-Hodgkin's lymphomas, cervical neuroblastoma, rhabdomyosarcoma, leukemia, histiocytosis-X, and others that are described in more detail elsewhere in this text.

INGUINAL HERNIA AND HYDROCELE

Inguinal hernia is a common finding in infants and children and represents the condition most frequently requiring surgical repair in the pediatric age group.[42] Persistence of all or part of the embryonic processus vaginalis (which follows the descent of the testis down to the scrotal sac) causes a variety of inguinal anomalies including scrotal hernia, distal obliteration with proximal hernia sac, communicating hydrocele (which is a hernia with a small connection to the peritoneal cavity), hydrocele of the spermatic cord, and hydrocele of the tunica vaginalis (Fig. 22). The incidence of inguinal hernia varies with gestational age from 9 to 11 per cent in preterm infants to 3.5 to 5 per cent in full-term infants. Inguinal hernia is more common in males than in females, has a definite familial tendency, and presents more frequently on the right side as a result of later descent of the right testis and delayed obliteration of the processus vaginalis. Clinical presentation is on the right side in 60 per cent of patients, on the left side in 30 per cent, and bilateral in 10 per cent. Bilateral inguinal hernias are more common in the preterm infant.[100] The major risk factor in inguinal hernia is the occurrence of bowel incarceration and possible strangulation. The rate of bowel incarceration is significantly higher in the premature infant and in infants in the first year of life (31 per cent) compared with the general pediatric age group (12 to 15 per cent).[43,97,100–109] Bowel obstruction, gonadal infarction, and intestinal gangrene requiring resection occur more commonly in the first 6 months of life as a result of incarceration.[97,100] It is often possible to safely reduce an incarcerated hernia in infants and convert an emergent problem that requires an immediate operation to an elective procedure.[42,43] Sedation, positioning, and gentle taxis to reduce the hernia is successful in 70 per cent. The postoperative complication rate is greater than 20 per cent

in incarcerated cases as compared with 1 to 2 per cent in elective procedures.[43,109] These observations suggest that the best time to repair an inguinal hernia in infancy is shortly after making the diagnosis and before complications occur. A number of recent trends have influenced the type of patients currently being referred for hernia repair. Advances in neonatal intensive care have led to the survival of many small premature infants who have a high incidence of inguinal hernia.[39,100] A significant number of these infants have been hospitalized for birth asphyxia, respiratory distress syndrome, apnea and bradycardia, and so on, and develop a symptomatic hernia in the neonatal intensive care unit. These infants should have hernia repair just prior to hospital discharge.[39,100] Recent information regarding depletion of germ cells and volume loss in the first 6 months of age in males with undescended testis has stimulated the performance of early orchiopexy at age 1 year. More than 90 per cent of these infants have an associated inguinal hernia that requires repair at the time of orchiopexy.[42] The use of the peritoneal cavity for fluid absorptive purposes in infants with hydrocephalus treated by ventriculoperitoneal shunts and continuous ambulatory peritoneal dialysis for chronic renal failure or metabolic derangements (hyperammonemia, lactic acidosis) cause increased intra-abdominal pressure leading to a high incidence of previously unrecognized inguinal hernia.[42,124,126] Recognition of these and other conditions (Table 5) associated with an increased incidence of inguinal hernia should allow early recognition and treatment prior to the development of serious complications.

The technical details of inguinal hernia repair in children have been previously published.[43] Most infants can be successfully managed by high suture ligation of the indirect hernia sac at the level of the internal ring with nonabsorbable suture. In some with a large internal ring, the transversalis fascia inferior to the internal ring is snugged to reduce the size of the excessively large opening without causing compression of the spermatic vessels. Contralateral exploration of the opposite groin is routinely performed in the first 3 years of life, in young females (who have a higher rate of bilaterality), in patients with ventriculoperitoneal shunts, and in children who present with a clinical hernia on the left side.[43,110] All full-term infants and older children without underlying illness may undergo hernia repair in an outpatient setting. Outpatient hernia repair in children is safe, effective, and well tolerated, avoids the psychological trauma of hospitalization, reduces the cross-infection rate, and leads to cost savings to the patient's family. Outpatient surgery centers for children require the availability of skilled pediatric anesthesia and nursing staff, a pleasant environment for children, appropriate-sized pediatric equipment and monitoring capability, and the ability to admit an infant postoperatively to a pediatric inpatient facility if necessary. There is still a need for some infants with symptomatic inguinal hernias to be admitted to the hospital. Infants with bronchopulmonary dysplasia, a history of prematurity (up to 6 months of age), a history of apnea or bradycardia, severe congenital heart disease, and seizure disorder should be admitted postoperatively for a one-night stay for monitoring purposes.[80,123]

In instances of communicating hydrocele, the child's parent often describes a changing size of the scrotal sac due to exchange of fluid between a narrow connection of the hydrocele and the peritoneal cavity. Communicating hydrocele is a misnomer since the pathologic process is that of a hernia that requires repair. A hydrocele of the spermatic cord often presents as a spherical mass in the inguinal canal. In most instances, the hydrocele has a small connection with the peritoneal cavity and should be treated by surgical excision and high ligation of the sac. In young females, this presents as a hydrocele in the canal of Nuck. Occasionally they have sliding hernias containing the ovary and fallopian tube. These should be repaired promptly because there is a risk of ovarian torsion in the inguinal canal.

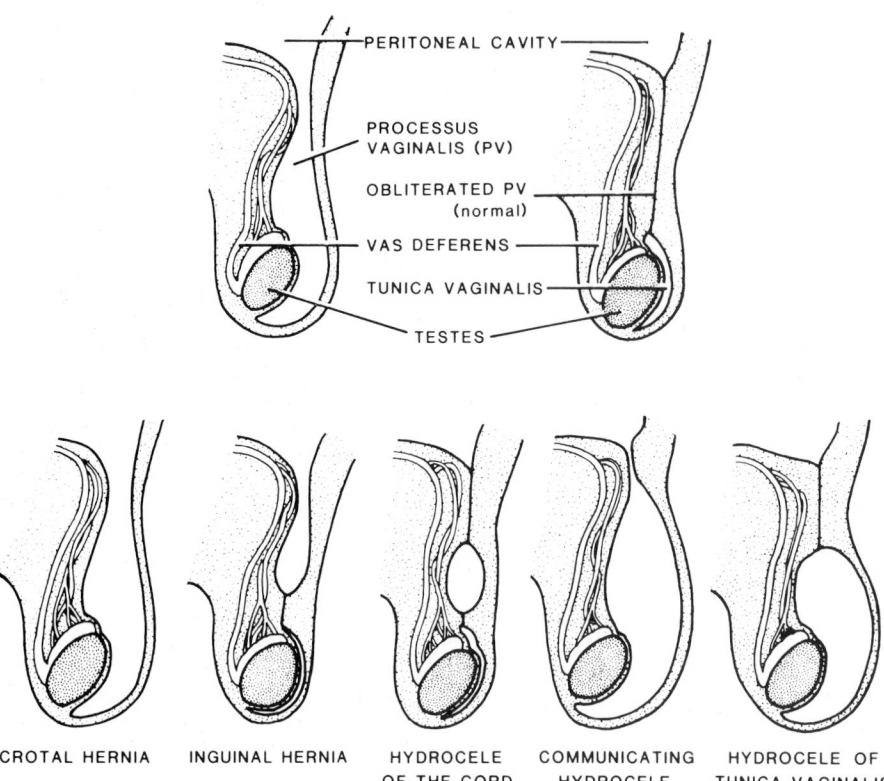

Figure 22. The upper portion of this illustration demonstrates fetal development of the processus vaginalis and normal full-term appearance following its obliterations. The lower illustrations indicate the common variants of inguinal canal anomalies in infants and children characterized by persistence of all or part of the processus. (From Grosfeld, J. L.: Current concepts in inguinal hernia in infants and children. World J. Surg., *13:*506, 1989.)

The hydrocele of the tunica vaginalis may spontaneously resolve in the first 6 months of life. If it persists beyond that time, there is probably a connection to the peritoneal cavity indicating that surgical intervention is warranted. Acquired hydroceles may develop in older children as a result of tumor, trauma, or inflammation and may require hydrocelectomy.

UMBILICAL HERNIA

Umbilical hernia is a defect of the umbilical ring. The sac has an inner lining of peritoneum that is adherent to the undersurface of the umbilical skin. Umbilical hernia is more common in females and black children. The natural history of umbilical hernia is spontaneous involution in 80 per cent of patients. The defect is usually less than 2 cm. Hernia defects greater than

TABLE 5. Conditions Associated with an Increased Incidence of Inguinal Hernia

Prematurity
Positive family history
Hydrops
Meconium peritonitis
Chylous ascites
Liver disease with ascites
Abdominal wall defects
Ambiguous genitalia
Hypospadias, epispadias
Exstrophy of bladder, cloaca
Cryptorchid testes
Cystic fibrosis
Connective tissue disorders
Ventriculoperitoneal shunt
Continuous ambulatory peritoneal dialysis
Hunter-Hurler syndrome
Mucopolysaccharidosis

Patients seen at the J. W. Riley Hospital for Children, Indiana University Medical Center, Indianapolis, IN.

From Grosfeld, J. L.: Current concepts in inguinal hernia in infants and children. World J. Surg., *13:*506, 1989.

2 cm. often do not close. Unlike inguinal hernias, the umbilical hernia rarely is associated with complications. As it is a low-risk lesion, it is reasonable to observe the umbilical hernia for 3 to 4 years in anticipation of spontaneous closure. In cases that persist for more than 4 years, an umbilical hernia repair should be performed with suture inversion of the undersurface of the umbilical skin for cosmetic purposes. If the patient requires a general anesthetic for repair of inguinal hernias, the umbilical hernia can be repaired simultaneously before 3 to 4 years of age.

UNDESCENDED TESTES

Undescended testis is observed in 1 to 2 per cent of full-term males. The actual incidence varies considerably with gestational age. Up to 30 per cent of preterm babies may have an undescended testis.[73] The cryptorchid testis is associated with both histologic and morphologic changes in the affected testis characterized by loss of volume and progressive germ cell depletion beginning at 6 months of age.[32] Other histologic changes occur including atrophy of Leydig cells, decreased tubular diameter, and reduced number of spermatogonia by 2 years of age. Since some undescended testes noted in premature infants eventually descend by 1 year of age, the author usually observes the infant until that time. The differential diagnosis includes "bashful" (retractile) testis, ectopic testis, and monorchism. The retractile testis can be brought into the scrotal sac on physical examination in a frog-leg position and is managed nonoperatively. Ectopic testis is usually detected in an aberrant location after exiting from the external ring at the time of inguinal exploration. Although some clinicians advocate therapy with human chorionic gonadotropin, the results have been discouraging and the response rate is least favorable between 1 and 2 years of age.[32] The author recommends early orchiopexy with dartos pouch fixation at 1 year of age.

TUMORS

During the past decade significant advances have been made in the management of infants and children with malignant solid tumors. Improved understanding of tumor behavior and response to combined modalities of treatment has led to improved survival in a number of patients with neoplasms. Many of these advances have been made possible by the development of cooperative study groups and multidisciplined care.

Wilms' Tumor

Wilms' tumor (nephroblastoma) is an embryonal tumor of renal origin. Approximately 500 new cases of this pediatric malignancy are seen in the United States annually.[45] Most are managed according to protocols of the National Wilms' Tumor Study Group (NWTS).[13,25] An abdominal mass is often detected by a parent while bathing the infant or child. Hematuria is noted in 10 to 15 per cent of patients, often after relatively minimal trauma to an unsuspected renal tumor. Hypertension is present in 20 per cent and is related to compression of the juxtaglomerular apparatus by the tumor. The majority of patients are diagnosed between 1 and 4 years of age. However, the tumor is noted in older children and occasionally adolescents or young adults. Wilms' tumor is more commonly observed in infants with sporadic aniridia, hemihypertrophy, Beckwith-Wiedemann syndrome, neurofibromatosis, and horseshoe kidney; in families with genitourinary anomalies; and as a hereditary factor associated with the eighth and eleventh chromosome.[45] On physical examination, the tumor presents as a round, smooth, and hard flank mass; the mass is usually nontender. Ultrasonography demonstrates a solid intrarenal lesion and also indicates whether the tumor has extended into the renal vein, inferior vena cava, or, occasionally, right atrium. The next diagnostic test obtained is computed tomography (CT) study of the abdomen with intravenous contrast.[22] This demonstrates a renal mass and a pyelogram effect indicating intrinsic distortion of the collecting system with medial displacement of the kidney. The CT study also separates the kidney from other organs (e.g., adrenal), indicates if the tumor involves the liver on the right or diaphragm on either side by direct extension, identifies the presence of enlarged and suspicious perirenal and para-aortic lymph nodes or a second tumor in the opposite kidney, and determines if the patient has liver metastases. A chest film and CT scan are obtained to determine lung metastases. Bone survey is obtained since patients with clear-cell histologic type of Wilms' tumor may have bone metastases, which is otherwise rare in patients with this neoplasm. Arteriograms and magnetic resonance imaging are rarely helpful in the preoperative evaluation of Wilms' tumor, and for most patients these tests are both unnecessary and unduly expensive.

The treatment of Wilms' tumor depends on the staging of the specific case by preoperative and postoperative evaluation of the extent of disease based on preliminary studies as outlined, the resectability of the primary tumor, the status of perirenal, capsular, and lymph node involvement, the local invasion of nearby organs and structures (e.g., liver, diaphragm, mesentery), the tumor histologic type, and the presence or absence of distant metastases or contralateral involvement (second Wilms' tumor). Operative management includes a carefully planned, well monitored radical resection of the affected kidney through a long transverse transabdominal incision under general endotracheal anesthesia.[44,45] The incision should be sufficiently large to examine both sides and remove the tumor without spillage. The opposite kidney and liver are first evaluated for possible tumor involvement. The colon attachment and mesentery are carefully separated from the tumor and moved medially. The duodenum and liver are carefully freed on the right side, and the splenic flexure of the colon is mobilized on the left. The spleen and pancreas are elevated and retracted anteriorly and superiorly on the left side, exposing the entire upper retroperitoneal space and diaphragm. When feasible, the hilum of the kidney is approached initially and the renal artery and vein are identified and divided. This controls blood loss during the re-

section and also theoretically reduces the risk of blood-borne and lymphatic metastases during the procedure. This may not always be possible, and mobilization of the tumor may be necessary in some instances to clearly identify the vascular pedicle without injury to other structures (e.g., superior mesenteric artery). The tumor is dissected free from the aorta, and the lymph node–bearing tissues in the renal hilum and ipsilateral para-aortic region are excised for staging purposes. The retrorenal fossa is freed, and any attachments to the diaphragm may require *en bloc* excision with the tumor. On the right side, direct extension of tumor into the liver also requires *en bloc* resection in 1.5 to 7 per cent of patients. The adrenal gland can be spared if the tumor is small or is located in the inferior pole; however, this organ must be excised if the primary lesion involves the superior pole of the kidney. In rare instances, the tumor may not be safely resected at the first procedure. Under these circumstances, a biopsy should be obtained to confirm the histologic type (which is inadequate with a needle biopsy) and the patient treated with two courses of chemotherapy to shrink the tumor. A successful second-look resection of the tumor has almost always been possible in the author's experience.[49]

The current staging system for Wilms' tumor is listed in Table 6. Following surgical excision, treatment depends on both stage and histologic type. The histologic evaluation of Wilms' tumor is accomplished in a central pathology center to confirm local impressions. Histologic type is divided into "favorable" (FH) and "unfavorable" (UH), which reflect both invasiveness of the tumor and response to therapy. Favorable lesions represent 89 per cent of the cases, whereas unfavorable cases occur in 11 per cent. The former is characterized by blastemal, epithelial, mixed, and even glomerular elements; the latter is further subgrouped into anaplastic (4.4 per cent), clear-cell (4 per cent), and rhabdoid (2.3 per cent). Anaplastic tumors are characterized by nuclear pleomorphism and extreme hyperdiploidy. Clear-cell tumors may involve bone and brain and appear to disseminate early, but their survival is altered (improved) by additional therapy given in the treatment program (e.g., doxorubicin). Survival at 2 years is 91 per cent but declines to 77 per cent at 4 years. Unfortunately, infants and children with rhabdoid tumors have aggressive disease with widespread metastases and frequently succumb early (within 1 to 2 years; 90 per cent relapse rate and 86 per cent mortality) despite multidrug treatment. Stage I and Stage II patients with FH are treated with actinomycin-D and vincristine in pulse courses and have a 95 per cent survival. Anaplastic tumors are rare under the age of 2 years. If an anaplastic tumor is completely resected and considered Stage I, the outcome is similar to Stage I infants with FH. In more advanced stages, however, anaplastic tumors have a 55 per cent relapse rate and 45 per cent mortality. The overall survival for patients with FH tumors is 90 per cent for all stages. The few patients with FH tumors who succumb are nonresponsive to treatment and have usually primitive blastemal tumors that are more invasive in nature.[137] In Stage I and Stage II, these tumors are more adherent to surrounding structures and tumor may be

TABLE 6. Current Staging for Wilms' Tumor

Group I	Tumor limited to the kidney and completely resected
Group II	Tumor extends beyond the kidney but is completely resected; capsule invasion, perirenal tissues may be involved
Group III	Residual nonhematogenous tumor confined to the abdomen, including tumor rupture (or biopsy) or peritoneal implants; lymph nodes involved
Group IV	Hematogenous metastases (lung, distant lymph nodes, brain)
Group V	Bilateral renal involvement

noted in intrarenal vessels. Patients with Stage III have an 80 per cent survival, and even in the presence of metastatic disease (Stage IV) 60 per cent survive.[25,45] Patients with lower-staged procedures are given three-drug chemotherapy with the addition of doxorubicin to the treatment protocol. Unresponsive patients are treated with second-phase drugs including ifosfamide and cis-platinum.

The treatment of pulmonary metastases remains controversial. Treatment with chemotherapy and whole-lung irradiation (1800 rads to each side) appears to be as effective as surgical excision of multiple metastases. The incidence of pulmonary relapse is quite low (7 per cent); however, 13 per cent acquire radiation pneumonitis as a complication of therapy. Another special circumstance is management of intracaval involvement, which occurs in 4 per cent of patients. Appropriate excision of the primary tumor and tumor thrombus when feasible is advised. The level of tumor thrombus is an important preoperative consideration (infrahepatic cava, 61 per cent; intrahepatic cava, 14 per cent; suprahepatic inferior vena cava or right atrium, 21 per cent). In the last cases, cardiopulmonary bypass should be an available surgical adjunct. Cardiopulmonary bypass has been used successfully by a number of investigators in the field to safely remove tumor thrombus from the right atrium and pulmonary artery.[45] The level of thrombus involvement does not affect outcome.

The overall survival is 88 per cent, 89 per cent, and 62 per cent for Stage II, Stage III, and Stage IV, respectively. The key indicator of survival is tumor histologic type. There may be an alternative method of therapy in massive involvement, using preoperative chemotherapy to shrink the tumor, which may make the resection safer. In Stage V disease (bilateral Wilms' tumor), a very conservative approach to therapy is recommended in an attempt to preserve renal parenchyma and avoid bilateral nephrectomy, the need for dialysis, and renal transplantation. Treatment options include bilateral heminephrectomy if feasible, initial bilateral biopsy, chemotherapy, avoidance of irradiation therapy and second-look or even third-look laparotomies to limit renal resection, or total nephrectomy on one side and partial nephrectomy on the other. In a relatively large group of NWTS patients, the 3-year survival was 76 per cent despite institutional variation in therapy. Currently, unless both tumors are small and allow bilateral partial nephrectomy, the author favors bilateral biopsy and chemotherapy at the onset of treatment. Fortunately, most patients have favorable histologic type (86 per cent). Ten per cent have unfavorable histologic type, and 4 per cent have discordant pathology with favorable on one side and unfavorable on the other. This observation indicates both kidneys must always be biopsied. The best prognosis in Stage V disease is age less than 3 years, favorable histologic type, negative lymph node involvement, and lower staging of the most advanced of the two renal lesions.

Mesoblastic Nephroma

Mesoblastic nephroma (renal embryoma) is a renal tumor that usually presents in infants less than 3 to 4 months of age.[18] The tumor is embryonic in nature and has been detected on prenatal ultrasound examination. The mass appears as a solid lesion with a concentric ring pattern. An abdominal CT examination with contrast shows a solid neoplasm (that occasionally contains calcium) with intrarenal distortion of the collecting system. The treatment of choice is nephrectomy with lymph node sampling since rarely the tumor appears malignant. More than 95 per cent of mesonephric nephromas are benign and require no other treatment.

Nephroblastomatosis

Nephroblastomatosis (nodular renal blastema) is a benign condition with subcapsular nests of primitive metanephric epithelial rests around the rim of the kidney. This condition may be multifocal and involve both kidneys. The nephrogenic rest may undergo sclerosis, involution, or hyperplastic overgrowth with tumor induction to a neoplastic rest that has the potential to progress to a Wilms' tumor (with mitosis) or an adenomatous rest (no mitosis). Nephroblastomatosis is therefore an accumulation of multiple nephrogenic rests. Ninety per cent of synchronous bilateral Wilms' tumors and 94 per cent of metachronous bilateral tumors contain areas of nephrogenic rests. The risk of a nephrogenic rest becoming malignant is 1 to 3 per cent.

Neuroblastoma

Neuroblastoma is an embryonal tumor of neural crest origin that may arise anywhere in the sympathetic nervous system including the neck (3 per cent), posterior mediastinum (20 per cent), pelvis (3 per cent), para-aortic paraspinal ganglia (24 per cent), and adrenal medulla (50 per cent).[40] This is the most common solid malignant tumor of infancy and occurs in 1 in 7000 to 10,000 live births. More than 50 per cent occur in the first 2 years of life and 90 per cent by 8 years. The tumor may be observed in patients with Hirschsprung's disease, fetal alcohol syndrome, and Beckwith-Weidemann syndrome and in mothers taking phenylhydantoin for seizures. The tumor should be classified as an APUD tumor since it secretes a number of hormones and other substances including vasoactive intestinal polypeptide, vasoactive substances such as catecholamines and their by-products (homovanillic acid [HVA], vanillylmandelic acid [VMA], and 3-methyltyrosine [3-MT], metanephrines, and dopamine), ferritin, and rarely acetylcholine. Symptoms vary according to tumor location and whether metastases have occurred. An abdominal mass is palpable in 50 per cent of patients and is firm, nodular, and somewhat tender. Respiratory distress (mediastinal tumor), Horner's syndrome (upper chest or neck lesion), proptosis or bilateral black eyes ("panda eyes") from orbital metastases, leg pain and refusal to walk because of bone metastases, hepatomegaly, and subcutaneous tumor nodules are other findings. Systemic manifestations such as anemia, failure to thrive, weight loss, and poor nutritional status may be observed in patients with bone marrow metastases and advanced disease. Paraplegia or the cauda equina syndrome are related to extradural extension of tumor. Hypokalemic watery diarrhea syndrome (due to vasoactive intestinal polypeptide secretion) and opsoclonus and nystagmus ("dancing-eye syndrome") may also be indicative of a neurogenic tumor.[129] Hypertension is noted in 20 to 35 per cent of patients due to release of catecholamines. Diagnosis is achieved with plain radiographic and CT examination of the area involved. Stippled calcification within the mass and paraspinal widening may also be noted. CT scans usually differentiate a renal tumor and neuroblastoma that either displaces the kidney downward (adrenal tumor) or laterally (paraspinal lesion).[40] Spinal involvement is best detected with a magnetic resonance imaging study. Bone survey and bone-seeking [99m]technetium scintiscan are useful in detecting bone metastases. Bone marrow aspirate may demonstrate the presence of tumor rosettes. A 24-hour urinary collection to measure urinary VMA, HVA, and metanephrines confirms elevated levels in more than 85 per cent of patients. Preoperative serum ferritin, neuron-specific enolase, coagulation profile, and complete blood count are obtained.

Therapy depends on the extent of disease as determined by preoperative clinical and operative staging. The most frequent staging system utilized has been the Evans system (Table 7). A new international staging system has recently been developed to allow comparison of data between groups and countries[120] (Table 8). Very few patients are classified as having Stage I (5 per cent); 25 per cent have Stage II; and the majority have advanced disease, with Stage III affecting 20 per cent and Stage IV or IV-S (with metastases) affecting 50 per cent. Complete surgical excision is the only treatment required for Stage I. In

TABLE 7. Staging of Neuroblastoma (Evans)

Stage	Description
I	Tumor is confined to organ of origin (totally excised)
II	Tumor extends beyond organ of origin but does not cross the midline; regional lymph nodes may be involved
III	Tumor extends beyond midline to encroach on tissues on opposite side (exclude overhanging tumor)
IV	Distant metastases (skeletal, other organs, soft tissues, distant lymph nodes)
IV-S	Localized primary tumor not crossing midline with remote disease confined to liver, subcutaneous tissues, and bone marrow, but without evidence of bone cortex involvement

patients with Stage II disease, surgical excision may also be reasonable if the tumor histologic type is favorable, DNA–flow cytometry shows an aneuploid tumor, and there are less than 3 copies of the N-*myc* oncogene.[84,116,118,127] Normal neuron-specific enolase levels and low serum ferritin levels are also useful determinants of the aggressive nature of the tumor.[40] If some of these tests are unfavorable (especially the N-*myc*), then aggressive chemotherapy programs are added. In Stage III, surgical therapy alone may be reasonable if total excision can be accomplished and all tumor markers are negative. However, at the initial operation, most Stage III cases are large, often unresectable neoplasms. Following a biopsy to evaluate histologic type, N-*myc* testing and DNA–flow cytometry, these patients are treated with aggressive programs of chemotherapy to shrink the tumor and, it is hoped, allow second-look resection prior to the development of metastases.[41,49] Unfortunately, many patients with Stage III develop metastases early and require the same type of aggressive treatment programs as infants and children with Stage IV (metastatic) disease. This includes multiple-drug chemotherapy programs (*cis*-platinum, doxorubicin, VP-16, and melphalan) combined with delayed primary tumor excision,[41] regional radiation therapy for residual nonresectable retroperitoneal disease, total-body irradiation or near-lethal melphalan therapy, and rescue with an autologous bone marrow

TABLE 8. Proposed International Staging System for Neuroblastoma

Stage	Description
I	Localized tumor confined to the area of origin; complete gross excision, with or without microscopic residual disease; identifiable ipsilateral and contralateral lymph nodes negative microscopically.
2A	Unilateral tumor with incomplete gross excision; identifiable ipsilateral and contralateral lymph nodes negative microscopically
2B	Unilateral tumor with complete or incomplete gross excision; with positive ipsilateral regional lymph nodes; identifiable contralateral lymph nodes negative microscopically
3	Tumor infiltrating across the midline with or without regional lymph node involvement; or unilateral tumor with contralateral regional lymph node involvement; or midline tumor with bilateral regional lymph node involvement
4	Dissemination of tumor to distant lymph nodes, bone, bone marrow, liver, and/or other organs (except as defined in Stage 4S)
4S	Localized primary tumor as defined for Stage 1 or Stage 2A, with dissemination limited to liver, skin, or bone marrow

From Smith, E. I., et al: Surgical perspective on the current staging in neuroblastoma: The International Neuroblastoma Staging System Proposal. J. Pediatr. Surg., 24:386, 1989.

transplant in which the marrow has been purged of potential neuroblasts with monoclonal antibodies. Operation in Stage IV permits evaluation of lymph node involvement and resection of the primary tumor, converts cases from a partial response to a complete tumor response at the local site, and determines if local irradiation is required for unresectable tumor. In some series, the only survivors with metastatic disease had the primary tumor resected. Treatment for Stage IV-S disease is controversial. Survival in these unusual cases with hepatic metastases, subcutaneous tumor nodules, and sometimes bone marrow metastases without bone cortex involvement is greater than 80 per cent even without treatment in some. Patients with IV-S with bone marrow metastases and those with more than 10 copies of the N-*myc* oncogene should be treated with chemotherapy. Patients with Stage IV-S with significant hepatomegaly may develop respiratory distress due to diaphragmatic elevation, which can be improved with radiation to the liver (600 to 1000 rads). The use of a temporary ventral hernia with Dacron-reinforced Silastic has been attempted in some; however, this is not routinely recommended.

The two key determinants of survival in instances of neuroblastoma have been the age of the patient and the stage of disease at diagnosis. In 266 children with neuroblastoma at the author's institution, survival of children less than 1 year was 76 per cent versus 32 per cent for those older than 1 year of age. Survival has been near 100 per cent for Stage I, 80 per cent for Stage II, 37 per cent for Stage III, a rather dismal 12 per cent for Stage IV, and 81 per cent for Stage IV-S. Survival for site was 100 per cent for both pelvic and neck primary tumors, 81 per cent for mediastinal lesions, and only 28 per cent for retroperitoneal cases. The overall survival was 44 per cent. However, 87 of 119 survivors had Stage I, Stage II, or Stage IV-S disease and 56 cases were less than 1 year of age. Children with vasoactive intestinal polypeptide secretion and opsoclonus/nystagmus have an excellent prognosis with more than 90 per cent of these patients surviving following tumor resection.[129] These data indicate that an improved prognosis can be anticipated in infants less than 1 year of age with Stage I, Stage II, and Stage IV-S, normal neuron-specific enolase and serum ferritin, favorable Shimada tumor histology,[118] aneuploid DNA–flow cytometry,[127] less than three copies of N-*myc*, primary tumors affecting the pelvis, neck, and mediastinum, and good nutrition. In contrast, a poor prognosis might be expected in children with Stage III and Stage IV, retroperitoneal tumors,[60] elevated HVA:VMA ratio, elevated neuron-specific enolase and serum ferritin levels, more than 10 copies of N-*myc*,[84,116] diploid DNA–flow cytometry, unfavorable Shimada tumor histology,[118] and malnutrition at diagnosis. An improved understanding of the immune aspects of neuroblastoma, screening programs for early detection of unsuspected disease in infancy (as practiced in Japan),[112] refinements in combined treatment programs (use of bone marrow transplant early in the treatment phase), and a more careful selection of patients for aggressive therapy based on age, stage, histology, tumor markers, DNA–flow cytometry, and the number of copies of N-*myc* may prove useful in reducing the mortality of this unusual and highly lethal pediatric cancer.

Rhabdomyosarcoma

Rhabdomyosarcoma is a highly malignant soft tissue sarcoma of infancy and childhood that can occur in many areas of the body including the head and neck, orbit, chest wall and mediastinum, respiratory tract, trunk and extremities, perianal region, retroperitoneum, bile duct, bladder and prostate, uterus, vagina, and paratesticular tissues.[48] The survival of infants and children with rhabdomyosarcoma depends on the site of occurrence, extent of disease (stage) and tumor histology.[48] The location of the primary tumor is often age-dependent with lower genitourinary, head and neck, perianal, and bile duct lesions more common in infancy and early childhood, whereas trunk, extremity, and uterine lesions are more commonly encountered in adolescents. Diagnostic work-up involves a CT scan of the involved region, which also assesses the extent of tissue involvement and local tumor spread. Ultrasonography is useful for a suspected bile duct lesion; cystoscopy and vaginoscopy are important in staging and acquiring a biopsy specimen in bladder or vaginal tumors. Magnetic resonance imaging is useful in evaluating possible spinal canal encroachment by a paraspinal tumor or muscle planes in extremity lesions. Since there are no known tumor markers for rhabdomyosarcoma, an accurate diagnosis is dependent on a tissue biopsy.

Staging is performed according to the Intergroup Rhabdomyosarcoma Staging System (Table 9). Accurate staging requires preoperative radiologic assessment and histologic evaluation of the surgical margins and lymph nodes as well as the tumor type. In a survey of 146 patients at the author's institution, 21 per cent had Stage I, 22 per cent Stage II, 28 per cent Stage III, and 29 per cent Stage IV disease at the time of diagnosis. The pathology of rhabdomyosarcoma has been in flux in the past few years. The commonly referred to cell lines are embryonal, alveolar, pleomorphic, and undifferentiated. Botryoid tumor refers to a physical appearance of grapelike clusters of an embryonal tumor growing into a cavity from the wall of the bladder, vagina, and bile duct. The undifferentiated tumors represents 15 to 20 per cent of rhabdomyosarcomas. Embryonal tumors have a favorable prognosis; alveolar tumors are considered unfavorable and have a very poor prognosis. Alveolar tumors are more commonly noted in the extremities. The nuclear characteristics of the tumor cells and the predominance of tumor subtype within a specific neoplasm determine the prognosis. Disease-free survival for favorable tumors is 65 per cent at 2 years but is less than 40 per cent for unfavorable lesions.

The most important part of therapy for rhabdomyosarcoma is resection of the primary tumor when possible. Patients with complete resection do better than those with gross residual disease, particularly in trunk and extremity tumors. Vincristine, actinomycin-D and cyclophosphamide (VAC) have been the chemotherapy agents commonly employed. Patients with Stage I with favorable histologic type require adjunctive chemotherapy without radiation. Doxorubicin is not additive when given with the VAC program in Stage III cases and may induce cardiotoxicity. Cis-platinum and VP-16 are added in recurrent or unresponsive cases. Local radiotherapy to the tumor bed is required in Stage II, Stage III, and Stage IV and instances of tumor relapse (4000 rads to be effective) and reduces the risk of local tumor recurrence. Some sites of primary tumor occurrence preclude a wide cancer resection (e.g., head and neck, pelvis), making adjunctive therapy (chemotherapy and radiation) the mainstay of treatment. For genitourinary tumors, initial biopsy is employed as primary treatment with chemotherapy in attempt to avoid pelvic exenteration.[61] Genitourinary lesions often are favorable histologic types and tend to stay localized for extended periods, making this approach reasonable. More localized resection of the primary tumor including partial cystectomy and partial vaginectomy has been successfully accomplished in some. Salvage cystectomy is possible in patients when relapse occurs. The survival for bladder and prostate tumors is 70 per cent.[61,82] These results, however, do not compare with the greater than 90 per cent survival noted in bladder/prostate tumors managed by anterior pelvic exenteration.[48] Patients with vaginal lesions have a greater than 90 per cent survival, but only 40 per cent of patients with uterine tumors survive.[62]

For patients with head and neck primary tumors, especially those with a parameningeal location (sinus, middle ear), craniospinal irradiation and intrathecal chemotherapy reduce the incidence of meningeal spread from 35 per cent to 6 per cent and increase survival. Unfortunately, this treatment caused late complications in survivors characterized by cognitive deficits. Craniospinal irradiation will be used only in known intracerebral lesions in the future. The overall survival for tumors of the head and neck is 60 per cent. Patients with orbital tumors have an excellent prognosis (greater than 90 per cent survival) with either primary chemotherapy or extirpation of the globe.

Survival in patients with extremity lesions has been adversely affected by attempts to treat these lesions with biopsy and primary chemotherapy (converting potential Stage I cases to Stage III) and the high incidence of alveolar histologic type (44 per cent). Patients with Stage III cases have a 35 per cent survival and high rate of local recurrence. Preoperative chemotherapy has been ineffective treatment. Optimal treatment involves early wide local excision, paying careful attention to the muscle compartments during the resection. Limb salvage is usually possible with survival greater than 70 to 75 per cent in Stage I and Stage II after appropriate chemotherapy (VAC) and radiation therapy in Stage II. If microscopic residual disease is noted on histologic evaluation of the initial specimen (Stage IIa), re-excision of the tumor site within 2 weeks of previous surgical therapy leads to a statistically improved survival.

Excellent survival is achieved in instances of paratesticular rhabdomyosarcoma (greater than 85 per cent). Most have favorable histologic type. The treatment of choice is an orchiectomy with high ligation of the spermatic cord on the affected side through an inguinal incision. The spermatic cord is controlled at the level of the internal inguinal ring prior to mobilizing the tumor and testis. If a biopsy has been done elsewhere through the scrotal sac, a scrotectomy should also be done at the time of definitive resection. Retroperitoneal exploration to evaluate for lymph node involvement (45 per cent) is performed for staging purposes. The fact that chemotherapy (VAC) is so effective suggests that radiation therapy may not be necessary for paratesticular tumors.

Although excellent results have been obtained for certain tumor sites, primary tumors affecting the chest wall, bile ducts, buttocks, and retroperitoneum have a poor prognosis. Infants with tumors involving the perianal area have fared well following abdominoperineal resection, permanent colostomy, chemotherapy, and irradiation. Recently, the author has treated an additional child with initial biopsy and chemotherapy with no evidence of tumor residual at 1 year.

A review of 3000 patients from Intergroup Rhabdomyosarcoma Study III (IRS) indicates that the overall 3-year survival was 70 per cent. The 5-year survival for the IRS-I study was only 55 per cent. Stage, site, histologic type, and tumor size were the main predicators of outcome. Although significant advances have been achieved in certain tumor sites, other locations remain a problem, and Stage IV has a continued dismal

TABLE 9. Current Staging for Rhabdomyosarcoma

Group I	Localized disease, completely resected, no lymph node involvement a. Tumor confined to the muscle or organ of origin b. Tumor infiltration outside this structure
Group II	Localized or regional disease with total gross resection a. Primary tumor grossly resected, with "microscopic residual" disease, regional nodes negative b. Completely resected primary tumor, i.e., no "microscopic residual" disease in which there is extension into an adjacent organ (no "microscopic residual") c. Resected primary tumor, with evidence of "microscopic residual" disease and positive nodes (all resected)
Group III	Incomplete resection or biopsy, with residual unresected disease (either primary tumor or regional nodes)
Group IV	Distant metastatic disease present at diagnosis (regional nodes excluded)

outcome. Pilot studies using more aggressive chemotherapy programs in conjunction with bone marrow transplantation (as currently employed in Stage IV neuroblastoma) and second-look procedures to accurately assess complete response to chemotherapy will be considered in a treatment plan for advanced cases of rhabdomyosarcoma in the future.

Hepatic Tumors

Liver tumors in children can be benign or malignant. Benign tumors include hemangioma, hemangioendothelioma, mesenchymal hamartoma, teratoma, and focal nodular hyperplasia. *Hemangioma* is the most frequently benign liver tumor in infancy. These lesions may be solitary and involve a single segment or lobe or present as multiple hemangiomatosis involving the entire liver.[9,21,122] On rare occasion, a large vascular malformation may rupture and cause hemoperitoneum. A dynamic CT scan with intravenous bolus contrast is usually diagnostic and shows a characteristic pattern of heterogeneous areas within the liver with increased filling and rapid emptying of the contrast. Liver hemangiomas follow the natural history of most hemangiomas—spontaneous involution. Unfortunately, some infants present with a syndrome of hepatomegaly, cutaneous hemangioma, and cardiac failure due to arteriovenous shunting within the liver. Treatment includes corticosteroids, diuretics, and digoxin. Continued symptoms may require more aggressive treatment. Hepatic resection may be possible for hemangiomas affecting a single liver segment or lobe. In some patients, hepatic artery embolization or ligation may be necessary. The mortality in these cases remains high (20 to 33 per cent). Malignant tumors include *hepatoblastoma* and *hepatoma.* The former is seen in infants in the first 3 years of life and the latter in older children and adolescents.

Liver tumors are more common in children with hemihypertrophy, the Beckwith-Wiedemann syndrome, Fanconi's disease, and cirrhosis due to a variety of conditions including cholestasis from the use of total parenteral nutrition in infancy, Type 1 glycogen storage disease, and hereditary tyrosinemia. The patient is usually not jaundiced. The main findings on physical examination are abdominal distention and a right upper quadrant mass that moves with respiration. Serum alpha-fetoprotein and ferritin levels may be elevated and can be used as tumor markers. Diagnosis can be achieved by observing a right upper quadrant mass sometimes containing calcium on plain abdominal films and CT scan of the abdomen with contrast. The CT scan usually outlines the site of the tumor, clarifies its relationship to the central structures, evaluates multicentricity (common in hepatoma patients) and involvement of the contralateral lobe, and often predicts resectability. An ultrasound study determines if the tumor is solid and detects extension into the hepatic veins or vena cava. Although an arteriogram was routinely obtained in every prospective candidate for liver resection in the past, a greater appreciation of the segmental anatomy and vascular variations has made this invasive test less necessary currently. The treatment of choice is complete resection of the tumor by lobectomy or trisegmentectomy. The availability of the CUSA ultrasonic dissector, the cell saver, and rapid autotransfusers have made hepatic resection a much safer and well controlled procedure. Recent data indicate that a biopsy and courses of preoperative chemotherapy (doxorubicin) in patients with very large primary tumors or those initially considered unresectable lead to significant reduction of tumor size and allow subsequent hepatic resection and long-term survival.

Malignant liver tumors are staged according to whether the tumor is completely resected (Stage I), the tumor is resected with microscopic residual disease (Stage II), there is unresectable tumor or gross residual disease (Stage III), and metastases are present (usually to the lungs—Stage IV). The best survival is achieved in patients with Stage I disease with a complete resec-

tion who receive chemotherapy (85 to 90 per cent). A new Intergroup Hepatoma Protocol has been developed to (1) evaluate the effectiveness of four short courses of doxorubicin in completely resected Stage I hepatoblastoma with fetal histologic type, and (2) compare the effects of *cis*-platinum and doxorubicin with *cis*-platinum, 5-fluorouracil, and vincristine in hepatoma and hepatoblastoma Stages I, II, III, and IV. In addition to infants with fetal histologic type, children with a fibrolaminar histologic type also have an improved prognosis. The overall survival for all patients with hepatoblastoma is 50 per cent but is only 15 per cent for hepatocarcinoma.

Teratomas

Teratomas are composed of tissues from all three germ layers (endoderm, ectoderm, and mesoderm). These lesions may be cystic or solid and occur along the para-axial tissues throughout the body including the brain, tongue, neck, anterior mediastinum, retroperitoneum, liver, gonadal tissues, and sacrococcygeal region. In the neonate, the sacrococcygeal area is the most common site of tumor occurrence. These tumors are often detected by prenatal ultrasound examination in both the cervical and sacral areas. In the latter instances, delivery by cesarean section may be necessary. In some cases arteriovenous shunting through the tumor causes a shocklike syndrome associated with severe metabolic acidosis and requires emergency resection in an attempt to salvage the infant. Sacrococcygeal tumors are much more common in females (4 : 1 ratio). A family history of twins is observed in 10 per cent of patients. Plain radiographs may demonstrate calcium within the tumor. An ultrasound examination may demonstrate extension of the tumor into the pelvis or abdomen and may also demonstrate that the bladder and rectum are displaced anteriorly and the ureters are partially obstructed causing hydroureter and hydronephrosis. Malignancy is rarely observed in the neonate. Elective resection should be performed in the first week of life. Long delays in recognition, diagnosis, and surgical excision may be associated with a higher rate of malignancy. Malignant teratomas are either endodermal sinus tumors (yolk sac tumors) or embryonal carcinomas. Serum alpha-fetoprotein and human chorionic gonadotropin levels may be elevated in instances of yolk sac tumor and can be used as tumor markers. The treatment of choice for sacrococcygeal teratoma is complete excision through a chevron-shaped buttocks incision with careful preservation of the rectal sphincter. The coccyx should always be resected with the tumor. Failure to do so leads to a 35 to 40 per cent tumor recurrence. During the dissection, early control of the midsacral vessels that supply the tumor is important and prevents significant hemorrhage, which is the most common operative complication. In instances of malignancy, a careful search for metastatic disease in the liver, lungs, and retroperitoneum with chest films and CT scan should be done. Malignant cases are treated with cisplatin and bleomycin. Radiation therapy is probably not indicated since these agents lead to an excellent tumor response. In instances in which the malignant tumor is not resectable, courses of chemotherapy may shrink the tumor, convert the tumor to a benign-appearing teratoma, and allow complete resection at a second-look procedure with gratifying survival in some cases.

SELECTED REFERENCES

Ashcraft, K. W., and Holder, T. M.: Pediatric Esophageal Surgery. Orlando, Grune & Stratton, 1986.
This is an excellent monograph concerning disorders of the esophagus in children. The section on embryology is quite thorough. The chapters present the various aspects of pediatric esophageal disease in great detail. The book is nicely illustrated and is a useful resource for the practicing surgeon.

Dehner, L.: Pediatric Surgical Pathology, 2nd ed. Baltimore, Williams & Wilkins, 1987.
This is a new edition of a fine publication concerning pediatric surgical pathology.

This text is very complete and well written. The content allows the reader to correlate the clinical aspects of the various pediatric disease states with an in-depth review of the pathologic findings.

Gross, R. E.: The Surgery of Infancy and Childhood. Philadelphia, W. B. Saunders Company, 1953.
This book was the most influential textbook of pediatric surgery for more than 2 decades. The content reflects the enormous personal experience of the late Robert E. Gross, one of the paternal figures of pediatric surgery at the Boston Children's Hospital. In addition to the historical significance as a reference source, the text is so well written it is worthwhile reading.

Hays, D. M.: Pediatric Surgical Oncology. Orlando, Grune & Stratton, 1986.
This monograph is an important resource for surgeons interested in pediatric surgical oncology. Each chapter is written by a contributing author who is an expert in the field. The rapid growth of information based on data accrued from cooperative multidisciplined tumor study group activities is carefully presented and highlights the current management of solid pediatric malignancies.

Jones, K. L.: Smith's Recognizable Patterns of Human Malformations, 4th ed. Philadelphia, W. B. Saunders Company, 1986.
This superb textbook is an easily readable repository of human malformations including developmental anomalies and intrauterine acquired conditions. The text is well written, is beautifully illustrated, and presents a concise review of the etiology, history, and prognosis for each syndrome.

Rogers, M. C.: Textbook of Pediatric Intensive Care, 2nd Ed. Baltimore, Williams & Wilkins, 1987.
This two-volume text is currently the most comprehensive resource concerning the rapidly expanding field of pediatric intensive care and critical care. The text exposes the reader to the mainstream concepts of intensive care practice in the pediatric setting.

Stephens, F. D., Smith, E. D., and Paul, N. W.: Anorectal Malformations in Children: Update 1988. (Birth Defects Foundation, Vol. 24.) New York, Alan R. Liss, 1988.
This is a new edition of the leading text describing the various types of congenital anorectal anomalies. The book includes the new "Wingspread Classification" of these complex defects and a detailed clinical presentation of current methods of diagnosis and treatment. The recommended surgical techniques are well described and illustrated.

Welch, K. W., Randolph, J. G., Ravitch, M. M., O'Neill, J. A., and Rowe, M. I. (Eds.): Pediatric Surgery, 4th ed. Chicago, Year Book Medical Publishers, 1986.
This two-volume textbook of pediatric surgery is the best comprehensive resource for information regarding patient care management. It is considered the major reference source currently available. The text covers all areas of pediatric surgical care and has numerous contributors who have written chapters in their areas of expertise.

REFERENCES

1. Adzick, N. S., Vacanti, J. P., Lillihei, C. W., et al.: Fetal diaphragmatic hernia: Ultrasound diagnosis and clinical outcome in 38 cases. J. Pediatr. Surg., 24:654, 1989.
2. Allam, B. F., Tillman, J. E., Thomson, T. J., Crossling, F. T., and Gilbert, L. M.: Effective intravenous cyclosporine therapy in a patient with severe Crohn's disease on parenteral nutrition. Gut, 28:1166, 1987.
3. Altman, R. P., and Margileth, A. M.: Cervical lymphadenopathy from atypical mycobacteria: Diagnosis and surgical treatment. J. Pediatr. Surg., 10:419, 1975.
4. Ashcraft, K. W., Holder, T. M., Amoury, F. A., et al.: Diagnosis and treatment of right Bochdalek hernia associated with Group B–streptococcal septicemia. J. Pediatr. Surg., 18:480, 1983.
5. Ashcraft, K. W., Holder, T. M., and Amoury, R. A.: The Thal fundoplication for gastroesophageal reflux. J. Pediatr. Surg., 19:480, 1984.
6. Axelrod, F. B., and Abubbrage, J. J.: Familial dysautonomia: A prospective study of survival. J. Pediatr., 101:234, 1982.
7. Bartlett, R. H.: Extracorporeal life support in neonatal respiratory failure. Surg. Rounds, 12:41, 1989.
8. Bartlett, R. H., Gazzaniga, A. B., et al.: Extracorporeal membrane oxygenation (ECMO) in neonatal respiratory failure: 100 cases. Ann. Surg., 204:236, 1986.
9. Becker, J. M., and Heitler, M. S.: Hepatic hemangioendotheliomas in infancy. Surg. Gynecol. Obstet., 168:189, 1989.
10. Bishop, H. C., and Koop, C. E.: Management of meconium ileus: Resection, Roux-en-Y anastomosis and ileostomy irrigation with pancreatic enzymes. Ann. Surg., 145:410, 1957.
11. Boix-Ochoa, J.: The physiologic approach to the management of gastric esophageal reflux. J. Pediatr. Surg., 21:1032, 1986.
12. Bradburn, N. C., and Schreiner, R. L.: Neonatal seizures. In Schreiner, R. L., and Bradburn, N. C. (Eds.): Care of the Newborn, 2nd ed. New York, Raven Press, 1988, pp. 153–157.
13. Breslow, N., Churchill, G., et al.: Prognosis for Wilms' tumor patients with nonmetastatic disease at diagnosis: Results of the 2nd National Wilms' tumor Study. J. Clin. Oncol., 3:521, 1985.
14. Brynskov, J., Freund, L., Rasmussen, S. N., Lauritzen, K., et al.: A placebo-

15. Canal, D. F., Vane, D. W., Goto, S., and Grosfeld, J. L.: Reduction of lower esophageal sphincter pressure with Stamm gastrostomy. J. Pediatr. Surg., 22:54, 1987.
16. Caniano, D. A., and Beaver, B. L.: Meconium ileus: A 15 year experience with 42 neonates. Surgery, 102:699, 1987.
17. Cates, M., Billmire, D. F., Bill, M. J., and Grosfeld, J. L.: Gastroesophageal dysfunction in Cornelia deLange syndrome. J. Pediatr. Surg., 24:248, 1989.
18. Chan, H. S. L., Cheng, M. Y., Mancer, K., et al.: Congenital mesoblastic nephroma: A clinicoradiologic study of 17 cases representing the pathologic spectrum of disease. J. Pediatr. Surg., 111:64, 1987.
19. Cheney, M., Rustad, D. G., and Lilly, J. R.: Choledochal cyst. World J. Surg., 9:244, 1985.
20. Cikrit, D., Mastandrea, J., West, K. W., Schreiner, R. L., and Grosfeld, J. L.: Necrotizing enterocolitis: Factors affecting mortality in 101 surgical cases. Surgery, 96:648, 1984.
21. Cohen, R. C., and Myers, N. A.: Diagnosis and management of massive hepatic hemangiomas in childhood. J. Pediatr. Surg., 21:6, 1986.
22. Cohen, M. D., Siddiqui, A., and Weetman, R. M.: A rational approach to the radiologic evaluation of children with Wilms' tumor. Cancer, 50:887, 1982.
23. Coran, A. G.: Perioperative care of the pediatric surgical patient. In Wilmore, D. W., Brennan, M. F., Harken, A. H., Holcroft, J. W., and Meakins, J. L. (Eds.): Care of the Surgical Patient. Vol. 1. New York, Scientific American, Inc., 1989, pp. 1–26.
24. Crombleholme, T. M., Harrison, M. R., Langer, J. C., and Longaker, M. T.: Biliary appendicoduodenostomy: A nonrefluxing conduit for biliary reconstruction. J. Pediatr. Surg., 24:665, 1989.
25. D'Angio, G. J., Evans, A. E., et al.: Results of the 3rd National Wilms' tumor study (NWTS-3): A preliminary report. Proc. Am. Assoc. Cancer Res., 153:177, 1987.
26. Dedinsky, G. K., Vane, D. W., Black, C. T., and Grosfeld, J. L.: Complications and reoperation after Nissen fundoplication in childhood. Am. J. Surg., 153:177, 1987.
27. deLorimier, A. A.: Congenital malformations and neonatal problems of the respiratory tract. In Welch, K. J., Randolph, J. G., Ravitch, M. M., O'Neill, J. A., and Rowe, M. I. (Eds.): Pediatric Surgery, 4th ed. Chicago, Year Book Medical Publishers, 1986, pp. 639–640.
28. deVries, P. A., and Cox, K. L.: Surgery of anorectal anomalies. Surg. Clin. North Am., 65:1139, 1985.
29. deVries, P. A., and Peña, A.: Posterior sagittal anorectoplasty. J. Pediatr. Surg., 17:638, 1982.
30. Ein, S. H., Mercer, S., Humphrey, A., and MacDonald, P.: Colon perforation during attempted barium enema reduction of intussusception. J. Pediatr. Surg., 16:313, 1981.
31. Ein, S. H., Shandling, B., Reilly, B. J., and Stringer, D. A.: Hydrostatic reduction of intussusception caused by lead points. J. Pediatr. Surg., 21:883, 1986.
32. Elder, J. S.: The undescended testis: Hormonal and surgical management. Surg. Clin. North Am., 68:983, 1988.
33. Evans, A. E., D'Angio, G. J., and Randolph, J. G.: A proposed staging for children with neuroblastoma. Cancer, 27:374, 1971.
34. Filston, H. C.: Head and neck: Sinuses and masses. In Holder, T. M., and Ashcraft, K. W. (Eds.): Pediatric Surgery. Philadelphia, W. B. Saunders Company, 1981, pp. 1062–1079.
35. Fonkalsrud, E. W., Berquist, W., Vargas, J., Turner, M. K., Ament, M. E., and Foglia, R. P.: Surgical treatment of gastroesophageal reflux syndrome in infants and children. Am. J. Surg., 154:11, 1987.
36. Forbes, D., Hodgson, M., and Hill, R.: The effects of gaviscon and metoclopramide in gastroesophageal reflux in children. J. Pediatr. Gastroenterol. Nutr., 5:549, 1986.
37. Forster, J. C.: The Surgical Diseases of Children. London, John W. Parker & Son, 1860.
38. Frietas, L., Gauthier, F., and Valayer, J.: Second operation for repair of biliary atresia. J. Pediatr. Surg., 22:857, 1987.
39. Groff, D., Nagaraj, H. S., and Peitsch, J. B.: Inguinal hernias in premature infants operated on before discharge from the neonatal intensive care unit. Arch. Surg., 120:962, 1985.
40. Grosfeld, J. L.: Neuroblastoma in infants and childhood. In Hays, D. M. (Ed.): Pediatric Surgical Oncology, Orlando, Grune & Stratton, 1986, pp. 63–85.
41. Grosfeld, J. L.: Operations for neuroblastoma. In Spitz, L., and Nixon, H. H. (Eds.): Operative Surgery (Pediatric Surgery), 4th ed. London, Butterworth & Company, 1988, pp. 478–487.
42. Grosfeld, J. L.: Current concepts in inguinal hernia in infants and children. World J. Surg., 13:506, 1989.
43. Grosfeld, J. L.: Groin hernia in infants and children. In Nyhus, L. M., and Condon, R. E. (Eds.): Hernia. Philadelphia, J. B. Lippincott Company, 1989, pp. 81–96.
44. Grosfeld, J. L.: Resection of Wilms' tumor. Surg. Rounds, 12:17, 1989.
45. Grosfeld, J. L., and Weber, T. R.: Surgical considerations in the treatment of Wilm's Tumor. In Gonzales-Crussi, F. (Ed.): Wilms' Tumor (Nephroblastoma) and Related Neoplasms of Childhood. Boca Raton, CRC Press, 1984, pp. 263–283.
46. Grosfeld, J. L., Weinberger, M., and Clatworthy, H. W., Jr.: Acute appendicitis in the first two years of life. J. Pediatr. Surg., 8:285, 1973.
47. Grosfeld, J. L., Ballantine, T. V. N., and Shoemaker, R.: Operative manage-

ment of intestinal atresia based on pathologic findings. J. Pediatr. Surg., 14:368, 1979.

48. Grosfeld, J. L., Weber, T. R., Weetman, R. M., and Baehner, R. L.: Rhabdomyosarcomas in childhood: Analysis of survival in 98 cases. J. Pediatr. Surg., 18:141, 1983.

49. Grosfeld, J. L., West, K. W., and Weber, T. R.: The role of second-look procedures in the management of retroperitoneal tumors in children. Am. J. Pediatr. Hematol. Oncol., 16:441, 1984.

50. Grosfeld, J. L., Rescorla, F. J., and West, K. W.: Short bowel syndrome in infants and children: Analysis of survival in 60 cases. Am. J. Surg., 151:41, 1986.

51. Grosfeld, J. L., Rescorla, F. J., West, K. W., and Vane, D. W.: Gastrointestinal injuries in childhood: Analysis of 53 cases. J. Pediatr. Surg., 24:580, 1989.

52. Grosfeld, J. L., Fitzgerald, J. F., Predaina, R., West, K. W., and Vane, D. W.: The efficacy of hepatoportoenterostomy in biliary atresia. Surgery, 106:692, 1989.

53. Gross, R. E.: The Surgery of Infancy and Childhood. Philadelphia, W. B. Saunders Company, 1953.

54. Guersant, P. L. B.: Notices sur la Chirurgie des Infants. Paris, Asselin, 1864.

55. Guo, J. B., Ma, X., and Zhou, Q.: Results of air pressure enema reduction of intussusception: 6,396 cases in 13 years. J. Pediatr. Surg., 12:1201, 1986.

56. Harberg, F. J., Senekjian, E. K., and Pokorny, W. J.: Treatment of uncomplicated meconium ileus via T-tube ileostomy. J. Pediatr. Surg., 16:61, 1981.

57. Harrison, M. R., Langer, J. C., Adzick, N. S., et al.: Correction of congenital diaphragmatic hernia in utero. V. Initial clinical experience. J. Pediatr. Surg., 25:47, 1990.

58. Hatch, E. I.: The acute abdomen in children. Pediatr. Clin. North Am., 32:1151, 1985.

59. Hatch, E. I., Naffis, D., and Chandler, N. W.: Pitfalls in the use of barium enema in early appendicitis in children. J. Pediatr. Surg., 16:309, 1981.

60. Hayes, F. K., Green, A., et al.: Surgicopathologic staging of neuroblastoma: Prognostic significance of regional lymph node metastases. J. Pediatr., 102:59, 1983.

61. Hays, D. M., Raney, R. B., and Lawrence, W.: Primary chemotherapy in the treatment of children with bladder-prostate tumor in the intergroup rhabdomyosarcoma study (IRS II). J. Pediatr. Surg., 17:813, 1982.

62. Hays, D. M., Shimada, H., Raney, R. B., et al.: Clinical staging and treatment results in rhabdomyosarcoma of the female genital tract among children and adolescents. Cancer, 61:1893, 1988.

63. Holder, T. M., Ashcraft, K. W., Sharp, R. J., and Amoury, R. A.: Care of infants with esophageal atresia, tracheoesophageal fistula, and associated anomalies. J. Thorac. Cardiovasc. Surg., 94:828, 1987.

64. Jolley, S. G., Leonard, J. C., and Tunell, W. P.: Gastric emptying in children with gastroesophageal reflux. II. The relationship to retching symptoms following antireflux surgery. J. Pediatr. Surg., 22:929, 1987.

65. Jolley, S. G., Tunell, W. P., Leonard, J. C., Hoelzer, D. J., and Smith, E. I.: Gastric emptying in children with gastroesophageal reflux. I. An estimate of effective gastric emptying. J. Pediatr. Surg., 22:923, 1987.

66. Karp, M. P., Cooney, D. R., Pros, G. A., Newman, B. M., and Jewett, T. C.: The nonoperative management of pediatric hepatic trauma. J. Pediatr. Surg., 18:512, 1983.

67. Karrer, F. M., and Lilly, J. R.: Corticosteroid therapy in biliary atresia. J. Pediatr. Surg., 20:593, 1985.

68. Karrer, F. M., Flannery, A. M., Nelson, M. D., McLone, C. G., and Raffensperger, J. G.: Anorectal malformations: Evaluation of associated spinal dysraphic syndrome. J. Pediatr. Surg., 23:45, 1988.

69. Kasai, M., Kimura, K., Asakura, Y., et al.: Surgical treatment of biliary atresia. J. Pediatr. Surg., 3:665, 1985.

70. Kelley, S. W.: Surgical Diseases of Children: A Modern Treatise on Pediatric Surgery. New York, E. B. Treat & Company, 1909.

71. Kimura, K., Nishijima, E., Muraji, T., et al.: A new surgical approach to extensive aganglionosis. J. Pediatr. Surg., 16:840, 1981.

72. King, D. R., Lobe, T. E., Haase, G. M., et al.: Selective management of the injured spleen. Surgery, 90:677, 1981.

73. Kogan, S. J.: The case for early orchiopexy. In King, L. R. (Ed.): Urologic Surgery in Neonates and Infants. Philadelphia, W. B. Saunders Company, 1988, pp. 396–416.

74. Kottmeier, P. K., Jongco, B., Velcek, F. T., and Klotz, D.: Absorptive function of the aganglionic ileum. J. Pediatr. Surg., 16:275, 1981.

75. Ladd, W. E., and Gross, R. E.: Abdominal Surgery of Infancy and Childhood. Philadelphia, W. B. Saunders Company, 1941.

76. Lemons, J. A., and Bradburn, N. C.: Temperature regulation. In Shreiner, R. L., and Bradburn, N. C. (Eds.): Care of the Newborn, 2nd ed. New York, Raven Press, 1988, pp. 42–46.

77. Lenaerts, C., Roy, C. C., Vaillancourt, M., Weber, A. M., Morin, C. L., and Seidman, E.: High incidence of upper gastrointestinal tract involvement on children with Crohn's disease. Pediatrics, 83:777, 1989.

78. Lennard-Jones, J. E.: Azopriothine and 6-mercaptopurine have a role in the treatment of Crohn's disease. Dig. Dis. Sci., 26:364, 1981.

79. Lilly, J. R., Karrer, F. M., Hall, R. J., Stellin, G. P., Vasquez-Estevez, J. J., Greenholz, S. K., Wanek, E. A., and Schroter, G. P.: The surgery of biliary atresia. Ann. Surg., 210:289, 1989.

80. Liu, L. M. P., Cote, C. J., Goudsouzian, N. G., and Ryan, J. F.: Life-threatening apnea in infants recovering from anesthesia. Anesthesiology, 59:506, 1983.

81. Livaditis, A.: Esophageal atresia: A method of bridging large segmental gaps. Z. Kinderchir., 13:298, 1973.

82. Loughlin, K. R., Retik, A. B., Weinstein, J., et al.: Genitourinary rhabdomyosarcoma in children. Cancer, 63:1600, 1989.

83. Mollard, P., Marechal, J. M., and Jaubert de Beaujen, M.: Surgical treatment of high imperforate anus with definition of the puborectalis sling by an anterior perineal approach. J. Pediatr. Surg., 13:499, 1978.

84. Nakagawara, A., Ikeda, K., Yokoyama, T., et al.: Surgical aspects of N-myc oncogene amplification of neuroblastoma. Surgery, 104:34, 1988.

85. Neuhauser, E. D.: Roentgen changes associated with pancreatic insufficiency in early life. Radiology, 46:319, 1946.

86. Noblett, H.: Meconium ileus. In Ravitch, M. M., Welch, K., Benson, C. D., Aberdeen, E. I., and Randolph, J. G. (Eds.): Pediatric Surgery, 3rd ed. Chicago, Year Book Medical Publishers, 1979, pp. 943–952.

87. Nomura, F., Hatano, H., Ohnishi, K., Akikusa, B., and Okuda, K.: Effects of anticonvulsant agents on halothane-induced liver injury in human subjects and experimental animals. Hepatology, 6:952, 1986.

88. Ohi, R., Hanamatsu, M., Modizuki, I., et al.: Progress in the treatment of biliary atresia. World J. Surg., 2:285, 1985.

89. Oldham, K. I., Guice, K. S., Kaufman, R. A., et al.: Blunt hepatic injury and elevated hepatic enzymes: A clinical correlation in children. J. Pediatr. Surg., 19:457, 1984.

90. Olsen, M. M., Luck, S. R., Lloyd-Still, J., and Raffensperger, J. G.: The spectrum of meconium disease in infancy. J. Pediatr. Surg., 17:479, 1982.

91. O'Neill, J. A., Templeton, J. M., Schaufner, L., Bishop, H. C., Ziegler, M. M., and Ross, A. J.: Recent experience with choledochal cyst. Ann. Surg., 205:533, 1985.

92. Orenstien, S. R., Lofton, S. W., and Orenstien, D. M.: Bethanechol for pediatric gastroesophageal reflux: A prospective, blind, controlled study. J. Pediatr. Gastroenterol. Nutr., 5:556, 1986.

93. Papaila, J. G., Vane, D. W., Colville, C., Berend, M., Mallik, G., Canal, D., and Grosfeld, J. L.: The effect of various types of gastrostomy on the lower esophageal sphincter. J. Pediatr. Surg., 22:1198, 1987.

94. Papaila, J. G., Wilnot, D., Grosfeld, J. L., Rescorla, F. J., West, K. W., and Vane, D. W.: Increased incidence of delayed gastric emptying in children with gastroesophageal reflux. Arch. Surg., 124:933, 1989.

95. Pearl, R. H., Wesson, D. E., Spence, L. J., et al.: Splenic injury: A five year update with improved results and changing criteria for conservative management. J. Pediatr. Surg., 24:121, 1989.

96. Peña, A.: Atlas of Surgical Management of Anorectal Malformations. New York, Springer-Verlag, 1989, pp. 1–95.

97. Puri, P., Guiney, E. J., and O'Donnell, B.: Inguinal hernia in infants: The fate of the testis following incarceration. J. Pediatr. Surg., 19:44, 1984.

98. Ramenofsky, M. L.: Pediatric abdominal trauma. Pediatr. Ann., 16:318, 1987.

99. Randolph, J. G., Newman, K. D., and Anderson, K. D.: Current results in repair of esophageal atresia with tracheoesophageal fistula using physiologic status as a guide to therapy. Ann. Surg., 209:526, 1989.

100. Rescorla, F. J., and Grosfeld, J. L.: Inguinal hernia repair in the perinatal period and early infancy. J. Pediatr. Surg., 19:832, 1984.

101. Rescorla, F. J., and Grosfeld, J. L.: Intestinal atresia and stenosis: Analysis of survival in 120 cases. Surgery, 98:668, 1985.

102. Rescorla, F. J., and Grosfeld, J. L.: Splenic and liver trauma in children. Indiana Med., 82:516, 1989.

103. Rescorla, F. J., Yoder, M. C., West, K. W., and Grosfeld, J. L.: Delayed presentation of a right sided diaphragmatic hernia and Group B streptococcal sepsis. Arch. Surg., 124:1083, 1989.

104. Rescorla, F. J., Grosfeld, J. L., West, K. W., and Vane, D. W.: Changing patterns of treatment and survival in neonates with meconium ileus. Arch. Surg., 142:837, 1989.

105. Reynolds, M., Luck, S. R., and Raffensperger, J. G.: The valved conduit prevents ascending cholangitis: A follow-up. J. Pediatr. Surg., 20:696, 1985.

106. Rickham, P. P.: Denis Brown: Surgeon. (Progress in Pediatric Surgery, Vol. 20. Rickham, P. P., Ed.) Berlin, Springer-Verlag, 1986, pp. 69–75.

107. Rosenstien, B. J.: Cystic fibrosis presenting with the meconium plug syndrome. Am. J. Dis. Child., 132:167, 1978.

108. Roshkow, J. E., Haller, J. O., Berdon, W. E., and Sane, S. M.: Hirschsprung's disease, Ondine's curse, and neuroblastoma—manifestations of neurocristopathy. Pediatr. Radiol., 19:45, 1988.

109. Rowe, M. I., and Chatworthy, H. W., Jr.: Incarcerated and strangulated hernias in children. Arch. Surg., 101:136, 1970.

110. Rowe, M. I., and Marchildon, M. G.: Inguinal hernia and hydrocele in infants and children. Surg. Clin. North Am., 61:1137, 1981.

111. Savin, R. A., and Clatworthy, H. W., Jr.: Appendiceal rupture: A continuing problem. Pediatrics, 63:36, 1979.

112. Sawada, T., Kidowaki, T., Sakamoto, I., et al.: Neuroblastoma: Mass screening for early detection and its prognosis. Cancer, 53:2731, 1984.

113. Schorr, R. M., Greaney, G. C., and Donovan, A. J.: Injuries of the duodenum. Am. J. Surg., 154:938, 1987.

114. Schwartz, M. Z.: An improved technique for circular myotomy in long gap esophageal atresia. J. Pediatr. Surg., 18:833, 1983.

115. Schwartz, M. Z., Tapper, D. M., and Solenberger, R. I.: Management of perforated appendicitis in children. Ann. Surg., 197:407, 1983.

116. Seeger, R. C., Brodeur, G. M., Sather, H., et al.: Association of multiple copies of the N-myc oncogene with rapid progression of neuroblastoma. N. Engl. J. Med., 313:1111, 1985.

117. Shaul, D. B., Schwartz, M. Z., Marr, C., and Tyson, K. R.: Primary repair without routine gastrostomy is the treatment of choice for neonates with esophageal atresia and tracheoesophageal fistula. Arch. Surg., 124:1188, 1989.

118. Shimada, H., Chatten, J., and Newton, W. A.: Histopathologic prognostic factors in neuroblastic tumors. J. Natl. Cancer Inst., 73:409, 1984.

119. Smith, E. D.: The bath water needs changing but don't throw out the baby: An overview of anorectal anomalies. J. Pediatr. Surg., 22:335, 1988.

120. Smith, E. I., Haase, G. M., Seeger, R. C., and Brodeur, G. M.: Surgical perspective on the current staging in neuroblastoma: The International Neuroblastoma Staging System Proposal. J. Pediatr. Surg., 24:386, 1989.

121. Spitz, L., Kiely, E., and Brerton, R. J.: Esophageal atresia: A five year experience with 148 cases. J. Pediatr. Surg., 22:103, 1987.

122. Stanley, P., Geer, G. D., Miller, J. H., Gilsanz, V., Landing, B. H., and Boechat, I. M.: Infantile hepatic hemangiomas—clinical features, radiologic investigation, and treatment in 20 patients. Cancer, 64:936, 1989.

123. Steward, D. J.: Preterm infants are more prone to complications following minor surgery than are fullterm infants. Anesthesiology, 59:304, 1982.

124. Stone, M. M., Fondalsrud, E. W., Salusky, I. B., Takiff, H., Hall, T., and Fine, R. N.: Surgical management of peritoneal dialysis catheters in children: Five-year experience with 1,800 patient-month follow-up. J. Pediatr. Surg., 21:1177, 1986.

125. Synn, A. Y., Mulvihill, S. I., and Fonkalsrud, E. W.: Surgical disorders of the pancreas in infancy and childhood. Am. J. Surg., 156:201, 1988.

126. Tank, E. S., and Hatch, E. I.: Hernia complicating chronic ambulatory peritoneal dialysis in children. J. Pediatr. Surg., 21:41, 1986.

127. Taylor, S. R., Blatt, J., Costantino, J. P., et al.: Flow cytometric DNA analysis of neuroblastoma and ganglioneuroma: A 10 year retrospective study. Cancer, 62:749, 1988.

128. Telander, R. L., and Deane, S. A.: Thyroglossal duct and branchial cleft cysts and sinuses. Surg. Clin. North Am., 57:779, 1977.

129. Telander, F. L., Smithson, W. A., and Groover, R. V.: Clinical outcome in children with acute cerebellar encephalopathy and neuroblastoma. J. Pediatr. Surg., 24:11, 1989.

130. Templeton, J. M., and O'Neill, J. A.: Anorectal malformations. In Welch, K., Randolph, J. G., Ravitch, M. M., O'Neill, J. A., and Rowe, M. I. (Eds.): Pediatric Surgery, 4th ed. Chicago, Year Book Medical Publishers, 1986, pp. 1022–1034.

131. Tunell, W. D., Austin, J. C., Barnes, P. A., and Reynolds, A.: Neuroradiologic evaluation of sacral abnormalities in imperforate anus complex. J. Pediatr. Surg., 22:58, 1987.

132. Vane, D. W., West, K. W., and Grosfeld, J. L.: Vitelline duct anomalies: Experience with 217 childhood cases. Arch. Surg., 122:542, 1987.

133. Vane, D. W., Grosfeld, J. L., West, K. W., and Rescorla, F. J.: Pancreatic disorders in infancy and childhood: Experience with 92 cases. J. Pediatr. Surg., 24:771, 1989.

134. Vasquez-Estevez, J. J., Stewart, B. A., Shikes, R. A., et al.: Biliary atresia: Early determination of prognosis. J. Pediatr. Surg., 24:48, 1989.

135. Vaughn, G. D., III, Frazier, O. H., Graham, D. Y., et al.: The use of pyloric exclusion in the management of severe duodenal injury. Am. J. Surg., 134:785, 1962.

136. Waterston, D., Bonham-Carter, R., and Aberdeen, E.: Oesophageal atresia and tracheoesophageal fistula: A study of survival in 218 infants. Lancet, 1:819, 1962.

137. Weeks, D. A., Beckwith, J. B., and Luckey, D. W.: Relapse-associated variable in Stage I favorable histology Wilms' tumor. Cancer, 60:1204, 1987.

138. West, K. W., and Grosfeld, J. L.: Postsplenectomy sepsis: Historical background and current concepts. World J. Surg., 9:477, 1985.

139. West, K. W., Stephens, B., Vane, D. W., and Grosfeld, J. L.: Intussusception: Current management in infants and children. Surgery, 102:704, 1987.

140. Winthrop, A. L., Wesson, D. E., and Filler, R. M.: Traumatic duodenal hematoma in the pediatric patient. J. Pediatr. Surg., 21:757, 1986.

141. Wurtz, F.: Practica der Wendartzney. Basel, 1563.

142. Ziegler, M. M., Ross, A. J., and Bishop, H. L.: Total intestinal aganglionosis: A new technique for prolonged survival. J. Pediatr. Surg., 22:82, 1987.

39

SURGICAL DISORDERS OF THE EARS, NOSE, PARANASAL SINUSES, PHARYNX, AND LARYNX

James B. Snow, Jr., M.D.

THE EARS

Progress in surgical therapy of the ear began in 1853 when Sir William Wilde of Dublin, father of Oscar Wilde, advocated a postauricular incision for the drainage of subperiosteal abscesses in acute mastoiditis. The next major advance occurred with Herman Schwartze's introduction in 1873 of the complete mastoidectomy. This operation gained great popularity because of its effectiveness in resolving acute mastoiditis. Emanuel Zaufal recognized that the operation did not solve the problem in the presence of a cholesteatoma and in 1890 described the radical mastoidectomy, in which the disease process in the middle ear, antrum, and mastoid cell area is exteriorized by removal of the posterior and superior portion of the bony canal wall. Bondy observed that removal of the tympanic membrane remnants and auditory ossicles was not always necessary to exteriorize cholesteatomas and in 1910 introduced the modified radical mastoidectomy, in which a cholesteatoma lateral to the ossicles could be exteriorized and the hearing preserved. In the 1930s Lempert popularized endaural incisions. The development of the binocular surgical microscope by Holmgren and improved illumination was followed by the introduction of tympanoplasty by Wullstein and Zöllner in the 1950s.[67] The next major advance occurred in 1952 when Rosen mobilized the stapes in a patient with otosclerosis.[48] Shea introduced stapedectomy in 1958 and brought a century of surgical therapy for the middle ear to a dramatic climax.[54] House later developed endolymphatic subarachnoid shunt surgery for Meniere's disease and translabyrinthine and middle cranial fossa approaches to the internal auditory meatus for removal of acoustic neurinomas, vestibular neurectomy, and vascular compression of the eighth nerve.[24-26,28] Several techniques have been developed for the implantation of electrodes into the inner ear, eighth cranial nerve, and brain stem auditory structures of the profoundly deaf.[27,36] Multichannel cochlear implants with complex speech processors that provide help with speech reading and some open-set understanding of speech are available for postlingually deaf adults and children.[9] Further development of auditory prostheses that allow more complete understanding of speech is the new frontier.

Anatomy of the Ear

The external auditory canal makes a slightly S-shaped curve. The outer third has a cartilaginous skeleton, and the inner two thirds has a bony skeleton. Sebaceous glands and hair are borne in the outer third. The plane of the tympanic membrane makes an angle of 55 degrees with the long axis of the external auditory canal. The tympanic membrane is divided into the pars tensa and the pars flaccida. The pars tensa is composed of three layers: the outer stratified squamous epithelium, which is continuous with the skin of the canal; the fibrous layer; and the inner mucous membrane, which is continuous with the rest of the mucous membrane of the middle ear. The fibrous layer thickens toward the periphery of the tympanic membrane to form the anulus tympanicus, which rests in the sulcus tympanicus, a groove in the most medial aspect of the canal. The fibrous layer ends at the anterior and posterior malleolar folds. The pars flaccida has only two layers, the stratified squamous epithelium laterally and the mucous membrane medially (Fig. 1). The long process of the malleus is embedded in the fibrous layer of the tympanic membrane, and the short process projects laterally. The head of the malleus articulates with the body of the incus. The lenticular process of the incus articulates with the head of the stapes. The footplate of the stapes articulates with the oval window (Fig. 2).

The middle ear space is irregular and compressed laterally. The part superior to the level of the tympanic membrane is the epitympanum, or attic. The mesotympanum lies directly medial to the tympanic membrane. The hypotympanum is inferior to the level of the tympanic membrane. The basal turn of the cochlea makes an impression on the medial wall of the middle ear termed the promontory. The tegmen, or roof, of the tympanum is opposite the middle cranial fossa. The tegmen tympani extends posteriorly to become the tegmen of the antrum and mastoid process. The middle ear communicates with the mastoid process through the antrum. All mastoid air cells communicate one through another with the antrum. Pneumatic cells also extend into the petrous pyramid from the antrum, attic, and hypotympanum. The floor of the middle ear is the roof of the jugular fossa.[4]

The cochlea makes two and three-quarters turns in the human. A cross section through the modiolus, or central bony framework, demonstrates in each turn the scala vestibuli, the scala media, and the scala tympani (Fig. 3). The scala vestibuli is separated from the scala media by Reissner's membrane. The scala media is separated from the scala tympani by the basilar membrane. The organ of Corti, with its hair cells and their supporting cells, rests on the basilar membrane. The hairs of the hair cells are in contact with the tectorial membrane. Dendrites of the first-order neurons, of which the cell bodies are in the spiral canal of Rosenthal in the modiolus, arborize around the base of the hair cells.

The axons terminate in the dorsal and ventral cochlear nuclei in the medulla. The pathway to the auditory cortex consists of at least four orders of neurons and includes the superior olivary complexes, the lateral lemnisci, the inferior colliculi, and the

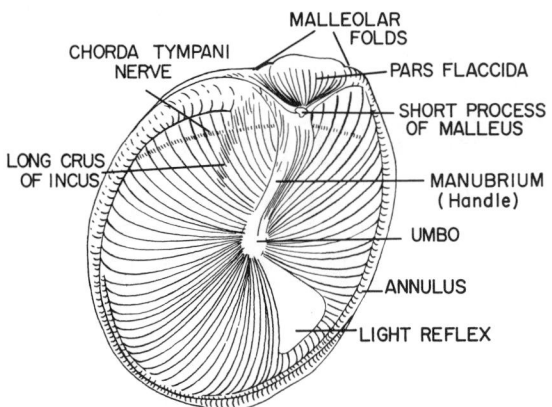

Figure 1. Landmarks of the right tympanic membrane. (From Saunders, W. H.: Ears, nose and throat. *In* Prior, J. H., and Silberstein, J. S.: Physical Diagnosis: The History and Examination of the Patient. St. Louis, C. V. Mosby Company, 1963.)

medial geniculate bodies. Crossing of the midline occurs at the level of the brain stem nuclei and the inferior colliculi. In man the auditory cortex lies in the posterior portion of the superior temporal gyrus in the sylvian fissure, which is termed Heschl's gyrus.

The saccule is spherical and is connected with the scala media through the canalis reuniens of Hensen (Fig. 4). The saccular duct joins the utricular duct to form the endolymphatic duct. The utricle is larger than the saccule and is ovoid. The utricle has five openings for the three ampullated ends of the semicircular canals, the crus simplex of the horizontal semicircular canal, and the crus commune of the superior and posterior semicircular canals. The endolymphatic duct extends through the vestibular aqueduct to the endolymphatic sac, which is located between sheaves of dura on the posterior surface of the petrous pyramid.

The membranous labyrinth contains endolymph. The space between the bony labyrinth and the membranous labyrinth is filled with perilymph. The perilymphatic space communicates with the subarachnoid space through the cochlear aqueduct, which enters the scala tympani. The endolymph is chemically similar to intracellular fluid, with a high K^+ concentration and a low Na^+ concentration, whereas the perilymph resembles ex-

tracellular fluid, with a low K^+ and a high Na^+. There is a resting direct current potential difference of 80 millivolts between the endolymph in the scala media and the perilymph, and the endolymph is positively charged relative to the perilymph.[47]

Physiology of the Ear

The external auditory canal maintains the temperature and humidity of the external environment of the tympanic membrane, and this environment varies very little regardless of the ambient temperature or humidity. The canal is self-cleansing. Debris is carried by the migration of a sheet of desquamated epithelial cells from the center of the tympanic membrane to its periphery and from the medial portion of the canal to its lateral extent.

AUDITORY FUNCTION. Sound waves impinging upon the tympanic membrane set the tympanic membrane in motion. Movement of the tympanic membrane then causes movement of the malleus, incus, and stapes. Movement of the stapes causes pressure changes in the fluid in the inner ear. These pressure changes cause deformation of the basilar membrane. A traveling wave is propagated in the basilar membrane from the base to the apex of the cochlea. Along the length of the basilar membrane, a point of maximal displacement occurs with each traveling wave. The location of the point of maximal displacement depends on the frequency of the stimulating tone. High-frequency tones cause maximal displacement near the base of the cochlea. As the frequency of the stimulating tone is decreased, the point of maximal displacement moves from the base to the apex.

Displacement of the basilar membrane causes movement of the organ of Corti and deformation of the hairs of the hair cells. As the hairs of the hair cells are bent away from the modiolus, a depolarization occurs within the hair cell. An alternating current potential known as the cochlear potential or cochlear microphonic occurs in response to stimulation of the hair cells. The cochlear potential faithfully reproduces the frequency and intensity of the acoustic stimulation through a wide intensity range. A chemical transmitter is released in the region of the boutons terminaux of the afferent eighth nerve fibers. This chemical transmitter initiates depolarization of the dendritic terminals of the afferent nerve fibers.

Trauma and Foreign Bodies

Blunt trauma to the pinna causes a subperichondrial hematoma. When bleeding occurs between the cartilage and the perichondrium, the pinna becomes a reddish purple shapeless mass. Because the perichondrium carries the blood supply to the cartilage, the cartilage undergoes avascular necrosis if the hematoma is present on both sides of the cartilage, and with time the pinna becomes shriveled. A hematoma may become organized and calcify, which produces the cauliflower ear characteristic of wrestlers and boxers. Treatment consists of incision for aspiration of the clot and approximation of the perichondrium to the cartilage by the use of closed suction drainage so that the cartilage and its blood supply are in contact.[12]

Lacerations of the pinna extending through skin, cartilage, and skin are repaired by suturing of the skin margins of the wound, external splinting of the cartilage of the pinna with a molded splint of cotton soaked in benzoin, and protective dressing. Sutures are not placed in the cartilage.

Perichondritis of the pinna causes accumulation of pus between the perichondrium and the cartilage and leads to avascular and septic necrosis of the cartilage. The infection persists for long periods. The treatment for perichondritis is wide incision for drainage and systemic antibiotic therapy. Often, perichondritis follows a gram-negative rod infection, and culture and sensitivities are of considerable importance. Incisions in the skin of the pinna on its lateral surface for drainage of hematomas

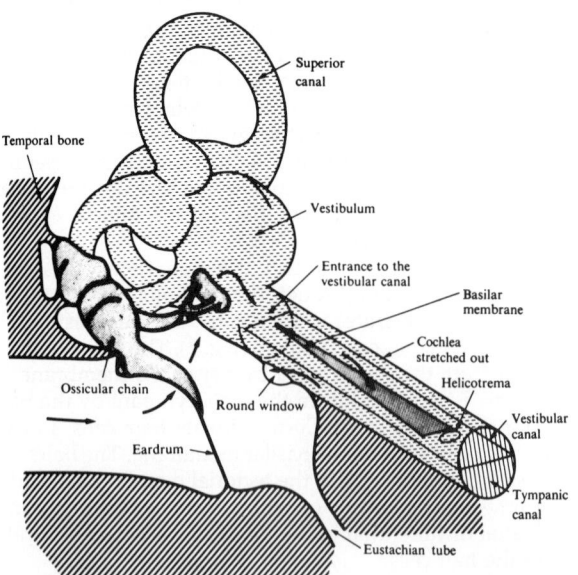

Figure 2. Functional diagram of the external, middle, and inner ear with the cochlea unrolled. (From von Békésy, G.: Cochlea mechanics. *In* Theoretical and Mathematical Biology, edited by Talbot H. Waterman and Harold J. Morowitz © 1965, Xerox.)

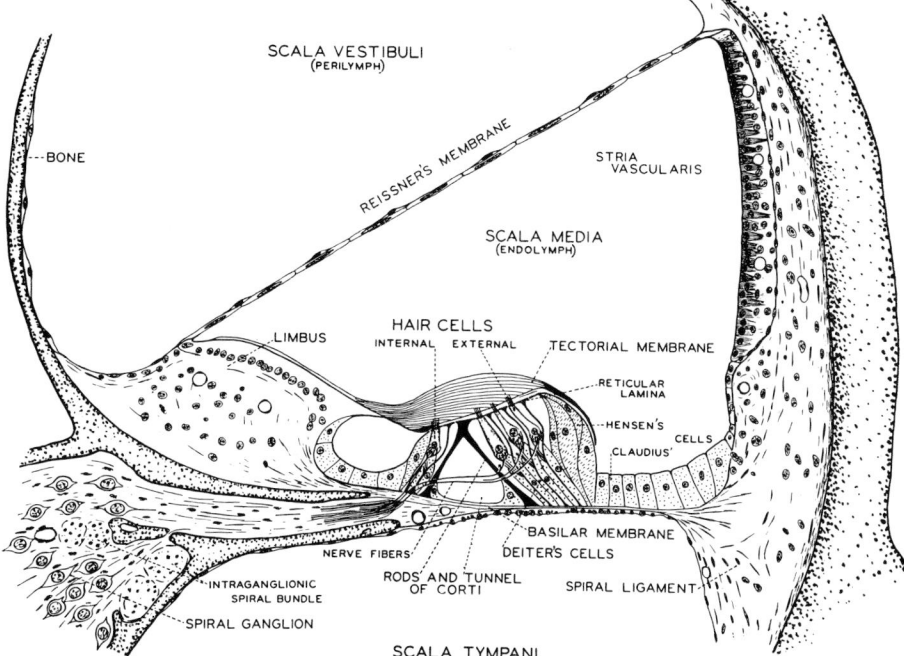

Figure 3. Cross section of a turn of the cochlea. (From Davis, H., et al.: Acoustic trauma in the guinea pig. J. Acoust. Soc. Am., 25:1180, 1953.)

and perichondritis should be made just anterior to the antihelix so that the scar is not visible on the lateral view of the ear.

Incision of superficial infections of the pinna is avoided for fear of initiating perichondritis.

Foreign bodies in the external auditory canal are a common problem. Beads, erasers, beans, and other objects may be inserted by children and their siblings into their ears. An insect may find its way into the ear canal and is particularly annoying to the patient until it is killed or removed. Foreign bodies are removed by passing a blunt hook deep to the foreign body for extraction (Fig. 5). A forceps is likely to push smooth foreign bodies ahead of it. If the foreign body is far medial, it is difficult to remove without injuring the tympanic membrane and ossicular chain. If a child is uncooperative or the mechanical problem is difficult, a general anesthetic is used for the removal of a foreign body. Metal and glass beads may be removed by irrigation, but care is used to be certain that the foreign body is not hygroscopic, like a bean, because swelling with the addition of water complicates removal. An insect is killed to give the patient immediate relief and facilitate its removal by filling the ear canal with mineral oil. The dead insect is removed with a forceps.

The force of blows to the mandible may be transmitted to the anterior wall of the external auditory canal, which is the posterior wall of the glenoid fossa. In fractures of the anterior wall of the canal, fragments may be displaced to such a degree that stenosis of the canal results. The displaced fragments are reduced or excised under general anesthesia.

The tympanic membrane may be perforated with twigs of a tree, cotton applicators, and other objects placed in the ear canal, missiles such as hot slag in welding, and a sudden overpressure in an explosion (acoustic trauma). Perforations of the tympanic membrane may be associated with dislocation of the ossicular chain. Vertigo or a sensorineural hearing loss suggests that a portion of an ossicle or a missile has been driven into the inner ear or that there is a fistula between the perilymphatic space of the vestibule and the middle ear.[55] These conditions require prompt exploration of the middle ear with an operative microscope and repair of the labyrinthine fistula. Most perforations of the tympanic membrane heal spontaneously in 6 weeks.

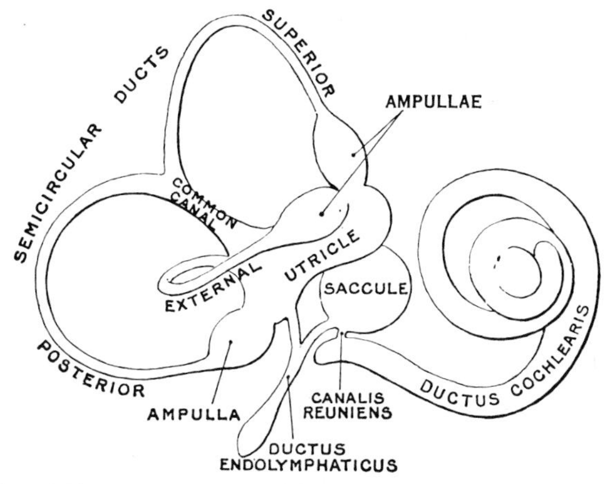

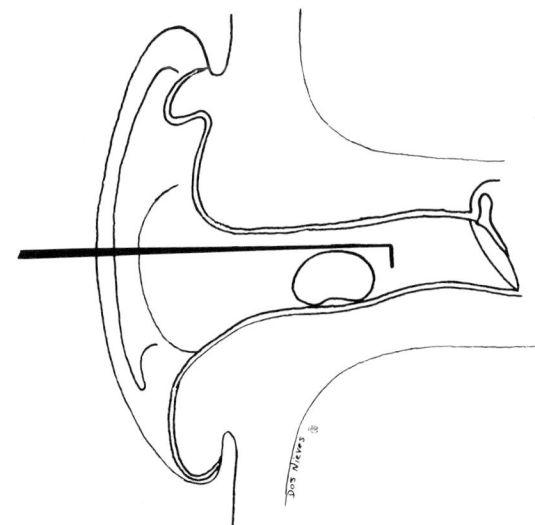

Figure 4. Membranous labyrinth. (After Goss, C. N. (Ed.): Gray's Anatomy of the Human Body, 27th ed. Philadelphia, Lea & Febiger, 1959.)

Figure 5. Technique for the removal of foreign bodies of the ear canal. The foreign body is raked out with a blunt Day hook.

Instrumentation to approximate the wound margins of the tympanic membrane should be performed under aseptic conditions and microscopic control. It is important to avoid infection during the healing period. The patient must be careful to avoid getting water in the ear. Topical applications have the risk of introducing microorganisms. Prophylactic antibiotic therapy in the form of oral penicillin for the first 7 days is recommended. If the perforation fails to heal or if there is a persisting conductive hearing loss suggesting discontinuity of the ossicular chain, the middle ear is explored and repaired.

FRACTURES OF THE TEMPORAL BONE. Basal skull fractures follow blunt trauma to the head, particularly to the occipital area. Basal skull fractures are in essence fractures of the temporal bone, and they are a frequent cause of profound sensorineural hearing loss. Bleeding from the ear following an injury to the skull is pathognomonic of a fracture of the temporal bone whether the bleeding is medial to an intact tympanic membrane, from the middle ear through a rupture of the tympanic membrane, or from a fracture line in the ear canal. Hemotympanum gives the tympanic membrane a blue-black color. Usually, there is a communication with the subarachnoid space through the fracture line. Often there is cerebrospinal fluid otorrhea. Cleaning of the ear canal should be avoided for fear of introducing microorganisms. The immediate danger to the patient is the development of meningitis. Therefore, prophylactic antibiotic therapy is initiated and continued for 7 to 10 days. More fractures of the temporal bone are longitudinal (80 per cent) than are transverse (20 per cent) to the long axis of the petrous pyramid. Longitudinal fractures extend through the middle ear into the ear canal and cause rupture of the tympanic membrane. Transverse fractures extend across the cochlea and fallopian canal to produce a profound, permanent sensorineural hearing loss and a facial paralysis.[59] These fractures are usually well demonstrated with computed tomography (CT). Approximately 35 per cent of longitudinal fractures produce a sensorineural hearing loss, and approximately 15 per cent produce facial paralysis. The fracture extending through the middle ear may cause a dislocation of the ossicular chain that requires subsequent repair. Persistence of a facial paralysis requires decompression of the facial nerve under certain circumstances.

PERILYMPHATIC FISTULAS. Strenuous physical exertion or abrupt changes in ambient atmospheric pressure as in flying or diving may cause a communication between the perilymphatic space in the inner ear and the middle ear through the footplate of the stapes or the round window membrane.[17] Perilymphatic fistulas also occur spontaneously. The patient may experience a popping sound or the feeling of an explosion in the ear at the onset. Tinnitus, a sensory hearing loss that may fluctuate, and persistent or intermittent vertigo may occur. Increasing and decreasing the pressure in the external auditory canal with a pneumatic otoscope may cause vertigo and nystagmus; this is known as a positive fistula test. The fistula may be found in an exploratory tympanotomy by observing the leak of perilymph through a defect in or around the footplate of the stapes or a laceration of the round window membrane. The fistula may be repaired with a graft of fibrous tissue.

Infectious Diseases

EXTERNAL OTITIS. Infection of the ear canal occurs in a diffuse form involving the entire canal, termed otitis externa diffusa, and a localized form due to furunculosis, termed otitis externa circumscripta. The diffuse form may be caused by a gram-negative rod such as *Escherichia coli*, *Pseudomonas aeruginosa*, or *Proteus* or by *Staphylococcus aureus*. Rarely a fungus may have a pathogenic role. Furunculosis is usually due to *S. aureus*.

Patients with diffuse external otitis complain of itching, pain, foul-smelling discharge, and loss of hearing if the canal becomes swollen or filled with purulent debris. Tenderness on traction of the pinna and on pressure over the tragus tends to distinguish it from otitis media. The skin of the external auditory canal appears red, swollen, and littered with moist purulent debris.

Treatment with topical antibiotics and corticosteroids is efficacious. Systemic therapy is rarely necessary unless there is a spreading cellulitis around the ear. Furuncles of the canal should be allowed to resolve because incision may cause perichondritis of the pinna.

MALIGNANT EXTERNAL OTITIS. An unusually virulent form of external otitis due to infection with *P. aeruginosa* occurs in diabetics, particularly elderly diabetics in poor metabolic control. It produces pain, purulent otorrhea, and hearing loss. Characteristically, the external auditory canal contains granulation tissue. There is destruction of the bone of the external auditory canal, and the osteomyelitis may spread along the base of the skull to the midline or even to the opposite side.[38] Facial paralysis often occurs owing to involvement of the fallopian canal. Its lethal potential follows the infection's ability to spread intracranially. Surgical intervention is of limited value. Therapy is based on the antibiotic sensitivities of the causative *Pseudomonas* organism and usually requires 6 weeks of intravenous administration of an aminoglycoside antibiotic and a semisynthetic penicillin. Careful control of the diabetes is an essential part of the treatment.

ACUTE OTITIS MEDIA. Acute otitis media is an infectious inflammatory process in the middle ear, usually secondary to an upper respiratory tract infection. It is the most common localized infection in children. Most children between 1 and 5 years of age have two or three episodes of acute otitis media each winter. Acute otitis media may be viral or bacterial. Viral otitis media may resolve, or the middle ear may be secondarily invaded by bacteria. In neonates, otitis media is caused by gram-negative enteric bacilli, especially *E. coli*, and *S. aureus*. In older infants and children under 15 years of age, acute suppurative otitis media is caused by group A beta-hemolytic streptococci, *Streptococcus pneumoniae*, *S. aureus*, *Branhamella catarrhalis*, and *Haemophilus influenzae*. In adults, streptococcal, pneumococcal, and staphylococcal infections are most common. Rarely *E. coli*, *Klebsiella pneumoniae*, and *Bacteroides* may produce acute otitis media in children.

Penicillin is the drug of choice for acute otitis media in patients over 14 years of age and adults. In those under 15 years of age, amoxicillin is preferred because of the frequency of *H. influenzae* infections. The treatment is continued for 12 days to ensure resolution and prevention of the sequelae of streptococcal infections.

A myringotomy is indicated when bulging of the tympanic membrane persists despite antibiotic therapy or when the pain and systemic symptoms and signs such as fever, vomiting, and diarrhea are severe. A large curvilinear incision is made parallel to the annulus in the inferior quadrants midway between the umbo and the canal wall (Fig. 6). The appearance and movement of the tympanic membrane, tympanometry, and the patient's hearing are followed until there is complete resolution. The management of incomplete resolution is discussed later under *Serous and Secretory Otitis Media*.

The infectious complications of acute otitis media are acute mastoiditis, petrositis, labyrinthitis, facial paralysis, conductive and sensorineural hearing loss, epidural abscess, meningitis, brain abscess, lateral sinus thrombosis, subdural empyema, and otitic hydrocephalus. The most common intracranial complication of acute otitis media is meningitis.

ACUTE MASTOIDITIS. In acute otitis media, the infection almost invariably extends through the mastoid antrum into the mastoid cells. However, the term *acute mastoiditis* is not used clinically until destruction of the bony partitions between the mastoid air cells has occurred. Progression of the acute infectious stages in the mastoid process is so regularly aborted by

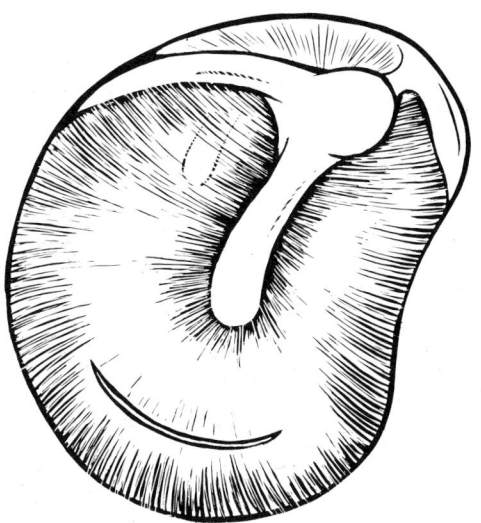

Figure 6. Myringotomy incision that occupies one fourth of the circumference of the tympanic membrane midway between the umbo and the annulus tympanicus.

antibiotic therapy that clinically apparent acute mastoiditis has become a rare condition. The responsible bacteria are the same as those responsible for acute otitis media.

Acute mastoiditis becomes clinically apparent 14 days or more after the onset of acute otitis media as one of the cortices of the mastoid process is destroyed. Usually associated with this destruction of the mastoid cortex is an exacerbation of the aural pain, fever, and otorrhea. The pain tends to be persistent and throbbing, and the discharge is usually creamy and profuse. Increasing hearing loss is characteristic of acute mastoiditis.

The lateral mastoid cortex is most frequently the first to be destroyed, and a postauricular subperiosteal abscess develops. The first signs are thickening of the postauricular tissue, reduced mobility of the skin over the mastoid cortex, and blunting of the postauricular crease. As pus exudes from the mastoid cortex deep to the periosteum, an erythematous, warm, tender, fluctuant postauricular mass develops, displacing the pinna laterally and inferiorly.

In acute otitis media, there is increased density of the mastoid air cells due to swollen mucous membrane and purulent fluid in the air cells on CT scanning of the temporal bones. In coalescent mastoiditis the partitions between the air cells become indistinct. The individual septa can no longer be seen as one air cell coalesces with another.

In early cases of acute mastoiditis in which there are postauricular signs of tenderness and edema but no fluctuant subperiosteal abscess, antibiotic therapy may effect complete resolution with spontaneous healing of the tympanic membrane, reventilation of the middle ear, and return of the hearing to the preinfection level.

In the presence of a subperiosteal abscess, complete exenteration of the mastoid air cells (Schwartze operation) should be performed. The operation should include inspection of a small area of the middle and posterior fossa dura to exclude an epidural abscess. The objective of the complete mastoidectomy is to drain the abscess in the mastoid air cells and antrum. Through-and-through drainage of the middle ear is provided by the myringotomy or perforation of the tympanic membrane anteriorly and through the antrum posteriorly. The goals of this operation are resolution of the infection, prevention of intracranial infectious complications, spontaneous healing of the perforation of the tympanic membrane, reventilation of the middle ear, and return of hearing to the preinfection level.

SEROUS AND SECRETORY OTITIS MEDIA. Serous and secretory otitis media are manifested as effusions in the middle ear. Such effusions follow incomplete resolution of acute otitis

media or eustachian tube obstruction due to inflammatory processes in the nasopharynx, allergic manifestations, hypertrophic adenoids, or benign or malignant nasopharyngeal neoplasms. Normally the middle ear is ventilated three to four times per minute as the eustachian tube opens during swallowing. If the patency of the eustachian tube is compromised, oxygen in the middle ear is absorbed by the blood in the vessels of the mucous membrane of the middle ear, and a relative negative pressure develops. At first there is mild retraction of the tympanic membrane. Soon a transudate of fluid occurs from the blood in the vessels in the mucous membrane of the middle ear. The presence of fluid in the middle ear may be recognized by an amber or dark gray color of the tympanic membrane, immobility of the tympanic membrane, a tympanogram indicating negative pressure in the middle ear, and conductive hearing loss.[58] Rarely an air-fluid level or bubbles of air may be observed through the tympanic membrane. Although there is usually little evidence of acute inflammation, pathogenic bacteria may be cultured from the middle ear in approximately half of children with effusions.[20] In adults the possibility of a malignant tumor of the nasopharynx must be excluded, requiring careful inspection and often biopsy of the nasopharynx.

Myringotomy for aspiration of the fluid and insertion of a tympanostomy tube for ventilation of the middle ear ameliorate the problem of eustachian tube obstruction regardless of the cause (Fig. 7). In children, thorough adenoidectomy is frequently a necessary part of the treatment. Allergic evaluation and management with either elimination of the allergen from the patient's environment or immunotherapy is helpful if there is an underlying allergic manifestation.

In children with middle ear effusions, initial treatment consists of antibiotic therapy appropriate for acute otitis media for 6 weeks. The antibiotic therapy may sterilize the middle ear as well as ameliorate the eustachian tube obstruction secondary to purulent rhinitis, sinusitis, or adenoiditis. It results in resolution of the middle ear effusion in one third to one half of the patients. Immunologic investigation is occasionally helpful. The Valsalva maneuver and politzerization are employed in the absence of tympanostomy tubes.

CHRONIC OTITIS MEDIA. Chronic otitis media means a permanent perforation of the tympanic membrane. Perforations follow acute otitis media, mechanical trauma, thermal and chemical burns, and blast injuries. Chronic otitis media can be divided into two major categories depending on the type of perforation present. There is a benign tubotympanic type, with a central perforation of the tympanic membrane, and a dangerous type, with a pars flaccida or marginal perforation.

A central perforation is one in which there is some substance of the tympanic membrane between the rim of the perforation and the bony sulcus tympanicus. These perforations follow

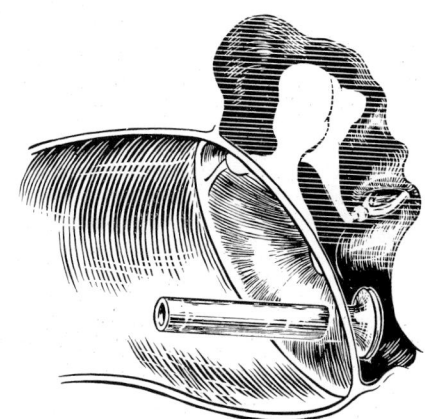

Figure 7. Tympanostomy tube placed through a myringotomy incision for ventilation of the middle ear in serous and secretory otitis media.

commonly from acute otitis media produced by relatively virulent microorganisms. Exacerbations of the chronic otitis media cause painless, purulent otorrhea, which may be foul-smelling and occur secondary to upper respiratory infections and when water gains access to the middle ear in bathing and swimming.

The middle ear can generally be repaired in chronic otitis media with a central perforation. A tympanoplasty provides sound protection for the round window and restores sound-pressure transformation to the oval window.[67] Wullstein categorized tympanoplastic procedures into five types (Fig. 8). The Type I tympanoplasty is applicable to the patient with a perforation of the tympanic membrane in which the ossicular chain is intact and mobile. The Type I tympanoplasty, sometimes termed a myringoplasty, restores the tympanic membrane by the use of a graft of soft tissue such as temporalis muscle fascia.[23] A Type II tympanoplasty is required if there has been greater damage to the middle ear. Disruption of the ossicular chain, which often occurs as a result of necrosis of the long process of the incus, must be repaired in addition to grafting of the tympanic membrane.[23] Often the remnant of the incus or the head of the malleus can be remodeled and repositioned for the purpose of re-establishing the continuity of the ossicular chain. Preserved homograft ossicles or alloplastic materials such as hydroxylapatite are also used for restoring the sound-

conducting mechanism.[19] A Type III tympanoplasty is required for a still more severely damaged middle ear in which the malleus and incus are not usable and only the stapes remains. Under these circumstances, the graft is placed in contact with the head of the stapes for the purpose of producing a columellar effect similar to the single middle ear ossicle or columella found in birds. Tympanoplasty Types I, II, and III include sound protection for the round window as well as sound-pressure transformation for the oval window. In more severe degrees of damage to the middle ear in which the superstructure of the stapes has been destroyed, only sound protection of the round window can be achieved by grafting from the promontory to the inferior remnant of the tympanic membrane. This Type IV tympanoplasty creates a small closed space that communicates with the eustachian tube and provides an air-filled cushion over the round window. A Type V tympanoplasty is utilized when the footplate of the stapes is fixed. It provides sound protection for the round window as in a Type IV tympanoplasty and fenestration of the horizontal semicircular canal for the admission of acoustic energy into the inner ear. This type of tympanoplasty is rarely used.

The dangerous type of chronic otitis media occurs with pars flaccida and marginal perforations. Pars flaccida perforations lead into the epitympanum and are termed attic perforations. Marginal perforations usually occur in the posterosuperior portion of the pars tensa. There is no substance of tympanic membrane between the periphery of the perforation and the bony sulcus tympanicus. The anulus tympanicus has been destroyed.

Theories of the pathogenesis of perforations of the pars flaccida include progressive retraction of the pars flaccida secondary to eustachian tube obstruction, rupture during acute otitis media, and hyperactivity of the basal layer of the epidermis of the pars flaccida due to long-standing inflammation in the middle ear. Each of these mechanisms may cause an invasive cholesteatoma.[49]

A cholesteatoma occurs when the middle ear is lined with stratified squamous epithelium. The stratified squamous epithelium desquamates in this closed space. The desquamated epithelial debris cannot be cleared and accumulates in ever enlarging concentric layers. This debris serves as a culture medium for microorganisms. Cholesteatomas have the ability to destroy bone, including the tympanic ossicles, probably because of the elaboration of collagenase.[1]

Pars flaccida and marginal perforations are very frequently associated with cholesteatomas. Those cholesteatomas arising in association with pars flaccida perforations are classified as primary acquired cholesteatomas and may develop as an integral part of the development of the perforation or from the migration of stratified squamous epithelium when perforation has occurred.

Marginal perforations are produced by acute otitis media with an especially virulent bacterium, particularly a group A beta-hemolytic streptococcus, or in association with other infectious diseases such as diphtheria, chickenpox, or measles. This necrotizing otitis media destroys large areas of the tympanic membrane, including the anulus tympanicus and the middle ear mucous membrane, as well as the ossicles and their vascular and ligamentous support. During the healing process, the remaining epithelium of the mucous membrane of the middle ear migrates to cover the denuded areas. Likewise, the stratified squamous epithelium of the ear canal migrates into the middle ear to re-epithelialize the denuded areas. When stratified squamous epithelium is established in the middle ear, it begins to desquamate, and a cholesteatoma results. Cholesteatomas developing by this mechanism are classified as secondary acquired cholesteatomas.

The presence of a cholesteatoma greatly increases the probability of the development of a serious complication such as a purulent labyrinthitis, facial paralysis, or intracranial suppura-

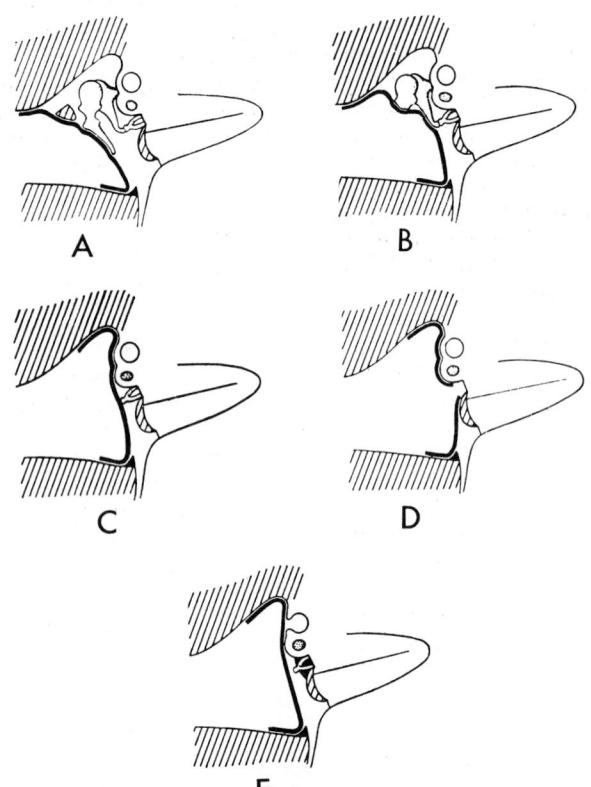

Figure 8. Five types of tympanoplasty: *A*, Type I: Perforation of the tympanic membrane repaired with soft tissue graft to the tympanic membrane remnants. *B*, Type II: Perforation of the tympanic membrane and discontinuity of the ossicular chain repaired by soft tissue graft to the tympanic membrane remnants and by rearrangement of the ossicles, bony graft, or prosthesis. *C*, Type III: Perforation of the tympanic membrane and destruction of the incus and malleus repaired by applying to the tympanic membrane remnants a soft tissue graft, which is placed in contact with the head of the stapes (columellar effect). *D*, Type IV: Perforation of the tympanic membrane with destruction of the superstructure (head, neck, and crura) of the stapes repaired by creating an air-filled space between the round window and the eustachian tube to provide sound protection for the round window. *E*, Type V: Perforation of the tympanic membrane with destruction of the stapedial superstructure and fixation of its footplate repaired by protecting the round window from sound and fenestrating the horizontal semicircular canal. (From Shambaugh, G. E., Jr.: Surgery of the Ear, 2nd ed. Philadelphia, W. B. Saunders Company, 1967.)

tions. Intracranial infections include meningitis, brain abscess, lateral sinus thrombosis, subdural empyema, and epidural abscess. Magnetic resonance imaging (MRI) readily allows identification and differentiation of these entities. The propensity of cholesteatomas to produce these complications stems from their ability to destroy bone and the persistence of infection in the area bearing cholesteatoma.

Cholesteatomas are usually recognized by the small bits of white, amorphous debris in the middle ear and by the destruction of the external auditory canal bone superior to the pars flaccida or marginal perforation. Cholesteatomas are often associated with aural polyps, which may conceal the epithelial debris and bone destruction. CT of the temporal bone may demonstrate destruction of bone due to the cholesteatoma. Destruction of the scutum of Leidy (lateral wall of the epitympanum) and enlargement of the antrum greater than 1 cm. in diameter can be considered evidence of cholesteatoma.

Cholesteatomas require surgical treatment. The objective of surgical therapy is to exteriorize the cholesteatoma and if possible remove it. In a radical mastoidectomy, the middle ear, including the attic and the antrum, and the mastoid air cell area are converted into one cavity that communicates with the exterior through the ear canal. If the cholesteatoma lies superficial to the remnants of the tympanic membrane and ossicles, a modified radical mastoidectomy can be performed (Fig. 9). The modified radical mastoidectomy spares the tympanic membrane remnants and ossicles and preserves the remaining hearing. Under favorable circumstances, the cholesteatoma can be completely removed and the middle ear reconstructed. Exteriorization or removal of the cholesteatoma greatly reduces the possibility of intracranial complications. The primary goal of

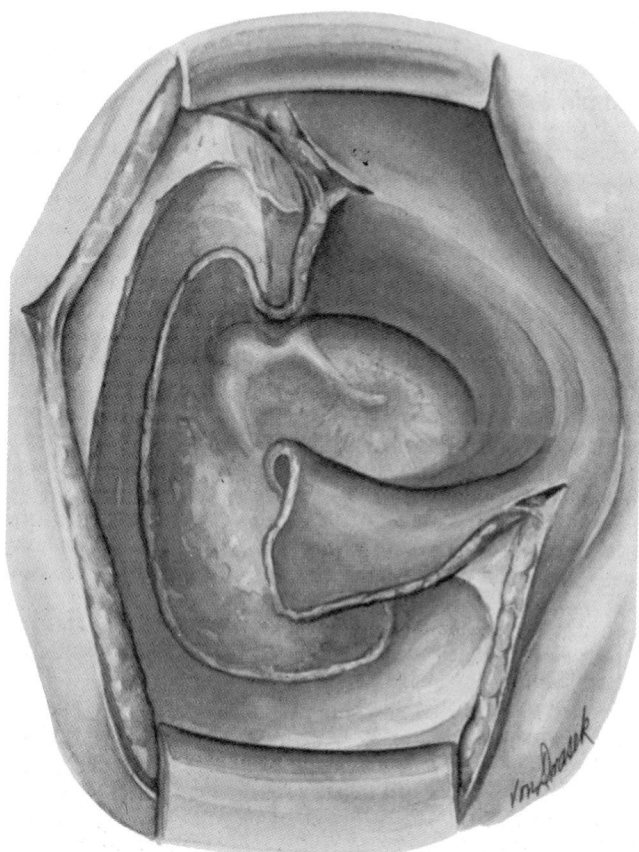

Figure 9. Modified radical mastoidectomy for exteriorizing cholesteatoma that is superficial to the remnants of the tympanic membrane and ossicles. The remnants of the tympanic membrane and ossicles are preserved. (From Shambaugh, G. E., Jr.: Surgery of the Ear, 2nd ed. Philadelphia, W. B. Saunders Company, 1967.)

operation for cholesteatoma is to make the ear safe, and the secondary goal is to maintain or improve the hearing.

Congenital Malformations

The auricle may stand out too far from the skull and be termed an outstanding ear, lop ear, or protruding ear. The basic deformity is a lack of development of the antihelix. This deformity can be corrected surgically by weakening the spring of the cartilage of the pinna so that an antihelical fold can be created. This deformity is ideally corrected at age 5 to 6 years.

Preauricular cysts and sinuses are fairly common and may be unilateral or bilateral. They are usually asymptomatic but may become infected and require incision and drainage and later excision. Complete excision is difficult because the ramification of these sinuses may be in proximity to the branches of the facial nerve. Excision is recommended only if recurrent infection has become a problem.

Severe congenital deformities of the ear are referred to as microtia and are frequently associated with urinary tract malformations. There may be major developmental defects in the pinna causing relatively small and misshapen external ears. With absence of a major portion of the auricular cartilage, surgical reconstruction rarely produces a satisfactory cosmetic result. An artistic prosthesis is the best solution to this cosmetic problem. Microtia is often associated with stenosis or atresia of the external auditory canal. These deformities are often associated with developmental abnormalities in the middle ear causing profound conductive hearing losses. The course of the facial nerve in the temporal bone may also be abnormal, and surgical repair of the sound-pressure transformation apparatus of the middle ear is hazardous.[52] In unilateral defects with normal hearing in the other ear, middle ear reconstruction is not recommended because of the danger of facial nerve injury. However, if there is a bilateral profound hearing loss, attempts at reconstruction should be made. A bone conduction hearing aid contributes to habilitation if surgical reconstruction is not feasible. Congenital malformations of the inner ear causing profound sensorineural hearing losses may or may not be associated with abnormalities of the external and middle ear. The evaluation of congenital malformation of the ear is facilitated by CT of the temporal bone.

Idiopathic Diseases

OTOSCLEROSIS. Otosclerosis is the most common cause of a progressive conductive hearing loss in the adult with a normal ear drum. Otosclerosis is a disease of the bone of the otic capsule with predilection for the anterior part of the oval window. Histologically, foci of otosclerosis demonstrate irregularly arranged, immature bone interspersed with numerous vascular channels. As the focus of the otosclerotic bone enlarges, it causes ankylosis of the footplate of the stapes and produces a conductive hearing loss. A second site of predilection is the posterior part to the oval window.

Otosclerosis tends to be familial. It is more common in women than in men. Approximately 10 per cent of the adult white population have foci of otosclerosis. Only 1 in 10 of these, or approximately 1 per cent of the white population, has clinical otosclerosis as evidenced by conductive hearing loss. Otosclerosis is rare in blacks, American Indians, and Japanese. It is common in Asiatic Indians. Otosclerosis also produces a sensorineural hearing loss when the focus is adjacent to the scala media. The conductive hearing loss becomes clinically evident in the late teenage and early adult years. The fixation of the stapes may progress rapidly during pregnancy. The conductive hearing loss can be corrected surgically in most instances. With microsurgical techniques, the superstructure (head, neck, and crura) of the stapes is removed and replaced with a prosthesis. A widely used prosthesis is one composed of a stainless steel wire and a Teflon piston. The wire, which is shaped like a shepherd's crook, is crimped around the long process of the incus, and the piston is placed through a hole created in the footplate of the stapes (Fig. 10). The sound conduction characteristics of this arrangement are excellent. The complication of a profound sensorineural hearing loss occurs in 2 to 4 per cent of patients. If a good initial hearing result is obtained, ordinarily a good result is maintained.

MENIERE'S DISEASE. Meniere's disease is characterized by hearing loss, tinnitus, and recurrent prostrating vertigo. The pathologic change in the inner ear is generalized dilation of the membranous labyrinth, or endolymphatic hydrops. Only one ear is involved in 85 per cent of patients with Meniere's disease. The sensorineural hearing loss is initially more severe in the lower frequencies than in the higher frequencies. The hearing tends to fluctuate. It is depressed after an attack of vertigo. The tinnitus has a low-pitched, roaring quality and is worse just before, during, or after an attack of vertigo. The attacks of vertigo occur suddenly, last from a few to 24 hours, and subside gradually. The attacks are associated with nausea and vomiting. The patient often has a full feeling or a pressure sensation in the affected ear. Over the course of many years, hearing loss progressively worsens.

Neither medical nor surgical therapy has been demonstrated to be effective in arresting the progression of the hearing disorder or preventing recurrent attacks of vertigo. There are a number of drugs that are effective in suppressing the vertigo and its side effects. Cholinolytic agents such as atropine and scopolamine reduce the autonomic side effects. Phenothiazines, antihistamines, and barbiturates are effective, and diphenhydramine is widely used. Perhaps the most effective agent in suppressing vertigo is diazepam.[35] A number of operations have been advocated for the treatment of the patient who is disabled by the frequency of the recurrent attacks of vertigo. Fick introduced the sacculotomy, in which the saccule is ruptured with a pick placed through the footplate of the stapes.[13a] Cody has advocated the placement of a stainless steel tack through the footplate of the stapes so that a sacculotomy is performed each time the membranous labyrinth begins to distend.[10] House has advocated the production of an artificial communication between the membranous labyrinth and subarachnoid space.[24] The middle cranial fossa approach for transection of the vestibular division of the eighth nerve is a logical approach to the control of vertigo in Meniere's disease, but it requires further evaluation.[25,63] A labyrinthectomy can be performed if the vertigo is sufficiently disabling and the hearing has degenerated to a useless level.

BENIGN PAROXYSMAL POSITIONAL VERTIGO AND NYSTAGMUS. Vertigo that occurs with changes in position may follow lesions in the inner ear, eighth nerve, brain stem, or cerebellum. Positional vertigo and nystagmus arising from the inner ear is termed benign paroxysmal positional vertigo and nystagmus. The patient experiences vertigo when lying on or rolling over onto the affected ear or when tilting the head back to look up. There is a latency of a few seconds after assuming the provocative position before the vertigo and nystagmus begin. The vertigo is characterized by an intense sensation of spinning, and the nystagmus is rotary and counterclockwise when the affected right ear is placed under and clockwise when the affected left ear is placed under. The quick component of the nystagmus is always toward the affected ear. The vertigo and nystagmus last less than 20 seconds, and the response fatigues with repeated assumption of the provocative position. Peripheral (inner ear) positional vertigo and nystagmus are distinguishable from central (brain stem or cerebellum) positional vertigo and nystagmus. In the central form, there is no intense subjective sensation of spinning, latency of response, or fatigability on repeated testing, and the nystagmus persists as long as the provocative position is maintained. There are no auditory symptoms or signs in benign paroxysmal positional vertigo and nystagmus that differentiate it from Meniere's disease and acoustic neurinomas.

The finding of basophilic calcium-containing concretions in the ampulla of the posterior semicircular canal has led some to refer to this condition as cupulolithiasis.[51] The patient should be advised to avoid the provocative position. The symptoms rarely last more than several weeks or months but may recur. If the condition persists for more than 1 year, the nerve to the posterior semicircular canal can be divided in the singular canal through the middle ear, providing relief of symptoms in 90 per cent of patients.[14]

BELL'S PALSY. Bell's palsy is a unilateral facial paralysis that develops suddenly and is accompanied by pain in the postauricular area. It is thought to be of viral etiology. All divisions of the nerve are paralyzed; this distinguishes the disease from a supranuclear lesion. The lesion is in the internal auditory meatus or the intratemporal course of the nerve. The initial pathologic changes are hyperemia and edema. The edema compresses the blood supply to the nerve because of the bony confines of the fallopian canal. A conduction block develops without death or degeneration of the axons. Release of the pressure on the nerve produces rapid recovery of function. This type of paralysis is termed neurapraxia. It should be differentiated from axonotmesis, in which the pressure on the nerve is sufficiently severe to cause death of the axons distal to the compression within a period of several days. Neurotmesis designates complete transection of the facial nerve. In neurapraxia the flow of axoplasm has been interrupted; with resumption of the flow of axoplasm, the function of the distal axon recovers.

Corticosteroid therapy is initiated as soon as possible after the onset of the paralysis and is continued for 10 days to minimize the inflammatory reaction.[2]

Nerve excitability testing or electroneurography is performed to determine whether neurapraxia or axonotmesis or neurotmesis exists.[15] As long as muscular contraction can be induced at approximately the same direct current stimulus intensity on the affected side as on the normal side with nerve excitability testing, the paralysis is probably a neurapraxia, and complete recovery may be anticipated. Loss of nerve excitability or 90 per cent or greater nerve degeneration found on electroneurography is an indication for decompression of the facial nerve by removing the bone of the fallopian canal. Approximately 85 per

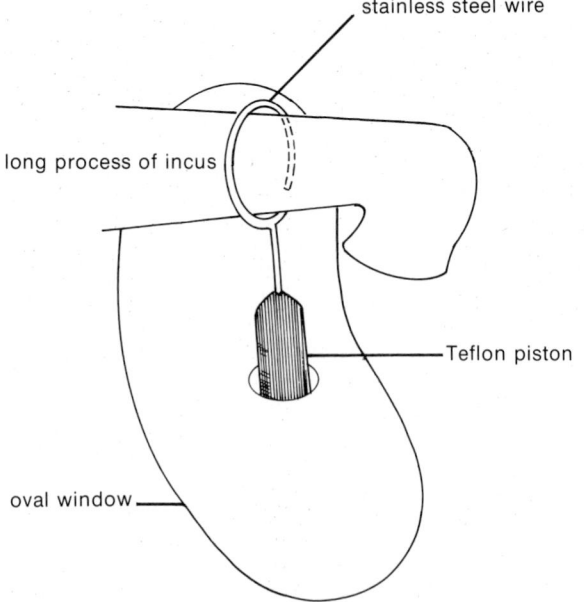

Figure 10. Stapedectomy with wire and Teflon piston prosthesis. The wire is crimped around the long process of the incus, and the Teflon piston is placed through a hole created in the fixed footplate of the stapes.

cent of all patients with idiopathic facial nerve paralysis recover spontaneously. If recovery has not begun at 3 weeks after the onset of the facial paralysis, the possibility of spontaneous recovery is greatly reduced. Ordinarily, facial nerve decompression is performed 3 weeks after the onset if there has been no recovery, or at any time when the nerve excitability deteriorates.

Neoplasms

Squamous cell and basal cell carcinomas frequently develop on the pinna of those who are exposed to the sun. Early lesions can be successfully treated with irradiation or cautery and curettage. Surgical excision of a V-shaped wedge or larger amounts of the pinna is required in more advanced lesions. Invasion of cartilage usually dictates against radiation therapy and makes surgical therapy the treatment of choice. Squamous cell and basal cell carcinomas also arise in the external auditory canal and under these circumstances require extensive resection in order to offer the best likelihood of cure. *En bloc* resection of the external auditory canal with sparing of the facial nerve is performed for lesions that are limited to the ear canal and have not invaded the middle ear.[11] Squamous cell carcinoma may arise in the middle ear. Persistent otorrhea of chronic otitis media predisposes to squamous cell carcinomas arising in the middle ear and the external auditory canal. Squamous cell carcinoma involving the middle ear requires resection of the temporal bone to obtain an adequate margin around the tumor. Preoperative or postoperative radiation therapy increases the likelihood of cure.

Ceruminomas arise in the outer third of the external auditory canal. Although these neoplasms appear to be benign histologically, they behave in a malignant manner and should be widely excised.

Chemodectomas arise in the middle ear. These nonchromaffin paragangliomas are termed glomus jugulare or glomus tympanicus tumors, depending on their site of origin. The glomus tympanicus tumor arises from the area of Jacobson's nerve in the tympanic plexus on the promontory of the middle ear. The glomus jugulare tumor arises from the glomus jugulare body in the jugular bulb. Both tumors consist of rich networks of vascular spaces surrounded by epithelioid cells. Usually the neoplasms grow slowly, and symptoms may not be evident until the neoplasm is quite large. Pulsatile tinnitus, facial nerve paralysis, otorrhea, hemorrhage, vertigo, and paralysis of cranial nerves IX, X, XI, and XII are often the presenting symptoms and signs. Characteristically, a red mass that pulsates and blanches with compression with a pneumatic otoscope can be seen in the ear canal or middle ear. The pulsation can also be demonstrated with tympanometry. There may be evidence of bone erosion in the mastoid process, middle ear, or petrous pyramid on CT. The extent of the lesion is best demonstrated with MRI with enhancement with gadolinium. Treatment consists of excision of the smaller neoplasms with or without a radical mastoidectomy. With large lesions, radiation therapy is the treatment of choice.

Acoustic neuromas represent approximately 7 per cent of all intracranial neoplasms. They arise twice as often from the vestibular division of the eighth nerve as from the auditory division. These neoplasms are derived from Schwann cells. Initially, they produce tinnitus and a neural hearing loss. The patient complains of unsteadiness or imbalance. True vertigo is not a common complaint. The hearing loss is predominantly a high-tone loss with greater impairment of the speech discrimination than would be expected with a cochlear lesion producing the same amount of pure-tone hearing loss. Loudness recruitment is absent. Tone decay is present. Decay of the acoustic reflex is pronounced. There is a decrement in speech discrimination with increasing intensity. The structure of the five waves in auditory brain stem responses is disrupted, the interwave latency is increased, and the interaural latency difference of the fifth peak is increased.[6] Hallpike caloric testing usually demonstrates canal paresis on the involved side.[7] Initially, the tumor is confined to the internal auditory meatus. As it increases in size, it projects into the cerebellopontine angle and begins to compress the cerebellum and brain stem. With the passage of time, the fifth and ultimately the seventh cranial nerves become involved. Papilledema is a late sign of acoustic neuromas. Early diagnosis is based on auditory findings suggesting a neural loss of hearing. Auditory brain stem responses have become the most effective means of differentiating sensory from neural hearing losses. Acoustic neuromas as small as 6 mm. can be visualized with MRI with enhancement with gadolinium. For the removal of small tumors, microsurgical approaches have been developed that utilize a translabyrinthine route if no useful hearing remains and a middle cranial fossa route for the preservation of the remaining hearing. Both routes allow preservation of the facial nerve. For very large neoplasms, the combined suboccipital and translabyrinthine approach offers the best likelihood of complete removal.[26] New closed skull radiation therapy through 201 sharply focused cobalt 60 sources (gamma knife) offers an alternative form of treatment for the elderly, those with bilateral acoustic neuroma, and those with tumors affecting the only hearing ear.[29]

THE NOSE AND THE PARANASAL SINUSES

In ancient India, adultery was punished by amputation of the nose. Suśruta (circa A.D. 1000) described the reconstruction of the nose with a pedicle flap from the cheek. Another ancient Indian method described the forehead flap. Tagliacozzi in Renaissance Italy developed the arm-to-nose pedicle graft. Sir William Ferguson in 1845 introduced an approach for tumors of the nose and paranasal sinuses. It included splitting of the lip in the midline as well as a horizontal incision along the inferior orbital rim to reflect the soft tissues of the face laterally. Ingals introduced nasal septal surgery by partial excision of the nasal septum for deviation of the septum in 1882. This operation was later improved by Krieg in 1899 and by Freer in 1902.

In 1903, Killian was the first to operate for an infection in the frontal sinus; in 1904, he refined the submucous resection of the nasal septum. Joseph, at the turn of the century in Berlin, developed techniques and principles upon which modern rhinoplasty is based.

Anatomy of the Nose and Paranasal Sinuses

The skeleton of the nose consists of the nasal bones, the ascending processes of the maxilla, the upper lateral cartilages, the lower lateral cartilages, and the septal cartilage. The nasal septum is the medial wall of each nasal cavity. The lateral wall of each nasal cavity provides the attachment for the three turbinates. The inferior turbinate is the largest of the three. It extends from far anterior in the nasal cavity to the choana. The middle turbinate is somewhat smaller. Although it extends to the choana, its anterior tip is 2 cm. posterior to the anterior tip of the inferior turbinate. Its attachment to the lateral wall of the nasal cavity is oblique from superior anteriorly to inferior posteriorly. The superior turbinate arises from the far posterosuperior portion of the lateral wall of the nasal cavity. Inferior to the inferior turbinate is the inferior meatus. The nasolacrimal duct opens into the inferior meatus. The middle meatus lies between the middle turbinate and the inferior turbinate. The ostia of the maxillary and anterior ethmoid cells and the nasofrontal duct are in the middle meatus. The superior meatus lies between the superior turbinate and the middle turbinate. The ostia of the posterior ethmoid cells are in the superior meatus. The ostium of the sphenoid sinus is in the posterior part of the superior meatus, the sphenoethmoid recess.

Trauma and Foreign Bodies

NASAL FRACTURE. The nose is a vulnerable leading part. Fractures of the nasal bones are the most common fractures of the facial bones. Fractures of the nose may involve the ascending processes of the maxillae and the nasal processes of the frontal bones as well as the nasal bones. A fracture of the nose is usually an open fracture. The skin of the dorsum of the nose may be lacerated, and the mucous membrane in the nasal cavity is generally torn. The most common deformity is a deviation of the nasal bones to the right with depression of the nasal bones on the left, characteristically occurring with a right hook. Fractures of the nose may be associated with septal fractures and hematomas.

Fractures of the nasal bones are generally associated with bleeding from the nose owing to the tear of the mucous membrane. A fracture should be suspected if blunt injury causes bleeding from the nose. Soft tissue swelling occurs fairly promptly and may tend to obscure the underlying bony deformity. Ecchymosis may spread into the upper and lower eyelids. The diagnosis can ordinarily be established by gentle palpation of the dorsum of the nose. Any deformity suggests a fracture. Radiographs of the nasal bones tend to confirm the diagnosis. Linear radiolucencies parallel to the long axis of the nasal bones are usually nutrient vessels. Radiolucencies transverse to the long axis of the nasal bones are usually fractures. Displacement of the bony fragments may be demonstrated; however, the degree of displacement is more readily determined by physical examination.

Fractures of the nasal complex are often associated with fractures of other facial bones, and a CT scan of the paranasal sinuses is obtained. Trauma to the facial bones is often associated with a cerebrospinal fluid rhinorrhea. After injury to the central portion of the face, the patient is specifically examined for cerebrospinal fluid rhinorrhea by having him tip his head forward and collecting any drainage from the nose. Cerebrospinal rhinorrhea requires prophylactic antibiotic therapy to prevent meningitis. The patient is instructed to avoid blowing the nose. In most cases cerebrospinal fluid rhinorrhea ceases spontaneously. The location of a cerebrospinal fluid leak may be determined with CT scanning with intrathecal iohexol. If the site of the suspected leak is not found in this manner, its presence or absence can be determined by the introduction of a radioactive isotope into the cerebrospinal fluid at lumbar puncture, and cotton pledgets placed in the nasal cavities are counted for radioactivity after several hours. If the rhinorrhea does not cease within 14 to 21 days, the dural leak is repaired through a frontal craniotomy or through a transethmoid approach to the roof of the nasal cavity.

Nasal fractures in adults may be reduced under local anesthesia. General anesthesia is necessary for the reduction of nasal fractures in children. The local anesthesia required is similar to that used for a rhinoplasty. Thorough anesthesia is necessary for a satisfactory reduction of the nasal bones. The fracture is manipulated into a good position by internal traction on the fracture fragments with a blunt periosteal elevator in association with external traction with the fingers. The need for internal and external splinting depends on the postreduction stability of the fracture.

If blunt trauma to the nose is neglected, it causes permanent deformity that ultimately requires septal surgery to improve the airway and rhinoplasty to improve the appearance of the nose.

Fractures of the nasal septum may be reduced at the same time as the reduction of the fracture of the nasal bones. Often these fractures are difficult to maintain in a position of good alignment and require a subsequent septoplasty or submucous resection of the nasal septum.

Septal hematomas lie between the quadrangular cartilage and the perichondrium. When the perichondrium has been elevated from both sides of the septal cartilage, the cartilage undergoes avascular necrosis. Septal hematomas frequently become infected, and abscess formation produces avascular and septic necrosis of the septal cartilage, which causes a saddle deformity of the nose. Septal hematomas are incised and drained as soon as the diagnosis is made. An incision in the mucoperichondrium over the anterior part of the hematoma allows access for aspiration. The perichondrium is placed in contact with the septal cartilage by packing the nasal cavity with petrolatum gauze.

Septal abscesses are located between the cartilage and the perichondrium. They may involve both sides of the cartilage. Septal abscesses are incised and drained under general anesthesia as soon as the diagnosis is established. Incisions are made bilaterally if there is pus on both sides of the septum. A small rubber drain is sutured to a lip of the wound until the drainage subsides. Vigorous systemic antibiotic therapy is employed.

DEVIATIONS OF THE NASAL SEPTUM. Deviations of the nasal septum may be caused by trauma or may occur as developmental abnormalities, particularly in individuals with highly arched palates. The nasal bones and septum are frequently fractured at the time of birth. This injury is of the greenstick type, and often it corrects itself. However, correction is usually simply accomplished by moving the nose digitally back toward the midline. Slight anterior traction is applied to the tip of the nose during this maneuver. No internal or external splinting is required.

Deviations of the nasal septum produce varying degrees of nasal obstruction and predispose the patient to sinusitis, particularly if the deviation tends to obstruct one of the ostia of the paranasal sinuses during acute inflammatory processes, and to epistaxis as a result of drying air currents over the deflected septum. The caudal edge of the nasal septum may be dislocated and produce an external deformity of the columella.

Deviations of the septum are corrected by septoplasty or submucous resection of the nasal septum. In these procedures, the mucoperichondrium is elevated from the cartilage. The deviated cartilage and bone are resected or remodeled to straighten the septum.

Perforations of the nasal septum may be secondary to nasal surgery or repeated trauma, as in picking the nose. In the past, perforations due to syphilis and tuberculosis were common. Perforations of the septum produce crusting around their margins and repeated epistaxis. Small perforations whistle. The crusting and bleeding can be controlled with the use of a Silastic septal button, which is shaped like a collar button. The post extends through the perforation, and the two flanges cover the perforation on each side of the nasal septum. Septal perforations are closed by the development of opposing mucoperichondrial flaps over free grafts of fascia.[13]

Rhinoplasty is performed for physiologic as well as cosmetic purposes. A deformed nose is usually associated with airway obstruction. The aims of rhinoplasty are to eliminate the airway obstruction and to correct the external deformity of the nose. Usually rhinoplasty is performed under local anesthesia. The surgical procedure is directed toward the cartilaginous and bony framework of the nose. The soft tissue of the nose conforms postoperatively to the modification of the bony and cartilaginous framework. Generally, modification of each element of the nasal skeleton is necessary for aesthetically pleasing results. Saddle deformities of the nose may be corrected by augmentation with autogenous bone or silicone rubber implants.

FOREIGN BODIES. Children put all manner of objects in their noses. Erasers, beans, buttons, pebbles, wool nap, paper, and sponge rubber are common foreign bodies. A foreign body in the nasal cavity produces a severe inflammatory reaction and causes a foul-smelling, bloody, unilateral discharge. Removal of the foreign body is facilitated by producing vasoconstriction anterior to it with a topical sympathomimetic amine such as phenylephrine. The foreign body is removed by placing a blunt hook posterior to it and raking it anteriorly. Attempts at grasping smooth, firm foreign bodies with forceps tend to push them farther posteriorly. General anesthesia is used if good cooperation from a child cannot be obtained by gentle reassurance.

If a foreign body dwells long in the nose, mineral salts are deposited on it and produce a rhinolith. The rhinolith tends to conform to the contour of the nasal cavity, and its removal is usually difficult.

Sinusitis

Acute rhinitis is the usual manifestation of a common cold. Acute sinusitis is usually initiated by an acute respiratory tract infection of viral etiology. Nearly all cases of acute sinusitis and most cases of chronic sinusitis respond well to antibiotic therapy. The complications of acute and chronic sinusitis often require surgical therapy, as does unresponsive chronic sinusitis. Complications of maxillary sinusitis are rare. Ethmoid sinusitis is frequently complicated in children by orbital cellulitis and abscess. Eighty per cent of all cases of orbital cellulitis are secondary to ethmoid sinusitis. In the patient who presents with erythema and swelling of the eyelids, proptosis, and displacement of the globe laterally and inferiorly, the source of the infection is sought by inspection of the nose for mucopus in the middle meatus and by CT scanning of the paranasal sinuses for ethmoid sinusitis. CT scanning of the orbits may allow differentiation of orbital cellulitis from orbital abscess. Ethmoid sinusitis and orbital cellulitis respond well to systemic antibiotic therapy. If the proptosis fails to subside or progresses, incision and drainage of the abscess, which is between the lamina papyracea and the orbital periosteum, is performed through a Killian incision that extends from the lateral aspect of the nose to the eyebrow. The orbital periosteum is elevated from the medial wall of the orbit so that the abscess cavity can be reached. The optic nerve tolerates 11 to 14 mm. of proptosis. The point at which extraocular motion is lost is also the limit of stretch of the optic nerve. Therefore, incision and drainage of an orbital abscess is performed prior to complete loss of extraocular motion to prevent permanent blindness.

Frontal sinusitis may cause intracranial complications such as meningitis, epidural abscess, subdural empyema, and brain abscess. In severe acute frontal sinusitis that fails to respond promptly to systemic antibiotic therapy, the floor of the frontal sinus is trephined through an incision just inferior to the medial part of the eyebrow. An opening of approximately 7 to 8 mm. is made, and a catheter is placed in the sinus to maintain drainage. Trephination is performed in an attempt to prevent the intracranial complications of frontal sinusitis.

Fractures of the frontal sinus lead to the development of mucoceles. Mucoceles follow duplication of the mucous membrane. They gradually enlarge and destroy the floor of the frontal sinus; and as they expand into the orbital cavity, they produce proptosis and inferior and lateral displacement of the eye. Mucoceles and other forms of chronic frontal sinusitis that do not respond to medical management can be managed surgically by an osteoplastic flap approach for obliteration of the frontal sinus (Fig. 11). The incision in the bone is made at the periphery of the frontal sinus, and the anterior wall is rotated inferiorly on the hinge of periosteum at the floor of the sinus. Infected mucous membrane is removed with a gas-driven burr under microscopic control, and the cavity of the frontal sinus is obliterated by the implantation of fat taken from the abdominal wall.

Approximately 25 per cent of cases of chronic maxillary sinusitis are secondary to a dental infection. In chronic maxillary sinusitis, radiographs of the apices of the teeth should be obtained to exclude the possibility of a periapical abscess.

Chronic maxillary sinusitis that does not respond to medical management may be controlled with the Caldwell-Luc operation, which is a maxillary sinusotomy performed through an incision in the canine fossa. The bone of the anterior wall of the maxillary sinus is resected to permit access to the interior of the sinus for removal of infected mucous membrane, cysts, and epithelial debris. Drainage of the maxillary sinus is improved by creating a nasoantral window in the inferior meatus.

Chronic ethmoid sinusitis is often associated with allergic

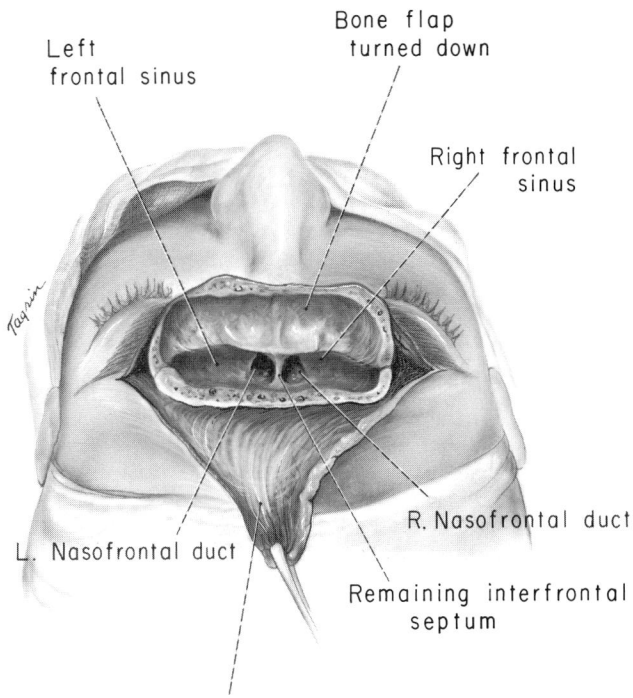

Figure 11. Approach to the frontal sinuses by the use of an osteoplastic flap for obliteration of the sinuses. (From Goodale, R. L., and Montgomery, W. W.: Technical advances in osteoplastic frontal sinusectomy. Arch. Otolaryngol., 79:522, 1964.)

rhinitis and the formation of nasal polyps. In those individuals in whom the formation of nasal polyps and the symptoms of ethmoid sinusitis cannot be controlled adequately by intranasal polypectomy and medical management including topical corticosteroid therapy and immunotherapy, an ethmoidectomy is indicated. Ethmoidectomy is performed intranasally with endoscopic guidance and through an external approach utilizing a Killian incision.[30] In the external ethmoidectomy, the orbital periosteum is elevated, and the lamina papyracea is removed for the purpose of giving access to the ethmoid air cells. Infected mucous membrane, polypoid tissue, and epithelial debris are removed. The anterior half of the middle turbinate is excised for creation of a large opening between the ethmoid air cells and the nasal cavity. In essence, an ethmoidectomy incorporates the ethmoid air cell area into the nasal cavity.

Chronic sphenoid sinusitis that does not respond to medical management may be controlled by an operation in which the sphenoid sinus is approached through an external ethmoidectomy. After an external ethmoidectomy has been accomplished, the anterior wall of the sphenoid sinus is resected to remove infected mucous membrane, polypoid tissue, and epithelial debris. The anterior and inferior walls of the sphenoid sinus are removed. In this way, the interior of the sphenoid sinus is incorporated in the posterior part of the nasal cavity and the nasopharynx, and in essence, the sphenoid sinus is eliminated as a separate entity.

Epistaxis

Bleeding from the nose is a common clinical problem. Ninety per cent of the time epistaxis occurs from a plexus of vessels in the anteroinferior part of the septum. In the other 10 per cent of cases nasal bleeding occurs from the posterior part of the nose, particularly from far posterior in the inferior meatus at the junction of the inferior meatus and the nasopharynx. It is from this area that individuals with arteriosclerosis and hypertension are likely to bleed. This type of bleeding may be difficult to control and is associated with a 4 to 5 per cent mortality. Mild epistaxis from the anterior part of the nasal septum is usually effectively controlled by steady pressure applied by squeezing the mobile portion of the nose between the index finger and thumb for 5 to 10 minutes. Treatment for epistaxis that is not controlled by this simple measure requires visualization of the bleeding point. The bleeding point can be controlled temporarily and anesthesia achieved with pressure applied over a cotton pledget impregnated with a vasoconstrictor and a topically active local anesthetic such as lidocaine. The bleeding point can be cauterized chemically or with electrocautery. Silver nitrate is preferred as the cauterizing agent, since it produces satisfactory intravascular coagulation without a severe burn of the mucous membrane. If the bleeding cannot be easily controlled with cautery or if the bleeding point cannot be visualized, strips of ½-inch petrolatum gauze are used for applying pressure to the bleeding point. Pressure is applied as atraumatically as possible. This method is preferred in a patient with a bleeding tendency because the periphery of a cauterized area may begin to bleed.

In order to pack the posterior part of the nasal cavity, the choana is obstructed with the balloon of a Foley catheter (Fig. 12) or a postnasal pack (Fig. 13). Although the Foley catheter is easier to insert, the gauze postnasal pack is more secure. The postnasal pack is made by folding and rolling 4- by 4-inch gauze squares into a tight pack and tying the pack with two strands of No. 2 black silk. The ends of one tie are oriented inferiorly, and the ends of the other tie are oriented superiorly. After topical anesthesia of the nose, nasopharynx, and pharynx has been induced, a catheter is introduced through the nasal cavity on the side of the bleeding and brought out through the mouth. The superiorly oriented ends of the tie are tied to the catheter, and the catheter is withdrawn from the nose as the pack is placed posterior to the soft palate into the nasopharynx. The inferiorly oriented ends of the tie are trimmed below the level of the soft palate so that they can be utilized in removing the pack. The superiorly oriented strands are held taut while the nasal cavity is firmly packed with petrolatum gauze. If the bleeding point is in the inferior meatus, this area is packed tightly. The superiorly oriented strands are tied over a roll of a 4- by 4-inch gauze square. The packing is left in place for 4 days. Prophylactic antibiotic therapy is indicated to prevent sinusitis and otitis media. Patients requiring postnasal packing generally have serious systemic vascular diseases. They have a low arterial P_{O_2} while the packing is in place and should be given supplemental humidified oxygen by mask.

An alternate method of treatment of patients with severe bleeding from the posterior part of the nose is ligation of the

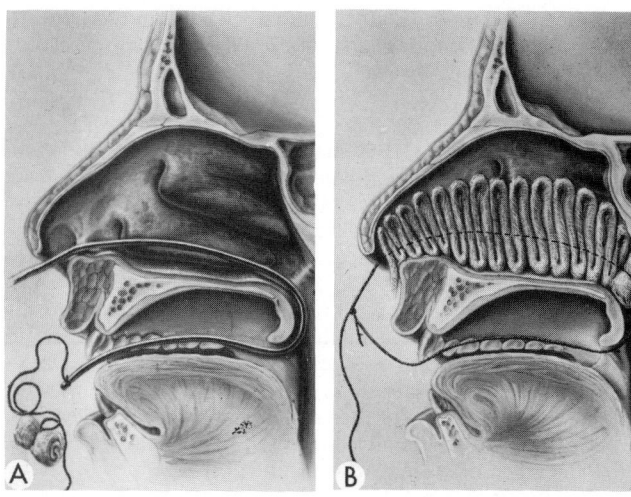

Figure 13. Packing of the nose for epistaxis with a postnasal pack and an anterior nasal pack. (From Boles, L. R., et al.: Fundamentals of Otolaryngology. A Textbook of Ear, Nose and Throat Diseases, 4th ed. Philadelphia, W. B. Saunders Company, 1964.)

internal maxillary artery (Fig. 14).[8] The artery is reached through the maxillary sinus. An incision is made in the canine fossa, and the anterior wall of the maxillary sinus is removed as in the Caldwell-Luc operation. The bone of the posterior wall of the sinus is removed, and the internal maxillary artery and its branches are gently dissected under microscopic control from the adipose tissue in the pterygomaxillary fossa. Metallic clips are placed on the internal maxillary artery as it enters the fossa and its major branches, the sphenopalatine and descending palatine arteries, as they leave the fossa. This method avoids nasal packing and the problems of hypoxemia associated with it, requires less hospitalization, and involves less discomfort for the patient.[16]

Severe epistaxis is often associated with pre-existing liver disease. Large amounts of blood may have been swallowed prior to the nasal packing. Blood is eliminated from the gastrointestinal

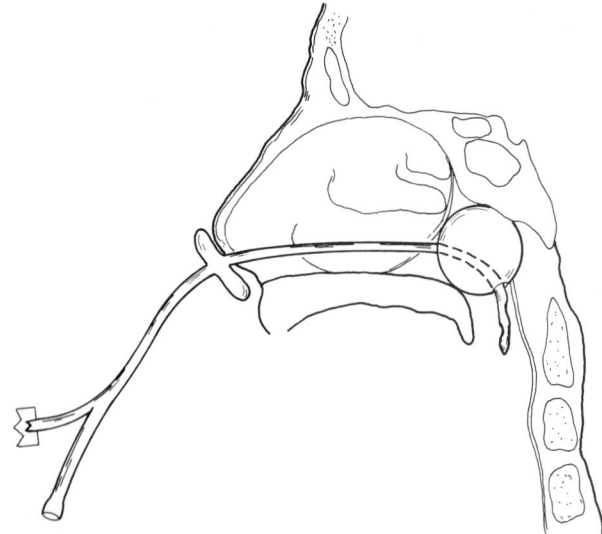

Figure 12. Use of a Foley catheter to obstruct the choana so that petrolatum gauze may be used to pack the nasal cavity tightly without prolapse of the packing in the nasopharynx.

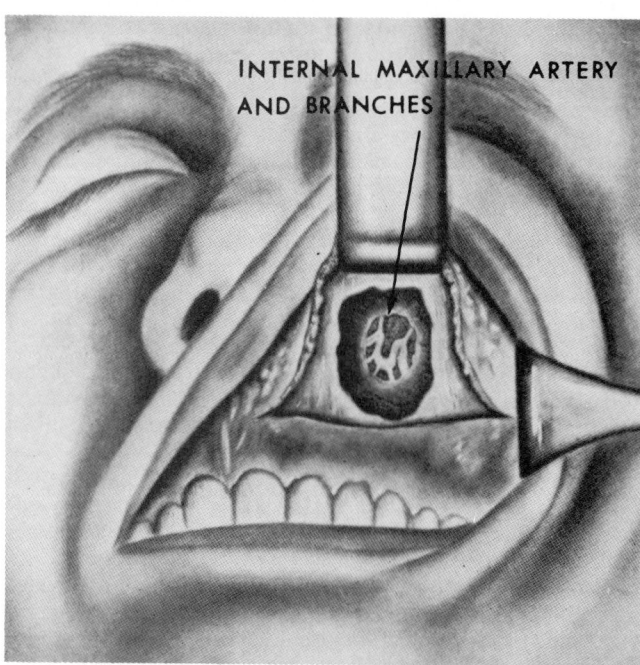

Figure 14. Approach through the canine fossa as in the Caldwell-Luc operation to ligate the internal maxillary artery. The anterior and posterior walls of the maxillary sinus have been removed to expose the artery. (From Chandler, J. R., and Serrins, A. J.: Transantral ligation of the internal maxillary artery for epistaxis. Laryngoscope, 75:1151, 1965.)

tract as promptly as possible by the use of cathartics and enemas. Sterilization of the gastrointestinal tract to prevent the breakdown of blood by microorganisms and the absorption of ammonia is indicated by the presence of liver disease.

Replacement of blood lost as a result of the epistaxis is carried out as indicated by the hemoglobin and hematocrit determinations as well as by the patient's vital signs.

A particularly debilitating form of epistaxis occurs in hereditary hemorrhagic telangiectasia (Rendu-Osler-Weber disease). Patients with this disease have frequent bleeding from the nose and gastrointestinal tract. Often the bleeding from the nose is sufficient to cause a chronic anemia that cannot be overcome by iron supplementation. A septal dermoplasty, in which the mucous membrane of the anterior portions of the nasal cavity is replaced with a split-thickness skin graft, is very effective in reducing the severity and frequency of the epistaxis so that the hemoglobin concentration may be brought to the normal level.[50]

Congenital Malformations

CHOANAL ATRESIA. Choanal atresia is a malformation in which the opening of the nasal cavity into the nasopharynx is obstructed by a partition of mucous membrane and bone. The malformation may occur unilaterally or bilaterally. If it occurs bilaterally, it produces respiratory distress in the neonate. Newborn infants are obligatory nasal breathers. If there is obstruction to the nasal airway, asphyxia occurs. The newborn presses his tongue against the roof of his mouth during the inspiratory effort. Fortunately, crying with its attendant mouth breathing often allows some ventilatory exchange. This diagnosis should be made in the delivery room. Choanal atresia should be considered in the infant who makes respiratory effort but fails to accomplish ventilatory exchange. The immediate solution to the problem is the insertion of an oral airway. The nursing care of the oral airway during the next 2 to 3 weeks must be extremely meticulous. After 2 to 3 weeks the newborn learns to breathe through his mouth, and the danger abates. Most experts advocate perforation of the atretic area in the neonatal period for the insertion of polyethylene tubes. This operation often fails to provide permanent improvement, and a better repair can be performed when the child is 4 to 5 years of age through a transpalatal approach (Fig. 15). With careful nursing supervision of the oral airway, a tracheotomy can be avoided in the neonatal period. The diagnosis is made by attempting without success to pass a catheter through the nose into the pharynx. The diagnosis is confirmed by instilling radiopaque dye into the nasal cavity and taking a lateral radiograph of the nasopharynx in the supine position. If choanal atresia is present, the dye pools

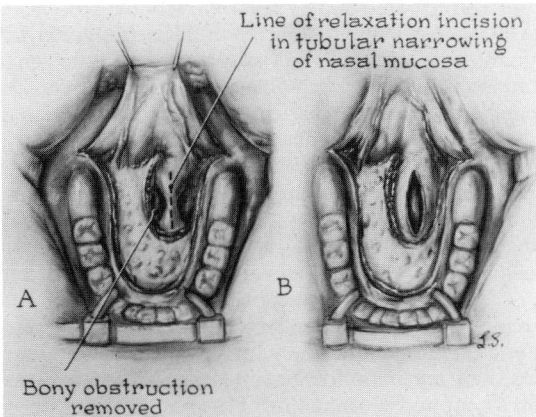

Figure 15. Transpalatal approach for repair of choanal atresia. (From Cherry, J., and Bordley, J. E.: Surgical correction of choanal atresia. Ann. Otol. Rhinol. Laryngol., 5:911, 1966.)

in the posterior part of the nasal cavity. The thickness, composition, and location of the atretic plate and the contour of the walls of the adjacent nasal cavities can be precisely determined with CT.

NASAL GLIOMAS, DERMOIDS, ENCEPHALOCELES, AND MENINGOCELES. Nasal gliomas and dermoids may present as a malformation of the dorsum of the nose evident at birth or as a mass in the nasal cavity. Nasal gliomas and dermoids often have intracranial connections that can be demonstrated with computed tomography. Under these circumstances, a frontal craniotomy is performed prior to the removal of the nasal glioma. Encephaloceles and meningoceles may present in the nasal cavity through defects in the cribriform plate. Clinically they have an appearance similar to that of a nasal polyp. Nasal polyps ordinarily arise from the middle meatus. If what appears to be a nasal polyp does not arise from the middle meatus, computed tomography with iohexol introduced into the cerebrospinal fluid is performed to exclude an encephalocele or meningocele.

Neoplasms

BENIGN NEOPLASMS OF THE NOSE AND PARANASAL SINUSES. Squamous cell papillomas occur in the nasal cavity and are thought to be caused by papovaviruses. Exophytic papillomas occasionally recur after excision but have a benign course. Inverted papillomas are invasive and behave in a locally malignant manner. They arise from the lateral wall of the nasal cavity and invade bone. Inverted papillomas require removal of a margin of normal tissue through a lateral rhinotomy. Fibromas, hemangiomas, and neurofibromas occur occasionally in the nasal cavity. Fibromas, neurolemmomas, and ossifying fibromas occur in the paranasal sinuses.[5]

MALIGNANT NEOPLASMS OF THE NOSE AND PARANASAL SINUSES. The most common malignant neoplasm occurring in the nose and paranasal sinuses is squamous cell carcinoma. Adenoid cystic carcinomas, adenocarcinomas (particularly in the ethmoid sinuses), mucoepidermoid carcinomas, malignant mixed tumors, lymphomas, fibrosarcomas, osteosarcomas, chondrosarcomas, and melanomas also occur in the nose and paranasal sinuses.[5] Metastatic tumors may involve the paranasal sinuses, and the most common neoplasm to metastasize to the paranasal sinuses is the hypernephroma.

Early squamous cell and basal cell carcinomas of the skin of the nose are treated with radiation therapy or cauterization and curettage. Larger carcinomas involving cartilage require excision. Nasal septal carcinomas often require sacrifice of the columella as well as adjacent structures.

A combination of radiation therapy and radical resection provides the best survival rates in carcinomas and sarcomas of the nasal cavities and paranasal sinuses. Malignant neoplasms of the lateral wall of the nose require lateral rhinotomy. Malignant neoplasms of the maxillary sinus require partial or radical maxillectomy.[34] A radical maxillectomy usually includes exenteration of the orbit. Malignant neoplasms of the ethmoid sinus require radical resection of the ethmoid complex, including exenteration of the orbit and partial maxillectomy. Malignant neoplasms of the frontal sinus and the sphenoid sinus are not satisfactorily resected and are usually treated with radiation therapy. Lymphomas limited to the nasal cavities or paranasal sinuses are treated with radiation therapy. Disseminated lymphomas require chemotherapy. Melanomas arising in mucous membrane are treated with surgical therapy and radiation therapy, with only rare success.

THE PHARYNX

Celsus is generally recognized as the first to describe tonsillectomy in his first-century *De medicina.* However, the Asiatic Indians frequently performed the operation 1000 years earlier.

Anatomy of the Pharynx

For descriptive purposes the pharynx can be divided into the nasopharynx, oropharynx, and hypopharynx. However, from a functional point of view, the pharynx remains united by the constrictors of the pharynx. They have a common insertion in the median pharyngeal raphe and form a musculomembranous tubular passage from the base of the skull to the opening of the esophagus. The lymphoid structures of the pharynx include the pharyngeal tonsil or adenoid, the palatine tonsils, the lateral bands, and the lingual tonsils.

Foreign Bodies

Foreign bodies of the pharynx are likely to be found in four locations: the palatine tonsils, the lingual tonsils, the valleculae, and the pyriform sinuses. Sharp foreign bodies, such as fish bones, are particularly likely to lodge in the palatine tonsils and the lingual tonsils. Smooth, small, oval foreign bodies, such as capsules, are likely to come to rest in the valleculae. Irregular sharp foreign bodies are likely to be retained in the pyriform sinuses. Rarely, foreign bodies are coughed into the nasopharynx and become trapped there. Radiopaque foreign bodies may be located in a lateral neck film. Foreign bodies in the palatine tonsil are removed by grasping the foreign body with a hemostat. Foreign bodies in the nasopharynx require general anesthesia for their removal. Foreign bodies of the hypopharynx are removed at direct laryngoscopy under local anesthesia.

Nasopharynx

THE ADENOIDS. Adenoid hypertrophy in childhood often leads to obstruction of the eustachian tubes and the choanae. This lymphoid hyperplasia may be physiologic or secondary to infectious and allergic manifestations. Obstruction of the eustachian tubes leads to serous or secretory otitis media, recurrent acute otitis media, and exacerbations of chronic otitis media. Obstruction of the choanae produces mouth breathing, a hyponasal voice, and rhinorrhea.

Recurrent serous or secretory otitis media is the most common indication for the removal of the adenoid tissue. An effusion in the middle ear in a child lasting 6 weeks or longer, occurring *de novo* or following acute otitis media, that does not respond to medical management responds regularly but not invariably to the use of myringotomies with the insertion of tympanostomy tubes. In patients with recurrent or persistent serous or secretory otitis media, adenoidectomy increases the likelihood of success.

Chronic otitis media in children is another indication for adenoidectomy. The procedure reduces the severity and frequency of exacerbations of chronic otitis media. It prepares the patient for subsequent mastoidectomy and tympanoplasty. Recurrent acute otitis media is a fairly frequent indication for these procedures. Many children between the ages of 1 and 6 years have two or three episodes of acute otitis media per year that completely resolve with antibiotic therapy. However, the child who is on antibiotic therapy for otitis media half of the time should be considered for this procedure. The duration of the pain, the presence of spontaneous perforation, the regularity with which myringotomy is required, and the associated systemic symptoms deserve consideration. Febrile convulsions with acute otitis media weigh heavily in favor of adenoidectomy, since antibiotic therapy ordinarily is not initiated prior to the convulsion.

Persistent nasal obstruction due to adenoid hypertrophy is a problem in which the age of the patient is considered as well as the severity, since lymphoid tissue reaches a relative and absolute maximum at puberty. Persistent and recurrent purulent rhinorrhea despite adequate antibiotic therapy is occasionally encountered in association with adenoid hypertrophy and chronic adenoiditis. Chronic sinusitis in children without an underlying immunologic or other defense mechanism defect such as agammaglobulinemia or hypogammaglobulinemia, cystic fibrosis, or Kartagener's syndrome is relatively rare but is rather regularly improved or eliminated by adenoidectomy.

An adenoidectomy is performed under general anesthesia. The adenoid tissue is sheared from the posterior nasopharyngeal wall with a guillotine-type adenotome placed posterior to the soft palate. The lymphoid tissue is removed superficial to the fascia of the superior constrictor of the pharynx without damaging the fascia or the underlying musculature.

TORNWALDT'S CYST. Cysts occasionally form in the region of the medial recess of the nasopharynx. These cysts become symptomatic when they become infected. There may be persistent purulent drainage that has a foul taste and odor. Symptoms of eustachian tube obstruction and sore throat may be prominent. Excision or marsupialization of the cyst with an adenotome is the treatment of choice.

BENIGN NEOPLASMS OF THE NASOPHARYNX. Juvenile angiofibromas are very vascular neoplasms that occur in pubescent males. They develop in the vault of the nasopharynx from the area of the basisphenoid and grow to a large size. Angiofibromas may extend into and obstruct the nasal cavity, and their extensions may develop parasitic attachments distant to their site of origin. They may encroach upon the paranasal sinuses, the orbit, and the intracranial cavity. Histologically, these neoplasms are composed of fibrous tissue and numerous thin-walled vessels without contractile elements. Angiofibromas tend to involute at maturity.

Epistaxis is the major problem with angiofibromas, and the magnitude of the bleeding can be very great. The neoplasms are red and quite firm. Those portions of the neoplasm that project into the airway often become ulcerated during upper respiratory tract infections and bleed from the ulcerated surface. Their surgical removal is necessitated by recurrent massive bleeding. The extent of the neoplasm can be determined with CT and angiography. The pterygomaxillary fissure is often widened on the sagittal plane of the computed tomography of the lateral part of the nasopharynx by the extension of the neoplasm into the infratemporal fossa. These neoplasms give a characteristic vascular pattern on angiography. The main blood supply is usually from the branches of the internal maxillary artery, although the branches of the internal carotid artery and the middle meningeal artery also may contribute. Usually, they are removed through a transpalatal approach. Often a lateral rhinotomy offers significant advantages. The blood loss during excision is often very great, and rapid blood replacement is required. Treatment with estrogens and embolization of the internal maxillary artery at angiography have been used to reduce the operative blood loss.[53] These neoplasms are responsive to radiation therapy. This is often the treatment of choice for the neoplasm that has invaded the orbit or the intracranial cavity or receives a large blood supply from intracranial vessels.

MALIGNANT NEOPLASMS OF THE NASOPHARYNX. Malignant neoplasms of the nasopharynx include squamous cell carcinomas, adenocarcinomas, adenoid cystic carcinomas, mucoepidermoid carcinomas, malignant mixed tumors, melanomas, chordomas, sarcomas including fibrosarcoma, rhabdomyosarcoma, liposarcoma and myxosarcoma, plasmacytomas, and lymphomas. Among children, lymphomas are the most common malignant neoplasms arising from and secondarily involving the nasopharynx. Among the carcinomas, lymphoepithelioma or squamous cell carcinoma is the most common type.

Carcinoma of the nasopharynx occurs at relatively young ages, and there is an unusually high incidence among the Chinese.[37] There are immunologic similarities among patients with Burkitt's lymphoma, carcinoma of the nasopharynx, and infectious mononucleosis. Elevated titers of anti–Epstein-Barr virus antibodies are present in 45 per cent of patients with Stage I carcinoma of the nasopharynx and 100 per cent of patients with

Stage V lesions.[22] The majority of patients with carcinoma of the nasopharynx present with nasal or eustachian tube obstruction. Obstruction of the eustachian tube may cause a middle ear effusion. The nasal obstruction may be associated with purulent, bloody rhinorrhea and frank epistaxis. The more dramatic symptoms following cranial nerve paralysis and cervical lymph node metastasis are, unfortunately, common presenting complaints. Metastasis tends to be limited to the neck until the late stages of the disease. A granular mass or ulcer may be seen in the nasopharynx. The palate may be deformed by the bulk of the nasopharyngeal mass, or its mobility may be limited by paralysis of the levator veli palatini. Not infrequently the neoplasm extends deep to the mucous membrane, appears only as a slight fullness, and produces no abnormality of the mucous membrane. It is this feature of carcinoma of the nasopharynx that makes biopsy through apparently normal mucous membrane occasionally fruitful.

The diagnosis is made by biopsy of the primary tumor. Adequate access to the nasopharynx ordinarily requires general anesthesia. General anesthesia also allows the opportunity to judge the extent of the primary lesion by palpation. Biopsy of the metastasis in the neck should be avoided until the nasopharynx has been inspected and palpated and any suspicious lesion has been biopsied. Biopsy of the cervical metastasis violates the integrity of the block of tissue that is removed in a radical neck dissection. It may cause implantation of the neoplasm in the skin and subcutaneous tissue. The necessity for demonstrating the neoplasm in the nasopharynx prior to treatment remains, even if a histologic diagnosis is obtained from biopsy of the cervical metastasis.

The treatment of choice for carcinoma of the nasopharynx is irradiation with a supervoltage source. The radiation should be delivered to the primary tumor-bearing area of the nasopharynx and to both sides of the neck whether there is clinically demonstrated metastasis or not. Surgery has no role in the initial therapy of carcinoma of the nasopharynx. Those cervical metastases that remain clinically palpable following radiation therapy or that subsequently become apparent should be eradicated by radical neck dissection. Generally, control of the metastatic lesions should be attempted only after there is evidence that the primary lesion has been controlled. The overall 5-year survival for carcinoma of the nasopharynx is approximately 35 per cent.

Oropharynx

PERITONSILLAR ABSCESS. Peritonsillar cellulitis and abscess are complications of acute tonsillitis in which the infection has spread deep to the tonsillar capsule. Pus forms between the tonsillar capsule and the superior constrictor of the pharynx, and the tonsil is displaced medially. The uvula becomes tremendously edematous and is displaced to the opposite side. The soft palate is very red and displaced forward. There is marked trismus due to irritation of the pterygoid muscles, and the head is held tilted toward the side of the abscess. It is painful for the patient to talk and to swallow. Swallowing is so painful that the patient drools. The breath is foul-smelling. The temperature is usually 38 to 40°C. Peritonsillar cellulitis or abscess is rare in children under the age of 10 to 12 years and is usually caused by a group A beta-hemolytic streptococcus or anaerobe. If a cellulitis without pus formation exists, it responds in a matter of 24 to 48 hours to penicillin therapy. If pus is present, it may resolve or require incision and drainage. The pus may be difficult to locate. Incision is performed as the mucous membrane overlying the pus assumes a pale yellow color. The patient is placed in the sitting position to avoid aspiration of the pus. Under topical anesthesia, the incision is made in the anterior pillar parallel to its free edge. The incision need only split the mucous membrane, and the pus is obtained by spreading gently with a hemostat. No drain is required because the abscess cavity is emptied by each swallow.

These abscesses tend to recur and are an indication for tonsillectomy, which is usually performed 6 weeks after the acute infection. At the time of tonsillectomy, 1 to 2 ml. of pus is often encountered between the capsule and the tonsillar fossa. This persistent abscess is the apparent reason for the recurrence of these abscesses. Some advocate that the tonsillectomy be performed within a day or two after the antibiotic therapy is initiated.

PARAPHARYNGEAL ABSCESS. Parapharyngeal abscess may occur in infants and young children as well as in adults. The abscess is usually secondary to streptococcal pharyngitis or tonsillitis. Pus forms in the parapharyngeal space secondarily from the breakdown of lymphadenitis. The pus is located lateral to the superior constrictor of the pharynx and adjacent to the carotid sheath. The tonsil and soft palate may be displaced medially, but there may be no inflammatory reaction in the pharynx. There is marked swelling in the anterior cervical triangle. Penicillin is the antibiotic of choice. Pus formation can be demonstrated with CT or MRI before the abscess becomes fluctuant. When pus formation has been demonstrated, the abscess is incised and drained. The abscess is not drained through the lateral pharyngeal wall because of the proximity of the internal carotid artery and the internal jugular vein. An incision is made parallel to the skin folds over the anterior border of the sternocleidomastoid muscle. The anterior border of the muscle is identified, and blunt dissection is carried toward the carotid sheath, where the pus is encountered. A drain is sewn in place and removed when the drainage subsides.

RETROPHARYNGEAL ABSCESS. Retropharyngeal abscess occurs in infants and young children and is rare after the age of 10 years. These infections are located between the constrictors of the pharynx and the prevertebral fascia. They are secondary to pharyngitis and are due to the breakdown of retropharyngeal lymphadenitis. Infants with retropharyngeal abscesses usually present with stridor and hyperextension of the neck. A lumbar puncture is the appropriate diagnostic procedure in a febrile infant who presents in opisthotonos. If the cerebrospinal fluid is normal, the possibility of a retropharyngeal abscess must be excluded. The diagnosis is made by palpating the posterior pharyngeal wall. The infant is held in the prone position for the examination so that if the abscess is ruptured during the examination, the pus flows out of the infant's mouth and is not aspirated. The abscess has a boggy fluctuant texture, and the bodies of the cervical vertebrae are not palpable. Inspection of the pharynx may not demonstrate the abscess because the whole posterior pharyngeal wall may be displaced forward and there may be no inflammatory reaction in the mucous membrane. The abscess can also be demonstrated by a radiograph of the lateral neck in which the posterior pharyngeal wall is displaced anteriorly or by CT of the neck. To maintain the airway, the child should be allowed to hyperextend the neck. A tracheotomy is rarely necessary. In addition to penicillin therapy, the posterior pharyngeal wall should be incised under general endotracheal anesthesia with the patient in the Rose position. The mucous membrane at the posterior wall of the pharynx is incised vertically. The incision need only split the mucous membrane. The pus is obtained by gently spreading a hemostat in the wound toward the retropharyngeal space. No drain is necessary because the abscess cavity tends to be emptied on swallowing.

TONSILLECTOMY. Recurrent acute bacterial tonsillitis caused by a group A beta-hemolytic streptococcus occurring three to four times during the year in children from 2 to 7 years of age can be adequately managed with penicillin or other appropriate antibiotics administered for 12 days. The rationale for this length of treatment is that a shorter period may not eliminate a streptococcal infection. In addition to inappropriate selection of antibiotics and inadequate duration of therapy, passage of the streptococcus among family members is a cause of failure in the medical management of tonsillitis. This situation requires simultaneous cultures of the entire family and simultaneous treatment of all carriers. Despite these precautions, in some patients tonsillitis repeatedly develops within a few days after the completion of adequate treatment. When this pattern cannot be altered by medical management, tonsillectomy is indicated.

Chronic tonsillitis with persistent sore throat, either briefly relieved or not at all relieved by antibiotic therapy, constitutes another indication for tonsillectomy. One peritonsillar abscess is an indication for tonsillectomy.

In adults, tonsillectomy is performed under local or general anesthesia. In children, general anesthesia is required. The technique involves an incision in the free edge of the tonsillar pillars. The dissection of the tonsil from the tonsillar fossa is performed in the plane between the tonsillar capsule and the superior constrictor muscle of the pharynx and is completed by closing a snare placed inferior to the lower pole of the tonsil. The objective is to remove the tonsil and its capsule intact and spare the musculature of the tonsillar fossa.

UVULOPALATOPHARYNGOPLASTY. Snoring is usually due to the vibration of the soft palate during respiration. Relaxation of the soft palate can also contribute to the airway obstruction in obstructive sleep apnea. Other contributing factors include the posterior displacement of the base of the tongue and collapse of the hypopharyngeal airway, of which obesity is a predisposing condition. It is important to differentiate obstructive from central sleep apnea by overnight evaluation in a sleep laboratory. Uvulopalatopharyngoplasty (UPPP) involves removing the uvula, approximately 1 cm. of the free edge of the soft palate, and the palatine tonsils if they have not previously been removed. The resulting scarring tends to stiffen the soft palate and is fairly reliable in reducing snoring but is less efficacious in relieving obstructive sleep apnea. With life-threatening obstructive sleep apnea, a tracheotomy is indicated.

CARCINOMA OF THE TONSIL. Carcinoma of the tonsil represents 1.5 to 3 per cent of all cancers and is second in frequency only to carcinoma of the larynx among malignant neoplasms of the upper respiratory tract. It is predominantly a disease of males, and smoking cigarettes and consumption of more than 100 ml. of ethanol per day are etiologic factors. Squamous cell carcinoma is the predominant histologic type. These carcinomas may be exophytic with superficial ulceration or deeply invasive. At times they present as lobulated submucosal masses. The neoplasm frequently extends into the base of the tongue. Carcinoma of the tonsil usually remains asymptomatic until it has reached considerable size. Sore throat is the most common presenting complaint, and pain often radiates to the ear on the same side. Not infrequently the patient presents with a metastatic mass in the neck as the first symptom. The diagnosis is established by biopsy of the primary lesion. Treatment requires combined radiation therapy and operation. Radiation therapy may be given preoperatively or postoperatively. If preoperative irradiation is utilized, 5000 rads are delivered to the primary lesion and both sides of the neck over a 5-week period. The patient is given a 6-week rest. The operation consists of radical resection of the tonsillar fossa, hemimandibulectomy, and radical neck dissection if there are palpable metastases. If postoperative irradiation is utilized, 6000 rads are delivered to the primary site and 5000 rads to both sides of the neck. The 2-year disease-free survival approximates 50 per cent.[39]

Hypopharynx

DIVERTICULUM OF THE HYPOPHARYNX. Pharyngoesophageal diverticula follow herniation of the mucous membrane of the hypopharynx through weak points in the inferior constrictor muscle; spasm of the cricopharyngeal muscle may have an etiologic role. They occur in the older age group. These pulsion diverticula usually occur on the left side. The sac lies between the prevertebral fascia and the left posterolateral wall

of the esophagus. Although the origin of the diverticulum is the hypopharynx, the esophagus is compressed by the diverticulum, and dysphagia and weight loss follow. During deglutition, the diverticulum fills with food and fluid. When the patient lies down, the diverticulum empties into the pharynx, and aspiration of food and fluid into the lower respiratory tract may occur and may cause recurrent and debilitating pneumonitis. The diverticulum is demonstrated with a barium swallow. Treatment consists of cricopharyngeal myotomy and excision of the diverticulum through a cervical incision or by endoscopic cautery of the party wall between the cervical esophagus and the diverticulum.

THE LARYNX

Caelius Aurelianus credits Asclepiades with having first employed tracheotomy in cynanche (probably diphtheria) in the century before the birth of Christ. In 1778, the French surgeon Pelletan performed a successful laryngofissure for the removal of a bolus of meat that had become entrapped between the vocal cords. In 1854, Manuel Garcia, a Spanish singing teacher, succeeded in observing his own larynx with two mirrors and the sun as a light source. In 1856, Türck and Czermak independently developed the laryngoscope in Vienna. After the development of the laryngoscope, peroral endolaryngeal surgery flourished in many centers. In the 1870s Bergman performed laryngotomies for removal of parts of the larynx involved with carcinoma. Billroth performed the first successful laryngectomy in 1873.

Anatomy of the Larynx

The skeleton of the larynx consists of the thyroid cartilage, the cricoid cartilage, the arytenoid cartilages with corniculate and cuneiform cartilages, and the epiglottis. Phylogenetically the arytenoid cartilages are the oldest elements of the laryngeal skeleton. This fact emphasizes the primeval role of the larynx as a sphincter rather than a conduit for air. The cricoid cartilage completely encircles the airway and maintains its patency. The arytenoid cartilages articulate with the cricoid cartilage. The true vocal cords are attached to the vocal processes of the arytenoid cartilages and to the isthmus of the thyroid cartilage. The superior surfaces of the true vocal cords are flat, and the inferior surfaces are concave. The inferior surfaces of the false vocal cords are flat, and the superior surfaces of the false vocal cords are convex. The true vocal cords and the false vocal cords make a double-layered sphincter. The configuration of the true vocal cords makes them a good barrier to the ingress of air and a poor barrier to the egress of air. The configuration of the false vocal cords makes them a poor barrier to the ingress of air and a good barrier to the egress of air. The true vocal cords can be regarded as an inlet valve and the false vocal cords as an outlet valve.

Physiology of the Larynx

The primary function of the larynx is that of a sphincter. During deglutition both the true vocal cord sphincter and the false vocal cord sphincter are closed, and the epiglottis is drawn posteriorly over the closed sphincter and serves as a watershed deflecting food and fluid into the pyriform sinuses. The larynx also serves as a sphincter during parturition, coughing, and defecation. At these times, it serves primarily as an outlet valve. In lifting heavy objects and climbing hand over hand as in climbing a tree, the pull of the shoulder girdles on the thorax tends to expand the thoracic cage. The larynx limits the ingress of air as an inlet valve and thereby stabilizes the thorax.

The larynx serves as the sounding source for speech. A fundamental tone is produced by the movement of the vocal cords, which is brought about by the flow of exhaled air past lightly approximated vocal cords. The fundamental tone and its overtones are modified into meaningful symbols or speech by articulators such as the pharynx, palate, tongue, teeth, and lips. Synchrony of the vibration of the two vocal cords exists normally at any given instant, but aperiodicity over time also occurs. The fundamental tone varies with the sex and age of the individual. Adult males produce a fundamental tone of 125 Hz., and adult females produce a fundamental tone of 250 Hz. In the healthy voice, the predominant overtones of these fundamental tones are partial and whole-number multiples of the fundamental tone. The predominance of harmonic overtones gives the voice a musical quality. The distribution of the harmonics gives the voice a timbre that is characteristic of that individual. In the healthy voice there are frequent changes in the frequency of the fundamental tone that provide it with a melodious quality. The normal speaker usually uses changes in frequency rather than changes in intensity for emphasis.

Pathophysiology of the Larynx

Various pathologic changes in the vocal cords cause the prominence of nonharmonic noise components in the voice. In contrast to the healthy musical voice, overtones that are not partial or whole-number multiples of the fundamental tone produce a noisy voice or hoarseness. Structural changes in the vocal cords cause greater aperiodicity and asynchrony of the vibration of the vocal cords. Aperiodicity and asynchrony disrupt the harmonic relationships of the voice by limiting the possibility of the occurrence of overtones that are partial and whole-number multiples of the fundamental tone. Characteristically, the abnormal voice is monotonous. A monotone may occur because of loss of flexibility in the frequency range of the larynx due to a disease process or it may be acquired as a habit, particularly in speakers who tend to use increases in intensity for emphasis rather than changes in frequency. Structural changes in the vocal cords often interfere with their approximation and result in air wastage, which gives the voice a breathy quality.

Structural Changes in the True Vocal Cords Secondary to Misuse and Abuse of the Voice

Abuse and misuse of the voice can cause structural changes in the true vocal cords.[61] Using the voice too loudly and too long produces acute and chronic changes in the true vocal cords. Prolonged use of intensity rather than frequency for emphasis, the employment of a monotone, the affectation of a frequency that is too low, and a very abrupt onset of high intensities (sharp glottal attack) produce structural changes in the true vocal cords.

POLYPS OF THE VOCAL CORDS. Polyps of the true vocal cords develop in response to using the voice too loudly and too long, as in the individual who must speak over a great deal of background noise in a factory or who demonstrates wares in a department store or barks at a circus or carnival. Chronic subepithelial edema develops in the lamina propia of the true vocal cords. Similar pathologic changes follow chronic allergic reactions and the chronic inhalation of irritants such as tobacco smoke and industrial fumes. Such polypoid swellings of the free edge of the true vocal cord interfere with the approximation of the true vocal cords and with the maintenance of periodicity and synchrony of the vibration of the vocal cords. They produce hoarseness and give a breathy quality to the voice. To restore the voice, polyps are removed with the use of an operation microscope at direct laryngoscopy with the patient under general anesthesia.

VOCAL NODULES. Vocal nodules are caused by using a fundamental frequency that is unnaturally low and using the voice too loudly and too long. Vocal nodules occur in children as well as adults and are likely to occur in robust, athletic boys 8 to 12 years of age who yell frequently. Men affect an unnaturally low pitch to give an air of authority; women do it to give an impression of sexiness; and young boys probably do it to iden-

tify with older males in the family or community. Vocal nodules are condensations of hyaline connective tissue in the lamina propria at the junction of the anterior one third and the posterior two thirds of the true vocal cord. These nodules produce hoarseness and give the voice a breathy quality. In adults, these lesions are removed at direct laryngoscopy to restore the voice. However, it is necessary to begin voice therapy prior to surgical therapy, because if the underlying misuse of the voice is not corrected, the nodules recur. In children, surgical removal is not usually necessary because the vocal nodules regress with voice therapy, which consists of voice rest, reduction in intensity and duration of voice production, and elevation of the pitch.

CONTACT ULCERS. Contact ulcers of the larynx are thought to follow misuse and abuse of the voice, particularly in the form of a sharp glottal attack, and reflux of gastric contents. They occur unilaterally or bilaterally over the vocal process of the arytenoid. The presence of these lesions causes mild pain on phonation and swallowing and varying degrees of hoarseness. The ulcers have a shaggy or granular base. Gastroesophageal reflux should be identified and managed if found on barium esophagography. Biopsy of these ulcers to exclude the possibility of carcinoma is done at direct laryngoscopy. Voice therapy to correct the underlying misuse of the voice is important. However, prolonged voice rest is required for contact ulcers to heal.

Trauma

Trauma has replaced infectious diseases such as diphtheria, streptococcal croup, syphilis, tuberculosis, rhinoscleroma, and typhoid fever as the most common cause of laryngeal stenosis. Automobile accidents in which the patient is thrown forward and the larynx is crushed between the cervical vertebrae and the object against which it decelerates are the single most important cause of laryngeal stenosis. Children may fracture the larynx by falling against the handlebars of a bicycle or riding a horse or bicycle under a taut line. Another cause of laryngeal stenosis is the high tracheotomy in which perichondritis of the cricoid cartilage follows pressure of the tube on the cartilage. Prolonged endotracheal intubation frequently causes subglottic stenosis, as do infectious processes.

Fractures of the thyroid cartilage may cause supraglottic, glottic, or transglottic stenosis. Individuals with long slender necks are more likely to sustain supraglottic injuries in which the hyoid bone is also fractured. The suprahyoid muscles are disrupted, and the thyrohyoid membrane is ruptured. Fracture of the cricoid cartilage causes subglottic stenosis. Fractures of the cricoid cartilage are more likely to occur in males with short, thick necks and are relatively rare in females. Often a blow to the neck spares the larynx but transects the trachea.

Patients with crush injuries of the larynx complain of pain on swallowing. Hoarseness may progress to aphonia. Hemoptysis is usually present. Progressive dyspnea due to upper respiratory obstruction is to be anticipated. Subcutaneous emphysema is usually present in fractures of the larynx or trachea. The laryngeal cartilages cannot be distinctly palpated, nor can the trachea, owing to soft tissue swelling. Lateral neck radiographs should be performed to exclude or demonstrate associated fractures or dislocations of the cervical vertebrae. On direct laryngoscopy, the laryngeal lumen appears disrupted or obliterated, and there may be exposed cartilage and lacerated mucous membrane. Vocal cord paralysis may be noted. A barium swallow is required to exclude a perforation of the hypopharynx or cervical esophagus if the patient's condition permits. CT scanning of the neck indicates the type and degree of injury.

In the initial management of the patient with a laryngeal fracture, a tracheotomy is performed and followed by direct laryngoscopy and tracheoscopy. Often, patients with multiple injuries are treated with a tracheotomy because of the upper airway obstruction, and the reason for the need for the tracheotomy is forgotten during the management of the thoracic and abdominal or perhaps intracranial injuries. The laryngeal trauma is rediscovered 10 or so days later when it appears that it would be appropriate to remove the tracheostomy tube. Evaluation of the larynx should be performed early for one to be certain that there has not been a fracture of the laryngeal cartilages that requires early repair.

The repair of the fracture is done through a transverse incision in the neck. To gain access to the interior of the larynx, a laryngofissure is performed by dividing the thyroid cartilage at its isthmus, or the fracture in the thyroid and cricoid cartilage is utilized. Mucous membrane lacerations are repaired, and the cartilages are returned to their normal alignment.[57] Internal splinting is maintained with a solid-core mold for as long as 6 weeks. Failure to reduce a dislocated or fractured cartilage causes laryngeal stenosis. Late repair of laryngeal stenosis can sometimes be accomplished by an arytenoidectomy. At other times a supraglottic partial laryngectomy is required to restore the airway and the functional integrity of the laryngeal sphincter.[42] A keel is often employed to repair the angle of the anterior commissure. Subglottic stenosis can be relieved by laser therapy or repaired by excision of the stenotic area and internal splinting for a period of 6 weeks or more.

In addition to external trauma, tracheal stenosis occurs secondary to pressure necrosis of the tracheal walls caused by the inflated cuff in prolonged endotracheal intubation. Tracheal stenosis also occurs secondary to tracheotomy, particularly when the wound becomes infected and there is cicatricial healing of large eroded tracheostomas. Tracheal stenosis may be managed by dilations, excision of the stenotic area with internal splinting for 6 weeks or more, or excision of the stenotic area with end-to-end anastomosis of the trachea. As much as 50 per cent of the length of the trachea can be resected and end-to-end anastomosis performed.[18]

Vocal Cord Paralysis

Vocal cord paralysis follows traumatic, infectious, and neoplastic involvement of the vagus and recurrent laryngeal nerves and degenerative neurologic disorders. Unilateral vocal cord paralysis produces hoarseness and aspiration. Bilateral vocal cord paralysis causes upper airway obstruction with little adverse effect on the voice. In unilateral vocal paralysis injection of Teflon paste at direct laryngoscopy lateral to the vocalis muscle causes medialization and augmentation of the paralyzed vocal cord so that the unaffected vocal cord can approximate with it. Teflon injection produces improvement of the voice and elimination of aspiration.[33] Similar results have been obtained with phonosurgical techniques in which the paralyzed vocal cord is moved toward the midline with the implantation of autografts lateral to the vocal cord.[31]

The upper airway obstruction caused by bilateral vocal cord paralysis usually requires a tracheostomy initially. Subsequent improvement in the airway can be obtained with an arytenoidectomy or a nerve-muscle transplant for reinnervation of the muscles that control the movement of the arytenoid cartilage.[66]

Foreign Bodies of the Larynx, Tracheobronchial Tree, and Esophagus

Foreign bodies are retained in the larynx because they are sharp and stick into the mucous membrane or are irregular and soft and are caught between the two vocal cords in laryngospasm. A frequently fatal laryngeal foreign body is a bolus of meat. The resulting laryngospasm completely occludes the larynx and makes a choking person mute. This "café coronary" may be distinguished from a myocardial infarct by the respiratory effort without exchange and the marked suprasternal, intercostal, and subxiphoid retraction. Death occurs rapidly unless an alternate airway is established or the foreign body is dislodged. As long as adequate respiratory exchange occurs, the choking individual should be allowed to employ protective re-

flexes to manage the problem. Maneuvers such as striking the choking individual on the back or turning a choking child upside down may make it more difficult for the choking individual to handle the problem successfully and may convert the situation into one that is less easily managed. If the choking individual is mute and makes no respiratory exchange, the Heimlich (abdominal thrust) maneuver should be attempted.[21] In this maneuver, the operator places his arms around the choking individual from behind, grasps the fist of one hand in the other hand, and brings both hands up in the subxiphoid area briskly to apply pressure to the diaphragm. The pressure increases the intrathoracic pressure and may expel the foreign body. Should this maneuver fail, an alternate airway must be established by the prompt performance of a tracheotomy. Even nonobstructing foreign bodies of the larynx induce a degree of laryngospasm that makes their removal difficult without general anesthesia, and a tracheotomy is often the first step in their removal, particularly subglottic foreign bodies such as sand or grass burrs. The site of the foreign body is exposed with a laryngoscope, and the foreign body is grasped, disengaged, and removed with alligator or other appropriate forceps.

Smooth objects such as nuts, kernels of corn, watermelon seeds, beans, peas, and plastic toys pass through the larynx into the tracheobronchial tree. At the onset, there is severe spasmodic coughing that continues for approximately 30 minutes. During this time, the foreign body migrates from one portion of the tracheobronchial tree to another. It more frequently comes to rest in the right bronchus because the right bronchus is larger than the left and makes less of an angle with the long axis of the trachea, and the carina is to the left of the midline of the tracheal lumen. As it finally comes to rest, the coughing subsides, and a latent period begins during which the patient is free of symptoms. The mistaken inference is often made by the family and the physician in attendance that the foreign body has been expelled. However, careful auscultation of the chest may demonstrate an expiratory wheeze and the signs of obstructive emphysema. The most common mechanism of the bronchial obstruction due to a foreign body is a one-way valve through which air may enter the bronchus distal to the foreign body during inspiration but which affords limited egress on expiration. This type of obstruction produces emphysema distal to the foreign body. The obstructive emphysema may become apparent radiographically only on expiration or fluoroscopy. The mediastinum shifts away from the obstructed lung, and the obstructed portion of the lung becomes radiolucent, compared with the normal lung. This type of partial obstruction of the bronchus is likely to occur with the aspiration of nuts. In the evaluation of a patient with a suspected nonradiopaque foreign body of the bronchus, comparison of inspiratory and expiratory chest films and fluoroscopy of the chest may demonstrate obstructive emphysema that would not be apparent on inspiration radiographs.

A foreign body that completely obstructs the bronchus causes the rapid development of a more serious pathophysiologic state. Complete atelectasis of the obstructed lung occurs as a result of absorption of the remaining air in the lung. The mediastinum shifts toward the atelectatic lung, and the remaining lung undergoes compensatory emphysema (Fig. 16). The atelectatic lung is useless as far as ventilatory exchange is concerned, and the efficiency of the emphysematous lung is greatly reduced. Rapid cardiorespiratory failure occurs unless the foreign body is removed. This type of complete bronchial obstruction is likely to occur with smooth hygroscopic foreign bodies, such as beans, that swell in the bronchus.

Vegetable foreign bodies are very poorly tolerated. Metallic and plastic foreign bodies that cause partial obstruction of the bronchus may be tolerated for long periods. Nuts, particularly peanuts, produce a very severe tracheobronchitis. After a latent period of 24 hours, the patient develops a cough productive of

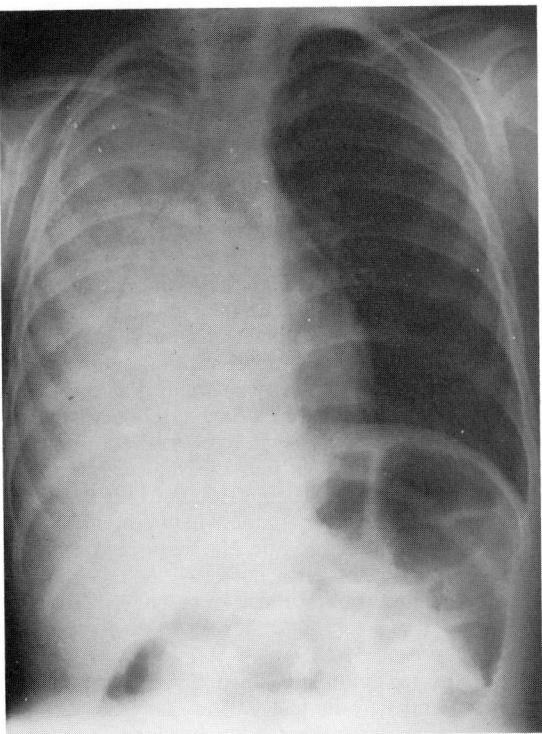

Figure 16. Posteroanterior radiography of the chest of a child with a pinto bean in the right bronchus. There is atelectasis of the right lung and compensatory emphysema of the left lung.

purulent sputum, and a febrile course begins. A long-indwelling foreign body of the bronchus may produce bronchiectasis, recurrent pneumonitis, lung abscess, and empyema. Tracheobronchial foreign bodies are removed with general anesthesia through an open bronchoscope with forceps designed specifically for each type of foreign body.

Foreign bodies of the esophagus are likely to lodge just below the cricopharyngeus muscle. Ninety-five per cent of esophageal foreign bodies are found in this location. Other locations are the gastroesophageal junction and the indentations of the esophagus caused by the left bronchus and the arch of the aorta. The constrictors of the pharynx are very strong and can propel almost any irregular object through the cricopharyngeus muscle. When the foreign body has passed the cricopharyngeus, the muscular activity is very weak, and progress occurs mainly by gravity. Therefore, irregular objects are brought to a very abrupt stop just below the cricopharyngeus muscle.

The symptoms of a foreign body of the esophagus are dysphagia and pain in the suprasternal area on swallowing. Bulky foreign bodies in the cervical esophagus may produce upper airway obstruction by extrinsic pressure through the membranous posterior wall of the trachea. Foreign bodies can be identified on a lateral neck film if they are radiopaque. If they are radiolucent, evidence of a foreign body may still be obtained, because the foreign body tends to hold the esophageal walls apart and air may be observed in the cervical esophagus. If the foreign body cannot be located on a lateral neck radiograph, posteroanterior and lateral chest films are obtained. If the foreign body cannot be located in this manner, an esophagogram may demonstrate it. A small pledget of cotton saturated with a solution of barium sulfate may hang on a sharp foreign body. A foreign body of the esophagus is removed under general anesthesia through an open esophagoscope. The foreign body is grasped, disengaged, and removed as a trailing foreign body or through the esophagoscope with a foreign body forceps appropriate to the object. The longer a foreign body remains in the esophagus, the greater the risk of perforation of the esophagus.

Perforation of the esophagus causes air and soft tissue swelling in the paraesophageal tissue that may be demonstrated on physical examination and radiographically.

Infectious Diseases

CROUP. There are two forms of croup, epiglottitis and laryngotracheobronchitis. Croup occurs primarily in children over 1 year and under 5 years of age. It may be viral or bacterial. Parainfluenza Type I is the most frequently isolated agent in viral croup. *Haemophilus influenzae* is the most frequently isolated agent in bacterial croup, but *Staphylococcus* and *Streptococcus* may also cause croup.

H. influenzae type B is the predominant microorganism in epiglottitis and frequently causes a bacteremia. Both epiglottitis and laryngotracheobronchitis may produce the rapid onset of upper respiratory obstruction with inspiratory stridor and suprasternal, supraclavicular, intercostal, and subxiphoid retractions. The voice may be hoarse, and the cough has a brassy quality with subglottic edema. The supraglottic swelling may be demonstrated on a lateral neck radiograph (Fig. 17).[46] In laryngotracheobronchitis, the major problem is subglottic edema.

Epiglottitis or supraglottic laryngitis is more likely to cause abrupt and complete airway obstruction. When the diagnosis of epiglottitis is made, nasotracheal intubation is performed and maintained for 48 hours until the supraglottic swelling subsides.[65] In laryngotracheobronchitis, the airway obstruction results in part from edema, but there are also tenacious mucoid secretions. Humidification of the inspired atmosphere liquifies the material, and the patient may cough it out to reduce the degree of airway obstruction. Antibiotic therapy is initiated at the onset of both diseases; amoxicillin is the drug of choice (pending blood culture and sensitivities) because the infection is frequently caused by *H. influenzae*. There is usually bacteremia when it is the causative microorganism. Corticosteroid therapy is controversial, but it may be initiated in an attempt to reduce the inflammatory swelling. If the degree of airway obstruction becomes severe in laryngotracheobronchitis, a tracheotomy is performed in preference to prolonged endotracheal intubation,

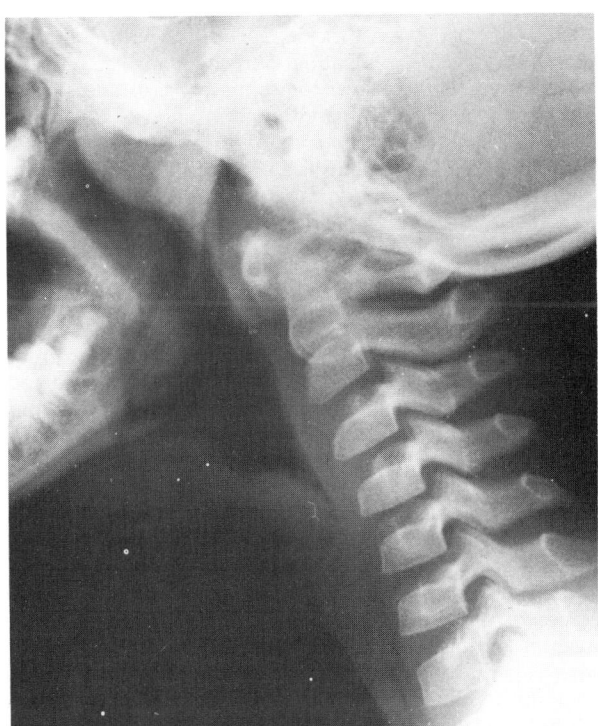

Figure 17. Lateral radiograph of the neck in a child with supraglottic laryngitis. Note the swelling of the epiglottis, aryepiglottic folds, and arytenoids.

because the rate of complications, such as laryngeal and subglottic stenosis, is quite high with prolonged endotracheal intubation in laryngotracheobronchitis. The decision regarding a tracheotomy depends on the evaluation of the amount of ventilatory exchange that is taking place, the degree of fatigue of the patient, and the respiratory and pulse rates. Development of cyanosis is a late sign, and the decision to perform a tracheotomy should be made prior to the advent of this ominous sign. Blood gas determinations are helpful, but the clinical situation may change very rapidly. If it appears that the ventilatory exchange is inadequate, the necessary ventilatory effort cannot be maintained, or there is a progressive increase in the pulse rate above 140 per minute, a tracheotomy is performed. The airway emergency is converted to an elective tracheotomy by insertion of an endotracheal tube or a bronchoscope. General anesthesia is induced, and the tracheotomy is performed in a relaxed patient under unhurried and ideal circumstances. This approach reduces the incidence of complications such as pneumothorax.

TRACHEOTOMY. The indications for tracheotomy form three broad categories: upper respiratory obstruction, inability to handle upper respiratory secretions, and inability to handle lower respiratory secretions. Among those causes of upper respiratory obstruction that frequently require tracheotomy are congenital malformations of the upper respiratory tract, laryngotracheobronchitis, diphtheria, foreign bodies, bilateral vocal cord paralyses, neoplasms of the larynx, postintubation edema, allergic reactions, and maxillofacial and laryngeal trauma. The importance of a tracheotomy in patients who are having difficulty managing upper respiratory secretions became well recognized during the polio epidemics. Neurologic problems other than infections, such as intracranial trauma and neoplasms, also lead to difficulty in managing upper respiratory secretions. Patients with ineffective respiratory effort on a neurologic or mechanical basis, chronic obstructive pulmonary disease, and parenchymal infections may have difficulty managing lower respiratory secretions. Many of these problems can be managed with endotracheal intubation on a short-term basis.

A tracheotomy has several advantages and disadvantages. It relieves upper respiratory obstruction and allows more effective access to the lower respiratory tract for suctioning the tracheobronchial tree. It decreases the dead space and reduces the work required for effective ventilation. A tracheotomy can readily be used as a route for the delivery of respiratory assistance. It eliminates the normal warming and humidification of the inspired air by bypassing the upper respiratory tract. A very serious disadvantage of the tracheotomy is the loss of an effective cough. It opens the lower respiratory tract to environmental pathogens and increases the vulnerability to *Pseudomonas* infections.

JUVENILE PAPILLOMAS OF THE LARYNX. Papillomas of the larynx are thought to be of viral etiology. Although these lesions may occur as early as 1 year of age, they more commonly make their appearance in the second or third year of life. Papillomas may recur promptly after excision. Exuberant growth from multiple sites in the larynx makes maintenance of an adequate airway difficult. Many children with laryngeal papillomas require a tracheotomy. The papillomas are periodically vaporized with a laser or removed gingerly at direct laryngoscopy under general anesthesia to maintain the voice and the airway.[64] Involution of the papillomas usually occurs at puberty.

Congenital Malformations

Congenital malformations of the larynx may produce varying degrees of airway obstruction. Among the well-recognized causes of laryngeal obstruction encountered in the immediate neonatal period are bilateral vocal cord paralyses and subluxation of the arytenoids secondary to traumatic delivery, laryngomalacia or the exaggerated infantile larynx, stenosis and atresia of the larynx, cysts, and subglottic hemangioma. Tracheal obstruction may be due to intrinsic tracheal lesions such as tracheomalacia, absence of tracheal rings, and tracheal stenosis or

to extrinsic tracheal compression from neoplasms of the thyroid, thymus, esophagus, and mediastinum and vascular rings. Tetany of the newborn with laryngospasm is usually recognized by other characteristics of this condition. Newborns with tracheoesophageal fistulas have respiratory distress due to aspiration, but usually no true airway obstruction.

In the delivery room, exposure of the vocal cords with a laryngoscope relieves the obstruction of an exaggerated infantile larynx, in which the flexible epiglottis and arytenoids prolapse into the glottis with inspiration. Inserting a laryngoscope does not relieve obstruction from bilateral vocal cord paralyses, stenosis, or subglottic hemangiomas. Insertion of a 3.5-mm. bronchoscope improves ventilation in these laryngeal lesions but does not relieve tracheal obstruction until the bronchoscope is passed beyond it. These maneuvers are of the utmost risk to a newborn and should not be undertaken unless the infant's exchange is inadequate for survival. In general, if the exchange is adequate, the infant should be managed expectantly in the neonatal period. Most forms of congenital stridor improve with time. Inappropriate instrumentation may convert a tolerable degree of airway obstruction into one requiring prolonged endotracheal intubation or a tracheotomy. A tracheotomy in a newborn is hazardous and difficult to manage.

Laryngoceles

Laryngoceles are epithelium-lined diverticula of the laryngeal ventricle and may be located internal or external to the laryngeal skeleton. An internal laryngocele may displace and enlarge the false vocal cord and may cause hoarseness and airway obstruction. External laryngoceles pass through the thyrohyoid membrane and present as a mass in the neck over the thyrohyoid membrane. The mass rises with the larynx on swallowing. Internal and external laryngoceles may coexist. Laryngoceles are more common in glassblowers, wind instrument musicians, and others who develop high intraluminal pressures. Initially, laryngoceles are filled with air and expand and collapse with changes in the intraluminal pressure. They are expanded during the Valsalva maneuver. They appear as smooth, ovoid, air-filled masses on CT scans of the neck. Laryngoceles may fill with mucoid fluid and become infected, under which circumstance the term *laryngopyocele* is appropriate. External laryngoceles are excised through a transverse cervical incision. The sac is dissected from surrounding tissue to its point of penetration of the thyrohyoid membrane. The sac is transected, and the mucous membrane of the ventricle is repaired. Internal laryngoceles are managed by the same approach but require extension of the dissection into the larynx through a thyrotomy.

Neoplasms

Benign neoplasms, including papillomas, fibromas, myxomas, chondromas, neurofibromas, hemangiomas, and so forth, may involve any part of the larynx, including the true vocal cords. Such lesions can ordinarily be removed at direct laryngoscopy with restoration of the voice, the airway, and the functional integrity of the laryngeal sphincter.

MALIGNANT NEOPLASMS OF THE LARYNX. The majority of malignant neoplasms of the larynx are squamous cell carcinomas. Squamous cell carcinomas of the larynx represent approximately 2 per cent of all cancer deaths. It is a disease mainly of males, with a sex ratio of 8 : 1. The peak incidence of carcinoma of the larynx is in the fifth and sixth decades of life. Laryngeal carcinoma occurs more commonly in individuals with a large ethanol intake. It rarely develops in an individual who does not smoke. Dysplasia follows the inhalation of irritants such as tobacco smoke that contain known potent carcinogens including 3,4-benzpyrene and other polycyclic aromatic hydrocarbons. It is a premalignant condition from which carcinoma may develop after a period of months or years.

Carcinoma may arise from the mucous membrane of any part

of the larynx; however, there is a predilection for the true vocal cords, particularly the anterior portions of the true vocal cords. The epiglottis, pyriform sinus, and postcricoid area also are common sites of origin of carcinoma. For purposes of clinical staging and end result reporting, carcinomas of the larynx can be divided into supraglottic, glottic, subglottic, and hypopharyngeal lesions.[3] Supraglottic lesions involve the epiglottis, aryepiglottic fold, and false vocal cords. Glottic lesions are limited to the area of the true vocal cords. Subglottic lesions include the glottic area as well as the subglottic area. Hypopharyngeal lesions may be divided into lesions of the pyriform sinus, postcricoid area, and posterior pharyngeal wall.

The natural history of the carcinoma varies considerably from one location to another. The early symptom of carcinoma of the true vocal cords is hoarseness. In any patient with hoarseness lasting 2 weeks, indirect laryngoscopy should be done. Any discrete lesions of the mucous membrane of the larynx should be biopsied. Carcinomas of the true vocal cord limited to the middle third of the true vocal cord and not impairing the mobility of the cord are treated with radiation therapy or cordectomy with an overall 5-year survival rate of 85 to 95 per cent. Because cordectomy causes permanent hoarseness and irradiation usually returns the voice to normal, radiation therapy is the treatment of choice. Cordectomy is reserved for the 5 to 15 per cent who have persistent carcinoma following radiation therapy. The likelihood of metastasis in early carcinoma of the true vocal cord is very slight.

The mobility of the vocal cord becomes impaired in more advanced carcinomas as a result of invasion of the intrinsic musculature and cartilage. With invasion of the intrinsic musculature, the rate of metastasis increases. With invasion of the thyroid cartilage, the rate of 5-year survival with radiation therapy decreases precipitously. Operation becomes the treatment of choice for lesions that involve the anterior commissure where cartilage is very early invaded and for larger glottic lesions in which the mobility of the true vocal cord is impaired. Often a vertical hemilaryngectomy can be performed to preserve the phonatory and sphincteric functions of the larynx.[40] In more advanced cases, total laryngectomy is required, and the laryngectomy may be combined with a radical neck dissection if palpable metastases are present.[60] In view of the fact that only 15 to 20 per cent of patients with glottic carcinomas have nonpalpable metastasis present at the time of initial treatment, a radical neck dissection is not performed electively.

Supraglottic carcinomas tend to be asymptomatic until they reach considerable size. They may produce hoarseness by secondary involvement of the vocal cords, or they may produce pain on swallowing as the first symptom. Often the pain radiates to the ears. Not infrequently, a patient with a supraglottic carcinoma presents with the chief complaint of a swelling in the neck that represents a metastasis. The chance of nonpalpable metastasis being present is 35 per cent. Early supraglottic carcinoma is successfully treated with radiation therapy, but in advanced lesions better survival rates are obtained with a combination of radiation therapy and surgical therapy.[43] Better local and regional control is obtained with postoperative radiation therapy than with preoperative radiation therapy.[32] The 2-year disease-free survival approximates 70 per cent. In many patients with supraglottic carcinomas, the neoplasm can be completely removed by supraglottic partial laryngectomy with preservation of the phonatory and sphincteric function of the larynx.[41] If the glottis is involved, a total laryngectomy is usually required. These procedures are often combined with a radical neck dissection if there are palpable metastases.

Subglottic lesions represent more advanced glottic carcinomas in which the neoplasm has secondarily invaded the subglottic area as well as the supraglottic area. Metastasis to the same side is present in 50 per cent of patients. Subglottic extension of the carcinoma requires a total laryngectomy and radical neck dissection with thyroid lobectomy on the same side. The overall 5-year survival rate for patients with glottic or subglottic carcinomas treated with total laryngectomy for all stages approximates 65 per cent.

Pyriform sinus carcinomas tend to remain asymptomatic for long periods of time. Often the patient presents with dysphagia and pain on swallowing that may radiate to the ear on the same side. Often the presenting complaint is a mass in the neck that represents a metastasis. A combination of preoperative or postoperative radiation therapy and operation yields better survival rates than operation alone. The results of preoperative and postoperative radiation therapy are equivalent in this site.[32] Depending on the location of the lesion in the pyriform sinus, a partial laryngectomy can sometimes be accomplished with preservation of the phonatory and sphincteric functions of the larynx. More often, a total laryngectomy is required. More extensive lesions require pharyngolaryngectomy with replacement of the pharynx with a free jejunal graft with microvascular anastomosis.[62] Either of these procedures is combined with a radical neck dissection if there are palpable metastases. The 5-year survival rate for all stages is 30 per cent.

Postcricoid carcinoma has a female predominance of 10 to 1. Women with the Plummer-Vinson syndrome have a predilection for the development of postcricoid carcinoma. The presenting complaint is usually pain on swallowing and dysphagia. Metastasis to both sides of the neck is common. A combination of preoperative or postoperative radiation and surgical therapy is usually employed, and the operation required is pharyngectomy, total laryngectomy, and, if there are palpable metastases, radical neck dissection on one side followed by radical neck dissection on the other side in approximately 6 weeks. The 5-year survival rate for all stages is 25 per cent.

A total laryngectomy requires the formation of a permanent tracheostomy in which the trachea is transected and anastomosed to the skin of the lower part of the neck. Rehabilitation of the postlaryngectomy patient requires the development of alaryngeal or esophageal speech. In this technique, the patient draws air into the esophagus during inspiration and gradually eructs the air through the cricopharyngeus muscle. The opening of the esophagus vibrates and serves as the sounding source. The sound is articulated by the pharynx, palate, tongue, teeth, and lips into speech. For those individuals who, because of age or other physical or emotional reasons, cannot develop alaryngeal speech, an electrolarynx can serve as the sounding source for modification by the articulators. The oscillator of the electrolarynx is placed in the submandibular area, and the sound is articulated into speech. Most individuals who require a laryngectomy may return to their former occupation.[45] With proper guidance in their rehabilitation, laryngectomees may resume all activities except swimming.

SELECTED REFERENCES

Alberti, P. W., and Ruben, R. J.: Otologic Medicine and Surgery. New York, Churchill Livingstone, 1988.
A complete encyclopedia of otology.

Ballenger, J. J.: Disease of the Nose, Throat, Ear, Head and Neck, 13th ed. Philadelphia, Lea & Febiger, 1985.
Part 6 provides a comprehensive discussion of peroral endoscopy.

Cummings, C. W., et al. (Eds.): Otolaryngology—Head and Neck Surgery. St. Louis, C. V. Mosby Company, 1986.
Excellent presentation of major concerns in head and neck oncology.

Goldman, J. L.: The Principles and Practice of Rhinology. New York, John Wiley and Sons, 1987.
A thorough discussion of many important topics in rhinology.

Paparella, M. M., Shumrick, D. A., Gluckman, J., and Meyerhoff, W. L.: Otolaryngology, 3rd ed. Philadelphia, W. B. Saunders Company, 1991.
A comprehensive compendium of otology, maxillofacial surgery, and head and neck surgery by many authorities.

Schuknecht, H. F.: Pathology of the Ear. Cambridge, Harvard University Press, 1974.
A comprehensive compendium of otopathology that incorporates much of the author's vast knowledge of otology.

Shambaugh, G. E., Jr., and Glasscock, M. E.: Surgery of the Ear, 3rd ed. Philadelphia, W. B. Saunders Company, 1980.
This textbook is a comprehensive source of information in operative otology. It is authoritative and well written.

Snow, J. B.: Introduction to Otorhinolaryngology. Chicago, Year Book Medical Publishers, 1979.
This textbook is concise, with an emphasis on basic concepts.

REFERENCES

1. Abramson, M., and Gross, J.: Further studies on a collagenase in middle ear cholesteatoma. Ann. Otol. Rhinol. Laryngol., *80:*177, 1971.
2. Adour, K. K., Byl, F. M., Hilsenger, R. L., Jr., Kahn, Z. M., and Sheldon, M. I.: The true nature of Bell's palsy. Analysis of 1,000 consecutive patients. Laryngoscope, *88:*787, 1978.
3. American Joint Committee for Cancer Staging and End-Results Reporting. Manual for Staging Cancer 1989. Chicago, American Joint Committee, 1989.
4. Anson, B. J., and Donaldson, J. A.: The Surgical Anatomy of the Temporal Bone and Ear. Philadelphia, W. B. Saunders Company, 1967.
5. Batsakis, J. G.: Tumors of the Head and Neck: Clinical and Pathologic Considerations. Baltimore, Williams & Wilkins, 1979.
6. Brackman, D. E.: Electric response audiometry in a clinical practice. Laryngoscope, *87*(Suppl.5):1, 1977.
7. Cawthorne, T., Dix. W. R., Hallpike, C. S., and Hood, J. D.: The investigation of vestibular function. Br. Med. Bull., *12:*131, 1956.
8. Chandler, J. R., and Serrins, A. J.: Transantral ligation of the internal maxillary artery for epistaxis. Laryngoscope, *75:*1151, 1965.
9. Clark, G. M., Shepherd, R. K., Franz, B. K., et al.: The histopathology of the human temporal bone and auditory central nervous system following cochlear implantation in a patient: Correlation with psychophysics and speech perception results. Acta Otolaryngol., Suppl. 448, 1988.
10. Cody, D. T. R., Simonton, K. M., and Hallberg, O. E.: Automatic repetitive decompression of the saccule in endolymphatic hydrops (Tack operation). Laryngoscope, *77:*1480, 1967.
11. Conley, J. J., and Novack, A. J.: The surgical treatment of malignant tumors of the ear and temporal bone. Arch. Otolaryngol., *71:*635, 1960.
12. Eliachar, I., Golz, A., Joachims, H. Z., and Goldsher, M.: Continuous portable vacuum drainage of auricular hematomas. Am. J. Otolaryngol., *4:*141, 1983.
13. Fairbanks, D. N. F.: Closure of large nasal septum perforations. Arch. Otolaryngol., *91:*403, 1970.
13a. Fick, I. A. van N.: Decompression of the labyrinth. Arch. Otolaryngol., *79:*447, 1964.
14. Gacek, R. R.: Singular neurectomy update. Ann. Otol. Rhinol. Laryngol., *91:*469, 1982.
15. Gantz, B. J., Amur, A., and Fisch, U.: Intraoperative evoked electromyography in Bell's palsy. Am. J. Otolaryngol., *3:*273, 1982.
16. Geroulis, A. T., and Powell, W. J.: Internal maxillary artery ligation for posterior epistaxis. Surg. Forum, *26:*531, 1975.
17. Goodhill, V., Harris, I., Brockman, S. J., and Hantz, D.: Sudden deafness and labyrinthine window ruptures. Ann. Otol. Rhinol. Laryngol., *82:*2, 1973.
18. Grillo, H. C.: Obstructive lesions of the trachea. Ann. Otol. Rhinol. Laryngol., *82:*770, 1973.
19. Grote, J. J.: Reconstruction of the middle ear with hydroxylapatite implants: Long-term results. Ann. Otol. Rhinol. Laryngol., *99*(Suppl. 144):12, 1990.
20. Healy, G. B., and Teele, D. W.: The microbiology of chronic middle ear effusions in children. Laryngoscope, *87:*1472, 1977.
21. Heimlich, H. J.: A life-saving maneuver to prevent food-choking. J.A.M.A., *234:*398, 1975.
22. Henle, W.: Elevated antibody titers to Epstein-Barr virus in nasopharyngeal carcinoma, other head and neck neoplasms and control groups. J. Natl. Cancer Inst., *44:*225, 1970.
23. Hough, J. V. D.: Tympanoplasty with the interior fascial graft technique and ossicular reconstruction. Laryngoscope, *80:*1385, 1970.
24. House, W. F.: Subarachnoid shunt for drainage of hydrops. Arch. Otolaryngol., *79:*328, 1964.
25. House, W. F.: Surgical exposure of internal auditory canal and its contents through middle cranial fossa. Laryngoscope, *71:*1363, 1961.
26. House, W. F.: Transtemporal bone microsurgical removal of acoustic neuromas. Arch. Otolaryngol., *80:*601, 1964.
27. House, W. F.: Cochlear implants. Ann. Otol. Rhinol. Laryngol., *27*(Suppl.):1, 1976.
28. Jannetta, P. T., Moller, M. D., and Moller, A.: Disabling positional vertigo. N. Engl. J. Med., *310:*1700, 1984.
29. Kamerer, D. B., Lunsford, L. D., and Moller, M.: Gamma knife: An alternative treatment for acoustic neurinomas. Ann. Otol. Rhinol. Laryngol., *97:*631, 1988.
30. Kennedy, D. W.: Functional endoscopic sinus surgery. Arch. Otolaryngol., *111:*643, 1985.
31. Koufman, J. A.: Laryngoplasty for vocal cord medialization: An alternative to Teflon. Laryngoscope, *96:*726, 1986.
32. Kramer, S., Gelber, R. D., Snow, J. B., Marcial, V. A., Lowry, L. D., Davis, L. W., and Chandler, R.: Combined radiation therapy and surgery in the management of advanced head and neck cancer: Final report of study 73-03 of the Radiation Therapy Oncology Group. Head Neck Surg., *10:*19, 1987.
33. Lewy, R. B.: Experience with vocal cord injection. Ann. Otol. Rhinol. Laryngol., *85:*440, 1976.
34. Martin, H.: Surgery of Head and Neck Tumors. New York, Harper & Row, 1957.
35. McCabe, B. F.: Central aspects of drugs for motion sickness and vertigo. Adv. Otorhinolaryngol., *20:*458, 1973.
36. Michelson, R. P., Merzenich, M. M., Schindler, R. A., and Schindler, D. N.: Present status and future development of the cochlear prosthesis. Ann. Otol. Rhinol. Laryngol., *84:*494, 1975.
37. Muir, C. S., and Shanmugaratnam, L.: Cancer of the Nasopharynx. Flushing, N.Y., Medical Examination Publishing Co., 1967.
38. Nadol, J. B.: Histopathology of Pseudomonas osteomyelitis of the temporal bone starting as malignant external otitis. Am. J. Otolaryngol., *1:*359, 1980.
39. Neal, L. C., Snow, J. B., and Seda, H. J.: An analysis of therapy for carcinoma of the tonsil. Trans. Am. Acad. Ophthalmol. Otolaryngol., *77:*97, 1973.
40. Ogura, J. H., and Biller, H. F.: Glottic reconstruction following extended frontolateral hemilaryngectomy. Laryngoscope, *75:*2181, 1965.
41. Ogura, J. H., and Dedo, H. H.: Glottic reconstruction following subtotal glottic-supraglottic laryngectomy. Laryngoscope, *75:*865, 1965.
42. Ogura, J. H., and Powers, W. E.: Functional restitution of traumatic stenosis of the larynx and pharynx. Laryngoscope, *74:*1081, 1964.
43. Ogura, J. H., Sessions, D. G., and Spector, G. J.: Conservation surgery for epidermoid carcinoma of the supraglottic larynx. Laryngoscope, *85:*1808, 1975.
44. Owens, E., and Telleen, C. C.: Speech perception with hearing aids and cochlear implants. Arch. Otolaryngol., *107:*160, 1981.
45. Ranney, J. L.: Rehabilitation through employment. Laryngoscope, *85:*674, 1975.
46. Rapkin, R. H.: The diagnosis of epiglottitis: Simplicity and reliability of radiographs of the neck in the differential diagnosis of the croup syndrome. J. Pediatr., *80:*96, 1972.
47. Rauch, S., and Rauch, I.: Physio-chemical properties of the inner ear especially ionic transport. *In* Keidel, W. D., and Neff, W. D. (Eds.): Handbook of Sensory Physiology, Vol. 1, Auditory System. New York, Springer-Verlag, 1974.
48. Rosen, S.: Mobilization of the stapes to restore hearing in otosclerosis. N.Y. J. Med., *53:*2650, 1953.
49. Ruedi, L.: Pathogenesis and treatment of cholesteatoma in chronic suppuration of the temporal bone. Ann. Otol. Rhinol. Laryngol., *66:*283, 1957.
50. Saunders, W. H.: Hereditary hemorrhagic telangiectasis. Its familial pattern, clinical characteristics and surgical treatment. Arch. Otolaryngol., *76:*245, 1962.
51. Schuknecht, H. F.: Cupulolithiasis. Arch. Otolaryngol., *90:*765, 1969.
52. Schuknecht, H. F.: Reconstructive procedures for congenital aural atresia. Arch. Otolaryngol., *101:*170, 1975.
53. Sessions, R. B., Wills, P. I., Alford, B. R., Harrell, J. E., and Evans, R. A.: Juvenile nasopharyngeal angiofibroma: Radiographic aspects. Laryngoscope, *86:*2, 1976.
54. Shea, J. J., Jr.: Fenestration of the oval window. Ann. Otol. Rhinol. Laryngol., *67:*932, 1958.
55. Silverstein, H., Fabian, R. L., Stool, S. E., and Hong, S. W.: Penetrating wounds of the tympanic membrane and ossicular chain. Trans. Am. Acad. Ophthalmol. Otolaryngol., *77:*125, 1973.
56. Snow, J. B.: Cranial and intracranial complications of otitis media. *In* English, G. M. (Ed.): Otolaryngology. Vol. 1. New York, J. B. Lippincott Company, 1988.
57. Snow, J. B.: Diagnosis and therapy for acute laryngeal and tracheal trauma. Otolaryngol. Clin. North Am., *17:*101, 1984.
58. Snow, J. B.: Introduction to Otorhinolaryngology. Chicago, Year Book Medical Publishers, 1979.
59. Snow, J. B.: Management and therapy of trauma to the external ear and auditory and vestibular systems. *In* Alberti, P. W., and Ruben, R. J. (Eds.): Otologic Medicine and Surgery. New York, Churchill Livingstone, 1988, pp. 1561–1576.
60. Snow, J. B.: Surgical management of head and neck cancer. Semin. Oncol., *15:*20, 1988.
61. Snow, J. B.: Surgical therapy for vocal dysfunction. Otolaryngol. Clin. North Am., *17:*91, 1984.
62. Snow, J. B.: Malignant neoplasms of the hypopharynx. *In* Cummings, C. W., et al. (Eds.): Otolaryngology—Head and Neck Surgery. Vol. 3. St. Louis, C. V. Mosby Company, 1986, pp. 2017–2028.
63. Snow, J. B., and Kimmelman, C. P.: Assessment of surgical procedures for Meniere's disease. Laryngoscope, *89:*737, 1979.
64. Strong, M. S., Vaughan, C. W., Healy, G. B., Cooperband, S. R., and Clemente, M. A. C. P.: Recurrent respiratory papillomatosis: Management with the CO₂ laser. Ann. Otol. Rhinol. Laryngol., *85:*508, 1976.
65. Tos, M.: Nasotracheal intubation in acute epiglottitis. Arch. Otolaryngol., *97:*373, 1973.
66. Tucker, H. M.: Long term results of nerve-muscle pedicle reinnervation for laryngeal paralysis. Ann. Otol. Rhinol. Laryngol., *98:*674, 1989.
67. Wullstein, H.: The restoration of function of the middle ear in chronic otitis media. Ann. Otol. Rhinol. Laryngol., *65:*1020, 1956.

40

THE MOUTH, TONGUE, JAWS, AND SALIVARY GLANDS

Milton T. Edgerton, M.D., Michael F. Angel, M.D., and Raymond F. Morgan, M.D., D.M.D.

HISTORICAL ASPECTS

There is evidence that surgical therapy was performed in and about the mouth as early as 3000 B.C.[33] On a wall of the tomb of Hesi-re at Saqqara in Egypt, near the ruins of ancient Memphis, was found a picture of a seated dentist with instruments in his left hand.[41] A Babylonian cuneiform inscription, dating from about 2000 B.C. and now preserved in the British Museum, exorcises the tooth worm (believed to be the cause of dental decay until the eighteenth century). The Edwin Smith Surgical Papyrus, now in the New York Academy of Medicine library and dating from Egypt in 1700 B.C., presents 27 head injury cases with descriptions of fractures and dislocations of the jaw and injuries to the lips and chin, generally providing diagnosis, treatment, and prognosis. From about the sixth century B.C. through the second century of the Christian era, the Greeks developed a system of medicine that was the basis of treatment in Europe until near the end of the fifteenth century. Hippocrates (born about 460 B.C.) is credited with having described a method for reduction of fractures of the lower jaw by binding together the firm teeth on each side of the break with linen thread or gold wire and supporting loose teeth by similar ligatures.[33] Celsus, a Roman of the first century, in his multivolume work, *De medicina*, described ulcers of the mouth, which the Greeks termed *aphthae*; small tumors of the gingiva, termed *parulides* by the Greeks; a method for extracting teeth with forceps; treatment for toothache; incision and drainage of abscesses; and reduction of fractures of the jaw using methods very similar to those of the Egyptians. Galen (A.D. 131–201) wrote voluminously, explaining all disease in the light of pure, dogmatic theory, and substituting a strict system of medical philosophy for the plain notation and interpretation of facts as taught by Hippocrates. His work was so well accepted as authoritative that "European medicine remained at a dead level for nearly fourteen centuries."[26]

After the death of the Prophet in A.D. 632, the religion of Mohammed spread east to Persia and west along both shores of the Mediterranean to Spain and north through central Europe. Parchments from libraries of overrun provinces traveled by ship and by camel to the various capitals, including Samarkand and Cairo, where they were translated into Arabic. Thus, Islamic and Arabic medicine was influenced by Galenic dogma.[33] Medicine in this period of the Dark Ages in Europe and the Mediterranean basin was mainly nonsurgical because of religious proscriptions against cutting human flesh. Most treatment consisted of experiments in chemistry and pharmacology. Cautery became extremely popular. In the twelfth century, with the dawning of the Renaissance, medicine again began to move forward. Theodoric, Bishop of Cervia (1205–1298), advocated that wounds should heal by primary intention. William, in his *Praecox totius medicinae*, in 1275, first described intermaxillary fixation. He advised not only binding together firm teeth adja-

cent to a fracture in the mandible but also binding them in contact with the corresponding teeth in the maxilla. Fallopius (1528–1562) adopted the term "hard" and "soft" palate and described the fifth, seventh, and ninth cranial nerves. Eustachius (1520–1574) published in 1563 *Libellus de dentibus*, the first treatise ever written on the anatomy of the teeth and containing the first description of the periodontal membrane.

The celebrated French surgeon Ambroïse Paré (1510–1590) described methods of transplanting and reimplanting teeth; he used obturators to close cleft or perforated palates, extracted teeth, drained dental abscesses, and set fractured jaws.[33]

In the seventeenth century, the specialties of dentistry and oral surgery began to develop. More than 100 works were published on dentistry.[14] Wilhelm Fabry (1556–1634) reported more than 600 cases, many of which concerned oral surgical problems of toothache to tumor. Jourdain-Berchillet (1734–1816) was trained in surgery but specialized in dentistry and oral surgery. In 1778, he published his major work, *Treatise on the Diseases and Essentially Surgical Operations of the Mouth*. In this, he described the treatment of abscesses, caries, and necrosis of the jaws, diseases of salivary glands and ducts, ramuli, calculi, various tumors, hemorrhages, and maxillary sinus problems. He thought that general surgeons needed more special dental knowledge and that dentists "lacked a sufficiently broad surgical view."

The effect of the elevator and depressor muscles on fragments in mandibular fractures was described by Chopart and Desault in 1779.[32]

In the nineteenth and twentieth centuries, because of advances in technology, all forms of surgery advanced exponentially. The rapid developments of asepsis, radiographic diagnosis, blood transfusions, antibiotics, and endotracheal anesthesia made possible the surgical management of lesions about the mouth.

Aseptic technique has been practiced rigorously and generally only in the twentieth century. Understanding of the germ theory of disease and its practical application began in the latter half of the nineteenth century, notably with Lister's (1827–1912) antiseptic technique. Principal advocates of the aseptic system were Macewen (1848–1924), a pupil of Lister, and von Bergmann (1836–1907), who introduced steam sterilization. Clean, white surgical gowns replaced the old frock coat at the operating table only in the 1880s, and rubber gloves were introduced by Halsted in 1890. Infection was so feared that a casual glance through any text on facial fractures antedating World War II reveals that open surgical reductions of mandibular fractures were avoided because of high risk. The introduction of antibiotics and chemotherapeutic agents altered the course of operative intervention.

The modern attempt to treat cancer of the head and neck by surgical excision probably began with Billroth's resection of the cervical esophagus and larynx on December 31, 1873.[22] Butlin, surgeon to St. Bartholomew's Hospital in London, in 1885 published a monograph entitled *Diseases of the Tongue*. Without any of the advantages of modern surgical therapy, Butlin courageously and repeatedly attempted by operation to control cancer of the tongue, even excising the mandible and portions of the soft tissues and lymphatics of the upper cervical region. He reported more than 100 cases, performing total glossectomy on many, and noted that in the early nineteenth century, in England alone, more than 750 people died each year from tongue cancer. Efforts to cure this type of cancer were minimal in America.

Butlin emphasized that "even the smallest, earliest, and most insignificant epithelioma of the tongue commonly produced cervical lymph node metastases," and therefore, he concluded, "the surgeon would still be needed for the treatment of the regional metastases even if other methods for controlling the primary lesion should appear."

Roentgen, in 1895, and the Curies, in 1898, introduced the use of the Roentgen ray and radium in the treatment of cancer. As is so often true with a new modality, enthusiasm and overtreatment led to discouraging results. Quinby, Janeway, and others contributed significantly to studies in the use of radiation.

In 1906, Crile presented a paper, "Excision of Cancer of the Head and Neck," in which he stated: "The operative treatment is hampered by tradition and conventionality, and the tragic ending of so large a proportion of these cases has held back lay and even professional confidence." He emphasized that fewer than 1 per cent of patients with head and neck cancer died of metastases to distant tissues, and he became convinced of the necessity of performing wider local excision and radical block dissection of the lymphatics of the neck. Crile was the first to describe staged, bilateral neck dissection. He was able to demonstrate in a personal series that the patient undergoing an *en bloc* neck dissection had a 25 per cent better chance of living for 3 years without disease than one treated only for the primary lesion.

In 1923, Brewer, of New York, presented statistics from several New York hospitals that indicated that the results of surgical treatment of cancer of the lip were far superior to those obtained with radium treatment. He thought that the treatment of cancer of the cheek by radium offered more promise. Gillies, in England, and Davis and Blair, in this country, emphasized the problems of deformity following treatment of head and neck cancer and developed techniques to reconstruct the face and jaws of these patients when the cancer was controlled. Reluctance to perform adequate surgical resections led to a disappointing number of cancer recurrences, and radiation therapy was reconsidered. Radium was used in the form of plaques and molds in the early 1920s; shortly thereafter, Evans and Cade, in Great Britain, reported the use of interstitial radium therapy for tongue cancer.

When the 200-kV. roentgen ray machine was developed, the therapeutic use of external radium became less popular. Coutard (1937) made an outstanding contribution to the treatment of head and neck cancer by demonstrating the value of fractionation of x-radiation over a period of approximately 3 weeks, thus greatly reducing damage to overlying normal structures and skin. During the early 1930s, irradiation treatment for oral cancer was very common in America, but gradually increasing numbers of cases of irradiation necrosis and of radioresistant tumors were encountered.

Later it was recognized that *new* malignancies — both carcinomas and sarcomas — were caused by the irradiation used in the treatment of the primary cancer. Just as surgeons had learned earlier that some tumors appeared to be inoperable, radiotherapists began to recognize that some of these tumors were not responsive to irradiation. Martin, MacFee, Ward, Brown, and Byars were beginning to salvage many patients previously deemed incurable by more radical excisions of the cancers. Discriminating radiotherapists began to realize that patients with thyroid cancer, salivary gland cancer, and cancers that had penetrated the jaw or facial bones were usually not candidates for irradiation treatment. It was recognized that many squamous cell cancers responded poorly, if at all, to irradiation.[22]

During World War II, striking improvements were made in maxillofacial surgery through the use of endotracheal anesthesia, more adequate blood transfusion with major operative procedures, and the advent of antibiotics as a prophylaxis against infection from bacteria in the oral cavity. These changes and new surgical skills learned in the care of the war-wounded contributed to a marked reduction in operative mortality in operations on the head and neck. It became increasingly clear that even wider local excisions of cancers of the oral cavity could be accomplished with low acceptable mortality; whether such radical excisions would improve the cure rates of head and neck cancer remained to be seen. Many surgeons treating head and neck cancer were trained in the use of modern reconstructive techniques by wartime experience; some enlarged the reasonable limits of resection of cancers. The concept of "excision in continuity" as previously advocated by Halsted in the treatment of cancer of the breast, and by Miles in abdominoperineal resection, was applied to oral and laryngeal cancer in the late 1940s. A larger number of patients were cured of their cancers. Of necessity more attention was focused on the resulting deformities among the salvaged patients. Plastic surgeons realized that they could contribute much to the rehabilitation of patients with head and neck cancer.[22]

In 1949, Baclesse advocated extending the total treatment time of fractionated external irradiation from 3 weeks to 2 or 3 months. With this extension, he reduced some of the severe acute irradiation reaction and allowed greater doses to be applied to the tumor. In 1938, after Paterson and Parker published their work on the use of low-intensity radium needles, the supervoltage machine was developed as a possible improvement in the method of administration. The radiologists of this period began to emphasize the importance of knowing the exact site of origin of a tumor rather than the amount of anatomic involvement. Nonetheless, results with radiation therapy in almost all clinics in America continued to be disappointing; and after 1945, physicians returned again to surgical therapy for primary treatment. In 1942, Wookey reported the use of combined surgical therapy and irradiation for the treatment of intraoral cancer, and Fletcher followed a similar program. Ward and Edgerton (1951) and others emphasized the value of preoperative irradiation in reducing exfoliation in many types of oral cavity cancer. Smith and Gehan (1959), at the National Clinical Center, in extensive wound-washing studies, demonstrated that preoperative irradiation reduces cell viability and makes seeding of surgical wounds with cancer cells much less common.

The use of appropriate methods of reconstructive surgery employed both at the time of tumor resection and in the days and weeks immediately after the operation has greatly reduced deformity and shortened hospital stay for many patients in recent years. Inevitably, new and complex methods of irradiation are continuously being developed, but each requires extensive adequate evaluation of true cure rates and untoward late effects. Chemotherapy to date has been disappointing in its effect on head and neck cancer and is not sufficiently successful for clinical use, except in conjunction with surgical therapy and irradiation.[22] When oral cavity cancer is confined to a local site and regional lymph nodes, *en bloc* surgical resection offers the most favorable method of providing maximal cure and minimal morbidity from treatment.

Treatment of lesions about the mouth, tongue, jaws, and salivary glands demands the attention of numerous medical, surgical, and paramedical disciplines in order to deliver optimal health care benefits to the patient. General practitioners, dentists, periodontists, orthodontists, oral surgeons, plastic surgeons, general surgeons, ear, nose, and throat surgeons, radiotherapists, chemotherapists, prosthetists, prosthodontists, speech therapists, social workers, and even cosmeticians may all have a role in the diagnosis, operation, reconstruction, and ultimate rehabilitation of patients undergoing treatment for lesions or disease in this area. Because of this, there is a growing tendency in major medical centers for the utilization of a combined cooperative multidisciplinary team approach to the management of complex lesions in the head and neck region.

In recent years, research in all fields of science has continued to yield improvement and modifications in the ability to diagnose and treat disease, trauma, and deformity of the mouth, tongue, jaws, and salivary glands. Developments in high-technology electronics have provided computers, scanners, nuclear fiberoptics, and lasers. Imaging by computed tomography (CT) and nuclear magnetic resonance (MRI) has greatly refined diagnostic capabilities. Reconstruction and repair have been greatly enhanced by the development of muscle and musculocutaneous flaps; established techniques of microsurgery and free flap transfers of skin, muscle, and bone have greatly augmented reconstructive procedures and have provided stronger and more reliable flaps. Flaps of appropriate size and thickness can be raised and transposed in fewer steps and with less morbidity now than a few years ago. Unfortunately, the basic mechanisms of control of cell replication are not understood, and treatment of cancer in the region of the mouth and jaws with wide ablative surgery must be continued until establishment of the cause and nature of cancer.

LIPS

Anatomy of the Lips and Tongue

In repose, the upper lip is slightly anterior to the lower lip because of the maxillary alveolar bony projection. The junction between the red-colored epithelium of the lips and the external surface of lip skin is the vermilion border. There are several surface landmarks of the upper lip; in the central lip are two columns bounding a central dimple, known as the philtrum. Inferior to the philtrum there is a gentle downward curving of the vermilion, which is termed the cupid's bow.

The lips have a complex anatomy. They also have a role in several important functions, including alimentation, facial expression, speech, and the erotic sensations involved in kissing. The major muscle of the lips is the orbicularis oris, which has two components. The deep fibers originate from each commissure and travel horizontally across the midline and, by contracting, allow the lips to seal the mouth. The superficial fibers originate from the muscles of facial expression. There are 13 pairs of these muscles, and they work in concert with the superficial fibers of the orbicularis to provide a multiplicity of facial expressions.

The blood supply of the lips is abundant, largely derived from three branches of the facial artery: the superior labial, the inferior labial, and the submental. The motor nerve supply is via branches of the facial nerve, whereas sensations to the upper lip are conducted by the infraorbital nerve (branch of maxillary division of the trigeminal nerve). Sensation to the lower lip is conducted through the mental nerve, a branch of the inferior alveolar nerve, which is a branch of mandibular division of the trigeminal nerve.

The tongue is a large structure (250 to 300 cu. cm.) that occupies a prominent position within the floor of the oral cavity. The anterior two thirds of the tongue can be readily examined when a patient opens his mouth. The posterior third of the tongue can be visually examined only with the use of a laryngeal mirror. The tongue is important in speech and in the propulsion of food into the pharynx. To achieve this, there is a complex synchronous interaction of both intrinsic and extrinsic lingual muscles.

The intrinsic muscles of the tongue allow reshaping and complex movements within the tongue, whereas the extrinsic muscles (genioglossus, hyoglossus, styloglossus, and palatoglossus) position the entire tongue within the mandibular arch.

Sensory innervation to the anterior two thirds of the tongue is via the lingual nerve (a branch of the trigeminal nerve). The sensation to the posterior third of the tongue is provided by the glossopharyngeal nerve. The hypoglossal nerve supplies motor innervation to both intrinsic and extrinsic muscles.

On the surface of the tongue are small, elevated, rounded prominences termed papillae. Within the papillae, there are individual taste buds, which allow perception of sweet, sour, bitter, and salty tastes. Taste to the anterior two thirds of the tongue is mediated via the chorda tympani nerve, a branch of the facial nerve, whereas taste to the posterior third is by a branch of the glossopharyngeal nerve.

Congenital Malformations and Developmental Anomalies

CLEFTS. The incidence of cleft lip with or without cleft palate is reported to be between 1 in 800 and 1 in 1300 live births. This variation is related to the racial and ethnic composition of the particular community. Cleft lip is eight times more frequent in whites than in blacks. The usual cleft lip represents a defect in skin, vermilion, muscle, and mucosa that courses vertically upward from the vermilion to the floor of the nose. These clefts may be complete or incomplete, unilateral or bilateral. They are caused by a lack of fusion of one (or both) lateral margin of the central prolabium with one (or both) of the two lateral mesodermal masses. These units of mesenchyme arise from migrating neural crest cells in the second week of life and normally fuse in the central lip regions of the embryo between the fourth and seventh weeks of embryonic life. Failure of normal fusion at this tripartite junction of mesodermal masses in the central upper lip leads to any of the aforementioned types of cleft. Aplasia or hypoplasia of the median mesodermal mass (which arises from the frontonasal process) causes the rare "midline" facial cleft of the upper lip.[54] This is much like the true midline "harelip" seen in rodents. Median clefts of the lower lip are extremely rare and represent a failure of the union of the lateral limbs of the mandibular arch at the ventral midline. They are frequently associated with a bony cleft in the midline of the mandible (in the region of the symphysis) and with a bifid tongue.

The most common type of cleft lip is associated with a cleft palate and occurs three times more frequently than cleft palate alone. Cleft lip alone is seen predominantly (2:1) with the male sex; cleft palate alone is twice as common in the female. Cleft lip with associated cleft palate occurs with equal frequency in males and females.

CLASSIFICATION. The usual type of vertical paramedian cleft is divided into two main categories: (1) clefts of the primary palate and (2) clefts of the secondary palate. The primary palate comprises the lip and alveolar ridge and is demarcated posteriorly by the incisive foramen (located in the midline, just behind the upper alveolar ridge). Posterior to the incisive foramen, the hard and soft palates compose the secondary palate. Clefts of the primary palate (lip or alveolus or both) may vary from an incomplete cleft, with only slight notching of the lip, to a complete cleft extending into the floor of the nose. Clefts of the primary palate may be unilateral or bilateral and may or may not be associated with clefts in the secondary palate. Clefts of the secondary palate (the hard and soft palate behind the incisive foramen) may also be incomplete or complete and may be unilateral or bilateral in the region of the hard palate.[29] A very mild form of clefting is seen in 3 per cent of the population and is manifested by a bifid or split uvula on oral examination. Multiple genes have a role in the transmission of cleft lip and palate.

TREATMENT. Clefts of the lip (primary palate) are usually closed surgically during the first 3 months of life. Some prefer to close the lip deformity within the first few days after birth in order to take advantage of passively transferred maternal immunity and allow the parents to take home a nearly normal child. Most prefer to delay operation until the child is 2 to 3 months of age, when structures are larger and anesthesia is safer. Some apply the "rule of tens"—that is, they delay closure of the lip until the child has reached a weight of 10 pounds and has a hemoglobin of 10 gm. or greater, which usually occur when the child is 10 weeks of age or older.

To avoid future deformity, closure of a cleft lip must be performed with meticulous accuracy with a fine-layered plastic closure. The defect in a cleft lip deformity involves not only a transverse gap in the soft tissues but also a loss of vertical length of the lip and an overall hypoplasia or deficiency of tissue. These two aspects of the deformity must be simultaneously corrected as the defect is surgically closed. In general, lateral lip tissue is obtained by modification of the Z-plasty principle with use of tissue from the lateral lip and cheek added to the cleft area. This increases the vertical length of the lip on the cleft side and helps to restore symmetry. Surgical repair is done by one of four basic methods. The first, the straight-line (Rose-Thompson) technique, is occasionally satisfactory for minimal incomplete clefts and modest notching of the lip.[51,60] In larger clefts, this procedure sacrifices too much normal tissue and may destroy the shape of the cupid's bow. Straight-line closures tend to contract, producing a postoperative notching deformity in the vermilion.[14] If this method of repair is used, vertical height may be gained by curving the skin incisions so that the lateral borders of the wound are shaped with their concavities toward the cleft.

Two techniques that are now commonly employed utilize the principle of the Z-plasty. These methods include the quadrilateral flap of Mirault and LeMesurier[35] and the triangular flap technique first described by Tennison[58] (Fig. 1). These may be considered variations of the Z-plasty with the adjacent sides of the cleft as the central limb of the Z-plasty. The techniques vary only in the positioning and lengths of the lateral limbs of the Z-plasty. Vertical height of the repaired side of the lip is provided by transverse incisions across both the lateral and the medial lip elements and rotation of the created flap; these transverse incisions correspond to the lateral limbs of the Z-plasty. In the rotation-advancement technique of Millard[42] (see Fig. 1), a curving incision in the noncleft side allows downward rotation of the philtral portion of the lip. Advancement of the flap from the cleft side into the space opened by this downward rotation places the scar along the line of the philtral ridge on the side of the cleft.

Bilateral clefts of the lip (primary palate) present an even more grotesque congenital deformity. The problems of surgical repair are frequently compounded by an elevated, protruding prolabium and premaxilla. These vestigial midline parts frequently appear to be suspended from the dome of the nose by a very short columella. The timing of surgical repair for bilateral clefts is essentially the same as for unilateral clefts. As in unilateral cleft repairs, very little or no tissue is discarded or excised in the repair. All of these patients suffer from a deficiency of tissue in the region of the upper lip, and great care must be taken to preserve every possible landmark of the normal lip elements. Meticulous repositioning and suturing of the muscles within the lip are essential. Occasionally, one must repair bilateral clefts in stages to allow muscular action of the repair side of the lip to mold the premaxilla inward toward the dental arch, thus facilitating a later closure of the opposite side of the lip. Surgical osteotomy and placement of the premaxilla into the alveolar arch may on occasion be necessary (Fig. 2) but should be done so as to avoid surgical injury to growth centers in the premaxilla and septum.

CONGENITAL SINUSES (MUCOUS PITS). These usually appear (Van der Woude's syndrome) as a symmetrically placed pair of dimples on the vermilion border of the lower lip, one on

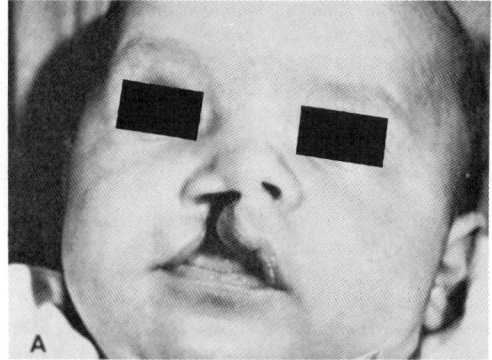
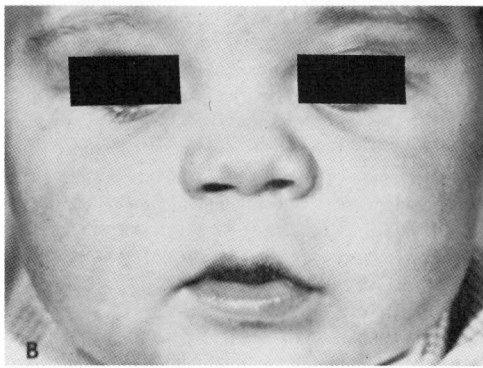

Figure 1. *A*, Complete cleft lip with some nostril distortion. *B*, Seven months after rectangular flap repair (LeMesurier). (From Musgrave, R. H. *In* Converse, J. M. (Ed.): Reconstructive Plastic Surgery, 2nd ed. Vol. 3. Philadelphia, W. B. Saunders Company, 1977.)

each side of the midline (Fig. 3). These slitlike pits are the external orifices of sinus tracts, which extend downward through the orbicularis oris muscle, to end blindly just beneath the mucosal surface of the lower lip or gingiva. They are lined with squamous cell epithelium, and numerous mucous glands empty into the lumen of the pits near their blind end. They are usually asymptomatic but cause vermilion deformity and are often associated with clefts of the secondary palate. Heredity is the most important etiologic factor.[61] The most effective treatment is precise surgical excision of the entire sinus tract after staining of the lumen by filling it with aqueous methylene blue dye. All attached mucous glands whose ducts drain into the sinus must be removed with the tract. If they are not, a mucoid cyst may form.

RETENTION CYSTS. Small retention cysts may involve the mucous glands of the lips. These are mucoceles, caused by obstruction of the ducts of the mucous glands. They appear as small, nontender masses filled with fluid. They are usually asymptomatic except for their annoying bulk. Treatment consists of surgical extirpation.

MACROSTOMIA. This is a rare form of lateral facial clefting characterized by lateral displacement of the oral commissure. The orbicularis oris muscle is incomplete at the site of the cleft. It occurs either unilaterally or bilaterally and is often associated with malformations of the maxilla and mandible and other deformities related to the second branchial arch.

MICROSTOMIA. Children born with extremely small mouths occasionally present major problems in feeding. Microstomia is usually associated with a small, retruded jaw (micrognathia). A small mouth opening rarely requires surgical intervention and is best left to enlarge by normal growth and development. Small dynamic circular splints effectively enlarge the mouth over a period of weeks.

MACROCHEILIA. This is enlargement of either the upper or lower lip caused by inflammatory, neoplastic, or congenital factors. A rare variety of macrocheilia is congenital double lip. This double lip deformity occurs most frequently in the upper lip.

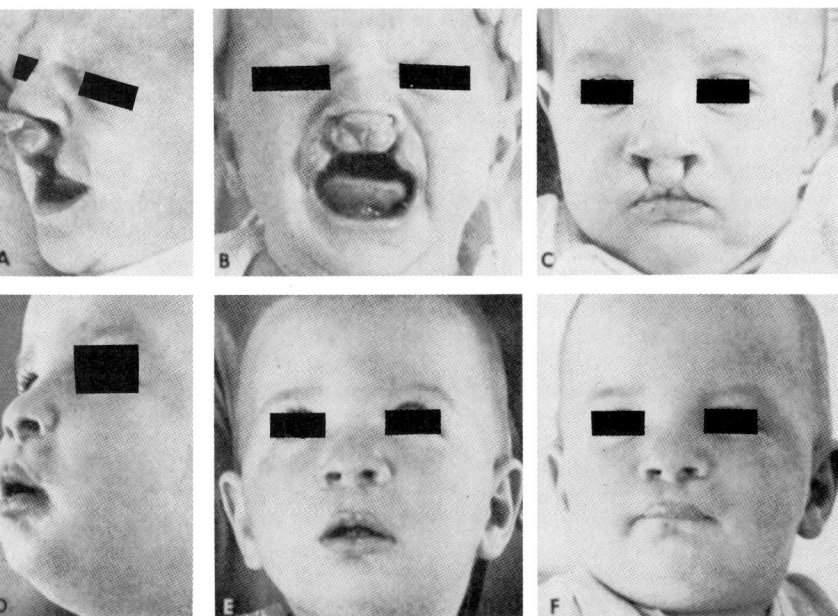

Figure 2. A and B, Bilateral complete cleft of lip with protruding premaxilla, absence of columella, side nostril flare, and small prolabium. C, The premaxilla has been returned into the alveolar arch, and lateral vermilion flaps have been attached to the prolabium for blood supply and cupid's bow. D to F, Forked flap from the prolabium has produced primary columella lengthening. Medical advancement of lateral triangular flaps has narrowed alar flares and incorporated the prolabium as a philtrum. (From Millard, D. R.: Transactions of the International Society of Plastic Surgeons, Second Congress. Edinburgh, E. & S. Livingstone, 1959.)

The deformity is not obvious when the mouth is closed; however, with the mouth open, a double vermilion is exhibited with a transverse furrow of varying depth between the reduplicated lips. The buccal portion of the double vermilion is usually loose and redundant. Treatment consists of transverse excision of the buccal redundancy with primary closure.[61] This is best accomplished by a zigzag (W-plasty) type closure to avoid a bandlike transverse scar in the lip.

PEUTZ-JEGHERS SYNDROME. Melanin-like spots of pigmentation on the lips may be associated with multiple intestinal polyposis. This syndrome was first described by Peutz in 1921 and explained in more detail by Jeghers and associates in 1949. The syndrome is congenital and inherited. The lip (and occasionally buccal) lesions are benign and are significant in calling attention to the possible presence of intestinal polyposis.[46] Bleeding and malignant change in the polyps may be seen. Proper recognition of the pathognomonic lesions on the lips may be lifesaving.

Injuries Due to Trauma

LACERATIONS. Lacerations of the lip frequently involve both the mucosal and the skin surfaces with division of the intervening musculature. Because of the circular and radial distribution of the perioral musculature, full-thickness lacerations tend to open widely whenever the muscle is divided. Because of this, inexperienced clinicians may suspect tissue loss when the defect is primarily a result of tissue retraction. In closing lacerations of the lip, it is important to reconstitute accurately both divided muscles and the vermilion-cutaneous junction. Even a slight disparity in reconstituting this line produces an obvious deformity. Therefore, appropriate lighting, assistance, and anesthesia are important in repair of lip lacerations. It is quite helpful to temporarily tattoo the vermilion-cutaneous junction on either side of a laceration with a 25-gauge needle dipped in aqueous methylene blue. The dye should be allowed to penetrate the skin along the vermilion edge on either side of the laceration prior to the infiltration of any local anesthetic that contains epinephrine. The first skin suture is usually placed exactly at the vermilion-cutaneous junction (Fig. 4). Local anesthetics and vasoconstrictors tend to blanch out the color differentiation between the vermilion and facial skin and when injected make the junction line difficult to recognize. Two marker

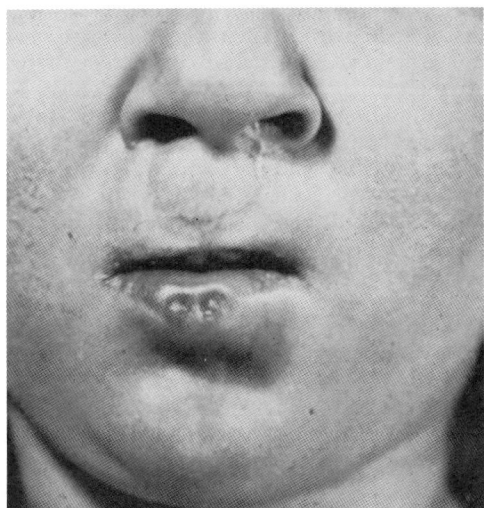

Figure 3. Congenital lip sinuses. The illustration shows bilateral, symmetrically situated sinus openings at the apices of a pair of nipple-like protrusions of the lower lip. Note the associated bilateral cleft lip, shown postoperatively. (From Wang, M. K. H., Macomber, W. B., Converse, J. M., and Wood-Smith, D.: In Converse, J. M. (Ed.): Reconstructive Plastic Surgery, 2nd ed. Vol. 2. Philadelphia, W. B. Saunders Company, 1977.)

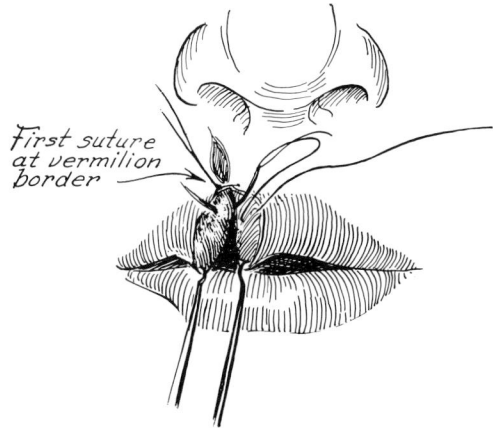

First suture at vermilion border

Figure 4. Repair of vertical lacerations of the vermilion-cutaneous margin. The first skin suture should be used for approximation of the conspicuous irregularity of the lip after healing occurs. (From Dingman, R. O.: In Converse, J. M. (Ed.): Reconstructive Plastic Surgery. Vol. 2. Philadelphia, W. B. Saunders Company, 1964.)

needle pricks with methylene blue prior to local anesthetic injection greatly simplify accurate alignment of the vermilion-cutaneous junction.

Through-and-through lacerations should be closed in layers with absorbable suture material in the muscle and subcutaneous tissues. Copious irrigation and complete hemostasis are essential. The skin can be closed with 5-0 or 6-0 silk or nylon; the mucosa is loosely closed with similarly sized silk, polyglycolic acid, or chromic gut.

The lips and most of the face are blessed with an excellent blood supply. Because of this, stellate lacerations with multiple tiny flaps of tissue usually heal quite well if accurately repaired. Relatively clean wounds of the lips and face can be closed primarily even up to 24 hours after injury. Very fine sutures and very few buried sutures are employed for repair of this type of laceration.

Because of the presence of Vincent's spirochetes, fusiform bacilli, and numerous pathogenic resident anaerobes in the human mouth, it is advisable to administer oral penicillin in therapeutic doses for several days following closure of any lip lacerations that involve the oral surface.[46] This is especially true if the tissues have been crushed during the injury.

BURNS. Thermal burns of the lips generally involve the exposed skin, vermilion, and mucosal surfaces. They are treated in much the same manner as are cutaneous burns elsewhere on the body, depending on the depth of burn injury. Topical antibiotic ointment therapy may be applied with care about the mouth and immediately relieves burn pain. It should be emphasized that the presence of a thermal burn about the mouth or nares should not be taken as an absolute indication for a tracheotomy. Certainly, burns in this area should alert the surgeon to the possible need for a tracheotomy, but routine tracheotomy for all patients with perioral burns is not only unnecessary but indeed contraindicated unless there are definite signs of upper airway obstruction or a definite history of the patient's confinement in a small space at the time of the burn.[43] Elevation of the head of the patient's bed, use of a croup tent, short courses of anti-inflammatory steroids, and use of prolonged endotracheal intubation further decrease the need for tracheotomy.

Burns of the inner surfaces of the lips, from the accidental ingestion of very hot liquids, are rarely deeper than second-degree. These are usually adequately managed by giving the patient a mild, orally administered analgesic. Alcoholic mouthwashes add further tissue injury and may be painful and irritating; topical opiates are rather ineffective and unnecessary.

One of the most frequently encountered chemical burns of the lips is that due to lye consumption in attempted suicides. This strong alkali penetrates the tissues of the lip, saponifies the fat, and reacts with tissue proteins to form soluble alkaline proteinate. The combination of lye with fats to form soaps produces an exothermic reaction and generates sufficient additional heat to damage surrounding tissue. The hygroscopic nature of lye produces cellular dehydration and cell death. If not removed, the soluble alkaline proteinates formed penetrate deeply into the tissues, where they cause delayed further injury and an increase in the depth of the burn wound.

The treatment of lye burns of the mouth should consist of early, copious, and *prolonged* irrigation with cold tap water. Water dilutes the injurious lye, washes away the noxious agent, and decreases the mass action and exothermic effect of the chemical reaction, thereby diminishing the inflammatory reaction. This is best done with a small rubber hose attached to a water faucet, so that large volumes of fresh, clean water can be used to irrigate the mouth continuously for at least 12 hours. The direct cooling of the tissues also reduces cell death. The irrigation should be initiated as rapidly as possible. Systemic steroids also are helpful in diminishing the inflammatory reaction, and penicillin should be administered as with any other burn. Attempts to chemically neutralize the lye are fraught with

many hazards and have proved to be inferior to simple water irrigation.[63]

Electrical burns of the lips are most frequently seen in small children, who are apt to chew on electrical cords or place the ends of extension cords in their mouths. Saliva creates a short circuit across the terminals within the plug, causing the electrical burn. Tissue destruction from an electric current is sudden and extensive. Deep coagulation necrosis is instantaneously produced by the extremely high temperature of an electrical arc. If the child is well grounded, the current flow through the body may, although quite rarely, cause cardiac arrest.

The initial treatment of electrical burns of the lips should be conservative and not unlike the treatment of any other form of burn. Antibiotics should be administered for 5 days. Débridement should be limited to the excision of obviously dead and necrotic tissue, done without anesthesia, and should produce no bleeding. This can be accomplished in the first few days after injury if the surgeon is experienced in the recognition of tissue necrosis associated with electrical currents. The wound should be allowed to heal spontaneously. Reconstructive efforts should be reserved until well after healing has occurred and after the scars have softened and matured. Delayed bleeding from the coronary labial arteries of the lips is frequently seen about 10 to 18 days after electrical burns. This is easily controlled with a hemostat and a simple catgut ligature. When it occurs, the wound should be débrided and skin closed to mucous membrane. This treatment reduces the danger of recurrent exsanguinating hemorrhage during sleep.

Superior results with greatly diminished contracture of electrically burned oral commissures have been obtained with the use of a smooth, curved acrylic splint shaped somewhat like a blunted bull's horn and attached to the ipsilateral maxillary teeth. With major destruction of tissue about the commissure, complex and extremely difficult reconstructive operations are required.

Infections

LABIAL ABSCESS OR CELLULITIS. The skin of the lips is well endowed with hair follicles, sweat glands, and sebaceous glands. Minor infections due to blockage of these openings in the skin that produce pustules or small abscesses are relatively common. Warm soaks and appropriate surgical drainage are usually adequate therapy. Numerous persistent or recurrent infections or those with surrounding cellulitis should be treated from the outset with appropriate antibiotics following culture. The usual offending organism is *Staphylococcus*. Larger abscesses can be drained through the buccal surface of the lips and cheeks so that visible external scars are avoided, following which a small drain should be sutured in the intraoral wound at two points and left in place for a minimum of 3 days. Cellulitis of the lips almost always indicates a streptococcal infection and usually responds to penicillin.

HERPETIC STOMATITIS. Herpetic stomatitis is a herpes simplex virus infection that presents as yellowish papulovesicular lesions, which may be discrete or occur in groups. Initially, a small vesicle appears and soon ruptures; a small ulceration then occurs. Symptoms consist of pain and burning in the region of the ulcer; the ulcer is particularly sensitive to touch. After a 10- to 12-day course, the lesion usually clears spontaneously.[4] Topical steroids such as triamcinolone and Orabase may speed symptomatic recovery. Early herpetic lesions may respond to topical 5-fluorouracil cream, but this has no efficacy when an ulcer has developed. Locally recurrent herpetic lesions may respond to subcutaneous injection of small amounts of triamcinolone at the site of recurrence; chronic cases respond to viral vaccines. Acyclovir has shown promise in the treatment of severe herpetic lesions in immunocompromised patients. Patients with a history of recurrent lesions are advised to avoid fatigue, exhaustion, and dehydration.

CANKER SORES. Canker sores occur on the buccal surface of the lips and are characteristically small, superficial ulcerations that are exquisitely tender and irritated by acid foods. They are usually surrounded by an inflammatory halo of erythema. These lesions are usually associated with gastrointestinal disorders, dehydration, or nutritional disturbances. They respond well to a bland diet, oral fluids, avoidance of acid foods and juices, and vitamin supplementation. Symptomatic relief may be obtained by holding promethazine (Phenergan) syrup in the mouth in the region of the lesion for 5 to 10 minutes before swallowing. One teaspoon of the syrup every 2 hours during waking hours is sufficient for most adults. Phenergan acts locally as a topical anesthetic and when swallowed has a systemic sedative effect. Tetracycline syrup, held in the mouth for its topical action and then swallowed, may also reduce the course of these lesions.

NOMA. Noma is a rapidly progressive gangrenous stomatitis that is rarely seen in well-nourished persons. It occurs in patients with general debility and metabolic dyscrasia. These lesions rapidly invade and destroy soft tissues about the mouth and face. The destruction may involve bone and frequently leads to death. Nomas are more common in children and occur after measles and other contagious diseases. They are initiated by anaerobic bacteria, among which are found fusospirochetal organisms.[28]

MONILIASIS. Moniliasis (thrush) is the most common fungal disease involving the oral cavity. Its incidence is increased in patients who are on antibiotic long-term therapy. The acute form produces multiple, white, adherent, curdlike patches, irregularly distributed over the mucosal surfaces. Inflammation and fissuring of the labial commissures and encrustations on the lip frequently accompany the intraoral lesions. The specific treatment agent is nystatin (Mycostatin).[4]

SYPHILIS. Syphilis, in its primary form, may produce a chancre on the lips. This is a foul, discharging, dirty ulcer without the surrounding characteristic hardness of carcinoma. Treatment is systemic antisyphilitic therapy. If suspected, a dark field examination of the ulcer shows *Treponema pallidum* and excludes cancer.

OTHER INFECTIONS. Other infrequently encountered infections involving the lips include actinomycosis, histoplasmosis, molluscum contagiosum, and lymphogranuloma venereum. A thorough history, culture, and biopsy usually establishes the correct diagnosis.

Benign Tumors of the Lips

Benign tumors may arise from any of the tissues forming the lips. Benign tumors may occur in the epithelium, dermis, fibrous tissue, fat, muscle, blood vessels, lymphatics, nerves, or specialized glands. Treatment of these lesions is usually surgical excision and microscopic examination for confirmation of the diagnosis and identification of the completeness of excision. Larger lesions require special reconstructive procedures and are best treated by plastic surgery techniques at the time of the initial excision.

NEVI. Nevi may be subdivided microscopically into three groups, based on the depth of penetration of nevus cells across the dermal-epidermal junction: (1) Intradermal nevi contain most of the nevus cells within the dermis. They are frequently raised above the skin surface, may contain hair, and demonstrate varying degrees of pigmentation. (2) Junctional nevi demonstrate the nevus cells to be concentrated at the junction between the dermis and epidermis. They are usually flat, do not contain hair, and may vary in the depth of their pigmentation. (3) Compound nevi demonstrate nevus cells distributed through both the dermis and the junctional zones. They may be elevated or sessile and may or may not contain hair. It is generally agreed that intradermal nevi almost never become malignant and that junctional nevi may become malignant with disturbing frequency. The exact incidence is not known. Compound nevi have been followed and reported to become malignant by several authors. Any nevus of the lip (or elsewhere) that demonstrates change in size or pigmentation, or in any way appears to be undergoing change by itching or bleeding, for example, should be surgically excised and biopsied. Similarly, any pigmented nevus that remains chronically irritated should be excised.

PAPILLOMAS. These are commonly termed skin tags, frequently observed about the face and neck and usually multiple. Microscopically, they appear to primarily follow epithelial hyperplasia. The matrix of the skin tag demonstrates a pattern of randomly arranged, delicate fibers that resembles the pattern of normal dermis. They vary in size but are usually less than 1 cm. in diameter. They are usually soft and have a pedicle of soft skin. Surgical excision is the treatment of choice.

FIBROMAS. These benign tumors arise in the deeper layers of the skin and contain mesodermal and, at times, epithelial elements. They may be classified as fibrolipoma, myofibroma, angiofibroma, or neurofibroma. Those with a gelatinous stroma are termed fibromyxomas. These tumors are rare but may occur on the lip. Treatment is by local surgical excision; fibromas rarely become malignant.

LIPOMAS AND MYOMAS. Lipomas and myomas rarely occur on the lips. These benign tumors are excised surgically for diagnosis and cure.

HEMANGIOMAS. Benign vascular malformations or hamartomas, hyperplasia, and vascular ectasias are quite common on the lips. Classification is critical to knowledge about prognosis and is based on the clinical characteristics and the histologic features of these angiomas. In general, they can be grouped into four categories: (1) juvenile capillary angiomas, (2) cavernous hamartomas, (3) telangiectases, and (4) arteriovenous malformations, which may be congenital or traumatic in origin and are progressive, dangerous, and may require extensive surgical excision.

JUVENILE CAPILLARY ANGIOMAS. The most common capillary angioma, often called a strawberry nevus, is usually present at or shortly after birth. It tends to be polypoid, raised, and bright red to purple in color, occasionally is bosselated, and involves the dermis and subcutis. Lesions that are superficial are bright red, those with deep components tend to be darker in color. They may grow at an alarming rate and are occasionally complicated by ulceration and infection. When they are untreated, spontaneous involution usually begins by the age of 2 or 3 years and is first noted by the appearance of patchy, pale areas, usually near the center of the lesion. Gradually, the tumor shrinks and involutes, losing its vascular color. When involution is complete, the site may appear normal or may show loose, wrinkled skin with slight atrophy and scarring and occasionally remaining telangiectatic vessels in the surrounding skin.[48]

Treatment of capillary hemangiomas in the past has consisted of cryotherapy, injection of sclerosing agents, surgical excision, x-ray or radium therapy, or no treatment at all. Most of the invasive methods of treatment have produced cosmetic results that are definitely inferior to those after natural involution. Uncomplicated capillary hemangiomas that do not disturb function, produce unusual deformity, or cause troublesome frequent bleeding are best followed conservatively. Most undergo natural involution with superior results. If the hemangioma continues to enlarge alarmingly, the involution process can frequently be dramatically initiated and hastened by the oral administration of prednisolone. This should be administered in high doses (beginning with at least 40 mg. every 2 days for 10 doses, and then a halving of the dose for each 10 successive administrations). This dosage has been free of complications when administered to otherwise healthy infants in whom there is no contraindication to this form of therapy.[20,54]

X-ray therapy, either as superficial irradiation or in the form of radium implantation, is unfortunately frequently advocated as a method for "inducing regression" of these nonmalignant lesions. Irradiation of benign disease is mentioned here only for the purpose of criticizing it. The late sequelae of radiation damage include atrophy, dermatitis, and scarring in surrounding normal tissue. Cessation of underlying bony growth and development, radionecrosis, and even late development of malignant neoplastic changes are also frequently seen. These complications present problems of much greater magnitude than those of the original lesion.

Argon laser treatment for superficial intradermal capillary hemangiomas (port-wine stains) has been demonstrated to be very effective. The blue energy beam from the argon laser is selectively absorbed by the red blood cells within the angioma. The adjacent endothelium of the capillaries is vaporized with little or no damage to the surrounding tissues.

The tunable-dye laser has recently been introduced and shows much promise in this area. It produces less skin scarring than does the argon laser and has the added advantage of being much less painful. This means that general anesthetics are not required with these multiple treatments — even with children.

The more common juvenile capillary angiomas must be treated by the laser very soon after appearance for control. They frequently arise shortly after birth as small, red, slightly elevated lesions on the skin and occasionally grow and spread over large areas with alarming speed; it is essential to be aware that early laser therapy of the small lesions can completely prevent this subsequent growth and spread while causing little or no damage to the adjacent normal tissues. If the lesion is allowed to enlarge and thicken prior to laser therapy, more damage and subsequent scarring result from laser treatment. Early eradication of the small capillary angiomas also prevents the subsequent development of a bulky cavernous component that frequently develops beneath these capillary lesions. These deeper vessels are largely beyond the reach of the laser. Effective laser treatment for juvenile capillary hemangiomas depends, therefore, on early recognition and diagnosis and prompt referral of these infants.

CAVERNOUS ANGIOMAS (CIRSOID HAMARTOMAS). These are tumor-like aggregates of larger dilated vessels or sinusoidal blood spaces in a fibrous stroma. They are usually not present at birth, but appear during early childhood. They extend into the subcutaneous tissue with poorly defined borders. Histologically, the vessels appear more mature and lack the angioblastic qualities of the capillary hemangioma. Also, unlike capillary hemangiomas, they show no tendency for involution and, indeed, usually show insidious, progressive enlargement. They may cause considerable pain when distended. Irradiation is contraindicated and has no more effect on the cavernous hemangioma than on the surrounding normal tissues. Interruption of feeding vessels, by ligation or by injection embolization, has been used with variable success. The vascular spaces are on the efferent side of the vascular bed and thus are not reached by emboli introduced through the regional arteries. Surgical resection and reconstruction provide the best results.[42] Sometimes multiple stages are required, and hemostasis may be very difficult to obtain during these operations.

TELANGIECTASES. Nevus flammeus (port-wine stain) is a macular, pink-to-purple vascular malformation that is frequently distributed along the course of sensory peripheral nerves. Most of these nevi are present at birth and do not grow or involute. They do not respond to irradiation, freezing, or surgical abrasion. Many are managed by the application of cosmetics to hide the discoloration, but this does not relieve the patient's "sense of deformity." Plastic surgeons now use more "color-matched" skin grafts from "blush" areas of the neck or scalp to replace these lesions on the lips and face.

Treatment of port-wine stains with the argon laser has also shown promise. Total eradication of these lesions has been

demonstrated in very few patients, but improvement has been noted in most. The tunable-dye laser has reduced the pain of laser treatments and made treatment practical in children without the need to resort to general anesthesia.

The venous varix (senile hemangioma, venous lake) may appear as a solitary, deep blue nodule on the lips. It resembles a blood blister but is not tense. It empties easily with pressure. These lesions tend to persist unless excised for cosmetic purposes.[42]

The Osler-Rendu-Weber syndrome (hereditary hemorrhagic telangiectasia) is characterized by discrete, red, small, superficial punctate telangiectatic lesions on the skin and oral mucous membranes. They may be flat or slightly raised and are seldom more than a few mm. in diameter. They are frequently accompanied by lesions on the fingers, face, and nasal mucous membranes. These lesions are prone to ulceration and hemorrhage and are frequently associated with arteriovenous fistulas in the lungs and vascular malformations of the liver. When seen on the lips, they should arouse suspicion and stimulate the search for the other facets of the syndrome. The lip lesions can be controlled by cautery or excision.[48]

LYMPHANGIOMAS. These growths of thin-walled, vascular spaces that contain lymph involve the lips, tongue, and cheeks, producing visible deformity. They show no tendency toward spontaneous involution, and they are not radiosensitive. Treatment, if indicated, is surgical; and if surgical therapy is incomplete, the lesions likely recur.[48] When they are large and associated with giantism and skeletal abnormalities, the condition is known as the Proteus syndrome.

PYOGENIC GRANULOMAS. These are localized, superficial polypoid masses of new capillaries within an edematous matrix, devoid of epithelium and grossly resembling polyps of granulation tissue. Despite the name, an infectious etiology for these lesions is not firmly established. These lesions may occur at any age, and symptoms of pain or tenderness are variable. They tend to bleed easily when traumatized. Treatment should be surgical excision, with microscopic confirmation of the diagnosis to exclude the presence of other lesions that may mimic pyogenic granuloma, i.e., Kaposi's disease and metastatic renal cell carcinoma.[48]

EPIDERMAL INCLUSION CYSTS (SEBACEOUS CYSTS). These occur commonly on the skin of the lips. They are more common in individuals with thick, oily skin. They follow occlusion of the drainage pores of the sebaceous glands, are usually firm and discrete, and usually contain a concentrated creamy paste of oil. Palpating the cyst and moving it beneath the skin frequently demonstrates traction umbilication of the skin at the site of the occluded pore. These cysts are best treated by excising a small, elliptical sliver of skin containing the punctum along with the entire wall of the underlying cyst.

KERATOACANTHOMAS. These common benign cutaneous tumors may arise from the hair follicles on the lips. Their rapid growth and histologic appearance may lead the surgeon, and occasionally the pathologist, to make a diagnosis of squamous carcinoma. Keratoacanthoma is, however, a benign tumor that has a self-limited course. If untreated, it may heal spontaneously but produce a cicatricial deformity of the lips. This tumor is limited to whites and has its highest incidence in individuals between the ages of 50 and 70. The etiology of keratoacanthoma is unclear. Actinic rays, chemical carcinogens, trauma, genetic factors, and viral infection may all have a role in its etiology. Clinically, the tumors may appear as dome-shaped buds with a pink to reddish hue. Later in the evolution of the tumor, the epithelium over the center of the dome deteriorates to reveal a central keratin plug. Ultimately, the keratin plug detaches, leaving a crater-shaped lesion. The lesion becomes ulcerated and then regresses completely, healing by scar formation. Treatment is by surgical excision with primary closure. The specimen must be submitted for accurate histopathologic diagnosis. Other methods of treatment such as curettage, cautery, diathermy, or x-ray therapy usually prove curative for kerato-acanthoma but prolong the healing process and make accurate pathologic diagnosis difficult or impossible. The excision of large keratoacanthomas may make it advisable to use pedicle flaps or skin grafts to reconstruct the lips.[27]

KERATOSES. These rough, scaly, slightly raised lesions occur on the skin surface or at the vermilion-cutaneous junction of the lips of elderly patients with fair skin who have been chronically exposed to solar radiation. If untreated, they may evolve to invasive squamous cell carcinomas of the lips. Chronic labial keratoses are best excised by a "lip shave" procedure with mucosal advancement. The full thickness of the skin should be excised, and the tissue should be examined microscopically.[22,56] When keratoses are white in color, they are usually called leukoplakia.

LEUKOPLAKIA. This condition commonly presents with slightly elevated white patches on the buccal mucosa, tongue, palate, or lip vermilion. Treatment initially consists of the removal of any possible mouth irritant, such as tobacco or snuff. General mouth cleanliness and hygiene should be encouraged, and any caries or rough teeth should receive prompt dental care. Daily abrasion with a stiff-bristle toothbrush resolves superficial problems. Recently, vitamin A has been found effective in reversing the epithelial changes in some patients. After these conservative measures have been employed, any persistent lesions should be excised and examined microscopically. This condition is definitely precancerous and should be treated promptly.[5]

Squamous Cell Cancer of the Lips

Nearly all "lip cancers" are epidermoid in type and arise at the skin-vermilion junction. Basal cell cancers and melanomas arising in the lips are considered elsewhere.

Lip carcinoma represents approximately 15 per cent of all malignant diseases of the head and neck and approximately 1 per cent of all cancers. These lesions mainly occur on the lower lip, and 87 per cent occur in males. They are rarely seen in individuals below the age of 40, and there is an increasing incidence with advancing age. Individuals with light-colored hair who tend to freckle (rather than tan) when exposed to sunlight appear to be highly susceptible. Carcinoma of the lip is rarely seen in blacks. There is a definite correlation between lip cancer and exposure to sunlight.[1] The incidence of these cancers gradually increases in susceptible individuals as the equator is approached from the extreme northern or southern latitudes. Individuals who spend most of their lives out of doors, or at higher elevations, where the effects of less filtered actinic irradiation are stronger, also are more susceptible to the development of lip cancer. Other factors that frequently occur in the histories of patients with lip cancer that have some etiologic significance include syphilis, prior gamma irradiation, excessive use of tobacco (particularly smoking of pipes with clay stems), and heavy alcohol consumption.

Diagnostic work-up for a suspected lip cancer should include biopsy of the lesion. Biopsies are 100 per cent accurate if positive.[7] If negative, they should be repeated. Bidigital examination of the floor of the mouth and the submental submaxillary triangles for metastatic disease should be done, and both sides of the entire neck should be carefully palpated for enlarged lymph nodes. A chest film may reveal metastases.

CLASSIFICATION. Clinically, lip cancer presents as one of two major types: (1) exophytic lesions, in which superficial proliferation predominates, and (2) endophytic lesions, in which invasion, ulceration, and early involvement of muscle, bone, and skin predominate (Fig. 5). Histologically, epidermoid carcinoma represents 99 per cent of all lip cancers[6] and is usually well differentiated. Basal cell carcinoma occasionally appears on the lips, but this more often than not can be demonstrated to

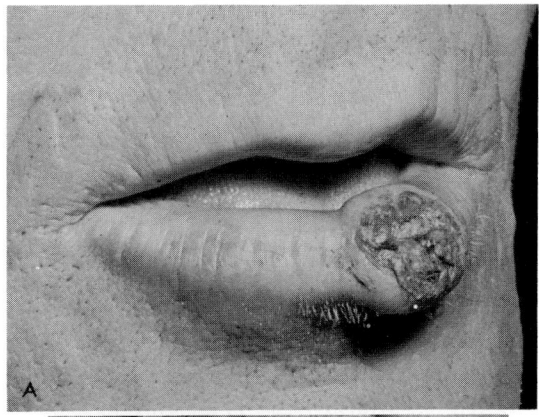
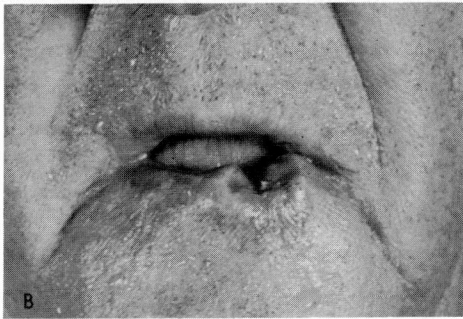

Figure 5. *A,* Exophytic carcinoma of lower lip with central ulceration and raised, rolled borders. *B,* Ulcerating carcinoma of lower lip with diffuse infiltration. (From Ackerman, L. V., and del Regato, J. A.: Cancer: Diagnosis, Treatment, and Prognosis, 4th ed. St. Louis, C. V. Mosby Company, 1970.)

be associated with basal cell carcinoma arising in the skin surrounding the lips. Melanoma is occasionally seen as a primary lip cancer.

The metastatic behavior of lip cancer is characterized by relatively late spread to regional lymph nodes except in the undifferentiated lesions. The most common metastatic route is to the facial and submental lymph nodes and the nodes that lie along the anterior portion of the submaxillary gland, with subsequent spread to the jugular chain. Late invasion of the mandible occurs most commonly via direct soft tissue extension, usually entering the mental foramen to reach the marrow cavity. Distant metastasis to the lungs and liver occurs late and is rare. When death occurs, it is usually due to uncontrolled growth of a metastatic tumor in the neck—and not to the effects of distant metastasis.

PRINCIPLES OF TREATMENT. The management of carcinoma of the lip must be individualized. Factors that enter into the decision include the following:

1. *The age of the patient.* Younger patients are more likely to have early metastases than older ones.[11]

2. *The reliability of the patient and the logistical practicality for close follow-up of the patient.* Patients in whom the potential for close follow-up appears dubious are better served by a "diagnostic" dissection and removal of the regional upper cervical lymph nodes at the time of initial resection of the lip primary. If the pathology report shows tumor in any of the nodes on either side of the neck, complete neck dissection is performed. Experience has shown that large recurrences may appear rapidly in the neck, and they are most difficult to treat. Withholding neck dissection until a suspicious (enlarged and firm) node is palpated in the neck is a dangerous policy.

3. *The nature of the lesion.* The endophytic, invasive type of carcinoma tends to metastasize much earlier than the exophytic type.[8] Even large exophytic cancers have a good prognosis if widely excised.

4. *The size of the lesion.* Lesions less than 1 cm. in size rarely

metastasize to the neck, and these smaller lesions can usually be managed by resection with margins of normal lip skin. Lesions larger than 1 cm. are much more likely to have spread to the regional nodes. The size of the lesion is usually correlated with duration on the lip; the longer a lesion has been present, the more likely that metastasis has occurred in the nodes in the neck.[11]

5. *The histologic gradation of the cell malignancy.* High-grade or undifferentiated carcinoma is more likely to develop early metastasis than are low-grade, well-differentiated tumors.

6. *Staging.* The presence of palpable enlarged or indurated nodes in the submental area or neck is a definite indication for radical neck dissection to remove regional nodes. Palpation of cervical nodes is a notoriously poor method for diagnosing cancer.

7. *Recurrent or persistent lesions.* Lesions that have previously been treated inadequately need wide re-resection of the lip with simultaneous cervical node dissection. If the primary tumor involves the skin of the chin, an *en bloc* resection may be indicated.

8. *The experience and ability of the surgeon.* Those who undertake to treat lip carcinoma should be thoroughly familiar with the techniques of neck dissection and should be competent in the planning, elevation, mobilization, and transportation of local flap tissue for immediate reconstruction. Excision of lip cancer is relatively easy, but reconstruction of the lips and commissures demands considerable skill and experience.

Small primary lip cancers of the well-differentiated type are adequately treated by local resection; the V-excision is a popular method that facilitates closure (Fig. 6). Surgical treatment of larger lip lesions in which adequate resection requires excision of more than half of the lip demands a thorough knowledge of many ingenious local and distant flap techniques that have been designed for lip reconstruction.[6] For larger, invasive lesions with a highly malignant histologic pattern, recurrent lesions, or lip cancers in patients in whom adequate follow-up is doubtful, a "diagnostic" bilateral supraomohyoid neck dissection is the treatment of choice. The morbidity and deformity from this operation are minimal, and 90 per cent of the patients are found to have only "inflammatory hyperplasia" of their nodes. These patients require no further surgical therapy. The remaining 10 per cent may require radical removal of lymph nodes.

Radiotherapy has many advocates as a primary modality in the treatment of lip cancer. A typical course of radiation therapy encompasses several weeks, with daily treatments five times a week, followed by disruption of the tumor, with ulceration and slow healing. In favorable lesions, the cure for radiation therapy is 80 to 90 per cent and approaches, but does not equal, that of surgical therapy.[25] However, radiation therapy leads to considerable morbidity, does not provide pathologic assessment of the margins of treatment, and is less effective than surgical therapy in control of the disease in the regional nodes. When cervical nodes are involved and contain a large volume of tumor cells,

radiation therapy is particularly ineffective. Prior radiotherapy also increases problems with wound healing if recurrence develops, and surgical therapy should be recommended.

Melanomas of the lip require wide, radical, surgical resection with *en bloc* dissection of the nodal drainage areas in the neck. Radiotherapy is not effective, and chemotherapy for this lesion has been disappointing.

ORAL CAVITY

Congenital Malformations and Developmental Anomalies

CLEFT PALATE. Clefts of the secondary palate, from the incisive foramen posteriorly to the tip of the uvula, develop during the seventh to twelfth weeks of embryonic life.[51] Normally, two lateral mesodermal palatal shelves develop and fuse in the midline during this time, separating the oral and nasal cavities. Prior to fusion, these shelves hang downward in a vertical position alongside the tongue. During the seventh week, as the mandible enlarges and the tongue descends into the oral cavity, they begin to fuse in the midline from anterior to posterior. The two parts of the soft palate are joined by the ninth week; the uvula is completed by the twelfth week. Insults to the developing embryo during this time may produce arrest in the developmental process, causing clefts of the secondary palate.[53] The defect may vary from total, complete, bilateral clefting of the hard and soft palate, with wide communication between the oral and nasal cavities, to a cleft manifested by only slight notching of the tip of the uvula (Fig. 7).

Occult submucosal clefts of the soft palate sometimes occur with an intact mucous membrane, but with lack of fusion of the muscle masses in the midline. These are usually associated with a notching of the posterior edge of the bony hard palate and a midline cleft of the uvula. Submucosal clefts quite often cause the child to have rhinolalia aperta, or typical "cleft palate speech."

TREATMENT. Clefts of the palate are repaired surgically when the child is between 1 and 2 years old. This operation requires the use of general endotracheal anesthesia, which is easier and safer when the child has reached this age. It is desirable to complete the palate repair by the time the child begins meaningful attempts at speech. If the repair is unduly delayed, the child develops faulty speech habits that are difficult to correct later with speech therapy.[14]

The operations utilized to repair a palatal cleft vary, but the older techniques are designed to close the medial cleft with the aid of bilateral relaxing incisions in the palatal mucoperiosteum. This allows the soft tissues of the hard and soft palates to be shifted to the midline and sutured to one another. In recent operations, lengthening or retrodisplacement of the levator muscles of the soft palate by local soft tissue flaps is emphasized. Elevation and mobilization of mucoperiosteal flaps from the oral surface of the hard palate allow both a pushing back and lengthening of the soft tissues. Pushing-back procedures

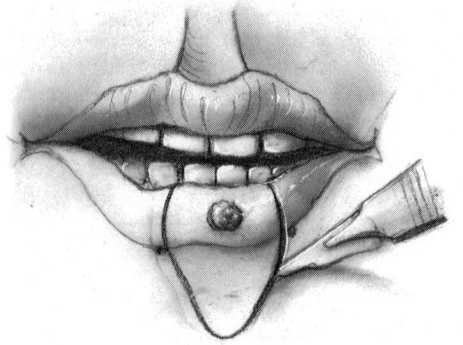
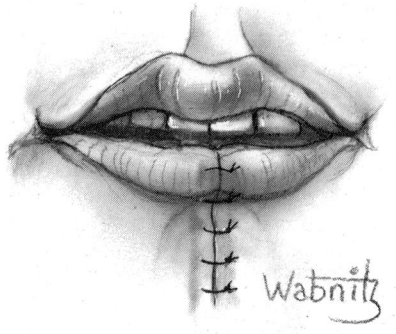

Figure 6. Small squamous carcinoma of lower lip treated by V-excision with direct closure. (From Lore, J. M., Jr.: An Atlas of Head and Neck Surgery, 2nd ed. Philadelphia, W. B. Saunders Company, 1973.)

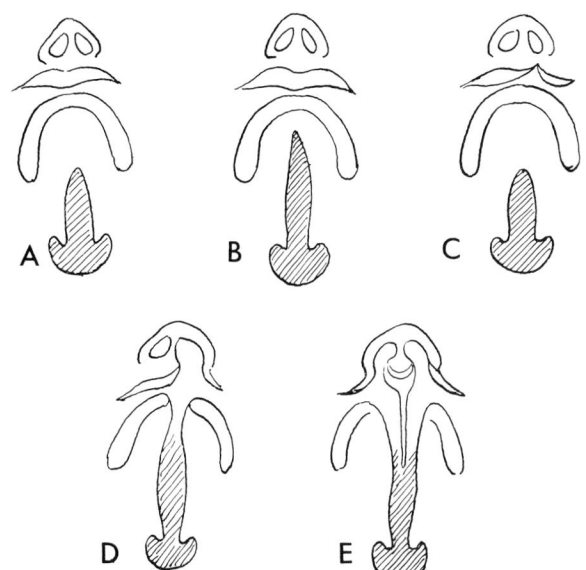

Figure 7. Classification of cleft palate (after Kernahan and Stark, 1958). The division between primary palate (prolabium, premaxilla, and anterior septum) and secondary palate is the incisive foramen. *A,* Incomplete cleft of the secondary palate. *B,* Complete cleft of the secondary palate (extending as far as the incisive foramen). *C,* Incomplete cleft of the primary and secondary palate. *D,* Unilateral complete cleft of the primary and secondary palate. *E,* Bilateral complete cleft of the primary and secondary palate. (From Converse, J. M. *In* Converse, J. M. (Ed.): Reconstructive Plastic Surgery. Vol. 3. Philadelphia, W. B. Saunders Company, 1984.)

require incisions in the mucous membranes on the nasal surface of the palate. These create open defects in the mucous membrane of the floor of the nose, which, if left to heal by cicatrization and epithelialization, contract and cause postoperative shortening of the palate, partially negating the pushing-back procedure. Operations incorporating island flaps, the Z-plasty principle, or flaps of pharyngeal mucosa have now been designed to close these defects on the nasal surface of the repaired palates.

Flaps of mucosa and muscle may be elevated from the posterior pharyngeal wall and attached to the posterior aspect of the soft palate to form a bridge of tissue across the velopharyngeal space. This reduces the velopharyngeal opening and provides a posterior point of fixation for the pushed-back palate. This procedure is known as a posterior pharyngeal flap. More intricate muscle-plasty operations may be used to selectively reposition the levator veli palatine muscles more posteriorly within the soft palate in order to obtain a better mechanical advantage for elevation of the dome of the soft palate during speech.[17]

Cleft palate surgery is *exacting* and *demanding.* Each patient's repair should be individualized.

PIERRE ROBIN SYNDROME. This congenital anomaly is characterized by a small mandible, retrodisplacement of the chin, and consequent posterior displacement and ptosis of the tongue into the hypopharynx, producing upper airway obstruction. It was described in 1923 by the French stomatologist Pierre Robin, who emphasized its frequent fatal termination.[50] Clefts of the secondary palate are found in 40 per cent of children with this syndrome. The exact etiology is unknown. Many believe the retrognathia is due to intrauterine pressure against the chin caused by sharp flexion of the head downward and forward, delaying anterior development of the mandible. The degree of airway obstruction varies from minimal to quite severe. Infants with greater degrees of airway obstruction expend all of their energy in breathing and cannot eat without choking. Without treatment, they rapidly die from exhaustion or sudden respiratory obstruction. Only the mildest forms should be treated by positioning (the child is maintained on his side or in a prone

position and is fed with the head held in a vertical, upright position) or by nasoesophageal tube feeding. If the child has even *one* well-documented episode of cyanosis, surgical intervention becomes urgent. Tracheotomy in the neonate has a high morbidity and may be avoided by several operations that relieve the obstruction by fixing the tongue forward to the lip, hypoplastic mandible, or hyoid by the use of adhesions, sutures, or strips of fascia.[18,32,36,44] The ultimate growth potential of these hypoplastic mandibles is unpredictable. Most develop to approximately normal size; others may require later secondary corrective surgery.

TORUS PALATINUS. This relatively common and usually insignificant lesion is an exostosis in the midline of the hard palate. It is occasionally seen in newborns but is more common after adolescence. Of major significance is that it is occasionally mistaken for a neoplasm. The enlarged nodule of bone is usually symmetrically distributed on both sides of the midline and is covered with normal mucosa. Excision is advised if there is chronic irritation of the overlying mucosa or if a full upper denture is to be worn.

RANULA. A ranula is a thin-walled, bluish retention cyst located beneath the tongue in the anterior floor of the oral cavity. It follows obstruction of a mucous gland or one of the sublingual salivary glands. Ranulas are filled with a thick, crystal-clear, mucoid fluid. They are soft and fluctuant but not painful, and they are usually unilateral and form slowly. They occasionally rupture spontaneously but then usually recur. Treatment consists of marsupialization of the cyst by excision of a generous segment of its anterior superior wall and suturing of the remaining posterior cyst wall to the mucous membrane of the floor of the surrounding oral cavity. Because of the thinness of the walls of these cysts, excision by enucleation is nearly impossible, and the attempt may lead to obstruction of the ipsilateral Wharton's duct.

Injuries

BURNS (THERMAL TRAUMA). Thermal and electrical burns are rarely seen within the oral cavity beyond the lips and tongue tip. Chemical burns of the oral, palatal, or lingual mucosa due to the accidental or suicidal ingestion of caustics or acids are occasionally seen. These should be immediately treated with copious and prolonged water irrigation, systemic steroids, elevation of the patient's head, nothing by mouth and parenteral alimentation, and penicillin. Rapidly developing edema may necessitate a tracheotomy; surgical therapy is reserved for late sequelae and contractures. The oral mucous membrane has a remarkable capacity for rapid healing.

LACERATIONS. Because of the extreme vascularity of the cheeks, tongue, and mouth, bleeding from lacerations is usually profuse. Hemorrhage is best controlled initially by digital pressure and packing. The application of multiple hemostats in deep lacerations of the cheeks and floor of the mouth to control bleeding in an emergency room is unnecessary and may frequently cause damage to branches of the facial, trigeminal, lingual, or hypoglossal nerve, or to one of the major salivary ducts. Local anesthetic agents containing vasoconstrictor pharmacologic agents (epinephrine 1 : 100,000) are recommended for use within the mouth. Adequate lighting, good assistance and anesthesia, and proper instruments are indispensable for efficient repair of intraoral lacerations. After hemostasis is obtained, the membranes are loosely approximated with a proper suture material. Plain catgut sutures rupture after a few days in the mouth and should not be used. Chromic catgut or polyglycolic acid sutures last for several weeks and do not require later removal. Silk sutures are excellent for repair of intraoral lacerations, but require subsequent removal. Monofilament nylon and wire sutures are stiff, bristly, and uncomfortable and should not be used within the mouth.

DISLODGED TEETH. Recently loosened or dislodged permanent teeth should not be discarded. They can be replaced in an intact alveolar bone socket and wired in place with a high percentage of tooth survival. If the root canal of the tooth is treated and filled prior to replacement or shortly thereafter, tooth survival approaches 95 per cent. These free dental grafts are exposed to a traumatized, contaminated oral cavity and should be protected with prophylactic penicillin therapy.

CHRONIC TRAUMA. Chronic trauma to the lining tissues of the oral cavity may induce reactive hyperkeratosis or leukoplakia. If prolonged, this may lead to dyskeratosis with dissolution of the epithelial basement membrane and even to the development of epidermoid cancer. Irritants such as smoke, snuff, chewing tobacco, strong condiments, alcohol, oral trauma from various dental sources, hot spicy foods, allergy, galvanism, and lesions secondary to avitaminosis A have all been incriminated in the development of oral leukoplakia. Reactive patches appear as grayish white plaques on the epithelial membrane. Initial treatment consists of identification and elimination of all irritant factors. If the lesion does not disappear within 2 weeks, it should be surgically excised and biopsied. The defect may be closed or grafted. Long periods of "watchful waiting" are definitely contraindicated and may allow the development of invasive carcinoma.

Infections Requiring Surgical Therapy

The greatest number of infections within the oral cavity are odontogenic in origin. Lacerations of the soft tissues or fractures of the maxilla or mandible represent only a small percentage of infections. Extension of infection from an obstructed salivary gland or blood-borne septic emboli from infection elsewhere in the body are unusual. Most oral cavity infections arise from periapical or periodontal infection. They may be associated with cysts, root fragments, or pericoronal pockets.

The bacteria found in infections of the oral cavity are characteristically mixtures of the same organisms that comprise the oral flora — unless the flora have been altered by previous antibiotic therapy. Nearly all are penicillin-sensitive. Fungal infections (i.e., actinomycosis) are slow in development and progression. Some are difficult to diagnose; biopsies and special culture techniques may be required.

Anatomically, bacterial infections of the oral cavity may extend into the sublingual area, the mental and submental areas, the buccal space, the submandibular or submaxillary areas, the pterygomandibular space, the peripharyngeal space, the zygomaticotemporal space, or the fascial planes of the neck. Massive infections may threaten the airway and necessitate a tracheotomy.

A much feared complication of maxillary or mandibular infection is cavernous sinus thrombophlebitis. Veins of the upper jaw drain via the anterior facial vein or pterygoid plexus into the ophthalmic veins and then into the cavernous sinus.

Septic phlebitis in the lower jaw may spread along the inferior dental vein into the pterygoid plexus and then by way of the ophthalmic veins or the vein of Vesalius to the cavernous sinus. Surprisingly, fatal cavernous sinus thrombosis arising from the infections in the lower jaw has been reported with twice the frequency of that arising from infections in the upper jaw.[5] Treatment is by massive intravenous doses of antibiotics and by anticoagulants. The causative abscess should, of course, be drained.

In general, the treatment of bacterial oral cavity infection consists initially of large doses of antibiotics. A high circulating antibiotic blood level is desirable prior to manipulation or drainage of the abscess. Relatively small collections such as gumboil or pericoronal abscess may be drained into the mouth. Larger abscess extensions require external incisions through a line of election beneath the mandible in a dependent position. Drainage is maintained by a rubber or gauze drain left in the wound for several days.

Benign Tumors of the Mouth

Nonmalignant tumors or abnormal growths within the soft tissues of the oral cavity arise most frequently from the gingival tissues or the mucoperiosteal membrane of the alveolar processes of the maxilla or mandible. These include fibromas, hyperplasia, pyogenic granulomas, hemangiomas, gingival hyperplasia caused by phenytoin, peripheral giant cell tumors, and neuromas. Second in frequency are the hyperplasias of the lining mucosa of the cheeks and lips from chronic trauma. Third in frequency are benign tumors found on or beneath the mucosa of the cheek; these include fibromas, fibropapillomas, lipomas, hemangiomas, mixed tumors, and traumatic neuromas. Fourth in the order of frequency are benign growths on the palate, including fibromas, fibropapillomas, acute inflammatory papillary hyperplasia, and mixed tumors. The least common site in the oral cavity for the occurrence of nonmalignant tumors is the floor of the mouth, where mixed tumors, myxofibromas, and dermoid cysts may be found.

Most benign tumors of the oral cavity are readily diagnosed by observation, palpation, and radiographic studies. When the diagnosis is not readily made by these means, biopsy is indicated. When diagnosed, all benign oral cavity tumors should be treated by simple surgical excision. Radiotherapy has no role in treatment, and excised surgical specimens should always be examined microscopically by a competent pathologist for confirmation of the diagnosis.

Malignant Neoplasms of the Soft Tissues of the Oral Cavity

SARCOMA. This rare neoplasm, which occurs on the lips and cheeks, may mimic a benign tumor. It usually appears as a firm growth with an intact mucosal covering and is frequently seen many (12 to 15) years after radiotherapy to an earlier squamous cancer of the area. Biopsy is usually diagnostic. Treatment is wide surgical excision. Most sarcomas are resistant to irradiation; neck dissection is only rarely indicated.

ADENOCARCINOMA. Adenocarcinomas occur in the mouth more frequently than sarcomas. They arise in *minor* salivary glands in the soft tissues of the oral cavity, and they often pursue a more malignant course than their counterparts that arise from the *major* salivary glands. Because of their submucosal location, they exfoliate few cells, and cytologic studies of oral cavity washings are of little help in diagnosis. Adenocystic carcinoma, sometimes referred to as cylindroma, shows a marked invasive tendency and characteristically spreads widely along nerve sheaths. There are frequent local recurrences of the tumor with time unless extremely wide resection is performed at the *initial* attempt at cure.

EPIDERMOID CARCINOMA. By far the most frequent malignant neoplasm of the oral cavity is squamous cell carcinoma. It constitutes 95 to 97 per cent of all malignant lesions. In 1968, carcinoma of the buccal cavity and pharynx represented 2 per cent of mortality from all forms of cancer in the United States. Carcinoma of the oral cavity is best considered anatomically by region and it is usually a disease of elderly white men, many of whom have a history of excessive use of tobacco or alcohol.

FLOOR OF THE MOUTH. Fifteen per cent of oral cavity cancers arise in the crescent-shaped area bounded anteriorly by the inferior dental arch and posteriorly by the inferior surface of the tongue.[1] Squamous cell carcinoma represents nearly all lesions located in this area; the average age for development of floor of the mouth carcinoma is 60 years. Ninety-seven per cent of carcinomas in this area occur in males,[7] although the male-to-female ratio has recently decreased. Moore and Catlin suggest that because of its dependent position the floor of the mouth has longer periods of contact with saliva that may be laden with topical carcinogens. This may lead to carcinoma. It often arises close to one of the submaxillary gland ducts (Wharton's). Patients may first be seen when they notice a submaxillary mass that is diagnosed as a duct obstruction or a nodal metastasis.

Carcinoma in this area usually presents as an infiltrative lesion with a fissure-like penetrating ulceration. Spread is rapid, involving the contralateral side of the floor of the mouth and the mandible. The tongue may be involved, and this may make it difficult to determine the exact origin of the tumor. Assessment of the extent and staging of the tumor are best done by bimanual palpation. Carcinoma of the floor of the mouth frequently presents with metastases already present in the submaxillary nodes. These are the primary drainage sites,[1] but subsequent spread to the deep cervical nodes is frequent. Biopsy is easily accomplished and is always indicated before instituting radical surgery or irradiation therapy. Radiographs of the mandible are indicated to determine bony involvement. CT scanning is helpful in assessing tumor extent and at times will detect nodal metastasis.

Treatment of carcinoma of the floor of the mouth must be varied according to the size and stage of the primary tumor. Smaller primaries away from the mandible are well controlled with either radiation therapy or surgical excision, but patient morbidity is less with surgery and cure rate may be somewhat higher. Larger primaries that encroach upon or involve the mandible are best treated by a composite resection of the floor of the mouth, partial mandibulectomy, and *en bloc* neck dissection. Regardless of the treatment of the primary lesion, a neck dissection with removal of cervical lymph nodes should be performed on the ipsilateral side of the lesion. When the tumor goes beyond the midline, or when positive nodes are found on the ipsilateral side, the neck dissection should be extended by adding a supraomohyoid dissection of the lymphatics of the contralateral side of the neck. Experience has shown that when neck dissection is not performed at time of treatment of the primary, in 50 per cent of all patients with carcinoma of the floor of the mouth nodal metastases will develop in the neck within the first year of follow-up.[38] Thus, treatment by neck dissection at the time of resection of the primary tumor is often advisable, even in the absence of clinically suspicious nodes. The prognosis for 5-year survival with no evidence of disease is 60 per cent in the absence of palpable nodes in the neck. The presence of positive nodes at the time of initial treatment reduces the incidence to 30 per cent.

BUCCAL MUCOSA. The lining of the cheeks extending from the upper to the lower gingivobuccal gutters and from the oral commissures posteriorly to the ascending ramus of the mandible gives rise to 10 per cent of oral cavity cancer. Cancer in this area is more frequent in the older age groups, with the mean age in the seventies. It is nine times as frequent in males as in females.[7] Certain chronic irritants such as the use of chewing tobacco or betel nut have been shown to be causative.[1] Carcinoma in this area is preceded by clinically detectable leukoplakia more frequently than is carcinoma in any other part of the oral cavity.[7] Squamous cancer in the buccal mucosa also tends to be better differentiated; it grows more slowly and has a lower rate of nodal metastasis than cancer of the floor of the mouth or tongue. Nodal metastases usually occur first in the submaxillary and upper cervical nodes (Levels I to III). The primary lesions are usually painless exophytic growths or ulcerations of the mucosa that develop in areas of leukoplakia or hyperkeratosis. Diagnosis is by direct inspection, bimanual palpation, and biopsy. Treatment for early lesions is surgical excision and reconstruction. Radiation therapy yields a somewhat lower cure rate. The exophytic, verrucous lesion offers a much more favorable prognosis than the deeply ulcerating endophytic type. Adequate surgical resection sometimes requires excision of the overlying skin of the external cheek, so that a through-and-through cheek defect is produced. Immediate flap reconstruction should be performed to reduce cosmetic deformity

and functional impairment, i.e., fistula, drooling speech, and eating problems, or trismus. For smaller lesions that involve only the mucosa, a thick skin graft, which may be secured by a tie-on bolus at the time of operation, is adequate reconstruction. For larger lesions such as those that involve the mandible or skin of the cheek, reconstruction by a pedicle and skin flap (from a cervical, deltopectoral, or forehead donor site) is usually indicated. In some patients with prior irradiation injury, a musculocutaneous major flap or even a free flap may be more appropriate. The determinate 5-year survival (all methods of treatment) is approximately 43 per cent.[1]

GINGIVAE AND HARD PALATE. Squamous carcinoma is surprisingly rare in the hard palate. It is also infrequent in the upper gingiva, but fairly common along the lower gingiva, where it represents 12 per cent of all oral cavity cancer.[7] There is no difference in the incidence between the sexes; the average age of patients with gingival carcinomas is 60. Characteristically, the tumor is a well-differentiated carcinoma in the molar area. Nodal metastases develop in 40 to 65 per cent of these patients.[22] Patients usually first complain of difficulty in wearing dentures or pain on mastication, or they may notice blood-streaked saliva. Biopsy and mandibular and maxillary radiographs are indispensable diagnostic procedures.

Surgical therapy is the preferred method for treatment for gingival and palatal carcinoma. All but the earliest gingival lesions involve bone, and cancer in bone is extremely difficult to cure with any form of irradiation.[17] Some surgeons precede operation for gingival carcinoma with a course of irradiation, believing that this reduces the incidence of tumor exfoliation and implantation.[33] Palatal carcinoma is usually of salivary gland origin and is relatively radioresistant. Because adequate excision of lower gingival carcinoma involves at least a rim mandibulectomy or partial mandibulectomy, the deep tissue planes of the upper portion of the neck must be opened. Thus, a neck dissection should be performed at least on the ipsilateral side at the time of resection of the primary tumor. In older patients, a tracheostomy is routinely performed to avoid low-grade anoxia and cardiac problems in the postoperative period. In surgical resections of palatal and upper gingival carcinomas, if there are no clinically palpable nodes in the neck, an expectant, careful follow-up without neck dissection is justified, although 5-year survival is only 25 to 35 per cent.

MALIGNANT NEOPLASMS OF THE TONGUE. Malignant neoplasms of the tongue usually arise from the mucosa and are mainly epidermoid carcinomas. Those of the posterior third of the tongue are similar to oropharyngeal lesions. Tongue carcinoma represents approximately 15 per cent of all cases of malignant disease of the head and neck. Eighty per cent of cases of tongue cancer occur in males.[21] Tongue carcinoma is unusual in individuals under age 40 and has a peak incidence in those around age 60. Chronic alcoholism, heavy use of tobacco, poor oral hygiene, syphilis, and the Plummer-Vinson syndrome are known etiologic factors. Premalignant changes of leukoplakia and erythroplasia frequently precede the development of tongue cancer. Clinically, carcinoma of the tongue usually presents as a chronic nonhealing, painless ulcer. Small lesions can be accurately assessed; however, as the lesion grows and infiltrates muscle, judgment of tumor extent becomes more difficult. Restriction of tongue movement is an indication of deep muscular invasion.

Early involvement of submaxillary and digastric nodes with metastases is frequently seen. Biopsy, cultures of the lesion, and radiographs of the mandible and chest are essential diagnostic aids. Ninety-five per cent of all malignant neoplasms of the tongue are epidermoid carcinoma.[1,7] Adenocarcinoma is occasionally seen. Sarcoma and metastatic carcinoma to the tongue from a distant primary are rare.

In the treatment of carcinoma of the tongue, it should be remembered that in *half of all patients with nonpalpable nodes in*

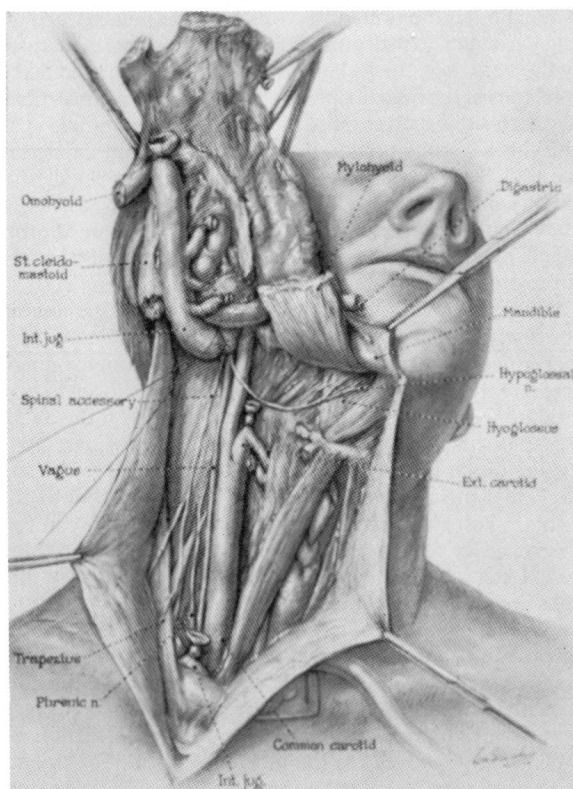

Figure 8. Drawing showing the extent of the usual radical neck dissection. The specimen is retracted superiorly. As is shown, resection of the posterior belly of the digastric muscle permits high ligation of the internal jugular vein and also facilitates dissection around the hypoglossal nerve. (From Edgerton, M. T., and DeVito, R. T. *In* Converse, J. M. (Ed.): Reconstructive Plastic Surgery. Vol. 3. Philadelphia, W. B. Saunders Company, 1964.)

the neck, metastasis to these nodes has already occurred at the time of diagnosis, regardless of the size of the primary lesion.[22] Therefore, resection of a tongue carcinoma should always include an *en bloc* neck dissection at least on the side of the lesion (Fig. 8). For many years, the senior author has routinely performed *bilateral* neck dissections (in two stages — or saving one internal jugular vein) in *all* patients with cancer of the tongue. This is justified when one realizes that 68 per cent of all patients with tongue cancer ultimately have *bilateral* affected cervical nodes.

In the case of larger primary lesions or lesions approaching or encroaching upon the midline, a staged, bilateral neck dissection is undertaken with even less hesitation. If the mandible is eroded by tumor or adherent to the primary, a composite resection, including hemiglossectomy, partial mandibulectomy, and neck dissection, is indicated. The treatment of lymph node metastasis in the neck is primarily surgical. The most frequent reason for failure in the treatment of tongue cancer is too limited a resection of the primary tongue lesion and failure to adequately clear the nodal drainage areas early in the course of the disease. The overall 5-year survival for carcinoma of the oral tongue is approximately 40 per cent and has improved in recent years with bolder resections of the tongue. Immediate flap reconstruction of the tongue and floor of the mouth with a cervical apron flap provides excellent function and leaves any tongue remnant mobile for speech and swallowing.[18]

OROPHARYNX. This region lies between the nasopharynx and the hypopharynx. It includes the soft palate, pharyngeal walls, tonsils, lingual tonsil (when present), and posterior third of the tongue. Carcinoma here occurs predominantly in males, with a peak incidence in those about 60 years old. The tonsil is the most common primary site, and carcinoma of the tonsil represents 10 per cent of all head and neck cancers.[7] Pain on swallowing, frequently referred to the ear (otalgia), is a common presenting complaint. An enlarging upper cervical mass (jugulodigastric lymph nodes) beneath the angle of the mandible is

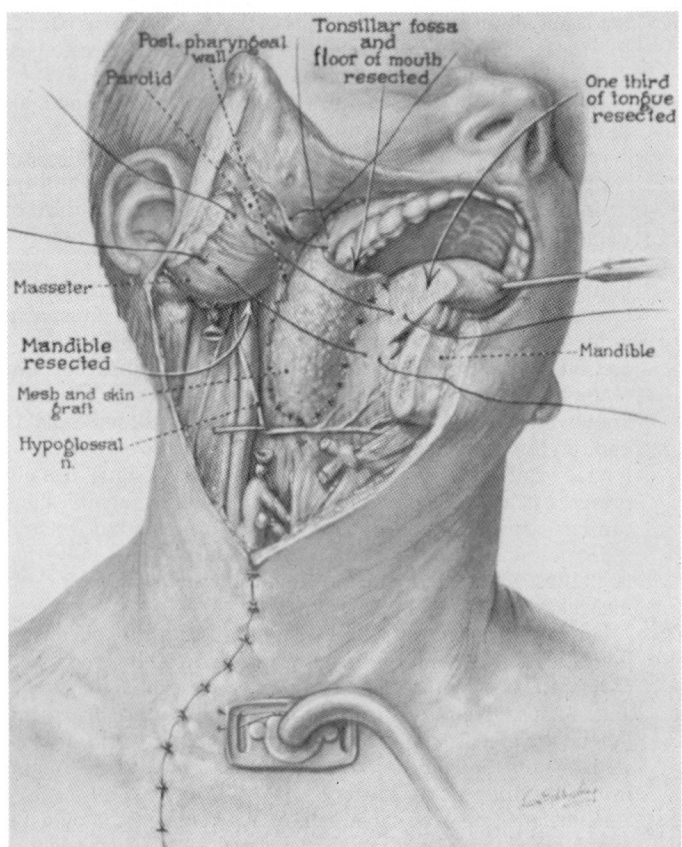

Figure 9. Drawing demonstrating the technique used for large posterior defects. The split-thickness skin graft is mounted on a framework of tantalum mesh and sutured into place. A vascular bed for the graft is provided by adjacent tissue such as a cervical flap or masseter muscle. A tie-on dressing is applied intraorally so that firm contact is maintained between the graft and its bed. (From Edgerton, M. T., and DeVito, R. T. *In* Converse, J. M. (Ed.): Reconstructive Plastic Surgery. Vol. 3. Philadelphia, W. B. Saunders Company, 1964.)

frequently noted. In addition to palpation, direct and indirect laryngoscopy is diagnostically useful. Histologically, carcinoma in this region is usually squamous cell carcinoma more undifferentiated than that found elsewhere in the oral cavity.[1] Lymphosarcoma also is frequently seen in this lymphoid-rich area of Waldeyer's ring.

The highest reported cure rates in the treatment of oropharyngeal carcinoma have been by radical surgical extirpation of the primary cancer, with a composite resection that includes a partial mandibulectomy and *en bloc* dissection of the neck with primary skin graft or flap (in the case of patients with prior irradiation of the area) reconstruction (Fig. 9). Some patients (especially those with lymphosarcomas) are treated by radiation therapy alone or by combinations of these modalities.[31] Oropharyngeal carcinomas frequently cross the midline in the areas of the soft palate and base of the tongue, making the operation less feasible and providing the indication for bilateral neck dissections in order to remove the most likely involved nodal drainage areas. The 5-year survival for patients with carcinoma of the oropharynx, presenting—as they usually do—with Stage 3 or Stage 4 disease, treated by any form of therapy, is distressingly low and averages approximately 20 to 30 per cent.[1]

HEAD AND NECK CANCER

Staging

Staging cancer is a means of attempting to standardize treatment and predict the probability of a patient's survival. The principal system used for head and neck cancer is the TNM system. The T is an indication of the size of the tumor; N, the extent of lymph node involvement; and M, the presence of metatastic disease. The criteria for each category using the guidelines of the American Joint Committee on Cancer are depicted in Table 1.[3] As can be seen, the size of the primary tumor and the presence of lymph node metastases are important quantities for staging.

There has been controversy surrounding this system, however, because of its lack of precision in defining prognosis for the individual patient. Current investigation of additional factors that may be important is currently under way. Histologically, the grade of tumor (nondifferentiated versus well differentiated), depth of invasion, and histologic evidence of vascular and neural invasion have all been found to affect overall outcome. Recently, the importance of "killer cell" activity and other parameters of immune response has been noted.[52] These and other avenues may provide better staging for these patients.

Neck Dissection

Head and neck cancer frequently leads to metastatic spread to regional lymph nodes. Removal of lymph nodes by neck dissection is required. Crile in 1906 first described and later Martin in 1931 championed an *en bloc* resection. This procedure involves complete removal of the primary tumor and the intervening lymphatic system between this primary and any metastatic neck disease. The lymph nodes of the neck are distributed over the surface of the submaxillary glands and along the jugular vein. Martin thought that in order to achieve complete removal of the cervical nodes, the submental and submaxillary glands, the jugular vein, and the sternocleidomastoid muscle had to be sacrificed along with the spinal accessory nerve. This is the classic "radical neck dissection."

Removal of the jugular vein and spinal accessory nerve in this operation causes significant morbidity. This is especially true when *bilateral* simultaneous neck dissections are performed, because sacrificing both internal jugular veins may cause severe facial edema. Another issue is whether an N_0 neck (i.e., without evidence of disease) should be subjected to a "prophylactic" radical neck dissection. It is now appreciated that certain

TABLE 1. Criteria for Staging Head and Neck Cancer (American Joint Committee on Cancer)

Primary tumor (T)

T_X: Minimal requirements to assess the primary tumor cannot be met
T_0: No evidence of primary tumor
T_{is}: Carcinoma *in situ*
T_1: Greatest diameter of primary tumor 2 cm. or less
T_2: Greatest diameter of primary tumor less than 4 cm.
T_3: Greatest diameter of primary tumor more than 4 cm.
T_4: Massive tumor more than 4 cm. in diameter with deep invasion to involve antrum, pterygoid muscles, base of tongue, skin of neck

Nodal Involvement (N)

N_X: Minimal requirements to assess the regional nodes cannot be met
N_0: No clinically positive node
N_1: Single clinically positive homolateral node 3 cm. or less in diameter
N_2: Single clinically positive homolateral node more than 3 cm. but less than 6 cm. in diameter or multiple clinically positive homolateral nodes, none more than 6 cm. in diameter
N_{2a}: Single clinically positive homolateral node more than 3 cm. but less than 6 cm. in diameter
N_{2b}: Multiple clinically positive homolateral nodes, none more than 6 cm. in diameter
N_{3a}: Clinically positive homolateral node(s), one more than 6 cm. in diameter
N_{3b}: Bilateral clinically positive nodes (in this situation, each side of the neck should be staged separately, i.e., N_{3b}: right, N_{2a}; left, N_1)
N_{3c}: Contralateral clinically positive node(s) only

Tumor Metastasis (M)

M_0: No metastases present
M_1: Metastases clinically demonstrable

Stage Grouping

Stage I: $T_1N_0M_0$
Stage II: $T_2N_0M_0$
Stage III: $T_3N_0M_0$
$\qquad T_1T_2T_3$; N_1M_0
Stage IV: T_4N_0 or N_1M_0
$\qquad$ Any T, N_2 or N_3, M_0
$\qquad$ Any T, any N, M_1

cancers (i.e., skin and thyroid) lead to early metastatic disease in areas that cannot be extirpated by the radical neck dissection.

As a result of controversy and clinical experience, the concept of the "modified" neck dissection has arisen. Unfortunately, the term *modified* is imprecise, because it is applied to almost *any* variance from the standard neck dissection. This variance includes anything from saving the eleventh cranial nerve to adding a subtotal parotidectomy to the procedure if indicated by the location of tumor.

The "functional" neck dissection is a modification of the radical neck dissection first championed by Boca. This procedure completely removes neck lymph nodes *and the submaxillary gland* while preserving the jugular vein and the eleventh nerve. The current indications for this procedure are controversial. Many suggest that it is an adequate means of managing an N_0 neck when the likelihood of cervical metastasis is not high.

Current efforts and long-term follow-up results are directed to better definition of the nomenclature and indications for various modified neck dissections. Many types of head and neck cancer are controlled in the neck regions by neck dissections that correlate with the biology of the tumor. For example, papillary thyroid cancer is rarely an indication for a classic complete radical neck dissection.

Reconstruction

In the 45 years since World War II, the most significant recent advance in treatment of patients with head and neck cancer has been the development of a series of new flaps and flap techniques that permit immediate reconstruction of the defect created by tumor removal. The concept of the myocutaneous circulatory unit, together with the parallel development of microsurgical techniques for free flap transfers, has provided further options for soft tissue reconstruction. These techniques allow the immediate transfer of large islands of full-thickness skin along with subcutaneous fat in single operations. Blood supply is based on direct perforating vessels from a subjacent muscle.[39] To a large extent, they reduced the need for lengthy, costly, and less reliable "delay" techniques, which were often necessary in earlier years in the preparation of random skin pedicle flaps for transfer.

Reconstruction of the oropharyngeal area often requires the replacement of multiple layers of tissue (intraoral mucosa, external skin, and even portions of the mandible). Flaps, in addition, need to be sufficiently thin to fit into this region without bulk that limits function.

Myocutaneous flaps such as the pectoralis major and trapezius flaps are useful in head and neck reconstruction. They, however, are often bulky, may cause tethering in the neck, and may leave some degree of donor site morbidity.

Several donor sites for microvascular free-flap transfer have been used.[45] Fasciocutaneous flaps such as the radial artery forearm flap or the lateral (tensor fascia lata muscle) leg flap allow the surgeon to transpose a large amount of relatively thin tissue to the oropharyngeal region. However, these flaps are sometimes still bulky and create substantial donor site morbidity. The jejunum has also been successfully transferred to reconstruct intraoral and pharyngeal regions, allowing the transfer of mucosa to line the upper gastrointestinal tract. A major disadvantage of this method, however, is that it requires entering the abdomen during the time of reconstruction.

Thus, although much progress has been made in reconstructing these defects over the past two decades, an active search for improved methods continues.

NON-MALIGNANT TONGUE LESIONS

Congenital Malformations and Developmental Anomalies

THYROGLOSSAL DUCT CYSTS. The pyramidal lobe of the thyroid gland arises from a median pharyngeal diverticulum during embryogenesis. The tongue, which develops later, surrounds the opening of this diverticulum at the foramen cecum. Normally the diverticulum becomes obliterated, and all but the lower portion is reabsorbed. Failure of obliteration of the diverticulum at any point along its course from the base of the tongue to the thyroid gland may cause formation of a thyroglossal duct cyst. This situation is very similar to the development of a hydrocele at any level of the spermatic cord and testicle. The hyoid bone develops after the diverticulum is formed and may pass behind, in front of, or around the diverticulum. Clinically, patients present with a midline cystic mass in the neck, which may steadily enlarge or fluctuate in size. These cysts usually appear before adulthood, and one third are seen in children under 10 years of age. The cysts are usually freely movable beneath the platysma and strap muscles and are not tender. If spontaneous perforation or previous surgical drainage of the cyst has occurred, a thyroglossal duct sinus tract may be present. Treatment is by total excision of the cyst and the entire thyroglossal duct tract. This may be facilitated by injecting the cyst with aqueous methylene blue dye. If infection is present, the cyst should be drained and excised several weeks later. Complete excision of the tract is essential and may require resection of the central portion of the hyoid bone. The tract must then be followed and completely removed through the base of the tongue.

LINGUAL THYROID. Failure of descent of the midline pharyngeal diverticulum or of the two lateral diverticula from the fourth pharyngeal pouches may cause thyroid tissue to remain in the base of the tongue. This is mentioned only to caution against resection of a mass of reddish brown thyroid tissue from the base of the tongue without first making sure that other thyroid tissue is present in its normal position beneath the strap muscles.

ANKYLOGLOSSIA. *Ankyloglossia* and *tongue-tied* are terms applied to a short lingual frenulum. If severe, this condition may cause an infant to have difficulty in nursing and may subsequently cause a speech impediment. The condition is readily treated by splitting the frenular band longitudinally, cutting one limb of a Z-plasty from each side, and transposing the two flaps. Local anesthesia is quite effective in children over the age of 8 years.

MEDIAN RHOMBOID GLOSSITIS. This condition, sometimes termed grooved tongue, follows embryologic failure of the lateral halves of the tongue to fuse before the tuberculum impar becomes interposed between them, just anterior to the circumvallate papillae. This leads to a rhomboid plaque of tissue that lies in the midline of the tongue immediately anterior to the circumvallate papillae. It produces no symptoms and should be recognized so that confusion with neoplastic lesions is avoided. This conditions requires no treatment.

Tongue Injuries Due to Trauma

Lacerations of the tongue bleed freely and may be difficult to expose for repair. Exposure may be facilitated by injection of local anesthetic into the tongue and passing a suture through the tip. The suture may then be used for retraction and tongue fixation. Lidocaine or procaine, containing 1:100,000 epinephrine, provides good anesthesia of adequate (90 minutes) duration and aids hemostasis. Larger bleeding vessels should be carefully grasped with hemostats and ligated with absorbable ligatures. The tongue mucosa should then be carefully approximated with silk or absorbable sutures. If catgut is used, the sutures may be placed in an inverted manner with the knots buried so that they have less tendency to untie prematurely with the constant motion of the tongue against the palate. The patient should be kept on a liquid diet for several days and advised to use a diluted mouthwash. Penicillin should be administered daily for 3 to 4 days.

Infections of the Tongue

SYPHILIS. Syphilis in the oral cavity is quite likely to involve the tongue and may present as a primary chancre or as a secondary gumma. Syphilitic glossitis is always associated with a positive serologic test for syphilis.[43] Because of numerous varieties of spirochetes normally in the mouth, darkfield examination may be misleading. Syphilitic ulcers of the tongue are frequent in the midline and near the base or tip of the tongue. They should always be biopsied to exclude a malignant neoplasm. Treatment consists of a complete course of antisyphilitic medication.

LICHEN PLANUS. This chronic disease may affect the skin and oral mucous membranes. It characteristically produces hyperkeratotic nodules with associated inflammatory changes. The lesions may appear white or bluish white and may be confused with leukoplakia. The bluish color of these white, often lacelike lesions is helpful in differentiating them from leukoplakia. Lichen planus has not definitely been associated with the development of malignant change. Spontaneous remissions may occur. Vitamin A therapy has been reported to be of value in treatment.

Benign Tumors of the Tongue

GRANULAR CELL MYOBLASTOMA. The myoblastoma is a benign, firm, usually small, spherical mass that may occur in the tongue. Although its designation implies an origin from muscle tissue, it is not invariably found in relation to striated muscle and is probably not histogenetically derived from muscle cells.

Myoblastomas probably arise from perineural fibroblasts; however, their origin remains debatable. They have no malignant potential and are readily cured by local surgical excision. When they occur submucosally, the overlying epithelium may undergo striking hyperplasia, sometimes simulating the development of carcinoma (pseudoepitheliomatous hyperplasia).[43]

LYMPHANGIOMA AND CAVERNOUS LYMPHANGIOMA. These are ecstasias of the lymph vessels. Many are present at birth as congenital collections of proliferation lymph vessels, quite like cavernous hemangiomas. When oral mucosa is involved, it shows tiny white and red tufts on the surface. This appearance is pathognomonic. Lymphangiomas may cause great enlargement of the tongue (macroglossia). Surgical excision and debulking of the tumor may be required to establish and maintain an airway, but some tongue should be left for speech, even if it contains residual lymphangioma. Use of the carbon dioxide laser scalpel in resection of these lesions greatly minimizes blood loss without adversely affecting healing at the resection margins.

AMYLOIDOSIS. This condition may present in the tongue and associated structures of the oral mucosa as submucosal, mainly perivascular deposits or as solitary multiple nodules. Macroglossia, often to a severe degree, may develop. With enlargement of the tongue, indentations of the teeth along the border become very prominent, and impaired mobility may be observed. The upper airway may become obstructed, and tracheostomy may be required. Ulcerations of the mucosa may also develop. Biopsy establishes the diagnosis. Surgical reduction of the huge tongue may greatly relieve some patients. Splitting of lip and chin with osteotomy of the mandible may provide better surgical exposure of the infiltrated tongue.

JAWS

The bony upper and lower jaws in the human are sometimes referred to as the upper maxilla and lower maxilla. Thus, when the two jaws are wired together after injury, the method is called intermaxillary fixation. More commonly, the lower maxilla is known as the mandible. The upper jaw, or maxilla, comprises several membranous bones fused together to form a single functioning unit. This includes two maxillary bones, two palatine bones, and laterally, the two zygomas that form the bony prominence of each cheek. The upper jaw is thus fixed to the base of the skull and the orbit. The external nose is attached to its anterior surface, the upper teeth emerge from its alveolar process, and the two antral cavities lie within this bony complex on either side of the nasal cavity.

The mandible is composed of heavy cortical bone arising from Meckel's cartilaginous anlage. It articulates with the base of the skull at each glenoid fossa to form the temporomandibular joints. These joints are located just anterior to each bony ear canal. Movements of the mandible are controlled by powerful muscles of mastication, and its rigid arch has a vital role as a base for movements of the tongue and elevation of the larynx in swallowing and speech. An intact arch of the mandible is critical for support of the tongue and maintenance of an adequate air passage into the trachea. Severe deformity of the mandible and chin can cause great psychologic damage to the patient.

Surgical conditions involving the jaws may be conveniently divided on the basis of etiology of deformity. Deformities may be congenital or developmental, traumatic, metabolic, infectious, or neoplastic.

CONGENITAL MALFORMATIONS AND DEVELOPMENTAL ANOMALIES

Maxilla

More than 100 syndromes involving abnormal development of the jaw have been described. Most may be greatly improved by surgical methods. Many constitute a part of the spectrum of conditions treated in the special field of craniomaxillofacial surgery.

HYPOPLASTIC CONDITIONS. These include "dishface" deformities associated with recession of the maxilla, lateral constrictions of the upper arch, and craniofacial dysostoses such as Crouzon's disease and Apert's syndrome (Fig. 10). Maxillary hypoplasias usually follow premature fusion of bony epiphyses and incomplete descent of the midface from the base of the skull. There is often an associated brachycephaly of the cranial bones and exorbitism, producing a frog-faced appearance.

Surgical correction is best accomplished by extensive osteotomies of the maxilla to bring the midface and nose forward and re-establish occlusion of the teeth. These techniques are performed in increasingly younger children (6 to 7 years of age) for improving airways, protecting the eye, helping mastication, aiding speech, and overcoming the sense of deformity before school age. Bone grafting to supplement depressed areas is often required. Recent use of small and malleable metallic (Vitallium) mini-plates has improved bone fixation.

HYPERPLASIA OF THE MAXILLA. Symmetrical or asymmetrical overgrowth of the upper jaw may occur, producing giantism or hypertrophy of the middle face. This giantism may follow congenital arteriovenous fistulas within the bone or the presence of plexiform neurofibromatosis associated with von Recklinghausen's syndrome. When the hyperplasia is symmetrical and involves the bone in the midline, it may be associated with ocular or orbital hypertelorism (Fig. 11). Paramedian clefting also produces hypertelorism. Most of these children have normal intelligence, and surgical correction is effected by doing geometric osteotomies in association with intracranial exposure to displace and protect the brain. This permits resection of excessive bone and translocation of the orbits, upper jaw, and nose as required.[23,51]

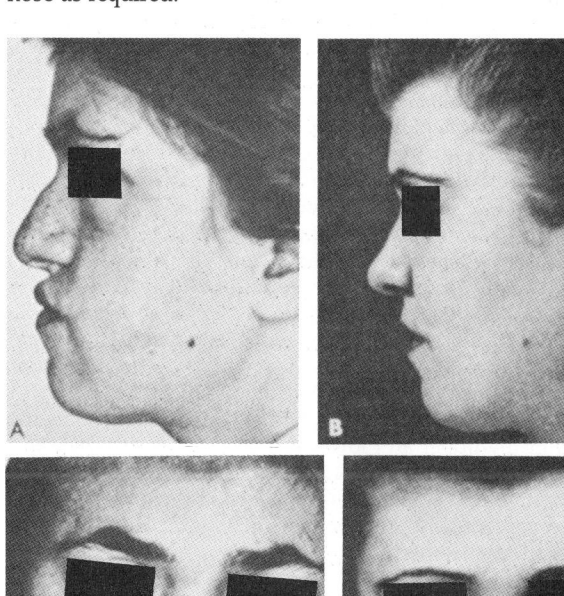
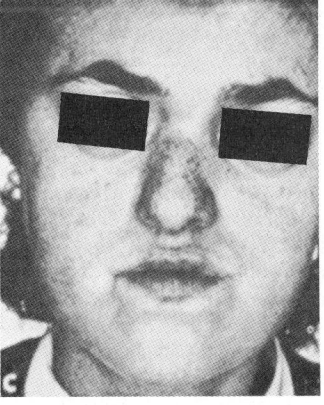
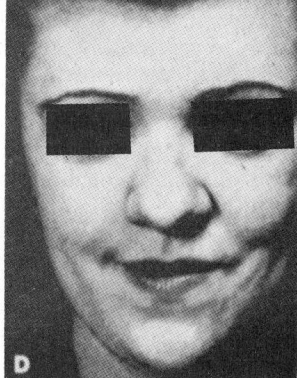

Figure 10. Surgical correction of Crouzon's disease by maxillary osteotomy and forward traction procedures. *A,* Before operation. *B,* After operation. *C,* Before operation. *D,* After operation. (From Gillies, H., and Harrison, S. H.: Br. J. Plast. Surg., *3:*123, 1950.)

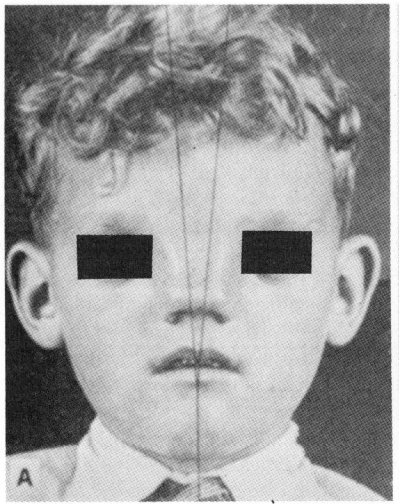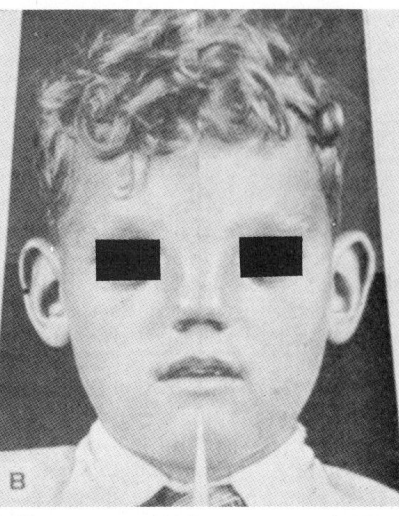

Figure 11. *A*, Hypertelorism and excessive width of the upper portion of the face. *B*, Same photograph as *A*, with central wedge removed as marked, showing a more normal head and face contour. (From Webster, J. P., and Deming, E. G.: Plast. Reconstr. Surg., *6*:1, 1950.)

Enlargement of the peripheral nerve that supplies an affected part is often seen in cases of giantism associated with neurofibromatosis. These patients should undergo surgical therapy at an early age, and total resection of the neurofibroma is both unnecessary and undesirable. Early partial nerve resection or nerve grafting may arrest the developing giantism and reduce the surgical procedure required later.

BONY CLEFTS OF THE MAXILLA. In addition to the common clefts of the upper lip and palate, patients may be seen with lateral facial clefts. These usually occupy an oblique position, radiating from the mouth in a caudal, lateral, or cephalic direction. They may open into the floor of the nose, or they may pass lateral to the nose to some point along the floor of the bony orbit. The antrum may be totally absent on one or both sides, and little bone is present beneath the eye to provide support for the globe. Rarely, patients with midline clefts of the upper or lower jaw are encountered. Some children are born with complete mandibular agnathia or absence of the premaxillary bone segment. These patients require complex surgical correction involving bone grafting and, at times, pedicle flap migration.

OTHER CONGENITAL SYNDROMES INVOLVING THE MAXILLA. These include the Byzantine arch of the hard palate with its extremely narrow and high vault. This high position of the bone causes obstruction of the nasal airway. The airway may be opened by surgical division of the bony palate, rapid orthodontic expansion of the upper jaw, and insertion of a stabilizing bone graft.

Children with one of the orofaciodigital syndromes (OFD I or II) often have constricting mucosal adhesions producing notches in the upper and lower alveolar processes. They also have lobulated tongues, small mandibles, cleft palates, and associated underdevelopment of the maxilla. Multiple reconstructive procedures on the tongue, lips, and palate are quite helpful to these children.

Mandible

HYPOPLASIA OF THE MANDIBLE (MICROGNATHIA). Micrognathia is probably most commonly seen with the Pierre Robin syndrome, consisting of symmetrical underdevelopment of the chin with breathing problems and associated clefts of the soft palate (present in 45 per cent of the patients). Other hypoplasias include asymmetrical underdevelopment of one side of the bony face and narrow lower arches with a "pointed chin," owing to lack of development of the symphysis. Lack of development of the mandibular condyles, bilaterally or unilaterally, may produce ankylosis. Very rarely, total absence (agnathia) of the lower jaw has been encountered. All of these conditions may be helped by appropriate reconstructive techniques involving osteotomies, maxillary orthopedics, bone and cartilage, and the use of implants of alloplastic materials.

HYPERPLASIA (PROGNATHISM). Mandibular overgrowth is most commonly symmetrical and causes the condition known as prognathism. This deformity usually does not become evident until late childhood or adolescence. With growth of the mandibular body and ramus, the chin and lip are carried forward to produce deformity and associated malocclusion of the teeth. Failure to correct this condition may cause a severe deformity and premature loss of dentition. Correction usually involves vertical or sagittal bilateral osteotomies of the ramus or body of the mandible with appropriate retropositioning of the chin to improve both appearance and occlusion (Fig. 12). The condition may be unilateral, bilateral, or involve simultaneous osteotomy of the maxilla to raise, lower, or tilt the occlusal plane.

Second Branchial Arch

Branchial arch anomalies produce characteristic deformities involving the middle and external ear, the mandible, the parotid gland, and at times the facial nerve. Unlike the case in Pierre Robin syndrome, the relative growth of the mandible is not expected to improve with growth and development. Instead, the deformity and the dental malocclusion become progressively more severe with increasing age. Such children often require serial augmentation of the affected mandible with bone grafts to increase length, width, and height of the jaw. Many require associated building up of the hypoplastic soft tissues in the overlying parotid region. If reconstruction is performed at an early age (the senior author does the first bone graft at 2 to 3 years of age), improved dental health and occlusion are maintained. The associated ear deformities require separate staged reconstructive techniques. In most such children middle ear reconstruction permits biaural hearing when external ear construction has been completed.

INJURIES

Most injuries to the jaw are secondary to mechanical trauma associated with falls, fights, or automobile accidents. The membranous bone that constitutes the support to the upper jaw has a great capacity to absorb force with deceleration injuries that cause blows to the face. This property of energy absorption has saved many lives by protecting the brain from lethal injury when the facial bones crumple from a severe blow.[57]

The muscles attached to the upper jaw are small and lack the strength and leverage of the muscles of mastication that insert on the mandible. Consequently, reduction of maxillary fractures does not require strong or prolonged fixation of the bone fragments after surgical reduction. The fractures usually occur in well-defined patterns located at weak points in the bones.[34] In contrast, fractures of the mandible are often accompanied by severe and increasing displacement as a result of the spasm and

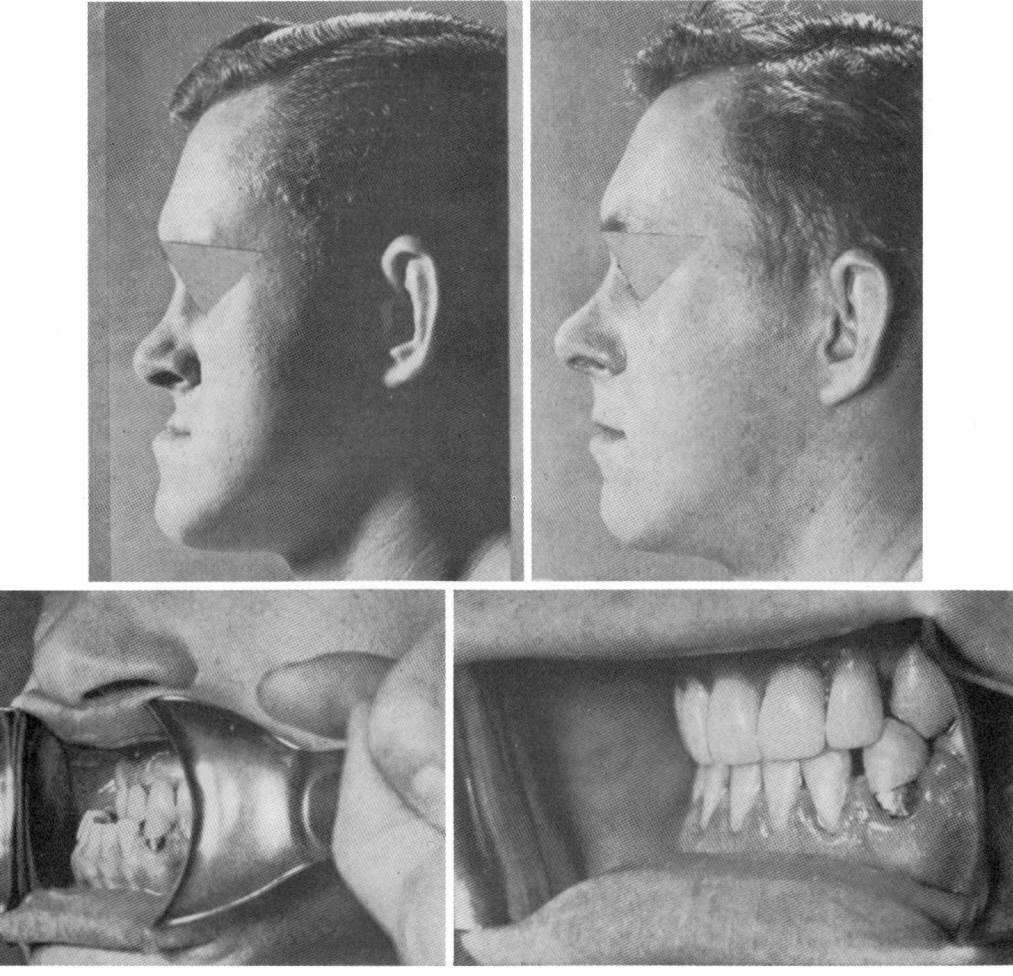

Figure 12. Surgically corrected prognathism. *Top left*, Preoperative lateral view. *Top right*, Postoperative lateral view. *Bottom left*, Preoperative malocclusion. *Bottom right*, Postoperative balanced occlusion. (From Archer, W. H.: Oral and Maxillofacial Surgery, 5th ed. Philadelphia, W. B. Saunders Company, 1975.)

pull of the strong muscles of mastication. Methods of mandibular fixation must thus be more secure and maintained for longer periods than in the case of fractures of the upper jaw.

MANDIBULAR FRACTURES

Diagnosis of fracture of the mandible is best made by physical examination. Point tenderness is usually found along the lower border of the mandible at the fracture line. Crepitus and movement of the bone fragments at this point are often noted (Fig. 13). The patient usually complains of an "abnormal" position of his teeth when he attempts to close his mouth. Numbness of the lower lip is present if the inferior alveolar nerve has also been damaged.

Several factors should be considered in judging the seriousness of the fracture and in planning the subsequent treatment. Different regions of the mandible may be fractured. The condyle, angle, ramus, symphysis, and parasymphysis are frequent sites. The orientation of the fracture line is also important. Certain fractures (with "favorable" lines of fracture) tend to be reduced by the surrounding muscles, whereas other "unfavorable" fractures are distracted by muscle spasm in the postinjury period.

Radiology is helpful in managing mandibular fractures. The most useful radiographic view is the circumferential panorex, which provides excellent visualization of the extent of most fractures and their displacements.

There are several methods of treating mandibular fractures. Simple intermaxillary wiring or elastic band fixation of the remaining teeth in the upper and lower jaws is a common means

of treating these fractures. A soft metallic bar is bent and applied to the remaining teeth in each fracture fragment of the upper and lower jaw. Small elastic bands are then looped over prongs on the arch bars and used to draw these fragments into position so that teeth mesh in their normal occlusional relationships (Fig. 14). When inadequate teeth remain for this type of stabilization, surgical open reduction may be required. The open reduction may be accomplished by either an intraoral or extraoral approach. The number of bone fragments and position of the fracture line dictate which route is chosen. For example, fractures at the angle of the mandible should have open reduction only by the extraoral route, whereas a fracture of the body of the mandible can be treated either intraorally or extraorally.

In performing a surgical open reduction, there are several useful means of fragment fixation. For many years, direct transosseous steel wire fixation has been used. In the 1980s, plastic and oral surgeons increasingly utilized mini-plates and screws made of various nonreactive materials (Vitallium, titanium, etc.) to treat complex mandibular fractures. Plastic surgeons have used open reduction increasingly, because this reduces the morbidity of mandibular fractures by eliminating or greatly reducing the period of required intermaxillary fixation.

If any patient with a jaw fracture has missing teeth that are unaccounted for at the time of initial examination, a chest film should be obtained for assurance that no teeth have been aspirated. Formerly, surgeons routinely recommended the extraction of all teeth whose roots lay within the fracture line of the jaw. It is now recognized that many of these teeth may be saved if the patient has maintained reasonable oral hygiene and if they are

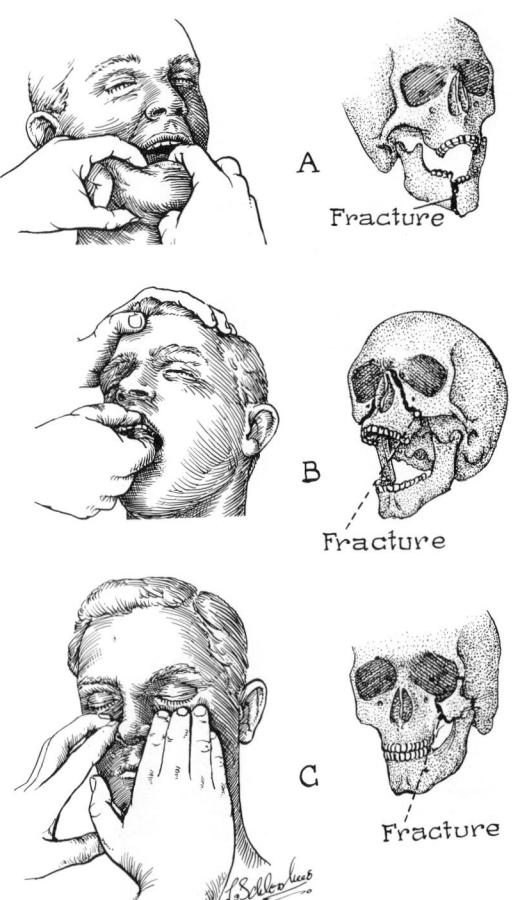

Figure 13. Manual examination for diagnosis of fractured bones of the face and jaws; careful examination with bimanual palpation reveals the majority of facial fractures. In *A*, a gentle rocking motion of the fingers reveals movement or pain at the site of fractures of the mandibular body or symphysis. In *B*, the top of the head is fixed, and an attempt is made to move the hard palate by grasping the upper central incisor teeth. Midface fractures often reveal slight movement or pain. In *C*, the examiner feels for symmetry of the infraorbital rim, or for a step or "notch" along the normal smooth lateral rim of the orbit. (From Edgerton, M. T. Fractures of the face and jaws. *In* Ballinger, W. F., II, Rutherford, R. B., and Zuidema, G. D. (Eds.): The Management of Trauma, 2nd ed. Philadelphia, W. B. Saunders Company, 1973.)

neither fractured nor grossly carious. Antibiotics are used to minimize abscess or osteomyelitis.

Elderly patients with fractures may frequently be edentulous. In such patients, immobilization by intermaxillary fixation of the prosthetic teeth in the patient's own dentures may be effective. The dentures are first fixed firmly to the upper and lower jaws by circumferential wiring or by wires placed in drilled holes in the bone. Fixation is often maintained for a longer period after fractures in an edentulous mandible, because the healing rate is often delayed when compared with that in a mandible with teeth and a larger cross section for bony contact.

External fixation devices for mandibular fractures were at one time popular. They are, however, cumbersome and often unnecessary because of other more sophisticated treatment modalities. They do have a place in compound injuries of the mandible such as gunshot wounds, where large segments of bone are missing. In patients with such injuries, an external device such as the Joe Hall Price splint can bridge this bony defect until a bone graft is added.

Under battlefield conditions, when instruments, wires, and time are all in short supply, the fractured lower jaw may be temporarily well splinted by use of a Barton head dressing. The gauze or Ace bandage goes from the vertex of the head to the occiput and then under the chin. It then repeats this order of wrapping four or five more times. This dressing avoids constriction of the airway in the upper neck.

FRACTURES OF THE MANDIBULAR CONDYLE. Most condylar fractures can be treated conservatively by simply restoring dental occlusion by elastic (rubber band) intermaxillary fixation for a 3-week period. Badly displaced fractures of the head of the condyle, especially in a young child, often require open reductions for lessening the likelihood of progressive unilateral growth arrest of one or both sides of the jaw. The external auditory canal should be carefully examined after condylar fracture; the condyle head may fracture the bony ear canal.

Temporomandibular Joint Dislocations

Dislocations of the temporomandibular joint usually occur when the head of the condyle comes forward through a tear in the anterior joint capsule. The lower jaw may be locked in an open-bite position with considerable pain and muscle spasm. Local injection with lidocaine and downward traction by firm thumb pressure on the molar teeth often reduce the dislocation. At times diazepam (Valium) is useful as a muscle relaxant, and general anesthesia is sometimes required. A history of recurrent

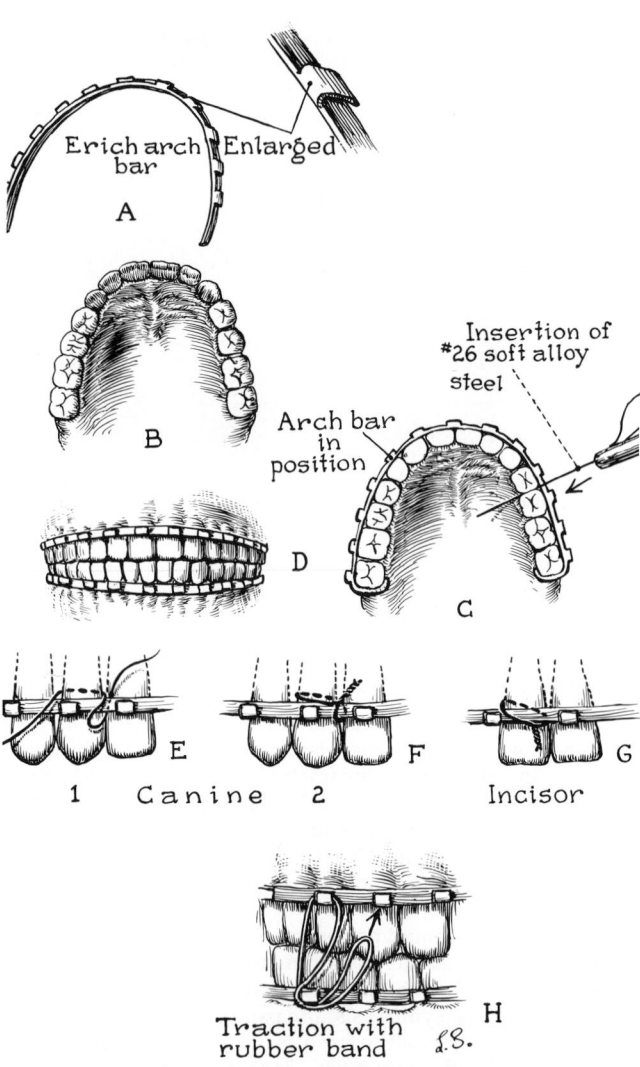

Figure 14. *A* to *D*, Method of applying soft metallic arch bars to the upper or lower jaw in preparation for the use of intermaxillary elastic band fixation of a fractured maxilla or mandible. The soft metal Erich bar is bent to fit against the dental arch and allowed to curve about the most posterior tooth. Soft steel wires are then passed about the necks of the molar teeth and about the bar to make the latter secure. *E* to *G* illustrate the variation in applying the wire when it is necessary to use a canine or incisor tooth as one point of fixation. This method prevents the tendency of such forces to slowly extract the anchored tooth. *H*, When the arch bars are properly attached, elastic bands may be applied to the metal hooks to bring the jaw fragments and teeth into satisfactory occlusion. (From Edgerton, M. T. Fractures of the face and jaws. *In* Ballinger, W. F., II, Rutherford, R. B., and Zuidema, G. D. (Eds.): The Management of Trauma, 2nd ed. Philadelphia, W. B. Saunders Company, 1973.)

dislocations is an indication for temporomandibular joint reconstruction with tendon or fascia lata.

Fractures of the Upper Jaw

Middle face fractures usually involve both maxillae and the paired palatine bones. In 1900, Le Fort[34] classified these fractures as follows (Fig. 15):

LE FORT I FRACTURES (TRANSVERSE MAXILLARY FRACTURE OF GUÉRIN). The fractured segment contains the upper teeth, the palate, lower portions of the pterygoid processes, and a portion of the wall of each maxillary sinus.

LE FORT II FRACTURES (PYRAMIDAL FRACTURES). These fractures also contain the nasal bones and the frontal processes of the maxilla. The malar bones are usually not displaced with this fracture. Significant widening of the inner canthi of the eyes and the bridge of the nose usually occurs with this fracture and there is often destruction of the ethmoid sinus cells.

LE FORT III FRACTURES (CRANIOFACIAL DISJUNCTION). The maxillas, nasal bones, and zygomatic compound are separated as a unit from the cranial attachments (Fig. 15).

Diagnostic features of the upper jaw fractures include malocclusion, open-bite deformity, and mobility of the upper jaw and hard palate (when the upper teeth are grasped between the examiner's thumb and index finger). Stereoscopic roentgenograms in the Waters position (Fig. 16) provide excellent visualization of midline fractures.

Diagnostic imaging has made important strides in the past decade. Computed tomography (CT) has enhanced understanding of facial fractures. Images can be viewed in multiple planes (axial and coronal), and, recently, three-dimensional image reconstructions are available. All of these techniques aid in accurate diagnosis and treatment.

Treatment of these fractures is best accomplished by direct surgical exposure. Through the use of techniques learned in the practice of craniofacial surgery, the entire facial skeleton can now be exposed by combining a full coronal (forehead flap reflecting) incision with subciliary muscle splitting incisions, and with upper buccal sulcus incisions. These incisions provide exposure that allows bone pieces to be accurately reduced and fixed with either wires or mini-plates. In severe injuries where much bone is missing, primary bone grafts may be harvested from ribs, iliac crest, or calvarium and used to bridge the gaps.

Fractures of the Zygomatic Compound

The malar bone is extremely dense, forming the prominence of each cheek. This bone is commonly fractured in conjunction with injuries to the upper jaw. The zygoma is often driven by an external blow into the antrum and beneath the orbit. There are six common types of zygomatic fractures based on the displacement of the bone. Each requires a different method of reduction (Fig. 17). These fractures tear the mucosa of the maxillary sinus and cause hematoma within the sinus cavity. The floor of the orbit may be displaced, causing injury to the globe or subse-

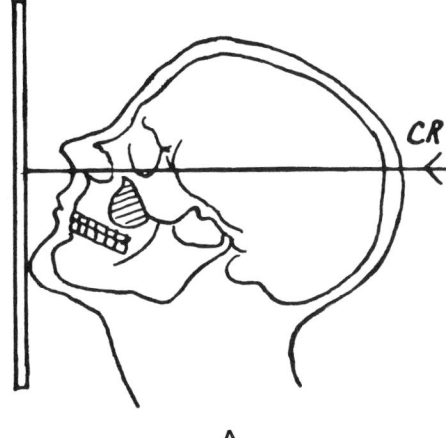

A

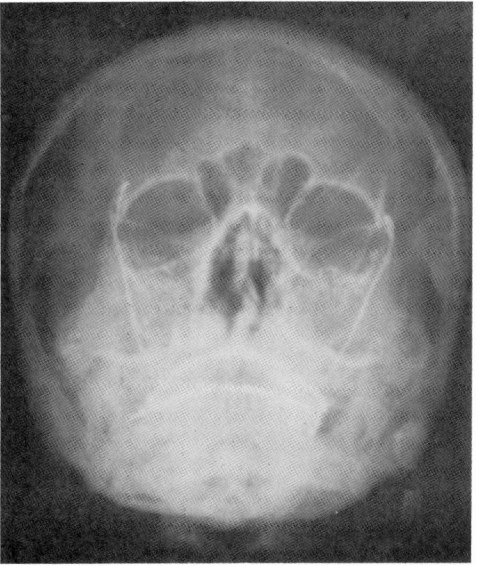

B

Figure 16. Waters position. Posteroanterior view for maxillary sinuses, maxilla, orbits, and zygomatic arches. This projection also may be helpful in demonstration of fractures of the nasal bones and nasal processes of the maxilla. In this view, the petrous ridges are projected just below the floors of the maxillary sinuses. *A,* Position of the patient in relation to the film in the central ray. *B,* Waters view showing internal wire suspension for fixation in features of the middle third of the face. (From Digman, R. O. *In* Converse, J. M. (Ed.): Reconstructive Plastic Surgery, 2nd ed. Vol. 2. Philadelphia, W. B. Saunders Company, 1977. *A* modified from Zizmor, J. *In* Kazanjian, V. H., and Converse, J. M.: The Surgical Treatment of Facial Injuries, 2nd ed. Baltimore, Williams & Wilkins, 1959.)

quent diplopia. Enophthalmos may appear as edema subsides after injury. The cheek bone is flattened, and the lateral palpebral ligament may be displaced downward. Often there is a laterally based subconjunctival hemorrhage, and the ipsilateral half of the upper lip is often numb because of injury to the infraorbital nerve. Irregularity of the bone may be felt by the examining finger when the rim of the orbit is palpated.

Treatment involves closed or open reduction to replace bony parts and fix them with either wires or mini-plates. Existing lacerations or a surgical incision within the "lines of skin relation" may be used for exposure. To reduce a zygomatic arch fracture, an incision can be made in the hair-bearing temple to allow an elevator to be passed beneath the depressed arch. The bone is then levered laterally into the normal position (Gillies' maneuver). If double vision is persistent after healing, it may be corrected by secondary repositioning of the bony walls of the orbit (or by insertion of an orbital implant) in approximately 80 per cent of patients.

Approximately 7 per cent of all patients with major fractures

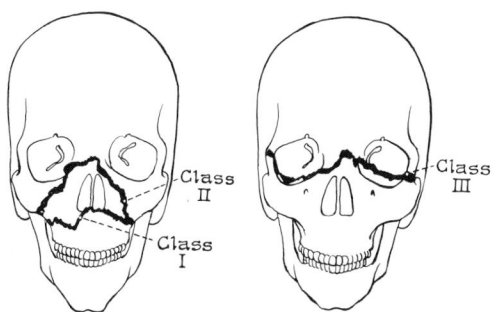

Figure 15. Diagram showing the usual lines of fracture in LeFort's Class I, II, and III fractures. (From Edgerton, M. T. Fractures of the face and jaws. *In* Ballinger, W. F., II, Rutherford, R. B., and Zuidema, G. D. (Eds.): The Management of Trauma, 2nd ed. Philadelphia, W. B. Saunders Company, 1973.)

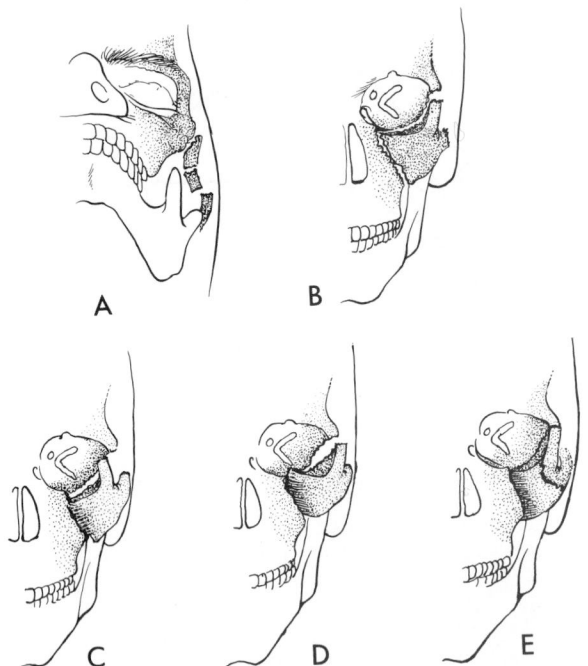

Figure 17. Simple classification of displaced fractures of the zygomatic compound. One in 20 fractures of the malar compound shows no significant displacement, and treatment is not required. One tenth involve the arch only (A), one third show inward or downward displacement without rotation (B), one tenth show medial rotation of the upper part of the zygoma toward the midline (C), one fifth are rotated laterally (D), and one fifth are complicated by additional fractures of the central heavy portion of the malar bone (E). These various types of fracture may be readily determined on examination and radiograph, and their recognition is of considerable help in planning operative reductions. (From Edgerton, M. T. Fractures of the face and jaws. In Ballinger, W. F., II, Rutherford, R. B., and Zuidema, G. D., (Eds.): The Management of Trauma, 2nd ed. Philadelphia, W. B. Saunders Company, 1973.)

of the upper and lower jaws have associated injury to the cervical vertebrae. Careful examination of the neck and radiographs are indicated in all such patients. It is imperative on initial examination to establish the presence of an adequate airway and exclude injuries to other organ systems. Visual acuity and the presence of diplopia should be recorded before treatment. The management of severe facial injuries often involves a multidisciplinary approach, as in severe trauma involving other parts of the body.

INFECTIOUS DEFORMITY OF THE JAWS

The most common problem associated with infection in the jaw bones follows diseased teeth. Root abscesses and secondary osteomyelitis often follow poor dental hygiene. This may cause chronic draining sinuses with pain, sequestration, and loss of bone. If infection is severe, nonunion of a fractured mandible may result. Treatment usually requires surgical débridement, removal of sequestra, adequate soft tissue closure with dependent drainage, and appropriate antibiotic therapy. If the upper jaw is involved, the infection may enter the antrum and require the surgeon to open and drain the sinus (preferably through a nasal antrostomy).

Chronic infections such as tuberculosis and actinomycosis must be recognized as diagnostic possibilities in patients with low-grade chronic drainage into the oral cavity or through the skin of the face or neck. They may be diagnosed only by appropriate stains, cultures, and biopsies of tissue. Syphilis of the jawbone is now quite rare but should be considered when associated defects in the bone and cartilaginous support of the nose and hard palate are also present.

In recent years, radio-osteonecrosis of the jaw has been seen in increasing numbers of patients after the treatment of cancer with various radiotherapy techniques. This is sometimes an inevitable complication of adequate radiation treatment of malignant disease. A characteristic of this type of bone necrosis and infection is the severe pain that accompanies it, *even in the absence of significant change on radiographic examination of the bone.* Treatment usually requires wide removal of the damaged bone, because spontaneous recovery with conservative management is nearly always prolonged and unpleasant. Spontaneous sequestration of dead bone is so delayed in such patients that surgical intervention at an early date is indicated. Gamma irradiation is very damaging to both normal and malignant living tissue!

DEFICIENCY STATES AND METABOLIC DERANGEMENTS INVOLVING THE JAWS

Surgical treatment is of considerable value for many patients with metabolic disorders of bone. This includes young patients with fibrous dysplasia involving, commonly, the maxilla or mandible. Such patients may have associated disorders involving the long bones of the extremities, and some have a sensorineural hearing loss. The extensive facial deformities may be corrected by surgical sculpturing of the involved bones. Radiation therapy should be avoided for such conditions.

Other patients may suffer from ossifying fibromas with localized enlargement of the upper or lower jaw, or they may experience a cyst formation in the jaws and facial bones associated with parathyroid adenomas. These hormone disorders produce giant cell tumors within the bones. In the mandible, such a condition may cause pathologic features. Bone grafting and cyst removal may be required.

BENIGN TUMORS OF THE JAWS

Most benign tumors of the upper and lower jaw may be readily excised surgically, when the diagnosis is established. Radiolucent lesions on radiographs often prove to be dental or root cysts. Radicular dentigerous cysts may cause considerable expansion of the alveolar cortex. Radiopaque benign tumors, such as cementomas, osteomas, odontomas, and torus palatinus tumors, are also quite common.

Fibromas and osteofibromas are frequently encountered. Most of these benign lesions may be removed by straightforward intraoral surgical techniques. If the resulting cavities are large and the mandibular bone has been weakened, the cavity may be filled with iliac crest bone chips to accelerate healing and provide strength. If bone grafting is used to fill the cavities, a flap of well-vascularized mucous membrane must be used to close the pocket and exclude oral cavity secretions in the postoperative period.

MALIGNANT TUMORS OF THE JAWS

ADAMANTINOMA (AMELOBLASTOMA). This interesting tumor appears to arise from the embryonic enamel organ of a tooth and may be found in either the upper or the lower jaw. It is a slow-growing, low-grade malignant tumor that is known to metastasize to the bones or lungs (perhaps by aspiration of tumor cells) at times. The histologic appearance is characteristic on biopsy, but local removal by curettage is commonly followed by recurrence. Wide excision of the lesion with bone grafting is the treatment of choice with larger lesions. Smaller lesions may be excised without grafting. Radiographs of these lesions show a characteristic radiolucent "soap bubble" appearance.

OSTEOGENIC SARCOMA. Osteogenic sarcoma may involve either the mandible or the upper jaw. The condition has a very grave prognosis but occasionally may be cured by extremely wide resection. Reconstruction of the jaw should be deferred for a reasonable period because of the high incidence of early local recurrence. Postoperative radiation therapy should be used if the surgical margins are in doubt after resection.

OSTEOCHONDROSARCOMA. This type of cancer may be seen to develop after a history of repeated removal of recurrent bony tumors by a pathologist diagnosed as "osteochondromas." With each successive recurrence, there may be a slight change in the histologic appearance of the tumor. Wide removal of this lesion at the first opportunity may prevent this progressive and ominous change in clinical character. This tumor is sometimes encountered in children. When the full-fledged sarcoma has developed, the cure rate without evidence of disease (WED) at 5 years is less than 20 per cent.

METASTATIC CARCINOMA. The mandible and, less commonly, the upper jaw may be the seat of occasional metastatic tumors. They usually arise from the breast, thyroid, or prostate. In some instances, the metastasis to the mandible may produce the first symptoms of the patient's disease. Biopsy usually provides the diagnosis. Hypernephromas may appear as metastatic lesions in the mandible years after the primary renal tumor has been removed. These may be solitary metastases.

BONE GRAFTING FOR JAW RECONSTRUCTION

Bone grafting to the jaw is commonly required in an effort to reconstruct the mandibular arch. Autogenous bone taken from the patient's iliac crest, rib cage, or, more recently, the skull is the most suitable donor material. Studies using radioactive material to label the cells of the bone graft suggest that some of the osteoblastic cells remain viable after transplantation to the jaw region. If bony union is established with the recipient bone, creeping replacement of the cells within the bone graft by those of the recipient bone appears to occur. A period of demineralization of the bone graft (clearly evident on radiographs) develops and reaches its peak approximately 6 months after operation. Subsequently, a healthy bone graft develops increased density and strength, manifested by greater radiodensity.

In cases of large bony defects or bone defects lying in radiated beds, the likelihood of successful bone graft healing is much reduced. In such patients, the use of vascularized bone grafts—i.e., bone transferred with an intact blood supply—produces excellent healing. Iliac crest, fibula, and radius are anatomically suitable sources for such a vascularized bone graft. Choice of site is determined by the size of the defect, requirements for concurrent soft tissue replacement, donor site morbidity, and the surgeon's judgment as to the wound healing capacity of the recipient defect.

SALIVARY GLANDS

The salivary glands are tubuloacinar glands arising from ectodermal and endodermal invaginations. They are described as major and minor glands. There are six major salivary glands consisting of three pairs, namely, the parotid, submandibular, and sublingual glands. There are numerous minor salivary glands located submucosally throughout the oral cavity and pharynx. These minor glands produce mucous or mixed mucoserous secretions, except for Ebner's posterior lingual gland, which produces a pure serous secretion similar to that from the parotid glands.

Samuel White of Hudson, New York, is credited with the first successful surgical removal of the parotid gland in 1808. Since that time, surgical therapy has been increasingly useful in treating problems of the salivary glands.

Trauma of the Salivary Glands

Mechanical injury to the face may cause division of parotid glandular tissue or transection of Stensen's duct. When the duct is divided, the two ends should be carefully identified and, after appropriate wound débridement, repaired over a small plastic catheter that emerges into the oral cavity. Closure of the skin over the injured glandular tissue is usually followed by satisfactory healing. Late complications of injury to the parotid gland may include the development of salivary-cutaneous fistulas or obstruction of the duct, with resulting enlargement of the gland. Chronic salivary fistulae that persist for more than 3 months may require reconstruction. Acute obstruction or ligation of the duct may lead to atrophy of the entire parotid gland on that side of the face. Contour reconstruction of the face by dermal grafts, synthetic implants, or flaps (pedicled or free tissue transfer) may be required after such an event.

Children suffering from cerebral palsy or other congenital syndromes or patients with damage to the tongue and lips after oncologic surgery may be troubled by chronic drooling. Posterior transplantation of Stensen's ducts to the pharynx is often helpful in this situation. Occasionally, submandibular glands are removed for further lessening of salivary flow.[13,62]

Deep injuries to the parotid gland commonly also divide one or more branches of the facial nerve. These nerves should be repaired within the first 3 days after injury while stimulation of the distal nerve end still produces a muscle contraction.

Infections of Salivary Glands (Sialoadenitis)

Mumps is an acute febrile illness of viral origin. It is one of the most common infections of the parotid gland. Treatment is symptomatic and recovery usually uneventful. Low-grade infection of the salivary glands by bacteria is usually self-limiting in the adult and responds well to broad-spectrum antibiotics. If, however, the salivary ducts are strictured or calculi are present, repeated attacks of obstruction and infection may occur that require surgical removal of the gland.

Acute suppurative parotitis occurs generally in either the very young or the elderly. Dehydration and poor oral hygiene are important contributing factors. If treated early, this disease often responds to conservative therapy with antibiotics, hydration, and sialagogues. As the disease progresses, however, it may lead to abscess formation and severe cellulitis. At this point, antibiotic therapy and surgical excision of necrotic tissue are often lifesaving.

Recurrent acute sialoadenitis may develop in some patients with reduced or thickened secretions. It is believed that infections are caused by bacteria that ascend the salivary ducts from the oral cavity. Ligation of the ducts produces relief of symptoms and good results in approximately 65 per cent of patients. Those who do not respond to this procedure may require parotidectomy or removal of the submandibular glands.

Metabolic Disorders

Calculi may form in the major salivary glands. They are thought to follow improper duct drainage and abnormal salivary pH within the oral cavity. Stones may be removed surgically, but prevention of further stone formation in such patients is difficult. Infection is often present in the ducts with calculi and thought to be a secondary phenomenon. Diagnosis of calculi can be made by palpation with a lacrimal probe or by an intraoral radiograph. When located, the calculus may usually be removed by intraorally incising the duct directly over the stone. Sometimes continued infection makes total removal of the gland necessary.

Chronic enlargement of the parotid glands follows a variety of conditions: endocrine problems (diabetes mellitus, gout), granulomatous lesions (sarcoidosis, actinomycosis), and malnutrition states (beriberi). Elderly patients frequently have reduced salivary flow with secondary paradoxical salivary gland enlargement. They frequently have xerostomia (dryness of the mouth). Sjögren's syndrome produces an enlargement of parotid and lacrimal glands with decreasing flow from these glands and resultant dryness of the mouth and eyes. It is often associated with rheumatoid arthritis or other connective tissue diseases. Treatment is symptomatic, and diagnostic studies are directed to assessment of associated connective tissue disease.

The parotid duct may sometimes be transplanted to the conjunctival sulcus if keratitis sicca endangers vision.

Salivary Tumors

Neoplasms of the salivary glands constitute approximately 5 per cent of all head and neck tumors. They are a major cause for salivary gland surgery. Approximately 70 per cent of salivary gland tumors occur in the parotid gland; and of these, 70 per cent are benign. Approximately 60 per cent of submandibular gland tumors, however, are malignant.

DIAGNOSIS OF PAROTID TUMORS. Most parotid tumors arise as slow-growing, firm, nodular masses that are sometimes mistaken for lymph nodes in the upper neck. They are usually painless, and fewer than 30 per cent of those that are malignant produce paralysis of one or more branches of the facial nerve.

In the parotid region, there are several other anatomic structures that can mimic a parotid tumor—the tip of the styloid process, the angle of the mandible, the head of the mandibular condyle, a hypertrophied masseter muscle, the transverse process of the atlas, or an intraparotid lymph node. Careful physical examination can usually separate these possibilities. In questionable cases, CT scanning and MRI may be of help. These imaging techniques can assess involvement of the deep lobe and the parapharyngeal space or detect deep cervical lymph nodes before they become clinically evident.

Biopsy is required before final commitment to a surgical plan is made. This can be done in several ways. Core-needle biopsy by a Silverman needle has been used in the past. Unfortunately, there are reports of microscopic nests of tumor implanted by this method. Fine-needle aspiration biopsy done with a 22-gauge needle is an inexpensive and rapid method for parotid mass diagnosis. The thin needle has a minimal risk of tumor implantation, but the specimen is small and requires a skilled pathologist. When the surgeon and pathologist are adept with the technique, the complications are minimal. Another satisfactory approach is a direct scalpel biopsy of the tumor under local anesthesia. The specimen is sent for frozen section. The modern cryostat now makes it possible for a competent pathologist to give a reliable frozen section diagnosis of most salivary tumors. In case of uncertainty after review of the frozen section diagnosis, the surgeon has the option of waiting for permanent sections. It is dangerous to do a superficial lobectomy *before* one is certain that the lesion is not malignant!

Certain clinical features make a malignancy more likely. Facial paralysis or paresis associated with a parotid tumor is an ominous sign indicative of a malignancy and poor prognosis. Spiro and associates found that a malignant parotid tumor, presenting with pain, had a poorer prognosis than pain-free malignancies (35 versus 68 per cent 5-year cures). Rapid enlargement of the tumor and the appearance of enlarged hard lymph nodes are further signs of malignancy.

Mixed tumors (pleomorphic adenomas) constitute approximately 70 per cent of all neoplasms of the parotid gland. Warthin's tumors are the next most common, followed by adenomas and oncocytomas. Malignant tumors can be classified as low-grade (acinic cell, mucoepidermoid [low-grade], and adenoid-cystic) and high-grade (adenocarcinoma, mucoepidermoid [high-grade], and squamous cell). This classification aids in assessing the speed of tumor growth and the type of surgical excision indicated.

In all benign parotid tumors and, indeed, with many of the smaller malignant tumors, great care should be taken to preserve branches of the facial nerve. The patient's lips and eyelids should be left in view during operation, and the anesthesiologist must avoid all drugs that produce muscle paralysis.

The technique of lateral lobectomy with facial nerve dissection is useful for tumors lying in the lateral lobe. For benign tumors and low-grade malignancy, this subtotal parotidectomy is both diagnostic and therapeutic. The authors do *not* recommend the use of faradic current nerve stimulators, because this method is less precise in localizing the nerve than simple mechanical stimulation with forceps and clamp. It also tends to fatigue the nerve more quickly than mechanical stimulation. Any failure of the electric charge also produces a dangerous false-negative response.

Most surgeons prefer to locate the facial nerve by first exposing the proximal part of the nerve at the stylomastoid foramen. The tumor and parotid gland are rolled forward as the branches of the nerve are exposed. Some inject the parotid duct with methylene blue at the beginning of the operation to help outline the nerve branches and ducts. Others find the resultant staining of the adjacent parotid gland undesirable. The operation is tedious and should be undertaken only by those very familiar with the anatomy of the region. Even with great gentleness, transient paralysis of the face is sometimes present after removal of a benign tumor. The patient should be warned of this possibility in advance and told that several months may be required for recovery of facial movements. Any identified surgical injury to a major branch of the facial nerve should be repaired immediately by suture or nerve grafting. After parotid resection with preservation of the facial nerve, approximately 50 per cent of patients develop abnormal sweating of the skin overlying the parotid region in response to eating and other stimulation. This condition is known as gustatory sweating or Frey's syndrome. It is believed to be due to injury of the branches of the auriculotemporal nerve with subsequent crossing of the sweat and salivary nerve fibers during regeneration following surgical therapy. It usually appears within 3 to 9 months after operation. Many patients find that these symptoms spontaneously improve. Frey's syndrome is rarely, if ever, seen in patients who have had total resection of the facial nerve along with parotidectomy for the removal of malignant parotid tumors.

The mixed tumor of the parotid recurs in progressively more malignant forms if any attempt is made to remove it by simple "enucleation" techniques. The tiny nests of tumor cells may be seen extending through and beyond the gross capsule of these tumors. *An abundant layer of normal parotid tissue must be removed around the margins of mixed tumors in order to produce a consistent cure.* The best opportunity for cure of this tumor is at initial surgical resection.

SURGICAL TREATMENT OF MALIGNANT SALIVARY TUMORS. Malignant parotid tumors may require, because of their size or location, deliberate removal of portions of the facial nerve, overlying adherent skin, portions of the mandible, segments of the external auditory canal, or an in-continuity removal of the lymph nodes of the neck. In some instances, the deep surface of the tumor may involve the wall of the internal carotid artery, requiring its resection and the use of a vein graft to re-establish circulation to that side of the brain. Cranial nerves such as the vagus or hypoglossal may be invaded by tumor; and if the patient has a history of pain in the face, the auriculotemporal nerve should be traced to the Gasserian ganglion and resected with a sample biopsy at that point.

Radical neck dissection of the regional cervical lymph nodes should be reserved for salivary tumors that are accompanied by enlarged and clinically palpable nodes, for large or rapidly growing primary tumors, and for smaller tumors that are diagnosed histologically as squamous carcinoma, malignant mixed tumor, adenoid-cystic carcinoma, or the high-grade variety of mucoepidermoid carcinoma. Lymph node metastasis to the neck is distinctly less common in the other histologic types of malignant parotid and submaxillary tumors.

USE OF IMMEDIATE RECONSTRUCTIVE TECHNIQUES AT THE TIME OF THE PAROTID GLAND TUMOR REMOVAL. *Surgical therapy continues to offer the best possibility of cure with most salivary gland tumors.* Approximately 50 per cent of the patients who undergo parotid resection remain free of disease. Approximately 800 deaths per year from salivary gland cancer are recorded in the United States. The most dramatic improvement in the treatment of salivary gland cancer in the past decade has been the increased use of immediate reconstructive techniques that make radical excisional surgery more acceptable to the patient.[30] Free skin grafts, rotation flaps, and microvascular transfers can be used to replace cutaneous defects. Occasionally, mandibular reconstruction is necessary.

If the facial nerve is divided, there are several means of reconstruction. When proximal and distal nerve segments remain, a nerve graft to bridge the defects is the best technique.[41] Other techniques involve anastomosing the proximal hypoglossal nerve to the distal branches of the seventh nerve to provide tone and some movement.[13] In addition, masseter and temporalis muscle transfers have been used.[40] Most recently, free tissue transfer of the gracilis muscle has been successfully used. Anderl and Terzis continue to report promising results from using crossed nerve grafts to bring fibers from the normal side of the face to the paralyzed side. No patient should suffer an uncorrected facial nerve paralysis whose prognosis for remaining life exceeds even 1 or 2 years. Several of these reconstructive procedures are best accomplished at the time of removal of the cancer.

SUBMAXILLARY GLAND TUMORS. Because of the deep location of the submaxillary gland and the high incidence of malignancy, lymph node dissection should be performed more often for submaxillary gland cancer than for parotid cancer. Often the mylohyoid muscle and portions of the mandible must be resected for adequate local tumor margins. At times, tumors of the submaxillary gland also require removal of the lingual and hypoglossal nerves for adequate margins.

MINOR SALIVARY GLAND TUMORS. The most frequent tumors of the minor salivary glands occur in the palate, and most of these are mixed tumors. When mixed tumors lie over the bony hard palate, it is sometimes wise to remove this bone *en bloc* with the tumor and immediately apply a split-thickness skin graft to the subjacent mucosa of the nasal floor. This prevents postoperative oronasal fistulas of the palate. *Almost 75 per cent of the salivary gland tumors in the palate prove to be malignant.* Patients with such tumors require full-thickness resections of portions of the hard and the soft palate. Although hard palate defects may be managed appropriately by the use of a dental prosthesis, defects involving the posterior border of the soft palate are often best managed by an immediate reconstruction, using a flap of mucosa and muscle from the posterior pharynx.

When a prosthesis is to be used for an expected defect in the hard palate, a preoperative dental impression of the palate and upper jaw should be made. Patients who remain well for several years after resection of a malignant tumor of the palate benefit from replacing the palatal prosthesis with a pedicle flap reconstruction of the palate. When the palate is reconstructed, oral hygiene and taste improve, and the patient does not have to rely on retaining good teeth to support the dental prosthesis for the remainder of his life.

USE OF RADIATION THERAPY FOR SALIVARY GLAND TUMORS. Surgical excision offers the best method for cure of most salivary tumors other than lymphomas or metastatic tumors. However, in certain circumstances postoperative radiation therapy appears to improve the cure rate. Such treatment is indicated if the surgeon believes that there is a likelihood of residual cancer after radical resection. If the pathologist reports "cancer extending to the margins of the resection," the surgeon may think that his surgical margin was too narrow. In such instances, postoperative cobalt therapy should be initiated as soon as satisfactory wound healing has been obtained. Other advanced parotid cancers that are clearly nonresectable may be controlled for many months by appropriate radiation therapy.[48]

CHEMOTHERAPY FOR SALIVARY TUMORS. In occasional circumstances, methotrexate or 5-fluorouracil therapy may produce limited regression of malignant neoplasms of the parotid or submaxillary gland. Such treatment, however, is often disappointing and serves primarily for late palliation, rather than for an improved cure rate. Perfusion of an advanced parotid tumor with cyclophosphamide (Cytoxan), administered by retrograde catheter in the superficial temporal artery, has produced marked regression in a few special tumors.

SELECTED REFERENCES

Anderson, R., and Hoopes, J. E.: Symposium on Malignancies of the Head and Neck. St. Louis, C. V. Mosby Company, 1975.
 A series of enlightening discussions of current thinking in the management of cancer in this area.

Bardwil, J. M., Luna, M. A., and Healey, J. E.: Salivary glands. *In* MacComb, W. S., and Fletcher, G. H.: Cancer of the Head and Neck. Baltimore, Williams & Wilkins, 1967, p. 357.
 A concise review of anatomy and more recent pathologic classifications of parotid tumors. The results reported with postoperative radiotherapy in selected cases are of interest.

Converse, J. M.: Kazanjian & Converse's Surgical Treatment of Facial Injuries, 3rd ed. Baltimore, Williams & Wilkins, 1974.
 A thorough and detailed compendium of treatment of all types of facial injuries, early and late, with clear, beautiful illustrations supporting an authoritative text.

Converse, J. M. (Ed.): Reconstructive Plastic Surgery, 2nd ed. Philadelphia, W. B. Saunders Company, 1977.
 A very thorough treatise covering the basic aspects of cleft lip and palate surgery. It is well illustrated and referenced and provides a lucid introduction to this subject in full.

Hanna, D. C.: Salivary gland tumors. *In* Gaisford, J. C. (Ed.): Symposium on cancer of the Head and Neck. Vol. 2. St. Louis, C. V. Mosby Company, 1969, p. 352.
 A sound review of the practical surgical management of parotid tumors, with emphasis on reconstructive techniques.

Suen, J. Y., and Myers, E. N.: Cancer of the Head and Neck. London, Churchill Livingstone, 1981.
 A broad general reference text on the subject of malignancy of the head and neck region by 54 contributors.

Thackray, A. C., and Lucas, R. B.: Tumors of the major salivary glands. *In* Atlas of Tumor Pathology. Second Series, Fascicle 10. Washington, D.C., Armed Forces Institute of Pathology, 1974.
 A thorough compendium on the classification, histology, and prognosis of salivary gland tumors.

REFERENCES

1. Ackerman, L. V., and del Regato, J. A.: Cancer: Diagnosis, Treatment and Prognosis, 4th ed. St. Louis, C. V. Mosby Company, 1970, pp. 183–354; 276–296.
2. Ackerman, L. V., and Wheat, M. W., Jr.: The implantation of cancer—an avoidable surgical risk? Surgery, 37:341, 1955.
3. American Joint Committee on Cancer: Staging of cancer of head and neck sites and of melanoma, Annual Report, 1983.
4. Archard, H. O.: Biology of the human oral integument. *In* Fitzgerald, T. B., et al. (Eds.): Dermatology in General Medicine. New York, McGraw-Hill Book Company, 1971, pp. 804–808.
5. Archer, W. H.: Oral and Maxillofacial Surgery, 5th ed. Philadelphia, W. B. Saunders Company, 1975, pp. 510–514; 899–917.
6. Bakamjian, V. Y.: Reconstructive use of flaps in cancer surgery of the head and neck. *In* Reviews in Plastic Surgery: General and Reconstructive. Amsterdam, Excerpta Medica, 1974.
7. Bales, H. W.: Head and neck tumors. *In* Clinical Oncology for Medical Students and Physicians: A Multidisciplinary Approach, 3rd ed. New York, American Cancer Society, 1970–1971, pp. 228–261.
8. Bardwil, J. M., Luna, M. A., and Healey, J. E.: Salivary glands. *In* MacComb, W. S., and Fletcher, G. H.: Cancer of the Head and Neck. Baltimore, Williams & Wilkins, 1967, p. 357.
9. Boca, E., Pignataro, O., Oldini, C., Cappa, C.: Functional neck dissection: An evaluation and review of 843 cases. Laryngoscope, 94:942, 1984.
10. Bochlogyros, P. N.: A retrospective study of 1521 mandibular fractures. J. Oral Maxillofac. Surg., 43:597, 1985.
11. Brown, J. B., and Freyer, M. P.: The Mouth, Tongue, Jaws and Salivary Glands. *In* Davis, L. (Ed.): Christopher's Textbook of Surgery, 9th ed. Philadelphia, W. B. Saunders Company, 1968, pp. 323–357.
12. Cohen, I. K., Holmes, E. C., and Edgerton, M. T.: Parotid duct transplantation for correction of drooling in patients with cancer of the head and neck. Surg. Gynecol. Obstet., 133:663, 1971.
13. Conley, J., and Baker, D. L.: Hypoglossal-facial nerve anastomasis for reinnervation of the paralyzed face. Plast. Reconstr. Surg., 63:63, 1979.
14. Converse, J. M. (Ed.): Reconstructive Plastic Surgery, 2nd ed. Philadelphia, W. B. Saunders Company, 1977, Chapters 38–53.

15. Diamant, H., and Salen, B.: Akut varig parotid opus. Med. (Stockholm), 9:56, 1964.
16. Dingman, R. P., and Natvig, P.: Surgery of Facial Fractures, Philadelphia, W. B. Saunders Company, 1964.
17. Douglas, B.: The treatment of micrognathia associated with obstruction by a plastic procedure. Plast. Reconstr. Surg., 1:300, 1946.
18. Edgerton, M. T., and Des Pres, J. D.: Reconstruction of the oral cavity in the treatment of cancer. Plast. Reconst. Surg., 19:89, 1957.
19. Edgerton, M. T.: Surgical correction of facial paralysis: A plea for better reconstruction. Trans. South. Surg. Assoc., 1966, p. 341.
20. Edgerton, M. T.: The treatment of hemangiomas (with special reference to the role of steroid therapy). Ann. Surg., 183:517, 1976.
21. Edgerton, M. T., and Dellon, A. L.: Surgical retrodisplacement of the levator veli palatini muscle. Plast. Reconstr. Surg., 47:154, 1971.
22. Edgerton, M. T., and Bull, J. C.: Surgery in head and neck tumors: Introduction. In Converse, J. M. (Ed.): Reconstructive Plastic Surgery, 2nd ed. Philadelphia, W. B. Saunders Company, 1977.
23. Edgerton, M. T., Unvarhelyi, G. B., and Knox, D. L.: The surgical correction of ocular hypertelorism. Ann Surg., 172:473, 1970.
24. Foote, F. W., Jr., and Frazelle, E. L.: Tumors of the major salivary glands. In Atlas of Tumor Pathology. Section IV, Fascicle II. Washington, D. C., Armed Forces Institute of Pathology, 1954.
25. Freund, R. H.: Principles of Head and Neck Surgery. New York, Appleton-Century-Crofts, 1967, p. 291.
26. Garrison, F. H.: An Introduction to the History of Medicine, 4th ed. Philadelphia, W. B. Saunders Company, 1929.
27. Ghadially, F. N.: Keratoacanthoma. In Fitzgerald, T. B., et al. (Eds.): Dermatology in General Medicine. New York, McGraw-Hill Book Company, 1971.
28. Glickman, I.: The oral cavity. In Robbins, S. L.: Textbook of Pathology, 3rd ed. Philadelphia, W. B. Saunders Company, 1967.
29. Grabb, W. C.: Rosentein, S. W., and Bzoach, K. R.: Cleft Lip and Palate. Boston, Little, Brown and Company, 1971.
30. Hanna, D. C.: Salivary gland tumors. In Gaisford, J. E. (Ed.): Textbook of Oral Surgery. Boston, Little, Brown and Company, 1968, pp. 1–8.
31. Jabaley, M. E.: Reconstruction of patients with oral and pharyngeal cancer. Curr. Probl. Surg., 14:12, 1977.
32. Lapidot, A., and Ben-Hur, N.: Fastening the base of the tongue forward to the hyoid for relief of respiratory distress in Pierre Robin syndrome. Plast. Reconstr. Surg., 56:89, 1975.
33. Leake, D.: History of oral surgery. In Gulanick, W. C. (Ed.): Textbook of Oral Surgery. Boston, Little, Brown and Company, 1968, pp. 1–8.
34. Le Fort, R.: Fractures de la machoire superieure. Cong. Intern. Med., Paris, 1900, pp. 275–278.
35. LeMesurier, A. B.: The quadrilateral Mirault flap operation for harelip, Plast. Reconstr. Surg., 33:26, 1964.
36. Lewis, S. R., Lynch, J. B., and Blocker, T. G., Jr.: The use of facial slings for tongue stabilization in the Pierre Robin syndrome. Plast. Reconstr. Surg., 42:237, 1968.
37. MacComb, W. S., Fletcher, G. H., and Healey, J. E., Jr.: Intraoral cavity. In MacComb, W. S., and Fletcher, G. H.: Cancer of the Head and Neck. Baltimore, Williams & Wilkins, 1967, pp. 89–151.
38. MacFee, W. F.: Carcinoma of the floor of the mouth: Clinical observations and surgical treatment. Ann. Surg., 149:172, 1959.
39. Mathes, S. J., and Nahai, F.: Clinical Atlas of Muscle and Musculocutaneous Flaps. St. Louis, C. V. Mosby Company, 1979.
40. May, M.: Methods of rehabilitation of paralyzed face. In Graham, M., and House, W. (Eds.): Disorders of the Facial Nerve. New York, Raven Press, 1983, pp. 519–522.
41. Miehlke, A.: Nerve grafting for restoration of lost facial expression. In Conley, J.: Cancer of the Head and Neck. Washington, Butterworths, 1967, p. 550.
42. Millard, D. R.: Refinements in rotation-advancement cleft lip technique. Plast. Reconstr. Surg., 33:26, 1964.
43. Moncrief, J. A.: Burns. In Schwartz, S. E., et al. (Eds.): Principles of Surgery. New York, McGraw-Hill Book Company, 1969, pp. 211–212.
44. Monroe, C. W., and Ogo, K.: Treatment of micrognathia in the neonatal period. Plast. Reconstr. Surg., 50:317, 1972.
45. O'Brien, B. McC., Morrison, W. A.: Reconstructive Microsurgery. New York, Churchill Livingstone, 1988.
46. Ochsner, A.: Diseases of the mouth. In Ochsner, A., and DeBakey, M. E. (Eds.): Christopher's Minor Surgery, 8th ed. Philadelphia, W. B. Saunders Company, 1959, pp. 270–283.
47. Proskauer, C., and Witt, F. H.: Bildeschichte der Zahnheilkunde. Cologne, Dumont, 1962.
48. Reed, R. J., and O'Quinn, S. E.: Vascular neoplasms. In Fitzgerald, T. B., et al. (Eds.): Dermatology in General Medicine. New York, McGraw-Hill Book Company, 1971, pp. 533–547.
49. Robbins, S. L.: Textbook of Pathology, 3rd ed. Philadelphia, W. B. Saunders Company, 1967, pp. 1313–1367.
50. Robin, P.: Backward lowering of the root of the tongue causing respiratory disturbances. Bull. Acad. Natl. Med., 89:38, 1923.
51. Rose, W.: Harelip and Cleft Palate. London, H. K. Lewis and Company, 1891.
52. Schantz, S. P.: Biological staging of head and neck cancer. Cancer Bull., 39:107, 1987.
53. Stark, R. B.: Pathogenesis of harelip and cleft palate. Plast. Reconstr. Surg., 13:20, 1954.
54. Stark, R. B.: Embryology of cleft lip and palate. In Converse, J. M. (Ed.): Reconstructive Plastic Surgery, 2nd ed. Philadelphia, W. B. Saunders Company, 1977.
55. Stewart, J. B., Jackson, A. W., and Chew, M. K.: The role of radiotherapy in the management of malignant tumors of the salivary glands. A.J.R., 102:100, 1968.
56. Stoll, H. L.: Squamous cell carcinoma. In Fitzgerald, T. B., et al. (Eds.): Dermatology in General Medicine. New York, McGraw-Hill Book Company, 1971, pp. 407–422.
57. Swearingen, J. J.: Tolerances of the Human Face to Crash Impact. Report from the Office of Aviation Medicine. Washington, D. C., Federal Aviation Agency, July 1965.
58. Tennison, C. W.: The repair of unilateral cleft lip by the stencil method. Plast. Reconstr. Surg., 9:115, 1952.
59. Tennison, P., Guiot, G., Rougerie, J., Delbet, P., and Pastoriza, J.: Osteotomies cranio-naso-faciales. Hypertelorisme. Ann. Chir. Plast., 12:103, 1967.
60. Thompson, J. E.: An artistic and mathematically accurate method of repairing the defect in cases of harelip. Surg. Gynecol. Obstet., 14:498, 1912.
61. Wang, M. K. H., and Macomber, W. B.: Deformities of the lips and cheeks. In Converse, J. M. (Ed.): Reconstructive Plastic Surgery, 2nd ed. Philadelphia, W. B. Saunders Company, 1977.
62. Wilkie, T. F.: Surgical treatment of drooling: Follow-up report of five years' experience. Plast. Reconstr. Surg., 45:549, 1970.
63. Wolfort, F. G., DeMeester, F., Knorr, N., and Edgerton, M. T.: Surgical management of cutaneous lye burns. Surg. Gynecol. Obstet., 131:873, 1970.
64. Zarem, H. A., and Edgerton, M. T.: Induced resolution of cavernous demangeomas following prednisolone therapy. J. Plast. Reconstr. Surg., 39:76, 1967.

41

NEUROSURGERY

I

HISTORICAL ASPECTS

Robert H. Wilkins, M.D.

The American student who is interested in the history of neurosurgery has a unique advantage. This specialty is of relatively recent origin and has been developed mainly in the English-speaking countries. For this reason, classic works in neurosurgery are usually obtainable and understandable.[7,8] In addition, there are several excellent reviews of neurosurgical history written in English.[2-6]

These reviews emphasize the fact that although the great majority of neurosurgical procedures have been developed recently, the history of trepanation dates back to the Neolithic period of the Stone Age. In widely separated geographic locations, archeologists have discovered human skulls containing craniectomy defects. Moreover, in many of these skulls there are evidences of healing along the bony edges, indicating that the *patient* survived the operation. The rationale for these procedures is not known, because there are no written records from this era, but it is conceivable that skull deformities, injuries, or headaches might have led to this drastic form of treatment.

The oldest known writing concerning surgical topics, the *Edwin Smith Papyrus,* is of special interest to the neurosurgeon. This treatise dates back to the seventeenth century B.C. and contains the first descriptions of the cranial sutures, the meninges, the external surface of the brain, the cerebrospinal fluid, and the intracranial pulsations. Brain injuries are related to changes in the function of other parts of the body, and hemiplegic contractures are well described. In addition, quadriplegia, urinary incontinence, and priapism are noted to occur in association with cervical vertebral dislocation. The Egyptian physicians of that period had a surprising knowledge of rudimentary neuroanatomy and neurophysiology, but their treatment of injuries of the central nervous system was only supportive. Significantly, trepanation is not mentioned in the *Edwin Smith Papyrus.*

The writings of Hippocrates contain the first recorded descriptions of trepanation, and his instruments and methods are very similar to their modern counterparts. In addition, Hippocrates considered other subjects of neurosurgical interest. He discussed epilepsy, the coexistence of spinal deformity with pulmonary tubercles, and the functional effects of compression of the spinal cord. He devised a method for reducing vertebral dislocations and described permanent and transient facial paralyses, sciatica, and the complex of headache, visual disturbance, and vomiting. The ability of Hippocrates as an observer is well demonstrated by his descriptions of aphasia, unconsciousness, respiratory and cardiac irregularity, carphologia, pupillary inequality, and ophthalmoplegia associated with cerebral disease. He realized that a blow on one side of the head occasionally is followed by convulsions or paralysis of the contralateral side of the body, and he recognized the poor prognosis of the patient with a head injury complicated by a dural lacera-

tion. These and other observations made the contributions of Hippocrates a beacon to surgeons for over 2000 years, until the development of anesthesia, asepsis, and the concept of cerebral localization in the nineteenth century established the foundation of modern neurosurgery.

The introduction of anesthesia and asepsis vastly increased the scope of surgical therapy in general and made brain surgery feasible. Such operations were not performed often, however, because of inability to locate lesions that did not involve the skull. The problem was resolved by the discovery of Bouillaud, Broca, Fritsch, Hitzig, Ferrier, and others that there is focal representation of bodily function in the brain. This third fundamental concept—cerebral localization—became an important part of the foundation upon which modern neurosurgery was established.

Another vital advancement made during the late nineteenth century was the development of the technique of osteoplastic craniotomy by Wagner, which was later facilitated by the use of Gigli's wire saw. The introduction of this technique permitted the exploration of relatively large areas of cortex and, in so doing, significantly extended the limits of brain surgery.

British surgeons were among the first to take advantage of these new developments, and they guided neurosurgery through its infancy in the last two decades of the nineteenth century. Macewen, professor of surgery at the University of Glasgow, and a powerful figure in international surgical circles, was a pioneer in surgical therapy of the central nervous system. Macewen was a pupil of Joseph Lister, and he strongly believed in Lister's principles of antisepsis. His phenomenal success in treating intracranial abscesses was rarely equaled after that time, despite the subsequent use of antibiotics, until the introduction of computed tomography scanning, which now allows earlier and more accurate treatment.

Godlee also applied Lister's principles of antisepsis to neurosurgery in 1884, when he became the first surgeon to resect an intracranial tumor that had been localized solely by neurologic means. Bennett was another pioneering British surgeon. In 1888, he introduced the operation of posterior rhizotomy for the relief of pain.

The most outstanding surgeon in this field at that time, however, was Horsley of London. He devoted the majority of his efforts to clinical and experimental neurosurgery with exceptional results. Although he made myriad contributions, Horsley is best remembered today as the first surgeon to remove a neoplasm from the spinal canal (1887) and the first to attempt retrogasserian neurotomy for tic douloureux (1890). He and Robert Clarke also described a stereotactic apparatus for intracranial procedures in 1908.

During the early development of neurosurgery, it was common for neurologists to diagnose the disease, devise the operation, and direct the surgeon in its performance. For example, Hughes Bennett localized the brain tumor that was removed in 1884 by Richman Godlee, and William gowers diagnosed the spinal tumor that was removed by Victor Horsley in 1887. In the United States, similar situations were encountered frequently. William Spiller, at the University of Pennsylvania, directed Charles Frazier in the performance of a successful retrogasserian neurotomy in 1901 and 10 years later directed Edward Martin in the performance of the first cordotomy. Similarly, Charles Dana at the Cornell University Medical College proposed posterior rhizotomy, as performed a short time later by William Bennett in London and Robert Abbe in New York. Two outstanding neurologists of a later generation, Otfrid Foerster in Germany and Clovis Vincent in France, actually became neurosurgeons to facilitate the procedures they recommended. Foerster independently devised the operation of cordotomy; he also performed classic studies of human cortical function and peripheral sensory innervation during operations that he performed to treat epilepsy or pain.

A host of general surgeons attempted neurosurgical procedures during the formative years at the turn of the century. Most were soon discouraged by the innumerable difficulties accompanying this type of surgical therapy. For example, more than 500 surgeons reported brain operations between 1886 and 1896, but the number fell below 80 between 1896 and 1906.

Fortunately, during this time a young surgeon at Johns Hopkins Hospital became interested in neurosurgery and decided to devote his full attention to it. With little assistance, Harvey Cushing advanced neurosurgery from its infancy through its childhood.[1] He standardized operative technique and, by applying the rigid principles of William Halsted to neurosurgical procedures, was able to reduce operative morbidity and mortality. Prior to this time, hemorrhage presented an almost insurmountable problem during brain surgery. In his typically thorough manner, Cushing mastered the techniques of compressing the scalp, waxing the diploë, and other approaches, and then introduced the vessel clips and electrocautery that have become indispensable in the control of intracranial and intraspinal bleeding.

Brain tumors also attracted Cushing's attention, and during the course of his career more than 2000 patients with brain tumors were seen in his clinic. With the aid of several brilliant assistants, such as Percival Bailey and Louise Eisenhardt, Cushing classified these tumors morphologically, described their biologic behavior, and formulated their surgical treatment. The standardization of technique and the classification of brain tumors were only two of Cushing's many contributions. There are few areas of modern neurosurgical interest that are not based to some extent on the important investigations of this one man.

Another such giant was Dandy. He worked with Cushing for a short time at Johns Hopkins before the latter moved to the Peter Bent Brigham Hospital. Dandy remained at Johns Hopkins, and before he finished his residency in surgery, he made two important discoveries. In association with Kenneth Blackfan, he established the modern concept of hydrocephalus and developed the operations of choroid plexectomy and third ventriculostomy for the relief of communicating and obstructive hydrocephalus. A few years later, in 1918 and 1919, he introduced pneumoventriculography and pneumoencephalography, which then proved to be of inestimable diagnostic value to neurosurgeons. As was true of Cushing, Dandy's contributions to neurosurgery were legion, and he profoundly influenced the subsequent course of modern neurosurgery.

A third such contributor was the Portuguese neurologist Antonio Egas Moniz. Moniz was unusually talented in a number of fields other than medicine, but he still found time to produce more than 300 medical publications. With neurosurgeon Pedro Manuel de Almeida Lima, he introduced the diagnostic technique of carotid arteriography in 1927 and initiated prefrontal lobotomy for psychiatric illness in 1936. For the latter work, Moniz received a Nobel Prize in 1949.

Despite the outstanding work of Cushing, Dandy, and Moniz, most advancements in neurosurgery have been made slowly by the patient efforts of many pioneers. The subsequent developments in the various areas of neurosurgery are outlined in the remainder of this chapter.

SELECTED REFERENCES

Walker, A. E.: History of Neurological Surgery. Baltimore, Williams & Wilkins, 1951.
  This book is the standard for history of neurosurgery, with 18 chapters on various aspects of the specialty by 12 contributors. It also contains 14 biographic sketches of pioneering neurosurgeons and a bibliography containing 2371 references.

Wilkins, R. H.: Neurosurgical Classics. New York, Johnson Reprint Corp., 1965.
  This is a collection of 52 of the most outstanding written contributions in the field of neurologic surgery. These have been compiled into 38 groups, each of which is accompanied by a commentary and a list of related references. The 15 works originally printed in other languages have been translated into English.

REFERENCES

1. Fulton, J. F.: Harvey Cushing. A Biography. Springfield, Ill., Charles C Thomas, 1946.
2. Green, J. R.: The concept of cerebral and spinal localization and the beginnings of neurological surgery. In Wilkins, R. H., and Rengachary, S. S. (Eds.): Neurosurgery Update I. New York, McGraw-Hill Book Company, 1990, pp. 3–11.
3. Horrax, G.: Neurosurgery: An Historical Sketch. Springfield, Ill., Charles C Thomas, 1952.
4. Sachs, E.: History and Development of Neurological Surgery. New York, Paul B. Hoeber, Inc., 1952.
5. Scarff, J. E.: Fifty years of neurosurgery, 1905–1955. Int. Abstr. Surg., 101:417, 1955.
6. Walker, A. E.: History of Neurological Surgery. Baltimore, Williams & Wilkins, 1951.
7. Wilkins, R. H.: Neurosurgical Classics. New York, Johnson Reprint Corp., 1965.
8. Wilkins, R. H.: History of neurosurgery. In Wilkins, R. H., and Rengachary, S. S. (Eds.): Neurosurgery. New York, McGraw-Hill Book Company, 1985, pp. 3–15.

II

NEURORADIOLOGY

William J. Meisler, M.D.

HISTORIC ASPECTS

Prior to the advent of computed tomographic (CT) scanning in 1974, the subspecialty of neuroradiology consisted primarily of the performance and interpretation of plain films of the skull, sinuses, and spine as well as cerebral and spinal angiography, myelography, and pneumoencephalography. CT totally revolutionized the diagnostic work-up of neurologic disease. In most instances, CT allows direct visualization of disease processes of the brain and spinal canal in a very simple manner with minimal risk to the patient. Because of this, pneumoencephalography, a very uncomfortable examination requiring a lumbar puncture with introduction of air into the cisterns and ventricles, became outmoded and the use of cerebral angiography became sharply circumscribed. The addition of magnetic resonance imaging (MRI) to the diagnostic evaluation of neurologic disease further refined and expanded noninvasive neurologic imaging; however, MRI has not had the revolutionary impact that CT scanning has had, inasmuch as MRI represents a refinement of the format introduced with CT, rather than a wholly different approach to neuro-imaging.

Today, diagnostic tests available to the surgeon in the evaluation of neurologic disease include CT; MRI; cerebral angiography; water-soluble myelography; and plain films of the skull, sinuses, and spine.

COMPUTED TOMOGRAPHY

CT is the recording of cross sections of variable thickness obtained by irradiation of the head or spine with the aid of computer enhancement. The study is performed by placing the patient on a table inside the CT scanning machine. The computer is then programmed to record cross sections of variable thickness. Scans can be obtained at direct axial (parallel to the base of the skull) or coronal (perpendicular to the base of the skull) planes. Manipulation of controls on the computer console allows visualization of tissues on a soft tissue or bone format (Fig. 1). The major advantage of computer enhancement is that it allows clear differentiation of soft tissues such as gray matter, white matter, and cerebrospinal fluid (CSF), which on routine radiography ("plain films") have the same radiographic density and therefore are indistinguishable.

In interpreting CT scans, particularly of the brain, it should be borne in mind that this involves an attempt not only to visualize the lesion itself but also to note how the surrounding soft tissues, particularly in the brain, are being affected by the abnormality. In addition, attempts should be made to localize as best as possible the position of the lesion in the brain or spine, for example, intra-axial (a lesion totally within the brain parenchyma or spinal cord) versus extra-axial (a lesion located outside of the brain parenchyma or spinal cord) lesions. A noncontrast examination of the brain that demonstrates an area of hyperdensity along the left convexity that is located outside of the brain, i.e., extra-axial, is depicted in Figure 2. The configuration is typical of a subdural hematoma. The hyperdensity reflects clotted blood, demonstrating that this hemorrhage is acute. However, it should also be observed that there is considerable shift of midline structures from left to right, indicating that the

subdural hematoma is causing a significant mass effect that ultimately may cause transtentorial herniation and the demise of the patient. When one considers that this information can be obtained within 15 minutes when the patient is placed on the CT scanner and that before CT scanning this abnormality would have required analysis by cerebral angiography, an invasive procedure with risk that can require as long as an hour or more to perform, the revolutionary impact that CT has had on imaging of the central nervous system is appreciated. A metastasis totally within the brain parenchyma, i.e., intra-axial, is demonstrated in Figure 3. Note that the total extent of the lesion is visible only after administration of intravenous iodinated contrast. Only the white matter edema, mass effect, and cystic portion of the lesion are visible on the non–contrast-enhanced study; but these findings can also be observed on the contrast study; and therefore the non–contrast-enhanced study is superfluous. Only when there is a question of hemorrhage or calcification is the non–contrast-enhanced study of aid in evaluation of tumor or abscess.

Any substance with a high water content on CT appears relatively lucent (such as CSF); therefore, any tissue with an abnormally high water content appears more lucent than normal on CT. This frequently can be observed on CT in two types of edema. Cytotoxic edema is increased intracellular water content related to cell death from ischemia, such as with infarction. This corresponds to a vascular distribution and may involve both the gray and white matter. White matter edema (also termed interstitial or vasogenic edema) reflects increased water content in the interstitium and is always confined to the white matter, which is less tightly packed than the gray matter. Interstitial edema usually is associated with a tumor, an abscess, a hematoma, or another mass.

An infarct appearing as a lucency on the CT scan indicates that there is increased water in the cells in the area of infarction. Because infarcts reflect vascular events, a lucency from infarction always corresponds to a vascular distribution. In considering infarction, small vessel territories such as the basal ganglia, thalamus, and internal capsule (areas usually affected by hypertensive and other small vessel diseases) must be distinguished from large vessel territories such as the cortex and subcortical white matter (areas frequently affected by embolic disease) for determination of the cause of infarction. Infarcts do not cause mass effect unless they are massive. When they have associated hemorrhage (usually these infarcts are of embolic origin), there may be areas of hyperdensity within the lucency of the infarct.

The differentiation between intra-axial and extra-axial lesions is extremely critical in the management of tumors (Figs. 2 and 3). Most extra-axial tumors are benign (usually meningiomas), and most intra-axial tumors are malignant (usually either primary brain tumors or metastatic disease). Many tumors cause associated white matter edema and mass effect. Indeed, the associated findings, rather than the lesion itself, may be responsible for the symptoms. Other masses such as abscesses can frequently appear identical to tumors and may require biopsy for differentiation from tumor and determination of the nature of the microorganism.

CT can be performed with or without iodinated contrast enhancement. A simple rule usually suffices for determining whether a contrast or noncontrast study should be performed: in most instances, in an acute situation a non–contrast-enhanced study is the best study; however, in a chronic situation a contrast-enhanced study is usually the only examination necessary.

In most acute situations, the reason for clinical concern is either intracerebral hemorrhage or infarction. On the non–contrast-enhanced study, hemorrhage appears hyperdense (white) and is usually very obvious. Contrast administration therefore is not necessary for visualization of hemorrhage; if only a contrast-enhanced study were performed, differentiation

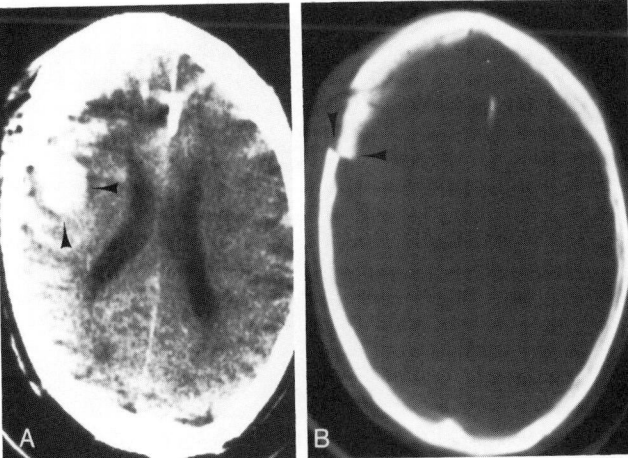

Figure 1. A, The quality of the noncontrast CT scan is degraded by patient motion but nevertheless demonstrates a right frontal hematoma (arrows). B, Same cut as A, with windows set for bone detail, demonstrates a depressed skull fracture (arrows) not at all apparent on the soft tissue windows.

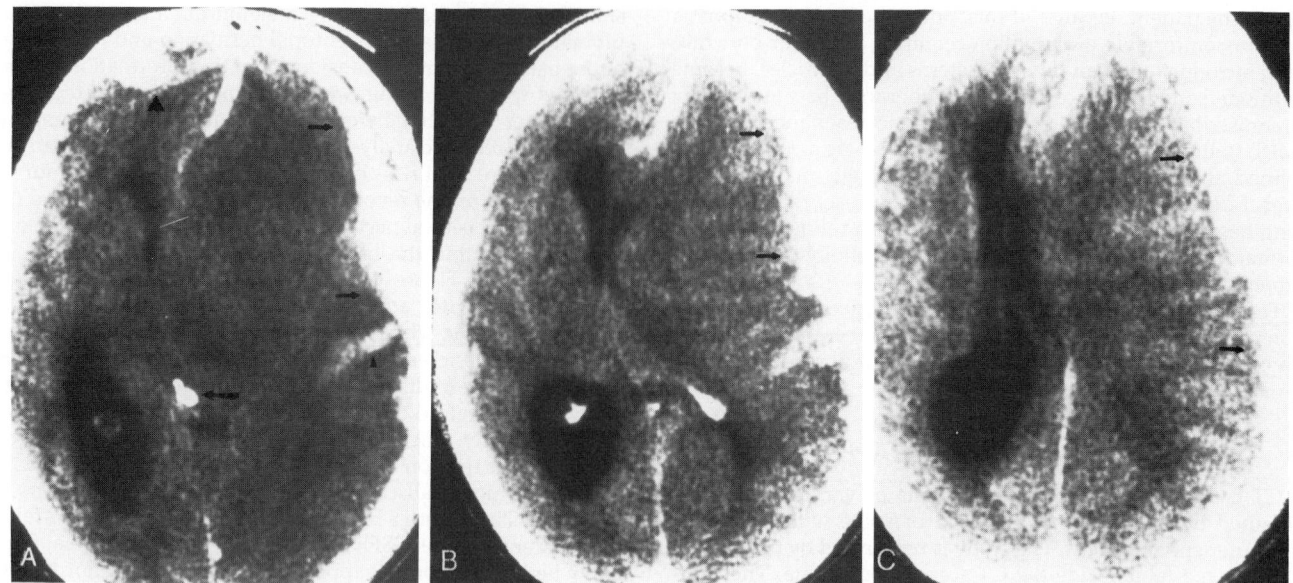

Figure 2. *A* to *C,* Noncontrast CT scan of the brain demonstrates an acute left-sided subdural hematoma (small arrows), which has caused a rightward shift across the midline below the falx. Note also the rightward shift of the normally midline calcified pineal gland (large arrow). There is also acute hemorrhage in the right frontal location (large arrowhead) and probably in the subarachnoid space (small arrowhead).

of whether the hyperdensity observed reflected hemorrhage or abnormal enhancement (which also appears hyperdense) would not be possible. Most *infarcts* appear as a lucency (darker gray or black) and do not show any contrast enhancement for 1 to 2 weeks. Therefore, any change that an infarct demonstrates acutely is apparent on the non–contrast-enhanced study.

In chronic neurologic disease, such as a tumor or an abscess, the total definition of disease can be obtained only on the contrast-enhanced study; rarely does a non–contrast-enhanced study add helpful information. The abnormal enhancement exhibited by tumors and abscesses that are intra-axial is the result of breakdown of the blood-brain barrier and not abnormally increased vascularity. Metastases and abscesses frequently appear as sharply marginated, noncalcified nodules or ring-enhancing lesions (usually reflecting central necrosis) with a large amount of white matter edema. They are often located more peripherally in areas supplied by the large vessels because they reflect embolic disease. Primary brain tumors tend to be less well marginated, irregularly enhancing lesions, with or without calcification and white matter edema, which may be central or peripheral. However, despite these differentiating features, it is

not always possible to confidently distinguish a primary brain tumor from metastasis or abscess.

CT scanning of the spine without contrast is most useful in examining lumbar disc disease, spinal trauma, and epidural hematoma. Disc herniations and degenerative changes are readily apparent on high-quality CT scanning of the lumbar spine. This is not the case, however, in evaluation of cervical and thoracic disc disease or of involvement of the intraspinal contents by tumor, whether from metastatic disease or primary tumors of the spinal sac contents. In these cases, opacification of the subarachnoid space on CT after intrathecal administration of water-soluble contrast via lumbar puncture is often necessary (the "CT-myelogram") (see Fig. 4).

Intravenous enhanced CT scanning of the spine may aid in differentiating herniated disc from scar material. A herniated disc is not enhanced; a scar is enhanced. Comparison of the non–contrast-enhanced and contrast-enhanced studies determines whether the suspected density observed on the non–

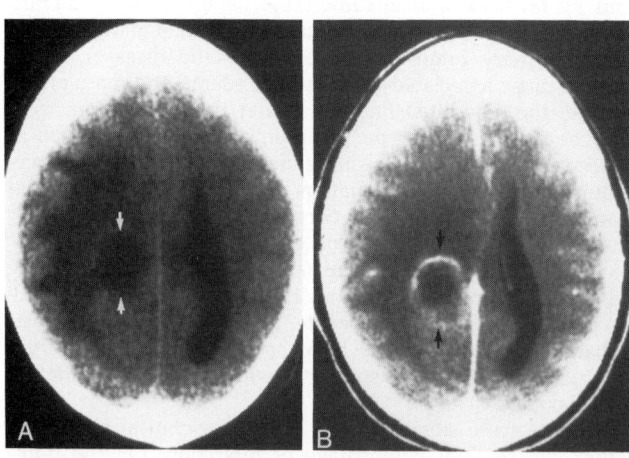

Figure 3. *A,* Noncontrast CT scan *(A)* demonstrates white matter edema in the right cerebrum with obliteration of the right lateral ventricle. The lesion causing the white matter edema is seen on the noncontrast study (arrows) but is demonstrated more clearly on the contrast-enhanced study (arrows, *B*).

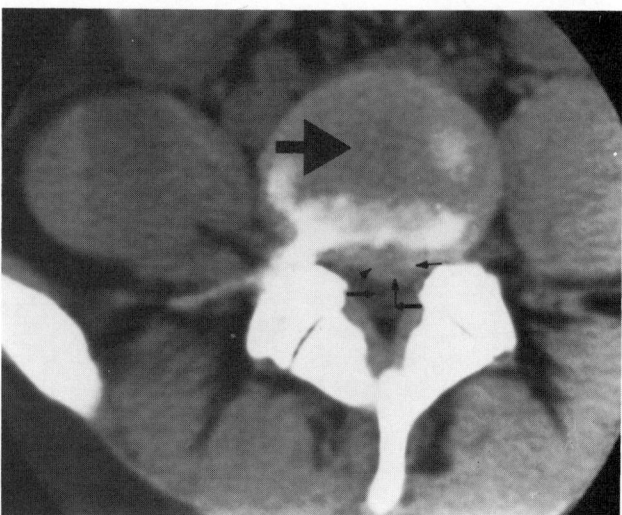

Figure 4. Noncontrast CT scan of the lumbar spine at the disc space nicely demonstrates the difference in CT density between the spinal sac filled with cerebrospinal fluid (medium arrows) and disc material (large arrow). The asymmetrical contours of the disc material (facing the spinal canal), centrally and to the left, represent a herniated disc (small arrows).

contrast-enhanced CT scanning of the spine is enhanced (scar) or not (herniated disc). Intravenous enhanced CT scanning of the spine is also useful in defining an epidural abscess in the spine.

The exact indications for CT scanning of the spine are being re-evaluated at present because of the introduction of MRI. In addition, CT scanning has been successfully applied in sinus disease, particularly for evaluation of tumors in this region and as an aid to endoscopic evaluation of the sinuses; lesions of the base of the skull, particularly tumors, temporal bone and inner ear lesions, and trauma; facial trauma; and laryngeal and other upper airway tumors, for location and staging.

MAGNETIC RESONANCE IMAGING

Images obtained with magnetic resonance reflect the individual magnetic properties of the tissues of the body, rather than their ability to attenuate irradiation. However, the cross-sectional format is identical to that of CT; and the nature of the changes, with regard not only to alteration of normal structures but also to abnormal contrast enhancement, are very similar. Thus, a tumor enhanced on CT scanning is enhanced with the same pattern on MRI. However, certain abnormalities are evident with MRI that are not observed on CT scans (and vice versa) because the information obtained by MRI and that by CT reflect different properties of the tissues of the body (in the case of CT, ability to absorb radiation energy; and in the case of MRI, the exposure of tissues to high magnetic fields). The two modalities therefore have different sensitivities for detecting disease.

There are two types of images traditionally included in an MRI examination. On T1 images CSF or water-type structures are fairly dark (hypointense) and fat is very bright (hyperintense). These sequences provide exquisite anatomic detail (Fig. 5). They also demonstrate abnormal contrast enhancement clearly on the contrast-enhanced sequences. T2 sequences demonstrate the water-related densities to be hyperintense and fat to be relatively hypointense. Anatomy on T2 sequences is less well demonstrated than on T1 sequences, but T2 sequences are more sensitive than T1 sequences in detecting focal abnormality. Contrast enhancement is poorly appreciated on T2 sequences.

The contrast used with MRI is gadolinium, a substance administered intravenously that affects the magnetic properties of the tissues (both normal and abnormal) that accumulate the contrast. Although the appearance is similar to that of iodinated contrast on CT, it should be remembered that gadolinium is totally different from iodinated contrast; it has no iodine and has very few of the systemic effects of iodinated contrast and is therefore much safer.

In many cases, MRI has proved superior to CT scanning in evaluation of disease of the central nervous system. For this reason, where MRI is available it has supplanted CT scanning for much routine evaluation of neurologic disease. However, the sheer volume of neurologic disease in conjunction with the limited availability of MRI indicates that CT scanning remains and will continue to be a very important method in the analysis of neurologic disease. CT also remains superior to MRI in evaluation of acute hemorrhage and thus is a better method of examination in cases involving acute trauma, subarachnoid hemorrhage, or other intracerebral hemorrhage. Calcification is poorly demonstrated on all sequences of MRI. Therefore, MRI has limited application in evaluation of bony (but not necessarily ligamentous or marrow) abnormality. In addition, for patients who have certain types of metal in their bodies (which may rotate because they are susceptible to the magnetic field and cause injury to the patient or significant artifact) or cannot cooperate sufficiently for the relatively long period of time required for MRI, CT scanning remains the better option.

More specifically, at present it can generally be stated that MRI is superior to CT in evaluation of disease at the base of the skull, particularly the sellar and cerebellopontine angle cistern regions (Figs. 6 and 7), and also for most tumors, multiple sclerosis, congenital abnormalities, and other lesions such as vascular malformations. CT scanning, however, is frequently superior to MRI in evaluation of acute trauma as well as disease processes requiring analysis with fine bone detail. In almost all cases involving spinal disease, MRI is superior to CT scanning except in evaluation of fractures.

In addition to being more sensitive than CT scanning, MRI provides unique information, not only because it allows imaging in planes not available to CT, particularly the sagittal plane, but also because it often demonstrates vascular structures much more clearly than CT and whether vessels are encased by surrounding masses. Because the indications for MRI versus CT are being evaluated, consultation with the radiologist is often useful in determining which examination is the most appropriate for each patient.

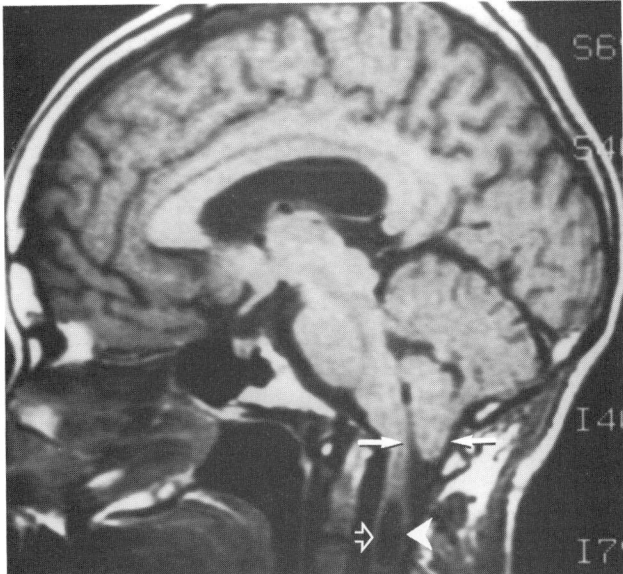

Figure 5. Sagittal off midline T1-weighted cut through the brain demonstrates herniation of the cerebellar tonsil (arrows) and a syrinx in the upper cervical cord (large arrowhead, posteriorly; open arrowhead, anteriorly) in this patient with a Chiari I malformation.

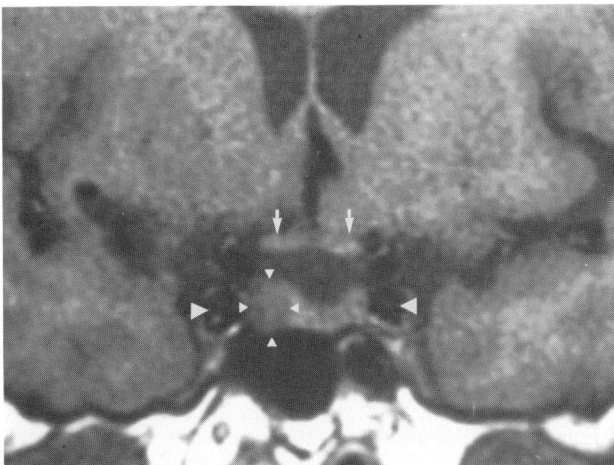

Figure 6. Coronal T1-weighted image through the region of the sella demonstrates a mass in the right pituitary fossa consistent with a pituitary microadenoma (small arrowheads). Note also the cavernous carotid arteries (large arrowheads) and the intracranial optic nerves (small arrows) above the suprasellar cistern.

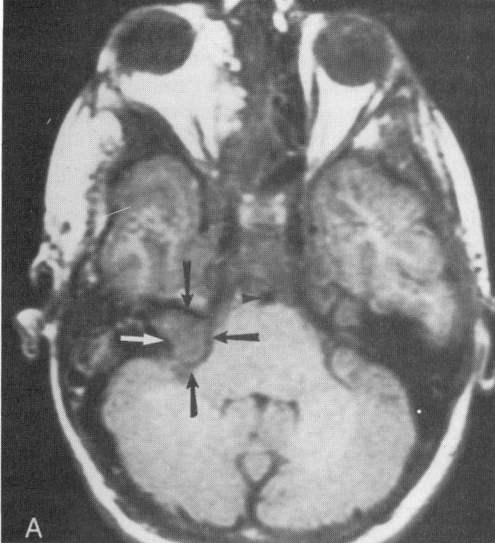

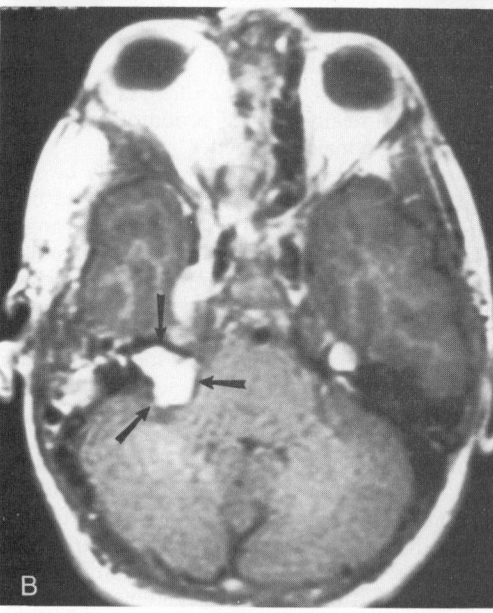

Figure 7. *A*, Noncontrast MRI of the brain at the level of the cerebellopontine angle cisterns reveals an isointense mass on the right in the region of the internal auditory canal (arrows). Note the typical lack of signal exhibited by flowing blood in the basilar artery (arrowhead). *B*, Contrast-enhanced examination at the same level as in *A* indicates that the mass is enhanced uniformly (arrows). This proved to be an acoustic neuroma.

CEREBRAL ANGIOGRAPHY

Cerebral angiography is an invasive procedure with small but ominous risks. The most worrisome complication of cerebral angiography is precipitation of a cerebral vascular accident related to dislodgment of embolic material at the time of catheterization of the great vessels of the neck. The risk for this procedure is 0.5 to 3 per cent, depending on the angiographer and the patient population. Fortunately, cerebral angiography is a relatively rare examination at present, because CT scanning and MRI have supplanted many of its former functions. Nevertheless, cerebral angiography remains an important or definitive examination in the following situations:

1. Detection and evaluation of intracerebral aneurysms.
2. Evaluation of arteriovenous malformations (usually initially detected on CT scanning or MRI).
3. Evaluation of vasculitis.

4. Detection of vessel displacement or encasement by tumor when not readily apparent on MRI.
5. Definition of superficial landmarks such as cortical veins for the purposes of neurosurgical procedures.
6. Evaluation of atherosclerotic disease of the carotid bifurcation and cavernous carotid artery.
7. Conditions requiring treatment by intravascular neurointerventional means such as embolization of vessels responsible for uncontrollable nosebleed or gluing of cerebral arteriovenous malformations (for more details see references).

There are two methods of imaging angiographic information at present. The "cut film" method employs routine radiographic film exposure and is employed when fine radiographic detail, such as in work-up for cerebral aneurysm, is required. "Digital" imaging utilizes computer-assisted enhancement of images when fine anatomic detail is not required, such as in work-up for carotid artery disease. "Cut film" imaging provides superior resolution and a larger field of view; "digital" images require less contrast and may be much more quickly performed. The determination of which type of imaging to employ is usually left to the discretion of the radiologist.

MYELOGRAPHY

Myelography was formerly the most important examination for evaluation of disease of the spine involving the central nervous system. This no longer prevails because of the superior analysis obtained with the use of noninvasive procedures such as CT scanning and MRI. In most cases, myelography is necessary only for evaluating diffuse disease of the subarachnoid space that may be difficult to discern on MRI or CT, such as diffuse subarachnoid seeding of tumor, and in cases where other modalities have not clearly answered the clinical questions. Even in the latter, myelography alone is rarely sufficient, and CT scanning of the spine in the region of interest is usually required after insertion of myelographic contrast (the CT-myelogram).

Two common indications for myelography prior to the advent of CT scanning were evaluation of lumbar disc disease and metastatic disease. In lumbar disc disease, myelography is not as accurate as CT scanning or MRI in detecting herniated discs and provides only limited information concerning the bony canal and essentially no information concerning ligamentous structures. In metastatic disease, myelography is most often employed to demonstrate a "block" that represents tumor invading the spinal canal to such an extent that contrast cannot flow freely throughout the subarachnoid space. However, MRI adequately demonstrates this lesion in a noninvasive manner with minimal discomfort for the patient. A myelogram may be required only when the exact level of involvement cannot be determined clinically, because it is often too time-consuming or difficult to use MRI for the entire spine.

PLAIN FILMS

CT scanning and MRI of the brain are so effective in demonstrating disease of the central nervous system that plain films are seldom of value in evaluation of intracerebral disease. Plain films are most useful in demonstrating fractures, particularly of the face, and sinus disease.

SUMMARY

Imaging of neurologic disease was greatly altered with the advent of CT scanning, which provided a quick, noninvasive, and much more accurate means of determining pathologic conditions in the central nervous system than did angiography, myelography, and pneumoencephalography. Further refinements have been obtained with MRI, and the indications for CT scanning versus MRI are being determined. However, in most cases MRI provides superior anatomic information as well as greater sensitivity for disease, whereas CT scanning is frequently superior for evaluation of acute neurologic events and bony problems. Angiography is reserved for specific diagnostic problems, such as evaluation of cerebral aneurysms, carotid artery disease, and vasculitis. Myelography is rarely indicated when CT scanning and MRI are available.

SELECTED REFERENCES

Brant-Zawadzki, M.: Magnetic Resonance Imaging of the Central Nervous System. New York, Raven Press, 1987.
Although this book was written several years ago when MRI was quite new, it remains an excellent introductory text to MRI because of the breadth of the thoughtfully written text and the high quality of the images.

Neuroradiology. Radiol. Clin. of North Am., 20 (1), 1982.
This volume is a group of articles on selected topics. While almost all the articles are well written and worth reading, the articles on intracranial hemorrhage and infarctions are classics.

Pomeranz, S.: Craniospinal Magnetic Resonance Imaging. Philadelphia, W. B. Saunders Company, 1989.
At present, this textbook probably represents the best single volume devoted to MRI of the brain and spine.

Taveras, J. M., and Wood, E. H.: Diagnostic Neuroradiology, 2nd ed. Baltimore, William & Wilkins, 1976.
As a general textbook on neuroradiology, this book is out of date because it does not include CT or MRI. However, it contains the best discussion of the interpretation of cerebral angiography in a single volume.

William, A., and Haughton, V.: Cranial Computed Tomography. St. Louis, C. V. Mosby Company, 1985.
Of the several textbooks available on head CT, this is the one most frequently read by radiology residents.

REFERENCES

1. Bergeron, R. T., Osborn, A. G., and Som, P. M.: Head and Neck Imaging Excluding the Brain. St. Louis, C. V. Mosby Company, 1984.
2. Brant-Zawadzki, M.: Magnetic Resonance Imaging of the Central Nervous System. New York, Raven Press, 1987.
3. CT of the Ear, Nose and Throat. Radiol. Clin. North Am., 22(1), 1984.
4. Enzmann, D. R.: Imaging of Infections and Inflammations of the Central Nervous System: Computed Tomography, Ultrasound and Nuclear Magnetic Resonance. New York, Raven Press, 1984.
5. Enzmann, D. R., De La Paz, R. L., and Rubin, R. L.: Magnetic Resonance of the Spine. St Louis, C. V. Mosby Company, 1990.
6. Gonzalez, C. F., Grossman, C. B., and Masdeu, J. C.: Head and Spine Imaging. New York, John Wiley & Sons, 1985.
7. Imaging in Neuroradiology. Radiol Clin. North Am., 26 (4 and 5), 1988.
8. Imaging in Ophthalmology. Radiol. Clin. North Am., 25 (3 and 4), 1987.
9. Lasjuanias, R. L., and Berenstein, A.: Surgical Neuroangiography. New York, Springer Verlag, 1987.
10. Latchaw, R. E.: Computed Tomography of the Head, Neck and Spine. Chicago, Year Book Medical Publishers, 1985.
11. Modic, M. T., Masaryk, T. J., and Ross, J. S.: Magnetic Resonance Imaging of the Spine. Chicago, Year Book Medical Publishers, 1989.
12. Neuroradiology. Radiol. Clin. North Am., 20(1), 1982.
13. Newton, T., and Potts, D. A.: Radiology of the Skull and Brain. St. Louis, C. V. Mosby Company, 1974.
14. Pomeranz, S.: Craniospinal Magnetic Resonance Imaging. Philadelphia, W. B. Saunders Company, 1989.
15. Primary Brain Tumors. Semin. Roentgenol., *19* (1 and 2), 1984.
16. Taveras, J. M., Ferrucci, J. T., Elliott, L. P., et al.: Radiology: Diagnosis, Imaging, Intervention. Vol. 3. Philadelphia, J. B. Lippincott Company, 1987.
17. Taveras, J. M., and Wood, E. H.: Diagnostic Neuroradiology, 2nd ed. Baltimore, Williams & Wilkins, 1976.
18. Valvassori, G. E., Buckingham, R. A., Carter, B. L., et al.: Head and Neck Imaging. New York, Thieme Medical Publishers, 1988.
19. Williams, A., and Haughton, V.: Cranial Computed Tomography. St. Louis, C. V. Mosby Company, 1985.

III

INTRACRANIAL TUMORS

Robert H. Wilkins, M.D.

Primary intracranial tumors arise from tissues of the brain or pituitary gland or their coverings.[3,11–13] Often, these lesions are not clearly separable into benign and malignant forms. Some histologically benign pituitary adenomas, for example, may invade the adjacent dura mater and bone, and grow into the cavernous sinus or the sphenoid sinus. Another example, the most histologically malignant of the astrocytomas, the glioblastoma multiforme, invades the brain locally but seldom spreads elsewhere.

Secondary intracranial tumors represent local extensions from regional tumors or metastases from a primary malignancy elsewhere in the body.[3,11–13] Examples of regional tumors that can extend intracranially are chordomas and glomus jugulare paragangliomas. In regard to metastatic tumors, different malignancies vary in their propensity to metastasize to the brain and pituitary gland. Melanoma is especially prone to spread in this way. However, because carcinoma of the lung and carcinoma of the breast are more common lesions, these usually represent larger percentages of intracranial metastases in reported series.

The most common location of brain tumors in childhood is below the tentorium, within the posterior cranial fossa. In contrast, the most common location of brain tumors in adult life is above the tentorium. Within the various intracranial locations, certain types of tumors occur more commonly than others, both in childhood (Fig. 1) and in adulthood (Fig. 2).

Symptoms and Signs

Intracranial tumors can present in several different ways. By their growth, they can cause an increase in intracranial pressure, either directly by the mass of the tumor or indirectly by obstructing the circulation of the cerebrospinal fluid and producing hydrocephalus. In addition, bleeding may occur into the tumor, with a sudden increase in its mass effect. The symptoms that may be produced by a generalized increase in intracranial pressure are headaches (especially prominent in the morning, with a dependent head position, or during straining), nausea, vomiting, and a reduction in the level of consciousness. Such a patient may exhibit papilledema and unilateral or bilateral abducens paresis. A generalized increase in intracranial pressure may be tolerated for a period of time, but with further tumor growth, brain herniation may occur, with a rapid decline in the patient's neurologic function. Herniation of the medial aspect of the temporal lobe over the edge of the tentorium with compression of the midbrain, downward brain stem displacement, or herniation of the cerebellar tonsils through the foramen magnum may cause a progressive loss of consciousness, an elevation of the systemic blood pressure with widening of the pulse pressure, and the development of bradycardia.

A second way in which an intracranial tumor may present is by the loss of function of the portion of the nervous system that is involved by the tumor. In contrast to the symptoms and signs

TOPOGRAPHIC DISTRIBUTION OF INTRACRANIAL TUMORS IN CHILDHOOD

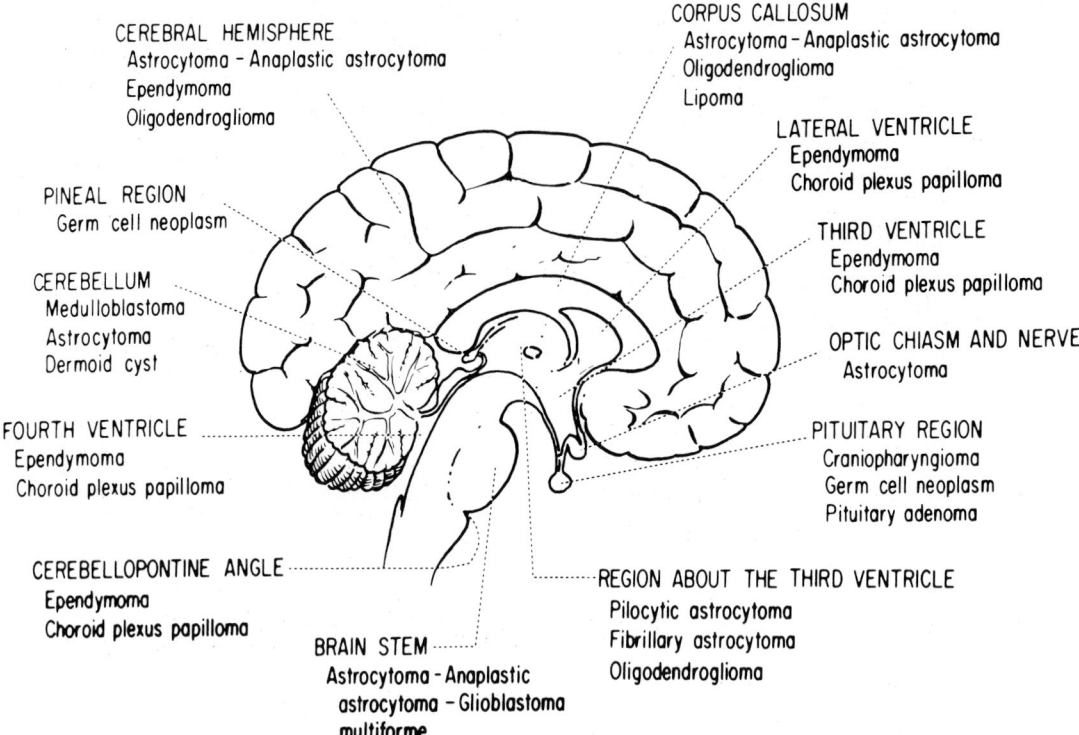

CEREBRAL HEMISPHERE
Astrocytoma – Anaplastic astrocytoma
Ependymoma
Oligodendroglioma

CORPUS CALLOSUM
Astrocytoma – Anaplastic astrocytoma
Oligodendroglioma
Lipoma

LATERAL VENTRICLE
Ependymoma
Choroid plexus papilloma

THIRD VENTRICLE
Ependymoma
Choroid plexus papilloma

PINEAL REGION
Germ cell neoplasm

OPTIC CHIASM AND NERVE
Astrocytoma

CEREBELLUM
Medulloblastoma
Astrocytoma
Dermoid cyst

PITUITARY REGION
Craniopharyngioma
Germ cell neoplasm
Pituitary adenoma

FOURTH VENTRICLE
Ependymoma
Choroid plexus papilloma

CEREBELLOPONTINE ANGLE
Ependymoma
Choroid plexus papilloma

REGION ABOUT THE THIRD VENTRICLE
Pilocytic astrocytoma
Fibrillary astrocytoma
Oligodendroglioma

BRAIN STEM
Astrocytoma – Anaplastic
astrocytoma – Glioblastoma
multiforme

Figure 1. The most common types of intracranial tumors in childhood, by location. (From Burger, P. C., Scheithaver, B. W., and Vogel, F. S.: Surgical Pathology of the Nervous System and Its Coverings, 3rd ed. New York, Churchill Livingstone, 1991.)

TOPOGRAPHIC DISTRIBUTION OF INTRACRANIAL TUMORS IN ADULTHOOD

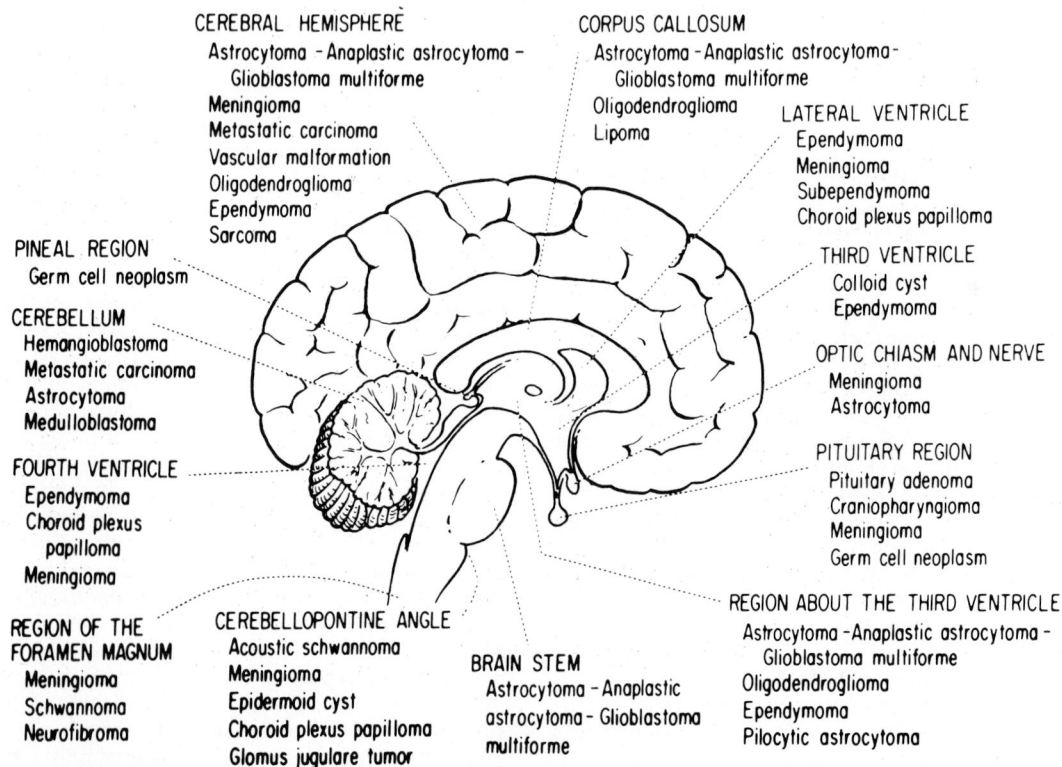

CEREBRAL HEMISPHERE
Astrocytoma – Anaplastic astrocytoma –
Glioblastoma multiforme
Meningioma
Metastatic carcinoma
Vascular malformation
Oligodendroglioma
Ependymoma
Sarcoma

CORPUS CALLOSUM
Astrocytoma – Anaplastic astrocytoma –
Glioblastoma multiforme
Oligodendroglioma
Lipoma

LATERAL VENTRICLE
Ependymoma
Meningioma
Subependymoma
Choroid plexus papilloma

PINEAL REGION
Germ cell neoplasm

THIRD VENTRICLE
Colloid cyst
Ependymoma

CEREBELLUM
Hemangioblastoma
Metastatic carcinoma
Astrocytoma
Medulloblastoma

OPTIC CHIASM AND NERVE
Meningioma
Astrocytoma

PITUITARY REGION
Pituitary adenoma
Craniopharyngioma
Meningioma
Germ cell neoplasm

FOURTH VENTRICLE
Ependymoma
Choroid plexus
papilloma
Meningioma

REGION OF THE
FORAMEN MAGNUM
Meningioma
Schwannoma
Neurofibroma

CEREBELLOPONTINE ANGLE
Acoustic schwannoma
Meningioma
Epidermoid cyst
Choroid plexus papilloma
Glomus jugulare tumor

BRAIN STEM
Astrocytoma – Anaplastic
astrocytoma – Glioblastoma
multiforme

REGION ABOUT THE THIRD VENTRICLE
Astrocytoma – Anaplastic astrocytoma –
Glioblastoma multiforme
Oligodendroglioma
Ependymoma
Pilocytic astrocytoma

Figure 2. The most common types of intracranial tumors in adulthood, by location. (From Burger, P. C., Scheithaver, B. W., and Vogel, F. S.: Surgical Pathology of the Nervous System and Its Coverings, 3rd ed. New York, Churchill Livingstone, 1991.)

caused by an increase in intracranial pressure, the symptoms and signs caused by the loss of function of a specific area of the nervous system often permit an accurate presumptive diagnosis based on the neurologic history and physical examination. For example, if a patient presents with a progressive unilateral hearing loss that was manifested initially by difficulty in understanding speech, and demonstrates a unilateral reduction in pure tone hearing with a disproportionate loss of speech discrimination, and an ipsilateral reduction in corneal sensation, the suspected diagnosis would be an acoustic neurinoma.

Finally, an intracranial tumor may be manifested by hyperactive function. The tumor itself can be the cause of this hyperfunction, such as a pituitary adenoma that overproduces one or more hormones or a choroid plexus papilloma that overproduces cerebrospinal fluid; or the tumor may stimulate seizures that arise from the adjacent or infiltrated brain.

Diagnosis

At times the presence, location, and type of intracranial tumor can be suspected from the patient's symptoms and signs. In this case, the diagnostic studies are tailored to confirm the suspicion and to facilitate treatment. Yet often the symptoms are vague and the signs are nonspecific, especially early in the course of the disease. In this circumstance, the initial diagnostic studies are more of a general or screening type.

At present, the most common screening examination is computed tomography (CT) scanning. Most intracranial tumors are demonstrated by such scanning, especially if scans made after the intravenous injection of an iodinated contrast agent (contrast-enhanced scans) are compared with analogous unenhanced scans. The bony structures forming the base of the skull are especially well demonstrated by CT scanning. However, these same bony structures are often the source of artifacts that degrade the images of the adjacent portions of the brain. Magnetic resonance imaging (MRI) does not demonstrate bony detail, but does provide excellent visualization of the brain at the cranial base and at the craniocervical junction. MRI also offers much clearer and more easily obtained coronal and sagittal views (Fig. 3). MRI does not expose the patient to x-rays, but the magnet may have adverse effects on certain metallic objects within a patient's body such as an implanted cardiac pacemaker, and this property as well as the claustrophobia that some

patients experience within the tight confines of the MRI device limit its applicability somewhat. Among other types of radiologic studies are those done for specific purposes rather than for screening. For example, cerebral angiography may be useful to determine the vascularity of the tumor and its effect on the major adjacent vessels; with very vascular tumors, preoperative embolization of the tumor at the time of angiography can be used to reduce the intraoperative blood loss. Plain roentgenograms of the skull and radionuclide brain scanning, which were of value before the introduction of CT scanning and MRI, are seldom employed now in the diagnosis of brain tumors.

In certain circumstances, other types of studies may have diagnostic value. Electroencephalography may be helpful in analyzing patients with seizure disorders. Detailed hormonal assays can be useful in assessing the nature of a pituitary or hypothalamic tumor and in guiding its medical management. A thorough ophthalmologic examination, including visual field testing, is important in the pre- and postoperative evaluation of patients with tumors involving, or adjacent to, the visual or ocular motor pathways. Careful evaluation with audiometry, auditory evoked potential testing, and electronystagmography is ordinarily helpful in the assessment and management of patients with tumors of the cerebellopontine angle or posterior skull base.

Preoperatively, the intracarotid injection of amobarbital sodium can be used to assess cerebral hemispheric dominance for speech. During the resection of a tumor, brain function can be tested directly (if the operation is done under local anesthesia and the patient is awake and cooperative) or indirectly by such techniques as electrical stimulation of the brain or cranial nerves (to determine areas important for motor function) or somatosensory and auditory evoked potential monitoring.

Lumbar puncture for examination of the cerebrospinal fluid has little role in the evaluation of intracranial tumors. This test usually does not provide significant diagnostic information, and it is dangerous in that it may precipitate brain herniation in a patient with a mass lesion.

Treatment

The mainstay of the treatment of intracranial tumors is surgical removal. The major advances that have been made in the past 2 decades in diagnostic and therapeutic technology have

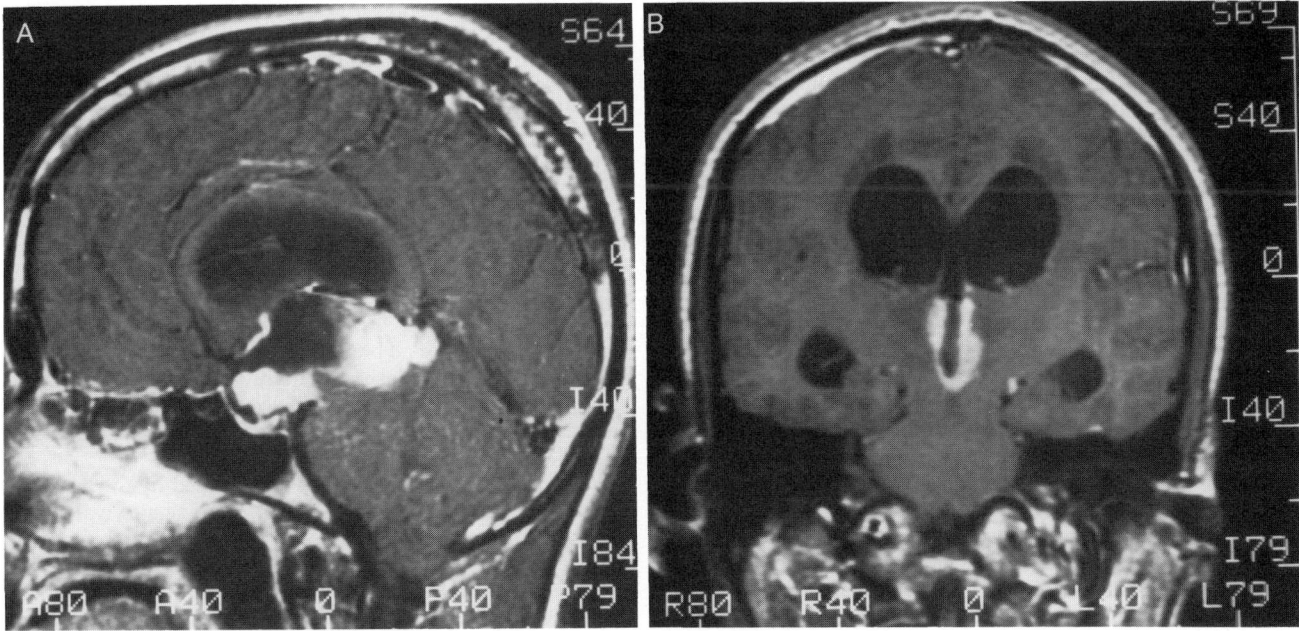

Figure 3. Sagittal (A) and coronal (B) magnetic resonance images, showing an enhancing germinoma in the pineal and suprasellar areas with spread along the walls of the third ventricle. Obstructive hydrocephalus is also demonstrated.

made this task easier and safer than ever before. With CT-guided or MRI-guided stereotactic techniques, tumors within the nervous system can now be biopsied through a burr hole, with low morbidity. The introduction of the operative microscope into neurosurgery and the development of neurosurgical microtechnique have permitted tumor exposure through a small cranial opening with the double aids of magnification and excellent illumination. The simultaneous evolution of bipolar electrical technology for tissue coagulation and cutting with the development of devices that employ laser energy, ultrasonic vibration, suction, or mechanical cutting to remove tissue permits the modern neurosurgeon to resect intracranial tumors more easily and safely.

The technological advances have brought about improvement in the prognosis for patients with certain types of intracranial tumors, such as meningiomas, pituitary adenomas, and neurinomas of the cranial nerves. However, they have not had a large impact on the gliomas, which in most instances cannot be cured by surgical resection.

TUMOR TYPES

Various schemes have been used over the years to classify intracranial neoplasms, and in large part these have been based on the presumed cell of origin. Among the tumors considered to arise from cells derived from the primitive neuroectoderm, the greatest number are attributable to the neuroglia and are called gliomas.

Intraparenchymal (Intra-axial) Brain Tumors

Among the primary tumors that arise within the brain, those of astrocytic, oligodendroglial, and ependymal origin are not divided sharply into benign and malignant forms, but rather represent gradations on a spectrum from slowly growing to rapidly growing neoplasms. Moreover, with time some tumors may shift from the benign end of the spectrum to the malignant end as the more aggressive cells replicate themselves to a greater extent than do the more indolent cells.

Brain tumors ordinarily exert their effects by progressive growth within one area of the brain, although some types such as medulloblastomas, ependymomas, and certain pineal tumors may spread via the cerebrospinal fluid through the ventricular system or the subarachnoid spaces. Intraparenchymal tumors of the brain rarely spread outside the confines of the cranial cavity and spinal canal unless an operative procedure has interfered with the normal meningeal barriers to such spread. Yet, even though these tumors grow focally and recur focally after surgical resection, with few exceptions they cannot be cured surgically.

ASTROCYTOMAS. Astrocytic neoplasms are the most common of the primary brain tumors. Among Zülch's personal series of 9000 intracranial tumors, 6.0 per cent were pilocytic astrocytomas, 6.6 per cent were astrocytomas, and 12.2 per cent were glioblastomas.[13] The peak age of occurrence for pilocytic astrocytoma is between 10 and 25 years, for astrocytoma between 30 and 50 years, and for glioblastoma multiforme between 50 and 70 years.

Astrocytic neoplasms of the cerebral hemisphere infiltrate the brain and have indistinct boundaries.[2] They tend to spread along white matter tracts and may cross the corpus callosum into the opposite hemisphere. The astrocytoma is more cellular than the normal brain and grows relatively slowly. The anaplastic astrocytoma is more cellular than the astrocytoma and has more of the cellular characteristics of malignancy; it also grows more rapidly. The most malignant form, the glioblastoma multiforme, exhibits additional histologic changes, including necrosis, neovascularity with endothelial proliferation, polymorphism, and hemorrhage.

Despite the many recent improvements in diagnostic, surgi-

cal, radiotherapeutic, and chemotherapeutic techniques, the prognosis for a patient with an astrocytic neoplasm of the cerebral hemisphere is poor. Even with the best current combination of these modalities, such tumors are seldom cured. Most patients with glioblastoma multiforme die within 1 year of diagnosis, and few survive beyond 2 years.[9]

The pilocytic astrocytoma in the region of the third ventricle has a benign histologic appearance and grows slowly, but because of its location it ordinarily cannot be cured, and the patient's life expectancy is usually less than 5 years from the time of diagnosis. Likewise, with few exceptions, astrocytic neoplasms arising within the brain stem cannot be cured, because of their location and their biologic behavior.

In contrast, astrocytomas of the cerebellum or optic nerve are usually amenable to surgical removal. There is a high probability of cure if the surgeon can remove the entire tumor mass. Why these tumors behave differently from the other astrocytomas is not well understood.

OLIGODENDROGLIOMAS. Oligodendrogliomas typically grow within the cerebral hemisphere, especially within the frontal, parietal, or temporal lobe. In Zülch's series of 9000 intracranial tumors, 9.6 per cent were oligodendrogliomas.[13] The peak age of occurrence is between 40 and 50 years.

Calcification within oligodendrogliomas is often sufficiently prominent to be detected radiographically. Histologically, oligodendrogliomas vary. In 1986, Ludwig and associates reported the largest clinicopathologic study of oligodendrogliomas to that date.[4] The tumors of 323 patients were graded A through D, based on the presence, absence, and degree of five criteria: cell density, nuclear : cytoplasmic ratio, pleomorphism, endothelial proliferation, and necrosis. Of the 323 tumors, 23 per cent were grade A, 49 per cent were grade B, 22 per cent were grade C, and 6 per cent were grade D. Patient age and tumor grade were related in that 68 per cent of the patients with grade A tumors were younger than 40 years at the time of diagnosis, whereas 83 per cent of the patients with grade D tumors were older than 40 years. The usual form of treatment was surgical resection and postoperative radiotherapy. Despite this, the median survival after diagnosis was as follows: grade A, 94 months; grade B, 51 months; grade C, 45 months; grade D, 17 months.

EPENDYMOMAS. Although intracranial ependymomas can occur throughout life, there is a peak incidence during childhood, at which time an infratentorial location is most common. In Zülch's series of 9000 intracranial tumors, ependymomas constituted 4.3 per cent.[13] Surgical resection and postoperative radiotherapy are the mainstays of treatment but seldom result in a cure. In a series from the author's institution, reported by Rawlings and associates, the median survival time from first symptoms was 36 months for 21 patients (mean age, 7 years) with infratentorial ependymomas and 92 months for 22 patients (mean age, 17 years) with supratentorial ependymomas.[7]

MEDULLOBLASTOMAS. The medulloblastoma is a malignant tumor occurring in early life, with a peak incidence between 7 and 12 years. It seldom occurs in individuals over the age of 40. Among Zülch's 9000 intracranial tumors, 4.2 per cent were medulloblastomas.[13] Medulloblastomas comprise approximately 20 per cent of all brain tumors of childhood and adolescence. Most medulloblastomas involve the cerebellar vermis and extend into the fourth ventricle. Occasionally, and especially in patients over 15 years of age, they lie primarily in a cerebellar hemisphere.

When medulloblastomas were first studied in an organized manner between 1925 and 1930, the average survival period was only 17 months.[13] With present-day treatment, the survival statistics have improved considerably. The current survival rates for patients of all ages are in the range of 40 per cent at 5 years and 20 per cent at 10 years, with a cure rate approaching 20 per cent. These figures are even better for those patients having gross total tumor removal and postoperative radiotherapy with at least 5200 rads directed to the posterior fossa.[12] However, the price paid for radiation therapy to the whole brain and spinal axis in young children is retardation of intellect, endocrine function, and skeletal growth.

PRIMARY LYMPHOMAS. Primary lymphomas constitute less than 2 per cent of primary brain tumors, but their frequency of occurrence is increasing beyond that which can be attributed to improved diagnostic capabilities.[6] They appear to be in some way related to immunosuppression and are encountered especially in the recipients of transplanted organs and in patients with the acquired immunodeficiency syndrome. The typical patient is a middle-age man with a single mass lesion within a cerebral hemisphere, but multiple tumors occur in about one fourth of patients. Conventional management consists of a biopsy for pathologic confirmation of the diagnosis followed by radiotherapy, with or without chemotherapy. The median duration of survival is less than 2 years, and the 5-year survival is less than 5 per cent.

HEMANGIOBLASTOMAS. Hemangioblastomas are uncommon vascular benign tumors that occur preferentially within the cerebellum and brain stem. A hemangioblastoma may develop as a solid small mass or as a mural nodule in the wall of a cyst. Occasionally, it may be seen as part of von Hippel–Lindau disease. If a hemangioblastoma is asymptomatic, it may be followed; if it is symptomatic, the treatment ordinarily consists of surgical excision, which is usually curative.

METASTATIC NEOPLASMS. The incidence of these tumors varies depending on the source of the material studied. The highest incidence would be expected if a pathologist with a special interest in the subject performed a prospective study of serially sectioned brains from patients dying at a cancer hospital. Neurosurgeons ordinarily only become involved with metastatic brain tumors if the diagnosis is not known, if the patient has a single brain lesion, or if it is thought that the removal of a metastatic tumor would provide significant palliation. Therefore, in surgical series of brain tumors, metastatic tumors comprise only a small segment, usually less than 5 per cent.

Lung, breast, skin (malignant melanoma), kidney, and the gastrointestinal tract are the most common primary sites of neoplasms that metastasize to the brain, contributing, respectively, approximately 35, 20, 10, 10, and 5 per cent of all metastatic neoplasms.[3] Metastatic tumors ordinarily affect older adults and are distributed throughout the brain in accordance with the arterial supply. Management consists of biopsy or surgical resection (depending on the location and nature of the lesion) followed by radiotherapy and/or chemotherapy (depending on the exact tumor type). The prognosis depends on many factors including the nature of the tumor, the completeness of the surgical resection, the sensitivity of the tumor to radiotherapy and chemotherapy, the status of the primary neoplasm, and the existence of other metastases.

Extraparenchymal (Extra-axial) Brain Tumors

MENINGIOMAS. These benign tumors comprise a significant proportion of the intracranial neoplasms seen by the neurosurgeon. In Zülch's series of 9000 intracranial tumors, 16.6 per cent were meningiomas.[13] Although they can arise from the meninges at any place, meningiomas favor certain locations such as the cerebral convexity, the parasagittal area, the floor of the anterior cranial fossa in the midline, the sphenoid wings, and the clivus. They ordinarily indent or surround neural structures rather than invade them, but they often extend through the dura mater into the adjacent bone of the skull.

Meningiomas typically occur in the second half of life, and they are more common in women than in men. Because of their focal and benign nature, they offer the potential for a surgical cure. Yet, the location of many of these lesions makes their exposure and removal a challenge for the neurosurgeon. This

problem as well as their tendency to involve adjacent bone, and the fact that multiple tiny meningiomas may also exist near the main tumor, all result in a high rate of recurrence. Even if the surgeon thinks that a complete removal has been achieved, there is approximately a 10 to 15 per cent recurrence rate by 5 years. However, a recurrent meningioma still ordinarily represents a focal benign neoplasm, and it can again be treated by surgical resection. Meningiomas are not very radiosensitive, so radiotherapy is usually reserved to treat certain inoperable lesions.

NEURINOMAS. Like meningiomas, these are benign tumors that constitute a significant portion of neurosurgical practice. Among 9000 intracranial tumors reported by Zülch, 8.7 per cent were neurinomas.[13] They typically form on sensory cranial nerves, in particular the acoustic nerve or, less frequently, the trigeminal nerve, and they usually appear in adult life.

If the surgeon can remove the tumor completely, which is usually the case, a cure can be achieved. The challenge is to excise the tumor without damaging adjacent structures such as the facial nerve. Radiotherapy ordinarily is not used, but, in certain unusual circumstances, small acoustic neurinomas are treated with a single treatment of focused high-energy radiation (stereotactic radiosurgery).

PITUITARY ADENOMAS. These benign tumors typically originate from the anterior lobe of the pituitary gland.[1,8] In Zülch's series of 9000 intracranial tumors, pituitary adenomas comprised 6.6 per cent.[13] They are typically a tumor that occurs in adult life.

If a pituitary adenoma overproduces one or more pituitary hormones, it may cause a recognizable clinical entity such as the syndrome of amenorrhea and galactorrhea (prolactin overproduction), acromegaly (growth hormone overproduction), or Cushing's disease (adrenocorticotropic hormone overproduction).[1] In this situation, a pituitary adenoma may be identified by the history and physical examination, the endocrine testing results, and the MRI and CT appearances while it is still smaller than 1 cm. in diameter (microadenoma) and still confined within the gland. This circumstance offers the possibility of surgical excision of the adenoma (by a transsphenoidal approach) without significant injury to the remainder of the gland and therefore the possibility of a return to a normal endocrine status.

If the tumor does not overproduce a hormone, it usually does not come to medical attention until it has grown sufficiently (macroadenoma) to cause headaches, visual loss (typically a bitemporal hemianopsia by distortion of the optic chiasm), hypopituitary hormonal dysfunction, or hyperprolactinemia from interference with normal hypothalamic-pituitary transmission of a prolactin inhibitory factor (dopamine). In this case, the tumor is still treated surgically but cannot be removed completely. Postoperative radiotherapy and lifelong hormone replacement are ordinarily necessary as well.

If a pituitary adenoma is small, it can be treated by stereotactic radiosurgery instead of transsphenoidal surgical excision. If it is overproducing prolactin, it can be treated medically with a dopamine agonist such as bromocriptine to reduce the size of the tumor and suppress its activity; such management does not result in a cure, however.

A high percentage of the tumors treated by the previously mentioned surgical and radiation techniques are brought under long-term control. The overall prognosis for these benign lesions is good.

OTHER TUMORS. There are several other types of extra-axial intracranial tumors, including epidermoid and dermoid tumors, teratomas, craniopharyngiomas, and pineal region tumors. Each has its own characteristics and forms of therapy. As with the meningiomas, neurinomas, and pituitary adenomas, many of these tumors are benign but are located in regions that are difficult to reach. They provide a challenge to the surgeon who wants to achieve total extirpation without an increase in neurologic dysfunction.

FUTURE DIRECTIONS

Further technical improvements could improve the outcome of patients with benign, extra-axial tumors but are unlikely to improve the prognosis of patients with primary intra-axial neoplasms. The future hope in the latter area, as well as the former, is that with an increased understanding of the molecular biology of intracranial tumors, some nonsurgical approach will be found to prevent or reverse their growth.[5,10]

SELECTED REFERENCES

Wilkins, R. H., and Rengachary, S. S. (Eds.): Neurosurgery. New York, McGraw-Hill Book Company, 1985, pp. 505–1038, 1084–1163.

Youmans, J. R. (Ed.): Neurological Surgery, 3rd ed. Philadelphia, W. B. Saunders Company, 1990, pp. 2967–3504.
These works contain numerous chapters about various intracranial tumors, with emphasis on their surgical management.

REFERENCES

1. Black, P. McL., Zervas, N. T., Ridgway, E. C., and Martin, J. B. (Eds.): Secretory Tumors of the Pituitary Gland. New York, Raven Press, 1984.

2. Burger, P. C., Dubois, P. J., Schold, S. C., Jr., Smith, K. R., Jr., Odom, G. L., Crafts, D. C., and Giangaspero, F.: Computerized tomographic and pathologic studies of the untreated, quiescent, and recurrent glioblastoma multiforme. J. Neurosurg., 58:159, 1983.

3. Burger, P. C., and Vogel, F. S.: Surgical Pathology of the Nervous System and Its Coverings, 2nd ed. New York, John Wiley & Sons, 1982.

4. Ludwig, C. L., Smith M. T., Godfrey, A. D., and Armbrustmacher, V. W.: A clinicopathological study of 323 patients with oligodendrogliomas. Ann. Neurol., 19:15, 1986.

5. McDonald, J. D., and Dohrmann, G. J.: Molecular biology of brain tumors. Neurosurgery, 23:537, 1988.

6. O'Neill, B. P., and Illig, J. J.: Primary central nervous system lymphoma. Mayo Clin. Proc. 64:1005, 1989.

7. Rawlings, C. E., III, Giangaspero, F., Burger, P. C., and Bullard, D. E.: Ependymomas: A clinicopathologic study. Surg. Neurol., 29:271, 1988.

8. Tindall, G. T., and Barrow, D. L.: Disorders of the Pituitary. St. Louis, C. V. Mosby, 1986.

9. Walker, M. D., Alexander, E., Jr., Hunt, W. E., MacCarty, C. S., Mahaley, M. S., Jr., Mealey, J., Jr., Norrell, H. A., Owens, G., Ransohoff, J., Wilson, C. B., Gehan, E. A., and Strike, T. A.: Evaluation of BCNU and/or radiotherapy in the treatment of anaplastic gliomas: A cooperative clinical trial. J. Neurosurg., 49:333, 1978.

10. Westphal, M., and Herrmann, H. D.: Growth factor biology and oncogene activation in human gliomas and their implications for specific therapeutic concepts. Neurosurgery, 25:681, 1989.

11. Wilkins, R. H., and Rengachary, S. S. (Eds.): Neurosurgery. New York, McGraw-Hill Book Company, 1985, pp. 505–1038, 1084–1163.

12. Youmans, J. R. (Ed.): Neurological Surgery, 3rd ed. Philadelphia, W. B. Saunders Company, 1990, pp. 2967–3504.

13. Zülch, K. J.: Brain Tumors: Their Biology and Pathology, 3rd ed. Berlin, Springer-Verlag, 1986.

IV ———————————————

SPONTANEOUS INTRACRANIAL AND INTRASPINAL HEMORRHAGE

Allan H. Friedman, M.D., and Robert H. Wilkins, M.D.

SPONTANEOUS SUBARACHNOID HEMORRHAGE AND INTRACRANIAL ANEURYSMS

Subarachnoid Hemorrhage

SYMPTOMS AND SIGNS. Characteristically, this type of bleeding has an explosive onset, causing severe headache, nausea, vomiting, and perhaps loss of consciousness, with or without a concomitant seizure.[6] These symptoms are most likely due to the sudden increase in intracranial pressure caused by a jet of arterial blood at a mean pressure of perhaps 100 to 150 mm. Hg spurting into a space filled with cerebrospinal fluid having a pressure of about 10 to 15 mm. Hg. Fortunately, the bleeding ceases after a small amount of blood has escaped, perhaps as a result of a transient muscular spasm in the walls of the arteries adjacent to the site of bleeding or because the local intracranial pressure transiently is equal to the arterial pressure. Then, as the blood induces a sterile meningitis over the ensuing hours, stiff neck, minor fever, and photophobia develop. In approximately one third of patients, a particularly severe headache may precede the dramatic onset of subarachnoid hemorrhage, indicating a "small leak" of subarachnoid blood.[13] Unfortunately, these warning events may go unrecognized.

The ictus itself may be precipitated by physical stress, but more than one third of patients sustain the subarachnoid hemorrhage during sleep. An unusually high number of patients who have experienced a subarachnoid hemorrhage are noted to be hypertensive when they are brought to the hospital. However, in many instances, this systemic arterial hypertension sim-

ply reflects a physiologic response to increased intracranial pressure.

Retinal hemorrhages may develop, because the blood in the subarachnoid spaces about each optic nerve compresses the central retinal vein at its exit from the nerve, causing retrograde venous distention back within the eye itself. Changes in the electrocardiogram, primarily involving altered and delayed ventricular repolarization, may occur in association with subarachnoid hemorrhage. Fluid and electrolyte disturbances are also common in patients with subarachnoid hemorrhage from a ruptured aneurysm. These and the electrocardiographic changes are thought to follow hypothalamic injury.[20]

Approximately 20 per cent of patients die within 24 hours of their first major subarachnoid hemorrhage, largely because of the damage sustained by the brain by intracerebral hemorrhage or by acutely increased intracranial pressure with cerebral herniation. The survivors frequently recover within a few days with little or no neurologic deficit, only to confront two more serious threats: cerebral arterial spasm and recurrent subarachnoid hemorrhage.

CEREBRAL ARTERIAL SPASM. Cerebral arterial spasm is demonstrated in cerebral arteriograms as a narrowing of previously normal arteries (Fig. 1).[20] This phenomenon is encountered in the arteriograms of at least 40 per cent of patients with subarachnoid hemorrhage from a ruptured aneurysm. It almost never appears until the third day after the bleeding episode and rarely has its onset after the tenth day. Once it occurs, it lasts for days to weeks. Cerebral arterial spasm is frequently associated with decreased blood flow through the involved arteries,[23] and

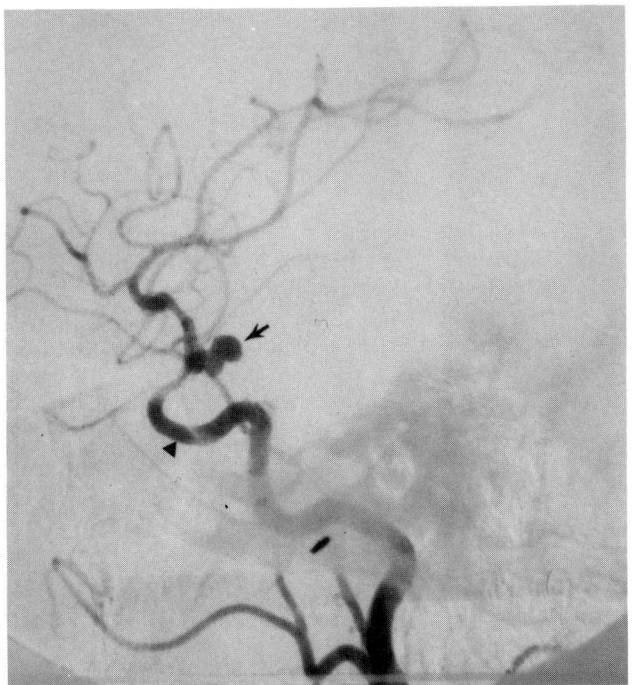

Figure 1. Angiographic demonstration of an aneurysm (dark arrow) of the internal carotid artery. Note the vasospasm of the internal carotid artery adjacent to the aneurysm.

depending on its severity, it may be manifested clinically as cerebral ischemia or infarction. Recent evidence indicates that the propensity of a patient for developing vasospasm is proportional to the amount of subarachnoid hemorrhage visualized on the computed tomographic (CT) scan.[7]

Intravascular volume expansion and systemic arterial hypertension are the most effective therapies for cerebral arterial spasm. Nimodipine appears to protect patients from stroke following a subarachnoid hemorrhage.[1,18]

ETIOLOGY. After the first bleeding episode, the patient's subsequent course depends a great deal on whether an aneurysm, arteriovenous malformation, or some other detectable lesion was responsible. In an extensive cooperative study involving 19 medical centers, the causes of spontaneous (i.e., nontraumatic) subarachnoid hemorrhage in 5834 patients were found to be intracranial aneurysm in 51 per cent, cerebral angiomatous malformation in 6 per cent, and both in 0.7 per cent. A small number of additional patients had hypertensive intracerebral hemorrhage, primary or metastatic brain tumor, cerebral embolus, blood dyscrasia, anticoagulation therapy, eclampsia, intracranial infection, spinal angiomatous malformation, or some other condition. Rarely subarachnoid hemorrhage occurs secondary to a dissecting aneurysm.[8] In the remainder, the etiology of the hemorrhage was never satisfactorily explained.

RECURRENT BLEEDING. The patients in whom arteriography of both carotid and both vertebral circulations is normal seldom have any recurrence of bleeding, and their prognosis is good. However, intracranial aneurysms have a high propensity for recurrent hemorrhage. One in 5 patients experiences a second bleeding episode during the 2 weeks following the initial hemorrhage,[12] and the second rupture has a mortality of approximately 50 per cent. The goal of surgical therapy is to prevent subsequent episodes of hemorrhage.

Antifibrinolytic agents have been shown to decrease the incidence of recurrent hemorrhage for the first 2 weeks following the rupture of an aneurysm.[12] Such agents are often employed by surgeons who delay intracranial surgery. Unfortunately, patients treated with these agents have a higher incidence of posthemorrhage stroke, which negates their beneficial effect.

The incidence of rehemorrhage from an arteriovenous malformation is much lower than that from an intracranial aneurysm. A recent study reports a rate of rebleeding of 6 per cent in the year following a hemorrhage from an arteriovenous malformation and a 3 per cent per year rate of hemorrhage in subsequent years.[9,21]

Cerebral Aneurysms

As stated earlier, cerebral arterial aneurysms (sometimes referred to as berry aneurysms) comprise slightly more than half of all cases of spontaneous subarachnoid hemorrhage. Unruptured congenital aneurysms appear to rupture at a rate of 1 to 2 per cent per year.[22] The propensity of an unruptured aneurysm to rupture is proportional to its size. Congenital cerebral aneurysms typically develop at vessel bifurcations and have been postulated to follow congenital deficiencies or degenerative changes in the vessel's wall. As the aneurysm enlarges, its internal elastic lamina frays apart, and its dome consists primarily of intima and the remaining adventitial connective tissue. The turbulent and irregular flow of the blood entering the aneurysm through its relatively narrow neck contributes to its enlargement, and also to the laminations of thrombus that are frequently deposited within its sac. These thrombi may be viewed as the body's attempts to obliterate the aneurysm. However, they are usually inadequate to prevent rupture of the aneurysm, especially after it becomes larger than 1 cm. in diameter.

Aneurysms usually come to clinical attention as the source of a subarachnoid hemorrhage, but they may also give rise to an intracerebral or subdural hematoma. Giant aneurysms (greater than 2.5 cm. in diameter) can present as a tumor mass causing clinically detectable dysfunction in the adjacent brain. An aneurysm of the internal carotid artery may compress the adjacent oculomotor nerve or optic nerve. Similarly, an aneurysm of the internal carotid artery that occurs within the cavernous sinus may compress the adjacent ipsilateral third, fourth, fifth, and sixth cranial nerves as it enlarges. If such an aneurysm ruptures, it causes a carotid cavernous fistula rather than a subarachnoid hemorrhage. Although this does not involve a serious threat to the patient's life, it may cause a series of disabling complications from an annoying bruit to bilateral blindness. Occasionally an aneurysm is detected on an angiogram or CT scan as an incidental finding.

Although they appear to be due to a congenital weakness of the arterial wall, cerebral aneurysms seldom rupture or otherwise make their presence known during childhood. Instead, they are one of the causes of "stroke," or "cerebrovascular accident," in the adult. Atherosclerosis, inflammation, and other pathologic processes may also involve the walls of a congenital aneurysm. Moreover, several other types of aneurysms may occur on the larger cerebral arteries and may be demonstrated angiographically. These include (1) fusiform atherosclerotic aneurysms or ectasias involving mainly the proximal internal carotid arteries or the vertebrobasilar complex; (2) mycotic aneurysms, usually involving the distal branches of the middle cerebral arteries; (3) dissecting aneurysms; (4) traumatic aneurysms; and (5) luetic aneurysms. However, these are unusual or rare forms of intracranial aneurysm, and a discussion of their pathogenesis and treatment is beyond the scope of this chapter.

Congenital berry aneurysms occur almost anywhere along the components and larger branches of the arterial circle of Willis, but especially at a few specific locations. Most of these aneurysms are located at the junction of the posterior communicating artery with the internal carotid artery (Fig. 1), at the junction of the anterior communicating artery with one of the anterior cerebral arteries (Fig. 2), or at the first major branches of the middle cerebral artery (Fig. 3). Another, less common, site is the terminal bifurcation of the basilar artery. Multiple aneurysms

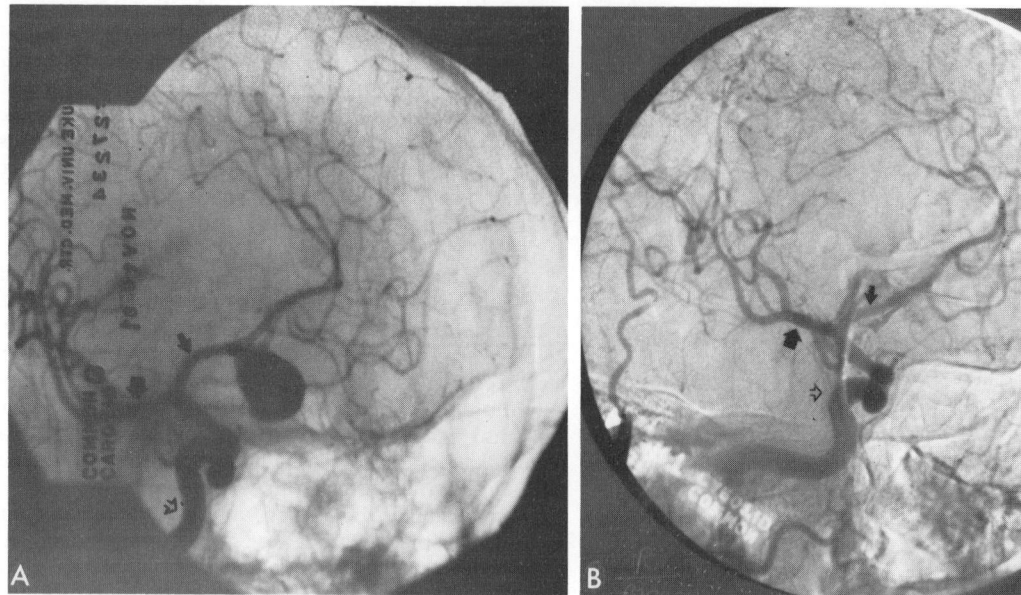

Figure 2. *A*, Oblique view of a right carotid angiogram demonstrating an aneurysm originating at the anterior communicating artery. *B*, The same angiographic view following surgical ligation of the aneurysm. Internal carotid artery, open arrow; middle cerebral artery, thick arrow; anterior cerebral artery, thin arrow.

can be found in approximately 20 per cent of patients with aneurysms.

Management of Subarachnoid Hemorrhage

In a patient suspected of having a spontaneous subarachnoid hemorrhage, the diagnosis should be verified by a CT scan (or lumbar puncture if the scan is negative). The CT scan, if positive, may demonstrate the location or even the source of the hemorrhage. If a lumbar puncture is done, a few milliliters of the bloody cerebrospinal fluid should be centrifuged, and the appearance of the supernatant fluid noted. Oxyhemoglobin appears in the cerebrospinal fluid a few hours after the hemorrhage and then bilirubin appears and persists for 2 to 3 weeks.[2]

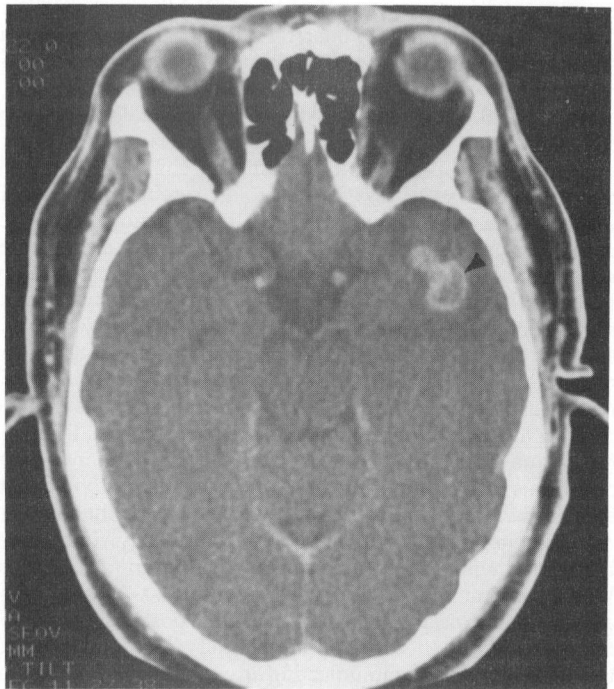

Figure 3. Iodine-enhanced computed axial tomogram (CT) of the brain demonstrating an aneurysm of the left middle cerebral artery (arrowhead). The large size of this aneurysm makes it visible on CT scan.

Therefore, during the first few days after the hemorrhage, the presence of xanthochromia in the supernatant demonstrates that bleeding has occurred and that the bloody cerebrospinal fluid is not the result of a traumatic lumbar puncture. Similarly, when cerebrospinal fluid is obtained 1 to 3 weeks after hemorrhage, the red blood cells are usually not present and xanthochromia may be the only proof that bleeding did occur. There may also be abnormally low cerebrospinal fluid sugar value, probably because of the obstruction by the blood of routes of entry of sugar from the bloodstream into the cerebrospinal fluid.

The patient should then be transferred as soon as possible to a neurosurgical center equipped to treat intracranial aneurysms. The patient is maintained at strict bed rest in peaceful surroundings to minimize the danger of rebleeding, and cerebral angiography is performed to visualize the cerebral arteries. If the angiogram is normal and focal hemorrhage has been identified on the CT scan, the angiogram should be repeated. When no source of hemorrhage can be identified, the patient is kept at bed rest for a 2-week period and then gradually returned to normal activities over the third week. Patients in whom a source for the subarachnoid hemorrhage cannot be found have a low incidence of recurrent hemorrhage, but they are at risk for developing vasospasm, hydrocephalus, and cognitive deficits.

Surgical Treatment of Aneurysms

If an aneurysm is demonstrated arteriographically, the neurosurgeon must then decide when and how to treat it. The definitive treatment is the surgical obliteration of the aneurysm. In the early days of aneurysm surgery, surgeons operated on ruptured aneurysms as soon as possible. At operation they often confronted a swollen brain and premature rupture of the aneurysm, and following the procedure, the patient often deteriorated from vasospasm. Soon it was noted that if surgical therapy was delayed until the third week after the initial hemorrhage, the surgical morbidity and mortality would be dramatically diminished. In many clinics, delayed surgical intervention became the standard method of therapy, with the patients being given antifibrinolytic agents while awaiting operation. Unfortunately, the patient is still exposed to the risk of a devastating recurrent hemorrhage or neurologic deficit secondary to vasospasm while awaiting surgical therapy. Although operative complications have decreased dramatically, studies have emphasized that patients who enter the hospital in relatively good condition following the rupture of an aneurysm have only a 50 per cent likelihood of leaving the hospital in good condition when surgical therapy is delayed. For this reason, many authorities now advocate a reassessment of early surgical intervention for the treatment of intracranial aneurysms.[11] At present, most patients who have survived their hemorrhage in good neurologic condition are operated upon within 3 days after hemorrhage.

An aneurysm is best treated by removing it from the cerebral circulation, while keeping the arteries from which it arises intact (Fig. 2). If the aneurysm is accessible surgically and has a definable narrow neck that involves only a short segment of its parent artery, this goal can be accomplished by placing a metal clip or ligature about its neck. Such procedures are attended by various hazards, such as the possible rupture of the aneurysm while it is being exposed. With experienced hands, using the operating microscope, controlled intraoperative hypotension, modern microsurgical instrumentation, and a wide array of removable aneurysm clips, the operative mortality should be less than 5 per cent.

Some authors advocate reinforcement of the aneurysm by wrapping it with strips of muscle, fascia, cloth, or other material or by coating it with plastic. However, unlike the cases in which just the neck of the aneurysm must be exposed to accept a clip or ligature, in these cases the entire aneurysm, including its previous point of rupture, must be dissected free of the surrounding tissue before it can be adequately reinforced.

A third technique, proximal artery occlusion, reduces the pressure and promotes thrombosis within the aneurysm. This is accompanied with the danger of distal cerebral ischemia and infarction, especially if such treatment is complicated by cerebral arterial spasm. Gradual occlusion of the common or internal carotid artery has frequently been employed for the treatment of giant aneurysms of the internal carotid artery. Proximal artery occlusion has also been employed in the treatment of giant aneurysms throughout the cerebral vasculature.[5] However, as surgical technology improves, "second best methods" such as proximal artery occlusion and aneurysm wrapping are employed less frequently.

Blood within the subarachnoid space from any cause obliterates the arachnoidal villi and other arachnoidal channels that are important in the normal absorption of cerebrospinal fluid. This frequently causes mild hydrocephalus for a few days or weeks until the blood has been absorbed. However, in some cases, the communicating hydrocephalus persists, and some type of shunt operation (e.g., ventriculo- or lumboperitoneal) may then be required.

Operative complications represent only a small portion of the morbidity and mortality associated with ruptured intracranial aneurysms. Of the 28,000 patients who are expected to suffer from the rupture of an intracranial aneurysm this year in the United States and Canada, the major causes of morbidity and mortality will be misdiagnosis, rebleeding, and vasospasm.[11]

While unruptured, an aneurysm can be treated with a morbidity and mortality of under 5 per cent. Once the aneurysm ruptures, its management mortality and major morbidity approaches 60 per cent. Since unruptured aneurysms of significant size have a propensity to rupture at a rate of 1 to 2.5 per cent per year, a patient with an aneurysm of more than 5 mm. in diameter and an expected longevity of more than a few years should be considered for surgical therapy.

SPONTANEOUS INTRACEREBRAL HEMORRHAGE

Congenital berry aneurysms usually bleed primarily into the subarachnoid space and rarely bleed into the cerebral substance. However, intracerebral hemorrhages are more commonly associated with hypertension, arteriovenous malforma-

tions, intrinsic clotting disorders, anticoagulants, brain tumors, or cerebral angiopathies.

Hypertensive Hemorrhage

Hypertensive intracerebral hemorrhages most frequently occur in the putamen, thalamus, cerebellum, or pons.[15] These hemorrhages follow bleeding from the small perforating arteries of the brain such as the thalamoperforating, lenticulostriate, or midline perforating basilar artery branches. Although these arteries can usually withstand high pressures, when subjected to long-standing hypertension, their walls undergo fibrinoid necrosis, and miliary microaneurysms known as Charcot-Bouchard aneurysms appear. Rebleeding seldom occurs, although patients may deteriorate days after the first hemorrhage from perihematoma edema.

Hypertensive hemorrhages most frequently originate in the putamen. Patients harboring a hematoma in the putamen typically experience a rapidly progressive hemiparesis, hemisensory loss, and hemianopsia contralateral to the hemorrhage. If the hemorrhage involves the dominant hemisphere, an aphasia is usually present. Patients suffering a thalamic hemorrhage usually manifest a hemisensory loss greater than their motor deficit. Small reactive pupils and downward eye deviation characteristically occur with this lesion.

Pontine hypertensive hemorrhages have a mortality of at least 75 per cent.[14] In fatal cases, the patients demonstrate small pupils, bilateral pyramidal signs, and a rapid loss of consciousness. In nonfatal cases, the patient may complain of headache, vertigo, and transient visual hallucinations and demonstrate bilateral pyramidal dysfunction and various abnormalities of conjugate eye movements.

Cerebellar hemorrhage characteristically presents with headache, dizziness, nausea, and vomiting. Examination may demonstrate an early inability to walk, appendicular ataxia, facial weakness, and paresis of conjugate gaze. Hemiparesis, sensory deficit, homonymous field defect, and aphasia are conspicuous for their absence. Deterioration occurs secondary to progressive brain stem compression. In a patient with a rapidly progressive syndrome, prompt recognition of the cerebellar hematoma clinically is imperative to permit evacuation of the clot before the condition ends fatally.[17]

The diagnosis of a hypertensive intracerebral hematoma is corroborated by CT scan (Fig. 4). Angiography is performed in equivocal cases to identify surgically remediable lesions.

The neurologic deficit developing from the tissue destroyed directly by hemorrhage cannot be reversed. Therapy is directed to controlling edema and reducing mass effect to prevent brain herniation. Increased intracranial pressure is treated vigorously with steroids, mannitol, hyperventilation, and furosemide.

Surgical therapy is routinely employed for the evacuation of cerebellar hematomas. Since the clot is quite tenacious, it cannot be simply evacuated through a burr hole with a needle and syringe. A suboccipital craniectomy and surgical evacuation of the hematoma with suction are required. When brain stem compression is allowed to progress to the point that the patient loses consciousness, the patient's prognosis drastically worsens.[17]

The indications for the evacuation of supratentorial hematomas is less clear. Surgical therapy is undertaken in patients in whom the primary neurologic deficit is secondary to increased intracranial pressure and the neurologic examination does not demonstrate signs of irreversible brain stem damage. Patients with massive intracranial hemorrhages and signs of irreversible brain stem damage are generally not treated surgically.

Angiomatous Malformations

Pathologists differentiate vascular malformations into four categories. Venous angiomas are characterized by an extensive network of veins separated by normal parenchyma. These lesions seldom bleed or give rise to clinical symptoms.

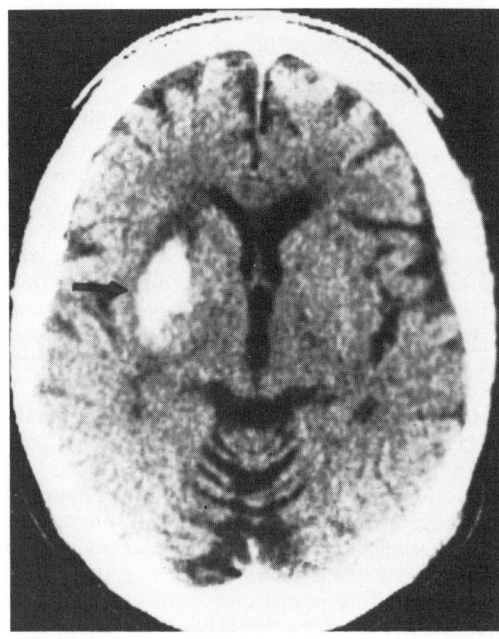

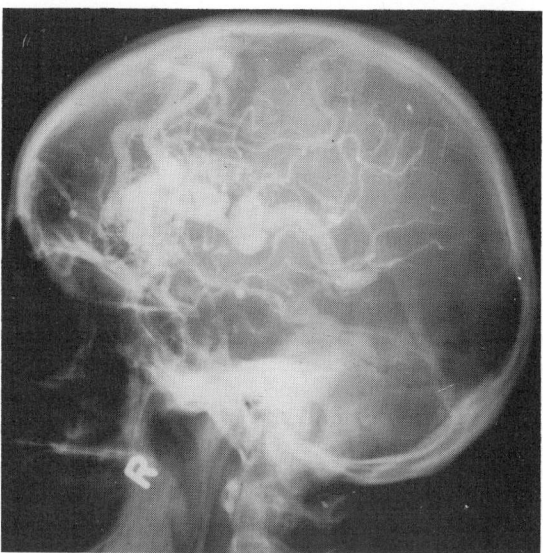

Figure 6. Arteriographic demonstration of an intracranial arteriovenous malformation.

Figure 4. Computed axial tomogram from a hypertensive patient who suffered a spontaneous intracerebral hemorrhage in the basal ganglia (arrow).

Telangiectasias (capillary angiomas) are generally benign lesions of the brain stem. Cavernous angiomas are typically developmental malformations within the brain substance that are poorly visualized by angiography. They are best demonstrated by magnetic resonance imaging (Fig. 5). Cavernous angiomas may manifest clinically as a growing mass, intracerebral hemorrhage, or intractable seizures. Symptomatic lesions are removed surgically.

Arteriovenous malformations are usually much larger, and most often can be visualized angiographically (Figs. 6 and 7). Many occur in the distribution of the middle cerebral artery. The superficial portions of the malformation may cover part of the cerebral surface, but the lesion frequently extends like a cone down to the ventricular surface. Therefore, the intracerebral hemorrhage that may occur from these lesions may spill into the subarachnoid space or the ventricular system. Unruptured arteriovenous malformations bleed at a rate of 2 to 3 per cent per year.[21]

In addition to bleeding, arteriovenous malformations may "steal" blood from the surrounding brain, and may cause a

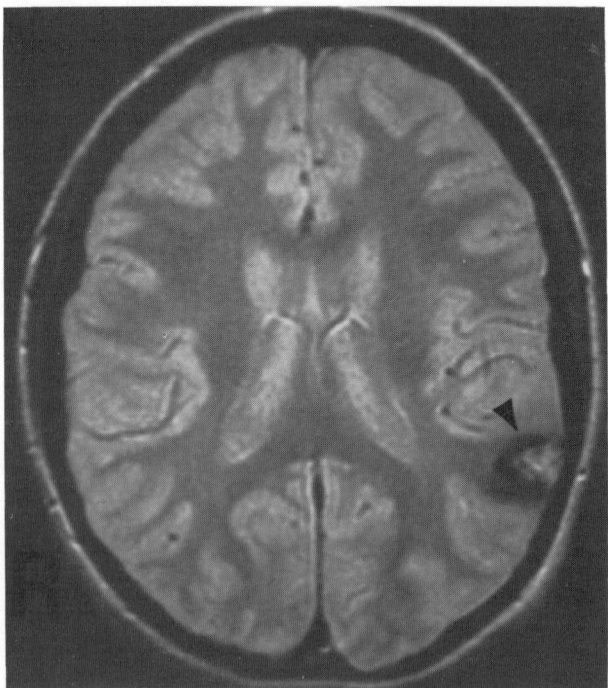

Figure 5. Magnetic resonance imaging scan demonstrating a left temporoparietal cavernous angioma. The black halo around the lesion is the result of previous hemorrhage.

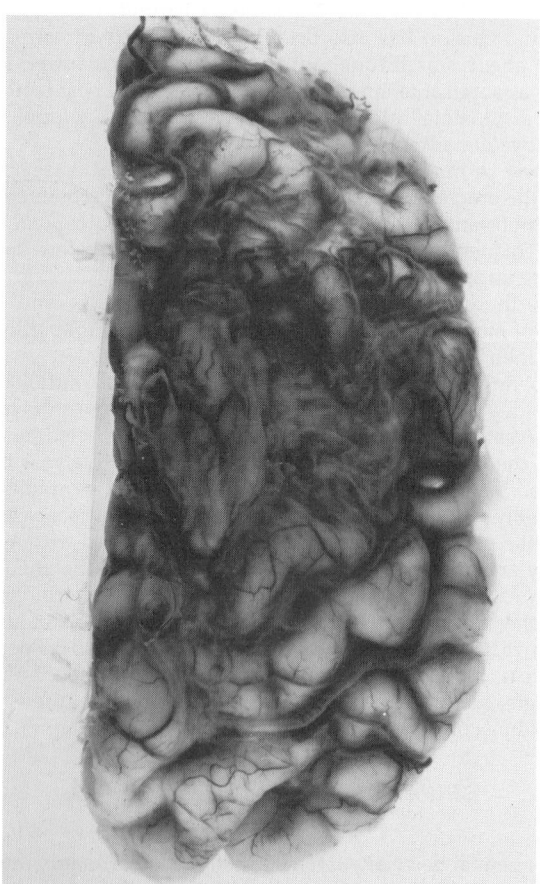

Figure 7. Superior aspect of the right cerebral hemisphere, showing a large arteriovenous malformation that had caused headaches and seizures during life.

significant increase in cardiac output. Likewise, patients with large arteriovenous malformations may have a variety of symptoms and signs aside from those directly related to bleeding, such as headaches, cranial bruits, convulsive seizures, mental deterioration, or a hemispheric neurologic deficit. Therefore, in contrast to intracranial aneurysms, arteriovenous malformations may frequently be diagnosed by angiography before they bleed. However, arteriovenous malformations tend to bleed earlier in life than aneurysms, with the peak incidence in individuals between 30 and 39 years of age.

Surgical treatment by occlusion of the ipsilateral carotid arteries or of the arterial branches directly feeding the arteriovenous malformation does not have lasting value since collateral feeding arteries quickly enlarge and the malformation persists. Repeated embolization of these malformations with glue or thrombogenic particles introduced through a percutaneously placed catheter or directly into the feeding arteries through a craniotomy has proved to be an effective method for reducing the size of the malformation. Unfortunately, only a small number of malformations can be totally obliterated by this technique. Recently several investigators have reported that focus radiation is effective in obliterating small arteriovenous malformations.[3,19] It is sometimes necessary to perform a craniotomy to evacuate an intracerebral hematoma even if the malformation cannot be resected.

The symptoms of untreated arteriovenous malformations tend to increase with time, and recurrent episodes of bleeding are common. The prognosis of lesions treated surgically depends upon the size and location of the malformation, and the extent of cerebral destruction from intracerebral hemorrhage, direct surgical trauma, and cerebral infarction due to arterial interruption.

Cerebral Arteritis

Intracerebral hematomas may occur in association with collagen vascular disease, methamphetamine abuse, or amyloid angiopathy. Amyloid angiopathy should be considered when a lobar hematoma occurs in a normotensive elderly individual. This entity may present with multiple discrete intracranial hemorrhages.

Clotting Disorders

Intracerebral hematomas may occur in association with primary hematologic disorders such as idiopathic thrombocytopenic purpura or hemophilia or as a complication of anticoagulant therapy. Surgical therapy for such a hematoma is hazardous when the patient's platelet count is below 50,000 cells per cu. mm. or the prothrombin time is prolonged.

SPONTANEOUS INTRASPINAL HEMORRHAGE

Angiomatous Malformations

Spinal arteriovenous malformations are best divided into those that are predominantly intramedullary, those that are extramedullary but intradural, and those that are extradural. The intramedullary malformations may be quite discrete, being fed by a small number of branches from the anterior spinal artery, or quite complex with large feeding vessels. The intradural extramedullary lesions usually consist of congeries of vessels on the dorsum of the spinal cord (Fig. 8). In some instances, these vessels are the draining veins from a dural fistula.[16]

Spinal arteriovenous malformations occasionally present with a subarachnoid hemorrhage or sudden infarction of the spinal cord. More frequently the patients present with a progressive myelopathy.

Myelography often reveals an expansion of the cord with an intramedullary lesion. Dilated tortuous vessels are commonly

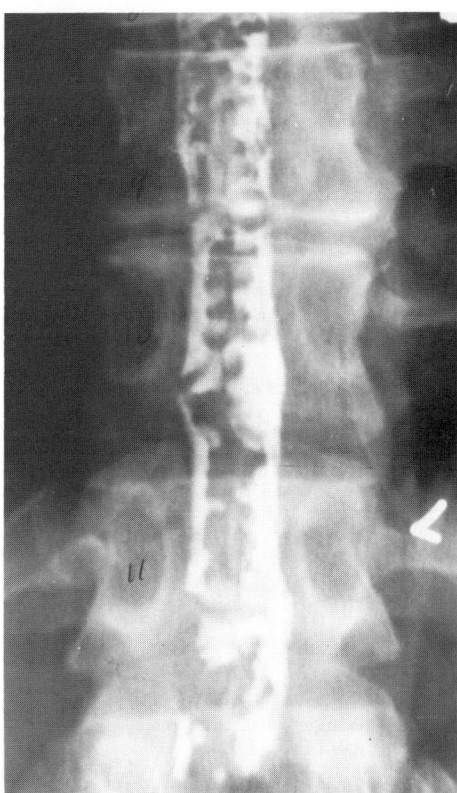

Figure 8. A low thoracic myelogram demonstrating the impression of a serpiginous vein of a spinal arteriovenous malformation.

visualized (Fig. 8). The malformation is best delineated by spinal angiography.

Because of the predictable progressive deterioration suffered by most patients, surgical resection is indicated. Good results are routinely reported in patients with extradural and intradural extramedullary lesions. Although encouraging results have been reported in the treatment of small intramedullary lesions, the larger lesions still remain a difficult challenge.

Neoplasms

Neoplasms of various types comprise a significant percentage of the cases of spontaneous spinal subarachnoid hemorrhage, so they must be considered in the differential diagnosis of these cases along with the angiomatous malformation.

Spinal Epidural Hematomas

Epidural spinal hemorrhage may occur spontaneously or be associated with anticoagulation, a bleeding diathesis, or spinal trauma. Patients suffering from a spinal epidural hemorrhage typically experience the sudden onset of back pain followed by paralysis and loss of sphincter control.

The diagnosis is made by myelography, which demonstrates an extradural mass, or by CT scan, which reveals an epidural high-density lesion compressing the spinal cord.[4] Rapid operative evacuation of the hematoma is imperative. Good results are most likely to occur when the patient still has demonstrable neurologic function below the level of the hematoma prior to operation.

SELECTED REFERENCES

Clinical Neurosurgery: Vol. 21, 1974; Vol. 24, 1977; and Vol. 26, 1979.
These volumes, the proceedings of the 1973, 1976, and 1978 annual meetings of the Congress of Neurological Surgeons, contain a number of chapters about various aspects of spontaneous intracranial hemorrhage.

Drake, C. G.: Management of cerebral aneurysm. Stroke, 12:273, 1981.
In this article, Drake reviews the history, epidemiology, and rationale for the treatment of intracranial aneurysms.

Kassell, N. F., Kongable, G. I., Torner, J. C., et al.: Delay in referral of patients with ruptured aneurysms to neurosurgical attention. Stroke, 16:587, 1985.
The pitfalls of diagnosing a subarachnoid hemorrhage are reviewed in this article as are the consequences of delayed diagnosis.

Wilkins, R. H.: Cerebral Vasospasm. New York, Raven Press, 1988.
This book contains the proceedings of the Third International Workshop on Cerebral Vasospasm.

Yasargil, M. G., Fox, J. L., and Ray, M. W.: The operative approach to aneurysms of the anterior communicating artery. Adv. Tech. Stds. Neurosurg., 2:114, 1975.
This is a classic article that explains the microsurgical approach to intracranial aneurysms.

REFERENCES

1. Allen, G. S., Ahn, H. S., Preziosi, T. J., et al.: Cerebral arterial spasm—A controlled trial of nimodipine in patients with subarachnoid hemorrhage. N. Engl. J. Med., 308:619, 1983.
2. Barrows, L. J., Hunter, F. T., and Banker, B. Q.: The nature and significance of pigments in the cerebrospinal fluid. Brain, 78:59, 1955.
3. Colombo, F., Benedetti, A., and Pozza, F.: Linear accelerator radiosurgery of cerebral arteriovenous malformations. Neurosurgery, 24:833, 1989.
4. Costabile, G., Husag, L., and Probst, C.: Spinal epidural hematoma. Surg. Neurol., 21:489, 1984.
5. Drake, C. G.: Giant intracranial aneurysms: Experience with surgical treatment of 174 patients. Clin. Neurosurg., 26:12, 1979.
6. Fisher, C. M.: Clinical syndromes in cerebral thrombosis, hypertensive hemorrhage, and ruptured saccular aneurysm. Clin. Neurosurg., 22:117, 1975.
7. Fisher, C. M., Kistler, J. P., and Davis, J. M.: Relation of cerebral vasospasm to subarachnoid hemorrhage visualized by computerized tomographic scanning. Neurosurgery, 6:1, 1980.
8. Friedman, A. H., and Drake, C. G.: Subarachnoid hemorrhage from intracranial dissecting aneurysm. J. Neurosurg., 60:325, 1984.
9. Graf, C. J., Perret, G. E., and Torner, J. C.: Bleeding from cerebral arteriovenous malformations as part of their natural history. J. Neurosurg., 58:331, 1983.
10. Juol, R., Fredriksen, T. P., and Ringkjob, R.: Prognosis in subarachnoid hemorrhage of unknown etiology. J. Neurosurg., 64:359, 1986.
11. Kassell, N. F., and Drake, C. G.: Timing of aneurysm surgery. Neurosurgery, 10:514, 1982.
12. Kassell, N. F., and Torner, J. C.: Aneurysmal rebleeding: A preliminary report from the Cooperative Aneurysm Study. Neurosurgery, 13:479, 1983.
13. Leblanc, R.: The minor leak preceding subarachnoid hemorrhage. J. Neurosurg., 66:35, 1987.
14. Nakajima, K.: Clinicopathological study of pontine hemorrhage. Stroke, 14:485, 1983.
15. Ojemann, R. G., and Heros, R. C.: Spontaneous brain hemorrhage. Stroke, 14:468, 1983.
16. Oldfield, E. H., DiChiro, G., Quindlen, E. A., Reith, K. G., and Doppman, J. L.: Successful treatment of a group of spinal cord arteriovenous malformations by interruption of dural fistula. J. Neurosurg., 59:1019, 1983.
17. Ott, K. H., Kase, C. S., Ojemann, R. G., and Mohr, J. P.: Cerebellar hemorrhage: Diagnosis and treatment. A review of 56 cases. Arch. Neurol., 31:160, 1974.
18. Pickard, J. D., Murray, G. D., Illingworth, R., et al.: Effect of oral nimodipine on cerebral infarction and outcome after subarachnoid haemorrhage: British aneurysm nimodipine trial. Br. Med. J., 298:636, 1989.
19. Steiner, L., Lindquist, C., and Steiner, M.: Radiosurgery in arteriovenous malformations of the basal ganglia. J. Neurosurg., 70:320A, 1989.
20. Wilkins, R. H.: Cerebral Arterial Spasm. Baltimore, Williams & Wilkins, 1980.
21. Wilkins, R. H.: Natural history of intracranial vascular malformations: A review. Neurosurgery, 16:421, 1985.
22. Winn, H. R., Almaani, W. S., Berga, S. L., Jane, J. A., and Richardson, A. E.: The long-term outcome in patients with multiple aneurysms: Incidence of late hemorrhage and implication for treatment of incidental aneurysms. J. Neurosurg., 59:642, 1983.
23. Yamakami, I., Isobe, K., Yamaura, A., Nakamura, T., and Makino, H.: Vasospasm and regional cerebral blood flow (rCBF) in patients with ruptured intracranial aneurysm: Serial rCBF studies with the xenon-133 inhalation method. Neurosurgery, 13:394, 1983.

V

CRANIOCEREBRAL INJURIES

Allan H. Friedman, M.D.

Accidental injury is the fourth leading cause of death in the United States and the leading cause of death in individuals between the ages of 1 and 44 years. Head injuries are present in more than 50 per cent of trauma-related deaths. An estimated 400,000 patients with head injuries are admitted to the hospital each year, and an even larger number are evaluated and treated in emergency rooms.[11] Because head injuries are so ubiquitous, their primary management should be understood by all physicians.

The final neurologic status of the patient who has sustained brain trauma is the sum of the irreversible damage acquired at the time of the initial injury and the damage that is the consequence of secondary insults. At the time of the initial injury, a portion of the brain may sustain irreversible damage and a second portion may sustain a lesser degree of damage, from which it will recover over a period of months. Secondary insults that cause worsening of the patient's neurologic deficits include (1) systemic disorders such as hypoxia or hypotension; (2) expanding intracranial mass such as a subdural, epidural, or, rarely, intraparenchymal hematoma; and (3) sustained raised intracranial pressure. Although several forms of intervention have been proposed to enhance the brain's normal repair processes, at this time the physician can do nothing either to replace those cells that have suffered a fatal injury or to accelerate the restoration of recovering tissue. The swift recognition or prevention of these secondary insults offers the best likelihood of improving the prognosis of the patient who has sustained a brain injury. It

is the physician's role in treating the patient with head injury to identify rapidly and to correct these injurious influences.[19]

Primary Brain Injuries[9]

At the time of the initial head injury, the brain may suffer contusion, laceration, and shearing injuries. These injuries follow local direct brain trauma and brain acceleration and deceleration relative to the skull. Local direct brain trauma occurs when a stationary skull is struck by an object. If the force is sufficient, the skull indents, directly striking the underlying brain. More deleterious are the injuries that follow acceleration or deceleration of the brain relative to the skull. At the time of impact, there is considerable movement of the brain relative to the skull. For example, when the skull is suddenly stopped by a windshield in an automobile accident, the brain continues to decelerate relative to the skull for approximately 20 msec. In a similar manner at the time of impact, the brain may experience linear or rotational acceleration with respect to the sagittal, lateral, or vertical axis of the skull. This acceleration causes contusion of the brain, shearing of axons, and tearing of bridging veins. These mechanisms are responsible for the damage the brain incurs in a closed head injury.

Contusions occur in regions where the moving brain abruptly strikes the fixed skull, or under areas of impact where the skull is sufficiently bent inward to strike the underlying brain. Areas of contusion are marked by hemorrhage, which frequently spreads under the pia, and by swelling and necrosis of underlying tissue. If the impact is sufficiently severe, the pia will be lacerated and the hemorrhage spills out into the subarachnoid or subdural space. After brain deceleration, areas of contusion tend to concentrate along the undersurface of the frontal lobes and the anterior poles of the temporal lobes where the brain is relatively confined by bone. The neurologic deficit produced coincides with the region of direct brain injury; a contusion of the motor strip, for example, may produce a contralateral hemiparesis. The contusion is clinically silent when restricted to portions of the brain that have no clinically demonstrable function, such as the anterior temporal lobes or the inferior aspect of the frontal lobes. These silent areas of contusion may become clinically significant days after the initial injury, as edema accumulates in areas where the blood-brain barrier has been destroyed and the swollen region begins to act as an intracranial mass. Occasionally a hematoma of significant size accumulates in an area of contusion 24 to 72 hours after the initial injury.[22] These delayed traumatic hematomas are most likely to occur in older patients and may be responsible for deterioration in neurologic function days after the initial injury.

Rotation of the brain within the skull may lead in tearing of axons within the white matter of the brain, causing diffuse axonal injury.[1] According to the theory of Ommaya and Gennarelli, mild injuries damage only subcortical axons, but increases in the rotational force involve progressively deeper areas of brain.[16] There is little cerebral swelling and no increased intracranial pressure associated with this form of brain injury. A computed tomographic (CT) scan made immediately following such an injury may demonstrate hemorrhage in the corpus callosum and the superolateral aspect of the brain stem, but the remainder of the brain appears relatively normal even though the patient may manifest severe neurologic damage. Months after the injury, the CT scan demonstrates that the bulk of the white matter is reduced. Magnetic resonance imaging demonstrates diffuse, small, focal abnormalities limited to white matter tracts.[8]

Children may demonstrate rapid neurologic deterioration and a concomitant increase in intracranial pressure in minutes to hours following a relatively mild head injury.[4] The clinical presentation can be mistaken as indicative of an enlarging intracranial mass. This increased pressure is thought to be secondary to vasodilation with concomitant increased intracranial blood volume. These children often develop grave neurologic signs, but with control of their intracranial hypertension, their neurologic outcome is far better than that of adults who manifest the identical clinical findings.

The neurologic deficit that follows a penetrating brain injury is manifested only by a loss of function of the brain that is directly injured. Delayed deterioration in the patient's neurologic status following such an injury occurs secondary to a complicating hemorrhage or an infection induced by debris pushed into the brain at the time of injury. For this reason, penetrating injuries should be rapidly cleansed of bone fragments and debris. High-speed missile wounds produce a shock wave that cuts a wider area of damage than the bullet tract itself.

Secondary Brain Injuries

Patients who have sustained head injuries must be monitored for factors that can produce further brain damage. Metabolic abnormalities are the most common secondary insults in patients who have suffered brain trauma. An evaluation of head trauma patients upon arrival to a university hospital emergency room demonstrated that approximately 35 per cent have a Po_2 less than 60 mm. water. Fifteen per cent have a systolic blood pressure less than 95 mm. Hg, and 10 per cent have a hematocrit of less than 30.[15] The unconscious patient has a diminution of the normal protective reflexes that may lead to mechanical obstruction of the oropharynx or to aspiration pneumonia. Pulmonary contusion, a flail chest, or, rarely, fat emboli or neuro-

genic pulmonary edema may further compromise the patient's oxygenation. Hypercapnia, although a rare concomitant of head injury alone, causes vasodilation and increased intracranial pressure. At the scene of the accident, the patient's mouth should be cleared of debris and hypoventilation should be treated by the placement of an oral airway and the institution of positive-pressure ventilation. In the emergency room, all patients who are not verbalizing or following commands should be intubated. Care should be taken not to flex the spine, as a concomitant spine injury may be present.

Hypotension is rarely a direct result of intracranial trauma and should alert the physician to the possibility of intra- or extracorporeal hemorrhage. A positive abdominal tap is reported to occur in 17 per cent of patients who have sustained severe head trauma.[5] Serious scalp bleeding may also cause major blood loss and can be controlled by applying pressure to the lacerations. Life-threatening dural sinus bleeding can be slowed by placing the patient in the reverse Trendelenburg position. In rare cases, hypotension may develop in infants with large intracranial hemorrhage or in patients with high cervical fractures that produce medullary compression. Hypotension occurring later during the hospitalization of a patient with head injury may reflect hemorrhage from gastritis or a gastrointestinal ulcer, infection with secondary gram-negative sepsis, myocardial infarction, or pulmonary embolism. Hypotension is particularly deleterious in the setting of increased intracranial pressure because it further diminishes cerebral perfusion. Mean arterial blood pressure should be restored quickly to at least 80 mm. Hg.

Increased intracranial pressure produces neurologic dysfunction by (1) decreasing cerebral blood flow and (2) causing transtentorial herniation.

Brain edema, an enlarging hematoma, or cerebrovascular engorgement can act as a supratentorial mass. An enlarging supratentorial mass is first partially compensated by the displacement of intracranial venous blood and cerebrospinal fluid out of the skull. When these buffering systems are exhausted, any further increase in mass results in a marked increase in intracranial pressure.

Intracranial pressure is frequently monitored in patients who have sustained a severe head injury. Since the venous outflow pressure in the brain approximates the intracranial pressure, the cerebral perfusion pressure is equal to the mean arterial pressure minus the intracranial pressure. With elevation of the intracranial pressure, the cerebral perfusion pressure becomes compromised. The cerebral blood flow is maintained constant when the decrease in cerebral perfusion pressure is small through reflexive lowering of the cerebral vascular resistance. With further decreases in the cerebral perfusion pressure, the cerebral blood flow diminishes. In clinical practice, all patients who have an intracranial pressure greater than 40 mm. Hg have a significantly diminished cerebral blood flow. If the intracranial pressure becomes equal to or greater than the systemic arterial pressure, brain death quickly ensues.

Intracranial pressure can be monitored by measuring the pressure in the epidural space, the subarachnoid space, or the intraventricular fluid. Normal intracranial pressure is less than 15 mm. Hg and becomes elevated with the appearance of an intracranial mass. The intracranial pressure is dynamic, and it is not unusual for a patient with a partially compensated intracranial mass to have a wave of pressure measuring 50 mm. Hg and lasting 5 to 20 minutes superimposed on a relatively normal pressure. Mortality is reduced without a concomitant increase in morbidity by aggressively lowering an increased intracranial pressure.[20] Methods used to lower intracranial pressure are outlined in Table 1.

An expanding intracranial mass not only causes a generalized increase in intracranial pressure but distorts and shifts the brain. Focal mass lesions can cause brain herniations under the falx

TABLE 1. Methods of Lowering Intracranial Pressure

Mechanical reduction of intracranial volume
   Decrease intracranial venous blood by elevating head of bed
   Drain cerebrospinal fluid through ventricular drain
   Remove intracranial mass
Induce vasoconstriction
   Hyperventilation to P_{CO_2} = 25 mm. Hg
   Sedation and paralysis
   Give intravenous barbiturates
Removal of intracerebral water using osmotic agents such as
   mannitol, urea, glycerol
Stabilization of membranes with steroids (steroids are rarely used in
   the treatment of head trauma)
Dehydration of brain with furosemide

cerebri, through the tentorial notch, or through the foramen magnum. The most common form of herniation, transtentorial herniation, follows a supratentorial mass crowding the supratentorial contents into the tentorial notch secondarily distorting the midbrain, third nerve, and posterior cerebral artery. Clinically, transtentorial herniation manifests as one of two clinical syndromes designated central and uncal herniation (Table 2).

Central herniation is most likely to occur following a nonfocal increase in the pressure above the tentorium as seen in a multicentric supratentorial brain injury. The earliest warning of impending central herniation is a progressive depression in the patient's level of consciousness, followed by reflex flexor posturing of the patient's upper extremities to a painful stimulus (decorticate posturing) and Cheyne-Stokes respirations. This is followed by a progressive rostral to caudal brain stem ischemia manifest as a sequential dysfunction of successively lower brain stem levels. Midbrain dysfunction is marked by decerebrate posturing (abnormal extensor response to pain), fixed midposition pupils, and hyperventilation. As lower elements of the brain stem fail, the patient becomes flaccid, develops spasmodic respirations, and loses the oculocephalic reflexes.

Uncal herniation is most likely to develop from a focal, laterally placed mass such as an epidural hematoma. Usually the examiner first notes a progressing contralateral hemiparesis. Early compression of the third cranial nerve causes myosis of the ipsilateral pupil followed by ptosis and a limitation of motion of the ipsilateral eye. As the midbrain is compressed, the patient loses consciousness, begins to hyperventilate, and develops bilateral decerebrate posturing. If the intracranial pressure is not reduced, the patient demonstrates signs characteristic of progressive rostral to caudal ischemia.

Patient Evaluation

After stabilization of the respiratory and cardiovascular systems, attention is turned to the central nervous system. Care is taken not to manipulate the neck prior to excluding cervical fractures. The initial examination must be recorded such that it may be compared with subsequent examinations in order to detect a deterioration in the patient's condition. The head is inspected for scalp lacerations, compound skull fractures, or signs of a basilar skull fracture. In the awake patient, a detailed neurologic examination should be performed with special attention to the abnormalities in mental status, asymmetries of pupillary size, unilateral weakness, changes in muscle tone, asymmetries of deep tendon reflexes, and the presence of pathologic reflex responses. In the uncooperative, stuporous, or comatose patient, the examiner must rely on the evaluation of reflexes to detect focal abnormalities in the nervous system. Special attention is placed on respiratory patterns, pupillary size and light response, oculocephalic reflexes, motor response to painful stimuli, and deep tendon reflexes.[7]

An assessment of mental status is particularly difficult to denote in such a way that the patient's condition can be conveyed from examiner to examiner. The Glasgow Coma Scale is a standardized method of measuring the severity of the patient's neurologic deficits with a high concordance among different observers and should be employed in measuring all patients who have sustained a head injury. The 15 point scale assesses the patient's neurologic responsiveness in three categories: eye opening, verbal response, and best motor response (Table 3).

Attention is then turned to the evaluation of the chest, abdomen, and extremities for other injuries. Many patients rendered comatose in an automobile accident have sustained other major injuries. The neurosurgeon must be aware of the presence of these injuries and their possible effect on the brain injury.

Mild nonpenetrating head injuries are associated with a transient disturbance in vision, a transient period of confusion, and a loss of memory for the moment of impact. With progressively greater degrees of brain injury, the patient remains confused for proportionately longer periods of time and demonstrates a longer period of memory loss. Antegrade memory loss is loss of memory for events that follow the accident and may be the only type of memory loss present in the milder head injuries. With more severe injuries, the patient may demonstrate retrograde memory loss, that is, the loss of memory of events that preceded the accident. As the degree of the brain injury increases, the patient experiences a period of loss of consciousness proportional to the magnitude of the injury. Concomitant with the initial impact, there may be a period of apnea and systemic arterial hypertension and occasionally a generalized seizure.

Patients with mild head injuries and a brief loss of consciousness are often expected to make an uneventful recovery. In fact, these patients are found to have a surprising degree of post-injury disability in the form of persistent headaches, memory deficits, and difficulties with activities of daily living that persist for months following the accident. One study documented that

TABLE 2. Signs of Transtentorial Herniation

	Level of Consciousness	Respiratory Pattern	Pupillary Size; Response to Light	Oculovestibular Reflex	Motor Response to Pain
Uncal Herniation					
Early oculomotor nerve compression	Normal to obtunded	Normal	Unilaterally dilated; fixed	Full, conjugate	Appropriate
Late oculomotor nerve compression	Normal to obtunded	Normal	Unilaterally dilated; fixed	Unilateral third nerve palsy	Appropriate
Midbrain compression	Comatose	Hyperventilation	Bilaterally midposition; fixed	Dysconjugate gaze	Decerebrate posturing
Central Herniation					
Early diencephalon compression	Obtunded	Deep sighs, yawns	Small; reactive	Conjugate	Appropriate
Late diencephalon compression	Barely arousable to comatose	Cheyne-Stokes respirations	Small; reactive	Conjugate without nystagmus	Cortical
Midbrain compression	Comatose	Hyperventilation	Midposition; fixed	Dysconjugate	Decerebrate

TABLE 3. Glasgow Coma Scale

Eye Opening

Spontaneous	E4
To speech	3
To pain	2
Nil	1

Best Motor Response

Obeys	M6
Localizes	5
Withdraws	4
Abnormal flexion	3
Extension response	2
Nil	1

Verbal Response

Oriented	V5
Confused conversation	4
Inappropriate words	3
Incomprehensible sounds	2
Nil	1

Coma Score = E + M + V.

TABLE 4. Basic Care of the Comatose Adult Patient

Position
  Elevate head 30 degrees
  Turn frequently
Respiratory Care
  Endotracheal intubation
  Controlled respiration
  Pulmonary toilet
Management of intracranial pressure as indicated
Nutrition: 2500 kcal./day
Intravenous fluid: 0.45% normal saline and 5% dextrose—125 ml./hr.
Medications
  Antacid therapy
  Seizure prophylaxis
Monitor
  Arterial blood pressure
  Arterial Po_2 and Pco_2
  Serum sodium, glucose
  Serum osmolarity

one third of patients who had sustained minor head injuries had not returned to gainful employment in the 3 months following the injury.[17] Patients who have sustained mild head injuries but have a severe headache, lethargy, or restlessness should be observed for 24 hours. If the patient shows any deterioration in neurologic status or demonstrates any signs of a focal neurologic lesion on examination, a CT scan of the brain should be obtained.[6]

Patients who have sustained a moderate head injury are likely to be lethargic, stuporous, or combative when they first regain consciousness. Ten to 15 per cent of patients entering the hospital with a moderate head injury are found to have a focal intracranial lesion. A CT scan of the brain is indicated in all patients with persistent lethargy. Nearly all patients who sustain an injury of this order of magnitude have persistent headaches, memory difficulties, and difficulties with activities of daily living months following the injury. Three months after a moderate head injury, two thirds of patients are still unemployed.[10]

A severe head injury is defined by a score on the Glasgow Coma Scale of eight or less. Forty per cent of patients who have sustained a severe brain injury harbor a focal intracranial mass lesion. Signs of severe neurologic dysfunction such as an abnormal motor response, abnormal oculocephalic reflexes, or bilateral fixed pupils indicate a brain stem injury.

Each of these abnormal brain stem reflexes can be demonstrated in approximately one third of severely injured patients and is associated with an increased mortality. Mortality has also been shown to be proportional to the patient's age. Other factors associated with a poorer outcome include the presence of a focal intracranial lesion, concomitant abdominal or chest injury, systemic arterial hypotension, and elevated intracranial pressure.[12]

A CT scan of the brain is indicated in all comatose patients. Frequent neurologic examinations are necessary to detect a change in the patient's neurologic status. Patients should be treated in an intensive care setting (Table 4).

Scalp and Skull Injuries

Scalp lacerations frequently occur at the site of impact. Because of the scalp's rich vascular supply, most uncomplicated lacerations can be closed after cleansing and débridement. If a portion of the scalp is lost, the deficit may be repaired by rotating a portion of scalp. A large scalp deficit requires a skin graft or vascularized free flap for repair.

Although indicative of a relatively severe cranial blow, skull fractures are conspicuous for their absence in patients who have sustained severe brain trauma. The fracture follows inbending or outbending of the skull beyond its elastic tolerance. The linear nondisplaced skull fracture in and of itself requires no special therapy but has stronger clinical implications when it extends into the air sinuses or base of the skull, crosses one of the meningeal arteries, is associated with an underlying dural tear, or underlies a scalp laceration.

Basilar skull fractures are difficult to detect on plain skull films. Because of the tenacity with which the dura adheres to the base of the skull, these lesions are frequently associated with a cerebrospinal fluid fistula. A basilar skull fracture of the anterior fossa should be suspected when the patient manifests the raccoon sign, periorbital ecchymosis limited at the edge of the orbit. A fracture involving the petrous portions of the temporal bone should be suspected either when the patient is found to have blood or cerebrospinal fluid behind the tympanic membrane, or when he demonstrates a Battle's sign with ecchymosis of the mastoid prominence. A basilar skull fracture should also be suspected when an air-fluid level is seen on the lateral skull film in the frontal, sphenoid, or mastoid sinus. Most traumatic cerebrospinal fluid fistulas subside spontaneously if the patient's head is maintained elevated at 30 degrees, but a persistent fistula places the patient at risk for recurrent episodes of meningitis. It should be noted that the leak may be only temporarily closed with brain and then may recur. If the leak persists longer than 10 days, craniotomy with reapproximation of the torn dura is indicated.

A linear fracture crossing the groove of the middle meningeal artery may be seen in patients with accumulating epidural hematoma. However, most patients with fractures in this location do not develop epidural hematomas, and some such hematomas are not accompanied by a skull fracture.

An infrequent complication of skull fracture seen exclusively in children is the progressive separation of the long edges of a seemingly benign linear skull fracture. The patient presents with a growing scalp mass or a dysfunction of the brain underlying the fracture. This type of fracture is always associated with an underlying dural tear. The most important aspect of the operative repair is the dural closure. A cranioplasty is usually performed.

If a hard blow is delivered to a small area of the skull, the fracture is comminuted and the portion of bone lying under the area of impact is depressed. Depressed skull fractures may be associated with an underlying dural tear or lacerated cerebral cortex. These lesions are associated with a higher incidence of brain laceration and posttraumatic epilepsy. Such fractures should be surgically repaired unless they are over a major dural sinus or the inward displacement of the bone fragments is less than the thickness of the skull.[2] A burr hole is placed next to the depressed fracture and the bone fragments are carefully eased from the underlying dura. Brain lacerations are débrided and dural tears are closed. The bone fragments may be cleansed and replaced.

Epidural Hematomas

The acute epidural hematoma usually follows arterial hemorrhage between the skull and the dura.[10] At the time of impact, a dural artery is torn, and the inbending of the skull initiates the stripping of the dura from the bone. Occasionally an epidural hematoma follows a torn venous sinus. Most frequently acute epidural hematomas occur in the temporal or temporoparietal region as a consequence of hemorrhage from one of the branches of the middle meningeal artery, but the hematoma can collect under the cranium in any location.

The clinical presentation is variable. The trauma responsible for an acute epidural hematoma may create an immediate neurologic deficit following direct brain injury. The hematoma manifests as an enlarging intracranial mass that eventually precipitates transtentorial herniation. The classic clinical presentation is that of a brief loss of consciousness secondary to the initial cerebral concussion followed by a lucid interval. The patient eventually lapses from the lucid interval into a coma after the epidural hematoma enlarges to a size sufficient to precipitate tentorial herniation and midbrain compression. This classic triphasic clinical pattern is seen in only 20 per cent of patients who have an epidural hematoma. More frequently, the initial concussion is insufficient to cause any loss of consciousness or it is so severe that the patient does not regain consciousness prior to the herniation. In either case, the "characteristic" lucid interval does not occur.

Although skull films frequently demonstrate a linear skull fracture, an epidural hematoma may accumulate without a concomitant fracture. The absence of a fracture is especially common in children. The CT scan demonstrates a biconvex high-density lesion that lies between the skull and the brain (Fig. 1).

The treatment for this lesion is early recognition and rapid surgical decompression. In the rapidly deteriorating patient who is suspected of harboring an epidural hematoma, a diagnostic burr hole is placed 1.5 inches above the zygoma on the side of the dilating pupil. Because of the jelly-like nature of the

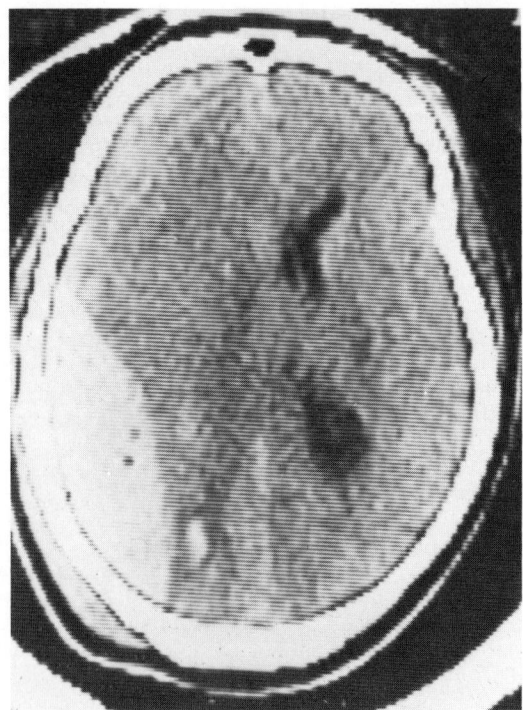

Figure 1. Computed axial tomogram of a patient who suffered a traumatic epidural hematoma. Note the shift of the ventricles off of the midline.

acute hematoma, a craniotomy must be performed to completely evaluate the mass. There is a strong correlation between the patient's preoperative level of consciousness and the outcome of therapy. With early diagnosis and rapid therapy, the mortality from this lesion approaches zero.[3]

Epidural hematomas occasionally accumulate in the posterior fossa secondary to bleeding from the transverse sinus or meningeal arteries.[23] The patient may present with signs of acute brain stem compression such as decerebrate rigidity and loss of consciousness, or a clinical pattern may slowly evolve that is characterized by altered mental status, headache, nausea, vomiting, and nystagmus prior to the patient's lapsing into unconsciousness. The posterior fossa epidural hematoma is frequently associated with an occipital skull fracture and is easily demonstrated on CT scan. Rapid surgical decompression is indicated.

Subdural Hematomas

Subdural hematomas are blood collections that occur in the plane between the dura and the arachnoid. Unlike epidural hematomas, subdural hematomas most commonly develop from ruptured veins. Anterior or posterior acceleration of the skull with respect to the brain causes traction on the veins that traverse the subdural cleft as they pass between the cerebral cortex and the dural venous sinuses. Cerebral atrophy is seen in chronic alcohol abusers and some elderly patients, and increases the size of the potential subdural space, thus enhancing this mechanism. Because of the lack of adhesions between the dura and the arachnoid, the venous blood spreads rapidly over the cerebral convexity. Rarely a subdural hematoma may develop from a bleeding cortical artery, a ruptured aneurysm, or a superficial arteriovenous malformation.[14]

Acute subdural hematomas present with signs of rapid increase in intracranial pressure and herniation. A moderate-sized subdural collection may be compensated for initially, but may become clinically symptomatic after edema accumulates.

A subdural hematoma may develop from oozing following a brain laceration. In these cases, the problem is usually the intrinsic brain injury and not the subdural blood collection. In comparison with a massive primary brain injury, a rim of subdural blood is not clinically significant. It is only when the hemorrhage is sufficiently extensive to serve as an intracranial mass that it is of clinical significance.

Less than 50 per cent of patients harboring a subdural hematoma have a skull fracture demonstrable on skull roentgenograms. An acute subdural hematoma appears as a high-density spread over the convexity of the cerebral cortex on CT scan (Fig. 2). A chronic subdural hematoma, in which the blood clot has lysed, appears as a biconvex low-density area lying between the skull and the compressed brain. A subdural hematoma of intermediate age or a subdural hematoma in an anemic patient may appear isodense with the adjacent brain and is detected by noting a shift of the ventricular system or the adjacent cortex.

The mortality associated with an acute subdural hematoma is 25 to 90 per cent. This high mortality is due to the frequency of concomitant direct brain injury. If the patient has no primary brain injury, the mortality from the subdural hematoma is a direct function of the patient's age, neurologic status, and delay from time of trauma to the surgical evacuation of the hematoma.[21] Although an acute subdural hematoma may first be detected through a diagnostic burr hole, its viscous nature necessitates a larger craniectomy or craniotomy for complete removal. Usually the subdural hematoma is evacuated through a question mark–shaped flap that begins at the ear and continues to the midline.

An amount of subdural blood insufficient to cause a mass effect may accumulate following minor trauma. This is especially prone to occur in patients with cerebral atrophy. Although small amounts of subdural blood are usually spontaneously reabsorbed, the hematoma may occasionally become encapsu-

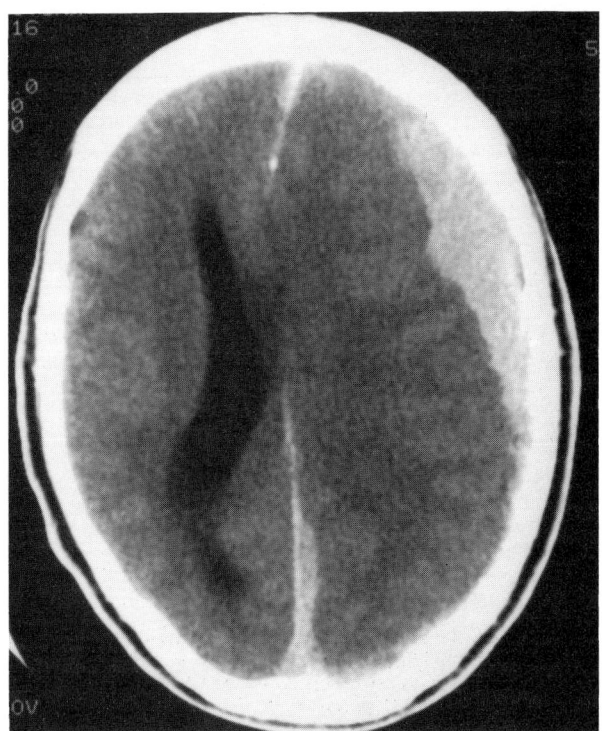

Figure 2. Computed axial tomogram of a patient who sustained a subdural hematoma from head trauma. The left subdural space in this photograph appears isodense as compared with the adjacent skull.

lated by a membrane of fibrous tissue and friable capillaries emanating from the dura mater.[13] Small recurrent hemorrhages from the thin-walled vessels within the membrane cause the collection of liquefied blood to enlarge. This chronic subdural hematoma may come to clinical attention months to years after the initial insult when it presents as an intracranial mass. The patient may complain of an altered mental status, headaches, seizures, or a focal neurologic dysfunction (i.e., hemiparesis, aphasia) reflecting the position of the brain compressed by the hematoma.

The content of a chronic subdural hematoma is a thin liquid that can be washed out through multiple burr holes. In children, the liquid can be removed via a needle placed in the anterior fontanelle. If the chronic subdural hematoma recurs after simple drainage, a craniotomy with partial removal of the enveloping membranes or a shunting of the subdural cavity into the pleural or peritoneal cavities may be necessary.

Delayed Complications

The likelihood of a patient's developing a seizure disorder following a head injury is proportional to the severity of the injury. It is estimated that 5 per cent of patients admitted to the hospital with a head injury develop a seizure disorder. Early epilepsy, penetration of the dura, intracranial hematomas, and depressed skull fractures all predispose the patient to a delayed seizure disorder.

Several vascular complications associated with head injuries produce symptoms. A traumatic carotid cavernous sinus fistula may present as an audible bruit, conjunctival edema, chemosis, impaired extraocular motion, or loss of visual acuity. Dissecting aneurysms present as a sudden stroke or transient ischemic episode. Rarely, a traumatic intracranial aneurysm ruptures in the weeks following a head injury.

SELECTED REFERENCES

Becker, D. P., Miller, J. D., Young, H. F., et al.: Diagnosis and Treatment of Head Injury in Adults: Neurological Surgery. Philadelphia, W. B. Saunders Company, 1982.
Becker and his colleagues have written a fine review on the clinical aspects of head injury. They neatly connect the physiologic rationale behind the treatment of brain injuries.

Clinical Neurosurgery: Vol. 29, 1982, and Vol. 34, 1988.
The proceedings of the 1981 and 1987 Congress of Neurological Surgeons contains several chapters reviewing the physiology and treatment of head trauma.

Plum, F., and Posner, J. B.: The Diagnosis of Stupor and Coma. Philadelphia, F. A. Davis Company, 1980.
This classic, now in its third edition, provides a detailed account of the assessment of the comatose patient.

REFERENCES

1. Adams, J. H., Graham, D. I., Murray, L. S., and Scott, G.: Diffuse axonal injury due to nonmissile head injury in humans. An analysis of 45 cases. Ann. Neurol., 12:557, 1982.
2. Braakman, R.: Depressed skull fracture: Data, treatment, and followup in 225 consecutive cases. J. Neurol. Neurosurg. Psychiatry. 35:395, 1972.
3. Bricolo, A. P., and Pasut, L. M.: Extradural hematoma: Toward zero mortality. A prospective study. Neurosurgery, 14:8, 1984.
4. Bruce, B. A., Alavi, A., Bilaniak, L., et al.: Diffuse cerebral swelling following head injuries in children: The syndrome of "malignant brain edema." J. Neurosurg. 54:170, 1981.
5. Butterworth, J. F., Maull, K. I., Miller J. D., and Becker, D. P.: Detection of occult abdominal trauma in patients with severe head injuries. Lancet, 2:759, 1980.
6. Feverman, T., Wackym, P. A., Gade, G. F., and Becker, D. P.: Value of skull radiography, head computed tomographic scanning, and admission for observation in cases of minor head injury. Neurosurgery, 22:449, 1988.
7. Friedman, A. H.: Head injuries: Initial evaluation and management. Postgrad. Med., 73:219, 1983.
8. Gentry, L. R., Godersky, J. C., and Thompson, B.: MR imaging of head trauma: Review of the distribution and radiopathic features of traumatic lesions. A.J.R., 150:663, 1988.
9. Hardman, J. M.: The pathology of traumatic brain injury. Adv. Neurol., 22:15, 1979.
10. Jamieson, K. G.: Epidural Haematoma: Handbook of Clinical Neurology. Vol. 24, Amsterdam, North-Holland Publishing Company, 1976.
11. Kalsbeck, U. D., Melaurin, R. L., Harris, B. S. H., et al.: The national head and spinal cord injury survey: Major findings. J. Neurosurg., 53(Suppl.):S19, 1980.
12. Klauber, M. R., Marshall, L. F., Luarssen, T. G., et al.: Determinants of head injury mortality: Importance of the low risk patient. Neurosurgery, 24:31, 1989.
13. Markwalder, T. M.: Chronic subdural hematomas: A review. J. Neurosurg., 54:637, 1981.
14. McDermott, M., Fleming, J. F. R., Vanderlinden, R. G., and Tucker, W. S.: Spontaneous arterial subdural hematoma. Neurosurgery, 14:13, 1984.
15. Miller, J. D., Sweet, R. C., Narayan, R., and Becker, D. P.: Early insults to the injured brain. J.A.M.A., 240:439, 1978.
16. Ommaya, A. K., and Gennarelli, T. A.: Cerebral concussion and traumatic unconsciousness: Correlation of experimental and clinical observations on blunt head injury. Brain, 97:633, 1974.
17. Rimel, R. W., Giordani, B., Barth, J. T., et al.: Disability caused by minor head injury. Neurosurgery, 9:221, 1981.
18. Rimel, R. W., Giordani, B., Barth, J. T., and Jane, J. A.: Moderate head injury: Completing the clinical spectrum of brain trauma. Neurosurgery, 11:344, 1982.
19. Rose, J., Valtonen, S., and Jennett, B.: Avoidable factors contributing to death after head injury. Br. Med. J., 2:615, 1977.
20. Saul, T. G.: Is ICP monitoring worthwhile? Clin. Neurosurg., 34:560, 1988.
21. Seelig, M., Becker, D. P., Miller, J. D., et al.: Traumatic acute subdural hematoma: Major mortality reduction in comatose patients treated within four hours. N. Engl. J. Med., 304:1511, 1981.
22. Young, H. A., Gleave, J. R. W., Schmidek, H. H., and Gregory, S.: Delayed traumatic intracerebral hematoma: Report of 15 cases operatively treated. Neurosurgery, 14:22, 1984.
23. Zuccarello, M., Pardatscher, K., Andrioli, G. C., et al.: Epidural hematomas of the posterior fossa. Neurosurgery, 8:434, 1981.

VI

INTRACRANIAL INFECTIONS

Robert H. Wilkins, M.D.

The number of patients with infections amenable to neurosurgical treatment is relatively small, but because of the wide variety of infectious agents and the different pathologic lesions they can incite, this area remains a challenge for the neurosurgeon.

Cranial Osteomyelitis, Epidural Abscess, Subdural Empyema[2,4,10]

A cranial bone may be the site of hematogenous spread of a bacterial infection from another area of the body, but more often it becomes involved by adjacent spread from an infected paranasal sinus, by a penetrating wound, or by an operative infection involving a craniotomy flap. Pott's puffy tumor is such a frontal osteomyelitis with marked overlying soft tissue swelling that is secondary to frontal sinusitis.

Treatment is centered around the surgical removal of the infected bone, with simultaneous treatment of any coexisting sinusitis. Appropriate systemic antibiotics are administered, and an adequate margin of normal bone is removed with the specimen to minimize the risk of recurrent infection. A cranioplasty may be performed later for cosmetic and protective reasons, but at least a year should be allowed to pass, during which there is no evidence of inflammation in the area, before the plate is inserted. Otherwise, this large foreign body serves as a focus for a further inflammatory response.

An epidural infection is usually a well-confined bacterial abscess associated with one or more of the previously mentioned infections, and it is drained at the same time the coexisting osteomyelitis or sinusitis is treated. A subdural infection, however, is usually a more widespread empyema rather than a localized abscess, since the developing infection easily dissects open the subdural space to cover the surface of an entire cerebral hemisphere. Subdural empyema may begin by the extension of infection through the dura mater from without or through the arachnoid from within, or it may result from the operative infection of a subdural hematoma. In any event, a subdural empyema is usually treated by immediate evacuation through multiple trephine openings or a craniotomy flap in order to avert death or serious neurologic morbidity. Drains are usually left in the subdural space, to be removed days later, after all drainage has ceased.

Meningitis[3,4,10]

Bacterial meningitis as such is not a surgical disease, and all but the most resistant or unusual forms usually respond to systemic antibiotics. However, if recurrent episodes of meningitis occur, the neurosurgeon may become involved in the search for and treatment of cerebrospinal fluid rhinorrhea, a midline cranial or spinal dermal sinus tract, or some other portal of entry for organisms into the central nervous system.

Also, in a certain number of patients recovering from meningitis, effusions develop in the subdural spaces over the cerebral hemispheres, or hydrocephalus occurs owing to the obstruction of subarachnoid pathways concerned with the normal absorption of cerebrospinal fluid. Subdural effusions ordinarily occur in infants and frequently may be cured by repeated aspiration with needle and syringe through the coronal suture. Rarely, unilateral or bilateral burr holes, craniectomies, or craniotomies are necessary for the evacuation of the effusions and perhaps the removal of coexisting subdural membranes that are formed by the same inflammatory process. Occasionally, the excessive fluid in the subdural space or ventricular system must be shunted into other areas of the body, such as the peritoneal cavity.

Encephalitis, Cerebritis, Brain Abscess[1,4,5,7-10]

The neurosurgeon may be deceived into exploring and resecting an area of severe viral encephalitis, thinking it is a malignant glioma. Herpes simplex, for example, may cause a necrotic and cystic mass in the temporal lobe that closely resembles a brain tumor. However, even if the correct diagnosis is suspected preoperatively, biopsy of the lesion may be of value for verification. Moreover, resection of such a lesion, or some type of decompressive operation, may also be necessary if steroids and other medical measures are inadequate to control the severe elevations of intracranial pressure that frequently accompany encephalitis.

The term "cerebritis" is usually reserved to describe the focal area of cerebral inflammation that immediately precedes the development of a brain abscess. Such areas of cerebritis may arise from:

1. Extension of an infection through the meninges. In this way, mastoiditis may lead to an abscess in the ipsilateral temporal lobe or cerebellar hemisphere, or frontal sinusitis may produce a frontal lobe abscess.

2. Hematogenous spread from some other site, especially from the lungs, pleura, or heart, or from other areas of the body via congenital heart defects that permit the paradoxical embolism of infected material. Brain abscesses that originate in this manner are distributed among the various areas of the brain in proportion to the vascular supply, so a large number occur in the territory of the middle cerebral arteries.

3. Inoculation through the meninges, as by a compound depressed skull fracture.

Typically, the patient with a brain abscess uncomplicated by meningitis has no systemic signs of infection, such as fever, tachycardia, or leukocytosis. The abscess presents clinically, and by electroencephalography, computed tomography, magnetic resonance imaging, and cerebral angiography as an intracranial mass that must be differentiated from a neoplasm, hematoma, or some other type of space-consuming lesion (Fig. 1).

A brain abscess may contain one or more of a variety of organisms. Aerobic bacteria are often found. In addition, anaerobic or microaerophilic bacteria (frequently) or fungi (occasionally) can be discovered if appropriate culture and staining techniques are employed. Even so, a significant percentage of brain abscesses are found to be sterile.

In the past, the preferred treatment of a brain abscess was total surgical excision. Now that such abscesses can be followed closely by computed tomography or magnetic resonance imaging, stereotactic aspiration and drainage are frequently employed, at least initially, to reduce the mass effect, provide information about the causative organism(s), and lower the risk of intraventricular rupture while the abscess is treated by the systemic administration of antibiotics. A patient with a brain abscess may also require treatment with a steroid medication to reduce reactive brain edema. No matter which operative tech-

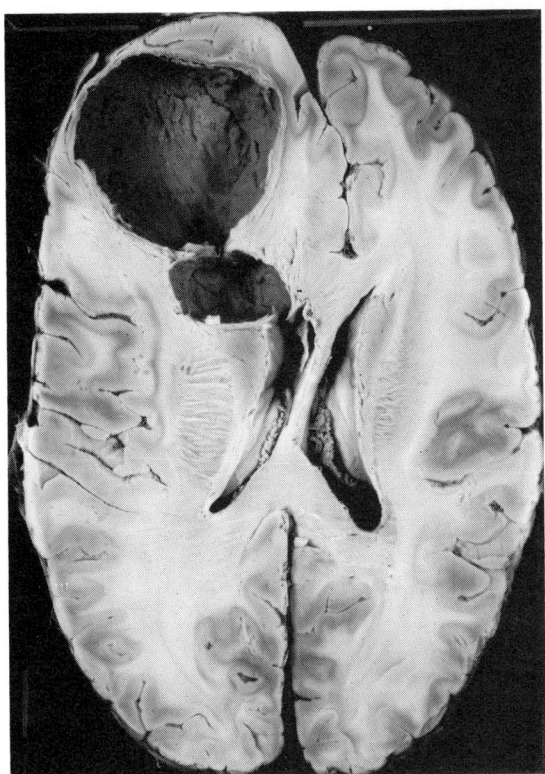

Figure 1. Brain abscess, left frontal lobe. A "daughter" abscess, posterior to the main lesion, had ruptured into the left lateral ventricle as the terminal event in this case.

nique is used, there is a high incidence of seizures among survivors of abscesses of the cerebral hemispheres, which justifies the prophylactic administration of anticonvulsants in most of these patients.

Other Types of Intracranial Infections[6,10,11]

Numerous organisms can cause lesions within the cranial cavity or spinal canal, varying from meningitis (at times accompanied by hydrocephalus) to one or more intraparenchymal granulomas or abscesses. In the setting of the acquired immunodeficiency syndrome (AIDS), lesions within the brain may be caused by the human immunodeficiency virus itself or by opportunistic organisms such as *Toxoplasma gondii, Cryptococcus neoformans,* and JC virus. The neurosurgeon's first task is often

to establish the diagnosis by a stereotactic or open biopsy. Then the condition is ordinarily treated with the appropriate systemic medication; however, in certain circumstances, the neurosurgeon may be called upon to insert an intraventricular catheter attached to a subcutaneous reservoir to facilitate intraventricular drug administration. The neurosurgeon may also be required to drain or excise a fungal abscess or to shunt hydrocephalus resulting from the basal meningitis associated with tuberculosis, sarcoidosis, or a fungal infection.

The parasitic infections, especially echinococcosis and cysticercosis, present a problem to neurosurgeons in some countries, and although they are being encountered more often in the United States, they are still seen too infrequently to justify further discussion here.

SELECTED REFERENCE

Wilkins, R. H., and Rengachary, S. S. (Eds.): Neurosurgery. New York, McGraw-Hill Book Company, 1985.
Part X of this textbook deals with infections of neurosurgical interest, in 14 categories (Chapters 242 through 255).

REFERENCES

1. Alderson, D., Strong, A. J., Ingham, H. R., and Selkon, J. B.: Fifteen-year review of the mortality of brain abscess. Neurosurgery, *8:*1, 1981.
2. Bannister, G., Williams, B., and Smith, S.: Treatment of subdural empyema. J. Neurosurg., *55:*82, 1981.
3. Dodge, P. R., and Swartz, M. N.: Bacterial meningitis—a review of selected aspects. II. Special neurologic problems, postmeningitic complications and clinicopathological correlations. N. Engl. J. Med., *272:*954, 1003, 1965.
4. Garvey, G.: Current concepts of bacterial infections of the central nervous system: Bacterial meningitis and bacterial brain abscess. J. Neurosurg., *59:*735, 1983.
5. Kim, J. H., and Gallis, H. A.: Antimicrobials for use in neurosurgical patients. *In* Wilkins, R. H., and Rengachary, S. S. (Eds.): Neurosurgery Update II. New York, McGraw-Hill Book Company, 1990.
6. Levy, R. M., and Rosenblum, M. L.: Neurosurgical aspects of human immunodeficiency virus-1 (HIV-1) infection. *In* Wilkins, R. H., and Rengachary, S. S. (Eds.): Neurosurgery Update II. New York, McGraw-Hill Book Company, 1990.
7. Mampalam, T. J., and Rosenblum, M. L.: Trends in the management of bacterial brain abscesses: A review of 102 cases over 17 years. Neurosurgery, *23:*451, 1988.
8. Schlitt, M. J., Morawetz, R. B., Bonnin, J. M., Zeiger, H. E., and Whitley, R. J.: Brain biopsy for encephalitis. Clin. Neurosurg., *33:*591, 1986.
9. Stephanov, S.: Surgical treatment of brain abscess. Neurosurgery, *22:*724, 1988.
10. Wilkins, R. H., and Rengachary, S. S. (Eds.): Neurosurgery. New York, McGraw-Hill Book Company, 1985 (see Part X, Infections).
11. Young, R. F., Gade, G., and Grinnell, V.: Surgical treatment for fungal infections in the central nervous system. J. Neurosurg., *63:*371, 1985.

VII _____

INTRASPINAL TUMORS

Robert H. Wilkins, M.D.

Intraspinal tumors can be divided into three groups according to location: extradural, intradural extramedullary, and intramedullary (Figs. 1 and 2). The neoplasms that occur in each of these three locations have clinical and radiologic characteristics that are different from those of the neoplasms in the other locations.

Extradural Neoplasms

Extradural (epidural) tumors are usually malignant.[1,2,6,7,9] The most common example is a metastasis to a vertebra from a

primary carcinoma of the lung, breast, or prostate. Other examples of malignant extradural spinal tumors are lymphoma and myeloma.

Typically, such a tumor begins within the vertebral bone and extends into the epidural space or begins within the epidural space. In either case, the tumor gradually compresses the spinal cord or cauda equina and interferes with the blood supply to this neural tissue. On plain roentgenograms, destruction of the pedicles may be apparent on the anteroposterior views and destruction and collapse of one or more vertebral bodies on the

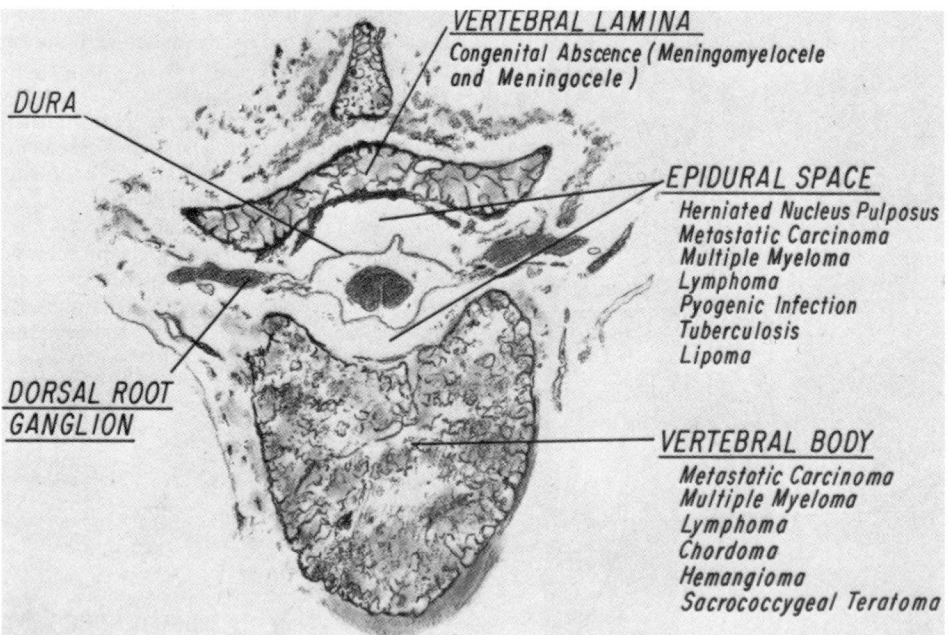

Figure 1. Topographic distribution of lesions of the spine and epidural space. (From Burger, P. C., and Vogel, F. S.: Surgical Pathology of the Nervous System and Its Coverings, 2nd ed. New York, John Wiley & Sons, 1982.)

lateral views. Metastases of this sort are usually lytic but may be blastic (especially those from prostatic carcinoma). Computed tomography (CT) scanning permits the identification of bony involvement, epidural tumor extension, and neural compro-

mise in the axial plane. Magnetic resonance imaging (MRI) permits similar identifications, but in sagittal and coronal planes as well as axial planes.[3]

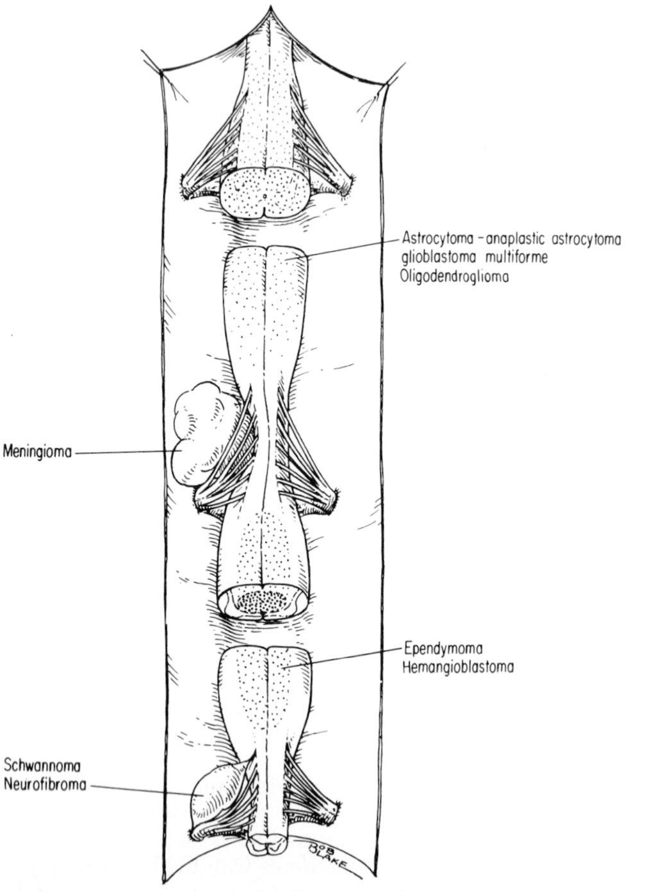

The most common location for an extradural neoplasm is in the thoracic area of the spine. The typical symptoms relate to the directions of tumor growth: the patient first develops back pain centered where the tumor involves the vertebral bone, then the patient experiences radicular pain and dysfunction (radiculopathy) extending around the trunk at the same level on one or both sides as the tumor involves the exiting spinal nerve roots, and finally the patient develops a progressive interference with spinal cord function (myelopathy) with eventual paraplegia.

If a patient presents with progressive back pain (and especially pain that is not improved by recumbency), radicular pain, and neurologic loss, the preliminary assessment should include plain roentgenograms and CT scanning or MRI (Fig. 3), or both. If such studies do not provide sufficient information, they can be supplemented by other studies such as radionuclide bone scanning and positive contrast myelography accompanied by postmyelographic CT scanning.

There are generally two treatment options, radiation therapy or surgical resection followed by radiation therapy. With either option, steroid administration is often advantageous; it can be given immediately and reduces the bulk of the tumor (and the degree of neural compression) temporarily while the primary treatment modality is being accomplished. Surgical resection prior to radiotherapy is usually preferred if the patient is not known to have a malignancy or if the loss of neurologic function is proceeding rapidly. The goals of surgical treatment are to establish the diagnosis, to decompress the spinal cord or cauda equina, and to stabilize that area of the spine if the tumor has produced instability. Ordinarily, the tumor cannot be removed entirely, and radiotherapy is required postoperatively. Depending upon the nature of the tumor, hormonal therapy or chemotherapy may also be beneficial.

Intradural Extramedullary Neoplasms

Tumors that occur within the spinal subarachnoid space are of two types. The first type are benign neoplasms that arise from the meninges (meningiomas) or the nerve roots (neurofibromas, schwannomas).[2,5,7,9] The second type are malignant tumors that have spread through the spinal subarachnoid space from a pri-

Astrocytoma - anaplastic astrocytoma glioblastoma multiforme Oligodendroglioma

Meningioma

Ependymoma Hemangioblastoma

Schwannoma Neurofibroma

Figure 2. Topographic distribution of the common neoplasms of the spinal meninges, spinal nerve roots, and spinal cord. (From Burger, P. C., and Vogel, F. S.: Surgical Pathology of the Nervous System and Its Coverings, 2nd ed. New York, John Wiley & Sons, 1982.)

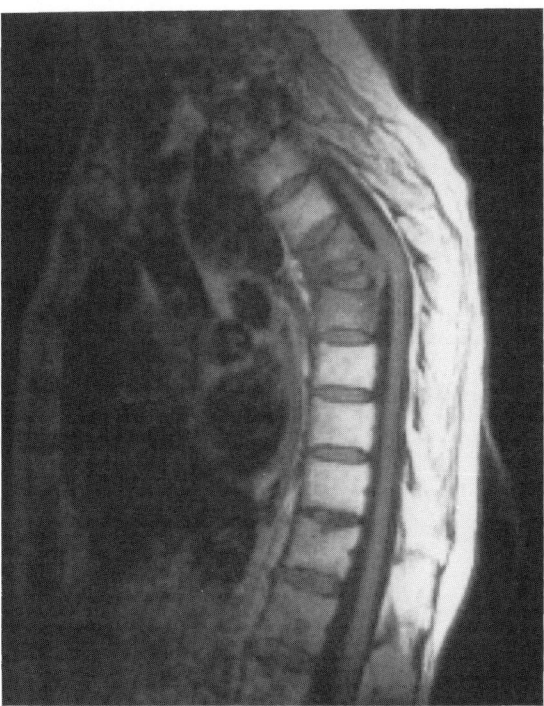

Figure 3. A sagittal magnetic resonance image of metastatic carcinoma of the breast in three contiguous thoracic vertebral segments, with vertebral marrow replacement, compression fracture, spinal angulation, and spinal cord compression. The epidural extension of the tumor anterior to the spinal cord is well demonstrated. (From Miller, K. D., Jr.: Magnetic resonance imaging of the vertebral column and spinal cord. *In* Wilkins, R. H., and Rengachary, S. S. (Eds.): Neurosurgery Update I. New York, McGraw-Hill Book Company, 1990, pp. 104–118.)

mary intracranial location (e.g., medulloblastoma, ependymoma, certain pineal region tumors), or from a malignancy elsewhere in the body (meningeal carcinomatosis). Fortunately, the first type is more common than the second.

Although nerve root tumors can arise at any spinal level, meningiomas rarely develop in the lumbar area. For reasons that are not clear, intraspinal meningiomas are ten times more frequent in women than in men. The patient with a meningioma, neurofibroma, or schwannoma usually presents with myelopathy (if the tumor is located above the level of the cauda equina) but may also exhibit a radiculopathy in the distribution of the involved nerve root or roots. A nerve root tumor occasionally extends along the nerve, with one end being within the dural sac, an isthmus extending through the intervertebral foramen (and enlarging it), and the other end being outside the spine; a tumor with this configuration is called a *dumbbell tumor.*

Except for the occasional demonstration of an enlarged intervertebral foramen, plain roentgenograms and CT scans are not usually of value in the diagnosis of intradural extramedullary tumors. Myelography and postmyelographic CT scanning and/or MRI with gadolinium enhancement are the most useful diagnostic studies. For meningeal carcinomatosis, the key diagnostic test is the cytologic examination of cerebrospinal fluid removed by lumbar puncture.

The treatment of intraspinal meningiomas, neurofibromas, and schwannomas is surgical excision, which may include excision of the involved portion of the dura mater (meningioma) or the involved nerve rootlets or root (neurofibroma, schwannoma). At the level of involvement, neurofibromas and schwannomas typically grow on the sensory (dorsal) root in preference to the motor (ventral) root, and it may be possible to spare motor function during tumor removal. However, such tumors may be part of a more widespread process, neurofibromatosis, in which case there will be similar tumors on other nerve roots and nerves. If the gross total removal of a solitary intraspinal meningioma, neurofibroma, or schwannoma can be

achieved, which is usually the case, the patient is ordinarily cured. For example, Solero and associates followed 156 patients for an average of 15 years after the removal of a spinal meningioma.[5] The rate of recurrence was only 6 per cent among the 150 patients who had gross total tumor removal.

Metastases within the subarachnoid space are not treated surgically. These are ordinarily managed with radiotherapy and hormonal or chemotherapy.

Intramedullary Neoplasms

This type of tumor develops within the spinal cord, enlarging it in a fusiform manner.[2,3,7,9] The patient experiences a progressive myelopathy, and the radiographic studies demonstrate evidence of spinal cord expansion. Although plain roentgenologic films and CT scans may show enlargement of the spinal canal, the MRI examination with gadolinium enhancement is the most useful test in demonstrating the tumor and any associated syrinx. Myelography and postmyelographic CT scanning may also be of value.

Intramedullary tumors are ordinarily treated surgically, through a laminectomy. If an ependymoma is encountered, it may be possible to excise it completely, with maintenance of the surrounding spinal cord. If only a partial resection can be achieved, radiotherapy can be given postoperatively. The outlook of the patient with an intraspinal ependymoma is significantly better than that of the patient with an intracranial ependymoma.[4]

As is true of most astrocytomas of the brain, an intramedullary astrocytoma ordinarily cannot be removed completely surgically. The decision about giving postoperative radiotherapy is based on the exact histology of the tumor, the degree of surgical resection, and the age of the patient. In contrast, the intramedullary hemangioblastoma is a benign tumor that can be cured by surgical excision, without the need for radiotherapy.

Intraspinal dermoid and epidermoid tumors are benign lesions that can be found within the subarachnoid space or the spinal cord, or both.[8] They are most common in the lumbosacral area, especially at the level of the conus medullaris. Either type of tumor can be associated with spinal dysraphism and in particular with a dermal sinus tract that opens onto the back, usually in the lumbosacral region. Lipomas are also benign spinal tumors that are often associated with spinal dysraphism. They can be found at any level from extradural to intramedullary and are most common in the lumbosacral region. These various benign tumors can be resected surgically, with the risks and difficulties of such treatment being related to the degree of involvement of the tumor with critical areas of the spinal cord and to the extent of any associated dysraphic changes.

Conclusions

The spread of malignant neoplasms into the spinal canal has a poor prognosis. The success of treatment is usually defined as either an improvement in neurologic function or the maintenance of ambulation during the patient's short remaining life span. However, many intraspinal neoplasms such as meningiomas, neurofibromas, schwannomas, dermoid tumors, epidermoid tumors, lipomas, hemangioblastomas, and ependymomas have a high potential for surgical cure. The recent remarkable advances in neuroradiologic and neurosurgical technology have enabled the neurosurgeon to achieve this potential to a greater degree than ever before, and at the same time have reduced the risks of such treatment and made it safer.

REFERENCES

1. Barcena, A., Lobato, R. D., Rivas, J. J., Cordobes, F., de Castro, S., Cabrera, A., and Lamas, E.: Spinal metastatic disease: Analysis of factors determining functional prognosis and the choice of treatment. Neurosurgery, 15:820, 1984.
2. Burger, P. C., and Vogel, F. S.: Surgical Pathology of the Nervous System and Its Coverings, 2nd ed. New York, John Wiley & Sons, 1982, pp. 553–568, 585–648.

3. Miller, K. D., Jr.: Magnetic resonance imaging of the vertebral column and spinal cord. *In* Wilkins, R. H., and Rengachary, S. S. (Eds.): Neurosurgery Update I. New York, McGraw-Hill Book Company, 1990, pp. 104–118.
4. Rawlings, C. E., III, Giangaspero, F., Burger, P. C., and Bullard, D. E.: Ependymomas: A clinicopathologic study. Surg. Neurol., 29:271, 1988.
5. Solero, C. L., Fornari, M., Giombini, S., Lasio, G., Oliveri, G., Cimino, C., and Pluchino, F.: Spinal meningiomas: Review of 174 operated cases. Neurosurgery, 125:153, 1989.
6. Vieth, R. G., and Odom, G. L.: Extradural spinal metastases and their neurosurgical treatment. J. Neurosurg., 23:501, 1965.
7. Wilkins, R. H., and Rengachary, S. S. (Eds.): Neurosurgery. New York, McGraw-Hill Book Company, 1985, pp. 1039–1069.
8. Wilkins, R. H., and Rossitch, E., Jr.: Intraspinal cysts. *In* Pang, D. (Ed.): Disorders of the Paediatric Spine. New York, Raven Press, 1990.
9. Youmans, J. R. (Ed.): Neurological Surgery, 3rd ed. Philadelphia, W. B. Saunders Company, 1990, pp. 3531–3592.

VIII

RUPTURED LUMBAR INTERVERTEBRAL DISC

Robert H. Wilkins, M.D.

Despite its common occurrence,[1-6,8-11] intervertebral disc rupture escaped clinical recognition until just over 50 years ago. Low back pain and sciatica had been discussed in medical treatises for centuries, but it was not until the publication by Mixter and Barr in the *New England Journal of Medicine* in 1934 that herniation of a lumbar intervertebral disc (formerly thought to be a rare result of severe spinal injury) was first linked clearly to the syndrome of low back pain and sciatica.[7] Today this is one of the most common conditions treated by neurosurgeons in the United States.

Normal Anatomy

The central portion of the intervertebral disc, the nucleus pulposus, is left as a remnant of the notochord as the spinal column is formed during embryonic life. It is ringed by the tough annulus fibrosus and is situated somewhat eccentrically toward the posterior aspect of the disc. It is bounded above and below by the cartilaginous plates covering the opposing surfaces of the two adjacent vertebral bodies. The nucleus pulposus is gelatinous in infancy but becomes more fibrous with age. The annulus fibrosus is supported anteriorly by the anterior longitudinal ligament and posteriorly by the posterior longitudinal ligament.

The bony arch that encircles the spinal canal posteriorly is formed by the two pedicles, the two transverse processes, the two laminae, and the spinous process. On each side of the midline, the laminal arches of adjacent vertebrae are connected by an elastic yellow ligament, the ligamentum flavum.

The tip of the spinal cord (conus medullaris) ends at the T12 or L1 level of the spinal canal. Caudal to the conus medullaris, the nerve roots of the cauda equina lie immersed in cerebrospinal fluid within the subarachnoid space, surrounded by concentric cylindrical sheaths, the arachnoid and the dura mater. The dural-arachnoidal sac usually ends at about the level of the first sacral vertebra. The space that surrounds the dura within the spinal canal, the epidural space, is filled with fat and is traversed by veins. The spinal nerves leave the dural sac in pairs, with one nerve on each side exiting at each vertebral level. Each nerve lies along the caudal border of the pedicle as it exits through the intervertebral foramen; in this position it lies between the intervertebral disc anteromedially and the facet joint posterolaterally (Fig. 1). The nerve roots, however, do not exit directly transversely. Each nerve root exits from the main dural sac and then lies immediately lateral to it for 1 to 2 cm. before it turns further laterally to leave the bony spinal canal about one vertebral level below where it left the dural sac. For example, the left L5 nerve root ordinarily leaves the dural sac at the level of the L4–L5 intervertebral disc (where it is most likely to be involved by a left-sided L4–L5 disc herniation), but it leaves the

bony spinal canal below the left L5 pedicle, opposite the L5–S1 disc (Fig. 2).

Clinicopathologic Features

Degenerative changes in an intervertebral disc can take two main forms: (1) the nucleus pulposus can herniate out of its normally confined space (soft disc protrusion), or (2) the entire disc can lose substance, with loss of disc height and the formation of osteophytes that project outward from the adjacent rims of the vertebral body above and the vertebral body below the involved disc (hard disc protrusion).

SOFT DISC PROTRUSION (HERNIATED NUCLEUS PULPOSUS, HERNIATED DISC, RUPTURED DISC). The nucleus pulposus can herniate superiorly or inferiorly through the confining cartilaginous plate into the cancellous bone of the adjacent vertebral body. These are called Schmorl's nodules and are incidental radiographic or postmortem findings.

The disc herniation that is important clinically begins with the development of a posterolateral or posterior fissure through the concentric rings of the annulus fibrosus. The nucleus pulposus may then begin to extend into this fissure (Fig. 3, top). The patient at this stage may experience low back pain and perhaps

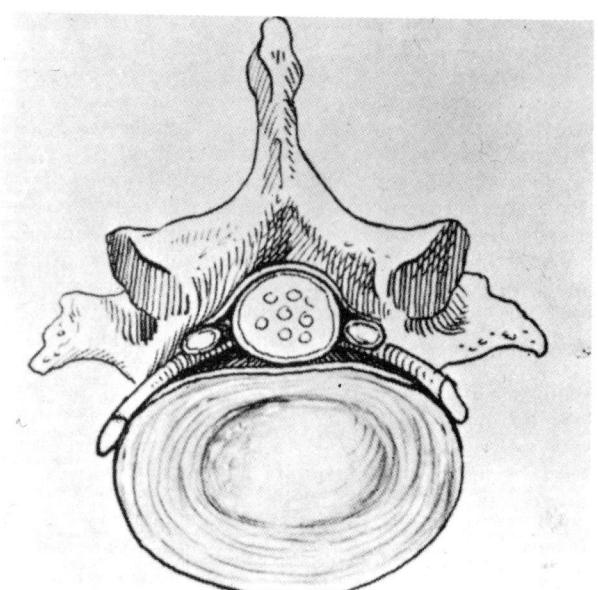

Figure 1. A lumbar vertebra, demonstrating the relationship of the exiting nerve root on each side to the intervertebral disc and the ipsilateral facet. (From Semmes, R. E.: Ruptures of the Lumbar Intervertebral Disc: Their Mechanism, Diagnosis, and Treatment. Springfield, Ill., Charles C Thomas, 1964.)

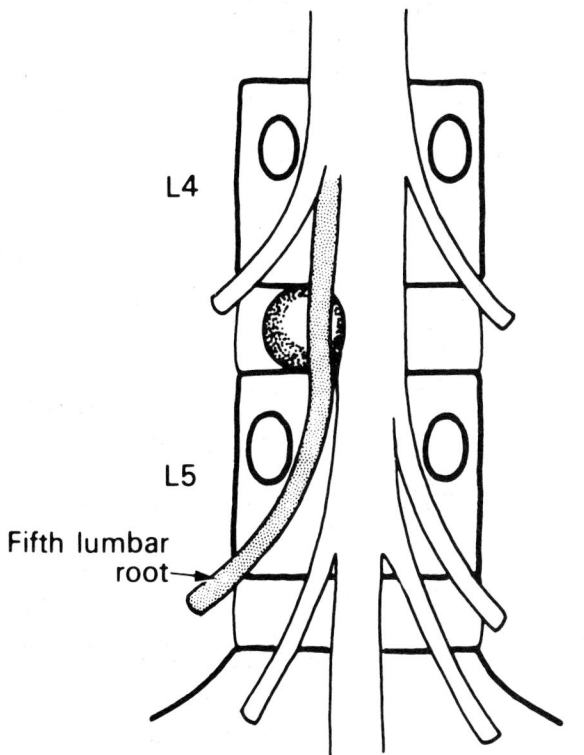

Figure 2. Herniation of the disc between the L4 and L5 vertebrae compresses the L5 nerve root. (From Macnab, I.: Backache. Baltimore, Williams & Wilkins, 1977.)

some referred pain into the buttock or hip on the affected side. Further protrusion of the nucleus pulposus may then occur, causing bulging of the outer layers of the annulus and of the posterior longitudinal ligament sufficient to pinch the adjacent nerve root between the protruding disc and the lamina or the intervertebral facet (Fig. 3, lower left). Finally, a fragment of the disc may actually be extruded completely through the remaining layers of the annulus fibrosus and posterior longitudinal ligament and become wedged anterior to the nerve root; this is referred to as a free fragment (Fig. 3, lower right). When the nerve root is compressed by a protruding or extruded disc, the patient develops radiating pain along the distribution of the sciatic nerve (sciatica) on the involved side in addition to low

back pain. The patient may also have neurologic deficits (hypesthesia, weakness, or reduction of the deep tendon reflex) in the distribution of the involved nerve root. This clinical pattern of radiating pain, perhaps with neurologic deficits, is referred to as a radiculopathy.

If the disc herniation is quite large or in the midline (posterocentral rather than posterolateral herniation), it may compress many of the nerves of the cauda equina still within the dural sac at that level. Such compression may cause low back pain, bilateral sciatica, and interference with urinary and anal sphincter function and with sexual function. The latter neurologic deficits are fortunately rare; of these unusual dysfunctions, urinary retention is the most likely to occur.

Approximately 95 per cent of lumbar disc herniations occur at the L5–S1 or L4–L5 level, with a slight numerical preponderance at one or the other level being reported by various authors. About 4 per cent occur at the L3–L4 level, and less than 1 per cent at the L2–L3 or L1–L2 level.

HARD DISC PROTRUSION (DEGENERATIVE DISC DISEASE WITH SPINAL OSTEOARTHRITIS, LUMBAR SPONDYLOSIS). Degeneration in a lumbar intervertebral disc with narrowing of the disc space and generalized bulging of the annulus fibrosus is frequently associated with the formation of osteoarthritic bony ridges (osteophytes) along the rims of the vertebral bodies adjacent to the involved disc. The posterior elements (laminae, facet joints, ligamenta flava) may become thickened, and osteophytes may project anteriorly from the facets. All of these changes tend to narrow the spinal canal (especially its lateral recesses) and the intervertebral foramina. Such narrowing may cause compression of an individual nerve root or multiple nerve roots of the cauda equina. The resulting symptoms and signs are similar to those caused by disc herniation but tend to be more gradual in onset and more protracted in course. If significant narrowing of the spinal canal occurs (acquired spinal stenosis), the cauda equina may be compressed when the lumbar spine is placed into certain positions, such as extension; when the patient walks, he may develop disagreeable paresthesias, numbness, or weakness in the lower extremities (neurogenic intermittent claudication).

Symptoms and Signs

The typical patient with a posterolateral lumbar disc herniation has intermittent low back pain for several weeks to several years and then develops sciatica as well. The pain is usually aggravated by back movement, by sitting or standing for long

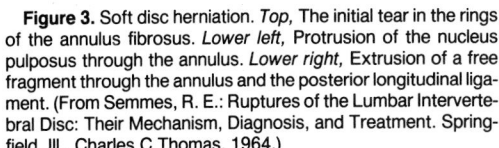

Figure 3. Soft disc herniation. *Top,* The initial tear in the rings of the annulus fibrosus. *Lower left,* Protrusion of the nucleus pulposus through the annulus. *Lower right,* Extrusion of a free fragment through the annulus and the posterior longitudinal ligament. (From Semmes, R. E.: Ruptures of the Lumbar Intervertebral Disc: Their Mechanism, Diagnosis, and Treatment. Springfield, Ill., Charles C Thomas, 1964.)

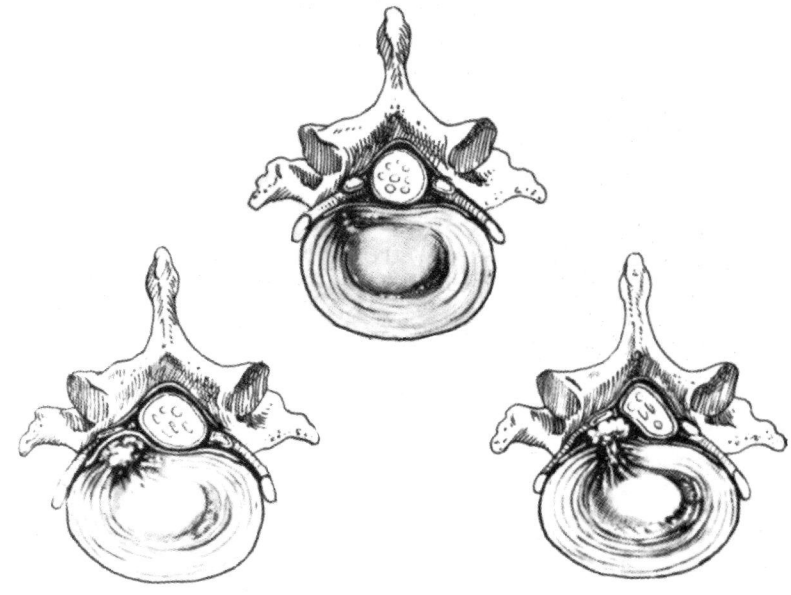

TABLE 1. Patterns of Neurologic Deficit Caused by Intervertebral Disc Herniation

Involved Disc	Involved Nerve Root	Reduced Neurologic Function		
		Sensory	Motor	Reflex
L3–L4	L4	Anterior thigh, anteromedial calf	Quadriceps femoris	Knee jerk
L4–L5	L5	Anterior calf, medial dorsum of foot, great toe	Foot dorsiflexors	Variable
L5–S1	S1	Lateral calf, lateral dorsum of foot, small toe	Foot plantar flexors	Ankle jerk

periods, by lifting an object from the bent position, and by coughing or straining. It ordinarily is relieved temporarily by bed rest; the most comfortable position is horizontal, usually on the side, with the hips and knees flexed. The patient may also notice tingling paresthesias or numbness in certain aspects of the involved leg and foot, weakness in some muscle groups in that limb (less frequent), or, rarely, urinary retention.

On physical examination the patient may demonstrate one or more of the following mechanical signs: lumbar scoliosis, paravertebral muscle spasm, tenderness over one or more of the lower lumbar spines, limitation by pain of low back motion (especially forward flexion), limitation by pain of straight leg raising on one or both sides, or the initiation or intensification of sciatic and back pain by the popliteal compression test. Neurologic deficits, if present, have a typical pattern for each of the commonly involved lumbar discs (Table 1).

Management

Roentgenograms are made of the lumbosacral spine and pelvis to assess disc narrowing and osteophyte formation, but especially to identify causes of back and leg pain other than disc disease, such as spinal or intraspinal neoplasms, infections, congenital malformations, and so forth. The initial treatment of the acute symptoms of lumbar disc disease consists of bed rest on a firm mattress, with medication to combat pain and muscle spasm as needed. Locally applied heat, anti-inflammatory medication, pelvic traction, or the use of a lumbosacral corset may also be helpful at times. If these measures give relief of the acute episode, recurrences may be minimized by a daily maintenance program of low back exercises and the avoidance of certain activities such as frequent bending at the waist, lifting heavy objects, and sitting in an automobile for prolonged periods. Anti-inflammatory medication may be beneficial over a prolonged period to reduce the discomfort of lumbar osteoarthritis.

If conservative measures fail to relieve the patient's pain or if the patient develops significant weakness or urinary retention, a more aggressive approach to treatment should be taken. The patient should have further diagnostic tests such as an electromyogram, a spinal computed tomography scan, or magnetic resonance imaging, or a lumbar myelogram (perhaps followed by a computed tomography scan while the contrast agent is still within the spinal canal). If all available evidence indicates that a soft or hard lumbar disc protrusion is present, it should then be treated surgically.

The aim of surgical treatment is to provide relief of existing nerve compression. The standard surgical treatment of a unilateral radiculopathy is via a partial hemilaminectomy. The surgeon makes a midline lower lumbar incision and retracts the paravertebral muscles away from the spine and laminae on the involved side. He then removes portions of one or two laminae and the attached ligamentum flavum to gain entrance into the lateral aspect of the spinal canal. After retracting the affected nerve root and exposing the disc herniation immediately anterior to it, the surgeon incises any remaining fibers of the posterior longitudinal ligament and annulus fibrosus and extracts as much of the degenerated disc material (mainly nucleus pulposus) as is feasible. The wound is then closed in anatomic layers. The same technique is used for decompression of a nerve root entrapped by the changes of spondylosis, except that no disc material is removed.

If there is a central or transverse disc herniation or if there is generalized spinal stenosis from spondylosis, the surgeon generally removes the spine, both laminae, the ligamenta flava, and perhaps portions of the facets at one or more levels to provide posterior decompression. Any disc herniation present is removed in the manner previously stated via an approach from one or both sides of the spinal canal.

The patient ordinarily leaves the hospital 3 to 6 days postoperatively and returns to work after another 4 to 6 weeks of recuperation at home. The patient is instructed in a maintenance program such as that mentioned earlier.

An alternative to open surgical treatment of a lumbar disc protrusion is the percutaneous removal of disc material (automated percutaneous lumbar discectomy) or the percutaneous injection of chymopapain, an enzyme that reduces the size of the disc. However, neither procedure can effectively treat a free-fragment disc extrusion.

Although a disc herniation usually can be managed effectively, with resolution or improvement of the symptoms and signs, the underlying (and poorly understood) biochemical abnormality that led to the herniation continues. Therefore, some of these patients are destined to have problems from disc disease at the same or a different spinal level at a later time.

SELECTED REFERENCES

Spurling, R. G.: Lesions of the Lumbar Intervertebral Disc. Springfield, Ill., Charles C Thomas, 1953.
  This helpful little book (148 pages) is based on an earlier monograph on the intervertebral disc by F. K. Bradford and R. G. Spurling, also published by the Charles C Thomas Company. Although it was written more than 35 years ago, it is concise, practical, and readable; it provides the basic information that underlies the present management of the ruptured lumbar intervertebral disc.

REFERENCES

1. Abdullah, A. F., Wolber, P. G. H., Warfield, J. R., and Gunadi, I. K.: Surgical management of extreme lateral lumbar disc herniations: Review of 138 cases. Neurosurgery, 22:648, 1988.
2. Camins, M. B., and O'Leary, P. F. (Eds.): The Lumbar Spine. New York, Raven Press, 1987.
3. Cauthen, J. C. (Ed.): Lumbar Spine Surgery: Indications, Techniques, Failures, and Alternatives, 2nd ed. Baltimore, Williams & Wilkins, 1988.
4. Dunsker, S. B.: Alternatives in the surgical treatment of herniated lumbar disks. Clin. Neurosurg., 35:459, 1989.
5. Frymoyer, J. W.: Back pain and sciatica. N. Engl. J. Med., 318:291, 1988.
6. Maciunas, R. J., and Onofrio, B. M.: The long-term results of chymopapain chemonucleolysis for lumbar disc disease: Ten-year follow-up results in 268 patients injected at the Mayo Clinic. J. Neurosurg., 65:1, 1986.
7. Mixter, W. J., and Barr, J. S.: Rupture of the intervertebral disc with involvement of the spinal canal. N. Engl. J. Med., 211:210, 1934.
8. Ramirez, L. F., and Thisted, R.: Complications and demographic characteristics of patients undergoing lumbar discectomy in community hospitals. Neurosurgery, 25:226, 1989.
9. Rothman, R. H., Simeone, F. A., and Bernini, P. M.: Lumbar disc disease. In Rothman, R. H., and Simeone, F. A. (Eds.): The Spine, 2nd ed. Philadelphia, W. B. Saunders Company, 1982, pp. 508–645.
10. Semmes, R. E.: Ruptures of the Lumbar Intervertebral Disc. Their Mechanism, Diagnosis, and Treatment. Springfield, Ill., Charles C Thomas, 1964.
11. Spurling, R. G.: Lesions of the Lumbar Intervertebral Disc. Springfield, Ill., Charles C Thomas, 1953.

IX

CERVICAL DISC LESIONS

Robert H. Wilkins, M.D.

Lesions of the cervical intervertebral discs are analogous to those that affect the lumbar discs. However, in the cervical region the anatomy is somewhat different (Figs. 1 and 2), and those differences introduce variations in symptoms, signs, and treatment.

Normal Anatomy

The cervical disc, like the lumbar disc, is composed of a tough outer anulus fibrosus and a softer inner nucleus pulposus and is separated by a cartilaginous plate from the vertebral body above it and by another such plate from the vertebral body below. However, the entire cervical disc is much smaller than a lumbar disc.

The spinal canal in the cervical area contains the spinal cord rather than the cauda equina, so a reduction in the size of the spinal canal by spondylosis or a midline disc herniation causes compression of the spinal cord rather than of the cauda equina, a more serious form of neurologic involvement with a worse prognosis. The nerve roots of the cauda equina are more resistant to compression than is the spinal cord and are more likely to recover after surgical decompression.

In addition, the cervical spine contains the joints of Luschka, which are not present elsewhere in the spine. These joints, one on each side of the disc, can give rise to bony spurs or ridges (osteophytes) as can the main facet joints (apophyseal or interpedicular joints) and the edges of the vertebral bodies adjacent to the intervertebral disc (which is a symphysis type of articulation between vertebral bodies). The exiting nerve root on each side travels between these joints (Fig. 1) and can be compressed by osteophytes extending into the intervertebral foramen from any or all of the three sources just mentioned (Fig. 2).

In the cervical area, the nerves exit transversely. There are seven cervical vertebrae and eight pairs of cervical nerves. The nerve root exiting on each side at the level of the intervertebral disc between the C7 vertebral body and the T1 vertebral body (the C7–T1 disc) is the C8 nerve root. The nerve root exiting on each side at the level of the C6–C7 disc is the C7 nerve root; the nerve root exiting on each side at the level of the C5–C6 disc is the C6 nerve root, and so on (Table 1).

Clinicopathologic Features

As with a lumbar disc, degenerative changes in a cervical intervertebral disc can take two main forms: (1) the nucleus pulposus can herniate out of its normal confined space (soft disc protrusion), or (2) the entire disc can lose substance, with loss of disc height and the formation of osteophytes that project outward from the adjacent rims of the vertebral body above and the vertebral body below the involved disc. The second process is often combined with osteoarthritis of the apophyseal joints and the joints of Luschka. The combination of degenerative disc disease and osteophyte formation is called spondylosis.

SOFT DISC PROTRUSION (HERNIATED NUCLEUS PULPOSUS, HERNIATED DISC, RUPTURED DISC). The pathologic process and the steps in the development of a cervical disc herniation are similar to those of a lumbar disc herniation. Cervical disc herniations are most frequent at the C6–C7 level but also occur at C5–C6 and to a lesser extent at C4–C5 and other levels.

With the usual posterolateral disc rupture, the patient experiences pain in the neck, and then as the nerve root is compressed, the patient develops pain radiating into the ipsilateral upper extremity and may also develop paresthesias, numbness, or weakness in an appropriate distribution (Table 1). The pain and paresthesias may be intensified by neck movement, especially by extension or by lateral flexion to the side of the herniation, and by coughing or straining. They may be improved by bed rest.

On examination, the patient frequently exhibits restriction of neck movement, especially extension. Downward head compression by the examiner increases the patient's radicular pain

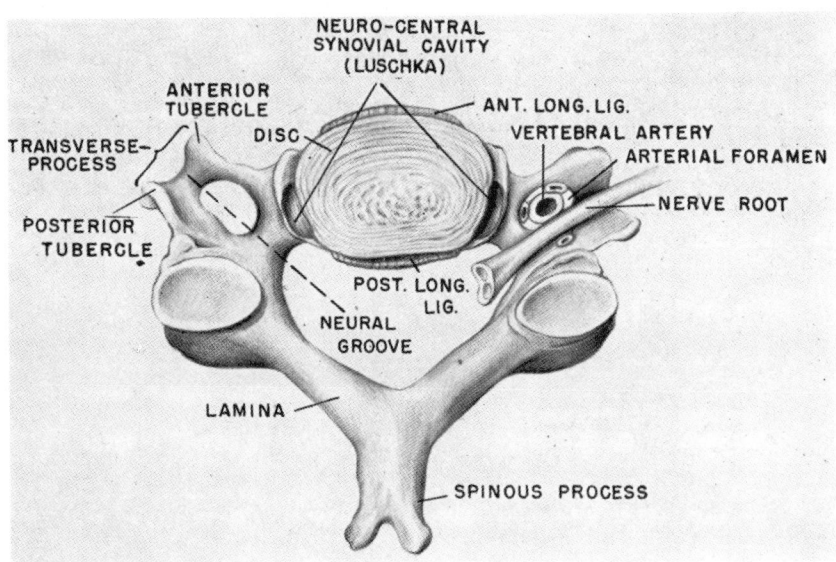

Figure 1. Semidiagrammatic representation of a vertebra from the midcervical region, viewed from above. (From Spurling, R. G.: Lesions of the Cervical Intervertebral Disc. Springfield, Ill., Charles C Thomas, 1956.)

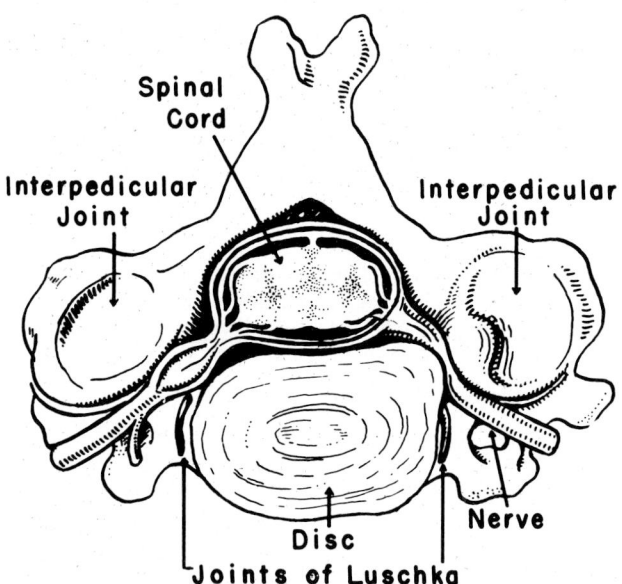

Figure 2. Mechanism of cervical nerve root compression by osteophytes extending into the intervertebral foramen. (From Spurling, R. G.: Lesions of the Cervical Intervertebral Disc. Springfield, Ill., Charles C Thomas, 1956.)

and paresthesias, especially if the neck is simultaneously flexed to the side of the involvement. Hypesthesia, weakness, or the reduction of a deep tendon reflex may be present and should provide a clue to the level of the disc rupture and nerve root compression (Table 1).

If the disc herniation occurs more toward the midline (i.e., a more direct posterior herniation), it compresses the spinal cord in addition to, or instead of, a nerve root. This produces cervical myelopathy manifested by lower motor neuron dysfunction (muscle weakness and hypotonia, reduction or loss of appropriate deep tendon reflexes, dermatomal sensory impairment) at the level of the compression and upper motor neuron dysfunction (spasticity, clonus, increased deep tendon reflexes, Babinski's sign, reduction of sensation) below that level. Loss of voluntary control of bowel, bladder, and sexual function may also develop.

HARD DISC PROTRUSION (DEGENERATIVE DISC DISEASE WITH SPINAL OSTEOARTHRITIS, CERVICAL SPONDYLOSIS). As in the lumbar area, these changes tend to narrow the spinal canal and the intervertebral foramina, which may result in the compression of one or more cervical nerve roots or of the spinal cord at one or more levels. The resulting symptoms and signs are similar to those caused by disc herniation but tend to be more gradual in onset and more protracted in course.

Management

Roentgenograms of the cervical spine are obtained to assess the presence and degree of spondylosis, but especially to iden-

tify a cause of neck and arm pain other than disc disease, such as a neoplasm or infection. The initial treatment of the patient with acute radiculopathy consists of bed rest, with medication for pain and muscle spasm. Locally applied heat may provide additional comfort. Intermittent cervical halter traction (e.g., 7 pounds starting at 30 minutes four times per day and increasing to 2 hours four times per day) is often beneficial as well, but the direction of traction must be comfortable. Traction with the neck extended may actually increase the pain. Anti-inflammatory medication may be of value over a prolonged period to reduce the discomfort of cervical spondylosis.

If these measures do not provide adequate pain relief, or if the patient shows evidence of spinal cord compression, a more aggressive approach should be taken. The patient should have further diagnostic tests. Although electromyography, plain computed tomography scanning, and magnetic resonance imaging may be useful, the best current study for assessing the presence and extent of cervical disc herniation or cervical spondylosis is the cervical myelogram followed by computed tomography scanning while the contrast material is still present in the cervical subarachnoid space.

Surgical treatment to provide nerve root decompression can be accomplished by a posterior approach through a hemilaminectomy (Fig. 3) or by an anterior approach through the intervertebral disc (Figs. 4 and 5).[1,3,4,6,8-11] The posterior procedure is a smaller operation that takes less time and does not require a bone graft. The results are good. For example, Henderson and associates reviewed the results of 736 consecutive patients treated by a posterior approach and followed for an average of 2.8 years; there was a 96 per cent incidence of relief of significant arm pain and/or paresthesias and a 98 per cent incidence of resolution of a preoperative motor deficit, with only a 1.5 per cent minor complication rate and a 3 per cent rate of recurrent radiculopathy.[3]

If a patient is being treated for the unusual circumstance of a single midline disc herniation with spinal cord compression, an anterior discectomy is the procedure of choice. Provided that the myelopathy is not too severe or too long-standing, improvement can be expected.

In contrast, the surgical treatment of spinal cord compression from spondylosis usually requires a larger operation, and the results are not as favorable.[1,2,4,5,7,9] If the operation is done via a posterior approach, it necessitates a full laminectomy (removal of the spinous process and the lamina on each side) at multiple levels. If an anterior approach is chosen, it involves either a discectomy/osteophytectomy at one or more levels or the resection of the central aspects of one or more vertebral bodies, usually with the insertion of a bone graft to ensure the postoperative maintenance of vertebral alignment and stability. These larger procedures carry additional risk, but more important, the results are less satisfactory. For example, reports of the treatment of cervical spondylotic myelopathy by anterior discectomy/osteophytectomy typically indicate neurologic improvement in only 40 to 75 per cent, with a significant percentage of patients showing further deterioration despite treatment.

TABLE 1. Patterns of Radiculopathy Caused by Cervical Disc Herniation or Osteophyte Formation

Involved Disc Level	Involved Nerve Root	Key Areas of Reduced Neurologic Function		
		Sensory	*Motor*	*Reflex*
C4–C5	C5	Deltoid area	Deltoid	—
C5–C6	C6	Thumb, index finger	Biceps	Biceps
C6–C7	C7	Index and long fingers	Triceps	Triceps
C7–T1	C8	Ring and small fingers	Grip	—

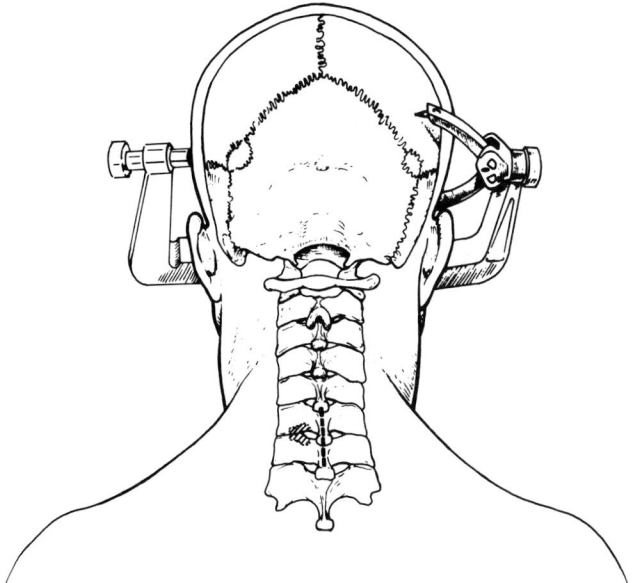

Figure 3. The posterior approach to a cervical nerve root decompression, in this case for the removal of a disc herniation at the C6–C7 level on the left. The dotted line shows the position of the skin incision and the oblique lines show the area of bone removal that exposes the left C7 nerve root and the disc herniation that is anterior to it. (From Wilkins, R. H., and Gaskill, S. J.: Cervical hemilaminectomy for excision of herniated disc. *In* Rengachary, S. S., and Wilkins, R. H. (Eds.): Neurosurgical Operative Atlas. Baltimore, Williams & Wilkins, 1991.)

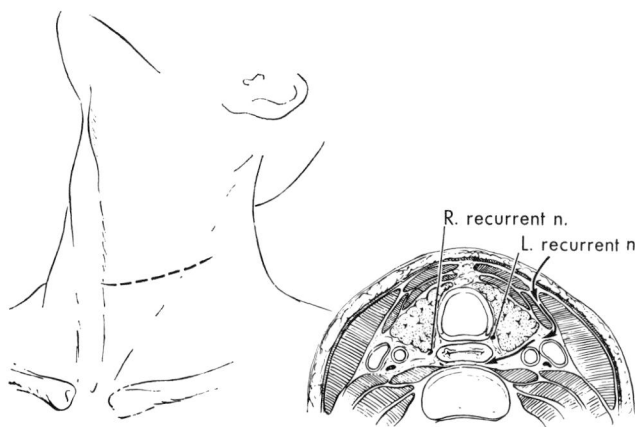

Figure 4. The anterior approach to the midcervical spine. A typical skin incision is shown on the left, and the route of approach is shown on the right. (From Aronson, N. I.: The management of soft cervical disc protrusions using the Smith-Robinson approach. Clin. Neurosurg., *20:*253, 1973.)

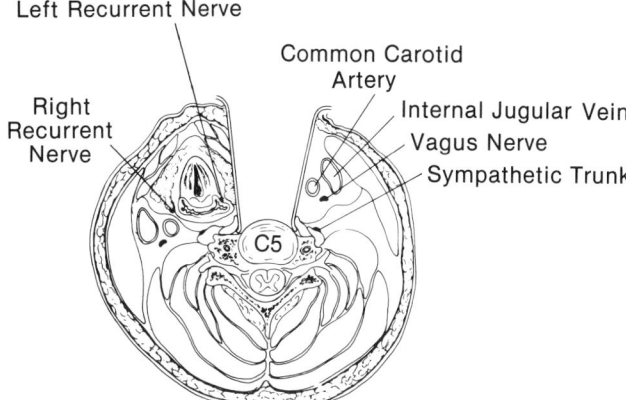

Figure 5. The anterior exposure of the midcervical spine. (From Tew, J. M., Jr., and Mayfield, F. H.: Complications of surgery of the anterior cervical spine. Clin. Neurosurg., *23:*424, 1976.)

REFERENCES

1. Collias, J. C., and Roberts, M. P.: Posterior operations for cervical disc herniation and spondylotic myelopathy. *In* Schmidek, H. H., and Sweet, W. H. (Eds.): Operative Neurosurgical Techniques: Indications, Methods and Results, 2nd ed. Orlando, Grune & Stratton, 1988, pp. 1347–1358.
2. Fager, C. A.: Results of adequate posterior decompression in the relief of spondylotic cervical myelopathy. J. Neurosurg., 38:684, 1973.
3. Henderson, C. M., Hennessy, R. G., Shuey, H. M., Jr., and Shackelford, E. G.: Posterior-lateral foraminotomy as an exclusive operative technique for cervical radiculopathy: A review of 846 consecutively operated cases. Neurosurgery, 13:504, 1983.
4. Hoff, J. T.: Cervical disc disease and cervical spondylosis. *In* Wilkins, R. H., and Rengachary, S. S. (Eds.): Neurosurgery. New York, McGraw-Hill Book Company, 1985, pp. 2230–2239.
5. Kojima, T., Waga, S., Kubo, Y., Kanamaru, K., Shimosaka, S., and Shimizu, T.: Anterior cervical vertebrectomy and interbody fusion for multi-level spondylosis and ossification of the posterior longitudinal ligament. Neurosurgery, 24:864, 1989.
6. Lunsford, L. D., Bissonette, D. J., Jannetta, P. L., Sheptak, P. E., and Zorub, D. S.: Anterior surgery for cervical disc disease. Part 1: Treatment of lateral cervical disc herniation in 253 cases. J. Neurosurg., 53:1, 1980.
7. Lunsford, L. D., Bissonette, D. J., and Zorub, D. S.: Anterior surgery for cervical disc disease. Part 2: Treatment of cervical spondylotic myelopathy in 32 cases. J Neurosurg., 53:12, 1980.
8. Raynor, R. B.: Anterior or posterior approach to the cervical spine: An anatomical and radiographic evaluation and comparison. Neurosurgery, 12:7, 1983.
9. Schmidek, H. H., and Smith, D. A.: Anterior cervical disc excision in cervical spondylosis. In Schmidek, H. H., and Sweet, W. H. (Eds.): Operative Neurosurgical Techniques: Indications, Methods and Results, 2nd ed. Orlando, Grune & Stratton, 1988, pp. 1327–1342.
10. Spurling, R. G.: Lesions of the Cervical Intervertebral Disc. Springfield, Ill., Charles C Thomas, 1956.
11. Wilkins, R. H., and Gaskill, S. J.: Cervical hemilaminectomy for excision of herniated disc. In Rengachary, S. S., and Wilkins, R. H. (Eds.): Neurosurgical Operative Atlas. Baltimore, Williams & Wilkins, 1991.

X

PERIPHERAL NERVE INJURIES

Robert H. Wilkins, M.D.

Anatomy and Pathophysiology

To correctly diagnose and treat peripheral nerve injuries, the surgeon must understand the anatomy and pathophysiology of peripheral nerves. The "wiring diagram" of the human body is complex,[2,8–10] in part because peripheral nerves contain varying proportions of motor, sensory, and sympathetic axons from diverse sources, and in part because of the mixing that occurs in the cervical, brachial, lumbar, and sacral nerve plexuses. In addition, the fascicles within a peripheral nerve divide and recombine along their course (funicular plexuses), and intercommunications between peripheral nerves (such as the ulnar and median nerves) are not uncommon. There also may be shared innervation by adjacent nerves and variations in nerve distribution in individuals. In assessing the patient with a peripheral nerve injury, the surgeon must bear in mind these facts about normal anatomy while evaluating the changes caused by the injury.

The axons within a peripheral nerve are myelinated to varying degrees, and each is maintained by its neuronal cell body and by the Schwann cells along its lengthy course. The proportions are such that if a typical 50 μ neuronal cell body were 6 feet tall, its axon would be 3 to 4 cm. in diameter and about 2 miles long.[1]

In the Sunderland classification[10] there are five degrees of nerve injury:

1. Physiologic loss of axonal conduction
2. Loss of continuity of the axons without interruption of their investing tissue, the endoneurium
3. Disruption of the endoneurium
4. Disruption of fascicles and their connective tissue sheaths, the perineurium
5. Disruption of continuity of the entire nerve, including its connective tissue sheath, the epineurium

Seddon[8] used only three terms to classify nerve injuries: neurapraxia, axonotmesis, and neurotmesis.

Neurapraxia is equivalent to first-degree nerve injury. Anatomic continuity is preserved, but there is selective demyelination of large nerve fibers that typically causes complete motor paralysis with very little muscle atrophy and considerable sparing of sensory and autonomic function. Electrical conductivity of the nerve distal to the lesion is preserved. Surgical repair is not necessary, and recovery is rapid (within days or weeks). Recovery does not depend on regeneration, and there is no orderly sequence in the recovery of innervation. The quality of recovery is excellent.

Axonotmesis is equivalent to Sunderland's second-degree nerve injury. Anatomic continuity of the nerve and the Schwann sheaths is preserved, but the axons are interrupted and must recover by axonal regeneration. There is complete motor, sensory, and autonomic paralysis and progressive muscle atrophy. Surgical repair is not necessary. Recovery occurs at the rate of about 1 mm. per day (1 inch per month); it occurs according to the order of innervation, and the quality of recovery is excellent.

Neurotmesis is a more severe injury. There is significant disorganization within the nerve or actual disruption of its continuity, which precludes recovery without surgical repair. Wallerian degeneration occurs. In association with this, there is gradual loss of electrical conductivity in the distal portion of the nerve over a period of up to 3 days. At 10 to 20 days, fibrillations in the denervated muscles may first be detected by electromyography. From the time of the injury there is complete motor, sensory, and autonomic paralysis and progressive muscle atrophy.

At 10 to 20 days, axonal sprouting begins.[1] If scar tissue blocks their entrance into the distal portion of the nerve, these sprouts coil into a disorganized, painful neuroma. In contrast, if the nerve has been repaired, axonal regrowth proceeds at the rate of about 1 mm. per day. After the initial lag of 10 to 20 days, there is usually a further delay in the forward progress of nerve restitution if the regenerating axons have to bridge a narrow gap (e.g., where a divided nerve has been reapproximated) and another delay at the end-organ before function resumes. The march of recovery occurs according to the order of innervation, and recovery is always imperfect.

The rate and success of nerve regeneration are influenced by several factors.[1,3-6,8,10,11] Patient age is important. The younger the patient, the faster and more complete is recovery. The nerve involved is also important. "Pure" motor or sensory nerves recover better than do mixed nerves. Recovery is better in the radial and musculocutaneous nerves than in the median nerve, and the tibial division of the sciatic nerve fares better than the peroneal division.

The level of the nerve injury and the duration of denervation also influence recovery significantly. If more than 12 months is required for regenerating axons to reach a denervated muscle, a significant degree of muscular atrophy has occurred and the muscle does not function. In contrast, sensory restitution may still be possible under these circumstances. Thus, from the standpoint of motor recovery, it is usually not worthwhile to suture the ulnar nerve near the axilla or the peroneal nerve above the midthigh; however, it may be worthwhile to suture the median nerve near the axilla or the tibial nerve above the midthigh to effect return of at least protective sensation.

Other factors that are significant in the rate and success of nerve recovery are the type of injury, the length of the defect in the nerve, the severity of associated injuries (to bones, blood vessels, muscles, tendons, and so forth), and the nature and timing of surgical treatment.

Diagnosis

A standard neurologic examination reveals the extent of the neurologic deficits following a peripheral nerve injury.[2,8,10] The examiner must not be deceived, however, by trick movements such as a movement that occurs when an uninvolved muscle or gravity compensates for a paralyzed muscle, a movement permitted by an accessory tendon slip or an anomalous muscle insertion or nerve supply, or a movement caused by strong contraction and sudden relaxation of an antagonist. Because of the overlap of sensory nerve distributions and the tendency for fibers to grow from adjacent nerves into a denervated area after injury, the sensory deficits may involve smaller areas than the examiner expects. Unless the injury is old and trophic changes in the affected limb have developed, autonomic changes may be subtle and may escape detection on routine testing. In a warm room, the examiner can map the pattern of sweating with a magnifying lens or an ophthalmoscope.

The Hoffmann-Tinel sign refers to the radiating tingling paresthesia that is felt in the cutaneous distribution of an injured nerve when the nerve is percussed lightly. If the distal aspect of the nerve is percussed progressively proximally, the level at which the sign is first elicited marks the most distal point of small fiber regeneration. The progress of nerve regeneration may thus be followed over a period of days to months by periodic charting of the location of the most distal point.

Causalgia is a unique pain syndrome that may accompany a partial injury to a mixed peripheral nerve (especially the median or sciatic nerve).[7] The constant burning pain is quite severe and may be intensified by various stimuli, including cutaneous stimuli in the affected area and loud noises. It may be improved to some extent by soaking the affected part in water. Autonomic and trophic changes are common. The condition is diagnosed by history and physical examination. Although improvement may eventually occur over 6 to 12 months without treatment, an early trial of medical management such as the administration of phenoxybenzamine, an alpha-adrenergic blocking agent, often provides some degree of relief. If a medical approach is unsuccessful, causalgia may often be improved or relieved by an appropriate sympathectomy, especially if one or more preoperative sympathetic blocks have provided temporary relief.

There are a variety of electrical examinations that may add significant diagnostic information to that gained from the history and physical examination. Electromyography shows changes of denervation (increased insertional activity, spontaneous fibrillation, positive waves, and absence of voluntary action potentials) and of early reinnervation (decreased insertional activity, decreased fibrillation, and nascent polyphasic potentials). Disappearance of fibrillations may antedate the reappearance of voluntary action potentials. Muscle contraction in response to electrical stimulation may precede voluntary recovery by weeks. Although electromyographic evidence of reinnervation may precede recovery, it does not guarantee recovery.

Other specialized testing for the evaluation of peripheral nerve injuries includes various tests of sweating, diagnostic anesthetic nerve blocks, and elicitation of the axon reflex by scratching the skin or injecting histamine.

Surgical Therapy

Since surgeons first began to repair injured nerves there has been controversy about the timing of such repair. For many years, delayed repair was favored; the rare exceptions involved clean lacerations made by sharp objects. With the recent development of microsurgery and replantation surgery, there has been increased interest in primary nerve repair at the time of injury.

The arguments in favor of primary repair are that the structures are easier to identify and mobilize in the absence of scar, the nerve ends have not retracted as much as they will in the ensuing weeks, and the greatest time is allowed for regeneration before irreversible muscle atrophy occurs. The arguments against primary nerve repair are that the damage to the nerve may be more extensive than is apparent initially, the epineurium and perineurium are delicate at this stage and difficult to suture, infection may occur from the initial wound contamination, emergency conditions may be suboptimal for a careful and tedious operation, and 4 to 6 weeks are required for the axons to cross the anastomosis because of the initial lag time.

With secondary repair at 3 to 8 weeks after injury, the extent of damage to the nerve can be better assessed and the correct amount trimmed off, the epineurium and perineurium are stronger and can be sutured more easily, optimal operating room conditions can be arranged, and there is no lag time for wallerian degeneration (the involved neurons are capable of immediately regenerating new distal segments, and the regenerating axons can penetrate the repair site before a significant amount of scar forms). Even if secondary nerve repair is the treatment selected, the initial wound should be explored to document the extent of injury, to treat conditions that require acute attention (e.g., arterial injury), to debride and cleanse the wound, and to tag any divided nerve ends so they can be found at later re-exploration or to loosely approximate the nerve ends with inert sutures to prevent their retraction.

If a clinically nonfunctioning nerve is in continuity when it is explored some weeks after the initial injury, the surgeon may find it helpful to electrically stimulate the nerve proximal to the injury and look distally for evidence of muscle contraction or transmission of nerve action potentials. If there is no evidence of transmission across the area of injury, the injured portion of the nerve should be excised and the cut ends of the nerve should be sutured together. If there is transmission across the area of injury, surgical treatment should be limited to an external neurolysis.

If the nerve was initially divided in the accident or is divided by the surgeon, it should be reapproximated carefully and without tension after each end has been trimmed back to healthy fascicles. To regain length so that the nerves can be sutured without tension, the nerve ends can be mobilized and rerouted, the adjacent joints can be flexed, and even a portion of the adjacent bone (e.g., humerus) can be removed if necessary. If the ends cannot be brought together even with these maneuvers, an interposed graft of an available cutaneous nerve, such as the sural nerve, can be used. Grafts of this type add another suture line that the regenerating axons must cross, and the results are not as good as with direct nerve reanastomosis.

SELECTED REFERENCES

Haymaker, W., and Woodhall, B.: Peripheral Nerve Injuries: Principles of Diagnosis, 2nd ed. Philadelphia, W. B. Saunders Company, 1953.
  This small book (333 pages) is a gem. It contains a wealth of material about the anatomy of peripheral nerves, the examination of the peripheral nervous system, and the causes and manifestations of peripheral nerve injuries. The last third of the book consists of a detailed analysis of injuries to each of the important nerve plexuses and peripheral nerves.
Sunderland, S.: Nerves and Nerve Injuries, 2nd ed. Edinburgh, Churchill Livingstone, 1978.
  This is the bible of peripheral nerve injuries. The book is large (1046 pages) and detailed. It is an excellent reference source.

REFERENCES

1. Ducker, T. B., Kempe, L. G., and Hayes, G. J.: The metabolic background for peripheral nerve surgery. J. Neurosurg., 30:270, 1969.
2. Haymaker, W., and Woodhall, B.: Peripheral Nerve Injuries: Principles of Diagnosis, 2nd ed. Philadelphia, W. B. Saunders Company, 1953.
3. Kline, D. G., Hackett, E. R., and Happel, L. H.: Surgery for lesions of the brachial plexus. Arch. Neurol., 43:170, 1986.
4. Kline, D. G., and Hudson, A. R.: Acute injuries of peripheral nerves. *In* Youmans, J. R. (Ed.): Neurological Surgery, 3rd ed. Philadelphia, W. B. Saunders Company, 1990, pp. 2423–2510.
5. MacKinnon, S. E., and Dellon, A. L.: Surgery of the Peripheral Nerve. New York, Thieme, 1988.
6. Omer, G. E., Jr., and Spinner, M. (Eds.): Management of Peripheral Nerve Problems. Philadelphia, W. B. Saunders Company, 1980.
7. Richards, R. L.: Causalgia, a centennial review. Arch. Neurol., 16:339, 1967.
8. Seddon, H.: Surgical Disorders of the Peripheral Nerves, 2nd ed. Baltimore, Williams & Wilkins, 1975.
9. Seletz, E.: Surgery of Peripheral Nerves. Springfield, Ill., Charles C Thomas, 1952.
10. Sunderland, S.: Nerves and Nerve Injuries, 2nd ed. Edinburgh, Churchill Livingstone, 1978.
11. Woodhall, B., and Beebe, G. W.: Peripheral Nerve Regeneration: A Follow-up Study of 3,656 World War II Injuries. (VA Medical Monograph.) Washington, DC, U. S. Government Printing Office, 1956.

XI

CONGENITAL ABNORMALITIES

W. Jerry Oakes, M.D.

Congenital abnormalities of the central nervous system are common clinical conditions, occurring in approximately 1 per cent of live births[21] and representing at least 72 per cent of fetal deaths before birth.[30] In the past several years, the outlook for patients with these lesions has significantly improved. Hydrocephalus can now be adequately controlled by the insertion of a valve-regulated shunt connecting the enlarged ventricular system with the peritoneal cavity or right atrium of the heart, which allows many patients to lead normal lives. More recently, severe cases of craniosynostosis with major involvement of the face and base of the skull have been significantly improved by craniofacial reconstructive surgery. Occult spinal cord abnormalities are now being recognized earlier in their clinical course, and operative correction is frequently recommended on a prophylactic basis to prevent major neurologic compromise. The progress that has been made on many diagnostic and therapeutic fronts justifies an optimistic viewpoint for patients with congenital abnormalities affecting the central nervous system.

Myelomeningocele and Encephalocele

Midline fusion defects of the central nervous system occur at a rate of 1 to 10 per 1000 live births, depending on the geographic area surveyed.[19] Their etiology is unknown, but a familial tendency has been noted. Affected families have defects in neural tube closure in 6.8 per cent of subsequent offspring.[20] With screening of maternal sera for alpha$_1$-fetoprotein combined with ultrasonography of the fetus, it is now possible to accurately identify more than 80 per cent of affected offspring prior to the twentieth week of gestation.[8] Therapeutic alternatives can then be discussed with the family and a decision made regarding interruption of the pregnancy. Those infants that are brought to term with reparable neural tube defects can be delivered in an institution equipped and prepared to close the defect immediately after delivery.

These lesions vary in severity from simple nonunion of the midline bony elements of the spine (spina bifida) or the skull (cranium bifidum) associated with normal neural formation and function to major anomalies of the brain and/or spinal cord or both associated with absence of the overlying skin, muscle, bone, and dura mater. The lesions may be covered by full-thickness skin, epithelialized leptomeninges, or arachnoid, or, more commonly, the exposed neural tissue may lie directly on the surface. Lesions over the spine that do not contain neural tissue but are simply cystic expansions of the leptomeninges through a mesodermal defect are termed *meningoceles* and occur very rarely.

Myelomeningoceles (spina bifida cystica) are complex congenital lesions that usually occur in the caudal third of the spine (Fig. 1). The malformed elements of the spinal cord are found on

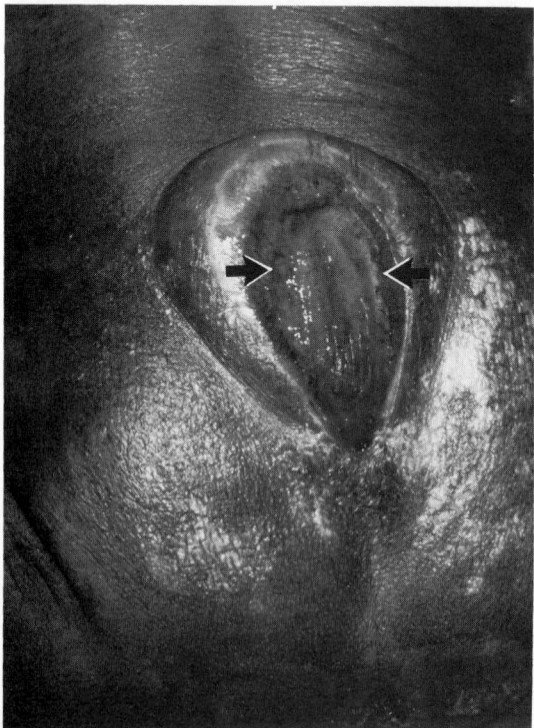

Figure 1. Infant with a lumbosacral myelomeningocele. Arrows point to the central area of the raised lesion representing the neural placode or malformed spinal cord.

or near the skin surface. The deformity, however, is not limited to the obvious spinal lesion but involves multiple areas of the central nervous system. The most frequently associated are hindbrain herniation anomalies grouped under the term Chiari II malformation. This group of anomalies is characterized by caudal displacement of the cerebellar vermis, lower brain stem, and fourth ventricle, kinking of the cervicomedullary junction, a beaklike deformity of the fused quadrigeminal plate, and aqueductal stenosis or forking causing hydrocephalus. These lesions represent the Type II Chiari malformation and are seen almost exclusively in association with a myelomeningocele.[28]

Encephaloceles are outpouchings of the leptomeninges associated with herniation of brain tissue into the sac. They characteristically occur in the midline of the occipital region, with the rare lesion being seen in the frontal or basal area. The size of the lesion is not a reliable indication of the quantity of neural tissue it contains and should not be used to advise a family about therapy or prognosis. Brain tissue contained within the encephalocele may appear amorphous and avascular. This tissue may be excised to allow adequate dural and skin coverage of the lesion during surgical closure; however, an attempt should be made to preserve viable tissue. Although the neurologic examination during the neonatal period may appear minimally abnormal, these children have a guarded prognosis owing to frequent mental, visual, and motor impairments that are more easily recognized with further growth.

In the evaluation of neonates with myelomeningoceles, attention should be given to the presence of spontaneous motor activity. Motor response to noxious stimuli is not a reliable indication of useful motor function and should not be equated with cortically mediated motor movement. Appreciation of pinprick, as judged by facial grimacing, and the presence of rectal tone should also be determined. During the initial assessment and prior to any decision regarding surgical therapy, tenuous lesions should be protected to avoid rupture, and those with exposed neural tissue should be kept moist with sterile saline-soaked sponges. The goals of closure of myelomeningoceles include (1) restoration of a watertight dural covering to prevent drying of delicate neural tissue, (2) closure of the skin to avoid infection, and (3) replacement of the neural elements within the spinal canal to prevent trauma. Postoperative patients are monitored for the development of meningitis and hydrocephalus.

The decision to recommend closure of a myelomeningocele or encephalocele is a complex medical, moral, and social problem. Opinions differ widely, ranging from a view that advocates repair of all lesions despite the degree of preoperative neurologic defect to a position that recommends repair based on a series of selection criteria. These criteria attempt to predict which individuals have the potential to become viable and productive members of society. What is becoming increasingly clear is that even patients with large myelomeningoceles can remain intellectually normal and continent of urine by means of intermittent catheterization.[25] With the prospect of normal intellectual function, urinary continence, and good upper extremity function, most families and surgeons are currently advising early closure of myelomeningoceles. Once aggressive treatment is begun, the patient's disability with regard to level of motor function, cranial nerve function, and cerebellar control should not decrease with time. Deterioration of function implies an ongoing process and demands evaluation.

Craniosynostosis

Premature closure of one or more of the cranial sutures (craniosynostosis) can cause an abnormal head shape. If the closure is restricted to a single suture, the condition is not usually associated with neurologic compromise and has cosmetic significance only.[31] As more sutures are involved, the growth of the brain becomes restricted. Mental retardation and blindness may result if operative treatment is inadequate or is performed too late to be effective.

The most common variety of craniosynostosis is isolated premature closure of the sagittal suture. In this condition, as in others, skull growth is exaggerated parallel to the involved suture and is restricted perpendicular to it. This causes a long, thin head (scaphocephaly), usually associated with a palpable ridge over the sagittal suture (Fig. 2). This condition is seen predominantly in males and is not associated with a neurologic deficit, either intellectual or physical. Therefore, surgical repair has primarily cosmetic indications. Patients who have a symmetric appearance of the head but a broad expansive forehead and shortening of the occipitofrontal diameter are termed brachycephalic. This condition is secondary to involvement of both coronal sutures as well as the frontosphenoidal sutures. Radiographic examination discloses a "tear drop" or harlequin deformity of the orbit bilaterally. Asymmetric flattening of a single supraorbital ridge with compensatory expansion of the contralateral forehead is seen with unilateral involvement of the coronal, frontosphenoidal, and, sometimes, frontoethmoidal sutures and is termed anterior plagiocephaly. The orbital deformity in this condition is unilateral. Trigonocephaly is premature fusion of the metopic suture and is characterized by a triangular deformity of the forehead with a palpable midline vertical ridge between the frontal bones. The orbits are hypoteloric. Flattening of one or both occipital regions results when the lambdoid suture is synostotic (posterior plagiocephaly).

In addition, there is a group of inherited disorders that involve not only the vault and skull base but also the face (Crouzon's syndrome) and the extremities (Apert's syndrome). These patients have a brachycephalic appearance combined with orbital and maxillary hypoplasia. Lesions causing alteration of the appearance of the orbits and face of necessity involve the sutures of the facial bones and skull base. Surgical therapy directed only at the simultaneously involved vault sutures may have little cosmetic effect on the facial deformity.[14]

It is believed that all primary craniosynostoses are present and recognizable at birth. Doubtful cases can be differentiated from skull molding secondary to passage through the birth canal by roentgenograms of the skull. Surgical correction of craniosynostosis should be advised for all patients with multiple suture involvement and for those with single suture involvement in whom the cosmetic appearance is deemed unacceptable. Patients treated by surgical release of the synostotic suture should be operated on within the first few months of life. After 1 year of age, simple suture release procedures produce minimal cosmetic improvement and are not advised. Surgical correction of major congenital anomalies that involve the skull base and face and that do not depend on the growing brain to reshape the skull can be performed at a later age.[7] Initial evaluation, however, should be done during the first few weeks of life to exclude the presence of restricted brain growth and secondary increased intracranial pressure. Early and more extensive bone removal of involved basal sutures in the patient with brachycephaly or plagiocephaly may eliminate the need for more involved procedures later in life.

Hydrocephalus

As further information becomes available, the production, reabsorption, and movement of cerebrospinal fluid (CSF) prove to be increasingly complex.[6] If the movement or bulk flow of CSF is restricted, intracranial pressure rises, the ventricular system dilates proximal to the obstruction to flow, and hydrocephalus ensues. Disturbances of flow are divided into two categories: (1) obstructions that occur within the ventricular system and cause internal, or noncommunicating, hydrocephalus, and (2) obstructions that occur outside the ventricular system, causing external, or communicating, hydrocephalus. There are rare instances in which hydrocephalus is not caused by alternations of CSF reabsorption or movement but is secondary to excessive CSF production. This occurs in the presence of a neoplasm of the choroid plexus, the tissue partially responsible for CSF pro-

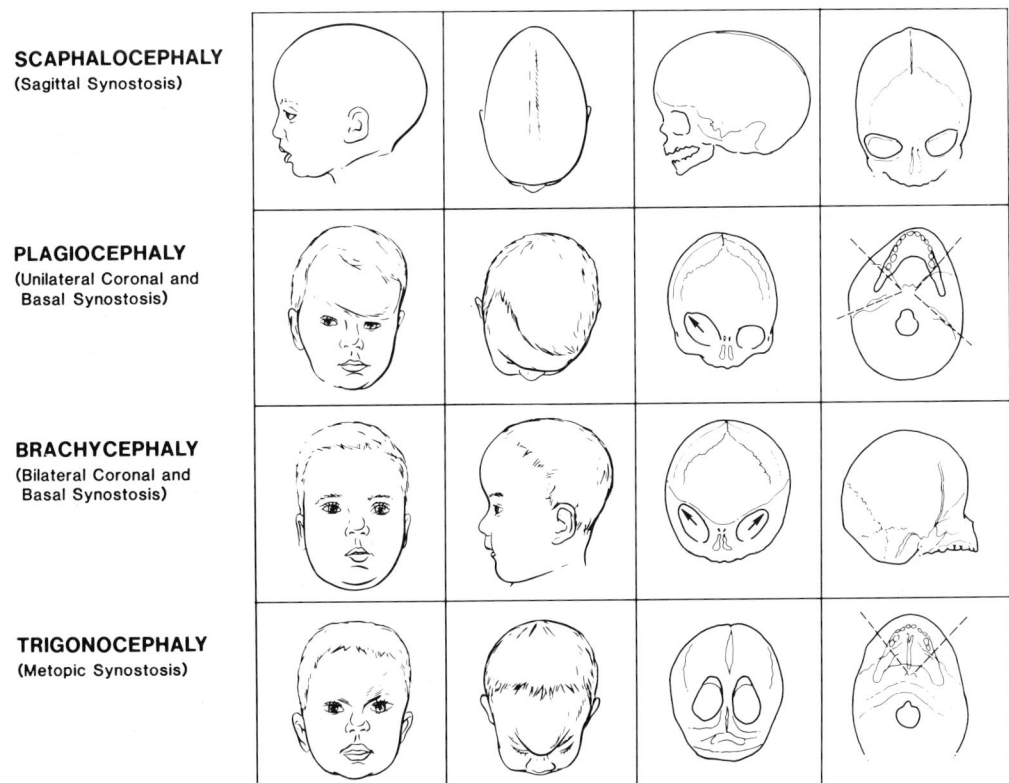

SCAPHALOCEPHALY
(Sagittal Synostosis)

PLAGIOCEPHALY
(Unilateral Coronal and Basal Synostosis)

BRACHYCEPHALY
(Bilateral Coronal and Basal Synostosis)

TRIGONOCEPHALY
(Metopic Synostosis)

Figure 2. Chart depicting the most common forms of craniosynostosis and their radiographic changes. (From Oakes, W. J., and Wilkins, R. H.: The newborn—Neurosurgical considerations. *In* Filston, H. C. (Ed.): Surgical Problems in Children: Recognition and Referral. St. Louis, C. V. Mosby, 1982.)

duction. In this unusual condition, CSF reabsorption and movement may be normal but cannot keep pace with the accelerated production by the neoplasm.[27] Internal hydrocephalus occurs when flow is restricted, usually at points of narrowing within the ventricular system. These points include the aqueduct of Sylvius, the two foramina of Monro, and the outlets of the fourth ventricle (the foramina of Luschka and Magendie). External hydrocephalus occurs by obstruction of flow at the level of the basal cisterns or at the point of reabsorption, that is, the arachnoid granulations.

Congenital hydrocephalus is a relatively common problem, with an incidence of 3 to 4 per 1000 live births.[27] In the vast majority of patients, the hydrocephalus is secondary to a benign process. Hydrocephalus frequently occurs in association with or following meningitis, myelomeningocele, or intraventricular or subarachnoid bleeding. An additional group of patients have no predisposing history and are found to have stenosis or atresia of the aqueduct of Sylvius.

Severe hydrocephalus in infancy is clinically obvious and is associated with macrocrania, prominence of the superficial scalp vessels, and bulging of the anterior fontanelle. If the condition is not treated, the patient may lose his upward gaze (sun-setting sign) and develop a spastic paraparesis secondary to stretching of the cortical leg fibers as they course over the expanded lateral ventricle. The diagnosis is confirmed by computed tomographic scanning or magnetic resonance imaging of the brain (Fig. 3).

Standard therapy is the insertion of a valve-regulated ventriculoperitoneal shunt. This has largely replaced ventriculoatrial shunting because of the ease of placement and the lower incidence of serious complications. The possible complications of shunt surgery are many, the most common being obstruction to flow through the shunting system and infection. Other complications include perforation of the abdominal wall or of an intra-abdominal hollow viscus by the peritoneal catheter, or clinical worsening of an inguinal hernia or hydrocele. Rapid and excessive decompression of a massively enlarged ventricular system may cause subdural hematoma formation. If ventriculoatrial shunting is performed, pulmonary emboli, shunt nephritis with renal failure, or actual perforation of the heart may be seen. During the postoperative follow-up, it is important to monitor the child's development and intellectual function as well as ventricular size in order to ensure adequate shunt function.[18]

Occult Spinal Dysraphism

The category occult spinal dysraphism encompasses lesions of the spine and spinal cord that are thought to date to within the first few weeks of embryonic life. Although their etiology is not proven, some investigators suggest that these lesions and spina bifida cystica (myelomeningocele) are both related to abnormal closure of the posterior neuropore. These lesions and myelomeningoceles frequently coexist, suggesting a common developmental origin. The clinical presentation and physical findings of patients with the various forms of occult spinal dysraphism are also similar.[1,17,23]

Dermal Sinus Tracts and Dermoid Tumors

These midline lesions occur primarily over the lumbosacral and occipital areas (Fig. 4). The tract may extend a variable distance from the skin to the underlying subcutaneous tissue, bone, or dura or into the nervous tissue. Occipital dermal sinus tracts course caudally from the skin defect to their eventual termination. At their deepest point of penetration, they may end in a dermoid tumor within the fourth ventricle.[35] Spinal dermal sinus tracts course cephalad and may be distinguished from pilonidal sinuses.[22] Ultimately, spinal dermal sinus tracts that extend within the dura may terminate in a dermoid tumor within the substance of the spinal cord. Either cranial or spinal sinus tracts may come to clinical attention in association with meningitis, with or without evidence of a mass lesion from abscess formation at the site of their termination. Ideally, all dermal sinuses should be recognized prior to the development of meningitis and excised in the neonatal period. Once infection has occurred, the tumor capsule and tract become densely adherent to the surrounding structures, making complete excision unlikely and therefore making recurrence common.[22] Any patient with multiple episodes of unexplained meningitis, particu-

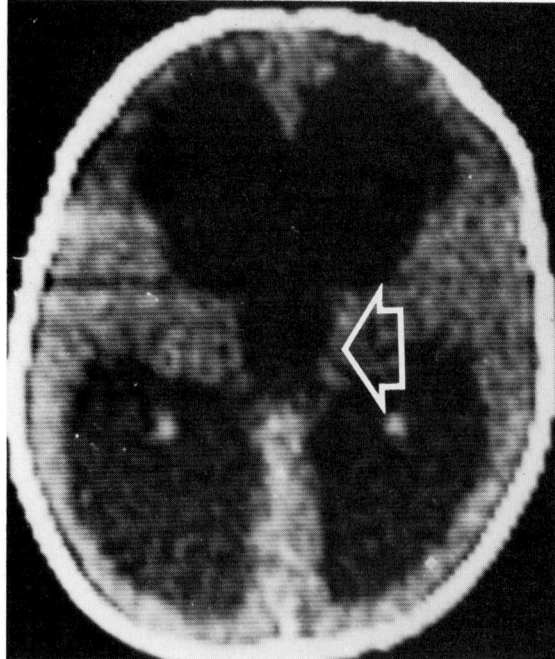

Figure 3. Computed tomographic brain scan of patient with hydrocephalus. Arrow indicates expanded third ventricle. Marked enlargement of the occipital horns is shown posterior and lateral to the third ventricle, with a central area of high attenuation representing the choroid plexus. Expanded frontal horns are anterior and lateral to the third ventricle.

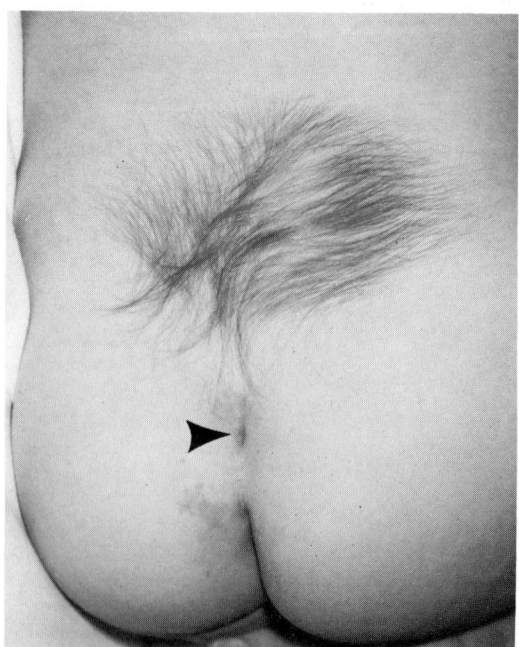

Figure 4. Photograph of an infant's back with a focal area of hirsutism and midsacral dermis sinus (arrowhead) that communicated with an intradural dermoid. Under the area of hirsutism the infant was found to have diastematomyelia with a fibrous median septum.

larly if it is secondary to *Staphylococcus aureus* infection, should be examined for the presence of a midline dermal sinus tract.

It is important to differentiate a significant dermal sinus tract that continues intradurally from the common and benign pilonidal sinus. Pilonidal sinuses occur over the coccyx and end blindly without reaching the subarachnoid space. In general, significant dermal sinus tracts occur over the midsacrum or above; those over the coccyx are generally benign.

Diastematomyelia with Median Septum

Separation of the spinal cord into two divisions by a sagittally oriented cleft (diastematomyelia) containing a bony, cartilaginous, or fibrous septum occurs most commonly near the lumbodorsal junction.[9,11] These patients may be brought to medical attention because of the overlying cutaneous stigmata of spinal dysraphism or because of the resultant neurologic damage to the spinal cord. The cutaneous signs include focal hirsutism (Fig. 4), midline capillary hemangiomas, dermal sinus tracts, and subcutaneous lipomas.[32]

The resulting neurologic abnormalities may be primarily orthopaedic, with scoliosis, kyphosis, or bony deformities of the leg or foot. The child may also present to the urologist with a neurogenic bladder or to the pediatrician with delay or abnormality of ambulation. Back pain and limited spinal mobility are occasional initial presenting symptoms, usually occurring in older children. Plain films of the spine are usually suggestive of a congenital bony abnormality, and myelography or magnetic resonance imaging is diagnostic (Fig. 5C). Elective removal of midline spurs or fibrous bands with their dural sleeves usually halts progressive neurologic deterioration and should be advised in all children once the diagnosis has been confirmed.[9] In those patients who are evaluated because of their overlying cutaneous abnormality, elective surgical therapy is also recommended prior to the development of a neurologic deficit.

Syringohydromyelia

Cystic dilation of the spinal cord (syringohydromyelia) has multiple causes, among which are congenital lesions sometimes associated with caudal displacement of the cerebellar tonsils (Type I Chiari malformation) or with myelomeningocele (Type II Chiari malformation). Spinal trauma (either mild or severe), spinal neoplasms, and arachnoiditis may also be associated with the development of syringohydromyelia.[3] This lesion, like diastematomyelia, can present with a urologic, orthopaedic, or neurologic syndrome. The diagnosis is easily confirmed by magnetic resonance imaging (Fig. 5). Therapeutic alternatives

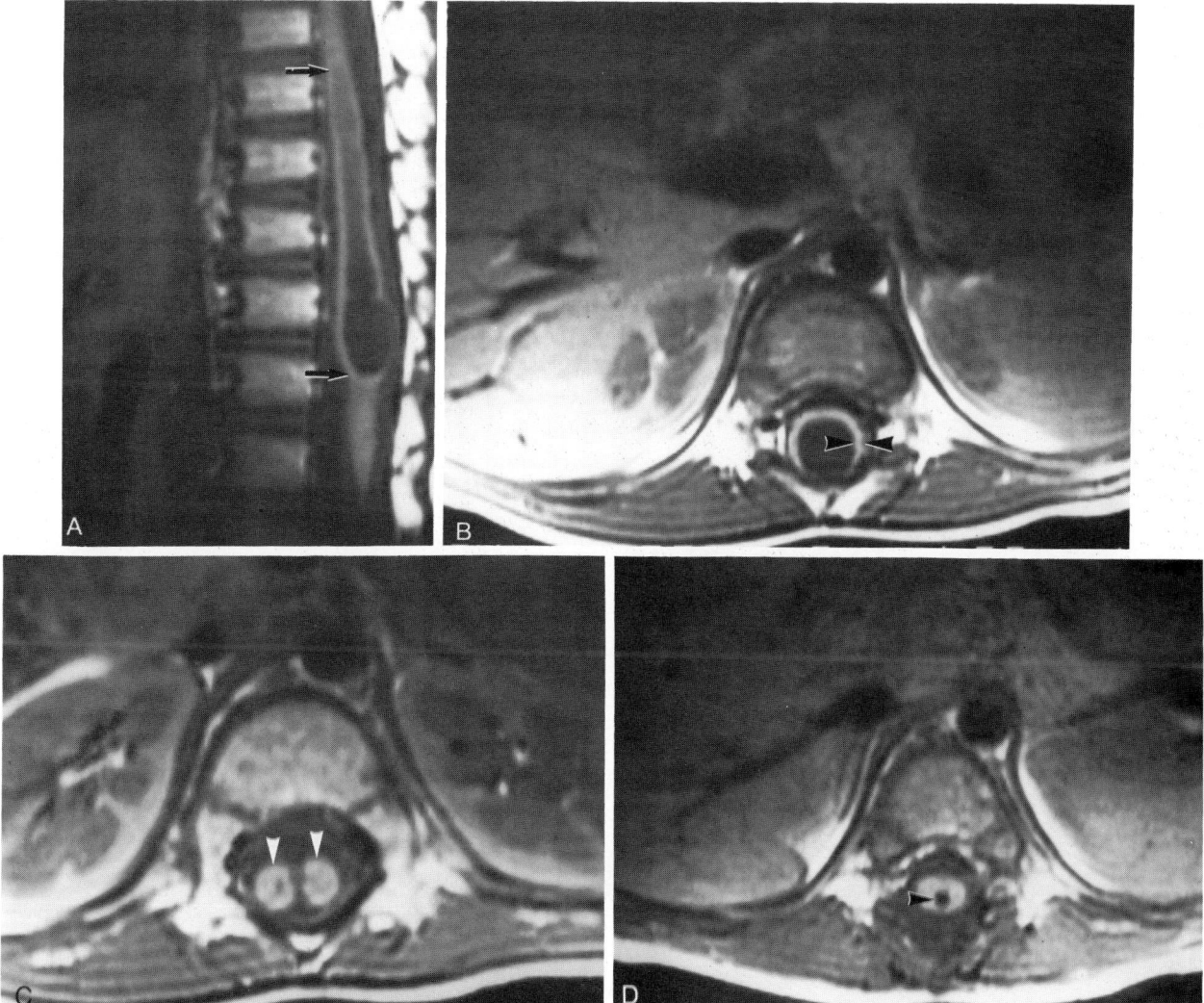

Figure 5. Three-year-old male with minimal evidence of neurologic difficulty and normal skin over the spine. Patient came to clinical attention because a routine abdominal radiograph for abdominal pain revealed mild increase in the interpeduncular distance. This subsequently led to magnetic resonance imaging (MRI) of the spine. *A,* Preoperative midsagittal MRI with T1 weighting. The large syrinx within the spinal cord is apparent (arrows). *B,* Axial image through the lower portion of the syrinx. The massive enlargement of the syrinx is surrounded by the rim of spinal cord (arrowheads). *C,* A somewhat caudal axial section below the syrinx demonstrating diastematomyelia with the two cut sections of the spinal cord seen on end (arrows). *D,* Postoperative axial MRI with total collapse of the syrinx cavity around a hollow tube (arrowhead) connecting the syrinx with the subarachnoid space.

include ventriculoperitoneal shunting when hydrocephalus coexists, drainage of the cystic cavity into the spinal subarachnoid space, obliteration of the opening of the syrinx at the caudal end of the fourth ventricle,[2,10] or establishment of a stent or conduit between the fourth ventricle and the spinal subarachnoid space. Reversal of a long-standing neurologic deficit is usually not possible, and stabilization of the pre-existing neurologic condition is a more realistic therapeutic goal. Postoperative magnetic resonance can easily document the collapse of the cyst.

Tethered Spinal Cord

Caudal displacement of the conus medullaris below the L1–L2 disc space after the age of 2 months is abnormal.[4] If seen in conjunction with an exaggerated horizontal angulation of the exiting nerve roots in addition to thickening and fatty infiltration of the filum terminale,[24] a tethered spinal cord is present. These children, like others with congenital abnormalities, are seen by multiple specialists because of a variety of complaints. The condition can be effectively treated by a limited laminectomy in the sacral region with sectioning of the thickened filum terminale.[15,16] This procedure is usually satisfactory in preventing progression of the neurologic symptoms; however, reversal of pre-existing neurologic deficits may not be possible, particularly if a disturbance of bladder function is present.

Neurenteric Cysts

These rare lesions may arise independently or in association with one of the other forms of spinal dysraphism. The cysts are lined by a variety of histologic tissue types, ranging from simple stratified epithelium to complex multilayered tissues representing all three embryonic germ layers.[34] They occur within the dura, outside the dura, or along the tract of their connection with the respiratory or gastrointestinal system. Congenital spinal deformities with clefts of the vertebral body are sometimes associated with these lesions. Their clinical presentation is that of a slowly progressive lesion compromising spinal cord function. Therapeutically, total surgical excision offers the best hope for alleviation of symptoms.

Lipomyelomeningocele

A lipomyelomeningocele can usually be diagnosed at birth by the presence of a subcutaneous lipoma over the lower spine (Fig. 6) in the lumbosacral area. Subcutaneous lipomas over the spine almost always terminate in a caudally displaced conus medullaris. The majority of patients are thought to be neurologically intact at birth and to lose neurologic function with time.[5,13] The rate of loss cannot be accurately predicted in any single individual; however, well-documented cases of loss of neurologic function within the first few weeks and months of life have been recorded. Early surgical resection of the lipoma not intimately involved with vital neural tissue and sectioning of the thickened filum terminale, if present, offers the best likelihood of maintaining normal neurologic function.[5,13,33] There is no cosmetic approach to the subcutaneous aspect of the lipoma without preparation and planning for an intradural exploration and spinal cord surgery.

SELECTED REFERENCES

Davson, H.: Physiology of the Cerebrospinal Fluid. Edinburgh, Churchill Livingstone, 1987.
The most comprehensive and authoritative reference to cerebrospinal fluid physiology. Also included are the changes seen in disease states.

Guthkelch, A. N.: Diastematomyelia with median septum. Brain, 97:729, 1974.
This comprehensive article outlines the natural history of a small group of patients with untreated diastematomyelia. The author gives strong support to the contention that these patients usually develop further neurologic difficulty and that early or prophylactic operation to prevent neurologic compromise is indicated.

James, C. C., and Lassman, L. P.: Spinal Dysraphism: Spina Bifida Occulta. London, Butterworth & Company, 1981.
A brief monograph that details the clinical presentation and operative results of a group of patients with occult spinal dysraphism. The monograph is particularly helpful because the authors have carefully followed many of their postoperative patients and include their long-term follow-up.

Lemire, J., Loeser, D., Leech, R. W., and Alvord, E. C., Jr.: Normal and Abnormal Development of the Human Nervous System. Hagerstown, Md., Harper & Row, 1975.
This text is a comprehensive review of intra- and extrauterine central nervous system development. The chapters are conveniently divided by anatomic region or structure. In addition to outlining the possible developmental abnormalities, the authors have included sufficient explanation of normal neural development to help the reader appreciate the complexity of many of the developmental anomalies.

McLaurin, R. L., Schut, L., Venes, J. L., and Epstein, F. (Eds.): Pediatric Neurosurgery, 2nd ed. Philadelphia, W.B. Saunders Company, 1989.
The current standard text in pediatric neurosurgery.

McLone, D.: Results of treatment of children born with a myelomeningocele. Clin. Neurosurg., 30:407, 1982.
The author reviews the outcome of 100 consecutively treated patients with myelomeningoceles. Follow-up was for 3.5 to 7 years. A 14 per cent mortality, usually from medullary compromise and a symptomatic Chiari malformation, is reported. Rates of urinary continence (87 per cent), normal intelligence (73 per cent), and community ambulation (54 per cent) were reported. This type of data supports an aggressive approach to the closure of myelomeningoceles.

REFERENCES

1. Anderson, F. M.: Occult spinal dysraphism, J. Pediatr., 73:163, 1968.
2. Ballantine, H. T., Jr., Ojemann, R. G., and Drew, J. H.: Syringohydromyelia. Prog. Neurol. Surg., 4:227, 1971.
3. Barnett, H. J. M., Foster, J. B., and Hudgson, P.: Syringomyelia. Philadelphia, W. B. Saunders Company, 1973.
4. Barson, A. J.: The vertebral level of termination of the spinal cord during normal and abnormal development. J. Anat., 106:489, 1970.
5. Chapman, P.: Congenital intraspinal lipomas: Anatomic considerations and surgical treatment. Childs Brain, 9:37, 1982.
6. Davson, H., Welck, K., and Segal, M. B.: Physiology of the cerebrospinal fluid. Edinburgh, Churchill Livingstone, 1987.
7. Epstein, F. J., Wood-Smith, D., Converse, J. M., Benjamin, M. V., Becker, M. H., and Ransohoff, J.: Radical one-stage correction of craniofacial anomalies. J. Neurosurg., 42:522, 1975.
8. Ferguson-Smith, M. A., May, H. M., Vince, J. D., Robinson, H. P., Rawlinson,

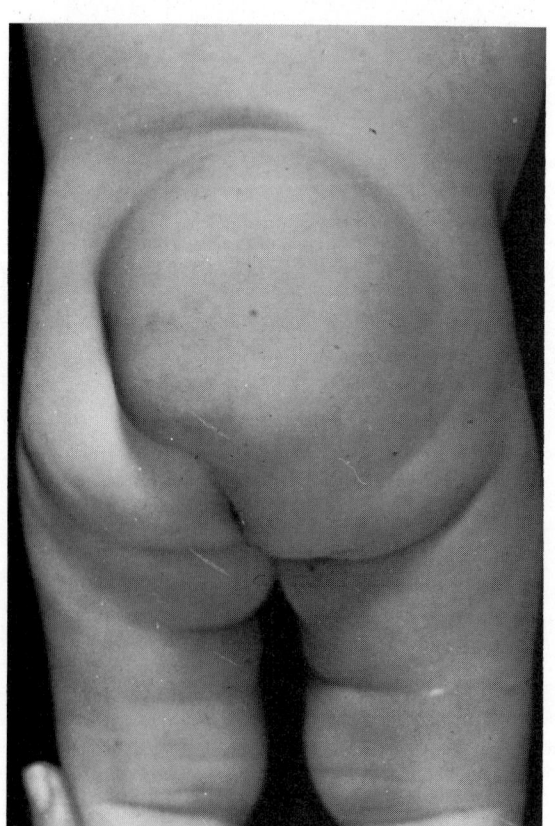

Figure 6. Large lumbosacral lipomeningocele.

H. A., Tait, H. A., Gibson, A. A. M., and Ratcliffe, J. G.: Avoidance of anencephalic and spina bifida births by maternal serum-alphafetoprotein screening. Lancet, 1:1330, 1978.

9. Guthkelch, A. N.: Diastematomyelia with median septum. Brain, 97:729, 1974.

10. Hankinson, J.: The surgical treatment of syringomyelia. Adv. Tech. Std. Neurosurg., 5:127, 1978.

11. Hendrick, E. G.: On diastematomyelia. Prog. Neurol. Surg., 4:277, 1971.

12. Hilal, S. K., Marton, D., and Pollack, E.: Diastematomyelia in children. Radiology, 112:609, 1974.

13. Hirsh, J. F., and Pierre-Kahn, A.: Lumbosacral lipomas with spina bifida. Childs Nerv. Syst., 4:354, 1988.

14. Hoffman, H. J., and Mohr, G.: Lateral canthal advancement of the supraorbital margin. J. Neurosurg., 45:376, 1976.

15. Hoffman, H. J., Hendrick, E. B., and Humphreys, R. P.: The tethered spinal cord: Its protean manifestations, diagnosis and surgical correction. Childs Brain, 2:145, 1976.

16. Holtzman, R. N. N., and Stein, B. M.: The tethered spinal cord. New York, Thieme-Stratton Inc., 1985.

17. James, C. C., and Lassman, L. P.: Spina Bifida Occulta: Orthopaedic Radiological and Neurosurgical Aspects. London, Butterworth & Company, 1981.

18. Keucher, T. R., and Mealey, J., Jr.: Long-term results after ventriculoatrial and ventriculoperitoneal shunting for infantile hydrocephalus. J. Neurosurg., 50:179, 1979.

19. Lemire, R. J., Loeser, J. D., Leech, R. W., and Alvord, E. C., Jr.: Normal and Abnormal Development of the Human Nervous System. Hagerstown, Md., Harper & Row, 1975.

20. Lorber, J.: The family history of spina bifida cystica. Pediatrics, 35:587, 1965.

21. Malpas, P.: The incidence of human malformations and the significance of changes in the maternal environment in their causation. J. Obstet. Gynaecol. Br. Commonw., 44:434, 1937.

22. Matson, D. D.: Neurosurgery of Infancy and Childhood. Springfield, Ill., Charles C Thomas, 1969.

23. McLaurin, R. L., Schut, L., Venes, J. L., and Epstein, F. (Eds.): Pediatric Neurosurgery, 2nd ed. Philadelphia, W.B. Saunders Company, 1989.

24. McLendon, R. E., Oakes, W. J., Heinz, E. R., Yeates, A. E., and Burger, P. C.: Adipose tissue in the filum terminale: A computed tomographic finding that may indicate tethering of the spinal cord. Neurosurgery, 22:873, 1988.

25. McLone, D.: Results of treatment of children born with a myelomeningocele. Clin. Neurosurg., 30:407, 1982.

26. Milhorat, T. H.: Hydrocephalus and the Cerebrospinal Fluid. Baltimore, Williams & Wilkins, 1972.

27. Milhorat, T. H.: Pediatric Neurosurgery. Philadelphia, F. A. Davis Company, 1978.

28. Oakes, W. J., Worley, G., Spock, A., and Whiting, K.: Surgical intervention in twenty-nine patients with symptomatic Type II Chiari malformations: Clinical presentation and outcome. Concepts Pediatr. Neurosurg., 8:76, 1988.

29. Peach, B.: Arnold-Chiari malformation. Arch. Neurol., 12:613, 1965.

30. Record, R. G., and McKeown, T.: Congenital malformations of the central nervous system. Br. J. Soc. Med., 4:183, 1949.

31. Shillito, J., Jr., and Matson, D. D.: Craniosynostosis: A review of 519 surgical patients. Pediatrics, 41:829, 1968.

32. Tavafoghi, V., Ghandchi, A., Hambrick. G. W., Jr., and Udverhelyi, G. V.: Cutaneous signs of spinal dysraphism. Arch. Dermatol., 114:573, 1978.

33. Villarejo, F. J., Blazques, M. G., and Gutierrez-Dias, J. A.: Intraspinal lipomas in children. Childs Brain, 2:361, 1976.

34. Wilkins, R. H., and Odom, L.: Tumors of the spine and spinal cord. Part II. In Vinken, P. J., and Bruyn, G. W. (Eds.): Handbook of Clinical Neurology. Vol. 20. Amsterdam, North-Holland Publishing Company, 1976, pp. 55–102.

35. Wright, R. L.: Congenital dermal sinuses. Prog. Neurol. Surg., 4:175, 1971.

XII

NEUROSURGICAL RELIEF OF PAIN

Blaine S. Nashold, Jr., M.D., and Eben Alexander III, M.D.

> Not everyone has a soul of fire. In actual human existence, even in the case of the great mystics, the struggle against pain exacts a high price.
>
> *Leriche*

Pain is not a simple sensory event but a complex physiologic phenomenon that involves the entire nervous system. Human beings differ remarkably in their individual reactions to pain and suffering, and when severe pain is unrelieved, a state of suffering intervenes that threatens the very existence of the individual. Understanding of the anatomy and the neurophysiology of pain perception in man has evolved slowly simply because pain is a private matter and direct observations in man have their limitations. It was stated that in order to relieve pain totally the nervous system must be destroyed, and yet it is known that section of the dorsal roots and spinal cordotomy, both time-honored neurosurgical operations, can relieve pain. Although the free endings of the C fibers are considered the primary receptors that signal pain, neurologic evidence indicates that there are free nerve endings also functioning as receptors for other types of painful perceptions. At the peripheral end, fine cutaneous afferent activity appears to be a necessary condition for the sensation of pain. Although the functional localization of pain is important, physiologic findings emphasize spatial and temporal mechanisms that are involved in the coding of sensory experience within the central nervous system.

The success of the spinal cordotomy in relieving pain is associated with the neuroanatomic organization of pain and thermal fibers in the lateral spinothalamic tract. Edinger described the spinothalamic tract in 1889, but its function was not known until 1905 when Spiller noted loss of pain and decrease in temperature sensation in a patient with a discrete tuberculoma in the anterior quadrant of the spinal cord.[14] Martin, in 1912, at the urging of Spiller, performed the first open thoracic cordotomy.[15] Although the lateral spinothalamic tract is of considerable importance in the transmission of painful and thermal sensation, neuroanatomic evidence indicates that additional pathways are available for the transmission of pain. The lateral spinothalamic tract is a phylogenetic recent pathway in man with its input directly into the sensory thalamus. Pain perception over the spinothalamic route has a rapid transit time to the thalamus where higher levels of integration occur through the thalamocortical connection. A definite topographic scheme of the body's image exists within the cord and thalamus, the input from the facial being medial to that of the body and the leg areas lateral to that of the body. Pain following electrical stimulation of the spinothalamic pathways in man is usually experienced by the patient as a sharp, well-demarcated painful sensation referred to a localized region of the body.

In contrast to this, the diffuse pain pathways appear to have multiple routes through the spinal cord with distribution to the midbrain, thalamus, and hypothalamus; these spinoreticular pathways are phylogenetically older than the newer lateral spinothalamic tract and have been designated as the paleothalamic system. They may be crossed or uncrossed tracts that are composed of short chains of the neurons that make synaptic connections at successive rostral levels in the central nervous system. Pain transmitted via these routes appears to be slower in transit to higher levels, and the sensation experienced by alert patients during stimulation is ill-defined and unpleasant, being diffusely localized to regions in the central parts of the body including the head, chest, and abdomen.

Pain can be considered as either a primary or secondary symptom. In most patients, it is a secondary symptom usually originating from some underlying pathologic cause, the correction of which relieves the pain. However, when the pathologic state cannot be eradicated, as may be the case in metastatic malignancy, the pain may be relieved by a specific neurosurgical operation.

Pain is the primary symptom that follows neurophysiologic and neuropathologic involvement of the pain pathways within the central nervous system. A painful dysesthesia occurring after a surgical cordotomy, tractotomy, or thalamotomy is an example of a primary central pain syndrome. Other examples include the pain of the thalamic syndrome or painful limb. Central pain syndromes often occur after trauma—vascular occlusion, tumor, degenerative disease of the central nervous system (multiple sclerosis), or infections (herpes zoster). The patient describes this type of pain as intense burning, crushing, or tearing and aggravated by the slightest sensory stimulation. An emotional upset intensifies the patient's pain, as can psychologic disturbance. These patients often become drug addicts and undergo permanent personality changes. Numerous theories have been proposed to explain central pain as the presence of highly irritable neurons at the site of the central nervous system injury involving the diffuse pain tracts, the diversion of noxious impulses from the spinothalamic tract into the paleothalamic system, or the possible release of the thalamus from higher cortical inhibition.

Neurosurgical treatment of central pain has not been completely successful, although midbrain tractotomy and thalamotomy have been used in a limited number of patients.

THE NEUROSURGICAL OPERATIONS FOR PAIN

The neurosurgeon must consider certain facts before recommending an operation to relieve pain. The neurosurgical operation must not be done as a last resort or in desperation. Most failures to relieve pain are due to delay in surgical treatment. The neurosurgeon should be consulted early and before the occurrence of drug addiction or prolonged suffering. Long-established pain leads to a state of suffering that should be avoided; ideally, benefit from operation should extend throughout the lifetime of the patient. Neurosurgical operations for the relief of pain can be divided into four types: (1) anatomic interruption of pathways serving pain or the destruction of sensory integration regions in the central nervous system (rhizotomy, cordotomy, tractotomy, thalamotomy, and cingulotomy); (2) sympathectomy for relief of causalgia and sympathetic dystrophy; (3) pituitary ablation to relieve generalized bone pain from metastatic tumors (breast, prostate) under hormonal influence; and (4) electroanalgesia to relieve pain by stimulation of peripheral nerves, dorsal columns, or central brain structures.

The simplest operation for pain relief is the section, avulsion, or alcohol injection of a peripheral nerve. It has the advantage of relieving pain originating in a small localized area. In trigeminal neuralgia, injection or avulsion of one of the peripheral branches of the fifth cranial nerve may provide several years of relief. When the pain recurs or involves large areas of the face, the gasserian ganglion may be sectioned, lightly traumatized by rubbing or using a vascular decompression technique, which adds additional long periods of relief. The disadvantage of sectioning of the peripheral nerve is the return of the pain with neural regeneration. The sensory loss from a dorsal rhizotomy involves a large area, but at least three or four nerve roots must be sectioned to produce an analgesic zone equal to the derma-

tome. The dorsal rhizotomy may be useful in relieving pain originating from the neck, shoulder, thorax, or abdominal wall, but it is usually unsuitable for pain that involves an entire arm or leg, since the sensory loss in these regions may often reduce the functional usefulness of the limb.

Tic douloureux or trigeminal neuralgia is a common symptom in the cause of facial pain. The discomfort is frequently described as a sudden lancinating pain that spreads into one or more of the representative divisions of the trigeminal nerve, more commonly in the lower face, often causing the patient to wince because of the severity—thus the term tic. These paroxysms usually continue for seconds to less than a minute, and although there is often an aching background sensation, onset is either spontaneous or due to stimulation of a "trigger zone" in the form of touching skin areas. Speaking, chewing, and talking may also activate the pain. It occurs most commonly in women, and 70 per cent of patients are 50 years of age at the onset of symptoms. Medical treatment is the first priority in these patients, using carbamazepine, phenytoin, or baclofen; but when medical treatment becomes ineffective, neurosurgical operation should be considered. In elderly patients, because the pain may be activated by chewing or talking, the individuals may be unable to eat and suffer severe dehydration requiring immediate attention to the intractable facial pain.

Percutaneous Radiofrequency Rhizotomy

One of the earliest surgical methods for management of trigeminal neuralgia is percutaneous radiofrequency lesions. Patients with multiple sclerosis as well as those infirm or over 70 years of age with pain in multiple divisions are especially suited to this procedure. Radiofrequency (RF) rhizotomy involves destruction of part of the trigeminal ganglion using heat from an electrode connected to an RF generator. The procedure is performed under local anesthesia and guided by electrical stimulation. Motor and sensory effects produced by stimulation may be helpful in precise placement of the lesion electrode in the trigeminal ganglion. Preliminary electrode placement is accomplished using roentgenograms or cinefluoroscopy.

The major advantages of the percutaneous technique include low morbidity and mortality with a high success rate. Patients who experience recurrence of pain are often improved by repeated lesions. One disadvantage of this method is reduction of corneal sensation with the possible development of keratitis. The patient must be forewarned of this. A cervical sympathectomy may have a protective effect on the cornea against the development of keratitis.[2]

In a recent review of percutaneous radiofrequency lesions of the gasserian ganglion performed between 1974 and 1984 in 89 patients for relief of trigeminal neuralgia, the average follow-up was 4.5 years and satisfactory pain relief was achieved in 69 per cent. Thirty patients had return of pain; recurrent neuralgia occurred in 46 per cent. Of those patients with a marked sensory deficit, the risk of recurrence was less. The postoperative complications included reduced or absent corneal reflex (18 patients), corneal keratitis (3 patients), and anesthesia dolorosa (2 patients). Age, sex, and duration of illness were unrelated to outcome.[11]

Glycerol Injection of the Gasserian Ganglion

Indication for percutaneous retroganglionic glycerol rhizotomy is similar to that for radiofrequency rhizotomy. Possible advantages are (1) significant reduction in facial deafferentation compared with the RF rhizotomy, (2) elimination of intraoperative sensory testing of RF lesion equipment leads to a simpler technique, and (3) intraoperative trigeminal water-soluble contrast cisternography allows precise anatomic location.[8] In one large series of patients with glycerol injection (552 total patients), 224 (59.1 per cent of those evaluated at 2 years) and 8 patients (8.1 per cent evaluated at 6 years) were pain-free after a single injection. Recurrence of pain occurred in 27 per cent of patients after 1 year and in 41 per cent after 2 years. Early recurrence of pain occurred in those patients who underwent a surgical procedure, compared with those patients treated with pharmacologic agents.

Microvascular Decompression for Relief of Trigeminal Neuralgia

Dandy was the first to suggest that vascular compression of the trigeminal nerve near the pons might be an etiologic cause for trigeminal neuralgia.[5] Later Janetta considered trigeminal neuralgia due to vascular compression of the trigeminal root entry zone in the pons and developed the microvascular decompression operation.[6]

Microsurgical decompression is appealing in that it addresses the possible cause of the disorder and does not rely on substantial ablation of part of the nervous system. However, it is a major cranial operation and is best performed on younger patients. Microvascular decompression is of no benefit in pain of anesthesia dolorosa or multiple sclerosis and should not be used in painful conditions of the trigeminal nerve due to peripheral involvement.

There are still dissenting views concerning the relevance of vascular compression in such entities as trigeminal neuralgia, hemifacial spasm, and glossopharyngeal neuralgia. After microvascular decompression, one third of the patients do not attain an optimal result, and the evidence used to support the hypothesis of microvascular crush including the neurophysiologic basis is believed to be insufficient and unconvincing by one author.[1] The therapeutic efficacy of "decompression" might actually consist of microtrauma to the nerve during operative manipulation, for pain is often relieved even after surgical exploration where no compressing structure is found.[1] Of some interest is an older operation of compression of the trigeminal nerve at the level of the gasserian ganglion through the dura propria, which is often followed by pain relief with minimal sensory changes.

Complications of microsurgical decompression include postoperative loss of hearing (23 per cent) and fusion of the middle ear (14 per cent). Forty patients were followed for an average period of 8½ years after 44 consecutive suboccipital craniotomies for trigeminal neuralgia. Among these, 36 had microvascular compression of the nerve. Of those undergoing the operation, 47 per cent experienced recurrence of neuralgic pain. In 31 per cent, pain recurrence was major and in 17 per cent it was minor. There was a strong statistical relationship between an operative finding of arterial cross-compression of the nerve and long-term complete pain relief rather than compression related to veins or bony structures. "There appears to be no point in time in the postoperative interval when the patient can be considered cured." Major recurrences average 3 per cent annually and minor recurrences 1 per cent annually.[4]

The most serious complications following microvascular decompression are intracerebral hematoma with acute hydrocephalus, cerebellar swelling, supratentorial subdural hematoma, status epilepticus, and infarction of the brain stem—all serious complications.

Another compressive technique that has not been widely used is balloon compression rhizolysis. A specialized balloon is inserted radiographically into the Meckel's cave and the balloon is inflated, producing compression on the nerve. In a group of 25 patients, there was immediate pain relief with minimal numbness in all three divisions and sparing of corneal sensation. Weakness of the ipsilateral muscles of mastication was noted transiently. The advantages of this operative procedure are the low rate of postoperative dysesthesia, minimal discomfort to the patient with a short operative time, minimal morbidity, no mortality, and minimal risk of loss of corneal sensation.

Open Trigeminal Rhizotomy

A partial section of the trigeminal nerve as it exits from the pons and posterior fossa is an alternative to microvascular decompression and was first performed by Walter Dandy. The trigeminal neuralgia was relieved by sectioning the lower third of the trigeminal nerve; no anesthesia dolorosa developed, and the patients experienced only minimal sensory loss. At times this partial section may be combined with vascular decompression. As with all manipulations of the trigeminal nerve, a few patients develop anesthesia dolorosa.

Trigeminal Nucleus Caudalis DREZ Lesions

Pain associated with posttrigeminal dysesthesia and anesthesia dolorosa has always been very difficult to control medically and surgically. Recently the DREZ (dorsal root entry zone) lesion technique has been applied to the trigeminal nucleus caudalis for pain relief. The trigeminal nucleus caudalis receives the majority of pain afferents from the face via the trigeminal nerve and can be lesioned at the cervicomedullary junction using a microsurgical technique and a special RF electrode. Best results are noted in patients with posttrigeminal dysesthesia and anesthesia dolorosa and postherpetic neuralgia. Although many of these patients have preoperative sensory loss following lesions of the caudalis nucleus, there is complete analgesia of all three divisions including the cornea. One of the major operative risks is the development of ipsilateral dysmetria in the arm or leg, which usually is transient and disappears within a short period of time. The caudalis DREZ lesion is used in those patients who have had previous multiple trigeminal operations to relieve pain and develop a serious dysesthesia.[3]

Miscellaneous Therapies

Use of electrical stimulation of the gasserian ganglion was proposed by Meyerson in 1980 and consists of chronic implantation of an electrode in the gasserian ganglion. Of 5 patients with trigeminal pain and partial sensory loss, 3 had relief of pain for a period of 2 years.[7]

Intractable pain of the head is one of the most difficult pain syndromes to treat. A number of specific neurosurgical operations are available, and careful patient selection is necessary for a successful result.

GENERALIZED SOMATIC AND VISCERAL PAIN

Spinal cordotomy remains the most useful operation for relief of widespread somatic and visceral pain (Fig. 1). It is especially helpful when pain originates from thoracic and abdominal regions. The surgical section is performed opposite the site of the pain in the anterolateral quadrant of the spinal cord at least six cord segments above the origin of the pain to allow some degree of postoperative regression of the sensory level. The analgesia following the cordotomy covers the opposite half of the body with the level beginning several segments below the cord section. For the most complete relief of pain, the entire lateral spinothalamic tract must be sectioned since an incomplete cut may lead to sparing of sensation in one region or another with persistence of the pain. An open surgical cordotomy has a mortality of 10 per cent. The cord section can be done at two different spinal levels—usually cervical (C1 to C3) and thoracic (T1 to T2). In the cervical operation, the analgesic level reaches the clavicle involving the arm to varying degrees, but the densest analgesia occurs over regions of the thorax, abdomen, and leg. A thoracic cordotomy produces contralateral analgesia beginning in the lower thorax (Fig. 2). A well-executed unilateral lumbar cordotomy should lead to good pain relief in 85 per cent

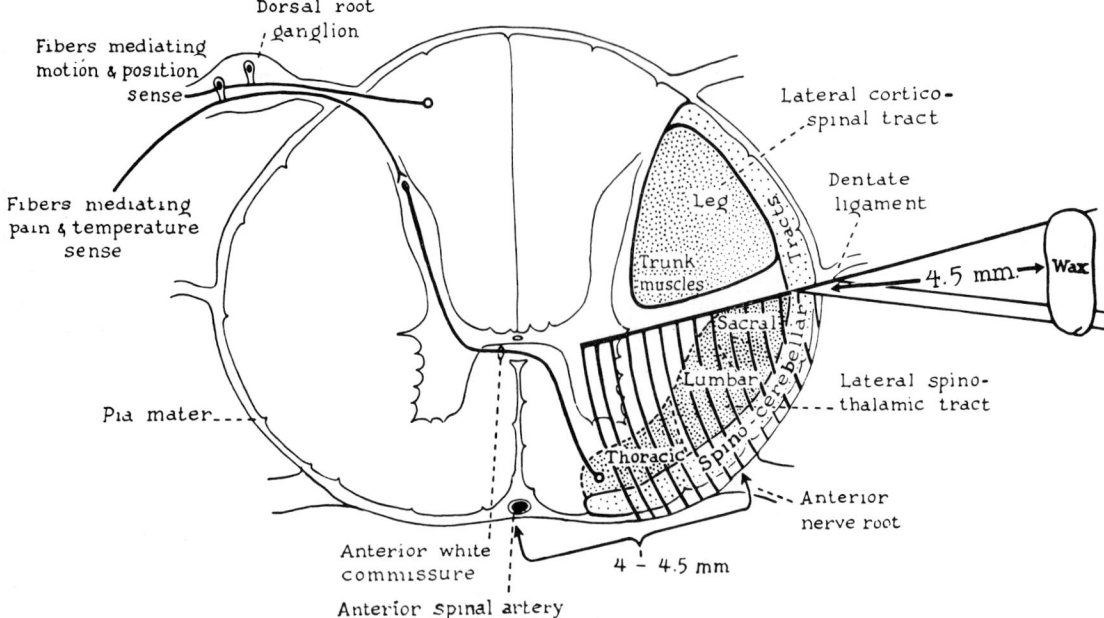

Figure 1. Cross-sectional drawing of thoracic cord showing extent of incision in anterolateral cordotomy. (From Kahn, E. A., Bassett, R. C., Schneider, R. C., and Crosly, E. C.: Correlative Neurosurgery. Springfield, Ill., Charles C Thomas, 1955.)

of patients, whereas with a high cervical cordotomy relief occurs in 50 per cent. After unilateral cordotomy, generally complications are few with normal bladder, bowel, and sexual functions. Postoperative complications such as ipsilateral hemiparesis or monoparesis can occur if the surgical incision involves a nearby corticospinal tract. A bilateral cordotomy performed either in the cervical or thoracic cord has high overall operative risk, and the postoperative risks are greater; most of these operations should be restricted to patients with widespread carcinoma whose life expectancy is limited. Bilateral cervical cordotomy at either level seriously interferes with bladder, bowel, and sexual functions.

Percutaneous spinothalamic cordotomy is a good technique for interrupting the pain pathways for somatic and visceral pain anywhere below the level of the mandible. This technique is best used in patients with unilateral pain who have malignant disease and are not expected to survive for more than 1 to 2

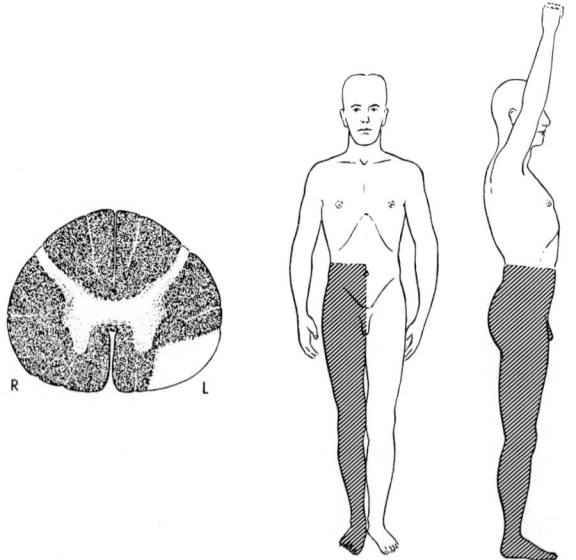

Figure 2. Extent of analgesia after thoracic cordotomy. Area of cord involved is shown in section on the left.

years. The reason for this stipulation is that there is a significant complication with anesthesia dolorosa in long-term survivors after cordotomy. Pain that is more lancinating or aching in quality has a higher response rate than that with burning or "crawling" dysesthesias. Ninety per cent of the former patients should respond to interruption of the lateral spinothalamic tract. Severe pulmonary dysfunction is a relative contraindication to cordotomy because of decrease in phrenic nerve function and the difficulty with sleep apnea after high cervical cordotomy.

Mullan and associates in 1963 introduced the percutaneous cervical cordotomy, and it has proved useful in patients who could not stand the operative rigors of an open cordotomy. The percutaneous cordotomy is done with local anesthesia under roentgenographic control guiding an RF needle into the anterolateral quadrant of the spinal cord between the first and second cervical vertebrae. Direction and depth of needle are controlled by roentgenograms, and electrical stimulation can be used to test the localization of the needle tip within the spinal cord tissue. The lateral spinothalamic tract can be coagulated unilaterally or bilaterally by means of a high-frequency electrical current. Such operations can be done rapidly by the experienced surgeon with a minimum of surgical trauma. It is, however, a blind operation, so the surgeon must exercise great care not to misplace the lesion and cause additional neurologic deficits. One risk of the percutaneous technique in the high cervical region may be interferrence with breathing, and after surgical therapy patients have died in their sleep because of respiratory failure. A percutaneous cordotomy is best suited for poor-risk patients with a short life expectancy. Long-term chronic pain is best not treated by percutaneous techniques because of the occurrence of postcordotomy dysesthesia and the risk of recurrence of the original pain, or a more serious risk of painful postoperative dysesthesia.

Pain involving overlapping areas of the head and neck or arm can be difficult to control by a single surgical operation owing to overlapping of the cranial and cervical nerves in the head and neck region. Stereotactic operations in the midbrain or thalamus have relieved these widespread cervical cranial pains. A stereotactic medullary tractotomy can be performed to selectively interrupt pain involving the individual divisions of the trigeminal nerve, although a caudalis DREZ procedure is probably preferable at this time. The first open surgical sections of the spinothalamic tract in the midbrain were performed by Walker in 1942, producing an analgesia in the opposite half of the body[3]; however, the open medullary or mesencephalic tractotomies were associated with a high mortality (7 per cent) and morbidity commonly. One serious problem is the risk of postoperative dysesthesia. Since 1947, using the human stereotactic instrument, Spiegel and Wycis and others have coagulated the mesencephalic pain tracts by introducing a small RF probe into the mesencephalon via a frontal burr hole (Fig. 3).[13] The mortality has been reduced to 1 per cent with good relief of pain, and although postoperative dysesthesia has occurred, this is less frequent. Postoperatively, there is usually loss of upward gaze and occasionally diplopia that may complicate the lesion. With improvements in the stereotactic technique, it is now possible to place lesions below the posterior commissure, which reduces the risk of ocular dysfunction, and successfully relieves pain of the thalamic syndrome.

Stereotactic lesions in the thalamus or the cingulum have been successfully employed to relieve widespread pain causing suffering. A unilateral thalamic lesion (center median or parafascicular nucleus or both) is often sufficient for relief of the pain of extensive carcinoma. The relief is thought to be due to interruption of the sensory integration at high levels in the central nervous system. A thalamic lesion does not alter the threshold for pain, and no analgesia occurs despite the relief of the patient's pain. An added risk of the thalamic operation may be an interference with memory or speech mechanisms. In some patients the relief of pain is short-lived.

When suffering is the most prominent clinical feature in a patient with intractable pain associated with maximal intake of narcotic drugs, it can best be relieved by a medial dorsal thalamic or cingulum gyrus lesion interrupting the cingulum bilaterally. The beneficial effect of the thalamic lesion is thought to be due to interruption of thalamofrontal connections, whereas the cingulate lesion exerts its effects by interfering with some circuits in the limbic system. Frontal leukotomy can no longer be recommended as an operation for the relief of pain.

Pain of Brachial and Lumbar Plexus Avulsion, Paraplegia, and Herpes

Intractable pain associated with avulsion injury to the brachial plexus has been refractory to treatment until the use of a new surgical procedure in which small thermal lesions are made in the injured dorsal root entry zone (DREZ). The operation has been designated the DREZ procedure. Pain can be significantly relieved in over 70 per cent of these patients.[10] Ten per cent of paraplegics develop intractable pain described as burning, crushing, or electrical in nature and involving the paralyzed limb. The onset of pain may be immediately after the injury or delayed for several years. When it is delayed in onset, the patient often has an intraspinal cyst observed on the computed tomography scan or magnetic resonance imaging of the injured spinal cord. The DREZ procedure has been successful in relieving this pain.

Herpes zoster is often followed by chronic pain syndrome in 10 per cent of patients and has been intractable to treatment. The patients are often elderly and rapidly become debilitated because of the pain. Therapeutic lesions involving the dorsal roots can relieve pain in approximately 50 per cent of these patients. One objection to this operation is a 5 per cent risk of ipsilateral leg weakness.

Painful Phantom Limb

The loss of an arm, leg, or breast can cause a phantom sensation. The neural substrate of one's conscious awareness of body image requires a period of learning—when the sensations of the body scheme are organized probably within the cortex. The individual with congenital absence of an arm or leg does not develop phantom sensation. After an amputation, phantom image appears to be fixed in the patient's awareness of the traumatic episode surrounding the loss of the limb and it appears to influence whether the individual may experience a phantom sensation. Normally the phantom sensation fades by retracting into the end of the stump, but the patient is often aware of the phantom limb and may be able to "move" the missing fingers or toes. Before an amputation, it is important that the surgeon forewarn the patient regarding the postoperative consequence of phantom sensation.

When the phantom sensation is accompanied with pain, surgical treatment may be necessary since the presence of the pain intensifies and prolongs the phantom sensation. When the pain is relieved, the phantom sensation fades. A painful phantom limb often follows a traumatic avulsion of the brachial plexus where the dorsal roots are disconnected from their attachment to the spinal cord. The arm becomes insensitive and flaccid. The pain is described as burning, tearing, or crushing and the intensity appears to heighten the patient's awareness of the phantom limb. Injury to the substantia gelatinosa in the spinal cord at the point where the dorsal roots exit may be the site of the origin for the phantom pain. A high cervical cordotomy, stereotactic mesencephalotomy, or thalamotomy has been reported to relieve phantom pain, whereas resection of an arm or leg area of the parietal sensory cortex relieves neither the pain nor the phantom sensation. Amputation of the arm after brachial avulsion does not relieve the pain. Recently successful relief of pain has followed the use of the DREZ lesion involving the dorsal roots of the phantom.

Surgical Sympathectomy for Relief of Causalgia and Sympathetic Dystrophy

Causalgia is a syndrome characterized by intense "burning pain" and autonomic dysfunction caused by partial injury to the large nerve trunk. The first detailed clinical description appeared in 1864 by Mitchell, Morehouse, and Keene, who exam-

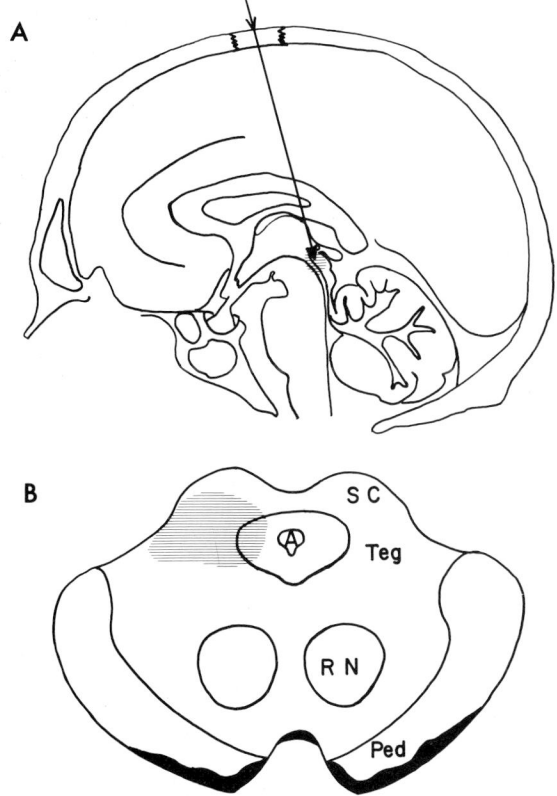

Figure 3. *A,* Sagittal section of brain shows target tract to midbrain. *B,* Cross section of mesencephalon at superior colliculus. Area of lesion is shown on the right.

ined Civil War veterans with gunshot wounds of the arm and leg that had injured major nerve trunks.[9] The etiology of this disorder is unknown, but the symptoms occur most often after injury to large peripheral nerves such as the brachial plexus or the median or sciatic nerves. Usually the nerve lesion is incomplete with partial sensory loss in the involved painful limb. The physiologic basis for the pain and its association with autonomic dysfunction are not understood. It has been postulated that the burning dysesthesia may be due to short-circuiting of C fiber impulses or the cross-circuiting of efferent sympathetic impulses via the peripheral nerves, which activate the pain fibers. When the pain persists for too long a time without relief, addiction and psychoneurosis may complicate treatment. The burning pain of causalgia usually involves the hand or foot. The skin may appear smooth with loss of hair, and vasomotor disturbance appears such as sweating involving the limb. The patient becomes irritable and protective of the injured limb. If the pain continues without relief, the patient may withdraw and react by avoiding bright lights and loud noises. The slightly emotional problem may aggravate the intractable pain. Some patients find temporary relief by bathing the involved extremity in tepid running water. Symptoms can be relieved temporarily by block of the sympathetic ganglion of the involved limb. Cure often results following sympathectomy.

Another group of painful disorders associated with autonomic dysfunction involves sympathetic disturbance occurring after trauma of a less specific nature in the extremity or joints. The pain is usually not as intense as causalgia, but there may be vasomotor disturbances such as vasospastic phenomenon, cyanosis, and trophic skin changes in the involved extremity. Diagnostic sympathetic block often relieves the symptoms, and surgical sympathectomy may be curative. Psychoneurosis is not uncommon and is often associated with personal problems associated with litigation and compensation claims. Ill-advised operation may magnify the entire symptom complex.

Relief of Pain by Pituitary Ablation

Intractable pain caused by metastasis from the bone and prostate dramatically subsides after ablation of the pituitary gland. The relief of pain was thought at one time to be related to the reduction or loss of the effect of the pituitary growth hormone, which has a direct stimulating effect on some of these tumors. It is now thought the effect is probably via the hypo-

thalamus and some alteration in the synthesis of polypeptides associated with the endorphins and enkephalins. Pain relief is immediate after the ablation procedure, and as the pain subsides, the tumor nodules also diminish in size and lesions in the bone observed on the roentgenogram often resolve with recalcification. Pituitary ablation should be considered after oophorectomy in women or following the removal of the gonads in men. Hypophysectomy exerts its best effects in the premenopausal woman, and the most satifactory results are noted if the pituitary gland is completely ablated, although the effect may be directly on the hypothalamus. Complete surgical removal of the pituitary can be accomplished through a frontal craniotomy, but more recently stereotactic ablations have been performed by introducing lesion probes into the sella turcica (Fig. 4). The overall operative risks are less following the stereotactic operation. The gland can be destroyed by freezing, heat coagulation, implanting radioactive yttrium, or injecting absolute alcohol. Postoperatively these patients must be maintained on hormone replacement often combined with vasopressin (Pitressin) if diabetes insipidus appears. Pituitary-hypothalamic ablation can be followed by many pain-free months during which time the patient's overall condition as well as life improves.

Relief of Pain by Electroanalgesia

In 1967 Wall and Sweet found that during stimulation of the peripheral nerves, pain sensation was reduced over the distribution area of the stimulated nerve.[17] They proposed that the electrical activation of A fibers of the peripheral nerves in some manner interfered with the perception of painful stimuli probably at the spinal cord level. Wall had already demonstrated in animals that when the activity of large A fibers in the peripheral nerves was increased by electrical stimulus, there occurred a concomitant inhibition of activity of the smaller pain fibers within the spinal cord.[16] Later, Shealy and associates noted that stimulation of the dorsal columns of the cat, which are composed entirely of large A fibers, reduced the animal's reaction to noxious stimuli.[12] The term *electroanalgesia* was coined, although the neurophysiologic mechanism responsible for pain relief was not known. Sweet originally employed the electrical stimulation technique to successfully relieve pain originating from an injured peripheral nerve. A pair of platinum electrodes is placed in contact with the nerve trunk above the level of the injury, and a miniature RF receiver attached to the stimulating

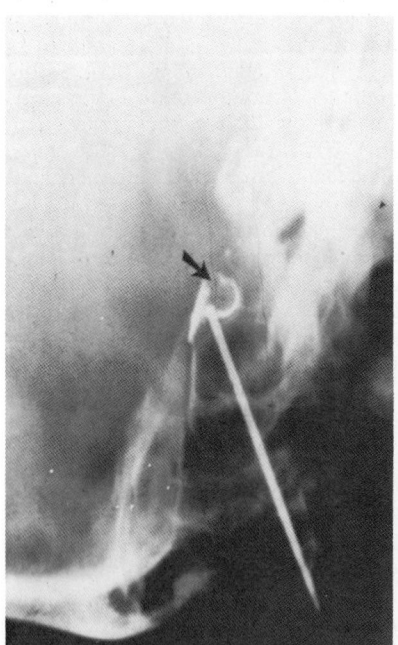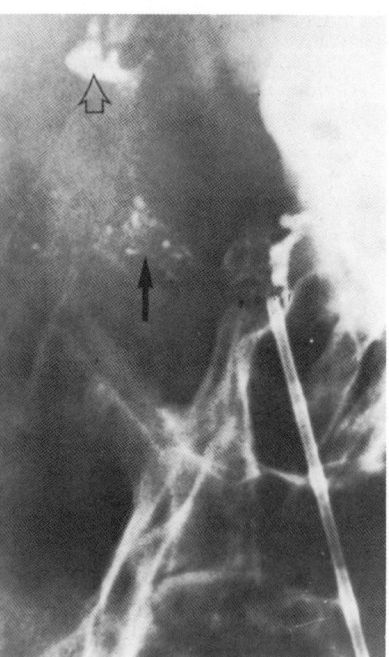

Figure 4. Alcohol injection in the pituitary gland to control pain of bone metastasis from prostate or breast cancer. Note radiopaque dye migration via the pituitary stalk into the hypothalamus. Pain relief is due to the hypothalamic lesion. (From Miles, J.: Pituitary destruction. *In* Wall, P. D., and Melzack, R.: Textbook of Pain. Edinburgh, Churchill Livingstone, 1984.)

platinum electrode is buried beneath the skin. The patient self-activates the painful nerve by electrical signal transmitted through the skin of the RF receiver by a small portable RF generator. The patient can vary the frequency or strength of the stimulating current in order to find a level of stimulation that relieves the pain. Later, in 1970, Shealy and Mortimer reported the implantation of stimulating electrodes to activate the dorsal columns of the spinal cord in patients with pain from widespread carcinoma.[12] The device can be inserted percutaneously or through a laminectomy in the cerivcal, thoracic, or lumbar areas, but always above the segmental level of the body from which the pain originates. Self-activation of the dorsal columns by the patient leads to experience of a paresthesia in the painful region with an associated reduction of pain. The technique has been used in a wide number of chronic pain problems with success. The greatest potential of electroanalgesia is based on the concept that the nervous system is not physically disrupted, but the "ongoing" neural activity related to pain perception is in some manner altered by the introduction of an extrinsic electrical impulse, thereby preserving the physical integrity of the central nervous system.

Three endogenous peptides having analgesic action have been isolated from the brain: beta-endorphin, methionine, and leucine-enkephalins. Electrical stimulation of the midbrain in both man and animals activates these opioid neurons and leads to reduction of experimental and pathologic pain. The neurophysiologic role of these opioid peptides in human pain syndromes remains to be elucidated and applied in clinical practice.

It is obvious that there are numerous options for the relief of pain, and the patient's pain syndrome must be analyzed prior to the application of any one of these special techniques.

SELECTED REFERENCES

Livingston, W. K.: Pain Mechanisms: A Physiologic Interpretation of Causalgia and its Related States. New York, Plenum Press, 1976.
An analysis of the central neurophysiologic concepts of pain.

Noordenbos, W.: Pain. Amsterdam, Elsevier Publishing Company, 1959.
Presents the concept of central pain phenomenon based on analysis of clinical pain syndromes. A landmark book on pain.

Spiller, W. G.: The occasional clinical resemblance between caries of the vertebral and lumbothoracic syringomyelia, and the location within the spinal cord of the fibres for the sensations of pain and temperature. Univ. Penn. Med. Bull., 18:147, 1905.

Sternbach, R. A.: Pain Patients. Traits and Treatment. New York, Academic Press, 1974.

Wall, P. D., and Melzack, R.: Textbook of Pain. Edinburgh, Churchill Livingstone, 1984.

White, J. C., and Sweet, W. H.: Pain and The Neurosurgeon. A Forty Year Experience. Springfield, Ill., Charles C Thomas, 1969.

REFERENCES

1. Adams, C. B.: Microvascular compression: An alternative view and hypothesis. J. Neurosurg., 70:1, 1989.
2. Adams, G. G., and Cullen, J. F.: Neuroparalytic keratitis and the effect of cervical sympathectomy following operative procedures for trigeminal neuralgia. Scott. Med. J., 32:86, 1987.
3. Bernard, E. J., Jr., Nashold, B. S., Jr., Caputi, F., and Moossy, J. J.: Nucleus caudalis DREZ lesions for facial pain. Br. J. Neurosurg., 1:81, 1987.
4. Burchiel, J. J., Clarke, H., Haglund, M., and Loesser, J. D.: Long-term efficacy of microvascular decompression in trigeminal neuralgia. J. Neurosurg., 69:39, 1988.
5. Dandy, W. E.: Concerning the cause of trigeminal neuralgia. Am. J. Surg., 24:447, 1934.
6. Jannetta, P. J.: Arterial compression of the trigeminal nerve in patients with trigeminal neuralgia. J. Neurosurg., 26(Suppl.):159, 1967.
7. Lazorthes, Y., Armenguad, J. P., and Da Motta, M.: Chronic stimulation of the gasserian ganglion for treatment of atypical facial neuralgia. PACE, 10:257, 1987.
8. Lunsford, L. D.: Trigeminal neuralgia: Treatment by glycerol rhizotomy. In Wilkins, R. H., and Rengachary, S. S. (Eds.): Neurosurgery. New York, McGraw-Hill, 1985, pp. 2351–2356.
9. Mitchell, S. W., Morehouse, G. R., and Keen, W. W.: Gunshot wounds and other injuries of nerves. Philadelphia, J. B. Lippincott Company, 1864, p. 164.
9a. Mullan, S., Harper, P. V., Hekmatpanah, J., Torres, H., and Dobbin, G.: Percutaneous interruption of spinal-pain tracts by means of a strontium[90] needle. J. Neurosurg., 20:931, 1963.
10. Nashold, B. S., Jr., Ostdahl, R. H., Bullitt, E., Friedman, A., and Brophy, B.: Drsal root entry zone lesions: A new neurosurgical therapy for deafferentation pain. In Bonica, J. (Ed.): Advances in Pain Research and Therapy. Vol. 5. New York, Raven Press, 1983, pp. 739–750.
11. Piquer, J., Joanes, V., Roldan, P., Barcia-Salorio, J. L., and Masbout, G.: Long-term results of percutaneous gasserian ganglion lesions. Acta Neurochir. Suppl. (Wien), 39:139, 1987.
11a. Saini, S. S.: Retrogasserian anhydrous glycerol injection therapy in trigeminal neuralgia: Observations in 552 patients. J. Neurol. Neurosurg. Psychiatry, 50:1536, 1987.
12. Shealy, C. N., Mortimer, J. T., and Hagsfors, N.: Dorsal column electroanalgesia. J. Neurosurg., 32:560, 1970.
13. Spiegel, E. A., Wycis, H. T., Marks, M., and Lee, A. J.: Stereotactic apparatus for operation on the human brain. Science, 106:349, 1947.
14. Spiller, W. G.: The occasional clinical resemblance between caries of the vertebral and lumbothoracic syringomyelia, and the location within the spinal cord of the fibres for the sensations of pain and temperature. Univ. Penn. Med. Bull., 18:147, 1905.
15. Spiller, W. G., and Martin, E.: The treatment of persistent pain of organic origin in the lower part of the body by division of the anterolateral column of the spinal cord. J.A.M.A., 58:1489, 1912.
16. Wall, P. D.: Control of impulses at the first central synapse in cutaneous pathways. In Eccles, J. C., and Schade, J. P. (Eds.): Physiology of Spinal Neurons. (Progress in Brain Research, Vol. 12.) New York, Elsevier, 1964.
17. Wall, P. D., and Sweet, W. H.: Temporary abolition of pain in man. Science, 155:108, 1967.

XIII

NEUROSURGICAL TREATMENT OF EPILEPSY

John J. Moossy, M.D., and Blaine S. Nashold, Jr., M.D.

Epilepsy is a common human ailment; as many as 1 in 100 persons may have an epileptic seizure at some time in life. However, a physician may consider the diagnosis of epilepsy only when the patient has had more than one seizure. A seizure is the result of an abnormal synchronous electrical discharge from a group of cortical neurons. The discharge causes some types of uncontrolled movement or behavior. Often the patient has an alteration in consciousness; however, in some types of epilepsy consciousness is not affected. A seizure may be the first manifestation of a structural abnormality in the brain, i.e., a tumor, vascular malformation, or abscess. In this section, only the treatment of those patients in whom the seizures are not a manifestation of disease, but represent the disease process itself, is discussed.

HISTORICAL ASPECTS

Epilepsy was described in the earliest medical treatises; the Hippocratic writings have excellent accounts of patients with tonic-clonic seizures. In the nearly 2500 years since Hippocrates, many have been interested in patients with seizures; the modern era of epileptology and the beginning of surgical treatment of medically intractable epilepsy began in the late nineteenth century. J. Hughlings Jackson is regarded as the seminal figure in establishing the modern interest in epilepsy. It is not surprising that one of the first persons successfully treated for epilepsy by surgical extirpation of the seizure focus was a patient referred by Jackson to Sir Victor Horsley in 1886. Jackson's patient was included with two others operated upon by Horsley in a report published in the *British Medical Journal* of October 9, 1886.[7] This paper marks the beginning of the modern era of surgical therapy for epilepsy. Since that auspicious beginning, many others have made important contributions. Early in this century, Foerster used electrical stimulation to map the brain of patients having resections for epilepsy.[4] Penfield and Jasper, in the 1930s, popularized the electroencephalogram (EEG) as a diagnostic test for localizing the seizure focus and electrocorticography (E cog) for intraoperative mapping of seizure foci to plan resections.[10] Van Wagenen and Herren, in 1940, devised and performed corpus callosum sections to control the spread of the epileptic discharge.[12] Krynauw, in 1950, introduced hemispherectomy to control seizures associated with infantile hemiplegia.[8]

CLASSIFICATION OF SEIZURES

The classification of seizures has been an area of repeated disagreement in the modern study of epilepsy. Disputes about the results of therapeutic trials arise from differences in nomenclature. The classification system of the International League Against Epilepsy, which emphasizes the differences between partial and generalized seizure types, has reduced the disagreements in this area (Table 1).[5]

TABLE 1. International Classification of Epileptic Seizures

I. Partial seizures (seizures beginning locally)
  A. Partial seizures with elementary symptomatology (generally without impairment of consciousness)
    1. With motor symptoms (includes jacksonian seizures)
    2. With special sensory or somatosensory symptoms
    3. With autonomic symptoms
    4. Compound forms
  B. Partial seizures with complex symptomatology (generally with impairment of consciousness; temporal lobe or psychomotor seizures)
    1. With impairment of consciousness only
    2. With cognitive symptomatology
    3. With affective symptomatology
    4. With "psychosensory" symptomatology (automatisms)
    5. With "psychomotor" symptomatology
    6. Compound forms
  C. Partial seizures secondarily generalized
II. Generalized seizures (bilaterally symmetric and without local onset)
  A. Absences (petit mal)
  B. Bilateral massive epileptic myoclonus
  C. Infantile spasms
  D. Clonic seizures
  E. Tonic seizures
  F. Tonic-clonic seizures (grand mal)
  G. Atonic seizures
  H. Akinetic seizures
III. Unilateral seizures (or predominantly unilateral)
IV. Unclassified epileptic seizures (resulting from incomplete data)

Adapted from Baker, A. B., and Joynt, R. J. (Eds.): Clinical Neurology, Vol. 3. Philadelphia, J. B. Lippincott Company, 1988, p. 14.

PATIENT SELECTION

The selection from the population of all patients with epilepsy of those who are candidates for surgical therapy requires careful thought and analysis. All patients who are seizure-free with medical therapy can be eliminated from consideration. The first criterion for considering surgical treatment, therefore, is that a patient has persistent seizures with a documented therapeutic level of one or more anticonvulsive drugs. Second, the seizure frequency interferes with that patient's normal existence. Third, the seizure focus can be localized and is unilateral. Fourth, the area of the brain to which the seizure focus is localized can be removed with little likelihood of a new neurologic deficit.

Most patients who fulfill these four criteria have partial complex seizures with a unilateral temporal lobe focus; this group represents about 80 per cent of patients who undergo surgical therapy for seizure control.[7] To identify patients who may benefit from surgical treatment, epilepsy centers have protocols. In order to enter any epilepsy surgery center protocol, the first and second criteria must be present. The protocol then determines whether the third and fourth criteria can be met, using techniques described later.

The first step in defining the site of origin of seizures in any patient suspected of having epilepsy is the scalp EEG. Electroencephalographic localization from external or scalp electrodes takes two forms. The standard EEG is performed in the outpatient setting with electrodes placed in a standard array (Fig. 1) and the patient is monitored for 1 to 2 hours. More prolonged monitoring with simultaneous videotaping of the patient provides better information about the onset of behavioral abnormalities in relationship to the abnormal electrical activity in the brain. Because of limitations of scalp EEG, video-monitored patients often require placement of depth electrodes for final determination of seizure origin. New adjuncts to the analysis of scalp EEG include computer-assisted analysis of the phase of interictal epileptiform potentials recorded from homologous contralateral brain regions.[2,3]

Recently, major advances have been made in analysis of patients with medically intractable epilepsy with the ability to image the brain using non-invasive, or minimally invasive, radiologic techniques. The advent of computed tomography (CT) in the mid 1970s increased the preoperative recognition of hamartomas, gliomas, gangliogliomas and vascular malformation in the temporal lobe, which were previously unsuspected preoperatively and found only in pathologic specimens.[2,3] In the mid 1980s, the clinical availability of magnetic resonance imaging (MRI) made possible the preoperative diagnosis of mesial temporal sclerosis (MTS),[2,3] one of the most common pathologic findings in large series of temporal lobe resections. Positron emission tomography (PET) provides preoperative physiologic data, including metabolic and blood flow information, that appear to have some predictive value in localizing abnormal areas of decreased brain metabolism that coincide with seizure foci[3] (Fig. 2).

Just as MRI and PET provide both anatomic and physiologic information upon intravenous injection of paramagnetic contrast and radionuclide, respectively, amytal angiography provides largely physiologic data using angiographic techniques. Since this is an invasive diagnostic test, it is reserved for those patients who have fulfilled the first three criteria to qualify for surgical therapy for seizure and is an exclusionary test. The test is performed using the selective injection of amytal into each internal carotid artery, followed by memory and speech testing. If the amytal angiogram reveals the location of memory or language to be in the site considered for resection, the patient is not a candidate for operative therapy, because the possible deficits from the planned resection would create an unacceptable alteration in the patient's neurologic condition.

Many centers routinely perform depth electrode (DE) EEG for

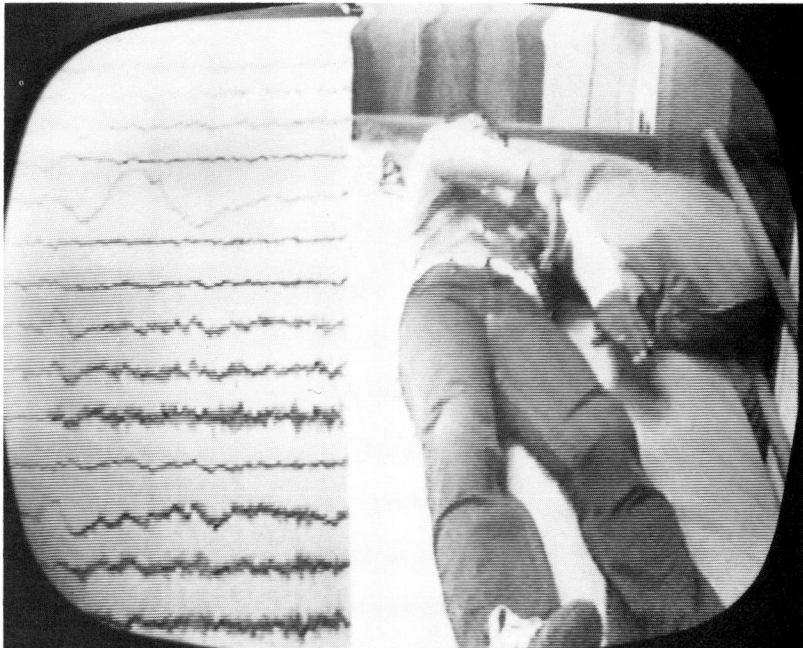

Figure 1. Split-screen monitoring of a patient during an epileptic seizure (on the right). The epileptic activity from the patient's scalp is seen on the left half of the TV screen.

final localization of the seizure focus; other centers reserve DE for those patients whose surface EEG does not provide clear lateralization. The insertion of depth electrodes is performed in the operating room, using stereotactic techniques (Fig. 3). The current methods for stereotactic localization of the amygdala and hippocampus, the medial structures of the temporal lobe, involve standard reference to the anterior and posterior commissures (AC-PC line), using positive contrast ventriculography or localization by CT or MRI images in conjunction with an imaging compatible stereotactic frame. A post-DE placement CT shows the electrodes in homologous positions in both temporal lobes (Fig. 4). Depth electrode placement is followed by chronic EEG recording with simultaneous videotaping. During this period of observation, seizures and their associated physical or behavioral manifestations are videotaped with on-screen

EEG recording from the depth electrodes to provide clear definition of the side of origin of the seizures. Some centers include frontal depth electrodes as part of the standard array. The target for the frontal electrodes is less well established than for the temporal electrodes but is designed to sample the orbitofrontal cortex.

Some centers in which surgical therapy is performed for epilepsy do not rely on depth electrode information; instead, these centers place subdural or epidural electrodes in strips or mat arrays for chronic surface electrocorticograms[6] (Fig. 5). In all the invasive recording techniques, the goal is to achieve a clear lateralization of seizure onset to guide the surgeon in choosing the site of resection. After this information has been obtained and the neurologist, neurosurgeon, and patient are satisfied that the site of seizures has been identified and is in an area that can be resected or severed, operation is recommended for seizure control (Fig. 6).

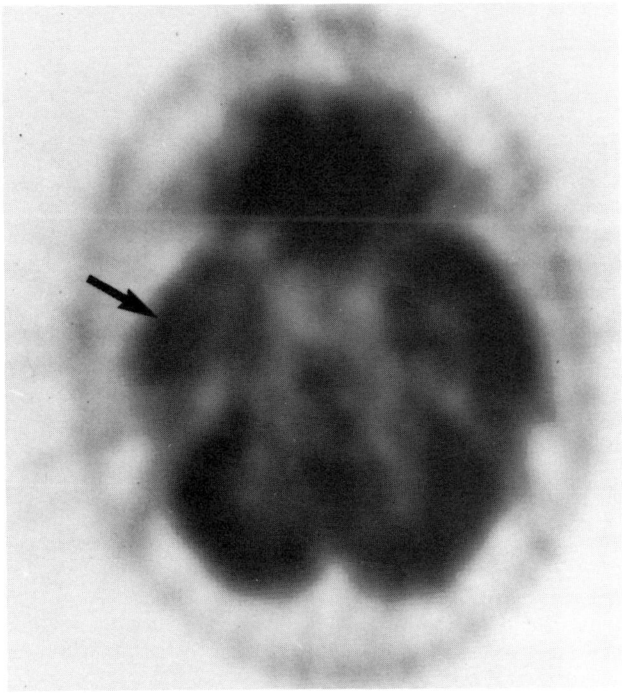

SURGICAL TREATMENT

Anterior temporal lobectomy is the most frequently performed operation for control of medically intractable epilepsy.

Figure 2. PET scan of a patient with temporal lobe epilepsy. Arrow indicates a hypodense temporal lobe on the side of the epileptic focus.

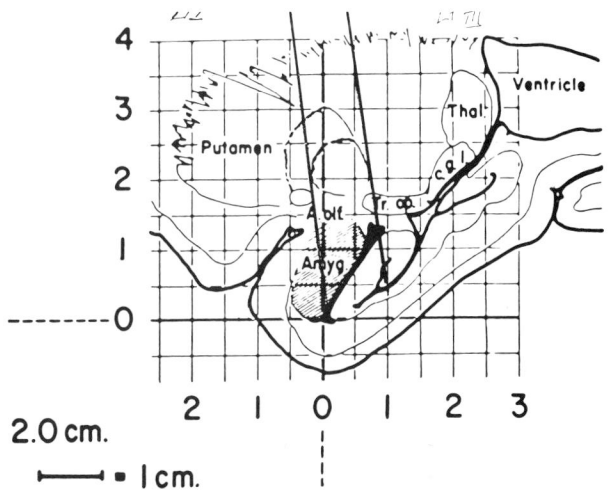

Figure 3. Schematic drawing of sagittal brain section showing the location of stereotactically implanted depth electrodes (see Fig. 4).

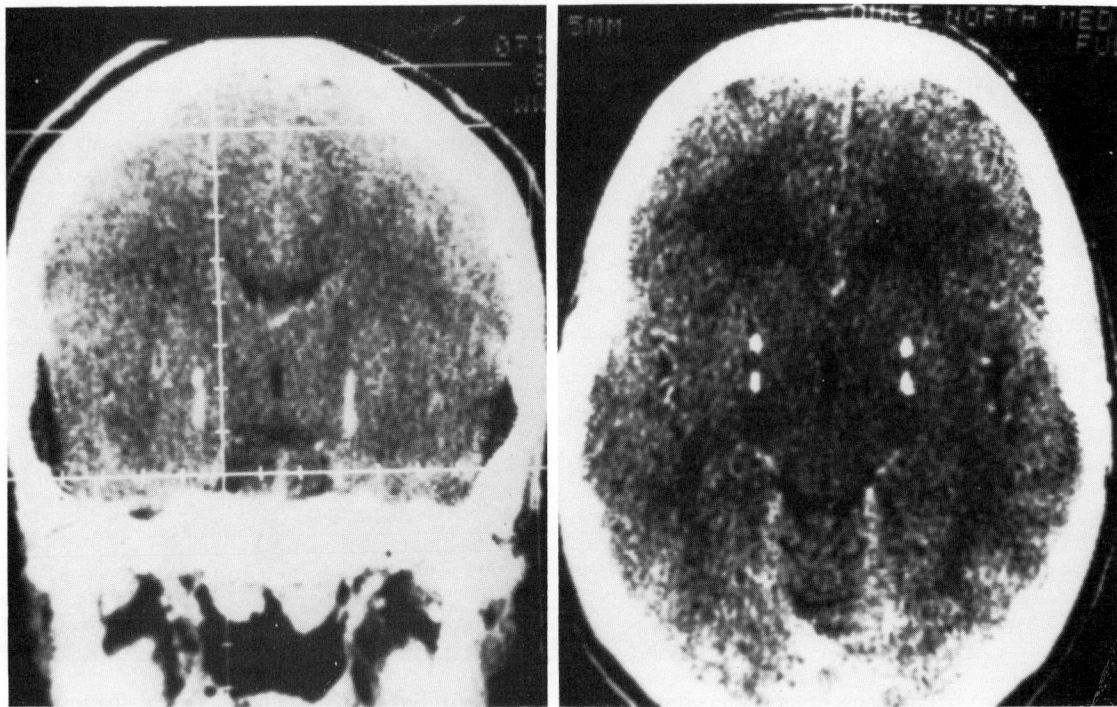

Figure 4. Scan showing bilaterally implanted depth electrodes in mesial temporal lobes.

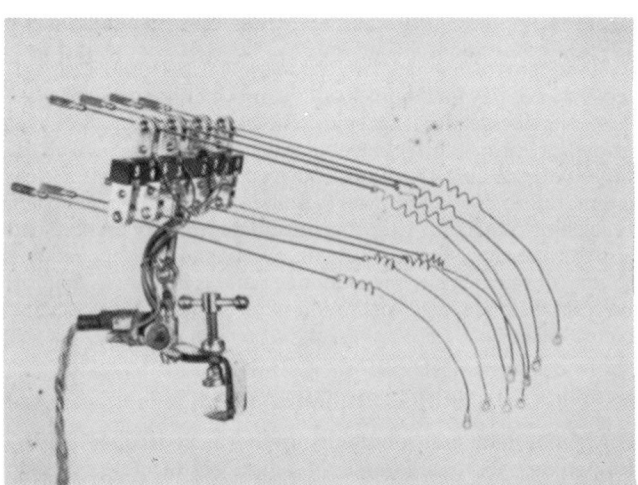

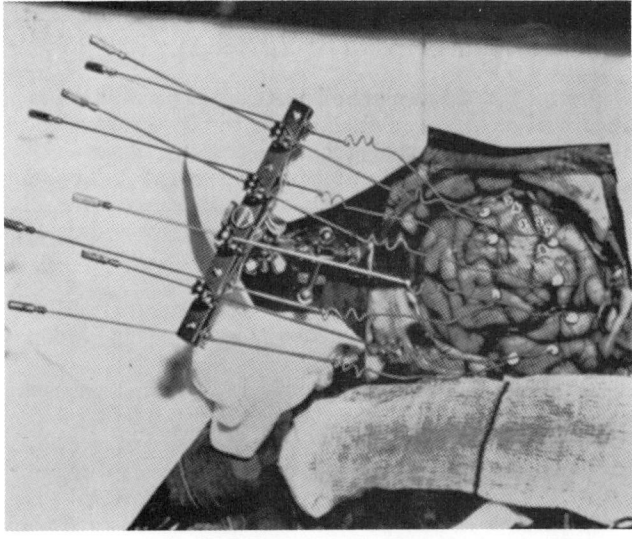

Figure 5. Electrodes used by Penfield and Jasper on the exposed brain. (From Penfield, W., and Jasper, H.: Epilepsy and the Functional Anatomy of the Human Brain. Boston, Little, Brown and Company, 1954.)

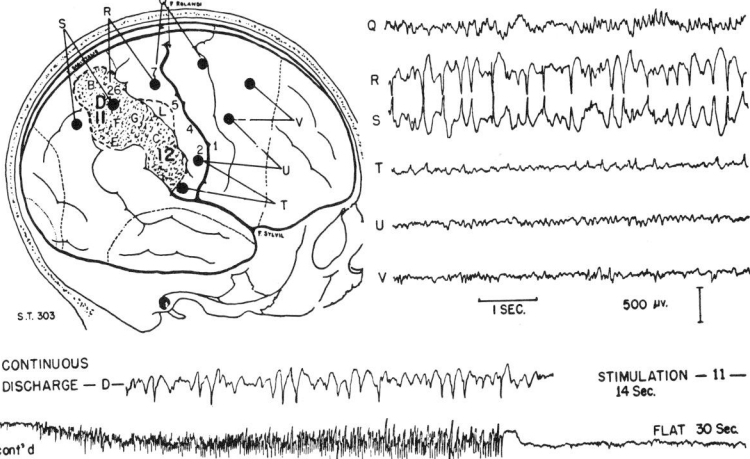

Figure 6. Focal cortical seizures from centro-parietal cortex. Note continuous after-discharge following electrical stimulation at *D*. (From Penfield, W., and Jasper, H.: Epilepsy and the Functional Anatomy of the Human Brain. Boston, Little, Brown and Company, 1954.)

The technique for removal of the temporal lobe has evolved during the last 50 years. Most surgeons performing an anterior temporal lobectomy for epilepsy first perform a standard frontotemporal craniotomy and open the dura over the surface of the temporal lobe. Some surgeons then perform electrocorticography to customize the area of resection to the patient's seizure focus. In most circumstances, the resection is limited to 5 to 7 cm. posterior to the tip of the temporal lobe. Many surgeons have begun to use the ultrasonic aspirator (CUSA) to minimize the manipulation outside the resection site. Others have instituted the use of the operating microscope for removal of the medial structures to assure complete resection of amygdala and hippocampus with minimal risk to adjacent structures.

For the patients in whom a unilateral frontal focus is found, a standard frontal craniotomy and frontal lobectomy are performed. The frontal lobectomy is limited posteriorly by the coronal suture and the frontal horn of the lateral ventricle. The medial structures of the orbitofrontal cortex are carefully removed to avoid injury to the optic apparatus or carotid complex.

Another operation in the armamentarium of neurosurgeons treating medically intractable epilepsy is corpus callosum section. The corpus callosum is the major white matter connection or commissure between the two cerebral hemispheres. Other commissures include the habenular commissure, the fornix, and the anterior commissure. Some or all of these have been sectioned at various times in the evolution of the sectioning of the corpus callosum for seizure control. Sectioning of the corpus callosum is a difficult operation. It remains a rarely used operative technique, and centers that perform this technique may use slightly different methods. The three common approaches are anterior section, posterior section, and complete section. When complete sectioning is performed, it may be done in a single operation or it may be staged. The postoperative study by Sperry of patients who had complete section of the corpus callosum was rewarded with the Nobel Prize in medicine in 1981.

Hemispherectomy for seizure control was introduced by Krynauw in 1950.[8] It remains a consideration for the treatment of intractable epilepsy associated with infantile hemiplegia and the Sturge-Weber syndrome. As with the other surgical techniques, hemispherectomy has undergone considerable refinement in the 40 years since its introduction. The early results of this operation were extraordinary, with 83 per cent of patients experiencing a reduction in seizure frequency.[9] However, analysis of the late morbidity and mortality showed a fatal complication, superficial cerebral hemosiderosis, in one fourth to one third of patients. Now hemispherectomy involves subtotal resection of the hemisphere, with complete separation from the other hemisphere by complete commissural sectioning. With this modification, seizure control is slightly less, with 68 per cent of the patients experiencing significantly fewer seizures.[11]

In addition to these four standard, although hardly universal, operations, a number of unusual procedures are used in the surgical treatment of epilepsy. Yasargil has advocated selective amygdala hippocampectomy with preservation of the temporal lobe cortex, using microsurgical techniques to resect only the medial structures.[2,6,9] Topectomy is performed in several centers for patients with parietal, occipital, and, occasionally, frontal seizure foci. Some centers still perform stereotactic interruption of pathways, using radiofrequency lesioning techniques. Stereotactic amygdalotomy has also been performed with variable results.

COMPLICATIONS

All intracranial surgical procedures are associated with complications. The rate and severity of complication must enter into the decisions regarding the benefits of the procedure in question. The complication rate from anterior temporal lobectomy has been low. In the largest centers, the mortality is 0 to 1 per cent. Major morbidity usually is limited to a contralateral hemiparesis in 3 to 6 per cent, with persistent weakness in less than 1 per cent. The most frequent persistent neurologic deficit is a superior homonymous quadrantanopsia, which is infrequently symptomatic. Rarely in dominant hemisphere resections, there are speech and language difficulties, usually described as dysphasia. There have been patients with memory difficulties (most complications related to memory are in patients whose care antedates the amytal test). As with any surgical procedure, a certain number of patients have postoperative infection (1.5 per cent), hemorrhage (0.01 per cent), and anesthetic complications (0.06 per cent).[2]

In patients undergoing frontal resection, the major morbidity is contralateral weakness and speech problems when the operation involves the dominant hemisphere. Cortical mapping of the motor strip and avoidance of the opercular gyri in the dominant hemisphere are the two best methods to minimize these complications. The frequency of these complications and perioperative mortality parallel that for temporal lobectomy.

The complications of hemispherectomy, i.e., the late morbidity and mortality from cerebral superficial hemosiderosis, may occur as long as 15 to 20 years after resection. Techniques used to avoid this complication have been employed for only 10 to 15 years, so there is still uncertainty regarding the frequency of this complication in this series. Other complications occur with comparable frequency to the two previously discussed procedures.

The complications of sectioning the corpus callosum have changed with advances in technique. The early operations were associated with a high rate of ventricular contamination and resultant meningitis, and postoperative hydrocephalus and hemorrhagic infarction occurred in a smaller percentage. The

TABLE 2. Operative Results for Epileptic Seizures

Classification	Hemispherectomy	Anterior Temporal Lobectomy	Extratemporal Resection	Corpus Callosum Section
Total patients	88	2336	825	197
Total centers	17	40	32	16
Seizure-free	68	1296	356	10
Per cent (range)	77.3 (0–100)	55.5 (26–80)	43.2 (0–73)	5.0 (0–13)
Improved	16	648	229	140
Per cent	18.2	27.7	27.8	71.0
Not improved	4	392	240	47
Per cent (range)	4.5 (0–33)	16.8 (6–29)	29.1 (17–89)	23.9 (10–38)

Adapted from Engel, J. (Ed.): Surgical Treatment of the Epilepsies. New York, Raven Press, 1987, p. 569.

most consistent neurologic consequences of callosal sectioning are not true complications but consequences of the procedure, which include mutism, left-sided apraxia that may resemble a hemiparesis, bilateral grasp reflexes, and bilateral Babinski signs.[2]

Complications of DE and subdural and epidural electrode mats or strips are rare. In 560 patients, Talairach reported three intracerebral hemorrhages (ICH) for DE.[2] Engel and associates reported two deaths from ICH in a series of 140 patients.[2] Minor complications, such as scalp infection, or more serious infection, such as meningitis, occurs in less than 1 per cent.[2] Subdural and epidural electrode arrays have been associated with scalp and bone flap infection but no reported cases of subdural or epidural empyema. Few postoperative hemorrhages have been reported.[2]

RESULTS

The goal of surgical therapy for medically intractable epilepsy is a reduction or elimination of seizures. Each procedure discussed in this section has a different effectiveness; the reliability of the data depends upon the frequency with which a procedure is performed. In a survey of centers performing surgical therapy for epilepsy, Engel recorded the results seen in Table 2.[2] From this, it can be seen that anterior temporal lobectomy for control of epilepsy is performed twice as often as any other operation; combined, the seizure-free and "improved" results for this procedure approach 85 per cent. The other operations, with the exception of hemispherectomy, have a lower success rate; however, as is obvious from this table and the foregoing discussion, hemispherectomy has limited application. In addition to seizure control, surgical therapy for seizure has important neurologic and neuropsychologic consequences. Analysis of results must consider these aspects of the patient's condition. Among the goals of surgical therapy is more normal socialization through reduction of seizure and anticonvulsant medications. Whether successful social integration is a result of alteration in seizures and medication or a more concerted effort by social services as a consequence of the epilepsy center involvement is difficult to predict from the reports available.

The pathologic findings of tissue removed in surgical therapy for epilepsy have largely been an analysis of the temporal lobes removed en bloc. Abnormal tissue has been found in most cases. Mesial temporal sclerosis appears to be the most frequent finding, ranging from 22 to 76 per cent in different centers, with the overall average about 60 per cent for all series reported.[1,2]

Next in frequency are tumors, usually low-grade glioma or ganglioglioma or extra-axial tumors such as meningioma, which constitute about 19 per cent. Hamartomas and heterotopia combined comprise about 18 per cent. Other findings include a combination of infection, vascular malformation, and unclassified abnormalities, such as gliosis.[2,6,9] Many theories exist regarding the pathogenesis of MTS and its causative role in epilepsy. Several investigators have suggested early life trauma, infection, and hypoxic ischemic insults as likely causes. No statistically significant correlation between these problems and MTS has been established.

In summary, there is a definite role for the surgical treatment of patients with medically intractable epilepsy. As with most operations, the preoperative evaluation and selection of appropriate candidates determine the success rate. The complication rate is acceptably low from the point of view of surgical morbidity and mortality. The assessment and perioperative care of these patients require the concerted efforts of a team of physicians and other personnel interested in the problems and care of patients with epilepsy.

REFERENCES

1. Engel, J.: Seizures and Epilepsy. Philadelphia, F. A. Davis Company, 1989, pp. 443–464.
2. Engel, J. (Ed.): Complications of surgical procedures in the diagnosis and treatment of epilepsy. In Surgical Treatment of the Epilepsies. New York, Raven Press, 1987.
3. Engel, J., Kuhl, D. E., Phelps, M. E., and Crandall, P. H.: Comparative localization of epileptic foci in partial epilepsy by PCT and EEG. Ann. Neurol., 12:529, 1982.
4. Foerster, O.: Zur operativen Behandlung der Epilepsie. Dtsch Z Nervenheilkd, 89:137, 1926.
5. Forster, F. M., and Booker, H. E.: The epilepsies and convulsive disorder. In Baker, A. B., and Joynt, R. J. (Eds.): Clinical Neurology, Vol. 3. Philadelphia, J. B. Lippincott Company, 1988, pp. 1–68.
6. Goldring, S.: Neurosurgical aspects of epilepsy in adults. In Youmans, J. R. (Ed.): Neurological Surgery, Vol 6. Philadelphia, W. B. Saunders Company, 1982, pp. 3910–3926.
7. Horsley, V.: Brain surgery. Br. Med. J., 2:670, 1886.
8. Krynauw, R. A.: Infantile hemiplegia treated by removal of one cerebral hemisphere. J. Neurol. Neurosurg. Psychiatr., 13:243, 1950.
9. Ojemann, G. A.: Surgical treatment of epilepsy. In Wilkins, R. H., and Rengachary, S. S. (Eds.): Neurosurgery, Part XIV. New York, McGraw-Hill Book Company, 1985, pp. 2517–2527.
10. Penfield, W., and Jasper, H.: Epilepsy and the functional anatomy of the human brain. Boston, Little, Brown and Company, 1954.
11. Rasmussen, T.: Hemispherectomy for seizures revisited. Can. J. Neurol. Sci., 10:71, 1983.
12. Van Wagenen, W. P., and Herren, R. Y.: Surgical division of commissural pathways in the corpus callosum. Arch. Neurol. Psychiatr., 44:740, 1940.

XIV

STEREOTACTIC NEUROSURGERY

Robert P. Iacono, M.D., and Blaine S. Nashold, Jr., M.D.

Rapid evolution of stereotactic methods has followed the development of computed brain imaging systems, allowing new application of therapeutic modalities to neurosurgery. These advances originated in 1906 when Horsley and Clarke reported the use of a stereotactic instrument for accurate insertion of probes into the cerebellar nuclei of animals, allowing them, and subsequently others, free anatomical access for neurophysiologic exploration of deep brain centers.[2,9] By 1950, Spiegel and Wycis and others had applied stereotactic technique to man[23,24] (Fig. 1) for the purpose of treating involuntary movement disorders and psychiatric disturbances for which no other therapy was then available.[13,23] It became relatively widely used in the 1960s following Cooper's serendipitous discovery of the globus pallidus and later the ventrolateral thalamus as a therapeutic target for the tremor and rigidity of Parkinson's disease.[3,8,22,23,35,37] However, following the development in 1970 of L-dopa therapy, the number of stereotactic procedures decreased abruptly.[4,18]

The advent of computed tomographic (CT) scanning and the availability of quality imaging techniques by 1980 were responsible for a rapid resurgence of interest in stereotactics. This was in part due to the natural motivation to access now visible, sometimes small, deep intracerebral lesions *seen* on CT scans and in part due to the format of CT scans, the planes, accuracy, and software available for stereotactic use. CT image localization was adapted to existing stereotactic frames, and then new instruments, the design of which was predicated on the scanning and computing capabilities of CT and magnetic resonance imaging (MRI) equipment, became available.[5,8]

Conventional Stereotactic Technique for Functional Neurosurgery

In conventional stereotactic surgery, the main intent is the highly accurate placement of lesions and sometimes electrodes for neurophysiologic purposes, requiring the use of a precision instrument that can direct a probe into deep brain targets with submillimeter accuracy. The intracerebral target is determined from the coordinates of a special stereotactic atlas of the human brain with sections in three planes (Fig. 2). Localization of the target is made from an outline of landmarks of the third ventricle (anterior and posterior commissures) seen on intraoperative films (Fig. 3). The position of the target can be calculated from measurements, and its coordinates can then be translated to adjustments of the stereotactic frame, which either directs the probe to the center of the frame (and therefore target) or directs the trajectory of the probe in the exact angles of the target.[13,22] Alternatively, scans taken with the patient's head in a CT-visible localizing stereotactic frame may be used to achieve targeting information[7,8] (Fig. 4). Following localization and probe insertion, anatomic variability errors are minimized by the use of electrophysiologic methods, by either stimulation or recording from the target area. Usually the patients are under local anesthesia so that their neurologic reactions can be monitored. For physiologic localization, electrical stimulation with variable frequencies produces a characteristic pattern of responses for each location that the experienced stereotactician can recognize. For example, stimulation in the ventrolateral region of the thalamus may arrest a symptomatic tremor,[13,22] in the hypothalamus, have profound autonomic effects,[12] or near the midbrain periaqueductal region, affect eye movements.[20,21] For localization of subnuclei of the thalamus, observation of neuronal unit discharges with a microelectrode has proved useful.[18] Moreover,

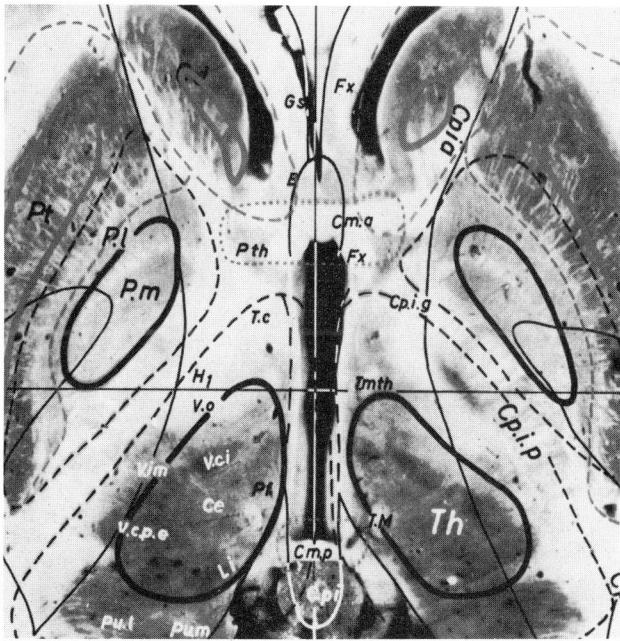

Figure 2. Stereotactic map of a horizontal section of the human brain through the diencephalon and basal ganglia showing the third ventricle (center) bordered by the anterior (Cm.a.) and posterior (Cm.p.) commissures. Note these positions are circled on Figure 3, which is a lateral (sagittal) view. Also note the position marked V.im of the left ventrolateral thalamus next to the internal capsule, which can be seen targeted by cursor coordinates in Figure 4. (From Schaltenbrand, G., and Waltren, W.: Atlas for Stereotaxy of the Human Brain, Plate 17. Chicago, Year Book Medical Publishers, 1977.)

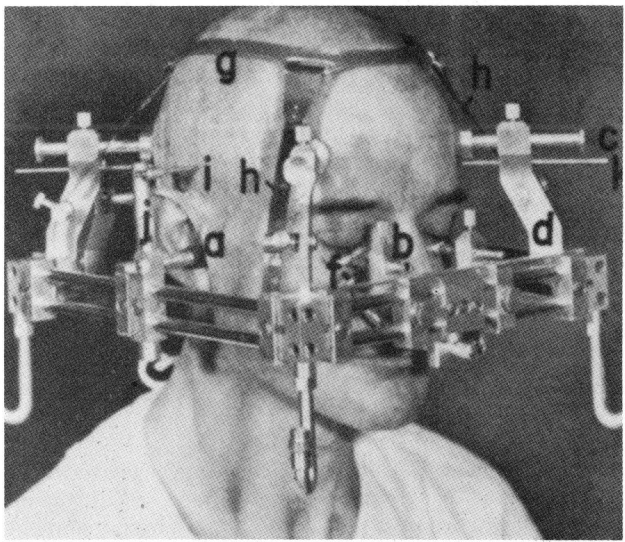

Figure 1. Human stereotactic instrument as devised by Spiegel and Wycis, showing base plate attached to patient's head. (From Spiegel E. A., et al.: Stereotaxic apparatus for operations on the human brain. Science, *106*:349, 1947.)

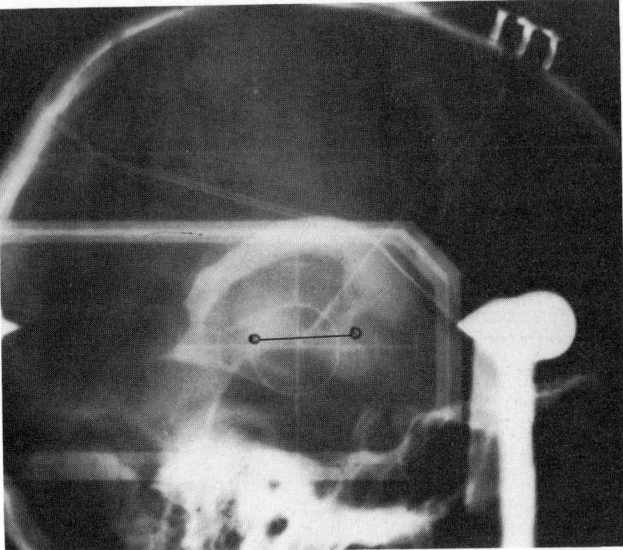

Figure 3. Positive contrast ventriculogram filmed in the Todd-Wells stereotactic frame showing the lateral projection of the third ventricles and anterior and posterior commissure landmarks (circled), as well as a stimulation electrode (deep brain stimulation, for pain) at the midpoint of the anterior-posterior commissure line in the hypothalamus.

evoked electrical responses produced by the stimulation of a peripheral nerve have been employed for localization within sensory areas of the central nervous system.[17,22]

The most ideal techniques for producing a therapeutic lesion in the central nervous system of man have been thermocouple-monitored radiofrequency thermal coagulation or freezing coagulation.[13]

Functional Stereotactic Surgical Indications

Current indications for functional stereotactic intervention remain patients with Parkinson's disease with hemiparkinsonism, severe tremor, or tremor without rigidity, levodopa-in-

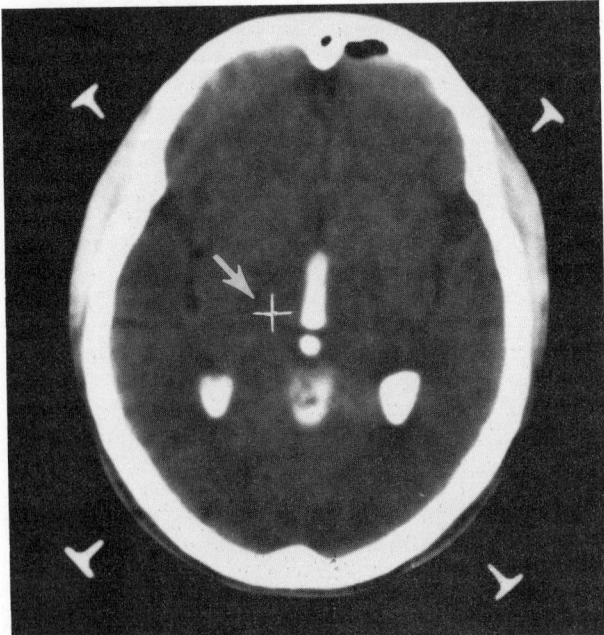

Figure 4. CT localization of the (V.im) ventral lateral nucleus of the thalamus (cursor). Note coordinates obtained with positive contrast in the third ventricle. CT gantry angle in the horizontal plane of the anterior and posterior commissures. The posterior commissure is visible. Treatment of Parkinson's tremor.[11]

duced dyskinesia, asymmetric symptoms, or unsatisfactory treatment with medication. Patients with persistent hemiballismus, although rare, and essential tremor may benefit from lesions designed to interrupt pallidothalamic pathways or tremor generators from the ventrobasal thalamus. Tremor or unilateral rigidity as the major disabling symptom can be permanently and reliably arrested by such a therapeutic lesion in the ventrobasal complex of the thalamus. Other hyperkinetic disorders such as athetosis, chorea, dystonia, and spasmodic torticollis may be successfully alleviated by similar stereotactic lesions, although the therapeutic target may differ.[8,13,18,22]

Stereotactic procedures have also been used for the treatment of psychiatric disorders recalcitrant to conventional therapy including obsessive-compulsive psychosis, oligophrenic aggressive or manic disorders, or paroxysmal behavioral outbursts, especially when associated with electroencephalographic abnormalities or seizures.[13,15,22,23] The use of stereotactic methods for the control of intractable pain has grown with understanding of neurophysiology and neuropharmacology. Placement of electrodes into the hypothalamus (Fig. 3) or into the periaqueductal-gray area of the upper midbrain can be effective treatment for pain of somatic origin. The pain relief, which lasts hours after a brief period of stimulation, is thought by some to be based on release of endorphin into the surrounding reticular areas of the brain.[8,10,12] For deafferentation or neurogenic pain, electrodes are usually placed within the sensory regions (ventroposterolateral, ventroposteromedial) of the thalamus or internal capsule.[8,22] Externally programmable, totally implanted generators (similar to cardiac pacemakers) are employed. This general method is referred to as stimulation-induced analgesia or deep brain stimulation. High-frequency intense stimulation may cause strong emotional responses, whereas low-intensity stimulation can be subliminal and still provide good analgesia.[10,12] Interestingly, lesions in some of these same areas may also provide pain relief, without producing any numbness on the surface of the body or decreased sensation in the affected area.[20,21]

The use of chronically implanted depth electrodes for diagnostic awake recording in complex-partial seizures often identifies deep epileptogenic foci, which may be followed by temporal lobectomy with marked improvement. Some successful attempts have also been made to use stereotactic lesions in order to interrupt pathways or structures thought to propagate seizures.[13,20,22,23]

Image-Guided and Computer-Simulated Stereotactic Principles and Methods

In the early 1980s, stereotactic neurosurgeons quickly modified their procedures and conventional stereotactic frames to couple with CT scan measurements of targets.[5,8] This transition has been followed by development of CT- and MRI-compatible stereotactic instruments with localizing attachments that are scanned after being placed on the patient's head. Because of the inherent compatibility of the cartesian coordinate system of the stereotactic method and the accurate orthogonal CT or MRI data, each point in the intracranial space can be co-defined. By use of the CT- or MRI-provided software for measurements or data collection, the target may be localized by measurement or computation (Fig. 4).[1,7,8,13]

Indications for CT-Guided Stereotactic Surgery

Numerous indications for CT- and MRI-guided stereotactic neurosurgery have developed in the decade since its introduction. These include biopsy of primary and metastatic tumors, drainage of abscesses and cysts, evacuation of intracerebral hematomas, tissue transplantation, endoscopy, implantation of multiple afterloading catheters for interstitial radiation (brachytherapy), or hyperthermia.[6,8,11,25] Localization for laser resection or for craniotomy and, finally, localization for linear accelerator or proton beam radiotherapy and focused gamma emission radiosurgery have all been applied using stereotactic instruments and principles.[6,8,14]

The most common stereotactic procedures are for biopsy of intraparenchymal mass lesions initially identified by CT or MRI studies. Large series have reported a diagnostic rate greater than 90 per cent. These procedures can be undertaken under local anesthesia and are especially appropriate to minimize morbidity, diminish postoperative convalescence in hospital, and end treatment delays for several groups of patients including those with primary malignant brain tumors. For benign lesions such as colloid cysts of the third ventricle, cyst aspiration may be curative, whereas aspiration of pus from an abscess followed by appropriate antibiotics often proves adequate therapy. Similarly, evacuation of intracerebral hematomas, with or without the instillation of urokinase, and serial drain aspiration is another common operation.[1,8,13]

Radiobrachytherapy via stereotactically implanted arrays of afterloading cannulas (Fig. 5), combined with geometrical dosimetry simulation for catheter placement and treatment planning (Fig. 6), is becoming increasingly important in the management of malignant gliomas.[6,8,16] From a radiobiological standpoint, large doses of radiation in the range of 60 Gy can be administered using ^{192}iridium to a target volume (e.g., incorporating a 1- to 2-cm. border around an enhancing tumor) delivering a protracted dose over 24 to 96 hours through cell cycle–sensitive phases (M, G2). Hyperthermia may be used in conjunction with brachytherapy by the use of ferromagnetic induction to heat metallic seeds implanted through the same array of catheters as the ^{192}iridium. Hyperthermia compensates for the shortcoming of radiation by being effective at low pH and during the radioinsensitive S-phase. In addition, there are roles for immunotherapy, chemotherapy, and phototherapy using stereotactic methods.[8,25]

Complications of these methods include intraparenchymal bleeding, infection, and increased neurologic deficits due to local damage or to exacerbation of mass effect.[19] An overall morbidity in the range of 5 per cent occurs, but can be expected

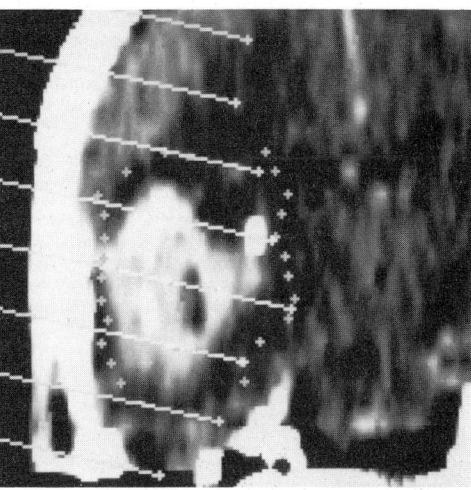

Figure 6. Computer three-dimensional simulation of a multiple catheter array for interstitial radiotherapy/hyperthermia treatment of a glioblastoma.[16,22,25]

to vary with the extent of the procedure and preoperative condition of the patient.[8] Preoperative evaluation of the patient should be as extensive as that for a craniotomy (which may follow on a routine or emergent basis) and include a bleeding time and coagulation studies. Attention to detail including scalp stitches to preclude cerebrospinal fluid leak should be emphasized. In patients with significant mass effect, care should be taken with regard to fluids and steroid doses.

Future Directions

The field of stereotactic technique is being widely incorporated into general neurosurgery and radiation therapy.[8] Stereotactic radiosurgery can deliver externally directed gamma radiation, particles such as protons, or x-rays produced by a linear accelerator to restricted volumes of intracranial lesions in such a way as to produce focal tissue destruction, the result of which is analogous to surgical resection. Pioneering work has been accomplished to extract tumor boundaries from CT and MRI data and allow the reconstructed target volume (tumor) to be resected by a stereotactically directed CO_2 laser, mechanically directed and computer monitored in three-dimensional space.[8,14] Stereotactic devices can be automatically robotically controlled, and stereotactic guiding systems have been developed using robotic arms for precise tumor resection during craniotomies.[8] By using computer graphics, spatial transformations make it possible to simulate target volumes and for multiple cannula trajectories (Fig. 6) in order to plan treatment volumes, rather than points.[16] In summary, future possibilities for stereotactic surgery based on computer technology are likely to further improve our access and treatment of difficult problems involving the central nervous system.

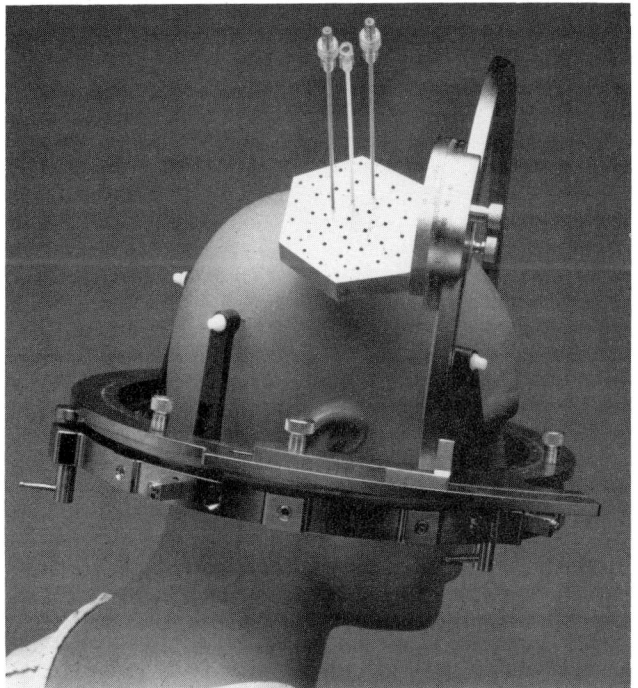

Figure 5. Brown-Roberts-Wells CT frame fixed to a manikin to demonstrate template and multiple catheter array for combination interstitial radiotherapy and hyperthermia for treatment of glioblastoma.[16,22,25]

SELECTED REFERENCES

Heilbrun, M. P. (Ed.): Stereotactic Neurosurgery. (Concepts in Neurosurgery, Vol. 2.) Baltimore, Williams & Wilkins, 1988.
  This monograph presents the theory and practice of modern stereotactic surgery in a clear and understandable manner. The 16 chapters are excellent in-depth contributions from many of the original innovators on every currently important area of stereotactics. The extensive number of illustrations and references, which are current and extremely useful, make this book a classic resource for everyone interested in stereotactics from medical students to practicing neurosurgeons.

Heilbrun, M. P., Roberts, T. S., Apuzzo, M. L. J., Wells, T., and Sabshin, J. K.: Preliminary experience with Brown-Roberts-Wells (BRW) Computerized Tomography Stereotaxic Guidance System. J. Neurosurg., 59:217, 1983.
  An important paper documenting one of the initial methods of application and results of CT-guided stereotactic surgery by the team responsible for the design, development, and popularization of a currently widely used system.

Kandel, E. I.: Functional and Stereotactic Neurosurgery. New York, Plenum, 1989.
This extensive new text reviews the anatomy and pathophysiology of all functional stereotactic neurosurgical problems in detail. The descriptions of the stereotactic methods and techniques used to solve these problems, including their historical development by the international figures involved, provides a fascinating and useful in-depth perspective of stereotactics.

Schaltenbrand, G., and Walker, A. E.: Stereotaxy of the Human Brain. Anatomical, Physiological and Clinical Applications, 2nd ed. New York, Georg Thieme Verlag/Thieme-Stratton, 1982.
This reference textbook contains the most rigorous information on the scientific rationale for stereotaxis. Much of the data presented on functional neuroanatomy and neurophysiology is based on human observations acquired during therapeutic procedures and as such cannot be found in standard neuroanatomy or physiology texts. An extremely important book for understanding accessible dimensions of the human brain.

REFERENCES

1. Apuzzo, M. L. J., and Sabshin, J. K.: Computed tomographic guidance stereotaxis in the management of intracranial mass lesions. Neurosurgery, 12:277, 1983.
2. Clarke, R. H., and Horsley, V.: On a method of investigating the deep ganglia and tracts of the central nervous system. Br. Med. J., 2:1799, 1906.
3. Cooper, I.S.: Clinical and physiologic implications of thalamic surgery for dystonia and torticollis. Bull. N.Y. Acad. Med., 41:870, 1965.
4. Gildenberg, P. L.: Survey of stereotactic and functional neurosurgery in the U.S. and Canada. Appl. Neurophysiol., 38:31, 1975.
5. Gildenberg, P. L., and Kaufman, H. H.: Direct calculation of stereotactic coordinates from CT scans. Appl. Neurophysiol., 45:347, 1982.
6. Gutin, P. H., Phillips, T. L., Ward, W. M., Leibel, S. A., Hosobuchi, Y., Levin, V. A., Weaver, K. A., and Lamb, S.: Brachytherapy of recurrent malignant brain tumors with removable high-activity iodine-125 sources. J. Neurosurg., 60:61, 1984.
7. Hariz, M. I., and Bergenheim, A. T.: A comparative study on the ventriculographic and CT-guided determination of brain targets in functional stereotactic surgery. J Neurosurg, 73:565, 1990.
8. Heilbrun, P. M. (Ed.): Stereotactic Neurosurgery. (Concepts in Neurosurgery, Vol. 2.) Baltimore, Williams & Wilkins, 1988.
9. Horsley, V., and Clarke, R. H.: The structure and functions of the cerebellum examined by a new method. Brain, 31:45, 1908.
10. Hosobuchi, Y.: Subcortical electrical stimulation for control of intractable pain in humans. J. Neurosurg, 64:543, 1986.
11. Iacono, R. P.: Multiple fetal brain transplantations for Parkinson's disease. Unpublished data.
12. Iacono, R. P., and Nashold, B. S., Jr.: Mental and behavioral effects of brain stem and hypothalamic stimulation in man. Hum. Neurobiol., 1:273, 1982.
13. Kandel, E. I.: Functional and Stereotactic Neurosurgery. New York, Plenum, 1989.
14. Kelly, P. J.: Stereotactic technology in tumor surgery. Clin. Neurosurg., 35:215, 1989.
15. Laitinen, L. V.: Psychosurgery today. Acta Neurochir. (Suppl.), 44: 158, 1988.
16. Lulu, B. A., Lutz, W., Stea, B., and Cetas, T. C.: Treatment planning of template-guided stereotactic brain implants. Int. J. Radiat. Oncol. Biol. Phys., 18:951, 1990.
17. Morioka, T., Shima, F., Kato, M., and Fukui, M.: Origin and distribution of thalamic somatosensory evoked potentials in humans. (Electroencephalography and Clinical Neurophysiology, 74:186.) Ireland, Elsevier Scientific Publishers, 1989.
18. Narabayashi, H., Maeda, T., and Yokochi, F.: Long-term follow-up study of nucleus ventralis intermedius and ventrolateralis thalamotomy using a microelectrode technique in parkinsonism. Appl. Neurophysiol., 50:330, 1987.
19. Nashold, B. S., Jr.: Operative complications due to stereotactic surgery. Confin. Neurol., 30:325, 1968.
20. Nashold, B. S., Jr., Wilson, W. P., and Boone, E.: Depth recording and stimulation of the human brain: Twenty year experience. In Rasmussen, T. (Ed.): Functional Neurosurgery. New York, Raven Press, 1979, pp. 181–195.
21. Nashold, B. S., Jr., Wilson, W. P., and Slaughter, D. G.: Stereotactic midbrain lesions for central dysesthesia and phantom pain. J. Neurosurg., 30:116, 1969.
22. Schaltenbrand, G., and Walker, A. E.: Stereotaxy of the Human Brain. Anatomical, Physiological and Clinical Applications. New York, Georg Thieme Verlag/Thieme-Stratton, 1982.
23. Spiegel, E. A., and Wycis, H. T.: Stereoencephalotomy. Part II. Clinical and Physiological Applications. New York, Grune & Stratton, 1962.
24. Spiegel, E. A., Wycis, H. T., Marks, M., and Lee, A. J.: Stereotaxic apparatus for operations on the human brain. Science, 106:349, 1947.
25. Stea, B., Cetas, T. C., Cassady, J. R., Guthkelch, A. N., Iacono, R., Lulu, B., Lutz, W., Obbens, E., Rossman, K., Seeger, J., Shetter, A., and Shimm, D. S.: Interstitial thermoradiotherapy of brain tumors: Preliminary results of a phase I clinical trial. Int. J. Radiat. Oncol. Biol. Phys, 19:1463, 1990.

42

FRACTURES AND DISLOCATIONS

GENERAL PRINCIPLES

John M. Harrelson, M.D., and John A. Feagin, M.D.

> There is no class of injuries which a practitioner approaches with more doubt and misgiving than fractures, or one which demands a greater amount of ready knowledge, self reliance, and consummate skill.
>
> *Samuel D. Gross, 1882*[1]

The treatment of fractures and dislocations requires a knowledge of the anatomy, physiology, and biomechanics of the musculoskeletal system. Although a fracture represents a disruption in the continuity of a bone, it also represents a major soft tissue injury. The surgeon must be aware of the soft tissue structures adjacent to a fracture site and be particularly alert for neurologic and vascular components of the injury. Because many fractures occur in a setting of violent trauma, complete evaluation of each patient is necessary, and the surgeon must be prepared to consider major injuries in other tissue systems.

Mechanism and Classification of Fractures

Sufficient force applied to a bone causes fracture. A single fracture line is referred to as a *simple* fracture. When multiple fracture lines and bone fragments exist, the fracture is said to be *comminuted.* Penetrating injury producing a fracture or fracture fragments protruding through the skin constitute an *open* fracture. When no such wound is present, the fracture is classified as *closed* (Fig. 1). These distinctions are important because open fractures are likely to be contaminated with pyogenic bacteria. The treatment and prognosis of open fractures are significantly different from those of closed fractures.

The force necessary to produce a fracture may be transmitted to the skeleton in a variety of ways. The direction and rate of application of the force govern, to some extent, the pattern of the fracture and the associated soft tissue injury. A bending moment applied to bone usually produces a simple transverse or oblique fracture line. When a direct blow or crushing force is applied to bone, a comminuted, open fracture often results, accompanied by severe soft tissue injury. Torque force applied to bone produces a spiral or oblique fracture. Compression forces applied along the longitudinal axis of the bone cause an impacted fracture at the junction between the metaphysis and the diaphysis where the cortex becomes thin, with the diaphyseal portion of the bone usually impacted into the metaphyseal fragment. Traction force applied to a bone may also produce fracture. Vigorous or violent muscle contraction may produce avulsion of portions of bone where major tendons attach.

Fractures in children deserve special consideration. The periosteum is extremely strong in children; children's bones are much more resilient and less brittle than those of adults. Bending moments applied to the bone of a child may cause a greenstick fracture, in which there is distraction of the cortex on the convex side and compression of bone on the concave side. There is angulation at the fracture site but no other displacement. Fractures may occur through the physeal plates and cause future growth disturbance. The parents accordingly should be cautioned. When fracture occurs entirely within the physeal plate and there is no displacement of the epiphysis relative to the metaphysis, anatomic reduction produces good results with no disturbance in growth. When the fracture line extends part way through the physeal plate and then through either the adjacent metaphysis or the epiphysis, accurate anatomic reduction is mandatory to avoid future growth disturbance. When compression forces have produced a fracture across the physeal plate, growth disturbance is a likely result.

More subtle trauma may also produce fractures. In the elderly patient with osteoporosis or in the patient with a metabolic bone-wasting disease, the activities of daily living may be sufficient to produce fracture in diseased bone. Such injuries are referred to as *pathologic fractures.* The most common causes of pathologic fracture are osteoporosis and metastatic carcinoma. Fracture may occur through a deposit of tumor or weakened bone. Healthy bone may fracture with the repetitive application of minor trauma. Such fractures are called *fatigue* or *stress* fracture and may be seen in the metatarsals after a long hike or in the tibia, fibula, femur, or other skeletal locations in individuals involved in regular athletic activities.

Acute Complications

Following fracture, bleeding from the bone ends and the adjacent soft tissues produces a rapidly enlarging hematoma that envelops the fracture site. Because most fractures occur following significant force, the bone ends are frequently displaced. This displacement is increased by the pull of those muscles that cross the fracture site and may further increase the extent of soft tissue injury.

The initial evaluation of the fracture patient requires a careful neurologic and vascular examination. The proximity of major nerves to bone makes them vulnerable to injury from adjacent fracture fragments. Direct arterial injury may also occur following penetration by a sharp bone fragment. More often, vascular insufficiency of a fractured limb is caused by swelling from the fracture hematoma with compression of adjacent vessels. Bleeding within a closed compartment may cause muscle ischemia progressing to eventual muscle necrosis. This situation particularly exists with bleeding into the anterior compartment of the leg or into the volar compartment of the forearm. The surgeon must be aware of these syndromes and be prepared to do a decompressive fasciotomy.

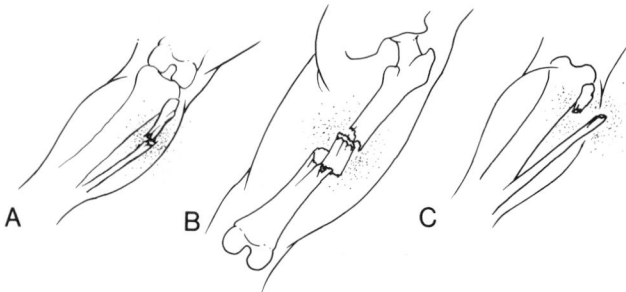

Figure 1. *A,* Closed simple fracture of the fibula. *B,* Closed, comminuted fracture of the femur. *C,* Open fracture of the fibula.

Adjacent organ injury may occur with certain fractures. Fractures of the rib cage may rupture the lung, produce lacerations of the liver, or penetrate the spleen. Fractures of the pelvis, particularly those in which there is disruption of the symphysis pubis, may rupture the bladder. Spinal fracture introduces the risk of injury to the spinal cord. Bleeding from spinal fractures into the retroperitoneal space may produce a temporary paralytic ileus. With fractures of the femur or pelvis or with multiple fractures, the hemorrhage at the fracture sites may be sufficient to produce hypovolemic shock.

In a small number of patients with fractures, the syndrome of *fat embolization* occurs. This respiratory complication is most frequently seen in patients who have been in hypovolemic shock. The earliest clinical signs of a developing syndrome are rising pulse and respiratory rates, and they may occur within the first 12 to 72 hours following injury. Tachypnea and dyspnea occur following decreasing pulmonary function. Petechiae over the chest and abdomen are a transient finding. Confusion and delirium progressing to coma without associated localized neurologic signs may ensue. These cerebral changes are the direct result of a decreasing arterial Po_2. Chest films in these patients demonstrate diffuse, patchy infiltrates throughout both lungs, the urine may show free fat particles, and the serum lipase may be elevated. Early recognition of a developing fat embolization syndrome is essential. The symptoms may be sudden in onset with rapid, fatal deterioration. A falling arterial Po_2 is a sensitive indicator of impending problems. Monitoring by pulse oximetry or the drawing of arterial blood gases daily for the first few days after injury in patients with major skeletal trauma allows early recognition and treatment. Large doses of corticosteroids, with supplemental oxygen administered by tent, intubation, or tracheostomy as necessary, are usually of value. A volume respirator may be necessary.

Fracture Reduction

Fractures are displaced as a result of etiologic trauma, the pull of muscles crossing the fracture site, or both. The first step in reducing a displaced fracture is to relieve the patient of pain, by either local anesthetic injection or systemic analgesics. It is then necessary to overcome the spasm of those muscles bridging the fracture site, allowing restoration of length of the fractured member and correction of angulation and rotation. The reduction of a fracture may be accomplished in several ways.

Manipulative reduction can be accomplished in fractures of the distal portion of the extremities, in which it is possible to manually overcome the pull of those muscles bridging the fracture site. When the fracture is more proximal (humerus, femur), muscle spasm is too great for manipulative reduction. In this situation, it may be necessary to apply continuous *traction* by inserting a transverse pin distal to the fracture site and placing the patient in bed with continuous pull on the pin. As muscle spasm is gradually overcome, length is restored and alignment is achieved. It is sometimes acceptable to use skin traction by applying strips of felt to the extremity with adhesive and attaching them to the appropriate amount of weight. Some fractures

are not appropriately treated by manipulative reduction or traction. Such fractures may require surgical therapy and *open reduction.* When open reduction is required, it is usually accompanied by some form of internal fixation of the fracture. Fractures that are inherently stable and in acceptable alignment require no reduction.

The goal of reduction is restoration of length of the extremity, correction of angulation and rotation, and apposition of the bone ends. Once reduction has been accomplished, fracture healing requires that the bone be immobilized.

Some fractures require excision of a portion of bone rather than reduction and immobilization. Comminuted fractures of the patella are appropriately treated by excision of the patella and repair of the patellar tendon rather than by attempts at reduction. Fractures of the radial head with severe comminution of the articular surface are best treated by excision of the radial head and replacement with a prosthesis. In both these situations, excision is performed to avoid a painful, irregular articular surface. *Prosthetic replacement* may be required in fractures of the neck of the femur in elderly patients. In this situation, the articular surface is not comminuted. Rather, healing is prolonged in these fractures and the circulation to the femoral head is disrupted. Rehabilitation of the elderly patient may be significantly shortened by prosthetic replacement.

Immobilization

Impacted fractures with inherent stability may require only a sling or soft dressing for comfort. Fractures requiring operative reduction because of instability or inability to achieve or maintain closed reduction also require internal fixation. Techniques of internal fixation are discussed in sections that follow. Most fractures of the extremities can be appropriately treated by plaster immobilization. Although the many advantages of plaster are well recognized, it should be borne in mind that improperly applied plaster may create more injury than it treats. The surgeon should be familiar with proper plaster technique. The cast should be appropriately padded and smooth on its inner surface and should not be constricting.

Because a bone participates in joint motion at both ends, it is necessary to immobilize the joint above and below the fracture site. Thus, forearm fractures require long-arm plaster immobilization of both the wrist and the elbow. Plaster maintains the reduction that has been achieved, provides rigid immobility, and relieves pain. A well-reduced, rigidly immobilized fracture should not require a significant amount of analgesic. Swelling occurs at a fracture site and, because a plaster cast is rigid, increasing pressure within the cast is heralded by increasing pain in the extremity and progressive numbness and diminished circulation of the digits. All patients with fracture are cautioned to watch for these signs; they should be examined promptly for assessment of the cast and the neurovascular status upon increasing pain, numbness, or diminished circulation of the digits.

Skeletal traction is used not only to achieve reduction of fractures but also to maintain relative immobilization of the fracture. The injured part is placed at rest either on an appropriate splint or on the bed while traction is being applied. Traction is continued until the fracture is stable enough to allow cast or brace immobilization.

Open Fractures

An open fracture should be treated as an emergency. Surgical débridement of the wound is required. Because open fractures usually follow more violent trauma, other major injuries may be present. When the patient has been fully evaluated and the condition is stable, *débridement* is performed in the operating room as a formal surgical procedure. All devitalized tissue is removed, with special attention given to devitalized muscle.

Macerated skin edges are débrided and the wound is thoroughly irrigated with saline-containing antibiotics. Fascia that is constricting should be released and bone ends, which may have embedded debris, are débrided by sharp dissection, with care taken to preserve nerves, vessels, and tendons. Repair of nerves and tendons in an open fracture wound is rarely indicated. Vessels require repair if the circulation to the extremity is in jeopardy. When débridement is completed, a decision must be made about stabilization of the fracture. Although some unstable fractures may require internal fixation devices, the immediate use of such devices is generally not desirable in a contaminated wound. Skeletal traction with a transverse pin placed at some distance from the fracture, cast immobilization with a window overlying the wound, or delayed internal fixation may be used. A decision must also be made regarding wound closure. When minimal penetration of the skin has occurred, no foreign body contamination is present, and no significant muscle injury is encountered, wound closure may be acceptable. If there is *any* question regarding viability of muscle tissue or degree of contamination, the wound should be dressed open. The morbidity from delayed closure at 3 to 5 days following débridement is minimal compared with the consequences of infection. Intravenous antibiotics are administered during débridement, and cultures of the wound should be obtained at the time of delayed closure. When extensive skin loss has occurred, split-thickness grafting or pedicle or free-flap grafting may be required.

Fracture Healing

Following fracture, a hematoma rapidly develops about the bone ends. As pressure from the hematoma increases, interstitial edema develops in the adjacent soft tissues, and there is some degree of venous congestion. Leukocytes invade the hematoma, producing a sterile traumatic inflammatory reaction. Primitive mesenchymal cells within the periosteum and the medullary canal differentiate into primitive osteoblasts and proliferate. These changes are appreciated microscopically at 48 to 72 hours. At this time, there is also development of early granulation tissue about the periphery of the hematoma. This granulation tissue contains other primitive cells from adjacent fascial planes, which also differentiate into osteoblasts. This proliferation of osteogenic cells and the early primitive bone that they produce constitute the *fracture callus*. If the fracture fragments are in apposition and rigidly immobilized, bone growth progresses until the two fracture fragments are united by a network of primitive new bone. As this bone matures, constant remodeling occurs and the trabeculae become oriented to the long axis of the bone.

If there is motion at the fracture site, the primitive mesenchymal cells may differentiate into chondroblasts. If the motion is not excessive or if the fracture site is subsequently rigidly immobilized, this cartilaginous tissue calcifies and is gradually replaced by new bone by the process of endochondral ossification. When distraction of the fracture fragments is present or when muscle is interposed between the fracture fragments, dense fibrous tissue develops between the bone ends. Again, if rigid immobilization is achieved, this fibrous tissue may ultimately be replaced by bone. If in the latter two situations rigid immobilization is not achieved, nonunion results. When motion is persistent at the fracture site, the differentiation of cartilage progresses. A cleft develops between the layers of cartilage covering each fracture fragment, and cells at the periphery of this cleft differentiate into synovial cells, producing a *pseudarthrosis*. If distraction at the fracture site is allowed to persist, a dense fibrous scar develops between the bone ends, producing a *fibrous nonunion*.

Compression of a fracture enhances fracture healing. This principle is used in treatment. Fractures of the tibial shaft may be treated in a walking cast, allowing the patient to bear weight across the fracture site. The compression principle also may be used with internal fixation devices.

Fracture healing is also affected by the available blood supply. In general, cancellous bone at the metaphyseal ends of long bones has a richer blood supply than the diaphysis; fractures in these areas heal more rapidly than shaft fractures. Long bones with more overlying muscle have a greater blood supply. The shaft of the femur, enveloped by muscle, has a better blood supply than the distal tibia, which is subcutaneous in one third of its circumference. Fractures of the tibial shaft traditionally are slower to heal.

Late Complications

The soft tissue injury that accompanies a fracture causes scarring of the adjacent muscles, ligaments, and tendons and produces limitation of motion of the joints adjacent to the fracture. Fractures occurring close to a joint produce more limitation of motion than fractures of the midshaft. Restoration of joint motion involves rehabilitation of the soft tissues. Physical therapy in the form of active and passive exercises may be necessary. Tendons may become adherent to the underlying bone, and subsequent surgical release may be necessary. Because of the muscle atrophy that follows inactivity, stasis edema is usually present after fracture and gradually diminishes as muscle tone and strength return.

Nonunion of a fracture, either as a pseudarthrosis or a fibrous nonunion, may develop for the reasons mentioned. When an established nonunion is present, operative intervention is usually indicated. Surgical removal of the fibrocartilage or scar tissue that has formed at the fracture site and apposition of fresh bone ends are necessary. It is desirable to bone graft the nonunion at the time of surgical therapy. Bone is obtained from the patient (autogenous) or from a donor (homologous). The bone graft serves as a mineral lattice for new bone formation and becomes incorporated in the fracture callus. It is gradually replaced by osteoclastic resorption and subsequent new bone deposition, a process known as "creeping substitution." In recent years, electrical stimulation of delayed union or nonunion by externally applied coils or implanted electrodes has resulted in healing without surgical intervention.

When a fracture heals with unacceptable angulation or rotation, a *malunion* has occurred. The disability from malunion may be immediately apparent (rotatory malalignment of a forearm fracture, which limits pronation and supination) or may not develop for some time (valgus malalignment of a distal tibial fracture producing subsequent degenerative arthritis of the ankle). Malunion may require surgical intervention. Osteotomy is performed at either the old fracture site or at a more appropriate level, and the angular or rotary deformity is corrected. In almost all fractures, some degree of shortening occurs. In the upper extremities, shortening is seldom noticeable and is rarely a functional disability. In the lower extremities, if shortening exceeds 0.5 inch, a shoe lift may be required. In children, fracture may cause stimulation of the physeal growth plates throughout the involved extremity, and overgrowth of that extremity may occur. In some fractures, there is loss of circulation to the involved bone, with subsequent *avascular necrosis*. This situation occurs in fractures of the femoral neck in the elderly patient, in fracture-dislocations of the talus in any age group, and in fracture through the waist of the carpal navicular bone. Avascular necrosis usually causes collapse of the articular surface of the involved bone and the development of subsequent degenerative arthritis.

Fractures that involve articular surfaces may eventually cause *traumatic arthritis*. Even with accurate anatomic reduction, the process of healing may produce irregularities on the cartilaginous surface, with in-growth of fibrous tissue, fracture callus, or both. Once the congruity of the joint has been lost, gradual deterioration usually occurs. The rate at which degenerative arthritis develops depends upon the degree of incongruity, the age and activity level of the patient, and the amount of injury to the articular surface at the time of fracture.

SUMMARY

The purpose of this section has been to emphasize the principles of fracture care and associated soft tissue management. Specific fracture treatments are discussed in sections that follow. The primary principles emphasized in this section were

1. An appreciation of fracture mechanics, and a description of the fracture—i.e., simple, comminuted, open, closed.

2. The evaluation and treatment of adjacent soft tissue injury to include vascular, nerve, ligament, muscle, fascia, and skin.

3. The avoidance of local wound complications by appropriate débridement, fasciotomy, immobilization, and antibiotics.

4. The avoidance of systemic complications by recognizing and treating associated injuries, hypovolemia, and fat embolization promptly and appropriately.

5. That open fractures are an emergency and require formal surgical debridement.

6. That fracture healing proceeds most expeditiously with compression and function.

7. That late complications, such as nonunion, malunion, or traumatic arthritis, may require reconstructive surgery, such as bone graft, osteotomy, or joint mobilization.

8. That new methods of fracture immobilization, such as improved intermedullary fixation, the AO system, and the Ilizarov system, require special skills but are based on the premise that constant compression and early function enhance healing. These methods extend the armamentarium of the fracture surgeon, particularly in the restitution of multiply injured patients.

SELECTED REFERENCES

Bick, E. M.: Primitive man and ancient practice. *In* Source Book of Orthopaedics. New York, Hafner Publishing Company, 1968.
   A superb historical perspective of fracture care referenced in a definitive text relating the development of the specialty of orthopaedics.

Chapman, M. W.: Operative Orthopaedics, Vols. 1–4. Philadelphia, J. B. Lippincott Company, 1988.
   A current and complete textbook of operative orthopaedics—well referenced.

Charnley, J.: The Closed Treatment of Common Fractures, 3rd ed. Baltimore, Williams & Wilkins, 1963.
   An unparalleled, historical classic, which provides an anatomic basis for nonoperative treatment of a selected group of fractures.

Evarts, C. M.: Surgery of the Musculoskeletal System, 2nd ed., Vols. 1–4. New York, Churchill Livingstone, 1989.
   An excellent reference for surgical treatment of the musculoskeletal system; includes diagnosis, treatment, pathophysiology, and appropriate references.

Muller, M. E., et al.: Manual of Internal Fixation; Techniques Recommended by the AO Group, 2nd ed. New York, Springer-Verlag, 1979.
   The techniques recommended by the AO Group (the Association for the Study of the Problems of Internal Fixation).

Rockwood, C. A., and Green, D. P.: Fractures in Adults, 2nd ed., Vols. 1 and 2. Philadelphia, J. B. Lippincott Company, 1984.
   The definitive fracture text for orthopedic surgery. An in-depth discussion of the diagnosis, treatment, pitfalls, and outcome of adult fractures. Excellent references. Each section includes the author's preferred method of treatment for that fracture. A very useful reference.

Rockwood, C. A., Wilkins, K., and King, R. E.: Fractures in Children. Vol. 3. Philadelphia, J. B. Lippincott Company, 1984.
   An excellent reference for children's fractures. Current standard of treatment and appropriate references.

REFERENCE

1. Gross, S. D.: A System of Surgery: Pathologic, Diagnostic, and Operative, Vol. 2, 6th ed. Philadelphia, Henry C. Lea's Son and Company, 1882, p. 894.

II

FRACTURES OF THE SPINE

William T. Hardaker, Jr., M.D., and William J. Richardson, M.D.

The diagnosis of fracture of the spine ("broken neck" or "broken back") is terrifying to the patient and the family. When the fracture is associated with concomitant spinal cord injury, it represents one of the most physically disabling and economically devastating conditions seen in modern medicine. Few events can be more tragic than a vigorous young adult who has been rendered para- or quadriplegic and will very likely remain forever dependent upon others for assistance in the activities of daily living.

Statistics regarding the precise incidence of spine injuries and their economic consequences are incomplete. Approximately 10,000 such injuries occur yearly within the the United States. Fifty per cent of these injuries occur in individuals 23 years of age or younger. The economic consequences of such injuries are enormous. The cost to society for the lifetime care of spinal cord–injured patients may approach 800 million dollars yearly. Although these figures represent estimates, they do not include the cost of care of people with spinal injuries without attendant cord injury.

Fortunately, although fractures of the vertebral column are common, less than 10 per cent of spine fractures are associated with neurologic deficit. Because the majority of spine fractures involve primarily the skeletal structures, proper treatment can often lead to an excellent prognosis. Patients who present complaining of pain or tenderness in the neck or back following injury must be suspected of having a fracture of the spine until proven otherwise. The attending physician should determine the neurologic involvement in the initial assessment, because early neurologic status greatly influences both the course of treatment and the prognosis.

Trauma may subject the vertebral column to one or combinations of violent force including flexion, extension, axial compression, rotation, and shearing. If these forces produce motion greater than the physiologic range of the spine, a fracture or dislocation occurs. The spinal cord usually terminates between L1 and L2. In the cervical and thoracic spinal canal, it occupies approximately 50 per cent of the available space. In the lumbar area, the cauda equina is the only neural element within the canal and therefore more free space surrounds the neural tube. The anatomic relationship of the vertebral supporting structures, the neural elements, and the types of forces producing the injury determines the amount of displacement, stability, and neurologic involvement within a given spinal injury.

THE CERVICAL SPINE

When a patient complains of pain in the neck after an injury, a fracture or dislocation of the cervical spine should be suspected.

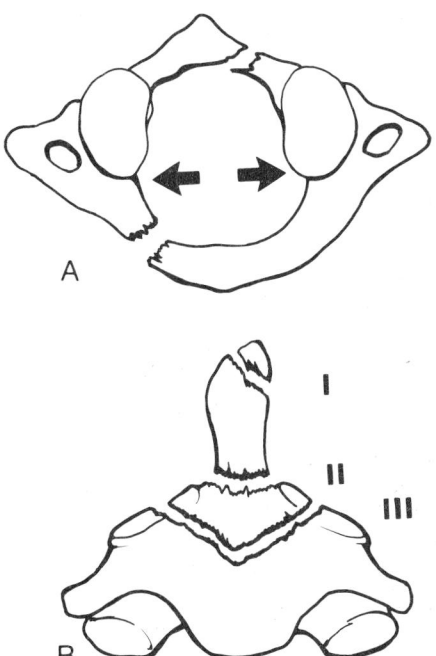

Figure 1. *A,* Jefferson fracture. Fractures of the arch of C1 are secondary to axial loads. The resultant of this force leads to expansion of the ring of C1 as indicated by the arrows, leading to a fracture of the narrow areas of the arch. *B,* Fractures of the odontoid may be Type I, oblique fracture of the tip of the odontoid process (dens); Type II, which occurs at the waist of the odontoid process; or Type III, which extends through the cancellous bone of the C2 vertebral body.

A careful history concerning the mechanism of injury is important. If tenderness is present about the cervical region, a complete neurologic examination is followed by cervical spine roentgenograms. The roentgenographic examination should define the fractures and determine if soft tissue swelling is present about the spinal column. Examination of plain films can often provide information on which to assess the stability of the spine. Plain films should include anteroposterior, lateral open-mouth odontoid, and trauma oblique views. The patient's head should not be moved for conventional oblique examinations. If these studies are negative, supervised general lateral flexion-extension views of the cervical spine may be obtained to exclude an unstable cervical spine secondary to soft tissue injury only. However, because of severe muscle spasm, this evaluation may be initially unreliable. If the patient has pain, tenderness, and decreased motion of the neck, or neurologic symptoms or signs, the cervical spine must be immobilized pending a more complete roentgenographic evaluation.

FRACTURE OF THE ATLAS (JEFFERSON'S FRACTURE). In 1920 Sir Geoffrey Jefferson described the mechanism of fracture of the first cervical vertebra. The injury occurs from an axial load on the top of the head. The resultant of the forces is exerted laterally on the ring of C1, and the arches fracture at the thinnest and weakest points (Fig. 1). Usually the spinal cord is not damaged, because the canal of the atlas is normally large, and, with fracture, the fragments spread outward to further increase the dimensions of the neural canal. The fracture can usually be diagnosed on the lateral cervical spine roentgenograms, but special plain films such as the submental vertex view may better delineate the injury. Computed tomography represents the best available roentgenographic study to evaluate the injury. If the results of the neurologic examination are normal, this injury can be managed in a four-poster brace (Fig. 2A). In situations of considerable instability, the halo-vest system is preferred (Fig. 2B).

FRACTURES OF THE ODONTOID. An understanding of the anatomic relationship of the first two cervical vertebrae is essential for a discussion of these injuries. Rotation of the atlas about the odontoid process of the axis represents about half of the rotatory movement of the head. The dens is held adjacent to the anterior arch of C1 by the transverse and alar ligaments. It is important to remember that the dens, spinal cord, and empty space each occupy approximately one third of the spinal canal at the arch of the atlas (the "rule of thirds"). On a lateral roentgenogram centered at C2, the predental space is 3 mm. or less in the adult. A predental space of greater than 5 mm. indicates rupture

Figure 2. *A,* A four-poster brace. The uprights and the chin piece and the occiput pad limit flexion and extension of the cervical spine, and the addition of the head band restricts rotation at C1–C2. The earlobe must be opposite the shoulder tip. *B,* Halo vest. The halo has four screws inserted into the outer table of the skull and provides very rigid external immobilization of the cervical spine. The halo may be used for cervical traction in the recumbent position or attached to a cast or body jacket lined with sheepskin. The patient may be ambulatory in the halo cast or vest.

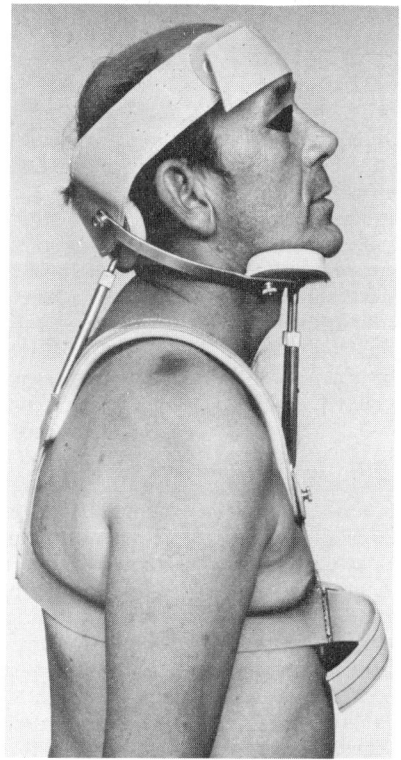

A

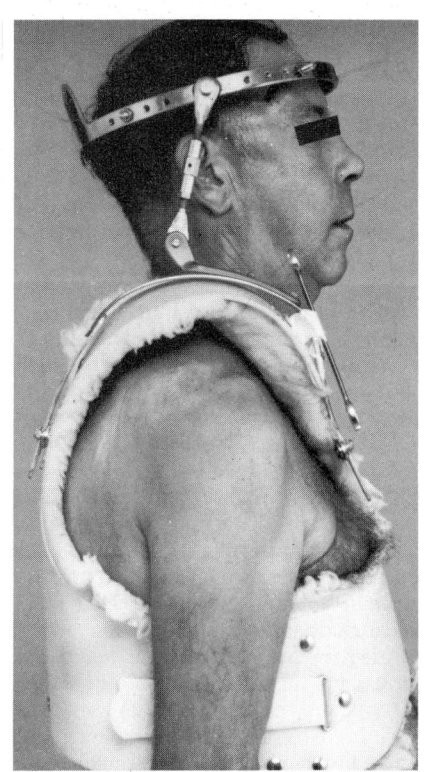

B

of the transverse ligaments, and a predental space of 12 mm. means that all ligaments about the dens have been ruptured.

Transverse or alar ligament ruptures are uncommon unless there are predisposing factors such as rheumatoid arthritis, posterior pharyngitis, or ankylosing spondylitis. If such a rupture occurs and the odontoid is intact, cervical myelopathy may be the presenting symptom.

Fractures of the odontoid (dens), however, occur relatively frequently and represent about 10 per cent of cervical spine fractures. Odontoid fractures as well as transverse ligament injuries occur following falls or blows to the head, in automobile accidents, and in sports such as gymnastics.

The diagnosis may be delayed because of difficulty in visualizing the dens on routine films. If the injured patient complains of neck or occipital pain or headaches, or has torticollis, the odontoid area should be examined thoroughly. Lateral views centered on the C2 vertebra and open-mouth views of the odontoid usually allow adequate visualization of the dens. However, tomograms in the anteroposterior and lateral views may be necessary to demonstrate the fracture.

Anderson and D'Alonzo have described three basic types of fractures based on the anatomic level of the injury. Type I fractures are oblique and occur at the extreme upper level of the odontoid process (dens). These injuries do not lead to gross instability of the first cervical vertebra in relation to the second. A hard cervical orthosis provides satisfactory stability of this fracture. Type II fractures occur through the junction of the odontoid process and the C2 vertebral body. Type II injuries are the most common odontoid fracture and should be considered unstable injuries. Type II odontoid fractures may have nonunion rates as high as 50 per cent if not treated effectively. Union occurs in most cases with prompt diagnosis, satisfactory reduction, and rigid external fixation. Operative arthrodesis using autogenous iliac bone grafts and wiring of C1 to C2 through a posterior approach is indicated if union is not achieved. Type III fractures extend through the cancellous bone of the C2 vertebral body. These injuries are rarely unstable and unite following 3 months of immobilization in a four-poster brace or halo-vest.

FRACTURE OF THE PEDICLES OF THE AXIS (HANGMAN'S FRACTURE). A fracture through the pedicles of C2 usually occurs from a severe extension injury, such as an automobile accident or fall. This injury has been labeled the "hangman's fracture" because autopsy studies have demonstrated that a long drop from a rope about the neck with a knot in the submental position produces a similar lesion. Frequently, the subjacent disc bond is broken, allowing varying degrees of anterior subluxation of C2 on C3 to occur. Cord compression is rare because the neural canal is enlarged with forward displacement of the body of C2. The posterior elements may rotate posteriorly, but generally remain in near anatomic alignment. Nonunion is uncommon in this fracture. If the injury is stable with little or no displacement, the four-poster brace is usually satisfactory treatment. In unstable circumstances, more rigid stabilization using the halo-vest may be required. Union usually occurs within 3 months with spontaneous anterior interbody fusion. Operative intervention to achieve stability is rarely required.

FRACTURES AND DISLOCATIONS OF C3 TO C7 VERTEBRAE. Fractures and dislocations of the lower cervical spine are common. The majority are caused by vehicular accidents, diving into shallow water, falls, and sports injuries. After the initial neurologic assessment, the patient with a suspected cervical spine injury should have completed roentgenograms. These should include study from the occiput down to the C7–T1 junction. Adequate roentgenographic studies in some obese or muscular patients may require traction on the patient's upper extremities, the swimmer's view, or tomography.

Fractures of the lower cervical spine may be stable or unstable and may involve injury to the spinal cord and/or nerve roots.

These fractures may follow the forces of flexion, extension, lateral bending, rotation, axial loads, or various combinations of these forces. The understanding of the mechanism of injury deduced from the analysis of the roentgenographic studies enables the physician to assess the stability of the cervical spine. Such information is paramount to selecting an appropriate method of treatment.

COMPRESSION FRACTURES OF THE CERVICAL VERTEBRAL BODIES. Compression fractures of the cervical vertebral bodies can follow flexion, axial loading, or coupling of these two forces. The injuries can range from very mild to severe in terms of neurologic involvement. If there is minimal comminution of the vertebral body and no dislocation of the facets, the fracture is usually stable. Rarely are such injuries associated with neurologic deficits. These injuries can be adequately stablized with minimal bracing such as a soft or hard cervical collar.

In contrast, comminuted "bursting" or "tear drop" fractures usually represent catastrophic injuries with a high association of significant spinal cord injury. These injuries are frequently caused by axial loading of the cervical spine with varying degrees of concomitant flexion. The fragments of the vertebral body are displaced posteriorly into the spinal canal, with resulting injury to the spinal cord. This fracture is grossly unstable and requires skull traction with the halo or similar device for reduction and then application of the halo-vest system for satisfactory stabilization. Immobilization may be necessary for 3 to 4 months. In patients with incomplete neurologic injury and evidence of compression of the neural elements, operative anterior decompression with interbody bone grafting may be indicated. Such decompressions should not be attempted until adequate external stabilization is provided by the halo-vest system or until posterior wire stabilization has been performed initially.

DISLOCATIONS OF THE CERVICAL SPINE. Dislocations of the cervical spine occur most commonly at the interspaces between C3 and C7. The C5–C6 level is most frequently involved. The injury is caused by a flexion-distraction force. These forces combine to dislocate the facet joints with concomitant failure of the disc bond and varying degrees of failure of the longitudinal cervical ligaments. One or both facets may dislocate and interlock. Associated fractures of the facets or other posterior elements may occur at the time of dislocation. These injuries may be associated with a variable degree of neurologic loss ranging from none to complete quadriplegia.

Because of supraimposition of the facet joints on lateral roentgenograms, dislocation of a single facet may be difficult to directly visualize. A 25 per cent anterior listhesis of a vertebral body on the body below in a neutral roentgenogram indicates probable fracture or dislocation of one of the posterior facet joints. An anteroposterior projection demonstrates displacement of the spinous processes from the midline as well as asymmetry of the uncovertebral joints serving to corroborate the diagnosis of unilateral facet dislocation. Trauma oblique roentgenograms further delineate the subluxation or dislocation.

Bilateral dislocation of the facets presents with forward subluxation of at least 50 per cent on the lateral roentgenogram (Fig. 3). In the anteroposterior view there is widening of the intervertebral disc space at the joint of Luschka.

Fractures and dislocations of the cervical spine are managed by prompt realignment. Many such dislocations can be reduced by serial traction under direct roentgenographic control and with concomitant serial neurologic examinations. Many dislocations reduce after brief periods of traction. Initially, 15 pounds of traction is applied and the weight is gradually increased, while monitoring the cervical spine with serial lateral roentgenograms or with direct C-arm radiographic visualization. The weight is increased by 5-pound increments. If reduction is not achieved with 35 to 40 pounds of weight and with adequate muscle relaxation, bony or soft tissue interposition should be suspected. Increasing the weight usually does not cause a physi-

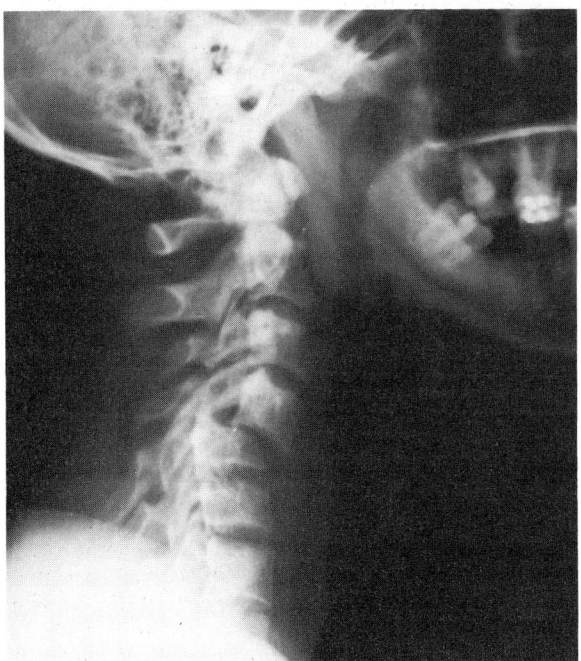

Figure 3. Bilateral facet dislocation of the cervical spine. This is a flexion-distraction injury and is often associated with complete quadriplegia at the level of the injury. Reduction is achieved by skull traction with tongs or halo. Surgical therapy may be necessary to achieve reduction and stabilization.

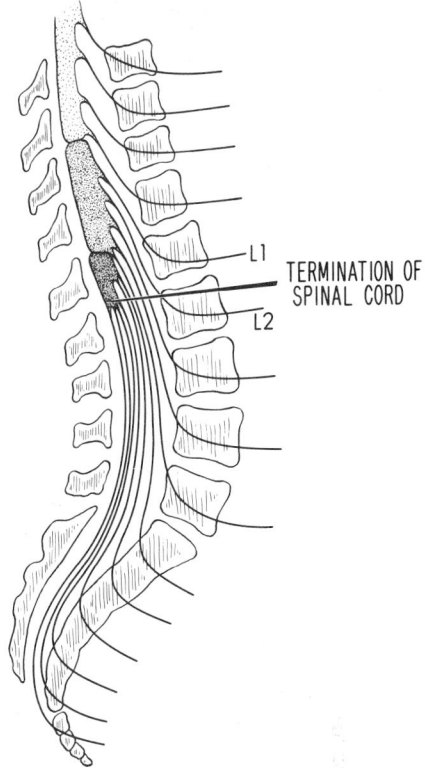

Figure 4. The spinal cord terminates at the L1 vertebra. The cauda equina, composed of spinal roots, is caudal to L1. These relationships are important in the diagnosis and treatment of fractures and fracture-dislocations of the thoracic spine, the lumbar spine, and the thoracolumbar junction.

ologic reduction and may produce cord or nerve root injury. Manipulation under general anesthesia is not recommended. If reduction with the patient awake cannot be achieved, operative reduction under direct vision followed by wire fixation and fusion using autogenous bone graft should be performed.

Following closed reduction, the patient should be maintained in the halo-vest. In dislocations with marked instability, early posterior wiring and autogenous bone grafting are recommended. In more stable situations, the patient may be maintained in the halo-vest until spontaneous fusion occurs. In some cases, however, such spontaneous arthrodesis does not occur, and late operative stabilization may be required.

FRACTURES OF THE POSTERIOR ELEMENTS. Lateral bending, tension, or compressive forces may cause mild fractures of a facet or pedicle. Avulsion fractures of the spinous processes are caused by sudden severe muscle contraction (clay shoveler's fracture) or by direct blows. These fractures are stable and are not associated with neurologic loss. They may be effectively managed by a soft collar until the patient is comfortable.

THE THORACOLUMBAR SPINE

It is important to recognize the relationship of the neural elements to the thoracolumbar skeletal structures when evaluating and treating injuries in this location. The spinal cord usually terminates at the lower margin of the L1 vertebra (Fig. 4). Caudal to L1, the spinal cord contains only spinal roots, the cauda equina. Whereas the spinal cord occupies nearly one half of the spinal canal in the thoracic area, the neural canal has considerable free space below L1. Fractures or dislocations of the lumbar area require considerably more displacement to injure the neural elements than do fractures in the thoracic spine. Moreover, the cauda equina consists of nerve roots that have a greater capacity for recovery following an injury than does the spinal cord. A bursting fracture in the cervical or thoracic region may cause devastating neurologic loss, whereas a similar fracture in the lumbar area may produce no permanent neurologic deficit. Because of the anatomic structure of the terminal cord and roots, spinal injuries caphalad to T10 involved only the

cord; from T10 to L1 involve both the cord and roots; and caudal to L1 involve only the roots. Individual spinal roots may be injured as they exit the intervertebral foramina by skeletal disruption. Because the sympathetic ganglia are located anterior and lateral to the vertebral bodies, fractures of the vertebral bodies or transverse processes frequently cause temporary paralytic ileus.

Diagnosis

The history of the mechanism of injury is helpful in the evaluation of the patient with a suspected thoracolumbar injury. Usually there is a clear history of sudden violence followed immediately by severe backache and muscle spasm. In the osteoporotic patient, a rather minimal incident such as bending, lifting an object, or a missed step may cause a compression fracture of the thoracic spine. However, most thoracolumbar fractures follow violent forces such as falls from heights, automobile collisions, or the fall of a heavy object onto the back.

Careful documentation of the onset of partial or complete loss of lower extremity motor or sensory function is essential for both management and determining prognosis. If a spinal injury is suspected, the patient should be initially examined in the position in which he is first seen. A brief neurologic examination to determine the motor and sensory status of the extremities should first be performed. The patient's clothing should be removed to allow a detailed inspection of the skin overlying the spine. If the patient is in the supine position, the examiner's hand may be gently positioned to palpate each spinous process for tenderness. The patient may then be gently rolled to the lateral position for inspection of possible swelling, abrasions, ecchymoses, or distortions such as spasm, a "step-off," or gibbus.

A complete neurologic evaluation is essential in all individuals with suspected spinal injuries. This should be performed prior to the roentgenographic studies. The intercostal and abdominal muscles sould be examined, and motor, sensory, and reflex testing of the extremities should be performed. The anal sphincter tone and bulbocavernosus reflexes must be included in the evaluation. In the sensory testing, particular attention should be given the perianal region because many spinal cord levels are represented in this small cutaneous area.

Complete loss of motor and sensory function, including perianal sensation, during the first 24 hours after injury indicates complete cord injury. The bulbocavernosus reflex usually recovers within the first 24 hours. Recovery of this reflex together with presence of complete anesthesia and paralysis is compelling evidence that the patient will not recover functional motor power of the lower extremity muscle groups innervated below the level of fracture.

Anteroposterior and lateral roentgenographic views generally demonstrate fractures of the vertebral body (Fig. 5). Computed axial tomography (CT) and water-soluble contrast agents greatly improve the ability to thoroughly evaluate fractures and dislocations in the thoracolumbar area. A CT scan provides an extremely accurate assessment of the degree of spinal canal compromise. In addition, a CT scan provides valuable data for suspected fractures of the posterior elements.

Myelography is not necessary in most cases of significant fracture-dislocation in which the results of the neurologic examination are consistent with the level of fracture. Metrizamide myelography is indicated, however, when there is no apparent fracture or dislocation and neurologic loss is present, or when the skeletal findings do not correlate with the neurologic findings.

Classification and Management

A spine fracture and dislocation is considered stable if the fragments are not likely to move when the spine is physiologi-

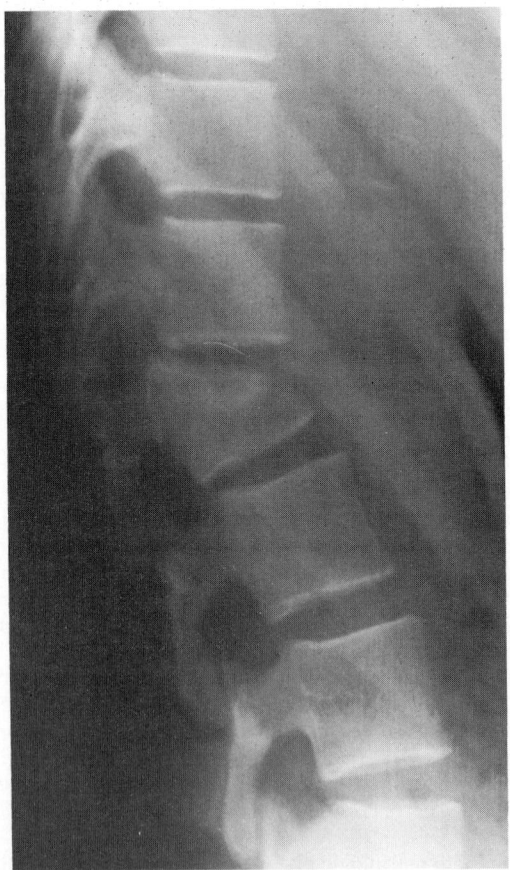

Figure 5. Burst fracture of T12 with anterior deformation, comminution, and retropulsion of bone fragments into the spinal canal.

cally loaded and possibly cause neural damage. Conversely, if movement and neural damage are likely, the injured spine is labeled unstable. The instability may be acute or chronic depending upon whether the displacement is immediately threatening or is a progressing deformity likely to occur during the extended healing process.

Denis developed a classification system for thoracolumbar spine injuries based on a "three-column" concept. In this system, the spine is divided into three longitudinal regions or columns: (1) the anterior column consisting of the anterior longitudinal ligament and the anterior half of the vertebral body including the annulus fibrosus; (2) the middle column consisting of the posterior half of the vertebral body, disc elements, and the posterior longitudinal ligament; and (3) the posterior column consisting of the supraspinous and intraspinous ligaments, spinous processes, laminal arch, pedicles, facet joints, and capsule.

Although references to such "columns" are anatomically imprecise, the terms are clinically useful in assessing the stability of the injured spine. In general, instability results when significant disruption is present in two of the three columns. Although classification into stable and unstable spine fractures and dislocations is not absolute, this scheme is practical from a management standpoint if the physician is cognizant that each injury must be individualized. A major goal of treatment is to maintain or achieve a painless functional back, which to a great degree means maintenance or restoration of spinal stability.

FLEXION INJURIES. Pure flexion injuries are the most common of all thoracolumbar skeletal fractures. Compression anteriorly with or without distraction of the posterior ligaments causes an anterior wedge compression fracture of the vertebral body (Fig. 6A). Most pure flexion injuries involve only the anterior column and, therefore, are acutely stable. Neurologic loss is uncommon. When there is greater than 50 per cent anterior wedging or with multiple contiguous anterior wedge compression fractures, progressive angulation may occur with time. This progressive, flexion angulation during the healing phase would be considered an example of chronic instability.

These fractures can be painful, especially at the level of the injury. Paralytic ileus secondary to hemorrhage of the sympathetic ganglion is common. The patient should be admitted to the hospital and placed at bed rest on a firm mattress, with analgesics and muscle relaxants. Because there is an increased incidence of thromboembolic disease in patients with thoracolumbar fractures, anticoagulation therapy is indicated. The patient should be encouraged to move about the bed and may become ambulatory in an appropriate orthosis as soon as he is comfortable (3 to 5 days). If the compression is mild, a three-point brace will be satisfactory. When wedging is greater than 50 per cent of the anterior body height, a modified polypropylene jacket may be necessary to prevent progressive angulation. In severe cases with major anterior column comminution and also significant posterior element disruption, posterior operative stablization using the Harrington or Cotrel-Dubousset instrumentation and autogenous iliac bone graft may be indicated.

LATERAL COMPRESSION INJURIES. Lateral compression forces may produce a lateral wedge fracture of the vertebral body (Fig. 6B). These fractures are relatively uncommon and usually stable. Neurologic deficit is also unusual. The initial symptoms are treated in a manner similar to anterior wedge compression fractures and orthotic management for comfort is all that is usually required.

AXIAL COMPRESSION INJURIES. Burst fractures result from axial compression of the spine frequently associated with varying degrees of flexion. These injuries, which most commonly occur at the thoracolumbar junction (Fig. 5), are characterized by circumferential expansion of the entire involved vertebra with failure of the anterior, the middle, and, in some cases,

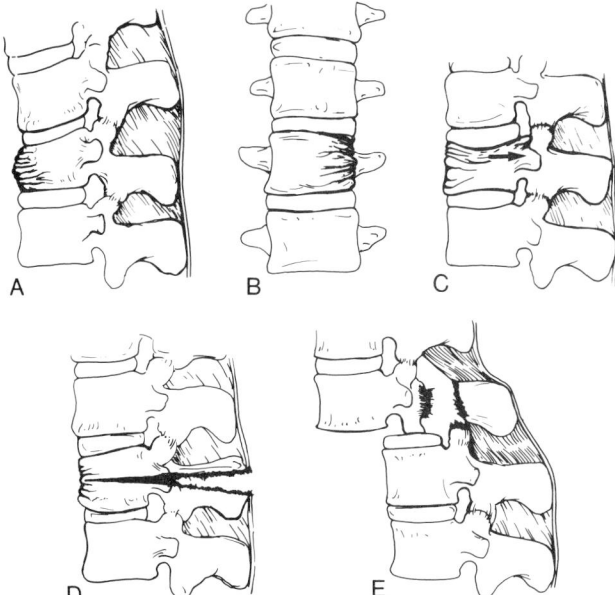

Figure 6. *A*, In an anterior wedge compression fracture, the posterior elements and ligaments generally remain intact. This fracture is usually stable, and neurologic loss is uncommon. *B*, A lateral wedge compression fracture of the vertebral body is a stable fracture and usually is not associated with neurologic loss. *C*, Burst fracture located at the thoracolumbar junction. These fractures are frequently unstable, and neurologic loss can follow posterior displacement or fractures into the spinal canal. *D*, A "chance" fracture is a horizontal splitting of the neural arch and vertebral body. This injury is secondary to a flexion-distraction force. Although three columns are involved, this injury is often clinically stable. *E*, A fracture-dislocation of the thoracolumbar spine. Severe anterior translation is present. The injury is grossly unstable and requires open reduction and internal stabilization is most cases.

the posterior spinal columns. Middle column failure in burst fractures causes retropulsion of the posterosuperior portion of the vertebral body into the spinal canal. With marked retropulsion, compression of the dural tube occurs often with associated neurologic deficit (Fig. 6C).

Radiographically, burst fractures can be recognized on the anteroposterior roentgenogram with widening of the interpedicular distance. Severe burst fractures are three-column injuries with fracture of the posterior elements as well. Dural tears are commonly associated with posterior element fractures.

Mild burst fractures with minimal anterior body deformation, minimal retropulsion of fragments into the spinal canal, no posterior element involvement, and minimal kyphotic angulation can be treated satisfactorily with a molded polypropylene body jacket. Healing of the fracture usually occurs within 3 to 5 months.

If there is incomplete neurologic involvement, usually from fragments impinging on the cauda equina, surgical management may be indicated. The goal of surgical therapy is to provide an environment for spinal cord recovery. Fundamental to this goal are (1) decompression of the spinal canal to remove impinging bone and disc fragments, (2) restoration of the normal alignment of the spine at the thoracolumbar junction, (3) immediate stabilization of the spine with restoration of the normal vertebral body height, and (4) long-term stabilization of the fracture site by means of a posterior spine fusion using autogenous iliac bone graft. At the time of surgical therapy, dural tears should be identified and repaired. Not infrequently portions of the cauda equina herniate through the dural defect, and, if not repaired, scarring and a chronic pain syndrome can ensue. When available, intraoperative somatosensory evoked potential monitoring is recommended.

Surgical procedures designed to decompress and stabilize thoracolumbar burst fractures can be performed through ante-

rior or posterior approaches. The major site of compression is anterior, and, for this reason, laminectomy does little to relieve traction or compression of the spinal cord over an anterior lesion. Indeed, laminectomy may add to the instability of the spinal column.

Anterior exposure of the vertebral body is gained by a transthoracic, transabdominal, or combined approach. Simple anterior fusion may be inadequate to prevent graft collapse and progressive angulation of the spine with weight-bearing. Anterior instrumentation or posterior Harrington instrumentation and fusion in a staged or combined procedure is usually required. Anterior decompression can also be achieved through a posterior lateral approach. Access is gained to the cephalad portion of the vertebral body through the pedicles. Transpedicular decompression is a technically demanding procedure, and meticulous attention to detail is necessary in order to achieve an adequate decompression without undue risk of further neurologic injury.

The Harrington distraction system has been a major contribution to the operative management of fractures and fracture-dislocations of the thoracolumbar spine. Using the principle of distraction and three-point bending, the Harrington or Cotrel-Dubousset instrumentation can effectively restore height and realign the spinal column. Realignment of the spinal column and restoration of height does not, in many cases, effectively decompress the spinal canal. The procedure should, therefore, be combined with definitive removal of bony and disc fragments under direct observation. Somatosensory evoked potentials are closely monitored during and following the realignment procedure.

FRACTURE-DISLOCATIONS. Fracture-dislocations always involve translation of one spinal motion segment or a portion of one spinal segment in relationship to the remaining spine. Translation may be anterior, posterior, or lateral but, by definition, always causes failure of all three columns. A variety of failure modes including shear, compression, tension, and also rotation can occur within the individual columns and various combinations of injury produce characteristic radiographic patterns.

In most cases, the radiographic appearance of these injuries represents the recoiled position of some, even greater, displacement at the time of injury. The shear mode of failure of fracture-dislocations often causes severe injury to the neural elements and complete paraplegia.

If the fracture occurs in the thoracic region, it may be relatively stabilized by the rib cage and heal without operative management. However, in the lumbar region, (Fig. 6E), these injuries are usually grossly unstable and great care must be exercised in managing these patients with such injuries. Operative reduction and internal fixation are the most reliable means of creating a stable environment for potential maximal neurologic return.

FLEXION-DISTRACTION INJURIES. Flexion-distraction forces classically occur in seatbelt injuries in which the individual is subjected to sudden deceleration and the torso is flexed forward over the restraining belt. Tension failure occurs in the posterior and middle columns. Failure of the anterior column also occurs. The mode of anterior column failure depends on the location of the fulcrum of rotation. If the fulcrum exists within the anterior column, compression failure of that column results. If the failure is anterior to the spine, tension failure of all three spinal columns occurs and the spine is literally pulled apart. These injuries may be associated with marked displacement and are usually very unstable. Open reduction with realignment and internal fixation is usually required in order to regain stability.

The "chance" fracture is a unique flexion-distraction injury in which there is a horizontal splitting of the neural arch, the pedicles, and the vertebral body (Fig. 6D).

SELECTED REFERENCES

Bohlman, H. H., and Eismont, F. J.: Surgical techniques of anterior decompression and fusion for spinal cord injuries. Clin. Orthop. Rel. Res., 154:57, 1981.
An excellent description of the rationale and indications for the anterior approach for decompression of spinal cord injuries.

Denis, F.: The three-column spine and its significance in the classification of acute thoracolumbar spinal injuries. Spine, 8:817, 1983.
A presentation of the three-column concept in the classification of thoracolumbar spine fractures.

Ferguson, R. L., and Allen, B. L.: A mechanistic classification of thoracolumbar spine fractures. Clin. Orthop. Rel. Res., 189:77, 1984.
A concise classification of thoracolumbar spine fractures based on modes of failure and their consequences to stability.

Flesch, J. R., Leider, L. L., Erickson, D. L., Chou, S. N., and Bradford, D. S.: Harrington instrumentation and spine fusion for unstable fractures and fracture-dislocations of the thoracic and lumbar spine. J. Bone Joint Surg. [Am.], 52:143, 1977.
A good description of spinal stabilization by early surgical therapy, which allows mobilization and rehabilitation and prevention of late deformity.

Holdsworth, F. W.: Fractures, dislocations, and fracture-dislocations of the spine. J. Bone Joint Surg. [Am.], 52:1534, 1970.
A classic description of spinal fractures and their management.

Kostuik, J. P.: Anterior spinal cord decompression for lesions of the thoracic and lumbar spine, techniques, and new methods of internal fixation, results. Spine, 8:512, 1983.
Surgical techniques of anterior decompression and instrumentation for spinal cord injuries.

McAfee, P. C., Yuan, H. A., and Lasda, N. A.: The unstable burst fracture. Spine, 7:365, 1982.
An excellent description of the posterolateral approach for decompression of fractures of the thoracolumbar junction.

Rockwood, C., and Green, D.: *Fractures*, Vol. II, Chapter 12. Philadelphia, J. B. Lippincott Company, 1975.
The chapters on cervical and lumbar spine injuries are thorough and well-illustrated and provide a foundation for the understanding of the management of trauma to the axial skeleton.

REFERENCES

1. Anderson, L. D., and D'Alonzo, R. T.: Fractures of the odontoid process of the axis. J. Bone Joint Surg. [Am.], 56:663, 1974.
2. Brashear, H. R., Venters, G. C., and Preston, E. T.: Fractures of the neural arch of the axis. J. Bone Joint Surg. [Am.], 57:879, 1975.
3. Chance, C. Q.: Note on a type of flexion fracture of the spine. Br. J. Radiol., 21:452, 1948.
4. Davies, W. E., Morris, J. H., and Hill, V.: Analysis of conservative management of thoracolumbar fractures and fracture-dislocations with neural damage. J. Bone Joint Surg. [Am.], 62:1324, 1980.
5. Dunn, H. K.: Anterior spine stabilization and decompression for thoracolumbar injuries. Orthop. Clin. North Am., 17:113, 1986.
6. Eismont, F. J., Green, B. A., Berkowitz, B. N., Montalvo, B. M., Quencer, R. M., and Brown, M. J.: The role of intra-operative ultrasonography in the treatment of thoracic and lumbar fractures. Spine, 9:782, 1984.
7. Erickson, D. L., Leider, L. L., and Brown, W. E.: One-stage decompression-stabilization for thoracolumbar fractures. Spine, 2:53, 1977.
8. Fielding, J. W., Cochran, G. V. B., Lawsing, J. F., and Hohl, N: Tears of the transverse ligament of the axis. J. Bone Joint Surg. [Am.], 56:683, 1974.
9. Gaines, R. W., Breedlove, R. F., and Munson, G.: Stabilization of thoracic and thoracolumbar fracture-dislocations with Harrington rods and sublaminal wires. Clin. Orthop. Rel. Res., 189:195, 1984.
10. Grundy, B. L.: Monitoring of sensory revoked potentials during neurosurgical operations: Methods and applications. Neurosurgery, 11:556, 1982.
11. Guttman, L.: Spinal Cord Injuries, Comprehensive Management and Research. Oxford, Blackwell Scientific Publications Ltd., 1973, p. 694.
12. Jefferson, G.: Fracture of the atlas vertebra: Report of four cases and review of those previously recorded. Br. J. Surg., 7:407, 1920.
13. Kaufer, H., and Hayes, J. T.: Lumbar fracture-dislocations. J. Bone Joint Surg. [Am.], 48:712, 1966.
14. Keene, J. S., Goletz, T. H., Lilleas, F., Alter, A. J., and Sackett, J. F.: Diagnosis of vertebral fractures: A comparison of conventional radiography, conventional tomography, and computed axial tomography. J. Bone Joint Surg. [Am.], 64:586, 1982.
15. Larson, S. J., Holst, R. A., Hemmy, D. C., and Sanes, A., Jr.: Lateral extracavity approach to traumatic lesions of the thoracic and lumbar spine. J. Neurosurg., 45:628, 1976.
16. McCraw, R. W., and Ruschi, R. N.: Atlanto-axial arthrodesis. J. Bone Joint Surg. [Br.], 55:482, 1973.
17. McEvoy, R. D., and Bradford, D. S.: The management of burst fractures of the thoracic and lumbar spine. Spine, 10:631, 1985.
18. Miller, C. A., Dewey, R. C., and Hunt, W. E.: Impaction fracture of the lumbar vertebra with dural tear. J. Neurosurg., 53:765, 1980.
19. Nash, C. L., Jr., Lorig, R. A., Schatzinger, L. A., and Brown, R. H.: Spinal cord monitoring during operative treatment of the spine. Clin. Orthop. Rel. Res., 126:100, 1977.
20. Riggins, R. S., and Krause, J. F.: The risk of neurologic damage with fractures of the vertebra. J. Trauma, 17:126, 1977.
21. Roberts, J. B., and Curtiss, P. H.: Stability of the thoracic and lumbar spine in traumatic paraplegia following fracture or fracture-dislocations. J. Bone Joint Surg. [Am.], 52:1115, 1970.
22. Schneider, R. C., and Kahn, E. A.: Chronic neurological sequelae of acute trauma to the spine and spinal cord. J. Bone Joint Surg. [Am.], 38:985, 1956.
23. Schneider, R. C., Livingstone, K. E., Cowe, A. J. E., and Hamilton, G.,: Hangman's fracture. J. Neurosurg., 22:141, 1965.
24. Smart, C. N., and Sanders, C. R.: Cost of Motor Vehicle–Related Spinal Cord Injuries. Washington, DC, Insurance Institute for Highway Safety, 1965.
25. Whitesides, T. E., Jr., and Shaha, S. G. A.: On the management of unstable fractures of the thoracolumbar spine. Spine, 1:99, 1976.

III

FRACTURES AND DISLOCATIONS OF THE SHOULDER, ARM, AND FOREARM

Robert D. Fitch, M.D.

Traumatic Anterior Dislocation of the Shoulder

The cumulative range of motion of the shoulder is greater than that of any other joint. This is due to the lack of bony and soft tissue constraints. The humeral head articulates with the glenoid, a shallow disc with a surface area one-third that of the humeral head. The range of motion of the shoulder is further augmented by the presence of a redundant joint capsule. These anatomic peculiarities render this joint susceptible to traumatic dislocation. Bony stability is provided by the glenoid medially and acromion superiorly, whereas the glenoid labrum, capsule, and rotator cuff musculature provide soft tissue constraint. Anatomically, the humeral head lies retroverted 35 degrees, and

the glenoid is anteverted 20 degrees. This in part is responsible for the more frequent occurrence of anterior dislocations, compared with posterior dislocations.

MECHANISM OF INJURY. Acute traumatic anterior dislocations occur as a result of forced abduction, extension, and external rotation of the shoulder. In most cases, the humeral head is levered over the rim of the glenoid and causes a tear or defect in the glenoid labrum (Bankart lesion).[3] With repetitive traumatic dislocations, a groove in the posterior portion of the humeral head (Hill-Sachs' lesion)[29] can occur.

CLINICAL FINDINGS. Traumatic dislocations most commonly occur in active adults. Children and adolescents are more likely to have an epiphyseal separation with the same mechanism.[47,67] Individuals with traumatic dislocations must be further differentiated from a group of habitual dislocators,[58] that is, those persons who can voluntarily dislocate their shoulders, as well as those with conditions associated with ligament laxity, such as the Ehlers-Danlos syndrome. Following a traumatic dislocation of the shoulder, the arm is held at the side. The acromion process is prominent, and the normal fullness of the shoulder is replaced by a concave contour just below the acromion. Evaluation must include complete neurologic and vascular examination, because injury to the brachial plexus (particularly the axillary nerve) or axillary artery can occur.[36,51,64] Radiographs should include anteroposterior and tangential scapular views. These confirm the position of the dislocation according to the anatomic site: subcoracoid, subglenoid, or (rare) intrathoracic. Displacement of the proximal humerus in the neonatal period may roentgenographically appear as a shoulder dislocation. However, in this age group, it is more likely to be the result of a traumatic separation of the proximal growth plate with displacement of the metaphysis anteriorly.[24] The diagnosis can be confirmed by arthrography or ultrasonography[10] if necessary.

TREATMENT. Reduction of the dislocation should be prompt. The longer the shoulder remains unreduced, the more muscle spasm there is to overcome. Reduction should be gentle; and unless it is done immediately after the injury, sedation is required. Occasionally, a general anesthetic is needed. Reduction is accomplished by longitudinal traction on the arm, with countertraction applied in the axilla. An alternative method is the Stimson technique[66] (Fig. 1). With this method, the patient is placed in the prone position, and the arm is allowed to relax. Progressive weight is added to the extremity, up to 15 to 20 pounds, followed by a waiting period of 15 to 20 minutes. Usually reduction is accomplished by this time. Following reduction, the neurovascular status to the extremity is again reassessed. The arm is then immobilized in a sling held in internal rotation for approximately 3 weeks. Protected range-of-motion exercises are then initiated, but excessive abduction and external rotation should be avoided for 3 months. Recurrence is a common complication in younger patients and is less common in individuals over 40 years of age. In these older patients, the

rotator cuff is frequently torn at the time of the traumatic dislocation.[26]

Recurrent Anterior Dislocations

Younger individuals are likely to have recurrent dislocations. After two or three recurrences, operative repair is usually indicated. Good results have been reported with many procedures. The Bankart operation repairs the torn capsule and labrum[2,3]; the Putti-Platt procedure[48] plicates the capsule and the subscapularis tendon. The subscapularis muscle insertion is transferred laterally in the Magnuson-Stack procedure[39] after the capsule is repaired. The Bristow procedure[28] transfers the coracoid process and the attached musculature is attached to the anterior rim of the glenoid.

A condition termed the "dead arm" syndrome is observed in patients suffering recurrent and transient anterior subluxation of the shoulder.[57] With elevation and external rotation of the shoulder a sudden incapacitating pain occurs which may or may not be associated with a sensation of instability. Arthrotomography[9] of the shoulder and recently diagnostic arthroscopy[34] have demonstrated defects and tears in the glenoid labrum, and this condition may warrant surgical repair.

Posterior Dislocations

These injuries are much less common than anterior dislocations, representing approximately 2 per cent of all glenohumeral joint dislocations.[55] This injury may occur as a result of a violent seizure or may be due to a direct anterior blow. As with anterior dislocations, the voluntary or habitual dislocation must be differentiated from that due to trauma. This condition can be overlooked initially because radiographic changes are subtle. Routine anteroposterior views may appear normal. A true anteroposterior radiograph of the glenoid demonstrates overlap of the humeral head and glenoid, and a transaxillary or transscapular lateral radiograph also clarifies the diagnosis. As with anterior dislocations, traction should allow reduction of the joint. Postreduction immobilization, however, is quite different, because with the arm in a sling, the position of maximal instability is reproduced. Rather, the arm should be immobilized in moderate abduction and external rotation.

Fractures of the Proximal Humerus

Fractures of the proximal humerus occur more frequently with advancing age. As with fractures of the proximal femur, loss of normal trabecular bone with aging makes this area more susceptible to injury. However, this fracture is observed in all age groups and merges with epiphyseal separation injuries of the proximal humerus, which occur in individuals prior to skeletal maturity. In the elderly patient, fractures may occur as a result of minor trauma, whereas fractures in younger individuals require considerable force, and fracture dislocations may occur. In this group of fractures, the prognosis depends upon the degree of displacement and the number of fracture fragments.

Although many classifications for this fracture have been proposed, that described by Neer[44] is the most widely accepted. This classification is based on the observation that fractures of the proximal humerus occur between all four of its major segments: (1) the articular segment or fracture occurring through the "anatomic neck," (2) fracture involving the greater tuberosity, (3) fracture involving the lesser tuberosity, and (4) fracture through the metaphyseal region or "surgical neck" (Fig. 2). The classification then identifies the fractures as one-, two-, three-, or four-part fractures, depending upon the number of segments displaced. One centimeter of separation or 45 degrees of angulation of any segment is considered a displaced fragment. Nondisplaced fractures are considered one-part fractures, even though a fracture line may exist between any number of these segments. For example, a three-part fracture is one in which two

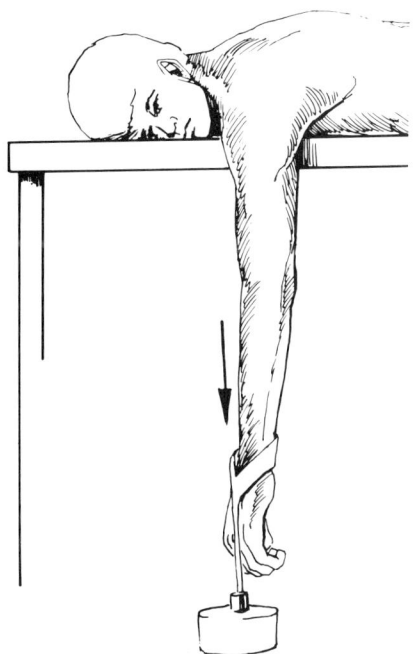

Figure 1. The modified Stimson technique of closed reduction. The amount of weight that is hung from the hand depends on the size of the patient. (From Rockwood, C. A., and Green, D. P.: Fractures. Vol. 1. Philadelphia, J. B. Lippincott Company, 1984, p. 750.)

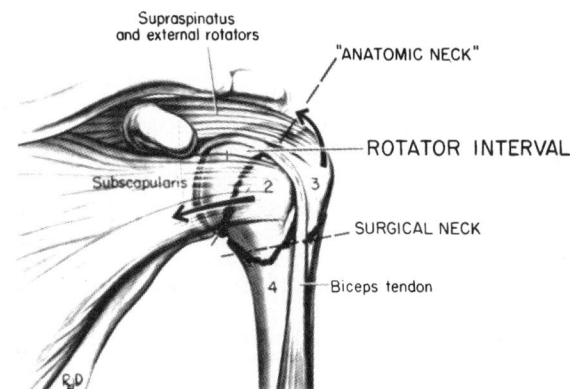

Figure 2. The classification of Neer is based on recognition of the four major fragments of proximal humeral fractures: (1) articular fragment, (2) lesser tuberosity, (3) greater tuberosity, and (4) shaft. (From Neer, C. S., II: Displaced proximal humeral fractures. I. Classification and evaluation. J. Bone Joint Surg. [Am.], 52:1077, 1970).

segments are displaced in relationship to the other two remaining segments.

MECHANISM OF INJURY. Most fractures occur as a result of a fall on the outstretched arm causing forced abduction, extension, and external rotation. Similarly, this mechanism of injury is responsible for most cases of fracture separation of the proximal humeral epiphysis. Proximal humeral fractures can also follow a direct blow to the lateral aspect of the shoulder.

CLINICAL FINDINGS. In older patients, only mild ecchymosis and swelling may be present. Clinically, attempts should be made to exclude humeral head dislocation or associated acromioclavicular separation. The vascular supply to the limb must be assessed, because axillary artery thrombosis or laceration can occur.[62] Neurologic examination excludes associated brachial plexus injury. A complete roentgenographic series is important in determining the severity of injury and the appropriate treatment. This consists of an anteroposterior view and a view tangential to the scapula. Often, an axillary view is unobtainable because of pain; a transscapular lateral view is performed in this case.

TREATMENT. A minimally displaced or impacted fracture without significant angulation is fortunately the most common injury, representing approximately 80 per cent of all proximal humeral fractures.[55] These fractures are usually stabilized by the intact rotator cuff and periosteum and are treated by external immobilization, consisting of a sling and swathe, or a commercially available shoulder immobilizer. Within 2 to 3 weeks, range-of-motion exercises can be initiated according to patient comfort. Pendulum exercises and passive range-of-motion exercises are followed by isometric exercises and finally by active exercises against resistance.

Two-part fractures usually involve either the greater or lesser tuberosity of the humerus or the surgical neck. If the greater tuberosity cannot be reduced and remains displaced more than 1 cm., open reduction and internal fixation is advisable because malunion in a displaced position interferes with abduction and external rotation of the humerus and may be painful. Separation of the lesser tuberosity usually requires no treatment other than immobilization. If significant angulation or displacement of the shaft is present, closed reduction should be performed. Open reduction is rarely necessary.

Three-part fractures usually cannot be reduced closed because of muscle forces acting on separate fragments. These fractures are best managed by open reduction and internal fixation with wire, screws, and intramedullary rods as needed.[25]

Four-part fractures involve loss of all soft tissue continuity to the articular fragment and therefore are associated with disruption of the blood supply and avascular necrosis of the segment.

Early surgical therapy with prosthetic replacement of the articular segment and reapproximation of the tuberosities is indicated and has been demonstrated to provide better results than open reduction and internal fixation of all fragments.[46,49,64]

Fractures of the proximal humerus can occur in the neonatal period or in infancy and can be confused with dislocation of the shoulder. A complete fracture separation of the proximal humerus in childhood is managed nonoperatively even if severe displacement remains following closed reduction, since angulation resolves as the bone remodels. In the adolescent, however, this fracture should not remain severely displaced, because the potential for remodeling is limited. An attempt at closed reduction should be made in severely displaced fractures; and if reduction cannot be maintained with the arm at the side, percutaneous pinning is preferable to placing the arm in a "Statue of Liberty" position in a spica cast.

Fractures and Dislocations of the Clavicle

The clavicle is an S-shaped bone that provides connection between the shoulder girdle and the axial skeleton. This bone structurally maintains shoulder separation. This is the first bone to ossify *in utero*; and ossification occurs, unlike that in other long bones, by intramembranous ossification. The clavicle is tubular in the proximal and middle segment and becomes flat laterally. Proximally it articulates with the sternum, and stability is maintained by a complex of capsule and sternoclavicular ligaments. Laterally articulation occurs with the acromion process of the scapula, and stability is by strong acromioclavicular and coracoclavicular ligaments.

The clavicle is one of the most frequently fractured bones. This injury is especially common in children. Sixty per cent of all clavicle fractures occur in children younger than 10 years of age.[47]

These fractures are divided by anatomic region (proximal one third, middle one third, and distal one third). Treatment is based on age, location of the fracture, and degree of displacement. Despite the proximity of the subclavian artery, pleura, and brachial plexus, injuries to these structures are uncommon.

MECHANISM OF INJURY. Fractures of the distal third of the clavicle follow a blow to the superior aspect of the shoulder. A similar mechanism is responsible for acromioclavicular separations with the force applied somewhat more posteriorly on the shoulder. Fractures of the middle third of the clavicle are usually the result of a shearing force, and proximal fractures most commonly follow direct trauma. Sternoclavicular dislocations may follow direct trauma or indirect forces applied through the clavicle to the ligamentous complex medially. Fractures of the clavicle may occur in the neonatal period as a result of traumatic delivery.

CLINICAL FINDINGS. Birth fractures may present as a pseudoparalysis of the limb, because the infant is reluctant to use the extremity because of pain. Often these fractures go unnoticed because they can be relatively asymptomatic. The only clue may be a prominence over the clavicle as callus begins to form. In these injuries an associated brachial plexus birth palsy must be excluded. Minimally displaced fractures in children may also be relatively asymptomatic, because the thick periosteal sleeve provides stability. In adolescents and adults the deformity is obvious. In acromioclavicular joint injuries tenderness is present over this joint, and subluxation with tenting of the skin may be present if sufficient ligamentous disruption has occurred. Sternoclavicular dislocations present as local pain in the region of the sternoclavicular joint. With an anterior dislocation, the proximal clavicle is prominent and palpable under the skin. Posterior dislocations may be more difficult to diagnose, but careful examination demonstrates a cavity where the clinician would expect to palpate the proximal clavicle.

Routine anteroposterior radiographs of the clavicle are sufficient for most fractures. Radiographic examination of the acromioclavicular joint may require stress films.[45] The diagnosis of sternoclavicular dislocations is difficult, however, and requires special techniques. Hobbs[31] and Rockwood and Green[55] have described a special radiographic view to delineate these dislocations. In the child or adolescent, a physeal injury of the proximal apophysis may stimulate a true sternoclavicular dislocation.[21]

TREATMENT. Most clavicular fractures require only symptomatic treatment. In infants, callus forms rapidly and pain subsides as stability occurs. Generally no immobilization is necessary. Support for the shoulder and arm can be provided with a stockinette bandage.

In children, anatomic reduction of the fracture is not necessary, because the potential for bone remodeling is great. Even in displaced distal third fractures of the clavicle, the coracoclavicular ligaments remain attached to the periosteum and remarkable remodeling occurs. Application of a figure-eight bandage and arm sling assists in comfort. Unlike other long bone fractures, a greenstick fracture should never be completed, because this may cause injury to the subclavian vessels or brachial plexus. Two to 3 weeks of immobilization are all that is required. In adults, displacement and angulation at the fracture results in some residual deformity as the remodeling potential has diminished. Although this deformity may cause no functional impairment, some cosmetic deformity is noted. Therefore, it is important to obtain reduction in displaced fractures. For middle third fractures, a figure-eight bandage is usually sufficient to restore length and alignment. For fractures of the lateral third, without significant disruption of the coracoclavicular ligament complex, a figure-eight dressing is all that is required. However, in severely displaced fractures with disruption of this ligament complex, the figure-eight dressing may not be sufficient for obtaining an acceptable reduction. In this instance, a modification of the Kenny-Howard splint,[19] which applies an upward pull on the elbow and a downward pull on the clavicle, may be indicated. With appropriate techniques, almost all fractures can be reduced acceptably.

Some authors recommend open reduction and internal fixation of selected clavicle fractures.[69] However, this method of treatment may be associated with increased incidence of nonunion.[58] This may be related to extensive periosteal stripping required for plating. If open reduction in severely displaced fractures of the middle and distal third of the clavicle is contemplated, intramedullary fixation is preferred.

Sprains of the acromioclavicular joint without significant displacement can be treated with a protective sling. Subluxation or complete dislocation of the acromioclavicular joint can be managed by application of the Kenny-Howard splint. This device applies an upward force to the elbow and a downward force to the distal clavicle, reducing the displacement. This splint should be worn for 6 weeks and requires frequent readjustments. Some authors make no attempt to reduce the subluxation of the distal end of the clavicle because long-term studies have demonstrated that these are rarely symptomatic. An arm sling is worn for 2 to 3 weeks until the discomfort subsides, and then active motion exercises of the shoulder are initiated. Rarely are open reduction and reconstruction of the acromioclavicular and coracoclavicular ligaments performed.[6,35]

Anterior dislocations of the sternoclavicular joint can usually be reduced by abduction and extension of the shoulders over a bolster, with application of direct posterior pressure over the proximal clavicle. Position is maintained with a figure-eight clavicle strap. For reduction of posterior dislocations, the shoulders are again extended over a bolster, and the proximal clavicle is pulled anteriorly, usually with a sterile towel clip. This can be done under local or general anesthesia.

COMPLICATIONS. The most frequent complication of clavicular fractures is malunion. Rarely do brachial plexus injuries and subclavian artery thrombosis occur.[20] Serious complications can be associated with posterior dislocation of the sterno-clavicular joint, which can cause compression of the vena cava,[68] trachea,[50] or brachial plexus.[40]

Nonunion of the clavicle is rare with closed methods of treatment. There is, however, a significant (3 to 4 per cent) incidence of nonunion of clavicle fractures treated by open reduction.[69] Brachial plexus symptoms can occur as a result of pressure on the brachial plexus from a hypertrophic nonunion.

Fractures of the Scapula

The scapula is a broad, flat bone that helps stabilize the shoulder girdle by providing contact with the ribs, around which it is supported by multiple muscle insertions. Medially it forms the glenoid, acromion process, and coracoid. Fractures of the scapula are relatively uncommon, usually involve the broad cancellous portion, and therefore heal quickly without residual disability. Fractures of the body of the scapula are the result of direct trauma. Because of the multiple muscles attached to the scapula, the fracture is usually not significantly displaced. Occasionally, fractures of the body can extend intra-articularly to involve the glenoid. Fractures of the acromion are usually a result of direct trauma, although there has been a case report of fracture due to muscle contracture.[54] Fractures of the coracoid process can occur as a result of either direct trauma or avulsion by the pull of the attached muscles.

TREATMENT. Most scapular fractures are managed by symptomatic relief, which includes an arm sling until pain subsides. Fractures that involve the neck of the scapula and/or glenoid should be assessed by tangential views in addition to the routine anteroposterior radiographs. Occasionally, computed tomography (CT) is indicated to delineate the intra-articular fractures involving the glenoid. In the rare case of significant displacement of an intra-articular fracture, open reduction may be indicated to re-establish joint congruity.[1]

Fractures of the Shaft of the Humerus

ANATOMY. The humeral shaft is cylindrical proximally and broadens distally. The major neurovascular structures are located medially except for the radial nerve, which courses laterally. The muscles of the arm and gravity act on midshaft fractures to produce shortening and varus angulation. In fractures below the insertion of the deltoid muscle, the proximal fragment is abducted by the deltoid while the biceps, triceps, and coracobrachialis adduct and shorten the distal fragment. In fractures above the insertion of the deltoid and below the insertion of the pectoralis major, the distal fragment is drawn into abduction by the deltoid while the proximal fragment is adducted by the pectoralis major. In fractures above the insertion of the pectoralis major, the distal fragment is held in alignment while the proximal fragment is abducted by the rotator cuff and internally rotated by the subscapularis.

MECHANISM OF INJURY. The majority of these fractures are caused by direct trauma or a fall on the arm. Bending moments cause transverse fractures, whereas torsional forces cause spiral fractures.

CLINICAL AND RADIOLOGIC FINDINGS. Pain, tenderness, and instability of the arm are obvious. Radial nerve involvement is relatively common and should be suspected in all cases.

TREATMENT. Open fractures are treated as emergencies with immediate débridement. Injuries to the vascular structures, either directly or indirectly, should likewise be treated as emergencies with appropriate arteriograms, internal injury exploration, and repair or grafting of the artery. Nerve trauma is usually treated by reduction of the fracture and not by immediate operation.

After emergency treatment has been administered, the principles of treatment to be considered are the method of initial immobilization and alignment of the fragment. After stability has occurred, in 5 to 6 weeks, shoulder and elbow motion should be initiated.

UNDISPLACED FRACTURES. These fractures can be treated by padding the axilla and wrapping the arm to the chest. Early protective motion is started in 2 to 3 weeks, and healing occurs in approximately 10 weeks. The arm only may be splinted, leaving the elbow mobile.

DISPLACED FRACTURES. Several methods have been used for the treatment of these fractures. The hanging arm cast[14,15,59] is a lightweight cast applied to the arm from just above the level of the fracture to the hand. A sling is placed under the involved axilla and over the opposite trapezius through a loop or rope fixed to the forearm cast.

The alignment of the fragments can be controlled by the length of the sling and the position of the hoop on the forearm cast, either dorsal or volar. This changes the rotation and angulation at the fracture site in three planes. During the first 3 weeks of treatment, the patient is kept in an upright or semirecumbent position because the weight of the arm and the cast provides traction and aligns the fracture. Periodic radiographs are necessary, and early shoulder motion is initiated. Pendulum exercises with the cuff still attached maintain shoulder motion. Finger and hand exercises are encouraged. More recently, some authors have found an increased incidence of nonunion of humeral shaft fractures treated with the hanging arm cast method.[27]

A coaptation splint[8,16,18] consists of a single 10- to 15-thickness splint applied from the axilla, around the elbow, and over the deltoid with light padding and nonelastic wrapping. This holds the fragments in alignment, and a sling is used for comfort. This has the advantage of allowing earlier elbow, wrist, and hand motion and often provides the patient more comfort initially than does the hanging cast. Adjustment of fracture alignment is more difficult.

Patients who have associated injuries or who are bedridden for other reasons can be treated by traction through an olecranon pin or by skin traction. Traction aligns the fragments, but care must be taken to prevent overpull of the fragment, pressure on the radial nerve, or injury to the ulnar nerve from the pin.

In fractures associated with vascular injury, rapid internal fixation of the fragments is done prior to repair of the vessels if the time interval from injury to repair is not greater than 4 hours.

In established nonunions or in fractures with soft tissue interposition, open reduction and fixation with metallic devices are necessary.[27]

The humerus is the common site of pathologic fractures caused by metastatic tumors, and these may be treated by local radiation and/or chemotherapy, and the fracture may heal. More commonly, however, there is a large defect in the bone with gross instability of the humerus. The patient is often uncomfortable, and open fixation is done followed by appropriate treatment of the tumor. Healing may be delayed in these patients. If there is extensive bone loss, methylmethacrylate supplements the metallic fixation.

PROGNOSIS. Nondisplaced and minimally displaced fractures heal in 6 to 10 weeks and allow early functional use of the arm for light activities. In severely displaced or comminuted fractures associated with neurovascular injuries, the prognosis is guarded. Associated fractures of the elbow or shoulder worsen the prognosis.

COMPLICATIONS. The radial nerve may be injured in open fractures or fractures at the junction of the middle and distal thirds of the humerus. At this point, the nerve is in proximity to the humerus. In most instances, the injury is a result of stretching or contusion, and function returns within several weeks to 6 months. It is safe to wait for at least 3 months to determine whether regeneration will occur.[59,60] The electromyogram demonstrates early regeneration. In open fractures involving the radial nerve or in fractures with soft tissue interposition, exploration of the radial nerve is indicated. Delayed suture is acceptable, but the decision depends upon the lesion.

Fractures of the Distal Humerus and Elbow

In this section, supracondylar fractures of the humerus, which represent 50 to 60 per cent of all fractures around the elbow, plus intra-articular fractures of the distal humerus, fractures of the radial head, and fractures of the olecranon are discussed. Fractures around the elbow are common in children and frequently lead to malunion, growth disturbance, or joint incongruity. Adult fractures around the elbow, especially distal humerus fractures, tend to be comminuted and intra-articular and may cause permanent stiffness and posttraumatic arthrosis.

ANATOMY OF THE ELBOW. The distal humerus, in the transition from diaphysis to epiphysis, becomes progressively broad and fan-shaped. The medial and lateral condyles of the humerus are separated by a thin membrane of bone that anatomically separates the coronoid fossa anteriorly and the olecranon fossa posteriorly. The lateral condyle consists of the lateral epicondyle (the origin of the extensor muscle mass) and the capitellum. The medial condyle is formed by the medial epicondyle (the origin of the flexor muscle mass) and trochlea. The capitellum laterally and trochlea medially are covered by hyaline cartilage and form the humeral portion of the elbow's articular surface. The trochlea has a central groove that is directed laterally in extension, and this determines the carrying angle (normal 7 to 15 degrees). The radial head articulates with the capitellum, and it is through this proximal radial-humeral joint that pronation and supination of the forearm occur. Flexion, extension, and rotation are dependent upon the congruity among the three articulations: the humeral-ulnar joint, radial-humeral joint, and radial-ulnar joint. Any disturbance in the anatomy of these articulations causes diminished elbow motion and function. When the elbow is flexed to 90 degrees, an isosceles triangle is formed posteriorly by the landmarks of the lateral epicondyle, the medial epicondyle, and the tip of the olecranon. Displaced fractures involving the elbow joint cause distortion of the relationship. The brachial artery and medial nerve pass anterior to the elbow joint and can be damaged by displaced fractures, particularly supracondylar fractures of the humerus. The ulnar nerve, which is behind the medial epicondyle in continuity with bone, is subject to early or late compression. The radial nerve courses laterally between the brachialis and brachioradialis, and, distal to the elbow, enters the supinator muscle mass.

Radiographic interpretation of anatomy is particularly difficult in children if the secondary centers of ossification have not yet begun to ossify. The capitellar secondary ossification centers should be present by 6 months of age. Radial head ossification is present at 4 to 5 years. Medial epicondylar ossification appears between 5 and 7 years, trochlear ossification between 8 and 9 years, and the lateral epicondyle ossification center at age 12 to 14 years.[13]

SUPRACONDYLAR AND INTERCONDYLAR FRACTURES

MECHANISM OF INJURY. Supracondylar fractures occur as a result of a fall on the outstretched arm or flexed elbow. Two types of supracondylar fractures are distinguished: the flexion type and the extension type. The most common by far is the extension injury. This occurs as a result of a fall on the outstretched arm, which causes a compression and hyperextension force applied indirectly to the distal humerus. On the lateral radiograph, the normal anterior tilt of the distal humerus is lost and there may be anterior angulation at the fracture site. Less commonly, compression and flexion forces cause a flexion type of injury. In this case, the fracture is angulated posteriorly, and there may be an increase in anterior displacement and angulation of the distal fragment.

Transcondylar and intracondylar fractures are observed in

adults, particularly in the elderly, related to significant trauma. Much comminution of the fragments is often noted.

CLINICAL FINDINGS. Pain and swelling are present. Neurovascular status must be carefully assessed, because arterial or neurologic injury can occur by laceration and direct or indirect compression.

Properly obtained radiographs are a very important aspect of initial evaluation. In children, comparison films of the uninvolved distal humerus and elbow are helpful. During interpretation, obvious findings such as degree of displacement and level and number of fracture fragments should be noted. In addition, particularly in children, subtle changes such as rotary malalignment and varus impaction should be sought. Measurement of Baumann's[5,22] angle on both the involved and uninvolved extremity may be a helpful guide in preventing varus malunion. In the anteroposterior radiograph, the presence of medial or lateral displacement should be recognized, because this must be corrected during treatment and should be a guide to positioning of the forearm.

TREATMENT. In children, undisplaced fractures are treated by immobilization of the arm with the elbow flexed to 90 degrees. The period of immobilization is approximately 3 weeks. However, care must be taken so that it is certain that an apparent nondisplaced fracture is not in fact a varus impacted fracture, which can cause the late complication of cubitus varus. Measurement of Baumann's angle may help in ensuring a normal carrying angle. Varus impacted fractures should be manipulated, and this usually can be done with sedation. In the significantly displaced supracondylar humerus fracture without neurologic deficit, a reduction with anesthesia is warranted. Reduction is performed by traction of the forearm with countertraction proximally. This maneuver is done with the elbow in slight flexion. Traction should never be applied with the elbow hyperextended, because this may cause further compression of the neurovascular structures anteriorly. The extension deformity of the distal fragment is then corrected by pressure applied posteriorly.

After this, any medial or lateral angulation is corrected. The elbow is then flexed to 90 degrees, and stability is tested. If this fracture is unstable with the elbow at 90 degrees, percutaneous pinning is recommended.[52] This is preferable to further flexion of the elbow for stability, because the latter may cause vascular embarrassment and lead to Volkmann's ischemic contracture. Initial displacement in the anteroposterior plane that is medial indicates that the medial periosteum is intact and the lateral periosteum is disrupted. Soft tissue should be tightened laterally by pronation of the forearm. This allows reduction to be maintained against the medial periosteal hinge. Conversely, if initial displacement is lateral, the medial periosteum is disrupted and the medial soft tissue should be tightened, which requires supination of the forearm.

In the severely swollen displaced supracondylar fracture without neurovascular compromise, preliminary side arm or overhead traction may be warranted. This can be provided by Dunlop's skin traction[22] or by olecranon pin traction. Attempts to obtain and maintain reduction in traction are worthwhile. If the fracture cannot be aligned with traction, an anesthetic and closed reduction with or without percutaneous pinning is indicated after the swelling has subsided.

Occasionally fractures cannot be reduced either by traction or by closed reduction because of soft tissue interposition. These fractures require open reduction and pinning. Likewise, in the case of neurologic deficit or vascular insufficiency, this fracture should undergo open reduction, and the involved structures should be explored.

Supracondylar fractures in adults are often comminuted and have intra-articular extension, and are usually best managed by open reduction and internal fixation for early range-of-motion exercises of the elbow.

COMPLICATIONS. The most serious complication is Volkmann's ischemia with subsequent contracture.[36] Varus, valgus, or rotary malunion do not remodel and persist. The most common malunion observed is that of cubitus varus (gun stock deformity; Fig. 3). If significant, this may require a corrective supracondylar valgus osteotomy.

PHYSEAL INJURIES. A variation of the supracondylar fracture in children is a transcondylar or transphyseal injury. The entire epiphysis of the distal humerus is displaced from the metaphysis, and the displacement can be anterior, posterior, or lateral, depending upon the applied forces. In young children, this injury may be undiagnosed or may be confused with an elbow dislocation. Diagnosis is made on the basis of the abnormal relationship between the distal humeral metaphysis and the proximal ulna and radius and preservation of a normal anatomic relationship between the capitellum and proximal radius. Radiographs should be examined closely for the presence of a small metaphyseal fragment arising from the distal humerus (Thurston Holland sign)[32] as a clue to the diagnosis. Normally, this injury can be managed by closed reduction, and reduction is usually stable. A posterior splint is then applied for 3 to 4 weeks.

LATERAL CONDYLE FRACTURES. This fracture is a significant fracture of childhood and deserves special consideration. This fracture may be misdiagnosed as a minor injury. The lateral condyle fracture is an intra-articular fracture, usually a Salter Type IV injury. Unlike most children's fractures, this fracture has a tendency to progress to nonunion (Fig. 4).[23] Even minimally displaced fractures may fail to unite if inappropriately managed. This injury usually occurs as a result of a fall on the outstretched arm with the elbow extended and the forearm abducted, leading to forces transmitted to the lateral condyle of the humerus through the radius. Displaced fractures must be treated by open reduction and internal fixation with smooth pins. Minimally displaced fractures, if determined radiographically to be not malrotated or significantly displaced, can be managed by plaster immobilization. However, if there is any question of malalignment, open reduction is indicated.

MEDIAL EPICONDYLE FRACTURES. This fracture is usually the result of a traction injury from the flexor origin. This may be an isolated injury or may be associated with dislocation of the elbow. Minimally displaced fractures require no treatment other than temporary immobilization; usually 3 weeks is sufficient. Fractures displaced more than 5 mm. warrant open reduction and internal fixation with pins. Pin placement should be under direct vision to avoid injury to the ulnar nerve.[30]

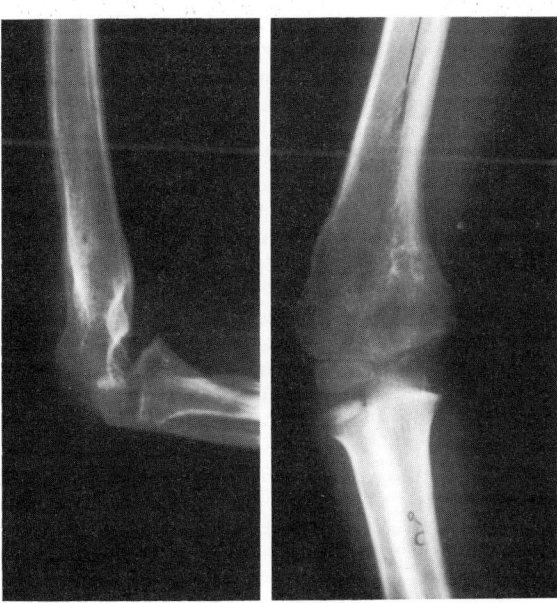

Figure 3. A malunion of a supracondylar humerus fracture has led to loss of the normal valgus carrying angle because of a varus malunion causing a gun stock deformity.

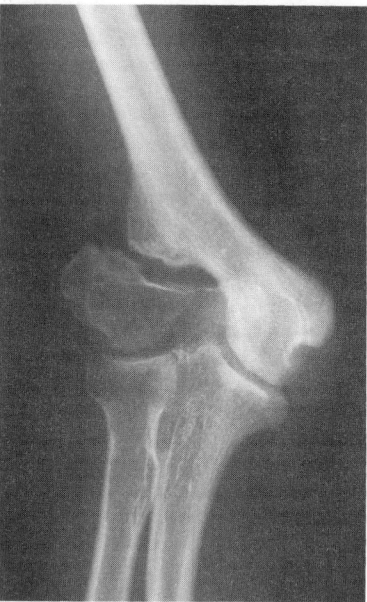

Figure 4. This elbow radiograph is of a 14-year-old girl with an old nonunion of a lateral condyle fracture. This has led to a cubitus valgus deformity, and the patient has developed tardy ulnar nerve symptoms.

DISLOCATIONS OF THE ELBOW. Posterior dislocation is caused by a fall on the outstretched arm, causing dislocation of the radius and ulna. Neurovascular structures are rarely affected, although arterial injury occurs occasionally. Anterior dislocations are caused by a blow on the flexed elbow. Dislocation of the radial head can occur as an isolated injury anteriorly or posteriorly. Dislocation of the ulna alone occurs rarely. Associated fractures of the coronoid process, medial epicondyle, or radial head may result when dislocation occurs.

CLINICAL FINDINGS. Elbow motion is limited. There is deformity, and the neurovascular structures are usually intact. Median nerve injury occasionally occurs.

TREATMENT. Gentle pull on the olecranon followed by flexion usually relocates the dislocation. After reduction, the elbow should be extended through a reasonable range of motion for testing stability. If the elbow is stable, immobilization is done for comfort, and motion exercises are initiated as soon as tolerated, preferably within the first week.

COMPLICATIONS. In simple dislocations, a functional range of motion usually results. Myositis ossificans, however, can produce mild or severe limitation of motion in a small percentage of patients. Neurovascular complications occasionally occur.

FRACTURES OF THE OLECRANON. The olecranon process constitutes the proximal ulnar articulation with the humerus and serves as a point of attachment for the triceps tendon. Because of the subcutaneous location on the extensor surface of the arm, it is susceptible to direct trauma. Fractures may also occur as a result of a traction-avulsion mechanism caused by the pull of the triceps tendon.

CLINICAL FINDINGS. There is swelling and tenderness in the region of the proximal ulna. Because of the subcutaneous location, the fracture site may be palpable. Ulnar nerve function should be carefully tested, because contusion neurapraxia can be associated with this injury. Anteroposterior and lateral radiographs should be assessed for the size of the olecranon fragment, the degree of comminution, and the amount of displacement.

TREATMENT. Undisplaced fractures are treated by splinting with the elbow in 60 degrees of flexion. Fractures with any significant displacement should be treated by open reduction with anatomic realignment of the articular surface when possible. Avulsion fractures usually involve only a small piece of the olecranon and can be excised or repaired. Comminuted fractures may be best managed by primary excision of the olecranon and triceps tendon repair. Internal fixation can be achieved by intramedullary screw fixation or a modified tension band wiring technique.

Achieving an anatomic reduction with rigid internal fixation allows early active motion and should diminish the delayed complications of limited motion and degenerative arthritis.[43]

FRACTURES AND DISLOCATION OF THE RADIAL HEAD. An isolated dislocation of the radial head in children or adults is uncommon. When a dislocation occurs, it is generally associated with a fracture of the proximal ulna (Monteggia's fracture dislocation).[12] In young children, subluxation of the radial head through the annular ligament is common and is referred to as a "pulled elbow" or "nursemaid's elbow." This is the result of forced distraction and pronation of the forearm.

Radial head fractures, however, are common in both children and adults. Because of the normal valgus carrying angle, a fall on the outstretched arm results in transmission of forces along the radius causing impaction of the radial head against the capitellum. This results in three patterns of fractures in children. The most common injury is a compression fracture through the metaphysis causing angular displacement. Less commonly, the injury causes a physeal plate fracture (Type I or II) and, rarely, in the adolescent, an intra-articular Type III fracture can occur. In adults, most fractures are intra-articular; therefore, it is important to determine the degree of displacement, depression, and the amount of articular surface involved.

CLINICAL FINDINGS. The diagnosis is made by noting direct tenderness over the radial head. There is pain and limited motion on pronation and supination of the forearm.

TREATMENT. The pulled elbow is often reduced by the time the child is examined by the physician or may be reduced when the arm is supinated for obtaining a radiograph. Flexion and supination of the forearm allow the radial head to slip back under the annular ligament, facilitating a reduction.

Nonarticular radial head fractures in children require only temporary immobilization for pain if angular displacement is less than 30 degrees. If angular displacement is greater than this, closed reduction should be attempted. Displaced epiphyseal fractures may require open reduction if a closed reduction fails to restore length and alignment. Radial head excision should never be performed in a child.

In adults, minimally displaced fractures require temporary immobilization until pain subsides. If the fragment involves more than 50 per cent of the articular surface and is comminuted, primary radial head excision is warranted. A silicone prosthesis may be a useful substitute if elbow instability is present. Articular fractures involving less than 50 per cent of the articular surface should be treated by temporary immobilization and early range-of-motion exercises to include pronation, supination, and elbow flexion and extension.

Fractures of the Shaft of the Radius and Ulna

The proximal and distal articulations of the radius and ulna allow the radius to rotate around the ulna, providing pronation and supination of the forearm. Proximally this rotation is permitted through the complex articulation at the radial-ulnar and radial-humeral joints. Distally the radial-ulnar relationship is maintained by the triangular fibrocartilage complex. The shaft of the radius and ulna is connected by the fibrous interosseous membrane, which serves as a hinge allowing the radius to rotate around the ulna. Distortion of the anatomy by fractures or dislocations alters the biomechanics of the forearm. A change in the normal interosseous membrane space causes limitation of pronation and supination. Distortion of the proximal or distal radial-ulnar joint similarly limits forearm rotation.

MECHANISM OF INJURY. Isolated fractures of the radius or ulna and both bone fractures of the shaft are usually due to a direct blow. A fall on the outstretched arm combined with a torsional stress may cause fracture of both the radius and ulna. Monteggia's fracture,[12] a fracture of the proximal ulna associated with radial head dislocation, may also be due to a fall on the outstretched arm and hyperpronation of the forearm. Similarly, the shaft of the radius may be fractured in the region of the distal third with subluxation of the distal ulna termed the Galeazzi[53] or Piedmont fracture.[33]

CLINICAL FINDINGS. Pain and deformity of the forearm are present. Evaluation of the neurovascular condition of the extremity must be made as well as the presence or absence of increased pressure within the muscle compartments of the forearm. Swelling within the tight muscle compartments of the forearm can cause occlusion of venous and arterial circulation and may cause Volkmann's ischemic contracture. Significant swelling of the forearm compartments associated with pain on passive extension of the fingers should call attention to this possibility.

Radiographs in forearm injuries should include views of the elbow and wrist and define the location of the fracture, the degree of comminution, any rotational deformity, and the presence of associated radial head or distal ulna subluxation or dislocation.

TREATMENT. A compartment syndrome should be recognized and treated expeditiously so that irreversible muscle necrosis is avoided. Forearm compartment fasciotomy and median nerve decompression should be performed.

In adults, displaced fractures of the shaft of the radius and ulna, fractures of the proximal ulna associated with radial head dislocation (Monteggia's lesion), and fractures of the radius associated with disruption of the distal radial ulnar joint (Piedmont fracture) are best managed by operative methods. With Monteggia's fracture, the radial head must be reduced and the fracture of the ulna stabilized. Both bone forearm fractures are best managed by compression plating of the radius and ulna to restore a normal interosseous space.[42]

Conversely, most forearm fractures in children can be managed by closed means. The thick periosteum makes reduction of the fractures more stable than those in adults, and the osteogenic potential in children allows excellent remodeling of angular deformities. However, rotational malalignment does not remodel and must be avoided during closed treatment of these fractures. Occasionally with a Monteggia's fracture dislocation, the radial head cannot be reduced because of a greenstick fracture of the proximal ulna or because of interposed tissue; and in this instance, open reduction of the fracture and dislocation is indicated.

COMPLICATIONS. The most serious complication in forearm fractures, neurovascular compromise and subsequent ischemic contracture, must be avoided. Nonunion of forearm shaft fractures occurs in 5 to 10 per cent of the cases in which closed treatment is used. Open treatment may be complicated by nonunion with or without infection. The most frequent complication is malunion and occurs more commonly with closed reduction of displaced fractures in adults. Malunion with compromise of the interosseous space causes limited pronation and supination. Other complications are elbow stiffness, finger stiffness, and reflex sympathetic dystrophy.

Fractures of the Distal Forearm

ANATOMY. The distal radius and ulna articulate with the proximal carpal row. The radial-ulnar articulation allows pronation and supination. The distal ulna is stabilized and covered by a sheet of ligament and cartilage termed the triangular fibrocartilage. The radial styloid extends distal relative to the ulnar styloid, creating an angle of approximately 15 degrees from a line perpendicular to the axis of the forearm. The distal radius normally has a volar angulation of 10 degrees.

MECHANISM OF INJURY. Fractures of the distal radius and ulna are common in children and adults. The injury occurs by a fall on the outstretched arm with forces transmitted through the carpus, causing either volar or dorsal displacement. In children, displacement may occur through the metaphysis or through the physeal plate. In adults, the fracture line is usually through the metaphysis, although intra-articular fractures may occur. In elderly patients, the dorsal cortex tends to become comminuted.

A Colles fracture[17] is a fracture of the distal radial metaphysis with dorsal displacement and volar angulation. A Smith fracture[60] is a fracture with volar displacement and dorsal angulation. Barton[4] described an intra-articular fracture of either the dorsal or volar lip of the distal radius.

CLINICAL FINDINGS. Pain, swelling, and deformity are present just proximal to the wrist. Often a "step-off" in the distal radius can be appreciated by palpation. Median nerve function should be tested because this nerve is susceptible to damage either by direct contusion or secondary compression.

TREATMENT. Nondisplaced or minimally displaced fractures are treated by immobilization for 3 to 4 weeks. Displaced fractures should be reduced with the patient under regional anesthesia. Occasionally epiphyseal injuries in children require a general anesthetic to obtain reduction without undue force. A Colles fracture is reduced by distraction, which allows disimpaction of the dorsal cortex and then flexion of the distal fragment and wrist to obtain reduction. The wrist should be immobilized in mild flexion and ulnar deviation for maintenance of reduction. Intra-articular fractures of the distal radius, if displaced, should be treated by open reduction. Severely comminuted fractures may best be managed by pins and plaster or application of an external fixator.[41]

COMPLICATIONS. In children, physeal plate injuries may cause permanent growth disturbance. Comminuted fractures may cause shortening of the distal radius, with incongruity of the distal radial-ulnar joint and subsequent limited motion and pain. Acute or late median nerve symptoms may occur.

Other complications include rupture of the extensor pollicis longus and reflex sympathetic dystrophy.

SELECTED REFERENCES

Bankart, A. S. B.: Pathology and treatment of recurrent dislocation of the shoulder joint. Br. J. Surg., 26:23, 1939.
This is a classic description of the pathology of shoulder dislocations and the description of a technique that is still considered to be one of the best methods of surgical repair.

Neer, C. S., II: Displaced proximal humeral fractures. I. Classification and evaluation. J. Bone Joint Surg. [Am.], 52:1077, 1970.
In this article, Neer describes a useful classification for proximal humerus fractures based on the number of fracture fragments and the amount of displacement.

Ogden, J. A.: Skeletal Injury in the Child. Philadelphia, Lea & Febiger, 1982.
This is an excellent reference text for fractures involving the immature skeleton.

Pirone, A. M., Graham, H. K., and Krajbich, J. I.: Management of displaced extension-type supracondylar fractures of the humerus in children. J. Bone Joint Surg. [Am.], 70:641, 1988.
These authors review the results of various methods of managing displaced supracondylar fractures of the humerus in children. They conclude that percutaneous pinning is the method that consistently provides the best results.

Rockwood, C. A., and Green, D. P.: Fractures. Philadelphia, J. B. Lippincott Company, 1984.
This textbook is a complete reference source. Two volumes cover adult fractures, and one volume is dedicated to pediatric fractures.

REFERENCES

1. Aulicino, P. L., Reinert, C., Kornberg, M., and Williamson, S.: Displaced intra-articular glenoid fractures treated by open reduction and internal fixation. J. Trauma, 26:1137, 1986.
2. Bankart, A. S. B.: Dislocation of the shoulder joints. *In* Robert Jones' Birthday Volume. A Collection of Surgical Essays. London, Oxford University Press, 1928.
3. Bankart, A. S. B.: Pathology and treatment of recurrent dislocation of the shoulder joint. Br. J. Surg., 26:23, 1939.

4. Barton, J. R.: Views in treatment of an important injury to the wrist. Med. Examiner, 1:365, 1838.
5. Baumann, E.: Bietage zur kenntnis der Frakturen am Ellbogengelenk. Unter besonderer Berucksichtigung der Spatfolgen. I. Allgemeines und Fractura supra condylica. Beitr. Klin. Chir., 146:1, 1929.
6. Bearden, J. M., Hughston, J. C., and Whatley, G. S.: Acromioclavicular dislocation: Method of treatment. J. Sports Med., 1:5, 1973.
7. Blazina, M. E., and Saltzman, J. S.: Recurrent anterior subluxation of the shoulder in athletes—a distinct entity. J. Bone Joint Surg. [Am.], 51:1037, 1969.
8. Bohler, L.: The Treatment of Fractures. Supplementary Volume. New York, Grune & Stratton, 1966.
9. Braunstein, E. M., and O'Conner, G.: Double contrast arthrotomography of the shoulder. J. Bone Joint Surg. [Am.], 64:192, 1982.
10. Broker, F. H. L., and Burbach, T.: Ultrasonic Diagnosis of Separation of the Proximal Humeral Epiphysis in the Newborn. J. Bone Joint Surg. [Am.], 72:187, 1990.
11. Browne, A. O., O'Riordan, M., and Quinlan, W.: Supracondylar fractures of the humerus in adults. Injury, 17:184, 1986.
12. Bryan, R. S.: Monteggia's fracture of the forearm. J. Trauma, 11:992, 1971.
13. Caffey, J. P.: Pediatric X-ray Diagnosis: A Textbook for Students of Pediatric Surgery and Radiology, 7th ed. Chicago, Year Book Medical Publishers, 1978.
14. Caldwell, J. A.: Treatment of fractures in the Cincinnati General Hospital. Ann. Surg., 97:161, 1933.
15. Caldwell, J. A.: Treatment of fractures of the shaft of the humerus by hanging cast. Surg. Gynecol. Obstet., 70:421, 1940.
16. Charnley, J.: The Closed Treatment of Common Fractures. Baltimore, Williams & Wilkins, 1961.
17. Colles, A.: On the fracture of the carpal extremity of the radius. Edinburgh Med. Surg. J., 10:182, 1814.
18. Connolly, J. F.: DePalma's Management of Fractures and Dislocations, 3rd ed. Philadelphia, W. B. Saunders Company, 1981.
19. Cox, J. S.: The fate of the AC joint in athletic injuries. Am. J. Sports Med., 9:1, 1981.
20. Tse, D. H. W., Slabaugh, P. B., and Carlson, P. A.: Injury to the axillary artery by a closed fracture of the clavicle. J. Bone Joint Surg. [Am.], 62:1372, 1980.
21. Denham, R. H., Jr., and Dingley, A. F., Jr.: Epiphyseal separation of the medial end of the clavicle. J. Bone Joint Surg. [Am.], 49:1179, 1967.
22. Dodge, H. S.: Displaced supracondylar fractures of the humerus in children: Treatment by Dunlop's traction. J. Bone Joint Surg. [Am.], 54:1408, 1972.
23. Flynn, J. C., and Richards, J. F., Jr.: Nonunion of minimally displaced fractures of the lateral condyle of the humerus in children. J. Bone Joint Surg. [Am.], 53:1096, 1971.
24. Halliburton, R. A., Barbour, J. R., and Fraser, R. L.: Pseudodislocation: an unusual birth injury. Can. J. Surg., 10:455, 1967.
25. Hawkins, R. J., and Kiefer, G. N.: Internal fixation techniques for proximal humeral fractures. Clin. Orthop., 223:77, 1987.
26. Hawkins, R. J., and Koppert, G.: The natural history following anterior dislocation of the shoulder in the older patient. J. Bone Joint Surg. [Br.], 64:255, 1982.
27. Healy, W. L., White, G. N., Mick, C. A., Brooker, A. F., and Weiland, A. J.: Nonunion of the humeral shaft. Clin. Orthop., 219:206, 1987.
28. Helfet, A. J.: Coracoid transplantation for recurring dislocation of the shoulder. J. Bone Joint Surg. [Br.], 40:198, 1958.
29. Hill, H. A., and Sachs, M. D.: A groove defect of the humeral head: A shoulder joint. Radiology, 35:690, 1940.
30. Hines, R. F., Herndon, W. A., and Evans, J. P.: Operative treatment of medial epicondyle fractures in children. Clin. Orthop., 223:170, 1987.
31. Hobbs, D. W.: Sternoclavicular joint: A new axial radiographic view. Radiology, 90:801, 1968.
32. Holland, C. T.: Radiographic note on injuries to the distal epiphyses of radius and ulna. Proc. World Soc. Med., 22:695, 1929.
33. Hughston, J. C.: Fracture of the distal radial shaft, mistakes in management. J. Bone Joint Surg. [Am.], 39:249, 1957.
34. Johnson, L. L.: The shoulder joint. An arthroscopist's perspective of anatomy and pathology. Clin. Orthop., 223:113, 1987.
35. Kennedy, J. C., and Cameron, H.: Complete dislocation of the acromioclavicular joint. J. Bone Joint Surg. [Br.], 36:202, 1954.
36. Kirker, J. R.: Dislocation of the shoulder complicated by rupture of the axillary vessels: Report of a case. J. Bone Joint Surg. [Br.], 34:72, 1952.
37. Lipscomb, P. R., and Burlson, R. J.: Vascular and neural complications in supracondylar fractures of the humerus in children. J. Bone Joint Surg. [Am.], 37:487, 1955.
38. Magill, H. K., and Aitken, A. P.: Pulled elbow. Surg. Gynecol. Obstet., 98:753, 1954.
39. Magnuson, P. B.: Treatment of recurrent dislocation of the shoulder. Surg. Clin. North Am., 25:14, 1945.
40. McKenzie, J. M. M.: Retrosternal dislocation of the clavicle: Report of two cases. J. Bone Joint Surg. [Br.], 45:138, 1963.
41. Mears, D. C.: External Skeletal Fixation. Baltimore, Williams & Wilkins, 1983.
42. Muller, M. E., Allgower, M., and Willenegger, H.: Manual of internal fixation, technique recommended by the AP-Group. New York, Heidelberg, Berlin, Springer-Verlag, 1970.
43. Murphy, D. F., Green, W. B., and Dameron, T. B.: Displaced olecranon fractures in adults. Clin. Orthop., 224:215, 1987.
44. Neer, C. S., II: Displaced proximal humeral fractures. I. Classification and evaluation. J. Bone Joint Surg. [Am.], 52:1077, 1970.
45. Neer, C. S., II: Fractures of the distal third of the clavicle. Clin. Orthop., 58:43, 1968.
46. Neer, C. S., II: Prosthetic replacement of the humeral head: Indications and operative technique. Surg. Clin. North Am., 43:1581, 1963.
47. Ogden, J. A.: Skeletal Injury in the Child. Philadelphia, Lea & Febiger, 1982.
48. Osmond-Clarke, H.: Habitual dislocation of the shoulder. The Putti-Platt operation. J. Bone Joint Surg. [Br.], 30:19, 1948.
49. Paquet, R., Des Marchais, J. E., and Benazet, J. P.: Evaluation of Neer prostheses for humeral fractures. J. Bone Joint Surg. [Br.], 62:128, 1980.
50. Paterson, D. C.: Retrosternal dislocation of the clavicle. J. Bone Joint Surg. [Br.], 43:90, 1961.
51. Penn, I.: The vascular complications of fractures of the clavicle. J. Trauma, 4:819, 1964.
52. Pirone, A. M., Graham, H. K., Krajbich, J. I.: Management of displaced extension-type supracondylar fractures of the humerus in children. J. Bone Joint Surg. [Am.], 70:641, 1988.
53. Rang, M.: Anthology of orthopaedics. Edinburgh, E. & S. Livingstone, 1968.
54. Rask, M. R., and Steinberg, L. H.: Fracture of the acromion caused by muscle force: A case report. J. Bone Joint Surg. [Am.], 60:1146, 1978.
55. Rockwood, C. A., and Green, D. P.: Fractures. Philadelphia, J. B. Lippincott Company, 1984.
56. Rowe, C. R.: An atlas of anatomy in treatment of mid-clavicular fractures. Clin. Orthop., 58:29, 1968.
57. Rowe, C. R.: Recurrent transient anterior subluxation of the shoulder, the "dead arm" syndrome. Clin. Orthop., 223:11, 1987.
58. Rowe, C. R., Pierce, D. S., and Clark, J. G.: Voluntary dislocations of the shoulder: A preliminary report on a clinical, electromyographic, and psychiatric study of 26 patients. J. Bone Joint Surg. [Am.], 55:445, 1973.
59. Scientific Research Committee, Pennsylvania Orthopaedic Society: Fresh midshaft fractures of the humerus in adults. Penn. Med. J., 62:848, 1959.
60. Seedon, H. J.: Nerve lesions complicating certain closed bone injuries. J.A.M.A., 135:691, 1947.
61. Smith, R. W.: A treatise on fractures in the vicinity in joints and on certain forms of accidental and congenital dislocations. Dublin, Hodges and Smith, 1854.
62. Smyth, E. H. J.: Major arterial injury in closed fracture of the neck of the humerus. Report of a case. J. Bone Joint Surg. [Br.], 51:508, 1969.
63. Stableforth, P. G.: Treatment of four-part proximal humeral fractures. J. Bone Joint Surg. [Br.], 63:288, 1981.
64. Stener, B.: Dislocation of the shoulder complicated by complete rupture of the axillary artery. J. Bone Joint Surg. [Br.], 39:714, 1957.
65. Stewart, M. J.: Fractures of the humeral shaft. In Adams, J. P. (Ed.): Current Practice in Orthopaedic Surgery. St. Louis, C. V. Mosby Company, 1964.
66. Stimson, L. A.: An easy method of reducing dislocations of the shoulder and hip. Med. Rec., 57:356, 1900.
67. Williams, D. J.: The mechanisms producing fracture-separation of the proximal humeral epiphysis. J. Bone Joint Surg. [Br.], 63:102, 1981.
68. Worman, L. W., and Leagus, C.: Intrathoracic injury following retrosternal dislocation of the clavicle. J. Trauma, 7:416, 1967.
69. Zenni, E. J., Krieg, J. K., and Rosen, M. J.: Open reduction and internal fixation of clavicular fractures. J. Bone Joint Surg. [Am.], 63:147, 1981.

IV _____

FRACTURE OF THE CARPAL SCAPHOID

Richard D. Goldner, M.D., and J. Leonard Goldner, M.D.

Because the scaphoid is the most frequently fractured carpal bone, the major emphasis of this section concerns injuries involving the carpal scaphoid.

WRIST MOTION. Wrist dorsiflexion and volar flexion occur at both the radial carpal and intercarpal joints. The relationships of the eight carpal bones are depicted in Figure 1. Physiologic movement of the wrist joint is an intercalated, smooth activity. The axis of normal carpal movement is in the neck of the capitate. At the radial carpal joint, the movement includes scaphoid, lunate, and triquetrum. The scaphoid bridges the proximal and distal carpal rows. The motion of dorsiflexion and volar flexion of the wrist joint occurs approximately half at the radial carpal and half at the intercarpal joints. The scaphoid moves through an arc of approximately 40 degrees and articulates with the radius, lunate, capitate, and trapezium through the entire arc of flexion and extension.

Wrist motion is initiated by muscles that insert into metacarpals. As the wrist rotates from neutral to ulnar deviation, the proximal carpal row dorsiflexes and the profile of the scaphoid appears longer; from neutral to radial deviation, the proximal carpal row volar flexes and the scaphoid appears foreshortened. For this reason, ulnar deviation radiographs are necessary for adequate visualization of the scaphoid. Because the scaphoid crosses both proximal and distal carpal rows, excessive dorsiflexion causes it to be pinned between the dorsal lip of the radius and the palmar sling of the strong radial capitate ligament. The scaphoid is the principal bony block to excessive dorsiflexion of the hand and wrist and is particularly susceptible to fracture during a fall on the outstretched hand.

History and Physical Examination

A careful history and detailed physical examination are crucial in diagnosing wrist injuries. The amount of force sustained during the injury and the position of the wrist and upper extremity while that force occurred should increase the physician's suspicion regarding significant carpal injury.

A force of 2000 pounds per square inch may be involved in causing the original fracture, although in other instances, a relatively "minor injury" may produce ligamentous injury without fracture. An apparently "minor injury," however, often is associated with a tremendous torque and twisting motion, and the patient may not appreciate the forces involved.

Examination of the patient with a carpal injury includes careful palpation to detect areas of tenderness, edema, or contusion; measurements of range of motion; motor and sensory assessment; and use of the Allen test to determine the integrity of the radial and ulnar arteries. The examiner should not overlook concomitant trauma such as anterior dislocation of the humerus or radial head fracture.

Clinical Assessment of the Painful Wrist

The most consistent sign of carpal injury is localized tenderness to digital pressure. Fracture of the carpal scaphoid produces tenderness to pressure in the anatomic "snuffbox" that is located between the extensor pollicis longus and extensor pollicis brevis–abductor pollicis longus compartments.

Radial and ulnar deviation results in pain on the radial side of the wrist. Stress must be applied, in certain instances, if the fracture is occult. Forced dorsiflexion is the most painful ma-

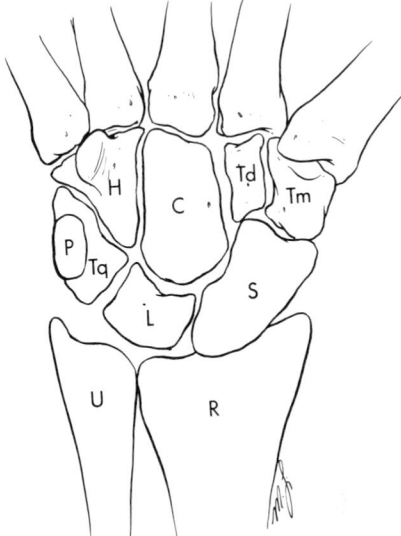

Figure 1. The carpal bones: scaphoid (S); lunate (L); triquetrum (Tq); pisiform (P), which is a sesamoid bone within the flexor carpi ulnaris; trapezium (Tm); trapezoid (Td); capitate (C); and hamate (H). Radius (R) and ulna (U) are noted. (From Goldner, R. D., Ugino, M. R., and Goldner, J. L.: Injuries to carpal bones. *In* Edlich, R. F., and Spyker, D. A. (Eds.): Current Emergency Medical Therapy. Norwalk, Conn., Appleton-Century-Crofts, 1984.)

neuver. If the patient is asked to supinate and the examiner attempts to pronate the hand and wrist against resistance, and vice versa, pain may be stimulated. Pain can be produced by having the patient put extreme pressure on the fingertips with the wrist in dorsiflexion.

SURFACE ANATOMY. Certain critical points that should be examined after known trauma to the hand are demonstrated in Figure 2, which demonstrates the outstretched hand with the possible lines of force that occur, depending upon how the individual breaks the fall. The lowest line of force may cause a Colles' fracture, whereas the upper line of force may cause a metacarpal fracture. The central force would be involved in a carpal injury.

Radiographic Findings

The initial radiographic examination of the patient with carpal injury should include at least anteroposterior (AP), lateral, and supination and pronation oblique views. The lateral view must be a "true lateral," with the wrist in neutral position, to demonstrate the linear relationship between the distal radius, lunate, and capitate.

In patients in whom a scaphoid fracture is suspected, and in whom the clinical findings are strongly positive, a projection in ulnar deviation and pronation (posteroanterior [PA], palm down) may demonstrate the scaphoid clearly and reveal an undisplaced fracture not evident on the other views. During the ulnar deviation maneuver, excessive stress should not be applied; otherwise, displacement of a nondisplaced scaphoid fracture may occur.

A simultaneous radial styloid fracture is relatively common with a carpal dislocation, and a patient with radial styloid fracture should have radiographs to exclude scapholunate dissocia-

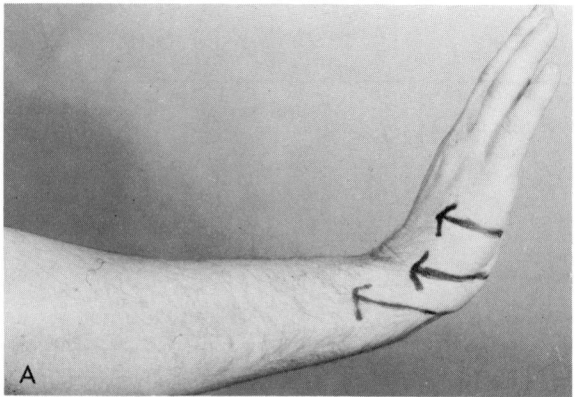

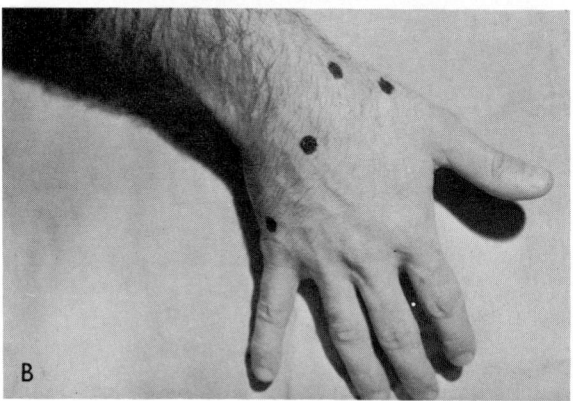

Figure 2. A, Position of the hand and forearm usually associated with a "fall on the outstretched hand." Arrows represent lines of force that might occur. B, The dots correspond to common areas of fracture of the hand: the base of the thumb metacarpal, the proximal carpal row, and the metacarpals.

tion (Fig. 3C). These radiographs should include anteroposterior (AP, supination, palm up) and clenched-fist AP views in addition to the true lateral.

SPECIAL ROENTGENOGRAPHIC CONSIDERATIONS. Radiographic projections at the time of original injury may not demonstrate a fracture because of impaction and absence of resorption. Decreased bone density at the fracture site and physiologic resorption demonstrate a fracture line evident on the radiograph obtained 10 to 14 days after injury. If the clinical findings are strongly suggestive of fracture, but routine radiographs are negative, special techniques and projections are con-

sidered: (1) a magnification radiograph that may demonstrate interruption of trabeculae, which implies an occult fracture; (2) PA and lateral tomograms or direct sagittal and transverse computed tomographic (CT) scans, which may demonstrate a fracture at a level deeper than that which the plain radiograph visualizes; (3) repeat stress radiographs in ulnar deviation after the wrist joint has been injected with a local anesthetic; (4) fluoroscopic visualization of the wrist movements after injection with a local anesthetic. If these special techniques do not detect a fracture, and if pain and tenderness persist, a technetium-99 bone scan a few weeks after trauma may detect the fracture that plain radiographs would not necessarily demonstrate.

There are numerous instances of "sprained wrists" treated by simple soft dressing with subsequent nonunion of the carpal scaphoid, which if treated originally for 8 to 10 weeks in an appropriate cast, probably would have united, with elimination of the impairment that occurs with nonunion of the scaphoid.

Treatment

The major problems that occur when managing the scaphoid fracture are lack of an early diagnosis and delayed initiation of appropriate treatment. If the initial radiographs are negative, but tenderness to pressure exists in the anatomic snuffbox, a cast should be applied in radial deviation and 10 degrees of flexion for immobilization of the thumb, including the proximal phalanx, the wrist, and the forearm. This cast is removed at 2 weeks, and the radiographs are repeated. Bone resorption occurring by that time usually allows the fracture line to be visible. If clinical findings persist, but the radiographs are negative, the special radiographs noted above or a technetium bone scan is obtained. The displaced, unstable scaphoid fracture usually does not heal with cast treatment and requires surgical treatment for internal fixation.

The major blood supply to the scaphoid is from the radial artery. Branches have been demonstrated at the palmar surface (tubercle), but the majority enter through the dorsal surface. The distal location of the major blood supply has been considered to be the cause of the high incidence of nonunion and aseptic necrosis of the proximal fragment. The blood vessels passing distal to proximal are interrupted when the scaphoid fracture occurs, and the proximal segment becomes temporarily ischemic. The location and obliquity of the fracture line influence the average healing time of a scaphoid fracture.

Fractures of the *distal third* constitute 10 per cent of the total number of scaphoid fractures and usually heal in approximately

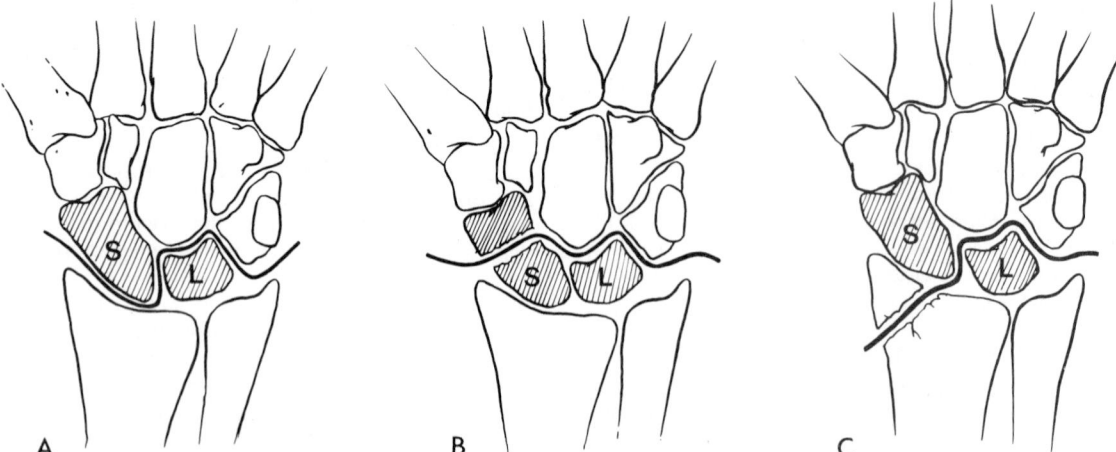

Figure 3. The scaphoid bridges the proximal and distal carpal rows. With a dislocation between these two rows, the scaphoid must either rotate or fracture. This produces (A) a perilunate dislocation, in which the remainder of the carpus dislocates around the lunate (L); (B) a transscaphoid perilunate dislocation, in which the distal half of the scaphoid (S) and the remaining carpus dislocate around the lunate; or (C) a transradial styloid perilunate dislocation, a fracture of the radial styloid with subsequent dislocation of it and the remaining carpus around the lunate. (From Goldner, R. D., Ugino, M. R., and Goldner, J. L.: Injuries to carpal bones. In Edlich, R. F., and Spyker, D. A. (Eds.): Current Emergency Medical Therapy. Norwalk, Conn., Appleton-Century-Crofts, 1984.)

8 weeks. Seventy per cent of scaphoid fractures involve the *middle third* of the bone, and the healing time at this location is generally 8 to 12 weeks, although many fractures may require 16 to 18 weeks. In approximately 30 per cent of the *middle third* fractures, aseptic necrosis of the proximal fragment develops because of the blood flow pattern. Fractures of the *proximal third* constitute approximately 20 per cent of scaphoid fractures, and this group heals more slowly than the others. Healing time is 10 to 20 weeks, averaging approximately 16 weeks. In most of the fractures of the proximal fifth of the scaphoid, aseptic necrosis develops.

The orientation of the fracture and the alignment of the fragments affect healing. Horizontal oblique and transverse fractures are more stable and heal more rapidly than vertical oblique fractures, which have a high longitudinal shear component and less stability than the horizontal fractures.

If the scaphoid fracture fragments are displaced or angulated, some degree of carpal instability exists. Displaced fractures with ligamentous injuries are treated in most instances under direct vision by open reduction and internal fixation. Fixation pins, a lag screw or the Herbert screw, are employed for the latter.

Nondisplaced fractures of the scaphoid and those fractures without evidence of ligamentous instability are adequately treated by external immobilization in a cast. However, there is no clear consensus concerning the necessity of a long arm versus a short arm cast in the treatment of the stable scaphoid fracture. Also, there is limited consensus concerning the extent of the thumb and the digits to be included. Most surgeons agree that at least the forearm and the proximal phalanx of the thumb should be included in the initial cast. For the nondisplaced, stable fracture, the authors favor a gauntlet-type short arm cast from the midpalmar crease, including the proximal phalanx of the thumb with the wrist in 10-degree flexion and radial deviation to provide compression and apposition of the fragments. This wrist position should allow anatomic alignment of the fracture fragments and should be documented by radiographs after the cast is applied. If a short arm cast is used and the patient is usually active, the cast should be changed every 10 to 14 days for the first 6 weeks, so that it remains firm both around the forearm muscles and at the wrist.

TECHNIQUE OF APPLYING THE CAST. The cast should be molded carefully and extended proximally over the muscles of the forearm, following the shape of the forearm (Fig. 4*A* and *B*). The cast should not be contoured circularly but should be molded in a quadrilateral shape. Minimal padding should be used throughout, so that when edema subsides, fixation is adequate and the proximal end of the cast is not hypermobile. The styloid process of the ulna and the radial styloid should be carefully padded for avoidance of cast pressure on the skin. The cast should be molded into the palm, and the fingers should be free at the metacarpophalangeal joints and distally. The proximal phalanx of the thumb should be in a position of abduction, so that the patient may write.

Differential Diagnosis

1. *Rotatory subluxation of the scaphoid,* or scapholunate dissociation, occurs because of a tear of the complex ligaments between the radius, scaphoid, and lunate (Fig. 5). When these ligaments are avulsed or ruptured, the relationship between the scaphoid-lunate and the scaphoid and trapezium is distorted. The patient complains of a "popping" and "clicking" in the wrist joint associated with pain and limited motion. The condition is not readily diagnosed unless suspected.

2. *Rupture of the flexor carpi radialis tendon* occurs from a fall on the outstretched hand, causing separation of the insertion of the flexor carpi radialis deep to the thenar muscles. A chip of bone may separate with the tendon, or, in patients older than 35 years of age, the tendon may rupture partially or completely. This tendon is also affected by collagen aging, and localized partial ruptures occur as a result of minimal trauma. Pain is detected over the scaphoid on the palmar surface of the wrist or

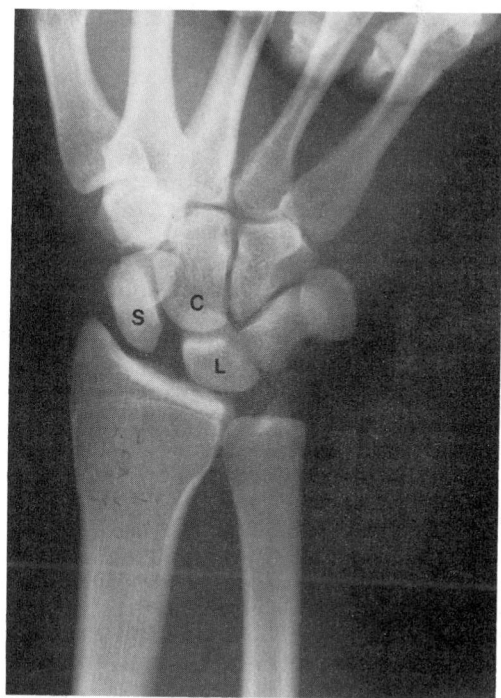

Figure 5. Clenched fist view in a patient with scapholunate dissociation demonstrating widening of the space between the scaphoid (S) and lunate (L) (Terry Thomas sign) and foreshortened appearance of the scaphoid. The AP view is taken with the forearm in supination (palm up), to demonstrate scapholunate dissociation. This diagnosis is made by the following roentgenographic findings: (1) distance between the scaphoid and lunate (scapholunate gap on the AP film greater than 2 mm. [Terry Thomas sign]); (2) foreshortened appearance of the abnormally palmar flexed scaphoid on the AP view; (3) cortical "signet ring" shadow, representing an axial projection of the abnormally oriented scaphoid; and (4) more vertical orientation at the scaphoid as demonstrated by the increased angle between the scaphoid and lunate on the true lateral x-ray (normal, 30 to 60 degrees; see Fig. 6). Those patients suspected of having scapholunate dissociation should have a compression stress view, which is performed by having the patient clench his fist for the AP film. This view often demonstrates scapholunate widening not seen on the static view. (From Goldner, R. D., Ugino, M. R., and Goldner, J. L.: Injuries of carpal bone. *In* Edlich, R. F., and Spyker, D. A. (Eds.): Current Emergency Medical Therapy. Norwalk, Conn., Appleton-Century-Crofts, 1984.)

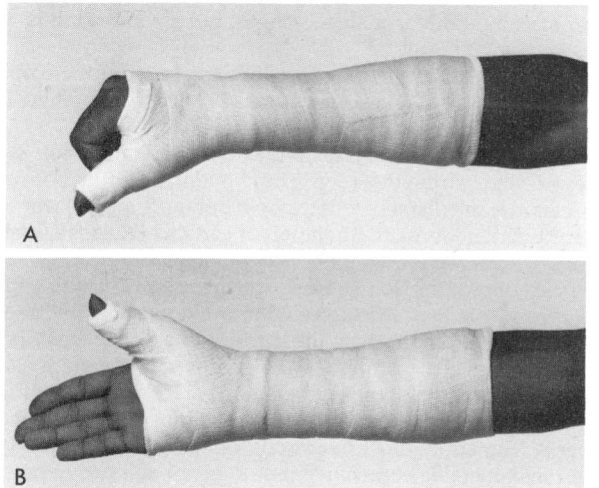

Figure 4. *A*, A well-fitting short arm cast is sufficient to immobilize stable, nondisplaced carpal scaphoid fragments. The contour of the forearm is used for molding of the plaster, thereby eliminating the need for cast above the elbow. *B*, In many instances, radial deviation and volar flexion give the best contact. The thumb metacarpal and proximal phalanx are included.

is present proximally along the course of the flexor carpi radialis tendon.

3. *A fracture of the styloid process of the radius* may result from a fall on the outstretched hand or a direct blow (see Figs. 2*B* and 3*C*). This site also coincides with the body of the scaphoid, and compression of the styloid process may cause pain at about the same location as does compression of the scaphoid.

4. *A trapezium fracture* following a direct blow of the fist or a fall on the radially deviated closed hand may resemble the findings associated with a fractured scaphoid. The swelling and pain are usually directly at the base of the thumb, rather than over the scaphoid; and the mechanism of injury is usually different.

5. *Extensor carpi radialis longus avulsion* from the base of the second metacarpal occurs as a result of a forceful injury with the hand in ulnar deviation or a direct blow or a downward stroke such as might occur while the individual is swinging a golf club and strikes the ground. There is pain around the anatomic snuffbox near the location that is painful when the carpal scaphoid is injured. However, the radiograph demonstrates no fracture, and the palmar aspect of the wrist is not painful.

6. *Extensor carpi radialis brevis tendon avulsion* may occur from a forceful palmar flexion injury of the wrist. Palpation dorsally causes pain at the base of the third metacarpal, more distal than that which would occur if the scaphoid were fractured, and the palmar aspect of the wrist is not painful.

7. *Osteochondral fracture of the distal radius* follows an injury similar to that which causes the scaphoid to fracture. The mechanism of injury, the radiographic findings, and the location of pain primarily on the dorsal and radial aspects of the wrist aid in differentiating this injury from the carpal scaphoid fracture.

8. *Lunate dislocation or fracture* causes pain on the dorsum of the wrist more to the center of the wrist area and less on the radial side. Neurologic assessment of the median nerve is essential because this nerve is frequently compressed with the lunate displacement. Wrist motion is limited, and the radiograph demonstrates distortion of the proximal carpal row. This malalignment in lateral carpal projection is diagnostic of lunate dislocation. The distal concavity of the lunate may be rotated 90 degrees and may be palmar to the capitate, rather than having its arc between the distal radius and the proximal capitate. The palmar lunate dislocation has been compared to a "spilled tea cup" (Fig. 6). AP radiographs of a dislocated lunate demonstrate a triangular or wedge shape rather than the usual quadrilateral appearance. Also, a more subtle sign of instability or subluxation of the lunate is elongation of the palmar lip when visualized on the AP radiograph.

Delayed Healing

In addition to osteonecrosis of the proximal pole, delayed union or nonunion is usually due to a late diagnosis with resultant lack of adequate immobilization or to malposition. A "sprained wrist" is not an acceptable diagnosis until a fracture of the carpal scaphoid has been excluded completely. When the diagnosis is established, but reduction is not anatomic, incomplete apposition of the fragments can cause nonunion. With certain complex injuries such as a transscaphoid perilunar dislocation (see Fig. 3*B*), open reduction and pin or screw fixation provide firm stabilization.

Pathologic Changes Associated with Nonunion or Malunion

Osteonecrosis of the fragment of the scaphoid proximal to the fracture occurs from inadequate blood supply and depends upon the anatomic composition of the scaphoid and the relationship of the fracture to the distal arterial inflow.

Traumatic arthrosis follows cartilage damage at the time of original injury, incongruity of cartilage surfaces secondary to malposition or malunion, or hypermobility from nonunion or ligament injury. Excision of one or both large fragments of a nonunited, displaced, painful scaphoid may produce satisfactory wrist function and motion for a few years, but the long-term follow-up generally has been unsatisfactory because of carpal bone migration, radial deviation of the hand, and subsequent traumatic arthrosis.

Reconstructive Procedures for Nonunion

Iliac crest bone grafting to bridge both proximal and distal segments of the scaphoid on the palmar surface as described by Russe has been 90 per cent successful in treating scaphoid nonunion. Also, internal lag screw fixation has been employed. Recently the development of the Herbert screw and jig has improved the fixation of the fragments and diminished the time that a cast is necessary for postoperative immobilization (Fig. 7*A* and *B*).

Another option for treatment of the established nonunion of the scaphoid *without a synovial pseudoarthrosis* or malposition is pulsing electromagnetic field treatments applied over a cast for at least 3 months.

Other Treatments Available When Bone Grafting Is Not Indicated

Proximal carpalectomy: If the proximal carpal row cannot be reconstructed, excision of these bones allows the radius to articulate with the capitate and provide reasonably good function, as long as the articular surfaces of the proximal capitate and the lunate fossa of the radius are healthy. Late carpalectomy for either nonunion or traumatic arthrosis may provide temporary relief of pain and reasonable strength, but a good result is not achieved consistently.

Radial styloidectomy: This procedure is selected if the scaphoid is healed but has an exostosis on its surface that impinges on the radial styloid.

Arthrodesis of the wrist: This procedure eliminates pain, provides excellent strength and grip, and maintains pronation and supination if the distal ulna is excised; but there are subsequent absent wrist motion and limitation of certain activities of daily living.

Silicone prosthesis: Replacement of the scaphoid with a silicone prosthesis that articulates with the lunate and the trapezium and is held in place by the surrounding capsule may provide a relatively painless wrist with fair strength and satisfactory range of motion for 5 to 7 years. Dislocation of the scaphoid prosthesis, despite careful technique, may occur in patients who apply repetitive strong forces to the wrist joint or who have unstable connective tissue. As an adjunctive procedure, intercarpal fusion such as that of the lunate, capitate, hamate and triquetrum may prevent the carpal bones from migrating and causing excessive stress to the silicone prosthesis.

Silicone breakage, fragmentation, and deposition in regional synovium and lymph nodes (silicone synovitis) occur occasion-

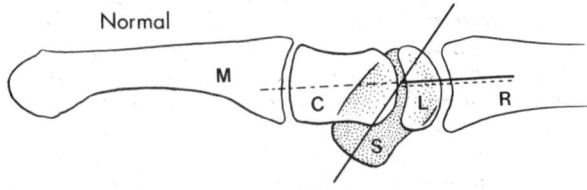

Figure 6. Diagram of a true lateral radiograph of the wrist. Lines are drawn through the longitudinal axis of the scaphoid (S), capitate (C), and radius (R) and through the midportion of the lunate (L). In a normal wrist in neutral position, the longitudinal axis of the center of the radius, lunate, capitate, and third metacarpal is, in general, linear. The normal angle between the scaphoid and lunate is 30 to 60 degrees. The normal angles between the capitate and lunate and between the radius and lunate are 0 to 15 degrees. (From Goldner, R. D., Ugino, M. R., and Goldner, J. L.: Injuries to carpal bones. *In* Edlich, R. F., and Spyker, D. A. (Eds.): Current Emergency Medical Therapy. Norwalk, Conn., Appleton-Century-Crofts, 1984.)

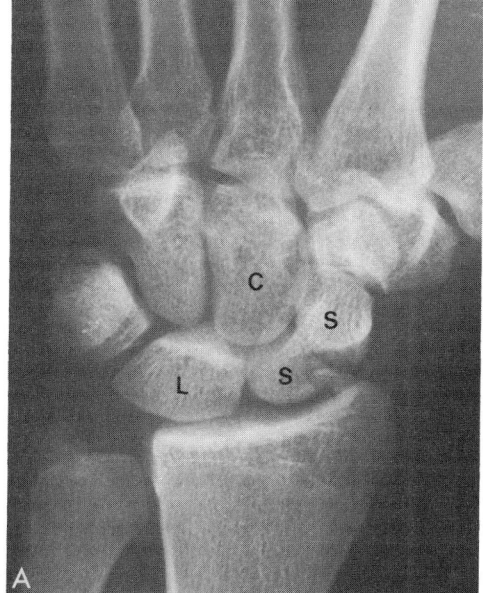

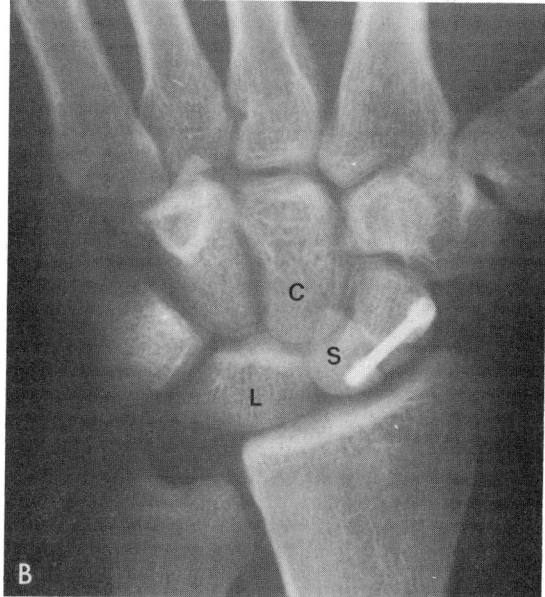

Figure 7. *A*, Fracture of the scaphoid with displacement and comminution. Closed reduction is not successful. *B*, Open realignment of the scaphoid through a palmar approach. The Herbert jig and screw were used for fixation.

ally. The incidence is low, and the condition can be managed by excision of the silicone and bone grafting or arthrodesis if wrist motion is not to be maintained. Use of tendon or fascial arthroplasty to replace the excised scaphoid in conjunction with intercarpal arthrodesis eliminates the possibility of silicone synovitis.

SELECTED REFERENCES

Dobyns, J. H., and Linscheid, R. L.: Fractures and dislocations of the wrist. *In* Rockwood, C. A., Jr., and Green, D. P. (Eds.): Fractures. Philadelphia, J. B. Lippincott Company, 1984, pp. 411–510.
This comprehensive chapter includes a historical prospective, alternate methods of treatment, and the authors' preferred method of managing fractures and dislocations of the wrist.

Green, D. P.: Carpal dislocations and instabilities. *In* Green, D. P. (Ed.): Operative Hand Surgery. New York, Churchill Livingstone, 1988, pp. 875–938.
Current concepts in anatomy, kinematics, diagnosis, and treatment of carpal dislocations and instabilities.

Linscheid, R. L., Dobyns, J. H., Beabout, J. W., and Bryan, R. S.: Traumatic Instability of the Wrist: Diagnosis, classification and pathomechanics. J. Bone Joint Surg. [Am.], *54*:1612, 1972.
These authors present a biomechanical background and classification of wrist instability after trauma. Difficulties associated with recognition of instability and treatment are emphasized.

Taleisnik, J.: Fractures of the carpal bones. *In* Green, D. P. (Ed.): Operative Hand Surgery. New York, Churchill Livingstone, 1988, pp. 813–841.
A well-illustrated chapter including diagnosis, radiographic evaluation, and methods of treatment of carpal fractures.

REFERENCES

1. Bora, W. F., Osterman, A. L., and Brighton, C. T.: The electrical treatment of scaphoid nonunion. Clin. Orthop., *161*:33, 1981.
2. Cooney, W. P., Dobyns, M. D., and Linscheid, R. L.: Fractures of the scaphoid: A rational approach to management. Clin. Orthop., *149*:90, 1980.
3. Cooney, W. P., Dobyns, J. H., and Linscheid, R. L.: Nonunion of the scaphoid: Analysis of the results from bone grafting. J. Hand Surg., *5*:343, 1980.
4. Gelberman, R. H., and Menon, J.: The vascularity of the scaphoid bone. J. Hand Surg., *5*:508, 1980.
5. Goldner, R. D., Ugino, M. R., and Goldner, J. L.: Injuries to carpal bones. *In* Edlich, R. F., and Spyker, D. A. (Eds.): Current Emergency Medical Therapy. Norwalk, Conn., Appleton-Century-Crofts, 1984, pp. 159–168.
6. Green, D. P.: The effect of avascular necrosis on Russe bone grafting for scaphoid nonunion. J. Hand Surg., *10*:1, 597, 1985.
7. Herbet, T. J., and Fisher, W.: Management of the fractured scaphoid using a new screw. J. Bone Joint Surg. [Br.], *66*:114, 1984.
8. Leslie, I. J., and Dickson, R. A.: The fractured carpal scaphoid. Natural history and factors influencing outcome. J. Bone Joint Surg. [Br.], *63*:225, 1981.
9. Mack, G. R., Bosse, M. J., Gelberman, R. H., and Yu, E.: The natural history of scaphoid nonunion. J. Bone Joint Surg. [Am.], *66*:504, 1984.
10. Mayfield, J. K., Johnson, R. P., and Kilcoyne, R. K.: Carpal dislocations: Pathomechanics and progressive perilunar instability. J. Hand Surg., *5*:226, 1980.
11. Palmer, A. K., Dobyns, J. H., and Linscheid, R. L.: Management of post-traumatic instability of the wrist secondary to ligament rupture. J. Hand Surg., *3*:507, 1978.
12. Taleisnik, J., and Kelly, P. J.: The extraosseous and intraosseous blood supply of the scaphoid bone. J. Bone Joint Surg. [Am.], *48*:1125, 1966.
13. Taleisnik, J.: The ligaments of the wrist. J. Hand Surg., *1*:110, 1976.
14. Watson, H. K., Goodman, M. L., and Johnson, T. R.: Limited arthrodesis. Part II. Intercarpal and radial carpal considerations. J. Hand Surg., *6*:223, 1981.
15. Swanson, A. B.: Silicone rubber implants for the replacement of the carpal scaphoid and lunate bones. Orthop. Clin. North Am., *1*:299, 1970.
16. Vender, M. I., Watson, K. H., Wiener, B. D., and Black, D. M.: Degenerative change in symptomatic scaphoid nonunion. J. Hand Surg., *12A*:514, 1987.
17. Zemel, N. P., Stark, H. H., Ashworth, C. R., Rickard, T. A., and Anderson, D. R.: The treatment of selected patients with an ununited fracture of the proximal part of the scaphoid by excision of the fragment and insertion of a carved silicone-rubber spacer. J. Bone Joint Surg. [Am.], *66*:510, 1989.

V

FRACTURES AND DISLOCATIONS OF THE HAND

Richard D. Goldner, M.D., and J. Leonard Goldner, M.D.

Hands are exposed to many forces that may cause bone or joint trauma. Fractures of the metacarpals and phalanges are estimated to comprise 10 per cent of all fractures that occur; of these, fractures of the distal phalanx are the most common, followed in order by fractures of the metacarpals, the proximal phalanges, and the middle phalanges.

The individual joints in each digit have a direct effect on the total function of the involved and the adjacent digits. An extension contracture of the metacarpophalangeal (MCP) joint limits the degree of flexion of the adjacent digits; if the MCP joint is held in flexion, the adjacent fingers cannot be extended completely. If the proximal interphalangeal (PIP) joint has been injured and fibrosis occurs, the fingertip cannot be flexed to the distal palmar crease. If the distal interphalangeal (DIP) joint has been affected by a ruptured extensor tendon, the distal phalanx remains in flexion and interferes with dexterity of the involved digit and usually the adjacent digits.

The avoidance of hand and finger injuries is a part of preventive medicine. Admonitions to children about placing their hands near sharp, moving objects and the same advice to adults working with machinery and participating in athletics are part of this effort to prevent soft tissue trauma, joint injuries, and fractures. When the injury occurs, the physician must be able to diagnose the pathologic process and provide patient care or direct the patient to an appropriate source of treatment.

FUNCTIONAL ANATOMY OF THE HAND

Functional anatomy of the hand must be understood in order to diagnose and treat bone and joint injuries of the hand. The distal transverse crease on the palmar aspect of the wrist corresponds to the carpal bones. The radial and ulnar arteries, median and ulnar nerves, and flexor tendons are frequently injured at that level.

The transverse crease in the distal palm corresponds to the MCP joints. The proximal crease of the fingers is located in the midportion of the proximal phalanx, the middle crease is opposite the PIP joint, and the distal crease is opposite the DIP joint. These joints are active in flexion and extension. The distal phalanx includes the pulp or pad of the finger, the fingernail (nail plate), the nail bed, the nail matrix (germinal layer), the attachment of the extensor tendon, and the insertion of the flexor profundus tendon.

The middle phalanx is located between the proximal and distal phalanges. Dorsally, it is covered by the extensor mechanism, and the flexor superficialis inserts on the palmar surface. The tendon of the flexor digitorum profundus passes palmar to the middle phalanx after passing through the superficialis chiasm.

The proximal phalanx articulates with the metacarpal head. The oblique fibers of the lateral bands and the intrinsic tendons cover it on the radial and ulnar surfaces. The flexor tendons are on the palmar surface. The extensor tendon covers the dorsum of the proximal phalanx but is not firmly adherent to bone at that level. The proximal phalanx is longer than the middle or distal phalanges.

The metacarpal head articulates with the proximal phalanx.

The large articular surface provides a wide range of flexion, extension, abduction, and adduction. The joint is stabilized by the extensor hood, the collateral ligaments, the dorsal capsule, and the palmar capsule.

The fourth and fifth metacarpals are mobile. The second and third metacarpals are relatively stable, and the first metacarpal is hypermobile when compared with the others. The first metacarpal has an epiphysis at its proximal end, as do the proximal phalanges of the fingers. The second through fifth metacarpals have an epiphysis at the distal end. Each tubular bone is divided anatomically into the base, shaft, neck, and head (articular).

The first ray or digit (thumb) has one metacarpal and two phalanges and independent intrinsic muscles as well as extensors and flexors (extensor and flexor pollicis longus). Stabilization of the thumb and the carpometacarpal joint is dependent on extrinsic and intrinsic muscles and tendons and the supportive ligaments.

As the fingers are flexed, their line of action converges, with the center of each nail pointing toward the scaphoid. Since none of the fingers is flexed in a straight line, the fingers should not be immobilized parallel to the long axis of the hand. In order to avoid malrotation, the proper position of digit immobilization is determined by observing the position of flexion in the normal, uninjured digits.

Splints, plaster, and dressings should hold the digits in the "intrinsic plus" position. This may include 60 to 80 degrees of flexion at the MCP joints, 10 to 20 degrees of flexion at the PIP joints, and 5 to 10 degrees of flexion at the DIP joints. With MCP joint flexion and interphalangeal (IP) joint extension, the collateral ligaments at the respective joints are elongated, thereby decreasing the likelihood of ligament contracture and subsequent joint stiffness. At times, however, the IP joint is immobilized in greater flexion to correct palmar angulation or to maintain proper rotational alignment.

Each finger has a flexor profundus tendon that inserts into the proximal segment of the distal phalanx, and a flexor superficialis tendon inserts into the middle phalanx. The thumb has a single flexor pollicis longus. These "extrinsic" muscles originate in the forearm.

The interossei that abduct and adduct the fingers and the lumbricals that assist in flexing the MCP joints and extending the IP joints originate within the hand and are termed intrinsic muscles. The thumb intrinsics include the opponens pollicis, abductor pollicis brevis, flexor pollicis brevis, and adductor pollicis.

The ulnar three fingers must be flexed and extended almost in unison. Full flexion of the index finger requires partial flexion of the long and ring fingers. Individual variations occur. The thumb may be flexed almost completely without simultaneous action of the adjacent fingers, although about 10 per cent of the population has a connection between the flexor digitorum profundus of the index finger and the flexor pollicis longus.

The extensor aspect of the hand contains the subcutaneous extensor digitorum communis tendons and the anatomic snuffbox, which is visible at the base of the thumb. The radial border consists of tendons of the extensor pollicis brevis and abductor pollicis longus; the ulnar border is the extensor pollicis longus.

Branches of the superficial radial nerve and the radial artery lie in the anatomic snuffbox. There are multiple skin creases over the finger joints so that skin stretches and is not excessively tense when all joints are flexed.

CLINICAL EXAMINATION OF THE HAND

The injured part may be examined before obtaining the history or after details concerning the injury have been elicited. A pattern of assessment should be followed consistently. This includes the patient's age, sex, occupation, and hand dominance and accurate data concerning the injury (when, where, how, why). What was the time interval between injury and examination? Who treated the injury initially, and what was this treatment? Was the injury in a dirty or clean environment? Was it a bite? Did it occur at work? What was the mechanism of injury (crush, direct blow, twist)? For example, was the ball that injured the hand large or small, and did it hit the tip or the middle of the finger? Was the thumb twisted in the loop of the ski pole, or was it caught on the rope attached to the boat that was pulling the water skier out of the water? Other factors to consider in determining the most appropriate treatment are associated diseases, patient motivation, and socioeconomic factors.

Initially, the resting position of the hand is observed. If a flexor tendon has been avulsed, the digit rests in more extension than usual. Also, the physician should refer to the wrist, thumb, and finger motion of the normal hand in both flexion and extension to perform a more meaningful assessment of the injured hand. Swelling may follow hemorrhage or extravasation of joint fluid or edema fluid and may be confused with prominence of a displaced segment of the articular surface of the involved bone.

The circulation is tested by compressing the distal pulp adjacent to the nail for capillary refill, observing the color of the digit, and comparing the surface temperature with that of the adjacent digits. Often, the digital artery compression test (Allen's) cannot be performed because of pain or swelling; therefore, capillary refill is particularly helpful. A pale finger is usually the result of diminished arterial blood flow. A blue finger indicates venous congestion. Elevating and lowering the extremity may provide information about venous and arterial flow. After a hand injury, all rings and jewelry should be removed immediately from the hand before increased swelling occurs and subsequent compression causes compromise of the digital arteries and nerves.

Sensitivity is tested by determining light touch, deep pressure, two-point discrimination, and sharp point. The sensory deficit may be profound if the digital nerve was lacerated completely or may be minimal if the nerve was contused by trauma. In an open fracture with sensory loss, the assumption is that the digital nerve has been lacerated or at least severely contused if a sensory deficit exists.

Motor function may be limited because of soft tissue injury, bone deformity, or pain. However, an attempt is made to determine active flexion and extension of the IP joints and of the MCP joints and rotation of the base of the thumb. Wrist motion is tested also.

Joint motion may be limited by intra-articular or extra-articular damage or by injury to the extensor or flexor tendons. The latter indirectly limits distal or proximal IP joint motion or both. Each joint is tested by isolating it from the adjacent joints. The patient voluntarily attempts to flex the DIP joint, the PIP joint, and the MCP joint. The examiner must differentiate rebound motion from voluntary motion. For example, if the distal phalanx is flexed actively, the tip rebounds to extension when the flexor is released. This implies that the extensors are functioning, but actually they may not be. Conversely, active digit extension may be possible, and rebound flexion occurs when the extensor muscle is relaxed. Intrinsic function producing exten-

sion of the IP joints should not be confused with extensor digitorum communis action causing extension of the IP joints when the MCP joints are held in 90 degrees of flexion.

The involved digit is examined carefully to determine the site of disruption of bone and soft tissue. Precise areas of tenderness are palpated, such as the central slip (dorsal), the collateral ligaments (radial and ulnar), the palmar plate (volar), and the flexor and extensor tendon insertions. Stability of the joint is determined. Alignment of the digits is noted, and any angular or rotational deformities are corrected, since slight metacarpal or phalangeal malrotation may cause significant digit overlap.

Open wounds should be assessed relative to the mechanism of injury. A foreign body should be expected in any open or penetrating injury. Many objects are not radiopaque, such as wood, clothing, some forms of glass, and certain plastics.

Open wounds are examined cautiously. Both sides of the hand are inspected. Swelling on the dorsum may follow penetration on the volar surface. The examiner should wear a mask, use sterile gloves and instruments, and do minimal probing until adequate peripheral anesthesia has been obtained and the patient is in a location where definitive treatment can be completed.

Generally, open wounds should be treated in an operating room where clean air and adequate assistance, instrumentation, and equipment are available; where the traffic is limited; and where the proper protection of the patient and medical personnel from airborne and other infections exists.

TERMINOLOGY

Terminology providing description of the alignment is as follows. *Dislocation* means that the articular surfaces are not opposed or congruous and that the restraining ligaments and probably the capsule have been partially or completely torn. *Subluxation* means a partial displacement of one side of the joint on the other, but with less severe distortion than a dislocation. Soft tissue interposition may prevent complete reduction in either instance. The term *reduction* refers to the action required to obtain anatomic alignment.

Fractures are described as stable, unstable, displaced, nondisplaced, impacted, comminuted, intra-articular, extra-articular, transverse, oblique, or spiral. Angulation may occur in any direction: dorsal, volar, radial, ulnar, or combinations. Malrotation may also occur. If there is no wound, the fracture is referred to as closed; if the skin is broken, the fracture is referred to as open.

RADIOGRAPHIC EXAMINATION

Radiographs determine the exact location of the fracture: articular surface, epiphysis, neck, metaphysis, shaft, or base of the digit. They indicate the type of fracture: complete, incomplete, transverse, oblique, spiral, or comminuted; they indicate position of the fractured bones, amount of displacement of one segment relative to the other, and angulation of the segments compared with a straight line and with apex of angulation either dorsal or volar. Correct rotation of the digit may be assessed radiographically by the relationship of proximal to distal fractured segment but is best determined clinically by comparison with adjacent digits.

Multiple radiographic views of the involved hand or digit are essential for an accurate diagnosis. The usual views are posteroanterior, pronation and supination oblique, and true lateral. True lateral exposures must be obtained of the individual digits rather than of the entire hand, since in the latter case, the digits are overlapping. The addition of a 10-degree supination film for the ulnar side of the hand and a 10-degree pronation film at the radial side of the hand provides additional information.

Magnification views and tomography are helpful in determining occult fractures of the metacarpals or the phalanges. Occasionally, an arthrogram is helpful in assessing capsular or ligamentous injury to the joint. The xeroradiogram may be useful in determining the presence of nonradiopaque foreign bodies such as glass or wood in soft tissues. Radiographs should be obtained prior to reduction of the fracture or the dislocation in the emergency room. If vascular supply is compromised by the dislocation, arrangements are made to obtain the radiograph immediately. Stress views taken with the joint forced opened in a direction away from the injured ligaments provide more information about the extent of the dislocated joint than does a plain exposure.

The postreduction or posttreatment radiograph is usually obtained through plaster or fiber-glass cast, an aluminum splint, or a hand dressing. A portable radiograph before the dressing is applied but after reduction is helpful when an intra-articular fracture is being manipulated prior to determination of whether open reduction is required. Correct rotation of the digit may be assessed radiographically by the relationship of the proximal to distal fractured segment but is best determined clinically by comparison with adjacent digits.

ANESTHESIA

Relief of pain associated with trauma is essential if diagnosis and treatment are to be successful. Sensory and motor examination must be completed, however, before a local or regional anesthetic is administered. Manipulation and realignment of a fractured phalanx requires relaxation of the extensor and flexor tendons of the forearm.

Fractures of the phalanx or an intra-articular injury in the digit may be managed by local infiltration or by digital nerve block using lidocaine without epinephrine in the metacarpal area. Digital block is accomplished by injecting the anesthetic agent into the web space, where there is adequate area for swelling, or dorsally on either side of the metacarpal neck with the needle being inserted palmarward toward the digital nerve. A circular injection at the base of the digit is not advisable, nor should epinephrine be used in a solution. In certain instances, median or ulnar nerve block at the wrist and superficial radial nerve injection at the level of the styloid process of the radius are most effective.

If open reduction is necessary, intravenous regional anesthesia or axillary block may be preferred, since this allows greater tolerance of the tourniquet. This can be supplemented with systemic analgesia.

Because of the occasional occurrence of pneumothorax, supraclavicular block should be avoided unless it is done by experienced personnel. With severe injuries that require extensive reconstruction or distant bone graft, nerve grafts, or soft tissue coverage, general anesthesia is preferred.

Complications associated with the use of local or regional anesthesia are rare, but they occur, and the physician must be prepared to manage the patient who develops syncope, hypotension, seizures, and anaphylactic reactions. This mandates that even with local infiltration, one must have oxygen, a positive-pressure bag, an airway, and intravenous medications immediately available. Intravenous regional anesthesia should not be used in children or adults unless the physician is prepared to leave the tourniquet elevated for approximately 45 minutes so that the anesthetic can be fixed in the tissues of the forearm.

OPEN WOUNDS

At the time of the initial wound excision, all tight fascial compartments must be opened, open joints irrigated, and circulation established. Meticulous excision of devitalized tissue and thorough irrigation are essential to prevent infection. If the wound has been caused by a high-velocity missile, severe crush, human or animal bite, or high-pressure injury, no primary effort is made to repair digital nerves or flexor tendons. If internal fixation is required, pins placed through the extensor retinaculum should be avoided because this compromises joint motion.

The open fracture should be managed with consideration to the blood supply of the digit, nerve and tendon injury, intrinsic muscle injury, and skin injury. Circulation should be restored as quickly as possible by direct repair of digital arteries, by vein grafts to segmentally damaged arteries and veins, or by releasing edematous soft tissue to decrease external pressure or vascular spasm. Digital nerves and lacerated flexor tendons do not always require primary repair. Open joints must be irrigated and properly dressed but can be maintained open for 24 to 48 hours covered with saline dressings without damage to the articular surfaces. Severe injuries are inspected again at 24 to 48 hours.

A stable skeleton decreases persistent irritation to the adjacent vascular structures and diminishes the possibility of infection in open wounds. However, elongation of the digit to its original length may again compromise the circulation. Bone angulations should be corrected early, but not at the risk of damage to adjacent soft tissues. The concept of treating open wounds open until such time that it is safe to close them with direct suture or additional skin, or by allowing secondary healing, eliminates many complications that occur in wounds treated by both the expert and less experienced personnel.

Antibiotics should be administered for contaminated wounds. First-generation cephalosporins are given for most open hand fractures. Antibiotic coverage for human bite wounds includes penicillin. When there has been extreme contamination such as from farm injuries, aminoglycosides such as tobramycin or gentamicin should be given with a cephalosporin and penicillin. All open fractures are considered tetanus-prone wounds, and the patient's tetanus immunization should be updated.

With crush injuries, one should maintain a high index of suspicion of the development of the compartment syndrome. Signs of pain with passive stretch in addition to paresthesias in the digit may be secondary to nerve compression or to the pain from fractures. However, the compartment syndrome should be considered when these symptoms are present. In assessing a crushed, swollen hand, compartment pressure determination is appropriate. If the compartment pressure is above 40 mm. Hg in a normotensive individual, compartment release is advocated. Fasciotomy of the intrinsic muscles of the hand may be accomplished through two dorsal longitudinal incisions between the second and third and the fourth and fifth metacarpals.

ANATOMIC REGIONS OF FRACTURES

Distal Phalanx and Distal Interphalangeal Joint

DISTAL PHALANX FRACTURE. The distal phalanx is frequently fractured by a crush from a hammer, a heavy object, or a door. The fracture is splinted for 10 to 14 days to decrease discomfort and allow healing. The fingernail may be elevated by hematoma that is trapped between the nail plate and nail bed and is very painful. It is released after the digit has been cleansed with soap and water and antiseptic by making a hole in the center of the nail plate with the round end of an open paper clip that has been heated in a flame or by a disposable ophthalmic cautery. If the nail bed has been lacerated, the nail plate should be removed and the laceration repaired with fine absorbable sutures.

OPEN FRACTURES OF THE DISTAL PHALANX. The most important aspect of the open fracture of the distal phalanx is the skin and soft tissue damage. Initial treatment consists of wound débridement. If the wound is grossly contaminated, it is treated open and closed at 3 to 5 days with a skin graft or shifting of local flaps if direct closure is not possible. If the wound is clean, or can be converted to a clean wound by débridement, immediate skin grafting or local flaps can be used to provide closure.

DORSAL AVULSION FRACTURES. A dorsal segment of bone is elevated when the extensor digitorum communis is avulsed by an acute flexion or hyperextension injury. The superior aspect of the articular surface may constitute part of the fragment after extensor tendon continuity is lost at the distal joint, and a "drop finger" or "mallet finger" occurs. If the fragment is small (less than 40 per cent, displaced less than 2 mm.), slight hyperextension with a dorsal aluminum splint on the distal and middle phalanges provides sufficient apposition to allow healing. If blanching of the skin or increased pain is noted, the phalanx should be placed in neutral position. The splint is used for a total of 8 to 12 weeks. Similar treatment but longer protective splinting is used for the mallet finger of tendon origin in which no fracture of avulsion is noted.

A fracture fragment attached to the extensor tendon should be treated as early as possible after the injury. Alignment and function can be obtained as late as 2 to 3 weeks after injury, but each week decreases the likelihood of maximal recovery. If the fracture fragment is displaced and greater than 40 per cent of the articular surface, with volar subluxation of the distal phalanx, open reduction with suture and pin or screw fixation may be necessary. This type of treatment is not often required.

AVULSION OF A FRAGMENT FROM THE FLEXOR SURFACE. This occurs when the flexor digitorum profundus is forcibly pulled from its distal phalangeal insertion such as when the digit is hyperextended as a result of a forcible blow or fall or from catching the digit (usually the ring) in a football jersey. Physical findings are swelling, the patient's inability to flex the distal joint, and a palpable palmar mass at the base of the finger or in the palm. Radiographs may show the bone fragment in the digit.

Operative treatment is required to reattach the flexor tendon to the point of avulsion. This is usually performed with a polypropylene suture through the distal end of the tendon and attached to the tendon just proximal to the bone fragment. The suture is brought through the distal phalanx on either side of the fingernail and is tied over a button on the dorsum of the nail. Two interrupted sutures are also placed through the tendon and the fragment into the adjacent soft tissues. A dorsal plaster splint is applied from the fingertip to the elbow. Although several postoperative rehabilitation protocols are available, the repair should be protected for 4 to 6 weeks. Early protected passive motion is recommended.

Middle Phalanx and Proximal Interphalangeal Joint

The extrinsic muscles such as the extensor digitorum communis, flexor digitorum profundus, and flexor digitorum superficialis all affect the position of the fragments after phalangeal fractures. The force of the initial injury directs the distal or proximal fragment either dorsal or palmar, and the natural pull of the attached tendons either aggravates this or neutralizes it, depending on the exact location of the fracture.

The intrinsic muscle attachments also affect the position of the fragments by extension of the lateral band mechanism across the proximal phalanx, onto the sides of the PIP joint, and over the dorsum of the middle phalanx to the insertion of the tendon into the distal phalanx. Active muscle contraction of the lumbricals and the interossei influences the position of the fragments and the deformity of the digit. Fractures through the distal portion (neck) of the middle phalanx are likely to have apex palmar angulation, because the proximal fragment is flexed by the superficialis tendon. A fracture through the proximal portion (base) of the middle phalanx is likely to have apex dorsal angulation caused by flexion of the distal fragment by the

superficialis and extension of the proximal fragment by the central slip of the extensor. Fractures through the middle two thirds may be angulated in either direction or not at all. Rotary deformities and radial and ulnar deviation may also depend on the intrinsic tendon pull as well as the force of the original injury.

Stable fractures can be immobilized initially in a splint followed by adjacent digit taping (buddy taping). Fractures that are stable after closed reduction are immobilized for approximately 3 weeks. Although the fracture may be protected for 6 to 8 weeks, gentle motion should be initiated at 3 to 4 weeks. Displaced, unstable fracture of the middle phalanx that cannot be reduced or maintained by external immobilization requires fixation either by percutaneous pins or by open reduction and internal fixation. Spiral and long oblique fractures are well suited for internal lag screw fixation.

The PIP joint is stabilized by the main and accessory collateral ligaments. Collateral ligament tears or avulsions cause temporary instability. Fragments of bone avulsed with the collateral ligaments may be detected radiographically. The palmar capsule prevents excessive hyperextension and limits malrotation. A tear of the capsule may occur either with or without the bone fragment attached to it.

A chip fracture at the PIP joint indicates either collateral ligament tear or marginal capsular avulsion; this is a relatively common injury. This radiographic finding may be a subtle suggestion of more extensive instability, but as long as the phalanx can be placed in anatomic alignment, in the position that decreases tension and stress on the collateral ligaments, adequate healing usually occurs. Large, displaced avulsion fractures with collateral ligament attached are repaired surgically.

A nondisplaced condylar fracture should be splinted for 2 to 3 weeks. These fractures are followed frequently because displacement may occur after motion has been initiated. Displaced condylar fractures often cannot be adequately reduced and held by closed methods. Open reduction corrects incongruity of the articular surfaces that if uncorrected would cause traumatic arthrosis.

DORSAL DISLOCATION OF THE PIP JOINT. Dislocations of the PIP joint are classified by the location of the middle phalanx in relation to the proximal (palmar, dorsal, lateral).

Dorsal dislocation of the middle phalanx with avulsion of the volar plate from the middle phalanx is a common injury. The PIP joint is swollen and may be mistaken for a "sprained finger." The lateral radiograph demonstrates displacement and often a small volar fragment from the proximal end of the middle phalanx. Treatment consists of regional metacarpal block; the elbow is flexed at right angles, the wrist is dorsiflexed, and traction in slight extension is applied to the digit and held for about 1 minute. As traction is exerted, flexion is continued to about 70 degrees while gentle but firm compression is applied over the dorsum of the middle phalanx. After reduction, the stability is tested with attention given to collateral ligament instability. Flexion is continued to about 70 degrees. A splint is then applied with the PIP joint flexed 20 to 30 degrees for 2 to 3 weeks. If the joint is completely stable, taping the involved digit to the adjacent one provides assistive motion and protects the joint.

Irreducible PIP joint dislocation may follow interposition of collateral ligament, lateral band, or volar plate. Late problems such as flexion contracture may be treated with dynamic splinting; hyperextension deformity with instability is treated by reattachment of the volar plate or by flexor digitorum superficialis tenodesis.

DORSAL FRACTURE DISLOCATION OF THE PIP JOINT. Dorsal dislocation of the middle phalanx with displaced fracture of the volar portion is a serious injury (Fig. 1). Fractures of greater than 40 per cent of the articular surface are usually unstable. If the fracture is reduced and is stable, it can be treated by a splint that blocks extension but allows flexion. The PIP

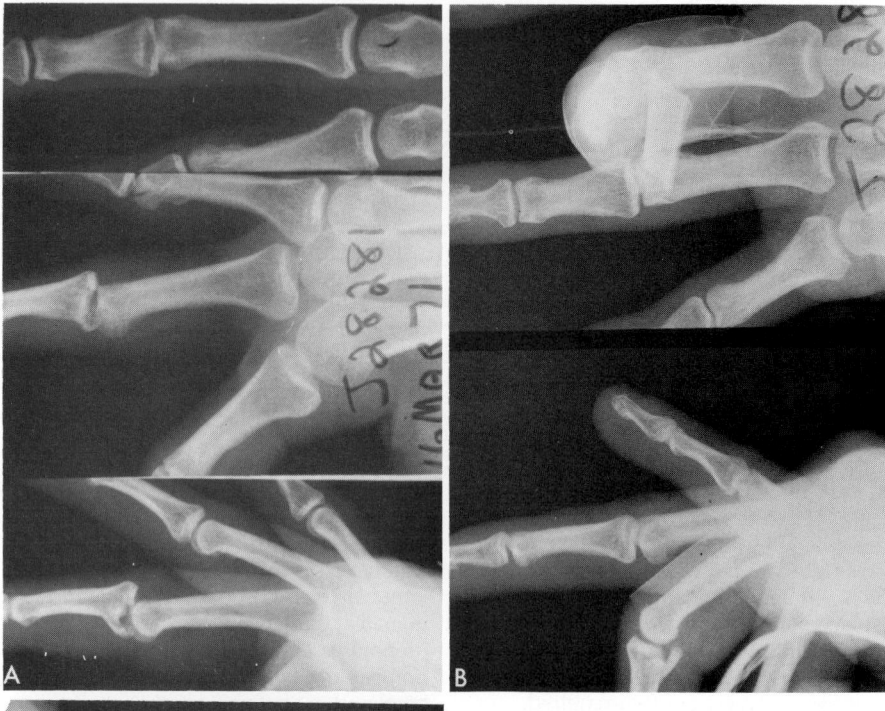

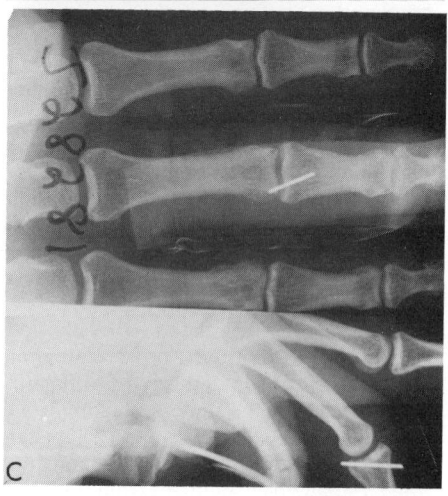

Figure 1. *A*, Proximal interphalangeal joint, dorsal fracture-dislocation with involvement of articular cartilage. Multiple views give a better representation of the fragments that are displaced. Both the dorsal capsule and the volar capsule are affected. *B*, The flexed lateral view shows where the volar capsule has been pulled off the proximal end of the proximal phalanx with a chip of bone, part of which is intra-articular. *C*, Fixation of the articular fragment with small fixation pins ensures articular congruity. However, cartilage damage and cartilage necrosis must be avoided in doing this kind of operation. The pins should not penetrate the joint, because this prevents early motion.

joint is blocked at 15 degrees short of the point of instability (approximately 40 degrees). The joint is then extended 25 per cent (10 degrees) each week. If reduction is not maintained and if the alignment of the joint cannot be re-established, an operative procedure is indicated. If the base of the middle phalanx is comminuted, options are to remove bone fragments surgically and advance the volar capsule into the defect or to apply a distraction-mobilization device to allow early motion.

PALMAR DISLOCATION OF THE PIP JOINT. Palmar dislocation of the middle phalanx may disrupt the central slip and dorsal capsule in addition to the palmar plate and one collateral ligament. This may cause a flexion deformity of the PIP joint and hyperextension of the DIP joint (boutonnière deformity). The central extensor mechanism is disrupted, and the lateral bands, which are normally dorsal to the axis of rotation of the PIP joint, slip palmar to that axis. Thus, the lateral bands, which normally extend the PIP joint, now flex the PIP joint and hyperextend the DIP joint. If PIP active extension is absent after reduction, the central attachment of the extensor tendon from the base of the middle phalanx has been disrupted. The PIP is then immobilized in extension for approximately 6 weeks with the DIP free to flex. Dorsal bone avulsion fractures from the middle phalanx with greater than 2 mm. displacement should be repaired.

LATERAL DISLOCATION OF THE PIP JOINT. Lateral PIP joint dislocation follows a lateral shear stress with collateral ligament disruption. The radial collateral is injured six times more frequently than is the ulnar. Associated avulsion of the palmar plate and extensor mechanism at the base of the middle phalanx is noted. This is diagnosed clinically by stress testing and radiographically by assessing joint asymmetry. Operative contrasted with nonoperative treatment depends on the degree of lateral instability and the severity of disruption of extensor mechanism.

Proximal Phalanx

Fractures of the proximal phalanx are divided into oblique and transverse types. *Oblique* fractures through the shaft usually include a rotary component. The distal fragment may be displaced radially or ulnarly, and the condylar segment may be displaced either superiorly or inferiorly. An alternative type of injury is a *transverse* fracture with resulting volar angulation. The interossei muscles flex at the proximal fragment, and the extensor central slip extends the distal fragment.

TRANSVERSE FRACTURE OF THE PROXIMAL PHALANX. A fracture through the midportion of the proximal phalanx with volar angulation presses the long flexor tendons and causes a flexion deformity at the PIP joint. Realignment of the

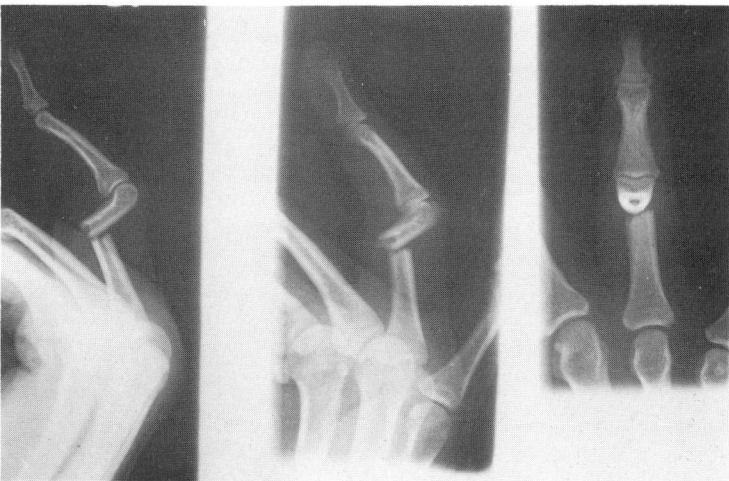

Figure 2. Fracture of proximal phalanx with apex volar angulation. Influence of the extensor tendon and intrinsic muscles affects the angulation.

fracture fragments restores active flexion at the proximal and distal interphalangeal joints, whereas persistent palmar angulation causes adherence of the flexor tendons to the periosteum and bone fragments during healing and produces a fixed flexion contracture of the PIP joint and often of the DIP joint.

A shaft fracture with palmar angulation of the fragments is shown in Figure 2. Treatment requires adequate relaxation of the extrinsic and intrinsic muscles, usually achieved by regional nerve block. Manipulation is performed by flexing the distal segment of the phalanx while countertraction is being applied to the proximal segment of the hand with the elbow flexed, the wrist dorsiflexed, and the MCP joint stabilized. Internal fixation, by percutaneous pins (Fig. 3) or after open reduction, is required if the alignment cannot be maintained by plaster splint.

OBLIQUE FRACTURE OF THE PROXIMAL PHALANX. For treatment of the oblique fracture, the distal fragment is derotated and the joints on either side of the phalanx are flexed. For dorsal angulation, the distal segment is extended and the MCP joint is flexed. When the angulation is palmar, the mobile distal fragment is placed in flexion, thereby bringing it into alignment with the proximal fragment. A dorsal plaster splint is usually sufficient to maintain reduction. The wrist is held in dorsiflexion, the MCP joints are flexed about 70 degrees, and the PIP and DIP joints are flexed slightly. Soft compressive material is

placed in the palm, and the rotation of the distal fragment is determined by the position of the fingernails when all joints are flexed. For fractures that can be reduced and held in a splint, immobilization for 3 weeks is necessary, after which several weeks of protected motion are required. An interval change of splint ensures maintenance of position. The oblique fracture of the proximal phalanx is likely to be unstable after closed reduction and often requires open reduction and internal fixation.

DORSAL COMPRESSION FRACTURE OF THE PROXIMAL PHALANX. Proximal dorsal compression injuries of the proximal phalanx result when the distal fragment is forced dorsally and the proximal fragment is stabilized by the collateral ligaments (Fig. 4). The dorsal cortex is compressed, and the angle between the articular surface and the shaft may be as much as 50 degrees. The muscle balance among the extensors, the flexors, and the intrinsic tendons is distorted. Edema on the dorsum of the digit causes additional deformity. A flexed position of the PIP joint occurs as a result of increased tension on the flexor digitorum superficialis. Radiographic diagnosis may be difficult because the anteroposterior film is misleading, since minimal radial or ulnar angulation occurs. The lateral view of the phalanges may be hidden by the adjacent digits, and the oblique view may not show the true extent of the deformity. A radiograph should be obtained with the digits in the position in which they are not overlapping completely, from both the radial and ulnar sides.

Treatment requires satisfactory regional block, counter- and straight traction, and a strong, forcible flexion manipulation that is done with the collateral ligaments under tension when the MCP joints are flexed. The thumb of the physician should be directly under the proximal fragment as the fulcrum, and the index finger compresses volarly on the distal fragment. Immobilization is maintained with the MCP joints and the IP joints in flexion.

INTERCONDYLAR FRACTURES OF THE PROXIMAL PHALANX. A condylar split fracture involving the distal end of the proximal phalanx is an intra-articular fracture. Collateral ligaments are attached to each of the condyles. Displacement of the condyles is demonstrated in Figure 5. Dorsal or palmar displacement of the condyles may complicate attempts at alignment.

To reduce an intercondylar fracture of the proximal phalanges of the finger, direct longitudinal traction is applied to tighten the collateral and the retinacular ligaments and approximate the condyles. When the fragments are replaced and the middle phalanx is flexed, the position may be maintained by a palmar aluminum splint. A short plaster cast, to which is incorporated a palmar aluminum splint, is applied to the hand, the wrist, and the lower forearm (Fig. 6). The involved digit is flexed at the MCP joint and the IP joint and held to the aluminum by

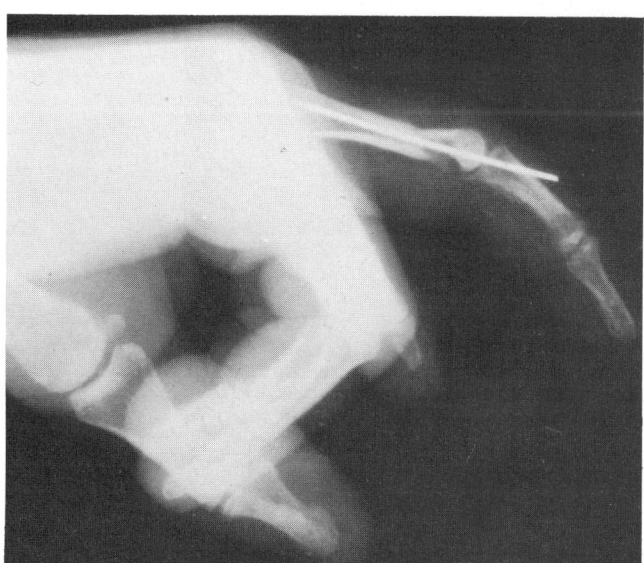

Figure 3. Pin fixation used to stabilize fracture of the proximal phalanx. The pin was placed across the joint. Limited motion due to arthrofibrosis resulted. *This procedure is not advisable.*

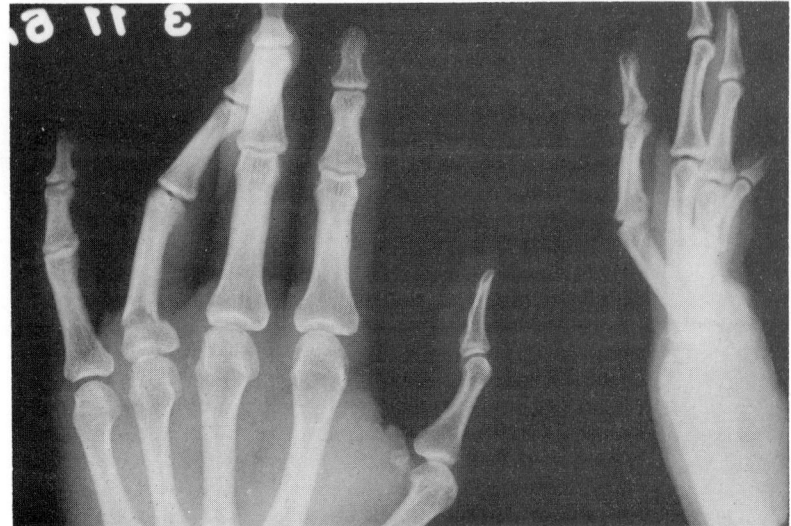

Figure 4. Fracture at the base of the proximal phalanx of the ring finger with malrotation, impaction, and apex volar angulation.

tape, which is wrapped in individual pieces, not under tension, and in such a way that each turn of tape overlaps the next most proximal turn to avoid edema. Rotation is corrected, and the nail plate is directed toward the radial aspect of the palm. The position is maintained for approximately 1 week, at which time the digit is retaped. Immobilization is continued for 3 weeks and the digit is protected for an additional 2 weeks, although an active range of flexion-extension is attempted several times a day.

If the condyles are malrotated and displaced greater than 2 mm., if adequate position cannot be obtained by manipulation, or if the reduction cannot be maintained, percutaneous pinning or open reduction with internal fixation of the condyles is performed. The latter procedure is usually necessary for fractures of one or both condyles of the proximal phalanx in order to prevent joint incongruity and angulation.

METACARPOPHALANGEAL JOINT DISLOCATION. Metacarpophalangeal joint dislocation follows a hyperextension force. The index finger is dislocated most frequently. If the palmar plate is avulsed from its origin and is trapped between the metacarpal head and the proximal phalanx, reduction is not possible by closed methods.

Open reduction can be accomplished through a palmar or dorsal approach. The palmar approach allows identification of the volar plate, the flexor tendons on the ulnar side, and the lumbrical on the radial side of the dislocated head. The radial digital nerve and artery to the index finger and the ulnar digital nerve and artery to the little finger are tethered over the metacarpal head and must be protected. Reduction is usually stable, and early motion with extension block splinting can be instituted.

Palmar MCP dislocation is uncommon and usually requires open reduction.

METACARPOPHALANGEAL JOINT COLLATERAL LIGAMENT INJURY. Metacarpophalangeal joint collateral ligament rupture in the digits may occur with forced abduction. This lesion most frequently affects the radial collateral ligament of the ulnar fingers but may also occur in the ulnar collateral ligament of the index finger. Discomfort to pressure is localized to the involved lateral aspect of the joint. The diagnosis is confirmed by stress radiographs. Treatment of acute injuries without ligament interposition consists of immobilization of the MCP joint in 30 degrees of flexion and slight overcorrection of the instability for 3 weeks with 3 additional weeks of buddy taping.

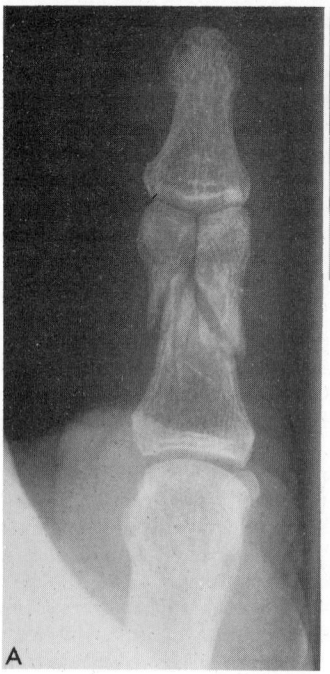

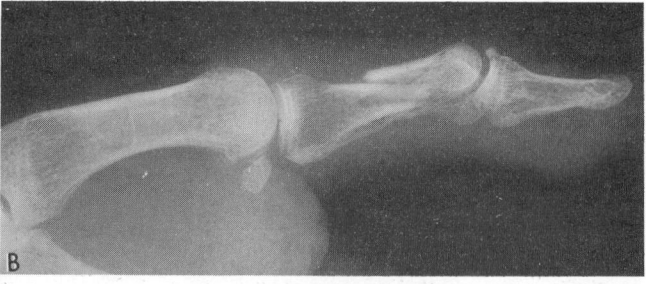

Figure 5. *A,* Fracture through the distal articular surface of the proximal phalanx. Closed manipulation and a dorsal plaster splint are occasionally sufficient for management of this injury. Internal fixation can be used if stability cannot be maintained or if intra-articular fragments cannot be aligned satisfactorily. *B,* Fracture of the proximal phalanx of the thumb with dorsal displacement of the distal fragment. An additional view is needed to determine if intra-articular injury has occurred.

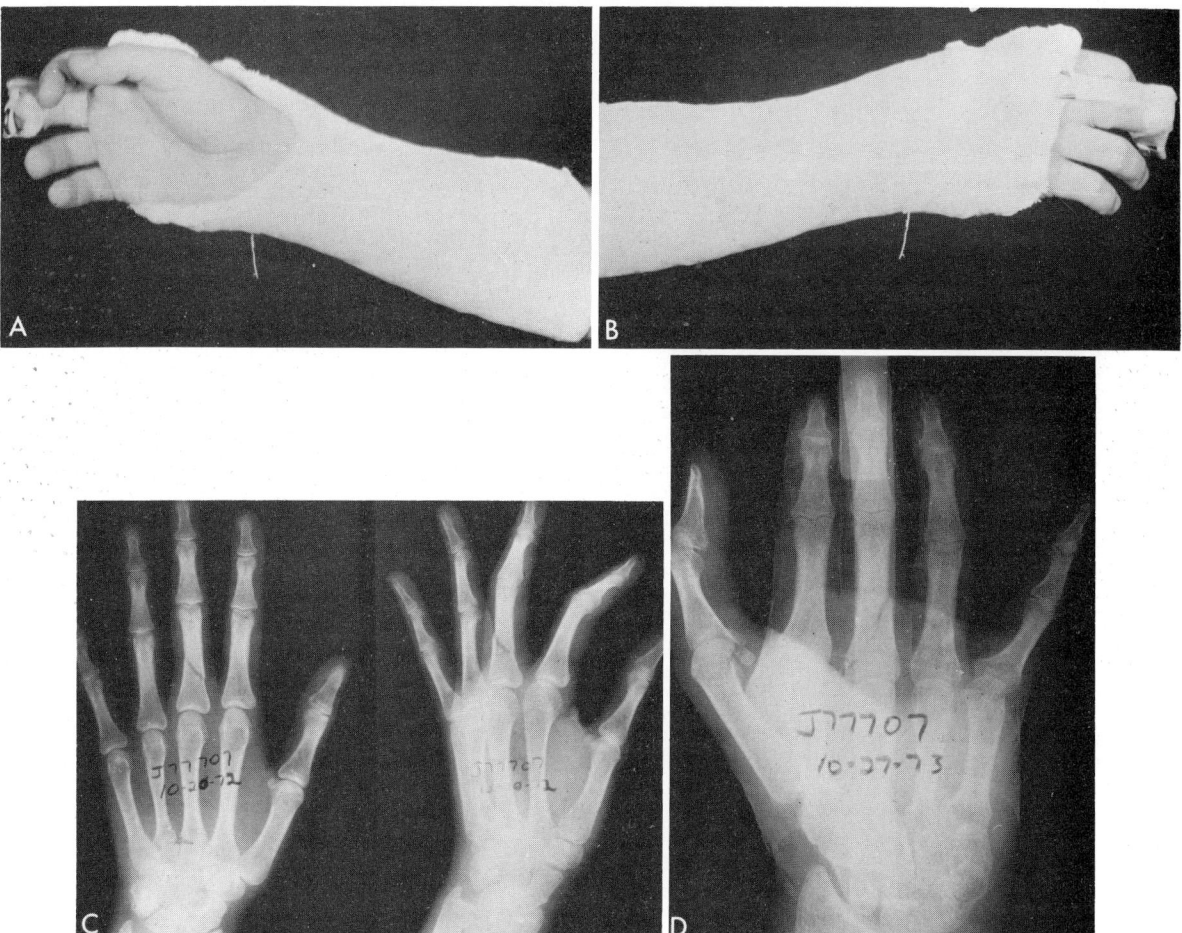

Figure 6. *A*, One method of managing phalangeal fracture. The plaster gauntlet serves as a base for the dorsal albumin splint. The tape immobilizes the digit for a few days, and the dorsal splint blocks extension. The digital fragment of the phalanx is held in flexion, and early active motion is encouraged. *B*, Other digits are freely movable. The splint can be adjusted and the digit visualized throughout the entire treatment. *C* and *D*, Long oblique fracture with malrotation, proximal phalanx. Pre- and postreduction and splinting. Open reduction and interfragmentary screw fixation allow anatomic alignment and early motion if the position cannot be maintained adequately in the splint.

Occasionally, an osteochondral fracture of the metacarpal head occurs and the segment is within the joint. If the avulsed chip of bone is displaced greater than 3 mm. or if the fragment involves greater than 20 per cent of the articular surface and is displaced, operative treatment is indicated.

EPIPHYSEAL INJURY. Management of a fracture involving the physis requires knowledge about the different zones of the physis (region from which the bone grows). If the fracture damages the physis, growth can cease or can occur in an irregular manner. If the fracture is through the junction of the metaphysis and the diaphysis, growth is not disturbed and healing occurs rapidly. Displaced fragments of the epiphysis are assessed by appropriate radiographic studies. Anatomic reduction should be attempted so that the physeal plate is anatomically aligned and cartilage fragments are undisplaced for uniform healing and growth (Fig. 7).

The Metacarpals

Metacarpal fractures are divided as follows: (1) fractures of the metacarpal *head,* with intra-articular involvement and dorsal or palmar angulation of the fragments; (2) fractures of the metacarpal *neck,* with dorsal or palmar angulation and with a rotary element; (3) *transverse* fractures through the shaft of the metacarpal; (4) *oblique* fractures through the shaft of the metacarpal; and (5) *dislocation* at the base of the metacarpals. Nondisplaced metacarpal fractures are treated closed and immobilized for 3 weeks followed by taping to the adjacent digit. Displaced fractures of the metacarpal head may require open

reduction and internal fixation with small screws or wires. Severely comminuted fractures limited to the metacarpal head distal to the collateral ligament should be treated with early protective motion. Large articular fragments with collateral ligament avulsion may require open reduction and internal fixation. The Brewerton radiograph view is obtained with the MCP joint flexed 65 degrees, the dorsum of the hand next to the plate, and the x-ray apparatus angled 15 degrees ulnar to radial. This helps to visualize fractures of the metacarpal head.

A fracture of the neck of the fifth metacarpal is a common injury caused by a direct blow. This is known as a boxer's fracture and occurs from a dorsal force applied directly to the metacarpal head. The head is displaced palmarward, the shaft bows dorsally, and the tip of the little finger rotates toward the radial side of the palm. Considerable soft tissue swelling usually occurs, and the alignment of the fragments cannot be determined from external examination. Radiographs show the angulation on the oblique and lateral views. Up to 40 to 45 degrees of dorsal angulation is acceptable in the fifth metacarpal, and approximately 30 degrees is acceptable in the fourth metacarpal; but in the index and long metacarpals, anatomic reduction is desirable because of the relative lack of mobility of the shaft. Angulation greater than 15 degrees is unacceptable secondary to the lack of compensatory carpometacarpal motion. Rotation alignment should be restored in all fingers.

Fractures with less than 15 degrees of angulation may be treated with an ulnar gutter splint for 10 to 14 days for the patient's comfort. Fifteen to 40 degrees of angulation is reduced

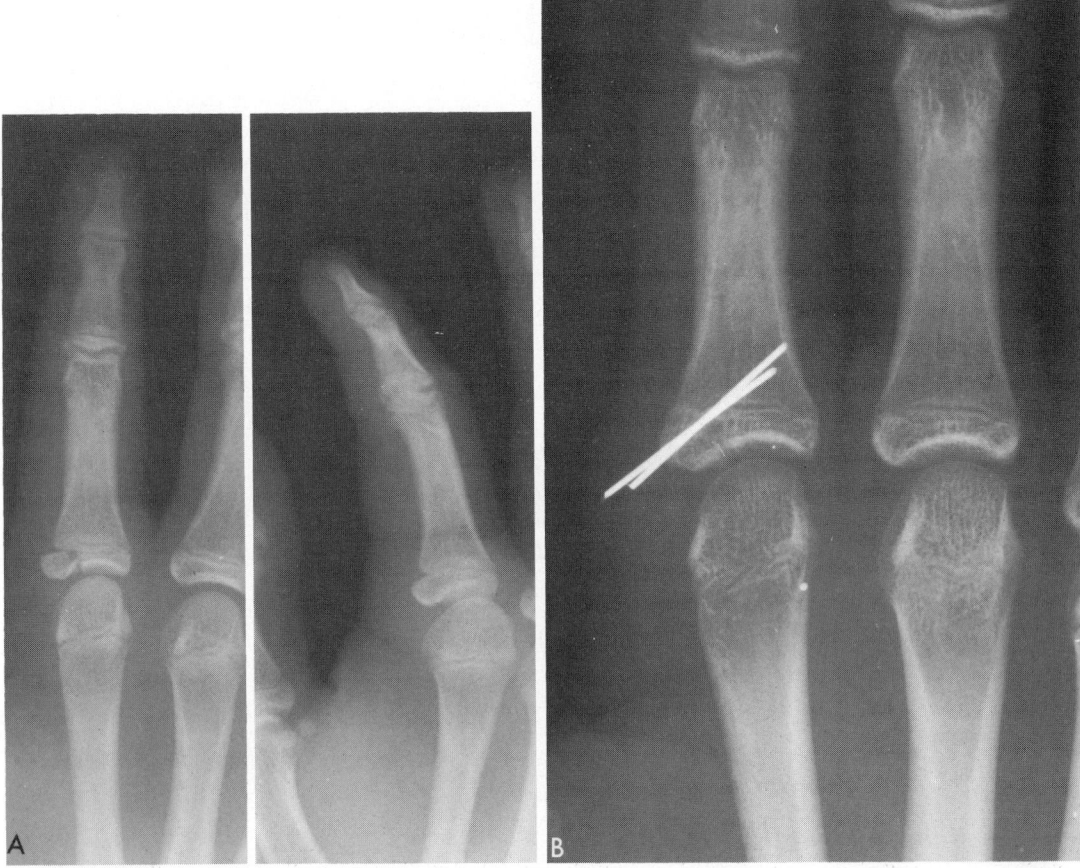

Figure 7. *A*, Intra-articular fracture of the proximal phalanx with osteochondral fracture attached to the collateral ligament. The lateral view shows probable rotation of the fragment. *B*, Open reduction and percutaneous pinning with 0.032 pins. The pins are subcutaneous and are left in place for approximately 3 weeks. Limited motion is initiated at 1 week, and active assistive motion is begun at 4 weeks.

and splinted for 3 weeks with the MCP joint flexed 50 to 70 degrees and the PIP joint flexed no more than 20 to 30 degrees.

For fractures with greater than 40 degrees of angulation, with palmar comminution of the neck and extensor lag, percutaneous pinning or occasionally open reduction and internal fixation may be necessary (Fig. 8).

Closed reduction can be achieved with MCP and PIP joints flexed to tighten the collateral ligaments. Momentary pressure is exerted dorsally on the 90-degree flexed proximal phalanx, and counterpressure is directed palmarward on the metacarpal shaft. It is not desirable to immobilize the fracture in this position, however, because secondary stiffness, malrotation, clawing, angulation, and skin problems may be greater than the functional loss that occurs with no treatment.

TRANSVERSE AND SHORT OBLIQUE METACARPAL SHAFT FRACTURES. *Transverse shaft fractures* are often caused by a direct blow with dorsal angulation secondary to exertion of palmar force by the interosseus muscles. The more proximal the fracture, the less the angulation. The intermetacarpal ligaments prevent shortening, and the interossei stabilize the digits. If the fracture is minimally displaced, it can be controlled with a well-molded short-arm cast for 4 to 6 weeks with the MCP joints flexed 60 degrees.

Indications for internal fixation include any persistent rotational deformity and uncorrected dorsal angulation greater than 10 degrees in the second or third metacarpal or greater than 20 degrees in the fourth or fifth metacarpal. Shortening more than 3 mm. or multiple displaced fractures usually require treatment of the adjacent soft tissues. Internal fixation of long oblique or spiral fractures with interfragmentary screw fixation controls

excessive shortening and angulation and allows early motion of the digits.

Malunion of a metacarpal fracture with dorsal angulation that disturbs the intrinsic balance and produces metacarpal head prominence in the palm and pain on gripping requires an osteotomy. Other complications are nonunion, MCP extension contractures, intrinsic muscle contractures, and tendon adhesions.

Long, oblique, or spiral metacarpal fractures, minimally displaced, are treated by splinting. Displaced fractures that are not able to be reduced adequately or that are unstable after reduction are best treated by lag screw fixation.

Dislocation at the metacarpal-carpal joint usually requires pin stabilization.

THUMB METACARPAL FRACTURES. Fractures at the base of the thumb are usually caused by a fall on the hand, a twisting mechanism that involves the projected thumb, or a direct blow of the fist against a firm object. Lesions are classified as follows: (1) *intra-articular fracture* through the proximal end of the metacarpal, leaving a fragment held by the intermetacarpal ligament, and the base of the metacarpal displaced laterally out of the joint by pull of the abductor pollicis longus (Bennett's fracture, Fig. 9A); simultaneously, the adductor pollicis pulls the proximal phalanx and distal metacarpal toward the palm and the proximal metacarpal away from its base; (2) a *comminuted intra-articular fracture* of the proximal end of the metacarpal (Rolando's fracture); and (3) *fracture through the metaphysis,* extra-articular, with angulation dorsal or volar. Other variations may occur.

Treatment of the displaced thumb fracture depends on the

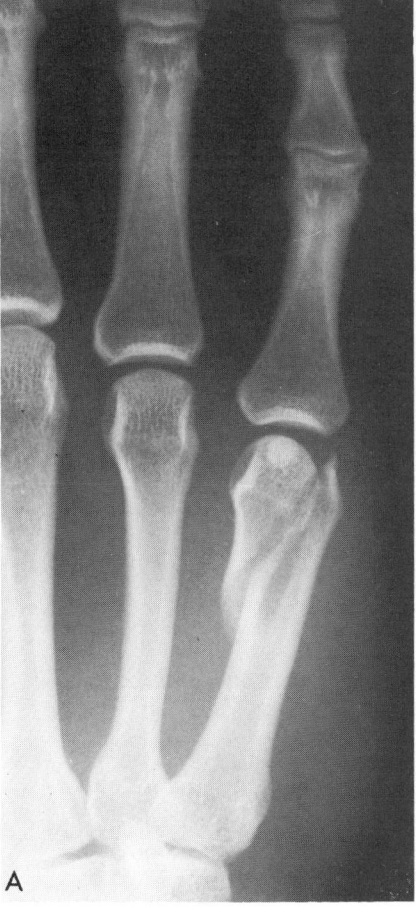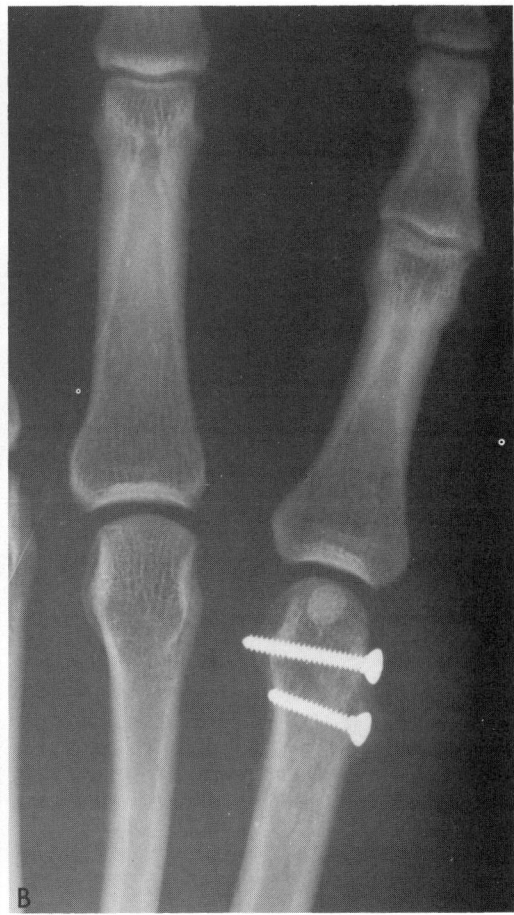

Figure 8. *A*, Spiral oblique intra-articular fracture with shortening and malrotation. The options for treatment are (1) manual traction and percutaneous pinning under image intensifier, (2) gauntlet plaster splint with aluminum extension on the volar aspect of the digit for slight traction and elongation of the fragments, and (3) open reduction and transfixation screw. *B*, In this instance, open reduction was selected, and anatomic alignment has been established.

type of injury. The *intra-articular fracture* with two segments (Bennett's) is managed as illustrated in Figure 9C. Force, directed inward, is applied at the base of the metacarpal. Traction is provided simultaneously, as is abduction and extension of the metacarpal head. A pin inserted percutaneously just distal to the articular surface of the first metacarpal and directed toward the base of the second metacarpal in line with the neck of the third metacarpal should allow the first metacarpal shaft, the fragment on the intermetacarpal ligament, and the base of the second metacarpal to be held adequately to maintain the reduction. This is followed by application of a light plaster splint or cast, which maintains the position described. The pin remains in place for 4 weeks, after which protected motion is initiated.

Open reduction and internal fixation is indicated if soft tissue is interposed between the fragments or if a large fragment is malrotated and prevents joint congruity.

The *comminuted fracture* at the base of the metacarpal (Rolando's) may be treated either by percutaneous pin fixation or by traction obtained by placing a transfixion pin through the base of the proximal phalanx or neck of the metacarpal. The authors seldom depend on the traction mechanism and prefer the direct plaster fixation or percutaneous pin. If the palmar and dorsal fragments are large and cannot be reduced anatomically, open reduction and internal fixation can be considered.

The fracture at the proximal metaphysis of the thumb metacarpal, which does not include the joint, is managed by manipulation, realignment, and plaster fixation, with the thumb in wide abduction and the MCP joint in flexion. Extra-articular fractures of the thumb metacarpal are reduced and placed in a short-arm–thumb spica cast for about 4 weeks. Twenty to 30 degrees of angulation usually causes no functional loss. If plaster immobilization is unsuccessful in treating an oblique fracture, percutaneous pinning or interfragmentary screw fixation is considered.

Injuries to the *MCP joint of the thumb* include chip fractures of the ulnar collateral ligament; the fragment is avulsed from the proximal phalanx or from the distal metacarpal. The ligament can also rupture in its central portion or pull from bone without a fracture. In addition to the collateral ligament injury, the palmar plate and the dorsal capsule are usually torn, causing the phalanx to displace palmarward and radially. In most instances, these injuries are detected by clinical examination (carpometacarpal flexion, MCP flexion with stress). The stress radiograph is not essential, but if there is any question about the extent of soft tissue injury, a stress radiograph under local or regional block is helpful.

If there is less than 30 degrees difference between the injured and uninjured thumb, incomplete tear is diagnosed. Treatment of an incomplete tear can be managed satisfactorily by application of a plaster or fiber-glass cast that holds the phalanx in the neutral adducted position and realigns the metacarpal and the phalanx. A cast is applied for a minimum of 4 weeks, and protection with hand-based splints is necessary for 4 additional weeks, during which time range of motion exercises are performed several times a day.

If there is greater than 30 degrees difference, complete tear is diagnosed and operative repair is usually indicated. When examination indicates that the collateral ligament is torn completely and could be caught outside the adductor aponeurosis and not heal (Stener), or when the individual is not willing to undergo 6 weeks of immobilization and still not be absolutely certain that stability is present, then open operation is recommended. *Displaced intra-articular fractures* involving more than 15 to 20 per cent of the articular surface and a small avulsion fracture displaced more than 5 mm. are relative indications for open reduction.

Dorsal subluxation of the proximal phalanx at the MCP level may cause a partial tear of the capsule and displacement of the

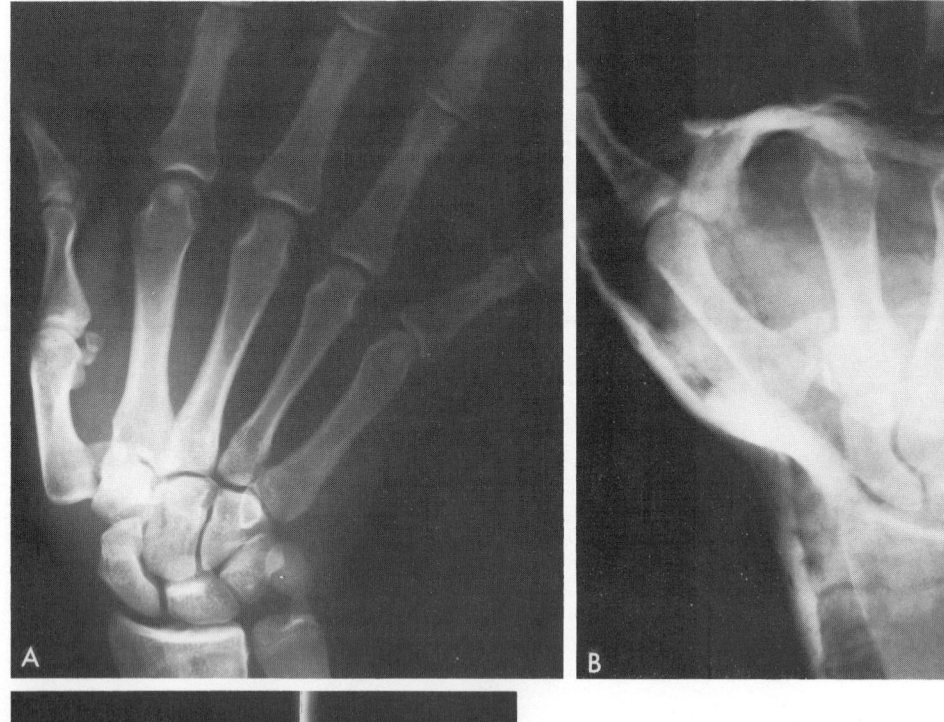

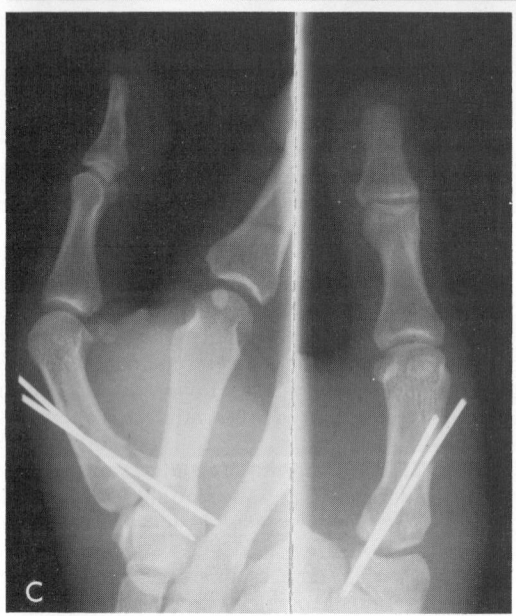

Figure 9. *A*, Bennett's fracture at the base of the first metacarpal. This involves the articular surface. The deformity is aggravated by pull of the abductor pollicis longus and the adductor pollicis. *B*, Realignment and reduction were attempted by extension traction. This is usually not successful if the metacarpal is displaced. The position for improving position is 45-degree abduction of the thumb from the palm rather than extension, external rotation. *C*, Anatomic position was regained by radial deviation and dorsiflexion of the hand and longitudinal traction abduction of the thumb. As traction was maintained, percutaneous 0.045 pins were inserted across the metacarpal and into the trapezium. At least two views are essential to document proper reduction. Pins are left in place for 4 weeks, and the thumb is protected for 6 weeks.

dorsal capsule and extensor mechanism. Relocation is not difficult, and immobilization in the flexed position is usually sufficient. A serious articular and vascular injury may occur with complete dislocation of the metacarpal head and displacement of the proximal phalanx. The head protrudes through a tear in the capsule, and the palmar plate may be interposed in the joint (Fig. 10). If a dislocation is unrecognized, vascular insufficiency may occur. Amputation has followed this type of injury as a result of inadequate early reduction or failure to recognize the dislocation, which can occlude the digital arteries. One must be prepared to proceed with an open operation if replacement of the fragments is not done with relative ease and without excessive manipulative forces.

GENERAL PRINCIPLES OF TREATMENT

Stable fractures (undisplaced or impacted) without angulation or rotation may be treated by taping the injured digit to the adjacent one and beginning early, protected, active motion.

Clinical and radiographic follow-up during the first several days is necessary. Joint dislocations require support after reduction to allow ligamentous healing for stability and to provide comfort. Less stable fractures often are treated by closed reduction and immobilization. However, if the patient is not willing to undergo several weeks of immobilization and when the fracture is unstable, open operation is recommended.

There are many instances, however, in which athletes have been treated by plastic tape and splint fixation with strong immobilization. This has allowed them to continue their athletic endeavors without the interruption of an operative procedure.

Aluminum splints, plaster casts or splints, or molded thermoplastic material provides support for certain fractures. A dorsal aluminum or plastic splint held by tape can be used for a mallet finger, for a dislocated joint, for a small chip fracture, and for a stable, oblique fracture. The splint need not be complicated, nor does it have to be padded extensively. It is usually applied without padding and can be bent to contour, but it must be narrower than the width of the finger. It should be firm enough to require

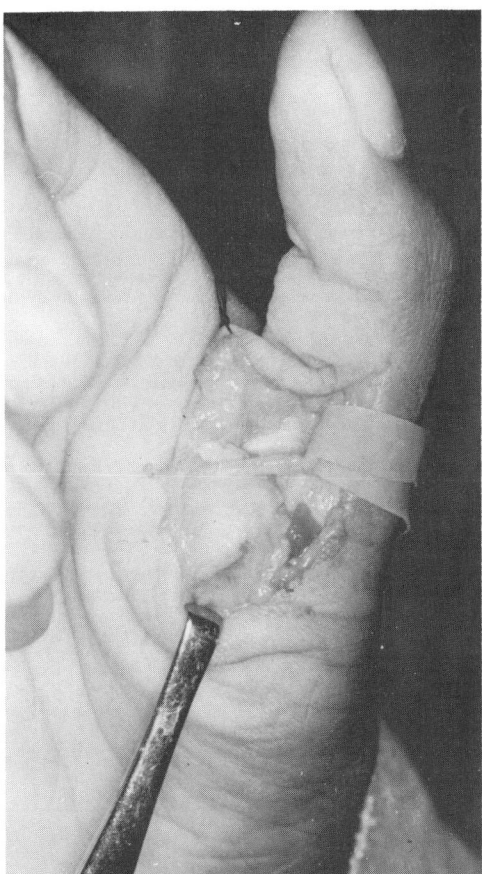

Figure 10. Dislocation of the metacarpophalangeal joint of the thumb with flexor tendon and capsule preventing relocation. Open operation is necessary.

bending with a lightweight pair of wire benders or the arms of a pair of bandage scissors. If the splint can be bent easily by the physician's fingers, it is not strong enough. When possible, a splint should be applied to the dorsal rather than the palmar surface of the digit so that the palmar tip of the finger can be used even with the splint applied. The end of the splint may be bent over the tip of the finger, depending on the type of injury that has occurred.

If a slight amount of elongation and traction of the fracture and the digit is needed, palmar or dorsal splints can be incorporated into a plaster gauntlet, and the digit can be held to the splint with tape after slight traction is applied and the splint is bent.

Plaster splints are useful and readily available for treatment of hand fractures. The position of the wrist, MCP joints, and IP joints determines the success of the plaster splint treatment. The wrist is dorsiflexed to stabilize the metacarpals and relax the extensor tendons. The MCP joint should be flexed at least 60 degrees to ensure proper rotation and to avoid contracture of the collateral ligaments. The IP joints should be extended or flexed, depending on the type of injury. Plaster splints can be about six thicknesses, covered by sheet cotton, and applied directly to the skin with a small amount of protective padding over the involved area. The bone prominences are padded with felt. The splint is applied when wet, and the hand and the digit are held in the appropriate position. The splints are then wrapped by narrow sheet cotton and then by bias-cut stockinette or more plaster. An uninvolved digit is usually included for additional protection. The hand should be elevated above the heart level for several days after the injury in order to decrease swelling. The initial plaster splint is often changed at 5 to 6 days when the swelling has decreased. Radiographs and clinical ex-

amination confirm adequate position of the fracture after changing of the splint or cast.

Prolonged periods of immobilization of fractures of the hand are not necessary. The radiograph is not a good guide to the length of time that the hand should be immobilized. Complete bone healing of hand fractures is not demonstrable by radiographs for approximately 5 months. With the exception of the mallet and boutonnière chip fractures, 3 to 4 weeks is usually sufficient time for immobilization of most fractures and ligamentous injuries. Protection is continued for an additional 3 to 4 weeks, but range of motion exercises are initiated promptly. Fractures of the midshaft region of the phalanges require protection for 5 to 7 weeks and middle phalanx fractures even longer.

Joint dislocations require support after reduction to allow ligamentous healing for stability and to provide comfort to the patient.

Fractures that are too unstable to be maintained by external immobilization usually require fixation of the fragments to allow healing with proper alignment and to permit early motion.

Open reduction is indicated in dislocations that are irreducible by closed means. Internal fixation, either percutaneous (K wires) or after open reduction (K wires, interosseous wiring, interfragmentary screws, mini plates and screws), is considered for irreducible or very unstable fractures, multiple-level fractures, displaced intra-articular fractures, and certain open hand injuries. External fixation with small threaded half-pins articulated with clamps and bars is used to stabilize fractures with extensive soft tissue injury. This provides access for wound care and maintains bone alignment even with extensive comminution or segmental bone loss. Certain severely comminuted and intra-articular fractures cannot be reconstructed adequately and are best treated by arthrodesis of the joint. During internal fixation of a fracture, effort is made to achieve stability of the fracture while deformities are corrected, including malrotation and angulation. Joints are not crossed by pins unless absolutely necessary.

Treatment of hand fractures is directed toward regaining flexible, properly aligned, strong digits with adequate vascular supply and sensibility. One common complication is decreased motion secondary to tendon adhesions or ligament and capsular contracture. This condition is often improved by active exercises and by dynamic splinting. Occasionally, however, these conditions require tendolysis or surgical release of joint capsules or ligaments. Malunion (malrotation, angulation) can be corrected by osteotomy, and nonunion can be corrected by bone grafting and rigid internal fixation if necessary. Infections may occur with open fractures or those fractures treated by open reduction and internal fixation. The infection is usually treated by surgical débridement and by antibiotics.

SELECTED REFERENCES

Dray, G. J., and Eaton, R. G.: Dislocations and ligament injuries in the digits. *In* Green, D. P. (Ed.): Operative Hand Surgery, 2nd ed. Vol. 1. New York, Churchill Livingstone, 1988, pp. 777–811.
This chapter provides detailed information, illustrations, and a comprehensive bibliography for treating dislocations and ligament injuries in the digits.

Green, D. P., and Rowland, S. A.: Fractures and dislocations in the hand. *In* Rockwood, C. A., and Green, D. P. (Eds.): Fractures in Adults, 2nd ed. Philadelphia, J. B. Lippincott Company, 1984, pp. 313–409.
These authors clearly detail the pathoanatomy, the various methods of treating, and the preferred method of managing fractures and dislocations of the hand. Illustrations, photographs, and an extensive bibliography strengthen this comprehensive chapter.

O'Brien, E. T.: Fractures of the metacarpals and phalanges. *In* Green, D. P. (Ed.): Operative Hand Surgery, 2nd ed. Vol. 1. New York, Churchill Livingstone, 1988, pp. 709–775.
This chapter provides detailed information, illustrations, and comprehensive bibliography for treating hand fractures.

REFERENCES

1. Belsky, M. R., Eaton, R. G., and Lane, L. B.: Closed reduction and internal fixation of proximal phalangeal fractures. J. Hand Surg., 9A:725, 1984.
2. Black, D. M., Mann, R. J., Constine, R. M., and Daniels, A. U.: The stability of internal fixation in the proximal phalanx. J. Hand Surg., 11A:672, 1986.
3. Black, D. M., Mann, R. J., Constine, R. M., and Daniels, A. U.: Comparison of internal fixation techniques in metacarpal fractures. J. Hand Surg., 10A:466, 1985.
4. Bowers, W. H.: The proximal interphalangeal joint volar plate. II: A clinical study of hyperextension injury. J. Hand Surg., 6:78, 1981.
5. Coonrad, R. W., and Goldner, J. L.: A study of the pathological findings and treatment in soft tissue injury of the thumb metacarpophalangeal joint. J. Bone Joint Surg. [Am.], 50:439, 1968.
6. Dabezies, E. J., and Schutte, J. P.: Fixation of metacarpal and phalangeal fractures with miniature plates and screws. J. Hand Surg., 11A:283, 1986.
7. Duncan, J., and Kettelkamp, D. B.: Low-velocity gunshot wounds of the hand. Arch. Surg., 109:395, 1974.
8. Eaton, R. G., and Malerich, M. M.: Volar plate arthroplasty of the proximal interphalangeal joint: A review of ten years' experience. J. Hand Surg., 5:260, 1980.
9. Fyfe, I. S., and Mason, S.: The mechanical stability of internal fixation of fractured phalanges. Hand, 11:50, 1979.
10. Goldner, J. L.: Trauma to the extensor mechanism at its attachment to the distal phalanx of the digits. In Current Practice in Orthopaedic Surgery. St. Louis, C. V. Mosby, 1964, pp. 143–152.
11. Hunter, J. M., and Cowen, N. J.: Fifth metacarpal fractures in a compensation clinic population. J. Bone Joint Surg. [Am.], 52:1159, 1979.
12. James, J. P.: Fractures of the proximal and middle phalanges of the fingers. Acta. Orthop., 32:401, 1962.
13. Kaplan, E. B.: Dorsal dislocation of the metacarpophalangeal joint of the index finger. J. Bone Joint Surg. [Am.], 39:1081, 1957.
14. Lister, G: Intraosseous wiring of the digital skeleton. J. Hand Surg., 3:427, 1978.
15. McCue, F. C., Honner, R., Johnson, M. C., Jr., and Gieck, J. H.: Athletic injuries of the proximal and interphalangeal joint requiring surgical treatment. J. Bone Joint Surg. [Am.], 52:937, 1970.
16. McElfresh, E. C., and Dobyns, J. H.: Intra-articular metacarpal head fractures. J. Hand Surg., 8:383, 1983.
17. McElfresh, E. C., Dobyns, J. H., and O'Brien, E. T.: Management of fracture-dislocation of the proximal interphalangeal joints by extension-block splinting. J. Bone Joint Surg. [Am.], 54:1705, 1972.
18. Neviaser, R. J., Wilson, J. N., and Lievano, A.: Rupture of the ulnar collateral ligament of the thumb (gamekeeper's thumb). Correction by dynamic repair. J. Bone Joint Surg. [Am.], 52:1357, 1971.
19. Peimer, C. A., Sullivan, D. J., and Wild, D. R.: Palmar dislocation of the proximal interphalangeal joint. J. Hand Surg., 9A:39, 1984.
20. Problem fractures of the hand and wrist. In Meals, R. A. (Ed.): Clinical Orthopaedics and Related Research. No. 214, January 1987.
21. Stark, H. H., Boyes, J. H., and Wilson, J. N.: Mallet finger. J. Bone Joint Surg., 44A:1061, 1962.
22. Stener, B.: Displacement of the ruptured collateral ligament of the metacarpophalangeal joint of the thumb. J. Bone Joint Surg. [Br.], 44:869, 1962.
23. Vanik, R. K., Weber, R. C., Matloub, H. S., Sanger, J. R., and Gingrass, R. P.: The comparative strengths of internal fixation techniques. J. Hand Surg., 9A:216, 1984.
24. Wehbe, M. A., and Schneider, L. H.: Mallet fractures. J. Bone Joint Surg. [Am.], 66:658, 1984.
25. Wilson, J. N., and Rowland, S. A.: Fracture-dislocation of the proximal interphalangeal joint of the finger. J. Bone Joint Surg. [Am.], 48:493, 1966.

VI

FRACTURES OF THE PELVIS, FEMUR, AND KNEE

Donald E. McCollum, M.D.

PELVIC FRACTURES

Pelvic fractures are associated with massive trauma and frequently follow automobile collision with pedestrians, a fall from a height, or ejection from an unprotected vehicle such as a motorcycle. In older patients with osteoporosis, fractures of the pelvis more commonly occur from minor injury such as a fall. Major pelvic fractures are life-threatening, and death occurs in as many as 20 per cent of patients. When the fractures are compound and associated with hemorrhage, mortality may be as high as 50 per cent. Many organ systems are involved in massive trauma causing pelvic fractures and may include retroperitoneal hemorrhage, neurologic changes from damages to the lumbosacral plexus and nerve roots, genitourinary damage, and damage to major arterial trunks. Pelvic injuries are also frequently associated with injury to internal organs, other skeletal injuries, and head injuries.

The pelvis is a rigid ring composed of the pubic rami, ischium, acetabulum, ilium, and sacrum joined by heavy ligaments at the symphysis and the sacroiliac joints. Disruption at one point does not necessarily produce instability; disruption at two points on the same side of the pelvis may allow displacement as the paravertebral muscles shorten. Either prolonged skeletal traction or open reduction with internal fixation is necessary for maintenance of the fracture in the position that can produce satisfactory results and function.

Classification of Fracture

Tile has classified pelvic injuries by the mechanism of injury: anteroposterior compression occurs when a patient is struck from the front by a car. There is disruption of the symphysis anteriorly and disruption of the anterior ligaments of the sacroiliac joint. The pelvis thus opens like an open book, leaving the posterior ligaments of the sacroiliac joint intact (Fig. 1C).

Lateral compression injuries result when a patient is struck from the side by a car. This injury may fracture one or both of the pubic rami, and there may be an associated fracture of the sacrum or the iliac wing. If the fracture of the pubic rami is impacted, as demonstrated in Figure 1A, and the ligaments of the sacroiliac joint are intact, the fracture may be stable and may be treated with bed rest.

Vertical shear fractures follow axial loading, as in a fall from a height. Anteriorly there may be fracture of one or both pubic rami or disruption of the symphysis pubis. There may be associated disruption posteriorly through the sacroiliac joint, through the ilium lateral to the sacroiliac joint, or through the sacrum medial to the sacroiliac joint. The vertical shear fracture is usually unstable and is difficult to treat with traction. Open reduction is generally indicated in this unstable fracture (Fig. 1D).

Minor fractures include fractures of the ilium, unilateral fractures of the pubic rami, and avulsion fractures at points of muscle attachment. Fractures of the anterosuperior spine occur in athletes by forcible contraction of the sartorius muscle. Treatment requires only bed rest with the hip in flexion for 10 days. The anteroinferior iliac spine is occasionally avulsed by forcible contraction of the rectus muscle, and treatment is similar. Sprinters may avulse the ischial tuberosity by forceful contraction of the hamstrings. Bed rest or crutches allow healing to occur spontaneously. Swelling of the thigh may be massive, and pain may be severe. The displaced avulsion fracture frequently

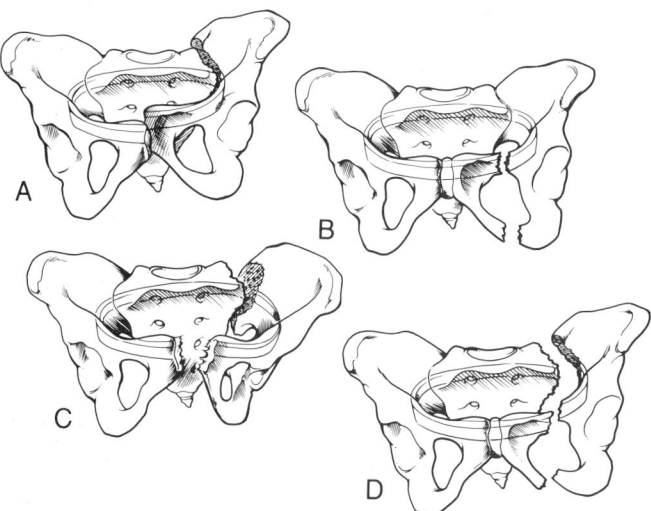

Figure 1. *A* and *B* are stable fractures, and *C* and *D* are unstable fractures. The lateral compression fracture in *A* impacts the symphysis. The ligaments of the posterior sacroiliac joint are intact, and the fracture is stable. In *B*, the ring is disrupted only on one side at the superior and inferior ramus of the pubis. The sacroiliac joint is intact, and the fracture is stable. In *C* the pelvis is opened as is a book. The symphysis is disrupted, and the anterior and posterior ligaments of the sacroiliac joint are disrupted. The fracture is unstable and is best treated by open reduction. In *D*, the fracture is caused by vertical shear and the ring is disrupted both anteriorly and posteriorly and the fracture is unstable. This fracture should be treated by open reduction and internal fixation anteriorly and posteriorly.

heals by fibrous union. The patient becomes asymptomatic after 1 or 2 years, but athletic ability is generally reduced.

Sacrum and Coccyx

Isolated fractures of the sacrum and coccyx are treated by bed rest until the patient is comfortable and can be mobilized with crutches. Frequently, after fractures of the sacrum, fibrosis may occur around the sacral nerve roots and produce persistent pain. Persistent coccygeal pain may be the result of traumatic arthritis of the sacrococcygeal joint or more commonly is due to muscular damage to the urogenital diaphragm. Surgical therapy is seldom indicated and frequently may contribute additional pain. Treatment of chronic coccygeal pain following injury should consist of a foam rubber coccygodynia pad, which relieves pressure on the coccyx, and analgesics and nonsteroidal anti-inflammatory drugs.

MAJOR FRACTURES OF THE PELVIS

Major fractures of the pelvis most frequently follow crush injuries to the passenger within an automobile or on a motorcycle, to the pedestrian struck by an automobile either from the front or the side, or to the patient falling from a height. These fractures are discussed separately because morbidity and mortality differ greatly. Spear found these fractures to be the third most common cause of death due to automobile accidents. They are frequently associated with other internal injuries to the urethra, bladder, and abdominal organs. The most common complication of this fracture is that of massive hemorrhage in the retroperitoneal space, which occurs from the plexus of veins and arteries lining the inner pelvic wall.

Treatment of the unstable pelvic fracture varies widely. Previous texts originally recommended manipulation of the fracture with the patient on his side, followed by application of a spica cast. The incidence of pelvic thrombophlebitis and pulmonary embolism is very high in patients with these fractures, and casts should be avoided if possible. Traction is seldom successful in reducing the unstable pelvic fracture and must be continued for at least 10 to 12 weeks for stability to continue. Most authors experienced in the treatment of pelvic fractures now agree that open reduction of the unstable pelvic fracture is man-

datory in order to achieve bony union in a satisfactory and functional position as quickly as possible. Persistent deformity can cause leg length inequality with difficulty in walking, pain in sitting, and difficulty with subsequent pregnancy.

Most pelvic injuries in which the ring is undisplaced are stable and can be treated closed by bed rest and ambulation after 3 weeks with crutches. Fracture of the anterior ramus and an undisplaced posterior ring are treated with bed rest until the patient is comfortable and can walk with crutches.

Emergency evaluation of a patient with a pelvic fracture must include all organ systems which frequently are involved. Careful neurologic evaluation should include evaluation of the obturator nerve, which supplies the adductor muscles; the sciatic nerve; and the lumbosacral plexus. Retroperitoneal bleeding may mimic gastrointestinal trauma, and peritoneal lavage may be necessary for excluding ruptured organs intraperitoneally. Careful examination of the rectum and vagina may reveal blood in either orifice and is presumptive evidence of an open fracture of the pelvis.

Emergency measures in the management of the patient with a pelvic fracture include wound packing to control bleeding and application of a compression suit for maintenance of blood pressure. In the event of an anteroposterior compression fracture, the volume of the pelvis is increased approximately four times. The use of an external fixator on the pelvis to close the symphysis and reduce the volume of the pelvis may be necessary to reduce retroperitoneal bleeding. After the application of an external fixator, if the blood pressure does not stabilize, ligation of the hypogastric artery must be considered by abdominal exploration.

Emergency radiographic evaluation should include an anteroposterior view and 40-degree caudad and cephalad projections of the pelvis. The caudad projection best defines the posterior lesions in the sacroiliac dislocation, and the cephalad view or the outlet view best demonstrates the cephalad or caudad displacement of both the anterior and posterior segments. When the acetabulum is involved, 45-degree oblique views of the acetabulum demonstrate disruption of the acetabulum and the sacroiliac joint. After the patient is stabilized, a computerized tomographic scan provides additional details.

Complications of Pelvic Fracture

HEMORRHAGE. Peltier found that the most common complication of pelvic fractures was massive hemorrhage. Bleeding may occur as mentioned from the laceration of hypogastric vessels by fractures extending into the sciatic notch. Shock occurs rapidly, as evidenced by decrease in vital signs, urinary output, central venous pressure, and an enlarging psoas shadow. Patients must be massively transfused for correction of shock and maintenance of urinary output. The use of a compression suit must be considered; and in the case of an anteroposterior compression fracture with widespread displacement of the symphysis, the application of an external fixator with closure of the symphysis decreases the volume of the pelvis, thus reducing retroperitoneal hemorrhage. If bleeding cannot be controlled, arteriography may be helpful in fractures that extend into the sciatic notch, the ilium, or the posterior ischium. If bleeding points can be demonstrated, hemorrhage can frequently be controlled by embolization with Gelfoam or an autogenous blood clot. Lacerations of the common iliac or external iliac artery are best treated open with ligation.

LOWER URINARY TRACT. The bladder rests against the pubic bones and when empty is seldom injured. As the bladder extends, it may fill most of the true pelvis and rise above the symphysis, where it becomes vulnerable to either intraperitoneal or extraperitoneal rupture. Injuries to the lower urinary tract (bladder and urethra) occur in 14 per cent of all pelvic fractures and must be detected by urethrogram, cystogram, and intravenous urogram.

If the injury occurs below the urogenital diaphragm, induration in the suprapubic region may be caused by perivesical hematoma. Extraperitoneal rupture of the bladder may present as a smooth, rounded mass above the pubis; whereas intraperitoneal rupture produces no palpable mass and no induration but produces ileus, abdominal rigidity, and rebound tenderness in the conscious patient.

If the injury occurs below the urogenital diaphragm, tenderness and swelling are usually found in the perineal area. Ecchymoses may be present in the skin of the perineum. Rectal examination must be done in all patients with pelvic fractures and may reveal hematoma, displacement of the prostate gland, or tenderness when disruption of the supramembranous urethra has occurred.

If the urethrogram demonstrates the urethra intact, retrograde cystography should be performed with a 14 or 16 French catheter, with injection of only 250 to 300 ml. of dye. The passage of a blind catheter without urethrography is condemned because it may enter and drain blood from the perivesical space, simulating extraperitoneal rupture of the bladder. Rupture of both bladder and urethra are surgical emergencies requiring immediate urinary diversion and repair.

RECTUM. The rectum lies directly on the sacrum, where it is well protected but may be lacerated by ischial or sacral fractures. Examination of the rectum for defects or fresh blood should be done in early pelvic fracture. The uterus, vagina, and vulva are rarely damaged, but compound fractures may extend into these structures.

NEUROLOGIC. The sciatic nerve is most frequently damaged by fractures of the pelvis extending into the ilium or into the sciatic notch, by fracture of the ischium with displacement, or by posterior dislocation of the hip. The peroneal division of the sciatic nerve is more often damaged than the tibial division. It can be recognized easily by failure to contract the hamstrings and dorsiflex the foot in the conscious patient or by failure to dorsiflex the foot in withdrawal in the semiconscious patient. The obturator nerve lies in the obturator canal on the medial aspect of the acetabulum and may be damaged by central dislocation of the hip. Paralysis of the obturator nerve can be recognized by inability to contract the adductor muscles and by irregular hypalgesia over the medial aspect of the thigh. The femoral nerve is seldom damaged directly by fractures of the pelvis but may be damaged by anterior dislocation of the hip. It more commonly is secondarily involved by compression from a hematoma, which often occurs after fracture around the pelvis and hip.

PULMONARY. In a review of 151 patients, Spear found the most common cause of death following pelvic fractures to be posttraumatic pulmonary insufficiency. This syndrome has been referred to by other authors as "shock lung." The respiratory distress syndrome can be recognized by a significant change in blood gases, with decreasing oxygen tension and rising carbon dioxide.

Because of damage to the retroperitoneal venous plexus, pelvic thrombophlebitis and pulmonary embolism constitute a major threat to these injured patients. Body casts are rarely indicated. Low-molecular-weight dextran may be used cautiously as prophylaxis against thromboembolic phenomena only after significant bleeding has ceased. Low-dose heparin has been shown to be ineffective, but aspirin has been demonstrated to be effective in preventing pulmonary embolism.

FAT EMBOLISM. Although fat embolism occurs more frequently in fractures of long bones, it is also observed as a complication of fractures of the pelvis. Forty-eight to 72 hours after injury, the patient becomes confused, there is a sudden drop in hemoglobin that is unexplained by blood loss, arterial oxygen saturation is decreased as measured by blood gases, and small petechiae appear on the conjunctiva and over the upper chest. The chest films may demonstrate hazy infiltrates throughout both lung fields. Fat globules are frequently present in the urine but are not diagnostic, because they are present with most major fractures. Prompt treatment by oxygen, blood replacement, and administration of albumin is necessary to prevent permanent brain damage.

ARTHRITIS. Traumatic arthritis frequently develops after acetabular fractures. Although function after treatment with prolonged traction is frequently much better than the radiologic appearance, after an undetermined number of years, the joint space begins to narrow, and the typical radiologic signs of posttraumatic arthritis develop. These are characterized by subchondral sclerosis and the development of cysts in the acetabulum and the femoral head. Range of motion gradually diminishes as pain increases. Such a complication in the adult is often managed best by total hip replacement. This procedure is seldom indicated in younger patients and is rarely indicated as a primary procedure.

Assessment of Stability of Pelvic Fractures

Stability of the pelvic fracture is influenced by bony deformity and by ligamentous injury. Pelvic instability is indicated by the amount of displacement of the posterior elements on either side of the sacroiliac joint. Displacement of the sacroiliac joint is a sign of instability. A fracture of the sacrum may be stable if minimally displaced. Any fracture or dislocation of the sacroiliac joint must be considered unstable. Fractures of the iliac wing when displaced are unstable. Anterior diastasis of the symphysis pubis when it exceeds 3 cm. is considered an unstable pelvic fracture. Diastasis of the pubic ramus does not usually occur when the rami on either side are fractured.

TREATMENT

The objective of treatment of fractures of the pelvis after the patient's general condition has stabilized is to achieve bony union in a functional position as quickly as possible. Deformities following pelvic fractures can cause leg length inequality, difficulty in walking, difficulty in sitting, and difficulty in subsequent pregnancy. Most fractures involving the pelvic ring are stable and can be treated by closed methods. Isolated fractures of the anterior ramus with an undisplaced posterior ring are stable and are best treated with bed rest until the patient is comfortable and then partial weight bearing. Serial radiographs are made for excluding subsequent further displacement.

Some fractures which are minimally displaced initially appear to be stable but are basically unstable fractures. Any fracture through the sacrum with disruption of the pubis must be considered an unstable fracture, and the treatment of choice is an open posterior reduction with plate fixation.

All unstable pelvic fractures are best treated by open reduction and internal fixation with plates or screws. Skeletal traction is not suitable for disruption of the sacroiliac joints, because nonunion and malunion are common. Open reduction is usually indicated when the acetabulum is involved.

Open reduction of pelvic fractures requires extensive specialized training and should not be attempted by surgeons who do not treat these injuries frequently. If a fracture requires open reduction, the patient should be referred to a trauma center.

Posterior Approaches

When the sacroiliac joint is involved, the most common approach is a vertical incision 2 cm. lateral to the posterosuperior spine, extending from the iliac crest to the sciatic notch. The short external rotators of the hip are mobilized to allow palpation inside the sciatic notch. The sacroiliac joint can be stabilized by two screws passing from lateral to medial from the ilium into the sacrum by means of radiographic control with the image intensifier. The sacroiliac joint, when disrupted, can be plated from the front. Fractures of the sacrum are best approached through a vertical incision posteriorly. The sacral nerve roots should be visualized and protected. The vertical fracture of the sacrum can be fixed with 6.5-mm. screws through the iliac wing into the S1 vertebral body. These may be augmented with a flexible plate extending from one iliac wing to the other just above the sciatic notch. Fractures of both sacroiliac joints are best fixed with long screws between the tables or by plates on the surface of the ilium. Special reduction forceps are necessary for the reduction of these fractures.

For open reduction of anterior lesions such as spread of the pubic symphysis or fracture of the pubic rami, a transverse incision is made 2 cm. above the symphysis. The linea alba is split between the two heads of the rectus abdominis, and the pubis is exposed by dissecting the rectus muscle from the symphysis. The spermatic cord is identified. The symphysis is then reduced by a special pointed reduction forceps, and the diaphysis is closed. The pubis is then stabilized with a six-hole 3.5-mm. curved plate, which is attached posterior to the rectus attachment (Fig. 2). If the spread of the symphysis is greater than 3 cm., the pelvis must be stabilized by fixing the posterior instability of the sacroiliac joint. If the lesion is unilateral, the patient can be mobilized with crutches after 1 week. If the sacroiliac

joint disruption is bilateral, gait training must be deferred for 6 weeks.

Acetabular Fractures

The radiographic evaluation of fractures of the acetabulum should include an anteroposterior view of the pelvis to demonstrate both hips and 45-degree oblique views of the acetabulum. If the patient's condition allows, a computerized tomographic scan is helpful in recognizing all the components of the fracture. The fracture may involve the posterior wall, the anterior wall, the posterior column, the anterior column, or any combination of these four elements of the acetabulum (Fig. 3). The goal of treatment is to stabilize the fracture in as near anatomic position as possible in order to prevent posttraumatic arthritis. Open reduction is indicated if displacement of the articular surface is greater than 2 mm. If the displacement is minimal and does not involve the weight-bearing surface, fracture of the acetabulum can be treated with traction; however, most displaced intra-articular fractures require open reduction (Figs. 4 and 5).

For exposure of the posterior wall of the acetabulum, the most frequently employed approach is the Kocher-Langenbeck, which provides access to the posterior acetabular wall and the ischial tuberosity (see Fig. 4). However, only the lower segment of the iliac wing is exposed. For exposure of the lateral aspect of the iliac wing and the roof of the acetabulum, the greater trochanter is osteotomized. For fractures involving the anterior acetabular wall and the anterior column, the preferred incision is the extended iliofemoral incision with the patient in the lateral position. The incision passes along the crest of the ilium and then downward over the anterolateral aspect of the hip joint in the interval between the sartorius and the tensor (see Fig. 4). The muscles are then elevated from the wing of the ilium and

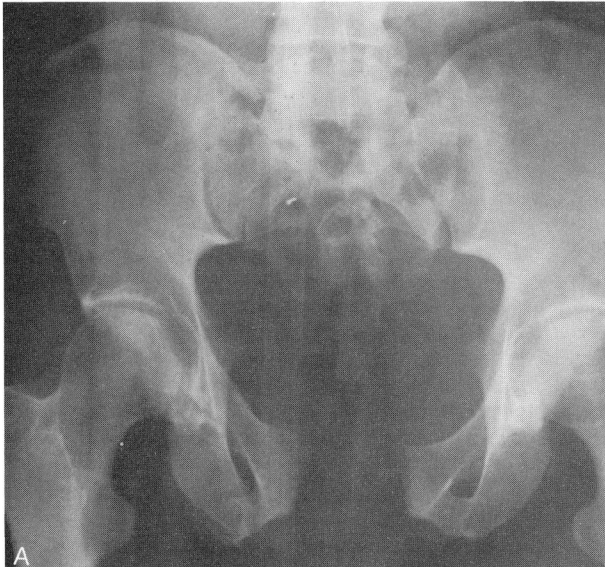

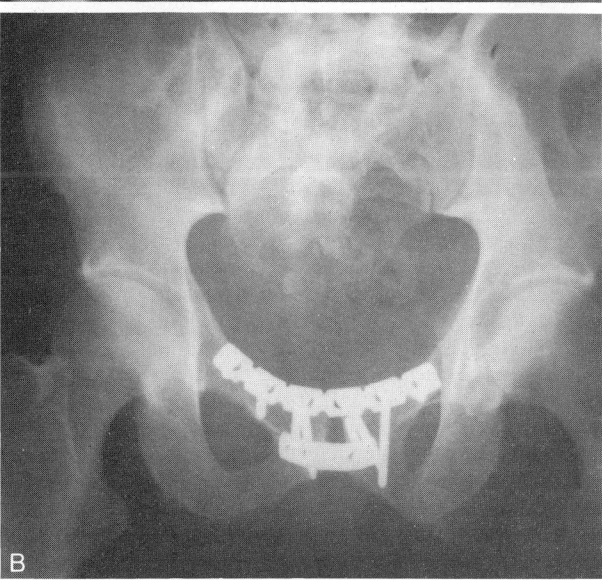

Figure 2. *A*, In this fracture the symphysis is spread 3 cm., and the left sacroiliac joint is disrupted. The posterior ligaments of the sacroiliac joint remain intact. *B*, The fracture is treated by open reduction and fixation with a six-hole plate and screws.

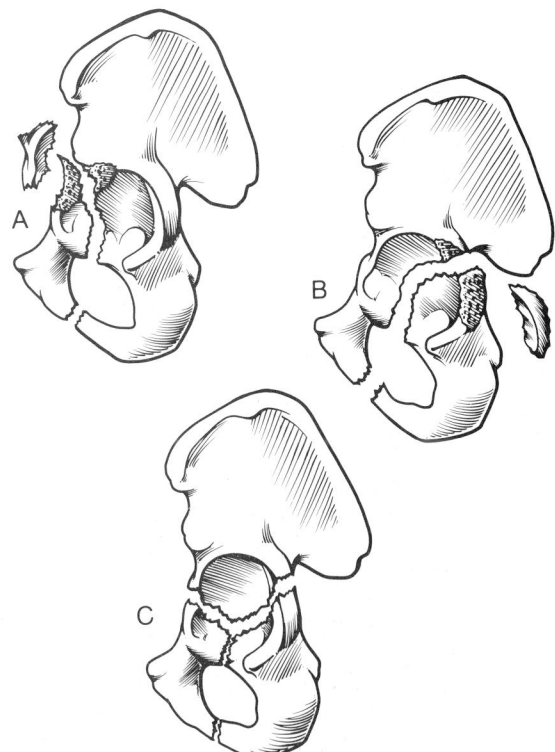

Figure 3. Fracture A involves the anterior column as well as the anterior wall. Open reduction and internal fixation are mandatory for restoration of anatomic alignment and painless function. In *B*, the posterior column (ischium) is fractured, as is the posterior wall. Open reduction and fixation of the posterior column with a plate and the posterior wall with lag screws are mandatory. In *C*, there is a combination of anterior column and posterior column fractures with a tranverse component through the acetabulum. Open reduction through both anterior and posterior approaches and fixation with plates are necessary.

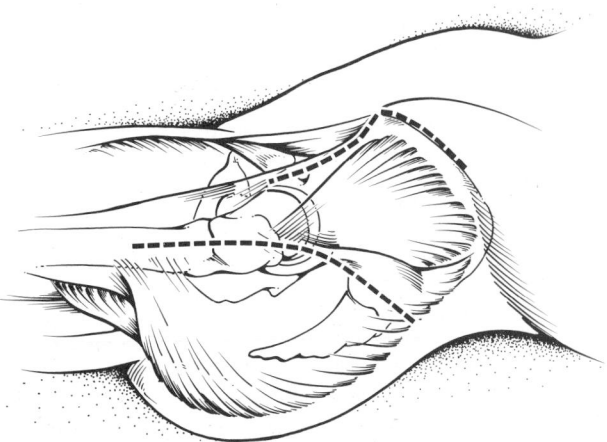

Figure 4. The anterior approach passes along the crest of the ilium and then curves downward between the sartorius and the tensor anteriorly. This affords wide exposure to the anterior column into the anterior wall of the acetabulum. The posterior approach (Kocher-Langenbach) passes across the trochanter, splits the gluteus maximus, and detaches the short external rotators for exposure of the posterior column and posterior wall of the acetabulum. If exposure of the ilium above the acetabulum is necessary, the greater trochanter must be removed.

the anterior column by subperiosteal dissection. For thorough visualization of the anterior column, it may be necessary to osteotomize the greater trochanter. The components of the fracture are reduced with pointed reduction forceps. The anterior column is usually secured with interfragmentary plates and then supplemented with screws.

Antibiotics should be administered preoperatively and continued for 48 hours postoperatively. Passive motion can be initiated in 72 hours, and crutch walking in 5 to 7 days. Weight bearing is withheld until evidence of healing occurs at approximately 6 weeks.

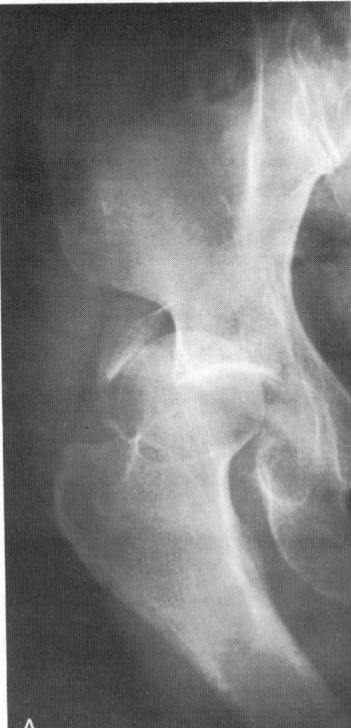
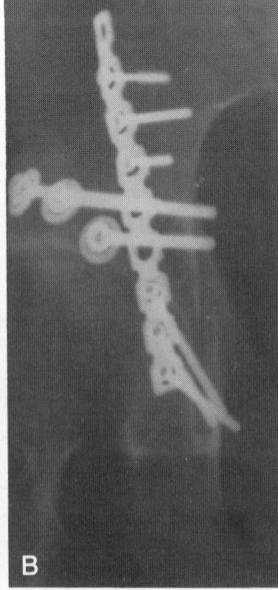

Figure 5. A and B, In this posterior fracture dislocation, the posterior wall is fractured, as is the posterior column separated from the ilium. The posterior column was repaired with a six-hole plate, and the posterior wall of the acetabulum was repaired with three screws. The fracture healed with good hip function within 6 weeks.

FRACTURES OF THE HIP AND UPPER FEMUR

Fractures of the proximal femur occur most commonly in elderly women but may occur at any age. Before the twentieth century, fracture of the femur was almost universally fatal because of pulmonary, renal, and cardiac complications. Survival was only slightly better when these elderly patients were treated by Whitman's method of closed reduction and cast immobilization, and the healing rate of 30 per cent was clearly unacceptable.

Progress in the treatment of this very common injury was made by Smith-Petersen in the 1930s when he developed the technique of open reduction and internal fixation with a tri-flanged nail. Advances have been rapid since then because of the addition of side plates, multiple pin fixation, and prosthetic replacement.

Classification

The most logical classification of hip fracture is one based upon prognosis. In any fracture, healing depends not only on fixation but, with more significance, on blood supply. Blood supply is marginal and more subject to damage in that portion of the femur that is intracapsular, which makes the prognosis for these fractures much worse than that for those that occur below the intertrochanteric line outside the capsule. Intracapsular fractures include fractures of the head of the femur, impacted subcapital fractures, and displaced subcapital and neck fractures. Because there is no periosteum on the femoral neck, healing is by endosteal callus. Fixation must be rigid and yet must allow impaction as the fracture line resorbs. The femoral head receives only a small amount of its blood supply from the pelvic side of the joint through the ligamentum teres. The major blood supply arises from the vascular ring at the base of the neck. The retinacular arteries pierce the capsule and course up the neck to enter the head in the subcapital area. These retinacular vessels may be damaged by torsion or fracture fragments or by intra-articular pressure from hematoma.

Fractures of the femoral head occur most often in posterior fracture dislocation of the hip. Either the central portion of the head is avulsed by the ligamentum teres or a quadrant of the head may be sheared off by the projecting lip of the acetabulum. This injury generally occurs when the knee strikes the dashboard of a car. The intra-articular fragments seldom heal, continue to cause pain, and cause traumatic arthritis. The treatment of choice is open reduction of the hip with removal of the loose fragments and repair of the capsule. If the dislocation is stable after repair, the patient can be mobilized rapidly on crutches. However, if manipulation allows redislocation, the patient should be maintained in simple traction for a period of 3 weeks to allow tissue healing.

Impacted subcapital fractures are relatively undisplaced fractures in which the neck of the femur is telescoped into the femoral head (Fig. 6). They may be impacted into either varus or valgus. Some believe that most impacted fractures are stress fractures. Large numbers of uniting trabecular fractures have been found in femoral necks of patients with senile subcapital fracture. The patient may present with minor groin pain with radiation to the knee. The initial films may not reveal the fracture line, and it frequently becomes visible only as the resorption phase of healing occurs. The elderly patient with hip pain must be treated for a fracture even though injury is not obvious on radiographs; otherwise, the undisplaced fracture may become displaced as demonstrated in Figure 7, which increases the likelihood of disruption of the blood supply to the femoral head.

The impacted valgus fracture is stable and may be managed conservatively by bed rest and skin traction for comfort; however, frequent radiographs are required for recognition and correction of progressive displacement of the head, which occurs as

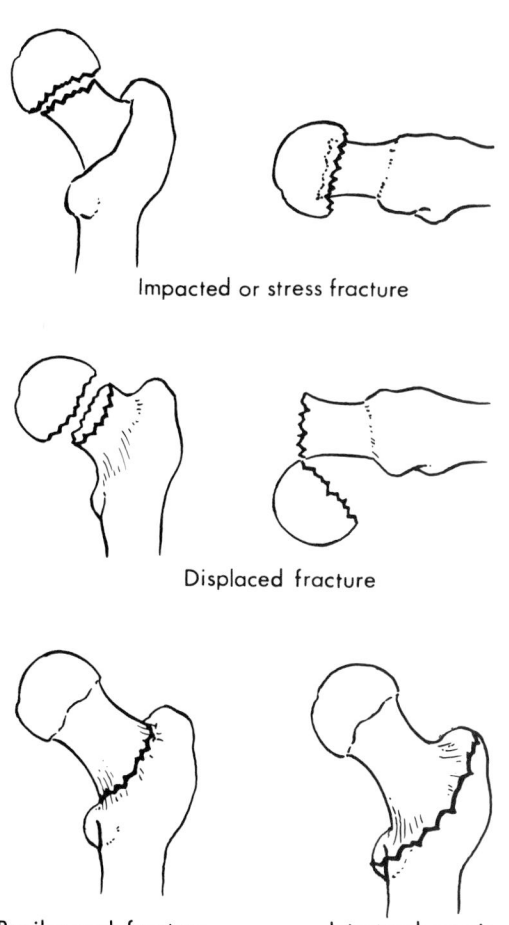

Impacted or stress fracture

Displaced fracture

Basilar neck fracture

Intertrochanteric fracture

Figure 6. The impacted subcapital fracture may heal without intervention, but there is a risk of the head slipping off of the neck during the healing period. In the younger patient, the displaced fracture should be reduced and fixed with multiple pins. In the older patient the displaced fracture is treated with prosthetic replacement. The basilar neck fracture and the intertrochanteric fracture must be fixed with a lag screw, which passes through the trochanter, into the neck and the head, and is attached to the femur by means of a side plate.

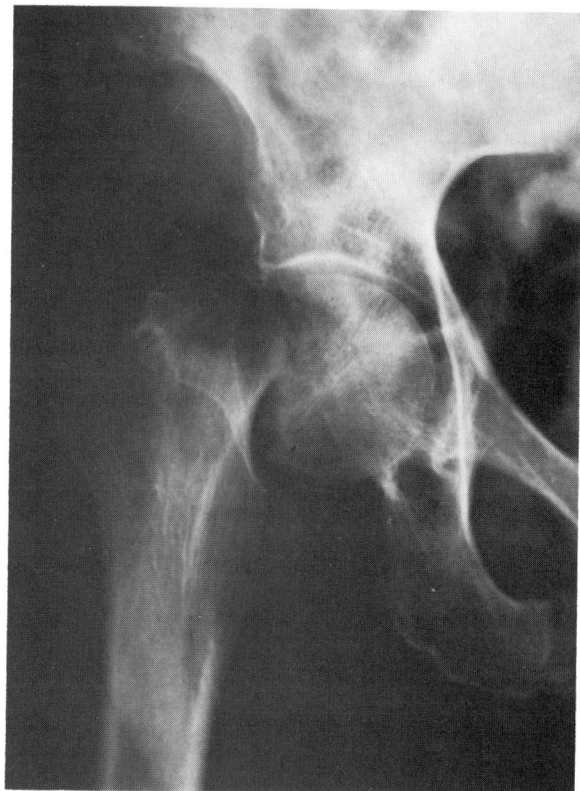

Figure 7. The displaced subcapital fracture in the elderly patient should be treated with prosthetic replacement, because nonunion and aseptic necrosis of the femoral head frequently occur.

the resorption phase of fracture healing occurs. Many apparently stable subcapital fractures have been allowed to slip into an unstable varus position despite bed rest with traction, and the safest course is application of several pins. Multiple pins destroy less of the endosteal blood supply to the femoral head and are less likely to disimpact or displace the head than insertion of a tri-flanged nail. Since only the metaphyseal and endosteal blood vessels are interrupted in the undisplaced subcapital fracture, the retinacular vessels remain intact. Healing usually occurs without difficulty if adequate immobilization by either closed or open means is maintained. Aseptic necrosis of the femoral head occurs less frequently after impacted fractures, but collapse of the head with recurrence of pain may develop as late as 5 or 6 years after the injury. Nevertheless, this relatively minor procedure provides several years of essentially normal function.

Displaced subcapital fractures and fractures of the neck of the femur are much more difficult to manage, and nonunion and avascular necrosis are much more frequent. In both of these fractures, bleeding occurs within the hip joint, and the resultant intracapsular pressure rapidly exceeds the pressure in capsular vessels, causing thrombosis. Displacement of the fragments destroys the metaphyseal and endosteal vessels, markedly reducing the blood supply to the femoral head. These fractures should be treated as emergencies; reduction should be accomplished with general or spinal anesthesia within 24 hours, and

fixation should be rigid. The rate of avascular necrosis increases with delay and even with immediate reduction approaches 25 per cent. When moderate displacement is present, reduction can be accomplished by gentle abduction and internal rotation. The Leadbetter maneuver described for more severe displacement is seldom necessary and may cause additional comminution of the neck. In younger patients, if anatomic reduction cannot be obtained by manipulation, the capsule should be opened anteriorly and the fragments reduced under direct vision. Although the rate of aseptic necrosis is high, the patient may remain asymptomatic for 6 or 7 years or more.

In young patients with good bone density, multiple-pin fixation is adequate and is preferable to a tri-flanged nail or lag screw, which is likely to displace the fracture or destroy more of the endosteal blood supply. The lower pins must rest on the inferior calcar femorale; otherwise, the varus deformity recurs as the pins settle through the hollow neck seeking support, allowing the head to displace inferiorly off the calcar. In older patients with osteoporotic bone or in fractures lower in the femoral neck, fixation between the head and shaft may require a side plate, as demonstrated in Figure 8. A guide pin is placed through the lateral cortex of the femur through the inferior aspect of the neck and into the head of the femur. The progress of the guide pin is followed by means of the image intensifier. When the guide pin is in a satisfactory position on both the anteroposterior and the lateral projection, a large screw is inserted over the guide pin through the lateral cortex of the femur through the neck and into the head. The side plate is then attached by means of a sleeve slipped over the shaft of the screw. The fracture is then impacted by means of an impacting screw, which shortens the screw into the sleeve of the side plate. Collapse at the fracture site as resorption occurs is provided by a Richards screw, and fixation is afforded by the side plate. Union of the displaced subcapital fracture may require 6 to 12 months before weight bearing can be allowed.

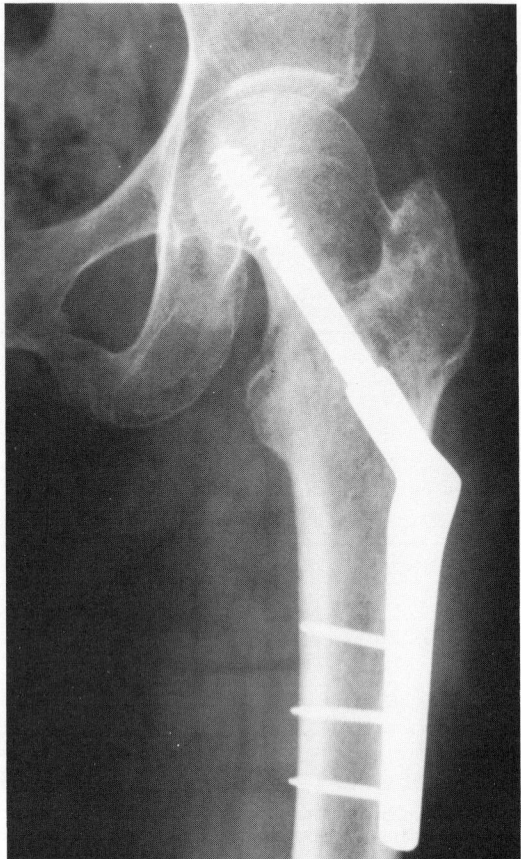

Figure 8. The Richards apparatus is the preferred method of treatment for basilar neck and intertrochanteric fractures. The fracture is impacted with a lag screw inserted through the side plate, and the side plate is fixed to the femur with multiple cortical screws. As the fracture heals, the nail telescopes, allowing impaction of the fracture to occur.

In the elderly or debilitated patient, reduction and fixation of a subcapital fracture should be done when possible, but if perfect reduction cannot be obtained, prosthetic replacement with a Moore prosthesis or the bipolar prosthesis is desirable for quicker mobilization of the patient. Prostheses should be used only as a last resort in younger patients because they eventually become painful and require further surgical therapy. Prosthetic replacement is most easily accomplished through a posterior approach, but in the uncooperative patient or the patient who tends to lie with the hip in flexion, an anterolateral approach prevents posterior dislocation. The uses of Enders nails, which are inserted through the distal femur and passed under radiographic control up into the neck of the femur and into the femoral head, allows subsequent deformity and poor fixation and is not recommended for fractures of the femoral neck.

Antibiotics should be continued for 48 hours, and the elderly patient should undergo anticoagulation either with Coumadin or salicylates.

Intertrochanteric fractures occur below the inferior attachment of the hip capsule, outside the vascular ring supplying the femoral neck and head. Blood supply is excellent, and aseptic necrosis occurs rarely. If adequate stability can be obtained, union in a functional position generally occurs. Thus, a functional classification of intertrochanteric fractures depends upon stability rather than blood supply.

Stability in intertrochanteric fractures requires both support along the medial calcar and a lateral buttress to prevent the femoral shaft from shifting medially where it tends to be drawn by the pull of the adductors. Muscle forces around the hip cause varus deformity at the fracture site and medial displacement of

the shaft. Boyd's classification into stable and unstable fractures is useful in determining the difficulty of fixation and prognosis (Fig. 9). Type I fracture is a linear break along the intertrochanteric line. Reduction is easily accomplished by abduction and internal rotation, and the fracture is stabilized firmly with a Richards screw and a side plate. The screw collapses as resorption occurs, and healing occurs in 12 weeks or less. Type II fracture is comminuted; the medial calcar is difficult to stabilize, and no lateral buttress is present. If fixation is attempted as for Type I fractures, the appliance bends or breaks, cuts out of the head, or allows the shaft to shift medially or to collapse into varus. Type III fracture is unstable and may be combined with Types I and II. Type IV fracture extends through the trochanter at least two planes and extends into the shaft. A special appliance such as the Zickel nail with additional circumferential wires around the subtrochanteric portion of the fracture is necessary to restore stability (Fig. 10).

Hip Fractures in Children

Intracapsular fractures in children are uncommon, but complications are common and include growth disturbance, avascular changes, nonunion, malunion, and partial ankylosis. For epiphyseal growth to continue, reduction must be anatomic and fixation secure. These goals can best be met by open reduction and internal fixation.

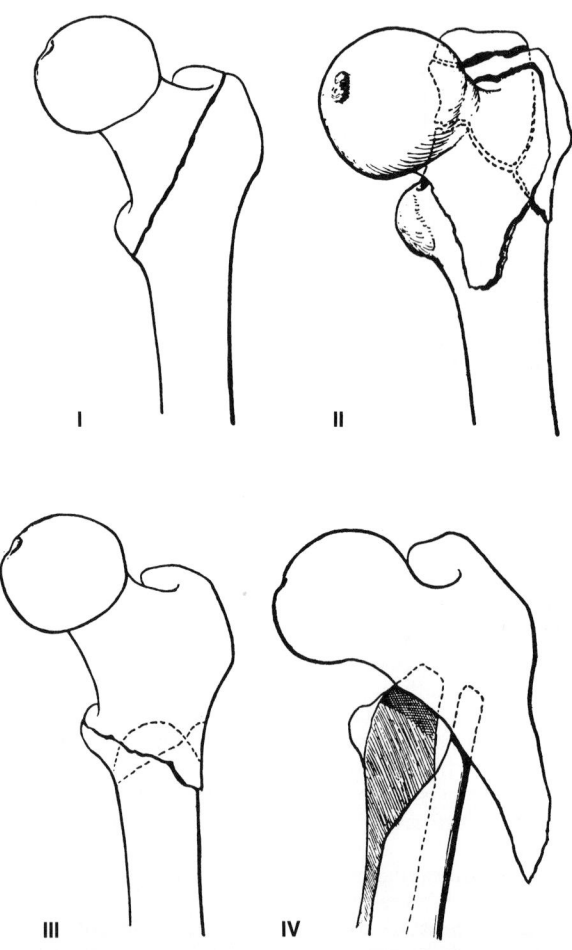

Figure 9. Intertrochanteric fractures. Type I is a stable fracture and can be fixed with a Richards screw and a side plate. Type II is an unstable fracture and may need an intramedullary component in the femur such as the Zickel nail. In Type III intertrochanteric fractures, the shaft tends to displace medially, carrying the Richards screw into the head of the femur. This fracture as well as Type IV may need to be fixed with an intramedullary appliance such as the Zickel nail. (From Boyd, H. B., and Griffin, L. L.: Classification and treatment of trochanteric fractures. Arch. Surg., *58:*854, 1949. Copyright 1949, American Medical Association.)

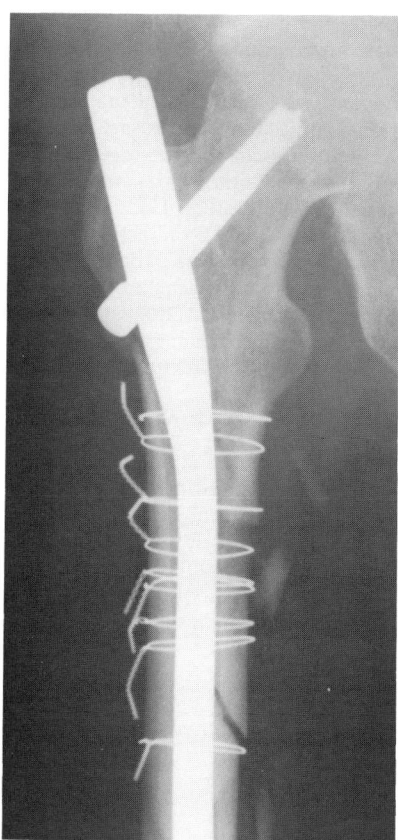

Figure 10. The Zickel nail is used for unstable intertrochanteric fractures or subtrochanteric fractures.

Transepiphyseal fractures may occur with severe trauma, or minor trauma may cause complete disruption of an epiphyseal line already weakened by chronic slipping capital femoral epiphysis (Fig. 11). Reduction should be accomplished by gentle abduction, internal rotation, and fixation by two or more parallel Knowles pins or screws.

Fractures of the neck of the femur produce a high incidence of avascular necrosis of the head of the femur in children. Minimal motion further destroys the metaphyseal and retinacular ar-

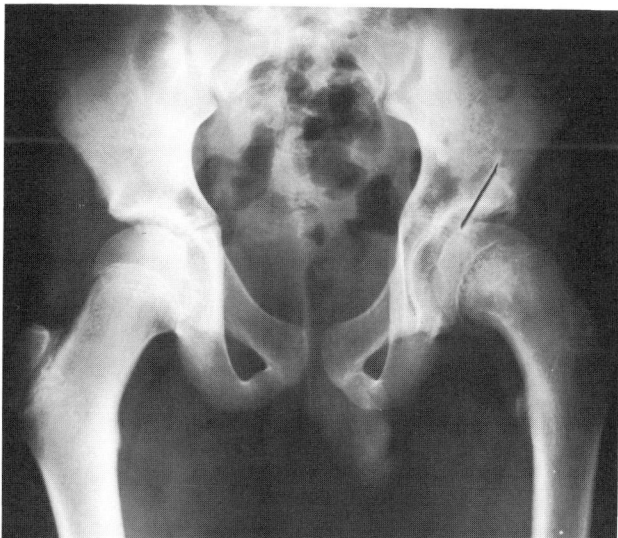

Figure 11. An acute slipped epiphysis may be superimposed on a chronic slipped capital femoral epiphysis in a teenager whose epiphyses are beginning to close. If the displacement is minimal, the capital femoral epiphysis should be fixed *in situ* with multiple pins. Manipulation may cause avascular necrosis.

teries and must be prevented by anatomic reduction and internal fixation. Multiple pins are easier to insert with power tools, because the neck of the femur in a growing child is very resistant. Nails should not be used, because they are likely to distract the fracture and destroy endosteal blood vessels. Immobilization of a neck fracture by plaster in a child is nearly impossible, and nonunion frequently results.

Intertrochanteric and subtrochanteric fractures in children are best managed with traction and plaster. In fractures below the lesser trochanter, the gluteus medius abducts the proximal fragment, and it is flexed by the iliopsoas muscle. In younger children the fracture may be reduced shortly after injury and the child immobilized in a body cast with the hip flexed and abducted, placing the distal fragment in line with the proximal one. The thick periosteum in younger children prevents marked displacement, and solid union occurs in 4 to 6 weeks. Bryant's traction is seldom necessary and requires constant nursing care. The combination of elevation of the extremity, extension of the knee producing tension in the popliteal artery, and compression of the calf by skin traction may cause gangrene of the extremity.

In the older child, subtrochanteric fractures are easily managed by 90-90 traction with a femoral pin which is maintained for 10 to 14 days for stability to occur, followed by plaster immobilization for 10 to 12 weeks.

Avulsion fractures of the lesser trochanter and less commonly the greater trochanter occur primarily in athletes. Open reduction is seldom necessary despite considerable displacement. Bed rest with simple Buck's extension or Russell's traction allows pain and muscle spasm to subside in 10 to 12 days, following which the patient can be mobilized comfortably on crutches.

FRACTURES OF THE FEMUR

Fractures of the femur can be divided into four areas: subtrochanteric, midshaft or diaphyseal, supracondylar, and condylar. Each level must be managed differently because the deforming forces acting on the fragments tend to produce different deformities and require different methods of fixation. Fractures in any of these areas may be either closed or open. Most open femoral fractures not due to gunshot wounds are compounded from within, when the femoral shaft penetrates the subcutaneous tissue and skin; as the deformity is corrected, the bone ends sink within the thigh, contaminating the deeper tissues. These sometimes small and benign-appearing wounds should be opened widely, and all traumatized tissue should be débrided thoroughly, irrigated copiously, and left open for secondary closure. Nothing is gained by débriding a compound wound and closing it. Necrotic tissue and hematoma provide an ideal culture medium for gas gangrene.

The patient with a fractured femur has undergone severe trauma and must be evaluated carefully. Loss of 2 to 3 units of blood within the thigh may not be apparent, and shock may ensue without warning. The hip and knee joints must be observed radiographically for detection of an associated hip dislocation or supracondylar fracture, if present. In fractures of the lower third of the femur, nerves and vessels lie close to the bone and can be damaged either by the initial injury or by faulty management.

In a younger child, reduction can often be obtained in the emergency room with the child under sedation and a 1½ body spica applied. The fracture of the femur in the younger child frequently heals within 8 to 12 weeks, but radiographs should be obtained weekly for certainty that displacement has not occurred.

Treatment of femoral fracture by means of traction followed by a cast brace was first recorded by Smith and was later popularized by Mooney. In this method the fracture of the shaft of the femur is maintained in balanced traction for approximately 10 days. At that time a lightly padded cast brace is applied over an elastic stump sock of Spandex. Total contact must be obtained; then a quadrilateral socket is molded to fit the proximal thigh. Polycentric hinges are applied to the knee, which is later windowed to allow knee motion. The fracture is stabilized by the hydrodynamic effect of the compressed thigh muscle. Early knee motion preserves function. Mooney found that in a review of 150 fractures all healed within 3½ months and knee motion was 80 per cent of normal on removal.

Other reports have documented considerable shortening following the cast brace treatment of fractures of the femoral shaft. Also in the adult several weeks of traction are frequently necessary before the cast brace can be applied. The technique is still useful for undisplaced supracondylar fractures of the femur in elderly patients, but generally the cast brace has been replaced by the use of the interlocking femoral nail in the treatment of fractures of the femoral shaft in adults (see Fig. 12).

Open Reduction of Femoral Shaft Fractures

The treatment of fractures of the shaft of the femur by skeletal traction and subsequent cast immobilization requires many weeks of hospital treatment; and the complications of acute respiratory distress syndrome, fat embolism, pulmonary embolism, and pneumonia can be decreased by early stabilization and rapid mobilization of the patient. This is best done by open reduction of shaft fracture and fixation with one of the various types of intramedullary nails. The external fixator with multiple pins above and below the fracture with the fracture stabilized by an outrigger is reserved primarily for compound fractures and for the severely injured patient. The use of the external fixator alone for fixation of femoral shaft fractures causes delayed union, nonunion, and poor restoration of knee motion. The external fixator should be used for compound fractures only until soft tissue healing occurs, and then open reduction and fixation with an intramedullary nail should be considered.

Compression plates can be used for fractures of the femur when other injuries are present either in the proximal aspect of the femur or in the supracondylar area, requiring other types of fixation. The disadvantage of the compression plate is that much subperiosteal stripping is necessary, and the plate must be long enough to engage eight cortices. As resorption occurs at the fracture site, the compression plate remains fixed and does not allow impaction of the fracture. Infection rates are much higher than with intramedullary fixation, plate failure is frequent, and stress fractures occasionally occur below the plate. In a patient with an ipsilateral fracture of the neck of the femur and shaft of the femur and a nail plate, a Richards apparatus with a long side plate may be used to fix the fracture of the proximal femur and the shaft of the femur.

The use of the Küntscher nail described in 1940 is useful in the patient with a transverse fracture in the proximal third to the middle third of the femur. Dissection is minimal, the union rate is high, and the infection rate is low. However, complications include malrotation, shortening, angulation of the rod, and fracture of the rod. For the comminuted fracture in the midshaft, additional cerclage wiring may be necessary.

Most fractures below the level of the lesser trochanter and above the level of the supracondylar area can be treated with the reamed interlocking nails. With this apparatus the femur is overreamed 1 to 2 mm. to allow for the anterior bow in the femur. A small incision is made over the greater trochanter and extended to the piriform sinus. A guide pin is inserted, and the fracture is reduced over the guide pin. A nail measured to the length of the opposite femur is inserted over the guide pin. One or two fixation screws are then passed from the greater trochanter through the nail into the lesser trochanter for fixation of the proximal fragment. After proper length has been maintained and the fracture reduced by traction, two additional screws are passed through holes in the distal nail, allowing constant internal distraction and maintenance of the length of

the femur. Using the interlocking nail, excellent results have been obtained in approximately 95 per cent of patients. Minimal shortening occurs, union rates are high, and infection rates are very low. The major disadvantage of the reamed interlocking nail is that special equipment is necessary. The procedure must be done on a fracture table, and the image intensifier must be used for insertion of the nail. Also, insertion of the interlocking nail requires special training (Fig. 12).

Preoperative antibiotics are administered and are continued for 48 hours postoperatively. The patient can walk in 48 to 72 hours, and early union of the fracture usually allows partial weight bearing at 6 to 8 weeks. The distraction screws should remain at least 6 months, at which time the distal screws can be removed for impaction of the fracture, if necessary.

SUPRACONDYLAR FEMORAL FRACTURES

Supracondylar femoral fractures may follow automobile dashboard injuries, a short fall from a standing position, or a free fall from a height. The more comminuted fractures are usually the result of a free fall or bumper injury. Contraction of the gastrocnemius pulls the distal fragment posteriorly (Fig. 13), but uncontrolled flexion does not occur unless there is overriding of the fragments. Treatment of this fracture with traction in 90 degrees of flexion produces varus angulation of the distal fragment and allows the shaft to shift forward. The most common residual deformity is that of varus and internal rotation of the distal fragment. This alignment occurs as the distal fragment

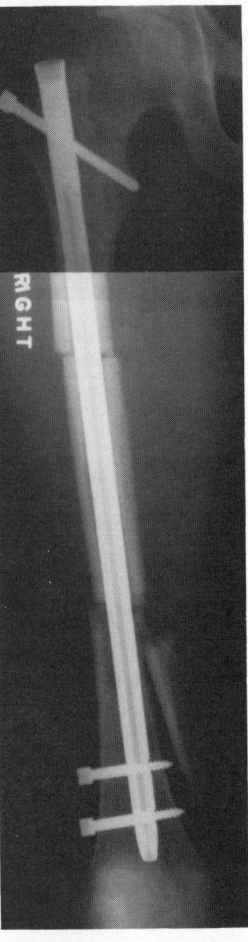

Figure 12. This composite radiograph of the femur demonstrates fixation of a segmental comminuted fracture of the femur with an interlocking nail. The proximal screw passes through the nail; and after the fracture is reduced with traction, the two additional interlocking screws are placed through holes in the distal portion of the nail to maintain continuous traction. Most fractures of the femur between the lesser trochanter and the adductor tubercle can be treated with this apparatus.

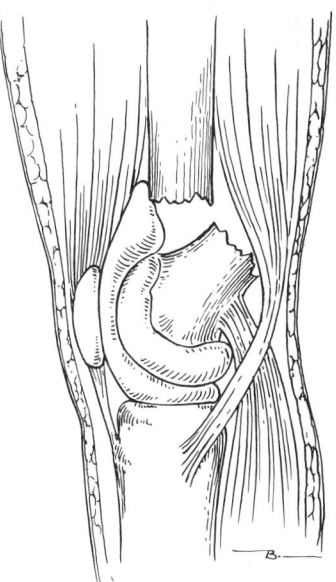

Figure 13. In the supracondylar fracture, the distal fragment of the femur is pulled posteriorly by the gastrocnemius. Complete displacement occurs when there is overriding of the fragments. Internal fixation is mandatory to restore early motion of the knee and healing of the fracture.

is held in neutral by traction applied through a pin in the tibia, and the proximal fragment externally rotates and angulates medially, producing a varus deformity. The fracture is best treated by open reduction, which allows early mobilization of the knee.

Supracondylar fractures frequently extend into the knee joint. Anatomic reduction and early mobilization are imperative for the avoidance of deformity and the preservation of motion. Functional bracing is not suitable for those fractures that extend into the joint. Appliances that are inserted in the femoral condyle, such as the Rush rod and the Enders rod, do not provide good stability and do not assure anatomic reduction of the intraarticular components of the fracture. In the unicondylar or intercondylar fracture, lag screws can be inserted between the condyles with the use of a guide wire. The best fixation device available at present is the AO condylar buttress plate, which is easier to apply than a nail plate. However, fixation is not absolutely rigid and the fracture must be protected postoperatively (Fig. 14).

FRACTURES OF THE PATELLA

The patella is vulnerable to injury, lying in its subcutaneous position on the hard surface of the femoral condyles. Fractures occur by direct injury to the knee from a direct blow or indirectly by contraction of the massive quadriceps muscle. Both mechanisms can occur simultaneously as the patient attempts to avoid falling by extending the knee; the patella separates, the knee collapses, and the patella strikes the ground.

Fractures due to direct injury are most often stellate, comminuted, and frequently compound. Displacement is usually minimal. Indirect fractures may occur in the upper, middle, or lower third and may be widely separated, indicating extensive tearing of the retinaculum. If the extensor retinaculum is torn, active extension of the knee is not possible and open reduction is mandatory.

Fractures of the patella are relatively easy to diagnose because of the subcutaneous position of the fragments. Effusion is usually marked, and ecchymosis is extensive. Extension may be limited by a tense effusion. If fragments are undisplaced, aspiration of hematoma and immobilization in a padded cylinder cast is sufficient treatment, and motion can be initiated at 3 to 4 weeks.

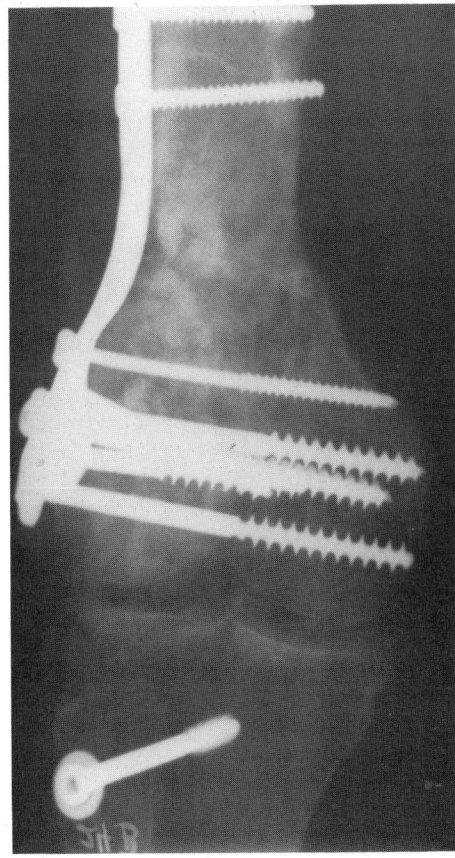

Figure 14. This comminuted supracondylar fracture in a young individual was treated with a condylar buttress plate, which is fixed to the shaft of the femur above and fixed to the condyles of the femur below with multiple screws. The screw in the tibia holds the tibial tubercle in place after it is removed to afford better exposure of the fracture. Early motion was begun and the fracture healed rapidly.

If the fracture fragments are separated and are approximately equal, open reduction and repair of the retinaculum are necessary. If the two fragments are approximately equal in size, the fragments are reduced and held in place by two longitudinal Kirschner wires and then a tension band is placed around the wires to maintain the reduction. It is frequently necessary to remove the tension band after the fracture is healed because of pain. Circumferential wiring is more difficult and accurate reduction is less certain than this method (Fig. 15).

In comminuted or stellate fracture with displacement, total patellectomy and repair of the retinaculum produce an excellent result without the almost certain complication of chondromalacia. Immobilization must be maintained for 4 weeks and forceful extension limited for another 4.

In fractures where the superior or inferior fragment constitutes less than one third of the patella, the smaller fragment should be excised and the remaining quadriceps or patellar tendon repaired with interrupted figure-eight nonabsorbable sutures. The knee is then immobilized in extension for 4 weeks in a cylinder cast. During this time full weight bearing is allowed. Activity is limited for another 4 weeks.

Fractures of the patella must be differentiated from a bipartite patella. When suspected, radiographs of the opposite knee may reveal the same condition. The fragments are surrounded by cortical bone with rounded margins, as compared with the jagged, sharp margins in a peripheral fracture.

DISLOCATION OF THE KNEE

Dislocations of the knee follow violent trauma, most commonly motorcycle accidents, bumper injuries, athletic injuries,

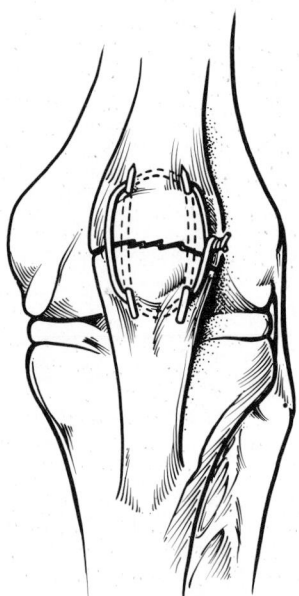

Figure 15. A preferred method of treating a transverse fracture of the patella is with the tension band technique. The fracture is reduced, two vertical Kirschner wires are placed across the fracture, and a circumferential wire is placed around the Kirschner wires and tightened to reduce the fracture completely. Early motion can begin 3 weeks after soft tissue healing has occurred.

or a fall from a height. The cruciate ligaments must be torn as well as the joint capsule. Displacement of the tibia may be anterior, posterior, lateral, or medial; but anterior dislocation is most common. Although partial disruption of major ligaments must be present for dislocation to occur, most dislocations are stable after reduction. Kennedy found both collateral ligaments to be intact at the time of delayed repair in six knees.

Most knee dislocations are easily reducible, and alignment may be normal by the time the patient arrives in the emergency room. Absence of deformity may be misleading, because severe vascular or nerve damage may be present. If the knee is still dislocated at the time of first examination, the deformity should be corrected as soon as possible by gentle longitudinal traction. The only knee deformity that does not reduce easily is the posterolateral dislocation. This injury can be recognized by the presence of a dimple over the medial joint line below the very prominent medial femoral condyle, which frequently projects through a buttonhole deformity in the medial capsule. The dimple is produced by invagination of the medial ligament into the joint. Open reduction must be done through a medial incision; the rent in the capsule is enlarged and alignment restored by gentle traction.

Most dislocations of the knee are stable after treatment with cast immobilization for 6 weeks. The greatest cause of morbidity from this injury is nerve and vascular damage. Goldner and Ford found peroneal palsy in half of their patients, and Shields found vascular damage in 40 per cent of 26 patients. The popliteal artery and vein are firmly fixed above and below the popliteal space, and hyperextension of the knee or anterior displacement of the tibia may either tear completely or produce enough intimal damage to cause thrombosis. Peripheral pulses must be assessed carefully on first examination and followed closely for several days. If pulses are diminished or there is any question about the continuity of vessels, immediate exploration of the popliteal space should be done. Arteriography is time-consuming and probably unnecessary, because vascular damage is always within a few inches of the joint line. Replacement by prosthetic artery or vein graft may be necessary.

Anterior or posterior compartment syndrome frequently follows knee dislocations and should be suspected when the patient continues to complain of severe pain in the leg after reduc-

tion. Pulses may be absent, but tissue ischemia can progress even though pulses are palpable. Normal tissue pressure is zero. As tissue pressure rises, tissue perfusion decreases significantly at a level 20 mm. below diastolic pressure. When it equals diastolic pressure, tissue perfusion ceases, although distal pulses may still be present. As it approaches systolic pressure, pulses disappear. When pain is persistent, tissue pressure should be measured by the method of Whitesides.

SELECTED REFERENCES

Boyd, H. B., and Griffin, L. L.: Classification and treatment of trochanteric fractures. Arch. Surg., 58:858, 1949.
This classic article analyzes 300 trochantric fractures and was one of the first to differentiate between stable and unstable trochanteric fractures. The use of an additional side plate to prevent medial migration of the femur was suggested for unstable Type III fractures.

d'Aubigne, R. M.: Management of acetabular fractures in multiple trauma. J. Trauma, 8:333, 1968.
This study analyzes 210 patients with acetabular fractures. The author emphasizes that fractures of the acetabulum are frequently overlooked because of other injuries. A classification based on prognosis of acetabular fractures is presented. Early surgical therapy and open reduction are advocated and have been demonstrated to produce better long-term results.

Dimon, J. H., and Hughston, J. C.: Unstable intertrochanteric fractures of the hip. J. Bone Joint Surg. [AM.], 49:440, 1967.
In an analysis of 302 trochanteric fractures, 140 were found to be unstable, most of them owing to comminution of the medial calcar with a large posterior fragment. A method of reduction by an osteotomy of the greater trochanter and shifting the shaft medially is described in order to prevent the late complications in unstable fractures.

Ford, G. L., and Goldner, J. L.: Dislocation of the knee joint. N.C. Med. J., 20:463, 1959.
This article, although it includes only 10 patients with dislocation of the knee, contains an excellent bibliography. Treatment by closed reduction and immobilization is advocated. The high incidence of circulatory and nerve palsy complications is emphasized.

Healy, W. L., and Booker, A. F.: Distal femoral fractures: comparison of open and closed methods of treatment. Clin. Orthop., 174:166, 1983.
Open reduction produced faster union, better range of motion, and lower incidence of complications.

Kyle, R. F., Gustilo, R. B., and Premer, R. F.: Analysis of six hundred twenty-two intertrochanteric hip fractures. J. Bone Joint Surg. [Am.] 321:216–221, 1979.
The sliding nail or screw was found to be superior to the rigid type, with a 90 per cent success rate.

McEachern, A. G., and Hayes Moore, G. H.: Stable intertrochanteric hip fractures: A misnomer? J. Bone Joint Surg. [Br.] 65:582, 1983.
Both stable and unstable fracture impact after fixation with the sliding nail. Success was greater with sliding than with fixed nails.

Mooney, V., Nickel, V. L., Harvey, J. P., and Snelson, R.: Cast brace treatment for fractures of the distal part of the femur. J. Bone Joint Surg. [Am.], 52:1563, 1970.
The technique described in this article has probably changed the management of fractures of the femur more than any other development in the past century. The techniques of applying the cast brace and of managing the patient are clearly outlined. Healing appears to be more rapid with a cast brace, and physiologic function is better maintained than with either treatment with prolonged traction or open reduction and internal fixation. Mean healing time for all fractured femurs was 14.5 weeks.

Neer, C. S., Grantham, S. A., and Shelton, M.: Supracondylar fracture of the adult femur: A study of 110 cases. J. Bone Joint Surg. [Am.], 49:591, 1967.
This analysis of 110 supracondylar fractures recommends the closed treatment of this injury. The most common deformity following supracondylar fracture is internal rotation and varus deformity, which can be prevented by placing the tibial pin used for traction in a position of external rotation. Prior to this article, most authors recommended that the supracondylar fracture be treated in a position of 90 degrees of flexion, which the author in this series has demonstrated actually aggravates the deformity by shifting the femoral shaft forward.

Balsano, N. A., and Reynolds, F. X.: Pelvic fractures. J. Trauma, 13:1011, 1973.
This comprehensive review of 273 fractures emphasizes the severity of pelvic fractures. The complications are clearly outlined, and their management is well discussed. Open reduction of pelvic fractures with massive bleeding is discouraged. Preferably, bleeding points should be localized by arteriography and hemorrhage controlled by the injection of autogenous blood clot unless major vessels are involved.

Swintowski, M. F., Hansen, S. T. Jr., and Kellon, J.: Ipsilateral fracture of the femoral neck and shaft: A treatment protocol. J. Bone and Joint Surg. [Am.], 66:260, 1984.
This article recommends screws for the neck and a retrograde rod form shaft.

REFERENCES

Fractures of the Pelvis

1. d'Aubigne, R. M.: Management of acetabular fractures in multiple trauma. J. Trauma, *8*:333, 1968.
2. Dunn, W., and Morris, H. D.: Fractures and dislocations of the pelvis. J. Bone Joint Surg. [Am.], *50*:1639, 1968.
3. Kadish, L. J., et al.: Angiographic diagnosis and treatment of bleeding due to pelvic trauma. J. Trauma, *13*:1083, 1973.
4. Malgaigne, J. F.: Treatise on Fractures. Philadelphia, J. B. Lippincott Company, 1859.
5. Miller, W. E.: Massive hemorrhage in fractures of the pelvis. South. Med. J., *56*:933, 1963.
6. Peltier, L. F.: Complications associated with fractures of the pelvis. J. Bone Joint Surg. [Am.], *47*:1069, 1965.
7. Reynolds, B. M., et al.: Pelvic fractures. J. Trauma, *13*:1011, 1973.
8. Schlonsky, J., et al.: Functional disability following avulsion fracture of the ischial epiphysis. J. Bone Joint Surg. [AM.], *54*:641, 1973.
9. Spear, C. V., et al.: Vascular and adjacent soft tissue injuries associated with fractures of the pelvis. South. Med. J., *68*:142, 1975.
10. Trunkey, D. D., et al.: Management of pelvic fractures in blunt trauma injury. J. Trauma, *14*:912, 1974.

Fractures of the Hip

11. Albright, J. P., and Weinstein, S. L.: Treatment for fracture complications. Arch. Surg., *110*:30, 1975.
12. Boyd, H. B., and Griffin, L. L.: Classification and treatment of trochanteric fractures. Arch. Surg., *58*:858, 1959.
13. Carnesale, P. G., and Anderson, L. D.: Primary prosthetic replacement for femoral neck fractures. Arch. Surg., *110*:27, 1975.
14. Coventry, M. B.: The treatment of fracture dislocation of the hip by total hip arthroplasty. J. Bone Joint Surg. [Am.], *56*:1103, 1974.
15. Dimon, J. H., and Hughston, J. C.: Unstable intertrochanteric fractures of the hip. J. Bone Joint Surg. [Br.], *49*:440, 1967.
16. DiStefano, V. J., Nixon, J. E., and Klein, K. S.: Stable fixation of the difficult subtrochanteric fracture. J. Trauma, *12*:1066, 1972.
17. Epstein, H. C.: Posterior fracture dislocation of the hip: Long term follow up. J. Bone Joint Surg. [Am.], *56*:1103, 1974.
18. Evarts, C. M., and Fail, E. J.: Prevention of thromboembolic disease after elective surgery of the hip. J. Bone Joint Surg. [Am.], *53*:1271, 1971.
19. Fielding, J. W.: Subtrochanteric fractures. Clin. Orthop., *92*:86, 1973.
20. Frankel, V. H., Burstein, A. H., Brown, R. H., et al.: Biotelemetry from the upper end of the femur (abstract). J. Bone Joint Surg. [Am.], *53*:1023, 1971.
21. Freeman, M. A., et al.: The role of fatigue in the pathogenesis of senile femoral neck fractures. J. Bone Joint Surg. [Br.], *56*:698, 1974.
22. Leadbetter, G. W.: A treatment for fracture of the neck of the femur. J. Bone Joint Surg. [Am.], *15*:931, 1933.
23. Lunceford, E. M.: Use of the Moore self locking vitallium prosthesis in acute fractures of the femoral neck. J. Bone Joint Surg. [Am.], *47*:832, 1965.
24. Mulholland, R. C., and Gunn, D. R.: Sliding screw fixation of intertrochanteric femoral fractures. J. Trauma, *12*:581, 1972.
25. Pankovich, A. M.: Primary internal fixation of femoral neck fractures. Arch. Surg., *110*:20, 1975.
26. Roberts, A., Rooney, T., Loupe, J., Roberts, F., et al.: A comparison of the functional results of anatomic and medial displacement valgus nailing of intertrochanteric fractures of the femur. J. Trauma, *12*:341, 1972.
27. Sarmiento, A.: The unstable intertrochanteric fracture: Treatment with a valgus osteotomy and I beam nail plate. J. Bone Joint Surg. [Am.], *52*:1309, 1970.
28. Shelton, M. L.: Subtrochanteric fractures of the femur. Arch. Surg., *110*:41, 1975.
29. Smith-Peterson, M. N., Cave, E. F., and Van Gorder, W.: Intracapsular fracture of the neck of the femur. Arch. Surg., *23*:715, 1931.
30. Welch, R. B., et al.: Total hip replacement as a salvage in traumatic lesions about the hip. Surg. Gynecol. Obstet. *140*:780, 1975.
31. Whitman, R.: A new method of treatment for fractures of the neck of the femur. Am. J. Surg., *36*:746, 1902.
32. Zickel, R. E.: A new fixation device for subtrochanteric fractures of the femur. Clin. Orthop., *54*:115, 1957.

Fractures of the Femur

33. Clawson, D. K.: Closed intramedullary nailing of the femur. J. Bone Joint Surg. [AM.], *53*:681, 1974.
34. Fitzpatrick, C. B.: The treatment of fractures of the shaft of the femur by closed intramedullary nailing. J. Bone Joint Surg. [Br.], *57*:255, 1975.
35. Kunscher, G.: Intramedullary surgical technique and its place in orthopedic surgery. J. Bone Joint Surg. [Am.], *47*:809, 1965.
36. Mooney, V., Nickel, V. L., Harvey, J. P., and Snelson, R.: Cast brace treatment for fractures of the distal part of the femur. J. Bone Joint Surg. [Am.], *52*:1563, 1970.
37. Neer, C. S., Granthan, S. A., and Shelton, M.: Supracondylar fracture of the adult femur: A study of 110 cases. J. Bone Joint Surg. [Am.], *49*:591, 1967.
38. Riggins, R. S., Garrick, J. G., and Lipscomb, P. R.: Supracondylar fractures of the femur. A survey of treatment. Clin. Orthop., *82*:32, 1972.
39. Shelton, M. L., Grantham, S. A., Neer, C. S., and Singh, R.: A new fixation device for supracondylar and low femoral shaft fractures. J. Trauma, *14*:821, 1974.
40. Stewart, M. J., Sisk, T. O., and Wallace, S. L.: Fractures of the distal third of the femur. J. Bone Joint Surg. [Am.], *48*:787, 1966.
41. Street, D. M.: One hundred fractures of the femur treated by means of the diamond shaped medullary nail. J. Bone Joint Surg. [Am.], *33*:659, 1951.

Fractures of the Knee

42. Ford, G. L., and Goldner, J. L.: Dislocation of the knee joint. N.C. Med. J., *20*:463, 1959.
43. Griswold, A. S.: Fractures of the patella. Clin. Orthop., *4*:44, 1954.
44. Kennedy, J. C.: Complete dislocation of the knee joint. J. Bone Joint Surg. [Am.], *45*:889, 1963.
45. Reckling, F. W., and Peltier, L. F.: Acute knee dislocations and their complications. J. Trauma, *9*:181, 1969.
46. Shields, L., Mital, M., and Cave, E. F.: Complete dislocation of the knee: Experience at the Massachusetts General Hospital. J. Trauma, *9*:192, 1969.
47. Taylor, A. R., Arden, G. P., and Rainey, M. H.: Traumatic dislocation of the knee: A report of 43 cases with special reference to conservative treatment. J. Bone Joint Surg. [Br.], *54*:96, 1972.
48. Whitesides, T. E., et al.: A simple method for tissue pressure determination. Arch. Surg., *110*:1311, 1975.

VII

FRACTURES OF THE TIBIA, FIBULA, ANKLE, AND FOOT

William E. Garrett, Jr., M.D., Ph.D., and L. Scott Levin, M.D.

FRACTURES OF THE TIBIA AND FIBULA

Historical Aspects

The tibia and fibula are two of the most frequently fractured long bones.[14,24] High-speed motor vehicular trauma causes many injuries producing open or "compound" fractures with soft tissue defects due to high-energy absorption. Treatment of fractures of the tibia and fibula has been the subject of much controversy for more than 2500 years. Hippocrates recognized in his treatise *Fractures*:[12] "Of the bones of the leg, the inner one, called the tibia, is the more troublesome to manage, and requires the greater extension; and if the broken bones are not properly arranged, it is impossible to conceal the distortion, for the bone is exposed and wholly uncovered with flesh; and it is much longer before patients can walk on the leg when this bone is broken [as compared with the isolated fibula fracture]." Three hundred years B.C., Hippocrates wrote about the treatment of open fractures with methods of reduction and stabilization using a device quite similar to the mechanical design of the twentieth-century external fixator introduced by Hoffman and

Vidal in the 1930s for management of the open tibia fracture. Ambroise Paré wrote on the treatment of open fractures, advocating débridement of exposed bone in compound fractures prior to reduction.[11]

Despite sound principles of treatment for lower extremity fractures recognized years ago, above-knee amputation rates for tibia fractures were as high as 62 per cent as reported by Malgaigne in the nineteenth century, 82 per cent during the Crimean War, and 54 per cent during the Civil War. Mortality from such fractures was as high as 76 per cent during the Franco-Prussian War (1870). Internal fixation for fractures was introduced at the turn of the century. The first record of tibial plate fixation was attributed to Hansman (1886). The use of plates for tibial fractures was popularized by Lane in 1894.[32] Lambotte introduced the term *osteosynthesis* to describe primary fracture healing (1907). This began the modern era of fracture care.

Despite introduction of the external fixator by Hippocrates and early success in Europe in the 1930s, the external fixator was condemned by the Surgeon General of the Army, Colonel Cleveland, in 1943, because of the high incidence of pin tract infections, osteomyelitis, and nonunion. Alternative methods of treatment were devised that included the iron nail (Hey Groves) and the more popular Küntscher nail (1940) that established the intramedullary technique of fracture fixation. In 1949 Robert Danis introduced the "coapter" as a method to fix long bone fractures with compressive forces that would serve to enhance stability of fixation. This led to the development of the A.O. group of Swiss surgeons (Association for the Study of Internal Fixation) who consolidated sound mechanical and biologic principles that enable effective treatment of open and closed fractures with internal and/or external fixation.[29] Despite the evolution of modern fracture care of the tibia, surgeons today still debate the best methods for treatment of the tibia.

Anatomy

The tibia is medial and stronger than the fibula. The upper end of the tibia is expanded particularly in the transverse axis to provide a bearing surface for the body weight transmitted through the femur. The upper tibia is divided into a medial and lateral condyle and has an anterior projection, the tibial tubercle, onto which the patellar tendon inserts. The lateral condyle articulates with the fibular head. The shaft of the tibia can be palpated along the medial subcutaneous border of the leg. The lower end of the tibia is slightly expanded and projects downward as the medial malleolus. The fibula can be divided into three regions: the head, the shaft, and the lateral malleolus. The two leg bones are connected by the interosseous ligament, a strong fascial band that supports the leg and serves as an origin for muscles of the anterior and posterior compartments.

Blood to the tibia and fibula is supplied by the popliteal artery, which branches into the anterior tibial, posterior tibial, and peroneal arteries. The posterior tibial nerve accompanies the posterior tibial artery and innervates the posterior compartment containing the gastrocnemius and soleus muscles superficially and the posterior tibial, flexor hallucis, and flexor digitorum longus muscles deeper. The nutrient artery to the tibia is derived from the posterior tibial artery. The anterior tibial nerve innervates the anterior compartment, which includes the anterior tibial, extensor hallucis longus, extensor digitorum longus, and peroneus tertius muscles. The lateral compartment includes the peroneus longus and brevis muscles innervated by the peroneal nerve.

Mechanism of Injury

Tibial fractures can be caused by high- or low-energy injury. Prognosis is determined by the initial energy absorbed, and not necessarily by the location of the fracture. Automobile-pedestrian accidents can impart up to 100,000 foot-pounds of energy to the victim in the bumper injury. These fractures are usually more comminuted than are low-energy injuries due to falls or skiing accidents that tend to produce torsional deformity and oblique fracture patterns. Gunshot or shotgun injuries often produce soft tissue defects dependent on muzzle velocity and range. Pathologic fractures due to tumor may occur in any region. Stress fractures, as a result of chronic cyclic loading of long bones that do not receive sufficient muscle support, particularly in athletes, can evade diagnosis, with radiographic findings not revealed until late in the course of the fracture. Fibular fractures are usually observed with tibial fractures if sufficient energy is imparted. The fibula may be fractured by direct blow, or the head may fracture with an isolated medial malleolar fracture ("Maisonneuve's fracture").

Classification of Fractures

Fractures of the tibia and fibula can be classified by anatomic region, whether they are open or closed, and by the fracture pattern or displacement. Tibial plateau fractures are commonly divided into six types according to Schatzker[38] (Fig. 1.) Type I is a wedge fracture of the lateral tibial plateau, usually occurring in young people. Type II is a wedge fracture combined with depression of the adjacent weight-bearing surface. Type III is a central lateral plateau depression fracture without a wedge fracture. Type IV is a medial tibial plateau fracture. Type V is a bicondylar fracture that consists of a wedge fracture of the medial and lateral plateau. Type VI fractures are the most complex fractures in that the metaphysis separates from the diaphysis of the tibia. An operative approach to Type V and VI fractures is generally required (Fig. 2). Tibial shaft fractures usually are classified into thirds with delays in healing observed commonly in the middle third and the region between the proximal and middle thirds. Open tibial fractures commonly involve the shaft. Gustilo and Anderson have classified open fractures into three categories that have significance regarding the incidence of fracture union and risk for infection and/or amputation. Grade I fractures are those that have perforation of the skin from the inside; wounds are less than or equal to 1 cm. Grade II open fractures are produced by outside to inside forces, with soft tissue injury being greater than 1 cm. Grade III injuries involve significant soft tissue damage. These are further classified as Grade IIIa, soft tissue injury without periosteal stripping or vessel damage; Grade IIIb, soft tissue damage with periosteal stripping; and Grade IIIc, major vascular injury and soft tissue damage. Difficult fractures involving the lower tibia are tibial plafond fractures occurring in the lower tibia and frequently extending into the ankle joint.

Physical Examination

Examination of patients with tibial and fibular fractures requires knowledge of topographic, vascular, and neural anatomy of the lower extremity. In severely injured legs, simply positioning the leg in proper anatomic alignment may restore absent pulses. All open wounds should be noted and covered with a sterile dressing. *All punctures and lacerations of the integument should be considered open fractures until proven otherwise in the operating room where irrigation and débridement of all open wounds is mandatory.*

Capillary refill, toe pulp turgor, and temperature should be assessed in addition to posterior tibial and dorsalis pedis pulses. If pulses are not palpable because of shock or vasoconstriction, a Doppler examination should be performed. Vascular injuries occur commonly above the trifurcation of the popliteal artery, and vascular injury should be suspected if fractures occur in this area.[23] If capillary refill is slow, or vessel damage is suspected, arteriography should be considered, particularly in cases of fracture-dislocation of the knee joint.

Palpation along the tibial crest may reveal a step-off or swelling that may represent a minimally displaced fracture. Exami-

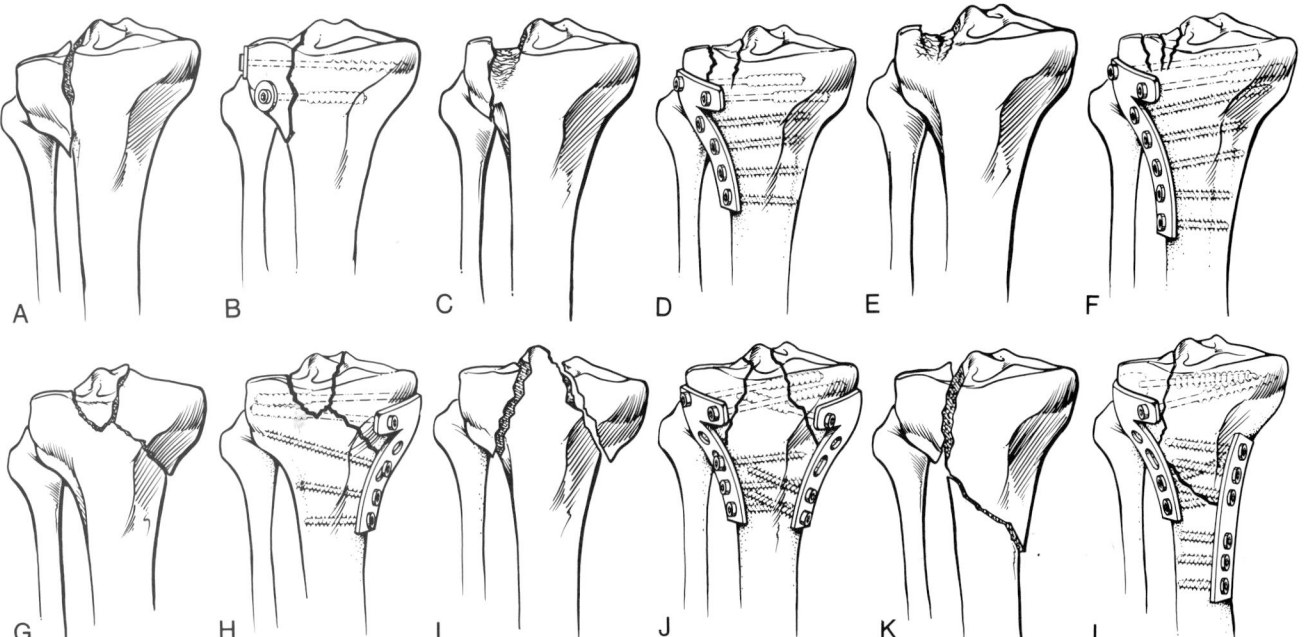

Figure 1. A and B, Type I tibial plateau fracture. C and D, Type II tibial plateau fracture. E and F, Type III tibial plateau fracture. G and H, Type IV tibial plateau fracture. I and J, Type V tibial plateau fracture. K and L, Type VI tibial plateau fracture. (From Schatzker, J., and Tile, M. (Eds.): The Rationale of Operative Fracture Care. New York, Springer-Verlag, 1985.)

nation of the ankle and knee joints when possible should be performed to exclude any associated ligamentous injury, such as in lateral tibial plateau fractures that often produce injury to the medial collateral ligament. Notice should be taken of any excessive varus or valgus angulation of the knee, which may suggest tibial plateau fracture.

A thorough sensory examination is required when one is evaluating tibial and fibular fractures. Proximal fibula fractures may cause peroneal nerve injury, with associated sensory and motor deficits. Anterior tibial nerve and deep peroneal nerve dysfunction may indicate the compartment syndrome, and, similarly, diminished sensibility to light touch on the plantar aspect of the foot suggests posterior tibial nerve compression.

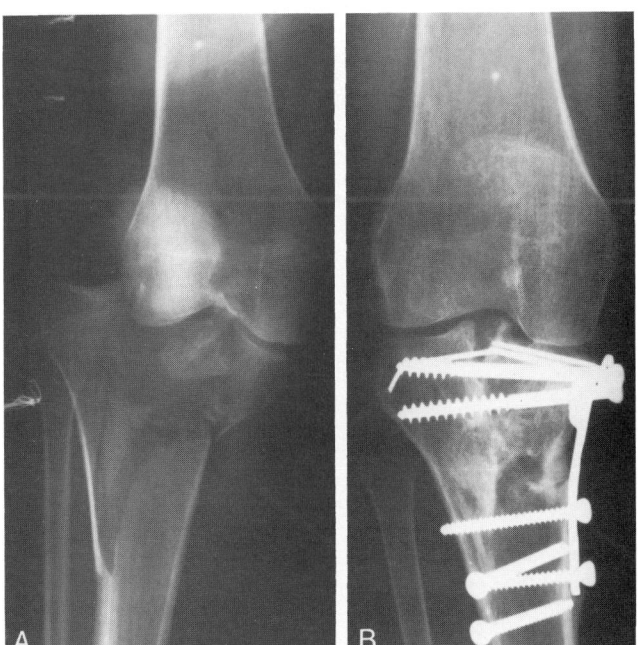

Figure 2. A and B, Type VI tibial plateau fracture. This patient was treated with open reduction and internal fixation using buttress plate and screws.

The compartment syndrome is defined as an increase in tissue pressure in the closed fascial compartments of the leg. It can occur in open or closed tibial fractures.[15,17,27] If intracompartment pressure exceeds capillary pressure, diminished tissue perfusion may cause anoxia and necrosis of tissue within the compartment. Signs include pain on passive stretching of muscles in the compartment, swollen compartments, diminished sensation, and motor weakness. A variety of methods may be used in measuring compartment pressure. Fasciotomy should be performed if clinical suspicion is high and pressures are elevated with respect to arterial pressure.

Radiographic Evaluation

Fractures involving the tibia and fibula should be visualized radiographically in the anteroposterior and lateral planes. It is imperative that the knee and ankle joint be visualized to avoid missing fractures that extend intra-articularly. Particularly in high-energy injuries, films of the ipsilateral femur and pelvis should be obtained to exclude the floating knee or pelvis injury. Forty-five–degree oblique radiographs may help in evaluating the tibial plateau. Tomography is helpful in fractures of the tibial plateau and plafond to define the extent of joint compression. Computed tomography with three-dimensional reconstruction has proved useful in planning open reduction and internal fixation of complex fractures.

Treatment

The principles of fracture care are classic, that is, reduction of the fracture, stabilization of the limb to allow fracture healing, and proper care of the soft tissue envelope.[28] The actual application of these tenets has changed several times in the last 50 years. Understanding the mechanism of injury and the deformities of length, angulation, rotation, and displacement (L.A.R.D.) enables the surgeon to obtain an acceptable reduction.

Treatment depends on the location of the fracture, whether it is open or closed, and the amount of displacement. This holds true for all fractures of the tibia and fibula.

Nondisplaced fractures of the tibia are traditionally treated with casting.[30] Long leg casts are used initially to control forces above the knee joint. When fractures become consolidated with early callus to ensure that they maintain their position, short leg casts are then used until the mechanical strength of the callus can support the patient. Disadvantages of cast treatment include the possibility of creating fracture disease; the term *fracture disease* refers to disuse osteoporosis, muscle wasting, joint stiffness, and posttraumatic dystrophy. Below-knee casts have been advocated by Sarmiento. The soft tissues act as hydrostatic supports for the bone in a total-contact patellar tendon–bearing cast.[37] Weight-bearing gradually increases as the fracture stabilizes.

The external fixator was employed infrequently during World War II. However, with improvement in materials, pins, and a better understanding of frame mechanics, it has been utilized for the majority of open tibial fractures where gross contamination or severe soft tissue injury precludes the judicious use of internal fixation.[4]

Fracture treatment is dependent on the anatomic location of the fracture, whether it is intra- or extra-articular, whether it is open or closed, and whether it is amenable to nonoperative or operative management that requires internal fixation, external fixation, or a combination of both.

Plating is indicated for the treatment of tibial fractures in specific instances such as preceding vascular repair or in fractures of the tibial plafond (Fig. 3).[9,26,34,35] It is a technically demanding procedure owing to the risk of soft tissue compromise and impairment of vascularity to underlying bone.[2] Plates are also used as buttress devices when open reduction with internal fixation is performed for tibial plateau fractures, when the articular surface is elevated, and when medial or lateral support is required.

Segmental fractures have been fixed with interfragmentary compression of large butterfly fragments, followed by the application of the plate as a neutralization device (Fig. 4). Advocates of open reduction believe that fracture disease is avoided and that early motion of joints and muscle units can be accomplished almost immediately with earlier functional return when compared with traction or casting.

Intramedullary devices may be used for stabilization of tibial shaft fractures.[8,25,33,42,44] These are usually reserved for fractures that are difficult to control with closed methods such as casting, or fractures that displace despite casting. They can be inserted with or without the locking screws that transfix the nail above and below the fracture to prevent shortening and to resist torque (Fig. 5). These devices (Fig. 6)[22] traditionally have required reaming of the medullary canal. There are more flexible intramedullary devices that can be inserted without reaming and stacked in the canal to provide internal splinting of the fracture. They are less stable devices than plates or reamed nails; however, their advantage is that the intramedullary blood supply is not disturbed as in conventional reaming. Currently, locked nonreamed nails that provide good stability without

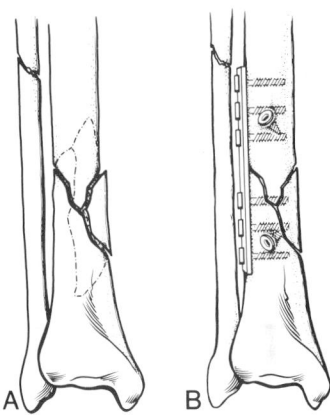

Figure 4. *A* and *B*, Schematic drawing of a tibial shaft fracture treated with open reduction and internal fixation using interfragmentary screw compression and a neutralization plate. (From Schatzker, J., and Tile, M., (Eds.): The Rationale of Operative Fracture Care. New York, Springer-Verlag, 1985.)

reaming are available but with slightly less bending resistance when compared with conventional Küntscher type devices. Most nailing is performed without opening the fracture, thereby reducing the risk of infection and vascular compromise to the fracture site.

The external fixator is commonly used to stabilize tibial shaft fractures. Whereas there is controversy surrounding its use, it does afford excellent access to soft tissue injuries that often accompany fractures of the tibial shaft. Its main purpose is to provide stability to the skeleton that allows the soft tissue to heal.[4,5] After the soft tissue envelope is restored, definitive treatment of the fracture can be undertaken. Often fractures involve bone loss that may require bone grafting, either vascu-

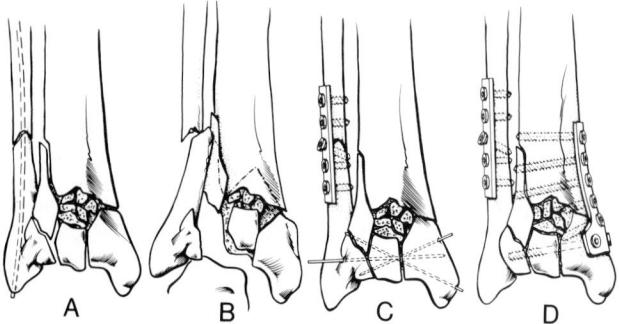

Figure 3. *A*, Schematic drawing of a fracture of the distal tibia at the ankle joint, also termed a pilon fracture. *B*, Temporary fibula fixation regaining length of the tibia-fibula complex. *C*, Rigid fixation of the fibula with temporary Kirschner wire fixation of the tibial plafond. *D*, Rigid fixation of the tibia using a buttress plate supplemented with bone grafting with restoration of the articular surface. (From Schatzker, J., and Tile, M., (Eds.): The Rationale of Operative Fracture Care. New York, Springer-Verlag, 1985.)

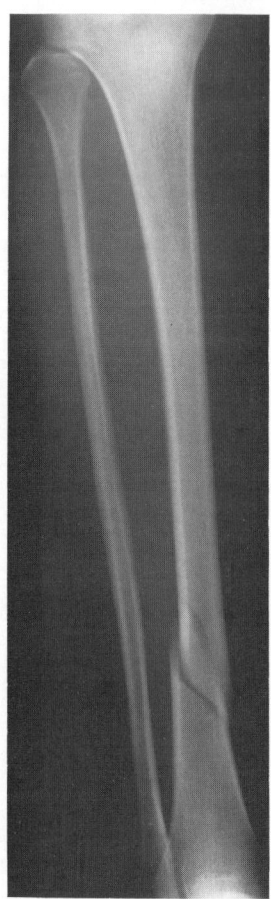

Figure 5. A closed oblique tibial fracture. Adequate closed reduction could not be maintained. The patient was treated with an intramedullary nail.

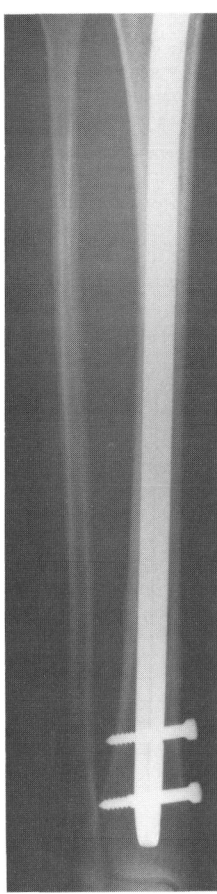

Figure 6. The fracture demonstrated in Figure 5 following closed reduction and intramedullary nailing. The screws shown in the distal tibia prevent shortening and rotational deformities.

larized (such as a free vascularized fibula) or nonvascularized (autogenous iliac crest).[41,46] The external fixator can be used as the definitive fracture treatment if there is evidence of callus formation and bone healing. When healing is not apparent, it should be removed and alternative methods of fracture fixation employed such as casting, use of a cast brace, or internal fixation. Conversion of open fractures treated initially with external fixation to internal fixation (plates or intramedullary nails) has a high risk of infection and should be reserved for select cases.

OPEN FRACTURES OF THE TIBIA AND FIBULA

These are usually high-energy injuries. The main treatment goal is to prevent acute and chronic infection. Management requires aggressive and thorough débridement of all nonvitalized tissue in the operating room with provisional or definitive fracture stabilization, depending on the nature of the fracture. *All* wounds are left open. Staged soft tissue reconstruction is then performed, which may include delayed wound closure, bone and skin grafting, local muscle flaps, or distant free tissue transfer for large defects.[6,16] Composite tissue transfer using techniques of microsurgery is highly effective in the treatment of these injuries. Entire muscles can be transferred for coverage and function. Bone with skin can be transplanted that provides structural stability as well as coverage.

Principles for coverage of open tibial shaft fractures suggest that the gastrocnemius muscle be used as a rotational flap for proximal-third soft tissue defects, the soleus for middle-third defects, and microsurgical free tissue transfer for distal-third soft tissue defects.[45] Godina was an advocate of early coverage of open extremity injuries. He treated 134 patients with free

tissue transfer within 72 hours of injury and had a 1.5 per cent infection rate.

Complications

Complications include delayed union and nonunion.[1] Nonunion usually is defined as a fracture that does not demonstrate healing by 6 months. However, this is a somewhat arbitrary definition, in that the condition of the soft tissue, comminution, and blood supply to bone all have a bearing on healing. Nonunions can be treated by a variety of bone grafting procedures, by increase in fracture stabilization, or by electrical stimulation, which remains controversial.[3] Bone augmentation includes corticocancellous grafts; free fibular microvascular transfers; fibular transpositions; deep circumflex iliac artery osteocutaneous composite transfers; bone substitutes such as calcium phosphate, allograft, or hydroxyapatite; and the Ilizarov method that transports bone segments by callus distraction.[6,18,31]

Infection is perhaps the most severe complication of tibial fractures and usually follows open injuries.[10,46] "Every man who develops separation has the right to ask his surgeon to justify it" (Alexis Carrel).[40] Current trends in aggressive management of soft tissue with early coverage of exposed implants and bone have reduced the incidence of infection-related morbidity and chronic osteomyelitis. One of the most unfavorable complications following open fracture of the tibia is the infected nonunion.[39] Treatment goals in this situation require first achieving union followed by eradication of the infection if possible.

Malunion is defined as a fracture that heals in a significantly nonanatomic position. In fractures of the tibial shaft, up to 5 degrees of varus or valgus deformity in the anteroposterior and lateral plane is acceptable. Internal rotation and external rotation of 5 degrees and 20 degrees are accepted. Shortening of 8 mm. or less is functionally insignificant. Other complications include venous stasis disease, traumatic arthritis, claw toes due to unrecognized posterior compartment syndrome, refracture, and amputation. The role of the arteriogram is to define injury, to detect any abnormal anatomy or pathologic conditions, and to help determine the possibility of repair of vessels.

Indications for primary amputation of mangled limbs are now evolving owing to the grave socioeconomic and personal consequences of limb salvage that often requires several years with results not equaling the gait and function of a conventional below-knee prosthesis.[7]

Primary amputation is still a treatment option for some open tibial fractures, and guidelines are now being set for indications for immediate amputation that include disruption of the posterior tibial nerve, more than 6 hours of warm ischemia, and segmental bone defects greater than 20 cm.[19,37]

FRACTURES OF THE FIBULA

Fractures of the fibula usually accompany fractures of the tibia and are usually not associated with the morbidity of tibial fractures. They heal rapidly. The fibula is important in providing a lateral buttress to the ankle joint and for optimal ankle function and requires accurate anatomic reduction. Proximal fibular fractures are indications that the medial malleolus may be injured and may involve injury to the peroneal nerve. Isolated fibular fractures produced by external direct blows can be treated with casting for comfort or protected weight-bearing until the fracture heals. Fractures of the fibula around the ankle are discussed in the next section.

FRACTURES AND FRACTURE DISLOCATIONS OF THE ANKLE

The ankle joint derives its stability and function from the precise alignment of osseous and ligamentous structures acting together as a functional unit. The distal fibula and the medial aspect of the tibia extend beyond the larger articulation of the tibia with the talus. These extensions, or the malleoli, give medial and lateral stability to the ankle joint, allowing flexion and extension of the hindfoot within the mortise. Strong ligamentous structures ensure the stability of the bones. The syndesmotic and tibiofibular ligaments hold the tibia and fibula together while medial and lateral ligaments extend from the respective malleoli to the hindfoot. The lateral malleolus extends farther than the medial malleolus for bone stability, and the medial ligament (or deltoid) provides stronger medial ligamentous stability. These structures have been considered together as a ring, displacement of the hindfoot being possible only when at least two breaks occur in the ring.

Ankle injuries are among the most frequent conditions treated in orthopedic surgery. Fractures may occur owing to several mechanisms of injury. Most frequently fractures involve *external rotation* of the foot in the ankle joint, which is most often due to an internal rotation or twisting of the leg on a foot fixed by weight-bearing. The fibula fractures in an oblique or spiral plane and is often displaced posteriorly. The medial malleolus or, frequently, the deltoid ligament may be injured. When the foot is everted at the time of injury, the fibula fracture is high and the damage to the interosseous ligament is greater than when the foot is inverted. When the mechanism of fracture is an *abduction* force, the medial malleolus fractures transversely or the deltoid tears first. The fibula then fractures low in an oblique plane or proximally following tear of the interosseous ligament. *Adduction forces* fracture the fibula or disrupt the lateral ligaments in combination with an oblique fracture of the medial malleolus without injuring the interosseous ligaments. Finally, *vertical compression* forces may disrupt the articular surface of the tibia and leave the malleoli uninjured. All of the fractures may be associated with an avulsion fracture of the posterior lip of the tibia.

Optimal treatment of ankle fractures should attain several goals. The talus must be located in its normal position in the ankle mortise. Even a slight amount of tilt or displacement can lead to early disabling arthritis. Joint congruity should be restored as with intra-articular fractures in general. If these requisites are not present initially, then reduction should be obtained by closed or open means. Closed reduction requires awareness of the mechanism of injury, since an opposite stress is used to hold the fractures stable. Immobilization should then follow until the bony and ligamentous injuries are healed. This usually requires 6 weeks or longer in an adult. Initially the cast is applied above the flexed knee to control rotational forces.

If the requisites for adequate treatment cannot be obtained by closed manipulation, open reduction and internal fixation techniques are employed. The procedure requires adequate reduction and stabilization of the fibular fracture. Screw fixation or plate and screw fixation is most commonly used. Fixation should be adequate to allow motion in order to prevent the need for casting and prolonged immobilization. The medial malleolus can usually be treated by screw or pin fixation. Oblique fractures of the tibia or fibula can be stabilized by interfragmentary screws. The screws are placed in a manner to allow compression between the fragments. Plates used for ankle fractures are neutralization plates; they hold the fracture stable after reduction, but they do not cause compression at the fracture site.

Ligamentous injuries should be considered and treated appropriately. The interosseous membrane may tear, leaving a diastasis between the distal tibia and fibula. Normal relationships must be re-established and maintained long enough to allow proper healing. Large associated fractures of the posterior lip of the tibia occasionally require fixation if the reduction of the malleoli and ligament stabilization do not achieve appropriate position of the fragment. Treatment following surgical therapy depends on the nature of the injury and the stability obtained. Total or partial immobilization for 4 to 8 weeks is

frequent. An advantage of surgical fixation is the avoidance of prolonged immobilization. This can allow better ankle and subtalar joint motion recovery and a shorter rehabilitation time.

FRACTURES OF THE FOOT

Fractures of the hindfoot are serious injuries that frequently result in significant functional disability. Chip fractures and small avulsion fractures of the talus are relatively common but do not cause substantial problems after the acute period. The most frequent major fracture of the talus is a transverse fracture through the neck of the bone, usually caused by forced hyperextension. Minimally displaced fractures of the talar neck can be treated by immobilization alone. Displaced fractures must be reduced for the best likelihood of a good result (Fig. 7). If closed means are unsuccessful, the fracture should be opened and reduced and held by internal fixation. Pins or longitudinal lag screws are used most often. Long-term results are related to the amount of displacement of the fracture. With displaced fractures or fracture-dislocations, there is a significant risk for avas-

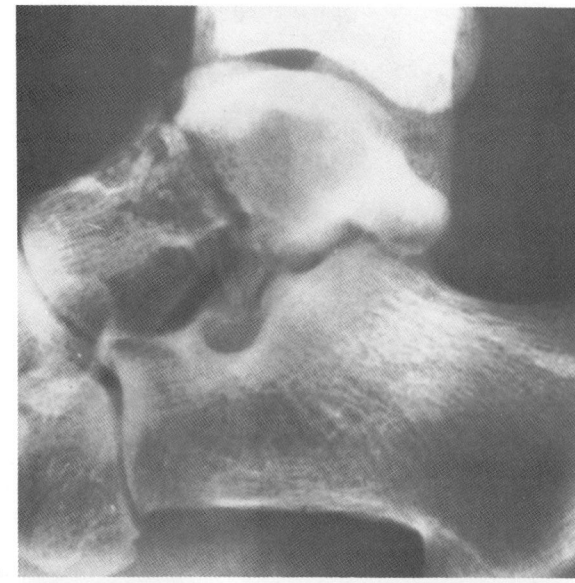

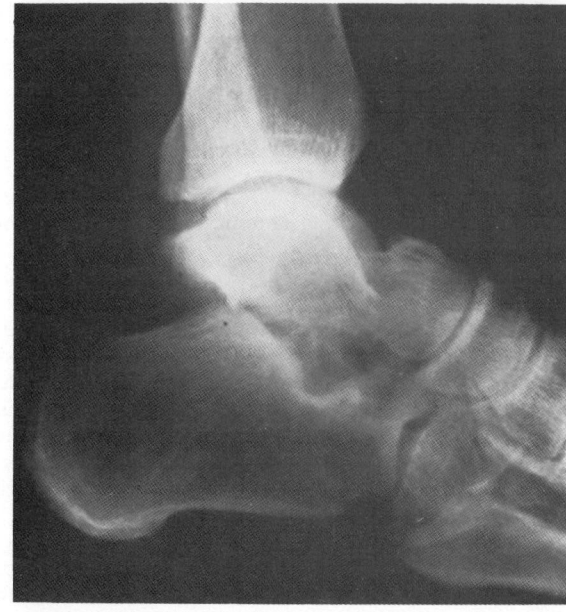

Figure 7. Fracture of the neck of the talus. *A*, Initial fracture line and the displacement. *B*, Satisfactory healing.

cular necrosis of the body of the talus. This may cause a poor result despite adequate stabilization and rehabilitation. The tenuous blood supply to the body may be interrupted by the fracture and cause eventual *collapse* of the body and disruption of the articular surfaces. Posttraumatic arthritis with or without avascular necrosis may ultimately require fusion of the ankle or subtalar joint. Additionally, there may be problems with skin necrosis and infection.

Fractures of the calcaneus can similarly cause persistent problems. Unfortunately, most fractures of the calcaneus involve the joint surface, and these fractures often have a poorer prognosis. Better definition of the fracture can be obtained with oblique radiographs. The mechanism of injury is most often a fall with compressive loading of the heel. The talus acts as a wedge and is driven into the calcaneus. The articular surface of the calcaneus is driven into the underlying cancellous bone, usually with some disruption of the articular cartilage. In addition, the body of the calcaneus is compressed downward and expanded outward, which causes shortening and widening of the bone (Fig. 8). Treatment options are many without consensus regarding the best methods for optimal results. Many accept nonanatomic alignment and begin early motion, avoiding weight-bearing until healing. There are also many who treat these fractures with operative reduction and internal fixation. The aim of operative treatment is to restore the calcaneus to its original height and width and to restore the articular surface to its anatomic position. Operative treatment should be for those with requisite experience and skill.

Fractures of the midfoot include fractures of the navicular, cuneiforms, and cuboid bones. These bones are often fractured as a result of crush injuries; many are quite severe. These severe injuries are often open and can ultimately cause significant disability. Isolated fractures of bones of the midfoot may occur. The navicular bone can be fractured in several ways. Cortical avulsion fractures, tuberosity, and body fractures may occur. In addition, stress fractures of the navicular can occur especially in endurance athletes.

Dislocations of the tarsometatarsal joints are usually the result of direct injury or twisting of the forefoot. This joint is known as Lisfranc's joint. The spectrum of dislocations of Lisfranc's joint ranges from complete dislocation of all five tarsometatarsal joints to the dislocation of one or two metatarsals. Occasionally, a divergent dislocation occurs, with dislocation of the first metatarsal medially and the other metatarsals laterally. Closed reduction of the dislocation is attempted by traction of the forefoot. If closed reduction is not possible, open reduction

and wire fixation may be necessary. Soft tissue damage may be extensive and must be recognized and treated. These injuries frequently cause persistent pain and arthrosis in the foot, necessitating special shoes or inserts.

Fractures of the metatarsals can involve the necks, shafts, or bases, depending on the direction of the force and the mechanism of injury. Fractures of the neck of the metatarsals can be impacted as the result of a direct longitudinal force, or they can be oblique as the result of indirect twisting forces. Anatomic reduction usually is not necessary unless the metatarsal heads are displaced into the plantar surface of the foot where future weight-bearing would be painful. Fractures of the shaft of the metatarsals can be transverse, oblique, or comminuted, depending on whether the trauma is direct or indirect. Fractures of the bases of the metatarsals, even when slightly displaced, usually produce no long-term ill effects and can be treated conservatively with a padded plaster cast. Avulsion of the styloid process at the base of the fifth metatarsal is the result of an inversion force, with avulsion following traction by the peroneus brevis tendon. Fractures of the diaphysis of the fifth metatarsal are considerably more difficult to treat because of their slower healing and potential for nonunion. These fractures may present as stress fractures or as pathologic fractures through a site of stress reaction in the bone. Immobilization and non–weight-bearing or open reduction and internal fixation are required. Stress and fatigue fractures of the metatarsals are common and should be suspected in any patient who presents with pain and puffiness in a foot following unaccustomed excess activity, such as walking or jogging. Such fractures are self-limited and treatment is creating comfort. The second metatarsal is most frequently involved.

Fractures of the phalanges usually do not require reduction unless badly deformed. Longitudinal traction on the toe usually reduces the fracture. The toe can be strapped to an adjacent toe for some degree of comfort. At times a shoe with a firm sole, a cast, or an orthosis may help provide pain relief.

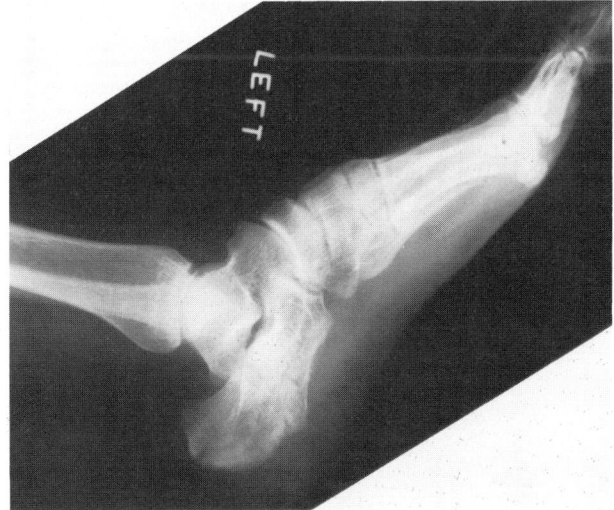

Figure 8. Calcaneus fracture. The fracture initially is depressed and involves the subtalar joint.

SELECTED REFERENCES

Bach, A. W., and Hansen, S. T.: Plate versus external fixation in severe open tibial shaft fractures: A randomized trial. Clin. Orthop. Rel. Res., 241:89, 1989.
Fifty-nine patients with Grade II or Grade III open tibial shaft fractures were randomized into external fixator or plate groups. Osteomyelitis was 19 per cent in the plate group and 3 per cent in the external fixation group.

Bassett, C. A. L., Mitchell, S. N., and Gaston, S. R.: Treatment of ununited tibial diaphyseal fractures with pulsing electromagnetic fields. J. Bone Joint Surg. [Am], 63:511, 1981.
The overall success rate in treating 127 ununited tibial diaphyseal fractures with pulsating electromagnetic fields was 87 per cent. The exact mechanism by which the fractures heal is unknown.

Blick, S. S., Brumback, R. J., Lakatos, R., Poka, A., and Burgess, A. R.: Early prophylactic bone grafting of high energy tibial fractures. Clin. Orthop. Rel. Res., 240:21, 1989.
Fifty-three high-energy tibial fractures were treated with early prophylactic posterolateral bone grafting performed at 10 weeks following injury and 8 weeks following soft tissue coverage. Seventy-nine per cent of the fractures were Grade III open fractures and 40 per cent had bone loss greater than 50 per cent of cortical circumference. Chronic osteomyelitis was 1.9 per cent.

Bone, L. B., and Johnson, K. D.: Treatment of tibial fractures by reaming and intramedullary nailing. J. Bone Joint Surg. [Am], 68:877, 1986.
One hundred twelve fractures were treated by intramedullary nailing. The main complication was infection, treated in six of seven patients successfully.

Bourne, R. B.: Pilon fractures of the distal tibia. Clin. Orthop. Rel. Res., 240:42, 1989.
Pilon fractures are categorized into Ruedi and Allgower Type I, Type II, and Type III. Type I and Type II had 80 per cent satisfactory function. In Type III only 32 per cent had satisfactory function. Seven per cent of tibial fractures are pilon type fractures.

DeLee, J. C., and Stiehl, J. B.: Open tibia fracture with compartment syndrome. Clin. Orthop. Rel. Res., 160:175, 1981.
Among 104 open tibial fractures, compartment syndromes developed in six.

Lange, R. H., Bach, A. W., Hansen, S. T., and Johansen, K. H.: Open tibial fractures with associated vascular injuries. Prognosis for limb salvage. J. Trauma, March:203, 1985.

This resulted in an ultimate amputation rate of 61 per cent (22 per cent primary, 39 per cent delayed).

McAndrew, M. T., and Brick, A. L.: Initial care of massively traumatized lower extremities. Clin. Orthop. Rel. Res., 243:20, 1989.

In a review of Grade IIIb and Grade IIIc injuries, the amputation rate was 35 per cent; 7 of 16, or 48 per cent, were infected. There were 8 infections in 19 patients. Seven of the limbs were salvaged. Eighty-eight per cent returned to their previous or a more vigorous occupation, and 12 of 16 patients became ambulatory within 1 year.

Wist, D. A.: Medullary nailing of acute shaft fractures. Clin. Orthop. Rel. Res., 212:1122, 1986.

One hundred and eleven tibial shaft fractures were treated with flexible intramedullary nailings. Advantages to this are less compromise to the medullary blood supply. There were four deep wound infections. Average healing time was 18.8 weeks, 5.4 per cent had delayed union, and there was 4.5 per cent incidence of angulatory malunion between 6 and 10 degrees.

REFERENCES

1. Bach, A. W., and Hansen, S. T.: Delayed union, nonunion, and malunion of the tibia shaft. *In* Evarts, M. (Ed.): Surgery of the Musculoskeletal System. Vol. 3, Section 8. New York, Churchill Livingstone, 1983, pp. 63–86.
2. Bach, A. W., and Hansen, S. T.: Plate versus external fixation in severe open tibial shaft fractures: A randomized trial. Clin. Orthop. Rel. Res., 241:89, 1989.
3. Bassett, C. A. L., Mitchell, S. N., and Gaston, S. R.: Treatment of ununited tibial diaphyseal fractures with pulsing electromagnetic fields. J. Bone Joint Surg. [Am], 63:511, 1981.
4. Behrens, F.: Unilateral external fixation for severe lower extremity lesions: Experience with the ASIF (AO tubular frame). *In* Feligson, D., and Pope, M. U. (Eds.): Concepts in Internal Fixation. New York, Grune & Stratton, 1982.
5. Behrens, F., Comfort, P. H., Searls, K., Dennis, F., and Young, J. T.: Unilateral external fixation for severe open tibial fractures: Preliminary report of a perspective study. Clin. Orthop. Rel. Res., 178:111, 1983.
6. Blick, S. S., Brumback, R. J., Lakatos, R., Poka, A., and Burgess, A. R.: Early prophylactic bone grafting of high energy tibial fractures. Clin. Orthop. Rel. Res., 240:21, 1989.
7. Bondurant, F. J., Cotler, H. B., Buckle, R., Miller, P., and Browner, B. D.: The medical and economic impact of severely injured lower extremities. J. Trauma, 28:1270, 1988.
8. Bone, L. B., and Johnson, K. D.: Treatment of tibial fractures by reaming and intramedullary nailing. J. Bone Joint Surg., 68A:877, 1986.
9. Bourne, R. B.: Pylon fractures of the distal tibia. Clin. Orthop. Rel. Res., 240:42, 1989.
10. Burgess, A. R., Poka, A., Brumback, R. J., and Bosse, M. J.: Management of open Grade III tibial fractures. Orthop. Clin. North Am., 18:85, 1987.
11. The apologies and treaties of Apologie. *In* Kuynes, G. (Ed.): Treaties of Ambroise Paré. Falcon Educational Books in London, Great Britain, 1951.
12. The Genuine Works of Hippocrates. Birmingham, Gryphon Editions, 1985.
13. Caudle, R. J., and Stern, P. J.: Severe open fractures of the tibia. J. Bone Joint Surg. [Am], 69:801, 1987.
14. Chapman, M.: Fractures of the tibia and fibula shaft. *In* Evarts, M. (Ed.): Surgery of the Musculoskeletal System. Vol. 3, Section 8. New York, Churchill Livingstone, 1983, pp. 5–62.
15. DeLee, J. C., and Stiehl, J. B.: Open tibia fracture with compartment syndrome. Clin. Orthop. Rel. Res., 160:175, 1981.
16. Ger, R.: Muscle transposition for treatment in prevention of chronic post-traumatic osteomyelitis of the tibia. J. Bone Joint Surg. [Am], 59:784, 1977.
17. Gershuni, D. H., Mubarak, S. J., Yaru, N. C., and Lee, Y. F.: Fracture of the tibia complicated by acute compartment syndrome. Clin. Orthop. Rel. Res., 217:221, 1987.
18. Hansen, L. W.: Posterior bone grafting of tibia for nonunion. J. Bone Joint Surg. [Am], 48:27, 1966.
19. Hansen, S. T., Jr.: The Type IIIc tibial fracture salvage or amputation. Editorial. J. Bone Joint Surg. [Am], 69:799, 1987.
20. Hechman, J. D.: Fractures and dislocations of the foot. *In* Rockwood, C. A., Jr., and Green, D. P. (Eds.): Fractures in Adults. Philadelphia, J. B. Lippincott Company, 1984.
21. Hohl, M.: Fractures and dislocations of the knee. *In* Rockwood, C. A., Jr., and Green, D. P. (Eds.): Fractures in Adults. Philadelphia, J. B. Lippincott Company, 1984.
22. Johnson, K. D.: Indications, instrumentation, and experience with locked tibial nails. Orthopaedics, 8:1377, 1985.
23. Lange, R. H., Bach, A. W., Hansen, S. T., and Johansen, K. H.: Open tibial fractures with associated vascular injuries. Prognosis for limb salvage. J. Trauma, March:203, 1985.
24. Leach, R. E.: Fractures of the tibia and fibula. *In* Rockwood, C. A., Jr., and Green, D. P. (Eds.): Fractures in Adults. Philadelphia, J. P. Lippincott Company, 1984.
25. Lerud, S. O., and Karistrom, G.: The spectrum of intramedullary nailing of the tibia. Clin. Orthop. Rel. Res., 212:101, 1986.
26. Mast, J. W., Spiegel, P. G., and Pappas, J. M.: Fractures of the tibial pylon. Clin. Orthop. Rel. Res., 230:68, 1988.
27. Matsen, F. A., III, Winquist, R. A., and Kurgmire, R. B.: Diagnosis and management of compartmental syndromes. J. Bone Joint Surg., 62A:286, 1980.
28. McAndrew, M. T., and Brick, A. L.: Initial care of massively traumatized lower extremities. Clin. Orthop. Rel. Res., 243:20, 1989.
29. Muller, M. E., Allgower, M., and Willenegger, H.: Manual of Internal Fixation. New York, Springer-Verlag, 1979.
30. Oni, O. O., Hui, A., and Gregg, P. J.: The healing of closed tibial shaft fractures: The natural history of union with closed treatment. J. Bone Joint Surg. [Br], 70:787, 1988.
31. Paley, D., Catagni, M. A., Argnanif, V. A., Benedetti, G. B., and Cattaneo, R.: Ilizarov treatment of tibial non unions with bone loss. Clin. Orthop., 241:146, 1989.
32. Rang, M.: Anthology of Orthopaedics. New York, Churchill Livingstone, 1966.
33. Rolando, P. K., Teynor, J., Nagano, J., and Gustilo, R.: Critical analysis of results of treatment of 201 tibial shaft fractures. Clin. Orthop. Rel. Res., 212:113, 1986.
34. Ruedi, T. P., and Allgower, M.: The operative treatment of intra-articular fractures of the lower end of the tibia. Clin. Orthop. Rel. Res., 138:105, 1979.
35. Ruedi, T., Webb, J. K., and Allgower, M.: Experience with a dynamic compression plate (DCP) in 418 recent fractures of the tibia shaft. Injury, 7:252, 1976.
36. Sarmiento, A.: Functional bracing of tibia fractures. Clin. Orthop. Rel. Res., 105:202, 1974.
37. Sarmiento, A., Sobol, P. A., Sew Hoy, A. L., Ross, S. D. K., Sacette, W. L., and Tarr, R. R.: Prefabricated functional braces for the treatment of fractures of the tibial diaphysis. J. Bone Joint Surg. [Am], 66:1328, 1984.
38. Schatzker, J., and McBroom, R. B.: Tibial plateau fracture of the Toronto experience. Clin. Orthop. Rel. Res., 138:94, 1979.
39. Seyfer, A.: Late results of free muscle flaps and delayed bone grafting in the secondary treatment of open distal tibial fractures. Plast. Reconstr. Surg., 83:77, 1989.
40. Shaw, W. (Ed.): Lower extremity reconstruction. (Clinics in Plastic Surgery.) Philadelphia, J. B. Lippincott Company, 1985.
41. Taylor, G. I., and Watson, M.: One stage repair of compound leg defects with free vascularized flaps of groin skin and iliac bone. Plast. Reconstr. Surg., 61:494, 1978.
42. Trafton, P. G.: Closed unstable fractures of the tibia. Clin. Orthop. Rel. Res., 230:58, 1988.
43. Wilson, F. C.: Fractures and dislocations of the ankle. *In* Rockwood, C. A., Jr., and Green, D. P. (Eds.): Fractures in Adults. Philadelphia, J. B. Lippincott Company, 1984.
44. Wist, D. A.: Medullary nailing of acute shaft fractures. Clin. Orthop. Rel. Res., 212:1122, 1986.
45. Wood, M. B., Cooney, W. P., and Irons, G. P.: Lower extremity salvage and reconstruction by free tissue transfer: Analysis of results. Clin. Orthop. Rel. Res., 201:1551, 1985.
46. Yaremchuk, J. M., Brumback, R. J., Manson, P. N., Burgess, A. R., Poka, A., and Weiland, A. J.: Acute and definitive management of traumatic osteocutaneous defects of lower extremity. Plast. Reconstr. Surg., 80:1, 1987.

VIII

AMPUTATIONS AND LIMB SUBSTITUTIONS

Frank W. Clippinger, M.D.

Amputation is one of the oldest surgical procedures known to man, existing before recorded history. Leprosy, ergotism, and punishment are no longer major causes of amputation in the Western world, but trauma, neoplasms, and dysvascular conditions are now so common that there are nearly 2 million amputees in the United States alone.[20,39]

Unlike much ablative surgery, amputation is followed by replacement with a prosthetic device that can restore a reasonable degree of function. However, the surgical loss is visible to all and, therefore, has an emotional component that does not exist in the same manner following gastrectomy, pneumonectomy, colectomy, and other procedures that cause as least as much inconvenience.[16]

For many years, amputation was performed with apology, a sense of failure, and a negative connotation to the patient. Recently there has been increasing media publicity featuring amputees who have "overcome their handicap" and are back in mainstream society or, at least, mainstream endeavors. There are organizations of amputee skiers and amputee golfers. Amputees are seen on the tennis court and running on the track. Whereas modern materials and techniques have made these endeavors easier, the potential for relatively normal existence has been present for many years. Publicity is removing some of the stigma.[33]

The surgeon's responsibility does not end when the wound is healed and the sutures have been removed. The patient must be guided through an emotionally difficult period, and to do so, the surgeon must be knowledgeable about prosthetic rehabilitation.

When timed properly and with consideration of physical restoration, amputation is not a destructive procedure. It is a form of reconstruction that may be elected whenever the outlook is such that a well-fitted prosthesis provides a better result for the patient than can be obtained in a reasonable length of time with further attempts at salvage.

LEVEL SELECTION

The older literature contains advice concerning selection of level or "site of election" for amputation.[22,23] It had been taught that partial foot amputation other than the transmetatarsal level, very long below-knee amputations, knee disarticulations, and elbow disarticulations are not advisable. These limitations were the result of extensive experience with wood and metal prostheses that today are rarely made (Fig. 1).

With total-contact molded plastic sockets, the only critical factor in determining the length of an amputation stump is the viability of skin.[13] Although it is true that supramalleolar, long below-knee, and knee and elbow disarticulations are more difficult for the prosthetist to fit and align, the longer lever arm and the greater surface area offer benefits to the amputee. In addition, good post-amputation reconstruction and better prostheses obviate many of the disadvantages of amputation through the mid- and hindfoot.

The dysvascular patient with actual or impending gangrene always presents a problem in selecting a level. There are no reliable clinical tests to make this determination and it becomes a matter of judgment. Radioactive isotope uptake, infrared pho-

tography, and skin temperature determinations provide information, but they are ordinarily insufficient. At this time, the best objective test is active bleeding of the skin at the time of amputation.[12,17,31,32,38]

The principle of amputating above the knee to be on the safe side if the femoral pulse is absent has not borne the test of time. Twenty-five years ago, the ratio of above-knee to below-knee amputations was 2:1. It is now well below 1:20. Above-knee amputation is done when gangrene is impending to the level of

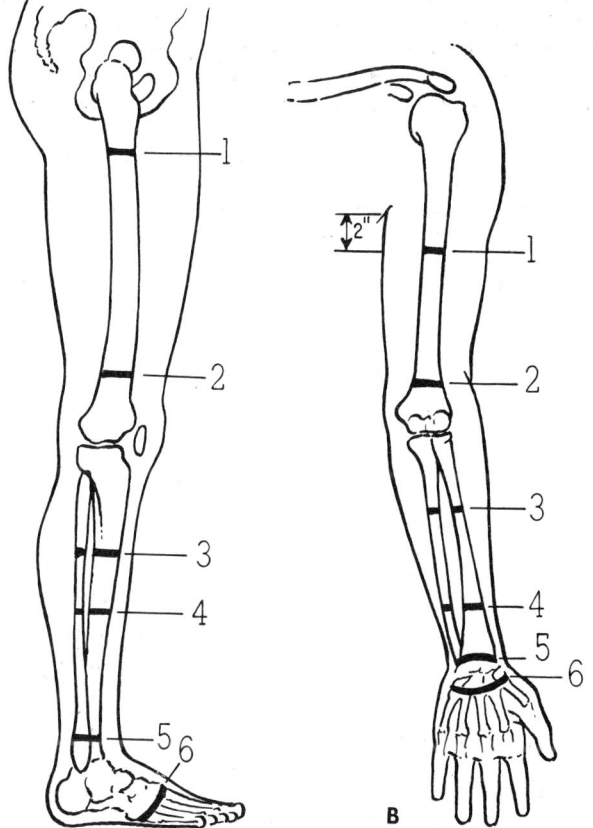

Figure 1. Traditional amputation levels. *A,* in the lower limb, amputation above 1 must be fitted with a hip disarticulation prosthesis because of the short stump. The area between 1 and 2 is fitted with the usual above-knee prosthesis with a quadrilateral socket and either pelvic band or suction suspension. Amputations between 2 and the knee joint do not have sufficient room in the prosthesis for a swing phase control knee mechanism and must be fitted with free-swinging outside joints. 3 and 4 are the conventional "sites of election" for below-knee amputations. Amputations between 4 and 5 are more difficult for the prosthetist but offer some advantage to the amputee. Amputations below 6 require little in the way of a prosthesis; a toe filler and a steel shank in the shoe usually suffice. *B,* Amputations through the upper limb above 1 require a modified socket over the shoulder, and active motion of the shoulder joint is not possible. Between 1 and 2, a conventional above-elbow prosthesis can be fitted. Between 2 and the elbow, an outside elbow joint must be used, but active humeral rotation is possible. Amputations through the forearm above 3 produce a very short forearm lever, and in some instances a geared elbow joint must be used to provide sufficient flexion of the forearm segment. Between 3 and 4, a conventional below-elbow prosthesis is used. Amputations below 4 allow some active pronation and supination. Transcarpal amputation (6) requires a prosthesis, but some hook function is provided by the stump alone.

the knee or in sudden catastrophic occlusion of the distal aorta or common iliac artery and attempted reconstruction failed to establish good blood flow.

It is extremely important to save the knee when possible. The presence of an active knee joint markedly decreases the physical impairment and may, in fact, determine whether an elderly patient can ambulate effectively with a prosthesis.[19,37]

SURGICAL PRINCIPLES

In considering surgical techniques, amputations can be divided into two types: elective procedures, in which there is some freedom in fashioning skin flaps and selecting the level; and urgent procedures for trauma, fulminating infection, and gangrene, in which the viability of muscles and the areas of healthy skin are important factors.

If infection is a distinct possibility, as in wet gangrene, osteomyelitis, or severe trauma, the amputation wound like all others in similar situations should be left open. Formerly, circumferential guillotine amputation was recommended in these patients because it could be performed rather rapidly with relative safety.[14] The guillotine procedure has a distinct disadvantage, however, in that it requires an extensive revision with significant shortening of the bone. An alternative is to fashion flaps in the usual manner but leave the wound open with the intent to perform a delayed primary closure at the appropriate time, usually 3 to 5 days later. If this is done, the flaps should be a little longer than normal because they have a tendency to swell to some extent and shorten. This may be prevented in some instances by one or two large through-and-through stay sutures from front to back preventing retraction of the skin but leaving the wound open sufficiently for proper drainage. A rigid postoperative dressing can be used. Skin traction may be helpful in young amputees, but when there is borderline circulatory status, this may produce a slough.

When infection is not a major hazard, a closed amputation may be planned. Skin flaps of equal length are appropriate for most amputations through the arm, forearm, or thigh. Muscle is tapered from the level of the bone to the end of the flap. A cylindrical stump is desirable if a total-contact socket is to be used in the prosthesis rather than the thin tapering contour thought to be an advantage in the open-end wood socket used in past years.

In the above-knee amputation, sagittal flaps have been advocated by some. The medial flap is made longer to allow preservation of the adductor muscle in an attempt to balance muscle power and prevent an abduction contracture.

It is the below-knee amputation in the dysvascular patient that presents the greatest possibility of failure.[4] If skin flaps of equal lengths are used, the most common site of a slough is the lateral half of the anterior flap. For this reason, in the dysvascular patient, the technique outlined by Burgess, which includes a long posterior flap, has had the highest success rate (Fig. 2).[5–7]

An anterior incision is made perpendicular to the tibia and extends two thirds of the distance posteriorly on the calf both medially and laterally. The posterior flap is cut relatively square and should be 1 to 1½ inches longer than the diameter of the calf at the level of the anterior incision. The anterior and lateral compartment muscles are divided at the level of the anterior incision. The posterior muscles are beveled from the posterior aspect of the tibia to the end of the flap and are not dissected from the subcutaneous tissue. Any questionable muscle can and should be resected. Although quite helpful, muscle is not mandatory for a functional amputation stump. The fibula is divided with a slight lateral bevel at or one half inch proximal to the level of the tibial section. This is longer than has been recommended in the past; but if a total-contact socket is used, the cylindrical shape of the stump that this provides is desirable. The tibia is divided with an anterior bevel. A power, hand, or

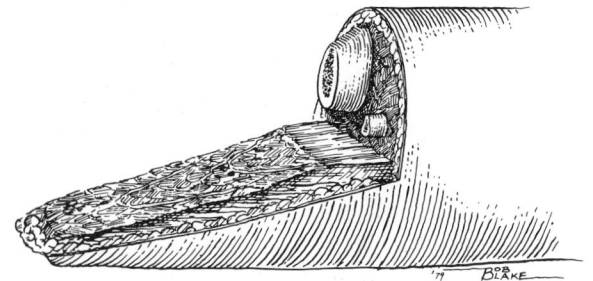

Figure 2. Below-knee amputation. A long posterior flap is used, and the posterior muscles are tapered from the posterior aspect of the bone to the end of the flap. The closure should not be tight, and "dog ears" should not be removed.

Gigli saw can be used, but if the last is selected, great care must be taken to avoid injury to the skin.

In amputations at or about the tibial tubercle, the fibula can be resected. If left in place, the proximal fibula has a tendency to angulate because there may be insufficient interosseous membrane remaining to hold it in position. An angulated fibula makes a bulge that is difficult to fit comfortably in the socket of the prosthesis. If the head of the fibula is removed, the lateral collateral ligament and biceps tendon should be reattached to the tibia and the peroneal nerve should be sectioned above the knee joint to prevent occurrence of a neuroma in a position where it is vulnerable to pressure against the prosthesis.

Some surgeons have advocated the creation of a synostosis between the tibia and fibula at all levels below the knee.[10] This may have some long-term advantages, but it prolongs the rehabilitation phase significantly.

The periosteum is not stripped from the bone proximal to the bone section as was formerly advocated, which can result in ectopic bone formation in some instances.[28] Large blood vessels are separated and doubly ligated for prevention of the possible formation of arteriovenous fistulas. Major nerves are indentified, pulled downward gently, and sharply sectioned, allowing them to retract above the level of the cut muscle. Excessive traction prior to section may cause a neuroma in continuity. A terminal neuroma should be expected, but it should be buried deep in soft tissue where it is not trapped in scar or irritated by the prosthesis. There is no known treatment for a cut nerve end to prevent the formation of a neuroma. A large vas concomitans can be cauterized or ligated; in a dysvascular patient, this is rarely a problem.

When there is no excessive bleeding, the wound may be closed by suturing the posterior deep fascia to the anterior fascia, thus bringing some muscle over the end of the bone, a "myofascial closure." The skin is closed with the desired suture, but the use of monofilament suture materials such as plastic and wire has been advocated because of lesser tendency to produce local tissue reaction. It should remembered, however, that these materials have a tendency to cut through skin in the presence of edema, and in addition, the cut ends of the suture may be uncomfortable to the patient.

The skin margins should be managed with meticulous care, particularly in patients with impaired circulation. The use of toothed thumb forceps should be avoided. There should be little or no tension on the skin. The presence of "dog ears" is not disadvantageous. These ordinarily disappear in several weeks and their removal may irrevocably impair the circulation to the flaps. Most major amputation wounds should be drained. A large hematoma can be catastrophic. Drains can be either Penrose or suction type and should be removed after 24 to 48 hours.

POSTOPERATIVE CARE

Immediate application of a prosthetic device at the time of amputation has been advocated in recent years (Fig. 3).[2,4,5,8] In

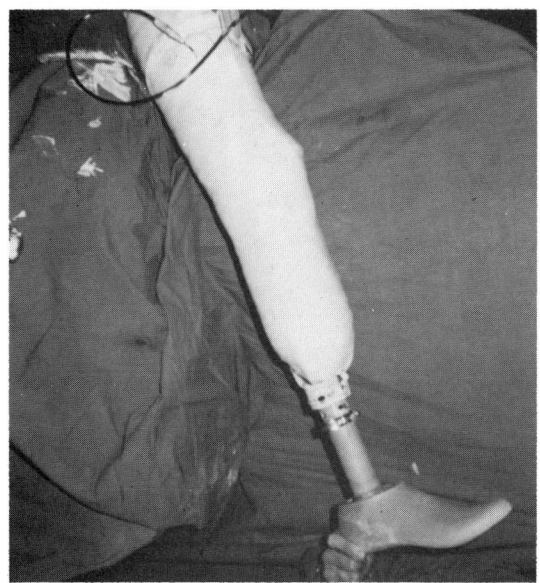

Figure 3. A long below-knee amputation with a rigid dressing and shin-foot unit applied in the operating room. Note the suction drainage tube. This is an excellent postoperative dressing, whether or not the shin-foot unit is used.

selected situations, this technique has some definite benefits to the amputee. This is especially true in amputations through the upper extremity wherein a terminal device and shoulder harness can be applied at the time of the amputation and the patient can immediately begin use of the extremity. This lessens the psychologic impact of the loss of the limb and initiates the rehabilitative phase immediately.

Whether or not a prosthetic device is actually used, the rigid dressing developed as part of this program has some very definite advantages. It has been claimed that healing of the wound is enhanced; however, edema and hematoma are controlled and the tissue is immobilized, decreasing some of the factors that complicate healing. Patients are more comfortable in this dressing and require less analgesic medication and for a shorter time than with the traditional bulky wrap.[5,36]

A rigid dressing is applied as follows. In the upper limb, the wound is covered with a light soft dressing over which is wrapped either sheet cotton or sterile knitted stump sock. Plaster is applied snugly and molded well with even compression.[8] Suspension is important, and the plaster should be well molded around the humeral epicondyles in the below-elbow amputation and should be suspended by a shoulder harness in the above-elbow level. If the dressing slips distally in the first 48 hours after the operation, it is important to replace it immediately because edema may occur very rapidly.

At the below-knee level, the technique developed by Burgess[6] is advised and, in essence, is as follows. A sterile dressing is applied and the distal end of the stump is covered with either two or three fluffed 4 by 4 gauze sponges or a polyurethane foam pad. A sterile knitted stump sock is pulled over the stump, and felt pads are used to enhance pressure on areas that tolerate it and relieve pressure in the areas between the pads such as over the crest of the tibia and the surface of the patella. The use of elastic plaster in the deeper layers of the cast makes it easier to apply even pressure and makes the plaster conform accurately to the shape of the stump. The cast is brought well above the knee level and is molded over the femoral condyles with the knee maintained in 5 to 10 degrees of flexion. An auxiliary suspension is added consisting of a strap incorporated in the cast and attached to a prefabricated waist belt. A similar dressing can be applied in an above-knee amputation, although it is much more cumbersome to do so because it has to be incorporated into a corset or extended around the pelvis as a spica to prevent the cast from loosening and shifting distally. If desired, a pylon fitting and prosthetic foot can be applied and the patient may begin touch-down weight-bearing the following day.

The drain in the wound is removed on the first or second day following amputation. The cast is left in place for 7 to 10 days unless the patient develops signs of wound complications such as fever, increasing white blood cell count, or significant pain, whereupon the cast should be removed and the wound inspected immediately. If the wound appears to be satisfactory at the end of a week, a removable prosthesis can be planned. Whether or not the immediate fitting technique has been used, either a preparatory or a definitive prosthesis can be made at that time, although it should be remembered that the muscles within the stump atrophy to some extent and a change of socket probably is necessary within several weeks.[18]

PROSTHETIC CONSIDERATIONS

Lower Extremity

BELOW-KNEE PROSTHESES. The most commonly prescribed prosthesis for the below-knee amputee is the PTB or patellar tendon–bearing limb. The interior of this socket contacts all surfaces of the stump, but with the weight borne mainly on the medial flare of the tibia, the shaft of the fibula, the patellar tendon, and the posterior surface of the calf. Pressure relief is provided for the subcutaneous crest of the tibia, the fibular head, and other tender areas. The socket may or may not be made with a removable insert composed of resilient foam material. Padding between the skin and the interior of the prosthesis is provided by the use of one or more cotton or wool stump socks.

The foot for this prosthesis is of the Solid Ankle Cushion Heel (SACH) type in which ankle motion is simulated by compressing a sponge rubber wedge in the heel. Several types of these feet incorporate a flexible keel that bends on weight-bearing and recoils as weight is removed, thus providing some push-off function. This feature is advantageous to very active amputees particularly in running, but the expense is greater than the conventional SACH foot and the durability thus far has not proved to be as great.[30]

There are several choices available to hold the prosthesis on, the simplest of which consists of a strap around the supracondylar area of the thigh with or without an additional elastic strap attached to a waist belt. While this holds the prosthesis in place, it allows some pistoning of the stump in the socket between stance and swing phase of gait. More secure is a sleeve of neoprene rubber rolled from the upper portion of the socket onto the thigh (Fig. 4). It has the disadvantage of being hot in some climates and irritating to the skin of some patients. The most secure suspension commonly used incorporates medial and lateral extensions on the socket that, in effect, clip over the condyles of the patient's femur. Although it must be adjusted very precisely for comfort and is not appropriate in an obese patient, this method of suspension nearly eliminates pistoning.

The prosthesis is aligned with the shin tilted 10 degrees forward when the shoe is flat on the floor. This places the knee into slight flexion at midstance and prevents it from being forced into recurvatum as weight is shifted to the forefoot.

ABOVE-KNEE PROSTHESES. There are several socket designs available for the above-knee amputee. For many years, the "quadrilateral socket," made for total contact or open-ended, has been used. This design accommodates various muscle groups at the hip level and, as the name implies, is relatively square in shape. Weight is borne on a shelf provided for the ischial tuberosity, which is held in place by forces from the anterior and lateral aspects of the socket.

An alternative is an "ischial containment" socket in which the ischium is not supported in the same manner but weight is

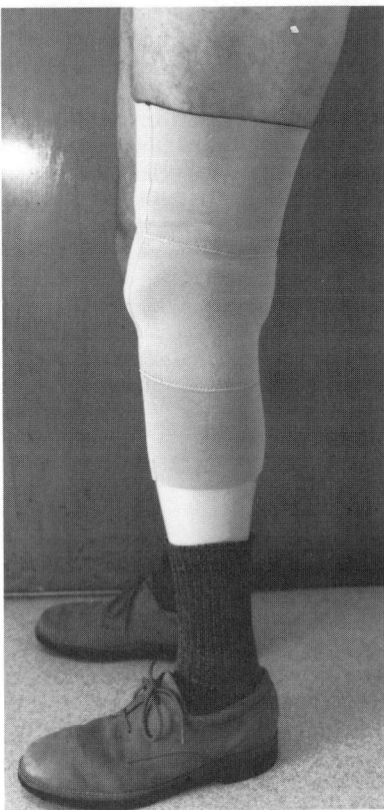

Figure 4. Elastic neoprene sleeve is effective for suspension of the patellar tendon–bearing prosthesis but may be uncomfortably hot and irritating to the skin.

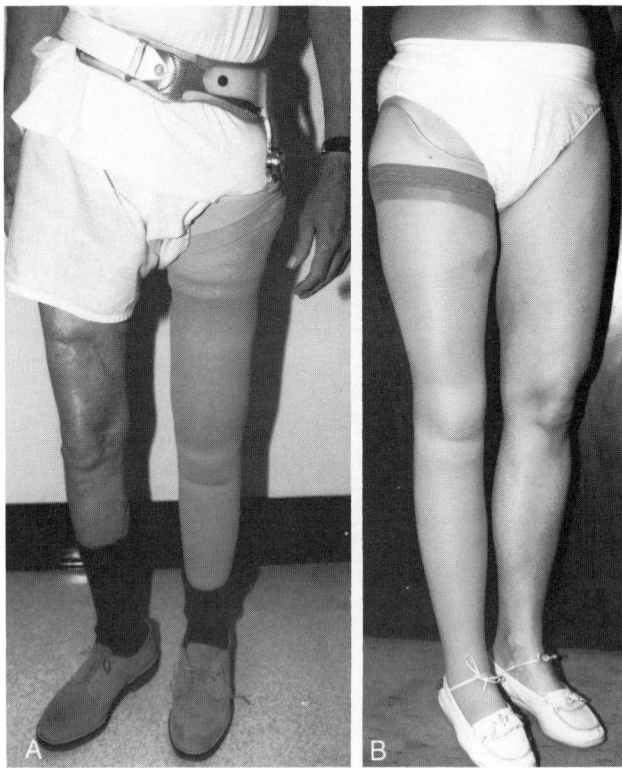

Figure 5. *A,* Suspension of above-knee prosthesis with hip joint and pelvic belt. *B,* Suspension of above-knee prosthesis with suction. The valve is hidden under the cosmetic cover, and the contours about the hip are quite cosmetic.

borne on the soft tissues in the proximal stump including the gluteus maximus muscle.[34] The thigh is adducted as much as is practical. The forces on the lateral thigh act as a counterforce across the hip joint; and, in addition, the lateral thigh becomes a weight-bearing surface. There are several types of this principle that have proved to be very comfortable in selected patients.[25] Variations of this socket may become more routine in the future.

The prosthetic knee must provide both stability in the stance phase of gait and flexibility in swing. Stance control is usually obtained by alignment of the prosthesis such that gravitational forces are anterior to the pivot point of a nonhyperextensible knee joint. In elderly amputees, patients with short stumps, and others with stability problems, a "stance control" knee is used. This automatically locks on weight-bearing and is free in swing phase of gait. In extreme situations, a mechanical, manually operated knee lock can be provided. With this, the knee is stiff and solid when the patient is walking but can be unlocked for sitting.

Control of the knee in swing phase of gait when the foot is off the ground is equally important. Either mechanical or hydraulic mechanisms are provided to damp out excessive heel rise and other physical characteristics of the pendulum that occur.

The foot-ankle complex for the above-knee amputee is the same as for the below-knee patients, with an additional choice of an articulated ankle. Whereas it would appear that the articulated ankle is more physiologic, it is actually less cosmetic and requires considerably more maintenance than the SACH type of components.

Two common methods of maintaining the prosthesis (Fig. 5) are the use of a hinged hip joint attached to a semirigid belt that suspends the prosthesis from the pelvis or a flexible belt known as a "Silesian bandage" with which the prosthesis is suspended from the contralateral iliac crest. A third mechanism is the "suction socket." This has a one-way valve incorporated in the

socket. It is worn without a stump sock and requires a very intimate air tight fit between the bare skin of the stump and the socket. Vacuum is produced during swing phase, which prevents the prosthesis from dropping off.

The suction socket is most effective in young active patients and is not very useful in the dysvascular or elderly patient with limited agility. Inguinal scarring from failed arterial surgery may prevent adequate suction to be attained.

Upper Extremity

Amputation of the upper extremity is usually necessitated by trauma, occasionally by malignancy, and rarely by peripheral vascular disease. The psychologic impact of these amputations is even greater than that of amputation of the lower extremity. The hand is used not only to manipulate the environment, but also to communicate and to express emotions.

It is most important to rehabilitate upper extremity amputees rapidly to decrease the emotional impact and to prove that life can go on in a relatively normal manner. Immediate postsurgical fitting of a prosthetic device has definite advantages.[26] It has not, however, been as successful in providing a replacement prosthesis for the upper extremity amputee as for the lower extremity amputee. Power and motion can be supplied in only a comparatively gross way, and cosmesis is obtained at the expense of function. The most functional terminal device is a hook, and this will remain true until some means of substitution for the complex action of the intrinsic muscles of the hand can be found.[3]

Cosmesis is important because the hand is always in public view, and some amputees are willing to sacrifice much function in order to obtain the best possible cosmetic replacement. Cosmetic gloves made of polyvinyl and similar materials incorporating normal skin creases, veins on the dorsum, and even hair have been available for years. Color matching is somewhat limited, however, not because it is difficult to reproduce skin tones but because the normal opposite hand continually changes shade with position, season, and other factors, and this cannot be reproduced.

Sensation is also an extremely important component of hand function. Surgeons involved in hand reconstruction are aware that no matter how well joint motion and finger function are restored, unless the hand retains significant proprioception and two-point discrimination, functional potential is never realized. Although there is some sensory feedback for the amputee from the prosthesis by means of pressure from the harness and the stump-socket interface, intrinsic sensation from the terminal device has not been possible. Current research efforts to provide this electrically by means of transducers in the terminal device that stimulate either nerves within the stump or skin elsewhere are promising, and it is hoped that this research leads to the development of practical sensory feedback mechanisms.[9]

CONTROL OF UPPER EXTREMITY PROSTHESES

Prostheses for the upper extremity consist of a hook or hand terminal device, a harness to supply force from proximal muscles, and appropriate segments between them including a socket for the stump. The socket is made of molded plastic from a cast of the stump and provides total contact with the skin. As in the lower limb, the socket may include a means of suspension. Ordinarily active control is provided only for the terminal device and elbow with other joint action being either passive or eliminated entirely.

Body Power

In the usual prosthesis, a harness made of web strap extends from the opposite axilla across the back of the shoulders to a cable that activates appropriate joints. A "Bowden cable," which includes a tubelike housing through which the cable slides in the manner of the throttle cable on a power lawn mower, has proved to be the most efficient transmission device. In the above-elbow prosthesis, the housing is omitted across the elbow joint, thus allowing the elbow to be moved. With the elbow in a locked position, further cable travel is transmitted then to the terminal device, thus activating it. Motion is initiated by the patient's either abducting his scapulae or flexing the shoulder on the prosthetic side. The elbow is locked by shrugging the shoulder, which pulls on a second cable that activates the elbow lock. Flexion and extension of the wrist are usually omitted, although there are prosthetic wrist units for special situations in which the wrist can be positioned in either flexed or extended modes. Pronation and supination are passive, and the desired position is preset by rotating the terminal device with the opposite hand (Fig. 6).

Electric Power

In recent years, other sources of force have been explored including myoelectric control.[1,15] In a myoelectric system, electrical potentials from active voluntary contraction of muscles in the stump are identified by electrodes in the socket, amplified, and used to control electric motors in the prosthesis. Opening and closing of the terminal device, pronation and supination, and elbow flexion and extension can be provided. The advantages of this type of system are that the harness is eliminated and the action is more natural. For example, for the below-elbow amputee, the residual finger flexors can be used to close the terminal device and the extensor mass to open it. Disadvantages include expense, the need for increased maintenance, the difficulty in waterproofing the system, and the loss of the sensory feedback the harness provides (Fig. 7).

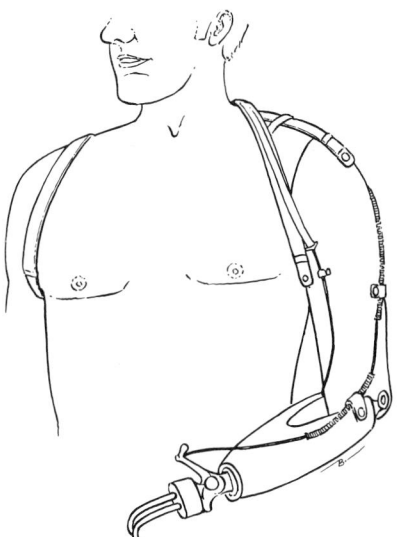

Figure 6. Prosthesis for the above-elbow amputee includes socket and arm segment, forearm, terminal device, harness, cable from harness that provides motion at the elbow and controls the terminal device, and control cable for the elbow lock.

Hybrid systems using the features of electric motors and body-powered mechanical switches are also practical, as would be expected.[29]

ONGOING PROBLEMS OF THE AMPUTEE

Loss of Socket Fit

In the early weeks after amputation, it is expected that the patient's stump will change in both size and shape.[27] Muscles that are not used atrophy, and the muscles in the stump for the most part act on the joint below. Most prostheses are worn with an interface of cotton or wool socks. Up to a point, fit can be maintained by adding additional socks or parts of socks. Liners, partial liners, and distal foam pads can be added by the prosthetist to help maintain the fit. The symptom of a malfitting socket is usually gradually increasing discomfort, often over bone prominences such as the fibular head or the anterior portion of the distal tibia anterior in the below-knee patient, or the ischial ramus in the above-knee patient. In the established amputee, gain or loss of weight can influence the fit, and for this reason the amputee should be counseled to maintain constant weight. In addition, excess fluid accumulation from renal or cardiac dysfunction may first be noted by the amputee in the fit of the limb.

Apparently the loss of total contact distally causing stretching of the skin over the end of the stump produces the same sensation as dropping into the socket, increasing contact pressure on the end of the stump. Very few amputees can distinguish the difference.

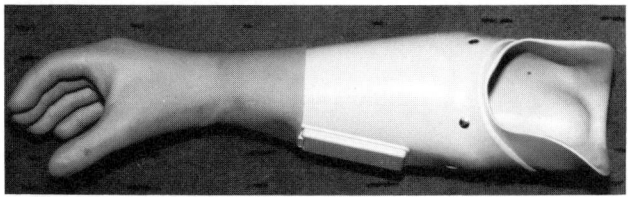

Figure 7. Myoelectric below-elbow prosthesis with cosmetic glove. Battery pack is on the volar surface of the forearm.

Neuroma

All peripheral nerves when divided attempt to regenerate; in the case of the amputee, this causes a tender ball-shaped mass of axons—an "amputation neuroma." This can be quite uncomfortable if it is trapped in scar or pinched between the soft tissues and the socket of the prosthesis.[21] The ulnar and peroneal nerves are frequently involved in painful neuromas.

Surgical excision of the neuroma is usually disappointing because another forms in the same area. It is better to do a more proximal neurectomy from the prosthetic socket such as in the upper popliteal space in the case of the peroneal nerve.

There is no treatment of the nerve at the time of amputation that has been effective in preventing amputation neuroma although many very innovative approaches have been devised. It is best to pull the nerve distally as far as practical and divide it sharply, allowing the cut end to retract into the soft tissues.

Phantom Limb

Phantom limb is a fixed central pain syndrome that does not relate to a specific neuroma or to the normal perception of the missing part that all amputees experience.[11,21,35] It is more common in the upper than in the lower extremity and is more common after trauma that included a stretch injury to peripheral nerves such as the brachial or lumbosacral plexus. It is also more common following amputations performed because of failure of multiple painful reconstruction attempts.

Phantom limb is a tragedy that is difficult to treat. It has physiologic and emotional aspects, and both must be addressed. In selected cases, implanted nerve stimulators may help, and destructive neurologic procedures such as tractotomies or dorsal root entry zone ablation may offer some relief.

Skin Lesions

The most frequent skin problems encountered are blisters or abrasions secondary to poor fit of the socket. Conventional local care of the lesion and attempts to regain a precise fit ordinarily solve the problem.

Because of limited ventilation, excess perspiration and local heat occur within the socket. Good personal hygiene is mandatory for the amputee. Stump socks should be changed daily and be clean and free of soap. Excessive perspiration can be controlled in some patients by the daily use of a spray antiperspirant on the stump. Despite this, some patients have problems with furuncles that occur in areas where there is both pressure and friction, such as the posterior socket brim in the below-knee amputee, and in the area of the ischial seat and the adductor longus tendon in the above-knee amputee. The treatment is local skin care, topical and/or systemic antibiotics when needed, and modification of that portion of the socket to decrease the pressure.[24]

A problem peculiar to amputees is "choked stump syndrome." This consists of a painful verrucous hyperplasia, often associated with cracking and weeping of the skin. Choked stump is the result of a combination of insecure suspension and lack of total contact distally. Circumferential pressure proximally contributes to distal edema, and the lack of suspension allows the skin to piston or slide on the underlying soft tissues, thus stretching the skin over the end of the bone with each step. Refitting the prosthesis usually solves the problem, and the skin changes gradually revert to normal.

REFERENCES

1. Agrew, J. P.: Functional effectiveness of a myoelectric prosthesis compared with a functional split-hook prosthesis: A single subject experiment. Prosthet. Ortho. Int. 5:92, 1981.
2. Berlemont, M., Weber, R., and Willot, J. P.: Ten years experience with immediate application of prosthetic devices to amputees of the lower extremity on the operating table. Prosthet. Orthot. Int., 3:8, 1969.
3. Billock, J. N.: Upper limb prosthetic terminal devices: Hands versus hooks. Clin. Prosthet. Orthot., 10:57, 1986.
4. Burgess, E. M.: General principles of amputation surgery. In American Academy of Orthopaedic Surgeons, Atlas of Limb Prosthetics: Surgical and Prosthetic Principles. St. Louis, C. V. Mosby, 1981, p. 14.
5. Burgess, E. M., Romano, R. L., and Zettl, J. H.: The management of lower extremity amputation. TR 10–6. Washington, D.C., U.S. Government Printing Office, 1969.
6. Burgess, E. M., Romano, R. L., Zettl, J. H., et al.: Amputation of the leg for peripheral vascular insufficiency. J. Bone Joint Surg., 53A:874, 1971.
7. Burgess, E. M., and Matson, F. A., III: Current concepts to review: Determining amputation level in peripheral vascular disease. J. Bone Joint Surg., 63A:1493, 1981.
8. Burkhalter, W. E., Mayfield, G., and Carmona, L. S.: The upper extremity amputee. Early and immediate postsurgical prosthetic fitting. J. Bone Joint Surg., 58A:46, 1976.
9. Clippinger, F. W., Avery, R., and Titus, B. R.: A sensory feedback system for an upper extremity amputation prosthesis. Bull. Prosth. Res., 10:22, 1974.
10. Deffer, P. A., Moll, J. H., and LaNoue, A. M.: The Ertl osteoplastic below knee amputation. J. Bone Joint Surg., 53A:1028, 1971.
11. DeGuiterrez-Mahoney, C. J.: The treatment of painful phantom limb. Surg. Clin. North Am., 28:401, 1948.
12. Dowd, G. S. E., Linge, K., and Bently, G.: Measurement of transcutaneous oxygen pressure in normal and ischemic skin. J. Bone Joint Surg., 65B:79, 1963.
13. Epps, C. H., Jr.: Amputation of the lower limb. In Evarts, C. M. (Ed.): Surgery of the Musculoskeletal System, 2nd ed. New York, Churchill Livingstone, 1990, p. 5139.
14. Epps, C. H., Jr., and Adams, J. P.: Wound management in open fractures. Am. J. Surg., 27:766, 1961.
15. Ferguson, S.: Electric power in upper limb prosthetics: The Michigan experience. Inter Clinic Information Bull., 18:1, 1983.
16. Friedman, L. W.: The Psychological Rehabilitation of the Amputee. Springfield, Ill., Charles C Thomas, 1978.
17. Gibbons, G. W., Wheelock, F. C., Siemtede, C., et al.: Noninvasive prediction of amputation level in diabetic patients. Arch. Surg., 114:1253, 1979.
18. Goldner, J. L., Clippinger, F. W., and Titus, B. R.: Use of temporary plaster or plastic pylons preparatory to fitting a permanent above knee prosthesis. Bull. Prosthet. Res., 87:107, 1970.
19. Gonzales, E. G., Corcoran, P. J., and Reyes, R. L.: Energy expenditure in below knee amputees: Correlation with stump strength. Arch. Phys. Med. Rehabil., 55:111, 1974.
20. Harisson, J.: The leg amputee: A clinical followup study. Acta Orthop. (Suppl.), 69:1, 1964.
21. Jensen, T. S., Krebs, B., Nielsen, J., et al.: Phantom limb, phantom pain, and stump pain in amputees during the first 6 months following limb amputation. Pain, 17:243, 1983.
22. Kirk, N. T., and Peterson, L. T.: Amputations. In Lewis, D.: Practice of Surgery. W. F. Pryor Company, 1963, p. 216.
23. Kostuik, J. P.: Indications, levels, and limiting factors in amputation surgery of the lower extremity. In Kostuik, J. P. (Ed.): Amputation Surgery and Rehabilitation: The Toronto Experience. New York, Churchill Livingstone, 1981.
24. Levy, S. W.: Skin problems of the leg amputee. Prosthet. Orthot. Int., 4:37, 1980.
25. Long, I. A.: Normal shape–normal alignment above knee prosthesis. Clin. Prosthet. Orthot. 9:9, 1985.
26. Malone, J. H., Childers, S. J., Underwood, J., et al.: Immediate postsurgical management of upper extremity amputations: Conventional, electronic, and myoelectric prostheses. Orthot. Prosthet., 35:1, 1981.
27. McCullough, N. C., III, Harris, A. R., and Hampton, F. L.: Below knee amputations. In American Academy of Orthopaedic Surgeons, Atlas of Limb Prosthetics. St. Louis, C. V. Mosby, 1981, p. 341.
28. McCullough, N. C., III, and Epps, C. H., Jr.: Principles of amputation surgery in vascular disease. In Evarts, C. M. (Ed): Surgery of the Musculoskeletal System, 2nd ed. New York, Churchill Livingstone, 1990, p. 5093.
29. Michael, J. W.: Upper limb powered components and controls: Current concepts. Clin. Prosthet. Orthot., 10:66, 1986.
30. Michael, J. W.: Energy storing feet: A clinical comparison. Clin. Prosthet. Orthot., 11:154, 1987.
31. Moore, W. S.: Determination of amputation level: Measurement of skin blood flow with xenon 133. Arch. Surg. 107:798, 1973.
32. Murdock, G.: Level of amputation and limiting factors. Ann. R. Coll. Surg., 40:204, 1967.
33. Riley, R.: The amputee athlete. Clin. Prosthet. Orthot., 11:109, 1987.
34. Sabolich, J.: Contoured Adducted Trochanteric–Controlled Alignment Method (CAT–CAM): Introduction and basic principles. Clin. Prosthet. Orthot., 9:15, 1985.
35. Schnell, M. D., and Bunch, W. H.: Management of pain in the amputee. American Academy of Orthopaedic Surgeons, In Atlas of Limb Prosthetics. St. Louis, C. V. Mosby, 1981, p. 464.
36. Shea, J. D.: Surgical techniques of lower extremity amputation. Orthop. Clin. North Am., 3:287, 1972.
37. Waters, R. L., Perry, J., Antonelli, D., et al.: Energy cost of walking of amputees: The influence of level of amputation. J. Bone Joint Surg., 58A:42, 1976.
38. White, R. A., Nolan, L., and Harley, D.: Noninvasive evaluation of peripheral vascular disease using transcutaneous oxygen tension. Am. J. Surg., 144:68, 1982.
39. Prevalence of Selected Impairments—United States–1972, Vital and Health Statistics. Series 10, Number 134. DHHS Publication (PHD), 81:1562, U.S. Department of Health and Human Services, 1981.

IX

INFECTIONS AND NEOPLASMS OF BONE

John M. Harrelson, M.D., and John J. Callaghan, M.D.

In discussing infections and neoplasms of bone, it is appropriate to combine the two because the clinical and radiographic presentation may be similar. The dictum that every suspected tumor should be cultured and every suspected infection be biopsied is definitely applicable to bone.

INFECTIONS OF BONE

Osteomyelitis is the general term used to denote infection of bone. Although the organisms responsible for soft tissue infections can also produce osteomyelitis, the majority of bone infections are the result of *Staphylococcus aureus.* The location, clinical presentation, and course of osteomyelitis vary with the offending organism and the age of the patient. *Staphylococcus* and other pus-forming bacteria usually produce an acute fulminating infection of bone, or "pyogenic osteomyelitis." Tuberculosis and other nonpyogenic organisms produce a less aggressive granulomatous type of infection. It is convenient to consider these two types of osteomyelitis separately.

Pyogenic Osteomyelitis

Suppurative infection of bone occurs in one of two ways. Blood-borne bacteria from an active focus of soft tissue infection (furuncle, upper respiratory infection, urinary tract infection) may lodge in bone and establish an abscess. This mechanism is referred to as "hematogenous osteomyelitis." More commonly observed in clinical practice today, bacteria may also reach bone from the external environment (penetrating wounds, open fractures, surgical incisions) and establish "exogenous osteomyelitis." Antibiotics have greatly reduced the incidence of both types of osteomyelitis and significantly improved prognosis. Prior to the antibiotic era, the mortality from pyogenic osteomyelitis was 20 to 30 per cent, and survivors could expect significant crippling effects of the disease. Today, death is rare and residual disability has been greatly minimized.

Hematogenous osteomyelitis is primarily a disease of childhood, occurring most frequently between the ages of 5 and 15. Males are affected three times more frequently than are females. In the growing child, the afferent arterial supply to bone enters through the nutrient artery and through small periosteal vessels penetrating the cortex. As these vessels reach the arteriolar level in the metaphysis at each end of the bone, they enter into numerous sinusoidal veins adjacent to the physeal plate in which flow is significantly diminished. These metaphyseal veins with sluggish blood flow provide an ideal location for the lodgment of bacteria and subsequent establishment of infection. Thus, hematogenous osteomyelitis in children is most frequently seen in the metaphyseal ends of long bones. The adjacent epiphysis has a separate blood supply, which enters through the joint capsule. The physeal plate has no traversing blood vessels and acts as a further barrier to the spread of infection from the metaphysis to the adjacent epiphysis and joint.

The femur, tibia, and humerus are most frequently affected, in that order. Other tubular bones and flat bones are less commonly involved. With bony maturity, ossification of the physeal plate occurs, and the circulation of the epiphysis and metaphysis merges. The characteristic of sluggish blood flow is lost. Thus, osteomyelitis in adults is less frequent and may occur at any point within a long bone.

Hematogenous osteomyelitis most frequently involves bone with a rich blood supply. Exogenous osteomyelitis is more common in those bones with the least soft tissue covering. Therefore, the tibia, with little soft tissue covering and often injured in high-speed trauma, is the most common bone involved in exogenous osteomyelitis.

PATHOLOGIC CONSIDERATIONS. As invading bacteria reach the metaphyseal veins and multiply, the initial host response is an infiltration of polymorphonuclear leukocytes. This combination of bacteria and leukocytes constitutes an abscess. As a result of the bacterial multiplication and interstitial edema, pressure increases within the rigid structure of the metaphysis, producing capillary destruction, thrombosis, loss of circulation, and subsequent death of the trabecular bone within the abscess. Increasing pressure produces localized pain.

In the early stages of the disease, infarction of a portion of the metaphysis does not produce any observable radiographic change. As the process continues, granulation tissue develops around the periphery of the abscess and with it there occurs osteoclastic resorption of the living bone in this area. The isolated necrotic bone within the abscess cavity is termed a *sequestrum.* Around the periphery of the granulation tissue, the host bone makes an effort to isolate the infectious process. New bone is deposited in this area and is termed the *involucrum.*

Because of the pain and subsequent diminished activity, disuse osteoporosis develops within the affected extremity. Increased circulation to the bone as a result of the infection accelerates the development of osteoporosis. Radiographs taken at 12 to 14 days following the onset of infection reveal a central area of increased radiodensity (sequestrum) surrounded by a zone of relative radiolucency (granulation tissue), which is surrounded by an area of increased radiodensity (involucrum). Generalized diminished radiodensity of the remainder of the long bone is the result of osteoporosis.

If the host is successful in repelling the infection at this stage, gradual obliteration of the abscess cavity with fibrous tissue occurs. This area is subsequently replaced by new bone, ultimately leaving no evidence of the infectious process. More frequently, the host is unable to contain the infection as an isolated abscess and continued growth of bacteria occurs. New areas of bone become involved as the process spreads outward toward the periosteum. Purulent material permeates through the haversian and Volkmann's canals of the cortex to the subperiosteal space. With increasing pressure, pus dissects along the subperiosteal plane, stripping the periosteum from the underlying cortex, interrupting blood supply, and extending the area of infarction. The subperiosteal spread of infection is limited at each end of the long bone by the adherence of the periosteum to the metaphyseal-physeal junction. The impermeability of the physeal plate prevents the spread of infection to the epiphysis. Thus, the entire shaft of the bone from one metaphysis to the other may be involved. From the inner surface of the elevated periosteum, osteoblasts begin to lay down new bone and form a periosteal involucrum (Fig. 1).

At this point, the infection may rupture through the periosteum into the adjacent soft tissues and ultimately to the skin, where it produces a draining sinus tract. Fragments of necrotic bone (sequestrum) may be extruded. If the sinus is large enough to extrude the entire sequestrum, subsequent healing may occur

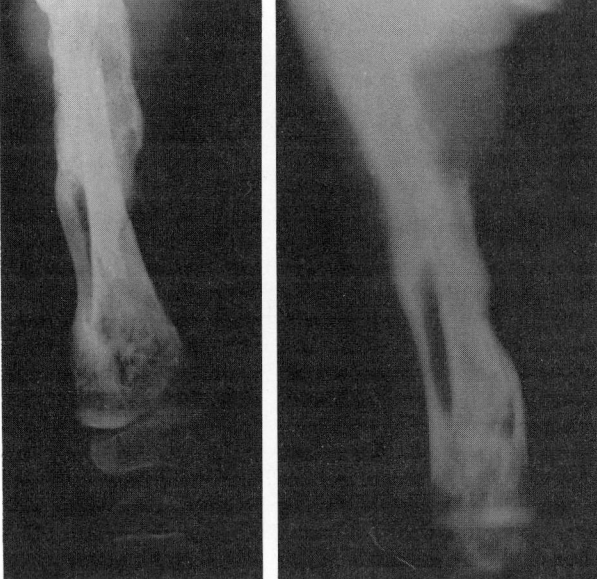

Figure 1. Notice the periosteal new bone (involucrum), which formed along the entire shaft of the femur. The central femoral cortex is necrotic and represents a sequestrum.

with obliteration of the abscess cavity by fibrous tissue. However, this situation rarely occurs, the sequestrum being too large for complete extrusion. Even with complete extrusion, the rigid nature of bone prevents collapse of the abscess cavity and greatly reduces the likelihood of total obliteration of the infection.

Adherence of the periosteum to the metaphysis and the impermeability of the physeal plate usually protect the adjacent joint from infection. In infants younger than the age of 12 months, there are vessels that traverse the physeal plate. Osteomyelitis in this age group may produce adjacent pyarthrosis. The hip joint, in any age group, is vulnerable to infection with osteomyelitis of the proximal femur, because the capital femoral epiphysis lies within the joint capsule. Metaphyseal infection of the proximal femur may permeate the outer cortex and enter the joint directly (Fig. 2).

CLINICAL CONSIDERATIONS. The onset of hematogenous osteomyelitis is usually abrupt, with fever, generalized malaise, and pain in the involved extremity. A history of preceding infection may be obtained. Early in the course of the disease, there may be generalized swelling of the extremity without erythema. A sterile sympathetic effusion of adjacent joints may be present. The patient is toxic and irritable, and manipulation of the extremity produces paroxysms of pain. Extremely gentle digital palpation along the course of the extremity usually localizes the infection.

Laboratory examination reveals a leukocytosis exceeding 15,000, mild to moderate anemia, and a markedly elevated erythrocyte sedimentation rate. In approximately 50 per cent of cases, blood cultures are positive. In the first 7 to 10 days of the disease, there are no evident radiographic bony changes, but subtle soft tissue changes can be recognized. As a result of inflammation and swelling of the extremity, the normal soft tissue shadows produced by muscle, fascial planes, and subcutaneous tissue are obliterated. This change is observed throughout the entire course of the involved long bone. Comparison radiographs of the opposite extremity may be helpful; within 10 to 14 days, bony changes are evident, consisting first of mottled lucency of the involved metaphysis followed by periosteal elevation and new bone formation.

Ewing's sarcoma and other neoplasms, acute rheumatic fever, leukemia, scurvy, acute septic arthritis, and acute juvenile

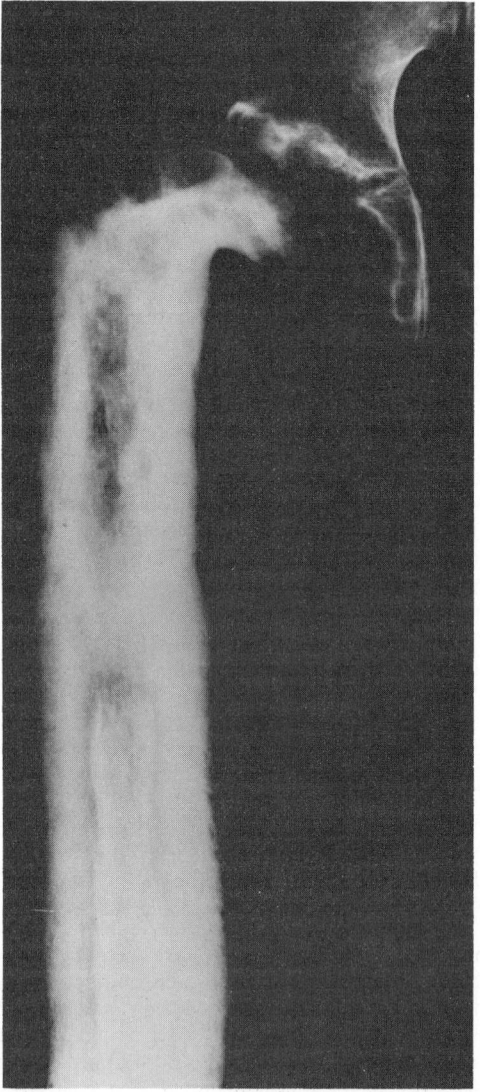

Figure 2. This child has osteomyelitis involving the entire femoral shaft. The central portion of the bone is the old femoral shaft, which is now necrotic and represents a sequestrum. Notice that the hip joint has been involved because the hip capsule extends beyond the capital femoral physeal plate.

rheumatoid arthritis may all mimic the clinical pattern of acute osteomyelitis. Careful examination of the involved extremity is required to distinguish acute osteomyelitis from acute pyarthrosis. In osteomyelitis, tenderness is usually located over the metaphysis of the long bone, and gentle manipulation allows motion of the adjacent joints. In contrast, acute pyarthrosis produces swelling localized at the joint level, and the patient cannot tolerate any joint motion. In acute rheumatic fever and acute juvenile rheumatoid arthritis, the tenderness is similarly located over the joint, and more than one joint may be involved.

Because of the widespread use of antibiotics, the pre-existing nidus of soft tissue infection may not be identified. When antibiotic therapy has been used for a preceding soft tissue infection, the subsequent clinical course of osteomyelitis may be considerably more benign and the true diagnosis may not be recognized until the infection is well established. In adults, osteomyelitis characteristically is more benign. Often the infection is limited to the metaphysis without spread to the subperiosteal space. Generalized toxicity is less, and symptoms are usually localized to the site of infection.

The organism most frequently encountered in hematogenous

osteomyelitis is *S. aureus* (90 per cent). In neonates and infants, *Streptococcus* may be the etiologic agent. These two bacteria produce the fulminating clinical presentation described. Less frequently, gram-negative organisms may produce osteomyelitis. In particular, *Salmonella* osteomyelitis may be a complication of sickle cell anemia and often involves the diaphysis of a long bone rather than the metaphysis. The gram-negative organisms characteristically produce a less virulent infection than gram-positive cocci.

Exogenous osteomyelitis is most frequently the result of open fracture. In that the infection follows contamination of an existing wound, any organism may be involved. If the fracture wound has been closed, the subsequent development of infection may produce the same symptoms as observed in hematogenous osteomyelitis, although to a lesser degree. Generally, the infection is limited to the site of injury and produces localized erythema and swelling. The continued multiplication of bacteria may cause spontaneous dehiscence of the wound with a discharge of purulent material. When the periosteum has been disrupted, as in the case of fracture, periosteal elevation is not seen as a result of infection. Rather, there is local destruction of bone at the fracture site. Aggressive multiple débridement, prophylactic antibiotics, and early muscular flap coverage of open fractures have markedly decreased the incidence of exogenous osteomyelitis.

TREATMENT. The treatment of acute hematogenous osteomyelitis begins immediately upon recognition. When blood cultures have been obtained, antibiotics are administered intravenously without awaiting the results of cultures. Because *S. aureus* is the most frequent offending organism, penicillin in combination with methicillin is used. Blood cultures do not always reveal the etiologic agent. If there are enough localizing physical findings or confirmatory radiographic changes, the subperiosteal space may be aspirated with a large-bore needle and material may be obtained for Gram stain and culture. Care must be taken not to contaminate an adjacent, sterile joint. If no material is obtained on penetration of the periosteum, the needle may be advanced through the cortex into the metaphysis and an aspirate may be obtained for culture.

The maintenance of fluid and electrolyte balance and the correction of an existing anemia with whole fresh blood are also necessary. Antipyretics are required to control fever, and anticonvulsants may be necessary. Immobilization of the involved extremity is accomplished by the use of bivalved plaster. Immobilization allows the extremity to rest and reduces muscle spasm and pain. Bivalved plaster is preferred in order to allow inspection of the extremity. In most instances, the administration of intravenous antibiotics produces improvement within 24 hours. If the patient's condition does not improve, surgical intervention is required.

The surgical principles in the treatment of osteomyelitis are the same as for the treatment of any soft tissue abscess and consist of incision and drainage. The surgical approach depends on both the location and the extent of infection. When possible, the incision should be placed to allow subsequent dependent drainage. If the infection is confined to the metaphysis without periosteal elevation and if the dissection of pus within the subperiosteal space has not occurred, a cortical window is created in the metaphysis, and the pus under pressure, together with the necrotic sequestrum, is removed. Care is taken not to damage the adjacent physeal plate. This procedure is termed *saucerization*. Care must also be taken not to strip the periosteum widely, because this interrupts the blood supply to the underlying cortex and allows extension of the infection. The wound is packed open to allow drainage, and the extremity is immobilized in plaster.

If the infectious process involves the majority of the shaft of the bone, a closed suction irrigation may be used. A cortical window is created in the same manner as just described, and two perforated polyethylene catheters are inserted into the medullary canal through separate stab wounds. The incision is then closed over drains.

Intravenous antibiotics are continued for a minimum of 2 weeks, followed by appropriate oral antibiotic therapy for an additional 4 weeks. Antibiotic treatment is discontinued when all clinical signs of infection are absent and the sedimentation rate returns to normal. When the acute infectious process is under control, the limb is removed from the bivalved plaster several times each day for gentle motion of adjacent joints. This prevents arthrofibrosis and maintains normal joint motion. The resumption of activity with the involved limb depends on the extent of bone destruction and the rate of healing. If a large area is involved, the return to full weight-bearing and normal activity may require many months in order to avoid pathologic fracture.

The best treatment of exogenous osteomyelitis is prevention. Open, contaminated fracture wounds should be débrided and packed open and closed as a delayed procedure in 2 to 5 days if there are no signs of infection. When a fracture wound has been closed and infection has developed, the wound must be opened widely and redébrided to allow complete drainage. Any nonviable bone at the fracture site is removed. Immobilization of the limb is mandatory. Adequate cultures are obtained and the appropriate antibiotics are selected, depending on bacterial sensitivity.

With the use of antibiotics, death is rare. The ultimate degree of disability depends on many factors. The location of infection, the extent of bony destruction, the involvement of adjacent joints, the virulence of the organism, and the rapidity with which treatment is initiated all affect the ultimate outcome. If the infection is successfully controlled by antibiotics or a combination of antibiotics and surgical therapy, ultimate eradication of the infection is possible. In some cases, it is not possible to eliminate the infection completely. When the extent of bony involvement is great and complete sequestrectomy is not possible, drainage sinus tracts may develop and indicate the initiation of chronic osteomyelitis. The infection may be quiescent for many months or years only to recur periodically with drainage, fever, and swelling. The sinus tract becomes lined with squamous epithelium and, in long-standing cases, may undergo metaplasia and develop squamous carcinoma within the tract. Chronic cases that cannot be adequately controlled by antibiotics and local measures may require amputation of the extremity and fitting with a prosthesis to eradicate the infection and provide better function.

Tuberculous Osteomyelitis and Pyarthrosis

Like hematogenous osteomyelitis, the incidence of skeletal tuberculosis decreased significantly in recent years. The development of effective antimicrobial agents was partly responsible. An improved standard of living that reduced overcrowding and malnutrition also contributed to the reduction of pulmonary (human type) tuberculosis. The identification of diseased cattle and the pasteurization of milk reduced the frequency of gastrointestinal (bovine type) tuberculosis. However, with the increased incidence of acquired immune deficiency syndrome, skeletal tuberculosis may be rising again.

Skeletal tuberculosis is the result of hematogenous seeding of tubercle bacilli from a pre-existing pulmonary or gastrointestinal focus. This organism most frequently involves the joints and adjacent bone rather than the metaphyseal area of long bones. The intervertebral discs of the lower thoracic and upper lumbar spine and the adjacent vertebrae are the most frequent sites of skeletal tuberculosis (approximately 30 per cent of all cases), the hip and knee joints being the next most frequently affected. Older statistics indicate that the majority of cases occur in children between the ages of 5 and 15 years. However, there appears to be a decline in the number of childhood cases and an increase in the incidence of skeletal tuberculosis in adults.

PATHOLOGIC CONSIDERATIONS. Following hematogenous inoculation, tubercle bacilli lodge in the subchondral bone of the epiphysis, in the joint capsule, or in the synovial membrane. The initial host response is an infiltration of lymphocytes, plasma cells, and monocytes. The histologic appearance of the tuberculous lesion in bone in every way resembles that observed in visceral tuberculosis. Histiocytes (epithelioid cells) appear and may aggregate to form Langhans' giant cells. There is considerable fibroblastic proliferation. Caseous necrosis surrounded by a granulomatous inflammatory response constitutes the classic tubercle. The destruction produced by granulomatous inflammation is characteristically slow. Within the joint, destruction tends to occur first at those areas where the joint surfaces are not in constant apposition. In the knee joint, this destruction occurs at the joint margins, producing a corner defect on radiography. In the hip joint, such lesions appear at the superior border of the femoral neck or in the inferior medial aspect of the joint away from the weight-bearing area. Erosion of articular cartilage in the weight-bearing area is a late development and represents the preservation of joint space observed on early radiographs. As the destruction proceeds, the joint becomes filled with caseous necrotic products and fragments of articular cartilage, material termed rice bodies because of its appearance. In some cases, the joint or disc space infection may erupt into the adjacent soft tissues, burrow along a fascial plane, and eventually penetrate the skin, producing a chronic draining sinus tract that exudes caseous necrotic material.

CLINICAL CONSIDERATIONS. The destruction of bone and articular cartilage by tuberculous infection is a slow process, and symptoms are correspondingly insidious in their development. The patient complains of a dull ache in the area of the affected joint, often worse at night than during the day. Because the skeletal lesion is preceded by a visceral infection, the patient often appears debilitated. A history of weight loss and easy fatigability may be obtained, as well as a history of close contact with a family member with known tuberculosis.

Spinal involvement with tuberculosis produces diminished motion at the thoracolumbar level and protective paraspinal muscle spasm, which holds the back hyperextended. When the tuberculous process has escaped the confines of the disc space and adjacent vertebrae, a large paraspinal abscess may result. As the spine becomes weakened, collapse of the vertebral column may occur, forcing the caseous necrotic debris into the spinal canal and producing neurologic deterioration ranging from paraparesis to complete paraplegia. Prior to the development of effective antituberculous drugs, this clinical pattern of spinal tuberculosis was more common. The paraspinal abscess, which develops around a focus of tuberculous infection, may extend for some distance beneath the paraspinal muscles and present as a mass in the buttock or medial thigh that represents a soft tissue extension of the paraspinal abscess beneath the psoas muscle. The mass characteristically does not produce overlying erythema and is known as a cold abscess.

The chief radiographic changes in tuberculous spondylitis is narrowing of the disc space at the affected level. The outlines of the adjacent end plates become smudgy in appearance. As the disease progresses, the interspace narrows and a kyphotic deformity develops. Destruction of the adjacent vertebral end plates follows. If a paraspinal abscess is present, it usually produces a soft tissue shadow on radiography. Calcification may occasionally be observed within the abscess.

In the extremities, there is mild synovial thickening and effusion, and increased local heat over the joint, but erythema is usually lacking. Mild limitation of motion, muscle atrophy, and a limp are present. There may be enlargement of the proximal regional lymph nodes.

Laboratory examination reveals a normal to slightly elevated white count, an elevated erythrocyte sedimentation rate, and mild anemia. The tuberculin skin test is usually positive. The patient should be questioned about previous bacille Calmette-Guérin vaccination. Synovial fluid from the involved joint is turbid, with a poor mucin clot and a lowered glucose level. The white cell count is elevated, with an increased number of mononuclear cells. The synovial fluid sediment should be examined for acid-fast bacilli and a portion should be retained for culture.

Radiographs of tuberculous diarthrodial joints demonstrate generalized osteoporosis with preservation of the joint space and distention of the joint capsule. The earliest bony changes consist of erosion of the joint margins at the point of capsular attachment to the epiphysis. Similar defects may occur within the epiphysis itself, and the infection may cross the physeal plate into the adjacent metaphysis. When the hip joint in children is involved, progressive capsular distention may interrupt the blood supply to the capital femoral epiphysis, causing its death and gradual disappearance (Fig. 3).

TREATMENT. The development of effective antituberculous drugs has radically altered the treatment of this disease. In the past, a patient's primary defense was his own immune system. If the lesion eventually showed signs of healing, arthrodesis of the joint was performed with the joint in the functional position. Today arthrodesis is less frequently required.

The initial treatment of skeletal tuberculosis consists of appropriate antituberculous drugs (isoniazid, rifampin, p-aminosalicylic acid (PAS), streptomycin, ethambutol) and protection of the involved joint. For spinal tuberculosis, the use of bed rest or plaster immobilization is recommended during the initial phase of chemotherapy. As healing occurs, gradual resumption of activity is allowed. Joints in the lower extremities are put at rest either by traction or by the use of bivalved plaster. Daily gentle range-of-motion exercises are performed to maintain joint function. If there is no significant evidence of healing after 6 to 8 weeks of antituberculous therapy, localized foci within the epiphysis may be carefully removed by curettage. Arthrodesis of the joint may still be required for excessive joint destruction.

Acute Pyogenic Arthritis

Joint infection with pyogenic organisms occurs as a result of hematogenous seeding of the joint, extension of adjacent osteomyelitis, or penetrating wounds of the joint. Hematogenous pyarthrosis is most commonly observed in children younger than 5 years of age. *S. aureus* is the most common etiologic agent, although *Haemophilus influenzae*, *Streptococcus*, gonococcus, and penumococcus may be etiologic. The condition is

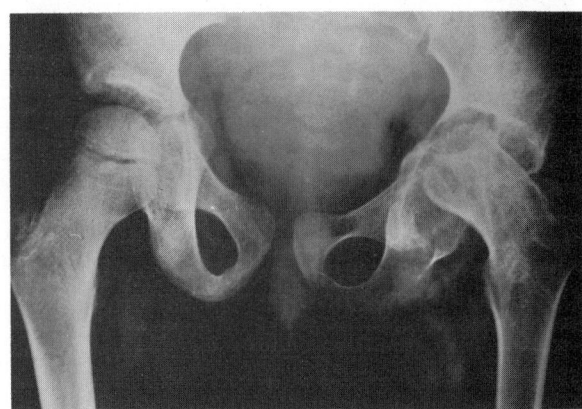

Figure 3. In this case of tuberculosis of the hip joint, the capital femoral epiphysis has been destroyed, probably owing to loss of blood supply. Notice the narrowing of the joint space and osteoporosis of the pelvis and femur on the involved side. There is very little reactive bone formation.

almost always monarticular. The hip joint is most frequently involved.

PATHOLOGIC CONSIDERATIONS. The infiltration of polymorphonuclear neutrophils following inoculation of the joint is similar to that of pyogenic infection elsewhere. The initial irritation of the synovial membrane causes an increased production of synovial fluid and effusion. As neutrophils and bacteria accumulate within the joint, the intra-articular pressure rises. The combination of toxic bacterial products, lysosomal enzymes, and increased pressure produces gradual destruction of the articular cartilage beginning in the weight-bearing portion of the articular surface. If the full thickness of the articular cartilage is destroyed in any area, infection may gain access to the underlying subchondral bone of the epiphysis. Rupture of the joint capsule due to increased pressure allows access to the adjacent soft tissues. The infection may rupture through the overlying skin and form a draining sinus tract.

CLINICAL CONSIDERATIONS. The onset of pyogenic arthritis is acute, with fever, irritability, and pain. In the early stages of infection, a limp may develop, which rapidly progresses to severe pain preventing ambulation. On examination, there is swelling, overlying erythema, and exquisite tenderness to direct palpation or any attempt at joint motion. Careful digital palpation without moving the affected joint aids in distinguishing metaphyseal osteomyelitis from acute pyarthrosis.

Laboratory studies demonstrate elevation of the white count and erythrocyte sedimentation rate. Aspiration of the involved joint under careful sterile conditions reveals a cloudy, turbid synovial fluid with a cell count ranging from 50,000 to 200,000 cells per cubic centimeter. These cells are at least 90 per cent polymorphonuclear neutrophils. The Gram stain shows organisms in approximately 50 per cent of patients. The joint fluid should be retained for aerobic and anaerobic culture. The blood cultures are frequently positive.

In the performance of joint aspiration, a large-bore needle should be used. Small-bore needles may become plugged with edematous synovium or proteinaceous debris within the joint and prevent retrieval of synovial fluid. Care should be exercised to avoid damage to the underlying epiphyseal bone or articular cartilage.

Radiographs in the early stages of septic arthritis reveal no bony change. There is distention of the joint capsule owing to increased pressure within the joint, and an abnormally widened joint space may be observed. In severe cases, there may be pathologic dislocation of the joint. With persistence of the infection in untreated or inadequately treated cases, destruction of the articular cartilage produces eventual narrowing of the joint space.

TREATMENT. Pyogenic arthritis is an emergency condition. When the diagnosis has been established, intravenous antibiotics are administered without awaiting the results of culture. A broad-spectrum antibiotic is selected and may be substituted, depending on the results of subsequent sensitivity testing. Supportive measures include fluid and electrolyte maintenance and the use of antipyretics. The affected joint must be put at rest to prevent further cartilage damage.

If the initial joint aspiration reveals a serosanguineous fluid,

the infection is in its early stages. In this situation, the joint may be irrigated with sterile saline and the patient observed during the first 24 hours of antibiotic therapy. Usually this treatment produces a marked improvement, with a fall in the temperature and diminished local symptoms. Reaspiration of the joint may be performed at intervals to confirm a reduction in the cell count. Repeat cultures are obtained on each aspiration to determine sterility. If improvement fails to occur, surgical incision and drainage of the joint are required.

If the initial joint aspiration produces thick pus, antibiotic therapy alone is unlikely to be adequate. At this stage, there is a thick edematous synovial membrane and a considerable amount of intra-articular necrotic debris, which prevents adequate antibiotic penetration. Surgical incision and drainage should be performed. Some believe that all infections of the hip joint should be drained primarily in addition to antibiotic therapy, since aspiration of the hip joint is difficult and the circulation to the capital femoral epiphysis is threatened by the increased intra-articular pressure. Active and passive joint exercises are initiated as soon as the infection is controlled in order to maintain normal joint function.

NEOPLASMS OF BONE

Primitive mesenchymal tissue produces cartilage, bone, fibrous tissue, and marrow elements, the four basic tissue components of the mature skeleton. From each of these tissue types, there may arise benign or malignant neoplasms. The skeleton may also be the site of neoplasms ordinarily associated with soft tissues. Hemangioma, hemangiosarcoma, lipoma, and liposarcoma may be rare primary bone tumors. Although only primary neoplasms of bone are discussed, metastatic disease from sarcomas and carcinomas to include breast, lung, thyroid, kidney, and prostate are the most common neoplasms to present in bone. The common benign and malignant primary skeletal neoplasms are listed in Table 1.

STAGING. Because the treatment of many skeletal neoplasms may involve radical surgical procedures and/or the use of chemotherapy and irradiation, accurate diagnosis is essential. In order to plan appropriate treatment, *staging* of skeletal lesions is necessary. Accurate determination of the anatomic site and aggressiveness (histologic grade, radiographic appearance) is mandatory.

A careful clinical history, physical examination, and biplane radiographs are the first steps in evaluation. In general, benign bone lesions can be staged by this initial evaluation. Aggressiveness of the lesion is primarily a radiographic assessment. Radionuclide scan, tomography, and computed tomography scanning may be required for accurate anatomic localization. Enneking has described a useful system for staging benign lesions: inactive lesions (Grade 1) tend to remain static or regress; active lesions (Grade 2) have a potential for continued local growth; and aggressive lesions (Grade 3) have a potential for rapid growth and further bone destruction.

Malignant bone lesions require more specific anatomic information; computed tomography scanning, angiography, and radionuclide scan are usually employed. It must be determined

TABLE 1. Common Skeletal Neoplasms

	Cartilage	Bone	Fibrous	Marrow
Benign	Osteochondroma Enchondroma Chondroblastoma	Osteoid osteoma Osteoblastoma	Nonossifying fibroma Giant cell tumor Desmoplastic fibroma	Eosinophilic granuloma
Malignant	Primary chondrosarcoma Secondary chondrosarcoma	Osteosarcoma Periosteal osteosarcoma	Fibrosarcoma Fibrous histiocytoma	Ewing's tumor Lymphoma Myeloma

TABLE 2. Staging Malignant Tumors (Enneking)

	Intracompartmental	Extracompartmental
Low-grade	Stage I, A	Stage I, B
High-grade	Stage II, A	Stage II, B

Stage III: any site, any grade, with metastases.

whether the lesion is restricted to the bone of origin (intracompartmental), whether it has invaded adjacent tissues (extracompartmental), and whether metastases are present. These anatomic data are obtained before biopsy is performed for histologic grading. By the Enneking staging system, intracompartmental lesions are designated by the letter A, extracompartmental lesions by the letter B, low-grade (histologically) by I, and high-grade by II. The Enneking staging system for malignant lesions is depicted in Table 2.

BIOPSY. Biopsy is performed only after anatomic staging is completed. Asymptomatic lesions that are clearly benign by radiographic evaluation may require no treatment. When biopsy of the lesion is required, several considerations should be borne in mind. Many skeletal neoplasms do not have a uniform histologic appearance. The biopsy specimen should therefore be sufficient to obtain representative material for histologic examination. Thus, needle biopsy is employed only in lesions that are difficult to approach surgically. The placement of the biopsy incision should take into consideration the possibility of future resection of the lesion and should allow complete removal of the biopsy site with the specimen. If the lesion is potentially malignant, it is inadvisable to exsanguinate the extremity with an Esmarch bandage before inflating the pneumatic tourniquet. In addition, careful hemostasis before wound closure is mandatory to avoid contamination of adjacent normal tissues by hematoma. The pathologist should be consulted prior to the biopsy and should be present in the operating room at the time of operation. The pathologist is thus aware of both the gross appearance of the lesion and the origin of the biopsy material relative to the radiographs. These procedures aid in making an accurate diagnosis and rendering future treatment.

TREATMENT. Four surgical procedures may be used in treating skeletal neoplasms. *Intralesional* removal involves curettage of the lesion from within. *Local resection* removes the lesion intact through the capsule or reactive tissues surrounding it. *Wide local excision* removes the lesion with a cuff of normal surrounding tissue. *Radical excision* removes the entire anatomic compartment in which the lesion arises and frequently requires amputation.

In general, Grade 1 benign lesions require no treatment if they are asymptomatic and require intralesional removal if they are painful. Grade 2 benign lesions have less likelihood of recurrence with local resection, and Grade 3 benign lesions are more appropriately treated by wide local excision. For malignant lesions, Stage IA lesions are adequately treated with wide local excision, whereas IB, IIA, and IIB lesions usually require radical excision.

TUMORS OF CARTILAGINOUS ORIGIN

Osteochondroma

The osteochondroma is the most common benign neoplasm of bone, composed of normal osseous and cartilaginous tissue, and is considered by some to be a hamartoma and not a true neoplasm. Occurring with equal frequency in males and females, the osteochondroma is usually discovered during the teenage years as a result of local mechanical symptoms. The metaphyseal end of long bones is the most common site, with 50 per cent occurring in the distal femur. Any bone may be involved, including ribs, pelvis, and vertebrae.

The radiographic appearance is that of a bony stalk arising from the metaphysis and usually pointing away from the adja-

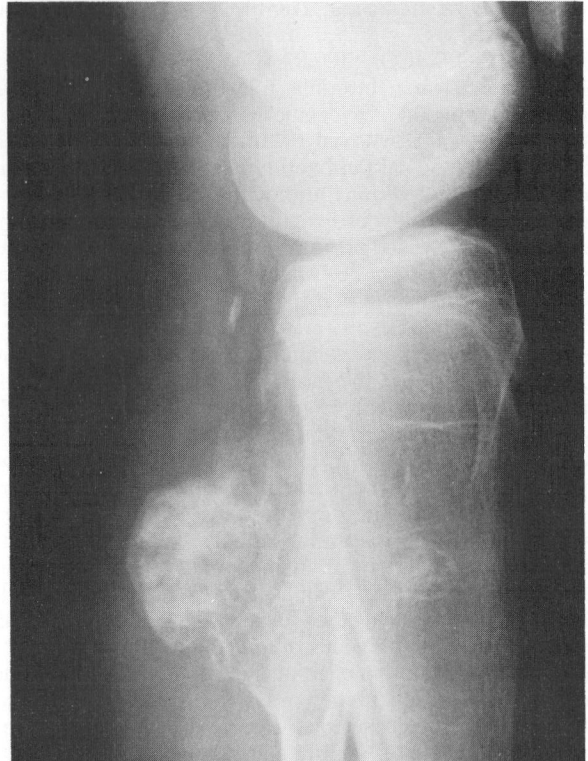

Figure 4. This child has multiple osteochondromatosis. Notice the lobulated bony stalk arising from the posterior portion of the fibula. This stalk is covered by a large cartilaginous cap not seen on radiographic examination.

cent epiphysis (Fig. 4). The end of this stalk is irregular and covered with a cartilaginous cap of varying thickness. Growth of the lesion ceases when growth of the adjacent epiphysis ceases. The bony stalk is in continuity with the underlying cortex of the long bone and is covered by a reflection of periosteum. The stalk may be thin with a pedunculated cartilaginous cap or broad and sessile with the cap closely adherent to the adjacent normal cortex.

Osteochondromas are probably the result of ectopic rests of epiphyseal cartilage. The junction between the cartilaginous cap and the underlying trabecular bone demonstrates endochondral bone formation like the epiphyseal plate, although less orderly. Grossly, the surface is lobulated, pearly white, and opalescent. Overlying the osteochondroma, a bursa is often found. Although osteochondromas are usually solitary, multiple osteochondromatosis is recognized as a familial disease.

The treatment of an osteochondroma depends on symptoms. If a lesion is producing mechanical difficulty adjacent to a joint, excision is indicated. As Grade 2 lesions, they may be cured by excision flush with the cortex of the underlying bone, with care taken to remove the periosteal envelope surrounding the bony stalk (local resection).

Malignant degeneration of osteochondromas may occur rarely in solitary osteochondromas and more frequently in multiple osteochondromas. Those lesions closer to the midline of the body (scapula and pelvis) are statistically more likely to undergo malignant degeneration. Evidence of growth of an osteochondroma (solitary or multiple lesions) after epiphyseal closure of the bone involved is an indication for removal. Malignant degeneration in these lesions occurs in the cartilaginous cap, and chondrosarcoma results. For this reason, careful radiographic follow-up of known osteochondromas is indicated.

Enchondroma

The enchondroma is a benign growth of hyaline cartilage within the medullary cavity of a bone. Like the osteochondroma, the lesion is considered to arise from ectopic cartilagi-

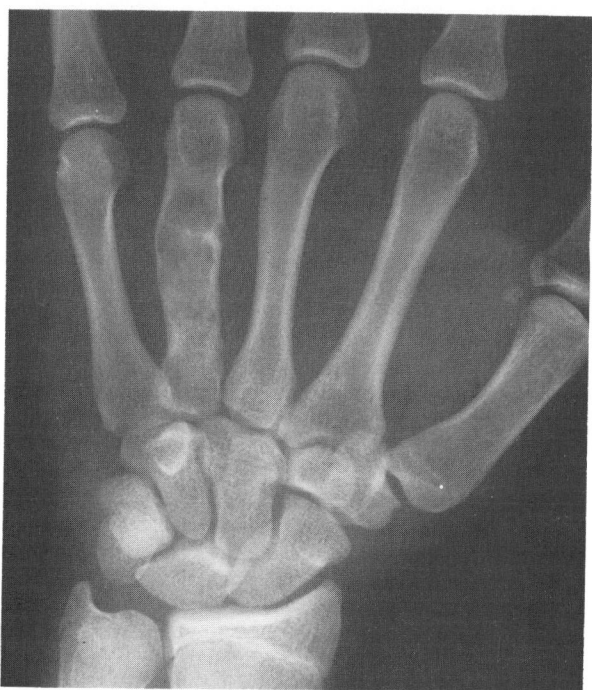

Figure 5. The lesion in the fourth metacarpal has expanded and thinned the overlying cortex. There is stippled calcification within the center of the lesion. This enchondroma was cured by curettage and bone grafting.

nous rests. Enchondromas have an equal gender distribution and most often occur in the phalanges, metacarpals, and metatarsals. They may appear in other long bones and in the pelvis, scapula, and ribs. Often they are discovered incidentally when radiographs are obtained for other reasons. When symptomatic, they present either as swelling of the bone involved, with mild tenderness, or as a pathologic fracture through an existing lesion.

Radiographically, the enchondroma produces a lucent defect, usually in the metaphyseal region of a long bone. The margins of the lesion are well defined, with sclerotic reactive bone (Fig. 5). The overlying cortex may be expanded and thinned. Varying degrees of stippled calcification may appear within the lesion.

Grossly an enchondroma is blue-white and translucent. On microscopic examination, lobules of hyaline cartilage with a mild degree of cellular atypia and a slight increase in cellularity compared with normal hyaline cartilage are observed.

The enchondroma, like the osteochondroma, has a malignant potential for degeneration to chondrosarcoma. Because these lesions are usually asymptomatic, any clinical evidence of recent growth or pain should raise suspicion of malignant degeneration. Radiographic evidence of erosion through the cortex by an enchondroma is a sign of malignant behavior.

Enchondromas may occur as multiple lesions in the same patient (Ollier's disease) and may be associated with multiple cavernous hemangiomas (Maffucci's syndrome). In multiple enchondromatosis, growth disturbance in early childhood may be the first manifestation of the disease. Distortion in both length growth and angular growth may be observed.

The likelihood of malignant degeneration in multiple enchondromatosis is higher than for the solitary lesion. Lesions located centrally (pelvis, scapulae, spine) are more likely to become malignant. Regular radiographic survey in patients with multiple lesions is required. For the symptomatic benign enchondroma, curettage and bone grafting are the treatments of choice. The rate of recurrence is low with adequate curettage.

Chondroblastoma

The chondroblastoma is a benign lesion of cartilaginous origin first identified as a separate entity in 1931 by Codman. Prior

to that time, it had been grouped with giant cell tumors of bone. The chondroblastoma occurs in the epiphyses of long bones, usually in the second decade of life, and is more frequent in males (2:1). The symptoms are variable but usually consist of the insidious onset of aching pain, usually at night, referred to the joint adjacent to the lesion. There may be some limitation of motion, mild effusion of the joint, and synovial thickening.

The radiographic appearance of this lesion is characteristic. Eccentrically placed within the epiphysis, it has a smooth border with only a slight sclerotic margin and may have central areas of stippling that represent calcification within the substance of the tumor. There may be involvement of the physeal plate and metaphysis adjacent to the lesion (Fig. 6). Grossly these lesions are gray to gray-yellow and gritty to the touch as a result of calcification. The articular surface of the adjacent joint may be penetrated by the tumor mass.

Histologically these lesions are highly cellular. The primary cell is usually described as polygonal in shape, with oval to round nuclei. In numerous areas of the tumor, these cells produce a chondroid matrix. Multinucleated giant cells can be found throughout the lesion and are usually in the more cellular areas of the tumor. Hypercellularity often leads to a mistaken diagnosis of malignancy, particularly chondrosarcoma. Reactive bone may be found in the periphery of these tumors, leading to the mistaken diagnosis of osteosarcoma. Areas of focal calcification may be observed throughout the tumor, particularly in areas where a rich chondroid matrix has been deposited.

Although generally considered a benign tumor, the chondroblastoma may behave aggressively (Grade 3), occasionally penetrating the joint surface or the cortex of the bone involved and invading the adjacent soft tissues. There are scattered reports of pulmonary metastases from chondroblastoma.

Conservative treatment in the form of curettage and bone grafting is indicated in less aggressive (Grade 2) lesions. Care must be taken to preserve the adjacent articular cartilage. When the epiphyseal plate is involved, epiphysiodesis may be required. Grade 3 lesions may require wide local excision. Irradiation has not proved beneficial.

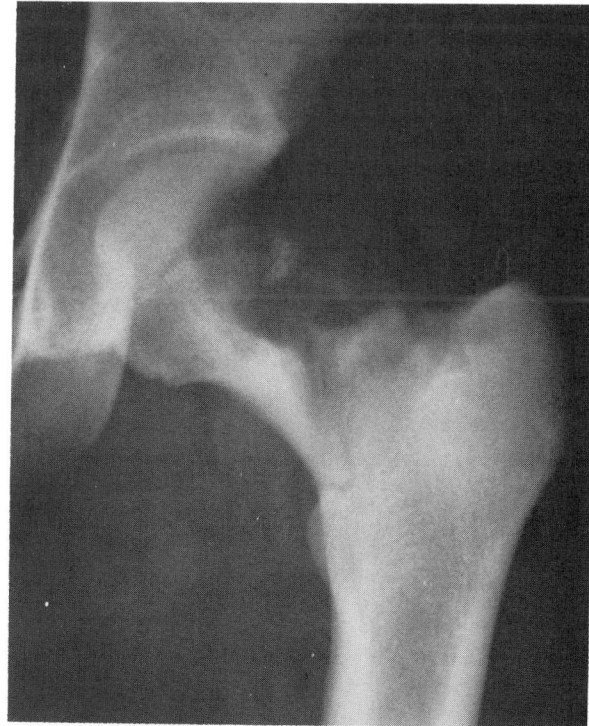

Figure 6. This rather aggressive chondroblastoma began in the epiphysis and subsequently has involved the superior femoral neck. Note the lack of sclerotic borders to the lesion. A pathologic fracture has occurred through the femoral calcar.

Chondrosarcoma

Malignant cartilaginous tumors may arise from pre-existing benign neoplasms of bone (secondary chondrosarcoma) or may arise *de novo* in bone (primary chondrosarcomas) and are the third most common primary malignant neoplasm of bone. The majority of chondrosarcomas are thought to be primary rather than secondary.

Chondrosarcoma demonstrates a slight male predominance and occurs most frequently in the fourth to sixth decades of life. In contrast to other malignant neoplasms of bone, which tend to occur in the peripheral skeleton, chondrosarcoma is most frequently encountered in the central flat bones (pelvis, scapula, sacrum), although any bone may be involved. Rarely are these tumors found in the small bones of the hand or foot or in the facial bones. The chondrosarcoma grows slowly, and patients with tumors of the extremity usually present with a history of local pain and swelling about the lesion that may have been present for months or years. Tumors within the pelvis grow silently without symptoms for a considerable period of time unless located near sensitive structures such as the sciatic or femoral nerves. There are no specific laboratory data that aid in the diagnosis of chondrosarcoma.

Radiographically this tumor demonstrates calcification occurring within the body of the tumor outlining a lobulated pattern. Calcification may be sparse and peripherally located or may be dense enough to obliterate the surrounding bone detail. Heavily calcified lesions are more differentiated. Poorly differentiated, more aggressive lesions tend to demonstrate less calcification and, when located centrally or within the pelvis, may be difficult to diagnose radiographically. Arteriography and computed tomography scanning are helpful in evaluating pelvic lesions, more for the anatomic information that they provide about the location of the tumor relative to other structures than for any specific information about malignancy. More aggressive tumors tend to be more vascular (Fig. 7).

On gross examination, the surface of a chondrosarcoma has a lobulated, cauliflower-like appearance. Malignant behavior is typified by invasion of adjacent muscles and entrapment of muscle fibers between lobules of tumor. Outgrowths of tumor may extend for some distance along a fascial plane. When previous needle biopsy has been performed, tumor may be found growing up the needle tract to the surface of the skin. On cut section, the surface is pearly white and opalescent. There may be areas of degeneration and liquefaction within the center of the tumor. Areas of calcification appear as dense, chalk-white areas on the cut surface.

The histologic appearance of the chondosarcoma is variable. Some lesions demonstrate well-differentiated hyaline cartilage with minimal cellular atypia, and the diagnosis of malignancy may be difficult. The radiographic appearance, the gross appearance, and the clinical behavior of the tumor must be considered in making the diagnosis. In lesions less well differentiated, the usual characteristics of malignancy appear. Variations in nuclear size and shape, hypercellularity, multiple nuclei per cartilaginous lacunae, and mitotic figures are seen. In some areas, reactive bone formation is encountered. It is important to determine whether this represents malignant bone formation or reactive bone formation, because the former implies a diagnosis of osteosarcoma with a more grave prognosis.

Most chondrosarcomas present as Stage IA lesions, and wide local excision is the treatment of choice. Because this tumor has a high incidence of local recurrence, meticulous technique should be used to avoid contamination of the operative field. Stage IB lesions may require amputation, which should include total removal of any previous biopsy site. Any biopsy of a suspected chondrosarcoma should be planned in such a way that the biopsy incision can be removed with subsequent definitive surgical therapy.

TUMORS OF OSSEOUS ORIGIN

Osteoid Osteoma

This benign Grade 1 lesion of bone was described by Jaffe in 1935 and is considered by some to be an inflammatory lesion. Most observers believe that this is a true benign neoplasm of bone. The osteoid osteoma is a solitary, exquisitely painful lesion. Bones of the lower extremity are most frequently affected, although almost any bone may be involved. This tumor generally occurs in the first and second decades of life and is more common in males.

The most common presenting symptom is pain, which may be described as mild to intense. The pain is of a persistent nature that is neither accentuated by activity nor relieved by rest or immobilization. Often the pain is totally relieved by the use of aspirin. In some patients, the pain may be increased by the use of alcohol.

Because these lesions are small and sometimes difficult to demonstrate on radiographs, many patients have consulted several doctors and are thought to have an emotional problem rather than true physical complaints. Also, these lesions may sometimes mimic other diseases. Osteoid osteomas of the vertebral arch may simulate intervertebral disc disease, including radiating leg pain.

The radiographic appearance of the osteoid osteoma depends on the location. When these lesions are located in cancellous bone, they present as a central radiolucent defect surrounded by a dense cloud of sclerotic bone. In lesions of long standing, the sclerosis may obscure the radiolucent center, or nidus, on routine films. Tomography may be required to identify the lesion. The osteoid osteoma may also be located in cortical bone. In this position, it produces thickening of the cortex, again with a radiolucent nidus.

The microscopic appearance of the osteoid osteoma is characteristic. Peripherally there is dense reactive new bone formation. The central nidus is composed of a fine network of close-packed trabeculae of partially mineralized osteoid. The surfaces of these trabeculae are usually lined with benign osteoblasts. In older lesions, mineralization of the nidus may be observed and usually begins centrally. The nidus is vascular, with numerous small capillary channels. Nerve endings have been demonstrated within the nidus.

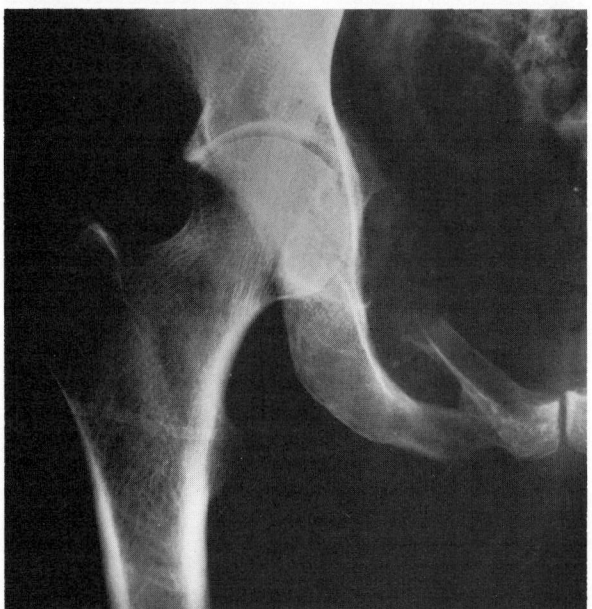

Figure 7. Chondrosarcoma. This lytic lesion has destroyed the pubic ramus from the level of the acetabulum to the midportion of the obturator foramen. There is minor stippling within the defect. This lesion was an aggressive chondrosarcoma.

The osteoid osteoma is completely cured by *en bloc* excision, which allows identification of the lesion and ensures complete removal. Because these lesions are small, radiographic control in the operating room may be required to ensure proper localization. In some locations, *en bloc* excision may not be feasible and curettage is necessary. Incompletely curetted lesions may recur.

Osteosarcoma

With the exception of multiple myeloma, osteosarcoma is the most common malignant primary neoplasm of bone. This tumor occurs with a frequency of approximately 1 in 100,000, or about 2000 cases per year in the United States. Osteosarcoma usually affects those in the second decade of life (mean age 15 years). Occurrence is in the metaphyseal ends of long bone; the distal femur is the most frequent site (30 per cent), followed by the proximal tibia and proximal humerus in that order. Any bone may be involved.

The most common presenting symptom is pain at the site of the tumor, which has been present for 1 or 2 months. There may be local swelling and some increased heat in the area. When the tumor is near a joint, there may be limitation of motion. A small percentage of patients present with a pathologic fracture as their initial complaint.

Radiographically there are areas of new bone formation and areas of lytic destruction. Within the metaphysis of a long bone, this tumor classically produces a "sunburst" appearance, which consists of trabeculae of bone oriented at right angles to the cortical surface beneath the periosteum. These trabeculae are mixed reactive and malignant bone. Some tumors may be almost purely lytic in nature, whereas others may produce abundant amounts of both malignant bone and surrounding reactive bone (Fig. 8).

On histologic examination, a disorderly deposition of osteoid surrounded by malignant osteoblasts is observed. Nuclear atypia and bizarre mitoses are noted. In addition to malignant bone, there may be areas of malignant cartilage and fibrous tissue. Despite the amount of these tissues present, if malignant bone is being produced, the lesion should be classified as an osteosarcoma.

The treatment of osteosarcoma has traditionally been amputation of the limb at a level above the tumor. It has been recognized that osteosarcoma may produce satellite lesions within the medullary canal of the bone involved proximal to the major lesion. These "skip lesions" are usually not seen on radiographs and are discovered only on pathologic examination of the specimen. For this reason, many believe that amputation should be performed through the joint above the bone involved. Others have followed the practice of amputation through the bone involved at a level proximal to the tumor. Although the incidence of skip lesions varies in different reports from 5 to 25 per cent, the overall survival figures for patients treated by disarticulation above the bone involved versus amputation through the bone involved do not vary significantly.

Older studies report a 5-year survival of 20 per cent with amputation. More recent figures have shown an increase in survival, which may be related to more sensitive techniques of detecting pulmonary metastases. Survival has not been improved by preamputation radiation.

With amputation as the only treatment, the average length of time between diagnosis and the development of pulmonary metastases is 6 months. The average length of time between diagnosis and death from metastases is 1 year. Approximately 80 per cent of those patients who die of their metastases do so within the first 2 years following diagnosis. Because osteosarcoma is known to invade blood vessels early in the course of development, it is assumed that pulmonary microemboli are already present at the time of diagnosis. It would further appear

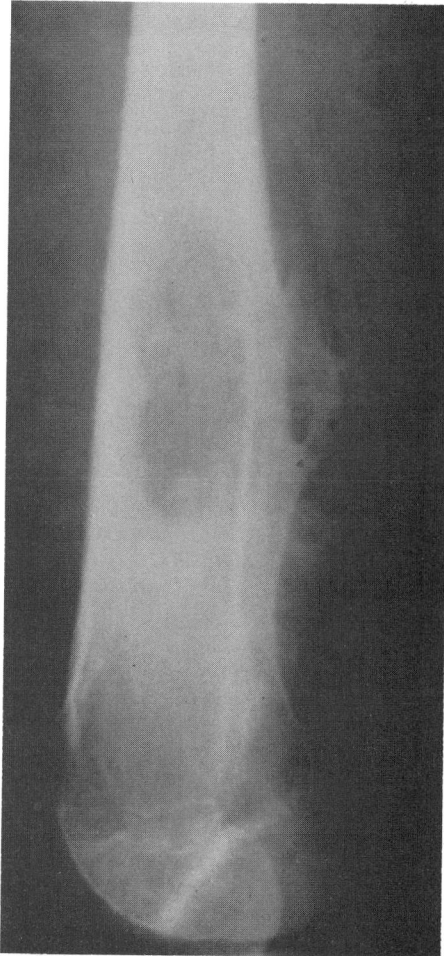

Figure 8. This lateral radiograph of the distal femur of a 14-year-old girl shows a central radiolucent defect in the femoral metaphysis, with periosteal elevation overlying the lesion. There has been erosion through the femoral cortex. Notice the "sunburst" appearance of the subperiosteal new bone along the posterior femoral cortex. This is the typical appearance of an osteosarcoma.

that approximately 20 per cent of patients have some innate resistance to their tumor or that their tumor is less virulent.

In recent years, adjunctive chemotherapy has been used as a means of treatment. Adriamycin, high-dose methotrexate, and *cis*-platinum have shown definite effects in the treatment of osteosarcoma. When these are used in combination with definitive surgical therapy, most current studies report a 50 per cent 5-year disease-free survival. Although initial protocols using adjunctive chemotherapy continue to use radical resection (amputation), the effect of presurgical chemotherapy on these lesions has led to a recent interest in limb salvage surgery (wide local excision) for these patients with similarly reported survival rates when compared with amputation. Pulmonary metastases tend to occur later and in fewer numbers in those patients treated with chemotherapy. Resection of pulmonary metastases has prolonged life in some patients, and, in a smaller number, it has apparently eradicated the disease.

TUMORS OF FIBROUS ORIGIN

Nonossifying Fibroma

This lesion is most likely not a true neoplasm but a focal developmental defect. Occurring primarily in children and located in the metaphysis of long bones, this lesion is also known as a benign metaphyseal cortical defect or fibrous cortical defect. These lesions are usually an incidental finding on radiographs obtained for other reasons. Rarely, they may be large

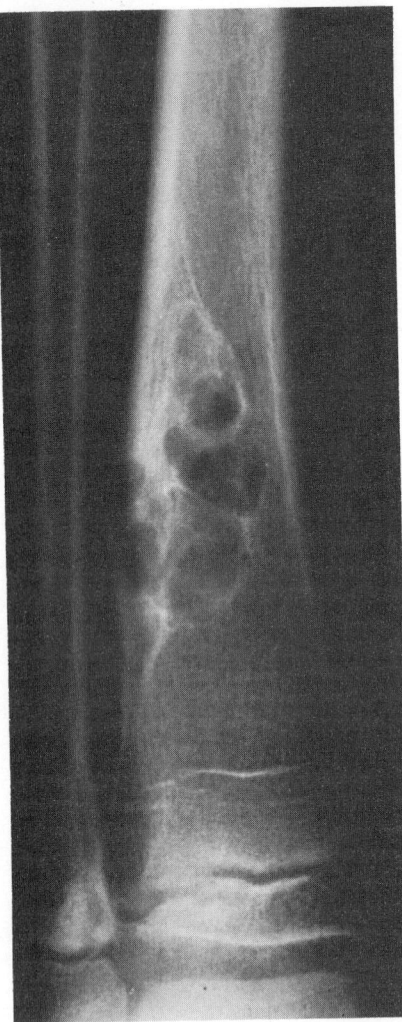

Figure 9. This eccentrically located metaphyseal lesion has smooth sclerotic borders on the medullary side and has expanded the overlying cortex. This appearance is typical of a nonossifying fibroma.

all other skeletal neoplasms. The presence of a radiolucent defect in an epiphysis strongly suggests the diagnosis of giant cell tumor. Beyond this, the appearance of this lesion may vary considerably. In slowly growing, less aggressive forms, the lesion presents as a radiolucent defect, usually eccentrically located within the bone involved with thinning and expansion of the overlying cortex. Thin bony septa within the center of the lesion produce a loculated appearance. There is usually extension into the adjacent metaphysis. In more aggressive tumors, rapid growth of the lesion may produce a poorly demarcated edge with little sclerotic bone peripherally. There may be penetration of the overlying cortex, with extension of tumor into the adjacent soft tissues.

Grossly, the tumor is red-gray in appearance with areas of soft yellow material representing lipid deposits and areas of brown-stained tissue indicating local hemorrhage. There may be areas of cystic degeneration.

It is the microscopic appearance of this tumor from which the name is derived. Numerous multinucleated giant cells are found within a fibrous stroma. Focal areas of hemorrhage and collections of lipid-filled histiocytes are seen. Reactive bone formation within the lesion (which produces the septa seen on radiographs) is common and must not be mistaken for malignant bone formation, leading to the erroneous diagnosis of osteosarcoma.

Approximately 10 per cent of giant cell tumors behave in a malignant manner. Within the basic histologic definition of this lesion, there may be considerable variation. Efforts have been made to grade this tumor on the basis of its fibrous stroma and on the number of giant cells present. In general, those tumors with poorly differentiated fibrous stroma have a higher likelihood of local recurrence and pulmonary metastasis than well-differentiated tumors, although the latter may occasionally show malignant behavior. Because the histologic appearance may vary from area to area within the same tumor, extensive sampling of the lesion is necessary and needle biopsy of the lesion is discouraged.

Curettage and bone grafting of this Grade 3 lesion cause a 20 to 40 per cent recurrence rate. When feasible, wide local resection of the tumor and bone grafting are desirable. There is no evidence that irradiation is of any therapeutic benefit. There is some evidence to suggest that irradiation may induce malignant change within these lesions. Recurrent, locally aggressive lesions may require amputation.

Fibrosarcoma

Fibrous tissue within the marrow cavity may produce primary fibrosarcoma of bone. This uncommon skeletal neoplasm is seen most frequently in the lower extremities (50 per cent), although almost any bone may be involved. There is a wide age distribution of this lesion, with the highest incidence in the third and fourth decades of life. Symptoms vary according to the location of the lesion and rate of growth.

Fibrosarcoma produces a variety of patterns radiographically, all of which basically involve destruction of bone. The lesion may be well circumscribed within the metaphysis, with thinning or penetration of the overlying cortex. If the growth is slow, there may be a thin sclerotic border. With more rapid growth, the border is usually ill-defined. In contrast to this "geographic" pattern of growth, this tumor may have radiographic signs of mottled destruction from permeative growth within the bone.

The microscopic appearance of bone is similar to that of its soft tissue counterpart. Malignant fibroblasts of varying degree of differentiation are observed. Multinucleated giant cells are present in some tumors. It may be difficult to distinguish this tumor from malignant fibrous histiocytoma. Many previously classified fibrosarcomas were probably malignant fibrous histiocytomas.

Fibrosarcomas are usually Stage IA lesions. Wide local exci-

enough to create pathologic fracture. The nonossifying fibroma occurs with equal frequency in males and females. The lower extremities are most often involved, and there may be multiple lesions.

The nonossifying fibroma is located eccentrically in the metaphysis of a long bone lying immediately beneath the cortex, which may be somewhat thinned. There is a distinct sclerotic margin to the intramedullary portion of the lesion. The central portion is relatively radiolucent and appears to be divided by bony septa (Fig. 9).

Grossly, the contents of a nonossifying fibroma are soft and yellow to brown. On histologic examination, swirls of fibrous tissue containing numerous multinucleated giant cells and lipid-filled histiocytes are observed. In lesions of considerable age, cholesterol clefts may be seen.

The natural history of the nonossifying fibroma is one of gradual healing as the patient matures (Grade 1). There is no indication for surgical therapy unless the lesion is demonstrated to be increasing in size and threatening to produce a pathologic fracture. Curettage and bone grafting are curative.

Giant Cell Tumor

This uncommon neoplasm arises in the third and fourth decades of life and is almost invariably found in the epiphyses of long bones, with subsequent involvement of the adjacent metaphysis. This anatomic location helps distinguish it from almost

sion is therefore the treatment of choice. When these lesions have violated the anatomic compartment and become Stage IB lesions, amputation may be required. Radiation therapy has not proved to be of benefit.

TUMORS OF MARROW CELL ORIGIN

Ewing's Sarcoma

This fortunately uncommon malignancy occurs most frequently in the first and second decades of life. It is included here as a tumor of marrow cell origin, although some believe that it arises from endothelial cells. Although almost any bone may be involved, long bones of the extremities are the most frequent site of Ewing's sarcoma.

Patient's present with complaints of local pain and swelling in the region of the tumor. There may be fever, leukocytosis, and an increased erythrocyte sedimentation rate. These findings, together with the early radiographic appearance of Ewing's sarcoma, may lead to a mistaken diagnosis of osteomyelitis. In some cases, the onset is less abrupt, and patients may present with a large local tumor mass that has been present for many months.

The radiographic appearance of Ewing's sarcoma in the diaphysis of a long bone is one of periosteal elevation or "onionskin" appearance as a result of permeation of the cortex by tumor. In this respect, the lesion may resemble osteomyelitis. In other locations, the radiographic changes are less distinct. In general, this tumor produces bone destruction of varying degrees. The changes may be slight, suggesting chondrosarcoma, or may be extensive and rapid, suggesting an osteolytic osteosarcoma. Grossly the tumor may be partially necrotic, resembling purulent exudate. Areas of hemorrhage may be seen. Microscopically the tumor is composed of uniform round cells gathered in nests or cords and separated by fibrous septa. They have a hazy appearance and indistinct cytoplasmic borders. Difficulty may arise in distinguishing this tumor from metastatic neuroblastoma, reticulum cell sarcoma of bone, and infection.

Histochemical staining for glycogen may aid in the differential diagnosis. Some Ewing's sarcomas contain glycogen on PAS staining or on electron microscopic examination, whereas glycogen is absent in reticulum cell sarcoma.

The 5-year survival rate for patients with Ewing's sarcoma treated by amputation of the limb involved is less than 10 per cent. At present, radiation therapy to the entire bone involved combined with chemotherapy has produced longer disease-free periods and higher survival rates.

Myeloma

This malignant neoplasm of marrow cell origin is the most common primary malignant neoplasm of bone. It is most often seen in the late decades of life and more frequently in males than in females. The disease may vary from a solitary lesion to widespread skeletal involvement.

The symptoms vary from local pain and discomfort to systemic symptoms of anemia, fever, hypercalcemia, and renal failure related to the extensive skeletal involvement and the abnormal production of immunoglobulins.

This neoplasm characteristically produces lytic destruction of bone. Usually there is a "punched-out" lesion with little or no accompanying sclerosis. The absence of reactive bone formation is borne out by the observation that the lesions of myeloma are often silent on a bone scan. Pathologic fracture may be seen as an initial finding.

The diagnosis of myeloma is made by marrow aspiration and the demonstration of abnormal plasma cells. In patients with disseminated disease, Bence Jones protein may be found in the urine in approximately 50 per cent. Serum electrophoresis demonstrates an abnormal amount of globulins. Urine electrophoresis is also helpful when the diagnosis is in doubt and may demonstrate abnormal proteins in patients with a normal serum electrophoretic pattern.

Microscopically, myeloma produces sheets of plasma cells. Usually these are fairly well-differentiated cells in which the eccentric nucleus and peripheral arrangement of chromatin within the nucleus can be identified. The more undifferentiated lesions may present a diagnostic problem in which the accessory laboratory data are helpful. With the exception of biopsy for diagnosis or the treatment of pathologic fracture, the treatment of myeloma is nonsurgical. Chemotherapy is the treatment of choice.

REFERENCES

1. Aegerter, E., and Kirkpatrick, J. A., Jr.: Orthopedic Diseases: Physiology, Pathology, Radiology, 4th ed. Philadelphia, W. B. Saunders Company, 1975.
2. Allen, A. R., and Stevenson, A. W.: A ten-year follow-up of combined drug therapy and early fusion in bone tuberculosis. J. Bone Joint Surg. [Am], 49:1001, 1967.
3. Barnes, R., and Catto, M.: Chondrosarcoma of bone. J. Bone Joint Surg. [Br], 48:729, 1966.
4. Boland, A. L.: Acute hematogenous osteomyelitis. Orthop. Clin. North Am., 3:275, 1972.
5. Clowson, D. K., and Dunn, A. W.: Management of common bacterial infections of bones and joints. J. Bone Joint Surg. [Am], 49:164, 1967.
6. Dahlin, D. C.: Bone Tumors, 3rd ed. Springfield, Ill., Charles C Thomas, 1978.
7. Dahlin, D. C., and Coventry, M. D.: Osteogenic sarcoma. A study of 600 cases. J. Bone Joint Surg. [Am], 49:101, 1967.
8. Dahlin, D. C., and Henderson, E. D.: Chondrosarcoma, a surgical and pathological problem. Review of 212 cases. J. Bone Joint Surg. [Am], 38:1025, 1956.
9. Dahlin, D. C., Cupps, R. E., and Johnson, E. W.: Giant cell tumor: A study of 195 cases. Cancer, 25:1061, 1970.
10. Enneking, W. F.: Principles of musculoskeletal pathology. Gainesville, Florida, W. F. Enneking, M. D., 1970.
11. Enneking, W. F.: Musculoskeletal Tumor Surgery. New York, Churchill Livingstone, 1983.
12. Enneking, W. F., and Springfield, D. S.: Osteosarcoma. Orthop. Clin. North Am., 8:785, 1977.
13. Hustu, H. O., Pinkel, D., and Pratt, C. B.: Treatment of clinically localized Ewing's sarcoma with radiotherapy and combination chemotherapy. Cancer, 30:1522, 1972.
14. Jaffe, H. L.: Metabolic, Generative, and Inflammatory Diseases of Bones and Joints. Philadelphia, Lea & Febiger, 1972.
15. Jaffe, H. L.: Tumors and Tumorous Conditions of the Bones and Joints, 2nd ed. Philadelphia, Lea & Febiger, 1961.
16. Jaffe, N.: Recent advances in the chemotherapy of metastatic osteosarcoma. Cancer, 30:1627, 1972.
17. Kelly, P. J., and Karlson, A. G.: Musculoskeletal tuberculosis. Mayo Clin. Proc., 44:73, 1969.
18. Marcove, R. C.: Chondrosarcoma: Diagnosis and treatment. Orthop. Clin. North Am., 8:811, 1977.
19. Morrey, B. F., and Peterson, H. A.: Hematogenous pyogenic osteomyelitis in children. Orthop. Clin. North Am., 6:935, 1975.
20. Morton, D. L.: Immunological aspects of neoplasia: A rational basis for immunotherapy. Ann. Intern. Med., 74:587, 1971.
21. Pritchard, D. J.: Granulomatous infections of bones and joints. Orthop. Clin. North Am., 6:1029, 1975.
22. Rhodes, K. H.: Antibiotic management of acute osteomyelitis and septic arthritis in children. Orthop. Clin. North Am., 6:915, 1975.
23. Rosen, G., Suwansirikul, S., et al.: High-dose methotrexate with citrovorum factor rescue and Adriamycin in childhood osteogenic sarcoma. Cancer, 33:1151, 1974.
24. Spjut, H. J., Dorfman, H. D., Fechner, M. D., and Akerman, L. V.: Tumors of Bone and Cartilage. Fasc. 5, 2nd ser. Washington, D.C., Armed Forces Institute of Pathology, 1971.
25. Stetson, J. W., DePone, R. J., and Southwick, W. O.: Acute septic arthritis of the hip in children. Clin. Orthop., 56:105, 1968.
26. Sweetnam, R., Knowelden, J., and Seddon, H.: Bone sarcoma—treatment by irradiation, amputation, or a combination of the two. Br. Med. J., 2:363, 1971.
27. Tachdjian, M. O.: Pediatric Orthopedics. Philadelphia, W. B. Saunders Company, 1972.
28. Waldvogel, F. A., Medoff, G., and Schwartz, M. N.: Osteomyelitis: A review of clinical features, therapeutic considerations, and unusual aspects. N. Engl. J. Med., 282:198, 260, 316, 1970.

X _____

THE HAND

1. TENDON INJURY AND REPAIR

*James A. Nunley, M.D., and
J. Leonard Goldner, M.D.*

Tendon continuity is necessary for transmission of force from the muscle bellies to the hand or digits. Each muscle tendon unit has a vascular supply, a nerve supply, and a gliding mechanism, all of which ensure good nutrition and smooth activity. Disruption of a tendon causes loss of motion of the digit and diminished grip or pinch. The severity of tendon injury varies according to the location of the loss of continuity, the mechanism of injury, the conditions that exist at the time of the injury, the particular tendon involved, and the anatomic location of the laceration in relationship to the muscle-tendon unit. A tendon laceration directly over a joint is more serious than is an injury at the musculotendinous junction. Maximal tendon function requires full-thickness skin coverage, epitenon and peritenon to protect the tendon from surrounding adhesions, and muscle bellies of adequate strength.

BIOMECHANICS OF HEALING TENDONS

The strength-duration curve shows that tendon healing is weak at 21 days but of sufficient strength to tolerate active contraction of the muscle. At 3 weeks, external elastic traction can be applied if the force is not excessive. At 3 months, moderate stress can be applied to the flexor tendon in both flexion and extension. At 8 months, full tensile strength has been recovered. The healing tendon forms a strong bond as fibroblasts realign, collagen matrices unite, blood vessels invade the area of healing, and fibroblasts migrate from the periphery to the centrum in order to establish a bond. The peripheral covering adheres to the tendon throughout its entire length early during the period of healing. A tenoma is formed, and this gradually matures. The degree of shortening or lengthening of the tendon should be within the limits of the tension-strength curve. If the tendon is shortened, too much stretch is applied to the muscle mass, and maximal strength is not obtained. A contracture results.

CLASSIFICATION OF TENDON INJURIES

In order to clarify the results of tendon repair, it is necessary to define the different anatomic regions of the flexor tendon so that injuries in different locations are readily compared.[1,2] The flexor system of the digits consists of two tendons for each finger and one for the thumb. The muscle bellies of these tendons originate from the distal humerus and the proximal ulna. The musculotendinous junction is located in the distal portion of the forearm from which the tendons pass to the wrist, through the carpal canal, and into the hand and digits. The flexor digitorum superficialis divides into two tendon slips within the palm and inserts on the middle phalanx of each digit. The flexor superficialis is intimately associated with the flexor profundus tendon. The flexor digitorum profundus and the flexor pollicis longus tendons insert on the base of the distal phalanges of the fingers and the thumb, respectively.

Zone System for Defining Tendon Injuries

The modified Verdan Zone System divides the entire length of the flexor tendons into five anatomic areas (Fig. 1).[10] Zone I extends from the flexor superficialis insertion to the tip of the finger and involves only the flexor digitorum profundus. The skin laceration may lie anywhere distal to the mid-finger crease. Zone II, which Bunnell termed "no man's land," begins proximal to the metacarpophalangeal joint and extends to the mid-portion of the middle phalanx. This corresponds to the distal palmar crease and the mid-finger crease. In this location, there are two flexor tendons tightly enclosed within an unyielding fibro-osseous canal, which is critical to the mechanical function of these tendons. Zone III extends from the base of the palm or the distal end of the transverse retinacular ligament to the transverse crease in the palm. In this location, the lumbrical muscle belly is firmly attached to the flexor digitorum profundus, and both lie deep to the flexor digitorum superficialis. Zone IV extends from the distal end of the transverse retinacular ligament to the proximal margin. The lumbrical muscle belly thins out in this location, and the flexor tendons to the fingers and the one to the thumb make a compact mass of collagen over which the median nerve passes. Zone V extends from the proximal transverse carpal ligament at the wrist to the musculotendinous junction of the flexor tendons in the distal third of the forearm. When correlating injury to end result, the most critical zone is Zone II.[3]

Flexor Retinaculum and Vincular Systems of Flexor Tendons

The complexity of early repair or late reconstruction of lacerated flexor tendons is best understood by having familiarity with the gliding and flexor retinaculum system and the intrica-

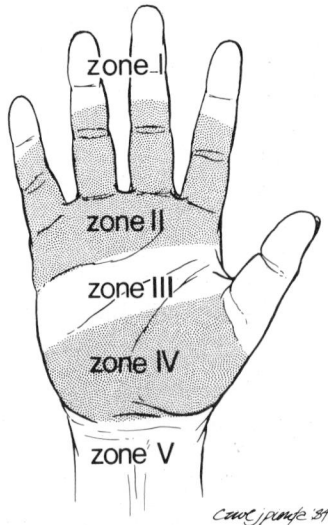

Figure 1. The hand zones are important in differentiating one tendon laceration from another and in determining how to treat single or double tendon lacerations that occur in the different zones. The annular ligaments vary according to the zones. They are most important in effecting postoperative function in Zone II. Zone I includes only the insertions of the flexor digitorum profundus, and Zone V contains median and ulnar nerves, median and ulnar arteries, the wrist flexor tendons, and all of the flexor digitorum profundus and flexor digitorum superficialis tendons.

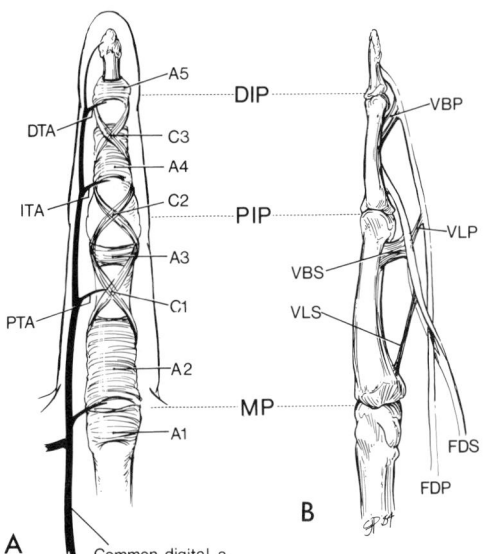

Figure 2. A, The annular ligaments covering the flexor tendons are represented by A1 – A2 as the proximal pulley. The A3 pulley is opposite the distal end of the proximal phalanx, and the A4 pulley is opposite the middle of the middle phalanx. The A2 and A4 pulleys are essential. The cruciate ligaments are thin and fill the intervals between the heavier annular ligaments. The blood supply from the common digital arteries sends branches to the vincula, which at each level supply major segments of the tendon. B, The lateral diagram shows the long and short vincula, VL and VB, and the flexor tendons and the relationship between vincula, the flexor tendons, and the adjacent joints. Function of the joints depends on the intact annular ligaments. DTA, distal tendon artery; PTA, proximal tendon artery; ITA, intermediate tendon artery; VBP, vincula brevis profundus; VBS, vincula brevis superficialis; VLP, vincula longus profundus; FDS, flexor digitorum superficialis; FDP, flexor digitorum profundus; VLS, vincula longus superficialis; A5, pulley annular ligament.

cies of blood supply as well as a knowledge of the biologic method of healing.

The flexor retinaculum system consists of a firm fibrous sheath lined by synovium that holds the flexor tendons close to bone. This strong constraint provides a straight mechanical advantage so that a large arc of motion occurs for a relatively small applied force. The entire digital sheath includes annular and cruciate ligaments that act as pulleys. The heavy annular ligaments are thicker and stronger than the thinner cruciate pulleys. Anatomic dissections have shown that preservation of the A2 and A4 pulleys is necessary for complete tendon excursion (Fig. 2).[3]

TENDON VASCULAR SUPPLY AND NUTRITION

Much information is available about the nutrition of flexor tendons. The vascular anatomy shows that each tendon receives its blood supply from segmental vessels arising from the surrounding peritenon and extending from the forearm to the midportion of the proximal phalanx. In the digits, however, blood supply reaches the flexor tendons through the vincula.[8] These are folds of mesotenon through which course the small vessels that penetrate the tendons. One short and one long vinculum supply each flexor digitorum superficialis and flexor digitorum profundus tendon (Fig. 2B). The vincula receive their blood vessels through the transverse communicating branches of the common digital artery located on the dorsal surface of the flexor tendons. The vincula provide the blood supply that participates in early healing of flexor tendons and that also serves as a rein to limit proximal retraction of a lacerated tendon.

Flexor Tendon Healing

Two forms of tendon healing occur within the *intrinsic* and *extrinsic* systems of the flexor tendons. (1) Intrinsic healing occurs without direct blood flow to the tendon. Animal models

have demonstrated that diffusion of synovial fluid around lacerated tendons allows intrinsic tendon healing without adhesion formation. The nutrition for tendon healing in that model comes indirectly from blood flow to the surrounding synovium. Moreover, the specimens that healed in a synovial pouch were not under stress.[8,9] (2) Extrinsic healing is known to occur by proliferation of fibroblasts from the peripheral epitenon. The fibrous proliferation forms a tenoma around the periphery of cut tendon ends and also invades the space between the tendon ends. Adhesions occur because of extrinsic healing of the tendon and limit tendon gliding within the fibrous and synovial sheaths. Both systems contribute to tendon healing and gliding. A healing tendon depends on nutrition from osmotic fluid high in protein and on granulation tissue that constitutes the tendon scar. The physiologic equilibrium between both systems allows healing without excessive scar.

TENDON REPAIR

Concepts Concerning When and How to Repair an Injured Tendon

The timing for and method of repairing a lacerated flexor tendon vary according to the existing conditions. There is agreement that either primary or delayed repair of all flexor tendons may be performed in Zones I, III, IV, and V. In Zone II, the options are primary repair of one or both lacerated flexor tendons, delayed repair, secondary repair, or tendon grafting 3 weeks or longer after injury.

Primary repair of a lacerated tendon is performed within 24 hours after injury. *Delayed repair* refers to a period of up to 1 week after the initial injury, during which time the initial wound heals and repair of the tendon is performed or delayed closure of the wound occurs and delayed repair of the tendon is performed at the same time as wound closure.[7] *Secondary repair* refers to any time longer than 1 week after the original injury when all wounds are healed and edema has subsided.

Primary repair of lacerated flexor tendons has several advantages compared with secondary repair: (1) accurate anatomic alignment, (2) no adhesions at the time repair is performed, and (3) no delay in initiation of recovery. Primary repair is appropriate if the surgeon is experienced in tendon repair, if the wound is exceptionally clean, and if there has been little or no crushing of the tendon or the surrounding tissues. The decision to perform delayed repair is made if the wound is contaminated, if trauma is severe, if the patient's general condition does not justify a prolonged operative procedure, and if the surgeon is not experienced in performing complicated tendon repair. The delay does not compromise the end result.

The delayed or secondary repair procedure involves initial wound exploration with excision of wound margins, removal of foreign material, and either primary or delayed wound closure at 3 to 5 days, depending on the mechanism of injury. The tendon may be repaired when delayed closure is occurring at 3 to 5 days after injury, or secondary repair may be performed at 3 to 6 weeks after wound healing has occurred. Delayed repair has several advantages compared with immediate repair: (1) risk of infection is diminished, (2) an experienced physician is available to perform the repair, and (3) multiple injuries such as fracture, vascular trauma, or nerve injury may be treated prior to the definitive tendon repair.

Examination Prior to Tendon Repair

Before repair of a lacerated tendon is performed, an accurate diagnosis must be made. The examiner determines if one, both, or neither of the flexor tendons is lacerated. The flexor digitorum superficialis is an isolated activator of the middle phalanx. Function of the superficialis is determined by holding the adjacent digits in extension so that the flexor profundi cannot

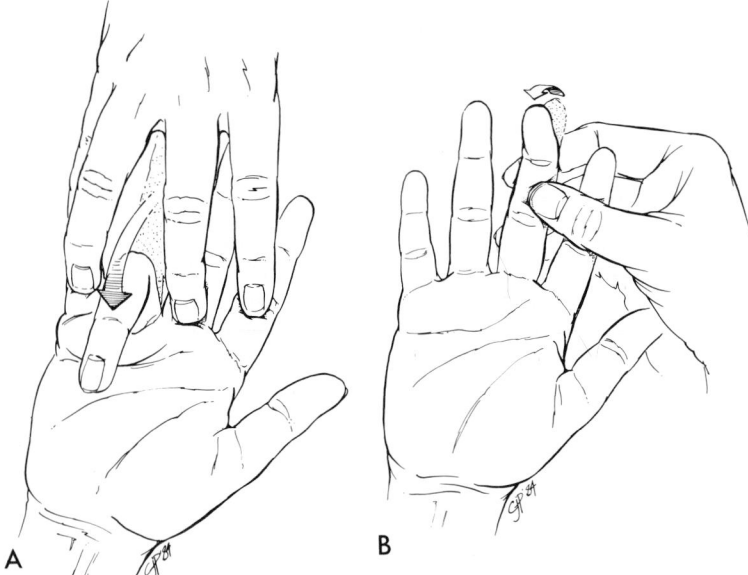

Figure 3. *A,* This technique is used to determine the strength of each individual flexor digitorum superficialis muscle. The adjacent digits are held in full extension to eliminate the action of the flexor digitorum profundus. The patient then voluntarily attempts to flex the proximal interphalangeal joint. Resistance is applied after flexion has occurred in order to determine the strength of the muscle. The distal phalanx of the same digit is tapped from the extensor side and the flexibility of the joint is determined. If there is no tension on the flexor digitorum profundus and if all of the action is through the flexor digitorum superficialis, then the differentiation of the two tendons in the digits is evident. *B,* A method of testing the strength of the flexor digitorum profundus of the long finger. The proximal interphalangeal joint is maintained in extension, as is the metacarpophalangeal joint. The patient is then asked to voluntarily flex the distal phalanx at the distal joint. Accurate testing of the ulnar three digits requires that the distal joints of the long, ring, and little fingers be flexed simultaneously, after which each digit is tested individually. The thumb and index finger may be tested individually in 85 per cent of the population and simultaneously in the remaining 15 per cent.

move. The patient is asked to voluntarily flex the involved digit at the proximal interphalangeal joint (Fig. 3*A*). This is an accurate test for the index and long fingers and usually for the ring finger. The little finger, however, should be tested by simultaneously flexing the ring finger, since the little finger occasionally has a single muscle belly with tendons to each of the digits.

An isolated laceration of the flexor digitorum profundus is determined by the examiner's holding all finger joints in extension except the distal joint and then asking the patient to flex the fingertips (Fig. 3*B*). The flexor digitorum profundus to the index finger shows isolated function in 85 per cent of the population, but simultaneous function with the flexor pollicis longus in only 15 per cent. The ulnar three digits act as a single unit and should be tested simultaneously.

Sensation, nail bed blanching, skin sweating, and temperature are determined before a decision is made about degree of tendon injury, since they may represent injury to neurovascular structures that require repair as well.

Technique of Flexor Tendon Repair

Anesthesia for flexor tendon repair depends on the age of the patient, the condition of the extremity, the emotional status of the patient, and the patient's preference (awake or not awake) as well as the surgeon's preference. The choices are general anesthesia, axillary nerve block, supraclavicular brachioplexus block, or intravenous regional anesthesia with double tourniquet. The extremity is exsanguinated with an Esmarch rubber bandage, and a pneumatic tourniquet is elevated to a pressure of 230 to 250 torr. The skin laceration is extended proximally and distally usually by zigzag extension. Medial or lateral digit incisions can be used if the repair is delayed. The lacerated flexor tendon ends are exposed, and the medial and lateral nerves and vessels are identified (Fig. 4). The lacerations of the flexor tendon and annular ligament are identified, and the edges are excised. All devitalized skin, fat, and fascia are removed. The wound is irrigated with antibiotic solution.

The severed distal stump of the tendon is then retrieved by flexing the middle or distal interphalangeal joints. At this time, the information previously obtained from the patient as to what position the fingers were in when the laceration occurred is valuable. If the fingers were flexed, the tendon was lacerated distal to the skin laceration. If the fingers were extended, the skin and tendon laceration coincide. The distal tendon is then held in maximal flexion with a straight Keith needle, which is passed directly through the skin, annular ligament, and flexor

tendons. The needle is usually dorsal to the neurovascular bundle. Proximally the lacerated tendon stump is identified by compressing the muscle belly and tendons from proximal to distal while the wrist and metacarpophalangeal joints are in flexion. The location of the proximal flexor tendon is affected by the condition of the vinculum. If the vinculum has been lacerated, the tendon retracts proximally. If the proximal tendon cannot be retrieved by joint flexion and compression, an Esmarch rubber roll is wrapped from the elbow distally to force the tendons into the wound. An additional method of extracting the tendon is to pass a thin bent suction catheter into the fibroosseous canal. Suction is applied as the wrist and fingers are flexed, and the tendon, if cut within 24 hours, may be retrieved. If the tendon cannot be retrieved by these techniques, a separate incision is made in the palm, proximal to the A1 pulley. The flexor tendons are identified and brought out by the silicone rod technique. A 4–0 silk suture is then placed in the tip of the tendon, and a silicone rod tendon is passed from distal to proximal. The silk suture is tied to the silicone tendon, which is pulled distally. The proximal tendon is then held in position by a Keith needle, and the cruciate and annular ligaments are opened and

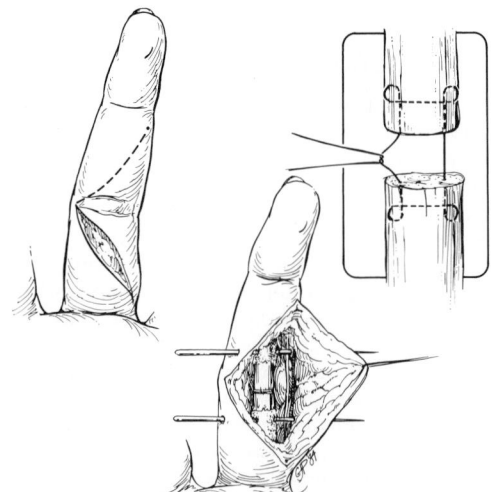

Figure 4. The zigzag incision on the volar surface allows exposure of the flexor tendons and annular ligaments. The nerves and vessels are on the radial and ulnar aspects of the tendons. This suture technique (Kessler) provides a strong grasp to the lacerated tendon ends. The major disadvantage is the knot between the tendon ends.

trimmed so that the suture line is not affected by the fibro-osseous canal. The vincula, if intact, are not removed since they bring blood to the tendon. Both ends of the tendon are held firmly, and the ends are sutured using nonabsorbable suture and circumferential reinforcing sutures. The tendons are brought together with minimal trauma.

SUTURE TECHNIQUES USED FOR FLEXOR TENDON REPAIR. Urbaniak and co-workers noted that the modified grasping suture (Kessler) (Fig. 4) and the figure-of-eight zigzag suture (Bunnell) were strongest at the time of initial repair. A modification of these (Goldner) (Fig. 5A and B) provided a crisscross without double knots and with good holding power. Suture material should be nonabsorbable and cause minimal reaction. The authors currently use 4–0 Ethibond (Ethicon, Johnson and Johnson), which satisfies all requirements. The modified Goldner or Kessler suture is used, and the knots are buried within the substance of the flexor tendon. A circumferential interrupted 6–0 nylon suture is used to smooth out the repair. The suture is placed at right angles to the fibers of the tendon, and the knot is buried (Fig. 5A and B). After tendon repair, the Keith needles are removed, and the digit is gently moved into flexion and extension to determine any binding of the suture lines on the annular ligaments. As much of the A2 and A4 pulleys (annular ligaments) is preserved as possible. Although closure of the annular ligament is desirable, stenosis must be avoided. A patch graft may be used to cover the tendon and fill the defect.

ZONE II LACERATION OF BOTH FLEXOR TENDONS. In Zone II injuries in which both flexor digitorum superficialis and flexor digitorum profundus tendons are lacerated, the authors believe that both flexor tendons should be repaired. A repaired flexor digitorum superficialis increases the strength of the digit, provides better and quicker flexion at the proximal interphalangeal joints, preserves the short vincula that provide blood supply to the flexor profundus, and acts as a pulley for the repaired profundus that provides improved excursion and strength. An intact functioning superficialis tendon has less tendency to hyperextension or excessive flexion of the proximal interphalangeal joint.

POST–TENDON REPAIR PROGRAM. In the operating

room, when the tendons have been sutured, the tourniquet is released and bleeding points are controlled. The wound is closed with interrupted sutures, the capillary return is noted, and if the skin edges are dusky or pale, corner sutures are not used. A compression dressing is applied, covering all areas of the skin and extending above the elbow. The wrist is held in 25 degrees volar flexion, the metacarpophalangeal joints at 60 degrees flexion, and the proximal and distal interphalangeal joints at 25 degrees flexion. A dorsal plaster splint is used for rigid immobilization, but no volar splint is used because if this slips distally there will be persistent traction on the repaired tendons and they will become separated. A drain may be inserted and is removed in 24 hours. The plaster is wrapped on with a bias-cut stockinette bandage rather than an elastic bandage, which tends to be wrapped too tightly and increases in tension as time passes. The arm is suspended by an external support without pressure or wrapping around the wrist.

Tetanus prophylaxis is administered if necessary; preoperative and postoperative antibiotics are used for 48 hours, and the operation is performed in a clean air environment.

Extent of Early Motion After Tendon Repair

There is a consensus that early but limited excursion of the repaired tendon diminishes peripheral adhesions during the postoperative healing period. However, the way to obtain this motion, the distance that the tendons are moved, and the frequency of motion are points about which there is no consensus. The frequency of rupture of repaired tendons following early forceful muscle contraction and passive motion has been as high as 35 per cent. Conversely, absolute immobilization causes peripheral adhesions that may require several months for stretching. Pulvertaft's study showed no difference between early motion or absolute immobilization at 6 months after operation. Current studies, however, suggest that limited motion is a compromise. The authors' postoperative program has included a few millimeters of passive assistive motion three times a day each day during the time that the extremity is in the cast. Duran and Houser[4] documented that 3 to 5 mm. of movement of the tendon at the suture line each day is sufficient to allow excursion of the fibroblastic scar during the healing period.

A study by Strickland indicated that active flexion and controlled extension, if carefully supervised, produced a greater range of motion and fewer ruptures. The actual difference at 1 year, however, was not determined. Kleinert and co-workers[7] recommended rubber band flexion and active extension early postoperatively. Flexion contractures and early ruptures are two of the complications that occur with this technique. However, if the procedure is well supervised, if the loop is placed on the proximal phalanx rather than on the fingernail, and if the proximal point of traction is in the midforearm, the technique has merit.

At 21 days, an active assistive exercise program is desirable, but the tendon should be protected for a minimum of 42 days. At that time, an outrigger splint is applied, and the patient is given specific exercises for elastic traction resistance against flexion, as well as Velcro splints at night to improve joint flexion and extension splints to stretch out the peripheral scar. The entire program of assistive flexion and extension must be performed meticulously, and the surgeon, patient, and therapist must be persistent. The greatest single complication associated with the vigorous postoperative therapy program is tendon rupture, which must be avoided. This is accomplished by a compromise between excessive exercise and no activity postoperatively.

Recently Gelberman and Nunley[5] have demonstrated in a prospective randomized series that continuous passive motion improves the results of Zone II flexor tendon repairs when compared with rubber band traction. The use of continuous passive

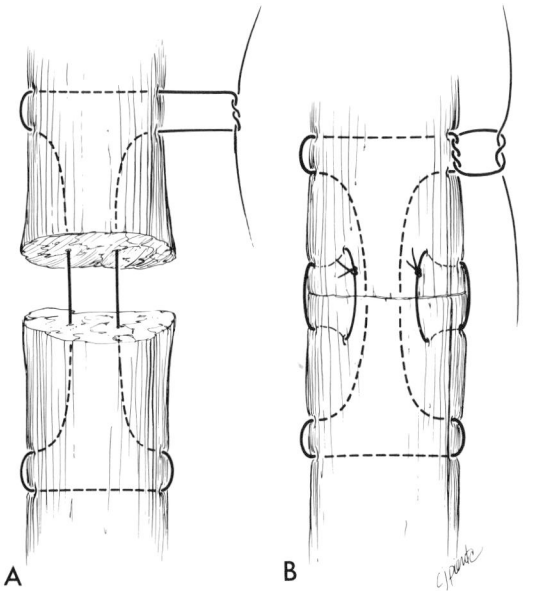

Figure 5. A, These structures are placed with either double-armed straight or curved needles. Minimal constriction is occurring. Because the blood supply is primarily on the dorsum of the tendon, the suture should be placed so that it bisects the tendon or is slightly toward the volar surface. Only one knot is used for each suture. There is an option for single or double placement of the sutures both proximally and distally. B, After the single or double sutures are placed, the reinforcing sutures are placed to secure the cut edges of the tendon.

motion in their series demonstrated the best results of tendon repairs to date.

Laceration of the flexor tendon at the wrist requires elbow flexion of 90 degrees for 21 days, wrist flexion of 45 degrees, metacarpophalangeal joint flexion of 30 degrees, and finger flexion of 20 degrees. Gradual extension is then allowed after 2 days, but the tendon is protected for 42 days.

Tendon Repair — Special Considerations According to the Anatomic Zone Involved

LACERATION OF FLEXOR PROFUNDUS DISTAL TO SUPERFICIALIS INSERTION IN ZONE I. The pathologic lesion may be a laceration or an avulsion from the distal phalanx.

MANAGEMENT OF AVULSION OF THE FLEXOR PROFUNDUS. The tendon retracts to the base of the digit or into the palm, depending on the force causing the avulsion; the vinculum prevents excessive retraction. Primary treatment is performed by isolating the tendon proximally and the phalanx distally and using a silicone flexible tendon as a guide to relocate the tendon to its usual position. A 3–0 Prolene suture is inserted into the distal end of the tendon as a double figure-of-eight, passed on either side of the phalanx through the periosteum, and tied over a rubber and plastic button insulator that is placed directly over the fingernail to avoid pressure on the tip of the digit (Fig. 6A and B). Delayed repair after 21 days is managed similarly. However, if the tendon has retracted into the palm, it may become adherent to itself after 7 days and cannot be used for replacement. It must then be excised and a free tendon graft used.

MANAGEMENT OF LACERATION OF THE FLEXOR PROFUNDUS. The skin laceration may not coincide with the point of tendon laceration. Primary repair is performed if the wound is clean or can be converted to a clean wound. If not, delayed repair is completed at 7 to 21 days or even as long as 6 weeks after the original laceration. The tendon is mobilized proximally, the annular ligaments are maintained, and the tendon is advanced distally and sutured to the distal stump by end-to-end suture or by advancement if the distal stump is 1 cm. long or less. *Advancement greater than 1 cm. causes contracture.*

LACERATION OF FLEXOR DIGITORUM PROFUNDUS AND SUPERFICIALIS IN ZONE II. Primary repair of both tendons is performed only under ideal circumstances. The wound must be clean, there should be no element of crush to soft tissues or bone, and the tendon sheath should be at least partially intact. The surgeon must be experienced in all aspects of tendon repair. Otherwise, the safest approach is delayed or secondary repair. Even at 3 to 6 weeks after the initial injury, an end-to-end suture of both tendons is possible, the alternative being a free tendon graft. If a crush injury occurred, a silicone rod may be inserted. The surgeon should be prepared for these options for either a primary or a delayed procedure.

The technique used in primary repair is critical. Both ends are retrieved, the annular ligament is trimmed, and the ends are held in place with Keith needles. The flexor digitorum superficialis (which is deep) is repaired initially using a Goldner suture technique (see Fig. 5A and B). The flexor digitorum profundus is then repaired end-to-end using 4–0 Ethibond suture with reinforcing peripheral sutures. An alternative technique is to use Prolene pull-out and circumferential sutures. A pull-out suture is placed over the middle phalanx, thereby obviating the need for extensive opening of the annular ligament or for extensive dissection in order to place the holding suture. Although closure of the annular ligament is desirable, in most instances it is not possible. As much of the proximal and middle pulleys as possible is left intact, and if a pulley requires splitting, it is left in place where it regenerates, or it is patched.

Lacerations of flexor tendons in Zone III (in the palm) involve injury to the lumbrical muscles as well as to the flexor tendons. A damaged lumbrical is either repaired or excised, depending on the severity of the injury and the location of the laceration. If

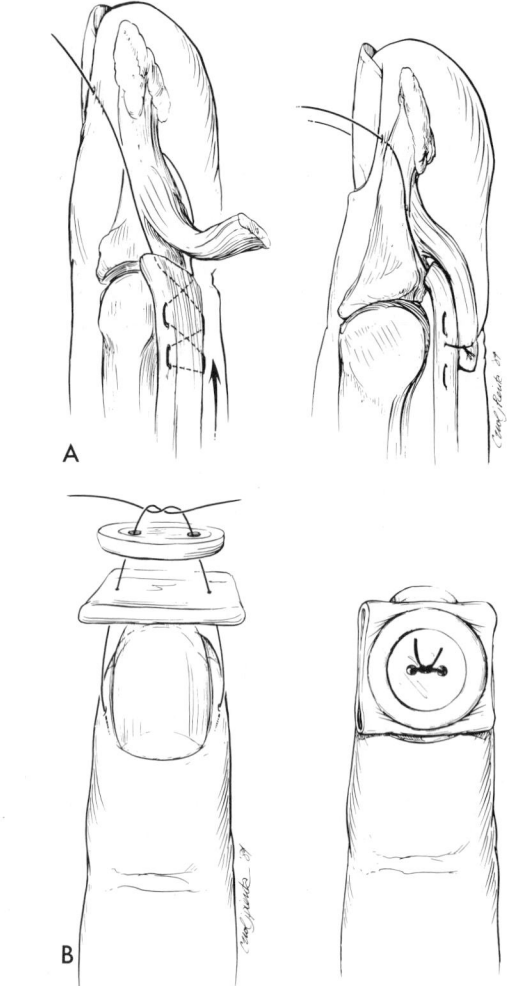

Figure 6. *A,* The technique for attaching the free tendon graft to bone and periosteum of the distal phalanx or to a remnant of lacerated flexor tendon. This technique is used for free graft or for an advancement of a previously lacerated tendon. The 3–0 Prolene suture is later extracted by cutting one segment of the suture distally and applying traction to the other. *B,* The pull-out sutures are placed adjacent to the nail plate as close as possible, or actually through the nail plate. A piece of firm rubber is applied against the nail plate, and a firm button prevents migration of the suture.

the lumbrical muscle is intact, it is left adjacent to the flexor digitorum profundus repair. It is *not* wrapped around the repaired flexor. A lumbrical contracture is avoided if this muscle is not tightened or manipulated excessively during the repair. Both tendons, if lacerated, are repaired by end-to-end sutures with circumferential reinforcement, as already described. *Excision of the superficialis tendon is therefore not advisable.*

LACERATION OF FLEXOR TENDONS IN ZONE IV (WITHIN THE CARPAL CANAL). Lacerations of the flexor tendons within the carpal canal are usually associated with partial or complete laceration of the median nerve. Nerve repair is performed as a primary procedure if the wound is clean and after meticulous excision of nonviable tissue has been accomplished. The median nerve is aligned by the proximal and distal central arteries, by fascicular topography, or by proximal and distal electrical stimulation if the procedure is performed within 48 hours after the initial injury. Delayed electrical stimulation is possible with the patient awake. The distal nerve, however, may not demonstrate the motor and sensory fibers by electrical stimuli.

NERVE INJURIES ASSOCIATED WITH FLEXOR TENDON LACERATION. Lacerations of the median or ulnar nerve in the carpal area or at the wrist or of the digital nerves in the palm may be repaired at the same time as the tendon repair is performed. Tension is removed from the nerve suture line by flexing the wrist 30 degrees and the metacarpophalangeal joints 60 degrees. The nerves should be repaired first and the tendons last. When the tendon ends are sutured together, the digit can be manipulated toward extension, provided the wrist is maintained in 30 degrees flexion. The combined nerve-tendon procedure can be safely delayed for 21 days if the original wound is contaminated, if crushing trauma has occurred, or if the initial wound is not excised within 24 hours after injury.[9]

If delayed repair is performed, there is clinical and experimental evidence to show that if Surgicel is wrapped around the nerve, adhesions between nerve and tendon are temporarily delayed. Occasionally, when an unusual amount of fibrosis exists, as noted in a delayed or secondary repair, a thin sheath of *silicone* is placed between the tendon and the nerve or between repaired tendons to prevent intertendinous adhesions. The silicone is removed several months later after healing has occurred and the range of motion has increased.

LACERATION OF FLEXOR TENDONS IN ZONE V (WRIST AND LOWER FOREARM LEVEL). Laceration of the flexor tendons proximal to the carpal canal may be associated with median or ulnar nerve injury and laceration of the radial or ulnar arteries. Primary repair of the arteries is usually indicated. If the wound is contaminated, the arteries are repaired, and delayed repair of nerve and tendons is planned. The wound is left open for 3 to 5 days, at which time delayed closure is performed. The decision is made at that time whether to proceed with nerve and tendon repair in 5 days or to wait 21 days. Repair of the lacerated mixed nerve is readily accomplished as a primary procedure when anatomic alignment of the nerve or electrical stimulation or both are used. However, delayed epineurial repair of nerves or tendons is safe, is acceptable, and provides excellent results.

The nerves are repaired with 7–0 nylon as holding tension sutures and 9–0 nylon interval sutures. The tendons are repaired with nonabsorbable 3–0 polyester sutures in adults and 4–0 polyester sutures in children. Supplemental 5–0 circumferential sutures are used to reinforce the repair. However, anatomic constriction and gliding problems are less evident at the wrist than in the digits. Peritendinous adhesions occur, and controlled motion and elastic traction 21 days after repair are important. When nerves and tendons are repaired simultaneously, the problem of adhesions must be recognized. Forceful stretching after 21 days may cause nerves to stretch at the suture line if the nerves are adherent to the adjacent tendons. Thus, the postoperative management must be gentle with use of elastic traction; forceful stretching must be avoided, and the program should be based primarily on the tensile strength of the nerve suture rather than of the tendon suture.

The wrist is maintained in volar flexion for 21 days and gradually brought to dorsiflexion during the subsequent 6 weeks. Tendon excursion is gradually increased with elastic traction and active exercise.

Technique of Free Tendon Grafting — Fingers or Thumb

A midlateral or midmedial skin incision is made to expose the tendon involved. The neurovascular structures are reflected volarly with the flap. The dorsal branch of the digital nerve is spared. An alternative method of exposure is a zigzag incision with a 45-degree angle and the base of the flaps as wide as possible. For the index finger, for example, the proximal incision extends from the radial aspect of the proximal finger crease to the ulnar aspect of the middle crease and the radial aspect of the distal crease and then to the ulnar aspect of the fingertip pad. The extension into the palm then follows the palmar creases. The tips of the flaps are rounded rather than pointed. The neurovascular structures are isolated with a rubber dam and re-

tracted medially and laterally (Fig. 7A and B). With the neurovascular structures and the flaps reflected, the annular ligaments are identified, and the proximal and distal ligaments are trimmed. The cruciate ligaments between the annular ligaments are opened so that the lacerated adherent tendons are retrieved and mobilized. As much of each annular ligament as possible is salvaged.

The distal stump of the profundus tendon is isolated and retracted so that a 6- to 10-mm. segment remains attached to the distal phalanx (see Fig. 6A). Proximally, the flexor digitorum profundus is identified at the base of the palm and cut back until healthy tendon is identified within the mass of the lumbrical. If it is fibrosed, the lumbrical is resected after it has been used to help identify the profundus. The flexor digitorum superficialis is removed at the wrist and may be used as a free tendon graft. This selection depends on the size of the profundus and the constriction of the annular ligaments in the digit.

The distal end of the free tendon graft is placed within the fibro-osseous canal from the tip of the finger to the base of the digit. Distally, the graft is held in place with a 3–0 Prolene pull-out suture tied over a button placed on the fingernail as described for Zone I flexor tendon repairs (see Fig. 6A and B). The remaining stump of the flexor digitorum profundus is sutured to the tendon graft with 4–0 nonabsorbable sutures. The distal incision is closed down to the base of the digit. Gentle

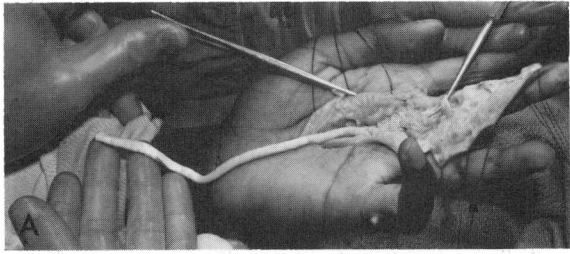

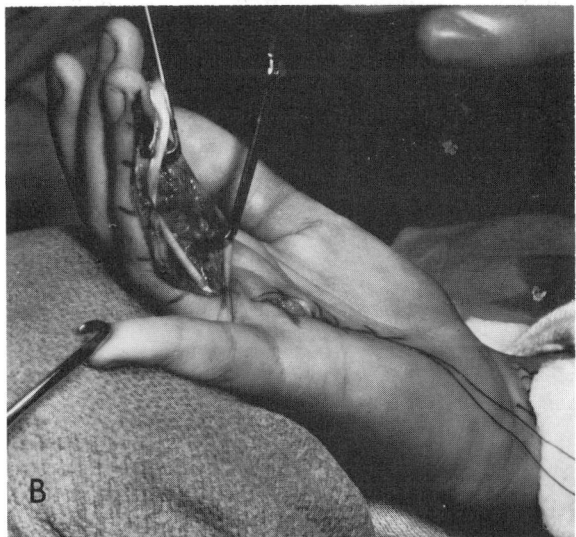

Figure 7. *A,* Free flexor tendon graft to the long finger is being completed. Original laceration was at the base of the digit, and attempted repair has failed. Three annular ligaments have been constructed. The flexor profundus proximally is being used as a motor, and the free tendon graft has been taken from the flexor digitorum superficialis. If excessive scarring is present, a silicone rod is inserted first and the flexor tendon is used later as an autogenous graft. *B,* A free tendon graft is being done to salvage a finger that has been affected by laceration through the proximal finger crease for which a repair had been attempted primarily. Fibrosis occurred, and an effort at a short tendon graft had failed. The entire digit has been opened, and annular ligaments have been reshaped and made more narrow. The free tendon graft extended from the fingertip to the base of the palm. A digital nerve laceration was repaired. Eventually the patient could flex the fingertip to within 1 cm. of the distal palm crease and extension was almost complete. (Reprinted with permission from Harper & Row from Surgery of the Hand, J. L. Goldner, 1970.)

traction is applied to the tendon, and the excursion and motion of the interphalangeal joints are tested.

An end-to-end or "buttonhole" suture is performed in the palm proximal to the annular ligament (A1 pulley). The tension of the final suture is determined by first observing the full excursion of the muscle belly of the flexor digitorum profundus by applying traction to the proximal tendon and measuring the distal and proximal excursion. The tendon graft is then sutured to the muscle belly, with the muscle belly at half resting length and under a sufficient amount of tension to cause the digit to be flexed at the metacarpophalangeal joint and at the proximal and distal joints approximately 10 degrees more than the normal resting position of the involved digit would be when the wrist is in neutral position. The resting attitude and position of the involved hand are used as a guide for determining the proper repair tension. The long finger, for example, is normally not flexed as much as the ring finger but is flexed more than the index finger. After the graft is in place, the long finger will be flexed approximately 5 degrees more than the adjacent ring finger and approximately 20 degrees more than the index finger.

Immobilization is completed by a compression dressing that extends from the fingertips to above the elbow. This is made by fluffing 2 by 2 inch gauze between the digits, with use of 4 by 4 inch gauze dressings for the palm and the back of the hand and the application of abdominal pads on the dorsal and volar aspects; the soft dressing is wrapped with 3-inch sheet cotton. A dorsal plaster splint extends 2 cm. beyond the fingertips to the olecranon process. A volar splint is *not* used, since this would cause undue tension on the flexor graft if the splint slipped. The plaster splint is then wrapped in place with a bias-cut stockinette in direct contact with the plaster so that it will not slip and will adhere to the plaster. The wrist is flexed 30 degrees, the metacarpophalangeal joints are flexed 60 degrees, and the interphalangeal joints are flexed 10 degrees. When this aspect of the dressing is applied, the elbow is included by posterior splints or U-shaped splints that hold the elbow at 90 degrees. This plaster is also wrapped on with a bias-cut stockinette. A segment of tubular stockinette is then placed from the axilla to the fingertips and form fit distally and cut to allow visualization of the fingers and the thumb. A second stockinette is then applied and is held to the arm by a bias-cut stockinette. The second stockinette is a suspension apparatus that is tied to an overhead pole with rope to provide constant elevation. Complete immobilization of the hand and forearm is maintained for 21 days, during which time the patient is shown how to flex the tips passively through a 5-mm. range of motion 10 times 3 times a day. Partial immobilization is then continued for an additional 21 days, after which assisted flexion and extension are initiated and an outrigger elastic splint is used.

Silicone as an Adjunct in Treatment of Tendon Repair and Tendon Fibrosis

Severe trauma, infection, or multiple tissue injuries may cause a fibrotic, adherent flexor tendon mechanism that adversely affects tendon gliding and digit function. The use of silicone sheeting, silicone rods, and, more recently, a permanent artificial silicone-Dacron tendon represents important advances in methods of reconstructing damaged flexor and extensor tendon complexes (Fig. 8). Attachment of the artificial tendon distally with a screw and proximally with Dacron ingrowth or bone-tendon junction is still under investigation.[6]

SILICONE ROD BEFORE FLEXOR TENDON GRAFTING. If the gliding surface of the involved digit is fibrotic and irregular, if annular ligaments require reconstruction because of damage to the major canals at the base of the finger, and if there is limited joint motion, a free tendon graft is usually not successful. A silicone rod (3 mm., 4 mm., or 5 mm.) provides an artificial tendon while pulleys are being reconstructed, joints are being

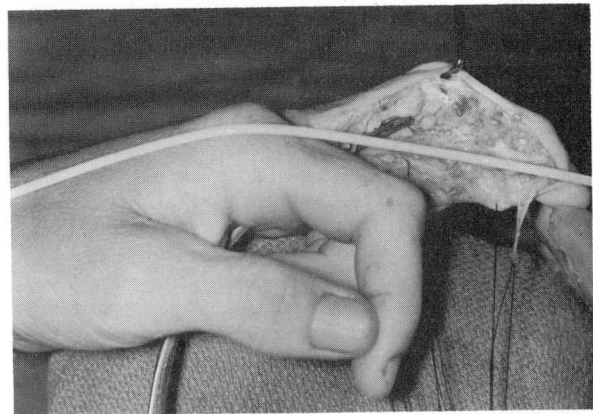

Figure 8. A flexor tendon injury caused severe fibrosis throughout the course of the tendon. The scarred tendon has been removed, annular ligaments have been reconstructed, digital nerve has been prepared for suture, and a silicone rod will be inserted into the digit from the tip to the wrist to act as a stimulus to pseudosheath formation. At a later time, the rod is removed and a biologic autogenous tendon graft is inserted.

mobilized, and a pseudosheath is forming. The rod orients collagen (Fig. 8).[6] The flexor tendon sheath is exposed through a midlateral or palmar zigzag incision that extends to the base of the palm. A second incision is made at the wrist, and both the flexor digitorum superficialis and the flexor digitorum profundus of the involved digit are isolated. The profundus is cut, and the distal segment within the base of the palm is usually bypassed. The segment from the palm to the digit is removed. The silicone rod is inserted from the wrist to the fingertip, where the end of the rod is attached by a Dacron suture to the remaining stump of the profundus and into the distal phalanx (see Fig. 6A and B).

The annular ligaments are reconstructed if they have been damaged. This is performed at the anatomic locations over the distal end of the proximal phalanx (A2) and over the middle of the middle phalanx (A4): Additional pulleys are made proximal to the metacarpophalangeal joint (A1), and cruciate ligaments are constructed to join the major A2 and A4 pulleys. The silicone rod is a structure over which the pulleys are formed; the distal end of the rod is attached to tendon and bone, but the proximal end moves freely so that passive motion forms an artificial fibrous synovium-lined sheath. The rod is ultimately in the same plane as the flexor digitorum profundus tendons.

The delay between the first-stage silicone rod insertion and the second-stage tendon insertion varies from 6 weeks to 6 months. The maximal range of passive motion must be recovered, and revascularization should be adequate in the sheath for tendon grafting. A segment of the extensor digitorum longus tendons from the second or third toe is selected as the graft, the involved hand digit is opened at the distal interphalangeal joint level where the pseudotendinous sheath and the silicone tendon are identified, and the tendons are exposed proximally at the wrist level. The silicone rod is identified proximal to the carpal canal, the free tendon graft is sutured to the proximal end of the silicone rod, the distal attachment of the rod is released, and traction is applied so that the free tendon graft enters the base of the palm, the mid-palm, and the digit as the silicone rod is removed distally. The free tendon graft is then attached distally to the remaining stump of the flexor digitorum profundus tendon or, if the stump is absent, directly into the distal phalanx with a 3–0 nonabsorbable pull-out suture. Proximally, the tendon graft is woven through the musculotendinous junction of the flexor digitorum profundus under sufficient tension to maintain the digit in slightly greater flexion than the adjacent digits when the wrist is at neutral position. The position for immobilization is 30 degrees wrist flexion, 60 degrees metacarpophalangeal joint flexion, and 10 degrees proximal and distal interphalangeal joint flexion. An oblique 0.045 fixation pin is drilled across the distal interphalangeal joint in a position of 10 degrees flexion. This prevents hyperflexion of the distal joint as the graft is maturing.

Five days after insertion of the graft, passive motion is initiated. Stress on the suture line is avoided for 21 days, at which time active motion is initiated. The pull-out suture is left in place for approximately 4 weeks, and an elastic outrigger to provide limited extension is first used at 6 weeks after the insertion of the graft. A protective night splint in alternate flexion and extension is applied from the dorsum of the digit. Active motion is initiated at the interphalangeal joints by use of a wooden block and plastic putty.

Permanent Artificial Tendon

A silicone rod reinforced with Dacron is now available as a controlled clinical research implement. This is useful in providing motion for a digit affected by extensive multi-tissue damage in which a two-stage reconstructive procedure is unlikely to succeed. The digit tolerates the artificial tendon without developing excess fibrous proliferation. However, if biologic collagen is inserted, adhesions may cause flexion contracture and loss of joint motion. The distal attachment of the artificial tendon is into bone with a screw or metallic fixation that is invaded by bone. Proximally, the attachment is completed by bone-tendon junction with Dacron for ingrowth. A small number of patients have been treated in this manner, and the results are improving as the quality of the artificial tendon and its mechanism of attachment to biologic tissue improve.

Silicone Tendons on the Extensor Aspect of the Hand

Severe damage to the dorsum of the hand may cause avulsion of the extensor tendons, damage to the extensor hood, and inability of the patient to actively elevate the digits, including the thumb. The skeleton is stabilized by pin fixation, the joints are mobilized, a split skin graft or pedicle skin graft is used to fill soft tissue defects, and autogenous tendons or fasciae latae or silicone tendons are then used, depending on the severity and extent of the previous injury. In many instances, silicone rods are inserted from the middle of the middle phalanx to the musculotendinous junction of the extensor digitorum communis. These tendons may be left in place for several weeks, and a pseudosheath forms around them. Occasionally, the pseudosheath acts as a tendon in itself, and the further addition of autogenous tendons can be delayed. In other situations, when greater strength and mobility are desired, the tendon graft is added through the pseudosheath in the same manner that the free tendon graft is used on the flexor surface. Combinations of silicone rods and silicone joints are now possible. A patient who has sustained a severe crushing injury to the metacarpophalangeal joint of the index finger and loss of the extensor tendon can be managed in this manner. Because of severe damage to the articular surfaces and because arthrodesis of that joint is not desirable, a silicone-Dacron joint is inserted to replace the damaged metacarpal head. The alternative to arthrodesis is resection, and the silicone-Dacron joint can be inserted for several years. If it fails to function mechanically, it can be resected, and the remaining pseudosheath provides a reasonably stable reaction. The combined tissue replacement also requires a silicone cord to replace the extensor tendon. The silicone rod serves as a replacement tendon for several months and eventually is replaced by an autogenous tendon graft.

REFERENCES

1. Boyes, J. H., and Stark, H. H.: Flexor-tendon grafts in the fingers and thumb. J. Bone Joint Surg. [Am.], 53:1332, 1971.
2. Bunnell, S.: Repair of tendons in the fingers and description of two new instruments. Surg. Gynecol. Obstet., 26:103, 1918.
3. Doyle, J. R., and Blythe, W. F.: Anatomy of the flexor tendon sheath and pulleys of the thumb. J. Hand Surg., 2:149, 1977.
4. Duran, R. J., and Houser, R. G.: Controlled passive motion following flexor tendon repair in zones two and three. In AAOS Symposium on Tendon Surgery in the Hand. St. Louis, C. V. Mosby, 1975, pp. 105–114.
5. Gelberman, R. H., Nunley, J. A., II, Osterman, A. L., Breen, T. F., Dimick, M. P., and Woo, S. L-Y.: Influences of the protected passive mobilization interval on flexor tendon healing: A prospective randomized clinical study. Clin. Orthop. Rel. Res., in press.
6. Hunter, J. M., and Salisbury, R. E.: Flexor-tendon reconstruction in severely damaged hands. J. Bone Joint Surg. [Am.], 53:829, 1971.
7. Kleinert, H. E., Kutz, J. E., Ashbell, T. S., and Martinez, E.: Primary repair of lacerated flexor tendons in "no man's land." J. Bone Joint Surg., 49A:577, 1967.
8. Potenza, A. D.: Tendon healing within the flexor digital sheath in the dog. J. Bone Joint Surg. [Am.], 44:49, 1962.
9. Urbaniak, J. R., and Goldner, J. L.: Laceration of flexor pollicis longus tendon: Delayed repair by advancement, free graft or suture. J. Bone Joint Surg. [Am.], 55:1123, 1973.
10. Vaughn-Jackson, O. T.: Rupture of the extensor tendons by attrition at the inferior radioulnar joint. J. Bone Jone Surg. [Br.], 30:528, 1948.

2. COMPRESSION NEUROPATHIES OF THE HAND AND FOREARM

Richard D. Goldner, M.D., and
J. Leonard Goldner, M.D.

The diagnosis of abnormal compression of the median, ulnar, or radial nerves may be easily missed even though these syndromes occur relatively frequently. The diagnosis may be unnecessarily delayed if the physician waits until muscle atrophy is obvious or until sensory deficits are profound. An early diagnosis is preferable to allow the surgeon to provide pain relief and to maintain complete motor power and full sensibility.

Clinical Investigation

An entrapped nerve is suspected if the patient complains of intermittent tingling, numbness, or functional impairment, and if the symptoms are recurrent and affect a particular anatomic area of the hand or forearm. Historical details such as occupation, physical activities that cause sensory changes, the occurrence of day or night paresthesias, the frequency of complaints, and information about temporary recovery are all helpful in making the proper diagnosis.

Examination consists of determining the patient's ability to recognize differences in light touch, sharp point, heat, cold, and static and dynamic two-point discrimination. Motor power of the hand and forearm muscles is tested manually while the examiner realizes that minimal substitution patterns affect the result. Adjunctive tests are helpful in establishing a diagnosis. These include the percussion test of the individual peripheral nerve from distal to proximal and from proximal to distal, the effect of wrist flexion or extension on paresthesias, and pain production. Other helpful methods of demonstrating changes in sensibility include the effects of a venous tourniquet on the arm, repetitive movement in the hand, and changes due to hand-held vibrating objects. Findings that may be related to the presence of focal nerve compression are unusual hypertrophy of muscles or the presence of an accessory muscle enlargement of the palmar wrist flexor tendon sheaths (a palmar wrist bulge), or specific bone or joint deformities.

Electrical Studies

Nerve conduction studies, particularly sensory latency, are helpful in localizing nerve compression lesions. Sensory conduction studies are more sensitive than is motor conduction velocity. The amplitude of action potentials also indicates alteration of participating motor nerve axons.

Other special studies, such as S wave, provide subtle information about alterations of conduction. An S wave occurs when action potentials travel from the point of stimulation of the peripheral nerve to the spinal cord and back to the muscle.

Electromyography detects abnormal electrical action potentials following disruption of motor axons and wallerian degeneration. The denervated muscle fibers become spontaneously active, producing fibrillation potentials and positive sharp waves approximately 10 to 20 days after nerve injury. This test assists in differentiating neuropathic muscle atrophy from myopathic atrophy.

If electrical studies do not confirm the clinical diagnosis of focal nerve compression, a lesion may be present but is affecting the nerve minimally or intermittently. Nonoperative treatment is usually indicated in this instance.

Differential Diagnosis

A focal nerve compression must be differentiated from a neuropathy associated with systemic disease such as diabetes mellitus, hypothyroidism, rheumatoid arthritis, acromegaly, heavy metal toxicity, or paresthesias due to certain medications.

Paresthesias may be caused by lesions proximal to the hand or wrist such as cervical root irritation or brachial plexitis. Also, a spinal cord tumor or syringomyelia may cause distal symptoms and signs that may resemble a nerve compression lesion.

Digital Nerve Compression in the Fingers or the Thumb

Compression of the digital nerves of the thumb by a bowling ball or harp string causes reactive perineural fibrosis. Thus, the patient's vocation or avocation must be determined in order to assess the cause of numbness, tingling, or paresthesias in the digits.

BOWLER'S THUMB. The edge of the hole in the bowling ball may irritate the ulnar or radial digital nerves of the thumb. The digital nerve nodule becomes painful to pressure and the distal skin is hypesthetic.

TREATMENT. Initially, bowling should be discontinued. After the initial irritation subsides, a protective thumb guard, a change of grip, and a rounded edge to the hole in the ball may prevent recurrence. Surgical treatment is usually not indicated.

HARP PLAYER'S THUMB. Strings of a musical instrument may irritate the ulnar or radial nerves of the strumming digit. Painful hyper- or hyposensitivity may occur. The digit should be rested and the strumming pattern changed.

TREATMENT. A surgical procedure is not indicated. An alteration of the instrument or in the mechanism of using it is recommended.

FINGER COMPRESSION. Digital nerve compression at the base of the finger by a palmar fibromatosis or a fascial band usually is recognized by history and examination.

TREATMENT. Surgical excision of the compressing tissue is indicated.

ARTHRITIC NODULES. Digital nerves in the distal segments of the fingers may be irritated by arthritic nodules. Hypesthesia or paresthesias are due to compression or tethering of the nerve and secondary vasospasm.

TREATMENT. Anti-inflammatory medication, avoidance of excessive trauma to the fingertips, and the passage of time usually provide spontaneous improvement.

Compression of the Median Nerve Within the Hand

The median nerve may be compressed in the palm secondary to direct trauma. Occasionally, the motor branch of the median nerve is compressed by a fascial ring that surrounds the nerve as it enters the thumb muscles.

TREATMENT. Avoid using the heel of the hand as a hammer; wear gloves while repetitively squeezing tools or instruments.

Surgical decompression is indicated when the lesion persists and when severity progresses after a reasonable period of observation.

Compression of the Median Nerve at the Wrist (Carpal Tunnel Syndrome)

The median nerve is compressed within the carpal canal formed by the transverse carpal ligament on the palmar surface and the carpal bones on the dorsal side (Fig. 1). The flexor tendons travel in the carpal canal with the median nerve.

Compression of the median nerve within or adjacent to the carpal canal is the most common neuropathy of the upper extremity. Women are affected more frequently than are men; the age range is wide but is usually between 40 and 60 years. The usual complaints are weakness or clumsiness of the hand and hypesthesia or paresthesias of the thumb, index, or long fingers aggravated by grasping with the digits while the wrist is flexed or occasionally even extended. Nocturnal or early morning numbness is a frequent complaint that is quickly relieved by the patient's shaking the hand or moving the fingers. Finger tingling may occur from vibrations that result while the individual is holding an electric razor or by repetitive rotatory and flexion extension movements of the fingers and hand. Cold intolerance may occur, and vague discomfort in the hand or forearm or retrograde sensations may be present. Other conditions such as rapid weight gain, fluid retention associated with pregnancy, or compression from tight watchbands or rubber gloves may initiate or aggravate the original symptoms.

Examination may demonstrate sensibility changes in the thumb, index, long, and radial aspect of the ring fingers in certain patients, whereas others may have changes in only one digit. Percussion of the median nerve at the wrist proximal to the flexor retinaculum, over the carpal ligament, or in the palm may cause paresthesias. Tingling may be produced or aggravated by wrist flexion (Phalen's test) for 20 or 30 seconds and occasionally by wrist hyperextension. A venous tourniquet applied around the arm at 60 mm. Hg may cause tingling in the fingers of the involved hand. *Thenar muscle atrophy and profound sensory deficit occur only in the advanced stages of nerve compression.* Many patients with mild median nerve compression have intermittent complaints but normal motor and sensory examination and electrical studies.

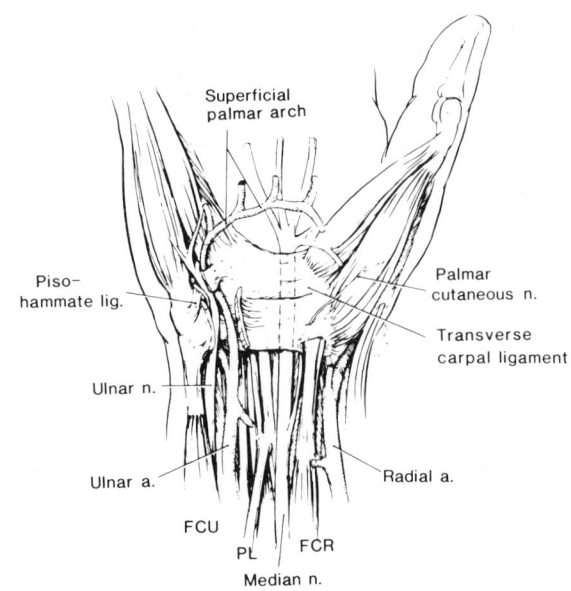

Figure 1. Volar aspect of wrist carpal tunnel showing flexor tendons to wrist and digits, course of median and ulnar nerves, and radial and ulnar arteries. (From Goldner, R. D.: Orthopedic Surgery Update Series, Vol. 3, Lesson 28, 1984.)

Factors that Contribute to Median Nerve Compression at the Wrist and in the Hand

1. Repetitive minor trauma such as grasping, squeezing, twisting, or hitting an object with the heel of the hand can produce symptoms of median nerve compression. If these actions are performed several hundred times a day, and if the frequency increases in an effort to increase production, median nerve compression may occur from tenosynovitis or trauma to the nerve from wrist flexion motions.

2. Synovial sheath hypertrophy of thumb and finger flexor tendons within the carpal canal may cause secondary median nerve compression.

3. Trauma to the heel of the hand often is not recognized by the patient.

4. A palmar mass such as a ganglion, aberrant calcification, uric acid crystals, or hypertrophic fat may increase the contents of the carpal canal and cause compression of the median nerve.

5. If the muscle bellies of the palmaris longus or flexor digitorum superficialis pass over or extend into the carpal canal, the median nerve may be compressed after vigorous hand activity or repetitive use. *These muscle variations are the most common causes of median nerve compression in young, active individuals.*

6. A mass in the carpal canal such as a neurofibroma, a neurilemoma, a lipohemangioma, or another rare lesion of the median nerve may cause symptoms and signs resembling a median nerve compression syndrome.

7. Dislocation of the carpal bones, particularly the lunate, or severe displacement of a Colles' fracture may cause immediate damage to the median nerve or delayed nerve compression of the median and the ulnar nerves.

8. After a partial digit amputation has occurred, the digital nerve may adhere to bone or tendon either distally or in the palm. This adherence may cause proximal tethering of the median nerve, particularly during dorsiflexion of the fingers or the hand, and may cause secondary paresthesias. Also, the lacerated flexor tendons may retract proximally and increase the soft tissue volume at the wrist. The combined tethering, the tenosynovitis, and the increased mass in the canal compress the median nerve.

9. Systemic conditions such as amyloidosis, Raynaud's syndrome, and myeloma may affect the median nerve at the wrist by formation of abnormal soft tissue lesions or vasospasm of the vessels of the hand or the median nerve.

Treatment of Median Nerve Compression at the Wrist

Initial treatment consists of splinting the wrist in neutral position at night, weight reduction if indicated, and decreasing the repetitive activities of the hand and wrist. Anti-inflammatory agents are useful in treating tenosynovitis, and a diuretic may assist in partially dehydrating synovial sheaths. A soluble corticosteroid mixed with 1 per cent lidocaine (1 ml. of steroid and 5 ml. of lidocaine) is injected into the tendon sheaths of the flexor digitorum profundus approximately 2 cm. proximal to the palmar flexor wrist crease and 1 cm. ulnarward to the palmaris longus. If the patient does not have a palmaris longus, the needle should be directed 1 cm. radial to the flexor carpi ulnaris at an angle of 30 degrees away from the ulnar nerve. The ulnar and median nerve should be avoided completely. Steroids should not be injected into or just adjacent to the median or ulnar nerve. The purpose of the injection is not to affect the median nerve directly, but to inject the anti-inflammatory medication into the flexor tendon sheaths to decrease synovitis and swelling.

These procedures reduce the symptoms in at least 40 per cent of patients who have mild compression lesions. Symptoms in individuals who have a moderate degree of compression are diminished but probably not eliminated. If symptoms worsen or demonstrate motor atrophy or more profound sensory change, surgical release is indicated.

NEUROLYSIS. Median nerve decompression is performed by incision of the transverse carpal ligament at the wrist from just proximal to the ligament to the midpalmar extension at the superficial palmar arch. This eliminates the external compression, aids regeneration of compressed motor and sensory fibers, and improves muscle strength of the thumb and sensibility of the digits. In the authors' experience, the incision should begin in line with the long axis of the ring finger in the transverse crease at the wrist, course obliquely within the skin crease at the base of the palm, and extend within or adjacent to the midpalmar crease to the level of the superficial palmar arch. This incision avoids the palmar cutaneous branch of the median nerve, allows proximal isolation of the nerve, and provides adequate visualization of abnormal muscles or proliferative flexor sheath synovium. The nerve is carefully isolated proximally and protected as the transverse carpal ligament is incised along the ulnar border. This avoids damaging the motor branch of the median nerve that supplies the thenar muscles. At the distal palm, the superficial palmar arch crosses volar to the nerve and must be protected. Incising the ligament over an instrument placed in the carpal canal helps to avoid damaging the median nerve. Epineurial splitting is done occasionally, and intraneurolysis is not recommended except in rare instances.

APPEARANCE OF THE MEDIAN NERVE AT OPERATION. The condition of the nerve reflects the severity of the compression lesion. The nerve may have the appearance of an isthmus with bulging masses both proximal and distal to the severe localized compression, or it may show only momentary obliteration of its vascular markings. The latter indicates minimal compression.

TENOSYNOVECTOMY ASSOCIATED WITH NEUROLYSIS. A tenosynovectomy may be desirable in patients with rheumatoid arthritis or other collagen diseases. The proliferating synovium may cause compression of the nerve even after the transverse carpal ligament has been incised. Also, the hypertrophy of the synovium may be causing tendon damage, and invasion of the tendon may cause tendon rupture.

BONE DEFORMITIES ASSOCIATED WITH NERVE COMPRESSION. If distal radial or carpal deformity persists, an osteotomy of the distal radius or reduction of the carpal bones may be performed in conjunction with median neurolysis.

RECURRENT MEDIAN NERVE SYMPTOMS. Recurrent median nerve symptoms may be due to (1) persistent compression of perineural fibrosis or prior trauma to the palmar cutaneous branch of the median nerve; (2) Prior incomplete neurolysis because of inadequate exposure through a short palmar incision; (3) Chronic tenosynovitis causing persistent median nerve compression; or (4) persistent pain due to prior damage to the median nerve from injection of steroid or other substance directly into the nerve.

Compression of the Median Nerve by the Pronator Teres

The median nerve may be compressed as it passes through or under the pronator teres and/or collagen bands proximal or distal to that muscle (Fig. 2). The syndrome includes forearm pain and numbness in the median nerve distribution, and it may coexist with median nerve compression at the wrist. Initial treatment of the syndrome is to diminish the repetitive activity that may be causing the complaints, diminish stress on the wrist as well, and be certain that the median nerve is not irritated more proximally.

Other *causes* of median nerve compression around the elbow and the forearm (Fig. 2) are (1) lacertus fibrosus; (2) the proximal edge of the origin of the flexor digitorum superficialis muscle after exercise or secondary to prior compartment syndrome; (3)

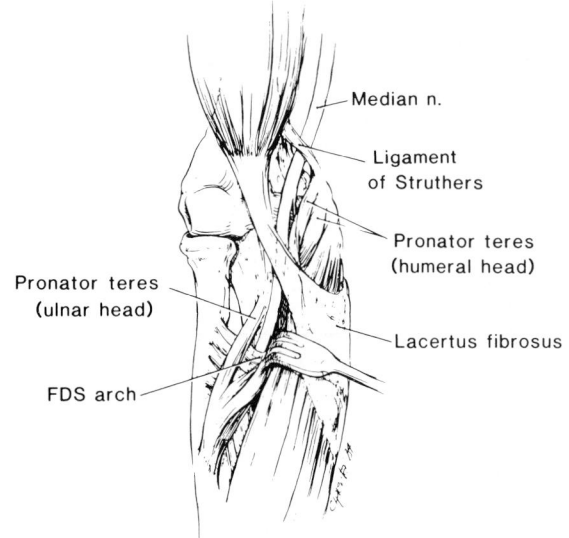

Figure 2. Diagram showing major points of possible median nerve compression. Above the elbow, the fibrous band from humeral shaft to the epicondyle (ligament of Struthers) may be associated with a supracondyloid process. Distally, the humeral head of the pronator radii teres may compress the nerve if the muscle is hypertrophied and subject to repeated contractions many times each hour. Distally, the ulnar head of the pronator may compress the median nerve. The fibrous bands of the pronator radii teres or a large pronator muscle and a combination of nerve tethering by both proximal and distal compression may result in pain, paresthesia, and even motor weakness. The flexor digitorum superficialis fascial arch may compress the median nerve if it is tethered or if the fascial band of the muscle is larger than average or is aggravated by repetitive activity. In the same way, the lacertus fibrosus may compress the median nerve in hyperextension, in direct extension, or in mid-flexion if the fibrous material shows minimal elasticity and if the contraction of the biceps is sufficient to shorten the lacertus. (From Goldner, R. D.: Orthopedic Surgery Update Series, Vol. 3, Lesson 28, 1984.)

accessory muscle masses from the pronator teres; or (4) a supracondyloid process from the distal end of the humerus to which is attached the ligament of Struthers.

Treatment of the elbow and forearm median nerve compression syndrome is initially nonoperative. If alteration of physical activity does not improve the syndrome, surgical release of the median nerve beginning proximal to the lacertus fibrosus and extending distally to the flexor digitorum superficialis is the treatment of choice.

Compression of the Anterior Interosseous Branch of the Median Nerve

The anterior interosseous nerve is a motor branch of the median nerve that is present in the proximal third of the forearm. It supplies the flexor pollicis longus, the flexor digitorum profundus of the index and long fingers, and the pronator quadratus. Specific causes of anterior interosseous nerve compression (Fig. 3) are (1) an enlarged bicipital tendon bursa that affects the motor aspect of the median nerve; (2) an aberrant or thrombosed radial artery in the midforearm; (3) the tendinous origin of the deep head of the pronator teres; (4) a fascial band at the origin of the flexor digitorum superficialis; and (5) compression within the deep palmar compartment from aberrant accessory muscles such as the flexor pollicis longus (Gantzer's) muscle, a palmaris profundus mass, or an enlarged flexor carpi radialis brevis.

Anterior interosseous nerve compression causes a vague pain in the proximal forearm that is aggravated by exercise and relieved by rest. The pinch between thumb and index finger is weak. Individual testing of the flexor pollicis longus and the flexor digitorum profundus of the index demonstrates these muscle bellies to be weak. There is no sensory deficiency. This syndrome must be differentiated from a rupture of the flexor pollicis longus or the index profundus tendons.

Tendon ruptures are usually determined by placing the digits

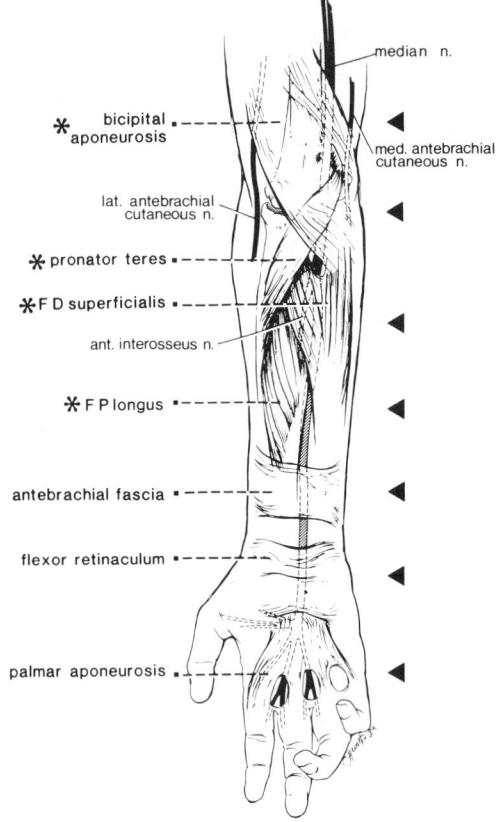

Figure 3. Composite diagram of multiple points of possible median nerve compression. The black points on the ulnar aspect of the elbow, forearm, and hand indicate sites of clinically recognized compression. The asterisks are adjacent to the names of structures that may cause compression of the median nerve, the lateral antebrachial cutaneous nerve, or the anterior interosseous nerve within the flexor pollicis (FP) longus. These points of compression are suspected by history and clinical examination and are usually documented by electrical studies. (From Bull. Hosp. Jt. Dis. Orthop. Inst. 44(2):201, 1984.)

in different positions and applying tension to the flexor tendons; by electrical stimulation that indicates whether the muscle belly is partially denervated; or by a succinylcholine test, which may demonstrate *more* fasciculations of the flexor pollicis longus if there is partial or complete denervation.

If symptoms persist after a reasonable period of observation, and depending on the other diagnostic studies, an operative procedure is performed isolating the median nerve proximal to the lacertus fibrosus and dissecting it distally through the pronator teres and distally to where the branches enter the flexor pollicis longus and flexor digitorum profundus of the index and long fingers. Electrical stimulation of the nerve during this decompression is helpful.

Ulnar Nerve Compression Within the Hand

HOOK OF THE HAMATE. Sensory branches of the ulnar nerve supply the palmar aspect of the little and one half of the palmar surface of the ring finger. The sensory and the motor branches are separate at this site. Degenerative arthrosis or trauma around the pisiform or the hook of the hamate may cause irritation or tethering of the sensory nerves and cause pain or paresthesias.

The sensory branch of the ulnar nerve within the ulnar canal (Guyon's) may be compressed. Repetitive trauma from a stapler or a bicycle handle may cause ulnar compression. Also, space-occupying lesions such as tumor, ganglion, lipoma, or anomalous muscles traversing the canal may cause nerve compression. External compression of the ulnar nerve by a heavy wrist watch band or by elastic garments may irritate the nerve.

TREATMENT. The diagnosis should be accurate. Daily activities should be investigated. Does the patient use the heel of the hand for a hammer, sleep on the palm, or use the hand repetitively on a chopping knife? When the diagnosis of nerve compression has been established, these movements should be discontinued and the patient observed. Electrical studies assist in establishing a baseline of muscle involvement, and nerve conduction velocities and especially sensory latencies are helpful in determining localization, gradual improvement, or regression.

If motor and sensory changes have occurred, the nerves should be decompressed and any subtle lesions removed.

Ulnar Nerve Compression at the Elbow

Ulnar nerve compression occurs within the cubital tunnel, or proximal or distal to it (Fig. 4). (1) A dense fascia over the flexor carpi ulnaris distally or the fibrous ridge of the interosseous membrane proximally may cause nerve irritation with repetitive motion. (2) Synovium or osteophytes within the cubital tunnel may irritate the nerve as a result of repetitive acute elbow flexion. (3) A synovial cyst arising from the elbow joint and extending into the canal may compress the nerve. (4) An ununited medial epicondyle of the humerus may irritate the nerve. (5) Repeated subluxation of the nerve as it moves across the medial epicondyle causes nerve compression. (6) Positional stress, such as prolonged elbow flexion during sleep or external pressure on the elbow during general anesthesia, or repetitive use of the flexed elbow against the mattress by the patient's changing position while on bed rest can cause ulnar nerve compression.

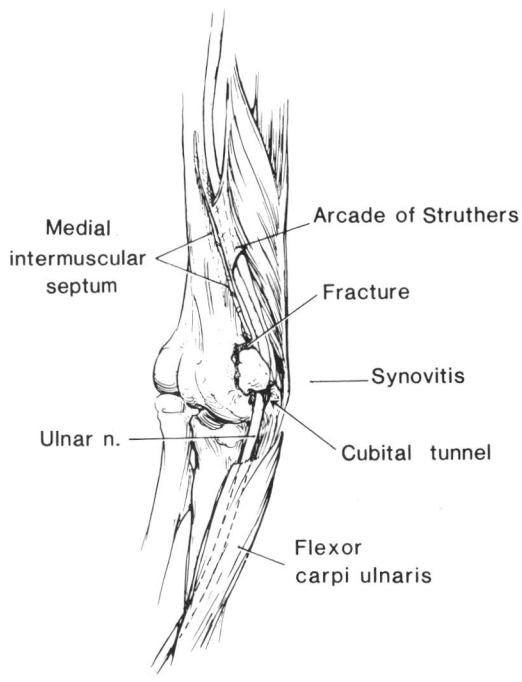

Figure 4. Ulnar nerve compression sites. The ulnar nerve is shown in the cubital tunnel. A fracture of the medial condyle, synovitis of the elbow joint, or compression by the arcade of Struthers may cause persistent compression of the ulnar nerve. The medial intermuscular septum may irritate the nerve proximal to the medial condyle. The nerve may slide anteriorly within the cubital tunnel, or it may be irritated by acute flexion of the elbow, which causes the nerve to displace forward. Synovitis of the elbow joint may cause indirect compression; fracture of the medial condyle affects the nerve because of condylar incongruity. The flexor carpi ulnaris covers the nerve as it enters the forearm. The fascial bands at the entrance of the nerve to the muscle may cause compression if the nerve is affected by progressive increase in muscle mass or decreased elasticity associated with aging. The nerve may migrate anteriorly from the cubital tunnel to directly over the medial epicondyle. The movement of the nerve during elbow flexion may result in chronic ulnar neuropathy. (From Goldner, R. D.: Orthopedic Surgery Update Series, Vol. 3, Lesson 28, 1984.)

(7) Other anatomic structures such as a fibrous arcade (arcade of Struthers) proximally or a combination of proximal tethering and distal muscle hypertrophy may irritate the nerve.

SYMPTOMS AND SIGNS. The symptoms of ulnar nerve compression at the elbow are aching or pain along the ulnar aspect of the proximal forearm and intermittent paresthesia, dysesthesia, or hyperesthesia of the little finger and the ulnar half of the ring finger. The patient usually complains that the "little finger is asleep." The heel of the hand may be "tingling."

Anatomic localization of the compressed nerve is determined by percussion of the nerve beginning distally and advancing proximally, by demonstrating hypermobility of the nerve over the medial epicondyle, or by persistent or intermittent tingling and numbness in the ring and little fingers after voluntary forced elbow and finger flexion.

Early or mild nerve compression causes no intrinsic atrophy, but prolonged nerve compression of a moderate or severe degree for several months causes atrophy of the hypothenar muscles and eventually the interossei muscles of the hand.

TREATMENT. The nonoperative treatment depends on an accurate diagnosis. The patient is advised to avoid resting the elbow on chair arms, table surfaces, and airplane armrests. If the elbow is acutely flexed during sleep, a splint is applied to prevent this. An elbow pad worn during the day may diminish direct contusion of the nerve and limit repetitive elbow flexion. Anti-inflammatory medications diminish connective tissue irritation and lessen the intensity of the complaints.

Surgical treatment is considered if one or more of the following is present: (1) hypesthesia and paresthesias persist for several months and are constantly uncomfortable; (2) rest, splinting, and other forms of treatment have not improved the persistent or progressive complaints after 3 months of observation; (3) atrophy of the intrinsic muscles of the hand is evident; or (4) electrophysiologic studies are positive in either motor or sensory conduction tests and abnormal action potentials are observed.

One method of surgical treatment is *subcutaneous transfer of the ulnar nerve anteriorly.* The important points to observe in order to prevent complications are (1) a long posterior medial incision for adequate exposure; (2) avoidance of the medial brachial and antebrachial cutaneous nerves; (3) adequate proximal dissection to incise the arcade of Struthers and the interosseous fibrous ridge; (4) distal mobilization of the nerve including cutting the nerve branch to the joint and opening the flexor carpi ulnaris fascia; (5) formation of a fat fascial flap that prevents the nerve from relocating; (6) consideration of medial epicondylectomy if the bone is prominent and the nerve is very loose; (7) avoidance of fascial compression of the nerve proximally and distally after the nerve is transferred; and (8) release of tourniquet, coagulation of bleeding points, and use of suction drainage.

Epineurial splitting is advisable if intrinsic atrophy is present or if sensory defect is dense. However, fascicular dissection is usually not advisable or necessary.

Alternative methods of managing the compressed ulnar nerve include the following: (1) The medial epicondyle of the humerus is excised without transferring the nerve anteriorly. This can be successful in some instances. (2) The nerve is placed anterior to the ulnar groove and within the forearm flexor muscles. This may be as successful as subcutaneous transfer, but the muscle tissue may eventually constrict or compress the nerve. (3) The nerve is placed deep to the forearm muscles not only to warm the nerve as in the case of leprosy but also to protect the nerve during forceful exercise.

Recurrent ulnar neuropathy after prior transfer requires special experience and pre-, post-, and intraoperative electrical studies. In addition to neurolysis, local protection of the nerve is beneficial by fat, muscle, fascicularized fascia, or circumferential vein graft at the time of the nerve decompression.

Figure labels: Medial intermuscular septum; Arcade of Struthers; Fracture; Synovitis; Ulnar n.; Cubital tunnel; Flexor carpi ulnaris

Compression Neuropathy of the Radial Nerve

With a complete radial nerve interruption (radial nerve palsy), there is no function of the muscles extending the wrist, thumb, or finger metacarpophalangeal joints. Anesthesia, hypesthesia, or paresthesia of the skin on the radiodorsal surface of the hand may occur. The radial nerve may be compressed by a displaced fracture of the distal third of the humerus or by prolonged external pressure associated with a "Saturday night palsy." The anatomic area of compression may be opposite the humeral midshaft in the radial groove or in the distal third of the humerus where the nerve courses from posterior to anterior. The radial nerve is directly adjacent to the humerus in the midshaft, and prolonged external pressure from the patient's head or a similar object compressing the nerve against bone may interrupt nerve conduction. If the patient has been asleep with the arm resting on the edge of a chair or bench, the nerve is also compressed.

The radial nerve injury associated with a proximal or midshaft fracture of the humerus usually follows trauma at the time of the injury. In 90 per cent of patients, these lesions recover spontaneously within 3 to 5 months after injury. The displaced distal oblique fracture of the humerus, however, occasionally may entrap the nerve between the fracture fragments and may require operative decompression.

Posterior Interosseous Nerve Compression

The common radial nerve lies between the brachioradialis and brachialis muscles. This nerve divides into the posterior interosseous branch, which enters the radial tunnel between the superficial and deep heads of the supinator muscle, and the superficial radial nerve, which innervates skin over the dorsal thumb, index, and dorsoradial hand. The posterior interosseous nerve supplies all of the radial nerve–innervated muscles except the brachioradialis, the extensor carpi radialis longus, and the extensor carpi radialis brevis. These muscles are innervated proximal to the origin of the posterior interosseous nerve. The posterior interosseous nerve may be compressed spontaneously in patients who perform repetitive pronation and supination several hundred times a day for months or years, or the lesion may occur between the radial head and the supinator after a fracture or dislocation of the proximal radius. Other causes are soft tissue tumor or synovial proliferation associated with rheumatoid disease.

Other points of nerve compression within the radial tunnel (Fig. 5) are (1) fibrous bands lying anterior to the radial head at the entrance of the radial tunnel; (2) a leash of vessels (radial recurrent artery) lying across the radial nerve and branching to the brachioradialis and extensor carpi radialis longus; (3) the proximal tendon margin of the extensor carpi radialis brevis compressing the posterior interosseous nerve and causing pain associated with "tennis elbow"; and (4) the arcade of Frohse, a ligamentous band spanning the posterior interosseous nerve as it enters the supinator muscle.

Symptoms may include aching of the extensor-supinator muscles and the entire dorsal forearm without muscle weakness (radial tunnel syndrome). If the lesion is confined to the posterior interosseous nerve but is not severe enough to cause motor weakness, pain without cutaneous sensory alteration may occur over the extensor muscle mass and is aggravated by forcible extension of the long finger against resistance when the wrist is held in neutral and the elbow is in a position of flexion from 45 to 90 degrees. Tenderness to digital compression is noted 4 cm. distal to the lateral epicondyle, and dorsal forearm pain is increased when the forearm is forcefully pronated and the wrist flexed. This condition can be confused with persistent lateral epicondylitis. This limited nerve compression does not cause motor weakness.

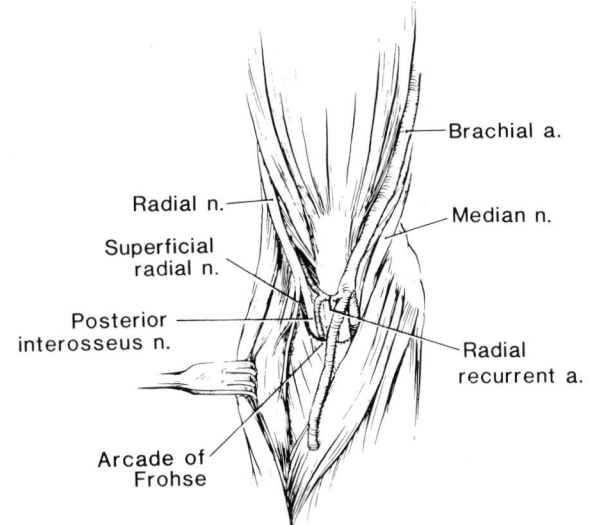

Figure 5. Diagram of the common radial nerve proximal to the elbow and lateral to the brachial muscle; the superficial radial nerve, which is primarily sensory; and the posterior interosseous nerve, which is almost entirely motor. This nerve enters the supinator muscle within which the condensed fascia (the arcade of Frohse) and blood vessels may cause compression of the tethered nerve. Also, the sensory component of the radial nerve may be compressed proximally or distally as the nerve emerges from under the brachioradialis tendon. (From Goldner, R. D.: Orthopedic Surgery Update Series, Vol. 3, Lesson 28, 1984.)

The clinical findings in an extremity with a complete posterior interosseous nerve lesion include active dorsiflexion of the hand in a position of radial deviation or by the proximally innervated extensor carpi radialis longus and brevis. The hand cannot be ulnarly deviated in extension because the extensor carpi ulnaris does not function. The thumb or fingers cannot be voluntarily extended at the metacarpophalangeal joints. Sensibility is intact since the compressive lesion is distal to the origin of the superficial radial nerve.

An incomplete lesion of the posterior interosseous nerve may cause lack of extension of only one or two digits at the metacarpophalangeal joint rather than all the muscles supplied by this nerve. The differential diagnosis of denervation versus tendon rupture or a conversion reaction must be considered.

TREATMENT. Management of this syndrome depends on the history, physical examination, and electrical studies. If the compressive lesion is localized proximal to the supinator and caused by the extensor carpi radialis brevis, a posterior interosseous neurolysis is performed through a dorsal lateral incision. If the muscle weakness is profound and the condition has persisted, operative treatment is indicated. The common radial nerve is isolated anterolaterally at the elbow, the dissection extends distally, and all anatomic areas of compression are released. The flattened area of the nerve may be recognized at the critical areas mentioned. The nerve is followed into the supinator muscle with the forearm supinated, and the muscle fibers are separated from the radius. The contour and density of the nerve are determined by direct examination, electrical stimulation is attempted proximally and distally and over the area of compression, and epineurial splitting is performed if necessary.

Results of treatment depend on the duration of compression and the severity of the nerve injury. If decompression is performed relatively early and repetitive physical activities are not resumed, improvement occurs. Reinnervation of the affected muscles may be determined by electrical studies 3 months after decompression and by clinical examination within 5 months after the operation. If improvement of muscle function does not occur within 1 year after nerve decompression, tendon transfers to replace the weak muscles should be considered.

Lesions Simulating Radial Nerve Palsy

Several conditions have an appearance similar to radial nerve injury. (1) Rheumatoid arthritis may cause rupture of the extensor digitorum communis tendons of the ring and little fingers and the extensor digiti quinti (Vaughn-Jackson syndrome). (2) Extensor pollicis longus tendon may separate by attrition or direct trauma after a distal radial fracture, or it may be ruptured by synovial invasion and erosion of collagen. (3) An incomplete radial nerve injury proximal to the elbow joint may be associated with neuralgic amyotrophy (Parsonage-Turner syndrome), usually causing pain and sensory diminution early in the onset of the syndrome. Asymmetrical weakness of the extensor muscles and diminished sensation along the course of the superficial radial nerve are noted. (4) Lead poisoning affects the radial nerve or the posterior interosseous branch. Symptoms are observed in children eating lead-based paint or inhaling burning battery fumes. An adult may develop lead poisoning from retained lead-based metals within a joint. (5) Diabetes mellitus or other neural toxic systemic diseases may cause altered conduction of the radial nerve.

Compression of the Sensory Component of the Radial Nerve

Hypesthesia or hyperesthesia on the dorsum of the thumb and/or the index finger may be related to compression of the cutaneous branch of the radial nerve at the point where the nerve exits beneath the brachioradialis and the shaft of the radius, or adjacent to an enlargement of the abductor pollicis longus annular ligament at the wrist. Also, direct trauma to the nerve at the wrist joint level or at the base of the thumb may affect sensory conduction of the radial nerve by primary compression. A careful history is important in establishing the diagnosis. For example, if the patient uses a tight bracelet, wears a heavy elastic watchband, or has been cutting with large dull scissors, the radial nerve may be compressed by external forces.

Clinical examination reveals an area of hyperesthesia or hypesthesia along the course of the nerve slightly proximal and always distal to the point of compression. The condition usually improves in time by eliminating the abnormal external compressive forces.

If the cutaneous symptoms persist, a neurolysis is performed from the proximal point of compression under the brachioradialis tendon, approximately 5 cm. proximal to the wrist joint, to the distal area of compression as determined by alteration of skin sensitivity and a positive percussion test.

Peripheral Nerve Repair

An extension of the management of focal peripheral nerve lesions, entrapment syndromes, or old nerve injury is a consideration of peripheral nerve management that may require resection and nerve repair to eliminate a damaged nerve segment. The concepts currently used in establishing continuity of lacerated nerves are (1) primary direct epineurial or fascicular sutures; (2) nerve grafts to bridge large gaps and provide continuity without suture line tension; and (3) bone shortening to perform direct epineurial suture.

The conditions that cause severe intraneural damage are prolonged localized nerve compression lesions, nerve segment damage due to local injection of a toxic agent, traumatic crushing of a nerve, or nerve compression by a bone fragment. Localized resection of a 2- to 3-cm. neuroma may be repaired by direct end-to-end suture with moderate mobilization of the nerve. This depends on the specific nerve and location of the defect. Defects that cannot be closed without tension after nerve mobilization usually require grafting. This decision depends on the length of the nerve gap, the ability of the adjacent nerve segments to be immobilized, and the diameter of the nerve segments.

EPINEURIAL REPAIR, END-TO-END. Epineurial or group fascicular repair is performed if the nerve gap allows end-to-end suture without tension. For example, a median nerve at the wrist with a total gap of 2 to 3 cm. after trimming and preparing for an end-to-end suture may require moderate mobilization of both proximal and distal segments after which an epineurial end-to-end suture may be performed without excessive tension. This would require the wrist to be in a position of flexion for several weeks.

NERVE GRAFTING. If the defect is greater than several centimeters, or when a full range of joint motion is desirable within 2 weeks after nerve repair, grafting of the defect should be considered. Nerve grafting requires a double suture line and each junction site may interfere with axon flow. Moreover, the nerve graft is temporarily ischemic unless a vascularized graft is performed, and nerve regeneration and ultimate function after grafting are slower than after end-to-end epineurial suture. However, the goal of the absence of tension on the suture line and the ability of nerve grafting to comprise large defects are strong indications for grafting in certain patients.

NERVE REPAIR TECHNIQUE. Adequate mobilization of both the proximal and the distal segments of the nerve should be accomplished without damage to the intrinsic blood supply of the nerve.

Mobilization may require transfer of the median nerve anterior to the pronator teres muscle in the upper forearm or transfer of the ulnar nerve anterior to the medial epicondyle. Mobilization of each of these nerves may be accomplished to gain 2 to 3 cm. of length without actually damaging the blood supply.

When the nerves are mobilized and the inherent elasticity is determined by gentle traction, a decision is made as to end-to-end epineurial or group fascicular repair or nerve grafting.

NERVE SUTURING PROCEDURE. (1) The nerve segment being prepared is stabilized with a nerve holder and cut carefully at right angles with a sharp knife. Cuts are made so that the nerve ends are trimmed back to healthy "pouting" fascicles. (2) Electrical stimulation, special nerve staining, and topographic alignment with magnification may be helpful in determining the proper orientation of the fascicles. Observation of peripheral vessels is helpful in aligning the fascicles. Adequate lighting and magnification in performing this maneuver are mandatory. Magnification may vary from 4 times for a large nerve to 10 times for a small nerve or graft. Topographic matching is attempted in order to bring proximal motor and sensory fibers to match with distal motor and sensory fibers. (3) Microneedle holders and small forceps are used to handle the epineurium and adjacent tissue with relatively atraumatic technique. (4) Sutures of 8-0 to 10-0 nylon are used to repair the nerve; the size of the suture depends on the size of the nerve and whether the repair is epineurial or group fascicular. Tension on the sutures should be sufficient to close the epineurium and prevent axons from escaping but not tight enough to wrinkle or cause malalignment of the fascicles.

The critical points to be remembered at the time of nerve repair are trimming of the nerve endings to nondamaged axons, adequate regional blood flow for nerve regeneration, anatomic topographic realignment of sensory and motor fascicles, apposition of nerve endings without tension, and adequate strength of apposition to avoid separation of the nerve segments.

SELECTED REFERENCES

Eversmann, W. W.: Entrapment and compression neuropathies. *In* Green, D. P. (Ed.): Operative Hand Surgery. New York, Churchill Livingstone, 1988, p. 1423.
  Current, well-illustrated discussion of entrapment and compression neuropathies of the upper extremity.

Spinner, M.: Management of nerve compression lesions of the upper extremity. *In* Omer, G. E., Jr., and Spinner, M. (Eds.): Management of Peripheral Nerve Problems. Philadelphia, W. B. Saunders Company, 1980, p. 569.

This small, clearly written text provides detailed anatomic and clinical information concerning peripheral nerves of the upper extremity.

REFERENCES

1. Bell, G. E., Jr., and Goldner, J. L.: Compression neuropathy of the median nerve. South. Med. J., *49*:966, 1956.
2. Blair, S. J.: Avoiding complications of surgery for nerve compression syndromes. Orthop. Clin. North Am., *19*:125, 1988.
3. Bolesta, M. J., Garret, W. E., Ribbeck, D. M., Glisson, R. R., Seaber, A. V., and Goldner, J. L.: Immediate and delayed neurorrhaphy in a rabbit model; a functional, histologic, and biochemical comparison. J. Hand Surg., *13A*:352, 1988.
4. Braun, R. M., Davidson, K., and Doehr, M. A.: Provocative testing in the diagnosis of dynamic carpal tunnel syndrome. J. Hand Surg., *14A*:195, 1989.
5. Eason, S. Y., Belsole, R. J., and Greene, T. L.: Carpal tunnel release: Analysis of suboptimal results. J. Hand Surg., *10B*:365, 1985.
6. Eversmann, W. W.: Entrapment and compression neuropathies. *In* Green, D. P. (Ed.): Operative Hand Surgery. New York, Churchill Livingstone, 1988, p. 1423.
7. Gelberman, R. H., Scabo, R. M., Williamson, R. V., and Dimick, M. P.: Sensibility testing in peripheral nerve compression syndromes. J. Bone Joint Surg., *65A*:632, 1963.
8. Gelberman, R. H., Aronson, D., and Weisman, M. H.: Carpal tunnel syndrome: Results of a prospective trial of steroid injection and splint. J. Bone Joint Surg., *62A*:1181, 1980.
9. Gelberman, R. H., Rydevik, B. L., Pess, G. M., Szabo, R. M., and Lundborg, G.: Carpal tunnel syndrome: A scientific basis for clinical care. Orthop. Clin. North Am., *19*:115, 1988.
10. Goldner, J. L.: Biological principles of repair and regeneration of nerve and tendon. South. Med. J., *64*:121, 1971.
11. Goldner, J. L.: Median nerve compression lesions, anatomical and clinical analysis. Bull. Hosp. J. Dis., *44*:199, 1984.
12. Goldner, J. L.: Function of the Hand Following Peripheral Nerve Injuries. Ann Arbor, Michigan, American Academy of Orthopaedic Surgeons, Instructional Course Lecture, Vol. X, 1953.
13. Goldner, R. D.: Nerve compressions in the upper extremity. Orthopaedic Surgery Update Series. Vol. 3, Lesson 28. Princeton, N.J., Bobbitt Publishers, 1984.
14. Goldner, R. D., and Koman, L. A.: Microsurgery of the hand. *In* Goldsmith, H. S. (Ed.): Practice of Surgery. Hagerstown, Md., Harper & Row, 1984, p. 1.
15. Groves, R. J., and Goldner, J. L.: Restoration of strong opposition after median nerve or brachial plexus paralysis. J. Bone Joint Surg., *57A*:112, 1975.
16. Kelley, J. M., and Goldner, J. L.: Radial nerve injuries. South. Med. J., *51*:873, 1958.
17. Lowry, W. E., Jr., and Follender, A. B.: Interfascicular neurolysis in severe carpal tunnel syndrome—a prospective, randomized, double-blind, controlled study. Clin. Orthop. Rel. Res., *227*:251, 1988.
18. McKinnon, S. E., and Dellon, A. L.: Experimental study of chronic nerve compression. Hand Clinics, *2*:639, 1986.
19. Ochoa, J., Fowler, T. J., and Gilliatt, R. W.: Anatomical changes in peripheral nerves compressed by a pneumatic tourniquet. J. Anat., *113*:433, 1972.
20. Osterman, A. L.: The double crush syndrome. Orthop. Clin. North Am., *19*:147, 1988.
21. Peimer, C.: Compression neuropathies in the upper extremities. Orthop. Rev., *16*:41, 1987.
22. Roles, N. C., and Maudsley, R. H.: Radial tunnel syndrome: Resistant tennis elbow as a nerve entrapment. J. Bone Joint Surg., *54B*:499, 1972.
23. Seddon, H. J.: Electrical Phenomena in Surgical Disorders of Peripheral Nerves. Baltimore, Williams & Wilkins, 1972, p. 577.
24. Seror, P.: Phalen's test in the diagnosis of carpal tunnel syndrome. J. Hand Surg., *13B*:383, 1988.
25. Seror, P.: Tinel's sign in the diagnosis of carpal tunnel syndrome. J. Hand Surg., *12B*:364, 1987.
26. Spindler, H. A., and Dellon, A. L.: Nerve conduction studies and sensibility testing in carpal tunnel syndrome. J. Hand Surg., *7*:260, 1982.
27. Spinner, M.: Management of nerve compression lesions of the upper extremity. *In* Omer, G. E., Jr., and Spinner, M. (Eds.): Management of Peripheral Nerve Problems. Philadelphia, W. B. Saunders Company, 1980, p. 569.
28. Sunderland, S.: Nerves and Nerve Injuries. New York, Churchill-Livingstone, 1978.
29. Szabo, R. M., and Gelberman, R. H.: The pathophysiology of nerve entrapment syndromes. J. Hand Surg., *12A*:880, 1987.
30. Urbaniak, J. R.: Nerve repair in the upper extremity. Orthopaedic Surgery Update Series. Vol. 1, Lesson 31. Princeton, N.J., Bobbitt Publishers, 1981.

43

REPLANTATION OF AMPUTATED LIMBS AND DIGITS

James R. Urbaniak, M.D.

Historical Aspects

The concepts of microsurgery and limb replantation developed in the early 1900s with the introduction of macrosurgical techniques for arterial and venous anastomoses in composite grafts and transplants. Hopfner, Carrel, and Guthrie began working on early animal limb replantation before 1905. However, it was not until the 1960s that Lapchinsky and Snyder succeeded in obtaining long-term results in dog replantations.

In 1922, Holmgren introduced the binocular operating microscope for middle ear surgery. The basic principles of anastomosing small vessels were described by Seidenberg and colleagues in 1958. The introduction of the operating microscope in 1960 by Jacobson and Suarez for the repair of small vessels had the greatest impact on the replantation of amputated hands and digits.

Microvascular surgery implies repair of small blood vessels (3 mm. or less in diameter), using an operating microscope, microsurgical instruments, and ultrafine suture material (usually approximately 20 μ in diameter). The $10-0$ (20μ) nylon or polypropylene suture, which is swedged on the needle of 50 to 130 μ in diameter, is essential in anastomosing small vessels of 1 mm. or less found at the base of an adult digit (Fig. 1).

Replantation is defined as reattachment of a part that has been completely severed, that is, there is no connection between the amputated part and the patient. *Revascularization* is the reattachment of a part of which some portion of the soft tissue (such as skin, nerves, or tendon) is still connected. Vascular repair is necessary to prevent necrosis of the partially severed distal limb. This may require repair of the arteries or the veins, or both.

Malt in 1962 first successfully replanted a completely amputated arm in a 12-year-old male. The first successful replantation of an amputated digit by microvascular technique was performed by Komatsu and Tamai in Nara, Japan, in 1965. Digit and hand replantation using microvascular anastomosis of small arteries and veins has become an effective method of reconstructing hands that have sustained complete or incomplete amputations.

Care of the Amputated Part

Amputated or devascularized tissue survives for approximately 6 hours if the part is not cooled. Cooling lessens the metabolic needs of the tissues, and an amputated part may be successfully restored 12 hours after severance if it is cooled. Because the digits essentially have no muscle tissue, they may be successfully replanted as long as 24 hours after amputation if they are cooled.

Because most replantations are performed in centers with experienced microvascular teams, the referring physician must be given clear instructions regarding preservation of the amputated part and the care of the injured patient. The amputated part should be placed into a plastic bag containing Ringer's lactate or saline solution; the plastic bag is placed on ice. The amputated part must not be allowed to come in direct contact with ice or to become frozen. The referring physician is instructed not to ligate or perfuse any of the vessels for fear of causing intimal damage. An alternative method of preserving the amputated part is to wrap it in a cloth or sponge moistened with Ringer's lactate or saline solution and place it in a plastic bag, which is put on ice.

Patient Selection

The decision of whether to replant an amputated part is not always easy. An experienced replantation team can restore almost any amputated part and have it remain viable. However, success in viability must not be misconstrued as success in useful function of the replanted extremity. Guillotine-type amputations are obviously ideal for replanting; however, this type of amputation is uncommon. Most amputated parts are avulsed or crushed, making reconstruction more complex and viability more difficult to achieve.

Candidates for replantation are selected according to the following priorities: (1) thumb, (2) multiple digits, (3) partial hand (amputation through the palm), (4) almost any part of a child, (5) wrist or forearm, (6) above-elbow amputation (only sharp or moderately avulsed), and (7) isolated digit distal to the superficialis insertion (distal to the proximal interphalangeal joint). This list is not necessarily in strict order of preference; however, if other factors are favorable, replantation should be attempted. The prime parts for replantation are thumbs, multiple digits, and the complete hand. Replantation of these parts provides the best results; however, replantation of the other parts listed generally produces better function than can be obtained by a prosthesis. In children an attempt should be made to replant almost any part, since if the replanted extremity survives, excellent function can be expected.

Type of injuries that are not favorable for replantation are (1) severely crushed or mangled parts, (2) amputations at multiple levels, (3) amputations in patients with other serious injuries or diseases, (4) amputations in which the vessels are arteriosclerotic, (5) amputations in mentally unstable patients, (6) more than 6 hours of ischemic time, (7) severely contaminated parts, and (8) an individual finger in the adult with the amputation proximal to the superficialis insertions (proximal to the proximal interphalangeal joint). Replantations of isolated fingers at the base (proximal to the superficialis insertion) generally produce a finger that "gets in the way" because of diminished tendon excursion. If the isolated finger is amputated distal to the proximal interphalangeal joint, the flexor superficialis tendon is still intact and replantation produces a functional digit with good tendon excursion. Selection is also influenced by the patient's

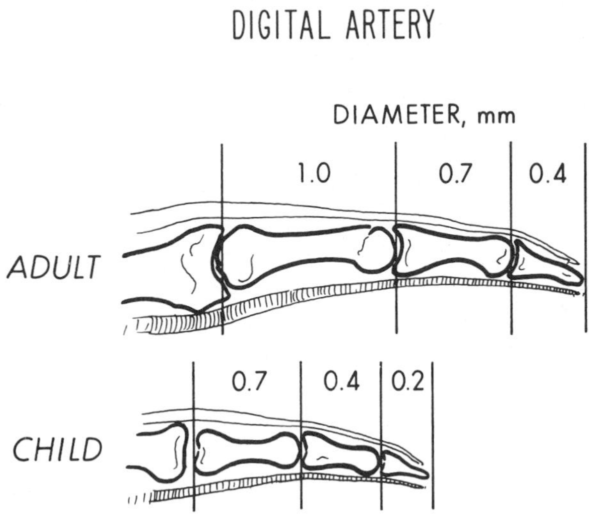

DIGITAL ARTERY

DIAMETER, mm

Figure 1. The comparative sizes of the human digital arteries in the adult and the child. Microsurgical anastomosis is possible in a vessel as small as 0.3 mm.

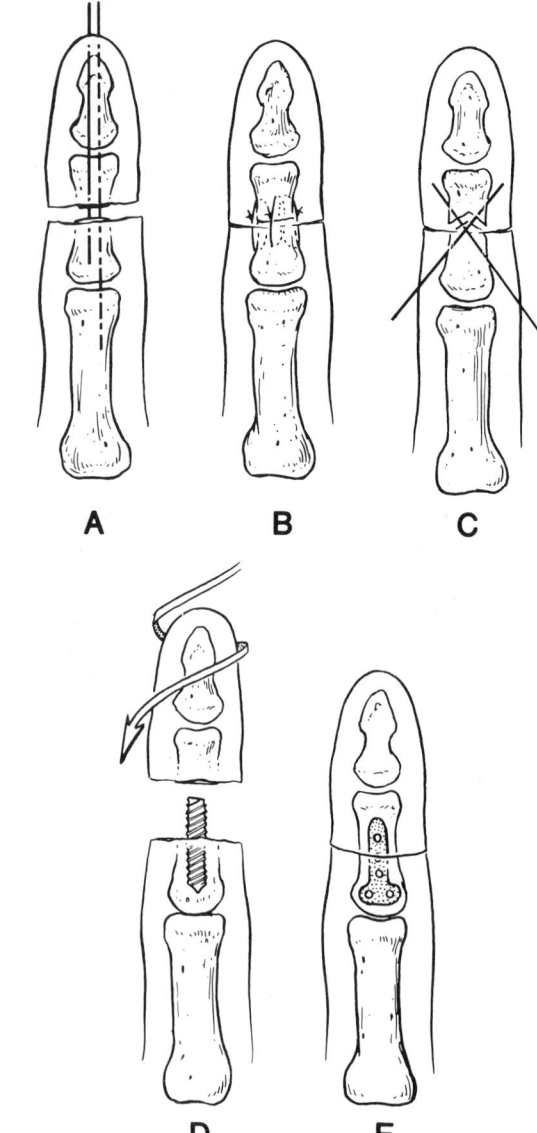

Figure 2. Methods of bone fixation. *A*, Intramedullary pins. *B*, Intraosseous wiring. *C*, Crossed pins. *D*, Intramedullary screw. *E*, Plate and screws. *A* is the preferred method. (From Goldner, R. D., and Urbaniak, J. R.: Replantation in the Upper Extremity. Orthopaedic Surgery Update Series, Vol. 2, Lesson 32, 1983.)

occupation, avocation, age, and sex. These contraindications to replantation are not absolute. Often the final decision cannot be made until the status of the damaged blood vessels is determined under the operating microscope.

Surgical Technique

When a patient with an amputated part arrives in the emergency room, the replantation team divides into two subteams. One team immediately takes the amputated part to the operating theater and prepares it for examination under the operating microscope. The vessels and nerves are located and labeled (with fine suture or hemaclips) under 10-power magnification. Microscopic evaluation determines the feasibility of restoration by revascularization. The other team assesses and prepares the patient for the operative procedure. Most replantations of upper extremity parts are performed under axillary block with a long-acting agent such as bupivacaine hydrochloride (Marcaine). General anesthesia is seldom indicated, and all the neural and vascular surgery is performed under the operating microscope.

The sequence of replantation of amputated digits or hands is as follows: (1) locate and tag the vessels and nerves, (2) shorten and fix the bone with an intramedullary pin, (3) repair the extensor tendons, (4) repair the flexor tendons, (5) repair the arteries, (6) repair the nerves, (7) repair the veins, and (8) obtain loose skin coverage (split-thickness graft if necessary) (Fig. 2).

The bone is shortened to allow normal intima to be attached to normal intima. Sometimes interposition vein grafts are necessary for arterial and/or venous repair when there is severe vascular damage. Usually two veins are repaired for each artery. An attempt is made to repair both digital arteries. Primary nerve grafts (from the medial antebrachial cutaneous nerve on the ipsilateral forearm) are used if the gap is large. None of the vascular or nerve repairs should be done under tension. *The most important factors in achieving permanent microvascular patency are easy coaptation of vessels with normal intima and the skill and expertise of the microsurgeon.*

Major Limb Replantation

Since most amputations of the upper extremity occur at the digit or hand level, emphasis has been placed on describing the reattachment at these levels. Major limb replantation implies replantation of limbs proximal to the wrist or of the lower extremity proximal to the ankle. Replantation of limbs amputated at or proximal to the wrist level or amputations of the lower extremity below or above the knee employ similar principles with minor modifications. The major differences are related to

the increased amount of muscle tissue involved. Because more muscle mass is involved, the duration of avascularity of the detached part is more critical.

Whereas amputated digits may be successfully replanted 24 hours after amputation, an arm amputated at the elbow is in jeopardy if it has been avascular for 10 or 12 hours even if it has been properly cooled. Extensive muscle débridement on both the detached part and the stump is essential to prevent myonecrosis with subsequent infection, which is the major problem in major limb replantation but is uncommon in digital reattachment. Rarely are major limbs cleanly severed, and, therefore, the muscle damage is usually quite severe.

In replantations proximal to the metacarpal level, immediate arterial inflow is necessary to prevent or diminish myonecrosis. If the amputated part and the patient arrive in the operating room more than 4 hours after injury, it is desirable to initiate immediate blood flow to the detached part. This is best accomplished by using some form of shunt, such as a Sundt or ventriculoperitoneal shunt, to obtain rapid arterial inflow from the proximal vessel to the detached part (Fig. 3). Shunting should be performed before bone fixation unless the bone can be rapidly

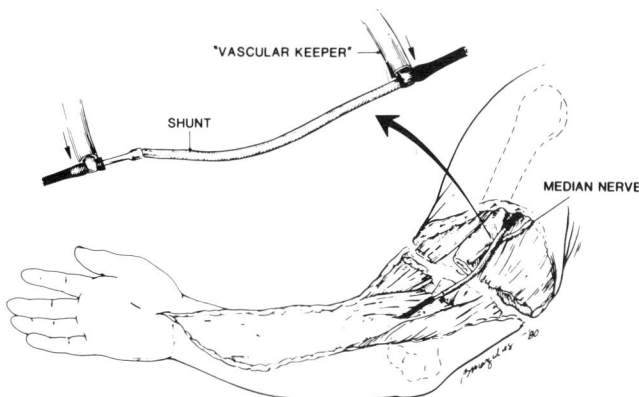

Figure 3. A Sundt shunt or a ventriculoperitoneal shunt is used to obtain rapid arterial inflow from the proximal vessel to the amputated part. (From Urbaniak, J. R.: Replantation. *In* Green, D. P.: Operative Hand Surgery, 2nd ed. New York, Churchill Livingstone, 1988, pp. 1105–1126.)

stabilized and early blood flow obtained. After the establishment of temporary blood flow, further débridement can be continued, the bone stabilized, the shunt removed, and a direct arterial repair or interposition vein grafting of the vessels performed.

Stable bone fixation is necessary for major limb replantation; however, the method should be rapid. Rigid plate and screw fixation of the long bones is preferable. As in digital replantation, bone shortening must be carefully planned relative to the type of injury and tissue damage. Usually the plate may be secured to the amputated part after the initial débridement and then fixed to the stump after blood flow has been established through shunts, particularly if the ischemic time has been prolonged.

In major limb replantation it is critical to perform the arterial anastomosis before the venous anastomosis. This sequence allows a physiologic washout of noxious agents such as lactic acid in the distal part. If this order is reversed, with the venous connection first, the return of toxic catabolites through the systemic circulation can cause serious consequences, even death. The administration of intravenous sodium bicarbonate before venous anastomosis is beneficial.

Extensive fasciotomies are always indicated in major limb replantations. *The two most common causes of failure in major limb replantation are myonecrosis with subsequent infection and failure to provide adequate decompression of the restored vessels.*

Meshed split-thickness skin grafts may be used to provide coverage over the exposed vessels. Other areas may be closed primarily or grafted several days later.

In replantations of major limbs, the patient should be returned to the operating room within 48 to 72 hours for evaluation of the state of muscle tissue. The dressing should be changed with the patient under general anesthesia or regional block, and any necrotic tissue must be further débrided for prevention of infection. In general, no anticoagulation is employed for major limb replantations. Whereas most patients with digital replantations are hospitalized for 6 or 7 days, those with major limb replantations require longer periods depending on the severity of the injury.

In major limb replantations, the likelihood for successful replantation ranks in the order of the wrist, the arm, and the distal forearm. The poorest results occur in the proximal third of the forearm, an area where the motor branches of the radial, median, and ulnar nerves enter the extrinsic musculature of the hand.

There are few indications for replantation of the lower extremity. The functional disability that follows a lower limb amputation is less than that sustained from an upper extremity amputation of a similar nature. Upper extremity prostheses poorly duplicate hand function; however, lower limb prostheses provide a stable stance and a functional gait.

In addition, the lower extremity injuries are usually caused by an extensive crush or avulsion mechanism and the skeletal shortening required to reapproximate undamaged tissue usually produces an unacceptable leg length discrepancy. It is usually prudent to revise the amputation of a lower extremity, sometimes using the amputated parts to serve as innervated free flaps to provide stump sensation and preserve more function, for example, preserving a below-knee amputation instead of an above-knee amputation. With the currently available lower extremity prostheses, considerable thought should be given before attempting replantation of the lower extremities even in rather cleanly severed limbs.

Postoperative Management

A careful postoperative regimen is paramount in achieving a high viability rate in replantation. Most patients receive some type of anticoagulation. Intravenous heparin at 1000 units per hour for approximately 7 days is usually administered. This is monitored by maintaining the activated partial thromboplastin time at one and one-half to two times normal. Low-molecular-weight dextran, aspirin, chlorpromazine, and dipyridamole

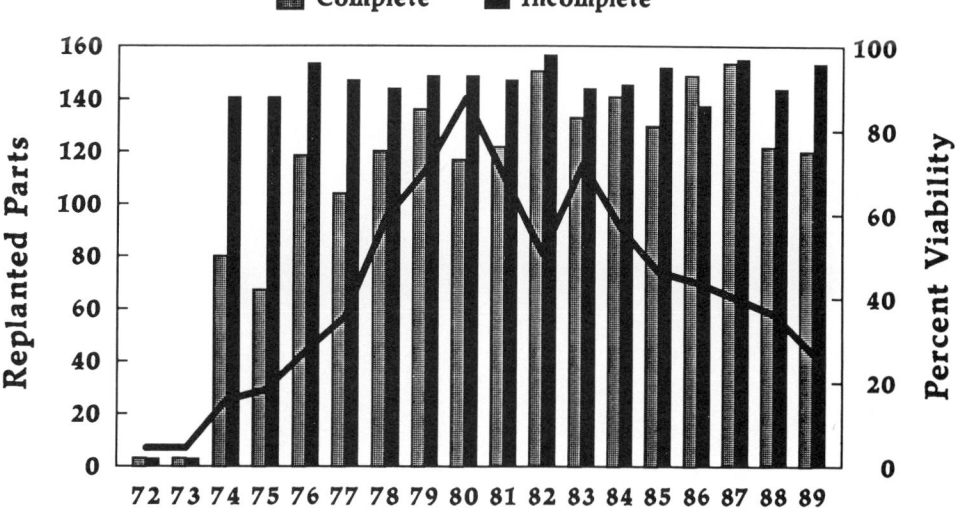

Figure 4. The 16-year Duke experience with more than 1200 attempted replantations. The vertical bars represent the success in viability, and the horizontal bar line represents the number of replantations each year.

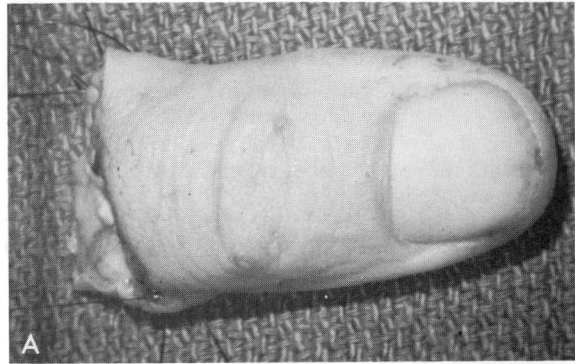

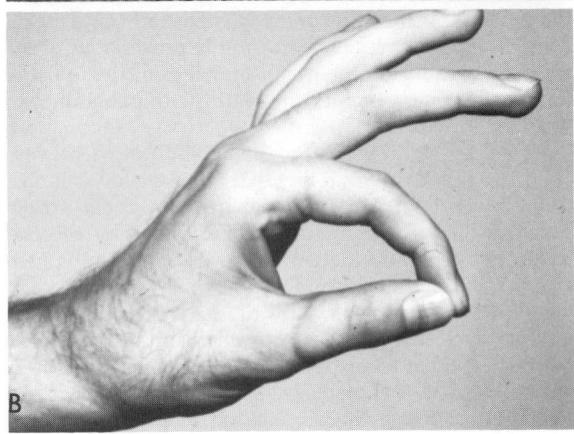

Figure 5. *A,* This clean thumb amputation was replanted in a 16-year-old male. *B,* Essentially normal sensibility, motor function, and pinch were achieved.

have all been used in difficult cases. Skin color, pulp turgor, capillary refill, and skin temperature are the most useful indicators for monitoring. In general, if the skin temperature of the replanted part, which is continuously monitored by a small surface probe taped to the digit, drops below 30° C., poor vascular perfusion of the digit is certain and a cause for the poor circulation must be found and corrected if possible. The dressing must be inspected for any constriction. Additional heparin may be indicated, and axillary or stellate blocks may be helpful. The hand may need to be elevated or depressed. Seldom is it necessary to return the patient to the operating room for a revision; however, if re-exploration is to be successful, it must usually be done within 24 to 48 hours after the primary procedure.

Results of Replantation

The Duke Orthopaedic Replantation Team has attempted revascularization or replantation of more than 1200 partial or total amputations from 1972 to 1989. Ninety-two per cent of the partial amputations have been successfully revascularized, and 77 per cent of the complete amputations have remained viable. The viability rates have improved with experience of the team (Fig. 4). Most major replantation centers are obtaining an approximately 80 per cent viability rate in complete replantations.

Recovery of sensibility in replanted digits is similar to results of repair of an isolated peripheral nerve. Cold intolerance is a problem in most patients, but this subsides in 1 to 2 years. Replanted thumbs provide the best functional results (Fig. 5). Strong pinch, adequate motion, excellent sensation, and almost normal appearance are to be expected. Replantation of digits distal to the superficialis insertions provide good appearance with excellent results, good pulp turgor, and nonpainful digits. Replantation of digits at the base of the finger (proximal to the superficialis insertion) produces good sensibility but usually poor functional motion. Replantations of multiple digits, partial hands (through the palm), or complete hands provide good sensibility and useful function (Fig. 6). Whereas amputations through the wrist or distal forearm provide good function of the hand, amputations at a more proximal level have varied results. Patients usually have weak pinch and grasp and poor sensibility. Amputations at the wrist or hand level seldom require addi-

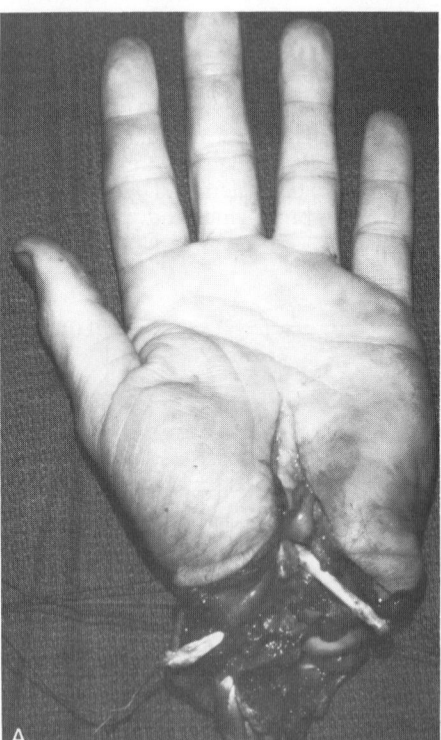

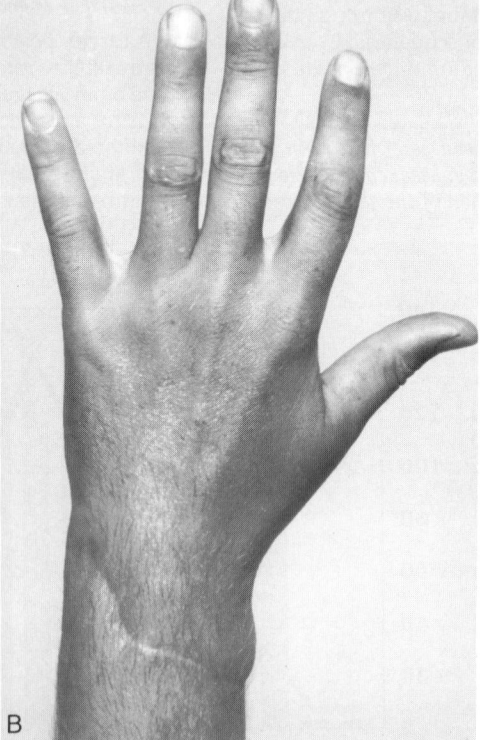

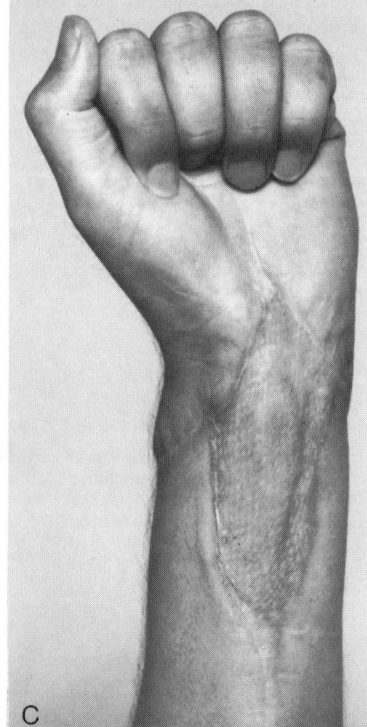

Figure 6. *A,* This 22-year-old male had replantation of a completely amputated hand. *B* and *C,* One year after replantation, he has nearly full flexion-extension of the hand. Intrinsic function has returned to the thenar and hyperthenar muscles. He has protective sensibility with a strong pinch and grip. (From Porubsky, G. L., and Urbaniak, J. R.: Limb and digital replantation. *In* Flye, M. W.: Principles of Organ Transplantation. Philadelphia, W. B. Saunders Company, 1989, pp. 453–477.)

tional secondary reconstructive procedures; however, amputations at a more proximal level, particularly above the elbow, usually require secondary nerve grafts and tendon or muscle transfers to achieve elbow and possibly digital flexion and extension.

SELECTED REFERENCES

Goldner, R. D., Fitch, R. D., Nunley, J. A., Aitken, M. S., and Urbaniak, J. R.: Demographics and replantation. J. Hand Surg., *12A*:961, 1987.
This is an excellent demographic study of more than 1200 replanted upper extremities.

Goldner, R. D., Stevanovic, M. V., Nunley, J. A., and Urbaniak, J. R.: Digital replantation at the level of the distal interphalangeal joint and the distal phalanx. J. Hand Surg., *14A*:214, 1989.
This study represents the largest collection of patients who have been followed after replantation of a single digit at or distal to the distal interphalangeal joint. This report documents the value of distal replantation as well as describing the microsurgical techniques.

Nunley, J. A., Koman, L. A., and Urbaniak, J. R.: Arterial shunting as an adjunct to major limb revascularization. Ann. Surg., *193*:271, 1981.
This article describes the method of temporary shunting to provide immediate perfusion into the amputated limb prior to reattachment. This innovation has significantly increased the viability rate and continues to be a vital step in major limb replantation.

Urbaniak, J. R.: Replantation. *In* Green, D. P. (Ed.): Operative Hand Surgery. New York, Churchill Livingstone, 1988, pp. 1105–1126.
This chapter provides a current detailed description of patient selection, technique, and expected results of digit, hand, and arm replantation.

Urbaniak, J. R., Roth, J. H., Nunley, J. A., Goldner, R. D., and Koman, L. A.: The results of replantation after amputation of a single finger. J. Bone Joint Surg. [Am], *67*:611, 1985.
This article is unique in that it is a study of a homogeneous group of patients with single digit amputation with no other hand injuries. It clearly defines criteria for patient selection for replantation based on the level of amputation.

REFERENCES

1. Beiber, E. J., Wood, M. B., Cooney, W. P., and Amadio, P. C.: Thumb avulsion: Results of replantation/revascularization. J. Hand Surg. [Am], *12*:786, 1987.
2. Gelberman, R. H., Urbaniak, J. R., Bright, D. S., and Levin, L. S.: Digital sensibility following replantation. J. Hand Surg. [Am], *3*:313, 1978.
3. Kutz, J. E., Jupiter, J. B., and Tsai, T.-M.: Lower limb replantation—a report of nine cases. Foot Ankle, *3*:197, 1983.
4. Russell, R. C., O'Brien, B. M., Morrison, W. A., et al.: The late functional results of upper limb revascularization and replantation. J. Hand Surg. [Am], *9*:623, 1984.
5. Stirrat, C. R., Seaber, A. V., Urbaniak, J. R., and Bright, D. S.: Temperature monitoring in digital replantation. J. Hand Surg. [Am], *3*:342, 1978.
6. Tark, K. C., Kim, Y. W., Lee, Y. H., and Lew, J. D.: Replantation and revascularization of hands: Clinical analysis and functional results of 261 cases. J. Hand Surg. [Am], *14*:17, 1989.
7. Urbaniak, J. R.: Replantation in children. *In* Serafin, D., and Georgiade, N. G. (Eds.): Pediatric Plastic Surgery. St. Louis, C. V. Mosby, 1984, pp. 1168–1187.
8. Urbaniak, J. R.: Digital replantation: A 12-year experience. *In* Urbaniak, J. R. (Ed.): Microsurgery for Major Limb Reconstruction. St. Louis, C. V. Mosby, 1987, pp. 12–21.
9. Urbaniak, J. R., Evans, J. P., and Bright, D. S.: Microvascular management of ring avulsion injuries. J. Hand Surg. [Am], *6*:25, 1981.
10. Urbaniak, J. R., Hayes, M. G., and Bright, D. S.: Management of bone in digital replantation: Free vascularized and composite bone grafts. Clin. Orthop., *133*:194, 1978.

44

THE SKIN

Functional, Metabolic, and Surgical Considerations

Donald Serafin, M.D.

All who study man are now reasonably clear that modern men of the most diverse types possess characters that stamp us all as of common ancestry, but with these common characters are interwoven others, some of which are clearly adaptations to diverse environments.[22]

H. J. Fleure
Professor of Geography and Anthropology
University College Wales, 1928

The evolution of *Homo sapiens* began approximately 15 million before present (MBP) in the open savannas of north central Africa.[9] Here, the last common ancestor of both apes and humans, *Dryopithecus*, evolved from forest living proto-monkeys and proto-apes. *Ramapithecus*, the suggested ancestor to humans, appeared later, from 14 to 9 MBP, moving from the forest into the open savannas, where human forms later evolved. In this same region *Australopithecus* also evolved at approximately 5 MBP. *Australopithecus*, of short stature (50 to 60 lbs.), living on the edge of the forest or out in the open plain, was able to run well enough to catch small prey. Although the color of his skin is unknown, it was probably quite dark and lightly covered with fine black hair. As hair became less dense, the sweat glands increased in number. This change sharply differentiated hominids from other primates. (Humans have approximately 2 to 5 million sweat glands in the skin, far more than any other primate.) The loss of hair and increase in the efficiency and number of sweat glands are thought to be related to an increasing need to sustain strenuous physical activity over prolonged periods of time.[9] As hominids moved from the protective forest to the open savannas, they became daytime hunters, generating an excessive amount of body heat in pursuit of their game. An efficient cooling mechanism was required and thus evolved. The dark melanin pigment protected these hominids from the deleterious effects of the sun.

Homo erectus appeared approximately 1.5 MBP in Africa, Europe, and Asia. This species was characterized by an enormous increase in body size as well as the brain. The skin was hairless and also quite pigmented.

Approximately 100,000 years ago *Homo sapiens* evolved. The Neanderthal was the earliest representative of the species. Approximately 75,000 years ago during the most recent glacial age (Würm), the world's climate changed significantly. Open grasslands and formerly wooded portions of Germany and northern France were transformed into tundra as a result of the scarcity of sunlight and the cold. During winter and in the higher latitudes melanin production in the skin decreased. The colder climes also necessitated the wearing of animal skins for warmth, further decreasing the area of skin to sun exposure. Lighter-skinned individuals evolved. The loss of skin pigment had sur-

vival function, however, permitting photosynthesis of vitamin D in the skin.[9] In the tropics a decrease of vitamin D production in pigmented individuals was not a serious problem because of intense and protracted sun exposure.

Geographic races evolved approximately 30,000 years ago, a relatively short evolutionary period. Differences in skin pigmentation and hair distribution are characteristic among the six major races.

It is apparent from the foregoing discussion that the skin is a highly complex organ whose adaptive and protective qualities not only ensured species survival but also contributed to the evolution of *Homo sapiens*.

The skin is an organ of astonishing complexity. It is the barrier between the relatively closed system of a human body and its external environment; it is strong, elastic, waterproof, protective, and self-repairing. Beyond this, it serves as a sense organ, an excretory organ, a heat control mechanism (involving hair and sweat glands), and the organ of individual identification. It responds to environmental stress, both directly (suntanning and healing) and indirectly (sweating).[9]

FUNCTIONS OF THE SKIN

BARRIER FUNCTION. Mammals distinguished themselves from lower phyla by maintaining a considerable degree of environmental dependence. This dependence is to a large extent permitted by the barrier function of the skin.[56] Interaction with the environment is possible, but its adverse effects are prevented from harming the organism. Thus, bacteria and other organisms, toxic chemicals, and gases have difficulty in penetrating the barrier. Previously, a barrier membrane was postulated to exist at the base of the horny layer. It is now believed that all of the cells of the stratum corneum fulfill this function. The thicker the stratum corneum, the better the barrier function. In addition, the gradient is increased from superficial to deep levels, where cells have increased cohesiveness.

The maintenance of an internal equilibrium and environment is also made possible by the impenetrable stratum corneum. In man, both diffusion and water loss are low and are inversely related to the thickness of this horny layer.

COMMUNICATION WITH THE ENVIRONMENT. The skin is a unique organ capable of performing simultaneously seemingly incongruous functions. Thus, while providing a barrier function, it must also provide continuous communication between the organism and its environment.[53] Most mammals, including humans, possess both glabrous and hairy skin, each with distinctive features. Glabrous skin is usually that portion that is in intimate contact with the environment and consequently is well-adapted for this function. By definition it is hairless and heavily keratinized. Its dermal-epidermal junction is corrugated and often labyrinthine, with a honeycombed appearance, permitting firm attachment to the underlying dermis.[53] Multiple subcutaneous septa analogous to Cooper's ligaments in the breast contribute to this anchoring function, lessening tangential shear stresses between the dermis and underlying bony architecture. Glabrous skin, topographically, is also organized into highly specialized papillary ridges and grooves[37] (Fig. 1). Sweat ducts located in the deep dermis empty through pores in the papillary ridges. This arrangement facilitates the grasping of smooth objects. Collagen anchoring fibers, associated with the dermal-epidermal ultrastructure, attach the limiting ridges of the epidermis (located beneath the papillary grooves) to the deep or reticular dermis. The limiting ridges and anchoring fibers stabilize the overlying epidermis. The intermediate ridge, located beneath the papillary ridge and between the limiting ridges, is associated with a complex network of nerve fibers and end organs. It acts as a magnifying lever for the transmission of pressure stimuli on the surface of the skin.

Sensory nerves are more complex in arrangement in glabrous skin, which also contains a greater proportion of myelinated fibers. These fibers, first-order afferents, are responsible for transmitting sensory stimuli to the brain. Finally, glabrous skin contains a large concentration of nonneural mechanoreceptors permitting fine tactile discrimination. A complex interrelationship with the papillary ridges, outlined previously, facilitates this discrimination.[10]

Hairy skin, in contrast to glabrous skin, contains fewer mechanoreceptors and a lower concentration of myelinated nerves. Hair functions to buffer the organism from tactile stimuli, thus buffering it from the environment. The dermal-epidermal junction is also relatively thin and somewhat flat, with poorly developed papillary ridges and grooves, reflecting its structural deficiency for tactile discrimination. Fibrous septa for attachment of

dermis to bone are absent, which causes skin laxity and permits tangential movement. A panniculus carnosus, present in most mammals, facilitates skin stretching and movement. Thus, nonglabrous skin is best suited to facilitate movement, but tactile discrimination is diminished.

Human skin is distinctive because its nakedness provides a large surface area to contact the environment. Numerous stimuli from the skin, especially from the glabrous prehensile hand, are transmitted to a large brain, permitting man's present eminence on earth.[56]

PROTECTION FROM MECHANICAL INJURY. The skin is a tough, relatively impenetrable, resilient structure that can withstand considerable mechanical injury. This property resides in the dermis and is made possible by collagen fibers, ground substance (mucopolysaccharides), elastin and reticulin, the noncellular components of the dermis. The dermis varies considerably throughout the body both in its thickness and in its composition, both cellular and noncellular elements. Viscoelastic properties characterize the dermis, which can be attributed to both its collagen content and the organization of its fibers and ground substance. When a force is applied to skin, it lengthens until the further application of increasing force does not cause more lengthening. If this force is increased even more, tensile strength is eventually exceeded and the skin ruptures. The ability to increase in length is related to the rearrangement of the randomly oriented collagen fibers to a more parallel configuration. Tensile strength is determined by collagen content and the degree and nature of binding.[49] Upon release of the force, collagen fibers resume their previous random organization, perhaps with the aid of the ground substance and elastin. This viscoelastic property permits flexibility over joints and accommodation to stretching.

The thickness of skin varies considerably in different areas — again reflecting its regional adaptation. Thus, on the back, the dermis is quite thick where it has a dual role in thermoregulation as well as protection from mechanical injury. Many sailors survived flogging only because of the thickness of the dermis on their backs.

Ground substance, composed of mucopolysaccharides, is the homogeneous medium in which collagen fibers are dispersed.[56] When a portion of skin is compressed, it becomes thinner directly under the force. Mucopolysaccharides function to distribute this force to the immediately surrounding area.

EPITHELIAL-MESENCHYMAL INTERACTION. The ability of one tissue to influence the growth and regeneration of another is well documented.[63] If an extremity of a young salamander is amputated, the limb regenerates distal to the site of amputation. If, however, the limb has been previously irradiated or if a major nerve supplying the limb transected, regeneration does not occur. Cell dedifferentiation, repression, an electrical biologic potential gradient, and inductive substances, including histones and RNA messenger, have all been implicated.[71]

Dermal mesenchyme has been demonstrated to be essential for the growth and regeneration of epithelium (inductive interaction is also quite probable).[56] In other experiments it has also been demonstrated that epidermis differentiates according to the site of origin of the dermis.[69]

Carcinogenesis has been described as uncontrolled multipolar regeneration. The modification of cell surfaces causes failure of cell aggregation. Cell contact is avoided, and repressive information cannot be transmitted.[63] Regeneration and uncontrolled cellular multiplication represent different but related events along the same continuum. In this context, it is interesting to speculate about the progressive loss of epithelial-mesenchyme interaction in chronic burn scars, previously irradiated skin, and chronic sun-exposed areas. Thus, dermal damage and repetitive trauma with accelerated epithelial proliferation can eventually cause uncontrolled cell growth, multiplication, and invasion.

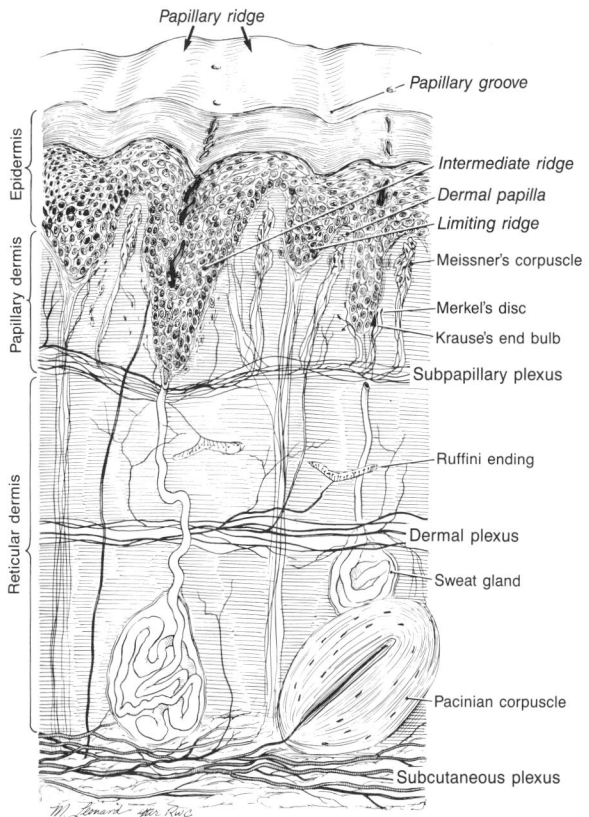

Figure 1. Cross section of glabrous skin. Note the intermediate ridge, which acts as a magnifying lever for the transmission of pressure stimuli on the surface of the skin.

TEMPERATURE REGULATION. Core body temperature, unless affected by disease, exercise, or alteration in metabolism, remains almost exactly constant at 98.6° F. (37° C.) Variation from this norm rarely exceeds ±1° F.

The importance of the skin in adaptation to adverse climatic conditions and its role in the evolution and survival of *Homo sapiens* was previously discussed. Intense energy expenditures necessitate an increased caloric intake. Conversely, the maintenance of a constant internal body temperature requires a mechanism to dissipate excessive energy into the environment. Heat is lost by radiation (60 per cent), evaporation (25 per cent), and conduction (15 per cent).[32] Heat dissipation by both radiation and conduction are influenced by (1) the degree of cutaneous blood flow and (2) ambient temperature and humidity. If environmental temperature exceeds body core temperature, loss of heat by radiation and conduction become less effective. Convection, or the movement of cooler air to displace warm air surrounding the body, augments the effects of conduction. Evaporative loss through sweating then becomes the most efficient mechanism for heat dissipation and survival.

Blood flow to the skin has both a nutrient and a thermoregulatory function. Local factors have a limited role in regulating cutaneous blood flow. The thermal regulation center is located in the preoptic portion of the anterior hypothalamus. Heating this area causes vasodilation and sweating, whereas cooling has an opposite effect. Sympathetic vasoconstriction mediated by the hypothalamus causes constant vasomotor tone. Extreme cold causes a further increase of vasomotor tone and a reduction of cutaneous flow. Blood flow values as low as 0.5 to 1.0 ml. per 100 ml. tissue can be demonstrated. This minimal flow is apparently sufficient to satisfy the metabolic tissue demands necessary for survival.[7] Increased vasomotor tone leads to closure of cutaneous precapillary sphincters throughout the body. Arteriovenous communications, concentrated in the face and distal palms and soles of the extremities, are also closed.[32] Glomus bodies, for sophisticated arteriovenous communication, are also found in these areas. Both are thought to mediate temperature and blood pressure changes by regulating and controlling blood flow into the subcutaneous venous plexuses. The mean cutaneous blood flow is 20 to 30 times greater than the minimal flow.[7] During periods of maximal exercise or intense heat, blood flow values are increased 100 times.[7] Vasomotor tone is decreased with opening of precapillary sphincters and arteriovenous communications. The subcutaneous venous lake then functions as a radiator, increasing heat loss into the environment.[32] Active vasodilatation is also thought to occur, but the exact mechanism remains obscure.

An increase in core body temperature also causes sweating,[32] with increased evaporation. It is estimated that 0.58 calorie of heat is lost for each gram of water that evaporates. In hot weather an unacclimatized person produces 1.5 liters per hour of sweat. Excessive sweating can cause loss of sodium and chloride equal to concentrations found in plasma. If sweating is minimal, then the concentrations of these ions are reduced because of removal from the precursor secretion. Other substances lost in reasonable quantities in the sweat include urea, lactic acid, and potassium.

ORGAN OF INDIVIDUAL IDENTIFICATION. In vertebrates, the skin has many functions, including that of individual identification. Appendages of the skin (i.e., hair and feathers) are important during mating with species preservation. They may also serve as camouflage, protecting the skin from predators in the environment. As indicated previously, races as well as individuals are distinguished primarily on the basis of their skin characteristics.

The competitive modern-day society is youth-oriented. A youthful appearance is desirable in order to enhance self-esteem as well as to augment other qualities in interpersonal relationships, in both private and public life. Redundant skin with loss of elasticity and removal of undesirable deposits of adipose tissue as a result of the aging process are frequently corrected in aesthetic surgery.

IMMUNOLOGIC FUNCTION OF THE SKIN. The skin has an important immunologic function that has only recently been characterized.[75,80] Three major epidermal cell populations are present that include keratinocytes (derived from ectoderm), melanocytes (neuroectoderm), and Langerhans cells (derived from mesenchyme). Langerhans cells represent approximately 2 to 4 per cent of the epithelial cell population and reside primarily in a suprabasal cell location.[73] These cells are derived from a mobile pool of bone-marrow precursor cells, where they enter the general circulation.[73] These cells then migrate to the epidermis. Unlike the stable keratinocyte population, Langerhans cells are mobile and transient. These cells are characterized by long dendritic processes that extend between the keratinocytes in three dimensions. The Langerhans cell population is constant for a given species and region.[2,81] These cells express Ia antigens and have receptor sites for the Fc portion of the IgG and complement components (C3).

Langerhans cells have been identified as being critical for the initiation of the cutaneous immune response.[8,54] Antigen, penetrating the epidermis, is taken up by Langerhans cells and processed. These immunologically active moieties are then presented to T lymphocytes, which are activated. As a consequence of their physical approximation, keratinocytes are stimulated to release interleukin-1, which influences the production of interleukin-2, further amplifying the T-cell response.

Langerhans cells are also known to induce the maturation of T lymphocytes into cytotoxic T lymphocytes.

Ultraviolet (UVB) light interferes with the immunologic function of epidermal cells by (1) affecting the processing of antigen by Langerhans cells and (2) altering the production of keratinocyte-derived factors required for T-cell proliferation.[74]

METABOLISM OF THE SKIN

CARBOHYDRATE. The epidermis is metabolically more active than the dermis. Qualitatively, pathways for glycolysis, oxidation, or other biosynthetic contributions do not differ from those in other tissues.[23] Numerous investigators have observed the preferential selection of the glycolytic pathway for energy production. At first inspection this is puzzling! The substrate glucose is readily available, as are other fuels. Certainly anaerobic glycolysis is not as energy-efficient as the tricarboxylic acid cycle, where 32 moles of adenosine triphosphate (ATP) are produced instead of two moles for each mole of glucose. Yet even in the presence of oxygen sufficiency, there is selective utilization of the glycolytic pathway with production of lactic acid. It is of historical interest to note that Baronio, an Italian physiologist in 1804, was the first investigator to successfully transplant cutaneous tissue. Partial-thickness skin grafts from the backs of sheep were totally separated from their blood supply and moved to an adjacent site. Subsequent investigators demonstrated that epidermal cell survival during the first 24 to 48 hours was indeed possible even with the limited oxygen available to inosculation. Thus, anaerobic glycolysis permitted successful transplantation. The selective use of the glycolytic pathway, even in the presence of an abundance of substrate glucose and oxygen, must then have survival value or provide additional essential function(s). Several explanations are possible. One of the most important functions of the skin is temperature regulation. This function is dependent, to a large extent, on blood flow. In an extremely cold environment, blood flow is reduced to values as low as 0.5 to 1 ml. per gm. of tissue. Under such conditions cell metabolism must be maintained despite limited oxygen availability in poorly perfused capillary beds. Another explanation may be related to ensuring cell maintenance, functioning, and growth of epidermal cells at an increased distance from blood supply. Thus, anaerobic glycolysis ensures survival in glabrous areas and in other regions (i.e., the back) with a thickened dermis. Finally, acid hydrolysates, e.g., lactic acid generated during anaerobic glycolysis, may have additional function, i.e., cornification.

PROSTAGLANDINS. Prostaglandins are ubiquitous throughout the body and are formed from essential fatty acids within or adjacent to cellular membranes.[62] Arachidonic acid in keratinocytes is metabolized to PGE_2 and $PGF_{2\alpha}$, each with opposite effects. PGE_2 and $PGF_{2\alpha}$ can be interconverted by the enzyme PGE_2 9-keto reductase, depending on local requirements.[62] Within 24 hours after exposure to ultraviolet light, PGE_2 is increased. Pain, erythema, and edema characterize the sunburn response. Vasodilation, keratinocyte stimulation, and interaction with leukocytes are present in varying degrees. Topical application of prostaglandin inhibitors (e.g., 2.5 per cent indomethacin) can prevent signs and symptoms, but damage to keratinocytes by the ultraviolet waves is unaltered. Thus, sunburn is a normal biologic defense mechanism employed against a potentially serious insult to the skin.

$PGF_{2\alpha}$ may function in resolving the inflammatory response evoked by PGE_2.[62] $PGF_{2\alpha}$ has been demonstrated to promote cutaneous vasoconstriction as well as to stimulate dermal reparative processes such as ground substance biosynthesis. In addition to these responses, prostaglandins in the skin influence epidermal maturation and have a role in regulating epidermal homeostasis, melanocyte function, hair, and sebaceous gland function.

PHOTOSYNTHESIS OF VITAMIN D. During the industrialization of northern Europe in the eighteenth century, rickets, a disease associated with skeletal deformities in children, appeared with increased frequency. Air pollution and the gathering of people to densely populated towns and cities led to a decrease in sun exposure. It was not until 1921, however, when Hess and Unger conclusively demonstrated that rickets was cured after simple exposure to sunlight.[35]

When 7-dehydrocholesterol is exposed to the ultraviolet rays of the sun (UVB, 295 nm.) the B-ring absorbs photons, which causes subsequent cleavage of the C_9-C_{10} bond, forming previtamin D_3.[48] Approximately 90 per cent of this conversion occurs in the stratum Malpighii. Melanin inhibits the transmission of radiation through the skin. Thus, penetration of UVB through Negroid epidermis is reduced approximately tenfold in comparison with that through the Caucasian epidermis. When previtamin D_3 is synthesized it is then converted by thermal isomerization to vitamin D_3.[48] The rate of conversion is controlled by the temperature of the environment, conversion being greatest at 37° C. Because of the proximity of the stratum Malpighii to the dermal blood supply, changes in environmental temperature in warm blooded animals have a limited influence on the thermal equilibration of previtamin D_3 to vitamin D_3. Vitamin D_3 is then translocated by a vitamin D binding protein (DBP) into the circulation, where it is taken to gastrointestinal mucosa to regulate the absorption of calcium and phosphorus.

The reason for the evolution of such an elaborate and unique cutaneous photoendocrine system for the purpose of controlling calcium and phosphorus metabolism remains an enigma. It is possible that, early in evolution, preD_3 or vitamin D_3, or one of their photoisomers or metabolites, performed an essential function for the skin in that only later in evolution did these 9,10-secosteroids also become important for development of a calcified skeleton.[48]

MELANIN PIGMENTATION. Skin color in humans is due largely to the content of melanin within keratinocytes. In the same species, the number of melanocytes is the same in any given region of skin regardless of the color of the individual.[21] Melanocytes, however, vary in numbers throughout the various regions of the body.[21]

In the skin, there appears to be a symbiotic relationship between the melanocytes and the keratinocytes. If, for example, the skin is exposed to ultraviolet light (UVA, UVB) the keratinocytes in the malpighian layer approach the melanocytes, which form dendritic processes that transfer melanosomes into the cytoplasm of the keratinocyte. Melanosomes contain the enzyme tyrosinase.[21] This enzyme converts tyrosine to an intermediate dopa and subsequently to melanin. It is the melanin within melanosomes that provides the dark pigmentation of the skin. Melanin protects the skin from the adverse effects of ultraviolet light by both absorption and scattering, these processes being influenced by the density in distribution of melanosomes. In pigmented races keratinocytes contain an increased number of melanosomes. In light-colored races, many of the melanosomes are only partially melanized, whereas others are partially degraded.[21] Melanogenesis is stimulated by exposure to ultraviolet radiation as well as a variety of endogenously secreted polypeptide and steroid hormones.

Ultraviolet light exposure is believed to be a principal etiologic factor in the development of human melanoma.[83] It is speculated that carcinogenic intermediates, which are generated during normal melanin synthesis (i.e., intermediates of the catechol type), could be increased by exposure to ultraviolet light. Catechols are also thought to be potent co-carcinogens in animal studies. Further discussion of malignant melanoma is available in other sections of this text.

MECHANISMS OF WOUND CLOSURE

AUTOGENOUS. The human organism cannot survive for prolonged periods of time if the protective barrier function of skin is lost. Open wounds following trauma or disease have to be closed for prevention of the ingress of bacteria and other organisms. Transudative and insensible fluid loss from the wound can rapidly lead to dehydration and death. Open wounds present over exposed tendon, bone, or joints rapidly result in desiccation, superimposed infection, necrosis, and loss of function.

The protective barrier function of skin must be replaced by wound coverage with viable epithelial cells. Dermis, devoid of epithelium, cannot alone replace this deficient barrier function. Epithelium alone lacks structural strength, blood supply, and innervation provided by the dermis. Epidermis can remain viable, however, without dermis. Eventually a substitute neodermis is formed by fibroplasia and angiogenesis.

When a wound is created, the organism attempts to close the wound to restore the protective barrier function. This is accomplished by (1) epithelialization and (2) wound *contraction* (Fig. 2). Within 24 hours after wounding, epithelial cells at the periphery of the wound begin multiplying and lose their cohesiveness to surrounding cells. These cells then begin to migrate toward areas devoid of epithelium utilizing the underlying clot with its fibrin strands as a lattice work. When one migrating cell meets another, movement stops by contact inhibition. Epithelial migration continues until the wound is completely resurfaced. In extensive wounds, devoid of viable epidermal structures, i.e., hair follicles and sweat glands, there are physical limitations for epithelial migration and survival. Wound contraction, mediated by myofibroblasts in 1 to 2 mm. of the wound margin, is another important mechanism employed by the organism to close an open wound. This is a centripetal process apparent 72 hours after wounding. The force of wound contraction is finite and is the resultant force of each individual myofibroblast (3.2×10^4 dynes per sq. cm.).[61] When this force becomes equal to forces resisting wound contraction, the process ceases. Thus, wounds overlying joints continue to contract, even at the expense of extreme flexion or extension of the joint. When fibrosis supervenes, joint mobility is lost and an irreversible joint *contracture* occurs.

WOUND CLOSURE OF SMALL DEFECTS. Small cutaneous

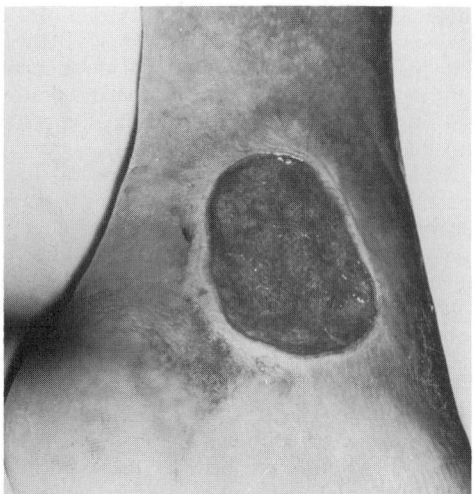

Figure 2. A stasis ulcer demonstrating mechanisms of autogenous wound closure — epithelialization and wound contraction.

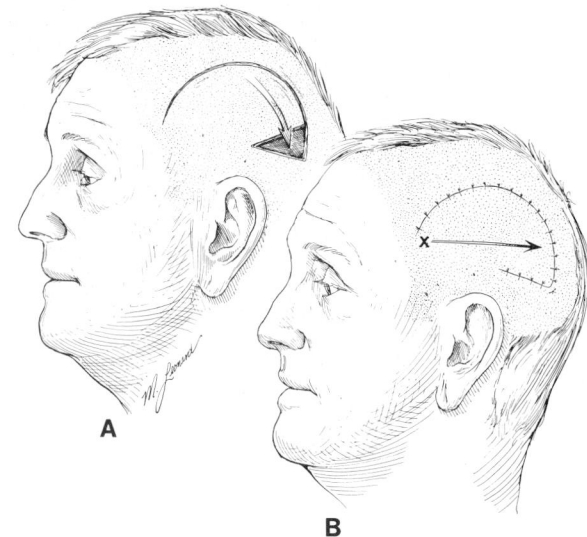

Figure 4. *A* and *B*, A rotation flap. Note that the radius of the arc of rotation is the line of greatest tension.

defects following trauma or disease can be closed by a variety of techniques employed to minimize scar contracture and to provide the optimal aesthetic result:

1. Excision and primary closure. A defect can be closed, utilizing the technique of simple wound edge approximation (Fig. 3). Several prerequisites apply: (1) the defect is small; (2) wound margins can be approximated with minimal tension; and (3) the incision, as much as possible, should parallel existing skin lines.

2. Local skin flaps. Local skin flaps, adjacent to a small tissue defect, are often employed in reconstruction because of similar skin characteristics (color, texture, thickness, and presence or absence of hair). Local flaps are random flaps (see later discussion) and are represented by two types (1) those that rotate about a pivot point and (2) advancement flaps. Flaps that rotate about a pivot point consist of (1) rotation (Fig. 4), (2) transposition (Figs. 5 and 6), and (3) interpolation. All have in common an arc of rotation whose radius is the line of greatest tension.[28]

Advancement flaps are flaps that are moved into a defect without rotation.[28].

SKIN GRAFTS. Autogenous wound healing by epithelialization and contracture has significant limitations both in the degree and the quality of wound closure. These mechanisms are totally inadequate in extensive full-thickness wounds devoid of epithelium and dermis.

Autogenous partial-thickness or full-thickness skin grafts can be employed for wound closure harvested from a more distant donor site, provided the recipient site (wound) can ensure the survival of the transplanted tissue. An absence of recipient site infection and an adequate blood supply encourage graft survival. Subcutaneous adipose tissue, granulation tissue, and viable paratenon have sufficient blood supply to ensure a "take" of the graft.

Skin grafts may be either full-thickness or partial-thickness, depending on whether part or all of the dermis is included.[52] Full-thickness grafts have the advantage of being thicker, providing a more durable wound cover and permitting less wound contracture. Disadvantages include (1) limited size, since the donor defect must be closed, and (2) poorer survival.

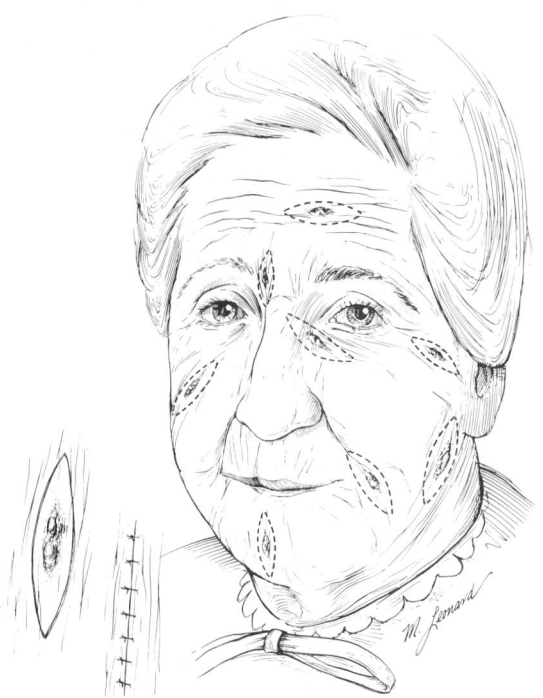

Figure 3. Lines of excision of a cutaneous lesion with primary wound closure. Note that the line of excision is placed parallel to existing skin tension lines.

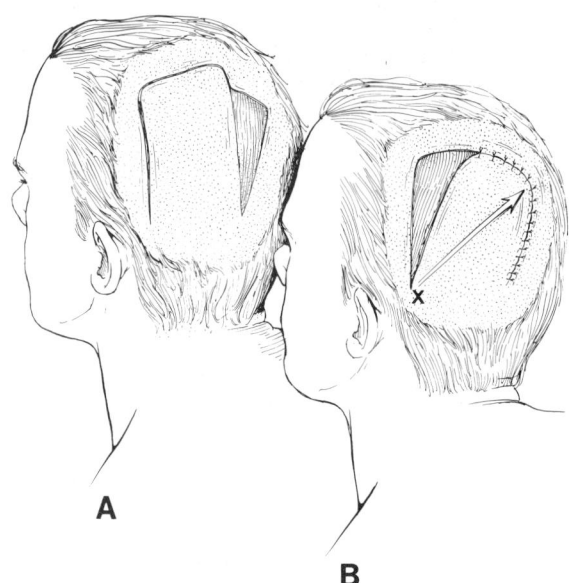

Figure 5. *A* and *B*, A transposition flap. Note the line of greatest tension.

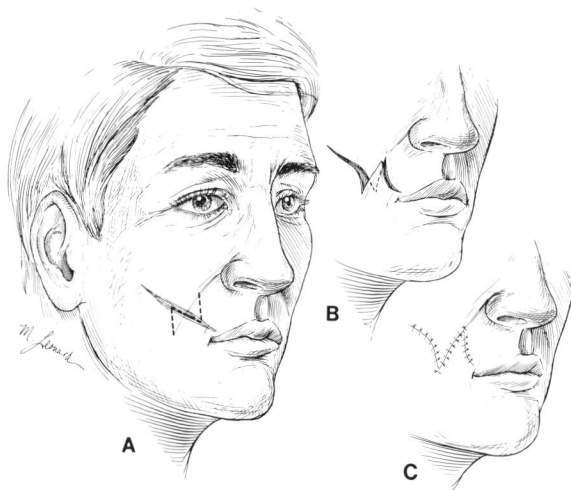

Figure 6. A to C, The various stages of a Z-plasty. Note that the scar is an unfavorable one because it lies perpendicular to the resting skin tension lines. The Z-plasty lengthens the scar and places a portion of it parallel to these lines, creating a more favorable scar.

Split-thickness skin grafts have many desirable qualities: (1) they can be harvested from a distant donor site with regeneration at this site of the missing epithelium; (2) a large area of split thickness skin can be harvested; and (3) survival following transplantation is good provided there is adherence to certain basic principles. Disadvantages are that (1) the quality of skin cover is not as good, and (2) wound contracture is greater because of the limited thickness of dermis. A split-thickness skin graft may vary in thickness from (1) 8 to 12/1000 of an inch to 12 to 16/1000 of an inch or 16 to 20/1000 of an inch, depending on the requirements of the recipient site[13] (Fig. 7).

FLAPS. Exposed bone devoid of periosteum or tendon devoid of paratenon requires an augmentation of existing blood supply, usually with a flap. A reasonable classification system of flaps can be formulated on the basis of the pattern of blood supply (Table 1). An in-depth review is not possible in this chapter, but excellent reviews are available.[14,27,51,66,70]

MICROCIRCULATION OF THE SKIN

The microcirculation consists of the terminal microscopic network of blood vessels, consisting of arterioles (50 to 100 μ), terminal arterioles (50 μ), capillaries (4 to 10 μ), postcapillary

TABLE 1. Classification of Flaps Based on Blood Supply

Random cutaneous
Axial cutaneous
Peninsular
Island
Vascularized
Random fasciocutaneous
Axial fascial or fasciocutaneous
Peninsular
Island
Vascularized
Muscle or musculocutaneous
Peninsular
Island
Vascularized

venules (8 to 30 μ), collecting venules (30 to 50 μ), muscular venules (50 to 100 μ), and arteriovenous anastomoses (10 to 30 μ)[66] (Fig. 8). Exchange of nutrients and gases and removal of metabolic waste occur at the capillary level. The entire cutaneous microcirculation participates in the regulation of blood flow necessary for temperature and blood pressure regulation. All of the microcirculation, except the capillaries, contains smooth muscle in various arrangements and concentrations whose function is to regulate local blood flow. Both arterioles and collecting veins contain terminal branches of the sympathetic nervous system.

Cutaneous blood flow is regulated by two mechanisms, extrinsic and intrinsic, the former predominating.[97] Extrinsic control is exerted in part by the sympathetic nervous system, and its mediator norepinephrine acts on alpha receptors. No beta receptors have been identified in skin. A sympathectomy causes cutaneous vasodilation. Within weeks, however, vasomotor tone returns (denervation hypersensitivity). Then, alpha receptors become sensitive to circulating catecholamines. The other known extrinsic control is hormonal. Physiologic levels of circulating epinephrine and norepinephrine can be demonstrated to exert their vasoconstrictive effect. Intrinsic control of cutaneous blood flow is incompletely understood. Tissue ischemia promotes an accumulation of tissue metabolites (i.e., Pco_2, lactate, and potassium) with a resulting decrease in vasomotor tone and resistance. Body tissues can also release vasoactive substances such as 5-hydroxytryptamine (serotonin), bradykinin, histamine, and prostaglandins in certain pathologic situations. The role and interrelationship of these substances in local regulation

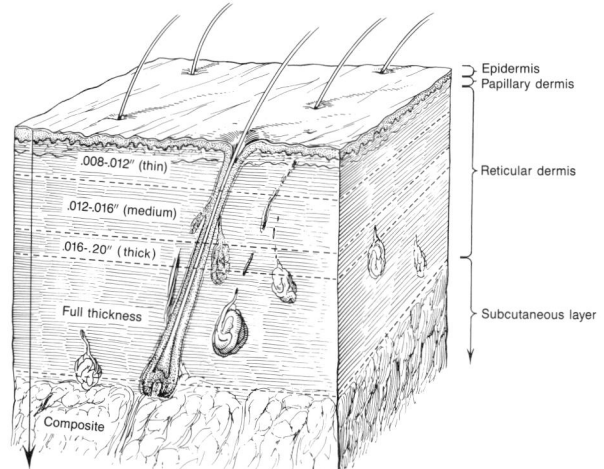

Figure 7. Cross section of skin indicating the varying thicknesses of skin grafts. Note that a full-thickness graft removes all of the epidermal appendages. Epithelialization is possible only from the periphery of the wound. Usually the donor site of full-thickness grafts are closed primarily.

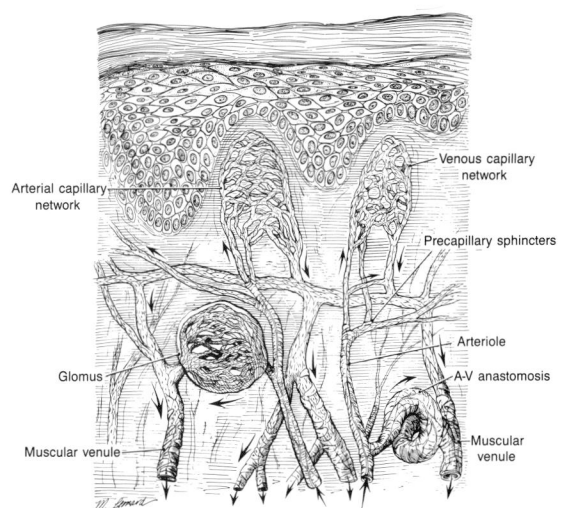

Figure 8. Microcirculation of the skin. Note the glomus body and AV anastomosis, which regulate blood flow to the surrounding capillary beds.

of physiologic blood flow is currently under active investigation. Myogenic autoregulation (contraction of smooth muscle in response to stretch and relaxation in response to nontension) is also incompletely understood.

In general, the microcirculation is concentrated in regions that are most active metabolically or where a specific function is to be served: (1) the subpapillary plexus is located at the dermal-epidermal junction following the contour of the rete ridges; (2) the dermal plexus is located throughout the reticular dermis with vertically angled communications to the subpapillary plexus; (3) skin appendages, i.e., sebaceous glands and hair follicles, contain an abundant microvasculature; and (4) the subdermal plexus, essential in thermal and blood pressure regulation, with its reservoir function, is located in the upper portion of the superficial cutaneous fascia.

MACROCIRCULATION OF SKIN FLAPS. Segmental arteries are branches from the aorta or its large tributaries (i.e., femoral or brachial arteries). They are usually located deep to muscle, frequently following intermuscular septa. These vessels are related to embryologic myotome segments and follow the migration of the specific muscle toward its final destination. Skin, directly over muscle, is perfused by musculocutaneous perforating arteries terminating in the subdermal plexus. These musculocutaneous perforating arteries arise from segmental arteries, which, while passing through the muscle, also send intramuscular branches before reaching their cutaneous destination. Perforating muscular arteries arise similarly but terminate in muscle. In areas of loose skin without underlying muscle mass (e.g., head and neck; over joints) direct cutaneous arteries arise from segmental arteries. They terminate (as do musculocutaneous perforating arteries) in the subdermal plexus. They are located immediately above the anterior muscle fascia but below the deep subcutaneous fascia.

Direct cutaneous arteries serve as the vascular basis for axial cutaneous and axial fasciocutaneous flaps. If the vascular pedicle is skeletonized to the cutaneous paddle (to permit insetting and facilitate transfer), an axial cutaneous island flap is created. If sufficient soft tissue is included with the vascular pedicle, a peninsular axial cutaneous flap is created (Fig. 9). If, however, the island vascular pedicle is transected and the cutaneous paddle transplanted to a more distant recipient site and revascularized, a vascularized axial cutaneous flap ("free flap") is created. Similar terminology is applied to axial fascial or axial fasciocutaneous flaps.

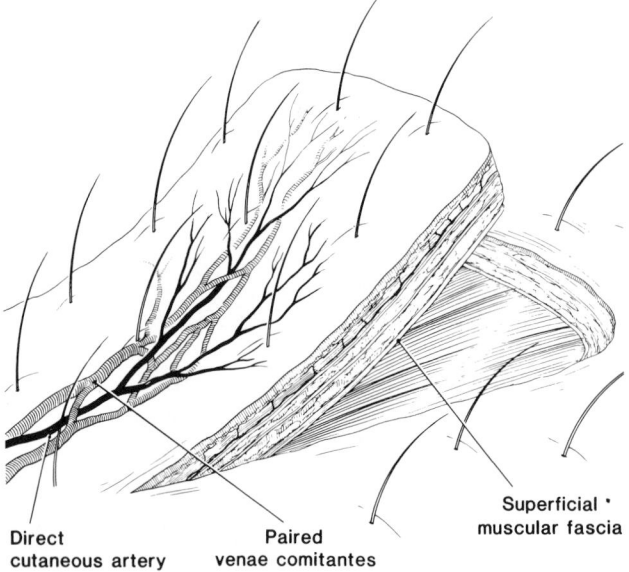

Figure 9. Peninsular axial cutaneous flap. Note that the vascular pedicle is not skeletonized. Blood flow to the flap is augmented by peninsular dermal and subcutaneous blood supply.

Direct cutaneous artery   Paired venae comitantes   Superficial muscular fascia

Random cutaneous or random fasciocutaneous flaps are characterized by the absence of a direct cutaneous artery supplying the flap. Lacking direct communication to the subdermal plexus, good flow and perfusion pressure are reduced, limiting the dimensions of the flap. The length of the flap can be increased if a *delay* procedure is first performed 1 to 2 weeks prior to transfer. The exact mechanism for the surgical delay phenomenon is not completely understood. An increase in perfusion pressure and/or a lack of vascular resistance, however, appears to be important.[34,41,53,65]

Muscle or musculocutaneous flaps are transferred with a dominant segmental vascular pedicle. As described for axial cutaneous flaps, these flaps can be transferred as peninsular or island flaps. They may also be transplanted as vascularized flaps, depending upon the limitations and requirements of the recipient site. During the past decade, transfer of muscle or musculocutaneous flaps and the transplantation of vascularized flaps have dramatically expanded the frontiers of reconstructive surgery.[51,70]

DECUBITUS ULCERS: PROPHYLAXIS AND MANAGEMENT

The incidence of pressure sores in patients with spinal injury varies from 25 to 35 per cent, and most occur below the waist. Death, usually from sepsis, occurs in 7 to 8 per cent of patients.[76]

Pressure sores result when excessive pressure is applied to a relatively small area over a prolonged period of time. Muscle is more susceptible to pressure necrosis than skin. Of interest is that all pressure areas noted during ambulation and when reclining in the supine and prone position are characterized by skin overlying bony prominences without muscle interpolation. Pressures in the supine position vary between 40 and 60 mm. Hg over the buttocks, sacrum, heels, and occiput.[46] In the prone position, pressure over the chest and knees is approximately 50 mm. Hg. While one is sitting, pressure over the ischial tuberosities develops to approximately 75 mm. Hg.

Pressure necrosis occurs when end arterial pressure of 32 mm. Hg is exceeded for a prolonged period. Application of pressure over a bony prominence initially increases the interstitial pressure. Subsequently, end-capillary venous pressure (12 mm. Hg) is exceeded with a further increase in tissue pressure by extravasation of fluid into the extravascular space. If the applied pressure is not relieved, end-capillary arteriolar pressure (32 mm. Hg) is exceeded, causing increased extravasation of fluid through the capillary walls with edema. Capillary perfusion ceases, with resulting ischemia.[43] Studies suggest that direct pressure (twice the end-capillary arteriolar pressure) of 70 mm. Hg applied for 2 hours' duration produces irreversible ischemia and tissue necrosis.

Prophylaxis

Prophylaxis against pressure sores is directed toward (1) patient education, (2) basic skin care, and (3) avoidance of excessive and prolonged pressure. Hospitalization and treatment costs of pressure sores are prolonged and excessive. Hospital admissions either with conservative or surgical treatment vary from 6 weeks to 6 months. Pressure ulceration can be reduced with appropriate education of patients and health care personnel. To be effective, these programs must be continuous, multidisciplinary, and directed to all facets of the patient's life. Psychologic counseling, education, and motivation must be included, as well as a return to employment. Treatment of spasticity must be effective to maximize rehabilitation and prevent pressure ulceration.

Basic skin care is essential. The skin should be kept dry and well-lubricated with creams. Prolonged moisture is avoided. Hyperemia over pressure areas must be noted and considered a potential area of future ulceration. Shear stress on the skin should be avoided. Particulate matter in the bed or chair as well as soiling from incontinence must be minimized. Wheelchairs with appropriate cushions must be provided and maintained in a functional condition. During waking hours, pressure should be relieved for 10 seconds every 10 minutes over weight-bearing bony prominences. Appropriate beds equipped with pressure and sheer stress relieving equipment is essential. Nursing personnel must be available to assist in turning, or special air flotation beds provided. High costs in providing this equipment and/or personnel would be offset by costs incurred during lengthy hospitalization. Prophylaxis is less costly and more effective than conservative or surgical treatment.

Avoidance of prolonged pressure is essential to prophylaxis. Various devices are available to diffuse localized pressure to a wider area. These weight dispersion devices are available for wheelchairs and beds. Despite design advances, only the recently developed air-flotation beds can reduce pressure below end-capillary arteriolar pressure (32 mm. Hg). During waking hours, pressure must be relieved by the patient as described previously. In addition, position should be changed every 2 hours, creating difficulty in social or employment environments.

Management

Nonoperative management of pressure ulcers should be provided to those areas of superficial ulceration or in those select cases of intractable failure to surgical management when all available flap options have been exhausted.

In a reported series, 50 to 80 per cent of pressure ulcerations (various locations and depth of involvement) healed without an operative procedure.[15] Nonsurgical management required hospitalization for 3 to 6 months. Unfortunately, the recurrence rate was 32 to 77 per cent, most recurring in the ischial area. Consequently, in an otherwise satisfactory surgical candidate, full-thickness ulceration should be treated by surgical intervention.

In partial-thickness loss, emphasis should be on limited debridement and the avoidance of infection. Obviously, all pressure should be avoided. The organisms most frequently cultured are both aerobic and anaerobic, most common being *Staphylococcus aureus*, *Proteus*, *Pseudomonas*, and *Bacteroides*. Silver sulfadiazine cream has proved to be the most effective in the topical treatment of these organisms. Penetration into an eschar is good, and wound desiccation is minimized.

Bacteremia is a serious consequence of pressure ulceration. Single anaerobes represent 50 per cent of cases, and polymicrobials represent 50 per cent.[24] Treatment is directed toward adequate débridement and drainage. Topical silver sulfadiazine cream and parenteral antibiotics consisting of clindamycin and aminoglycosides are administered.

Surgical management is reserved for treatment of all full-thickness skin defects greater than 2.0 cm. in diameter. Often two stages are required, the first consisting of débridement and application of topical antibiotics until a wound quantitative tissue sample reveals bacterial counts of less than 10^3 organisms. The second stage consists of wound closure.

Various options in wound closure techniques are available. Simple ulcer excision and closure may be possible, but usually the size of the defect and location preclude the use of this method. For example, an ischial ulcer may appear suitable for excision and closure. When the hip is flexed 90 degrees, however, excessive tension is placed on the suture line, with resulting wound dehiscence.

Wound closure with a split-thickness skin graft also has limited applicability. This method is reserved for pressure sores of limited size and depth in areas where pressure can be minimized postoperatively (e.g., occiput, thorax).

Wound closure by a cutaneous flap or musculocutaneous flap is the most commonly employed reconstructive method. Prior to the popularization of muscle flaps by Ger in 1971,[40] wound closure of large pressure sores was effected by large rotation advancement flaps often preceded by a delay procedure. This method of wound closure remains popular today for large pressure ulcers of limited depth (e.g., occipital, sacral, and trochanteric). If designed appropriately, recurrent ulceration can be closed by rotating and advancing a previous cutaneous flap.

Musculocutaneous flaps popularized by Mathes and Nahai in 1979 further expanded cutaneous areas previously not available for decubitus closure.[51] Ulcers of considerable depth could be obturated by the muscle bulk. Pressure could be diffused to a wider area. Well-vascularized muscle, in addition, provided optimal healing of a contaminated wound.

Muscle, however, is less resistant to pressure necrosis than skin. Consequently, long-term effects and incidence of recurrent ulceration remain to be documented. Certainly, for the short-term results, reconstructive options have been increased by their employment.

Ischiectomy, trochanterectomy, and amputation are additional surgical options that can be considered. Removal of a bony prominence, in part or totally, serves to reduce a localized protruding portion of bone and redistribute the pressure to a wider surrounding area. Balance, however, is often affected with increased pressure transmitted to other areas (ischium, pubis) and subsequent ulceration. Obviously, removal is recommended if the protruding segment is infected (osteomyelitis).

Amputation, either partial or complete, may be a viable option in patients with recurrent disease. A portion of the amputated extremity (e.g., plantar foot flap, thigh flap) can be employed for decubitus closure. Again, careful planning is required so that balance can be maintained. Other factors being equal, a paraplegic is much more mobile with bilateral above- or below-knee amputations. This treatment option, however, is usually resisted by most paraplegics.

Finally, there is a definite role for urinary and fecal diversion procedures. Self-care is facilitated and moisture, a contributing factor for ulceration, is eliminated.

TUMORS AND CYSTS OF THE EPIDERMIS

Tumors of the epidermis may be further divided into surface tumors of the epidermis and tumors of the epidermal appendages. Both benign and malignant tumors occur (Table 2).

Benign Tumors

A thorough discussion of each entity as well as a differential diagnosis is beyond the scope of this chapter. For an in-depth discussion, the reader is referred to a standard text by Lever[44] and a pictorial atlas by Kopf.[42] Only the more common lesions with specific interest to the surgeon are discussed.

LINEAR EPITHELIAL NEVI. Linear epithelial nevi consist of papillomatous hyperkeratotic papules that can be located anywhere on the body. All three types are present at birth or appear in early childhood.[44] Differentiation must be made between these and other papillomas, e.g., seborrheic keratosis, solar keratosis, and verruca vulgaris, all of which show hyperkeratosis. These lesions, because of their papillomatous growth, can be easily irritated. The topical application of liquid nitrogen (cryotherapy) may be useful in treatment.

SEBORRHEIC KERATOSIS. These common lesions occur everywhere except on the soles and palms (Fig. 10). Although dominantly inherited, these lesions do not appear before middle age. The lesions are raised and pigmented and often have a verrucous surface that is friable and easily scraped off. Size may vary from several millimeters to centimeters. Like other papillomatous lesions, seborrheic keratoses are easily irritated, with subsequent secondary infection. In addition, large lesions in exposed areas are conspicuous and unattractive. Rarely, differential diagnosis between pigmented basal cell epithelioma and

TABLE 2. Tumors of the Surface Epidermis

Benign tumors
    Localized linear epidermal nevus
    Inflammatory linear epidermal nevus
    Systematized linear epidermal nevus
    Oral epithelial nevus
    Seborrheic keratosis
    Clear cell acanthoma
    Epidermal, pilar, and dermoid cysts
    Steatocystoma multiplex
    Warty dyskeratoma
    Keratoacanthoma
Precancerous tumors (located largely *in situ*)
    Solar keratosis
    Leukoplakia
    Oral florid papillomatosis
    Bowen's disease
    Erythroplasia of Queyrat
Carcinomas
    Squamous cell carcinoma
    Paget's disease

From Lever, W. F., and Schaumburg-Lever, G.: Histopathology of the Skin, 6th ed. Philadelphia, J. B. Lippincott Company, 1983, p. 472.

malignant melanoma must be made. Cryotherapy is the treatment of choice. These lesions respond rapidly to this method without residual scarring. Hypopigmentation, seen initially, after treatment becomes more normal in time.

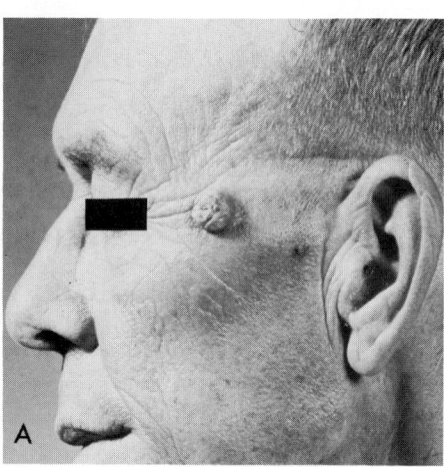

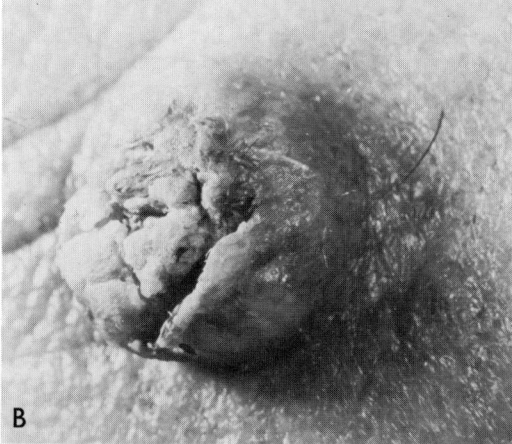

Figure 10. *A* and *B*, Seborrheic keratosis. Note that the lesion is raised and pigmented. It often contains a verrucous surface.

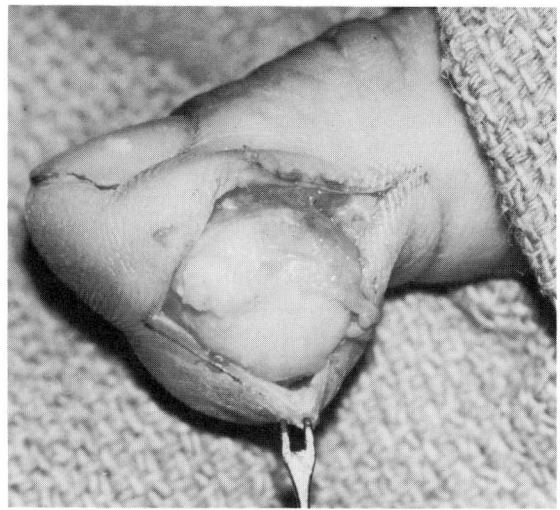

Figure 11. Epidermal inclusion cyst of the finger.

EPIDERMAL CYSTS, PILAR CYSTS, AND DERMOID CYSTS. These cysts are slow-growing, round, firm, intradermal or subcutaneous tumors (Fig. 11). They may vary in size from 1 to 5 cm., when growth usually ceases. These lesions are quite common and occur on the face, scalp, neck, and trunk. The lesions are frequently solitary. In Gardner's syndrome, however, numerous cysts occur on the scalp and face.[79] Histologically, epidermal cysts have a wall composed of true epidermis, as seen on the skin surface and on the infundibulum of the hair follicle. The cyst is filled with keratinaceous material in layers. Close inspection sometimes reveals a small dimple representing the site of origin and attachment to the infundibulum. These cysts, when subjected to trauma, may rupture, which leads to a foreign-body reaction with multinucleated giant cells. Malignant degeneration is rare.[44] Treatment consists of an elliptical surgical excision with approximation of all tissue layers. The line of excision should parallel skin tension or wrinkle lines (see Fig. 3). Pilar cysts are clinically indistinguishable from epidermal cysts. They are much less common, however, and the majority of pilar cysts occur on the scalp. Dermoid cysts are usually present at birth and are the result of the sequestration of epidermal cells along lines of embryologic closure.[44]

KERATOACANTHOMA. Clinically and histologically, this benign lesion must be differentiated from a squamous cell carcinoma. It usually occurs on an older person as a single lesion. The lesion is raised, 1 to 2 cm. in diameter, with a characteristic horn-filled crater. The majority of solitary lesions arise from exposed areas. The lesion begins with hyperplasia of one or more adjoining hair follicles and with squamous metaplasia of the attached sebaceous glands.[44] Keratoacanthomas are characterized by rapid growth, often reaching full size within a few weeks. Involution spontaneously occurs within a few months and is complete often by 6 months. It is doubtful that malignant degeneration occurs. When the lesion occurs on the lips, differentiation from squamous carcinoma may be difficult. Treatment consists first in establishing a diagnosis. This is done by history and by biopsy, which should include a segment of adjoining normal skin. If the lesion is small, an excisional biopsy is sufficient. In large lesions, involving cosmetically vital structures (e.g., eyelid, nose), incisional biopsy and observation are indicated. The scar following involution can later be revised.

Premalignant Tumors

SOLAR KERATOSIS. These lesions may be single or, more often, multiple on sun-exposed areas in middle-aged, fair-complexioned individuals (Fig. 12). Prolonged exposure to sunlight and environmental carcinogens are predisposing factors. Le-

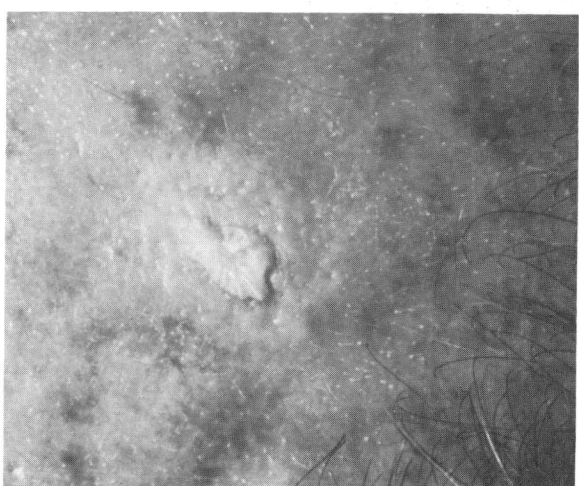

Figure 12. Solar keratosis of the temporal region. Note the formation of a cutaneous horn. (Courtesy of J. Lamar Callaway, M.D., James B. Duke Professor Emeritus of Dermatology, Duke University Medical Center, Durham, North Carolina.)

sions are characterized by hyperkeratosis, often marked as in a cutaneous horn, and measure usually less than 1.0 cm. in diameter.[44] Histologically, anaplasia of the nuclei in the lower dermis without invasion of the basement membrane is characteristic. It has been estimated that squamous carcinoma develops from solar keratoses in 20 per cent of patients.[57] It is of interest that when squamous carcinoma arises from solar keratosis, metastasis is rare, occurring in only 0.5 per cent of patients.[47] Lesions both large and small are treated with cryotherapy or topical 5-fluorouracil (5-FU) (Efudex). Persistent lesions, following nonsurgical treatment, should be treated with excisional biopsy. Invasion through the basement membrane into the dermis should be determined. The prognosis after treatment is quite good.

LEUKOPLAKIA. Leukoplakia is a premalignant condition occurring on oral or rectal mucosa and on the vulva (Fig. 13). It is manifested by raised, whitish, either single or confluent lesions, which may be extensive. Histologically, anaplasia of the basal layers is characteristic. This feature distinguishes leukoplakia from leukokeratosis, both of which appear identical clinically.[44] Chemical irritation, i.e., tobacco or mechanical irritation, i.e., dental irritation, are predisposing factors. Whereas leukokeratosis reverts to normal when the irritant is removed, leukoplakia does not. Squamous cell carcinoma can develop from leukoplakia. Unlike that originating from solar keratoses, these inva-

sive malignancies have a much greater tendency to metastasize. Diagnosis is often difficult because large areas may be involved with the presence of a gradation of histologic changes. Other nonmalignant conditions such as lichen planus and candidiasis must be excluded. Treatment is directed to removal of the irritant and biopsy of residual areas of leukoplakia. Small areas may be excised, but large areas require close observation and biopsy of those areas demonstrating signs of rapid proliferation. Cryotherapy may have a role in management. Wide excision and grafting is rarely indicated.

BOWEN'S DISEASE. The lesion is frequently solitary and is manifested by a slowly enlarging erythematous patch of skin with a sharp but irregular outline (Fig. 14); crusting is frequently noted in the center. When this lesion occurs on exposed areas, it is thought to be secondary to prolonged sun exposure. On nonexposed areas, it may be secondary to arsenic ingestion. When lesions occur on the glans penis, the vulva, or the oral mucosa, it is referred to as erythroplasia of Queyrat.[44] Histologically, the lesion is an intraepithelial squamous cell carcinoma. The epidermis is thickened, but the basement membrane is intact. Cells show parakeratosis with atypia. Individual cell keratinization is a common feature. Treatment consists of excision. Large lesions require a skin graft. Squamous cell carcinoma develops after many years in 11 per cent of patients.[29] When invasion has occurred, however, the likelihood of regional and visceral metastases is quite high.[29] Bowen's disease occurring in nonexposed areas is associated with an increased incidence of visceral cancer. Thus, thorough patient evaluation is mandatory.

Carcinoma

SQUAMOUS CELL CARCINOMA. Squamous cell carcinoma can arise from the skin or from the oral and rectal mucosa. Predisposing factors include sun exposure, chemical ingestion, chronic infection, chronic irritation, and irradiation. The rate of metastases varies according to the predisposing factors. It was stated previously that a squamous cell carcinoma arising from a solar keratosis has a low propensity to metastasize (0.5 per cent).[47] This is compared with 2 per cent of all squamous carcinomas of the skin.[19] Squamous cell carcinoma arising from a long-standing sinus tract in an area of osteomyelitis has a much higher rate of metastases, 31 per cent.[68] The rate of metastases is also high in those squamous cell cancers arising from a previously irradiated area, 20 to 26 per cent.[36] Squamous carcinoma arising from the oral mucosa, lips, rectal mucosa, glans penis, and vulva, also has a high rate of metastases.[44] It is also of interest that carcinoma arising from apparently uninvolved skin also has a high rate of metastases, 18 per cent.[30] This

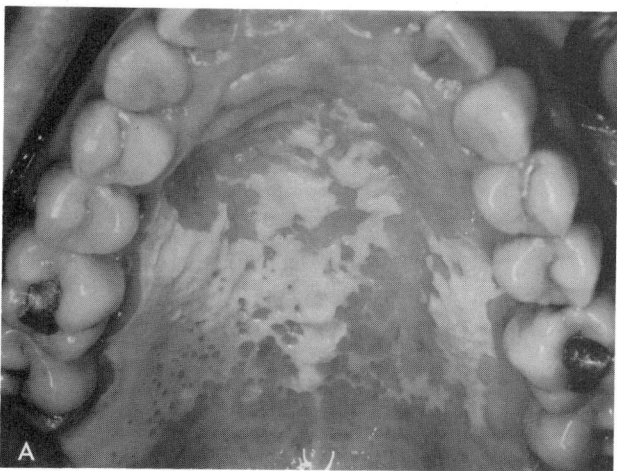
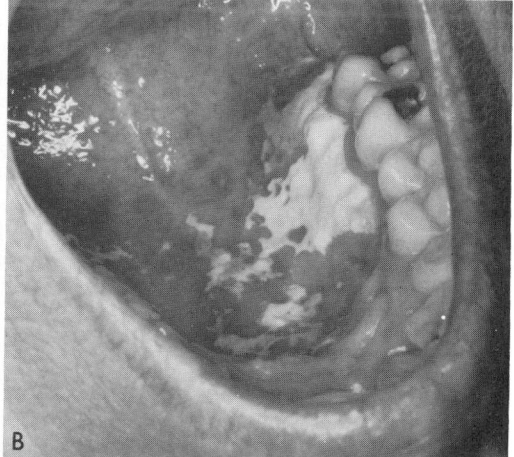

Figure 13. *A* and *B*, Leukoplakia of leukokeratosis, both of which appear identical clinically. Note that leukokeratosis reverts to normal when the irritant is removed; leukoplakia does not. (Courtesy of John C. Angelillo, M.D., D.D.S., Chief, Section of Oral Surgery, Duke University Medical Center, Durham, North Carolina.)

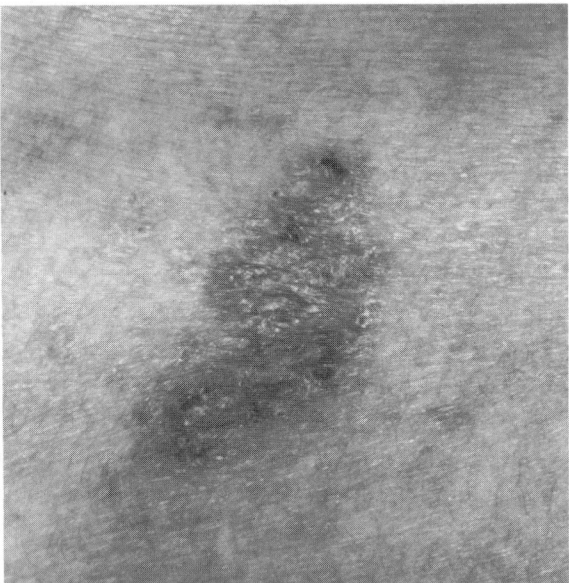

Figure 14. Bowen's disease. Note the sharp but irregular outline of lesion with central crusting. (Courtesy of J. Lamar Callaway, M.D., James B. Duke Professor Emeritus of Dermatology, Duke University Medical Center, Durham, North Carolina.)

suggests that genetic determinants of carcinogens, not yet identified, have a significant role in the histogenesis of this disease.

In 1932, Broder introduced a system of classification for squamous cell carcinoma determined by the degree of differentiation, manifested by keratinization.[5] In a Grade I lesion, more than 75 per cent of cells are differentiated; in Grade II lesion, 50 per cent; in Grade III, more than 25 per cent; and in Grade IV, less than 25 per cent. Recent investigators use this system but, in addition, include the degree of atypia and the degree of invasion into underlying tissue in the most undifferentiated section of the specimen in their system or grading. Thus, Grade IV cancers with atypia, penetration into dermis, and a poor inflammatory response have a much greater propensity for regional and distant metastases.

Treatment is dictated by the location, predisposing factors, and degree of differentiation. Thus, a squamous cell carcinoma arising from an area of solar elastosis can be excised. Depending on the quality and mobility of adjacent skin, the defect can be closed primarily or grafted. Usually, flap reconstruction is reserved until later, when margins are secure and there is no evidence of recurrence after adequate follow-up. Obviously, when bone, tendons, or nerves are exposed at a recipient site not suitable for grafting, immediate flap reconstruction is indicated.

A more aggressive approach is certainly indicated in squamous carcinoma arising from a chronic focus of osteomyelitis, a chronic burn scar (Marjolin's ulcer), or previously irradiated areas. It has been postulated that a squamous cell carcinoma arising in such locations is relatively isolated from both the cellular and humoral immunity of the host.[4,16] Blood flow is reduced and lymphatics are discontinuous. Recurrence after incomplete excision is often rapidly invasive. Treatment consists of wide surgical excision. A regional lymph node dissection, even if discontinuous, is usually recommended.

A similar aggressive approach is recommended for tumors arising from mucosa, lips, and vulva (Fig. 15). Wide excision with control of the primary lesion and regional node dissection is appropriate treatment. Radiation may be primary or adjunctive. For an in-depth review, the reader is referred to existing texts.[1]

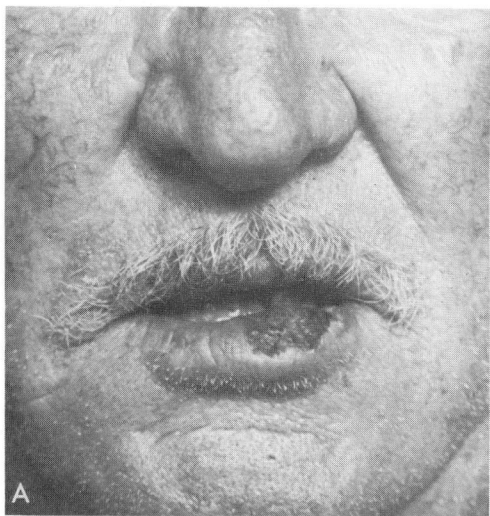
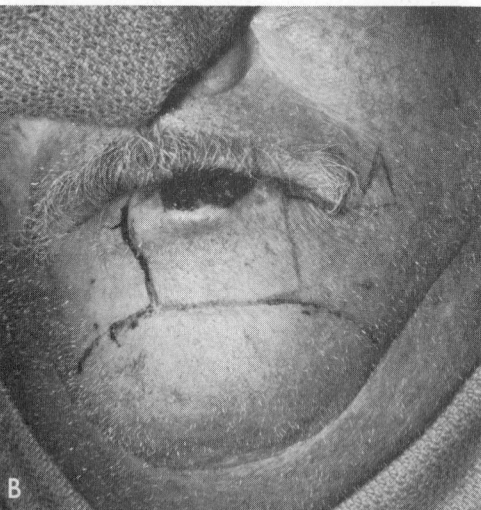
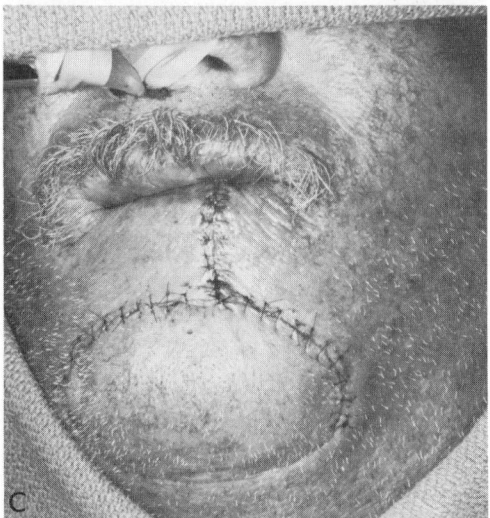

Figure 15. *A to C,* Well-differentiated squamous cell carcinoma arising from the lower lip vermilion. Treatment consists of wide excision with immediate reconstruction by adjacent soft tissue advancement flaps.

TUMORS OF THE EPIDERMAL APPENDAGES

Tumors of the epidermal appendages are classified by Lever according to (1) their degree of differentiation and (2) the specific epidermal appendage from which differentiation was di-

TABLE 3. Classification of Benign Appendage Tumors

	Hair Differentiation	Sebaceous Differentiation	Apocrine Differentiation	Eccrine Differentiation
Hyperplasias (hamartomas)		Nevus sebaceus Sebaceous hyperplasia Fordyce condition	Apocrine nevus	Eccrine nevus
Adenomas	Trichofolliculoma Dilated pore Pilar sheath acanthoma Multiple fibrofolliculomas Multiple trichodiscomas	Sebaceous adenoma Hidradenoma papilliferum Apocrine syringocystadenoma papilliferum Tubular apocrine adenoma Erosive adenomatosis of the nipple	Apocrine hidrocystoma Syringoma Eccrine syringocystadenoma papilliferum	Eccrine hidrocystoma
Benign epitheliomas	Trichoepithelioma Desmoplastic trichoepithelioma Trichoadenoma Generalized hair follicle hamartoma Pilomatricoma Proliferating trichilemmal tumor Trichilemmoma Tumor of the follicular infundibulum	Sebaceous epithelioma	Apocrine cylindroma (Apocrine chondroid syringoma)	(Eccrine cylindroma) Eccrine poroma Mucinous syringometaplasia Eccrine spiradenoma Clear cell hidradenoma Eccrine chondroid syringoma
Primordial epitheliomas*	Keratotic basal cell epithelioma	Cystic basal cell epithelioma	Adenoid basal cell epithelioma	Basal cell epithelioma with eccrine differentiation

*See text concerning classification.
From Lever, W. F., and Schaumburg-Lever, G.: Histopathology of the Skin, 6th ed. Philadelphia, J. B. Lippincott Company, 1983, p. 523.

rected.[44] This classification also recognizes three types of carcinomas: (1) carcinoma of sebaceous glands, (2) carcinoma of apocrine glands, and (3) carcinomas of eccrine glands[45] (Table 3). Because basal cell tumors are composed of immature, rather than anaplastic, cells, Lever believes that this entity should be included with benign lesions. Thus, the term *epithelioma*, rather than *carcinoma*, is employed. Other authors, however, consider basal cell tumors to be carcinomas.[17,20]

Hamartomas are composed of mature structures with an abnormal morphologic relationship to other structures in the organ in which it occurs. Adenomas and benign epitheliomas are thought to arise from pluripotential cells that have already undergone a significant degree of appendage differentiation. The latter is considered to represent a lesser degree of differentiation. Primordial epitheliomas are also thought to arise from pluripotential cells but at a stage where little or no differentiation has occurred.

A complete discussion of all tumors of epidermal appendages is beyond the scope of this text. The reader is therefore referred to other sources.[17,23,45] Only the primordial basal cell epithelioma/carcinoma is discussed. For clarity, only the term *carcinoma* is used.

Basal Cell Carcinoma

As indicated, basal cell carcinomas are considered to be derivatives of pluripotential cells. In the present schema, they are the least differentiated epidermal appendage tumors. Reported cases of regional node and visceral metastases have occurred, some in cachectic patients; this is not completely understood. Perhaps immune deficiency states exist in this small group of patients. Basosquamous carcinoma with metastases has also been reported, providing some credence to the hypothesis that basal cell carcinoma and squamous cell carcinoma exist at either end of a spectrum of invasiveness.

Basal cell carcinomas almost always occur on hair-bearing skin, almost never on glabrous skin. Sufficient evidence exists that demonstrates a close relationship to sun exposure and subsequent development of basal cell carcinoma. Of interest is a postulated stromal factor(s) that apparently exerts some control over the epithelial element. Basal cells, when autotransplanted, do not grow unless some stromal connective tissue is included.[78] The rarity of a basal cell carcinoma occurring on glabrous skin has been explained by the absence of a stromal factor(s). The converse is true in a morphea-like basal cell carcinoma where the epithelial appendage element appears to stimulate excessive connective tissue proliferation. Needless to say, much remains to be understood.

Most basal cell carcinomas are undifferentiated. Sections consist of palisading basal cells with uniform, elongated nuclei and very little cytoplasm. When basal cell carcinomas are more differentiated, they assume characteristics of epidermal appendages. Thus, those tumors with differentiation toward hair structures are termed keratotic; toward sebaceous glands, cystic; and toward apocrine or eccrine glands, adenoid basal cell carcinomas.[44]

Clinically, there are five common forms of basal cell carcinoma: (1) noduloulcerative, (2) pigmented, (3) sclerosing or morphea-like, (4) superficial, and (5) fibroepitheliomas.

NODULOULCERATIVE BASAL CELL CARCINOMA. This form is characterized by a waxy, nodular lesion, often with telangiectasia and an ulcerated center (Fig. 16).

PIGMENTED BASAL CELL CARCINOMA. This form has an appearance similar to that of the noduloulcerative form but is pigmented. Pigmentation leads to the ability of the tumor cells to accept only a small amount of melanin in melanosomes from melanocytes (Fig. 17). Differentiation must be made from seborrheic keratosis and nodular malignant melanoma.

SCLEROSING BASAL CELL CARCINOMA. Connective tissue proliferation characterizes the histology of this variant. Closely packed tumor cells are noted, often presenting in sheets within the dense stroma. Because the tumor cells may appear to be isolated from other clusters by the connective tissue, surgical

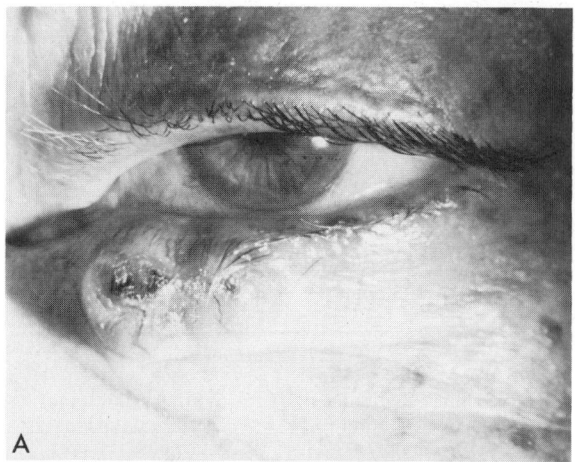

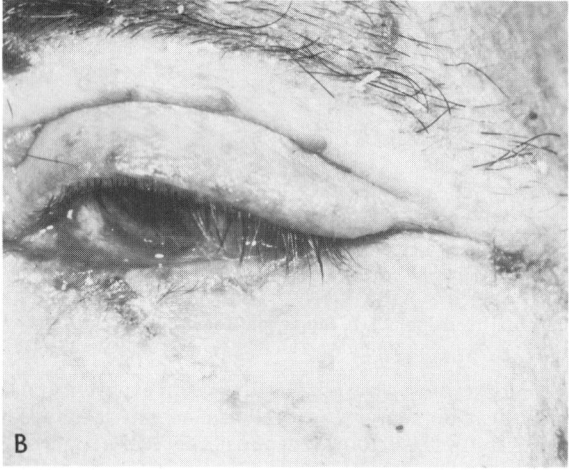

Figure 16. *A* and *B*, Noduloulcerative basal cell carcinoma, preoperatively and after excision and primary closure.

margins may be difficult to obtain unless the involved area is widely excised.

SUPERFICIAL BASAL CELL CARCINOMA. This form is characterized by a raised, scaly, erythematous plaque surrounded by a thin pearly border. Central crusting is often present. Whereas the other forms more commonly occur on the head and neck, this variant occurs predominantly on the trunk.

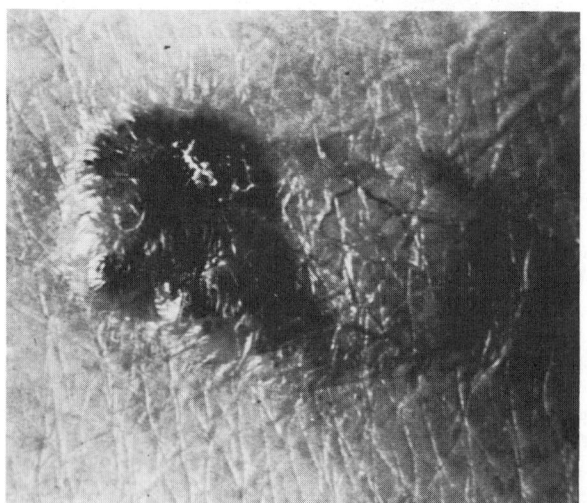

Figure 17. Pigmented basal cell carcinoma. Note how clinically this lesion resembles a nodular melanoma. (Courtesy of J. Lamar Callaway, M.D., James B. Duke Professor Emeritus of Dermatology, Duke University Medical Center, Durham, North Carolina.)

Superficial basal cell carcinomas often appear to casual inspection as dermatitis, with resultant delays in diagnosis and treatment. For this reason, lesions may become quite large. Treatment dictates wide excision, and often grafting if primary closure cannot be accomplished.

FIBROEPITHELIOMA/CARCINOMA. The form is often discrete and pedunculated and frequently occurs on the back.

TUMORS OF VASCULAR TISSUE

Cutaneous Vascular Lesions

Considerable confusion exists in the medical literature regarding the classification of tumors of vascular tissue. In recent years, a nomenclature has evolved that distinguishes between hemangiomas and vascular malformations. This new system has been adopted by most authorities because of its direct relevance to treatment of these lesions.[58]

HEMANGIOMAS. Hemangiomas are considered to be the most common and rapidly growing tumor of infancy. Approximately 2.6 per cent of newborns are afflicted.[38] This incidence increases significantly during the first postnatal year, but the majority appear during the second to fourth week of life.

Hemangiomas are characterized by an initial phase of rapid proliferation, followed by a protracted period of involution. Clinically, hemangiomas arising in the papillary dermis may be first represented by a macular patch. This macular patch then becomes bright red with an exfoliative growth. Hemangiomas arising in the reticular dermis tend to be bluer in appearance, with growth directed into the subcutaneous tissue. Hemangiomas are more common in the head and neck region. Histologically, endothelial proliferation characterizes the lesion. An increased number of mast cells are noted during the proliferative period of growth falling to normal levels with involution. Mast cells are not increased in vascular malformations.[26] There are also significant *in vitro* differences between hemangiomas and vascular malformations. Hemangiomas in tissue culture readily demonstrate endothelial proliferation and the formation of capillary tubules. Tissue culture of extracts from vascular malformations are difficult to obtain and do not form tubules.[59]

Treatment is determined by both the location and growth characteristics of the hemangioma. Smaller lesions involving the tip of the nose or the eyelid can be excised (Fig. 18). Larger lesions should be approached with patience and caution, because involution is possible in at least 90 per cent of cases. If the lesion is extensive and wide excision would produce an unsatisfactory aesthetic result, patient observation is recommended. Troublesome bleeding should be managed conservatively when possible.

Disseminated intravascular coagulation has been associated with very large lesions (Kasabach and Merritt syndrome).[40] After involution, excessive fibrofatty tissue may be elliptically excised along lines parallel to relaxed skin tension lines. Systemic steroids have been advocated for treatment of rapidly proliferating lesions. This treatment modality appears to be more efficacious at less than 6 months of age, but successful reports in older children have been described.[84] Recently, elevated serum estradiol and increased tissue estrogen receptors have been demonstrated in infants with hemangiomas. Similar findings were not noted in vascular malformations.[67] Future treatment possibilities with monoclonal antibodies directed at these receptor sites are intriguing.

VASCULAR MALFORMATIONS. Vascular malformations represent defects in morphogenesis. These malformations are present at birth and growth is commensurate with that of normal adjacent structures. In contradistinction to hemangiomas, proliferation and involution do not occur. Receptor sites have not been demonstrated. Growth of tissue explants in tissue cultures is difficult to obtain. There is also a failure to form vascular

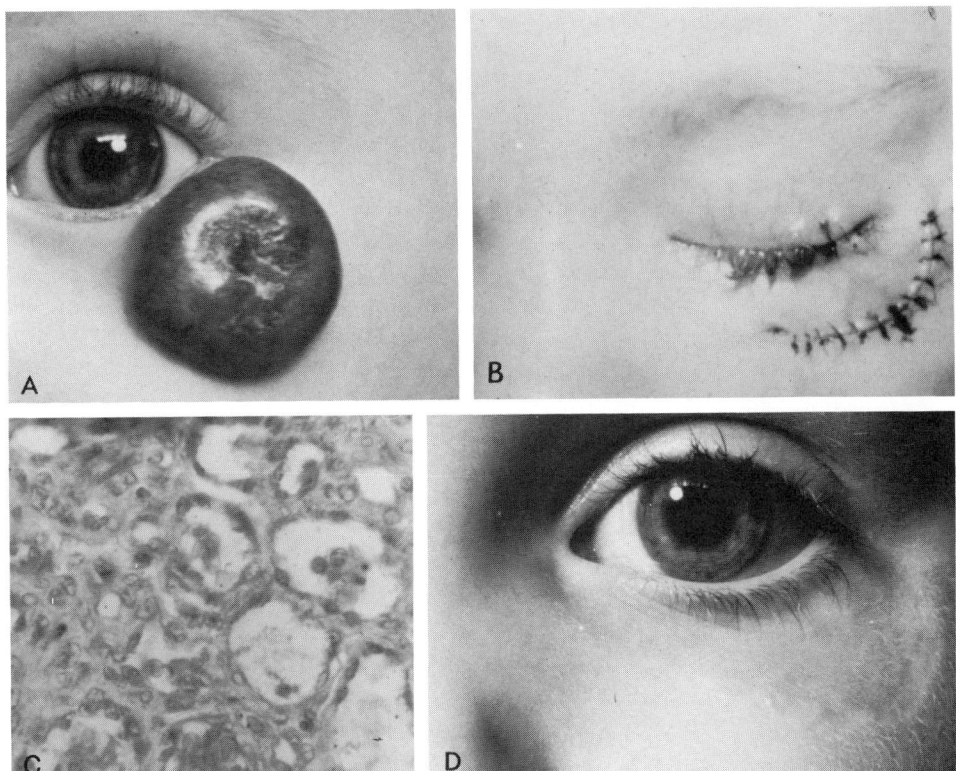

Figure 18. *A*, Hemangioma first noted in infancy with involvement of left lower eyelid. *B*, Intraoperative photographs following excision and primary closure. *C*, Hematoxylin and eosin preparation. Magnification, ×40. Note vascular spaces lined by plump and immature endothelial cells. *D*, Late postoperative photograph approximately 6 years after surgery.

tubules. Lymphatic, venous, and arterial vascular malformations may occur. It is not unusual for a given vascular malformation to contain all three histologic types. Lymphatic vascular malformations are common in the head and neck region and axilla. Venous and arterial malformations tend to predominate in the extremities. Fortunately, most vascular malformations are lymphatic or venous. Arterial vascular malformations are frequently associated with an increase in morbidity and mortality. Hemodynamically, active vascular malformations can expand with alterations in blood flow and pressure. Expansion may be related to hormonal alteration associated with growth and development, previous surgical therapy, or trauma. An abnormality of coagulation parameters may also be present in patients with vascular malformations. Mature vascular endothelium confined to the dermis is commonly referred to as a port-wine stain. Lesions occurring in the head frequently follow the trigeminal nerve distribution. Histologically, these lesions contain mature vascular endothelium. Venous malformations occurring in deeper tissues were previously described as cavernous hemangiomas. In current terminology this lesion is described as a venous vascular malformation. Vascular malformation containing predominantly lymphatic tissue in the head and neck were previously referred to as lymphangiomas or cystic hygromas (Fig. 19A, B). Again, in current terminology this entity is a lymphatic vascular malformation.

Treatment is dictated by the degree of symptomatology associated with the lesion and its location. Excision is recommended if adjacent vital structures are not jeopardized. Lymphatic malformations are characterized by repeated episodes of infection that should be treated with antibiotics. Obstruction to the upper airway may occur in large lesions involving the head and neck. Venous malformations are characterized by repeated episodes of venous thrombosis associated with pain and inflammation. Malformations containing an arterial component are particularly hazardous and difficult to treat (Fig. 20). Hemodynamic alterations may occur with heart failure. Embolization techniques associated with extirpative surgery have been employed successfully in some centers. Incomplete excision may actually increase the severity and the progression of the malformation.

Kaposi's Sarcoma

In 1872, Moritz Kaposi described 6 patients, primarily elderly men, with bluish-red nodules predominantly on the feet. Lesions were characterized by the proliferation of blood vessels, dermal hemorrhage, and hemosiderin deposition (Fig. 21).[39] This classic description of the disease was noted to occur predominantly in males in the sixth to eighth decade of Jewish and Italian ancestry. Prior to 1981, the annual incidence in the United States was between 0.02 and 0.6 per 100,000, with an expected 100 new cases each year.[64] In 1981, the Centers for Disease Control (CDC) reported the outbreak of an aggressive form of Kaposi's sarcoma in young homosexuals in New York, Los Angeles, and San Francisco.[11] The subsequent increase of newly reported cases has reached epidemic proportions, doubling every 6 months, with reported fatalities in 21 per cent of patients.[12] These patients demonstrating manifestations of Kaposi's sarcoma were also noted to have an acquired immunodeficiency syndrome (AIDS). With this recognition, more aggressive forms of Kaposi's sarcoma were found in other patients with immunodeficiency states. Thus, renal transplant patients have a 400 to 500 per cent greater incidence of Kaposi's sarcoma than noted in the general population.[33] Regression of the tumor has been noted when the immunosuppressive agents have been withdrawn. The acquired immune deficiency state has also been noted (in addition to homosexuals) in heroin addicts, hemophiliacs, and Haitian refugees. In addition, Kaposi's sarcoma has been found to be endemic in the Northeast Congo and Northwest Uganda,[77] representing approximately 10 per cent of malignancies reported in these areas.

CLINICAL SUBTYPES. Four distinct clinical subtypes of the disease are recognized: (1) nodular, (2) florid, (3) infiltrative, and (4) generalized lymphadenopathy with visceral involve-

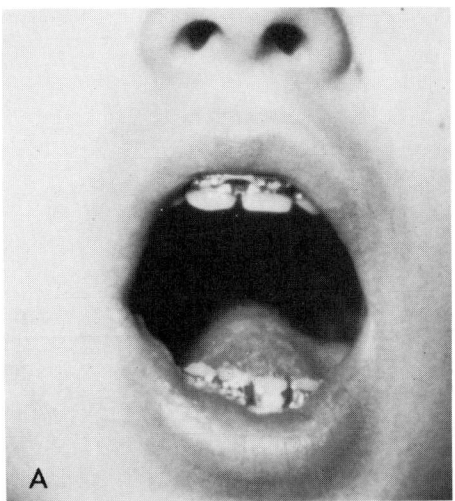

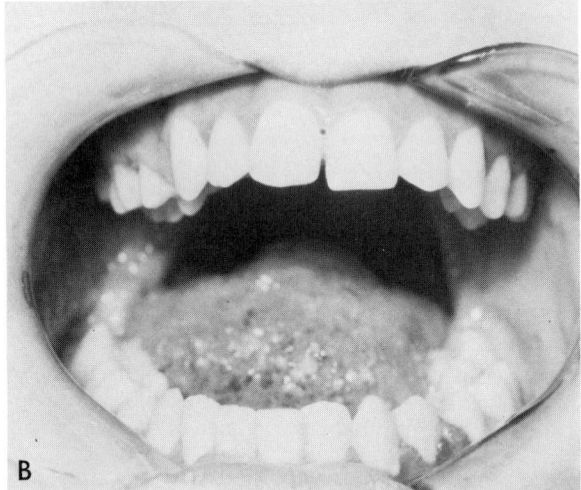

Figure 19. *A,* Vascular malformation (primarily lymphatic). Note asymmetry of right lower jaw as a result of the lymphatic vascular malformation and compensatory asymmetric mandibular growth. *B,* Intraoral photograph of same patient demonstrating capillary component primarily involving the tongue.

nant in behavior. In addition, various combinations of the clinical subtypes may also occur, often in atypical locations. Thus, nodular manifestations are noted to occur more frequently on the upper half of the body and oral cavity. In addition, the occurrence of generalized lymphadenopathy and gastrointestinal disease is more common.

PATHOPHYSIOLOGY. Early investigations of the immune system of patients with the classic nodular form of Kaposi's sarcoma often did not reveal any abnormality. With the identification of Kaposi's sarcoma in patients with AIDS, however, an immunologic basis has been provided for the pathogenesis of this type of cancer as well as others. An alteration of cell-mediated immunity has been conclusively demonstrated. This is manifested by a decreased number of T-helper/inducer lymphocytes, an increased number of T-suppressor/cytotoxic lymphocytes, and a decreased *ratio* of T-helper to T-suppressor lymphocytes. Decreased reactivity in mixed lymphocyte culture is also noted.[72]

Epidemiologic evidence derived from homosexuals contracting AIDS has provided strong evidence for an infectious agent.[18] This is further supported by the endemic occurrence of Kaposi's sarcoma in equatorial Africa. The cytomegalovirus (CMV) has been identified in some cell cultures. In addition, CMV antigens have been identified in a large number of patients. It is theorized that to develop Kaposi's sarcoma both immunocompromise and CMV infection have to be present. Infections with a CMV may suppress the immune system, but the virus also functions as an oncogenic virus. It is of interest that CMV has been demonstrated to have a tropism for endothelial cells.[82] A genetic predisposition for the disease has also been demonstrated. A significant elevation of the frequency of the HLA-DR5 alleles has been found both in homosexual and nonhomosexual men.[50] The DR5 group has also been identified with highest frequencies in blacks, Italians, and Jews, those individuals originally noted to be susceptible to the classic form of the disease. It is also of considerable interest that the HLA-DR5 antigen present on vascular endothelium has also been demonstrated on tumor cells. This finding supports the concept

ment. In its mildest least lethal subtype, bluish red raised nodular lesions are noted to occur predominantly on the lower extremities. Associated edema and hemosiderin deposition are also noted. This is the classic presentation of the disease and prior to 1981 represented approximately 85 per cent of patients. Histologically, the lesions are characterized by irregular vascular sinuses both lined and unlined by endothelial-like cells, which are noted to surround the vascular spaces and infiltrate into the adjacent collagen bundles and spindle-like cell formations containing vascular slits. This observation and immunohistochemical techniques have recently provided strong evidence that the vascular endothelial cell is the cell of origin of Kaposi's sarcoma.[60]

Other subtypes include the florid type and the infiltrative type. The former is characterized by exophytic ulceration, whereas the latter is deeply invasive into underlying structures. A similar histologic presentation is noted with the predominance of endothelial-like cells, collagen bundles, and spindle cell proliferation. Plasma cell infiltrates are common. When ulceration occurs, signs of acute inflammation are also present.

The generalized type, uncommon before 1981, has become more prevalent. It is usually associated with a poor prognosis and fatality. Cutaneous lesions may be absent. This type is characterized by lymph node involvement. Mucosal, gastrointestinal, and pulmonary disease may also be present.

Kaposi's sarcoma, occurring in AIDS patients, is more fulmi-

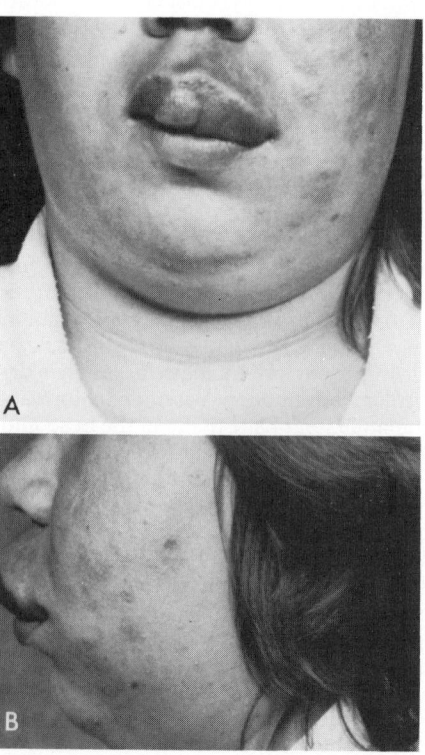

Figure 20. *A* and *B,* Combined arterial and venous vascular malformation. Prominent bruit and thrill noted in the upper lip.

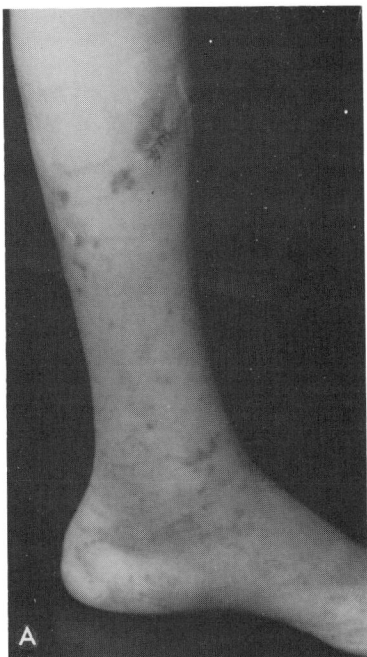

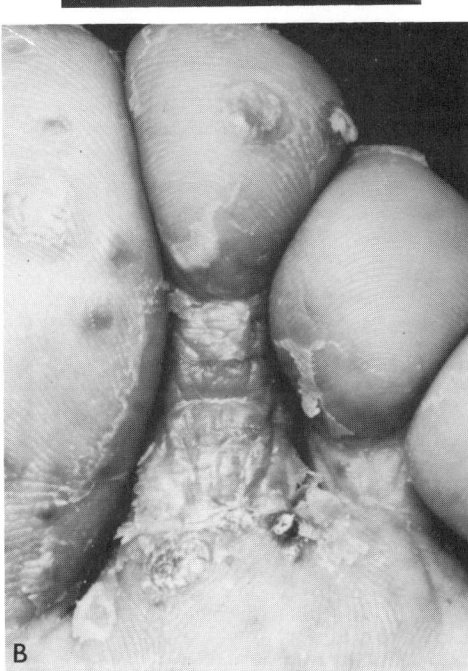

Figure 21. *A* and *B,* Classic form of Kaposi's sarcoma. Note presence of bluish-red nodules located primarily on the distal portion of the lower extremity. (Courtesy of J. Lamar Callaway, M.D., James B. Duke Professor Emeritus of Dermatology, Duke University Medical Center, Durham, North Carolina.)

SELECTED REFERENCES

Converse, J. M. (Ed.): Reconstructive Plastic Surgery, 2nd ed. Philadelphia, W. B. Saunders Company, 1977.
This is a multi-authored text in six volumes. It is a reference source for plastic and reconstructive surgeons.

Goldsmith, L. A. (Ed.): Biochemistry and Physiology of the Skin. New York, Oxford, Oxford University Press, 1983.
This is a textbook written for dermatologists and other specialists with a specific interest in the biochemistry and physiology of the skin.

Lever, S. F., and Schaumburg-Lever, W. F.: Histopathology of the Skin, 7th ed. Philadelphia, J. B. Lippincott Company, 1990.
This text, which is in its seventh edition, is written for dermatologists, dermopathologists and other specialists as well as students who have an interest in the pathology of skin lesions.

Mathes, S. J., and Nahai, F.: Clinical Atlas of Muscle and Musculocutaneous Flaps. St. Louis, C. V. Mosby, 1979.

Mathes, S. J., and Nahai, F.: Clinical Applications for Muscle and Myocutaneous Flaps. St. Louis, C. V. Mosby, 1982.
These two textbooks, written in 1979 and 1982, consider didactically and diagrammatically the clinical applications for musculocutaneous flaps. The atlas is useful in understanding the necessary steps during transfer of muscle or musculocutaneous flaps.

Montagna, W., and Parakkal, P. F.: The Structure and Function of the Skin, 3rd ed. New York, Academic Press, 1974.
This is a classic text concerned primarily with both the structure and function of the skin. Comparative physiology is also presented.

Peacock, E. E., Jr.: Wound Repair, 3rd ed. Philadelphia, W. B. Saunders Company, 1984.
This text is written primarily for plastic and reconstructive surgeons. It contains an extensive discussion of the physiology and biochemistry of wounds and tissue repair.

Rose, S. M.: Regeneration: Key to Understanding Normal and Abnormal Growth and Development. New York, Appleton-Century-Crofts, 1970.
This text was written in an effort to compile current thinking on regeneration. Although still valuable, the text is now 20 years old and lacks recent information. It is recommended, however, as an introductory text for all students.

Serafin, D., and Buncke, H. J., Jr.: Microsurgical Composite Tissue Transplantation. St. Louis, C. V. Mosby, 1979.
This is a multi-authored text edited in 1979. It discusses the physiology of autogenous composite tissue transplantation with an in-depth discussion on the effects of ischemia and hypoxia of composite tissue. It is useful for all specialists with an interest in reconstructive microsurgery.

REFERENCES

1. Batsakis, J. G.: Tumors of the Head and Neck: Clinical and Pathologic Considerations, 2nd ed. Baltimore, Williams & Wilkins, 1979.
2. Bergstresser, P. R., Fletcher, C. R., and Streilein, J. W.: Surface densities of Langerhans cells in relation to rodent epidermal sites with special immunologic properties. J. Invest. Dermatol., 74:77, 1980.
3. Borkovic, S. P., and Schwartz, R. A.: Kaposi's sarcoma. Am. Fam. Phys. 26:133, 1982.
4. Bostwick, J., Pendergrast, W. J., and Vasconez, L.: Marjolin's ulcer: An immunologically privileged tumor? Plast. Reconstr. Surg., 57:66, 1976.
5. Broders, A. C.: Practical points on the microscopic grading of carcinoma. N.Y. J. Med., 32:667, 1932.
6. Browning, Robert: Andrea del Sarto, 1855, l. 97.
7. Burton, A. C.: Special features of the circulation of the skin. *In* Montagna, W., and Ellis, R. A. (Eds.): Advances in the Biology of Skin, Blood Vessels and Circulation, Vol. 2. Oxford, Pergamon Press, 1961, p. 117.
8. Burger, R., and Shevach, E. M.: Monoclonal antibodies to guinea pig Ia antigens: II. Effect on alloantigen-, antigen- and mitogen-induced T lymphocyte proliferation in vitro. J. Exp. Med., 152:1011, 1980.
9. Campbell, B. G.: Humankind Emerging. Boston, Little, Brown, 1976.
10. Cauna, N., and Ross, L. L.: The fine structure of Meissner's touch corpuscles of human fingers. J. Biophys. Biochem. Cytol., 8:467, 1960.
11. Centers for Disease Control: Kaposi's sarcoma and *Pneumocystis* pneumonia among homosexual men — New York City and California. M.M.W.R., 30:306, 1981.
12. Centers for Disease Control: Update on acquired immune deficiency syndrome (AIDS) — United States. M.M.W.R., 31:507, 1982.
13. Chang, W. H. J.: Fundamentals of Plastic and Reconstructive Surgery. Baltimore, Williams & Wilkins, 1980.
14. Converse, J. M. (Ed.): Reconstructive Plastic surgery, 2nd ed. Philadelphia, W. B. Saunders Company, 1977.
15. Conway, H., and Griffith, B. H.: Plastic surgery for closure of decubitus ulcers in patients with paraplegia: Based on experience with 1000 cases. Am. J. Surg., 91:946, 1956.
16. Crawley, W. A., Dellon, A. L., and Ryan, J. J.: Does host response determine the prognosis of scar carcinoma? Plast. Reconstr. Surg., 62:407, 1978.

of a genetic predisposition as well as an endothelial origin for the tumor cells.[55]

TREATMENT. Treatment is determined by the extent of the disease. Localized indolent disease is best treated by local radiotherapy or the intralesional injection of vinblastine. More aggressive localized disease can be treated with local radiotherapy or intravenous vinblastine chemotherapy. Disseminated indolent disease is usually treated with intravenous vinblastine, whereas disseminated aggressive disease often requires multiple-agent intravenous chemotherapy and immunomodulation therapy. The combination of agents most frequently used consists of doxorubicin (Adriamycin), bleomycin (Blenoxane), and vinblastine. Immunomodulation consists of the administration of monoclonal antibodies directed to T-suppressor cells.[3]

17. Domonkos, A. N., Arnold, H. L., Jr., and Odom, R. B.: Andrews' Diseases of the Skin, 7th ed. Philadelphia, W. B. Saunders Company, 1982.

18. Drew, W. L., Conant, M. A., Miner, R. C., et al.: Cytomegalovirus and Kaposi's sarcoma in young homosexual men. Lancet, 2:125, 1982.

19. Epstein, E., Epstein, N. N., Bragg, K., and Linden, G.: Metastases from squamous cell carcinoma of the skin. Arch. Dermatol., 97:245, 1968.

20. Fitzpatrick, T. B., Arndt, K. A., Clark, W. H., Van Scott, E. J., and Vaughan, J. H.: Dermatology in General Medicine. New York, McGraw-Hill, 1971.

21. Fitzpatrick, T. B., Szabo, G., and Wick, M. M.: Biochemistry and physiology of melanin pigmentation. In Goldsmith, L. A. (Ed.): Biochemistry and Physiology of the Skin. New York, Oxford University Press, 1983, p. 687.

22. Fleure, H. J.: The Characters of the Human Skin in Their Relations to Questions of Race and Health. The Chadwick Trust First Lecture in Memory of Sir Malcolm Morris, M.D. London, Oxford University Press, 1927.

23. Freinkel, R. K.: Carbohydrate metabolism of epidermis. In Goldsmith, L. A. (Ed.): Biochemistry and Physiology of the Skin. New York, Oxford University Press, 1983, p. 329.

24. Galpin, J. E.: Sepsis associated with decubitus ulcers. Am. J. Med., 61:346, 1976.

25. Ger, R.: The surgical management of decubitus ulcers. Surgery, 69:106, 1971.

26. Glowacki, J., and Mulliken, J. B.: Mast cells in hemangiomas and vascular malformations. Pediatrics, 70:48, 1982.

27. Grabb, W. C., and Myers, M. B. (Eds.): Skin Flaps. Boston, Little, Brown, 1957.

28. Grabb, W. C., and Smith, J. W. (Eds.): Plastic Surgery, 3rd ed. Boston, Little, Brown, 1979.

29. Graham, J. H., and Helwig, E. B.: Bowen's disease and its relationship to systemic cancer. Arch. Dermatol., 80:133, 1959.

30. Graham, J. H., and Helwig, E. B.: Cutaneous premalignant lesions. In Advances in Biology of the Skin. Vol. 7, Carcinogenesis. New York, Pergamon Press, 1966.

31. Gore, R.: The once and future universe. National Geographic, 163:704, 1983.

32. Guyton, A. C.: Textbook of Medical Physiology, 7th ed. Philadelphia, W. B. Saunders Company, 1986.

33. Harwood, A. R., Osoba, D., Hofstader, S. L., et al.: Kaposi's sarcoma in recipients of renal transplants. Am. J. Med., 67:759, 1979.

34. Hendel, P. M., Lilien, D. L., and Buncke, H. J.: A study of the pharmacologic control of blood flow to acute skin flaps using xenon washout: Parts I and II. Plast. Reconstr. Surg., 71:387, 1983.

35. Hess, A. F., and Unger, L. J.: Cure of infantile rickets by sunlight. J.A.M.A., 77:39, 1921.

36. Hueper, W. C.: Occupational tumors and allied diseases. Springfield, Ill., Charles C Thomas, 1942.

37. Jabaley, M. E.: Recovery of sensation in flap and grafts. In Tubiana, R. (Ed.): The Hand. Philadelphia, W. B. Saunders Company, 1979.

38. Jacobs, A. J.: The incidence of birthmarks in the neonate. Pediatrics, 58:218, 1976.

39. Kaposi, M.: Idiopathisches multiples pigmentsarkom der Haut. Arch. Dermatol. Syphilol. 4:265, 1872.

40. Kasabach, H. H., and Merritt, K. K.: Capillary hemangioma with extensive purpura: Report of a case. Am. J. Dis. Child., 59:1063, 1940.

41. Kerrigan, C. L.: Skin flap failure: Pathophysiology. Plast. Reconstr. Surg., 72:766, 1983.

42. Kopf, A. W., Bart, R. S., and Andrade, R.: Atlas of Tumors of the Skin. Philadelphia, W. B. Saunders Company, 1978.

43. Kosiak, M.: Etiology and pathology of ischemic ulcers. Arch. Phys. Med. Rehab., 40:62, 1959.

44. Lever, W. F., and Schaumburg-Lever, G.: Histopathology of the Skin, 5th ed. Philadelphia, J. B. Lippincott Company, 1975.

45. Lever, W. F., and Schaumburg-Lever, G.: Histopathology of the Skin, 6th ed. Philadelphia, J. B. Lippincott Company, 1983.

46. Linden, O., Greenway, R. M., and Plazza, J. M.: Pressure distribution on the surface of the human body. I. Evaluation in lying and sitting positions using a "bed of springs and nails." Arch. Phys. Med. Rehab., 46:378, 1965.

47. Lund, H. Z.: How often does squamous cell carcinoma of the skin metastasize? Arch. Dermatol., 92:635, 1965.

48. Maclaughlin, J. A., and Holick, M. F.: Photobiology of vitamin D_3 in the skin. In Goldsmith, L. A. (Ed.): Biochemistry and Physiology of the Skin. New York, Oxford University Press, 1983.

49. Madden, J. W., and Peacock, E. E.: Studies on the biology of collagen during wound healing and dynamic metabolism of scar collagen and remodeling of dermal wounds. Ann. Surg., 174:511, 1971.

50. Marmor, M., Friedman-Kien, A. E., Laubenstein, L., et al.: Risk factors for Kaposi's sarcoma in homosexual men. Lancet, 1:1083, 1982.

51. Mathes, S. J., and Nahai, F.: Clinical Atlas of Muscle and Musculocutaneous Flaps. St. Louis, C. V. Mosby, 1979.

52. McGregor, I. A.: Fundamental Techniques of Plastic Surgery. Edinburgh, Churchill Livingstone, 1972, p. 56.

53. Milton, S. H.: The effects of delay on the survival of experimental pedicle skin flaps. Br. J. Plast. Surg., 22:244, 1969.

54. Mizel, S. B., and Ben-Zui, A.: Studies on the role of lymphocyte activating factor (interleukin 1) in antigen induced lymph node lymphocyte proliferation. Cell. Immunol., 54:382, 1980.

55. Modlin, R. L., Crissey, J. T., and Rea, T. H.: Kaposi's sarcoma. Int. J. Dermatol., 22:443, 1983.

56. Montagna, W., and Parakkal, P. F.: The Structure and Function of the Skin, 3rd ed. New York, Academic Press, 1974.

57. Montgomery, H., and Dörffel, J.: Verruca senilis und keratoma senile. Arch. Dermatol., 166:286, 1932.

58. Mulliken, J. B.: Cutaneous vascular lesions of children. In Serafin, D., and Georgiade, N. G. (Eds.): Pediatric Plastic Surgery. St. Louis, C. V. Mosby, 1984.

59. Mulliken, J. B., Zetter, B. R., and Folkman, J.: In vitro characteristics of endothelium from hemangiomas and vascular malformations. Surgery, 92:348, 1982.

60. Nadji, M., Morales, A. R., Ziegles Weissman, J., et al.: Kaposi's sarcoma: Immunohistologic evidence for an endothelial origin. Arch. Pathol. Lab. Med., 105:274, 1981.

61. Peacock, E. E., Jr.: Wound Repair, 3rd ed. Philadelphia, W. B. Saunders Company, 1984.

62. Penneys, N. S.: Prostaglandins and the skin. In Current Concepts. The Upjohn Company, Kalamazoo, Mich., 1980, p. 11.

63. Rose, S. M.: Regeneration: Key to Understanding Normal and Abnormal Growth and Development. New York, Appleton-Century-Crofts, 1970.

64. Safai, B., and Good, R. A.: Kaposi's sarcoma: A review and recent developments. CA, 31:2, 1981.

65. Sasaki, G. H., and Pang, C. Y.: Experimental evidence for involvement of prostaglandins in viability of acute skin flaps: Effects on viability and mode of action. Plast. Reconstr. Surg., 67:335, 1981.

66. Sasaki, G. H., and Pang, C. Y.: Vascular considerations in reconstructive surgery. In Current Concepts. The Upjohn Company, Kalamazoo, Mich., 1982.

67. Sasaki, G. H., and Pang, C. Y.: Role of hormone in the pathogenesis of infant skin strawberry hemangiomas. Presented at the twenty-seventh annual meeting of the Plastic Surgery Research Council, March 16, 1982, San Diego.

68. Sedlin, E. D., and Fleming, J. L.: Epidermoid carcinoma arising in osteomyelitic foci. J. Bone Joint Surg., 45:827, 1963.

69. Sengel, P.: The determination of the differentiation of the skin and the cutaneous appendages of the chick embryo. In Montagna, W., and Lubitz, W. C., Jr. (Eds.): The Epidermis. New York, Academic Press, 1974.

70. Serafin, D., and Buncke, H. J., Jr.: Microsurgical composite tissue transplantation. St. Louis, C. V. Mosby, 1979.

71. Spirin, A. S.: On "masked" forms of messenger RNA in early embryogenesis and in other differentiating systems. Curr. Top. Dev. Biol., 1:1, 1966.

72. Stahl, R. E., Friedman-Kien, A., Dubin, R., et al.: Immunologic abnormalities in homosexual men: Relationship to Kaposi's sarcoma. Am. J. Med., 73:171, 1982.

73. Stingl, G., Katz, S. I., Clement, L., Green, I., and Shevach, E. M.: Immunologic functions of Ia-bearing epidermal Langerhans cells. J. Immunol., 121:2005, 1978.

74. Stingl, L. A., Sander, D. N., Jijima, M. Wolff, K., Pehamberge, H., and Stingl, G.: Mechanism of UV-B-induced impairment of the antigen presenting capacity of murine epidermal cells. J. Immunol., 130:1586, 1983.

75. Stingl, G., Tamaki, K., and Katz, S. I.: Origin and function of epidermal Langerhans cells. Immunol. Rev., 53:149, 1980.

76. Tebbetts, J. B.: Pressure sores. Selected Readings in Plastic Surgery, 2(39):1, 1984.

77. Templeton, A. C.: Kaposi's sarcoma. Pathol. Annu., 16:315, 1981.

78. Van Scott, E. J., and Reinertson, R. P.: The modulating influence of stromal environment on epithelial cells studied in human autotransplants. J. Invest. Dermatol., 36:109, 1961.

79. Weary, P. E., Linthicum, A., Cawley, E. P., et al.: Gardner's syndrome. Arch. Dermatol., 90:20, 1964.

80. Wolff, K., and Stingl, G.: The Langerhans cell. J. Invest. Dermatol., 80:175, 1983.

81. Wolff, K., and Winkelmann, R. K.: Quantitative studies on the Langerhans cell population of guinea pig epidermis. J. Invest. Dermatol., 48:504, 1967.

82. Wong, T-W., and Warner, N. I.: Cytomegalic inclusion disease in adults. Arch. Pathol., 74:403, 1962.

83. Yaspa, S. H.: Cutaneous carcinogenesis: Natural and experimental. In Goldsmith, L. A. (Ed.): Biochemistry and Physiology of the Skin. New York, Oxford University Press, 1983, p. 1115.

84. Zarem, H. A., and Edgerton, M. T.: Induced resolution of cavernous hemangiomas following prednisolone therapy. Plast. Reconstr. Surg., 39:76, 1967.

I ——————————————————————————————————————

PILONIDAL CYSTS AND SINUSES

Onye E. Akwari, M.D.

Few conditions for which definitive cure is usually achieved have been debated as actively as pilonidal disease. Now over 150 years since Herbert Mayo[33] reported the case of a young woman with a hair-containing sinus in the sacrococcygeal region, controversy persists. In 1847, Anderson published *Hair Extracted from an Ulcer*,[2] which was followed in 1854 by Warren's report of incision and drainage of a sacrococcygeal abscess with extraction of a hair ball.[43] In 1880, Hodges introduced the term *pilonidal* (*pilus*, "hair," *nidus*, "nest") and proposed a theory of congenital origin of the disease.[24] Embryologic and autopsy studies by Mallory[30] found subcutaneous squamous epithelium-lined spaces in the tissues removed from the region of the sacrum and coccyx, which led some to conclude that a congenital origin was the primary and essential anatomic factor in the development of the clinical and pathologic entity.[11]

Since Patey and Scharff[37] reopened the debate concerning pathogenesis in 1946 the evidence has weighed heavily in favor of an acquired nature for all but the rare case of sacrococcygeal pilonidal disease. These investigators believed that the friction produced by the natal cleft was probably responsible for producing the sinus. Brearley[8] postulated that the hair becomes clustered in a drill-like form that enters the skin and that shedding causes the hairs to be drawn further into the sinus, thus increasing its depth. In 1959, Palmer[36] postulated that stretching of the integument at puberty, which was associated with rapid growth (particularly of the gluteal muscles), produced distention of hair follicles, sebaceous glands, and apocrine glands and sufficient spreading of their cutaneous orifices to allow the insinuation of foreign substances. There is growing evidence that these tiny midline holes or pits, sometimes termed sinuses, which are observed in the cleft of nearly all patients with pilonidal disease, are the source of the disease. It appears that these holes or pits represent distorted hair follicles that have enlarged. The pulling forces and the vacuum effect created in this area by gravity and by motion of the gluteal folds have been measured by Brearley and appear to be responsible for enlarging the follicles. The ingestion of hair by an existing pilonidal cavity was cleverly demonstrated by Page in 1969.[35] Thus, the emerging evidence is that enlarged hair follicles appear first and the ingested hair is a secondary invader that prolongs disease and interferes with healing. These are the primary elements of Boscom's attractive hypothesis (Fig. 1) of the evolution of pilonidal cysts from hair follicles, which offers a reasonable explanation for the fact that hair, which until now was considered the single source of pilonidal disease, is found in only one half of the patients.[5] In the other half, the follicles fill with keratin that becomes infected and ruptures into the deeper fat.

Although pilonidal disease most commonly occurs in the region of the sacrococcygeal junction, it has been reported in the umbilicus, the axilla, the clitoris, the interdigital webs of barber's hands, the interdigital web of the foot of a worker in a hair mattress factory, the sole of the foot, and the anal canal. A recent report describes periareolar pilonidal abscesses in a hairdresser. Pilonidal sinuses containing wool, grass, animal hair, and hair of a color different from the patient's hair color have all been reported.[12,15,17,21,37,42]

The condition was formerly thought to be common among army personnel (hence the name "jeep disease")[10]; however,

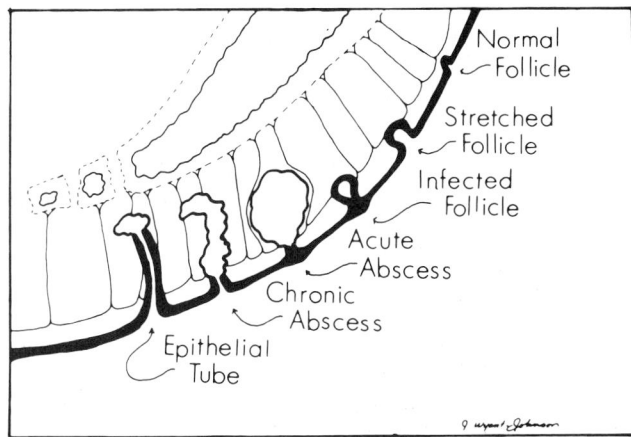

Figure 1. The stages of pilonidal disease (from top to bottom): (1) Normal follicle. (2) Follicle distended with keratin. Fibrous strands suspend follicle and skin from sacrum. (3) Infection of the distended follicle; edema closes the mouth of the follicle. (4) Rupture of infected follicle into fat, creating an acute pilonidal abscess. (5) Chronic pilonidal abscess. The ruptured follicle, which is now open at both ends, forms the mouth of the abscess. (6) Epithelial tube. Epithelium from the ragged end of a ruptured follicle has grown down the wall. (Adapted from Bascom, J.: Surgery, 87:567, 1980.)

such a predilection has not been demonstrated with certainty in the recent literature. The ratio of males to females in patients with pilonidal disease coming for treatment varies from 3 : 1 to 7 : 1. A survey of 31,497 male and 21,367 female students without symptoms observed at the University of Minnesota revealed 365 pilonidal sinuses among the males and only 24 among the females. The average age of both groups was 21 years. The affected students were more likely to be significantly overweight (45 per cent : 26 per cent).[14] From his clinicopathologic study of 354 patients observed at the Mayo Clinic, Franckowiak derived a hypothetical pilonidal habitus: ". . . the robust, fat, plethoric type of male with a narrow pelvis, a deep sulcus between prominent folds of the thick buttocks, an excessive glandular activity, and susceptibility to staph infection."[15]

In an early adolescent age group recently studied by Galladay and Wagner at the University of Arkansas, the male-female ratio was approximately 1 : 4 or 5. Goligher[18] has suggested that women may be affected at an earlier age because of development of large buttocks, which may predispose to early onset of stresses in the natal cleft conducive to manifestation of the disease.

CLINICAL FINDINGS

Presentation

Patients with pilonidal disease may seek advice about asymptomatic pits or pores in the natal cleft. Tenderness after physical activity or following a long drive that requires the patient to sit for a prolonged duration are common presentations. A tender or nontender nodule may be palpable. Twenty per cent of such patients seek care for the severe pain and tenderness of an acute abscess. Eighty per cent of patients with pilonidal disease present with moisture and drainage and occasional bleeding. They have usually not experienced previous difficulty, since the

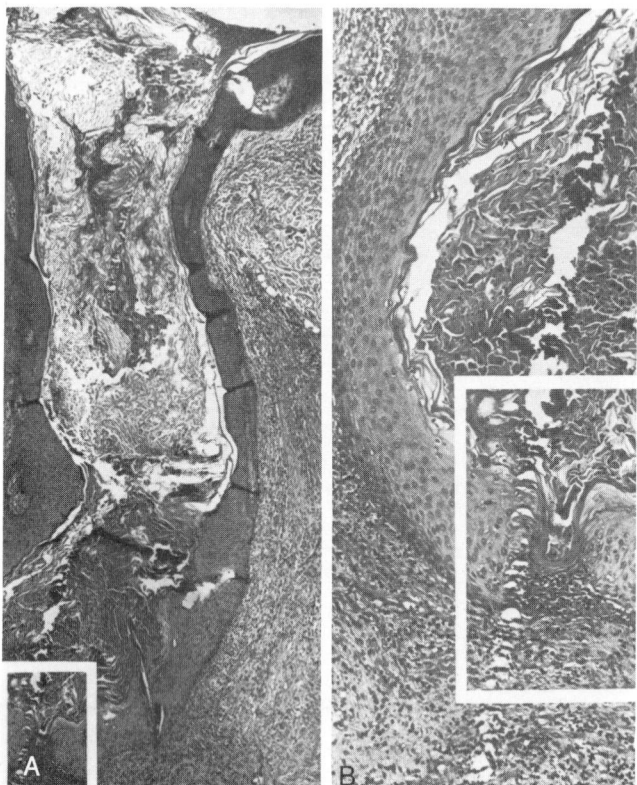

Figure 2. *A,* Early pilonidal disease. Section of a hole or pit from midline skin overlying a pilonidal abscess. This distended hair follicle is breaking out. Keratin is being evacuated. Inflammatory cells are gathering to meet the challenge and eventually form a pilonidal abscess. Original magnification, ×25. *B,* Magnification (×100) of area of hair follicle break-out and the resulting inflammatory response. See *A.* (From Bascom, J.: Pilonidal disease: Long-term results of follicle removal. Dis. Col. Rectum, *26:*800, 1983.)

lesion is usually asymptomatic until the affected follicle becomes infected and ruptures into the surrounding tissues[5] (Fig. 2). The findings of acute suppuration, tenderness, pain, swelling, and heat are similar to those of acute abscesses in other locations. In general, there is minimal cellulitis and induration surrounding the pilonidal abscess. Systemic reaction to the abscess is infrequent; but occasionally fever, leukocytosis, and malaise are found.

Because the abscess of an infected pilonidal cyst may be located deep to relatively thick skin, it enlarges rapidly and only rarely ruptures spontaneously. The abscess can extend in any direction but only infrequently extends to the perianal area. With enlargement of the abscess, tortuous, and usually multiple, sinuses develop external to the postsacral fascia. The inflammatory process may subside early or may progress until relief is obtained—usually by surgical means and rarely by spontaneous drainage. After drainage has occurred, the purulent discharge may cease completely, but more commonly it recurs intermittently with drainage from one or more sinuses[12,15,22] as the disease enters its chronic phase.

PATHOLOGY

The earliest stages of pilonidal *sinuses* demonstrate variously sized enlarged hair follicles in otherwise normal skin. Each follicle holds a single hair shaft surrounded by rings of keratin. The acute pilonidal *abscess* contains pus under pressure and a wall of edematous fat. Polymorphonuclear cells predominate. The chronic abscess has a wall of fibrous tissue lined by granulation tissue of capillaries, lymphocytes, and giant cells. The cavity is laden with *Staphylococcus aureus* and other organisms, including anaerobes (particularly *Bacteriodes* species).[31,32]

Infiltration of hair occurs in one half of the specimens. No hair follicles have ever been found in the sinus tracts; this observation provided an early clue that hair found therein was of extraneous origin. Chronic abscesses of long duration begin to receive a thin and flat lining of epithelium that grows into the cavity from the skin surface, thus forming a cyst. Epithelial tubes or epidermal inclusion cysts may follow but are uncommon. Indolent wounds that fail to heal after surgical procedures resemble chronic abscesses.[7]

DIFFERENTIAL DIAGNOSIS

The diagnosis is usually apparent; however, the possibility of other conditions should be considered, including perianal abscesses arising from the posterior midline crypt, hidradenitis suppurativa, and a simple carbuncle or furuncle. Some other focus of infection, such as osteomyelitis, may produce a sinus in this area, but this is not common. If a probe inserted in the sinus follows a course away from the anus, this may be considered indicative of a pilonidal sinus. Care must be taken to exclude a complicated anal fistula, which may angulate posteriorly before passing into a retrorectal abscess. In this situation thorough examination of the anal cavity usually discloses the point of origin.

Rarely, pilonidal disease and anal fistula coexist. It should be understood that they arise independently and develop into the combined disorder because the anal fistula has extended posteriorly and has involved the pilonidal cyst or sinus. Most such patients have had previous operations, and it is likely that the surgeon connected the two pathologic processes by incision. However, well-documented instances of pilonidal cysts with the fistulous tract situated inside the anal canal have been reported.[1] In the pediatric and adolescent age group, coccygeal sinuses (congenital skin adherence to the coccyx) and sinuses overlying the sacrum in which there is pigmented and hairy skin have been mistaken for pilonidal disease. The sacral sinus is associated with a great risk of incurring meningitis in early life, but fortunately meningitis is easily distinguishable from pilonidal disease.

TREATMENT

There is a growing consensus that management of pilonidal disease should involve conservative approaches, since these approaches have yielded satisfactory results and lower recurrence rates.[25,39] Treatment in an outpatient setting has gained acceptance and is widely practiced.

Acute Pilonidal Abscess

In a prospective study of 73 patients, Jensen and Harling[26] considered the results of simple incision and drainage of a first-episode acute pilonidal abscess with special emphasis on cure rate and recurrence rate among patients with healing *per primam.* The abscesses were incised with a cruciform incision and the four corners of the cruciform incision excised to allow adequate drainage. The wound was not curetted. The patients shaved the area around the wound and were examined every 2 weeks for 12 weeks. Their treatment relieved symptoms, and all patients returned to work immediately after treatment. They demonstrated convincingly that healing *per primam* occurred in 58 per cent of the patients within 10 weeks of treatment. Twenty-one per cent with healing *per primam* developed recurrence of their pilonidal abscess during the prospective follow-up period of 36 to 84 months; therefore they had a constant cure rate of 76 per cent after 18 months.[26] The best results were in patients with few pits and lateral tracts, whereas patients who developed recurrences had developed excessive granulation tissue and required later definitive surgical treatment. The decision to offer definitive treatment should be deferred for at least

10 weeks, and those patients with pits and lateral tracts should probably be selected for treatment using a more definitive procedure[27] that includes evacuation of hair and curetting of granulation tissue with wide exposure of the posterior wall of the abscess cavity. Some have advocated the use of sclerosing solutions such as phenol, silver nitrate, or Mousel's solution; but their use is probably not necessary and may be harmful.[6] With careful follow-up and local care, including careful shaving of hair, hot tub baths, and use of Water Pik irrigation, healing by secondary intention is generally complete in 2 weeks and recurrence is unusual.[25,39] Antibiotics are not generally indicated, unless the patient has a medical condition such as rheumatic heart disease or is immunosuppressed.

Some clinicians have advocated aspiration of the abscess or a small lateral incision for evacuation of the acute abscess and appropriate antibiotic coverage, which is adjusted according to the results of bacteriologic culture, to control the acute process. An early date is then scheduled for outpatient excision of the cyst with curettage of the pits. This approach, although attractive, remains to be proved by wider experience.

CHRONIC PILONIDAL DISEASE

Eighty per cent of patients with pilonidal disease present with a chronic abscess and no history of a prior clinically apparent acute stage. Marks and others[9,31,32] have demonstrated the central role of infection, particularly infection by anaerobic bacteria, in the extreme difficulties of wound healing that are often associated with chronic pilonidal disease. Therefore initial treatment involves providing an oral pain medication and an antibiotic regimen that is particularly directed against *Staphylococcus* and *Bacteriodes* species. After administering local or regional anesthesia to the patient, the chronic abscess is opened widely by a long incision that lies parallel to and 2 cm. to one side of the midline. Avoidance of the midline "ditch" containing the pits and sinuses is increasingly advocated.[27] The abscess cavity is scrubbed free of hair; this process removes portions of the cyst wall impregnated with hair (Fig. 3). In the rare patient with very long-standing disease, the abscess wall is covered with surface epithelium that has grown into the cavity. At this stage, it is no longer a chronic abscess; it becomes an epithelial inclusion cyst that is therefore excised. The lateral incision is left

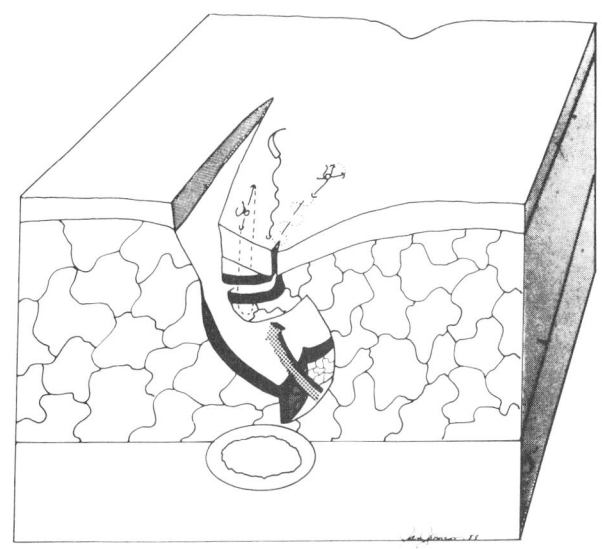

Figure 4. After procedures outlined in Figure 3, the lateral wound is left open to drain, but the midline wounds are sutured. Healing is enhanced by collapsing portion of the wall of the clean cavity against the underside and floor of the cavity.

widely open to permit drainage, whereas all small holes from the midline skin are excised with minimal tissue loss (Fig. 4). The visible holes that represent enlarged follicles must be completely excised if recurrence is to be avoided.

Occasionally, multiple cavities may appear under insignificant-appearing follicles. The amount of uninvolved tissue excised is kept to a minimum. The tiny midline openings are carefully closed with nonabsorbable suture material. Primary healing is aided by collapsing a portion of the "far wall" of the abscess against the underside of the closure (Fig. 4). The loose stitch of nonabsorbable suture material that holds this flap in place is removed in approximately 1 week.

Antibiotics are continued for 24 hours. The patient is instructed to shower daily and is taught about local cleansing and care of the wound with frequent changes of absorbent cotton dressings. Half of the patients return to work the following day, and disability rarely exceeds 4 days for the other half. All wounds are usually found to be closed by the sixth postoperative week. In a few patients, a midline hole remains open or a new one appears. These patients require a weekly shave and/or daily packing with cotton gauze and an occasional silver nitrate cauterization of granulation tissue. A rare patient may return years after surgical therapy with an inclusion cyst.

Although a randomized trial comparing excision and excision with suture with and without antibiotics,[28] and another comparing excision with marsupialization and phenolization[13] have recently been reported, the results confirm only the correctness of the present trend toward more conservative approaches. Asymptomatic patients who have sinuses that are dry and have never been painful should be observed.

RECURRENT PILONIDAL DISEASE

It is evident from the proliferation of procedures advocated for pilonidal disease that no failure-proof operation has yet been discovered. All of the following procedures have been associated with significant failure rates: excision and packing with healing by open granulation[32]; marsupialization, which was championed by Buie[2,10,13]; excision and closure[28]; injection[4,23]; destruction of the tract[16]; irradiation[40]; and various plastic tissue flap rotational procedures[3,41] and grafting.[20] Although the recurrence rate in some series is reasonably low, the procedures involved are long and complex, require prolonged hospitalization, or may cause potentially more morbidity than the

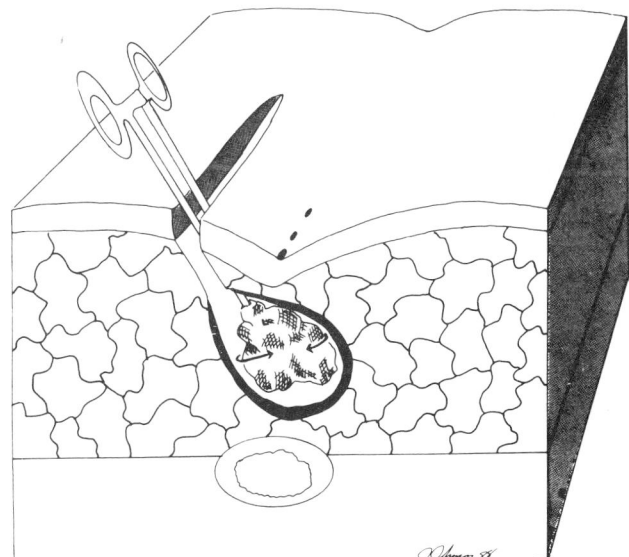

Figure 3. Principles of treatment of pilonidal abscess include (1) adequate incision *lateral* to the midline, (2) removal of hair and granulations, and (3) conservative removal of the midline holes and pits that sustain the abscess, minimizing tissue loss. (After Boscom, J.: Pilonidal sinus. *In* Sazio V. W. (Ed.): Current Therapy in Colon and Rectal Surgery. Toronto, B. C. Decker, 1990, p. 34.)

disease itself. Beginning with the identification of infection as an important common denominator in the failure of these approaches,[9,31,32] future investigation of those factors that delay wound healing has been emphasized. Marks and others have identified basic principles, including wound reshaping to facilitate better drainage of pockets of uneradicated infection and the early use of specific antibiotic treatment, as being important to the achievement of cure in these patients.

After formal conservative primary treatment, most recurrences develop in the inferior portion of the scar. A blind cavity or sinus tract is frequently encountered through a midline opening. The posterior wall of the tract should be exposed and scraped free of granulation tissue, and the edges of the tract should be débrided. The epithelialized posterior wall of the tract should be left intact. Hot baths and Water Pik irrigation that is performed at least once daily keep the wound clean. Granulation tissue is removed, and the wound is cauterized with silver nitrate when the patient returns for weekly visits. The healing time averages 3 to 4 weeks, depending on the size of the wound.

Surgical débridement and retailoring of the wound[6] for better drainage and for elimination of loculations may be necessary in the rare patient, but they should probably not be performed until local measures have been exhausted. Rarely, malignant degeneration occurs in these lesions.[19,29,38] Verrucous carcinoma (giant condyloma acuminatum)[34] developing within the pilonidal sinus has been described.

SELECTED REFERENCES

Boscom, J.: Pilonidal disease long-term results of follicle removal. Dis. Colon. Rectum, 26:800, 1983.
The author describes the results of therapy based on his hypothesis, which implicates hair follicles in the etiology of pilonidal disease. Very convincing histopathologic support for the hypothesis is presented as the author describes the stages of development of a pilonidal cyst from a hair follicle. The theory implicates hair as a confounding "secondary invader" and provides ready explanation for the fact that hair, until recently considered the single source of the disease, is found in only one half of the patients.

Hurst, D. W.: The evolution of management of pilonidal sinus disease. Can. J. Surg., 26:603, 1984.
An early advocate of conservative treatment, Hurst outlines a practical approach to pilonidal disease based on a comprehensive 10-year review of 72 consecutive patients who were successfully treated as outpatients, with the use of local anesthesia.

REFERENCES

1. Accarpio, G., Davini, M. D., Fazio, A., Senussi, O. H., and Yakubovich, A.: Pilonidal sinus with an anal canal fistula. Dis. Col. Rectum, 31:965, 1988.
2. Anderson, A. W.: Hair extracted from an ulcer. Boston Med. Surg. J., 36:74, 1847.
3. Azab, A. S., Kamal, M. S., and EL Bassyoni, F.: The rationale of using the Rhomboid fasciocutaneous transposition flap for the radical cure of pilonidal sinus. J. Dermatol. Surg. Oncol., 12:1295, 1986.
4. Biegeleisen, H. I.: Sclerotherapy for pilonidal cysts—sclerosing method of treatment. Arch. Surg., 37:112, 1938.
5. Boscom, J.: Pilonidal disease: Long-term results of follicle removal. Dis. Col. Rectum, 26:800, 1983.
6. Boscom, J.: Repeat pilonidal operations. Am. J. Surg., 154:118, 1987.
7. Boscom, J.: Pilonidal sinus. In Sazio, V. W. (Ed.): Current Therapy in Colon and Rectal Surgery. Toronto, B. C. Decker Inc., 1990.
8. Brearley, R.: Pilonidal sinus: a new theory of origin. Br. J. Surg., 43:62, 1955.
9. Brook, I., Anderson, K. D., Controni, G., and Rodriquez, W. J.: Aerobic and anaerobic bacteriology of pilonidal cyst abscess in children. Am. J. Dis. Child., 134:679, 1980.
10. Buie, L. A.: Jeep disease (pilonidal disease of mechanized warfare). South. Med. J., 37:103, 1944.
11. Chamberlain, J. W., and Vawter, G. F.: The congenital origin of pilonidal sinus. J. Pediatr. Surg., 9:441, 1974.
12. Culp, C. E.: Pilonidal disease and its treatment. Surg. Clin. North Am., 47:1007, 1967.
13. Duchateau, J., DeMol, J., Bosten, H., and Allegaert, W.: Pilonidal sinus excision-marsupialization-phenolization? Acta Chir. Belg., 85:325, 1985.
14. Dwight, R. W., and Maloy, J. K.: Pilonidal sinus experience with 449 cases. N. Engl. J. Med., 249:926, 1953.
15. Franckowiak, J. J.: The etiology of pilonidal sinus. University of Minnesota, unpublished thesis, 1960.
16. Gage, A. H., and Dutta, P.: Cryosurgery for pilonidal disease. Am. J. Surg., 133:249, 1977.
17. Gannon, M. X., et al.: Periareolar pilonidal diseases in a hairdresser. B.M.J. 297:1641, 1988.
18. Goligher, J. C.: Surgery of the Anus, Rectum and Colon, 3rd ed. Springfield, Ill., Charles C Thomas, 1975.
19. Gupta, S., Kumar, A., Khanna, A. K., and Khanna, S.: Pilonidal sinus epidermoid carcinoma: A clinicopathologic study and a collective review. Curr. Surg., 38:374, 1981.
20. Guyuron, B., Dinner, M. I., and Dowden, R. V.: Excision and grafting in treatment of recurrent pilonidal sinus disease. Surg. Gynecol. Obstet., 156:201, 1983.
21. Hanley, P. H.: Symposium: The dilemma of pilonidal disease. Dis. Colon. Rectum, 20:278, 1977.
22. Hanley, P. H.: Acute pilonidal disease. Surg. Gynecol. Obstet., 150:9, 1980.
23. Hegge, H. G. J., Vos, G. A., Patka, P., and Hoitsma, H. F. W.: Treatment of complicated or infected pilonidal sinus disease by local application of phenol. Surgery, 102:52, 1987.
24. Hodges, R. M.: Pilonidal sinus. Boston Med. Surg. J., 103:456, 1880.
25. Hurst, D. W.: The evolution of management of pilonidal sinus disease. Can. J. Surg., 27:603, 1984.
26. Jensen, S. L., and Harling, H.: Prognosis after simple incision and drainage for a first-episode acute pilonidal abscess. Br. J. Surg., 75:60, 1988.
27. Karydakis, G. E.: New approach to the problem of pilonidal sinus. Lancet, 2:1414, 1973.
28. Kronborg, O., Christensen, J., and Zimmermann-Nielsen, C.: Chronic pilonidal disease: A randomized trial with a complete 3-year follow-up. Br. J. Surg., 72:303, 1985.
29. Lineaweaver, W. C., Brunson, M. B., Smith, J. F., Franzini, D. A., and Rumley, T. O.: Squamous carcinoma arising in a pilonidal sinus. J. Surg. Oncol., 27:239, 1984.
30. Mallory, F. B.: Sacro-coccygeal dimples, sinuses and cyst. Am. J. Med. Sci., 103:263, 1892.
31. Marie, T. J., Aylward, D., Keer, E., and Haldene, E. V.: Bacteriology of pilonidal cyst abscesses. J. Clin. Pathol., 31:909, 1978.
32. Marks, J., Hughes, L. E., Harding, K. G., Campbell, H., and Ribeiro, C. D.: Pilonidal sinus excision—healing by open granulation. Br. J. Surg., 72:637, 1985.
33. Mayo, H.: Observations on Injuries and Diseases of the Rectum. London, Burgess and Hill, 1833.
34. Norris, C. S.: Giant condyloma acuminatum (Buschke-Lowenstein tumor) involving a pilonidal sinus: A case report and review of the literature. J. Surg. Oncol., 22:47, 1983.
35. Page, B. H.: The entry of hair into a pilonidal sinus. Br. J. Surg., 56:32, 1969.
36. Palmer, W. H.: Pilonidal disease: a new concept of pathogenesis. Dis. Col. Rectum, 2:303, 1959.
37. Patey, D. H., and Scharff, R. W.: Pathology of postanal pilonidal sinus: Its bearing on treatment. Lancet, 2:484, 1946.
38. Puckett, C. L., and Silver, D.: Carcinoma developing in pilonidal sinus: Report of two cases and review of the literature. Am. Surg., 39:151, 1973.
39. Salvati, E. P.: Symposium on outpatient anorectal procedures, Pilonidal Disease. Can. J. Surg., 28:225, 1985.
40. Smith, R. M.: Roentgen irradiation as an adjunct to surgical treatment of pilonidal cyst. Am. J. Roentgenol., 38:308, 1937.
41. Toubanakis, G.: Treatment of pilonidal sinus disease with the Z-plasty procedure (modified). Am. Surg., 52:611, 1986.
42. Walsh, T. H., and Mann, C. V.: Pilonidal sinuses of the anal canal. Br. J. Surg., 70:23, 1983.
43. Warren, J. M.: Abscess containing hair on the nates. Am. J. Med. Sci., 55:113, 1854.

45

GYNECOLOGY
The Female Reproductive Organs

Charles B. Hammond, M.D.

Gynecology is that branch of medicine which concerns diseases of the female reproductive system. In practice, however, it includes multiple other areas of interest that are common to any surgical specialty. Of particular interest are the closely proximate structures of the pelvis, such as the urinary system and the bowel, as well as remote, hormonally responsive structures such as the breast and even bone.

HISTORICAL ASPECTS

The art and practice of gynecology date from antiquity, when most thinking and practices of gynecology were vested in superstition and based on empirical observation. Rules concerning menstruation and sexual conduct are recorded in the Bible, Leviticus 15:19-32. Soranus, Hippocrates, and Galen taught about diseases of the uterus and observed mental attitudes and traits in women that they related to the uterus and its humors. The visible events of female physiology were so steeped in folklore and myth that it was not until the emergence of scientific medicine in the Middle Ages that gynecology actually profited from objective observation of the human body. Gynecology advanced as medical science as a whole prospered, but at perhaps a slower pace because of the persistence of the fantasies surrounding human reproduction, many of which remain in the twentieth century.

Modern gynecologic surgery dates from 1809, when Ephraim McDowell of Kentucky performed the first ovariotomy for a large ovarian cyst. The operation was a success and established the foundation for abdominal and pelvic surgery. Many others provided significant discoveries: In 1817, Langenbeck reported the first vaginal hysterectomy. Semmelweiss, in 1840, applied hypochlorite to all instruments, towels, and containers used during delivery and required thorough hand washing with soap, warm water, and hypochlorite rinse. His seminal work reduced the mortality of puerperal fever and introduced the concept of chemical antisepsis 20 years before Lister's first publication promulgating carbolic acid spray, and 50 years before Lister capitulated completely to the concept of preventative antisepsis. In 1842, Long and, in 1846, Morton introduced ether anesthesia. In 1849, Mattauer and, in 1852, Sims described successful closure of vesicovaginal fistula, a common complication of obstructed labor at that time. In 1860, Hodge described the vaginal pessary for support of the prolapsed uterus. In 1861, Pasteur noted that living organisms led to fermentation and tissue destruction. In 1867, Freund performed the first successful abdominal hysterectomy for cancer of the uterus. In 1884, Tait reported excellent success with abdominal operation for ruptured ectopic pregnancy. In 1895, Röntgen discovered x-rays. In 1898, the Curies discovered radium; Kelly described the operative cure of bladder and urethral prolapse and published a two-volume text of operative gynecology.

The twentieth century began with Wertheim describing a radical operation for cancer of the cervix and Landsteiner discovering the major human blood groups. In 1903, Cleaves first treated with radium a patient with cancer of the cervix. In 1908, Hitschmann and Alder demonstrated the cyclic physiologic changes of endometrium. In 1921, Sampson described pelvic endometriosis and published his theory of "retrograde menstruation." In 1923, Allen and Doisy isolated estrogen. In 1928, Aschheim and Zondek discovered human chorionic gonadotropin. In 1929, Allen and Corner isolated progesterone. In 1935, Stein and Leventhal described the polysystic ovary syndrome. In 1936, Hamblen first induced human ovulation with gonadotropins of nonhuman primates, and Colebrook and Kenny first used antibiotics (sulfanilamides) to treat human puerperal infections. In 1941, Papanicolaou and Traut published the classic monograph on vaginal cytology for cancer screening. In 1949, Barr discovered the sex chromatin body, and Li, Simpson, and Evans isolated human follicle-stimulating hormone. In 1951, Brunschwig reported exenterative pelvic surgery for advanced or recurrent cervical cancer. In 1956, Li, Hertz, and Spencer first cured metastatic choriocarcinoma with chemotherapy, and Tijo and Levan identified the normal human karyotype as 46 chromosomes. In 1958, Gemzell reported successful ovulatory induction with human gonadotropins, and Pincus introduced oral contraceptives. Ultrasonography and laparoscopy became necessary approaches in the 1970s in the assessment of obstetric and gynecologic patients. Rather amazingly, in 1978, the first child was born from *in vitro* fertilization.

In the 1980s, many further advances have served to expand gynecologic practice. Gonadotropin-releasing hormone analogues are available for medical therapy of selected patients with leiomyoma and endometriosis. Operative laparoscopy and hysteroscopy, with and without laser, have become increasingly important means for the surgical approaches to many problems. Magnetic resonance imaging (MRI) and computed tomography (CT) are increasingly important in the noninvasive evaluation of disease. Tumor markers (i.e., CA125, CEA) are being further used to aid diagnosis of malignancy, while understanding of receptor physiology allows further hormonal manipulation and novel therapeutic approaches. Menopause and other types of hormonal deprivation have been identified as major health problems for an aging population, and methods of safely replacing deficient hormones for these patients have been developed. Sexually transmitted infectious diseases have rapidly become one of the major problems for the 1990s and beyond—*Chlamydia*, herpes simplex, the papillomavirus, and the human immune deficiency virus (HIV) all pose threats for women and have yet to yield to present therapy as major risks to health, reproduction, and even to life.

These accomplishments, plus many others, have enabled gynecology to become a broadly based discipline. Although this chapter is not intended to be a complete treatise on the diagnosis and management of gynecologic disorders, it is hoped that it

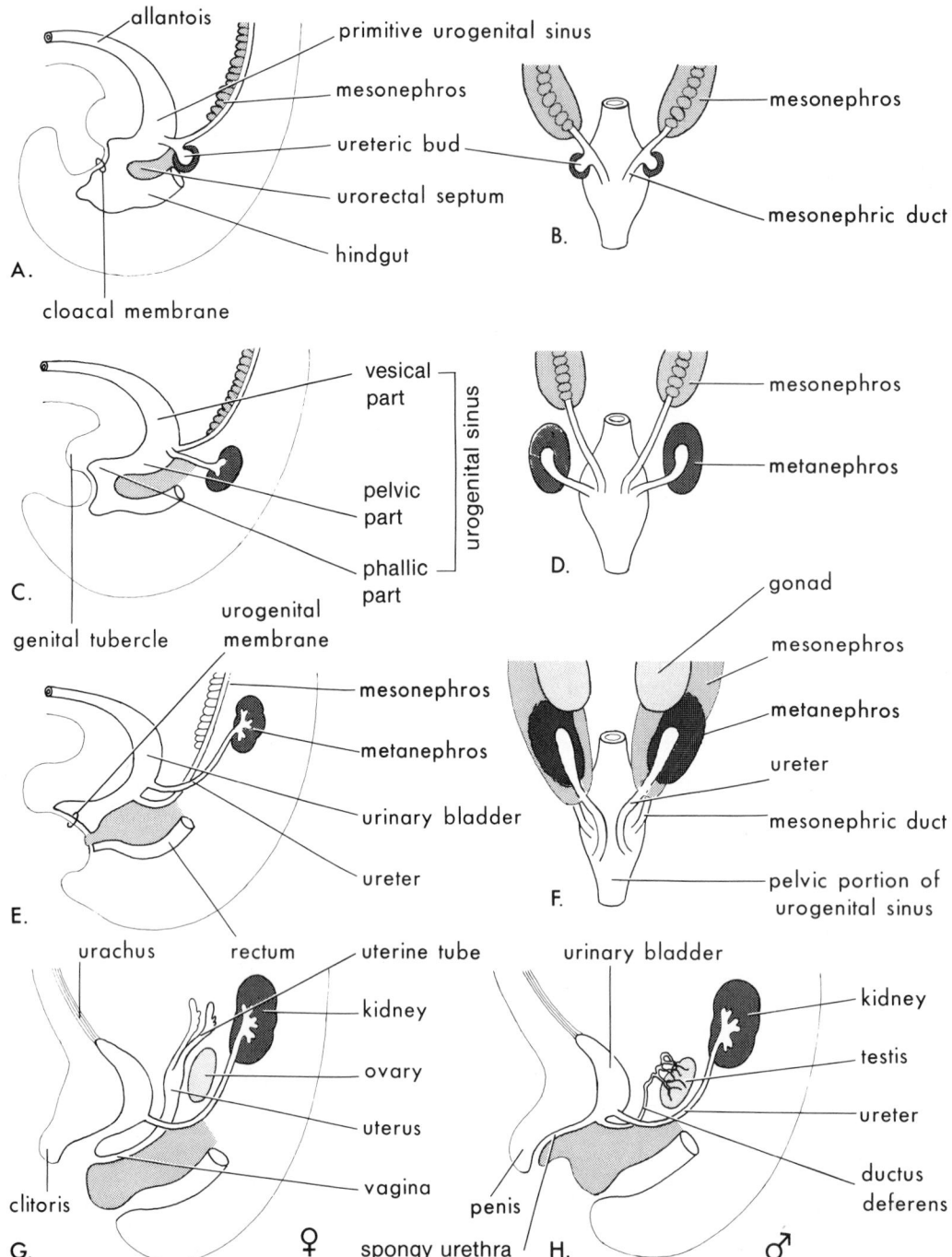

Figure 1. Graphic development of the urinary system in the male and female. Diagrams showing (1) division of the cloaca into urogenital sinus and rectum, (2) absorption of the mesonephric ducts, (3) development of the urinary bladder, urethra, and urachus, and (4) changes in the location of the ureters. *A*, Lateral view of the caudal half of 5-week-old embryo; *B, D,* and *F,* dorsal views; *C, E, G,* and *H,* lateral views. The stages shown in *G* and *H* are reached at about 12 weeks. (From Moore, K. L.: The Developing Human: Clinically Oriented Embryology, 3rd ed. Philadelphia, W. B. Saunders Company, 1982.)

will provide a summation of the current and accepted knowledge of the specialty. Ideally, it will stimulate the reader to in-depth study regarding specific problems.[14]

EMBRYOLOGY AND ANATOMY

A knowledge of embryology is necessary for proper understanding of gynecology, particularly as it relates to such problems as congenital malformations, hermaphroditism, endocrine interrelationships, and generative neoplasms. The external genitals develop from the genital tubercle, a group of cells found at the caudal end of the body. In the fourth week after fertilization, the genital tubercle develops at the ventral tip of the cloacal

membrane. Two sets of lateral structures, the labioscrotal swellings and urogenital folds, develop soon after. The genital tubercle elongates to form a phallus in both males and females. By the end of the sixth week, the cloacal membrane is joined by the urorectal septum, which divides the cloaca into the urogenital sinus and the anal canal–rectum. The cloacal membrane is then divided into the ventral urogenital membrane and the dorsal anal membrane, both of which then rupture, opening the vulva and the anal canal. With the opening of the urogenital membrane, a urethral groove forms on the undersurface of the phallus, completing the undifferentiated portion of external genital development.

Androgens produced by the testes are responsible for masculinization of the undifferentiated external genitalia. In the absence of androgens, feminization of these structures occurs. The embryonic phallus does not demonstrate rapid growth and becomes the clitoris. Urogenital folds do not fuse except in front of the anus and become the labia minora. The labioscrotal folds do fuse anteriorly and in the area of the perineal body and become the labia majora. As the urogenital sinus unfolds, it joins the müllerian tubercle, developing cephalad as the upper vagina. At this stage the urethra acquires a separate orifice.

The internal reproductive structures and the lower urinary tract develop by the growth and resorption of primordial ductal systems (Fig. 1). The urogenital ridge is formed on each side of the posterior body cavity. From these primordial cells develop the ovaries, the wolffian ducts and bodies, and the müllerian ducts. The müllerian ducts develop into the fallopian tubes, uterus, cervix, and upper vagina. To form these latter three structures, the müllerian ducts must fuse in the midline, and aplasia of one duct or failure of fusion may result in congenital malformations. The ovaries develop from coelomic epithelium covering the surfaces of the wolffian bodies. This epithelium forms early into a sex gland anlage, and at this stage histologic sexual differentiation is not evident. When ovarian development occurs, primordial follicles appear and remain inactive until gonadotropic stimulation begins. The wolffian ducts are the forerunner of the male reproductive system and undergo regressive changes in the female that cause them to become vestigial. Remnants of the wolffian ducts persist in the normal female as ductal structures that may become manifest clinically as Gartner's duct cysts (usually seen in the vagina), parovarian cysts, and the hydatid of Morgagni.

The External Genitalia (Fig. 2)

The female external genitals, or vulva, include the mons veneris, which is a fat pad over the pubic symphysis into which the labi majora blend. It is covered with skin that contains sweat glands and hair follicles. The labia majora are the most lateral structures of the external genitalia and do not acquire full growth until puberty. After menopause, atrophy may occur. These structures are covered with skin that contains sweat glands, hair follicles, and sebaceous and sudoriferous glands beneath the squamous epithelium. The underlying tissue is adipose, and the round ligaments of the uterus insert into the upper ends of the labia majora. The labia minora are medial to the majora and are covered with skin containing sweat glands but no hair follicles. The labia minora extend from the clitoris posteriorly and continue to the perineum. Anteriorly they pass over the top of the clitoris to form the prepuce and join below the clitoris to form the frenulum. Growth and configuration of the labia minora are influenced by estrogen. The clitoris is composed of two roots that traverse the pubic rami to unite beneath the symphysis in the clitoral body and terminate in the upper portion of the glans, which is exposed. The covering of the glans is modified cutaneous tissue. The clitoris contains two corpora cavernosa and is erectile.

The urethral meatus is situated below the clitoris and above the vaginal orifice. Lateral to this meatus open Skene's ducts, which lead from paraurethral glands. Bartholin's glands are located at 4 and 8 o'clock at the vulvovaginal orifice and are compound racemose glands that connect to the surface by a single tubule lined by transitional epithelium. The gland acini are lined by a single layer of cuboidal epithelium. In its normal state the gland usually cannot be seen or palpated. The hymen divides the external and internal genitalia and may be a fibrous structure. The aperture varies greatly in size and shape and may on occasion be imperforate.

The Muscles and Fascia of the Perineum (Fig. 3)

The superficial fascia of the perineum consists of outer and deep layers, both continuous with the layers of the anterior

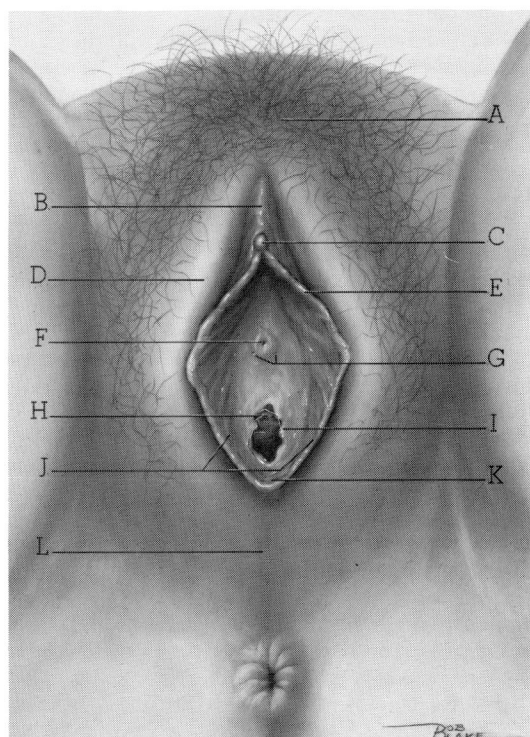

Figure 2. The external genitalia. *A,* Mons pubis. *B,* Prepuce. *C,* Clitoris. *D,* Labia majora. *E,* Labia minora. *F,* Urethral meatus. *G,* Skene's ducts. *H,* Vagina. *I,* Hymen. *J,* Bartholin's glands. *K,* Posterior fourchette. *L,* Perineal body.

abdominal wall; the outer layer is called Cruveilhier's fascia and is continuous with Camper's fascia of the anterior abdominal wall; the deep layer of the superficial perineal fascia is called Colles' fascia and is continuous with Scarpa's fascia of the ab-

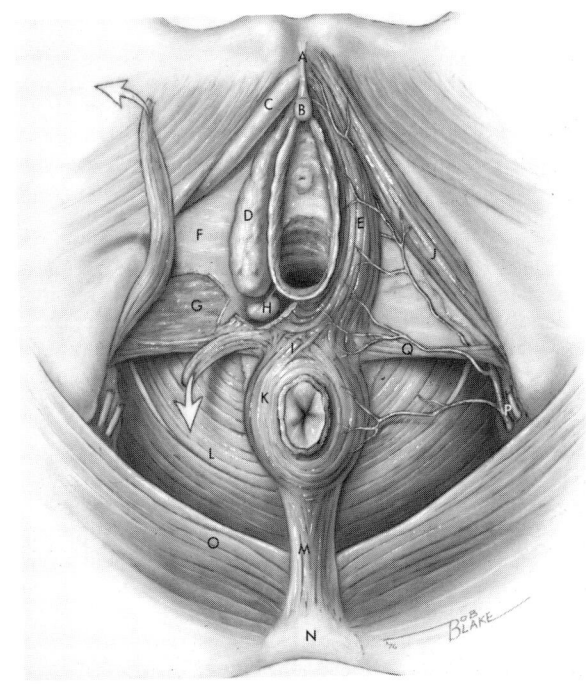

Figure 3. The muscles and fascia of the perineum. *A,* Suspensory ligament of clitoris. *B,* Clitoris. *C,* Crus of clitoris. *D,* Vestibular bulb. *E,* Bulbocavernosus muscle. *F,* Inferior fascia of urogenital diaphragm. *G,* Deep transverse perineal muscle. *H,* Bartholin's gland. *I,* Perineal body. *J,* Ischiocavernosus muscle. *K,* External anal sphincter. *L,* Levator ani muscle. *M,* Anococcygeal body. *N,* Coccyx. *O,* Gluteus maximus muscle. *P,* Pudendal artery and vein. *Q,* Superficial transverse perineal muscle.

domen. The outer layer of superficial fascia forms the greater part of the labium majus and is continuous with the superficial fascia of the thigh. The deep layer of superficial fascia, Colles' fascia, is a strong membrane adding support to the urogenital structures. This fascia is firmly attached laterally to the medial surface of the thigh, being continuous with the fascia that covers the saphenous vein opening. It becomes attached to the deep fascia along the posterior border of the superficial transverse perineal muscle and blends on either side into the medial raphe of the perineum.

The deep perineal fascia consists of obturator fascia, infra-anal fascia, and fascia of the bulbocavernosus, ischiocavernosus, and transverse perineal muscles. The obturator fascia forms the lateral wall of the ischiorectal fossa and meets the infra-anal fascia deep in the fossa. The infra-anal fascia is the fascia of the levator ani and coccygeus muscles. The deep transverse perineal muscle is covered on both sides by fascia, and the three structures constitute the urogenital diaphragm. The urethra and vagina perforate this diaphragm, which stretches as a wall across the space between the ischiopubic rami. The deep layer rests between the deep transverse perineal muscle and the pubococcygeal portions of the levator ani sling.

The perineal muscles divide into deep and superfical portions, sphincter urethrae, and bulbocavernosus and ischiocavernosus muscles. The superficial transverse perineal muscles arise from the ischial tuberosity on either side and insert into the central perineal tendon. They blend with the anal sphincter muscle and with fibers from the bulbocavernosus muscles. The bulbocavernosus muscles surround the vaginal orifice and have a sphincteric contractile effect arising anteriorly from the clitoris and inserting posteriorly into the perineal body. The ischiocavernosus muscles arise from the medial borders of the ischial rami and clitoris and course posteriorly and laterally to insert into the ischial tuberosity. The sphincter muscle of the urethra is attached to the periurethral structures and fans laterally on either side to attach to the pubic rami. The deep transverse perineal muscle lies below the superficial muscle and attaches in the midline of the perineal body.

The Internal Genitalia (Fig. 4)

THE VAGINA. The vagina is a muscular tube lined with stratified squamous epithelium that is histologically similar to the mucosa of the cervix and vulva. It does not contain glands or hair follicles, but individual cells produce mucus. The superficial layer is not keratinized. During menstrual life the vagina has transverse folds called rugae. After menopause, in the absence of estrogen, the vaginal walls become thin and atrophic, reflecting the lack of estrogen as seen in the childhood years. The adult vagina measures 12 to 13 cm. in depth, and in nulliparous women there is coaptation of the anterior and posterior walls. The vaginal axis is toward the sacral promontory, and the cervix is suspended at the upper end, surrounded by the anterior, posterior, and lateral fornices. The upper two thirds of the vagina is supported by the paravaginal fascia and the paracervical tissues, the lower one third by the perineal body.

THE CERVIX. The inferior portion of the uterus, the cervix, is a fibromuscular organ covered with stratified squamous epithelium. The portio vaginalis of the cervix arises in the vaginal fornices and ends at the external cervical os at the entrance of the endocervical canal. This squamocolumnar junction is the most common site of origin of squamous cell carcinoma. The endocervical canal is lined by columnar epithelium, and racemose glands, lined with similar epithelium, are found in the fibromuscular stroma. Such glands, if obstructed, may form nabothian cysts on the cervical surface. The nulliparous cervical os is round, but parturition changes this to a horizontally flattened orifice. The cervix is the second most common site of genital malignancy in women.

THE UTERUS. The uterus is a hollow, fibromuscular-walled organ between the bladder and rectum and consists of the cervix

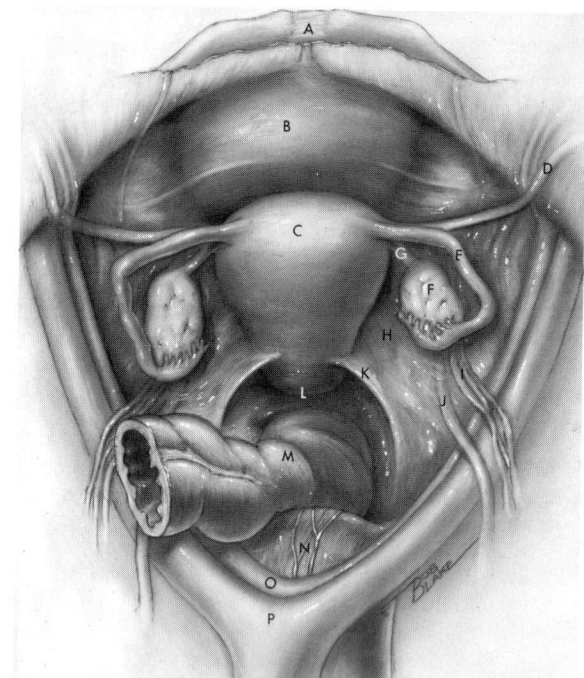

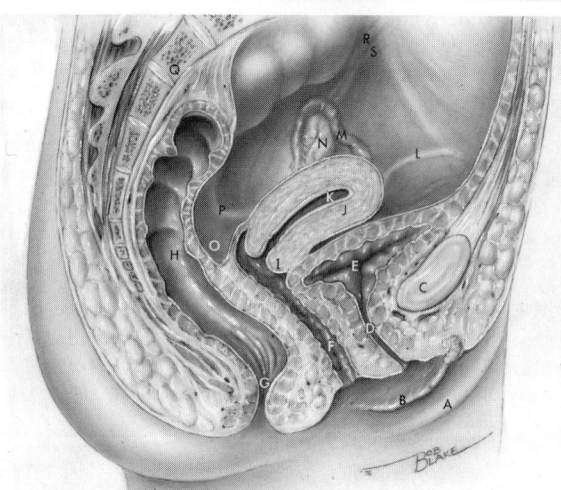

Figure 4. The internal genitalia. *Front view:* A, Symphysis pubis. B, Bladder. C, Corpus uteri. D, Round ligament. E, Fallopian tube. F, Ovary. G, Utero-ovarian ligament. H, Broad ligament. I, Ovarian artery and vein. J, Ureter. K, Uterosacral ligament. L, Cul-de-sac. M, Rectum. N, Middle sacral artery and vein. O, Vena cava. P, Aorta. *Side view:* A, Labium majus. B, Labium minus. C, Symphysis pubis. D, Urethra. E, Bladder. F, Vagina. G, Anus. H, Rectum. I, Cervix uteri. J, Corpus uteri. K, Endometrial cavity. L, Round ligament. M, Fallopian tube. N, Ovary. O, Cul-de-sac. P, Uterosacral ligament. Q, Sacrum. R, Ureter. S, Ovarian artery and vein.

and fundus. The organ is pear-shaped, and in nonpregnant women measures approximately 8 cm. in length and weighs 30 to 100 gm. The fallopian tubes and the cervical canal communicate with the uterine cavity, which is lined by the endometrium. The endometrium proliferates in response to estrogen, becomes secretory with progesterone, and bleeds as it sloughs when hormonal support is withdrawn or inadequate. The uterine fundus is covered by peritoneum except in the lower anterior portion, where the bladder is contiguous with the lower uterine segment and the peritoneum is reflected, and laterally where the folds of the broad ligament are attached. The uterus is supported by condensations of endopelvic fascia and fibromuscular tissue laterally at the base of the broad ligaments. The round ligaments provide support laterally and the uterovesical fold, anteriorly. Neither of these last two structures provides major uterine support.

THE OVIDUCTS. The fallopian tubes arise from the superior portion of the lateral borders of the uterus, superior to the attachment of the round ligaments, and are patent. The distal ends, the fimbriae, open into the abdominal cavity and the proximal ends into the uterine cavity. The tubes are lined by a single layer of low columnar epithelium, some ciliated, arranged in a branching or "frond" pattern. This structure is divided into interstitial, isthmic, ampullar, and fimbriated portions. The wall is thin, with two muscular layers and an outer layer of peritoneum within the upper borders of the broad ligament.

THE OVARIES. The normal ovary is a white, almond-shaped structure measuring 2 by 3 by 3 cm. and is located on the posterior surface of the broad ligament and inferior to the fallopian tube. The nerves, lymphatics, and blood vessels enter the ovary at the point of attachment to the broad ligament, the hilus. Lateral support of the ovary is provided by the infundibulopelvic ligament, which extends to the pelvic side wall, and medial support is to the uterus by the utero-ovarian ligament. The ovary has a cortex and a medulla. Germinal epithelium, a single layer of cuboidal cells, covers condensed fibrous tissue called the tunica albuginea. Follicles originate within the ovarian cortex and are composed of the basic embryonic complement; no new follicles are formed after birth. The medullary portion of the ovary is occupied by blood vessels, lymphatics, nerves, and connective tissue and contains remnants of wolffian body precursors. The ovary is an endocrine and a generative organ. Parafollicular granulosa cells produce estrogen and, after ovulation and corpus luteum formation, progestins. Androgens are produced by stromal cells, particularly in the hilus.

THE URINARY SYSTEM. The kidneys and ureters arise from the metanephros and a diverticulum from the wolffian duct in both sexes. The ureters vary from 28 to 34 cm. in length, the right about 1 to 2 cm. shorter than the left. The ureter is not of uniform caliber. The abdominal part of the ureter lies behind the peritoneum on the medial part of the psoas muscle and is crossed obliquely by the ovarian vessels. It enters the pelvis by crossing either the termination of the common iliac vessels or the commencement of the external iliac vessels. The pelvic ureter courses at first downward on the lateral wall of the pelvis, then medially and forward toward the lateral aspect of the cervix, about 1.5 cm. from the exterior of the cervix. In this course, it is accompanied by the uterine artery. The uterine artery then crosses over the ureter and ascends between the leaves of the broad ligament to enter the uterus laterally. The blood supply of the ureter arises from branches of the renal, ovarian, hypogastric, and inferior vesical arteries.

In the female, the uterus, cervix, and upper vagina are behind the bladder, which is separated from the uterus by the vesico-uterine fold. Below this peritoneal fold the bladder is connected to the cervix and upper vagina by areolar tissue. The bladder is stabilized by ligamentous attachments at its inferior portion or base, near the exit of the urethra, and at the vertex. The remainder is free to move. The basal attachment is to the internal investing layer of deep fascia on the pubic bone by strong fibrous bands. The arterial supply of the bladder is the superior, middle, and inferior vesical arteries, derived from the anterior hypogastric artery, the obturator and inferior gluteal arteries, and the uterine and vaginal arteries.

The female urethra is a narrow membranous canal about 4 cm. long, extending from the internal to the external urethral orifice. It is placed behind the symphysis, embedded in the anterior vaginal wall, and its direction is obliquely downward and forward. The resting diameter is about 6 mm. The urethra perforates the fasciae of the urogenital diaphragm, where it acquires longitudinal folds. Many small paraurethral glands open into the urethra.

The Blood Vessels of the Pelvis (Fig. 5)

The ovarian arteries arise from the front of the aorta just below the renal arteries. The left ovarian vein empties into the

left renal vein; the right ovarian vein empties into the vena cava just inferior to the renal vein. The ovarian vessels follow a downward course and pass between the layers of the infundibulopelvic ligament and the broad ligament to reach the ovary. Small branches divide to supply the ureter and fallopian tube. The main branches unite with the uterine vessels on the side of the uterus, and small branches supply the round ligaments.

The iliac vessels originate as the common iliac arteries from the aorta at the L4 vertebral level and slightly to the left of midline. Each is about 5 cm. long and, just below the S1 level, divide into the internal iliac (hypogastric) artery and the external iliac artery. The common iliac veins closely follow the arteries and join inferiorly and to the right of the aorta to form the vena cava. The external iliac vessels lie on the lateral walls of the pelvis above the psoas muscles, behind the peritoneum, to pass beneath the inguinal ligaments through the femoral canal to become the femoral artery and vein. The inferior epigastric vessels arise from the external iliac vessels immediately superior to the ligament. The hypogastric (internal iliac) vessels pass inferiorly and posteriorly along the border of the great sciatic notch. The hypogastric vessels are 3 to 4 cm. in length before they divide into anterior and posterior branches. The anterior branch provides the main blood supply to the bladder and forms the middle hemorrhoidal, obturator, internal pudendal, inferior gluteal, uterine, and vaginal arteries. The uterine artery arises from the anterior branch of the hypogastric artery and passes medially on the levator ani muscle toward the junction of the cervix and the uterus. At the level of the internal os, the vessels turn superiorly and follow a tortuous route between the leaves of the broad ligament to join the ovarian arteries. An inferior branch of the uterine artery turns inferiorly on either side to form the cervical arteries. The vaginal artery arises from the hypogastric artery below the level of the uterine artery and sends branches to the vagina, bladder, and rectum. The internal pudendal artery is the most caudal extension of the hypogastric

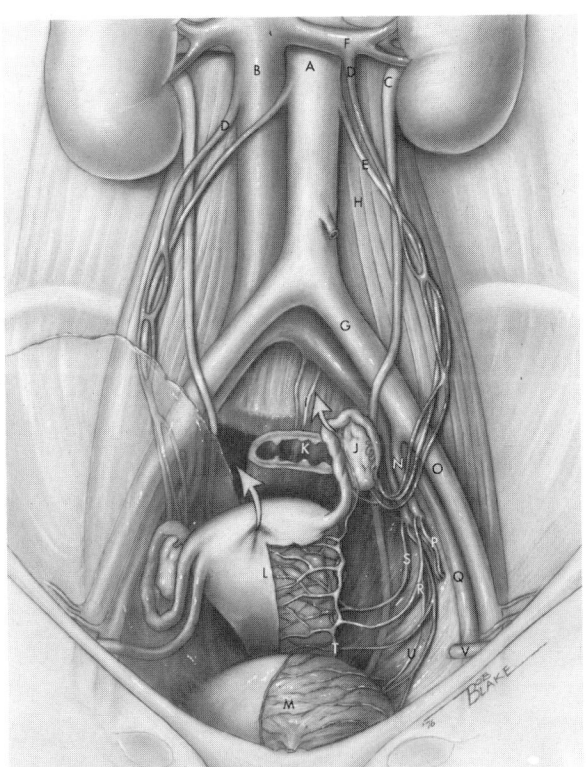

Figure 5. Blood supply of the pelvis. *A*, Aorta. *B*, Inferior vena cava. *C*, Ureter. *D*, Ovarian vein. *E*, Ovarian artery. *F*, Renal vein. *G*, Common iliac artery. *H*, Psoas muscle. *I*, Middle sacral artery. *J*, Ovary. *K*, Rectum. *L*, Corpus uteri. *M*, Bladder. *N*, Internal iliac (hypogastric) artery, anterior branch. *O*, External iliac artery. *P*, Obturator artery. *Q*, External iliac vein. *R*, Uterine artery. *S*, Uterine vein. *T*, Vaginal artery. *U*, Superior vesicle artery. *V*, Inferior epigastric artery.

artery and supplies the internal genital organs. This vessel emerges from the pelvis between the piriformis and coccygeus muscles, crosses the ischial spine, and passes through the lesser sciatic foramen to enter the perineum. The artery traverses the lateral wall of the ischiorectal fossa and supplies the erectile tissue of the vulva.

The Lymphatics of the Pelvis (Fig. 6)

The lymphatics of the pelvis parallel the vascular channels. The external iliac nodes are interposed in the drainage pattern of the deep inguinal nodes, the fundus of the bladder, and the uterus, cervix, and upper vagina. The external iliac and hypogastric drainage occurs via the common iliac nodes. The hypogastric nodes surround the hypogastric vessels and receive drainage from the cervix, uterine fundus, upper vagina, bladder, urethra, and lower ureter. The obturator nodes reside in the obturator fossa, lateral to and surrounding the obturator nerve, and receive channels from the cervix, uterus, and part of the buttocks. The sacral nodes receive branches from the cervix and uterus and reside in the sacral concavity. The rectal lymphatics course posteriorly to the sacral nodes also. The vulvar drainage takes place via subcutaneous ascending lymphatics to the superficial and deep inguinal nodes and femoral nodes, which also receive the lymphatics from the lower portions of the vagina and urethra. The lower extremity lymphatics lead to the femoral and inguinal nodes. Cross drainage in this region may occur via Cloquet's node (femoral canal) to deep nodes of the pelvis.

The Nerve Supply of the Pelvis

The sacral plexus arises from the fourth and fifth lumbar and the first four sacral cord segments. The pudendal nerve originates from the second, third, and fourth sacral segments. The plexus rests in the hollow of the pelvis over the piriformis muscle. The branches of the plexus contain fibers of sympathetic and parasympathetic nerve trunks. The parasympathetic fibers are efferent preganglionic to the pelvic viscera and afferent from the pelvic organs. The sympathetic fibers arise from the hypogastric sympathetic plexus. The levator ani, coccygeus, and sphincter ani muscles receive branches from the pudendal plexus. The pudendal nerve leaves the pelvis through the greater sciatic foramen, crosses the ischial spine, and re-enters the pelvis via the lesser sciatic foramen. It accompanies the pudendal vessels and sends branches to the sphincter ani muscle and sensory fibers to the labia majora, while another branch supplies the perineal muscles. The dorsal nerve of the clitoris also arises from the pudendal nerve.

PHYSIOLOGY AND ENDOCRINOLOGY

The interactions of physiologic and endocrinologic mechanisms cannot be separated in any adequate summary of the function of the female genital system. Numerous workers have identified the interrelationships among the central nervous system, hypothalamus, pituitary, ovary, and other endocrine systems. Dependence on estrogen and progesterone of the pelvic structures, breasts, skin, other organs, and many metabolic processes has been demonstrated.[16]

HYPOTHALAMUS, PITUITARY, AND GONADOTROPINS. The hypothalamus serves as the primary control center for the reproductive endocrine system. This system is essentially dormant until late childhood, when activation begins and certain hypothalamic cells become capable of releasing short-chain peptides to the anterior pituitary via the hypophyseal portal system. With the discovery of gonadotropin-releasing hormone (Gn-RH) by Schally and Guillemin, followed shortly thereafter by the synthesis of this compound, many new understandings of the hypothalamic control of gonadotropin secretion became possible. In experimental animals and in humans, these humoral agents, or releasing factors, cause the anterior pituitary to produce and release follicle-stimulating hormone (FSH) and luteinizing hormone (LH). Physiologic, pathologic, and even psychologic problems can alter these interrelationships.[17,18]

The pituitary gonadotropins, FSH and LH, are necessary for normal ovarian function and, via the hypothalamus, are in turn regulated through feedback mechanisms from ovarian estrogen and progesterone (Fig. 7). FSH arises from the anterior pituitary, is transmitted through the blood, and stimulates maturation of the ovarian follicle and parafollicular cells to produce estrogen. FSH, which can occasionally be found in small amounts in young girls, increases nocturnally just prior to puberty, and is found in large quantities in mature women. After the ovarian failure of menopause, there is a sharp rise in FSH as the hypo-

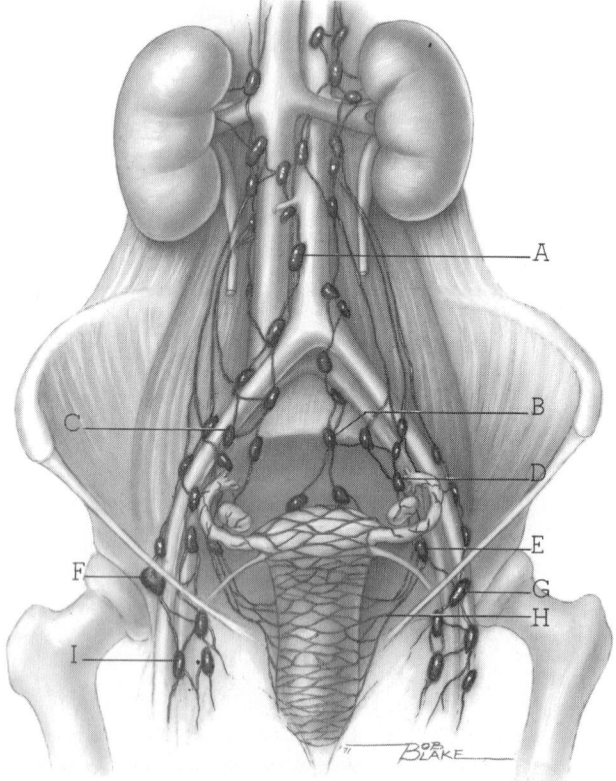

Figure 6. Lymphatics of the pelvis. *A*, Aortic. *B*, Sacral. *C*, Common iliac. *D*, Hypogastric. *E*, Obturator. *F*, Deep inguinal. *G*, Cloquet's node. *H*, Parametrial. *I*, Superficial inguinal.

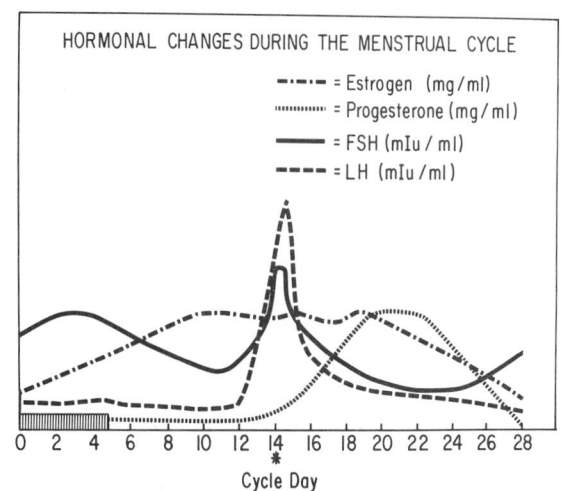

Figure 7. Hormonal changes during the menstrual cycle. Menses, days 0–5; ovulation, day 14.

thalamus attempts to correct resultant hypoestrogenism. In ovulating women, FSH is elevated during the follicular phase of the cycle, then rises sharply at midcycle. FSH levels are relatively low during the luteal phase of the cycle. LH complements FSH secretion, and the two provide a synergistic effect on ovarian function. LH levels are relatively low during the follicular and luteal phases of the menstrual cycle but rise sharply for a 72-hour span surrounding ovulation. LH, acting on the FSH-stimulated follicle, can cause ovulation. LH also stimulates the interstitial cells of the ovary and may be an integral part of corpus luteum maintenance. Still another ovarian hormone, inhibin, is not yet fully characterized but appears to be a true ovarian secretory product. It appears that inhibin participates in regulation of FSH, in addition to estrogen, but its precise mechanisms are still being elucidated. Excessive amounts of sex steroid hormones, estrogen, progesterone, or androgens, inhibit hypothalamic control of pituitary secretion.

NEUROTRANSMITTERS. Much work has been done during the last decade to study mechanisms of control of release of hypothalamic Gn-RH, as well as the pituitary gonadotropins LH and FSH. The amplitude and frequency of the pulsatile release of Gn-RH not only are regulated by the feedback of two ovarian steroids, estradiol and progesterone, as well as by gonadotropins through the hormonal input pathway, but are also modulated by several neurotransmitters and neuromodulators within the brain through a neural input pathway.

The most important neurotransmitters involved in reproductive endocrinology are two catecholamines, dopamine and norepinephrine, as well as an indolamine, serotonin (Figs. 8 and 9). All three are monoamines. Dopamine is a neurotransmitter itself, as well as the precursor of another neurotransmitter, norepinephrine. Dopamine, in addition to stimulating prolactin-inhibiting factor and thus decreasing prolactin release, acts in the median eminence and appears to inhibit the release of Gn-RH. Several studies have demonstrated that dopamine inhibits LH secretion in humans. The role of norepinephrine is less clear; however, it may stimulate the release of Gn-RH. Epinephrine has little effect on reproductive hormone release. Serotonin has not been shown to affect Gn-RH release, but it does stimulate the release of prolactin.

NEUROMODULATORS

OPIOIDS. Receptors for opioid peptides are present in the brain. There are three subgroups of opioids: enkephalins, en-

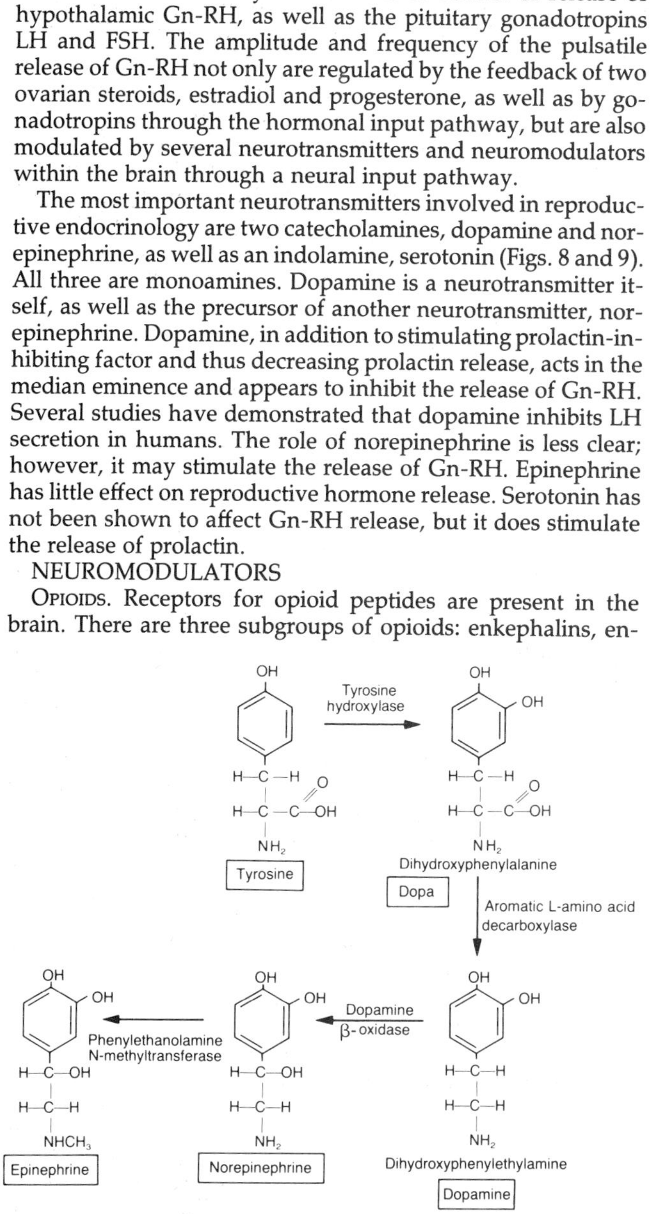

Figure 8. Metabolic pathways of dopamine, norepinephrine, and epinephrine synthesis. (From Kletzky, O. A., and Lobo, R. A.: Reproductive neuroendocrinology. *In* Mishell, D. R., Jr., and Davajan, V. (Eds.): Infertility, Contraception and Reproductive Endocrinology, 2nd ed. Oradell, N. J., Medical Economics Books, 1986.)

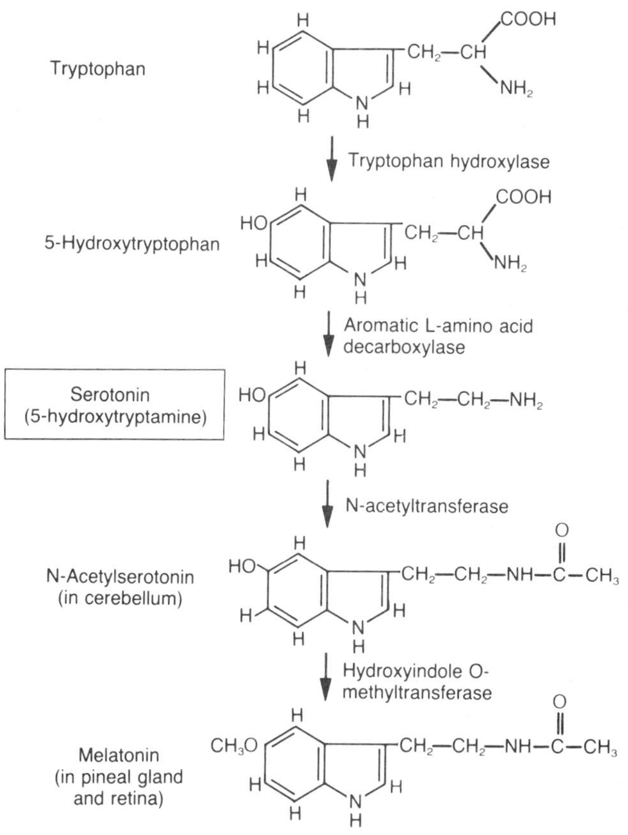

Figure 9. Metabolic pathways of serotonin synthesis. (From Kletzky, O. A., and Lobo, R. A.: Reproductive neuroendocrinology. *In* Mishell, D. R., Jr., and Davajan, V. (Eds.): Infertility, Contraception and Reproductive Endocrinology, 2nd ed. Oradell, N. J., Medical Economics Books, 1986.)

dorphins (alpha, beta, gamma), and dynorphins. The concentrations of endorphins are approximately 1000 times higher in the pituitary than in the hypothalamus. Infusion of beta-endorphin results in an increase of prolactin and a decrease of LH.

PROSTAGLANDINS. Hypothalamic levels of prostaglandins may modulate the release of Gn-RH. Infusion of prostaglandin E_2 significantly increases Gn-RH levels in portal blood.

CATECHOL ESTROGENS. The compounds 2-hydroxyestradiol and 2-hyroxyestrone, as well as their 3-methyl derivatives, are present in the hypothalamus and are postulated to act as neuromodulators by altering the function of catecholamines.

OVARIAN FUNCTION. During infancy and childhood, the ovary is dormant, owing to low gonadotropin production, but it is capable of being stimulated if these hormones are present. The beginning of puberty and the age of menarche vary considerably among individuals, but the usual age for the first menstrual period is from 12 to 15 years. The early menstrual periods are usually irregular and anovulatory. Later, regular ovulatory cycles usually ensue. At puberty there is a spurt in somatic growth. Later in adolescence, higher levels of estrogen result in epiphyseal plate closure.

Before puberty, the primordial follicles develop in the deeper portions of the ovary, and after puberty, the maturing follicle migrates to the surface of the ovary. After achieving full maturation, the graafian follicle ruptures, and the ovum is extruded into the peritoneal cavity, usually around the fourteenth day of the cycle. With rupture of the follicle, the corpus luteum is formed. It persists for 14 days in a normal cycle. Should pregnancy occur, the corpus luteum will persist for approximately 12 weeks before beginning regression. After ovulation, the corpus luteum shows hypertrophy and vascularization of the theca lutein cells. The granulosa cells about the follicle become enlarged and polyhedral and are transformed into lutein cells.

Progesterone, produced in small amounts just prior to ovulation, is now produced in large amounts. About 4 days before menses, the corpus luteum regresses and loses the ability to produce progesterone unless human chorionic gonadotropin from pregnancy sustains corpus luteum function.

Menopause occurs with waning of ovarian function, usually between 46 and 53 years of age. With intrinsic failure of the ovary, there is atresia of the follicles and failure of estrogen production, which is at first sharp but later becomes more gradual, with a minimal amount of estrogen production extending for several additional years. With decline of estrogen, the breasts atrophy, the pelvic structures become smaller, and the vaginal mucosa becomes thin and smooth.

ESTROGEN. Many studies have demonstrated that oophorectomy performed on the immature female is followed by persistent infantile characteristics of genital tissues. If the gonads are removed from a mature female animal, the uterus and breasts atrophy. The human ovary produces estradiol-17β, the most potent naturally occurring estrogen, and estriol. These estrogens are produced primarily in the theca interna cells. Preadolescent girls and women beyond the menopause secrete little estrogen. The adult cycling woman produces 10 to 55 μg. of the various estrogens each day, with a low level during menses, which increases steadily until ovulation. After ovulation there is a slight decline, then significant levels persist until 2 to 3 days prior to menses. The placenta and adrenal glands also produce estrogens.

The estrogens are lipids with the same phenanthrene nucleus as the other steroids, from which they are distinguished by a phenolic ring A. In addition to natural estrogens, chemicals with estrogenic activity have been synthesized. These include diethylstilbestrol, hexestrol, dienestrol, and, most recently, a group of ethinyl-17α steroids. The various estrogens are rapidly metabolized by the liver and are conjugated with glucuronic and sulfuric acid. These conjugated compounds are excreted 60 per cent in urine and 40 per cent in bile and feces and by other routes.

The principal physiologic function of estrogen is stimulation of growth of the endometrium, the myometrium, other tissues of müllerian origin, the vulva, and the breast. Estrogen is responsible for uterine and tubal contractility and is the feminizing hormone that at puberty brings about the secondary sex characteristics: mammary growth, primarily of ductal tissue, and the adult female fat pad distribution. A variety of metabolic processes are also influenced by estrogen, notably plasma protein production, bone matrix stabilization, and lipid metabolism.

PROGESTERONE. Progesterone is the other steroid hormone produced by the ovary. The corpus luteum begins to secrete this hormone just before ovulation and throughout the luteal phase of the cycle. The placenta and adrenal glands also produce progesterone. It is synthesized in the body from cholesterol via pregnenolone and is converted by the ovary to estrogens and small amounts of testosterone. The production rate of progesterone from the ovary and adrenal glands of a normal adult female is approximately 3 mg. per 24 hours during the follicular phase of the cycle and 22 mg. per 24 hours during the luteal phase. Progesterone is readily synthesized for both oral and parenteral use. Natural progesterone is deactivated by gastric secretions. Synthetic progestins are abundantly available and are useful for treating menstrual disorders, endometriosis, and inhibition of ovulation.

Progesterone is essential for the maintenance of pregnancy; initially it is produced by the corpus luteum and later by the placenta. It has not been of major use as a drug for quieting uterine activity or labor. There is some evidence that progesterone reduces tubal activity. Progesterone is responsible for the acinar and lobular development in the breast and characteristic changes seen in cervical mucus and in cervical and vaginal cy-

tology. Progesterone is thermogenic, and basal body temperatures are 0.2 to 0.8° F. higher in the latter half of the ovulatory cycle.

GENITAL STRUCTURES. The female genitalia are responsive to estrogen.[2] In the child, these structures are immature and thin and begin to mature only with pubescence and the onset of ovarian function. The vulva is thin and not prominent. The vaginal epithelium, which is quite thick at birth because of maternal gestational hormones, rapidly regresses to thin membrane and is pH neutral. With puberty the vagina thickens, glycogen storage increases, and pH becomes more acid. The cycling woman's vagina normally contains diphtheroids and Döderlein's bacilli, which aid normal vaginal secretion and acidity. After menopause, the vagina again becomes thin and loses the normal rugal pattern, and pH slowly rises. Exfoliated vaginal cells may be stained and microscopically examined for histologic changes that occur with the varying hormonal patterns.

The cervix of the child is disproportionately larger than the fundus, but after puberty this ratio is reversed. As in the vagina, the cervical epithelium undergoes cyclic changes during the menstrual cycle, but these are less than those seen in the endometrium. The racemose glands of the endocervix are dormant in children but initiate secretion of mucus after puberty. Under the dominance of estrogen, the cervical mucus increases, is thin and watery, and forms a "fern" pattern when dried. When progesterone is present, cervical mucus is opaque, thick, and tenacious and does not "fern." After menopause, cervical mucus production declines as estrogen production declines.

The myometrium of the adult woman normally undergoes spontaneous rhythmic contractions. The uteri of castrates lose this rhythmicity. Hypertrophy of myometrium occurs when higher levels of estrogen are present, and uterine atrophy occurs after menopause. The endometrium reflects generally the levels of estrogen and progesterone. Estrogen causes proliferation of the endometrium and its vascular channels. Progesterone transforms proliferative into secretory endometrium with glandular and stromal features that promote possible implantation. Endometrial biopsy is a simple office procedure that may allow precise interpretation of ovarian hormonal production.

The fallopian tube epithelium also reflects ovarian hormonal changes through cyclic modification, maturation, and regression changes. The tubal musculature possesses an intrinsic peristaltic action believed to aid tubal transport. The action of cilia of certain tubal cells may also be involved in transport. Estrogen appears to influence these activities.

Of recent interest have been studies of the impact of chronic hypoestrogenism (menopause, castration, other causes) upon maintenance of bone density (osteoporosis) and upon arteriosclerotic cardiovascular diseases, particularly coronary artery disease. It now appears that replacement of estrogen is the most potent prophylaxis to retard the development of age-related osteoporosis and fracture, as well as providing a significant benefit upon these cardiovascular diseases, probably through beneficial modulation of plasma lipids.[16]

THE GYNECOLOGIC HISTORY AND EXAMINATION

An adequate history remains a prerequisite for intelligent diagnosis and treatment. All elements of a general medical history are essential to adequate evaluation of pelvic complaints. This gynecologic history should include:

Present illness: A chronologic story of the patient's problem, relating symptoms, signs, dates, effects of other organ function, and prior investigation or therapy.

Menstrual pattern: Age at onset of menses; frequency, duration, and amount of flow; menstrual irregularities; date of the first day of the two most recent episodes of menstrual bleeding;

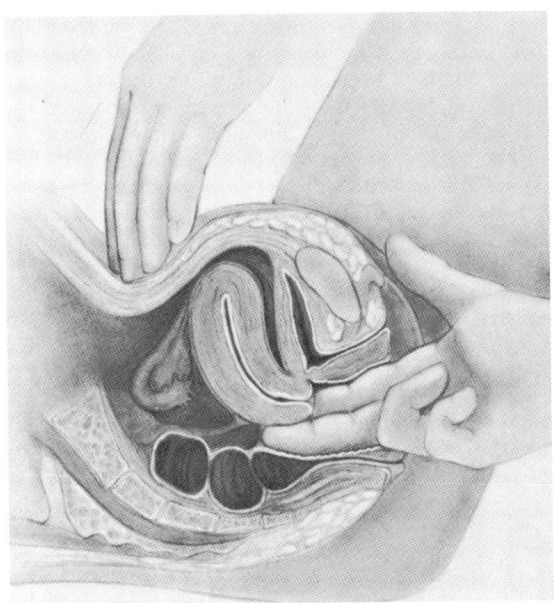

Figure 10. Bimanual pelvic examination. The examiner inserts two fingers into the vagina and places the other hand on the lower abdomen. The structures of the pelvis are then outlined between the two hands. (From Nelson, J. H., Jr.: Atlas of Radical Pelvic Surgery. New York, Appleton-Century-Crofts, 1969.)

history of pain with menses and its location, character, and duration; any vaginal bleeding between periods or any contact such as douching or coitus; and any other major physiologic or pathologic changes associated with menses.

Vaginal discharge: Amount, type, color, relation to menses, itching, and previous vaginal infections and therapy.

Obstetric history: Each pregnancy should be listed chronologically with comments about duration, complications, delivery, and the puerperium.

Marital history: The dates of marriages, contraceptive techniques and duration of use, frequency of coitus, and dyspareunia.

Other factors: Sensations of pressure, incontinence, urinary symptoms, bowel complaints, pelvic or abdominal surgery including findings and complications, and a thorough general and endocrine systems review.

The normal woman dislikes a pelvic examination and presents herself for examination with reservation. Gentleness, privacy, and dignity are necessary, and a female chaperon should always be present for assistance, patient reassurance, and protection from possible legal embarrassment. Each step in the pelvic examination should be explained briefly to the patient to gain her confidence and cooperation. The pelvic examination is done with the patient in the lithotomy position with the legs placed in stirrups. Before being placed on the table, the patient should empty her bladder. The chaperon aids in positioning of the patient and drapes her.

The first part of the pelvic examination consists of inspection of the external genitalia for evidence of infection, neoplasia, hypertrophy, atrophy, or trauma. Specific note is made about skin texture, hair patterns, clitoral size, Skene's ducts, and Bartholin's glands. The groin should be examined. The speculum examination is next, and a variety of instruments of different sizes and shapes are available. There is no substitute for adequate equipment and lighting. The instrument should be at approximately body temperature and lubricated slightly. The vaginal wall and cervix should be inspected for size, shape, and evidence of atrophy, infection, trauma, bleeding, or neoplasia. Specimens can be obtained for cancer cytologic study, hormonal interpretation, and bacteriologic examination. The vagina should be inspected again during withdrawal of the specu-

lum, particularly the anterior and posterior surfaces, which may have been covered initially by the blades of the speculum. The patient then performs the Valsalva maneuver while the support of the bladder, rectum, and uterus is visualized, and note is made of any stress incontinence.

The examiner then proceeds to the bimanual part of the examination, introducing the first two fingers of one hand into the vagina and palpating above the symphysis with the other hand (Fig. 10). The physician attempts to determine the consistency, size, shape, and mobility of the uterus. After the uterus is palpated, the adnexal regions are felt. Next, it is important to palpate the parametrial and paracervical areas. Finally, a combined rectovaginal examination should be done. In children and virgins, a rectal examination may be all that is possible because of the intact hymen. A child's small speculum or Kelly cystoscope may aid visualization, and appropriate smears should be obtained.

LABORATORY AND CLINICAL TESTS

CYTOLOGIC STUDIES. Approximately 20 per cent of cases of cancer in women arise in the genital tract. The most useful techniques for the early detection of genital malignant diseases are the pelvic examination and Papanicolaou studies.[5] It should be routine to utilize these techniques for all women when they become sexually active or by 18 years of age and at least at yearly intervals thereafter. Not only can early malignancy be detected, but also premalignant changes may frequently be discovered. Malignant and preinvasive lesions arising from the genital organs exfoliate tumor cells, which may traverse the intermediate structures and collect in the vaginal pool and on the surface of the cervix. Malignant cells from the vagina and the cervix will be present in 90 per cent of patients with these lesions. If the tumor is of the vulva, it may be missed unless the external genitals are carefully examined and direct scrapings obtained from suspicious areas. For endometrial or uterine smears, best results are achieved by passing a fine probe, sound, or small brush into the uterine cavity and obtaining direct smears. Malignant tumors of the tubes or ovaries rarely exfoliate cells that can be collected on routine pelvic examinations.

Exfoliated cells are collected by aspiration or gentle scraping and are evenly spread onto glass slides, then immediately fixed in an equal solution of ether and 95 per cent alcohol. Deeper scraping may yield basal cells of different cytologic patterns, which may confuse the unwary cytologist. Delay in fixation may allow drying and cytologic alteration. After fixation and Papanicolaou staining, slides should be studied microscopically by an experienced cytologist for cytologic changes compatible with malignancy.

Papanicolaou cervical cytology offers a high degree of accuracy, but can be no better than the material collected. If gross infection or blood and mucus are present, care must be exercised to provide sufficient material for study. Such cytologic studies should be used in the detection of premalignant disease of hidden or occult malignant disease and for follow-up of patients after treatment of malignant disease. *Cytologic studies should rarely if ever be used as an indication for surgical or irradiative therapy;* rather, they should lead the examiner to diagnostic surgical studies to provide adequate tissue for histopathologic diagnosis.

Vaginal material obtained for study of the etiology of vaginal infection is mixed with saline, placed on a slide, and microscopically examined for the presence of *Trichomonas vaginalis* or *Candida albicans* (Fig. 11). Cultures may be required for positive identification of vulvovaginal fungi.

CERVICAL STUDIES. While Papanicolaou cytology is the major approach in the screening for premalignant cervical or vaginal neoplasia, other techniques may also be of use. Gross visualization of the cervix is mandatory, and any suspicious

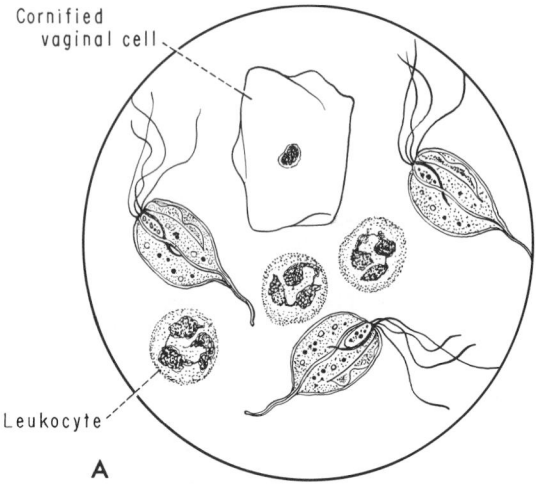

Cornified
vaginal cell

Leukocyte

A

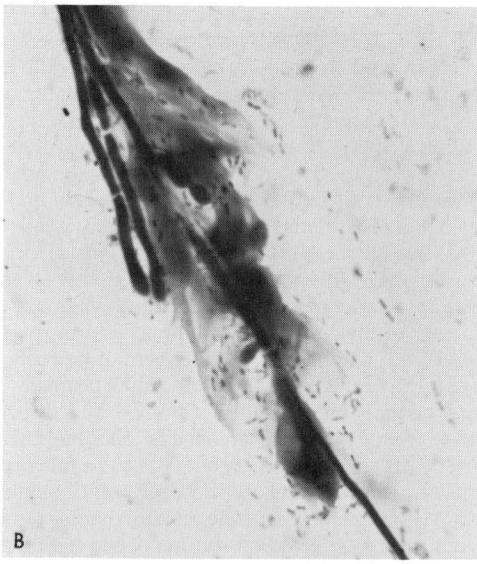

B

Figure 11. Preparations of vaginal secretions, showing in A, trichomonads, about one half the size of a cornified vaginal cell but larger than leukocytes, and B, the fiber-like mycelia of *Candida albicans*. (From Kistner, R. W.: Gynecology: Principles and Practice. Chicago, Year Book Medical Publishers, 1964. Used by permission.)

areas should be biopsied, usually without anesthesia. The cervix may be painted with an iodine solution, such as Schiller's stain, with which normal cells rich in glycogen stain darkly, whereas neoplastic cells do not take the stain. This technique, as well as colposcopy or colpomicroscopy (microscopic visualization of the cervix *in situ*), can serve to direct biopsies for histologic diagnosis. Endocervical curettage should also be used with this technique. If abnormal Papanicolaou smears have been reported, use must be made of either multiple biopsies or cold-knife conization of the cervix, which removes the exocervix, including the squamocolumnar junction, and the endocervical canal. The important fact is not to overlook the diagnosis of invasive carcinoma. Presumption of a benign or premalignant diagnosis on the basis of cytology alone may result in a patient with occult invasive carcinoma receiving inadequate therapy.

The colposcope (Hinselman, 1924) and the colpomicroscope (Antoine, 1954) have more recently become most valuable means in the evaluation of suspected neoplastic genital lesions. Magnification, coupled with various staining techniques, allows an accurate *in vivo* analysis of genital neoplasia and enables the examiner to direct biopsies to suspicious lesions that might not be noted during a nonmagnified evaluation.

Cervical smears and cultures are quite important for the diagnosis of gonorrhea and chlamydia, but all too often negative results are obtained because of faulty technique. To properly obtain cervical cultures, a vaginal speculum is inserted and the cervix is wiped clean with cotton swabs. Through compressive force of the blade of the speculum on the anterior and posterior cervix, the mucus of the endocervical glands is "milked" into the endocervical canal. A sterile culture swab is introduced into the endocervical canal, with care not to contaminate the swab with other vaginal secretions. One such swab is spread on a slide, dried, stained with Gram's stain, and examined under high microscopic power for the classic gram-negative intracellular diplococci. Another swab is immediately placed onto Thayer-Martin medium and then incubated in carbon dioxide for culture identification. One should never inform a patient that she unequivocally has gonorrhea on the basis of a smear, although therapy can be initiated. Diagnosis of this disease without culture identification may be fraught with legal hazard. In similar manner, cultures for chlamydia can be made. The presence of herpes virus should be ascertained by opening vulvar or vaginal "blisters" and, after mild abrasion, placing swabs in appropriate transfer media.[6]

ENDOMETRIAL STUDIES. The endometrial biopsy is used to study hormonal effects, fertility, and ovulatory factors, and on occasion to aid in the diagnosis of malignancy. The procedure is done without anesthesia, and discomfort is minimal. By the insertion of a fine curette, several samples of endometrium can be obtained for histopathologic examination. If the diagnosis for suspected neoplasia is negative, however, an indicated dilatation and curettage with or without hysteroscopic guidance should seldom be replaced by endometrial biopsy, since the tissue sampled by curettage is considerably greater and diagnosis more accurate. Endocrine changes are reflected quite adequately through such endometrial biopsy techniques, and by timing the biopsy to the latter half of the menstrual cycle, the presence of progesterone and ovulation can be detected.

PREGNANCY TESTS. Pregnancy may be determined by a variety of tests that detect the presence of human chorionic gonadotropin (hCG). Most immunologic tests give a positive result with a concentration of 20 to 40 mI.U. per ml. Such concentrations are usually achieved just prior to or near the time of the first missed menstrual period. Highly specific radioimmunoassays for the beta subunit of hCG can be even more sensitive and specific. Quantified levels of hCG are now readily available and are particularly useful in monitoring for ectopic gestation or other abnormal pregnancies.

OTHER STUDIES. Several other diagnostic tests should be mentioned. Hysterosalpingography is a technique by which a cannula attached to the cervix allows the uterine cavity and fallopian tubes to be filled with radiopaque dye. By appropriate roentgenologic techniques the endometrial cavity and tubes can be outlined quite adequately. Laparoscopy is a technique by which the pelvic viscera can be directly visualized by a transperitoneal route and with a minimum of morbidity.[8]

Hysteroscopy has become an increasingly useful technique in the assessment of intrauterine structures and pathology. This technique, which can be done under local anesthesia, offers an enhanced view of the endometrial cavity. Operative capabilities with the hysteroscope are now available. An additional technique that has received increasing usage in this specialty is ultrasonography, particularly transvaginal probe ultrasound. Through the use of real-time or sector scanning techniques, pelvic pathology can be clearly demonstrated in a significant percentage of patients. This can be particularly useful in discerning the presence of a mass in a patient in whom examination was difficult, confirming the presence of an intrauterine pregnancy, or discerning the general characteristics of an adnexal mass as solid, cystic, or mixed. CT, MRI, fine-needle aspirates (directed by ultrasound), and culdocentesis are other useful techniques.

CONGENITAL ANOMALIES

Imperforate Hymen

An imperforate hymen may lead to retention of mucus or blood, causing hematocolpos, hematometrium, hematosalpinx, and even hematoperitoneum. Such defects are rarely recognized until after puberty and the onset of menses and may present as primary amenorrhea, pelvic pain, or a palpable abdominopelvic mass. Diagnosis is based on careful examination of the external genitals, which reveals a bulging hymen without communication with the vagina and a fluctuant pelvic mass that lies anterior to the rectum. Pelvic ultrasonography may be a particularly useful study. With adequate surgical drainage, the distended structures will promptly return to normal.

A transverse vaginal septum is rare but may present in similar manner to that of imperforate hymen. A vertical vaginal septum occurs with failure of müllerian fusion. In both cases, the septum can be partial or complete. Therapy, if necessary at all, is surgical excision.

Defects of Müllerian Fusion

Other defects in müllerian fusion can present a spectrum of congenital anomalies. As one tube and half of the uterine fundus, cervix, and upper vagina arise from each müllerian duct, improper fusion can result in duplication of part or of all of the system. One abnormality is uterus didelphys, with two vaginas, cervices and uteri, each with a separate tube and ovary. Such patients can present with pelvic pain due to obstruction of outflow of blood from one uterine horn, with an intra-abdominal crisis if pregnancy occurs in a rudimentary horn that cannot expand properly, or with an undiagnosed pelvic mass. Therapy, if indicated, is surgical excision or reconstruction.

Dysgenesis

A variety of defects of the female genital tract are due to hypoplasia or aplasia of its various components. Such defects may occur either primarily or as secondary underdevelopment because of lack of estrogen. Congenital absence of both ovaries is rare, but absence of one tube or ovary at birth is not unusual. There are cases of complete absence of the vagina, usually associated with absence of the uterus, and congenital absence of the uterus despite a normal vagina. In these patients, the testicular feminizing syndrome should be suspected, in which case the gonads are testicular, yet secondary sexual characteristics are feminine as the patient lacks the ability to respond to androgen. Most of these patients present with primary amenorrhea. Jacobs has shown that 40 per cent of patients with primary amenorrhea have demonstrable chromosomal abnormalities or sex inversions of some type. Karyotypic studies are therefore important.[11]

In patients with vaginal agenesis, a normally functional vagina can be surgically created by dissection of the potential space between the bladder and rectum, or in some, by progressive dilatation. Skin grafting may be required. Such reconstruction should be delayed until the individual is mature and ready for coitus, as repetitive dilatation is mandatory to retain patency. If the primary defect is due to ovarian abnormalities, replacement of estrogen provides a growth stimulus to the genital structures. In patients with testicular feminization, the intra-abdominal gonad should be removed in late adolescence because of the high rates of malignancy during the third and fourth decades of life. In such patients, the excision of the gonads and the vaginoplasty can often be done as combined procedures. A male pseudohermaphrodite has testes with the genitalia of a female.

During evaluation of patients with congenital anomalies of the female genital system, one should always evaluate the urinary system. Associated urinary tract anomalies are quite common, occurring in as many as 50 per cent of patients with müllerian malformations.[9]

Wolffian Duct Persistence

Other congenital anomalies of the female genital system consist of those derived from remnants of the mesonephric duct or the wolffian duct and body, which normally regress during female genital development. The most common of these is the parovarian cyst, which arises from the upper wolffian duct and may grow to be as large as 20 cm. No symptoms are specific to a parovarian cyst to differentiate it from an ovarian cyst. The treatment is surgical excision, with preservation of the tube and ovary. A similar cyst, the hydatid of Morgagni, may also develop near the distal end of the fallopian tube. Significant enlargement of these cysts is rare, and only under unusual circumstances is their removal mandatory. Similarly, the wolffian system may give rise to Gartner's duct cysts. As the lower portion of the wolffian duct courses along the lateral vaginal wall, remnants persist and may later form this tubular cystic tumor mass. Only if dyspareunia develops because of excessive size is surgical excision indicated. Finally, remnants of the mesonephric system may remain in the cervix, broad ligament, and ovarian hilus and rarely may develop into bizarre varieties of malignant neoplasms. These include clear cell tumors, adenocarcinomas, and mixed tumors.

THE VULVA

The gynecologist faces an exceptional variety of problems in the area of female external genitalia. Trauma, allergy, inflammatory conditions, infections, degenerative changes, and neoplasia give rise to disorders ranging from minor annoyances to major hazards to life.

An important precept in the evaluation and management of any noted abnormality of the vulva is to be absolutely sure to exclude neoplasia. Punch biopsy with local anesthesia should be done at any time a suspicious or unusual vulvar lesion is noted.

The vulva is rich in pigment, which increases in pregnancy. Vitiligo of the vulvar skin is no different from the same lesion in other locations, nor does it require treatment. Vitiligo should not be confused with leukoplakia, in which the skin is whitish, but thickened and leathery. Various skin eruptions involving the body as a whole may affect the vulva and appear as do other lesions elsewhere on the body. Varicose veins of the vulva are often found in association with varicosities of the lower extremities, and pregnancy may cause further hypertrophy. Therapy consists of lower extremity and vulvar support and ligation or injection in the nonpregnant patient. A severe direct blow to the vulva may be complicated by subcutaneous hematoma formation. Such a hematoma may dissect widely beneath the fascia of the vulva, and surgical evacuation is often necessary. It is frequently difficult to isolate bleeding points, and packing may be required. Vulvar lacerations should be cleansed and sutured as lacerations elsewhere on the body.

Glandular Lesions

The vulvar glands are subject to a variety of disorders. Skenitis usually occurs as a consequence of gonococcal infection. In the acute phase, the exudate may be expressed from ductal orifices, and the patient often has dysuria and other symptoms of urethral irritation. In chronic infections, secondary organisms are usually present, and on occasion these glands may become abscessed and require surgical drainage. Antibiotic therapy is indicated for both acute and chronic infections. Infections and cysts of Bartholin's glands are common. A Bartholin's abscess should be treated with heat until fluctuant and then sharply incised on the mucocutaneous junction between the vagina and vulva. Often, a small inflatable Worde catheter may be inserted. If drained by incision, the margins of the incision are marsupialized with interrupted sutures of fine chromic catgut. Bartholin's abscesses may occur initially from gonococcal infection, but more commonly other organisms are also involved. Antibiotic therapy is indicated in cases of significant cellulitis or systemic symptoms, but drainage remains the treatment of choice. Bartholin's cysts may be marsupialized or excised, but the latter procedure is usually associated with significant blood loss. Small asymptomatic Bartholin's cysts usually require no treatment unless biopsy is necessary to exclude malignancy. The vulva is also a common site of sebaceous cysts. These may be removed if they become greatly enlarged or secondarily infected. Rarely, one may find vulvar apocrine tumors (hidradenomas) as raised, red, sessile masses less than 5 cm. in diameter. These are treated by wide local excision.

Vulvitis

Vulvar irritation occurs from a variety of causes: allergic, infectious, degenerative, or neoplastic. Pruritus accompanied by vaginal infection or vulvar skin change suggests allergy as the underlying cause. Usually the sensitivity is due to undergarments made of synthetic fibers or washed with harsh detergents. Other contact irritants can include soaps, vaginal lubricants or sprays, rubber condoms, and spermicidal foams or jellies. Other causes of vulvar irritation include pediculosis pubis or mechanical irritation from obesity, clothing, or menstrual pads. Intestinal parasites may remain on the vulva and cause irritation. Systemic diseases such as Hodgkin's disease, diabetes mellitus, leukemia, congestive heart failure, and anemia may cause vulvar irritation. Inadequate nutrition, poor hygiene, and vitamin deficiencies also have been associated with vulvar irritation. The basic principles of management of a patient with vulvitis are to search thoroughly for a diagnosis, treat any specific infectious disease, investigate possible allergies, and then keep the area clean and dry and avoid trauma from scratching, harsh soaps, drugs, ointments, or rubbing with a towel.

The most common cause of vulvar irritation is an infectious vulvovaginitis caused by either *Candida albicans* or *Trichomonas vaginalis* or both. The vulva appears swollen and red and may be excoriated and secondarily infected. Mycotic vulvovaginitis is a common problem among diabetic patients, oral contraceptive users, and persons receiving systemic antibiotics. Diagnosis is based on fresh-preparation identification of yeast of *Trichomonas* (see Fig. 11). Therapy is discussed in the section dealing with vaginitis. For both types of infection, immediate relief is obtained by additional use of topical creams containing hydrocortisone or miconazole, as well as by following the general instructions for nonspecific vulvitis.

Follicular vulvitis may occur, and penicillin treatment and local therapy are recommended. Finally, condylomata acuminata, or venereal warts, occur as a presumed infectious vulvitis of viral origin (human papilloma virus, HPV). Many different subtypes of HPV have been involved in pelvic infection. HPV types 16 and 18 may also be associated with premalignant and malignant lesions of the female genital tract. Such lesions are associated with an irritating vaginal discharge. These benign epithelial neoplasms may be few or many, in some cases even covering the entire perineum and extending onto the vagina or cervix (Fig. 12). Therapy is topical use of podophyllin or trichloroacetic acid. On occasion one may use 5-fluorouracil. Cautery is used for the more extensive forms of the disease but requires an anesthetic. Cryosurgery, laser therapy, and even interferon have all been used with increasing success in difficult cases of venereal warts.

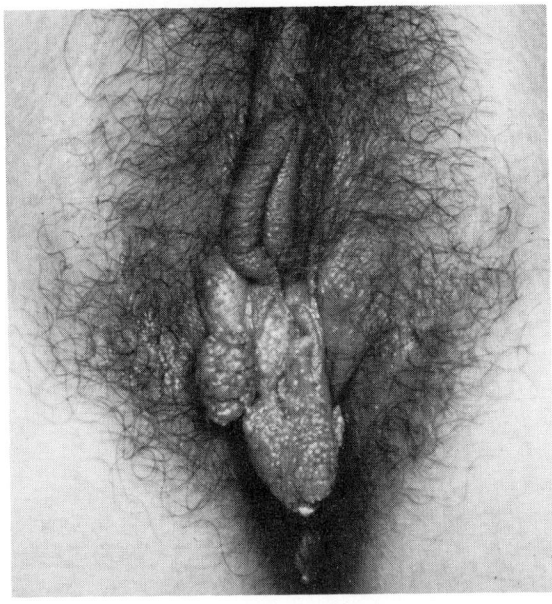

Figure 12. Condylomata acuminata. These growths may appear anywhere on the vulva. They may be either broad and confluent or papillary. (Courtesy of Mr. C. P. Jones.)

Recently, a near-epidemic of sexually transmitted vulvovaginitis has occurred, caused by herpes progenitalis (h. simplex, Type II). This infection is characterized by vesicular eruptions that are extremely painful and often are secondarily infected when the patient is seen. Current therapy includes warm baths in water containing potassium permanganate, drying, and systemic analgesics. The duration of this infection is usually limited to 1 to 2 weeks, but it may recur. The antiviral agent acyclovir will reduce the severity of primary herpetic infections. Other data suggest that chronic acyclovir use may reduce the frequency and severity of recurrences. To date, however, there is no permanent cure, and approximately 20 per cent of patients with a primary herpetic lesion will develop recurrent episodes.

Other venereal diseases may present as vulvar lesions. These include the primary chancre of syphilis or the moist, grayish patches (condylomata lata) of secondary syphilis. After dark-field examination for diagnosis, therapy consists of penicillin or its substitute. Granuloma inguinale is a rare infectious disease of the vulva caused by the Donovan bacillus. A scraping of the serpiginous lesion may reveal the intracellular Donovan body. Tetracycline and aminoglycosides are the most useful agents for this disease. Lymphogranuloma venereum is a disease of viral origin, associated frequently with inguinal adenitis, multiple draining sinuses, and rectal stricture. The diagnosis is made by the Frei skin test. Erythromycin and tetracycline are useful, as are the sulfonamides. Chancroid is caused by the gram-negative Ducrey's bacillus. It appears as a small papule 2 to 4 days after exposure, and afterward becomes an indurated and punched-out lesion with soft edges and a purulent surface. Inguinal adenitis, often suppurative, is a frequent occurrence. Chancroid is treated with sulfonamides, although other broad-spectrum antibiotics may be useful.

Degenerative Diseases of the Vulva

There are three degenerative diseases of the vulva, all occurring most frequently after menopause. All result in itching, pain, dyspareunia, and frequent secondary infection. These diseases are more commonly seen after bulbar irradiation or premature menopause. The incidence of vulvar carcinoma is increased with these lesions, and biopsy should be employed when necessary to exclude neoplasia. Papanicolaou cytology of scrapings is of aid.

Kraurosis vulvae is a disease in which the vulva appears shrunken and dried. *Leukoplakia,* another degenerative vulvar disease, presents initially as a hypertrophic lesion and later as an atrophic problem. The skin is whitened and leathery. *Lichen sclerosis et atrophicus* may be difficult to differentiate from either kraurosis or leukoplakia. This is a slowly changing, chronic, localized lesion but, unlike the other two problems, tends to involve the skin of the thighs. In all three lesions an intense pruritus frequently occurs, and excoriation with secondary infection is often noted. Approximately 50 per cent of vulvar carcinomas are found in areas of these degenerative lesions, and both cytologic smears and biopsy should be frequently used. Treatment of these three lesions is symptomatic, with relief of pruritus a primary goal. Systemic estrogens may offer limited aid. Local excision is frequently necessary, and with more extensive lesions simple vulvectomy may rarely be required. Topical 2 per cent testosterone ointment may be of some benefit.

Carcinoma in situ *of the Vulva*

Bowen originally described a preinvasive cancer of the skin of the vulva, and others have noted a high incidence of this disease associated with previous sexually transmitted diseases. Carcinoma *in situ* of the vulva (vulvar intraepithelial neoplasia, VIN-III) may appear in a woman who has leukoplakia, kraurosis vulvae, or lichen sclerosis et atrophicus, with or without pruritus. The diagnosis should be made only after adequate histologic study shows the criteria of intraepithelial changes characteristic of epidermoid carcinoma, but without invasion. Treatment should be simple vulvectomy in most instances. In patients with carcinoma *in situ* of the vulva, up to 35 per cent may have a second malignant genital lesion. In approximately 15 per cent of patients with either intraepithelial or invasive carcinoma of the vulva, carcinoma of the vagina or cervix later develops. Thus, patients with carcinoma *in situ* of the vulva should be carefully followed.

Carcinoma of the Vulva (Fig. 13)

Vulvar cancers constitute about 3.5 per cent of all genital cancers, and the peak incidence occurs in the seventh decade of life. DiSaia and Creasman reported that among patients with vulvar cancer, 20 per cent were between 20 and 50 years old, 26 per cent were in the sixth decade, and 40 per cent were in the 61- to 70- year age range. In approximately half the patients, the cancer develops in areas of pre-existing leukoplakia, kraurosis

vulvae, or lichen sclerosis et atrophicus; others report a high incidence of syphilis and other vulvar venereal diseases among these patients. Most patients with vulvar carcinoma complain of a mass on the vulva or perineum, ulceration or vulvar irritation, or pruritus. Bleeding and pain may be additional findings. Any firm tumor or ulceration must be biopsied, and the biopsy should include the primary lesion and some adjacent normal tissue. There is an average delay by the patient of 20 months from discovery of some vulvar abnormality to examination and treatment.

Carcinoma of the vulva is usually squamous (95 per cent) but adenocarcinoma, melanocarcinoma, basal cell carcinoma, and Paget's disease are reported. Squamous cancer may arise anywhere on the vulva, but lesions of the labia majora or labia minora are most frequent. Most squamous cancers of the vulva are rather well differentiated. Adenocarcinoma of the vulva usually arises from Bartholin's glands but may develop from paraurethral glands or embryonic cell nests. Melanocarcinoma is an infrequently found vulvar cancer, as is Paget's disease, a slowly spreading ulcerative eczematoid lesion of the vulvar skin that is thought to be an adenocarcinoma of the apocrine sweat glands of that region. Basal cell carcinoma of the vulva is most frequently seen on the labium majus but may appear on other structures. Microscopically, basal cell carcinoma shows extensive proliferation of the cells of the basal layer of the epidermis, which invade the dermis beneath and usually present as a crater-like ulcer. Unlike other varieties of vulvar cancer, basal cell carcinoma usually does not metastasize but grows deeply into underlying or adjacent tissues. Some basal cell cancers have squamous cell carcinoma elements.

Vulvar cancer tends to spread by local extension and lymphatic metastasis. The frequency and sites of metastasis depend upon the size, location, and differentiation of the vulvar lesion. Of patients in whom the primary lesion is less than 1.5 cm. in diameter, approximately 12 per cent have positive lymph nodes. However, if the vulvar lesion measures 1.5 to 3.0 cm. in diameter, the incidence of lymph node metastasis is 45 per cent. Way found lymph node metastasis in 62 per cent of patients with anaplastic cancer, but if the primary tumor was well differentiated, the incidence of lymphatic metastasis was only 35 per cent. The primary lymphatic drainage of the vulva is via superficial inguinal lymph nodes of that side. From there, the lymphatics drain via Cloquet's node to the external iliac nodes and up the aortic chain. Contralateral vulvar drainage may occur, however, even from well-lateralized lesions. The upper vulvar areas, principally around the clitoris, may drain directly to Cloquet's node, which then may be involved with tumor while the superficial inguinal nodes are negative. Vulvar lesions in the perineal, Bartholin's, or posterior fourchette areas may involve the rectovaginal septum, rectum, or vagina and may metastasize via the deep pelvic nodes. Way has demonstrated the difficulty of detecting inguinal node metastases by palpation, as many enlarged nodes will not contain metastases, whereas nodes normal to palpation may have tumor cells when microscopically examined. In general, however, if the primary vulvar lesion is small and the superficial inguinal lymphatics and Cloquet's node are negative for malignancy, it is unlikely that the deeper nodes will be involved. Metastasis may also occur to the skin of the thigh, pubis, and groin and to the bladder, urethra, upper vagina, or rectovaginal septum. Blood-borne metastases are unusual.

The treatment of vulvar cancer is surgical.[15] Radiotherapy has been of little use for primary or recurrent disease and is contraindicated because of the risk of extensive vulvar necrosis. Basal cell carcinoma and Paget's disease of the vulva should be treated with wide and deep local excision of the tumor, and if it is large, hemivulvectomy should be done. Removal of regional lymph nodes is not indicated. The prognosis is generally excellent, but these patients should be followed closely for local

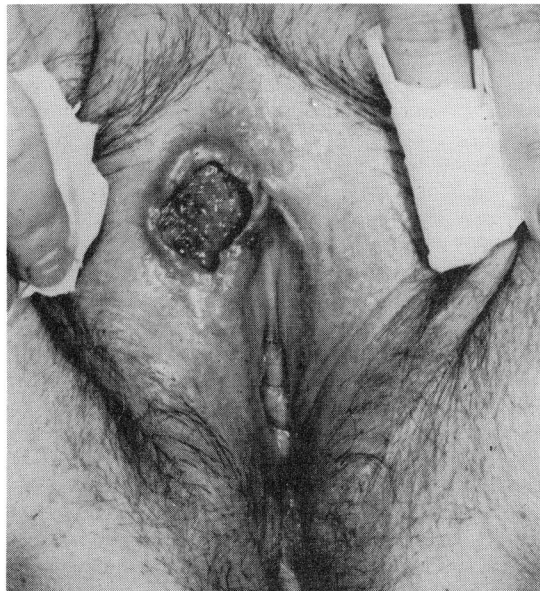

Figure 13. Carcinoma of the vulva. (Courtesy of Mr. C. P. Jones.)

recurrence. *Operations such as local excision, hemivulvectomy, and simple vulvectomy have proved, in general, to be inadequate therapy for vulvar cancer.* Most investigators have outlined appropriate therapy as including at least a block dissection of the vulva, in continuity, removing the skin, subcutaneous tissues, and lymphatic tissues of the groin, vulva, and perineum as one specimen. Controversy exists as to whether all patients should also have retroperitoneal node dissection to include removal of the femoral, iliac, and obturator nodes. These procedures are usually done as a one-stage operation, but may be divided, with the deep node dissection performed later. Utilizing the radical vulvectomy and node dissections, one can expect a 5-year cure rate of over 80 per cent in patients without positive nodes and a 5-year survival of 47 per cent even in patients with positive inguinal nodes. Overall, the 5-year cure rate after surgical therapy of cancer of the vulva is approximately 60 per cent. If the vulvar lesion involves the vagina, rectum, or urethra, then pelvic exenteration may be the operation of choice. Recurrence of surgically treated vulvar cancer may occur at the skin margins of the primary operation or in the skin of the groin. Distant metastases may also develop. Treatment of recurrent vulvar cancer with local excision or chemotherapy may provide palliation. Irradiation to the vulva is usually very toxic and is rarely indicated.

THE VAGINA

The stratified squamous epithelium of the vagina is histologically similar to epithelium of the cervix and the skin of the vulva and responds to estrogen by proliferation. The vagina of the child and that of the postmenopausal woman are similar in that the epithelial layer is quite thin, is easily traumatized, and is subject to a variety of infections. The normal adult vagina contains diphtheroids, Döderlein's bacilli, and anaerobic streptococci. This flora converts glycogen of vaginal cells to lactic acid, which maintains the vagina with an acid pH and enhances normal secretions.

Vaginitis

Vaginal inflammation can occur from protozoan, fungal, bacterial, or viral infection and also from deficiencies of estrogen. *Trichomonas vaginalis* is a common protozoan organism causing pruritus, tenderness, and dyspareunia. *Trichomonas* vaginitis is characterized by a foamy, greenish-yellow vaginal exudate; the vaginal walls are erythematous and tender. The diagnosis of this infection is made by high-power microscopic examination of fresh preparations of the vaginal discharge and identification of the flagellated, motile organisms, which are the size of leukocytes (see Fig. 11). There is uncertainty about the epidemiology of *Trichomonas* vaginitis, but it is seen most commonly among sexually active women. The male sexual partner may harbor these organisms without symptoms and promptly reinfect the woman who has been treated successfully. This infection is also frequently seen in chronically ill and debilitated women and in women with other pelvic infections. Current therapy consists of oral metronidazole (Flagyl) for both sexual partners.

Candida albicans is probably the most frequent and bothersome cause of vaginitis. The wide use of antibiotics and oral contraceptives predisposes to this fungal infection, as does diabetes mellitus. Symptoms are vaginal discharge, vulvar and vaginal irritation, and itching. Inspection reveals a "curdy" white vaginal exudate, intense vaginal erythema, and a white, watery discharge. Diagnosis is made from fresh preparations of vaginal discharge, which microscopically reveals the mycelia as thread-like fibers or budding forms (see Fig. 11). Cultures on Sabourad's medium may be necessary to identify the etiology of low-grade vaginitis. Therapy consists of the intravaginal application of the synthetic imidazoles — miconazole (Monistat), clotrima-

zole (Lotrimin), or butoconazole (FemStat). There is a tendency for vaginal moniliasis to recur, and in these patients one should consider evaluation for diabetes mellitus. If such a patient is taking oral contraceptives, their use may have to be temporarily terminated until the infection is controlled.

Vaginal irritation can occur in the patient with insufficient estrogen to maintain normal vaginal thickness. Infection of this thin, atrophic, easily traumatized vagina is often nonspecific and caused by a variety of usually nonpathogenic bacteria. Treatment is replacement of systemic or topical estrogen. In some women, there exists a nonspecific bacterial infection, now thought sexually transmitted, which most likely appears to be a symbiotic infection between anaerobic bacteria and *Gardnerella*. Both organisms conribute to produce clinical symptoms. This infection, now termed *bacterial vaginosis,* is confirmed by "clue cells" on wet preparations and is best treated with metronidazole or cephadine. Concurrent treatment of the male partner remains controversial.

Herpes simplex virus may result in an intense, painful vaginitis that is associated with a granular surface and vesicular eruptions. The diagnosis is made clinically and by serial serum antibody determinations. Fresh preparations of ulcerations, stained as for a Papanicolaou slide, may show classic inclusion bodies that are highly suggestive but not diagnostic of herpes. Therapy is supportive, but, fortunately, the episode usually terminates within 2 to 3 weeks. The antiviral agent acyclovir may reduce the severity of primary infections but is rarely indicated. More recent studies have suggested that chronic acyclovir therapy may reduce the frequency and severity of recurrent episodes after the primary infection.

Gonorrhea is an occasional cause of vaginitis in the child. The diagnosis is made by smear and culture, and therapy with penicillin is recommended. Children with vaginitis should be examined for intestinal parasites and intravaginal foreign bodies. Rarely do these three causes of childhood vaginitis produce similar problems in the adult.

Dysplasia and Intraepithelial Carcinoma of the Vagina

Dysplasia of the vaginal epithelium may be the source of abnormal genital smears even if the cervix is normal or absent. Treatment consists of excision or cryosurgery to remove abnormal epithelium. Intraepithelial carcinoma may also develop, most commonly in patients treated previously for other lower genital tract cancers. These lesions may occur at the apex of the vagina in patients after hysterectomy or may be multifocal in areas remote from the vagina apex. As in dysplasia, intraepithelial carcinoma of the vagina causes no specific symptoms. Diagnosis is suspected from genital cytology and colposcopy and confirmed by biopsy. Therapy can be by irradiation or surgical treatment, either excision or partial or total colpectomy. The frequency of these lesions justifies the close follow-up suggested for patients, even adequately treated, who have had other lower genital tract cancers. Results of therapy are excellent.

Carcinoma of the Vagina

Primary carcinoma of the vagina is a rare lesion, and most are epidermoid in variety. Postcontact bleeding is the usual presenting complaint. Many patients with invasive vaginal carcinoma have previously had other preinvasive or invasive epidermoid lesions of the lower genital system. Primary vaginal cancer may occur in any location, but the prognosis is considerably more grave if the lesion is situated anteriorly.

The current classification of primary vaginal cancer (International Federation of Gynecology and Obstetrics) includes Stage I, limited to the vaginal mucosa; Stage II, subvaginal tissue involved, but not to the pelvic wall; Stage III, tumor extending to the pelvic wall or to the symphysis, but not fixed to the symphysis; and Stage IV, tumor fixed to the symphysis, outside the pelvis, or proved by biopsy to involve the bladder or rectum. Treatment may be by irradiation or surgical therapy. Rutledge's review of radiation therapy of primary vaginal carcinoma describes the type of treatment, varied according to the location of the vaginal lesion. In general, it consists of 3000 to 5000 rads of external irradiation followed by 3000 to 5000 rads of intravaginal radium by sources specifically designed to deliver the radiation to the primary lesion. He reports survivors as follows: Stage I, 16 of 22 patients; Stage II, 19 of 25 patients; Stage III, 3 of 14 patients; Stage IV, 3 of 16 patients. Complications of therapy are relatively low but include radiation cystitis and proctitis. Individualization of therapy was recommended. Exenterative surgery may be used as primary therapy or therapy for recurrence. Results of primary surgical therapy are not as good as those achieved with irradiation, and the operative and postoperative morbidity and mortality are significant.

The vagina may also be the site of other histologic types of cancer, including melanocarcinoma, sarcoma, and mesonephric adenocarcinoma. Melanomas of this organ have an extremely poor prognosis, regardless of the therapy utilized. Only 3 of 30 patients reported in the literature have survived 5 years or longer. Surgical therapy should be radical and usually exenterative and should include removal of the regional lymph nodes. Sarcoma of the vagina, the so-called sarcoma botryoides, is most frequently seen in children, and the prognosis is grave. Irradiation is ineffective, and radical surgery is of only limited success. These tumors are thought to be of mixed mesodermal origin. Primary vaginal adenocarcinoma, while rarely seen in the past, is more common now in women who were exposed to diethylstilbestrol *in utero*. These tumors usually become symptomatic shortly after puberty. Older women may occasionally have similar lesions from mesonephric remnants or paraurethral glands. Treatment is usually exenteration or irradiation.

DEFECTS OF PELVIC SUPPORT

The major support of the uterus and vagina is provided by the cardinal ligaments, condensations of endopelvic fascia at the bases of the broad ligaments. The round, broad, and uterosacral ligaments are more important in maintaining uterine position than in providing support. Support from the vaginal side of the bladder and rectum is provided by the pubocervical fascia, which is not true fascia but condensed connective tissue in the vesicovaginal and rectovaginal septum. The distal vagina is also supported by the perineal body. Overdistention of these supporting structures, usually by childbirth, may give rise to a variety of defects in pelvic support. Frequently, these defects cause few symptoms until atrophy after menopause results in further weakness. Such defects include cystocele, urethrocele, rectocele, enterocele, and uterine descensus (Fig. 14).

Cystocele and Urethrocele; Stress Urinary Incontinence

A cystocele is a herniation of the anterior vaginal wall with secondary relaxation, descent, and protrusion of the bladder floor into the vaginal introitus. A cystocele is usually accompanied by some degree of uterine descensus or rectocele. The classic symptoms of cystocele are vaginal protrusion and recurrent cystitis, which occurs because of incomplete bladder emptying. A large cystocele may be relatively asymptomatic. Surgical repair is indicated not for the size of the cystocele but rather for its symptoms. A common problem associated with cystocele is urethrocele, and together they may produce flattening of the vesical neck, predisposing to stress urinary incontinence. Stress incontinence can be identified by observation of bladder support during the Valsalva maneuver. If pressure and elevation lateral to the urethrovesical junction inhibit the incontinence (Marshall test), good results can be expected from surgical repair. Such

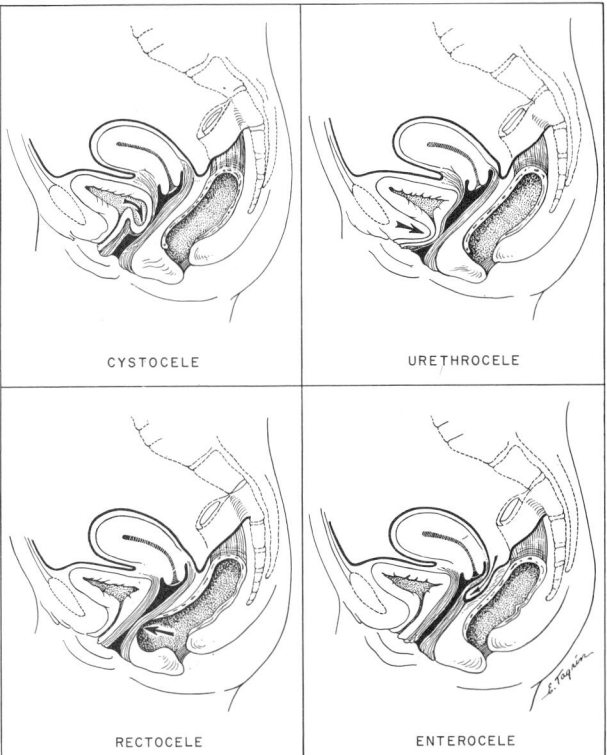

Figure 14. Diagrammatic representation of the four most common types of pelvic floor relaxation: cystocele, urethrocele, rectocele, and enterocele. Arrows depict sites of maximal protrusion. (From Kistner, R. W.: Gynecology: Principles and Practice. Chicago, Year Book Medical Publishers, 1964. Used by permission.)

supporting surgical therapy should be postponed until childbearing has been completed, since delivery after repair usually will be accompanied by return of the defect. The primary surgical repair is usually anterior colporrhaphy, frequently performed with vaginal hysterectomy.[3] This operation includes separation of the overlying vaginal mucosa from the bladder and urethra, followed by plication of the pubocervical fascia beneath these organs before reclosure of the vaginal mucosa. Elevation and narrowing of the urethrovesical neck denote success of the procedure. Anterior colporrhaphy provides successful repair in approximately 85 per cent of patients with stress urinary incontinence. Such procedures as the retropubic Marshall-Marchetti-Krantz cystourethropexy or the suburethral sling techniques may also offer good results for selected patients.

Rectocele

Rectocele is protrusion of the rectal wall toward the vaginal canal. In this condition, the paravaginal tissue which is normally interposed between the vagina and rectum becomes attenuated and lacerated, usually during delivery. Symptoms of rectocele are vaginal protrusion and sacculation of the rectal wall when fecal material is propelled into the anal canal. Defecation may require digital pressure to the posterior vaginal wall to force the feces from the sacculation back into the ampulla. Such problems may be reduced by posterior colpoperineorrhaphy, by which the rectovaginal fascia is rebuilt and the pubococcygeus and lower levator ani muscles are joined. Most patients with rectocele also have some associated cystocele or uterine descensus. Thus, vaginal hysterectomy and anterior colporrhaphy often should be combined with the posterior repair for best results. In addition, combined repairs may be mutually supporting, as the posterior repair may provide extra support for cystourethrocele. Nonoperative treatment is usually unsuccessful.

Enterocele

Pelvic enterocele is a herniation of the peritoneum of the cul-de-sac with invagination of the sac into the rectovaginal septum. A sliding hernia may develop in this space, usually created by labor, delivery, or vaginal hysterectomy. An enterocele of considerable size may exist without symptoms, but most provoke pelvic pressure, pain, and posterior vaginal protrusion. Enterocele may be difficult to separate from rectocele, but combined rectovaginal examination, or examination with the patient in the standing position, will usually clarify the problem. Enterocele may be surgically repaired by vaginal or abdominal approaches, but the gynecologist usually utilizes the former to allow repair of other associated defects.[10] From either approach, surgical repair of enterocele consists of plication of the uterosacral ligaments and obliteration of the cul-de-sac. If there is accompanying rectocele, it also should be repaired.

Prolapse of the Uterus

Uterine prolapse, or procidentia and uterine descensus, occurs when the uterus and its adjoining structures herniate through the vaginal canal. Prolapse is described as first, second, or third degree in severity, the last being protrusion of the entire uterus from the vagina, with the entire vagina everted as a consequence. Although congenital weakness of the supporting tissues may occasionally cause uterine prolapse, the most frequent cause is childbirth. The signs of uterine prolapse are protrusion of the cervix or uterus through the introitus. Prolapse frequently is associated with cystocele or rectocele, and these defects may cause presenting symptoms. Symptoms include backache, significant pelvic pressure, and ulceration or bleeding of the prolapsed structures. Uterine prolapse cannot be cured by nonoperative means but some patients can be supported by a pessary if surgical therapy is not feasible. Uterine prolapse is best approached vaginally for surgical repair, since abdominal procedures are usually inadequate. Successful procedures include vaginal hysterectomy and repair of the pelvic diaphragm, procedures that preserve the uterus while resupporting these structures, and rarely total colpocleisis if coital function is never again anticipated.

BENIGN DISEASES OF THE CERVIX

The portio vaginalis of the normal cervix is covered with squamous epithelium that is similar to that of the vagina. In the nulliparous woman, the external cervical os is a centrally located, small, round opening connecting with the endocervical canal. After childbearing, the external os is longitudinally flattened. Mucus-secreting columnar epithelium lines the endocervical canal, and its junction with the squamous epithelium of the portio cervicis is the squamocolumnar zone.

Cervicitis

Cervical infection, in one form or another, is one of the most frequently encountered gynecologic lesions. Acute cervicitis is rarely seen except in gonorrhea, in patients with acute vaginitis from *Trichomonas vaginalis* or *Candida albicans*, in patients with puerperal endometritis, or in patients with retained vaginal foreign bodies. The cervix is erythematous and edematous, and leukocytic infiltration is prominent. Pain and tenderness are rarely prominent symptoms, but a purulent discharge is frequently seen. Diagnosis is made by appropriate smears and cultures (see Laboratory Tests), and therapy with topical or systemic antibiotics usually is curative.

In chronic cervicitis, the cervical mucus is mucopurulent and profuse. The histologic changes seen in chronic cervicitis are variable and are present to some extent in nearly all women. Cellular changes, such as metaplasia, epidermization, and hyperplasia of the basal cells, are frequently seen. Often seen are erosions or eversions of the cervix. An erosion is a true ulcer of the cervix, whereas the eversion is formed by columnar epithelium of the endocervical canal proliferating downward, forming a lowered squamocolumnar line. Orifices of the cervical mucus-secreting glands may become obstructed to form nabothian cysts. A mucopurulent discharge may be the only symptom of chronic cervicitis, although postcontact bleeding, infertility, and, rarely, pain may occur. Diagnosis is based on cytology and biopsy, but one must remember that while cervical cytologic studies are very effective in the discovery of early cervical cancer with an intact surface epithelium, they are much less reliable when an erosion is present. Colposcopy, colpomicroscopy, and iodine staining may be of aid in localizing areas for biopsy. Any suspicious or eroded area should be biopsied before treatment. Therapy of chronic cervicitis is usually by electrodesiccation, ultrarefrigeration (cryosurgery), laser, or silver nitrate. Cautery should include the involved exocervix and endocervical canal and rarely requires an anesthetic. These methods destroy the infection of the columnar area and allow the squamous epithelium to grow over the area. Repeated cautery, surgical conization, and, on occasion, even hysterectomy (if childbearing is ended) may be necessary for severe chronic cervicitis.

Cervical Polyps

Polyps may arise from the endocervix and are rarely malignant. The usual symptom is postcontact bleeding. They appear as single or multiple cherry-red growths protruding from the external cervical os. Such polyps may be removed by biopsy or dilatation and curettage, with cauterization of the pedicle. One must not overlook uterine or other cervical causes of the abnormal bleeding, which may be the symptom of other, more severe, pelvic disease.

CANCER OF THE CERVIX

Invasive carcinoma of the cervix is now the second most common pelvic malignancy and comprises 15 per cent of cancers of women. It is estimated that 10,000 women die in the United States each year from these neoplasms. It is encouraging that during the past 20 years, primarily through early detection, the death rate from cervical cancer has declined from 21.8 to 11.5 per 100,000 population. Invasive carcinoma of the cervix should be a preventable disease, as regular examinations and frequent use of today's diagnostic techniques should enable detection of nearly all patients with preinvasive cervical carcinoma, a totally curable disease.

The average age of occurrence of carcinoma of the cervix is 49 years, with the majority of patients between 35 and 55 years of age. However, many workers have reported cervical cancer in women as young as the teens and as old as the eighth decade. Much has been written about the etiology of cervical carcinoma. Epidemiologic studies show peak occurrences among women of low socioeconomic status, those who begin coitus and childbearing at an early age, and those with multiple sexual partners. Heredity appears to have a small role. The theory of a viral relationship has been advanced, suggesting that a virus transmitted though intercourse may be at least partially responsible for cervical cancer.

Preinvasive Carcinoma or Carcinoma in Situ of the Cervix

Bowen in 1912 described a preinvasive malignant lesion of the skin, and in the same year others described preinvasive carcinoma of the cervix. Thirty years later it was described as a precursor to invasive carcinoma. It remained for Papanicolaou and Traut, in 1941, to develop the cytologic evaluation of exfoliated cells that suggests the need for biopsy and adequate tissue study. Histopathologically, carcinoma *in situ* consists of cellular

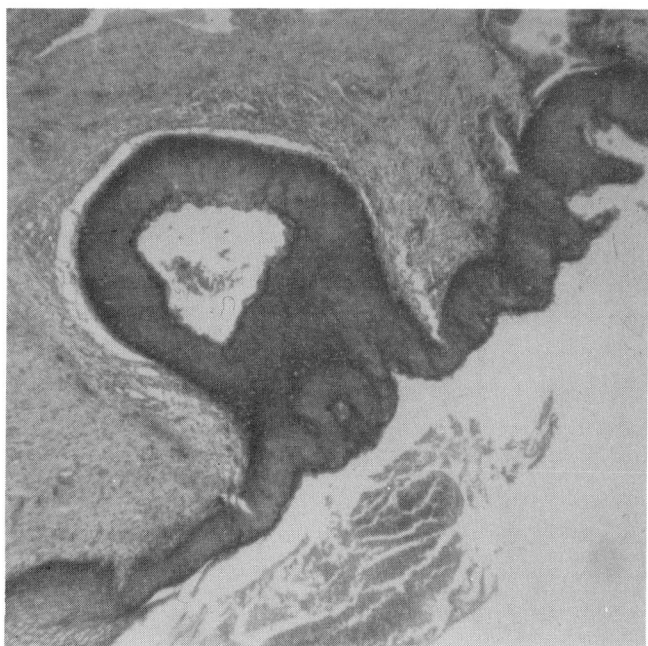

Figure 15. Carcinoma *in situ* of the cervix. Note sharp demarcation between normal and malignant epithelium (lower border) and the glandular epithelial involvement. (Courtesy of Dr. D. E. D. Jones.)

changes in the squamous epithelium of the cervix that are compatible with cancer, but evidence of invasion in the underlying stroma is absent. Glandular epithelial replacement by neoplastic cells may be mistaken for invasion, and it is important that this differentiation be made. Other benign conditions that may confuse diagnosis are atypical basilar hyperplasia or the metaplasia and hyperplasia of glandular elements frequently seen in pregnancy. The peak incidence of carcinoma *in situ* is at approximately 35 to 40 years of age. *There are no gross lesions or symptoms of carcinoma* in situ *of the cervix.* The use of Papanicolaou cytology screening and adequate biopsy techniques is discussed in the Laboratory Tests section of this chapter. The diagnosis of carcinoma *in situ* is made by histologic review of biopsy specimens (Fig. 15).

Many patients with dysplasia or carcinoma *in situ* of the cervix are now being treated with electrocautery, cryosurgery, or cone biopsy. Close follow-up after therapy is warranted, with repeat cytologic studies used frequently. If the lesion has been eradicated, as demonstrated on Papanicolaou stain smears and colposcopy, follow-up alone is indicated.

Treatment for extensive or recurrent carcinoma *in situ* of the cervix may be abdominal or vaginal hysterectomy, with excision of 2 to 3 cm. of upper vagina. The tubes and ovaries are usually left in place in younger women. Radical hysterectomy and pelvic lymph node dissection are not indicated. Results of therapy are uniformly good, and 5-year survival approaches 100 per cent. Radiation therapy is rarely indicated for carcinoma *in situ*. Since carcinoma *in situ* is a disease of younger women, the question of allowing continued reproduction prior to hysterectomy has been raised. If the patient has normal smears after conization and desires to have more children, she is allowed to do so and deliver vaginally. If the smears remain positive after conization, hysterectomy is usually suggested at that time. If abnormal smears are detected during pregnancy, cervical conization is used for diagnosis, or quadrant biopsy is used later in pregnancy and when no obvious lesion is present. If carcinoma *in situ* only is detected, the pregnancy is allowed to continue with vaginal delivery. If invasive carcinoma is present, appropriate therapy is begun immediately.

Microinvasive Cancer of the Cervix (Stage IA1)

There has been considerable debate as to both the diagnosis and the treatment of microinvasive carcinoma of the cervix, a condition in which carcinoma *in situ* exists and less than 3 mm. of invasion is present. Data showing lack of nodal metastasis have led to treatment of patients as if the lesions were only carcinoma *in situ*. Results of this treatment in microinvasive cancer of the cervix are equally as good as those of full radical surgery or irradiation, and morbidity has been much less.

Carcinoma of the Cervix

Approximately 95 per cent of cervical cancers are squamous, the remaining 5 per cent usually being adenocarcinoma. Most often the adenocarcinoma arises from the mucus-secreting epithelium of the cervix, but, rarely, adenocarcinoma may arise in mesonephric duct remants. Squamous cell, or epidermoid, carcinoma of the cervix usually arises at the squamocolumnar junction. Varying degrees of microscopic differentiation are found. A halo of carcinoma *in situ* is frequently found around the invasive cancer or on the vagina.

There are no symptoms of early carcinoma of the cervix; the first symptoms of bleeding, usually postcontact, or a bloody discharge do not begin until ulceration is present. More advanced cervical cancers cause symptoms referable to invasion of adjacent organs (bladder, rectum, ureter) or to distant metastasis. Pain is usually a sign of advanced cervical cancer.

Although cytologic findings and clinical appearance may strongly suggest carcinoma of the cervix, the diagnosis can be made only by histopathologic study. In the presence of an obvious exophytic lesion, as is found in more than 80 per cent of patients with even early cervical cancer, tissue may be easily obtained by punch biopsy. If the lesion is endophytic, or if the punch biopsy shows carcinoma *in situ* (or less), conization may be mandatory to fully evaluate abnormal cytologic studies. Broken and ulcerated epithelium and proliferating tissue that bleeds easily upon touch are most valuable clinical signs, particularly when such lesions involve the squamocolumnar junction. Colposcopy and staining techniques may aid direction of biopsies. Even if Papanicolaou smears are benign, the presence of an ulcerated lesion or exophytic cervical growth warrants biopsy.

If treatment of cervical cancer is adequate, the single most important factor in prognosis is the extent of disease when therapy is begun. For this reason, each patient should have a careful pelvic examination, cystoscopy, proctoscopy, intravenous pyelography, roentgenograms of the chest and possibly a pelvic CT or MRI scan so that the extent of the disease may be established. Staging of cervical cancer is arrived at entirely by clinical evaluation and is made before treatment is initiated (Fig. 16). Such staging should not be changed at a later time. The author currently utilizes the classification for clinical staging of cervical carcinoma provided in 1985 by the Cancer Committee of the International Federation of Gynecology and Obstetrics:

Stage I
  Carcinoma is strictly confined to cervix (extension to corpus should be disregarded)
  IA   Preclinical carcinoma
  IA1 Minimal microscopically evident stromal invasion
  IA2 Microscopic lesions no more than 5 mm. in depth measured from base of epithelium, either surface or glandular, from which it originates, and horizontal spread not to exceed 7 mm.
  IB   All other cases of Stage I; occult cancer should be marked "occ"
Stage II
  Carcinoma extends beyond cervix but has not extended to pelvic wall; it involves vagina, but not as far as lower third
  IIA No obvious parametrial involvement
  IIB Obvious parametrial involvement

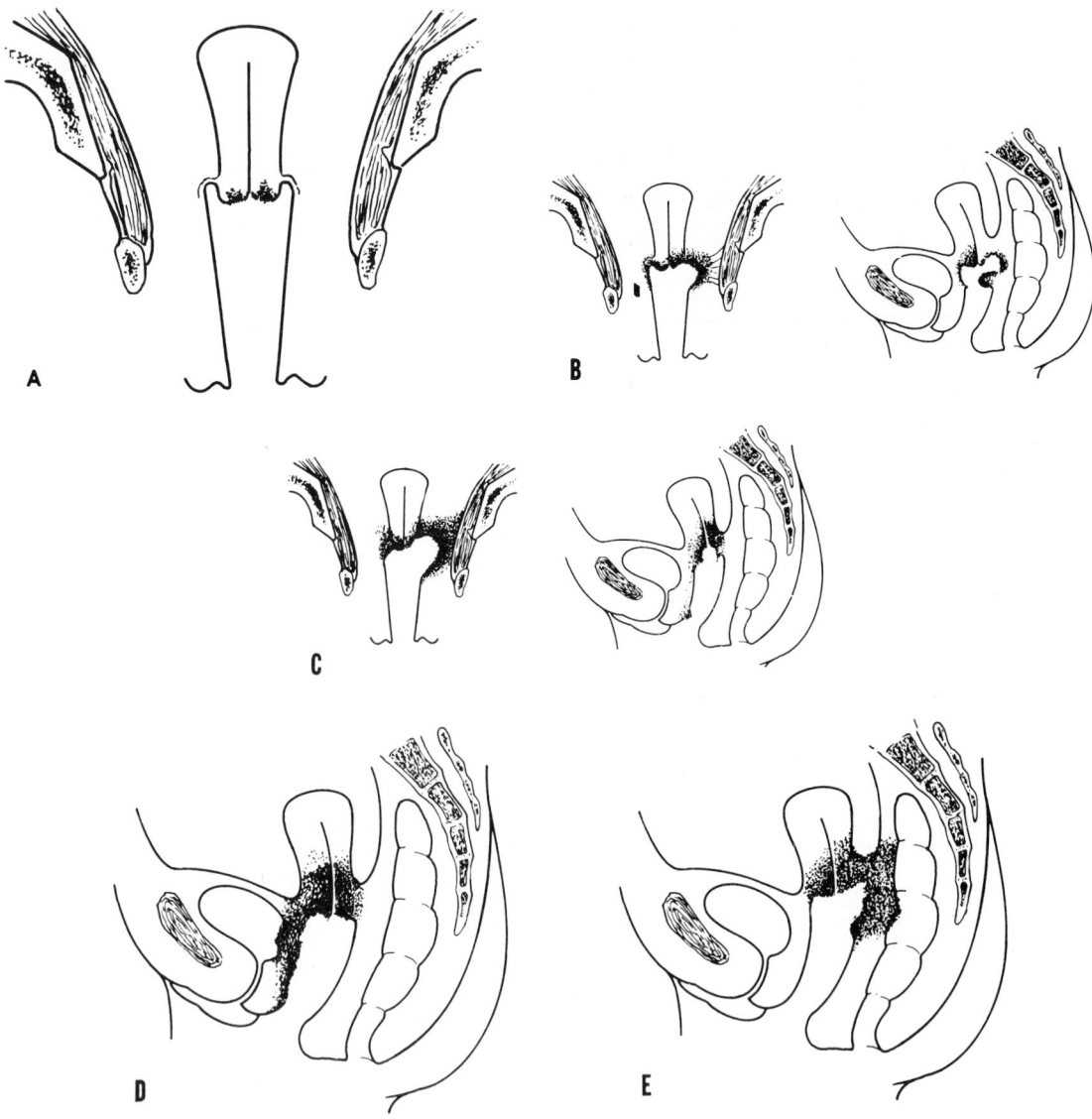

Figure 16. Stages of carcinoma of the cervix. *A*, Stage I: the cancer is confined to the cervix. *B*, Stage II: the cancer is confined to the parametrium on one or both sides and is not fixed to either pelvic wall, or the cancer involves the upper one third of the vagina. *C*, Stage III: the cancer has spread to one or both pelvic walls or has invaded the lower third of the vagina. *D* and *E*, Stage IV: the cancer involves the bladder or the rectum, or it has spread beyond the pelvis. (From Taylor, E. S.: Essentials of Gynecology, 4th ed. Philadelphia, Lea and Febiger, 1969.)

Stage III

    Carcinoma has extended to pelvic wall; on rectal examination there is no cancer-free space between tumor and pelvic wall; tumor involves lower third of vagina; all cases with hydronephrosis or nonfunctioning kidney should be included, unless they are known to be due to another cause

    IIIA   No extension to pelvic wall, but involvement of lower third of vagina

    IIIB   Extension to pelvic wall, or hydronephrosis or nonfunctioning kidney due to tumor

Stage IV

    Carcinoma has extended beyond true pelvis or has clinically involved mucosa of bladder or rectum

    IVA   Spread of growth to adjacent pelvic organs

    IVB   Spread to distant organs

Although clinical staging is done before therapy, it is useful to understand the significance of such staging on disease spread. The most common method of tumor spread, and the most frequent cause of patient death, is direct extension of cervical cancer to involve the vagina, uterus, parametrium, pelvic side wall, ureter, bladder, and rectum. More than 50 per cent of patients who die with cervical cancer die of ureteral obstruction and uremia. Fistula formation from the ureter, bladder, and rectum is rather frequent, and bleeding may be a serious complication. Carcinoma of the cervix also has a propensity for lymphatic metastasis. Lymphatic drainage of the cervix is via the hypogastric and obturator lymph chains to the iliac and then the aortic nodal systems. Vertebral lymphatic metastases may also occur. Morton and others have shown lymph node metastases in the following percentages of clinically staged cases of cervical carcinoma: Stage I, 15.5; Stage II, 31.9: Stage III, 46.7; and Stage IV, 80.8. In addition to the clinical staging, the size of the primary cervical lesion has also been shown to influence the frequency with which lymph node metastases are found: less than 1 cm., rare metastases; 1 to 3 cm., 17 per cent with metastases; greater than 3 cm., 52 per cent with lymph node metastases. These latter two factors of lymphatic node metastasis are variable and of little predictive value in the therapy of a given patient.

Other studies have shown that lymphatic spread beyond the pelvic nodal chains is present in more than 40 per cent of patients who die of cervical cancer. Autopsy data demonstrate distant metastases in many patients dying of carcinoma of the cervix, and nearly every organ may be involved. The most common sites of distant metastases include liver, 16 per cent; lung, 14 per cent; vertebrae, 9 per cent; and other bony metastases, 9 per cent.

TREATMENT OF CERVICAL CANCER. Carcinoma of the cervix can be effectively treated by surgical therapy or irradiation, *but treatment does not include simple hysterectomy or nonindividualized radiotherapy*. No other major lesion requires more critical selection of techniques and methods of therapy. The present operation for cancer of the cervix (Stages I and IIA) is an extended or radical hysterectomy (Wertheim) that removes the parametrial tissues, the upper third of the vagina, and perhaps the adnexa, and a pelvic node dissection that removes the iliac, hypogastric, ureteral, obturator, and lower aortic lymph nodes. The radical operation for cancer of the cervix has two primary disadvantages. First, there is a 7 to 8 per cent incidence of ureteral or bladder fistula; and second, few surgeons are qualified to undertake the operation and perform it satisfactorily. Certain patients with Stage IV carcinoma, those with only rectal or bladder involvement, may be candidates for primary surgical therapy by pelvic exenteration. The results of primary surgical treatment for cervical cancer show 5-year survivals of Stage I, 78 per cent; Stage II, 53 per cent; Stage III, 31 per cent; and Stage IV, 19 per cent. The operative mortality should be under 1.0 per cent, and a significant rate of postoperative urinary fistulas occur. Most gynecologists now reserve the primary surgical treatment of carcinoma of the cervix for those operable patients with smaller Stage I or early Stage II lesions.

Many clinics favor primary radiation treatment of cancer of the cervix, especially those staged beyond IIA. The purpose of therapy is to deliver to the lesion and to areas of possible pelvic spread sufficient radiation to destroy the cancer and still not cause irreparable damage to surrounding tissues. Most therapists employ a combination of external supervoltage therapy, such as from cobalt-60, linear accelerators, and the betatron megavoltage units, as well as brachytherapy and intravaginal, contracervical, and intracervical irradiation with radium or cesium. Usually external radiotherapy is initially delivered in a dosage of 4000 to 6000 rads to the entire pelvis over a 4- to 6-week course. This is followed by one or two interval applications to deliver 4000 to 6000 rads to the primary cervical lesion. Stage I and II disease tend to receive the higher dose by radium; in Stage III and IV disease, the higher dose is usually administered by external cobalt-60. Total dosage administered by the two routes approximates 10,000 rads. As in surgical therapy, the prognosis with primary radiation therapy for carcinoma of the cervix varies with the clinical stage present at the time therapy is begun. The usually accepted figures for 5-year survival with this type of treatment are for Stage I, 86.4 per cent; Stage II, 60.0 per cent; Stage III, 26.3 per cent; and Stage IV, 8.8 per cent.

Regardless of the type of therapy utilized, patients with carcinoma of the cervix must be followed frequently and regularly. One speaks optimistically of 5-year "cures," but in significant numbers of patients, recurrent disease develops 10 to 20 years later, or they later have other malignant lesions of the genital tract. Follow-up should include frequent cytologic study and appropriate biopsy. Secondary treatment for therapeutic failures, with surgical therapy or additional irradiation, has provided limited success. Chemotherapy has been of palliative aid only.

BENIGN UTERINE DISEASE

Various benign uterine diseases occur, including leiomyoma uteri, adenomyosis, endometrial hyperplasia, and polyps. Abnormal bleeding, uterine enlargement, and pain are the usual symptoms associated with these diseases, but the primary difficulty is to achieve an accurate diagnosis.

Leiomyoma Uteri

Uterine leiomyomas, also called myomas, fibromyomas, or fibroids, are the most common cause of benign uterine enlargement and are seen in 20 per cent of women, with a higher incidence in blacks. Leiomyomas originate from the smooth muscle cells of the myometrium and vary in size from microscopic to large enough to fill the entire abdomen. Such tumors may be single but are more often multiple. On cut section these solid tumors have a white, glistening appearance with a characteristic whorl pattern. There is no true capsule; compressed peripheral fibers from a pseudocapsule are seen. Microscopically, smooth muscle cells are arranged in interlacing muscle bundles, interspaced with varying amounts of connective tissue and hyaline material. Such tumors may be submucous, intramural, subserous, pedunculated, parasitic, cervical, or interligamentous (Fig. 17).

The symptoms of leiomyoma vary according to location. Some may produce severe complaints; others, none at all. The three most common symptoms are abnormal bleeding, pain, and uterine enlargement. Abnormal bleeding, usually cyclic but profuse and prolonged, is most frequently due to submucous

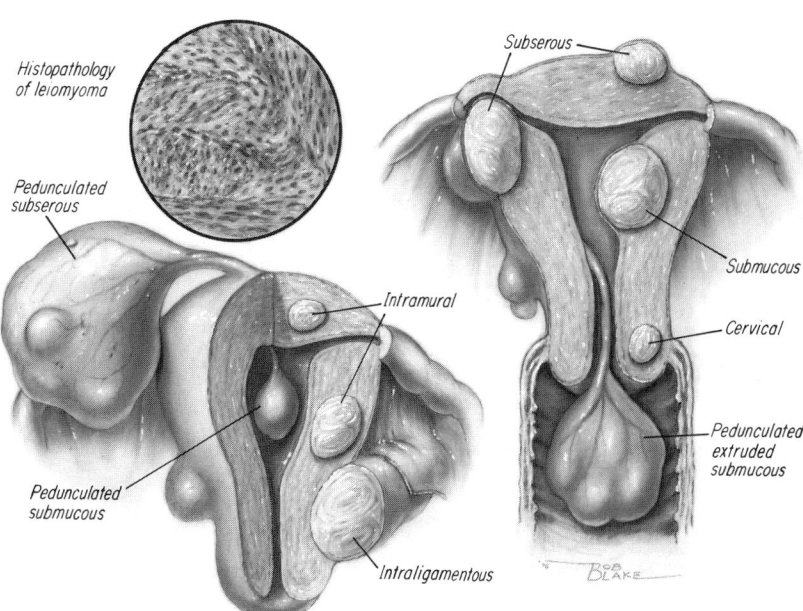

Figure 17. Leiomyomata uteri.

Histopathology of leiomyoma

Pedunculated subserous

Pedunculated submucous

Intraligamentous

Intramural

Subserous

Submucous

Cervical

Pedunculated extruded submucous

tumors that distort the overlying endometrium and interfere with normal hemostatic mechanisms. Occasionally a submucuous or cervical myoma may be extruded and also cause abnormal bleeding. Abnormal bleeding is the most common indication for hysterectomy for leiomyoma, but caution must be taken to exclude other causes, as a malignant lesion may coexist with myoma. Often a curettage may be mandatory to make this differentiation. Rapid enlargement is another symptom of concern in patients with leiomyoma; 1 to 2 per cent of such tumors may undergo sarcomatous change or degeneration of other nonmalignant varieties. Estrogen, including the synthetic estrogens of oral contraceptives, may cause enlargement of myomas. Myomas tend to regress after menopause, and any enlargement of these tumors demands prompt removal of the uterus. Slow enlargement of leiomyomas during the menstrual years frequently occurs with a minimum of symptoms. Surgical removal is not mandatory for slow growth or moderate size unless other symptoms occur. Pelvic pressure, frequency of urination, and sciatic or hip pain from pressure on pelvic nerves can be symptoms of uterine leiomyoma. Tenderness in a myoma is usually caused by degeneration or by impairment of the blood supply. Cystic changes and calcification can follow degeneration. Significant pain or tenderness usually warrants hysterectomy. Infertility is not infrequently seen in patients with myomas, nor is abortion, but in the former it is not known whether the infertility or the myoma is primary. The increased rate of abortion is attributed to poor uterine distensibility and compression. While uterine myomas are usually recognized without difficulty in the operating room, their preoperative diagnosis may be quite difficult, especially if the myoma primarily involves one of the adnexa.

The treatment of leiomyoma demands individualization for each patient. Some tumors require no treatment if small and asymptomatic, and only semiannual examination is warranted. If a young patient who desires further childbearing has symptomatic leiomyomas, then myomectomy may be a useful surgical procedure. For larger or more symptomatic myomas in a woman who has completed her reproduction, hysterectomy is the treatment of choice.

Recent work has focused upon medical treatment of leiomyoma with gonadotropin-releasing hormone analogue (Gn-RH-A). Significant size reduction has been made, presumably due to the acute hypoestrogenism that occurs with such therapy. However, regrowth rapidly occurs after treatment ceases, and this has not become a significant management method for long-term use. The attendant amenorrhea with Gn-RH-A treatment may allow rebuilding of hemoglobin prior to anticipated conservative surgical therapy or hysterectomy.

Adenomyosis

Invasion of the myometrium by endometrium, adenomyosis, is a frequent cause of uterine enlargement and pain. Grossly, the uterus is enlarged, fibrotic, and thickened, and on cut section the areas of endometrial growth and loculated menstruation may be quite apparent.

The classic symptoms and signs of adenomyosis are acquired dysmenorrhea occurring in the 35- to 40-year age group, menstrual irregularities with cyclic, prolonged, and profuse flow, and an enlarged, tender uterus. Treatment is hysterectomy, although hormonal suppression (pseudopregnancy regimen with estrogen and progesterone) may provide relief without removal of the uterus.

Endometrial Hyperplasia and Polyps

Hyperplasia of the endometrium, causing abnormal uterine bleeding, is a common problem of women. Women near menopause or, less frequently, in early adolescence are most frequently affected. The basic problem is anovulation and failure of corpus luteum formation without production of progester-

one. Continued stimulation of the endometrium by estrogen brings about proliferation, overgrowth, and hyperplasia of the endometrium. Areas of thickened endometrium may form polyps. Cycles become irregular, with intervals of amenorrhea associated with other intervals of intermenstrual spotting or bleeding. Pelvic examination is usually nonrevealing, and curettage produces copious amounts of endometrial scrapings. Microscopic examination shows hyperplasia of the epithelium and stroma. The cells lining the glands are nonsecretory, and the stroma often contains cells with frequent mitotic figures. Cystic changes of the glands may be present.

Curettage is useful in diagnosis and for treatment, as it removes the hypertrophied endometrium and leaves a fresh surface for endometrial regeneration. Because of the frequency of recurrence of hyperplasia, the administration of cyclic progesterone often aids in prevention of recurrence and promotes cyclic menses. If endometrial hyperplasia recurs, it may proceed to atypical or adenomatous hyperplasia and then to carcinoma *in situ*, which may lead to endometrial cancer. Recurrent abnormal bleeding requires repeated curettage for diagnosis and proper therapy.

Adenomatous hyperplasia is diagnosed when there is marked proliferation, with the glands being closely packed and the stroma quite dense and hyperplastic. This adenomatous pattern closely resembles adenocarcinoma and is thought to be a precancerous lesion. Diagnosis of this lesion is by curettage. While cyclic progesterone is of aid for most patients, hysterectomy is probably the treatment of choice for the older patient who has completed her reproduction.

MALIGNANT DISEASES OF THE UTERUS

Adenocarcinoma of the Endometrium

Adenocarcinoma of the endometrium, now the most prevalent gynecologic cancer, is seen most commonly among postmenopausal women. The peak incidence occurs in the 50- to 70-year age group, but one must suspect the condition as early as the third decade if there is menstrual irregularity. Postmenopausal bleeding is the cardinal symptom of endometrial cancer and must be considered as due to malignancy until proved otherwise. Prolonged, profuse, or irregular bleeding may occur in the premenopausal woman. Papanicolaou cytologic study may yield negative results, as the exfoliated cells may not reach the vaginal pool. Cervical stenosis with secondary hematometrium or pyometrium is frequently present and can be identified by passage of an endocervical probe. Fractional curettage is the diagnostic method of choice, and only in this manner can the diagnosis be established as well as the degree of cervical involvement, an important factor influencing therapy. Histologically, adenocarcinoma of the endometrium has wide variations in differentiation and in stromal invasion by the glandular epithelial cells, and, finally, there is a highly undifferentiated type in which neither glandular nor stromal elements can be identified.

The etiology of endometrial cancer is unknown. There does appear to be a relationship to prolonged estrogenic stimulation, as in patients with estrogen-producing ovarian tumors. Newer studies also suggest a higher incidence of endometrial adenocarcinoma in women given high-dose estrogen replacement therapy for menopausal symptoms. Still other studies suggest that the sequential addition of progesterone to estrogen therapy significantly reduces the increased risk seen in patients who receive estrogen alone. Other frequently associated findings in patients with endometrial adenocarcinoma are obesity, diabetes, hypertension, and low parity.

Endometrial cancer is usually a polypoid lesion growing into the endometrial cavity, and only late in the disease does myometrial or cervical involvement occur (Fig. 18). Uterine size is

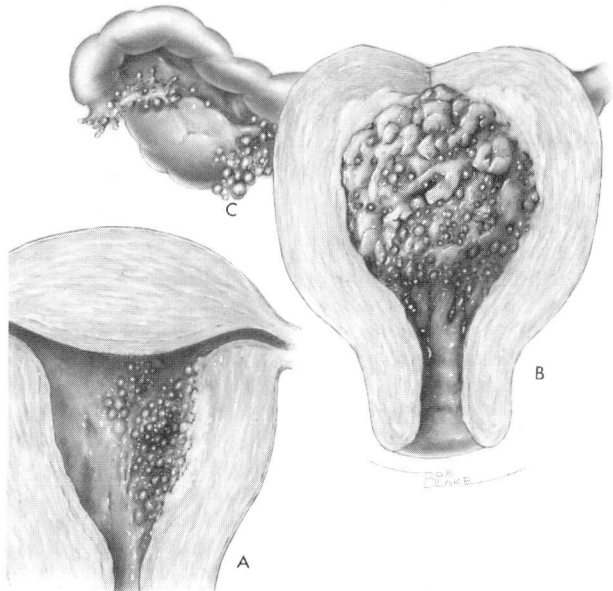

Figure 18. Carcinoma of the endometrium. *A*, Stage I. *B*, Stage III, myometrial invasion plus. *C*, Ovarian extension of metastases.

usually normal to slightly increased in women with early cancer of the endometrium. Uterine enlargement and menstrual irregularity occur in advanced disease or disease associated with hematometrium or leiomyoma. In addition to direct extension to adjacent structures, adenocarcinoma of the endometrium may spread through the extensive lymphatic anastomosis at the upper uterus between the tube and ovary. Thus, the tubes and ovaries are frequent sites of early metastases. In addition to this direct lymphatic extension of endometrial cancer, these tumors may spread by regional and distant lymph node metastasis to the pelvic and aortic nodal chains. The incidence of such lymph node metastasis is rare when only the uterine fundus is involved (2 per cent) but is frequent if the primary lesion is near the cervical junction (50 per cent). Hematogenous dissemination may also occur; the most frequent sites are the peritoneal surfaces, lungs, liver, and skin. Local recurrence in the apex of the vagina, vaginal walls, and perineum occurs in 10 per cent of patients who have been treated for endometrial cancer.

The usual clinical staging of endometrial cancer includes Stage 0, preinvasive carcinoma or carcinoma *in situ* of the endometrium; Stage I, in which the growth is confined to the uterine body; Stage II, in which the carcinoma involves the corpus and the cervix; Stage III, in which the tumor extends outside the uterus but not outside the true pelvis; and Stage IV, in which the carcinoma has extended outside the true pelvis or has involved the mucosa of the rectum or bladder. The location of the primary neoplasm in the uterus, the degree of anaplasia of the cells, and the gross size of the uterus influence the prognosis and the effectiveness of treatment.

The treatment of adenocarcinoma of the endometrium is primarily surgical. Survival for patients with cancer spread beyond the uterus is poor, regardless of whether surgical therapy, irradiation, or a combination of the two methods is used. Approximately 30 per cent of patients with recurrent or metastatic adenocarcinoma of the endometrium benefit from large doses of parenteral progesterone (Megace or Depo-Provera)—usually those with tumors that are well differentiated histologically. Other forms of chemotherapy have been of little aid. External pelvic radiotherapy or transvaginal irradiation and intravaginal radium may provide palliation for locally recurrent adenocarcinoma of the endometrium.

The prognosis for adenocarcinoma of the endometrium is generally good, but results of larger series are frequently diffi-

cult to compare owing to differences in tumor size, differentiation, stage, and type of treatment. Of those patients selected for surgical therapy because of an operable lesion, with or without preoperative irradiation, approximately 60 per cent survive 5 years.

Sarcoma of the Uterus

Sarcomas may arise from the endometrium, myometrium, cervix, uterine blood vessels, or a leiomyoma. These diseases are most frequently seen in the fifth decade; a rare sarcoma of the cervix, sarcoma botryoides, is seen in infants. The incidence of corpus sarcoma is much higher than that of sarcoma of the cervix. As all elements of the uterus are mesodermal in origin and ectodermal rests may be present, mixed tumors may occur. A wide spectrum of histopathologic types can be found. Rapid uterine enlargement is a prominent sign of uterine sarcoma, and abnormal bleeding may or may not be present. Pain, anemia, and weight loss are late symptoms. Pulmonary metastases frequently occur early. Surgical excision of the uterus, tubes, and ovaries is the recommended treatment for sarcoma of the uterus. The prognosis after treatment varies with the type and extent of the original tumor. The sarcomas arising in myomas generally appear to be of low grade and thus have a relatively good prognosis, with 45 to 50 per cent of patients with operable lesions surviving. There are very few survivors among patients with the other types of uterine sarcoma despite appropriate surgical therapy for patients with operable lesions. Radiotherapy may offer benefit. The author is currently exploring a combination approach, with extirpative surgical therapy and combination chemotherapy, followed by external pelvic irradiation. The initial results are encouraging but warrant further investigation.

PELVIC INFECTION

Acute Pelvic Infection

Acute pelvic infection (pelvic inflammatory disease [PID]) may occur after pelvic surgery or result from other causes, but by far the most frequent causes are gonorrhea and chlamydial infection. The initial symptoms of acute PID usually occur within 3 to 6 days after inoculation and consist of urethritis, skenitis, bartholinitis, cervicitis, and vaginal discharge. Tubal involvement is often a later symptom and usually does not occur until after a menstrual period. At this time, the organisms spread rapidly from the endocervix and across the endometrium, and involve the endosalpinx. The major infection and damage occur in the fallopian tube. The tube becomes acutely inflamed and edematous, and its lumen fills with a purulent exudate. The tubular, peritubular, ovarian, and pelvic peritoneal surfaces are rapidly involved. Secondary infection with anaerobic bacteria is common. Pelvic abscess may develop.

The signs and symptoms of acute pelvic infection are those of pelvic peritonitis with bilateral lower abdominal pain and tenderness, temperature of 38 to 39° C., and signs of peritoneal irritation with direct and rebound tenderness and muscle spasm. On pelvic examination, one may be able to express pus from the paraurethral glands or cervix. Exquisite tenderness is present with cervical manipulation and in the adnexal areas, and there is a thickened, doughy feeling in the tubular areas. Bilaterality of pain is an important point in differentiating acute pelvic infection from appendicitis, and the fever associated with PID is usually higher. The diagnosis of acute pelvic infection is made by cervical smear and culture (see Laboratory Tests).

Therapy is based on the degree of peritonitis and fever. If significant peritonitis is present or the temperature is greater than 38.5° C., hospitalization is indicated and intravenous antibiotic therapy recommended. For women with more serious episodes of pelvic infection, several therapeutic regimens are presently recommended. Included are doxycycline, 100 mg. intravenously every 12 hours plus cefoxitan, 2.0 gm. intravenously every 6 hours. An alternative therapy includes clindamycin, 600 mg. intravenously every 6 hours, plus gentamicin or tobramycin, 2.0 mg. per kg. intravenously, then 1.5 mg. per kg. intravenously every 8 hours for patients with normal renal function. Finally, the regimen of doxycycline, 100 mg. intravenously every 12 hours, plus metronizadole, 1 gm. intravenously every 12 hours, can be used. This intensive treatment, plus analgesia, elevation of the head to encourage pelvic localization of pus, and parenteral fluid replacement, is continued until the acute symptoms have subsided; then oral therapy is begun and continued for at least a week. If the presenting symptoms are not severe, one can treat the patient entirely as an outpatient.

The patient with relatively asymptomatic gonorrhea can be treated with aqueous procaine penicillin G, 4.8 million units intramuscularly in divided doses at two sites, preceded by probenecid, 1 gm. by mouth. Alternatives to this therapy include oral ampicillin or amoxicillin, 3.5 gm., and probenecid, 1.0 gm., or tetracycline hydrochloride, 500 mg. four times a day for 5 days. An alternative regimen is a single intramuscular dose of spectinomycin, 2.0 gm., preceded by probenecid, 1.0 gm. by mouth. Approximately a week after the therapy is completed, a follow-up culture for "test of cure" should be done. The patient should be examined twice weekly to follow her progress and exclude pelvic abscess. Surgical therapy is not indicated for acute pelvic infection unless pelvic abscess drainage is required. If the abdomen is opened for other preoperative diagnoses but acute pelvic infection is found, no further operative procedure is indicated and the abdomen is closed and antibiotics are initiated. If significant pelvic contamination with pus is present, cul-de-sac drains are inserted.

Pelvic Abscess

This condition may follow acute pelvic infection, pelvic surgery, septicemia, puerperal endometritis, appendicitis, or peritonitis of any cause. The abscess may be localized in the cul-de-sac or between the leaves of the broad ligament, or it may be tubo-ovarian in location. If gonorrhea is the primary etiology, the purulent exudate usually does not contain the organism, since it is short-lived in such conditions. Secondary organisms such as colon bacilli and anaerobic organisms such as *Bacteroides*, streptococci, and staphylococci may be present in large quantities. The signs and symptoms of pelvic abscess are elevation of temperature and pulse, pelvic or lower abdominal pain, and leukocytosis. If the abscess is anteriorly placed, as in an interligamentous pelvic abscess, one may discover a tender, fluctuant mass on abdominal examination. Pelvic examination is usually quite helpful. A cul-de-sac abscess bulges into the posterior vaginal fornix and displaces the cervix anteriorly. Interligamentous abscesses may bulge into the lateral fornix and displace the cervix to one side.

Treatment of pelvic abscess consists of surgical drainage. Posterior colpotomy is performed to drain a pelvic abscess localized in the cul-de-sac; loculations are digitally opened, and large drains are left indwelling. Antibiotics should be used after surgical drainage. Other pelvic abscesses may be drained vaginally but may require anterior extraperitoneal drainage or abdominal exploration for removal of involved structures and drainage. If a pelvic abscess ruptures intra-abdominally, there is significant morbidity and mortality from disseminated infection. In that event, the uterus, tubes, and ovaries should be removed and adequate drainage and antibiotic coverage instituted.

Chronic Pelvic Infection

Included among chronic pelvic infections are chronic salpingo-oophoritis, pyosalpinx, hydrosalpinx, and tubercular salpingitis. Chronic salpingo-oophoritis is one of the major complications of gonorrhea. The patient may have few complaints. Since the endosalpinx was intensely involved in the acute infection, the tube may be agglutinized. Pyosalpinx is one of the chronic destructive lesions of gonorrhea in which the tube is dilated, closed, and filled with pus. Hydrosalpinx results from pyosalpinx in which the purulent material is replaced by a serous fluid. Chronic oophoritis may develop after ovarian surface involvement, and often the tube and ovary are involved in a single inflammatory process. The classic pattern of chronic pelvic infection is one of quiescent intervals interspaced with episodes of more acute inflammation. After the initial infection, usually gonococcal, anaerobic organisms invade and involve these tissues. Tuberculous salpingitis is now a rare problem in the United States, and the process usually involves the endometrium and adjacent structures as well. The dense adhesions of pelvic viscera to bowel and omentum are outstanding features of this disease, and these structures may be covered with a caseous exudate.

Chronic pelvic infection may be treated medically or surgically. The important elements of medical therapy are rest, heat, and antibiotic therapy. Sedation and analgesia usually are required. Oral metronidazole, doxycycline, or tetracycline are the appropriate antibiotics utilized with modest increase of pain and symptoms from chronic pelvic infection. Those patients who have recurrent pain or abnormal uterine bleeding from reduced ovarian function caused by chronic pelvic infection are often difficult to relieve of symptoms.

This disease is a common gynecologic complaint, and surgical therapy is often required. The only cure for chronic, recurrent pelvic infection is surgical removal of the uterus, tubes, and ovaries. Surgical therapy should always be delayed, if possible, until maximal medical control has been obtained. Estrogen replacement is indicated for the younger woman if both ovaries are removed.

BENIGN DISEASES OF THE OVARY

Benign ovarian tumors may be solid or cystic and may represent a "functional" process or neoplasia. Although these growths are usually small, they may persist or become massively enlarged. The judgment about the necessity of surgical removal should be based on size, duration, or symptoms; the interval of persistence of the smaller lesions; and the age of the patient. Most classifications of such benign tumors include ovarian cysts, nonneoplastic and neoplastic, and solid ovarian tumors.

Many investigators report that more than 90 per cent of ovarian growths discovered in women less than 30 years old are benign. In the 30- to 50-year age group, 80 per cent are benign. After 50 years of age, approximately half of such ovarian growths are malignant. Other investigators report the likelihood of the various benign ovarian growths, excluding the frequently seen follicular and corpus luteum cysts, as endometrial cysts, 33 per cent; simple cysts, 26 per cent; serous and mucinous cystadenomas, 19 per cent; dermoids, 15.2 per cent; others, 2 per cent. The most frequent sign of benign ovarian growths is slow abdominal enlargement. Other symptoms are pain and tenderness from torsion of the pedicle and interference with the blood supply. Less than 10 per cent of such growths are associated with aberrations in the menstrual cycle. Amenorrhea or irregular bleeding may accompany follicular or corpus luteum cysts, polycystic ovaries, or endometrial cysts. Unless quite large, most benign ovarian tumors rarely cause pressure on adjacent pelvic structures. Most commonly, such ovarian growths are asymptomatic and discovered on routine pelvic examination.

The benign, nonneoplastic ovarian cysts are usually of "functional" origin. The follicular cyst represents failure of a developing follicle to rupture or regress and rarely exceeds 8 cm. in diameter. Corpus luteum cysts occur from hemorrhage into the corpus luteum; these blood-filled cysts have the yellow granular color of the normal corpus luteum, whereas the follicular cyst is filled with clear fluid. Both usually regress over a 4- to 8-week period. The theca lutein cyst and the luteoma of pregnancy are also functional cysts resulting from the high levels of circulating chorionic gonadotropin of normal pregnancy and trophoblastic disease. They regress after pregnancy is terminated. Germinal inclusion cysts occur in the cortex of the ovary and represent inward growth of the germinal epithelium that has undergone cystic change. These cysts are thought to be the origin of the neoplastic serous cystadenoma. Polycystic ovaries are enlarged with multiple small follicular cysts and luteinization of the stroma and have a thickened capsule. The etiology is unknown but may relate to tonic elevation of luteinizing hormone.

The benign neoplastic ovarian cysts are most frequently the endometrial cyst or "chocolate" cyst of pelvic endometriosis (Fig. 19) or the simple cyst. These may achieve large size, especially the latter. Serous and mucinous cystadenomas arise from neoplastic changes in germinal epithelium and often reach considerable size. These cystic tumors are multilocular, have smooth capsules, and usually replace the entire ovary. Histologic examination reveals an adenomatous pattern or tall columnar cells producing mucin, respectively. The benign teratoma, or dermoid cyst, is a common ovarian tumor, benign in more than 99 per cent of patients. The gross appearance is that of a smooth-coated, gray tumor that usually replaces the ovary. Microscopically, ectodermal and mesodermal structures are found with hair, teeth, bone, and cartilage present. Approximately 25 per cent of dermoids are bilateral, and thus if one ovary is involved, the other should be carefully inspected.

The solid benign ovarian tumors include the Brenner tumor, which is thought to arise from Walthard inclusion rests in the cortex of the ovary. This tumor grossly resembles the ovarian fibroma, another benign solid tumor. Ovarian fibromas are occasionally the cause of Meigs' syndrome with concomitant sympathetic pleural effusion and ascites. Other solid ovarian tumors include the rare androgen-producing Leydig cell tumor, or hilus cell tumor, and the neuroma, angioma, papilloma, and fibroadenoma. The most important decision facing the surgeon who finds a solid ovarian tumor is to differentiate benign from malignant.

The treatment of benign ovarian growths is primarily surgical removal with conservation of all possible normal ovarian tissue. The functional cysts, follicular and corpus luteum, should regress in a relatively short interval and do not require removal unless rupture and hemorrhage have occurred. These are frequently found during surgical therapy for other reasons and do not require treatment. The majority of the other benign cystic and solid ovarian tumors usually replace or destroy any remain-

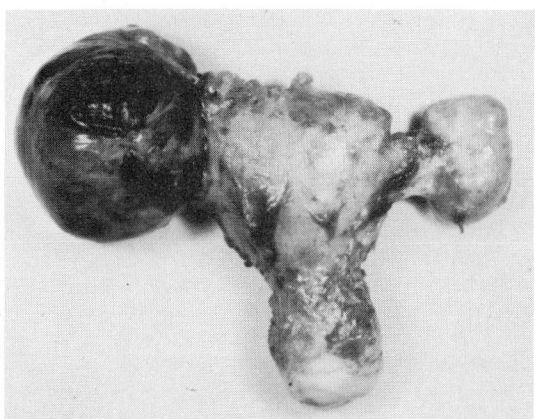

Figure 19. Endometrioma ("chocolate cyst") of ovary with attached hysterectomy specimen.

ing ovarian tissue in the involved gonad, and oophorectomy, preserving the tube, is often indicated. Endometrial or "chocolate" cysts are an exception, and after all involved ovarian tissue is resected, one attempts to leave even a small amount of normal ovarian tissue for future fertility. In any event, bilateral oophorectomy is rarely indicated in the young woman unless one is *certain* that malignancy is present. If there is any doubt, the abdomen should be closed even if reoperation is needed at a later date. In general, it has been thought that if an undiagnosed ovarian mass is larger than 6 cm. or if it persists without diminution in size for longer than 3 months, exploration should be done. Acute torsion or significant hemorrhage may require immediate operative intervention.

OVARIAN CANCER

The incidence of cancer of the ovary varies considerably in different reports because of the wide range of criteria accepted for making this diagnosis. Among the adenomatous tumors, there is a broad group of borderline cases. Most series report that ovarian cancer comprises 4 to 6 per cent of all cases of malignant disease in women. Most investigators report incidences of histologic types as serous cystadenocarcinoma, 60 per cent; pseudomucinous carcinoma, 15 per cent; solid undifferentiated adenocarcinoma, 10 per cent; granulosa cell carcinoma, 6 per cent; dysgerminoma, 2 per cent; and other rare types (arrhenoblastoma, teratoma, mesonephroma), 7 per cent. The ratio of benign ovarian tumors to malignant ovarian tumors is 4 to 1, until the peak incidence of ovarian cancer at 40 to 60 years of age, when the ratio is 1 to 1.

The International Federation of Gynecology and Obstetrics has adopted the following clinical classification, based on clinical studies and surgical exploration, for staging primary carcinoma of the ovary. Further modification and expansion of this basic staging occurred in 1985.

Stage I
Growth limited to the ovaries
Stage II
Growth involves one or both ovaries with extension of the cancer to other areas within the pelvis
Stage III
Growth involves one or both ovaries with widespread intraperitoneal metastasis to the abdomen
Stage IV
Growth involves one or both ovaries with distant metastasis outside the peritoneal cavity

Several factors need to be emphasized in regard to ovarian cancer. First, the delay in diagnosis is reprehensible: 50 per cent of ovarian cancers are neglected by the patient and 25 per cent by the physician, who does not examine the patient in more than 60 per cent of cases. Second, 30 to 50 per cent of ovarian cancers are inoperable at the time of diagnosis, and in only 20 per cent can the tumor be entirely removed surgically. Third, only 11 per cent of patients have suspicious or positive Papanicolaou cytologic findings. Fourth, as expected, the survival is greater the earlier the stage of the disease at the time of diagnosis. As the overall survival of patients with ovarian cancer has improved only slightly in the past 25 years, earlier diagnosis is mandatory.

Ovarian cancer occurs more frequently in white women, and the mean age at diagnosis is 51 years. Fifty-eight per cent of patients are postmenopausal. Childbearing may have some effect in reducing the likelihood of ovarian cancer. It is suggested that a family history of cancer, exposure to pelvic irradiation, and previously existing benign ovarian tumors may increase the likelihood of development of cancer of the ovary.

SIGNS AND SYMPTOMS. The signs and symptoms of ovarian cancer may be only those of an enlarging tumor in the pelvis. Parker reported that 56 per cent of patients complained of pain and 46 per cent of abdominal swelling. He also reported that 31 per cent had experienced at least a 10-pound weight change, usually loss, and 22 per cent had either abnormal or postmenopausal bleeding. There may be ascites with unilateral or bilateral pleural effusion. Anemia is frequently seen in advanced disease. Pelvic examination may reveal firm, nodular implants of metastatic tumor in the cul-de-sac and pelvic viscera. As noted, often there are no early symptoms of ovarian cancer. Every woman should have an annual pelvic examination before age 40 years and more frequently thereafter.

DIAGNOSIS. The diagnosis is made histopathologically, and the differential diagnosis between benign and malignant ovarian tumors cannot be made until operation. The gross examination of the tumor at operation is usually helpful, since papillary growths on the surface of a cystic or semicystic tumor or papillations on the inside of the tumor are suggestive of malignancy (Fig. 20). Solid ovarian tumors that are lobulated or have hemorrhagic areas in the capsule are usually malignant. Peritoneal cell washings should be obtained with any suggestive ovarian tumor. Recent work has centered on evaluation of tumor "markers" for ovarian cancer. Although not highly accurate for diagnosis, if present they may have a useful role (CA 125, CEA).

TREATMENT. The reader is referred to the many excellent reviews on the various types of therapy for ovarian cancer. Results of all therapy, however, remain poor, and various proponents report limited success with a variety of therapeutic regimens. There is general agreement that total abdominal hysterectomy, bilateral salpingo-oophorectomy, and omentectomy should be performed, even if some tumor is left behind. The abdomen, including the diaphragm, should be carefully inspected and appropriate lymph node sampling performed. The surgeon should routinely obtain peritoneal washings for cytology upon entering the abdomen of patients suspected of having ovarian cancer. As the 5-year survival for Stage I ovarian cancer is only 66 per cent, and only 20 percent of patients explored have disease as limited as Stage I, most investigators believe supplemental therapy is mandatory for all patients with ovarian cancer. Radiotherapy and chemotherapy have both been used with moderate palliative success. Total pelvic and abdominal irradiation, intraperitoneal radioisotopes, alkylating agents, and combination chemotherapy are of significant palliative aid in nearly half of patients so treated.

MALIGNANT TROPHOBLASTIC DISEASE

Malignant gestational trophoblastic diseases are relatively rare cancers of women but are of major importance. Even if metastases are present, essentially all patients with these tumors can be cured. It is tragic for a woman to have an erroneous diagnosis of "anaplastic metastatic cancer" made and the diagnosis of trophoblastic malignancy overlooked. As these tumors frequently present with the symptoms of metastases, it is useful for any physician who treats women of reproductive age to be aware of the patterns of these diseases.

Malignant trophoblastic disease may follow any type of pregnancy, including abortion or term live birth, although more than half the tumors occur after hydatidiform mole. Tissue diagnoses include invasive mole (chorioadenoma destruens), choriocarcinoma, and anaplastic trophoblastic tissue. Irregular uterine bleeding is a common presenting sign, but patients present with amenorrhea, uterine rupture, or the sequelae of distant metastasis to the lung, vagina, brain, bowel, kidney, or elsewhere. The anaplastic pattern of the placental trophoblasts, with or without preservation of the pattern of the villus, may be seen histologically. Fortunately, all these tumors produce a hormone identical to human chorionic gonadotropin (HCG), which can be measured by sensitive radioimmunologic techniques. The finding of a suspicious metastic lesion, with or without pelvic symptoms, should lead to HCG testing. If the HCG level is elevated and normal pregnancy can be excluded, one should strongly suspect malignant trophoblastic disease.

Considerable assistance for physicians treating patients with suspected malignant trophoblastic disease can be obtained from any of the several trophoblastic disease centers in the United States.[7] Treatment consists of intensive chemotherapy with methotrexate or actinomycin D, given alone or in combination with surgical therapy or irradiation. With appropriate and intensive therapy, essentially all patients with these diseases can be cured, even when metastases are present.

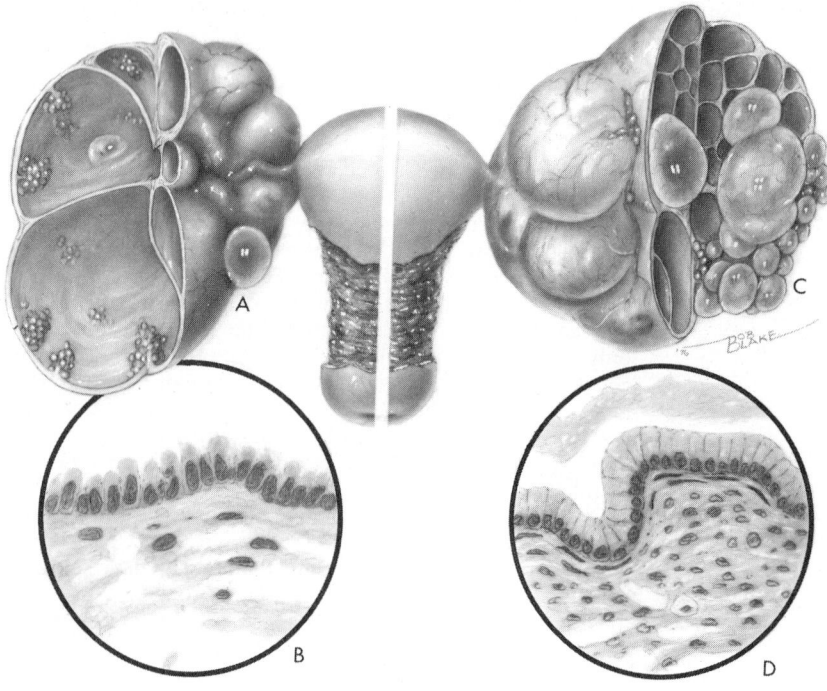

Figure 20. Ovarian carcinoma. *A*, Cystic, papillary. *B*, Microscopic view of *A*. *C*, Pseudomucinous. *D*, Microscopic view of *C*.

AMENORRHEA

Amenorrhea is defined as the absence of menses at the time a woman should be menstruating and may be classified as primary or secondary. Most investigators believe a patient should be without menses for at least 6 months before the diagnosis of amenorrhea is made. Amenorrhea occurs physiologically in pregnancy and lactation. Menstruation is based on the interaction of the central nervous system, hypothalamus, pituitary, ovary, uterus, with other glands and their hormones (see Physiology and Endocrinology).

Primary amenorrhea, in which the patient has never had menses, occasionally may be due to abnormalities of the central nervous system or the pituitary gland but much more commonly occurs from gonadal, adrenal, or uterine defects. Most girls begin menses by 18 years of age, and failure of menstruation by this age warrants careful examination, chromosomal testing, hormonal assays, and, on occasion, visualization of the gonad. Gonadotropin assays frequently provide the appropriate direction for further study, since these levels are increased in cases of ovarian failure or abnormal function and are usually reduced with central nervous system or pituitary gland diseases. Congenital absence of the uterus always, and endometrial disease frequently, result in amenorrhea although gonadotropins are normal.

Secondary amenorrhea, or cessation of menses, may be due to a variety of problems. However, the most common cause of absence of menses is pregnancy. Space-occupying lesions of the central nervous system, hypothalamus, or pituitary result in absence or low levels of gonadotropins and amenorrhea. Pituitary tumors or infarction can also yield similar results. Skull films, visual field examinations, appropriate imaging, and hormonal studies may aid in making these diagnoses. However, one must always remember that the symptom of amenorrhea may precede the diagnosis of such lesions by a span of years, and prolonged follow-up is mandatory.

Psychiatric illnesses may interfere with gonadotropin release and result in amenorrhea. Ovarian problems, such as polycystic ovaries and premature ovarian failure, may cause secondary amenorrhea, and in these patients gonadotropins are normal and elevated, respectively. Acquired failure of endometrial responsiveness also may cause secondary amenorrhea, as can significant dysfunction of the thyroid or adrenal glands. Treatment is based on the appropriate diagnosis.

ECTOPIC PREGNANCY

An ectopic pregnancy is one in which the ovum implants and develops outside the normal location, the uterine cavity. Ninety-five per cent of ectopic pregnancies are tubal, with the greatest percentage of these occurring in the dilated ampulla, that portion of the distal tube immediately proximal to the fimbriated end. Less common sites of ectopic pregnancy are abdominal, ovarian, and interligamentary (Fig. 21). Abdominal ectopic pregnancy usually occurs after tubal abortion, with secondary reimplantation elsewhere in the abdominal cavity. The incidence of all types of ectopic pregnancy is increasing and is approximately 3 in 100 births.

Despite the fact that the ovum is implanted outside the uterine cavity, the uterine endometrium is converted into a decidua similar to that of normal pregnancy. The size and consistency of the uterus also change in ectopic pregnancy. The cervix and body of the uterus soften, and the corpus may enlarge to a size compatible with a 6- to 8-week intrauterine pregnancy. All these changes are due to the production of placental hormones from the ectopic embryo. As ectopic placental function declines, as usually occurs in tubal pregnancy, the hormonal support declines and irregular uterine bleeding begins. The decidua is

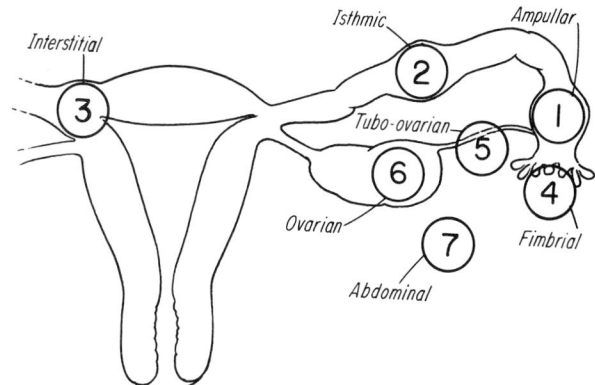

Figure 21. Ectopic pregnancy. Diagram shows the various implantation sites, numbered in order of decreasing frequency of occurrence.

usually discharged in fragments, but may on occasion be expelled intact as a decidual cast.

The duration and eventual outcome of tubal ectopic pregnancy are determined primarily by the area of tube involved. If the ovum implants in the relatively large ampullary region of the tube, the pregnancy usually continues longer than one in the narrow isthmus. Local bleeding from trophoblastic invasion continues and increases, and blood dissects the ovular sac from the tubal wall. With complete separation, the ovular sac is usually extruded from the end of the tube, and unless a major vessel is involved, bleeding is terminated. More often, however, the process is prolonged, and repeated bleeding episodes yield a pelvic hematoma. In other areas of the tube, the tubal wall is less distensible and the lumen narrower, and tubal rupture is inevitable as the trophoblasts invade and blood collects. Episodic pregnancies in the narrow isthmic segment usually rupture in 6 to 8 weeks, whereas those in the interstitial portion, where the tube traverses the uterine wall, continue for 14 to 16 weeks before rupture. Rupture is usually into the peritoneal cavity and is accompanied by sudden and significant bleeding. Tubal pregnancies may regress spontaneously, with the ovum either dying at an early age or being extruded from the tubal ostium without significant bleeding.

The classic symptoms of ectopic pregnancy are a history of infertility or pelvic disease, light vaginal bleeding within 2 to 4 weeks after the first missed period, and sharp and fleeting lower abdominal pain. Eventually the patient experiences sudden severe abdominal pain and shock as the tube ruptures. On examination, one usually notes the signs of early pregnancy such as cyanosis and softening of the cervix and uterine enlargement. The most important pelvic finding prior to tubal rupture is a unilateral tender mass. In patients with pelvic hematoma, the cul-de-sac may be "doughy" and distended. Signs of peritoneal inflammation may be present. Fever is a rare finding, but progressive anemia is frequently observed. Newer, more sensitive pregnancy tests are positive in most patients with unruptured tubal pregnancy.

The diagnosis of an unruptured tubal pregnancy is not difficult to make when classic symptoms are present but, unfortunately, the symptoms are frequently atypical and the pelvic findings misleading. A high index of suspicion is the most valuable adjunct. Culdocentesis, or large-gauge needle perforation of the cul-de-sac, may reveal considerable dark old blood and strongly suggest pelvic hematoma. Laparoscopy may allow visualization of the ectopic pregnancy. Although it is usually possible to diagnose tubal pregnancy with reasonable accuracy, problems such as uterine abortion, salpingitis, appendicitis, or ruptured corpus luteum or follicular cysts may produce signs and symptoms causing confusion in diagnosis. In uterine abortion, the period of amenorrhea is usually longer, the amount of vaginal bleeding is greater, and pain is less severe, more midline, and cramping in nature. No adnexal mass or tenderness is present. Salpingitis and appendicitis usually present with signs of infection and without prior amenorrhea or irregular bleeding. Ruptured cysts, particularly those of the corpus luteum, usually are not associated with prolonged amenorrhea. Follicular cysts tend to rupture at midcycle. In both varieties, an occasional patient may require surgical exploration for control of hemorrhage.

The diagnostic armamentarium for the assessment of ectopic pregnancy has recently changed dramatically. When this diagnosis is suspected, a sensitive pregnancy test should be done to determine whether HCG is present. If positive, a quantified assay should be obtained. If the HCG titer is in excess of 4000 mI.U. per ml., an intrauterine pregnancy, if present, should be seen by ultrasonography, preferably by the more sensitive vaginal probe technique. The finding of an intrauterine pregnancy in such a setting likely excludes the ectopic pregnancy in all but the very rare patient who might have simultaneous intrauterine and ectopic pregnancies. Failure to note an ectopically placed pregnancy with ultrasonography is not diagnostic of the absence of that problem. Likewise, if the HCG titer is less than 4000 mI.U. per ml., an intrauterine pregnancy may not be apparent with even well-done ultrasound examination. In patients in whom the initial value of HCG is less than 4000 mI.U. per ml., every-other-day assays should be done. In normal gestations, HCG doubles every 48 hours during this portion of pregnancy. If this doubling is not observed, the diagnosis of an abnormal pregnancy—either a missed abortion, an incomplete abortion, or possibly an ectopic gestation—is supported. All these studies should be utilized in the subtle case.

Treatment of ectopic pregnancy is surgical therapy.[13] In patients who desire preservation of childbearing ability, one often can salvage even the involved fallopian tube by "milking out" the ectopic gestation from the ampulla of the tube, performing a linear salpingostomy with removal of the ectopic pregnancy, and, after achievement of hemostasis with ultrafine suture, leaving the tube *in situ*. Occasionally, a tube may be so destroyed that it cannot be salvaged and must be removed. Rarely is removal of the ovary a necessary part of this procedure. Finally, if hemostasis cannot be obtained after linear salpingostomy, segmental resection of the fallopian tube can be accomplished, leaving the proximal and distal portions of the normal tube *in situ*. It is inappropriate to attempt reanastomosis at the time of extirpation of the segment of tube, but such microscopic reanastomosis may be done at a later date. Even if the ectopic pregnancy is in the remaining fallopian tube of a patient who has previously had the other tube removed, it may be inappropriate to perform a hysterectomy at the time of removal of the only remaining fallopian tube. With the newer technologies of *in vitro* fertilization and embryo transplant, pregnancy may be possible for this patient even without fallopian tubes.

Prompt blood replacement and surgical intervention are mandatory, but the patient's condition should be stabilized prior to operation if at all possible. General anesthesia should be used. Abdominal pregnancy is treated by removal of the fetus and ligation of the umbilical cord near its insertion into the placenta. Owing to the intense vascularity of the placenta, it is usually best to leave this *in situ*. Prognosis with prompt management is good, and mortality from ectopic pregnancy has been reduced to 1 to 2 percent. Recurrence of ectopic pregnancy in the remaining tube occurs in about 10 per cent of patients.

SURGICAL DISEASE IN PREGNANCY

The pregnant woman is subject to all the surgical diseases of the nonpregnant patient. Often, however, the diagnosis and management of such patients must be modified to allow for the

physiologic changes that normally occur or to manage concerns generated about a second patient, the fetus.[4] Added to these physiologic changes are the mechanical alterations associated with the enlarging uterus. Close collaboration between obstetrician, anesthesiologist, and surgeon is necessary if tragic consequences to the mother and child are to be avoided. This section can review only general concepts regarding common surgical diseases and pregnancy. It is to be hoped that the presentation of these concerns will stimulate the reader to consult the expanding literature on these topics. For further details, the reader is referred to the texts listed at the end of this chapter.

General Considerations, Including Anesthesia

Many remarkable physiologic changes occur in pregnant women, involving respiratory, circulatory, hepatic, renal, and gastrointestinal functions and acid-base balance. Most of the changes are induced by endocrinologic substances produced from the placenta and by the mechanical effects of the enlarging uterus.

RESPIRATION. There is a progressive increase in minute ventilation, which, near term, is at a peak level of about 50 per cent above normal. This effect is primarily through an increase in tidal volume and, to a much lesser extent, through a rise in respiratory rate. Consequently, alveolar ventilation is increased about 70 per cent above normal at term. These changes are associated with a reduction in alveolar and arterial carbon dioxide tension to about 32 mm. Hg and an increase in oxygen tension to 95 to 105 mm. Hg. There is a progressive decrease in expiratory volume and residual volume, and consequently the functional residual capacity decreases to about 20 per cent below that in the nonpregnant state. There is little or no change in vital capacity, maximal breathing capacity, or other pulmonary function parameters. Other physiologic changes occurring in pregnancy include edema and erythema of the nasopharynx, larynx, trachea, and bronchi. Chest films show increased lung markings, which may be of a degree to simulate the features of mild congestive failure.

CIRCULATION. Cardiac output increases progressively during pregnancy, reaching a maximum of 30 to 50 per cent greater than normal by the seventh to eighth month, then falling to more normal levels during the thirty-sixth to fortieth week. Cardiac rate increases progressively until the last trimester, when it is approximately ten beats per minute above the nonpregnant level. Arterial blood pressure decreases slightly during pregnancy, while venous blood pressure is normal in the lower extremities, where it becomes progressively increased as pregnancy advances. Hypotension may occur when the gravid patient assumes a supine position with concomitant venocaval obstruction. Operative positioning may thus be of major importance. The changes in arterial and venous pressure induced by pregnancy and the changes in the supine position may markedly influence anesthetic management. Vasomotor block, inherent in spinal and peridural anesthesia, often deprives the patient of the compensatory vasoconstriction and usually results in a much greater fall in arterial pressure than occurs in the nonpregnant state.

The increase in cardiac work is not a transient occurrence associated with activity but is maintained throughout the day. Although these increases are well tolerated by patients with normal hearts, they may present an excessive strain in patients with a low myocardial reserve and may precipitate pulmonary decompensation.

HEMATOLOGIC CHANGES. There is a progressive increase in plasma volume, a lesser increase in red cell volume, and an intermediate increase in total blood volume. A resultant hemodilution occurs. There is an increase in total plasma protein, fibrinogen, and sedimentation rate. The oxygen and carbon dioxide dissociation curves of maternal blood are shifted to the right, while those of fetal blood are shifted to the left. During pregnancy, a significant decrease in cholinesterase activity may occur and may result in a prolonged paralysis and apnea following the administration of succinylcholine.

ACID-BASE BALANCE. The total base decreases from the normal nonpregnant level of about 155 mEq. per liter to about 148 mEq. per liter. This is reflected in the decline of plasma sodium and a corresponding decrease in potassium, calcium, and magnesium. There is a commensurate total amnion diminution. As noted previously, Pco_2 decreases to about 32 mm. Hg, and the plasma buffer base decreases fro 47 to 42 mEq. per liter. In most patients, blood pH remains unchanged at 7.40.

OTHER PHYSIOLOGIC CHANGES. Pregnancy is associated with a diminution of gastric and intestinal motility, a relative hyperchlorhydria, and a slight delay in emptying time of the stomach. These changes are exaggerated by sedatives, general anesthetics, and labor. Regurgitation of acid stomach contents is a particular hazard of general anesthesia in the pregnant patient. Although some of the liver function tests are deranged during normal pregnancy, it appears that the liver is capable of functioning without difficulty in the normal individual. Hepatic blood flow is normal.

During pregnancy, there is a gradual dilatation of the urinary collecting system and a progressive increase in glomerular filtration rate, affecting renal plasma flow, filtration fraction, and tubular capacity for the rate of absorption.

A number of endocrinologic changes occur in pregnancy. Notable are hyperplasia of the thyroid and parathyroid glands, hypertrophy of the pituitary gland to nearly twice its normal size, enlargement of the adrenal glands with increased plasma levels of glucocorticoids, and a threefold increase in aldosterone secretion. During pregnancy, there is a progressive increase in basal metabolic rate, in oxygen consumption, in retention and storage of water, protein, and minerals, in retention of salts, and in acquisition of fat.

ANESTHETIC MANAGEMENT. The objective of surgical anesthesia for the gravida is to prevent pain and emotional stress and to provide the surgeon with optimal operating conditions without undue risk to the mother and child. The ideal anesthetic for every surgical operation has not yet been developed, and the type of anesthesia must be selected for the needs of the individual patient. Preanesthetic medication in the form of a sedative, such as a barbiturate or an ataractic, is frequently utilized. If the patient is to receive a general anesthetic, it may be desirable to give atropine to reduce secretions within the respiratory tract.

Induction of general anesthesia should begin with the administration of 100 per cent oxygen for at least 3 minutes prior to the induction. In maintaining anesthesia, the concentration of oxygen in the anesthetic mixture should never be less than 35 per cent. Every precaution should be taken to avoid respiratory obstruction and hypoventilation, and often an endotracheal tube and assisted or controlled ventilation will be needed. If regional anesthesia is to be utilized, it is especially important that this procedure not be initiated unless all materials needed to treat cardiovascular and respiratory complications are ready for immediate use. The incidence and magnitude of arterial hypotension may be minimized by the prophylactic administration of 500 to 1000 ml. of lactated Ringer's solution. If hypotension develops, it should be treated promptly. Of the many vasopressors available, ephedrine is perhaps the best, since it has the least effect on uterine circulation. Obviously, in late pregnancy, the first maneuver is to displace the uterus to one side or to tilt the table to relieve venous compression.

General anesthesia is perhaps the most hazardous of the techniques of emergency surgical anesthesia, mainly because of the danger of aspiration of gastric contents. Pneumonia, cardiac arrest, and respiratory failure are also particular hazards. Again, the use of adequate preanesthetic oxygenation and the prompt placement of an endotracheal tube minimize these risks.

The Acute Abdomen in Pregnancy

As noted previously, a complex series of changes occur in pregnancy, and these may modify the manifestations of intra-abdominal disease processes. The continued growth of the uterus produces mechanical displacement of the gastrointestinal tract and a diminished motility. The stomach assumes a more horizontal position and comes to lie in the left upper quadrant beneath the diaphragm. Gastric emptying time is delayed and near term may be more than twice normal. Gastroesophageal regurgitation is common. Normally, the small intestine is displaced upward during pregnancy, with little alteration in its function. In the presence of incarcerated hernia or adhesion, however, the enlarging uterus may compound the obstructive process.

Since *acute appendicitis* is one of the most common and one of the most serious surgical complications of pregnancy, the anatomic changes in this area deserve particular attention. The colon is displaced by the enlarging uterus, so that the transverse colon deviates upward and the ascending and descending segments are displaced toward the flanks. The cecum and the base of the appendix rise from the iliac fossa and are displaced laterally, so that by the sixth month they are situated at the level of the iliac crest; at term the appendix is well up in the right upper quadrant, near the base of the liver.

The most frequent presenting symptoms in the pregnant patient with an acute abdomen are abdominal pain, nausea and vomiting, abdominal distention, and shock. Each of these may be attributable to or associated with the pregnancy or may herald the onset of an acute, nonobstetric emergency. In the assessment of a pregnant patient with a suspected acute abdomen, the usual signs of intra-abdominal disease remain valid—in particular, indications of generalized peritonitis, separate from uterine or adnexal tenderness *per se*. With recognition of the changing anatomic relationships of the abdominal contents occurring in pregnancy, one may usually rely on traditional symptoms and findings for acute appendicitis, cholecystitis, peptic ulcer disease, intestinal obstruction, and intra-abdominal hemorrhage. Radiologic and laboratory techniques generally retain their usefulness, although the relative leukocytosis and other hematologic changes seen in normal pregnancy may be confusing.

In general, laparotomy incisions heal well during pregnancy. The choice of an incision is dictated by the stage of pregnancy and the nature of the problem, with the anatomic variations of pregnancy borne in mind. For acute appendicitis, a right lower quadrant, muscle-splitting incision is appropriate; in biliary tract disease, a high subcostal incision is usually desirable. Long vertical incisions may be indicated for intestinal obstruction. In all these procedures, adequate exposure is of paramount importance. The abdominal incision may be closed in the usual manner, preferably with interrupted sutures. If drainage or exteriorization is necessary, it is usually advisable to perform it through a separate stab incision.

In addition to the supportive postoperative measures usually employed, the following points should be emphasized in the care of the pregnant surgical patient: adequate efforts to ensure oxygenation and maintenance of an airway with supplemental oxygen as needed; accurate monitoring of blood volume and transfusion as necessary to maintain an adequate level; careful evaluation of fluid and electrolyte balance; adequate sedation to minimize the likelihood of premature labor (newer studies suggest prophylactic tocolysis may be of significant benefit); continuous gastrointestinal decompression; careful attention to an indwelling Foley catheter and the urinary retention to which the enlarged uterus predisposes; and careful attention to the extremities, particularly if varicosities are present. The incidence of phlebitis is considerably increased during pregnancy, because of venostasis. Unless specifically indicated, early ambulation is not advisable, nor is routine antibiotic prophylaxis indicated. Again, recent studies are exploring the use of tocolytic agents to reduce premature labor, and the practitioner would be well advised to consider these new approaches as they become further defined.

Cardiovascular Surgery in Pregnancy

The gestational changes of significance in cardiovascular disease have been mentioned earlier. In addition to the physiologic changes, there are anatomic changes with special relationships to the cardiovascular system. During pregnancy and the puerperium, there is a general loosening of the ground substance of connective tissue, affecting the vascular system by reducing the tensile strength of blood vessels. The local anatomic change of importance in vascular disorders is the enlargement of the uterus, which results in compression of the vascular structures of the pelvis, obstructing venous return from the legs and setting the stage for venous thrombosis and its sequelae.

ACQUIRED HEART DISEASE. Surgical treatment of acquired heart disease in pregnancy was first reported in 1952 by Cooley and Chapman. Within a short time, mitral valvulotomy during pregnancy was being performed in many centers, and by the mid-1950s sufficient data had accrued to indicate that mitral commissurotomy could be done during pregnancy with a relatively low risk of harm to the mother or fetus. It should be emphasized that optimal medical management should precede the decision for operation. The operative risk to the pregnant patient in general is no greater than that to the nonpregnant patient. With increasing severity of disease, the risk of death increases in both the nonoperated and the operated patient. Candidates for operation during pregnancy are Class III and IV patients with mitral stenosis and those patients with mitral stenosis who during a previous pregnancy experienced an acute episode of cardiac decompensation. In addition, any patient who has sustained a systemic embolus associated with mitral valve disease should be considered for surgical intervention.

As to the timing of cardiac operation, commissurotomy is best done during the first trimester of pregnancy when the cardiac load has not yet increased appreciably. A contraindication to mitral commissurotomy is the presence of mitral insufficiency or coexisting aortic stenosis. These lesions are not now considered correctable by the technique of closed heart surgery. Closed mitral commissurotomy is unnecessary in asymptomatic patients but is an effective alternative to protracted bed rest and congestive heart failure in patients with functional limitations who become pregnant. Maternal and fetal mortality are lower in such patients operated on by the technique of closed commissurotomy than in the unoperated patient. There are fewer data regarding open mitral operations than for closed mitral commissurotomies. Although a definitive statistical statement cannot be made at this time, published data indicate a favorable trend.

In an effort to provide optimal correction in patients whose valves were not amenable to closed or open heart reconstruction, newer techniques of valvular surgical repair have allowed restoration of cardiac function. To date, there are relatively few reports of mitral valvular replacement procedures in pregnant women. It remains difficult to separate the hazards of anticoagulation from those of the surgical procedures in the long-term management of these gravidas.

VENOUS THROMBOSIS AND PULMONARY EMBOLISM. In pregnancy, as in the nonpregnant state, venostasis is a most controllable factor in preventing venous thrombosis and pulmonary embolism. Pregnant women are susceptible to venostasis in the lower extremities, as the gravid uterus interrupts flow through segments of the iliac veins and inferior vena cava. The primary means of alleviating venostasis is elastic compression of the legs, and it is thought that effective elastic compression should be used in all patients with varicose veins or a

history of thrombophlebitis. Anticoagulation is important in limiting extension of thrombosis. The means of anticoagulation remains of great concern, however, as fetal hemorrhage and teratogenicity have been reported in patients treated with the coumarins. Because heparin does not cross the placental barrier, its use is advisable in the interval prior to delivery. In general, heparin anticoagulation does not appreciably increase the blood loss associated with normal vaginal delivery (excluding bleeding from sites lacerated by trauma or episiotomy).

Venous thrombosis may be complicated by pulmonary embolism, and such embolism must be suspected as the cause of pleuritic chest pain or unexplained hemoptysis. Appropriate treatment is adequate heparinization with general supportive management for 10 to 14 days. At that time, the decision must be made to change to a coumarin anticoagulant or to continue the heparinization for the remainder of the pregnancy and puerperium. If pulmonary embolism recurs during heparin anticoagulation, ligation of the inferior vena cava and left ovarian veins by the transperitoneal route should be considered. Pulmonary embolectomy should be reserved for those patients in clinical shock with the appropriate clinical features and suggestive right-sided cardiac catheterization studies. In general, the usual diagnostic studies for pulmonary embolus are allowable in the pregnant patient.

VARICOSE VEINS. Varicosities in pregnancy are a significant problem and usually have a fairly distinct pattern. They appear during the second or third month of pregnancy and become progressively larger until the last trimester. They may be unilateral or scattered over both lower extremities. Susceptible women have progressively larger varicosities with each successive pregnancy.

Many reports have described the surgical injection treatment of varicose veins during pregnancy. Many workers believe that pregnancy is no contraindication to injection or surgical therapy when such treatment is indicated. Others, however, believe that it is technically difficult to perform an adequate operation during pregnancy and that the danger of postoperative thrombosis and embolism is great. Before initiation of any therapy for varicose veins during pregnancy, several factors should be considered: (1) many of the dilated veins recede spontaneously after delivery; (2) although it is technically feasible to correct varices surgically, pregnancy often produces such distortion of the veins that the procedure can be difficult; (3) superior treatment is usually achieved when varices are treated in the postpartum state; and (4) in practically all cases, effective compression of the varicosities with elastic supports during pregnancy controls all symptoms and prevents complications.

Because elastic supports are effective, their use has become standard therapy for the enlarged varicosities in pregnancy. Elastic bandages are usually recommended to compress all varices from the time they appear until after delivery. The rubberized elastic bandages are considered preferable to rubber stockings to ensure adequate tension and compression. If there are large vulvar varices, a vulvar compressive support is available. In addition to elastic support, the patient is instructed to avoid prolonged standing. Frequent elevation of the legs and leg exercises have also been of help.

Trauma in Pregnancy

Trauma is responsible for a significant percentage of nonobstetric maternal deaths in the United States. Traumatic injury during pregnancy ranges from insignificant to catastrophic.

EFFECT OF TRAUMA IN PREGNANCY. For many years there was thought to be a significant causal relationship between maternal injury and interruption of pregnancy. More current data, however, suggest that perinatal mortality does not appear appreciably increased in cases in which the mother has sustained noncatastrophic abdominal trauma during pregnancy. Yet even maternal injury that is less than catastrophic can alter the course of a pregnancy and jeopardize the fetus. The fetus in later pregnancy can be injured *in utero* as a result of blunt or penetrating trauma. The placenta, cord, or membranes can be damaged. Maternal injury can cause severe alterations in maternal homeostasis and severely compromise the fetus. Abruptio placentae and psychologic shock secondary to maternal trauma appear to have nonspecific roles.

MATERNAL INJURY. Blunt injury is the most common form of abdominal trauma currently seen. It most frequently results in damage to a solid viscus, which is relatively thick and sustains injury either from direct blows to the abdomen or by contrecoup action. The spleen is the most commonly injured organ in pregnant women, followed by the liver and kidney. The pregnant uterus occupies a middle position between solid and hollow viscera. Rupture can occur, usually in the fundal portion.

Penetrating wounds of the abdomen and pregnant uterus have resulted from a variety of instruments. With penetrating wounds, unlike blunt trauma, of the pregnant abdomen multiple organ injury is the rule. The frequency with which an organ is injured is in direct proportion to the space it occupies in the abdomen. With increasing duration of gestation, the uterus tends to displace the small bowel into a smaller space in the upper abdomen and acts as a protective shield for other viscera. The mortality of penetrating wounds of the abdomen in pregnant patients is related to the number of organs injured. Only about one third of the patients who have sustained gunshot wounds in the pregnant uterus, however, have had other associated visceral injury. A review of gunshot wounds to the pregnant uterus revealed a perinatal mortality rate of 70 per cent. Approximately half the infants sustained wounds that could have contributed to their demise; the remainder died as a result of premature delivery, often performed unnecessarily during the acute care of the mother.

DIAGNOSIS AND TREATMENT OF ABDOMINAL TRAUMA. As with any injured patient, those conditions that interfere with vital functions or threaten life require immediate attention. Hypotension and hypoxia must be corrected. Both experimental studies and clinical experience have shown that maternal shock has a deleterious effect on the fetus. The effect appears related to the period of gestation, since the fetus is better able to tolerate maternal hypotension in early pregnancy. The fetus becomes anoxic during periods of maternal hypotension as a result of decreased uterine blood flow. The mother responds to hemorrhage by attempting to maintain her blood pressure by decreasing perfusion of the uterine vascular bed.

As a result of the physiologic changes of pregnancy, the pregnant patient is better able to tolerate acute blood loss than is the nonpregnant one. Clinical signs and symptoms of blood loss may not appear in the obstetric patient until there has been a 30 to 35 per cent reduction in blood volume. This would suggest that maternal blood pressure and pulse are not satisfactory parameters of fetal well-being. Adequate circulating blood volume, therefore, must be maintained, and therapy should be directed to restoring both maternal and fetal homeostasis. After emergency measures to control bleeding, restore blood volume, and maintain respiration have been instituted, diagnostic procedures must be accomplished systematically to spare the fetus unnecessary and hazardous exposure to radiologic and invasive procedures.

Roentgenograms have been proved useful in the care of accident victims with fractures and chest injuries, and contrast studies are essential in determining urinary tract status. The value of routine radiographic studies in abdominal trauma is limited. Arteriography is finding increased application in the detection of splenic, hepatic, and renal injuries. Roentgenograms must be used selectively during pregnancy, and their use should be supervised in order to reduce the hazard to the fetus. The fetus can be further protected by proper shielding and appropriate radiographic techniques.

Other hematologic studies, including leukocyte count, may be utilized in the assessment of the patient with abdominal trauma; the physician should exercise caution, however, because the normal leukocyte count in pregnancy is increased and may approach 20,000 in the last trimester. Central venous pressure studies may be of use, but several investigators have shown a progressive fall in central venous pressure during pregnancy, with an average of 3.8 cm. H_2O in the third trimester in normal patients.

In general, conservatism may be recommended in patients with blunt abdominal trauma, and a conservative approach to penetrating abdominal trauma is receiving increased attention. The conservative approach is utilized when signs or symptoms do not definitely indicate visceral injury; these patients are observed closely for the presence of bowel sounds, direct or rebound tenderness, and abdominal rigidity. If blood is found in the peritoneum on paracentesis or in the urine, feces, or gastric aspirates, or if there is a worsening of vital signs, laparotomy is indicated.

FRACTURES. Fractures comprise 10 per cent of accidental injuries during pregnancy. It has been suggested that fracture healing is less effective during pregnancy, but studies have not supported this contention. In general, these studies indicate that changes in the healing strength of fractures parallel those of connective tissue alterations, which become progressively greater in later pregnancy and are probably hormone related.

Fractures need have no deleterious effect on pregnancy, but their management is somewhat modified by the pregnancy and anticipated delivery. The number of roentgenograms taken should be limited and the abdomen and pelvis shielded whenever practical to reduce the radiation hazard to the fetus.

Generally, simple fractures of the extremities present no problems in management. Internal fixation is preferable to prolonged traction in complicated fractures. Vertebral fractures that are stable require only bed rest and need no special attention in the pregnant patient. Fracture-dislocations requiring open reduction and spinal fusion do present significant problems. An abdominal window must be cut and the cast changed frequently to allow space for the growing uterus. Vaginal delivery is not contraindicated in stable fractures, but in patients with unstable fractures, abdominal delivery should be considered. Pelvic fractures, commonly seen since the advent of widespread automotive travel, now constitute a large percentage of fractures in women. Most pelvic fractures do not interfere with vaginal delivery, since distortions of the diameters of the birth canal are rare. Vaginal delivery usually can be anticipated in most cases of pelvic fracture after 8 weeks. In unhealed fractures with separation or displacement, the patient should be delivered by cesarean section.

HEAD INJURIES. In general, the management of the pregnant patient with a head injury is no different from that of the nonpregnant patient. Immediate concerns include stabilization of the patient, evaluation of the patient's vital systems, assessment of the degree of damage incurred, and appropriate neurologic and other specific recommendations regarding the gestational status beyond support and maintenance of the patient.

SELECTED REFERENCES

The following texts are among those used in the preparation of this chapter. For further details and factual information about gynecology, the reader is referred to them.

1. Danforth, D. L., and Scott, J. R. (Eds.): Obstetrics and Gynecology, 5th ed. Philadelphia, J. B. Lippincott Company, 1986.
2. DiSaia, P. J., and Creasman, W. T.: Clinical Gynecologic Cancer, 2nd ed. St. Louis, C. V. Mosby Company, 1984.
3. Droegemueller, W., Herbst, A. L., Mishell, D. R., and Stenchever, M. A. (Eds.): Comprehensive Gynecology. St. Louis, C. V. Mosby Company, 1987.
4. Gusberg, S. B., Shingleton, H. M., and Deppe, G. (Eds.): Female Genital Cancer. New York, Churchill Livingstone, 1988.

5. Nichols, D. H., and Randall, C. L.: Vaginal Surgery, 2nd ed. Baltimore, Waverly Press, 1983.
6. Rosenwaks, Z., Benjamin, F., and Stone, M. L. (Eds.): Gynecology. New York, Macmillan Company, 1987.
7. Speroff, L., Glass, R. N., and Kase, N. G.: Clinical Gynecologic Endocrinology and Infertility, 4th ed. Baltimore, Williams & Wilkins, 1989.
8. Sweet, R. L., and Gibbs, R. S.: Infectious Diseases of the Female Genital Tract. Baltimore, Williams & Wilkins, 1985.

REFERENCES

Barber, H. R. K., and Graber, E. A.: Surgical Disease in Pregnancy. Philadelphia, W. B. Saunders Company, 1974.
This text is now somewhat out of date, but there are many very useful points in considering the surgical diseases that may occur during pregnancy. Of particular interest are the physical findings and clinical observations in various disease states.

Bongiovanni, A. M. (Ed.): Adolescent Gynecology. New York, Plenum Publishing Corporation, 1983.
This text provides useful information for physicians who deal with pelvic problems in the child and adolescent woman. Special needs and disease states are appropriately presented.

Buchsbaum, J. J., and Schmidt, J. D. (Eds.): Gynecologic and Obstetric Urology, 2nd ed. Philadelphia, W. B. Saunders Company, 1982.

Cunningham, F. G., MacDonald, P. C., and Gant, N. F.: Williams' Obstetrics, 18th ed. Norwalk, Conn., Appleton and Lange, 1989.
This classic textbook has become the standard text for obstetrics. It provides much information regarding anatomy, genetics, and physiologic changes during pregnancy. Obstetric and medical complications, as well as those requiring surgical intervention, are fully covered.

Case, N. G., and Weingold, A. B. (Eds.): Principles in the Practice of Clinical Gynecology. New York, John Wiley and Sons, 1983.
An excellent standard text of gynecology with authoritative essays by experts in the various fields. The section on genetics is quite good, as is that on basic physiology.

Duenhoelter, J. H.: Greenhill's Office Gynecology, 10th ed. Chicago, Year Book Medical Publishers, 1983.
This is an excellent textbook of outpatient gynecologic evaluation and therapy. It is easily readable and useful to the practitioner in the ambulatory setting.

Hammond, C. B. (Ed.): Trophoblastic disease. Obstet. Gynecol. Clin. North Am., 15:1, 1988.
This monograph provides detailed information on the diagnosis and management of patients with trophoblastic disease. This once-fatal malignancy is now highly curable with appropriate chemotherapy.

Hulka, J. F.: Textbook of Laparoscopy. Orlando, Fla., Grune and Stratton, 1985.
Laparoscopy has rapidly become a major diagnostic method in gynecologic practice. Hulka's text is beautifully illustrated and provides a thorough and complete overview of laparoscopic technology.

Jones, H. W., Jr., and Rock, J. A.: Reparative and Reconstructive Surgery of the Female Genital Tract. Baltimore, Williams & Wilkins, 1983.
An excellent textbook of reconstructive structures. It is recommended to all who are involved in infertility surgical therapy or who perform conservative operations upon the woman still desirous of pregnancy.

Mattingly, R. F., and Thompson, J. D.: TeLinde's Operative Gynecology, 6th ed. Philadelphia, J. B. Lippincott Company, 1985.
This is the classic surgical text in gynecology. It provides excellent illustrations and a thorough text. It is believed a new edition will be published in early 1990.

Miller, O. J.: The sex chromosome anomalies, Part 2. Am. J. Obstet. Gynecol. 90:1078, 1964.
This classic article is one of the first detailed summaries of chromosomal aberrations that can result in gonadal and extragonadal defects. The article is commended for its clarity and completeness.

Parker, R. T. (Ed.): Woman: The Climacteric and Beyond. Clin. Obstet. Gynecol., 29:1, 1988.
Menopause is a phenomenon seen with increasing frequency in an aging population. Many diseases are now evident, and special requirements for care exist in the surgical as well as medical management of these patients.

Reyniak, J. V., and Lauersen, N. (Eds.): Principles of Microsurgical Techniques in Infertility. New York, Plenum Publishing Corporation, 1982.
This text provides capable descriptions of microsurgical technique, results, and problems.

Speert, H.: Obstetric and Gynecologic Milestones. New York, Macmillan Company, 1958.
This book, subtitled "Essays in Eponymy," explores the discoveries and men who have contributed to this specialty. It is recommended to all practitioners of this area of medicine and to any student of medical history.

Way, S.: Carcinoma of the vulva. Am. J. Obstet. Gynecol., 79:692, 1960.
The names of Taussig, Basset, Twombly, Collins, and others all come to mind during any discussion of vulvar cancer. Way must certainly be included among those who have made major contributions to the knowledge of these diseases and their surgical treatment. This article summarizes his experiences and is the classic.

Williams, R. H. (Ed.): Textbook of Endocrinology, 6th ed. Philadelphia, W. B. Saunders Company, 1981.
This classic textbook on human endocrinology considers much about human reproduction and endocrinology. It is concise, yet provides detailed information regarding the physiology and biochemistry of this system.

Yen, S. S. C., and Jaffe, R. B.: Reproductive Endocrinology, 2nd ed. Philadelphia, W. B. Saunders Company, 1984.
This detailed book provides excellent material regarding gynecologic endocrinology at both the basic and the clinical levels. The reader is referred to it for further details of these problems.

Young, D. D., and Ehrnhardt, A. A. (Eds.): Psychosomatic Obstetrics and Gynecology. New York, Appleton-Century-Crofts, 1980.
Patients are seen with increasing frequency with psychosomatic or biobehavioral gynecologic complaints. This text provides a starting point in the assessment of the problems of such patients.

46

THE URINARY SYSTEM

David F. Paulson, M.D.

ANATOMY[7]

The kidneys and ureters are paired structures. The kidneys are responsible for the formation of urine, and the ureters are responsible for conduction of the formed urine into the single midline bladder. The paired kidneys each are about 9 to 15 cm. long, 4 to 5 cm. wide, and approximately 3 cm. thick (Fig. 1). The paired kidneys lie on each side of the vertebral column between the parietal peritoneum and the fascia and the musculature of the posterior abdominal wall. They are embedded in a variable amount of fat and surrounded by a special layer of fascia (Gerota's fascia) (Fig. 2). The kidneys lie on the side of the psoas muscles; and for this reason they are not parallel, the upper poles being approximately 2 cm. from the midline and the lower poles approximately 3.5 cm. from the midline. The anterior relationships of the two kidneys vary somewhat between individuals; however, an awareness of the structures overlying the kidneys when they are approached from the ventral surface is necessary for the surgeon in order that damage to these structures be avoided (Fig. 3). The kidney may be approached from a transabdominal transperitoneal route, through a flank incision that enters directly into the retroperitoneal space, displacing the peritoneal envelope anteriorly, or through a posterior incision that provides ready access into the renal pelvis.

EMBRYOLOGY OF THE URINARY SYSTEM[7,8,16,17]

The adult human kidney develops progressively as three distinct entities: pronephros, mesonephros, and metanephros (Fig. 4). The pronephros is the most primitive form of renal development and disappears completely by the fourth week of embryonic life. The embryonic mesonephros corresponds to the mature excretory organ of higher fish and amphibians. It is the principal excretory organ during the fourth to eighth week of embryonic life, but it gradually disintegrates, although parts of its ductal system remain associated with the male reproductive organs. The final phase in the development of the nephric system originates from both the intermediate mesoderm and the mesonephric duct. The joining of the ureter, which arises from the wolffian duct, with the mesoderm of the nephrogenic cord is necessary for the final development of the collecting tubules and functioning nephrons. The development begins in the 5- to 6-mm. embryo with a budlike outgrowth from the mesonephric duct. This ureteral bud grows cephalad and collects mesoderm from the nephrogenic cord of the intermediate mesoderm. This mesoderm with the metanephric cap migrates progressively cephalad, and during this migration the metanephric cap becomes larger and undergoes internal differentiation. As the kidney matures, it migrates upward from the region of the fourth to the first lumbar vertebra and progressively rotates so that the originally dorsal border becomes the convex lateral border. The ureter (metanephric duct) develops as a hollow outgrowth (ureteric bud) from the inferior end of the mesonephric duct. This metanephric duct grows cephalad, its blind end expanding to form the renal pelvis. As this primitive renal pelvis comes in

contact with the undifferentiated metanephrogenic mass at the caudal end of the urogenital ridge, it branches into primary tubules that in turn branch to form secondary tubules. The secondary tubules then form tertiary tubules and the branching goes on until approximately 12 generations of tubules are formed. The primary tubules develop into the major calyces of the adult kidney; the tubules of the second through the fourth generation fuse to form the minor calyces, those of the fifth order form the papillary ducts, and the higher orders form the several generations of collecting tubules. Each blind-ending collecting tubule develops into a secretory tubule with its associated Bowman's capsule and glomerulus.

During its formation by the union of the ureteric bud and the nephrogenic tissue, the kidney progressively migrates out of the pelvis and into the upper portion of the retroperitoneum. Renal ectopia, or the location of a kidney in a fixed position below its normal adult level, must be viewed as a failure of normal ascent. The kidney may fail to leave the true pelvis, or it may remain at any higher level in its retroperitoneal ascent. As the kidney ascends, it is supplied by progressively cephalad arteries. If the kidney fails to reach its normal adult position, it often retains an anomalous blood supply that arises from the aorta or its branches below the level of the definitive renal arteries. Moreover, as a kidney undergoes cephalad migration, it undergoes a "rotation" so that the renal pelvis, which in the embryo faces ventrally, comes to face medially with the major calyces projecting laterally. Ectopic kidneys, which have failed to ascend to the normal position, frequently fail to undergo rotation and their pelves still face forward.

Abnormal development of the kidneys leads to development of abnormalities that may make clinical care of the patient difficult. Failure of the metanephros to ascend properly leads to an "ectopic" kidney. The ectopic kidney may be on the proper side or it may be on the opposite side (a cross-ectopy) with or without fusion to the contralateral renal mass. Failure of the kidney to rotate during ascent produces a malrotated kidney. Fusion of the paired metanephric masses in the pelvis prior to ascent leads to various abnormalities, the most common being a "horseshoe kidney."

During development, the cloaca also undergoes subdivision, which changes the relationships of the mesonephric ducts and the ureter, and they come to have separate openings rather than a common one. As the cloaca is divided by the urorectal septum, the ureter migrates to empty into the larger ventral derivative of the cloaca, which becomes the urinary bladder. Growth of the bladder then leads to an absorption of the lower ends of the two mesonephric ducts so that these ducts and ureters open separately into the bladder. Further growth results in additional separation between the openings of the ureters and the mesonephric ducts and occurs in such a manner that the openings of the ureters remain some distance apart on the posterior wall of the bladder, while the openings of the mesonephric ducts are shifted farther distally into the urogenital sinus. Once this has been accomplished, the urinary ductal system in the male is completely separated from the genital ductal system.

The ureteral bud that arises from the mesonephric duct may

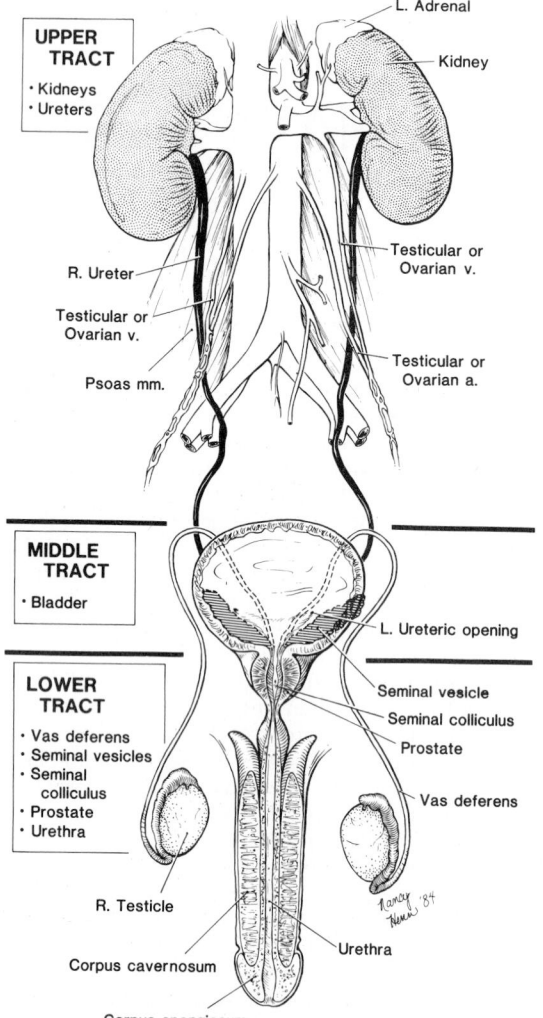

Figure 1. Anatomy of the male genitourinary tract. The upper and middle tracts have urologic function only. The lower tract has both genital and urinary functions.

bifurcate, causing a bifid ureter at varying levels. An accessory ureteral bud may develop from the mesonephric duct, thereby forming a duplicated ureter. If the ureteral buds are close together on the mesonephric duct, they will open near each other in the bladder. When this occurs, the main ureteral bud, which is the first to appear, and the most caudal of the mesonephric ducts will reach the bladder first and then move upward and laterally and will be followed later by a second accessory bud. When this occurs, the main ureteral bud drains the lower portion of the kidney, the lower ureteral bud draining the upper

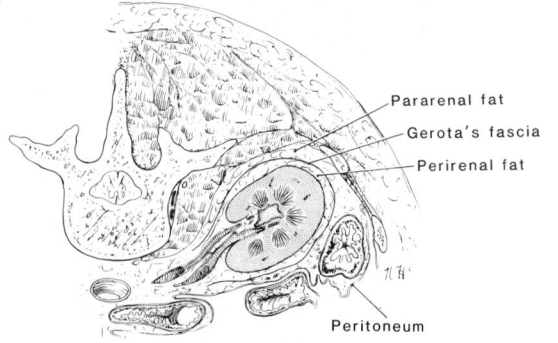

Figure 2. Diagram of the renal fascia in a cross section through the posterior abdominal wall.

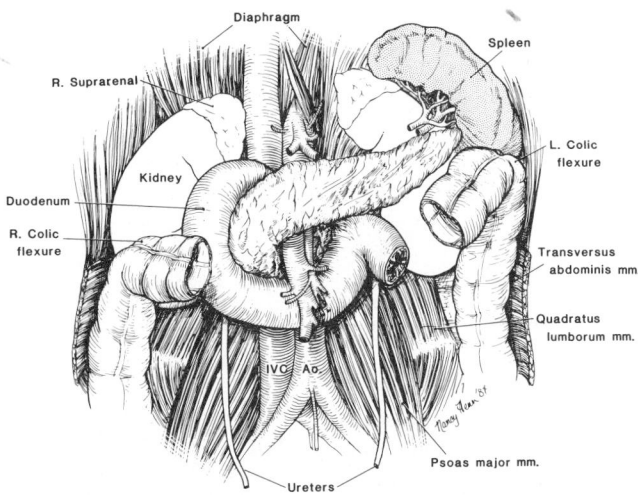

Figure 3. Some relations of the kidneys, anterior view. Compare with Figure 2.

portion of the kidney. The two ureteral buds will have reversed their relationship as they move from the mesonephric duct to the urogenital sinus. This is the reason double ureters always cross (the Weigert-Meyer law). Failure of development of a ureteral bud leads to the production of a solitary kidney with a hemitrigone in the bladder.

PHYSIOLOGY OF THE URINARY TRACT[2,14]

The kidney is divided into a cortex and medulla. The cortex contains glomeruli and portions of the tubules and is located peripherally. The medulla, located centrally, is composed primarily of the remaining portions of the tubules and the collecting ducts (Fig. 5). Urine formation is initiated by filtration, which is accomplished within the glomerulus. The composition of the glomerular filtrate within the tubules is altered by reabsorption of specific solutes and water and by the secretion of specific substances.

SIGNS AND SYMPTOMS OF UROLOGIC DISEASE

Frequently pain is the initial indication of disease involving the urinary tract. Renal pain, ureteral pain, and bladder pain have distinct characteristics, and a careful history often suggests the diagnosis and directs the attention of the surgeon to a specific anatomic site (Table 1). Renal pain may be dull and aching in character, localized to the flank. In contrast, it may be sharp, localized in the flank, or radiate into the lower abdomen or the buttocks. It may be episodic, appearing in waves, or it may be persistent and may produce loss of appetite with nausea and vomiting. Renal pain, when dull in character, often indicates a long-standing process such as chronic infection or a slowly growing tumor. With severe renal discomfort, the patient tends to be restless and may hold his flank in an attempt to minimize the discomfort.

Ureteral pain may cause flank discomfort and may be associated with severe abdominal pain, nausea, and vomiting. As the clot or calculus moves distally in the ureter, the pain radiates from the flank to the lower abdomen and may radiate into the scrotum or the labia majora, or occasionally into the thigh. A calculus in the lower ureter, or at the ureterovesicle junction, may cause urinary frequency with urgency and painful urination.

Bladder pain is usually dull and aching in nature, localized to the suprapubic area. When it is accompanied by an acute infection, the pain is severe and precipitates a desire to void.

Figure 4. Schematic representation of the development of the nephric system. Only a few of the tubules of the pronephros are seen in the fourth week, while the mesonephric tissue differentiates into mesonephric tubules that progressively join the mesonephric duct. The first sign of the ureteral bud from the mesonephric duct is seen. At 6 weeks, the pronephros has completely degenerated and the mesonephric tubules start to do so. The ureteral bud grows dorsocranially and has met the metanephrogenic cap. At the eighth week, there is cranial migration of the differentiating metanephros. The cranial end of the ureteric bud expands and starts to show multiple successive outgrowths.

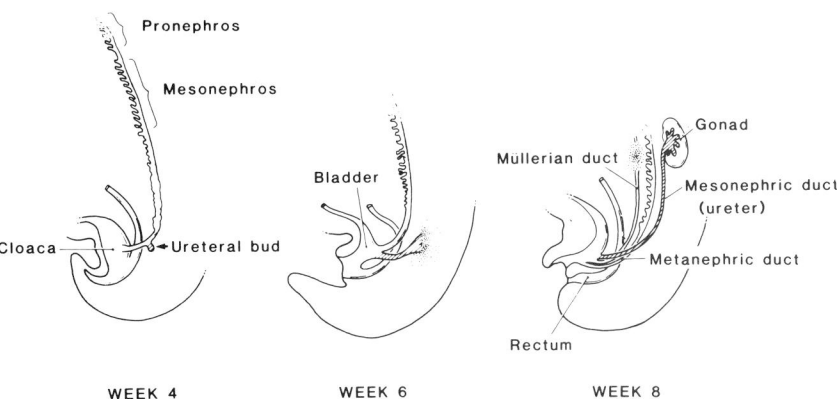

EVALUATION OF THE PATIENT WITH URINARY TRACT DISEASE

Physical Examination

Patients who present with the signs and symptoms of urinary tract disease, or present with disordered urinary renal function, deserve a complete evaluation that consists of a physical examination, laboratory studies to determine the degree of renal functional impairment, and imaging studies that permit definition of the anatomy of the urinary tract. Patients with urologic complaints should have a complete physical examination. Inspection of the abdomen may disclose a lower midline mass when the bladder is full and flattening rather than accentuation of the transverse lower abdominal crease. In adults, neither the distended bladder nor the hydronephrotic kidney is easy to define. However, in the child, the bladder is an intra-abdominal organ and is readily palpated and ballotted. Similarly, the child's kidney is easily palpated and transilluminated. To palpate the kidney, the patient should be supine and the physician should place one hand posteriorly on the flank and press with another hand anteriorly on the abdomen. Careful observation of any alteration in the position of the mass as the patient breathes or moves from a supine to a lateral or erect posture may identify the nature of the mass. When the kidney is tense or inflamed, sudden pressure in the costovertebral angle may produce pain.

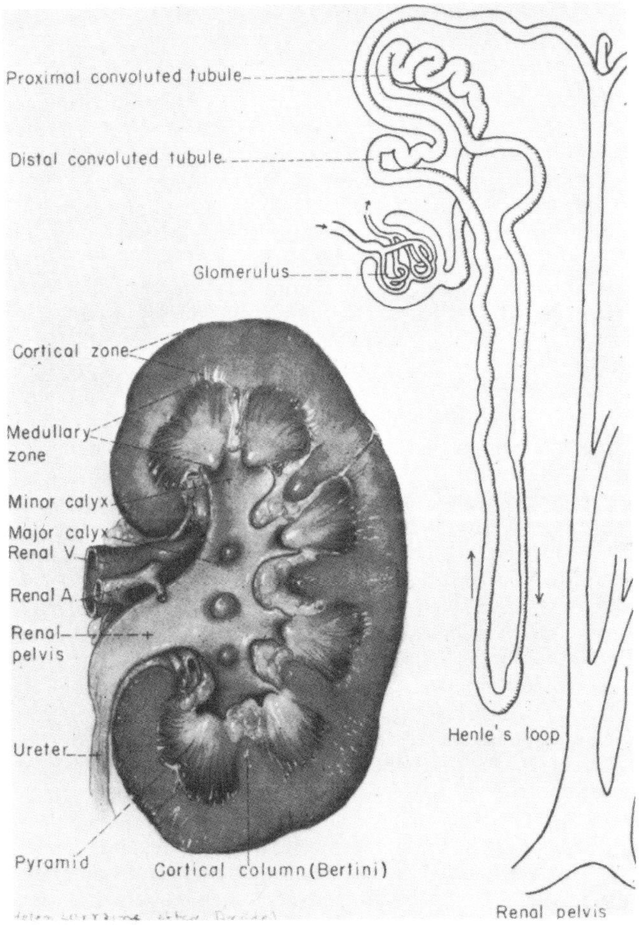

Laboratory Studies

After completion of the physical examination, the physician should obtain laboratory studies that further define the nature of the abnormality.

URINALYSIS.[6] Care should be taken to obtain the urine without contamination by the foreskin in the male or the vulva and labia in the female. It is best to discard the first portion of the voided stream, since this may contain urethral contaminates. The midportion of the stream usually reflects the pathologic process ongoing within the bladder. The third portion of the urinary stream may be discarded. In the male, the foreskin should be stripped from the glans penis and the glans cleansed with either saline or zephrine. In the female, the labia should be separated and the female instructed to initiate voiding and then to collect the midportion of the urinary stream in a wide-mouth container.

The urine should be analyzed for (1) specific gravity, (2) pH, (3) protein, (4) sugar, (5) acetone, (6) red blood cells, (7) white blood cells, (8) bacteria, (9) casts, and (optional studies) bilirubin, osmolality, and cytologic findings.

EVALUATION OF THE RENAL FUNCTION. It is necessary that the clinician determine the renal function of each patient with urinary tract disease. An evaluation of the total renal function is achieved by determining endogenous wastes in the blood such as urea or creatinine and the excretion of these substances in the urine. The serum creatinine level is a better indication of renal function than is the blood urea nitrogen. Both substances are excreted by glomerular filtration; however, the amount of urea that is available for excretion is quite variable. After hemorrhage, there may be excessive protein breakdown with a marked increase in the total urea production, while creatinine production is essentially constant. The creatinine clearance test is a ready measure of glomerular filtration rate. The measured excretion of specifically administered substances such as inulin or *para*-aminohippurate measures specific aspects of the renal function. Inulin clearance measures primarily glomerular filtration; *para*-aminohippurate, secreted by the proximal tubule, is primarily a measure of renal plasma flow. All of the excretory

Figure 5. Cross section of kidney showing gross anatomic relationships. *Inset:* Diagrammatic representation of the nephron shown joining a collecting duct. (From Dodson, A. I.: *In* Campbell, M. F. (Ed.): Urology. Philadelphia, W. B. Saunders Company, 1954.)

TABLE 1. Signs and Symptoms of Urologic Disease

Sign or Symptom	Definition	Disease Process
Hematuria	Blood in the urine (gross or microscopic)	Malignancy, calculus, iatrogenic injury, infection, trauma, foreign body
Pneumaturia	Air (gas) in the urine	Fistula between bowel and urinary tract, iatrogenic injury, infection
Pyuria	Pus in the urine	Infection
Nocturia	Awakening at night to void	Infection, obstruction (incomplete voiding), neurologic disease, metabolic disorder (diabetes mellitus, diabetes insipidus), congestive heart failure, renal failure, excessive fluid intake
Frequency	Voiding more than three to five times daily	Infection, obstruction, neurologic disease, metabolic disorder, excessive fluid intake, functional disease, psychogenic disorder
Polyuria	Greater than normal urine volume	Metabolic disease (diabetes mellitus, diabetes insipidus, adrenal insufficiency, etc.), renal disease, excessive fluid intake
Oliguria	Volume less than 400 ml. daily	Renal disease, cardiovascular disease, toxic drug effect
Anuria	No urine output	Obstruction, calculous disease, renal failure
Urgency	Precipitous desire to void	Infection, calculous disease, malignancy, idiopathic, neurogenic disease
Dysuria	Painful voiding	Infection, malignancy, calculus
Hesitancy	Delay and difficulty in beginning to void	Obstruction, neurogenic disease
Incontinence	Involuntary loss of urine	Anatomic loss of bladder support (stress incontinence), fistula, loss of sphincter control (urgent or iatrogenic)

tests (creatinine clearance, inulin clearance, and *para*-aminohippurate clearance) depend on a complete urine collection for accuracy.

IMAGING THE ANATOMY OF THE URINARY TRACT[11]

Imaging of the Urinary Tract

Multiple methods are now available to image the urinary tract. Whereas in years past, most of the imaging studies permitted only a structural or anatomic evaluation of the urinary tract, many of the imaging studies now also provide an assessment of function. Current methodology includes excretory urography with nephrotomography, retrograde ureteropyelography, retrograde cystography, arteriography, venography, digital venous arteriography, computed axial tomography, ultrasonography, radioisotope renography, and magnetic resonance imaging. Each of these studies provides different pieces of information that can be used to compile a complete understanding of the urinary tract pathology.

Excretory urography is dependent on renal function and visualizes the urinary tract by concentration of an intravenous injection of organic iodine within the urinary tract. The contrast material is excreted primarily by renal function and is concentrated as the glomerular filtrate is reabsorbed. The kidney and its collecting system become radiopaque as the x-rays are absorbed by the iodinated agent (Fig. 6). Increasing the amount of the iodinated contrast material that is delivered to the patient or dehydrating the patient to increase absorption of water from the

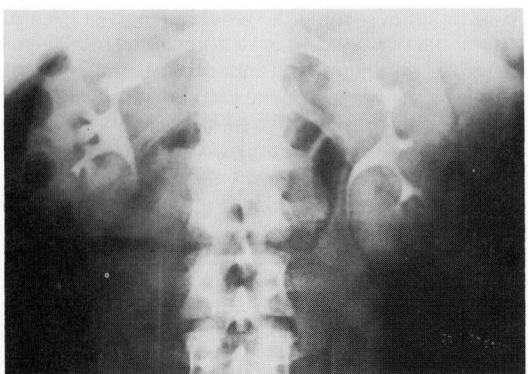

Figure 6. The iodinated contrast agent is excreted and appears in the collecting system. Note that the renal outline of the left kidney is sharp and distinct. The collecting system is delicate and shows no evidence of obstruction.

glomerular filtrate improves visualization. Excretory urography should be the first imaging study chosen for evaluation of the urinary tract. Excretory urography is specifically indicated when the suspected diagnosis is a space-occupying lesion of the kidney such as a cyst or tumor, pyelonephritis, hydronephrosis, hypertension, or urinary tract calculi. Since the ability to visualize the kidney and urinary tract is dependent upon renal function and the ability of the kidney to concentrate, the quality of the urinary tract imaging may be markedly diminished in the patient with compromised renal function. Excretory urograms may be contraindicated if there is any evidence of hypersensitivity to iodinated contrast materials or to foods or substances containing iodine. This contraindication is waived if this history is noted and the patient is appropriately prepared with steroids and antihistamines prior to injection of the contrast agent. Excretory urography is best avoided during pregnancy.

Retrograde ureteropyelograms require specific training in urologic instrumentation and are utilized when excretory urography fails to provide adequate visualization of the collecting system and ureter. Retrograde ureteropyelograms are indicated in patients in whom the excretory renograms do not provide adequate ureteropelvic detail, in patients in whom renal function is impaired to the point where it is anticipated that excretory urography will be inadequate, or when it is necessary to assess the level or degree of ureteral obstruction. They also may be utilized in patients who have a stated history of sensitivity to iodinated contrast agents.

Cystograms are performed by instilling the radiopaque contrast material into the bladder through the urethra. Roentgenograms are then taken to define the contour of the bladder. Cystography is indicated in patients with neurogenic bladder, in patients who are suspected of having pelvic trauma sufficient to rupture the bladder, and in patients who have recurrent infections or in whom a fistula in between the bladder and bowel or other pelvic organ is suspected. Cystography should be avoided during acute urinary tract infection since instillation of the contrast material under pressure may precipitate systemic infection by forcing bacteria into the lymphatics and venules of the bladder or kidney.

Arteriography permits visualization of the main renal artery(ies) and/or its branches. Arteriography is dependent upon the delivery of a specific volume of iodinated contrast material into the renal arterial system and is independent of renal function. Renal arteriography is indicated whenever a vascular malformation, malignancy, or renovascular hypertension is suspected. Since most primary renal tumors are hypervascular, they are readily identified. Renal angiography may produce transient depression in renal function, particularly in patients who already have compromised renal function.

Digital venous angiography is a new technology that utilizes computer-enhanced imaging of the renal vasculature following a venous injection of contrast material. This provides visualization of the arterial system of the kidney, but not in detail compatible with that of a direct arterial injection.

Venacavography is performed by the injection of iodinated contrast material into the vena cava. Venography is important to outline enlarged retroperitoneal structures that may impinge upon the vena cava or displace the vena cava, or to define extension of tumor from the renal vein into the vena cava itself.

Computed axial tomography utilizes technology in which the x-ray tube and the detection system are on opposite sides of the patient. During the conduct of this study, they rotate around the patient, recording information about the internal structure of the thin transverse cross section through which the x-ray beam crosses. A computer then "reconstructs" the cross-sectional image as an array or grid of individual picture elements. The image bears a resemblance to a transverse anatomical section. The approximate density of any tissue within the image can be determined. The computed axial tomograph provides information distinct from that obtained by the arteriogram or the excretory urogram. Its primary value is in determining the relationship of normal or abnormal anatomic structures to contiguous structures.

Ultrasonography uses vibrational energy generated at a frequency above the level of human hearing to produce information about the urinary tract. The primary advantage of ultrasonic scanning is that it is independent of renal function. Ultrasonography permits identification of solid and cystic masses within the kidney and identification of calculi.

Radioisotopic techniques permit the clinician to evaluate both anatomic structure and function of the kidney without distorting normal physiologic processes. The radiopharmaceuticals used to evaluate the kidney function do not impose the hypertonic or chemical stress associated with intravenous iodinated contrast material, and the low iodine content of the iodinated radiopharmaceuticals is not associated with any hypersensitivity risks. These pharmaceuticals are detected externally so that instrumentation may be avoided. The radiotracers provide information concerning renal position, anatomy, and function (Table 2). In the radionuclide renogram, computer analysis of the critical areas is produced as a function of time following injection of the radiopharmaceutical. There are essentially three portions of the curve: a vascular phase, a functional phase, and a drainage phase. An analysis of the differential occurrence of these three portions of the radioisotopic renogram provides a differential assessment between the renal and ureteral function on both the right and the left sides.

Magnetic resonance imaging permits the physician to image both bony and parenchymal structures in transverse and sagittal planes utilizing information derived from hydrogen nuclei. Because hydrogen nuclei contain an odd number of nucleons, they demonstrate a property called spin, and each nucleon generates a magnetic field similar to that of a small bar magnet. Although normally oriented in a random manner to each other, in the presence of a strong, external magnetic field, the protons become oriented in either a parallel or antiparallel direction. From this new state of equilibrium, the protons can be deflected either 90 or 180 degrees from the magnetic field by an applied radiofrequency pulse that causes the protons to resonate in a higher state of energy. Termination of the radiofrequency pulse allows the protons to return to the previous equilibrium, and the

TABLE 2. Radiopharmaceuticals for Urologic Diagnosis

Radiopharmaceutical	Usual Dose (μCi)	Radiation-Absorbed Dose (Rads) From Usual Doses		Usual Scintiphoto Exposure Time and Imaging Time Post Dose	Use
		Renal	Whole Body		
^{99m}Tc-Fe ascorbate DTPA ^{99m}Tc glucoheptonate ^{99m}Tc methylsuccinate	20,000	1.0	0.008	Serial: 4-sec. photos at 0–30 sec.; static: 2- to 4-min. photos at 30 min.	Localized in renal cortex by deposition and retention in renal tubular cells; uptake is proportionate to regional renal blood flow; rapid serial photos show renal blood flow distribution
^{99m}Tc-(Sn)-DTPA	20,000	0.1	0.030	Serial: 1- or 2-min. photos at 0–20 min. or longer; also useful to image blood flow	Excreted solely by glomerular filtration; useful for function imaging, but cortical definition versus background less than with other ^{99m}Tc agents
Sodium iothalamate (^{125}I)	50	Negligible	0.00015	Not useful for imaging	Glomerular filtration rate measurement
^{99m}Tc-(Sn)-DTPA	1000	0.03 (bladder)	0.001	Static views during filling of bladder, 6-sec. images during voiding	Direct radionuclide cystography to detect and measure reflux
Sodium iodohippurate (^{131}I)	200	0.080	0.0042 (assumes normal clearance)	2- to 10-min. photos (depending on renal function): 0–30 min. for normal function to 1–2 hours for poor function	Excreted by tubular function (like para-aminohippurate); 70–80% extraction causes rapid clearance in normal tissue; prolonged cortical transit time occurs in ischemic or other forms of tubular damage with increased water reabsorption
Sodium iodohippurate (^{123}I)	2000	0.01	0.0005	Serial images for 30 min. or longer for poor function	Excreted by tubular function; same uses as for ^{131}I-iodohippurate

From, Smith, D. R.: General Urology, 10th ed. Los Altos, Lange Medical Publishers, 1981; p. 103.

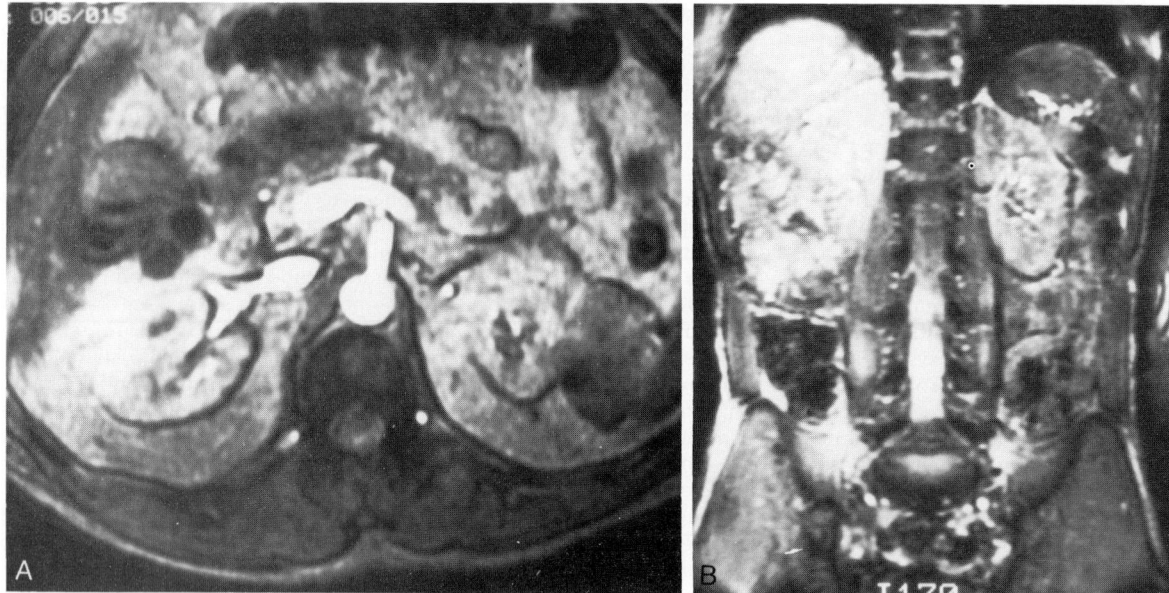

Figure 7. *A*, Magnetic resonance imaging transverse section at the level of the kidneys, demonstrating a large left renal cancer and a normal right kidney. Note that the vascular structures are white on this T3 weighted image. *B*, The image has been oriented at a coronal section, again demonstrating a large left renal cancer with a normal right renal unit. Note that the blood flow through the large left renal kidney causes this mass to be white in nature on the T3 weighted image.

absorbed energy is emitted as a radiofrequency that can be received by a detecting coil within the scanner. A computer processes the acquired information by a complex technique known as Fourier transformation, and an image is constructed from a set of encoded signals. In this manner, transverse, sagittal, and coronal views may be obtained.

Magnetic resonance imaging allows one to also determine flow patterns within vascular structures, permitting accurate determination of the vasculature supplying tumors or occluded by tumors. Magnetic resonance imaging has proved to be of great value in the staging of renal and prostatic malignancy (Figs. 7 and 8).

NONSURGICAL DISEASES OF THE URINARY TRACT

Nonsurgical diseases of the kidney can be divided into those medical renal diseases that may produce complications in the management of the patient undergoing surgical therapy and

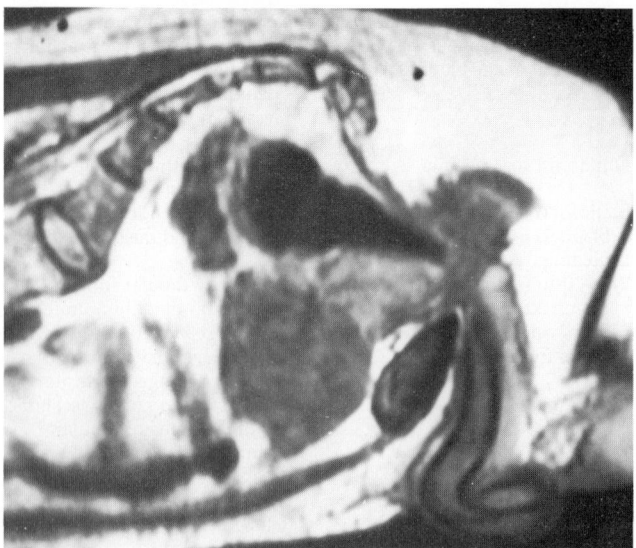

Figure 8. Sagittal section of the pelvis demonstrating the air-filled rectum posteriorly, the fluid-filled bladder anteriorly, and a large prostatic carcinoma.

those disease processes that may result from or be a concomitant of a surgical procedure. Most of the medical renal diseases produce specific alterations in the urinalysis and in the serum biochemical profile, which are indicators that the etiologic disease process must be identified prior to operation. Frequently the abnormalities produced by these disease processes cannot be reversed and the patient must be supported throughout the pre-, inter-, and postoperative surgical period by a coordinated effort of surgeon and nephrologist.

Renal Obstruction and Renal Parenchymal Failure

Postrenal obstruction may occur in a patient with bilateral renal calculi or a single kidney and calculus obstruction. It also is seen in patients with retroperitoneal fibrosis, in patients with retroperitoneal malignancies, or in patients who have unanticipated surgical occlusion of the ureters. *Acute intrarenal obstruction* occurs when the collecting tubules are blocked by crystals, debris, or Bence-Jones protein. Certain drugs such as the sulfonamides and methotrexate have been known to produce acute crystalluria with obstruction if administered in excessive dosages. Acute obstructive oxaluria can be seen after anesthesia with methoxyflurane or in patients who ingest ethylene glycol, commonly used in antifreeze. Acute uric acid nephropathy may be precipitated by use of cytotoxic drugs that cause nuclear lysis.

Surgical patients may be susceptible to gram-negative sepsis, particularly while undergoing hepatobiliary or colonic surgery. Moreover, there are certain specifically used drugs that are nephrotoxic and produce tubular necrosis (Table 3).

Renal parenchymal failure occurs with rapidly progressive glomerulonephritis, acute interstitial nephritis, or the toxic nephropathies. These processes are not readily correctable upon diagnosis; however, the etiology should be established in order that patients not be subjected to other procedures that may exacerbate their renal failure.

Urinary Tract Infection

The patient who presents with an acute urinary tract infection usually has symptoms related to the site and severity of the infection. The most frequent urinary tract infection is "cystitis," an infection within the bladder. Patients with cystitis present with urinary frequency, painful urination, urgency, suprapubic pain, and hematuria. Pyelonephritis occurs when the infection

TABLE 3. Common Nephrotoxins

Antibiotics	Aminoglycosides, cephalosporins, polymyxins, amphotericin, co-trimoxazole
Heavy metals	Mercury, arsenic, *cis*-platinum
Solvents	Carbon tetrachloride
X-ray contrast media	
Miscellaneous	Paraquat, paracetamol, *Amanita phallodes*

involves the kidney. "Acute pyelonephritis" is accompanied by flank pain, fever, chills, and occasionally nausea and vomiting. Acute pyelonephritis differs from acute cystitis in that most patients with bacterial cystitis do not have chills and fever. The diagnosis of the urinary tract infection is supported by urinalysis and confirmed by a positive urinary culture. The urine in a patient with an acute urinary tract infection yields an increased number of white cells. In the uncentrifuged urine specimen, 10 white blood cells per high-power field is indicative of an infection. The presence of bacteria in the wet smear or Gram stain of the urine supports the diagnosis. It should be recognized that the patient who is maintaining a high fluid volume and voiding frequently may have a urinalysis that appears normal but that on culture demonstrates bacteria. In the catheterized urine specimen, the presence of any pathogenic bacteria in the cultured specimen is indicative of infection. However, when the specimen is a midstream voided specimen, it currently is thought that the colony count must exceed more than 100,000 organisms per milliliter in order to confirm a urinary tract infection. Catheterized urine specimens are appropriate in the patient with a symptomatic and suspected urinary tract infection, since the introduction of a new infection in the patient already infected is unlikely.

Most urinary tract infections in nonhospitalized patients are ascending infections and occur by entrance of bacteria along the urethra into the bladder. This concept supports the observation that the incidence of urinary tract infections is greater in the female with the short urethra than in the male whose urethra is much longer. Pyelonephritis usually results from the ascent of bacteria from the bladder up the ureter to the kidney. However,

hematogenous spread of infection from other sites to the kidney can occur. The most commonly encountered organisms and the drug of choice are listed in Table 4. Dosages of the commonly used drugs and their side effects are given in Table 5.

Gram-Negative Septicemia[4]

The most serious accompaniment of an infection of the urinary tract is the production of gram-negative septicemia. Gram-negative septicemia may produce two distinctly different hemodynamic events. It is necessary that the physician recognize the differences between hypodynamic and hyperdynamic septic shock, since the management is different (Table 6). In both instances, identification of the organism involved and delivery of organism-specific antibiotics is the fundamental basis of treatment. In the patient with gram-negative shock whose intravenous pressure is low, fluids for intravascular expansion should be given rapidly to restore intravascular volume and pressure. When the hematocrit is decreased, intravascular volume should be expanded with whole blood. If central venous pressure rises, indicating progressive myocardial failure, a cardiac glycoside or isoproterenol is a suitable drug. Isoproterenol, a beta-adrenergic agent, increases the force of contraction of the heart while relaxing the smooth muscles of the splanchnic bed to cause vascular dilation. In hypodynamic shock, peripheral resistance is increased, and isoproterenol aids in shunting circulation back into the capillary bed, relieving tissue anoxia and helping to correct acidosis. The alpha-adrenergic blocking agents, such as phenoxybenzamine, relax arterioles and venules to enhance the circulation. As this occurs, intravascular volume may be depleted and further vascular expansion may be necessary. The use of corticosteroids to reduce peripheral resistance and increase cardiac output has been advocated, but their benefit is unproven. Associated abnormalities that accompany septic shock, such as acidosis and hyperkalemia, should be treated as recognized. The acidosis may be corrected with bicarbonate, and acute hyperkalemia may be managed by the simultaneous administration of glucose and insulin to increase potassium uptake by the cells.

TABLE 4. Choices of Drugs for Microorganisms Commonly Encountered in Infections of the Urinary and Genital Tracts

	Drug(s) of Choice	Alternative Drug(s)
Gram-Positive Cocci		
Staphylococcus aureus (β-lactamase-producing)	Nafcillin or cephradine*	Vancomycin
Staphylococcus (non-β-lactamase-producing)	Penicillin G	Erythromycin
Streptococcus, group D		
Streptococcus faecalis (also *Streptococcus faecium*, enterococci)	Ampicillin plus gentamicin†	Penicillin G plus amikacin
Streptococcus bovis	Penicillin G	Vancomycin
Streptococcus, group B	Ampicillin	Cephalexin*
Gram-Negative Cocci		
Gonococcus	Penicillin G plus probenecid	Tetracycline
Gonococcus (β-lactamase-producing)	Spectinomycin	Cefoxitin plus probenecid
Gram-Negative Rods		
Escherichia coli	Sulfonamide or ampicillin	Gentamicin or probenecid
Klebsiella sp.	Gentamicin	Cefamandole
Enterobacter sp.	Gentamicin	Cefamandole
Proteus mirabilis	Ampicillin	Gentamicin
Proteus vulgaris and others	Gentamicin or amikacin	Cefoxitin or chloramphenicol
Pseudomonas aeruginosa	Gentamicin plus carbenicillin	Polymyxin or colistimethate
Serratia sp.	Co-trimoxazole and polymyxin	Gentamicin or amikacin
Haemophilus vaginalis	Metronidazole	Tetracycline
Chlamydiae (*Chlamydia trachomatis*)	Tetracycline	Erythromycin
Mycoplasmas (*Ureaplasma urealyticum*)	Erythromycin	Tetracycline

* Or other oral cephalosporin.
† Or amoxicillin.

TABLE 5. Antimicrobials Often Used in Urology

Drug	Route	Daily Adult Dose	Daily Pediatric Dose	Untoward Effects
Soluble sulfonamide (sulfisoxazole, trisulfapyrimidines)	Oral	1 gm. 4 times	100–150 mg./kg.	Rashes, fever, nausea, vomiting, diarrhea, arthritis, stomatitis, thrombocytopenia, hemolytic or aplastic anemia, granulocytopenia, hepatitis, vasculitis, Stevens-Johnson syndrome, psychosis, etc.; crystalluria and hematuria rare
Trimethoprim	Oral	100 mg. twice	15–30 mg./kg.	
Trimethoprim-sulfamethoxazole (co-trimoxazole)	Oral	4 tablets	Trimethoprim, 15 mg./kg., and sulfamethoxazole, 150 mg./kg.	
Ampicillin	Oral	2–4 gm.	50–100 mg./kg.	Hypersensitivity: rashes, fever, anaphylaxis, dermatitis, serum sickness, nephritis, eosinophilia, vasculitis, hemolytic anemia, granulocytopenia; nausea, vomiting, diarrhea especially with oral penicillins; CNS toxicity with very large doses and renal insufficiency
	IV	2–10 gm.	100–300 mg./kg.	
Amoxicillin	Oral	0.75–1.5 gm.	20–40 mg./kg.	
Carbenicillin	Oral	1.5–3 gm.	50–70 mg./kg.	
	IV	30 gm.	100–600 mg./kg.	
Ticarcillin	IV	200–300 mg./kg.	200–300 mg./kg.	
Nafcillin	Oral	2–4 gm.	50–100 mg./kg.	
	IV	3–12 gm.	100–200 mg./kg.	
Dicloxacillin	Oral	1–2 gm.	25–50 mg./kg.	
Penicillin V or G	Oral	1.6–3.2 million units	0.05–0.1 million units/kg.	
Penicillin G	IV	1.2–20 million units	0.05–0.3 million units/kg.	
Cefazolin	IV	3–6 gm.	25–100 mg./kg.	Same as with penicillins
Cephalothin	IV	3–12 gm.	60–100 mg./kg.	
Cefoxitin	IV	3–12 gm.	?	
Cefamandole	IV	2–10 gm.	50–150 mg./kg.	
Cephalexin	Oral	1–4 gm.	25–50 mg./kg.	
Cephradine	Oral	1–4 gm.	25–50 mg./kg.	
Tetracycline	Oral	1–2 gm.	20–40 mg./kg.	Fever, rashes, anorexia, nausea, diarrhea, yellow mottling of teeth and bones, liver damage, vestibular reactions, renal tubular damage
Oxytetracycline	Oral	1–2 gm.	20–40 mg./kg.	
Doxycycline	Oral	200 mg.	2.5–4 mg./kg.	
Minocycline	Oral	200 mg.	2.5–4 mg./kg.	
Chloramphenicol	Oral	1–3 gm.	50 mg./kg.	Anorexia, nausea, diarrhea, aplastic anemia (rare), gray syndrome in neonates
	IV	2–4 gm.	50–100 mg./kg.	
Erythromycin	Oral	1–2 gm.	30–50 mg./kg.	Anorexia, nausea, diarrhea, cholestatic hepatitis as a hypersensitivity reaction
Gentamicin	IM or IV	3–5 mg./kg.	3–5 mg./kg.	Nephrotoxicity and ototoxicity
Tobramycin	IM or IV	3–5 mg./kg.	3–5 mg./kg.	
Amikacin	IM or IV	15 mg./kg.	15 mg./kg.	
Kanamycin	IM or IV	15 mg./kg.	15 mg./kg.	
Polymyxin B	IV	2.5 mg./kg.	1.5–2.5 mg./kg.	Paresthesias, dizziness, nephrotoxicity.
Colistimethate	IM	2.5–5 mg./kg.	2.5 mg./kg.	
Nitrofurantoin	Oral	200–400 mg.	5–7 mg./kg.	Nausea, vomiting, rashes, pulmonary infiltrates, rare neurotoxicity
Methenamine hippurate	Oral	2 gm.	75 mg./kg.	Vesical irritation
Methenamine mandelate	Oral	4 gm.	75 mg./kg.	
Nalidixic acid	Oral	4 gm.	30–60 mg./kg.	Rashes, gastrointestinal disturbances, visual and CNS disturbances, photosensitization (rare)
Oxolinic acid	Oral	4 gm.	—	

THE KIDNEYS

RENAL CALCULI

The calcium oxalate calculus is the most common urinary stone in the United States, 33 per cent of recovered stones being pure calcium oxalate. Approximately 34 per cent of all stones are mixtures of calcium oxalate and phosphate; approximately 15 per cent are magnesium ammonium phosphate, 6 per cent pure calcium phosphate, 8 per cent uric acid, and 3 per cent cystine. Conditions that promote an alkaline pH of the urine (urinary tract infections, metabolic disease such as hyperparathyroidism, renal tubular acidosis, and medullary sponge kidney) predispose to an increased incidence of calcium phosphate stones. Discussion of the etiology and medical prevention of each specific type of stone is beyond the scope of this chapter. Nonetheless, the goal of each physician who treats the patient with renal calculous disease should be to attempt to (1) identify the chemical composition of the stone, (2) initiate therapy designed to remove the stone, (3) establish medical therapy designed to prevent recurrence of the stone, and (4) control any associated urinary tract infection.

Diagnostic Studies

An *intravenous pyelogram* should be obtained in all patients who present with the symptoms (flank pain; cramping, abdominal discomfort radiating to the groin, scrotum, or labia; microscopic hematuria) of urinary calculi. The plain scout film of the intravenous pyelogram identifies the location of the stone and directs the form of intervention. The intravenous pyelogram also reveals whether the stone is obstructing, or partially obstructing, and identifies any anatomic condition that produces stasis (such as ureteropelvic junction obstruction, pyelonephric scarring, or calyceal diverticulum), which will promote stone formation (Fig. 9).

TABLE 6. Findings in Patients with Gram-Negative Septicemic Shock

	Circulatory States	
	Hypodynamic	Hyperdynamic
Arterial blood pressure	↓	↓
Pulse rate	↑	↑
Central venous pressure	↓	↑
Urine flow	↓	↓
Hematocrit	↑	May be normal
With arterial blood samples, the following are measured:		
Cardiac index	↓	↑
Blood gases		
Po₂	↓	↓
Pco₂	↓	↓
Blood lactate	↑	↑
Blood pH	↓	Normal or ↑

Surgical Management

The presence of a calculus in the urinary tract is not an indication for open surgical therapy. Prior to this date, many calculi in the urinary tract were observed only, either because they were asymptomatic or because they were of small enough size that spontaneous passage through the urinary tract was a high likelihood. However, in today's high-technology world, methods exist for the nonsurgical removal of many of these calculi either by ultrasonic energy delivered through a hollow probe or by extracorporeal shock waves focused through a fluid medium on the offending calculi in such a way as to initiate dissolution of the calculus itself. It is axiomatic that all calculi producing obstruction, intractable pain, persistent urinary tract infection despite appropriate antibiotic therapy, or progressive renal deterioration should be removed. Only when there is an associated anatomic abnormality within the kidney, such as outflow obstruction at the ureteropelvic junction, such that this obstruc-

tion will promote future stone formation by promoting stasis, is it necessary to proceed with surgical exploration for removal of the stone with simultaneous correction of the defect. There are instances in which the amount of stone burden is such that open surgical removal is necessary; however, almost all stones can be managed by a combination of percutaneous ultrasonic lithotripsy and extracorporeal shock wave lithotripsy. Although previous texts dealing with the urinary system have devoted considerable space to the open surgical removal of calculi of the urinary tract, these operative procedures are of historical interest and are not included in this discussion.

Use of Ultrasonic Lithotripsy and Extracorporeal Shock Wave Lithotripsy

ULTRASONIC LITHOTRIPSY. By use of a piezoceramic crystal to generate a high-frequency sound wave vibration (2300 to 2700 Hz.), acoustic energy is transmitted via an acoustic horn that focuses the sound wave longitudinally down a rigid-hollow steel rod, concentrating the energy at the end of the rod. The renal stone is broken when the probe end contacts the stone as the end of the probe strikes the stone several thousand times per second, essentially battering the stone until it fractures. Fluid circulates through the ultrasound probe, and, with the circulation of this fluid, the small stone pieces are removed as they are created. Access to the stone in the kidney occurs by making a puncture wound in the skin and placing a long sharp probe through the renal substance itself, into the collecting system. Through this hollow needle is passed a guidewire, over which are passed either hollow dilating probes of increasing size or a dilating balloon. Once access to the kidney has been created by progressive dilation, the rigid uretero-scope is passed through the flank and renal substance, and the stone is visualized. The ultrasound probe is then inserted and the stone is fragmented. Both stone and associated blood fragments are suctioned away (Fig. 10). Using this technique, stones of various size can be fragmented and removed from the kidney without the necessity for open surgery.

EXTRACORPOREAL SHOCK WAVE LITHOTRIPSY. Extracorporeal shock wave lithotripsy is based on the principle that shock waves, generated in a fluid medium, can be focused through that fluid medium and through the human body to impact and destroy calculi within the urinary tract. Currently, the shock waves are generated either by an underwater spark discharge unit in which a capacitor stores electrical energy that is released within a microsecond, or by the simultaneous discharge of thousands of piezoelectrodes, similarly activated by an electrical discharge. This discharge gives rise to a shock wave in the surrounding fluid, which then propagates concentrically in a manner similar to sound waves in air, expanding from its origin until it hits a solid structure. To transfer the pressure of these shock waves to the renal calculus, the shock wave created by the underwater spark discharge unit is focused using a rota-

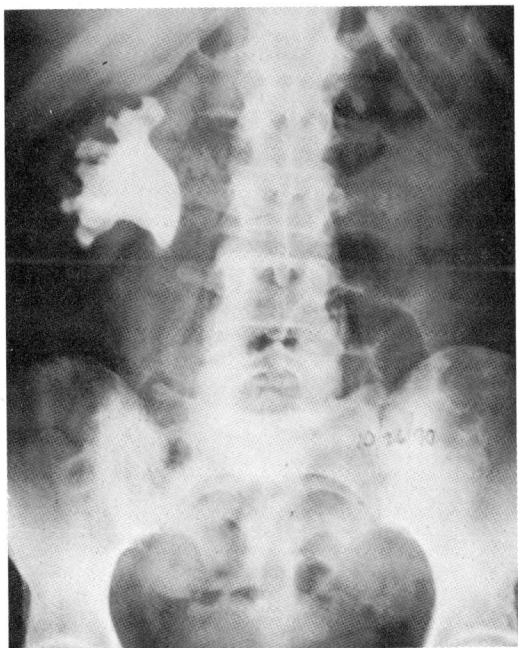

Figure 9. KUB view demonstrating large right staghorn calculus. While many surgeons may favor an anatrophic nephrolithotomy for removal of this calculus, it is feasible to remove calculi like this through an extended pyelolithotomy. The rather short unobstructed infundibula seen in this case make removal of the calculus through an extended pyelolithotomy possible. (From Paulson, D. F.: Genitourinary Surgery. New York, Churchill Livingstone, 1983, p. 62.)

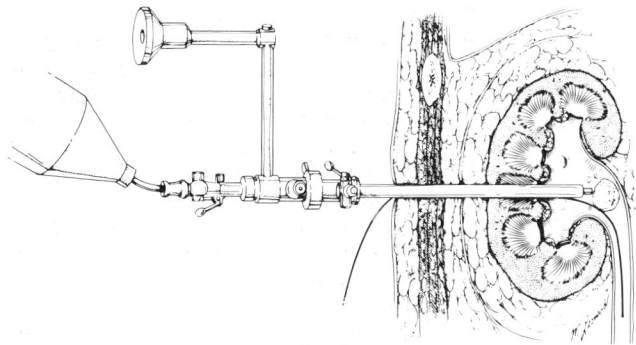

Figure 10. A percutaneous nephroscope has been placed through the body wall and the kidney. The stone that lies within the collecting system of the kidney can be visualized and destroyed by ultrasound waves.

tionally specific semi-ellipsoid whose walls are placed around the first geometric focus of the geometric configuration to direct the shock wave energy in a singular path. The electrode within the semi-ellipsoid and the patient are positioned so that the second geometric focus positioned by the shape of the ellipsoid is at the center of the calculus. Thus, reflection of waves from the ellipsoid walls transfers the maximal energy from the spark gap electrode to the center of the calculus itself. Shock waves generated by the piezoelectrode are focused on the stone without use of the semi-ellipsoid, but by specific focusing of the piezoelectrode crystals. The energy delivered by the spark gap generator and the area of entry of the energy through the patient's body are such that general anesthesia is required for pain relief during the treatment. However, with the piezoelectrode shock wave lithotriptors, the entry point of the shock wave is so diffuse that the treatments can be delivered without anesthesia, the patient essentially walking in, lying down on the instrument, and being able to arise after the treatment and walk from the treatment facility. It is currently thought that approximately 75 to 80 per cent of all patients with renal calculi can be managed by extracorporeal shock wave lithotripsy, and nearly all patients can be managed by a combination of extracorporeal shock wave lithotripsy and percutaneous ultrahydraulic lithotripsy. Thus, open stone surgery for the management of renal calculous disease has become largely an item of historical interest.

Metabolic Evaluation of the Patient with Recurrent Calculi

The patient who presents with recurrent stone disease should be evaluated to determine if there is a correctable metabolic cause for the stone formation. Initially the physician should obtain a complete blood count; an SMA-12 including serum calcium, phosphorus, uric acid, creatinine, blood urea nitrogen, total protein with albumin:globulin ratio, and alkaline phosphatase; and measurement of serum electrolytes. A 24-hour urine collection should be obtained for calcium, uric acid, oxalate, mean pH, sodium concentration, and total volume. This 24-hour urine sample should be obtained on a random diet. A second set of serum samples is obtained at the conclusion of the 24-hour urine collection. The patient should then be placed on a restrictive calcium-sodium diet of approximately 400 mg. of calcium daily and 100 mg. of sodium. A second 24-hour urine is then collected for uric acid, creatinine, oxalate, calcium, sodium, pH, volume, and cyclic adenosine monophosphate (cyclic AMP). A third set of serum samples is then collected for the previous studies plus a serum parathormone test. Patients with uric acid calculi, cystine stones, or struvite calculi with an associated urinary tract infection do not require this detailed metabolic evaluation. Although most calcium stone-formers respond to thiazide diuretics, it is important to determine the etiology of recurrent stone formation. It should be possible to establish the cause in more than 80 per cent of calcium stone formers. Hypercalciuria is defined as the urinary calcium level that exceeds 200 mg. per 24 hours on a restricted calcium and sodium diet. An excretion of greater than 4 mg. calcium per kg. for 24 hours on a random diet is also considered excessive. Patients with normal serum calcium values who are hypercalciuric are categorized in the "idiopathic" hypercalciuric group and may be further subdivided into those with absorptive hypercalciuria and those with renal hypercalciuria.

A detailed outpatient evaluation of the hypercalciuric stone-forming patient should be done. A fasting 2-hour urine sample is obtained after an overnight fast, with a 4-hour urine sample then obtained following the administration of 1 gm. of calcium by mouth. These two urine samples then are analyzed for creatinine, calcium, and cyclic AMP. To promote diuresis, 600 ml. of distilled water is ingested at the beginning of the test, followed by 300 ml. at the time of calcium ingestion, with an additional

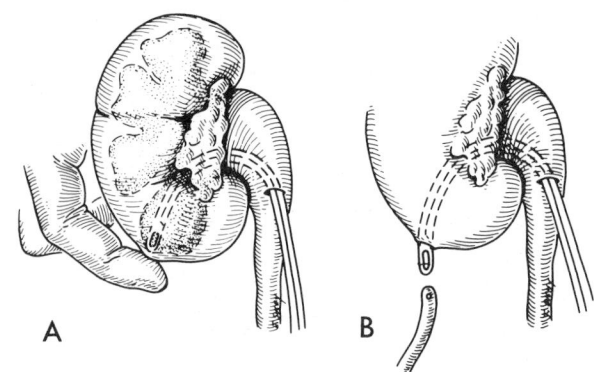

Figure 11. *A,* A sharply curved stone forceps was introduced into the interior calix through an opening in the renal pelvis and guided to the thinnest point of the parenchyma. *B,* The end of the clamp is pushed through the renal parenchyma, and a small (No. 12 or 14 Fr) red rubber catheter is tied to the end of the clamp. (From Paulson, D. F.: Genitourinary Surgery. New York, Churchill Livingstone, 1983, p. 37.)

300 ml. 2 hours later. A high excretion of calcium during the fasting state represents either impaired tubular absorption of calcium or excessive mobilization of calcium from bone. Intestinal calcium absorption can be assessed by renal calcium excretion after the calcium load. Fasting urinary calcium and cyclic AMP are increased in renal hypercalciuria caused by renal leak and in secondary hyperparathyroidism. Patients with absorptive hypercalciuria have a normal calcium excretion in the fasting state with an elevated urine calcium following an oral calcium load.

SURGICAL MANAGEMENT OF RENAL OBSTRUCTION[5]

Occasionally the renal outflow tract may be obstructed by stone, tumor, or an iatrogenic complication of other surgical therapy. When this occurs, drainage of the obstructed kidney must be accomplished. Current technology allows this to be accomplished either via an open surgical procedure or with a closed percutaneous technique. The preferred method today is to drain the upper tract using percutaneous techniques except when other events prompt open surgical exposure of the kidney (Figs. 11 and 12).

RENAL INFECTIONS[5]

Severe infections of the kidney are not common today except in the immunosuppressed patient, in the patient with diabetes mellitus, or with other significant renal disease. These infections may be occult and go unrecognized until severe life-threatening symptoms appear. The perinephric abscess, a potentially fatal

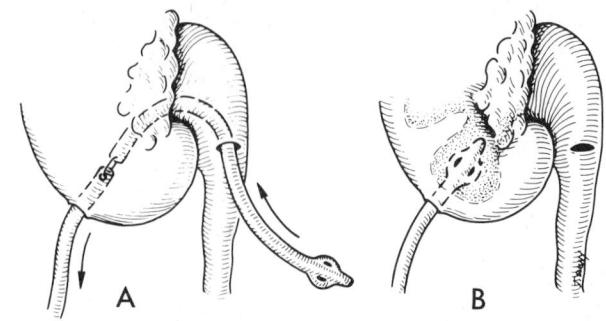

Figure 12. *A,* The external or distal end of a Malecot catheter is then sutured through the drainage end of the red Robinson catheter. A No. 16 or 18 Malecot catheter is usually suitable. *B,* The red Robinson catheter is then carefully withdrawn, pulling the Malecot catheter after it. The drainage end of the Malecot catheter is carefully positioned in the inferior calix. The opening in the renal pelvis is then closed and drained and red rubber drains are also usually passed through a separate stab wound in the skin. (From Paulson, D. F.: Genitourinary Surgery. New York, Churchill Livingstone, 1983, p. 38.)

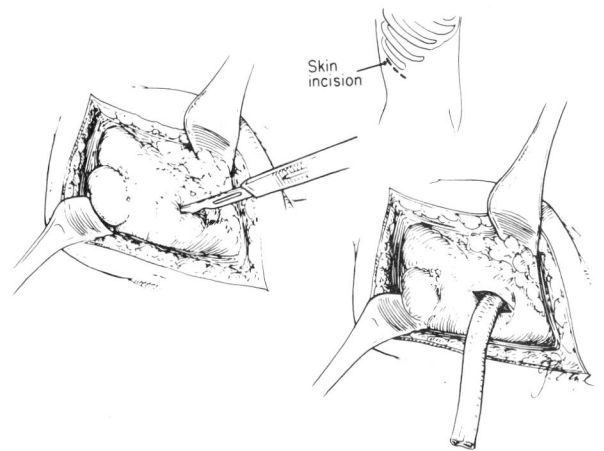

Figure 13. When exploring and draining an abscess or swelling in the kidney, it is important that the body cavities (intrathoracic and intraperitoneal) not be opened and violated. A small incision directly over the suspected area usually suffices, preferably a subcostal or posterior incision. The affected area is opened widely and drained with soft rubber drains. Cultures for anaerobic and aerobic bacteria should always be obtained. The skin incision may be closed, but in widespread infection it is best left open with packing, to be closed by secondary intention. (From Paulson, D. F.: Genitourinary Surgery. New York, Churchill Livingstone, 1983, p. 39.)

process, usually arises from rupture of a renal abscess but can be secondary to hematogenous dissemination from another site or from pyelonephritis. Patients may appear with pyelonephritis or fever of undetermined origin. They frequently have diabetes mellitus or an antecedent history of recurrent urinary tract infection. The symptomatic presentation is with fever, abdominal or flank pain, and abdominal tenderness. When the diagnosis is suspected, blood and urine cultures should be obtained; blood cultures will be positive in approximately 40 per cent of patients, with urine cultures positive in 80 per cent of patients. The organisms identified from these sites frequently are identical to the organisms isolated from the perinephric abscess with the predominant organisms being *Escherichia coli, Proteus* species, and *Staphylococcus aureus.* Imaging studies may assist in diagnosis. The patient with a perinephric abscess usually has immobility of the kidney and the renal shadow does not move with inspiration or expiration. There is a tendency to develop scoliosis as the patient splints toward the involved side. Loss of the psoas shadow may occur. Ultrasonography and the gallium scan may assist diagnosis. Occasionally, percutaneous aspiration or lavage confirms the diagnosis. The treatment of a perinephric abscess is incision and drainage or nephrectomy (Fig. 13).

RENAL ADENOCARCINOMA[10]

This malignancy is the most common malignancy involving the kidney. It is most common in the fifth decade of life with the incidence three times higher in males than in females. These tumors are of tubular origin. Antibodies specific for microvilli of the convoluted proximal tubular cells cross-react with cells of both renal adenomas and renal adenocarcinomas. Renal adenomas can be segregated from renal adenocarcinomas on the basis of size; lesions less than 2 cm. are termed adenomas, with lesions larger than 2 cm. being termed adenocarcinomas. Whether renal adenomas are small renal carcinomas that have the potential for growth and subsequent metastases is debated. Three cell types can be identified: (1) the clear cell carcinoma composed of large polyhedral cells with distinct margins and clear to lightly vacuolated cytoplasm. The cytoplasm is clear because it contains large amounts of triglycerides and phospholipids that are removed during histologic processing, thus providing the "empty cell" appearance. (2) Granular cells are smaller in size and are round or cuboidal. With progressive anaplasia they become more irregular in shape. (3) Sarcomatoid tumors are composed of spindle-shaped cells resembling a fibrosarcoma. The cells often are arranged in papillary or tubular structures. Mitotic cells are rare.

Signs and Symptoms of Renal Adenocarcinoma[10]

Renal carcinoma may present with a wide variety of symptomatic patterns (Table 7). The symptom complex of reversible hepatosplenomegaly with hepatic dysfunction in the absence of liver metastases has been identified in some 10 per cent of patients. The liver function parameters improve with disappearance of the hepatosplenomegaly following nephrectomy. Hypertension occurs in 14 to 40 per cent of patients.

Evaluation of Renal Mass Lesions[9,10]

Symptomatic or asymptomatic renal mass lesions of renal parenchyma should be evaluated by a series of sequential steps (Fig. 14). With a systematic approach to identification of renal mass lesions, 85 per cent can be correctly identified by a combination of only two sequential examinations. Seventy per cent of all mass lesions identified by nephrotomography in the asymptomatic patient are benign renal cysts; only 5.5 per cent are

TABLE 7. Presenting Symptom, Laboratory Abnormality, or Abnormality on Physical Examination and its Relation to Survival Rate in 309 Consecutive Patients Undergoing Nephrectomy for Renal Cell Carcinoma

Presenting Symptom, Abnormal Laboratory Finding, or Abnormality on Physical Examination	Number of Patients and Percentage of Total (309)	Number of Patients Surviving 5 Years
Classic triad (gross hematuria, abnormal mass, pain)	29 (9%)	9 (of 29) 31%
Hematuria	183 (59%)	74 (of 183) 40%
Pain	127 (41%)	56 (of 127) 44%
Abdominal mass	139 (45%)	49 (of 139) 35%
Fever	21 (7%)	8 (of 21) 38%
Weight loss	85 (28%)	29 (of 85) 39%
Anemia	64 (21%)	24 (of 64) 38%
Erythrocytosis	10 (3%)	4 (of 10) 40%
Hypercalcemia	11 (3%)	4 (of 11) 35%
Acute varicocele	7 (2%)	3 (of 7) 43%
Tumor calcification on roentgenogram	39 (13%)	18 (of 39) 46%
Symptoms from metastases	31 (10%)	1 (of 31) 3%
Cancer, an incidental finding (silent)	20 (7%)	13 (of 20) 65%

Modified from Skinner, D. G., Colvin, R. B., Vermillion, C. D., et al.: Diagnosis and management of renal cell carcinoma: A clinical and pathologic study of 309 cases. Cancer, *28:*1165, 1971.

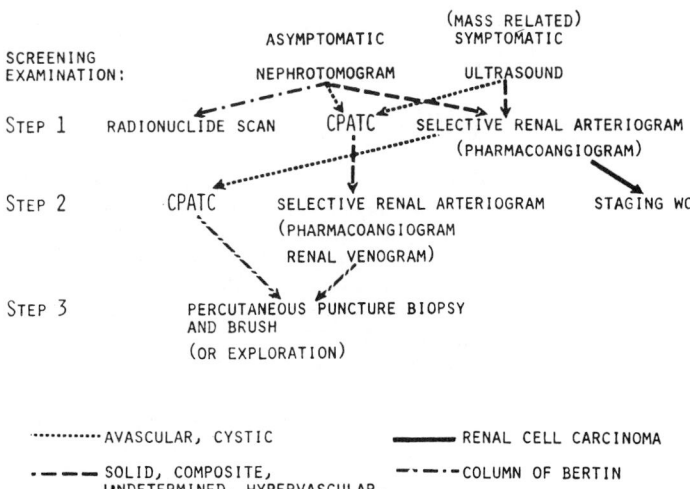

Figure 14. Steps in evaluating renal mass lesions. (CPATC, computed axial tomography.) (From Paulson, D. F.: Genitourinary malignancies. *In* Devita, V. T., Hellman, S., and Rosenberg, S. A. (Eds.): Cancer: Principles and Practice of Oncology. Philadelphia, J. B. Lippincott Company, 1982, p. 734.)

malignant neoplasms. The most frequent asymptomatic renal neoplasm is metastatic tumor, with carcinoma of the breast being most common. Only 2.2 per cent of asymptomatic space-occupying lesions of the kidney are renal cell malignancies.

The renal cyst presents a sharply defined interface against adjacent renal parenchyma. The lesions are thin-walled in those areas that project outside of the renal border. Ultrasonography may confirm the lesion as being cystic or solid. The benign cyst contains fluid that is clear, lightly straw-colored, and low in fat, protein, lactic acid dehydrogenase, and amylase content. Cystic tumors have a darker, cloudy cystic fluid that is high in fat, protein, and lactic acid dehydrogenase. When the urea nitrogen content of the cyst fluid is greater than 40 mg. per 100 ml., the cyst has a tendency to reform. A cyst fluid pressure of less than 8 cm. H_2O is an indicator that the cyst will possibly regress if it is treated by aspiration alone. Should the opening pressure be greater than 16 cm. H_2O, the cyst is likely to reform following aspiration. If the intravenous pyelogram by bolus tomography demonstrates a hypervascular or mottled appearance, or if ultrasound is indeterminate or represents a solid lesion, the patient should undergo angiography or computed axial tomography. Approximately 85 per cent of renal cell carcinomas are hypervascular by angiography and can be diagnosed with accuracy by selective renal artery angiography.

A more accurate method for evaluating renal cell masses is the use of computed axial tomography. Computed axial tomography allows the determination of the extension of disease to associated structures, the presence or absence of associated adenopathy, and the definition of the density of the lesion. Magnetic resonance imaging is very useful in identifying the extent of associated vascular extension and is superior to venacavography in determining the degree of tumor thrombus extension into the vena cava and the level of such extension.

From a practical standpoint, once the renal mass lesion is

identified by nephrotomography, most physicians move directly to computed axial tomography to evaluate the nature of the mass lesion. Computed tomography is much more accurate in evaluating the lesion than is a combination of ultrasonography and angiography.

Staging of Renal Adenocarcinoma[9]

Malignancies of the urinary tract are staged according to the anatomic distribution of disease. Currently, two staging systems exist for identification of the anatomic distribution of renal cell malignancies (Table 8).

Surgical Therapy of Renal Adenocarcinoma[10,15]

The treatment of renal cell carcinoma is based on the anatomic extent of disease with treatment directed toward surgical removal of the kidney and associated tumor, the adrenal gland, the surrounding perinephric fat, and Gerota's fascia along with the regional lymph nodes. Surgical removal of the kidney can be conducted through either one of several incisions: transabdomi-

TABLE 8. Comparison of the Two Classification Systems for Staging of Renal Cell Carcinoma

	TNM(1978)	Robson
Small tumor, no enlargement of kidney	T_1	A
Large tumor, cortex not broken	T_2	A
Perinephric or hilar extension	T_3	B
Extension to neighboring organs	T_4	D
Nodal invasion	N_+	C
Renal vein involved	V_1	C
Vena cava involved	V_2	C
Distant metastases	M_+	D

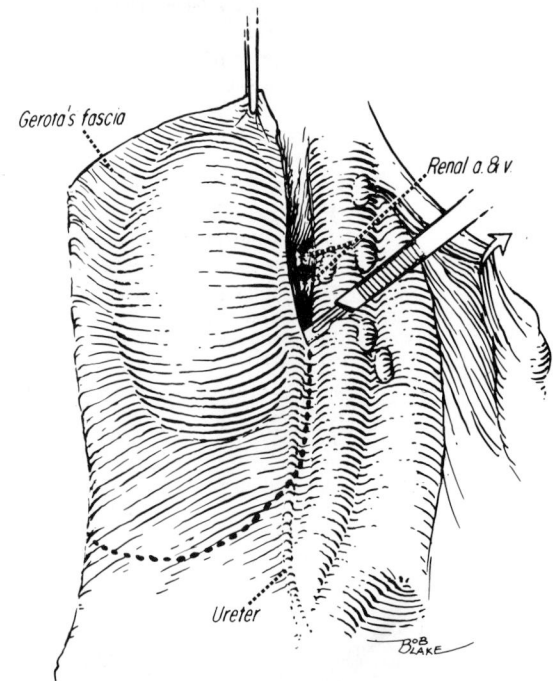

Figure 15. Radical nephrectomy. Kidney is removed within its investing fascia. (From Paulson, D. F.: Genitourinary malignancies. *In* Devita, V. T., Hellman, S., and Rosenberg, S. A. (Eds.): Cancer: Principles and Practice of Oncology. Philadelphia, J. B. Lippincott, 1982, p. 737.)

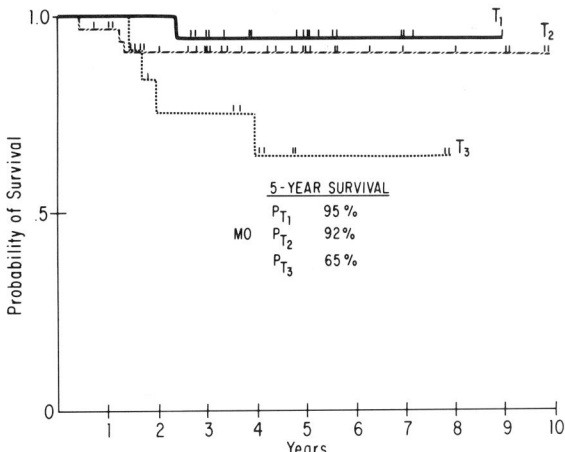

Figure 16. Survival of the nonmetastatic patients staged with the TNM classification. (From Selli, S., et al.: Stratification of risk factors in renal cell carcinoma. Cancer, 52:399, 1983.)

nal, modified flank, full flank, or thoracoabdominal. Irrespective of the incision utilized to gain access to the tumor, once the incision has been made, early control of the vascular supply of the tumor should be established to reduce the possibility of tumor dissemination with dissection and to permit mobilization of the renal mass with minimal blood loss (Fig. 15). Surgical therapy is effective in controlling renal adenocarcinoma when the disease is confined to the kidney itself, or when it has extended minimally outside the renal capsule. Surgical therapy is not effective once the disease has extended to adjacent structures or to regional lymph nodes, or when it has invaded the renal vein or vena cava. When the tumor is confined to the renal substance beneath the capsule itself, survival rates greater than 90 per cent in 10 years can be expected (Fig. 16).

The survival benefits of regional lymphadenectomy have not been established despite the occurrence of nodal spread in approximately 22 per cent of patients. Node dissection may be performed in continuity with nephrectomy or after the renal mass has been removed. The dissection should include a minimal distance of 4 to 6 cm. above and below the renal vessels along with lymphatic drainage posterior to the aorta and vena cava. The profuse lymphatic drainage, the difficulty in removing all involved nodes, the frequency with which local nodes are bypassed with drainage directly to the cisterna chyli, and the frequency with which blood-borne metastases occur all militate against a therapeutically successful lymphadenectomy.

The benefit of surgical removal of the primary renal lesion with concomitant metastatic disease is controversial. Whereas it has been argued that removal of the primary renal malignancy may provide control of symptoms such as fever, pain, hematuria, anemia, and hypercalcemia and that it may reduce the likelihood of further dissemination of disease, there is no evidence that removal of the primary tumor will promote spontaneous regression of metastases or that removal of the primary renal malignancy will improve the response of metastatic disease to either hormonal manipulation or the chemotherapy.

Renal Trauma

Renal trauma may be classified as either blunt (nonpenetrating) or penetrating. Both blunt and penetrating trauma can be divided into two major classifications, those that involve the parenchyma and those that involve the renal pedicle. Patients with nonpenetrating injury who have microscopic hematuria are no longer thought to be candidates for intravenous pyelography. The incidence of identifying abnormalities requiring treatment is so low as to cause many clinicians to reject this study in this specific population. However, patients who have gross hematuria or who have penetrating injuries must be evaluated to determine the extent of the genitourinary injury. Much

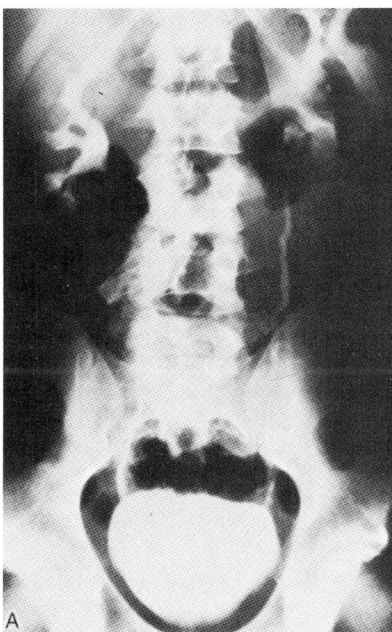
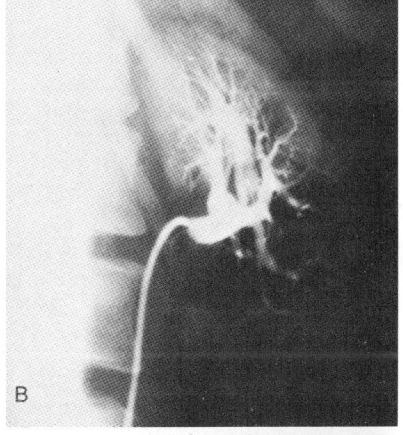
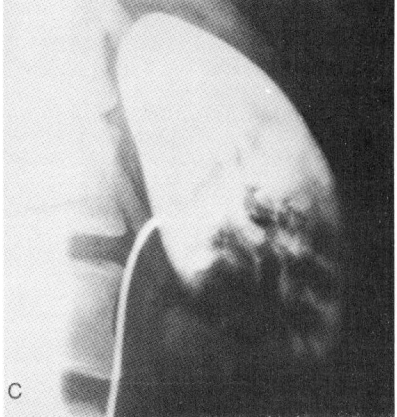

Figure 17. *A,* Intravenous pyelogram of a 26-year-old male with a fracture of the left kidney caused by a horseback riding accident. Intravenous pyelogram shows rather vague filling of the lower pole of the left kidney with evidence of extravasated contrast. (Note accentuation of left psoas margin secondary to extravasated urine.) *B,* Selective renal angiogram showing poor perfusion of the left lower pole. *C,* Delayed angiogram, nephrogram phase, showing disrupted parenchymal lower pole with deep laceration. (From Paulson, D. F.: Genitourinary Surgery. New York, Churchill Livingstone, 1983, p. 111.)

debate exists as to the optimal study. In patients who have blunt trauma, fracture of the lower ribs, fracture of the transverse vertebral processes, or scoliosis on the routine abdominal film should prompt urologic evaluation. An obliterated psoas margin or renal outline may indicate the presence of a large retroperitoneal perirenal hematoma. Unexplained ileus or abdominal pain also should raise the possibility of either retroperitoneal or renal injury. The patient who has sustained blunt renal trauma with gross hematuria or who has penetrating trauma and who presents with any of the signs or symptoms of vascular instability is currently thought to be an optimal candidate for computed axial tomography with contrast to determine the extent of the lesion and any associated perirenal hematuria. This study also allows the clinician to determine the bilaterality of renal function and the amount of gross urinary extravasation (Fig. 17). Any patient demonstrating nonvisualization should undergo renal angiography to assess injury to the renal vasculature.

Blunt renal trauma can be classified according to the severity of injury (Fig. 18). The most common form of blunt renal injury is renal contusion. Patients with renal contusion need no specific therapy other than observation for 48 to 72 hours. They may return to normal activity when the hematuria clears. Parenchymal lacerations that extend no deeper than the cortex may be treated nonsurgically with bed rest and broad-spectrum antibiotics. Patients who have a major parenchymal laceration may be treated conservatively; however, this patient population, when so treated, has a high incidence of infection, abscess formation, renal atrophy, hypertension, and secondary hemorrhage. Thus, it is thought that patients who have the more significant parenchymal lacerations should undergo surgical exploration and primary repair of these injuries.

When the decision is made to explore the patient with blunt renal trauma, the primary surgical principle focuses on wide exposure and early vascular control, especially in patients with persistent hemodynamic instability. This is best done through a transabdominal, transperitoneal approach. Gerota's fascia is left intact until the renal artery and vein are controlled. If Gerota's fascia is incised prior to vascular control, the tamponading effect of the fascia is lost and massive, life-threatening bleeding may occur. Once the renal vasculature is controlled, Gerota's fascia can be incised, the perirenal hematoma evacuated, and the renal injury assessed with intent to repair. Blunt trauma to

the renal pedicle usually is produced by deceleration injury as the more mobile kidney moves away from the stationary aorta. As this occurs, the media and adventitia stretch because of their elasticity; however, the intima, not as elastic as the other components of the vessel, tears. This intimal disruption leads to subsequent dissection and thrombosis. Salvage depends upon early recognition, usually identified by failure of visualization on bolus nephrotomography with perfusion failure confirmed by renal angiography.

Penetrating renal injuries are associated with other intra-abdominal injuries in 80 per cent of all patients. Thus, with the exception of superficial stab wounds, it is recommended that patients who have penetrating injuries near the kidney have an intravenous pyelogram and be considered for surgical exploration. The principles for evaluation and management are similar to those that exist in blunt renal trauma.

THE URETER

The ureters convey urine from the renal pelvis to the bladder. They lie protected in the fibrofatty tissue of the retroperitoneum and their integrity can be threatened by a variety of congenital, inflammatory, traumatic, or neoplastic diseases or iatrogenic injury. The ureters lie in the retroperitoneal space and are adherent to the posterior peritoneum. As they descend, they cross the common iliac vasculature to enter the true pelvis. The ureters then arc along the sacral promontory before converging toward the bladder trigone. The left ureter passes behind the pelvic mesoncolon and the right behind the root of the mesentery. In the male, the ureters cross the vas deferens ventrally to enter the wall of the bladder superior to the prostate and seminal vesicles; in the female, the ureters cross dorsally behind the uterine arteries and pass near the uterine cervix before entering the bladder.

The principles of management of ureteral injury include (1) gentle manipulation of ureteral tissue with noncrushing instruments or traction sutures to prevent damage to delicate ureteral vasculature, (2) adequate wound drainage at the site of ureteral repair to remove any urine that may leak through the site of repair and inhibit the healing process, and (3) the use of absorbable suture material, because the use of nonabsorbable suture material provides a nidus that promotes the deposition of urinary salts and formation of calculi.

Ureteral injury or disease often is defined by the intravenous pyelogram, which permits visualization of the course of the ureter and identification of obstruction or deviation. When visualization of the ureter is not complete, cystoscopy and retrograde bulb occlusive ureteropyelography are required.

Calculous obstruction of the ureter is common, particularly in the more arid climates of the sunbelt. Open ureterolithotomy was at one time thought to be indicated by the following specific clinical situations: (1) a ureteral calculus greater than 1 cm. in diameter in a patient with a normal-sized ureter or in an individual who has not previously passed ureteral calculi; (2) sepsis associated with hydronephrosis secondary to obstruction by the calculus; (3) a jagged hooked calculus that has impaled the ureteral mucosa and will not pass spontaneously; (4) a calculus in the upper ureter that remains stationary for at least 2 weeks with hydronephrosis and hydroureter; and (5) symptoms of increasing pain uncontrolled by oral pain medications, progressive nausea and vomiting, or associated fever in a patient with obstructing urinary calculus. Nonetheless, these clinical situations that were once thought to mandate open ureterolithotomy may now be managed by a combination of ureteroscopy and basket extraction of the stone under direct vision, ureteroscopy with ultrasonic fracture of the stone followed by basket extraction of the fragments, or a percutaneous nephroscopy with basket extraction from above.

The ureteroscope may be passed through the urethra,

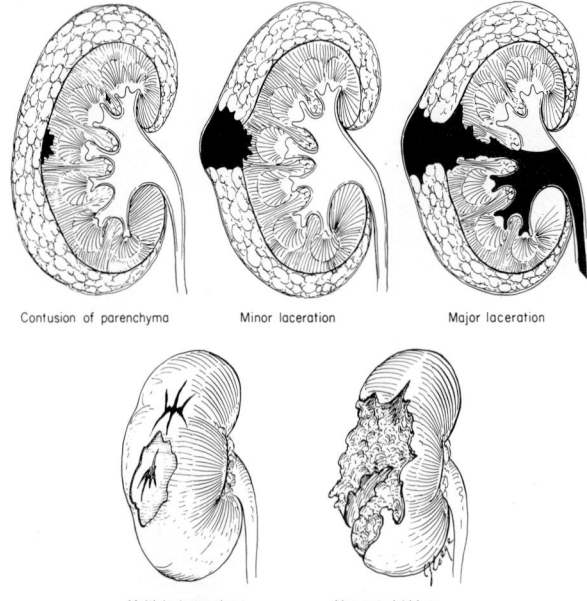

Contusion of parenchyma   Minor laceration   Major laceration

Multiple lacerations   Macerated kidney

Figure 18. Categories of renal trauma. (From Paulson, D. F.: Genitourinary Surgery. New York, Churchill Livingstone, 1983, p. 112.)

through the ureteral orifice, and up the ureter all the way to the renal pelvis (Fig. 19). Using different lens systems, the entire ureter and renal collecting system may be viewed. Passage of the ureteroscope requires initial passage of floppy-tipped guidewire catheters through the ureteral orifice and up the ureter into the renal pelvis. The ureterovesical junction and distal ureter then are dilated to a caliber that will accept the ureteroscope. Then, under direct vision, the ureteroscope is passed over the working guidewire. Once the stone is visualized, it may be basketed under direct vision or fractured with the ultrasonic probe if it is too large for primary removal. Using this technique, the majority of ureteral calculi may be removed without resorting to surgical incision.

When these methods of nonsurgical intervention do not allow removal of the stone, or when such technology results in damage to the ureter without removal of the stone, it may be necessary to proceed to an open surgical procedure both to remove the stone and to correct the ureteral injury. The ureter is divided into three segments: upper third, middle third, and lower third. The surgical approach to the ureter depends upon the anatomic site of the pathologic process. The upper ureter is best exposed through the anterior half of a full flank incision; the midportion may be exposed through a Gibson, muscle-splitting, or hockey-stick incision; the lower ureter is best approached through a midline infraumbilical incision, through a Pfannenstiel incision, or through an extension of the Gibson incision with division of a portion of the rectus muscle.

Renal pelvic or ureteropelvic stones also may be removed through a posterior lumbotomy incision. The patient is placed prone or semiprone with the anterior rib cage elevated on blanket rolls. A vertical skin incision is made 2 cm. medial to the lateral edge of the sacrospinalis muscle with the incision extended to the level of the twelfth rib superiorly and downward toward the iliac crest. This posterior approach produces minimal postoperative pain. In addition, there is seldom postoperative adynamic ileus. No major muscle bundles are divided, and the patient often is ambulatory within 24 hours after operation. Alternatively, a muscle-splitting incision may be utilized for upper ureteral calculi through a posterior flank approach.

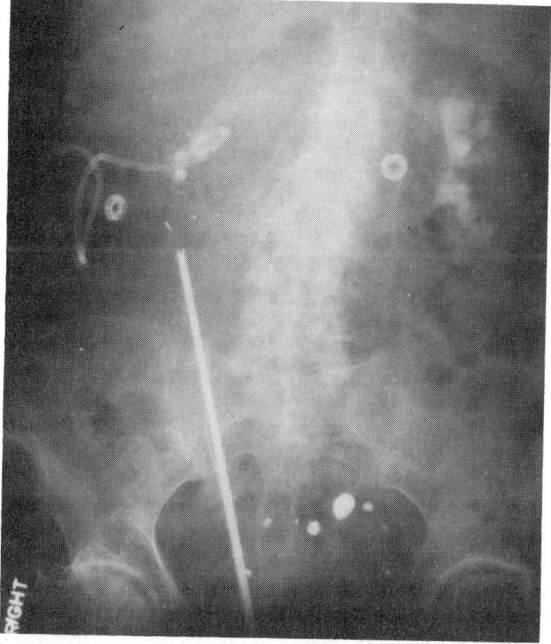

Figure 19. Urethrorenoscope in place, having been passed through the urethra and across the bladder up the ureter. The stone basket has engaged a fragment of stone in the upper ureter and the fragment will be extracted. (Provided by Dr. John L. Weinerth, Division of Urology, Duke University Medical Center, Durham, North Carolina.)

URETERAL OBSTRUCTION SECONDARY TO MALIGNANT OR NONMALIGNANT DISEASE[13]

The ureter may be obstructed secondary to malignant or nonmalignant disease and the obstruction may be unilateral or bilateral. When bilateral, frequently it is associated with progressive loss of renal function. When unilateral, it frequently is not associated with any specific symptomatic presentation. In patients with known malignancy, a persistent urinary tract infection, proteinuria, or hematuria should suggest the possibility of retroperitoneal involvement. Any slow progressive rise in serum creatinine or deterioration of renal function should be viewed with alarm. Early diagnosis is promoted by careful attention to these nonspecific signs and symptoms.

Obstruction of the ureter is best delineated initially by ultrasonography, intravenous pyelography with nephrotomography, or computed axial tomography. Ultrasonography may suggest ureteral or renal pelvic enlargement and is a recommended initial study. Once ureteral or renal pelvic dilation is identified, the intravenous pyelogram with nephrotomography may further define the lesion. In those patients who have marked dilation of the upper urinary tract secondary to involvement of the middle to lower ureter and in whom a retrograde ureteropyelogram is not possible, percutaneous puncture of a dilated collecting system with antegrade pyeloureterography may identify the site of obstruction and the nature of the pathologic process. The computed axial tomogram also shows the obstruction and may identify any surrounding anatomic disease. In patients with known malignancy, the surgeon must be certain that he is dealing with obstruction secondary to recurrent malignancy, since fibrosis from previous surgical therapy or radiation therapy may mimic malignancy. In previous years, ureteral obstruction required either cutaneous ureterostomy or open nephrostomy. Today, current methods effect relief of the obstruction without open surgical intervention. In the patient with unilateral or bilateral obstruction, internal drainage can be established using a "double-J" Silastic catheter. These catheters may be inserted transurethrally from below or percutaneously from above. In either instance, a guidewire is passed through the urethral lumen and a soft Silastic catheter is threaded over the guidewire and manipulated in place using a "pusher" catheter. When the pusher catheter and guidewire are withdrawn, the preformed curves appear at either end of the indwelling ureteral stent, holding it in place. The Silastic indwelling catheters may be left in place for 6 to 12 months with minimal encrustation. They may be removed transurethrally and replaced without difficulty.

Percutaneous Nephrostomy

When a transluminal ureteral catheter cannot be placed, a percutaneous nephrostomy tube can be placed without the necessity for open surgical intervention. When the renal collecting system is markedly dilated, the percutaneous tube may be placed blindly as described by Goodwin. However, using ultrasonography or computed axial tomography, the dilated collecting system can be visualized and a guidewire passed into the collecting system under direct vision. Over the guidewire a series of dilating catheters can be passed to progressively dilate the tract to a 9 Fr. catheter, after which an 8.5 Fr. pigtail catheter can be inserted over the guidewire and passed into the renal pelvis to facilitate drainage. These techniques permit relief of obstruction and the placement of percutaneous catheters and indwelling stents in patients with a variety of obstructing lesions. They permit the physician to stabilize renal function and to approach definitive treatment under optimal physiologic conditions.

URETERAL REPLACEMENT[13]

In certain clinical situations precipitated by malignant or nonmalignant disease, it may be necessary to replace the ureter

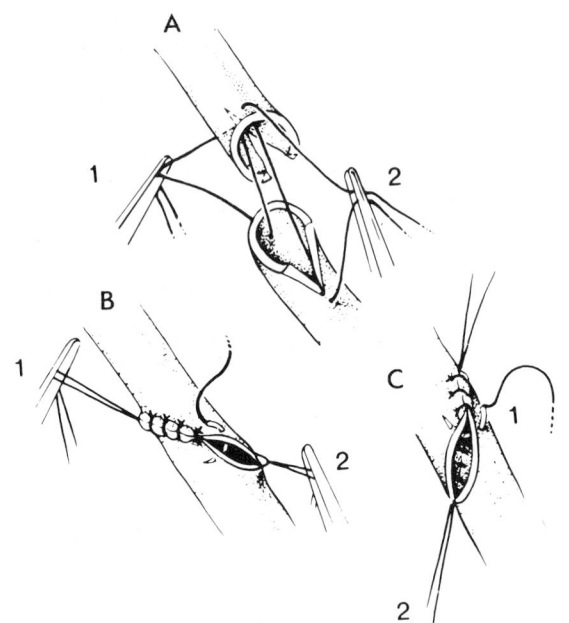

Figure 20. Technique for oblique spatulated end-to-end ureteroureterostomy. *A*, Initial suture placement. *B*, 90-degree rotation for closure of one wall. *C*, 180-degree rotation in the opposite direction to close the other wall. (From Paulson, D. F.: Genitourinary Surgery. New York, Churchill Livingstone, 1983, p. 179.)

either in part or *in toto*. Various surgical maneuvers have been developed for ureteral replacement. When the distal third of the ureter must be replaced, ureteroneocystostomy, with either a psoas hitch or bladder flap, may be the treatment of choice. When there is a small segmental defect of the ureter, ureteroureterostomy may be the simplest and best procedure. When there is destruction of the major portion of any one ureter, transureteroureterostomy may be appropriate (Fig. 20). When there is involvement of all or most of one ureter, replacement with a segment of ileum may be considered. Autotransplantation with ureteroneocystostomy or vesicopyelostomy is an alternative procedure.

CARCINOMA OF THE URETER AND RENAL PELVIS[10]

Carcinoma of the renal pelvis constitutes 5 per cent of all renal carcinomas. Ninety per cent of all carcinomas of the renal pelvis are transitional cell tumors with the remaining being either squamous cell carcinomas or adenocarcinomas. About 25 per cent of all patients who have a single pelvic transitional cell tumor develop malignancy at some other site in their urinary tract at a future date. Patients who have multiple upper tract tumors of transitional cell origin have a 50 per cent probability of the delayed appearance of invasive malignancy. Transitional cell carcinomas spread by direct extension and by blood and lymphatic embolization. The malignant transitional cells are shed into the urine where they can be identified by Papanicolaou's smear of the voided urine. Eighty to 90 per cent of all patients with renal pelvic tumors have either gross or microscopic hematuria. Pain precipitated by ureteropelvic junction obstruction secondary to the tumor mass produces a symptom complex similar to renal calculus disease. The diagnosis is suggested by the appearance of a defect in the collecting system or in the renal pelvis by excretory pyelography (Table 9). The classical surgical treatment of the renal pelvic tumors is nephroureterectomy with excision of the ureteral orifice and surrounding bladder. Removal of the entire ureter is recommended since approximately one fifth of all patients who have a residual portion of the ureter develop tumor in the ureteral remnant. There

TABLE 9. Differential Diagnosis of Cancer of the Renal Pelvis

Intrinsic Lesions
Calculus
Blood clot
Cholesteatoma
Malacoplakia
Inflammatory lesions of urothelium (pyelitis cystica, etc.)
Benign ureteropelvic junction obstruction
Benign (connective tissue) tumors of renal pelvis
Renal cell carcinoma
Suburothelial hemorrhage

Extrinsic Lesions
Vascular impressions
Parapelvic cyst

Modified from Fraly, E. E.: *In* Skinner, D. G., and deKernion, J. B. (Eds.): Geritourinary Cancer. Philadelphia, W. B. Saunders Company, 1978.

are no data to indicate that lymph node dissection at the level of the renal hilum provides enhanced disease control.

Carcinoma of the ureter is usually a transitional cell tumor. The characteristic ureteral dilation associated with ureteral tumors was described by Bergman and is said to distinguish ureteral tumors from ureteral calculi (Fig. 21). The dilation that accompanies the ureteral tumor is the response of the ureter to accommodate a slowly expanding tumor mass and reflects the absence of renal spasm initiated by the presence of an irritating calculus. The differential diagnosis of the radiographic abnormalities associated with ureteral tumors includes nonopaque calculi, blood clots, ureteritis cystica, ureteral varicosities, extraluminal malignancy with ureteral compression, periureteral fibrosis, and endometriosis. The diagnosis is suggested by the radiographic characteristics of the lesion in association with hematuria but is confirmed by the presence of urinary cytologic findings compatible with malignancy.

Treatment of ureteral tumors has traditionally been nephroureterectomy with removal of the entire renal unit and ureter. There is, however, a current argument to preserve the renal unit through local resection of the malignancy only. The relative advantages and disadvantages of these two philosophies remain undefined. However, the argument for less than nephroureterectomy springs from an interpretation that the salvage rate in patients with ureteral tumors is dependent more on the biological aggressiveness of the tumor rather than on the aggressiveness of the surgical therapy that is chosen. It would appear that patients with high-grade lesions or lesions that have penetrated into or through the ureteral wall have little chance for cure even with the most radical surgical therapy, whereas patients with low-grade lesions have an excellent chance of cure

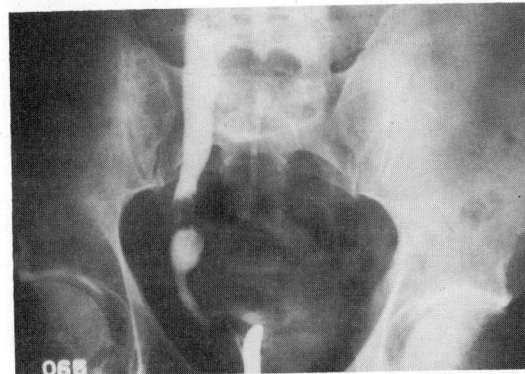

Figure 21. Retrograde ureteropyelogram showing ureteral dilation about a filling defect in the lower ureter. (From Paulson, D. F.: Genitourinary malignancies. *In* Devita, V. T., Hellman, S., and Rosenberg, S. A. (Eds.): Cancer: Principles and Practice of Oncology. Philadelphia, J. B. Lippincott Company, 1982, p. 744.)

TABLE 10. Correlation of Survival Rate with Pathologic Characteristics
of Ureteral Cancer

	Five-Year Survival Rate (%)	
	Bloom and Associates (1970) (54 Patients)	Batata and Associates (1975) (41 Patients)
Histologic Grade		
I	83.0	78.0
II	52.0	50.0
III	18.0	0
IV	12.0	0
Pathologic Stage		
0, A	62.0	91.0
B	50.0	43.0
C	33.3	23.0
D	0	0

Modified from Bloom, P. A., et al.: J. Urol., *103*:590, 1970; Batata, M. A., et al.: Cancer, *35*:1626, 1975; Richie, J. P.: *In* Skinner, D. G., and deKernion, J. B. (Eds.): Geritourinary Cancer. Philadelphia, W. B. Saunders Co., 1978.

with only a regional resection. Preservation of the renal unit allows use of nephrotoxic chemotherapeutic agents should the patient subsequently present with metastatic disease. The survival of patients with ureteral malignancy is influenced by the grade and stage of the tumor (Table 10).

THE URINARY BLADDER[3]

The urinary bladder can be carefully assessed by radiographic, physiologic, and endoscopic examination prior to the initiation of any therapeutic modality. This allows the surgeon to carefully select and plan appropriate treatment for a variety of disease processes. An awareness of the anatomy and physiology of the bladder is essential before undertaking any operative procedure since the objectives of surgical therapy should be resolution of the disease processes and restoration of normal storage and voiding function. The bladder in the adult lies in the true pelvis below the peritoneal cavity. It functions as a urinary reservoir and is under volitional control. The area surrounding the bladder contains loose areolar tissue, fat, and a plexus of veins that drain the pelvis, bladder, and anterior perineum. The bladder is covered superiorly by a reflection of the peritoneum. The arterial supply of the bladder is from the internal iliac artery with three arterial branches called the superior, middle, and inferior vesical arteries. In the female, the uterine and vaginal vessels may have contralateral branches that anastomose with the vesical blood supply. The arterial blood supply is not constant and there are many variations. The veins of the bladder do not travel with the arteries. They tend to be short and unite to form the plexus of Santorini anteriorly and the pudendal plexus inferiorly. These two venous plexi, which have numerous interconnection, communicate with the veins of the perineum and the dorsal vein of the penis or clitoris. The bladder receives innervation from both sympathetic and parasympathetic autonomic nerves. The sympathetic preganglionic nuclei are in the first and second lumbar segments and possibly the twelfth thoracic spinal cord segment. This sympathetic outflow proceeds through either the inferior mesenteric ganglia or the inferior hypogastric plexus. If the outflow is via the inferior mesenteric ganglia, fibers proceed down the aorta to the iliac vasculature and then follow the ureters before fanning out to enter the bladder. When the outflow is via the inferior hypogastric plexus, the fibers leave the ganglia in the lower pelvis and immediately fan out to enter the bladder. Although the course of the preganglionic sympathetic fibers is variable, the postganglionic fibers enter the bladder posterolaterally with the arteries and branch out to include the entire bladder. Parasympathetic

preganglionic cell nuclei are in the second, third, and fourth sacral segments of the spinal cord and travel with the nervi erigentes or pelvic splanchnic nerves to enter the bladder in the same manner as the sympathetic fibers. Postganglionic cells arise in the wall of the urinary bladder proper. Afferent sensory fibers from the bladder can exit along either sympathetic or parasympathetic pathways.

The primary function of the bladder is to store urine until volitional voiding is prompted. In its simplest terms, bladder dysfunction can be segregated into disorders of storage and disorders of emptying. The disease processes that produce these disorders can be identified by a combination of contrast studies and urodynamic evaluation. Urodynamic evaluation is a physiologic study that determines the neuromuscular response of the bladder to filling and emptying. The urodynamic evaluation of the bladder consists of (1) a cystometrogram with a coordinated electromyographic evaluation of the urinary sphincter, (2) urethral pressure profile, and (3) urinary flow rate. Cystometrography is performed to determine bladder capacity, the presence of voluntary or involuntary contractions of the detrusor, and the compliance of the bladder (the ability of the detrusor muscle to stretch with filling), and to evaluate the integrity of the afferent (sensory) limbs of the detrusor reflex arc. The normal bladder fills to a volume of 400 ml. with no increase in pressure, no uninhibited contractions, and normal bladder wall compliance. At this volume, the patient states that the bladder feels full; when the patient is asked to void, there is a spiking increase in intravesical pressure and a coincidental relaxation of the sphincter mechanisms. When rising intravesical pressure overcomes falling urethral resistance, voiding begins and the bladder empties. By measuring the electrical activity of the distal sphincter mechanisms during bladder filling and voiding, vesicosphincter dyssynergia (failure of sphincter relaxation during detrusor contraction) may be identified. If uninhibited contractions of the detrusor muscle occur during periods of electrical sphincter silence, the patient leaks urine involuntarily. The urethral pressure profile is used to determine functional length, resting pressure, and maximal pressure (in response to stress) of the sphincteric mechanisms. A normal urethral pressure profile shows an increase in pressure at the bladder neck, which normally corresponds to pressure exerted by the proximal urethral sphincter. Maximal pressure is recorded at the level of the distal urethral sphincter and is approximately 70 to 90 cm. of water. The functional urethral length is the distance from the rise in pressure at the bladder neck to the point in the distal urethra where intraurethral pressure falls below intravesical pressure. In normal males without benign prostatic hypertrophy this

TABLE 11. Drugs Affecting Urinary Control

I. Therapy to facilitate bladder emptying	*II. Therapy to facilitate urine storage*
A. Increase intravesical pressure	A. Inhibit bladder contractility
1. External compression	1. Pharmacologic manipulation
2. Promotion or initiation of reflex contractions	a. Anticholinergic agents
a. Trigger zones or maneuvers	b. Beta-adrenergic stimulation
b. Bladder training, tidal drainage	c. Musculotropic relaxants
3. Pharmacologic manipulation	d. Membrane stabilizers
a. Parasympathomimetic agents (acetylcholine-like agents, anticholinesterases)	2. Interruption of innervation
b. Blockers of inhibition (alpha-adrenergic blockage?)	a. Subarachnoid block
4. Electrical stimulation	b. Sacral rhizotomy
a. Directly to the bladder	3. Bladder distention
b. To the spinal cord or nerve roots	4. Cystolysis
	5. Electrical stimulation of the pelvic floor
B. Decrease outlet resistance	B. Increase outlet resistance
1. At the level of the bladder neck	1. At the level of the bladder neck
a. Incision of the bladder neck	a. Alpha-adrenergic stimulation; beta-adrenergic blockage?
b. Y-V plasty of the bladder neck	b. Mechanical compression
c. Pharmacologic manipulation (alpha-adrenergic blockade, beta-adrenergic stimulation?)	2. At the level of the distal mechanism
2. At the level of the distal mechanism*	a. Alpha-adrenergic stimulation (smooth muscle), beta-adrenergic blockade?
a. External sphincterotomy	b. Mechanical compression
b. Urethral overdilation	c. Electrical stimulation of the pelvic floor
c. Pudendal nerve interruption	
d. Pharmacologic inhibition	
(1) External sphincter/pelvic floor (striated muscle relaxant, mono- and polysynaptic spinal cord reflex inhibition)	
(2) Proximal urethra (alpha-adrenergic blockade, beta-adrenergic stimulation.)	
e. Psychotherapy, biofeedback	
C. Circumvent problem	C. Circumvent problem
1. Intermittent catheterization	1. Intermittent catheterization
2. Urinary diversion	2. Urinary diversion

* Includes the smooth muscle of the proximal urethra and the striated musculature of the external urethral sphincter.
Reprinted from Wein, A. J.: Pharmacology of the bladder and ureter. *In* Stanton, S. L., and Tanagho, E. A. (Eds.) Surgery of Female Incontinence. Berlin, Springer-Verlag, 1980.

length is 2.5 to 4 cm. Urinary flow rates are physiologic, noninvasive, and informative. The volume of urine voided, voiding time, peak flow rate, and average flow rate are the usually determined parameters. A peak flow rate greater than 25 ml. per second is consistent with an unobstructed flow, provided the patient voids in less than 15 seconds. Peak flow rates below 10 ml. per second are consistent with obstruction, either functional or secondary to benign prostatic hypertrophy or to stricture of the outflow passage. Although no absolute recommendations can be made as to the appropriate management of the various disorders of storage and emptying, when no specific anatomic defect that requires surgical correction can be identified, it may be possible to enhance emptying or facilitate storage by pharmaceutical manipulation (Table 11).

BLADDER FISTULA[3]

Disorders of storage are occasioned by fistula between the bladder and either the small or large bowel (enteric fistula), the vagina, the uterus, or the skin. Vesical fistulas are usually of inflammatory, neoplastic, iatrogenic, or traumatic origin or secondary to radiation.

Vesicoenteric Fistula

Fifty per cent of all vesicoenteric fistulas are secondary to sigmoid diverticulitis. Colorectal malignancy represents approximately 16 to 20 per cent of all enteric fistulas with 12 to 15 per cent of fistulas associated with Crohn's disease. Primary bladder malignancy is the cause of about 5 per cent of all vesicoenteric fistulas. Pneumaturia and fecaluria are classic symptoms of the vesicoenteric fistula. Pneumaturia is not pathognomonic of an enteric fistula, since gas per urethra may result from fermentation of diabetic urine, from urinary tract infection by gas-producing organisms, or from urinary tract instrumentation. However, pneumaturia is the presenting symptom in two thirds of patients who present with a vesicoenteric fistula. Fecaluria is diagnostic of a vesicoenteric fistula; however, it occurs in only 20 to 50 per cent of all patients. The differential diagnosis of vesicoenteric fistula should include recurrent urinary tract infections and interstitial cystitis. The diagnosis usually is established by cystoscopic examination of the bladder. However, contrast studies (intravenous pyelography, upper gastrointestinal or barium enema) may be necessary to identify the fistula. When a fistula is suspected but cannot be confirmed, the urine should be examined for barium after barium contrast studies of the bowel or for the appearance of charcoal granules in the urinary sediment after oral administration of charcoal.

Surgical repair may require resection of the offending bowel segment and bladder *en bloc* with primary restitution of the bowel and primary closure of the bladder. When possible, omentum should be interposed over the surface of the bladder closure to ensure against recurrence of the fistula and a breakdown of the closure.

Vesicovaginal Fistula

Vesicovaginal fistulas are commonly seen as a complication of unattended childbirth. Today, in most of the civilized world, approximately 90 per cent of vesicovaginal fistulas are secondary to gynecologic procedures. The remaining patients develop these fistulas as a consequence of urologic surgery, extensive pelvic trauma, or complications of internal or external radiotherapy for pelvic malignancies, or by direct extension of a malignant process (most commonly squamous cell carcinoma of the cervix). The signs and symptoms of a vesicovaginal fistula depend upon its size and location. Patients with small fistulas may have the intermittent appearance of a watery vaginal discharge and appear to void normally, whereas patients with large fistulas have total urinary leakage through the vagina with no urethral voiding. Small fistulas located high in the vaginal vault may leak only when the bladder is full, whereas those located farther distally in the bladder base may leak constantly. Most patients complain of a malodorous watery vaginal discharge. When the fistula is secondary to recent vaginal or pelvic surgery, it usually becomes evident between 5 and 14 days postoperatively.

Identification of a vesicovaginal fistula may be difficult. Urinary leakage through the vagina may initiate from the ureter(s), bladder, or any of these three structures. Diagnostic evaluation should include an intravenous urogram with special attention to the lower ureters. The vagina should be viewed on lateral films for the appearance of intravaginal contrast material. Cystography usually adds little to the diagnosis. The use of intravesical dye may assist in localization and diagnosis. A clean vaginal tampon should be placed in the vagina and methylene blue instilled in the bladder. The patient then is asked to retain the methylene blue within the bladder and be ambulatory for several hours. The patient then returns, a catheter is passed, and the bladder is drained. The tampon is removed. The presence of methylene blue on the upper end of the tampon confirms the diagnosis of a vesicovaginal fistula. If the test is negative, the sequence of events is repeated following intravenous injection of indigo carmine. If staining of the tampon occurs after a negative intravesical methylene blue test, a ureterovaginal fistula is suggested.

Small vesicovaginal fistulas that occur after either vaginal or pelvic surgery may close spontaneously if the bladder urine is diverted by use of a Foley catheter. Larger fistulas may require surgical intervention for closure. Although it has been recommended that repair be delayed 4 to 6 months after the appearance of the fistula to allow tissues to soften and mature and become less inflamed, and thus enhance the possibility of repair, recent studies have demonstrated that immediate surgical closure of uncomplicated vesicovaginal fistulas that occur following hysterectomy or related procedures in otherwise healthy women may be accomplished with a high degree of success and thus spare the patient the prolonged morbidity and mental anguish of vaginal leakage. Vesicovaginal fistulas may be closed either perineally via a transvaginal route or suprapubically via a transvesical route. The principles of surgical closure are similar: (1) total separation of the tissues comprising the wall of the vagina and the wall of the bladder; (2) sharp excision of the fistulous tract between the two structures; (3) closure of the defect in the vagina and the bladder with absorbable suture material with nonopposed, nonoverlapping suture lines; and (4) where possible, interposition of alternative tissue (a myocutaneous gracilis flap or omentum) between the two suture lines.

Disorders of Storage[3,19]

Disorders of storage may occur when an inadequate bladder volume exists and may require bladder augmentation to increase bladder volume. Currently, intestinal segments utilizing ileum, cecum, or sigmoid colon are utilized to increase bladder capacity (Fig. 22). Use of these bowel segments to augment bladder capacity and facilitate storage is contraindicated only in patients who have bladder outlet obstruction, an antecedent history of vesical malignancy, or borderline renal function with creatinine clearances of less than 40 to 50 ml. per minute.

A second disorder of storage is urinary incontinence secondary to damage of the sphincteric mechanisms that provide the resistance to bladder emptying. Total incontinence is the continuous leakage of urine with the bladder functioning only as a

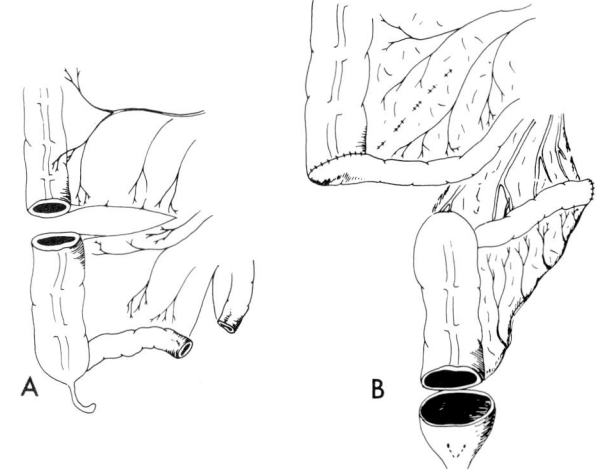

Figure 22. Ileocecal cystoplasty. *A,* The ascending colon is divided at a point just below the right colic artery. If it is intended to employ the distal ileum for ureteral anastomosis, an appropriate length of ileum is selected and its mesentery divided, taking care to ensure a good blood supply to the isolated ileocecal segment from the ileocolic artery. *B,* The isolated segment is rotated 180 degrees on its vascular pedicle, bringing the open end of ascending colon in apposition with the bladder remnant. Care should be taken that this rotation does not interfere with good vascular flow to and from the rotated segment. (From Paulson, D. F.: Genitourinary Surgery. New York, Churchill Livingstone, 1983, p. 252.)

urinary conduit. In total incontinence, there must be incompetence of both the proximal and distal urethral sphincter mechanisms. This may be either neurologic or iatrogenic. Stress urinary incontinence refers to the intermittent leakage of urine associated with sudden increases in intra-abdominal pressure.

Incontinence occurs when there has been a disruption of the sphincter mechanism. In males, this is most usually postsurgical, although it can be posttraumatic. In females, loss of closing urethral pressure occurs with loss of pelvic floor support and shortening of total urethral length. In males, the internal or proximal urethral sphincter routinely is destroyed by prostatectomy. The distal urethral mechanism, consisting of smooth muscle and fibroelastic tissue representing the intrinsic portion of the distal urethra as well as the surrounding skeletal muscle of the pelvic floor, is routinely undamaged during either transurethral or open prostatectomy. However, when the anatomy is such that the surgical procedure carries through both sphincter mechanisms, or when a previous disease process, trauma, or surgical intervention has destroyed either the internal or the distal urethral sphincter, then either transurethral resection or open prostatectomy has a high likelihood of leaving the patient without urinary control in the postoperative period. When urodynamic studies demonstrate that anatomic incontinence is present in the male, then it may be necessary to surgically intervene to increase urethral closing pressure.

A single operative procedure is currently in vogue to increase intrinsic urethral closing pressures. This operative procedure utilizes a volitionally controlled occlusive device to provide increase in outflow obstruction to a point at which this obstruction is greater than the voiding pressure created by the bladder. The volitionally controlled occlusive device or the artificial inflatable sphincter functions in a more physiologic way, and the total closing pressure can be regulated so that regional tissue ischemia does not occur.

The techniques that have been devised for control of urinary incontinence in the female in the presence of a supple, compliant, and nonhostile reservoir consist primarily of urethral lengthening procedures. These may be done transvaginally or suprapubically. The surgical principle to be followed in each of these procedures is to increase urethral length and thus enhance urethral closing pressure.

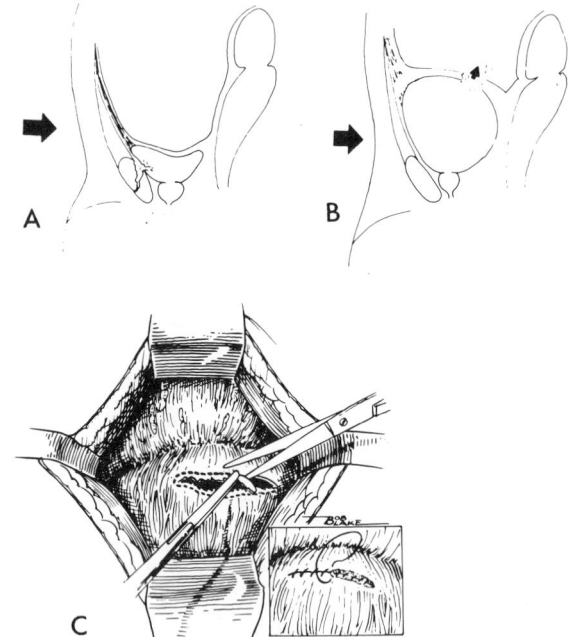

Figure 23. Types of bladder wall disruption associated with blunt lower abdominal trauma. *A,* When blunt injury results in pelvic fracture, associated bladder perforation is usually extraperitoneal and caused by mechanical perforation of the bladder by a bony spicule. *B,* If the bladder is full, the sudden increase in intravesical pressure may result in a disruption of bladder wall integrity at the dome, resulting in intraperitoneal extravasation. *C,* Limited debridement of edges of bladder rupture. (From Paulson, D. F.: Genitourinary Surgery. New York, Churchill Livingstone, 1983, p. 222.)

Vesical Trauma[3]

Trauma to the bladder can be divided into (1) trauma with and without pelvic fracture, (2) penetrating injuries, either high- or low-velocity, and (3) iatrogenic trauma. Each requires identification and repair. Blunt trauma without pelvic fracture damages the bladder only if the bladder is full. Rupture of the bladder either with or without pelvic fracture may be either extraperitoneal or intraperitoneal (Fig. 23). The patient who has lower abdominal trauma with or without bony fracture or who has penetrating trauma to the lower abdomen should have cystography to determine the nature and extent of the bladder rupture, followed by surgical exploration, identification of the traumatized site, sharp excision of the devitalized tissue, and primary repair using either a two- or three-layer closure. It is not necessary to drain the bladder with a suprapubic tube unless there has been severe bladder trauma and the likelihood of primary healing is diminished.

CARCINOMA OF THE BLADDER[10]

Ninety per cent of bladder malignancies are transitional cell tumors, reflecting their origin from the transitional cells that line the bladder. Squamous cell carcinoma comprises approximately 6 to 8 per cent of bladder tumors, with only 2 per cent being adenocarcinomas. Tumors are graded on a scale of 1 to 4 dependent upon the degree of cellular atypia and nuclear abnormalities in association with the number of mitotic figures. The anatomic distribution of disease may be identified by one of several staging systems (Tables 12 and 13).

Clinical Presentation and Diagnosis

Hematuria occurs in 75 per cent of all patients with carcinoma of the bladder. Approximately 30 per cent of patients may have an associated urinary tract infection and the presenting symptom complex is frequently dismissed as "hemorrhagic cystitis." Bladder irritability alone is a presenting symptom in 30 per cent

of patients and is thought to be associated with muscle invasion. A presumptive diagnosis of transitional cell carcinoma of the bladder may be supported by urinary cytologic studies but is confirmed by cystoscopic examination and transurethral biopsy of the suspected area.

Treatment Considerations

Treatment of transitional cell carcinoma is directed to removal of the offending malignancy with treatment based on the anatomic distribution of disease. Tumors that have not invaded through the lamina propria, Stage 0 tumors, may be controlled by transurethral resection or fulguration or by intravesical drugs that promote removal of the malignancy (Tables 14 and 15). Whether the drugs placed within the bladder produce their ef-

TABLE 12. TNM Classification

Primary Tumor (T)
The suffix "m" should be added to the appropriate T category to indicate multiple lesions. Papilloma is classified as "GO."

T_x — Minimum requirements cannot be met
T_0 — No evidence of primary tumor
T_{is} — Sessile carcinoma *in situ*
T_a — Papillary noninvasive carcinoma
T_1 — On bimanual examination, a freely mobile mass may be felt; this should not be felt after complete transurethral resection of the lesion and/or if there is papillary carcinoma without microscopic invasion beyond the lamina propria
T_2 — On bimanual examination there is induration of the bladder wall, which is mobile; there is no residual induration after complete transurethral resection of the lesion and/or there is microscopic invasion of superficial muscle of bladder
T_3 — On bimanual examination there is induration, or a nodular mobile mass is palpable in the bladder wall that persists after transurethral resection
T_{3a} — Microscopic invasion of deep muscle
T_{3b} — Invasion through the full thickness of bladder wall
T_4 — Tumor fixed or invading neighboring structures and/or there is microscopic evidence of invasion of the prostate and in the other circumstances listed below at least muscle invasion
T_{4a} — Tumor invading substance of prostate, uterus, or vagina
T_{4b} — Tumor fixed to the pelvic wall and/or infiltrating the abdominal wall

Nodal Involvement (N)
The regional lymph nodes are the pelvic nodes just below the bifurcation of the common iliac arteries. The juxtaregional lymph nodes are the inguinal nodes, the common iliac, and the para-aortic nodes.
N_x — Minimum requirements cannot be met
N_0 — No involvement of regional lymph nodes
N_1 — Involvement of a single homolateral regional lymph node
N_2 — Involvement of contralateral bilateral or multiple regional lymph nodes
N_3 — There is a fixed mass on the pelvic wall with a free space between this and the tumor
N_4 — Involvement of juxtaregional lymph nodes
Note: Subsequent data regarding the histologic assessment of the regional lymph nodes may be added to the N category thus: N− for nodes with no microscopic evidence of metastases, or N+ for those with microscopic evidence of metastasis, for example, N0+.

Distant Metastasis (M)
M_x — Not assessed
M_0 — No (known) distant metastasis
M_1 — Distant metastasis present
Specify _____
Specify sites according to the following notations:
Pulmonary—PUL	Bone Marrow—MAR
Osseous—OSS	Pleura—PLE
Hepatic—HEP	Skin—SKI
Brain—BRA	Eye—EYE
Lymph Nodes—LYM	Other—OTH

Note: Add + to the abbreviated notation to indicate that the pathology (p) is proved.

TABLE 13. Staging of Bladder Cancer

	Jewett and Strong (1946)	Jewett (1952)	Marshall (1952)	TNM (1974) Clinical (T)	TNM (1974) Pathologic (P)
0 Confined to mucosa			0	$T_0N_xM_0+$	$P_0N_0M_0$
Ps Carcinoma *in situ*				T_{is}	P_{is}
A Infiltration of submucosa	A	A	0	$T_1N_xM_0$	$P_1N_0M_0$
B Infiltration of:					
Superficial muscle +		B_1	B_1	$T_2N_xM_0$	$P_2N_0M_0$
Deep muscle	B	B_2	B_2	$T_{3a}N_xM_0$	$P_{3a}N_0M_0$
Perivesical infiltration	C	C	C	$T_{3b}N_xM_0$	$P_{3b}N_0M_0$
Prostate				$T_{4a}N_xM_0$	$P_{4a}N_0M_0$
Uterus/vagina				$T_{4b}N_xM_0$	$P_{4b}N_0M_0$
Adjacent organ			D_1		
				Pelvic abdominal wall	
Nodes + (pelvic only)			D_1	$T_{(any)}N_xM_0$	$P_{(any)}N_{1-3}M_0$
Distant metastases, or Nodes + (above aortic bifurcation)			D_2	$T_{(any)}N_xM_{1a-d}$	$T_{(any)}N_4M_{1a-d}$
Pelvic, abdominal wall fixation					

T, primary tumor; N, nodal involvement; M, distant metastases; x, cannot be assessed.

fect by interdicting cell metabolism or whether these agents produce their effect through intravesical cauterization that promotes sloughing of the offending malignant mucosa is unknown. Nonetheless, these intravesical agents rid the patient of tumor with varying effectiveness. It should be recognized that irrespective of treatment, patients with tumors that do not penetrate through the lamina propria have less than a 7 per cent chance of ever dying of their malignancy. Once the tumor penetrates through the lamina propria (Stage A), the patient has a 30 per cent chance of succumbing to malignancy. The chance of death from the submucosally invasive tumor is a function of the pathologic grade of the malignancy, which seemingly reflects the biological aggressiveness of the disease.

There is currently controversy as to whether intravesical chemotherapy is appropriate for disease that penetrates through the lamina propria or whether these patients should be treated more aggressively with wide local transurethral resection, with aggressive partial cystectomy, or with total cystectomy and urinary diversion (Table 16). Disease that penetrates into the muscle of the bladder is best managed by either partial or total removal of the bladder. The role of partial removal of the bladder (segmental cystectomy) in the management of this disease is controversial. Segmental cystectomy is no longer recommended because of high intravesical recurrence in the residual bladder. This probably reflects the biological nature of the disease rather than the surgical procedure itself. Patients who have no evidence of atypia or carcinoma *in situ* at other sites within the bladder either adjacent to or distant to the offending invasive malignancy may be appropriate candidates for partial cystectomy. However, the selection of patients for partial cystectomy is complicated by the tendency of the entire urothelial surface of the bladder to show premalignant change even in the presence of an isolated tumor.

TABLE 14. Response Rates after Treatment with Intravesical Therapy

Drug	Number of Patients	CR (%)	PR (%)	Total (%)
Thio-TEPA	420	29	29	47
Doxorubicin	521	38	35	64
Mitomycin C	170	48	26	75
Bacille Calmette-Guérin (BCG)	70	56	18	70

CR, complete response; PR, partial response.

Radical cystectomy is advised for patients whose tumors demonstrate muscle invasion and in current practice may very well be advised for patients who have high-grade disease that penetrates the lamina propria. Radical cystectomy in the male includes the bladder, prostate, seminal vesicles, and the immediate adjacent perivesical tissues; in women, radical cystectomy includes the bladder, uterus, tubes, ovaries, anterior vagina, and urethra. Pelvic lymphadenectomy is advocated by some; however, the poor survival identified when pelvic node metastasis exists makes the potential benefit of this additional procedure questionable. The value of preoperative radiotherapy prior to cystectomy is no longer questioned. However, the debate over the value of preoperative radiation therapy has been replaced by a debate over preoperative chemotherapy, currently called neoadjuvant chemotherapy. The purpose of the preoperative chemotherapy is to reduce the volume of disease within the bladder and also control any metastatic sites. However, no data exist to support the rationale for preoperative chemotherapy, and the current practice is to ablate the primary tumor by surgical removal of the bladder and associated structures and to secondarily treat metastatic disease with multiagent *cis*-platinum–based chemotherapy when such disease appears.

Results of Treatment[10]

The survival rates appear dependent more on the grade, stage, and cell type of the tumor rather than on maneuvers that occur at the time of removal (Tables 17 and 18).

For radical cystectomy, the patient is best approached through a lower abdominal midline incision. Following bladder removal, urinary diversion must be accomplished. The necessity for an effective and satisfactory bladder substitute has led to the development of multiple procedures to produce adequate drainage of urine. Initial attempts involved anastomosing the ureters to the sigmoid colon, to rely upon the intact anal sphincter to control both urinary and fecal streams. Ureterosigmoidostomy was popular until the early 1950s. However, the reflux of high-pressure colonic contents up the low-pressure ureter produced frequent upper urinary tract infections with coliform bacteria. Subsequent technological improvements led to the development of an anti-refluxing anastomosis between the ureter and the colon, which obviated the problem of reflux of colonic contents into the upper urinary tract. Nonetheless, even with the utilization of the anti-reflux anastomosis, the ureterosigmoidostomy has continued to be plagued with the electrolyte abnormalities of hyperchloremic acidosis occasioned

TABLE 15. Dosages Currently Used for Intravesical Therapy

Drug	Dosage	Frequency
Thio-TEPA	30–60 mg./30–60 ml. H_2O	Every week × 4; every month × 12
Doxorubicin	50 mg./50 ml. saline	Every week × 4; every month × 12
Mitomycin C	40 mg./40 ml. H_2O	Every week × 4; every month × 6–12
Bacille Calmette-Guérin (BCG)	120 mg. Pasteur strain 600 mg. Tice strain	Every week × 6; then at 3, 6, and 12 months

TABLE 16. Phase Specificity of Drugs Used Intravesically in Bladder Carcinoma

Drug	Molecular Weight	Cell Cycle	Mechanism of Action	Absorption*
Epodyl	252	Cell cycle–independent	Alkylating agent	Minimal
Mitomycin C	334	Cell cycle–independent	Alkylating agent	Minimal
Doxorubicin	544	Cell cycle–independent	Intercalates DNA	11%
Thio-TEPA	188	Cell cycle–independent	Alkylating agent	74%
Cis-platinum	300	Cell cycle–independent	Alkylating agent	25%
Bleomycin	1400	Action in G2 and M	DNA scission	13%
5-Fluorouracil	130	Action in S-phase	Antimetabolite	28%
Methotrexate	472	Action in S-phase	Antimetabolite	15%
VM–26	656	Action in S-phase	Metaphase arrest Premitosis block	—

* Relative absorption percentages are based on animal studies with intraperitoneal administration. Jones, R. B., et al.: Cancer Chemother. Pharmacol., 1:161, 1978.

From Lamm, D. L.: Intravesical therapy of superficial bladder cancer. AUA Update Series, Lesson 20, Vol. II, 1983.

TABLE 17. Patient Survival Following Cystectomy and Preoperative Radiotherapy

Series	Stage B_1		B_2	C	D_1	D_2	No Tumor	Operative Mortality		Number of Rads
Reid	28/43	(64%)	38/92	(34%)	5/24	(25%)		13%	(135)	2000
Whitmore	4/9	(44%)	8/18 (45%)	2/8 (25%)	2/9 (22%)	1/16 (6%)	10/19	11%	(119)	4000
Whitmore	8/16	(50%)	9/14 (64%)	6/12 (50%)	3/12 (21%)	116 (6%)	2/4	9%	(86)	2000
Vanderwerf Messing	10/21	(48%)	24/54	(44%)	2/7	(29%)				4000
Wallace			34/98	(33%)				7%	(77)	4000
Miller			18/35	(51%)						5000
Totals	50/89	(56%)	139/331	(42%)	14/84	(17%)	12/23			

TABLE 18. Patient Survival Following Cystectomy Alone

Series	Stage B_1		B_2		C		D_1	D_2	Operative Mortality
Whitmore	18/30	(60%)	8/31	(26%)	2/19	(16%)	2/16	0/18	14%
Riches			3/33	(9%)	1/28	(4%)			12%
Jewett	2/4	(50%)	2/12	(16%)	5/45	(12%)			
Bowles and Cordonnier	11/17	(63%)	5/10	(50%)	4/20	(20%)	0/3		5%
Pearse	7/14	(50%)	5/12	(42%)	2/15	(13%)	0/11		19%
Totals	38/65	(58%)	20/65	(30%)	14/125	(11%)			
Subtotal			B_2C 34/190	(18%)					

by the absorptive characteristics of the colon and the recently described increased incidence of colonic malignancy in patients in whom there is a progressive series of technological maneuvers for urinary diversion. In conduit diversion, a segment of either large or small bowel is selected and is used merely as a conduit to establish rapid transit of urine to the body surface where the urine is collected in a plastic collecting bag. This method adheres to the principle of separation of urine and fecal streams. The conduit diversion uses distal ileum, but a large bowel segment also can be utilized. The primary consideration in creation of a large or small bowel conduit is that the bowel tube be created sufficiently short to function merely as a conduit and not as a reservoir. The continent reservoir utilizes either large or small bowel and provides an internal storage device that is drained by intermittent catheterization of an external stoma created at the skin surface. The continent diversion attempts to create this internal reservoir utilizing a nonrefluxing cutaneous stoma catheterized at intermittent intervals by the patient.

An alternative to the continent diversion is orthotopic bladder replacement in which an internal reservoir utilizing either large or small bowel is created and anastomosed to the native urethra at the level of the perineal diaphragm (Fig. 24). Such a maneuver allows the patient to void volitionally through the normal urinary tract. Modification of the cystectomy in order to preserve the nerves that innervate blood supply to the corpora cavernosa also permits these patients to be sexually active fol-

lowing removal of the bladder and prostate. The persistent infection of urine retained within this internal pouch and the probability of recurrent stone formation within this pouch are such that the long-term consequences of this form of diversion are not yet established. However, the internal reservoirs that provide volitional control of the urinary stream are much desired by many patients.

The need to remove the urethra in males who undergo radical cystectomy currently is being debated. Approximately 7 per cent of all males who undergo radical cystectomy eventually develop a malignancy in the residual urethra. However, this figure may triple when diffuse carcinoma in situ exists within the bladder or prostatic urethra or when the primary tumor is at the level of the bladder neck. It is therefore recommended that patients with this form of malignancy undergo a simultaneous in-continuity urethrectomy. Patients whose urethras are not removed should have follow-up urethral cytologic studies obtained either by urethral lavage or by direct swabbing of the retained urethra.

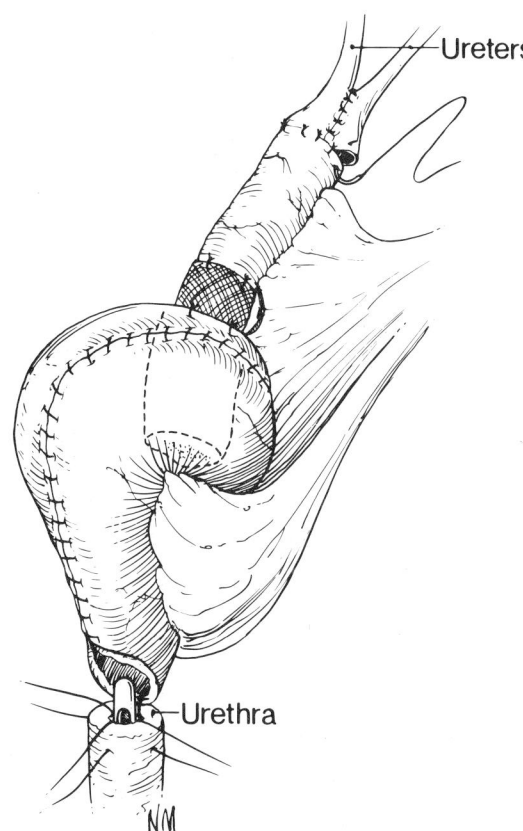

Figure 24. The open lower end of the pouch is approximated to the pelvic floor so that the length of the afferent ileal limb necessary for ureteroileal anastomosis without tension can be ascertained and any redundant ileal limb excised. A Wallace-type spatulated stented end-to-end ureteroileal anastomosis is performed. The urethral anastomosis is now performed between the membranous urethra and the residual opening at the inferior aspect of the pouch using interrupted sutures. A No. 20 to 24 Fr. Foley catheter inserted per urethra across the anastomosis completes pouch construction. (Provided by Dr. George D. Webster, Division of Urology, Duke University Medical Center, Durham, North Carolina.)

SELECTED REFERENCES

Chisholm, G. D., and Williams, D. I.: Scientific Foundations: Urology, 2nd ed. London, William Heinemann Medical Books, Ltd., 1982.
    This text is appropriately titled. The goal of the editor was to describe particularly the pathophysiology of the disease processes of the various organ systems and the newer aspects of the histopathology and oncology. The text deals specifically with disorders of the urinary tract with specific attention to the surgical aspect of urologic disease. The goal of the contributors was to establish a scientific foundation for the practice of urological surgery, and this has been accomplished with clarity. The contributors clearly establish the scientific basis for treatment and provide information that can be integrated with the doctor's traditional concern for the total care of the individual patient.

Devita, V. T., Hellman, S., and Rosenberg, S. A.: Cancer: Principles and Practice of Oncology, 2nd ed. Philadelphia, J. B. Lippincott Company, 1985.
    This is a magnificent textbook divided into two specific sections. The first section deals with the principles of oncology and covers in detail aspects of the cause and evolution of malignant disease as a biologic phenomenon and the essential principles that serve as the underpinning for modern cancer diagnosis and treatment. The second section, the practice of oncology, deals with the management of specific cancers themselves, the complications that malignant diseases produce, and the difficulties of therapy. The two chapters on urologic malignancy within this text are clear and concise and provide an up-to-date statement of the theory and practice of urologic oncology. Amply referenced, the chapters on urologic malignancy provide a ready reference source for the individual who wishes to expand his fund of knowledge by accessing original articles. This text is strongly recommended to individuals who wish to explore more fully malignant urologic disease.

Glenn, J. F., and Graham, S. D.: Urologic Surgery, 4th ed. Philadelphia, J. B. Lippincott Company, 1990.
    This text is a fine atlas of urologic surgery with 100 chapters by 100 different contributors. This is the fourth edition of this textbook, and an attempt is made by the various authors to make current recent advances in urologic surgery and in the parasurgical areas. This fourth edition details advances in the surgical techniques necessary for the surgical management of urologic disease. It provides ample and detailed descriptions of the surgical procedures and their conduct. It is strongly recommended for the individual who wishes to know in detail the methodology for the surgical management of urologic disease.

Paulson, D. F.: Genitourinary Surgery. New York, Churchill Livingstone, 1983.
    This unique text has a limited number of contributors. The goal of the editor was to identify individuals with recognized expertise in a single organ system and to have them present their philosophy of management of anatomic disease. The text is structured to present the normal anatomy and physiology of the kidney, ureter, and bladder and to identify abnormalities in development and other pathophysiologic processes that involve these organ sites. This has been accomplished well by each of the contributors. The narrative was structured so that the reader will be able to follow the surgical methodology of each expert as he considers the appropriate surgery of the diseased organ and the rationale for the specific bias of that author. Special care has been taken by the contributors to provide a series of illustrations that describes, step by step, the technique of surgical control.

Walsh, P. C., Retik, A. B., Stamey, T. A., and Vaughan, E. D.: Campbell's Urology, 6th ed. Philadelphia, W. B. Saunders Company, 1991. In press.
    This three-volume text has been the standard referenced text in urologic surgery. It contains approximately 86 chapters written by recognized authors from the various disciplines. The book is heavy in detail regarding the normal and abnormal anatomy and physiology. Each chapter is well referenced in order to assist the interested student in expanding his fund of knowledge.

REFERENCES

1. Amend, W. J. C., and Vincenti, F. G.: Oliguria; acute renal failure. *In* Smith, D. R. (Ed.): General Urology, 10th ed. Los Altos, Lange Medical Publications, 1981, pp. 446–449.
2. Barratt, T. M.: Fundamentals of renal physiology. *In* Chisholm, G. D., and Williams, D. I. (Ed.): Scientific Foundations: Urology, 2nd ed. London, William Heinemann Medical Books, Ltd., 1982, pp. 21–31.
3. Benson, M., and Olsson, C. A.: The bladder. *In* Paulson, D. F. (Ed.): Genitourinary Surgery. New York, Churchill Livingstone, 1983, pp. 209–312.
4. Charlton C. A. C.: Gram-negative septicaemia. *In* Chisholm, G. D., and Williams, D. I. (Eds.): Scientific Foundations: Urology, 2nd ed. London, William Heinemann Medical Books, Ltd., 1982, pp. 212–216.
5. deKernion, J. B., and Smith, R. B.: The kidney and adrenal glands. *In* Paulson, D. F. (Ed.): Genitourinary Surgery. New York, Churchill Livingstone, 1983, pp. 1–154.
6. Hodson, C. J.: Hypertension of renal origin. *In* McLaren, J. W. (Ed.): Modern Trends in Diagnostic Radiology. New York, Hoeber, 1960.
7. Hollingshead, W. H. (Ed.): Anatomy for Surgeons, 2nd ed. Vol. 2, The Thorax, Abdomen, and Pelvis. New York, Harper & Row, 1971.
8. Moffat, D. B.: Development of the urogenital system in the male. *In* Chisholm, G. D., and Williams, D. I. (Eds.): Scientific Foundations: Urology, 2nd ed. London, William Heinemann Medical Books, Ltd., 1982, pp. 344–356.
9. Paulson, D. F.: Prognostic factors predicting treatment response. World J. Urol., World J. Urol., 2:99, 1984.
10. Paulson, D. F., Anderson, T., and Perez, C. A.: Genitourinary malignancy. *In* Devita, V. T., Hellman, S., and Rosenberg, S. A. (Eds.): Cancer: Principles and Practice of Oncology. Philadelphia, J. B. Lippincott Company, 1982, pp. 731–785.
11. Powell, M. R., and Barnett, C. A.: Radioisotopic kidney stones. *In* Smith, D. R. (Ed.): General Urology, 10th ed. Los Altos, Lange Medical Publications, 1981, pp. 101–115.
12. Rees, A. J.: Pathophysiology of acute renal failure. *In* Chisholm, G. D., and Williams, D. I. (Eds.): Scientific Foundations: Urology, 2nd ed. London, William Heinemann Medical Books, Ltd., 1982, pp. 81–88.
13. Richie, J. P.: The ureter. *In* Paulson, D. F. (Ed.): Genitourinary Surgery. New York, Churchill Livingstone, 1983, 155–208.
14. Scott, F. B., and Attia, S. L.: Urodynamics. *In* Devine, C. J., and Stecker, J. F. (Eds.): Urology in Practice. Boston, Little, Brown & Company, 1978, pp. 113–122.
15. Selli, C., Hinshaw, W. M., Woodard, B. H., and Paulson, D. F.: Stratification of risk factors in renal cell carcinoma. Cancer, 52:899, 1983.
16. Tanagho, E. A.: Anatomy of the genitourinary tract. *In* Smith, D. R. (Ed.): General Urology, 10th ed. Los Altos, Lange Medical Publications, 1981, pp. 1–13.
17. Tanagho, E. A.: Embryology of the genitourinary system. *In* Smith, D. R. (Ed.): General Urology, 10th ed. Los Altos, Lange Medical Publications, 1981, pp. 14–26.
18. Tanagho, E. A.: Nonspecific infections of the urinary tract. *In* Smith, D. R. (Ed.): General Urology, 10th ed. Los Altos, Lange Medical Publications, 1981, pp. 153–198.
19. Webster, G. D.: Female urinary incontinence. *In* Glenn, J. F. (Ed.): Urologic Surgery. Philadelphia, J. B. Lippincott Company, 1983, pp. 665–680.

47

THE MALE GENITAL SYSTEM

John L. Weinerth, M.D.

HISTORICAL ASPECTS[42,48,76]

The development of genitourinary surgery constitutes an important and provocative chapter in surgical history. Numerous and sometimes extensive descriptions of genital afflictions can be found in Egyptian, Indian, Chinese, and Middle Eastern literature thousands of years B.C. Primarily descriptive, these writings were often fanciful, but occasionally incisive insights to the pathophysiology of the problems were noted. Anatomic interest in the lower urinary tract and male genital system grew rapidly in early Greece; Hemophilus, cofounder of the School of Alexandria, identified and named the prostate, indicating the gland that guards or stands before the bladder. Early Roman medicine continued more careful anatomic descriptions, but after Galen, it was not until the time of Vesalius that a more modern approach to anatomy, specifically of the genitourinary system, was available. However, during this entire period a preoccupation with lower urinary tract stone disease brought about the development of many instruments and techniques for traversing the urinary tract for the relief of urinary retention or the removal of bladder and urethral calculi. Some vague concepts regarding the reproductive function of the genitourinary tract existed in early times, but more comprehensive understanding had to wait until the Renaissance with progressive development into the twentieth century.

Diagnostic evaluation of the lower genitourinary tract evolved with endoscopic techniques; in 1879, Nitze developed the cystoscope employing Edison's incandescent bulb. Discovery of the roentgen ray in 1895 added another modality of diagnosis, and radiographic contrast material such as collodion silver, introduced by von Lichtenberg in 1906, prompted further urographic evaluation of the urinary tract. Excretory urography utilizing sodium iodine was discovered by Rowntree and associates in 1923. Swick, working in von Lichtenberg's laboratories in 1929, introduced a new substance, "uroselectan," a pyridine ring iodine compound, which enhanced successful excretory definition of the urinary tract.

The surgical treatment of genital problems and specifically the prostate was rudimentary before the late 1800s. Textbooks before that period dealt extensively with kidney disorders, stones, inflammatory conditions of the bladder, urethral abnormalities, and other urologic difficulties, but operative maneuvers on the large prostate were rudimentary. Although somewhat historically controversial, Sir Peter Fryer, of London, claimed first total prostatic enucleation on November 21, 1900. Shortly before the turn of the century, Hugh H. Young accomplished successful "operative removal of the enlarged prostate that was causing obstruction to urination." Perineal prostatectomy was probably first accomplished in this country by Goodfellow in 1891. In 1909, Young designed the urethral cold punch for the excision of median bars and contractures of the prostatic orifice and, with subsequent development, was the forerunner of modern transurethral prostatic resection with improvement and modifications made by Davis, Stern, and McCarthy, among others.

During the last 50 years, the modern perception of disorders of the male genitourinary system has been based on the advanced understanding of the physiology of the genital system, the endocrinology of sexual disorders, and the biochemistry of diseases of the prostate, seminal vesicles, and external genitalia. Recognition of the biochemical, neurologic, and hormonal capabilities of the male genital system have permitted accurate diagnosis and definitive therapy in a wide range of conditions including carcinoma of the prostate, testicular tumors, infertility, sexual function, and urinary obstructive disease. In addition, the development of microsurgical techniques has allowed reconstructive processes on very small structures within the male genitourinary system; the explosion and technology with endoscopic instruments, now with very small calibers and the capability for flexibility, have increased the diagnostic and therapeutic capabilities of the urologist.

ANATOMY[27,35,37,43,63,81]

Unlike in the female, parts of the male genital system are conjoined with regard to sexual and excretory functions, specifically the prostate and the urethra. The components of the male genital tract are the prostate gland, seminal vesicles, Cowper's glands, glands of Littre, the penis with its incorporated urethra, and the scrotum containing the testes, epididymides, vasa deferentia, and spermatic vessels. The male genitourinary system functions for the purposes of copulation, reproduction, hormone production, and urinary excretion (Fig. 1).

The prostate gland, seminal vesicles, Cowper's glands, and glands of Littre produce secretions that serve to lubricate the system and provide a vehicle for storage and passage of spermatozoa. In addition, secretions of the seminal vesicles as a base and enzymes from the prostate gland and Cowper's glands conjoin to produce coagulation and subsequent liquefaction of the ejaculate. The penis is composed of two vascular erectile bodies. The corpora cavernosa also incorporate the corpus spongiosum, which contains the male urethra. The paired testes produce both male hormones, predominantly testosterone, and spermatozoa, the former in the interstitial cells and the latter in the seminiferous tubules. The epididymides, lying in intimate contact with the testes, serve as an area of maturation and storage of sperm, which are further transported along the efferent tract composed of the vasa deferentia and the ejaculatory ducts, emptying into the posterior urethra at the verumontanum of the prostate.

TESTES. The testes are the central organs of male reproduction, two in number, ovoid in form, averaging 4 to 5 cm. in length and 2.5 to 3.5 cm. in width in the normal adult male. On the posterolateral surface of the testes, the epididymides are intimately attached to the surface and connected only via the tiny efferent ductules at the head of the epididymis to the interior portion of the testes. This is also the location of the terminal portions of the spermatic cord. The factors that control the descent of the testes from the abdominal cavity into the scrotum are probably mostly hormonal, but there may be some anatomic

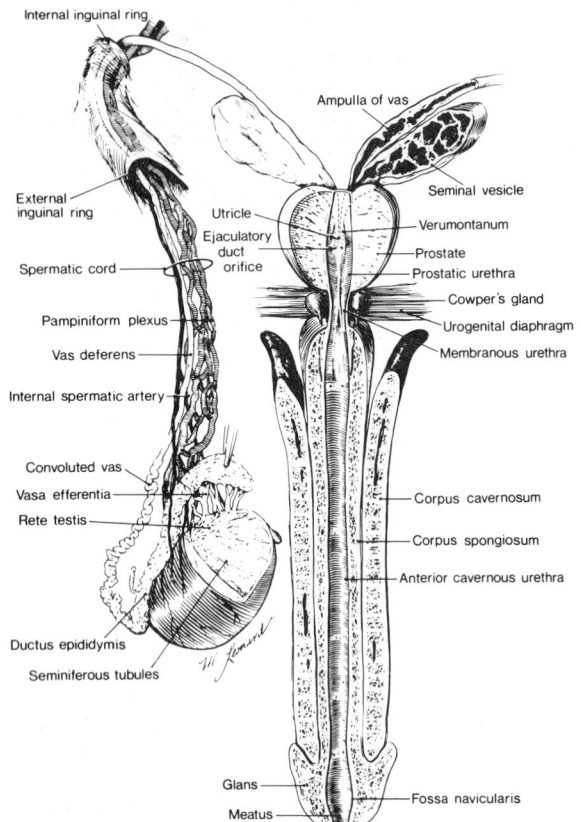

Figure 1. Schematic representation of the male genital system.

Histologically, there are two principal portions of the testis: the seminiferous tubules, which are responsible along with the Sertoli cells for spermatogenesis, and the interstitial or Leydig cells, which elaborate androgenic hormones, predominantly testosterone. Spermatogenesis appears to require relative hypothermia; seminiferous tubule function may be impaired in the cryptorchid or maldescended testis, whereas hormonal function may be unimpaired even in the intra-abdominal undescended testicle.

EPIDIDYMIDES.[16,27] The epididymides are coiled structures each containing a single epididymal tubule 12 to 19 feet long and attached to the posterior lateral surface of each testis. The actual connection between the testis and the epididymis is the efferent ductules resting on the superior extremity of the testicle, whereas the body of the epididymis is along the midportion of the testicle and the tail of the epididymis is attached to the inferior extremity of the testis. The medial surface of each epididymis attaches to the terminal portions of the spermatic cord through which the blood, nerve, and lymphatic supply are received. After the spermatozoa pass from the rete testis via the dozen or more tiny tubular efferent ducts into the epididymis, they progressively pass through the entire length of the epididymis, undergoing maturation and finally storage in the more distal portions. From the tails of the epididymides, sperm are transmitted into the vasa deferentia, which are direct continuations of the duct of the epididymides, passing up the spermatic cord, across the inguinal canal, and then retroperitoneally to the ampulla of the seminal vesicles with which they conjoin to form an ejaculatory duct on each side. The ejaculatory duct then empties directly into the prostatic urethra. The principal blood supply for the epididymis is from the internal spermatic artery, which also supplies the testis, but the deferential artery arising from the superior inferior vesicle artery follows the course of the vas deferens and provides some vascular supply to the epididymis. Venous drainage corresponds to the arterial supply, and the lymphatic drainage of the epididymis parallels that of the testis. The prime function of the epididymis is not only as a conduit for spermatozoa but also for biochemical and functional maturation and ultimate storage. Sperm recovered from the tail of the epididymis have exhibited a greater degree of maturation and fertilizing capacity than sperm recovered directly from the head or body of the epididymis.

VAS DEFERENS. The vas deferens is an easily discernible structure within the scrotum and spermatic cord since it is a heavily muscled tubular structure that aids in the transportation of the spermatozoa via contractions regulated by the autonomic nervous system. It has two main portions, namely, the straight portion that starts at about the level of the upper pole of the testicle and ends at the ejaculatory duct, and a second portion, called the convoluted vas, that joins the straight portion to the epididymal tubule at the lower pole of the testis.

SPERMATIC CORD. The spermatic cord, suspending each testicle and its attached epididymis, is comprised of the vas deferens, the internal spermatic artery, the external spermatic artery, the pampiniform plexus of veins, the lymphatic drainage system of the contents of the scrotum, and the autonomic nerve supply to the testicle. In addition, the cord is surrounded by fibers of the cremasteric muscle, which assist by contraction and relaxation in the maintenance of optimal testicular temperature as well as provide testicular retraction with sexual excitation or in the primitive fright reaction.

The spermatic cord joins as a single unit at the internal ring of the inguinal canal. The spermatic vessels, the spermatic nerves, and the spermatic veins coming from higher retroperitoneal positions and the vas deferens with its artery coming from a more inferior retroperitoneal position join at the internal ring and are then surrounded by the cremasteric muscle to extend into the scrotum where all components terminate into the testicle and epididymis.

considerations associated with the poorly defined gubernaculum testis. The descent occurs predominantly during the later phase of gestation but may continue into early childhood. The peritoneum anterolateral to the testis invaginates into the scrotum, and following the descent of the testicle this processus vaginalis is obliterated, leaving two layers of peritoneum around most of the testicle to become the tunica albuginea investing the testicle itself and the tunica vaginalis providing a potential cushioning space around the testis.

Since the testis arises from portions of the wolffian body on the genital ridge in proximity to the kidney, it is not surprising that the major blood supply of the testis arises from the aorta just below the renal arteries. Further blood supply follows the course of the vas deferens and may be sufficient to maintain testicular viability in instances where the internal spermatic artery is divided. A third vascular supply, the external spermatic artery, a branch of the epigastric artery, probably forms during descent. Venous drainage of the testis is through multiple veins of the pampiniform plexus to the spermatic vein, usually single, emerging from the upper end of the cord, then following the internal spermatic artery through the retroperitoneum. On the right, the spermatic vein empties into the vena cava below the right renal vein; on the left, the spermatic vein empties into the left renal vein. Increased hydrostatic pressure, particularly on the left, may result in dilation of the pampiniform venous plexus, producing a varicocele. The lymphatic drainage of the testis is through the spermatic cord and the inguinal canal and then to the common iliac and periaortic nodes, which communicate across the midline at the level of the kidneys and also communicate with the mediastinal and supraclavicular chains. Testicular nerves derive from the aortic and renal plexuses, which in turn communicate with the solar plexus. Traumatic injuries of the testicle may produce acute abdominal pain because of these interdigitating pathways, and in a like manner, intra-abdominal disease may cause referred pain to the testes.

SCROTUM. The scrotal sac, consisting of two lateral compartments fused in the midline and denoted by the median raphe, encloses the testes, epididymides, and terminal portions of the spermatic cords. The dartos, consisting of elastic fibers, connective tissue, and smooth muscle fibers, is intimately attached to the corrugated skin of the scrotum, rich in sebaceous glands, and provides muscular contraction of the scrotal sac in response to temperature changes or sexual excitation. The principal function of the scrotum is to aid in temperature control of the testes for optimal spermatogenesis, which takes place at temperatures several degrees lower than in the intra-abdominal cavity. The alternate contraction and relaxation of the scrotum in conjunction with a similar but separate contraction and relaxation of the cremasteric muscles of the spermatic cord allows maintenance of testicular temperature within a narrow and precise range. The blood supply of the scrotum comes from the deep pudendal branches of the femoral artery and branches of the internal pudendal artery. The lymphatics of the scrotal halves anastomose freely, surround the penis, and drain to the inguinal and femoral nodes. There are no connections between the lymphatics of the scrotum and the testes; the scrotal lymphatics do not accompany the pudendal vessels.

SEMINAL VESICLES.[10,20,41,57] The seminal vesicles are paired, monotubular, convoluted structures lying beneath the base of the bladder and trigone. Posteriorly they are invested by Denonvilliers' fascia, which separates them from the anterior wall of the rectum; in addition, one leaf of Denonvilliers' fascia separates the most cephalad portion of the seminal vesicles from the bladder. The two seminal vesicles fuse immediately with the ampullae of the vasa forming the ejaculatory ducts that open into the prostatic urethra at the level of the verumontanum. The seminal vesicles secrete a mucoid vehicle for the spermatozoa and also elaborate the body's only source of fructose, used as an essential nutrient for maintenance of spermatozoal viability. The muscular component of the seminal vesicle is contractile during ejaculation, expelling its contents through the ejaculatory ducts into the posterior urethra.

PROSTATE GLAND.[10] The prostate is a fibromuscular glandular organ that surrounds the vesicle neck and the proximal portion of the male urethra. The prostate of a normal young adult male is approximately 20 gm., consisting of two portions: an anterior (inner) group of glands intimately associated with the urethra, and a posterior (outer) portion of more fibromuscular character. Embryologically the gland derives from five to seven epithelial evaginations of the posterior urethra producing alveolar glands emptying into the urethra.

Normal prostatic function is dependent upon androgens, principally testosterone, which is metabolized to dihydrotestosterone and other substances of similar androgenicity within the prostate. The prostate itself is capable of elaborating specific enzymes, principally lactic acid dehydrogenase and acid phosphatase. The interrelated physiologic and endocrinologic functions of the prostate are necessary for normal reproductive function.

The inferior vesicle and internal pudendal arteries provide the blood supply to the prostate, entering the gland posterolaterally at the vesicle neck. Venous drainage of the prostate is complex and diffuse, with plexuses over the anterior and lateral portions of the gland that drain into the internal iliac veins. The nerve supply is both secretory and motor, derived from the sympathetic fibers of the hypogastric plexus as well as the sacral plexus. Intercommunicating lymphatics of the prostate, bladder, seminal vesicles, vasa deferentia, and rectum provide drainage into both the internal and external iliac systems as well as the sacral promontory nodes.

The difference in origin of the two portions of the prostate gland, namely, the anterior (inner) and posterior (outer) glands, has considerable surgical importance. The anterior (inner) portion, consisting of the periurethral glandular structures, gives rise to the hyperplasia and hypertrophy of benign enlargement in bladder neck obstruction in older men. The posterior segment, however, a musculoglandular structure, is the most frequent origin of prostatic carcinoma. Operations that deal with benign hyperplasia and hypertrophy leave the posterior (outer) portion of the gland behind.

The gland is supported anteriorly by the puboprostatic ligament, inferiorly by the genitourinary diaphragm (external urinary sphincter), and posteriorly by the rectal wall, which is separated from the prostate by an obliterated pelvic reflection of the peritoneum called Denonvilliers' fascia. The urinary sphincters are located at either end of the prostate with one at the vesicle neck and the other at the external muscular sphincter in the urogenital diaphragm.

MALE URETHRA. The male urethra consists of two major portions, the posterior urethra and the anterior urethra, each with two subdivisions. Beginning most proximally at the bladder neck, the posterior urethra consists of the prostatic portion and the membranous urethra. The prostatic urethra is analogous to the entire urethra of the female and is liberally invested with periurethral glands. The verumontanum opens in the floor of the prostatic urethra proximal to the apex of the prostate gland. The membranous urethra lacks periurethral glands, although Cowper's glands are located in the urogenital diaphragm lateral to the membranous urethra, the site of external or voluntary sphincteric action. The prostatic and membranous portions of the urethra are relatively fixed by the puboprostatic ligaments and the inherent stability of the urogenital diaphragm, whereas the urethra distal to the urogenital diaphragm is relatively mobile.

The anterior urethra includes the bulbous or perineal portion of the urethra, beginning at the urogenital diaphragm and extending to the penoscrotal junction, and the distal penile or pendulous urethra. The bulbous urethra exhibits a larger caliber than the remainder of the male urethra and is richly invested with periurethral glands. The penile or pendulous portion of the anterior urethra begins at the penoscrotal junction and extends distally to the external urethral meatus, just proximal to which is a bulbous enlargement, the fossa navicularis, which has a nozzle-like effect that produces a unified urinary stream.

COWPER'S GLANDS.[26] Cowper's glands (also called bulbourethral glands of Cowper) are small, paired glands lying between the layers of the urogenital diaphragm at the junction of the bulbous and membranous portions of the urethra. The ducts of the glands may be as long as 1.5 to 2 cm. and empty distally into the bulbous urethra traversing the corpus spongiosum. The secretions from this gland not only act as a lubricant but also may have factors that aid in seminal fluid coagulation after ejaculation.

PENIS.[56] The penis serves the dual function of copulation and excretion of urine. It consists of two parallel erectile compartments known as the corpora cavernosa, which are situated dorsolaterally, and the corpus spongiosum, which invests the urethra ventrally terminating distally in the erectile glans penis. Each corpus cavernosum and the corpus spongiosum are enveloped in fascial sheaths; in addition, all three corpora are surrounded by the dense fibrous Buck's fascia. The principal blood supply of the penis is through the dorsal arteries that course over the superior portion of the corpora cavernosa, lying deep to Buck's fascia, and being derived initially from the internal pudendal arteries, branches of the internal iliac artery. An additional branch of the internal pudendal artery enters the crura on each side of the corpora cavernosa, traversing it lengthwise.

The venous drainage is through the dorsal veins, the superficial dorsal vein emptying into the saphenous vein, and the deep dorsal vein emptying into the prostatic plexus known as the plexus of Santorini. Penile erection is induced by the engorgement of the erectile tissues of the corpora, principally the corpora cavernosa. The exact mechanisms of erection are not fully understood, but the competence of the pelvic blood supply and autonomic nervous system is essential for complete erection. The corpora cavernosa take origin from the ischial pubic rami as the crura, then fuse in the perineum. Further fixation of the penis is provided by the suspensory ligament, which connects the root of the penis to the underside of the pubis.

In addition, the erectile mechanisms respond to both psychic and tactile stimuli, which produce engorgement of the corpora cavernosa and to some extent the corpora spongiosum. Neurophysiologic studies indicate that there is a center localized to the medial frontal lobe that is a positive locus for penile erection. Certain anterior thalamic nuclei and mammillary bodies may also be involved.

Lymphatic drainage of the penis is abundant. The lymphatics from the shaft of the penis, the corpora cavernosa, and the skin pass through the superficial and deep inguinal nodes communicating with the iliac nodes. Lymphatic drainage of the glans penis parallels that of the urethra to the subinguinal, external iliac, and deep pelvic nodes; lymphatics from the urethral mucosa drain to the hypogastric nodes. The skin of the penis differs considerably from other skin of the body in its paucity of sebaceous glands, its elasticity, and the extensive blood supply.

TESTIS

Function and Infertility[3,54,61,63,68,69]

The testes have two primary functions: the production of the major male sex hormone, testosterone, and the production of spermatozoa. Biochemical activity within the testicle having to do with the production of testosterone and other androgens is extremely complex but is regulated in part through a feedback mechanism of the hypothalamus and pituitary gland via release of a luteinizing hormone. The production of testosterone and its release into the male environment enables the growth of secondary sex organs, maintains male body habitus, and is essential for sexual and reproductive function. The production of spermatozoa by the testis is also influenced by pituitary hormones, namely, follicle-stimulating hormone, in a similar feedback mechanism. Adequate function of the cells of the seminiferous tubules, including the Sertoli cells, is essential for the production of adequate numbers and quality of the spermatozoa necessary for fertility.

Infertility, therefore, can be the consequence of disturbance in either one or both of the primary testicular functions. The inability of a couple to produce offspring is termed infertility or sterility. It is estimated that up to 10 to 15 per cent of marriages in this country are initially barren, approximately half of this number responding to various therapeutic measures.

Infertility may be attributed to the male in as many as 50 per cent of these barren marriages. Adequate evaluation of the marital unit for infertility demands assessment of the male partner and a thorough evaluation of the possible factors involved. Infertility and sterility should not be confused with impotence, the latter term applying to the inability to achieve or sustain satisfactory erection for intercourse. The principal cause of male infertility is a spermatogenic defect estimated to comprise 95 per cent of cases of male infertility or sterility. Most males with such spermatogenic defects produce sperm in some quantity although there are usually diminished numbers of sperm, and those produced are of inadequate quality, exhibiting malformations and diminished motility. Oligospermia, by definition, indicates a sperm count of less than 20 million per milliliter, and under such circumstances fertilization is difficult. The principal causes of defective spermatogenesis include congenital inadequacy of the seminiferous tubules; testicular damage as a consequence of pyogenic infection, mumps orchitis, trauma, or infarction; chromosomal abnormalities such as Klinefelter's syndrome; hormonal defects as in hypopituitarism; varicocele;

and cryptorchidism. Other causes of oligospermia may relate to the transport of spermatozoa. Chronic prostatitis and seminal vesiculitis may result in fibrosis and impede transport and delivery of sperm. Infection spreading into the vasa deferentia may induce fibrosis and stricture even to the point of total occlusion. Abnormal fructose metabolism in the seminal vesical may predispose to inadequate storage capacity, inadequate spermatozoa nutrition, and diminished numbers of spermatozoa available for fertilization.

Azospermia, complete absence of spermatozoa in the ejaculate, may be caused by total occlusion of the sperm transport system, vasa, seminal vesicles, or ejaculatory ducts. Congenital absence of the vas and seminal vesicles may occur as an isolated anatomic defect, and congenital absence of the vas is usual in males with cystic fibrosis. In addition, an infection such as gonococcal epididymitis and vasitis may cause complete stenosis and azospermia. Complete nonresponsiveness of the germinal epithelium as in primary gonadal failure may also produce a form of azospermia despite elevated follicle-stimulating hormone levels. Trauma to the vasa in the course of an inguinal hernia operation or orchidopexy certainly may result in complete obstruction.

In some patients, infertility may be due to mechanical factors with no defects in spermatogenesis or delivery of spermatozoa. Surgical therapy of the vesicle neck, particularly transurethral resection, open wedge resection, or plastic reconstruction, or treatment of a congenital contracture may result in inability of the vesical neck to close with ejaculation, causing the ejaculate to pass in a retrograde fashion into the bladder rather than out through the urethra.

Physical examination of the infertile male should include careful and painstaking examination of the genitalia, particularly to ensure the testes are of normal size and consistency, the epididymides and vasa are present, and there is no evidence of chronic inflammatory disease of the external genitalia. Prostatitis should be excluded by digital examination, prostatic massage, and examination of the prostatic fluid. Appropriate cultures constitute the basis for antibiotic therapy, sometimes effective in alleviating chronic inflammatory processes as the cause of infertility. Other diagnostic modalities, such as cystourethroscopy and radiographic studies of the ejaculatory ducts, vasa, and seminal vesicles, are occasionally helpful to identify obstructive problems in the transport system.

Laboratory studies helpful in the evaluation of infertility include complete semen analyses, usually obtained after a 3-day absence from sexual activity, collected in a glass container. The same sample can also be tested for fructose, the absence of which would suggest either obstruction of the seminal vesicles or their absence. Serum levels of luteinizing hormone, follicle-stimulating hormone, and testosterone are helpful to identify pregonadal, gonadal, and postgonadal reasons for infertility.

Occasionally scrotal exploration and testicular biopsy may be indicated; the identification of normal architecture of the seminiferous tubules and normal spermatogenesis strongly suggests the possibility that an obstructive or inflammatory phenomenon is being overlooked, whereas inadequacy of the spermatogenic element suggests congenital or hormonal defects.

In the case of mechanical obstruction, new microsurgical techniques have been of considerable help. Epididymal inflammatory lesions may be bypassed by vasoepididymostomy. Vas ligation or stricture may be treated by reanastomosis of the vas. Results have been encouraging. Measures used in oligospermia include the administration of clomiphene citrate, gonadotropins, treatment of hypothyroidism, and scrotal hypothermia.

Orchidopexy cannot be expected to improve spermatogenesis if the patient is beyond the age of 12 years. More recently, high ligation of the internal spermatic vein has been advocated in the treatment of oligospermia associated with a varicocele, although the final rationale is still unclear. It is suggested that the varicocele causes defective spermatogenesis on the basis of increased intrascrotal temperature and the possible backflow of inhibiting adrenal hormones from the adrenal and renal veins down the left spermatic vein. A high inguinal division of the left spermatic vein occasionally may result in an increased sperm count and often results in improved sperm motility. Pregnancy rates have been reported as high as 44 per cent after patients have undergone treatment for varicocele. Generally a figure of 30 per cent is more widely accepted.

Congenital Anomalies[53]

The most common congenital anomalies of the testes relate to anomalous location, although congenital absence of one or both testes may be observed. The testes develop within the abdominal cavity, differentiating from the primitive gonadal ridge in the early weeks of fetal life. Normally, the testis begins its migration and descent through the inguinal canal at the end of the first trimester of gestation, but various mechanical and hormonal events may impede or alter normal descent. The gubernaculum, previously thought to provide a fibroelastic cord for guidance of the testis into the scrotal compartment, probably adds little mechanical assistance in this process. It appears most likely that the inherent functions of the testis itself are primarily responsible for the necessary ductal differentiation and descent.

ANORCHISM. The classic experiments of Jost indicate that the primitive gonad must differentiate as a testis in order to produce androgens, which are the stimulus to normal male (wolffian) ductal development. In the complete absence of testes, female (müllerian) ductal development differentiates in feminine configuration. However, one testis may fail to develop, occasionally in association with ipsilateral agenesis of kidney and ureter; monorchism is seen most often on the right and is termed the right-sided syndrome. Rare individuals are seen who exhibit no evidence of viable testicular tissue, although the external genitalia are fully differentiated in masculine configuration. In these cases, internal male ductal structures, the vasa deferentia, can be identified, usually extending to the internal inguinal ring and terminating blindly in fibrous tissue. These individuals are apparently normal males, although with a completely empty scrotum; puberty is delayed and incomplete with persistent elevation of gonadotropin levels and inadequate plasma testosterone levels. It is postulated that these patients with complete anorchism did indeed have normal testes at an early stage of gestation, but that sometime after the sixteenth week of fetal life the testes atrophied, possibly because of mechanical torsion or other interference with testicular blood supply in the course of the descent. Surgical exploration is required to establish a diagnosis, and a gratifying therapeutic response to continuing exogenous testosterone therapy is observed: sexual maturation, cessation of growth, increased libido, and masculine redistribution of body fat and muscle mass are concomitants to treatment.

CRYPTORCHIDISM.[28,29,35,36] The term *cryptorchidism*, derived from the Greek *cryptos*, or hidden, should be reserved for those testes that are truly obscure, usually within the abdominal cavity and not palpable on examination. Testes lying in the course of normal descent in the inguinal canal or in ectopic locations can usually be palpated and are not truly hidden. Cryptorchid or intra-abdominal testes are observed unilaterally or bilaterally in 1 to 10 per cent of male infants. Again, the cause of cryptorchidism is obscure, but a selective hormonal deficiency of the testis is suspected as a factor in such failure of descent. Occasionally, a truly cryptorchid testis will descend spontaneously at puberty or in response to parenteral chorionic gonadotropin therapy, but this is not usual and surgical exploration with orchidopexy generally is required. The cryptorchid abdominal testis fails in its spermatogenic function, although it may secrete adequate amounts of androgens. Spermatogenic failure is progressive, and transposition of an intra-abdominal

testis to the scrotum should be accomplished before the age of 2 years to ensure production of normal quantity and quality of spermatozoa. In cases of unilateral cryptorchidism, the matter of surgical exploration is less critical, but in bilateral cryptorchidism early surgical intervention is necessary. Exploration may be accomplished through an extraperitoneal inguinal incision, but more adequate exposure is obtained through an abdominal approach, particularly if bilateral cryptorchidism exists. Cryptorchid testes are usually found retroperitoneally deep within the pelvis and in proximity to the internal inguinal ring but may be located almost anywhere within the lower abdomen, even in the renal fossa. It is necessary to isolate the testis with its vas and vessels, mobilizing these structures completely. When the spermatic artery is short, it may be possible to bring the testis through the abdominal wall at Hesselbach's triangle, rather than through the inguinal canal, which necessitates a more devious course. Finally, since the testis may derive some blood supply from the small vessels coursing along the vas deferens, it may be feasible to divide the spermatic vessels and depend upon this collateral blood supply, permitting scrotal placement of the testis. When it is impossible to bring the testis to a palpable location within the scrotum or low in the inguinal canal, it is generally thought best to remove the testis, since there is a very high incidence of carcinoma in abdominal testes, the incidence perhaps being as much as 20 times greater than that of carcinoma in a normally undescended testis. When cryptorchidism is diagnosed after the age of 10 or 12 years, orchiectomy may be the preferred treatment, since such testes rarely exhibit normal function despite adequate scrotal placement. In carefully chosen patients, translocation of the testicle by complete division of the vessels and microsurgical reanastomosis of the artery and vein using the inferior epigastric artery may allow the salvage of a testicle with placement in the scrotum where it might otherwise be surgically impossible to perform an orchidopexy.

INCOMPLETE DESCENT. Incomplete descent or maldescent of the testis is the term reserved for those cases in which the testis is arrested at some point in its normal course of descent and is palpable on careful examination. The usual sites of arrest are at the internal inguinal ring, within the inguinal canal, or at the external ring. Most often, there is an associated congenital indirect inguinal hernia, since the processus vaginalis has not been obliterated at its proximal extent; there is potential for inguinal hernia, and the accumulation of normal peritoneal fluid dependently within the processus vaginalis produces a communicating hydrocele. Since function of a testis in the inguinal region is less compromised than that of the abdominal cryptorchid testis, treatment may depend on other associated factors. The presence of overt hernia prompts earlier surgical correction, and bilateral maldescent constitutes cause for earlier surgical intervention. Some authorities recommend the use of chorionic gonadotropin in dosages of up to 500 units 3 times weekly for 6 weeks as a stimulus to testicular descent, but in the truly arrested testis, such treatment is generally ineffective. Further prolonged chorionic gonadotropin therapy may lead to premature pubescence and growth arrest. A brief course of chorionic gonadotropin therapy may, however, be employed in preparation before orchidopexy and herniorrhaphy, since such stimulation may improve the vascular supply and augment the potential for surgical success. Exploration is accomplished through a high inguinal incision, exposing the entire cord to the internal inguinal ring. The testis and cord are completely freed from the surrounding structures; the patent processus vaginalis is identified, opened, stripped from the cord, and excised, so that the neck of the peritoneal sac is closed, and the spermatic vessels are carefully dissected extraperitoneally in order to afford maximal cord length. The testis is then positioned and fixed within the scrotum using a variety of techniques.

HYPERMOBILE TESTIS. In many young males thought to

have cryptorchidism, the testis or testes are merely highly mobile, retracting into the inguinal canal in an inaccessible position owing to hyperactivity of the cremasteric muscle. The simplest means of evaluation is to have the patient sit in a tub of hot water for up to 15 minutes; hypermobile testes descend into the scrotum and are normally palpable under such conditions. At puberty, hypermobile testes tend to situate normally within the scrotum; there is rarely any associated hernia, and surgical therapy can be avoided.

ECTOPIC TESTIS. Occasionally, one or both testes may undergo vicarious excursion in the course of descent, coming to lodge in ectopic positions. The exact cause of such wandering ectopia is obscure but must relate to mechanical factors. Favorite sites of testicular ectopia are symphyseal, prepubic, femoral, crural, penile, or perineal positions. Surgical correction should be accomplished for cosmetic reasons as well as to ensure normal testicular function and patient comfort.

Trauma

Surprisingly, the testes are relatively protected against trauma despite their external position. The primitive cremasteric reflex causes retraction of the testes to a protected inguinal position under extreme stress. Even in instances of avulsion of skin of the genitalia, the testes, appendages, and cords are usually undisturbed, remaining inviolate within their fascial coverings. Blunt external trauma may result in testicular hemorrhage and infarction, usually requiring surgical intervention. Penetrating wounds should be treated by surgical exploration. Torsion of the spermatic cord may occur as a result of external trauma, compromising blood supply and threatening viability of the testis, but such torsion is usually of spontaneous variety. Surgical intervention in instances of testicular trauma should be accomplished promptly, since the operative risk is minimal and early surgical repair can prevent subsequent infarction, atrophy, and loss of testicular function.

Infections[46]

Pyogenic infections of the testis are almost always secondary to spread of infection through the male ductal system, the vas deferens, and the epididymis. Chronic urinary tract infection, particularly suppurative prostatitis and seminal vesiculitis, predisposes to the spread of bacteria via the vas into the epididymis and the testis. It is rare to observe pyogenic orchitis without associated epididymitis, whereas epididymitis may occur with almost no involvement of the associated testis. In rare instances, systematic bacteremia may result in embolic metastatic foci of infection within the testis.

Orchitis may result from viral infection in association with mumps, usually will not after the patient has reached pubescence. Mumps orchitis produces severe local inflammatory reactions with excess accumulation of fluid within the compartment of the tunica vaginalis, the acute hydrocele of mumps. Supportive treatment is generally indicated, and aspiration of the hydrocele is avoided, since there is a risk of introducing bacteria and initiating a secondary infection that can result in testicular atrophy. Mechanical support of the scrotum with an adhesive bridge, bed rest, analgesics, and antipyretics constitute the first line of treatment. Smallpox, varicella, measles, influenza, and other similar infections may occasionally induce a secondary orchitis.

Tuberculous orchitis is almost always secondary to tuberculous epididymitis, the primary focus within the urinary tract generally being within the kidneys, sometimes in the prostate. Genitourinary tuberculosis is responsive to intensive antituberculous medical management, and surgical therapy is reserved for advanced cases of localized tuberculosis. Syphilitic gummas may occur within the testis, and surgical removal is almost always required, since chronic draining fistulas generally occur.

Fungus infections such as blastomycosis and actinomycosis of the testis are rarely observed but usually necessitate orchiectomy and continuing medical management.

The patient with an acute testicular infection is quick to appear for examination and treatment, since the condition is exquisitely painful. Orchitis must be differentiated from testicular tumor with hemorrhage and from torsion of the spermatic cord, both conditions demanding immediate surgical intervention.

Testicular Tumors[13,39,40,82]

Neoplasms of the testis itself are almost universally malignant, with the only exception being rare fibromas of the tunica vaginalis and pure Leydig cell tumors, which are usually benign. In contrast, extratesticular tumors within the scrotum are almost always benign, such as the adenomatoid tumors of the epididymis and cord. Because of this sharp distinction in the potential of neoplasms within the scrotum, diligent physical examination is necessary in distinguishing the site of origin of a scrotal mass.

Malignant neoplasms of the testes may be of germinal or nongerminal origin; nongerminal tumors arise from the interstitial cells and are known as interstitial cell tumors, Leydig cell tumors, or androblastomas. These are relatively rare tumors, producing excessive quantities of androgenizing hormones, which may cause virilism and precocious puberty in young males, impotence and gynecomastia in adults, and feminizing changes in the male that are analogous to those alterations observed with ovarian arrhenoblastomas in the female. Interstitial cell tumors of the testis must be differentiated from adrenal rest tumors, cells of adrenal origin being of very similar histologic character. It has been suggested that many cases of testicular tumors identified as interstitial cell neoplasms may indeed have represented unrecognized rests of hyperplastic adrenal tissue.

The malignant germinal tumors of the testis arise from the totipotential cells of seminiferous tubules and constitute a serious threat to the male population, representing 2 per cent of all malignant tumors, the dominant cause of death from genitourinary malignant disease in the younger adult male population. Testicular tumors are seen in all ages but predominate in individuals between the ages of 20 and 35 years. Germinal testicular tumors are categorized according to degree of cellular differentiation, which parallels malignant potential.

SEMINOMA. The most common of testicular malignant lesions, comprising approximately 40 per cent of germinal tumors, seminomas are uniform in gross and histologic appearance and are characterized by slow growth and late invasion. Metastatic spread is via the testicular lymphatics and predominates in the iliac, aortic, and renal hilar nodes. Because of the relatively slow growth of these tumors, they may be appreciated and removed surgically prior to the development of metastases. Metastatic seminoma of moderate tumor burden confined to the abdominal lymph nodes is responsive to radiation therapy, with 5-year survival rates in the range of 90 per cent. Other patients with more metastatic extension should receive multiagent chemotherapy in the same manner as for nonseminomatous tumors. In such patients, combination chemotherapy may still bring about complete remission in at least two thirds of the patients.

EMBRYONAL CARCINOMA. Of somewhat more malignant potential, embryonal carcinoma may also be seen in the younger age group and is usually thought to be the most common testicular tumor of childhood. The histologic pattern of embryonal carcinoma is of a less differentiated form than that of seminoma, and invasion and metastases occur earlier in the course of the disease. Because of relatively rapid growth of the tumor, hemorrhage and necrosis are common. Metastases to the abdominal lymphatics and the lungs may occur as an early event.

CHORIOCARCINOMA. Fortunately, pure choriocarcinomas represent only a small number of the germinal cell tumors. The tumor is extremely invasive, with trophoblasts invading the venous system early in the course of the disease. Metastasis may be both blood-borne and via lymphatics and has usually occurred by the time of diagnosis. Unlike choriocarcinoma in the female, which responds well to methotrexate, choriocarcinoma in the male is best treated with other agents such as *cis*-platinum, bleomycin, and additional agents. The prognosis for these patients is usually far worse than for other patients because of the advanced stage at time of diagnosis.

DIAGNOSIS AND MANAGEMENT. The earliest symptom of testicular tumor is a mass in the testicle, unfortunately unrecognized by most patients until there is associated pain, usually of a dull aching character. Hemorrhage within the testicle may follow minimal trauma, suggesting that traumatic injury is related to the tumor, which is probably not the case. Some of the more malignant tumors may produce hormones, measured as gonadotropins, which induce gynecomastia. In other instances, the more malignant tumors, relatively small in the primary location, may induce an abdominal mass as an early manifestation of disease.

The successful treatment of testicular tumors demands scrupulous physical examination, a high index of suspicion, and the willingness to accomplish prompt inguinal exploration when the diagnosis is suggested. The typical testicular neoplasm is stony hard in character with a suggestion of weightiness on palpation. When the suspicion of testicular tumor is raised, extensive laboratory evaluation should be deferred, with the exception of drawing serum for beta-subunit human chorionic gonadotropin and alpha-fetoprotein, which are important tumor markers, and surgical exploration should be accomplished as a primary event. The approach is through a high inguinal incision, exposing the spermatic cord at its emergence from the internal inguinal ring where it is isolated. Rubber-shod clamps are applied, and the testicle with its surrounding attachments can be mobilized for inspection and biopsy. If diagnosis of testicular neoplasm is confirmed, high inguinal orchiectomy is accomplished, removing the entire cord with the involved testicle, and leaving the stump of the cord within the retroperitoneum.

After orchiectomy, further diagnostic studies may be undertaken. Computed tomography of the chest, abdomen, and pelvis is generally the diagnostic imaging modality of choice and the basis for following the patient with regard to success of therapy. Beta-subunit human chorionic gonadotropin and alpha-fetoprotein should be determined after orchiectomy for comparison with the preoperative values. Elevations of gonadotropins are observed most commonly with choriocarcinoma, less frequently with embryonal carcinoma or teratocarcinoma, and only occasionally with pure seminoma. Bone survey and bone scan may exclude skeletal metastases, a relatively uncommon event in most testicular tumors, the metastatic pattern being lymphatic and visceral.

Further treatment of testicular tumors following orchiectomy is dictated by the results of evaluation and by the philosophy of the urologic surgeon. In most instances, it is thought that abdominal node dissection is of little value when pulmonary metastases have been demonstrated. If no pulmonary metastases are detected, radical retroperitoneal node dissection usually through a transabdominal approach and less commonly through thoracoabdominal exposures is advocated as an effective modality in the staging and control of the malignant process. Since metastatic seminoma is highly radiosensitive, many authorities question node dissection in treatment of seminoma. Although it may be pointed out that any seminoma may contain a microscopic focus of more malignant germinal elements and that metastases may reflect embryonal carcinoma, teratocarcinoma, or even choriocarcinoma, which may not respond favorably to radiation therapy, multiagent chemotherapy protocols rather than retroperitoneal node dissection appear to be the treatment of choice for this disease.

Because of these considerations, it is the usual practice to accomplish transabdominal radical retroperitoneal lymph node dissections in all instances of nonseminomatous testicular tumors except when very large masses of nodes are discovered by computed tomography or there is tumor in the lung.

Few patients with extensive abdominal tumor burdens or pulmonary metastases will more than likely undergo cyclical chemotherapy using multiple agents and then undergo retroperitoneal lymph node dissection and possible thoracotomy if the computed tomography scans are still positive or if there is suspected residual tumor once the tumor markers have normalized.

The efficacy of surgical node dissection has been elaborated irrespective of ancillary radiation therapy or chemotherapy. When node dissection is accomplished and there is no histologic evidence of metastatic disease, no further treatment is given. Survival in this group of patients irrespective of the histologic classification of the primary tumor is extremely good. However, when positive nodes are identified or removed at dissection, adjunctive therapy is indicated with chemotherapy depending on the cell type demonstrated in the nodes and the primary lesion.

A variety of chemotherapeutic agents have been developed over the last few years, resulting in dramatic responses. Historically, the antitumor agents have included actinomycin D, methotrexate, and chlorambucil. Some activity has also been noted with vinblastin. *Cis*-platinum, bleomycin, and vinblastine, with the addition of etoposide are now considered to be the primary therapeutic agents.

The ultimate prognosis in testicular malignant disease depends upon the stage of the disease at diagnosis, the histologic character of the tumor, and the vigor with which therapeutic measures are pursued. With the advent of combination surgical, radiation, and chemotherapeutic regimens, the outlook for patients with testicular carcinoma is extremely optimistic. The follow-up should extend over a minimum of 5 years with regular and periodic examinations, monitoring of serum beta-subunit human chorionic gonadotropin and alpha-fetoprotein, chest roentgenograms, and other indicated modalities of evaluation in the hope of identifying recurrence of disease and initiating appropriate new therapeutic maneuvers.

SPERMATIC CORDS AND TUNICS

The entire spermatic cord is subject to inflammatory diseases, usually the result of trauma or pyogenic bacteria termed funiculitis, occasionally seen with scrotal inflammation or epididymitis. Neoplasms of the spermatic cord are extremely rare, but sarcoma, usually rhabdomyosarcoma, and both invasive and metastatic malignant lesions from other structures may involve the cord. Benign tumors of the cord include adenomatoid tumors, lipoma, fibroma, and cysts, particularly hydrocele of the cord, a remnant of the processus vaginalis. However, the principal abnormality of the cord is torsion.

Torsion[24,33,34,62]

Torsion of the spermatic cord is probably the result of an abnormally high attachment of the tunica vaginalis around the terminal cord, allowing the testicle to twist freely within the compartment, the so-called bell clapper deformity (Fig. 2). When rotation of the testicle on the end of the cord exceeds 90 degrees, there may be compromise of the blood supply, which causes exquisite pain and results in gangrene and subsequent atrophy of the testicle unless the torsion is treated immediately.

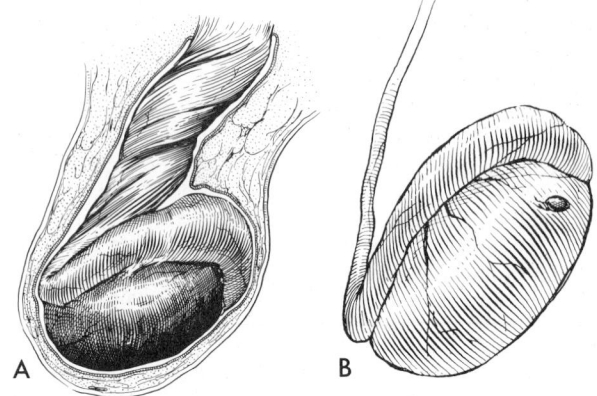

Figure 2. Torsion of the testis (A) is the result of twisting of the spermatic cord, usually within the tunica vaginalis; the appendix testis may also become twisted (B).

Incomplete torsion may result in partial strangulation, the effects of which may be overcome if surgical intervention is accomplished within about 12 hours, whereas severe torsion with total compromise of the blood supply results in loss of testes unless surgical therapy is effected within about 4 hours.

Torsion is usually seen in young males and most often occurs spontaneously, even during sleep. Physical and sexual activity may predispose to torsion and aggravate it by contraction of the cremasteric muscle. There is a rapid onset of severe pain and swelling accompanied by nausea, vomiting, abdominal pain, and even occasionally fever.

On examination, the involved testicle appears to ride rather high in the scrotal compartment and have a horizontal orientation. The differential diagnosis is between torsion and epididymitis, and it should be remembered that epididymitis is almost always accompanied by evidence of prostatitis and pyuria. With torsion, the entire testicle and appendages are involved in the swelling process, whereas with epididymitis the prominent induration is within the epididymides and not the testes; however, after a relatively short time this differentiation can often not be made.

Torsion must always be suspected with acute onset of scrotal pain, and prompt surgical intervention is required. Any delay in operation diminishes the prospects for salvage of the testicle. Nuclear blood flow scans and detection of testicular blood flow by a Doppler stethoscope have been used to differentiate epididymitis from torsion of the testicle, but it should be remembered that false-negative studies have been reported, and any question about the diagnosis should prompt surgical exploration.

When torsion is treated on one side, the contralateral scrotum should also be explored; the tunica vaginalis should be opened and inverted around the testis as with hydrocele repair, and any additional defect such as deficient attachment of the epididymis to the testis should be surgically corrected.

The appendix epididymis and the appendix testis (hydatid of Morgagni) are vestigial remnants of ducts attached to the head of the epididymis and to the superior pole of the testis, respectively. These small cystic structures may be twisted, producing acute and severe pain with generalized scrotal edema. Little permanent damage or disability is incurred by torsion of these appendages, but because of diagnostic confusion, it is often advisable to explore the scrotum when any doubt exists. Occasionally it is possible to make the diagnosis without exploration if the process is very localized and the small area of tenderness can be seen as a "blue dot" through the scrotal skin.

VAS DEFERENS[19,70,80]

The vasa deferentia are the conduits for spermatozoa from the epididymis to the seminal vesicles and prostate. Thus, normal vasa are necessary to human reproduction. Since a single testis is capable of producing sufficient numbers of sperm for purposes of fertilization, a single, normal, intact vas is all that is necessary to ensure the reproductive capacity of the male. The most common anomaly of the vas is congenital absence, seen almost universally in males with cystic fibrosis. There are other isolated instances of unilateral duct failure with the absence of the vas deferens. Discovery of bilateral vas absence should alert the clinician to the possibility of other wolffian duct abnormalities such as renal agenesis or renal ectopia.

While the vas is responsible for transit of the spermatozoa, it also serves as a conduit for retrograde passage of bacteria and infection of the epididymis and testicle, usually associated with prostatic infection, infected urine, or extremely high urinary outflow pressures.

Division of the vas for the purpose of sterilization, vasectomy, is the most popular means of elective sterilization at the present time. Millions of men have undergone vasectomy in the past few years, and most of these operations are being accomplished as an outpatient procedure. Although vasectomy is very simple, it must be remembered that spermatozoa distal to the point of ligation and stored within the seminal tract and prostate may remain viable for many weeks.

Spermatozoa disappear from the ejaculate at a rate of 50 to 70 per cent of the remaining sperm with each ejaculation, and most sexually active males have emptied all viable spermatozoa from the seminal tract after ten or more ejaculations. Microscopic examination of a freshly collected specimen of ejaculate should be accomplished 6 to 8 weeks after the procedure. The patient should not be pronounced surgically sterile until a negative specimen of ejaculate has been carefully examined. Such elective vasectomy is gaining legal as well as public acceptance. It is incumbent upon the urologic surgeon to ensure that the legal aspects are met in performance of sterilization operations. Optimally, a conference with both patient and spouse is arranged, and a waiting period may be required before the procedure is done. It must be made clear that a follow-up examination of the ejaculate is essential, since not all spermatozoa are cleared from the seminal tract at a predictable rate. It should also be explained to the couple that vasectomy must be considered a permanent sterilization measure despite the fact that there are increasing successes in utilizing microsurgical reconstruction of the vasa. Even with excellent technical success rates of greater than 95 per cent in terms of returning sperm to the ejaculate using microsurgical vasovasostomy techniques, the actual pregnancy rate may approximate only 50 per cent.

SEMINAL VESICLES[10,49]

Abnormalities of the seminal vesicles are relatively uncommon. Rarely, one of the seminal vesicles may be congenitally absent or exhibit cystic anomalies, usually associated with the ipsilateral absence of kidney and ureter. Occasionally, with ureteral duplication, one of the ureters will empty into the seminal vesicle, causing symptoms. Because of the secluded and protected location of the seminal vesicles, they are infrequently involved in trauma.

The most common clinical problems related to the seminal vesicles are those of inflammation and involvement by malignancy, owing to the intimate connection of the seminal vesicles with the prostate and the base of the bladder.

Chronic lower urinary tract infection may cause seminal vesiculitis, usually seen in association with chronic prostatitis and obstruction of the ejaculatory ducts at the ampullae. This may predispose to an abscess of the seminal vesicle, although this is rare. A diagnosis of such inflammatory disease is made by digital examination; the dilation and induration of the seminal vesicles can be readily appreciated, whereas the normal seminal vesicles are very difficult to palpate. A massage and stripping of the seminal vesicles produces purulent debris, confirming the diagnosis. Occasionally, pelvic computed tomography in association with vasography identifies an abnormal seminal vesicle.

Primary carcinoma of seminal vesicles is extremely rare. The surgical approach to seminal vesicles may be perineal, retropubic, transvesicular, or transperitoneal, the method selected depending upon the original diagnosis; benign cysts of the seminal vesicle are best approached abdominally, whereas removal of the entire seminal vesicles with the prostate may be most readily accomplished by perineal exposure. If the seminal vesicles alone are to be removed, leaving the prostate undisturbed and intact, a transvesicle, transtrigonal exposure may be most appropriate.

COWPER'S GLANDS

Under normal circumstances, Cowper's glands are not palpable, but occasionally infection may occur, usually secondary to urethritis, predisposing to enlargement that is palpable on rectal examination *distal* to the prostate in the genitourinary diaphragm in a paraurethral position. Dilated Cowper's ducts and dilated Cowper's glands may be demonstrated by retrograde urethrography, especially in association with stricture or urethral inflammatory disease. Treatment is usually conservative, although transurethral or perineal incision and drainage may be required. Carcinoma of the Cowper's glands is extremely rare but produces perineal pain, difficult urination, and a stony hard mass that presents rectally and perineally. Rectal fistulas may occur, and radical surgical therapy is indicated for cure.

EPIDIDYMIDES

FUNCTION AND INFERTILITY[27,60]

The epididymides are more than simply transport tubules. The epididymis, which if dissected free is approximately 4.5 meters long, gradually increases in its lumen from the head of the epididymis to the tail of the epididymis where it connects with the convoluted portion of the vas. An excellent review of the present knowledge and physiology of the epididymis has been presented by Howards. It appears that not only is there a storage factor in the epididymis, but there is also a maturation phase changing physiologic conditions within the epididymal tubules. During ejaculation, sperm are actually brought from the very distal epididymis through the vas to the posterior urethra in the process called emission. Ejaculation then delivers the bolus of the semen from the posterior urethra to the outside.

The genital abnormalities of the epididymis include total absence with or without the absence of the associated vas. In addition, there may be defects in the fusion of the epididymis and the testis as well as defects in fusion of the epididymis and the vas despite what appears by physical examination to be an entirely normal system. The incidence of epididymal defects appears to be higher in undescended testes. They may take the form of an extremely elongated epididymis, detached epididymis, or disruption of continuity.

Specific trauma to the epididymis is rare but certainly accompanies testicular injuries. The most common problem with the epididymis is infection, particularly after puberty, but occasionally it is seen in a prepubescent male, usually with chronic urinary tract infection, obstructed urethra, or high voiding pressure.

Acute nonspecific epididymitis is nongonococcal and nontuberculous, secondary to suppurative infection that usually has its origin in the prostate and seminal vesicles and then spreads in a retrograde manner to the epididymis.

Hematogenous and lymphatic spread of infection from a distant focus may occur but is probably quite rare. The inflammation is diffuse throughout the epididymis and may or may not involve the testicle, depending upon the severity.

The patient complains of severe pain and swelling with chills, fever, and other systemic symptoms that may include headache, nausea, and vomiting. Symptoms of urinary tract infection such as frequency, urgency, burning, dysuria, pyuria, and hematuria may be present. The epididymis and surrounding structures, including the spermatic cord, may be thickened by edema, swollen, and exquisitely tender to palpation. It is important to differentiate testicular swelling from epididymitis, since a mass in the testicle always suggests testicular tumor, and to differentiate acute epididymitis from torsion of the spermatic cord; torsion demands immediate surgical exploration, whereas epididymitis is treated by conservative measures.

In the very early phases of epididymitis, this distinction may be quite easy to make, but once the epididymitis has progressed to the point of causing inflammation of the surrounding tissue, distinction from torsion may be very difficult, and since torsion of the testicle can lead to total destruction, exploration may be required to make the correct diagnosis. Other conditions that may confuse the diagnosis include inguinal hernia with or without trapped bowel and an acute hydrocele.

Treatment of epididymitis consists of bed rest, elevation and support of the scrotum, application of cold packs, antipyretics, anti-inflammatory agents, and appropriate antimicrobial agents, sometimes administered intravenously. Occasionally, suppurative epididymitis may localize into an abscess and drain spontaneously; usually surgical intervention should be avoided unless testicular abscess develops.

Acute epididymitis then progresses to some degree of chronic epididymitis continuing over a period of several weeks, finally resolving and often leaving an epididymis that is indistinguishable from a normal epididymis after a period of several months. In past years, acute epididymitis was a common concomitant of all forms of prostatic surgery. However, utilization of routine preoperative vas ligation has been extremely effective in preventing such epididymal infections, and now, even without vas ligation, the utilization of preoperative, intraoperative, and postoperative broad-spectrum antibiotics diminishes the propensity for such a disabling infection.

Chronic epididymitis is usually the sequel of acute epididymitis but may arise insidiously with few localizing symptoms except the sensation of epididymal enlargement and slight tenderness. The demonstration of an associated prostatic infection is an adjunct to differential diagnosis, but tumor must always be suspected when there is a relatively painless chronic enlargement of the epididymis. Fortunately, however, the most common neoplasms of the epididymis are benign and include adenomatoid tumors, leiomyomas, and cysts.

A spermatocele is a diverticulum of the epididymis, containing cloudy fluid with spermatozoa, unilocular or multilocular, often confused with hydrocele since both a spermatocele and hydrocele can be transilluminated. Differential diagnosis of spermatocele and hydrocele is aided by the localization of the mass: hydrocele generally surrounds the testis, whereas the spermatocele is more eccentric in location and can often be palpated in direct conjunction with the epididymis and is often tender.

Other epididymal abnormalities are less common. Gonococcal epididymitis, once seen with relative frequency, is less common now, although certainly gonorrhea continues to exist in epidemic proportions. It is probable that earlier treatment of gonococcal urethritis diminishes the tendency to the development of subsequent gonococcal prostatitis, seminal vesiculitis, vasitis, and epididymitis. Similarly, tuberculous epididymitis is extremely rare today. Caseation necrosis may ensue, often involving the scrotal wall and skin with ulceration and fistula formation. In such cases, epididymo-orchiectomy with excision of the involved portion of the scrotal wall is usually necessary despite the use of newer antituberculous drugs. Other granulomatous reactions in the epididymis may be observed in association with syphilis or as a consequence of escape of spermatozoa with development of a sperm granuloma, sometimes painful and requiring excision. This is occasionally seen after bilateral vasectomy for voluntary sterilization.

Varicocele[54]

Varicocele is the term applied to dilation and tortuosity of the veins of the pampiniform plexus, most commonly observed on the left (Fig. 3). It has been stated that a varicocele may be an indicator of a left renal tumor, since the left spermatic vein system drains into the renal vein and obstruction at that point could produce dilation of the veins of the left cord; however, varicocele is uncommonly found to be associated with a renal tumor. Most varicoceles are idiopathic, although there may be a defect in the valve system of the spermatic vein, particularly on the left where the vein takes a longer course. Varicoceles rarely cause symptoms, but there may be a heavy, dragging, aching sensation in the scrotal compartment. Discomfort or infertility may prompt surgical repair, accomplished by varicocelectomy, which is a dissection and ligation of the multiple venous chan-

nels of the cord, or by high ligation of the spermatic vein through an incision at the level of the internal inguinal ring, giving ready access to the single vein. Following such ligation, venous collateral circulation is assumed by the deep pelvic venous system.

Hydrocele

The tunica vaginalis, derived from the peritoneum as the processus vaginalis at the time of testicular descent, is a secretory membrane. Fluid is generated by the serous surface of the tunica vaginalis, fluid formation being enhanced by inflammation or trauma. Fluid within the tunica vaginalis is resorbed at a constant rate through the extensive venous and lymphatic systems of the spermatic cord. Hydrocele, the excessive accumulation of this serous fluid, results when there is increased production or decreased resorption, the latter condition usually being idiopathic.

Congenital hydrocele may result from failure of obliteration of the processus vaginalis, and fluid formed within the peritoneal cavity may gravitate into the tunica vaginalis. Such congenital hydroceles may fluctuate in size, depending upon position of the child, and there may sometimes be an associated palpable inguinal hernia; whether a hernia exists or not, the potential for herniation is present. Occasionally, spontaneous closure of the processus vaginalis occurs during infancy and surgical intervention may be unnecessary. Even in instances of complete obliteration of the processus vaginalis along the spermatic cord, there may be excessive accumulation of fluid in the tunica vaginalis in the newborn, sometimes requiring aspiration or early surgical intervention for fear of mechanical compression and compromise of testicular viability. Congenital hydrocele, particularly with associated hernia, demands surgical repair, accomplished through a high inguinal incision, giving access to the internal inguinal ring, at which point the hernia sac or processus vaginalis is ligated.

In older individuals, hydrocele is frequently the result of epididymo-orchitis or trauma. If there is active pyogenic infection, the hydrocele may become infected, demanding surgical incision and drainage. Compromise of venous and lymphatic return along the cord may occur with a large inguinal hernia or as a result of herniorrhaphy with fibrosis of the inguinal canal obstructing venous and lymphatic drainage. Large intra-abdominal and pelvic masses may similarly compromise return and predispose to hydrocele. Although small hydroceles may require no treatment, the edema may assume such proportions as to cause severe discomfort and interfere with physical and sexual activity. Hydrocelectomy is accomplished by scrotal exploration with excision of redundant tunica vaginalis and retroversion of the remaining sac around the testes, epididymis, and terminal portion of the cord. A permanent cure may be expected by this procedure. Aspiration and injection of sclerosing materials is condemned because of the risk of infection.

INGUINAL LYMPHATICS[45]

The superficial and inguinal lymphatic intervals constitute the principal drainage system for the external genitalia. There is interdigitation of lymphatic drainage between the superficial inguinal nodes and the deep inguinal groups, which communicate with the hypogastric and iliac nodes. Lymphatics of the penis, penile skin, and scrotum drain to the superficial inguinal group; drainage from the urethra is to the inguinal and hypogastric nodes, and that from the glans penis is to the external iliac group. Inflammatory lymphadenitis occurs with many infections of the external genitalia and is usually treated conservatively with antimicrobial agents, bed rest, and other supportive measures. Suppuration may necessitate incision and drainage. Inguinal buboes may result from chancroid, the soft chancre that usually occurs primarily on the corona of the glans penis.

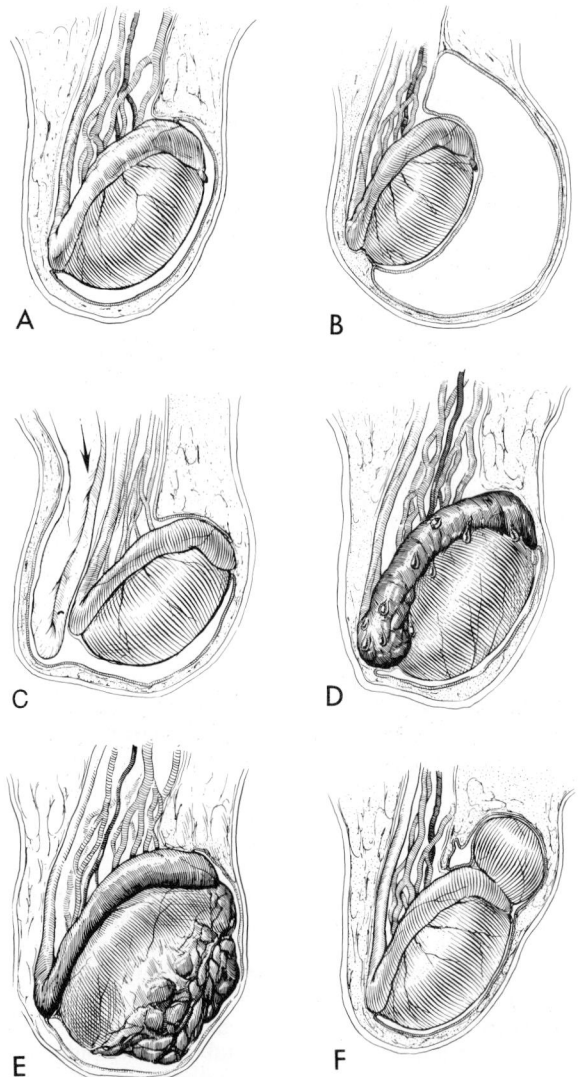

Figure 3. Common scrotal masses can be differentiated with knowledge of normal anatomy *(A)* as compared with *(B)* hydrocele of the tunica vaginalis, *(C)* inguinal hernia penetrating the scrotal compartment, *(D)* epididymitis causing induration and enlargement of the epididymis but not the testis, *(E)* testicular tumor causing an irregular mass intrinsic to the testis, and *(F)* spermatocele or epididymal cyst arising extrinsic to the testis.

Lymphogranuloma Venereum

Probably of viral origin although possibly due to L-forms, lymphogranuloma is also known as lymphopathia venereum and lymphogranuloma inguinale. Transmission of infection is by sexual intercourse, either genital or anal. Severe adenitis is sometimes associated with elephantiasis of the genitalia. Diagnosis is established by an intradermal Frei test and complement fixation, although these are not positive early in the course of the disease. There may be spontaneous remission, but therapy is usually effective with sulfadiazine, tetracyclines, and chloramphenicol. Surgical excision of the involved node groups may be required, particularly if secondary infection supervenes.

Granuloma Inguinale

Granuloma inguinale is a superficial ulcerative skin lesion associated with inguinal adenitis, due to the encapsulated gram-negative Donovan body, which is transmitted by sexual contact and is related to the Friedländer and *Klebsiella* groups of organisms. Granuloma inguinale is seen more commonly in the South and among the black population. Multiple painless granulomatous lesions cause extensive scarring, which may necessitate surgical excision. Streptomycin and tetracyclines are effective in controlling the infectious process.

PROSTATE GLAND
CONGENITAL ANOMALIES

Complete absence of the prostate gland in an otherwise normal male has not been observed. However, failure of normal development and maturation of the prostate may be associated with the intersex states and male gonadal failure. Congenital contracture of the vesical neck at the point of juncture of prostate and bladder may cause severe urinary obstruction. Congenital valves of the prostatic urethra — mucosal folds that may be diaphragmatic or alar — occur relatively frequently and cause profound obstructive uropathy in some cases. Congenital müllerian cysts predispose to obstruction and infection, presenting as midline masses beneath the gland and base of the bladder; treatment is by open surgical removal.

TRAUMA[79]

Fracture of the bony pelvis may often result in laceration and transection of the membranous urethra just distal to the prostate, and urinary extravasation as well as bleeding may displace the prostate and bladder superiorly. Occasional penetrating wounds of the prostate due to gunshot wounds or perineal straddle injuries have been reported. The most common cause of prostatic injury is inexpert urethral instrumentation, generally in the course of urethral dilation in treatment of stricture, although injury at the time of rectal surgery is occasionally encountered. The usual concomitant of prostatic injury is damage to the external urinary sphincter, which lies in proximity to the distal portion of the gland, with fibrosis and stricture. Another major complication of prostatic trauma is impotence.

Prostatic Infections[18,38]

Prostatic infections constitute a significant fraction of urologic practice. Infectious agents that may involve the prostate gland include the spectrum of gram-negative organisms, gram-positive cocci, gonococci, various mycotic organisms, mycobacteria, trichomonads, *Chlamydia*, and *Candida* species. The ascending transurethral route of infection is usual, and exogenous infection is enhanced by urethral abnormalities. Hematogenous and lymphatic routes of access to the prostate as well as descending infection from the upper urinary tract have been described, especially with tuberculosis.

ACUTE PROSTATITIS. Suppurative acute prostatitis may be seen from pubescence throughout the life span. The organisms most commonly involved are the gram-negative group, principally *Escherichia coli.* Acute gonococcal prostatitis is relatively uncommon, but the involvement of the periurethral glands by gonorrhea predisposes to inflammation and stricture, which invite secondary gram-negative infection in the prostate. Both bacteriostasis and a bactericidal effect of prostatic fluid have been demonstrated, indicating that there are natural defense mechanisms inherent in the prostate gland. Simple prostatic congestion may predispose to acute prostatitis.

Symptoms include urgency, frequency, dysuria, perineal aching, rectal discomfort, and even chills and fever with bacteremia. Edema may predispose to acute urinary retention. Examination discloses an exquisitely tender prostate that is diffusely indurated and enlarged. Urinalysis usually reveals pyuria, and often the offending organisms can be cultured. Prostatic massage should be accomplished most gently if at all, seeking to avoid bacteremia. Prostatic secretions are filled with purulent debris, and the stained smear may reveal bacteria.

Instrumentation should be avoided in the acute phase of prostatitis unless there is associated urinary retention that demands catheterization. Vigorous antibiotic therapy with a broad-spectrum agent should be initiated, pending culture and sensitivity studies. Bed rest, intermittent hot sitz baths, antipyretics, and restriction of sexual activity are necessary supportive measures. Antibiotic therapy should be continued for not less than 2 weeks, followed by a course of supplemental chemotherapeutic agents in association with follow-up examination and prostatic massage.

PROSTATIC ABSCESS. Prior to the era of antibiotic therapy, prostatic abscesses were frequent sequelae of acute prostatitis, but they are encountered less frequently today. Surgical drainage of prostatic abscess is required and may be accomplished by transurethral incision and resection, perineal incision and drainage, aspiration, or massage. Transrectal drainage of prostatic abscess is effective and is attended by surprisingly few complications, spontaneous healing of both the prostate and the rectal wall occurring in the majority of cases.

CHRONIC PROSTATITIS. Chronic inflammation of the prostate gland may ensue as a sequel of acute prostatitis or may occur as a complication of prostatic enlargement and obstruction. Presenting symptoms usually consist of dull aching perineal discomfort with minimal but recurring symptoms of lower urinary tract irritation, frequency, and urgency with symptoms of fullness and irritability. Occasionally, urethral discharge occurs. Many patients may have chronic prostatitis without symptoms. Chronic prostatitis predisposes to associated urethritis, cystitis, vasitis, epididymitis, and even orchitis.

On examination, the prostate gland may be essentially normal in size and consistency, enlarged and boggy, or irregularly indurated and tender to palpation. Urinalysis may reveal red cells, white cells, and bacteria or may be entirely within normal limits. Prostatic secretions, elicited by gentle massage accomplished by a sweeping motion of the examining finger over the lobes of the prostate from lateral to medial, followed by antegrade stripping of the prostatic urethra in the midline, contain pus cells with or without demonstrable bacteria. Normal prostatic secretions contain few white blood cells in the cellular elements of prostatic secretion, but greater numbers of pus cells, and particularly leukocytes, trapped in mucoid clumps confirm the diagnosis of chronic prostatitis.

The treatment of chronic prostatitis is often less than satisfactory. Antimicrobial agents may or may not be effective, and unless the symptoms are extremely severe and a positive culture can be elicited, antibiotics are usually avoided. Regular and periodic prostatic massage is probably the most beneficial modality of treatment and must be accomplished over periods of several weeks or months. Hot sitz baths may offer symptomatic relief, and regular sexual intercourse will encourage normal drainage of inspissated secretions. Anti-inflammatory agents may be of some help in selected patients. Surgical intervention is not often indicated, but prolonged and severe chronic prostatitis may lead to fibrosis, scarring, contracture of the vesical neck, and prostatic calculi; these conditions sometimes require intervention by transurethral prostatic resection. Calculi may occur in the glandular acini and ducts of the prostate gland, most often as the result of chronic inflammatory reaction with cellular necrosis, inspissation of debris, and deposition of calcific deposits. Whereas prostatic calculi may be scattered through the gland, they most often occur near the periphery of the prostate, lying in a cleavage plane between the adenomatous periurethral glands and the fibromuscular capsule; the stony hard induration produced may be mistaken for prostatic carcinoma. Bacteria may be trapped in the interstices of prostatic calculi, contributing to perpetuation of prostatitis. Treatment is dictated by the clinical course: if the patient is asymptomatic and the urine is negative, no treatment is required, but associated obstructive or irritative symptoms, persistent urinary infection, or severe pain may necessitate prostatectomy, accomplished transurethrally or by open surgical procedure.

TUBERCULOUS PROSTATITIS. Tuberculosis of the prostate gland does not occur as an isolated entity. Genitourinary tuberculosis is always secondary to a primary infection, either pulmonary or gastrointestinal. Tubercle bacilli are transmitted hematogenously, usually to the kidney and thence to the ureter, bladder, prostate, and other genitourinary organs. Digital examination of the prostate may disclose stony hard induration, reminiscent of carcinoma or prostatic calculi. The diagnosis is established by demonstration of tubercle bacilli in the urine or by prostatic biopsy. Medical management is indicated, employing various combinations of effective antituberculous drugs.

GRANULOMATOUS PROSTATITIS. Chronic prostatitis may predispose to a severe multifocal, abacterial inflammatory process that is thought to be due to extravasation of prostatic excretions into the interstitium of the prostate gland, initiating the histiocytic granulomatous reaction. Examination of the prostate reveals irregular induration that mimics prostatic carcinoma. Prostatic biopsy is needed to determine the diagnosis and exclude the possibility of carcinoma. Once the diagnosis is histologically established, treatment includes prostatic massage and elimination of any associated bacterial infection, although occasionally a prostatectomy may be required if outlet obstruction is present.

MISCELLANEOUS PROSTATIC INFECTIONS. Other inflammatory processes in the prostate gland are encountered less frequently. Blastomycosis and actinomycosis have been reported as causes of chronic prostatitis, and treatment of these conditions may require surgical extirpation of the prostate gland. Moniliasis involving the urethra and prostate is usually alleviated by simple urinary acidification with concomitant treatment of the involved sexual partner. *Trichomonas vaginalis* may infest the prostate gland and produce symptoms and findings similar to those of chronic nonspecific prostatitis, the diagnosis being established by identification of trichomonads in the urine or prostatic secretions. A 10-day course of antitrichomonad chemotherapy for both sexual partners usually eradicates the infestation. *Chlamydia* has been identified as an infecting organism by cell culture methods. Tetracycline derivatives are usually the treatment of choice.

Benign Prostatic Hyperplasia[22,77]

Benign prostatic overgrowth is the most common cause of bladder outlet obstruction in men over 50 years of age. Although exact mechanisms of prostatic hyperplasia are incompletely appreciated, it is recognized that adolescent development of the glandular acini and the fibromuscular matrix of the prostate is stimulated by gonadotropins and the androgens of the interstitial cells of the testes. After the age of 60, androgen production diminishes and glandular hypertrophy and hyperplasia of the prostate occur, progressing with advancing age. Typically the glandular elements surrounding the prostatic urethra centrally—analogous to the periurethral glands of the female urethra—undergo spheroidal proliferation. The true acinar glands of the prostate and the fibromuscular capsule of the gland are displaced peripherally and compressed as the adenomatous hyperplasia progresses. A lobular pattern of growth is observed, the hyperplastic process involving the two lateral lobes of the gland and the median lobe.

As the enlargement progresses, the prostatic urethra may become elongated and the caliber of the prostatic portion of the urethra may actually increase. However, the adenomatous process causes compression of the prostatic urethra, restricting the free flow of urine, sometimes associated with actual mechanical intrusion of a median lobe at the vesical outlet. Mechanical pressure phenomena then may include upward displacement of the base of the bladder, fishhooking of the lower ureters due to trigonal displacement, hypertrophy of the bladder wall with trabeculation, cellule formation, and even diverticula of the bladder. Complete bladder outlet obstruction may result in decompensation of the detrusor muscle and total urinary retention.

The symptoms of benign prostatic hyperplasia are those of mechanical obstruction and the consequences of urinary stasis. In the early stages of prostatic enlargement, the patient complains of diminished size and force of the urinary stream, and as obstruction progresses, there is increasing frequency of urination, probably owing to pressure of the enlarging gland beneath the trigone of the bladder. Nocturia is a similar index of the mechanical pressure of the enlarging prostate. It should be noted that nocturia normally occurs in older patients, both men and women, partially as a result of the inability of the kidney to concentrate urine, with resultant excretion of larger nocturnal volumes. However, nocturia more than once or twice nightly in the elderly male suggests mechanical pressure of prostatic enlargement as well as the possibility that the bladder is emptying incompletely with each voiding. Later, the patient with prostatic obstruction may note hesitancy and intermittency of the urinary stream, occasioned by intermittent fluttering occlusion of the prostatic urethra by the hypertrophic lateral lobes. Terminal dribbling suggests both residual urine and pooling of urine within the prostatic urethra.

Urinary bleeding may first bring the patient to the attention of the physician. Hematuria may result from prostatic enlargement with engorgement of the small mucosal vessels covering the adenomatous gland, ruptured as a consequence of straining to urinate. With progressive residual urine, infection may occur with purulent cystitis. Similarly, vesical stasis of urine can predispose to the formation of bladder calculi with severe symptoms of dysuria and stranguria. Occasionally, patients may have few symptoms of bladder outlet obstruction, the syndrome of so-called silent prostatism. Residual urines of 1000 ml. or more may produce a palpable lower abdominal mass before the patient experiences any particular symptoms, and it is not uncommon to observe bilateral hydroureteronephrosis and evidence of impending renal failure with azotemia and electrolyte imbalance.

The diagnosis of prostatic hypertrophy with bladder outlet obstruction is suggested by the history and is confirmed by careful physical and ancillary examinations. Rectal examination reveals varying degrees of prostatic enlargement, most often symmetric with the prostate rubbery in consistency. As enlargement progresses, the gland protrudes posteriorly, compressing the anterior rectal wall and sometimes producing symptoms of constipation. The size of the gland may bear little relationship to the degree of symptomatic difficulty incurred by the patient, a small gland often completely obstructing the bladder outlet, whereas a large prostate three or four times normal size may produce few if any obstructive symptoms. Palpation of the distended bladder suggests incomplete emptying with significant residual urine. Cystourethroscopy confirms the presence of prostatic enlargement and permits assessment of the degree of occlusion of the bladder neck or prostatic urethra, and the degree of bladder trabeculation and cellule or diverticulum formation. Azotemia may occur insidiously with bladder outlet obstruction, and the usual measurements of blood urea nitrogen, serum creatinine, and creatinine clearance provide indices of renal functional capacity. Thorough urodynamic study confirms both the absence of primary bladder or neurologic problems and the presence of outlet obstruction. Occasional secondary bladder instability is also demonstrated by these studies.

Conservative and medical measures of managing benign prostatic enlargement with bladder outlet obstruction are generally unsuccessful. Prostatic massage and urethral dilation are of little value unless there is demonstrated substantial congestion and stricture formation, respectively. Anticholinergic drugs and antihistamines should be avoided since they may precipitate urinary retention. Occasionally, estrogens in low dosage may induce minimal improvement in the urinary stream, presumably through the mechanism of some prostatic shrinkage, but in general hormonal measures have been ineffective in benign prostatic hypertrophy.

The decision for surgical intervention in benign prostatic enlargement is reached after evaluation of a variety of factors. Indications for surgical therapy include residual urine of more than 100 ml., particularly when there is associated azotemia of any degree; persistent or recurrent urinary infection refractory to usual therapeutic methods; gross hematuria on more than one occasion; acute urinary retention; or chronic urinary retention with overflow dribbling. To these classic indications for operative intervention, most urologic surgeons add the factors of patient comfort and desire for surgical therapy, nocturia more than two or three times nightly interfering with rest, and diurnal urinary frequency. The patient may be significantly concerned about the prospects of urinary retention, or it may be suspected that the enlarged prostate may be compromising sexual function, as it sometimes does.

There are four standard surgical procedures for removal of the obstructing enlarged portion of the prostate gland (Fig. 4). None of these procedures constitutes total prostatectomy; all are designed for removal of the adenomatous hyperplastic portion

of the gland, lying centrally and periurethrally. Therefore, these procedures should most properly be termed prostatic adenectomy rather than prostatectomy since the true prostate, compressed laterally into a fibromuscular and acinar surgical capsule, is retained after removal of the central adenomatous elements and may be the source of later carcinoma of the prostate.

SUPRAPUBIC PROSTATECTOMY.[47] Historically, the suprapubic or transvesical method of enucleating the prostatic adenoma was the first to be generally employed. Although utilized with less frequency today, this procedure still constitutes a fundamental method of surgical treatment in benign prostatic hyperplasia. A suprapubic incision, either vertical or transverse, gives access to the anterior surface of the bladder, which is then opened to give exposure of the vesical neck and the underlying prostate. From inside the bladder, the mucosa surrounding the bladder neck is incised and the adenomatous elements are removed by the establishment of a cleavage plane between the benign prostatic hypertrophy and the peripheral surgical capsule. Re-epithelialization occurs by growth of mucosa into the prostatic fossa from the trigone and bladder neck as well as from the membranous urethra below. Foley catheter drainage as well as suprapubic drainage is established, and the catheter is removed between 5 and 9 days postoperatively. Surgical mortality of 1 to 5 per cent is generally recognized, and the morbidity of suprapubic prostatectomy tends to be somewhat higher than that incurred with the other operative approaches to benign prostatic hyperplasia. However, suprapubic or transvesical prostatectomy remains a useful procedure, particularly when there is a very large median lobe, intrusion of the prostate well within the bladder cavity, or bladder diverticulum.

PERINEAL PROSTATECTOMY.[6] Perineal enucleation of the hyperplastic prostate was popularized at the turn of the century by Young. Perineal prostatectomy is particularly suitable to the large, low-lying prostate. The patient is placed in the extreme lithotomy position, giving access to the perineum, where a transverse incision in the shape of an inverted U is made anterior to the rectum. The rectum is separated from the posterior aspect of the prostate. The prostatic capsule is incised, and sharp and blunt dissection is employed to free the adenoma from the interior of the prostatic surgical capsule. The adenoma is amputated from the urethra distally and at the bladder neck. Hemostasis is effected with absorbable suture material at the vesical neck. A Foley catheter is inserted into the bladder through the urethra, and the capsulotomy opening is closed to re-establish continuity. A rubber wick or drain is employed in the perineal incision. Catheter drainage is generally maintained for 7 to 10 days. The perineal procedure carries a lower mortality and morbidity than suprapubic prostatectomy, but hospitalization is usually somewhat longer. The procedure offers the advantage of good control of bleeding, and it is thought that the extreme lithotomy position promotes venous return and minimizes operative vascular complications.

TRANSURETHRAL PROSTATIC RESECTION.[6,17] The emergence of endoscopic transurethral resection was dependent upon the development of adequate lens systems, the incandescent bulb and later fiberoptics, the refinement of electrical current for purposes of cutting and coagulation, and the ingenious combination of these advances into instruments satisfactory for surgical purposes. Transurethral prostatectomy has become the most commonly employed form of surgical treatment of benign prostatic hyperplasia with obstruction. Endoscopic resection of the enlarged prostate is most suitable in the smaller prostatic adenomas, those under 40 or 50 gm. in total resectable weight. It is better to resect the smaller fibrotic glands than to attempt difficult open surgical enucleative procedures.

The patient is placed in the lithotomy position, and the urethra is calibrated with progressive urethral sounds. The resectoscope sheath is introduced into the bladder, and the working

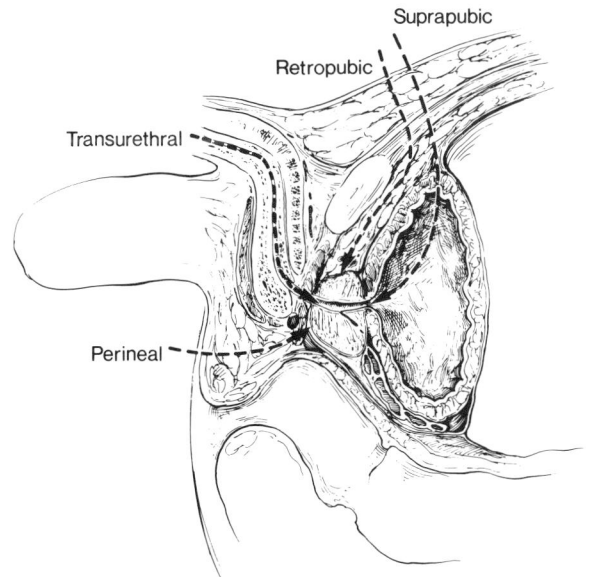

Figure 4. The prostate gland before basic surgical enucleative procedures for benign prostatic hypertrophy: perineal prostatectomy, suprapubic prostatectomy, retropubic prostatectomy, and transurethral resection of the prostate.

element is positioned. Under direct vision, the wire loop is employed to cut away fragments of the obstructing adenoma. These fragments are subsequently evacuated from the urinary bladder. Constant irrigation is required, employing a nonelectrolytic isotonic irrigant of satisfactory optical properties. An isotonic solution must be employed, since fluid extravasated into the circulation may cause hemolysis with subsequent acute tubular necrosis. The electrical current passed through the wire loop may be modified as a high-frequency, high-amplitude cutting current or as a low-frequency, low-amplitude coagulating current for control of bleeding. Hemostasis is ensured, and a balloon catheter is left indwelling for 3 or 4 days. Operative mortality is minimal, usually only 0.1 to 0.5 per cent; hospitalization is generally a matter of a week or less; and morbidity and complications are minimal in patients properly selected for transurethral prostatic surgery.

RETROPUBIC PROSTATECTOMY.[67] The retropubic route to prostatic enucleation was popularized by Millin and is ideally suited to the rather high-lying larger gland with little if any intravesical component. The patient is operated on in the supine position, and a transverse suprapubic incision is preferred. The anterior surface of the prostate is exposed, and the surgical capsule is incised transversely. Under direct vision, enucleation of the adenomatous portion of the gland is initiated by sharp dissection and completed bluntly. After the adenoma is removed, the catheter is passed through the urethra and the prostatic capsule closed. The procedure is modified by some surgeons who prefer to employ a vertical capsulotomy, extending the incision superiorly on the anterior surface of the bladder to gain added exposure of the bladder neck and the interior of the bladder. There are no contraindications to such an incision, which transects the region of the vesical neck, and exposure may be improved by this approach, particularly when there is a median lobe extending intravesically. In general, only a single urethral catheter is employed, and this is usually removed 5 to 7 days postoperatively. Problems of postoperative urinary incontinence are minimal with retropubic prostatectomy, morbidity is approximately equivalent to that of transurethral resection, although hospitalization may be somewhat longer, and the operative mortality is only slightly greater than that of transurethral resection, considerably less than that reported with suprapubic prostatic enucleation.

Long-term complications following prostatic surgery for benign adenomatous hyperplasia are relatively minimal. Since the surgical capsule is retained, sexual potency is usually unaltered, sometimes even improved, by these enucleative procedures. Urinary incontinence may occur as a permanent result of any form of prostatectomy for benign enlargement, but tends to be more prevalent after perineal prostatectomy and transurethral resection. Even here, the incidence of true and total urinary incontinence is minimal, probably no more than 1 per cent. The retained surgical capsule may afford an opportunity for regrowth of further adenomatous tissue. A small percentage of patients who undergo transurethral resection may have recurrent prostatic obstruction at a later date, necessitating another operative intervention, whereas recurrent adenomatous obstruction is seen with less frequency after the open procedures.

Occasionally a fibrotic process can involve the entire vesical neck without significant benign prostatic hypertrophy but causing the same outlet obstruction. This may occur with or without surgical procedures involving the prostate or vesical neck. Treatment of this bladder neck contracture can be treated both by open means such as a Bradford-Young YV-plasty, or probably much more simply by a transurethral incision of the bladder neck down through the scar tissue to the muscle, which then allows complete opening of the vesical neck and relief of obstruction.

Carcinoma of the Prostate[8,12,15,50,51,65,66,74]

Adenocarcinoma of the prostate is the most common malignant disease of men. The incidence of cancer has increased. Cancer of the prostate is now the most prevalent cancer in men by the most recent American Cancer Society Statistics. It barely exceeds cancer of the lung with 21 per cent of all cancers in males. Autopsy studies have established the fact that prostatic carcinoma, occult or overt, is present in about 15 per cent of men over the age of 50. It is estimated that the prevalence of prostatic carcinoma may be up to 48 cases per 100,000 population at the present time, and as the geriatric population increases, so must an increase in prevalence be expected. Squamous cell carcinoma of the prostate remains a relatively rare occurrence, and sarcoma of the prostate, still rarer, is generally seen only in the first two decades of life.

The etiology of prostatic carcinoma remains unknown, and although carcinoma of the prostate frequently coexists with benign prostatic hypertrophy, they are not believed to be causally related. There are no definite carcinogens known to be responsible for prostatic carcinoma; a viral etiology has been suggested but to this point there is no verification. There also appears no correlation with chronic prostatitis and prostatic calculi with ultimate development of prostatic carcinoma. It is quite possible that alterations in the estrogen-androgen balance and metabolic alterations in the prostate have a role, but the exact clinical significance of these changes remains to be established. Sexual activity is apparently not a factor, since prostatic carcinoma has been observed in both celibate groups and in men with histories of excessive sexual activity.

Prostatic carcinoma most often has its origin in glandular acini of the peripheral group of glands located in the posterior and posterolateral regions of the prostate. It appears that adenocarcinoma of the prostate does originate in glands that are metabolically and biologically active, although the acinar elements of the fibromuscular surgical capsule of the peripheral prostate are often of an atrophic nature. There are variations in biologic activity of prostate cancers among those individuals in whom the malignant lesion is peripheral as opposed to those who have a more centrally located paraurethral tumor, suggesting that different groups of glandular elements within the prostate may given rise to tumors of varying malignant potential.

One of the unique qualities of prostatic carcinoma is that many tumors produce an enzyme, acid phosphatase, that can be detected in the serum of patients with metastatic disease or at least a very large local lesion. Serum acid phosphatase has many sources, but the addition of tartrate to the serum inhibits over 90 per cent of the prostatic contribution and thereby separates the prostatic acid phosphatase from the total acid phosphatase. Since acid phosphatase is richly concentrated in normal prostatic tissue, prostatic examination or massage may elevate the serum level for up to 36 hours after rectal examination. Normal levels of serum acid phosphatase do not exclude prostatic carcinoma, since patients with small local lesions may not exhibit acid phosphatase elevation, prostatic tumors of low order of metabolic activity or great dedifferentiation may not produce such elevations, and even patients with advanced osteoblastic metastatic disease may on occasion display normal serum acid phosphatase values.

The prostate gland is also known to be the source of fibrinolytic factors. Normal seminal fluid has significant fibrinolytic activity, possibly enhancing motility of the sperm, attributed to the release of fibrinolytic activators from prostatic epithelium. Plasminogen, the precursor of plasmin, is a fibrinolytic protease found in many tissues including the prostate. In prostatic carcinoma, increased fibrinolytic activity predisposes to spontaneous bleeding and hemorrhage, particularly after prostatic surgery. Prostatic carcinoma may predispose to increased production of plasminogen, although the source of fibrinolytic activity in the blood of patients with prostatic carcinoma has not yet been identified.

Unfortunately, early symptoms of prostatic carcinoma are lacking. Since the majority of prostatic tumors occur in the periphery of the gland, encroachment on the urethra is a late manifestation of the disease. Irritative obstructive symptoms therefore do not signal the presence of the cancer, and it is only in advanced prostatic carcinoma that the lower tract symptoms occur. Occasionally, the patients may present with bone pain, usually lumbosacral, as a manifestation of metastatic disease long before local urologic symptoms occur. At the present time there are no satisfactory screening methods for prostatic carcinoma other than routine and regular rectal examination.

In essence, the diagnosis of prostatic carcinoma must be based upon suspicion. Every man over the age of 50 should have a regular rectal examination, and the findings of areas of induration and irregularity should suggest the diagnosis. Characteristically, prostatic carcinoma is stony hard in consistency and must be differentiated from focal tuberculosis, granulomatous prostatitis, and prostatic calculi. The isolated prostatic nodule must be regarded with the highest suspicion and the appropriate diagnostic maneuvers undertaken, including serum acid phosphatase determination, prostatic specific antigen, skeletal bone films, and radionuclide bone scan, but most important, an appropriate form of biopsy. In advanced cases of local disease there is usually little doubt as to the diagnosis. The prostate becomes nodular and irregular with extension of the indurated process beyond the confines of the gland, culminating in fixation of the prostate to the surrounding pelvic structures. At this stage of the disease, the patient often is experiencing significant symptoms, although they may not be local urinary tract symptoms.

Definition of the stage of prostatic disease is aided by ancillary clinical and laboratory determinations. A long bone survey may disclose metastatic lesions. As an adjunct to the bone survey, which may be negative, radionuclide bone scans are helpful in demonstrating tumor metastases. Serum acid phosphatase determination constitutes a necessary step in diagnostic evaluation, since an elevated acid phosphatase certainly suggests metastatic disease, precluding cure by local therapy, be it either radical prostatic surgery or radiation therapy. Prostatic ultrasonography has recently been developed as a technology useful for the staging of prostatic cancer patients and possibly for screening of selected populations of male patients.

Occasionally intravenous urography and cystourethrography are useful in evaluating degrees of lower tract obstruction or obstruction of the ureters by advanced carcinoma.

The metastatic patterns of carcinoma of the prostate are unique and interesting. The most common manifestations of metastatic disease are bony lesions in the sacrum and lumbar spine, although it is thought that earlier metastases occur at the regional lymph nodes, supporting the rationale of staging pelvic lymphadenectomy to assess the obturator, hypogastric, and iliac nodes for the presence of disease as a method of establishing extent and anatomic stage of prostatic carcinoma. Paradoxical metastases to the brain and skull with no intervening metastatic lesions in the lung or other bones may occur via Batson's plexus, the spinal venous system that communicates directly with the periprostatic veins. Pulmonary lesions may be isolated nodular metastatic defects but are more often of an interstitial pattern or diffuse multiple seedlike lesions reminiscent of miliary tuberculosis. In advanced stages of the disease, metastatic adenocarcinoma of the prostate may be observed in nearly every organ, including such unlikely sites as the testes, the skin of the scrotum, and the adrenal glands.

Prostatic carcinoma can metastasize by local extension, hematologic dissemination, or lymphatic invasion and may occur early even with a very small lesion, although generally the size of the primary lesion correlates with the degree of metastatic extent of the disease. The treatment of prostatic carcinoma at the present time is selected on the basis of accurate anatomic definition of the stage of the disease. It is the general belief that local disease that has not escaped the confines of the prostate is best treated by surgical extirpation. The potential for surgical cure of early carcinoma of the prostate was clearly demonstrated shortly after the turn of the century. Radical prostatectomy involving removal of the entire prostate and the seminal vesicles can constitute cure only when the malignant process is confined to the prostate with no contiguous or distant spread. It is estimated that as many as 10 per cent of the patients presenting with prostatic carcinoma are in such an early stage amenable to cure by radical surgical therapy. In general, the indications for radical prostatectomy include the isolated and localized prostatic malignant process, anticipated life expectancy of 10 years or more, good general health in the patient with no other life-threatening ancillary disease, and the absence of indication of metastatic disease evaluated by bone survey, radionuclide bone scans, multiple serum acid phosphatase determinations, and negative pelvic lymphadenectomy.

Prostatectomy can be accomplished in the classic perineal procedure or by the retropubic approach, during which both pelvic lymphadenectomy and radical prostatectomy can be accomplished at the same time if the surgeon is willing to base surgical decisions on frozen section. Complications of radical prostatectomy include impotence, a small percentage of urinary incontinence, occasional rectal injury, and a surgical mortality of approximately 1 per cent. However, the efficacy of radical prostatectomy, given accurate tumor staging, is apparent in various reports; Dees recorded a 60 per cent 10-year survival following radical perineal prostatectomy as compared with a 22 per cent 10-year survival with palliative therapy and a 30 percent 10-year survival with hormonal manipulation measures.

The use of radiation therapy for the curative treatment of local disease is attractive and some evidence is available that suggests equivalent survivals for surgical versus radiation therapy for localized prostatic carcinoma. There are a number of studies in which external beam radiation therapy was used with various doses and fields, as well as interstitial radiation therapy with iodine-125 seed implantation. Careful follow-up is needed with regard to specific anatomic tumor staging, disease control failure, patient morbidity, and ultimate survival before these studies can be matched with a surgical series. Radiation therapy, however, does have an important role in the management of bone pain from metastatic disease and may offer palliation for patients with large local disease who are not candidates for radical surgical procedures. The attractiveness of radiation therapy for the management of local disease creates hope that the precise place of this modality in the treatment of carcinoma of the prostate will be clearly defined in the near future.

Observations by Huggins and associates more than 40 years ago led to the recognition of the androgen dependency of a large percentage of prostatic tumors and the therapeutic response of these tumors to estrogen administration. These observations and subsequent investigations demonstrated the efficacy of hormonal management and provided the basis for the first genuinely effective chemotherapeutic approach to malignant disease. Whereas hormonal manipulation cannot effect cure of prostatic carcinoma, excellent prolonged tumor control can be achieved. The administration of exogenous estrogens, bilateral orchiectomy, pituitary ablation, use of androgen synthesis inhibitors, or antiandrogens may affect androgen-dependent tumors. The most efficacious method is bilateral orchiectomy or the use of exogenous estrogens such as diethylstilbestrol. However, there is recent evidence that the use of combination drugs such as leuprolide and flutamide may be equivalent to orchiectomy and flutamide.

If exogenous estrogens such as diethylstilbestrol are considered, doses of diethylstilbestrol should be carefully managed since doses as small as 1 mg. per day do not produce anorchic levels of serum testosterone, but it is clear that doses as large as 5 mg. per day may have an adverse effect on the cardiovascular system. Therefore, the present recommended dose of diethylstilbestrol is approximately 3 mg. per day, but the long-term effects on the cardiovascular system have not been established. It is thought by a number of investigators that hormonal treatment, because of its potential side effects, should be withheld until the patient becomes symptomatic, since it appears that on a statistical basis longevity is not particularly affected by adjunctive therapies and therefore they should be reserved for symptomatic states. A new area of adjunctive therapy is the use of multiple chemotherapeutic agents. A number of drugs including 5-fluorouracil, estramustine phosphate, and cis-platinum have been used in various protocols with some success in terms of partial objective and subjective responses. Major effects of these drugs are bone marrow suppression, gastrointestinal toxicity, and nephrotoxicity. Considering the rapid development of new chemotherapeutic agents, this is an area that may have the greatest impact over the next 10 years on the treatment of metastatic prostatic carcinoma and even as an adjunctive treatment for localized disease.

In summary, the treatment of carcinoma of the prostate is dependent primarily on establishment of correct anatomic definition of the disease. Disease that is confined to the single organ site of the prostate is best controlled at present by radical surgical removal. Disease outside of the prostate should be treated depending on the patient's symptoms or physiologic abnormalities caused by the tumor. The timing of the treatment remains a controversy. At the present time it appears reasonable to withhold adjunctive therapy, including androgen deprivation, until the rate of the disease progression is identified or the patient becomes symptomatic from malignant disease.

MALE URETHRA

Congenital Abnormalities[78]

Congenital abnormalities in the male urethra can occur anywhere: the bladder neck, prostatic urethra, membranous urethra, bulbous urethra, pendulous urethra, or meatus. The most common distal abnormality is urethral meatal stenosis, which can usually be recognized by inspection and is suspected when the urinary stream is of poor caliber. Such stenoses may predispose to infection and be associated with enuresis. Simple meatotomy usually cures the stenosis. Other congenital strictures can be seen in the bulbous or pendulous urethra but are usually uncommon. Open surgical repair is preferred in longer strictures, whereas lesser areas of involvement can be satisfactorily handled by internal urethrotomy. In the area of the bulbous and membranous urethra, there are also occurrences of diverticula, which may be a source of infection or, by a flap-valve effect, obstruction. Open surgical incision in primary repair of the urethra is necessary. Occasionally, duplication of the anterior urethra, either incomplete or complete, occurs with subsequent symptoms of potential obstruction, infection, or double stream.

In the area of the prostatic urethra, congenital valves occur, usually causing severe obstructive uropathy with decompensation of the urinary bladder, hydroureteronephrosis, infection, and renal insufficiency unless prompt and adequate treatment is instituted. Valves are mucosal or fibrous folds obstructing urethral urinary flow, usually in the distal portion of the prostatic urethra at the level of the verumontanum, and occur in several configurations. Transurethral electroresection or destruction by fulguration is most often employed and is much

preferable to the older retropubic transprostatic open exposure. The spectrum of secondary problems associated with urethral valves is wide but may be so severe that temporary or permanent urinary diversion is required.

Another anomaly of the urethra is called hypospadias, which involves varying degrees of failure of complete development of the distal urethra. The urethra may terminate just proximal to the glans (glanular hypospadias), at some point along the penile shaft (penile hypospadias), at the anterior margin of the scrotum (penoscrotal hypospadias), or in the perineum with a bifid scrotum (perineal hypospadias). Associated with this defect is a severe ventral curvature of the penis, or chordee, which results from a fibrous band occurring in the projected course of the urethra. The embryologic defect is a failure of closure of the urethral groove. In extreme cases, particularly if there is associated bilateral testicular maldescent, the configuration of the genitalia may be so ambiguous that an intersex state results.

Early and accurate diagnosis is imperative. Almost all degrees of hypospadias demand surgical repair, for cosmetic as well as functional reasons. A variety of operative procedures are available depending on the severity of the defect and may involve single- or multiple-stage urethroplasties. The principal difficulty encountered in surgical repair of hypospadias with surgical chordee relates to achieving adequate penile straightening, which is imperative before urethral reconstruction is effected. The commonly employed techniques of urethroplasty involve construction of a skin tube from the original orifice to the coronal margin or the tip of the glans. Since hypospadias and chordee are universally associated with splaying of the glans and a hooded redundant dorsal foreskin, the glans can be reconstructed in conjunction with the urethroplasty, and the redundant dorsal foreskin can be mobilized and brought ventrally as a neourethra. The operative complications of urethroplasties of all types include fistula and stricture, both of which may be managed by relatively minor secondary surgical procedures.

Epispadias is the failure of development of the anterior wall of the urethra and concomitant failure of dorsal fusion of the penile corpora. Complete vesical exstrophy, a rare condition, is always associated with epispadias; epispadias alone with some degree of urinary continence is more commonly seen, although still infrequently. The urethral opening may lie anywhere from the vesical neck to the glans, but if it is distal to the prostatic urethra, urinary continence and control may be satisfactory. The severe cosmetic deformity and the associated difficulty in controlling the urinary stream demand surgical correction, usually accomplished in infancy. Plastic reconstruction and lengthening of the penis, closure and ventral inversion of the urethra, and reconstruction of the bladder neck is often satisfactory. Unless there is a complete failure of urinary control, urinary diversion is not necessary and with newer artificial urinary sphincters may never be necessary. While early repair is desirable, the child is usually better able to cooperate in achieving urinary control after the age of 3.

Trauma[11,52,79]

Traumatic injury of the urethra commonly occurs in association with pelvic fractures but also can occur with injuries to the perineum, gunshot or stab wounds, or iatrogenic injury from instrumentation. Shearing injuries induced by external forces during blunt trauma cause rupture at the urogenital diaphragm in the region of the membranous urethra. Urinary extravasation is noted, often with extensive pelvic hemorrhage. The prostate and bladder may be displaced superiorly, well away from the distal urethra. Urethral catheterization is often impossible, and many centers contraindicate it under such circumstances since a partial tear could be converted to a complete tear if undue force is used. Depending on the circumstances, either open surgical repair or temporizing suprapubic urinary diversion should be accomplished promptly. The diagnosis of urethral rupture must be suspected in every instance of pelvic injury, and unless the patient is able to void clear urine in a normal manner, a retrograde urethrogram should be obtained in an aseptic technique to determine the patency and competence of the urethra. If the urethra is normal, a catheter can be passed to obtain a cystogram, but if not, the bladder should be assessed either by the cystogram phase of an intravenous pyelogram or at open surgical therapy. Untreated urethral rupture, whether partial or complete, can result in urethral stricture and possible urinary incontinence.

Penetrating injuries of the urethra are also observed, most commonly due to shotgun or stab wounds. Immediate urethral reconstruction and urinary diversion by suprapubic cystostomy is appropriate. Similarly, straddle injuries to the perineum may cause urethral rupture on the ventral surface, which usually demands prompt surgical intervention and urethral stenting with a fenestrated catheter for a period of at least 7 to 10 days. Iatrogenic perforation or rupture of the urethra may occur in the course of instrumentation, cystoscopy, or urethral dilation. Preexisting urethral strictures due to trauma or gonococcal urethritis predispose to difficult instrumentation and potential perforation of the urethra, often followed by the establishment of a urethral diverticulum or false urinary passage. Periurethral abscesses and attendant complications may ensue unless urethral injury is recognized and promptly treated. In the event of iatrogenic injury, suprapubic cystostomy or urinary diversion should be performed together with administration of antibiotics.

Infections[14,32]

The urethra is subject to both gonococcal and nonspecific infections. Abnormalities of the urethra such as urethral stenosis, acquired stricture, urethral diverticulum, or other structural abnormalities predispose to the development of urethritis and complicate management. Often it is necessary to correct the anatomic abnormalities and treat the infection simultaneously in order to achieve maximal control of the infectious process.

Acute gonococcal urethritis results when gonococci are introduced into the urethra, finding an appropriate milieu in the relatively hypoxic recesses of the periurethral glands. Squamous cells are relatively resistant to infection so that the fossa navicularis is rarely involved. Infestation of the periurethral glands tends to lead to microabscesses, which may extend into the tissues of the corpus spongiosum. Characteristic symptoms of gonococcal urethritis include dysuria, frequency, and urethral discharge that is usually creamy white in character, exhibiting the typical gram-negative diplococci on the stained smear. Specific gonococcal cultures of the urethral discharge confirm the diagnosis. Treatment of acute gonococcal urethritis is through the use of penicillin, ampicillin, or relatively large doses of the tetracyclines. The rapid development of resistant organisms prompts perusal of the most up-to-date Centers for Disease Control bulletin.

Secondary associated gram-negative infections may demand adjunctive antibiotic therapy. Untreated acute gonococcal urethritis may lead to urethral stricture through the mechanism of fibrosis and cicatrix formation, and such gonococcal strictures then predispose to the development of posterior urethritis, prostatitis, and epididymitis, which may be refractory to general methods of management.

The term *nonspecific urethritis* refers to urethral infections in which no evidence of gonorrhea can be found. Nonspecific urethritis can be due to bacteria, virus, *Chlamydia*, or a fungus. The typical complaint of the patient with nonspecific urethritis is the clear mucous urethral discharge, particularly in the early morning, associated with some degree of urinary frequency and burning discomfort on urination. Prostatitis may or may not accompany the urethritis. Treatment is usually with one of the tetracycline derivatives.

Urethral Malignant Disease[5,11,21,55,64]

Carcinoma of the male urethra is rare, with less than 1000 cases being documented in the English literature. Those malignant lesions occurring in the distal penile portion of the urethra are most often squamous cell carcinoma, whereas the more proximal tumors are transitional cell lesions. Symptoms of urethral malignant disease are hematuria, dysuria, frequency, and possible ultimate urinary retention. The diagnosis is established by endoscopic visualization of the lesion and appropriate biopsy either cystoscopically or by open biopsy of a palpable lesion. Spread of the malignancy is by lymphatics of the corpus spongiosum into the deep pelvic nodes and by venous channels. Since the diagnosis is usually established late in the course of the disease, the prognosis is poor despite radical surgical intervention. Depending on the location of the lesion, partial urethrectomy with or without penectomy may be effective as well as possible anterior exenteration and lymphadenectomy. Radiation therapy and chemotherapeutic measures are presently unproven as effective therapeutic modalities, but the development of new chemotherapeutic agents or combinations of agents may be helpful in the future. Since a high percentage of patients with carcinoma of the urethra give a history of previous venereal disease or urethral stricture, any stricture that fails to respond to appropriate therapy should be thoroughly investigated.

PENIS

Congenital Anomalies[2]

It is fortunate the congenital anomalies of the penis (other than hypospadias) are rare, since abnormalities of the genitalia may be the cause of severe anxiety and psychologic stress not only to the patient but to the parents of the newborn male as well. Rare anomalies of the penis include duplication (double penis), complete transposition of the penis and scrotum, and congenital absence of the penis in an otherwise normal male. The last condition is probably best treated by sex conversion operative procedures, since there are no adequate surgical methods for reconstruction of a satisfactory erectile phallus. A persistently small penis despite normal growth in an otherwise normal male is called microphallus, and this can be treated medically, with fair success.

The most common congenital curvature of the penis is chordee, the fibrous band along the ventral aspect of the penis that is usually associated with hypospadias, the congenital defect of the distal urethra. Epispadias, congenital absence of the upper portion of the urethra, causes dorsal deflection and curvature of the penis. In addition, abnormalities of the investing Buck's fascia may cause asymmetry with various lateral deviations. There is also an entity known as torsion, in which the actual defect is in the investing skin and can be corrected by rotation of penile skin.

The normal foreskin of the penis provides a covering for the glans, the redundant portion of the foreskin being termed the prepuce. In many newborn infants, the prepuce cannot be retracted satisfactorily; infection and inflammatory reaction may result as well as edema, fibrosis, and scarring, preventing retraction of the foreskin, or phimosis. Obstruction to urination may occur, and urinary infection can result. Moreover, such chronic inflammation is thought to predispose to penile malignancy. In the past, prophylactic infant circumcision has been widely practiced, although in the most recent years, universal necessity for such a routine circumcision has been questioned.

When phimosis leads to one of the above-mentioned complications, a dorsal slit of the foreskin may be required as an emergency measure, and circumcision should be accomplished at an appropriate time. Very often, phimosis is accompanied by meatal stenosis, and a urethral meatotomy may be performed at the time of circumcision. If the contracted foreskin becomes retracted and trapped proximal to the glans, severe swelling and even necrosis of the glans may ensue, a condition known as paraphimosis. Emergency surgical intervention is necessary if the paraphimotic prepuce cannot be reduced manually; dorsal slitting of the constricted foreskin is the procedure of choice.

Penile Trauma[25,52]

Trauma to the penis is relatively uncommon but can cause total sexual disability. In pelvic fracture, rupture of the urethra causes extravasation of blood and urine in the penile tissues; treatment is immediate correction of the urethral rupture. In the erect state, the penis is subject to dislocation or even fracture, the latter condition being rupture of one or both of the corpora cavernosa with severe bleeding and hematoma. Immediate surgical intervention is required to repair the laceration in the investing fascia.

Rupture of the veins of the penis may produce severe hemorrhage, and subcutaneous hematoma is usually best managed by urethral catheter drainage and compression dressings. Laceration of the penile skin and the glans are not uncommon as a consequence of masturbation, manipulation, or sexual activity, and the frenulum of the penis occasionally tears with sexual intercourse. Avulsion of the penis and scrotal skin may result when clothing is caught in various types of machinery, the loose integument of the genitalia being avulsed rather readily. Split-thickness skin grafts to the penile shaft take well, and the cosmetic and functional results of such repairs are satisfactory providing all distal loose skin is débrided at the time of the split-thickness grafting.

Complete traumatic amputation, whether intentional or unintentional, has occasionally been seen. It is treated by complete reanastomosis of all structures including arteries, nerves, veins, and corporal bodies as well as the urethra by microsurgical techniques.

Penile Infections[44,45]

The penis is subject to infectious involvement by various venereal diseases as well as other pathogenic bacteria and viruses. The abundant blood supply of the penile skin predisposes to excellent healing of such lesions. However, furunculosis of the penis may lead to severe cellulitis and even infection of the erectile corpora of the penis, cavernositis, most frequently due to urethritis of gonorrheal or nongonorrheal origin. Incision and drainage with appropriate antibiotic therapy constitute the treatment of choice.

Inflammation of the glans penis and the prepuce constitutes balanoposthitis, most frequently the result of retained secretions and bacterial infection underneath the redundant prepuce, particularly when phimosis is present. Local irritative symptoms vary according to the severity of the infection, and it is thought that such chronic infections may predispose to squamous cell carcinoma of the penis. Dorsal slitting of the foreskin, local measures, and antifungal agents are employed initially. After the inflammation has resolved, elective circumcision should be seriously considered.

Condyloma acuminatum is a cauliflower-like growth known as venereal wart, occurring singly or multiply on the prepuce and glans penis, and within the urethra itself. The lesions are of viral origin, usually associated with poor hygiene, and may be transmitted from one sexual partner to another. In cases of redundant foreskin, circumcision may be helpful in preventing recurrence, although in the past the topical application of 20 to 25 per cent podophyllum in benzoin on superficial lesions on several successive occasions has been helpful. There appears to be an increased use of 5-fluorouracil cream for lesions on the glans or intraurethrally. Occasionally the venereal warts may achieve such size that surgical excision is necessary. In advanced cases the differential diagnosis lies between condylomata acuminata and carcinoma of the penis.

Herpes progenitalis may appear as small reddened areas on the glans penis and dorsal surface of the penile shaft, which become vesiculated, rupturing to leave superficial ulcerations or foci of secondary infection. These may be very small lesions; in some cases, depending on the hematologic state of the patient, the lesions may become extensive and debilitating. Small lesions, a common viral infection, are best managed by local cleansing and application of drying agents such as cornstarch or baby powder. On larger lesions, in addition to older therapies of anti-inflammatory agents, L-lysine, and idoxuridine, the treatment of choice is one of the newer antiviral agents, acyclovir.

The principal venereal diseases (other than herpetic lesions) to involve the penis itself are syphilis and chancroid. The primary lesion of syphilis is an ulcer or chancre, craterlike in appearance, usually appearing around the corona of the glans penis. Dark-field smear of the lesion reveals *Treponema pallidum*. Similar chancres may be caused by sporotrichosis and tularemia, but these lesions do not usually involve the penis. The penile lesion of chancroid is a soft ulcerated area, again usually on the distal portion of the penis, later associated with inguinal buboes. Gonorrhea does not produce external penile lesions, the primary involvement being of the urethra and periurethral glands. Granuloma inguinale and lymphogranuloma venereum involve the inguinal lymphatics.

Penile Malignant Disease[58]

Cancer of the penis is a rare tumor in the United States. It has a much higher incidence in populations in which circumcision and personal hygiene are not well established. The most common form of cancer of the penis is squamous cell carcinoma, although basal cell carcinoma and melanoma have been described. Benign lesions such as nevi, hemangiomas, and papillomas are readily managed by local excision. Squamous cell carcinoma constitutes a more difficult challenge and is generally seen associated with chronic balanoposthitis from lack of circumcision, although occasional cases of penile carcinoma have been reported in circumcised individuals. The lesion is frequently initially ignored by the patient or is hidden by the foreskin and possible phimosis. Treatment of the primary lesion is dependent on the extent identified at presentation and the status of the regional nodes. The Jackson classification defines Stage I, limited to the glans and prepuce; Stage II, invasion involving the shaft or corpora but without nodal or distant node metastases; Stage III, tumor confined to the shaft but with proven regional node metastases; and Stage IV, tumor invasive from the shaft with inoperable regional node metastases or with distant metastases.

Unfortunately, this classification does not allow cross-comparison of results of different series, and a TNM classification is now under consideration for more accurately assessing the extent of the patient's disease at time of diagnosis. Clearly, the lower the stage of tumor, the better the cure and survival rate that will ensue, and this declines with increasing staging.

Diagnosis is established by biopsy. Treatment consists of partial or total penectomy; a proximal tumor-free margin of at least 1.5 cm. is desirable. Inguinal node dissection with excision of both superficial and deep inguinal nodes is advocated when clinically palpable nodes persist after amputation. Lymphadenopathy may result from secondary infection seen in most advanced penile carcinoma. Radiation therapy in squamous cell carcinoma of the penis is ineffective for large primary lesions but may be employed in the treatment of known lymph node metastatic disease; the primary lesion should always be treated surgically. Chemotherapeutic efforts have been attempted with bleomycin either locally or systemically, or in conjunction with other agents for very small lesions and carcinoma *in situ*, or as an adjunct to systemic disease. The use of *cis*-platinum and methotrexate has been tested with some reasonable results; however, overall, with the exception of very small glandular lesions, the results have not been encouraging.

Special Conditions

Certain peculiar disorders of the penis or of penile function deserve special consideration, particularly since etiologic factors remain obscure in these disorders.

PEYRONIE'S DISEASE.[30,75] A localized induration of the fibrous investments of the penile shaft was first described by the French surgeon Peyronie more than 100 years ago. Despite adequate description and an abundance of clinical observation, the etiology of the condition is unknown. A firm fibrotic thickening of the fascia of the corpora cavernosa is observed, usually involving the dorsolateral aspects of the penile shaft or the intracavernous septum between the corpora cavernosa, histologically similar to keloid or Dupuytren's contracture. The fibrous plaques may be painless, but there is often compromise of erectile capacity of the penis with deviation of the penis on erection and pain as a consequence of this derangement.

Patients usually note the lesion by self-examination, and they may have experienced significant deviation of the penis that interferes with intromission and coitus. Progression is slow, and spontaneous remissions are observed. Treatment has been generally unsatisfactory, and recurrence, after local excision, has been noted. Therapy that has been used in the past includes vitamin E, potassium *para*-aminobenzoate (Potaba), systemic steroid therapy, local injection of high-dose corticosteroids, radiation, and ultrasound therapy. Since the disease appears to remit, there is no clear evidence in any of these modalities of an advantage over time for natural resolution. However, if the patient is totally disabled and has long-term resistant disease, excision of the plaque with skin grafting with or without the insertion of penile prostheses has been advocated.

When the diagnosis of Peyronie's disease has been established, it is perhaps most important to reassure the patient that the process is not malignant and that in many cases the disease process is self-limiting with slow, if any, progression, and perhaps resolution. Often anti-inflammatory agents alleviate some of the discomfort associated with the plaque in most patients, and although there is some penile deviation, sexual disability is unusual.

PRIAPISM.[4,30] Prolonged pathologic and painful erection of the penis is termed priapism, in recognition of the Greek god of sexual excess, Priapus. Pelvic venous thrombosis predisposes to priapism, and such thrombosis is observed with various metastatic malignant diseases, leukemia, pelvic trauma, sickle cell disease or trait, trauma to the corpora, or spinal cord injury. In the majority of patients, no definite etiologic factor can be identified, and both local and neurovascular abnormalities have been incriminated as possible causes. Prompt recognition and therapy are essential, since prolonged unrelieved priapism almost inevitably leads to subsequent permanent impotence from fibrosis of the corpora cavernosa.

Immediate sedation and analgesia sometimes relieves priapism, and continuous spinal anesthesia has been advocated as occasionally effective in the early hours of the condition. Classic treatments consist of insertion of large-bore needles for aspiration and detumescence; but unless pelvic venous congestion is relieved simultaneously, the turgidity recurs. Thrombosis of the corpora occurs late in the course of priapism; accordingly, venous bypass operations have included the corporosaphenous vein shunt, unilaterally or bilaterally, and the cavernosa-spongiosum shunt, unilaterally or bilaterally. More recently, the primary choice has been the creation of a fistula between the corpora cavernosa and corpus spongiosum, opening the tunica between these bodies via incision through the glans penis since the corpus spongiosum is rarely obstructed in priapism.

IMPOTENCE.[31,59,72,73] Although it is recognized that the aging process diminishes not only the libido but the capacity of erection as well, many men remain potent throughout their lifetime. Potency in the elderly male may be related to psychologic factors as much as to general health. Disease processes may well affect the ability of any male to be potent, and they should be carefully elicited. Arteriosclerotic cardiovascular disease may compromise circulation to the corpora, and in addition, many of the drugs used to treat hypertension and cardiovascular disease may have a secondary effect on the ability to maintain an erection. Diabetes and other systemic disorders producing generalized neuropathies may diminish ability for erection. Impotence may be one of the earliest signs of the Leriche syndrome, thrombotic obstruction of the iliac arteries, and the condition may be relieved by appropriate vascular surgery. Spinal cord injuries may impair the capacity for erection as may prostatic surgery, particularly perineal prostatic surgery, which apparently compromises the pudendal nerves in some men undergoing such surgical treatment for benign prostatic enlargement. It should be noted that the vast majority of potent males who undergo prostatectomy remain potent postoperatively irrespective of the surgical method employed. Radical prostatectomy for malignant disease usually results in impotence; there are recent reports of modifications of the perineal prostatectomy that may leave the patient potent, although the long-term results as a cure of cancer have not yet been assessed.

Finally, certain drugs may impair erections and produce impotence, presumably by the adrenergic blocking effect of the medication. Despite knowledge of this spectrum of potential causes of impotence, a large number of males who are otherwise healthy and who complain of isolated problems of impotence must be suspected of having idiopathic or psychologic difficulties. Psychologic consultation is mandatory when the various physical causes of impotence have been eliminated. The use of nocturnal penile tumescence studies has been helpful in distinguishing some patients with purely psychologic reasons for impotence from those with physiologic causes.

EJACULATORY DISORDERS.[4] One of the most distressing sexual disabilities of the young or middle-aged male may be premature ejaculation. Intromission may be scarcely achieved before ejaculation occurs, terminating the sexual act to the frustration of the patient and the partner. Certain organic and psychic factors can be incriminated: chronic prostatitis can increase irritability and predisposition to ejaculation, and long abstinence with attendant sexual excitation can initiate premature ejaculation. In most cases, however, the problem relates to inadequate sexual technique in the marital unit, and careful consultation and counseling may aid in overcoming premature ejaculation.

Another disorder of sexual function is retrograde ejaculation, occasionally seen as a consequence of neuromuscular disturbance of the vesical neck secondary to diabetes, spinal cord injury, and other causes of neuropathy, but most often due to surgical alteration of the vesical neck. Prostatectomy by open and endoscopic means, transurethral resection of the bladder neck, vesical outlet reconstructive procedures, and even retroperitoneal surgery with autonomic nerve damage may diminish the capacity for closure of the bladder neck, an essential ingredient in normal ejaculation, with consequent retrograde flow of ejaculate into the bladder. When such a surgical abnormality is incurred, little can be done to overcome retrograde ejaculation. In some patients, a trial of alpha-adrenergic drugs such as ephedrine or phenylpropanolamine may be administered to facilitate closure of the bladder neck. In some instances, gradual narrowing of the bladder neck over a period of a year or two after prostatectomy promotes more normal ejaculation. Retrograde ejaculation in no way diminishes sexual gratification, but it may, of course, be the cause of infertility, since the sperm are deposited in the bladder rather than being expelled through the urethra.

INTERSEX STATES[2,9,23]

The intersex state is that congenital condition in which there is ambiguity of the external genitalia or inadequate and incomplete differentiation in gonadal and ductal structures. The most common mode of presentation of the intersex patient is by request for sexual differentiation in the neonatal nursery. Ambiguity of the external genitalia necessitates prompt and definitive assignment of sex, reassurance of parents, and early mobilization of medical and surgical measures required to establish the appropriate sex of the child. On occasion, the intersex patient may be seen rather late, often because of microphallus, undescended testes, labial fusion, or clitoral hypertrophy noted as late as pubescence. The interested reader is referred to a number of definitive texts and monographs dealing with the various types of intersex states.

True Hermaphroditism

The true hermaphrodite is an individual with gonadal tissue of both sexes, manifesting as ovary and testis, ovary and ovotestis, testis and ovotestis, or two ovotestes. In such instances, relatively rare, ductal development may also be ambiguous, with male wolffian ductal structures ipsilateral to the testicular tissue and feminine müllerian ductal structures ipsilateral to the gonad with ovarian differentiation. Chromosomes are generally normal in number, and buccal smear reveals XX or XY patterns. The dominant gender role, as dictated by external genital development, should be pursued and supported by medical and surgical measures. When the external genitalia exhibit severe ambiguity, it is generally best to seek a feminine role for the patient, removing male gonadal tissue and ductal structures, effecting reduction phalloplasty if necessary, and constructing a vagina when the patient reaches marriageable age if there is no vaginal canal present. As for other forms of the intersex state, satisfactory cosmetic and functional results may be achieved with the external genitalia, restoring the patient to a fully satisfactory male or female role as the conditions warrant. Endocrine abnormalities usually do not coexist, but complete removal of gonadal tissue, as in instances of bilateral ovotestes, may demand lifelong supportive endocrine therapy in the form of appropriate estrogens or androgens.

Adrenogenitalism

The adrenogenital syndrome may occur in males or females, more commonly the latter. Congenital adrenal hyperplasia with excessive production of androgenizing steroid precursors, such as the 17-ketosteroids and pregnanetriol, results from one of several basic enzymatic defects within the gland, compromising the capability of the adrenal to synthesize cortisone and cortisol. Deficiencies of corticosteroids prompt excessive production of andrenocorticotropic hormone by the pituitary, stimulating the already hyperplastic adrenal glands to still further production of androgenizing precursors. The usual enzymatic defect is a deficiency of 11-beta-hydroxylase or 21-hydroxylase. Associated hypertension may be observed, and one third or more of children so affected may exhibit a salt-losing tendency with severe vomiting and dehydration, often mistaken for the syndrome of pyloric stenosis. In the male, precocious puberty is observed as a result of the androgenizing influence: early appearance of pubic hair, growth of genitalia to adult proportions, increased muscle mass, and early epiphyseal closure leading to the terms *infant Hercules* and *macrogenitosomia praecox*. In the female, similar androgenizing changes occur with hypertrophy of the clitoris to the point that it simulates a penis, growth of pubic hair, fusion of the labia in the midline obscuring the urethra and the vaginal introitus behind the single perineal opening or urogenital sinus, and other stigmata including acne, hirsutism, voice changes, and the musculoskeletal changes also seen in the male. Adrenogenitalism is the most common cause of intersex, girls so affected presenting at birth with ambiguous genitalia. The diagnosis is established by demonstration of a normal female chromatin pattern (XX) and an evaluation of urinary 17-ketosteroids and 17-hydroxycorticoids. Accurate assessment of urinary

steroids may be accomplished in the first week of life, and appropriate definition of sex is essential during the neonatal period if subsequent emotional trauma is to be avoided. Urologic investigation of the female with adrenogenitalism should include cystourethroscopy through the urogenital sinus; introduction of the examining instrument into the vaginal introitus will permit identification of a cervix, almost certain evidence that there is a normal uterus. Once the diagnosis is established, appropriate exogenous cortisone therapy should be initiated, suppressing further pituitary activity and diminishing endogenous adrenal output of androgens. When adequate control is effected, surgical correction of the external genitalia can be accomplished; subtotal phallectomy and labioplasty result in a satisfactory cosmetic appearance of the external female genitalia. Pubic hair, seen in the older patients with adrenogenitalism, may be removed periodically with one of the liquid depilatories. Abdominal exploration is unnecessary when appropriate diagnostic measures have been accomplished, and adrenal surgery is undesirable since adequate suppression can be achieved by medical management.

The Male Intersex

Differentiation of the external genitalia to a completely masculine configuration is apparently dependent on the fetal testes elaborating testosterone or some other substance, sometimes referred to as müllerian-inhibiting factor. If the fetal testes fail before genital differentiation has been completed during the first trimester of gestation, ambiguous external genitalia result. Occasionally, mechanical developmental defects may be responsible for genital ambiguity in the male, and often such genital abnormalities are associated with congenital deformities of the gastrointestinal system as well. The most common ambiguity of the male external genitalia is the association of cryptorchidism or incomplete testicular descent with perineal hypospadias and severe penile chordee. A male chromatin pattern (XY) can be demonstrated, and there are no associated endocrinopathies. Cystourethroscopic evaluation is helpful, since identification of a verumontanum is evidence of normal internal male ductal structures. Release of chordee and bilateral orchidopexy can be accomplished at an early age, and urethroplasty should be effected before the child reaches school age.

Maternal Virilization

In the past, it was common practice to treat abortion and habitual abortion with androgenizing drugs such as testosterone. Even though this mode of therapy is less frequently employed today, occasional instances of virilization of females are still observed. The administration of androgenizing agents to the mother has little or no effect on the male fetus, although there may be some precocious genital growth. In the female, the clitoris may be stimulated to considerable enlargement, assuming penile proportions. Some degree of labial fusion may also be observed, although usually the urogenital sinus is not fully formed and the urethra and vaginal introitus can be visualized. Since the influences are terminated at the end of gestation, there is no progression of the deformity. External genital reconstructive procedures are effected as with adrenogenitalism, but no continuing therapy is necessary.

Gonadal Dysgenesis

The dysgenetic testis results in varying degrees of ambiguity of the external genitalia. In males with dysplastic testes, diagnosis may not be suspected until a normal age of pubescence, at which time failure of development of secondary sex characteristics points to testicular inadequacy, as with Klinefelter's syndrome. The diagnosis of gonadal dysgenesis should be approached with caution, since delayed pubescence may be a simple genetic characteristic, not indicative of any serious underlying disease process. In the male child approaching puberty with small penis and testes, gonadal dysgenesis should be suspected, but the diagnosis is dependent on testicular biopsy and should be confirmed by complete endocrine evaluation. Gonadotropins become elevated at puberty, inducing increase in testosterone production. Measurement of urinary gonadotropins and plasma testosterone is effective in defining hypogonadal states; persistent elevation of gonadotropins with inadequate levels of testosterone supports the diagnosis of hypogonadism. Management is by medical measures.

SELECTED REFERENCES

Chisholm, G. D., and Williams, D. I.: Scientific Foundations: Urology, 2nd ed. London, William Heinemann Medical Books Ltd., 1982.
This outstanding text deals with much of the physiology, endocrinology, and embryology of urology. This book deals primarily with the scientific foundations of urologic practice and, as such, treats extensively the scientific basis of urology, which is missing or dealt with in cursory manner in most surgical texts.

Federman, D. D.: Abnormal Sexual Development: The Genetic and Endocrine Approach to Differential Diagnosis. Philadelphia, W. B. Saunders Company, 1967.
The complexities of sexual differentiation in the intersex states are fully presented in this compendium. The normal process of sexual differentiation is emphasized, and the chromosomal and endocrinologic abnormalities associated with intersex are elaborated. A rational approach to the diagnosis and treatment of intersex patients is presented.

Gillenwater, J. Y., Grayhack, J. T., Howards, S. S., and Duckett, J. W.: Adult and Pediatric Urology. Chicago, Year Book Medical Publishers, 1987.
This new two-volume compendium of adult and pediatric urology provides an excellent updating of current knowledge in both adult and pediatric urology. New sections have been added on specialized subjects such as gynecology, laser therapy, new imaging technologies, and new treatments for stone disease. The text also has a second advantage in that the Yearbook of Urology, published by Year Book Medical Publishers, will be used as a yearly update and be fashioned as a supplement to this textbook. It is well worth perusing and recommended as a long-term addition to any urologic library.

Glenn, J. F., and Graham, S. D. (Eds.): Urologic Surgery, 4th ed. Philadelphia, J. B. Lippincott Company, 1990.
This text provides an excellent descriptive and artistic presentation of the vast variety of surgical techniques and procedures used in the treatment of urologic disease. The history, methods of diagnosis, indications, and complications of surgical therapy are also well documented. This is an excellent reference text for all forms of urologic surgery.

Walsh, P. C., et al. (Eds.): Campbell's Urology, 5th ed. Philadelphia, W. B. Saunders Company, 1986.
This last edition far surpasses any effort made in the past for complete description of all areas of urology including physiology, embryology, diagnosis, and treatment. It constitutes one of the most exhaustive treatments of urologic surgery and its associated medical subspecialties. Excellent bibliographies with each subsection are up-to-date and pertinent.

REFERENCES

1. Allen, T. D.: Disorders of the male external genitalia. *In* Kelalis, P. P., and King, L. R. (Eds.): Clinical Pediatric Urology. Philadelphia, W. B. Saunders Company, 1976, p. 636.
2. Allen, T. D.: Disorders of sexual differentiation. *In* Kelalis, B. P., King, L. R., and Belman, A. B. (Eds.): Clinical Pediatric Urology, 2nd ed. Philadelphia, W. B. Saunders Company, 1985, p. 904.
3. Belker, A. M.: Vasovasostomy and vasoepididymostomy. AUA Update Series, 2:1, 1981.
4. Benson, G. S., and McConnell, J.: Erection, emission and ejaculation: Physiological mechanisms. *In* Lipschultz, L. I., and Howards, S. S. (Eds.): Infertility in the Male. New York, Churchill Livingstone, 1983, p. 165.
5. Berger, R. E.: Sexually transmitted diseases. *In* Walsh, P. C., Gittes, R. E., Perlmutter, A. D., and Stamey, T. A. (Eds.): Campbell's Urology, 5th ed. Philadelphia, W. B. Saunders Company, 1986, p. 900.
6. Brendler, H. B.: Perineal prostatectomy. *In* Glenn, J. F. (Ed.): Urologic Surgery, 3rd ed. Philadelphia, J. B. Lippincott Company, 1983, p. 867.
7. Bright, T. C., and Peters, P. C.: Injuries of the external genitalia. *In* Walsh, P. C., Gittes, R. E., Perlmutter, A. D., and Stamey, T. A. (Eds.): Campbell's Urology, 4th ed. Philadelphia, W. B. Saunders Company, 1979, p. 931.
8. Catalona, W. J., and Scott, W. W.: Carcinoma of the prostate. *In* Walsh, P. C., Gittes, R. E., Perlmutter, A. D., and Stamey, T. A. (Eds.): Campbell's Urology, 5th ed. Philadelphia, W. B. Saunders Company, 1986, p. 1463.
9. Churchill, B. M., and McLorie, G. A.: Intersex. *In* Gillenwater, J. Y., et al. (Eds.): Adult and Pediatric Urology. Chicago, Year Book Medical Publishers, 1987, p. 1916.
10. Coffey, D. S.: The biochemistry and physiology of the prostate and seminal vesicles. *In* Walsh, P. C., Gittes, R. E., Perlmutter, A. D., and Stamey, T. A.
11. Corriere, J. N.: Trauma to the lower urinary tract. *In* Gillenwater, J. Y., et al. (Eds.): Adult and Pediatric Urology. Chicago, Year Book Medical Publishers, 1987, p. 450.
12. Dees, J. E.: Radical perineal prostatectomy for carcinoma. J. Urol., 104:160, 1970.
13. Donohue, J. P.: The testis. *In* Paulson, D. F. (Ed.): Genitourinary Surgery. New York, Churchill Livingstone, 1983, p. 655.
14. Dunlop, E. M. C.: Chlamydial infection. *In* Chisholm, G. D., and Williams, I. (Eds.): Scientific Foundations of Urology, 2nd ed. London, William Heinemann, Ltd., 1982, p. 227.
15. Ercole, C. J., et al.: Prostatic specific antigen and prostatic acid phosphatase in the monitoring and staging of patients with prostatic carcinoma. J. Urol., 141:1181, 1987.
16. Ewing, L. L., and Chang, T. S. K.: Physiology of male reproduction: The testis, epididymis and ductus deferens. *In* Walsh, P. C., Gittes, R. E., Perlmutter, A. D., and Stamey, T. A. (Eds.): Campbell's Urology, 5th ed. Philadelphia, W. B. Saunders Company, 1986, p. 215.
17. Fair, W. R.: Transurethral prostatic resection. *In* Glenn, J. F. (Ed.): Urologic Surgery, 3rd ed. Philadelphia, J. B. Lippincott Company, 1983, p. 891.
18. Fowler, J. E.: Prostatitis. *In* Gillenwater, J. Y., et al. (Eds.): Adult and Pediatric Urology. Chicago, Year Book Medical Publishers, 1987, p. 1220.
19. Fuchs, E. F., and Alexander, N. J.: Immunologic considerations before and after vasovasostomy. Fertil. Steril., 40:497, 1983.
20. Goldwasser, B., Weinerth, J. L., and Carson, C. C.: Ejaculatory duct obstruction: A case for aggressive diagnosis and treatment. J. Urol., 134:964, 1985.
21. Grabstald, H.: Tumors of the urethra in men and women. Cancer, 32:1236, 1973.
22. Grayhack, J. T., and Kozlowski, J. M.: Benign prostatic hyperplasia. *In* Gillenwater, J. Y., et al. (Eds.): Adult and Pediatric Urology. Chicago, Year Book Medical Publishers, 1987, p. 1062.
23. Griffin, J. E., and Wilson, J. D.: Disorders of sexual differentiation. *In* Walsh, P. C., Gittes, R. E., Perlmutter, A. D., and Stamey, T. A. (Eds.): Campbell's Urology, 5th ed. Philadelphia, W. B. Saunders Company, 1986, p. 1819.
24. Hahn, L., Nodel, M., Gitter, M., et al.: Testicular scanning: A new modality for the preoperative diagnosis of testicular torsion. J. Urol., 113:60, 1975.
25. Hopkins, S. C., and Grabstald, H.: Benign and malignant tumors of the male and female urethra. *In* Walsh, P. C., Gittes, R. E., Perlmutter, A. D., and Stamey, T. A. (Eds.): Campbell's Urology, 5th ed. Philadelphia, W. B. Saunders Company, 1986, p. 1449.
26. Hopkins, S. C., and Grabstald, H.: Tumors of the male urethra. *In* Walsh, P. C., Gittes, R. E., Perlmutter, A. D., and Stamey, T. A. (Eds.): Campbell's Urology, 5th ed. Philadelphia, W. B. Saunders Company, 1986, p. 1458.
27. Howards, S. S.: The epididymis: Sperm maturation and capacitation. *In* Lipschultz, L. L., and Howards, S. S. (Eds.): Infertility in the Male. New York, Churchill Livingstone, 1983, p. 121.
28. Klauber, G. T., and Sant, G. R.: Disorders of the male external genitalia. *In* Kelalis, B. P., King, L. R., and Belman, A. B. (Eds.): Clinical Pediatric Urology, 2nd ed. Philadelphia, W. B. Saunders Company, 1985, p. 825.
29. Kogan, S. J.: Cryptorchidism. *In* Kelalis, B. P., King, L. R., and Belman, A. B. (Eds.): Clinical Pediatric Urology, 2nd ed. Philadelphia, W. B. Saunders Company, 1985, p. 864.
30. Krane, R. J.: Sexual function and dysfunction. *In* Walsh, P. C., Gittes, R. E., Perlmutter, A. D., and Stamey, T. A. (Eds.): Campbell's Urology, 5th ed. Philadelphia, W. B. Saunders Company, 1986, p. 700.
31. Krane, R. J. (Ed.): Impotence. Urol. Clin. North Am., 15:1, 1988.
32. Krieger, J. N.: Urethritis in men: Etiology, diagnosis, treatment and complications. *In* Gillenwater, J. Y., et al. (Eds.): Adult and Pediatric Urology. Chicago, Year Book Medical Publishers, 1987, p. 1343.
33. Lavy, B.: The diagnosis of torsion of the testicle using the Doppler ultrasonic stethoscope. J. Urol., 113:63, 1975.
34. Leape, L. L.: Torsion of the testis: Invitation to error. J.A.M.A., 200:93, 1967.
35. Martin, D. C., and Menck, H. R.: The undescended testis: Management after puberty. J. Urol., 114:77, 1975.
36. Martin, D. L., and Salibian, A. H.: Orchiopexy using microvascular surgical technique. J. Urol., 123:435, 1980.
37. Mawhinney, M. G.: Male accessory sex organs and androgen action. *In* Lipschultz, L. I., and Howards, S. S. (Eds.): Infertility in the Male. New York, Churchill Livingstone, 1983, p. 135.
38. Meares, E. M.: Prostatitis and related disorders. *In* Walsh, P. C., Gittes, R. E., Perlmutter, A. D., and Stamey, T. A. (Eds.): Campbell's Urology, 5th ed. Philadelphia, W. B. Saunders Company, 1986, p. 868.
39. Morse, M. J., and Whitmore, W. F.: Neoplasms of the testis. *In* Walsh, P. C., Gittes, R. E., Perlmutter, A. D., and Stamey, T. A. (Eds.): Campbell's Urology, 5th ed. Philadelphia, W. B. Saunders Company, 1986, p. 1535.
40. Mostofi, F. K.: Testicular tumors: Epidemiologic, etiologic and pathologic features. Cancer, 32:1186, 1973.
41. Murphy, G. P., and Gaeta, J. F.: Tumors of the testicular and adnexal structures and seminal vesicles. *In* Walsh, P. C., Gittes, R. E., Perlmutter, A. D., and Stamey, T. A. (Eds.): Campbell's Urology, 5th ed. Philadelphia, W. B. Saunders Company, 1986, p. 612.
42. Murphy, L. J. T.: The History of Urology. Springfield, Ill., Charles C Thomas, 1972.
43. Netter, F. H.: Atlas of Human Anatomy. Summit, N.J., Ciba Geigy Corp., 1989, plates 334–357.

44. Nickel, W. R., and Plum, R. T.: Other infections and inflammations of the external genitalia. *In* Walsh, P. C., Gittes, R. E., Perlmutter, A. D., and Stamey, T. A. (Eds.): Campbell's Urology, 4th ed. Philadelphia, W. B. Saunders Company, 1979, pp. 640, 670.

45. Nickel, W. R., and Plum, R. T.: Visible lesions of the male genitalia. *In* Walsh, P. C., Gittes, R. E., Perlmutter, A. D., and Stamey, T. A. (Eds.): Campbell's Urology, 5th ed. Philadelphia, W. B. Saunders Company, 1986, p. 946.

46. Nickel, W. R., and Plum R. T.: Cutaneous disease of external genitalia. *In* Walsh, P. C., Gittes, R. E., Perlmutter, A. D., and Stamey, T. A. (Eds.): Campbell's Urology, 5th ed. Philadelphia, W. B. Saunders Company, 1986, p. 975.

47. O'Conor, V. J., Jr.: Suprapubic prostatectomy. *In* Glenn, J. F. (Ed.): Urologic Surgery, 3rd ed. Philadelphia, J. B. Lippincott Company, 1983, p. 853.

48. Osborne, E. D., Sutherland, C. G., Scholl, A. J., and Rowntree, L. G.: Roentgenology of urinary tract during excretion of sodium iodide. J.A.M.A., *80*:368, 1923.

49. Palmer, J. M.: Surgery of the seminal vesicles. *In* Walsh, P. C., Gittes, R. E., Perlmutter, A. D., and Stamey, T. A. (Eds.): Campbell's Urology, 5th ed. Philadelphia, W. B. Saunders Company, 1986, p. 2847.

50. Paulson, D. F.: Carcinoma of the prostate: The therapeutic dilemma. Annu. Rev. Med., *35*:341, 1984.

51. Paulson, D. F.: Treatment selection in the patients with prostatic cancer. *In* Paulson, D. F. (Ed.): Prostatic Disorders. Philadelphia, Lea & Febiger, 1989, 287–304.

52. Peters, P. C., and Sagalowsky, A. I.: Genitourinary trauma. *In* Walsh, P. C., Gittes, R. E., Perlmutter, A. D., and Stamey, T. A. (Eds.): Campbell's Urology, 5th ed. Philadelphia, W. B. Saunders Company, 1986, p. 1192.

53. Prentiss, R. J.: Anomalies of the male genitalia. *In* Amar, A. D., et al. (Eds.): Encyclopedia of Urology. Berlin, Springer-Verlag, 1968, p. 287.

54. Pryor, J. L., and Howards, S. S.: Varicocele in infertility. Urol. Clin. North Am., *14*:499, 1987.

55. Ray, B., Canto, A. K., and Whitmore, W. F.: Experience with primary carcinoma of the male urethra. J. Urol., *117*:591, 1977.

56. Redman, J. F.: Anatomy of the genitourinary system. *In* Gillenwater, J. Y., et al. (Eds.): Adult and Pediatric Urology. Chicago, Year Book Medical Publishers, 1987, p. 3.

57. Redman, J. F.: Anatomy of the genitourinary system. *In* Gillenwater, J. Y., et al. (Eds.): Adult and Pediatric Urology. Chicago, Year Book Medical Publishers, 1987, p. 45.

58. Schellhammer, P. F., and Grabstald, H.: Tumors of the penis. *In* Walsh, P. C., Gittes, R. E., Perlmutter, A. D., and Stamey, T. A. (Eds.): Campbell's Urology, 5th ed. Philadelphia, W. B. Saunders Company, 1986, p. 1583.

59. Schlegel, P. M., and Walsh, P. C.: Neuroanatomical approach to radical cystoprostatectomy with preservation of sexual function. J. Urol., *138*:1402, 1987.

60. Scorer, C. G., and Farrington, G. H.: Congenital anomalies of the testis. *In* Walsh, P. C., Gittes, R. E., Perlmutter, A. D., and Stamey, T. A. (Eds.): Campbell's Urology, 4th ed. Philadelphia, W. B. Saunders Company, 1979, p. 1561.

61. Sherins, R. J., and Howards, S. S.: Male infertility. *In* Walsh, P. C., Gittes, R. E., Perlmutter, A. D., and Stamey, T. A. (Eds.): Campbell's Urology, 5th ed. Philadelphia, W. B. Saunders Company, 1986, p. 640.

62. Skoglund, R., McRoberts, J., and Radge, H.: Torsion of the spermatic cord: A review of the literature and analysis of 70 new cases. J. Urol., *104*:604, 1970.

63. Spark, R. F.: Anatomic and developmental considerations. *In* The Infertile Male: The Clinician's Guide to Diagnosis and Treatment. New York, Plenum Medical Book Company, 1988, p. 15.

64. Spaulding, J. T., and Grabstald, H.: Surgery of penile and urethral carcinoma. *In* Walsh, P. C., Gittes, R. E., Perlmutter, A. D., and Stamey, T. A. (Eds.): Campbell's Urology, 5th ed. Philadelphia, W. B. Saunders Company, 1986, p. 291.

65. Stamey, T. A., and Kabalin, J. M.: Prostatic specific antigen and the diagnosis and treatment of adenocarcinoma of the prostate. J. Urol., *141*:1070, 1989.

66. Stamey, T. A., et al.: Prostatic specific antigen in the diagnosis and treatment of adenocarcinoma of the prostate. II. Radical prostatectomy treated patients. J. Urol., *141*:1076, 1989.

67. Straffon, R. A.: Retropubic prostatectomy. *In* Glenn, J. F. (Ed.): Urologic Surgery. Philadelphia, J. B. Lippincott Company, 1983, p. 861.

68. Swerdloff, R. S., and Boyers, S. P.: Evaluation of the male partner of the infertile couple. J.A.M.A., *247*:2418, 1982.

69. Swerdloff, R. S., and deKretser, D. M.: Endocrine evaluations of the infertile male. *In* Lipschultz, L. I., and Howard, S. S. (Eds.): New York, Churchill Livingstone, 1983, p. 207.

70. Tailly, G., Vereecken, R. L., and Verduyn, H.: A review of 357 bilateral vasectomies for male sterilization. Fertil. Steril., *41*:424, 1984.

71. Tanagho, E. A.: Anatomy of the lower urinary tract. *In* Walsh, P. C., Gittes, R. E., Perlmutter, A. D., and Stamey, T. A. (Eds.): Campbell's Urology, 5th ed. Philadelphia, W. B. Saunders Company, 1986, p. 65.

72. Tanagho, E. H., Lue, T. F., and McClure, R. D. (Eds.): Contemporary Management of Impotence and Infertility. Baltimore, Williams & Wilkins, 1988.

73. The Medical Newsletter on Drugs and Therapeutics: Drugs that cause sexual dysfunction. Med. Lett., *25*:73, 1983.

74. Veterans Administration Cooperative Urological Research Group: Treatment and survival of patients with cancer of the prostate. Surg. Gynecol. Obstet., *124*:1011, 1967.

75. Vinson, G. S., and Boileau, M. A.: The penis: Sexual function and dysfunction. *In* Gillenwater, J. Y., et al. (Eds.): Adult and Pediatric Urology. Chicago, Year Book Medical Publishers, 1987, p. 1407.

76. von Lichtenberg, A., and Swick, M.: Klinische Prufung des Uroselectans. Klin. Wochenschr., *8*:2089, 1921.

77. Walsh, P. C.: Benign prostatic hypertrophy. *In* Walsh, P. C., Gittes, R. E., Perlmutter, A. D., and Stamey, T. A. (Eds.): Campbell's Urology, 5th ed. Philadelphia, W. B. Saunders Company, 1986, p. 1248.

78. Waterhouse, K.: Anomalies of the urethra. *In* Amar, A. D., et al. (Eds.): Encyclopedia of Urology. Berlin, Springer Verlag, 1968, p. 242.

79. Webster, G. D.: The urethra. *In* Paulson, D. F. (Ed.): Genitourinary Surgery. New York, Churchill Livingstone, 1983, p. 399.

80. Weinerth, J. L.: Long-term management of vasovasostomy patients. Fertil. Steril., *41*:623, 1984.

81. Weiss, H. D.: Physiology of human penile erection. Ann. Intern. Med., *72*:793, 1972.

82. Whitmore, W. F., and Morse, M. J.: Surgery of testicular neoplasms. *In* Walsh, P. C., Gittes, R. E., Perlmutter, A. D., and Stamey, T. A. (Eds.): Campbell's Urology, 5th ed. Philadelphia, W. B. Saunders Company, 1986, p. 2933.

83. Zorgniotti, A. W., and Sealfon, A. I.: Scrotal hypothermia: New therapy for poor semen. Urology, *23*:439, 1984.

48

DISORDERS OF THE LYMPHATIC SYSTEM

Ralph G. DePalma, M.D.

The lymphatic system is an intriguing part of the vascular system, yet surgical therapy for it is underdeveloped, and the functions of the lymphatic system and its diseases are incompletely understood. Primary disorders of the lymphatic system amenable to direct surgical intervention are uncommon, although effective treatment exists for certain patients with particularly challenging problems.

Historical Aspects

Aristotle and the anatomists Herophilos and Erasistratos are said to have observed aspects of the lymphatic system between 348 and 250 B.C. Knowledge about these recordings is hearsay; none of the works of the Alexandrian School of Medicine come directly to us. In the sixteenth century, Vesalius, professor of anatomy and surgery at Padua, named the thoracic duct *vena alba thoracis* because of its contents of milky fluid; his contemporary Eustachius also described the equine thoracic duct. In 1627, Aselli of Pavia illustrated lymphatics in the mesentery of fed dogs (Fig. 1). Aselli noted the relationship of these structures to intestinal absorption, noting that puncture of the vessels yielded "white liquid-like milk or cream." He traced the vessels into the abdominal receptaculum chyli but mistakenly concluded that the lymphatics ended in the liver. The Parisian Pecquet observed in 1651 that the intestinal "lacteals" emptied into the receptaculum chyli, thence drained into the thoracic duct, eventually emptying into "the whirlpool of the heart." Pecquet also confirmed his observations about the lacteals in a criminal autopsied after a large meal. Rudbeck of Uppsala described liver lymphatics as "vasa serosa"; in 1653, Bartholin named the vessels "lymphatics," and George Jolyffe, an Englishman, also recognized that vessels known as lymphatics were widely distributed throughout the body and conducted an "aqueous humor."[24]

Aselli's observations were published about the time of William Harvey's classic description of the circulation, *De Motu Cordis.* However, Harvey never considered the lymphatics important. He believed that "lymphatics arose occasionally and by accident and proceeded from too ample a supply of nourishment." After the observations of the seventeenth century, lymphatic anatomy and circulation remained a matter of conjecture for over 100 years. The next discoveries about the lymphatic system occurred in the Hunterian Anatomic School in the eighteenth century. These resulted from the work of two talented anatomic assistants, William Hewson and William Cruikshank, and William Hunter, the physician director of this school. Hewson, after resigning from the Hunterian School, published an important anatomic treatise in 1774 entitled *The Lymphatic System in the Human Subject and in Other Animals.*[24] This book was dedicated to Benjamin Franklin of Philadelphia who, just prior to the American Revolution, mediated a dispute between Hewson and Hunter. The young anatomist had sought permission from Hunter to retain his personal anatomic dissections and was refused.

William Hunter[27] assessed his own contribution, stating, "I think I have proved that the lymphatic vessels are the absorbing vessels, all over the body; that they are the same as the lacteals; and that these altogether with the thoracic duct constitute one great and general system dispersed through the whole body for absorption; that this system only does absorb and not the veins; that it serves to take up and convey whatever is to make or to be mixed with the blood from the skin, from the intestinal canal and from all the internal cavities or surfaces whatever." While neither modest nor generous, Hunter was a forceful man. He said, "If we mistake not, in a proper time it [the lymphatics] will allow to be the greatest discovery both in physiology and pathology that anatomy has suggested, since the discovery of the circulation." Surgical therapy of the lymphatic system has yet to fulfill this Hunterian prophecy as it has for the heart and arteries; however, an understanding of processes involved in the generation of infection, along with interventions to control HIV and other immune deficiency states, might still fulfill this prophecy.

In the nineteenth century, the role of the lymphatics was illuminated by Claude Bernard's global concept of a mammalian requirement for maintenance of a constant *internal milieu* bathing all cells.[4] By the late nineteenth century, Starling had clarified the relationship between the hydrostatic pressure of the blood in the capillaries and the colloid osmotic pressure of the plasma proteins.[53] The Starling hypothesis, along with previous insights about capillary circulation, led to a theory of capillary exchange with oncotic pressure of plasma proteins as the main driving force within capillaries thought to be relatively impermeable to protein.

In the twentieth century, from 1930 to 1941, Drinker and colleagues measured protein flux from the capillaries to the tissues, showing that blood capillaries were leakier than hitherto believed. These workers solidified the physiologic concept of lymphatic capillaries as vessels serving to return protein molecules to the central circulation. Relationships between a blood capillary, the interstitium, and a lymphatic capillary are shown in Figure 2. The diagram illustrates the concept that interstitial pressure may be negative or vary. The magnitude of interstitial pressure varies in different organs and tissues and increases with movement, which, in turn, stimulates lymph flow.

When excess protein is trapped in the interstitial spaces, the protein-laden interstitium attracts water. Subcutaneous interstitial fluid aspirated under conditions of lymphatic obstruction in the extremities exhibits protein concentrations greater than 1.0 to 1.5 gm. per 100 ml.[12] Whereas Starling believed that capillaries leaked small amounts of protein, Drinker and colleagues and later Landis[34] showed this leakage to be considerable, substantiating the role of lymphatic capillaries as vessels that return blood protein molecules from the periphery to the central circulation.

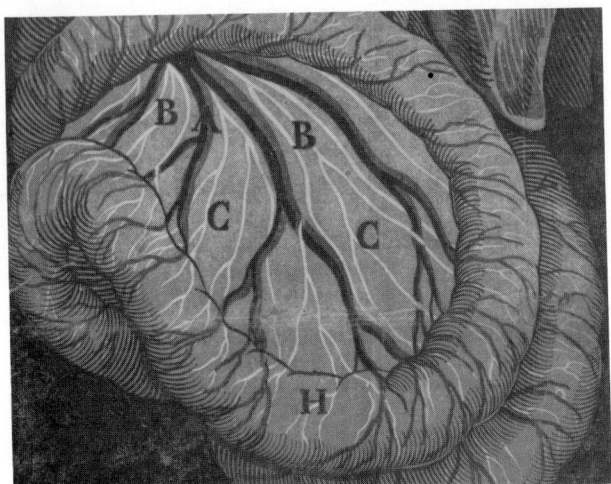

Figure 1. First illustration of the lymphatic system, showing engorged lacteals in a dog after feeding. (From Aselli, G.: De Factibus sive Lacteis Venis, Quarto Vasorum Mesarai Corum Genere Novo Invento. Milano, J. B. Bieldellium, Mediolani, 1627. Original at Harvard's Frances A. Countway Library of Medicine. Courtesy of Dr. Mitchell Kanter.)

Anatomic and Histologic Aspects

In understanding lymphatic structure and function, a teleologic view stated by Mayerson[36] is useful: "In the mammal it became necessary to evolve a closed high pressure system with conduits of diminishing thickness carrying blood and oxygen to thin walled capillaries. But here nature ran into a snag: the high pressures made the capillaries leaky and fluid and various substances left the blood stream. It now became necessary to evolve a drainage system to clear the tissue spaces of substances which had leaked out of the blood capillaries and which could not be reabsorbed directly into the blood stream."

Embryology

Sabin gathered embryologic evidence showing that lymphatics develop in close relationship to venous structures.[48] Huntington believed that systemic lymphatics developed from fusion of perivenous mesenchymal clefts.[28] Lymphatic vessels generally course parallel with major veins, and when obstructed in the adult state, variable direct lymphatic venous connections develop.[5] This suggests a venous origin of otherwise unused channels. By the sixth week of gestation, the lymphatic system of human embryos is seen in the form of paired jugular lymph sacs in the neck and iliac sacs in the lumbar region. By the eighth week, a retroperitoneal lymph sac appears at the root of the mesentery, and the cisterna chyli develops dorsal to the abdominal aorta. Subsequently, the jugular lymph sacs are linked with

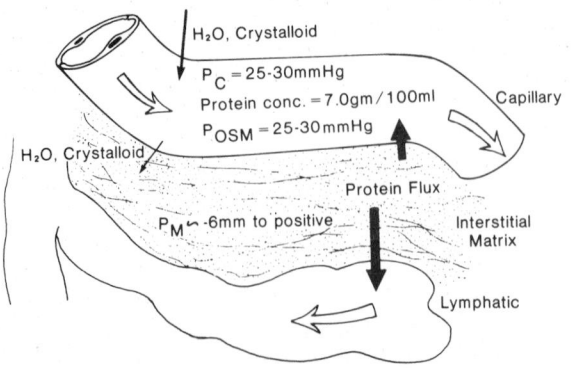

Figure 2. Diagrammatic representation of relationships between a blood capillary, the interstitium, and a lymph capillary. Heavy arrows indicate protein flux. (PC = capillary pressure, Posm = osmotic pressure, Pm = matrix pressure)

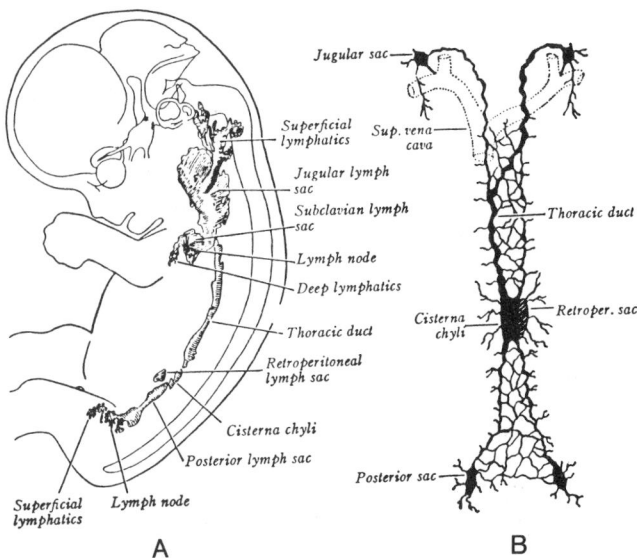

Figure 3. Development of lymphatic vessels in humans. A, Profile reconstruction of the primitive lymphatic system in a 9-week embryo. (After Sabin,[48] × 3.) B, Diagram in ventral view of emergence of the thoracic duct and main lymphatic ducts from the lymphatic plexus. (From Arey, L. B.: Developmental Anatomy. Philadelphia, W. B. Saunders Company, 1975, with permission.)

the cisterna chyli to produce paired thoracic ducts. Early there are numerous anastomoses across the midline between the paired thoracic ducts. However, in most individuals the inferior portion of the right lymphatic duct merges via a cross connection at the level of the fourth to the sixth vertebra to form a dominant left thoracic duct that drains into the left subclavian vein at the root of the neck. A right lymphatic duct or, more commonly, several lymphatic ducts persist on the right side. The human lymphatic system at 9 weeks of gestation is shown in Figure 3.

Primary lymphatic disorders are mainly developmental abnormalities consisting of hypoplasia or absence of lymph nodes and ducts. In some cases, inguinal lymph nodes are fibrotic, and conducting lymph vessels of the lower extremities are absent or hypoplastic. Rarely, hyperplasias with valvular incompetence occur. Abnormal growth of primitive lymph sacs in the area of the jugular buds causes multilocular lymph cysts called cystic hygromas, which are commonly seen in children in the neck, axilla, and mediastinum. Hyperplasia of lymphatic capillaries often combines with a variety of congenital vascular tumors.

General Anatomy

The lymphatic system accommodates overflow of protein, water, and electrolytes from the blood capillaries. Anatomically, the lymphatics are highly developed in mammals because of the high-pressure arterial circulation that provides varying blood flows to different organs and tissues. Lymphatic capillaries transport lymph to valved collecting vessels; the arrangement of the lymphatics varies from organ to organ. Interposed lymph nodes act as mechanical filters and are sites of immunologic responses. Other lymphoid organs include the adenoidal tonsillar complex, the pulmonary lymphatics, the spleen, the thymus, and the intestinal lymphatics, such as Peyer's patches.

Lymphatic capillaries consist of single layers of flat endothelial cells, slightly larger and thinner than those of the blood capillaries. The permeability of lymphatic capillaries to large molecules and cells is due to the absent or vestigial basement membrane. Under usual conditions of histologic fixation, lymph capillaries are not visible, but with special efforts, lymphatic networks can be distinguished from blood capillaries. The lymph capillaries tend to end blindly in rounded ends, consistent with their drainage function. Lymph vessels are no-

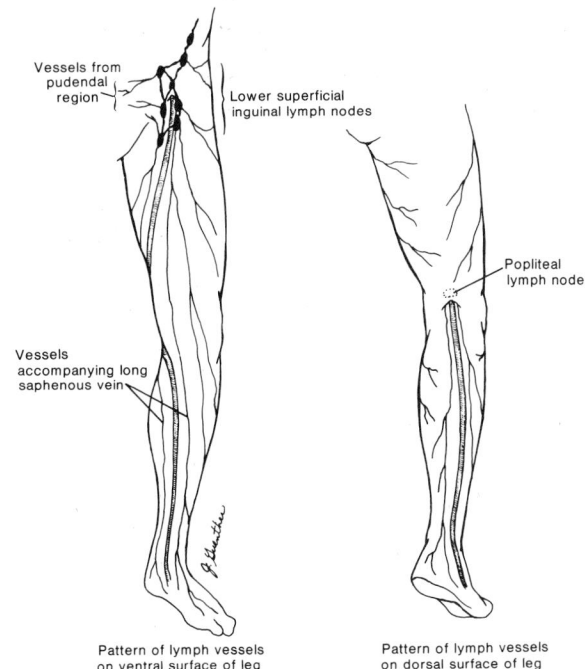

Figure 4. Diagram of superficial (subcutaneous) lymph vessels and nodes of the lower extremity.

tably absent from the cornea, the central nervous system deep to the meninges, cartilage, and tendon. Lymphatics exist in the intermuscular fascia, but not in muscle bundles.

There are no lymphatics in the epidermis of the skin. Fixed macrophages (Langerhans' cells) in the epidermis do enter the lymphatic circulation, comprising an immune arc, of which the afferent limb ends in the regional nodes.[6] The rich lymphatic network[26] just beneath the superficial dermis contains abundant lymphatic capillaries without valves. These drain into the valved channels of the deep dermis and subcutaneous tissue. Because lymphatic disorders often involve the extremities, the anatomy of the lymphatics of the upper and lower extremities is important. The lymphatics of the upper and lower extremities are characterized by dermal plexi, collecting channels, and superficial lymphatic trunks that parallel veins superficial to the muscular fascia (Figs. 4 and 5). Some of the afferent trunks pass through a small number of popliteal and epitrochlear nodes distally; most pass into the inguinal and axillary nodes proxi-

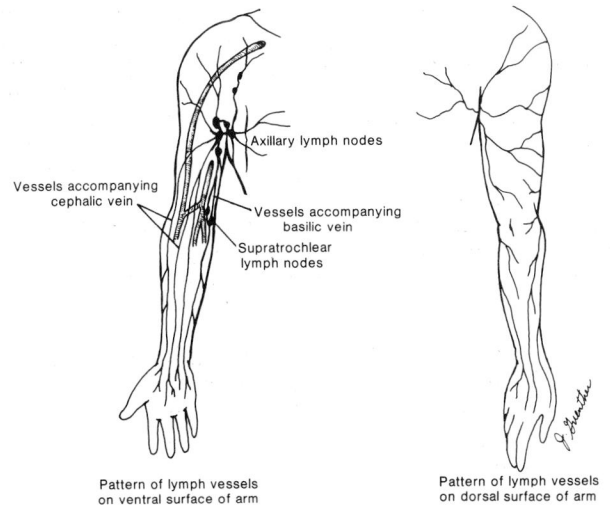

Figure 5. Diagram of superficial (subcutaneous) lymph vessels and nodes of the upper extremity.

mally. Large efferent trunks then arise from inguinal and axillary nodes to course retroperitoneally or in the upper extremity in close relationship with major vessels. A sparse, separate deep lymphatic system of the intramuscular fascia in humans is believed to communicate only under abnormal conditions[35] with the functional superficial network.

The valves of the collecting lymphatics help maintain prograde lymphatic drainage. Collecting ducts exhibit an endothelial layer covered by connective tissue containing both elastic and muscular elements. The larger ducts are supplied by vasa vasora. The lymphatic collecting duct walls also contain well-developed basement membranes. Probably owing to muscular elements, these vessels contract rhythmically to aid in lymph propulsion. Muscular and respiratory activity also contributes to proximal lymph flow. Although abundant collaterals exist, extensive loss of lymph nodes and collecting channels leads to obstruction. Valvular incompetence causes lymph reflux when the channels are distended.

LYMPH NODES. It is estimated that 500 to 1000 lymph nodes exist in individual humans.[17] These are accumulations of lymphatic tissue varying in size from a millimeter to more than 2 cm. Nodes are located along the course of the lymphatic vessels; their contents pass through the regional nodes to the main drainage systems of the thoracic and right lymphatic ducts. Lymph nodes in health are usually not palpable, although nodes enlarge transiently with heavy exercise in young athletes. Lymph nodes are round or kidney-shaped structures, with a hilus on one side containing an efferent lymphatic along with blood vessels. Afferent lymphatics enter the node at multiple sites over its convex surface (Fig. 6.). When lymph nodes or vessels are excised, regeneration proceeds by vascular budding or sprouting to produce continuation of lymph flow. Lymphatic vessels do not regenerate when node-bearing areas are destroyed by radiation and operative excision. Lymphatic regeneration is severely restricted by scar tissue.[18]

Anatomic knowledge of the location and distribution of lymph nodes is critical in understanding the natural history of malignant tumors and lymphomas affecting almost every part of the body. This detailed anatomy is considered with each organ system and in chapters dealing with the treatment of Hodgkin's disease and lymphomas. The large collecting ducts of the thorax and abdomen, important conduits for large volumes of lymph, are shown in Figure 7.

Basic Science Aspects

The drainage concept of the lymphatic system simplifies an understanding of the physiology of obstructive lymphatic disorders. However, the lymphatic system performs myriad additional functions: it removes macromolecules and foreign substances from tissues and participates in the clearing of debris from areas of tissue injury; lymph flow increases particularly in scald injuries.[1] T-cell lymphocytes have a dual role in wound healing with early stimulatory effects and a late counter-regulatory role that may limit fibroplasia and contribute to orderly wound repair.[2] The lymphatic system regulates tissue fluid volume and pressure, protecting the circulating blood volume by volume repletion to compensate hypovolemia. In a 24-hour period, the volume of lymph returned to the central circulation approximates the plasma volume. Lymphocytes and other cells enter the central circulation by its channels, along with proteins and other large molecules. Chylomicrons and lipoprotein complexes also enter the bloodstream via the lymphatic system. Thus, the lymphatics comprise an additional circulatory system managing enormous volumes of fluid, fat, protein, and cells. The blind-ended villous lymphatics of the intestine selectively absorb cholesterol, long chain fatty acids, and triglycerides, accounting for the milky appearance of intestinal lymph or chyle. Regional lymph flow and its composition from various organs varies considerably, depending on organ function. Small

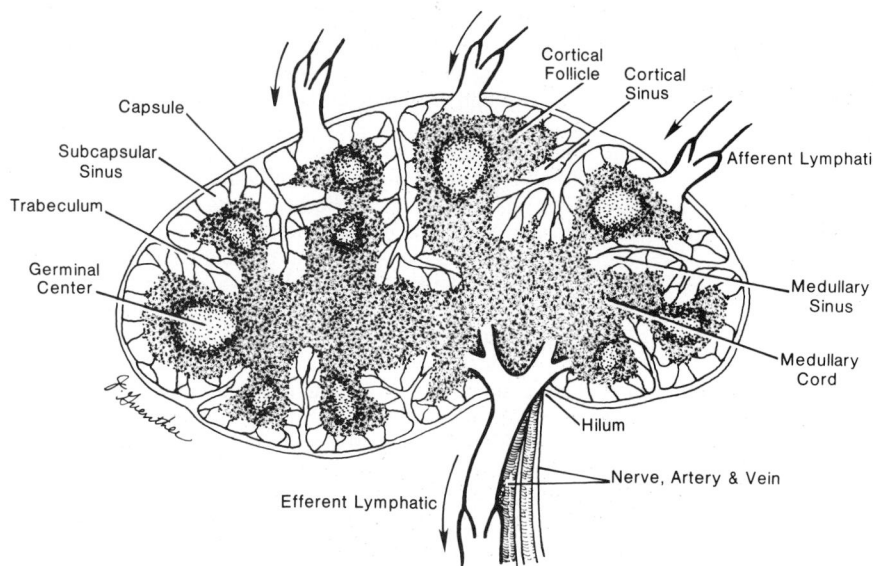

Figure 6. Diagram of an idealized typical lymph node. Note multiple afferent ducts and the single efferent duct. The "traffic area" for migrating cells is in the periphery of the node.

amounts of transudative fluid from serous cavities are also continuously absorbed.

Lymphocytes with distinct immunologic functions originate in the central lymphatic organs.[58] The circulation of lymphocytes is illustrated in Figure 8, which is adapted from Roitt and associates.[47] Animal experiments and studies on congenitally athymic patients show that lymphocytes derived from the thymus, or T cells, mediate cellular immunity. Neonatal thymectomy results in continuance of a receptor repertoire of early postnatal life that correlates with later organ-specific autoimmune disease in experimental animals.[52] A second class of lymphocytes, the B cells, is generated independently of the thymus. These cells produce antibodies mediating humoral immunity. A third division of heterogeneous lymphocytes, known as null or non-B, non-T types, is a source of extramedullary hematopoiesis, or it can form specialized cytotoxic cells that kill target cells in either the presence or absence of specific antibodies. The different types of lymphatic cells had been identified largely by surface markers.[38] Overall, on this basis there are probably now more than 38 types of lymphatic cells, which now also can be classified on the basis of nuclear DNA. Cohen and Jaffe provided a recent review of T- and B-cell derivation.[10] Thus, all lymphocytes, derived from a specialized, architecturally arranged system, are intimately involved with immune competence as well as immunologic tolerance, a process in which limits are placed on lymphocytic responses to inherent antigens.[41]

Clinical correlates of disordered lymphatic drainage function are commonly observed. For example, in acute pulmonary edema, regional lymph flow increases from six- to eightfold. Even when the hemodynamic abnormality is reversed, trapped protein clears rather slowly from the lung parenchyma; thus interstitial edema detected radiographically persists. An uncontrolled lymphatic leak from the thoracic or other major lymphatics causes hypoproteinemia, malnutrition, and loss of immune competence within days or weeks. In an interesting early effort to enhance renal transplantation, controlled thoracic duct drainage was used by Starzl and associates in 40 patients.[54] With drainage of a daily average of 1.88 ± 0.19 (SE) $\times 10^9$ cells and 4.7 liters of lymph for about 2 months, cellular and humoral immunity was suppressed in most patients.

Lymph nodes are primary filters for trapping foreign protein and viral and bacterial particles and are sites of important first encounters with the immune system. It is interesting that malnutrition results in lymphatic atrophy, particularly of the thymus, which probably relates to immunologic deficiencies in malnutrition and severe injury.

To illustrate the role of lymphatics in circulatory homeostasis, it is useful to consider thoracic duct lymph composition and

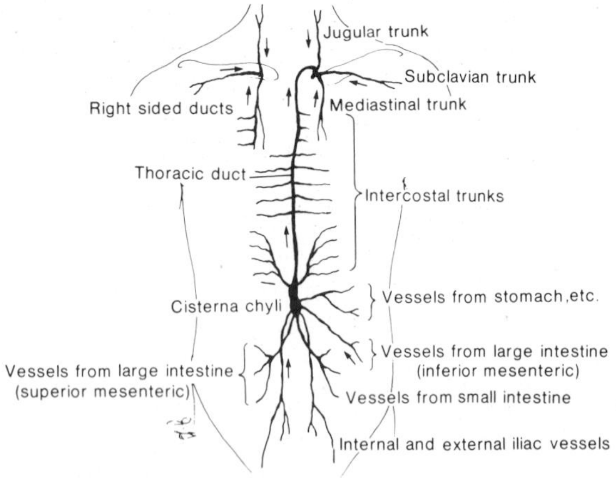

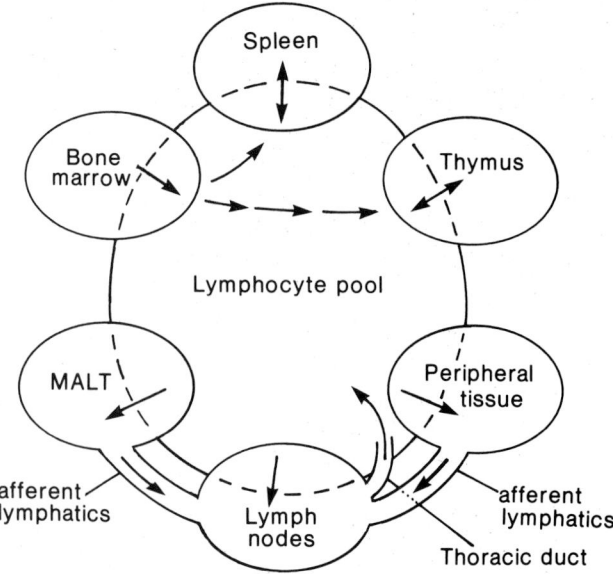

Figure 7. Diagram of main collecting lymph channels of the abdomen and thorax. Note multiple right lymphatic ducts.

Figure 8. Circulation of lymphocytes. (Adapted from Roitt, I., Brastoff, J., and Male, D.: Immunology. St. Louis, C.V. Mosby, 1985, with permission.)

flow in a 70-kg. man at bed rest. If thoracic duct lymph flow approximates 2 liters daily, with an average protein concentration of 4.8 gm. per dl., the average daily protein turnover of intravascular plasma proteins within the lymphatic system is about 40 per cent, approaching about 50 per cent of total protein turnover in active people. In hepatic cirrhosis, the flow and volume of thoracic duct lymph is three to six times greater.[16]

Lymphatic vessels readily absorb particulate matter from their surrounding interstitial milieu, including chylomicrons, red cells, bacteria, viruses, and foreign protein selectives such as snake venom. Red cells enter the peripheral lymphatic capillaries during heavy exercise and also appear in the thoracic duct in pathologic conditions, such as hepatic cirrhosis and endotoxic shock. In these circumstances, red cells traverse liver lymphatics, then drain into the thoracic duct lymph. The peritoneal lymphatics also absorb intact erythrocytes. Once macromolecules or cells enter collecting lymphatics, there is little exchange with the blood until the lymph enters the venous system.

Within lymph nodes in experimental animals, there is no exchange with the blood of molecules greater than molecular weight 2300. In a variety of circumstances, labeled soluble antigens or homologous cells are recovered intact from the efferent lymph node ducts.[49] Migrating cells pass through "traffic areas" in lymph nodes, away from the germinal centers.[19] Cells destined to remain in the node become distributed throughout the superficial and the deep cortex. The proportion of blood-borne versus lymph-borne lymphocytes entering and leaving the node varies, depending on whether the node is a peripheral or a central one. Less than 10 per cent of the cells leaving peripheral nodes reach the node in the lymph; 90 per cent arrive via the bloodstream.

VISUALIZATION OF LYMPHATICS

Even in the current era of high technology, it is technically difficult to visualize lymphatics. One of the challenges in studying lymphatics is simply finding them. In early cadaver dissections, mercury injections delineated the lymphatics. Dyes and India ink were later injected into living tissues to identify lymphatic ducts to be cannulated *in vivo*. Feeding of cream or milk rapidly renders visible the intestinal lacteals and the major abdominal and thoracic duct systems. Hudack and McMaster used intradermal patent blue violet dye injections in 1933 to demonstrate the minute lymph vessels in skin.[26] Subsequently, Kinmonth in 1951 extended the use of patent blue violet dye (molecular weight, 1158) in a 10 per cent solution for intradermal injection.[31] Currently, 1 per cent isosulfan blue (Lymphazurin: Hirsch Industries, Cherry Hill, N.J.) can be used. Normally, a small blue wheal occurs and extends proximally up to 8 cm.; in lymphedema, a large network of dilated dermal lymphatics is seen. Dye injections are used to visualize large ducts and with lymphangiography to locate peripheral lymphatics suitable for cannulation.

Servelle reports performing the first lymphangiogram in 1943, using Thorotrast.[51] For modern lymphangiography, lipiodol, an oil-soluble medium made from poppy seed oil containing 30 per cent iodine, is used. This radiopaque medium opacifies lymphatic ducts and lymph nodes. In contrast to water-soluble angiographic contrast media, lipiodol remains in nodes for long periods after lymphangiography. With the use of lipiodol, lymphomatous deposits within central lymph nodes as well as peripheral nodes and lymphatic networks are visualized. When lymphatic visualization is necessary, lymphangiography is an important clinical procedure, which, however, has certain disadvantages. The viscid oil requires slow automatic injection; excess doses may cause pulmonary edema or, rarely, cerebral oil embolism; and the contrast medium can damage lymphatic ducts. Lymphangiography may precipitate lymphangitis and lead to worsening of lymphedema.

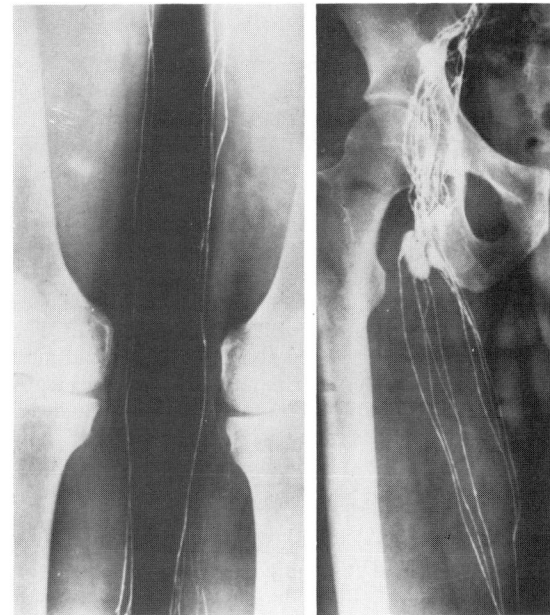

Figure 9. Normal lower extremity lymphatics on lymphangiogram. (From Browse, N. L.: Normal lymphographic appearances: Lower limb and pelvis. *In* Kinmonth, J. B. (Ed.): The Lymphatics. London, Edward Arnold Publishers, 1982, with permission.)

Normal lower extremity lymphatics as visualized lymphangiographically are illustrated in Figure 9. Using this method, Kinmonth[31] and Browse and associates made landmark contributions to the diagnosis and treatment of lymphatic disease. The performance of lymphangiography requires skill to isolate the lymphatic ducts for prolonged injection and patience to follow the progress of the oil into the proximal collecting sys-

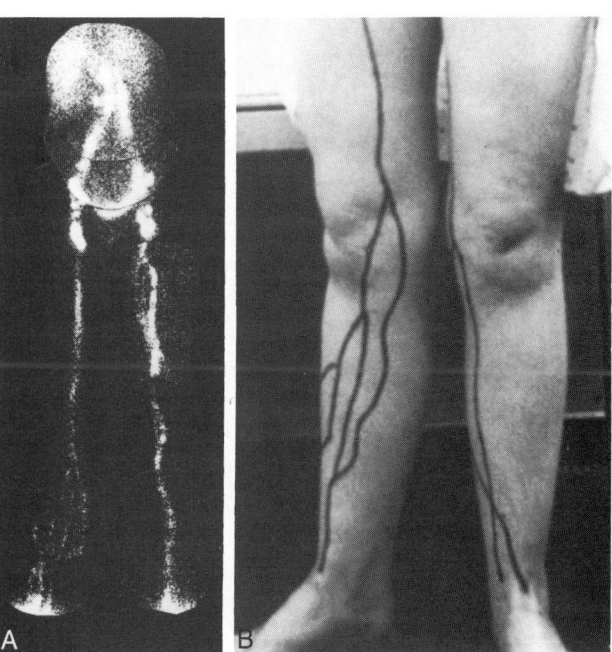

Figure 10. *A*, Lymphoscintiscan 3 hours following intradermal injections of 1 mCi (per injection site) of technetium-99 N antimony trisulfide colloid at sites overlying the first and fifth metatarsals. This is a 38-year-old woman with lymphedema praecox and multiple episodes of cellulitis of the right lower extremity. Note abdominal distal lymphatics and normal proximal drainage. *B*, Photograph of same patient with course of lymphatics as marked. (Courtesy of William D. Kaplan, M.D., Dana Farber Cancer Institute, Boston, Mass. Reproduced with permission from DePalma, R. G., and Kanter, M.: Structure and function of the lymphatics. *In* Giordano, J. M., Trout, H. H., III, and DePalma, R. G. (Eds.): The Basic Science of Vascular Surgery. Mt. Kisco, N.Y., Futura Publishing, 1988.)

tems. The maximal adult dose of lipiodol by the bipedal route should not exceed 12 ml.

Complications of lymphangiography led to the development and use of radionucleotide imaging. Radiopharmaceuticals of appropriate size are absorbed by the lymphatics and can be scanned using a standard gamma camera. Currently, for lymphoscintigraphy, the preferred compound is technetium-99 antimony sulfide colloid. With a particle size of 4 to 11 microns, this compound yields images within 3 hours of subcutaneous injection. Although anatomic definition is much less compared with a lymphangiogram, lymphoscintigraphy is sufficient to demonstrate lymphatic channels and sites of obstruction, as shown in Figure 10. Stewart, with the group from St. Thomas Hospital in London, quantified decreasing uptakes of radioisotope in ilioinguinal nodes in extremities with varying degrees of lymphedema. This group still recommends lymphangiography when direct lymphatic surgery is to be considered.[56]

LYMPHEDEMA

Primary lymphedemas are diagnosed in the absence of acquired diseases damaging the lymphatic system. Most commonly, the condition affects the lower limbs. Edema may be present at birth or begin later in life. The usual clinical pattern is onset of lymphedema at the time of puberty. Most patients are women. Lymphedema presenting at birth is *lymphedema congenita* (Fig. 11). When the swelling begins before the age of 35 years, as is most common, the term *lymphedema praecox* is used. Lymphedema beginning after the age of 35 years is called *lymphedema tarda*. Milroy's disease is an eponym often misapplied in cases or primary lymphedema.[37] True Milroy's disease is a congenital familial lymphedema recently shown to result from vertical autosomal inheritance of a single gene.[50] Men are affected as frequently as women. Milroy's disease is rare, comprising less than 2 per cent of primary lymphedemas. When

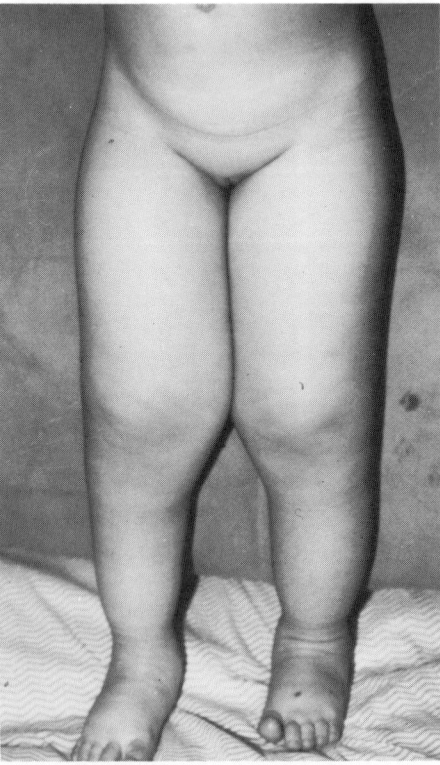

Figure 11. Congenital familial lymphedema of the left lower extremity in an 18-month-old child, a patient of Dr. J. Leonel Villavicencio. Edema was present at birth and increased with walking.

lymphedema appears in a single limb, the most important differential diagnoses include lymphoma, malignancy involving iliac and lumbar lymph nodes, and venous occlusion.

In primary lymphedemas, lymphangiography nearly always documents defective lymphatic development. Female patients of all age groups comprise 63 to 77 per cent of these cases. Swelling often begins spontaneously but can be precipitated by trauma, pregnancy, and other events, including infection, insect bites, or episodes of lymphangitis and cellulitis. A surgical cause of acceleration of congenital lymphedema is excision of a benign groin tumor with a preoperative diagnosis of lipoma or fibroma. In these instances, the "tumor" consists of fibrous tissue, deformed nodes, and lymphatic collaterals. Kinmonth describes ten such cases, stressing the importance of proper recognition of a groin mass as an abnormal lymphatic channel. Prior lymphangiography should be considered when unusual groin masses are encountered in young individuals. Differentiation from inguinal hernia should not be difficult on clinical examination. Primary lymphedemas are also associated with developmental deformities, including gonadal dysgeneses such as Turner's syndrome. Certain individuals with megalymphatics exhibit patches of blood capillary angiomas of the skin; some exhibit overgrowth of bones of the involved limb.

Using lymphographic classification, hypoplasia of the lymphatics exists in 90 per cent of these patients. Most involve the distal rather than the proximal lymphatics, making surgical treatment less likely to succeed. Unilateral or bilateral hyperplasia exists in only 10 per cent of patients. Megalymphatics can cause incompetence of the distal lymphatic valves. A diffuse increase in the size and number of the lymphatics of both lower limbs, with hyperplasia of the abdominal vessels and nodes, can lead to chylous reflux lymphedema and, rarely, chronic lymphatic skin leaks.

Secondary lymphedemas are due to trauma and wounds involving the lymph pathways, malignant disease, filariasis, infections and inflammations, and radiation. Ulceration is rare in lymphedema; however, a common cause of lymphedema is chronic venous ulceration leading to episodes of lymphangitis that obliterate normal lymph channels. Patients prone to recurrent attacks of lymphangitis are best treated with intermittent long-term antibiotic therapy used at the first sign of infection. A spectacular type of lymphedema occurs in filarial infection with *Wuchereria bancrofti* or *malaysii*, one of the most common tropical diseases of the world. In this type of lymphedema, adult worms lodge in the lymph nodes and vessels, eventually leading to grotesque swelling termed *elephantiasis* (Fig. 12). The skin of these extremities is often affected by filiform verrucae and hyperkeratosis. The disease is transmitted by a mosquito bite; microfiliaria are inoculated and then develop into adult filaria within regional nodes and vessels.

Lymphedema of the upper extremity was commonly secondary to radical mastectomy, which removes the axillary nodes en bloc. Defects in healing and concomitant infection and fibrosis lead to obliteration of remaining lymphatics. A lesser incidence of lymphedema occurs with modified radical mastectomy, possibly due to uneventful healing of thicker skin flaps and less interference with collateral lymphatic ducts satellite to the cephalic vein.

CONSERVATIVE TREATMENT. To plan treatment, it is important to discern the rate of progression of primary lymphedema. In most cases, a prognosis of the eventual extent of limb swelling can be estimated within the first year of symptoms.[60] Treatment is conservative; overall, only 15 per cent of patients eventually require surgical therapy. Late prognosis is determined by the location of hypoplastic lymphatics. Severe lymphedema seldom develops in patients with distal hypoplasia and adequate pelvic lymph nodes. Operations to reconstitute lymphatic drainage are not possible in these cases since the lym-

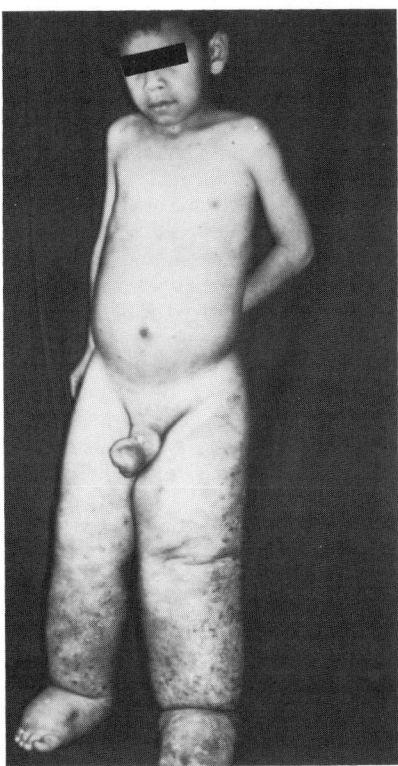

Figure 12. Secondary lower extremity and genital lymphedema caused by filariasis. Patient of Dr. Manuel Valdez and Dr. J. Leonel Villavicencio, Institute de Infermedades Tropicales, Mexico, D. F.

phatics in the leg are sparse. However, the ultimate prognosis is favorable, massive swelling does not occur, and conservative treatment controls edema. Proximal obstructive hypoplasia has more severe consequences; many of these patients develop severe whole limb edema; a higher proportion with this type of involvement later need surgical treatment.

Lymphedema is best treated by rigorous nonoperative measures. These have the goals of minimizing the risk of infection and reducing the subcutaneous fluid volume. The most trivial skin complications are treated to prevent infection, which might further damage lymph channels. The patient should be fitted with graduated compression support stockings (40 to 60 mm. Hg pressure at the ankle) after the limb has achieved maximal reduction using elevation and sequential pneumatic compression.[46] Support stockings must be replaced every 3 to 4 months if they are to yield effective compression. The support stockings are removed at night, and the patient must sleep with the bed raised to keep the legs above the level of the right atrium. This is best accomplished by placing 10- to 12-inch blocks under the foot of the bed; pillows are ineffective as the legs slip off them during the night.

Modern devices that use sequential pneumatic compression are particularly useful for control of lymphedema;[46] although home use is possible, the initial period of treatment often requires 1 to 3 days of hospitalization. Diuretics are not prescribed unless, in women, excess fluid is retained in the premenstrual period. Eczema is treated with triamcinolone, 0.05 to 0.1 per cent, and fungal lesions must be treated with specific agents. Occasionally, lymph-producing fistulas and vesicles appear. These sometimes require excision. Secondary lymphedema demands specific therapy for the underlying disease process. Filariasis is treated with diethylcarbamazine; rare secondary lymphedemas due to tuberculosis or lymphogranuloma venereum are treated with appropriate antibiotic therapy. Massive lymphedema can ensue as a result of venous occlusion, and

secondary lymphedema is worsened by venous ulceration. The goal here is healing of the ulceration so that this portal of entry of infection does not further compromise remaining lymphatic drainage.

SURGICAL TREATMENT. Operations for treatment of lymphedema are divided into two general categories: excisional or physiologic. Excisional operations remove excess skin and subcutaneous tissue and are based on the principle that the subfascial tissues are unaffected by lymphedema. Currently, these operations offer one solution to the problem of massive limb enlargement. An alternative to surgical therapy is hospitalization and intensive therapy with sequential compression. Major excisional procedures are summarized in Figure 13. Among these excisional operations, the procedure first described by Charles (Fig. 13A) employs free skin grafts to cover the lower leg after excision of lymphedematous tissue.[8] This operation is applicable when local skin is in poor condition and not suitable for flaps, as is common in tropical lymphedemas. The other reducing operations elevate thick flaps with good blood supply, then underlying lymphedematous tissue is excised. Servelle stresses the need for preoperative venography to assure normal venous drainage.[51] Limb reduction is usually first done on the medial side. Kinmonth's modification of Homan's procedure is most commonly used (Fig. 13B). In Thompson's operation, of historical interest, wide excision of the subcutaneous tissues, with a dermal flap buried in a muscular compartment in the direction of lymph flow, was employed. It is now believed that the excisional component of this procedure is its major benefit.

The second operative principle aims to provide or enhance lymph drainage. Attempts have been made to create artificial lymph channels through subcutaneous tissues, using nonabsorbable thread such as Prolene or other material. These operations do not have a convincing history of success. Other procedures attempt to link subcutaneous tissues to the deep lymphatics (e.g., the Thompson principle) or to attach lym-

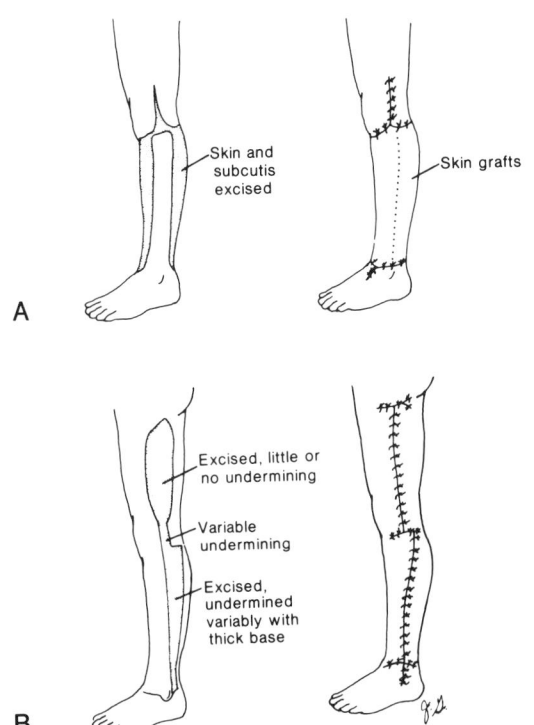

Figure 13. Excisional operations for reduction of lymphedematous lower limbs. A, The Charles operation. B, Kinmonth's modification of Homan's procedure (see text).

phatic-bearing pedicles, such as omentum[22] or small bowel, to the root of the affected limb.[29] Finally, direct lymphovenous shunts have been described,[15] but their efficacy and long-term patency have yet to be proved.

To achieve adequate lymphatic drainage, the proximal and distal anatomy of the veins and lymphatics must be suitable. Therefore, both venography and lymphangiography are indicated preoperatively. Kinmonth and associates described an opened defunctionalized small bowel pedicle to construct a lymphatic anastomosis with inguinal nodes.[33] The small bowel pedicle is isolated and stripped of mucosa. Patency of these enteromesenteric bridges was proved by lymphography. This operation is not suitable for most patients with primary lymphedema because adequate lymphatics must exist distally in the leg.

Since lymphovenous shunts develop naturally, another evolutionary approach creates anastomoses between lymphatics and veins. Nielubowicz and associates first used lymphoidal venous shunts and reported postoperative patency using lymphography.[40] These operations involve sectioning a node[39] or sectioning and removing the lymph node pulp under magnification.[9] The node capsule with its afferent lymphatics is then sutured into a vein. Direct lymphatic vein anastomoses also have been performed. In the rare case of hyperplastic lymphatics with reflux, the saphenous vein has been sutured to dilated inguinal or external iliac megalymphatics. Preserving the saphenous valve at its entrance to the common femoral vein prevents blood reflux. While chyle was seen to flow into lymphaticovenous anastomoses at the time of these operations, follow-up has not convincingly demonstrated patency in the opinion of this author.

The opportunity to perform and observe long-term results of lymphovenous anastomoses is limited by the rarity of these disease entities, along with the problems related to repeated visualization. Lymph nodal venous shunt, direct lymphaticovenous shunts, and small bowel pedicle grafts are more applicable to cases of secondary lymphedema rather than to primary lymphedema because of anatomic limitations previously considered. Microsurgical techniques of lymphovenous anastomosis have been described by Degni[15], Cordiero[11] in Sao Paulo, Brazil, and more recently by Huang and associates[25] in China. From these reports it is also not proved that these anastomoses remain patent. Because of the lack of an objective method to show late patency, Gloviczki and co-workers performed an experimental study in dogs showing lymphovenous shunt patency in two of six animals at 8 months.[21] They concluded that patency rates are low but are objectively demonstrable. Another microsurgical approach, described by Baumeister and associates, used autogenous transplantation of lymphatic collectors.[3]

Lymphedema of the arm following radical mastectomy is a distressing problem. Conscientiously applied conservative measures can usually control the swelling. In 1979, direct microlymphaticovenous anastomoses and resectional surgery were described to treat upper extremity lymphedema.[43] The proponents of this approach avoid preoperative lymphography, which they believe obliterates usable ducts. Since the last edition of this chapter, no follow-up to demonstrate patency of this procedure is available. Therefore, the applicability of direct lymphaticovenous anastomoses as a standard operation is open to question. Current therapy for lymphedema remains conservative, with use of reduction procedures in extreme cases and then only after prolonged sequential compression.

LYMPHANGITIS AND LYMPHADENITIS

Lymphangitis is an inflammation of the peripheral lymphatics, which appears as erythematous streaks progressively coursing toward regional lymph nodes. As infection ascends, brawny distal edema develops because of coagulation of lymph within the vessels. Lymphangitis is most frequently caused by hemolytic streptococci but can also occur with staphylococcal infections. Irritative lymphangitis can also be provoked by lymphangiography.[42] With ascending lymphangitis, there is usually little pus; incision is contraindicated, unless a distal purulent accumulation, such as a paronychia or an infected blister, exists.

Lymphangitis is treated with rest to decrease lymph flow, local heat, elevation of the extremity, and specific antibiotics. Since beta-hemolytic streptococci are the common infecting organisms, penicillin is first employed until cultures show another etiology. Many decades ago, serious epidemics of invasive streptococcal infection occurred in the form of an acutely spreading cellulitis and lymphangitis known as erysipelas. This clinical pattern is now rarely seen. With onset of erysipelas, there is bacteremia with severe systemic symptoms of chills, fever, and generalized aching. The cellulitis coalesces, rapidly extending to uninvolved skin.

Enlargement of the regional lymph nodes draining areas of infection is an almost universal reaction to sepsis. Common regional viral lymphadenopathies include granuloma venereum, cat scratch fever, and cytomegalovirus infections. Human immunodeficiency virus infection has emerged as a common cause of lymphadenopathy and will be discussed further. Among the chronic indolent adenopathies are tuberculosis and fungal infections such as sporotrichosis or toxoplasmosis. When acute suppuration of lymph nodes occurs, the surgeon must seek the infecting agent among a vast number of organisms. Certain adenopathies require special consideration. An uncommon acute adenopathy requiring early diagnosis is *Pasteurella pestis* infection. The disease still occurs in the United States and is transmitted by flea bites from infected rodents. The initial flea bite is rarely visible; however, the inflamed regional lymph nodes present a striking appearance, with a hemorrhagic edematous zone or skin surrounding the suppurating nodes. These lesions are termed buboes; acute adenopathies with this appearance should be viewed suspiciously. The treatment of choice, pending culture verification, is tetracycline and streptomycin. Tularemia causes an acute regional adenitis and is due to handling infected animals. Exquisitely tender and purulent lymph nodes with overlying cellulitis result.

Acute and chronic cervical lymphadenitis secondary to infection are among the most common disorders of childhood. In most cases a diagnosis can be made by carefully collating clinical data. Because of the widespread use of antibiotics, patients present with chronic, indurated, nonfluctuant lymph nodes. In young adults, chronic cervical lymphadenopathy is also not an uncommon finding, and it is often difficult to delineate precisely a primary focus of infection. Before excising lymph nodes, the patient must be examined completely, with emphasis on foci of infection or tumors of the head and neck. Computed axial tomography is also useful in seeking mediastinal involvement. If a focus of infection is detected, antibiotic therapy and the observation of regression of adenopathy suffice. There has been a trend toward delayed use of cervical lymph node biopsy when malignancy is improbable, because so many of these nodes simply exhibit reactive hyperplasia. When the abnormal nodes are supraclavicular in location, prompt excisional biopsy is recommended.

Persistent generalized adenopathy may be caused by HIV infection, presenting as a prodrome of acquired immunodeficiency syndrome.[7] The syndrome is defined as lymphadenopathy of at least 3 months' duration involving two or more extrainguinal sites and absence of other illness or drug use causing lymphadenopathy. Here serologic testing for HIV infection rather than biopsy should be chosen. Lymph nodes or any tissue obtained from cases of HIV infection require special handling. Lymph node excision may be requested for diagnosis of *Mycobacterium avium* infection, which may require specific therapy.

Fine needle aspiration is often preferable to biopsy for initial diagnosis of cervical lymphadenopathy.[22,44,59] This procedure minimizes the necessity for open biopsies. Whenever there is a need for lymph node excision, the involved nodes should be excised by an incision in the skin lines. When anterior cervical nodes appear to be matted, extensive, or adherent to vessels and deep structures, excision is more safely done under general anesthesia. Posterior cervical nodes can be more easily removed under local anesthesia. Lymph node biopsy requires meticulous attention to hemostasis; all lymphatic ducts should be ligated with absorbable suture material. Fresh nodes should be delivered immediately to the pathologist after obtaining appropriate cultures, including bacterial, acid-fast, and fungal cultures. A smear for bacteria and touch preparations of the sectioned node to diagnose certain types of lymphoma are also useful. The remaining material is sectioned by the pathologist and fixed for microscopic examination. Under no circumstances should excised lymph nodes be placed directly in formalin.

TUMORS OF LYMPH VESSELS

Benign lymphatic tumors appear often, commonly in the area of the jugular buds in the neck, and also in the axilla, shoulders, and groin. Simple pathologic classification of these tumors is difficult; most are of developmental origin and are noted at birth or soon after. These are classified as (1) simple and capillary lymphangiomas, (2) cavernous lymphangiomas, and (3) cystic hygromas.

Among the first type, diffuse or localized lymphangiomas affecting the skin appear as vesicles typically localizing on the inner side of the thigh, the axilla, or the shoulder. If lymphangiography reveals that the lesion is separate from the main lymphatic system, it can be excised. Diffuse and cavernous lymphangiomas often involve the face and mouth to cause enlargement of the lips and alarming swelling of the tongue. On occasion, these tumors in children demand emergency operation to maintain the airway. Pathologically, cavernous lymph spaces are found interspersed among muscle fibers.

The most common lymphangioma, cystic hygroma, exhibits large, cystlike cavities containing clear, watery fluid. The lesion, which is seen in infants, usually can be transilluminated. Occasionally, hemorrhage within the cyst renders the mass tense and opaque. Most cystic hygromas present in the neck; 20 per cent are observed in the axillary region (Fig. 14) and the remaining 5 per cent are seen in the mediastinum, retroperitoneum, pelvis, and groin. Two or three per cent of the cervical hygromas have mediastinal extensions extending as far as the diaphragm.

After assessing the extent of the lesion, cystic hygromas are best treated by operative excision.[23] In the neck, they are removed by means of a transverse incision and general endotracheal anesthesia. The cysts are entwined with vital structures and require careful dissection to remove the lobules. Cyst walls appear in juxtaposition to the carotid artery, jugular vein, brachial plexus, vagus nerves, and other deep structures. Cystic hygroma is not a malignant neoplasm, but a development anomaly related to the jugular lymphatic buds. Normal anatomy must not be sacrificed at operation. When a macroscopically identifiable cyst wall is dissected, recurrence is rare.

LYMPHANGIOSARCOMA. This rare malignant tumor occurs in long-standing cases of primary or acquired lymphedema of the extremities. Lymphangiosarcoma was first reported in the arm by Lowenstein in 1906[13] and later in a lymphedematous leg by Kettle in 1918.[30] The description of Stewart and Treves, emphasizing its usual occurrence in postmastectomy lymphedema, was published in 1948.[55] This tumor in-

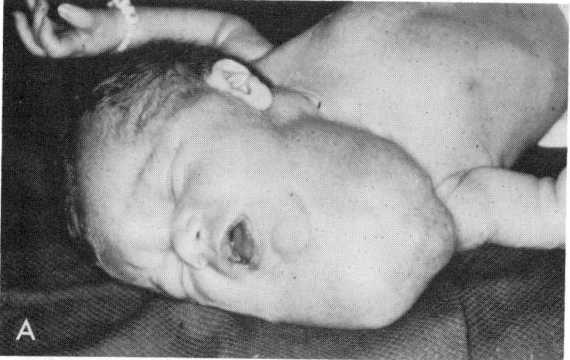
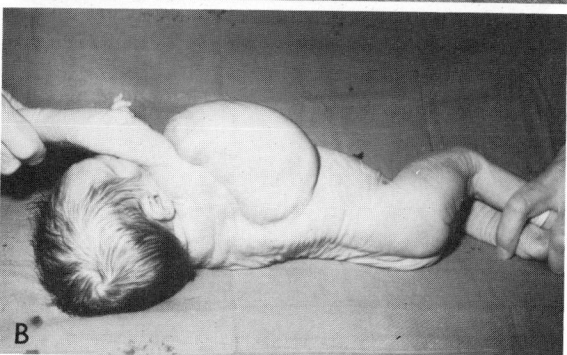

Figure 14. Cystic hygromas of the neck *(A)* and axilla *(B)* in infants. (Courtesy of Dr. Judson G. Randolph, Children's Hospital National Medical Center, Washington, D.C.)

volves either upper or lower lymphedematous extremities, but most commonly it involves the upper extremity. The malignancy first appears as a bruise mark, a purplish discoloration, or a tender skin nodule in the chronically lymphedematous extremity. Typically, early lesions appear first on the anterior surface of the extremity, progress to ulcers with crusting, and then to necrosis that extends to involve the skin and subcutaneous tissue. The lesion progresses and metastasizes widely. The tumor mass is composed of neoplastic endothelial cells sometimes exhibiting poorly defined lymph spaces. There are no reports of effective therapy; the tumors are uniformly fatal.

CHYLOUS EFFUSIONS AND LYMPHATIC LEAKS

Chylous effusions and lymphatic leaks occur for a variety of reasons. Their most common causes are trauma, malignant disease, primary lymphatic deformities due to hyperplasia or megalymphatics, and filariasis. As previously emphasized, chronic chyle loss threatens nutrition and immune competence. Intravenous alimentation and oral feeding with medium chain triglycerides are needed until the chyle leaks can be stopped. Various types of chylous effusions and lymphatic leaks are summarized in Table 1.

In addition to those listed in Table 1, lymph also leaks through vesicles of the extremities and scrotum in certain instances of developmental lymphangiomas. Patients with congenital lymphatic skin lesions exhibit a pink patch or a capillary angioma. Patients with cutaneous vesicles discharging chyle also exhibit lymphedema praecox, with incompetent megalymphatics in the abdomen and limb. When megalymphatics continue to drain, the basic pathology is dilated incompetent lymph pathways located proximal to the leak. Abnormal thoracic duct anatomy appears to be a factor in some of these cases. Surgical operations to divide and ligate incompetent abdominal lymph pathways are facilitated by preoperative milk ingestion on the day before operation or by preoperative injection.

TABLE 1. Chylous Effusions and Lymphatic Leaks

Chylous Ascites
Primary fistulas
Primary lymphatic disease
Secondary
    Malignancy
    Postradiation obstruction
    Postoperative

Exudative Enteropathies

Chylothorax
Trauma
Malignancy
Primary disease of lymph vessels
Filariasis
Subclavian vein thrombosis
Secondary to chylous ascites

Chyluria
Megalymphatics with urethral and vesical fistulas
Filariasis

Chylopericardium
Postoperative
Congenital

Chylometrorrhea

Lymphoceles
Primary
Postoperative

Chylous ascites is usually secondary to malignancy, commonly lymphoma. Primary fistulas or primary lymphatic disease in young children also causes intraperitoneal chyle accumulation. When a lymphatic fistula is found, closure of the fistula with nonabsorbable sutures is indicated. Chylous ascites is also encountered rarely after abdominal operations. Following distal splenorenal shunt and with other secondary types of chylous ascites, otherwise uncontrollable by direct surgical therapy, Leveen peritoneal venous shunts are useful for returning the peritoneal lymph accumulation to the central circulation. Exudative enteropathy due to congenital intestinal lymphatic leaks can be diagnosed when hypoproteinemia is combined with abnormal lymphography. Chyle leaks from the duodenal lumen have been documented by duodenoscopy and also occur from other areas of the upper small bowel.[32]

The most common chylous effusion is chylothorax; it is usually due to trauma or neoplasm. These effusions also can be initiated by penetrating or crushing wounds, or they can follow surgical procedures. The existence of a chylothorax should be established promptly, since death can ensue if the leak is not controlled. Chest films show an unencapsulated pleural effusion which, when aspirated, is creamy and opalescent. It separates upon standing into three layers. Microscopic examination of the fluid shows a predominance of lymphocytes. The culture is sterile due to the bacteriostatic characteristics of lymph. Chylothorax secondary to trauma responds favorably to nonoperative measures; however, treatment must not be delayed because of the debilitating effects of continued chyle loss. In simple trauma, the leak is usually controlled by re-expansion of the lung with restoration of normal intrathoracic pressure. If lymphatic accumulation continues, the site of injury is visualized either by lymphography or by preoperative milk and cream feeding, and the injured thoracic duct is then ligated at thoracotomy. Rarely, chylous effusions appear in the chest secondary to chylous ascites. This occurrence represents transudation of lymph through abnormal lymphatic connections in the diaphragm.

Chyluria, or urinary chyle excretion, is a striking clinical syndrome in which the urine is milky. It is usually due to filariasis but occasionally relates to congenital megalymphatics that leak into the urethra or the bladder. Chylopericardium is extremely rare; two of the spontaneous instances described in the literature were associated with lymphangiomas of the mediastinum.[14] Cases of chylous pericardium have been reported following cardiac surgery.[45] These respond to drainage of the pericardial cavity, the oral administration of medium-chain triglycerides, and intravenous alimentation to compensate the protein loss. Another very rare syndrome is the loss of chyle per vagina, or chylometrorrhea, which is associated with megalymphatics. The treatment of chylometrorrhea is either hysterectomy or ligation of the megalymphatics.

Lymphoceles occasionally present in the groin as primary complications of developmental lymphatic disease and, as mentioned, must not be excised. Postoperative lymphoceles in the femoral triangle are among the most common lymph collections now encountered. These are due usually to disruption of nodes and lymphatics when a vascular graft has been placed in this area. Lymphoceles also occur in the subclavian and supraclavicular areas. The sterile lymph effusion does not require open drainage; in fact, open drainage is contraindicated as this will cause infection of the vascular graft. Repeated aspirations and application of pressure dressings for several weeks generally resolve this problem. Postoperative lymphoceles can be avoided by meticulous dissection, approaching the femoral arteries laterally to avoid lymph nodes and trunks, minimizing the use of cautery, and ligation of lymphatic tributaries.

SELECTED REFERENCES

DePalma, R. G., and Kanter, M.: Structure and function of the lymphatic system. *In* Giordano, J. M., Trout, H. H. III, and DePalma, R. G. (Eds.): The Basic Science of Vascular Surgery, Mt. Kisco, N.Y., 1988, pp. 31–65.
A recent summary of historical and basic science information compiled by a vascular and plastic surgeon. The chapter contains 124 references and includes details on lymphatic structure and the function and anatomy of the peripheral and central lymphatic organs.

Drinker, C. K., and Yoffey, J. M.: Lymphatics, Lymph and Lymphoid Tissue: Their Physiological and Clinical Significance. Cambridge, Mass., Harvard University Press, 1941.
This classic volume summarizes the life work of two pioneer scientists in lymphatic physiology and delineates capillary and lymphatic circulation. Chapters on physiology and practical considerations provide important historical insights into the pathophysiology of lymphatic disorders.

Kanter, M. A.: The lymphatic system: An historical perspective. Plastic Reconstr. Surg. 79:131–139, 1987.
This review traces the history of the lymphatics with emphasis on visualization. It contains valuable illustrations of concepts of gross anatomy.

Kinmonth, J. B.: The Lymphatics: Surgery, Lymphography and Diseases of the Chyle and Lymph Systems, 2nd ed. London, Edward Arnold, 1982.
This book is founded on the clinical work of the Surgical Professional Unit at St. Thomas's Hospital and that of St. Bartholomew's in London. It contains chapters by Professor N. L. Browse, Mr. J. M. Edwards, Mr. B. T. Jackson, and Dr. J. S. MacDonald. It reflects a life work and authoritative contributions based on a large clinical experience in lymphatic disorders. The latest techniques for operative treatment and for lymphography are discussed. This comprehensive volume remains an invaluable aid for the practitioner wishing to learn about treatment of lymphatic disorders. It also presents a lucid classification of the mixed vascular tumors and their relation to the lymphatics.

Miller, A. J.: Lymphatics of the Heart. New York, Raven Press, 1982.
This book views the lymphatic system of the heart, based on the hypothesis that these are integral to normal cardiac function. In addition, it is a valuable source of historical, physiologic, and pathologic summaries of the lymphatic system in general. Lymphatic occlusion of the heart may result in fibroelastosis; the role of the lymphatics in normal cardiac physiology is summarized from an experimental point of view.

Servelle, M.: Klippel and Tranaunay's syndrome: 768 operative cases. Ann Surg., 201:365, 1985.
Servelle, M.: Surgical treatment of lymphedemas: A report of 652 cases. Surgery, 101:485, 1987.
These two articles by Professor Servelle represent the largest number of personally observed cases by a single worker for these two interrelated conditions. The second article contains detailed descriptions of operative ablative techniques.

Wolfe, J. H. N.: Diagnosis and classification of lymphedema. Chapter 146, pp. 1450–1462; Wolfe, J. H. N.: Treatment of lymphedema. Chapter 147, pp. 1463–1474; and Wolfe, J. H. N., and Futrell, J. W.: The management of lymphedema. Chapter 145, pp. 1440–1449. In Rutherford, R. B. (Ed.): Vascular Surgery. Philadelphia, W. B. Saunders Company, 1984.

These chapters are authoritative summaries of the management, pathophysiology, diagnosis, and treatment of lymphedema by two surgeons with clinical experience in this field. Limb reducing operations are particularly well summarized, and the discussion of conservative management is comprehensive.

REFERENCES

1. Arturson, G., and Soeda, S.: Changes in transcapillary leakage during healing of experimental burns. Acta Chir. Scand., *133*:609, 1967.
2. Barbul, A., Shawe, T., Rotter, S. M., Efron, J. E., Wasserkrug, H. L., and Badawy, S. B.: Wound healing in nude mice: A study on the regulatory role of lymphocytes in fibroplasia. Surgery, *105*;764, 1989.
3. Baumeister, R. G., Siuda, S., Bohmert, H., and Moser, E.: A microsurgical method for reconstruction of interrupted lymphatic pathways: Autologous lymph-vessel transplantation for treatment of lymphedemas. Scand. J. Plast. Reconstr. Surg., *20*:141, 1986.
4. Bernard, C.: Leçons sur les Phenomenes de la Vie Communs aux Animaux et aux Vegetaux, Vol. 1. Paris, J. B. Bailliere et Fils, 1878.
5. Blalock, A., Robinson, C. S., Cunningham, R. S., and Gray, M. E.: Experimental studies of lymphatic blockage. AMA Arch. Surg., *34*:1049, 1937.
6. Breathnach, S. M.: Centenary review: The Langerhans cells. Br. J. Dermatol. *119*:463, 1988.
7. Centers for Disease Control: Classification system for human T-lymphotropic virus Type III/lymphadenopathy-associated virus infections. Mort. Morbid. Weekly Reports, *35*:334, 1986.
8. Charles, H.: In a System of Treatment, Vol. 3. London, Churchill, 1912.
9. Clodius, L.: The experimental basis for the surgical treatment of lymphedema. In Clodius, L. (Ed.): Lymphedema. Stuttgart, Georg Thieme, 1977.
10. Cohen, P. J., and Jaffe, E. S.: Current methods used in the diagnosis and classification of malignant lymphomas. Updates Oncol., *1*:1, 1987.
11. Cordiero, A. K.: Novas tecnicas de anastomose linfovenoa para tratamento cirurgico do linfedma de membros inferiores e linfedma de membro superior pos mastectomia. Maternidad Infancia *34*:211, 1975 (Brazil).
12. Crockett, D. J.: The protein levels of edema fluid. Lancet *1*:1179, 1956.
13. Danese, C. A., Grisham, E. O., and Dreiling, D. A.: Malignant vascular tumors of the lymphedematous extremity. Ann. Surg., *166*:245, 1967.
14. Daniel, T. G., and Bressie, J. L.: Chyloperiocardium. J. Thorac. Cardiovasc. Surg., *51*:408, 1969.
15. Degni, M.: New technique of lymphatic-venous anastomosis for the treatment of lymphedema. Vasa, *3*:479, 1974.
16. Dumont, A. E., and Mulholland, J. H.: Hepatic lymph in cirrhosis. Prog. Liver Dis., *2*:427, 1965.
17. Ehrich, W. E.: The role of the lymphocyte in the circulation of lymph. Ann. N.Y. Acad. Sci., *46*:823, 1946.
18. Eloesser, L.: Obstruction of lymph channels by scar. J.A.M.A., *81*:1867, 1923.
19. Fahy, V. A., Gerber, H. A., Morris, B., Trevella, W., and Zukoski, C. F.: The function of lymph nodes in the formulation of lymph. In Trnka, Z., and Cahill, R. N. P. (Eds.): Lymphoid Tissue. Basel, Karger, 1980, pp. 82–99.
20. Feldman, P. S., Kaplan, M. J., Johns, M. E., and Cantrell, R. W.: Fine needle aspiration in squamous cell carcinoma of the head and neck. Arch. Otolaryngol., *104*:735, 1983.
21. Gloviczki, P., Hollier, L. H., Nora, F. E., and Kaye, M. P.: The natural history of microsurgical lymphovenous anastomoses: An experimental study. J. Vasc. Surg., *4*:148, 1986.
22. Goldsmith, H. S.: Long-term evaluation of omental transposition for chronic lymphedema. Ann. Surg., *180*:847, 1974.
23. Grosfeld, J. L., Weber, T. R., and Vane, D. W.: One-stage resection for massive cervicomediastinal hygroma. Surgery, *92*:693, 1982.
24. Hewson, W.: The Lymphatic System in the Human and Other Animals. London, J. Johnson, 1774.
25. Huang, G-K., Ru-Qi, H., Long-Zhao, L., Yao-Liang, S., Tie-De, L., and Gong-Ping, P.: Microlymphaticovenous anastomosis in the treatment of lower limb obstructive lymphedema: Analysis of 91 cases. Plast. Reconstr. Surg., *76*:671, 1985.
26. Hudack, S. S., and McMaster, P. D.: The lymphatic participation in human cutaneous phenomena. J. Exp. Med., *57*:751, 1933.
27. Hunter, W.: Two Introductory Lectures in His Last Course of Anatomic Lectures at His Theatre in Windmill Street. London, J. Johnson, 1784.
28. Huntington, G. S.: The Anatomy and Development of the Systemic Lymphatics in the Domestic Cat. Philadelphia, Wistar Institute Press, 1911.
29. Hurst, P. A., Kinmonth, J. B., and Rutt, D. L.: A gut and mesentery pedicle for bridging lymphatic obstruction. J. Cardiovasc. Surg., *19*:589, 1978.
30. Kettle, E. H.: Tumors arising from endothelium. Proc. Roy. Soc. Med., *11*:19, 1918.
31. Kinmonth, J. B.: Lymphangiography in man. Clin. Sci., *11*:13, 1951.
32. Kinmonth, J. B., and Eustace, P. W.: Gut protein loss in lymphedema. Proc. Roy. Soc. Med., *68*:673, 1975.
33. Kinmonth, J. B., Hurst, P. A. E., Edwards, J. M., and Rutt, D. L.: Relief of lymph obstruction by use of a bridge of mesentery and ileum. Br. J. Surg., *65*:829, 1979.
34. Landis, E. M.: Capillary permeability and the factors affecting the composition of the capillary filtrate. Ann. N.Y. Acad. Sci., *46*:713, 1946.
35. Malek, P., Belan, A., and Kocandrle, U. L.: The superficial and deep lymphatic system of the lower extremities and their mutual relationship under physiological and pathological conditions. J. Cardiovasc. Surg., *5*:686, 1964.
36. Mayerson, H. S.: The lymphatic system with particular reference to the kidney. Surg. Gynecol. Obstet., *116*:259, 1963.
37. Milroy, W. F.: Chronic hereditary edema. JAMA, *91*:1172, 1928.
38. Moretta, L., Mingari, M. C., Moretta, A., and Fauci, A. S.: Human lymphocyte surface markers. Semin. Hematol., *19*:273, 1982.
39. Nielubowicz, J., and Olszewski, W.: Surgical lymphaticovenous shunts in patients with secondary lymphedema. Br. J. Surg., *55*:440, 1968.
40. Nielubowicz, J., Olszewski, W., Muszynski, M., and Sawicki, J.: Late results of lymphovenous anastomosis. J. Cardiovasc. Surg. (Torino), *14*:113, 1973.
41. Nossal, G. J. V.: Immunologic tolerance: Collaboration between antigen and lymphokines. Science, *245*:147, 1989.
42. O'Brien, B. M., Das, S. K., Franklin, J. D., and Morrison, W. A.: Effect of lymphangiography on lymphedema. Plast. Reconstr. Surg., *68*:922, 1981.
43. O'Brien, B. M., and Shafiroff, B. B.: Microlymphaticovenous and resectional surgery in obstructive lymphedema. World J. Surg., *3*:3, 1979.
44. Oertel, Y. C.: Fine needle aspiration: A personal view. Lab. Med., *13*:343, 1982.
45. Pugliese, P., Santi, C., and Eufrate, S.: Isolated chyloperiocardium after successful correction of total anomalous pulmonary venous drainage. J. Cardiovasc. Surg., *25*:75, 1984.
46. Richmond, D. M., O'Donnell, T. F., Jr., and Zelikovski, A.: Sequential pneumatic compression for lymphedema: A controlled trial. Arch. Surg., *120*:1116, 1985.
47. Roitt, I., Brastoff, J., and Male, D.: Immunology. St. Louis, C.V. Mosby, 1985.
48. Sabin, F. R.: The Origin and Development of the Lymphatic System. Baltimore, The Johns Hopkins Press, 1912.
49. Sabiston, D. C., Archer, G. W., and Blalock, A.: Fate of cells in passage through lymphatics and lymph nodes. Ann. Surg., *158*:570, 1963.
50. Salem, A. H., Mulhim, A. M., Grant, C., and Khwaja, M. S.: Milroy's disease in a Saudi family. J. R. Coll. Surg. Edinb. *31*:143, 1986.
51. Servelle, M.: Surgical treatment of lymphedema: A report on 652 cases. Surgery, *101*:485, 1987.
52. Smith, H., Chen, I.-M., Kubo, R., and Tung, K. S. K.: Neonatal thymectomy results in a repertoire enriched in T cells deleted in adult thymus. Science, *245*:749, 1989.
53. Starling, E. H.: On the absorption of fluid from the connective tissue spaces. J. Physiol. (London), *19*:312, 1986.
54. Starzl, T. E., Weil, R., Koep, L. J., McCalmon, R. T. Jr., Terasaki, P. I., Iwaki, Y., Schroter, G. P., Franks, J. J., Subryan, V., and Halgrimson, C. G.: Thoracic duct fistula and renal transplantation. Ann. Surg., *190*:474, 1979.
55. Stewart, F. S., and Treves, N.: Lymphangiosarcoma in post mastectomy lymphedema. Report of 6 cases in elephantiasis chirurgica. Chirurgien Cancer, *1*:64, 1948.
56. Stewart, G., Gaunt, J. I., Croft, D. N., and Browse, D. L.: Isotope lymphography: A new method of investigating the role of the lymphatics in chronic limb edema. Br. J. Surg., *72*:906, 1985.
57. Thompson, N.: The surgical treatment of chronic lymphedema of the extremities. Surg. Clin. North Am., *47*:445, 1967.
58. Vogler, L. B., Grossi, C. E., and Cooper, M. D.: Human lymphocyte subpopulations. In Brown, E. G. (Ed.): Progress in Haematology, Vol. XI. New York, Grune and Stratton, 1979, pp. 1–46.
59. Weymuller, E. A., Kiviat, N. B., and Duckert, J.: Aspiration cytology: An efficient and cost-effective modality. Laryngoscope, *93*:561, 1983.
60. Wolfe, J. H. N., and Kinmonth, J. B.: The prognosis of primary lymphedema of the lower limb. Arch. Surg., *116*:1157, 1981.

49

VENOUS DISORDERS

M. Wayne Flye, M.D., Ph.D.

The pathophysiology of venous disease is in many respects more complex than that of arterial disease. With the exception of aneurysm formation, obstruction is responsible for nearly all the physiologic aberrations characteristic of arterial disease. Venous pathophysiology, however, involves both obstruction and valvular insufficiency.[16] Moreover, the disability from venous disease includes not only regional problems but also those that follow the escape of thrombi into the pulmonary circulation.[33] Together with the copious network of venous collaterals, the low intraluminal pressure, the collapsible nature of the venous wall, and the intermittency of venous flow, definition of the features of venous pathophysiology provide a real challenge.

Varicose veins with their associated symptoms and complications constitute the most common vascular disorder of the lower extremities.[55] More than 20 million people in the United States alone are reportedly significantly affected. Most of these individuals have either symptoms or complications from chronic venous insufficiency, and a substantial number suffer the disability and resulting economic hardship. Of all the earth's mobile creatures, only man, with his penchant for standing erect, is afflicted by this abnormal condition. In the upright position, blood from the leg must be returned to the heart against gravity. The delicate valves in the venous system interrupt the column of blood from ankle to atrium, which if unopposed would potentially exert a pressure at the ankle of 110 to 120 mm. Hg. Even modest motion, however, such as shifting weight, contracts the calf muscles, which forces blood toward the heart in the valved venous system.[20] No description of varicosities in horses, dogs, cats, or other four-legged animals has been recorded.

The term *varicose* is derived from the Latin word meaning "dilated." It implies a dilated, tortuous, and elongated vein. Although varicosities may occur in any venous system, including the lower esophageal area, the anorectal area, and the spermatic cord, they most frequently occur in the lower extremity. They range widely in size from tiny cutaneous spider bursts to large protruding veins that may be confined to localized areas or may widely involve the venous system. Incompetence of venous valves predisposes to the development of varicosities. Although Fabricius' description of these venous valves in 1574 was instrumental in the elucidation by William Harvey of the blood circulation, their importance in the integrity of the venous system was not recognized for almost another 400 years.[22]

HISTORICAL ASPECTS

Varicosities have long been recognized as an important and commonplace venous disorder. Hippocrates discussed their treatment at length 2500 years ago and noted "that it was better not to stand in the case of an ulcer on the leg." Over the intervening centuries, numerous modes of therapy, including puncture, avulsion, excision, cautery, ligation, resection, injection, and stripping, were advocated with variable degrees of success. John Gay in the 1800s recognized that lower extremity ulcer-

ation was usually due to more than just the presence of varicose veins. Although current methods, surgical as well as nonsurgical, have proved generally therapeutic, the search for an effective means of prevention and the perfect cure for this common malady continues.

Sclerotherapy of varicose veins began in Europe soon after Pravaz devised the hypodermic syringe in 1851. Injection therapy had become widely accepted in most European countries as the best form of treatment after Linser of the Tubingen Clinic in 1911 discovered that bichloride of mercury used as a sclerosing agent was less toxic when injected intravenously than were previously used agents. It soon became evident that although the incidence of side effects was low, the recurrence rate was very high after sclerotherapy. This occurred particularly when the valves were also incompetent and the varicosities would not remain occluded in the presence of nature's efforts to canalize the thrombosed veins.

Although early practitioners had performed ligation or local excision of varicose veins, it was not until the advent of general anesthesia and aseptic surgical therapy that a more extensive and definitive operation could be undertaken with success. In 1884, Madelung of Germany, in a radical surgical procedure, excised the greater saphenous vein through a long incision over the medial aspect of the leg and thigh. Although this formidable procedure was associated with a high morbidity and mortality, it remained the most favored of the early operations for varicose veins.

In 1905, Keller, in the United States, first reported the removal of varicose veins without extensive incisions. A wire was passed through the lumen of the saphenous vein, and the vein was pulled or stripped by inverting the vein on itself. Homans, in 1916, emphasized that ligation of the saphenofemoral junction was a vital step in the prevention of recurrence of varicosities, since tributaries to a patent proximal saphenous segment would often allow refilling of distal varicosities. Linton,[18] in the late 1930s, emphasized the pathologic contribution of incompetent perforating veins to venous insufficiency and devised an operation to separate the deep and superficial venous systems by dividing these perforating veins.

Surgical treatment by venous stripping and excision now offers the best long-term prognosis in the treatment of superficial varicosities if the deep venous system is patent. However, for patients in poor general health or for those with trivial or cosmetic problems, other alternatives are often employed. Sclerotherapy, external elastic support, periodic leg elevation, and exercise all have a role.

ANATOMIC AND PHYSIOLOGIC CONSIDERATIONS

The primary and most obvious function of the venous system is the return of blood to the heart from the capillary beds. In addition, veins have a predominant role in regulating vascular capacity. They also assist the return of blood to the heart during exercise by serving as part of the peripheral pump mechanism.

Functioning together with the capillaries, they also help with thermoregulation.

Anatomy of the Veins

Veins possess muscle and collagen but have considerably less elastic tissue than arteries. The smooth muscle is arranged both circularly and longitudinally. In general, the amount of circularly arranged muscle reflects the pressure in that particular vein. As is expected, there is more muscle present in veins of the lower extremity than in those of the chest. Unlike arteries, veins are divided into a superficial and a deep system. The superficial veins are large, relatively thick-walled muscular structures that are located just under the skin. Among the superficial veins are the greater and lesser saphenous veins of the leg (Fig. 1), the cephalic and basilic veins of the arm, and the external jugular veins of the neck. The deep veins, in contrast, are thin-walled and less muscular. These deep veins, unlike the superficial veins, are protected by the muscles and deep fascia, accompany the arteries, and bear the same names as the arteries they parallel (Fig. 2). The cross-sectional area of these veins is approximately three times that of the adjacent artery.

As part of the deep venous system, large, very thin-walled veins are located within the skeletal muscle and are referred to as *sinusoids.* They serve a particularly important function as part of the "bellows" of the muscle pump mechanism during exercise. The soleal sinusoids of the lower leg empty into the posterior tibial vein, and the gastrocnemius sinusoids empty into the popliteal vein.

Perforating veins connect the deep and superficial systems by passing through the fascial layer that invests the deep system (Fig. 3). Of particular importance in the pathophysiology of lower leg venous stasis are a series of approximately six medial calf perforators that join the posterior tibial vein to the greater saphenous vein. This area is most susceptible to venous hypertension and the development of ulceration. In the posterior calf, the superficial system is connected indirectly with the deep system via the large intramuscular sinusoids.

The most important anatomic and functional feature of veins is the presence of delicate but extremely strong bicuspid valves. An expanded sinus at the site of each valve allows the valves to open widely without making contact with the wall. Thus, when venous flow begins to reverse, rapid valvular closure is permitted. The deep veins contain more valves than the superficial veins. Whereas there may be 9 to 19 valves in the distal posterior tibial or anterior tibial vein, the number decreases more proximally so that the common iliac and vena cava usually have no

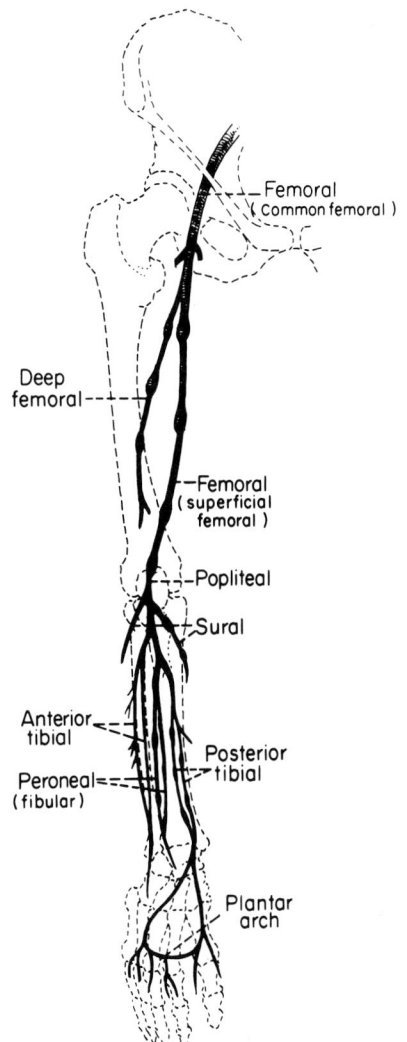

Figure 2. Deep venous system of the lower extremity that parallels the arterial supply. (From Juergens, J. L., Jr., Spittell, J. A., Jr., and Fairbairn, J. F., II: Peripheral Vascular Disease. Philadelphia, W. B. Saunders Company, 1980.)

valves. Valves are present in venules as small as 0.15 mm. in diameter. In all areas of the legs and arms, valve cusps are oriented to direct flow of blood centrally and to prevent reflux. Although valves in perforating veins usually permit blood to flow only from the superficial to the deep venous system, valves in the foot, in contrast, allow flow from the deep to the superficial system. This may exacerbate the venous hypertension and stasis changes that occur around the ankle with venous insufficiency.

The veins of the lower extremity are part of the postcapillary blood reservoir, which holds approximately 70 per cent of the total blood volume. The venous system, however, is not merely a passive conduit, because the total potential venous volume is far from filled owing to some veins that are always either partially or completely collapsed. Because of a great venous capacitance, large fluctuations in venous volume are possible with little change in central venous pressure. When veins are sufficiently filled to assume a circular cross section, the venous smooth muscle contractile state has an important role in regulating venous tone and volume and serves to regulate cardiac output. Regulation of hydrostatic pressure in the capillaries and regulation of temperature via the cutaneous veins are other functions of the venous system. It is estimated that 80 per cent of an increase in venous pressure is transmitted to the capillaries, whereas only approximately 10 per cent of an increase in

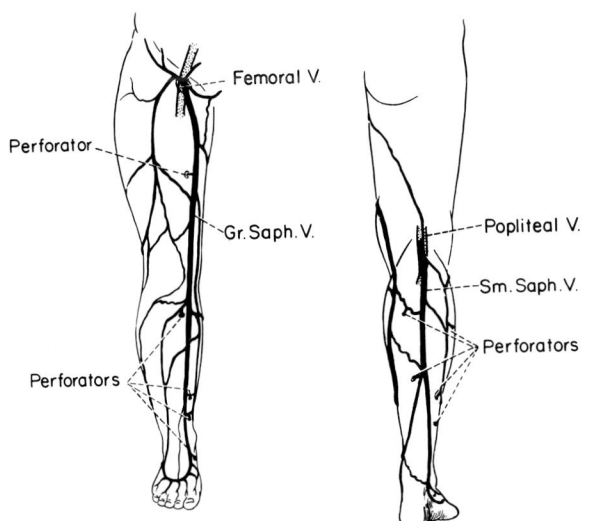

Figure 1. Greater and smaller saphenous superficial veins of the lower extremity and the perforating veins that communicate with the deep veins.

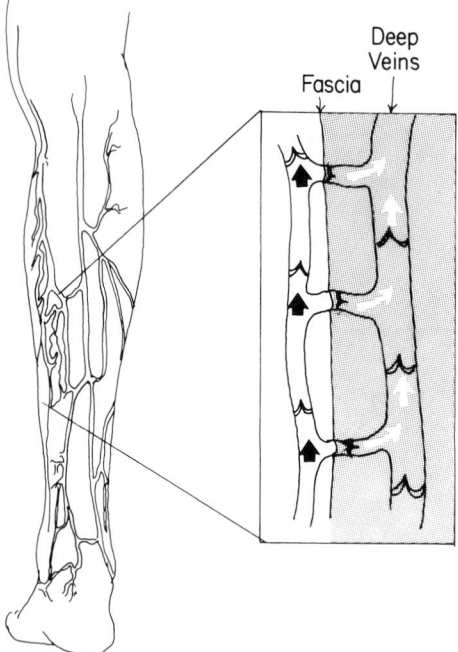

Figure 3. Direction of blood flow in the transfascial perforating veins between the superficial and deep venous systems. (From Burnham, S. J.: Operative treatment for varicose veins. *In* Rutherford, R. B. (Ed.): Vascular Surgery, 2nd ed. Philadelphia, W. B. Saunders Company, 1984, p. 1348.)

arterial pressure is reflected as an increase in capillary hydrostatic pressure.[38]

Venous Pump

When skeletal muscles contract, blood is forced from the intramuscular and surrounding veins and propelled toward the heart. As a consequence of this pumping action, venous pressures in the dependent portion of the leg are lowered, venous congestion is relieved, edema is reduced, and blood flow through exercising muscles is facilitated[6,62] (Fig. 4).

The components of the venous pump are the skeletal muscle, the intramuscular venous sinusoids, and the superficial and deep veins. This venous mechanism is most highly developed in the calf, where the soleal and gastrocnemius sinusoids compose

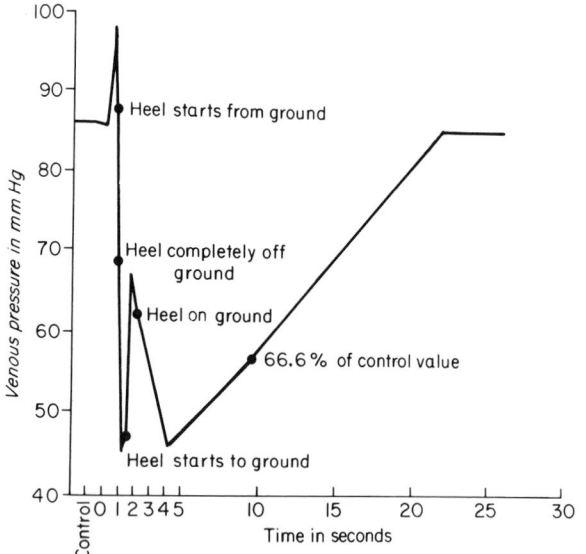

Figure 4. Pressure changes that occur in the deep venous pump of the lower extremity with each step.

the major bellows of the muscle pump. Contraction of the calf muscles produces pressures in excess of 200 mm. Hg, which is sufficient to compress the intramuscular veins even in the standing position. With each muscle contraction, blood is therefore propelled centrally.

Although higher pressure is generated in the deep venous system during muscle contraction, valves in the connecting perforating veins prevent reflux flow from the deep to the superficial system.[40] The proper function of the venous pump depends on the presence of these competent venous valves, particularly in the upright position. This valved venomotor pump mechanism is presumably an evolutionary adaptation to man's assumption of the upright position, because, if a normal individual were to stand motionless for a sufficient period of time, venous pressures at the ankle would stabilize in the range of 80 to 100 mm. Hg and swelling and petechiae would appear. Competent venous valves normally prevent reflux of blood, and the venous pressure is reduced following venous emptying by muscle contraction.[36] With even modest activity of the calf muscles, such as occurs in intermittently shifting one's weight, this pressure is transiently reduced to 20 to 30 mm. Hg. Venous pressure again rises when the collapsed veins are refilled by inflow from capillaries or communicating veins.[41]

When venous valves are incompetent, the resulting hydrostatic column of blood is longer and there is immediate retrograde venous filling with muscle contraction. The venous pressure of the lower leg therefore remains high. This predisposes to the development of dependent edema. According to the Starling concept, return of fluid escaping from the arteriolar end of a capillary to the circulation at the venular end is facilitated by lower venous pressures. In the normal situation, the little swelling that accumulates during the day usually disappears overnight when the body is horizontal. In the abnormal state, greater edema formation resolves more slowly and predisposes the body to chronic changes.

TREATMENT OF VARICOSE VEINS

Operation may be performed for cosmetic reasons or to relieve symptoms, but it should be intended to correct abnormal venous hemodynamics. Little more than visual inspection is required for diagnosis of varicose veins. Before they can be treated intelligently, however, the surgeon should be aware of the functional status of the deep iliofemoral vein and perforating vein valves. The ideal patient for varicose vein surgery is one who has patent deep veins and competent valves in the deep and perforator systems. The next most suitable patient is one who has a patent deep venous system with competent deep valves but incompetent perforator valves. When the perforating veins are ablated along with superficial venous stripping, good results can be expected. Patients with incompetence of all or most deep and perforator venous valves should not be considered for simple vein stripping because recurrence of varicosities is likely. Venous valve reconstruction or transposition may prove to be a logical choice for these patients to restore deep venous valvular competency. Patients with deep vein obstruction, regardless of the condition of their venous valves, are poor candidates for superficial ligation and stripping because stripping the superficial vein may remove the major patent collateral vein and cause a precipitous worsening of the venous outflow problem.

Venous Assessment

Prior to operative treatment, the patency of the deep venous system and valvular competence should be determined. In fact, the deep system is usually patent if there is no history of deep venous thrombosis.[30] Historically, the *Perthes test*, or some variant, has been used in assessing deep venous patency. With this test, superficial varicosities are compressed by wrapping the

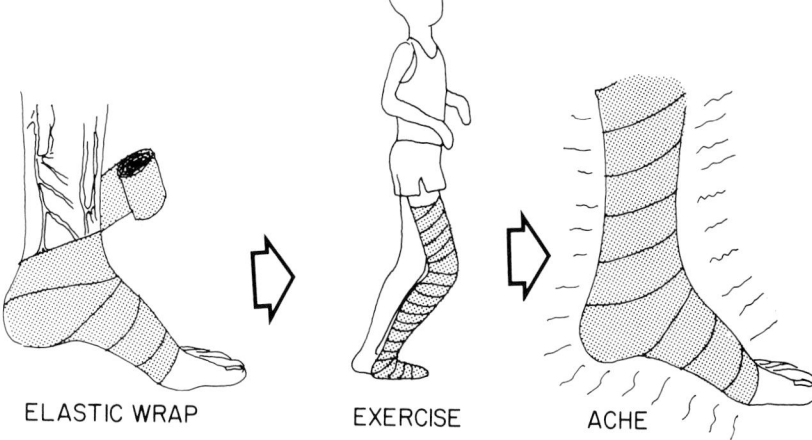

Figure 5. Perthes' test for deep venous occlusion. (From Burnham, S. J.: Operative treatment for varicose veins. *In* Rutherford, R. B. (Ed.): Vascular Surgery, 2nd ed. Philadelphia, W. B. Saunders Company, 1984, p. 1348.)

ELASTIC WRAP   EXERCISE   ACHE

extremity with elastic bandages. Increasingly severe crampy pain during exercise suggests a deep venous obstruction, if arterial occlusive disease has been excluded (Fig. 5). Other noninvasive methods can be used to detect deep venous thrombosis. These methods include venous plethysmography and Doppler flow detection. Doppler flow studies are preferable because they can detect not only deep venous thrombosis but also postthrombotic venous collateral veins and postphlebitic valvular insufficiency (Figs. 6 and 7).

The retrograde-filling test described by Brodie in 1846 and by Trendelenburg in 1890 (*Brodie-Trendelenburg test*) was the first scientific attempt to evaluate valve function.[11] With the patient in the supine position, the leg to be examined is elevated approximately 30 to 45 degrees for the purpose of ensuring maximal venous drainage. An elastic tourniquet is adjusted around the thigh just below the saphenofemoral junction to occlude the superficial veins. The patient is allowed to stand while the pattern of superficial venous refill is noted. In the normal limb, venous refill is incomplete at 30 seconds, and removal of the tourniquet does not cause rapid retrograde filling. Rapid venous refilling on release of the tourniquet suggests incompetent valves in the saphenous system. Filling of the superficial veins prior to release of the tourniquet indicates that incompetent valves are also present in some of the perforating veins.

Measurement of ambulatory venous pressures by direct venous cannulation has been used to refine such physiologic measurements (Fig. 8). Different forms of plethysmography have also been used noninvasively to obtain similar information that is based on volume changes rather than on pressure changes. The photo-cell plethysmograph is particularly applicable because it primarily reflects changes in subcutaneous blood volume that is primarily venous and not arterial.[43,47]

Treatment of Superficial Varicose Veins

Both surgical and nonsurgical methods are used in the management of superficial varicose veins. In general, the surgical removal of incompetent veins is the more definitive treatment because the results are more satisfactory and lasting. Nonsurgical methods are generally reserved for patients with medical contraindications to surgical treatment, deep venous insufficiency, or very minimal varicosities. These nonsurgical methods include sclerotherapy, elastic support,[48] periodic elevation of the lower extremity, and exercise of the leg muscles. Normal prominent superficial veins should not be disturbed or destroyed. Before any treatment is advised, the severity of the varicose problem must be carefully assessed.

SURGICAL TREATMENT. The philosophy in the treatment of varicose veins has changed from "radical" to "selective" in

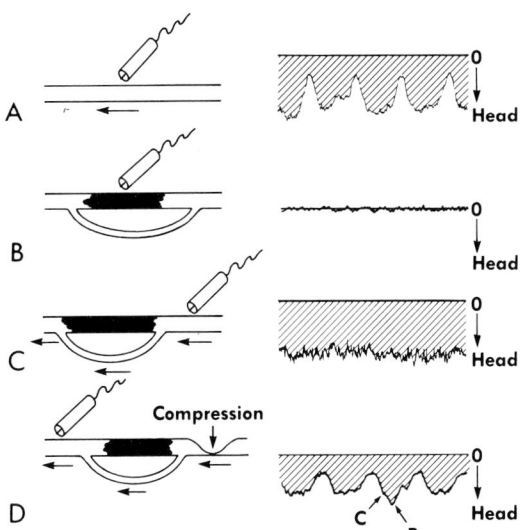

Figure 6. Doppler examination of an occluded vein (C, compression; R, release). *A*, Normal vein. *B*, Probe over the occluded segment. *C*, Below the occluded segment with collateral flow. *D*, Above the occluded segment. (From Sumner, D. S.: Evaluation of venous circulation with the ultrasonic Doppler velocity detector. *In* Rutherford, R. B. (Ed.): Vascular Surgery, 2nd ed. Philadelphia, W. B. Saunders Company, 1984, p. 187.)

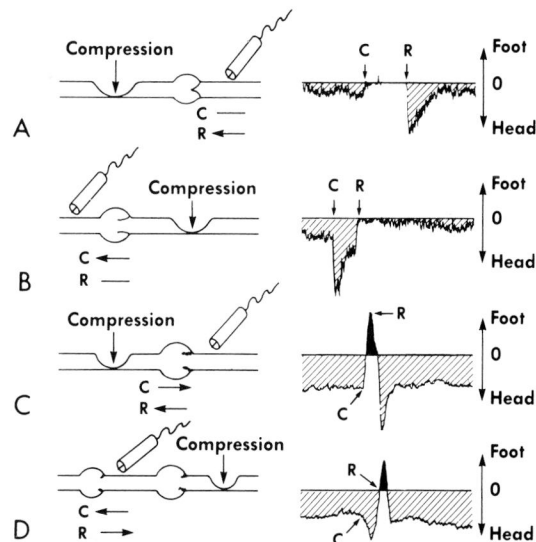

Figure 7. Doppler detection of venous valvular insufficiency. Normal venous valve. *A*, Retrograde. *B*, Antegrade. *C*, Incompetent venous valve. *D*, Retrograde antegrade. (From Sumner, D. S.: Evaluation of venous circulation with the ultrasonic Doppler velocity detector. *In* Rutherford, R. B. (Ed.): Vascular Surgery, 2nd ed. Philadelphia, W. B. Saunders Company, 1984, p. 187.)

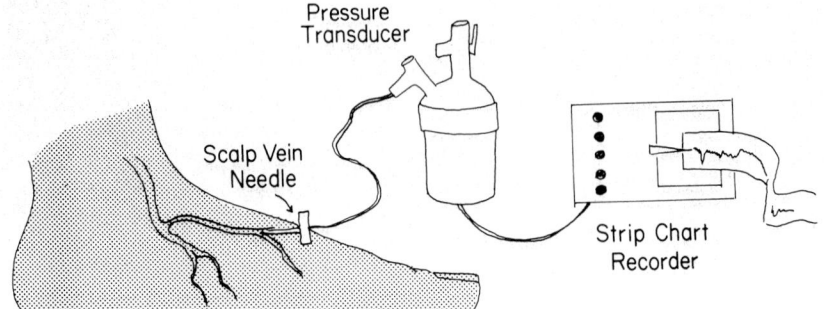

Figure 8. Direct measurement of ambulatory venous pressure in the foot. (From Burnham, S. J.: Operative treatment for varicose veins. In Rutherford, R. B. (Ed.): Vascular Surgery, 2nd ed. Philadelphia, W. B. Saunders Company, 1984, p. 1348.)

order to preserve the saphenous vein for reconstructive vascular procedures. Increased sophistication in localizing abnormal venous physiology justifies more limited procedures. Surgical management of varicose veins involving the superficial venous system is based on the premise that the removed varicosity cannot recur. Removal of symptomatic malfunctioning superficial veins restores the venous circulation to a more normal state and provides relief of symptoms. Surgical therapy may also prevent progressive breakdown and incompetence of more distal but still normal tributaries of the saphenous system. However, surgical therapy of superficial veins is not usually indicated unless definite venous incompetency and reflux are demonstrated by clinical examination.

General indications for surgical treatment are symptoms of aching, heaviness, and cramps; complications of venous stasis such as pigmentation, dermatitis, induration, superficial ulceration, and thrombosis of varicosities; large varicosities subject to trauma; cosmetic concern; and need for prophylaxis in younger patients. Surgical treatment is not required for those patients who obtain relief by elastic stocking support, and it should be recommended only for those patients who are in satisfactory general condition.

The objectives of surgical treatment are to relieve symptoms, to alleviate stasis complications, to restore normal venous physiology, and to improve cosmetic appearance. All incompetent superficial veins and perforators should be thoroughly removed for prevention of the tendency toward recurrence. Veins in which there is a potential for the development of varicosities should also be removed; particular attention should be directed to the smaller dilated tributaries in the thighs, legs, and feet. Special care should be taken neither to damage nor to destroy normal competent greater or lesser saphenous veins, because they may be needed for surgical bypass operations in the future.

OPERATIVE TECHNIQUE. One of the most important steps in the surgical procedure is the preoperative marking of veins. This must be done carefully and accurately with an indelible skin pencil. It is best accomplished while the patient stands on a platform in front of a movable light source. By inspection and palpation, all varicosities, including the main saphenous channel, tributaries, and incompetent perforating veins, are marked. Particular attention should be focused on the identification of tortuous tributaries and perforating veins within fascial defects (Fig. 9).

At the time of operation, general, spinal, or epidural anesthesia is administered. Each leg is prepared with a suitable antiseptic solution and draped from the ankle to the umbilicus. Venous bleeding may be minimized by elevating the legs at an angle of 15 to 20 degrees during the operation.

If the saphenous vein is not directly involved with the varicosities, it may be preserved by removing only the varicose vein.[31] When a classic high ligation and stripping of the saphenous vein is performed, the operation should follow a systematic plan that includes: (1) high ligation at the saphenofemoral or saphenopopliteal junction; (2) insertion of a stripper into

the greater or lesser saphenous vein; (3) removal of tributaries; (4) resection of incompetent perforating veins; (5) stripping of the saphenous veins; and (6) closure (Fig. 10).

A groin incision is made just below the inguinal fold and medial to the femoral arterial pulse. The incision should be cosmetic but generous enough to allow dissection of the superficial tributaries that enter close to the saphenous bulb. The tributaries vary widely in number and distribution, but the classic physiologic formation includes the medial and lateral femoral cutaneous tributaries and the superficial external pudendal, circumflex iliac, and inferior epigastric branches. Removal of these tributaries decreases the risk of recurrence and facilitates precise transfixion ligation of the saphenous vein at its junction with the deep femoral vein.

A small transverse incision is made over the distal greater saphenous vein just anterior and proximal to the medial malleolus. This segment of venous anatomy is consistent in its location on all patients and can be identified even in the morbidly obese. A distal ligature is placed, and the flexible intraluminal stripper is passed proximally. The stripper may encounter obstruction caused by tortuosity of the varicosities or by angulation at the sites of perforating veins. Transcutaneous palpation of the tip allows cutdown at these sites and manipulation of the stripper. Caution is needed because the stripper may enter the deep venous system through one of these connections. The tip of the stripper is brought out through the saphenous vein in the groin incision and anchored to the saphenous vein with a ligature. The stripper is left in place until just before closure. Care is taken to avoid damage to the saphenous nerve, which lies adjacent to the saphenous vein from the level of the ankle to the knee.

Although most tributaries have already been identified by the

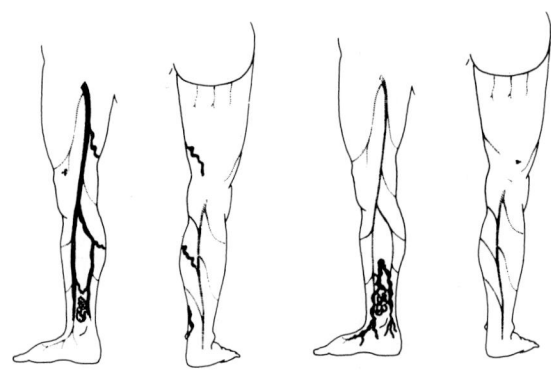

GROSS GREAT SAPHENOUS INCOMPETENCE   **INCOMPETENT ANTERO - MEDIAL PERFORATORS**

Figure 9. Patterns of superficial venous varicosities in the greater and lesser saphenous veins.

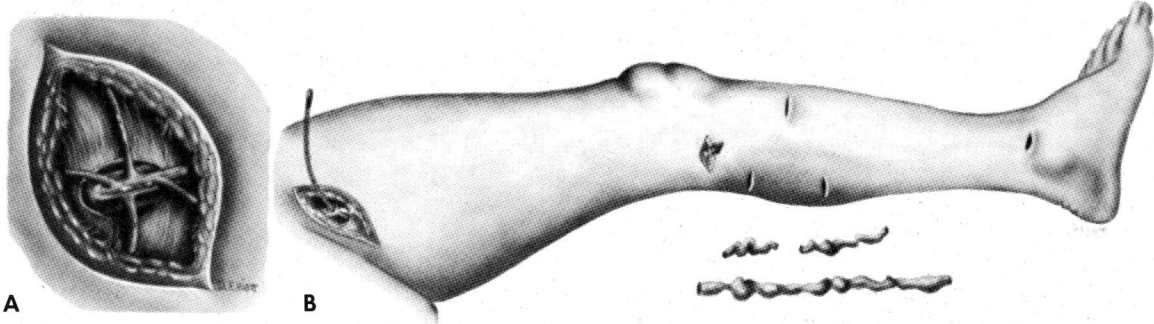

Figure 10. Technique of greater saphenous vein ligation and stripping. *A*, Groin incision exposes the junction of the greater saphenous and femoral veins. Four major branches of the saphenous vein require ligation and division. *B*, Incision at the knee and ankle allow stripping of the saphenous vein. Varicose tributaries are removed by additional incisions (From Schwartz, S. I.: Principles of Surgery. New York, McGraw-Hill, 1969.)

preoperative marking, additional ones may be found during the operation. The tributaries are exposed through multiple, small transverse incisions and are removed by either stripping or excision. Because many of the perforating veins do not directly join with the saphenous vein, they are often not eliminated by mere stripping of the saphenous vein. Perforating veins should, therefore, be ligated individually at the point where they emerge through the deep fascial layer. The more important ones are found on the medial distal third of the lower leg. Associated incompetent perforating veins are found more commonly in the postphlebitic leg and in recurrent varicose conditions.

Stripping of the saphenous vein should be the last step before closure in order to minimize bleeding. All incisions are closed with absorbable subcutaneous and subcuticular sutures and are reinforced with sterile wound closure tapes. The assistant applies firm compression over the course of the stripper (with the leg elevated) while it is gently but forcefully removed via the lower incision from the proximal to the distal location. Compression is maintained while the ankle incision is closed. The leg is then placed in an elastic wrap bandage with sterile gauze pads over the incisions. Adhesive tape placed in a spiral over the elastic wrap prevents bunching of the wrap into tourniquets at the knee and ankle. The patient is encouraged to ambulate on the first postoperative day. On the second day, bandages are removed for inspection of wounds prior to discharge. Ambulation is permitted only with elastic external support for the first 10 to 14 days. Continued use of support stockings is not necessary in patients who achieve a normal venous reflux time after operation.

When performed as a separate procedure, operation on the lesser saphenous system is most easily accomplished with the patient in the prone position. When this operation is combined with a procedure on the greater saphenous system, the patient is in a supine position and the incision is made while the leg is elevated. A small transverse incision is made just below the popliteal skin fold, and the lesser saphenous vein is doubly ligated at its junction with the popliteal vein. The distal lesser saphenous vein is exposed by an incision just posterior to the lateral malleolus. Interjoining tributaries between the greater and lesser saphenous veins and incompetent perforating veins are excised before the lesser saphenous vein is stripped. Care is taken to preserve the sensory sural nerve, which lies adjacent to the saphenous vein from the level of the ankle to the midcalf region.

UNSATISFACTORY SURGICAL RESULTS. The results of surgical treatment may be unsatisfactory because of inaccurate preoperative assessment, incomplete operative treatment, or inadequate follow-up.

Inaccurate assessment can be caused by attributing venous incompetency to the wrong saphenous vein (greater instead of lesser or vice versa), by overlooking either important tributaries or incompetent perforating veins, or by failing to recognize con-

comitant deep venous insufficiency. An accurate diagnosis depends on exact preoperative marking of all faulty superficial veins.

Incomplete operative treatment is the leading cause of unsatisfactory results. Limiting the operation to the strippable veins, neglecting to excise tortuous branches, and failing to resect incompetent perforating veins are considered major surgical errors. Recurrent varicose veins most often are represented by larger tributaries over the medial and lateral aspects of the thigh and leg that had not been removed because the original operation was limited to stripping only the main saphenous vein. Stripping alone also fails to remove incompetent perforating veins, which should be ligated and resected individually. Parallel or duplicate saphenous channels must be recognized as a possible cause of recurrence. Smaller varicosities, for which further operation is usually not necessary, sometimes develop as a true recurrence after an adequate and complete operation.

Inadequate follow-up may cause unsatisfactory long-term results. Because there is an intrinsic weakness of the superficial veins and a propensity for further varicosity development, periodic follow-up examinations are advisable after operation for uncomplicated primary varicose veins. For patients with stasis problems or with postphlebitic conditions in which superficial vein surgery does not restore normal venous physiologic character, follow-up examinations are most important and should be performed at frequent intervals.

In the early postoperative period, small varicosities can be extirpated under local anesthesia in the outpatient clinic or injected with a sclerosing solution. The Mayo Clinic reports satisfactory surgical results (excellent or good) in 94 per cent of patients after 5 years, and in 85 per cent after 10 or more years. The surgical recurrence rate remains low many years after an adequate operation.

NONSURGICAL TREATMENT. The aim of sclerotherapy is to inject a small volume of an effective sclerosant into the vein's lumen in order to destroy the venous intima. If compression is not then applied, a large thrombus forms, which soon recanalizes. This process may cause destruction of valves, so that the venous pathologic character is actually worsened. However, if the sclerosant is injected into an empty vein and external compression is maintained until permanent fibrosis has obliterated the lumen, good results may be obtained.

Three per cent sodium tetradecyl sulfate (Trombovar, Sotradecol, S.T.D.) has been found to be an effective and safe sclerosing agent. Using disposable 2- or 3-ml. syringes fitted with 25-gauge 16-mm. needles, 0.5 ml. of the sclerosant is injected into the empty vein at each of the "points of control." These "points of control" are sites at which incompetent perforating veins join the superficial veins. The nearer the injection is made to the perforating vein, the more certain are the results. Repeated injections may be used for residual veins.

When larger veins are treated, the leg is elevated to an angle of 45 degrees and the segment of vein is isolated by pressure from the operator's index and ring fingers. As the injection is made, the top of the middle finger is placed over the tip of the needle so that one can monitor the injection and ensure that there is no perivenous leak of sclerosant. Cotton balls are then placed over each injection site, and the leg is firmly bandaged with 7.5-cm. cotton crepe, followed by 10-cm. crepe with limited stretch (Elastocrepe). This bandage must be smoothly applied, with steadily reducing pressure up the leg. Finally, these bandages are covered by a length of flesh-colored elasticized tubular stockinette (Tubigrip) size D.

The patient is instructed to walk immediately and to increase the distance daily. After 3 weeks, the legs are examined and rebandaged. After 6 weeks (less for smaller veins), the bandages are removed, and the patient wears two-way stretch elastic stockings during the day for at least 4 more weeks.

The enthusiasm for sclerotherapy varies, but many authorities do not use this means of treatment as the primary treatment for incompetent varicose veins. They believe that it has many disadvantages, in contrast to the advantages of surgical treatment. The recurrence rate is high, even after relatively few years. Hobbs reported a recurrence rate of 29.5 per cent with sclerotherapy versus 7 per cent with surgical therapy at 3 years.[20] This is a problem particularly when sclerotherapy is used for veins of large caliber.

Sclerosing solutions can be dangerous for patients with an allergic condition. An inflammatory reaction can cause local pain, and periphlebitis can sometimes be quite disabling. Repeated courses of massive injection therapy have been known to produce chronic swelling of the leg from inadvertent sclerosing damage of an otherwise normal deep venous system.

Less controversial is the use of sclerotherapy for small prominent venules causing cosmetic concern or for minor varicosities unsuitable for surgical removal. Small recurrent varicosities following surgical therapy are often treated by this method.

DEEP VENOUS DISEASE

Whereas superficial venous thrombosis is usually a benign self-limiting disease, involvement of the deep venous system is a major cause of morbidity and mortality.[4] Any venous system may be involved. The incidence of venous thrombosis in all surgical patients is between 40 and 50 per cent in older patients undergoing operation. In the United States, Hume and associates[22] estimated that at least 140,000 fatal and 400,000 nonfatal cases of pulmonary embolism occur each year. This subject as well as deep venous thrombosis are discussed in Chapter 50.

SUPERFICIAL VENOUS THROMBOSIS

Unlike deep venous thrombosis, the clinical diagnosis of superficial thrombophlebitis is usually easily made. The physical finding of a linear indurated, tender subcutaneous venous cord with local erythema is common. This type of thrombophlebitis most commonly occurs at the site of an intravenous infusion as a result of the drugs administered or because of the intraluminal catheter itself. This condition also frequently occurs in the greater saphenous system below the knee in patients with varicose veins.[59] If there is no predisposing cause in the superficial venous system, Doppler examination may occasionally be necessary to exclude the presence of associated deep venous thrombosis.

Septic phlebitis usually occurs in association with infection of an intravenous cannula that is inserted for long-term administration of fluids or medications. Removal of the cannula and administration of systemic antibiotics are usually effective treatment. However, purulence within the vein or suppurative thrombophlebitis is a more lethal condition that is often asso-

ciated with generalized septicemia. Treatment requires that all of the involved vein be immediately and completely excised. The wound is packed open for later closure, and appropriate systemic antibiotics should always be administered.

Mondor's disease, spontaneous thrombophlebitis of the superficial veins of the breast and anterior chest wall, is a rare condition. This self-limited condition usually involves a vein in the anterolateral aspect of the upper portion of the breast or in the region extending from the submammary fold toward the costal margin and epigastrium.

Migratory thrombophlebitis is repeated thrombosis in superficial veins that occurs at varying sites but most commonly in the lower extremity. No definite etiologic factor has been confirmed; however, in 1856, Trousseau reported an association with carcinoma. This has been noted to be especially prevalent with carcinoma of the tail of the pancreas.

TREATMENT. The treatment of superficial venous thrombosis depends on its etiology, extent, and symptoms. Localized thrombophlebitis usually requires a mild analgesic, such as aspirin, and activity may be continued. More severe thrombophlebitis with increased pain and redness should be treated with bed rest, elevation, and hot compresses.[2] On resolution of symptoms, the patient begins ambulation while wearing elastic stockings. Antibiotics are usually not necessary unless the process is suppurative, in which case both antibiotics and adequate drainage are indicated.

Surgical intervention is rarely indicated in nonsuppurative superficial venous thrombosis unless the process continues to worsen despite adequate nonoperative management, the inflammatory reaction is very severe, or a varicose vein is involved that eventually requires stripping. This disease rarely causes pulmonary embolism. Also, deep venous thrombosis rarely develops in association with superficial venous thrombosis; but superficial involvement frequently occurs in patients with deep venous disease, especially in those with ankle ulceration.

Chronic Venous Insufficiency

The edema that immediately follows deep venous thrombosis is purely obstructive in origin and quickly subsides with bed rest and anticoagulants as venous collaterals develop. Cessation of edema should not lull the physician into inadequately treating the underlying thrombophlebitis. If the deep venous system is allowed to recanalize eventually, the delicate valves will remain imprisoned laterally in organized thrombosis. The resulting patent but valveless deep venous system then transmits the gravitational pressure of the blood column unimpeded from the level of the heart to the ankles.[5] This is the central predisposing feature in the pathophysiology of the postphlebitic state.[19]

However, valvular incompetence alone is not sufficient to produce serious stasis sequelae; it must occur with incompetent perforator veins through which the high deep venous pressure in the ambulatory state is transmitted to the superficial tissues.[13] The location of these perforating veins determines the predilection of stasis changes and ulcers for the area extending from the malleoli up the lower half of the leg (Fig. 11). These perforators may have been involved in the initial thrombosis or may become incompetent by dilatation caused by the back pressure of the valveless deep venous system.[42] Within 10 years of untreated thrombophlebitis, 75 per cent of patients have advanced stasis changes and 50 per cent have had stasis ulcers.[5]

The high ambulatory venous pressure within the calf muscle pump is transmitted through communicating veins to the superficial veins within the skin and subcutaneous tissues of the calf. This distends the local capillary bed and widens the endothelial pores, thus allowing large molecules to escape into the intestinal fluid (Fig. 12). The most important molecule, fibrinogen, polymerizes to form insoluble fibrin. The accumulating

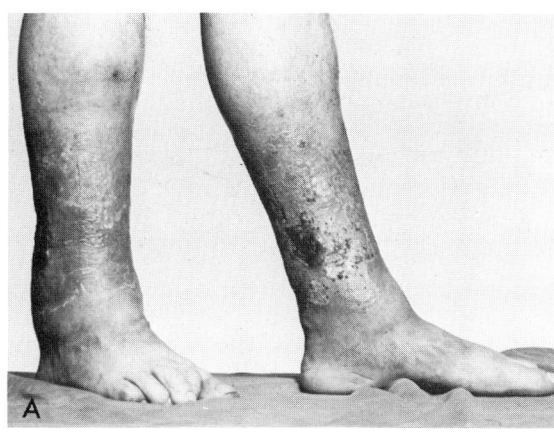

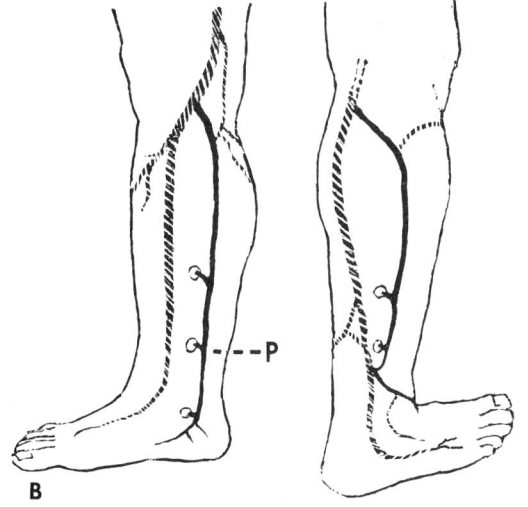

Figure 11. Chronic venous stasis changes usually occur in the lower half of the leg (*A*) where incompetent perforating (P) veins are located (*B*). From Rutherford, R. B., and Johnson, G., Jr.: Nonoperative management of chronic venous insufficiency. *In* Rutherford, R. B. (Ed.): Vascular Surgery, 2nd ed. Philadelphia, W. B. Saunders Company, 1984, p. 1395.)

fibrin cannot be removed because of inadequate blood and tissue fibrinolysis.[8] This accumulation acts as a barrier to diffusion of oxygen and other nutrients; and thick, hard, tender subcutaneous tissue (liposclerosis) develops. These changes of stasis dermatitis (brawny edema, subcutaneous fibrosis, pigmentation, and cutaneous atrophy) may cause tissue death and ulceration.[9] Although varicosities are frequently associated with these changes, the opposite is not true; uncomplicated varicose veins are rarely associated with ulcers.

Postphlebitic Syndrome

The hemodynamics of the arterial circulation are dominated by the pumping function of the heart and are relatively simple to understand. In contrast, the hemodynamics of venous return from the lower limbs against gravity are dominated by the pumping function of the calf muscle contraction and are more complicated.[50] In limbs with primary varicose veins, the calf muscle functions like a heart with a normal stroke volume but with an increased preload because of reflux.[12] In limbs with deep venous disease, the calf muscle functions like a heart with a reduced stroke volume because of the destruction and reduction of the volume of the deep veins of the calf, the increased afterload owing to high outflow resistance caused by venous obstruction, and the increased preload as a result of venous reflux.[12,50]

The patient with postphlebitic syndrome has little if any venous pressure reduction during exercise.[49] In contrast, pressure in normal patients not only rapidly decreases with exercise but also requires several minutes to rise after exercise has been discontinued.[3] The changes in venous pressure in patients with primary varicose veins are between these two extremes (Fig. 13).

In chronic venous insufficiency, when the deep venous hypertension is finally transmitted into the superficial veins and tissues, edema recurs in the patient who is in an upright position for any significant period of time.[37] The edema associated with peripheral venous disease, even in the acute stage, does not "pit" readily. In the chronic stage, it is frankly "brawny" and is associated with characteristic skin changes caused by chronic venous hypertension. Unfortunately, these changes are subtle and gradual at first, and the patient accepts a degree of swelling, discoloration, and aching in the involved leg. It is often not until some minor trauma leading to a skin break occurs that an actual stasis ulcer develops.[1,51]

Treatment of chronic venous insufficiency should begin as soon as the diagnosis has been made. The patients must understand that the damage to the leg is directly proportional to the swelling that they allow to occur. They must also understand that their wearing of good custom-fitted elastic stockings whenever they are out of bed is not sufficient and must be combined with periods of elevation of the ankles above the heart level during the day. It is rarely necessary for a patient to wear stockings above the knee, because ulceration does not occur above the knee; the higher stockings are so uncomfortable that most patients do not wear them for any extended period of time. The frequency of daily leg elevation must be individualized according to the rapidity of edema formation. If scrupulously followed, these measures control stasis sequelae in 100 per cent of patients. Unfortunately, patients who believe that they are doing well are less attentive to this chronic problem.

Figure 12. Venous hypertension and distention causes extravasation of large molecules into the surrounding soft tissue. Accumulation blocks diffusion and predisposes to ulceration. (From Browse, N. S., and Burnand, K. G.: The cause of venous ulceration. Lancet, 2:243, 1982.)

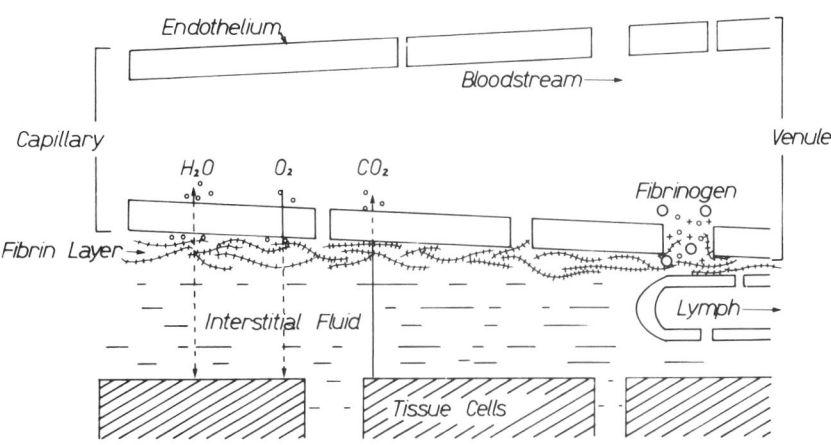

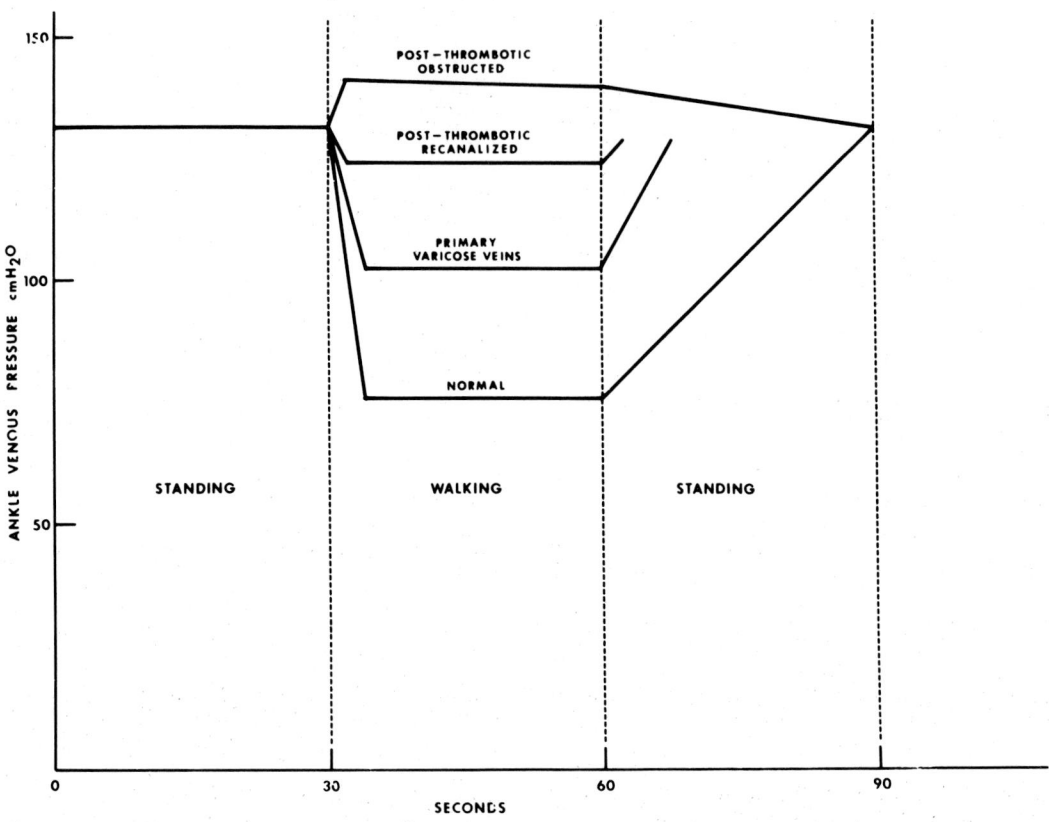

Figure 13. Ambulatory venous pressure in patients with postthrombotic obstructed veins, postthrombotic recanalized veins, primary varicose veins, or normal deep veins. (From Smith, D. E.: Surgical management of chronic obstructive venous disease of the lower extremity. *In* Rutherford, R. B. (Ed.): Vascular Surgery, 2nd ed. Philadelphia, W. B. Saunders Company, 1984, p. 1414.)

In those patients in whom stasis ulcers develop, periodic application of Unna's paste boots is the mainstay of ambulatory treatment. This consists of a gauze dressing impregnated with gelatin, zinc oxide, and calamine, which is applied from the toes to knee after the ulcer has initially been cleansed and wrapped with an Ace bandage. Weekly reapplication of these compressive "boots" combined with elevation of the legs for at least 20 minutes several times each day allows healing of the stasis ulcer. Excision of the ulcer and skin grafting should be necessary only for large ulcerations.

SURGICAL MANAGEMENT. While 90 per cent of venous stasis ulcers can be managed nonoperatively, those patients who cannot or will not follow this postphlebitic routine should be evaluated for an operative procedure[10] (Table 1).

Linton developed subfascial ligation of incompetent perforators for the treatment of stasis dermatitis and ulceration.[18,34] He ligated and stripped all superficial varicosities, ligated the superficial femoral vein, subfascially ligated and divided all medial communicating (perforating) veins, and excised a strip of posterior calf fascia.[23] With increasing experience, Linton found that removal of all superficial varicosities and complete subfascial ligation of all incompetent perforating veins were essential in this operation (Fig. 14). Following this procedure the ulcer recurrence is 2 to 43 per cent.[25]

Noninvasive techniques and phlebography have made it easier to detect the contribution of incompetent superficial, perforating, or deep veins to the pathologic process.[7,58] Surgical therapy must be directed toward these abnormal veins.[10] The three major medial posterior arch vein perforators described by Cockett and Jones are especially important.[12] In addition, if there is incompetence of the superficial veins, they should be stripped in combination with ligation of the incompetent perforators. If proximal deep venous occlusion is present, it must be relieved before the incompetent perforators are ligated.

Both the calf muscle pump ejection fraction and the degree of deep venous reflux determine the propensity for venous stasis ulceration to occur. A poor ejection fraction is the primary cause of ulceration in limbs with minimal reflux. A good ejection fraction, however, significantly reduces the incidence of ulceration in limbs with marked reflux. Air-plethysmographic measure-

TABLE 1. Comparison of Clinical, Hemodynamic, and Anatomic Results
of Venous Reconstruction

| Type of Procedure | Number of Limbs | Healing of Ulcer (%) | | Hemodynamic Improvement (%) | Anatomic Potency (%) |
		Early	*Late*		
Valvuloplasty	93	84	63	93	88
Venous segment transfer	26	65	—	71	80
Femoral vein transfer	67	82	66	67	95
Popliteal vein transfer	10	100	100	30	100

Adapted from O'Donnell, T. F., et al.: Clinical hemodynamic and anatomic follow-up of direct venous reconstruction. Arch. Surg. 122:474, 1987.

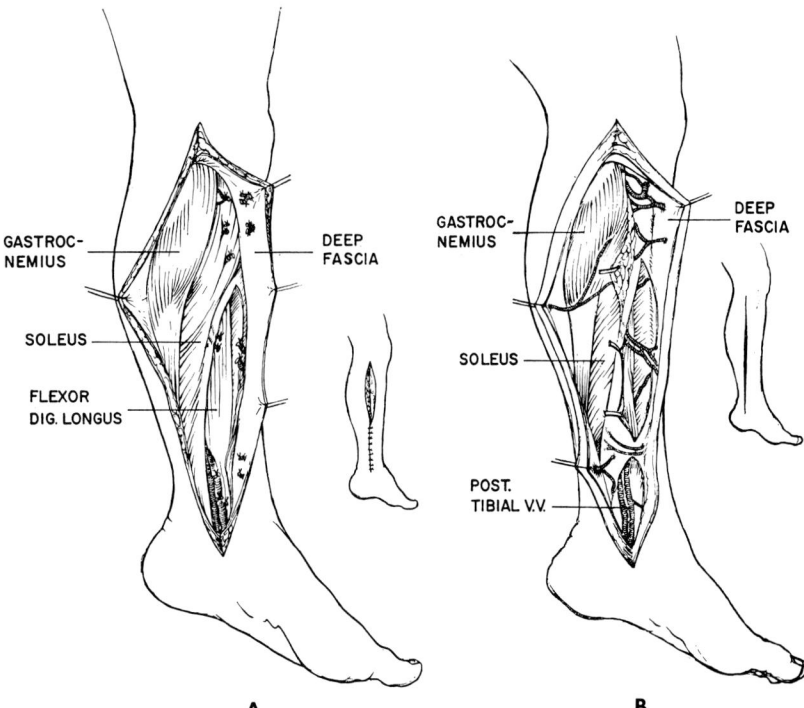

Figure 14. Linton's subfascial approach to the division of perforating veins in the medial compartment of the leg. The deep fascia is incised and undermined, and all perforators are divided. The largest number of perforators are found near the attachment of the fascia to the edge of the tibia. (From Barker, W. F.: Surgical Treatment of Peripheral Vascular Disease. New York, McGraw-Hill, 1962.)

ments have been found to identify the predominant hemodynamic factor or factors (ejection fraction, reflux, or both).[11] Only if there is marked deep venous reflux will venous valvular reconstruction improve the abnormal venous hemodynamics.

CROSS-FEMORAL VENOUS BYPASS. The saphenous vein has been used to bypass segmental venous occlusion of the iliofemoral or femoropopliteal veins. For iliofemoral occlusion, the contralateral saphenous vein is passed suprapubically and anastomosed to the affected side (Palma or Dale procedure).[14,45] A temporary arteriovenous fistula distal to the anastomosis may ensure patency. When occlusive disease is limited to the femoropopliteal veins, the obstructed segment can be bypassed by anastomosis of the saphenous vein to the popliteal tibial trunk at the level of the knee (Husni or May procedure).

If there is isolated iliac venous compression and entrapment by the right common iliac artery, this may be decompressed by completely mobilizing the arteries overlying the veins. Division of the right common iliac artery and reanastomosis behind the left common iliac vein may be necessary to prevent recompression of the vein.[15]

VENOUS VALVULOPLASTY. Occasionally, chronic venous insufficiency is caused by primary valvular incompetence. Descending venography demonstrates the contrast agent regurgitating through a prolapsing valve cusp.[6] Direct repair of these incompetent valves and ligation of any associated incompetent perforators have controlled induration and ulceration in 90 per cent of the patients so treated.[28,29,44]

VENOUS VALVE TRANSPOSITION OR TRANSPLANTATION. In those patients in whom the valves of the superficial femoral and popliteal veins have been destroyed by thrombophlebitis, a competent valvular system can be produced by transposition of a proximal venous segment containing a valve.[24] This is anastomosed to the incompetent superficial femoral or profunda femoris vein. Free transplantation of venous valves is used infrequently because of the need for autogenous veins elsewhere and their propensity for thrombosis.[56] When employed, distal arteriovenous fistulae and postoperative anticoagulation[17,26] are thought to improve patency.[57]

In some but not in all cases of venous reconstruction, the initial physiologic response has been favorable. The ambulatory venous pressure has decreased and the plethysmographic trac-

ings have normalized. However, data from follow-up studies of many of the patients have demonstrated a disappointing return to the previously abnormal hemodynamic state, particularly when there is residual incompetence of the perforating veins or of the superficial venous systems. Such physiologic monitoring is essential for understanding of the results of venous surgery and for the design of better operations and better patient selection.[21,27]

EXTERNAL POPLITEAL VALVE. In an effort to control deep venous reflux caused by incompetence of the popliteal veins without venous invasion, a technique has been developed to produce a valvelike external compression of the popliteal vein by an implanted silicone tendon[46] that is attached to the gracilis muscle. During walking, the popliteal vein becomes patent during contraction of the calf muscles when the knee is extended and the gracilis is relaxed. The popliteal vein is closed during relaxation of the calf muscles when the foot is off the ground, because the knee is flexed and the gracilis muscle is contracted. Thus, the "valve" effect prevents or minimizes reflux in the deep veins during relaxation of the calf muscles.

Thrombosis of Other Deep Veins

AXILLARY SUBCLAVIAN VEIN OCCLUSION. The axillary-subclavian vein occupies a unique position in the thoracic outlet at the junction of three major anatomic regions of the body: the neck, the shoulder girdle, and the thorax. In this position it is subject to pivotal motion and segmented stress between relatively stationary veins at either end. Motion subjects this vein to stretching and shearing trauma that may induce an inflammatory reaction in the wall of the vein.

A number of factors may cause external compression and stasis of blood flow in the axillary-subclavian vein, including an anomalous subclavius or anterior scalene muscle, congenital fibromuscular bands, callus from a fractured clavicle or first rib, or narrowing of the costoclavicular space from depression of the shoulder girdle while lifting or working overhead.

The frequent association of thrombosis of the axillary-subclavian vein with exertion has led to the phrase "effort vein thrombosis" (Pagen-Von Schroetter syndrome).[53] This syndrome typically develops as an abrupt swelling of the upper extremity. Even with early medical treatment complete resolution occurs in only 15 to 30 per cent of patients, and most patients have residual symptoms or impaired use of the arm. Pulmonary embolism is not as rare as it was originally thought to be. Adams and DeWeese found that it occurred in 12 per cent of their patients.[1] Symptomatic thrombosis of the subclavian vein, although not common, has also been noted with the use of permanent transvenous pacing electrodes and with the use of the Swan-Ganz catheter in the coronary care setting.[60]

Superior Vena Caval Obstruction

Invasive malignant tumors, usually anaplastic lung cancers, are the most common cause of the distinctive "superior vena caval syndrome." Occasionally, primary thrombosis, a chronic fibrosing mediastinitis, or a granulomatous lesion may be responsible. Depending on the rapidity of the development of vena caval obstruction, there are varying degrees of edema of the neck, head, and arms, with evidence of venous stasis. Acute obstruction of the superior vena cava, as during a thoracic operation, can produce fatal cerebral edema within a few minutes. When obstruction develops slowly, collateral circulation develops and the symptoms are mild (Fig. 15).

Malignant involvement of the superior vena cava precludes curative surgical resection; however, significant palliation can be obtained with intensive radiation therapy. Symptoms in benign obstructions usually improve or subside completely as collateral circulation develops. Attempts to reconstruct the occluded superior vena cava have frequently been unsuccessful. The most favorable graft is a spiral or panel composite autogenous vein, which creates a graft of a sufficiently large diameter.

Inferior Vena Caval Obstruction

Anatomically, the inferior vena cava may be divided into three parts. The lower third extends from the confluence of the iliac veins that form the cava to the renal veins. The middle third extends from the renal veins to the hepatic veins, and the upper third extends from the hepatic veins to the right atrium. Obstruction of the inferior vena cava most commonly occurs by extension of pelvic and thigh vein thrombosis. Rapid blood flow from the renal veins usually halts the thrombus at this level. However, if the renal veins are involved, the nephrotic syndrome may result. If renal vein obstruction is bilateral and acute, renal failure may ensue. If it is unilateral or slowly progressive, pain, hematuria, and proteinuria may result. If adequate collateral circulation develops, these findings may be reversible (see Fig. 15). If the upper third of the inferior vena cava is involved and the hepatic veins are occluded, portal hypertension and the Budd-Chiari syndrome cause ascites, hepatomegaly, and hepatic decompensation.

Renal carcinoma is the second most common cause of caval obstruction, which usually occurs by invasion rather than from external compression. Other causes include hepatomegaly secondary to a variety of hepatic diseases, ascites, primary leiomyosarcoma, retroperitoneal fibrosis, congenital membranes, hypercoagulable states, and expanding or leaking abdominal aortic aneurysms. In children, the causes of inferior vena caval obstruction are specific for this age group and include right-sided Wilms' tumor, adrenal carcinoma, neuroblastoma, hepatoma, and multicystic kidney. The site and extent of obstruction is determined by venography.

The treatment for inferior vena caval obstruction varies according to the underlying cause, location, and extent of the process. Thrombectomy and fibrinolytic therapy have occasionally been used for a benign process. Radiation therapy and/or chemotherapy are indicated when a malignant disease is involved. When the Budd-Chiari syndrome of the membranous type occurs, dilatation of the hepatic vein membrane via the femoral vein or the transcardiac route may be effective. When more diffuse hepatic vein involvement occurs, a mesocaval shunt can decompress the portal system; when obstruction of the vena cava occurs, the liver may be replaced with a transplanted liver.

SUMMARY

Prevention of initial venous thrombosis by preventive measures more easily avoids the sequelae of deep venous thrombosis and prevents possibly fatal pulmonary embolism. However, venous diseases that do occur continue to incapacitate patients and cause death. The venous problems that arise are primarily managed nonoperatively. Nevertheless, there is now a definite role for surgical management of many of these disorders, and the indications for operative intervention have become clearer.

SELECTED REFERENCES

Christopoulos, D., Nicolaides, A. N., Cook, A., et al.: Pathogenesis of venous ulceration in relation to the calf muscle pump function. Surgery, 106:829, 1989.

An increase in the incidence of venous stasis ulceration occurs with increasing reflux and decreasing calf muscle pump ejection fraction as measured by air plethysmography. The residual volume fraction, which expresses the combined effect of venous reflux and ejection fraction with rhythmic exercise, demonstrated a good correlation with the incidence of ulceration and the measurements of ambulatory venous pressure.

Schanzer, H., and Pierce, E. C., II: A rational approach to surgery of the chronic venous stasis syndrome. Ann. Surg., 195:25, 1982.

Because different mechanisms are responsible for the production of the chronic venous stasis syndrome, no single method of treatment is satisfactory for the entire population. Ambulatory venous pressure and ascending and retrograde phlebography were measured in 49 patients with chronic venous stasis for determination of the specific venous abnormality. Significant improvement in the ambulatory venous pressure was obtained postoperatively when one of the following surgical procedures was correctly chosen: ligation of perforators, superficial femoral valvuloplasty, segmental venous transposition, ligation of the superficial femoral vein, cross-femoral venous bypass, or high ligation and stripping of the long saphenous vein.

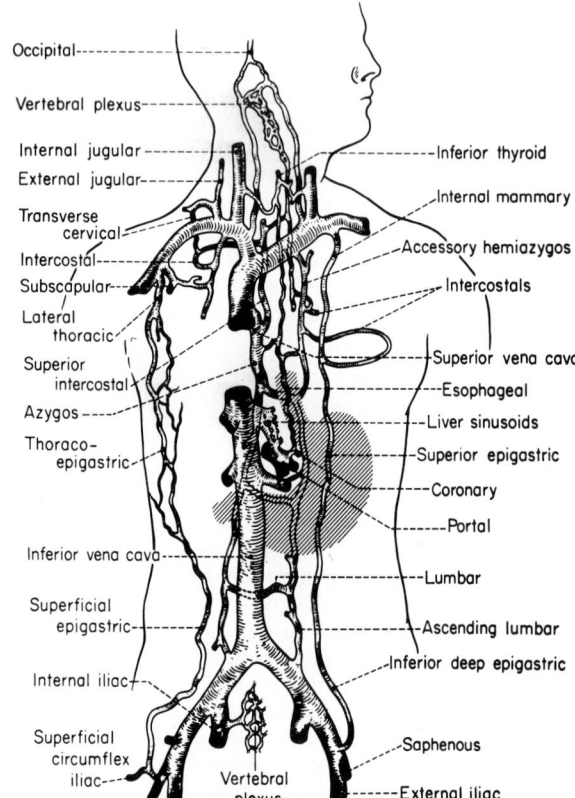

Figure 15. Diagrammatic representation of the main collateral channels by which blood may return to the heart in the event of either superior or inferior vena caval obstruction. (From Juergens, J. L., Jr., Spitzel, J. A., Jr., and Fairbairn, J. F., II: Peripheral Vascular Disease. Philadelphia, W. B. Saunders Company, 1980.)

Labels in figure:
Occipital — Vertebral plexus — Internal jugular — External jugular — Transverse cervical — Intercostal — Subscapular — Lateral thoracic — Superior intercostal — Azygos — Thoraco-epigastric — Inferior vena cava — Superficial epigastric — Internal iliac — Superficial circumflex iliac — Vertebral plexus

Inferior thyroid — Internal mammary — Accessory hemiazygos — Intercostals — Superior vena cava — Esophageal — Liver sinusoids — Superior epigastric — Coronary — Portal — Lumbar — Ascending lumbar — Inferior deep epigastric — Saphenous — External iliac

REFERENCES

1. Adams, J. T., and DeWeese, J. A.: "Effort" thrombosis of the axillary and subclavian veins. J. Trauma, 11:923, 1971.
2. Adar, R., and Salzman, E. W.: Treatment of thrombosis of veins of the lower extremities. N. Engl. J. Med., 292:348, 1985.
3. Barnes, R. W., Collicott, P. E., Mozersky, D. J., Sumner, D. S., and Strandness, D. E., Jr.: Noninvasive quantitation of venous hemodynamics in postphlebitic syndrome. Arch. Surg., 107:807, 1973.
4. Barnes, R. W., and Miller, E. V.: Late venous hemodynamics following thrombectomy for iliofemoral venous thrombosis. Vasc. Surg., 12:228, 1978.
5. Bauer, G.: A roentgenological and clinical study of the sequels of thrombosis. Acta Clin. Scand., 74:1, 1942.
6. Bentley, G. P., Hill, P. L., deHass, H. A., Mistry, F., and Kakkar, V. V.: Radionuclide venography in the management of proximal venous occlusion: A comparison with contrast venography. Br. J. Radiol., 52:289, 1979.
7. Bettmann, M. A.: Noninvasive and venographic diagnosis of deep vein thrombosis. Cardiovasc. Intervent. Radiol., 11:S15, 1988.
8. Browse, N. L., and Burnand, K. G.: Hypothesis: The course of venous ulceration. Lancet, 2:243, 1982.
9. Burnand, K., Clemenson, G., Morland, M., Jarrett, P. E. M., and Browse, N. L.: Venous lipodermatosclerosis: Treatment by fibrinolytic enhancement and elastic compression. Br. Med. J., 280:7, 1980.
10. Burnand, K. G., O'Donnell, T. F., Thomas, M. L., and Browse, N. L.: Relation between postphlebitic changes in the deep veins and results of surgical treatment of venous ulcers. Lancet, 1:936, 1976.
11. Christopoulos, D., Nicolaides, A. N., Cook, A., Irvine, A., et al.: Pathogenesis of venous ulceration in relation to the calf muscle pump function. Surgery, 106:829, 1989.
12. Cockett, F. B., and Jones, D. E. E.: The ankle blow-out syndrome. Lancet, 1:17, 1953.
13. Cockett, F. B.: Ulcers of the leg. Adv. Surg. 12:327, 1978.
14. Dale, W. A., and Harris, J.: Cross-over vein grafts for iliac and femoral venous occlusion. Ann. Surg., 168:319, 1988.
15. Eriksson, I.: Reconstructive venous surgery. Acta Clin. Scand. Suppl., 544:69, 1988.
16. Flanigan, D. P., Goodreau, J. J., Burnham, S. J., Bergan, J. J., and Yao, J. S. T.: Vascular laboratory diagnosis of clinically suspected acute deep vein thrombosis. Lancet, 2:331, 1978.
17. Foster, J., Cikrit, D., Walker, N., and Silver, D.: The heparin-induced thrombocytopenic syndrome.: An update. Surgery, 102:763, 1987.
18. Halliday, P.: The place of subfascial ligation of perforating veins in the treatment of the postphlebitic syndrome. Br. J. Surg., 58:104, 1971.
19. Hoare, M. C., Nicolaides, A. N., Miles, C. R., Skull, K., Jury, R. P., Needham, T., and Dudley, H. A. F.: The role of primary varicose veins in venous ulceration. Surgery, 92:450, 1982.
20. Hobbs, J. T.: Management of varicose veins. Surg. Annu., 12:184, 1980.
21. Hull, R., Taylor, D. W., Hirsh, J., Sackett, D. L., Power, P., Turpie, A. G. G., and Walker, I.: Impedance plethysmography: The relationship between venous filling and sensitivity and specificity for proximal vein thrombosis. Circulation, 58:898, 1978.
22. Hume, M., Sevitt, S., and Thomas, D. P.: Venous Thrombosis and Pulmonary Embolism. Cambridge, Mass., Harvard University Press, 1970.
23. Hyde, G. L., Litton, T. C., and Hull, D. A.: Long-term results of subfascial vein ligation for venous stasis disease. Surg. Gynecol. Obstet., 153:683, 1981.
24. Johnson, N. D., Queral, L. A., Flinn, W. R., Yao, J. S., and Bergan, J. J.: Late objective assessment of venous valve surgery. Arch. Surg., 116:1461, 1981.
25. Johnson, W. C., O'Hara, E. T., and Corey, C.: Venous stasis ulceration: Effectiveness of subfascial ligation. Arch. Surg., 120:797, 1985.
26. Kapsch, D. N., Adelstein, E. H., Rhodes, G. R., and Silver, D.: Heparin-induced thrombocytopenia, thrombosis, and hemorrhage. Surgery, 86:148, 1979.
27. Killewich, L. A., Martin, R., Cramer, M., Beach, W., and Strandness, D. E., Jr.: Pathophysiology of venous claudication. J. Vasc. Surg., 1:507, 1984.
28. Kistner, R. L.: Primary venous valve incompetence of the leg. Am. J. Surg., 140:218, 1980.
29. Kistner, R. L.: Surgical repair of the incompetent femoral vein valve. Arch. Surg., 110:1336, 1975.
30. Kakkar, V. V., and Lawrence, D.: Hemodynamic and clinical assessment of therapy for acute deep vein thrombosis. Suppl., Symposium on Deep Venous Thrombosis. Am. J. Surg., 150:54, 1985.
31. Large, J.: Surgical treatment of saphenous varices with preservation of the main great saphenous trunk. J. Vasc. Surg., 2:886, 1985.
32. Laster, J., Cikrit, D., Walker, N., and Silver, D.: The heparin-induced thrombocytopenic syndrome: An update. Surgery, 102:763, 1987.
33. Lewis, C. E., Jr., Mueller, C., and Edwards, W. S.: Venous stasis on the operating table. Am. J. Surg., 124:780, 1972.
34. Linton, R. R.: Postphlebitic ulceration of the lower extremity: Its etiology and surgical treatment. Ann. Surg., 138:415, 1953.
35. Marciniak, E., Garley, C. H., and DeSimone, P. A.: Familial thrombosis due to antithrombin III deficiency. Blood, 43:219, 1974.
36. Mason, R., and Giron, F.: Noninvasive evaluation of venous function in chronic venous disease. Surgery, 91:312, 1982.
37. McEnroe, C. S., O'Donnell, T. F., and Mackey, W. C.: Correlation of clinical findings with venous hemodynamics in 386 patients with chronic venous insufficiency. Am. J. Surg., 156:148, 1988.
38. McLachlin, A. D., McLachlin, J. A., Jory, T. A., and Rawling, E. G.: Venous stasis in the lower extremities. Ann. Surg., 152:678, 1980.
39. Moser, K. M., Brach, B. B., and Dolan, G. F.: Clinically suspected deep venous thrombosis of the lower extremities. A comparison of venography, impedance plethysmography, and radiolabeled fibrinogen. J.A.M.A., 237:2195, 1977.
40. Nicolaides, A., Hoare, M., Miles, C., Schull, K., and Fernandes e Fernandes, J.: The value of ambulatory venous pressure in the assessment of venous insufficiency. Vasc. Diag. Ther., 3:41, 1982.
41. Nicolaides, A. N., and Zukowski, A. J.: The value of dynamic venous pressure measurements. World J. Surg., 10:919, 1986.
42. O'Donnell, T. F., Jr., Burnand, K. G., Clemenson, G., Thomas, M. L., and Browse, N. J.: Doppler examination vs. clinical and phlebographic detection of the location of incompetent perforating veins. Arch. Surg., 112:31, 1977.
43. O'Donnell, T. F., Abbott, W. M., Athanasoulis, C. A., Millan, V. G., and Callow, A. D.: Diagnosis of deep venous thrombosis in the outpatient by venography. Surg. Gynecol. Obstet., 150:69, 1980.
44. O'Donnell, T. F., Mackey, W. C., Shepard, A. D., and Callow, A. D.: Clinical hemodynamic and anatomic follow-up of direct venous reconstruction. Arch. Surg., 122:474, 1987.
45. Palma, E. C., and Esperon, R.: Vein transplants and grafts in the surgical treatment of the post-phlebitic syndrome. J. Cardiovasc. Surg., 1:94, 1960.
46. Psathakis, N. D., and Psathakis, D. N.: Surgical treatment of deep venous insufficiency of the lower limb. Surg. Gynecol. Obstet., 166:131, 1988.
47. Randhawa, G. K., Dhillon, J. S., Kistner, R. L., and Ferris, E. B.: Assessment of chronic venous insufficiency using dynamic venous pressure studies. Am. J. Surg., 148:203, 1984.
48. Roberts, V. S., Sabri, S., Beeley, A. H., and Cotton, L. T.: The effect of intermittently applied external pressure on the haemodynamics of the lower limb in man. Br. J. Surg., 59:223, 1972.
49. Schanzer, H., and Pierce, E. C., II: Pathophysiology evaluation of chronic venous stasis with ambulatory venous pressure studies. Angiology, 33:183, 1982.
50. Schmidt, C., Schmitt, J., and Scheffmann, J.: Haemodynamics of the postphlebitic syndrome. Int. Angiol., 6:187, 1987.
51. Schull, K. C., Nicolaides, A. N., Fernandes e Fernandes, J., Miles, C., Horner, J., Needham, T., Cooke, E. D., and Eastcott, H. H. G.: Significance of popliteal reflux in relation to ambulatory venous pressure and ulceration. Arch. Surg., 114:1304, 1979.
52. Simmons, A. V., Sheppard, M. A., and Cox, A. F.: Deep venous thrombosis after myocardial infarction: Predisposing factors. Br. Heart J., 35:623, 1973.
53. Sottiurai, V. A., Towner, K., McDonnel, A. E., and Zarins, C. K.: Diagnosis of upper extremity deep venous thrombosis using noninvasive technique. Surgery, 91:582, 1982.
54. Steele, P. P., Weily, H. S., and Genton, E.: Platelet survival and adhesiveness in recurrent venous thrombosis. N. Engl. J. Med., 288:1148, 1973.
55. Sumner, D. S.: Venous dynamics-varicosities. Clin. Obstet. Gynecol., 24:743, 1981.
56. Taheri, S. A., Lazar, L., and Elias, S.: Status of vein valve transplant after 12 months. Arch. Surg., 117:1313, 1982.
57. Taheri, S. A., Pendergast, D. R., Lazar, E., Meenaghan, M. A., et al.: Vein valve transplantation. Am. J. Surg., 150:201, 1985.
58. Takeri, S. A., Sheehan, F., and Elias, S.: Descending venography. Angiology 34:299, 1983.
59. Thomas, D. P.: Overview of venous thrombogenesis. Sem. Throm. Hemo. 14:1, 1988.
60. Tilney, N. L., Griffiths, H. J. G., and Edwards, E. A.: Natural history of major venous thrombosis of the upper extremity. Arch. Surg., 101:792, 1970.
61. Whitehead, S., Lemenson, G., and Browse, N. L.: The assessment of calf pump function by isotope plethysmography. Br. J. Surg., 70:675, 1983.
62. Young, A. E., Henderson, B. A., and Philips, D. A.: Impedance plethysmography: Its limitations as a substitute for phlebography. Cardiovasc. Radiol., 1:233, 1978.

50

PULMONARY EMBOLISM

David C. Sabiston, Jr., M.D.

Pulmonary embolism is a common complication; and despite an improved understanding of its pathogenesis, diagnosis, and management, it remains a frequent and often fatal disorder. Although it is a well recognized postoperative surgical problem, most patients with this disorder are not surgical patients and experience development of pulmonary embolism secondary to a serious medical disorder such as congestive heart failure, cerebrovascular accidents, chronic pulmonary disease, systemic infections, or carcinomatosis, among many others. For this reason, it occurs more often on the medical, rather than on the surgical, service. Nevertheless, is continues as a very significant postoperative complication; surgeons should be constantly aware that it may be a lurking problem in all patients, especially in older patients. The annual incidence of pulmonary embolism in the United States is estimated to be in excess of 600,000, with some 200,000 deaths (Fig. 1).[11] It is interesting that in routine autopsies in patients over the age of 40, two thirds have either gross or microscopic evidence of pulmonary emboli. Although in many patients pulmonary embolism is found *incidentally* at death, in many it either *contributes* to, or is actually the principal *cause* of, death.

HISTORICAL ASPECTS

Laennec described pulmonary embolism as "pulmonary apoplexy" in a treatise on the diagnosis of diseases of the lung and heart.[22] He differentiated the lesion caused by pulmonary embolism from other pulmonary disorders causing hemoptysis. Cruveilhier said "all arterial branches which led to those lesions were filled with clots that branched according to the vascular tree."[10] Despite these descriptions, neither of these investigators sought the *origin* of the thrombi and viewed them as arising as a *primary process* in the pulmonary arteries. Rokitansky confirmed Laennec's findings in 1842 and introduced the term *hemorrhagic infarct*.

The famed pathologist Rudolph Virchow introduced the *embolic* concept of this disorder. He stated:

In the peripheral veins the danger proceeds chiefly from the small branches. By no means rarely do these become quite filled with masses of coagulum. As long, however, as the thrombus is confined to the branch itself, so long as the body is not exposed . . . only the greater number of the thrombi in the small branches do not content themselves with advancing up to the level of the main trunk, but pretty constantly new masses of coagulum deposit themselves from the blood upon the end of the thrombus layer after layer; the thrombus is prolonged beyond the mouth of the branch into the trunk in the direction of the current of blood, shoots out in the form of a thick cylinder farther and farther, and becomes continually larger and larger. From a lumbar vein, for example, a plug may extend into the vena cava as thick as the last phalanx of the thumb. These are the thrombi that constitute the source of real danger; it is in them that ensues the crumbling away which leads to secondary occlusion in remote vessels.[37]

Virchow also observed two types of thrombus in the pulmonary arteries in such patients: first, the embolus that arises as a thrombus in a systemic vein and, after being dislodged from its site of origin, is swept into the venous circulation, through the heart, and into the pulmonary arteries. Second is the thrombus that occurs *in situ* into the pulmonary artery distal to the occluding embolus as a result of stagnant blood flow in that vessel. Responding to critics of his newly announced pathogenesis of pulmonary embolism and wishing to prove the embolic doctrine, Virchow inserted pieces of rubber and venous thrombi recovered from humans at autopsy into the jugular veins of dogs. When the animals were sacrificed, the emboli were found in the pulmonary arteries. An essential part of Virchow's studies concerned the identification of the assumed embolic particle with the apparent structure from which it had been detached. Embolism alone did not explain the development of a hemorrhagic infarct; and because he frequently found occluding emboli in pulmonary branches without an infarct, he considered the problem of infarction of pulmonary tissue difficult to explain. In 1872 Cohnheim provided additional basic data, particularly the importance of pulmonary congestion and left ventricular failure in the development of *hemorrhagic* infarction. He also recognized that not all patients with pulmonary embolism have concomitant pulmonary infarction and that concomitant congestive heart failure is an important aspect of infarction.

The concept of *acute cor pulmonale* led to an understanding of pulmonary embolism through its physiologic features. It was apparent that pulmonary embolism was not exclusively a postoperative surgical complication, but occurred even more frequently in cardiac and other debilitated patients as a sequel of many chronic illnesses. The diagnosis of embolism is often missed by the clinician and also, to a lesser degree, by the pathologist. An important clinical and pathologic feature is the observation that many patients with pulmonary embolism do *not* have evidence of infarction. It is currently thought that only 10 per cent or fewer of emboli are associated with true *infarction*. This fact makes it even more important that a firm clinical diagnosis be made before the onset of treatment and demonstrates the need for accurate diagnostic assessment, including pulmonary arteriography and scanning. Although knowledge of the pathogenesis of thrombosis was evolving, scant attention was given the basic features of venous thrombosis. Virchow concluded that primary thrombosis of the systemic veins was caused by three factors (Virchow's triad): (1) stasis of blood flow, (2) injury to the vein, and (3) a state of hypercoagulability, factors still regarded as being very important in the pathogenesis of venous thrombosis. Once the concepts of the pathophysiology of venous thrombosis and pulmonary embolism were recognized, accurate diagnosis became paramount for therapy; pulmonary scanning, pulmonary arteriography, and magnetic resonance imaging are now recognized as the primary diagnostic techniques.

In 1908 Trendelenburg first performed pulmonary embolectomy, describing emergency thoracotomy and removal of the emboli in three patients. The longest survivor lived for 37 hours and ultimately died of hemorrhage from an internal mammary artery. Kirschner did the first successful pulmonary embolectomy in 1924 with a long-term survivor, and the first successful

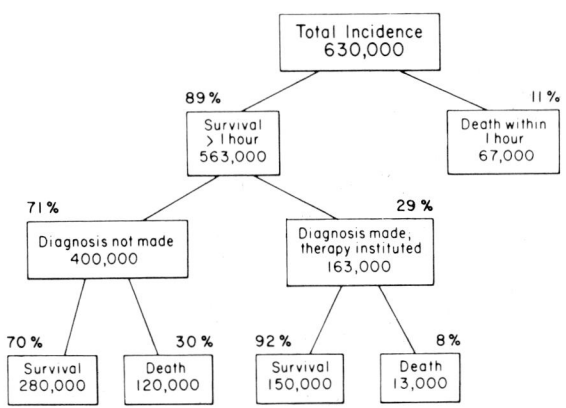

Figure 1. Annual incidence of pulmonary embolism in the United States showing the subsequent course of this complication with deaths and survivors. (From Dalen, J. E., and Alpert, J. S.: Natural history of pulmonary embolism. Prog. Cardiovasc. Dis., 57:259, 1975.)

pulmonary embolectomy using cardiopulmonary bypass was performed by Sharp in 1962.[34] As a medical student, McLean discovered heparin in 1916[27]; and its value in the management of thromboembolism was confirmed by Murray et al.[29] in 1937 and later extended.[9]

PATHOGENESIS OF VENOUS THROMBOSIS

Venous stasis is the most important feature predisposing to venous thrombosis. Radiopaque contrast medium injected into the deep veins of the leg may take surprisingly long to clear when the postoperative patient remains flat in bed with little movement due to pain. Moreover, Allison[2] showed that in *postoperative* patients, who are apt to remain still, radiopaque dye may linger in the calf veins for as long as 25 minutes after injection. Similarly, patients ill for any reason are less likely to move the extremities, predisposing to intravenous thrombosis. The venous sinuses of the veins are especially vulnerable to stasis and thrombosis. Platelets become adherent at these sites; and a thrombus develops and enlarges by successive deposition of aggregated platelets, leukocytes, and fibrin (Fig. 2). Propagation of the thrombus may then follow upstream, or the process may spread retrograde (Fig. 3).

Trauma or injury following a surgical procedure is known to

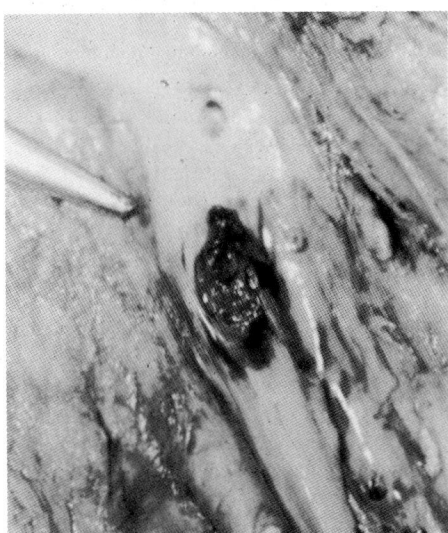

Figure 2. A primary thrombus forming in the valve pocket at the mouth of the deep femoral vein. (From Hume, M., Sevitt, S., and Thomas, D. P.: Venous Thrombosis and Pulmonary Embolism. Cambridge, Mass., Harvard University Press, 1970.)

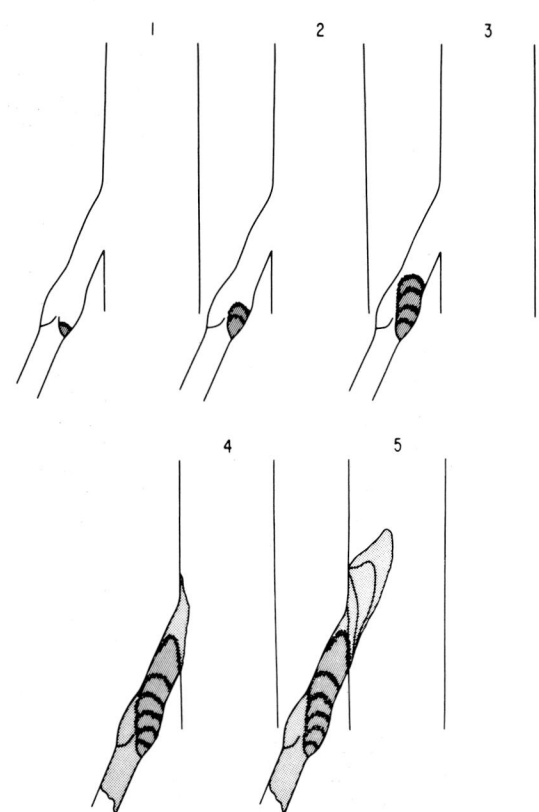

Figure 3. Illustration showing propagation of deep thrombus arising in a valvular pocket with deposition of successive layers and ultimate extension of the nonadherent red thrombus into the lumen of a larger parent vein. (From Cox, J. L., and Sabiston, D. C., Jr.: Phlebitis, thrombosis, and pulmonary embolism. In Condon, R. E., and DeCosse, J. J. (Eds.): Surgical Care: A Physiologic Approach to Clinical Management. Philadelphia, Lea & Febiger, 1980.)

be associated with an increased incidence of venous thrombosis. Hypercoagulability has been defined as "the existence of an excessive amount of activity of one or more procoagulant substances or a decrease in anticoagulant factors."[8] Thus during pregnancy, when thrombosis is more prevalent, the concentrations of fibrinogen, prothrombin, factor VII, Stuart factor, Christmas factor, and antihemophilic factor are elevated,[1] and the risk of venous thrombosis is increased.

PATHOLOGIC ASPECTS

Pulmonary emboli are frequently present in the lungs at routine autopsy. This is emphasized by evidence that old or fresh pulmonary emboli are found in 64 per cent of those over the age of 40. Moreover, the clinical diagnosis is frequently not established, and embolism is often first recognized at autopsy. The *physiologic* changes after embolism are primarily the result of the mechanical factor of arterial occlusion. This is demonstrated in the classic pathologic studies of Gorham[15,16] of 100 consecutive patients with fatal pulmonary emboli, 85 of whom had emboli in *both* pulmonary arteries (Fig. 4). Among the 100 patients, only 15 had emboli restricted *solely* to one lung; 12 of these were more than 54 years of age, an age group with an appreciable incidence of underlying cardiac and respiratory disease. Moreover, in patients with massive pulmonary embolism in whom embolectomy is done, it is usual to find emboli in more than one pulmonary artery.[32] Other observations have shown that a marked reduction in pulmonary blood flow with other causes, including arterial ligature, intravascular balloons, and pulmonary resection, is surprisingly well tolerated.[5] After injection of experimental pulmonary emboli, reduced function of the embolized lung comes immediately, but pulmonary function

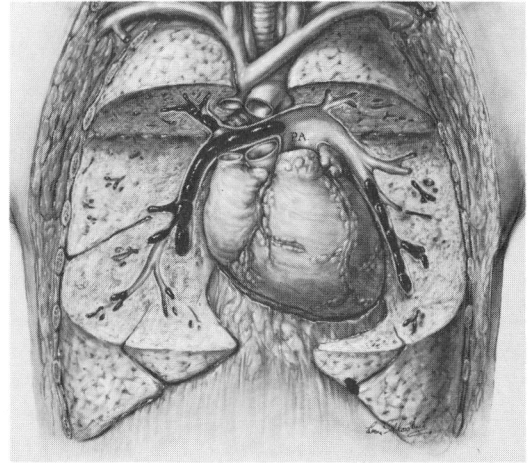

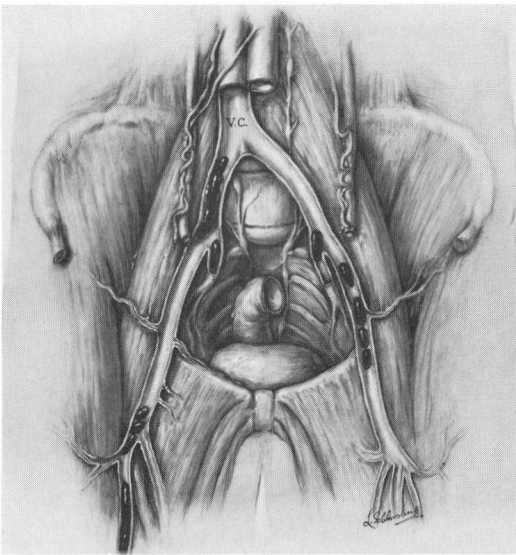

Figure 4. Illustration of the findings in a patient with massive pulmonary embolism at the time of postmortem examination. Multiple thrombi are present in the iliofemoral system. The right pulmonary artery and its branches are totally occluded by emboli. The left lower lobar pulmonary artery is also occluded. Under these circumstances, the entire output of the right ventricle must pass through the left upper lobe, which greatly increases pulmonary resistance and right ventricular work. The sudden development of this degree of pulmonary arterial occlusion produces a clinical state of severe shock, since the left ventricle receives a much diminished amount of blood to supply the systemic arterial circulation. In otherwise normal patients, 50 per cent or more of the pulmonary arterial circulation must be occluded before serious cardiovascular manifestations are produced. (From Sabiston, D. C., Jr.: Pathophysiology, diagnosis and management of pulmonary embolism. Adv. Surg., 3:351, 1968.)

returns almost to normal within several weeks.[32] Marked histologic changes occur in these thrombi, with intravascular resolution and the ultimate disappearance of most of them. This resolution can be confirmed by serial pulmonary radioactive scans, arteriograms, and pulmonary function studies as well as gross and microscopic evaluation.

Whether anticoagulants or fibrinolysins are used, the resolution of large pulmonary emboli is the usual course of events (Fig. 5). Such observations have shown convincingly that the natural history of pulmonary embolism in most patients is *spontaneous resolution*.[32] This concept has become increasingly significant in a more complete understanding of the principles of diagnosis and management.

Although pulmonary embolism usually occurs in adults, it has also been reported in children. In one study of children at autopsy, the incidence was approximately 1 per cent and was usually a secondary manifestation of a serious illness such as respiratory infection, phlebitis, systemic infection, or heart dis-

ease.[19] Although rarely diagnosed before death in childhood, the clinical manifestations are similar to those in adults. Emboli found at postmortem examination as a cause of death are generally 1 to 1.5 cm. or more in diameter, providing evidence of having arisen in sizable veins. Their length ranges up to 50 cm. or more, and they often fragment into smaller pieces. The *right* pulmonary artery is more commonly involved than the left, and the *lower* lobes more often than the upper lobes. Emboli originate primarily in the systemic venous circulation, and the prevailing evidence indicates that most of these thrombi arise in the iliac and femoral veins.

When an embolus passes through an intracardiac defect such as a patent foramen ovale, atrial septal defect, or ventricular septal defect with embolization of a systemic organ, it is termed a *paradoxical embolus.* This is likely to occur with right atrial and right ventricular hypertension, and many paradoxical emboli can be diagnosed during life.

The iliofemoral and pelvic veins are commonly the sites of major thrombi, but other sources include the inferior vena cava, the subclavian, axillary, and internal jugular veins, and the cavernous sinuses of the brain (Table 1). As many as 20 per cent of pulmonary emboli arise from sources other than veins drained by the inferior vena cava. Emboli due to *neoplasms* should also be considered in the differential diagnosis. Renal cell carcinoma is known for its ability to metastasize early, and involvement of the renal vein and inferior vena cava by renal cell carcinoma by direct extension causing pulmonary embolism occurs in 10 to 54 per cent of patients with this disorder.[3] Primary pulmonary neoplasms can mimic pulmonary embolism. *Cardiac tumors* arising in the right atrium and right ventricle may be the site of extensive pulmonary emboli, as can *missiles* such as bullets embolizing the pulmonary arteries. The clinical manifestations of missiles lodging in the pulmonary arteries are usually related to complications including erosion of the vessel, infarction of the distal lung, sepsis, and pulmonary vascular thrombosis. Among 18 cases, there were 7 deaths (37 per cent), all occurring in patients who did not undergo removal of the missiles. Therefore, removal of a missile embolus is recommended.

Asymptomatic pulmonary embolism in postoperative patients is frequent. Ventilation and perfusion scans and arteriograms often show patterns strongly suggesting pulmonary embolism. It is now thought that asymptomatic pulmonary embolism is a common postoperative event.

PREDISPOSING FACTORS

The patient's *age* is an important factor, because pulmonary embolism primarily affects the middle-aged and elderly (Fig. 6). Inactivity, bed rest, and reduced exercise are well-established causes of pulmonary embolism and cause a twofold or greater incidence. Cardiac disorders, especially congestive heart failure or atrial fibrillation, are particularly conducive to the development of pulmonary embolism. Acute myocardial infarction may be complicated by an increase in deep venous thrombosis, and the same occurs after cerebrovascular accidents. *Cancer*, particularly carcinoma of the pancreas and prostate and carcinomatosis, is associated with a higher incidence of pulmonary embolism.

Radioactive scanning of the lower extremities often demonstrates deep venous thrombosis in 54 per cent of patients with hip fractures after operation, 50 per cent following prostatectomy, and 28 per cent of general surgical patients over the age of 40. Pregnancy increases the risk of pulmonary embolism, because pressure from the gravid uterus may retard venous flow from the legs and pelvis. Postpartum infection may also give rise to septic thrombophlebitis and embolism, and oral contraceptives have a positive association with the occurrence of pulmonary embolism.

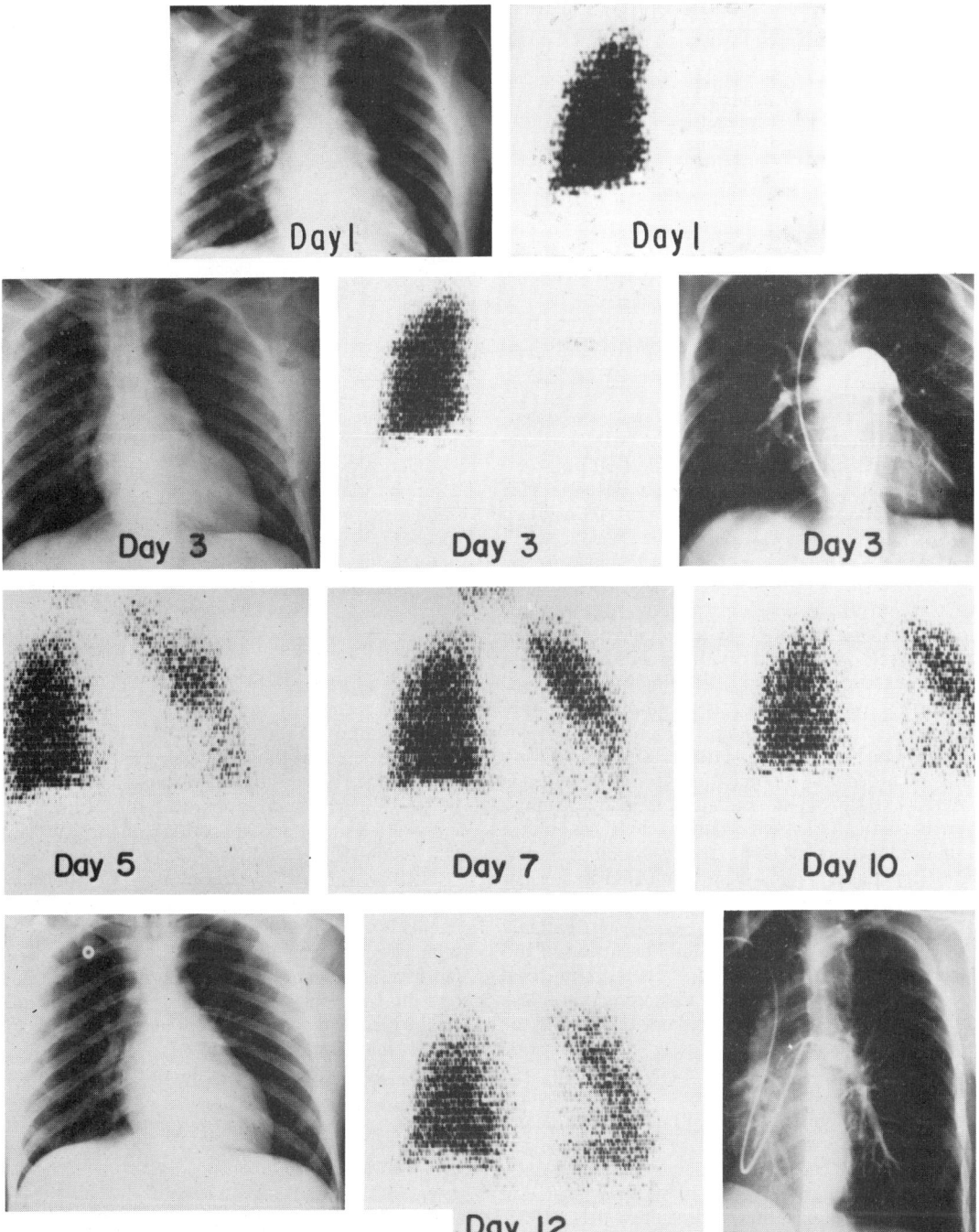

Figure 5. Serial chest films and scans following a massive pulmonary embolus to the left pulmonary artery in a 25-year-old woman after a pelvic operation. On the fifth postoperative day, discomfort was noted in the left chest, with dyspnea. A plain chest film taken on this day (day 1) showed diminished vascular markings (Westermark's sign). A radioactive pulmonary scan showed no evidence of pulmonary flow to the entire left lobe. Beginning on the third day after the embolus, the scan and arteriogram both show evidence of flow to the left lung. In subsequent scans and pulmonary arteriograms, resolution of the thrombus occurred, with progressively increasing amounts of flow by the twelfth day.

PHYSIOLOGIC RESPONSES

A primary feature of pulmonary blood flow is the *low* vascular resistance that enables flow in the vascular bed to be increased severalfold with minimal elevation of pulmonary arterial pressure. The occasional finding of a small pulmonary embolus in a patient after sudden death has been cited as evidence that occlusion of a relatively small pulmonary artery can produce death, presumably as a result of reflex mechanisms. Currently, such an explanation is rarely tenable.

The physiologic changes following pulmonary embolism are related to the *size* of the emboli and can be divided into those that produce *microembolism* (obstruction of terminal small arteries and arterioles) and those that produce *macroembolism* (occlusion of the large pulmonary vessels). Considerable reduction in the diameter of the main pulmonary artery or the primary branches (at least 50 per cent) is required to reduce pulmonary blood flow significantly or to produce pulmonary hypertension. Experimental thrombi of larger diameter produced in the inferior vena cava and embolized to either the right or the left pulmonary artery 10 to 14 days later produce minimal cardiovascular and respiratory responses. Specifically, occlusion of

TABLE 1. Site of Origin of Venous Thrombi*

References	Cases with Thrombosis at Necropsy	Per Cent of Cases with Thrombi in				
		Iliac Veins	Femoral Veins	Popliteal Veins	Soleal Veins	Any Deep Calf Vein
Rossle	94	—	49	—	—	92
Neumann	100	—	22	—	—	87
McLachlin and Paterson	34	9	82	—	—	41
Gibbs	149	—	42	—	—	65
Sevitt and Gallagher	81		70	33	67	74
Roberts	58	14	43	41	86	95

* From Hume, M., Sevitt, S., and Thomas, D. P.: Venous Thrombosis and Pulmonary Embolism. Cambridge, Mass., Harvard University Press, 1970.

one pulmonary artery causes insignificant changes in the central venous pressure, right ventricular pressure, pulmonary arterial pressure, systemic arterial pressure, cardiac output, total oxygen consumption, and the electrocardiogram despite occlusion of half of the pulmonary arterial circulation. From these studies, it is concluded that this type of embolism produces few circulatory effects that can be attributed specifically to reflex action.

If one lung is normal, or nearly normal, removal of the opposite lung is relatively well tolerated. Tidal volume and oxygen consumption at rest after resection of a lung change only to a small degree.[6] Similarly, ligation of one pulmonary artery or occlusion by an intraluminal balloon is accompanied by few cardiodynamic changes. Patients tolerate balloon obstruction of pulmonary flow to one lung for up to 2 hours[5]; and even during exercise with similar occlusion, pulmonary arterial pressure is increased only 12 to 50 per cent, whereas cardiac output may increase as much as threefold. Such occlusion closely simulates the obstruction produced by large pulmonary emboli. It should be emphasized that these studies were conducted in normal subjects, and the presence of underlying cardiac or respiratory insufficiency will alter this response appreciably. In patients with heart disease, exercise during unilateral occlusion of the right or left pulmonary artery by a balloon catheter produces a sharp elevation in pulmonary arterial pressure. Resection of less than one lung is followed by only minor changes in the pulmonary arterial pressure, whereas removal of greater amount of pulmonary tissue produces elevated pulmonary arterial pressure.

Clearly mechanical factors are the most important in determining cardiodynamic effects of pulmonary embolism; nevertheless, *reflex* effects may cause bronchoconstriction.[18] Moreover, tachypnea, pulmonary hypertension, and systemic hypotension can follow embolization with *small* particles (100 μ or less). However, it is currently thought that such is infrequent as a clinical problem, although it does occur after massive blood transfusion, during which platelet, leukocyte, and fibrin emboli may occlude the pulmonary microcirculation. Embolization with larger particles requires considerably more blockage of the pulmonary arterial system to produce significant effects. Most believe that *arterial* emboli produce pulmonary hypertension by mechanical obstruction, whereas bronchoconstriction and vasoconstriction are produced by *arteriolar* embolism and are largely mediated by reflex changes.

INCIDENCE

Of the approximately 200,000 in whom pulmonary embolism develops each year,[11] approximately 10 per cent die within the first hour and the remaining 90 per cent survive for 1 hour or longer. In most of the latter (70 per cent), the diagnosis is not made, and in this group, the mortality is 30 per cent. Among the 30 per cent who survive for more than 1 hour and in whom a diagnosis is made and appropriate therapy is started, the mortality is only 8 per cent (see Fig. 1).

The risk of death due to pulmonary embolism after surgical procedures in a collected series was 0.11 per cent. There has been a progressive increase in the incidence of death from pulmonary embolism and infarction in the United States, and similar data have been reported from England and Germany. Factors cited as being responsible for the increase in cases include (1) the increasing age of the population, (2) larger numbers and greater magnitude of operative procedures, (3) increased recognition, and (4) the use of birth control agents.

DIAGNOSIS

Clinical Manifestations

The establishment of a clinical diagnosis of pulmonary embolism may be difficult because of its similarity to a number of other cardiorespiratory disorders. Dyspnea, chest pain, hemoptysis, and hypotension are classic but are not sufficiently specific to finalize a definite diagnosis. The following should be emphasized: (1) many patients have underlying cardiac disease; (2) dyspnea and tachypnea are the most frequent clinical findings; (3) accentuation of the pulmonary second sound is common. The more classic signs of hemoptysis, pleural friction rub, gallop rhythm, cyanosis, and chest splinting are present in only a quarter or less of patients; and (4) clinical evidence of venous thrombosis is the exception and occurs in only one third of patients. The symptoms in 1000 consecutive patients at the Duke University Medical Center are shown in Table 2.[12]

Special Examinations

In acute pulmonary embolism and in the absence of other lung disease, the plain chest film is most often within normal limits. Diminished pulmonary vascular markings at the site of the embolus may be present (Westermark's sign).[38] The *ECG* is

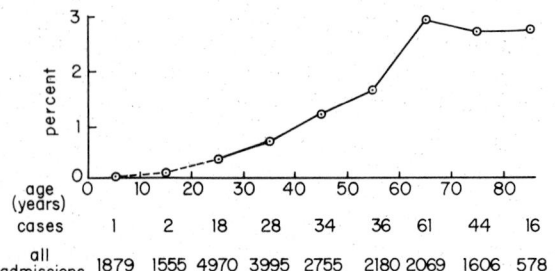

Figure 6. Graph showing the relationship of age to occurrence of thromboembolism. The ordinate represents the percentage of all hospital admissions in which a diagnosis was made clinically or at necropsy. The abscissa indicates age by decade. (From Hume, M., Sevitt, S., and Thomas, D. P.: Venous Thrombosis and Pulmonary Embolism. Cambridge, Mass., Harvard University Press, 1970.)

TABLE 2. Clinical Manifestations in 1000 Patients with Pulmonary Embolism at the Duke University Medical Center

	Per Cent
Symptoms	
Dyspnea	77
Chest pain	63
Hemoptysis	26
Altered mental status	23
Dyspnea, chest pain, hemoptysis	14
Signs	
Tachycardia	59
Recent fever	43
Rales	42
Tachypnea	38
Leg edema and tenderness	23
Elevated venous pressure	18
Shock	11
Accentuated P_2	11
Cyanosis	9
Pleural friction rub	8

not specific, but changes can be confirmatory. It is probable that not more than 10 to 20 per cent of patients subsequently proven to have pulmonary embolism show any ECG changes; and of these, a smaller number show diagnostic abnormalities.[23] ECG alterations include disturbances of rhythm (atrial fibrillation, ectopic beats, heart block), enlargement of P waves, S-T segment depression, and T-wave inversion (particularly in leads III, aVF, V_1, V_4, and V_3). The most common abnormality is S-T segment depression, a result of myocardial ischemia from reduced cardiac output and arterial pressure as well as increased right ventricular pressure. *Impedance plethysmography* is a noninvasive method for assessment of the presence of proximal venous thrombosis, but it is mainly insensitive in calf vein thrombi.

RADIOACTIVE PULMONARY SCANNING. Sabiston and Wagner[30,31] introduced radioisotope *perfusion pulmonary scanning*, and it remains the most frequently employed technique in the diagnosis of pulmonary embolism (see Fig. 5). The principal method is measurement of intravenous injected particles such as technetium 99m that become lodged in the pulmonary capillary bed.

Definitions commonly used for ventilation/perfusion scans concern the *probability* of embolism. For example, *high probability* indicates segmental or greater perfusion defects with a normal ventilation scan (V/Q mismatch); *moderate probability* indicates multiple subsegmental perfusion defects with a normal ventilation scan or segmental perfusion defects without a ventilation scan performed; *indeterminate probability* signifies chronic obstructive pulmonary disease (COPD) on a chest film or an abnormal chest film in regions of perfusion defects; *intermediate probability* means moderate or indeterminate probability scans; and *low probability* means subsegmental perfusion defects without a ventilation scan performed or matched perfusion and ventilation defects.

Venograms may be useful in establishing a definitive diagnosis of deep venous thrombosis. It is of special significance in patients in whom the diagnosis is in doubt or when a vena caval procedure is being considered. Fibrinogen scans, although sensitive in the detection of the development of the new thrombi in the extremities, are less accurate in detecting thrombi in the iliofemoral and pelvic regions owing to the background of radioactivity in the urinary bladder. *Magnetic resonance imaging* is now recognized to be a very reliable method of diagnosing venous thrombosis and is quite useful in demonstration of the pelvic veins. A schematic outline of a plan to be followed in

establishing the diagnosis of pulmonary embolism is shown in Figure 7.[14]

The most definitive method of diagnosis of pulmonary embolism is pulmonary arteriography. It is important to recognize the appearance of the normal pulmonary angiogram to permit appropriate interpretation of morphologic and physiologic changes. The arteries in the lower areas of the lung are normally larger because of a greater volume of pulmonary tissue. In most patients who survive the initial attack, the obstruction in the pulmonary arteries involves lobar or segmental branches. The defect should remain constant on several successive films in the series, and the flow may be sluggish, which is shown by a small pool of contrast medium that may persist in the artery above the obstruction after the venous phase of the angiogram. When pulmonary arteriography is done later in the course of embolism, contrast medium may pass around the obstruction, causing delayed opacification of the artery distally. The pattern in some areas may show avascular segments that represent the result of unresolved thromboembolism. Oblique views of the pulmonary arteriogram should be obtained for maximal visualization and more accurate diagnosis.

MANAGEMENT

It is important to emphasize that the single most important feature to be established prior to the onset of therapy of pulmonary embolism is an unequivocal diagnosis. The most reliable means of achieving this are pulmonary scanning and arteriography. Because scanning is a simple, safe, and reliable technique,

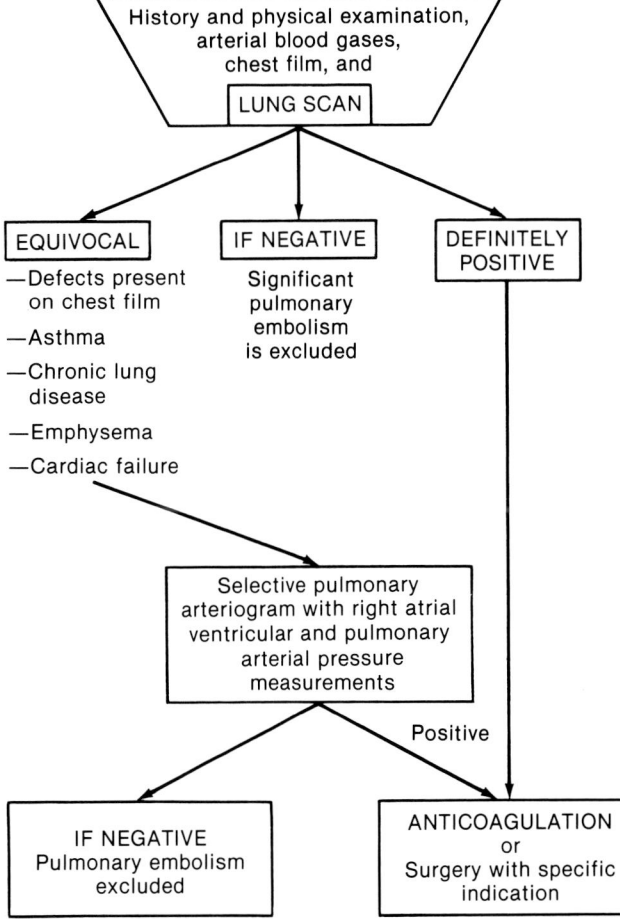

Figure 7. Schematic outline of the plan to be followed in establishing the diagnosis of pulmonary embolism. (Redrawn from Duranceau, A., Jones, R. H., and Sabiston, D. C., Jr.: The diagnosis of pulmonary embolism. Compr. Ther., 2:6, 1976.)

it is generally performed initially. It must be emphasized that if the pulmonary scan is to be used for definitive diagnosis, a concomitant plain chest film must show a normal pulmonary appearance in the area in which the scan demonstrates pulmonary arterial occlusion.

Prevention

Prophylaxis is an important aspect of postoperative cure, because the incidence of pulmonary embolism can be predicted to be appreciable. Nevertheless, no proven method or combination of methods has been found that causes complete prevention of thromboembolism. Several factors are considered of importance, including physical activity and elevation of the lower extremities for gravity drainage of venous return.[26] Some consider compression of the legs by stockings and prophylactic anticoagulation to be useful, but both remain controversial. Early ambulation and resumption of physical activity after operation or bed rest for any reason has long been recommended. In a study evaluating the role of exercise, postmortem vein dissections showed that thrombi were found in only 18 per cent of patients who had exercised before death, compared with 53 per cent in controls (nonexercised and nonambulatory).

Antiplatelet Hyperaggregability Agents

Much emphasis is given a group of nonsteroidal anti-inflammatory drugs, including aspirin and dipyridamole, which have been shown to inhibit the platelet-release reaction, secondary ADP-induced platelet aggregation, and adherence to collagen when tested *in vitro*. Among those receiving aspirin, 12.5 per cent had venous thrombosis; whereas those in the control series had a 20.4 per cent incidence, as shown by scans.[7] The use of dipyridamole in the treatment and prevention of postoperative thrombosis is less effective. The role of 1.2 gm. of aspirin daily as a preventive measure was compared with that of warfarin in a group of patients having elective hip replacement. Aspirin was as effective as warfarin in preventing clinically diagnosed venous thrombosis and pulmonary embolism. In this study, the incidence in the treated group receiving aspirin was 9 per cent, compared with 35 per cent in a previously studied control group. Studies of the overall effectiveness of antiplatelet drugs in the prevention of venous thrombosis and pulmonary embolism are continuing, because absolute certainty concerning their use has not yet been established.

In some patients prophylactic anticoagulation has proved beneficial, especially after trauma and in orthopedic disorders, including fracture of the hip. The concept of "low-dose heparin" as a prophylactic measure was introduced in 1966 but remains controversial.[33] The usual recommendation is an initial dose of 5000 units subcutaneously every 8 to 12 hours until the patient is fully ambulatory. Routine coagulation tests are prolonged minimally, if at all, with a low risk of bleeding. The protection, if any, may be in its potentiation of a naturally occurring plasma inhibitor of activated factor X.

A large number of trials with low-dose heparin given surgical patients postoperatively have been reported using ^{123}I-labeled fibrinogen scanning or venography, or both, for demonstration of development of venous thrombosis. With some exceptions, these studies have generally indicated a decrease in the occurrence of deep venous thrombosis, compared with that in controls. Although it appears that the incidence of deep vein thrombosis is reduced, it has been difficult to firmly conclude that low-dose heparin is effective in the *prevention of postoperative pulmonary embolism*. The most quoted of these studies are included in a multicenter clinical trial involving more than 4000 patients.[20] In a reassessment of this often cited multicenter study, Mitchell says that if the patient asks, "Will low-dose heparin increase my chances of surviving an operation?" we can only give the answer dreaded by pollsters: "We don't

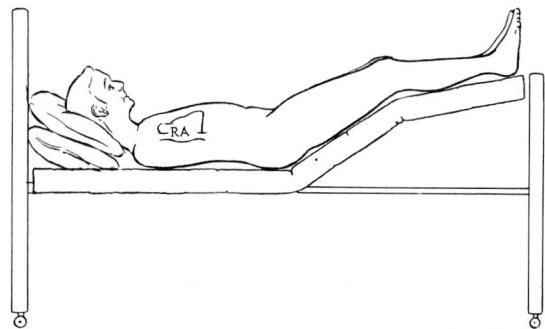

Figure 8. Correct position for lower extremities in prophylaxis of pulmonary embolism. Note the additional break at the knee. It is important that the level of the veins in the lower extremities be above the mean level of the right atrium (RA).

know."[28] In addition, another randomized study of a series of patients over 40 following intraperitoneal procedures under general anesthesia lasting more than 30 minutes indicated that calf vein thrombosis was reduced by low-dose heparin but that proximal vein thrombosis and pulmonary emboli, which were detected by chest films, pulmonary function tests, and perfusion scanning, were *not* reduced.

Although low-dose heparin is recommended by some to prevent thromboembolism, it is now much less frequently used. Moreover, there is evidence that it has limited or inadequate value after prostatectomy, after myocardial infarction, and in major orthopedic procedures, particularly repair of femoral fractures and reconstructive surgery of the hip and knee. Low-dose heparin prophylaxis is also inadequate for patients with an active thrombotic process. It should be emphasized that one serious complication of heparin is *disseminated intravascular coagulation* (DIC), in which platelets aggregate and cause arterial thrombi, which may lead to gangrene of the extremities and other serious thrombotic problems.[25]

ELEVATION OF LEGS. Elevation of the legs with flexion of the knee as depicted in Figure 8 causes rapid runoff of the blood in the veins of the leg and thigh due to gravity. This is a simple, effective, and broadly applicable prophylactic measure.

Medical Management

ANTICOAGULANTS. The management of venous thrombosis and pulmonary embolism is primarily by anticoagulant therapy. Heparin should be administered intravenously by constant infusion. Blood coagulation is affected by heparin in at least two ways: (1) by preventing the activation of factor IX (Christmas factor) by factor XI (thromboplastin antecedent) in the early coagulation sequence, and (2) by acting as a potent antithrombin in the presence of heparin cofactor. Therefore, it inhibits both the intrinsic and extrinsic coagulation mechanisms. In its antithrombin effects, heparin inhibits the conversion of fibrinogen to fibrin by thrombin and, in high doses, prevents the action of thrombin on platelets. Heparin is excreted mainly in the urine, and awareness of the patient's renal status is important. In addition, the enzyme heparinase is present in the liver, the site of some degradation.

Heparin should be administered in a concentration designed to prolong the partial thromboplastin time (PTT) to 1½ to 2½ times the upper limit of normal. Heparin prevents both extension of the thrombus in the venous system and the formation of *distal in situ* thrombi in the pulmonary arteries. It is best administered by continuous intravenous infusion. The *duration* of heparin therapy depends on the individual patient, but 5 to 10 days is generally appropriate. This approximates the time necessary for thrombi to become adherent to the venous wall. The continuous intravenous infusion provides a more stabilized level of anticoagulation and a lower incidence of hemorrhage.

Oral coumarin anticoagulation is customarily begun several days before the cessation of heparin therapy to allow time for adequate prolongation of the prothrombin time. Delayed postoperative hemorrhage may occur in patients receiving heparin therapy for pulmonary emboli, particularly those with recent prosthetic arterial grafts. There may be a continuous lysis and resorption of old thrombus and replacement with new thrombus in arterial prosthesis suture lines until it is sealed by regeneration of new intima. Thus, patients have had serious hemorrhage occurring as long as 1 month after the placement of aortic arterial grafts when maintained on heparin therapy.

The coumarin drugs have an indirect and delayed action on the blood clotting mechanism. These agents act on the liver and inhibit the production of four of the factors involved in the transformation of prothrombin to thrombin: factors XII, IX, and X and prothrombin itself. The sum of these effects produces "hypoprothrombinemia." These agents are rapidly absorbed from the gastrointestinal tract and are concentrated primarily in the liver. Although short-acting, sodium warfarin is one of the more commonly used coumarin drugs, with only a slight cumulative effect. The average loading dose on the first day is 15 to 30 mg. and on the second day, 10 to 20 mg. The maximal effect is usually reached in 1½ to 2 days, and the average daily maintenance dose is usually between 5 and 10 mg. (range, 2 to 20 mg.). The duration of coumarin therapy is controversial, but most believe it should be continued for at least 6 weeks, whereas others advocate treatment up to 6 months or longer. However, local responses and subsequent course of the patient are the primary indications for the continuance of anticoagulation. The recovery time required after maximal effect is 2 to 4 days. Administration of vitamin K counteracts the effect of the coumarin and should be used if bleeding occurs.

THROMBOLYTIC AGENTS. Much effort has been directed toward identification of appropriate thrombolytic agents in the treatment of venous thrombosis and pulmonary embolism. Plasminogen is the inactive precursor of plasmin, the active fibrinolytic enzyme. Normally plasminogen is present in the blood and tissues; and exercise, stress, and shock cause plasminogen to be activated to plasmin by a labile activator present in many tissues, especially in venous endothelium. Plasmin activity in the bloodstream is prevented by inhibitors, both an antiactivator and antiplasmins. Two thrombolytic agents, streptokinase and urokinase, have been studied extensively. Both act by transforming plasminogen to plasmin. Streptokinase is a soluble product of the metabolism of *Streptococcus pyogenes* (Lancefield group A) and is available in a highly purified form. Because patients with previous streptococcal infections may be allergic to streptokinase, it can produce toxic reactions (pyrexia, dyspnea, tachycardia, and anaphylaxis). Urokinase is a strong thrombolytic agent found in human urine. To study its effects, the National Heart, Lung, and Blood Institute conducted a national cooperative study, and the results showed that urokinase combined with heparin therapy, compared with heparin alone, significantly accelerated the *resolution* of pulmonary thromboemboli at 24 hours, as shown by pulmonary arteriograms, pulmonary scans, and right-sided heart pressure measurements. However, *no significant differences* in recurrence rate of pulmonary embolism or in the 2-week mortality were noted. Bleeding was a prominent complication and occurred in 45 per cent of patients receiving urokinase and heparin, compared with 27 per cent of those given heparin alone.

To determine the long-term effects of thrombolytic treatment of acute and massive embolism, seven patients with this problem underwent pulmonary angiography with pressure measurements before and after treatment with intrapulmonary infusion of urokinase (average dose, 1724 units per kg. per hr.) and heparin (average dose, 17 units per kg. per hr.). The treatment was monitored by daily measurement of pulmonary arterial pressure and was continued until the pressure had normalized (average, 6 days later). The patients later had pulmonary angiographic examinations and right-sided heart catheterization at rest and during bicycle exercise as well as phlebography of the deep veins of both legs. The pulmonary angiograms showed massive obstruction before therapy with improvement occurring within 6 days after treatment. The mean pulmonary arterial pressure declined from an average of 37 ± 9 to $13 \pm$ mm. Hg after 6 days and to 15 ± 3 mm. Hg after 15 months. No recurrence of pulmonary embolism was observed. In six of seven patients at rest and during bicycle exercise in the supine position, mean pulmonary arterial pressure and total pulmonary resistance remained within normal limits. Over the short term, all patients showed clinical signs of deep venous thrombosis. Fifteen months later, four patients had normal deep veins, and three had phlebographic signs of old thrombosis. Thus, after thrombolytic treatment of acute massive pulmonary embolism, normal pulmonary arteriograms were obtained in six of seven patients studied. Moreover, the reserve capacity of the pulmonary vasculature that was assessed during heavy exercise was normal.

The role of streptokinase therapy in the routine management of deep venous thrombosis in the lower extremities was evaluated in a retrospective study of phlebographic results and therapeutic complications. Among 108 patients with phlebographically verified deep venous thrombosis treated with streptokinase, total or partial thrombolysis was demonstrated angiographically in 60 (55.6 per cent). However, three died during treatment, each from pulmonary embolism, and six developed clinical signs suggestive of pulmonary embolism. Major bleeding complicated the therapy in 16 patients (14.8 per cent). Allergic reactions to streptokinase occurred in 22 patients, and 1 had anaphylactic shock. The authors concluded that streptokinase was effective in the management of deep venous thrombosis, but complications were significant.

An example of a massive embolus in the right pulmonary artery from an indwelling catheter in the right atrium in a child receiving total intravenous hyperalimentation was shown in the chest film with marked oligemia of the entire right lung (Westermark's sign). The pulmonary radioactive scan showed no perfusion of the right lung, and the pulmonary arteriogram demonstrated total occlusion of the right pulmonary artery. After 24 hours of intravenous streptokinase, the pulmonary scan returned to normal. Clinical evidence further emphasizes the importance of considering all the systemic veins and the right heart as potential sources of pulmonary emboli.

The effects of recombinant tissue plasminogen activator (rTPA) have also been evaluated, and this agent is now available for general use. In a study using rTPA, Goldhaber and associates[14] reviewed a group of patients with angiographically documented pulmonary embolism. All had segmental or proximal pulmonary arterial obstruction within 5 days of the onset of symptoms or signs. The dosage consisted of 50 mg. of rTPA every 2 hours, followed by repeat angiography, and, if necessary, an additional 40 mg. every 4 hours. Thirty-four of the 36 patients had angiographic evidence of clot lysis by 6 hours. Of these patients, clot lysis was slight in 4, moderate in 6, and marked in 24. The fibrinogen levels decreased 30 per cent from baseline at 2 hours and 38 per cent from baseline at 6 hours. There were only two major complications. In a cooperative study for evaluation of intrapulmonary and intravenous administration of rTPA, the results indicated that pulmonary arterial infusion of rTPA does not offer a significant benefit over the intravenous route and suggested that a prolonged infusion of rTPA over 7 hours (100 mg.) is superior to a single infusion of 50 mg. over 2 hours. The contraindications to thrombolytic therapy can be divided into those that are *firm* and those that are *relative. Firm contraindications* include internal bleeding (recent or active), recent neurosurgery, cranial trauma, and a history of hemorrhagic stroke. *Relative contraindications* include a recent surgical procedure (within 7 to 10 days), cardiopulmonary resuscitation (within 7 to 10 days), and the presence of coagulopathy.

Surgical Management

Although anticoagulant therapy for pulmonary embolism is most often successful, there are cases in which it fails, and the role of surgical management should then be considered individually for each patient.

VENOUS THROMBECTOMY. Although the direct removal of venous thrombi was previously recommended, it is now rarely done because of the high incidence of recurrent postoperative thrombosis. One rare indication for thrombectomy, however, is phlegmasia cerulea dolens with secondary arterial spasm. Even though venous thrombosis may recur after thrombectomy, patency of the venous lumen may persist sufficiently long to relieve the arterial spasm and prevent a gangrenous limb. Systemic heparin is indicated to prolong venous patency.

INTERRUPTION OF THE INFERIOR VENA CAVA. Interruption of the vena cava was previously recommended for selected patients with pulmonary embolism but is seldom performed today.[35] Moreover, it does not necessarily prevent subsequent embolism, because evidence of recurrent pulmonary embolism is reported in as many as 20 per cent of patients after ligation.

USE OF TRANSLUMINAL FILTERS. Several procedures designed to simplify caval interruption have been developed, with emphasis on reducing postoperative morbidity and mortality. One device is a filter designed to trap large emboli arising from the branches of the inferior vena cava. A cone-shaped stainless steel umbrella that causes minimal reduction in venous flow has been designed by Greenfield and Michna and can be inserted under local anesthesia through the femoral or jugular vein (Fig. 9).[17] Of importance is the principle of fixation of the filter, which is achieved by hooks that grasp the wall of the inferior vena cava. This is designed to prevent proximal migration, and the filter becomes even more securely fixed when emboli become trapped. Occasionally, distal migration to the bifurcation of the inferior vena cava occurs, the struts may protrude through the caval wall, and thrombus may also form on the filter. The most serious complication of the filter is its migration into the iliac

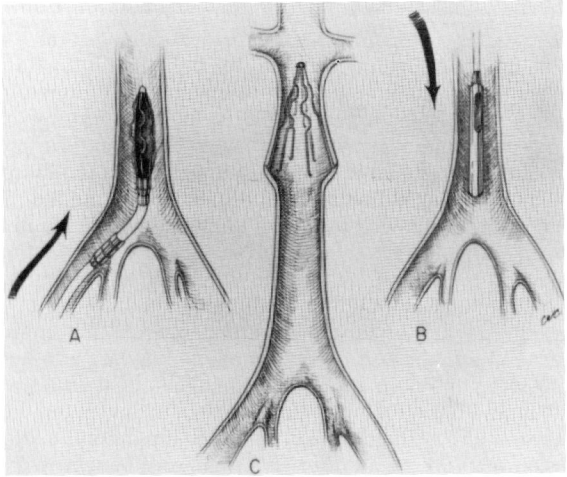

Figure 9. Insertion of the cone filter is accomplished by a carrier catheter inserted from the femoral vein *(A)* or retrograde from the jugular vein *(B)*. To avoid misplacement into the right renal vein, the jugular inserter should be passed down to the level of the pelvis and then withdrawn to the level of L3 for discharge *(C)*. Fixation is automatic, as the limbs spring open and the recurved hooks engage the wall of the inferior vena cava. (From Greenfield, L. J.: Pulmonary embolism: Diagnosis and management. Curr. Probl. Surg., *13*(4):1, 1976.)

vein, renal vein, right atrium, right ventricle, or pulmonary artery, and such migration may end fatally. Additional complications reported with these intraluminal devices include misplacement, retroperitoneal hemorrhage, perforation of the duodenum and of the ureter, and development of a thrombus proximal to the umbrella, producing recurrent emboli. The filter may stimulate distal thrombosis in the vena cava, and late occlusion may occur.

PULMONARY EMBOLECTOMY. In 1908, Trendelenburg performed the first pulmonary embolectomy and described three patients having the procedure. The longest survivor lived for 37 hours and ultimately died of hemorrhage from an internal mammary artery. In 1924, Kirschner performed the first successful pulmonary embolectomy with long-term survival.[21] Nevertheless, more patients have succumbed from this approach than have survived it, because significant brain damage due to cerebral hypoxia after interruption of the circulation was common. In a collective review, 22 patients managed by Trendelenburg's technique were reported.[4] Most had postoperative brain damage caused by both pre-existing hypoxia before embolectomy and that occurring after the procedure. Only 3 of the 22 patients were long-term survivors. In 1960, a significant advance was made by Allison in doing a pulmonary embolectomy on a young athlete with massive pulmonary embolism secondary to traumatic thrombophlebitis. With total body hypothermia (20° C.), the chest was opened and both venae cavae were occluded. The pulmonary artery was opened, a massive embolus was removed, the pulmonary arteriotomy was closed, the caval occlusion was released, and the normal circulation was re-established. With the brain and heart protected by hypothermia while the circulation was temporarily occluded, the patient made a good recovery.

In 1961, Sharp was the first to perform pulmonary embolectomy using extracorporeal circulation.[34] This technique is now preferred, since it permits continuous perfusion of the entire body with concomitant oxygenation while the emboli are safely removed from the pulmonary arteries. Massive pulmonary emboli may cause sudden death; but it has long been recognized that many patients, even those with massive embolism, survive for a period of minutes or hours. The protocols of 52 patients with fatal pulmonary embolism were reviewed, and two groups were identified: (1) those in good general condition before the embolism and (2) those who had serious underlying or terminal illnesses and in whom pulmonary embolism was a more serious complication. Among the patients previously in good condition, 55 per cent lived longer than 2 hours and 48 per cent survived for 8 or more hours. However, among those with terminal illnesses, only 32 per cent lived for 2 hours.[13] These data clearly emphasize the fact that a serious underlying illness gravely affects prognosis.

The indications for emergency pulmonary embolectomy are *persistent and refractory hypotension* despite maximal resuscitation in a patient with massive embolism clearly *documented* by either a pulmonary scan or pulmonary arteriogram. The immediate treatment of these patients includes systemic heparinization and administration of vasopressors, inotropic agents, and endotracheal oxygen. Every effort should be made to manage the patient by this approach. Many patients previously thought to require embolectomy now respond favorably, without the need for operation. Depending on the severity of the clinical condition, 1 or 2 hours may be taken in an effort to restore acceptable cardiopulmonary function. If this approach is effective in maintaining a blood pressure of 80 mm. Hg or more, as shown by a continuous intra-arterial recording, embolectomy may be deferred, particularly if acceptable renal and cerebral function is maintained. The pulmonary scan and the emboli removed from a patient with massive pulmonary embolism and intractable shock are shown in Figure 10. Such a patient is appropriate for the procedure, because all attempts to correct the

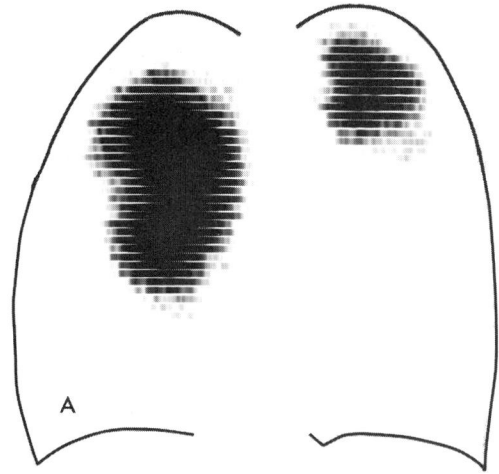

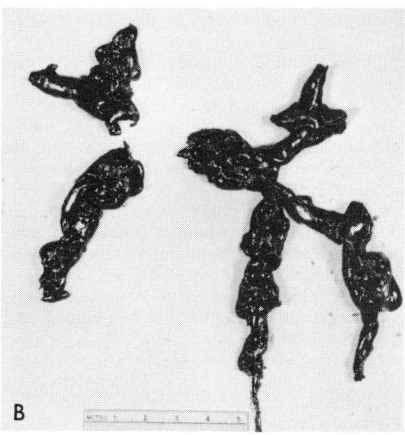

Figure 10. Illustration from a patient with massive pulmonary embolism on the twelfth postoperative day following an orthopedic operation and accompanied by intractable shock. *A,* The pulmonary scan shows massive occlusion of the right lower and middle lobar pulmonary arteries as well as nearly all of the pulmonary arterial circulation of the left lung. *B,* Emboli removed from both pulmonary arteries at the time of embolectomy. (From Sabiston, D. C., Jr.: Pathophysiology, diagnosis and management of pulmonary embolism. Adv. Surg., *3:*351, 1968.

severe state of hypotension failed despite vigorous resuscitative therapy.

That *small* numbers of pulmonary emboli in the presence of pre-existing cardiac and pulmonary insufficiency can produce serious cardiovascular manifestations is illustrated in Figure 11. Admitted for an ophthalmic procedure under local anesthesia, this 72-year-old man had a history of hypertensive cardiovascular disease and chronic respiratory insufficiency due to emphysema. Postoperatively, he was found in a state of cardiovascular collapse. A pulmonary scan showed evidence of obstruction to the pulmonary arterial flow in the left lower lobe. Under usual circumstances, this relatively small number of emboli would not produce serious cardiopulmonary symptoms. In this patient, however, a persistent state of profound hypotension ensued that could not be corrected by vigorous resuscitative management. The presence of pre-existing cardiac and respiratory insufficiency obviously augmented the effects of this amount of obstruction. Ultimately, it was necessary to remove the emboli by using cardiopulmonary bypass. All emboli were confined to the left lower lobe pulmonary artery. The patient made an uneventful recovery.

TECHNIQUE. A median sternotomy provides excellent exposure of the pulmonary artery for pulmonary embolectomy. Once the pericardium is opened, cardiopulmonary bypass is established. The main pulmonary artery is exposed and incised

and is usually free of emboli, although partial obstruction may be present. Using forceps, the emboli are removed from the right and left pulmonary arteries and their major branches. A Fogarty catheter is passed into the pulmonary arterial branches for removal of smaller emboli. Finally, the entire pulmonary arterial tree is irrigated with saline. During this portion of the procedure, gentle compression of both lungs with the hand directs peripheral emboli toward the central arteries for more effective aspiration. The pulmonary artery is closed and cardiopulmonary bypass is gradually discontinued, allowing the heart and lungs to resume normal function.

When severe cardiovascular collapse is present, the patient can be supported by partial cardiopulmonary bypass by means of a circuit from femoral vein to femoral artery for immediate resuscitation. If extracorporeal circulation is not available, a right or left thoracotomy with exposure of the most severely involved pulmonary artery can be done with the side of predominant occlusion as determined by the scan or arteriogram. An anterior thoracotomy in the third interspace is appropriate for exposure of either the right or left pulmonary artery. The artery can then be dissected, occluded, and opened distally for removal of emboli while the normal circulation and pulmonary function in the opposite lung continue; successful results with this technique have been described. One of the complications that has been reported to follow pulmonary embolectomy is *massive endobronchial hemorrhage.* Successful management of this complication has been achieved by the use of an endotracheal tube for selective collapse of the lung and entrapment of the bleeding into either the right or left main bronchus.[24] *Reperfusion pulmonary edema* after pulmonary artery thromboendar-

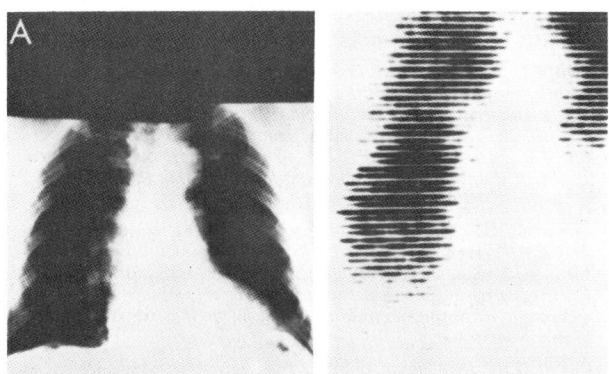

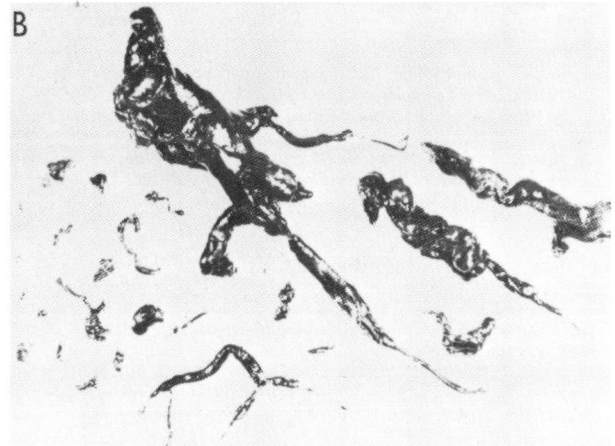

Figure 11. *A,* Chest film from a postoperative patient with pre-existing cardiac and respiratory insufficiency. Pulmonary emboli are present in the left lower lobe. The patient was in severe and refractory shock. *B,* Emboli removed from the left lower lobe pulmonary artery at embolectomy. The result was that the patient's signs and symptoms improved, and he made an uneventful recovery. (From Sabiston, D. C., Jr., and Wolfe, W. G.: Pulmonary embolectomy. *In* Moser, K. M., and Stein, M. [Eds.]: Pulmonary Thromboembolism. Chicago, Year Book Medical Publishers, 1973.)

terectomy has been described and may be a serious complication, often requiring prolonged mechanical ventilation. The syndrome is a cause of hypoxemia postoperatively with local pulmonary infiltrates.

RESULTS. Among 24 patients undergoing open pulmonary embolectomy with extracorporeal circulation, 17 (71 per cent) had acute pulmonary embolism after a surgical procedure.[36] In the remaining seven patients (29 per cent) the embolism was secondary to a chronic medical disorder. The interval between clinical manifestations of acute pulmonary embolism and the embolectomy varied between 8 to 36 hours, and a definitive diagnosis of pulmonary embolism was made in each patient by pulmonary arteriography. All were in a state of shock, with an arterial oxygen tension less than 65 mm. Hg and the presence of acidosis. The definitive indication for embolectomy was occlusion of the right or left pulmonary artery. In the last 2 years of the study, the operative mortality in 17 patients was 23 per cent.

SELECTED REFERENCES

Goldhaber, S. Z. (Ed.): Pulmonary Embolism and Deep Venous Thrombosis. Philadelphia, W. B. Saunders Company, 1985.
This is an updated monograph that is quite complete and highly recommended to students wishing to consult an authoritative and considerably detailed series of presentations on all aspects of this subject.

Goldhaber, S. Z., Vaughan, D. E., Markis, J. E., et al.: Acute pulmonary embolism treated with tissue plasminogen activator. Lancet, 2:886, 1986.
An important series of patients managed with rTPA.

Gorham, L. W.: A study of pulmonary embolism. Parts I and II. Arch. Intern. Med., 108:8, 189, 1961.
These companion papers emphasize the gross pathology of pulmonary embolism. Special emphasis is given the fact that in most patients with fatal embolism a substantial amount of the pulmonary arterial bed is occluded, generally more than half. This is one of the best pathologic studies in the literature.

Makhoul, R. G., Greenberg, C. S., and McCann, R. L.: Heparin-associated thrombocytopenia and thrombosis: A serious clinical problem and potential solution. J. Vasc. Surg., 5:522, 1986.
This reference provides an excellent presentation of heparin-associated thrombocytopenia and thrombosis (HATT). The pathogenesis, diagnosis, and management are discussed including high incidence of amputation of extremities.

Marshall, R., Sabiston, D. C., Jr., Allison, P. R., Bosman, A. R., and Dunnill, M. S.: Immediate and late effects of pulmonary embolism by large thrombi in dogs. Thorax, 18:1, 1963.
In this experimental study, a variety of physiologic measurements were determined following pulmonary embolism. The study emphasized the paucity of changes that occur when only one pulmonary artery is occluded and illustrates the wide margin of pulmonary reserve.

Sabiston, D. C., Jr., and Wagner, H. N., Jr.: The diagnosis of pulmonary embolism by radioisotope scanning. Ann. Surg., 160:585, 1964.
In this paper the original experimental and clinical studies introducing the technique of radioactive pulmonary scanning are described.

Sabiston, D. C., Jr., and Wolfe, W. G.: Experimental and clinical observations on the natural history of pulmonary embolism. Ann. Surg., 168:1, 1968.
In this paper the natural history of pulmonary emboli in the experimental animal and man is discussed. The gross and microscopic features and their changes with the passage of time are illustrated. The gradual resolution of the emboli and final disappearance in most instances are confirmed by serial scans and pulmonary arteriograms.

REFERENCES

1. Alexander, B., Meyers, L., Kenny, J., et al.: Blood coagulation in pregnancy. Proconvertin and prothrombin, and the hypercoagulable state. N. Engl. J. Med., 254:466, 1956.
2. Allison, P. R.: Pulmonary embolism and thrombophlebitis. Br. J. Surg., 54:466, 1967.
3. Arkless, R.: Renal carcinoma: How it metastasizes. Radiology, 84:496, 1965.
4. Benichoux, R.: The surgical treatment of massive pulmonary embolism: Report of 22 cases of Trendelenburg's operation. J. Int. Chir., 11:464, 1951.
5. Brofman, B. L., Charms, B. L., Kohn, P. M., et al: Unilateral pulmonary artery occlusion in man. Control studies. J. Thorac. Surg., 34:206, 1957.
6. Burnett, W. E., Long, J. H., Norris, C., et al.: The effect of pneumonectomy on pulmonary function. J. Thorac. Surg., 18:569, 1949.
7. Clagett, G. P., Schneider, P., Rosoff, C. B., and Salzman, E. W.: The influence of aspirin on postoperative platelet kinetics and venous thrombosis. Surgery, 77:61, 1975.
8. Coon, W. W., and Coller, F. A.: Some epidemiologic considerations of thromboembolism. Surg. Gynecol. Obstet., 109:487, 1959.
9. Craoord, C., and Jorpes, E.: Heparin as a prophylactic against thrombosis. J.A.M.A., 116:2831, 1941.
10. Cruveilhier, J.: Anatomie Pathologique de Corps Humain. Paris, J. B. Bailliere, 1829, p. 42.
11. Dalen, J. E., and Alpert, J. S.: Natural history of pulmonary embolism. Prog. Cardiovasc. Dis., 17:259, 1975.
12. Duranceau, A., Jones, R. H., and Sabiston, D. C., Jr.: The diagnosis of pulmonary embolism. Compr. Ther., 2:6, 1976.
13. Flemma, R. J., Young, W. G., Jr., Wallace, A., et al.: Feasibility of pulmonary embolectomy. Circulation, 30:234, 1964.
14. Goldhaber, S. Z., Vaughan, D. E., Markis, J. E., et al: Acute pulmonary embolism treated with tissue plasminogen activator. Lancet, 2:886, 1986.
15. Gorham, L. W.: A study of pulmonary embolism. Part I. Arch. Intern. Med., 108:8, 1961.
16. Gorham, L. W.: A study of pulmonary embolism. Part II. Arch. Intern. Med., 108:189, 1961.
17. Greenfield, L. J., and Michna, B. A.: Twelve-year clinical experience with the Greenfield vena caval filter. Surgery, 104:706, 1988.
18. Gurewich, V., Sasahara, A. A., and Stein, M.: Pulmonary embolism, bronchoconstriction and response to heparin. In Sasahara, A. A., and Stein, M. (Eds.): Pulmonary Embolic Disease. New York, Grune & Stratton, 1965.
19. Jones, R. H., and Sabiston, D. C., Jr.: Pulmonary embolism in childhood. Monogr. Surg. Sci., 3:35, 1966.
20. Kakkar, V. V., et al.: Prevention of fatal postoperative pulmonary embolism by low doses of heparin: An international multicentre trial. Lancet, 2:45, 1975.
21. Kirschner, M.: Ein durch die Trendelenburgsche Operation geheilter Fall von Embolie det Arterien pulmonalis. Arch Klin. Chir., 133:312, 1924.
22. Laennec, R. T. H.: De l'auscultation mediate. Paris, Brossen et Chaude, 1819.
23. Littmann, D.: Observations on the electrocardiographic changes in pulmonary embolism. In Sasahara, A. A., and Stein, M. (Eds.): Pulmonary Embolic Disease. New York, Grune & Stratton, 1965.
24. Lyerly, H. K., Reves, J. G., and Sabiston, D. C., Jr.: Management of primary sarcomas of the pulmonary artery and reperfusion of intrabronchial hemorrhage. Surg. Gynecol. Obstet., 163:291, 1986.
25. Makhoul, R. G., Greenberg, C. S., and McCann, R. L.: Heparin-associated thrombocytopenia and thrombosis: A serious clinical problem and potential solution. J. Vasc. Surg., 5:522, 1986.
26. McLachlin, A. D., McLachlin, J. A., Jory, T. A., and Rawling, E. G.: Venous stasis in the lower extremities. Ann. Surg., 152:678, 1960.
27. McLean, J.: The thromboplastin action of cephalin. Am. J. Physiol., 41:250, 1916.
28. Mitchell, J. R. A.: Can we really prevent postoperative pulmonary emboli? Br. Med. J., 1:1523, 1979.
29. Murray, G. D. W., Jacques, L. B., Perrett, T. S., and Best, C. H.: Heparin and thrombosis of veins following injury. Surgery, 2:163, 1937.
30. Sabiston, D. C., Jr., and Wagner, H. N., Jr.: The diagnosis of pulmonary embolism by radioisotope scanning. Ann. Surg., 160:585, 1964.
31. Sabiston, D. C., Jr., and Wagner, H. N., Jr.: The pathophysiology of pulmonary embolism: Relationships to accurate diagnosis and choice of therapy. J. Thorac. Cardiovasc. Surg., 50:339, 1965.
32. Sabiston, D. C., Jr., and Wolfe, W. G.: Experimental and clinical observations on the natural history of pulmonary embolism. Ann. Surg., 168:1, 1968.
33. Sharnoff, J. G.: Results in the prophylaxis of postoperative thromboembolism. Surg. Gynecol. Obstet., 123:303, 1966.
34. Sharp, E. H.: Pulmonary embolectomy: Successful removal of a massive pulmonary embolus with the support of cardiopulmonary bypass: A case report. Ann. Surg., 156:1, 1962.
35. Silver, D., and Sabiston, D. C., Jr.: The role of vena caval interruption in the management of pulmonary embolism. Surgery, 77:1, 1975.
36. Tschirkov, A., Krause, E., Elert, O., and Satter, P.: Surgical management of massive pulmonary embolism. J. Thorac. Cardiovasc. Surg., 75:730, 1978.
37. Virchow, R.: Die Cellularpathologie in ihrer Begrudung auf physiologische und pathologische Gewebelehre. Berlin, A. Hirschwald, 1858.
38. Westermark, N.: On the roentgen diagnosis of lung embolism. Acta Radiol., 19:357, 1938.

I

CHRONIC PULMONARY EMBOLISM

H. Kim Lyerly, M.D., and David C. Sabiston, Jr., M.D.

Pulmonary embolism usually presents as an acute clinical problem but may present with *chronic* manifestations as a characteristic syndrome. Most pulmonary emboli eventually resolve spontaneously as a result of naturally occurring fibrinolytic systems in the body.[12,13] In some patients, owing to inadequate fibrinolysis or recurrent episodes of embolism, emboli gradually accumulate in the pulmonary arterial system. This may ultimately cause pulmonary hypertension and produce symptoms of progressive respiratory insufficiency, hypoxemia, and right ventricular failure.[12,35,41,45] In most patients, medical management of these disorders is unsatisfactory, and clinical studies in this group have revealed a poor prognosis.[28,38,44,53] Those thought to have pulmonary hypertension secondary to chronic pulmonary emboli should undergo pulmonary angiography for documentation of emboli, determination of anatomic distribution of emboli, and a recording of pulmonary artery pressure. Determining the presence of elevated pulmonary artery pressures is important, because it has been demonstrated that the natural history of this syndrome is related to the magnitude of the pulmonary arterial hypertension. If the mean pulmonary artery pressure is more than 30 mm. Hg, survival at 5 years is only 30 per cent. In those patients with mean pressure greater than 50 mm. Hg, only 10 per cent were alive at 5 years (Fig. 1). Fortunately, it is now established that pulmonary embolectomy in patients with proximal pulmonary arterial obstruction is likely to produce relief of respiratory insufficiency, with reduction in pulmonary hypertension and improvement of right-sided heart failure.

Historical Aspects

Hart first suspected chronic pulmonary embolism (CPE) in 1916; Molle, in 1920. Ljungdahl described two patients, one 38 and the other 51, with chronic symptoms of dyspnea, cyanosis, and palpitations.[26] Both ultimately died of right-sided heart failure; and chronic pulmonary arterial obstruction was present at autopsy, with dilatation of the proximal main pulmonary artery. The bronchial circulation was increased, and adequacy of the collaterals was demonstrated by the absence of pulmonary in-

farction. Ljungdahl thought it likely that obstruction was due to pulmonary emboli, rather than the previously held view that in patients with cor pulmonale the process was caused by primary thrombosis of the pulmonary artery.

Several years later, Brenner described a systematic study of the pulmonary vasculature and attributed numerous changes in the pulmonary vessels to pulmonary embolism.[4] In the last century, Virchow suspected that pulmonary infarction did not occur in most patients after pulmonary embolism because bronchial collateral circulation was adequate.[50] Blalock confirmed these observations in 1948 by detecting bright red arterial blood in pulmonary vessels distal to chronic emboli, and collateral perfusion by bronchial arteries was demonstrated angiographically by Viamonte in 1964.[48]

Carroll described the clinical features of CPE and made a premortem diagnosis of the syndrome.[6] The diagnosis in this patient was confirmed at thoracotomy by opening the pulmonary artery and demonstrating the chronic emboli by biopsy. Several early surgical attempts to remove emboli were made; however, the first successful embolectomy for recurrent pulmonary emboli was performed by Allison in 1958.[2]

Fleishner reviewed the clinical and diagnostic aspects of chronic recurrent pulmonary emboli and emphasized the radiolucency of the vascular markings that were sometimes apparent on chest films.[18] Cabrol and colleagues recommended a lateral thoracotomy in order to easily approach the distal pulmonary arterial branches.[5] Daily and associates reported bilateral thromboendarterectomy by means of a median sternotomy and extrapericardial dissection of the pulmonary arteries.[11] Cardiopulmonary bypass was conducted with deep hypothermia and intermittent circulatory arrest in performing pulmonary thromboendarterectomy. Chitwood and colleagues emphasized the importance of bronchial arteriography and the need to identify obstructing lesions in the proximal pulmonary arterial system.[7]

Clinical Presentation

Patients with the syndrome of CPE have a history of exertional dyspnea progressing to severe respiratory insufficiency for several months to years. They may also complain of recurrent episodes of thrombophlebitis, hemoptysis due to the presence of large bronchial collaterals, and chest pain (Table 1). Physical findings include signs of severe pulmonary hypertension, often combined with evidence of right ventricular failure, and may be manifested as an increased pulmonary second sound, a systolic murmur, hepatomegaly, and an S3 or S4 gallop. Other physical findings may include pulmonary rales, jugular venous distention, cyanosis, and clubbing of the fingers

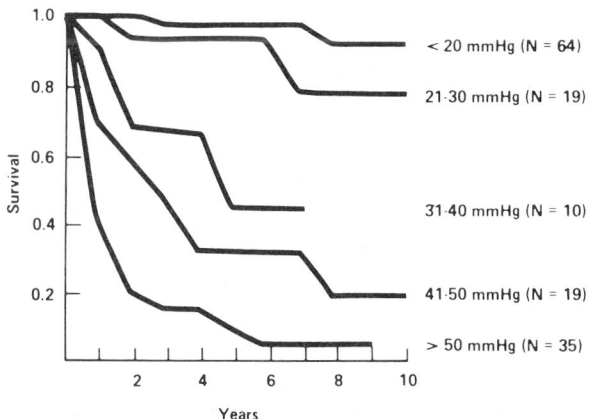

Figure 1. Survival in patients with pulmonary hypertension resulting from chronic recurrent emboli. Groups of patients are compared at different mean pulmonary artery pressures. (Modified from Riedel, M., Stanek, V., Widimsky, J., et al.: Long-term follow-up of patients with pulmonary thromboembolism. Chest, *81:*151, 1982.)

TABLE 1. Symptoms of Patients with Chronic Pulmonary Emboli (*n* = 49)

Symptom	% Afflicted
Dyspnea — exertion (45)	92
Thrombophlebitis (27)	55
Dyspnea — progressive (40)	82
Hemoptysis (13)	27
Chest pain (12)	24
Fatigue (12)	24

TABLE 2. Physical Findings in Patients with Chronic Pulmonary Embolism (n = 49)

Physical Finding	% Afflicted
Increased P2 (29)	59
Cardiac murmur (22)	45
Hepatomegaly (13)	27
S3 or S4 gallop (13)	27
Pulmonary rales (12)	24
Jugular venous distention (11)	22
Cyanosis (2)	4
Clubbing (1)	2

(Table 2). A recent report of CPE mimicking pulmonary artery agenesis (PAA) describes patients with PAA who underwent thrombectomy for suspected CPE.[31] Clues in the differentiation of CPE from PAA include history of deep venous thrombosis, cardiac flow murmur, signs of pulmonary hypertension, and areas of ventilation-perfusion mismatch discovered in the opposite lung in patients with CPE.

Radiographic Studies

Chest films show a dilated pulmonary artery and oligemic pulmonary fields in approximately 50 per cent of patients. Right ventricular enlargement is present in 68 per cent and pleural effusion in approximately one third of patients (Table 3). A typical preoperative chest film is shown in Figure 2. Although some patients with CPE have been described as having a normal chest film, this is probably unusual. In the authors' series, all plain films revealed abnormalities, including cardiomegaly (84 per cent), right-sided heart enlargement (55 per cent), enlargement of the pulmonary artery (43 per cent), azygos vein enlargement (27 per cent), chronic volume loss (24 per cent), atelectasis or effusion (22 per cent), and pleural thickening (12 per cent).[56] Embolic involvement of the right lung was present in 96 per cent of patients and of the left lung in 80 per cent. Bilateral emboli were present in 85 per cent.

Arterial blood gases at room air revealed evidence of severe respiratory insufficiency, with hypoxemia and arterial oxygen tension (Pa_{O_2}) values of 55 to 60 mm. Hg and an arterial carbon dioxide tension (Pa_{CO_2}) of approximately 30 mm. Hg. The pH showed mild respiratory alkalosis (pH = 7.5). Hypoxemia is a consequence of a ventilation-perfusion mismatch abnormality amplified by a lowered mixed venous P_{O_2}.[25]

The electrocardiogram usually suggests the presence of chronic cor pulmonale and includes right-axis deviation and right ventricular hypertrophy. S-T segment and T wave changes are present in approximately one third of patients, and somewhat fewer have right bundle branch block.

Peripheral venography demonstrates venous thrombosis in patients and indicates the source of the emboli. Magnetic resonance imaging provides more accurate delineation of pelvic vein thrombosis than venography and is more reliable as well as noninvasive.

TABLE 3. Chest Film Findings in Patients with Chronic Pulmonary Embolism (n = 49)

Finding	% Afflicted
Cardiomegaly (41)	84
Right-sided heart enlargement (27)	55
Enlargement of pulmonary artery (21)	43
Azygos vein enlargement (13)	27
Chronic volume loss (12)	24
Atelectasis (11)	22
Effusion (8)	16
Pleural thickening (6)	12

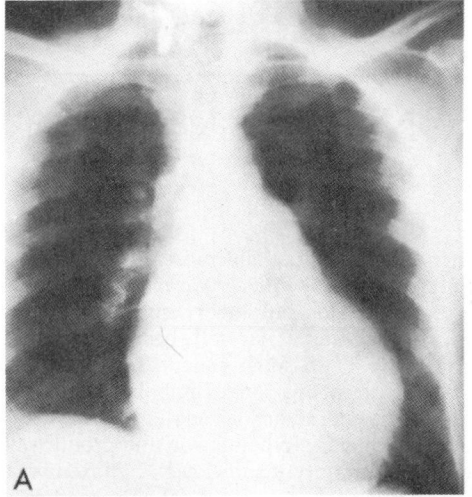

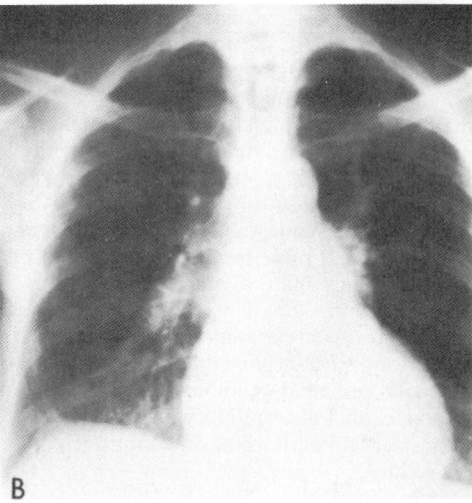

Figure 2. The anteroposterior chest film is shown before *(A)* and after *(B)* embolectomy of the right lower lobe pulmonary artery for chronic pulmonary emboli. Note an increase in parenchymal flow to the right lower lobe after operation. Also note the decrease in the size of both the right main pulmonary artery and the cardiac silhouette after embolectomy. (From Chitwood, W. R., Jr., Lyerly, H. K., and Sabiston, D. C., Jr.: Surgical management of chronic pulmonary embolism. Ann. Surg., *201*:11, 1985.)

Ventilation and perfusion radionuclide scans obtained during evaluation are consistent with pulmonary emboli, and perfusion defects correspond to oligemic regions on the plain film and arteriogram. Perfusion defects are usually noted bilaterally.

Pulmonary arteriography usually shows emboli in both lungs, with 55 to 75 per cent of the total pulmonary blood flow obstructed. Pulmonary hypertension was present in all 48 patients with chronic pulmonary emboli evaluated in the series at the Duke University Medical Center. The systolic pressure was 75.0 ± 8.0 mm. Hg, distolic pressure was 26.0 ± 3.0 mm. Hg, and mean pressure was 42.0 ± 5.0 mm. Hg.

Pulmonary angioscopy may permit more accurate definition of the proximal extent of organized thrombus in the major pulmonary arteries if doubt remains after angiography. Angioscopy differentiates thromboemboli from tumor and fibrosing mediastinitis from congenital absence of a pulmonary artery.[33] Further preoperative studies include a thoracic aortogram or selective bronchial arteriography to demonstrate dilated and tortuous bronchial vessels (Fig. 3). The bronchial circulation is often considerably dilated and communicates by collaterals with the distal pulmonary arteries. In patients in whom selective bronchial arteriograms were obtained, patency of the distal pulmonary arteries was shown in all except one patient. When

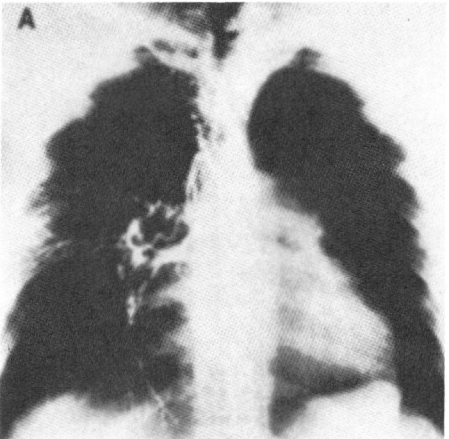
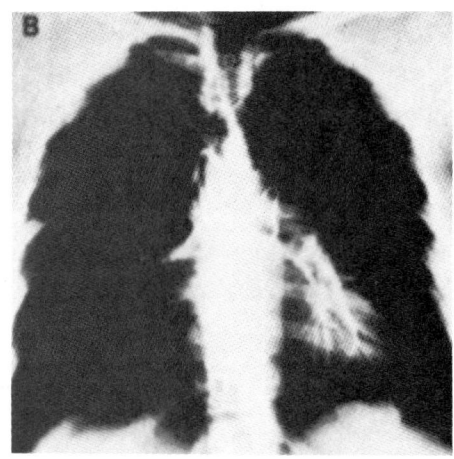

Figure 3. *A*, A selective bronchial arterial injection showing dilated bronchial collaterals on the right supplying the distal pulmonary parenchyma. *B*, A later phase of the same injection in which collaterals from the right side supply the distal pulmonary parenchyma in the left lower lobe. The left lower lobe pulmonary artery was noted to have a total proximal obstruction on the pulmonary arteriogram. (From Chitwood, W. R., Jr., Lyerly, H. K., and Sabiston, D. C., Jr.: Surgical management of chronic pulmonary embolism. Ann. Surg., *201*:11, 1985.)

patent distal pulmonary arteries are present, the prognosis is favorable because it can be established preoperatively that the distal pulmonary arterial bed is patent and removal of the proximal thrombus produces increased pulmonary arterial blood flow.

Right ventricular function may be assessed by first-pass radionuclide angiography, which shows severe chronic pulmonary arterial obstruction with a significant delay in arrival of the tracer. The mean resting ejection fraction for patients in the series was 23.5 ± 2.2 at rest and 28.0 ± 2.0 with exercise.

A thorough preoperative evaluation is necessary before suitability for operation in individual patients can be determined. The most appropriate candidates for pulmonary embolectomy are those with severe respiratory insufficiency and a low Pao_2 and those in whom enlarged bronchial vessels can be demonstrated by arteriography. A number of patients with this syndrome are unsuitable for embolectomy. The most common contraindication is distal pulmonary emboli that diffusely involve

the small pulmonary arteries, and these are not amenable to surgical removal (Fig. 4).[7] Other contraindications include severe cardiac failure and massive obesity. The majority of these patients are disabled and are assigned a New York Heart Association (NYHA) class of IV.

Surgical Management

Pulmonary embolectomy may be performed on one or both pulmonary arteries. In a number of patients, the pulmonary artery is occluded unilaterally and there are few if any proximal emboli in the contralateral lung. These patients usually improve dramatically after embolectomy. In patients who have primarily unilateral involvement, either a right or left anterior thoracotomy can be done when there is proximal occlusion of the vessel. In patients with bilateral pulmonary emboli or in those with involvement of the main pulmonary artery, extracorporeal circulation is generally indicated. However, cardiopulmonary bypass may be associated with bleeding complications due to the need for anticoagulation.

When extracorporeal circulation is used, the venous cannula can be placed in either the right atrium or the outflow tract of the right ventricle. Involvement of the main pulmonary artery

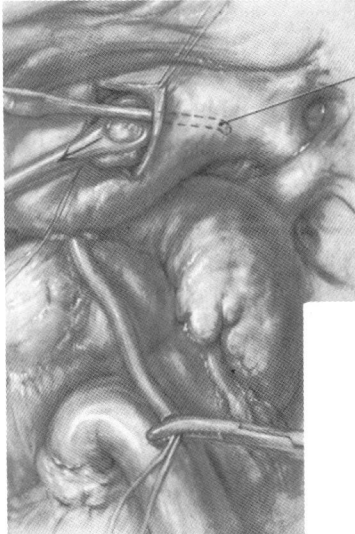

Endarterectomy instrument dissecting thrombus from intima left pulmonary artery

Figure 4. A pulmonary arteriogram from the patient demonstrates multiple peripheral filling defects. Organized emboli can be seen within the proximal right pulmonary arteries *(A, arrows)*. In the left lower lobe, a calcified embolus is present *(B, arrow)*. (From Chitwood, W. R., Jr., Lyerly, H. K., and Sabiston, D. C., Jr.: Surgical management of chronic pulmonary embolism. Ann. Surg., *201*:11, 1985.)

Figure 5. *A*, After occlusion of the proximal pulmonary artery by the tape when the patient is on cardiopulmonary bypass, an incision is made into the main pulmonary artery for removal of the chronic embolus. The thrombus is densely adherent to the wall of the pulmonary artery and requires exacting and tedious dissection. As much of the thrombus is removed through this incision as possible preparatory to a counterincision in the distal left pulmonary artery. (From Wolfe, W. G., and Sabiston, D. C., Jr.: Pulmonary embolism. *In* Ebert, P. A. [Ed.]: Major Problems in Clinical Surgery. Vol. 25. Philadelphia, W. B. Saunders Company, 1980.)

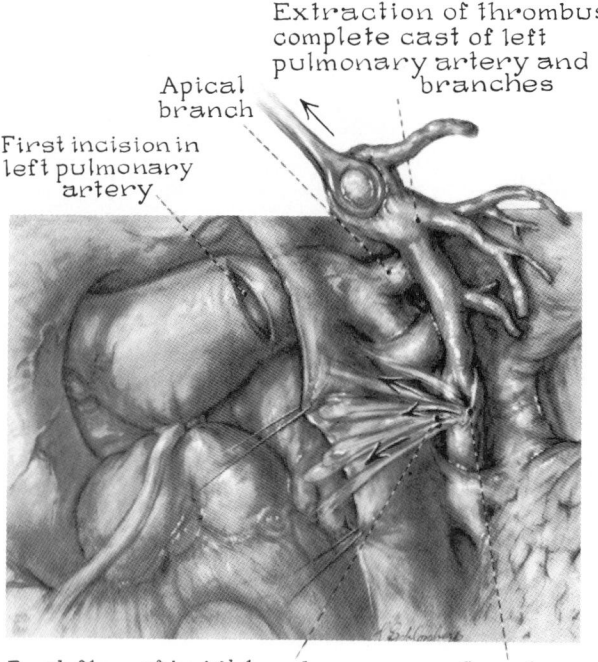

Extraction of thrombus—
complete cast of left
pulmonary artery and
branches

Apical
branch

First incision in
left pulmonary
artery

Backflow of bright red
blood from distal branches
left pulmonary artery

Counter
incision

Figure 6. Through a counterincision in the distal left pulmonary artery, the branches of the chronic embolus are removed (as shown). Actually, the chronic embolus has formed a cast of the pulmonary arterial tree. After the cast has been removed a large amount of back-bleeding occurs. The retrograde blood flow is bright red, which indicates that its source from the bronchial circulation is supplied by the aorta. The arteriotomies are closed. (From Wolfe, W. G., and Sabiston, D. C., Jr.: Pulmonary embolism. *In* Ebert, P. A. [ed]: Major Problems in Clinical Surgery. Vol. 25. Philadelphia, W. B. Saunders Company, 1980.)

and the left pulmonary artery and its branches is shown in Figure 5. These emboli are densely adherent to the wall of the pulmonary artery, and great care must be taken in the dissection. All distal emboli should be removed until there is adequate back-bleeding of bright red blood. It is often preferable to close the arteriotomy with a pericardial patch to prevent constriction of the lumen. It is usually necessary to make a counterincision in the distal pulmonary artery to remove completely the adherent emboli in the secondary and tertiary branches of the pulmonary arteries (Fig. 6). Typical specimens removed at operation are shown in Figure 7.

Satisfactory distal back-bleeding can usually be predicted in advance from the information gained by the thoracic aortogram with selective injection of the bronchial arteries. These arteries are often dilated and tortuous and fill the distal pulmonary arterial circuit in a retrograde manner.

Postoperative Complications

Postoperative complications include right ventricular failure in patients with long-standing cor pulmonale and pulmonary hypertension. One patient in the authors' series died of this cause 3 days after operation despite removal of the chronic pulmonary emboli. Another complication that has been described is the hemorrhagic lung syndrome.

After embolectomy and after re-establishment of pulmonary blood flow, massive parenchymal and *intrabronchial hemorrhage* ("postperfusion bleeding") may occur during or after cardiopulmonary bypass. Successful management of this complication can be achieved by the use of a Carlens (Broncho-Cath) catheter for tracheal intubation.[27] A Fogarty catheter is inserted to occlude the right or left mainstem bronchus and tamponade the blood within the lumen until appropriate blood coagulation can be achieved. The bleeding usually ceases when protamine is

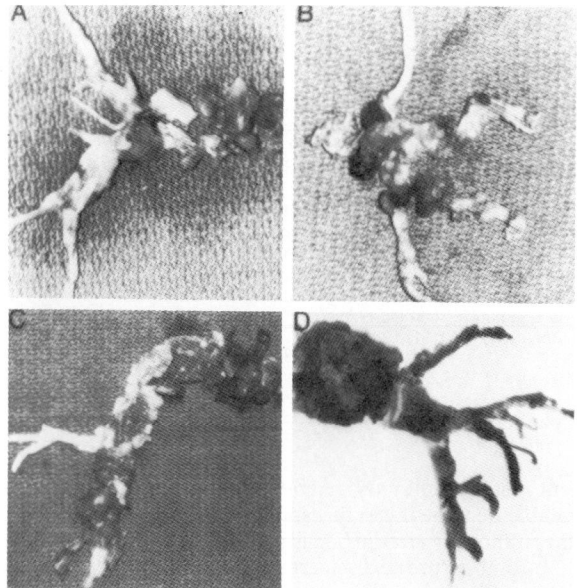

Figure 7. Chronic emboli removed from four patients undergoing pulmonary embolectomy. Patients (specimens shown in *A* to *C*) had embolectomy via thoracotomy and localized lobar pulmonary artery occlusion. One patient (specimen shown in *D*) required cardiopulmonary bypass because of very proximal pulmonary artery involvement. Note the tenacious fibrotic material extended into the segmental vessels. In most patients, distal branches could be embolectomized. (From Chitwood, W. R., Jr., Lyerly, H. K., and Sabiston, D. C., Jr.: Surgical management of chronic pulmonary embolism. Ann. Surg., *201*:11, 1985.)

injected to counteract the heparin used during cardiopulmonary bypass.

Other postoperative complications include phrenic nerve paresis following use of deep hypothermia and psychiatric disturbances that are usually transient.

Postoperative Results

Embolectomy for chronic pulmonary embolism generally causes a decrease in pulmonary artery pressures along with an increase in Pa_{O_2} toward normal (Fig. 8). In this series, 22 patients had embolectomy. Long-term follow-up data show that the NYHA functional class of most patients changed dramatically, moving from Class III or IV to Class I in most cases and in others to Class II, only one patient showing a change from Class IV to Class III postoperatively (Fig. 9). These data, combined with that of other similar series in the literature, indicate favorable results. A long-term follow-up arteriogram is shown in Figure 10.

Arterial Blood Gases (N=17)

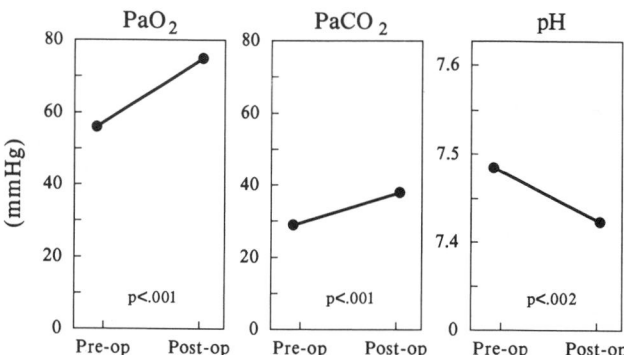

Figure 8. In the present series, arterial blood gases are shown before and after embolectomy. All values were statistically significant ($p < 0.05$). (From Lyerly, H. K., and Sabiston, D. C., Jr.: Chronic pulmonary embolism. *In* Sabiston, D. C., Jr., and Spencer, F. C.: Surgery of the Chest, 5th ed. Philadelphia, W. B. Saunders Company, 1990.)

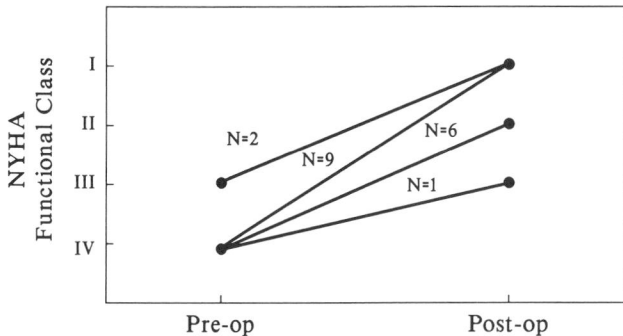

Figure 9. Preoperative and postoperative functional class of 13 patients having successful pulmonary embolectomy (NYHA = New York Heart Association). (From Lyerly, H. K., and Sabiston, D. C., Jr.: Chronic pulmonary embolism. *In* Sabiston, D. C., Jr., and Spencer, F. C.: Surgery of the Chest. Philadelphia, W. B. Saunders Company, 1990.)

In contradistinction, those patients found unsuitable for embolectomy have a poor prognosis. In this group, 3 of 11 patients died, and the majority of the survivors are currently disabled at rest.

DISCUSSION

Most patients with pulmonary embolism have an active fibrinolytic system responsible for the rapid resolution of pulmonary emboli. Therefore, most pulmonary emboli present as acute clinical problems. Experimental studies have shown that by 21 days after embolism major perfusion defects are usually resolved almost completely.[55] Clinical studies using pulmonary scans and arteriograms have shown that complete resolution of pulmonary emboli may occur as early as 8 to 14 days after the clinical event, although in some patients this response may be delayed for several months and may uncommonly persist for months, especially in the presence of congestive heart failure.[13,42,46,51] In most patients, the natural fibrinolytic sequences occur with resolution of the emboli and few if any long-term symptoms or residual effects.

A few patients may develop recurrent pulmonary emboli. As many as 16 per cent of patients with pulmonary emboli have been shown to have continued pathologic evidence of emboli as a long-term phenomenon, although most of these chronic changes do not produce pulmonary hypertension.[19] In one series, 22 per cent of patients had findings of unresolved emboli, and in only 2 per cent did chronic cor pulmonale actually

develop.[36] In this small group, recurrent attacks of pulmonary emboli without resolution led to a syndrome of chronic pulmonary hypertension and ensuing complications.

Failure of the emboli to resolve is thought to be the result of inadequate fibrinolysis. Deficiencies of coagulation inhibitors cause an inability to regulate intravascular clot formation. Antithrombin III (AT-III) is a protein essential for coagulation hemostasis. It is released during coagulation and inactivates thrombin and other serine proteases.[9] Patients with deficiencies of AT-III have a hypercoagulable state clinically manifested by recurrent thrombosis and pulmonary emboli. Deficiencies of activated protein C, which inhibits factors V and IV, and protein S, which serves as a cofactor for activated factor C, have also been reported to lead to an increased incidence of thromoembolism.[8,22] In addition to inadequate fibrinolysis, embolization of previously organized thrombi that are resistant to resolution may be another cause of chronic pulmonary emboli, but this has not been proved.

Adequate anticoagulation in patients with chronic emboli decreases the number of recurrent episodes of emboli to the pulmonary circulation. Despite anticoagulation, a few patients continue to have showers of emboli in the absence of significant resolution, which may proceed to major pulmonary arterial obstruction. Pulmonary hypertension is present in 0.5 to 0.4 per cent of these patients.[15,24,45]

In the presence of chronic pulmonary hypertension, the actual role of thromboembolism is controversial. Although repeated pulmonary embolism is thought to be the usual underlying cause, there is little clinical evidence to support this theory.[37] Studies of the endothelium of the pulmonary vasculature have shown that permutations of the normal endothelium can create a procoagulant environment that could lead to the development of thrombus *in situ* at the level of the large or smaller pulmonary vessels. Some patients develop proximal pulmonary thromboemboli, which may cause retrograde propagation of the thrombi after the initial pulmonary embolism. Other patients present with unexplained pulmonary hypertension secondary to thrombotic occlusion of the pulmonary microvasculature. A perfusion pulmonary scan shows abnormalities that should provide the correct clinical diagnosis and confirmatory evaluation. Thromboendarterectomy in selected patients provides dramatic clinical improvement in those with proximal thromboemboli. Vasodilators may be effective in some patients with obstruction at the arteriolar level. Both groups should be treated with chronic warfarin anticoagulant therapy to protect against progression of thromboembolism.

Medical management of chronic pulmonary emboli includes

Figure 10. *A,* Pulmonary arteriogram in a patient before embolectomy. *B,* Six years after right lower lobe embolectomy. Note the continued perfusion of the right lower lobe after embolectomy. (From Chitwood, W. R., Jr., Lyerly, H. K., and Sabiston, D. C., Jr.: Surgical management of chronic pulmonary embolism. Ann. Surg., *201:*11, 1985.)

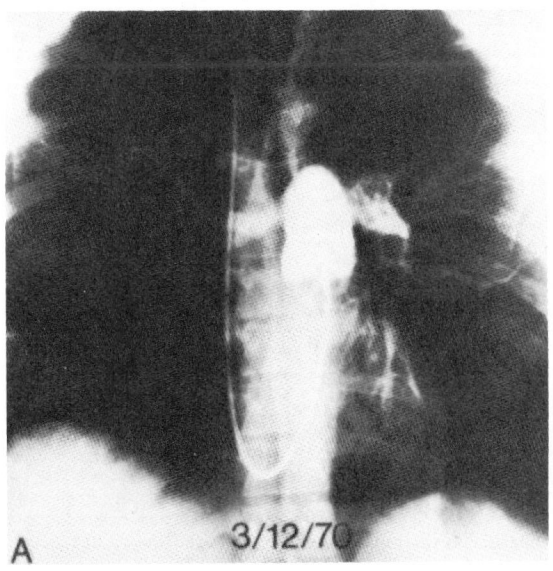
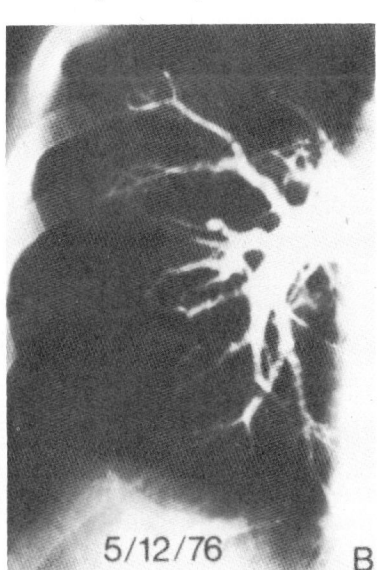

a number of fibrinolytic and vasodilating agents, although they are thus far mainly ineffective.[14,34,39,40] Plasminogen activation has been shown to provide local thrombinolysis of relatively old thrombi in peripheral veins and may lead to the future resolution of chronic pulmonary emboli.[52] However, the organized emboli with ingrowth of fibroblasts may be resistant to any form of thrombolytic therapy.

A group of patients were reported with pulmonary embolectomy for chronic pulmonary emboli. In Group A (n = 16), myocardial protection consisted of single-dose crystalloid cardioplegia followed by pericardial irrigation with cold saline. Extrapericardial dissection of the pulmonary arteries was performed. In Group B (n = 7), the treatment was the same as for Group A except for the substitution of saline slush contained in a laparotomy pad for iced saline. In Group C (n = 18), myocardial protection was achieved by single-dose blood cardioplegia followed by the application of a specially designed cooling jacket to the right and left ventricles. Another modification was the use of intrapericardial dissection of the pulmonary arteries with extension of the dissection into the hilar tissues without entrance into either pleural cavity. The hospital mortality of the groups was as follows: Group A, 18.7 per cent; Group B, 14.3 per cent; and Group C, 5.5 per cent (no statistically significant difference). However, some significant differences ($P < 0.05$) among the groups were observed: phrenic nerve paresis occurred in 5 of 7 (71 per cent) Group B patients, but none in Group A or C; and patients in Group B required ventilatory support for 32.2 days, compared with 8.4 days for Group A and 6.2 days for Group C. The time spent in the intensive care unit was 36 days for patients in Group B, compared with 13 days for patients in Group A and 10.3 days for patients in Group C. Pulmonary vascular resistance decreased 59 per cent (649 versus 259) intraoperatively in 13 patients in Group C. These authors believe that simultaneous bilateral pulmonary thromboendarterectomy by means of a median sternotomy, cardiopulmonary bypass, deep hypothermia with circulatory arrest, and modified methods of myocardial preservation and intrapericardial dissection of the pulmonary arteries constitutes the optimal surgical procedure.

In summary, selected patients with symptoms of severe respiratory insufficiency, hypoxemia, and pulmonary hypertension with proximal pulmonary arterial occlusion and adequate bronchial collateral circulation with minimally impaired right ventricular function are appropriate candidates for surgical embolectomy. However, patients with this syndrome and with distal pulmonary emboli in the small arterial branches with patent proximal vessels, as well as patients with severe right ventricular failure and massive obesity, are generally unsuitable for surgical management. Long-term follow-up of patients with operable pulmonary emboli shows favorable respiratory and cardiodynamic changes. These patients have relief of incapacitating symptoms and maintain clinical improvement for prolonged periods.

SELECTED REFERENCES

Cabrol, C., Cabrol, A., Acar, J., et al.: Surgical correction of chronic postembolic obstructions of the pulmonary arteries. J. Thorac. Cardiovasc. Surg., 76:620, 1978.
  This article reports a relatively large series of patients with chronic pulmonary embolism managed by embolectomy. Discussion is directed toward diagnosis, details of surgical management, and the results.

Chitwood, W. R., Jr., Lyerly, H. K., and Sabiston, D. C., Jr.: Surgical management of chronic pulmonary embolism. Ann. Surg., 201:11, 1985.
  This is a report of the experience of a large series of patients in the United States on surgical management of chronic pulmonary embolism. The clinical manifestations, management, and results are evaluated in detail.

REFERENCES

 1. Abrams, M. L.: Angiography in pulmonary embolism. In Greenspan, R. H. (Ed.): Abrams Angiography. Boston, Little, Brown and Company, 1983, p. 803.

 2. Allison, P. R., Dunnill, M. S., and Marshall, R.: Pulmonary embolism. Thorax, 15:273, 1960.
 3. Benaim, R., Calvo, G., Fischler, M., and Chiche, P.: Les thromboembolies subaigues ou chroniques de l'artè pulmonaire: La place due traitement fibrinolytique. Ann. Med. Interne, 127:767, 1978.
 4. Brenner, O.: Pathology of the pulmonary circulation. Arch. Intern. Med., 56:1189, 1935.
 5. Cabrol, C., Cabrol, A., Acar, J., et al.: Surgical correction of chronic postembolic obstruction of the pulmonary arteries. J. Thorac. Cardiovasc. Surg., 76:620, 1978.
 6. Carroll, D.: Chronic obstruction of major pulmonary arteries. Am. J. Med., 9:175, 1950.
 7. Chitwood, W. R., Jr., Lyerly, H. K., and Sabiston, D. C., Jr.: Surgical management of chronic pulmonary embolism. Ann. Surg., 201:11, 1985.
 8. Comp, P. C., and Esmon, C. T.: Recurrent venous thromboembolism in patients with a partial deficiency of protein S. N. Engl. J. Med., 311:1525, 1984.
 9. Cosgriff, T. M., Bishop, D. T., Hershgold, E. J., et al.: Familial Antithrombin III deficiency: Its natural history, genetics, diagnosis and treatment. Medicine, 62:209, 1983.
10. Couves, C. M., Makai, S. S., Sterns, L. P., et al.: Hemorrhagic lung syndrome. Ann. Thorac. Surg., 15:187, 1973.
11. Daily, P. O., Dembitsky, W. P., Peterson, K. L., and Moser, K. M.: Modifications of techniques and early results of pulmonary thromboendarterectomy for chronic pulmonary embolism. J. Thorac. Cardiovasc. Surg., 93:221, 1987.

12. Dalen, J. E., and Alpert, J. S.: Natural history of pulmonary embolism. Prog. Cardiovasc. Dis., 17:259, 1975.
13. Dalen, J. E., Banas, J. S., Jr., Brooks, H. L., et al.: Resolution rate of acute pulmonary embolism in man. N. Engl. J. Med., 280:1194, 1969.
14. Dash, H., Ballentine, N., and Zelis, R.: Vasodilators ineffective in secondary pulmonary hypertension. N. Engl. J. Med., 303:1062, 1980.
15. deSoyza, W. D., and Murphy, M. L.: Persistent post-embolic pulmonary hypertension. Chest, 62:665, 1972.
16. Dor, V., Jourdan, J., Schmitt, R., et al.: Delayed pulmonary thrombectomy via a peripheral approach in the treatment of pulmonary embolism and sequelae. Thorac. Cardiovasc. Surg., 29:227, 1981.
17. Elliott, J. A.: Fatal massive haemoptysis after embolectomy for chronic pulmonary embolism. Thorax, 35:705, 1980.
18. Fleishner, F. G.: Recurrent pulmonary embolism and cor pulmonale. N. Engl. J. Med., 276:1213, 1967.
19. Freiman, D. G., Suyemoto, J., and Wessler, S.: Frequency of pulmonary thromboembolism in man. N. Engl. J. Med., 272:1278, 1965.
20. Garvey, J. W., Wisoff, G., and Voletti, C.: Haemorrhagic pulmonary edema: Post-pulmonary embolectomy. Thorax, 31:605, 1976.
21. Goodwin, J. F., Harrison, C. V., and Wilcken, D. E. L.: Obliterative pulmonary hypertension and thromboembolism. Br. Med. J., 16:701, 1963.
22. Griffin, J. H., Bezeaud, A., Evatt, B., and Mosher, D.: Functional and immunologic studies of protein C in thromboembolic disease. Blood, 62:1, 1983.
23. Gurewich, V., Thomas, D. P., and Rabinov, K. R.: Pulmonary embolism after ligation of the inferior vena cava. N. Engl. J. Med., 274:1350, 1966.
24. Hollister, L. E., and Cull, V. L.: The syndrome of chronic thrombosis of the major pulmonary arteries. Am. J. Med., 21:312, 1956.
25. Kapitan, K. S., Buchbinder, M., Wagner, P. D., and Moser, K. M.: Mechanisms of hypoxemia in chronic thromboembolic pulmonary hypertension. Department of Medicine, UCSD Medical Center, San Diego, California. June, 1988 and November 1988.
26. Ljungdahl, M.: Bibt es eine chronische embolistierung der lungen arterie? Dtsch. Arch. Klin. Med., 120:1, 1928.
27. Lyerly, H. K., Reves, J. G., and Sabiston, J. D., Jr.: Primary sarcomas of the pulmonary artery and management of intrabronchial hemorrhage. Surg. Gynecol. Obstet., 163:291, 1986.
28. McIntyre, K. M., and Sarahara, A. A.: The hemodynamic response to pulmonary embolism in patients without prior cardiopulmonary disease. Am. J. Cardiol., 28:288, 1971.
29. Mills, S. R., Jackson, D. C., Older, R. A., et al.: The incidence, etiologies, and avoidance of the complications of pulmonary angiography in a large series. Radiology, 136:295, 1980.
30. Mills, S. R., Jackson, D. C., Sullivan, D. C., et al.: Angiographic evaluation of chronic pulmonary embolism. Radiology, 136:301, 1980.
31. Moser, K. M., Olson, L. K., Schlusselberg, M., Daily, P. O., and Dembitsky, W. P.: Chronic thromboembolic occlusion in the adult can mimic pulmonary artery agenesis. Chest, 95:503, 1989.
32. Moser, K. M.: Pulmonary Vascular Disease. New York, Marcel Dekker, 1979.
33. Moser, K. M., Daily, P. A., Peterson, K., Dembitsky, W., Vapnek, J. M., Shure, D., Utley, J., and Archibald, C.: Thromboendarterectomy for chronic, major-vessel thromboembolic pulmonary hypertension: Immediate and long-term results in 42 patients. Ann. Intern. Med., 107:560, 1987.
34. Olukotun, A. Y.: Vasodilator therapy for pulmonary hypertension (letter). N. Engl. J. Med., 302:1261, 1980.
35. Owen, W. R., Thomas, W. A., Castleman, B., and Bland, E. F.: Unrecognized emboli to the lungs with subsequent cor pulmonale. N. Engl. J. Med., 249:919, 1953.
36. Parakos, J. A., Adelstein, S. J., Smith, R. E., et al.: Late prognosis of acute pulmonary embolism. N. Engl. J. Med., 289:55, 1973.
37. Rich, S., Levitsky, S., and Brundage, B. H.: Pulmonary hypertension in chronic pulmonary thromboembolism. Ann. Intern. Med. 108:425, 1988.
38. Riedel, M., Stanek, V., Widimsky, J., and Prerovsky, I.: Long-term follow-up

of patients with pulmonary thromboembolism: Late prognosis and evaluation of hemodynamic and respiratory data. Chest, *81*:151, 1982.

39. Rubin, L. J., and Peter, R. H.: Oral hydralazine therapy for primary pulmonary hypertension. N. Engl. J. Med., *302*:69, 1980.

40. Ruskin, J. N., and Hutter, A. M.: Primary pulmonary hypertension treated with oral phentolamine. Ann. Intern. Med., *90*:772, 1979.

41. Sabiston, D. C., Jr., Wolfe, W. G., Oldham, H. N., et al.: Surgical management of chronic pulmonary embolism. Ann. Surg., *185*:699, 1977.

42. Sasahara, A. A., and Hyers, T. M.: Urokinase pulmonary embolism trial: A national cooperative study. Circulation, *47*:38, 1973.

43. Silver, D., and Sabiston, D. C., Jr.: The role of vena caval interruption in the management of pulmonary embolism. Surgery, *77*:1, 1975.

44. Sutton, G. C., Hall, R. J. C., and Kerr, I. H.: Clinical course and late prognosis of subacute massive, acute minor, and chronic pulmonary thromboembolism. Br. Heart J., *39*:1135, 1977.

45. Tilkian, A. G., Schroeder, J. S., and Robin, E. D.: Chronic thromboembolic occlusion of main pulmonary artery or primary branches: Case report and review of the literature. Am. J. Med., *60*:563, 1976.

46. Tow, F. R., and Wagner, H. N., Jr.: Recovery of pulmonary arterial blood flow in patients with pulmonary embolism. N. Engl. J. Med., *276*:1053, 1976.

47. Utley, J. R., Spragg, R. G., Long, W. B., and Moser, K. M.: Pulmonary endarterectomy for chronic obstruction: Recent surgical experience. Surgery, *92*:1096, 1982.

48. Viamonte, M.: Selective bronchial arteriography in man. Radiology, *83*:830, 1964.

49. Viamonte, M., Parks, R. E., and Smoak, W. M., III: Guided catheterization of the bronchial arteries. Radiology, *85*:205, 1965.

50. Virchow, R.: Uber die standpunkte in der wissenschaftlichen medcin. Virchows Arch. [A], *1*:1, 1847.

51. Wagenvoort, C. A., and Wagenvoort, N.: Pathology of Pulmonary Hypertension. New York, John Wiley & Sons, 1977, p. 143.

52. Weimar, W., Stibbe, J., van Seyen, A. J., Billau, A., DeSomer, P., and Collen, D.: Specific lysis of an ileofemoral thrombus by administration of extrinsic (tissue-type) plasminogen activator. Lancet, *2*:1018, 1981.

53. Wilhelmsen, L., Hagman, M., and Werko, L.: Recurrent pulmonary embolism: Incidence, predisposing factors, and prognosis. Acta Med. Scand., *192*:565, 1972.

54. Wolfe, W. G., and Sabiston, D. C., Jr.: Radioactive ventilation scanning in the diagnosis of pulmonary embolism. J. Thorac. Cardiovasc. Surg., *55*:149, 1968.

55. Wolfe, W. G., and Sabiston, D. C., Jr.: Pulmonary Embolism: Major Problems in Clinical Surgery. Philadelphia, W. B. Saunders Company, 1980.

56. Woodruff, W. W., III, Hoeck, B. E., Chitwood, W. R., Jr., et al.: Radiographic findings in pulmonary hypertension from unresolved embolism. A.J.R., *144*:681, 1985.

51

FAT EMBOLI SYNDROME

Joseph A. Moylan, M.D.

Posttraumatic respiratory insufficiency, along with sepsis, remains the leading cause of morbidity and mortality following severe injury. During the first week following major trauma, the causes of posttraumatic respiratory insufficiency include pulmonary contusion, fat emboli syndrome, and shock lung. Complications of fat emboli syndrome were first described in 1862, when Bergmann reported a triad of confusion, dyspnea, and petechiae following long bone fractures.[5] Dennis, in his book *Systems of Surgery*, emphasized fat emboli as a major cause of death, particularly in the first 3 days after injury.[10] A variety of therapies have been suggested, beginning with ethyl alcohol[13] and ranging to the present-day administration of steroids.[1] The importance of the morbidity and mortality resulting from this postinjury complication was highlighted by military conflict, from World War I through the Korean War.[17,25,29] Some series describing civilian trauma have reported incidences of this syndrome as high as 80 per cent,[26] although most reports have documented the incidence at approximately 35 per cent.[9]

Pathophysiology of Fat Embolism

Two major theories about the pathophysiology and classification of fat embolization have been promulgated. The mechanical theory offered by Gauss[12] in 1924 has many supporters, including Morton and Kendall,[20] and Arnim and Grant.[2] This thesis supports mobilization of fat from the marrow at the site of a fracture, which produces ischemia and hemorrhagic changes due to temporary occlusion of the pulmonary circulation. Pathologic and animal studies have demonstrated gross fat particles in the pulmonary capillaries.

The physiochemical theory, proposed by Lehmann and Moore, suggests that neutral fat stores in the marrow cavity release free fatty acids (FFAs) that are shown to have a toxic effect in a variety of tissues, especially the lung.[16] Refinement of the theory by Peltier showed that free fatty acids, which derive from either hydrolysis of neutral fats by lipase or mobilization of fat stores by catecholamines, produce alterations in the capillary alveolar membrane as well as changes in lung surfactant production.[24] The end results of the phenomenon are hemorrhage, edema, and alveolar collapse. A correlation between elevated free fatty acids and the severity of the fat emboli syndrome has been documented in the literature[22] (Table 1).

Classification and grading of fat emboli syndrome have been attempted both clinically and pathologically. One method is the respiratory distress index (RDI):

$$RDI = \frac{Po_2}{Fio_2} (VF + PF)$$

$$VF = 1 \text{ (without mechanical ventilation)}$$
$$= 1.5 \text{ (with mechanical ventilation)}$$

$$PF = 0 \text{ (PEEP = less than 5 cm. } H_2O)$$
$$= 0.5 \text{ (PEEP = greater than 5 cm. } H_2O).$$

A method of grading the impact of severity of the fat emboli syndrome has been described.[21] Correlation between increasing levels of free fatty acids and the severity of pulmonary dysfunction has been statistically documented. The grading of chest films and other parameters has not been satisfactory in describing the severity of this disease process. Pathologically, reliable grading of fat emboli has not been established. Attempts to classify embolic phenomena by size and distribution have been met with marked variance, making this method ineffective. Use of a quantitative image analysis of size and location of fat emboli is promising; however, further work in this area is needed.[7]

Experimentally, unbound free fatty acids have been shown to produce significant pulmonary decompensation in a variety of animal models. Studies with oleic acid by Kreis and associates[15] and others by Cahill and colleagues[8] have produced both radiologic and physiologic abnormalities following administration. In clinical studies, the use of albumin as a method for binding free fatty acids has been shown to be effective in decreasing their levels, particularly during the second and third day after injury[21] (Table 2).

Diagnosis

The fat emboli syndrome involves changes in the cerebral, pulmonary, and cutaneous organ systems. Patients exhibit hypoxia, confusion, and petechiae. Classically, petechiae are found over the upper extremities and chest, particularly in the axillary areas, conjunctiva, and uvula. Cerebral signs include confusion, agitation, or stupor, and even coma. Respiratory abnormalities begin with tachypnea and may progress to profound hypoxia and cardiac arrest (Fig. 1).

The peak incidence of respiratory insufficiency for pulmonary embolization is on the second to fourth day after injury. Other causes, such as contusion and shock lung, either precede or follow this time period. There is no predilection for development of this morbid complication based on age or sex; however, the percentage is higher in male patients due to the higher frequency of occupational and recreational exposure to multisystem trauma.

The diagnosis is made using a combination of laboratory and clinical parameters. Clinical indicators include a history of skeletal trauma, the presence of posttraumatic shock, respiratory

TABLE 1. FFA Inverse Relationship to the Respiratory Distress Index (RDI)*

FFA (mmol./L.)	RDI	FFA (mmol./L.)	RDI
88	3.0	175	1.6
110	1.8	185	2.1
134	2.8	198	1.8
165	3.2	235	1.0
166	3.2	321	1.7
173	4.1	352	1.7
		360	1.4
		384	1.5

* $p < 0.01$.

TABLE 2. FFA Levels in Patients With and Without Albumin Administration

Postoperative Day	Serum FFA (4 mmol./L.) (Mean ± SEM)				
	1	2	3	4	5
No albumin (n = 24)	356 ± 34	356 ± 31	280 ± 33	271 ± 38	239 ± 37
Albumin (n = 20)	354 ± 62	301 ± 48	260 ± 34	222 ± 30	153 ± 16

distress, change in cerebral function, and appearance of petechiae in classic distribution. A number of laboratory tests provide additional confirmation. Chest films demonstrate bilateral fluffy densities similar to those found following congestive heart failure with pulmonary edema (Fig. 2). Although the initial chest film may be abnormal in only 30 per cent of the patients with respiratory distress, over the subsequent 24 hours almost all patients develop radiologic abnormalities.

Another important laboratory test is the arterial Po_2. An arterial Po_2 of less than 60 mm. Hg on room air is highly suggestive of respiratory distress and, when coupled with a positive history and chest film, is indicative of the fat emboli syndrome. This laboratory test is also valuable for following the course of the disease. Initially, the pH may be increased and the Pco_2 slightly decreased secondary to hyperventilation; however, further deterioration may produce serious hypoxia, hypercapnia, and respiratory acidosis.

Fat globules found in the urine were initially thought to be syndrome-specific; however, further investigations have shown that most patients with major trauma involving long bones have urinary fat globules whether or not they develop the fat emboli syndrome.[19] However, the absence of fat in the urine makes the diagnosis of fat emboli unlikely.

Electrocardiographic changes are usually nonspecific and include prominent S waves in lead 1, prominent Q waves in lead 3, ST segment depression, and right axis strain, all indicative of increasing pulmonary resistance.

Thrombocytopenia, hypofibrinogenemia, and prolongation of the partial thromboplastin time have been reported in patients with the fat emboli syndrome. These changes, however, are not disease specific and may relate more to the primary problem of multisystem injury in major trauma.[18] Other serum tests, such as serum lipase or tributyrinase levels, do not appear to correlate well with either elevated free fatty acid levels or progressive respiratory failure.[14,23] On an experimental basis, serum free fatty acid levels correlate very well with increasing severe pulmonary insufficiency. Unbound free fatty acids appear to reach their nadir at approximately 48 hours after injury, which correlates well with the onset of the fat emboli syndrome.

Prevention and Treatment

Recent clinical experience has shown that the incidence of fat emboli syndrome can be reduced and prevented by careful stabilization of fractures and the treatment of shock. The use of air splints at the scene of the accident and early operative intervention with intramedullary nailing and fracture plating have decreased the incidence of complications associated with the fat emboli syndrome.[18,30] The aggressive treatment of hypovolemic shock has also contributed to reduced incidence. The use of albumin to bind circulating free fatty acids has been particularly beneficial in the first 24 to 72 hours in reducing the incidence of posttraumatic respiratory distress secondary to this complication. Other agents, such as alcohol[20] and heparin, have never been effective and actually may produce significant complications, such as bleeding with heparin administration.

The role of corticosteroids remains controversial. In the late 1960s, steroids were thought to be effective in minimizing the morbidity and mortality of fat emboli syndrome.[3] Some have suggested the use of prophylactic steroids in high-risk groups of patients.[27] Some side effects of steroids, including stress bleeding and increased infection due to suppression of immune competence, have made this prophylactic use questionable. Recent double-blind studies with high-dose methylprednisolone in patients with the respiratory distress syndrome from a variety of causes, including fat emboli, have not shown a beneficial influence on outcome.[6]

Ventilatory support, using a volume respirator with an endotracheal tube and positive end-expiratory pressure (PEEP), remains a primary therapy in stabilizing or reversing posttraumatic pulmonary distress syndrome. PEEP produces an increase in the functional residual capacity and a decrease in pulmonary shunting.[4]

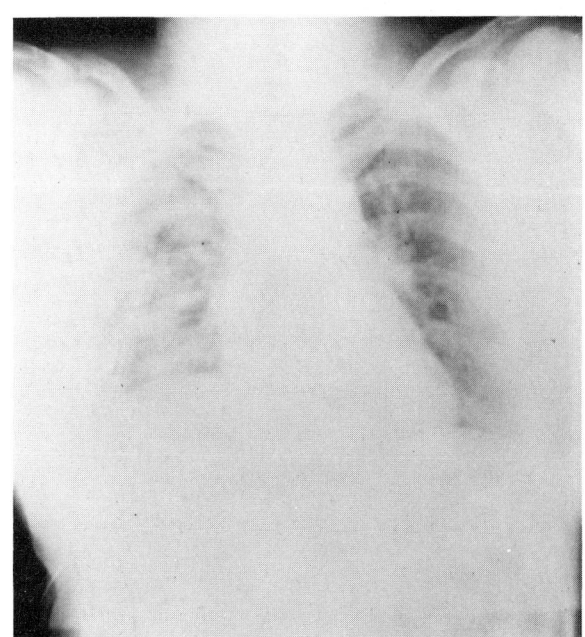

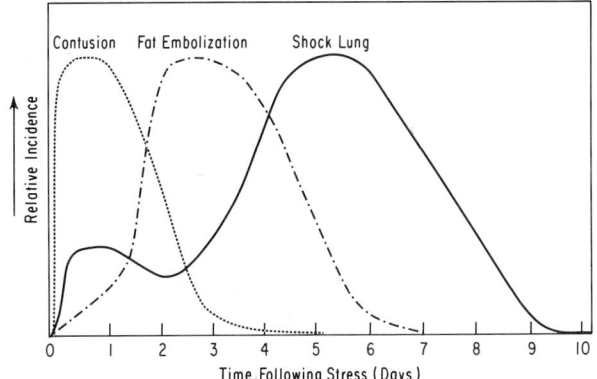

Figure 1. The peak incidence of respiratory insufficiency for fat embolism is between 2 and 4 days after injury. Pulmonary contusion is functionally significant in the first day following chest trauma, and shock lung presents later in the course.

Figure 2. Diffuse, fluffy infiltrate at 72 hours after injury. Patient had progressive hypoxia during the preceding 12-hour period.

With increased attention to the diagnosis and prevention of fat emboli, the high mortality and morbidity associated with this complication of major injury have been markedly reduced. However, vigilance for the development of this posttraumatic syndrome, despite good therapy, is mandatory.

SELECTED REFERENCES

Evarts, C. M.: The fat embolism syndrome: A review. Surg. Clin. North Am., 50:493, 1970.

Peltier, L. F.: The diagnosis and treatment of fat embolism. J. Trauma, 11:661, 1971.

Both references discuss the historical background, the clinical presentation, and the course of fat embolism, with one emphasizing the mechanical theory of the syndrome and the other the physiochemical. Laboratory evaluation and treatment modalities are discussed.

Moylan, J. A., and Evenson, M.: Diagnosis and treatment of fat embolism. Annu. Rev. Med., 28:85, 1977.

A complete review, including basic science and the clinical approach to the patient with fat emboli, with emphasis on prognosis and treatment.

REFERENCES

1. Alho, A., Saikkon, K., Eerola, P., and Koskinen, M.: Corticosteroids in patients with a high risk of fat embolism syndrome. Surg. Gynecol. Obstet., 147:358, 1978.
2. Arnim, J., and Grant, R. E.: Observations on gross pulmonary fat embolism in man and in the rabbit. Can. J. Surg., 9:286, 1966.
3. Ashbaugh, D. G., and Petty, T. L.: The use of corticosteroids in the treatment of respiratory failure associated with massive fat embolism. Surg. Gynecol. Obstet., 123:493, 1966.
4. Ashbaugh, D. G., and Petty, T. L.: Positive end-expiratory pressure: Physiology, indications and contraindications. J. Thorac. Cardiovasc. Surg., 65:165, 1973.
5. Bergmann, E. B.: Ein Fall todlicher fetlenbolic. Berl. Klin. Wochenschr., 1873, p. 10385.
6. Bernar, G. R., Luce, J., Sprung, C. L., Rinaldo, J. E., Tate, R. M., Sibbaild, W. J., Kariman, K., Higgins, S., Bradley, R., Metz, C. A., Harris, T. R., and Brigham, K. L.: High-dose corticosteroids in patients with adult respiratory distress syndrome. N. Engl. J. Med., 317:1565, 1987.
7. Bunai, Y., Yoshimi, N., Komorija, H., Iwasa, M., and Ohya, I.: An application of a quantitative analytical system for grading pulmonary fat emboli. Forensic Sci. Int., 39:263, 1988.
8. Cahill, J. M., Daly, B. F. T., and Byrne, J. J.: Ventilatory and circulatory response to oleic acid embolus. J. Trauma, 14:73, 1974.
9. Chan, K. M., Tham, K. T., Chiu, H. S., Chow, Y. N., and Leung, P. C.: Post-traumatic fat embolism—its clinical and subclinical presentations. J. Trauma, 24:45, 1984.
10. Dennis, F. S.: Systems of Surgery, Vol. 1. Philadelphia, Lea Brothers & Company, 1895, p. 533.
11. Fenger, C., and Salisbury, J. H.: Diffuse multiple capillary fat embolism in the lungs and brain is a fatal complication in common fracture: Illustrated by a case. Chicago Med. J. Examiner, 39:587, 1879.
12. Gauss, H.: The pathology of fat embolism. Arch. Surg., 9:593, 1924.
13. Hermann, L. G.: Effect of dextrose alcohol mixture upon pulmonary fat embolism. Proc. Soc. Exp. Biol. Med., 30:588, 1932–1933.
14. Herndon, J. H., Riseborough, E. J., and Fischer, J. E.: Fat embolism, a review of current concepts. J. Trauma, 11:673, 1971.
15. Kreis, W. R., Lindenaur, S. M., and Dent, T. L.: Corticosteroids in experimental fat embolization. J. Surg. Res., 14:238, 1973.
16. Lehmann, E. P., and Moore, R. M.: Fat embolism, including experimental production with trauma. Arch. Surg., 14:621, 1927.
17. Malloy, T. B., Sullivan, E. R., Burnett, C. H., et al.: The general pathology of traumatic shock. Surgery, 27:627, 1950.
18. Manning, J. B., Bach, A. W., Herman, C. M., and Carrico, C. J.: Fat release after femur nailing in the dog. J. Trauma, 23:322, 1983.
19. Morton, K. S.: Fat embolism: Incidence of urinary fat in trauma. Can. Med. Assoc. J., 74:441, 1956.
20. Morton, K. S., and Kendall, M. J.: The failure of intravenous alcohol in the treatment of experimental pulmonary fat embolism. Can. J. Surg., 9:286, 1966.
21. Moylan, J. A.: Fat emboli syndrome. *In* Sabiston, D. C., Jr. (Ed.): Textbook of Surgery: The Biological Basis of Modern Surgical Practice. Philadelphia, W. B. Saunders Company, 1986, p. 1768.
22. Moylan, J. A., Evenson, M. E., and Birnbaum, M.: Fat emboli syndrome. J. Trauma, 16:339, 1976.
23. Peltier, J. F.: Fat embolism: The prophylactic value of a tourniquet. J. Bone Joint Surg., 38A:385, 1956.
24. Peltier, L. F.: Fat embolism: The toxic properties of neutral fat and free fatty acids. Surgery, 40:665, 1956.
25. Scully, R. E.: Fat embolism in Korean battle casualties; Its incidence, clinical significance and pathologic aspects. Am. J. Pathol., 32:379, 1956.
26. Sevitt, S.: Fat embolism. London, Butterworths, 1962.
27. Shier, M. R., Wilson, R. F., James, R. E., et al.: Fat embolism prophylaxis: A study of four treatment modalities. J. Trauma, 17:721, 1977.
28. Stitt, R. W., and Adler, F.: The effects of corticosteroids on lung surfactant activity in experimentally produced fat embolism in rats. Surg. Forum, 28:492, 1977.
29. Sutton, G. E.: Pulmonary fat embolism and its relation to traumatic shock. Br. Med. J., 2:368, 1918.
30. Talucci, R. D., Manning, J. B., Lampard, S., Bach, A., and Carrico, C. J.: Early intramedullary nailing of femoral shaft fractures. Am. J. Surg., 146:107, 1983.
31. Zenker, F. A.: Bertrage zur normalen und pathologischen. Anatomie der Lunger. Dresden, Braunsdorf, 1862.

52

DISORDERS OF THE ARTERIAL SYSTEM

I

INTRODUCTION

David C. Sabiston, Jr., M.D.

The history of surgery is in large part a record of its technical advances, and the development of surgical control of the *arterial* system represents one of the most important of its achievements. Of significance is the fact that within the past several decades vascular surgery has reached a high level of accomplishment. Direct operations on arteries and the use of autografts, arterial prostheses, and extracorporeal circulation form the basis for many brilliant surgical procedures.

Hemostasis is recorded in ancient Chinese literature where bandaging and use of styptics were advocated. During the era of Hippocrates, ligation of vessels was rarely practiced, and amputations were done only through a gangrenous extremity at a site where the vessels were thrombosed to assure that significant bleeding did not occur. Celsus recommended amputation at the line of demarcation, but again most of the vessels at this level were thrombosed. At that time he advocated limited use of ligatures of Celtic linen. In about A.D. 100, Archigenes was more daring and advanced the scope of amputation significantly by proposing that it be performed for "gangrene, necrosis, cancer, and certain callous tumors." Antyllus contributed by recommending surgical treatment of aneurysms by proximal ligation of the arteries. Despite these advances, the ligature was rarely used for amputations and then only as a last resort, preference being given to the hot, searing cautery for achieving hemostasis.

Paré rediscovered the ligature and used it, rather than the hot iron, to control hemorrhage in amputating the leg of an officer wounded at the siege of Danvilliers in 1552. This procedure prompted Paré to state, "I dressed him and God healed him. He returned home gaily with a wooden leg saying that he had got off cheaply without being miserably burned to stop the bleeding." This operation initiated the beginning of the standard use of the ligature to control arterial bleeding, and Paré deserves great credit for reintroducing a forgotten principle. An excellent account of the historical facts concerning control of bleeding and the development of ligatures is found in *The History of Hemostasis* by Harvey.[11]

To William Hunter is due recognition for his dissections of aneurysms and recommendations for proximal arterial ligature to control them. He also was the first to recognize that an *arteriovenous* aneurysm represented a direct communication between an artery and vein and was not a simple arterial aneurysm. In the next century, Matas first advocated endoaneurysmorrhaphy in the treatment of arterial aneurysms.[12] Another major advance was made by Carrel with the contribution of anastomosis of arteries.[4–6] It was for this and pioneering work in the transplantation of organs that Carrel was awarded the Nobel Prize in 1912. Goyanes was the first to successfully use a venous autograft to replace a popliteal aneurysm in 1906.[10] The following year Lexer inserted a segment of saphenous vein for reconstruction of an axillary-brachial aneurysm following trauma. The first successful venous autograft in the United States was by Bernheim in replacement of a popliteal aneurysm.[2] In discussing the paper, Halsted called it the "ideal operation" for this lesion. Despite these important early contributions, venous autografts were rarely employed until they were used in the Mobile Army Surgical Hospitals in the Korean conflict. At that time venous autografts were used in the management of arterial wounds, especially those in the lower extremities in which gangrene would have occurred, requiring amputation unless venous autografts were inserted to restore arterial continuity.

Brooks reported the use of intra-arterial injection and published beautiful arteriograms utilizing this technique in 1924.[3] In 1927, Moniz used intra-arterial injection of thorium dioxide to outline the cerebral vessels,[13] and dos Santos and associates injected contrast medium directly into the aorta.[14] An aortic abdominal aneurysm was successfully removed and replaced by an arterial homograft for the first time by Dubost in 1951.[8] Later thoracic aneurysms were successfully attacked by DeBakey[7] and Bahnson,[1] and these procedures were greatly augmented by the introduction by Gibbon of successful extracorporeal circulation in 1953.[9] The introduction of prosthetic arterial substitutes began in 1952 when Voorhees and Blakemore first used Vinyon-N; additional study with other materials led to the present-day use of Dacron and Gore-Tex.

SELECTED REFERENCES

Edwards, W. S.: Alexis Carrel's contributions to thoracic surgery. Ann. Thorac. Surg., *35*:111, 1983.

Edwards, W. S.: Alexis Carrel: A century later. Arch. Surg., *124*:1014, 1989.
  The first of these articles is a concise review of Alexis Carrel's contributions to thoracic surgery. The same author updated this subject in the second paper cited above.

Harrison, L. H., Jr.: Historical aspects in the development of venous autografts. Ann. Surg., *183*:101, 1976.
  This is a very commendable and detailed description of the early use of venous autografts by Goyanes, Lexer, Bernheim, and others. These contributions are described and related to other associated achievements.

Harvey, S. C.: The History of Hemostasis. New York, Paul B. Hoeber, 1929.
  This excellent monograph concisely describes the history of surgical approaches to control bleeding and the development of ligatures. It is fascinating and makes excellent reading for all who desire a thorough understanding of this subject.

REFERENCES

1. Bahnson, H. T.: Definitive treatment of saccular aneurysms of the aorta with excision of sac and aortic sutures. Surg. Gynecol. Obstet., *96*:382, 1953.

2. Bernheim, B. M.: The ideal operation for aneurysm of the extremity: Report of a case. Bull. Johns Hopkins Hosp., 27:93, 1916.
3. Brooks, B.: Intra-arterial injection of sodium iodide. J.A.M.A., 82:1016, 1924.
4. Carrel, A.: La technique operatoire des anastomoses vasculaires et la transplantation des visceres. Lyon Med., 98:859, 1902.
5. Carrel, A.: Suture of blood-vessels and transplantation of organs. Nobel Lecture, 1912. In Nobel Lectures in Physiology-Medicine. Vol. 1, New York, American Elsevier Publishing Company, 1967, p. 442.
6. Carrel, A., and Guthrie, C. C.: Uniterminal and biterminal venous transplantations. Surg. Gynecol. Obstet., 2:266, 1906.
7. DeBakey, M. E., and Cooley, D. A.: Successful resection of aneurysm of thoracic aorta and replacement by graft. J.A.M.A., 152:673, 1953.
8. Dubost, C. Allary, M., and Oeconomos, N.: Resection of an aneurysm of the abdominal aorta: Reestablishment of the continuity by a preserved human arterial graft, with results after five months. Arch. Surg., 64:405, 1952.
9. Gibbon, J. H., Jr.: Application of a mechanical heart and lung apparatus to cardiac surgery. Minn. Med., 37:171, 1954.
10. Goyanes, D. J.: Substitution plastica de las arterias por las venae, ó arterioplastia venosa, aplicada, como neuvo metodo, al tratamiento de los aneurismas. El Siglo Medico, Sept. 1, 1906, p. 346; Sept. 8, 1906, p. 561.
11. Harvey, S. C.: The History of Hemostasis. New York, Paul B. Hoeber, 1929.
12. Matas, R.: An operation for the radical cure of aneurysm based upon arteriorrhaphy. Ann. Surg., 37:161, 1903.
13. Moniz, E.: Injections intracarotidiennes et substances injectables opaques aux rayons. X. Presse Med., 2:969, 1927.
14. dos Santos, R., Lamas, A., and Caldas, J.: L'arteriographie des membres, de l'aorte et des ses branches abdominales. Bull. Soc. Nat. Chir., 55:587, 1929.

II

ANATOMY

David C. Sabiston, Jr., M.D.

The arterial system is designed to deliver blood from the heart to the tissues. Arteries may be categorized as (1) large, (2) medium-sized, and (3) small. Arteries less than 100 μ in diameter are termed *arterioles*. The histologic characteristics of the arterial wall are largely dependent upon the size of the vessel. The *large* arteries must withstand the greatest stress and pressure and therefore contain considerable *elastic tissue* in their walls. The *medium-sized* arteries have less elastic tissue and more *smooth muscle*. At the level of the arteriole, elastic tissue is scant or absent. *Collagen* is present in all parts of the arterial system, the collagen ratio becoming dominant as the arteries become smaller.

The principles of *collateral circulation* are of primary importance in all aspects of medicine, particularly in surgery. All organs have some degree of collateral circulation, although it varies greatly in different tissues and organs. The subclavian artery usually can be ligated safely in the first portion, as in the performance of a subclavian-pulmonary anastomosis for congenital cyanotic heart disease (Blalock's operation), since the collateral circulation around the shoulder is excellent. It is rare for ischemic symptoms to follow ligation of the subclavian at this site, and, indeed, with the passage of time a pulse frequently reappears in the radial artery as additional collateral circulation develops. Moreover, three of the four major arteries of the stomach (the left and right gastric and left and right gastric epiploic) can be ligated without significant ischemia. With a number of other arteries the extensiveness of collaterals varies considerably, ligation producing no ill effects in some

patients and ischemic symptoms in others. Finally, some arteries, such as the coronary, renal, and retinal arteries, have a very inadequate natural collateral circulation. Acute occlusion of these vessels is usually followed by serious changes of ischemia or infarction, and such arteries are referred to as "end-arteries."

The *natural* collateral circulation of tissues and organs is important in the sequence of events following acute occlusion. In addition, the *time* involved in occlusion of an artery is of considerable significance. For example, with *slow, progressive* occlusion of an artery there is ample time for collateral vessels to develop and become larger. Generally, as a smaller vessel is subjected to a need for increased flow (primarily due to a pressure gradient), the vessel is apt to become thin-walled and *tortuous*. The latter characteristic is easily demonstrated by arteriography, as in chronic occlusion of the abdominal aorta (Leriche's syndrome). Under these circumstances, adequate arterial collaterals develop that join the branches above the occlusion with the iliac and femoral systems distally. It is surprising that *total* occlusion over a period of time of the entire abdominal aorta may produce minimal symptoms in some patients, whereas in others it produces the characteristic symptoms of intermittent claudication and impotence. Nevertheless, in the Leriche syndrome, it is rare to note gangrene until late in the disease, whereas *acute* occlusion of the abdominal aorta usually produces disastrous effects with acute appearance of severe ischemia and gangrene of the lower extremities if untreated.

III

PHYSIOLOGY OF THE ARTERIAL SYSTEM

Richard L. McCann, M.D.

> Everywhere he feels his heart because its vessels run to all his limbs.
>
> *The Ebers Papyrus, Chapter XX*

The arterial system is an intricate structure that functions not only to passively distribute blood to all the tissues of the body but also to regulate distribution of blood flow to different vascular beds during diverse physiologic conditions. In this section, the unique structural properties of the arterial system that allow it to perform these important functions are reviewed and the effects of arterial disease upon these functions are examined.

HISTORICAL ASPECTS

The brilliant proof by William Harvey (1578–1657) that blood continuously circulates within a contained system provided one of the most significant scientific achievements of all time. Harvey was educated at Cambridge and at Padua, which was the most important center for medicine at that time. After studying anatomy with Fabricius, he returned to England in 1602 and became court physician to two monarchs and was elected to the London College of Physicians. Harvey performed anatomic dissections, made physiologic observations in both humans and animals, and also produced quantitative experimental data, a remarkable achievement for the time. He reasoned that the human heart contained two ounces of blood; and using the pulse rate, he calculated the amount of blood pumped in a 24-hour period. Because this sum was a huge quantity, he deduced that it was far too much volume for the body to produce continuously and therefore proposed that the circulation of blood was in a closed system. Harvey could not see them, but postulated the existence of connections between arteries and veins, which he termed *porosities carnis* (porosities of the flesh). Malpighi (1628–1694), 4 years later, actually observed the passage of blood through capillaries in the lung of the frog, supplying the missing element in the investigations of Harvey.

ANATOMIC AND HISTOLOGIC ASPECTS

The arterial vessels can be divided into several categories. The large elastic arteries, principally the aorta and its major named branches, contain a high proportion of elastin fibers to allow increments in blood volume and to store the kinetic energy generated by the pumping action of the heart. The elastic recoil of these vessels helps promote continued distribution of the blood during diastole. The elastic vessels branch into the muscular arteries, which contain a higher proportion of smooth muscle cells in their walls. This large amount of muscular tissue is important in the function of these vessels, which is to regulate relative blood flow to various vascular beds by controlling vessel diameter. The greatest degree of regulation of blood flow occurs at the local level by the arterioles. These vessels are 20 to 50 μ in diameter and consist of a single layer of vascular smooth muscle cells. Small changes in the caliber of these vessels cause large changes in total peripheral resistance.

Progressing from the aorta to the capillaries, several general changes occur in the circulatory system. These are as follows: (1) individual vessel diameter decreases, but net vascular cross-sectional area progressively increases; (2) elasticity of arterial walls decreases, and muscular construction increases; (3) neural innervation becomes maximal at the arteriolar level; (4) velocity of blood flow steadily decreases; and (5) a major pressure drop occurs across the arteriolar vessels. As these changes occur, the role of the arterial vasculature progresses from one of major systemic hemodynamic modulation to one of fine regulation of flow distribution in accord with regional metabolic demand. These relationships are illustrated graphically in Figure 1.

PRIMARY FACTORS GOVERNING FLOW IN THE ARTERIAL SYSTEM

Blood flow in the arterial circulation is described by the physical laws of fluid dynamics. Understanding these and their application to the complex physiologic changes that may occur in both normal and pathologic conditions provides a better understanding of the abnormalities that are associated with arterial disease.

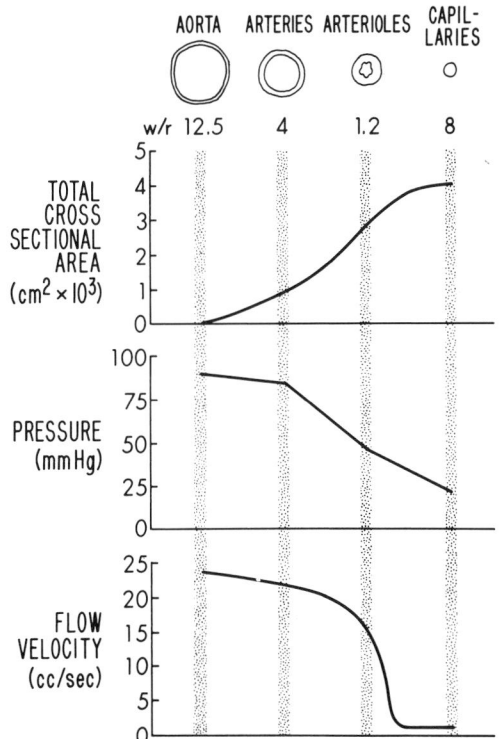

Figure 1. Profile of changes in ratio of wall thickness (w) to radius (r), total vascular cross-sectional area, pressure, and blood flow velocity as flow progresses from the aorta to the peripheral vascular bed. The most prominent changes occur at the arteriolar level.

BASIC LAWS OF FLUID DYNAMICS APPLIED TO THE ARTERIAL SYSTEM

The motion of blood in the arterial system is best understood by considering the total energy involved. The pumping action of the heart imparts potential and kinetic energy to the blood through several mechanisms. The most important of these is the potential energy stored as the intravascular pressure due to the blood volume contained within the elastic confines of the vascular tree. There is also potential energy that is due to hydrostatic forces associated with gravity, that is, the weight of the blood. Because there are no valves in the peripheral arterial system, the pressure at any point is influenced by the height of the column of blood between it and the reference point, which is usually taken to be the level of the right atrium. For example, in the erect 6-foot man, there is a distance of approximately 120 cm. between the ankle and the heart. A column of blood this high exerts a pressure equivalent to 93 mm. Hg. Thus, the pressure at the ankle would be increased by that amount in the erect individual. This has clinical importance, for example, in the patient with a critical stenosis in the vascular supply to the foot. Such a patient may have adequate flow when erect when the driving pressure is high; but when there is loss of the hydrostatic component by assumption of the recumbent position, as at night during sleep, flow may be reduced below a threshold, and overt vascular insufficiency and pain may result. Assuming the erect position again will often improve flow sufficiently to alleviate the symptoms. These are illustrated diagrammatically in Figure 2, showing that the pumping action of the heart imparts the intravascular hydrostatic pressure. The pressure due to elastic recoil of the arterial tree is responsible for only a small increment in normal persons, on the order of 5 to 10 mm. Hg. The hydrostatic pressure due to the weight of the blood is significant and may be calculated as follows:

$$P = \rho gh \qquad (1)$$

HEIGHT
cm

PRESSURE
mmHg

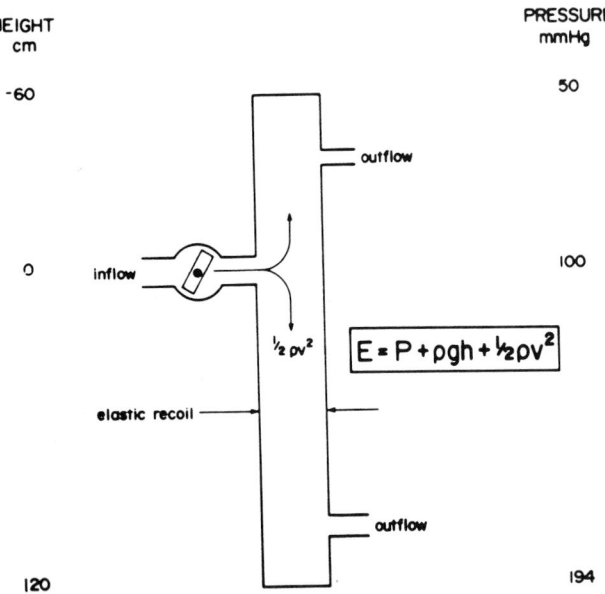

-60

50

outflow

0   inflow

100

½ρv² $E = P + \rho g h + \frac{1}{2}\rho v^2$

elastic recoil

120

outflow

194

Figure 2. Diagrammatic representation of the vascular system. Energy is provided by the cardiac muscular pump, which produces the intravascular pressure, and pressure due to the elastic recoil of the vessel wall. Addition (or subtraction) of pressure is also due to the hydrostatic component contributed by the weight of the column of blood and its distance from the reference point.

where ρ = density (for blood 1.056 gm. per cu. cm.), g = acceleration of gravity (980 cm. per second per second), and h = height. Thus, for a height of 120 cm., the hydrostatic pressure increment is P = (1.056 gm. per cu. cm.)(980 cm. per sec.²)(120 cm.) = 124,186 dynes (sq. cm.) and since 1 mm. Hg exerts a force of 1330 dynes per sq. cm. [(13.6 gm. per cu. cm.)(980 cm. per sec.²)], P = 124,186 dynes per sq. cm. per 1330 dynes per sq. cm. per mm. Hg = 93 mm. Hg.

Thus, the total energy is described as the sum of the energy of the intravascular pressure, the hydrostatic pressure, and the kinetic energy less any energy losses.

ENERGY LOSSES

The arterial system is not ideal, in that energy is lost in the transit of blood from one point to another. Energy losses occur primarily in two forms, viscous and inertial. Viscous losses are the result of friction within the flowing blood due to intermolecular attractions between the fluid layers. The relative viscosity of protein containing plasma, compared with water, is 1.8, whereas whole blood has a viscosity of 3.5. Thus, hematocrit is the critical factor in determining the viscosity of whole blood, which increases exponentially with the hematocrit. Viscosity is also dependent upon flow rate. At high flow rates viscosity actually decreases, because the red blood cells migrate to the center of the bloodstream and the less viscous plasma remains near the vessel wall. Viscous energy losses are expressed by Poiseuille's law. This states that the pressure gradient across a uniform cylinder is related to the fluid flow, the cylinder length, and fluid viscosity and is inversely proportional to the fourth power of the radius. This can be expressed as

$$P_1 - P_2 = \frac{Q 8 L \eta}{\pi r^4} \qquad (2)$$

where Px = pressure at a point, Q = flow, L = length, η = viscosity, and r = radius. It must be recognized that in strict terms Poiseuille's law applies only to nonpulsatile laminar flow in rigid straight cylinders. These conditions are not met in bio-

logic systems but are a reasonable approximation. This formula can be solved for flow:

$$Q = \Delta P \frac{\pi r^4}{8 L \eta} \qquad (3)$$

Because flow varies as the fourth power of the radius and linearly with length, it is the radius of a stenosis that primarily influences flow at the site of an obstruction. Moreover, for any given pressure gradient, flow changes will be exponentially related to the radius. This is the reason that flow changes are small until a vascular stenosis produces 70 to 80 per cent narrowing of the cross-sectional area.

Inertial energy losses also occur and are proportional to the specific gravity of blood and its velocity as

$$E = k \frac{1}{2} \rho V^2 \qquad (4)$$

where k is a constant, ρ = density of the fluid, and v = velocity.

Thus, energy losses due to inertia are proportional to acceleration and deceleration, changes in the lumen diameter, and changes in the direction of flow. In areas of vessel stenosis, rapid velocity changes occur in proportion to the degree of narrowing of the vessel lumen. At these locations, considerable inertial energy losses occur that are related to the marked decrease in flow that can occur. Turbulent flow depletes energy and dissipates it as heat. Reynold's equation describes the ratio of the inertial forces acting on the fluid with respect to the viscous forces. Reynold's number is defined as

$$Re = \frac{\rho \bar{v} d}{\eta} \qquad (5)$$

where ρ = density, $\bar{v}$ = kinetic viscosity (η/ρ), d = diameter, and η = viscosity. Turbulent flow occurs when the Reynold's number exceeds 2000 and indicates that inertial disturbances may disrupt the laminar flow and produce disorganized motion and loss of energy.

THE EFFECT OF VASCULAR STENOSIS

A critical stenosis is defined as the degree of narrowing of a vessel that is required to produce a measurable reduction in pressure or reduction in flow of the blood through it. A critical stenosis is generally accepted to become hemodynamically significant when a diameter reduction of 50 per cent occurs. This corresponds to a reduction in vessel cross-sectional area of 75 per cent. This simplified concept of critical stenosis is complicated by considerations of flow velocity and inertial energy. As shown by Poiseuille's law, energy losses at the site of a stenosis are related to the fourth power of the radius and the first power of the length. From this it can be seen that a short stenosis with marked reduction in diameter is more important than a stenosis over a longer segment with a more modest reduction in vessel diameter. Energy losses also increase in relation to the flow rate. Thus, stenoses that may produce no or only a modest pressure drop at low flow rates may become "critical" at higher flow rates. A clinical example of this phenomenon is stenosis in the iliac artery, which often produces only a modest decrease in pressure in the leg at rest. However, during exercise, when the flow rate increases, the stenosis may become critical and produce a marked reduction in pressure distally.

In addition, there are entry and exit inertial losses that occur as primary sources of energy loss. Thus, two stenoses in tandem have a greater effect than a single stenosis, the length of which is the sum of the lengths of the tandem stenoses. Therefore, multiple stenoses in series are additive, and several subcritical stenoses may become the equivalent of a critical stenosis and produce a significant decrease in flow. A corollary to this is that bypass of only a single stenosis in a series may improve the flow only modestly. Also, if two unequal stenoses exist, the one producing the greater diameter reduction is the more critical, and failure to correct it may result in absence of improvement.

RESISTANCE

The concept of hemodynamic resistance is helpful in understanding the physiology of arterial disease. By analogy to Ohm's law, resistance is defined as the ratio between the pressure drop between two points along a circuit and the flow between the two points. However, unlike the electrical analog, the resistance in a hydrodynamic circuit is not constant. Energy losses occur, due to turbulence, acceleration, and other forces, thus leading to an increase in resistance as flow velocity increases. It follows that Poiseuille's law increasingly underestimates energy losses as flow and/or velocity increases (Fig. 3). The practical significance of this is that resistances that may be insignificant at low flow rates become critically significant as flow rates are increased, for example, during the demands of exercise.

In the normal limb, resistance is very low in the large axial vessels. The major site of peripheral resistance exists in the muscular runoff bed. This high resistance is remarkably variable and is used to control the blood flow to muscular beds during exercise. When obstruction occurs in the major axial vessels in the course of the development of atherosclerosis, flow is forced to proceed through smaller collateral vessels. Collateral vessels characteristically have a smaller diameter, usually 1 to 2 mm. If we recall the Poiseuille relationship, it can be seen that it would require thousands of these collaterals to reduce the segmental resistance to that of a major axial vessel with a diameter of 8 to 10 mm. Resistance in these vessels is relatively fixed, compared with that in the vascular runoff bed. This is illustrated in Figure 4 along with the electrical analog of the hemodynamic circuit. Study of this illustration helps one to understand the phenomenon of intermittent claudication. In this condition, blood flow to the limb is satisfactory at rest when the peripheral resistance in the muscular bed is naturally high. Under the demands of exer-

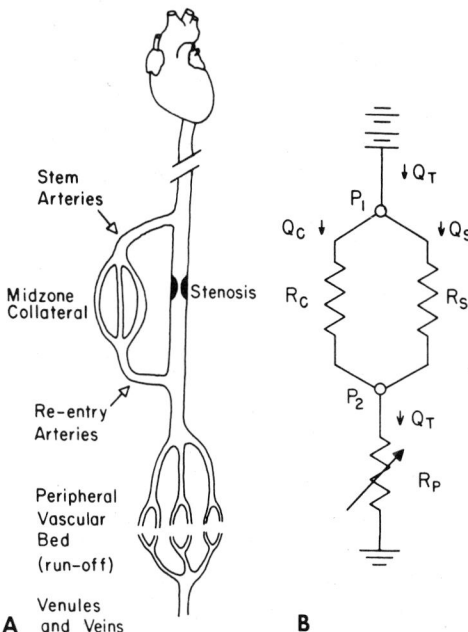

Figure 4. *A*, The major components of an arterial circuit containing a stenotic major artery. *B*, An electric analog of this circuit. The battery at the top represents the potential energy source, that is, the heart; ground potential, at the bottom, indicates the central vein. QT is total flow, QC is collateral flow, and QS is flow through the stenotic artery. Resistances are c, collateral; s, stenotic artery; and r$_p$, peripheral runoff bed. R$_c$S are relatively fixed; r$_p$ is variable. (From Sumner, D. S.: Essential hemodynamic principles. *In* Rutherford, R. B. (Ed.): Vascular Surgery, 3rd ed. Philadelphia, W. B. Saunders Company, 1989, p. 25.)

cise, the resistance in the muscular runoff bed decreases sharply. However, because of the fixed obstruction proximally, flow cannot increase to maintain pressure, and the pressure distally in the limb falls precipitously with the onset of symptoms, which occur as muscular pain. This drop in ankle pressure with exercise is a characteristic of peripheral vascular obstructive disease and is shown in Figure 5. This illustration shows the normal resting blood flow to the extremity to be approximately 3.5 ml. per 100 gm. per minute. The ankle pressure is only

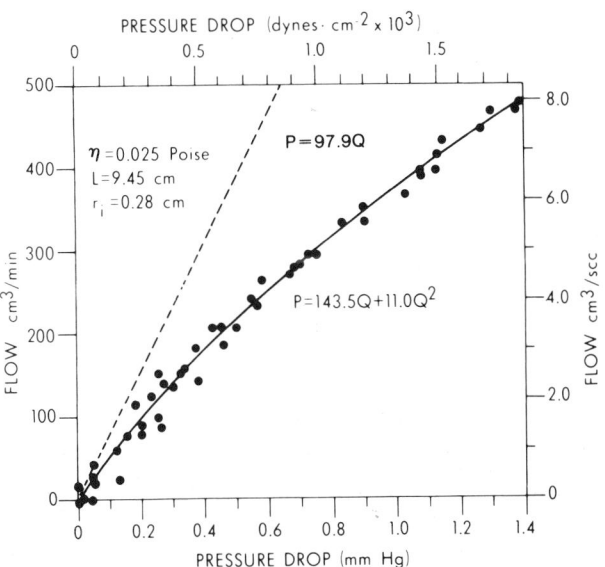

Figure 3. Pressure drop experimentally determined across a 9.5-cm. length of canine femoral artery at various flow rates. This is compared with the theoretic pressure drop as predicted by Poiseuille's law. Flow rate is varied by constricting a distally located arteriovenous fistula. Note that the line that fits the experimental data best has both a linear and a squared term, corresponding to Poiseuille's law, plus kinetic energy losses. Note also that the pressure flow curve predicted from Poiseuille's law predicts much less energy loss than actually is the case. (From Sumner, D. S.: Essential hemodynamic principles. *In* Rutherford, R. B. (Ed.): Vascular Surgery, 3rd ed. Philadelphia, W. B. Saunders Company, 1989, p. 22.)

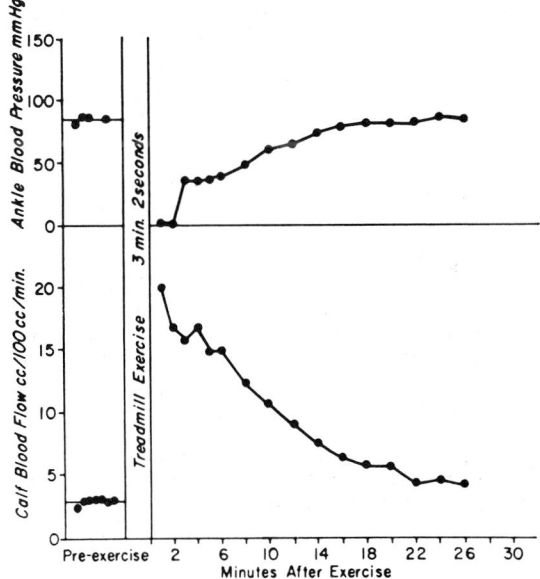

Figure 5. Ankle blood pressure and calf blood flow before and after exercise in a patient with stenosis of the superficial femoral artery. (From Sumner, D. S., Strandness, D. E., Jr.: Essential hemodynamic principles. Surgery 65:763, 1969.)

modestly reduced at 90 mm. Hg at rest. After exercise on the treadmill, however, blood flow increases dramatically in response to the demands of exercise and reduction in the resistance vessels of the calf muscles. Concomitantly there is a marked drop in blood pressure measured at the ankle. Over time these values return to resting levels as the limb recovers.

These concepts help to explain the nature of intermittent claudication. With the demands of exercise, blood flow in the limb increases 5- to 10-fold. One can understand that symptoms would appear much earlier in the course of the disease during periods of exercise or high demand. When flow is high, it requires only a modest degree of stenosis to become critical in terms of limitation of flow augmentation. In order for symptoms to occur at rest and viability of the limb to be in jeopardy, the stenosis must progress to a point at which the flow is 5 or 10 times less than normal. This correlates with the clinical observation that intermittent claudication or inadequate flow during

exercise occurs much more frequently and usually many years in advance of disease that produces such critical stenosis that viability of the limb is jeopardized.

SELECTED REFERENCES

Giordano, J. M., Trout, H. H., and DePalma, R. G. (Eds.): The Basic Science of Vascular Surgery. Mt. Kisco, Futura Publishing Company, 1988.
This excellent volume outlines the basic scientific underpinnings of modern vascular surgery. Many contributors are outstanding authorities in their fields. Of particular relevance to this section is the chapter on the hemodynamics of arterial blood flow, which is an excellent and concise description of this subject.

Sumner, D. S.: Essential hemodynamic principles. *In* Rutherford, R. B. (Ed.): Vascular Surgery, 3rd ed. Philadelphia, W. B. Saunders Company, 1989.
This is a definitive chapter by the acknowledged authority on biophysical properties of the peripheral arterial circulation. Both theoretic and experimental concepts that contribute to the understanding of arterial physiology in the normal and diseased vasculature are thoroughly covered.

IV

ARTERIAL SUBSTITUTES

Gregory L. Moneta, M.D., and John M. Porter, M.D.

The explosive growth in arterial surgical procedures over the last 40 years has in large part been dependent upon the increased use of arterial substitutes. It has been estimated recently that in the United States alone over 350,000 synthetic arterial grafts are implanted each year, while the annual use of peripheral autogenous vein grafts exceeds 200,000 per year.[15] This large annual use of arterial grafts clearly indicates that the development of optimal arterial substitutes is of great clinical importance. A critical review of the results of arterial grafting at present leads to the conclusion that the ideal arterial substitute has not yet been developed.

The optimal arterial substitute should (1) be strong, inexpensive, and capable of lifetime use by the patient; (2) be easily and permanently attachable to the host vessel; (3) be biocompatible with the host and have a nonthrombogenic luminal surface; (4) resist infection; (5) be readily available in appropriate sizes; (6) remain patent without subsequent intervention; and (7) have viscoelastic properties similar to those of a normal artery. Moreover, an ideal vascular graft should not (1) leak blood or serous fluid with restoration of flow; (2) degenerate chemically or physically with time; (3) incite an abnormal proliferative response from the native vessel or the surrounding tissue; (4) promote thrombus formation or be a source of embolic material; (5) occlude when flexed; or (6) damage blood components. No currently available arterial substitute approaches these requirements; hence the large amount of clinical and basic research devoted to the evaluation and development of vascular grafts.

HISTORICAL ASPECTS

In 1906, Carrel and Guthrie first reported succsful implantation of venous autografts into the arterial system of dogs.[19] They observed that venous autografts underwent rapid structural change, consisting primarily of a marked thickening of connective tissue in the adventitia and media, and also noted that better results were obtained when the caliber of the vein and the artery to which it was anastomosed were similar. This soon was followed by the clinical use of the popliteal vein for arterial reconstruction after popliteal aneurysm excision by Goyanes in

1906.[46] The first use of a saphenous vein graft in popliteal artery reconstruction after aneurysm excision in the United States was by Bernheim in 1915.[10]

The first successful arterial allograft was reported by Hoepfner in 1903.[57] Carrel performed a series of experimental arterial autografts and allografts several years later, accompanied by detailed microscopic studies.[18] He found that fresh arterial autografts functioned well and remained microscopically normal during several month's observation. He also performed studies with viable, refrigerated allografts and nonviable, preserved allografts. Carrel noted progressive arterial allograft wall thickening and hyalinization, depending generally upon the type of preservative used and the duration of refrigeration. Nonviable grafts killed by heat, formalin, or glycerin showed rapid degeneration accompanied by significant host fibrous reaction.

The monumental work of Carrel and Guthrie established the feasibility of arterial and venous autografts and allografts early in this century. Not until almost 50 years later, however, was widespread clinical application of arterial reconstruction feasible. The pioneering work of Murray[76] in the intraoperative use of heparin and the work of Moniz[75] and dos Santos, and colleagues[34] in establishing the technique of arteriography then combined with the concept of arterial substitutes to initiate the modern era of clinical vascular grafting.

EVALUATION OF ARTERIAL SUBSTITUTES

Patency is the most important endpoint in the evaluation of the clinical performance of any arterial substitute. It is critical to distinguish between primary and secondary patency. Primary patency is that achieved without additional graft-directed surgical procedures. Secondary patency refers to grafts that have been maintained patent by one or more additional graft-directed procedures, such as thrombectomy, anastomotic revision, and so on. If a later operation involves only the inflow or outflow of the graft and not the graft or the anastomosis, the graft may still be regarded as primarily patent. Both primary and secondary patency rates are important. Primary patency assesses the natural history of the graft, whereas secondary patency assesses the success of the clinical follow-up program to detect and correct failing grafts. Clearly, primary patency is of the greatest importance in assessing the true value of the graft itself.

Ideally, criteria for patency should be uniformly accepted and clearly stated. It is especially important that life table analysis be used to display patency rates. Unfortunately, many reports of arterial substitutes have not employed uniform methods of obtaining and reporting data. Primary and secondary patency rates are frequently confused, especially in older publications. However, standards for reports considering lower extremity revascularization now exist.[95] This will undoubtedly enhance future ability to critically evaluate published reports on the use of arterial substitutes.

In the following sections, the available arterial substitutes, including allografts, xenografts, and prosthetic grafts are reviewed.

ALLOGRAFTS

Arterial Allografts

Arterial allografts were the first widely used arterial substitute. Gross and associates reported the use of viable arterial allografts in patients in 1948.[49] Early results were encouraging, and it soon was recognized that tissue viability was not essential for successful grafting provided the vessels were properly preserved. This realization, in combination with increasing demand for allografts, led to the establishment of human arterial banks in the early 1950s, freeze-drying being the most popular method of allograft preservation.

Widespread clinical use of arterial allografts in the early 1950s caused a rapid increase in knowledge of the biology and natural history of this type of arterial substitute. Arterial allografts rapidly lose endothelium. A platelet-fibrin coagulum forms on the exposed basement membrane and slowly undergoes fibrous organization. This process begins in anastomotic sites and is frequently incomplete in the central area of the allograft, leaving this area covered with only a fibrin coagulum prone to ulceration. Allograft walls become less cellular with time. Progressive thinning of the wall, with loss of collagen and fragmentation of elastic fibers, frequently occurs after several years. Similar degenerative changes affect both muscular and elastic arterial allografts but occur much more rapidly with the former. Thus, allografts of the aorta, composed predominantly of collagen and elastin, were associated with fewer complications (thrombosis, calcification, aneurysm formation, rupture) and longer graft function than femoral artery allografts, which contained a large component of smooth muscle and elicited a more prominent rejection reaction.[32] However, with the exception of short segment repairs for aortic coarctation, even aortic allografts gave disappointing long-term results; several reports described a very high closure rate after only a few years, occasionally accompanied by dilatation and/or rupture.[68,101,116]

Because of the high incidence of complications, arterial allografts have been abandoned clinically in favor of more satisfactory arterial substitutes. Allografts, however, occupy an important place in the history of vascular surgery. The modern era of vascular grafting began with the successful clinical use of arterial allografts by Gross and associates.[49] The aortic allograft was the arterial substitute used by Oudot and Beaconsfield[83] for the first aortic resection and replacement for occlusive disease, and by DuBost and colleagues[36] for the first excision and grafting of an abdominal aortic aneurysm. Recent studies in animal models suggest that the immunologic rejection process that contributes to the degeneration of these grafts may be modified with low doses of cyclosporin-A.[98] Such studies raise the intriguing possibility of new applications for these grafts in the future.

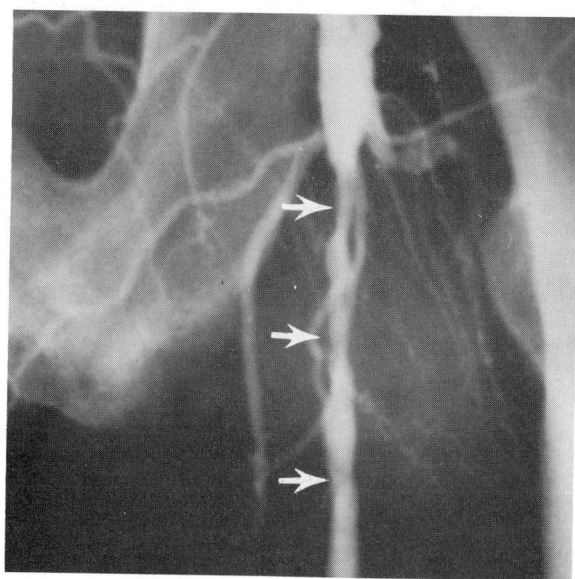

Figure 1. Angiogram of a femoropopliteal venous allograft in a patient 1 year after implantation. Diffuse stenosis of the proximal portion of the allograft is present (arrows). The graft subsequently thrombosed. Pathologic examination revealed diffuse fibrous thickening of all layers of the graft wall, accompanied by a striking mononuclear and giant cell infiltration.

Saphenous Vein Allografts

Saphenous vein allografts from human cadavers generally have proved unsatisfactory in clinical practice. Initial encouraging reports were rapidly overwhelmed by studies demonstrating a high failure rate in the first postoperative year and a large incidence of late aneurysmal degeneration.[78,79,112,120]

Like arterial allografts, venous allografts are normally antigenic and elicit an immunologic rejection response by the host (Fig. 1).[3] Microscopic analysis of failed saphenous vein allografts reveals areas of wall necrosis and intimal disruption.[84,125] Cryopreservation alone does not alter allograft immunogenicity, and the suggestion by some that cryopreservation may enhance vein allograft function has not been confirmed.[94] However, the ability to preserve veins coupled with advances in immunosuppression may eventually lead to establishment of practical antigen-defined allograft vein banks. Currently, however, saphenous vein allografts have no significant clinical application. The only vascular allograft that has been widely employed is the umbilical vein allograft described next.

Umbilical Vein Allografts

These grafts have been used primarily for lower extremity revascularization and were developed as an alternative to autogenous vein. The grafts are prepared from human umbilical cords that are subjected to glutaraldehyde tanning and multiple ethanol extractions and are externally reinforced with a Dacron mesh tube (Fig. 2). The resulting conduit has a bursting pressure

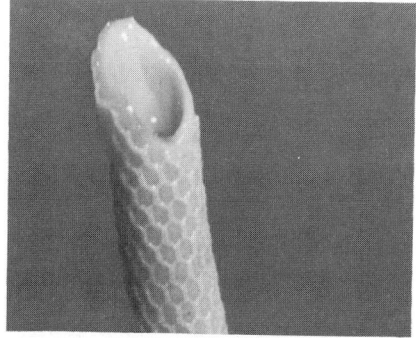

Figure 2. An umbilical vein graft. Note the external Dacron mesh.

approaching 1000 mm. Hg and is essentially nonantigenic.[27] The largest clinical experience by far has been accumulated by Dardik and co-workers, who reported primary patency rates of 70 to 50 per cent at 1 and 5 years for femoropopliteal grafts and 50 and 25 per cent at 1 and 5 years for femorotibial grafts.[28] These results, however, are distinctly inferior to patency rates for saphenous vein autografts in the same locations. Randomized prospective evaluation of umbilical vein grafts compared with polytetrafluoroethylene (PTFE) grafts (discussed later) has indicated comparable patency rates for both grafts when used as below-knee femoropopliteal bypasses.[39]

Umbilical vein grafts have several disadvantages that have precluded their widespread clinical use. The grafts exhibit degenerative changes over time and are prone to the development of aneurysms, which have occurred in a distressingly large number of these grafts.[44] In addition, they are technically difficult to implant, and the intima is easily damaged by clamps or attempts at thrombectomy. At present, umbilical vein grafts have no well-defined place in the modern practice of vascular surgery, and they are being used with decreasing frequency.

XENOGRAFTS

Unmodified arterial xenografts were used clinically in the early 1950s. These grafts elicited a prominent host immunologic reaction, leading to severe damage to the graft wall. Their use was associated with a high incidence of thrombosis and rupture, and it soon became obvious that unmodified arterial xenografts were not suitable for clinical use.

Rosenberg and associates produced modified xenografts by treating bovine carotid arteries with the proteolytic enzyme ficin, followed by tanning with dialdehyde starch. The result was an almost nonantigenic, collagenous tube devoid of smooth muscle and elastic tissue but possessing the same tensile strength as a normal artery.[91]

Modified xenografts were used frequently as arterial substitutes in vascular surgery from the mid 1960s to the mid 1970s but did not produce satsifactory clinical results, particularly in infrainguinal reconstructions. When used in the femoropopliteal position, these grafts were plagued by a tendency to perioperative thrombosis and exhibited poor long-term patency rates of approximately 40 per cent at 3 to 6 years following implantation. In addition, aneurysms occurred in 3 to 6 per cent of grafts, usually several years after graft placement.[26,92] These figures represent aneurysm formation in all implanted grafts. The incidence of aneurysm formation in grafts which remained patent was probably considerably higher, because many grafts thrombosed later. Moreover, clinical use of these grafts was associated with an unacceptable infection rate of 3 to 7 per cent, several times that seen in other arterial substitutes. Nevertheless, bovine xenografts have proved to function satisfactorily as hemodialysis access shunts and remain the preferred conduit for dialysis access in some centers. They have no other well-defined role in vascular surgery presently.

AUTOGRAFTS

Arterial Autografts

The clinical use of arterial autografts was introduced by Wylie in 1965.[126] Proponents of autografts cite numerous advantages of this vascular substitute, including retention of viability associated with the maintenance of an intact intrinsic blood supply during grafting, absence of aneurysmal degeneration, resistance to infection, preservation of normal flexibility at points of joint motion, and possession of growth potential when used in pediatric patients. The obvious disadvantage is lack of availability and length of arteries usable for autografting.

Detailed studies by Berger and colleagues,[9] Geiringer,[43] and

others have clearly shown that the innermost 300 to 500 μ the arterial wall are nourished by luminal diffusion. The outer layers of the arterial wall are nourished by a complex vasa vasorum system that is derived primarily from the very proximal portions of arterial side branches. If the proximal side branches are excised or damaged during preparation of the autograft, spotty arterial wall necrosis may develop in the part of the arterial wall more than 500 to 600 μ from the lumen (Figs. 3 and 4).

The clinical use of arterial autografts is restricted primarily to coronary artery bypass grafting, renal artery bypass in children, and arterial substitutes in infected surgical fields. Radial arteries have been used as free grafts in coronary bypass surgery, but unfortunately their use has been largely unsuccesful due to early graft closure associated with florid intimal proliferation.[25] Currently, however, the internal mammary artery is frequently used as a conduit in coronary bypass surgery and appears to provide patency rates superior to those of saphenous vein grafts.[72]

There is general agreement that children who require renal artery reconstruction are best served by arterial autografting. The internal iliac artery has proved to be a suitable conduit, and its use obviates the high incidence of late aneurysmal graft dilatation so frequently seen in this age group when saphenous vein grafts are used. Iliac artery autografts have also proved remarkably effective in a limited number of adult patients undergoing renal vascular surgery. In a primarily adult population, Stoney and associates have reported only two arterial autograft occlusions in 86 patients undergoing renovascular surgery with follow-up extending to 16 years.[113] Use of the internal iliac artery, however, is limited in the adult population by the frequent involvement of this artery with advanced atherosclerosis. The external iliac artery may also be used as an arterial autograft but generally requires prosthetic replacement of the autograft donor site.

Arterial autografts are occasionally used to bridge short arterial defects in infected or contaminated surgical fields that preclude use of synthetic grafts. Atherosclerotic arteries may be endarterectomized and used as either autogenous bypass con-

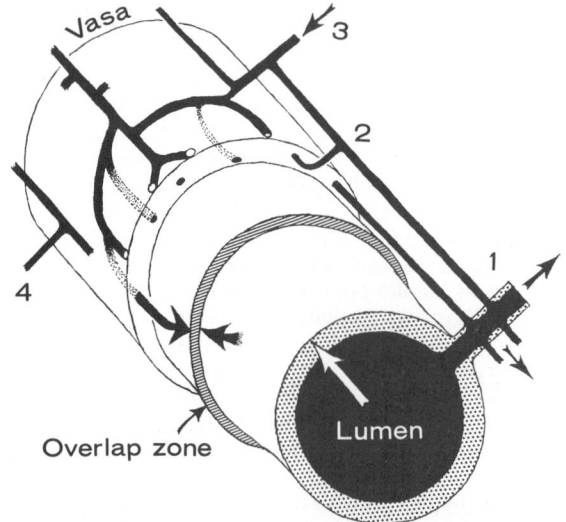

Figure 3. Diagrammatic conception of nutrition to the thoracic aortic wall. Luminal diffusion serves the inner portion of the wall. Vasa vasorum serve the outer portion. A narrower zone, the overlap zone, is served by both mechanisms. At 1, an intercostal artery emerges. This in turn gives off branches that travel in the outer medial layer of the wall, as well as along the adventitia. At 2, branches from the adventitial system traverse into the outer media. At 3, connections may occur at adventitial vessels other than those derived from intercostals. At 4, an adventitial vessel derived from the "nonintercostal" system. (From Berger, K., Sauvage, L. R., Wood, S. J., and Sameh, A. A.: Endarterectomy and other surgical injuries to vascular walls. Pacific Med. Surg., 75:367, 1967.)

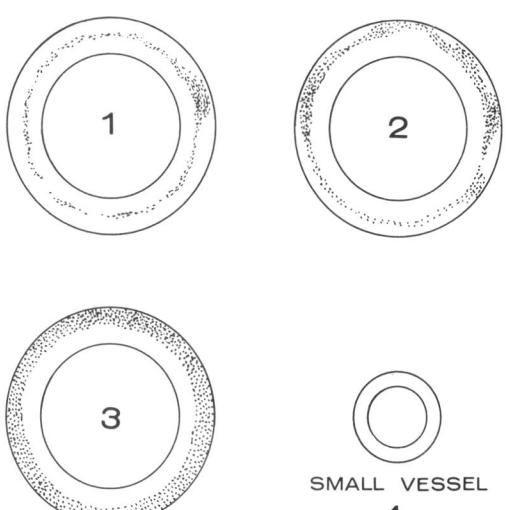

Figure 4. Diagrammatic summary of luminal diffusion and vasa vasorum zones of influence as observed in canine experiments. Necrosis is indicated by stippled areas. 1, Results from minor trauma exemplified by aortic-aortic anastomoses, namely, freeing of the vessel ends necessary for sewing them together. This is judged to be an example of overlap zone damage. 2, Irregular necrosis of outer wall following removal of thoracic aortic segment with only intercostals ligated. 3, Necrosis of the outer wall following removal of aortic segment, plus excision of intercostal ostia. In all three instances, the viable luminal diffusion zone remains at about the same order of thickness. 4, Full wall viability of a small transected and reanastomosed vessel, the wall thickness of which falls within the diffusion zone distance. (From Berger, K., Sauvage, L. R., Wood, S. J., and Sameh, A. A.: Endarterectomy and other surgical injuries to vascular walls. Pacific Med. Surg.,75:367, 1967).

duits or, more frequently, as patch grafts. These technical adjuncts are primarily employed in the management of traumatic wounds or infected prosthetic grafts. Unfortunately, the use of endarterectomized arteries as autografts has been associated with a disturbing incidence of fibrointimal hyperplasia leading to graft failure.

Venous Autografts

The routine clinical use of venous autografts began with the pivotal clinical report of a femoropopliteal bypass by Kunlin in 1949.[64] Since that time, venous autografts have proved to be the most successful and clearly the most clinically important small caliber arterial substitute. They are the preferred graft for infrainguinal arterial reconstruction. Greater saphenous vein, lesser saphenous vein, cephalic vein and basilic vein, as well as superficial femoral and internal jugular vein, have all been used as bypass conduits.

GREATER SAPHENOUS VEIN. Greater saphenous vein autografts are by far the most widely used autogenous vascular graft in modern vascular surgery and are currently the standard with which all other small caliber arterial substitutes are compared. Over 200,000 peripheral vascular operations using saphenous vein autografts are performed in the United States annually.[15]

The normal greater saphenous vein averages 70 to 80 cm. in length in adult men. It begins at the medial malleolus at the junction of the medial marginal and internal malleolar veins. This vein is quite superficial in the leg but lies close to the deep fascia in the thigh. It exists as a single vessel in the thigh in 75 per cent of patients; contains 8 to 12 bicuspid valves, mainly below the knee; and averages 5.5 mm. in diameter. The luminal surface consists of a monolayer of endothelial cells. The media is composed of an inner layer of longitudinally arranged smooth muscle cells and an outer layer of circumferentially oriented smooth muscle cells. The outer adventitial layer is composed of a loose mixture of collagen and elastic tissue.

The saphenous vein has been used as a replacement for small and medium-sized arteries in all parts of the body, with most being used for coronary artery bypass grafts and for lower extremity bypass of occluded superficial femoral, popliteal, and tibial arteries. Other less frequent uses include upper extremity bypass and visceral and renal artery bypass. The coronary, visceral, and renal results are described in other sections of this book and generally have been excellent.

Lower extremity bypasses using autogenous saphenous vein may be performed using one of the two basic techniques. An appropriate length of vein may be removed from either the ipsilateral or contralateral lower extremity; reversed in direction to permit arterial flow in the direction of the venous valves; and sutured in place, usually in an end-to-side configuration. Alternatively, an intact ipsilateral vein of adequate quality may largely be left in its anatomic position and the valves destroyed by means of one of a variety of intraluminal devices, followed by similar proximal and distal arterial anastomoses. This has been termed the *in situ* saphenous vein bypass technique. Both techniques are currently widely employed and generally produce similar results.

Reversed femoropopliteal saphenous vein autograft primary patency has ranged from 80 to 90 per cent at 1 year to 55 to 86 per cent at 5 years and 38 to 46 per cent at 10 years (Fig. 5).[33,115,118] Reversed saphenous vein grafting to tibial arteries produces a patency about 10 to 15 per cent lower than femoropopliteal grafting at all time intervals.[117] Exhaustive analysis of variables affecting femoropopliteal patency indicates that patency is higher when bypass surgery is performed for claudication rather than limb salvage and generally is higher with a widely patent popliteal and tibial artery outflow tract. A patent outflow tract, however, is not an absolute requirement for long-term patency. Mannick and co-workers have reported an intermediate-term patency rate of 65 per cent when bypassing to an isolated popliteal segment without demonstrated angiographic patency of the popliteal artery trifurcation vessels.[74] Both continued cigarette smoking and the use of a small vein (less than 4 mm. after gentle distention) decrease long-term patency. Curiously, vein graft patency appears to be slightly higher in diabetic pateints.[118] The role, if any, of antiplatelet drugs in enhancing vein graft patency is unclear.[45]

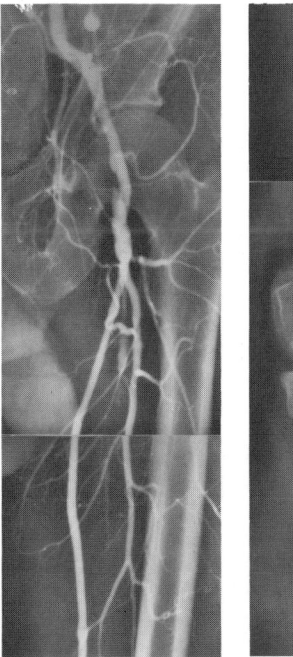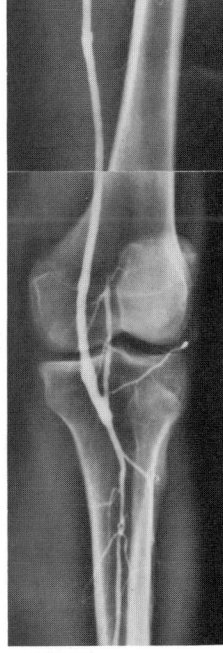

Figure 5. Angiogram of a well-functioning femoropopliteal venous autograft 2 years after implantation. Normal slight graft dilation at the site of the venous valves is still present.

Large modern series of *in situ* vein bypasses initially suggested patency rates with this technique superior to those with the reversed vein technique.[66] Modern series of reversed vein bypasses, however, have demonstrated similar or superior patency rates to *in situ* bypasses in grafts to the popliteal and tibial arteries.[118] In fact, it has been suggested that because a high percentage of *in situ* bypasses must undergo secondary operations to maintain graft patency, primary patency[61,65] actually may be better with reversed rather than *in situ* grafts. Clearly reversed vein grafting is applicable to larger numbers of patients, because many individuals do not have an intact ipsilateral saphenous vein, which is, of course, mandatory for *in situ* bypasses.

ALTERNATIVE VENOUS AUTOGRAFTS. Recently, interest has been rekindled in the use of venous conduits other than the greater saphenous vein for lower extremity bypass. As many as 20 to 30 per cent of patients do not possess an adequate greater saphenous vein for arterial grafting.[37,117] The vein is anatomically too small in 5 to 10 per cent of patients and is unavailable or unusable in another 10 to 20 per cent of patients because of prior removal, phlebitis, or varicosities. In such patients, alternate veins have been used for arterial grafting, including the lesser saphenous, basilic, cephalic, and superficial femoral.[63] Various venous segments also may be joined with venovenostomies for achieving an autogenous conduit of adequate length.[117]

Although the long-term effectiveness of these alternate conduits has been questioned,[99] several recent publications suggest they can serve as quite acceptable arterial substitutes. Harris and associates[55] reported 3 year patency rates of 82 and 65 per cent using cephalic vein bypasses to the below-knee popliteal and tibial arteries, respectively. The superficial femoral vein has been used as a femoropopliteal bypass conduit with a primary patency rate of 82 per cent at 3 years.[100] Some workers report surprisingly little postoperative morbidity with the use of the superficial femoral veins as a bypass graft, but most surgeons are reluctant to use it because of concern of postoperative edema. Other investigators have also found alternative vein sources to be satisfactory conduits in the lower extremity.[117]

PATHOLOGY OF VENOUS AUTOGRAFTS. Early postoperative vein graft failure can usually be attributed to technical flaws in the performance of the operative procedure or the presence of an unrecognized hypercoagulable state. Late failures may result from progression of atherosclerotic disease above or below the vein graft. It is quite clear, however, that the vein graft itself is subject to a number of pathologic alterations that may contribute to occlusion of the bypass.

Carrel first noted that veins implanted into the arterial system that remain patent invariably undergo significant thickening.[19] This process, which has been erroneously termed "arterialization" of vein grafts, results from medial and subintimal fibrous hyperplasia, often in combination with fibrin deposition on the intimal surface.[107] The result is a variable thickening of the vein wall that may be minimal and remarkably localized or involve the entire vein graft to the point of diffuse obliteration of the lumen.

Szilagyi and colleagues, in a landmark review of the clinical outcome of peripheral arterial saphenous vein bypass grafting, found that marked fibrointimal hyperplasia occurred in 8 per cent of vein grafts.[114] It is interesting that this process has been implicated as the cause of failure in 15 to 30 per cent of aortocoronary grafts occluding during the first year.[110] A search for the cause and prevention of the fibrointimal hyperplasia routinely affecting venous autografts continues to be the focus of intense investigation.

Fibrointimal hyperplasia follows the stimulation of normal quiescent myointimal and medial smooth muscle cells into actively proliferating secretory myofibroblasts. A number of factors appear important in stimulating this proliferative process.

The predominant current theory regards fibrointimal hyperplasia as a response to vein injury occurring during and following vein grafting. Without doubt, veins are mechanically injured during removal and storage preparatory to arterial grafting. In addition, the vein wall is rendered ischemic during its dissection because of disruption of the vasa vasorum. Electron micrographs after vein harvest frequently have shown massive areas of endothelial denudation and medial injury. Although there appears to be general agreement on the importance of gentle vein harvest techniques and avoidance of excessive hydrostatic venous distention, there is little agreement on the optimal media in which to store veins for reversed bypass between harvest and arterial grafting. Some have found minimal endothelial disruption with storage in chilled autogenous blood. Others have recommended placing the vein in tissue culture media at 37°C. with added papaverine. Many surgeons simply leave the vein in a heparinized saline solution for the short time period between vein excision and implantation.[71,108]

In addition to the actual vein harvest, other mechanical factors may be important in inciting fibrointimal hyperplasia. These include increases in shear forces and venous wall stress induced by arterial pressure and compliance mismatch at anastomotic sites. The potential importance of the latter is suggested by the observation that failed saphenous vein grafts frequently have prominent fibrointimal hyperplasia at the distal anastomosis.[109] Recent animal studies, however, have suggested that while compliance mismatch may contribute to graft thrombosis,[1] there does not appear to be any significant difference in distal anastomotic fibrointimal hyperplasia in compliant versus noncompliant grafts.[81]

Endothelial damage appears to be the final common pathway in the production of fibrointimal hyperplasia. Whereas in the past the endothelium was regarded merely as an inert, nonthrombogenic surface lining, it is now clear that these cells are very active biochemical factories capable of responding to injury and producing a variety of substances involved in the regulation of vascular wall function.

Platelets, endothelium, smooth muscle cells, and macrophages all can produce similar growth factor proteins that can induce smooth muscle cell proliferation.[93,102] Endothelial cells also produce growth-inhibiting factors (heparan sulfate), which suggests that endothelial cells may be capable of modulating various mitogens capable of stimulating fibrointimal hyperplasia.[20] The mechanisms by which alterations in cellular interactions and growth factor production combine to produce fibrointimal hyperplasia, leading to a failing or failed vascular graft are currently the focus of intense investigation with important clinical implications.

A number of other pathologic changes have been noted in vein grafts. Clamp trauma may produce localized stenoses associated with transmural fibrosis. This has been reported in 4 per cent of lower extremity vein grafts.[114] About 9 per cent of vein grafts develop localized stenosis following fibrosis of the venous valves or suture narrowing caused by improper stuture ligation of venous side branches. Significant vein graft arteriosclerosis occurs after variable periods in approximately 7 per cent of aortocoronary grafts and 15 per cent of lower extremity grafts, causing localized stenosis in about 7 per cent of the latter.[31,114] Arteriosclerotic venous aneurysms develop in 3 to 8 per cent of lower extremity vein grafts.[114] The incidence of nonatherosclerotic vein graft dilation or aneurysm formation varies significantly with the location of the graft and the age of the patient. Stanley and colleagues noted that although one third of aortorenal vein grafts become ectatic, actual aneurysmal degeneration occurs in only 1.5 per cent of adult patients. In pediatric patients, however, the incidence of aneurysmal degeneration with similar grafts is 20 per cent, a finding that has led to the current preference for arterial autografts in pediatric patients who require renal artery reconstruction.[111]

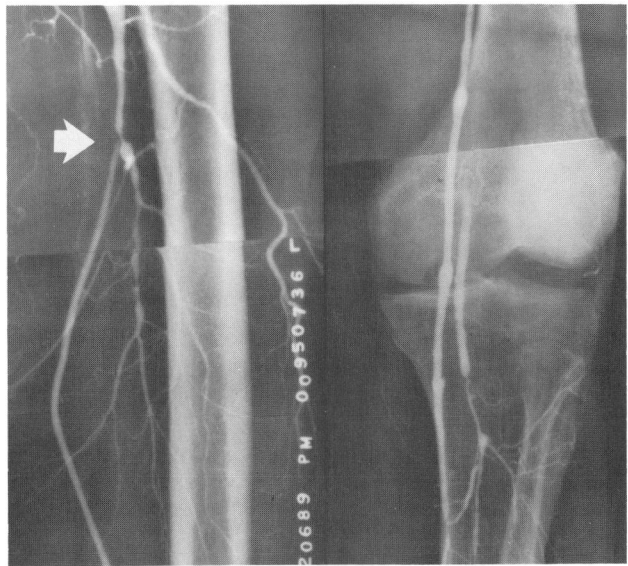

Figure 6. This high-grade stenosis (arrow) of a venous autograft was suggested by a duplex determined low graft flow velocity.

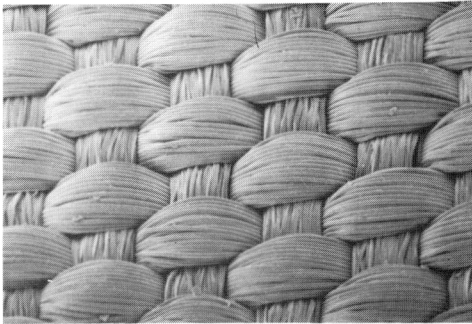

Figure 7. Close-up photograph (×50) of a woven Dacron prosthetic vascular graft. This graft is relatively impervious to blood because of the tightness of the weave.

About one third of vein grafts in clinical use eventually develop recognizable structural defects.[114] Many of these defects, if not corrected, may lead to failure of the graft. In the past, this has led some surgeons to recommend routine postoperative angiography at 1- to 2-year intervals.[35,114] Currently, however, it appears that noninvasive determination of blood flow velocity within the graft, by means of duplex ultrasound, is quite accurate in predicting subsequent graft thrombosis. Patients with graft flow velocities below about 45 cm. per second should undergo angiography for locating a potentially correctable lesion. (Fig. 6).[4]

PROSTHETIC GRAFTS

Textile Grafts

The development of prosthetic arterial grafts was stimulated by the observation by Voorhees in the early 1950s that silk threads in the canine vascular system become covered with a glistening, endothelium-like cellular coating.[15] The hypothesis was then proposed that a fine mesh fabric would cause similar healing and thus function as a satisfactory arterial subsitute. Voorhees and associates subsequently described successful replacement of arteries in animals with a porous textile graft made from the nylon derivative, Vinyon "N."[123] Two years later the same graft was successfully implanted in humans.[11] The field of prosthetic vascular grafting has since achieved enormous clinical and laboratory importance.

COMPOSITION AND FABRICATION. Both the material and its method of fabrication are important in the manufacturing of prosthetic arterial substitutes. Materials such as nylon, Orlon, Ivalon, and Marlex have all proved disappointing primarily because of loss of tensile strength and kinking. The only textile materials thus far that have proven to function satisfactorily are Dacron and Teflon, neither of which loses significant tensile strength even after many years of implantation.

Dacron and Teflon grafts are manufactured by weaving or knitting multifilament texturized yarns (Figs. 7 and 8). Each process has advantages and disadvantages. Woven grafts must be tightly interlaced to prevent slippage and fraying of the yarn. This compact structure of the graft causes small interstices and low porosity. These grafts leak minimally at the time of implantation but are somewhat stiff and slightly more difficult to manage. In addition, the tight configuration of the graft theoretically reduces the potential for development of a living neointima by connective tissue ingrowth through the graft interstices (see the following).

Knitted grafts are softer and more compliant than woven grafts. The knit can be varied. The looser the knit, the more elastic and more porous the graft. They have been widely used in vascular surgical operations below the diaphragm because of excellent handling characteristics, including softness and lack of fraying at cut ends.

Knitted grafts in clinical use are quite porous, between 1200 and 1900 ml. per cm. per minute and, therefore, must be preclotted prior to implantation. (Porosity for graft applications is defined as the amount of water that will pass through 1 sq. cm. of graft wall per minute under a hydrostatic driving pressure of 120 mm. Hg.) A sample of the patient's blood is forced repeatedly through the graft interstices. This causes platelet-fibrin deposition in the interstices, which renders the graft temporarily impervious to blood. After implantation, this platelet-fibrin material is slowly replaced by fibrous ingrowth from the host. Porous grafts must be used with great caution in patients with platelet or coagulation defects. Under these circumstances, the necessary initial coagulum may never properly form, and the patient may bleed excessively through the graft interstices. A tightly woven graft is preferred in this setting. Woven grafts are also generally preferred in repairs of the intrathoracic aorta to limit hemorrhage through the graft interstices, especially in operations requiring full heparinization and cardiopulmonary bypass.

Innovative manufacturing modifications have been superimposed on the basic concepts of knitted and woven textile grafts. Velour surfaces can be added to the inside, outside, or both sides of knitted or woven grafts. Velour surfaces have loops of yarn extending almost perpendicular to the fabric surface (Fig.9).[67,96] Various porosities and thicknesses are possible. The velour surfaces improve the handling characteristics of woven grafts and provide a scaffold for fibroblast ingrowth, leading to firm graft adherence to surrounding tissue. The velour concept is widely

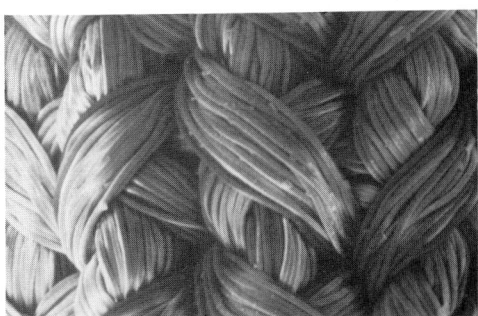

Figure 8. Close-up photograph (×50) of a knitted Dacron prosthetic vascular graft. The large openings between the knitted yarns make this graft relatively permeable to blood, and the graft must be preclotted before use in order to fill the interstices with fibrin.

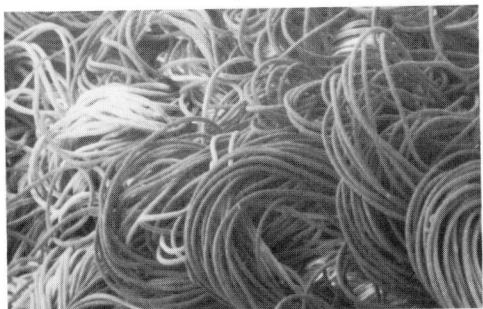

Figure 9. Photograph (×50) of the external surface of a woven double velour Dacron graft. The striking difference in the surface texture compared with that of a standard knitted or woven Dacron prosthesis (Figs. 7 and 8) is obvious. The velour configuration promotes rapid fibrous anchoring of the graft to surrounding tissues.

accepted, and a large percentage of textile vascular grafts in current use have a velour surface.

Most textile grafts in clinical use are also crimped to impart greater flexibility without kinking.[38] Although widely employed, this process has several potential disadvantages. Crimping diminishes luminal diameter, increases the thickness of the graft material, and may cause deposition of thrombogenic fibrin in the crimped areas.[60] Recent evidence suggests that it is possible to manufacture externally supported grafts that avoid kinking with angulation and yield results equal or superior to these obtained with crimped grafts. These grafts have an incompressible large fiber wound around and adherent to the external surface.

CLINICAL APPLICATIONS OF TEXTILE GRAFTS. The knitted Dacron graft has been the most frequently used prosthetic arterial graft during the past 25 years, although the woven graft is currently approaching it in popularity. In recent years, the majority of knitted grafts used have been those with a velour surface. Woven Dacron grafts have traditionally been used primarily in those settings in which interstitial bleeding would present major problems. The addition of velour surfaces to woven Dacron grafts has prompted widespread application of woven grafts. Textile-fabricated Teflon grafts are presently used by only a few surgeons but generally appear to function satisfactorily, especially in large artery applications.[12]

Textile grafts function most satisfactorily when used for arterial replacement proximal to the inguinal ligament (Figs. 10 and 11). Five-and 10-year patencies have been reported as high as 91 and 66 per cent, respectively, for aortofemoral bypass.[13,73,85] Axillofemoral bypass patency has been in the range of 75 to 77 per cent at 5 years, and femorofemoral bypass patency at 5 years has similarly been 75 to 80 percent.[14,54,59,70,105] Textile grafts have usually produced patency results distinctly inferior to that of the saphenous vein when used for bypass below the inguinal ligament. In the most favorable reports, Dacron bypass to the popliteal artery has produced a 5-year patency in the range of 50 per cent, about 20 to 30 per cent lower than comparable vein

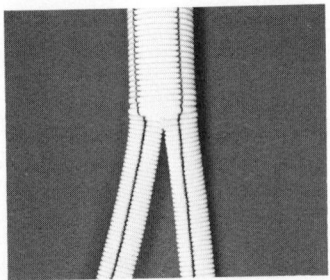

Figure 10. Photograph of a standard knitted Dacron bifurcation graft. The crimp pattern is clearly seen. The strips aid the surgeon in proper graft positioning and diminish the likelihood of unrecognized axial rotation of the graft limb when placed in the aortofemoral position.

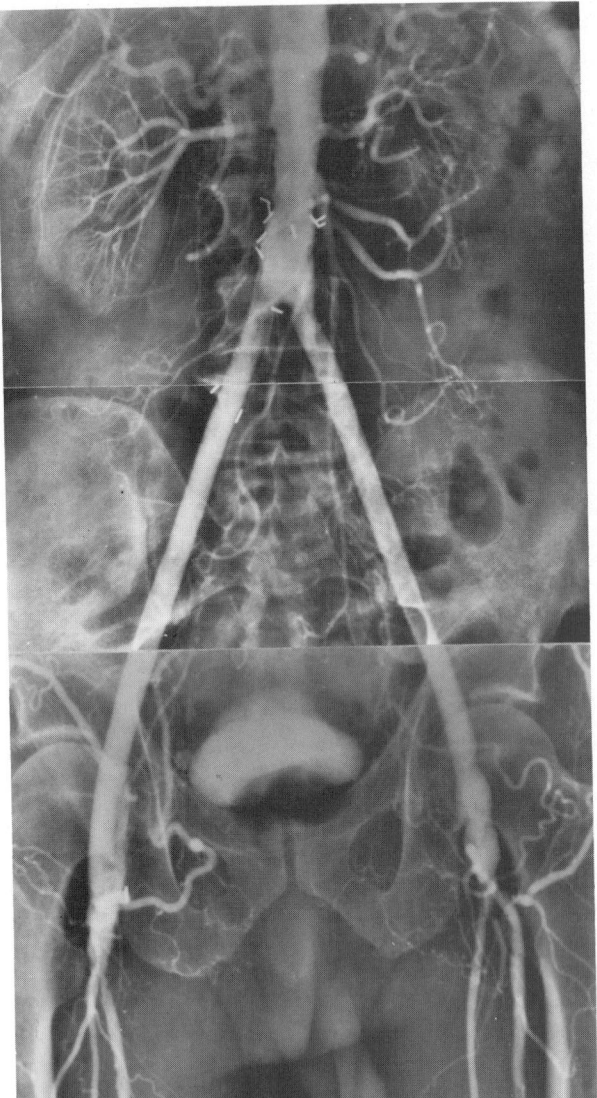

Figure 11. Angiogram of an aortofemoral knitted bifurcation Dacron graft. The graft extends from the infrarenal aorta to the common femoral arteries.

bypass series.[88] The textile grafts have produced low patency results when used to bypass arteries distal to the popliteal artery; therefore, their clinical use in this setting is not recommended.

Polytetrafluoroethylene (PTFE) Grafts

PTFE is a fluorocarbon polymer formed into sheets by a unique paste extrusion process. PTFE is not a textile but rather a semi-inert polymer consisting of solid nodes of PTFE with interconnecting small fibrils.[16] The intranodal distance can be varied in the manufacturing process and is about 40 μ for grafts in clinical use (Fig. 12). The graft has a highly electronegative surface charge and is thus hydrophobic and resistant to thrombosis. The grafts are coated with a thick outer wrap of PTFE, added for avoidance of aneurysm formation, which occurred frequently with early clinical use of unwrapped grafts.[17] PTFE grafts are available with external ring supports for avoidance of compression in subcutaneous locations and kinking with angulation. Wall thickness may be varied, with thin-walled grafts preferred for infrainguinal bypasses. Thick-walled grafts function well as hemodialysis shunts and, in most centers, have replaced bovine grafts as the preferred material for hemodialysis access when creation of a native fistula is not possible.

CLINICAL APPLICATIONS OF PTFE GRAFTS. Although

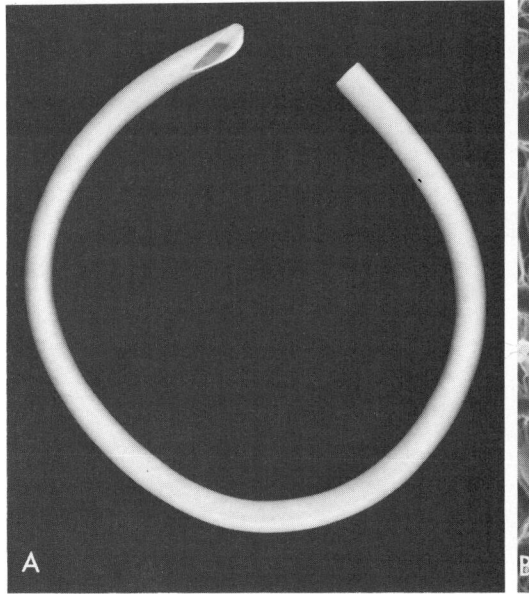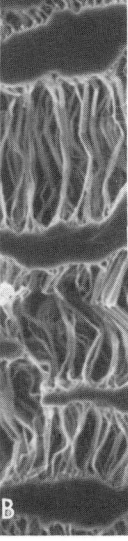

Figure 12. *A*, Photograph of a PTFE graft; *B*, photomicrograph (×1000) of PTFE graft. The dark areas are PTFE nodes interconnected by many PTFE fibrils. Average internodal distance in grafts in clinical use now is 40 μ.

available in a wide variety of sizes and configurations suitable for nearly any arterial reconstructive procedure, PTFE grafts have been used most widely as a substitute for autogenous vein in infrainguinal bypasses. Initial reports of patency rates similar to those of saphenous vein grafts have since been modified by larger series with longer postoperative follow-up.[6,50,80,86] Cumulative patency of PTFE grafts used in the above-knee femoropopliteal position is about 75 per cent at 1 year and 55 per cent at 5 years. These results, at least in the short-term, are sufficiently close to those reported in certain series of saphenous vein grafts to prompt some workers to conclude that PTFE grafts should serve as the initial conduit for above-knee femoropopliteal bypass, especially in pateints with a limited life expectancy.[86] PTFE grafts, however, have performed poorly in comparison with saphenous vein when used as bypass conduits to the below-knee popliteal and tibial arteries or in situations with poor distal runoff.[6,50,128] Although some have reported 50 to 60 per cent intermediate patency of PTFE grafts performed for limb salvage,[47] others have concluded that when such grafts must be anastomosed to tibial arteries, the results are so poor that primary amputation should be strongly considered.[30] Despite these considerations, PTFE grafts are widely employed as the prosthetic arterial substitute of choice for infrainguinal bypass when autogenous vein is not available. Recent evidence suggests that the patency of PTFE grafts may be extended through the use of routine warfarin anticoagulation.[40] Although PTFE grafts are easily thrombectomized, it now appears that thrombosis of established infrainguinal PTFE grafts is best treated by placement of a new conduit.[119]

Prosthetic Graft Healing

Shortly after prosthetic graft implantation, a thin layer of fibrin is deposited on the luminal surface. In grafts with high flow, the thickness stabilizes at about 1 mm. and is well tolerated. In a low-flow environment, however, the fibrin layer frequently continues to increase in thickness, proceeding to luminal occlusion.

In the experimental animal, the fibrin layer is progressively organized, causing development of a lining consisting of fibroblasts, myofibroblasts, and fibrocollagenous connective tissue. The graft lining then becomes connected to the perigraft tissue by ingrowth through the interstices of the fabric.[124] Prosthetic

graft healing refers to the development of a living neointima inside the graft, connected to an external fibrous capsule around the graft by means of connective tissue ingrowth through graft interstices. "Well-healed" grafts offer the possibility of decreased thrombogenicity and increased resistance to infection.

The extent of graft healing is related to both the host species and the graft itself. With respect to the graft, the quality of healing reflects both the porosity of the graft and the thickness of the graft wall. Healing is favored by increased porosity and decreased wall thickness. Additional healing may occur at the graft margins by means of endothelial ingrowth from the host vessels. Healing by this mechanism is limited to the few centimeters adjacent to the anastomosis.

Complete graft healing routinely occurs in animal models when thin, porous grafts are used. However, such grafts, when implanted in patients, never develop a complete living neointima. An extremely important clinical study by Sauvage and associates in 1972 first clearly demonstrated that prosthetic grafts in humans do not develop a living neointimal lining but rather maintain a permanent lining composed primarily of compacted fibrin.[8] These investigators later described detailed studies of prosthetic grafts removed from 64 patients months to years after implantation. The results clearly showed that human beings have very limited abilities to organize fibrin deposits on the luminal surface of grafts, in sharp contrast to experimental animals. A small zone of luminal healing occurs adjacent to suture lines, but otherwise the graft is typically lined with compacted fibrin even years after implantation. Only 2 of the 64 grafts showed significant luminal healing, and even then endothelial cells could not be identified. Although Sauvage's studies involved primarily fabric grafts, recent work suggests a similar situation with PTFE grafts.[70]

The concept of limited graft healing in humans is supported by platelet survival and localization studies. Several investigators have correlated platelet survival and platelet-graft deposition with healing of the graft lumen. In the totally healed grafts of animals, both platelet survival and platelet-graft deposition return to normal. Harker and colleagues have shown that humans with aortic prostheses have shortened platelet survival for 9 months after graft implantation but have increased platelet deposition upon the graft for at least 120 months.[52,53] Thus, one is forced to conclude that a large majority of prosthetic arterial grafts in man, unlike those in the experimental animal, never develop an organized internal lining and remain permanently lined with compacted fibrin. The relevance to man of animal-derived optimal graft design characteristics must be regarded as uncertain.

Complications of Prosthetic Grafting

The most frequently observed prosthetic graft complications include anastomotic neointimal hyperplasia, graft infection, graft failure caused by fiber disruption or stretching, perigraft seromas, and development of anastomotic false aneurysms.

NEOINTIMAL HYPERPLASIA. This process is similar to that described for saphenous vein grafts and is present at both proximal and distal anastomoses. The distal anastomotic process appears clinically to be the more significant and is frequently implicated as a cause of prosthetic graft failure. Both textile and PTFE grafts are affected. The aforementioned hypothetic etiologic factors for neointimal hyperplasia associated with saphenous vein grafts probably also apply to prosthetic grafts. As with saphenous vein grafts, antiplatelet drugs are frequently prescribed for patients with prosthetic grafts, in an effort to reduce the magnitude of anastomotic fibroplasia. However, the evidence for the efficacy of this treatment is weak.[45] Use of antiplatelet agents, specifically aspirin, however, is clearly indicated in patients with peripheral vascular disease since these agents have been shown to decrease significantly overall cardiovascular-associated morbidity and mortality.[2]

GRAFT INFECTION. Infection is one of the most feared complications of prosthetic grafting. *Staphylococcus aureus, Staphylococcus epidermidis,* and *Escherichia coli* are the most frequently isolated organisms. The incidence is about 1.5 to 2.5 per cent; it is slightly lower when the graft is completely intra-abdominal and higher when a groin anastomosis is present. Aortic graft infections currently are associated with an operative mortality of 10 to 25 per cent and an amputation rate of 15 to 20 per cent.[90,129] Even infrainguinal graft infections are associated with very high mortality and amputation rates.[62] Graft infection may be decreased by careful patient selection, meticulous preparation of sites for surgical incision, and preoperative use of prophylatic antibiotics, usually a cephalosporin.[58] Actual bonding of antibiotics to prosthetic grafts is possible and is being currently evaluated in animal models.[5,104]

In a large majority of cases, an infected arterial graft must be removed for control of infection. Anecdotal reports of successful treatment of graft infection by local drainage and antibiotic irrigation without graft removal appear the exception. The basic principle of infected graft treatment remains graft excision and revascularization through a clean field. It appears that both mortality and amputation rates can be improved if the revascularization is performed first, followed by removal of the infected prosthetic graft.[90] Staging the operation in this manner lessens the complications of prolonged distal ischemia. On occasion, revascularization through the contaminated field may be successful if entirely autogenous tissue is used.

GRAFT FAILURE. Two distinct types of Dacron graft failure have been described. The first consists of a gradual, diffuse graft dilatation, which was observed frequently with the ultralightweight knitted Dacron in widespread use in the early 1970s.[23,77,82] The dilatation was caused by expansion of the knit rather than elongation or weakening of individual fibers. These diffusely dilated grafts frequently caused no trouble but on occasion were associated with delayed graft rupture or diffuse interstitial bleeding.[7,127] The ultralightweight method of fabrication has been abandoned by all manufacturers.

The second type of graft failure follows specific defects, such as a dropped stitch in the manufacturing process, or fiber degeneration. This type of defect usually causes localized holes and leaks, with the potential for false aneurysm formation (Fig. 13).

ANASTOMOTIC FALSE ANEURYSMS. An anastomotic aneurysm follows a partial or total separation of the prosthetic graft from the host artery. These are termed false aneurysms, because the blood is contained by the nonelastic surrounding fibrous capsule rather than the true vessel wall. The natural history of an anastomotic aneurysm is progressive expansion, with an eventual serious complication of rupture, thrombosis, or embolism. The incidence of false aneurysm with prosthetic grafting is estimated to be at least 3 per cent. Both Dacron and PTFE grafts are affected, although there is suggestive evidence that the incidence may be less with PTFE grafts.[87]

Because a prosthetic arterial anastomosis is forever dependent upon the anastomotic suture line, many false aneurysms in the past resulted from degeneration and fragmentation of silk sutures used for construction of the anastomosis. Since the recognition of this problem, silk sutures are no longer used for arterial anastomoses. The exact cause of currently encountered false aneurysms is unclear. Frequently, the suture line and sutures are found intact, with the aneurysm occurring through a tear in the host artery adjacent to the suture line. Obvious clinical infection can be implicated in only a small percentage of cases. Recent work, however, has suggested that with rigorous culture techniques infectious organisms can be demonstrated in a large number of false aneurysms.[119] Whether these subclinical infections are the actual cause of the false aneurysms or merely incidental findings is unknown. Other suggested etiologies of false aneurysms include shallow suture placement or arterial

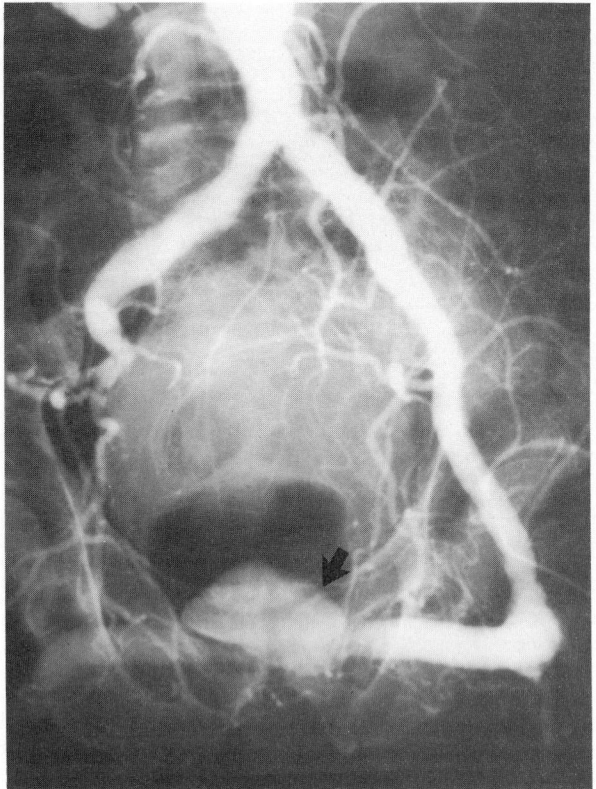

Figure 13. A defective knitted Dacron prosthesis resulted in this false aneurysm (arrow) of the mid-portion of a femorofemoral graft.

degeneration associated with hypertension. Several interesting studies have suggested that anastomotic aneurysms may follow graft-artery compliance mismatches accentuated by graft dilation.[21,41] With rare exception, anastomotic aneurysms should be repaired when discovered. The usual repair consists of a graft-artery reanastomosis, frequently with the insertion of a short additional piece of graft material.

PERIGRAFT SEROMA. A perigraft seroma is a sterile collection of clear fluid within a nonsecretory pseudomembrane surrounding a prosthetic vascular graft. It usually occurs in association with extra-anatomic bypasses, i.e., an axillofemoral or femorofemoral graft. The incidence is probably around 2 per cent, occurring with both Dacron and PTFE grafts. The etiology is unknown but may relate to relative fibroblast inhibition, with failure of the graft incorporation into surrounding tissues.[106] Treatment has included observation alone, multiple aspirations, graft removal, injection of perigraft sclerosing agents, excision of the fibrous pseudocapsule, or intraperitoneal drainage.

Graft Modifications and Experimental Arterial Substitutes

A number of modifications of knitted Dacron grafts have been proposed to eliminate the need for preclotting by rendering the grafts temporarily impervious to blood while maintaining desirable handling properties. Cooley and associates have described soaking knitted Dacron grafts in the patient's own plasma, followed by steam autoclaving for 3 to 5 minutes.[24] Other investigators have used albumin to temporarily coat knitted grafts.[29] These grafts require special packaging and must be rehydrated prior to implantation but do handle somewhat better than standard low-porosity woven arterial substitutes. Finally, Dacron grafts may be impregnated with bovine Type I collagen.[89] The grafts are leakproof and handle essentially the same as standard knitted grafts. Crosslinking of the collagen during the manufacturing process appears to eliminate the normal thrombogenicity of collagen, and the grafts appear no more prone to thrombosis than a standard preclotted, knitted prosthesis. The ultimate clinical usefulness of many of these modifications of knitted grafts is unknown; new woven double velour grafts are less expensive, easily preclotted, and handle nearly as well as standard knitted grafts.

Bovine carotid xenografts have been modified with a combination of amino acid carboxylation and glutaraldehyde tanning. The negative luminal electrical charge imparted by this process supposedly makes the grafts relatively resistant to thrombosis.[97] Despite encouraging preliminary reports several years ago, no controlled clinical information has subsequently been reported. These grafts must therefore be regarded as experimental and of unproved clinical efficacy. The same applies to autogenous fibrocollagenous tubes formed over silicone mandrils,[51] pyrolytic carbon-coated grafts,[103] polyurethane grafts of various configurations,[42] and combinations of Dacron and PTFE.[48]

Many studies have been published over the last 10 to 15 years with respect to endothelial seeding of small caliber synthetic vascular prostheses. The presence of a living neointima composed of viable endothelial cells, it is hoped, would cause improved patency of prosthetic infrainguinal bypasses. The research is complex, with problems in harvesting viable endothelial cells, optimizing methods of seeding and cellular attachment to the graft, tracking of cells from harvesting to healing, and documenting normal function of seeded endothelial cells. Nevertheless, the field is now moving into its first significant clinical trials and will bear watching over the next 5 to 10 years.

OVERVIEW

Arterial grafting is of critical importance in modern vascular surgery. Available evidence clearly indicates that large artery bypass is best accomplished with textile-fabricated Dacron grafts or with PTFE grafts. For small artery bypass below the inguinal ligament, no arterial prosthesis has matched the performance and patency of autogenous saphenous vein grafts. To date, no arterial prosthesis 4 mm. or smaller in diameter has produced satisfactory clinical patency. Various prosthetic grafts to the above-knee popliteal artery have approached intermediate-term vein bypass patency results, athough none appears as good as vein. No prosthetic graft has approached saphenous vein results for bypass to the below-knee popliteal artery or to the tibial arteries.

Research activity in graft design and fabrication presently is directed toward the development of a satisfactory prosthetic graft for small artery bypass. Most investigators believe that a satisfactory small artery prosthesis requires luminal healing and compliance characteristics considerably superior to grafts in present use, undoubtedly accompanied by improved understanding of the processes of atherosclerosis, thrombosis, and arterial healing.

SELECTED REFERENCES

Berger, K., Sauvage, L. R., Rao, A. M., and Wood, S. J.: Healing of arterial prostheses in man: Its incompleteness. Ann. Surg., 175:113, 1972.
This article reports detailed pathologic observations on arterial prostheses removed from patients. It is of pivotal importance in emphasizing the marked differences between humans and the experimental animal in the healing of prosthetic arterial grafts.

Sawyer, P. N., (Ed.): Modern Vascular Grafts. New York, McGraw-Hill Book Company, 1987.
A multiauthored text containing literature reviews of various grafts by noted authorities.

Stanley, J. C., (Ed.): Biologic and Synthetic Vascular Prostheses. New York, Grune & Stratton, 1982.
This well-edited book reports the proceedings of a symposium on vascular grafts held in 1982. Although now slightly dated, it remains the most thorough and well-referenced resource book available on arterial grafting.

Szilagyi, D. E., Elliott, J. P., Hageman, J. H., Smith, R. F., and Dall'Olmo, C. A.: Biologic fate of autogenous vein implants and arterial substitutes. Ann. Surg., 178:232, 1973.
The authors present detailed clinical, angiographic, and pathologic follow-up information of a personal series of 377 autogenous vein bypass grafts. This excellent reference clearly documents the long-term performance of autogenous vein grafts in humans.

Wesolowski, S. A., and Dennis, C.: Fundamentals of Vascular Grafting. New York, McGraw-Hill Book Company, 1963.
This monograph contains a summary of most of the important history, experiments, and clinical fundamentals of prosthetic vascular grafting.

Wright, C. B., (Ed.): Vascular Grafting. Boston, John Wright Co., 1983.
A multiauthored book with wide variations between chapters. Certain chapters are of remarkable quality, such as that on femoropopliteal grafting by Lynch and Hobson.

REFERENCES

1. Abbott, W. M., Megerman, J. M., Hasson, J. E. , L'Italien, G., and Warnock, D. F.: Effect of compliance mismatch on vascular graft patency. J. Vasc. Surg., 5:376, 1987.
2. Antiplatelet Trialists Collaboration: Secondary prevention of vascular disease by prolonged antiplatelet treatment. Br. Med. J., 296:320, 1988.
3. Axthelm, S. C., Porter, J. M., Strickland, S., et al.: Antigenicity of venous allografts. Ann. Surg., 189:290, 1978.
4. Bandyk, D. F., Cato, R. F., and Towne, J. B.: A low flow velocity predicts failure of femoropopliteal and femorotibial bypass grafts. Surgery, 98:799, 1985.
5. Benvenisty, A. I., Modak, S., Ahlborn, T. N., et al.: Prevention of vascular prosthetic infection with silver-containing antibiotics using model of direct bacterial contamination. Surg. Forum, 36:433, 1985.
6. Bergan, J. J., Veith, F. J., and Bernhard, V.M. Randomization of autogenous vein and polytetrafluoroethylene grafts in femoral distal reconstruction. Surgery, 92:921, 1982.
7. Berger, K., and Sauvage, L. R.: Late fiber deterioration in Dacron arterial grafts. Ann. Surg., 193:477, 1981.
8. Berger, K., Sauvage, L. R., Rao, A. M., and Wood, S. J.: Healing of arterial prostheses in man: Its incompleteness. Ann. Surg. 175:118, 1972.
9. Berger, K., Sauvage, L. R., Wood, S. J., and Sameh, A. A.: Endarterectomy and other surgical injuries to cardiovascular walls. Pacific Med. Surg., 75:367, 1967.
10. Bernheim, B. M.: The ideal operation for aneurysm of the extremity. Report of a case. Bull. Johns Hopkins Hosp., 27:93, 1916.
11. Blakemore, A., and Voorhees, A. B., Jr.: The use of tubes constructed of Vinyon "N" cloth in bridging arterial defects. Experimental and clinical. Ann. Surg., 140:324, 1954.
12. Boyd, D. P., and Midell, A. I.: The use of Teflon in artery surgery. Surg. Clin. North Am., 53:351, 1973.
13. Brewster, D. C., and Darling, R. C.: Optimal methods of aortoiliac reconstruction. Surgery, 84:739, 1978.
14. Brief, D. K., Brener, B., and Alpert, J.: Crossover femorofemoral grafts followed up five years or more: An analysis. Arch. Surg., 110:1294, 1975.
15. Callow, A. D.: Historical overview of experimental and clinical development of vascular grafts.In Stanley, J. (Ed.): Biologic and Synthetic Vascular Prostheses. New York, Grune & Stratton, 1982, p. 11.
16. Campbell, C. D., Brooks, D. H., and Bahnson, H. T.: Expanded microporous polytetrafluoroethylene as a vascular conduit. In Sawyer, P. N., Kaplitt, M. J. (Eds.): Vascular Grafts. New York, Appleton-Century-Crofts, 1978, p. 335.
17. Campbell, C. D., Brooks, D. H., and Webster, M. W.: Aneurysm formation in expanded polytetrafluoroethylene prostheses. Surgery, 79:491, 1976.
18. Carrel, A.: Results of the transplantation of blood vessels, organs, and limbs. J.A.M.A. 51:1162, 1908.
19. Carrel, A., and Guthrie, C.: Uniterminal and biterminal venous transplantations. Surg. Gynecol. Obstet. 2:226, 1906.
20. Castellot, J. J., Addonizio, M. L., Rosenberg, R., and Karnovsky, M. J.: Cultured endothelial cells produce a heparin-like inhibitor of smooth muscle cell growth. J. Cell. Biol., 90:372, 1981.
21. Clagett, G. P., Salander, J. M., and Eddleman, W. L.: Dilatation of knitted Dacron aortic prostheses and anastomotic false aneurysms: Etiologic considerations. Surgery, 93:9, 1983.
22. Clowes, A. W., Kirkman, T. R., and Reidy, M. A.: Mechanisms of arterial graft healing. Rapid transmural capillary ingrowth provides a source of intimal endothelium and smooth muscle in porous PTFE prostheses. Am. J. Pathol., 123:220, 1986.
23. Cooke, P. A., Nobis, P. A., and Stoney, R. J.: Dacron aortic graft failure. Arch. Surg., 108:101, 1974.
24. Cooley, D. A., Romagnoli, A., Milam, J. D., and Bossart, M.I.: A method of preparing woven Dacron aortic grafts to prevent interstitial hemorrhage. Bull. Texas Heart Inst., 8:48, 1981.
25. Curtis, J., Stoney, W. S., Alford, W. C., Burrus, G. R., and Thomas, C. S.: Intimal hyperplasia. Ann. Thorac. Surg., 20:628, 1975.
26. Dale, W. A., and Lewis, M. R.: Further experience with bovine arterial grafts. Surgery, 80:711, 1976.

27. Dardik, H., Ibrahim, I. M., Sussman, B. C., Kahn, M., and Dardik, I.: Glutaraldehyde-tanned umbilical vein grafts. *In* Stanley, J. (Ed.): Biologic and Synthetic Vascular Prostheses. New York, Grune & Stratton, 1982, p. 445.

28. Dardik, H., Miller, N., Dardik, A., Ibrahim, I. M., Sussman, B. C., Berry, S. M., Wolodiger, F., Kahn, M., and Dardik, I.: A decade of experience with the glutaraldehyde-tanned human umbilical cord vein graft for revascularization of the lower limb. J. Vasc. Surg., 7:336, 1988.

29. DeBakey, M., Noon, D., Edwards, W., Evan, W., and Vermilion, B.: Bard albumin-coated DeBakey Vasculour-II vascular prosthesis. Data on file. Bard Implant Division, C. R. Bard Inc., Box M, Billerica, Mass. 08121.

30. Dennis, J. W., Littooy, F. N., Greisler, H. P., and Baker, W. H.: Secondary vascular prcedures with polytetrafluoroethylene grafts for lower extremity ischemia in a male veteran population. J. Vasc. Surg., 8:137, 1988.

31. DePalma, R. G.: Atherosclerosis in vascular grafts. Atherosclerosis Rev., 6:147, 1979.

32. Deterling, R. A., and Clauss, R. H.: Long-term fate of aortic arterial homografts. J. Cardiovasc. Surg., 11:35, 1970.

33. Deweese, J. A., and Rob, C. G.: Autogenous venous grafts ten years later. Surgery, 82:775, 1977.

34. Dos Santos, R., Lamas, A., and Pereira-Caldas, J.: L'arteriographie des membres de l'aorte et de ses branches abdominales. Bull. Soc. Natl. Chir., 55:587, 1929.

35. Downs, A. R., and Morrow, I. M.: Angiographic assessment of autogenous vein grafts. Surgery, 72:699, 1972.

36. Dubost, C., Allary, M., and Deconomos, N.: Resection of aneurysm of the abdominal aorta. Reestablishment of continuity by a preserved human arterial graft with results after five months. Arch. Surg., 64:405, 1952.

37. Edwards, W. S., Hodefer, W. F., and Mofashemi, M.: The importance of proper caliber of lumen in femoropopliteal artery reconstruction. Surg. Gynecol. Obstet., 122:37, 1966.

38. Edwards, W. S., and Tapp, J. S.: Chemically treated nylon tubes as arterial grafts. Surgery, 38:61, 1955.

39. Eickhoff, J. H., Broome, A., Ericsson, B. F., Hansen, H. J. B., Kordt, K. F., Mouritzen, C., Kvernebo, K., Norgren, L., Rostad, H., and Trippestad, A.: Four years' results of prospective, randomized clinical trial comparing polytetrafluoroethylene and modified human umbilical vein for below-knee femoropopliteal bypass. J. Vasc. Surg., 6:506, 1987.

40. Flinn, W. R., Rohrer, M. J., Yao, J. S. T., McCarthy, W. J., III, Fahey, V. A., and Bergan, J. J.: Improved long-term patency of infragenicular polytetrafluoroethylene grafts. J. Vasc. Surg., 7:685, 1988.

41. Gaylis, H.: Pathogenesis of anastomotic aneurysms. Surgery, 90:509, 1981.

42. Geeraert, A. J., and Callaghan, J. C.: Experimental study of selected small caliber arterial grafts. J. Cardiovasc. Surg., 18:155, 1977.

43. Geiringer, E.: Intimal vascularization and atherosclerosis. J. Pathol. Bacteriol., 63:201, 1951.

44. Giordano, J. M., and Keshishian, J. M.: Aneurysm formation in human umbilical vein grafts. Surgery, 91:343, 1982.

45. Gloviczki, P., and Hollier, L. H. Can graft occlusion be prevented by drugs? *In* Greenhalgh, R. M., Jamieson, C. W., Nicolaides, A. N. (Eds.): Vascular Surgery; Issues in Current Practice. London, Grune & Stratton, 1986, pp. 37–48.

46. Goyanes, J.: Nuevos trabajos de cirugia vascular, substitucios plastic de las arterias por las venas o arterioplastia venous applicada, como nuevo metoclo, al tratamiento de las aneurismas. Siglo Med., 53:546, 1906.

47. Graham, L. M., and Bergan, J. J.: Expanded polytetrafluoroethylene vascular grafts: Clinical and experimental observations. *In* Stanley, J. C. (Ed.): Biologic and Synthetic Vascular Prostheses. New York, Grune & Stratton, 1982, pp. 563–586.

48. Greisler, H.P., Dennis, J. W., Schwarez, T. H., Klosak, J. J., Ellinger, J., and Kim, D. U. Plasma polymerized tetrafluoroethylene/polyethylene terephthalate vascular prostheses. Arch. Surg., 124:967, 1989.

49. Gross, R. E., Hierwitt, E. S., Bill, A. H., Jr., and Pierce, E. C.: Preliminary observations on the use of human arterial grafts in the treatment of certain cardiovascular defects. N. Engl. J. Med., 239:578, 1948.

50. Hallett, J. W., Jr., Brewster, D. C., and Darling, R. C.: The limitations of polytetrafluoroethylene in the reconstruction of femoropopliteal and tibial arteries. Surg. Gynecol. Obstet., 152:819, 1981.

51. Hallin, R. W., and Sweetman, W. R.: The Sparks mandril graft. Am. J. Surg., 132:221, 1976.

52. Harker, L.A., and Hanson, S. R.: Graft thrombus formation, detection, and resolution. *In* Stanley, J. (Ed.): Biologic and Synthetic Vascular Prostheses. New York, Grune & Stratton 1982, p. 101.

53. Harker, L. A., Slichter, L. J., and Sauvage, L. R.: Platelet consumption by arterial prostheses: The effects of endothelialization and pharmacologic inhibition of platelet function. Ann. Surg., 186:594, 1977.

54. Harris, E. J., Jr., Taylor, L. M., Jr., McConnell, D. B., Moneta, G. L., Yeager, R. A., and Porter, J. M.: Improved modern results of axillobifemoral bypass using externally supported PTFE. J. Vasc. Surg., 12(4):416, 1990.

55. Harris, R. W., Audros, G., Dulawa, L. B., Oblath, R. W., et al.: Successful long-term limb salvage using cephalic vein bypass grafts. Ann. Surg., 200:785, 1984.

56. Harrison, J. H., Jr.: Synthetic materials as vascular prostheses. Am. J. Surg., 95:16, 1958.

57. Hoepfner, E.: Über Gefassnaht, Gefasstransplantionen und Replantation von amputierten Extremitaten. Arch. Klin. Chir., 70:417, 1903.

58. Kaiser, A B., Clayson, K. R., and Mulherin, J. L.: Antibiotic prophylaxis in vascular surgery. Ann. Surg., 188:283, 1978.

59. Kalman, P. G., Hosang, M., Johnston, K. W., and Walker, D. M.: The current role of femorofemoral bypass. J. Vasc. Surg., 6:71, 1987.

60. Kenney, D. A., Berger, K., Walker, M. W., and Sauvage, L.: Experimental comparison of the thrombogenicity of fibrin and PTFE flow surfaces. Ann. Surg., 191:355, 1980.

61. Kent, K. C., Whittemore, A. D., and Mannick, J. A.: Short-term and mid-term results of an all-autogenous tissue policy for infrainguinal reconstruction. J. Vasc. Surg., 9:107, 1989.

62. Kikta, M. J., Goodson, S. F., Bishars, R. A., Meyer, J. P., Schuler, J. J., and Flanigan, D. P.: Mortality and limb loss with infected infrainguinal bypass grafts. J. Vasc. Surg., 5:566, 1987.

63. Klaysod, K. R., Edwards, W. H., and Allen, T. R.: Arm veins for peripheral arterial reconstruction. Arch. Surg., 111:1276, 1976.

64. Kunlin, J.: Le traitement de l'arterique obliterante par la greffe veinense. Arch. Mal. Coeur, 42:371, 1949.

65. Leather, R. P., Shah, D. M., Chang, B. B., and Kaufman, J. L.: Resurrection of the *in situ* saphenous vein bypass: 1000 cases later. Ann. Surg., 308:435, 1988.

66. Leather, R. P., Shah, D. M., and Karmody, A. M.: Infrapopliteal arterial bypass for limb salvage—increased patency and utilization of the saphenous vein used "in situ". Surgery, 90:1000, 1981.

67. Lindenauer, S. M., Lavanway, J. M., and Fry, W. J.: Development of a velour vascular prosthesis. Curr. Top. Surg. Res., 2:491, 1970.

68. Linton, R. R.: Discussion of paper by DeBakey, M. E., Crawford, E. S., Cooley, D. A., and Morris, G. C.: Surgical considerations of occlusive disease of the abdominal aorta and iliac and femoral arteries: Analysis of 803 cases. Ann. Surg., 148:306, 1958.

69. LoGerfo, F. W, Corson, J. D., and Mannick, J. A.: Improved results with femoropopliteal vein grafts for limb salvage. Arch. Surg., 112:567, 1977.

70. LoGerfo, F. W., Johnson, W. C., and Corson, J.: A comparison of the late patency rates of axillobilateral femoral and axillounilateral femoral grafts. Surgery, 81:33, 1977.

71. LoGerfo, F. W., Quist, W. C., Catelmo, W. L., and Handenschild, C. C.: Integrity of vein grafts as a function of initial intimal and medial preservation. Circulation, (II)63:117, 1983.

72. Lytle, B. W., Loo, F. D., Cosgrove, D. M., Ratliff, N. B., Easley, K., and Taylor, P. C.: Long-term (5 to 12 years) serial studies in internal mammary artery and saphenous vein coronary bypass grafts. J. Thorac. Cardiovasc. Surg., 89:248, 1985.

73. Malone, J. M., Moore, W. S., and Goldstone, J.: The natural history of bilateral aortofemoral bypass grafts for ischemia of the lower extremity. Arch. Surg., 110:1300, 1975.

74. Mannick, J. A., Jackson, B. T., Coffman, J. D., and Hume, D. M.: Success of bypass vein grafts in patients with isolated popliteal artery segments. Surgery, 61:17, 1967.

75. Moniz, E.: L'encephalographic arterielle, son importance dans la localisation des tumeurs cerebrales. Rev. Neurol. (Paris), 2:72, 1927.

76. Murray, G. D. W.: Heparin in thrombosis and blood vessel surgery. Surg. Gynecol. Obstet., 72:340, 1941.

77. Nunn, D. B., Freeman, M. H., and Hudgins, M. S.: Postoperative alterations in size of aortic Dacron grafts. Ann. Surg., 189:741, 1979.

78. Ochsner, J. L.: Discussion. *In* Williams, G. M., et al. (Eds.): Rejection and repair of endothelium in major vessel transplants. Surgery, 79:694, 1975.

79. Ochsner, J. L., DeCamp, P. T., and Leonard, G. L.: Experience with fresh venous allografts as an arterial substitute. Ann. Surg., 173:933, 1971.

80. O'Donnell, T. F., Farber, F. P., Richmond, D. M., Deterling, R. A, and Callow, A: Above-knee polytetrafluoroethylene bypass graft: Is it a reasonable alternative to the below-knee reversed autogenous vein grafts? Surgery, 94:26, 1983.

81. Okuhn, S. P., Connelly, D. P., Calakos, N., Ferrell, L., Man-Xiang, P, and Goldstone, J.: Compliance mismatch alone cause neointimal hyperplasia? J. Vasc. Surg. 9:35, 1989.

82. Ottinger, L. W., Darling, R. C., Wirthlin, L. S., et al.: Failure of ultralight-weight knitted Dacron grafts in arterial reconstruction. Arch. Surg., 111:146, 1976.

83. Oudot, J., and Beaconsfield, P.: Thrombosis of aortic bifurcation treated by resection and homograft replacement: Report of five cases. Arch. Surg., 66:365, 1953.

84. Perloff, L. J., Reckard, C. R., Rowlands, D. T., Jr., and Barker, C. F.: The venous homograft: An immunological question. Surgery, 72:961, 1972.

85. Piotrowski, J. J., Pearce, W. H., Jones, D. N., Whitehill, T., Bell, R., Patt, A., and Rutherford, R. B.: Aortobifemoral bypass: The operation of choice for unilateral iliac occlusion? J. Vasc. Surg., 8:211, 1988.

86. Quinones-Baldrich, W. J., Busuttil, R. W., Baker, J. D., Vescera, C. L., Ahn, S. S., Machleder, H. I., and Moore, W. S.: Is the preferential use of polytetrafluoroethylene grafts for femoropopliteal bypass justified? J. Vasc. Surg., 8:219, 1988.

87. Quinones-Baldrich, W. J., Ziomek, S., Henderon, T., and Moore, W. S.: Primary anastomotic bonding in polytetrafluoroethylene grafts? J. Vasc. Surg., 5:311, 1987.

88. Reichle, F. A.: Criteria for evaluation of new arterial prostheses by comparing vein with Dacron femoropopliteal bypasses. Surg. Gynecol. Obstet., 145:714, 1978.

89. Reigel, M. M., Hollier, L. H., Pairolero, P. C., and Hallett, J. W., Jr.,: Early experience with a new collagen-impregnated aortic graft. Am. Surg., 54(3):134, 1988.

90. Reilly, L. M., Stoney, F. J., Goldstone, J., and Ehrenfeld, W. K.: Improved management of aortic graft infection: The influence of operation sequence and staging. J. Vasc. Surg., 5:421, 1987.

91. Rosenberg, N., Gauhran, E. R. L., Henderson, J., Lord, G. H., and Douglas, J. F.: The use of segmental arterial implants prepared by enzymatic modifications of heterologous blood vessels. Surg. Forum, 6:242, 1956.

92. Rosenberg, N., Thompson, J. E., and Keshishian, J. M.: The modified bovine arterial graft. Arch. Surg., 111:222, 1976.

93. Ross, R., Raines, E. W., and Bowen-Pope, D. F.: The biology of platelet-derived growth factor. Cell, 46:155, 1986.

94. Brockbank, K. G. M., Donovan, T. J., Ruby, S. T., Carpenter, J. F., Hagen, P.-O., Woodley, M. A.: Functional analysis of cryopreserved veins. J. Vasc. Surg., 11:94, 1990.

95. Rutherford, R. R., Flanigan, D. P., Gupta, S.K., Johnston, K. W., Karmody, A., Whittemore, A. D., Baker, J. D., and Ernst, C. B.: Suggested standards for reports dealing with lower extremity ischemia. J. Vasc. Surg., 4:80, 1986.

96. Sauvage, L. R., Berger, K. E., Wood, S. J., Yates, S. G., Smith, J. C., and Mansfield, P. B.: An external surface for porous arterial prostheses. Surgery, 70:940, 1971.

97. Sawyer, P. N., Stanczewski, B., and Mistry, F. D.: Current appraisal of negatively charged glutaraldehyde-tanned grafts. In Stanley, J. C. (Ed.): Biologic and Synthetic Vascular Prostheses. New York, Grune & Stratton, 1982, p. 467.

98. Schmitz-Rixen, T., Megerman, J., Colvin, R. B., Williams, A. M. and Abbott, W. M.: Immunosuppressive treatment of aortic allografts. J. Vasc. Surg., 7:82, 1988.

99. Schulman, M. L., and Badhey, M. R.: Late results and angiographic evaluation of arm veins as long bypass grafts. Surgery, 92:1032, 1982.

100. Schulman, J. L., Badhey, M. R., and Yatco, R.: Superficial femoropopliteal veins and reversed saphenous veins as primary femoropopliteal bypass grafts: A randomized comparative study. J. Vasc. Surg., 6:1, 1987.

101. Schuster, S. R., and Gross, R. D.: Surgery for coarctation of the aorta. J. Thorac. Cardiovasc. Surg., 43:54, 1962.

102. Schwartz, S. M., Campbell, G. R., and Campbell, J. H.: Replication of smooth muscle cells in vascular disease. Circ. Res., 58:427, 1986.

103. Sharp W. V.: Update on carbon-coated grafts. In Sawyer, P. N. (Ed.): Modern Vascular Grafts. New York, McGraw-Hill Book Company, 1987, p. 215.

104. Shue, W. B., Worosilo, M. S., Donetz, A. P., Trooskin, S. Z., Harvey, R. A., and Greco, R. S.: Prevention of vascular prosthetic infection with an antibiotic-bonded Dacron graft. J. Vasc. Surg., 8:600, 1988.

105. Silverman, S. H., Brown, P. B., Simms, M. H., Downing F. A., and Slaney, G.:Primary and secondary vascular reconstruction by femorofemoral bypass. Br. J. Surg., 76:416, 1989.

106. Sladen, J. G., Mandl, M. A. J., Grossman, L., and Denegri, J. F.: Fibroblast inhibition: A new treatable cause of prosthetic graft failure. Am. J. Surg., 149:587, 1986.

107. Sottiurai, V. S., and Batson, R. C.: Ultrastructural studies of arterial grafts. In Bergan, J. J., Yao, J. S. T. (Eds.): Evaluation and Treatment of Upper and Lower Extremity Circulatory Disorders. New York, Grune & Stratton, 1984, p. 371.

108. Sottiurai, V. S., Stanley, J. C., and Fry, W. J.: Ultrastructure of human and transplanted canine veins: Effects of different preparation media. Surgery, 93:28, 1983.

109. Sottiurai, V. S., Yao, J. S. T., Flinn, W. R., and Batson, R. C.: Intimal hyperplasia and neointima: An ultrastructural analysis of thrombosed grafts in humans. Surgery, 93:809, 1983.

110. Spray, T. L., and Roberts, W C.: Fundamentals of clinical cardiology: Changes in saphenous veins used as aortocoronary bypass grafts. Am. Heart J., 94:500, 1977.

111. Stanley, J. C., Ernst, C. B. and Fry, W. J.: Fate of 100 aortorenal vein grafts: Characteristics of late graft expansion, aneurysmal dilation, and stenosis. Surgery, 74:931, 1973.

112. Stephen, M., Sheil, A. G. R., and Wong, J.: Allograft vein arterial bypass. Arch. Surg., 113:591, 1978.

113. Stoney, R. J., DeLuccia, N., Ehrenfeld, W. K., and Wylie, E. J.: Aortorenal arterial autografts. Arch. Surg., 116:1416, 1981.

114. Szilagyi, D. E., Elliott, J. P., Hageman, J. G., Smith, R. F., and Dall'Olmo, C. A.: Biologic fate of autogenous vein implants and arterial substitutes. Ann. Surg., 178:232, 1973.

115. Szilagyi, D. E., Hageman, J. G., Smith, R. F., et al.: Autogenous vein grafting in femoropopliteal atherosclerosis: The limit of its effectiveness. Surgery, 86:836, 1979.

116. Szilagyi, D. E., McDonald, R. T., Smith, R. F., et al.: Biologic fate of human arterial homografts. Arch. Surg. 75:506, 1957.

117. Taylor, L. M., Jr., Edwards, J. M., Phinney, E. S., and Porter, J. M.: Reversed vein bypass to infrapopliteal arteries. Ann. Surg., 205:90, 1987.

118. Taylor, L. M., Edwards, J. M., and Porter, J. M.: Present status of reversed vein bypass: Long-term results of a modern series. J. Vasc. Surg., 11:193, 1990.

119. Tollefson, D. F., Bandyk, D. F., Kaebnick, H. W., et al.: Surface biofilm disruption: Enhanced recovery of microorganisms from vascular prostheses. Arch. Surg., 122:38, 1986.

120. Tice, D. A., and Santoni, E.: Use of saphenous vein homograft in arterial reconstruction: A preliminary report. Surgery, 67:493, 1970.

121. Tice, D. A., and Zerbino, V.: Clinical experience with preserved human allografts for vascular reconstruction. Surgery, 72:260, 1972.

122. Veith, F. J., Ascer, E., Gupta, S. K., Sprayregen, S., Collier, P., and Wengerter, K. R.: Management of the occluded and failing PTFE graft. Acta Chir. Scand. [Suppl], 538:117, 1987.

123. Voorhees, A. B., Jr., Jaretzki, A., III, and Blakemore, A. H.: The use of tubes constructed from Vinyon "N" cloth in bridging arterial defects. Ann. Surg., 135:332, 1952.

124. Wesolowski, S. A., and Dennis, C.: Fundamentals of Vascular Grafting. New York, Blakiston Division, McGraw-Hill Book Company, 1963.

125. Williams, G. M. ter Haar, A., Krajewski, D., Parks, L. C., and Roth, J.: Rejection and repair of endothelium in major vessel transplants. Surgery, 78:694, 1975.

126. Wylie, E. J.: Vascular replacement with arterial autografts. Surgery, 57:14, 1965.

127. Yashar, R. A., Richman, M. H., and Dyckman, J.: Failure of Dacron prostheses caused by structural defect. Surgery, 84:659, 1978.

128. Yeager, R. A., Hobson, R. W., and Lynch, T. G.: Analysis of factors influencing patency of polytetrafluoroethylene prosthesis. J. Surg. Res., 32:409, 1982.

129. Yeager, R. A., Moneta, G. L., Taylor, L. M., Jr., Harris, E. J., Jr., McConnell, D. B., and Porter, J. M.: Improving survival and limb salvage in patients with aortic graft infection. Am. J. Surg., 159:466, 1990.

V

ANEURYSMS

David C. Sabiston, Jr., M.D.

An aneurysm is the dilatation of an artery full of spiritous blood.

Fernel, 1581

An aneurysm is a localized or diffuse dilatation of an artery. Most aneurysms are designated as *true* aneurysms and contain all three layers of the arterial wall (intima, media, and adventitia). *False aneurysm* ("pulsating hematoma") is the term applied when only the adventitia is present, as is often the situation after traumatic rupture of an artery with subsequent aneurysmal for-

mation. It is further helpful to classify aneurysms as *saccular* or *fusiform*. Saccular aneurysms usually arise from a distinct portion of the wall and have a mouth, whereas fusiform aneurysms involve the total circumference of the artery and represent a diffuse dilatation. Aneurysms tend to occur at certain anatomic sites; the most common locations are shown in Figure 1.

Aneurysms may be either *congenital* or *acquired*, the latter being much more frequent than the former. Acquired aneurysms may be caused by arteriosclerosis, trauma, infection (mycotic), syphilis, or medial cystic necrosis. Although aneurysms were once untreatable, nearly all can be managed now by surgical means. Moreover, the results are usually highly satisfactory.

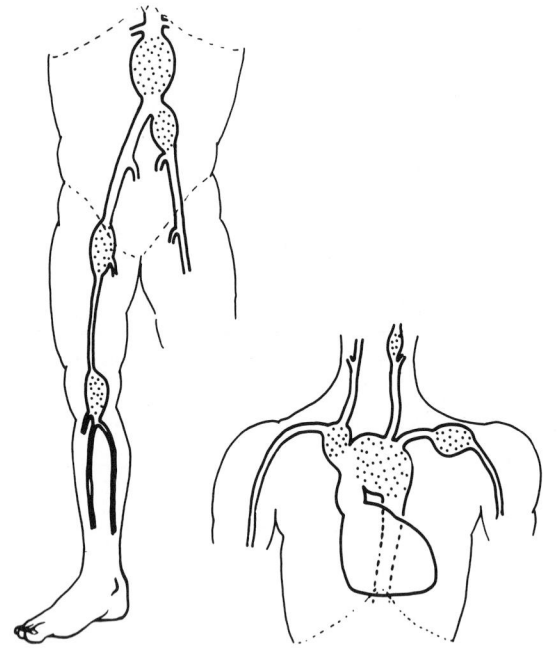

Figure 1. Common anatomic sites of arterial aneurysms. (From Ludbrook, J., and Elmsile, R. G.: An Introduction to Surgery: 100 Topics. New York, Academic Press, 1971.)

1. ANEURYSMS OF THE SINUS OF VALSALVA

Frederick L. Grover, M.D., and
John H. Calhoon, M.D.

Sinus of Valsalva aneurysms are dilatations of the aortic sinuses of Valsalva that may rupture into cardiac chambers or the pericardium. These aneurysms occur secondary to acquired or congenital disease.

Acquired Aneurysms of the Sinus of Valsalva

Causes of acquired sinus of Valsalva aneurysms include subacute bacterial endocarditis,[19] Marfan's syndrome, chronic dissection of the aorta and other degenerative lesions of the aortic root,[5,22] atherosclerosis,[13] and syphilis.[12,24] Those aneurysms associated with endocarditis are repaired usually at the time of aortic valve replacement and most commonly involve one sinus. The usual repair is by incorporating the mouth of the aneurysm with the valve sutures, thus obliterating the orifice, or by patching the orifice of the aneurysm.[19] Artherosclerotic aneurysms are usually repaired with a Dacron patch.[13] Those aneurysms caused by cystic medial necrosis or degenerative lesions of the aortic root usually require total replacement of the aortic root and valve by a composite graft, with implantation of the coronary arteries (Bentall or Cabrol procedure)[5,9,22] (Fig. 1). This can now be accomplished with a 5 per cent operative mortality rate and a 3-year actuarial survival of 81 to 88 per cent.[22]

Acquired aneurysms are also discussed in other sections of this chapter.

Congenital Aneurysms of the Sinus of Valsalva

HISTORICAL ASPECTS. The first described case of congenital sinus of Valsalva aneurysm was reported in 1835 by Hope in a patient whose condition was diagnosed at autopsy.[20] The first patient diagnosed during life by aortography was reported in 1953,[15] and the first surgical correction was performed by Lillehei and co-workers in 1956.[23] Since then, numerous reports of

surgical corrections of ruptured sinus of Valsalva aneurysms have been made. The incidence varies from 0.23 to 0.69 per cent of all cardiac procedures.[2,24]

ETIOLOGY AND PATHOPHYSIOLOGY. Abbott believed that congenital aneurysms were caused by an abnormal fusion of the aortic-pulmonary septum with the ventricular septum.[1] Venning postulated that the aneurysms were due to elastic tissue defects in the sinuses.[31] Edwards and Burchell demonstrated that the essential pathology was a separation between the aortic media and the heart at the anulus fibrosus of the aortic valve.[14]

Congenital aneurysms frequently rupture into an intracardiac chamber, producing a sudden left-to-right shunt.[2,6,8,11,24,25,29,32] The most common sinus involved is the right sinus, which usually ruptures into the right ventricle and less frequently into the right atrium. The noncoronary sinus is the next most frequent site, and it usually ruptures into the right atrium. Unusual reports of rupture of the left sinus into all four chambers and the pulmonary artery have been made. Nowicki and associates, in a collective review of 119 patients, noted that the right sinus was

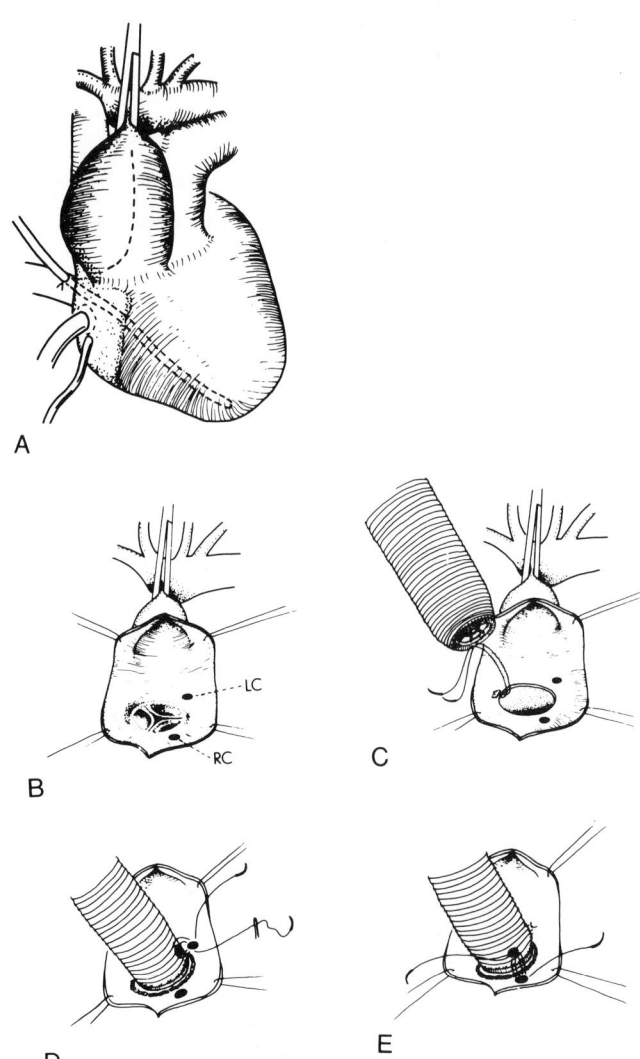

Figure 1. Insertion of a valved conduit into the aortic root (Bentall procedure). *A and B,* The aorta is opened longitudinally following institution of cardiopulmonary bypass and cross-clamping of the aorta. *C,* The valve conduit is sutured to the aortic valve anulus following removal of the aortic valve. *D and E,* The left and right coronary ostia are reimplanted into the sides of the graft. Following this, the distal anastomosis is performed to the aorta and the graft wrapped with residual aneurysm tissue. (From Kouchoukos, N. T., Karp, R. B., Lell, W. A.: Replacement of the ascending aorta and aortic valve with a composite graft: Results in 25 patients. Ann. Thorac. Surg., *24:*142, 1977.)

the origin of the fistula in 67 per cent of patients, the noncoronary in 25 per cent, and the left coronary sinus in 8 per cent.[26] The anatomic location of the fistulas in these patients is demonstrated in Figure 2. Taguchi and colleagues developed 16 anatomic classifications based on the sinus involved and the location of the fistula.[28]

Associated intracardiac defects are frequently present, the most common of which is ventricular septal defect. Another problem is aortic regurgitation, which is most common in those patients who have a ventricular septal defect. Nowicki and associates found that 33 per cent of patients had ventricular septal defects, and 8 percent had an aortic valve abnormality.[26]

CLINICAL PRESENTATION. The majority of patients are asymptomatic until the fistula ruptures. With rupture, the usual symptoms are dyspnea, palpitation, and chest pain. The symptoms are sometimes associated with dizziness, peripheral edema, and orthopnea. A precordial thrill with a continuous murmur may be heard, loudest over the second to fourth intercostal spaces to the left of the sternal border for those that communicate with the right ventricle, and over the right third and fourth intercostal spaces for those that rupture into the right atrium. Pulse pressures are increased, and the murmur of aortic regurgitation may be present. Approximately one third of patients have a sudden onset of symptoms, sometimes associated with strenuous activity. Patients whose fistulas rupture into the pericardium present in cardiogenic shock with signs of cardiac tamponade.[8,11,21,26,32] Other diseases that may have a similar clinical presentation and are to be considered in the differential diagnosis are patent ductus arteriosus, aortopulmonary window, coronary artery–cameral fistula, and ventricular septal defect with aortic insufficiency.

Nonruptured aneurysms can rarely cause symptoms because of compression of adjacent structures. Obstruction of the right ventricular outflow tract produces an elevated jugular venous pulse and a systolic murmur increasing with inspiration and hepatomegaly secondary to tricuspid insufficiency.[16] There are reports of aneurysms causing acute myocardial infarction or unstable angina secondary to coronary artery compression.[18] In addition, left ventricular obstruction has occurred when the right coronary sinus of Valsalva protrudes into the left ventricle[17]; ventricular tachycardia[27] and heart block[3] have also been reported.

Chest films usually reveal increased pulmonary vascular markings, with enlargement of the right side of the heart and prominence of the main pulmonary arteries.[26] Common electrocardiographic changes are left ventricular hypertrophy, right ventricular strain, axis shift, and biventricular hypertrophy.[8,11,24,26,32] By using two-dimensional and Doppler echocardiography techniques, it is possible to visualize the defect along with the aneurysm and to identify a fistula, if present, in well over 80 per cent of patients.[8,10] Cardiac catheterization is also very helpful in delineating the anatomy of the aneurysm and identifying and quantifying the shunt. In the review of Nowicki and associates, the left-to-right shunt ranged from 1.2:1 to 5:1 liters per minute, with a mean of 2.2.[26]

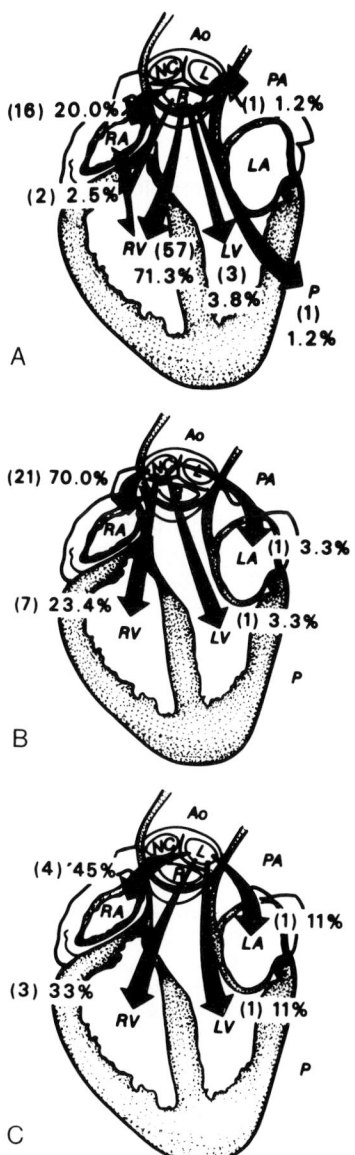

Figure 2. Origins and terminations of congenital sinus of Valsalva–cardiac fistulas in 119 patients. The chamber of termination for aortocameral fistulas is shown in *A* from the right sinus (80 patients); *B,* the noncoronary sinus (30 patients); and *C,* the left sinus (9 patients). (From Nowicki, E., Aberdeen, E., Friedman, S., and Rashkind, W.: Congenital left aortic sinus–left ventricle fistula and review of aortocardiac fistulas. Ann. Thorac. Surg., *23*:378, 1977.)

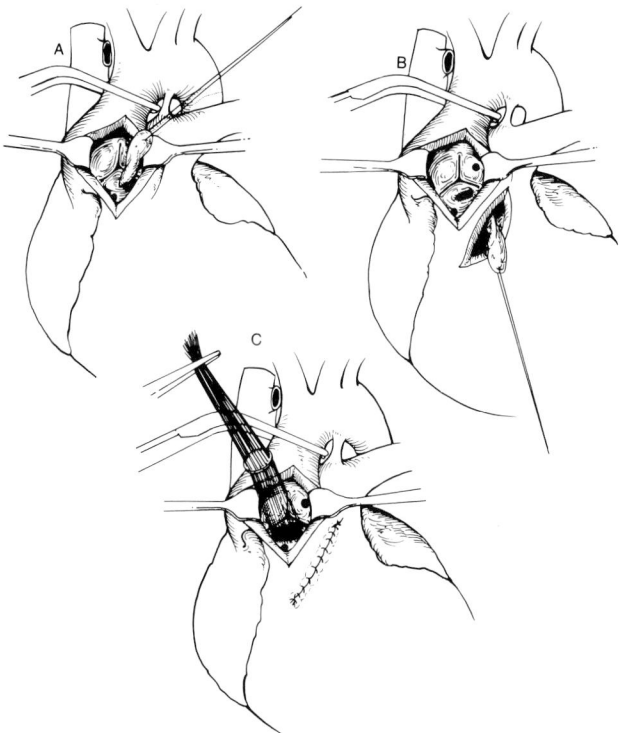

Figure 3. Repair of fistula from right sinus of Valsalva aneurysm into the right ventricle. The combined aortic and ventricular approach is shown, in which the fistula is identified from each end. The aortic opening is closed with a prosthetic patch and the cardiac end is closed separately. (From Arciniegas, E.: Pediatric Cardiac Surgery. Chicago, Year Book Medical Publishers, Inc., 1985, p. 383.)

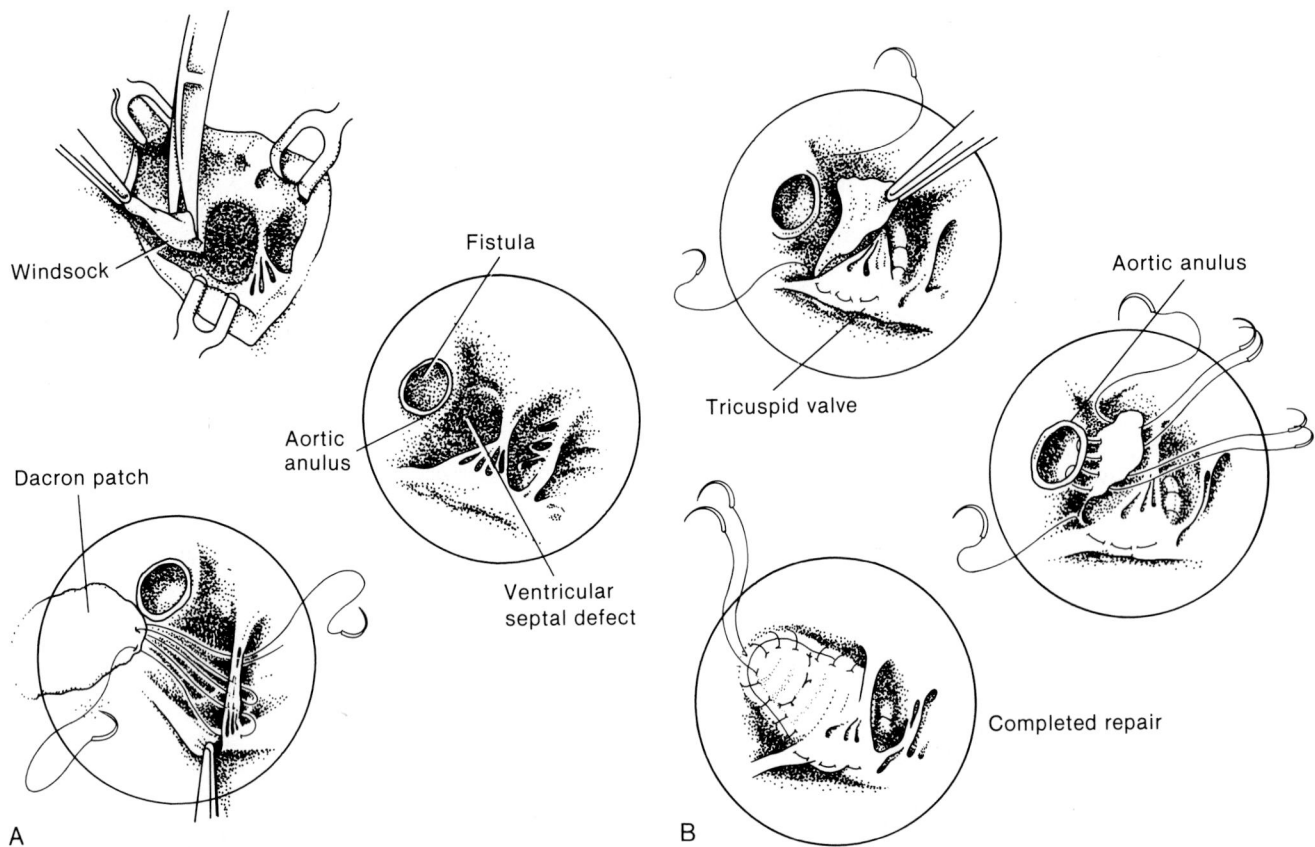

Figure 4. Closure of combined fistula and ventricular septal defect through right ventriculotomy. *A,* The windsock deformity is excised, the fistula and VSD identified, and a common patch sutured to the inferior wall of the ventricular septal defect. *B,* The patch is tacked to the septal-anulus tissue between the VSD and the orifice of the fistula and then also sewn over the fistula. This technique closes both orifices without allowing communication between the two. (From Doty, D. B.: Cardiac Surgery, Chicago. Year Book Medical Publishers, Inc., 1985.)

TREATMENT. The presence of a fistula involving the sinus of Valsalva is considered an indication for operation because of progressive heart failure that can lead to death.[2,8,24,26,32] If severe heart failure is present, urgent operation should be undertaken. Patients with a nonruptured aneurysm of the sinus of Valsalva should be managed conservatively if they are asymptomatic but followed closely with serial echocardiography because of the possibility of developing symptoms due to compression or later rupture.[26]

The fistula can be approached via the chamber into which it ruptures[6,8,11] or through the aorta.[26] Most investigators now recommend a dual approach via the aorta and the chamber of entry of the fistula[4,6–8,24,29,32] (Fig. 3). Right ventricular fistulas can also be approached through the pulmonary artery.[2,12] The advantage of the aortocameral approach is that the fistula can be probed from the aorta into the chamber involved and closed at both its origin and termination, with an apparent decrease in recurrent fistula. The aortic valve can be inspected and protected from improperly placed sutures, which could distort the valve and create aortic insufficiency. The aortic valve can also be evaluated for insufficiency, which, if present, can be repaired, using Trusler's technique[30] or replaced if necessary. The ventricular septum can be carefully inspected for the presence of a ventricular septal defect (VSD), which, if present, can be closed with a common patch covering the defect and the fistula, the patch tacked to the septum between the ventricular septal defect and fistula for elimination of communication between the two (Fig. 4). Small defects can be closed primarily.[6,11,29]

RESULTS. Nowicki and associates noted an operative mortality of 12.7 per cent, a failure to close the fistula in 1.6 per cent, and a good result in 85.7 per cent of patients.[26] Seventy per cent of the patients who died had an associated cardiac abnormality.

Much of the mortality was in the early years, more recent series reporting a mortality of 0 to 13 per cent with an almost negligible reoperation rate.[2,6,24,29] Actuarial survival at 25 years has been reported at 86 per cent.[2] Reoperation is rarely required for progression of aortic regurgitation, for recurrent fistula, or for a residual ventricular septal defect.

SELECTED REFERENCES

Barragry, T., Ring, W., Moller, J., and Lillehei, C.: Fifteen- to thirty-year follow-up of patients undergoing repair of ruptured congenital aneurysms of the sinus of Valsalva. Ann. Thorac. Surg., 46:515, 1988.
This report reviews the long-term results of repair of ruptured congenital aneurysms of the sinus of Valsalva and includes the first patient to undergo operative correction. Although the series is small, it reveals how surgical techniques for this entity have evolved over the past 35 years and illustrates the marked improvement in surgical and long-term results in recent years. Many of the important concepts in the treatment of this condition are reviewed.

Chih, P., Heng, T., Chun, C., and Chieh-Fu, L.: Surgical treatment of the ruptured aneurysm of the aortic sinuses. Ann. Thorac. Surg., 32:162, 1981.
This article reports the largest single institutional experience in the surgical treatment of ruptured aneurysm of the sinus of Valsalva. The report originates from the Shanghai Chest Hospital and reviews the higher incidence of this entity in the Oriental population; patient characteristics, including symptomatology, associated defects, diagnostic studies, and operative technique; and early and late results.

Edwards, J., and Burchell, H.: The pathological anatomy of deficiencies between the aortic root and the heart, including aortic sinus aneurysms. Thorax, 12:125, 1957.
This classic report concerns the anatomy of the aortic sinuses, the pathologic anatomy of those lesions that lie at the aortic root, and the deficiencies between the aortic media and the heart. It not only is a detailed pathophysiologic study of historical importance but also remains the most important pathologic paper describing these abnormalities.

Kouchoukos, N., Karp, R., Blackstone, E., Kirklin, J., Pacifico, A., and Zorn, G.: Replacement of the ascending aorta and aortic valve with a composite graft. Ann. Surg., 192:403, 1980.

This is a detailed review of one institution's experience in replacing the ascending aorta and aortic valve with a composite graft using the Bentall technique. The study includes 86 patients, of whom 44 underwent operation for anuloaortic ectasia, 31 for aortic dissections, 8 for aneurysms of the sinus of Valsalva following a suprasinus of Valsalva graft replacement of the ascending aorta, 2 for leutic aortitis, and 1 for poststenotic dilatation. The authors report a remarkable 5 per cent hospital mortality for this group of patients, with no deaths among those with anuloaortic ectasia, only one death in the chronic dissection group (3 per cent), two deaths in acute dissection (25 per cent), and one other death. In addition, there is a careful statistical analysis of preoperative and intraoperative risk factors, morbidity, the incidence of reoperation, and long-term survival.

Nowicki, E., Aberdeen, E., Friedman, S., and Rashkind, W.: Congenital left aortic sinus–left ventricle fistula and review of aortocardiac fistulas. Ann. Thorac. Surg., 23:378, 1977.

This paper offers a very thorough review of 175 cases of aortocardiac fistulas from sinus of Valsalva aneurysms that were published in the English literature from 1839 to 1972. The authors very carefully review patient characteristics, symptomatology, physical findings, diagnostic studies, the anatomic location and frequency of each of the subgroups of fistulas, the techniques of surgical resection, and short- and long-term results.

REFERENCES

1. Abbott, M.: Clinical and developmental study of a case of ruptured aneurysm of the right anterior aortic sinus of Valsalva. Contrib. Med. Biol. Res., 2:899, 1919.
2. Abe, T., and Komatsu, S.: Surgical repair and long-term results in ruptured sinus of Valsalva aneurysm. Ann. Thorac. Surg., 46:520, 1988.
3. Ahmad, R., Sturman, S., and Watson, R.: Unruptured aneurysm of the sinus of Valsalva presenting with isolated heart block: Echocardiographic diagnosis and successful surgical repair. Br. Heart J., 61:375, 1989.
4. Barragry, T., Ring, W., Moller, J., and Lillehei, C.: Fifteen- to thirty-year follow-up of patients undergoing repair of ruptured congenital aneurysms of the sinus of Valsalva. Ann. Thorac. Surg., 46:515, 1988.
5. Bentall, H., and DeBono, A.: A technique for complete replacement of the ascending aorta. Thorax, 23:338, 1968.
6. Bonfils-Roberts, E., DuShane, J., McGoon, D., and Danielson, G.: Aortic sinus fistula — surgical considerations and results of operation. Ann. Thorac. Surg., 15:492, 1971.
7. Bosher, L., Jr.: The combined surgical approach (transaortic and transatrial) for the correction of congenital aortic sinus fistula into the right atrium. J. Thorac. Cardiovasc. Surg., 50:243, 1965.
8. Burakovsky, V., Podsolkov, V., Sabirow, M., Nasedkina, A., Alekian, B., and Dvinyaninova, N.: Ruptured congenital aneurysm of the sinus of Valsalva: Clinical manifestations, diagnosis, and results of surgical correction. J. Thorac. Cardiovasc. Surg., 95:836, 1988.
9. Cabrol, C., Pavie, A., Gandjbakhch, I., Villemot, J., Guiraudon, G., Laughlin, L., Etievent, P., and Cham, B.: Complete replacement of the ascending aorta with reimplantation of the coronary arteries. J. Thorac. Cardiovasc. Surg., 81:309, 1981.
10. Chiang, C., Lin, F., Fang, B., Kuo, C., Lee, Y., and Chang, C.: Doppler and two-dimensional echocardiographic features of sinus of Valsalva aneurysm. Am. Heart J., 116:1283, 1988.
11. Chih, P., Heng, T., Chun, C., and Chieh-Fu, L.: Surgical treatment of the ruptured aneurysm of the aortic sinuses. Ann. Thorac. Surg., 32:162, 1981.
12. DeBakey, M., Diethrich, E., Liddicoat, J., Kinard, S., and Garrett, H.: Abnormalities of the sinuses of Valsalva: Experience with 35 patients. J. Thorac. Cardiovasc. Surg., 54:312, 1967.
13. DeBakey, M., and Lawrie, G.: Aneurysm of sinus of Valsalva with coronary atherosclerosis: Successful surgical correction. Ann. Surg., 189:303, 1979.
14. Edwards, J., and Burchell, H.: The pathological anatomy of deficiencies between the aortic root and the heart, including aortic sinus aneurysms. Thorax, 12:125, 1957.
15. Falholt, W., and Thomsen, G.: Congenital aneurysm of the right sinus of Valsalva, diagnosed by aortography. Circulation, 8:549, 1953.
16. Gibbs, J., Reardon, M., Strickman, N., DeCastro, C., Gerard, J., Rycyna, J., Hall, R., and Cooley, D.: Hemodynamic compromise (tricuspid stenosis and insufficiency) caused by an unruptured aneurysm of the sinus of Valsalva. J. Am. Coll. Cardiol., 7:1177, 1986.
17. Heydorn, W., Nelson, W., Fitterer, J., Floyd, G., and Strevey, T.: Congenital aneurysm of the sinus of Valsalva protruding into the left ventricle: Review of diagnosis and treatment of unruptured aneurysm. J. Thorac. Cardiovasc. Surg., 71:839, 1976.
18. Hiyamuta, K., Ohtsuki, T., Shimamatsu, M., Ohkita, Y., Terasawa, M., Bekki, H., Toshima, H., Utsu, F., Ohishi, K., Koga, M., and Nagayama, K.: Aneurysm of the left aortic sinus causing acute myocardial infarction. Circulation, 67:1151, 1983.
19. Holmes, E., Bredenberg, C., and Brawley, R.: Aneurysm of the sinus of Valsalva resulting from bacterial endocarditis. Ann. Thorac. Surg., 15:628, 1973.
20. Hope, J.: A Treatise of Diseases of the Heart and Great Vessels, 3rd ed. London, John Churchill, 1839, pp. 432–444.
21. Killen, D., Wathanacharoen, S., and Pogson, G., Jr.: Repair of intrapericardial rupture of left sinus of Valsalva aneurysm. Ann. Thorac. Surg., 44:310, 1987.
22. Kouchoukos, N., Karp, R., Blackstone, E., Kirklin, J., Pacifico, A., and Zorn, G.: Replacement of the ascending aorta and aortic valve with a composite graft. Ann. Surg., 192:403, 1980.
23. Lillehei, C., Stanley, P., and Varco, R.: Surgical treatment of ruptured aneurysms of the sinus of Valsalva. Ann. Surg., 146:459, 1957.
24. Mayer, E., Ruffmann, K., Saggau, W., Butzmann, B., Bernhardt-Mayer, K., Schatton, N., and Schmitz, W.: Ruptured aneurysms of the sinus of Valsalva. Ann. Thorac. Surg., 42:81, 1986.
25. Meyer, J., Wukasch, D., Hallman, G., and Cooley, D.: Aneurysm and fistula of the sinus of Valsalva: Clinical considerations and surgical treatment in 45 patients. Ann. Thorac. Surg., 19:170, 1975.
26. Nowicki, E., Aberdeen, E., Friedman, S., and Rashkind, W.: Congenital left aortic sinus–left ventricle fistula and review of aortocardiac fistulas. Ann. Thorac. Surg., 23:378, 1977.
27. Raizes, G., Smith, H., Vlietstra, R., and Puga, F.: Ventricular tachycardia secondary to aneurysm of sinus of Valsalva. J. Thorac. Cardiovasc. Surg., 78:110, 1979.
28. Taguchi, K., Sasaki, N., Matsuura, Y., and Uemura, R.: Clinical studies: Surgical correction of aneurysm of the sinus of Valsalva: A report of forty-five consecutive patients, including eight with total replacement of the aortic valve. Am. J. Cardiol., 23:180, 1969.
29. Tanabe, T., Yokota, A., and Sugie, S.: Surgical treatment of aneurysms of the sinus of Valsalva. Ann. Thorac. Surg., 27:133, 1979.
30. Trusler, G., Moes, C., and Kidd, B.: Repair of ventricular septal defect with aortic insufficiency. J. Thorac. Cardiovasc. Surg., 66:394, 1973.
31. Venning, G.: Aneurysms of the sinuses of Valsalva. Am. Heart J., 57:69, 1951.
32. Verghese, M., Jairaj, P., Babuthaman, C., Sukumar, I., and John, S.: Surgical treatment of ruptured aneurysms of the sinus of Valsalva. Ann. Thorac. Surg., 41:284, 1986.

2. TRAUMATIC ANEURYSMS OF THE AORTA

Walter G. Wolfe, M.D.

It is amazing that any patient survives traumatic rupture of the aorta. In those who do, survival is dependent on the formation of a false aneurysm contained by the adventitia and the support of mediastinal structures. Such an aneurysm may rupture within minutes or persist for a prolonged period. In some patients who initially survive without evidence of aortic injury, an unsuspected aneurysm may be discovered or may rupture suddenly months or even years later. In a review of 296 fatal cases of injury of the aorta, approximately 13 per cent of the patients survived initially,[22] a finding confirmed in another study.[27] It was apparent that sudden death did not occur in all patients, with some 20 per cent surviving longer than 30 minutes after injury.

Incidence

The incidence of traumatic rupture of the aorta has increased markedly with the development of high-speed vehicles, and posttraumatic aneurysms now represent the most common thoracic aortic aneurysm in the younger age group (Fig. 1). The number of traffic accidents each year and the number of individuals sustaining thoracic injuries have risen sharply; and acute aortic rupture occurs in 15 to 20 per cent of individuals killed in vehicular accidents. Therefore, a history of sudden deceleration injury should immediately arouse the suspicion of acute aortic transection.

Improved methods of treating injuries and improved medical care of the injured have increased survival at the accident site.[6] The care of these patients is complicated by the fact that many suffer from multiple injuries,[4,30] a factor that increases mortality. Because significant thoracic injury is often present without external evidence of an obvious superficial wound, attention is concentrated on problems that are apparent.

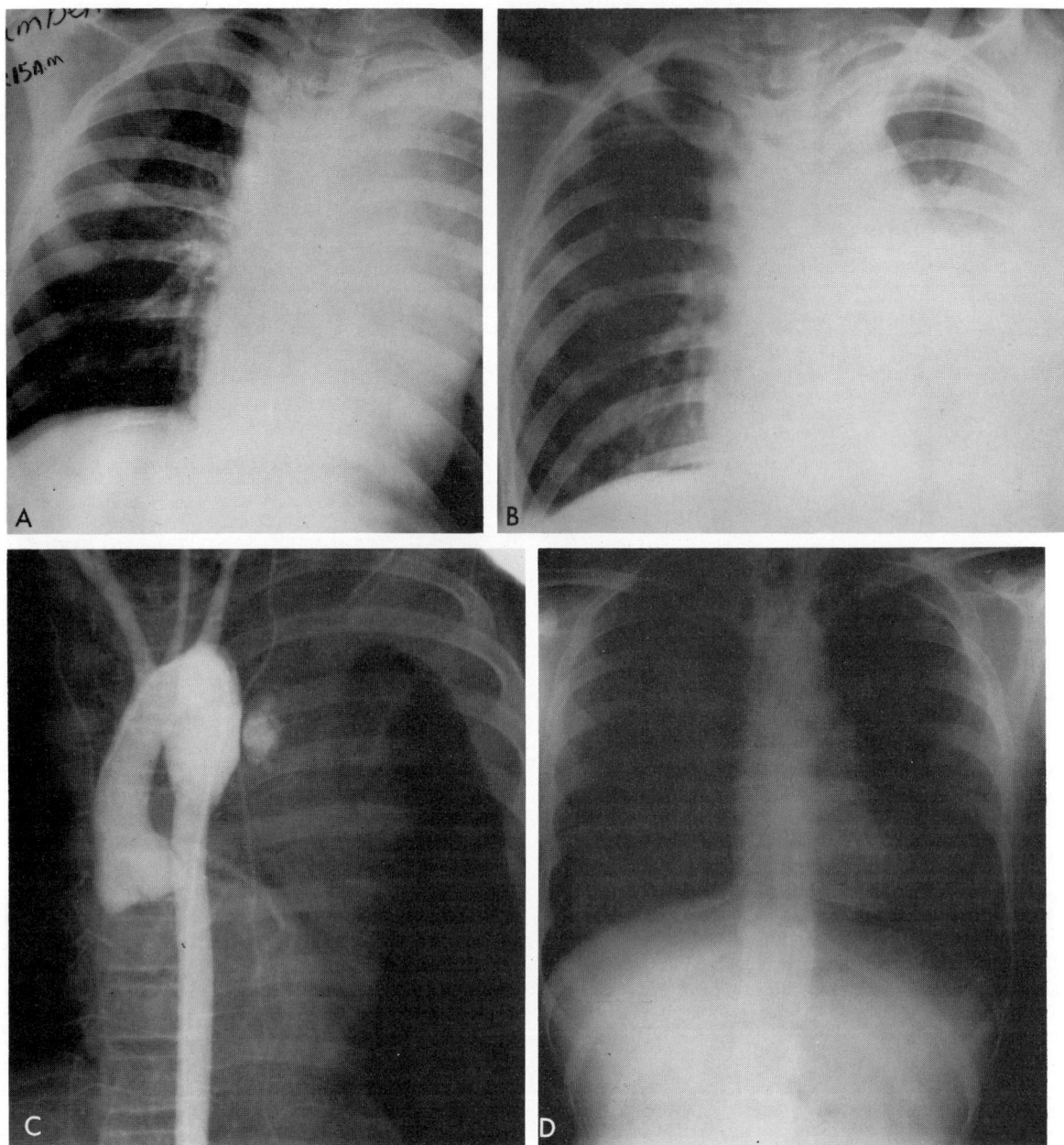

Figure 1. *A*, Chest film shows a large mediastinal hematoma in a 14-year-old boy after an accident involving a motorbike. Following chest x-ray examination at his local hospital, he was transferred. *B*, Chest film taken upon admission to the emergency room shows progression of the hematoma and pleural effusion in the left side of the chest indicative of rupture. *C*, Aortogram demonstrating the pleural effusion and mediastinal hematoma as well as a complete transection of the aorta and mediastinal extravasation of contrast material. *D*, Radiograph 2 years following repair of the thoracic aorta with a Dacron graft.

Methods of Injury

Prior to high-speed travel, direct blows to the thoracic cage were common, but serious associated injuries were seldom seen. Such blows may produce rib or sternal fractures; pulmonary contusion and fractured ribs may secondarily cause pulmonary laceration with subsequent pneumothorax and hemothorax. Compression injuries of the chest, another common form of trauma, may cause rupture of the diaphragm, fractured ribs, and contusions of the lung. High-speed automobile accidents produce deceleration injuries, which are also seen in airplane or train accidents as well as in falls from appreciable heights and compression by heavy objects.[4,9,22]

In general, such an injury is related to direct contact between the thoracic cage and a hard object, for example, the steering column or dashboard in a car. This type of injury follows rapid deceleration of the body and continued movement of the inter-

nal organs. The suspended heart and great vessels continue to travel, and tears occur at various attachments of fixed points within the chest.

The pathogenesis of thoracic aortic injury was first defined by Rindfleisch[26] in 1893. He surmised that the aortic arch and great vessels have relatively fixed attachments, whereas the heart and descending thoracic aorta are mobile. Sudden deceleration of the body at the time of impact with differential rates of deceleration of the thoracic organs, the thoracic aorta, and the great vessels can cause a tear involving the intima, the intima and media, or the entire wall. This tear is usually transverse and may be partial or complete. The average age of these patients is in the third decade, and atherosclerosis is seldom a factor in the aortic injury. Since the adventitia provides 60 per cent of the tensile strength of the thoracic aorta, survival of the patient depends on the continuity of this layer. The mechanism of aortic rupture with deceleration is related to different deceleration rates be-

TABLE 1. Site of Injury

Isthmus
Arch
Ascending aorta
Descending thoracic aorta
Abdominal aorta
Multiple sites

TABLE 2. Associated Thoracic Injuries

Rib fractures
Sternal fractures
Thoracic vertebral fractures
Clavicular fracture
Scapula fracture
Pneumothorax
Hemothorax
Cardiac injury

tween fixed and mobile parts. Thus, in violent deceleration, the relatively free descending thoracic aorta snaps forward at a rate different from the fixed portion of the aorta. Such unequal forces subject the aorta to stretch, torsion, and shearing stress with rupture at fixed points. An alternative interpretation is avulsion of the heart and aortic arch from the aorta at the ligamentum, which occurs as the heart is projected forward and upward in a violent deceleration. Therefore, the most frequent site of damage of the aorta is at its isthmus,[5,22,27,29] that is, the segment just distal to the left subclavian artery at the ligamentum arteriosum (Table 1). Injuries to the ascending aorta and aortic vessels are more likely to follow direct trauma than deceleration, and with such injuries it is common to find fractures and fracture-dislocations in the region of the anterior chest wall overlying these vessels. This includes fracture of the first rib, fracture of the clavicle, and dislocation of the clavicle.

Falls from heights landing feet first may rupture the descending aorta by avulsion of the junction of the fixed aortic arch with the mobile heart, and such tears are usually associated with aortic valvular injury.

Pathologic Findings

Traumatic rupture of the aorta has the appearance of an incised wound extending transversely or spirally. It may be partial or complete and involve the entire aortic wall. There is usually no evidence suggestive of existing disease such as medial necrosis, atheroma, or syphilitic aortitis, and the histologic appearance of the aorta in these patients, many of whom are young, is usually normal.

It has been shown that a pressure between 1000 and 3000 mm. Hg is required to rupture the aorta. If complete rupture of all layers occurs, immediate exsanguination is likely, but if the adventitia remains intact, 15 to 20 per cent of patients survive the initial injury. In those who reach the hospital alive, the intima and media are usually ruptured and continuity is retained by intact adventitia. Although this adventitia may contain the aortic pressure, rupture usually follows. If the diagnosis is not made in the acute situation and the patient survives, a chronic false aneurysm develops,[5] which may enlarge, rupture spontaneously, or later be demonstrated radiographically as a calcified aneurysm.

Although it is not unusual for these patients to have other major injuries, many patients sustaining rupture of the aorta have no other apparent injury. In those with severe associated injuries, it is not surprising that the aortic damage is often initially overlooked, and, unfortunately, rupture of the traumatic aneurysm may be fatal.

Associated Injuries

There may be no external manifestations of a severe closed-chest injury; however, associated injuries may be obvious (Tables 2 and 3). These include serious head injuries, closed and compound fractures, hematuria from pelvic fractures or bladder and kidney injuries, and intra-abdominal bleeding from visceral trauma. Although associated thoracic injuries such as pneumothorax or hemothorax call attention to a chest injury coupled with fractured ribs, the involvement of the thoracic spine with these associated injuries confuses the situation, and the medias-

tinal changes seen on the chest film may be thought to be related to such injuries.

Management of associated injuries may be lifesaving in the resuscitative period. However, once stabilized, all severely injured patients should have adequate evaluation of the mediastinum and thoracic aorta if any abnormalities are present on the chest film.[3,4,6,14,21,30]

Clinical Presentation

Few conditions are of such sudden onset as the catastrophic outcome characteristic of traumatic rupture of the thoracic aorta. The single most important factor in considering the diagnosis of acute traumatic rupture is awareness of its occurrence in those involved in violent accidents that include sudden deceleration regardless of external evidence of injury. The spectrum of the initial presentation ranges from no evidence of external injury in a stable and otherwise healthy-appearing patient with only minor complaints to the multiple injuries of a patient with evidence of two or three life-threatening problems, including head injuries or intra-abdominal bleeding. It should be emphasized that there is a twofold increase in acute aortic transections in patients who are ejected from the vehicle, which explains the high incidence of aortic transection in patients thrown from motorcycles.[15,16]

Diagnosis

The diagnosis of acute aortic transection is made by the history of a violent, sudden, decelerating accident. The physical findings in this setting may be entirely negative but often include a history of severe chest pain, hypertension in the upper extremities, evidence of blood loss, and shock; in addition, a harsh systolic murmur may be present in the precordium or posterior scapular area.[21,28] The patient may present with anuria and may be paraplegic (Fig. 2). More often, in those surviving acute transection, pulses may be equal. A very important radiographic finding is widening of the mediastinum, often with blunting of contour of the aortic knob.[3,12,21] Clearly, widening does not always indicate transection of the aorta, and there are instances of transection without this finding. Also, in acutely injured patients, the anteroposterior chest film frequently demonstrates a widened mediastinum. Therefore, posteroanterior chest films should be obtained if possible. The chest film may also demonstrate deviation of the trachea to the right, pleural effusion, and depression of the left main stem bronchus. There may also be associated rib fractures and pneumothorax along with contusion of the lungs. In the presence of any of these findings or if there is suspicion of transection of the aorta, an

TABLE 3. Extrathoracic Injuries

Facial lacerations
Facial fractures
Head injuries
Liver, spleen, pancreas injury
Bladder injury
Pelvic fracture
Kidney contusion and laceration
Dislocated hip
Long bone fracture

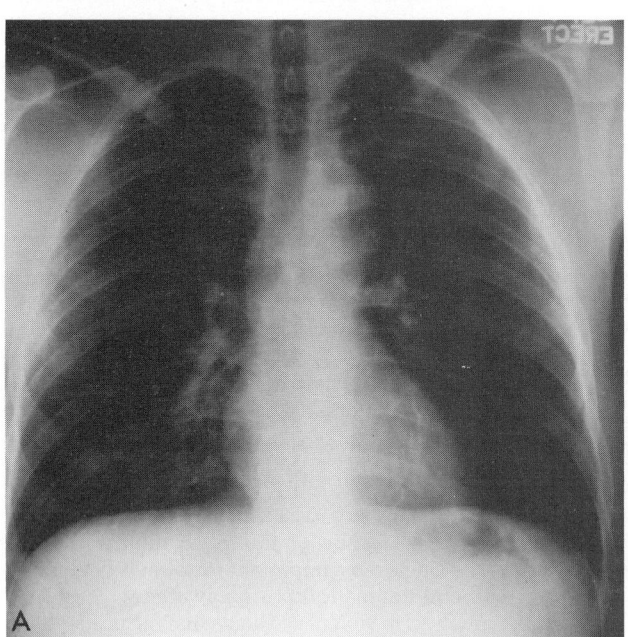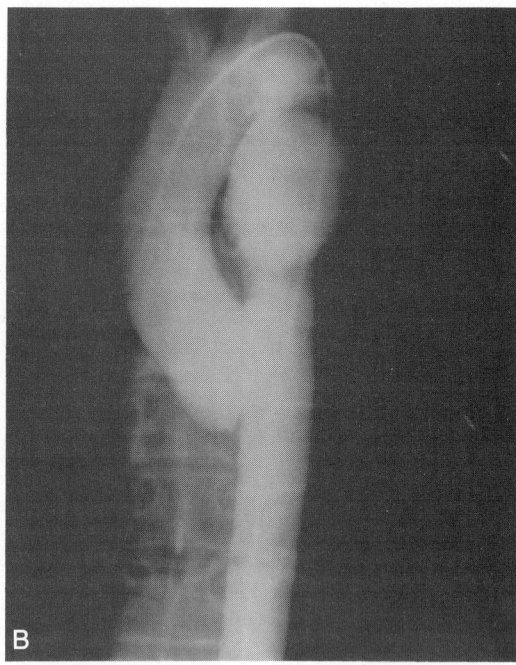

Figure 2. *A*, Chest film of a young man whose injuries in a severe auto accident resulted in paraplegia. This film shows a subtle widening of the mediastinum. He was admitted for evaluation and myelogram 4 years after the accident. *B*, Aortogram demonstrating chronic false aneurysm secondary to aortic transection.

aortogram must be obtained.[3,12,17,21] Although this may lead to more frequent aortograms with a lower incidence of positive findings, the high mortality associated with a failure to diagnose makes the procedure justifiable. In the presence of first rib fracture, significant sternal injury, or posteriorly displaced clavicular fractures, aortography is generally indicated.

Management

Approximately 80 per cent of patients with traumatic rupture of the aorta succumb before reaching the hospital.[22,27] Without treatment, the majority of survivors dies of secondary hemorrhage within the next 2 weeks. A small number survive and develop chronic aneurysms, and many future complications. For these reasons, early repair should be performed in most patients with acute traumatic rupture of the aorta.

When the diagnosis is established, preparation for operation should be made immediately.[12,24] Resuscitation and supportive measures are initiated; other critical injuries may require prior or simultaneous treatment.[2] The operation is complicated by the need to cross-clamp the aorta in the region of or above the subclavian artery and at the same time prevent left ventricular strain as well as provide protection for the viscera and the spinal cord from ischemia.

In the first report of successful repair of traumatic rupture of the aorta, it was noted that following cross-clamping of the aorta of a 30-year-old man without bypass support for a period of 17 minutes, during which a 3-mm. tear was closed at the isthmus, the heart became grossly distended, the electrocardiographic pattern became bizarre, and the systolic blood pressure rose to 200 mm. Hg. Thus, this simple approach is inadequate.

There is current evidence that if the operation is performed very expeditiously, bypass support is not necessary.[1,11] Many, however, believe it is preferable to give more attention to possible renal damage or the risk of paraplegia in these patients. Although paraplegia may be part of the process itself, reduction in arterial blood flow through the main branch of the anterior spinal artery supplying the spinal cord as it originates in the region of the lower thoracic and upper lumbar segmental vessels may produce spinal cord ischemia and can often be avoided. Since cardiac dilation and strain and ischemia to the visceral vessels as well as paraplegia may occur, careful consid-

eration must be given to these complications if operation is undertaken without bypass.[2,4,7,19,20,31]

For correction of rupture of the descending thoracic aorta, a left lateral thoracotomy is performed with entry into the chest through the fourth or fifth interspace. The mediastinal structures must be dissected, care being taken to preserve the vagus, phrenic, and recurrent laryngeal nerves. Proximal and distal control must be obtained without entering the hematoma. Although hypothermia alone was initially used, this was rapidly supported by cardiopulmonary bypass or left heart bypass. A troublesome complication of these types of bypass is postoperative bleeding secondary to the necessity of total-body heparinization. Femoral vein to femoral artery bypass with a pump oxygenator can also be used for partial cardiopulmonary support, but again systemic heparinization is required.

Recently, left atrial to descending aorta or femoral artery bypass has been greatly improved and can support the distal circulation without the use of heparin; it is probably the preferred method of bypass today.

The second method is the use of heparin-bonded shunts from the ascending aorta proximal to the aneurysm to the lower thoracic aorta or the femoral artery (or from the left ventricle to the femoral artery). The aorta should be clamped between the carotid and subclavian artery and the hematoma opened, and the aorta repaired either primarily or with the use of a Dacron graft. In most instances, primary repair is not feasible and the use of a graft is mandatory, since repair of the aorta may place undue tension on the suture line. A Carlen double-lumen endotracheal tube is usually used, with selective ventilation of the right lung and collapse of the left lung making exposure and dissection much easier.[17,18,31]

It is clear that these lesions can be safely operated on today with simple clamping of the aorta, pharmacologic support, and efforts to lower the left ventricular pressure with nitroprusside. Crawford and Rubio[11] and Appelbaum and colleagues[1] have both presented data emphasizing the safety of this technique; they believe that the incidence of paraplegia is no greater in those patients managed with bypass or a shunt and that operative time and blood loss are usually less with this direct approach.

As soon as the operative repair is completed, the chest is

closed and ventilatory support continued as necessary, depending on associated lung and other chest injuries as well as nonthoracic injuries. Long-term results have been excellent following repair of transection; in fact, the morbidity and mortality are usually related to other injuries rather than to the transection itself.

MANAGEMENT OF CHRONIC TRAUMATIC ANEURYSMS OF THE AORTA. Only 2 per cent of patients with acute transection of the aorta survive to develop chronic aneurysms.[5,13] Symptoms of such lesions include chest pain, hoarseness, cough, and dysphagia. In some patients, the lesion is found on routine roentgenogram as an enlarging aortic shadow. In general, the patient with chronic aneurysm shows evidence of instability with the passage of time, usually due to increasing size of the aneurysm. When a chronic traumatic aneurysm of the aorta is diagnosed, operative correction is recommended. This recommendation is based on the fact that over half of these patients ultimately show instability; in addition, there are no criteria to predict which aneurysms will remain stable. The majority of these lesions occur in young, healthy individuals; the operative mortality is low, and the results are quite successful.

MORTALITY AND MORBIDITY. The mortality for management of acute transections is less than 10 per cent, and the deaths are usually related to associated injuries. In many series of chronic transections with aortic aneurysms, the mortality is less than 5 per cent.[5,11,13,31] The primary complications include recurrent laryngeal nerve injury and reoperation for bleeding. There is risk of a false aneurysm at the suture line, which is unusual, and phrenic nerve injury has been reported. In general, the morbidity in the management of these patients is related to the associated injuries and not to the operative procedure itself in either the acute or the chronic form of aortic aneurysm.

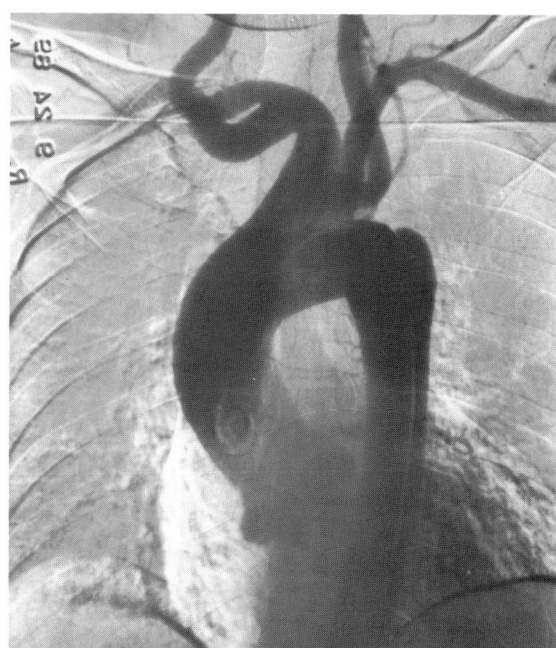

Figure 4. Aortogram demonstrates a transection of the ascending aorta with aortic insufficiency as well as transection at the isthmus. The patient's injuries were successfully managed approaching the ascending aorta through a median sternotomy first, and then the descending aortic tear was repaired via a left thoracotomy.

MANAGEMENT OF ASCENDING AORTIC INJURY. The diagnosis of ascending aortic transection should be suspected in patients who have a fracture of the first rib.[9,25] Mediastinal widening is usually evident on the chest film. A powerful and unique force is required for fracture of the first rib, and this force is transmitted throughout the thorax. Therefore, not only may transection of a bronchus or of the ascending aorta be present, but also transection at the aortic isthmus may occur. The diagnosis is confirmed by arteriography (Fig. 3).

Management of ascending aortic injuries involving the aorta at its attachment to the heart or the great vessels is accomplished through a median sternotomy. Full heparinization and cardiopulmonary bypass are usually required, although heparinized shunts may be utilized in some patients with great vessel injury.[9] Repair is accomplished with grafting of the ascending aorta or primary repair, depending on the extent of injury. Injury to the aortic valve may be such that valve replacement may be necessary (Fig. 4).

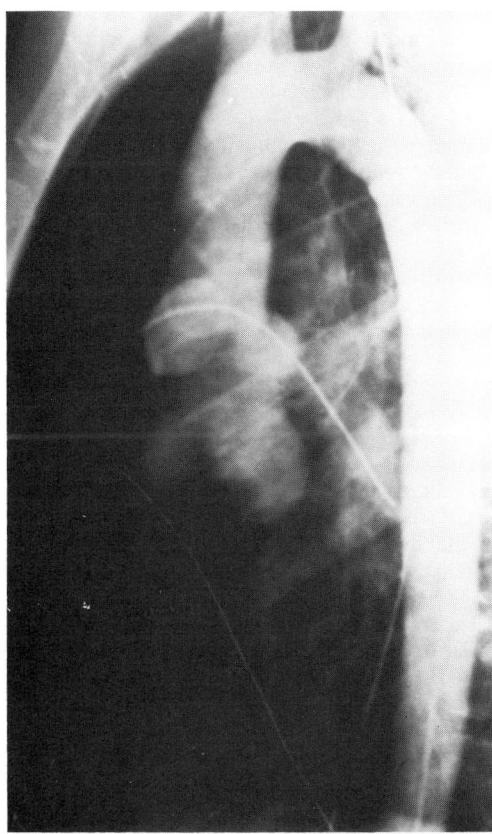

Figure 3. Films from a 20-year-old male involved in a motorcycle accident. He suffered a closed head injury, transection of the ascending aorta, and compound fractures of the left femur and tibia. The aortic injury was repaired successfully with primary suture through median sternotomy using cardiopulmonary bypass and cardioplegic arrest.

SELECTED REFERENCES

Bennett, D.E., and Cherry, J.K.: The natural history of traumatic aneurysms of the aorta. Surgery, 61:516, 1967.
The incidence of chronic aneurysm following transection, the site, the time of death, and the prognosis of chronic aneurysms are discussed with excellent references to the world literature.

Freed, T. A., Neal, M. P., Jr., and Vinik, M.: Roentgenographic findings in extracardiac injury secondary to blunt chest automobile trauma. Am. J. Roentgenol., 104:424, 1968.
This thorough discussion of the diagnosis of traumatic injury of the aorta emphasizes the importance of routine chest films and arteriography in the diagnosis.

Kirsh, M. M., Behrendt, D. M., Orringer, M. B., Gago, O., Gray, L. A., Jr., Mills, L. J., Walter, J. F., and Sloan, H.: The treatment of acute traumatic rupture of the aorta. A ten year experience. Ann. Surg., 184:308, 1976.
This is one of the largest series published and thoroughly reviews the management of this problem and associated injuries.

Parmley, L. F., Mattingly, T. W., Manion, W. C., and Jahnke, E. J.: Nonpenetrating traumatic injury of the aorta. Circulation, 17:1086, 1958.
This classic reference to the pathology, clinical aspects, and management of nonpenetrating injuries of the aorta should be read by any surgeon involved with this problem.

Peyton, R. B., and Wolfe, W. G.: Traumatic thoracic aneurysm. *In* Moylan, J. A. (Ed.): Trauma Surgery. Philadelphia, J. B. Lippincott Company, 1988.
This chapter reviews traumatic thoracic aortic injuries and illustrates technical features involved in the repair of these injuries.

Spencer, F. C., Guerin, P. F., Blake, H. A., and Bahnson, H. T.: A report of fifteen patients with traumatic rupture of the thoracic aorta. J. Thorac. Cardiovasc. Surg., 41:1, 1961.
This article of an early series of 15 cases, 7 acute and 8 chronic, reviews the early problems with this lesion.

REFERENCES

1. Appelbaum, A., Karp, R. B., and Kirklin, J. W.: Surgical treatment for closed thoracic aortic injuries. J. Thorac. Cardiovasc. Surg., 71:458, 1976.
2. Aronstam, E. M., Gomez, A. C., O'Connell, T. J., Jr., and Geiger, J. P.: Recent surgical and pharmacologic experience with acute dissecting and traumatic aneurysms. J. Thorac. Cardiovasc. Surg., 59:231, 1970.
3. Attar, S., Ayella, R. J., and McLaughlin, J. S.: The widened mediastinum in trauma. Ann. Thorac. Surg., 13:435, 1972.
4. Ayella, R. J., Hankins, J. R., Turney, S. Z., and Cowley, R. A.: Ruptured thoracic aorta due to blunt trauma. J. Trauma, 17:199, 1977.
5. Bennett, D. E., and Cherry, J. K.: The natural history of traumatic aneurysms of the aorta. Surgery, 61:516, 1967.
6. Bodily, K., Perry, J. F., Jr., Strate, R. G., and Fischer, R. P.: The salvageability of patients with post-traumatic rupture of the descending thoracic aorta in a primary trauma center. J. Trauma, 17:754, 1977.
7. Burnsed, D. W., Weiss, J. B., Campbell, G. S., and Williams, G. D.: The relative merits of the heparin-bonded shunt vs. femorofemoral bypass for aortic arch injury. Surgery, 78:176, 1975.
8. Cammack, K., Rapport, R. L., Paul, J., and Baird, W. C.: Deceleration injuries of the thoracic aorta. Arch. Surg., 79:244, 1959.
9. Castagna, J., and Nelson, R. J.: Blunt injuries to branches of the aortic arch. J. Thorac. Cardiovasc. Surg., 69:521, 1975.
10. Connors, J. P., Ferguson, T. B., Roper, C. L., and Weldon, C. S.: The use of TDMAC-heparin shunt in replacement of the descending aorta. Ann. Surg., 181:735, 1975.
11. Crawford, E. S., and Rubio, P. A.: Reappraisal of adjuncts to avoid ischemia in the treatment of aneurysms of descending thoracic aorta. J. Thorac. Cardiovasc. Surg., 66:693, 1973.
12. DeMeules, J. E., Cramer, G., and Perry, J. F., Jr.: Rupture of aorta and great vessels due to blunt thoracic trauma. J. Thorac. Cardiovasc. Surg., 61:440, 1971.
13. Fleming, A. W., and Green, D. C.: Traumatic aneurysms of the thoracic aorta. Ann. Thorac. Surg., 18:91, 1974.
14. Freed, T. A., Neal, M. P., Jr., and Vinik, M.: Roentgenographic findings in extracardiac injury secondary to blunt chest automobile trauma. Am. J. Roentgenol., 104:424, 1968.
15. Gazzaniga, A. B., Khuri, E. I., Mir-Sepasi, H. M., and Bartlett, R. H.: Rupture of the thoracic aorta following blunt trauma. Arch. Surg., 110:1119, 1975.
16. Greendyke, R. M.: Traumatic rupture of aorta. J.A.M.A., 195:119, 1966.
17. Kirsh, M. M., Behrendt, D. M., Orringer, M. B., Gago, O., Gray, L. J., Jr., Mills, L. J., Walter, J. F., and Sloan, H.: The treatment of acute traumatic rupture of the aorta. A 10 year experience. Ann. Surg., 184:308, 1976.
18. Kirsh, M. M., Kahn, D. R., Crane, J. D., Anastasia, L. F., Lui, A. H., Moores, W. Y., Vathayanon, S., Bookstein, J. J., and Sloan, H.: Repair of acute traumatic rupture of the aorta without extracorporeal circulation. Ann. Thorac. Surg., 10:227, 1970.
19. Krause, A. H., Ferguson, T. B., and Weldon, C. S.: Thoracic aneurysmectomy utilizing the TDMAC-heparin shunt. Ann. Thorac. Surg., 14:123, 1972.
20. Lawrence, G. H., Hessel, E. A., Sauvage, L. R., and Krause, A. H.: Results of the use of the TDMAC-heparin shunt in the surgery of aneurysms of the descending thoracic aorta. J. Thorac. Cardiovasc. Surg., 73:393, 1977.
21. Marsh, D. G., and Sturm, J. T.: Traumatic aortic rupture: Roentgenographic indications for angiography. Ann. Thorac. Surg., 21:337, 1976.
22. Parmley, L. F., Mattingly, T. W., Manion, W. C., and Jahnke, E. J., Jr.: Nonpenetrating traumatic injury of the aorta. Circulation, 17:1086, 1958.
23. Passaro, E., and Pace, W. G.: Traumatic rupture of the aorta. Surgery, 46:787, 1959.
24. Pickard, L. R., Mattox, K. L., Espada, R., Beall, A. C., Jr., and DeBakey, M. E.: Transection of the descending thoracic aorta secondary to blunt trauma. J. Trauma, 17:749, 1977.
25. Richardson, J. D., McElvein, R. B., and Trinkle, J. K.: First rib fracture: A hallmark of severe trauma. Ann. Surg., 181:251, 1975.
26. Rindfleisch, W.: Zur Entshung und Heilung des Aneurysmsma dissecans aortae. Arch. Pathol. Anat., 13:374, 1893.
27. Spencer, F. C., Guerin, P. F., Blake, H. A., and Bahnson, H. T.: A report of fifteen patients with traumatic rupture of the thoracic aorta. J. Thorac. Cardiovasc. Surg., 41:1, 1961.
28. Symbas, P. N.: Great vessel injury. Am. Heart J., 93:518, 1977.
29. Symbas, P. N., Tyras, D. H., Ware, R. E., and Diorio, D. A.: Traumatic rupture of the aorta. Ann. Surg., 178:6, 1973.
30. Turney, S. Z., Attar, S., Ayella, R., Crowley, R. A., and McLaughlin, J.: Traumatic rupture of the aorta. A five year experience. J. Thorac. Cardiovasc. Surg., 71:727, 1976.
31. Wolfe, W. G., Kleinman, L. H., Wechsler, A. S., and Sabiston, D. C., Jr.: Heparin-coated shunts for lesions of the descending thoracic aorta. Arch. Surg., 112:1481, 1977.

3. DISSECTING ANEURYSMS OF THE AORTA

Walter G. Wolfe, M.D.

Historical Aspects

In 1761, Morgagni described the clinical course and pathologic findings in three patients with aortic dissection in whom the condition was fatal. Since then the grave prognosis of this disease has become well recognized. His description was quite succinct:

. . . the blood forcing its way by degrees obliquely through the wall and coming out under the external coat of the artery, first by drawing it from the internal coats then by raising it as to a large kind of ecchymoses.[18]

Throughout the nineteenth and first half of the twentieth century the true incidence of aortic dissection was not realized. In 1934, Shennan was able to collect only 300 cases from the world literature during the previous 150 years.[2] The term *dissecting aneurysm* was first used by René Laennec in 1819.[13] Although it has been retained, it is clearly a misnomer, since in an acute dissection a hematoma is present that dissects between the vessel layers for a varying length of the aorta and is not an aneurysm in the usual meaning of the term. The first correct clinical diagnosis was made by Swain and Lathrop in 1855, and more than a century passed before the correct diagnosis could be made in more than one quarter of patients. Subsequently, the term *intramural hematoma* was proposed to distinguish aortic dissections from other, more classic forms of aneurysms. Although Shennan's report exhaustively documented the clinical and pathologic features of aortic dissections and clarified the probable pathogenesis, recognition of dissection during life remained infrequent and treatment continued to be symptomatic.[2]

The astonishingly high mortality of aortic dissection treated with the early forms of medical therapy was emphasized in 1958 by Hirst and colleagues in a review of 505 dissections accumulated over a 21-year period.[10] In this series, the mortality was 50 per cent at 4 days, 75 per cent at 2 weeks, and 90 per cent after 3 months. Their review also emphasized the protean manifestations of acute dissections, the infrequency of correct antemortem diagnosis (only 40 per cent), and the progressive increase in incidence of dissection to approximately 1 in 360 autopsies.

The availability of angiography during the past 20 years has sharply increased the ability to establish a clinical diagnosis, which is now generally greater than 90 per cent. Until 1955 surgical treatment of aortic dissections had been confined to local fenestration procedures, the results of which were poor.[6,23] During the past 20 years, since DeBakey, Cooley, and Creech reported early successful experiences with surgical management,[6] the treatment of aortic dissection has evolved rapidly, and by 1965 the surgical mortality was 21 per cent.[7]

Classification and Incidence

DeBakey classified aortic dissections into Type I, Type II, and Type III (Fig. 1) and urged emergency surgical intervention as the treatment of choice for nearly all patients. During the early 1970s, this original classification was reduced to two groups, those involving the ascending aorta and those originating in the

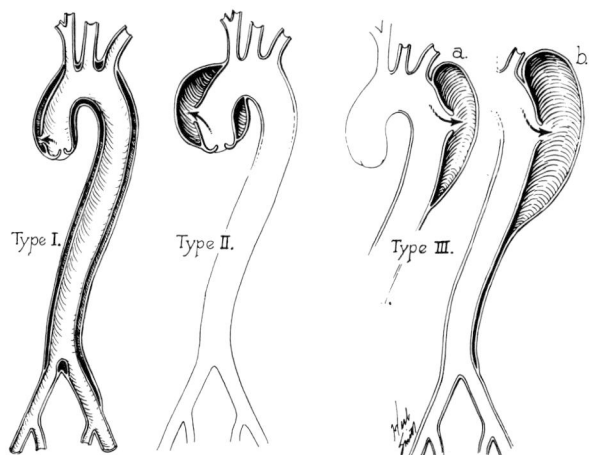

Figure 1. DeBakey's classification of dissecting aortic aneurysms: Type I, Type II, and Type III. (From DeBakey, M. E., Henly, W. S., Cooley, D. A., et al.: Surgical management of dissecting aneurysms of the aorta. J. Thorac. Cardiovasc. Surg., 49:130, 1965.)

descending aorta.[1,3,7] This was the result of evolving attitudes toward surgical therapy as well as the fact that only 10 per cent of patients have involvement limited to the ascending aorta. Moreover, the clinical problems encountered in the patients with ascending versus descending dissections, the presence of hypertension, and the pathophysiologic aspects leading to the patient's death are somewhat different. Ascending and descending dissections should also be categorized as to whether they are acute or chronic. Ascending dissections can be termed Type A and descending lesions Type B. Type C indicated fatal, inoperable dissections.[1] The incidence of acute aortic dissection is two to three times more frequent than that of ruptured abdominal aortic aneurysms.

Acute aortic dissection is the most common catastrophic event involving the aorta.[22] There are approximately 60,000 patients who have dissecting aneurysms in the United States annually.[22] Aortic dissections are three times more frequent in males; however, 50 per cent of the dissections seen in females under the age of 40 occur in pregnancy.[14] Acute dissection occurs most frequently between the ages of 45 and 70; the incidence appears to be greater in patients with Marfan's syndrome or congenital heart disease, such as coarctation of the aorta or bicuspid aortic valve disease.[16] A history of hypertension is present in approximately 80 to 90 per cent of patients. It is clear that the incidence of hypertension is over 95 per cent in patients with descending dissections.[5]

Etiology and Pathophysiology

The aorta maintains a flexible blood flow pattern required for organ support under many different conditions and is subjected to 3 billion pulsations during an average life span. Unfortunately, there are several serious disease processes that have the potential to weaken the aortic wall. Although syphilitic aortitis has almost disappeared, atherosclerosis remains very common. In dissecting aneurysms, as in other diseases affecting the aortic wall, the underlying defect is the destruction of the medial layer that contains the elastic fibers. Although medial necrosis is associated with Marfan's syndrome, the relationship of this lesion to aortas with dissection or to aging without dissection is unknown. Hypertension, atherosclerosis, coarctation, epinephrine-induced dissection, and endocrine factors may cause medial necrosis. The epinephrine effect that produces a hyperkinetic heart may be important even though hypertension is not present. Pregnancy may incite the hypertension and hyperkinetic heart, and these responses may represent dissections in these patients. Trauma may also cause dissection. Medial necrosis is seen in congenital vessel anomalies in addition to Mar-

fan's syndrome. Since, in most patients, acute aortic dissection occurs in the well-defined region of the aortic media, it may also be associated with necrosis, hemorrhage, or degenerative changes in this layer.

The aortic wall is elastic and constantly expanding during the pressure pulse wave and serves to dampen the suddenness of the compression wave. This is accomplished by the circumferential placement of intermingled collagen fibers and smooth muscle cells in the tunica media, which are arranged in laminar layers between layers of elastin fibers. The elastin allows expansion of the wall by its rubber-like nature, and muscle cells act as shock absorbers contracting in response to the acceleration of the systolic pulse. Collagen provides tensile strength to the wall and protection from rupture should high tension develop.

Another major stress acting on the inner aortic wall is longitudinal shear. Viscous blood flows through the aorta and places a considerable and continuous shearing force along the wall in the direction of flow. The high-risk shear points of the aorta are often most affected by proliferative changes in early atherosclerosis.

Most dissections occur in the inner one third to one half of the aorta wall. When medial degeneration of the wall of the thoracic aorta has occurred, the likelihood of dissection is increased by the diminished cohesiveness of the layers of the aortic wall. Medial necrosis leads to decreased intimal adherence, and specific mechanical factors may or may not cause dissection. Repeated motion of the aorta related to the beating heart causes flexion stresses, most marked in the ascending aorta and in the first portion of the descending aorta. This stress occurs some 35 to 40 million times per year. Along with this repeated motion of the aorta, patients with aortic stenosis, bicuspid aortic valves, and pure Marfan's syndrome have a greater risk of dissection. Hemodynamic forces in the bloodstream related to the pulse wave propagated by each cardiac systole act upon the wall of the aorta and, most markedly, the proximal aorta. The combination of factors eventually leads to an intimal tear, following which there is a propagation of a dissecting hematoma of varying depth and length into the media of the aortic wall.

Most commonly, however, tears originating in the ascending aorta proceed along the entire length of the aorta, whereas those that originate distal to the left subclavian dissect distally into the descending thoracic aorta and abdominal aorta (Fig. 2). This hematoma dissects and commonly re-enters the lumen of the aorta. Multiple entry and re-entry points are seen throughout the aorta. Ascending dissection may proceed retrograde to involve coronary arteries and pericardium and to rupture into the mediastinum, leading to death. Dissection back toward the coronaries and aortic valve frequently produces aortic insufficiency, a situation that is poorly tolerated and is associated with cardiac failure and pulmonary edema.[1,11] Those descending dissections that rupture into the pleural cavity are usually fatal.

The surgical approach to aortic dissection is based on the pathogenesis of this lesion.[28] An acute aortic dissection involving the ascending aorta usually affects the entire aorta. Only some 10 per cent of the patients have involvement limited to the ascending aorta or the aortic arch. As the dissection advances distally, the visceral vessels are involved in varying degrees, as are the arteries to the brain. Usually, the noncoronary cusp becomes incompetent as the dissection proceeds toward the anulus, and this cusp prolapses into the left ventricle to produce acute aortic insufficiency (Fig. 3). Other cusps in spiraling dissections are usually spared as the coronaries anchor the media, intima, and adventitia in this area and protect them from separation. If the dissection involves a coronary artery, sudden death is likely as a result of myocardial ischemia. Blood may enter the pericardium and cause tamponade or rupture into the mediastinum, either of which may lead to sudden death.

Dissections that involve the descending aorta with the point of origin distal to the subclavian artery may proceed to the

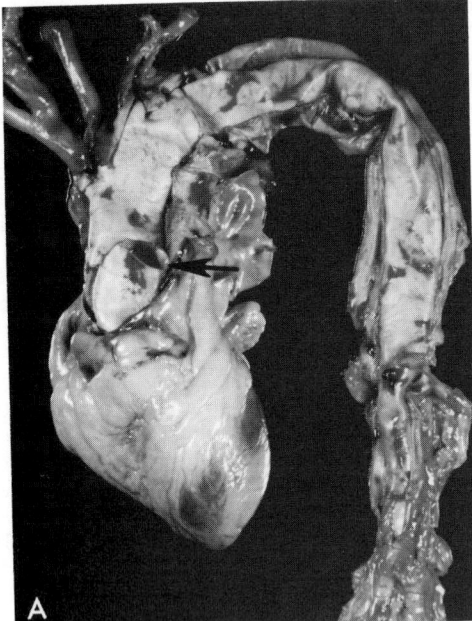

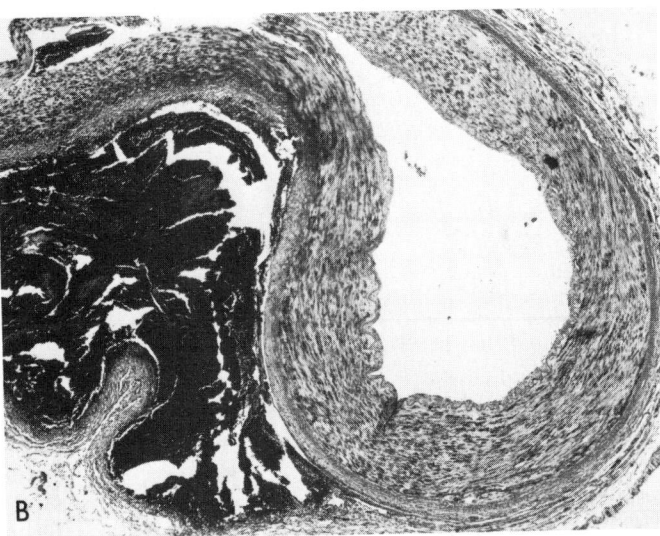

Figure 2. *A*, Pathologic specimen demonstrating an intimal tear in the ascending aorta distal to the aortic valve. The dissection involves the entire aorta. *B*, Example of the hematoma in the false lumen compressing the true lumen of a renal artery.

subclavian artery and head vessels and often progress distally for the length of the aorta. Again, multiple re-entry points are not uncommon and the visceral vessels may be involved to varying degrees, these vessels originating from either the true or the false lumen of the aorta (Fig. 4).

Acute dissection of the ascending aorta usually produces aortic insufficiency and entry of blood into the pericardium, causing tamponade (Fig. 5). Varying degrees of coronary as well as cerebral insufficiency may also occur (Fig. 6). Many times, the blood flow to the visceral organs is spared through perfusion of the false lumen as the aortic dissection advances. It is not uncommon for one renal artery to be perfused by the true lumen

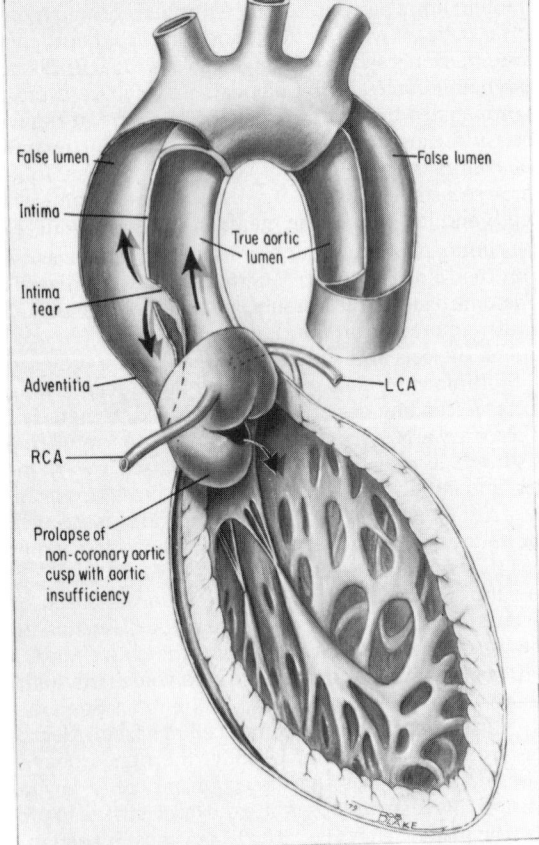

Figure 3. Illustration of the pathophysiologic mechanism of acute ascending dissection. The intimal tear originates above the aortic valve, and the dissection proceeds down the thoracic aorta and into the abdominal aorta. Mechanisms of aortic regurgitation in this situation were produced by circumferential widening of the aortic root and separation of the aortic cusp. There may be displacement of the aortic cusp substantially below the level of the anulus produced by the pressure of the dissecting hematoma. At times there may be actual disruption of the annular leaflet support leading to a flail cusp.

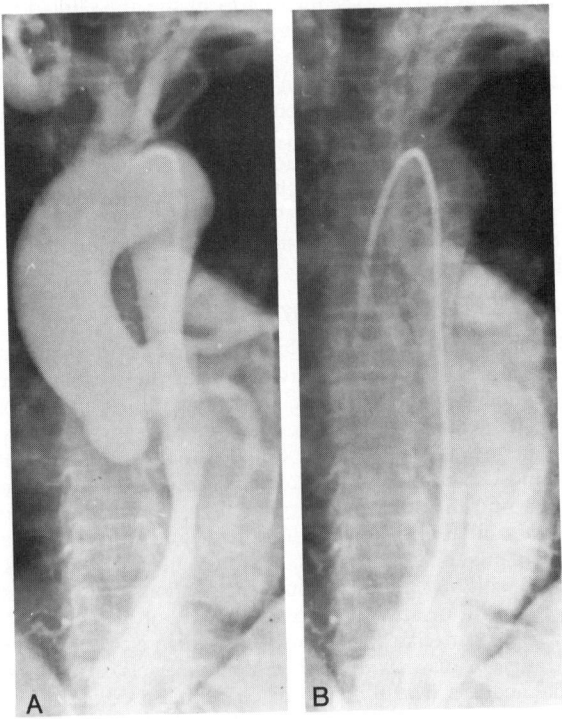

Figure 4. *A*, Example of a descending dissection showing marked compression of the thoracic aorta, normal aortic cusps, arch, and head vessels with marked compression of the descending thoracic aorta continuing on into the abdominal aorta. *B*, Late film shows opacification of the false channel.

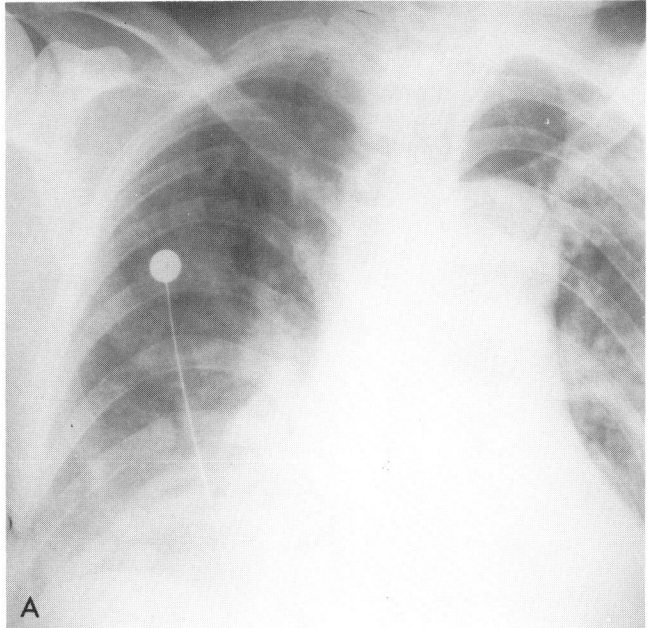

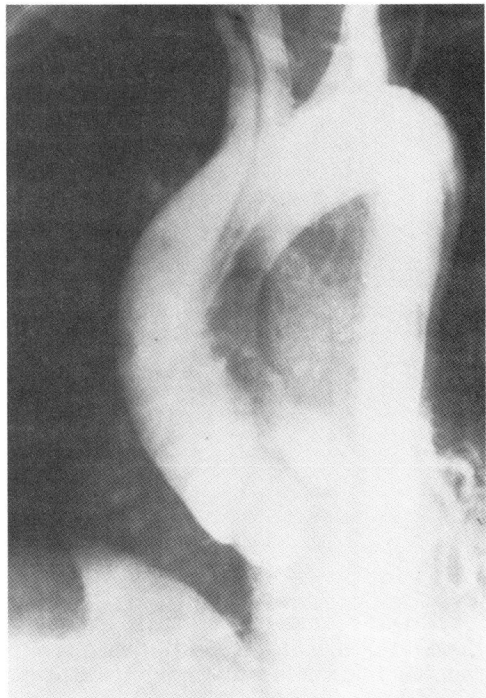

Figure 6. Arteriogram revealing ascending dissection with marked involvement of the innominate and arch vessels. The dissection continues distally into the abdominal aorta.

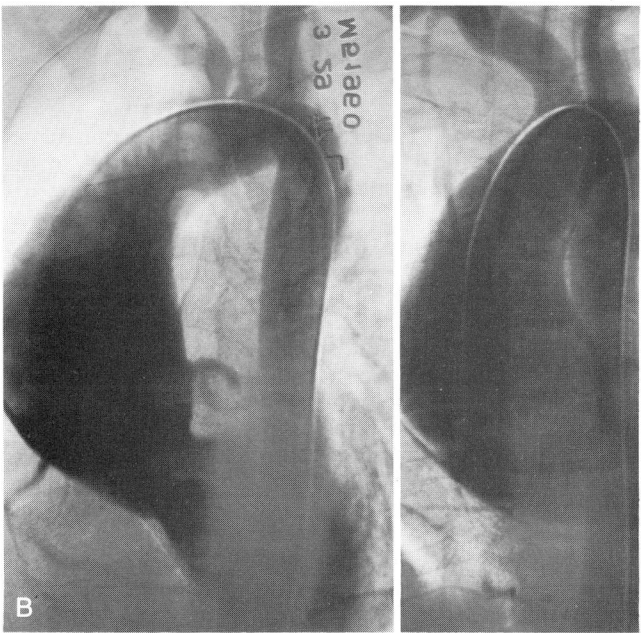

Figure 5. *A*, Chest film of a patient with acute ascending dissection illustrating massive pulmonary edema produced by aortic insufficiency. *B*, Arteriogram demonstrating aortic valve incompetence and filling of ventricle with contrast material.

and the other by the false lumen (Fig. 7). In both ascending and descending aortic dissections, the extremities may be involved, producing varying degrees of vascular insufficiency.

Clinical Presentation

Pain is the most frequent symptom of patients presenting with acute aortic dissection. It is best described as catastrophic chest pain, so severe that the individual almost immediately seeks medical attention. Although many terms are used to describe this pain, including "tearing," "throbbing," or "ripping," the onset is almost always sudden. After the initial episode, the pain may be confined to the chest or may be substernal, in the back, along the route of the aorta, in the abdomen, or in a combination of these sites. Many times, the pain radiates into

the upper or lower extremities. The point to be emphasized is the fact that the pain is catastrophic and may take one of several forms. Unless the history and physical examination are carefully considered, the correct diagnosis may not be made.

Ninety-two per cent of patients with catastrophic pain were seen in the Duke Emergency Clinic. The pain was described as being located in the back, chest, or abdomen; 30 per cent presented with extremity pain. Neurologic deficit was present in 30 per cent, and 25 per cent had nausea and vomiting. Dyspnea is not uncommon, and pulmonary edema may be present. Many patients may be normotensive or hypotensive in the aftermath of the acute episode, or this finding may be the result of pericardial tamponade.

PHYSICAL EXAMINATION. Frequently, the seriously ill patients present with shock despite previously known hypertension. Examination of the chest may reveal pulmonary edema, diminished heart sounds, and a murmur of aortic insufficiency. Examination may demonstrate a differential blood pressure and pulse in the upper extremities or diminished or differential pulses in the legs. The patient who presents with both catastrophic chest pain and diminished pulses must be immediately considered to have had an aortic dissection. Neurologic findings are clearly related to the degree of dissection and to involvement of the arch vessels involved in the cerebral blood supply.

The differential diagnosis in this group of patients includes myocardial infarction, rupture of the sinus of Valsalva, cerebrovascular accident, acute surgical abdomen, pulmonary embolism, arterial thrombosis or embolism of the aortic bifurcation, or occlusion of the peripheral arteries. There may be a variety of murmurs and bruits varying from that of aortic insufficiency to those over major branches of the aorta such as the carotid or renal arteries. Most significant is the difference in blood pressure that may be seen between two upper extremities. The patient may appear to be in shock while the pressure in the opposite extremity shows marked hypertension. When the condition is suspected, the patient is immediately prepared for arteriography to achieve an objective diagnosis.

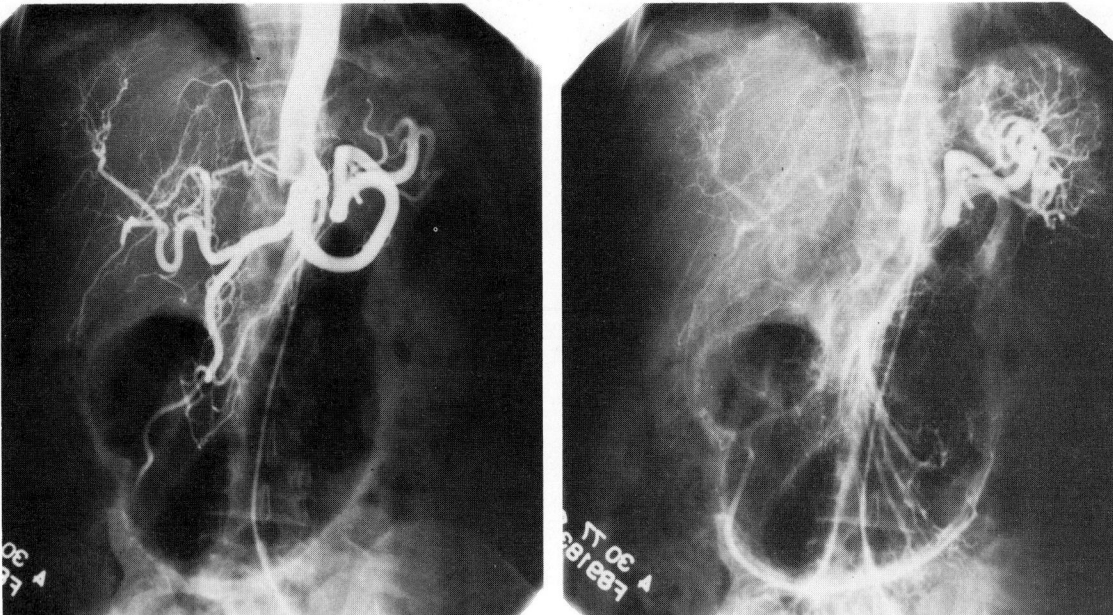

Figure 7. Abdominal aortogram revealing the celiac axis originating from the true lumen and no filling of either renal vessels or distal visceral vessels from the true lumen. Late film shows filling of the superior mesenteric vessels from the false lumen.

Diagnosis

Since severe chest pain is the common presenting symptom, the primary problem is that of differentiating acute dissection from acute myocardial infarction. The accessory clinical findings are important. Electrocardiographic abnormalities include left axis deviation, left ventricular hypertrophy, ischemic changes of varying degrees, conduction defects, and dysrhythmias. However, in none was the electrocardiogram diagnostic of acute myocardial infarction. In contrast, chest roentgenography yielded what was considered to be a normal chest film in only 10 per cent of patients. The remainder had a dilated aorta, a widened mediastinum with cardiomegaly, pulmonary edema, or a mass effect with or without pleural effusion. Therefore, the plain chest film is of critical importance, and a normal film in this group of patients is extremely unusual.

Mediastinal widening is highly suggestive but not necessarily diagnostic of aortic dissection, since tumors can produce a similar change. Calcium in the wall of the aorta, with obvious widening beyond the calcium, is also suggestive but again is not diagnostic. Patients presenting with a combination of chest pain and abnormal chest film should have aortography. If this study reveals splitting of the contrast column, distortion of the contrast column, or aortic insufficiency, the test is positive. If a computed tomogram has been obtained, an aortogram may still be necessary to define the origin and extent of the dissection (Fig. 8).

In the majority of patients the aortogram localizes the origin of the dissection either distal to the left subclavian artery or in the ascending aorta. When the diagnosis has been confirmed, determination of whether the dissection is ascending or descending is important in deciding the type of management.

SURVIVAL OF UNTREATED DISSECTION. The lethality of this condition makes early diagnosis and appropriate therapy mandatory. This is emphasized by Hirst's review, in which the 15-minute mortality was approximately 20 per cent. At 24 hours, 40 per cent of the patients had died, and by 48 hours the death rate was 50 per cent. At 2 weeks, only 20 per cent of the untreated patients were alive; only 10 per cent were alive at 1 year (Fig. 9). Therefore, a high index of suspicion is imperative in this group of patients.

Management

Wheat and colleagues[26] pioneered modern pharmacologic hypotensive therapy for acute dissecting aneurysms of the aorta. They reduced both mean and systemic arterial pressure and dp/dt through the administration of trimethaphan, reserpine, and guanethidine. The goal was conversion of all acute aortic dissections to subacute or chronic status. Then, after careful evaluation, treatment by elective operation was reserved for any complications that arose. They initiated this therapy for all patients with dissection, and early results showed an impressive 1-year survival of 84 per cent. Nevertheless, there are clearly serious limitations to nonoperative therapy.[7,25] Although many authorities originally employed pharmacologic therapy and reserved a surgical approach for patients with localized rupture, tamponade, or associated severe aortic insufficiency, it became evident that adoption of nonsurgical management did not ensure the high 1-year survival that was initially attained.[4,15] One substantial advantage of induced hypotensive therapy is that it can be instituted in a community hospital following the initial diagnosis of dissecting aneurysm, with subsequent stabilization and transport to a cardiovascular surgical center.

Complications of an antihypertensive regimen, however, have included drug sensitivity and aggravation of concomitant renal failure. Sensitivity to drugs varies in each patient; trimethaphan may cause respiratory arrest, and the cerebral effects of reserpine are common. Nitroprusside has replaced these agents in the management of acute aortic dissection because of its effectiveness in lowering blood pressure, ease of administration, and rapid control.[19] However, some question has arisen as to its effectiveness in protecting against continued dissection despite lowering of the arterial pressure following the effect of increased aortic dp/dt. It is currently believed that intravenous nitroprusside is the agent of choice in controlling blood pressure in acute aortic dissection. Propranolol and methyldopa may be administered simultaneously, and when pressure is controlled, the nitroprusside may be slowly discontinued. Although lowering of the blood pressure is mandatory in these patients, urinary output must also be carefully monitored and maintained. It is important that physicians managing acute aortic dissection be familiar with the use of antihypertensive drugs in this group of

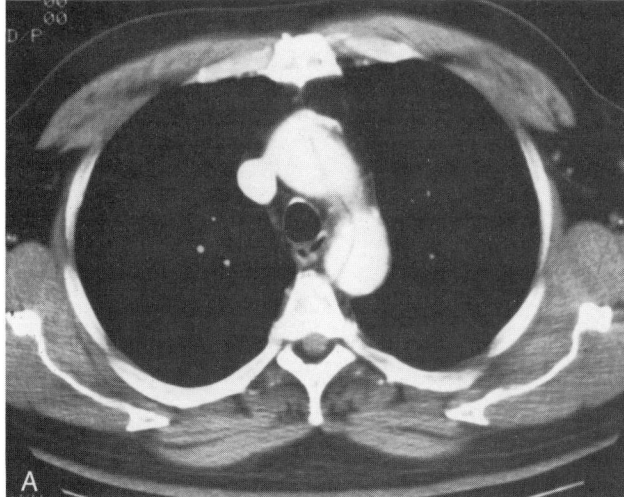

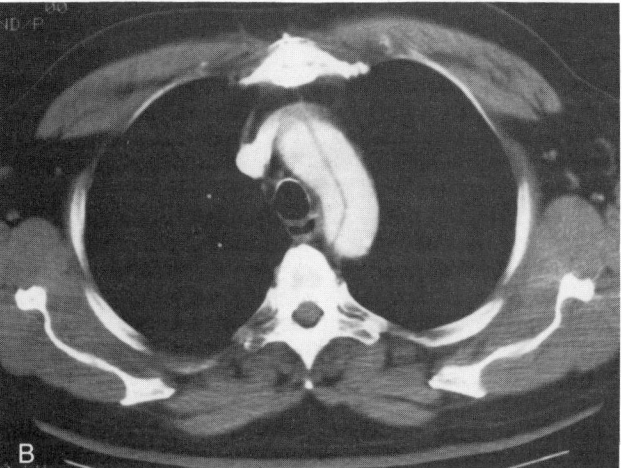

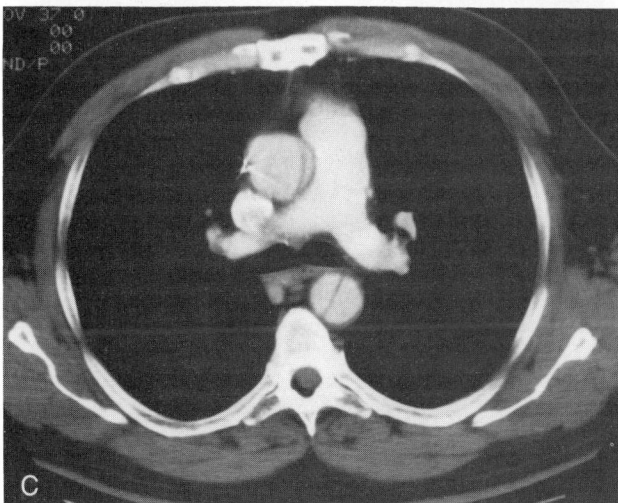

Figure 8. *A* to *C*, Computed tomography slices of a patient with a Type I dissecting aortic aneurysm demonstrating the dissection in the ascending aorta, arch, and descending aorta.

troprusside) before and during aortography. During this time, all necessary preparations for operation can be made. Aortography should confirm the diagnosis of either an ascending or a descending dissection, at which point therapy, whether definitive or expectant, is chosen.

ASCENDING DISSECTIONS. Nearly all patients with ascending aortic dissection should be managed surgically immediately after the diagnosis is established. Acute aortic dissection of the ascending aorta almost invariably involves the entire aorta, except in 10 per cent of patients (Fig. 10), in whom the involvement is limited to the ascending aorta or the aortic arch. Dissection begins proximal in the ascending aorta and continues around the arch to the iliac arteries. The visceral vessels are involved to varying degrees, as are the head vessels. The early causes of death in these patients are pericardial tamponade, rupture into the mediastinum, or acute aortic insufficiency with cardiac and renal failure. These are basically mechanical problems, and therefore surgical correction is mandatory.

Although the first successful treatment of dissecting aneurysm of the aorta using the fenestration operation was reported by DeBakey and colleagues in 1955,[6] this operation is now rarely used. DeBakey's group reported the most successful results with surgical therapy of the dissecting aneurysm in 179 patients, with a survival of 79 per cent.[7] The most favored operative approach at present is a median sternotomy with cardiopulmonary bypass. Cannulation is made through the femoral artery; most patients have bloody fluid within the pericardium that may produce tamponade. The goal of the operation, then, is to correct the aortic insufficiency, either with aortic valve replacement or more often with resuspension of the aortic valve, and to graft the ascending aorta directing the blood into the true lumen with obliteration of the false lumen, thereby providing protection from rupture into the mediastinum or pericardium.[27,30] When the operation is completed and cardiopulmonary bypass is discontinued, heparin is reversed with protamine, and antihypertensive therapy is instituted (usually with nitroprusside). Propranolol, methyldopa, or hydralazine to control the blood pressure is then administered; most normotensive patients are given propranolol.

DESCENDING AORTIC DISSECTION. Dissections confined to the descending aorta can usually be carefully moni-

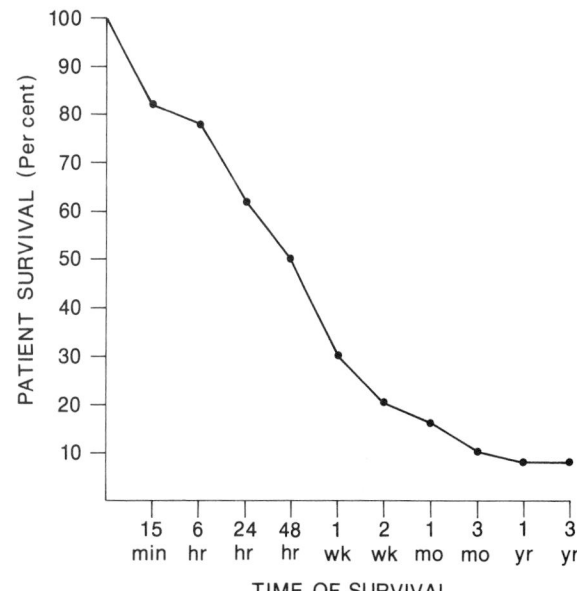

Figure 9. Graph indicating survival of patients with *untreated* acute dissecting aneurysms. (Adapted from Anagnostopoulos, C. E., et al.: Am. J. Cardiol., *30*:263, 1972.)

patients, since their roles in acute management and in the postoperative period are of great importance.

The consensus concerning the principles of management of acute aortic dissections has evolved from the collective experience of the past 20 years.[1,3,7,12,19,24] After the initial presentation and diagnosis, time should be devoted to stabilization of the patient and utilization of antihypertensive therapy (usually ni-

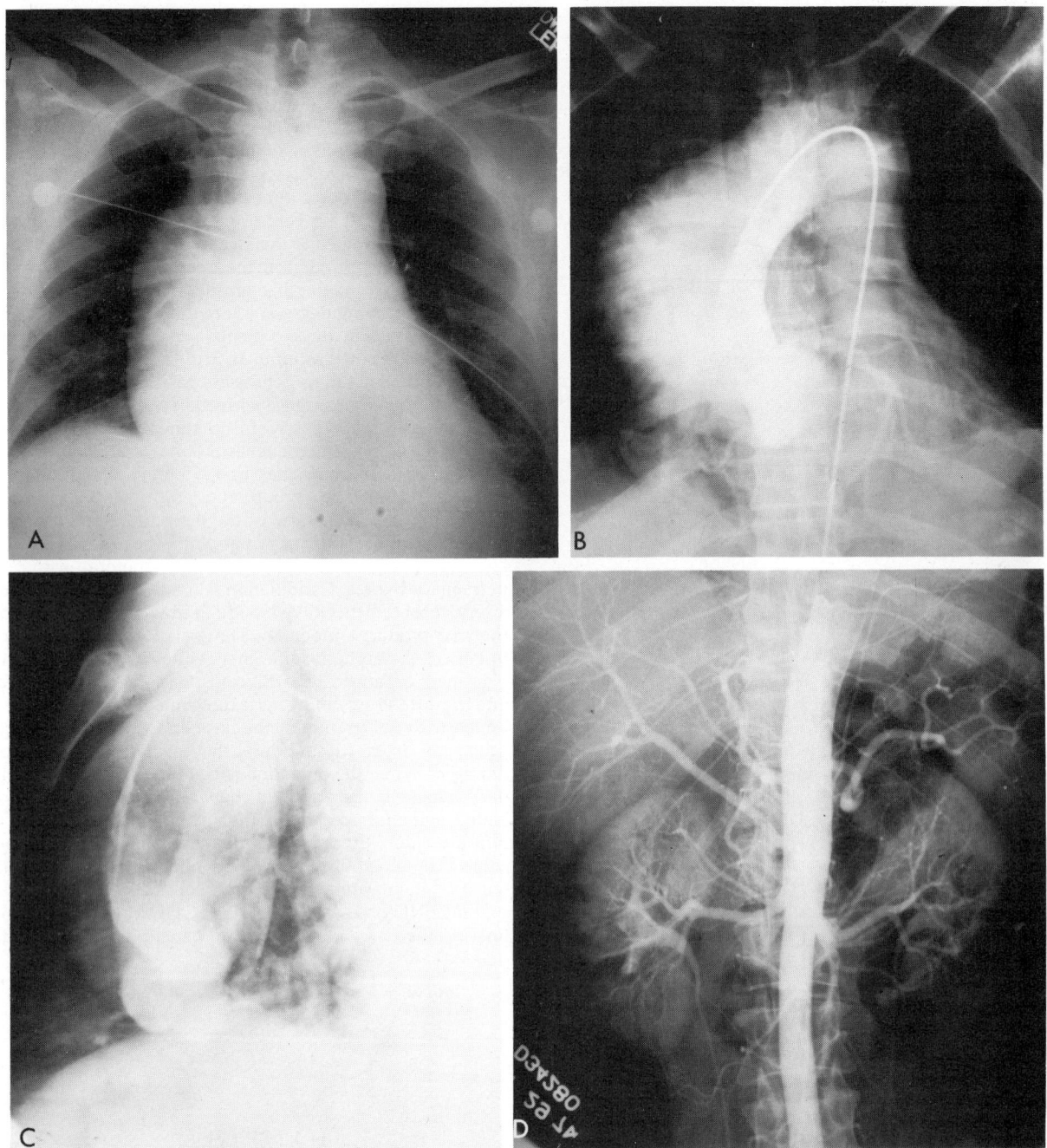

Figure 10. *A*, Chest film in a patient with an acute ascending dissection showing marked widening of the mediastinum without evidence of pulmonary edema. *B*, The aortogram shows an ascending dissection (Type II); the dissection does not involve the arch or descending thoracic abdominal aorta. *C*, Lateral view revealing the true and false lumens. *D*, Abdominal aortogram shows normal abdominal aorta and normal placement of the visceral vessels. Postoperative chest film reveals a Starr-Edwards prosthesis. A graft was inserted in the ascending aorta.

tored. The life-threatening nature of descending aortic dissection is determined by, first, rupture into the pleural space, and, second, involvement of the visceral vessels. After the diagnosis has been confirmed and hypotensive therapy instituted, monitoring under close observation is imperative. Indications for immediate operative intervention include failure to control hypertension, continued pain, expansion of the aneurysm, or signs or symptoms of rupture such as pleural effusion, development of a neurologic deficit, or evidence of compromise of major visceral vessels or arteries to the lower extremities.

By use of a left lateral thoracotomy and either partial cardiopulmonary bypass or a heparin-bonded shunt, a graft is inserted into the thoracic aorta, obliterating the false lumen and redirecting blood flow into the true aortic lumen. In the absence of any of the previously mentioned indications, operation can be postponed. With the passage of time, edema around the aorta clears, and the development of fibrosis transforms initially friable adventitia of the aorta into less fragile tissue. The patient should be discharged from the hospital on antihypertensive therapy. These patients should be followed carefully by their personal physicians to be certain that the arterial blood pressure is maintained in an acceptable range. If with the passage of time there is enlargement of the thoracic aneurysm observed on the chest film, the patient must be considered a candidate for resection and grafting. It appears that approximately one third of these patients ultimately require operation, usually for an enlarging aneurysm. Late surgical procedures on descending aortic dissections are associated with a low mortality.[20,21]

For postoperative patients, effective treatment consists of stringent control of the arterial blood pressure to protect suture lines as well as the diseased aorta. Careful attention is paid to respiratory function, gradual progressive ambulation, and careful monitoring of renal function. After discharge, follow-up of blood pressure is essential to achieve satisfactory long-term results in these patients.

TREATMENT OF CHRONIC DISSECTIONS. Chronic dissection of the aorta can best be defined as the patient who has survived 2 or more weeks after the acute episode. In patients with ascending dissection seen during this period, urgent therapy is usually indicated. Surgical treatment is directed toward the complications of dissection (i.e., progressive aortic insufficiency and heart failure or, again, expanding and enlarging aneurysm of the ascending aorta, or continuing pain that has not been controlled by appropriate antihypertensive therapy). An operative approach for these patients is similar to that described for acute dissection, but a far greater number of individuals with chronic dissection and aortic insufficiency require valve replacement, since resuspension of the aortic valve has not been satisfactory. The ascending aorta is grafted, and blood flow is directed into the true lumen.

Patients with chronic descending aortic dissection usually present with an enlarging aneurysm or back pain or both and require surgical therapy. Operative management is a left thoracotomy and the use of a heparinized shunt both to decompress the left side of the heart while the descending aorta is occluded and to perfuse the lower body. The shunt can be inserted into the ascending aorta, into the subclavian artery, or into the apex of the left ventricle and then placed distally into the femoral artery.[29] The graft is inserted so that the flow of blood into the distal aorta is directed into the true lumen, with concomitant obliteration of the false lumen.

Long-term Follow-up

DeBakey and colleagues reviewed their 20-year experience,[8] and patients have been followed at Duke University Medical Center over 5 years.[30] Long-term survivors can be classified in two groups, those with DeBakey Type II dissections and those with DeBakey Type IIIA lesions. In each group the disease process is localized and can be completely removed surgically. The DeBakey Type I lesion, which begins in the ascending aorta, and Type IIIB involve nearly total dissection of the aorta, including involvement of the visceral vessels, and therefore the prognosis is poorer for both surgical and medical management of these patients. The other classifications that have been suggested are helpful in distinguishing surgical versus medical management for dissecting aneurysms, that is, surgical management for almost all dissecting aneurysms that originate in the ascending aorta (DeBakey Type I and Type II), and initial medical therapy for descending aneurysms (DeBakey Type III). It is clear that more than 95 per cent of patients with Type III descending dissection aneurysms are hypertensive contrasted with only 50 per cent of those with ascending dissections (Type I and Type II). It also follows that the best results from therapy occur in patients with localized dissection (DeBakey Type II and Type IIIA). As stated earlier, surgical therapy in ascending dissections is performed to correct the aortic insufficiency that commonly accompanies it and to prevent rupture into the pericardium and mediastinum. However, in descending dissections (DeBakey Type III), the indication for surgical intervention is impending rupture or continued pain. There are patients with chronic enlargement who require operation. The best long-term results occur in those patients with DeBakey Type IIIA lesions with the dissection localized to the thoracic aorta. As many as one fourth to one third may eventually require surgical management after successful medical therapy. The usual indication is an enlarging thoracic aortic aneurysm.

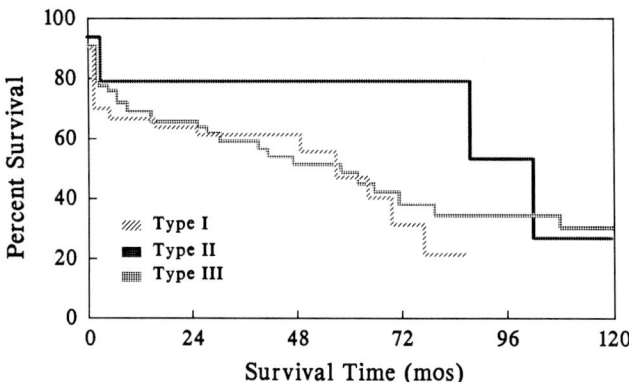

Figure 11. The 10-year survival at Duke University Medical Center for Type I, Type II, and Type III dissecting aneurysms.

Mortality

The mortality of untreated aortic dissections is catastrophic, making immediate therapy of some type mandatory. Initially, antihypertensive pharmacologic therapy is generally employed. Although the early survival with antihypertensive therapy in Wheat's series was approximately 86 per cent, it is now apparent that drug therapy alone (unless there are extenuating circumstances) should not be undertaken for long-term management of acute ascending dissections.[26] The control of descending dissections, however, is quite different.

The surgical mortality in acute ascending dissections should be between 10 and 20 per cent, with long-term survival approaching 60 per cent. In patients with descending aortic dissections, the mortality for those in the surgical series and those managed with antihypertensive therapy is essentially the same. It is apparent that some patients with descending aortic dissections who are successfully managed with antihypertensive therapy will later be managed operatively for the reasons previously described, the most common indication being an expanding thoracic aneurysm. The operative mortality is less than 10 per cent and the long-term outlook excellent.[21]

The ultimate prognosis of these patients is clearly related to the severity of the disease in the aorta and to the visceral involvement at the time of acute dissection. The survival over a 10-year period is shown in Figure 11.

SELECTED REFERENCES

Anagnostopoulos, C. E.: Acute Aortic Dissections. Baltimore, University Park Press, 1975.
  This monograph is a thorough review of the problem of dissecting aneurysms of the aorta.

Appelbaum, A., Karp, R. B., and Kirklin, J. W.: Ascending versus descending aortic dissections. Ann. Surg., 183:296, 1976.
  This article summarizes the surgical experience with dissecting aneurysms and indicates the importance of early surgical management.

Crawford, E. S., Svensson, L. G., Coselli, J. S., Safi, H. J., and Hess, K. R.: Aortic dissection and dissecting aortic aneurysms. Ann. Surg., 208:254, 1988.
  This is one of the most recent articles that summarizes one of the largest series of dissecting aneurysms in the literature.

Crawford, E. S., and Crawford, J. L.: Diseases of the Aorta. Tracy, T. M. (Ed.). Baltimore, Williams & Wilkins, 1984.
  This classic is the state-of-the-art atlas for the surgical treatment of aneurysmal aortic disease.

DeBakey, M. E., McCollum, C. H., Crawford, E. S., Morris, G. C., Jr., Howell, J., Noon, G. P., and Lawrie, G.: Dissection and dissecting aneurysms of the aorta: Twenty-year follow-up of five hundred twenty-seven patients treated surgically. Surgery, 92:1118, 1982.

4. ANEURYSMS OF THE THORACIC AORTA

Walter G. Wolfe, M.D.

The thoracic aorta is composed of the ascending thoracic aorta, the aortic arch, and the descending thoracic aorta that ends the diaphragmatic hiatus. Aneurysms of the ascending aorta may include the aortic valve, the sinuses, and the ascending aorta proper up to the innominate. The arch of the aorta includes the great vessels (the innominate, carotid, and subclavian) and ends in the area of the ligamentum. The descending thoracic aorta can be defined anatomically as that portion of the thoracic aorta from the subclavian to the diaphragm. Histologically, the aorta is composed of three layers, the intima, media, and adventitia. The intima is important since the etiologic factor of many thoracic aneurysms is atherosclerosis. The media is important because of the degenerative nature of cystic medial necrosis and its involvement in patients as well as in dissecting aneurysms. The adventitia is important because it is a strong supportive tissue that may protect patients from sudden death secondary to rupture into the mediastinum or free pleural space, which may be seen in dissecting aneurysms and/or traumatic transected aortas following high-speed automobile accidents.

Historical Aspects

Surgical therapies for thoracic aneurysms were attempted in the twentieth century[1] and Bahnson repaired a thoracic aneurysm in 1953,[2] although it was not until 1956 that successful excision and replacement was done by Cooley and DeBakey.[6] Since then, there have been advances in the management of thoracic aortic aneurysms and treatment methods that are now well established, such as cardiopulmonary bypass and deep hypothermia for ascending aneurysms and arch aneurysms, direct clamping of the descending thoracic aorta, or use of other bypass techniques.[7,8,23,30] With refinement in techniques, the mortality for surgical therapy of the thoracic aorta is 5 to 10 per cent. The most serious complications that may occur following resection of arch aneurysms or descending thoracic aneurysms are significant central nervous system defect or, as in the descending thoracic aorta, paraplegia.

Etiology

The etiology of thoracic aortic aneurysms includes atherosclerosis, cystic medial degeneration, myxomatous degeneration, dissection, infection, trauma, and post-stenotic dilatation. In this country today, syphilitic aortitis is unusual as a cause of thoracic aneurysms. Cystic medial necrosis was described by Erdheim in 1929,[17] and this finding is one of the prominent features in patients with Marfan's syndrome. The incidence of thoracic aneurysms increases with age. In the aging aorta, cystic medial necrosis is seen almost routinely and it may accompany degenerative changes seen with atherosclerosis. Atherosclerosis that causes occlusion of the vasa vasorum produces medial necrosis and subsequent aneurysm formation. Aneurysm formation can be classified as either localized, as seen in saccular aneurysms, or fusiform, which produces a more generalized aneurysm.

Presentation

Presenting symptoms of thoracic aneurysm depend on the area of the thoracic aorta involved. In general, compression, pressure, and chest pain are the main presenting symptoms. Many times, a routine chest film reveals an asymptomatic thoracic aneurysm. Patients may experience hoarseness and superior vena caval syndrome. Cough and dyspnea from tracheobronchial obstruction may occur, and hemoptysis is a very serious sign usually indicating erosion into the trachea, main

REFERENCES

1. Anagnostopoulos, C. E.: Classification. *In* Anagnostopoulos, C. E. (Ed.): Acute Aortic Dissections. Baltimore, University Park Press, 1975.
2. Anagnostopoulos, C. E.: History. *In* Anagnostopoulos, C. E.: Acute Aortic Dissections. Baltimore, University Park Press, 1975.
3. Appelbaum, A., Karp, R. B., and Kirklin, J. W.: Ascending versus descending aortic dissections. Ann. Surg., 183:296, 1976.
4. Daily, P. O., Trueblood, H. W., Stinson, E. B., Wuerflein, R. D., and Shumway, N. E.: Management of acute aortic dissections. Ann. Thorac. Surg., 10:237, 1970.
5. Dalen, J. E., Alpert, J. S., Cohn, L. H., Black, H., and Collins, J. J.: Dissection of the thoracic aorta. Am. J. Cardiol., 34:803, 1974.
6. DeBakey, M. E., Cooley, D. A., and Creech, O., Jr.: Surgical considerations of dissecting aneurysm of the aorta. Ann. Surg., 142:587, 1955.
7. DeBakey, M. E., Henly, W. S., Cooley, D. A., Morris, G. C., Jr., Crawford, E. S., and Beall, A. C., Jr.: Surgical management of dissecting aneurysms of the aorta. J. Thorac. Cardiovasc. Surg., 49:130, 1965.
8. DeBakey, M. E., McCollum, C. H., Crawford, E. S., Morris, G. C., Jr., Howell, J., Noon, G. P., and Lawrie, G.: Dissection and dissecting aneurysms of the aorta: Twenty-year follow-up of five hundred twenty-seven patients treated surgically. Surgery, 92:1118, 1982.
9. Harris, P. D., Bowman, F. O., Jr., and Malm, J. R.: The management of acute dissections of the thoracic aorta. Am. Heart J., 78:419, 1969.
10. Hirst, A. E., Jr., Johns, V. L., Jr., and Kime, S. W., Jr.: Dissecting aneurysm of the aorta: A review of 505 cases. Medicine, 37:217, 1958.
11. Hume, D. M., and Porter, R. R.: Acute dissecting aortic aneurysms. Surgery, 53:122, 1963.
12. Kidd, J. N., Reul, G. J., Jr., Cooley, D. A., Sandiford, F. M., Kyger, E. R., and Wukasch, D. C.: Surgical treatment of aneurysms of the ascending aorta. Circulation, 54:III-111, 1976.
13. Laennec, R. T. H.: Trait de l'Auscultation Mediate. Brosson, J. A., and Chaude, J. S., Paris, 1819, p. 441.
14. Mandel, W., Evans, E. W., and Walsford, R. L.: Dissecting aortic aneurysm during pregnancy. N. Engl. J. Med., 251:1059, 1954.
15. McFarland, J., Willerson, J. T., Dinsmore, R. E., Austen, W. G., Buckley, M. J., Sanders, C. A., and DeSanctis, R. W.: The medical treatment of dissecting aortic aneurysms. N. Engl. J. Med., 286:115, 1972.
16. McKusick, V. A.: Cardiovascular aspects of Marfan's syndrome: A heritable disorder of connective tissue. Circulation, 11:321, 1955.
17. Miller, D. C., Stinson, E. B., Oyer, P. E., Rossiter, S. J., Reitz, B. A., Griepp, R. B., and Shumway, N. E.: Operative treatment of aortic dissections. Experience with 125 patients over a sixteen-year period. J. Thorac. Cardiovasc. Surg., 78:365, 1979.
18. Morgagni, G. B.: De Sedibus et Causis Morborum per Anatomen Indagitis (Venetiis, 1761): The Seats and Causes of Disease Investigated by Anatomy, Vol. 1. Translated by Alexander, A. London, A. Miller, and T. Cadele, 1769, pp. 802–808.
19. Palmer, R. F., and Lasseter, K. C.: Sodium nitroprusside. N. Engl. J. Med., 292:294, 1975.
20. Parker, F. B., Jr., Neville, J. F., Jr., Hanson, E. L., Mohiuddin, S., and Webb, W. R.: Management of acute aortic dissection. Ann. Thorac. Surg., 19:436, 1975.
21. Reul, G. J., Jr., Cooley, D. A., Hallman, G. L., Reddy, S. B., Kyger, E. R., and Wukasch, D. C.: Dissecting aneurysm of the descending aorta. Arch. Surg., 110:632, 1975.
22. Sorenson, H. R., and Olsen, H.: Ruptured and dissecting aneurysms of the aorta. Acta Chir. Scand., 128:644, 1964.
23. Warren, W. D., Beckwith, J., and Muller, W. H., Jr.: Problems in the surgical management of acute dissecting aneurysm of the aorta. Ann. Surg., 144:530, 1956.
24. Wheat, M. W., Jr.: Treatment of dissecting aneurysms of the aorta. Ann. Thorac. Surg., 12:582, 1971.
25. Wheat, M. W., Jr., Harris, P. D., Malm, M. R., Kaiser, G., Bowman, F. O., Jr., and Palmer, R. F.: Acute dissecting aneurysms of the aorta. J. Thorac. Cardiovasc. Surg., 58:344, 1969.
26. Wheat, M. W., Jr., Palmer, R. F., Bartley, T. D., and Seelman, R. C.: Treatment of dissecting aneurysm of the aorta without surgery. J. Thorac. Cardiovasc. Surg., 50:364, 1965.
27. Wolfe, W. G.: Acute ascending aortic dissection. Ann. Surg., 192:658, 1980.
28. Wolfe, W. G., and Moran, J. F.: The evolution of medical and surgical management of acute aortic dissection. Circulation, 56:503, 1977.
29. Wolfe, W. G., Kleinman, L. H., Wechsler, A. S., and Sabiston, D. C., Jr.: Heparin-coated shunts for lesions of the descending thoracic aorta. Arch. Surg., 112:1481, 1977.
30. Wolfe, W. G., Oldham, H. N., Rankin, J. S., and Moran, J. F.: Surgical treatment of acute ascending aortic dissection. Ann. Surg., 197:738, 1983.

stem bronchus, or lung tissue. Specifically, aneurysms in the ascending aorta may produce aortic insufficiency leading to cardiac failure and angina.

Diagnosis

Although aortic aneurysms may be diagnosed on the plain chest film, the specific location of the aneurysm and the structures involved must be located using aortography. Computed tomography and now magnetic resonance imaging can be helpful in making specific anatomic diagnoses. Aortic aneurysms may also be detected by echocardiography and standard cardiac catheterization. In general, aortography including the entire thoracic aorta is the diagnostic procedure of choice in individuals with thoracic aortic aneurysms.

Prognosis

The natural history of abdominal aortic aneurysms was well described by Estes.[18] One study indicated the seriousness of thoracic aortic aneurysms and the risk of rupture in this group of patients.[4] Consequently, a much more aggressive approach is taken toward thoracic aortic aneurysms with resection and grafting of the aneurysms always being recommended unless there are extenuating circumstances that make the risk of operation prohibitive. Rupture is the most common cause of death in these patients. Documented enlargement of an aneurysm is a clear indication for operation. MacDonald and colleagues believe that aneurysms of the ascending aorta over 5 cm. should be managed surgically even if they are asymptomatic.[25] Although the age of the patient and other clinical information must be evaluated before recommending an operation, the presence of an aneurysm and knowledge of the natural history (i.e., rupture and death) demand that strong consideration be given to resection in almost every case.

ASCENDING AORTIC ANEURYSMS

Aneurysms of the ascending aorta are almost always degenerative with a high incidence of medial necrosis or myxomatous degeneration being present. The process may include the aortic root, the anulus, and the aortic leaflets. The diagnosis of ascending aortic aneurysms is suggested by prominence of the ascending aorta on the chest film and by the finding of a murmur of aortic insufficiency. Again, aortography is used to confirm the diagnosis. Treatment is basically resection and grafting of the ascending aorta with the other involved structures being managed separately or at the same time, as in the Bentall operation described later.

Aneurysms involving the sinus of Valsalva often rupture into one of the chambers of the heart (Fig. 1). Aneurysms originating from the right coronary sinus are common and may follow endocarditis, but in the Oriental race there is evidence that this aneurysm may be congenital and that infectious processes are secondary.[26,29] Right coronary sinus aneurysms may be asymptomatic until they rupture into the mediastinum or into a cardiac chamber, most frequently the right ventricle or the right atrium. Aneurysms of the left coronary sinus are relatively uncommon.

Anuloaortic ectasia is another common condition of the ascending aorta and can be seen with Marfan's disease (Fig. 2). Anuloaortic ectasia involves dilation of both the sinuses and the anulus of the aorta, usually often accompanied by aortic insufficiency. Therapy in this case is resection and grafting of the aneurysm, replacement of the aortic valve, and reimplantation of the coronary arteries.[19] This operation is named the Bentall procedure after the article by Bentall and DeBono in 1968 describing the technique for replacement of the ascending aorta and valve with a composite graft.[3]

Using homografts and cardiopulmonary bypass, Cooley, DeBakey, and Bahnson developed the early techniques for resection of ascending aortic aneurysms. By 1958, synthetic grafts

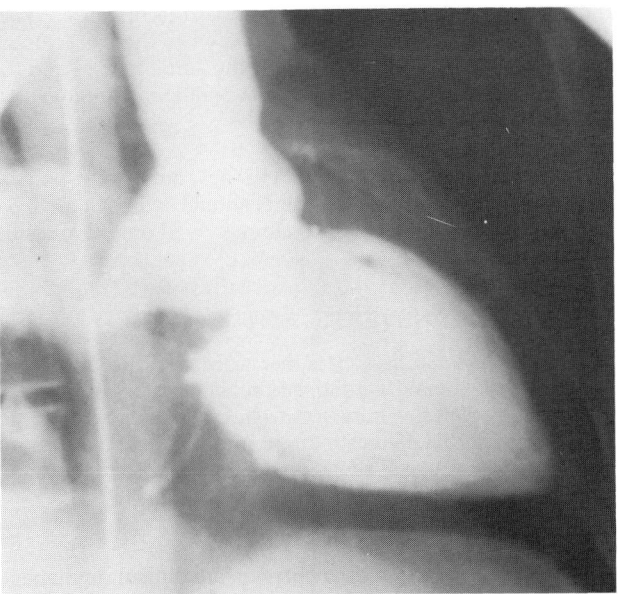

Figure 1. Aortogram demonstrates a sinus of Valsalva aneurysm and fistula that enters into the right atrium via the atrial septum. The lesion is repaired by approaching through both an aortotomy and an atriotomy.

were used for most aortic operations.[29] Development of prosthetic heart valves in the early 1960s was a major advance in managing the valvular component of aneurysms in the ascending aorta. Currently, woven Dacron grafts are used, in the ascending aorta, arch, or descending thoracic aorta. Recently, frozen homografts have been used as in the Bentall operation. The frozen homograft may be the graft of choice in mycotic aneurysms in which the etiology is related to infectious complications.

Technical Points

Aneurysms of the ascending aorta with or without aortic ectasia are managed using cardiopulmonary bypass and resection

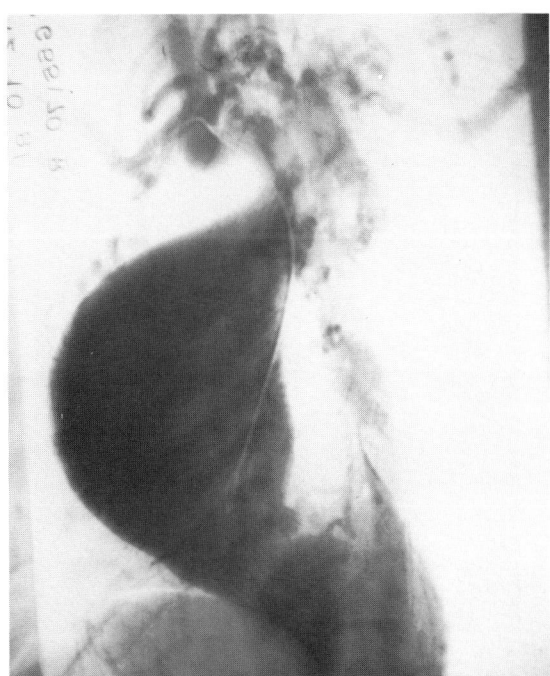

Figure 2. A large ascending aortic aneurysm with 4+ aortic insufficiency. Repair here is with the use of a composite graft with aortic valve replacement, reimplantation of the coronaries, and grafting of the ascending aorta, a Bentall operation.

and grafting of the aneurysms as standard techniques. Hypothermic circulatory arrest may be added when the aorta close to the innominate artery is involved. If the aortic sinuses and the aortic valve are involved, the Bentall operation is employed.[3,22]

Results

The results of surgical treatment of these aneurysms are generally excellent. Mortality in general should be less than 10 per cent, and serious complications are rare.[22,26] Long-term results have been excellent.

TRANSVERSE AORTIC ARCH

The transverse aortic arch is that segment of the aorta from which the innominate, carotid, and subclavian vessels arise. As mentioned earlier, these aneurysms have a tendency to rupture into the pericardial mediastinum or into the pleural space and can compress airways, the pulmonary artery, and the great veins. The diagnosis is made with aortography (Fig. 3).

Treatment

Patients with aortic arch aneurysms are difficult to manage. In general, the operation is performed through a median sternotomy on cardiopulmonary bypass with deep hypothermic circulatory arrest.[9,11,12,14,20] and a rectal temperature of 12° to 16°C. The aneurysm is resected and the segment reconstructed usually with a Dacron graft, reinserting the brachiocephalic vessels usually as a button. When the arrest time is below 45 minutes, the incidence of central nervous system complications is less than 10 per cent. In some cases, selected perfusion of the cerebral vessels can be performed under cardiopulmonary by-

pass. In 1957, DeBakey and colleagues first successfully replaced an aneurysm involving the ascending and transverse arch with aortic homograft, using total cardiopulmonary bypass with innominate and left carotid artery perfusion.[16] Griepp and associates used cardiopulmonary bypass and total-body hypothermia with cerebral circulatory arrest to simplify the aortic reconstruction described.[20]

Results

Results of therapy of arch aneurysms in most series have a mortality of 10 to 15 per cent with significant neurologic complications occurring in another 10 per cent. Crawford and Crawford present one of the largest series and the best results in the management of this complex problem with an overall survival of approximately 90 per cent.[10]

DESCENDING THORACIC AORTA

The descending thoracic aorta is that segment of the aorta from the left subclavian artery to the diaphragm (Fig. 4). The etiology is most commonly atherosclerosis, and the incidence of aneurysm in this area is second only to that seen in the infrarenal abdominal aorta. Patients with untreated aneurysms of the descending thoracic aorta usually die from rupture into the pleural space.[4] Perhaps 80 per cent of these patients die within 5 years if untreated. Aneurysms of the descending thoracic aorta compress and erode adjacent structures including the spine, airway, lung, and esophagus. Patients may present with hoarseness, chest pain, cough, or hemoptysis as well as dysphagia. All of these symptoms represent late manifestations and serious complications of the aneurysm.

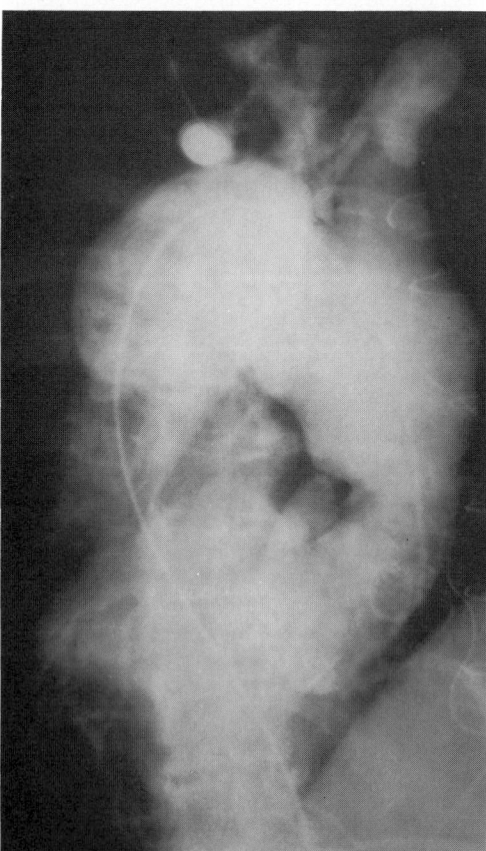

Figure 3. An aneurysm involving the aortic arch and extending down into the proximal descending thoracic aorta. The operation in this case is done through a left thoracotomy with cardiopulmonary bypass and profound hypothermia so that the graft can be placed in the arch and then down through the descending thoracic aorta.

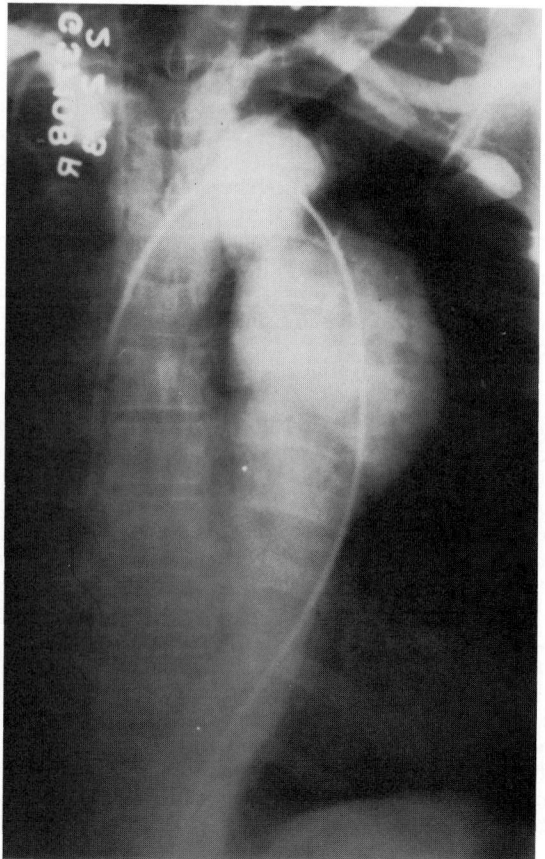

Figure 4. Aortogram demonstrates a standard descending thoracic aortic aneurysm originating below the subclavian artery. Approach is through a left thoracotomy with the use of a Dacron graft to replace the aneurysm segment.

Diagnosis

The diagnosis can be made by a plain chest film or computed tomographic scan. However, aortography is the best method of evaluating the entire aorta to demonstrate the extent of the disease and its relationship to the subclavian and arch vessels.

Treatment

The treatment is resection and grafting of the aneurysmal segment. The first successful segmental resection of the thoracic aorta was done by Alexander and Byron, who removed a segment involved with congenital coarctation and poststenotic aneurysm.[1] Shumacker[27] treated a similar case by end-to-end anastomosis in 1948, and Gross[21] and Swan[28] and their colleagues contributed to the management of these lesions using homografts to replace sections of the thoracic aorta. Lam and Arom[24] were the first to segmentally replace the descending thoracic aorta for acquired disease using a homograft to replace the syphilitic aneurysm of the descending thoracic aorta. Interestingly, an intraluminal shunt was used in this patient but partial paraplegia occurred and remains one of the most dreaded complications of operations on the thoracic aorta. In 1953, DeBakey and Cooley[15] successfully replaced a thoracic aortic aneurysm with an aortic homograft without using shunts or bypass.

Today these aneurysms are most commonly replaced with synthetic grafts made from woven Dacron. The patient may be operated on using partial femorofemoral bypass and a pump oxygenator with or without profound hypothermia (Crawford). Heparin-bonded shunts may be inserted to bypass the aneurysm from the ascending aorta, left ventricle, or subclavian artery to the distal circulation via the aorta or femoral artery. Finally, the Biomedicus pump can be used for left heart bypass from the left atrium to the distal aorta.[5] These techniques have been developed in an attempt to reduce complications of clamping of the descending thoracic aorta, such as left ventricular strain and renal or spinal cord ischemia. Although shunting methods and cardiopulmonary bypass improve cardiac hemodynamics and protect the viscera from ischemia (i.e., the gut and kidneys), no system completely prevents development of paraplegia with replacement of long segments of the thoracic aorta. Whereas aneurysms of the descending thoracic aorta in many instances are managed with clamping and supplemented vasodilation, the majority of surgeons continue to use some method of shunting with the belief that the incidence of paraplegia can be avoided.

Results

Aneurysms of the descending thoracic aorta can be treated with a mortality of less than 10 per cent and the incidence of paraplegia approximately 5 per cent.[14] The leading cause of death in operated patients is coronary artery disease, with renal insufficiency also being a serious postoperative complication. Lower limb neurologic disturbance (i.e., paraplegia) is still the most catastrophic complication involving surgical procedures on the thoracic aorta. Other complications include recurrent laryngeal nerve injury, bleeding, and infection. Long-term survival is excellent with the 5-year survival approaching 70 per cent.[10]

SELECTED REFERENCES

Crawford, E. S., and Crawford, J. L.: Diseases of the Aorta. Tracy, T. M. (Ed.). Baltimore, Williams & Wilkins, 1984.
This classic is the state-of-the-art atlas for the surgical treatment of aneurysmal aortic disease.

Crawford, E. S., Coselli, J. S., and Safi, H. J.: Partial cardiopulmonary bypass, hypothermic circulatory arrest, and posterolateral exposure for thoracic aortic aneurysm operation. J. Thorac. Cardiovasc. Surg. 94(6):824, 1987.
This article describes a unique and important technique in the management of arch and descending thoracic aortic aneurysms.

REFERENCES

1. Alexander, J., and Byron, F. X.: Aortectomy for thoracic aneurysm. Univ. Mich. Hosp. Bull., 9:101, 1943.
2. Bahnson, H. T.: Definitive treatment of saccular aneurysms of the aorta with excision of sac and aortic suture. Surg. Gynecol. Obstet., 96:383, 1953.
3. Bentall, H., and De Bono, A.: A technique for complete replacement of the ascending aorta. Thorax, 23:338, 1968.
4. Bickerstaff, L. K., Pairolero, P. C., Hollier, L. H., Melton, L. J., Van Peenen, H. J., Cherry, K. J., Joyce, J. W., and Lie, J. T.: Thoracic aortic aneurysms: A population-based study. Surgery, 92:1103, 1982.
5. Carlson, D. E., Karp, R. B., and Kouchoukos, N. T.: Surgical treatment of aneurysms of the descending thoracic aorta: An analysis of 85 patients. Ann. Thorac. Surg., 35:58, 1983.
6. Cooley, D. A., and DeBakey, M. E.: Resection of entire ascending aorta in fusiform aneurysm using cardiac bypass. J.A.M.A., 162:1158, 1956.
7. Cooley, D. A., and DeBakey, M. E.: Surgical considerations of intrathoracic aneurysms of the aorta and great vessels. Ann. Surg., 135:660, 1952.
8. Cooley, D. A., DeBakey, M. E., and Morris, G. C.: Controlled extracorporeal circulation in surgical treatment of aortic aneurysms. Ann. Surg., 146:473, 1957.
9. Cooley, D. A., Ott, D. A., Frazier, O. H., and Walker, W. E.: Surgical treatment of aneurysms of the transverse aortic arch: Experience with 25 patients using hypothermic techniques. Ann. Thorac. Surg., 32:260, 1981.
10. Crawford, E. S., and Crawford, J. L.: Diseases of the Aorta. Tracy, T. M. (Ed.). Baltimore, Williams & Wilkins, 1984.
11. Crawford, E. S., and Saleh, S. A.: Transverse aortic arch aneurysm: Improved results of treatment employing new modifications of aortic reconstruction and hypothermic cerebral circulatory arrest. Ann. Surg., 194:180, 1981.
12. Crawford, E. S., Saleh, S. A., and Schuessler, J. S.: Treatment of aneurysms of transverse aortic arch. J. Thorac. Cardiovasc. Surg., 78:383, 1979.
13. Crawford, E. S., Stowe, C. L., Crawford, J. L., Titus, J. L., and Weilbaecher, D. G.: Aortic arch aneurysm: A sentinel of extensive aortic disease requiring subtotal and total aortic replacement. Ann. Surg., 199:742, 1984.
14. Crawford, E. S., Walker, H. S. J., III, Saleh, S. A., and Normann, N. A.: Graft replacement of aneurysm in descending thoracic aorta: Results without bypass or shunting. Surgery, 89:73, 1981.
15. DeBakey, M. E., and Cooley, D. A.: Successful resection of aneurysm of thoracic aorta and replacement by graft. J.A.M.A., 152:673, 1953.
16. DeBakey, M. E., Crawford, E. S., Cooley, D. A., and Morris, G. C., Jr.: Successful resection of fusiform aneurysm of aortic arch with replacement by homograft. Surg. Gynecol. Obstet., 105:657, 1957.
17. Erdheim, J., Jr.: Medionecrosis aorte idiopathica apitca. Virchows Arch. Pathol. Anat., 276:187, 1930.
18. Estes, J. E., Jr.: Abdominal aortic aneurysm: A study of one hundred and two cases. Circulation, 2:258, 1950.
19. Gott, V. L., Pyeritz, R. E., Magovern, G. J., Jr., Cameron, D. E., and McKusick, V. A.: Surgical treatment of aneurysms of the ascending aorta in the Marfan syndrome. Results of composite-graft repair in 50 patients. N. Engl. J. Med., 314:1070, 1986.
20. Griepp, R. B., Stinson, E. B., Hollingsworth, J. F., and Buehler, D.: Prosthetic replacement of the aortic arch. J. Thorac. Cardiovasc. Surg., 70:1051, 1975.
21. Gross, R. E., Hurwitt, E. S., Bill, A. H., and Pierce, E. C.: Preliminary observation in the use of human arterial grafts in the treatment of certain cardiovascular defects. N. Engl. J. Med., 239:578, 1948.
22. Kouchoukos, N. T., Karp, R. B., Blackstone, E. H., Kirklin, J. W., Pacifico, A. D., and Zorn, G. L.: Replacement of the ascending aorta and aortic valve with a composite graft. Ann. Surg., 192:403, 1980.
23. Krause, A. H., Ferguson, T. B., and Weldon, C. S.: Thoracic aneurysmectomy utilizing the TDMAC-heparin shunt. Ann. Thorac. Surg., 14:123, 1972.
24. Lam, C. R., and Arom, H. H.: Resection of descending thoracic aorta for aneurysm: Report of use of homograft in case and experimental study. Ann. Surg., 134:743, 1951.
25. McDonald, G. R., Schaff, H. V., Pyeritz, R. E., McKusick, V. A., and Gott, V. L.: Surgical management of patients with the Marfan syndrome and dilatation of the ascending aorta. J. Thorac. Cardiovasc. Surg., 81:180, 1981.
26. Sakakibara, S., and Konno, S.: Congenital aneurysm of the sinus of Valsalva: Anatomy and classification. Am. Heart J., 63:405, 1962.
27. Shumacker, H. B., Jr.,: Coarctation and aneurysm of aorta: Report of case treatment by excision and end to end suture of aorta. Ann. Surg., 127:655, 1948.
28. Swan, H., Maaske, C., Johnson, M., and Grover, R.: Arterial homografts: Resection of thoracic aortic aneurysm using sternal human arterial transplant. Arch. Surg., 61:732, 1950.
29. Taguchi, K., Sasaki, N., Matsuura, Y., and Uemura, R.: Surgical correction of aneurysm of the sinus of Valsalva. A report of forty-five consecutive patients including eight with total replacement of the aortic valve. Am. J. Cardiol., 23:181, 1969.
30. Wolfe, W. G., Kleinman, L. H., Wechsler, A. S., and Sabiston, D. C., Jr.: Heparin-coated shunts for lesions of the descending thoracic aorta. Arch. Surg., 112:1481, 1977.

5. ANEURYSMS OF THE CAROTID ARTERY

Richard H. Dean, M.D.

Extracranial aneurysms of the carotid artery are extremely uncommon. Although the widespread use of cerebral arteriography probably has led to an increase in the discovery of carotid artery aneurysms over the last 25 years, McCollum and associates reported performing only 28 operations for carotid artery aneurysms among 8500 operations for aneurysms at all sites over a 21-year period.[8] Owing to the rarity of carotid aneurysms, details regarding their etiology, most common locations, natural history, presenting symptoms, and treatment cannot be discerned from any one surgeon's experience. Instead, collective reviews of reported cases are needed to provide those details.

The most frequent site of carotid artery aneurysms is the common carotid artery, particularly its bifurcation. The middle and distal portions of the internal carotid artery are the next most common sites. Aneurysms at the bifurcation are usually fusiform, whereas those located in the internal carotid artery are usually saccular. Atherosclerosis is responsible for 46 per cent to 70 per cent of all carotid artery aneurysms.[10] Trauma and previous carotid artery surgery are less common causes. Although syphilis was the most common cause 50 years ago, it is a rare cause today.

Natural History

Since most carotid artery aneurysms are identified because of the presence of symptoms, the true risk associated with the presence of an aneurysm is poorly defined. Nevertheless, it would appear that their natural history is generally unfavorable. In a 1937 collective review, Shipley and associates found a 71 per cent mortality among 41 patients treated expectantly.[11] That review demonstrated that aneurysms may present with rupture, cerebral embolization, thrombosis, or expansion onto adjacent structures with pressure symptoms. Zwolak and associates underscored the frequency of embolization in their review, which reported a stroke rate of 50 per cent for atherosclerotic aneurysms followed without operation.[14] In contrast, some small, posttraumatic, distal internal carotid artery aneurysms have been demonstrated to regress spontaneously. Therefore, therapy must be individualized, the major objective being prevention of the neurologic sequelae of the embolization of clot fragments from the aneurysm wall. Occasionally, progressive enlargement of the aneurysm may produce pressure on the vagus, the glossopharyngeus, the hypoglossus, or the sympathetic nerves in the region and thus cause dysfunction of any of these nerves.

Clinical Manifestations

The clinical presentation of carotid artery aneurysms varies according to their location and size. Distal internal carotid artery aneurysms may be completely hidden. In contrast, almost every common carotid artery and bifurcation aneurysm is first discovered as a pulsatile mass just below the angle of the mandible. Occasionally, an aneurysm may present as a pulsatile mass in the tonsillar fossa or oropharynx without external manifestation. With either presentation, the aneurysm may have associated symptoms of pain and tenderness or they may be completely asymptomatic. Distal internal carotid artery aneurysms may produce recurrent facial pain, fifth or sixth cranial nerve palsy, deafness, or even a Horner's syndrome when they compress adjacent structures at the base of the skull. Even Raeder's paratrigeminal syndrome, the combination of intermittent facial pain and oculosympathethic paresis, has been caused by aneurysms situated at the base of the skull.[7]

The most common serious risks associated with carotid artery aneurysms are transient ischemic attacks and stroke.[9] Most such central nervous system defects are caused by embolization of laminated thrombus lining the wall of the aneurysm. Less commonly, cerebral symptoms are caused by diminished flow through the carotid artery secondary to its compression by the mass of an adjacent saccular aneurysm.

Although common in reports during the late nineteenth and early twentieth centuries, rupture of carotid artery aneurysms is rare today. When rupture does occur, it is manifested by hemorrhage from the pharynx, ear, or nose and may lead to death by suffocation.

Differential Diagnosis

Elongation with kinking of the carotid artery is the most frequently found lesion masking as a carotid artery aneurysm. Usually, this lesion presents as a pulsatile mass at the base of the right side of the neck, typically in hypertensive elderly women. This mass is easily distinguished from an aneurysm by the fact that the pulsation is along the long axis of the vessel. A prominent carotid artery bifurcation in a patient with a thin neck, carotid body tumors, enlarged lymph nodes, branchial cleft cysts, or other masses that overlie and transmit the carotid pulse can be mistaken for an aneurysm. Usually, careful palpation discriminates between these entities and a true aneurysm of the carotid bifurcation.

Duplex sonography with B-mode imaging usually confirms or excludes the presence of an aneurysm of the extracranial carotid artery. Nevertheless, high internal carotid artery aneurysms cannot be diagnosed accurately by this method because of the limitations in visualizing that region. Computed tomography and magnetic resonance imaging are useful substitutes for B-mode imaging for the diagnosis of such lesions located high in the neck.[4]

Angiography remains the definitive diagnostic test on which to base therapy, even when the diagnosis has been established by one of the noninvasive methods. Visualization of the entire length of both extracranial and intracranial components of the carotid artery and the vertebrobasilar system is required for any treatment strategies to be adequate. Examples of saccular and fusiform aneurysms of the carotid artery are depicted in Figures 1 and 2.

Treatment

Sir Astley Cooper introduced the operative treatment of carotid artery aneurysms by ligating one such aneurysm in 1805.

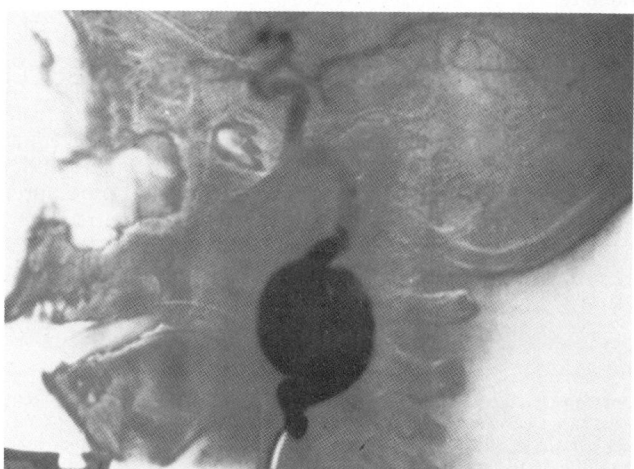

Figure 1. Carotid arteriogram showing typical appearance of an internal carotid artery aneurysm. (From Stoney, R. J., and Qvarfordt, P. G.: Accessible and inaccessible aneurysm of the extracranial carotid artery. *In* Moore, W. S. (Ed.). Surgery for Cerebrovascular Disease. New York, Churchill Livingstone, 1987, pp. 567–577.)

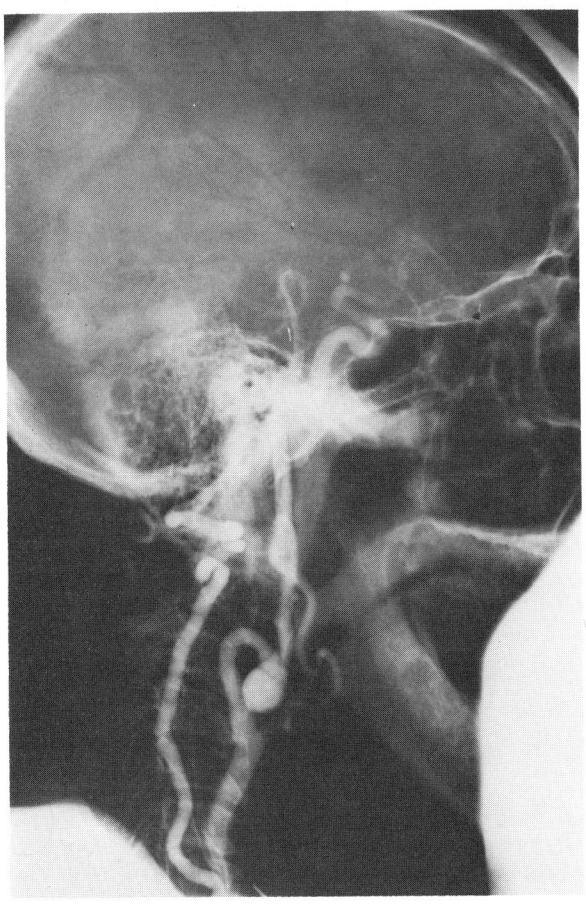

Figure 2. Carotid arteriogram showing distal internal carotid saccular aneurysm. (Courtesy of George Plum, M.D.)

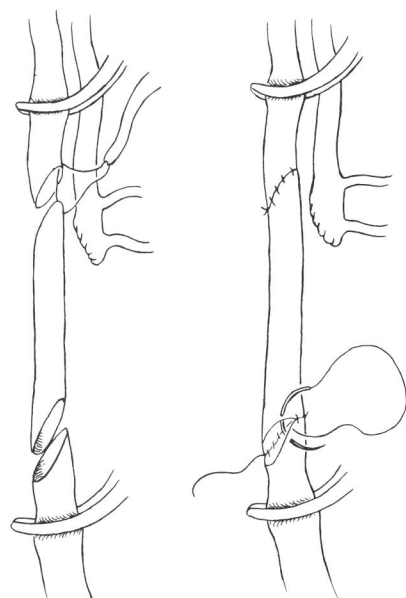

Figure 3. Drawings depicting technique of interposition grafting over a temporary shunt. (From Moore, W. S.: Reoperative carotid artery surgery. *In* Bergan, J. J., and Yao, J. S. T. (Eds.): Techniques in Arterial Surgery. Philadelphia, W. B. Saunders Company, 1990, pp. 206–213.)

Although that patient died in the immediate postoperative period, a second patient treated similarly in 1808 survived for 13 years.[1] Proximal ligation of the aneurysm remained the only treatment for the next 150 years, even though it was associated with a high rate of postoperative stroke and death. Even with that high morbidity and mortality, Winslow could report in 1926 that the 71 per cent death rate from observational management alone was reduced to 30 per cent following ligation of the aneurysm.[13]

Dimtza reported the first successful resection of an internal carotid artery aneurysm with reanastomosis.[3] Since most such aneurysms are associated with an elongated, tortuous vessel, this technique can be employed in about 50 per cent of patients. Most other aneurysms are now treated by resection and interpositional placement of either a saphenous vein graft or a polytetrafluoroethylene graft. Occasionally, saccular aneurysms can be treated by resection and lateral arteriorrhaphy or patch angioplasty.

The techniques for resection of the aneurysm and re-establishment of cerebral perfusion have been well described.[5,8,12,14] Through the use of electroencephalography, stump pressure measurements, or test clamping of the carotid artery using regional anesthesia, the need for temporary shunting can be identified. When a neurologic deficit is produced by test cross-clamping or electroencephalographic monitoring or when the distal stump pressure is lower than 50 mm. Hg, resection, reanastomosis, or graft interposition is performed over a temporary shunt (Fig. 3). Using these techniques of cerebral protection, as well as intraoperative heparin anticoagulation and modern anesthetic techniques, the operative mortality should be no higher than 1 per cent and permanent neurologic deficits should be less than 5 per cent.

Occasionally, resection of the aneurysm is impossible owing to its distal location at the base of the skull. In this instance, ligation of the internal carotid artery remains the only therapeutic option. If test clamping of the vessel is tolerated, ligation can be performed at a single stage. If cross-clamping cannot be tolerated, extracranial-to-intracranial bypass using a microvascular technique can provide improved collateral perfusion to allow ligation.[6] Gradual occlusion (over several days) using a Crutchfield clamp also continues to be useful.[2] With either technique, anticoagulation for 10 days to 2 weeks is necessary to reduce the frequency of propagation of the distal clot into the collateral cerebral circulation.

SELECTED REFERENCES

Hardin, C. A.: Surgical treatment of extracranial carotid aneurysms with excision and arterial restoration. Vasc. Surg., 7:247, 1973.
This is a detailed review of the literature with analysis of 64 cases of carotid aneurysm treated by excision and arterial restoration, with a breakdown showing the various methods of cerebral protection used during operation.

Goldstone, J.: Aneurysms of the extracranial carotid artery. *In* Rutherford, R. B. (Ed.): Vascular Surgery, 3rd ed. Philadelphia, W. B. Saunders Company, 1989, p. 1418.
This review of the literature provides a complete résumé of the causes, clinical presentation, differential diagnosis, and treatment of carotid artery aneurysms.

Zwolak, R. M., Whitehouse, W. M., Jr., Knake, J. E., Bernfeld, B. D., Zelenock, G. B., Cronenwett, J. L., Erlandson, E. E., Kazmers, A., Graham, L. M., Lindenauer, S. M., and Stanley, J. C.: Atherosclerotic extracranial carotid artery aneurysms. J. Vasc. Surg., 1:415, 1984.
This is an extensive review of the literature together with an analysis of a personal experience with 52 carotid aneurysms, 24 of which were atherosclerotic. Characteristics of this particular group are described in detail.

REFERENCES

1. Cooper, A.: Account of the first successful operation performed on the common carotid artery for aneurysm in the year 1808 with the postmortem examination in the year 1821. Guy's Hosp. Rep., 1:53, 1836.
2. Crutchfield, W. G.: Instructions for the use in the treatment of certain intracranial vascular lesions. J. Neurosurg., 16:471, 1959.
3. Dimtza, A.: Aneurysms of the carotid arteries. Report of two cases. Angiology, 7:218, 1956.
4. Duvall, E. R., Gupta, K. L., Vitek, J. J., Stanley, R. J., Luna, R. F., and Howieson, J.: CT demonstration of extracranial carotid artery aneurysms. J. Comput. Assist. Tomogr., 10:404, 1986.

5. Hardin, C. A.: Surgical treatment of extracranial carotid aneurysms with excision and arterial restoration. Vasc. Surg., 7:247, 1973.
6. Krupski, W. C., Effeney, D. J., and Ehrenfeld, W. K.: Fibromuscular dysplasia, aneurysms and spontaneous dissection of the carotid artery. In Bergan, J. J., and Yao, J. S. T. (Eds.): Cerebrovascular Insufficiency. New York, Grune & Stratton, 1983, p. 369.
7. Goldstone, J.: Aneurysms of the extracranial carotid artery. In Rutherford, R. B. (Ed.): Vascular Surgery, 3rd ed. Philadelphia, W. B. Saunders Company, 1989, p. 1418.
8. McCollum, C H., Wheeler, W. G., Noon, G. P., and DeBakey, M. E.: Aneurysms of the extracranial carotid artery. Twenty-one years' experience. Am. J. Surg., 137:196, 1979.
9. Rhodes, E. L., Stanley, J. C., Hoffman, G. L., Cronenwett, J. L., and Fry, W. J.: Aneurysms of extracranial carotid arteries. Arch. Surg., 111:339, 1976.
10. Rittenhouse, E. A., Radke, H. M., and Sumner, D. S.: Carotid artery aneurysm. Review of the literature and report of a case with rupture into the oropharynx. Arch. Surg., 105:786, 1972.
11. Shipley, A. M., Winslow, N., and Walker, W. W.: Aneurysm in the cervical portion of the internal carotid artery. An analytical study of the cases recorded in the literature between August 1, 1925 and July 31, 1936. Report of two new cases. Ann. Surg., 105:673, 1937.
12. Welling, R. E., Taha, A., Goel, T., Cranley, J., Krause, R., Hafner, C., and Tew, J.: Extracranial carotid artery aneurysms. Surgery, 93:319, 1983.
13. Winslow, N.: Extracranial aneurysm of the internal carotid artery. History and analysis of cases registered up to August 1, 1925. Arch. Surg., 13:689, 1926.
14. Zwolak, R. M., Whitehouse, W. M., Jr., Knake, J. E., et al.: Atherosclerotic extracranial carotid artery aneurysms. J. Vasc. Surg., 1:415, 1984.

6. CAROTID BODY TUMORS

Richard H. Dean, M.D.

The carotid body is derived from both mesoderm and elements of the third branchial arch and neural crest ectoderm. It is a pinkish-gray structure, 3 to 4 mm. in size, and located within the adventitial layer of the posteromedial aspect of the common carotid bifurcation. Only very rarely is it involved in the medial layer. Tumors arising from this body were termed chemodectomas originally, but they actually arise from paraganglionic cells and thereby should be classified as paragangliomas.

Normally, the cells of the carotid body sense changes in Po_2, Pco_2, and pH. In this regard, an unusually high incidence of carotid body tumors has been reported in individuals living at altitudes between 6900 and 14,000 feet, suggesting that chronic stimulation by chronic hypoxia may have a role in carotid body cell hyperplasia.[8]

The malignant potential of carotid body tumors is disputed, and reported figures range from 2.6 per cent to 50 per cent.[1,6,15,16] Standard pathologic criteria for malignancy do not correlate well with the biologic behavior of the tumor. The metastatic rate of these tumors is approximately 5 per cent.[9,15] Regional lymph nodes are the most common site of metastatic spread.

Epidemiologic studies suggest that two types of carotid body tumors are seen. The first is a randomly occurring sporadic type, which has a 5 per cent incidence of bilaterality.[11,15] The second has an autosomal dominant pattern of familial occurrence, which is less common and has a 32 per cent incidence of bilaterality.[7,14]

Clinical Presentation

Most commonly, a carotid body tumor presents as a painless, palpable mass over the carotid bifurcation region of the neck. Invasive and large benign tumors may produce associated hoarseness, dysphagia, stridor, or tongue weakness. Cranial nerve involvement has been estimated at 20 per cent; most frequently, the vagal and hypoglossal nerves are involved.[3] Although dizziness is frequently described by the patient, it is rarely associated with identifiable cerebral ischemia. Hypertension is found in about 6 per cent of patients[15] and has been associated with catecholamine secretion from the tumor in rare

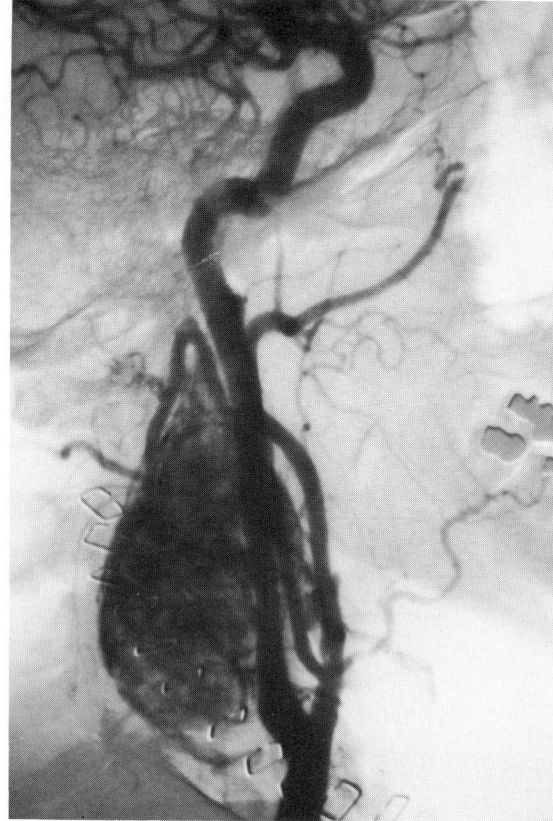

Figure 1. Characteristic arteriographic appearance of a carotid body tumor. Note the dramatic vascularity of the tumor. (From Hallett, J. W., Jr.: Carotid body tumor resection. In Bergan, J. J., and Yao, J. S. T. (Eds.): Techniques in Arterial Surgery. Philadelphia, W. B. Saunders Company, 1990.)

cases.[5] The differential diagnosis includes branchial cleft cyst, carotid artery aneurysm, enlarged lymph nodes, and metastatic tumor.

Diagnosis

The definitive study for diagnosis of carotid body tumors is selective bilateral cerebral arteriography. Characteristically, these tumors appear as a hypervascular oval mass widening the angle of the carotid bifurcation (Fig. 1). Although the location of the mass can be identified with computed tomography, arteriography additionally identifies the sources and extent of "nonbifurcation" blood supply. In addition, arteriography is required to define the presence and need for treatment of concomitant atherosclerotic disease of the carotid artery bifurcation.

Treatment

Current treatment of carotid body tumors is primarily operative, with excision of the tumor and maintenance of the integrity of carotid flow. The most important advancement in surgical therapy of these tumors has been recognition of and dissection along the subadventitial plane, which almost always allows complete removal of the tumor while maintaining carotid artery integrity (Fig. 2).

When there is deeper involvement of the carotid bifurcation wall or when combined endarterectomy of the carotid bifurcation is necessary, full-thickness excision of the base of the tumor with vein or synthetic patch closure of the defect facilitates the operation. Rarely, an interposition graft for replacement of the entire carotid bifurcation is necessary. When carotid artery cross-clamping is required, one should monitor cerebral function and be prepared to use an indwelling carotid shunt to maintain cerebral perfusion during the procedure.

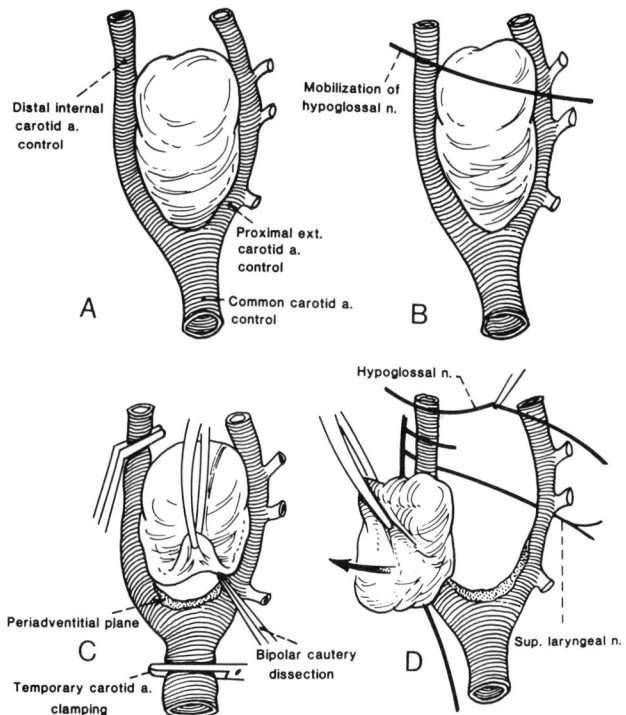

Figure 2. Artist's drawing of the technique of subadventitial resection of a carotid body tumor. (From Hallett, J. W., Jr., et al.: J. Vasc. Surg., 7:284, 1988, with permission from C. V. Mosby.)

When the tumor is very large, invasive, or malignant, the carotid artery may have to be sacrificed. If the artery is already occluded, this poses no hazard. If the artery is patent, carotid circulation may be restored by means of an arterial graft, using a shunt for cerebral protection. If no distal artery is available for anastomosis, attempts at resection should probably be abandoned unless the pressure in the carotid stump is higher than 65 mm. Hg, under which circumstance carotid ligation without reconstruction usually can be performed safely. For the rare tumor that is unresectable, radiation therapy may be of some value.[15,17]

Seldom should simple excision of the tumor be associated with cerebral morbidity or mortality. In 1962, Rush[13] reported a mortality of 1.5 per cent and a 2.9 per cent incidence of hemiplegia. In several more recently reported series, which included cases of carotid replacement, there was no associated mortality or cerebral morbidity.[2,4,10,12,17]

SELECTED REFERENCES

Connell, J.: Carotid body tumours. Aust. N.Z. J. Surg., 47:495, 1977.
  This article describes the details of the author's technique for simplified and safe removal of carotid body tumors, together with results of an extensive personal experience.

Hallett, J. W., Jr., Nora, J. D., Hollier, L. H., Cherry, K. J., Jr., and Pairolero, P. C.: Trends in neurovascular complications of surgical management for carotid body and cervical paragangliomas: A fifty-year experience with 153 tumors. J. Vasc. Surg., 7:284, 1988.
  This article summarizes 50 years of experience in surgical management of carotid body tumors. It provides an up-to-date consideration of the technical problems with resection of all varieties of these tumors.

Rush, B. F., Jr.: Current concepts in the treatment of carotid body tumors. Surgery, 52:679, 1962.
  This is a review of the subject up to 1962, with emphasis being placed on the natural history of untreated tumors and the mortality and morbidity associated with various types of surgical therapy.

Westbrook K. C., Guillamondegui, O. M., Medellin, H., and Jesse, R. H.: Chemodectomas of the neck. Selective management. Am. J. Surg., 124:760, 1972.
  This article clearly outlines signs and symptoms, the usefulness of angiography, indications for surgical therapy, and results of treatment in the authors' large series.

REFERENCES

1. Chambers, R. G., and Mahoney, W. D.: Carotid body tumors. Am J. Surg., 116:554, 1968.
2. Connell, J.: Carotid body tumours. Aust. N.Z. J. Surg., 47:495, 1977.
3. Davidge-Pitts, K. J., and Pantanowitz, D.: Carotid body tumors. Surg. Annu., 16:203, 1984.
4. Dent, T. L., Thompson, N. W., and Fry, W. J.: Carotid body tumors. Surgery, 80:365, 1976.
5. Fries, J. G., and Chamberlin, J. A.: Extra-adrenal pheochromocytoma: Literature review and report of a cervical pheochromocytoma. Surgery, 63:268, 1968.
6. Gaylis, H., and Mieny, C. J.: The incidence of malignancy in carotid body tumours. Br. J. Surg., 64:885, 1977.
7. Grufferman, S., Gillman, M. W., Pasternak, L. R., Peterson, C. L., and Young, W. G., Jr.: Familial carotid body tumors: Case report and epidemiologic review. Cancer, 46:2116, 1980.
8. High-altitude chemodectoma (editorial). Lancet, 1:1493, 1973.
9. Irons, G. B., Weiland, L. H., and Brown, W. L.: Paragangliomas of the neck: Clinical and pathologic analysis of 116 cases. Surg. Clin. North Am., 57:575, 1977.
10. Lees, C. D., Levine, H. L., Beven, E. G., and Tucker, H. M.: Tumors of the carotid body. Experience with 41 operative cases. Am. J. Surg., 142:362, 1981.
11. McIlrath, D. C., and ReMine, W. H.: Carotid-body tumors. Surg. Clin. North Am., 43:1135, 1963.
12. Morris, G. C., Jr., Balas, P. E., Cooley, D. A., Crawford, E. S., and DeBakey, M. E.: Surgical treatment of benign and malignant carotid body tumors. Clinical experience with sixteen tumors in twelve patients. Am. Surg., 29:429, 1963.
13. Rush, B. F., Jr.: Current concepts in the treatment of carotid body tumors. Surgery, 52:679, 1962.
14. Rush, B. F., Jr.: Familial bilateral carotid body tumors. Ann. Surg., 157:633, 1963.
15. Shamblin, W. R., ReMine, W. H., Sheps, S. G., and Harrison, E. G., Jr.: Carotid body tumor (chemodectoma). Clinicopathologic analysis of ninety cases. Am. J. Surg., 122:732, 1971.
16. Staats, E. F., Brown, R. L., and Smith, R. R.: Carotid body tumors, benign and malignant. Laryngoscope, 76:907, 1966.
17. Westbrook, K. C., Guillamondegui, O. M., Medellin, H., and Jesse, R. H.: Chemodectomas of the neck. Selective management. Am. J. Surg., 124:760, 1972.

7. SUBCLAVIAN ARTERY ANEURYSMS

David C. Sabiston, Jr., M.D.

Aneurysms of the subclavian artery are usually due to atherosclerosis, but trauma is also a cause. Poststenotic dilatation may cause an aneurysm in the thoracic outlet syndrome. If thrombosis is present, there may be subsequent emboli in the arteries of the arm and hand. The lesions may be either intrathoracic (often asymptomatic) or supraclavicular (presenting as a pulsating mass). In a series of 31 patients with subclavian-axillary aneurysms, the lesion was located on the right side in 20 patients and on the left in 10; 1 patient had bilateral aneurysms. It is interesting that mural thrombi were present in 25 of the 31 patients; and of these, 23 presented with upper extremity pain. Thromboembolism occurred in five of the patients, and two had rupture of the aneurysm, followed by one death. A pulsatile mass was palpable in 20, including 8 patients who were asymptomatic. The etiology was atherosclerosis in 12, trauma in 10, and poststenotic dilatation secondary to thoracic outlet obstruction in 6. At follow-up, there were no recurrences, and no further complications appeared.[8] Treatment consists of excision with restoration of arterial continuity, but occasionally tangential aneurysmorrhaphy may be appropriate. Rarely, ligation of the artery proximally and distally with excision of the aneurysm can be performed if there is sufficient collateral circulation. However, excision with restoration of arterial continuity is the most desirable operation. This condition is also presented in the section on the thoracic outlet syndrome, in which subclavian-axillary aneurysms are often seen.

For references, see page 1757.

8. VISCERAL ARTERIAL
ANEURYSMS

David C. Sabiston, Jr., M.D.

Visceral arterial aneurysms are more common than usually appreciated. Although these aneurysms may be asymptomatic, they can be catastrophic. The fact that the condition is not rare is emphasized in a series of 45 patients with splanchnic arterial aneurysms seen in one center during a 12-year period. The most important visceral arterial aneurysms are those of the splenic, celiac, hepatic, superior mesenteric, and renal arteries. Similar aneurysms have also been reported of the gastroduodenal, pancreaticoduodenal, and gastroepiploic arteries. Selective arteriography of the visceral circulation has greatly aided the diagnosis of aneurysms of these arteries (Figs. 1 and 2), and a number have been discovered by this means when it is being performed for other reasons.

Splenic Artery Aneurysms

Splenic aneurysms are the most common of the visceral arterial aneurysms and constitute about two thirds of all lesions in this group. In 1770, Beaussier[1] was the first to describe a splenic artery aneurysm, and since then many have been reported. They are most commonly found in females, and rupture of the aneurysm during *pregnancy* is a recognized complication. The most common cause is medial degeneration of the arterial wall, usually inducing a saccular aneurysm, which may contain calcium in the wall. Forty-five per cent of women with these aneurysms have had six or more pregnancies.[10] Splenic artery aneurysms may also be caused by fibromuscular dysplasia with involvement of the renal arteries. Atherosclerosis is also a cause of visceral aneurysms. Congenital aneurysms are rare and when present, usually multiple. Mycotic lesions usually follow sepsis, often with splenic emboli, after subacute bacterial endocarditis.

The clinical manifestations of splenic artery aneurysms vary considerably, and many patients are asymptomatic. The most common complaint is vague pain in the left upper quadrant with radiation to the left subscapular region. In expanding aneurysms, the symptoms may be more prominent and become acute with rupture. The diagnosis is most often made by the discovery of a calcified lesion on abdominal films and proof by arteriography (Fig. 3). Physical findings are uncommon, although rarely a tender, pulsatile mass can be palpated in the left upper quadrant.

The risk of rupture of splenic aneurysms is difficult to assess, but some reports stress a high likelihood.[7] Among 40 ruptured splenic artery aneurysms, 10 were fatal (25 per cent).[10] Operation should be recommended for most splenic artery aneurysms, especially during pregnancy, in view of the risk of rupture, because mortality is high (68 per cent in one group of 65 patients).[10] Other complications caused by splenic artery aneurysms include portal hypertension and rupture into the stomach.[4] The surgical procedure of choice is excision of the splenic artery with splenectomy or, if possible, preservation of the spleen.[4]

Celiac Artery Aneurysms

Celiac aneurysms are relatively uncommon and are arteriosclerotic, congenital, mycotic, or traumatic in origin. The clinical manifestations are primarily those of vague abdominal discomfort, most previously reported cases having been recognized at rupture. Excision of the aneurysms with restoration of continuity either directly or with an interposed graft is the treatment of choice. In one report of 14 cases managed surgically, 13 had a good result.[6]

Hepatic Artery Aneurysms

A hepatic artery aneurysm was first described by Wilson[13] in 1819, and the etiology includes arteriosclerosis, infection (mycotic), trauma, medial degeneration, and rarely periarteritis nodosa. The most prominent clinical manifestation is right upper quadrant or epigastric pain, frequently similar to gallbladder disease. Hematemesis or melena may follow erosion of the aneurysm into the gastrointestinal tract, as may fever and jaundice. Free rupture into the peritoneal cavity is the most serious complication, and only 5 survivors after this complication have been reported.[10]

When diagnosed, surgical extirpation is indicated. Most of these aneurysms are discovered incidentally at operation. Eighty per cent are extrahepatic and can be identified during abdominal operation, whereas 20 per cent lie within the liver and are not easily discovered.[12] The procedure of choice is excision of the aneurysm. If the aneurysm is located proximal to the gastroduodenal artery, the lesion may simply be excised with

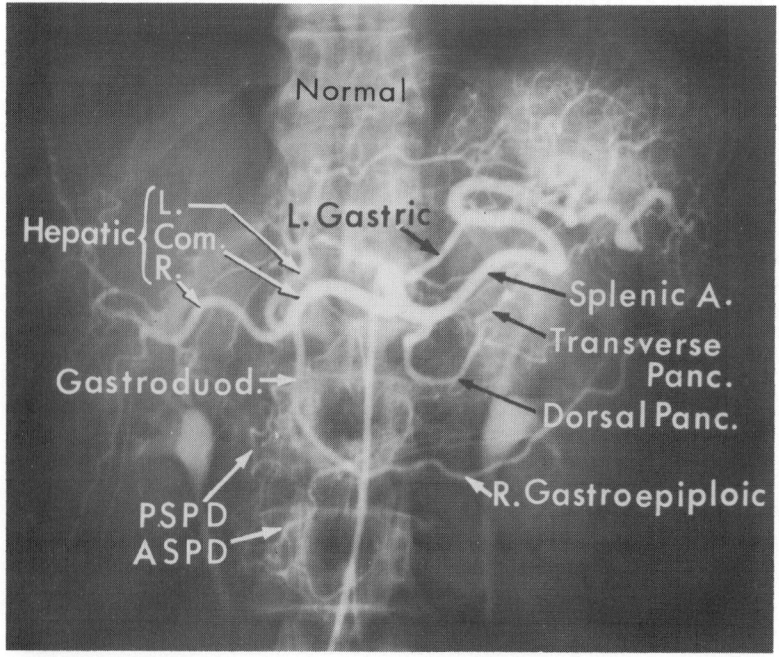

Figure 1. Selective injection of the celiac axis demonstrating normal anatomy. PSPD: posterior-superior pancreaticoduodenal artery; ASPD: anterior-superior pancreaticoduodenal artery. (Courtesy of Dr. Irwin Johnsrude.)

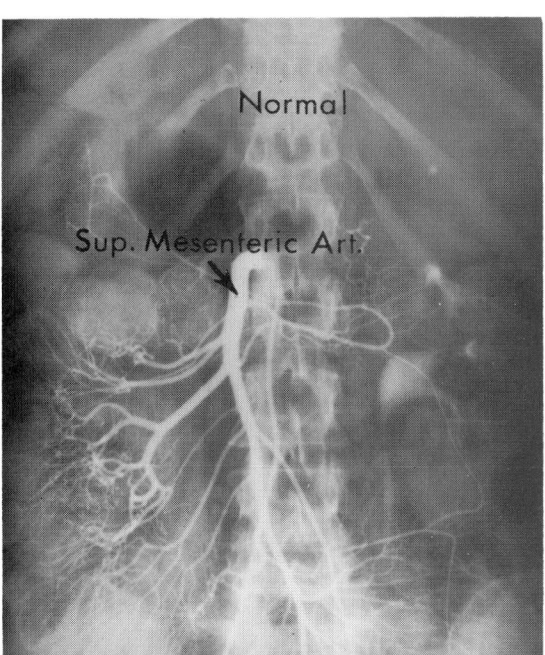

Figure 2. Selective injection of superior mesenteric artery demonstrating normal anatomy. (Courtesy of Dr. Irwin Johnsrude.)

distal ligation, because the collateral circulation through the gastroduodenal artery to the liver is excellent. If the aneurysm involves the hepatic artery distal to the gastroduodenal branch, preservation of arterial continuity to prevent liver necrosis is best managed by aneurysmorrhaphy or the use of a venous graft.

Gastroduodenal Artery Aneurysms

With the advent of wider use of arteriography, gastroduodenal arterial aneurysms are more frequently discovered. Acute pancreatitis may cause enzymatic destruction of the aneurysmal wall with rupture and ensuing hemorrhage.[5] It is usually preferable to excise these aneurysms when they are discovered.

Aneurysms of the Superior Mesenteric Artery

Superior mesenteric arterial aneurysms are often mycotic (57 in one series); atherosclerosis, trauma, and medial degeneration are other causes. In particular, this lesion should be suspected in patients with subacute bacterial endocarditis in whom abdominal pain develops in association with an expanding, tender mass. A high percentage of these lesions rupture. The first successful treatment was performed in 1949.[2] Since then, a number have been successfully managed by excision.[10]

Aneurysms of the Gastroduodenal and Pancreaticoduodenal Arteries

Aneurysms of the gastroduodenal and pancreaticoduodenal arteries are rare, aneurysms of the gastric and gastroepiploic arteries being more common. The majority present with rupture either into the peritoneal cavity or into the upper gastrointestinal tract, presenting with massive bleeding. Ligation of the aneurysm or partial gastric resection has been accomplished in some 30 per cent.

Aneurysms of the Renal Arteries

Although once considered rare, aneurysms of the renal arteries are being recognized with increasing frequency since the first description in 1770. These lesions constitute approximately 1 per cent of all aneurysms and occur most frequently in patients with hypertension. They are located in the main renal artery or the bifurcation of the primary branches in approximately 60 per cent (Fig. 4). Approximately 15 per cent of the aneurysms are intrarenal, and in about a quarter calcification is present in the wall. Most of the lesions are due to atherosclerosis or medial necrosis, and occurrence distal to a renal arterial stenosis is not uncommon. Saccular aneurysms are the most frequent, and the primary risk is rupture. The clinical manifestations include the symptoms of hypertension, especially headache. Less common are symptoms of upper abdominal and flank pain. A bruit may be present over the flank, and hematuria may also occur. A palpable mass is rare (in less than 10 per cent of cases). The diagnosis is made by arteriography.

The management of renal artery aneurysms includes careful demonstration of the size, type, and location of the aneurysm by arteriography. Rupture is an absolute indication for emergency operation. The majority, aneurysms without calcification, are

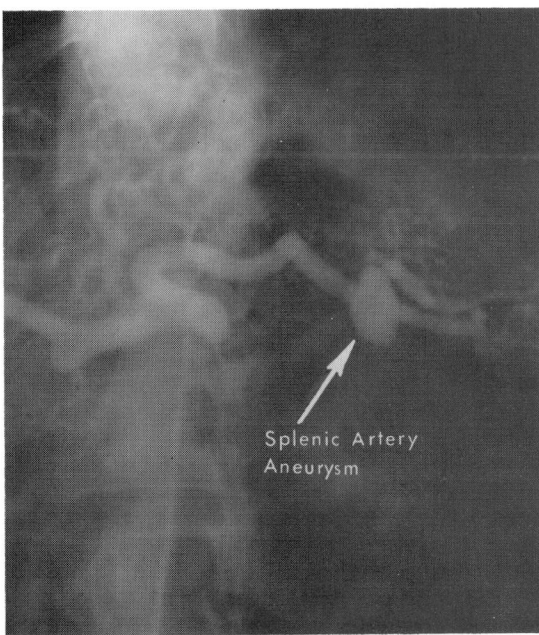

Figure 3. Splenic artery aneurysm demonstrated by selective arteriographic injection into the celiac axis. (Courtesy of Dr. Irwin Johnsrude.)

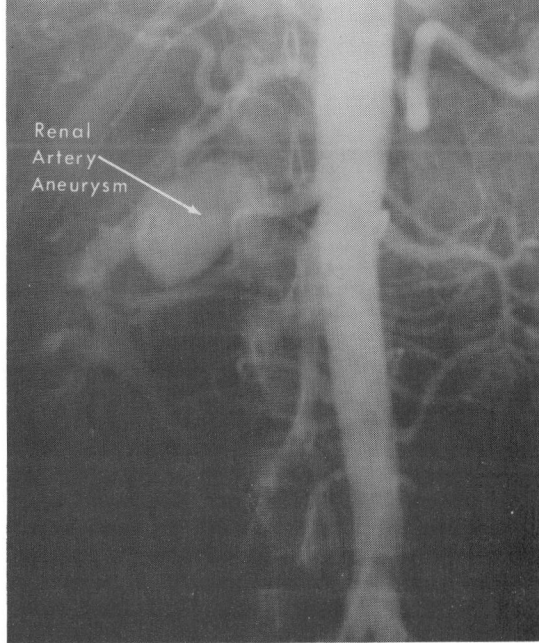

Figure 4. Aneurysm of the right renal artery. (Courtesy of Dr. Irwin Johnsrude.)

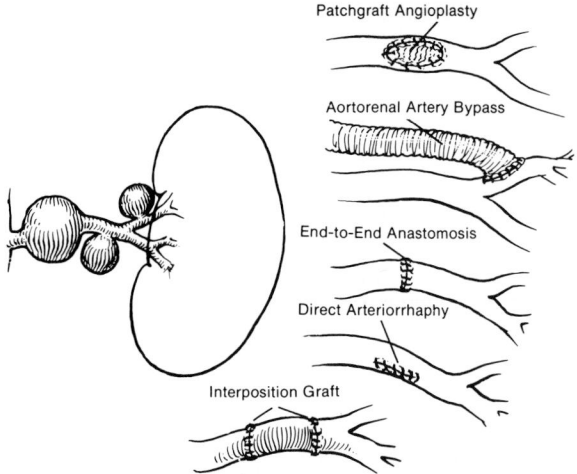

Figure 5. Surgical techniques employed in excision of renal artery aneurysms with preservation of the kidney. (From DeBakey, M. E., Lefrak, E. A., Garcia-Rinaldi, R., and Noon, G. P.: Aneurysm of the renal artery. Arch. Surg., *106*:438, 1973, with permission of authors and publisher.)

more prone to rupture. For those aneurysms that are calcified, opinion is divided concerning management, since they are less apt to rupture, but there is no doubt that they may. At present, the majority favor operation for these lesions, and it is usually possible to preserve the kidney. In a series of 72 patients, solitary aneurysms occurred in 53 and multiple lesions in 19. Arteriosclerotic changes were present in nearly 30 per cent, and fibrodysplasia was an associated finding in 27 of the 72 patients; 57 of the group were hypertensive. Two patients experienced frank aneurysmal rupture, and rupture occurred into the renal veins twice. Aneurysmectomy was performed in 31 of the 72 patients; and nephrectomy, either partial or total, was the procedure in 17. In this series, the authors recommended operation for most lesions 1.5 cm. in diameter or greater. It was also emphasized that in many instances renal artery stenosis is present, requiring correction for associated hypertension.[9] A renal artery aneurysm has also been removed successfully from a solitary kidney. In operative correction of these defects, emphasis is placed on a vascular reconstructive approach, making every effort to avoid nephrectomy (Fig. 5).[3] Among a series of 8525 patients undergoing renal angiography, 83 had renal artery aneurysms, of which 6 were bilateral and 11 multiple. Sixty-nine were not treated, and there were no deaths due to rupture of the aneurysm in a mean follow-up of 4 years. Fourteen patients underwent surgical correction.[11]

SELECTED REFERENCES

Stanley, J. C., Rhodes, E. L., Gewertz, B. L., Chang, C. Y., Walter, J. F., and Fry, W. J.: Renal artery aneurysms: Significance of macroaneurysms exclusive of dissections and fibrodysplastic mural dilations. Arch. Surg., *110*:1327, 1975.
In this review, the experience with 72 patients with renal artery aneurysms is presented. The majority of the patients were managed surgically, and the indications for operation and results are reviewed. This represents an unusually large series of patients from a single clinic.

Stanley, J. C., Thompson, N. W., and Fry, W. J.: Splanchnic artery aneurysms. Arch. Surg., *101*:698, 1970.
A very good review of splanchnic aneurysms. The natural history, diagnosis, management, and results are described.

REFERENCES

1. Beaussier, M.: Sur un aneurisme de l'artere splenique dont les parois se sont ossifiees. J. Med. Toulous., *32*:157, 1770.
2. DeBakey, M. E., and Cocley, D. A.: Successful resection of mycotic aneurysms of superior mesenteric artery: Case report and review of the literature. Am. Surg., *19*:202, 1953.
3. DeBakey, M. E., Lefrak, E. A., Garcia-Rinaldi, R., and Noon, G. P.: Aneurysm of the renal artery: A vascular approach. Arch. Surg., *106*:438, 1973.
4. de Vries, J. E. Schattenkerk, M. E., and Malt, R. A.: Complications of splenic artery aneurysm other than intraperitoneal rupture. Surgery, *91*:200, 1982.
5. Eckhauser, F. E., Stanley, J. C., Zelenock, G. B., Borlaza, G. S., Freier, D. T., and Lindenauer, S. M.: Gastroduodenal and pancreaticoduodenal artery aneurysms: Complication of pancreatitis causing spontaneous gastrointestinal hemorrhage. Surgery, *88*:335, 1980.
6. Haimovici, H. Sprayregen, S., Eckstein, P., and Veith, F. J.: Celiac artery aneurysmectomy: Case report with review of the literature. Surgery, *79*:592, 1976.
7. Owens, J. C., and Coffey, R. J.: Aneurysm of the splenic artery, including a report of six additional cases. Int. Abstr. Surg., *97*:313, 1953.
8. Pairolero, P. C., Walls, J. T., Payne, W. S., Hollier, L. H., and Fairbairn, J. F., II: Subclavian-axillary artery aneurysms. Surgery, *90*:757, 1981.
9. Stanley, J. C., Rhodes, E. L., Gewertz, B. L., Chang, C. Y., Walter, J. F., and Fry, W. J.: Renal artery aneurysms: Significance of macroaneurysms exclusive of dissections and fibrodysplastic mural dilations. Arch. Surg., *110*:1327, 1975.
10. Stanley, J. C., Thompson, N. W., and Fry, W. J.: Splanchnic artery aneurysms. Arch. Surg., *101*:689, 1970.
11. Tham, G., Ekelund, L., Herrlin, K., Lindstedt, E. L., Olin, T., and Bergentz, S-E.: Renal artery aneurysms: Natural history and prognosis. Ann. Surg., *197*:348, 1983.
12. Weaver, D. H., Fleming, R. J., and Barnes, W. A.: Aneurysm of the hepatic artery: The value of arteriography in surgical management. Surgery, *64*:891, 1968.
13. Wilson, J.: Lectures on the Blood, and on the Anatomy, Physiology, and Surgical Pathology of the Vascular System of the Human Body. Read before the Royal College of Surgeons, London, 1819.

9. AORTIC ABDOMINAL ANEURYSMS

David C. Sabiston, Jr., M.D.

One of the most common and most dangerous of arterial aneurysms is that encountered in the abdominal aorta. Although recognized for many years, it was not until 1951 that the first aortic abdominal aneurysm was successfully resected by Dubost and replaced with an aortic homograft.[10] Aortic abdominal aneurysms have since been resected with an appreciable extension of life.

Pathologic Aspects

More than 95 per cent of abdominal aortic aneurysms are due to atherosclerosis. Rarely trauma, syphilis, mycotic infection, or Marfan's syndrome may be responsible. The majority of the atherosclerotic aneurysms occur in the sixth and seventh decades. *Inflammatory* aneurysms have also been noted to have distinctive clinical and physical characteristics that separate them from typical atherosclerotic aneurysms. They appear to occur in 7 to 10 per cent of patients undergoing aneurysmectomy. In one series of 19 patients with this problem, 63 per cent were symptomatic, and all exhibited dense periaortic inflammation. Adjacent structures most frequently involved were the duodenum, left renal vein, and ureter.[27]

Natural History

The natural history of untreated abdominal aortic aneurysms is of much practical significance, especially in discussing with the patient the course of the disorder in relation to therapy to delineate the role of surgical treatment. Prior to the advent of surgical therapy, Estes published a classic study of the natural history of abdominal aneurysms in 102 patients seen at the Mayo Clinic.[12] In this group, 64 patients died, and in 63 per cent death was due to rupture. Only 67 per cent of these patients survived 1 year, 49 per cent survived 3 years, and 19 per cent survived 4 years. Similar findings were reported by Schatz[30] and Klippel (Fig. 1).[20] In another study, emphasis was placed upon patients with *symptomatic* aortic abdominal aneurysms. Thirty per cent of these patients had died within 1 month after onset of symptoms, 74 per cent had died by 6 months, and 80 per cent had died at 1 year.[14] Thus, the survival in this group was found to be much lower than that in a group of patients in

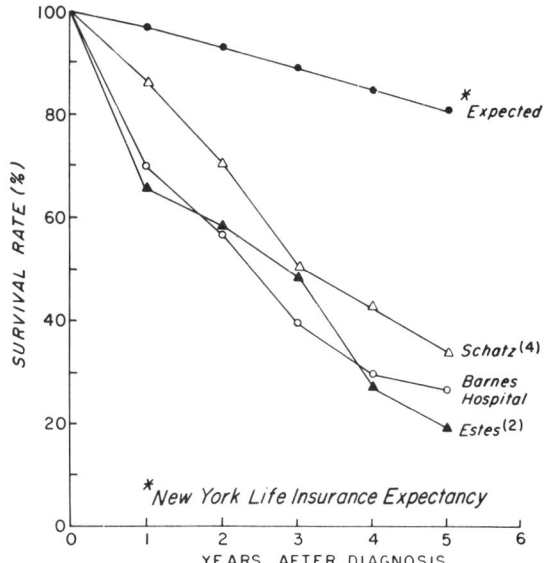

Figure 1. The natural history and survival rates among patients with *untreated* abdominal aortic aneurysms. (From Klippel, A. P., and Butcher, H. R., Jr.: The unoperated abdominal aortic aneurysm. Am. J. Surg., *111:*629, 1966.)

whom aneurysms were asymptomatic. In the group in whom rupture of the aneurysm did not occur, other causes of death included coronary, cerebral, and renal complications of atherosclerosis (Fig. 2). Hypertension was present in 47 per cent of the patients.

Clinical Manifestations

The majority of abdominal aortic aneurysms are discovered at the time of routine examination and are *asymptomatic.* In the remainder, abdominal symptoms range from vague discomfort in the epigastrium to excruciating pain. Severe pain in the flank or back suggests leakage or rupture of the aneurysm and is usually accompanied by signs of blood loss.

Physical examination shows the presence of a pulsating mass. The smallest aneurysms are approximately 4 cm. in diameter, but the size may range upward to 20 cm. or more, and they may be tender on palpation. Fortunately, more than 95 per cent of abdominal aortic aneurysms arise below the level of the renal arteries, the inferior mesenteric artery being the only important vessel arising from the aneurysm. Generally, the latter is either completely occluded or severely stenotic, in which case the development of a prominent collateral circulation via the distal branches of the inferior mesenteric artery is stimulated. A careful bilateral examination of the femoral, popliteal, dorsal pedal, and posterior tibial pulses should be done, particularly in reference to possible postoperative changes.

Diagnostic Studies

Plain films of the abdomen frequently show calcification in the wall of the aneurysm, often best observed in the lateral view (Fig. 3). The "eggshell" appearance is essentially diagnostic. The use of lateral films has also been helpful in those instances in which the calcification in the aortic aneurysmal wall is not clear on the AP abdominal films. Ultrasonography has become particularly useful and is a very simple, noninvasive technique that allows an accurate diagnosis and also provides information concerning the size and location of the aneurysm (Fig. 4). Moreover, it is quite helpful in following the progress of small aneurysms in patients who are not surgical candidates owing to specific medical contraindications.[22] Computed tomography is also valuable in the diagnosis and is a technique which allows delineation of the aortic lumen and intra-aneurysmal thrombus by the addition of contrast enhancement. It is helpful in following

the size of small aneurysms in patients not considered ideal surgical candidates (see Fig. 4).[15] Arteriography is a very useful method of objective diagnosis and in addition provides much accessory information of value (see Fig. 4). With modern techniques, this procedure has become quite safe, and it is probably wise to obtain an arteriogram in most patients with a suspected or actual diagnosis of aortic abdominal aneurysm, particularly those in whom operation is planned.[6] Important surgical findings include suprarenal extension of the aneurysm; demonstration of stenotic lesions in the renal arteries, superior mesenteric artery, or celiac axis; the presence of thrombus in the aneurysm; and patency of the inferior mesenteric artery.[6] Arteriography is also of aid in the patient with a pulsating abdominal mass in whom a neoplasm or cyst must be seriously considered in the differential diagnosis. Arteriography is essential for evaluation of the distal circulation in patients who have evidence of obstruction in the iliac, femoral, or popliteal arteries, because additional procedures may be required for these lesions.

Complications

The complications that may be associated with untreated aortic abdominal aneurysms are largely dependent upon the size of the aneurysm. In a collective survey, patients with aneurysms less than 7 cm. in diameter had a lower mortality from rupture (4 to 18 per cent), whereas in those with aneurysms greater than 7 cm. in diameter mortality was 72 to 83 per cent.[2] For these reasons, some believe that for asymptomatic aneurysms less than 7 cm. in diameter, observation without operation may be permissible. However, should symptoms appear, operation is indicated.

Although it is clear that rupture is the most frequent and serious complication of aortic abdominal aneurysms, there are additional hazards, including (1) distal embolization of the peripheral arterial system by thrombi originating in the aneurysm,[24] (2) sudden complete thrombosis,[19] (3) infection, particularly with gram-negative organisms and staphylococci,[18] (4) chronic consumption coagulopathy,[34] (5) aortic-intestinal fistula,[23] and (6) the development of an arteriovenous fistula from erosion of the aortic abdominal aneurysm into the inferior vena cava.[26] In this situation, hematuria frequently occurs and may be a sign of this complication.[5] Congestive heart failure may appear and require emergent operation.

Cholelithiasis can be present concomitantly with an aortic abdominal aneurysm; in one series of 865 patients, 42 (5 per cent) had this combination.[28] Although in that series simultaneous aneurysmectomy and cholecystectomy were advised provided no contraindications existed, this nevertheless remains a controversial subject and most surgeons prefer to perform aortic aneurysmectomy without an additional procedure that could potentially introduce infection into the graft. Of the 18 patients with gallstones in that series, 11 had aneurysmectomy without cholecystectomy and 13 had cholecystectomy only. For those in whom the gallbladder was removed at the time of aneurysmectomy, there was one instance of prosthetic

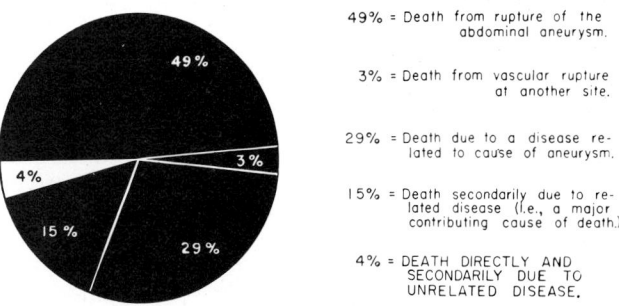

49% = Death from rupture of the abdominal aneurysm.

3% = Death from vascular rupture at another site.

29% = Death due to a disease related to cause of aneurysm.

15% = Death secondarily due to related disease (i.e., a major contributing cause of death.)

4% = DEATH DIRECTLY AND SECONDARILY DUE TO UNRELATED DISEASE.

Figure 2. Cause of death in 68 patients with an untreated abdominal aneurysm. (From Gliedman, M. L., Ayers, W. B., and Vestal, B. L.: Aneurysms of the abdominal aorta and its branches. Ann. Surg., *146:*207, 1957.)

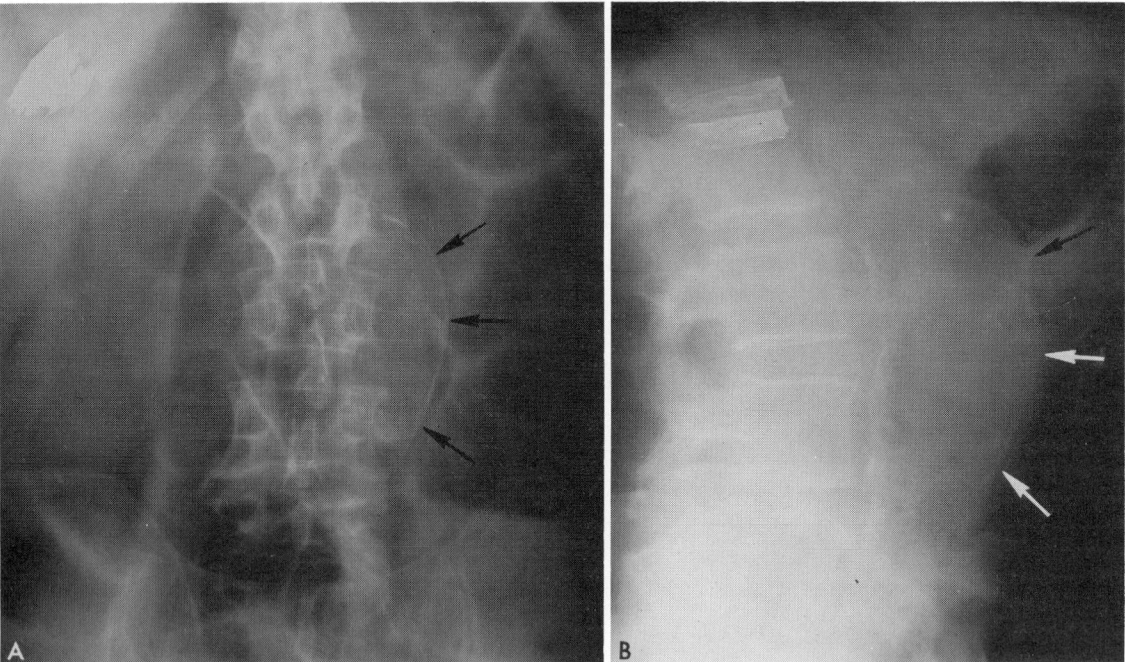

Figure 3. *A*, Plain film of abdomen of a patient with an abdominal aortic aneurysm. Note the calcium in the wall of the aneurysm outlining its border ("eggshell"). *B*, Lateral film showing calcified wall of the aneurysm.

infection that occurred in a patient in whom the graft was not retroperitonealized prior to cholecystectomy; this patient also had drainage of the liver bed and a gastrostomy. It was interesting that of the 11 patients who underwent aneurysmectomy only, 9 subsequently experienced an episode of acute cholecystitis in the mean follow-up period of 2.9 years. Two patients had acute cholecystitis in the immediate postoperative period, 1 of whom died of biliary sepsis. It is difficult to be certain whether or not a combined procedure should be recommended, and the issue remains controversial.

Treatment

Most abdominal aortic aneurysms should be managed by excision and restoration of arterial continuity with a prosthetic graft. Rarely, as already mentioned, those with small aneurysms and those who are poor risks may be observed if asymptomatic. However, the majority of aneurysms should be excised.

OPERATIVE TECHNIQUE. Operation for excision of abdominal aortic aneurysm is best accomplished through a midline incision extending from the xiphoid process to the symphysis pubis, which provides excellent exposure. The abdominal aorta is mobilized proximally so that an arterial clamp can be placed across it for total occlusion (Fig. 5). Similarly, the iliac arteries are clamped below. The inferior mesenteric artery is ligated at its origin from the aneurysm and divided. The anterior portion of the aneurysmal sac, including any thrombus present, is then removed. Much of the aneurysmal sac is usually left in place to prevent unnecessary dissection and for use in wrapping around the prosthetic graft to separate it from the duodenum. The lumbar vessels entering the aneurysm are susceptible to retrograde bleeding, which is controlled with transfixion ligatures. A preclotted, straight prosthetic graft of woven Dacron is inserted, and a bifurcation graft is reserved for iliac arteries involved in the aneurysm (Fig. 6).[9] Prophylactic antibiotics are administered several hours preoperatively and for several days after operation. The results of operation have been highly gratifying.

Certain special features of the operative approach deserve emphasis. During the procedure, it is possible to dislodge thrombi from the aortic aneurysm, which may embolize distally

and cause arterial obstruction. Therefore, it is important to demonstrate good back-bleeding from both iliac arteries and to determine the presence of pulses in the femoral, popliteal, posterior tibial, and dorsal pedal arteries at the end of the procedure. Should discrepancy occur in postoperative pulses, compared with those present preoperatively, arterial embolectomy should be considered, by the Fogarty technique. Anomalies are also important and include the presence of a retroaortic left renal vein in approximately 5 per cent of patients. Therefore, the left renal vein should be identified routinely in its normal anterior position; if it is not present, care must be taken to prevent injury to it in gaining proximal control of the abdominal aorta. The inferior vena cava may be transposed and found to the left of the aorta. In some instances, there is a duplication of the inferior vena cava, which represents a persistent left inferior vena cava. The vena cava may cross the aorta in the region of the renal vessels and constitute a circumaortic renal collar.[4] If the latter is present, division of the left inferior vena cava provides adequate exposure. Although the inferior mesenteric artery can usually be ligated without concern, since its proximal portion is already occluded, in a small number of patients (1 to 2 per cent) serious ischemia of the sigmoid colon can result. Determination of inferior mesenteric arterial stump pressure has been advocated.[11] If ischemia of the colon develops, the inferior mesenteric artery should be anastomosed to the graft whenever possible. If this is not possible, the colon may be exteriorized (Mikulicz) with resection in several days after the wound has sealed to reduce the likelihood of infection of the graft with later closure of the colostomy. In one series, in 7 patients with ruptured aortic abdominal aneurysms who underwent aneurysmectomy, postoperative ischemic colitis developed. This emphasizes the high incidence of this complication in patients with rupture, and in this series 6 of the 7 patients died.[38] The cause is undoubtedly the prolonged hypotension which occurs with ruptured aneurysms prior to the time they are corrected. A fiberoptic colonoscopy is helpful in making the diagnosis as well as examination of the stool for occult blood. Patients with a horseshoe kidney associated with aortic abdominal aneurysm have been reported and present special operative problems.[3] Occasionally in patients with previous abdominal procedures who may have ex-

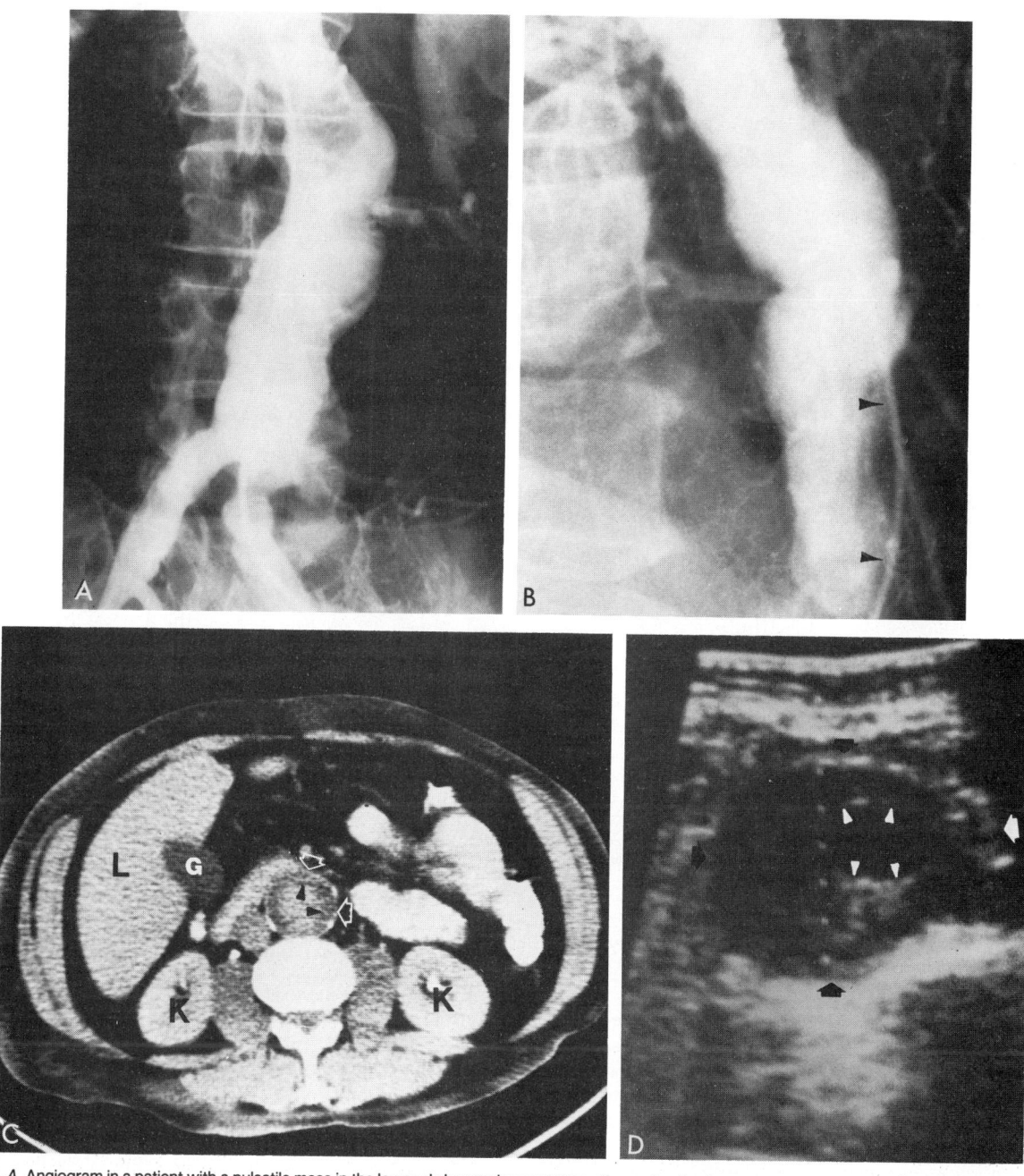

Figure 4. *A,* Angiogram in a patient with a pulsatile mass in the lower abdomen demonstrates atherosclerotic changes and mild aneurysmal dilatation of the abdominal aorta. There is some irregularity noted along the lumen of the common iliac arteries. The outer wall of the vessel is not demonstrated, as only the patent portion of the lumen can be opacified with this study. *B,* Cross-table lateral view demonstrates stretching of a peripheral vessel (arrowheads) by a mass in the vicinity of the common iliac artery. *C,* Computed tomographic scan in a patient with an abdominal aortic aneurysm following intravenous contrast injection demonstrates the opacified lumen of the aorta (arrowheads define the outer limit of the aortic lumen). The outside wall of the aorta (open arrows) is calcified. The space between the lumen (arrowheads) and the aortic wall (open arrows) represents a clot in the aorta. The scan also demonstrates the liver (L), gallbladder (G), and kidneys (K). *D,* Cross-sectional ultrasonogram through the right common iliac artery demonstrates the vessel to be markedly dilated (arrows indicate outside diameter of vessel) and the lumen to be filled with a considerable amount of clot around the patent central lumen (arrowheads indicate margin of patent lumen). The distance between arrowheads and arrows represents clot-filled lumen. This case illustrates both the ability of ultrasound to define the entire thickness of a vessel and its use in defining a clot within a vessel. Arteriography is limited to opacification of the patent vessel lumen.

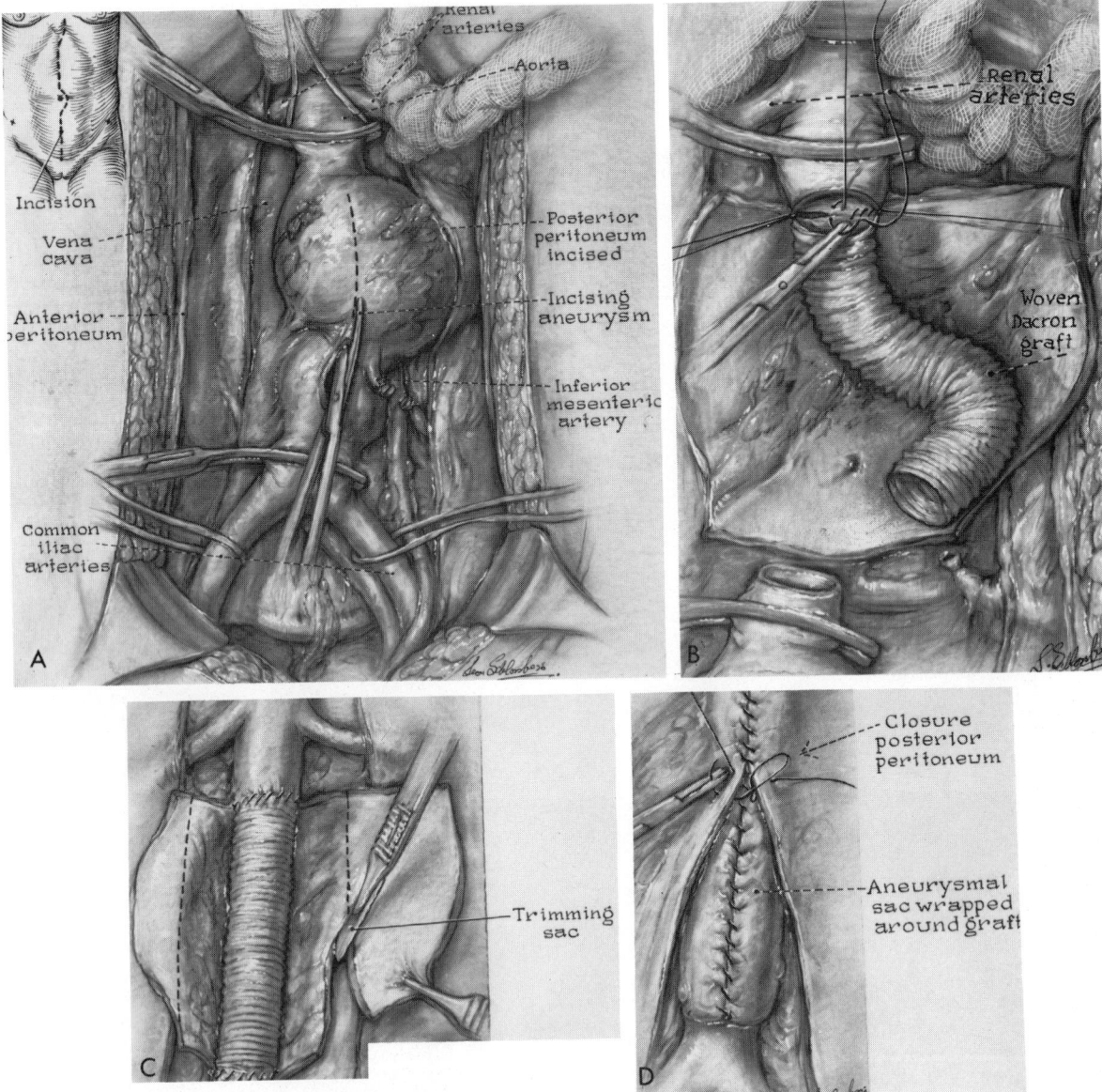

Figure 5. *A*, The retroperitoneal tissues are opened and the aneurysm exposed. A tape is passed proximally around the aneurysm just below the origin of the renal arteries. The inferior mesenteric artery, which is usually obliterated at its origin, is ligated and divided. Tapes are passed around both common iliac arteries distally. Vascular occlusion clamps are placed across the abdominal aorta just above the aneurysm and also just below it. The aneurysm is then incised. *B*, The thrombus in the aneurysm, if present, is removed, and the excess aneurysmal sac is trimmed away. A woven, preclotted Dacron graft is then inserted and sutured end-to-end. *C*, The graft is shown in place with closure of the remaining aneurysmal wall around it. *D*, The posterior peritoneum is then closed.

tensive adhesions, a retroperitoneal approach[32] can be utilized through the left flank. Some have emphasized that pulmonary complications, ileus, and pain are reduced with this approach (Fig. 7).[33]

Rarely, aortic aneurysms are extensive and involve the lower thoracic aorta; these thoracoabdominal aneurysms pose difficult problems in surgical treatment. The celiac axis, superior mesenteric artery, and renal arteries may arise from the aneurysm. Therefore, surgical correction requires extensive dissection and mobilization, with tedious restoration of blood flow to each of these critical vessels. By total resection of the aneurysm and stepwise insertion of appropriate grafts, these lesions can be successfully treated (Fig. 8).[8]

The transfusion of large amounts of stored blood may have deleterious effects owing to its increased affinity for oxygen, together with unknown effects of hemorrhage, which decreases the arterial oxygen concentration.[37] As a guide to the intraoperative replacement of fluid and blood, the preoperative insertion

of a Swan-Ganz catheter for continuous registration of pulmonary arterial pressures is helpful and is very frequently, if not routinely, used.[39] It is clearly recommended in patients with a history or suspicion of cardiac problems (Fig. 9).

In the patient presenting with a ruptured aortic abdominal aneurysm, an emergency operation should be undertaken immediately. The blood loss should be replaced rapidly; and as soon as the abdomen is entered, it is essential first to control the hemorrhage by proximal compression of the aorta. Large amounts of blood may be necessary in the resuscitation of these patients, and appropriate attention must be given the temperature of the infused blood as well as the administration of calcium. In those recovering from the immediate operative procedure, the effects of renal ischemia due to reduced perfusion associated with the low cardiac output state following rupture constitute the major cause of late death. Renal failure appearing postoperatively in these patients is usually associated with an unfavorable prognosis. However, aggressive management, in-

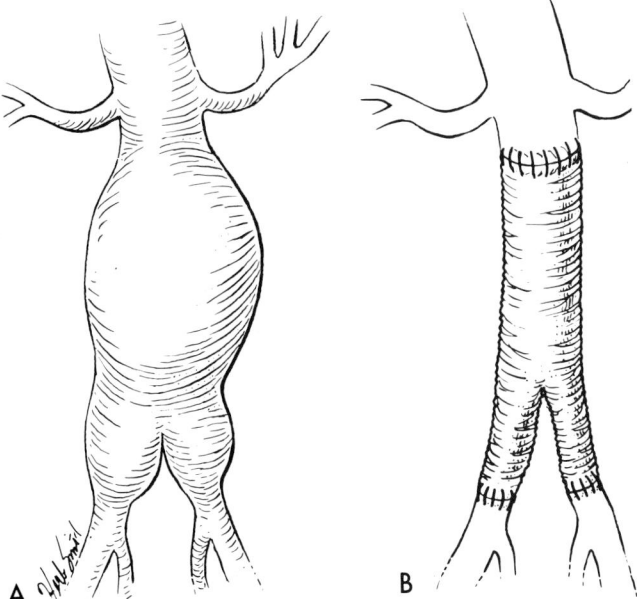

Figure 6. *A,* Characteristic type of arteriosclerotic aneurysm arising just below the renal arteries and involving both common iliac arteries. *B,* Treatment by resection and replacement with bifurcation Dacron graft. (From DeBakey, M. E., Crawford, E. S., Cooley, D. A., Morris, G. C., Jr., Royster, T. S., and Abbott, W. P.: Aneurysm of the abdominal aorta: Analysis of results of graft replacement therapy one to eleven years after operation. Ann. Surg., *160:*622, 1964.)

cluding the use of early hemodialysis, often necessary for a number of weeks, may reduce the mortality and allow ultimate recovery of renal function.[7] The results after ruptured aortic aneurysms have steadily improved, and lower mortality figures have resulted.[31] Myocardial infarction may also occur, precipitated by hypotension. The mortality varies between 30 to 50 per cent in operations for ruptured abdominal aortic aneurysms.[21]

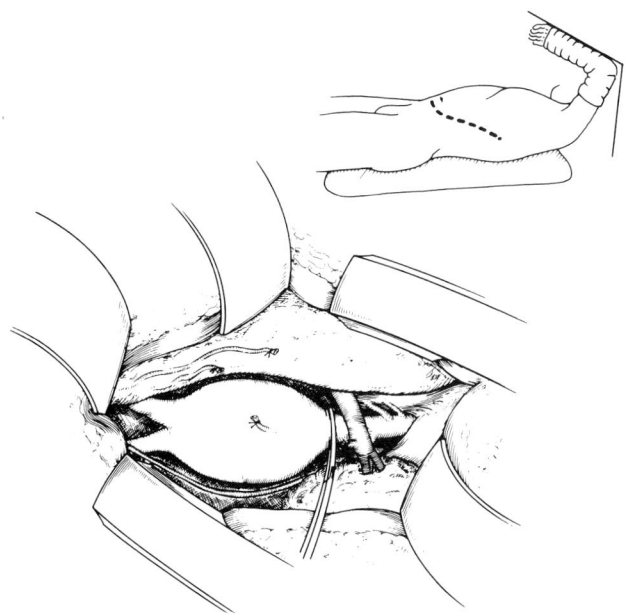

Figure 7. Retroperitoneal exposure of an infrarenal abdominal aortic aneurysm. Note that ligation of the gonadal vein and inferior mesenteric artery provides excellent access to the neck of the aneurysm as well as to the right common iliac artery. (From Sicard, G. A., Allen, B. T., Munn, J. S., and Anderson, C. B.: Retroperitoneal versus transperitoneal approach for repair of abdominal aortic aneurysms. Surg. Clin. North Am., *69:*795, 1989.)

Postoperative Complications

Aortic abdominal aneurysmectomy is recognized to be a major operative procedure, and a number of specific postoperative complications may occur. One of the most serious of these complications is acute myocardial infarction. Today every effort is made to prevent this problem, either by preoperative correction of the myocardial insufficiency or careful monitoring during the operative procedure. In a recent series of 246 patients with aortic abdominal aneurysms, severe surgically correctable coronary artery disease (CAD) was documented in 78 patients (32 per cent), and 70 underwent myocardial revascularization prior to aortic aneurysmectomy. The mortality for the CAD procedure was 5.7 per cent. The authors concluded that data support the conclusion of selected patients who require elective resection of aortic abdominal aneurysms also warrant myocardial revascularization to enhance perioperative risk and late survival.[17] Fortunately the majority of patients recover without significant problems and are often discharged from the hospital within a week. Abdominal distention, usually due to postoperative paralytic ileus, may occur and is usually self-limited. Although some routinely use a nasogastric tube for several days postoperatively, this has proved unnecessary, because at least three fourths of patients never require it. However, if distention occurs or if a distended stomach or bowel is demonstrated on physical examination or the abdominal film, insertion of a nasogastric tube is indicated for immediate decompression and removal or maintenance until the distention is relieved and peristalsis returns.

Bleeding from the graft may occur at the suture line or through the interstices of the graft. Continuous measurement of the abdominal girth postoperatively is useful, in addition to the usual measures for identification of reduced blood volume. Blood replacement may suffice if bleeding is minimal, but re-exploration should be performed if bleeding persists. Particular attention should be given the arterial circulation to the lower extremities, because emboli and thrombi may occur as a result of the operation or during the postoperative period.

Infection of the graft, especially at the suture lines, is a very serious complication[16] but, fortunately, is rare and occurs in 1 per cent or less in most series. Infection is particularly hazardous, because management is directed toward removal of the graft with occlusion of the terminal aorta by monofilament sutures or wire staples. Restoration of blood flow from an uninfected proximal area to the femoral vessels below, such as axillobifemoral grafting, is indicated (Fig. 10).[29] Unless a procedure of this magnitude is undertaken, ultimate massive hemorrhage from the infected anastomotic site usually follows. Thrombi in an abdominal aortic aneurysm are sometimes infected with various organisms, and in previous reports positive cultures have been found in 10 to 15 per cent. In one study, 14 per cent had positive cultures, but only rarely were specific antibiotics other than the routine prophylactic regimen given. There was no evidence of early or late prosthetic graft sepsis, and the conclusion was drawn that a positive result of culture may not imply clinical infection at the time of operation and that prolonged postoperative organism-specific antibiotic therapy does not appear necessary in patients who simply have a positive culture and no other clinical data to support the diagnosis of infection.[25]

Rupture of the proximal suture line of the anastomosis into the duodenum or intestine also occurs and presents an equally serious complication. Occasionally, chronic bleeding occurs in such a communication, allowing time for appropriate diagnosis and elective operation. In other instances, bleeding is sudden and massive, requiring emergency operation for control of the hemorrhage, closure of the duodenal or intestinal communication, and removal of the graft with appropriate reconstitution of blood flow through a noninfected area to the lower extremities.

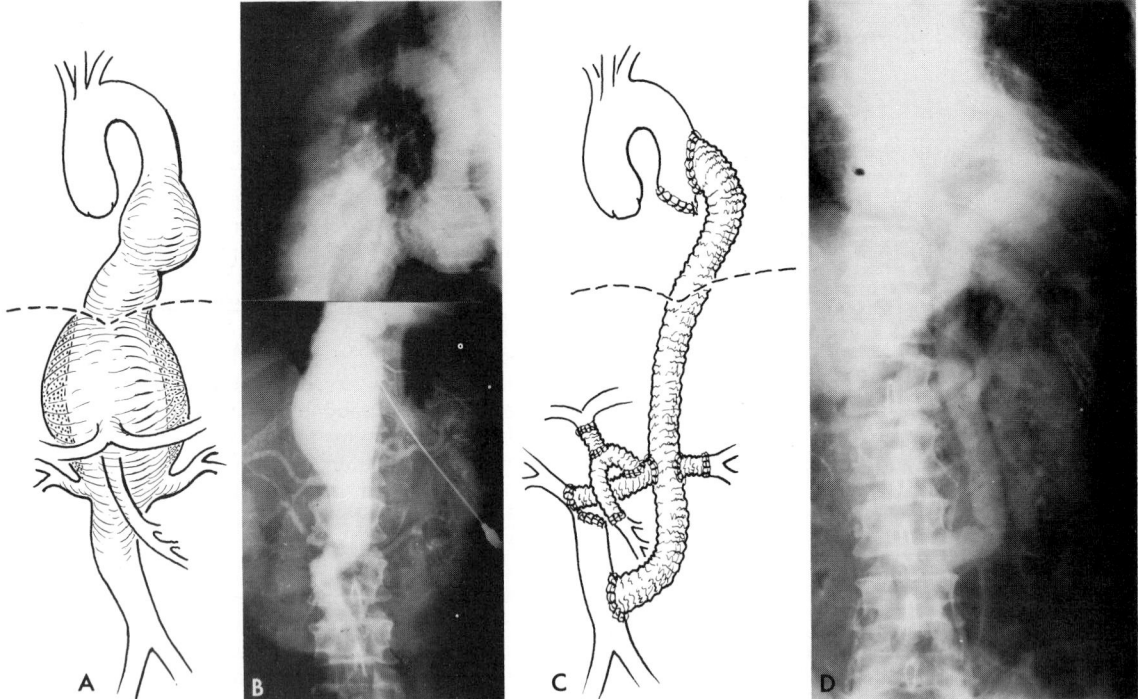

Figure 8. *A,* Drawing; and *B,* aortogram before operation, demonstrating arteriosclerotic thoracoabdominal aortic aneurysm in a 54-year-old male. *C,* Drawing illustrating method of resection and graft placement. *D,* Aortogram after operation, showing satisfactory function of graft replacements. Patient remains well 5 years after operation. (From DeBakey, M. E., Crawford, E. S., Garrett, H. E., Beall, A. C., Jr., and Howell, J. F.: Surgical considerations in the treatment of aneurysms of the thoraco-abdominal aorta. Ann. Surg., *162:*650, 1965.)

False aneurysms also occur at the suture lines and may become manifest by pain or a pulsatile mass. In such instances, an appropriate diagnosis can be established by arteriography, whereas in other instances the first sign of such an aneurysm may be rupture.

Changes in sexual function are of considerable importance after resection of abdominal aortic aneurysms, and retrograde ejaculation has been reported in as many as two thirds of patients.[36] Loss of potency also occurs in as many as a third of patients, and these complications appear to be related to the extensiveness of dissection of the enteric sympathetic plexus, which lies along the lower abdominal aorta on its left side and near the inferior mesenteric artery. If these are left undisturbed, interference with sexual function is minimized (Fig. 11).

Although infrequent, spinal ischemia may follow abdominal aortic surgery.[13] This complication appears to be somewhat more common in association with *ruptured* aortic abdominal aneurysms, perhaps aggravated by the associated hypotension. However, rupture is not a prerequisite, and the phenomenon occurs after elective operations. The classic anterior spinal artery syndrome is characterized by paraplegia, rectal and urinary incontinence, and loss of pain and temperature sensation below the lesion, but with sparing of vibration and proprioceptive sense. Patients sustaining neurologic deficits in the lower extremities after abdominal aortic procedures commonly have loss of posterior column modalities.

Results

Previously the mortality was appreciable,[2] but it has diminished in recent years and is now 5 per cent or less in most centers.[35] The mortality is primarily due to associated lesions of atherosclerosis that complicate the postoperative recovery, in-

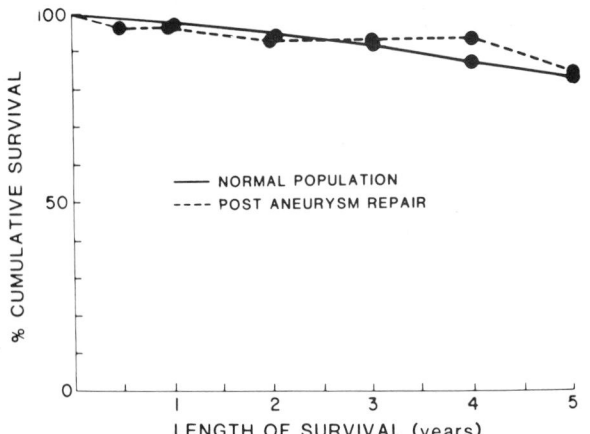

Figure 9. Five-year cumulative survival curve for 110 consecutive patients operated on for infrarenal abdominal aortic aneurysms compared with a similar curve for nonsurgical, age- and sex-adjusted populations derived from HEW life table statistics. The observed difference was not statistically significant (p = 0.157). (From Whittemore, A. D., Clowes, A. W., Hechtman, H. B., and Mannick, J. A.: Aortic aneurysm repair: Reduced operative mortality associated with optimal cardiac performance. Ann. Surg., *192:*414, 1980.)

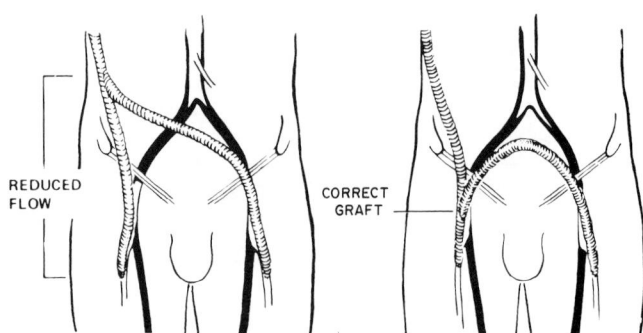

Figure 10. Optimal configuration of contralateral limb. *Left,* Diagrammatic representation of incorrect "bifurcation" limb to contralateral artery, which subjects the distal portion of main limb to a sudden drop in flow. *Right,* Correct axillobilateral femoral bypass configuration, allowing the main limb to have the benefit of higher flow throughout the entire length. (From Ray, L. I., et al.: Axillofemoral bypass: A critical reappraisal of its role in the management of aortoiliac occlusive disease. Am. J. Surg., *138:*117, 1979.)

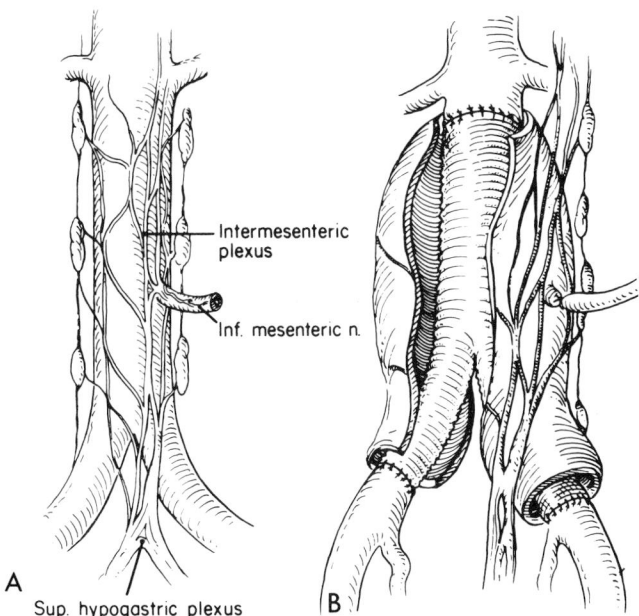

Figure 11. *A,* Normal sympathetic anatomy of distal abdominal aorta. *B,* Method of aortic aneurysmectomy preserving sympathetic plexi critical to normal sexual function. (From Weinstein, M. H., and Machleder, H. I.: Sexual function after aortoiliac surgery. Ann. Surg., *181:*787, 1975.)

cluding myocardial infarction, cerebrovascular lesions, and hypertensive cardiovascular renal disease. The long-term results of resection of abdominal aortic aneurysms were evaluated in a recent study. The 5-year survival was 72 per cent, and for those under age 70 at the time of operation, the 5-year survival probability was 79 per cent. These outstanding results were believed to be due to accomplishments following an aggressive policy of screening for and selectively treating coronary disease and carotid stenosis preoperatively and utilization of such intraoperative adjuncts as routine Swan-Ganz monitoring, autologous blood transfusion with the cell saver, and the frequent use of tube grafts.[1]

SELECTED REFERENCES

Crawford, E. S.: Thoraco-abdominal aortic aneurysms involving renal, superior mesenteric, and celiac arteries. Ann. Surg., *179:*763, 1974.
In this review, the management of 23 consecutive patients with thoracoabdominal aortic aneurysms, including those of renal, superior mesenteric, and celiac arteries, is presented. Emphasis is placed upon surgical technique, which depended upon the anatomic location of the aneurysm. A number of excellent illustrations are included and demonstrate the surgical procedures required. Of the 23 patients, 22 survived and did well for periods of up to 13 years, indicating the feasibility of the extensive operations required in the management of these lesions.

DeBakey, M. E., Crawford, E. S., Cooley, D. A., Morris, G. C., Jr., Royster, T. S., and Abbott, W. P.: Aneurysm of abdominal aorta: Analysis of results of graft replacement therapy one to eleven years after operation. Ann. Surg., *160:*622, 1964.
Long-term follow-up of the fate of patients with removal of abdominal aortic aneurysms is presented in this paper. The favorable prognosis following operation is emphasized.

Estes, J. E., Jr.: Abdominal aortic aneurysm: A study of one hundred and two cases. Circulation, 2:258, 1950.
This is an often quoted study of the follow-up of a large group of patients with aortic abdominal aneurysms prior to the advent of surgical treatment.

Pierce, G. E. (Guest Editor): Abdominal Aortic Aneurysms. Surg. Clin. North Am., 69(4), August 1989.
This is an updated review of the incidence, diagnosis, and management of abdominal aortic aneurysms. Considerable attention is given special preoperative, intraoperative, and postoperative complications. It is a valuable reference source for the entire field.

Thompson, J. E., Hollier, L. H., Patman, R. D., and Persson, A. V.: Surgical management of abdominal aortic aneurysms: Factors influencing mortality and morbidity: A 20-year experience. Ann. Surg., *181:*654, 1975.
The authors review a personal experience in a large group with aortic abdominal

aneurysms undergoing elective resection over a 20-year period. The mortality diminished from 17 per cent during the first 7 years of the study to 5.5 per cent in the 1968–1974 period. Reasons for the diminishing mortality are presented.

REFERENCES

1. Bernstein, E. F., Dilley, R. B., and Randolph, H. F. III: The improving long-term outlook for patients over 70 years of age with abdominal aortic aneurysms. Ann. Surg., 207:318, 1988.
2. Bernstein, E. F., Fisher, J. C., and Varco, R. L.: Is excision the optimum treatment for all abdominal aortic aneurysms. Surgery, 61:83, 1967.
3. Bietz, D., and Merendino, K. A.: Abdominal aortic aneurysm and horseshoe kidney. Ann. Surg., 181:333, 1975.
4. Brener, B. J., Darling, R. C., Frederick, P. L., and Linton, R. R.: Major venous anomalies complicating abdominal aortic surgery. Arch. Surg., 108:159, 1974.
5. Brewster, D. C., Ottinger, L. W., and Darling, R. C.: Hematuria as a sign of aortocaval fistula. Ann. Surg., 186:766, 1977.
6. Brewster, D. C., Retana, A., Waltman, A. C., and Darling, R. C.: Angiography in the management of aneurysms of the abdominal aorta: Its value and safety. N. Engl. J. Med., 292:822, 1975.
7. Chawla, S. K., Najafi, H., Ing, T. S., Dye, W. S., Javid, H., Hunter, J. A., Goldin, M. D., and Serry, C.: Acute renal failure complicating ruptured abdominal aortic aneurysm. Arch. Surg., 110:521, 1975.
8. Crawford, E. S.: Thoraco-abdominal and abdominal aortic aneurysms involving renal, superior mesenteric, and celiac arteries. Ann. Surg., 179:763, 1974.
9. DeBakey, M. E., Crawford, E. S., Cooley, D. A., Morris, G. C., Jr., Royster, T. S., and Abbott, W. P.: Aneurysm of the abdominal aorta: Analysis of results of graft replacement therapy one to eleven years after operation. Ann. Surg., 160:622, 1964.
10. Dubost, C., Allary, M., and Oeconomos, N.: Resection of an aneurysm of the abdominal aorta: Reestablishment of the continuity by a preserved human arterial graft, with results after five months. Arch. Surg., 64:405, 1952.
11. Ernst, C. B., Hagihara, P. F., Daugherty, M. E., and Griffen, W. O., Jr.: Inferior mesenteric artery stump pressure: A reliable index for safe IMA ligation during abdominal aortic aneurysmectomy. Ann. Surg., 187:641, 1978.
12. Estes, J. E., Jr.: Abdominal aortic aneurysm: A study of one hundred and two cases. Circulation, 2:258, 1950.
13. Ferguson, L. R. J., Bergan, J. J., Conn, J., Jr., and Yao, J. S. T.: Spinal ischemia following abdominal aortic surgery. Ann. Surg., 181:267, 1975.
14. Gliedman, M. L., Ayers, W. B., and Vestal, B. L.: Aneurysms of the abdominal aorta and its branches. A study of untreated patients. Ann. Surg., 146:207, 1957.
15. Gomes, M. N., Schellinger, D., and Hufnagel, C. A.: Abdominal aortic aneurysms: Diagnostic review and new technique. Ann. Thorac. Surg., 27:479, 1979.
16. Hardy, J. D., and Conn, J. H.: Infected arterial grafts. In Hardy, J. D. (Ed.): Critical Surgical Illness. Philadelphia, W. B. Saunders Company, 1971.
17. Hertzer, N. R., Young, J. R., Beven, E. G., O'Hara, P. J., Graor, R. A., Ruschhaupt, W. F., and Maljovec, L. C.: Late results of coronary bypass in patients with infrarenal aortic aneurysms. Ann. Surg., 205:360, 1987.
18. Jarrett, F., Darling, R. C., Mundth, E. D., and Austen, W. G.: Experience with infected aneurysms of the abdominal aorta. Arch. Surg., 110:1281, 1975.
19. Johnson, J. M., Gaspar, M. R., Movius, H. J., and Rosental, J. J.: Sudden complete thrombosis of aortic and iliac aneurysms. Arch. Surg., 108:792, 1974.
20. Klippel, A. P., and Butcher, H. R., Jr.: The unoperated abdominal aortic aneurysm. Am. J. Surg., 111:629, 1966.
21. Lawrence, M. S., Crosby, V. G., and Ehrenhaft, J. L.: Ruptured abdominal aortic aneurysm. Ann. Thorac. Surg., 2:159, 1966.
22. Leopold, G. R., Goldberger, L. E., and Bernstein, E. F.: Ultrasonic detection and evaluation of abdominal aortic aneurysms. Surgery, 72:939, 1972.
23. Levy, M. J., Todd, D. B., Lillehei, C. W., and Varco, R. L.: Aorticointestinal fistulas following surgery of the aorta. Surgery, 120:992, 1965.
24. Lord, J. W., Jr., Rossi, G., Daliana, M., Drago, J. R., and Schwartz, A. M.: Unsuspected abdominal aortic aneurysms as the cause of peripheral arterial occlusive disease. Ann. Surg., 177:767, 1973.
25. McAuley, C. E., Steed, D. L., and Webster, M. W.: Bacterial presence in aortic thrombus at elective aneurysm resection: Is it clinically significant? Am. J. Surg., 147:322, 1984.
26. Mohr, L. L., and Smith, L. L.: Arteriovenous fistula from rupture of abdominal aortic aneurysm. Arch. Surg., 110:806, 1975.
27. Moosa, H. H., Peitzman, A. B., Steed, D. L., Julian, T. B., Jarrett, F., and Webster, M. W.: Inflammatory aneurysms of the abdominal aorta. Arch. Surg., 124:673, 1989.
28. Ouriel, K., Ricotta, J. J., Adams, J. T., and DeWeese, J. A.: Management of cholelithiasis in patients with abdominal aortic aneurysm. Ann. Surg., 198:717, 1983.
29. Ray, L. I., O'Connor, J. B., Davis, C. C., Hall, D. G., Mansfield, P. B., Rittenhouse, E. A., Smith, J. C., Wood, S. G., and Sauvage, L. R.: Axillofemoral bypass: A critical reappraisal of its role in the management of aortoiliac occlusive disease. Am. J. Surg., 138:117, 1979.
30. Schatz, I. J., Fairbairn, J. F., II, and Juergens, J. L.: Abdominal aortic aneurysms: A reappraisal. Circulation, 26:200, 1962.
31. Schumacker, H. B., Jr., Barnes, D. L., and King, H.: Ruptured abdominal aortic aneurysms. Ann. Surg., 177:772, 1973.
32. Shepard, A. D., Scott, G. R., Mackey, W. C., O'Donnell, T. F., Jr., Bush, H. L.,

and Callow, A. D.: Retroperitoneal approach to high-risk abdominal aortic aneurysms. Arch. Surg., 121:444, 1986.

33. Sicard, G. A., Allen, B. T., Munn, J. S., and Anderson, C. B.: Retroperitoneal versus transperitoneal approach for repair of abdominal aortic aneurysms. Surg. Clin. North Am., 69:795, 1989.

34. Siebert, W. T., and Natelson, E. A.: Chronic consumption coagulopathy accompanying abdominal aortic aneurysm. Arch. Surg., 111:539, 1976.

35. Thompson, J. E., Hollier, L. H., Patman, R. D., and Persson, A. V.: Surgical management of abdominal aortic aneurysms: Factors influencing mortality and morbidity: A 20-year experience. Ann. Surg., 181:654, 1975.

36. Weinstein, M. H., and Machleder, H. I.: Sexual function after aortoiliac surgery. Ann. Surg., 181:787, 1975.

37. Weisel, R. D., Dennis, R. C., Manny, J., Mannick, J. A., Valeri, C. R., and Hechtman, H. B.: Adverse effects of transfusion therapy during abdominal aortic aneurysmectomy. Surgery, 83:682, 1978.

38. Welling, R. E., Roedersheimer, L. R., Arbaugh, J. J., and Cranley, J. J.: Ischemic colitis following repair of ruptured abdominal aortic aneurysm. Arch. Surg., 120:1368, 1985.

39. Whittemore, A. D., Clowes, A. W., Hechtman, H. B., and Mannick, J. A.: Aortic aneurysm repair: Reduced operative mortality associated with optimal cardiac performance. Ann. Surg., 191:414, 1980.

10. FEMORAL ARTERY ANEURYSMS

William J. Fry, M.D.

Artherosclerotic femoral artery aneurysms are uncommon and have been a problem in surgical care for many years. John Erichsen stated in his text *The Science and Art of Surgery*, published in 1877, "It occasionally, though rarely, happens that a varicose aneurysm is formed in the groin or upper part of the thigh." He further stated, "The treatment of this disease is exceedingly unsatisfactory. Of four cases in which the external iliac artery was tied, a fatal termination occurred in every instance." Bernheim, in his textbook *Surgery of the Vascular System*, published in 1913, reported 66 cases of femoral artery aneurysm with a recovery rate of 92 per cent. He used the method advocated by Halsted of gradual occlusion of the external iliac artery in an effort to stimulate collateral circulation. Using this technique, followed by endoaneurysmorrhaphy after the method of Matas, he was able to achieve a very satisfactory cure rate, with a 6.3 per cent incidence of amputation.

The most common etiologic factor in the development of femoral artery aneurysm is atherosclerosis. With the advent of peripheral vascular reconstructive surgical techniques, an increased incidence of false aneurysms associated with aortofemoral bypass has been seen. The incidence and etiologic factors, as well as the method of management, are well outlined by Szilagyi and associates. The third most common type of femoral artery aneurysm is that associated with trauma, secondary to either penetrating or blunt injury. The common sequela of trauma in the femoral area is disruption of the femoral artery. A high incidence of false aneurysm and arteriovenous fistula formation is seen after penetrating wounds of the groin. Bacterial aneurysms are increasing. These are, by and large, due to bacteria resistant to the usual antibiotics. In the past, they were almost always the result of *Salmonella* infection. Recently, bacterial aneurysms are being seen secondary to coagulase-positive *Staphylococcus* infections that are methicillin-resistant. Sepsis associated with femoral artery aneurysms has become more common and is related to the increase in the drug culture. Not only are these aneurysms difficult to treat, but the risks of associated acquired immune deficiency syndrome must be borne in mind. The infection may be so extensive and the patient so debilitated that ligation and debridement may be the therapy of choice.

False aneurysms of the femoral artery and its branches may occur after cardiac catheterization or angiography. These le-

sions if left unattended may pose a severe problem with distal embolization, occlusion of the femoral vein, or femoral nerve compression. They should be repaired as soon as the diagnosis is made. Duplex scanning can be very helpful in differentiating a false aneurysm from a hematoma.

The diagnosis of femoral artery aneurysm is usually self-evident on thorough physical examination. The palpation of a smooth, dilated femoral artery with expansile pulsations is, in most instances, sufficient to make the absolute diagnosis. In an occasional patient because of obesity, scar tissue formation, or heavy musculature, some doubt may be present after careful physical examination. In such instances, the use of ultrasound scanning is helpful in making the diagnosis and delineating the size of the femoral artery aneurysm.

Whenever a femoral artery aneurysm is suspected or diagnosed on physical examination, a complete arteriogram of the abdominal aorta and iliac, femoral, and tibial vessels should be obtained. It has been found that 85 per cent of patients with a femoral artery aneurysm have some other associated aneurysm within the arterial tree. The majority of these were associated aortoiliac artery aneurysms. Seventy-two per cent of atherosclerotic femoral artery aneurysms were found to be bilateral.

The natural history of untreated atherosclerotic femoral artery aneurysms is unknown. In bland femoral artery aneurysms, serious limb-threatening complications occur in only 3 per cent of the aneurysms that were followed an average of 52 months. Symptomatic aneurysms may occlude or embolize with resulting ischemia of the lower extremity. Spontaneous rupture of an atherosclerotic femoral artery aneurysm is a rare event. Because of the musculofascial compartment surrounding the common femoral artery, exsanguination is an unusual sequela. Tamponade usually occurs with marked ischemia of the distal portion of the involved extremity. Most femoral artery aneurysms are lined with laminated thrombus. The thrombus may lyse and portions may be carried distally, forming embolic occlusion in the popliteal or tibial vessels. Careful examination of the patient with a femoral artery aneurysm usually demonstrates the presence of multiple, small petechial hemorrhages in the distal portion of the extremity. These are secondary to microemboli from the interior of the aneurysmal sac.

Cutler and Darling classified femoral artery aneurysms, and this was further modified by Barker. The classification is shown in Table 1.

The techniques of reconstruction of the femoral artery after aneurysmectomy are shown in Figure 1. The preference, whenever possible, is to use autologous tissue, either artery or vein. When this is not possible because of previous vein stripping or marked disparity in size, the author does not hesitate to use a Dacron or polytetrafluoroethylene prosthesis. The disadvantages of using a Dacron prosthesis over a joint, with subsequent angulation, thrombus formation, and eventual occlusion, are well known. The author has not experienced problems in the reconstruction of femoral artery aneurysms, primarily because the prosthesis is usually very short and therefore not subject to

TABLE 1. Types of Femoral Artery Aneurysms

Type I	Terminating proximal to the orifice of the superficial and deep femoral arteries
Type II	Involving the superficial and deep femoral arteries
Type III	A. Femoral artery aneurysm with occlusion of the superficial femoral artery
	B. Femoral artery aneurysm with occlusion of the deep femoral artery
Type IV	Aneurysms of the deep femoral artery
Type V	Aneurysms of the superficial femoral artery

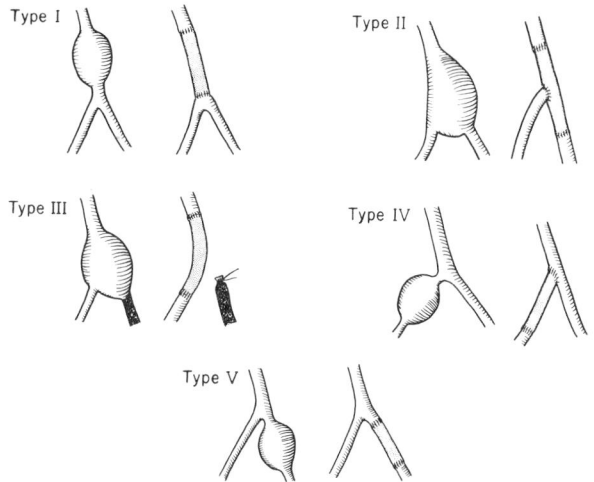

Figure 1. Methods of reconstruction of femoral artery aneurysms.

the buckling seen in longer prostheses. Another disadvantage to the use of a prosthesis in the groin is the hazard of infection. The skin over the groin is exceedingly difficult to clean, and the likelihood of bacterial contamination at the time of operation is always a hazard. Meticulous cleansing of the groin, utilizing a technique of shaving the skin immediately before the operation, combined with prophylactic antibiotics has made the incidence of graft infection relatively low (1.23 per cent). The difficulties with a cloth prosthesis in the area of the groin have led Stoney and associates to use a portion of autologous iliac artery with the substitution of the prosthesis replacing this within the abdomen. The author has not generally subscribed to this technique because it increases operative time, and with a relatively low incidence of graft infection, it has not been thought universally indicated.

The results of arterial reconstruction of the femoral artery are excellent with a mortality approaching zero. Cutler and Darling reported a series of 63 arteriosclerotic aneurysms treated surgically with a zero operative mortality. In addition, they demonstrated the superiority of vein graft replacement, which has a 100 per cent long-term patency rate, versus a 94 per cent patency rate using a Dacron prosthesis. The numbers, however, are so small that it is not statistically significant. A similar trend has been noted in a small series.

All patients, after repair of a femoral artery aneurysm, should be followed closely. This is particularly true in those patients who have a Dacron prosthesis. The incidence of false aneurysm formation at the suture line and secondary infection, although low, may be life- or limb-threatening if unrecognized for a long period of time. Because of the propensity of arterial aneurysms to develop at other sites, careful periodic examination is important.

REFERENCES

1. Barker, W. F.: Peripheral Arterial Disease. Philadelphia, W. B. Saunders Company, 1975.
2. Cutler, B. S., and Darling, R. C.: Surgical management of arteriosclerotic femoral aneurysms. Surgery, 74:764, 1973.
3. Dent, T. L., Lindenauer, S. M., Ernst, C. B., and Fry, W. J.: Multiple arteriosclerotic arterial aneurysms. Arch. Surg., 105:338, 1972.
4. Fry, W. J.: Vascular prosthesis infections. Surg. Clin. North Am., 52:1419, 1972.
5. Fry, W. J., and Lindenauer, S. M.: Infection complicating the use of plastic arterial implants. Arch. Surg., 94:600, 1967.
6. Stoney, R. J., and Wylie, E. J.: Arterial autografts. Surgery, 67:18, 1970.
7. Szilagyi, D. E., Smith, R. F., Elliott, J. P., Hageman, J. H., and Dall'Olmo, C. A.: Anastomotic aneurysms after vascular reconstruction: Problems of incidence, etiology and treatment. Surgery, 78:800, 1975.
8. Szilagyi, D. E., Smith, R. F., Elliott, J. P., and Vrandecic, M. P.: Infection in arterial reconstruction with synthetic grafts. Ann. Surg., 176:321, 1972.

11. POPLITEAL ARTERY ANEURYSMS

William J. Fry, M.D.

The treatment of popliteal aneurysms has been a challenge to skilled surgeons for more than 2000 years. The first recorded operation for popliteal aneurysm was by Antyllus, a Greek surgeon, in the second century. He ligated the popliteal artery proximal and distal to the aneurysm and incised and packed the aneurysmal sac. John Hunter, in 1785, ligated the superficial femoral artery in a coachman with a large popliteal artery aneurysm. The leg survived and the coachman returned to his occupation, only to succumb to pneumonia 4 months after the operative procedure. Desault, the French surgeon, preceded Hunter by 7 months in the performance of this operation. His operation was not based on the recognition of collateral circulation as was Hunter's. Limb salvage rates utilizing the hunterian principle were as high as 87 per cent. Rudolph Matas advocated endoaneurysmorrhaphy for the therapy of popliteal aneurysms. He first performed this operation in 1888 and in 1920 reported a series of 154 popliteal aneurysms treated by this technique. The operative mortality was 0.6 per cent, and the amputation rate was 5.2 per cent. The results represented a remarkable achievement in the days preceding arteriography, antibiotics, and adequate anesthesia.

Etiologic factors causing popliteal aneurysm formation are the same as those delineated in the section on femoral artery aneurysms. The majority of popliteal aneurysms seen today are secondary to atherosclerosis. The incidence of aneurysm secondary to bacterial invasion of the arterial wall is slightly higher in the popliteal area than it is in the femoral artery. As with infected femoral aneurysms, the methicillin-resistant *Staphylococcus* organism has an important role.

The diagnosis of a popliteal artery aneurysm is most commonly made by physical examination. The findings of an aneurysm in the popliteal space are sometimes subtle and may be overlooked by the inexperienced. Popliteal artery aneurysms seldom involve the distal popliteal artery. They more commonly present opposite the joint space. Physical findings may be masked in the heavily muscled lower extremity. Ultrasound scanning is a readily available, noninvasive diagnostic procedure that serves as a good screening technique for making the diagnosis of popliteal aneurysm when there is some question on physical examination.

Arteriography, as with femoral artery aneurysms, is mandatory. Popliteal aneurysms are bilateral in 47 per cent of patients. In addition, 78 per cent of patients with popliteal aneurysms have another aneurysm somewhere in the arterial tree. The majority, 64 per cent, are located in the abdominal aorta or iliac arteries. Popliteal artery aneurysms are often associated with distal occlusive disease (Fig. 1). The laminated thrombus within the wall of the aneurysm forms the nidus for distal embolization. Constant trauma secondary to motion of the knee joints adds to fragmentation of the intraluminal thrombus. Accurate arteriography to delineate the outflow tract is always necessary prior to any operative approach in the treatment of a popliteal artery aneurysm.

The most common sequela of the untreated popliteal artery aneurysm is distal arterial occlusion. Careful examination of the distal extremity in the patient with a popliteal artery aneurysm almost always reveals areas of petechial hemorrhage secondary to small emboli. As the laminated thrombus collection progresses with the aneurysmal sac, the following may occur: (1) extensive embolization, which may occlude the outflow tract; (2) laminated thrombus, which may occlude the orifices of the

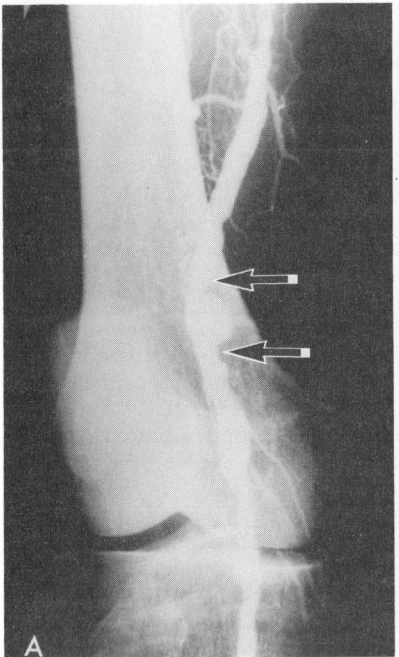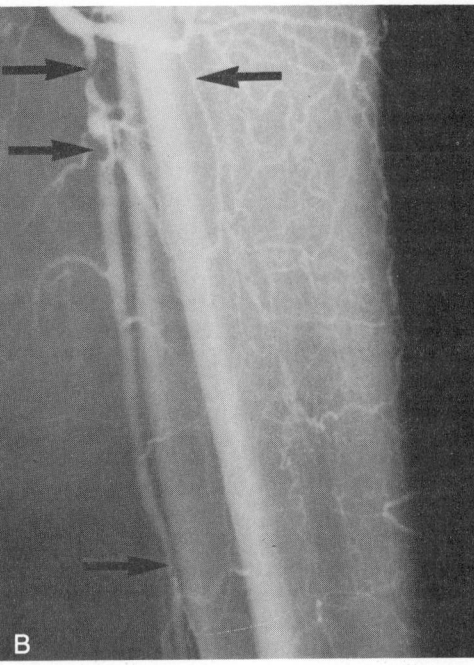

Figure 1. *A,* Arteriogram demonstrating laminated clot in the lumen of a popliteal aneurysm. *B,* Outflow arteriogram in patient shown in *A* shows multiple areas of distal occlusion secondary to embolization of laminated thrombus from popliteal aneurysm.

popliteal trifurcation; and (3) complete thrombosis of the aneurysm. These possibilities are limb-threatening, and the possibility of arterial reconstruction to maintain viability of the extremity may be compromised.

Popliteal aneurysm rupture is not a common occurrence. As with femoral artery aneurysms, the patient is not likely to exsanguinate because of the strong musculofascial compartment surrounding the popliteal artery. Rupture usually tamponades, and the resulting ischemia to the distal leg is severe. Attempts at arterial reconstruction after rupture are difficult as is the ability to restore viability. Large popliteal aneurysms may cause chronic or acute venous obstruction. Thrombophlebitis is not an uncommon finding with the acutely expanding popliteal artery aneurysm.

The author has used the medial approach to popliteal artery aneurysms as described by Szilagyi in 1959 (Fig. 2). The utilization of an autogenous saphenous vein is preferred. The arterial reconstruction used routinely in the management of popliteal aneurysms is depicted in Figure 3. It is important not to excise the popliteal artery aneurysm because damage to the popliteal vein invariably occurs. By trapping the aneurysms as illustrated

and utilizing a proximal and distal end-to-end anastomosis, the author has been able to restore blood flow with excellent long-term results.

The posterior approach has two disadvantages: the dissection required is much more extensive than in the medial approach, and there are marked limitations in the access of the superficial femoral artery and distal tibial vessels.

Experience in the therapy of popliteal aneurysms at the Cleveland Clinic reveals the continued preference for the use of autogenous saphenous vein as a replacement for the popliteal artery aneurysm. Their experience shows a continued lower failure rate with saphenous vein over either polytetrafluoroethylene or Dacron. Their long-term amputation rate with all forms of therapy was 6 per cent. The Cleveland experience emphasizes the danger of concomitant heart disease in patients with popliteal aneurysms, there being 15 per cent better survival in patients without aneurysms than in those with successfully repaired popliteal aneurysms. Szilagyi reported a long-term follow-up with 50 popliteal aneurysms treated by surgical therapy. He has treated 30 patients with an autologous saphenous vein and 20 with a Dacron prosthesis and has a cumulative patency

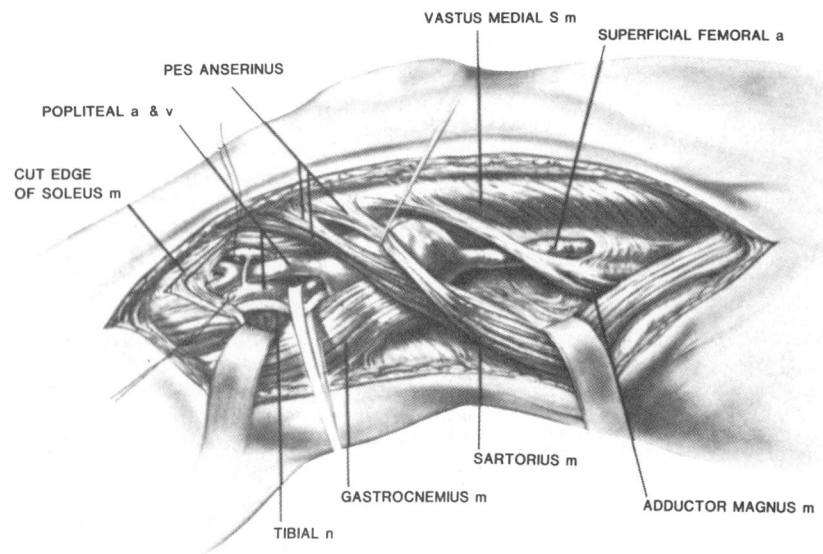

Figure 2. Anatomy of the medial approach to the distal superficial femoral artery and popliteal artery. (From Szilagyi, D. E., Schwartz, R. L., and Reddy, D. J.: Popliteal arterial aneurysms: Their natural history and management. Arch. Surg., *116:*724, 1981.)

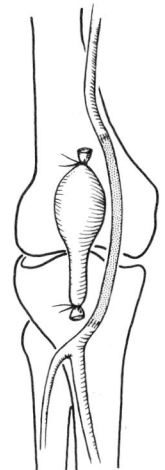

Figure 3. Preferred technique in therapy for popliteal artery aneurysm.

rate of 60 per cent at 5 years and 28 per cent at 10 years. In this series, there were no late amputations secondary to graft failure. These results emphasized that atherosclerotic popliteal artery aneurysms are part of the pathologic process of systemic atherosclerosis and that continued progression of the disease ulti-

mately may cause graft occlusion. One cannot help but question the role that Dacron prosthesis has in the high rate of occlusion. The use of the saphenous vein has allowed an 82 per cent patency rate after 5 years.

As for any patient who has had an operative procedure for aneurysmal disease, the patient who has had repair of a popliteal artery aneurysm should be followed indefinitely. The evidence of multiplicity of aneurysms as well as the ever-present hazard of occlusion of either a saphenous vein or a prosthetic graft replacement makes it mandatory to follow these patients very carefully.

REFERENCES

1. Anton, G. E., Hertzer, N. R., Bevin, E. G., O'Hara, P. J., and Krajewski, L. P.: Surgical management of popliteal aneurysms. J. Vasc. Surg. 3:125, 1986.
2. Dent, T. L., Lindenauer, S. M., Ernest, C. B., and Fry, W. J.: Multiple arteriosclerotic arterial aneurysms. Arch. Surg., 105:338, 1972.
3. Edmunds, L. H., Jr., Darling, R. C., and Linton, R. R.: Surgical management of popliteal aneurysms. Circulation, 32:517, 1965.
4. Evans, W. E., Conley, J. E., and Bernhard, V.: Popliteal aneurysms. Surgery, 70:762, 1971.
5. Gifford, R. W., Jr., Hines, E. A., Jr., and Janes, J. M.: An analysis and follow-up study of one hundred popliteal aneurysms. Surgery, 33:284, 1953.
6. Szilagyi, D. E., Whitcomb, J. G., and Smith R. F.: Anteromedial approach to the popliteal artery for femoropopliteal arterial grafting. Arch. Surg., 78:647, 1959.
7. Szilagyi, D. E., Schwartz, R. L., and Reddy, D. J.: Popliteal arterial aneurysms. Arch. Surg., 116:724, 1981.

VI

THROMBO-OBLITERATIVE DISEASE OF THE AORTA AND ITS BRANCHES

David C. Sabiston, Jr., M.D.

Atherosclerosis is the most frequent cause of occlusive disease of the major branches of the aorta. Certain arterial anatomic sites are especially susceptible to development of stenosis or total occlusion and the most common site is at the origin of the vessels where turbulence is present (Fig. 1).[5] When branches of the aortic arch (innominate, carotid, subclavian) become stenotic or occluded, the symptoms produced are causes by ischemic disturbances due to reduction in blood flow.

Clinical Manifestations

The site and extent of a large series of arterial occlusive lesions are shown in Table 1.[1] The symptoms are dependent upon the nature and extent of the obstruction. Moreover, the natural development of collateral circulation that follows arterial occlusion and the volume of blood flow through the collaterals are of prime importance. The symptoms and the distribution of symptoms are shown in Table 2.[1] The diagnosis is confirmed by arteriography, which shows the lesion and the collateral channels around it.

Surgical Management

The surgical management of patients with occlusive disease is primarily accomplished by bypass grafts (Fig. 2).[1] The results of surgical bypass are favorable, as shown in Table 3.[1] In this series, obstruction was incomplete in 168 and complete in 244 of the arteries involved. Regardless of the extent of obstruction, the occlusive process was segmental in almost every instance. The surgical treatment often is a bypass graft, and endarterectomy is only rarely applicable.

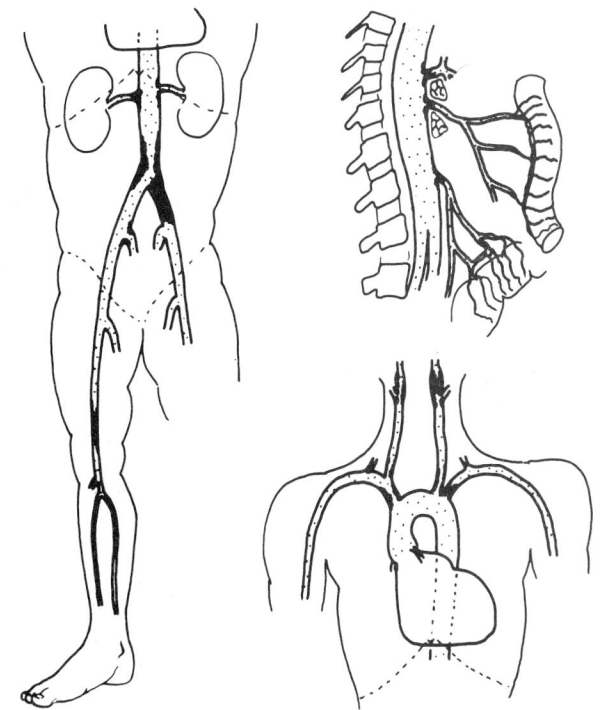

Figure 1. Anatomic sites particularly apt to become stenotic or occluded by atherosclerosis. (From Ludbrook, J., and Elmslie, R. G.: An Introduction to Surgery: 100 Topics. New York, Academic Press, 1971.)

TABLE 1. Location and Extent of 412 Lesions in 299 Patients

Location	Extent of Obstruction		
	Incomplete	Complete	Totals
Innominate artery	40	26	66
Right common carotid artery	5	19	24
Right subclavian artery	30	29	59
Left common carotid artery	24	37	61
Left subclavian artery	69	133	202
Total	168	244	412

From Crawford, E. S., DeBakey, M. E., Morris, G. C., Jr., and Howell, J. F.: Surgical treatment of occlusion of the innominate, common carotid, and subclavian arteries: A 10 year experience. Surgery *65*:17, 1969.

TABLE 2. Symptoms of Occlusion (299 Patients)

Type of Symptom	No. of Patients	Per Cent
Neurological only	97	32
Neurological and upper extremity ischemia	124	42
Upper extremity ischemia	63	21
Systolic ear noise	3	1
No symptoms	12	4
Total	299	100

From Crawford, E. S., DeBakey, M. E., Morris, G. C., Jr., and Howell, J. F.: Surgical treatment of occlusion of the innominate, common carotid, and subclavian arteries: A 10 year experience. Surgery *65*:17, 1969.

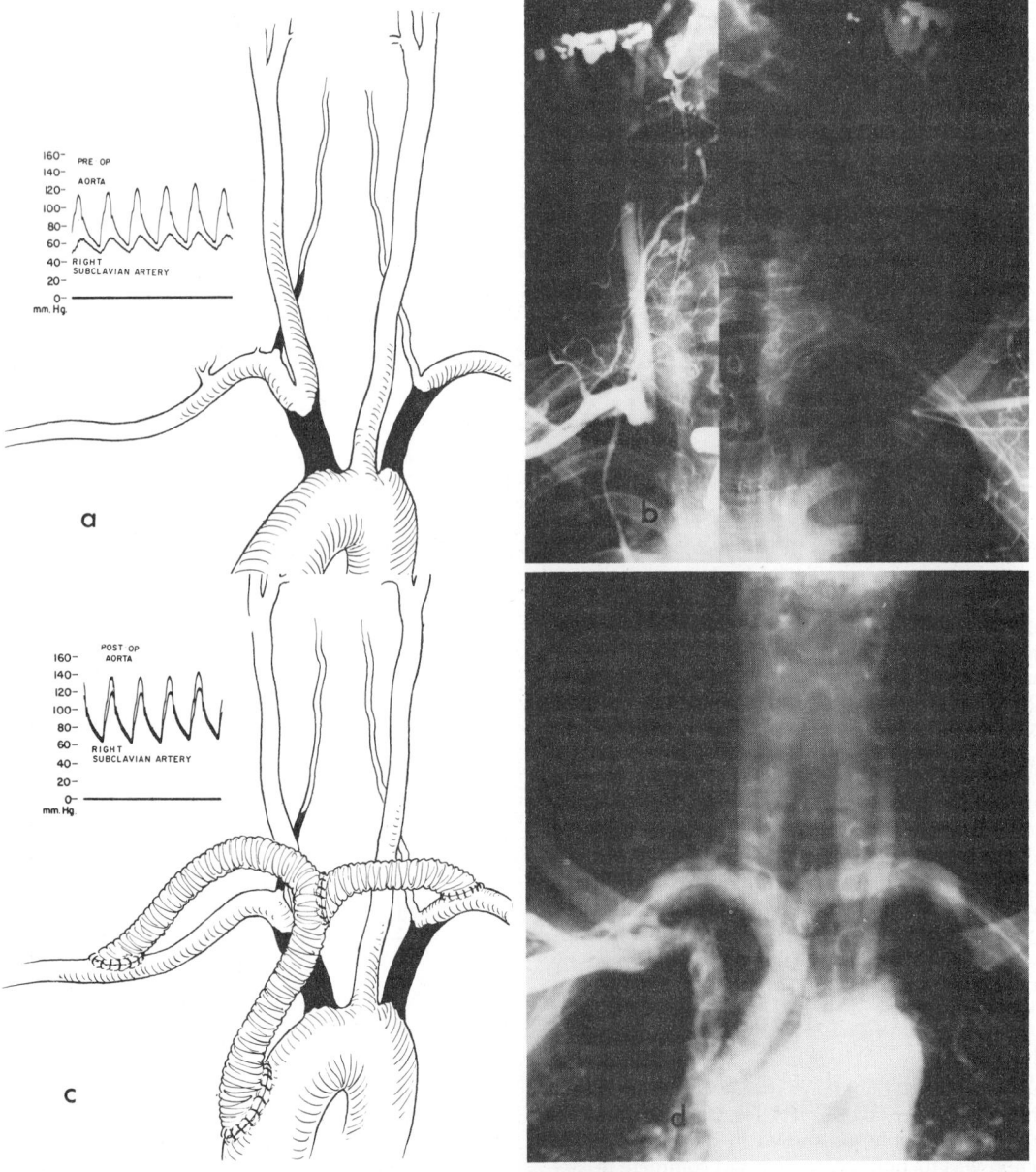

Figure 2. Patient with obstruction of innominate and left subclavian arteries, causing cerebral arterial insufficiency, and obstruction of the abdominal aorta and iliac arteries, causing both intermittent claudication and ischemic lesions of the feet. The patient was treated first at one operation by ascending aortobilateral subclavian bypass graft, and at a second operation by bilateral aortoexternal iliac artery bypass graft, relieving all symptoms. Diagram *(a)* and arteriogram *(b)* with pressure recording made before bypass show location and extent of innominate and subclavian lesions. Diagram *(c)* and aortogram *(d)* made 3 years after operation and pressure recordings made at operation after bypass show grafts in place and functioning.

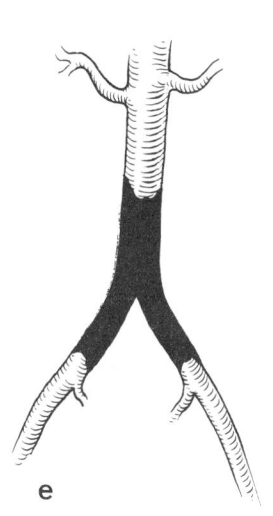

e

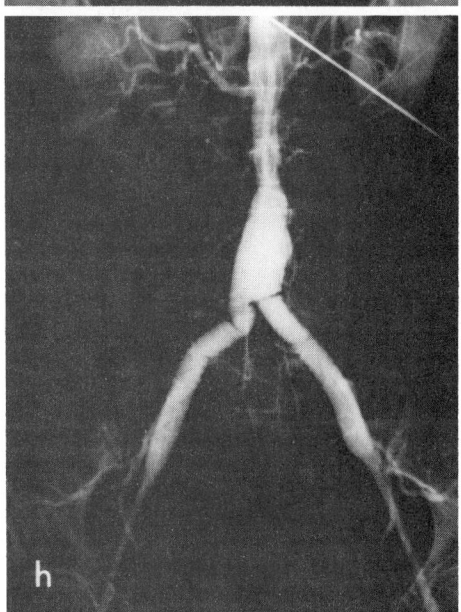

f

Figure 2. *Continued* Diagram *(e)* and aortogram *(f)* made before operation show location and extent of aortoiliac obstruction. Diagram *(g)* and aortogram *(h)* made 3 years after operation show graft in place and functioning. The patient is alive and well 5 years after operation. (From Crawford, E. S., DeBakey, M. E., Morris, G. C., Jr., and Howell, J. F.: Surgical treatment of occlusion of the innominate, common, carotid, and subclavian arteries: A 10-year experience. Surgery, *65:*17, 1969.)

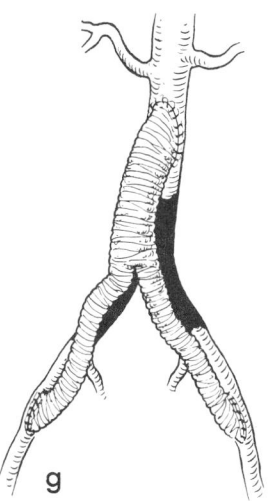

g

h

TABLE 3. Functional Results in 299 Patients with Occlusion of Great Vessels of the Aortic Arch

Time of Follow-up	Asymptomatic, Improved		Unimproved		Worse		Dead	
	No.	Per Cent	No.	Per Cent	No.	Per Cent	No.	Per Cent
Immediate	268	89.6	10	3.3	5	1.7	16	5.4
Late	274	91.6	3	1.0	6	2.0	43	14.4

From Crawford, E. S., DeBakey, M. E., Morris, G. C., Jr., and Howell, J. F.: Surgical treatment of occlusion of the innominate, common carotid, and subclavian arteries: A 10 year experience. Surgery, *65:*17, 1969.

1. TAKAYASU'S ARTERITIS

David C. Sabiston, Jr., M.D.

Takayasu's disease, described by a Japanese ophthalmologist in 1908,[7] is a nonspecific arteritis affecting the thoracic and abdominal aorta and its major branches. Although uncommon in the United States, it is often seen in the Orient and usually attacks young females. It has also been described in older women and males as well, and the natural history of the disorder has been carefully documented.[4] The arteritis involves all layers of the arterial wall, with proliferation of connective tissue and degeneration of the elastic fibers, and may also involve the pulmonary arteries. Granulomatous lesions may be present with associated fusiform or saccular aneurysms. Three types of this disorder are now recognized (Fig. 1).[2]

The clinical manifestations of Takayasu's arteritis are at first generalized and include fever, malaise, arthritis, and arthralgia. Pericardial pain, tachycardia, and vomiting may also occur. It has been suggested that the disorder may be an autoimmune disease,[6] and steroids may be beneficial. The later manifestations are those of ischemia of both the cerebral and upper extremity circuits. Surgical treatment of Takayasu's arteritis has often proved disappointing, because the endarterectomy site and grafts are apt to reocclude later. Operation is occasionally recommended for patients with disabling symptoms.[3]

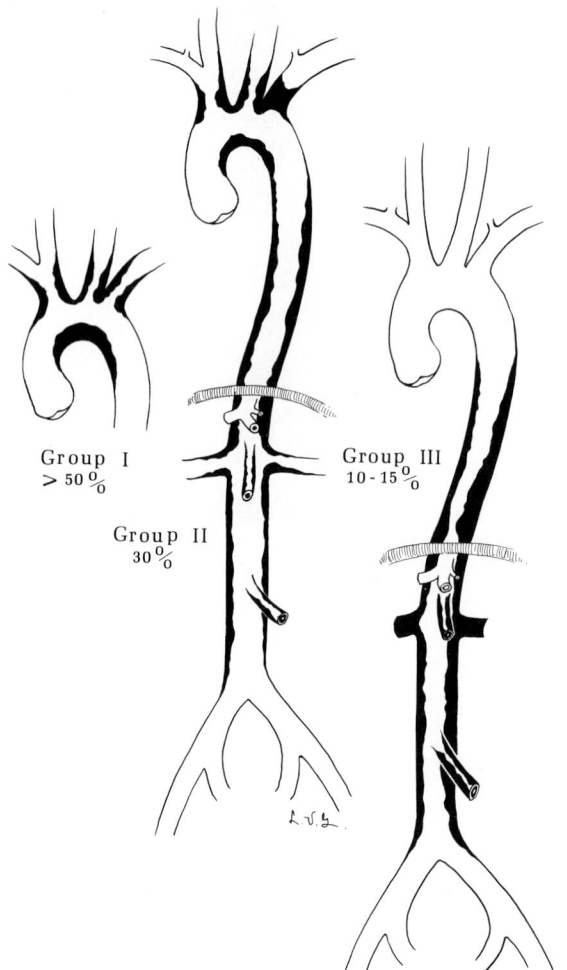

Group I
> 50%

Group II
30%

Group III
10 - 15%

Figure 1. Clinical subdivisions of Takayasu's arteritis. The panarteritis may be localized to the aortic arch and great vessels (Group 1), the distal thoracoabdominal aorta (Group III), or the entire aorta (Group II). (From Edmunds, L. H., Jr.: Trauma and occlusive disease. *In* Strandness, D. E., Jr. (Ed.): Collateral Circulation in Clinical Surgery. Philadelphia, W. B. Saunders Company, 1969.)

REFERENCES

1. Crawford, E. S., DeBakey, M. E., Morris, G. C., Jr., and Howell, J. F.: Surgical treatment of occlusion of the innominate, common carotid, and subclavian arteries: A 10 year experience. Surgery, *65*:17, 1969.
2. Edmunds, L. H., Jr.: Trauma and occlusive disease. *In* Strandness, D. E., Jr. (Ed.): Collateral Circulation in Clinical Surgery. Philadelphia, W. B. Saunders Company, 1969.
3. Ekestrom, S., and Hansson, L. O.: Surgical treatment of "pulseless disease." Acta Chir. Scand., *128*:127, 1964.
4. Ishikawa, K.: Natural history and classification of occlusive thromboaortopathy (Takayasu's disease). Circulation, *57*:27, 1978.
5. Ludbrook, J., and Elmslie, R. G.: An Introduction to Surgery: 100 Topics. New York, Academic Press, 1971.
6. Nakao, K., Ikeda, M., Kimata, S., Niitani, H., Miyahara, M., Ishimi, Z., Hashiba, K., Takeda, Y., Ozawa, T., Matsushita, S., and Kuramochi, M.: Takayasu's arteritis. Clinical report of eighty-four cases and immunological studies of seven cases. Circulation, *35*:1141, 1967.
7. Takayasu, M.: Case of queer changes in central blood vessels of retina. Acta Soc. Ophthal. Jap., *12*:2554, 1908.

2. CAROTID ARTERY OCCLUSIVE DISEASE

Richard H. Dean, M.D.

In 1856, Savory described the autopsy findings of an extracranial internal carotid artery occlusion and bilateral subclavian occlusions in a woman with hemiplegia and dysesthesia—the first description of a link between stroke and extracranial carotid artery disease.[14] In 1914, Ramsey Hunt correlated the relationship between partial carotid artery occlusion and what he termed "cerebral intermittent claudication."[6] Further evolution in the understanding and management of extracranial cerebrovascular disease came with the use of carotid angiography in the diagnosis of carotid artery occlusion by Moniz, reported in 1927.[10] Although reports of the association between extracranial carotid disease and stroke continued to appear, acceptance of its relative importance and enthusiasm for pre-emptive management of the carotid disease awaited popularization of carotid endarterectomy during the late 1950s and early 1960s.

Natural History

There are approximately 500,000 new strokes in the United States each year; the direct and indirect cost of these is about 8 billion dollars a year.[16] Initial mortality from stroke is estimated to be between 20 and 30 per cent.[12] The natural history of atherosclerotic occlusive disease of the extracranial carotid artery remains controversial.

In a recent report by Roederer and associates, 167 asymptomatic patients with cervical bruits were followed with serial duplex scanning regardless of the degree of the stenosis at the time of presentation.[13] Ten patients (6 per cent) became symptomatic during follow-up; the development of symptoms was accompanied by disease progression in 8 of those patients. By life-table analysis, the annual rate of symptom occurrence was 4 per cent; however, the presence of progression to 80 per cent stenosis was highly correlated with either total occlusion of the internal carotid artery or the development of new symptoms. Thus, 89 per cent of the symptoms were preceded by disease progression to a greater than 80 per cent stenosis. Progression to this extent was an important warning observation because the risk of ischemic symptoms or development of internal carotid occlusion was 35 per cent within 6 months and 46 per cent at 12 months. Conversely, only 1.5 per cent of the lesions that remained in a less than 80 per cent category developed such a complication. These data suggest that careful follow-up with repeated noninvasive evaluation is of great assistance in determining the appropriate management of the asymptomatic carotid lesion.

Other studies have suggested that the composition of the plaque influences the risk of stroke due to carotid artery lesions. In an analysis of 297 carotid arteries examined prospectively in asymptomatic patients, Johnson and colleagues concluded that patients with stenosis greater than 75 per cent at the time of the initial study were at higher risk of developing symptoms ipsilateral to the lesion than were patients without significant narrowing.[7] However, even patients with less than 75 per cent stenosis were at greater risk if their associated plaques were less organized, that is, soft. Plaque organization was determined by B-mode ultrasound, and plaques were classified as soft, calcified, or dense. A definite trend toward higher risk was seen in plaques of lower density.

Moreover, it has been shown that the development of transient ischemic attacks (TIAs) also places patients at a higher risk of developing a stroke. In the Mayo Clinic population study,[15] 118 patients with TIAs were followed as a control group without therapy. The stroke rate at 1, 3, and 5 years was 23 per cent, 37 per cent, and 45 per cent, respectively. Most permanent deficits occurred during the first year. This rate represents a 16-fold increased risk of stroke when compared with an age- and sex-adjusted population without TIAs. Some series[5,9] have reported lower figures, but the average reported in the literature is 30 per cent to 35 per cent at 5 years, or 10 per cent the first year, and 6 per cent each year thereafter.

Pathogenesis of Transient Ischemic Attacks and Stroke

Three causes of TIAs and stroke stem from occlusive disease of the extracranial carotid artery. These are thrombosis of the carotid artery, flow-related ischemic events, and embolization from the atherosclerotic lesion in the carotid artery.

Thrombosis of the internal carotid artery is the terminal event of progressive enlargement of the atherosclerotic lesion at the carotid artery bifurcation. If the distal propagation of the thrombus stops at the ophthalmic artery and remains stable, the event of total occlusion may be silent if collateral flow is sufficient. If the thrombus progresses beyond the ophthalmic artery into the middle cerebral artery, a hemispheric event varying from a TIA to a profound stroke occurs.

Flow-related ischemic events were once considered the most common cause of cerebral symptoms in conjunction with carotid artery disease. Although transient decreases in cerebral perfusion through a stenotic carotid artery can produce symptoms, the occurrence is rare. Owing to the rich collateral pathways for cerebral perfusion through the circle of Willis (Fig. 1) and the contralateral carotid artery and transcranial external-to-internal carotid artery connections, cerebral perfusion is rarely diminished to a critical level despite the presence of a severe carotid artery stenosis.

Cerebral embolization from the carotid artery lesion is the single most common cause of cerebral ischemic events. Embolization from the atherosclerotic plaque may occur by either of two mechanisms. First, the irregular surface of the plaque is thrombogenic and can accumulate platelet aggregates. If these platelet aggregates become large and embolize to an important cerebral branch, symtoms are produced. Second, as the atherosclerotic plaque becomes more advanced, it may undergo central degeneration. When this occurs, the plaque may rupture spontaneously, discharging its contents into the lumen, with subsequent embolization. In both of these instances, the type, severity, and permanency of the cerebral event is determined by the size and eventual location of the embolus.

Clinical Manifestations

The clinical presentations of carotid artery occlusive disease can be categorized into three general groups: asymptomatic lesions; lesions producing TIAs; and those lesions that have produced cerebral infarction.

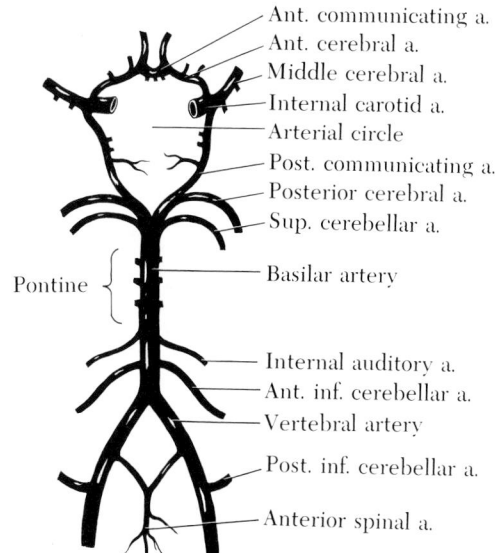

Figure 1. Diagram showing the most common configuration of the terminal branches of the vertebral and internal carotid arteries and their interconnections to form the circle of Willis. (From Wylie, E. J., and Ehrenfeld, W. K.: Extracranial Occlusive Cerebrovascular Disease. Philadelphia, W. B. Saunders Company, 1970.)

Asymptomatic patients are those who have a hemodynamically significant lesion or nonocclusive ulcerated lesion of the carotid artery but no history of cerebral symptoms. The presence of a bruit in an asymptomatic patient does not define this group, Kartchner and McRae[8] finding that less than one third of patients with a cervical bruit had a hemodynamically significant lesion of the carotid artery by noninvasive criteria. Therapeutic intervention may be indicated in certain of these asymptomatic patients with high-grade lesions.

By definition, TIAs are temporary neurologic deficits lasting for less than 24 hours and followed by complete recovery. In the area supplied by the carotid artery, they are usually discrete motor and/or sensory dysfunctions. Contralateral facial, arm, and/or leg motor weakness and sensory loss are the classic presentations. Since the left hemisphere is dominant in 95 per cent of the population, left hemispheric TIAs may also cause either receptive or expressive aphasia.

Probably the most classic TIA of carotid artery origin is transient loss or blurred vision (amaurosis fugax) in the ipsilateral eye (Fig. 2). It is classically described as a curtain being drawn down over the eye or as a quadrant field defect and is caused by embolization to the retinal branches of the ophthalmic artery, the first major intracranial branch of the internal carotid artery.

The first clinical manifestation of carotid artery disease may be a permanent neurologic deficit or stroke. Depending on the area of cerebral cortex affected, the defect may range from minimal with ultimate recovery of the lost function to massive leading to death.

Diagnostic Evaluation

A number of noninvasive diagnostic studies have been advocated in the preliminary evaluation of patients suspected of having cerebrovascular disease. The role of the respective diagnostic studies is dependent on the clinical presentation of the patient. Currently, evaluation of the asymptomatic patient with a cervical bruit is best achieved by duplex scanning of the carotid artery. Through the combination of B-mode imaging of the vessel to identify the presence of lumen-narrowing plaques and pulse Doppler sampling of velocity spectra, a relatively accurate assessment for identification of hemodynamically significant disease can be obtained. If duplex scanning defines the bruit arising from an external carotid lesion or a mild or moderate

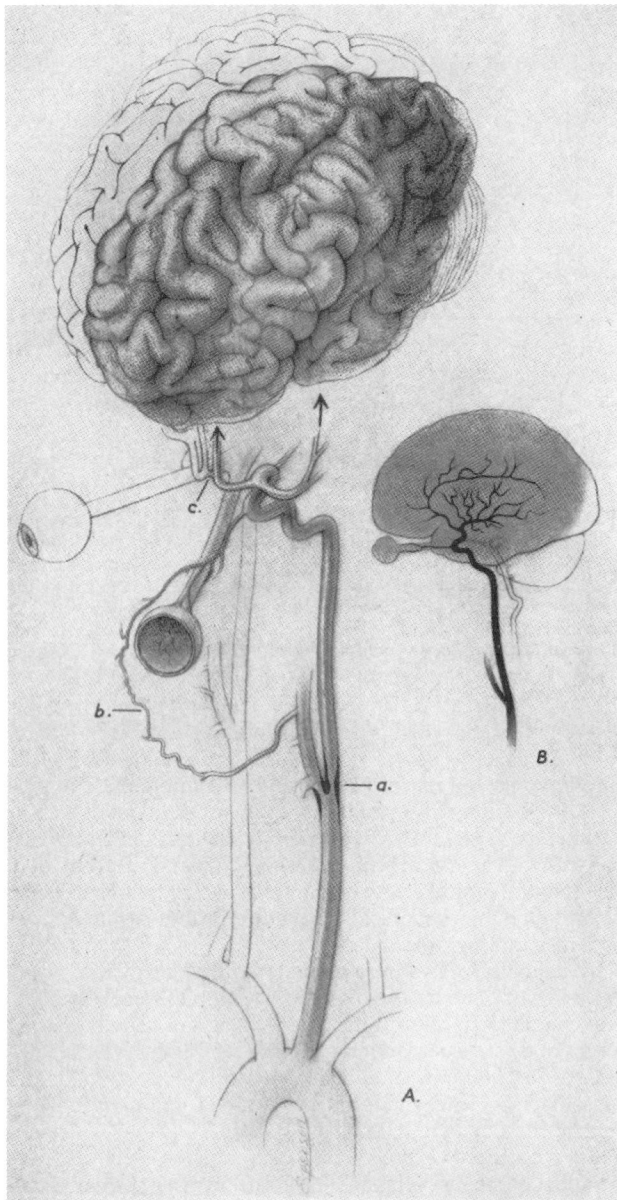

Figure 2. Atheromatous retinal embolus lodged at a bifurcation. (From Hoyt, W. F.: Some neuro-ophthalmological considerations in cerebral vascular insufficiency: Carotid and vertebral artery insufficiency. Arch. Ophthalmol., *62:*262, 1959.)

tem by subclavian inspection to visualize the origin and intracranial portions of the vertebral and basilar arteries.

Computed tomographic (CT) scanning of the head should be performed in all patients with cerebral symptoms. Intracranial space-occupying lesions such as neoplasms, vascular malformations, or subdural hematomas enter into the differential diagnosis of patients with even the most convincing symptoms of transient cerebral ischemia. CT scanning is a quick, noninvasive means of excluding alternative disease during patient diagnostic examinations.

The patient who presents with a TIA actually may have suffered a small cerebral infarction. CT scanning identifies an unsuspected cerebral infarction and establishes a baseline status before operative intervention.

Moreover, patients who present with a clinically overt cerebral infarction should have a CT scan to document infarct size and to differentiate between an ischemic and a hemorrhagic infarction. A hemorrhagic infarction is visible promptly on CT scan, whereas an ischemic infarction may take several days of evolution before its low-density mass is visualized. Data from CT scans are necessary in determining the proper timing of operative management following acute stroke in patients who have experienced a good neurologic recovery.

Operative Management

The first carotid artery operation for occlusive disease was performed in 1951 but was not reported until 1955. In that report, by Carrea, Molins, and Murphy,[2] an atherosclerotic carotid bifurcation was resected with reanastomosis of the internal carotid to the external carotid artery. The first successful carotid reconstruction, performed by DeBakey and colleagues, was not reported until 1959.[3] The first report of carotid endarterectomy appeared in *Lancet* in November 1954. That article by Eastcott, Pickering, and Rob[4] called the world's attention to the feasibility of managing this cause of TIAs.

Currently, carotid endarterectomy is indicated for treatment of patients with hemispheric TIAs and of patients with either retained or regained significant residual functional cortex after a completed stroke associated with carotid bifurcation occlusive disease. Although use of prophylactic carotid endarterectomy for asymptomatic patients remains debatable, it is probably indicated for patients with severe stenosis (greater than 80 per cent) and complexly ulcerated plaques.

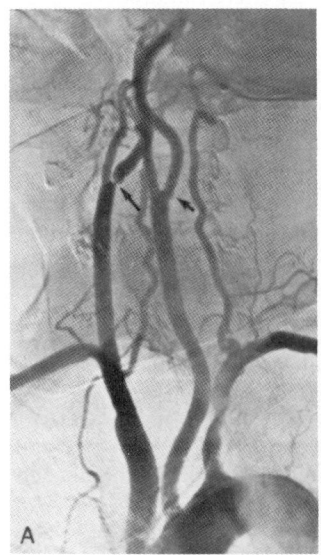
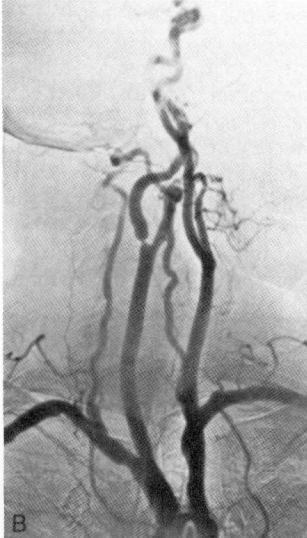

Figure 3. Arteriogram showing typical severe right internal carotid artery stenosis at its origin (long arrow). The left internal carotid artery has mild disease (short arrow). This particular study is a subtraction of an arch aortogram shown in the right posterior oblique (*A*) and left posterior oblique (*B*) projections. (From Gomes, A. S.: Aortic arch studies and selective arteriography. *In* Moore, W. S. (Ed.): Surgery for Cerebrovascular Disease. New York, Churchill Livingstone, 1987.)

internal carotid lesion, no further diagnostic evaluation is necessary and the patient should have a serial follow-up program of semiannual repeat scans. In contrast, if a severe lesion of the carotid bifurcation or the internal carotid artery is diagnosed, arteriography should be undertaken to determine more precisely the necessity of operative intervention.

Although duplex scanning may be performed in patients presenting with cerebral symptoms, it should not be used to determine the need for arteriography. Standard four-vessel carotid arteriography should be used in the evaluation of all patients presenting with TIAs or prior ischemic stroke in whom residual hemispheric function either remains or has been regained. The safest and most complete study is threefold: (1) assessment of the brachiocephalic trunks by intra-arterial digital subtraction arch aortography using the Seldinger technique from a femoral artery entrance site; followed by (2) selective cannulation and inspection of the carotid arteries for observation of both the extracranial and intracranial carotid arteries (Fig. 3); followed by (3) assessment of the vertebrobasilar sys-

The technique of carotid endarterectomy is relatively simple but requires precision if the results are to be favorable. The important landmarks of the exposure are depicted in Figure 4. Technical details of the dissection are discussed elsewhere.[11]

Operative techniques to optimize cerebral perfusion during carotid cross-clamping vary according to the preference of the surgeon. Options include routine use of a shunt, selective use of a shunt based on a certain stump pressure or a change in electroencephalogram, and performing the operation under local anesthesia using a shunt if neurologic changes develop. Many cerebrovascular surgeons, including the author, have now begun using the last-named option in patients with the usual variety of carotid lesion.

Although some surgeons routinely use a patch to close the arteriotomy following completion of the endarterectomy, implementation of microvascular techniques and magnification allows most arteriotomies to be closed primarily.

Current results of carotid endarterectomy should include less than a 5 per cent combined cerebrovascular morbidity and operative mortality. Most current series have combined morbidity and mortality in the asymptomatic patient group of less than 3 per cent. Obviously, the preoperative neurologic status of the patient affects the incidence of immediate perioperative events as well as the late results. Bernstein and colleagues[1] reported a series of 456 carotid endarterectomies in patients followed for 1 and 11 years, with an average follow-up of 45.3 months. Operated asymptomatic patients had a 1.6 per cent incidence of TIAs and a 3.2 per cent incidence of stroke on late follow-up. Those operated on because of TIAs had a 19.5 per cent and 5.2 per cent incidence of recurrent TIAs or stroke, respectively. Patients with a permanent neurologic deficit preoperatively had an incidence of TIAs of 7.9 per cent, and 11 per cent developed a stroke during late follow-up.

Certainly many issues regarding the necessity for evaluation of and intervention in patients with cerebrovascular disease remain controversial. The role of intervention for asymptomatic lesions is currently being investigated with a prospective randomized multicenter trial; antiplatelet therapy is being recommended by some physicians for even symptomatic disease. Until proven otherwise, however, carotid endarterectomy remains the treatment of choice for symptomatic carotid artery disease and severe asymptomatic lesions.

SELECTED REFERENCES

Moore, W. S.: Surgery for Cerebrovascular Disease. New York, Churchill Livingstone, 1987.
This book provides a detailed description of cerebrovascular disease by multiple authors considered to be experts in the field. It includes excellent chapters that discuss the natural history of cerebrovascular disease and stroke. In addition, detailed descriptions of the indications for and techniques of operative intervention are included.

Moore, W. S., and Quiñones-Baldrich, W. J.: Extracranial cerebrovascular disease. *In* Moore, W. S. (Ed.): Vascular Surgery, 2nd ed. Orlando, Grune & Stratton, 1986, pp. 621–680.
This review of extracranial cerebrovascular disease summarizes historical advances and provides an excellent summation regarding the current state of knowledge and controversy surrounding treatment of cerebrovascular disease. It also includes discussion of vertebrobasilar insufficiency and emergency management of stroke in progress.

Roederer, G.O., Langlois, Y. E., Jager, K. A., Primozich, J. F., Beach, K. W., Phillips, D. J., and Strandness, D. E., Jr.: The natural history of carotid arterial disease in asymptomatic patients with cervical bruits. Stroke, 15:605, 1984.
This report provides an excellent examination of factors influencing the subsequent incidence of symptoms in patients who present with asymptomatic carotid artery disease. It emphasizes the value of serial monitoring of patients with mild and moderate disease.

REFERENCES

1. Bernstein, E. F., et al.: Influence of preoperative factors on late neurologic events after carotid endarterectomy. International Vascular Symposium Programs and Abstracts. New York, Macmillan, 1981, p. 460.
2. Carrea, R., and Murphy, M. M.: Surgical treatment of spontaneous thrombosis of the internal carotid artery in the neck: Carotid-carotideal anastomosis. Report of a case. Acta Neurol. Latinoam., 1:71, 1955.
3. De Bakey, M. E., Crawford, E. S., Cooley, D. A., and Morris, G. C., Jr.: Surgical considerations of occlusive disease of innominate, carotid, subclavian, and vertebral arteries. Ann. Surg., 149:690, 1959.
4. Eastcott, H. H. G., Pickering, G. W., and Rob, C. G.: Reconstruction of internal carotid artery in a patient with intermittent attacks of hemiplegia. Lancet, 2:994, 1954.
5. Hass, W. K., and Jonas, S.: Caution falling rock zone: An analysis of the medical and surgical management of threatened stroke. Proc. Inst. Med. Chic., 33:80, 1980.
6. Hunt, J. R.: The role of the carotid arteries in the causation of vascular lesions of the brain, with remarks on certain special features of the symptomatology. Am. J. Med. Sci., 147:704, 1914.
7. Johnson, J. M., Kennelly, M. M., Decesare, D., Morgan, S., and Sparrow, A: Natural history of asymptomatic carotid plaque. Arch. Surg., 120:1010, 1985.
8. Kartchner, M. M., and McRae, L. P.: Noninvasive evaluation and management of the "asymptomatic" carotid bruit. Surgery, 82:840, 1977.
9. Loeb, C., Priano, A., and Albano, C.: Clinical features and long-term follow-up of patients with reversible ischemic attacks (RIA). Acta Neurol. Scand., 57:471, 1978.
10. Moniz, E.: L'encéphalographie artérielle, son importance dans la localisation des tumeurs cérébrales. Rev. Neurol. (Paris), 48:72, 1927.
11. Moore, W. S.: Technique of carotid endarterectomy. *In* Moore, W. S. (Ed.): Surgery for Cerebrovascular Disease. New York, Churchill Livingstone, 1987, pp. 491–502.
12. Moore, W. S., and Quiñones-Baldrich, W. J.: Extracranial cerebrovascular disease. *In* Moore, W. S. (Ed.): Vascular Surgery, 2nd ed. Orlando, Grune & Stratton, 1986, pp. 621–680.
13. Roederer, G. O., Langlois, Y. E., Jager, K. A., Primozich, J. F., Beach, K. W., Phillips, D. J., and Strandness, D. E., Jr.: The natural history of carotid arterial disease in asymptomatic patients with cervical bruits. Stroke, 15:605, 1984.
14. Savory, W. S.: Case of a young woman in whom the main arteries of both upper extremities and of the left side of the neck were throughout completely obliterated. Med.-Chir. Tr. Lond., 39:205, 1856.
15. Whisnant, J. P., Matsumoto, N., and Elveback, L. R.: The effects of anticoagulant therapy on the prognosis of patients with transient cerebral ischemic attacks in a community. Rochester, Minnesota, 1955–1969. Mayo Clin. Proc., 48:844, 1973.
16. Zarins, C. K., Giddens, D. P., and Glagov, S.: Atherosclerotic plaque distribution and flow velocity profiles in the carotid bifurcation. *In* Bergan, J. J., and Yao, J. S. T. (Eds.): Cerebrovascular Insufficiency, 1st ed. New York, Grune & Stratton, 1983, pp. 19–30.

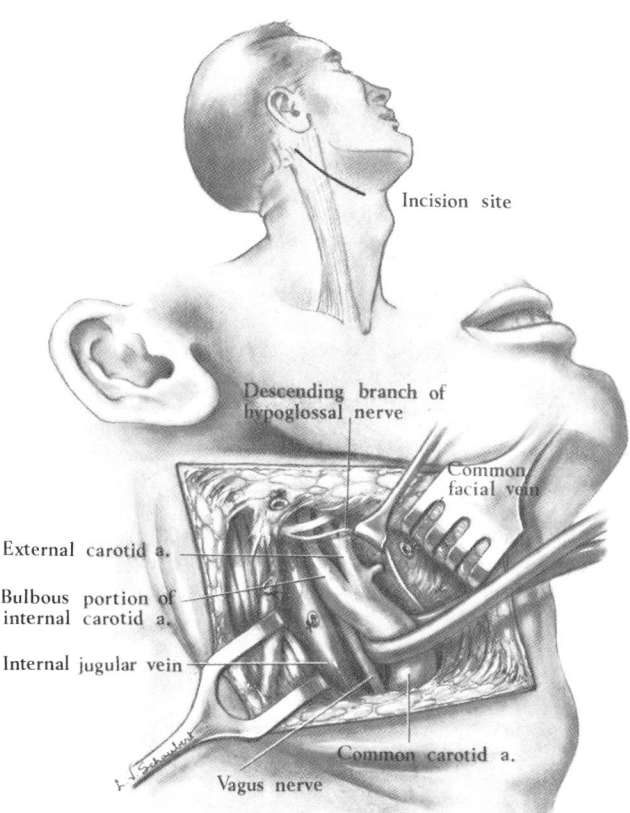

Figure 4. Incision site and exposure of the carotid bifurcation area. (From Wylie, E. J., and Ehrenfeld, W. K.: Extracranial Occlusive Cerebrovascular Disease. Philadelphia, W. B. Saunders Company, 1970.)

Incision site

Descending branch of hypoglossal nerve

Common facial vein

External carotid a.

Bulbous portion of internal carotid a.

Internal jugular vein

Common carotid a.

Vagus nerve

3. SUBCLAVIAN STEAL SYNDROME

John A. Mannick, M.D.

The subclavian steal syndrome occurs when there is reversal of flow in the ipsilateral vertebral artery distal to a stenosis or occlusion of the proximal subclavian or, more rarely, the innominate artery. Because of the lowering of pressure in the subclavian artery distal to the obstruction, blood flows up the vertebral artery on the unaffected side, into the basilar artery, and down the vertebral artery on the affected side to supply collateral circulation to the subclavian artery and its subsidiary arterial systems (Figs. 1 and 2). Thus, blood supply is presumably "stolen" from the basilar artery; and, at least theoretically, blood supply to the brain stem may be compromised.

Contorni[6] is credited with reporting the first angiographic visualization of subclavian steal in 1960; however, the potential clinical significance of this problem was not widely appreciated until the report of Reivich and his co-workers,[35] who in 1961 described two patients with clinical signs of cerebral vascular insufficiency and reversal of flow through the vertebral artery secondary to subclavian obstruction. In this report, reversal of flow was demonstrated not only by angiography but by the use of the electromagnetic flowmeter at the time of surgical correction of the subclavian lesion. In an editorial discussing the report of Reivich and associates, Fisher introduced the term "subclavian steal syndrome." Since that time, numerous reports have appeared in the literature describing patients who were found to have subclavian steal by angiography.* However, there has been considerable variation in the authors' assessment of the clinical significance of the phenomenon.

Clinical Evaluation

Classically, the subclavian steal syndrome should be suspected in a patient who manifests symptoms of vertebral-basilar arterial insufficiency and is found on examination to have a difference in brachial systolic blood pressure of at least 30 mm. Hg between the two arms and in whom there is a bruit at the base of the neck or in the supraclavicular area on the affected side. The cause of proximal subclavian obstruction is arteriosclerosis in the great majority of instances. The left subclavian artery is involved in a greater percentage of cases (about 70 per cent) than the right.[12] The neurologic symptoms reported in patients with this syndrome most commonly include vertigo, limb paresis, and paresthesias. Bilateral (cortical) visual disturbances, ataxia, syncope, and dysarthria occur somewhat less frequently. The symptoms have been encountered initially as transient ischemic attacks of cerebral ischemia in the majority of patients. However, a number of instances in which the symptoms progressed to complete stroke have been reported.[12,35] In patients with innominate artery stenosis, any neurologic manifestations of subclavian steal may be obscured by those caused by concomitant carotid insufficiency.

North and associates in 1962 reported that symptoms of cerebral ischemia were produced by exercise of the affected arm in six of seven patients they encountered with subclavian steal.[37] However, it is now apparent, from a review of the reported clinical experience with patients with this phenomenon, that, paradoxically, only a few have manifested neurologic symptoms in response to exercise of the involved arm, which would be expected to increase the demand for collateral blood flow.

The diagnosis of subclavian steal is made by retrograde catheter angiography. A number of reports have indicated that it is

---

* See references 2,4,7–9,14,16,19–23,26,29,31,32,36,37,39, and 41–44.

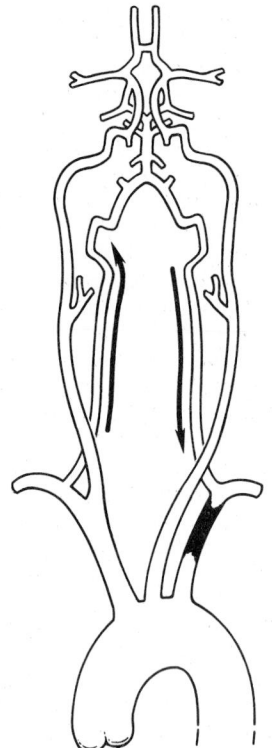

Figure 1. Diagram of the pattern of flow in the subclavian steal syndrome. Note the retrograde flow in the vertebral artery on the side of the lesion (after Weilbaecher).

possible to obtain an angiographic picture falsely suggestive of subclavian steal by pressure injection of contrast material through a catheter located in the vertebral artery itself or in the subclavian artery near the vertebral origin.[11,33,40] The force of the injection apparently alters hemodynamics so that contrast material may be forced up one vertebral artery and down the other even in the absence of any subclavian obstruction. Therefore, the angiographic diagnosis of true subclavian steal requires that the phenomenon be apparent on films obtained with the contrast medium injected into the aortic root.

The variable hemodynamic effects of a proximal subclavian occlusion must be appreciated for appropriate evaluation of the significance of subclavian steal in an individual patient. Although the retrograde flow rate in the ipsilateral vertebral artery has been shown by direct measurement to be as high as 120 ml. per minute,[35] in some patients with subclavian occlusion the simplistic assumption that the cerebral circulation is deprived of this quantity of blood is not necessarily valid. Since flow in the major arteries is limited much more by the peripheral resistance in the arteriolar bed supplied by these vessels than by the intrinsic resistance of the major vessels themselves, it is at least theoretically possible that a normal vertebral artery, on the side opposite the subclavian lesion in a patient with the subclavian steal phenomenon, could supply adequately the posterior cerebral circulation as well as the arm on the affected side. Moreover, the basilar circulation can draw on both internal carotid arteries for collateral supply through the circle of Willis.

Cerebral Blood Flow with Subclavian Occlusion

Conflicting experimental evidence has been reported concerning the effect of proximal subclavian occlusion on cerebral blood flow. Reivich and associates[35] and Sammartino and Toole[38] measured flow in the vertebral and carotid arteries of dogs subjected to unilateral proximal subclavian artery occlusion and observed reversal of flow in the ipsilateral vertebral

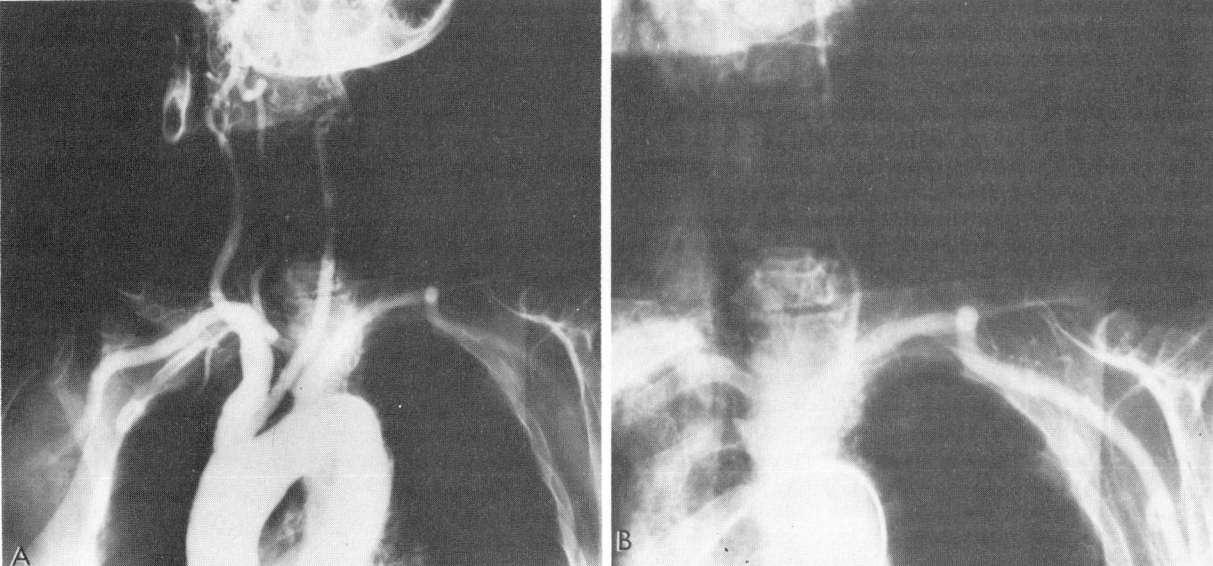

Figure 2. Early (A) and late (B) films of an angiogram of the aortic arch in a patient with the subclavian steal syndrome. In the early film, a stenosis of the origin of the left subclavian artery is seen. In the late film, there is retrograde flow of contrast material down the left vertebral artery, filling the left subclavian artery.

artery, which increased as the affected limb was exercised. They reported that the compensatory increase in forward flow through the other major arteries supplying the brain was insufficient to compensate for the flow lost through the steal phenomenon, and therefore concluded that there was a net deficit in cerebral blood flow. However, in similar studies Eklof and Schwartz failed to observe a net change in cerebral blood flow with proximal subclavian artery occlusion and reversal of ipsilateral vertebral artery flow.[10] Powers and associates studied the effect in monkeys of subclavian steal on cortical blood flow, measured by thermistor-tipped probes implanted in the brain substance and on auditory function in the awake state in the same animals.[34] After subclavian artery ligation and the production of a subclavian steal, these workers observed a 10 per cent decrease in total cerebral blood flow and a 20 to 70 per cent decrease in blood flow to the brain stem. Although subclavian steal failed to induce gross neurologic deficit in these experiments, measurable decreases in auditory discriminatory function in the awake state in these animals was noted after production of the subclavian steal. Auditory function reverted to normal after correction of the subclavian steal. Handa and associates studied cerebral blood flow in monkeys with an electromagnetic flowmeter and found that subclavian artery occlusion and reversal of flow in the ipsilateral vertebral artery were accompanied by a compensatory increase in flow in the remaining three arteries supplying the brain, and that there was a 6 per cent average decrease in total cerebral blood flow and no evidence of neurologic abnormality.[17]

Early reports suggested that subclavian steal was associated with disabling neurologic symptoms in most patients in whom it was encountered,[20,26,31,35] whereas increasing clinical experience led a number of observers to conclude, along with Ehrenfeld and co-workers,[9] that "the presence of subclavian steal is probably an asymptomatic lesion in most patients." With the realization that subclavian steal could occur, it was feared that this problem would appear in patients who had undergone the Blalock-Taussig operation for palliation of the tetralogy of Fallot, since proximal subclavian artery ligation was an integral part of this procedure. A report by Folger and Shah[14] suggested that some patients who had undergone the Blalock-Taussig procedure had symptoms suggestive of vertebral-basilar insufficiency; however, the most prominent symptom was severe headache in these patients, a complaint not commonly ob-

served in most other patients with the subclavian steal syndrome.[12]

Solti and associates concluded that total cerebral blood flow, as measured by isotope dilution, was significantly lower in patients with the subclavian steal syndrome than in a control group of patients of approximately similar age and sex.[42] They also reported an increase in cerebral blood flow following correction of the lesion in symptomatic patients. However, no mention was made in their report of other associated extracranial lesions of the cerebral arterial supply in the patients they studied. In an early report, Mannick and associates had suggested that the subclavian steal phenomenon was more likely to cause significant neurologic symptoms in patients with disease in other arteries supplying the brain.[26]

Considerable data have resulted from the report of the Joint Study of Extracranial Arterial Occlusion, in which 168 patients with the subclavian steal syndrome from 24 reporting institutions were evaluated.[12] More than 80 per cent of these 168 patients had disease involving one or more of the other vessels supplying the brain. Only 50 patients had subclavian disease only or subclavian and vertebral artery disease. There was a 25 per cent incidence of significant complications following operation, with an 8 per cent surgical mortality in those patients in whom the lesion was surgically corrected. It is of interest that in 34 patients treated medically or in those receiving no treatment at all, the three (9 per cent) who suffered strokes had associated carotid disease. Of the 130 surgically treated patients, 20 had strokes at operation or during the follow-up period (15 per cent). Of the nine asymptomatic patients in whom subclavian steal was discovered incidentally in this study, none developed neurologic symptoms during the follow-up period. Patients with subclavian artery disease alone did not have strokes during the follow-up period, whether they were treated medically, surgically, or not at all.

It appears reasonable to conclude, therefore, that the subclavian steal phenomenon may frequently be a clinically asymptomatic lesion but can produce or contribute to symptoms of cerebrovascular insufficiency when it exists in conjunction with other lesions of the extracranial cerebral arterial supply, particularly carotid bifurcation lesions. Whether or not the subclavian steal phenomenon produces symptoms in a given individual probably depends upon (1) the size of the vertebral artery on the uninvolved side and whether or not it is free from disease; (2)

the anatomy of the circle of Willis, which may have considerable individual variation; (3) the amount of collateral circulation from other sources (particularly the costocervical and thyrocervical trunks[3,30]) that develops to supply the arm of the affected side; and (4) the presence of other lesions in the cerebral arterial supply.

Surgical Correction

In patients in whom the subclavian steal syndrome appears to be responsible for symptoms of vertebral-basilar insufficiency in the absence of other lesions in the extracranial cerebral arterial circulation, surgical correction of the lesion appears warranted and can result in amelioration of symptoms, although surgical therapy cannot justifiably be urged for the prevention of stroke under these circumstances, since subclavian steal alone does not appear to cause stroke.[12] When the subclavian steal syndrome occurs in association with other extracranial arterial lesions, it is evident that the other significant lesions should be repaired as well. It appears likely that concomitant correction of the subclavian steal syndrome in certain of these patients should be undertaken; however, there are a number of reports of symptomatic relief in patients with subclavian steal in whom only the other arterial lesions were corrected.[9,12]

A variety of surgical procedures[5,7–9,13,15,19,22–24,35–37] have been recommended for correction of the subclavian steal, ranging in complexity from simple ligation of the vertebral artery on the affected side,[43] first performed by Rob in 1960,[37] to aorta-to-subclavian artery bypass graft, or subclavian endarterectomy by the mediastinal or transthoracic route. Frequently employed is the common carotid-to-subclavian artery bypass graft performed through a cervical incision. This procedure was once believed to have the potential hazard of stealing blood from the internal carotid circulation;[18] however, experimental observations[1,25] and widespread clinical application of this operation have demonstrated that significant reduction of internal carotid flow does not occur unless there is concomitant stenosis of the proximal common carotid artery. Under such circumstances, this operation is clearly not advisable. When it is normally patent, the common carotid artery apparently has the capacity in humans to supply both the brain and the arm without any drop in pressure distal to the origin of the carotid-to-subclavian artery bypass graft. Many surgeons in the late 1960s adopted this procedure as the method of choice for correction of the subclavian steal syndrome, to avoid the impressive morbidity and mortality[7,12] reported with intrathoracic operations for the correction of lesions of the origins of the brachiocephalic vessels, including the subclavian arteries. However, at least one more recent report[8] suggests that intrathoracic operations to correct the subclavian steal syndrome may have no greater mortality, and perhaps somewhat increased durability, than the carotid-to-subclavian bypass. Nevertheless, the latter operation clearly remains the standard at the present time.

The operative approach for performing a carotid-to-subclavian artery bypass is through a transverse incision placed at the base of the neck (Fig. 3). The clavicular portion of the sternocleidomastoid muscle is divided, exposing the scalene fat pad, which is swept inferiorly to expose the phrenic nerve and the anterior scalene muscle. The phrenic nerve is carefully freed and gently retracted medially. The scalene muscle is divided, exposing the fascia overlying the subclavian artery. The subclavian artery can then be freed from the origin of the vertebral artery to or slightly beyond the lateral border of the first rib. The common carotid artery is nearby, beneath the sternocleidomastoid muscle, and is freed from its companion structures for about 2 inches. Under systemic heparinization, a graft of autogenous saphenous vein, knitted Dacron, or polytetrafluoroethylene (PTFE) is sutured end-to-side to the common carotid artery. One recent report suggests that prostheses give better long-term results in this position than vein grafts.[45] An internal

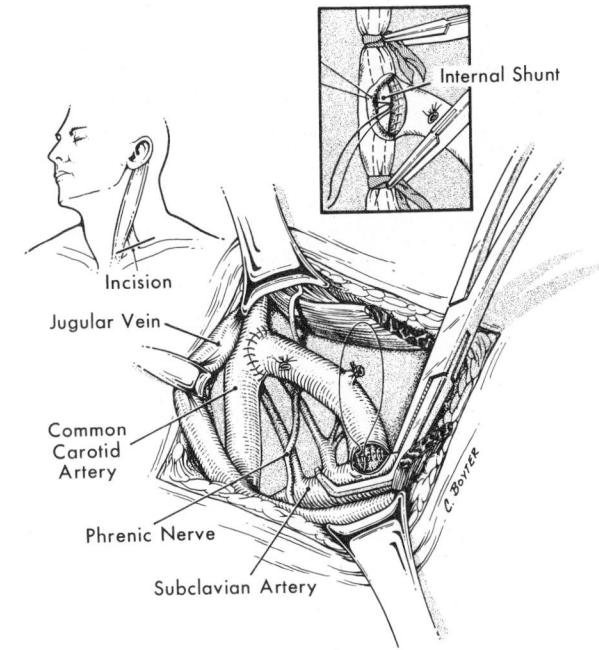

Figure 3. Diagrammatic illustration of the technique of carotid-to-subclavian bypass grafting. The incision is placed at the base of the neck. The clavicular portion of the sternocleidomastoid muscle is divided, exposing the anterior scalene muscle and phrenic nerve. The phrenic nerve is carefully spared and the anterior scalene is divided, exposing the fascia overlying the subclavian artery, which can be freed from the vertebral origin laterally beyond the margin of the first rib. The common carotid artery is exposed through the same incision as it lies beneath the sternocleidomastoid muscle posteromedial to the jugular vein. A graft of autogenous saphenous vein is sutured end-to-side to the common carotid artery. An internal shunt (inset) may be used to preserve flow in the carotid artery while the anastomosis is performed. The shunt is removed just before completion of the suture line. The vein graft is then trimmed to size and sutured end-to-side to the subclavian artery.

shunt may be employed, if desired, to permit carotid flow to continue while the anastomosis is performed. The distal end of the graft is then attached in a similar end-to-side manner to the exposed portion of the subclavian artery.

Embolic phenomena associated with proximal subclavian artery stenosis or occlusion appear to be uncommon. When distal embolization does occur, however, a carotid-to-subclavian bypass, which leaves the lesion in place, is a less desirable operation than alternative procedures that eliminate the source of emboli from the arterial circulation. A variation of the carotid-to-subclavian bypass recommended by Mehigan and associates[27] and others is probably the procedure of choice in such patients. In this procedure, called subclavian-carotid transposition, the subclavian artery is divided just distal to its proximal stenosis or occlusion. The proximal end is oversewn, and the distal end is sutured end-to-side to the common carotid artery, which thus acts as a new innominate artery perfusing the sub-

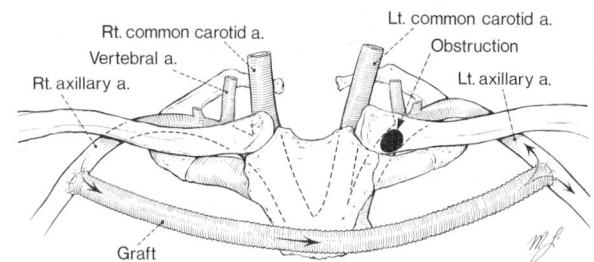

Figure 4. Axilloaxillary bypass graft for subclavian steal syndrome. The graft is passed subcutaneously in the anterior chest wall with end-to-side anastomosis of the graft to each axillary artery. (From Myers, W. O., Lawton, B. R., Ray, J. F., III, Kuehner, M. E., and Sautter, R. D.: Axillo-axillary bypass for subclavian steal syndrome. Arch. Surg., *114:*394, 1979.)

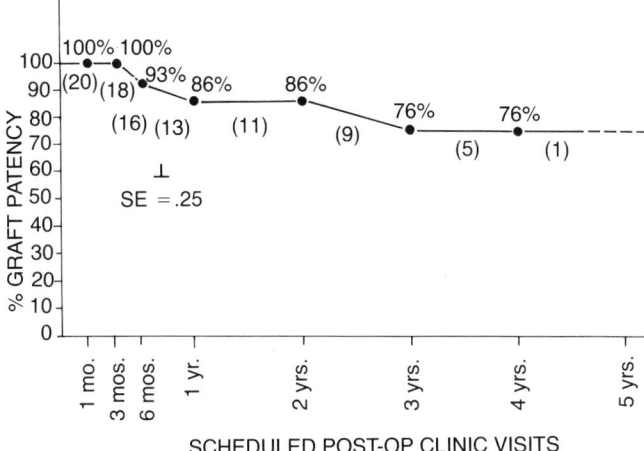

SCHEDULED POST-OP CLINIC VISITS

Figure 5. Life-table method gives an expectation of an 86 per cent graft patency at 1 year and a 76 per cent patency at 3 years. (From Myers, W. O., Lawton, B. R., Ray, J. F., III, Kuehner, M. E., and Sautter, R. D.: Axillo-axillary bypass for subclavian steal syndrome. Arch. Surg., *114*:394, 1979.)

clavian and vertebral systems. This procedure has the advantages of not requiring a graft and of eliminating any possibility of embolization of arteriosclerotic debris or thrombus from the diseased proximal subclavian artery into the vertebral circulation. It has the disadvantage of requiring much more extensive mobilization of the subclavian artery than the carotid-to-subclavian artery bypass graft.

To avoid the potential hazard of operating on the common carotid artery, several investigators have proposed alternative methods of correction of the subclavian steal syndrome through the use of the subclavian-to-subclavian artery bypass graft,[13,15] performed through two supraclavicular incisions, or the axillary-to-axillary bypass graft,[24] performed through two infraclavicular incisions. This procedure is currently favored by some surgeons (Fig. 4), and the patency of this graft in long-term studies has been favorable (Fig. 5).[28] Each procedure has the potential advantage of restoring normal hemodynamics in the patient with the subclavian steal syndrome without even temporarily interrupting the cerebral blood supply.

The subclavian-to-subclavian artery graft has the disadvantages of requiring much more extensive dissection than the carotid-to-subclavian bypass and of subjecting the patient to the potential hazard of bilateral phrenic nerve palsy. The axillary-to-axillary bypass graft again entails more extensive dissection than the carotid-to-subclavian bypass and requires the prosthesis to lie in a very exposed, superficial position between the skin and the sternum as it crosses the midline.

The results of corrective operative procedures have been excellent in terms of reversal of the hemodynamic abnormalities of the subclavian steal. Relief of associated cerebral symptoms has been achieved in 75 to 80 per cent of those patients operated on as well.[12] The operative mortality rate for carotid-to-subclavian artery bypass was reported at approximately 5 per cent in several large early series,[7,12] a figure that is surprisingly high, considering that carotid endarterectomy, a procedure of comparable magnitude performed in a similar patient population, has an operative mortality rate in the 1 per cent range. Fortunately, more recent publications have suggested that mortality from carotid-subclavian bypass by experienced surgeons is nearly nonexistent.

SELECTED REFERENCES

Crawford, E. S., Stowe, C. L., and Powers, R. W., Jr.: Occlusion of the innominate, common carotid and subclavian arteries: Long-term results of surgical treatment. Surgery *94*(5):781, 1983.

This recent report of the experience of the senior author with reconstructions for obstruction of the brachiocephalic arteries in 142 patients over a 23-year period points out that transthoracic and extrathoracic operations in recent years have carried an equally low mortality. In fact, 89 per cent of all patients survived operation, including early deaths when new techniques were being applied. Nevertheless, for single-vessel occlusions on one side of the neck, the authors still prefer the simplicity of the carotid-subclavian bypass and report that extrathoracic operations were performed in this large series in 69 per cent of their patients. Eighty-three per cent of the patients remained asymptomatic over a follow-up period that averaged 7.5 years.

Ehrenfeld, W. K., Chapman, R. D., and Wiley, E. J.: Management of occlusive lesions of the branches of the aortic arch. Am. J. Surg., *118*:236, 1969.
This in relatively early report from a group with wide experience in peripheral arterial surgery, the authors concluded that obstruction of the subclavian artery appeared to be better tolerated than obstruction of the other arteries supplying the brain, and that the presence of subclavian steal was probably an asymptomatic lesion in most patients. Of 157 patients with occlusive lesions of the major branches of the aortic arch, 50 per cent were free of significant symptoms from the onset or were made so by a carotid bifurcation endarterectomy.

Fields, W. S., and Lemak, N. A.: Joint study of extracranial artery occlusion. JAMA, *222*:139, 1972.
This is an excellent review of the fate of 168 patients with the subclavian steal syndrome, who were treated both medically and surgically in a large number of hospitals. The results of the study suggest that subclavian steal alone rarely, if ever, causes strokes and that symptomatic patients with subclavian steal are likely to have associated disease of the extracranial arteries. There was a relatively high incidence of complications (25 per cent) and mortality (8 per cent) following surgical correction of the subclavian steal.

Mehigan, J. T., Buch, W. S., Tipkin, R. D., and Fogarty, T. J.: Subclavian-carotid transposition for the subclavian steal syndrome. Am. J. Surg., *136*:15, 1978.
This paper was one of the first to describe the direct anastomosis of the divided distal subclavian artery to the side of the common carotid artery to correct cerebral symptoms of the subclavian steal syndrome and to relieve symptoms of arm claudication, often associated with proximal subclavian occlusive disease. The technique as described has the advantage of not requiring a graft to correct the subclavian steal and of eliminating the possibility of embolization of clot or atherosclerotic debris from the proximal subclavian stenosis, which theoretically can occur after repair of the subclavian steal by carotid-subclavian bypass.

Reivich, M., Holling, H. E., Roberts, B., and Toole, J. F.: Reversal of blood flow through the vertebral artery and its effect on cerebral circulation. N. Engl. J. Med., *265*:878, 1961.
This is the classic report describing the subclavian steal syndrome clinically and experimentally. Two patients were studied who had neurologic symptoms and reversal of flow in the left vertebral artery secondary to proximal subclavian stenosis, as demonstrated by angiography. Reversal of flow in the ipsilateral vertebral artery was demonstrated for the first time in the human at the time of operation in one of these patients by application of an electromagnetic flowmeter to the subclavian artery distal to the vertebral origin. The authors also report animal studies in which reversal of vertebral flow was demonstrated following subclavian artery occlusion. In the animal experiments, they concluded that total cerebral blood flow was markedly diminished by the subclavian steal.

REFERENCES

1. Barner, H. B., Kaiser, G. C., and Willman, V. L.: Hemodynamics of carotid-subclavian bypass. Arch. Surg., *103*:248, 1971.
2. Berger, R. L., Sidd, J. J., and Ramaswamy, K.: Retrograde vertebral-artery flow produced by correction of subclavian steal syndrome. N. Engl. J. Med., *277*:64, 1967.
3. Bosniak, M. A.: Cervical arterial pathways associated with brachiocephalic occlusive disease. Am. J. Roentgenol., *91*:1232, 1964.
4. Bryant, L. R., and Spencer, F. C.: Occlusive disease of the subclavian artery. JAMA, *196*:123, 1966.
5. Clark, K., and Perry, M. O.: Carotid vertebral anastomosis: An alternate technic for repair of the subclavian steal syndrome. Ann. Surg., *163*:414, 1966.
6. Contorni, L.: Il circolo collaterale vertebraovertebrale nella obliterazione dell'arterio subclavia all sua origine. Minerva Chir., *15*:268, 1960.
7. Crawford, E. S., DeBakey, M. E., Morris, G. C., Jr., and Howell, J. F.: Surgical treatment of occlusion of the innominate, common carotid, and subclavian arteries: A 10 year experience. Surgery, *65*:17, 1969.
8. Crawford, E. S., Stowe, C. L., and Power, R. W., Jr.: Occlusion of the innominate, common carotid, and subclavicular arteries: Long-term results of surgical treatment. Surgery, *94*:781, 1983.
9. Ehrenfeld, W. K., Chapman, R. D., and Wylie, E. J.: Management of occlusive lesions of the branches of the aortic arch. Am. J. Surg., *118*:236, 1969.
10. Eklof, B., and Schwartz, S. I.: Effects of subclavian steal and compromised cephalic blood flow on cerebral circulation. Surgery, *68*:431, 1970.
11. Ethier, R.: Observations on retrograde vertebral artery blood flow. Am. J. Roentgenol., *91*:1245, 1964.

12. Fields, W. S., and Lemak, N. A.: Joint study of extracranial arterial occlusion. JAMA, 222:1139, 1972.
13. Finkelstein, N. M., Byer, A., and Rush, B. F., Jr.: Subclavian-subclavian bypass for subclavian steal syndrome. Surgery, 71:142, 1972.
14. Folger, G. M., Jr., and Shah, K. D.: Subclavian steal, in patients with Blalock-Taussig anastomosis. Circulation, 31:241, 1965.
15. Forestner, J. E., Ghosh, S. K., Bergan, J. J., and Conn, J., Jr.: Subclavian-subclavian bypass for correction of the subclavian steal syndrome. Surgery, 71:136, 1972.
16. Gonzalez, L. L., Wiot, J. F., and Boyd, A. D.: Retrograde flow in the vertebral artery. Arch. Surg., 91:185, 1965.
17. Handa, J., Yoshida, K., and Meyer, J. S.: Hemodynamic effects of subclavian and innominate artery ligation. Surgery, 59:1069, 1966.
18. Harper, J. A., Golding, A. L., Mazzei, E. A., and Cannon, J. A.: An experimental hemodynamic study of the subclavian steal syndrome. Surg. Gynecol. Obstet., 124:1212, 1967.
19. Hewitt, R. L., Weichert, R. F., III, and Drapanas, T.: Centrifugal cerebral ischemia. Arch. Surg., 101:155, 1970.
20. Irvine, W. T., Luck, R. J., and Jacobey, J. A.: Reversed blood-flow in the vertebral arteries causing recurrent brain-stem ischaemia. Lancet, 1:994, 1965.
21. Janeway, R., Conrad, M., and Toole, J.: Chronic reversal of vertebral artery flow. Neurology, 15:430, 1965.
22. Killen, D. A., Foster, J. H., Gobbel, W. G., Jr., Stephenson, S. E., Jr., Collins, H. A., Billings, F. T., and Scott, H. W., Jr.: The subclavian steal syndrome. J. Thorac. Cardiovasc. Surg., 51:539, 1966.
23. LeVeen, H. H., Piccone, V. A., Jr., Diaz, C., Christoudias, G., Slade, W., and Norstrand, I.: A simplified correction of subclavian steal syndrome. Surgery, 72:299, 1974.
24. Lord, R. S. A., and Ehrenfeld, W. K.: Carotid-subclavian bypass: A hemodynamic study. Surgery, 66:521, 1969.
25. McDowell, H. A., Jr.: Surgical correction of vertebral steal followed by contralateral retrograde vertebral flow. Ann. Surg., 168:154, 1968.
26. Mannick, J. A., Suter, C. G., and Hume, D. M.: The "subclavian steal" syndrome: A further documentation. JAMA, 182:254, 1962.
27. Mehigan, J. T., Buch, W. S., Pipkin, R. D., and Fogarty, T. J.: Subclavian-carotid transposition for the subclavian steal syndrome. Am. J. Surg., 136:15, 1978.
28. Myers, W. O., Lawton, B. R., Ray, J. F., III, Kuehner, M. E., and Sautter, R. D.: Axillo-axillary bypass for subclavian steal syndrome. Arch. Surg., 114:394, 1979.
29. Najafi, H., Dye, W. S., Javid, H., Hunter, J. A., Ostermiller, W. E., and Julian, O. C.: Carotid bifurcation stenosis and ipsilateral subclavian steal. Arch. Surg., 99:289, 1969.
30. Newton, T. H., and Wylie, E. J.: Collateral circulation associated with occlusion of the proximal subclavian and innominate arteries. Am. J. Roentgenol., 91:394, 1964.
31. North, R. R., Fields, W. S., DeBakey, M. E., et al.: Brachial-basilar insufficiency syndrome. Neurology, 12:810, 1962.
32. Piccone, V. A., Jr., Karvounis, P., and LeVeen, H. H.: The subclavian steal syndrome. Angiology, 21:240, 1970.
33. Pineda, A., and Smith, J. L.: True and false subclavian steal syndromes. Collateral circulation of the true subclavian steal syndrome demonstrated by angiography. Arch. Surg., 92:258, 1966.
34. Powers, S. R., Jr., Roe, G. M., and Creel, W.: The relation between regional cerebral blood flow and cerebral function. Surgery, 61:74, 1967.
35. Reivich, M., Holling, H. E., Roberts, B., et al.: Reversal of blood flow through the vertebral artery and its effect on cerebral circulation. N. Engl. J. Med., 265:878, 1961.
36. Resnicoff, S. A., DeWeese J. A., and Rob, C. G.: Surgical treatment of the subclavian steal syndrome. Circulation, 41 and 42 (Suppl. 2):147, 1970.
37. Rob, C.: Technique of surgical therapy. In Millikan, C. H., Siekert, R. G., and Whisnant, J. P. (Eds.): Cerebral Vascular Diseases, Third Conference. New York, Grune & Stratton, 1961, p. 112.
38. Sammartino, W. F., and Toole, J. F.: Reversed vertebral artery flow. Arch. Neurol., 10:590, 1964.
39. Santschi, D. R., Frahm, C. J., Pascale, L. R., and Dumanian, A. V.: The subclavian steal syndrome. J. Thorac. Cardiovasc. Surg., 51:103, 1966.
40. Shockman, A. T.: Retrograde vertebral artery flow as an artifact of technique. Am. J. Roentgenol., 91:1258, 1964.
41. Siekert, R. G., Millikan, C. H., and Whisnant, J. P.: Reversed blood flow in the vertebral arteries. Ann. Intern. Med., 61:64, 1964.
42. Solti, F., Iskum, M., Papp, S., Turbok, E., and Nagy, J.: The regulation of cerebral blood circulation in subclavian steal syndrome. Circulation, 42:1185, 1970.
43. Vogt, D. P., Hertzer, N. R., O'Hara, P. J., and Beven, E. G.: Brachiocephalic arterial reconstruction. Ann. Surg., 196:541, 1982.
44. Yum, K. Y., and Myers, R. N.: Vertebral artery ligation. Arch. Surg., 98:199, 1969.
45. Ziomek, S., Quinones-Baldrich, W. J., Busuttil, R. W., Baker, J. D., Machleder, H. I., and Moore, W. S.: The superiority of synthetic arterial grafts over autologous veins in carotid-subclavian bypass. J. Vasc. Surg., 3:140, 1986.

4. THROMBOTIC OBLITERATION OF THE ABDOMINAL AORTA AND ILIAC ARTERIES (LERICHE SYNDROME)

David C. Sabiston, Jr., M.D.

Thrombotic obliteration of the aortic bifurcation was first described by Leriche in 1923.[3] An excellent summary appeared in English in 1948.[4] Leriche emphasized that the disorder is a chronic one and is associated with a specific symptom complex. Typically, the condition affects men 35 to 60 years of age.

Clinical Manifestations

The symptoms characteristic of thrombotic occlusion of the terminal aorta include (1) extreme liability to fatigue of both lower limbs, which Leriche described as a weariness, rather than the typical intermittent claudication; (2) symmetrical atrophy of both lower limbs without trophic changes of the skin or nails; (3) pallor of the legs and feet; and (4) inability to maintain a stable erection due to inadequate arterial flow to the penis from hypogastric arterial obstruction, thus reducing the blood flow through the internal pudendal artery and its blood flow to the corpora cavernosa. The physical findings include absence of pulses in the abdominal aorta and in arteries distally. The changes in arterial pressure are shown in Figure 1.[7] Distal sites of segmental occlusion produce a further fall in arterial pressure, and ischemic ulceration may appear.

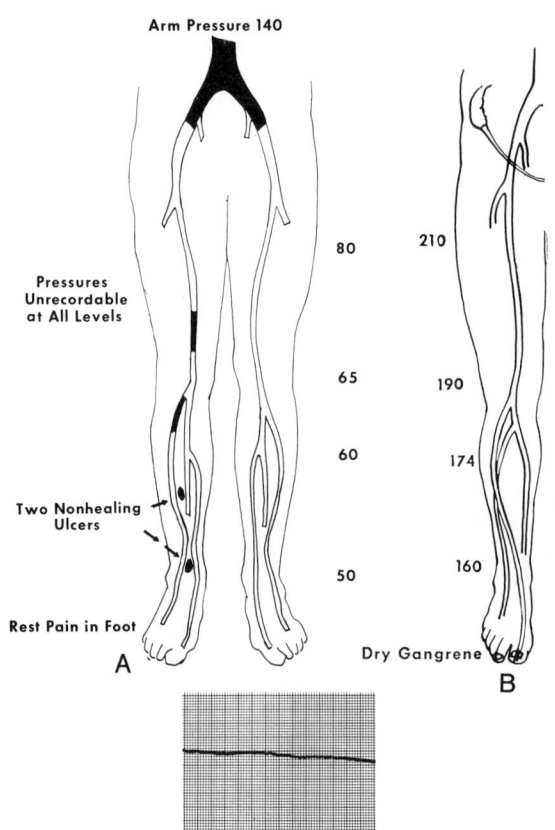

Figure 1. The extensive aortoiliac occlusion, combined with the superficial femoral artery and anterior tibial artery occlusion, reduced limb blood pressures below recordable levels. *B*, The normal ankle pressure of 160 mm. Hg and absent digit pulses placed the arterial occlusion between the ankle and digits. (From Strandness, D. E., Jr.: Collateral Circulation in Clinical Surgery. Philadelphia, W. B. Saunders Company, 1969.)

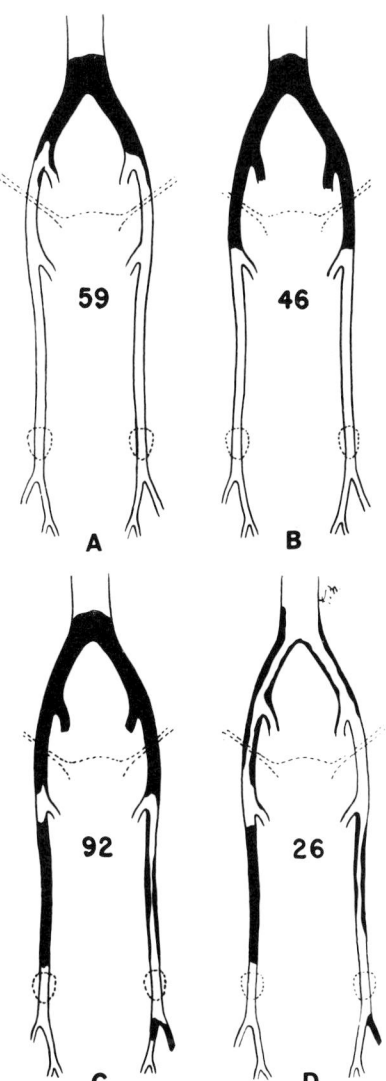

Figure 2. Classification of extent of involvement in a series of patients with aortoiliofemoral arterial occlusive disease. (From Perdue, G. D., Long, W. D., and Smith, R. B., III: *Perspective concerning aortofemoral arterial reconstruction.* Trans. South. Surg. Assoc., *82:*330, 1970.)

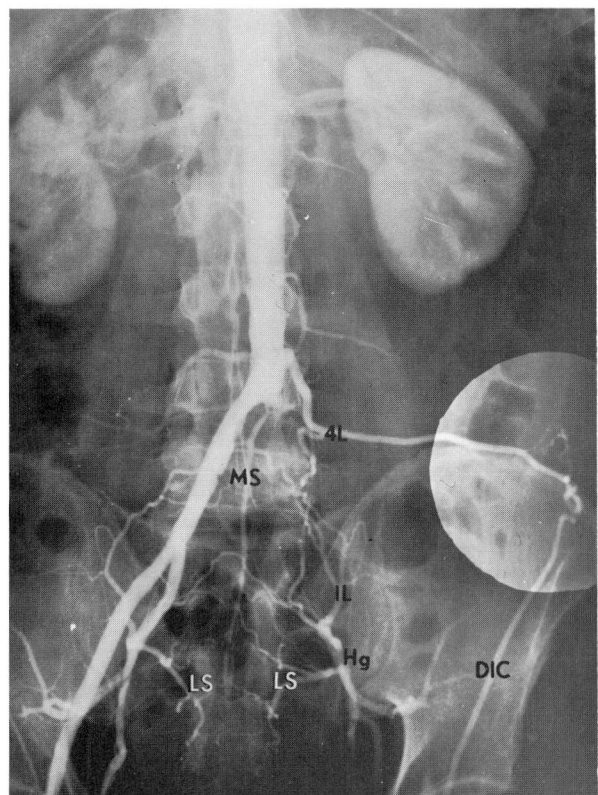

Figure 3. A 43-year-old male with left intermittent claudication. The fourth lumbar (4L) is the origin of a pathway to the femoral via the deep iliac circumflex (DIC) and to the hypogastric (Hg) via the iliolumbar (IL). The middle sacral (MS) and lateral sacral (LS) contribute to a transpelvic anastomosis to the hypogastric (Hg). (From Friedenberg, M. J., and Perez, C. A.: *Collateral circulation in aortoiliofemoral disease: As demonstrated by a unilateral percutaneous common femoral artery needle injection.* A. J. R., *94:*145, 1965.)

Leriche emphasized that the disorder was often well tolerated for 5 and even 10 years but usually ended in gangrene of one or both legs. The usual pathologic finding is atherosclerosis of the arterial wall with superimposed thrombosis. The lumen usually narrows over a period of months such that acute symptoms are not likely to occur.

The diagnosis is confirmed by arteriography showing occlusion of the terminal abdominal aorta and often of one or both common iliac arteries (Fig. 2).[1,5] The occlusion may involve any portion of the abdominal aorta from the renal arteries distally. The collateral circulation around the arterial blockage is shown in Figure 3.[2]

It is quite important that patients cease smoking after bypass grafts are performed. The evidence is clear that thrombosis of grafts is appreciably increased by continuance of smoking.[6] The relationship showing percentage of graft occlusion according to the smoking history is shown in Figure 4.

Surgical Management

Although thromboendarterectomy with direct reconstitution of flow is appropriate in a few patients, the majority with occlusion of the abdominal aorta are managed by bypass grafts from the aorta to the iliac or more often the common femoral arteries

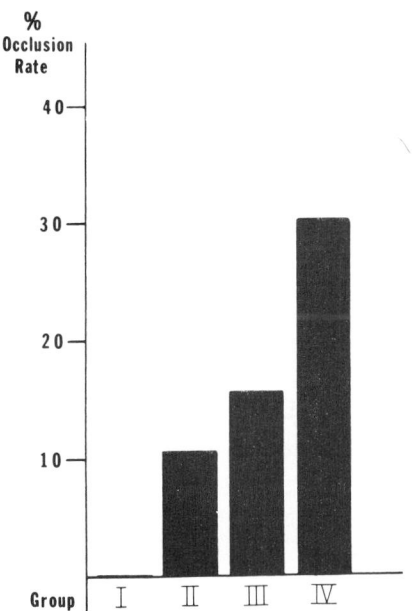

Figure 4. Occlusion rate of prosthetic grafts inserted for Leriche syndrome according to smoking history. Group I: Patients who did not smoke either before or after operation. Group II: Patients who were cigarette smokers before operation but ceased smoking postoperatively. Group III: Patients who were cigarette smokers preoperatively and who continued to smoke following operation up to one pack daily. Group IV: Patients who remained heavy smokers following operation, using more than a pack of cigarettes daily. (From Robicsek, F., Daugherty, H. K., Mullen, D. C., Masters, T. N., Narbay, D., and Sanger, P. W.: *The effect of continued cigarette smoking on the patency of synthetic vascular grafts in Leriche syndrome.* J. Thorac. Cardiovasc. Surg., *70:*107, 1975.)

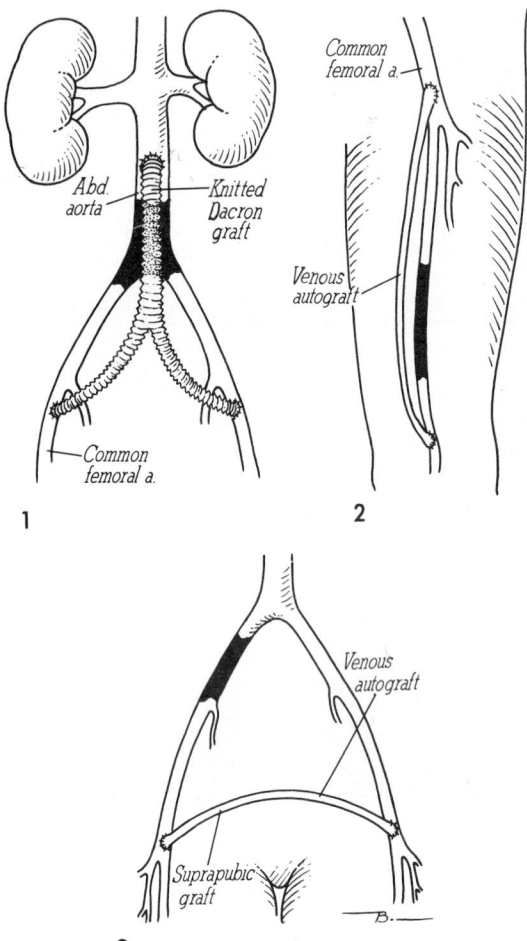

Figure 5. Diagrammatic illustration of various bypass grafts. *1*, For occlusion of the abdominal aorta, a bypass graft placed proximal to the occlusion can be inserted distally into each of the common femoral arteries in the groin. *2*, For occlusion of the superficial femoral artery, a venous autograft may be placed from the common femoral artery above to the femoral or popliteal artery distal to the obstruction. *3*, For unilateral iliac arterial occlusion, a suprapubic graft can be placed from one common femoral artery to the other in a subcutaneous suprapubic tunnel. Generally, under these circumstances a venous autograft is preferable to a plastic prosthesis, although the latter can be employed.

(Fig. 5). It may be necessary to perform a thromboendarterectomy distal to the renal arteries to permit a patent lumen for the proximal anastomosis. However, it is important to minimize dissection in this region for preventing damage to the sympathetic and parasympathetic nerves. This helps to prevent postoperative retrograde ejaculation.

SELECTED REFERENCES

Foster, J. H.: Arteriography. Cornerstone of vascular surgery. Arch. Surg., *109:*605, 1974.
  In this essay, the development of arteriography from its origin to the present is reviewed. Of particular significance is the fact that the author advocates more extensive use of arteriography.
Strandness, D. E., and Sumner, D. S.: Hemodynamics for Surgeons. New York, Grune & Stratton, 1975.
  This is an excellent and quite thorough monograph concerning the hemodynamics of the vascular system. The determinants of cardiac output and arterial and venous flow as well as a variety of physical and physiologic aspects of the entire field are discussed. In addition, a number of clinical problems are used as examples illustrating the basic physical and physiologic principles.

REFERENCES

1. Foster, J. H.: Arteriography. Cornerstone of vascular surgery. Arch Surg., *109:*605, 1974.

2. Friedenberg, M. J., and Perez, C. A.: Collateral circulation in aortoilio-femoral occlusive disease: As demonstrated by a unilateral percutaneous common femoral artery needle injection. A.J.R., *94:*145, 1965.
3. Leriche, R.: 3° Sympathectomie. Des obliterations arterielles hautes (obliteration de la terminaison de l'aorte) comme causes des insuffisances circulatoires des membres inferieurs. Bull. Mem. Soc. Chir. Paris, *49:*1404, 1923.
4. Leriche, R., and Morel, A.: The syndrome of thrombotic obliteration of the aortic bifurcation. Ann. Surg., *127:*193, 1948.
5. Perdue, G. D., Long, W. D., and Smith, R. B., III: Perspective concerning aortofemoral arterial reconstruction. Trans. South. Surg. Assoc., *82:*330, 1979.
6. Robicsek, F., Daughterty, H. K., Mullen, D. C., Masters, T. N., Narbay, D., and Sanger, P. W.: The effect of continued cigarette smoking on the patency of synthetic vascular grafts in Leriche syndrome. J. Thorac. Cardiovasc. Surg., *70:*107, 1975.
7. Strandness, D. E., Jr.: Chronic arterial occlusion. *In* Strandness, D. E., Jr. (Ed.): Collateral Circulation in Clinical Surgery. Philadelphia, W. B. Saunders Company, 1969.

5. ILIAC ARTERIAL OCCLUSION

David C. Sabiston, Jr., M.D.

The iliac arteries may be individually stenosed or occluded. The symptoms are usually those of claudication of the hip and thigh associated with diminished or absent pulses in that extremity. Arteriography is diagnostic. When symptoms are unilateral, involvement of the opposite leg can often be seen on the arteriogram. Indeed, symptoms may appear in the opposite leg following operation when the patient is able to exercise sufficiently. Bypass grafts from the aorta above to the common femoral artery below are usually indicated.

6. FEMOROPOPLITEAL AND FEMOROINFRAPOPLITEAL BYPASS

Richard L. McCann, M.D.

Historical Aspects

The present capability to revascularize the ischemic lower extremity is based on many experimental and clinical contributions that began with the first successful vascular anastomosis by Eck in 1877. In the first decade of the twentieth century, Alexis Carrel established the principles of vascular anastomosis by painstaking research in animals.[5] His work allowed the subsequent successful application of vascular surgery to man. Carrel emphasized delicate handling of vascular tissues and meticulous coaptation of flow surfaces by suturing with fine needles and lubricated sutures. He also demonstrated the feasibility of transplanting a segment of vein into the arterial circulation. For these achievements, Carrel was awarded the Nobel Prize for Physiology and Medicine in 1912. Important clinical advances soon followed. Goyanes is credited with the first successful application of vein grafting in man. In 1906, he used a segment of popliteal vein to bridge the defect created by resection of a syphilitic popliteal artery aneurysm. Six months later, Lexer reported a second case of arterial replacement, this time using a saphenous vein graft. It is interesting to note that both of these clinical surgeons were familiar with, and gave credit to, the pioneering experimental work of Carrel.[13] Fifty-one cases of vein grafts for trauma were reported by Weglowski from military casualties in World War I. Except for the discovery of heparin by Howell and McLean in 1916,[7] the treatment of obstructive peripheral vascular disease did not advance again until after World War II when Dos Santos reported the use of femoral endarterectomy. Also at this time, Jean Kunlin of Paris reintroduced the bypass principle first proposed by Jeger in 1913. In his 1949 paper, Kunlin[17] credits Carrel, Lexer, and Dos Santos for providing the foundation upon which his own achievement rested. The ingenious concept that it was not necessary to resect an obstructed artery but merely bypass it with end-to-side anastomoses proximal and distal to the occluded segment has remained an important principle in vascular surgery and has been expanded to encompass nearly all segments of the vascular tree. Dale, in 1963, first demonstrated the feasibility of placing vein grafts to the small tibial vessels in the calf.[8]

The first arterial substitutes to be used were biologic grafts obtained from cadavers. Fresh and later preserved human vessels were used to revascularize the lower extremity, but these have continued to be plagued by rapid degeneration.

After 2 ½ years of work in animals, Blakemore and Voorhees introduced the first synthetic arterial substitute in man in 1953.[3] The original fabric, "vinyon N," soon was replaced with the use of nylon, Orlon, Teflon, and Dacron. The last fabric became the preferred one. Although effective in large vessels, fabric grafts were found to be less suitable as substitutes for smaller arteries, especially when long grafts crossing joint lines were needed. Attempts to improve the performance of these grafts by "seeding" them with viable endothelial cells have been made but without clear-cut success to date. The use of expanded polytetrafluoroethylene tubes in the femoropopliteal position in man was reported in 1975.[4] This material has become the most frequently used arterial substitute when autogenous saphenous vein is not available.

The treatment of vascular stenoses and obstructions by catheter dilation techniques was reported by Dotter and Judkins in 1964.[10] Subsequently Grüntzig popularized the balloon dilation catheter technique for treatment of peripheral vascular stenosis.[12] More recently miniature cutting devices mounted on angiographic catheters have been used to obliterate arterial stenosis in the lower extremities.[24] Application of these catheter techniques to peripheral vascular disease continues to expand.

Thus, the current practice of revascularization of the ischemic lower extremity has developed both from the experimental laboratory and from clinical contributions. A firm basis has been established upon which it is expected that future developments and improvements will occur.

CLINICAL EVALUATION

An accurate diagnosis of the presence of vascular disease as well as its location and severity can often be made after completing a comprehensive history and physical examination. Patients with peripheral vascular disease usually complain of pain. Careful analysis of the location, quality, intensity, and factors that aggravate and relieve the pain yields important information. Ischemic pain has a characteristic quality that is unlikely to be confused with other conditions. The term claudication (from the Latin verb *claudicatio*, to limp) is applied to the cramping pain felt in specific muscle groups when nutritive blood flow is inadequate to meet the metabolic demands of exercise. The distance walked before onset of this pain is strikingly reproducible, and the pain is promptly relieved simply by cessation of ambulation. Claudication of the buttock and thigh muscles is indicative of aortoiliac obstruction, whereas calf claudication usually indicates femoral artery disease. When blood flow is inadequate to meet metabolic requirements at rest, continuous pain may be described. This pain is usually felt in the toes and feet. It is often prominent at night. With assumption of the recumbent position, there is a decrease in the driving pressure proximal to a vascular obstruction because of absence of the hydrostatic component of pressure. This may cause the flow across a stenosis to decrease below a threshold value and awaken the patient with pain.

Patients often discover that restoring a hydrostatic pressure component by hanging the foot over the bed or by standing relieves the pain. Rest pain is an ominous symptom and demands prompt evaluation not only because of the considerable discomfort for the patient but because it indicates such severe vascular compromise that the involved limb may soon progress to frank gangrene in the absence of intervention.

Ischemic ulceration refers to localized skin necrosis that is associated with arterial insufficiency and fails to heal after a period of 6 weeks. It may be observed anywhere but is usually found on the plantar surface of the foot or between the toes. This type of lesion occurs not so much from infarction of the skin as from local trauma that in the well-vascularized extremity would be minor. In the severely ischemic limb, reparative and healing processes are so impaired that even minor lesions fail to heal and often progress. The end stage of vascular insufficiency is frank tissue infarction or gangrene. If this is associated with infection, emergency treatment may be required to eliminate the source of systemic sepsis.

Other historical aspects in the initial clinical evaluation may aid in the management of the vascular patient. It is important to note the presence of vascular disease in other systems. Atherosclerosis is a systemic disorder, and overt manifestations of concomitant cerebrovascular or coronary artery disease may influence the management of lower extremity ischemia. It would be unwise, for example, to perform a major operative procedure to alleviate claudication at 100 yards if the patient remained severely limited by angina or shortness of breath. The importance of associated coronary and cerebrovascular disease in the patient with lower extremity ischemia cannot be overemphasized. In one major long-term study, 75 per cent of the patients with infrainguinal reconstructions were dead by 10 years, and most all deaths were from myocardial infarction or cerebrovascular accident.[9]

The presence of other conditions associated with vascular disease such as diabetes and hypertension must be noted. The social history is also of great importance. Patients who continue to use tobacco have inferior results and every effort should be made to induce these patients to cease.[1] In the patient with claudication, it is important to record the desired or necessary life-style. Claudication at 100 yards is obviously of greater significance to a patient who is required to walk to earn a living, such as a postman, than it is to an older retired patient whose life may be limited very little by having to rest after walking 100 yards.

Physical Examination

The physical examination often confirms the suspicions raised by the history. Inspection of the limb may reveal muscular atrophy; skin changes associated with vascular insufficiency include a thin, brittle, shiny texture, and often the nails are thick and opaque. Hair may be absent or thinned over the toes and feet. Pallor may be present particularly with elevation of the legs to 60 degrees for 1 to 2 minutes. This is usually associated with rubor when the feet are then placed in a dependent position. Rubor is thought to be due to cutaneous reactive vasodilation in response to chronic ischemia. Pallor of elevation and rubor of dependency are signs of advanced vascular insufficiency and are seldom seen if only claudication is present. Palpation of the extremities is important, searching for temperature changes and examining the pulses. An appreciation of the pulse amplitude and duration and the presence of turbulent flow may be obtained. Proximal obstruction affects the distal pulses not only by a decrease in the mean pressure but also by a decrease in the perceived pulse amplitude because the pulse pressure is narrowed distal to a site of obstruction. Palpation of the pulses is best made by a warm hand in a warm room. In the obese patient, external rotation of the hip may aid in palpation of the femoral pulse. The popliteal pulse is often difficult to palpate in the obese patient even by the experienced examiner. In fact, a prominent and easily palpable popliteal pulse should raise the question of a popliteal aneurysm. The dorsalis pedis and posterior tibial pulses are usually not palpable in patients with lower limb ischemia owing to proximal obstruction. It should be remembered that in up to 10 per cent of normal extremities one of these ankle pulses may be absent owing to anatomic variation in vascular supply to the foot. If ankle pulses are present, the effect of exercise should be noted, because if these pulses are not diminished directly following exercise, the diagnosis of vascular insufficiency is in doubt. Another important aspect of the vascular examination is an evaluation of the saphenous vein. The patient is asked to stand, and the vein is observed and palpated beginning at the medial malleolus and proceeding proximally. This is especially important when a long bypass to the tibial vessels is contemplated.

Auscultation for bruits should be performed over the femoral area and also over the abdomen to detect the presence of potentially limiting iliac and distal aortic lesions. The vascular examination also includes palpation for the presence of an abdominal aortic aneurysm, auscultation for a carotid bruit, and a search for cardiac disease. The general examination may also disclose other disease that may influence the management of the vascular patient, such as orthopedic or pulmonary conditions.

Vascular Laboratory

Noninvasive vascular laboratories have become common. Although these examinations have many limitations, they may be useful in evaluating the patient with lower extremity ischemia, particularly in quantification of disability and localization of the site of obstruction. The three most useful examinations are determinations of segmental Doppler pressures, pulse volume recordings, and response to standardized exercise.

The Doppler instrument is a velocity detector and not a flowmeter. It contains a piezoelectric crystal that when electrically excited emits a narrow ultrasound beam. The beam travels through a coupling gel and passes through the skin and tissues to an underlying blood vessel. The sound beam is then reflected by the moving red blood cells within the vessel lumen, and in this reflection the frequency of the sound waves is shifted (the Doppler shift) in proportion to the velocity of the blood. The reflected sound waves are sensed by a second crystal, and the shift in frequency is processed as an audible or analog signal. Commercial Doppler units are available with emitting frequencies of 3.5 to 10 megacycles per second. Because the depth of penetration of the sound waves is inversely proportional to the emitted frequency, the higher frequency units are most useful for examination of the relatively superficial vessels of the lower extremity.

Doppler examination of the lower extremity vessels can be used to determine the presence or absence of detectable flow within a vessel. It requires a flow velocity of 5 cm. per second to obtain a reliable signal in most commercially available units. The quality of the signal may also provide additional information. The normal arterial signal is triphasic. This corresponds to the rapid flow during systole, the initial reversal of flow in diastole, and the gradual return of forward flow during the late phase of diastole. When listening to a vessel distal to a site of obstruction, the signal first becomes biphasic, and as the degree of obstruction increases, the signal becomes uniphasic with no or little variation between systole and diastole. This corresponds to the dampening of the velocity profile across the site of obstruction (Fig. 1).

By inflation of appropriately sized blood pressure cuffs placed on the thigh, below the knee, and above the ankle and listening with the Doppler unit over a distal artery, segmental pressures can be obtained. A drop in pressure across a segment suggests the presence of a stenosis. Pressure values may be standardized by comparing the observed values with the brach-

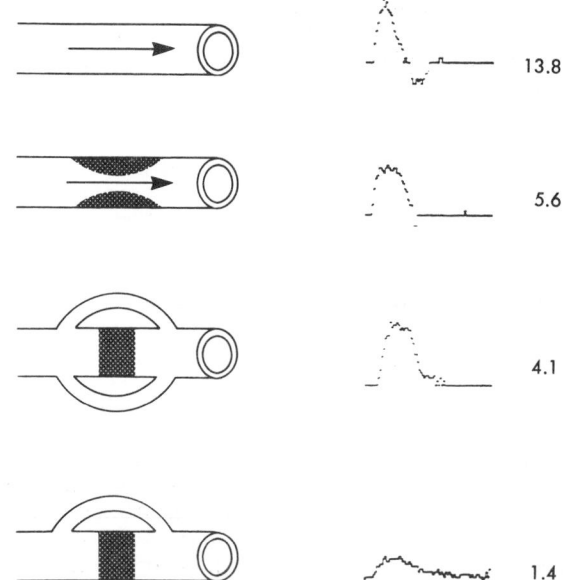

Figure 1. Progressive dampening of Doppler velocity waveform by proximal arterial stenosis. (From Johnson, K. W.: Doppler signal processing and waveform analysis: Problems and solutions. *In* Bernstein, E. F. (Ed.): Noninvasive Diagnostic Techniques in Vascular Disease. St. Louis, C. V. Mosby, 1982.)

ial pressure, for example, the ankle/brachial index. Simultaneously, recordings of the pulse volume can be obtained by using the cuffs as volume plethysmographs. The response of these parameters to exercise yields an evaluation of the functional significance of a stenosis. Exercise produces vasodilation in the distal vascular bed. If inflow is restricted by a proximal stenosis, the pressure in the distal bed falls. Practically, the degree and duration of the fall in ankle/brachial pressure index following a standardized (10 per cent grade, 2 m.p.h., 5 minutes) walking exercise is recorded. An added benefit of this test is a comparison of the exercise limitations imposed by lower limb vascular insufficiency with those of concomitant pulmonary, orthopedic, or cardiac disease. An example of a complete noninvasive laboratory examination report is shown in Figure 2.

A number of other techniques have utilized sophisticated new technology for noninvasive evaluation of patients with peripheral vascular disease. Among these are the use of an oxygen electrode coupled directly to the skin to measure transcutaneous oxygen tension ($tcPo_2$). This test purports to measure the metabolic state of the limb rather than specific hemodynamic variables. However, oxygen tension in the skin does not decrease until ischemia is far advanced, and thus this examination has limited usefulness in the patient with claudication. Similarly, a relative index of cutaneous blood flow at any site on the limb can be obtained with the laser Doppler. The principle used in this instrument is identical to that used in ultrasonic velocity detectors except that a laser beam is substituted for the sound beam. Because the incident laser beam intersects the cutaneous microvasculature at multiple angles and multiple levels, the frequency shift is a composite of various intercepts and angles. Thus, the frequency shift is averaged over a considerable area and specific quantitative information is not derived. Nevertheless, the information derived may be clinically useful particularly when only qualitative information is needed that can be compared over time such as before and after a revascularization. Perhaps the most promising new development in noninvasive vascular diagnosis is the recent technical improvements in and thus increased popularity of duplex scanning. Sophisticated, modern duplex ultrasound scanning instruments are able to simultaneously display a real-time image of the vessel structure as well as directionally segregated flow events within the lumen. This permits identification of areas of stenosis, identifi-

Peripheral Arterial Exam

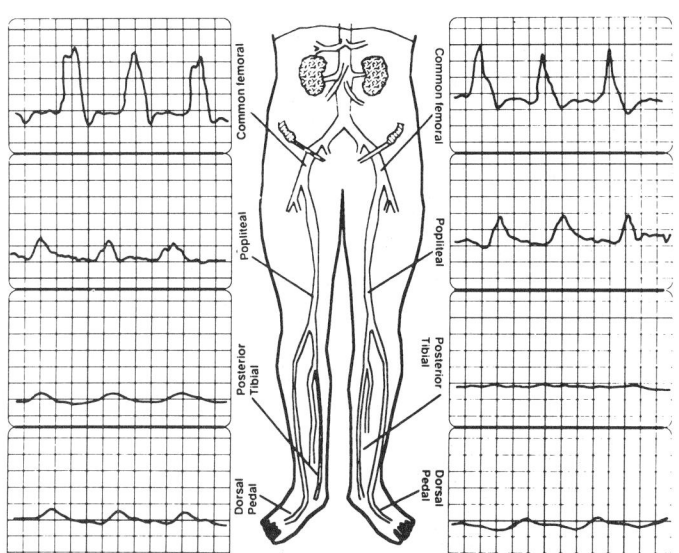

Resting Segmental Blood Pressures:

	RIGHT		LEFT	
	Pressure	Leg/Arm Ratio	Pressure	Leg/Arm Ratio
Arm	168		168	
Upper thigh	124	.74	127	.76
Above knee	99	.59	115	.68
Below knee	88	.52	100	.59
Ankle D.P.	82	.48	80	.48
P.T.	82	.48	74	.44
Toe	60	.36	66	.39

Treadmill: 1.5 mph at 0% grade.

Stopped arbitrarily; no discomfort at 5:00 (202 meters)

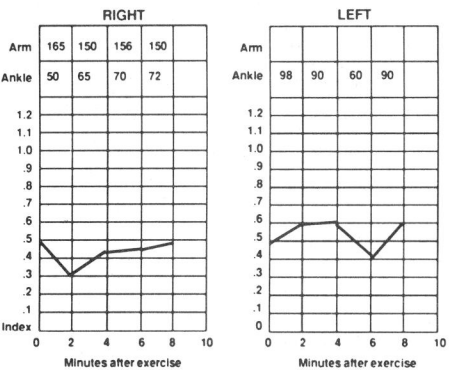

	RIGHT			
Arm	165	150	156	150
Ankle	50	65	70	72

	LEFT			
Arm				
Ankle	98	90	60	90

Minutes after exercise

Figure 2. Information obtained from standard noninvasive peripheral arterial examination provides complete assessment of lower extremity circulation. (From Taylor, L. M., Jr., and Porter, J. M.: Natural history and nonoperative treatment of chronic lower extremity ischemia. *In* Rutherford, R. B. (Ed.): Vascular Surgery, 3rd ed., Philadelphia, W. B. Saunders Company, 1989.

cation of areas of turbulence due to vessel wall irregularity, and visualization of flow disturbances such as stenotic jets. As technology and computer integration of the available images and data increase, advances and improvements are certain to occur.

The noninvasive vascular laboratory examination should not be used alone. Rather it is used to complement the information obtained from the history and physical examination and helps to establish a baseline for future comparison. This evaluation is useful whether the patient is treated medically or has an operation. In addition, these tests form an objective and semiquantitative method of following the success of revascularization procedures and may be helpful in detecting problems in the postoperative period at an early stage when they may still be corrected (Fig. 3).

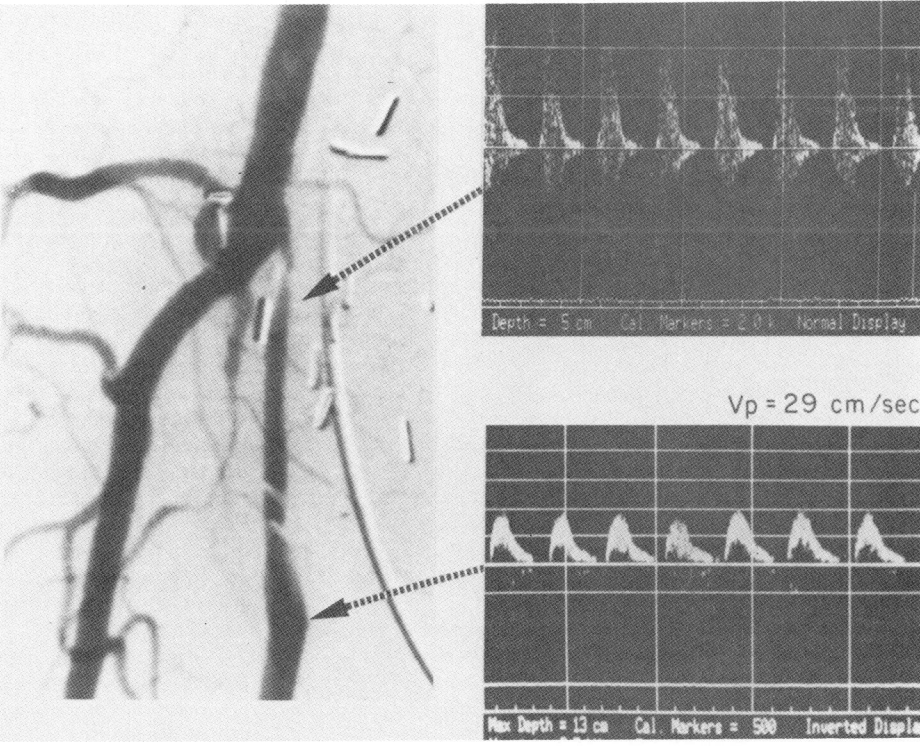

Figure 3. Use of duplex scan in postoperative surveillance detects graft stenosis before it progresses to graft thrombosis and while revision and graft salvage are possible. (From Bandyk, D. F.: Perioperative use of duplex scan. *In* Bergan, J. S., and Yao, J. S. T. (Eds.): Arterial Surgery: New Diagnostic and Operative Techniques. Orlando, Grune & Stratton, 1988.)

Indications for Surgical Intervention

Treatment decisions in patients with vascular insufficiency of the lower extremity are based on an analysis of the potential risks and benefits. The goals of therapy are prevention of limb loss, relief of pain, maintenance of bipedal gait, and avoidance of disability.

Studies of the natural history of intermittent claudication have shown that patients with this as the sole manifestation of lower limb ischemia have a low risk of limb loss. In fact, over 75 per cent of these patients remain stable or even improve with conservative management alone.[15,20] The amputation rate is less than 7 per cent in patients treated medically and followed up to 8 years. Nonsurgical management consists of cessation of smoking, control of weight, and a graduated exercise program. The importance of abstinence from tobacco cannot be overemphasized. Men who smoke are nine times more likely to develop intermittent claudication than are nonsmokers. Importantly, patients who stop smoking less frequently have progression of disease from claudication to rest pain, require fewer bypass operations, and experience a significantly reduced amputation and mortality.[14] Although tobacco smoke produces demonstrable changes in vascular endothelial cell function and metabolism, as well as alteration of blood viscosity, platelet function, and the coagulation mechanism, the exact process by which it exerts its deleterious effect on the development and progression of atherosclerosis remains undetermined.[6] It is important to note that the risk of limb loss in patients with chronic lower extremity ischemia who ceased smoking has been found to be reduced in many studies.[6] Conversely, it has been demonstrated that continued smoking following surgical lower extremity revascularization causes dramatically reduced limb salvage rate.[1]

It has been demonstrated in a number of longitudinal studies that a program of regular walking exercise leads to a measurable improvement in walking distance in patients with intermittent claudication. The mechanism responsible for this improvement is not fully understood. The assumption that exercise leads to stimulation of the development of natural collaterals has not been supported by objective data examining exercise-induced changes in blood flow. Rather it is now thought that improved performance following exercise is due to adaptive changes in

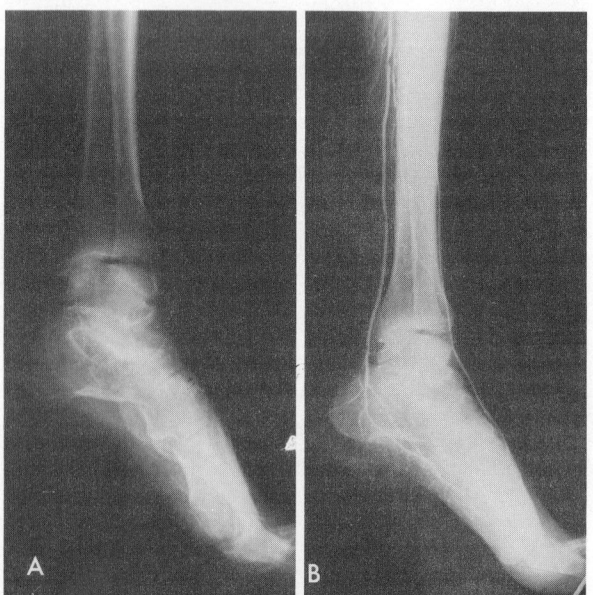

Figure 4. *A,* Preoperative arteriogram shows only faint visualization of the distal leg and foot vessels. *B,* Improved visualization of the distal vessels of the same patient by direct injection at operation. This visualization allowed subsequent femoral to posterior tibial bypass. (From Flanigan, D. F., Williams, L. R., Keith, J., Schuler, J. J., and Behrend, J. A.: Prebypass operative arteriography. Surgery, 92:627, 1982.)

the muscle enzyme systems leading to more efficient oxygen extraction and utilization.

Thus, initial recommendations for the patient presenting with intermittent claudication include strong encouragement to *completely* discontinue the use of tobacco, to participate in a regular exercise program of at least one hour's duration daily, of walking to the point of claudication, resting, and then continuing again for another cycle, and to control weight to minimize the amount of work required. Adherence to this advice often leads to a doubling or greater of claudication distance and may be the only treatment required.

In patients in whom nonsurgical treatment fails to alleviate the disability imposed by intermittent claudication and in whom symptoms interfere with gaining a livelihood or impose an intolerable limitation of life-style, surgical treatment can be offered with the understanding that the goal is improvement in exercise capacity rather than salvage of the limb. In contrast, patients with rest pain, ischemic ulcerations, or limited gangrene are generally candidates for vascular reconstruction because the threat of limb loss is much greater. In patients who present with gangrene, the necrotic tissue must be limited to the toes or distal metatarsal level. If the tissue remaining following debridement of the necrotic tissue is insufficient to function as a weight-bearing surface, the patient is more likely to maintain independent mobility and bipedal gait with amputation and a leg prosthesis.

Arteriography

Arteriography is necessary only if it has been decided that revascularization is indicated. It is used to determine if balloon dilation or other catheter-related treatment is feasible and in surgical patients to confirm the adequacy of inflow at the femoral level and to select the sites for the proximal and distal anastomoses. The entire vascular tree from the distal aorta to the foot should be visualized. Biplane views are occasionally helpful and may reveal lesions not seen with a single projection. Inadequate visualization of the distal vascular bed may be due to the small amount of contrast material reaching the leg if the obstructive process is severe. Reactive hyperemia induced by inflation of blood pressure cuffs placed around the thighs and inflated for several minutes before injection may be helpful. If doubt remains concerning optimal placement of the distal anastomosis, prebypass intraoperative arteriography with direct injection may be of benefit in selected cases (Fig. 4).

Adequate visualization of the entire arterial system of the lower extremity ensures that a bypass graft will not be placed proximal to a tandem stenosis, which might jeopardize long-term patency of the graft.

PERCUTANEOUS METHODS OF TREATMENT

A number of catheter-based treatment options are now available for treatment of patients with peripheral vascular obstructive disease in the lower extremities. The first of these to be widely introduced was balloon catheter dilation introduced by Grüntzig in 1974 following the successful coaxial dilation achieved by Dotter and Judkins a decade earlier. Dilation achieves an enlarged lumen by the mechanism of intimal fracture and stretching of the remaining vessel wall. This is a traumatic procedure and, as might be expected, causes a high rate of thrombosis if attempted over long vessel segments.[2] It succeeds quite well for stenoses and even occlusions that are less than 10 cm. in length that cause claudication, but the results with more severe disease that threatens limb survival has not been as favorable (Fig. 5).

In an attempt to improve the modest results achieved with balloon dilation, other catheter-based techniques have been introduced that attempt not only to stretch the vessel but to actually effect removal of plaque material. These include laser sys-

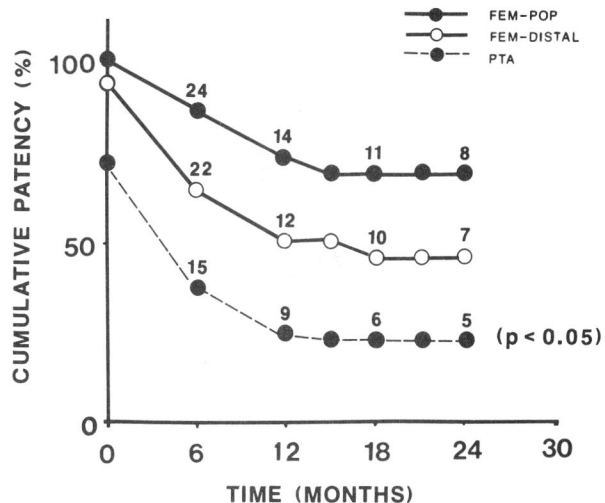

Figure 5. Cumulative patency of bypasses and percutaneous transluminal angioplasty by life-table method. Limbs at risk noted at each interval. (From Blair, J. M., Gewertz, B. L., Moosa, H., Lu, C. T., and Zarins, C. K.: Percutaneous transluminal angioplasty versus surgery for limb-threatening ischemia. J. Vasc. Surg., 9:698, 1989.)

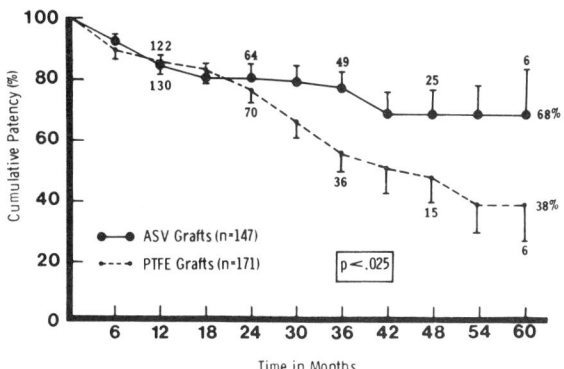

Figure 6. Cumulative life-table primary patency rates for all randomized bypasses performed to popliteal artery with autologous saphenous vein (ASV) and polytetrafluoroethylene (PTFE) grafts. Number with each point indicates number of patent grafts observed for that length of time. Standard error of each point is shown. (From Veith, F. J., Gupta, S. K., Ascer, E., et al.: Six-year prospective multicenter randomized comparison of autologous saphenous vein and expanded polytetrafluoroethylene grafts in infrainguinal arterial reconstructions. J. Vasc. Surg., 3:104, 1986.)

tems and mechanical atherectomy devices. Neither of these approaches has yet been shown to be clearly superior to traditional balloon angioplasty, and neither has been successful in the treatment of long and severe obstructive lesions that threaten limb viability, which remain best treated by surgical bypass.

SURGICAL LOWER EXTREMITY REVASCULARIZATION

Severe lower extremity ischemia due to femoral, popliteal, and tibial atherosclerosis is most frequently treated surgically by bypass grafting. Other options may be appropriate in highly selected cases. Endarterectomy may be used for localized disease in the superficial femoral artery, but it is unusual for the disease to be confined to a short segment of the vessel.[16] When the origin of the major collateral vessel in the thigh, the profunda femoris, is stenotic, flow through this system may be improved by patch profundaplasty. Profundaplasty has been shown to be effective in treating claudication but is much less successful in treating limb-threatening ischemia in which improved blood flow to the foot must be achieved.[29]

Bypass procedures are usually performed under general or regional anesthesia. Continuous epidural blockade is favored by many surgeons and anesthesiologists because distal procedures may require considerable time, and this method of anesthesia minimizes time constraints while providing effective analgesia with minimal cardiovascular stress. It is important to bear in mind that atherosclerosis is a systemic disorder and nearly all of these patients have some degree of associated coronary or cerebrovascular disease. In fact, when vigorously searched for, up to 40 per cent of patients undergoing lower extremity revascularization are found to have episodes of myocardial ischemia in the perioperative period.[21] As many as 5 per cent experience myocardial infarction, and half of these may be fatal.

Technique for Bypass Procedures

Successful bypass surgery for limb ischemia requires mature surgical judgment and meticulous attention to technical details. Surgical candidates are selected on the basis of clinical presentation and undergo arteriography to determine the optimal site for placement of the proximal and distal anastomoses. These sites are selected to allow unobstructed flow distally to the foot if

possible. If an adequate distal vessel is not visualized and the need for revascularization is clear, exploration and direct operative arteriography may reveal a patent distal vessel suitable for anastomosis. The proximal anastomosis is usually to the common femoral artery, but more distal sites of origin for the bypass have been used when the proximal superficial femoral artery is unobstructed.[23,26]

Choice of Graft Material

In recent years, there has been considerable debate regarding the most appropriate graft material. Whereas some continue to manifest enthusiasm for the synthetic graft, particularly for reconstructions to the popliteal artery,[18,24] it has clearly been shown in well-controlled randomized trials that the autogenous venous grafts provide the highest long- and short-term patency rates for lower extremity revascularization.[22,30,31] In a large multicenter trial, it was found that autogenous saphenous vein and polytetrafluoroethylene grafts to the popliteal artery yielded similar patency rates for the first 24 months postoperatively but diverged significantly thereafter.[30] At 5 years postoperatively, the patency rate for autogenous veins was 68 per cent compared with 38 per cent for the synthetic grafts (Fig. 6). In addition, the patency of synthetic grafts to vessels distal to the popliteal was worse in this study, with a long-term patency rate of 12 per cent. Therefore, it appears reasonable to recommend that prosthetic material be reserved

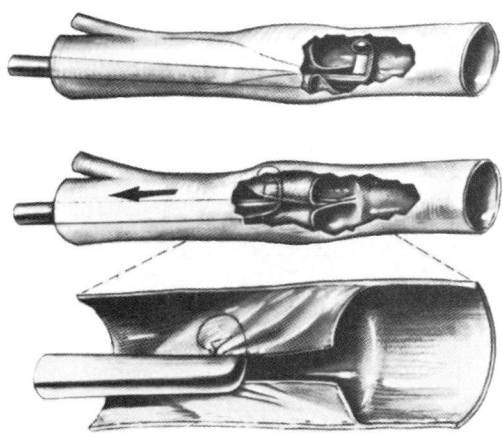

Figure 7. Valvulotome inserted through a side branch to cut the venous valve for an "*in situ*" vein graft. (From Leather, R. P., and Shah, D. M.: *In situ* saphenous vein arterial bypass. *In* Rutherford, R. B. (Ed.): Vascular Surgery, 3rd ed. Philadelphia, W. B. Saunders Company, 1989.)

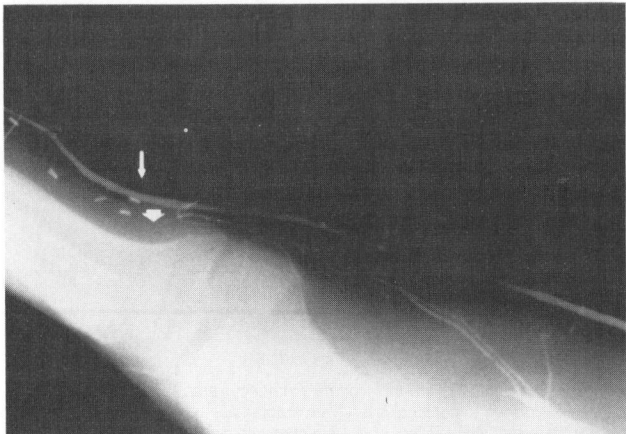

Figure 8. Operative arteriogram of *in situ* femoropopliteal saphenous vein graft (small arrow); large arrow points to residual arteriovenous fistula from a vein branch that requires ligation before wound closure.

for proximal lower extremity reconstruction only, and only in those cases in which autogenous vein is not available or in which survival beyond 2 years is not expected.

With respect to autogenous venous grafts, two opposing groups have been established. In the late 1970s, Leather and associates reintroduced the *in situ* saphenous vein graft.[19] In this technique, only the proximal and distal saphenous vein segments are mobilized for the proximal and distal anastomoses. The intervening graft may or may not be exposed, but in either case the vein is not dissected free from its bed. Valves may be rendered incompetent by a variety of valvulotomes introduced through the open end of the graft or through side branches (Fig. 7). The side branches of the saphenous vein must be ligated to prevent the occurrence of arteriovenous fistula postoperatively (Fig. 8). The advantages purported for this technique are that it allows the use of smaller veins and that it allows anastomosis of the largest end of the vein graft to the largest artery, and the smallest end of the vein graft to the smaller distal vessel. Excellent patency and limb salvage have been achieved with this technique (Fig. 9). However, comparable concurrent series using the more traditional reversed saphenous vein graft have also shown dramatic improvements in patency and limb salvage compared with results achieved a decade ago (Fig. 10).[28] The few randomized studies that have been published have suggested comparable results with modern techniques of vein harvesting when the graft is harvested and reversed or used *in situ*.[32] This is probably due to the now recognized importance of graft spatulation, gentle vein handling, and avoidance of overdistention and prolonged storage in unphysiologic solutions (Fig. 11). Moreover, the vein utilization is comparable or even higher using the reversed technique because an inadequate

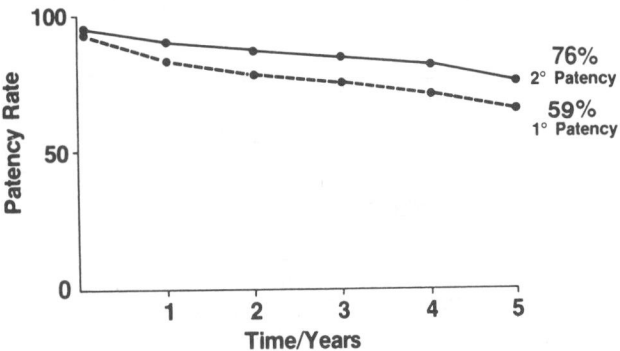

Figure 9. Primary and secondary patency rate for a large series of *in situ* grafts. (From Leather, R. P., Shah, D. M., Change, B. B., and Kaufman, J. L.: Resurrection of the *in situ* vein bypass. 1,000 cases later. Ann. Surg., *208*:434, 1988.)

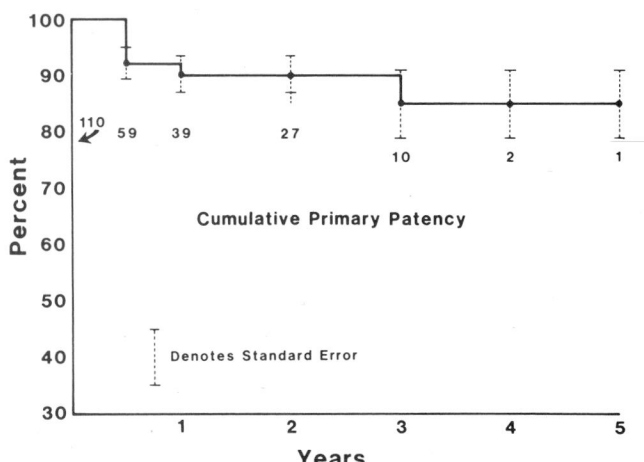

Figure 10. Life-table primary and secondary patency for a large series of reversed saphenous bypass grafts. Long-term results in this modern series are comparable to those achieved with the *in situ* technique. (From Taylor, L. M., Jr., Edwards, J. M., Phinney, E. S., and Porter, J. M.: Reversed vein bypass to infrapopliteal arteries: Modern results are superior to or equivalent to *in situ* bypass for patency and vein utilization. Ann. Surg., *205*:90, 1987.)

length of vein can be augmented by splicing additional segments harvested from the opposite leg or from the arm. Segments from the greater and lesser saphenous vein, the major tributaries, and the cephalic and basilic veins in the arm can all be used when necessary to achieve a graft of sufficient length.[27]

POSTOPERATIVE CARE

The elderly patient population and the systemic nature of the atherosclerotic process dictate careful intraoperative and postoperative monitoring. This frequently includes an arterial pressure line and a urethral catheter. Heparin administered intraoperatively is not continued postoperatively except in unusual circumstances. Routine completion intraoperative arteriography is employed to detect unsuspected technical faults or distal thromboembolism prior to complete wound closure.

Constant surveillance is maintained through periodic follow-up of all patients with lower extremity bypasses. This includes periodic noninvasive examinations and serial determinations of extremity blood pressures in order to detect any threat to the continued patency of the graft. More recently, duplex scanning has been used in postoperative graft surveillance with success.[11]

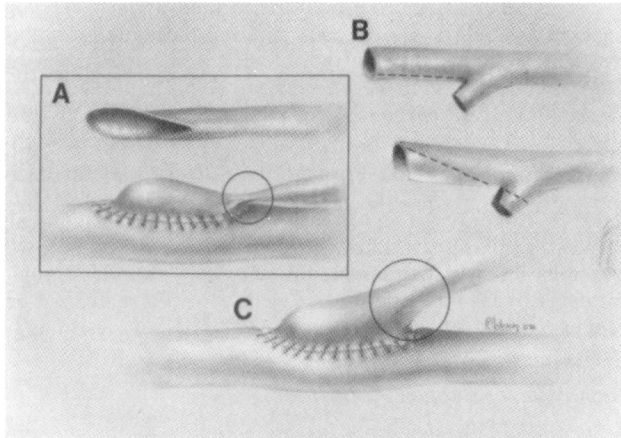

Figure 11. *A*, Preferred technique for proximal anastomosis. *B*, Conventional end-to-side anastomosis is prone to constriction at point of origin. *C*, Incorporation of adjacent side branch into anastomotic origin prevents constriction. (From Taylor, L. M., Jr., Edwards, J. M., Phinney, E. S., and Porter, J. M.: Reversed vein bypass to infrapopliteal arteries: Modern results are superior to or equivalent to *in situ* bypass for patency and vein utilization. Ann. Surg., *205*:90, 1987.)

Liberal use of angiography is employed to detect acquired graft stenoses or other potential graft problems prior to complete graft thrombosis. Correction of these defects may extend and improve long-term results.

RESULTS

Improvement in patency rates and limb salvage in patients treated for lower extremity peripheral vascular obstructive disease has been one of the most dramatic improvements in vascular surgery in the last decade. Compared with 75 per cent and 50 per cent, 1- and 5-year patency rates 10 years ago, today's results demonstrate 90 per cent 1-year and 70 per cent multi-year patency rates with limb salvage 5 per cent to 10 per cent higher. These improvements have been achieved by an increased appreciation for the fragility of the saphenous vein and the importance of gentle technique in preparation for use by either the *in situ* or reversed technique, and by the increased appreciation of the clear superiority of autogenous venous grafting over synthetic or modified biologic grafts. Technical advances including improved coaxial fiberoptic lighting and optical magnification likely have also had a role in this improvement. Because of these improved results, it appears more reasonable to offer treatment to patients not with minor but with disabling claudication who previously were untreated. Whether these patients are treated with catheter techniques or even with bypass surgery, they can be offered a reasonable likelihood of improved life-style with only a small risk.

SELECTED REFERENCES

Harrison, L. H.: Historical aspects in the development of venous autografts. Ann. Surg., 183:101, 1986.
This is an excellent brief review of the early experimental and clinical experience with autogenous vein grafts in the arterial circulation.

Leather, R. P., Shah, D. M., Chang, B. B., and Kaufman, J. L.: Resurrection in the *in situ* saphenous vein bypass — 1000 cases later. Ann. Surg., 208:435, 1988.
This is a careful analysis of over 1000 cases of in situ saphenous vein bypass grafting by the most vocal proponent of this procedure. It demonstrates excellent long-term patency rates and limb salvage with observation periods up to 5 years.

Taylor, L. M., Jr., Edwards, J. M., and Porter, J. M.: Present status of reversed vein bypass: Long-term results of a modern series. J. Vasc. Surg., 11:193, 1990.
This is a detailed analysis of over 500 reversed vein grafts by the strongest proponent of this procedure. It demonstrates over 75 per cent 5-year patency with 92 per cent limb salvage, clearly comparable to the results achieved with in situ bypass grafting.

Veith, F. J., Gupta, S. H., Ascer, E., et al.: Six-year prospective multicenter randomized comparison of autologous saphenous vein and expanded polytetrafluoroethylene grafts in infrainguinal arterial reconstructions. J. Vasc. Surg., 3:104, 1986.
This is the largest randomized trial comparing autogenous saphenous vein with synthetic polytetrafluoroethylene (PTFE) grafts for infrainguinal arterial reconstruction. It is a well-controlled study of a difficult topic and conclusively demonstrates the superiority of the autogenous venous graft for lower extremity reconstructions by careful analysis of patency rates over time.

REFERENCES

1. Ameli, F. M., Stein, M., Provan, J. L., and Prosser, M.: The effect of postoperative smoking on femoropopliteal bypass grafts. Ann. Vasc. Surg., 3:20, 1989.
2. Blair, J. M., Gewertz, B. L., Moosa, H., Lu, C. T., and Zarins, C. K.: Percutaneous transluminal angioplasty versus surgery for limb-threatening ischemia. J. Vasc. Surg., 9:698, 1989.
3. Blakemore, A. H., and Voorhees, A. B.: The use of tubes constructed from vinyon "N" cloth in bridging arterial defects: Experimental and clinical. Ann. Surg., 140:324, 1954.
4. Campbell, C. D., Brooks, D. H., Webster, M. W., and Bahnson, H. T.: The use of expanded microporous polytetrafluoroethylene for limb salvage; a preliminary report. Surgery, 79:485, 1976.
5. Carrel, A.: The surgery of blood vessels, etc. Johns Hopkins Hosp. Bull., 18:18, 1907.
6. Couch, N. P.: On the arterial consequences of smoking. J. Vasc. Surg., 3:807, 1986.
7. Couch, N. P.: About heparin, or whatever happened to Jay McLean? J. Vasc. Surg., 10:1, 1989.
8. Dale, W. A.: Grafting small arteries. Arch. Surg., 86:22, 1963.
9. DeWeese, J. A., and Rob, C. G.: Autogenous venous grafts ten years later. Surgery, 82:775, 1977.
10. Dotter, C. T., and Judkins, M. P.: Transluminal treatment of arteriosclerotic obstruction: Description of a new technique and a preliminary report of its application. Circulation, 30:654, 1964.
11. Green, R. M., McNamara, J., Ovriel, K., and DeWeese, J.: Comparison of infrainguinal graft surveillance techniques. J. Vasc. Surg., 11:207, 1990.
12. Grüntzig, A., and Kumpe, D. A.: Technique of percutaneous transluminal angioplasty with the Gruntzig balloon catheter. A. J. R., 132:547, 1979.
13. Harrison, L. H.: Historical aspects in the development of venous autografts. Ann. Surg., 183:101, 1976.
14. Hughson, W. G., Mann, J. I., and Garrod, A.: Intermittent claudication: Prevalence and risk factors. Br. Med. J., 1:1379, 1978.
15. Imparato, A. M., Kim, G. E., Davison, T., and Crowley, J. G.: Intermittent claudication: Its natural course. Surgery, 78:795, 1975.
16. Inahara, T., and Scott, C. M.: Endarterectomy for segmental occlusive disease of the superficial femoral artery. Arch. Surg., 116:1547, 1981.
17. Kunlin, J.: La traitement de l'arterite obliterance par la greffe veineuse. Arch. Mal. Coeur, 42:317, 1949.
18. Laurendeau, F., and Lassonde, F.: Above-knee femoropopliteal reconstruction with polytetrafluoroethylene: A good alternative to saphenous vein bypass. Can. J. Surg., 32:48, 1989.
19. Leather, R. P., Shah, D. M., Chang, B. B., and Kaufman, J. L.: Resurrection of the *in situ* saphenous vein bypass — 1000 cases later. Ann. Surg., 208:435, 1988.
20. McAllister, F. F.: The fate of patients with intermittent claudication managed nonoperatively. Am. J. Surg., 132:593, 1976.
21. McCann, R. L., and Clements, F. M.: Silent myocardial ischemia in patients undergoing peripheral vascular surgery; incidence and association with perioperative cardiac morbidity and mortality. J. Vasc. Surg., 9:583, 1989.
22. Michaels, J. A.: Choice of material for above-knee femoropopliteal bypass graft. Br. J. Surg., 76:7, 1989.
23. Najmaldin, A., Clifford, P. C., Chant, A. D., and Webster, J. H.: Inflow site: Its effect on femoropopliteal and distal graft patency. Br. J. Surg., 75:434, 1988.
24. Newman, G. E., Miner, D. G., Sussman, S. K., Phillips, H. R., Mikate, E. M., and McCann, R. L.: Peripheral artery atherectomy: Description of technique and report of initial results. Radiology, 169:677, 1988.
25. Quiñones-Baldrich, W. J., Busuttil, R. W., Baker, J. D., Vescera, C. L., Ahn, S. S., Machleder, H. I., and Moore, W. S.: Is the preferential use of polytetrafluoroethyline grafts for femoropopliteal bypass justified? J. Vasc. Surg., 8:219, 1988.
26. Rosenbloom, M. S., Walsh, J. J., Schuler, J. J., Meyer, J. P., et al.: Long-term results of infragenicular bypasses with autogenous vein originating from the distal superficial femoral and popliteal arteries. J. Vasc. Surg., 7:691, 1988.
27. Taylor, L. M., Jr., Edwards, J. M., and Porter, J. M.: Present status of reversed vein bypass: Long-term results of a modern series. J. Vasc. Surg., 11:193; 1990.
28. Taylor, L. M., Jr., Edwards, J. M., Phinney, E. S., and Porter, J. M.: Reversed vein bypass to infrapopliteal arteries: Modern results are superior to or equivalent to *in situ* bypass for patency and vein utilization. Ann. Surg., 205:90, 1987.
29. Towne, J. B., Bernhard, V. M., Rollins, D. L., and Baum, P. L.: Profundaplasty in perspective: Limitations in long-term management of limb ischemia. Surgery, 90:1037, 1981.
30. Veith, F. J., Gupta, S. K., Ascer, E., et al.: Six-year prospective multicenter randomized comparison of autologous saphenous vein and expanded polytetrafluoroethylene grafts in infrainguinal arterial reconstructions. J. Vasc. Surg., 3:104, 1986.
31. Veterans Administration Cooperative Study Group 141: Comparative evaluation of prosthetic, reversed, and *in situ* vein bypass grafts in distal popliteal and tibial-peroneal revascularization. Arch. Surg., 123:434, 1988.
32. Watelet, J., Cheysson, E., Poels, D., et al.: *In situ* versus reversed saphenous vein for femoropopliteal bypass: A prospective randomized study of 100 cases. Ann. Vasc. Surg., 1:441, 1986.

7. PERCUTANEOUS TRANSLUMINAL ANGIOPLASTY

R. Duane Davis, Jr., M.D.

Since the performance of the first successful percutaneous transluminal angioplasty (PTA) by Dotter and Judkins in 1964,[16] the technique of PTA has become an established procedure in the treatment of obstructive disorders in the arterial and venous circulation. With increased experience using PTA, improved clinical results and decreased morbidity have been obtained. Increasing numbers of clinical problems have been successfully treated using PTA. In certain clinical settings, PTA has become the treatment modality of choice. However, in the majority of circumstances, PTA is an adjunctive treatment to existing vascular surgical techniques.

HISTORICAL ASPECTS

In 1964, Dotter and Judkins first reported an initial series of 11 patients with atherosclerotic vascular obstruction treated by a percutaneous technique involving the transluminal serial passage of increasingly larger coaxial catheters (coaxial technique). Their initial experience with PTA was serendipitous and occurred during the performance of abdominal aortography, during which the passage of the diagnostic catheter dilated a right iliac artery stenosis. Subsequently, they performed the first intentional PTA in an elderly woman with gangrenous toes who had refused amputation. The severe stenosis of the right superficial femoral artery was successfully dilated with immediate restoration of circulation to the foot. An arteriogram obtained 3 weeks later documented continued patency (Fig. 1), and the patient remained ambulatory, with healing of the ischemic skin changes. Despite initial successes, concern arose regarding potentially serious complications, primarily the risk of thromboemboli due to the sheering forces on the vessel wall during passage of the dilating catheters. Such concern prevented a wider acceptance of angioplasty in North America, although further clinical experience was continued in Europe by Zeitler, van Andel, Porstmann, and Grüntzig. In 1968, Staple, with subsequent alterations by van Andel, modified the initial Dotter catheters and developed a series of graduated catheters with long, tapering tips. These had the advantage of decreasing the forward shearing force and increasing the radially directed compressive force (Fig. 2).

In 1972, Grüntzig introduced the double-lumen balloon catheter and 2 years later successfully applied it to the treatment of obstructive lesions of the iliac and femoral arteries[26]; obstructions of the renal and coronary arteries subsequently were managed successfully.[27,28] Grüntzig's catheters consisted of a polyethylene inner catheter with an outer layer of polyvinyl chloride molded to form a balloon at the tip of the catheter. The balloon could be inflated to a predetermined diameter, and because of limited linear-volume characteristics, it would not overinflate by more than 2 mm. greater than its determined size. The double-lumen balloon catheter's small diameter in the deflated state allowed a much smaller arteriotomy. The catheter's fixed size and shape in the inflated state applied only a centrifugal force to the vessel lumen, thus avoiding the shear stresses intrinsic to the coaxial technique. Theoretically, this decreased the risk of embolic complications.

Following Grüntzig's pioneering work, PTA gained wide acceptance, and its application has been extended to an increasing number of vascular problems. Continued technical advances have been made in instrumentation. The polyvinyl chloride balloons have been replaced by polyethylene chloride and polytetrafluoroethylene balloons, which are stronger and have higher tensile and yield strength characteristics. These characteristics prevent overdistention and therefore decrease the risk of arterial rupture. The development of balloons that can withstand higher pressures without deformation has enabled dilation of previously resistant vascular stenosis. The introduction of recanalization devices has enabled reperfusion of totally obstructed arterial segments and continues to alter the clinical utility of PTA.

TECHNIQUE

A series of arteriograms are required to define the arterial anatomy and the proximal and distal circulation prior to consideration of angioplasty. Because lesions are frequently underestimated on single-plane angiograms, particularly lesions in the aorta and iliac vessels, which are frequently eccentric and posterior in location, oblique and lateral views are needed to com-

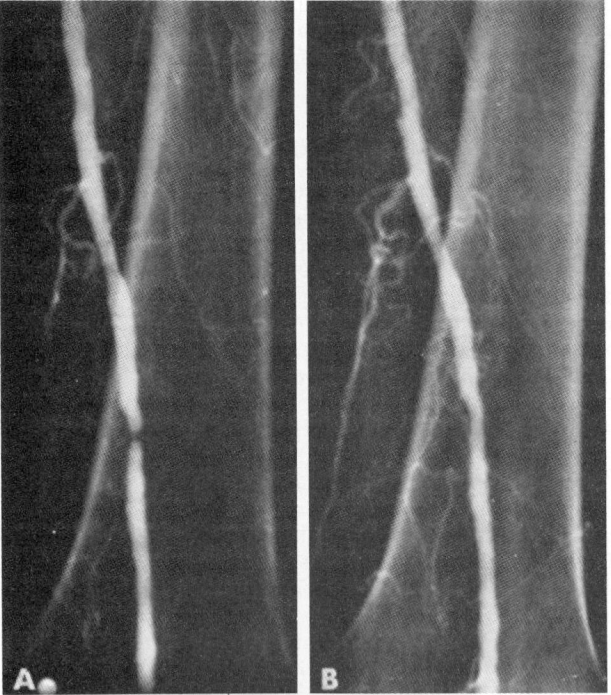

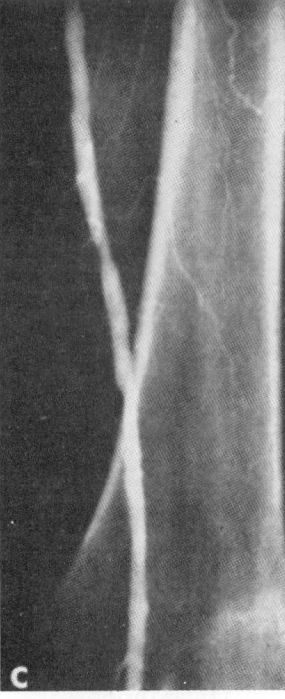

Figure 1. The first reported percutaneous angioplasty of a superficial femoral artery stenosis using coaxial catheters. *A*, Tight stenosis of the superficial femoral artery at the level of Hunter's canal. *B*, Immediately after dilation, which was associated with improvement in the patient's clinical status. *C*, Three weeks after PTA, the vessel lumen remains patent. (From Dotter, C. T., and Judkins, M. P.: Transluminal treatment of arteriosclerotic obstruction. Description of a new technic and report of its application. Circulation, *30*:654, 1964.)

pletely evaluate the exact nature of the lesions. Such thorough evaluation is necessary to enable an accurate assessment of the feasibility of PTA. Physiologic measurements, such as the pressure gradient across the lesion (10 to 15 mm. Hg is considered significant), are useful in evaluating the clinical significance of the lesion.

Using local anesthesia, a needle is introduced into an appropriate vessel, usually the femoral artery, although the axillary artery is sometimes preferred, depending on anatomic consider-

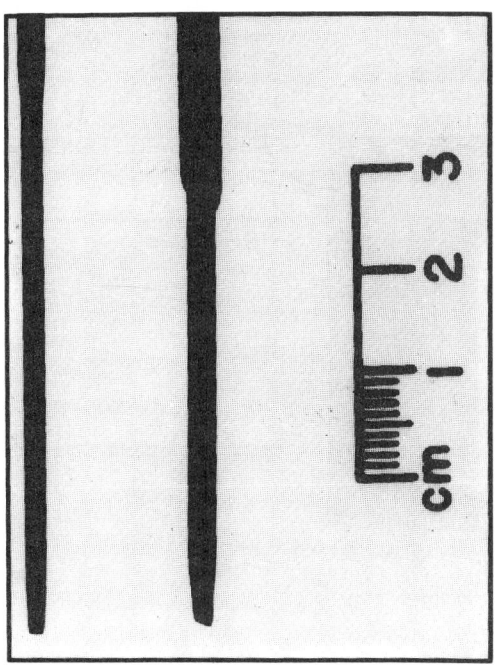

Figure 2. *Left*, a 12-French Dotter catheter system. The 12-French catheter is advanced over the inner 8-French catheter through the stenosis. *Right*, a 7-French Staple–van Andel tapered dilation catheter. (From Tegtmeyer, C. J.: Percutaneous transluminal angioplasty. Curr. Prob. Diagn. Radiol., *16*:75, 1987.)

ations. The approach to the lesion may be antegrade or retrograde through the ipsilateral femoral artery to the lesion or retrograde through the contralateral femoral artery. A catheter (usually a 5-French, but occasionally a 7-French) is introduced into the lumen and advanced under fluoroscopic visualization to a site near the stenosis or obstruction. A guidewire is then passed through the true lumen of the stenotic lesion or through the potential lumen of a complete obstruction. There are many types of guidewires with differing physical properties, as well as the ability to steer the tip of the wire. The selection depends on the local anatomy of the vasculature, nature of the stenosis, and characteristics of the lumen. In addition, there are numerous techniques to cross the lesion.[6,31] Passage of the guidewire is usually the limiting factor in the technical success of PTA. Subintimal passage of the wire and perforation of the vessel wall are potential complications that occasionally necessitate emergency surgical intervention, but such events are usually avoided by termination of the procedure. Subintimal passage and vessel perforation are more likely to occur when the vessel is occluded. However, in such circumstances, an adverse outcome is unlikely because of the prior presence of occlusion. After the guidewire and subsequently the catheter have been passed across the lesion, the initial guidewire is usually removed and an exchange guidewire with a flexible tip and stiffer body is placed, which enables easier catheter changes and minimizes vessel trauma. The angiocatheter is withdrawn and the balloon catheter is passed over the guidewire across the lesion. The size of the balloon chosen is approximately 10 to 20 per cent greater than the native lumen. Because of the magnification intrinsic to most angiography, an estimate of native lumen size by measuring proximally and distally to the lesion in the unaffected portion of the vessel approximates the appropriate-sized balloon catheter. Angioplasty catheters are available with balloon sizes of 2 to 20 mm. in inflation diameter and 2 to 10 cm. in length with catheter sizes of 2.9-French to 9-French. The lowest profile catheters have markedly improved the success with which small arteries can be dilated, such as the coronary and infrapopliteal vessels.

The balloon is inflated to a pressure of 4 to 10 atmospheres with a dilute contrast solution that allows accurate visualization of the balloon catheter in relation to the stenosis. The duration and frequency of inflation of the balloon depend on the vascular bed being treated and the resultant increase in arterial diameter. In organs that tolerate ischemia less well, the balloon is inflated for a shorter period. Continuous measurement of inflation pressure is necessary to limit complications related to vessel trauma and balloon rupture. Patients experience mild to moderate pain during balloon inflation; however, the pain should abate rapidly after balloon deflation and disappears usually within a minute. Continued intense pain after balloon deflation is indicative of arterial rupture or occlusion. Similarly, severe pain during inflation is often indicative of the use of a too-large balloon catheter. After dilation, an arteriogram is obtained to assess the immediate results. Care must be taken during repeat angiography, avoiding the angioplasty site with the contrast dye injection to minimize the risk of raising an intimal flap. In addition, physiologic measurements, particularly the pressure gradient across the stenosis, are useful in evaluating the result. Detailed descriptions of the technique of PTA can be found in several reports.[63]

The use of anticoagulants has remained controversial and is not standardized. A bolus of heparin (2500 to 7500 units) is usually administered after the stenotic area is traversed with the guidewire. When treating arteries that have a greater risk of spasm, such as the renal, brachiocephalic, popliteal, tibial, and peroneal arteries, vasodilators such as nifedipine, verapamil, nitroglycerin, and papaverine have been employed. Nifedipine in 10-mg. doses orally or sublingually and verapamil in 2.5-mg. doses administered intravenously, often in conjunction with nitroglycerin in 100- to 200-mg. doses, have been useful intraarterially, as either a prophylactic or therapeutic measure. Lidocaine is frequently used in conjunction with contrast agent injections to minimize spasm. The use of non-ionic contrast media may also be beneficial. Anticoagulation after PTA also varies. Heparin, coumadin, aspirin, and dipyridamole have all been used. Most authors recommend an antiplatelet regimen of aspirin with or without dipyridamole.

PATHOPHYSIOLOGY

When a balloon catheter is positioned across a stenotic lesion, a controlled injury is produced in the distended vessel wall, allowing a persistent increase in the luminal area. The precise nature of the structural changes in the arterial wall that occur at the site of dilation has been controversial. Dotter initially proposed that the increase in the luminal size was due to remodeling and lateral displacement of the atheromatous plaque. The metaphor he frequently used was that of snow underfoot. However, most studies have demonstrated that compaction is of limited importance. A mechanical study estimated that the contribution of compaction was 1 per cent of the overall increase in luminal surface area, whereas extrusion of fluid from the plaque represented approximately 6 to 12 per cent of the increase in luminal area. The majority of the increase (87 to 93 per cent) was due to plaque and arterial wall disruption.[37] The increased luminal area following dilation is associated with disruption of the intima near the edges of the plaque, separation of the edges of the plaque from the media, stretching of the media and adventitia, and often rupture of the media (Fig. 3).[43] Separation of the intima from the media occurs at the internal elastic membrane. The plaque separation extends from the lateral aspects of the plaque circumferentially toward the thickest portion of the plaque. This plaque separation also extends axially along the plaque within the vessel (Fig. 4). Plaques rarely become completely detached from the media, remaining adherent near the thickest portion of the plaque where shear and tangential stresses are the least. The plaques also remain attached to the media proximally and distally to the region of dilation. These attachments between the plaque and media explain the low incidence of clinically significant distal embolization with PTA.

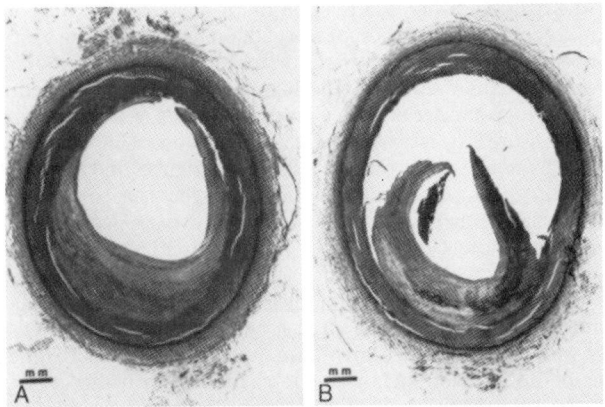

Figure 3. Histologic sections from adjacent vessel segments containing an obstructive atherosclerotic plaque. *A*, Nondilated segment. *B*, Dilated segment in which the plaque edges are separated from the media; however, the plaque is not disturbed. Although the lumen is increased in the dilated segment, lumen contour is distorted, assuming a "mushroom-shaped" contour. (From Lyon, R. T., Zarins, C. K., Lu, C. T., et al.: Vessel, plaque, and lumen morphology after transluminal balloon angioplasty. Arteriosclerosis, 7:310, 1987.)

With concentric plaques, the disruption occurs in the region of the thinnest portion of the plaque where shear and tangential stresses are greatest (Fig. 5). In addition, following the separation of the plaque from the media, the luminal circumference

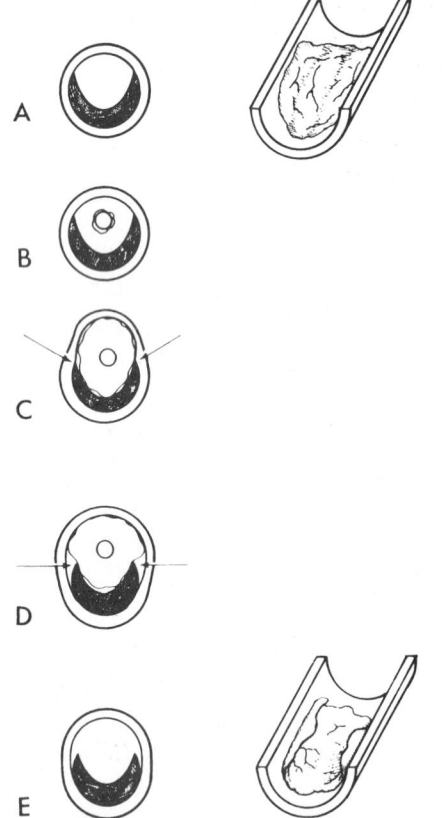

Figure 4. The physical mechanism of transluminal angioplasty. Mechanism of disruption that occurs during transluminal angioplasty. *A*, Cross-sectional view of an artery with an eccentric plaque. *B*, Deflated balloon catheter placed across the lesion. *C*, Partial inflation of the balloon causes deformation of the relatively normal artery wall, whereas the stiffer plaque retains its initial shape. Arrows point to the junction of the plaque and arterial wall and indicate regions where disruption starts. *D*, Full inflation of the balloon causes additional disruption of the plaque and artery. The tears have extended circumferentially along the plaque/artery border (arrows). *E*, Postdilation results show an enlarged lumen following disruption of the plaque and artery. (From Kinney, T. B., et al.: Transluminal angioplasty: A mechanical-pathophysiological correlation of its physical mechanisms. Radiology, 153:85, 1984.)

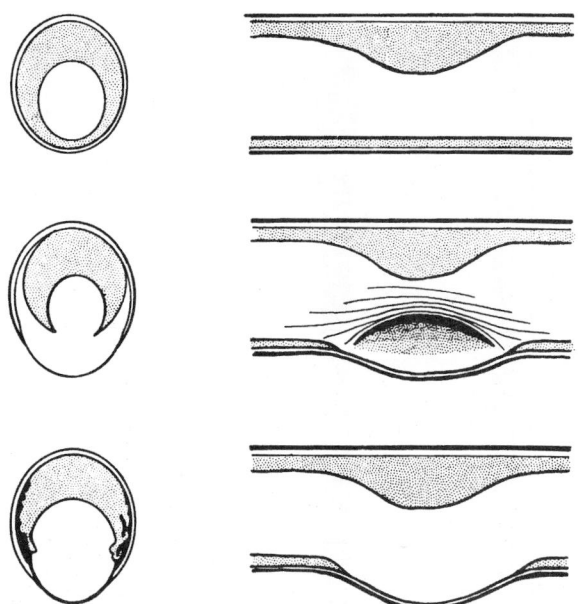

Figure 5. Disruption of intima and medial layers after balloon dilation. Increase in lumen size is reflected by bulging of remaining medial and adventitial fibers opposite the plaque. Remodeling occurs with time, as the irregular lumen surface changes to a rounded, smooth contour. (From Zarins, C. K., Chien-Tai, L., Gewertz, B. L., et al.: Arterial disruption and remodeling following balloon dilatation. Surgery, 92:1093, 1982.)

becomes more dependent on the media and adventitia. The increase in effective radius corresponds to an increase in the tangential tension in the medial and adventitial layers, which tends to maintain vessel patency. The plaque itself does not appear to undergo compression, fragmentation deformation, herniation into the media, or remodeling. The resulting separation of the relatively rigid, cohesive plaque from the underlying arterial wall frequently appears as dissection and local flaps on arteriography. Intimal remodeling, however, occurs rapidly as

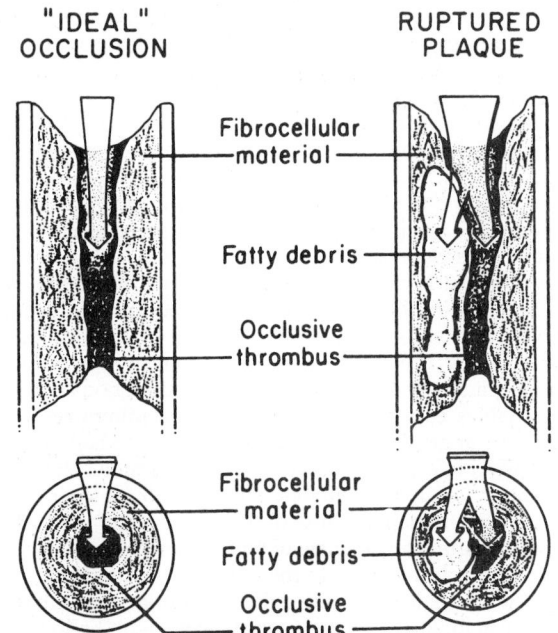

Figure 6. Pathways of recanalization in occluded vessels. In an "ideal" occlusion, a small, fresh central thrombus surrounded by a firmer fibrocellular narrowing provides the pathway of least resistance. When occlusion follows rupturing of an atherosclerotic plaque, the soft atheromatous debris may provide less resistance than the occlusive thrombus. (From Sanborn, T. A.: Recanalization of arterial occlusions: Pathological basis and contributing factors. J. Am. Coll. Cardiol., 13:1559, 1989.)

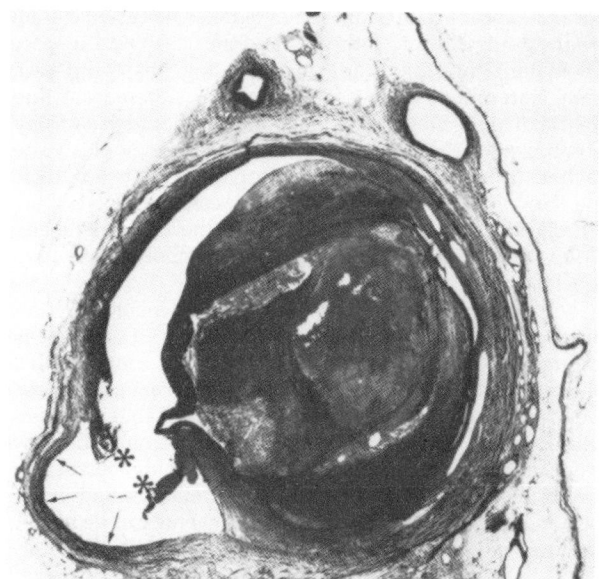

Figure 7. Histologic cross-section of a long-standing superficial femoral artery occlusion after PTA. The guidewire and balloon catheter passed in a plane between the plaque and media, producing an extensive cleavage plane as the arterial wall was stretched away from the plaque. This caused rupture of the media (*) and stretching of the adventitia (arrows) to enlarge the lumen. (From Lyon, R. T., Zarins, C. K., Lu, C. T., et al.: Vessel, plaque, and lumen morphology after transluminal balloon angioplasty. Arteriosclerosis, 7:310, 1987.)

the channels following separation become shorter and the vessel lumen regains its smooth contour. Arteriograms obtained during the weeks following PTA fail to demonstrate the ragged appearance typical of the immediate post-PTA arteriogram.

In contrast to dilation of a stenotic atherosclerotic lesion, often other mechanisms are utilized in recanalization of arterial occlusions. In circumstances in which a recent occlusion with fresh thrombus occurs, the guidewire or other catheter devices usually pass through the thrombus, and the increase in luminal area occurs through the mechanisms previously described. However, as the thrombus becomes more organized, it becomes more resistant to instrument passage, which frequently leads to traversing the vessel wall. Often the passage is in the layer between the plaque and the arterial wall.[43] Similarly, in the setting of obstruction secondary to a ruptured plaque, subintimal passage of the instrument is frequent (Fig. 6)[54] and success depends on re-entrance into the true lumen. Vessel perforation can easily occur in these settings. PTA most often does not disrupt the plaque, but causes atrophy or rupture of the media and stretching of the adventitia (Fig. 7).

COMPARISON OF SURGICAL MANAGEMENT WITH PTA

PTA has many inherent advantages as well as disadvantages compared with surgical revascularization. With the technical simplicity of PTA, and the need for only local anesthesia and mild sedation, the hospital stay, cost of the procedure, morbidity, and lost productivity all are reduced greatly. In addition, PTA can be applied to patients whose general medical condition would otherwise contraindicate surgical intervention. Complications of PTA, however, may lead to operative therapy on an emergency rather than elective basis with attendant increase in risk.

The transluminal approach avoids the disruption of local nerves, lymphatics, and blood vessels inherent in any surgical procedure. Because of the lack of postoperative fibrotic changes, PTA can be repeated easily. Also, when the procedure is technically unsuccessful, the patient is only rarely in a more unfavorable position than before PTA. In one series of 204 patients

undergoing PTA for peripheral vascular disease, 14 required subsequent operative therapy. Of these, six were treated with the vascular procedure required if PTA had not been attempted, four required a modified vascular procedure but without adverse effect, and three patients required operations to treat complications of PTA (two operative closures of the arteriotomy site, one embolectomy) which were less extensive than would have been required for surgical revascularization.[53] Because PTA is usually performed in patients with generalized atherosclerosis, an added advantage is the preservation of the saphenous vein for future use as a conduit for coronary or other organ revascularization. PTA of iliac vessels avoids the risk of impotence following disruption of autonomic nerves during aortofemoral grafting.

Technical considerations limit the spectrum of disease for which PTA is an effective modality of therapy. Ideal patients for treatment using PTA are those with short stenotic lesions less than 5 cm. in length; the best results occur from treatment of the shortest lesions. Although total occlusions and multiple stenoses have been treated successfully, there are fewer technical successes, less long-term patency, and a greater number of complications. The localized nature of angioplasty indicates that the patient is susceptible to recurrence of symptoms owing to progression of disease elsewhere in the vessel, whereas surgical revascularization with bypass grafts circumvents long segments of the vessel. Angioplasty appears to have a fixed restenosis rate that is dependent on the vascular system being treated. In the coronary circulation, the restenosis rate appears to be 30 per cent at 6 months of follow-up regardless of the postangioplasty pharmacologic regimen. In larger arteries, such as the iliac arteries, the rate of restenosis is much lower (approximately 10 per cent). When compared with surgical bypass grafting, angioplasty is less durable. Thus, patients treated with PTA require subsequent procedures more often than do those treated with surgical revascularization. However, patency rates for both treatments appear to be dependent on similar patient variables including the severity of vascular disease in the run-off vessels and the presence of associated risk factors such as smoking, hypertension, and diabetes mellitus.

Comparison of results using bypass grafting with those using PTA is complicated by differences between authors in defining success. A variety of modalities are used by authors to determine patency following PTA, including clinical information, noninvasive vascular studies, and angiography to determine patency, each of which provides different information. In patients who have undergone PTA of an iliac artery stenosis, the use of thigh:brachial pressure ratio is a reliable indicator of continued patency, whereas the ankle:brachial pressure ratio is a better indicator of clinical success. In addition, most series report patency rates only in patients who have a successful dilation. The determination of initial technical success also varies between authors with regard to the degree of residual stenosis and hemodynamic gradient. Further complicating comparisons is the lack of randomized studies and the use of retrospective comparisons between patient groups who are not comparable in the extent and severity of disease.

COMPLICATIONS

PTA is associated with a complication rate of 1 per cent to as high as 33 per cent, the average being approximately 5 to 10 per cent. The number and extent of complications are dependent on the vascular bed being treated, the severity and diffuseness of the atherosclerotic disease process, the experience of the investigator, and the diligence with which complications are reported. Mortality occurs in 0 to 2 per cent of patients and usually reflects the extent of atherosclerosis in other vascular beds, particularly the coronary circulation. Diffuse thromboemboli with mesenteric occlusion can complicate PTA, particularly the renal and mesenteric arteries, causing death. Complications of PTA can be categorized to those occurring at the puncture site, those at the angioplasty site, those distal to the angioplasty site, and those systemic in nature (Table 1).

Puncture site complications include hematoma, thrombosis, false aneurysm, infection, and arteriovenous fistula. The most common complication, hematoma formation, occurs most frequently in association with obesity, hypertension, and anticoagulation use. Significantly, femoral artery punctures above the inguinal ligament may cause retroperitoneal hematomas, the diagnosis of which requires a high index of suspicion. Hematomas occurring after axillary artery access can cause brachial nerve injury.

Angioplasty site complications include subintimal dissection, perforation, rupture, occlusion of adjacent or branch vessels, spasm, and thrombosis. Subintimal passage of the guidewire or catheter occurs most frequently when treating occlusions or complex stenotic lesions. Dilations of subintimal passages are prone to early thrombosis, usually within the first 48 hours. Subintimal passage of the guidewire usually necessitates termination of the procedure and may cause vessel occlusion. Optimally, the PTA procedure should be postponed for 4 to 6 weeks. Perforation of the vessel occurs most often when attempting to pass the lesion with the guidewire. These events are usually self-limiting if the procedure is terminated, especially when treating peripheral vessels below the inguinal ligament. Retroperitoneal vessels, such as the iliac and renal arteries, are more likely to continue to bleed because of the low tamponading pressure within the retroperitoneum and, therefore, often require surgical correction. Rupture of the artery is reported and is associated with persistent pain. Bleeding can usually be controlled by reinflating the balloon, which may seal the rupture site. Occlusion of branch vessels and collaterals occurs if the intimal fracture created by PTA extends into the branch orifice. Unless these vessels can be protected by placement of a separate wire in the orifices to allow PTA of the branch vessel if an occlusion develops, angioplasty is contraindicated when the stenosis occurs adjacent to a significant branch vessel. Vasospasm may complicate PTA of renal, brachiocephalic, popliteal, and infrapopliteal vessels, predisposing these vessels to occlusion. Pharmacologic treatment with calcium channel blockers,

TABLE 1. Complications of PTA

Puncture site
  Hemorrhage
  Hematoma
  Thrombosis
  False aneurysm
  Brachial plexus injury
  Arteriovenous fistula
  Infection
Angioplasty site
  Perforation
  Rupture
  Subintimal dissection
  Thrombosis
  Spasm
  Occlusion of adjacent/branch vessels
Distal
  Embolization
  Spasm
Systemic
  Renal insufficiency
  Hemorrhagic shock
  Contrast allergy
  Anemia
  Hypotension (PRTA)

Modified from Tegtmeyer, C. J.: Percutaneous transluminal angioplasty. Curr. Probl. Diagn. Radiol., 16:75, 1987.

lidocaine, and nitroglycerin, the avoidance of vascular trauma with the guidewire and catheters, and the use of non-ionic contrast material are important in preventing this complication. Conversion of a stenotic lesion to an occlusion may be due to subintimal dissection or dilation, intimal flap, spasm, or the thrombogenic nature of the vessel wall at the angioplasty site. If adequate collaterals exist, elective surgical repair is usually possible. However, sudden occlusion of vessels supplying tissue that tolerates ischemia poorly, such as the kidney and heart, requires emergency treatment using thrombolytic agents and surgical revascularization.

Complications distal to the site of dilation include embolization and spasm and occur in 1 to 5 per cent of angioplasties, although PTA of iliac occlusions has been associated with embolic rates as high as 40 per cent.[52] Emboli from atheromatous plaques probably occur more often than those that are detected clinically. However, diffuse emboli, typically from patients with severe atherosclerosis of the aorta undergoing percutaneous renal transluminal angioplasty (PRTA), may cause bowel infarction and can be fatal. Most embolic events can be managed conservatively, but many require surgical embolectomy or revascularization to prevent sequelae. Trauma to the distal vessel by the guidewire or catheter can induce vascular spasm, emphasizing the importance of atraumatic technique.

Systemic complications include renal insufficiency or allergic reactions due to the contrast agent, hypotension due to hemorrhage or PRTA, and anemia associated with hemorrhage. Renal insufficiency can occur in as many as 26 per cent of patients undergoing PRTA for renovascular hypertension, with 13 per cent requiring dialysis.[9] This complication can be minimized by maintaining patient hydration. In patients without renovascular disease, renal insufficiency occurs in less than 5 per cent.

Balloon rupture is less common with the newer balloons, but it can cause vessel wall damage and predisposition to thrombosis, distal embolization, and increased puncture site complications because of the increased difficulty in removing the balloon through the existing arteriotomy site.

LESIONS AMENABLE TO PTA

Following Grüntzig's introduction of the balloon catheter, the number and variety of vessels subjected to PTA increased dramatically. Theoretically, any vessel of sufficient size to allow atraumatic passage of a balloon catheter is suitable for PTA. However, the risk of embolization of atheromatous material to the brain has greatly limited the application of PTA in the treatment of cerebrovascular obstructions. The largest experience has been in the treatment of peripheral vascular disease. Criteria for selection of patients with peripheral vascular disease for PTA should be similar to the criteria used in selecting patients for surgical revascularization. Tegtmeyer recommends PTA in the following clinical situations: the presence of intermittent claudication when the patient's life-style is adversely affected by the symptoms; the presence of rest pain; the presence of ischemic ulceration, poor wound healing after a surgical procedure, and impending or overt gangrenous changes. He recommends PTA as an adjunct to surgical therapy in the following circumstances: correction of iliac obstruction to provide adequate inflow prior to femoropopliteal bypass or femorofemoral bypass; prior to amputation as an attempt at limb salvage or to decrease the level of amputation; correction of postoperative stenoses in bypass grafts; and correction of stenoses in the native vessels when symptoms are present and the graft is threatened after bypass surgery.[63]

ILIAC ARTERIAL OBSTRUCTION

The best results and longest experience with PTA have been in the treatment of stenosis of the iliac arteries (Fig. 8). Technical

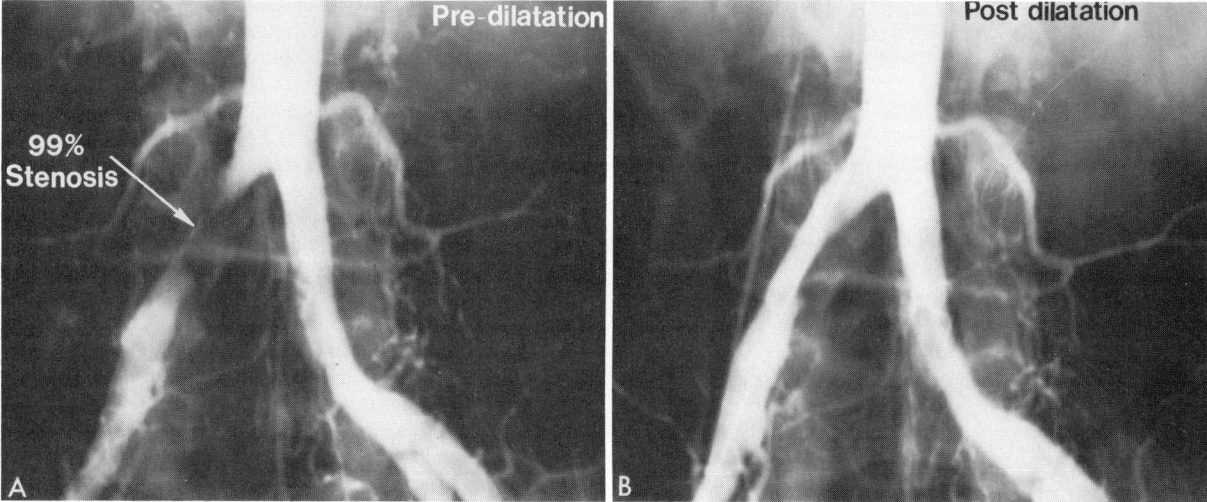

Figure 8. Arteriogram of a 68-year-old man with two-block claudication and a necrotic foot ulcer. *A*, Aortofemoral arteriogram demonstrates a 99 per cent stenosis of the right common iliac artery. *B*, PTA of the iliac artery provided marked improvement in the lumen diameter. The patient was relieved of his claudication and healed the ulcer. Symptoms recurred 15 months later. Arteriogram revealed restenosis of the right common iliac artery. Repeat PTA was successful, and the patient has remained asymptomatic.

success has been achieved in 85 to 95 per cent in most series. Long-term patency of successful dilations is reported in 86 to 100 per cent at 1 year, 78 to 100 per cent at 2 years, 78 to 89 per cent at 3 years, and 47 to 85 per cent at 5 years (Table 2). Although there is reasonable correlation between the quality and durability of the angioplasty result and the improvement in clinical and hemodynamic status of the patient,[31,36] this is not a direct correlation. In a series of 984 PTAs using a definition of clinical success that required the patient's clinical grade to improve by at least one level (asymptomatic, mild claudication, disabling claudication, rest pain, and ulceration or gangrene) and improvement of one of the vascular laboratory measurements (ankle:brachial ratio increases by at least 0.10, monophasic Doppler frequency analysis becomes biphasic or triphasic, Doppler pulsatility index increases greater than 20 per cent, or treadmill exercise distance doubles), continued success at 3 and 5 years was 65 and 60 per cent, respectively, for PTAs of the common iliac arteries and 50 and 48 per cent, respectively, for PTAs of the external iliac arteries.[31] An improved clinical outcome is dependent on multiple factors: (1) patients whose clinical indication for PTA is claudication versus limb-threatening ischemia; (2) focal disease versus diffuse stenosis or occlusion; (3) absence of diabetes mellitus; (4) good peripheral run-off; (5)

cessation of smoking; and (6) good technical result as determined by less than 30 per cent residual stenosis and pressure gradient less than 10 mm. Hg.[8,31,62,66,68] Whereas PTA of iliac artery stenosis has become an accepted procedure, PTA of iliac artery occlusions remains less established. PTA of iliac occlusions has a higher incidence of embolic complications, a lower rate of technical success (33 to 88 per cent), and a lower patency rate (50 to 100 per cent at 3 to 5 years).[31,52,61] Although the introduction of various recanalization devices may alter the efficacy of treating iliac occlusions, short occlusions in nontortuous iliac arteries allow reasonable results.

PTA of the iliac artery has been used as an adjunct to surgical therapy. In patients with inflow and outflow disease, PTA of focal iliac stenosis in conjunction with distal bypass has been successful. Similarly, in patients with bilateral iliac disease and one vessel containing a lesion ideally treated with angioplasty, PTA can be combined with femorofemoral artery bypass with good long-term patency.[62] Aortobifemoral grafting, which requires an abdominal incision with a greater morbidity and mortality, can be avoided.

The surgical treatment of iliac occlusive disease using aortofemoral grafting has been associated with a primary success rate of 92 to 100 per cent; cumulative patency rates are reported to be 94 to 98 per cent after 1 year, 90 to 97 per cent after 2 years, and 80 to 90 per cent after 5 years (mortality between 3 and 6 per cent).[40,68,69] PTA patency rates compare favorably with these surgical results. In a prospective, randomized series of patients with occlusive vascular disease who were thought to be candidates for either PTA or elective surgical revascularization, the 3-year survival rate as defined by freedom from study-related deaths, amputation, and intervention failure was 81 per cent for the surgical group and 67 per cent for the PTA group. However, the major difference between the groups was due to the decreased technical success rate in the PTA group. In patients with a technically successful procedure, the 3-year survival was 81.8 per cent for surgical therapy and 73.1 per cent for the PTA group. The hemodynamic benefit was similar between the 2 groups. The baseline ankle:brachial index was 0.50 in both groups and increased by 0.32 with surgical therapy and 0.28 with PTA, which was stable at 3 years (a 0.28 increase with surgical therapy and a 0.30 increase with PTA).[69] In a retrospective comparison between PTA and aortofemoral bypass, PTA was found to be less durable owing to recurrence or progression of disease within the iliac vessels. Late failure occurred in 36 per cent of PTA patients and 8 per cent of the surgical patients.[40]

TABLE 2. Iliac Artery PTA

Author	Patients	Technical Success	Patency Rate		
			1-yr.	2-yr.	5-yr.
Zeitler et al.	782	85%			
Johnston et al.					
Common iliac	376	91%	80%	70%	58%
External iliac	222	91%	73%	62%	47%
Schneider et al.	200	93%			85%
Spence et al.	160	92%	93%	87%	
Gallino et al.	153	95%			50%
Kadir et al.	141	96%	91%	89%	
Katzen	102	95%		93%	
Cambria et al.	94	89%	50%		
Wilson et al.	81	89%	74%	71%	61%
Samson et al.	69	88%	86%	78%	
Grüntzig et al.	64	92%		87%	
Fradet et al.	60	95%			
Waltman et al.	54	89%	100%		
Schwarten	50		89%		

FEMOROPOPLITEAL ARTERIAL OBSTRUCTION

Since Dotter's initial dilation of a superficial femoral artery stenosis, obstructive vascular disease of the femoropopliteal system has been most frequently treated with PTA. Initial technical success has been reported to be 70 to 96 per cent, with 1-year patency rates of 54 to 90 per cent, and 3-year patency rates of 43 to 84 per cent (Table 3). Because of the straight course of the femoral artery, treatment of femoral artery occlusions is more effective than treating those of the iliac artery. Although the technical success rate of dilating occlusions is only mildly less than treating stenoses, the long-term patency rates are poor (57 per cent at 2 years).[37] Clinical and hemodynamic success is significantly related to technical success and continued patency; however, the association is not absolute. Using a definition of clinical success as previously outlined (improvement of patient's clinical grade by at least one level [asymptomatic, mild claudication, disabling claudication, rest pain, and ulceration or gangrene] and improvement of one of the vascular laboratory measurements [ankle : brachial ratio increases by at least 0.10, monophasic Doppler frequency analysis becomes biphasic or triphasic, Doppler pulsatility index increases greater than 20 per cent, or treadmill exercise distance doubles]), in a series of 253 patients who underwent femoropopliteal PTA, success at 3 years and 5 years was approximately 50 and 40 per cent, respectively.[31] Better patency rates, as well as clinical success, are significantly associated with the following factors: (1) shorter stenosis or occlusion (greater than 10 cm. occlusions associated with poor results); (2) single versus multiple lesions; (3) open distal circulation (two- and three-vessel run-off associated with significantly better results); (4) absence of diabetes mellitus, hypertension, or continued tobacco use (greater adverse effect than with iliac disease); and (5) treatment of earlier stage of disease (claudication versus limb salvage).[11,62,66,68] Although technical success, hemodynamic improvement, and clinical success rates are significantly lower when treating patients for limb salvage, reasonable results can still be obtained. In a series of 27 patients with threatened limbs and considered to have a high risk for operative therapy, limb salvage at 2 years was 47 per cent.[47]

Comparisons between surgical bypass and PTA of the femoropopliteal system is difficult because of the differences in patient populations treated with respect to clinical variables. Femoropopliteal bypass using saphenous vein has an initial success rate of 85 to 90 per cent, with 1-year patency rates of 61 to 100 per cent, 2-year patency rates of 60 to 85 per cent, and 5-year patency rates of 55 to 80 per cent.[68] In a randomized series of patients undergoing femoropopliteal bypass using either saphenous vein or polytetrafluoroethylene, the patency rates using polytetrafluoroethylene were 75 per cent at 2 years and 38 per cent at 5 years.[65] Similar to PTA, patency rates are significantly affected by distal run-off and the indication for surgical therapy (claudication versus limb salvage).

In a prospective, randomized series of 98 patients with femoropopliteal disease undergoing either PTA or surgical revascularization, the 3-year survival of study-related deaths, amputation, and intervention failure for surgical therapy and PTA was 65.3 per cent and 59 per cent, respectively.[69] However, if only technically successful PTAs were considered, the cumulative survival was 65.3 per cent for surgical therapy and 75.7 per cent for PTA. In a nonrandomized, retrospective comparison of PTA and surgical therapy for limb-threatening ischemia, the 2-year patency rate for PTA was 18 per cent. Limb salvage after 2 years was 78 per cent; however, 59 per cent of the PTA patients underwent a secondary procedure. Two-year patency of femoropopliteal bypasses was 68 per cent with a limb salvage of 90 per cent.

Although comparisons of PTA and surgical revascularization are difficult, bypass procedures using saphenous vein appear to have better long-term patency and clinical benefit than does PTA, particularly in patients with impaired outflow and increasing ischemia. However, PTA patency rates are comparable to or better than those using synthetic graft material for bypass. In addition, PTA is easier to repeat than surgical revision of a failed graft. Also, PTA preserves the saphenous vein for possible use as a conduit for coronary or other vascular revascularization.

INFRAPOPLITEAL ARTERIAL OBSTRUCTION

Until recently PTA of infrapopliteal vessels was fraught with complications, primarily concerning vascular spasm and subsequent thrombosis. This risk has been greatly reduced through the use of aggressive pharmacologic treatment of vasospasm with calcium channel blockers and nitroglycerin in conjunction with anticoagulation, specifically systemic heparin and pretreatment with aspirin. More important, the development of small-bore, low-profile angioplasty catheters and steerable small-caliber guidewires (0.015- to 0.018-inch wire) for coronary artery angioplasty has allowed relatively atraumatic placement of these catheters into the infrapopliteal vasculature. Because complications may result in limb loss, PTA of infrapopliteal vessels has been limited to patients with threatened extremities.[7,58,63] In a series of 98 patients treated for limb-threatening ischemia, technical success was 97 per cent (100 per cent in treating stenoses, 88 per cent in treating obstructions)

TABLE 3. Femoral Artery PTA

Author	Patients	Technical Success	Patency Rate 1-yr.	2-yr.	5-yr.	Complications
Schneider et al.	682	88%			68%	
Gallino et al.	329	97%			58%	
Johnston et al.	284	89%	60%	52%	40%	
Krepel et al.	129	84%	77%		70%	
Spence et al.	122	84%	80%	75%		
Waltman et al.	98	84%				
Samson et al.	89	92%	50%	50%		25%
Greenfield	70	81%	89%	84%		11%
Propst et al.	57			70%		
Kaufman et al.	55	96%				
Neiman et al.	54	76%				
Wilson et al.	49	78%	62%	59%	59%	38%
Cambria et al.	48	96%	50%			
Martin et al.	46	74%	57%	57%		

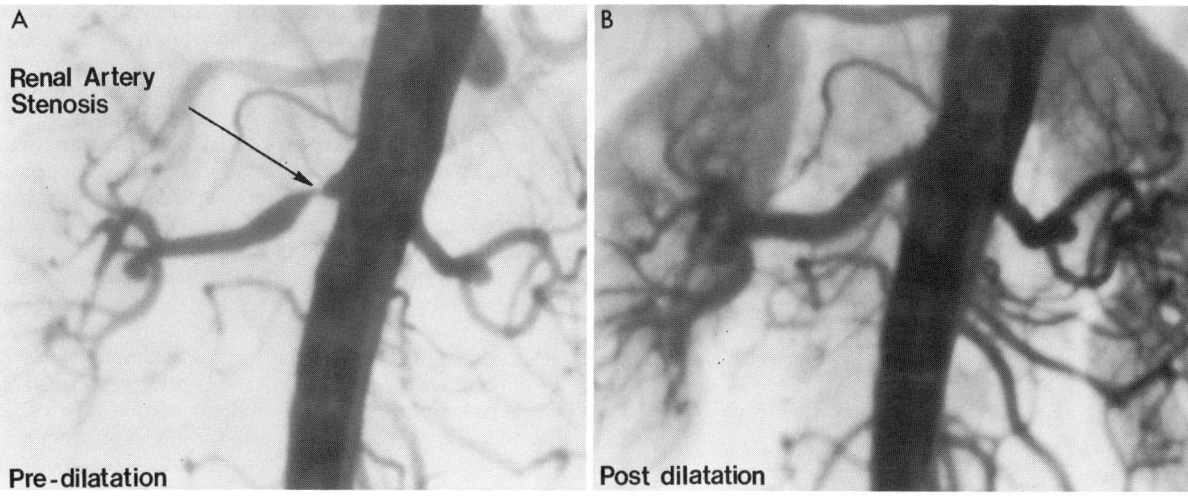

Figure 9. Arteriogram of a 44-year-old woman with multiple emergency room visits for uncontrolled hypertension. Her admission systolic and diastolic blood pressures ranged from 140 to 170 and 90 to 110 mm. Hg, respectively, on a three-drug regimen. *A*, Renal arteriogram demonstrates a 90 per cent stenosis of the right renal artery. *B*, Postdilation arteriogram demonstrates marked improvement of the arterial stenosis. After PTA, the patient was normotensive off all medications.

with a 2-year cumulative limb salvage rate of 86 per cent.[58] However, clinical success in 50 to 60 per cent is more typical.[7,63] Aggressive treatment of thrombosis following PTA with thrombolytic agents in patients with this complication allowed surgical revascularization without untoward sequelae.[58] Results in femorotibial bypass vary widely, and series report 5-year patency rates for saphenous vein bypass of 12 to 85 per cent.[4] Using the reversed saphenous vein as a conduit for infrapopliteal bypass, Taylor reported a patency rate of 85 per cent and a limb salvage rate of 93 per cent at 5 years. Comparison between PTA and surgical revascularization is particularly difficult because of the lack of data concerning treatment using the newer catheters and guidewires. Specifically, there are no series reporting long-term patency. However, PTA is a viable option in treating limb-threatening ischemia in infrapopliteal vessels, especially in patients with increased operative risk and short segment occlusive lesions.

RENAL ARTERIAL OBSTRUCTION

The large number of patients with renovascular hypertension and the reported increase in survival of patients treated with revascularization compared with medical management have led to considerable interest in renal artery PTA (PRTA). Ten to 15 per cent of adults in the United States have hypertension. Of these 23 million individuals, approximately 4 per cent have potentially correctable renovascular hypertension. In patients with accelerated or malignant hypertension, the incidence of a renovascular etiology is 30 per cent, and when present in conjunction with renal insufficiency, the incidence approaches 45 per cent.[34,44]

In 1978, Grüntzig reported the first successful treatment of renovascular hypertension using PRTA.[28] Since then, numerous series have documented the feasibility of using PRTA to treat renovascular hypertension (Fig. 9, Table 4). PRTA has also been used to preserve renal function that has been compromised by renal artery stenosis.[45,64] Ideal lesions treated by PRTA include atherosclerotic lesions that are short, located in the main renal artery and not contiguous with the renal artery ostium, and stenoses due to fibromuscular dysplasia that do not involve the branch vessels (in 30 per cent of patients, branch vessels are involved). PRTA of these lesions is associated with the greatest technical success and clinical benefit, the lowest restenosis rates, and the fewest complications. In contrast, PRTA of atherosclerotic ostial lesions is less often technically successful, is more prone to restenosis, and provides less clinical benefit.[9,29,45,61] The ostial lesions are usually secondary to atherosclerotic plaques of the aorta. The technical difficulties encountered may be partially explained by the increased number of elastic fibers in the aorta relative to the renal artery and the longitudinal orientation of the elastic fibers and plaque to the dilating force of the balloon (Figs. 10 and 11). Occlusions of the renal artery have been successfully dilated, although with a much lower rate of technical and clinical success than dilation of stenoses. Only patients whose occlusions occur in nontortuous arteries in whom the proximal and distal artery can be identified

TABLE 4. Renal Artery PTA

Author	Patients	Technical Success	Effect on Hypertension			
			Cure	Improved Blood Pressure	Benefit Rate	Failure
Klinge et al.	213	73%	16%	64%	80%	20%
Cananello et al.	100	73%	4%	39%	43%	57%
Tegtmeyer	98	97%	26%	67%	93%	7%
Sos et al.	82	56%	28%	23%	51%	49%
Geyskes et al.	70		22%	45%	66%	34%
Schwarten	70	93%			71%	29%
Colapinto et al.	68	85%	18%	56%	74%	26%
Hayes et al.	55	69%			26%	74%
Total	756	77%	18%	52%	67%	33%

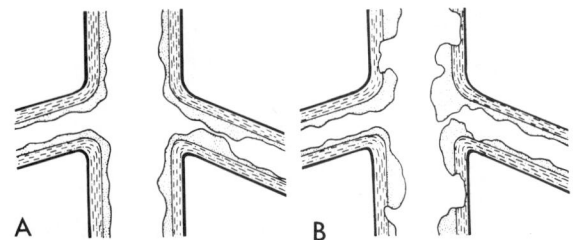

Figure 10. Lesions compromising renal blood flow. *A,* Renal artery lesion. Obstructing lesion lies within the confines of the renal artery. *B,* Aortic lesion. Large atherosclerotic plaques of the aorta encroach on the renal artery ostium, hindering blood flow. (From Cicuto, K. P., McLean, G. K., Oleaga, J. A., et al.: Renal artery stenosis: Anatomic classification for percutaneous transluminal angioplasty. A.J.R., *137:*601, 1981.)

angiographically and in whom the size of the kidney warrants attempted salvage should undergo PRTA.[63]

The indications for PRTA should be similar to those used for surgical intervention and include sustained hypertension, usually of a severe nature that is poorly controlled medically, and evidence of renal artery stenosis by angiographic and hemodynamic data. The role of abnormal renal vein renin values in patients with unilateral renal artery stenosis (abnormal is defined as 1.3 to 1.5 times the value from the kidney without an arterial stenosis) in selecting patients in whom PRTA may have clinical benefit is controversial. Although patients with abnormal renin values appear to have a higher rate of clinical success following technically successful PRTA, a significant proportion of patients without lateralizing renin values have clinical benefit, particularly those patients on beta-blockers or converting enzyme inhibitors at the time of evaluation.

The likelihood of technical success is dependent on the nature and etiology of the lesion. Angioplasty of stenoses caused by fibromuscular dysplasia is technically successful in approximately 87 to 100 per cent of patients (Table 5). In comparison, angioplasty of atherosclerotic stenoses is technically successful in 37 to 90 per cent of patients (Table 6). The technical success rate treating nonostial atherosclerotic lesions is higher and is 72 to 79 per cent compared with ostial lesions in which technical success is achieved in 62 to 66 per cent.[9,29]

Clinical benefit from PRTA is also lesion dependent. Patients with renovascular hypertension due to fibromuscular dysplasia are cured in 57 per cent (range 33 to 62 per cent) and improved in 27 per cent (range 29 to 66 per cent) for an overall improvement rate of 84 per cent. Treatment of atherosclerotic renovascular hypertension using PRTA cures approximately 22 per cent (range 4 to 41 per cent), and improves 39 per cent (range 19 to 61 per cent), for an overall improvement rate of 61 per cent. Clinical results are better in patients with nonostial stenoses with

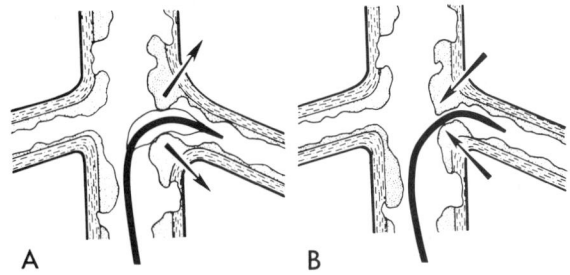

Figure 11. Displacement of aortic plaques rather than compression. *A,* Balloon catheter inflated in an area of narrowing. Large aortic plaques are displaced (arrows) rather than compressed because of the abundant elastic tissue underlying the diseased aortic intima and the orientation of the elastic and collagenous fibers of the aortic wall. *B,* After balloon deflation, aortic plaques return to original location (arrows). Although slight alteration of the plaque surface may occur, the stenosis remains relatively unchanged. (From Cicuto, K. P., McLean, G. K., Oleaga, J. A., et al.: Renal artery stenosis: Anatomic classification for percutaneous transluminal angioplasty. A.J.R., *137:*601, 1981.)

improvement observed in 42 to 86 per cent, as compared with patients with ostial stenoses in whom improvement is found in only 21 to 46 per cent.[9,29] Treatment of unilateral renal artery stenosis is associated with better clinical results than is treatment of bilateral stenoses or renal artery stenosis in a solitary kidney.[9] Using PRTA in the treatment of renal artery stenosis in a series of patients with progressive azotemia was successful in improving renal function in 43 per cent of patients (greater than 20 per cent decrease in serum creatinine).[45] Patients with bilateral renal artery stenoses had the best results (improvement in 61 per cent). The least improvement occurred in patients with serum creatinine that was greater than 4.0 mg. per 100 ml. (improvement in 14 per cent).

Restenosis after PRTA occurs in approximately 5 per cent of fibromuscular dysplasia lesions and between 15 and 25 per cent of atherosclerotic lesions. Restenosis occurs most commonly after dilation of ostial lesions and can occur as often as 74 per cent.[29] However, 50 to 75 per cent of restenosis can be redilated with clinical benefit in approximately 50 per cent of patients.[9,11,21,56]

Mortality associated with PRTA is approximately 1 per cent, but mortality up to 7.3 per cent has been reported.[29] Most deaths occur in patients with diffuse atherosclerotic disease, and myocardial infarction is the most common cause of death. Diffuse atherosclerotic emboli causing bowel infarction and peripheral ischemia as well as retroperitoneal hemorrhage are other common causes of mortality. Complications are more frequent than when performing PTA in other vascular beds, 5 to 33 per cent, the average being 7 to 10 per cent when treating fibromuscular dysplasia lesions and 15 to 25 per cent treating atherosclerotic lesions. The most common complications are renal insufficiency, renal artery dissection and perforation, renal artery emboli as well as other atheromatous emboli, myocardial infarction, and local complications at the femoral artery puncture site. Approximately 2 to 5 per cent of patients require operative intervention, sometimes as an emergency. Following complications involving the renal artery or its branches, such as perforation and thrombosis that require surgical intervention, a reasonable likelihood of renal salvage is possible with immediate surgical revascularization, although a more complex vascular procedure is often necessary. In these cases, the perivascular inflammatory response to PTA complicates the technical aspects of surgical revascularization. Because of these complications and the need for prompt intervention to optimize the clinical results, PRTA should be limited to centers with adequate surgical facilities to manage the complications.

Comparison of surgical revascularization versus PRTA in the treatment of renovascular hypertension is complicated by the lack of control trials and the differences in patient characteristics between series treated by PRTA and operative therapy. The National Cooperative Study on Renovascular Hypertension reported an overall surgical benefit of 78.7 per cent with a mortality of 5.9 per cent.[18] However, more recent reports utilizing better patient selection as well as improved technique and perioperative care have reported mortality of approximately 2 per cent and clinical benefit in 90 to 97 per cent. Forty to 72 per cent of the patients were cured of hypertension, and improved blood pressure control occurred in an additional 25 to 52 per cent (Table 7). Although cure of hypertension is less common, the comparable success using PRTA in patients with fibromuscular dysplasia (84 per cent benefit rate) and in patients with nonostial atherosclerotic lesions (benefit rate 70 per cent), coupled with the procedure's lower morbidity, mortality, expense, and lost productivity time, allows it to be an initial approach in these patients. Rarely does an unsuccessful angioplasty prevent or complicate a later surgical revascularization. However, the majority of patients with renovascular hypertension have atherosclerotic lesions that are not ideal for PRTA, and frequently

TABLE 5. PRTA Treatment of Stenosis due to Fibromuscular Dysplasia

| Author | Patients | Technical Success | Effect on Hypertension | | | Follow-up (mo.) Mean (range) |
			Cure	Improved Blood Pressure	Benefit Rate	
Klinge et al.	52	71%	35%	51%	86%	6
Sos et al.	31	87%	51%	29%	80%	16 (4–40)
Tegtmeyer et al.	21	100%	62%	38%	100%	11.5 (1–30)
Martin et al.	11	73%	45%	9%	54%	13 (4–25)
Grim et al.	10	90%	50%	40%	90%	6.8 (1–14)
Beebe et al.	9	89%	33%	56%	89%	23
Mahler et al.	6	100%	67%	33%	100%	19 (6–39)
Hayes et al.	6	50%			50%	13
Total	146	82%	46%	40%	84%	

Modified from Flechner, S. M.: Percutaneous transluminal dilatation. A realistic appraisal in patients with stenosing lesions of the renal artery. Urol. Clin. North Am., 11:515, 1984.

these are the patients with diffuse atherosclerosis and other medical conditions that increase the risk of operative intervention. PRTA in these patients is associated with fewer technical successes, less clinical benefit, and more complications that limit the overall utility of the angioplasty.

RENAL TRANSPLANT ARTERIAL OBSTRUCTION

Renovascular hypertension due to renal graft artery stenosis occurs in 4.9 to 7.1 per cent of patients who have undergone renal artery transplantation.[15,24] Treatment using PTA is technically successful in 84 to 90 per cent. Clinical success as determined by improvement of blood pressure control on the same or less medications occurs in 74 to 76 per cent of patients. Restenosis was present in 21 per cent of successfully dilated arteries at 1 year.[15] In a nonrandomized, retrospective study comparing PTA with saphenous vein bypass, PTA had a higher rate of initial failure (18 per cent versus 6 per cent) and a higher rate of control of hypertension (85 per cent versus 74 per cent).[15] However, because of the relative ease and better tolerance of the procedure in the immunosuppressed host with similar control of hypertension, PTA is the initial procedure of choice in most of these patients.

COARCTATION OF THE AORTA

PTA has been successfully applied to the treatment of both native and restenosis aortic coarctations (Fig. 12).[1,3,5,10,14,51] The first PTA of an aortic coarctation was reported in 1982,[59] and since then over 200 cases have been reported. Early technical success with significant gradient reduction and enlargement of the aorta at the coarctation site is generally accomplished. However, follow-up of patients indicates that significant problems with recoarctation and aneurysm formation at the angioplasty site ensue. Mortality is very rare and is associated with aortic perforation at the angioplasty site secondary to catheter manipulation without a guidewire in place across the coarctation site. Morbidity is primarily associated with arterial puncture site complications and includes bleeding and thrombosis. Cerebrovascular accidents have been reported.[3,14] Unlike surgical repair of aortic coarctation, PTA treatment has a much lower incidence of paradoxical hypertension (range of 0 to 21 per cent).[10,14] This appears to be due to the absence of activation of the renin-angiotensin and catecholamine axes.[10]

Long-term follow-up of PTA treatment of coarctations has demonstrated recurrences and aneurysms, which may be a late complication of the procedure. Although the majority of pa-

TABLE 6. PRTA Treatment of Stenosis due to Atherosclerosis

| Author | Patients | Technical Success | Effect on Hypertension | | | Follow-up (mo.) Mean (range) |
			Cure	Improved Blood Pressure	Benefit Rate	
Klinge et al.	134	74%	10%	68%	77%	6
Cananello et al.	100	73%	4%	39%	43%	29 (6–72)
Hayes et al.	55	69%			22%	
Schwarten et al.	54	89%	41%	46%	87%	5.3 (1–12)
Sos et al.	51	37%	14%	19%	33%	16 (4–40)
Beebe et al.	38	53%	11%	21%	32%	22
Flechner et al.	27	48%	7%	41%	48%	6.8 (2–15)
Grim et al.	16	100%	6%	43%	49%	9.8 (3–24)
Martin et al.	15	87%	13%	27%	40%	13 (4–24)
Tegtmeyer et al.	13	84%	23%	61%	84%	3.5 (0.5–10)
Total	503	70%	13%	45%	59%	

Modified from Flechner, S. M.: Percutaneous transluminal dilatation. A realistic appraisal in patients with stenosing lesions of the renal artery. Urol. Clin. North Am., 11:515, 1984.

TABLE 7. Surgical Therapy for Renovascular Hypertension

| Author | Patients | Effect on Hypertension | | | Failure | Mortality Rate |
		Cure	Improved Blood Pressure	Benefit Rate		
Novick et al.	78	40%	51%	91%	0	2%
Foster et al.	502	47%	14%	61%	0	6%
Laroche et al.	12	25%	75%	100%	0	0%
Libertino et al.	210	72%	25%	97%	0	2%

tients treated by PTA continue to have a good hemodynamic and angiographic result at follow-up, a proportion have significant gradients across the coarctation site (27 to 35 per cent gradients greater than 20 mm. Hg).[3,5,51] Since all patients studied were within 30 months of PTA in these series, the true long-term results regarding recurrent stenosis have not been determined. Factors identified as being significantly associated with a recurrent stenosis are as follows: (1) age less than 12 months at the time of PTA; (2) diffuse versus discrete coarctation; (3) smaller diameter at the coarctation site (less than 3.5 mm. before dilation); (4) smaller diameter after PTA (less than 6 mm.); and (5) larger gradient across the coarctation (greater than 50 mm. Hg).[3,14,51] Patients with recoarctation have been treated successfully with a second PTA or with surgical repair without apparent added morbidity.[5,51] Especially in the neonatal population with congestive heart failure associated with aortic coarctation, PTA has been successfully used in temporizing these patients and deferring operative intervention until a more fa-

vorable time. The patient population with the best long-term results following PTA appears to be those treated for recurrent stenosis after end-to-end surgical anastomosis.

Aneurysm formation occurs as a late complication of PTA. The incidence of this complication varies considerably between reported series and is 0 to 55 per cent (Table 8).[5,10,14,51] The reported incidence depends on the length of follow-up, the completeness with which the patients within a series are studied, and the technique utilized for PTA, particularly the balloon size and dilation pressure. Since most series report data from patients in the first 2 years after PTA, the long-term incidence of aneurysm formation remains to be determined. Because a successful dilation of a coarctation requires a controlled injury to the aorta manifest by intimal and medial tears, an uncontrolled injury with transmedial tears may occur, causing aneurysm formation. This appears to be associated with the use of oversized balloons or balloon overdistention. Another factor in the development of post-PTA aneurysms may be associated with the

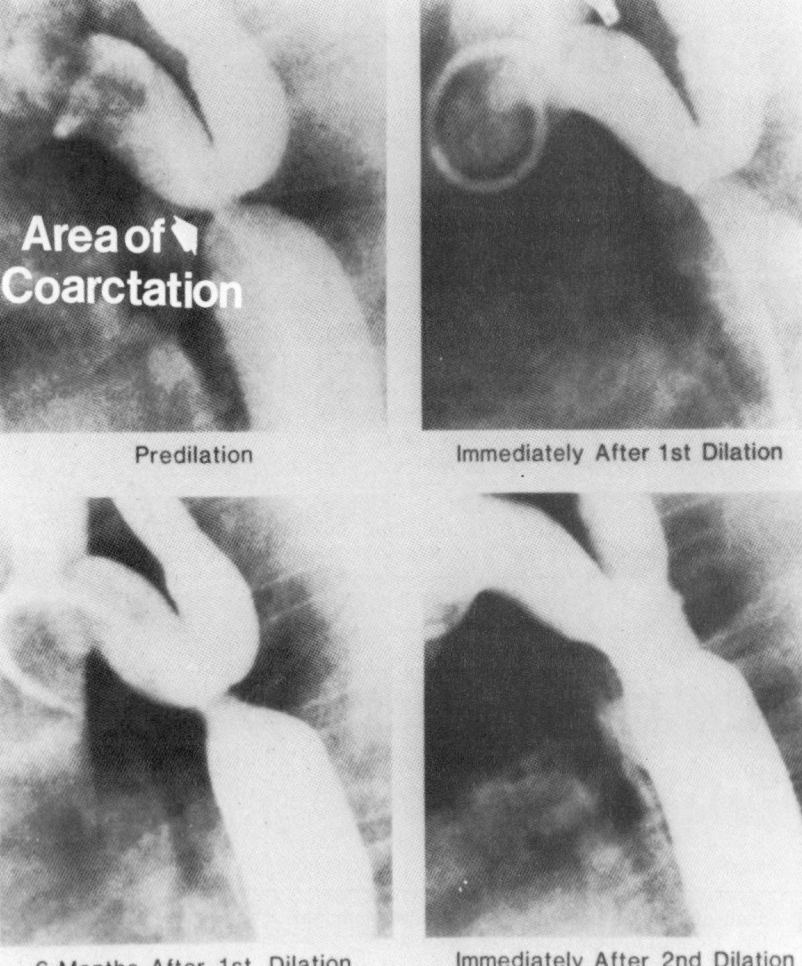

Figure 12. Aortic coarctation in a 6-year-old after surgical correction with end-to-end anastomosis. *A,* Before PTA, the diameter at the stenosis was 2.3 mm. and was associated with a gradient of 67 mm. Hg. *B,* After initial dilation using an 8-mm. balloon, the lumen diameter increased to 5.4 mm. with a residual gradient of 49 mm. Hg. *C,* Six months after initial PTA, the vessel lumen was 5.2 mm. with a gradient of 28 mm. Hg. *D,* After repeat PTA with a 12-mm. balloon, the vessel diameter increased to 9.3 mm. and the gradient had decreased to 8 mm. Hg. At follow-up 3 months later, the gradient was zero. (From Lock, J. E., Bass, J. L., Amplatz, K., et al.: Balloon dilation angioplasty of aortic coarctation in infants and children. Circulation, *68:*114, 1983.)

TABLE 8. Treatment of Aortic Coarctation Using PTA

Author	Number of Patients	Technical Success	Recoarctation	Aneurysm Formation	Follow-up Mean (Range) (mos.)
Beekman et al.	26	79%	29%	7%	15.3 (12–26)
Rao et al.	20	85%	35%	0%	11.6 (6–30)
Brandt et al.	11		27%	36%	10 (6–12)
De Lezo et al.	28			6%	
Choy et al.	8	88%	17%		
Attia and Lababidi	8	100%	0%	0%	12
Total	101	86%	25%	9%	

nearly uniform presence of cystic medial necrosis in the coarctation segment. In a pathologic study of 33 specimens excised at the time of operative repair, all exhibited degrees of cystic medial necrosis, whereas two thirds exhibited severe cystic medial necrosis.[30] Interestingly, the dilation of restenosis after surgical treatment of aortic coarctation is not associated with aneurysm formation.

Balloon angioplasty is a viable treatment of native and restenosis coarctation of the aorta. Immediate benefit after PTA is almost uniform with minimal mortality. Critically ill infants can often be treated with PTA, allowing time for a more opportune definitive therapy. PTA should probably be considered the treatment of choice for restenosis coarctation; however, the optimal clinical use of PTA for native coarctation remains to be defined, depending on the true long-term incidence of restenosis and aneurysm formation.

CEREBROVASCULAR ARTERIAL OBSTRUCTION

Because of the risk of embolization to the cerebral circulation with resulting ischemic stroke, experience with PTA of the cerebrovascular circulation has not increased relative to other vascular systems. However, nonatherosclerotic obstructions and stenoses of the subclavian arteries have been successfully dilated with an acceptable morbidity and clinical benefit. Although large series of patients are not available, treatment using PTA in symptomatic patients with obstruction of the common and internal carotid arteries by fibromuscular dysplasia has been documented (Fig. 13).[60] The low incidence of cerebral ischemia associated with these procedures reflects the decreased risk of embolization with fibromuscular dysplasia lesions. Angioplasty has been performed using the transfemoral approach as well as an operative approach through the common carotid artery after obtaining proximal and distal control of the carotid arteries.[60] This latter approach allows back-bleeding after performing the angioplasty to further minimize the risk of cerebral embolization. Similarly, inflammatory lesions of the brachiocephalic vessels, which also have an inherently lower risk of embolization, have been treated with PTA.

Treatment of atherosclerotic obstructions of the carotid, innominate, and vertebral arteries has been reported.[32] In some of these patients, attempts to protect the cerebral circulation by inflating a second balloon distal to the stenosis has been employed. Lesions at high risk for embolization have reportedly been avoided by means of scintigraphy for identifying those plaques that contain thrombus.[32] Although these series report technical success rates between 80 and 90 per cent, with low morbidity and good clinical response, the small number of patients reported in each series, as well as the lack of detailed analysis and long-term follow-up, emphasizes caution with regard to PTA of cerebrovascular atherosclerotic lesions. PTA of these vessels should be considered investigational until the risks are better defined. Particularly, PTA of the basilar artery, because of the large number of branches to the brain stem that can

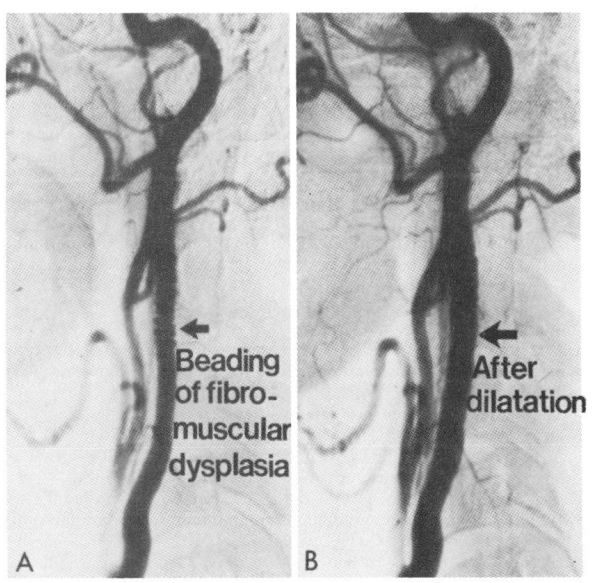

Figure 13. Transluminal angioplasty of a stenosis due to fibromuscular dysplasia. *A*, Carotid arteriogram demonstrates the typical "beaded" appearance of fibromuscular dysplasia. *B*, After dilation, resolution of the previously stenotic area. (From Garrido, E., and Montoya, J.: Transluminal dilatation of internal carotid artery in fibromuscular dysplasia: A preliminary report. Surg. Neurol., *16*:470, 1981.)

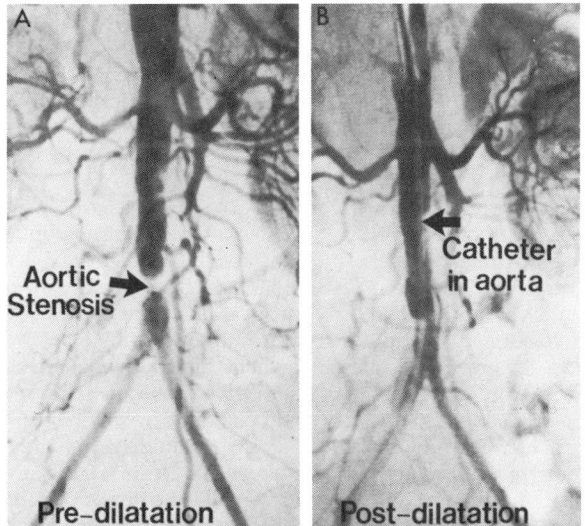

Figure 14. PTA of an abdominal aortic stenosis. *A*, Concentric hourglass stenosis of the infrarenal aorta. Lumen diameter was 4 mm. with a gradient of 10 mm. Hg. *B*, Following PTA, the lumen diameter was 9 mm. and the pressure gradient was zero. Patient was asymptomatic at 6-month follow-up. (From Heeney, D., Bookstein, J., Danield, E., et al.: Transluminal angioplasty of the abdominal aorta. Radiology, *148*:81, 1983.)

be occluded by the dilation, appears to have an increased intrinsic risk of stroke. The abdominal aorta may also be dilated (Fig. 14).

A greater experience in dilating atherosclerotic lesions of the subclavian arteries has been accumulated. Because blood flow does not reverse within the vertebral artery for 35 to 40 seconds after dilating a proximal subclavian artery obstruction, patients with the subclavian steal syndrome have been successfully treated with PTA.[32,67] Technically successful dilation of nonostial stenoses occurs in 85 to 95 per cent.[32,67] In a series of 22 patients who underwent subclavian artery PTA, the patency rate at 4 years was 80 per cent.[67] In two of the largest series, embolic complications occurred in 8 per cent of patients (4 of 49) with one transient ischemic attack, one stroke, and two emboli to the extremity. PTA of the subclavian artery has been used prior to and following coronary revascularization using the internal mammary artery with success. Temporary, but not long-term, success has been associated with the use of PTA prior to axillofemoral artery grafting.

HEMODIALYSIS ACCESS FISTULA OBSTRUCTION

The most common problems occurring in hemodialysis fistulas are graft thrombosis or inadequate dialysis that is usually due to venous outflow stenosis (70 per cent), arterial inflow stenosis (15 per cent), or a combination (15 per cent).[22] PTA of these stenoses has been used successfully in a number of different centers.[6,12,13,22] The early technical success is approximately 80 to 90 per cent. However, long-term patency has been fair with patency rates of 41 to 62 per cent at 6 months, 31 to 45 per cent at 1 year, and 24 per cent at 2 years.[12,13,22] Repeated PTA has maintained some grafts for more than 5 years. The advantages of PTA treatment of hemodialysis fistula stenosis include the following: (1) preservation of the existing dialysis site, potentially adding longevity to the graft and preserving other sites for future use; (2) the use of later surgical revision, when necessary, was not compromised; and (3) the grafts could continue to be used for dialysis without maturation delays. In a prospective, randomized study of 43 patients with venous outflow stenosis, the fistulas treated by surgical revision had a significantly better long-term patency than those treated with PTA.[6] The median survival in the surgical group was 12 months compared with 4 months in the PTA group. In addition, all long-term patency greater than 2 years was in the surgical revision group. In contrast, a nonrandomized, retrospective study found the opposite conclusion, with patency rates significantly better in the PTA group. The patency at 1 year in the surgical group was only 19 per cent compared with 31 per cent using PTA.[12]

SUMMARY

PTA, introduced in 1964 by Dotter and Judkins and popularized by Grüntzig, has become an established and effective technique in the treatment of vascular occlusive disease. Its role should not be considered competitive, but rather complementary to surgical therapy. Because results using angioplasty are lesion dependent, being most useful in the treatment of discrete stenoses and occlusions, optimally PTA should be used when such favorable anatomy is present. The more frequent morphologic characteristics of diffuse, long, or multiple lesions and nondiscrete occlusions are better treated with surgical revascularization. In addition, PTA can be applied to patients whose attendant risk with operation is great. Angioplasty can be used in a variety of clinical settings as an adjunct to surgical techniques to simplify arterial reconstruction or salvage existing grafts with occlusive lesions. Optimal care of the patient with vaso-occlusive disease requires close cooperation between the angiographer and surgeon to enable proper treatment selection

and management of the potentially catastrophic complications that may occur following angioplasty.

SELECTED REFERENCES

Dotter, C. T., and Judkins, M. P.: Transluminal treatment of arteriosclerotic obstruction. Description of a new technic and a preliminary report of its application. Circulation, 30:654, 1964.
This is the original article describing the use of PTA in the treatment of obstructive vascular disease. The authors report their initial experience treating 11 patients, 6 of whom had marked improvement in symptoms and peripheral blood flow.

Flechner, S. M.: Percutaneous transluminal dilatation. A realistic appraisal in patients with stenosing lesions of the renal artery. Urol. Clin. North Am., 11:515, 1984.
Excellent discussion of the role of PTA in the treatment of renovascular hypertension. A summary of results achieved treating atherosclerotic and fibromuscular stenoses is presented. Comparison of PTA, surgical, and medical therapy in the treatment of renal artery stenosis is made.

Johnston, K. W., Rae, M., Hogg-Johnston, S. A., Colapinto, R. F., Walker, P. M., Baird, R. J., Sniderman, K. W., and Kalman, P.: Five-year results of a prospective study of percutaneous transluminal angioplasty. Ann. Surg., 206:403, 1987.
This paper presents the most accurate clinical results using PTA for the treatment of occlusive vascular disease of the lower extremity. Life-table analysis of the 984 patients treated with PTA is utilized. Predictors of success are discussed.

Ritter, S. B.: Coarctation and balloons: Inflated or realistic? J. Am. Coll. Cardiol., 13:696, 1989.
Editorial review regarding the role of PTA in the treatment of native coarctation of the aorta. Issues of recoarctation, aneurysm formation, and hemodynamic results are discussed with literature references.

Tegtmeyer, C. J.: Percutaneous transluminal angioplasty. Curr. Probl. Diagn. Radiol., 16:75, 1987.
Excellent review of the technique of PTA with regard to the different vascular systems. Results with PTA in the treatment of occlusive disease in the different vascular systems from the author's experience as well as representative series from the literature are presented.

REFERENCES

1. Attia, I. M., and Lababidi, Z. A.: Early results of balloon angioplasty of native coarctation in young adults. Am. J. Cardiol., 61:930, 1988.
2. Beebe, H. G., Chesboro, K., Merchant, F., and Bush, W.: Results of renal artery balloon angioplasty limit its indications. J. Vasc. Surg., 8:300, 1988.
3. Beekman, R. H., Rocchini, A. P., Dick, M., Snider, R., Crowley, D. C., Serwer, G. A., Spicer, R. L., and Rosenthal, A.: Percutaneous balloon angioplasty for native coarctation of the aorta. J. Am. Coll. Cardiol., 10:1078, 1987.
4. Bernhard, V. M.: Bypass to the popliteal and infrapopliteal arteries. In Rutherford, R. B. (Ed.): Vascular Surgery. Philadelphia, W. B. Saunders Company, 1989.
5. Brandt, B., Marvin, W. J., Rose, E. F., and Mahoney, L. T.: Surgical treatment of the aorta after balloon angioplasty. J. Thorac. Cardiovasc. Surg., 94:715, 1987.
6. Brooks, J. L., Sigley, R. D., May, K. J., Jr., and Mack, R. M.: Transluminal angioplasty versus surgical repair for stenosis of hemodialysis grafts. A randomized study. Am. J. Surg., 153:530, 1987.
7. Brown, K. T., Schoenberg, N. Y., Moore, E. D., and Saddenkni, S.: Percutaneous transluminal angioplasty of infrapopliteal vessels: Preliminary results and technical considerations. Radiology, 169:75, 1988.
8. Cambria, R. P., Faust, G., Gusberg, R., Tilson, M. D., Zucker, K. A., and Modlin, I. M.: Percutaneous angioplasty for peripheral arterial occlusive disease. Arch. Surg., 122:283, 1987.
9. Cananello, V. J., Millan, V. G., Spiegel, J. E., Ponce, S. P., Kopelman, R. I., and Madias, N. E.: Percutaneous transluminal renal angioplasty in management of atherosclerotic renovascular hypertension: Results in 100 patients. Hypertension, 13:163, 1989.
10. Choy, M., Rocchini, A. P., Beekman, R. H., Rosenthal, A., Dick, M., Crowley, D., Behrendt, D., and Snider, A. R.: Paradoxical hypertension after repair of coarctation of the aorta in children: Balloon angioplasty versus surgical repair. Circulation, 75:1186, 1987.
11. Colapinto, R. F., Stronell, R. D., Haries-Jones, E. P., Gildimer, M., Hobbs, B. B., Farrow, G. A., Wilson, D. R., Morrow, J. D., Logan, A. G., and Birch, S. J.: Percutaneous transluminal dilatation of the renal artery: Follow-up studies on renovascular hypertension. Am. J. Roentgenol., 139:727, 1982.
12. Dapunt, O., Feurstein, M., Rendl, K. H., and Prenner, K.: Transluminal angioplasty versus conventional operation in the treatment of haemodialysis fistula stenosis: Results from a 5-year study. Br. J. Surg., 74:1004, 1987.
13. Davis, G. B., Dowd, C. F., Bookstein, J. J., Maroney, T. P., Lang, E. V., and Halasz, N.: Thrombosed dialysis grafts: Efficacy of intrathrombic deposition of concentrated urokinase, clot maceration, and angioplasty. A.J.R., 149:177, 1987.
14. De Lezo, J. S., Sancho, M., Pan, M., Romero, M., Olivera, C., and Luque, M.: Angiographic follow-up after balloon angioplasty for coarctation of the aorta. J. Am. Coll. Cardiol., 13:689, 1989.

15. De Meyer, M., Pirson, Y., Dautrebande, J., Squifflet, J. P., Alexandre, G. P., van Ypersele, de Strihou, C.: Treatment of renal graft artery stenosis. Comparison between surgical bypass and percutaneous transluminal angioplasty. Transplantation, 47:784, 1989.
16. Dotter, C. T., and Judkins, M. P.: Transluminal treatment of arteriosclerotic obstruction. Description of a new technic and a preliminary report of its application. Circulation, 30:654, 1964.
17. Flechner, S. M.: Percutaneous transluminal dilatation. A realistic appraisal in patients with stenosing lesions of the renal artery. Urol. Clin. North Am., 11:515, 1984.
18. Foster, J. H., Maxwell, M. H., Franklin, S. S., Bleifer, K. H., Trippel, O. H., Julian, O. C., DeCamp, P. T., and Varody, P. T.: Renovascular occlusive disease: Results of operative treatment. J.A.M.A., 231:1043, 1975.
19. Fradet, G., Lidstone, D., Herba, M., Chiu, R. C. J., and Blundell, P. E.: Percutaneous transluminal angioplasty of iliac arteries: The importance of functional studies. Can. J. Surg., 27:359, 1954.
20. Gallino, A., Mahler, F., Probst, P., and Nachbur, B.: Percutaneous transluminal angioplasties of arteries of the lower limb. Circulation, 70:619, 1984.
21. Geyskes, G. G., Puylaert, C. B. A. J., Oei, H. Y., and Dorhout Mees, E. J.: Follow-up study of 70 patients with renal artery stenosis treated by percutaneous transluminal dilatation. Br. Med. J., 287:333, 1983.
22. Glanz, S., Gordon, D. H., Butt, K. M., Hong, J., and Lipkowitz, G. S.: The role of percutaneous angioplasty in the management of chronic hemodialysis fistulas. Ann. Surg., 206:777, 1987.
23. Greenfield, A. J.: Femoral, popliteal and tibial arteries: Percutaneous transluminal angioplasty. Am. J. Roentgenol., 135:927, 1980.
24. Greenstein, S. M., Verstandig, A., McLean, G. K., Dafoe, D. C., Burke, D. R., Meranze, S. G., Naji, A., Grossman, R. A., Perloff, L. J., and Barker, C. F.: Percutaneous transluminal angioplasty. The procedure of choice in the hypertensive renal allograft recipient with renal artery stenosis. Transplantation, 43:29, 1987.
25. Grüntzig, A.: Percutaneous transluminal angioplasty. Am. J. Roentgenol., 136:216, 1981.
26. Grüntzig, A., and Hopff, H.: Perkutane Rekanalisation chronischer arterieller Verschlusse mit einen neuen Dilatationskatheter. Dtsch. Med. Wochenschr., 99:2502, 1974.
27. Grüntzig, A., Vetter, W., Meir, B., Kuhlman, U., Lutolf, U., and Siegenthaler, W.: Treatment of renovascular hypertension with percutaneous transluminal dilation of a renal artery stenosis. Lancet, 1:801, 1978.
28. Grüntzig, A. R., Myler, R. K., Stertzer, S., Kaltenbach, M., and Turinu, M. I.: Coronary percutaneous transluminal angioplasty: Preliminary results. Circulation, 1:263, 1978.
29. Hayes, J. M., Risius, B., Novick, A. C., Geisinger, M., Zelch, M., Gifford, R. W., Vidt, D. G., and Olin, J. W.: Experience with percutaneous transluminal angioplasty for renal artery stenosis at the Cleveland Clinic. J. Urol., 139:488, 1988.
30. Isner, J. M., Donaldson, R. F., Fulton, D., Bhan, I., Payne, D. D., and Cleveland, R. J.: Cystic medial necrosis in coarctation of the aorta: A potential factor contributing to adverse consequences observed after percutaneous balloon angioplasty of coarctation sites. Circulation, 75:689, 1987.
31. Johnston, K. W., Rae, M., Hogg-Johnston, S. A., Colapinto, R. F., Walker, P. M., Baird, R. J., Sniderman, K. W., and Kalman, P.: Five-year results of a prospective study of percutaneous transluminal angioplasty. Ann. Surg., 206:403, 1987.
32. Kachel, R., Endert, G., Basche, S., Grossmann, K., and Glaser, F. H.: Percutaneous transluminal angioplasty (dilatation) of carotid, vertebral, and innominate artery stenoses. Cardiovasc. Intervent. Radiol., 10:142, 1987.
33. Kadir, S., White, R. I., Kaufman, S. L., Barth, K. H., Williams, G. M., Burdick, J. F., O'Mara, C. S., Smith, G. W., Stonesifer, G. L., Ernst, C. B., and Minken, S. L.: Long-term results of aortoiliac angioplasty. Surgery, 94:10, 1983.
34. Kaplan, N. M.: Renal vascular hypertension. In Kaplan, N. M. (Ed.): Clinical Hypertension. Baltimore, Williams & Wilkins, 1986, pp. 317–344.
35. Katzen, B. T.: Percutaneous transluminal angioplasty for arterial disease of the lower extremities. Am. J. Roentgenol., 142:23, 1984.
36. Kaufman, S. C., Barth, K. H., Kadir, S., Williams, G. M., Smith, G. W., Stonesifer, G. L., Leand, P. M., Adams, P. E., Wenham, F., and White, R. I.: Hemodynamic measurements in the evaluation and follow-up of transluminal angioplasty of the iliac and femoral arteries. Radiology, 142:329, 1982.
37. Kinney, T. B., Chin, A. K., Rurik, G. W., Finn, J. C., Shoor, P. M., Hayden, W. G., and Fogarty, T. J.: Transluminal angioplasty: A mechanical-pathophysiological correlation of its physical mechanisms. Radiology, 153:85, 1984.
38. Klinge, J., Mali, W. P. T. M., Puijlaert, C. B. A., Geyskes, G. G., Becking, W. B., and Feldberg, W. A. M.: Percutaneous transluminal renal angioplasty: Initial and long-term results. Radiology, 171:501, 1989.
39. Krepel, V. M., van Andel, G. P., van Erp, W. F. M., and Breslau, P. J.: Percutaneous transluminal angioplasty of the femoropopliteal artery: Initial and long-term results. Radiology, 156:325, 1985.
40. Kwasnik, E. M., Sioufti, S. Y., Jay, M. E., and Khuri, S. F.: Comparative results of angioplasty and aortofemoral bypass in patients with symptomatic iliac disease. Arch. Surg., 122:288, 1987.
41. Laroche, G. P., Oachance, J. G., and Lebel, M.: Renal revascularization as treatment for malignant hypertension. Can. J. Surg., 23:329, 1980.
42. Libertino, J. A., and Zinmun, L.: Renal revascularization using aortorenal saphenous vein bypass grafting. Surg. Clin. North Am., 60:487, 1980.
43. Lyon, R. T., Zarins, C. K., Lu, C. T., Yang, O. F., and Glagov, W.: Vessel, plaque and lumen morphology after transluminal balloon angioplasty. Arteriosclerosis, 7:306, 1987.
44. Madias, N. E.: Renovascular hypertension. AKF Nephrology Letter, 3:27, 1986.
45. Martin, L. G., Casarella, W. J., and Gaylord, G. M.: Azotemia caused by renal artery stenosis: Treatment by percutaneous angioplasty. A.J.R., 150:839, 1988.
46. Martin, E. C., Fankuchen, E. I., Karlson, K. B., Dolgin, C., Collins, R. H., Voorhees, A. B., Jr., and Casarella, W. J.: Angioplasty for femoral artery occlusion: Comparison with surgery. Am. J. Roentgenol., 137:915, 1981.
47. Milford, M. A., Weaver, F. A., Lundell, C. J., and Yellin, A. E.: Femoropopliteal percutaneous transluminal angioplasty for limb salvage. J. Vasc. Surg., 8:292, 1988.
48. Neiman, H. L., Bergan, J. J., Yao, J. S., Brandt, T. D., Greenberg, M., and O'Mara, C. S.: Hemodynamic assessment of transluminal angioplasty for lower extremity ischemia. Radiology, 143:639, 1982.
49. Novick, A. C., Khauli, R. B., and Vidt, D. G.: Diminished operative risk and improved results following revascularization for atherosclerotic renovascular disease. Urol. Clin. North Am., 11:435, 1984.
50. Probst, P., Cerny, P., Owens, A., and Mahler, F.: Patency after femoral angioplasty: Correlation of angiographic appearance with clinical findings. Am. J. Roentgenol., 140:1227, 1983.
51. Rao, P. S., Thapar, M. K., Kutayli, F., and Carey, P.: Causes of recoarctation after balloon angioplasty of unoperated aortic coarctation. J. Am. Coll. Cardiol., 13:109, 1989.
52. Ring, E. J., Freiman, D. B., McLean, G. K., and Schwarz, W.: Percutaneous recanalization of common iliac artery occlusions: An unacceptable complication rate? Am. J. Roentgenol., 139:587, 1982.
53. Samson, R. H., Sproyregen, S., Veith, F. J., Scher, L. A., Cupta, S. K., and Ascer, E.: Management of angioplasty complications, unsuccessful procedures and early and late failures. Ann. Surg., 199:234, 1984.
54. Sanborn, T. A.: Recanalization of arterial occlusions: Pathological basis and contributing factors. J. Am. Coll. Cardiol., 13:1558, 1989.
55. Schneider, E., Grüntzig, A., and Bollinger, A.: Langzeitergebnisse nach perkutaner transluminaler Angioplastie (PTA) bei 882 konsekutiven Patienten mit ilikalen und femoropoplitealen Obstruktionen. Vasa, 11:322, 1982.
56. Schwarten, D. E.: Transluminal angioplasty of renal artery stenosis: 70 experiences. Am. J. Roentgenol., 135:969, 1980.
57. Schwarten, D. E.: Percutaneous transluminal angioplasty of the iliac arteries: Intravenous digital subtraction angiography for follow-up. Radiology, 150:363, 1980.
58. Schwarten, D. E., and Cutcliff, W. B.: Arterial occlusive disease below the knee: Treatment with percutaneous transluminal angioplasty performed with low-profile catheters and steerable guide wires. Radiology, 169:71, 1988.
59. Singer, M. I., Rowen, M., and Dorsey, T. J.: Transluminal aortic balloon angioplasty for coarctation of the aorta in the newborn. Am. Heart J., 103:131, 1982.
60. Smith, L. L., Smith, D. C., Killeen, J. D., and Hasso, A. N.: Operative balloon angioplasty in the treatment of internal carotid artery fibromuscular dysplasia. J. Vasc. Surg., 6:482, 1987.
61. Sos, T. A., Pickering, T. G., Phil, D., Sniderman, K., Saddekni, S., Case, D. B., Silane, M. F., Vaughan, E. D., Jr., and Laragh, J. H.: Percutaneous transluminal renal angioplasty in renovascular hypertension due to atheroma or fibromuscular dysplasia. N. Engl. J. Med., 309:274, 1983.
62. Spence, R. K., Freiman, D. B., Gatenby, R., Hobbs, C. L., Barker, C. R., Berkowitz, H. D., Roberts, B., McClean, G., Oleaga, J., and Ring, E. J.: Long-term results of transluminal angioplasty of the iliac and femoral arteries. Arch. Surg., 116:1377, 1981.
63. Tegtmeyer, C. J.: Percutaneous transluminal angioplasty. Curr. Probl. Diagn. Radiol., 16:75, 1987.
64. Tegtmeyer, C. J., Kellum, C. D., and Ayers, C.: Percutaneous transluminal angioplasty of the renal artery. Results and long-term follow-up. Radiology, 153:77, 1984.
65. Veith, F. J., Gupta, S. K., Ascer, E., et al.: Six-year prospective multicenter randomized comparison of autologous saphenous vein and expanded polytetrafluoroethylene grafts in infrainguinal arterial reconstruction. J. Vasc. Surg., 3:104, 1986.
66. Waltman, A. C., Greenfield, A. J., Novelline, R. A., Abbott, W. M., Brewster, D. C., Darling, R. C., Moncure, A. C., Ottinger, L. W., and Athanasoulis, C. A.: Transluminal angioplasty of the iliac and femoropopliteal arteries. Current status. Arch. Surg., 117:1218, 1982.
67. Wilms, G., Baert, A., Dewaele, D., Vermylen, J., Nevelsteen, A., and Suy, R.: Percutaneous transluminal angioplasty of the subclavian artery: Early and late results. Cardiovasc. Intervent. Radiol., 10:123, 1987.
68. Wilson, A. R., and Fuchs, J. C. A.: Percutaneous transluminal angioplasty. The radiologist's contribution to the treatment of vascular disease. Surg. Clin. North Am., 64:121, 1984.
69. Wilson, S. E., Wolf, G. L., and Cross, A. P.: Percutaneous transluminal angioplasty versus operation for peripheral arteriosclerosis. Report of a prospective randomized trial in a selected group of patients. J. Vasc. Surg., 9:1, 1989.
70. Zeitler, E., Richter, E. I., Roth, F. J., and Schoop, W.: Results of percutaneous transluminal angioplasty. Radiology, 146:57, 1983.

8. ARTERIAL INJURIES

Robert J. Freeark, M.D.,
William H. Baker, M.D., and
John J. Klosak, M.D.

HISTORICAL REVIEW

Arterial injuries date to the earliest conflicts and endeavors of mankind. Primitive caregivers charged with the task of preventing exsanguination were limited by a lack of fundamental knowledge concerning the function of the vascular system and the lack of suitable instruments and materials. They were rarely successful in preserving life. Cautery was the mainstay of treatment for arterial bleeding. Pouring boiling liquid on the injury and manual compression of the site were common methods used to stop bleeding. Both of these practices were frequently followed by disfigurement, amputation, sepsis, and death.

Ambroise Paré, during the sixteenth century, is reputed to be the first to use ligatures to control arterial bleeding in war injuries. Although Eck and Murphy[24] performed vascular anastomosis in the nineteenth century and Carrel, Guthrie[3] and others[11,28] performed arterial surgery in the early twentieth century, the amputation rate for significant arterial injury was as high as 50 per cent until the end of World War II.[7] Improvements in limb salvage awaited additional clinical experience and the development of antibiotics, fluid administration, blood transfusion, and rapid evacuation of the injured before being successfully applied in the Korean War experience.[13]

Currently in the United States, the two leading causes of arterial injury are urban violence and automobile accidents. Penetrating injuries, once almost exclusively caused by knives, are increasingly due to gunshot wounds. High-speed automobile accidents propel both occupants and pedestrians in a manner that may tear an artery, stretch it beyond its limits of elasticity, or disturb its layers as a result of direct impact or associated bone fractures. These injuries are to an increasing extent being treated in centers in which there are skills and facilities available for early diagnosis and definitive treatment. There remain, however, a distressing number of arterial injuries occurring in the home, on the athletic field, or at work that are unrecognized by the physician. Leg amputations of high-school athletes with knee injuries and deformed and functionless hands of children with elbow fractures are clear evidence for the need for greater awareness of these injuries. (See Table 1 for a list of specific arterial injuries.)

MECHANISMS OF INJURY

Arterial injury can be divided into three categories: penetrating, blunt, and deceleration. Knife wounds with low energy transect vessels much as a surgical scalpel. Gunshot wounds, often due to urban violence, produce a much more devastating injury with a direct correlation between the kinetic energy of the projectile and resultant tissue destruction. Kinetic energy varies as the square of the velocity of the projectile; thus, more devastating injuries occur by increasing the velocity rather than the mass of the bullet. A high-velocity projectile causes cavitation in soft tissues and impact injury to bone. The involved arteries are frequently destroyed and/or thrombosed for several centimeters beyond the path of penetration, requiring extensive débridement of devitalized tissues.

Blunt trauma causes arterial injury from one of two mechanisms. Compressive forces can damage the arterial wall directly, or rapid deceleration, as occurs when an automobile impacts on a stationary object, can stretch an artery and cause an intimal tear since the intima is the least elastic layer of the arterial wall. Blood dissects under this flap, frequently causing thrombosis of the vessel.[5] Several points in the arterial system are relatively fixed and nonmovable. The ligamentum arteriosum is one such point just distal to the origin of the left subclavian artery joining the aorta to the pulmonary vessels. With rapid deceleration, the proximal aortic arch moves violently forward and the distal descending aorta remains relatively stationary, producing a shearing force that disrupts the vessel at the fixed point. Other fixed points include the distal cervical internal carotid artery where it enters the skull, the proximal ascending aortic root, and branches of the thoracic or abdominal aorta.

PATHOPHYSIOLOGY

Three basic patterns of arterial injury are depicted in Figure 1. This simple classification provides a basis for understanding the pathogenesis, clinical characteristics, and method of diagnosis in the various types of arterial injury.

Completely Severed Artery

The completely severed artery is commonly encountered in penetrating wounds such as those inflicted by knives, missiles, or surgical instruments. The severed ends characteristically constrict and retract into the adjacent tissue, often leaving a considerable distance between them. Bleeding usually arrests spontaneously owing to the "tourniquet" effect of vasoconstriction and the development of a firm thrombus in each of the two ends. These clots tend to propagate distally until flow is restored by collateral circulation. The thrombus that occludes the severed ends can be likened to a cork in a wine bottle owing to the narrowing following vasoconstriction. Disruption of the entire wall and loss of blood flow in a major artery cause immediate disappearance of distal pulsations, which is the usual basis for the diagnosis of this type of injury.

The degree of ischemia that follows complete severance of a major artery varies with the site of interruption, the number, size, and condition of the collateral vessels, and the demands of the supplied tissues. A severed carotid artery may cause irreversible damage of the involved cerebral hemisphere in a matter of minutes, whereas severance of a superficial femoral artery in the upper thigh may cause only muscle pain (claudication) during later exercise. For most major extremity arteries, the skin at some point distal to the injury is pale or mottled in color and cool to the touch when compared with the uninvolved side. In addition, there may be loss of sensation, especially to light touch, or a feeling of numbness and tingling (paresthesias). Impairment of arterial supply to sensory nerves usually causes a stocking or glovelike loss of sensation in the involved skin, whereas loss of motor nerve function causes varying degrees of paralysis. In general, because of collateral circulation, the five Ps (pulselessness, paresthesias, paralysis, pallor, and pain) are noted at least one major joint below the site of arterial severance. The signs of ischemia are not always immediately apparent and may not develop until propagation of distal clot obliterates a large collateral; therefore, the loss of distal pulses is the earliest and at times the only sign of this type of arterial injury.

Whereas most completely severed arteries stop bleeding spontaneously, exceptions occur. Certain arteries (e.g., the intercostal and common iliac arteries) are surrounded by structures that either prevent their retraction into adjacent soft tissue or provide little compression of the severed ends. In patients with atherosclerosis, sufficient vasoconstriction does not always occur, and in patients with clotting disorders, the anticipated clot may not form or may dissolve spontaneously. Under each of these circumstances, completely severed arteries may bleed excessively or recurrently.

Partially Severed Artery

Severance or disruption of only a portion of the arterial wall is perhaps the most important arterial injury to recognize and

TABLE 1. Specific Arterial Injuries

Artery	Common Mechanisms of Injury	Possible Sequelae	Special Considerations
Common carotid[10,12]	Penetrating wounds of neck, blunt trauma to neck	Airway obstruction due to hematoma, cerebral ischemia, carotid jugular fistula	Treatment controversial; if neurologic deficit is present: if minor deficit, repair; if major or fixed deficit, ligation may be advisable
Internal carotid	Penetrating wounds	Cerebral ischemia	Similar to common carotid
Vertebral	Penetrating wounds	Cerebral ischemia—may bleed massively	Exposure and repair difficult; surgical or radiologic occlusion usually well tolerated
Innominate	Penetrating wounds of neck and chest, tracheostomy tube erosions	Cerebral and arm ischemia, innominate arteriovenous fistulas	Ideally preserve innominate vein, right carotid, and vertebral artery flow
Subclavian	Fractures of clavicle and first rib, penetrating trauma, iatrogenic (needles, catheters, thoracic outlet surgery)	Intrathoracic bleeding, brachial plexus symptoms from compression, hematoma, or associated injury	Proximal occlusions may steal vertebral flow for arm
Axillary	Fractures, dislocation of humerus, penetrating wounds	Gangrene—rare	Repair desirable
Brachial	Catheter injuries, fracture and dislocation of elbow, especially in children	Gangrene—rare; ischemic symptoms may result (Volkmann's ischemic contracture)	Repair desirable
Ulnar[41]	Lacerations, inadvertent injection into anomalous artery	Gangrene may follow injections of thiopental and other drugs	May ligate; heparin used for injection injuries
Thoracic aorta	Blunt (rapid deceleration), fractures of sternum, clavicle, and first and second ribs	Exsanguination; false aneurysm just distal to left subclavian	Angiography for mediastinal widening, tracheal shift, or diminished pulses
Abdominal aorta	Blunt, penetrating	Visceral or lower extremity ischemia	Repair or prosthetic graft replacement
Common and external iliac	Blunt, penetrating	Lower extremity ischemia	Repair
Internal iliac, gluteal[22,37]	Pelvic fractures	Pelvic hematoma, false aneurysms	Ligation or angiographic embolization
Renal	Blunt trauma—renal pedicle injury	Hematuria, renal ischemia	Early diagnosis important; unilateral nonvisualization on intravenous pyelogram requires angiography
Celiac, superior and inferior mesenteric[19]	Penetrating trauma, iatrogenic (surgery)	Variable—may cause intestinal ischemia	Repair superior mesenteric; may ligate celiac, inferior mesenteric if necessary
Common femoral	Penetrating, blunt, iatrogenic (catheters, aortic balloon pumps), anterior dislocation of femur	Leg ischemia	Repair
Superficial femoral[15]	Fractures of femur, esp. junction of middle and lower thirds; penetrating wounds	Leg ischemia (may be minimal)	Repair
Profunda femoris[35]	Penetrating wounds, surgery (hip fractures)	Valuable collateral for later life	No distal pulse point; preserve if feasible
Popliteal[16,31]	Fractures of tibial plateau, dislocation of knee, surgery of knee joint	Amputation likely without prompt and expert repair	Repair; venous repair also advisable
Anterior tibial	Fracture of tibial shaft	Anterior compartment ischemia	Repair
Posterior tibial	Dislocation of ankle, fracture of tibial shaft	Loss of artery—usually well tolerated if anterior tibial intact; posterior compartment hypertension may occur	Repair if feasible

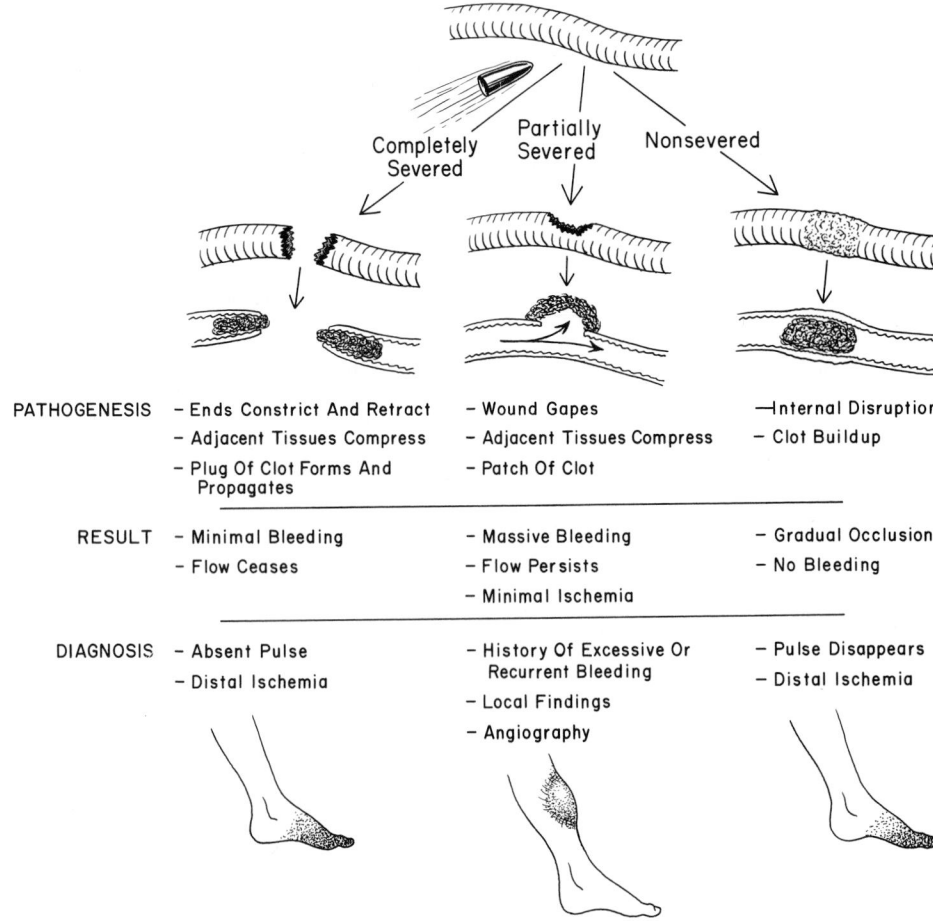

PATHOGENESIS
- Ends Constrict And Retract
- Adjacent Tissues Compress
- Plug Of Clot Forms And Propagates

- Wound Gapes
- Adjacent Tissues Compress
- Patch Of Clot

- Internal Disruption
- Clot Buildup

RESULT
- Minimal Bleeding
- Flow Ceases

- Massive Bleeding
- Flow Persists
- Minimal Ischemia

- Gradual Occlusion
- No Bleeding

DIAGNOSIS
- Absent Pulse
- Distal Ischemia

- History Of Excessive Or Recurrent Bleeding
- Local Findings
- Angiography

- Pulse Disappears
- Distal Ischemia

Figure 1. The three basic patterns of arterial injury. Careful and repeated examinations of the site of injury and the distal extremity will usually establish the need for treatment.

understand. This injury commonly produces serious or recurrent bleeding and is the forerunner of both false aneurysms and arteriovenous fistulas (Fig. 2). A wide variety of penetrating objects may be responsible, including knives, missiles, drill points, needles, and catheters used in angiographic and cardiovascular monitoring techniques. Occasionally, partial severance occurs in association with closed injuries, usually as a result of bone fragments that lacerate a portion of the adjacent arterial wall.

The partially severed artery differs profoundly from the completely severed artery in many important respects. Since a portion of the arterial wall remains intact, constriction of the artery may cause retraction of the opened portion of the arterial wall, causing the arterial wound to gape. Blood loss may actually be increased in this type of injury, causing more rapid exsanguination. More often the overlying muscles and skin tamponade the blood loss, particularly when the patient is hypotensive. This containment may be only a temporizing measure. The hematoma may increase gradually in size, particularly after the patient's blood volume has been restored and the blood pressure normalized. When the hematoma is carefully examined, it often has a pulsatile quality in appearance, since it communicates directly with the arterial lumen. Delayed or recurrent bleeding is a hallmark of the partially severed vessel. The blood clot that covers the arterial defect is more of a "patch" than a "plug" although it occasionally protrudes into the lumen (Fig. 2).

The arterial lumen initially is seldom narrowed by partial severance. Blood flow is maintained distally and pulses may be palpated. End-organ ischemia is absent. These lesions are notoriously difficult to diagnose and are recognized only by a physician with increased awareness of their possibility.

If the injury goes unrecognized, the course of events is highly variable. Minimal wounds may heal much like the wounds that

occur with diagnostic arterial punctures. However, the patient may present several days after the injury with discomfort in the region of the hematoma as it expands and stretches the overlying soft tissues. The mass may be warm and tender and the overlying skin erythematous. The mistaken impression that an abscess has developed at the site of penetration may be disas-

FATE OF PARTIALLY SEVERED ARTERY

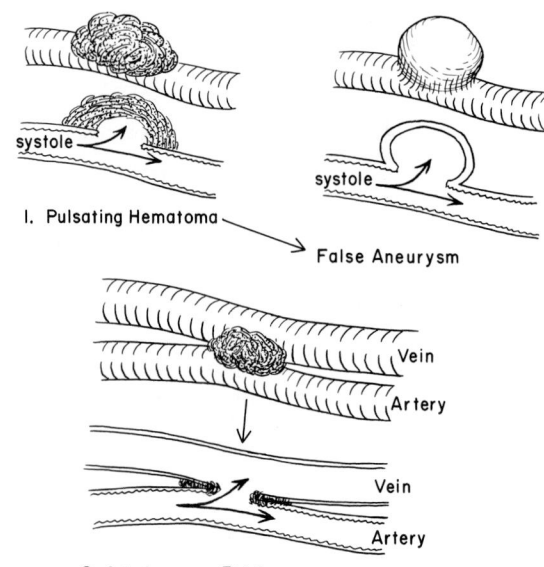

Figure 2. Partially severed arteries and those disrupted at their origin give rise to excessive or recurrent bleeding and the late development of false aneurysms or arteriovenous fistulas.

CAUSES OF INTERNAL OCCLUSION

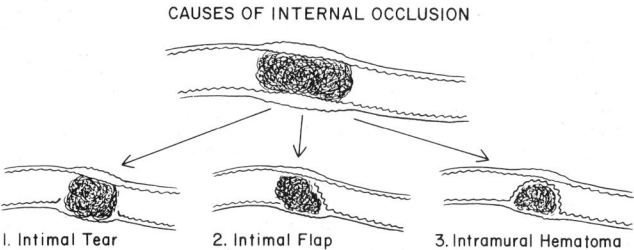

1. Intimal Tear   2. Intimal Flap   3. Intramural Hematoma

Figure 3. Mechanisms of occlusion in injuries in which the outside wall of an artery is intact (nonsevered artery).

trous if incision and drainage are attempted. The damaged intima may dissect some hours after injury, causing a delayed arterial occlusion. A late complication that occurs after internal resorption of the hematoma is a false aneurysm. Arteriovenous fistulas can occur if both the artery and vein are injured.

Nonsevered Artery

This third category of arterial injury is commonly seen when a blunt force or excessive stretch is applied to the arterial wall (Fig. 1). A similar injury may follow the passage of a high-velocity missile adjacent to the vessel that causes intimal damage without actually severing the vessel's outer circumference. This form of injury is characterized by reduction or loss of flow through the artery but without external bleeding. Patients with blunt injury often have a normal examination initially, but signs of ischemia and loss of pulses develop over a variable period of time. This injury emphasizes the need for repeated evaluations of the arterial circulation in the injured patient.

This delayed obliteration of the arterial lumen may result by one of several mechanisms (Fig. 3). The roughened or torn arterial intima attracts platelets and fibrin as part of the normal healing mechanisms. An excessive collection of blood elements results in a traumatic thrombosis. On occasion, the flow of blood may elevate the torn distal end of the intima, creating a subintimal dissection and lifting an intimal flap that occludes the distal lumen. Moreover, even though the inner and outer coats of the artery remain intact, an intramural hematoma may form that obliterates the lumen of the artery.

Recognition that one or more of the preceding mechanisms is usually responsible for the loss of blood flow and disappearance

of distal pulses has largely eliminated the concept of arterial "spasm" as a cause of arterial insufficiency. Although circular muscle fibers may contract segmentally or peripherally to narrow the arterial lumen and diminish blood flow, this phenomenon rarely obliterates pulses or causes ischemia. Spasm cannot be assumed unless angiographic evidence is irrefutable.

RECOGNITION OF ARTERIAL INJURY

History

The mechanisms of injury and the exact time and site at which it was sustained are helpful clues in the recognition of arterial injury. The magnitude of a blunt force or the length of the knife blade and its direction and depth of penetration in stab wounds are important. The number and direction of bullets fired may be of benefit in assessing patients with missile injuries. The extent of bleeding, the methods used to control hemorrhage, and the amount of blood loss after injury should be ascertained from the patient or knowledgeable individuals in attendance. The patient may be aware of coolness, paresthesias (numbness or tingling), loss of sensation, or severe pain in the extremity with arterial insufficiency. All too often, however, the symptoms of ischemia are masked by the presence of other injuries.

Examination

The injured patient should be fully disrobed to allow examination of all possible sites of injury and to permit a comparison with uninjured body parts. A patient with a thready radial pulse in an uninjured arm can at best have a thready pulse in an injured extremity. The examination should include an assessment of the entire arterial system including the presence and quality of all pulses of the neck, groin, and upper and lower extremities. In addition, auscultation is required for the presence or absence of bruits, especially in the area of suspected injury. The presence or suspicion of a fracture or dislocation requires a specific evaluation of adjacent vessels (Table 2). The extremity distal to the site of injury should be examined for pulse deficits or signs of ischemia. Fortunately, a proximal tourniquet is rarely applied by modern emergency medical technologists. If applied, its effect must be taken into consideration during the examination.

TABLE 2. Vascular Injury Accompanying Skeletal Trauma

Bone Injury	Vascular Injury	Associated Findings
Fracture of first and second ribs	Transection of thoracic aorta	Widened mediastinum
Fracture of clavicle and first rib	Laceration and contusion of subclavian artery or vein; false aneurysm	Diminished pulse or blood pressure in involved arm
Dislocation of shoulder	Thrombosis of axillary artery	Diminished or absent distal pulse
Fracture of humeral shaft	Laceration of brachial artery	Diminished or absent distal pulse
Supracondylar fracture of humerus	Obstruction of brachial artery	Compartment hypertension of forearm (Volkmann's phenomenon)
Dislocation of elbow	Disruption of brachial artery	Absent radial pulse
Fracture of ribs	Laceration of intercostal artery	Hemothorax
Fracture of pelvis	Laceration of superior gluteal artery	Massive pelvic hematoma
Anterior dislocation of hip	Femoral artery contusion	Diminished or absent distal pulse
Fracture of hip	Deep femoral artery injury during operative repair	Excessive bleeding with no pulse deficit
Fracture of femoral shaft (mid or lower third)	Occlusion and laceration of femoral artery	Loss of distal pulsations; cold foot with loss of pulsation; cold foot with bleeding
Supracondylar fracture of femur	Laceration of popliteal artery or vein	Bleeding with diminished foot pulses
Dislocation of knee	Disruption and thrombosis of popliteal artery or vein	Diminished pulses with cold foot
Fracture of proximal tibia	Disruption of thrombosis of popliteal artery or vein	Diminished pulses with cold foot
Fracture of tibial shaft	Transection of anterior or posterior tibial artery	Diminished pulses with cold foot; compartmental hypertension
Dislocation of ankle	Transection and thrombosis of tibial arteries	Diminished pulses

It is also important to recognize that many arteries do not have a distal point for palpating pulsations. The common and internal carotid, internal iliac, profunda femoris, and peroneal arteries defy evaluation by this means. Other arteries such as the renal or mesenteric vessels can be assessed only by radiologic means or direct examination.

The temperature, color, degree of venous distention, and quality of pulses should be noted and compared with the uninjured extremity. In an ischemic extremity, distal motor function is first affected. For example, the intrinsic muscles of the hand cease to function before the extensors and flexors of the wrist. Loss of sensation to cotton touch or pinprick should be noted. In the case of a specific nerve injury, the loss of sensation follows the anatomic route of that nerve. Ischemic extremities have a stocking or glove type pattern. If examination of the distal extremities shows definite evidence of arterial injury, angiography or operative repair or both are done as soon as possible. It is both unwise and unnecessary to inspect directly the area of injury since it risks contamination and rebleeding in a patient who will most certainly require operative repair.

However, the wound of a patient without obvious arterial injury may be gently explored under sterile conditions. A mask and sterile gloves are worn. If arterial injury is suspected, a blood pressure cuff should be applied proximally for use as an immediate tourniquet should bleeding recur. The missile track is gently probed with a finger. The relationship of the wound or missile track to the major vessels should be noted. If a large hematoma is present, the exploration should be completed in the operating room. Since the probing finger may excite arterial bleeding, this examination should not be done unless plans for operative control have been made.

The diagnosis of arterial injury is obvious in a patient with loss or diminution of pulses distal to the site of injury, particularly when signs and symptoms of distal ischemia are present. Interestingly, several studies have indicated that as many as 25 per cent of injured peripheral arteries have had palpable pulses on initial presentation,[34] and thus palpable pulses by no means exclude significant proximal arterial injury. In a patient with palpable pulses, the physician should maintain a high clinical suspicion of arterial injury when there is (1) a history of massive external bleeding from a penetrating wound, particularly when clinical shock is present or multiple transfusions have been required to stabilize the patient; (2) a history of recurrent bleeding; (3) rapid expansion of a large pulsatile hematoma; (4) presence of systolic or continuous bruit in the region of an injury; (5) marked venous distention of the injured extremity; or (6) wound or missile track adjacent to a major vessel. In these circumstances, diagnosis of arterial injury must be excluded by either arteriographic study or operative exploration. In those patients whose injuries preclude this approach, close clinical observation is required should delayed bleeding and/or ischemia occur. Observation of distal pulses may be unreliable because nursing personnel and house officers have a varying ability in this regard. Doppler ultrasound, when used with an ordinary blood pressure cuff, can be used to obtain a blood pressure except under the most difficult of circumstances. The pressure in the injured extremity should be the same as in the uninjured extremity. Any deterioration of this ratio indicates increasing arterial compromise.

Angiographic Study

Angiograms are available in most hospitals. A needle is inserted into an upstream artery, iodine-containing contrast material is injected, and films are taken of the area of interest. Using the Seldinger technique, a peripheral artery is cannulated and a catheter manipulated to study the area of interest. Some trauma surgeons advocate a single injection to be performed in the operating room, whereas other surgeons transport the pa-

tient to the radiology suite where multiple films, usually of higher quality, can be obtained.

Arteriography by necessity delays the surgical treatment of the truamatized patient. In patients with threatened uncontrolled exsanguination, immediate operative control of hemorrhage is indicated and angiography is not performed. If distal ischemia is present and the site of injury is obvious, arteriography is not required to plan the surgical procedure. If ischemia is not present, arteriography may provide a more precise diagnosis, but it is not required. If the site of injury is not obvious (multiple fractures, multiple sites of penetrating injury), arteriography may be necessary to guide the surgeon to the proper injured area. Regardless of the circumstances, the patient must be accompanied by a member of the trauma team in the event clinical deterioration suddenly occurs and prompt treatment is required. In the unstable patient, control of exsanguinating hemorrhage is of prime importance. An operative arteriogram can always be obtained.

ANGIOGRAPHIC FINDINGS. The angiographic findings in patients with aterial injury vary with the type of injury sustained. Completely severed arteries and complete occlusions arising from injuries in continuity show a sudden arrest of the column of contrast material (Fig. 4). In some patients, the collateral circulation may be sufficient to permit re-entry of dye into the more distal portions of the main artery, creating an angiographic gap at the site of injury. Although such collateral flow may be sufficient to prevent the development of signs of ischemia at rest, it rarely maintains a palpable distal pulse.

Angiographic studies of partially severed arteries may demonstrate the escape of contrast material from the arterial lumen. It is important to remember that the amount of contrast material outside the vessel may be relatively small in patients with a large hematoma because the palpable mass is composed largely of clot surrounding the arterial defect. In some patients, the resultant hematoma may actually protrude into the lumen and appear

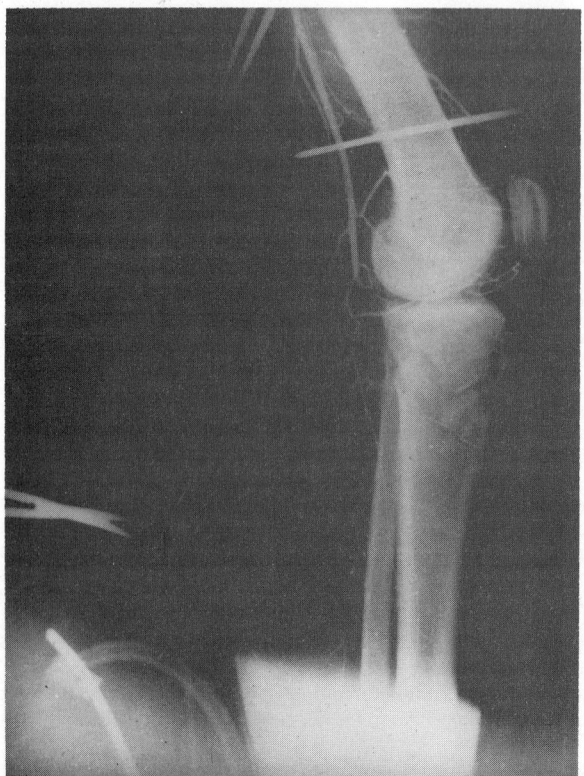

Figure 4. Arteriogram confirming complete occlusion of the popliteal artery associated with fracture of the tibial plateau. A fracture of the femur (not shown) and a pin previously placed for skeletal traction were other possible causes for the cold foot and loss of pulses in this patient.

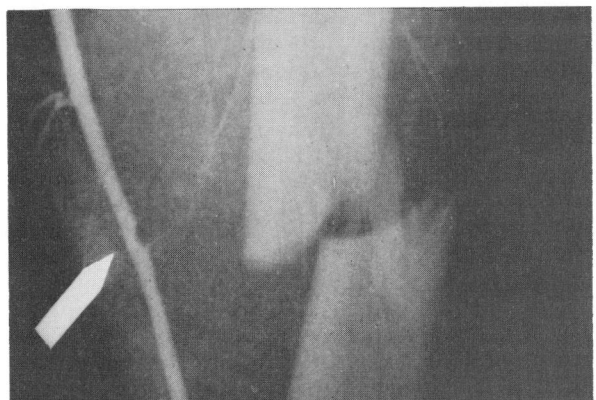

Figure 5. Femoral arteriogram in a patient with a closed fracture of the femur. Note the small filling defect at site of injury where sharp bone fragments had severed 60 per cent of the circumference of the arterial wall. Compare with Figure 6, as both are examples of angiographic evidence of partially severed arteries.

as a filling defect not unlike an arteriosclerotic plaque (Fig. 5). Any distortion of the normally smooth column of dye in the vicinity of the injury should be viewed with suspicion. In patients who develop arteriovenous fistulas, the visualization of the adjacent venous system as well as the sac of the false aneurysm or fistulous track confirms the diagnosis.

Patients with a pulse deficit on physical examination usually have an angiographic pattern of acute occlusion. Prior to the complete loss of arterial flow, the site of injury in nonsevered arteries may be noted as an asymmetric narrowing, a filling defect, or a point at which there is a sudden change in the diameter of the arteries. In the rare circumstance of arteriospasm causing a pulse deficit, the artery may be symmetrically narrowed and the entire distal arterial tree may appear markedly constricted. A smooth lumen is maintained, however, and complete interruption of arterial flow does not occur.

Doppler Ultrasonic Flow Studies

The transcutaneous Doppler ultrasound flow detection technique has proved to be a valuable addition to the management of arterial injuries.[42] An ultrasound beam up to 10 mHz. emitted from a ceramic crystal is coupled to the skin with a gel and then passed through an underlying blood vessel. Based on the "Doppler effect," ultrasound reflected from moving red cells in the blood vessel is shifted in frequency by an amount proportional to the flow velocity of the red cells. Both audible signals and waveform recordings are available for evaluation of accessible arteries. Using the ultrasound probe as a stethoscope, systolic pressure of the forearm and ankle can be recorded by placing a sphygmomanometer cuff on the extremity. The return of flow signals in the radial or posterior tibial artery during deflation of the cuff indicates the level of systolic pressure. Since collateral flow may provide an audible signal even in the presence of arterial interruption, the adequacy of collateral flow may be assessed by measuring the systolic pressure in these arteries. If no signal is audible, prompt arterial repair is indicated to prevent limb loss, whereas any audible signal is a good prognostic sign. A systolic pressure of approximately 60 mm. Hg (or 50 per cent of the pressure in the contralateral normal limb) usually indicates adequate collateral flow to maintain tissue viability. Knowledge of this status of collateral flow is helpful in determining the exact priority of arterial repair in patients with multiple injuries. In addition, the Doppler flow detection technique is of value in the determination of arterial patency when pulse examination is in doubt or when swelling or edema precludes reliable palpation of distal pulses. The technique is also useful in the detection of venous injuries and has been found to be of value in monitoring the patency of both arterial and venous reconstructions during the postoperative period.

TREATMENT

Emergency Treatment

The proper application of firm pressure over a site of arterial bleeding is the best method for its temporary control. Attempts to find the artery or control bleeding with clamps and/or ligatures usually dislodge clots and risk damage to adjacent neurovascular structures. Even well-applied but traumatic clamps may damage enough artery to convert a simple end-to-end reconstruction into a replacement graft. Proximal tourniquets other than inflatable blood pressure cuff are rarely effective and usually only increase venous bleeding. Tourniquets that are inflated above arterial pressure cause ischemic pain and are not well tolerated by patients. Severe skeletal deformities with vascular compromise should be corrected and aligned as best as possible. The injured extremity should be splinted and kept level during transport. The use of inflatable splints to immobilize extremity fractures or the use of military antishock trousers (MAST) or "G suit" in patients with hypotension should be recognized as potentially harmful to extremities with arterial injuries. Fortunately, these devices are usually removed after stabilization of the patient. Arterial injuries, particularly associated with hemorrhage or to a lesser degree ischemia, should receive high priority of treatment. On occasion, other life-threatening injuries may require more immediate attention (restoration of airway, control of internal bleeding, intracranial hematoma). If the surgeon believes that limb loss is more likely because of these necessary delays in establishing arterial flow, the feasibility of simultaneous treatment should be considered.

Patients with partially severed arteries who are no longer bleeding and who have no evidence of distal ischemia have less emergent but nonetheless urgent problems. These pulsating hematomas are subject to recurrent bleeding. Delay of repair of large arteriovenous fistulas may cause acute near-lethal congestive heart failure. Thus, these patients should be treated as soon as possible following diagnosis and localization of their injury. Experience has shown that these early repairs are more easily accomplished than are delayed repairs, and patient safety is enhanced.

Operative Repair

All major arterial injuries should be repaired when diagnosed, provided the tissues that they supply are viable, the general condition of the patient is satisfactory, and the risks of infection are not great. Notable exceptions include the carotid injuries in a patient with a major fixed neurologic deficit and delayed renal pedicle injuries. In injuries to the extremities, the presence of distal cutaneous gangrene or stony hard musculature makes the benefits of revascularization questionable, but successful repair may preserve the viable tissues and permit amputation at a lower level.

Operative repair should be undertaken promptly by a surgeon skilled in the techniques of emergency vascular surgery. Assuming hemorrhage is under control, the urgency of repair is directly related to the degree of ischemia. Re-establishment of arterial flow within 4 to 6 hours after arterial injury minimizes the possibility of permanent ischemic change. Although every hour of delay may diminish success, there is no absolute period beyond which repair is contraindicated.

Although the techniques of operative repair vary, local considerations are outlined in Table 1 and illustrated in Figure 6. In general, treatment proceeds as follows.

1. Treat hypovolemia and shock by controlling external blood loss and restoring blood volume. Ensure an adequate airway and respiratory mechanism. Establish the presence and extent of all injuries and determine their priority of repair.

2. Initiate antibiotic and tetanus prophylaxis when indicated and arrange for assistants, equipment, arteriography, and the

VASCULAR TRAUMA

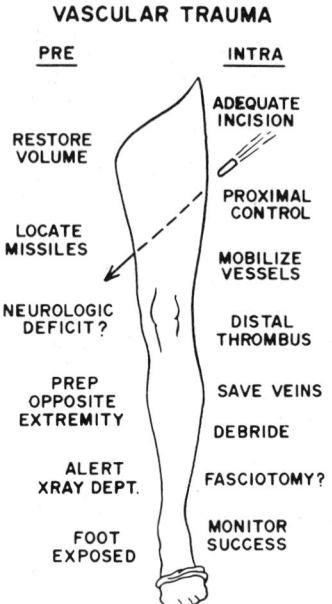

Figure 6. Important considerations prior to and during the operative treatment of a vascular injury to the lower extremity.

immediate availability of an adequate supply of type-specific and matched whole blood.

3. Prepare a wide operative field and an uninvolved lower extremity for ready access to the saphenous vein, the best and safest arterial substitute for all but the largest arteries. In an extremity injury, the entire limb and proximal torso should be prepared to ensure access to all involved vessels and the operative evaluation of distal pulses by palpation or arteriography.

4. Localize the site of arterial injury by the location of the wound missile track, pulse deficits, or arteriography.

5. The usual incisions should be utilized for exposure of blood vessels. Sometimes the wound forces an eclectic skin incision. In these cases, the usual anatomic planes are developed so that unnecessary injury to associated structures is avoided. Proximal control is always obtained prior to entering the field of injury. In the case of groin, neck, or shoulder wounds, this may necessitate entering the abdomen or thorax.

6. Obtain control of the artery distal to the presumed site of injury to minimize the loss of blood by back-bleeding. If the site of injury is inadvertently entered prior to control, balloon catheters of the Fogarty type[9] may be inflated to control both proximally or distally. In the case of an aortic wound, a Foley catheter with a large balloon may be required.

7. Inspect or palpate the site of injury and determine the need for repair.

8. Proximal and distal controls should be obtained at least 2 to 3 cm. from the site of injury so that the intima can be examined. In both penetrating and blunt trauma, the intima may be damaged beyond the obvious site of injury. This damaged intima requires resection.

9. Remove the proximal clot by flushing and the distal clot by milking the vessel, squeezing the distal limb, or passing a Fogarty balloon catheter.[9]

10. Systemic heparinization is usually not employed in the multiply injured patient. In single wounds of the extremity requiring extensive reconstruction, the benefits probably justify the risk. In most instances local heparinization with dilute heparinized saline (100 units per ml.) is enough to discourage local clot formation.

11. Prior to anastomosis, determine the need for graft replacement by estimating the amount of difficulty in approximating the severed ends. In general, 1 to 2 cm. of artery wall may be resected without graft replacement. This is especially true in

some older patients with redundant arteries and in younger patients who have healthy elastic arteries. Arterial anastomosis should not be performed under tension, but it is important not to interpret the retraction "gap" as a loss of arterial substance in making this decision.

12. Repair the injured artery using interrupted or continuous fine monofilament sutures. Smaller arteries and veins may be constricted using continuous suture techniques. In children, an interrupted suture repair is preferred to ensure circumferential growth.

13. Reversed saphenous vein is the graft material of choice. Prosthetic graft material is avoided if possible because of risk of infection. In addition, late graft failure is thought to be increased when prosthetic material is used in the extremity. Prosthetic material, however, is the preferred graft material within the thorax and abdomen. Again, its use must be balanced against the threat of infection and the severe consequences of an infected prosthetic graft.

14. Prior to completion of the repair, the arteries are fore-bled and back-bled. These final sutures are tied and flow is restored. Pulses in the distal extremity should be palpable.

15. If distal pulses are not restored or the quality of arterial flow is unsatisfactory, a cause for these findings must be ascertained. If the repair is not adequate, it must be redone. If no cause is seen, an operative arteriogram that includes not only the operative site but also the distal circulation is obtained. The surgeon must assume that there is a mechanically correctable cause of this problem. The surgeon cannot assume that spasm exists unless mechanical causes have been excluded.

16. The wound should be thoroughly débrided and explored, and other injuries should be identified and repaired as necessary. Drains are occasionally employed for a period of 24 to 48 hours. Every effort is made to cover the repaired artery with viable muscle and fascia. Skin closure is dictated by the nature of the injury and risk of infection.

17. If systemic heparinization has been employed, its effects usually disappear over the several hours required to complete the operation, and neutralization is not required. Dressings and splints should be well padded to protect anesthetic ischemic tissue. They should be applied in such a manner to allow inspection of toes or fingers for capillary circulation, easy palpation of distal pulses, assessment of the musculature of the distal extremity, and ready access to the operative wound should bleeding occur. Any constriction of the limb should be avoided, and immobilization of fractures should be achieved by either skeletal traction, posterior molds, or operative fixation (see later discussion).

POSTOPERATIVE CARE

Following repair, every effort should be made to maintain an effective circulating blood volume and hematocrit levels. Maintenance of a satisfactory perfusion pressure is confirmed by systemic blood pressure and urinary output monitoring. Systemic anticoagulation is not required to ensure arterial patency and may be detrimental to other injuries.

Pulses distal to the site of arterial repair should be evaluated at hourly intervals by digital palpation or Doppler ultrasonic flow technique. Decreasing pulses and lowered ankle/arm indices indicate thrombosis of the arterial repair. Re-exploration is indicated under these circumstances. Signs of compartmental compression syndromes and myoglobinuria should also be promptly treated.

SPECIAL PROBLEMS

Iatrogenic Arterial Injury

Currently, a very common form of arterial injury occurs after the diagnostic or therapeutic insertion of a needle or catheter into an artery. Coronary arteriograms performed via the brachial artery at the elbow may cause a thrombosis rate as high as 25 per cent.[25] Most thromboses involve the use of a large catheter in a small artery. Many of these injuries are benign and are unrecognized. Severe ischemia with gangrene of the finger is a rare complication. However, a significant number of patients experience pallor, coldness, numbness, or paresthesias. Depending on their occupation, many patients note diminished exercise tolerance in the forearm and hand. Cold intolerance is also increased after injury.

Additional examples of iatrogenic arterial injury include thrombosis of the radial artery following arterial blood sampling or pressure monitoring.[14] Such injuries have caused the loss of digits and the entire hand even when the ulnar artery was present. This is most likely to occur in patients with an incomplete palmar arch. Identification of these patients is possible prior to arterial cannulation by use of the Allen test. The subclavian and carotid arteries are occasionally injured during attempts to insert central venous catheters, during performance of brachial plexus or stellate ganglion anesthetic blocks, or in the course of surgical procedures to correct the thoracic outlet syndrome. Injuries to the common femoral artery and its immediate branches are also observed following catheterization of these vessels for a variety of angiograms including coronary arteriography. The large diameter of these vessels makes thrombosis much less likely, but when it occurs it is more likely to be associated with ischemic signs and symptoms. Withdrawal of the catheter may cause distal embolization of thrombus that is best treated by thrombolytic therapy. Bleeding after catheter withdrawal is usually controlled by direct pressure for 10 to 15 minutes. Late bleeding may be associated with false aneurysm formation. Arteriovenous fistulas have been reported after these studies.

The complications of transaxillary arteriography require a special note. The axillary artery is enclosed with the axillary vein and multiple nerves in a relatively inelastic neurovascular bundle. Relatively small amounts of bleeding within the sheath may cause a nerve compression syndrome. Unrecognized nerve compression may produce permanent neurologic sequelae. Therefore, special attention must be paid to patients following transaxillary arterial punctures with hourly evaluation of strength and sensation. Patients who have relatively minor complaints, particularly if they are new or increasing in severity, are operatively explored.

Current practice requires prompt exploration of the site of the catheterization in any patient with continued bleeding, the loss of distal pulses, or the development of neurologic sequelae. Bleeding is ordinarily easily controlled with one or two sutures in the anterior puncture site. The arteries should always be explored on the posterior aspect to ensure that a second site of bleeding is not overlooked. Thrombosed arteries are opened through either a transverse or longitudinally oriented arteriotomy. The intima must be inspected circumferentially to ensure that it has not been disrupted or dissected. The thrombus is extracted using a balloon catheter. If the posterior wall of the artery is extensively damaged, an arterial resection may be required. In small arteries opened via a longitudinal arteriotomy, a patch angioplasty may be required to ensure the closure does not compromise the lumen of the explored artery.

Drug Abuse

An increasing number of arterial injuries are a consequence of the recent surge of drug abuse.[41] Addicts who have progressively obliterated their venous channels or inexperienced "first timers" may accidentally inject a variety of pharmacologic agents and particulate matter into arteries, with resultant ischemia and gangrene of the distal extremity. The mechanism of the ischemic changes is unclear. Although true vasospasm has been shown to be unlikely, sympathectomy has been employed as

treatment. Anticoagulants and rheologic agents such as dextran are recommended but are unproven methods of treatment. Exclusion of other causes of vascular injury in drug abusers is also important. The most devastating complication in these patients is local infection at the site of injection causing infected false aneurysms. Although some may be repaired *in situ* with autogenous tissue, other aneurysms are so extensive and infected with such virulent organisms to require excision and extra-anatomic bypass, if possible.

Compartment Hypertension

Edema of or hemorrhage into the tight osseofascial compartment of the leg, thigh, and forearm may cause a marked increase in intracompartmental tissue pressure.[26] The possibility of compartmental hypertension is especially great following a delayed arterial repair. During the period of ischemia, functional arterial integrity is damaged. After reconstruction and restoration of normal pressures, edema forms in the surrounding tissues. As tissue pressures increase, venous flow is first compromised. The resulting venous hypertension causes an increase in the formation of the edema. These cascading events continue with resultant nerve and muscle dysfunction. Arterial flow to the muscles of the compartment usually ceases when the tissue pressure rises to within 10 to 20 mm. of diastolic arterial pressure. Higher levels of intracompartmental pressure cause obliteration of flow in the major arteries with reduction in distal pulses. Loss of audible Doppler flow distally is the last late finding.

A similar course has been described following venous occlusion, direct muscle trauma, vigorous exercise, deep burns, and application of MAST suits or as a result of hemorrhage within a closed fascial space. The forearm and calf are most frequently involved. The involved compartment becomes firm to palpation, and loss of muscle function soon becomes apparent. Loss of cutaneous sensation may result when sensory nerves that pass through the compartment are subjected to increased pressure. In the lower extremity, loss of sensation may be noted in the web space at the base of the first and second digits or on the plantar surface of the foot. Distal arterial pulsations are maintained until the more advanced stages of the condition occur. The end result of severe untreated compartmental hypertension is the loss or replacement of ischemic muscle with fibrous tissue causing deformity and loss of function.

Since early recognition of the syndrome permits treatment before irreversible damage has occurred, recent interest has centered on direct measurements of intracompartmental pressure by means of pressure transducers or a simple mercury manometer in line with an 18-gauge needle and plastic tubing containing air and fluid. In susceptible patients, direct or continuous measurements of the pressures in each of the muscular compartments should be made percutaneously in both extremities.[17,40] When the syndrome of significant compartmental hypertension is clinically or manometrically confirmed, it should be treated by an incision to release the trapped contents of the involved compartments (Fig. 7). The marked improvement in arterial flow that may follow fasciotomy in a patient with the anterior compartment syndrome is depicted in Figure 8. Complete fasciotomy is a prophylactic operation. Delayed fasciotomy that exposes ischemic or necrotic muscle to hospital bacteria may induce uncontrollable infection and amputation.

Volkmann's ischemic contracture is a special syndrome of compartmental hypertension that develops in some children with supracondylar fractures of the humerus. Pain develops in the muscles of the forearm, with or without evidence of overt arterial injury. This pain is usually increased by efforts to extend the fingers. The radial pulse may or may not be diminished. This clinical condition must be promptly investigated. All constricting bandages or plaster should be removed and the fracture reduced by the use of skeletal traction or open reduction. The failure to obtain prompt relief of symptoms despite these ma-

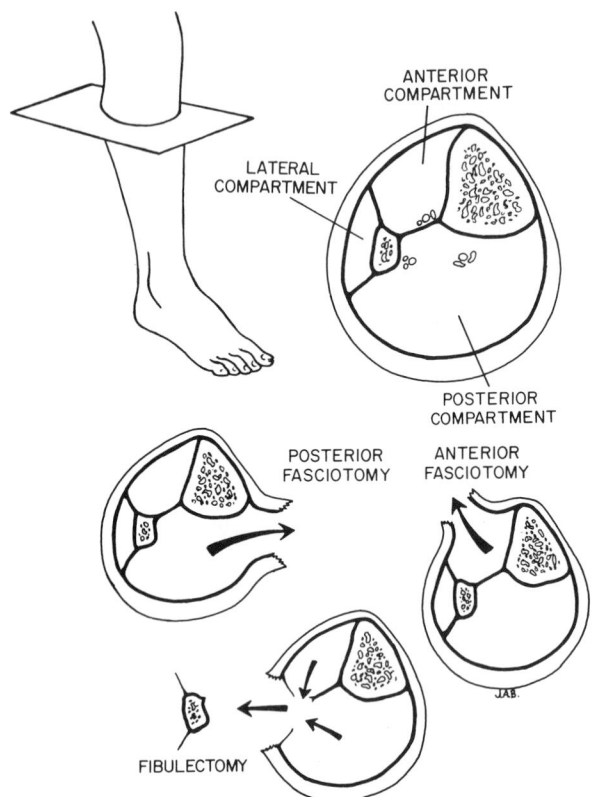

Figure 7. Diagram of the right calf, illustrating the muscular compartments and sites of incision to provide decompression when a rise in compartmental pressure occurs.

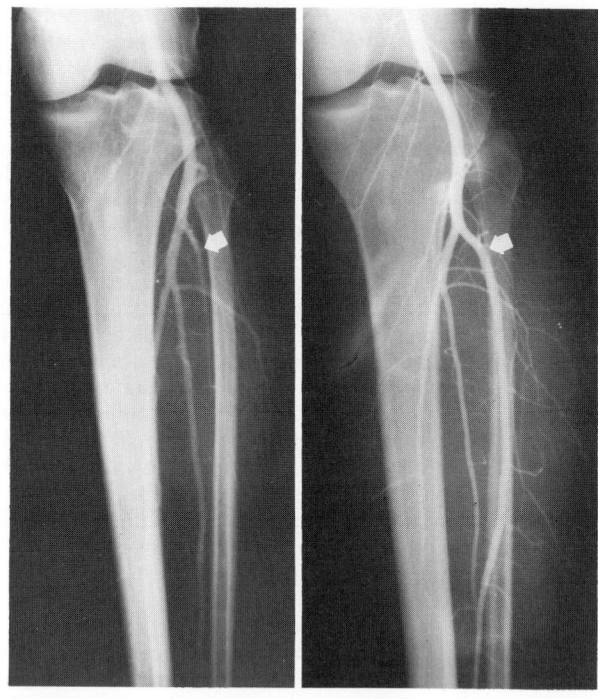

Figure 8. Pre- and postoperative femoral arteriograms in a patient with an anterior compartment syndrome secondary to femoral artery occlusion of over 6 hours duration. The very small (occluded) anterior tibial artery (arrows) is much enlarged following artery fasciotomy.

neuvers requires exploration of the brachial artery, evacuation of the hematoma, and fasciotomy of the forearm musculature.

VENOUS INJURIES

The safety of and need for repairing venous injuries is being increasingly appreciated.[31,32] The ligation of major veins not only impairs venous return and contributes to the late development of chronic venous insufficiency but acutely causes venous hypertension and may jeopardize the success of arterial reconstruction by contributing to the development of compartmental hypertension.

Chronic venous insufficiency is increased in those patients who have venous ligation as opposed to trauma victims who have had venous repair. The principles involved are the same as with arteries. Small stitches using fine monofilament suture material are required to produce the least venous constriction. Replacement of veins in the periphery is usually performed with saphenous vein taken from a contralateral or uninjured extremity. The use of a distal arterial venous fistula to keep these sites open is usually not employed in the trauma victim. Although thrombosis at the site of repair may commonly occur, most authorities believe that even a temporary flow achieved by venous reconstruction is beneficial to the total circulation and outweighs the risks involved. Reports of pulmonary embolism from these thrombi are rare. Postoperatively, elevation of the extremity is usually employed. Fasciotomy is prophylactically employed if there is an excessive delay in repair. Postoperative anticoagulants and dextran may be used depending on the extent of the original injury.

Reconstruction of the inferior and superior vena cava is especially difficult. Most superior vena cava injuries are lethal. Control may require the use of cardiopulmonary bypass. The inferior vena cava is more easily controlled in its infrarenal portion. The retrohepatic portion may require the use of a Shrock tube.[36]

Replacement of the superior vena cava is usually performed with prosthetic material. Associated injuries involving the bowel and its contents may preclude the use of prosthetic material for repair of the inferior vena cava.

INJURIES TO THE AORTIC ARCH AND ITS BRANCHES

Arterial injuries in the upper chest pose particular difficulties in diagnosis and surgical repair. Approximately one third of these patients are hemodynamically unstable on admission and require immediate surgical intervention to control hemorrhage. This hemorrhage may reside in the thorax or in the mediastinum or present as cervical bleeding, depending on the mode of injury. Compromise of the trachea is common.

Mortality in excess of 50 per cent has been reported with injuries of the thoracic aorta. When blunt trauma is the mechanism of injury, only 15 per cent of the patients survive the initial insult to reach medical care.[18] Aortography is indicated in all hemodynamically stable patients suspected of having an aortic injury. Emergency thoracotomy without angiography is reserved for the unstable patient with uncontrolled hemorrhage. With blunt trauma, a high clinical suspicion is necessary to diagnose the injury. Fifty per cent of the patients who reach the hospital with a blunt thoracic aortic injury have no external evidence of trauma to the chest. A widened mediastinum observed on the chest film in a patient with an appropriate mechanism of injury suggests aortic disruption. The authors recommend aortography to exclude this lesion. Computed tomography (CT) has been suggested in the past to screen high-risk patients for angiography. A recent prospective study from Louisville found only a 55 per cent sensitivity and 65 per cent specificity for contrast-enhanced CT, and thus concluded there is no role for CT in the management of this injury.[21]

Knowledge of thoracic anatomy is essential for the proper planning for surgical intervention. The ascending aorta, aortic arch, proximal innominate, and common carotid arteries are best approached via a median sternotomy. The incision can be extended appropriately over the clavicle or into the neck. The left subclavian artery, however, is quite posterior in the upper mediastinum and is best exposed through a left third interspace anterior thoracotomy. Distal control of the subclavian arteries may require clavicular excision.

Cardiopulmonary bypass is required for ascending aortic and aortic arch reconstructions. In general, carotid shunts are not used unless both carotids or the aortic arch is being repaired. The operative repair of the descending thoracic aorta is via a generous left posterolateral thoracotomy. Placement of the proximal vascular clamp produces a marked elevation in cardiac afterload. This is usually managed pharmacologically, although left atrial to femoral bypass and a "Gott" shunt from the subclavian artery to the descending thoracic aorta have been employed for this purpose. The most dreaded complication is postoperative paraplegia. This complication has not been reduced by either technique. Recently cerebospinal fluid drainage has been used to improve spinal cord perfusion. In addition naloxone and intrathecal papaverine have been used with some success.[1,38] In general, suture repair of the descending aorta is impossible, and replacement grafting of a short segment is required.

CEREBROVASCULAR INJURY

Ninety-five per cent of carotid arterial injury is secondary to penetrating trauma with over 80 per cent of these due to gunshot wounds. The injury is frequently associated with concomitant injury of the esophagus, pharynx, or respiratory tract. The location of the neck injury in hemodynamically stable patients without an expanding neck hematoma should alter the preoperative work-up. The authors find it helpful to divide the neck into three zones as originally described by Monson and Freeark.[23] Zone I extends from the sternal notch to the clavicles; Zone II extends from the clavicles to the angle of the mandible; Zone III extends from the angle of the mandible to the base of the skull. Proximal and distal control of the arterial system is somewhat more hazardous in Zone I and Zone III. Thus, in the stable patient who is not bleeding, the authors routinely perform angiography to identify vascular injuries prior to surgical therapy. In Zone II, exploration may be performed without angiography since arterial injuries in this location are readily controlled and repaired.

A neurologic deficit should suggest the location of an arterial injury. The presence of Horner's syndrome suggests an internal carotid artery injury in the mid neck or a subclavian/vertebral injury at the base of the neck. Cerebral symptoms may be due to either a carotid injury or an intracerebral pathologic process.

The operation is commenced with control of the airway. If extensive hematoma is present, tracheostomy is required. The chest and mediastinum are prepared in the operative field such that rapid sternotomy can be performed if needed. An incision is made that parallels the anterior border of the sternocleidomastoid muscle. Proximal carotid control is first achieved followed by distal control. The need for heparinization is debated. Certainly in the multiple trauma or head-injured patient its use is hazardous. Arterial repair is performed with either a primary anastomosis or an interposition graft. Autogenous vein is the graft of choice.

Hemorrhage is an obvious indication for operation regardless of neurologic status. Patients with intimal flaps and/or nonoccluding thrombus who are neurologically intact are reconstructed; a good outcome is anticipated. A more controversial management problem involves the neurologically impaired patient with a carotid injury. Patients with mild to moderate deficits are reconstructed. In a patient with a severe deficit, most surgeons repair a carotid if prograde flow is present. If the carotid is thrombosed, there is concern that restoration of flow may contribute to brain edema and worsening of the patient.

Contrariwise, there are isolated cases of neurologic recovery in comatose patients after restoration of internal carotid flow.[2,33] Thus, the treatment of the unconscious patient remains controversial. CT and magnetic resonance imaging have not clarified this dilemma.

INTRA-ABDOMINAL VASCULAR INJURY

Abdominal vascular injuries are usually discovered at the time of emergency laparotomy. Exploration of midline hematomas is mandated to prevent the late sequelae of unrecognized aortic injury. Prior to exploration of these hematomas, proximal control is advisable. In patients with precarious vital signs and a tense abdomen, control of the thoracic aorta at the level of the diaphragm through a low thoracic incision is advocated as a preliminary maneuver. When the abdomen is entered, proximal control of the arota is obtained at the lowest possible level. Patients with prolonged hepatic and renal ischemia do poorly. Exploration of the upper abdominal aorta may be facilitated by the retroperitoneal approach from the left side.[19]

Repair of intra-abdominal vascular injuries may require the use of the saphenous vein. Thus, one or both thighs should always be included in the preoperative preparation and draping. It is preferable to obtain saphenous vein in almost all cases of a contaminated abdomen rather than use prosthetic material.

RENAL ARTERY INJURY

Renal arterial trauma is uncommon with approximately 75 per cent of injuries secondary to blunt injury.[4] The mechanism of injury is usually a deceleration force with the relatively mobile kidney pulling away from the fixed aorta. The diagnosis is usually established in the multiple trauma patient by CT or intravenous pyelography, which demonstrates a nonfunctioning kidney. Arteriography is usually recommended in the stable patient if time permits.

The kidney tolerates warm ischemia poorly. If the renal artery is occluded and collateral circulation is poor, probable irreversible renal damage occurs by 90 minutes. The management of these patients is controversial; the authors, however, routinely explore patients who can obviously tolerate laparotomy and in whom early (hours) restoration of flow can be anticipated. There are isolated reports of salvage of renal function many days to years after renal artery occlusion.[5,39] but in general these reports represent incomplete occlusion or occlusion of a stenotic lesion with well-developed collaterals. In the patient with abrupt complete renal artery occlusion without pre-existing stenosis, the salvage rate of kidneys is dismal.[6] Dean in a recent editorial suggested that a less aggressive approach toward attempted retrieval of renal function is appropriate especially when there is no visualization of the distal arteries (i.e., no collateral flow) on arteriography.

Renal artery exploration is usually performed via a midline laparotomy to allow examination of the intraperitoneal organs. The small bowel is packed to the right and dissection performed at the base of the mesentery where the origin of the involved renal artery is controlled at the aorta. Alternatively each kidney can be exposed with anterior reflection of the colon. Dissection of the artery is extended distally past the injured segment. This segment is marked by a bluish discoloration of the wall secondary to the dissection. A longitudinal arteriotomy is made in the proximal artery and extended distally to normal lumen. The injured segment is resected. With mobilization of the kidney, a primary anastomosis is usually possible. If tension prohibits a primary anastomosis, a bypass graft is indicated. In the pediatric population, care must be used not to utilize saphenous vein since a high incidence of late aneurysmal degeneration occurs and most authors prefer hypogastric artery. Polytetrafluoroethylene or Dacron is suitable in adults if contamination is absent.

POPLITEAL ARTERY INJURY

In a significant number of knee dislocations, spontaneous reduction occurs, and the radiograph reveals only soft tissue swelling. Early after injury, flow may be maintained in the injured popliteal artery. Thus, close observation or arteriography is recommended for all patients with either anterior or posterior dislocations of the knee. This injury is especially dangerous because swelling associated with knee dislocation often obliterates the precarious collateral circulation around the knee. Immediate operative repair is mandatory.[16] Confirmation by arteriography is usually unnecessary, but if deemed advisable, it can be performed on the operating table just prior to exploration of the popliteal vessels. Every effort should be expended to restore flow in the distal arteries as soon as possible from the time of injury.

The operative incision should be extended well up into the medial thigh for proximal control and distally into the calf to aid exposure and facilitate clot removal from the main branches of the popliteal artery. The incision also serves to decompress the muscles of the medial compartment of the leg. If the patient's condition, other injuries, or orthopedic consideration significantly delays immediate arterial reconstruction, a temporary shunt can be employed betweeen the severed ends to maintain flow.[8]

Definitive arterial repair often requires a vein graft utilizing the saphenous vein from the opposite extremity. The popliteal vein should be inspected and if thrombosed or disrupted should also be repaired.

Because of the importance of the popliteal artery to the viability of the foot, both dorsalis pedis and posterior tibial pulses should return promptly; if not, a completion arteriogram should be obtained. Postoperatively, careful monitoring of the distal pulses, preferably with the use of Doppler-derived pressures, should be done as with any arterial reconstruction. Any loss of pulses or signs of ischemia should be immediately evaluated for the possibility of occlusion of the repair or the development of a compartmental syndrome and appropriate treatment instituted.

VASCULAR AND ORTHOPEDIC INJURIES

The important association of arterial injuries with open or closed fractures and dislocations is outlined in Table 2.[12,15,20,27] Recognition of the vascular injury is often obscured by the difficulties of examining the painful, swollen extremity that accompanies bone injury. More often than not, however, it is the failure to assess the status of the distal extremity or to appreciate the significance of a large hematoma, recurrent bleeding, and distal ischemia that causes delay in recognition of arterial injury. A distressing preoccupation with bone abnormalities observed on radiologic study is all too common in the care of extremity injuries and must be avoided to prevent the tragic consequences of overlooked arterial injury.

The methods of diagnosis and principles of repair are similar to those for other arterial injuries, except for the problem of achieving stabilization of the fracture fragments adjacent to the arterial repair. Both the orthopedic and vascular surgeon prefer to stabilize the bones prior to arterial repair. This operative sequence provides a stable environment in which to perform arterial reconstructive surgery. To reverse the operative sequence invites disruption of the artery during orthopedic manipulation.

However, this operative sequence promotes an increase in the ischemia time that may not be tolerated in a truly compromised limb. Thus, the following plan has evolved. Patients with an arterial injury but with a warm pink foot are treated in the preferred manner. Patients who have a severely ischemic foot have the orthopedic stabilization performed prior to arterial repair only in those instances in which orthopedic stabilization can be achieved within a relatively short (60 minutes) time. If stabilization requires a prolonged length of time and there has

been some delay in reaching the operating room, arterial repair is accomplished first.

When venous injuries are encountered, they are of course repaired concomitantly. The combination of arterial injury, venous injury, and soft tissue injury associated with fracture make these patients especially prone to develop compartmental syndromes. Constricting bandages are avoided. Plaster casts are split longitudinally so that they do not contribute to development of compression. Prophylactic fasciotomy is recommended if severe trauma exists, particularly if a delay in restoration of flow has occurred.

SHOTGUN WOUNDS

Arterial injuries arising from shotgun wounds pose unique clinical problems. In close-range injuries (those in which the gun muzzle is adjacent to the area of injury), the amount of destruction to adjacent nerves, veins, and soft tissues often precludes successful restoration of function. Wide débridement of devitalized tissue including skin and muscle is required, and the remaining arterial ends usually have to be bridged by a long segment of reversed saphenous vein. The exposed arterial anastomoses and graft must be covered with viable tissue to prevent drying and disruption, and this often necessitates the transfer of adjacent uninvolved muscle or skin. The risk of infection is high, and the deleterious effects of bacteria on the suture lines and graft must be carefully monitored.

Shotgun wounds received at some distance from the gun muzzle (i.e., greater than 7 meters) cause minimal tissue damage, but the multiple pellets scattered beneath the skin may penetrate arteries over long distances and in multiple locations. Liberal use of arteriography is advisable to detect sites of injury and their late sequelae.

INTERVENTIONAL RADIOGRAPHY

Improved techniques of interventional radiography have widened the armamentarium used in the treatment of vascular injuries. The ability to guide an arterial catheter into nearly every artery and its main branches permits the skilled radiologist to arrest bleeding or occlude false aneurysms by embolization techniques or the inflation of small detachable balloons. This method has proved particularly effective in controlling bleeding from severed branches of the internal iliac artery that are often responsible for the massive blood loss accompanying pelvic fractures.[22,29] Difficulties with identifying and controlling vascular injuries at the time of laparotomy and the lack of serious sequelae from distal embolization of this artery have made this the preferred method of control of this arterial injury. Similar applications have occasionally been utilized in injuries involving arteries to the abdominal viscera (e.g., traumatic hemobilia) and intra- and extracerebral vessels.

LATE SEQUELAE OF VASCULAR INJURY

Failure to recognize the existence of a vascular injury may cause acute or chronic ischemia. The most tragic examples are the young men and women who sustain orthopedic injuries. Their fractures and dislocations are realigned but nonetheless amputation results. In some patients, amputation is avoided but chronic ischemia causes intermittent claudication, ischemic rest pain, or Raynaud's phenomenon. Delayed arterial repair may cause ischemic neuropathy. This neuropathy is in a glove or stocking distribution and usually improves over months.

As noted previously, partially severed arteries and those in which a major branch is completely detached at its junction with a main artery often develop a false aneurysm (Fig. 6). Although initally this may present as a pulsating hematoma, eventually the hematoma undergoes organization with fibrous tissue replacement and the formation of a very thick walled sac.

Since this wall is composed of fibrous tissue elements not derived from the artery and, as such, lacks elastic fibers, the continued expansion of this "false" aneurysm is inevitable. The distal extremity or organ supplied is seldom ischemic and distal pulses are usually maintained unless thrombus within the aneurysm has embolized. The patient usually presents with a pulsating mass or because of signs or symptoms of compression on adjacent structures. Auscultation reveals a systolic bruit, and a systolic thrill may be palpable. Treatment is usually advisable and consists of surgical excision of the aneurysm with restoration of arterial flow. Under special circumstances, angiographic embolization or thrombosis of aneurysms is occasionally undertaken. Compression of the fistula on physical examination slows the heart rate (Branham's sign). In large fistulas, high-output cardiac failure may occur.

It is important to auscultate areas of old injury or operation in any patient with unexplained heart failure to detect these lesions and correct the underlying cardiac problem. Treatment is surgical and requires permanent obliteration of the fistula, usually by excision of the involved segment of artery with restoration of arterial flow and ligation or repair of the adjacent vein.

SELECTED REFERENCES

Eastcott, H. H. G.: Arterial Surgery, 2nd ed., chapter 13. Philadelphia, J. B. Lippincott Company, 1973.
This is an outstanding chapter by a British author in an excellent text of vascular surgery, which reviews many fine details of diagnosis and treatment of a wide variety of arterial injuries.

Hardy, J. D., Seshadri, R., Neeley, W. A., and Berry, D. W.: Aortic and other arterial injuries. Ann. Surg., 181:640, 1975.
This is an extensive review of 360 arterial injuries encountered at one center during an 18-year period. Over 85 per cent were the result of penetrating wounds, while the majority of blunt injuries were associated with fractures and dislocations. Major veins were involved in 20 per cent. An excellent discussion regarding management of the more complicated injuries to the aortic arch and carotid, popliteal, and renal arteries is included. The principles of management and the controversies surrounding ancillary measures are well presented.

Perry, M. O.: The Management of Acute Vascular Injuries. Baltimore, Williams & Wilkins, 1981.
A personal perspective of the approach to vascular trauma based on an extensive civilian experience.

Rich, N. M., and Spencer, F. C.: Vascular Trauma. Philadephia, W. B. Saunders Company. 1978.
A comprehensive review of vascular trauma by military-oriented surgeons.

Rich, N. M., Hobson, R. W., and Collins, G. J.: Traumatic arteriovenous fistulae and false aneurysms. Surgery, 78:817, 1975.
This review of 558 injuries in the Vietnam War provides a comprehensive but retrospective review of the diagnosis and treatment of this complication of arterial severance. It is hoped that the 7 per cent incidence will diminish as partial severance is recognized and repaired primarily.

REFERENCES

1. Acher, C. W., and Wynn, M. M.: Naloxone and spinal fluid drainage as adjuncts in the treatment of thoroco-abdominal and thoracic aneurysms. Presented at the 47th Annual Meeting, Central Surgical Association, 1990.
2. Brown, M. F., Graham, J. M., Feliciano, D. V., et al.: Carotid artery injuries. Am. J. Surg., 144:748, 1982.
3. Carrel, A., and Guthrie, C. C.: Uni-terminal and bi-terminal venous transplantation. Surg. Gynecol. Obstet., 2:266, 1906.
4. Cass, A. S.: Management of renal artery injuries from external trauma. J. Urol., 138:266, 1987.
5. Cosby, R. L.: Traumatic renal artery thrombosis. Am. J Med., 81:890, 1988.
6. Dean, R. H.: Management of renal artery trauma. J. Vasc. Surg., 8:89, 1988.
7. DeBakey, M. E., and Simeone, F. A: Battle injuries of the arteries in World War II. Ann. Surg., 123:534, 1946.
8. Eger, M., Goleman, L., Goldstein, A., and Hirsch, M.: The use of a temporary shunt in the management of arterial injuries. Surg. Gynecol. Obstet., 132:67, 1971.
9. Fogarty, T. H., et al.: A method for extraction of arterial thrombi. Surg. Gynecol. Obstet., 116:241, 1963.
10. Fry, R. E., and Fry, W. J.: Extracranial carotid artery injuries. Surgery, 88:581, 1980.
11. Goyanes, D. J.: Substitucion plastica de las arterias por las venas o arterioplastica venosa, aplicada, como neuvo metodo, al tratamiento de las aneurismas. El Siglo Medico, Sept. 8, 1906, pp. 346, 561.

12. Hardy, J. D., Seshadri, R., Neeley, W. A., and Berry, D. W.: Aortic and other arterial injuries. Ann. Surg., 181:640, 1975.
13. Hughes, C. W.: Arterial repair during the Korean War. Ann. Surg., 147:555, 1958.
14. Johnson, F. E., Sumner, D. S., and Strandness, D. F., Jr.: Extremity necrosis caused by indwelling arterial catheters. Am. J. Surg., 131:375, 1976.
15. Koostra, G., Schnipper, J. J., Boontje, A. H., Klasen, H. J., and Binnendijk, B.: Femoral shaft fracture with injury of the superficial femoral artery in civilian accidents. Surg. Gynecol. Obstet., 142:339, 1976.
16. Lim, L. T., Michuda, M. S., Flanigan, D. P., and Pankovitch, A.: Popliteal artery trauma. Arch. Surg., 115:1307, 1980.
17. Matsen, F. A., Mayo, K. A., Sheridan, G. W., and Krugmire, R. B., Jr.: Monitoring of intramuscular pressure. Surgery, 75:702, 1976.
18. Mattox, K. L.: Approaches to trauma involving the major vessels of the thorax. Surg. Clin. North Am. 69:77, 1989.
19. Mattox, K. L., McCollum, W. B., Beall, A. C., Jr., Gordan, G. L., Jr., and DeBakey, M. E.: Management of penetrating injuries of the suprarenal aorta. J. Trauma, 15:808, 1975.
20. McNamara, J. J., et al.: Management of fractures with associated injury in combat casualties. J. Trauma, 13:17, 1973.
21. Miller, F., Richardson, D. J., Hallis, T., Cryer, H., and Willary, S.: Role of CT in diagnosis of major arterial injury after blunt thoracic trauma. Surgery, 106:596, 1989.
22. Miller, W. F.: Massive hemorrhage in fractures of the pelvis. South. Med. J., 56:933, 1963.
23. Monson, D. O., Saletta, J. D., and Freeark, R. J.: Carotid vertebral trauma. J. Trauma, 9:987, 1969.
24. Murphy, J. B.: Resection of arteries and veins injured in continuity—end-to-end suture. Exp. Clin. Res. Med. Rec., 51:73, 1897.
25. Nicholas, G. G., and Demuth, W. E.: Long term results of brachial thrombectomy—following cardiac catheterization. Ann. Surg., 183:436, 1976.
26. Patman, R. D., and Thompson, J. E.: Fasciotomy in peripheral vascular surgery: Report of 164 patients. Arch. Surg., 101:663, 1970.
27. Pradham, D. J., Jauanteguy, J. M., Wilder, R. J., and Michelson, E.: Arterial injuries of the extremities associated with fractures. Arch. Surg., 105:582, 1972.
28. Pringle, J. H.: Two cases of vein grafting for the maintenance of direct arterial circulation. Lancet, 1:1795, 1913.
29. Rich, N. M.: Vascular trauma in Viet Nam. J. Cardiovasc. Surg., 2:368, 1970.
30. Rich, N. M., and Spencer, F. C.: Vascular Trauma. Philadelphia, W. B. Saunders Company, 1978.
31. Rich, N. M., Hobson, R. W., Collins, G. J., and Anderson, C. A.: The effect of acute popliteal venous interruption. Ann. Surg., 183:365, 1976.
32. Rich, N. M., Hughes, C. W., and Baugh, J. H.: Management of venous injuries. Ann. Surg., 171:724, 1970.
33. Robbs, J. V., Hum, R. R., Rajaruthman, P., et al.: Neurologic deficits and injuries involving the neck arteries. Br. J. Surg., 70:220, 1983.
34. Saletta, J. D., and Freeark, R. J.: The partially severed artery. Arch. Surg., 96:198, 1968.
35. Saletta, J. D., and Freeark, R. J.: Injuries to the profunda femoris artery. J. Trauma, 12:778, 1972.
36. Schrock, T., Blaisdell, F. W., and Mathewson, C., Jr.: Management of blunt trauma to the liver and hepatic veins. Arch. Surg., 96:698, 1968.
37. Smith, K., Ben-Menachen, Y., Kuke, J. H., and Hill, G. L.: The superior gluteal: An artery at risk in blunt pelvic trauma. J. Trauma, 16:273, 1976.
38. Svensson, L. G., Grum, D. F., Bednarski, M., Cosgrove, D., and Loop, F. D.: Appraisal of cerebrospinal fluid alterations during aortic surgery with intrathecal papaverine administrator and cerebrospinal fluid drainage. J. Vasc. Surg., 2:423, 1990.
39. Weisman, S., et al.: Traumatic renal artery occlusion: Is late reconstruction advisable? J. Urol., 137:727, 1987.
40. Whitesides, T. E., Jr., Haney, T. C., Harada, H., Holmes, H. E., and Morimoto, K.: A simple method for tissue pressure determination. Arch. Surg., 110:1311, 1975.
41. Wright, C. B., Lamoy, R. E., and Hobson, R. W., II: Hemodynamic effects of intra-arterial injection of drugs of abuse. Surgery, 79:425, 1976.
42. Yao, S. T.: Experience with the Doppler ultrasound flow velocity meter in peripheral vascular disease. In Gillespie, J. (Ed.): Modern Trends in Vascular Surgery, London, Butterworth, 1970.

9. ACUTE ARTERIAL OCCLUSION

Thomas J. Fogarty, M.D.

Reference to occlusion of the arterial circulation was first made by Harvey in 1628.[17] Labey[18] has been credited with the first successful surgical removal of an arterial embolus in 1911. The isolation of heparin by Murphy and Best in 1938 provided the surgeon a means to prevent thrombosis during the repair and manipulation of blood vessels. Review of the surgical literature indicates that the operative approach to acute arterial occlusion was limited by the inability of the surgeon to remove simply and effectively the embolus and distally propagated thrombus. Some of the methods employed included retrograde flushing with saline, the application of suction catheters, vein strippers, and local removal through multiple arteriotomies. None of these surgical techniques were particularly effective in reducing the high morbidity and mortality.

The introduction of the balloon catheter technique[14] in 1963 dramatically simplified the technical aspects of surgical therapy for acute arterial occlusion. Advances in the field of open-heart surgery have eliminated some of the sources of arterial emboli and further reduced mortality by making possible correction of the cardiac disorder.

PATHOLOGY

The primary source of acute arterial occlusion is embolization from the heart due to underlying cardiac disease. Today, the primary cardiac disorder is atherosclerotic heart disease, the manifestations of which include myocardial infarction, atrial fibrillation, congestive heart failure, and ventricular aneurysm. The decline in prevalence of rheumatic heart disease has led to a decreased incidence of acute occlusion due to embolization from mitral stenosis.[1,26] Acute occlusions may also be of thrombotic origin, prompted by chronic degenerative atherosclerotic disease of the periphery.

Regardless of the source or histologic structure of an embolus, it is the location and secondary events following the impaction that determine the viability of an extremity. Following occlusion, a softer coagulum of blood forms in areas of decreased flow. Linton[20] has emphasized that this propagation of thrombus distal to the embolus is of major importance in the outcome of the disease process (Fig. 1).

Compromised oxygenation of tissue at the site of the occlusion leads to an anaerobic cellular metabolism whereby tissue becomes acidotic. Elevated concentrations of potassium ions, lactic acid, P_{CO_2}, and the intracellular enzymes creatine phosphokinase (CPK) and lysozymes are released into the bloodstream and interstitial tissues. The ischemic state affects the neural tissue, which induces the symptoms of localized pain and paresthesia. Uncontrolled, muscle swelling and rigor follow. Tissue necrosis typically occurs after 6 to 12 hours of significant ischemia. Further propagation of the distal clot can eventually lead to venous thrombosis. Another feature thought to be

of significance is the small vessel thrombosis in the distal vascular bed in which *vasospasm* may be a feature contributing to further occlusion. In one series, vasodilator therapy by intra-arterial instillation of 0.5 mg. of reserpine was found to significantly decrease recurrent limb ischemia requiring reoperation.[2]

Failure to recognize and to remove atraumatically the distally propagated thrombus may cause less complete restoration of circulation and possibly amputation. Surgeons have often relied upon the presence or absence of back-bleeding from the peripheral arterial bed as a guide to distal patency. Repeated clinical observations have confirmed that back-bleeding is an unreliable guide to distal patency. Discontinuous thrombotic material is present in approximately one third of the cases (Fig. 2). Under these circumstances, back-bleeding may be quite forceful, despite the presence of additional distal thrombotic material. The presence of adequate collateral vessels causes significant bleeding from the distal segment despite the fact that the more peripheral arterial bed may be totally occluded. Failure to recognize this circumstance causes less than complete restoration of the circulation. For this reason, routine distal exploration with balloon catheters should be performed independently of the status of the back-bleeding.

The majority of surgically treatable emboli lodge in the lower extremities. Incidence of impaction is highest in the femoral arterial bed, with frequent occurrence in the iliac, aortic, and popliteal areas as well. Emboli in the renal, mesenteric, brachial, and cerebral arteries are less common, but not unusual.

Arterial emboli most commonly occur in the elderly, seriously ill patient with multiple systemic diseases. Prolonged periods of surgical manipulation and general anesthesia have been considered valid deterrents to operative intervention in such patients. This has been particularly true when the clinical finding indicated that conservative measures might preserve life at the cost of limb loss or impairment of function. In patients undergoing arterial embolectomy, a significant percentage similarly succumb or require amputation prior to discharge. The reason for this morbidity and mortality was the presence of preoperative life-threatening cardiac and other diseases in many of these patients.[22] In a series of more than 400 peripheral arterial embolectomies, the overall operative mortality was 10 per cent, again relating to pre-existing disease. Limb salvage rate was 90.5 per cent and the amputation rate 9.5 per cent.[24] The balloon catheter technique is an operative procedure designed to avoid general anesthesia, reduce surgical trauma, and effectively remove all thrombotic material in a simple manner, regardless of its anatomic location.

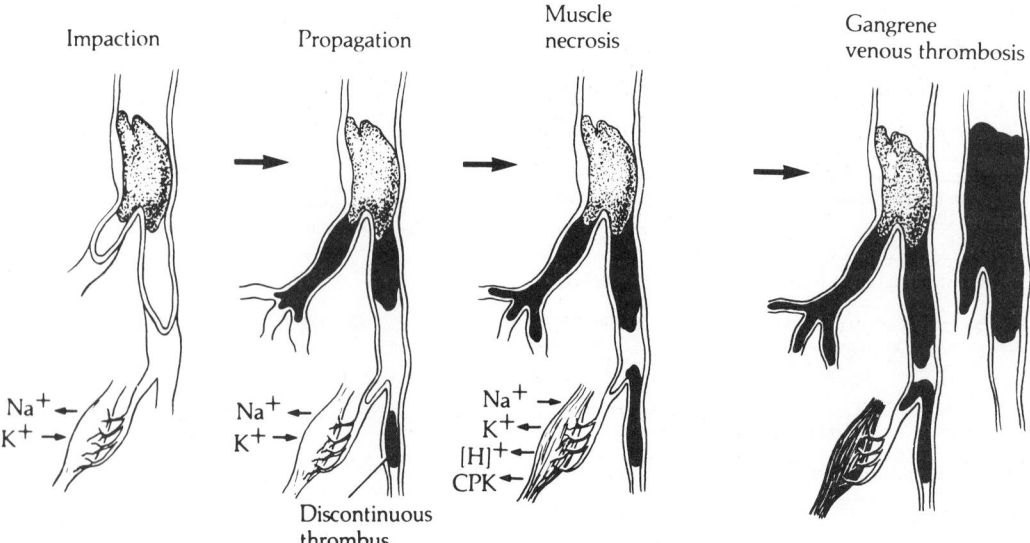

Figure 1. Progression of acute embolic arterial occlusion and its impact on adjacent tissue.

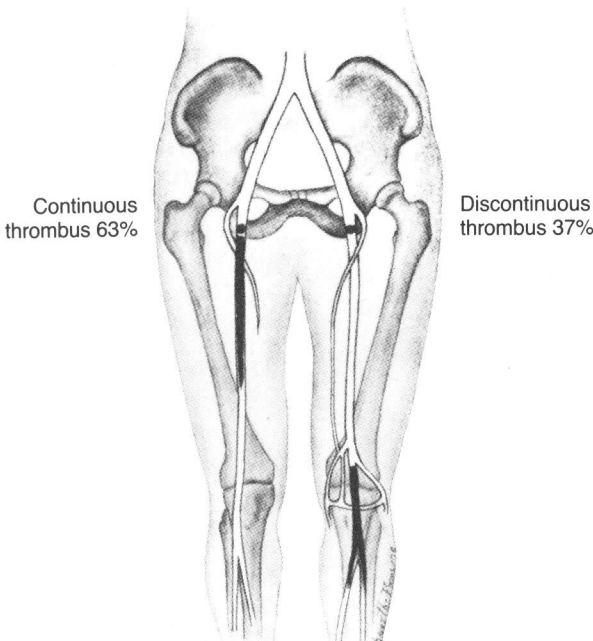

Continuous
thrombus 63%

Discontinuous
thrombus 37%

Figure 2. Incidence of discontinuous propagation of thrombus.

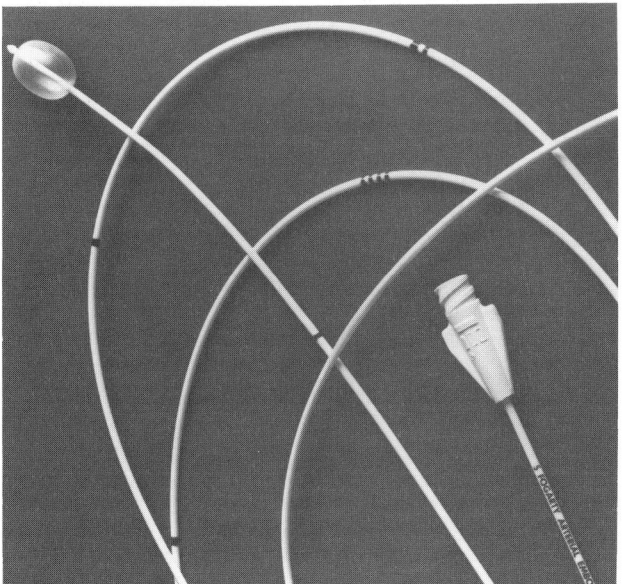

Figure 3. Fogarty catheter for extraction of arterial emboli and thrombus. Depth markings on catheter body indicate distance of balloon from arteriotomy.

PREOPERATIVE EVALUATION AND CARE

Patients presenting with an acute embolic occlusion should be assumed to have significant underlying heart disease. The sources of arterial emboli in a series of 300 patients are listed in Table 1. The large number of patients presenting with atherosclerotic heart disease reinforces the concept that the heart is the site of underlying pathologic change. Evaluation of cardiac function should proceed simultaneously with examination of the peripheral vasculature. Digitalis, antiarrhythmic agents, morphine, diuretics, and heparin are drugs basic to patient care. Utilization of these agents when indicated should not delay surgical intervention.

Noninvasive Doppler ultrasound techniques and pressure and waveform measurements are useful in the preoperative setting. They can be performed typically in 5 to 10 minutes. These procedures are helpful in differentiating occlusions of embolic origin from those of thrombotic origin in patients with underlying vascular disease. They also provide a useful preoperative benchmark against which postoperative results may be compared.

Appropriate therapy is initiated while emergency preparation for operation is accomplished. The presence of congestive heart failure, cardiogenic shock, and significant arrhythmias requires intensive care unit monitoring. Placement of a central venous catheter is required in the majority of patients. In addition to allowing rapid administration of drugs and fluids, this permits monitoring of central venous pressures. Central placement of catheters represents a convenient means for the intravenous administration of heparin. Cannulation of the internal jugular vein as advocated by Daily[7] is simple and has been free of

significant complication. Monitoring of the pulmonary artery pressure should be utilized in those patients who present with hemodynamic instability.

In the presence of an embolus to a lower extremity, the possibility of simultaneous emboli to mesenteric or renal arteries should always be entertained. Hematuria or abdominal complaints indicative of a possible occlusion require preoperative visualization of these vessels. Involvement of more than one extremity occurs in approximately 10 per cent of patients, and this fact should be emphasized. When the diagnosis of an acute arterial occlusion has been made, heparin should be administered immediately and preparation for operation initiated.

INSTRUMENTATION

The balloon embolectomy catheter was developed with specific adaptations in its construction for safe, effective extraction of arterial emboli. It consists of a hollow, pliable body in graduated sizes for use in major vessels of any caliber. At its proximal portion the syringe fitting provides the means for fluid exchange into a soft, distensible balloon located at the distal tip of the instrument (Fig. 3). The catheter is inserted into the acutely occluded vessel as far as possible. The balloon is inflated and withdrawn in the inflated position (Fig. 4). By a mechanism of fluid displacement, the balloon maintains uniform, even contact with the vessel wall as it proceeds through areas of narrowing (Fig. 5). This mechanism allows removal of thrombotic ma-

**TABLE 1. Source of Arterial Embolus
in 300 Consecutive Patients**

Atrial fibrillation	231
Atherosclerotic heart disease	183
Rheumatic heart disease	48
Acute myocardial infarction	50
Atherosclerotic plaque	7
Unknown	12

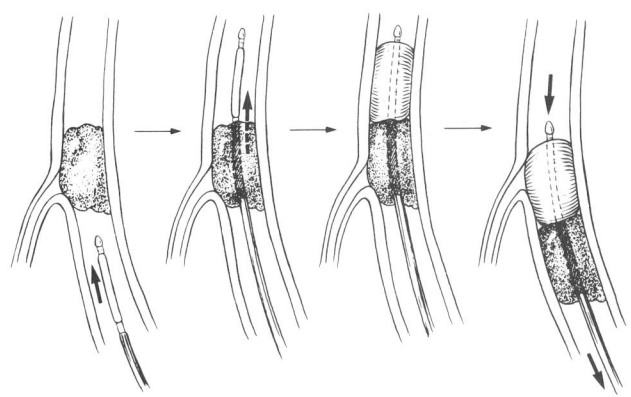

Figure 4. Technique of balloon catheter embolectomy.

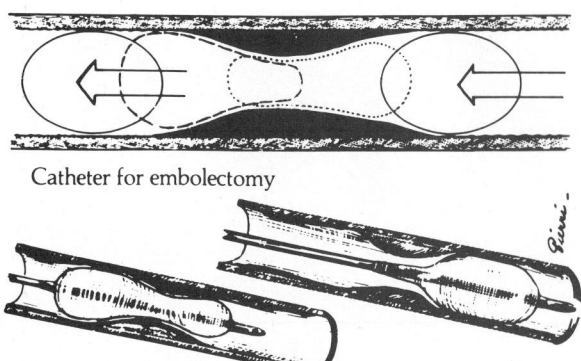

Figure 5. Compliant nature of fluid-filled latex balloon for embolectomy.

terial distal to stenotic areas. One surgeon manipulates both the syringe and the catheter during withdrawal. In this way it is easy to judge the amount of traction required for extraction of the occluding material as well as the quantity of fluid necessary to effect alternate inflation and deflation as the instrument proceeds through areas of atherosclerotic narrowing or vessels of increasing or decreasing diameter.

The concept of a balloon catheter for embolectomy has remained basically the same since its introduction. There have been minor changes in the instrument directed to increasing its effectiveness and reducing the incidence of complications. A variety of balloon configurations and catheter materials have been evaluated. Although double-lumen catheters and spiked balloon catheters appeared to offer improvements, significant disadvantages have been associated with their use. The utility and effectiveness of the instrument are related to its simplicity. Attempts to incorporate nonessential refinements have thus far not proved advantageous or practical.

One area of design improvement that has shown promise, however, is that for the removal of adherent thrombotic material. In recent years, there has been a significant increase in acute thrombotic episodes contrasted to embolic occlusions. Thrombotic pathologic processes have a higher incidence of more adherent thrombus. A special spiral balloon embolectomy catheter (Fig. 6) has been found to have significant utility in these situations. The catheter is inserted in a straight collapsed configuration. Once beyond the thrombus, it can be actuated into a corkscrew type configuration; withdrawing the instrument in the corkscrew shape increases traction on the clot but minimizes shear forces on the arterial wall.

With the increase in the number of patients with aortofemoral grafts, there is a concurrent increase in the number of late graft failures. A common failure mode of these grafts is the development of a thick pannus at anastomotic suture lines that extends into the graft proper. This pannus and associated thrombus can be very adherent and can be removed by a variable diameter thrombectomy catheter (Fig. 7). Utilization of this technique

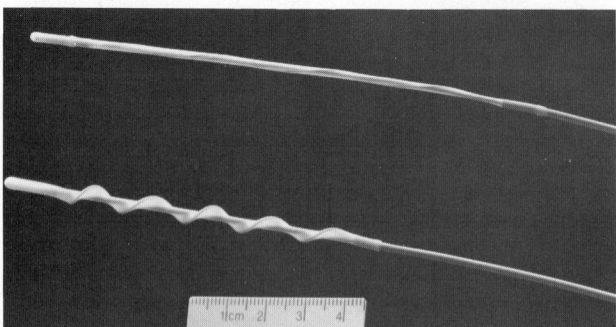

Figure 6. Spiral balloon embolectomy catheter. Working end demonstrated in expanded and collapsed positions.

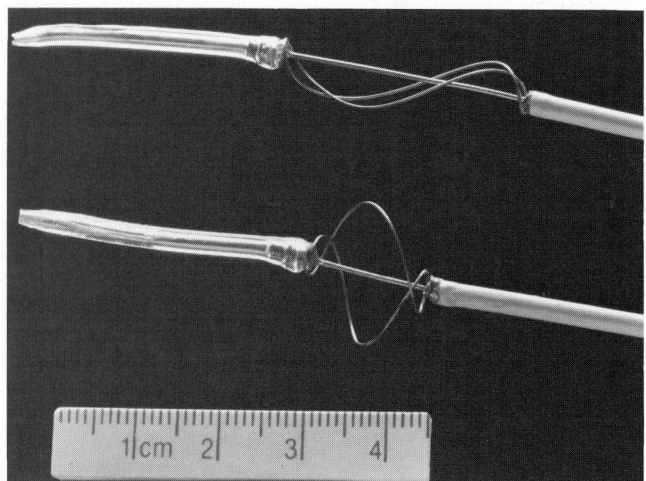

Figure 7. Variable diameter thrombectomy catheter. Working end demonstrated in expanded and collapsed positions.

and instrument has avoided major abdominal surgery in the debilitated and very elderly, a patient population who appear particularly susceptible to graft occlusions.

Complications secondary to the use of embolectomy and thrombectomy catheters have been those common to all catheter techniques and have included plaque dissection, catheter tip separation, and vessel perforation. Vessel rupture can occur if the balloon of the instrument is overdistended in small vessels. Experience and a realization of the limitations of the instrument are the most significant factors in reducing the incidence of complications.[11]

OPERATIVE PROCEDURE

The experience with acute peripheral arterial embolization has clearly indicated that successful management of these patients is related to well-defined factors. From a technical standpoint, it must be recognized that there are varying degrees of difficulty encountered in the attempt to re-establish the peripheral circulation. Patients with advanced ischemia with extensive distal propagation of the thrombus and those having significant chronic occlusive disease present the most difficult problems. A careful history and physical examination allow identification of these situations.

Preparation

The procedure is initiated with local anesthesia. An anesthetist should be in attendance to monitor vital signs and administer a general anesthetic if it becomes necessary. The extremity should be surgically prepared from the toes to the nipple line. A bilateral inguinal approach is utilized for aortic emboli, and both extremities are prepared. An iliac embolus requires bilateral preparation. The possibility of dislodging a high iliac embolus with occlusion of the opposite extremity exists. This has not occurred in the author's experience, but the possibility is always anticipated by preparation of the opposite extremity so that the pulses may be externally palpated at the time of operation. Intraoperative arteriographic equipment should be readily available for visualization of the extremities during the procedure.

Technique

The approach to embolic occlusion regardless of the anatomic location has been through a femoral incision (Fig. 8). The common femoral artery, superficial femoral artery, and deep femoral artery are isolated and occluded with cushioned atraumatic occluding instruments. The arterial incision is made in relation

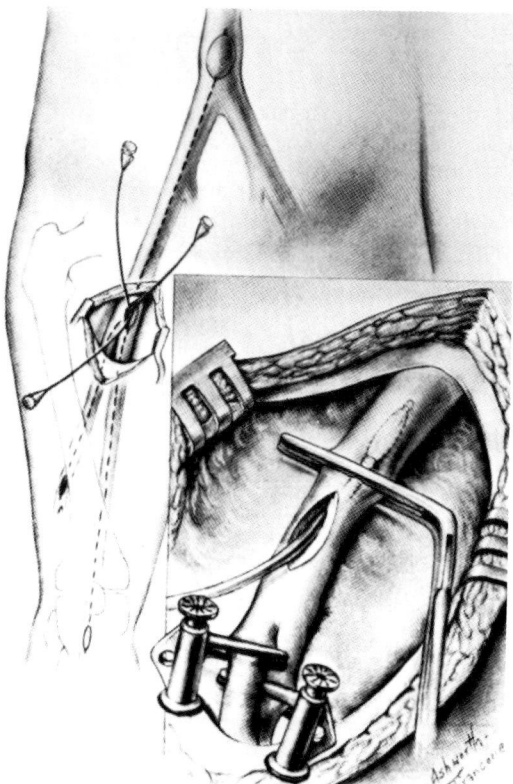

Figure 8. Balloon catheter extraction in the iliofemoral system via femoral incision. Use of padded clamps minimizes arterial trauma during instrumentation.

to the orifice of the superficial femoral artery and deep femoral artery. A distal exploration is initially performed and catheters should be routinely placed in the superficial and deep femoral arteries. An open deep femoral circulation is capable of providing the margin necessary to maintain viability in many patients with advanced ischemia or in those who had prior chronic occlusion of the superficial femoral system. Recovery of embolic material from the deep femoral artery, even in the presence of a patent common femoral artery, has been frequent in the author's experience. The 2-French and 3-French catheters are most commonly employed for exploration of the deep femoral system, whereas 3-French and 4-French catheters have been found suitable for exploration of the femoropopliteal systems.

If there is uncertainty about adequate distal clot removal, the vessel should be visualized. At this institution, the author visualizes the vessel via operative arteriography and, more recently, via angioscopy. Angioscopy has been found to be a valuable complement to operative arteriography for documenting clot removal. With the proper angioscopy equipment, one can quickly become proficient in its use. The author uses an angioscopy system that employs a pressure-modulated irrigation system and also a digitized image storage and retrieval mechanism.[5] These features make the system expedient in the operative setting and minimize the amount of irrigation fluid that is infused into the patient.

Angioscopy allows directional access to the tibial vessels and minimizes the need for distal incisions. Following removal of the thrombotic material, copious irrigation of the distal arterial system should be done with a heparinized saline solution.

In the presence of advanced ischemia, the simultaneous presence of major venous occlusion demands consideration. In a personal series of 300 patients, 8 per cent were found to have concomitant major venous occlusion.[15] The majority of the patients in this group had advanced ischemia with extensive distal propagation of clot on the arterial side. In this situation the vein is explored before the arterial circulation is re-established, and

large venous thrombi are removed by means of venous thrombectomy catheters.[12] Prior to suture closure of the vein, the arterial circulation is re-established. After removal of the arterial occlusions, the distal arterial system is irrigated with 200 to 300 ml. of a heparinized saline solution. The distal venous clamp is removed to allow smaller thrombi to be flushed out during this irrigation. The artery is closed first. The vein is flushed again after re-establishment of the arterial circulation. The venotomy is closed last.

There has been reference in the literature to delaying surgical intervention in patients who present with advanced ischemia.[4] The author has not employed this delayed approach and believes that advanced ischemia secondary to acute embolic occlusion represents a surgical emergency. In these patients, heparin is employed at the time of operation and in the immediate postoperative period.

In those situations in which it is recognized that heparin should be employed in the immediate postoperative period, in this hospital it has been the policy to anticipate the possible complications of hemorrhage and hematoma at incisional sites and to employ vacuum-type drainage.

Swelling of a revascularized, ischemic extremity can assume considerable proportions and requires treatment. Massive swelling that may embarrass arterial inflow is observed most frequently in those patients who present with advanced ischemia prior to surgical intervention. Capillary damage causing fluid exudation into ischemic tissues is a factor in this swelling. Obstruction of the venous outflow tract aggravates the problem. Failure to immediately control this edema may cause reocclusion of the arterial inflow. Fasciotomy has been required in 10 per cent of the patients who present with acute embolic occlusion. Initial decompression is accomplished through small skin incisions as described by Rosato.[25] If immediate improvement is not obtained by this limited fasciotomy, the skin incisions should be extended and the deeper fascial compartments widely opened. Radical decompression requiring fibular resection is rarely necessary in patients who have acute embolic occlusion. Patman and Thompson[23] have provided an excellent review of the technique and indications for fasciotomy.

Immediately following restoration of arterial continuity in extremities with advanced ischemia, significant alterations in electrolytes and acid balance may occur.[10] The venous efflux of ischemic extremities following restoration of arterial continuity was studied in 10 patients (Table 2). These data clearly indicated that following successful restoration of the circulation, there was a sudden return of very acidotic blood with a high potassium content to the heart. This metabolic effect in conjunction with pooling of blood in the revascularized extremity can cause significant hypotension. In 8 of the 10 patients studied, adverse effects were associated with clamp release, in the form of significant electrocardiographic changes or hypotension, or both. The necessity of using buffering agents and antiarrhythmic agents should be anticipated at the time of clamp release. Electrolytes

TABLE 2. Mean Values of Biochemical Determinations on Venous Efflux of Ischemic Extremity Before and After Restoration of Flow

Ten Patients	pH	PO_2	PCO_2	K	CPK
System venous blood before embolectomy	7.38	38.2	36.4	4.3	77
Venous blood from ischemic leg before embolectomy	7.31	19.3	45.8	4.7	200
Venous blood from ischemic leg 5 minutes after restoration of flow	6.80	34.8	77.3	7.2	653.4

should be closely followed in the postoperative period. A high creatine phosphokinase level noted in the venous efflux indicates significant muscle damage. Haimovici has described the adverse systemic effects that may occur following revascularization of the extremity presenting with advanced ischemia.[16]

EMBOLIC OCCLUSION IN THE PRESENCE OF SIGNIFICANT CHRONIC OCCLUSIVE DISEASE

A careful history and examination of the uninvolved extremity afford a reliable assessment of the peripheral circulation prior to the acute episode. The patient's general condition, prior level of activity, and extent of the pathologic change encountered at the time of operation all have an important role in determining the extent of the surgical procedure. In general, it is advisable to attempt initially only return of the circulation to its acute preocclusive state. Definitive reconstructive procedures are delayed until a more critical evaluation of the patient is possible. Major reconstructive procedures may be indicated, however, if the general condition is favorable when the patient is first observed. Definitive procedures may be performed, particularly if one is concerned about the viability of the extremity and if the patient was active prior to the acute occlusion. Elderly patients in poor general condition are poor candidates for major reconstructive procedures. Local angioplasty of the deep femoral system in these situations is simple and quick and can be done under anesthesia. Frequently it provides the margin necessary to maintain viability. Reconstructive procedures performed in conjunction with arterial embolectomy in a series of 300 patients are listed in Table 3.[15] Localized endarterectomy and femorofemoral jump grafts are simple and can be done under local anesthesia. In 15 cases the procedure was performed at the time of initial exploration, and in 14 it was performed as a second procedure during the initial hospital stay. In a total of 21 cases sympathectomy was performed; in 12 it was done in conjunction with a reconstructive procedure.

Adjunctive dilation[13] and/or atherectomy can be employed at the time of thrombectomy or embolectomy. This approach reduces the magnitude of the operation in the elderly and very ill patient and is being utilized with increasing frequency.

UPPER EXTREMITY EMBOLI

The management of emboli in the upper extremity is identical to that described for the lower extremity. Proximal subclavian artery emboli can be simply removed under local anesthesia by retrograde extraction. It should be borne in mind, however, that if the embolus appears to reside close to the origin of the cranial vessels, fragmentation of the embolus may occur during withdrawal, causing central nervous system ischemia. Thus far, this has not occurred in the author's experience, but the possibility should be anticipated. If there is serious doubt as to the exact location of the embolus relating to the orifices of the carotid and vertebral vessels, preoperative radiographic visualization should be performed.

The possible morbidity associated with upper extremity emboli should not be underestimated. Baird and Lagos noted in their study that more proximal emboli cause significantly more ischemia than do the more distal brachial occlusions.[3]

TABLE 3. Reconstructive Procedures Performed at the Time of Arterial Embolectomy

Common and deep femoral endarterectomy	14
Femorofemoral crossover graft	7
Iliac endarterectomy	3
Aortofemoral endarterectomy	3
Aortofemoral graft	2

RENAL, MESENTERIC, AND CAROTID ARTERY EMBOLI

The principles of management of emboli to these areas are similar to those described for management of peripheral arterial emboli. It should be borne in mind, however, that the external support provided by adjacent tissue is significantly less with vessels supplying the viscera and the brain than with the vessels of peripheral vasculature. Considerable care should be taken in introducing the catheter into these vessels. The 2-French and 3-French catheters are of appropriate size for distal exploration of these vessels, and the catheters are provided with a very flexible tip, which significantly diminishes the possibility of perforation of the vessel. Only gentle inflation and traction should be used in removing emboli located in these areas.

Unless emboli to the internal carotid system are observed within the first few hours of onset, surgical intervention should not be considered. Hemorrhagic infarction represents a frequent and often fatal complication when attempts are made to remove emboli to the cerebral circulation, especially when they are undertaken after a considerable lapse of time.

POSTOPERATIVE CARE AND MANAGEMENT

The value of heparin postoperatively has been well documented.[9] The indications should be individualized for each patient. The possible presence of simultaneous venous thrombosis and embolization following acute myocardial infarction represent indications for heparinization in the postoperative period.

The specific aspects of postoperative care obviously concern the underlying pathologic condition responsible for the embolus, the presence or absence of significant cardiac impairment, and the presence or absence of associated diseases. Concern with the status of the peripheral vasculature should not impair the management or care of these other critical disorders. Peripheral embolization following myocardial infarction should immediately direct one's attention to the underlying cardiac lesion. Catheterization of the left side of the heart and coronary artery visualization may be indicated in order to define whether a correctable cardiac lesion is present. The presence of significant valvular heart disease obviously deserves diagnostic investigation and surgical correction.

MORBIDITY AND MORTALITY

The aim of surgical intervention for arterial emboli is to restore the peripheral circulation to its preocclusive state. Evaluation of results is based on restoration of pulses, relief of symptoms, and return of normal color and temperature. It is sometimes difficult to assess results in those patients in whom the condition of the extremity prior to the acute occlusion was unknown. Conditions such as mental confusion, or concurrent illness obviously preclude evaluation by exercise tolerance. Evaluation of therapy is best determined by mortality and the amputation rates. The possibility of maintaining a viable, functional extremity following acute arterial occlusion should exceed 90 per cent. The possibility of a successful procedure obviously concerns the presence or absence of advanced ischemia. The condition of the extremity and not the duration of occlusion represents the primary determinant of operability. Reference to Table 4 indicates that even after prolonged periods of occlusion, successful surgical intervention is possible. Even in the presence of established gangrene, a lower level of amputation can often be achieved following successful embolectomy.

Failure of the initial exploration after an apparent success is an indication for re-exploration. The most common cause for failure concerns technical factors, which on occasion can be corrected if recognized. The possibility, however, of re-embolization to the same extremity should not be overlooked. Its documented occurrence should reinforce a second-look attitude.[14]

TABLE 4. Time Interval in Relation to Advanced Ischemia

Age of Embolus	Number of Emboli	Advanced Ischemia*	Amputations
1–24 hours	193	24	3
24–48 hours	57	21	3
2–90 days	80	39	10

* Advanced ischemia: early rigor or gangrene.

A constant physical finding that should be cause for considerable concern after an apparently successful embolectomy is the presence of a water-hammer type pulse. An apparently stronger than normal pulse has, in the author's experience, been associated with a high incidence of reocclusion. Under these circumstances, obstruction is present at the small artery and arteriolar level. Re-exploration should include copious distal irrigation in conjunction with venous exploration.

The mortality associated with acute arterial occlusion has, in the author's experience, been unrelated to surgical intervention. The causes of death in a series of 300 consecutive patients with acute arterial occlusion are listed in Table 5. All deaths were related to cardiovascular dysfunction. Seventy-seven per cent of the patients died as a direct result of a cardiac disease. It would appear from this study and from the reviews by Levy,[19] Thompson,[27] and Connett[6] that the mortality associated with arterial embolism concerns the underlying cardiac disorder. These findings reinforce the contention that the recognition and correction of the cause for embolism should represent a very important aspect of the care of these patients. It is only through aggressive treatment of the underlying lesion that mortality can be improved. With the increasing success of coronary artery surgery, patients in whom emboli develop after myocardial infarction deserve consideration for coronary visualization. The timing of such studies should concern the general condition of the patient. Revascularization or aneurysmectomy, if indicated, should be done as soon as possible. The number and types of associated cardiac procedures performed in a group of 300 patients who had peripheral arterial emboli are listed in Table 6. Half of these procedures represented emergency situations and were performed at the time of arterial embolectomy. The remaining half were semiurgent, and all were accomplished within 1 month from the time of acute occlusion.

THROMBOLYTIC AGENTS

Thrombolytic agents have been employed for the treatment of acute arterial occlusion for more than 25 years. The agents that have received the most widespread clinical use are streptokinase and urokinase. Streptokinase is a bacterial protein purified from beta-hemolytic streptococci. It combines with plasminogen through an intermediary complex to form plasmin. Because it is a foreign protein, it induces an antibody response that must be overcome by relatively large dose levels. Urokinase, however, is a naturally occurring human enzyme, produced

TABLE 5. Morbidity and Mortality in 300 Patients, 330 Embolectomies

Limb salvage	95%
Patient survival	84%
Cause of death	
Myocardial infarction	20
Congestive heart failure	16
Pulmonary embolus	5
Massive cerebrovascular accident	4
Renal failure	2

TABLE 6. Associated Cardiac Procedures

Replacement of S-E ball valve	
Aortic	2
Mitral	3
Replacement of mitral valve	
Ruptured papillary muscle	4
Rheumatic	12
Resection of ventricular aneurysm	5
Repair of infarct, ventricular septal defect	1

by the kidney. It combines with plasminogen to form plasmin as well, but does so without intermediary steps. Urokinase requires smaller doses because it is not antigenic and also because it converts plasminogen to plasmin more efficiently than does streptokinase. When formed, plasmin degrades fibrin to effect fibrinolysis.

Although originally administered systemically, lytic agents are currently delivered directly to the occlusive site via an infusion catheter or needle to reduce the systemic exposure to the lytic agent. In recent years, urokinase has been favored over streptokinase because of its lower complication rate and improved efficacy.[21] The major disadvantage of urokinase when compared with streptokinase is cost.

The primary complication of lytic agents is hemorrhage, which can manifest in the form of bleeding at wound sites, hematomas of varying severity, stroke, and myocardial infarction. Other concerns regarding the use of lytic therapy are the uncertain duration of therapy (up to 72 hours of infusion[8]), the extremity's tolerance of prolonged ischemia during therapy, and the risk of additional embolization from a cardiac source. Concern over the systemic complications from streptokinase and urokinase has led to the development of lytic agents that convert plasminogen to plasmin specifically at the clot site and not elsewhere in the circulation. Two such fibrin-specific lytic agents are tissue plasminogen activator (tPA), a naturally occurring protein produced in significant amounts via recombinant DNA technology, and pro-urokinase, a naturally occurring precursor to urokinase produced in quantity from modified human renal cells. Both of these substances are currently under clinical investigation to determine their safety and efficacy for peripheral arterial occlusion.

Despite the considerable interest in thrombolytic agents during the last 2 decades, intra-arterial dissolution of thrombotic material has yet to have a major role in the treatment of acute arterial occlusion in the periphery. Time delay to reperfusion, cost, multiple angiograms, and the potential for hemorrhage have limited the application of these agents. Heparinization with surgical balloon embolectomy remains the most effective form of treatment for acute arterial occlusion.

Recognition and appropriate surgical management of the more difficult technical problems associated with acute arterial occlusion cause a decreased morbidity. The mortality associated with embolic episodes is due primarily to severe underlying disorder.

SELECTED REFERENCES

Blaisdell, F. W., Steele, M., and Allen, R. E.: Management of acute lower extremity arterial ischemia due to embolism and thrombosis. Surgery, 84:822, 1978.
Despite an impression to the contrary, a recent survey demonstrates that the current mortality for acute arterial ischemia approximates 25 per cent in the lower extremities. Much of this apparently concerns toxins and procoagulants released from the ischemic tissue. In this series, the authors recommend selective management for acute arterial ischemia in an attempt to minimize the mortality and maximize the number of viable limbs.

Boley, S. J., et al.: An aggressive roentgenologic and surgical approach to acute mesenteric ischemia. Surg. Ann., 5:355, 1973.
The article represents a view of the entire spectrum of mesenteric ischemia. A plan of diagnosis and therapy is outlined. The article emphasizes an aggressive diagnostic and therapeutic approach as the means of decreasing morbidity and mortality.

Fogarty, T. J., Daily, P. O., Shumway, N. E., and Krippaehne, W.: Experience with balloon catheter technic for arterial embolectomy. Am. J. Surg., 122:231, 1971.

The authors report a series of 330 embolic occlusions occurring in 300 patients. The paper emphasizes the necessity of identifying high-risk areas in terms of morbidity and mortality. An aggressive overall approach to the medical and surgical problems is presented.

Patman, R. D., and Thompson, J. E.: Fasciotomy in peripheral vascular surgery. Arch. Surg., 101:663, 1970.

The authors review their personal experience with 164 patients who required fasciotomy. The indications for fasciotomy and the technique employed are presented. Fasciotomy, performed correctly and with proper indications, is a valuable procedure that can increase limb salvage and decrease morbidity. The paper is well written, and a variety of clinical situations that may require fasciotomy are detailed.

Tawes, R. L., Jr., Harris, E. J., Brown, W. H., et al.: Arterial thromboembolism: A 20-year perspective. Arch. Surg., 120:595, 1985.

The authors review their experience in 739 patients with lower extremity thromboembolism. They detail the factors that have contributed to their overall 12 per cent mortality and 95 per cent limb salvage rate. They stress the importance of prompt diagnosis and treatment, postoperative heparinization, and the necessity of viewing thromboembolism within the context of the underlying cardiovascular disease process.

REFERENCES

1. Abbott, W. M., Maloney, R. D., McCabe, C. C., et al.: Arterial embolism: A 44 year perspective. Am. J. Surg., *143:* 460, 1982.
2. Arneklo-Nobin, B., Norgren, L., and Johansen, K.: The beneficial effects of intra-arterial reserpine after upper-extremity embolectomy: A prospective randomised trial. Eur. J. Vasc. Surg., 2:305, 1988.
3. Baird, R. J., and Lagos, T. Z.: Emboli to the arm. Ann. Surg., 160:905, 1964.
4. Blaisdell, F. W.: Discussion of Levy, J. R., and Butcher, H. R.: Arterial emboli: An analysis of 125 patients. Surgery, 68:973, 1970.
5. Chin, A. K., and Fogarty, T. J.: Computerized digital angioscopy. *In* White, G. H., and White, R. A. (Eds.): Angioscopy: Vascular and Coronary Applications. Chicago, Year Book Medical Publishers, 1989, pp. 203–209.
6. Connett, M. C., Murray, D. H., Jr., and Wenneker, W. W.: Peripheral arterial emboli. Am. J. Surg., *148:*14, 1984.
7. Daily, P. O., Griepp, R. B., and Shumway, N. E.: Percutaneous internal jugular vein cannulation. Arch. Surg., 101:534, 1970.
8. Dardik, H., Sussman, B. C., Kahn, M., et al.: Lysis of arterial clot by intravenous or intra-arterial administration of streptokinase. Surg. Gynecol. Obstet., 158:137, 1984.
9. Elliott, J. P., Jr., Hageman, J. H., Szilagyi, D. E., et al.: Arterial embolization: Problems of source, multiplicity, recurrence, and delayed treatment. Surgery, 88:833, 1980.
10. Fisher, R. D., Fogarty, T. J., and Morrow, A. G.: Clinical and biochemical observations of the effect of transient femoral artery occlusion in man. Surgery, 68:323, 1970.
11. Fogarty, T. J.: Complications of arterial embolectomy. *In* Beebe, H. G. (Ed.): Complications in Vascular Surgery. Philadelphia, J. B. Lippincott Company, 1973, pp. 95–102.
12. Fogarty, T. J.: Surgical management of acute vascular occlusion. *In* Cooper, P., and Nyhus, L. M. (Eds.): Surgery Annual. New York, Appleton-Century-Crofts, 1970, pp. 207–221.
13. Fogarty, T. J., Chin, A. K., Olcott, C., IV, et al.: Combined thrombectomy and dilation for the treatment of acute lower extremity arterial thrombosis. J. Vasc. Surg., 10:530, 1989.
14. Fogarty, T. J., Cranley, J. J., Krause, R. J., et al.: A method for extraction of arterial emboli and thrombi. Surg. Gynecol. Obstet., 116:241, 1963.
15. Fogarty, T. J., Daily, P. O., Shumway, N. E., and Krippaehne, W.: Experience with balloon catheter technic for arterial embolectomy. Am. J. Surg., 122:231, 1971.
16. Haimovici, H.: Myopathic-nephrotic-metabolic syndrome associated with massive acute arterial occlusions. J. Cardiovasc. Surg., 14:589, 1973.
17. Harvey, S.: Exercitatio anatomica de motu cordis et sanguinis in animalibus (an English translation by Chauncey D. Leake). Springfield, Ill., Charles C Thomas, 1931, p. 37.
18. Labey: cited by Mosney, M., and Dumont, N. J.: Embolie fémorale au cours d'um rétrécissement mitral pur. Artériotomie. Guérison Bull. Acad. Med., 66:358, 1911.
19. Levy, J. F., and Butcher, H. R.: Arterial emboli: An analysis of 125 patients. Surgery, 68:968, 1970.
20. Linton, R. R.: Peripheral arterial embolism. A discussion of the postembolic vascular changes and their relation to the restoration of circulation in peripheral embolism. N. Engl. J. Med., 224:189, 1941.
21. Motarjeme, A.: Thrombolytic therapy in arterial occlusion and graft thrombosis. Semin. Vasc. Surg., 2:155, 1989.
22. Murie, J. A., and Mathieson, M.: Arterial embolectomy in the leg: Results in a referral hospital. J. Cardiovasc. Surg., 28:184, 1987.
23. Patman, R. D., and Thompson, J. E.: Fasciotomy in peripheral vascular surgery. Arch. Surg., 101:663, 1970.
24. Panetta, T., Thompson, J. E., Talkington, C. M., Garrett, W. V., and Smith,

B. L.: Arterial embolectomy: A 34-year experience with 400 cases. Surg. Clin. North Am., 66:339, 1986.
25. Rosato, F. E., Barker, C. F., Robert, B., and Danielson, G. K.: Subcutaneous fasciotomy. Description of a new technique and instrument. Surgery, 59:3, 1966.
26. Tawes, R. L., Jr., Harris, E. J., Brown, W. H., et al.: Arterial thromboembolism: A 20-year perspective. Arch. Surg. 120:595, 1985.
27. Thompson, J. E., Sigler, L., Raut, P. S., et al.: Arterial embolectomy: A 20-year experience with 163 cases. Surgery, 67:212, 1970.

10. ARTERIOVENOUS FISTULAS

H. Kim Lyerly, M.D., and David C. Sabiston, Jr., M.D.

Arteriovenous fistulas form a fascinating group of congenital and acquired lesions of variable etiology, anatomic distribution, and clinical presentation.[15] They are also associated with numerous pathophysiologic changes both at the local site and systemically. Collectively they represent some of the most challenging diagnostic and therapeutic problems in medicine.

In 1758, William Hunter first recognized that an arteriovenous aneurysm was characterized not only by the aneurysm but also by a direct communication between the involved artery and the accompanying vein.[19] Before this observation, such lesions were interpreted as simple aneurysms, whereas Hunter designated these as *aneurysms by anastomosis* and placed emphasis on the communication between the two vascular systems.

An arteriovenous fistula can be defined as a connection, other than the capillary bed, between the arterial and venous systems. This definition encompasses a vast array of conditions including some occurring in the normal development of the circulation, congenital malformations, acquired lesions, and iatrogenic shunts.[49] A classification based on the etiology of the fistula is helpful and is shown in Table 1.

CLASSIFICATION OF ARTERIOVENOUS COMMUNICATIONS

The two major types of arteriovenous fistulas are *congenital* and *acquired.* Among congenital communications, the terms cirsoid aneurysms and cavernous angiomas have also been used. Congenital lesions may have single or multiple communications and are respectively denoted as arteriovenous fistulas or arteriovenous malformations.

Lesions with a single communication usually represent normal fetal communications that fail to resolve or represent developmental abnormalities. Lesions with multiple communications usually represent persistent communications that normally

TABLE 1. Classification of Abnormal Arteriovenous Communication

Congenital	Acquired
Single fistula	Single fistula
Multiple fistula—	Surgical
arteriovenous malformation	Pathologic
Hemangiomas	Aneurysm
	Iatrogenic
	Infection
	Neoplasia
	Spontaneous
	Traumatic
	Tumor-associated communications
	Vascular tumors
	Tumors associated with shunting

exist during the early phase of the development of the arterial and venous systems. Both arteries and veins differentiate from a common capillary plexus during embryologic development. Thus, if failure occurs in differentiation of the common embryologic analog into arteries and veins, a multitude of communications may result between them. *Hemangiomas* are multiple abnormal venous malformations that do not have high-pressure arterial communications. *Acquired* lesions usually have a single communication and are termed arteriovenous fistulas; frequently they consist of a distinct communication between an artery and a vein bypassing the capillary bed. The causes of acquired arteriovenous fistula are shown in Table 1. Other acquired arteriovenous communications include vascular tumors such as angiosarcoma, glomus tumor or hemangiopericytoma, and tumors associated with shunting such as hepatoma or hypernephroma. In this section, arteriovenous fistulas and arteriovenous malformations are primarily presented.

PATHOPHYSIOLOGY

Abnormal arteriovenous communications produce pathophysiologic changes locally, but often, especially in larger fistulas, the most significant and pronounced changes involve the body as a whole. The pathophysiologic changes are most impressive in fistulas in which enormous amounts of arterial blood pass directly into the venous circulation. A number of important systemic physiologic changes occur in an attempt to compensate for a major circulatory abnormality.[43]

The local features characteristic of a direct communication between the arterial and venous systems are demonstrated by the presence of a *thrill* at the site of the lesion, especially if it is located near the surface. On auscultation, a *bruit* that continues through most if not all of the cardiac cycle is audible. An aneurysm or arterial and venous dilation is often seen or palpated. Large draining veins are also present, visible if they are subcutaneous, or apparent on angiography in the more deeply located fistulas. Angiography demonstrates dilated arteries, rapid filling of veins, and tortuous arterial collaterals. Dilated arteries and veins may also be demonstrated by ultrasonic determination, and the addition of Doppler color-flow imaging allows detection of small fistulas not only by direct detection of the anatomic defect but also by the turbulent flow in the vein from the jet of blood from the arterial side of the fistula (Fig. 1).[41]

The magnitude of systemic symptoms is generally related to the size of the fistula and its proximity to the heart. These changes are maximal in fistulas involving a large artery that conducts massive amounts of blood flow. Under these circumstances, much blood is shunted through the fistula because the venous side offers very little peripheral resistance. With large volumes of flow of blood being shunted directly into the venous circulation, a sequence of events follows that is directly related to the volume of blood flowing through the fistula (Figs. 2 and 3). The cardiac output increases, the heart rate rises, and the diastolic arterial pressure diminishes, usually with an increase in systolic pressure. The cardiac and pulmonary pressures also change with increases in ventricular end-diastolic pressure, right and left atrial pressures, and pulmonary wedge pressure (Table 2). The blood and plasma volume increases to compensate for the increased volume of blood in the venous circulation. Moreover, with the high cardiac output, the heart increases in size, particularly the atrial and ventricular cavities, and ultimately cardiac hypertrophy results. A large fistula may ultimately cause congestive heart failure, and if the fistula is acute with a large volume of blood through it, the heart may not be able to compensate adequately, which would cause pulmonary edema and death. It is interesting that experimental and clinical studies have indicated that digitalis preparations are largely ineffective in the management of high-output cardiac failure.[40] All of these features can be dramatically illustrated experimen-

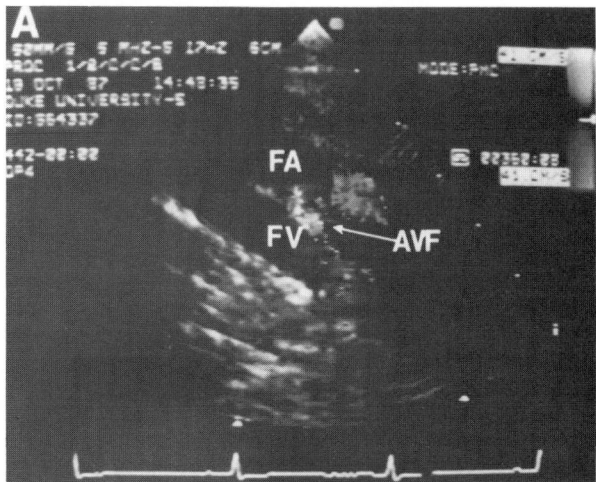

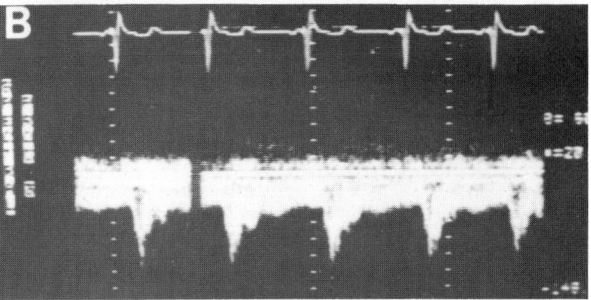

Figure 1. Color-flow imaging (*A*, reproduced in black and white) and pulsed wave Doppler recording (*B*) of a patient with a right femoral arteriovenous fistula. Color-flow examination shows flow going from the femoral artery to the femoral vein. Doppler recording shows high-velocity systolic flow away from the transducer and lower velocity diastolic flow also going away from the transducer. AVF, arteriovenous fistula; FA, femoral artery; FV, femoral vein. (From Sheikh, K. H., Adams, D. B., McCann, R., Lyerly, H. K., Sabiston, D. C., Jr., and Kisslo, J.: Utility of Doppler color flow imaging for identification of femoral arterial complications of cardiac catheterization. Am. Heart J., *117*:623, 1989.)

tally after creation of large fistulas and determination of physiologic measurements.[38]

In the presence of a high cardiac output due to the fistula, the oxygen saturation in the mixed venous blood of the right heart is greatly increased because much of the blood bypasses the capil-

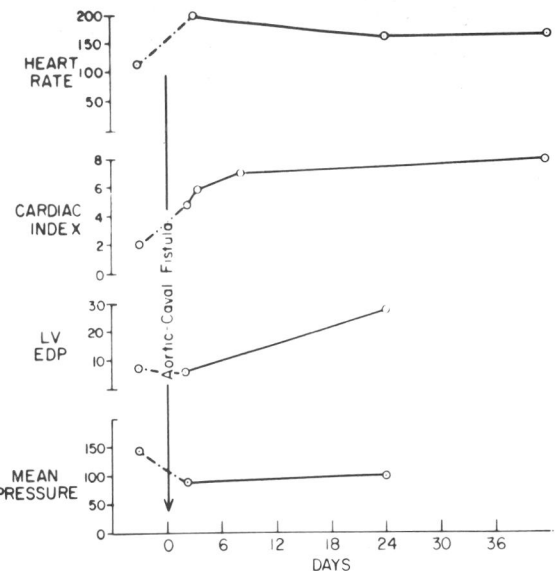

Figure 2. Changes in heart rate, cardiac index, left ventricular end-diastolic pressure, and mean arterial pressure in an experimental animal with a large aorto-caval fistula.

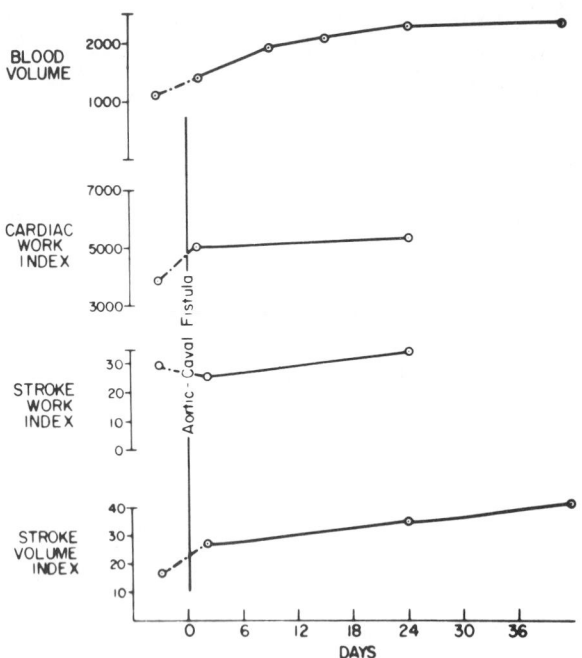

Figure 3. Changes in blood volume, cardiac work index, stroke work index, and stroke volume index in an experimental animal with a large aortocaval fistula.

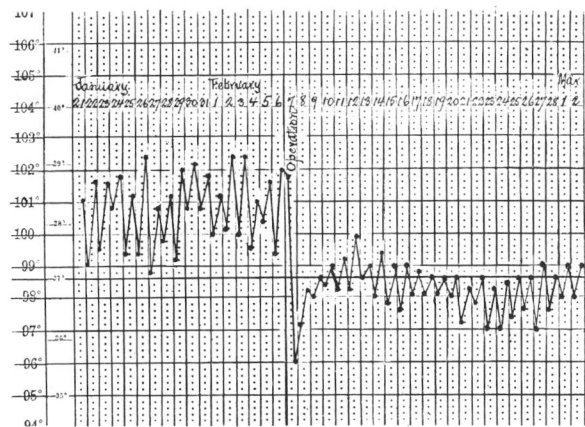

Figure 4. Condensed temperature chart, showing the maximal and minimal temperature each day before and after operation. The temperature, varying from 99° to 102.4° F., fell to subnormal on the day of operation and after a slight postoperative rise settled permanently at the normal level. (From Rienhoff, W. F., Jr., and Hamman, L.: Ann. Surg., 102:905, 1935.)

lary bed. The central venous pressure is usually increased. Of considerable importance is the anatomic site of the fistula and the systemic circulation because the diameter of the involved vessel is of crucial importance. For example, much more blood flows through a fistula of a specific size from an artery with a large diameter than from one with a smaller diameter. It has been shown experimentally that small aortic fistulas can produce severe symptoms when they are centrally located near the heart, for example, between the ascending aorta and the pulmonary artery, or the superior vena cava contrasted with similar, more distal shunts such as between the abdominal aorta and the vena cava or the iliac or femoral vessels.[39] Structural changes in the vascular wall are also created by hemodynamic disturbances associated with arteriovenous fistulas. In large fistulas, the venous wall becomes thin, closely simulating the sac of a false aneurysm. The walls of small fistulas may become thickened and assume the appearance of an artery. Thrombi are also apt to form in the dilated parts of these fistulas and may harbor bacterial organisms. Arteriovenous fistulas may be associated

with the development of bacterial endocarditis. In fact, the first patient ever cured of a chronic bloodstream infection (*Streptococcus viridans*) before the introduction of antibiotics was managed by surgical closure of an iliac arteriovenous fistula. After closure, the bloodstream infection disappeared, and the patient remained cured (Figs. 4 and 5).[36] Until that time, all such illnesses had ended fatally.

An aneurysmal dilation is usually present at the site of the fistula involving both the artery and vein caused by the turbu-

TABLE 2. Manifestations of Arteriovenous Fistula

Systemic

Pulse rate	↑	Diastolic arterial pressure	↓
Cardiac output	↑	Peripheral resistance	↓
Blood volume	↑		
Cardiac size	↑		

Local
Thrill
Continuous murmur
Increased arterial collaterals
Aneurysmal formation
Diminished pulse rate with occlusion

Physiologic changes occurring in the circulation with an arteriovenous fistula are most marked in the presence of a large fistula. These changes may be minimal to absent with a small fistula. Late manifestations of a large fistula include congestive heart failure, pulmonary edema, and death in untreated patients.

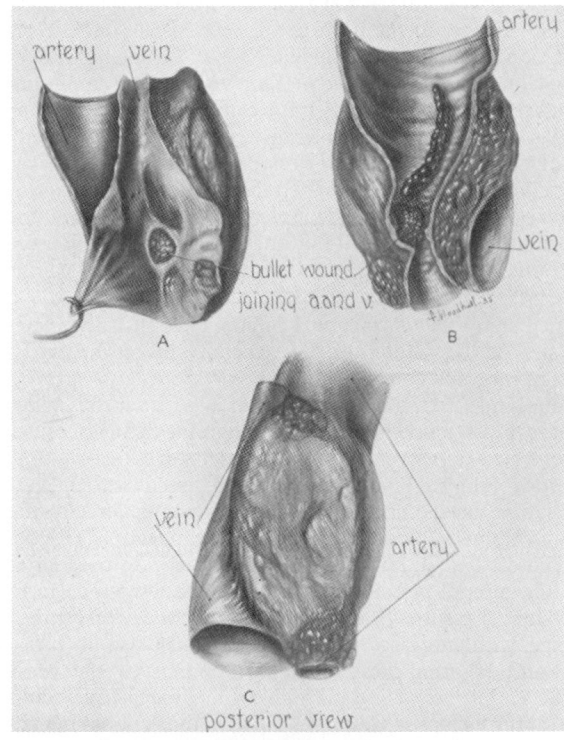

Figure 5. Drawings of specimen. *A*, Venous side of arterial venous aneurysm showing vegetation in the opening between the external iliac vein and aneurysm sac. The upper or proximal portion of the vein has been cut across on the bias, giving the false impression that the lumen of the vein is narrowed in this drawing. *B*, Arterial side of specimen revealing the openings into aneurysmal cavity filled with vegetations and the protruding thrombus, which points cephalad. The dilated proximal portion of the artery is shown in the upper portion of the illustration. The external iliac artery of normal size is shown below. Along the right margin of the artery is the dark calcified wall of the aneurysm. The external iliac vein is on the opposite side lying directly behind the artery. *C*, Posterior view of the encysted varicose aneurysm. (From Rienhoff, W. F., Jr., and Hamman, L.: Ann. Surg., 102:905, 1935.)

lence that occurs in the presence of the high to low pressure interface within the fistula. In response to the low distal arterial pressure beyond the site of the fistula, an extensive collateral circulation develops connecting the arteries above the fistula with those below. These collaterals become greatly dilated and tortuous and deliver considerable blood distally as a result of a large pressure gradient (Fig. 6). This collateral circulation can become massive and often causes an increase in temperature in both skin and muscle. When the fistulas occur in an extremity, the limb may increase in length, a fact that has been confirmed by both experimental and clinical observations.[20,21] An explanation for this increased bone growth is probably the result of the 1 or 2° C. elevation of the local temperature and resultant increase in metabolism. Typical changes in the arterial and venous pressures beyond the fistula are shown in Figure 7.[40]

Other diagnostic measures employed in evaluating arteriovenous fistulas include measurement of venous oxygen tension in the limb with the suspected fistula. Oxygenated arterial blood passing through the fistula then flows into the venous side with a high oxygen saturation unlike normal venous blood.

Cardiac output may be increased in patients with arteriovenous fistulas, and compression of the fistula, which diminishes the flow through the fistula, is followed by a diminished heart rate (Branham's or Nicoladoni's sign) and a lower cardiac output.

In 1875, Nicoladoni described a patient with an arteriovenous fistula in whom compression of the fistula (with cessation of flow through it) caused a decrease in the pulse rate from 96 to 64 per minute.[30] Matas termed this the "Branham bradycardic reaction," and it has since borne that name (Fig. 8).[4,18]

Angiography is the standard diagnostic study in the evaluation of an arteriovenous fistula. In acquired fistulas, a single communication often occurs at the site of the fistula and can be localized either by direct visualization of the communication or by the initial venous opacification at the site of the fistula (Fig. 9). Congenital lesions with multiple communications often have a radiologic appearance that is much more complicated. Indirect signs of an abnormal arteriovenous communication, including increased flow in the afferent arteries, decreased flow in the peripheral arteries, and rapid venous filling, are usually present. However, the multiple communications may not be

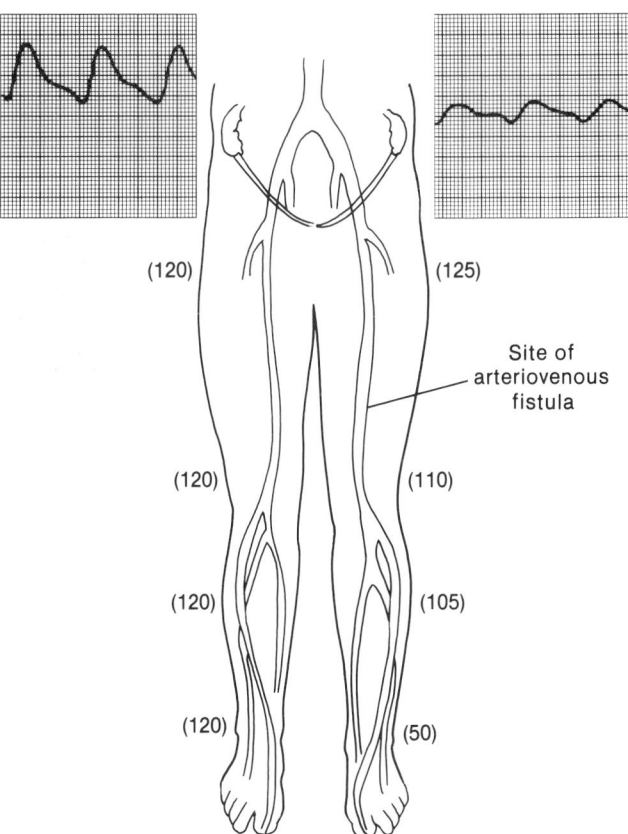

Figure 7. Plethysmographic record of a 35-year-old man with a traumatic superficial femoral arteriovenous fistula. Digit pulse contours are abnormal on the left, and there is a significant depression of the ankle pressure (50 mm. Hg) distal to the fistula. (Redrawn from Strandness, D. E., Jr. (Ed.): Collateral Circulation in Clinical Surgery. Philadelphia, W. B. Saunders Company, 1969.)

visible because they are often of microscopic size, and overlying opacified arteries and veins add to the complexity of the radiographic pattern. Selective angiography of the afferent artery or arteries may be helpful in delineating the extent of the fistula. Sometimes localized dilated contrast-filled spaces indicate the site of the fistula with some precision. On other occasions, small fistulas are revealed as faint, diffuse opacifications between major arterial and venous channels. Other indications may include abnormal vessels arising from the parent artery, horizontal branches connecting parallel veins, and venous retia. Be-

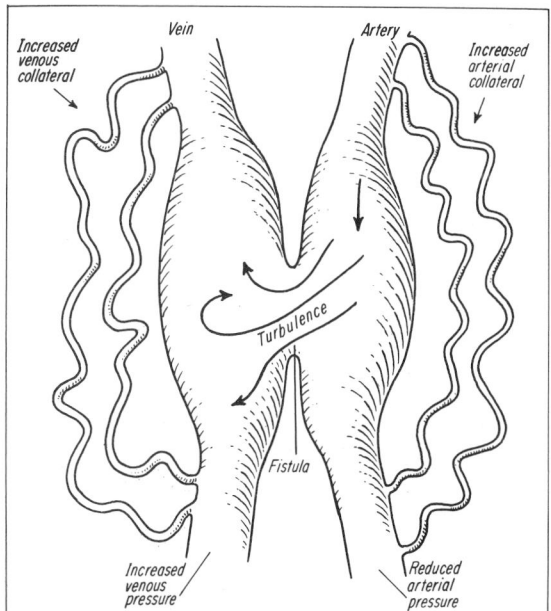

Figure 6. Diagrammatic illustration of the local changes that occur in the presence of an arteriovenous fistula. The changes shown are proportional to the *size* of the fistula. In a small fistula, these changes may be quite minimal.

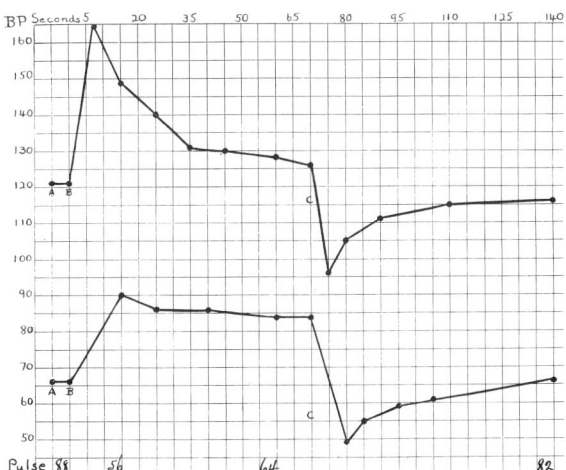

Figure 8. Demonstration of the Nicoladoni-Branham sign. Fluctuations in systemic blood pressure (left arm). *A*, Fistula open. *B*, Fistula closed by digital compression. *C*, Fistula reopened. (From Holman, E.: Abnormal Arteriovenous Communications. Springfield, Ill., Charles C Thomas, 1968.)

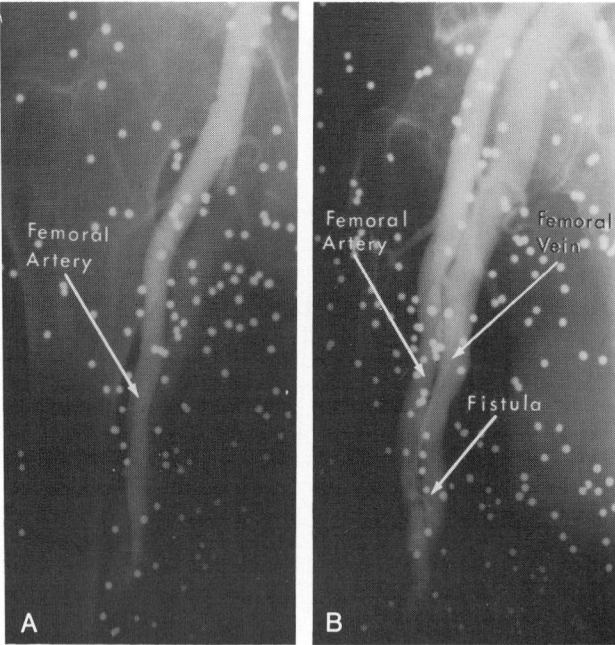

Figure 9. *A*, Femoral arteriogram in a patient with a gunshot wound of the thigh and a femoral arteriovenous fistula. *B*, The site of the fistula is seen with rapid filling of the proximal femoral vein without filling distally.

TABLE 3. Ten-Year Experience in Incidence of Congenital and Acquired Arteriovenous Fistulas

	Congenital	Acquired
AV fistulas of the extremities	80	17
Aorta–inferior vena cava fistulas	0	7
Pulmonary AV fistulas	47	0
Renal AV fistulas	0	6
AV fistulas of the portal system	0	1
AV fistulas of the neck and face	11	4
Pelvic AV fistulas	1	5
AV fistulas of the chest wall	0	2
Total	139	42

Adapted from Gomes, M. M. R., and Bernatz, P. E.: Arteriovenous fistulas: A review and ten-year experience at the Mayo Clinic. Mayo Clin. Proc., 45:81, 1970.

cause radiopaque media tend to fill the most proximal fistulas and those with the greatest volume of flow, smaller and more distally located communications may escape detection. This is particularly unfortunate in congenital arteriovenous malformations because of a tendency in the lesions for multiple communications.

Ultrasonic imaging has also been used to identify arteriovenous fistulas.[10,46] Although ultrasound may not be expected to reveal the actual fistula, the detection of aneurysms may call attention to a previously unsuspected fistula as well as determining the diameter and morphologic features of the proximal vessels.[41] Color-flow imaging may also reveal patterns suggestive of increased turbulence at sites of increased flow.

Computed tomography (CT) and magnetic resonance imaging (MRI) may be used to demonstrate the location and extent of arteriovenous communications, including the involvement of specific muscle groups and bone.[7] Deep intramuscular lesions have a mottled appearance, and administration of contrast during CT scanning causes an enhancement that depends on the rate of arteriovenous shunting and the degree of cellularity of the lesion. Offsetting the desirable features of the CT scan are the need for intravenous contrast and the lack of an optimal protocol for its administration. MRI has distinctive advantages over CT in evaluating congenital vascular malformations since there is no need for contrast and the anatomic extent is more clearly demonstrated.[32] Longitudinal as well as transverse sections may also be obtained in the flow patterns, and the arteriovenous malformation may be characterized. MRI can identify high-flow vascular spaces and their feeding arteries and draining veins.[27] By use of other MRI techniques, such as even echo rephasing, vessels with slow flow can be identified. In addition, MRI can identify hemorrhage into soft tissue because of the difference in signal intensity between blood and stromal tissue.

TYPES OF ARTERIOVENOUS COMMUNICATIONS

Congenital arteriovenous communications of the extremities are quite common, especially in the legs, and varicose veins often result (Table 3).[15,48] Hemangiomas may involve a consid-

erable part of the extremity and introduce serious cosmetic and physiologic problems. Congenital arteriovenous communications have been reported in all organs of the body and are frequently difficult to manage because multiple communications exist between arteries and veins. Treatment by local interruption or arterial repair is rarely feasible. Often the dilated arteries and veins encompass muscle and bone with extensive involvement of subcutaneous tissues and skin that makes *en bloc* resection impossible. Although surgical therapy has a role in specific types of arteriovenous communications, especially in localized lesions in which complete excision can be accomplished, some are too extensive for appropriate and complete surgical excision. For these, palliative surgical procedures are used to control disabling ulceration and infection or life-threatening hemorrhage. Ligation of major feeding arteries is not recommended because distal ischemia may result and the intravascular access required to allow embolization becomes limited. Alternative techniques of closure include selective intra-arterial embolization of autologous clot, wire coils, plastic balloons, or transcatheter coagulation.[14,23,25,34,35] Staged treatment with intervals between embolization allows portions of major malformations to be obliterated and repeated treatments performed in persistent areas. Each of these techniques has been reported with success in closing some of these fistulas that would be difficult, if not impossible, to manage surgically. Often this combination of embolization followed by surgical excision is effective in managing these difficult malformations. Other types of therapy include injection of sclerosing solutions or irradiation.

Some congenital fistulas are difficult to understand embryologically, such as those between the internal mammary artery and the pulmonary vessels.[37] Although such shunts may be small, closure of these lesions is nevertheless recommended owing to potential complications. Congenital pulmonary arteriovenous fistulas are common and are frequently multiple.[29] These are usually seen as well-circumscribed lesions on the chest film; if large, they may be accompanied by cyanosis due to the right-to-left shunting. The symptoms include exertional dyspnea, easy fatigability, cyanosis, and clubbing of the fingers. Approximately 10 to 15 per cent occur in children. Complications of these lesions include cerebrovascular accidents, brain abscesses, hemoptysis, and intrapleural rupture.[50] A continuous bruit with systolic accentuation during deep inspiration is heard in approximately two thirds of patients. Pulmonary arteriography confirms the diagnosis. Hereditary telangiectasis (Rendu-Osler-Weber disease) is quite common and may be familial in origin. These patients also have a tendency to develop additional fistulas with the passage of time. Management of pulmonary arteriovenous fistulas is primarily surgical, and because only the lesion requires removal, most can be managed by either

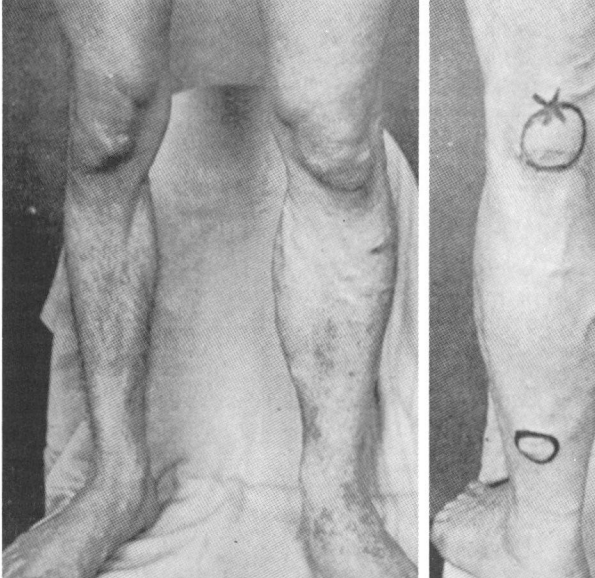

Figure 10. Appearance of patient with a left popliteal arteriovenous fistula of 25 years' duration located at X. Pulsating veins are circled. The palpated diameters of both femoral arteries are shown. (From Holman, E.: Abnormal Arteriovenous Communications. Springfield, Ill., Charles C Thomas, 1968.)

local or wedge resection. In the presence of bilateral fistulas, the site of major involvement is usually treated and the remaining one approached only if necessary. Some patients have also been managed by selective arterial embolization.[47] Penetrating pulmonary injuries can also produce this type of arteriovenous fistula, which should be surgically corrected.[44]

Venous malformations commonly referred to as hemangiomas represent a specific type of lesion composed of large venous spaces under low pressure with no clinical or angiographic evidence of significant arteriovenous shunting. They may occur anywhere in the body. When close to the skin surface, they may have a distinct bluish coloration, and the overlying skin may be thin, even to the extent that ulceration and spontaneous bleeding occur. Venous lesions are often asymptomatic but may be disfiguring in a large exposed area. Localized symptomatic lesions may be treated by excision, although, as previously mentioned, they may be more extensive than is evident clinically. Considerable cosmetic deformity may follow excision. Embolization of arterial branches supplying the lesion has been attempted with disappointing results, as might be anticipated on the basis of the fact that the lesion does not contain significant arteriovenous communications. Direct puncture followed by sclerosis with absolute alcohol has been much more effective, with marked shrinkage of the lesion in many patients. Currently, the tunable dye laser has produced dramatic results in some of these patients.

Acquired fistulas are most frequently found in the extremities and are often secondary to penetrating trauma with accompanying varices, edema, and pigmentation. Unlike congenital communications, a single or limited number of abnormal communications exist that can be demonstrated by angiography or color-flow Doppler. Vascular insufficiency of digits and ulceration may also be present in the more severe forms. A palpable thrill and an audible coarse machinery-like bruit are usually present at the site of the fistula. The affected extremity is generally warmer than is the control, and compression of the fistula usually causes a diminished heart rate and an increase in diastolic arterial pressure. A patient with a popliteal aneurysm and arteriovenous fistula is shown in Figure 10.

Iatrogenic fistulas can follow a number of surgical procedures, including operations on the kidney and intervertebral discs. Disc procedures may be associated with fistulas in the iliac vessels or with aortocaval fistulas.[22] Iatrogenic fistulas following thyroid procedures, coronary artery bypass grafting, distal splenorenal shunt, small bowel resection, Fontan's operation, and pelvic surgery have each been described.[11,12,16,28,33,51] Cardiac catheterization and percutaneous transhepatic variceal embolization for bleeding varices have been complicated by arteriovenous fistulas.[3,17] Renal arteriovenous fistulas after nephrectomy are usually large communications, and cardiac failure is not uncommon.[26] Increasing numbers of fistulas are observed after percutaneous biopsy or cardiac catheterization. Fistulas may also be present after *in situ* femoropopliteal bypass grafting if venous tributaries of the saphenous vein are not ligated.

Atherosclerosis of the wall of an aneurysm can also erode into accompanying veins, the prominent example being that of an aortocaval fistula from an abdominal aortic aneurysm (Fig. 11).[1] Such a lesion may place a patient precipitously in congestive

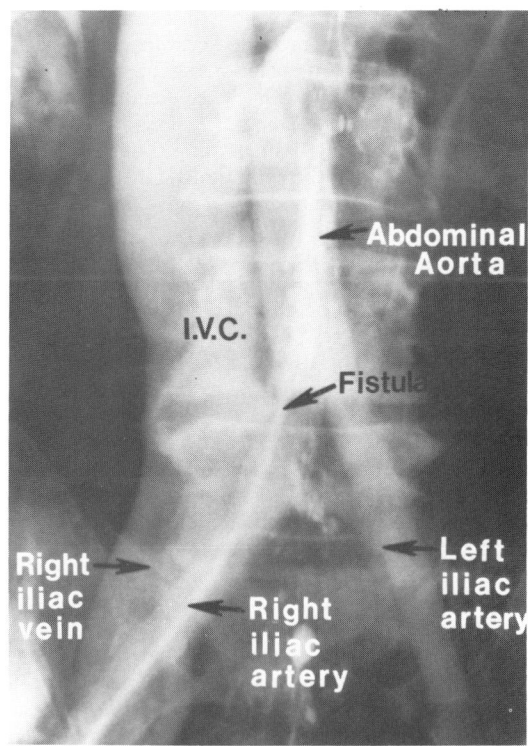

Figure 11. Arteriovenous fistula between the abdominal aorta and the right common iliac vein due to erosion by atherosclerosis.

heart failure and require an emergent surgical procedure. In a series of six patients from the University of Iowa, symptoms of an abdominal bruit, widened pulse pressure, venous hypertension, edema, arterial insufficiency, and congestive heart failure were present in three.[13] Proximal and distal control of the aorta allows the artery to be opened and the fistula controlled by a finger placed on the communication. Compression with sponge sticks proximal and distal to the fistula allows repair of the vein. After the vein is repaired, the preferred method for restoring arterial continuity is with a graft. Aortocaval fistulas of neoplastic origin have also been reported.[8]

In current practice, the most common acquired arteriovenous fistula is that associated with vascular access to permit renal dialysis in the management of renal insufficiency. Problems associated with this type of fistula are discussed in Chapter 18. Arteriovenous fistulas have also been surgically constructed to increase blood flow and patency to a vascular anastomosis, such as venous reconstruction procedures.[9,24]

MANAGEMENT OF ARTERIOVENOUS COMMUNICATIONS

Since most arteriovenous fistulas are potentially symptomatic, closure of the communication is generally recommended. Early surgical attempts to correct these lesions consisted primarily of ligation of the involved artery proximal to the fistula.[6] Whereas the threat of rupture of a classic arterial aneurysm might be diminished by ligating the artery proximally, this approach in the presence of an arteriovenous fistula is apt to end disastrously because it is quite likely to be followed by gangrene of the extremity. Gangrene can result because blood reaching the distal extremity by arterial collaterals is apt to drain retrograde through the fistula directly into the venous system, thus depriving the limb of adequate distal arterial blood flow. The first successful treatment of an arteriovenous fistula was proximal and distal ligation of both the artery and the vein.[31] This quadripolar ligation corrected the fistula and was not followed by peripheral vascular insufficiency of the limb, owing to the large number of arterial collaterals that had been formed as a result of the fistula.

Currently, management includes accurate diagnosis and determination of the extent of the lesions. Acute fistulas with high flow causing cardiovascular collapse or distal ischemia require urgent repair, whereas long-standing lesions with extensive involvement of surrounding tissue require thoughtful preoperative planning. The site of the communication should always be carefully localized by arteriography; however, CT scanning, MRI, and color-flow Doppler imaging are becoming increasingly utilized to diagnose arteriovenous communications. The ideal surgical management usually includes direct closure of the fistula with restoration of arterial and venous continuity.[2,5] However, when this is not possible, quadripolar ligation is acceptable when sufficient arterial collateral circulation to adequately supply the tissues distally exists. Although gangrene usually does not occur, intermittent claudication frequently results despite collateral circulation. However, in the majority of patients, it is possible to close the fistula without need for amputation. Complete excision is reserved for fistulas involving small nonessential arteries, such as the radial or ulnar arteries when adequate collaterals are present.

Rarely, small fistulas have been known to close spontaneously.[42] In congenital forms, excision of diffuse malformations may not be possible, as stated previously. The complex communications seen with congenital arteriovenous malformations often require a multidisciplinary approach including selective intra-arterial embolization in conjunction with surgical therapy. Asymptomatic lesions may not require treatment[45]; nevertheless, a fistula represents a hazard. Absolute indications for treatment include hemorrhage, secondary ischemic complications, and congestive heart failure from arteriovenous shunting; relative indications include pain, nonhealing ulcers, functional impairment, and cosmetic deformity. If treatment is required, careful planning is mandatory. Patients with symptomatic lesions thought to be resectable should undergo surgical excision, since complete removal provides the best likelihood for cure. This is more suitable for superficial lesions on the trunk, scalp, face, and extremities, and the goal of surgical therapy should be complete excision of the lesion. Ligation of feeding vessels is only temporarily effective, and the rapid recruitment of collateral channels makes further treatment, especially embolization, difficult or impossible. Resection of large lesions may be associated with significant blood loss, and preoperative embolization may facilitate surgical resection and reduce operative blood loss.

Transcatheter embolization has a significant role in the treatment of many malformations. Numerous embolic materials have been developed, from simple Gelfoam pledgets to complex systems employing microcatheters and detachable balloons. Embolization procedures must be carefully planned, and a detailed, selective angiographic examination must be made initially for determining which vessels supply the lesion, likely sources of collateral resupply, and routes of venous drainage. Embolization is then performed as a separate procedure, usually under general anesthesia. Secondary feeder arteries are embolized first for conversion of the lesion into one supplied by a single vessel. The primary feeding vessel is then selectively catheterized and embolized with the goal of penetration and obliteration of the lesion. Complex lesions may require multiple-stage embolization procedures because of limitation in anesthetic time as well as the volume of contrast material that can be safely administered. Complications of embolization include tissue necrosis, inadvertent embolization of normal tissues, and passage of embolic materials through arteriovenous communications causing pulmonary embolization. Recurrences after proximal ligation or embolization are extremely difficult to treat owing to the recruitment of multiple new sources of blood supply to the lesion.

SELECTED REFERENCES

Gomes, M. M. R., and Bernatz, P. E.: Arteriovenous fistulas: A review and ten-year experience at the Mayo Clinic. Mayo Clin. Proc., 45:81, 1970.
A large series of patients with congenital and acquired arteriovenous fistulas is presented over a 10-year period at the Mayo Clinic. It is a valuable reference and provides data on the large number of specific types of the lesions.

Holman, E.: Abnormal Arteriovenous Communications. Springfield, Ill., Charles C Thomas, 1968.
This is a classic and is an often cited authoritative reference on the subject of arteriovenous fistulas. All aspects of these lesions are considered from both the physiological and clinical viewpoints. It deservedly won the author the prestigious Samuel D. Gross Prize.

Tan, O. T., Sherwood, K., and Gilchrest, B. A.: Treatment of children with port-wine stains using the flashlamp-pulsed tunable dye laser. N. Engl. J. Med., 320:416, 1989.
Thirty-five children, 3 months to 14 years of age, with disfiguring port-wine stains were treated with a flashlamp-pulsed tunable dye laser. All had complete clearing of the stains after an average of 6.5 laser treatments to each lesional area.

REFERENCES

1. Baker, W. H., Sharzer, L. A., and Ehrenhaft, J. L.: Aortocaval fistula as a complication of abdominal aortic aneurysms. Surgery, 72:933, 1972.
2. Beall, A. C., Jr., Diethrich, E. B., Morris, G. C., Jr., and DeBakey, M. E.: Surgical management of vascular trauma. Surg. Clin. North Am., 46:1001, 1966.
3. Bedell, J. E., Keller, F. S., and Rosch, J.: Iatrogenic intrahepatic arterial-portal fistula. Radiology, 151:79, 1984.
4. Bramman, F.: Das arteriell-venous Aneurysma. Arch. Klin. Chir., 33:1, 1886.
5. Branham, H. H.: Aneurismal varix of the femoral artery and vein following a gunshot wound. Int. J. Surg., 3:250, 1890.
6. Breschet, G.: Memoire sur les aneurysmes. Mem. Acad. R. Med. (Paris), 3:101, 1883.
7. Cohen, J. M., Weinreb, J. C., and Redman, H. C.: Arteriovenous malformations of the extremities: MR imaging. Radiology, 158:475, 1986.

8. Crawford, E. S., Turell, D. J., and Alexander, J. K.: Aorto-inferior vena caval fistula of neoplastic origin. Circulation, 27:414, 1963.
9. Dardik, H., Sussman, B., Ibrahim, I. M., Kahn, M., Svoboda, J. J., Mendes, D., and Dardik, I.: Distal arteriovenous fistula as an adjunct to maintaining arterial and graft patency for limb salvage. Surgery, 94:478, 1983.
10. Daxini, B. V., Desai, A. G., and Sharma, S.: Echo-Doppler diagnosis of aortocaval fistula following blunt trauma to abdomen. Am. Heart J., 118:843, 1989.
11. Decker, D. G., Fish, C. R., and Juergens, J. L.: Arteriovenous fistulas of the female pelvis. A diagnostic problem. Obstet. Gynecol., 31:799, 1968.
12. Diehl, J. T., and Beven, E. G.: Arteriovenous fistulas of the mesenteric vessels. Report of a case and review of the literature. J. Cardiovasc. Surg., 23:334, 1982.
13. Doty, D. B., Wright, C. B., Lamberth, W. C., et al.: Aortocaval fistula associated with aneurysm of the abdominal aorta: Current management using autotransfusion techniques. Surgery, 84:250, 1978.
14. Gomes, A. S., Mali, W. P., and Oppenheim, W. L.: Embolization therapy in the management of congenital arteriovenous malformations. Radiology, 144:41, 1982.
15. Gomes, M. M. R., and Bernatz, P. E.: Arteriovenous fistulas: A review and ten-year experience at the Mayo Clinic. Mayo Clin. Proc., 45:81, 1970.
16. Gonzalez, E. M., Garcia, I. G., Blanch, G. G., Garcia, I. L., and Gonzalez, J. S.: Left gastric arteriovenous fistula after selective distal splenorenal shunt. Surgery, 93:510, 1983.
17. Hansbrough, J. F., Narrod, J. A., and Rutherford, R.: Arteriovenous fistulas following central venous catheterization. Intensive Care Med., 9:287, 1983.
18. Holman, E.: Abnormal Arteriovenous Communications. Springfield, Ill., Charles C Thomas, 1968.
19. Hunter, W.: The history of an aneurysm of the aorta, with some remarks on aneurysms in general. Med. Observ. Inquir., 1:323, 1757.
20. Janes, J. M., and Jennings, W. K., Jr.: Effect of induced arteriovenous fistula on leg length: 10-year observations. Mayo Clin. Proc., 36:1, 1961.
21. Janes, J. M., and Musgrove, J. E.: Effect of arteriovenous fistula on growth of bone: An experimental study. Surg. Clin. North Am., 30:1191, 1950.
22. Jarstfer, B. E., and Rich, N. M.: The challenge of arteriovenous fistula formation following disk surgery: A collective review. J. Trauma, 16:726, 1976.
23. Kerber, C. W., Freeny, P. C., Cromwell, L., et al.: Cyanoacrylate occlusion of a renal arteriovenous fistula. Am. J. Roentgenol., 128:663, 1977.
24. Levin, P. M., Rich, N. M., Hutton, J. E., Barker, W. F., and Zeller, J. A.: A role of arteriovenous shunts in venous reconstruction. Am. J. Surg., 122:183, 1971.
25. McAlister, D. S., Johnsrude, I., Miller, M. M., Clapp, J., and Thompson, W. M.: Occlusion of acquired renal arteriovenous fistula with transcatheter electrocoagulation. Am. J. Roentgenol., 132:998, 1979.
26. McCutcheon, F. B., and Hara, M.: Arteriovenous fistula following nephrectomy. J. Cardiovasc. Surg., 8:253, 1967.
27. Mills, C. M., Brant-Zawadzki, M., and Crooks, L. E.: Nuclear magnetic resonance: Principles of blood flow imaging. A.J.R., 142:165, 1984.
28. Moore, J. W., Kirby, W. C., Madden, W. A., and Gaither, N. S.: Development of pulmonary arteriovenous malformations after modified Fontan operations. J. Thorac. Cardiovasc. Surg., 98:1045, 1989.
29. Moyer, J. H., Glantz, G., and Brest, A. N.: Pulmonary arteriovenous fistulas. Physiologic and clinical considerations. Am. J. Med., 32:417, 1962.
30. Nicoladoni, C.: Phlebarteriectasie der rechten oberen Extremitat. Arch. Klin. Chir., 18:252, 1975.
31. Norris, G. W.: Varicose aneurism at the bend of the arm: Ligature of the artery above and below the sac; secondary hemorrhages with a return of the aneurismal thrill on the tenth day; cure. Am. J. Med. Sci., 5:27, 1843.
32. Pearce, W. H., Rutherford, R. B., Whitehill, T. A., et al.: Nuclear magnetic resonance imaging: Its diagnostic value in patients with congenital vascular malformations of the limbs. J. Vasc. Surg., 8:64, 1988.
33. Przybojewski, J. Z.: Iatrogenic aortocoronary vein fistula. S. Afr. Med. J., 62:908, 1982.
34. Ramchandani, P., Goldenberg, N. J., Soulen, R. L., and White, R. I., Jr.: Isobutyl 2-cyanoacrylate embolization of hepatoportal fistula. Am. J. Roentgenol., 140:137, 1983.
35. Ricketts, R. R., Fink, E., and Yellin, A. E.: Management of major arteriovenous fistulas by arteriographic techniques. Arch. Surg., 113:1153, 1978.
36. Reinhoff, W. F., Jr., and Hamman, L.: Subacute Streptococcus viridans septicemia cured by the excision of an arteriovenous aneurism of the external iliac artery and vein. Ann. Surg., 102:905, 1935.
37. Robinson, L. A., and Sabiston, D. C., Jr.: Syndrome of congenital internal mammary-to-pulmonary arteriovenous fistula associated with mitral valve prolapse. Arch. Surg., 116:1265, 1981.
38. Sabiston, D. C., Jr., Theilen, E. O., and Gregg, D. E.: Physiologic studies in experimental high output cardiac failure produced by aortic-caval fistula. Surg. Forum, 6:233, 1956.
39. Scott, H. W., Jr., and Sabiston, D. C., Jr.: Surgical treatment for congenital aorticopulmonary fistula. J. Thorac. Surg., 25:26, 1953.
40. Shadle, O. W., Ferguson, T. B., Sabiston, D. C., Jr., and Gregg, D. E.: The hemodynamic response to lanatoside C of dogs with experimental aortic-caval fistulas. J. Clin. Invest., 36:335, 1957.
41. Sheikh, K. H., Adams, D. B., McCann, R., Lyerly, H. K., Sabiston, D. C., Jr., and Kisslo, J.: Utility of Doppler color flow imaging for identification of femoral arterial complications of cardiac catheterization. Am. Heart J., 117:623, 1989.
42. Shumacker, H. B.: Arterial aneurysms and arteriovenous fistulas. Spontaneous cures. In Elkin, D. C., and DeBakey, M. E. (Eds.): Surgery in World War II:

43. Sumner, D. S.: Arteriovenous fistula. Physiology and pathological anatomy. In Strandness, D. E., Jr. (Ed.): Collateral Circulation in Clinical Surgery. Philadelphia, W. B. Saunders Company, 1969.
44. Symbas, P. N., Goldman, M., Erbesfeld, M. H., and Vlasis, S. E.: Pulmonary arteriovenous fistula, pulmonary artery aneurysm, and other vascular changes of the lung from penetrating trauma. Ann. Surg., 191:336, 1980.
45. Szilagyi, D. E., Elliot, J. P., DeRusso, F. J., et al.: Peripheral congenital arteriovenous fistulas. Surgery, 57:61, 1965.
46. Tafreshi, M., Steinbaum, S., Scarlett, K., and Alexander, L. L.: Ultrasonic demonstration of arteriovenous fistulas. J. Clin. Ultrasound, 12:299, 1984.
47. Taylor, B. G., Cockerill, E. M., Manfredi, F., and Klatte, E. C.: Therapeutic embolization of the pulmonary artery in pulmonary arteriovenous fistula. Am. J. Med., 64:360, 1978.
48. Tice, D. A., Clauss, R. H., Keirle, A. M., and Reed, G. E.: Congenital arteriovenous fistulae of the extremities: Observations concerning treatment. Arch. Surg., 86:460, 1963.
49. Trout, H. H., McAllister, H. A., Giordano, J. M., et al.: Vascular malformations. Surgery, 97:36, 1985.
50. Waldhausen, J. A., and Shumacker, H. B., Jr.: Pulmonary arteriovenous fistulae. Heart Bull., 14:57, 1965.
51. Webster, M. W.: Arteriovenous fistula following thyroidectomy. J. Cardiovasc. Surg., 23:515, 1982.

Vascular Surgery. Washington, D.C., Office of the Surgeon General, Department of the Army, 1955.

11. THROMBOANGIITIS OBLITERANS (BUERGER'S DISEASE)

H. Brownell Wheeler, M.D.

In 1908, Leo Buerger published clinical and pathologic observations on young men with severe ischemia of the extremities.[2] These patients were addicted to cigarette smoking and often had migratory superficial phlebitis. Buerger called the syndrome "thromboangiitis obliterans" because the acute histologic features were characterized by thrombosis in both arteries and veins and were associated with a marked inflammatory response. The condition became more commonly known as "Buerger's disease," a term often used inappropriately for peripheral arterial insufficiency of any cause. Most patients who were considered to have Buerger's disease actually suffered from arteriosclerosis, as became clear with the advent of angiography. In reality, the classic syndrome described by Buerger is an uncommon but dramatic form of peripheral vascular disease.

CLINICAL MANIFESTATIONS

Thromboangiitis obliterans typically occurs in heavy smokers who started smoking at an early age. The disease begins in young adult life, usually between 20 and 35 years of age. Originally, thromboangiitis obliterans was thought to occur only in men; but several cases in women have been reported in recent years, perhaps coincidental with the increase in women smokers.[11] The diagnosis of thromboangiitis obliterans should be considered in any young smoker with peripheral ischemia, particularly if the upper extremities are involved or if there is a history of migratory superficial phlebitis. The ischemic areas are usually sharply demarcated, with relatively good circulation in adjacent tissues. The pain is often excruciating. Associated symptoms include cold sensitivity, Raynaud's phenomenon, and peripheral neuropathy. Foot claudication is particularly characteristic.[8] Exacerbations with smoking and remissions following abstinence from tobacco are typical of thromboangiitis obliterans. The disease has been described in patients who chew tobacco[20] as well as those who smoke it. The disease has been reported infrequently in nonsmokers.[26] Careful clinical evaluation is necessary to exclude other causes of peripheral ischemia, especially arteriosclerosis and autoimmune disease.

Physical examination reveals involvement of small and medium-sized arteries. Forearm, calf, or digital arteries may be

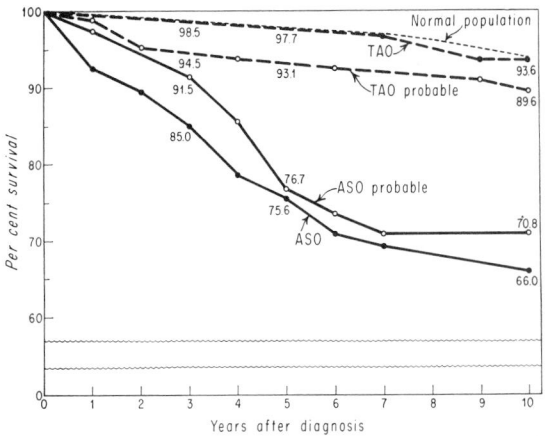

Figure 1. Widely differing 10-year survival rates in Buerger's disease (TAO) and arteriosclerosis (ASO). Confirmed cases of Buerger's disease show no significant difference from the normal population. (From McPherson, J. R., Juergens, J. L., and Gifford, R. W.: Ann. Intern. Med., *59:*288, 1963.)

occluded; the femoral and brachial arteries are usually not involved. The absence of a radial pulse, a positive Allen's sign, indicating ulnar artery occlusion, and superficial phlebitis may be clues to the diagnosis. Digital plethysmography is often helpful in determining the presence of small vessel disease. Small vessel occlusions are characteristic of thromboangiitis obliterans, but atypical for arteriosclerosis.[17] Serologic tests should be obtained to exclude autoimmune diseases, such as lupus erythematosus, which may be associated with peripheral arterial thrombosis.

Arteriography early in the disease usually reveals segmental obliteration of arteries, especially the medium-sized arteries of the forearm and calf, with a strikingly normal appearance of the remaining vessels. Digital arteries are frequently involved.[6] The irregular plaques characteristic of arteriosclerosis are conspicuously absent. Collateral circulation in chronic cases is unusually well developed and is often described as "tree roots" or "spider legs" in appearance. In about 25 percent of cases, a characteristic "corkscrew" appearance of collateral vessels is observed, presumably due to greatly dilated vasa vasorum in the occluded artery. An unusual corrugated or rippled appearance of an ar-

tery may sometimes be seen, resembling the stem of a gooseneck lamp.[23] This finding has been attributed to severe vasospasm.

The clinical course of Buerger's disease is protracted and painful, but relatively benign. If a patient ceases smoking, prolonged remission usually occurs. Most patients seem addicted to tobacco and continue to smoke despite all advice. They have repeated attacks and may require multiple amputations, but life-endangering complications are infrequent. Long-term life expectancy is only slightly less than that of the general population, unlike patients with comparable degrees of peripheral ischemia due to arteriosclerosis,[16,21] as shown in Figure 1. There is occasional involvement of the mesenteric or cerebrovascular circulation. Resection of ischemic or infarcted bowel may be required. In later life, patients with Buerger's disease often develop arteriosclerosis.

PATHOLOGY

In the acute stage, thrombosis occurs in arteries and veins of medium to small size. Digital vessels are commonly involved, unlike arteriosclerosis.[4] Dense aggregates of polymorphonuclear leukocytes are seen within the thrombus. There is an associated panvasculitis, but the elastic lamina remains intact.[30] Unlike arteriosclerosis or periarteritis nodosa, the disease does not cause necrosis of the arterial wall. Later, microabscesses are observed, and giant cells appear within the granulation tissue. The thrombus is organized, and recanalization of the lumen may occur, as shown in Figure 2. Older lesions show chronic inflammatory infiltrates or extensive fibrosis, which may involve peripheral nerves, as well as arteries and veins. There is considerable variability in histologic findings, depending upon the state of the disease observed.[12] The most characteristic changes are seen early in the pathologic process, but the timing of amputations for ischemic gangrene usually does not permit observation of the early phases of the disease.

ETIOLOGY

The striking association with cigarette smoking suggests a strong etiologic relationship, but a specific cause for thromboangiitis obliterans has never been demonstrated. An interaction of multiple etiologic factors is likely. Patients with Buerger's

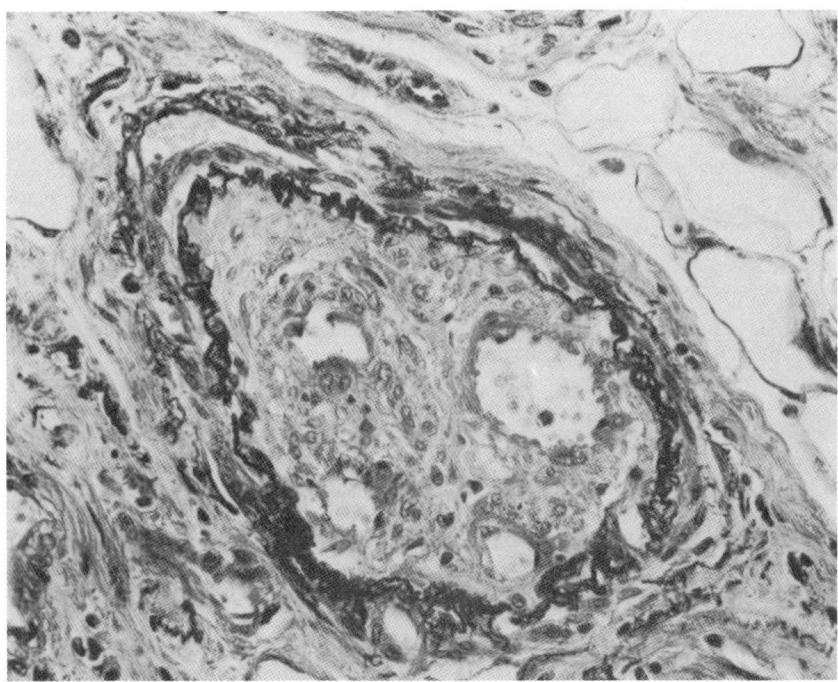

Figure 2. Chronic, well-organized arterial thrombosis in a 30-year-old man with Buerger's disease. Unlike arteriosclerosis, there is no degeneration or calcification in the vessel wall. The elastic lamina is intact, and the lumen has been partially recanalized. It would be unusual for arteriosclerosis to involve such a small artery (1 mm.). Van Giesen-elastic stain. ×570. (Courtesy of the Rev. Robert W. Bain, M.D., Department of Pathology, St. Vincent Hospital, Worcester, Mass.)

disease usually come from lower socioeconomic groups and often have poor hygiene and a history of chronic fungal infection or cold injury.[7] Fibrinogen levels may be elevated, blood viscosity may be increased,[27] and a hypercoagulable state has been postulated. Hyperaggregability of platelets has been reported during acute attacks. Familial predisposition has been reported, as well as a greater prevalence of specific leukocyte antigens, although others have failed to confirm this finding.[18] A genetic factor is also suggested by the fact that blacks are rarely affected, whereas the disease is common in Asia. Jewish men were originally reported to be particularly susceptible to the disease, although later studies failed to support any such predisposition. Autonomic overactivity is suggested by the association with severe peripheral vasospasm and hyperhidrosis. Any factor that causes vasospasm, thrombosis, or local inflammation may contribute to the development of the syndrome in a susceptible individual.

An autoimmune etiology of the disease has been postulated, based on the finding of both antibodies and lymphocyte-mediated sensitivity to collagen in thromboangiitis obliterans.[1,25] Antibodies to rickettsial organisms have been reported in patients with thromboangiitis obliterans, as have circulating immune complexes.[5] It appears increasingly likely that some immunologic process, typically initiated in response to cigarette smoking, has a major role in Buerger's disease.[29]

INCIDENCE

The frequency with which the diagnosis of Buerger's disease is made depends on the criteria used in establishing the diagnosis. Based on radiographic criteria, Buerger's disease is uncommon. When the diagnosis is based solely on the histologic findings originally described by Buerger, even large teaching hospitals rarely make the diagnosis. Some investigators have even doubted the existence of Buerger's disease. However, the occurrence of an infrequent but highly characteristic clinical syndrome has never been in doubt among clinicians who have cared for such patients.[15,16]

DeBakey and Cohen did a statistical analysis of 936 World War II veterans in whom the diagnosis of Buerger's disease was made during the years 1942 to 1948.[3] Extrapolating from their data, the authors estimated the minimal incidence in the United States at seven or eight cases per 100,000 white males 20 to 44 years of age; however, most experienced vascular surgeons believe that the incidence of Buerger's disease has decreased markedly since World War II. The prevalence of thromboangiitis obliterans at the Mayo Clinic declined from 104/100,000 patient registrants in 1947 to 9.9 in 1976, but there has been a slight upward trend in recent years (12.6 in 1986, 13.5 in 1987).[13] The incidence was 24 per cent of all young adults (age 35 or under) presenting at the Mayo Clinic with lower-limb ischemia from 1953 to 1981.[22]

In a recent retrospective review of 100 patients with ischemic finger ulcerations, thromboangiitis obliterans proved to be the final diagnosis in 9 per cent.[17] In another study of 700 patients with small vessel arterial disease, thromboangiitis obliterans was the final diagnosis in 3.7 per cent.[18] At present, thromboangiitis obliterans constitutes less than 1 per cent of all patients presenting initially with severe peripheral ischemia in the United States. In Israel and Eastern Europe, the corresponding incidence is approximately 5 per cent, whereas in Japan it has been reported to be 16 per cent. Patients with Buerger's disease are observed much more frequently in Asia, even in populations where arteriosclerosis is rare.

MANAGEMENT

The major problem in treating patients with Buerger's disease is the management of pain, which is often excruciating. Narcotics are usually necessary but must be used cautiously because of the frequency of drug addiction. Peripheral or sympathetic nerve blocks may provide temporary pain relief, especially when the disease is accompanied by severe vasospasm. Cervical or lumbar sympathectomy may benefit such patients. Relief of pain sometimes necessitates amputation, even if tissue necrosis has not occurred.

Every effort should be made to have the patient stop smoking, because indefinite remissions often follow abstinence from cigarettes. No specific medication has found wide acceptance, although anticoagulants, dextran, phenylbutazone, pyridinolcarbamate, inositol niacinate, and steroids have all been recommended. More recently, prostaglandin therapy (PGA$_1$)[24] and defibrotide[28] have been advocated, as well as agents to prevent platelet aggregation. Severe hand ischemia due to acute thrombosis in thromboangiitis obliterans has been dramatically improved by intra-arterial infusion of urokinase, followed by small-vessel balloon catheter angioplasty and anticoagulation.[10]

Arterial reconstruction is usually impossible because of the distal nature of the disease, but it should be considered in segmental proximal occlusions. Arterial reconstructions for Buerger's disease have a higher failure rate than comparable reconstructions for arteriosclerosis. Microvascular transplantation of free omental grafts to areas not amenable to arterial reconstruction has been successfully employed,[19] as have pedicled omental grafts.[9,14] When gangrene occurs, amputation at the lowest possible level is indicated. In this disease, unlike arteriosclerosis, it is often possible to do digital amputations with satisfactory healing.

SELECTED REFERENCES

Hagen, B., and Lohse, S.: Clinical and radiologic aspects of Buerger's disease. Cardiovasc. Intervent. Radiol., 7:283, 1984.
This article provides a comprehensive description of the angiographic signs of thromboangiitis obliterans with excellent illustrations of pedal and carpal angiograms.

Lie, J. T.: Thromboangiitis obliterans (Buerger's disease) revisited. Pathol. Annu., 23:257, 1988.
This review article describes the pathology of thromboangiitis obliterans in detail and contains many excellent photomicrographs. There is also a lengthy bibliography.

McKusick, V. A., Harris, W. S., Ottesen, O. E., Goodman, E. M., Shelley, W. M., and Bloodwell, R. D.: Buerger's disease: A distinct clinical and pathologic entity. J.A.M.A., 181:5, 1962.
This classic article makes a convincing case that Buerger's disease is a distinct clinical and pathologic entity, not merely arteriosclerosis in a younger age group. The conclusions are based on arteriographic study of all four extremities in 12 patients with Buerger's disease, as well as histopathologic study of biopsy and amputation specimens from 10 patients. No evidence of arteriosclerosis was observed in any of these patients, and angiographic and histopathologic findings consistent with Buerger's disease were documented. The authors also examined 28 additional patients and performed 24 angiograms in a Korean hospital. The findings were similar to those of American patients and are of particular interest because of the rarity of arteriosclerosis in young Korean men.

Mills, J. L., Friedman, E. I., Taylor, L. M. Jr., and Porter, J. M.: Upper extremity ischemia caused by small artery disease. Ann. Surg., 206:521, 1987.
This article documents the various causes of upper extremity ischemia in 100 patients. Buerger's disease constituted only 9 per cent of the population studied. The diagnostic evaluation of the patients with upper-extremity ischemia is thoroughly discussed, especially with respect to autoimmune disease.

Mills, J. L., Taylor, L. M. Jr., and Porter, J. M.: Buerger's disease in the modern era. Am. J. Surg., 154:123, 1987.
The authors reviewed over 700 patients with small artery disease and identified 26 patients who met rigid criteria for the diagnosis of thromboangiitis obliterans. There was a 31 per cent amputation rate in the lower extremity, but no patient lost further tissue after cessation of smoking. Current medical management and prognosis are well documented.

Ohta, T., and Shionoya, S.: Fate of the ischemic limb in Buerger's disease. Br. J. Surg., 75:259, 1988.
This article reports the long term follow-up in 328 patients with thromboangiitis obliterans. The prognosis was relatively benign, with a much higher survival rate than observed in patients with arteriosclerosis. There was only a 3.9 per cent incidence of major amputation, although minor digital amputations were common. The disease was often self-limited, especially in older patients, and sometimes improved even though the patient continued smoking.

REFERENCES

1. Adar, R., Papa, M. Z., Halpern, Z., Mozes, M., Shoshan, S., Sofer, B., Zinger, H., Dayan, M., and Mozes, E.: Cellular Sensitivity to Collagen in Thromboangiitis Obliterans. N. Engl. J. Med. 308:1113, 1983.
2. Buerger, L.: Thromboangiitis obliterans: A study of the vascular lesions leading to presenile spontaneous gangrene. Am. J. Med. Sci., 136:567, 1908.
3. DeBakey, M. D., and Cohen, B. M.: Buerger's Disease: A Follow-up Study of World War II Army Cases. Springfield, Ill., Charles C Thomas, 1963.
4. Dible, J. H.: In Cameron, R., and Wright, G. P. (Eds.): The Pathology of Limb Ischemia. St. Louis, Warren H. Green, 1966, p. 79.
5. Gulati, S. M., Saha, K., Kant, L., Thusoo, T. K., and Prakash, A.: Significance of circulatory immune complexes in thromboangiitis obliterans (Buerger's disease). Angiology, 35(5):276, 1984.
6. Hagan, B., Lohse, S.: Clinical and radiologic aspects of Buerger's disease. Cardiovasc. Intervent. Radiol., 7(6):283, 1984.
7. Hill, G. L., Moelino, J., Tumewu, F., Brataamadja, D, Tohardi, A.: The Buerger syndrome in JAVA. Br. J. Surg. 60:606, 1973.
8. Hirai, M., and Shionoya, S.: Intermittent claudication in the foot and Buerger's disease. Br. J. Surg., 65:210, 1978.
9. Hoshino, S., Nakayama, K., Igari, T., and Honda, K.: Long-term results of omental transplantation for chronic occlusive arterial diseases. Int. Surg., 68:47, 1983.
10. Lang, E. V., and Bookstein, J. J.: Accelerated thrombolysis and angioplasty for hand ischemia in Buerger's disease. Cardiovasc. Intervent. Radiol., 12:95, 1989.
11. Lie, J. T.: Thromboangiitis obliterans (Buerger's disease) in women. Medicine (Baltimore), 66:65, 1987.
12. Lie, J. T.: Thromboangiitis obliterans (Buerger's disease) revisited. Path. Annu., 23:257, 1988.
13. Lie, J. T.: The rise and fall and resurgence of thromboangiitis obliterans (Buerger's disease). Acta. Pathol. Jpn., 39:153, 1989.
14. Maurva, S. D., Singhal, S., Gupta, H. C., Elhence, I. P., Sharma, B. D.: Pedicled omental grafts in the revascularization of ischemic lower limbs in Buerger's disease. Int. Surg., 70:253, 1985.
15. McKusick, V. A., Harris, W. S., Ottesen, O. E., Goodman, E. M., Shelley, W. M., and Bloodwell, R. D.: Buerger's disease: A distinct clinical pathologic entity. J.A.M.A. 181:5, 1962.
16. McPherson, J. R., Juergens, J. L., and Gifford, R. W.: Thromboangiitis obliterans and arteriosclerosis obliterans: Clinical and prognostic differences. Ann. Intern. Med., 59:288, 1963.
17. Mills, J. L., Friedman, E. I., Taylor, L. M. Jr., and Porter, J. M.: Upper extremity ischemia caused by small artery disease. Ann. Surg., 206:521, 1987.
18. Mills, J. L., Taylor, L. M., Jr., and Porter, J. M.: Buerger's disease in the modern era. Am. J. Surg., 154:123, 1987.
19. Nishimura, A., Sano, F., Nakanishi, Y., Loshino, I., and Kassi, Y.: Omental transplantation for relief of limb ischaemia. Surg. Forum, 28:213, 1977.
20. O'Dell, J. R., Linder, J., Markin, R. S., and Moore, G. F.: Thromboangiitis obliterans (Buerger's disease) and smokeless tobacco. Arthritis Rheum., 30:1054, 1987.
21. Ohta, T., and Shionoya, S.: Fate of the ischaemic limb in Buerger's disease. Br. J. Surg., 75:259, 1988.
22. Pairolero, P. C., Joyce, J. W., Skinner, C. R., Hollier, L. H., and Cherry, K. J., Jr.: Lower limb ischemia in young adults: Prognostic implications. J. Vasc. Surg., 1:459, 1984.
23. Schatz, I. J., Fine, G., Eyler, W. R.: Thromboangiitis obliterans. Br. Heart J., 28:84, 1966.
24. Shionoya, S.: What is Buerger's disease? World J. Surg., 7:544, 1983.
25. Spittel, J. A.: Thromboangiitis obliterans: An autoimmune disorder? N. Engl. J. Med., 308:1157, 1983.
26. Stojanovic, V. K., Marcovic, A., Arsov, V., Bujanic, J., and Lolina, S.: Clinical course and therapy of Buerger's disease. J. Cardiothorac. Surg., 14:5, 1973.
27. Szendro, G., Golcman, L., and Cristal, N.: Study of the factors affecting blood viscosity in patients with thromboangiitis obliterans: A preliminary report. J. Vasc. Surg., 7:759, 1988.
28. Ulutin, O. N.: Clinical effectiveness of defibrotide in vaso-occlusive disorders and its mode of actions. Semin. Thromb. Hemost., 14(Suppl):58, 1988.
29. Vermylen, J., Blockmans, D., Spitz, B., and Deckmyn, H.: Thrombosis and immune disorders. Clin. Haematol. 15:393, 1986.
30. Williams, G.: Recent views on Buerger's disease. J. Clin. Pathol., 22:573, 1969.

12. RAYNAUD'S SYNDROME

*James M. Edwards, M.D., and
John M. Porter, M.D.**

Raynaud's syndrome defines a condition characterized by episodic attacks of vasospasm causing closure of the small arteries and arterioles of the distal parts of the extremities in re-

sponse to cold exposure or emotional stimuli. The fingers and hands are most frequently involved, although in many patients the toes and feet may be similarly affected. Classically, the episodes consist of intense pallor of the distal extremities followed by cyanosis and rubor upon rewarming with full recovery requiring 15 to 45 minutes. A large number of patients, however, develop only pallor or cyanosis during episodes and it is now clear that the classic tri-color pattern occurs only in a small number of patients. In recent years, a number of patients have been recognized who complain of cold hands without digital color changes and who have abnormal arteriographic and blood flow findings identical to those of patients with classic digital color changes, thus leading to the suggestion that digital color change may not be essential for the diagnosis.

HISTORICAL ASPECTS

Few topics exist in the field of vascular disease about which there has been more confusion and controversy than Raynaud's syndrome. In 1862 Raynaud described a clinical condition consisting of episodic digital pallor and cyanosis induced by cold or emotional stress.[49] Based entirely on the presence of a normally palpable radial pulse in most patients, he hypothesized an overactivity of the sympathetic nervous system that induced episodic arterial spasm. The digital gangrene present in many of Raynaud's original patients was erroneously ascribed to the accompanying vasospasm, a condition now known not to cause gangrene. Raynaud's primary vasospastic hypothesis was challenged at the turn of the century by Hutchinson, who observed that small arterial occlusive diseases might have a primary role in the production of cold or emotionally induced episodic digital vasospasm and indeed may have been responsible for the symptoms observed in many of Raynaud's original patients. He suggested that episodic digital ischemia did not represent a single disease, but rather a clinical sign common to diseases of diverse etiologies and that cold-induced episodic digital ischemia is present to some degree in many normal people.[23,24]

A milestone in the evolution of the understanding of Raynaud's syndrome occurred in 1932 with the publication of Allen and Brown's observations on the frequent presence of associated diseases.[1] They proposed division of the syndrome into Raynaud's disease, a benign idiopathic form of intermittent digital ischemia occurring in the absence of associated diseases, and Raynaud's phenomenon, a similar symptom complex occurring in association with one or more of a variety of systemic diseases. They described specific diagnostic criteria for the classification of patients with Raynaud's syndrome into one of the two categories. This report stimulated subsequent investigation of the clinical significance of Raynaud's syndrome, which continues to the present. Shortly after the publication of this influential paper, Lewis and Pickering reported that most of their patients with Raynaud's syndrome appeared to have the idiopathic form and subsequently had a benign clinical course.[34] This position was eventually challenged by Gifford and Hines[16] and deTakats and Fowler,[8] who emphasized that associated connective tissue disorders may not become apparent for years after the onset of Raynaud's syndrome.

There now appears little justification for attempting a rigid separation of Raynaud's disease from Raynaud's phenomenon. With the passage of time, the incidence of primary Raynaud's disease decreases as some associated disease process is found in more and more patients. It appears reasonable to refer to the condition as Raynaud's syndrome and to recognize that patients with this condition have an increased lifelong risk for the devel-

* Supported by Grant RR00334 from the General Clinical Research Centers branch of the Division of Research Resources, National Institutes of Health, and Grant 8839 from the Medical Research Foundation of Oregon.

opment of associated disease processes, especially autoimmune disease.

PATHOPHYSIOLOGY

The pallor in the early stage of Raynaud episodes is initiated by severe spasm of the arteries and arterioles, which causes cessation of capillary perfusion. After some minutes, the capillaries and probably the venules dilate, both from hypoxia and the accumulation of the metabolic products of regional anaerobic metabolism. This is followed by a slight relaxation of the arteriolar spasm with the entry of a trickle of blood into the dilated capillaries, where it rapidly becomes desaturated, producing cyanosis. Rubor results from the entry of increasing amounts of blood into dilated capillaries. The episode terminates with the entry of a normal volume of blood through the relaxed arterioles and the return of the dilated capillaries to normal.

An attempt to understand the mechanism of vasoconstriction that occurs during an episode of Raynaud's phenomenon has interested investigators for more than a century. Raynaud's suggestion that the episodes represented sympathetic nervous system hyperactivity was largely disproved by the methodical observations of Lewis in the 1920s and 1930s.[33,34] He concluded that the digital arteries in this condition close completely on exposure to cold and that this closure is responsible for the clinical symptoms. Based upon failure to prevent cold-induced vasospasm by digital nerve conduction anesthesia, Lewis proposed the theory of local vascular wall hyperresponsiveness to cold exclusive of sympathetic innervation, a condition he termed "local vascular fault."

A number of indirect measurements of blood flow and pressure in the hand and fingers have been obtained both at normal and cool temperatures by numerous investigators.[7,20,41] These studies have shown that patients with Raynaud's syndrome have considerably decreased hand and finger blood flow at room temperature and an additional decrease with cooling to a critical level of 18° to 20° C., at which digital artery closure occurs and digital flow abruptly ceases.

Considerable published information indicates that patients with Raynaud's syndrome may be divided into two distinct pathophysiologic groups, obstructive and spastic.[37,46,58] Patients with obstructive Raynaud's syndrome have a significant obstruction of the palmar and digital arteries caused by one of a variety of diseases, two of the more frequent being chronic arteritis associated with autoimmune disease and arteriosclerosis. To experience a Raynaud episode, the patient must have sufficiently severe arterial obstruction to cause significant reduction in resting digital artery pressure, a condition that requires obstruction of both arteries of a single digit. The quantitative relationship between arterial obstruction and Raynaud episodes has been described in a series of detailed studies by Hirai.[20] Available evidence suggests that in such patients a normal vasoconstrictive response to cold is sufficient to overcome the diminished intraluminal distending pressure and cause arterial closure. This theory predicts that all patients with arterial obstruction of the hand sufficient to cause resting digital hypotension experience cold-induced Raynaud episodes. In the authors' experience this appears to be true.

Patients with spastic Raynaud's syndrome do not have significant palmar-digital artery obstruction and accordingly have normal digital artery pressure at room temperature. Arterial closure in these patients is caused by the markedly increased force of cold-induced arterial spasm. Sir Thomas Lewis studied this event exhaustively and after repeatedly observing that both autonomic and somatic nerve blocks did not alter the episodes, concluded that the abnormality producing the spastic Raynaud episodes lay not in the sympathetic nervous system, but in the artery itself, a condition he termed local vascular fault. In the

succeeding 65 years, the nature of the local fault has never been defined.

A number of studies have suggested altered adrenoceptor activity in patients with spastic Raynaud's syndrome. Coffman and Cohen found decreased digital nutritive blood flow in patients with Raynaud's syndrome that was increased after treatment with the sympathetic blocking drug reserpine.[7] Early work in the authors' laboratory showed a marked reduction in cold-induced digital artery vasospasm after the intra-arterial administration of reserpine.[52] Jamieson and associates suggested that patients with Raynaud's syndrome may possess abnormal adrenergic receptors that become increasingly sensitive to stimulation after cold exposure.[25]

In recent years, knowledge of human adrenergic receptor function has increased markedly with the characterization of the alpha$_1$- and alpha$_2$-adrenoceptors. The alpha$_2$-adrenoceptors, which were initially thought to be presynaptic and inhibitory, are now known to occur both pre- and postsynaptically and may be facilitative as well as inhibitory.[32,39] Alpha$_2$-adrenoceptors are present in a pure population on human platelets.[39] Although the precise relationship between platelet adrenoceptor activity and that of arteries has not been established, a clear precedent exists for a direct relationship between blood cell and peripheral adrenoceptors in biologic systems. A study of alpha$_2$-adrenoceptor numbers on platelets from normal individuals, patients with spastic Raynaud's syndrome, and patients with obstructive Raynaud's syndrome by radioimmunoassay has been performed in the authors' laboratory.[29] The results of this assay are presented in Figure 1 and show a marked elevation of alpha$_2$-adrenoceptor activity in spastic Raynaud's patients. The same laboratory has presented confirmation of this finding as well as preliminary data that suggest there may be a factor in the blood of patients with spastic Raynaud's syndrome that interferes with the alpha$_1$-adrenoceptor assay.[10] In addition, a series of experiments was conducted during which normal whole platelets were incubated with serum from patients with spastic Raynaud's syndrome. Subsequent measurement of platelet alpha$_2$-adrenoceptor levels revealed a decrease in levels by approximately 15 to 20 per cent when compared with those in incubation with normal serum or assay buffer alone. The hypothesis advanced, and which is now being studied, is that there is a factor in the blood of patients with vasospastic Raynaud's syndrome that binds to alpha$_2$-adreno-

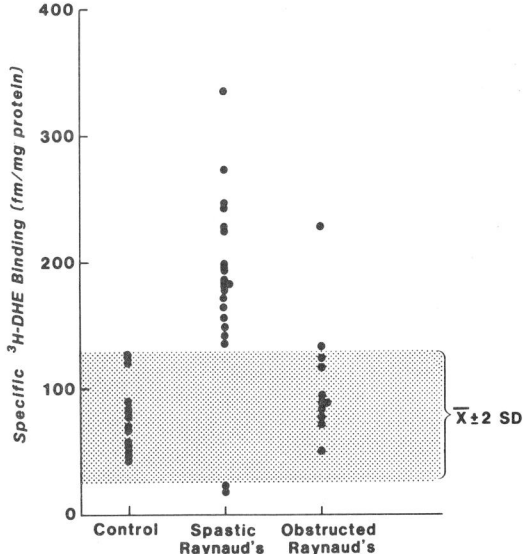

Figure 1. Range of alpha$_2$-adrenoreceptor concentrations from patients with Raynaud's syndrome. (From Keenan, E. J., and Porter, J. M.: Alpha-2 adrenergic receptors in platelets from patients with Raynaud's syndrome. Surgery, 94:204, 1983.)

ceptors that causes a compensatory increase in numbers of adrenoceptors with a resulting hypersensitivity to normal stimuli. If confirmed by others, increased alpha$_2$-adrenoceptor activity may prove to be the local vascular fault hypothesized by Lewis over 50 years ago.

An abnormality in presynaptic beta receptors has recently been advanced as a cause of Raynaud's syndrome.[3,4] This has been reported by only one group and awaits further confirmation.

The role of the sympathetic nervous system is unclear. In a series of papers by Lafferty and associates, abnormalities in the thermoregulatory response in patients with Raynaud's syndrome have been demonstrated by means of a test termed "thermal entrainment."[9,31] In this test the blood flow patterns in one hand are measured while the contralateral hand is alternately dipped in baths of hot and cold water. There are clear differences in blood flow responses demonstrable between normals and controls. The obvious way to explain contralateral changes in blood flow is through the function of the sympathetic nervous system, although no research has been done to prove or disprove this hypothesis.

Thus, the pathophysiology of Raynaud's syndrome and the role, if any, of the sympathetic nervous system are unclear.

EPIDEMIOLOGY

The incidence of Raynaud's syndrome in the general population is not known with certainty. Several small studies indicate a remarkable incidence of about 20 to 25 per cent in the cool, damp climates of Copenhagen, Denmark, and Portland, Oregon.[42,43] It is currently unknown whether cool, damp environmental conditions increase the true incidence of Raynaud's syndrome or merely make the underlying abnormality clinically apparent.[21]

Of considerable interest is the prevalence of Raynaud's syndrome in certain occupational groups, especially those who use vibrating tools or experience chronic cold exposure. This has received considerable attention in recent years, because of both the impaired life-style of the patients and the potential impact of this finding on industrial compensation claims. The incidence of digital ischemia among chainsaw operators and miners using vibrating equipment ranges from 40 to 90 per cent, the wide variation in incidence being generally related to the length of exposure.[6,18,59] A 50 per cent incidence of Raynaud's syndrome has been reported among food workers who work in cold areas.[35] The pathophysiologic mechanism underlying Raynaud's syndrome of occupational origin is unknown, because neither detailed sequential digital hypothermic tests nor angiography has been performed routinely. Available evidence suggests that the cases of short duration are probably vasospastic, whereas those of long standing may be primarily obstructive.

Women constitute 70 to 90 per cent of most reported patient series with Raynaud's syndrome.[56] Typically, younger women present with spastic Raynaud's syndrome, and idiopathic Raynaud's without associated disease is most common in this age and sex group. Some patients initially found to have no associated disease eventually are shown to have an autoimmune disorder, although the frequency of this occurrence remains unknown. Older men who develop Raynaud's syndrome usually have the obstructive variety associated with digital artery occlusion, usually due to atherosclerosis.

ASSOCIATED DISEASES

Raynaud's syndrome has been observed in association with a wide variety of disorders.[1,2,8,44,47,59] A general classification of these conditions appears in Table 1. Although in the past, this array of apparently unrelated clinical entities obscured under-

TABLE 1. Disorders Associated with Raynaud's Syndrome

I. Immunologic and connective tissue disorders
  A. Scleroderma
  B. Mixed connective tissue disease
  C. Systemic lupus erythematosus
  D. Rheumatoid arthritis
  E. Dermatomyositis
  F. Polymyositis
  G. Hepatitis B antigen–induced vasculitis
  H. Drug-induced vasculitis
  I. Sjögren's syndrome
II. Obstructive arterial diseases
  A. Arteriosclerosis
  B. Thromboangiitis obliterans
  C. Thoracic outlet syndrome
III. Environmental conditions
  A. Vibration injury
  B. Direct arterial trauma
  C. Cold injury
IV. Drug-induced Raynaud's syndrome without arteritis
  A. Ergot
  B. Beta-blocking drugs
  C. Cytotoxic drugs
  D. Birth control pills
V. Miscellaneous
  A. Vinyl chloride disease
  B. Chronic renal failure
  C. Cold agglutinins
  D. Cryoglobulinemia
  E. Neoplasia
  F. Neurologic disorders
    1. Central nervous system
    2. Peripheral nervous system
  G. Endocrinologic disorders

standing of the nature of Raynaud's syndrome, it now appears clear that all these conditions produce either spastic or obstructive arterial phenomena or a combination. A detailed characterization of the associated diseases noted in the first 615 patients with Raynaud's syndrome examined at this institution appears in Table 2.[12] Truly idiopathic Raynaud's syndrome occurred in 54 per cent of patients, although the precise pathophysiologic relationships between the associated conditions and Raynaud's syndrome are not clear. In recent years, the number of patients with idiopathic Raynaud's syndrome has increased in the authors' clinical practice in comparison with previous experience. In 1976, in a group of 100 patients, only 19 per cent were given a diagnosis of idiopathic Raynaud's syndrome.[44] The percentage of patients with idiopathic Raynaud's syndrome has steadily increased since then. The increase in the proportion of patients presenting to this clinic with idiopathic Raynaud's syndrome has become much more rapid in the last 5 years. The authors' only explanation for the change is that their interest in digital ischemia has become well known and has resulted in referral of increasing numbers of minimally symptomatic patients. Such patients are clearly less likely to have associated diseases than patients with severe vasospastic or obstructive symptoms.[12]

The data describing the percentage of patients presenting with Raynaud's syndrome who have an associated disease have been derived from tertiary referral centers. The obvious requirement for entry into such studies was that the patient have Raynaud's symptoms of sufficient severity to seek treatment. Although most of the published data clearly indicates that 70 per cent of this group has some associated disease process, this association in all likelihood does not apply to the minimally symptomatic individuals in the population who have never sought medical care. In these individuals, the incidence of Raynaud's syndrome unassociated with other disease processes must be much higher.

TABLE 2. Associated Diseases

Associated Disease	Number of Patients	Total
Connective tissue disorders		163 (27%)
Scleroderma	10	
PSS	56	
RA	15	
Sjögren's	11	
MCTD	14	
UCTD	16	
Misc/Unknown CTD	41	
Other associated disease		116 (19%)
Atherosclerosis	23	
Cancer	8	
Buerger's	10	
Frostbite/cold exp	7	
Carpal Tunnel	6	
Hypothyroid	6	
Vibration	7	
Acromegaly	2	
Erythromelagia	6	
Hypersens Angiitis	11	
Hematologic abnl	4	
Art/nerve trauma	2	
Neuropathy	6	
Misc	18	
No disease	336	336 (54%)
		615

CLINICAL DESCRIPTION

Most patients with spastic Raynaud's syndrome are women in whom the age of onset is typically under 30 years. Both hands are affected equally, and frequently the thumbs are spared. Although most patients have a mild associated vasospastic involvement of feet and toes, only about 10 per cent of patients have primary lower extremity involvement. Obstructive Raynaud's syndrome appears to be about equally distributed between men and women, and the symptomatic onset occurs after age 40. The lower extremities are infrequently involved. A striking difference from the vasospastic variety is that the area of involvement is frequently limited to one or several fingers and frequently affects only one hand.

Most episodes of digital vasospasm are induced by environmental cold exposure, although emotional stimuli such as fear or anger may also produce episodes in about half the patients. The required stimulus may be as mild as a draft from an air conditioner or hand immersion in tap water. At the beginning of an episode, the patient usually experiences blanching or cyanosis of one or several fingers that may extend proximally to the metacarpophalangeal junction or even to the wrist. An episode is usually associated with an uncomfortable sensation of numbness. Severe pain is rare. The initial pallor or cyanosis persists for as long as the cold exposure continues and is followed by a gradual return to normal color 15 to 30 minutes after entering a warm area. Fingertip ulceration occurs only in the presence of widespread palmar or digital artery obstruction. Ischemic ulceration is never caused by vasospasm alone.

PATIENT EVALUATION

Historical information should be sought regarding symptoms of connective tissue disease, including arthralgia, dysphagia, skin tightening, xerophthalmia, or xerostomia. Symptoms of large vessel occlusive disease, exposure to trauma or frostbite, drug history, and history of malignancy should also be sought. The skin of the hands and fingers should be inspected for ulceration or fingertip hyperkeratotic areas suggesting healed ulcers. The hand and fingers should be examined for evidence of skin thinning, tightening, sclerodactyly, or telangectasias, all of which may suggest associated autoimmune disease. The peripheral pulse status should be carefully noted, and special attention should be directed toward signs and symptoms of nerve compression syndrome. Carpal tunnel syndrome is seen with surprising frequency in Raynaud's patients, affecting about 15 per cent of these individuals.[47] Patients who present with the sudden onset of digital ischemia should be questioned about coagulation abnormalities and a history of previous thrombotic episodes. It should be noted that the physical examination is frequently completely normal in patients with Raynaud's syndrome. The diagnosis is made primarily from the history.

ANCILLARY EVALUATION

Hand arteriography was formerly used frequently at this institution in the evaluation of patients with Raynaud's syndrome. A detailed technique of cryogenic arteriography provided important anatomic, pathophysiologic, and diagnostic information.[52] Representative arteriograms can be seen in Figures 2 and 3. Increasingly sophisticated vascular laboratory techniques have largely replaced arteriography in the routine evaluation of patients with Raynaud's syndrome, and arteriography is now recommended infrequently and only then to exclude a surgically correctable proximal arterial lesion.[2] Currently, at this institution arteriography is obtained only in patients presenting with unilateral ischemic digital ulceration, because in a small percentage of these patients these ulcers develop as a result of embolization from a surgically correctable proximal arterial lesion.

The vascular laboratory has been of great help in objectively establishing the diagnosis of Raynaud's syndrome and allows a separation of spastic from obstructive Raynaud's syndrome. The change in digital blood pressure related to finger temperature is shown diagrammatically in Figure 4 for three groups: normal individuals, patients with vasospastic Raynaud's syndrome, and patients with significant digital artery obstruction. Normal individuals show only a modest digital pressure drop with decreasing temperature. Patients with vasospastic Raynaud's syndrome show a similar curve until a critical temperature is reached, at which time abrupt arterial closure occurs. Patients with severe arterial obstruction parallel normal but with a much lower pressure, with closure occurring at about 20 to 30 torr.

The first vascular laboratory test used widely for objective diagnosis of Raynaud's syndrome was the measurement of fingertip temperature recovery after digital ice-water exposure (Fig. 5).[47] Although normal individuals and patients with Raynaud's syndrome usually have similar resting digital temperatures and similar temperature drops after ice-water exposure, the time required for a return of digital temperature to normal averages 5 to 10 minutes in normal individuals and is prolonged to more than 20 minutes in most Raynaud's patients. Increasing experience has revealed that although this test is 100 per cent specific, it is only about 50 per cent sensitive and thus is insufficiently accurate for clinical use.

In recent years, the digital blood pressure response to 5 minutes of digital occlusive hypothermia as described by Nielsen and associates has proved to be quite accurate in the vascular laboratory diagnosis of Raynaud's syndrome.[41] In an evaluation of 100 patients at this institution, the test was found to be 87 per cent specific and 90 per cent sensitive, yielding an overall accuracy of 92 per cent.[15] Currently this is the diagnostic test of choice in those occasional patients in whom a test is necessary. As noted previously, the diagnosis is usually established by the clinical history. However, the use of an objective test is most helpful in certain patient groups, including those in whom the diagnosis is in doubt, epidemiologic study groups, and those

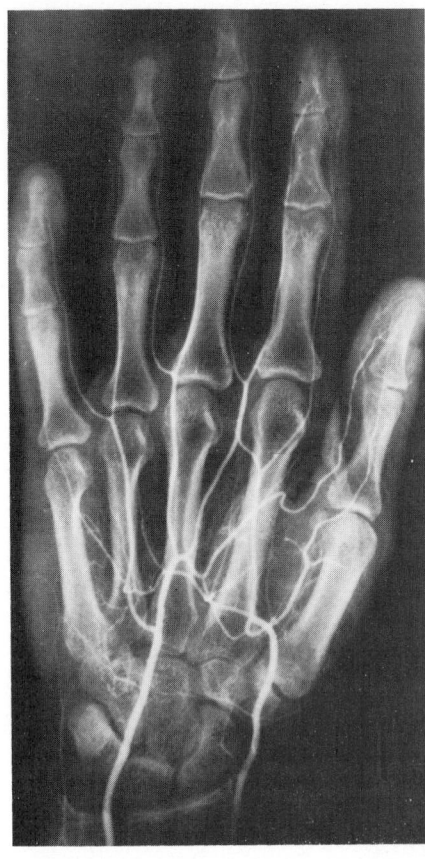
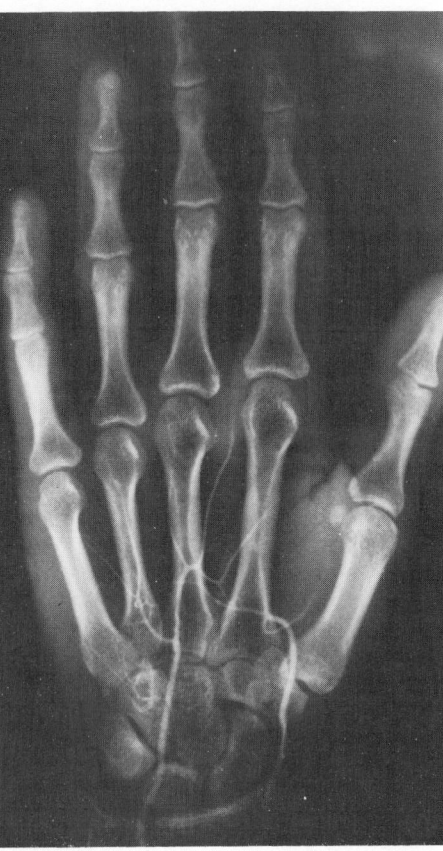

Figure 2. *Left,* Hand arteriogram in patient with Raynaud's symptoms at room temperature. Significant vasospasm is present. *Right,* Same patient after ice-water exposure for 30 seconds. A marked increase in vasospasm is present.

with pending litigation in whom historical accuracy is uncertain.

Digital photoplethysmography with digital blood pressure determination has become as accurate as arteriography in the detection of significant digital artery obstruction.[22] A finding of an obstructive digital plethysmographic waveform with a digital pressure of more than 10 torr below brachial pressure establishes the diagnosis of significant digital artery obstruction.[22]

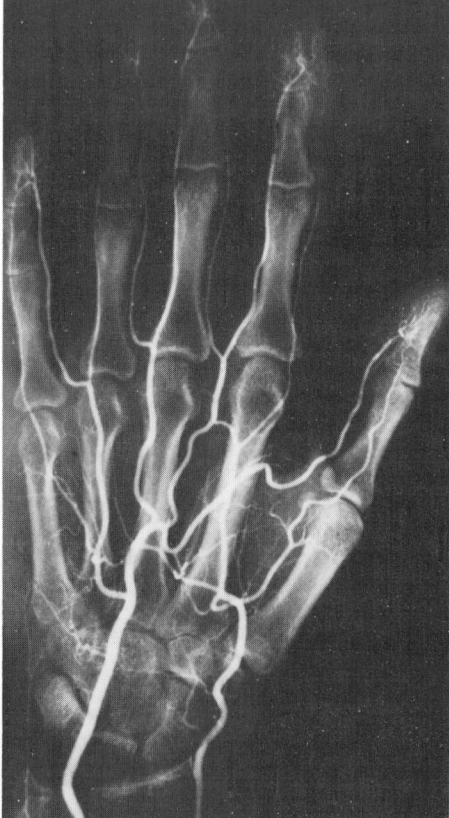
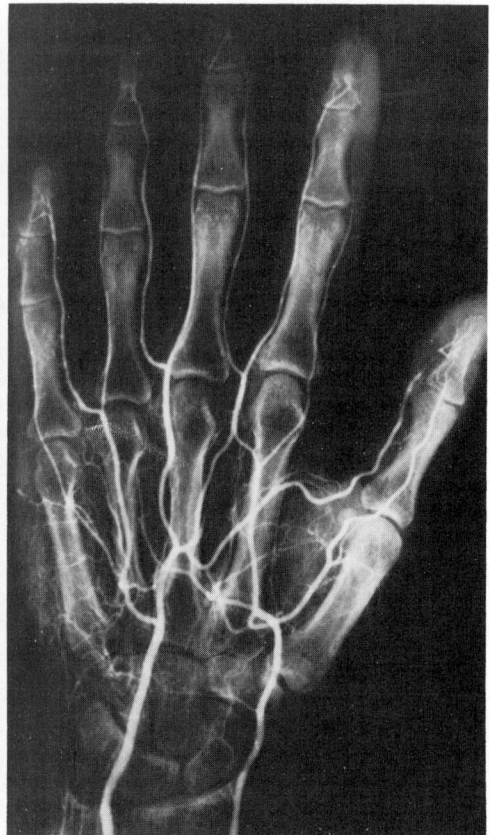

Figure 3. *Left,* Same patient as in Figure 2, 48 hours after sympathetic blockage, in this case accomplished by the intra-arterial injection of reserpine. A significant decrease in resting vasospasm is apparent. *Right,* After ice-water exposure. The vasoconstrictive response to cold is markedly diminished by sympathetic blockade.

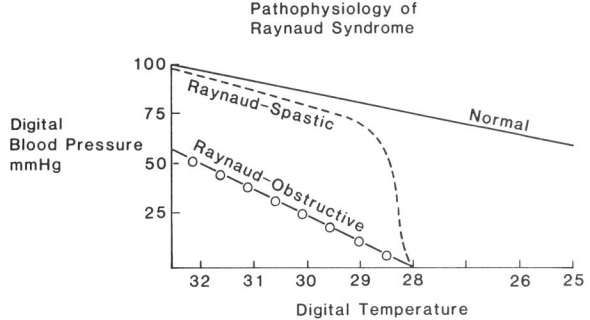

Figure 4. Alterations in digital blood pressure with decreasing digital temperature. See text.

This, combined with the digital hypothermic blood pressure test described above, allows accurate characterization of obstructive or spastic Raynaud's syndrome.

The extent of laboratory evaluation varies somewhat, depending on the findings of the history and physical examination. Minimal evaluation includes a hand roentgenogram for calcinosis or tuft resorption, hemogram, sedimentation rate, rheumatoid factor, and antinuclear antibody to aid in the diagnosis of any associated autoimmune disease. Additional information such as protein electrophoresis and antibodies to a variety of nuclear antigens may subsequently be obtained. Upper extremity nerve conduction testing should be considered if there is any clinical suspicion of carpal tunnel syndrome. Cases with a history of the sudden onset of digital occlusion should be evaluated for hypercoagulable states. The authors' current screening test consists of antithrombin III, protein S, and protein C levels as well as screening for the presence of lupus inhibitor and anticardiolipin antibodies.

TREATMENT

Satisfactory results have been reported with many agents empirically selected on the basis of the presumed pathophysiology of Raynaud's syndrome. Unfortunately, objective evaluation of every form of treatment including surgical sympathectomy has been made impossible by largely anecdotal reports and lack of controlled studies. Nearly every type of treatment has been used successfully in at least one study population. Few, if any, agents currently used have been subjected to rigorous randomized, double-blind trials with parallel-group placebo control.

Most patients with Raynaud's syndrome have only mild symptoms that respond well to simple conservative treatment, including the wearing of warm clothes and gloves and cold and tobacco avoidance. Patients who work in cold areas may not respond to any treatment until their occupational exposure is reduced. Because of the adverse digital circulatory effects of

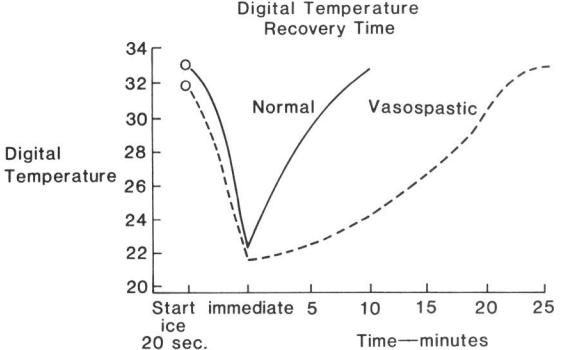

Figure 5. Digital temperature after cold exposure. The recovery time for patients with Raynaud's syndrome is markedly prolonged compared with normal individuals.

ergotamine tartrate and beta-adrenergic blocking drugs, equally effective alternative treatment should be sought in patients with Raynaud's syndrome.[14,19,40]

While a variety of vasodilator agents have been used in the pharmacologic treatment of patients with Raynaud's syndrome, it has been the authors' experience that only about 10 per cent of patients with Raynaud's syndrome require any treatment beyond cold and tobacco avoidance. The primary difficulty with evaluation of the benefit of pharmacologic therapy in Raynaud's syndrome has been the lack of objective methods of assessing drug response. Currently no vascular laboratory test allows an objective assessment of drug benefit. It is unknown whether this reflects an actual absence of objective drug benefit or an insensitivity of the currently available vascular laboratory tests. Unfortunately, in the absence of adequate methodology, the assessment of efficacy of any drug devolves to the patient's subjective impression of benefit, an assessment that may be markedly affected by such variables as environmental temperature, the patient's emotional state, or concomitant medications.

Many patients require pharmacologic therapy only in winter months. One of the most widely used agents in the past was reserpine.[7,47] Intra-arterial administration of reserpine appeared beneficial on occasion but is no longer available, having been removed from the market by the manufacturer. The intravenous tourniquet-controlled Bier block injection has proved to be useful in the treatment of certain patients because it provides a 2- to 3-day regional medical sympathectomy.[60] Although reserpine is no longer available, guanethidine is available on an experimental basis and may be similarly effective. In the past, guanethidine was found to be the most effective oral medication for the symptomatic treatment of Raynaud's syndrome.[47] A number of other adrenergic blocking drugs, including alpha-methyl-dopa, priscoline, tolazoline, phenoxybenzamine, and prazosin, have been used occasionally with anecdotal good results.

Other vasodilators have proved unsuccessful in the treatment of Raynaud's syndrome.[45] The beta-stimulating drugs have been ineffective, the two most widely used being nylidrin and isoxsuprine. The topical vasodilators papaverine and niacin as well as the topical application of nitroglycerin have been generally ineffective. The antifungal drug griseofulvin was initially thought to be helpful, but recent experience has not confirmed the early reports.

The calcium channel–blocking agents represent compounds that are finding wide clinical application. Nifedipine is the most potent peripheral vasodilator in this group and has been moderately effective in the treatment of Raynaud's syndrome, producing clinical improvement in 50 to 60 per cent of patients studied.[28,55,57] Headache is a frequently encountered side effect and is of sufficient severity to cause discontinuation of the drug in 10 to 20 per cent of patients. At present, nifedipine is the first-line drug for Raynaud's syndrome. Patients with spastic Raynaud's syndrome are more likely to respond than those with obstructive Raynaud's syndrome.

A variety of new drugs and unconventional treatments have been proposed for Raynaud's syndrome. Beta-blockers, which have been implicated in the causation of drug-induced Raynaud's syndrome, have been suggested for the treatment of Raynaud's syndrome in combination with a calcium channel blocker.[5] The authors have limited experience with this combination, but several patients who have failed to respond to a calcium channel blocker alone have had a beta-blocker (atenolol, 50 mg. per day) added with good results. Prostaglandin E_1 appeared to be beneficial in a number of anecdotal reports, but a randomized, double-blind, placebo-controlled study failed to show benefit. Ketanserin is a selective serotonin-2 receptor blocker that has been reported useful in the treatment of obstructive Raynaud's syndrome, particularly that seen in association with scleroderma.[30,51] Plasmapheresis has been attempted on occasion, as have agents that reduce blood viscosity, fibrinogen concentration, and platelet activity, with varying results.[50] These treatments have been of no benefit in the authors' experience. Treatment of associated autoimmune diseases does not appear to benefit Raynaud's syndrome.

SURGICAL THERAPY

In a very small number of patients with Raynaud's syndrome, there is a proximal cause of upper extremity arterial insufficiency, sometimes associated with distal emboli to the palmar and digital arteries. The occasional patient with Raynaud's syndrome associated with subclavian, axillary, or brachial obstruction from arteriosclerosis, emboli, thoracic outlet syndrome, aneurysm, or trauma is an appropriate subject for vascular surgery and generally may expect satisfactory results.[36,53]

For the past half century, one of the frequent treatments for Raynaud's syndrome has been upper extremity sympathectomy. The typical postoperative course is that the patient experiences a few months of good results followed by a gradual recurrence of symptoms.[45] It is unknown whether this represents an incomplete initial sympathectomy due to anatomic vagaries in the nerve distribution of the upper extremity or the development of receptor hypersensitivity to circulating catecholamines. Sympathectomy produces occasional anecdotal good long-term results, but in general these have been limited to patients with mild Raynaud's syndrome of the spastic variety. This is the same group of patients who respond best to pharmacologic treatment. There is general agreement that upper extremity sympathectomy is of little or no benefit in patients with Raynaud's syndrome who have associated connective tissue disease.[17,27] At present, the modest surgical risk, expense, and mediocre long-term results of thoracic sympathectomy for Raynaud's syndrome constitute overwhelming arguments against its use; the procedure is not recommended. In contrast, lumbar sympathectomy for lower extremity Raynaud's syndrome yields excellent long-term results.[26] The reason for the difference between the results of upper and lower sympathectomy is unknown.

In the treatment of patients with Raynaud's syndrome, one occasionally encounters patients with painful digital ulceration. This almost always implies widespread palmar and digital arterial obstruction, since ischemic ulceration does not result from vasospasm. The authors have achieved a healing rate of 85 per cent in a group of 100 such patients after scrubbing of the ulcer

with soap and water, antibiotics as selected by culture, and conservative débridement.[11,38,48] These results are equal to the healing rate achieved after thoracic sympathectomy and once again emphasize the critical lack of data supporting thoracic sympathectomy for either vasospasm or ischemia. A representative photograph of a painful digital ischemic ulcer that healed with conservative treatment is shown in Figure 6.

Recently, some surgeons advocated digital periarterial sympathectomy as an improved method of sympathectomy.[13,61] Proof that this procedure produces results superior to randomized nonoperative therapy is conspicuously lacking. Direct microvascular bypass of occluded segments of palmar and digital arteries has been reported in recent years with occasional relief of symptoms.[54] These have been carefully selected cases, primarily traumatic in etiology, in patients with normal vessels elsewhere. There appears little likelihood that these techniques are of benefit in patients with generalized small vessel disease.

OVERVIEW

Raynaud's syndrome is the symptomatic expression of episodic digital vasospasm that has multiple causes and can be seen in association with a myriad of apparently unrelated disorders. Most patients exhibit variable degrees of both vasospasm and palmar-digital arterial occlusions, although most cluster toward one end of the spectrum. Abnormal hemorrheologic parameters have been an inconsistent finding.

An objective evaluation of both medical and surgical treatments is hampered by a lack of controlled trials, poor definition of patient groups for the purpose of comparing results, variable follow-up, and a total unavailability of generally applied and accepted objective tests of digital blood flow and digital artery closure characteristics. Conservative treatment consisting of cold and tobacco avoidance is adequate for the majority of patients with mild to moderate symptoms. About 10 per cent of patients with Raynaud's syndrome have sufficiently severe and frequent or prolonged episodes to require drug therapy. Generally favorable anecdotal results have been achieved in about half of these patients after a variety of pharmacologic treatments. The authors' current preference is the use of nifedipine 10 mg. three times daily. The bias remains with conservative therapy even in the difficult group of patients with severe pain or persistent digital ischemia with localized gangrene. Constant and meticulous attention to the fundamental principles of con-

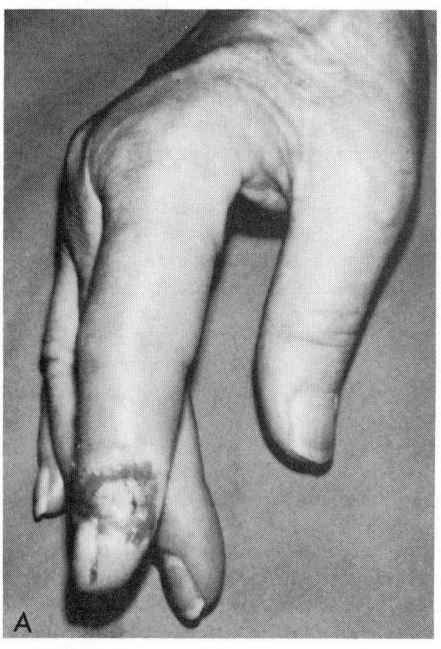
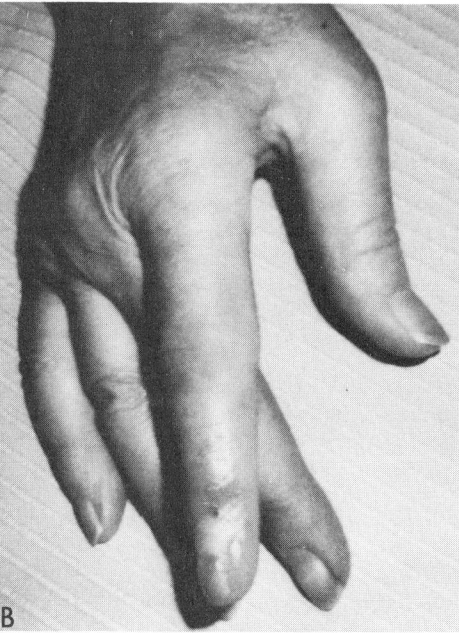

Figure 6. *A*, Painful digital ischemic ulcer in patient with scleroderma and massive digital artery obstruction. *B*, Total healing after 4 weeks of soap and water scrubs and antibiotics. Such healing with conservative treatment only may be expected in 85 per cent of patients with digital ischemic ulcers.

servative therapy, including cessation of tobacco use and gentle cleansing and débridement of ulcers, leads to gratifying results in most patients.

While upper extremity sympathectomy undoubtedly causes dramatic improvement in occasional patients, the result in any single patient is quite unpredictable and usually disappointing. Sympathectomy appears to have its best long-term results in those mildly symptomatic patients who need it least. Similarly, it is difficult to believe that digital artery sympathectomy or hand artery microvascular repair will be of any widespread use. Lumbar sympathectomy should be considered in the few patients who present with primary lower extremity Raynaud's syndrome and whose symptoms cannot be controlled by conservative measures and medical therapy.

SELECTED REFERENCES

Brotzu, G., Falchi, S., Mannu, B., Montisci, R., et al.: The importance of presynaptic beta receptors in Raynaud's disease. J. Vasc. Surg., 9:767, 1989.

In this article the authors suggest that the underlying pathophysiologic abnormality in Raynaud's syndrome is an abnormality in the presynaptic beta-adrenoceptor, rather than in alpha-adrenoceptors. This article is the third in a series, and in it the authors present the results of a trial of the use of beta-blockers in the treatment of Raynaud's syndrome. Although the authors conclude that the beta-blocker-treated group had superior results, the reader is cautioned that no test for Raynaud's syndrome has yet proved to objectively demonstrate benefit of treatment; thus the improvement noted is based on subjective criteria.

Edwards, J. M., Phinney, E. S., Taylor, L. M., Jr., Keenan, E. J., and Porter, J. M.: Alpha-2 adrenoreceptor differences in vasospastic and obstructive Raynaud's syndrome. J. Vasc. Surg., 5:38, 1987.

The authors describe abnormalities in platelet alpha₂-adrenoceptor levels in patients with Raynaud's syndrome. The number of measurable receptors in patients with vasospastic Raynaud's syndrome is significantly elevated over those seen in normal controls and patients with obstructive Raynaud's syndrome. Additionally, a series of experiments in which normal platelets are incubated in the serum from patients with Raynaud's syndrome is described. A decrease in measurable platelet alpha₂-adrenoceptor levels is noted, from which the authors hypothesize the possibility of a serum receptor–blocking substance.

Mills, J. L., Friedman, E. I., Taylor, L. M., Jr., and Porter, J. M.: Upper extremity ischemia caused by small artery disease. Ann. Surg., 206:521, 1987.

One hundred patients with ischemic digital ulceration are described in this article. The healing rate with local wound care and conservative débridement was 85 per cent. The authors conclude that the healing rate of digital ulcerations with conservative therapy is equal to or better than that reported after thoracic sympathectomy; thus sympathectomy should not be a routine adjunctive treatment of digital ulceration.

REFERENCES

1. Allen, E. V., and Brown, G. E.: Raynaud's disease: A critical review of minimal requisites for diagnosis. Am. J. Med. Sci., 183:187, 1932.
2. Blunt, R. J., and Porter, J. M.: Raynaud's syndrome. Semin. Arthritis Rheum., 10:282, 1981.
3. Brotzu, G., Carboni, M. G., Falchi, S., Montisci, R., and Petruzzo, P.: The role of presynaptic beta-receptors in Raynaud's disease. Artery, 13(2):77, 1985.
4. Brotzu, G., Susanna, F., Roberto, M., and Palmina, P.: Beta-blockers: A new therapeutic approach to Raynaud's disease. Microvasc. Res., 33:283, 1987.
5. Brotzu, G., Falchi, S., Mannu, B., Montisci, R., et al.: The importance of presynaptic beta receptors in Raynaud's disease. J. Vasc. Surg., 9:767, 1989.
6. Chatterjee, D. S., Petrie, A., and Taylor, W.: Prevalence of vibration-induced white finger in fluorspar mines in Weardale. Br. J. Indust. Med., 35:208, 1978.
7. Coffman, J. B., and Cohen, A. S.: Total and capillary fingertip blood flow in Raynaud's phenomenon. N. Engl. J. Med., 285:259, 1971.
8. deTakats, G., and Fowler, E. F.: Raynaud's phenomenon. J.A.M.A., 179:99, 1962.
9. de Trafford, J. C., Lafferty, K., Kitney, R. I., Cotton, L. T., and Roberts, V. C.: Modelling of the human thermal vasomotor control system and its application to the investigation of arterial disease. Proc. I.E.E., 129:A646, 1982.
10. Edwards, J. M., Phinney, E. S., Taylor, L. M., Jr., Keenan, E. J., and Porter, J. M.: Alpha-2 adrenoreceptor differences in vasospastic and obstructive Raynaud's syndrome. J. Vasc. Surg., 5:38, 1987.
11. Edwards, J. M., Harker, C. T., Taylor, L. M., Jr., and Porter, J. M.: Small artery disease of the upper extremity. In Machleder, H. I. (Ed.): Vascular Disorders of the Upper Extremity, 2nd ed. Mt. Kisco, New York, Futura Publishing Company, 1989, pp. 103–130.
12. Edwards, J. M., and Porter, J. M.: Associated diseases with Raynaud's syndrome. Vasc. Med. Rev., 1:51–58, 1990.
13. Flatt, A. E.: Digital artery sympathectomy. J. Hand Surg., 5:550, 1980.
14. Folich, E. D., Tarayi, R. C., and Duston, H. P.: Peripheral arterial insufficiency:

15. Gates, K. H., Tyburczy, J., Zupan, J., Baur, G. M., and Porter, J. M.: The non-invasive quantification of digital vasospasm. Bruit, 8:34, 1984.
16. Gifford, R. W., Jr., and Hines, E. A., Jr.: Raynaud's disease among women and girls. Circulation, 16:1012, 1957.
17. Hall, K. V., and Hillestad, L. K.: Raynaud's phenomenon treated with sympathectomy: A follow-up study of 28 patients. Angiology, 11:186, 1960.
18. Harris, E. J., Edwards, J. M., Taylor, L. M., and Porter, J. M.: Vibration arterial trauma. In Flanigan, D. P. (Ed.): Civilian Vascular Trauma. Philadelphia, Lea & Febiger, in press 1990.
19. Henry, L. G., Blackwood, J. S., Couley, J. E., et al.: Ergotism. Arch. Surg., 110:929, 1975.
20. Hirai, M.: Cold sensitivity of the hand in arterial occlusive disease. Surgery, 85:140, 1979.
21. Holling, H. E.: Digital ischemia. In Holling, H. E. (Ed.): Peripheral Vascular Disease: Diagnosis and Management. Philadelphia, J. B. Lippincott Company, 1972, pp. 137–161.
22. Holmgren, K., Baur, G. M., and Porter, J. M.: The role of digital photoplethysmography in the evaluation of Raynaud's syndrome. Bruit, 5:19, 1981.
23. Hutchinson, J.: Inherited liability to Raynaud's phenomenon with great proneness to chilblains — gradual increase of liability to paroxysmal and local asphyxia — acrosphacelus with scleroderma — cheeks affected. Arch. Surg., 4:312, 1893.
24. Hutchinson, J.: Raynaud's phenomenon. Med. Press Circ., 123:402, 1901.
25. Jamieson, G. G., Ludbrook, J., and Wilson, A.: Cold hypersensitivity in Raynaud's phenomenon. Circulation, 44:254, 1971.
26. Janoff, A. J., Phinney, E. S., and Porter, J. M.: Lumbar sympathectomy for lower extremity vasospasm. Am. J. Surg., 150:147, 1985.
27. Johnson, E. N., Summerly, R., and Birnstingl, M.: Prognosis in Raynaud's phenomenon after sympathectomy. Br. Med. J., 1:962, 1965.
28. Kahan, A., Weber, S., Amor, B., et al.: Nifedipine and Raynaud's phenomenon (Letter). Ann. Intern. Med., 94:546, 1981.
29. Keenan, E. J., and Porter, J. M.: Alpha-2 adrenergic receptors in platelets from patients with Raynaud's syndrome. Surgery, 94:204, 1983.
30. Kirch, W., Linder, H. R., Hutt, J. H., Ohnhaus, E. E., and Mahler, F.: Ketanserin versus nifedipine in secondary Raynaud's phenomenon. Vasa, 16:77, 1987.
31. Lafferty, K., de Trafford, J. C., Roberts, V. C., and Cotton, L. T.: Raynaud's phenomenon and thermal entrainment: An objective test. Br. Med. J., 286:90, 1983.
32. Langer, S. Z.: Presynaptic regulation of catecholamine release. Biochemistry, 23:793, 1974.
33. Lewis, T.: Experiments relating to the peripheral mechanism involved in spastic arrest of the circulation in the fingers, a variety of Raynaud's disease. Heart, 15:7, 1929.
34. Lewis, T., and Pickering, G. W.: Observations upon maladies in which the blood supply to digits ceases intermittent or permanently, and upon bilateral gangrene of the digits: Observation relevant to so-called "Raynaud's disease." Clin. Sci., 1:327, 1934.
35. MacKiewisz, A., and Piskorz, A.: Raynaud's phenomenon following long-term repeated action of great differences of temperature. J. Cardiovasc. Surg., 18:151, 1977.
36. McNamara, M. F., Takaki, H. S., Yao, J. S. T., et al.: A systematic approach to severe hand ischemia. Surgery, 83:1, 1978.
37. Mendlowitz, M., Naftchi, N.: The digital circulation of Raynaud's disease. Am. J. Cardiol., 4:580, 1959.
38. Mills, J. L., Friedman, E. I., Taylor, L. M., Jr., and Porter, J. M.: Upper extremity ischemia caused by small artery disease. Ann. Surg., 206:521, 1987.
39. Motulsky, H. F., and Insel, P. A.: Adrenergic receptors in man. N. Engl. J. Med., 307:18, 1982.
40. Muller-Schweinitzer, E.: Responsiveness of isolated canine cerebral and peripheral arteries to ergotamine. Arch. Pharmacol., 292:113, 1976.
41. Nielson, S. L., and Lassen, N. A.: Measurement of digital blood pressure after local cooling. J. Appl. Physiol., 43:907, 1977.
42. Olsen, N., and Nielsen, S. L.: Prevalence of primary Raynaud's phenomenon in young females. Scand. J. Clin. Lab. Invest., 37:761, 1978.
43. Porter, J. M.: Unpublished data, 1984.
44. Porter, J. M., Bardana, E. J., Baur, G. M., Wesche, D. H., et al.: The clinical significance of Raynaud's syndrome. Surgery, 80:756, 1976.
45. Porter, J. M., and Rivers, S. P.: Management of Raynaud's syndrome. In Bergan, J. J., and Yao, J. S. T. (Eds.): Evaluation and Treatment of Upper and Lower Extremity Vascular Disorders. Orlando, Grune & Stratton, 1984, pp. 181–202.
46. Porter, J. M., Rivers, S. P., and Anderson, C. J.: Evaluation and management of patients with Raynaud's syndrome. Am. J. Surg., 142:183, 1981.
47. Porter, J. M., Snider, R. L., Bardana, E. J., et al.: The diagnosis and treatment of Raynaud's phenomenon. Surgery, 77:11, 1975.
48. Porter, J. M., and Taylor, L. M.: Limb ischemia caused by small artery disease. World J. Surg., 7:326, 1983.
49. Raynaud, M.: On Local Asphyxia and Symmetrical Gangrene of the Extremities. Selected Monographs. London, New Sydenham Society, 1888.
50. Rivers, S. P., and Porter, J. M.: Treatment of Raynaud's syndrome. In Bergan, J. J. (Ed.): Arterial Surgery. Edinburgh, Churchill-Livingstone, 1984, pp. 185–202.
51. Roald, O. K., and Seem, E.: Treatment of Raynaud's phenomenon with ketan-

A complication of beta-adrenergic blocking therapy. J.A.M.A., 208:2471, 1969.

serin in patients with connective tissue disorders. Br. Med. J. [Clin. Res.], *289(6445)*:577, 1984.

52. Rosch, J., and Porter, J. M.: Cryodynamic hand angiography in the diagnosis and management of Raynaud's syndrome. Circulation, *55*:807, 1977.

53. Schmidt, F. E., and Hewitt, R. L.: Severe upper limb ischemia. Arch. Surg., *115*:1188, 1980.

54. Silcott, G. R., and Polich, V. L.: Palmar arch arterial reconstruction for the salvage of ischemic fingers. Am. J. Surg., *142*:219, 1981.

55. Smith, D. C., and McKendry, R. J.: Controlled trial of nifedipine in the treatment of Raynaud's phenomenon. Lancet, *2*:1299, 1982.

56. Spittell, J. A.: Raynaud's phenomenon and allied vasospastic conditions. *In* Fairbairn, J. F., Juergens, J. L., Spittell, J. A. (Eds.): Peripheral Vascular Diseases. Philadelphia, W. B. Saunders Company, 1972, pp. 387–419.

57. Stone, P. H., Autman, E. J., and Muller, J. E.: Calcium channel blocking agents in the treatment of cardiovascular disorders. Part II. Hemodynamic effects and clinical applications. Ann. Intern. Med., *93*:886, 1980.

58. Sumner, D. S., and Strandness, D. E.: An abnormal finger pulse associated with cold sensitivity. Ann. Surg., *175*:294, 1972.

59. Taylor, W., and Pelmear, P. L.: Raynaud's phenomenon of occupational origin: An epidemiological survey. Acta Chir. Scand. (Suppl.), *465*:27, 1976.

60. Taylor, L. M., Rivers, S. P., Keller, F. S., Porter, J. M., et al.: Treatment of finger ischemia with Bier block reserpine. Surg. Gynecol. Obstet., *154*:39, 1982.

61. Wilgis, E. F. S.: Evaluation and treatment of chronic digital ischemia. Ann. Surg., *193*:693, 1981.

13. CIRCULATORY PROBLEMS OF THE UPPER EXTREMITY

Donald Silver, M.D.

Arterial Insufficiency

Approximately 1 per cent of patients with peripheral vascular disorders have symptoms of upper extremity ischemia.[7] However, 17 per cent of patients studied angiographically had a greater than 30 per cent stenosis of the innominate and subclavian arteries.[4] The low frequency of symptoms in upper extremities with arterial stenoses is related to the rich collateral network, the small muscle mass, and the intermittent work requirements of the upper extremities.

Arterial flow to the upper extremity may be reduced by atherosclerotic stenoses or occlusions, thromboembolism, trauma, tumor, inflammatory processes (e.g., Takayasu's arteritis, Buerger's disease, and the like), and compression of the subclavian-axillary arteries in the region of the thoracic outlet. Atherosclerotic or embolic occlusions and aneurysms occur less frequently in the upper extremities than in the lower extremities, whereas vasospastic disorders and arteritis occur more frequently. Symptomatic atherosclerotic occlusions most commonly involve the subclavian or innominate arteries. Axillary and brachial arterial atherosclerotic occlusions are the next most frequent. The small arteries of the hands and fingers, in addition to being involved with atherosclerotic occlusions, are most often affected by vasospastic disorders, frostbite, drugs (e.g., ergot), hematologic disorders (e.g., thrombocytosis, polycythemia), and distal embolization.

Traumatic injuries to the upper extremity arteries occur about one fifth as often as do injuries to the arteries of the lower extremities.[3] Penetrating arterial injuries occur slightly more often in the upper extremities (53 per cent),[12] whereas vascular injuries from blunt trauma, usually associated with fractures or dislocation, occur most often in the lower extremities (89 per cent).[3] The injured arteries may be partially or totally disrupted or compressed. If the intima is torn by the sudden stretching of an artery, blood flow may lift the intima and produce a dissection, or "intimal flap" obstruction. Penetrating wounds to the arteries frequently penetrate adjacent veins and may produce arteriovenous fistulas.

Emboli are an increasingly common cause of arterial insufficiency, with 3 to 5 per cent of all arterial emboli lodging in the upper extremities. Emboli usually lodge at sites of arterial bifur-

cation or reduction of arterial diameters, with the majority of the emboli lodging in the axillary and brachial arteries.[2] A single embolus to the palmar or digital arteries is not likely to cause significant symptoms, but repeated embolization to these vessels may lead to ulceration and digital gangrene. Since most emboli arise in the heart, the incidence of thromboembolic occlusion of the upper extremity parallels the increasing number of geriatric patients with their cardiac problems. Brachial and axillary cardiac catheterizations also cause thrombotic occlusions of the respective arteries in approximately 0.5 per cent of the cases.[13]

The subclavian or axillary arteries or both may be compressed as they course through the thoracic outlet and (1) may be asymptomatic; (2) may cause intermittent ischemia or symptoms similar to those seen in Raynaud's syndrome; (3) may develop poststenotic aneurysmal dilatation; and (4) when there is major compression or embolization of a mural thrombus, may cause significant ischemia of the distal portion of the extremity.

Arteritis is being recognized with increased frequency as a cause of upper extremity and hand ischemia. The larger proximal arteries may be obstructed by idiopathic medial arteriopathy, giant cell arteritis or idiopathic arteritis, whereas the palmar and digital arteries are more frequently affected by collagen-related vasculitis (Fig. 1). The diagnosis may require arterial biopsy for confirmation. Management includes specific treatment of the identified arteritis with steroids and, at times, immunosuppression. If significant ischemia of the fingers and/or hand persists, arterial bypass, usually with a vein graft, is indicated. The graft should not be placed in a portion of the arteries involved with the inflammatory process.

A careful history and physical examination, supplemented by appropriate roentgenograms and angiograms, should document the site and extent of an arterial occlusion and provide some indication of the etiology of the insufficiency.

Asymptomatic or minimally symptomatic arterial occlusions usually require no therapy other than prolonged "antiplatelet therapy," e.g., 325 mg. of aspirin twice daily, to reduce the

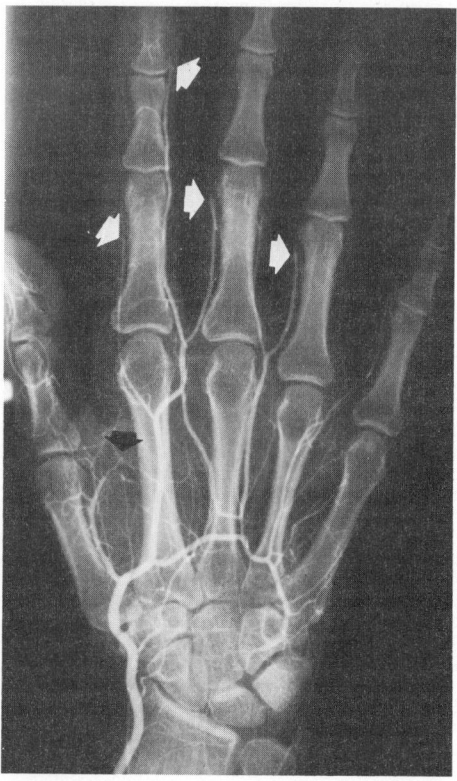

Figure 1. Arteriogram with magnification in a patient with scleroderma and Raynaud's phenomenon. Note absence of ulnar artery and superficial palmar arch. Several digital arteries are occluded (arrows).

incidence of thrombosis. The patient should be instructed to avoid injury to the ischemic parts and to use skin creams to keep the skin pliable. Symptomatic occlusions are treated according to the etiology, i.e., an embolus can usually be extracted using local anesthesia and an embolectomy catheter; compression in the thoracic outlet should be relieved, when necessary, with repair or replacement of the damaged artery; vein grafts may be utilized to bypass chronic occlusions; and vein patches may be utilized to enlarge short areas of stenoses. Infusions of fibrinolytic agents have restored patency to vessels obstructed by thromboembolism. The infusion is maintained until lysis occurs, but rarely longer than 3 to 4 days, and is followed with anticoagulant therapy. Causes of the thromboembolism should be corrected to prevent recurrences. If the source of the embolus can not be eliminated, long-term anticoagulation with warfarin is required. Innominate and subclavian artery occlusions can be readily bypassed with extrathoracic grafts with a low mortality, lasting patency, and relief of symptoms.[5] Traumatic vascular injuries usually require prompt angiography and restoration of flow, because frequently there has not been a previous stimulus to collateral development.

Principles of repair of traumatic vascular injuries include reducing associated dislocations, stabilizing associated fractures, and débridement of the injured artery with an end-to-end repair or an interposition vein graft. All associated significant venous injuries should also be repaired, either primarily or with a vein graft.

Venous Insufficiency

The manifestations of venous insufficiency include edema, distention of superficial veins, tightness, aching, a reddish blue discoloration, and pain. Edema of the upper extremity from venous insufficiency is most often caused by occlusion of the axillary, subclavian, or innominate veins, or the superior vena cava. More distal venous occlusions rarely produce significant edema or chronic symptoms.

Tumors, mediastinal fibrosis, and trauma are the traditional causes of thrombosis in the large central veins. However, indwelling catheters for central cardiovascular monitoring, intravenous nutrition, or chemotherapy are producing increasing numbers of thromboses of these veins. Thromboses of the distal veins most often follow intravenous infusions.

Thrombosis of the axillary or subclavian vein that occurs after effort or strain[9] has been called "effort thrombosis." This thrombosis occurs in the dominant arm of a young or middleaged healthy individual. It usually occurs immediately after the effort, but onset may be delayed several hours. A history of effort or strain with the arm abducted can be obtained in most patients. Many of the cases of effort thrombosis were probably caused by compression of the axillary vein by the pectoralis minor tendon, by the costocoracoid ligament, or between the clavicle and first rib and therefore could be considered manifestations of the thoracic outlet syndrome.

Some patients in whom edema develops after effort do not have demonstrable thrombosis of veins. Their phlebograms usually demonstrate areas of compression of the axillary and subclavian veins in the area of the thoracic outlet. The edema, which primarily follows chronic compression and secondarily the patient's efforts, may be effectively treated by eliminating the site(s) of venous compression.

The presence and extent of venous thrombosis should be documented by phlebography. When proximal venous obstructions are present, the distal venous pressures, with the patient supine and the extremity at the right atrial level, are elevated above the normal pressure of 8 to 12 cm. of saline.

Management of the patient with venous obstruction without thrombosis includes eliminating the cause of the obstruction. For those patients with the thoracic outlet syndrome, this includes improvement of posture, avoiding positions of hyperabduction, and, if symptoms persist, offering a scalenectomy and/

or first rib resection with, frequently, division of the pectoralis minor tendon. Those patients who present with acute thrombotic obstruction of their axillary-subclavian veins should receive fibrinolytic therapy, e.g., urokinase, streptokinase, or tissue plasminogen activator, to restore patency of the veins. The fibrinolytic therapy is followed by heparin for a few days and then by long-term anticoagulation with warfarin until the causes of the compression can be eliminated.

Many patients with thromboses of the veins in the upper extremities are treated with elevation and heparin (provided there are no contraindications) in sufficient amounts to prolong the activated partial thromboplastin time to twice the control. Heparin is given as a constant infusion for 8 to 10 days; it is continued for a longer period if symptoms persist or the edema does not resolve. After the acute process is controlled, the patient is maintained on self-injected subcutaneous heparin, 5000 units every 8 hours, or warfarin for 3 to 4 months to allow recanalization to occur.

Although thrombectomy must be employed to reduce the sequelae of venous thromboses,[8] most vascular surgeons use thrombectomy only if fibrinolytic agents or elevation and anticoagulation fail to restore the circulation and tissue perfusion remains altered, with gangrene imminent. Symptoms caused by proximal thrombotic obstructions can be relieved with saphenous vein bypasses of the obstruction, e.g., axillary-jugular bypass, brachial-subclavian bypass, and the like.

Lymphedema

Primary lymphedema of an upper extremity is extremely rare. Secondary lymphedema has occurred in up to 10 per cent of women who have had radical mastectomies, frequently with radiation, for breast cancer and is a potential complication of any axillary dissection. The incidence of lymphedema of the upper extremity has decreased with the advent of less radical resections for breast cancer.

Most often lymphedema can be controlled with elevation, elastic sleeves, salt restriction, good skin care, and prompt management of infection. Lymphedema resistant to these simple measures most often can be controlled by frequent use, 2 to 6 times a day, of a lymphedema pump. Uncontrollable edema is usually treated with operative procedures for improving lymph flow and/or reducing the size of the extremity.

Causalgia

In 1872, Mitchell coined the term "causalgia" to describe the burning, agonizing pain and vasomotor disturbances that occur in 2 to 5 per cent of patients after peripheral nerve injuries.[10] The pain of causalgia varies in intensity and is exacerbated by touching or moving the involved body part, changes in temperature, pressure changes, or local irritants. The pain may become so agonizing that complete cessation of motion of the involved extremity ensues.

Sympathetic blockade is an excellent diagnostic and therapeutic procedure, because it usually provides complete relief from pain and allows the use of the previously guarded limb. The vasomotor changes also are usually completely relieved by the blockade. In a few patients, lasting relief is provided by a single sympathetic blockade; other patients require repeated blocks to obtain complete relief. However, if sympathetic blocks provide only temporary relief, operative sympathetic denervation should be performed with the expectation that symptoms will be relieved. Active physical therapy is an important part of the postsympathectomy management.[11]

Posttraumatic Reflex Dystrophy

In some patients, causalgia-like pain develops following an injury to the soft tissues and/or a bone of the extremity in which there is no demonstrable nerve damage. In addition to the pain, there may be edema, vasomotor disturbances, soft tissue dystrophy, and atrophy of bone in the region or distal to the injury.

The process may follow minimal trauma, such as a sprain, or an infection and occasionally occurs after thrombophlebitis, burns, spinal anesthesia, or herniation of a nucleus pulposus. The syndrome has also been described after angina, myocardial infarction, stroke, and vascular disorders. The process is called post-traumatic reflex sympathetic dystrophy, or Sudeck's atrophy because of the description of bone atrophy by Sudeck in 1900.[16]

Treatment consists of treating the local injury with supportive measures: local heat, analgesics, and so forth. Sympathetic blockade may be necessary to control the pain before physical therapy is initiated and may have to be repeated several times. Early sympathetic blockades and physical therapy are the mainstays of therapy. The majority of patients recover completely with these supportive measures. However, if the supportive measures do not completely relieve the symptoms, medical treatment with alpha-adrenergic blocking agents or surgical sympathetic denervation of the involved extremity is indicated. Physical therapy is a very important adjunct to sympathetic denervation.[11]

Acrocyanosis

Acrocyanosis is characterized by painless coldness and cyanosis of the distal portions of the extremities. It is caused by constant spasm of the small arteries in response to an overactive vasomotor system. The condition should be easily differentiated from Raynaud's disease by careful history and physical examination. Treatment consists only of protection from cold in mild cases or sympathectomy, which usually provides complete relief from symptoms in severe cases.

Erythromelalgia

Erythromelalgia is characterized by a burning sensation in the extremities that is associated with local warmth and a reddish or cyanotic color of the skin of the affected part. It occurs most often in middle-aged men and women during times of exposure to increased heat and/or activity. It may be primary or secondary, occurring in patients with hypertension, myeloproliferative disorder, diabetes, or gout. Treatment of secondary erythromelalgia should be directed toward eliminating the underlying disorder. Treatment of primary erythromelalgia is symptomatic: local cooling and reduction of body temperature. Aspirin has been beneficial in relieving symptoms in patients with erythromelalgia and thrombocythemia.[6] Chemical sympathetic blockade may temporarily alleviate the symptoms. Surgical sympathectomy of the involved extremity provides favorable-to-excellent relief of symptoms.[14,17]

SELECTED REFERENCES

Rich, N. M., and Spencer, F. C.: Vascular Trauma. Philadelphia, W. B. Saunders Company, 1978.
   This comprehensive text of vascular trauma has several nicely written and illustrated chapters devoted to trauma of the vessels of the upper extremity.

Rutherford, R. B.: Vascular Surgery, 3rd ed. Philadelphia, W. B. Saunders Company, 1989.
   This comprehensive text of vascular surgery, which belongs in the library of all vascular surgeons, clearly defines many of the vascular disorders affecting the upper extremities.

REFERENCES

1. Adams, J. T., DeWeese, J. A., Mahoney, E. B., and Rob, C. G.: Intermittent subclavian vein obstruction without thrombosis. Surgery, 63:147, 1968.
2. Bernstein, E. J.: What's new in upper extremity ischemia. In Najarian, J. S., and Delaney, J. P. (Eds.): Advances in Vascular Surgery. Chicago, Year Book Medical Publishers, 1983, p. 435.
3. Bishara, R. A., Pasch, A. R., Lim, L. T., et al.: Improved results in the treatment of civilian vascular injuries associated with fractures and dislocations. J. Vasc. Surg., 3:707, 1986.
4. Fields, W. S., and Lemak, N. A.: Joint study of extracranial arterial occlusion. JAMA, 222:1139, 1972.
5. Finkelstein, N. M., Byer, A., and Rush, B. F., Jr.: Subclavian-subclavian bypass for the subclavian steal syndrome. Surgery, 71:142, 1972.
6. Harrison, R., Letz, G., Pasternak, G., et al.: Fulminant hepatic failure after occupational exposure to 2-nitropropane. Ann. Intern. Med., 107:466, 1987.
7. Jones, T. W., Thomas, G. I., and Edmark, K. W.: Thoracocervical occlusive disease. Am. Surg., 33:535, 1967.
8. Mahorner, H., Castleberry, J. W., and Coleman, W. O.: Attempts to restore function in major veins which are the site of massive thrombosis. Ann. Surg., 146:510, 1957.
9. Matas, R.: On so-called primary thrombosis of the axillary vein caused by strain. Am. J. Surg., 24:642, 1934.
10. Mitchell, S. E.: Injuries of Nerves and Their Consequences. Philadelphia, J. B. Lippincott Company, 1872.
11. Painter, P., and Blackburn, G.: Exercise for patients with chronic disease. Postgrad. Med., 83:185, 1988.
12. Pasch, A. R., Bishara, R. A., Lim, T. L., et al.: Optimal limb salvage in penetrating civilian vascular trauma. J. Vasc. Surg., 3:189, 1986.
13. Ross, R. S.: Cooperative study on cardiac catheterization. Arterial complications. Circulation, 37(Suppl. 3):67, 1968.
14. Shumacker, H. B., Jr.: Sympathetic denervation of the extremities. Curr. Probl. Surg., July 1965.
15. Snider, R., Porter, J. M., and Eidemiller, L. R.: Axillary-axillary artery bypass for the correction of subclavian artery occlusive disease. Ann. Surg., 180:888, 1974.
16. Sudeck, P.: Über die acute entzudliche Knochenatrophie. Arch. Klin. Cir., 62:147, 1900 (cited in Allen, E. V., Baker, N. W., and Hines, E. A., Jr.: Peripheral Vascular Diseases, 3rd ed. Philadelphia, W. B. Saunders Company, 1962, p. 459).
17. Telford, E. D.: Discussion on peripheral vascular lesions. Proc. R. Soc. Med., 37:621, 1944.

14. VISCERAL ISCHEMIC SYNDROMES: OBSTRUCTION OF THE SUPERIOR MESENTERIC ARTERY, CELIAC AXIS, AND INFERIOR MESENTERIC ARTERY

John J. Bergan, M.D.

Interference with the blood supply to specific organs produces a constellation of symptoms that may be described as a syndrome. This is true of the renal arterial bed, the cerebral arterial bed, and the intestinal blood supply. When visceral ischemia is produced, the syndrome may be either acute or primarily a chronic illness.

Chronic Visceral Ischemia

Symptoms of chronic visceral ischemia were recognized in the early part of the current century, but surgical recognition began in the mid-1930s with the landmark presentation by Dunphy.[17] His review of autopsy cases at the Peter Bent Brigham Hospital emphasized that chronic, recurrent abdominal pain might precede fatal intestinal infarction. Not until 20 years later was revascularization for intestinal angina suggested and then accomplished.[31,40]

The most common cause of chronic occlusion of the unpaired vessels to the intestines is atherosclerosis. In addition, the celiac axis may be markedly narrowed by the arcuate ligament or low-lying crura of the diaphragm. Because collateral circulation is well developed throughout the stomach and small bowel, severe stenosis or actual occlusion of one, or sometimes two, mesenteric arteries is well tolerated. Major collateral blood flow develops through the anterior and posterior pancreatoduodenal arteries, which form arcades with other unnamed vessels on the anterior and posterior surfaces of the head of the pancreas.

Two major points of collateralization of the superior mesenteric artery are of importance. The first is through arcades of the proximal jejunum, which connect to the celiac circulation through the aforementioned rich arterial blood supply. Inferiorly is the second collateral of importance. Here, the superior mesenteric artery collateralizes with the inferior mesenteric artery through the arc of Riolan and the ascending branch of the left colic artery, which takes its origin from the inferior mesenteric artery.

RARE CAUSES OF ISCHEMIA. Although atherosclerotic occlusion of the origins of the three named intestinal vessels is the most common form of chronic intestinal ischemia encountered by surgeons, it is necessary to consider other elements in the differential diagnosis. These include polyarteritis nodosa,[30] Kawasaki's syndrome,[23] drug abuse arteritis (amphetamine),[13] and Cogan's syndrome.[26]

Other rare causes of chronic intestinal ischemia include idiopathic aneurysm formation, allergic vasculitis, radiation arteritis, rheumatoid arteritis, systemic sclerosis, and lupus erythematosus.[44] Fibromuscular hyperplasia of the celiac axis and superior mesenteric artery has been reported,[38] as has mesenteric artery stenosis due to methysergide.[9]

An important cause of chronic intestinal ischemia leading to mesenteric infarction is the condition of intimal hyperplasia of visceral arteries leading to thrombosis in young women taking oral contraceptives and indulging in heavy cigarette smoking.[25] In these patients, the oral contraceptive contains a high concentration of estrogens and progestogens. Most important, the risk from these compounds increases with long-term use but not with age of the patient.

Peristalsis has a great influence upon mesenteric blood flow. This is important in understanding the origin of pain in intestinal ischemia. During intestinal contraction, arterial inflow decreases; during relaxation, blood flow increases. Strong contractions markedly decrease arterial inflow, especially those producing an intraluminal pressure of 30 mm. Hg or greater. Occlusions of intestinal arteries at their origins decrease distal perfusion pressure. During peristalsis, arterial inflow is decreased further as the extraluminal pressure exceeds perfusion pressure. The normal response of intestinal musculature to ischemia is intense spasm, which, in turn, further reduces arterial flow. The patient's interpretation of these events is a nauseating cramp or diffuse abdominal pain.

CLINICAL FINDINGS. The only constant finding in patients with symptomatic chronic intestinal ischemia is weight loss.[6] Because the first successful cases of intestinal revascularization emanated from the Nutrition Clinic of the Massachusetts General Hospital, malabsorption studies in the past have dominated clinical investigations of chronic intestinal ischemia. These studies showed that chronic intestinal ischemia was not associated with malabsorption of fat, nitrogen, total solids, d-xylose, carotene, vitamin B_{12}, or various radiolabeled substances.

Careful clinical observation of affected patients shows that the pain intensity after they eat is sufficiently great that caloric intake is decreased. Such food habits are known as "the small meal syndrome" or "food fear." Clinically, this is referred to as "postprandial pain." The natural history of this syndrome correlates well with Dunphy's 1936 observations.[17] Pain-free intervals that occur between meals shorten until aching abdominal pain is almost constant, and this is followed by intestinal infarction.

Various intestinal symptoms have been ascribed to chronic intestinal ischemia, but these are inconstant. Patients may exhibit diarrhea or constipation.[35] Occult blood may or may not be present in the stool. In contrast, coronary arterial occlusive disease is commonly found and peripheral atherosclerotic occlusive disease seen.

It is of fundamental importance to appreciate that a patient's appearance as a result of severe, chronic weight loss mimics malignant cachexia. Therefore, investigations of severe weight loss and abdominal pain that fail to reveal pancreatic carcinoma, gastric carcinoma, or chronic penetrating duodenal ulcer should lead the thoughtful physician to the diagnosis of chronic intestinal ischemia.

Endoscopy, performed to aid diagnosis of obscure abdominal pain and weight loss, may reveal superficial gastric or duodenal ulceration. This must not be considered as the cause of the pain and weight loss, and other investigations must be pursued.

If the combination of weight loss, absence of malignant disease, and presence of symptomatic arteriosclerotic occlusive disease suggests chronic visceral ischemia, duplex ultrasound scanning of the intestinal arteries can be accomplished.[27] Such examinations are accurate, revealing, and highly acceptable to the patient.

Ultimately, angiography confirms the clinical diagnosis and findings of ultrasound duplex scanning. Lateral films during aortic injection best demonstrate the obstructive lesions at the origin of the mesenteric vessels. Anteroposterior projections demonstrate the arc of Riolan connection (Figs. 1 and 2) of superior mesenteric arterial branches to the inferior mesenteric artery arcades. This connection elongates and dilates because of increased wall shear stress in response to increased blood flow. This elongated, tortuous vessel has been named the "meandering mesenteric artery."

Traditionally, chronic mesenteric ischemia has been thought to occur only with two or more intestinal artery occlusions. Nevertheless, single occlusions, such as celiac axis crus compression, may produce all the manifestations of chronic intestinal ischemia and will respond to arterial reconstruction.

SURGICAL CORRECTION OF CHRONIC VISCERAL ISCHEMIA. Many differing surgical techniques have evolved and have been advocated to correct visceral arterial obstructive disease, although no single technique has emerged to be definitive.[14,21,22,24,37] Although these disparate operations have included open endarterectomy, reimplantation of visceral vessels, bypass operations from the infrarenal aorta to visceral arteries or from the suprarenal aorta to visceral arteries, as well as bypasses from the iliac artery, certain trends can be detected. These are that multiple intestinal artery reconstructions are more effective than single reconstructions, and that a supraceliac origin of reconstructions may be superior to other bypass techniques. Thromboendarterectomy is important historically, but it demands a thoracoabdominal approach in which the aorta is cross-clamped above and below the major visceral arteries. In this procedure, a U-shaped aortotomy is created surrounding the orifices of the celiac axis and superior mesenteric artery. The atheroma is removed by means of an extraction and eversion endarterectomy, which may be combined with renal thromboendarterectomy.[42] Most surgeons favor aortovisceral bypass techniques, not endarterectomy. In these, autogenous vein or prosthetic grafts can be used alternatively. A transabdominal approach is used, and the better of the two segments of the aorta, either above the celiac axis or below the renal arteries, is used for graft origin. An undiseased aortic segment, usually superior to the celiac trunk, is absolutely necessary for graft origin.[46] Results of reconstruction for chronic visceral ischemia are generally favorable; however, the greatest number of failures is reported with superior mesenteric artery endarterectomy or mesenteric artery reimplantation.[36]

Celiac Artery Compression

Special mention must be made of this particular entity. Angiographic findings indicate that the celiac artery is frequently compressed by bands originating from the diaphragmatic crura.[23] Patients thus affected rarely have symptoms but do demonstrate an epigastric bruit. However, when collateral circulation to the celiac territory is inadequate, symptoms of intestinal ischemia may manifest as postprandial pain and severe weight loss. This syndrome was first suggested in 1965[16] but eventually was refuted by follow-up of the original group of

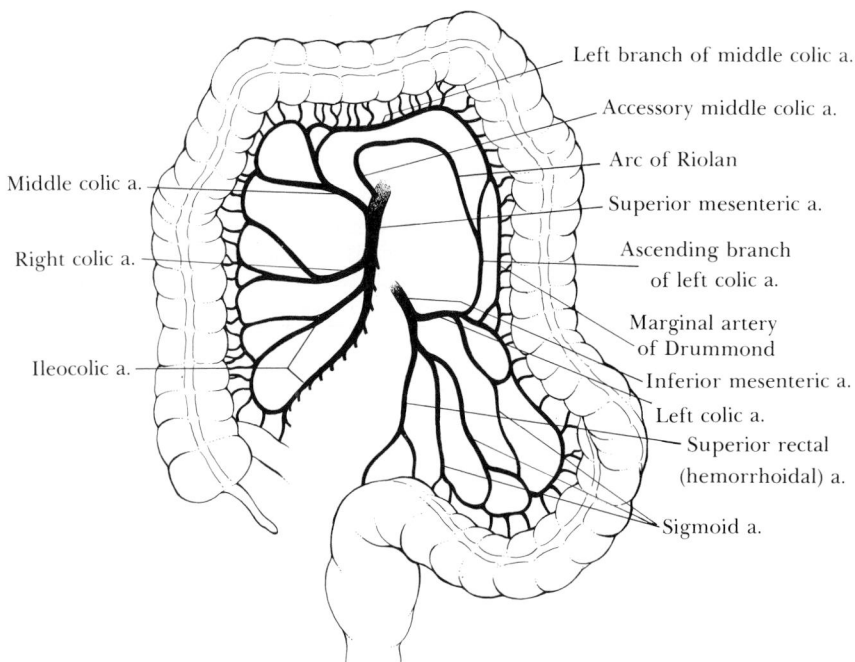

Left branch of middle colic a.

Accessory middle colic a.

Arc of Riolan

Superior mesenteric a.

Ascending branch
   of left colic a.

Marginal artery
   of Drummond

Inferior mesenteric a.

Left colic a.

Superior rectal
   (hemorrhoidal) a.

Sigmoid a.

Middle colic a.

Right colic a.

Ileocolic a.

Figure 1. This diagram illustrates the normal anatomy of the superior and inferior mesenteric arterial arborizations. The arc of Riolan is indicated separate from the marginal artery of Drummond. (From Ruzicka, F. F., Jr., and Rossi, P.: Normal vascular anatomy of the abdominal viscera. Radiol. Clin. North Am., 8:3, 1970.)

treated patients.[20] Since that time, it has been recognized that young women with nonspecific intestinal complaints and weight loss may show a deficient collateral bed upon selective mesenteric arteriography. In these patients, reconstruction of the celiac artery may relieve symptoms.

Acute Mesenteric Infarction

As an appreciation has developed of the differences between embolic occlusion of the mesenteric artery and thrombotic occlusion of mesenteric arteries, it has become increasingly possible to achieve accurate diagnosis of mesenteric infarction. Accurate diagnosis means that precise surgical therapy allows salvage of ischemic gut and eventually decreases mortality of this dangerous condition. From the 1895 report of Elliott[18] to 1950, the only treatment for intestinal infarction was resection.[33] The modern era of vascular surgery after 1950 was characterized by rapid advances in revascularization of chronic and acute ischemia of the extremities. However, intestinal revascularization did not advance, and even in the late 1980s the mortality in treating this condition remained over 85 per cent.[45] Now, the principle of revascularization of acutely ischemic in-

testine prior to resection has been established. Therefore, an aggressive diagnostic approach is justified.[7] Further decreases in mortality depend upon a thorough understanding of the pathophysiology of acute mesenteric infarction.

PATHOPHYSIOLOGY. Clinically, all forms of acute mesenteric arterial occlusion produce the same effects. These are severe abdominal pain commonly disproportionate to physical findings, profound leukocytosis generally in excess of 14,000 leukocytes per cu. mm., except in aged patients unable to mount such a leukocytosis, and gut emptying characterized by vomiting and defecation.[1] Later, all such patients manifest melena coincident with peritonitis and subsequent death.[5]

Grossly, the first changes that occur are an intense muscular contraction of the smooth muscle of the bowel, with the appearance of accordion-pleats and bluish white rippling of the seromuscular surfaces.[3] As necrosis of the intestine proceeds from the mucosa outward to involve the seromuscular layers, a peritoneal reaction occurs and the clinical state becomes that of a desperate illness, with gross intestinal distention, ileus, exquisite tenderness, and a characteristic fetid odor on the breath. Anxiety, restlessness, air hunger, and cyanosis appear as the

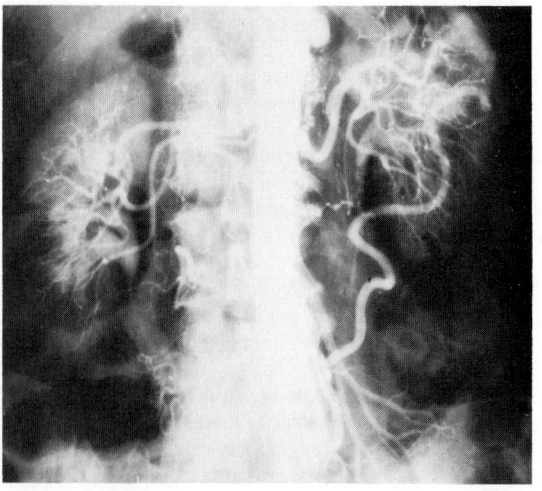

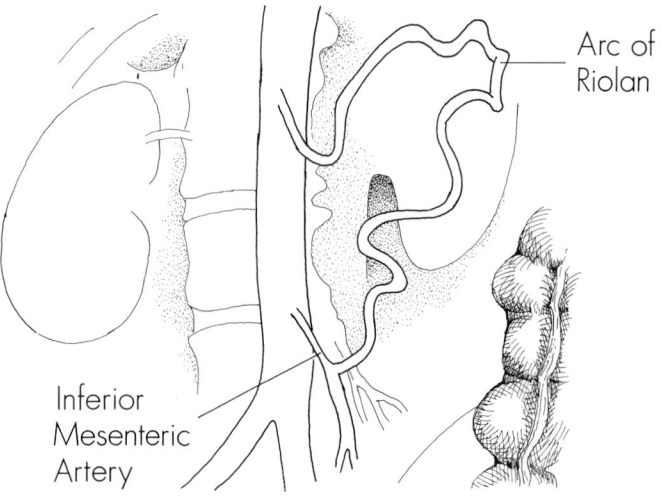

Arc of
Riolan

Inferior
Mesenteric
Artery

Figure 2. The arc of Riolan is an important collateral vessel to the superior mesenteric vascular bed. Its appearance on an anteroposterior abdominal angiogram is an indication of mesenteric artery occlusion.

patient becomes profoundly acidotic, anuric, and dehydrated. Multiorgan and multisystem failure ensues. No specific serum diagnostic studies are helpful. Serum inorganic phosphate elevations, reported by some, occur only when the patient is in renal failure.[32]

When acute intestinal ischemia occurs, Bulkley has described the situation as "... a balance between aggressive luminal toxins including acid, digestive enzymes, bacteria, and bacterial endo- and exotoxins pitted against the gastrointestinal mucosal barrier."[10] Bulkley further suggests that the damage observed subsequent to the ischemic interval is in excess of that to be expected from ischemia alone and postulates that reperfusion injury has a strong part in the failure of intestinal revascularization to salvage gut and the patient. It is hypothesized that toxic free radical metabolites of oxygen, triggered by the generation of superperoxide from activated xanthine oxidase at the time of reperfusion, are responsible for much of the injury that follows ischemia. Bulkley also suggests that treatment of this reperfusion injury may be a substantial contribution to therapy of multiple organ failure in these patients.

Electron microscopic changes occur within 10 minutes of arterial occlusion, but more than 30 minutes of total ischemia is required for extensive abnormalities to occur.[12] Mitochondria are the first organelles to show damage. Fluid begins to accumulate in the infranuclear portion of the cells, and these cells begin to show a washed-out appearance.[8] The simultaneous development of intracellular fluid leads to epithelial slough.

If the cell is to survive this insult, a conversion from aerobic to anaerobic metabolism is mandatory. After brief ischemia, changes in the rough and smooth endoplasmic reticulum are seen. The smooth endoplasmic reticulum is primarily responsible for maintaining a high concentration of glucose-6-phosphatase, but it is the rough endoplasmic reticulum that is concerned with reconstituting amino acids into proteins. Lysosomal membranes remain intact, and this is indicated clinically by failure to demonstrate such enzymes in the circulating blood until bowel necrosis occurs.[43] Ultimately, when lysosomal membranes rupture, autolytic enzymes are released that, by injuring adjacent cells, lead to a vicious cycle of continuing intestinal death.

Much later, gross signs of hemorrhage into the mesentery are seen, and the well-known clinical features of hemorrhagic infarction are manifest. The bowel wall becomes swollen and infiltrated with blood, and the mucosa becomes necrotic. Purulent peritonitis develops; histologically, the pattern is that of hemorrhagic necrosis, extensive submucosal edema, and cellular digestion from the luminal surface outward. Simultaneous with this is increased permeability of the intestinal wall to bacteria and a bidirectional flow of fluid producing massive intraluminal loss of plasma and fluid.[39]

Finally, successful revascularization of bowel is dependent upon knowledge that the pathophysiologic changes just cited affect the mucosa of the bowel far more than the seromuscular layers. Clinically, the appearance of the small bowel may be deceptive. The bowel may appear nonviable even though revascularization allows return of viability and eventual regeneration of mucosa.[15]

Superior Mesenteric Artery Embolization

Superior mesenteric artery embolization remains the most common cause of surgically treatable intestinal infarction.[34] The diagnostic triad consists of (1) severe abdominal pain in a patient with (2) a cardiac lesion that might produce embolization, followed by (3) gut emptying, vomiting, and defecation. To this can be added the history of a previous embolic event, present in more than one third of patients, and the severe leukocytosis referred to earlier. Thus, a clinical diagnosis of mesenteric embolus can be made without sophisticated testing.

The cardiac lesion responsible for embolization is atheroscle-rosis in two thirds of patients, rheumatic heart disease in patients seen in the remote past, and cardiomyopathy of atherosclerotic or alcoholic origin in recent times.

Diagnostic confirmation by angiography is recommended. Ultrasound duplex scans are flawed by the presence of intestinal gas. On the angiogram, the embolus is found distal to the origin of the mesenteric artery, where a classic mercury meniscus sign may be seen. In this location, a number of proximal collateral channels progressing to the jejunum are identifiable. Occasionally, these jejunal arteries and arcades may provide a spontaneous bypass of the embolic occlusion and a cure of the acute ischemia. This should not be anticipated.

SURGICAL TREATMENT. A standard vascular exposure of the abdominal contents is utilized and the bowel inspected. The upper portion of jejunum in the region of the ligament of Treitz may be found to be normal, with pulsatile arcade vessels. Variable lengths of distal intestine are ischemic; initially, these are gray; later, they are dark and hemorrhagic (Fig. 3). The mesenteric artery is palpated in the mesentery of the small bowel, and the point of cessation of pulsations becomes a focus of surgical exposure. When the mesenteric artery is freed of investing tissues and under control, a transverse arteriotomy and embolectomy with a Fogarty catheter can be done.[2]

Following restoration of blood flow, pulsations return in marginal vessels, and, after an appropriate period of time, judgment is made regarding whether or not intestine should be resected. Aids to assess bowel viability are numerous and include Doppler examination and intravenous fluorescein.[11]

A second-look procedure to ensure maintenance of bowel viability is an important consideration in acute intestinal revascularization. The decision for a second-look procedure must be made at the time of the primary operation, because no clinical findings assist in judgment later. Following abdominal closure, vigorous resuscitative efforts must continue, with restoration of blood and fluid volume and correction of acidosis.

Vigorous resuscitation should allow continual improvement in the patient's physical condition from the time of primary and secondary surgical therapy. Frequently, patients exhibit deterioration in their physical condition because of repetitive embolization, recurrent mesenteric infarction, or dehiscence of bowel anastomosis. Therefore, rapid return to the operating room and/or repeat aortography may be required in the early postoperative period.[28]

Acute Mesenteric Artery Thrombosis

It would be illogical to assume that patients with mesenteric artery embolization would have premonitory intestinal symptoms. In contrast, patients with acute mesenteric artery thrombosis are those in whom postprandial pain and profound weight loss may have occurred. This is important because unlike superior mesenteric artery embolization, the syndrome of acute mesenteric artery thrombosis has an insidious onset with progressively worsening steady or colicky abdominal pain. This is the pain of intestinal spasm, and initially the pain is disproportionate to the physical findings. Fully half of such patients give a history of prior intestinal ischemia manifested by weight loss; pain; and perhaps altered bowel habits, including constipation from lack of eating and diarrhea from an increase in velocity of intestinal motility. Many such patients have manifestations of other atherosclerotic occlusive disease, including extremity ischemia and ischemic brain and heart disease.

Following the development of constant abdominal pain with or without gut emptying, the syndrome progresses and is characterized by systemic hypovolemia; hemoconcentration; interstitial fluid extravasation into the splanchnic bed; and, as the bowel dies, abdominal distention, further vomiting, and bloody diarrhea.[29] As the syndrome progresses, profound leukocytosis is seen. Fever and other signs of sepsis indicate the onset of

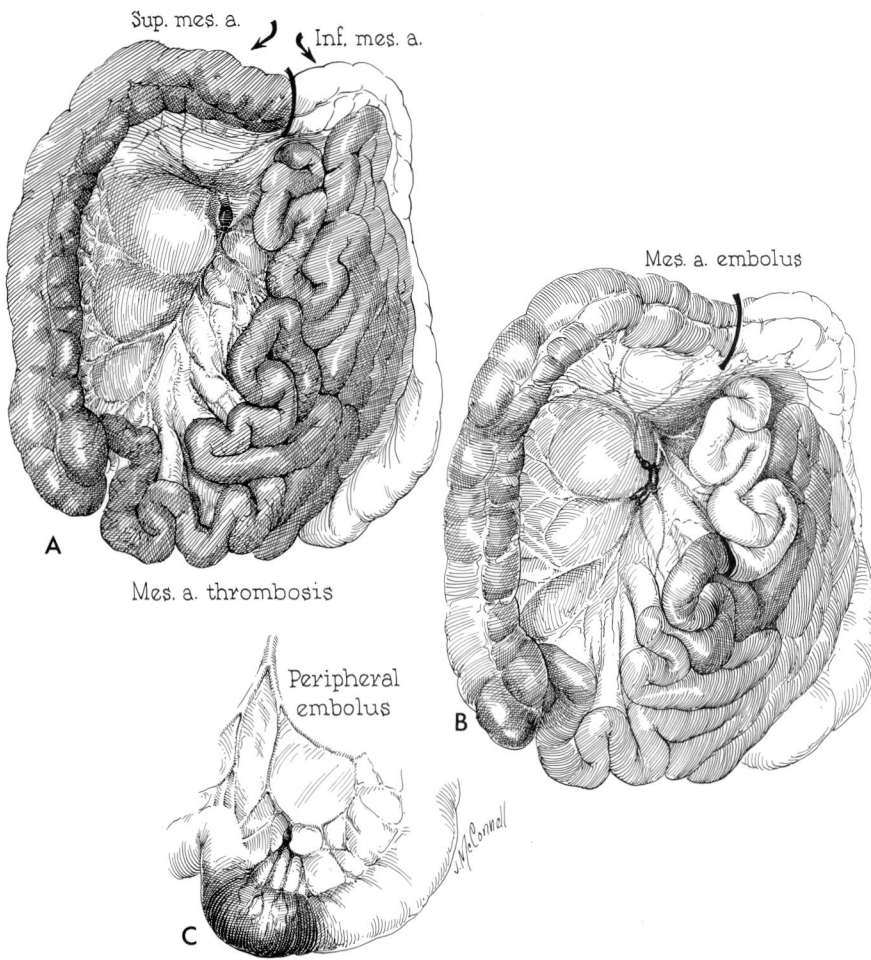

Mes. a. thrombosis

Peripheral embolus

Figure 3. This diagram illustrates differences seen at operation between patients with superior mesenteric artery thrombosis and those with mesenteric artery embolization. Notice the sparing of the upper jejunal arterial supply in mesenteric embolization, and how this area is infarcted when the superior mesenteric artery is occluded by atherosclerotic thrombosis. Segmental infarction of bowel may also occur when emboli lodge in peripheral mesenteric branches. (From Bergan, J. J.: Recognition and treatment of intestinal ischemia. Surg. Clin. North Am., 47:109, 1967.)

peritonitis. A plain film of the abdomen exposed at this time may show dilated bowel loops and later may show gas in the portal venous arborization.

Whenever the diagnosis is suspected, aortography should be performed unless the patient is moribund. *Survival is dependent upon swift action.* If mesenteric artery thrombosis is present, a sharp cutoff of the superior mesenteric artery is seen within 1 cm. of its origin. The celiac axis may or may not be occluded and, similarly, the inferior mesenteric artery may not be visualized. If the main trunks, the celiac axis, superior mesenteric artery, and inferior mesenteric artery are seen to be patent, the diagnosis of nonorganic intestinal infarction should be entertained as described next.

SURGICAL TREATMENT. Even in the late 1980s, results of pure resectional therapy for intestinal infarction approached the 85 to 100 per cent mortality of reports in the 1950s. A limited degree of success and improvement in results has been achieved with preliminary revascularization of the gut, followed by limited intestinal resection.[4] The same options in therapy exist for relief of acute mesenteric artery thrombosis as for chronic occlusion of mesenteric vessels. However, in the acute situation, thromboendarterectomy is too traumatic to the frail, dying patient. It may also be too time-consuming. Therefore, aortomesenteric grafting is favored, the grafts having a supraceliac origin (Fig. 4).

Following revascularization, the need for intestinal resection and a second-look procedure is decided upon as described earlier. As in surgical therapy for mesenteric embolus, the need for a second-look procedure must be determined at the time of the first operation. Judgment must be exercised with regard to performing double-grafting to the celiac axis and superior mesenteric artery, as the magnitude of the operative procedure contemplated must meet the needs of the desperately ill patient

being treated. The revascularization may allow short lengths of small bowel to be preserved and prevent the short-gut syndrome.[41] One of the major causes of death following resectional therapy for mesenteric infarction has been intestinal fistula formation. Therefore, revascularization is done to allow healing of the anastomosed bowel ends.

Nonorganic Intestinal Infarction

When the syndrome of abdominal pain, gut emptying, and leukocytosis with or without severe rebound tenderness and guarding has led to mesenteric arteriography and no organic occlusion of the mesenteric vessels is seen, the diagnosis may be nonorganic intestinal infarction. In this situation, a vicious cycle has been initiated by sepsis, cardiac failure, profound aortic valvular insufficiency, head injury, or other cause. In this cycle, vasoconstriction in the mesenteric arterial bed is induced by the remote stimulus. Resultant bowel ischemia allows bacterial

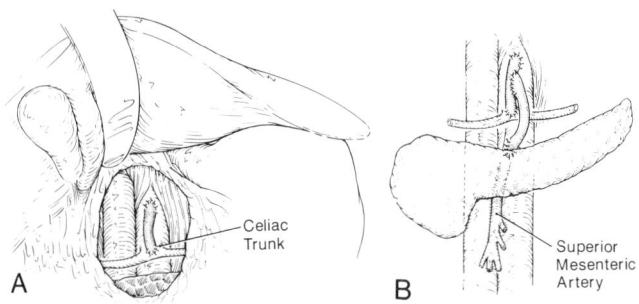

Figure 4. These diagrams illustrate use of the supraceliac aorta in revascularization of the celiac axis and superior mesenteric arterial territories. Note that single (A) or double grafts (B) may be utilized.

penetration of the mucosa and subsequent sepsis and hypovolemia with decreasing cardiac output, causing sympathetic stimulation that perpetuates the worsening cycle of intestinal ischemia. Clinically, the symptoms are those of acute intestinal ischemia, as described earlier. Before contemplation of surgical therapy, an aortogram will show the characteristic changes of nonorganic intestinal infarction. Segmental spasm of the peripheral branches of the mesenteric bed may be the only indication. Changes in the caliber of the vessel, especially with smooth margins and symmetrical involvement, indicate spasm, as opposed to the irregular margins and sharp cutoffs at bifurcations of vessels that are characteristic of thrombosis or embolization.

THERAPY. Treatment of nonorganic bowel infarction should be directed to the underlying cause, with proper attention given to cardiac decompensation, cardiac afterload reduction, and maintenance of fluid and blood volume. If the diagnosis has been made by aortography, the arterial catheter can be placed in the superior mesenteric artery and carefully controlled infusions of vasodilators, including papaverine or glucagon, administered. Such patients must be monitored carefully and laparotomy performed if signs of peritonitis signal development of gut necrosis.

Inferior Mesenteric Artery Occlusion

Ischemic colitis is discussed elsewhere in this text because it has little to do with occlusion of the inferior mesenteric artery. Instead, severe colonic ischemia due to occlusion of the inferior mesenteric artery occasionally attends aortic surgery and occurs following major alterations of blood flow to hemorrhoidal vessels and branches of the left colic artery. Only rarely does intestinal necrosis follow occlusion of the inferior mesenteric artery. This occurs when the superior mesenteric artery has occluded and the inferior mesenteric artery has become the sole supply to the midgut. Rare cases of colonic gangrene have been reported in which the inferior mesenteric artery has been demonstrated to have been the only vessel occluded. The subject of inferior mesenteric artery occlusion is best discussed as a complication of aortic surgery.[19]

SELECTED REFERENCES

Bergan, J. J., and Yao, J. S. T.: Chronic intestinal ischemia. In Rutherford, R. B. (Ed.): Vascular Surgery, 3rd ed. Philadelphia, W. B. Saunders Company, 1989.
A complete historical and recent exposition of the syndromes of chronic intestinal ischemia.

Boley, S. J., Sprayregen, S., Siegelman, S. S., et al.: Initial results from an aggressive roentgenological and surgical approach to acute mesenteric ischemia. Surgery 82:848, 1977.
Aggressive diagnostic approaches to acute mesenteric ischemia have been advocated by this group, and their report is an important one.

Bulkley, G. B.: Mediators of splanchnic organ injury. In Marston, A., Bulkley, G. B., Fiddian-Green, R. G., and Haglund, U. H. (Eds.): Splanchnic Ischemia and Multiple Organ Failure. St. Louis, C. V. Mosby Company, 1989, p. 183.
Future therapies in acute intestinal ischemia may depend upon concepts cited by Bulkley and colleagues.

Dunphy, J. E.: Abdominal pain of vascular origin. Am. J. Med. Sci., 192:109, 1936.
The classic article in which intestinal infarction was related to premorbid symptomatology.

Ernst, C. W.: Occlusion of the inferior mesenteric artery. In Rutherford, R. (Ed.): Vascular Surgery, 3rd ed. Philadelphia, W. B. Saunders Company, 1989.
A complete treatise on inferior mesenteric artery occlusion is found in this reference.

Lilly, M. P., Harward, T. R. S., Flinn, W. R., et al.: Duplex ultrasound measurement of changes in mesenteric blood flow. J. Vasc. Surg., 9:18, 1989.
Methods of ultrasound scanning in patients suspected of having chronic visceral ischemia are described in this key article.

Lindblad, B., and Hakansson, H.: Rationale for second-look operation in mesenteric vessel occlusion. J. Acta Chir. Scand., 153:531, 1988.
Aggressive postoperative care of patients may include multiple second-look procedures as described in this presentation.

Rheudasil, J. M., Stewart, N. T., Schellack, J. V., et al.: Surgical treatment of chronic mesenteric arterial insufficiency. J. Vasc. Surg., 8:495, 1988.
Modern techniques of revascularization in intestinal ischemia are described.

Shaw, R. S., and Maynard, E. P.: Acute and chronic thrombosis of the mesenteric arteries associated with malabsorption. N. Engl. J. Med., 258:874, 1958.
Successful mesenteric revascularization was performed in a patient being treated for malabsorption. This report led to futile studies of malabsorption in patients with chronic visceral ischemia.

REFERENCES

1. Bergan, J. J.: Recognition and treatment of superior mesenteric artery embolisation. Geriatrics 24:118, 1969.
2. Bergan, J. J.: Operative procedures in acute mesenteric infarction. In Bergan, J. J., and Yao, J. S. T. (Eds.): Operative Techniques in Vascular Surgery. Orlando, Fla., Grune and Stratton, 1980.
3. Bergan, J. J.: Unexpected vascular problems at laparotomy. In Probl. Gen. Surg., 1:190, 1984.
4. Bergan, J. J., Dean, R. H., Conn, J., Jr., and Yao, J. S. T.: Revascularization in treatment of mesenteric infarction. Ann. Surg., 182:430, 1975.
5. Bergan, J. J., Haid, S. P., and Conn, J., Jr.: Systemic effects of intestinal revascularization. Am. J. Surg., 117:235, 1969.
6. Bergan, J. J., and Yao, J. S. T.: Chronic intestinal ischemia. In Rutherford, R. B. (Ed.): Vascular Surgery, 3rd ed. Philadelphia, W. B. Saunders Company, 1989.
7. Boley, S. J., Sprayregen, S., Siegelman, S. S., et al.: Initial results from an aggressive roentgenological and surgical approach to acute mesenteric ischemia. Surgery, 82:848, 1977.
8. Brown, R. A., Chiu, C., Scott, H. J., et al.: Ultrastructural changes in the canine ileal mucosal cell after mesenteric arterial occlusion. Arch. Surg., 101:290, 1970.
9. Buenger, R. E., Hunter, J. A.: Reversible mesenteric artery stenoses due to methysergide maleate. JAMA, 198:558, 1966.
10. Bulkley, G. B.: Mediators of splanchnic organ injury. In Marston, A., Bulkley, G. B., Fiddian-Green, R. G., and Haglund, U. H. (Ed.): Splanchnic Ischemia and Multiple Organ Failure. St. Louis, C. V. Mosby Company, 1989, p. 183.
11. Bulkley, G. B., Zuidema, G. D., and Hamilton, S. R.: Intraoperative determination of small intestinal viability following ischemic injury. Ann. Surg., 193:628, 1981.
12. Chiu, C. H., Scott, H. J., and Gurd, F. N.: Circulatory collapse following the restoration of blood flow to the occluded superior mesenteric artery. Surg. Forum, 21:47, 1970.
13. Citron, B. P., Halpern, M., McCarron, M., et al.: Necrotizing angiitis associated with drug abuse. N. Engl. J. Med., 283:1003, 1970.
14. Croft, R. J., Menon, G. P., and Marston, A.: Does intestinal angina exist? A critical study of obstructed visceral arteries. Br. J. Surg., 68:316, 1981.
15. Dumont, A. E., Tice, D. A., and Mulholland, J. H.: Arteriosclerotic occlusion of the superior mesenteric artery. Ann. Surg., 154:833, 1961.
16. Dunbar, J. D., Molnar, W., Beman, F. F., and Marable, S. H.: Compression of the celiac trunk and abdominal angina: Preliminary report of 15 cases. Am. J. Roentgenol., 95:731, 1965.
17. Dunphy, J. E.: Abdominal pain of vascular origin. Am. J. Med. Sci., 192:109, 1936.
18. Elliott, J. W.: Operative relief of gangrene of intestines due to occlusion of mesenteric vessels. Ann. Surg., 21:9, 1895.
19. Ernst, C. W.: Occlusion of the inferior mesenteric artery. In Rutherford, R. (Ed.): Vascular Surgery. Philadelphia, W. B. Saunders Company, 1989.
20. Evans, W. E.: Long-term evaluation of the celiac band syndrome. Surgery, 76:867, 1974.
21. Hertzer, N. R., Beven, E. G., and Humphries, A. W.: Chronic intestinal ischemia. Surg. Gynecol. Obstet., 145:321, 1977.
22. Jaffe, M. S.: Status of abdominal visceral circulation via superior mesenteric prosthesis. Am. J. Surg., 121:736, 1971.
23. Kawasaki, T., Kosaki, F., Okawa, S., et al.: A new infantile acute febrile mucocutaneous lymph node syndrome. Pediatrics, 54:271, 1974.
24. Kieny, R.: Indications and results of surgical reconstructions of arteriosclerotic intestinal arteries. Observations on 30 patients. Vasa, 3:179, 1974.
25. Lamy, A. L., Roy, P. H., Morissette, J. J.: Intimal hyperplasia and thrombosis of the visceral arteries in a young woman. Surgery, 103:706, 1988.
26. LaRaja, R. D.: Cogan syndrome associated with mesenteric vascular insufficiency. Arch. Surg., 111:1028, 1976.
27. Lilly, M. P., Harward, T. R. S., Flinn, W. R., et al.: Duplex ultrasound measurement of changes in mesenteric blood flow. J. Vasc. Surg., 9:18, 1989.
28. Lindblad, B., and Hakansson, H.: Rationale for second-look operation in mesenteric vessel occlusion. J. Acta Chir. Scand., 153:531, 1988.
29. Marston, A.: Causes of death in mesenteric arterial occlusion. I. Local and general effects of devascularization of the bowel. Ann. Surg., 158:952, 1963.
30. McCauley, R. L., Johnston, M. R., and Fauci, A. S.: Surgical aspects of systemic necrotizing vasculitis. Surgery, 97:104, 1985.
31. Mikkelsen, W. P.: Intestinal angina. Its surgical significance. Am. J. Surg., 94:262, 1957.
32. Mosley, J. G., and Marston, A.: Acute intestinal ischemia. In Marston, A., Bulkley, G. B., Fiddian-Green, R. G., and Haglund, U. H. (Eds.): Splanchnic Ischemia and Multiple Organ Failure. St. Louis, C. V. Mosby Company, 1989.
33. Ottinger, L. W., and Austen, W. G.: A study of 136 patients with mesenteric infarction. Surg. Gynecol. Obstet., 124:251, 1967.

34. Paes, E., Vollmar, J. F., and Hutschenreiter, S., et al.: Der mesenterial Infarkt. J. Chirurg., *59*:828, 1988.
35. Palmer, W. L.: Clinical features of mesenteric artery insufficiency. J. Tennessee Med. Assoc., *59*:152, 1966.
36. Rheudasil, J. M., Stewart, N. T., Schellack, J. V., et al.: Surgical treatment of chronic mesenteric arterial insufficiency. J. Vasc. Surg., *8*:495, 1988.
37. Ricotta, J. J., and Williams, G. M.: Endarterectomy of the upper abdominal aorta and visceral arteries through an extraperitoneal approach. Ann. Surg., *192*:633, 1980.
38. Ripley, H. R., and Levin, S. M.: Abdominal angina associated with fibromuscular hyperplasia of the celiac and superior mesenteric arteries. Angiology, *17*:297, 1966.
39. Schennach, W., and Dorfmann, A.: Problem of acute obstruction of the mesenteric arteries. Thoraxchirurgie, *20*:457, 1972.
40. Shaw, R. S., and Maynard, E. P.: Acute and chronic thrombosis of the mesenteric arteries associated with malabsorption. N. Engl. J. Med., *258*:874, 1958.
41. Sitges-Serra, A., Mas, X., Roqueta, F., et al.: Mesenteric infarction: An analysis of 83 patients with prognostic studies and 44 cases undergoing massive small bowel resection. Br. J. Surg., *75*:544, 1988.
42. Stoney, R. J., and Schneider, P. A.: Technical aspects of visceral artery reconstruction. *In* Bergan, J. J., and Yao, J. S. T. (Eds.): Techniques in Arterial Surgery. Philadelphia, W. B. Saunders Company, 1990.
43. Vyden, J. K.: The systemic effects of acute superior mesenteric vascular insufficiency. *In* Boley, S. J. (Ed.): Vascular Disorders of the Intestines. New York, Appleton-Century-Crofts, 1971.
44. Williams, L. F., Jr.: Vascular insufficiency of the intestines. Gastroenterology *61*:757, 1971.
45. Wilson, C., Gupta, R., Gilmour, D. G., et al.: Acute superior mesenteric ischaemia. Br. J. Surg., *74*:279, 1987.
46. Yao, J. S. T., and Bergan, J. J.: Operative procedures in visceral ischemia. *In* Bergan, J. J., and Yao, J. S. T. (Eds.): Techniques in Arterial Surgery. Philadelphia, W. B. Saunders Company, 1990.

15. THE SURGICAL MANAGEMENT OF RENOVASCULAR HYPERTENSION

J. Caulie Gunnells, Jr., M.D., and Richard L. McCann, M.D.

The observation that obstructive lesions of the renal arteries produce hypertension is firmly established. Hypertension produced in this manner is referred to as renovascular hypertension and is the most common form of potentially curable high blood pressure. It is generally accepted that renovascular hypertension is usually relatively difficult to control by medical means and that patients with this disorder are at potential risk for irreversible renal damage if inappropriate pharmacologic modalities are utilized in the attempt to control blood pressure. More important, if the mechanical obstruction producing the hypertension is progressive, the inexorable loss of renal function is all too often an untoward and irreversible effect of inappropriate and untimely evaluation and treatment. Mechanical intervention utilizing revascularization techniques, by either surgical bypass or balloon angioplasty, provides a very appropriate and effective relief of this hypertension and as well often leads to preserved or improved renal function. In addition, occasionally a severely damaged kidney cannot be effectively revascularized, and removal of the involved kidney may be equally successful in controlling severe hypertension and preserving function of the contralateral kidney.

Systemic arterial pressure is controlled by a number of factors, including cardiac output, peripheral vascular resistance, and blood volume along with the activity of the renin-angiotensin-aldosterone system together with the integrating function of the sympathetic nervous system. Among the features determining the mechanisms underlying certain forms of renal and renovascular hypertension is the critical interplay between the renin-angiotensin-aldosterone cascade, together with its important effect on vascular resistance as well as its influence on the volume within the vascular tree. These actions are manifested through the potent vasoconstrictor angiotensin II, producing increased vascular resistance, and the action of aldosterone produced and released from the angiotensin II–stimulated adrenal gland, with its resultant action on the kidney leading to sodium retention and potassium excretion.

There are a number of specific causes for arterial hypertension. Among the forms of hypertension that are surgically correctable are those associated with coarctation of the aorta, pheochromocytoma, Cushings's syndrome (adrenal hyperplasia, cortical adenoma or carcinoma), primary aldosteronism (adenoma), and unilateral renal parenchymal disease. In addition, and more important, renovascular hypertension is, as mentioned earlier, the most common form of hypertension amenable to surgical therapy. This form of hypertension may be caused by any lesion that produces a significant obstruction to renal arterial blood flow, either unilaterally or bilaterally. The majority of patients with this disorder have atherosclerotic lesions or dysplasia involving the renal arteries. The most common form of dysplasia is fibromuscular.[22] Among other lesions that produce diminished renal arterial blood flow and may be associated with hypertension are renal artery aneurysms,[4] emboli, polyarteritis nodosa,[7] arteriovenous fistulas,[33] traumatic vascular injuries, radiation,[40] and a variety of extrinsic lesions that may compress the renal vascular supply, including neoplasms (metastatic or primary) and retroperitoneal fibrosis.

PHYSIOLOGIC ASPECTS

As stated earlier, occlusive lesions of the renal arteries are well recognized as a cause of sustained diastolic hypertension. The incidence of renal arterial lesions and coexistent hypertension has not been established with confidence. Estimates suggest their presence is less than 5 per cent to as much as 20 per cent or more of the adult hypertensive population in the United States. It is difficult to determine the true incidence with accuracy because of wide variability in the criteria for selecting patients for clinical investigation leading to the anatomic and functional diagnosis of renovascular hypertension.

The now famous experiments of Goldblatt approximately one half century ago, in which hypertension was produced by unilateral narrowing of the renal artery, clearly documented the role of the ischemic kidney in the production of hypertension.[15] In the Goldblatt experiment, unilateral renal arterial clamping caused transient hypertension, whereas sustained or persistent elevation in arterial pressure required constriction of both renal arteries or clamp restriction of one main renal artery with the removal of the contralateral kidney. This clamping of only one renal artery and removing the opposite kidney—one-kidney, one-clip Goldblatt hypertension—produced a form of high blood pressure that was characterized by volume expansion, and the blood pressure in this setting was maintained by an entirely different mechanism than in the two-kidney, one-clip Goldblatt hypertension model. This latter animal model is the experimental counterpart of renovascular hypertension in man that is recognized today. With understanding of the renin-angiotensin-aldosterone system in the functional maintenance of this vasoconstrictor form of hypertension produced by this model, the excess renin production by the ischemic kidney is thought to be largely responsible for the changes leading to the increased blood pressure observed clinically. The renal pressor mechanism initiated by renal ischemia, now known as the renin-angiotensin-aldosterone cascade, was first described by Tigerstedt and Bergman in 1898[45] and later amplified by Page and Corcoran,[34] Braun-Menendes,[2] and Helmer[21] following the classic anatomic experiments of Goldblatt. The commonly accepted relationship of this important homeostatic control mechanism of the renin cascade is outlined in Figure 1 along with markers indicating the various sites at which this cascade may

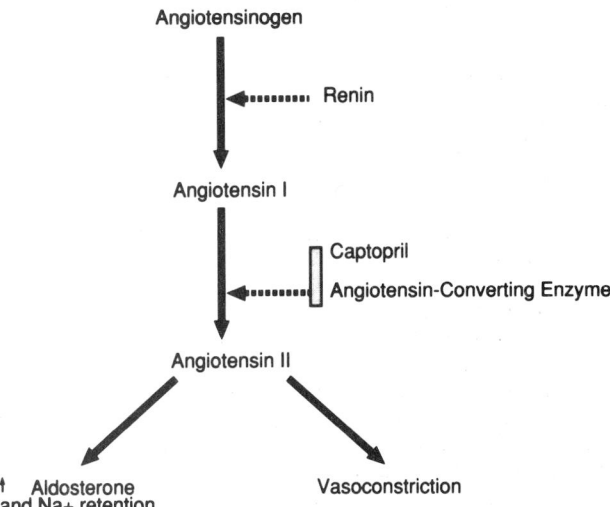

Figure 1. The renin-angiotensin system. (From Nally, J. V.: The captopril tests: A new concept in detecting renovascular hypertension? Cleve. Clin. J. Med., 56:395, 1989.)

be interrupted in order to further understand its mechanisms and participation in various clinical hypertensive states.

The recent introduction of the very important class of pharmacologic compounds known as angiotensin-converting enzyme inhibitors has greatly expanded understanding of the renin cascade and added to the diagnostic accuracy of patient evaluation for the presence of renovascular hypertension and the selection of candidates for further investigation leading to definitive invasive therapy.[13,19,30,31,44,46] In this cascade, renin is produced in excess from an ischemic kidney and released into the circulation where it reacts with renin substrate, an alpha₂ globulin produced by the liver. This enzymatic reaction cleaves off the decapeptide angiotensin I, which has little physiologic activity. Angiotensin I, in the presence of converting enzyme, is rapidly converted to the potent octapeptide angiotensin II. The effector limb of this cascade, angiotensin II, elicits two physiologic actions: (1) as a potent vasoconstrictor and (2) as a stimulator of the adrenal gland to produce and release aldosterone, thus indirectly increasing total vascular volume. The variable combination of these two actions leads to the hypertension initiated by the excess renin production by an ischemic kidney. The widespread availability of laboratory techniques to measure levels of plasma renin activity in both peripheral and renal venous blood, along with the appropriate utilization of angiotensin-converting enzyme inhibitors to enchance or augment renin secretion, has contributed greatly to the evaluation of patients suspected of having renovascular hypertension.

In man, convincing evidence has accumulated that in most patients with renovascular hypertension there does exist a role for the renin-angiotensin cascade as a major pathogenic mechanism. It is generally agreed that measurement of one or more of the compounds involving the renin cascade provides useful information in the diagnostic evaluation and treatment of a patient suspected of having renovascular hypertension produced by one or more of the lesions previously noted in unilateral or bilateral locations within the renal circulation.

PATHOLOGIC OBSERVATIONS

The most common cause of renovascular hypertension is atherosclerosis, which is the etiologic basis of the lesions in two thirds of the patients with this disorder. The lesions are most apt to occur near the origin (ostial) of the renal vessels from the aorta and are at times segmental, usually less than a centimeter in length. Males, and often patients in the older age group, are more commonly affected, and bilateral lesions are present in approximately one third of these patients.

Fibrous and fibromuscular dysplasia cause renovascular hypertension; these mural dysplasias may be classified according to the site and type of involvement (intimal, medial, or adventitial). The most commonly encountered is termed medial fibromuscular dysplasia or hyperplasia and occurs most often in young women.[22] The microscopic lesions consist of a thickening of the media with separation and distortion of the muscle fibers by a degenerative process involving myxomatous fibrous tissue. The lesions are apt to be multiple, and the term *microaneurysms* has been used to describe the appearance of serially constricted lesions interspersed with areas of greater diameter. On angiography this produces a corrugated effect termed the "string of beads" phenomenon (Fig. 2).

Other vascular lesions, including aneurysms (congenital and acquired), arteriovenous malformations, renal artery dissections, renal artery thrombosis, and emboli to the renal parenchyma, have been associated with, or productive of, renovascular hypertension and constitute an important reservoir of patients who profit from angiographic study to define the particular site, cause, and extent of vascular involvement necessary prior to any operative or angioplastic intervention.

In addition, a new group of vascular lesions—a special form of renovascular hypertension, namely, atheroembolic renal disease in association with renal artery stenosis[28]—has recently surfaced as an important consideration for surgical intervention. Renal cholesterol embolization may be an unsuspected cause of renal failure, particularly in the elderly and in patients with diffuse abdominal atherosclerosis in association with renal artery stenosis. Only recently has the close association of renal failure, renal arterial stenosis, and cholesterol emboli, leading to renal failure or an acute exacerbation of chronic renal insufficiency and hypertension, been considered a surgically approachable disease. However, the concomitant development of cholesterol emboli involving the renal circulation may contribute to hypertension as well as to compromised renal function, and this can be exacerbated or magnified in the presence of renal artery stenosis. The association of significant renal artery stenosis and its pivotal role in or contribution to progressive renal failure, usually noted in association with cholesterol em-

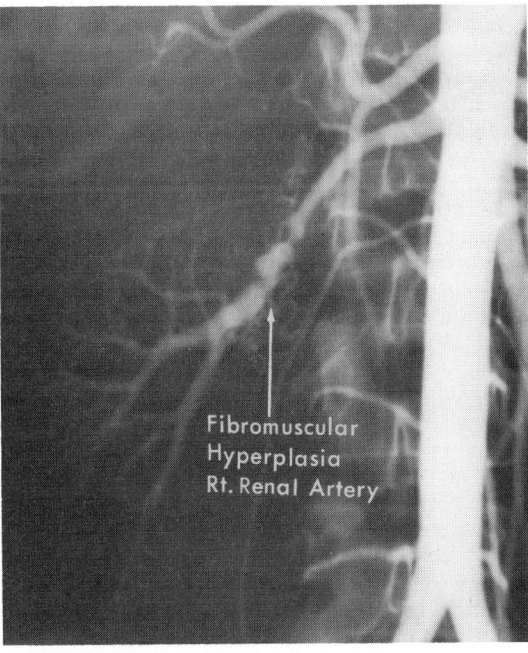

Figure 2. Arteriogram demonstrating fibromuscular dysplasia of the right renal artery producing hypertension. Note the characteristic "scalloping."

boli, is being recognized with considerable frequency. There are increasing reports of this association along with the successful intervention after angiographic and biopsy demonstration of the coexistent abnormalities. This constitutes a very important reservoir of patients who may benefit in two ways from correction of renovascular hypertension, that is, a reduction in blood pressure and preservation or improvement of renal function.

CLINICAL MANIFESTATIONS

Experience has demonstrated that there are a number of important clinical diagnostic features associated with renovascular hypertension. However, the choice as to which patients should be evaluated for the presence of renovascular hypertension remains controversial.[41] This problem was emphasized most recently in an editorial by Pauker and Kopelman.[35] These workers have correctly referred to this dilemma as a "which hunt"— which patients, which tests, which etiology, and which therapies. Important clinical diagnostic features include the sudden or abrupt onset of hypertension, often prior to the age of 35 or after the age of 55 and in the absence of a family history of hypertension.[26] In addition, there may be the onset or worsening of hypertension following an episode of flank pain. Another important feature may be the unexplained development or existence of accelerated or malignant hypertension at any age. It should be emphasized that patients with renovascular hypertension often have what may be called "significant" levels of high blood pressure, namely, those patients with sustained, severe diastolic hypertension (greater than 115 mm. Hg) or, as previously noted, accelerated or malignant hypertensive disease.[5] Rarely do patients with functionally significant renovascular hypertension have mild levels of blood pressure. Other features that may be of importance are patients who exhibit antihypertensive drug failure and/or intolerable side effects of drug therapy; escape from previous control, particularly in patients in the older age group; and patients with deteriorating renal function despite good blood pressure control.

It is well known there are serious limitations insofar as the medical history and physical examination are concerned in detection of renovascular hypertension. However, physical examination may reveal the most important diagnostic feature associated with this entity, namely, an abdominal bruit located in the epigastrium or in either upper abdominal quadrant. This finding is present in some 50 to 80 per cent of patients with renovascular hypertension, whereas it occurs in less than 5 per cent of those patients with essential hypertension. Patients with fibromuscular hyperplasia are more apt to have bruits than are those with atherosclerotic lesions. Moreover, in fibromuscular disease, the bruits are soft, to-and-fro or continuous, whereas higher pitched systolic bruits are more characteristic of atherosclerotic disease.

Other clinical features that have been emphasized and described in a large matched group of patients with proved renovascular hypertension, as compared with a similar group of patients with essential hypertension, indicated that in those patients with renovascular hypertension there is a duration of hypertension of less than 1 year, a higher incidence of spontaneous, nondiuretic-induced hypokalemia, and the presence of proteinuria.[26] Patients exhibiting all of these historical findings are relatively rare, but when several of these findings are present, they demand strong consideration for further investigation to establish a diagnosis of functionally significant renovascular hypertension. However, it is important to remember that all patients with significant hypertension must be initially considered as suspect for renovascular disease, and this high level of suspicion must be borne constantly in mind. Timely application of appropriate studies must be instituted if one is to detect a higher incidence of renovascular hypertension in the large number of patients with primary hypertension who present for clinical evaluation.

At the outset, it is important to recognize that a general medical evaluation is necessary and that attention should be given to the presence or absence of coexistent systemic diseases; emphasis must also be placed on a careful assessment of overall general health in addition to specific attention to the presence or absence of involvement of other vascular beds, including the cerebral, coronary, and peripheral circulations.[32]

LABORATORY EXAMINATIONS

The initial studies of importance include a urinalysis with culture, serum creatinine determination, chest roentgenography, electrocardiography, serum potassium determination, and measurements of plasma renin activity, in both the peripheral and renal venous blood. The recent availability of angiotensin-converting enzyme inhibitors and their ability to increase the value of plasma renin measurements have greatly augmented the value of laboratory evaluations using renin measurements.[29–31] In addition, the extension of using converting enzyme inhibition in the performance of radioisotope studies has attracted new emphasis and interest in this particular technique as a screening test for renovascular disease.[11,31,41,48] It has been emphasized by Wilcox[48] and associates that there are three aspects of response to angiotensin-converting enzyme inhibitors that may be helpful in evaluating patients for renovascular hypertension: (1) the drugs may increase plasma creatinine during administration, and when this occurs, it strongly suggests renovascular disease, particularly in patients with bilateral renal artery stenosis or arterial stenosis of a solitary kidney; (2) the exaggerated rise in plasma renin activity following an oral dose of a converting enzyme inhibitor also suggests the presence of renovascular hypertension; and (3) the previously mentioned converting enzyme inhibitor–induced changes in the radionuclide renogram may support the diagnosis after other preliminary studies have been performed and may also indicate the site of the functional stenosis.

The recent availability of digital subtraction venous angiography as an outpatient procedure has brought a great deal of attention and wide application of this technique in searching for patients with renovascular disease, thereby avoiding the usual necessity for hospital admission when using a standard renal arteriogram to visualize the renal vascular anatomy.[3,8,38,49]

RENIN ACTIVITY MEASUREMENT. In the hypertensive patient in whom there is suspected renovascular hypertension, the presence of an increased peripheral plasma renin activity suggests that unilateral renal arterial disease may be present and that it is producing a hormonally dependent form of hypertension.[9,12,18,23,25,27] However, peripheral venous plasma renin measurements may be quite variable and they may be elevated in a significant number of patients with the high renin variety of primary hypertension and may also be entirely normal in some 25 per cent of patients with subsequently proven, functionally significant renal artery stenosis. Unstimulated peripheral measurements of plasma renin activity as an indicator of the presence of renal artery stenosis were not considered reliable until the availability of captopril stimulation, which was used to differentiate these various subsets of patients undergoing investigation as to the etiologic basis or mechanisms of their hypertension. The captopril stimulation of peripheral plasma renin activity uses the angiotensin-converting enzyme inhibitor as a pharmacologic probe into the mechanism of the hypertension in the patient under investigation.[12,30,46] In preparing for such investigation, the patient should maintain a normal dietary sodium intake and also should not receive diuretic drugs for a minimum of 72 hours (preferably 2 weeks) before the test, and if possible, other hypertensive drugs other than beta-blockers should also be withdrawn 2 to 3 weeks before the test, since they may also depress the response of the renin cascade to captopril administration.[30,46] At the outpatient clinic, baseline blood pressures are taken in order to establish a mean baseline blood pressure value, and a venous blood sample is drawn for the measurement of plasma renin activity, after which captopril (a 50-mg. tablet) is crushed and diluted in 10 to 30 ml. of water and administered orally. Blood pressure is measured at 10 to 15-minute intervals over a 90-minute period of time. At the end of this time, blood pressure is again measured, and a repeat venous blood sample is drawn for the measurement of the stimulated peripheral venous renin activity. Two aspects of the test are utilized in evaluating the patient's response. In those patients with renovascular hypertension, the induced fall in blood pressure after administration of captopril is greater than in patients with essential hypertension, but this is less reliable than the response of the plasma renin activity. A more reliable differentiating point between the presence of essential versus renovascular hypertension is related to the degree to which the administered captopril enhances the rise in plasma renin activity. The criteria for a positive response have varied from investigator to investigator; however, the results of Muller[30] and colleagues have been most useful and they have proposed three criteria for a positive captopril test to distinguish between patients with renovascular hypertension and those with essential hypertension. Renovascular hypertension is considered to be present if one or more of the following conditions are met: (1) stimulated renin activity is 12 ng per ml per hour or more; (2) the absolute increase in plasma renin activity is 10 ng per ml per hour or more and the percentage increase in plasma renin activity is 150 per cent or more; or (3) the percentage increase in plasma renin activity is 400 per cent or more if the baseline plasma renin activity is less than 3 ng per ml per hour.[30,46] Representative results of renin measurements following the oral administration of captopril in a number of patients with proven forms of hypertension are depicted in Figure 3.[46] These data clearly indicate the efficacy and usefulness of this particular test as a screening maneuver in order to select patients for further study.

RENAL VEIN RENIN MEASUREMENTS. The accuracy and diagnostic significance of renal vein renin measurement have considerable importance and it is now the major preoperative diagnostic maneuver in patients with renovascular hypertension in order to establish the functional significance of the anatomic defect(s).[18] The accuracy and diagnostic significance of renal vein renin measurements have also been improved by the concomitant acute administration of captopril, utilizing the principles and action of this particular agent in a manner similar to that outlined in the peripheral plasma renin measurements.[19,36,44,46] The use of this agent magnifies the difference in renal vein renin activity in patients with functionally significant renal artery stenosis. Measuring renal vein renin following the administration of captopril may minimize false-negative ratios previously seen in patients who subsequently may have responded well to surgical therapy. Patients with hypertension and normal renal arteries only rarely exhibit a renal vein renin ratio greater than 1.5 to 2:1, whereas in patients with functionally significant renal stenosis, renal vein renin concentrations are at least 1.5 to 2 times higher in renal venous blood of the involved or affected kidney than in the renal effluent of the contralateral venous drainage.[18] The results of renal vein renin measurements in a group of patients assessed before and after the use of captopril are outlined in Figure 4, again demonstrating the usefulness of this particular technique in patients with renovascular disease.[46]

RADIOISOTOPE RENOGRAPHY. Prior to the advent of agents such as converting enzyme inhibitors, the use of radioisotope renography was thought by many investigators to provide little additional information before the consideration of more invasive type studies such as renal angiography. Radionuclide renal studies were at that time associated with a high incidence of false-negative and false-positive results, limiting their diagnostic usefulness except possibly in the preliminary investigation of those patients who exhibited an allergy to iodinated contrast media. However, the application and appreciation of captopril-induced changes in the renogram proved quite helpful in suspecting and confirming the diagnosis of renovascular hypertension.[11,13,31,41,48] The rationale for the captopril stimulation in radionuclide studies is related to the functional activity of the angiotensin II–dependent action on efferent arteriolar resistance that causes a reduction in transcapillary

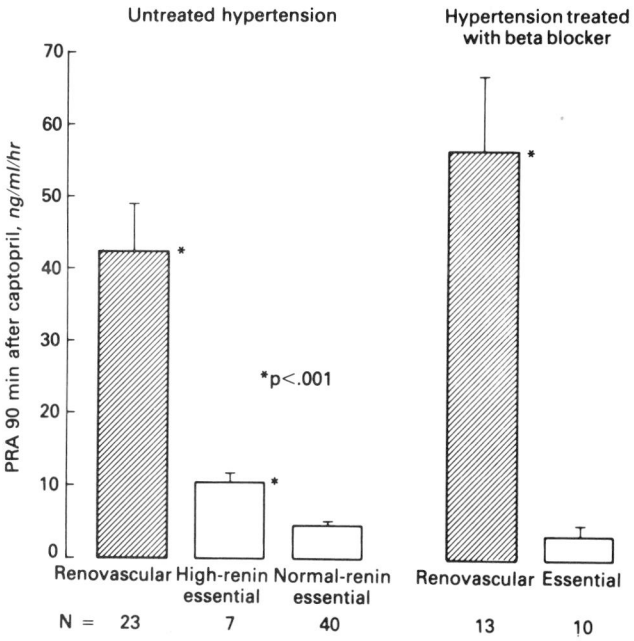

Figure 3. Levels of peripheral vein plasma renin activity in hypertensive patients after a single dose of captopril. (From Case, D. B., et al: Physiologic effects and diagnostic relevance of acute converting enzyme blockade. In Laragh, J. H., Buhler, F. R., and Seldin, D. W. (Eds.): Frontiers in Hypertension Research, New York, Springer-Verlag. 1982, p. 546.)

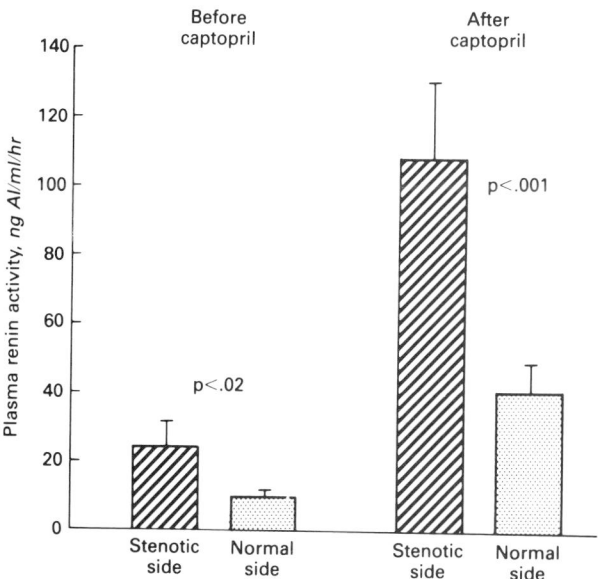

Figure 4. Levels of renal vein renin activity in patients with renovascular hypertension before and after captopril. (From Vaughan, E. D.: Clinical evaluation for renovascular hypertension and therapeutic decisions. Urol. Clin. North Am., 11:393, 1984.)

forces driving glomerular filtration, thereby reducing renal function of the kidney distal to renal arterial stenosis. This decrement in individual kidney function may be noninvasively assessed using two-dimensional radionuclide studies.[11,31]

Depending on the label and compound utilized, assessment of individual kidney function is possible using this noninvasive technology as well as the capability of measuring renal blood flow (^{131}I-Hippuran). Utilizing technetium-labeled diethylenetriaminepentacetic acid (DTPA), a measurement of glomerular filtration can be obtained at the time of the radionuclide angiogram since DTPA is excreted by the kidneys solely by way of glomerular filtration. Abnormalities in the conventional renogram suggesting the presence of renovascular disease include a reduction in kidney perfusion and size as well as a delay in the uptake and excretion of the radioactive label. The captopril-induced changes in the renogram that have been suggested as diagnostic criteria for the stenotic kidney include a reduction/delay in DTPA uptake of the stenotic kidney and a delay in the time of maximal activity of the labeled substance as well as the delay in the ^{131}I-Hippuran washout. It has been suggested that both DTPA- and ^{131}I-labeled studies be performed in order to detect the maximal changes in renovascular disease after captopril administration. The alterations in the renogram before and after the administration of DTPA with the associated time-activity curves are shown in Figure 5.[31] Utilizing similar studies, the nephrology group at the University of Florida[48] have gathered data relative to the usefulness of these studies in the screening evaluation for renovascular hypertension. They have suggested that there is a 20 per cent incidence of false-positive tests and that the sensitivity of the test is 93 to 100 per cent with a specificity of approximately 80 per cent in the population in whom they have studied and applied these techniques.

INTRAVENOUS UROGRAPHY. Minute sequence intravenous urography is a simple and widely available test and continues to be a very good anatomic screening maneuver for the presence of unilateral main stem renovascular hypertension. The usefulness of this test is related to its widespread availability and the facts that it can be performed utilizing conventional radiographic equipment, that it requires only a minimal exposure to contrast media and that it is relatively inexpensive and when properly interpreted correlates well with conventional angiography and the response to surgical intervention. A recent review and comparison of a number of radiographic techniques in the detection of renovascular hypertension by Del Greco and associates has again emphasized the value of minute sequence

intravenous urography by comparing this study with conventional radionuclide renography and digital subtraction venous angiography.[20] However, minute sequence intravenous urography yields a false-positive result in approximately 10 per cent of patients and a false-negative result in a similar percentage of the patients studied. The urogram has important diagnostic limitations in detecting segmental or branch arterial lesions, bilateral renal arterial disease, and bilateral parenchymal renal disease of unequal severity in certain congenital anomalies of the kidney.

DIGITAL SUBTRACTION VENOUS ANGIOGRAPHY. The recently introduced digital subtraction angiography as a method of directly imaging the renal arteries has proved to be a useful examination in the evaluation of renovascular hypertension.[3,8,38,49] It appears to be more sensitive than minute sequence urography in detecting renal arterial lesions, avoids arterial puncture, and reduces the need for hospitalization that is present with conventional angiography. In many areas it has become the technique of choice as a screening radiographic procedure to survey patients for the presence of main stem renal artery disease. It has a number of negative features, such as the requirement of special costly equipment to do the procedure that is not widely available in all centers, the necessity to inject large amounts of contrast media, the requirement for good cardiac function, and the fact that even with this technique there is a relatively high incidence of false-negative and false-positive results. In addition, the field visualized is relatively small, and adequate detail in the secondary and tertiary vascular branches cannot be appreciated. Clearly, significant lesions may occur in these locations and may be overlooked by this technique. Moreover, this technique is significantly more expensive than are other conventional screening techniques and does not avoid the subsequent need for conventional angiography to those patients with positive studies who subsequently are to undergo revascularization, nephrectomy, or angioplasty.

RENAL ARTERIOGRAPHY. The definitive study for the anatomic localization of a renal artery lesion is renal angiography.[10,16,23,39] This study is indicated in patients judged to be eventual candidates for surgical or balloon angioplasty therapy in whom preliminary results have suggested renovascular hypertension. The percutaneous retrograde transfemoral technique is widely used in the performance of "flush" aortography and in conjunction with selective renal arterial injections of contrast media adds diagnostic precision and greater vascular detail. In addition to demonstrating the main renal arteries, the study provides important additional information, including the

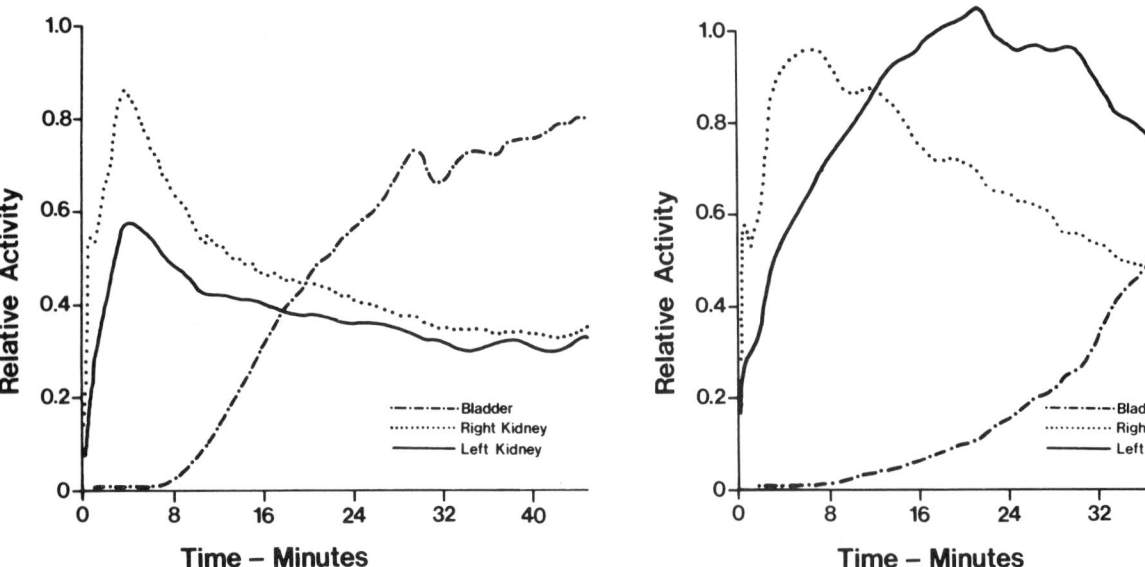

Figure 5. ^{99m}Tc-DTPA time-activity curves in a patient with unilateral left renal artery stenosis: Baseline on the left and after captopril stimulation on the right. (From Nally, J. V.: The captopril tests: A new concept in detecting renovascular hypertension? Cleve. Clin. J. Med., 56:395, 1989.)

extent of post-stenotic dilation, the presence of collateral circulation, and the visualization of other vessels that may be used for vascular repair, and makes possible the evaluation of the extra- and intrarenal arterial anatomy as well. After establishing the presence of a vascular lesion, it is then necessary to pursue further studies to determine whether the observed lesion is functionally responsible for the hypertension; this then leads to the measurement of renal venous plasma renin activity as previously described.

RENAL FUNCTION STUDIES. In addition to obtaining anatomic evidence, assessing the functional integrity of the kidneys is also of importance. Unfortunately, evaluation of total function often fails to reflect the presence of anatomic lesions that produce hypertension. This inadequacy and the lack of the wide availability of plasma renin measurements in the past led to the development of differential renal function studies to estimate the degree of functional alteration produced by unilateral renal ischemia. However, the high incidence of technical failure, postprocedural complications, unreliability in the presence of segmental or bilateral lesions, and otherwise unexplained false-positive and false-negative results have led to the rejection of this technique by most clinicians.

TREATMENT

The treatment of the patient with renovascular disease has two related goals. The first is amelioration (but not necessarily cure) of hypertension to prevent the long-term deleterious effects of elevated blood pressure on target organ systems such as the eye, the cerebral and coronary circulations, and the kidneys. A second goal of the treatment of patients with renovascular disease of preservation and occasionally improvement in renal function.

The surgical management of the hypertensive patient with renal artery stenosis requires experienced clinical judgment. There remains no unequivocal test that predicts the response to anatomic correction of renal artery stenosis. Patients with lateralizing renin ratios have a high probability of benefit from correction of unilateral renal artery stenosis, but even in patients with nonlateralizing renin ratios, up to 57 per cent may benefit from surgical therapy.[1]

Whereas medical therapy may obviate the risk of operation, it requires a high degree of patient compliance, constant medical supervision, and lifelong antihypertensive medication. Another consideration is that although medical therapy may be effective in controlling systemic blood pressure regardless of the cause, it is less effective than restoration of renal blood flow in terms of long-term preservation of renal function. In one study, 41 per cent of patients with renovascular disease treated medically had significant loss of renal mass determined radiographically or significant decline in renal function despite adequate control of blood pressure.[6]

Correction of Renal Artery Stenosis

PERCUTANEOUS TRANSLUMINAL ANGIOPLASTY. Balloon catheter techniques for dilation of renal artery stenosis were introduced by Grüntzig in 1978.[17] This technique requires passage of a guidewire under fluoroscopic control from a peripheral site across the stenosis in the renal artery. A balloon dilating catheter is passed over the guidewire and positioned within the area of stenosis and inflated to produce a controlled disruption of the arterial wall (Fig. 6). Completion angiography is usually performed to assess the immediate results.

The results of percutaneous balloon angioplasty of renal artery stenosis must be considered separately in the two principal disease entities causing renal artery stenosis. In patients with fibromuscular disease, particularly of the medial fibroplasia type, balloon angioplasty has a high rate of success and recurrence is particularly uncommon. The experience with athero-

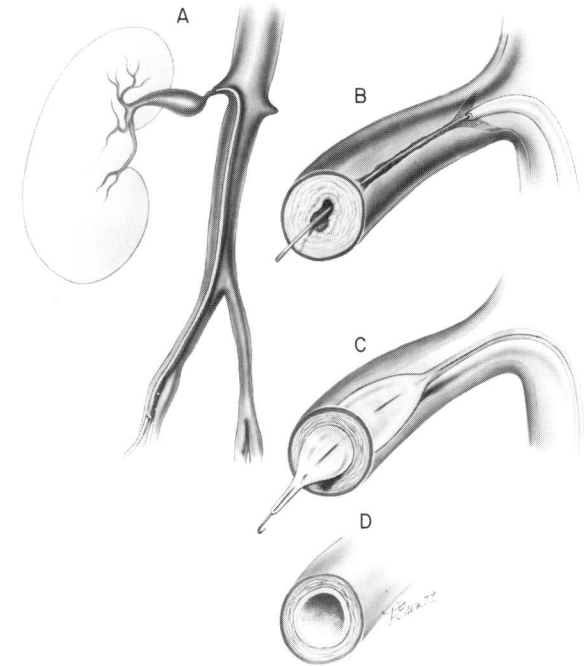

Figure 6. The technique of renal artery dilation with the dual-lumen balloon catheter system, using the femoral approach. *A,* The stenotic right renal artery is catheterized selectively. *B,* The guidewire is advanced through the stenosis. *C,* The selective catheter is exchanged for the dilation catheter and the balloon is inflated, dilating the stenosis. *D,* The obstruction is relieved. (From Tegtmeyer, C., Dyer, R., Teates, C., et al.: Percutaneous transluminal dilatation of the renal arteries: Techniques and results. Radiology, *135:*591, 1980.)

sclerotic disease has not been as favorable. In a recent series, only 34 per cent of patients with atherosclerotic obstructions of the renal artery were thought to be cured or improved after a mean follow-up of just 22 months.[1] Balloon dilation is much less successful if the renal artery stenosis is caused by plaques in the aortic wall, which encroach upon the ostium of the renal vessel. These so-called ostial lesions can be successfully dilated only 20 per cent of the time and many believe their presence is a relative contraindication to the use of balloon dilation.

The rate of major complications from percutaneous balloon dilation of the renal arteries has been reported between 10 and 21 per cent.[1,47] These include, in addition to puncture site complications common to angiography, uncontrolled renal artery dissection causing renal infarction, contrast-induced renal insufficiency, and renal artery rupture. Several deaths have also been reported.[47]

Surgical Therapy

NEPHRECTOMY. Simple nephrectomy may be the appropriate procedure for patients with severe hypertension when the involved kidney has been so severely affected that it contributes little to total renal function. A renal length of less than 7 cm., complete renal artery occlusion with infarction, and severe arteriolar nephrosclerosis are indications for nephrectomy, especially if the opposite kidney is normal or reconstructible. In selected instances, a partial nephrectomy may be performed for localized infarctions, noncorrectable branch lesions, segmental renal hypoplasia, and intrarenal aneurysms and arteriovenous malformations when these are associated with hypertension.

In some patients, total renal artery occlusion may be of gradual onset, allowing maintenance of renal viability through development of collateral circulation from lumbar, ureteral, capsular, or mesenteric vessels. Factors suggesting potential salvage of the kidney with revascularization include urographic visualization of the kidney, renal length of 9 cm. or more, retrograde filling of the distal arterial tree, and lateralizing renal vein renin

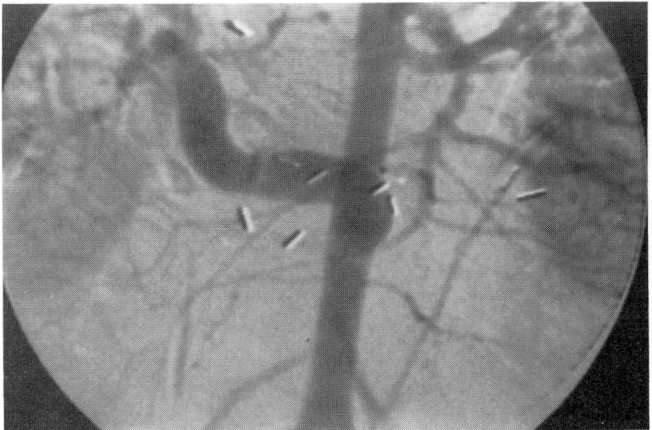

Figure 7. Aorta to right renal artery saphenous vein bypass graft done in an 11-year-old child. Routine follow-up angiography performed 1 year postoperatively demonstrates uniform expansion of the saphenous vein graft, which, despite its enlargement, continues to function well, and the patient remains normotensive with normal renal function.

assay. Intraoperative renal biopsy may be helpful in these cases because severe obliteration of all or most of the glomeruli indicates an unsalvageable kidney. Although selected studies have shown occasional improvement in renal function by revascularization of small atrophic kidneys, this is an unusual occurrence and should be reserved for the circumstance in which the alternative is chronic dialysis.

REVASCULARIZATION. A variety of operative techniques can be used to correct stenosis or occlusion of the renal arteries. The proper choice among these is based on the nature of the renal artery lesion, the presence or absence of associated aortic atherosclerotic disease, and the experience and preference of the surgeon treating the patient.

AORTORENAL BYPASS GRAFTS. Aortorenal bypass is the technique most frequently selected for surgical correction of renal artery stenosis. In most patients, the autogenous saphenous vein is the graft material of choice. Late follow-up of these grafts has sometimes demonstrated a tendency for uniform graft expansion. In extreme cases, this may progress to aneurysmal proportions. This phenomenon is particularly prevalent in children (Fig. 7), in whom many advocate the use of autogenous arterial grafts for renal artery reconstruction. The internal iliac artery is often chosen because it is of appropriate size, and since the pelvis is well supplied with collaterals, it can be removed with little hazard. Synthetic grafts have been used successfully, particularly when the distal renal artery is large owing to post-stenotic dilation.[24] However, long-term results have favored use of autogenous tissue grafts. It is important to spatulate the graft when attaching it to the thick-walled aorta to ensure an adequate orifice for inflow into the graft. This technique often is facilitated by incorporating a large side branch of the vein in the spatulation to increase the size of the orifice.

USE OF BRANCHES OF THE CELIAC AXIS TO REVASCULARIZE THE KIDNEYS. A more difficult group of patients to treat are those with severe atherosclerotic disease of the wall of the aorta in combination with renal artery stenosis. These patients are recognized by the appearance of marked irregularity of the aortic wall on angiography. If there is marked luminal stenosis or aneurysm formation, consideration should be given to replacement of the aorta and simultaneous revascularization of the kidneys with vein autografts taking origin from the Dacron tube. If there is no intrinsic indication for aortic replacement, however, and if the lateral aortogram shows a widely patent celiac axis, then consideration can be given to using branches of the celiac axis for revascularization of the kidneys alone. On the left side, the splenic artery may be divided distally and rotated inferiorly to form an anastomosis with the left renal

artery (Fig. 8). This procedure has the advantage of requiring only a single vascular anastomosis but does require a nearly normal splenic artery. The spleen may be left in place and is adequately nourished through the short gastric vessels. Splenic vessels that are extremely tortuous and with calcium in the walls may not rotate inferiorly without kinking. In this instance, if the lumen is of satisfactory caliber, the vessel can be used to supply blood to the left kidney using an interposition vein graft between the two vessels. On the right side, the hepatic or gastroduodenal artery serves as a convenient origin for a short vein graft to the right renal artery (Fig. 9). These techniques are particularly well suited for a staged approach to the surgical management of bilateral renal artery disease.

BENCH WORK SURGERY. Disease of the small branch vessels may now be treated by "bench work surgery." In these procedures, the vascular supply to the kidney is divided, and the organ can be completely removed from the body or left attached by only the ureter. The kidney is flushed with cold solution and is kept cold by packing in ice slush while delicate vascular repair of the branch vessels is performed, usually with the aid of optical magnification or even an operating microscope. When repaired, the kidney can be reimplanted into its original position or autografted to the pelvis using the iliac vessels for anastomoses. Using these techniques, the incidence of nephrectomy for "unreconstructible branch renal arterial disease" is steadily diminishing.

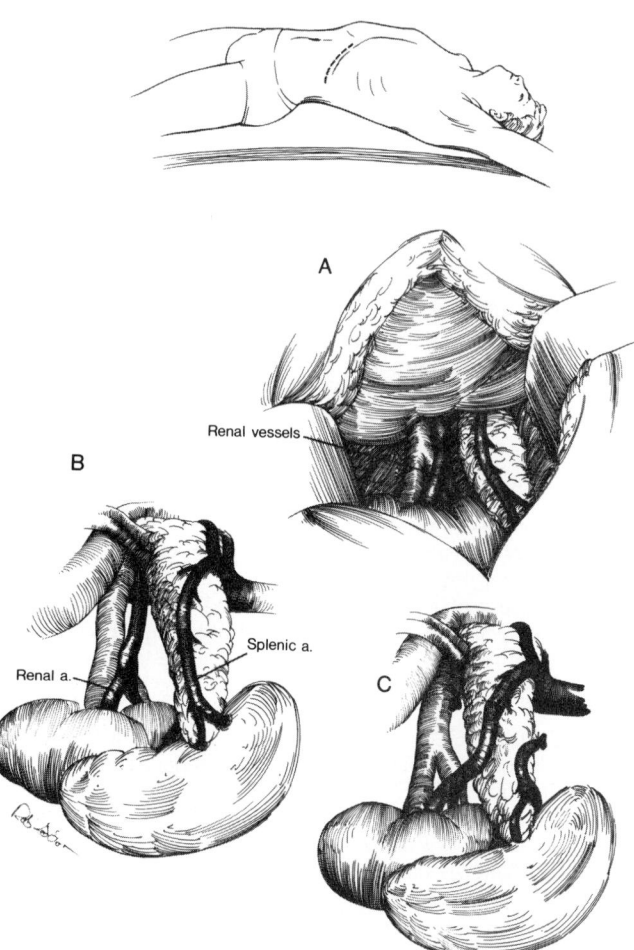

Figure 8. Technique of splenic to renal artery bypass. Inset shows the left subcostal incision. *A*, Retroperitoneal exposure of the renal artery and vein and the splenic artery on the inferior margin of the pancreas. *B*, The relationship between the renal artery and splenic artery is illustrated. *C*, The completed anastomosis is shown. The splenic artery should be kept as short as possible to prevent kinking. The spleen may be left in place since it is adequately nourished by the short gastric vessels.

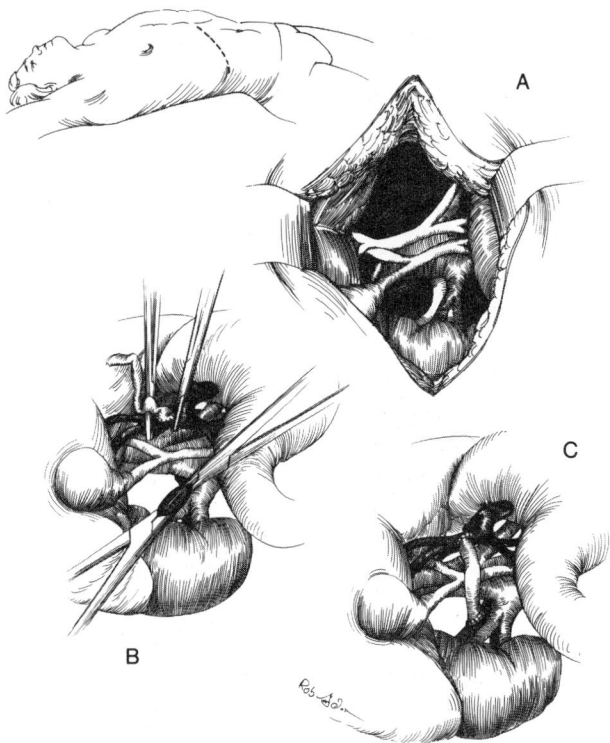

Figure 9. Technique of hepatic to right renal artery bypass. Inset shows the right subcostal incision. *A*, Exposure of the hepatic artery in the hepatoduodenal ligament. *B*, The proximal anastomosis is being placed on the common hepatic artery. *C*, The completed short vein graft in "H" configuration between the hepatic and the renal vessels.

RESULTS. Benefit from operative intervention in renovascular hypertension is directly related to accurate identification of surgical candidates and skilled performance of appropriate vascular reconstruction. Attention to these aspects in recent years has yielded improved long-term results. Most series report 70 to 90 per cent long-term improvement with 1 to 2 per cent operative mortality.[49] Mortality occurs almost exclusively in patients with widespread systemic atherosclerotic disease who require aortic or other arterial reconstruction in addition to renal revascularization.

SELECTED REFERENCES

Beebe, H. G., Chesebro, K., Merchant, F., and Bush, W.: Results of renal artery balloon angioplasty limit its indications. J. Vasc. Surg., 8:300, 1988.
This study carefully documents the results of 83 renal artery lesions in 55 patients who underwent percutaneous transluminal angioplasty for fibromuscular and atherosclerotic lesions. Careful documentation of the long-term results show that excellent response is obtained in patients with fibromuscular disease. In contrast, patients with atherosclerotic disease had a satisfactory result only 34 per cent of the time.

Dean, R. H.: Renovascular hypertension. (Current Problems in Surgery, Vol. 22.) Chicago, Year Book Publishers, 1985.
This is a review article discussing in some detail patient selection, diagnostic procedures, and treatment for patients with renovascular hypertension.

Kaplan, N. M.: Clinical Hypertension, 4th ed. Baltimore, Williams & Wilkins, 1986, pp. 317–344.
An excellent book that is well organized and presents a practical approach to the overall problem of hypertension, with a special reference to renovascular disease.

Novic, A. C., Ziegelbaum, M., Vidt, D. G., Gifford, R. W., Pohl, M. A., and Goormastic, M.: Trends in surgical revascularization for renal artery disease: Ten years experience. J.A.M.A., 257:498, 1987.
This study of 361 patients documents the increasing tendency to use surgical renal artery revascularization for preservation of renal function in elderly patients with systemic generalized atherosclerosis. The clinical results demonstrated with surgical revascularization are excellent in properly chosen patients with severe renal artery disease.

Working Group on Renovascular Hypertension: Detection, evaluation and treatment of renovascular hypertension: Final report. Ann. Intern. Med., 147:820, 1987.
This is a recent definitive report providing guidelines for the diagnosis and treatment of renovascular hypertension. They conclude that catheter arteriography remains the preferred procedure for the diagnosis of renovascular hypertension and recommend it when clinical evaluation strongly suggests the presence of renal artery stenosis.

REFERENCES

1. Beebe, H. G., Chesebro, K., Merchant, F., and Bush, W.: Results of renal artery balloon angioplasty limit its indications. J. Vasc. Surg., 8:300, 1988.
2. Braun-Menendes, E., Fasciolo, J. C., Lelior, L. F., Munoz, J. M., and Taquini, A. C.: Renal Hypertension. Translated by L. Dexter. Springfield, IL, Charles C Thomas, 1946.
3. Clark, R. A., and Alexander, E. S.: Digital subtraction angiography of the renal arteries: Prospective comparison with conventional arteriography. Invest. Radiol., 18:186, 1983.
4. Cummings, K. B., Lecky, J. W., and Kaufman, J. J.: Renal artery aneurysms and hypertensive retinopathy. J. Urol., 109:144, 1973.
5. Davis, B. A., Cook, J. E., Vestal, R. E., and Oates, J. A.: Prevalence of renovascular hypertension in patients with a Grade III or IV hypertensive retinopathy. N. Engl. J. Med., 301:1273, 1979.
6. Dean, R. H., Kieffer, R. W., Smith, B. M., Oates, J. A., Nadeau, J. H., Hollifield, J. W., and Dupont, W. D.: Renovascular hypertension: Anatomic and renal function changes during drug therapy. Arch. Surg., 116:1408, 1981.
7. Dornfeld, L., Ledky, J. W., and Peter, J. B.: Polyarteritis and intrarenal renal artery aneurysms. J.A.M.A., 215:1950, 1971.
8. Dunnick, N. R., Ford, K. K., Johnson, G. A., and Gunnells, J. C.: Digital intravenous subtraction angiography for the investigation of renovascular hypertension: A comparison with hypertensive urography. South. Med. J. 78:690, 1985.
9. Dzau, V. J., Gibbons, G. H., and Levin, D. C.: Renovascular hypertension: An update on pathophysiology, diagnosis and treatment. Am. J. Nephrol., 3:172, 1983.
10. Eyler, W. R., Clark, M. D., Garman, J. E., Rian, R. L., and Meininger, D. C.: Angiography of the renal areas including a comparative study of renal artery stenosis in patients with and without hypertension. Radiology, 78:879, 1962.
11. Gates, G. F.: Glomerular filtration rate: Estimation from fractional renal accumulation of 99mTC-DTPA (stannous). Am. J. Radiol., 138:565, 1982.
12. Gaul, M. K., Linn, W. D., and Mulrow, C. D.: Captopril-stimulated renin secretion in the diagnosis of renovascular hypertension. Am. J. Med., 80:633, 1986.
13. Geyskes, G. G., Oei, H. Y., Puylaert, C. B. A. J., and Mees, E. J.: Renovascular hypertension identified by captopril-induced changes in the renogram. Hypertension, 9:451, 1987.
14. Geyskes, G. G., Puylaert, C. B. A. J., Oei, H. Y., and Mees, E. J.: Follow-up study of 70 patients with renal artery stenosis treated by percutaneous transluminal dilation. Br. Med. J., 287:333, 1983.
15. Goldblatt, H., Lynch, J., Hanzal, R. F., and Summerville, W. D.: Studies in experimental hypertension. I. The production of persistent elevation of systolic blood pressure by means of renal ischemia. J. Exp. Med. 59:347, 1934.
16. Grim, C. E., Luft, F. C., Weinberger, M. H., and Grim, C. M.: Sensitivity and specificity of screening tests for renal vascular hypertension. Ann. Int. Med., 91:617, 1979.
17. Grüntzig, A., Kuhlman, K., Velter, W., Liefalf, K., Meyer, B., and Siengenthaler, W.: Treatment of renal artery stenosis. Lancet, 1:801, 1978.
18. Gunnells, J. C., Jr., McGriffin, W. L., Jr., Johnrude, I., and Robinson, R. R.: Peripheral and renal venous renin activity in hypertension. Ann. Intern. Med., 71:555, 1969.
19. Haber, E.: The renin-angiotensin system and hypertension. Kidney Int., 15:425, 1979.
20. Havey, R. J., Krumlovsky, E., Del Greco, F., and Martin, H. G.: Screening for renovascular hypertension. Is renal digital-subtraction angiography the preferred noninvasive test? J.A.M.A., 254:388, 1985.
21. Helmer, O. M.: Presence of renin in plasma of patients with arterial hypertension. Circulation, 25:169, 1962.
22. Hunt, J. C., Harrison, E. G., Jr., Kincaid, O. W., Bernatz, P. E., and Davis, G. D.: Idiopathic fibrous and fibromuscular stenoses of the renal arteries associated with hypertension. Mayo Clin. Proc., 37:181, 1962.
23. Krakoff, L. R., and Perla, C.: Screening for renovascular hypertension. J. Cardiovasc. Med., 8:555, 1983.
24. Lawrie, G. M., Morris, G. C., Jr., Glaeser, D. H., and DeBakey, M. E.: Renovascular reconstruction: Factors affecting long-term prognosis in 919 patients followed up to 31 years. Am. J. Cardiol., 63:1085, 1985.
25. Marks, L. S., Maxwell, M. H., Varady, P. D., Lupu, A. N., and Kaufman, J. J.: Renovascular hypertension: Does the renal vein renin ratio predict operative results? J. Urol., 115:365, 1976.
26. Maxwell, M. H., Bleifer, K. H., Franklin, S. S., and Varady, P. D.: Cooperative study of renovascular hypertension: Demographic analysis of the study. J.A.M.A., 220:1195, 1972.
27. Maxwell, M. H., Marx, L. S., Lupu, A. N., Cahill, P. J., Franklin, S. S., and Kaufman, J. J.: Predictive value of renin determinations in renal artery stenosis. J.A.M.A., 238:2617, 1977.

28. Meyrier, A., Buchet, P., Simon, P., Pernet, M., Rainfray, M., and Callard, P.: Atheromatous renal disease. Am. J. Med., 85:139, 1988.

29. Miamori, I., Yasuhara, S., Takeda, Y., Koshida, H., Ideda, M., Nagai, K., Odamoto, H., Morise, R., Takeda, R., and Aburano, T.: Effects of converting enzyme inhibition on split renal function in renovascular hypertension. Hypertension, 8:415, 1968.

30. Muller, F. B., Sealey, J. E., Case, D. B., Atlas, S. A., Pickering, T. G., Pecker, M. S., Preibisz, J. J., and Laragh, J. H.: The captopril test for identifying renovascular disease in hypertensive patients. Am. J. Med., 80:633, 1986.

31. Nally, J. V.: The captopril tests: A new concept in detecting renovascular hypertension? Cleve. Clin. J. Med., 56:395, 1989.

32. Novick, A. C., Straffon, R. A., Stewart, B. H., Gifford, R. W., and Vidt, D.: Diminished operative morbidity and mortality in renal revascularization. J.A.M.A., 246:749, 1981.

33. Oxman, H. A., Sheps, S. G., Bernatz, P. E., and Harrison, E. G., Jr.: An unusual case of renal arteriovenous fistula—fibromuscular dysplasia of the renal arteries. Report of a case. Mayo Clin. Proc., 48:207, 1983.

34. Page, I. H., and Corcoran, A. C.: Hypertension: Review of humoral pathogenesis and clinical treatment. Adv. Intern. Med., 1:183, 1942.

35. Pauker, S. G., and Kopelman, R. I.: Screening for renovascular hypertension: "A which hunt." Hypertension, 14:258, 1989.

36. Pickering, T. G., Sos, T. A., Vaughan, E. D., Case, D. B., Sealey, J. E., Harshfield, G. A., and Laragh, J. H.: Predictive value and changes of renin secretion in hypertensive patients with unilateral renovascular disease undergoing successful renal angioplasty. Am. J. Med., 76:398, 1984.

37. Rosenthal, J. T., Libertina, J. A., Zinman, L. N., Breslin, D. J., Swinton, N. W., Jr., and Christlieb, A. R.: Predictability of surgical cure of renovascular hypertension. Ann. Surg., 193:448, 1981.

38. Smith, C. W., Winfield, A. C., Price, R. R., Harding, D. R., Tucker, S. T., Witt, W. S., and Hollifield, J. W.: Evaluation of digital venous angiography for the diagnosis of renovascular hypertension. Radiology, 144:51, 1982.

39. Sos, T. A., Pickering, T. G., Sniderman, K., Saddekni, S., Case, D. B., Silane, M. F., Vaughan, E. D., Jr., and Laragh, J. H.: Percutaneous transluminal renal angioplasty in renovascular hypertension due to atheroma or fibromuscular dysplasia. N. Engl. J. Med., 309:274, 1983.

40. Staab, G. E., Tegtmeyer, C. J., and Constable, W. C.: Radiation-induced renovascular hypertension. Am. J. Roentgenol., 126:634, 1976.

41. Svetky, S. E., Himmelstein, S. I., et al.: Prospective analysis of strategies for diagnosing renovascular hypertension. Hypertension, 14:247, 1989.

42. Tegtmeyer, C. J., Dyer, R., Teates, C. D., Ayers, C. R., Carey, R. M., Wellson, H. A., Jr., and Stanton, L. W.: Percutaneous transluminal dilatation of the renal arteries: Techniques and results. Radiology, 135:589, 1980.

43. Tegtmeyer, C. J., Teates, C. D., Crigler, N., Gandee, R. W., Ayers, C. R., Stoddard, M., and Wellons, H. A., Jr.: Percutaneous angioplasty in patients with renal artery stenosis: Follow-up studies. Radiology, 140:323, 1981.

44. Thibonnier, M., Joseph, A., Sassano, P., Guyenne, T. T., Corvol, P., Ranaud, A., Seurot, M., and Gaux, J. X.: Improved diagnosis of unilateral renal artery lesions after captopril administration. J.A.M.A., 251:156, 1984.

45. Tigerstedt, R., and Bergman, P. B.: Niere und Kreislauf: Skand. Arch. Physiol., 8:223, 1898.

46. Vaughan, E. D.: Renovascular hypertension. Kidney Int., 27:811, 1985.

47. Weibull, H., Bergqvist, D., Jonsson, K., Carlsson, S., and Takolander, R.: Analysis of complications after percutaneous transluminal angioplasty of renal artery stenosis. Eur. J. Vasc. Surg., 1:77, 1987.

48. Wilcox, C. S., Williams, C. M., Smith, T. B., Frederickson, E. D., Wingo, C., and Bucci, C. N.: Diagnostic use of angiotensin-converting enzyme inhibitors in renovascular hypertension. Am. J. Hypertens., 34:S138, 1988.

49. Wise, K. L., McCann, R. L., Dunnick, N. R., and Paulson, D. F.: Renovascular hypertension. J. Urol., 140:911, 1988.

VII

VENOUS INJURIES

Norman M. Rich, M.D.

> Simple ligation of injured veins is the classic method of management . . . Lateral suture repair is preferred to ligation . . . Grafts to bridge venous defects are not advocated.
>
> —*M. R. Gaspar and R. L. Treiman, 1960*

> Initially, when we started the Vietnam Vascular Registry we felt that the greatest interest would come from management of arterial injuries. We more or less pushed venous injuries to the background. But in the last year we have become more interested in repair of venous injuries and feel that this area needs to be pursued with great vigor.
>
> —*N. M. Rich, C. W. Hughes, and J. H. Baugh, 1970*

These two quotations identify and emphasize important changes that have occurred in the management of injured veins, particularly during the past 25 years. In contrast to the management of injured arteries, in which repair, rather than ligation, has been widely and enthusiastically practiced in the years since the Korean conflict, the same approach has not been widely developed for the management of venous injuries. It is ironic that Murphy made the following statement in 1897 when he described the first successful clinical end-to-end anastomosis of an artery: ". . . closure of wounds in the veins by suture is now an acceptable surgical practice."[29]

Two major concerns prevented the development of repair of injured veins: (1) the belief that there would be an increased incidence of thrombophlebitis, and (2) the fear of pulmonary embolism. Morton, Southgate, and DeWeese summarized the general concern in 1966 when they stated: "Whether or not concomitant venous injuries should be repaired remains a point of contention."[29] It is recognized that many injured veins can be ligated with few or no immediate problems and no recognized long-term disability. Until the last 25 years, the effectiveness of venous repair remained uncertain. Thrombosis was recognized to be much more common in the lower-pressure venous system, compared with the good results achieved following repair of arterial injuries. Also, in contrast to arterial repair, in which simple palpation of a peripheral pulse is usually adequate to determine success or failure, effectiveness of venous repair is more difficult to evaluate because there is no simple method for determining the patency of a venous reconstruction. Acute venous hypertension in the extremities following ligation of major veins, particularly in the lower extremities, may contribute to an increased amputation rate.[33] In addition, the degree of disability from chronic venous insufficiency is not recognized by many.[30] This disability may not become evident for months or even 5 to 10 years following injury.[28]

It has been recognized and documented throughout history that important surgical progress has occurred during periods of armed conflict when surgeons are required to treat large numbers of patients with similar injuries within a relatively short period of time. This corollary between military surgery and vascular surgery has been particularly noteworthy in the nineteenth and twentieth centuries. An analysis that included the importance and effectiveness of repair of venous injuries during the American experience in Southeast Asia was started at Walter Reed Army Medical Center in 1966 as the Vietnam Vascular Registry. A preliminary report from the Vietnam Vascular Registry demonstrated a significant incidence of venous injuries: 27 per cent (Table 1).[32] An early report emphasized the need for the repair of injured veins,[26] and a more aggressive

TABLE 1. Incidence of Venous Trauma:
Preliminary Vietnam Vascular Registry
Report (500 Patients)

Total vascular injuries	718
Venous injuries	194 (27.0%)
Isolated	28 (14.4%)
Combined	166 (85.6%)

Modified from Rich, N. M., and Hughes, C. W.:
Vietnam Vascular Registry: A preliminary report.
Surgery, 62:218, 1969.

approach for the repair of injured veins, particularly in lower extremity venous trauma, was advocated in 1974.

Venous repair may be particularly important in large-caliber lower extremity veins, specifically the popliteal vein (Fig. 1). Venous repair may be necessary in the presence of massive soft tissue injury and is mandatory in replantation of extremities. Repair of injured large-caliber veins should be considered routinely in an attempt to prevent acute or chronic venous insufficiency. Important central veins, such as the portal vein, the superior mesenteric vein, and the vena cava, should be included. Lateral suture repair of a lacerated vein is frequently the most rapid and safest method of halting hemorrhage. Although the general status of the patient with multiple injuries must be considered, it is often possible to repair veins by end-to-end anastomosis and by interposition grafts, including compilation and spiral venous grafts. The challenge of obtaining successful venous reconstruction remains. A major obstacle is identifica-

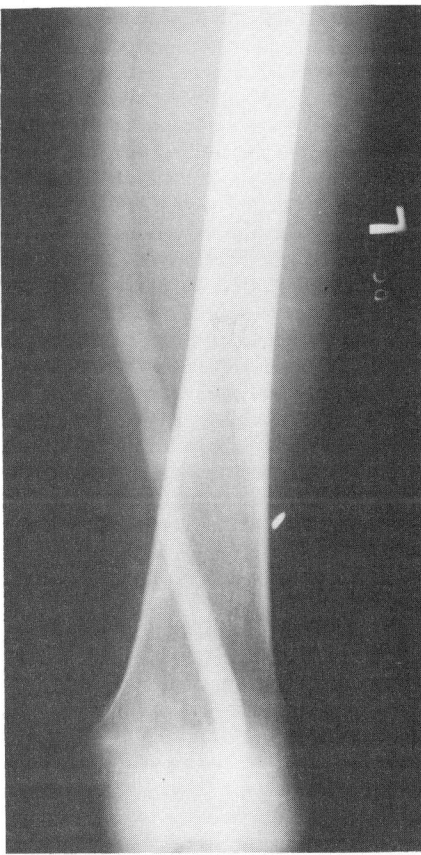

Figure 1. Venogram demonstrating patency of the popliteal vein at its junction with the superficial femoral vein. Note the metallic fragments that caused the injury. The vein had been repaired by lateral suture 3½ years earlier in Vietnam. Repair of concomitant venous injuries is advocated as one of the methods that will help lower the relatively high amputation rate associated with popliteal artery trauma. (From Rich, N. M., Jarstfer, B. S., and Geer, T. M.: Popliteal artery repair failure; Causes and possible prevention. J. Cardiovasc. Surg., 15:340, 1974.)

tion of the ideal vein substitute that will have a high degree of success with long-term patency in the venous system, where the pressure is lower than in the arterial system.

Recent studies have provided data that allay the fear of a higher incidence of venous thrombosis and pulmonary embolization following repair of injured veins.[24] Although this is a possible hazard, the dangerous sequence has been surprisingly absent. It is conceivable that small emboli may not be recognized clinically; however, the absence of clinically detectable pulmonary emboli has been uniformly documented both in the Vietnam Vascular Registry and in previous reports by others.[34] Civilian experience in the past decade has corroborated the previously cited military experience in some aspects; however, the difference in wounds in civilian practice also has been emphasized in a variety of experiences and results.[1–7,13,18,21,35,37]

Historical Aspects

The development of vascular surgery has been detailed in recent excellent reviews. Although Travers and Guthrie are given credit for successfully closing small venous lacerations, Schede is generally recognized for performing the first successful lateral suture repair in humans. In 1882, he repaired a laceration of the femoral vein and advocated this procedure in the clinical situation. The Russian surgeon Eck made an important contribution in experimental vascular surgery in 1877 with the first successful experimental anastomosis of two vessels with lateral communication between the portal vein and the inferior vena cava. Kummel is credited with performing the first clinical end-to-end anastomosis of a vein when he repaired the femoral vein in 1889. Carrel and Guthrie are recognized for their many outstanding contributions to the basic principles of vascular surgery.[29] The clinical use of lateral suture repair of venous lacerations in World War I was reported by Goodman in 1918. He described five patients with vascular lacerations, in four of whom a lateral suture repair involving two popliteal and two superficial femoral veins was done. The defects ranged from 5 to 20 mm. in length. The results are unknown because there was no follow-up evaluation. The importance of venous repair was minimized by the proposal of Makins in 1917 that the concomitant vein should be ligated when an arterial injury was treated by ligation. It was later found that the results reported by Makins to support this hypothesis had no statistical significance. Data from World War II by DeBakey and Simeone in 1946 demonstrated that there was no benefit from ligation of the concomitant vein with arterial injuries. During the Korean conflict, repair of injuries of major veins was again undertaken in selected patients and summarized by Hughes in 1959[29]:

> Most venous injuries were treated by ligation, resulting in various degrees of venostasis. Although some patients were symptomatic after ligation of a major vein, severe venostasis resulted in instances of limb loss. To eliminate these complications, two investigators began to repair major veins . . . some were known to have thrombosed later but without complications.

Although some surgeons are aware of the details of the controversy in the early part of this century regarding the concept of elective ligation of the accompanying vein when an injured artery was ligated, there is a startling and bizarre aspect to the management of vascular trauma that is not generally remembered. The approach to the management of venous injuries in the mid nineteenth century included ligation of the concomitant artery. Gensoul in 1833 supposedly was the first to describe venous engorgement as a dangerous problem that would result when only the femoral vein was ligated in an extremity.[29]

In considering experimental work that contributed to the development of venous reconstruction in the mid twentieth century, Johns re-established experimental studies on suture and nonsuture methods of venous anastomosis in 1947. As might be anticipated, some of the best early results were obtained in

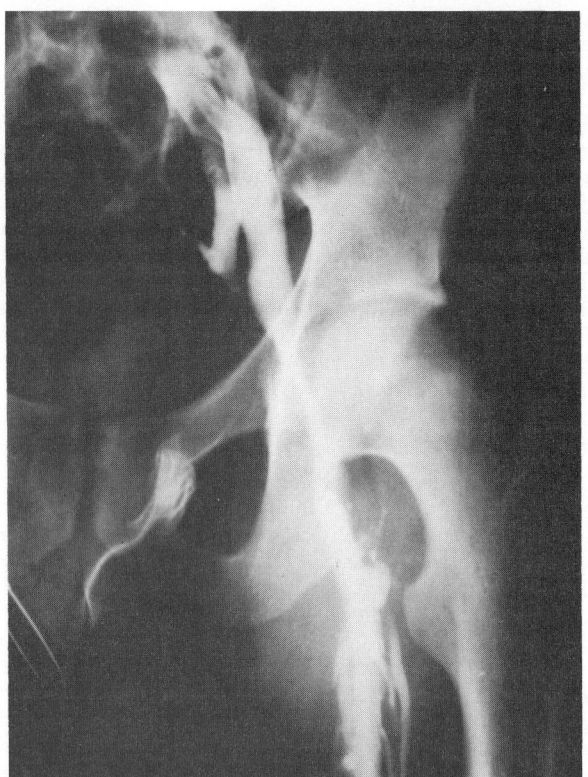

Figure 2. Clinical success is demonstrated angiographically by the patent compilation vein graft used to repair an injured common femoral vein. (Courtesy of Dr. William G. Sullivan. From Rich, N. M., and Spencer, F. C.: Vascular Trauma. Philadelphia, W. B. Saunders Company, 1978.)

reconstruction of the superior vena cava.[23] Favorable results have also been obtained in reconstruction of the portal vein.[13] There was less early success, however, with attempted repair and reconstruction of the abdominal inferior vena cava and the peripheral venous system.

Despite the large number of conduits that have been used in the venous system, no uniform degree of success has been established for any of these. A variety of techniques and adjunctive measures have also been utilized, but no uniformly associated high degree of patency has been established (Fig. 2).

Generally, the clinical progress has been more limited, and there has been less experience compared with the previously outlined experimental work. Similar to the experimental experience, the best early results have occurred in direct venous reconstruction of the superior vena cava. Additional details regarding the relatively extensive experience during the Vietnam War follow. Also, the crossover saphenofemoral bypass by Palma in the late 1950s has been demonstrated to be of value by

Dale and others in the United States in the treatment of patients with iliofemoral venous occlusion.

Incidence of Venous Injuries

Because many surgeons have considered venous injuries to be unimportant and have not reported many of them, their true incidence is undetermined. This is particularly true when venous injuries are associated with arterial injuries, with the emphasis usually being given to arterial repair. In an analysis of the data in the Vietnam Vascular Registry, numerous cases were found in which venous trauma was not documented in the records; however, this documentation was possible through retrospective analysis. Considering the many reports that have originated from the civilian community in the past 25 years regarding the repair of injured arteries, there is, in contrast, a marked paucity of papers specifically addressing the management of venous injuries.

As previously identified, there is one notable exception in the report by Gaspar and Treiman.[10] In a group of 228 patients with vascular injuries at the Los Angeles County General Hospital over a period of 10 years, 51 patients (about 22 per cent) had venous injuries. The superficial femoral vein was most frequently injured (nine cases). Injuries to an inferior vena cava and an internal jugular vein each occurred eight times, and seven injuries of the brachial veins were noted. In 1966, an additional 40 patients were added to the original series in a supplementary report by Treiman and associates.

The frequency of venous injuries in the different anatomic locations is outlined in Table 2. There are also recent reviews.[1–6,14,17,19,32,34] Agarwal and colleagues reported in 1982 a retrospective analysis of 115 patients with venous injuries managed at the Lincoln Hospital in New York City during a 7-year period.[1] Hardin and associates reported 83 patients with 86 venous injuries whose records were reviewed retrospectively in the Tulane University Hospital.[14] During a 4-year period (1979 to 1983), Hobson and colleagues reported a series of 81 venous injuries that were treated surgically. Thirty per cent, or 24 cases, involved femoral veins—9 of the common femoral and 15 of the superficial femoral vein.[17] Meyer and colleagues identified 36 patients with major extremity venous injuries, with 34 also having major arterial injury.[20] Aitken and co-workers reviewed the cases of 26 patients with lower limb venous trauma.[2]

During the Korean conflict, the first major interest in identifying the frequency of venous injuries in military trauma was established. An analysis of 180 acute vascular injuries showing that major veins were involved in approximately 40 per cent of the total is presented in Table 3. There were 71 major venous injuries and 79 major arterial injuries.[18a] The preliminary Vietnam Vascular Registry report, which included approximately 25 per cent of the patients with venous trauma, is shown in Table 4. There were only 28 isolated venous injuries, emphasizing that the majority of venous injuries were combined with adjacent

TABLE 2. Incidence of Venous Injuries in Los Angeles

Vein	Number (1948–1958)	Number (1958–1963)	Total (1948–1963)	Per Cent
Axillary-brachial	8	5	13	14.1
Innominate-subclavian	3	5	8	8.7
Superior vena cava	1	0	1	1.1
Inferior vena cava	8	4	12	13.0
Iliac	7	4	11	12.0
Femoral	11	6	17	18.5
Other	14	16	30	32.6
Total	52	40	92	100.0

Modified from Treiman, R. L., Doty, D., and Gaspar, M. R.: Acute vascular trauma. A fifteen year study. Am. J. Surg., *111*:469, 1966.

TABLE 3. Incidence of Acute Vascular
Trauma in Korean Casualties

Vessel	Number	Per Cent
Major arteries	79	43.9
Major veins	71	39.4
Minor arteries	30	16.7
Total	180	100.0

Modified from Hughes, C. W.: Acute vascular trauma in Korean War casualties: Analysis of 180 cases. Surg. Gynecol. Obstet., *99*:91, 1954.

arterial injuries. The interim Vietnam Vascular Registry report documented a concomitant venous injury incidence of approximately 38 per cent of cases with acute major arterial trauma.[26]

Etiology

Although an endless variety of wounding agents has been identified as the etiologic factor in venous trauma, specific documentation in published reports is very limited. In the civilian report by Gaspar and Treiman, sharp instruments were responsible for the largest number of injuries: 23, or approximately 44 per cent.[10] Venous injuries caused by missiles were almost equal to those caused by sharp instruments; only nine injuries were produced by blunt instruments. One iatrogenic laceration of the inferior vena cava occurred during abdominoperineal resection.

The number of iatrogenic injuries to the venous system has increased during the past 25 years as a result of the rapid development of vascular and cardiac angiography and catheterization. The reported cases of catheters that have been lost in the venous system are too numerous to review, emphasizing that this possibility must be fully appreciated. Thrombosis, sepsis, and phlebitis have also complicated the use of indwelling catheters. Iatrogenic venous injuries have been associated with the majority of major operations at one time or another. Inadvertent injury to the common femoral vein during stripping of the greater saphenous system, usually resulting from failure to recognize the common femoral vein, has been a published surgical error. An unusual example of iatrogenic venous trauma is the

TABLE 4. Location and Management of Concomitant Venous Injuries Associated with Arterial Injuries in the Vietnam Vascular Registry

Location	Arteries	Concomitant Veins	Ligation	Repair
Neck				
Carotid	50	14	10	4
Chest				
Innominate	3	1	0	1
Subclavian	8	4	1	3
Upper extremity				
Axillary	59	20	18	2
Brachial	283	54	42	12
Abdomen and pelvis				
Abdominal aorta	3	1	0	1
Common iliac	9	6	6	0
External iliac	17	5	3	2
Lower extremity				
Common femoral	46	17	8	9
Superficial femoral	305	139	83	56
Popliteal	217	116	82	34
Total	1000	377	253	124

Modified from Rich, N. M., Hughes, C. W., and Baugh, J. H.: Management of venous injuries. Ann. Surg., *171*:724, 1970.

report by Zabin[38] in 1950 of an accidental tear of the inferior vena cava complicating cholecystectomy.

Fractures have been associated with venous injuries. The potentially lethal exsanguinating hemorrhage from venous trauma associated with pelvic fractures remains a challenge for surgeons.

In military casualties, as might be expected, fragments and high-velocity missiles are responsible for most venous injuries. In an analysis of 1000 acute major arterial injuries in soldiers in Vietnam, which included 377 concomitant venous injuries, 60 per cent were produced by fragments from an assortment of exploding devices and 35 per cent by bullets.[26]

Pathophysiology

Most venous injuries that have been repaired have been lacerations. Despite the rather limited statistics, it is recognized that high-velocity missiles, as in military casualties, can be responsible for transection of veins. Considering the anatomic proximity of veins and arteries in most areas of the body, the possibility of concomitant arterial injuries should be suspected when a venous injury is found (Table 5).

Pertinent experimental research deserves mention. An immediate decrease in femoral arterial blood flow was demonstrated as part of the evaluation of the hemodynamics of acute venous occlusion in the experimental model. It was demonstrated that femoral venous ligation in the canine hindlimb resulted in a 50 to 75 per cent reduction in femoral arterial blood flow, with a marked increase in femoral venous pressure as well as in peripheral resistance.

As with arterial injuries, most venous injuries occur in the extremities (Table 5). Many veins are vulnerable to injury owing to their relatively superficial location. In contrast to the bright red, spurting blood of an arterial injury, there is usually dark, steady bleeding from a venous injury. In a closed wound, a massive hematoma may develop. It may not be possible to differentiate the etiology of such a hematoma from trauma to multiple small vessels or from arterial trauma. Consequently, many venous injuries are first recognized at the time of surgical exploration. It is particularly important to emphasize that acute venous insufficiency may develop within the first 12 to 24 hours following trauma. Massive edema and a cool, bluish extremity are the principal clinical findings. The clinical pattern of chronic venous insufficiency, a familiar one because of the frequency of thrombophlebitis in surgical patients, includes edema, varices, brown pigmentation of the skin, and stasis ulcers.

Diagnostic Considerations

As previously outlined, Doppler ultrasound may be useful as a diagnostic approach in the management of venous disease. Numerous clinical studies have a documented variation in the accuracy of the Doppler technique. In the early experience in the Vietnam Vascular Registry follow-up, the Doppler tech-

TABLE 5. Frequency of Concomitant Venous Injuries Associated with Acute Arterial Trauma

Artery	Number	Venous Injuries	Per Cent
Axillary	59	20	33.8
Brachial	283	54	19.0
Iliac	26	11	42.3
Common femoral	46	17	36.9
Superficial femoral	305	139	45.5
Popliteal	217	116	53.5
Total	936	357	37.9

Modified from Rich, N. M., Hughes, C. W., and Baugh, J. H.: Management of venous injuries. Ann. Surg., *171*:724, 1970.

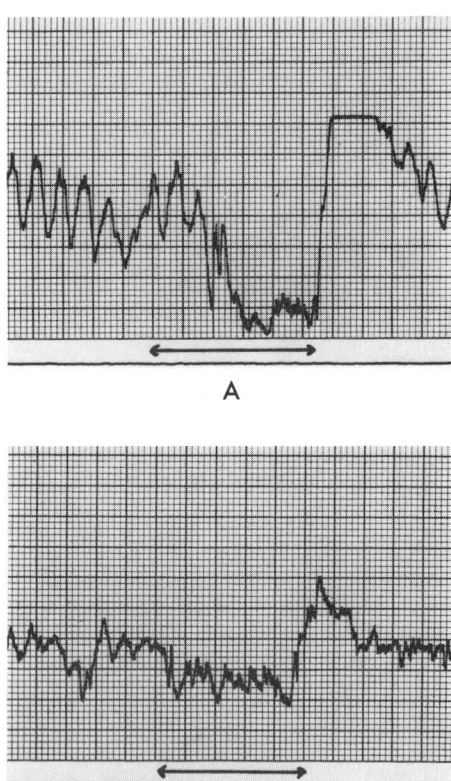

Figure 3. *A*, Normal depression with rapid elevation with the Vaughn maneuver is recorded with the Doppler over the right common femoral vein. *B*, In contrast, the characteristic flow pattern was absent when the Doppler was placed over the left common femoral vein above the occluded femoropopliteal veins. (From Rich, N. M., Hughes, C. W., and Baugh, J. H.: Management of venous injuries. Ann. Surg., *171:*724, 1970.)

nique was of value in determining patency of venous repairs, particularly in the lower extremities (Fig. 3).

Impedance plethysmography, phlebography, and radionuclide studies have also had a degree of success in diagnosing venous occlusions. The phlebograph has been used in the long-term follow-up at Walter Reed Army Medical Center for patients who had previous venous injuries. Whereas roentgenograms may be of value in identifying offending missile injuries or associated fractures, phlebography is the ultimate diagnostic means of determining the location and extent of venous injury, with or without associated thrombus formation. Gerlock and associates have provided valuable information in performing phlebograms in patients with venous injuries.[12]

Surgical Management

General considerations for management of injured patients should be of primary concern. Rapid assessment of multiple injuries with the establishment of priorities is mandatory. Shock is common with major venous injuries, particularly when active hemorrhage is unabated. Concomitant arterial injuries may be part of the multiple-injury complex and can contribute to exsanguinating hemorrhage. Hemorrhage from injured veins can usually be controlled by judicious pressure or packing, except with penetrating injuries of the body cavities. This approach also helps prevent the entrance of air into the venous system. In some patients, particularly those with penetrating injuries of the body cavities, immediate operation may be necessary to control profound shock from exsanguinating hemorrhage. Shock should be treated by rapid infusion of whole blood and appropriate electrolyte solutions. Broad-spectrum antibiotics should be given routinely.

The principles of elective surgical procedures should be fol-

lowed in the management of the injured patient who has sustained venous trauma. Elective incisions, usually longitudinal along the course of the vein, help in providing adequate exposure for proximal and distal control of the vein to halt the venous hemorrhage. A frequent question is raised regarding whether an arterial or a venous injury should be repaired first. Normally, the injured artery should be repaired first to minimize anoxia in the distal extremity. In some instances, however, it may be more expeditious to repair the venous injury first, usually by lateral suture, to establish hemostasis and provide better exposure of the arterial injury. Copious irrigation with saline solution is useful for both visualization and removal of foreign material. Adequate wound débridement is essential, as is the removal of nonviable tissue following trauma.

Bleeding can usually be controlled temporarily with digital pressure until blood clot and foreign debris have been irrigated from the wound. The digital pressure can be augmented by stick sponges. A combination of encircling tapes around the vein, both distal and proximal to the area of injury, and a proximal temporary tourniquet afford simple, atraumatic control of hemorrhage. This is usually preferable to vascular clamps, particularly when the exposure is limited. With tangential injuries to large veins, however, a partial occluding vascular clamp may be used. This approach avoids the necessity of wider mobilization of the vein and also permits the flow of venous blood to continue unabated.

A venous injury can be managed by at least five different methods. In order of popularity, they are (1) ligation, (2) lateral suture repair, (3) end-to-end anastomosis, (4) venous patch graft, and (5) venous replacement graft.[31]

Ligation, as mentioned, has been used for many injured veins. Nevertheless, lateral suture repair has been used increasingly. Most clinical data at present are concerned with techniques of lateral suture repair. Although the other methods of repair are theoretically satisfactory and there are anecdotal cases, few data are available for estimating the degree of success of venous reconstruction, particularly with venous replacement grafts, inserted for injuries in different parts of the body.

Before repair is begun, the vein should be explored both proximally and distally for thrombi. A balloon catheter is most useful, although difficulty may be encountered occasionally during retrograde insertion because of competent venous valves. Gentle manipulation is necessary to avoid perforation. If thrombus is present, it can be expressed by gentle pressure peripherally toward the area of venous injury. If thrombus is present or if venous occlusion is necessary for more than a few minutes, heparin can be administered either locally or systemically to help prevent additional propagation of thrombus.

Meticulous technique is mandatory during venous reconstruction.[31] Both experimentally and clinically, experience has demonstrated that this meticulous technique is more critical in the management of injured veins than of injured arteries. Obviously, venous repairs have a greater tendency to thrombose. A fine synthetic vascular suture on a small needle minimizes bleeding. When a continuous suture is used, less tension is applied than in arterial anastomoses in order to avoid circular constriction. Leaving the loops of a continuous suture somewhat loose may create a few leaks, but bleeding usually stops with mild pressure.

The apparent simplicity of venous repair often deceives the inexperienced operator, who may think the problem is simpler than the more complex arterial repair with associated pulsatile hemorrhage and threatened viability of the extremity. With lateral suture repair, as with arterial repairs, the principal consideration is avoidance of undue constriction of the venous lumen. Occasionally, autogenous venous patches may be useful in preventing constriction. When the repair cannot be done by lateral suture, reconstruction by end-to-end anastomosis or by insertion of a vascular graft can be considered if the patient's general

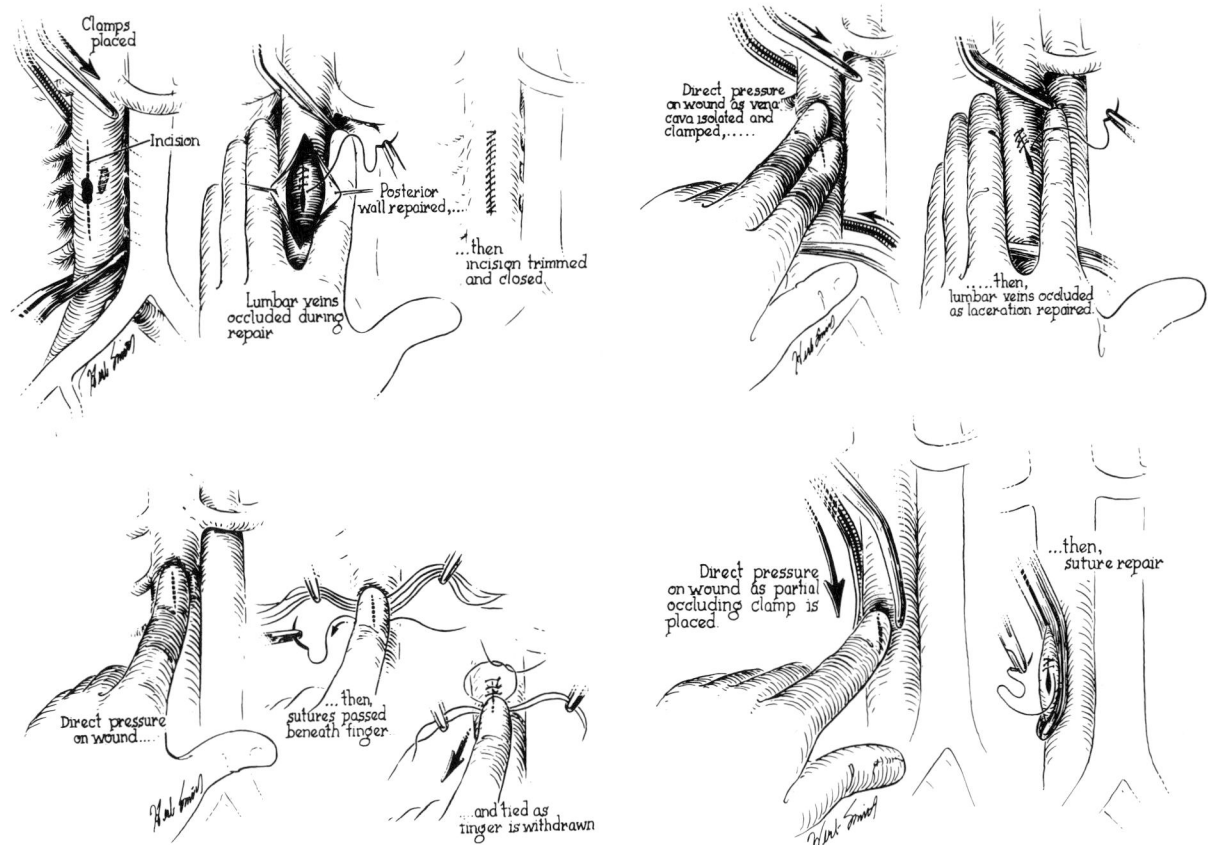

Figure 4. The management of vena caval injuries is outlined in these composite drawings. These methods can be utilized in injuries to large caliber veins. (From Quast, D. C., Shirkey, A. L., Fitzgerald, J. B., Beall, A. C., Jr., and DeBakey, M. E.: Surgical correction of injuries of the vena cava; An analysis of sixty-one cases. J. Trauma, 5:3, 1965.)

condition is stable. To date, autogenous venous grafts are the only satisfactory grafts. Synthetic grafts have had the most successful application in repair of large veins, such as the superior or inferior vena cava. If there is great disparity between the size of the vein and the size of the venous replacement segment, turbulence and eddying result and contribute to thrombus formation.

Specific mention is made of injuries of the venae cavae because no acceptable autogenous vein grafts are available for the large-caliber cava. Good results have been obtained by making composite grafts, such as those espoused by Doty and associates in 1976.[8] Quast and co-workers in 1965 outlined a number of techniques that can be considered for lacerations in the vena cava (Fig. 4).[23] Similar approaches can be utilized for other injuries of large-caliber veins. Schrock and colleagues[35a] in 1968 and Bricker and colleagues in 1971 described an internal vena caval shunt to maintain venous return during repair with the shunt introduced through the right atrium; however, the clinical experience with this approach is limited.

Operative phlebography is an adjunctive measure that may be of value after reconstruction, because palpation of distal pulses is not possible then, as it is after arterial reconstruction. A phlebogram performed in the operating room can help outline a stenotic area at the repair site or residual thrombus within the venous lumen.

Postoperative Care

Specific attempts should be made after the operation to minimize or eliminate edema of the involved extremity. This is particularly true when large veins, such as the vena cava, have been ligated. Early and vigorous postoperative care to prevent massive edema should be initiated as soon as possible, including elevation of the legs and careful wrapping of them or use of

elastic support hose when the patient is ambulatory. Disability from chronic venous insufficiency can be greatly minimized by early effective use of elastic support. This requires frequent inspection and periodic adjustment of both the type and the degree of support. These factors are probably mismanaged more often than any other form of supportive care in patients with chronic venous insufficiency.

Results

In a summary of the experience in the Korean conflict, Hughes[18a] reported that all 20 venous repairs were performed by lateral suture except for one end-to-end anastomosis. In Vietnam, approximately one third of the venous injuries were repaired. This was confirmed by both the initial and the interim Registry reports. Interest was concentrated particularly on major veins in the lower extremities, and 85 per cent of the repairs were performed by the lateral suture technique. As experience increased, however, end-to-end anastomosis and autogenous venous grafts were used more frequently. Follow-up phlebograms (Figs. 5 and 6) demonstrate the success of the various techniques that were employed. Sullivan and co-workers performed perhaps the most significant study on the management of injuries of the popliteal vein at the Twelfth Evacuation Hospital in Vietnam.[36] There were 27 injuries to the popliteal vein among 35 popliteal vascular injuries, and 21 of the 27 venous injuries were repaired. Phlebograms performed on 11 patients within the first 72 hours after operation showed patent repair in 8. Success included patency of an autogenous venous graft in the popliteal vein. Probably of greatest importance was the finding that massive edema did not occur in any of the 21 patients who had primary repair of the venous injury, which contrasted with severe venous insufficiency and morbidity in 4 patients in whom the popliteal vein was ligated. It is

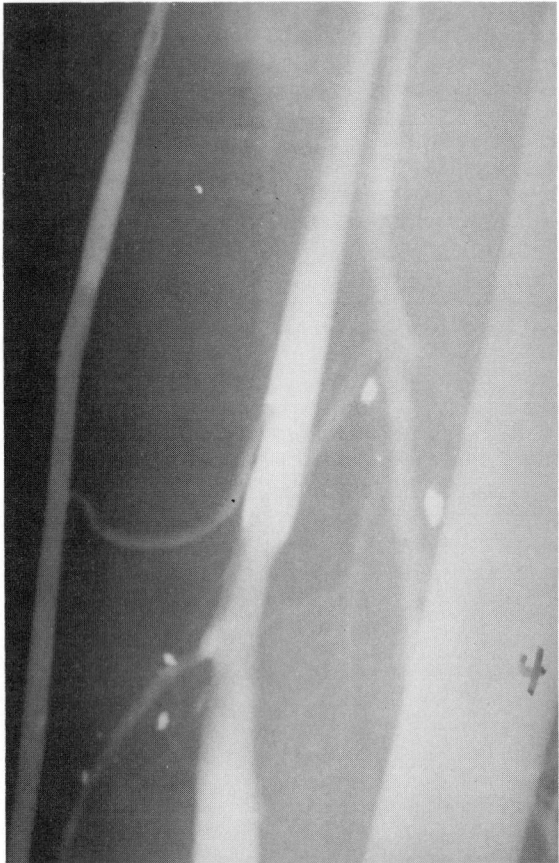

Figure 5. Patency of the superficial femoral vein is demonstrated by phlebography approximately 1 month after repair in a 20-year-old Vietnam casualty who developed a superficial femoral arteriovenous fistula from multiple fragment wounds. (From Rich, N. M., Hughes, C. W., and Baugh, J. H.: Management of venous injuries. Ann. Surg., *171*:724, 1970.)

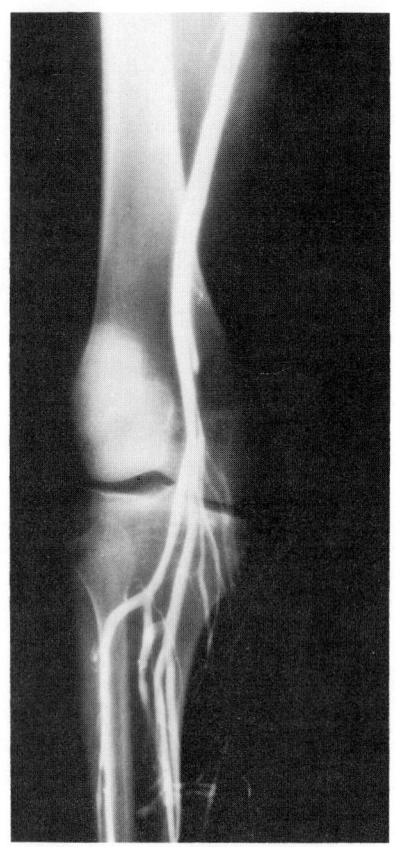

Figure 6. The distal superficial femoral vein in this patient was repaired with an autogenous greater saphenous vein patch graft. This venogram shows successful repair and patency of the vein at the junction with the popliteal vein. (From Rich, N. M., Hughes, C. W., and Baugh, J. H.: Management of venous injuries. Ann. Surg., *171*:724, 1970.)

remarkable that no known cases of pulmonary emboli were recognized after venous repair in the initial Vietnam series, which included 124 reconstructions.[26] In the later long-term follow-up, nonfatal pulmonary emboli have been seen infrequently. There is no statistically significant difference between these findings and those in patients who have had ligation of venous injuries.

One study from the Vietnam Vascular Registry evaluated the long-term follow-up of 110 patients with isolated popliteal venous trauma with the adjacent popliteal artery intact. Nearly an equal number were either ligated or repaired. Thrombophlebitis and pulmonary embolism were not significant complications in this series. Only one pulmonary embolus occurred after ligation of an injured popliteal vein. There was a significant increase, however, in edema in the involved extremity following ligation of the popliteal vein, as contrasted to the involved extremity following repair of the injured popliteal vein (Table 6). A second important study involved the 10-year follow-up of 51 Vietnam casualties whose lower extremity venous injuries were repaired by autogenous interposition venous grafts.[27] Only 1 patient (2 per cent) developed thrombophlebitis in the postoperative period, and this was transitory (Table 7). Of particular significance is the relatively low edema rate of approximately 12 per cent, as contrasted to the 51 per cent rate of edema following ligation of the popliteal veins.

In the civilian community, Gaspar and Treiman in 1960 documented lateral suture repair of 10 venous lacerations, representing only one fifth of the 52 venous injuries encountered.[10] Six of these ten injuries were located in the inferior vena cava. All but

one of the patients recovered, apparently with good results from the venous reconstruction. In the remaining patients, 27 ligations were performed, with good results in 21. Six could not be evaluated because of three deaths from associated injuries and three amputations due to concomitant arterial injuries. For various reasons, the venous injury was not treated in 15 patients, 8 of whom subsequently developed arteriovenous fistulas. In the supplemental report published by Treiman and associates in 1966, repair was utilized in approximately 50 per cent of a total of 92 venous injuries.

Agarwal and associates, in their report of 115 civilian venous injuries, disclosed a total mortality of 15 per cent.[1] In their experience, retrohepatic caval injury was uniformly fatal. They also documented that ligation of injured veins in upper extremities was not associated with any specific morbidity; however, ligation of larger-caliber lower extremity veins resulted in edema in 50 per cent of the patients, compared with edema in only 7 per cent of the patients who underwent repair of lower extremity veins.

TABLE 6. Incidence of Edema Following Ligation and Repair of Injured Popliteal Veins

Management	Number	With Edema	Per Cent
Ligation	57	29	50.9
Repair	53	7	13.2

Modified from Rich, N. M., Hobson, R. W., II, Collins, G. J., Jr., and Andersen, C. A.: The effect of acute popliteal venous interruption. Ann. Surg., *183*:365, 1976.

TABLE 7. Complications of Venous Repair Using Autogenous Venous Grafts (51 Patients)

Complication	Number	Per Cent
Thrombophlebitis	1	2.0
Pulmonary embolism	0	0.0
Amputation	0	0.0
Death	0	0.0
Edema		
None	34	66.6
Early	11	21.6
Residual	6	11.8
Total	51	100.0

From Rich, N. M., Collins, G. J., Jr., Andersen, C. A., and McDonald, P. T.: Autogenous venous interposition grafts in repair of major venous injuries. J. Trauma, 17:512, 1977.

Hobson and colleagues managed femoral venous injuries by lateral venorrhaphy in 10 cases (42 per cent), venous patch angioplasty in 5 cases (21 per cent), end-to-end anastomosis in 4 cases (17 per cent), interposition autogenous saphenous vein grafts in 3 patients (12 per cent), and ligation in 2 cases (8 per cent).[18] They excluded one early death from associated injuries and one superficial femoral venous injury managed by ligation without postoperative complications, reporting that 17 of 23 femoral venous repairs (74 per cent) were judged patent postoperatively, with 13 confirmed by venography and 4 by noninvasive testing. They believe that adjuvant use of intermittent pneumatic calf compression and low-molecular-weight dextran had some benefit in maintaining patency of the femoral venous repairs. Edema was treated in 6 of 8 patients (75 per cent) by ligation or was complicated by postoperative occlusion in their patients with femoral venous trauma.[18]

Additional evaluation of the management of injured veins in the civilian population will provide valuable information. A recent example is the valuable contribution by Phifer and colleagues, who evaluated the long-term patency of venous repairs with six femoral venous reconstructions.[22] Follow-up venography at 6 to 20 years demonstrated venous patency and functional valves in asymptomatic patients and no clinical evidence of venous insufficiency in all but 1 patient.[22] Mullins and colleagues from Detroit,[21] as well as Timberlake and co-workers from New Orleans,[37] have had varying results without identifying significant edema in civilian injuries following lower extremity venous ligation. Meyer and colleagues from Chicago reported a 61 per cent success rate in maintaining patency of lower extremity venous repair.[20] Aitken and colleagues made a long-term clinical and physiologic assessment of lower limb vein trauma; and their recommendation is, "Vein ligation should be avoided unless another life-threatening injury demands priority."[2] Although the final answer is not available at this time, it is obvious from both civilian and military experience that some patients, who may be difficult to identify at the time of injury, will have the sequelae that might be anticipated from interruption of the lower extremity venous return if ligation is performed. Even from the more recent civilian reports with contrary views, repair of venous injuries has been advocated. Additional studies, such as that identified by Aitken and co-workers, will provide additional data; however, those patients with lower extremity edema following ligation of injured veins attest to the challenge for some patients and their surgeons.

SELECTED REFERENCES

Aitken, R. J., Matley, P. J., and Immelman, E. J.: Lower limb vein trauma: A long-term clinical and physiological assessment. Br. J. Surg., 76:585, 1989.
This recent study reports long-term clinical and physiologic assessment of lower limb venous trauma with the recommendation that "Vein ligation should be avoided unless another life-threatening injury demands priority."

Bergan, J. J., and Yao, J. S. T. (Eds.): Venous Problems. Chicago, Year Book Medical Publishers, 1978.
The proceedings of a symposium in honor of Dr. Geza de Takats provided an opportunity to document the experience of a number of scientists and clinical investigators regarding the complex problems of venous disease and injury.

Hobson, R. W., 2d, Howard, E. W., Wright, C. B., Collins, G. J., and Rich, N. M.: Hemodynamics of canine femoral venous ligation; Significance in combined arterial and venous injuries. Surgery, 74:824, 1973.
One of numerous important contributions from investigators at Walter Reed Army Institute of Research, this study defines and elaborates the pathophysiology associated with acute venous interruption. This helps corroborate clinical observations.

Hobson, R. W., 2d, Rich, N. M., and Wright, C. B. (Eds.): Venous Trauma; Pathophysiology, Diagnosis and Surgical Management. Mount Kisco, N.Y., Futura Publishing, 1983.
This monograph provides the most recent review of the management of patients with injured veins.

Meyer, J., Walsh, J., Schuler, J., et al.: The early fate of venous repair following civilian vascular trauma; A clinical, hemodynamic, and venographic assessment. Ann. Surg., 206:458, 1987.
Early fate of venous repair after civilian vascular trauma is reviewed from a major trauma center. A patency rate of 61 per cent was documented.

Rich, N. M., Hughes, C. W., and Baugh, J. H.: Management of venous injuries. Ann. Surg., 171:724, 1970.
As a preliminary report from the Vietnam Vascular Registry based on American experience in Southeast Asia (1965–1969), this clinical study emphasizes the need for repair of injured veins.

Rich, N. M., Hobson, R. W., 2d, Collins, G. J., Jr., and Anderson, C. A.: The effect of acute popliteal venous interruption. Ann. Surg., 183:365, 1976.
This clinical study of Vietnam casualties provides long-term follow-up that emphasizes the contrasting results of ligation of injured veins (followed by a 51 per cent incidence of disabling edema) and the improved results following repair of injured popliteal veins (with residual edema of less than 15 per cent).

Rich, N. M., and Spencer, F. C.: Vascular Trauma. Philadelphia, W. B. Saunders Company, 1978.
This extensive review of civilian and military arterial and venous injuries provides additional references as well as information on venous injuries.

Rich, N. M.: Management of venous trauma. Surg. Clin. North Am., 68:809, 1988.
This recent review emphasizes differences between civilian and military experiences.

REFERENCES

1. Agarwal, N., Shah, P. M., Clauss, R. H., Reynolds, D. M., and Stahl, W. M.: Experience with 115 civilian venous injuries. J. Trauma, 22:827, 1982.
2. Aitken, R. J., Matley, P. J., and Immelman, E. J.: Lower limb vein trauma; A long-term clinical and physiological assessment. Br. J. Surg., 76:585, 1989.
3. Barkun, J. S., Terazza, O., Daignault, P., et al.: The fate of venous repair after shock and trauma. J. Trauma, 28:1322, 1988.
4. Bishara, R. A., Shuler, J. J., Lim, L. T., et al.: Results of venous reconstruction after civilian vascular trauma. Arch. Surg., 121:607, 1986.
5. Blumoff, R. L., Powell, T., and Johnson, G., Jr.: Femoral venous trauma in a university referral center. J. Trauma, 22:703, 1982.
6. Borman, K. R., Jones, G. H., and Snyder, W. H., III.: A decade of lower extremity venous trauma: Patency and outcome. Am. J. Surg., 154:608, 1987.
7. Brigham, R. A., Eddleman, W. L., Clagett, G. P., and Rich, N. M.: Isolated venous injury produced by penetrating trauma to the lower extremity. J. Trauma, 23:255, 1983.
8. Doty, D. B., and Baker, W. H.: Bypass of superior vena cava with spiral vein graft. Ann. Thorac. Surg., 22:490, 1976.
9. Fried, G., Salerno, T., Burke, D., Brown, H. C., and Mulder, D. S.: Management of the extremity with combined neurovascular and musculoskeletal trauma. J. Trauma, 18:481, 1978.
10. Gaspar, M. R., and Treiman, R. L.: The management of injuries to major veins. Am. J. Surg., 100:171, 1960.
11. Gerlock, A. J., and Muhletaler, C. A.: Venography of peripheral venous injuries. Radiology, 133:77, 1979.
12. Gerlock, A. J., Jr., Thal, E. R., and Snyder, W. H., III.: Venography in penetrating injuries of the extremities. Am. J. Roentgenol., 126:1023, 1976.
13. Graham, J. M., Mattox, K. L., and Beall, A. C., Jr.: Portal venous system injuries. J. Trauma, 18:419, 1978.
14. Haimovici, H., Hoffert, P. W., Zinicola, N., and Steinman, C.: An experimental and clinical evaluation of grafts in the venous system. Surg. Gynecol. Obstet., 131:1173, 1970.
15. Hardin, W. D., Jr., Adinolfi, M. F., O'Connell, R. C., and Kerstein, M. D.: Management of traumatic peripheral vein injuries: Primary repair or vein ligation. Am. J. Surg., 144:235, 1982.
16. Hiratzka, L. F., and Wright, C. B.: Experimental and clinical results of grafts in the venous system: A current review. J. Surg. Res., 25:542, 1978.

17. Hobson, R. W., 2d, Rich, N. M., and Wright, C. B. (Eds.): Venous Trauma; Pathophysiology, Diagnosis and Surgical Management. Mount Kisco, N.Y., Futura Publishing, 1983.

18. Hobson, R. W., Yeager, R. A., Lynch, T. G., et al.: Femoral venous trauma: Techniques for surgical management and early results. Am. J. Surg., 146:220, 1983.

18a. Hughes C. W.: Arterial repair during the Korean War. Ann. Surg., 147:555, 1958.

18b. Hughes, C. W.: Acute vascular trauma in Korean War casualties: Analysis of 180 cases. Surg. Gynecol. Obstet., 99:91, 1954.

19. Jacobson, J. H., and Haimov, J.: Venous revascularization of the arm: Report of three cases. Surgery, 81:599, 1977.

20. Meyer, J., Walsh, J., and Schuler, J., et al.: The early fate of venous repair following civilian vascular trauma; A clinical hemodynamic and venographic assessment. Ann. Surg., 206:458, 1987.

21. Mullins, R. J., Lucas, C. E., Ledgerwood, A. M.: The natural history following venous ligation for civilian injuries. J. Trauma, 20:737, 1980.

22. Phifer, T. J., Gerlock, A. J., Rich, N. M., and McDonald J. C.: Long-term patency of venous repairs demonstrated by venography. J. Trauma, 25:342, 1985.

23. Quast, D. C., Shirkey, A. L., Fitzgerald, J. B., Beall, A. C., Jr., and DeBakey, M. E.: Surgical correction of injuries to the vena cava; An analysis of sixty-one cases. J. Trauma, 5:1, 1965.

24. Rich, N. M.: Principles and indications for primary venous repair. Surgery, 91:492, 1982.

25. Rich, N. M.: Management of venous trauma. Surg. Clin. North Am., 68:809, 1988.

26. Rich, N. M., Baugh, J. H., and Hughes, C. W.: Acute arterial injuries in Vietnam: 1,000 cases. J. Trauma, 10:359, 1970.

27. Rich, N. M., Collins, G. J., Andersen, C. A., and McDonald, P. T.: Autogenous venous interposition grafts in repair of major venous injuries. J. Trauma, 17:512, 1977.

28. Rich, N. M., Collins, G. J., Jr., Andersen, C. A., McDonald, P. T., and Ricotta, J.

J.: Venous trauma: Successful venous reconstruction remains an interesting challenge. Am. J. Surg., 134:226, 1977.

29. Rich, N. M., Hobson, R. W., 2d, and Wright, C. B.: Historical aspects of direct venous reconstruction. In Bergan, J. J., and Yao, J. T. S. (Eds.): Symposium on Venous Problems in Honor of Geza de Takats. Chicago, Year Book Medical Publishers, 1977.

30. Rich, N. M., Hobson, R. W., 2d, Wright, C. B., and Fedde, C. W.: Repair of lower extremity venous trauma: A more aggressive approach required. J. Trauma, 14:639, 1974.

31. Rich, N. M., Hobson, R. W., 2d, Wright, C. B., and Swan, K. G.: Techniques of venous repair. In Swan, K. G., Hobson, R. W., 2d, Reynolds, D. G., Rich, N. M., and Wright, C. B. (Eds.): Symposium on Venous Surgery in the Lower Extremities. St. Louis, Warren H. Green Publishers, 1975, pp. 243–256.

32. Rich, N. M., and Hughes, C. W.: Vietnam Vascular Registry: A preliminary report. Surgery, 62:218, 1969.

33. Rich, N. M., Jarstfer, B. S., and Geer, T. M.: Popliteal artery repair failure: Causes and possible prevention. J. Cardiovasc. Surg., 15:340, 1974.

34. Rich, N. M., and Spencer, F. C.: Vascular Trauma. Philadelphia, W. B. Saunders Company, 1978.

35. Richardson, J. B., Jr., Jurkovich, G. J., Walker, G. T., Nenstiel, R., and Bone, E. G.: A temporary arteriovenous shunt (Scribner) in the management of traumatic venous injuries of the lower extremity. J. Trauma, 26:503, 1986.

35a. Schrock, T., Blaisdell, F. W., Mathewson, C., Jr.: Management of blunt trauma to the liver and hepatic veins. Arch. Surg., 96:698, 1968.

36. Sullivan, W. G., Thornton, F. H., Baker, L. H., LaPlante, E. S., and Cohen, A.: Early influence of popliteal vein repair in the treatment of popliteal vessel injuries. Am. J. Surg., 122:528, 1971.

37. Timberlake, G. A., O'Connell, R. C., and Kerstein, M. D.: Venous injury: To repair, to ligate, the dilemma. J. Vasc. Surg., 4:533, 1986.

38. Treman, R. L., Doty, D., and Gaspr, M. R.: Acute vascular trauma: A fifteen-year study. Am. Surg., 111:469–73, 1966.

39. Zabin, A.: Cholecystectomy complicated by hemorrhage from the inferior vena cava. N.Y. J. Med., 50:1500, 1950.

53

DISORDERS OF THE LUNGS, PLEURA, AND CHEST WALL

I ——————————————————————————————————————

ANATOMY

Walter G. Wolfe, M.D.

Malpighi, in the seventeenth century, demonstrated that the trachea terminated in dilated vesicles and not in porous parenchyma. By inflating and then drying a lung, he demonstrated that membranous vesicles formed from the ends of the trachea, which terminated "in spaces and unequal vesicles."[1] These observations made it clear for the first time that air passes from the trachea in and out of the sacs in the lung and provided the anatomic basis for true conception of the respiratory process. In 1880 Aeby published a treatise that was the first work of any consequence devoted to analysis of the branching of the bronchial tree.[5] Nine years later, Ewart, a pathologist, recognizing that the human lung must be divided into yet smaller regions than lobes, described nine bronchial distributions.[5]

In 1932 Kramer and Glass,[21] to better localize lung abscess, established smaller and more accurate units within the lobes, which they named *bronchopulmonary segments*. Brock[7,8] developed the clinical aspects of these segments, and Churchill and Belsey[10] established the principle of the bronchopulmonary segments as surgical units. The importance of segmental anatomy was illustrated by Churchill and Belsey's observation that 80 per cent of patients with bronchiectasis in the left lower lobe also had involvement of the lower portion of the upper lobe. They named this segment the *lingula*. In 1943 the decisive studies of Jackson and Huber[16,17] on the branching of the bronchopulmonary segments were reported and established the terminology accepted today.

While bronchial anatomy was of importance, development of microscopic anatomy allowed the lung to be studied as a physiologic unit. Malpighi described microscopic anatomy of the alveolus and used the terms "pulmonary artery" and "pulmonary vein." In 1733 Hales referred to the closed connections between artery and veins described by Malpighi as "capillary vessels."[31] The century-old question of whether alveoli of the mature lung were lined by continuous epithelium or whether the alveolar capillaries as viewed with the conventional light microscope were nakedly exposed to inspired air was resolved with electron microscopic studies of Low,[25,26] when he demonstrated a complete epithelial lining covering each alveolar surface. Electron microscopic study of the lung combined with physical and chemical studies of pulmonary tissue continues to complete and clarify the anatomy of the lung.

EMBRYOLOGY

The primordia of the principal respiratory organs appear as a medial longitudinal groove in the ventral wall of the pharynx.[1,12] The tube is lined with endoderm from which the epithe-

lium of the respiratory tract develops. The cephalic part of the tube becomes the larynx, followed by the trachea; and from its caudal end, two lateral outgrowths arise, the left and right lung buds. From these, the bronchi and lungs develop. The right and left lung buds are initially symmetrical. Their ends, however, soon become lobulated, three lobules appearing on the right and two on the left. During the course of development, the lungs migrate caudally so that by the time of birth, the bifurcation of the trachea is opposite the fourth thoracic vertebra. As the lungs grow, they project into that part of the coelom that ultimately forms the pleural cavities.

The pulmonary arteries form from the sixth arch.[1] Each pulmonary artery is closely related to the main stem bronchus and provides an arterial partner for each new bronchial ramification. As the airway-artery pairs enter first the lobe, then the segments, and finally lobules of developing lung tissue, they assume a central location in each and project branches toward the particular subdivision of the lung. As the veins develop, they receive tributaries from the pleura and the rich vascular networks developing about the growing tips of the respiratory tree. They arch across the base of the secondary lobules toward the periphery, where they turn into the planes of connective tissue that separate adjacent pulmonary lobules. Interlobular veins unite to form and serve as tributaries to intersegmental veins, which, near the pulmonary hilus, combine in most cases into the superior and inferior pulmonary veins.

ANATOMY

The respiratory system consists of the nose, nasal passages, nasopharynx, larynx, trachea, bronchi, and lungs. The respiratory tree functions proximate to the thorax and its bony and muscular components as well as to the pleura, pleural cavity, and mediastinum. The influence of pathologic changes in associated structures on the function of the respiratory system is important, and one should be familiar with these anatomic relationships and the "topographic anatomy" of the thorax (Fig. 1).[12,38]

CHEST WALL AND PLEURA. Beneath the skin and subcutaneous tissue, the chest wall is covered by the pectoralis muscles anteriorly, and posterolaterally the latissimus dorsi and serratus anterior muscles are encountered. In an anterior thoracotomy, the fibers of the pectoralis major may be split, exposing the intercostal muscles. However, in the standard posterolateral thoracotomy, the latissimus dorsi is divided, and then the serratus anterior is divided or split. From the standpoint of chest wall mechanics and involvement of chest wall muscles, an ante-

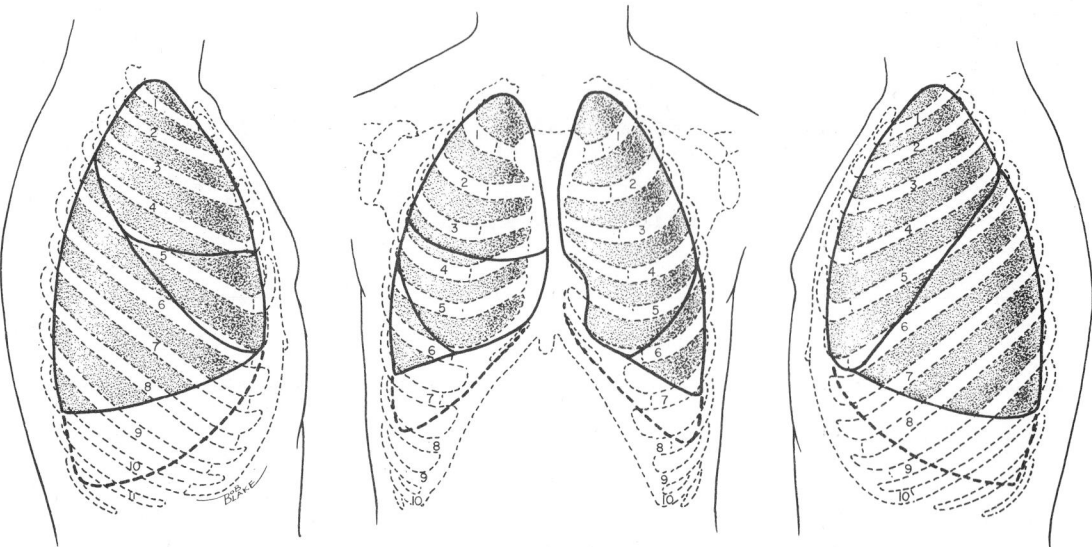

Figure 1. The relationships of the pleural reflections and the lobes of the lung to the ribs. The topographic anatomy and the relationship of the fissures of the lobes to ribs in inspiration and expiration are important in evaluation of the routine posteroanterior and lateral chest film.

rior thoracotomy is usually better tolerated. However, exposure and control of thoracic structures many times is best through the posterolateral approach, which is the standard thoracotomy incision.

There are 12 pairs of ribs, 7 of which are termed true ribs, where the cartilage articulates with the sternum, and the lower 5, false ribs, which are not connected directly to the sternum. The eleventh and twelfth ribs are termed floating ribs because they are not attached anteriorly. The sternum is divided into the manubrium, the body, and the xiphoid. The clavicle articulates with the sternum and the first costal cartilage. This is an important relationship, because a posterior dislocation of the clavicle can cause respiratory distress secondary to compression of the trachea by the head of the clavicle.

Muscles associated with the intercostal space are the external, internal, and transversus thoracic muscles. There are 11 intercostal spaces containing a vein, an artery, and a nerve, which course along the lower edge of each rib. All of the intercostal spaces are wider in the front than posteriorly, the widest being the third.

The parietal pleura is divided into four parts: costal, cervical, diaphragmatic, and mediastinal. The costal pleura lines the ribs, cartilages, and vertebral bodies and is the thickest portion of the parietal pleura. The visceral pleura covers the lungs so firmly that it is not possible to strip it from the lung tissue under normal circumstances.

The internal mammary artery and vein rise from the first portion of the subclavian artery opposite the thyrocervical trunk and descend along the sternum to anastomose with the superior epigastric artery. The lymphatics in the chest wall and their drainage patterns are important and are discussed in the section on carcinoma of the breast.

Trachea

The entrance to the trachea is guarded by the larynx. It functions to prevent aspiration and as the organ of phonation and has an important role in production of the cough. The mucous membrane lining of the larynx is covered by ciliated epithelial cells and a few goblet cells. The epithelial surfaces in contact with food are covered by stratified squamous epithelium.[13] Except for the cricothyroid muscle, which is innervated by the external laryngeal branch of the superior laryngeal nerve, the larynx receives both motor and sensory innervation by way of the vagal accessory complex of nerve fibers. The intrinsic muscles of the larynx receive their motor innervation by way of the inferior laryngeal branch of the recurrent vagus nerve.[12]

The trachea is a fibromuscular tube 10 to 12 cm. in length and varying from 13 to 22 mm. in width, supported laterally and ventrally by approximately 20 U-shaped hyaline cartilages. The trachea originates at the level of the cricoid cartilage and descends through the superior aperture of the thorax and the superior mediastinum to its bifurcation at the level of the sternal angle (lower border of the fourth thoracic vertebra). Here it divides into the right and left primary bronchi. The spur formed at the point of bifurcation is termed the carina. Half of the trachea lies in the neck and the other half within the thorax.[12,20]

The dimensions of the trachea are constantly changing with the movement of the head and neck. It is attached to a movable structure at both ends, namely, the larynx cranially and the pericardial sac and diaphragm caudally. During forced expiration, especially when the glottis is suddenly opened as in coughing, the trachea is markedly narrowed. In young subjects the lumen may be reduced to one-tenth its original size. Prior to cough, the bifurcation may ascend as much as 5 cm.[20]

The mucous membrane of the trachea rests on elastic lamina propria, beneath which is the submucosa. These layers are supported by another fibrous coat containing cartilage and smooth muscle. The dorsal membranous wall is fibromuscular. Smooth musculature elsewhere in the respiratory tree disposes in a helical arrangement about the airways; however, in the trachea it lies only in its dorsal wall. The submucosa varies in thickness, with the thinnest portion on the inner surface of the cartilage and the thicker, more loosely organized portion present on the muscular wall. In addition to blood vessels, nerves, and lymphatics, this layer contains the secretory portions of the mucous and serous glandular units. The trachea is lined with pseudostratified columnar ciliated epithelium containing goblet cells.[13] Near the basement membrane the formative cells may differentiate into new ciliated cells or goblet cells.

Bronchi

At its termination, the trachea divides into the right and left principal bronchi. The right bronchus is 12 to 16 mm. in diameter; the left, 10 to 14 mm. The combined cross-sectional area exceeds that of the trachea. The right main bronchus deviates less from the axis of the trachea than does the left; this explains why foreign objects entering the trachea more often lodge in the right bronchus or one of its branches.[12,20]

Within a primary lobe, the secondary bronchus soon divides into tertiary branches, which are remarkably constant in number and distribution. The segment of a lobe, aerated by a tertiary bronchus, is usually well delineated from adjoining segments

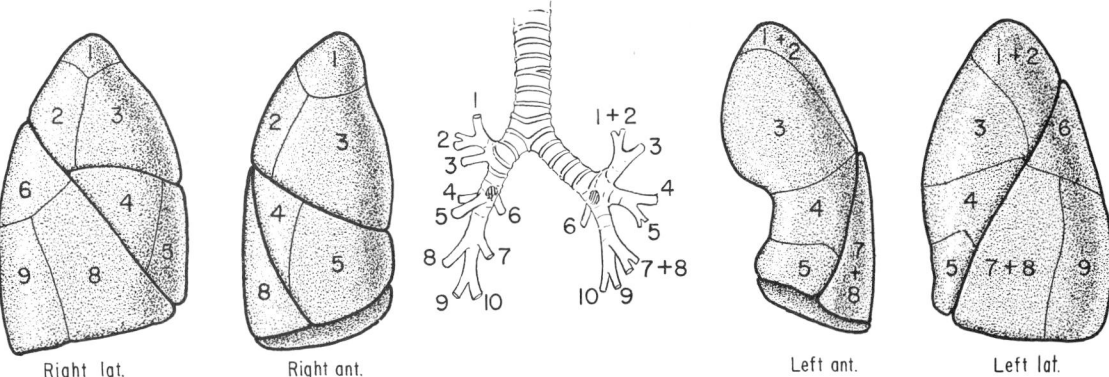

Figure 2. Segments of the pulmonary lobes. (Modified from Jackson, C. L., and Huber, J. F.: Dis. Chest, 9:319, 1943.)

by nearly complete planes of connective tissue. Knowledge of segmental anatomy is of great practical importance in radiology, bronchoscopy, and pulmonary surgery. Through painstaking anatomic studies of Jackson and Huber[16,17] and others, the description of the segments of the pulmonary lobes has been completed (Fig. 2). Each segment is identified by its position in the lobe of the lung, and the corresponding segmental bronchus is named for the segment it supplies (Fig. 3). A lobar abnormality, the azygos lobe, is illustrated in Figure 4. During fetal development the precursor of the azygos vein, the posterior cardinal vein, penetrates the right upper lobe, drawing with the azygos vein four layers of pleura. This traps a part of the right upper lobe between this fissure and the mediastinum, creating the azygos lobe. It is ventilated by the apical or posterior segmental bronchus of the right upper lobe and is perfused by a corresponding pulmonary artery.

In the human lung, bronchial branches usually arise from bifurcations, and although the resulting branches are smaller than the parent stem, their total cross-sectional area is always greater by approximately six fifths. Structurally, large bronchi do not differ markedly from the trachea. Medium bronchi are distinguished by the large plates of cartilage, by the musculature, and by their relative abundance of glands. The most peripheral airways containing cartilage are the terminal bronchi. The smaller bronchi have fewer glands and are distinguished by rich venous plexuses between the muscular and cartilaginous fibrous layers. The effect of bronchial muscle contraction on venous and lymphatic channels probably has an important role in propelling the vascular fluids toward the hilus of the lung. Also, these rich venous networks are thought to be an important factor in the warming of air en route to the pulmonary parenchyma (Fig. 5).[20]

The mucous membrane of the bronchial mucosa is composed of an epithelium, a basement membrane, and richly vascular

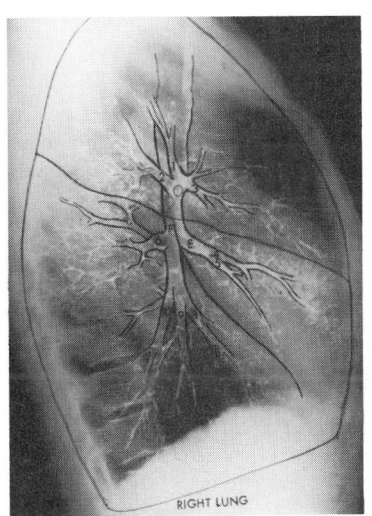
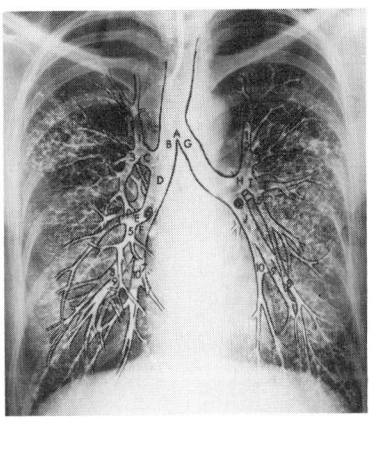
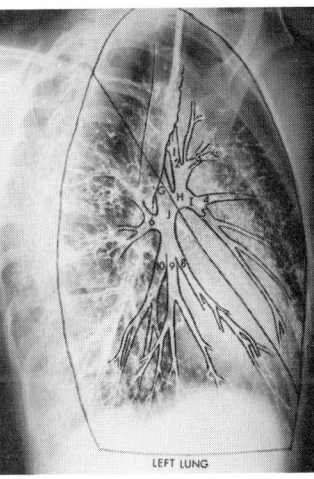

Figure 3. Normal bronchogram. The major bronchi are indicated by the letters: segmental bronchi are numbered. Key for Figures 2 and 3:

Right	
1. Apical	⎫
2. Posterior	⎬ upper lobe
3. Anterior	⎭
4. Lateral	⎫ middle lobe
5. Medial	⎭
6. Superior	⎫
7. Medial (basal) RLL	⎪
8. Anterior basal	⎬ lower lobe
9. Lateral basal	⎪
10. Posterior basal	⎭

Left	
1–2. Apical posterior	⎫
3. Anterior	⎬ upper lobe
4. Superior of lingula	⎪
5. Inferior of lingula	⎭
6. Superior	⎫
7.	⎪
8. Anterior-medial basal	⎬ lower lobe
9. Lateral basal	⎪
10. Posterior basal	⎭

A. Carina
B. R. main stem bronchus
C. RUL bronchus
D. Bronchus intermedius
E. RLM bronchus

F. RLL bronchus
G. L main stem bronchus
H. LUL bronchus
I. Lingula bronchus
J. LLL bronchus

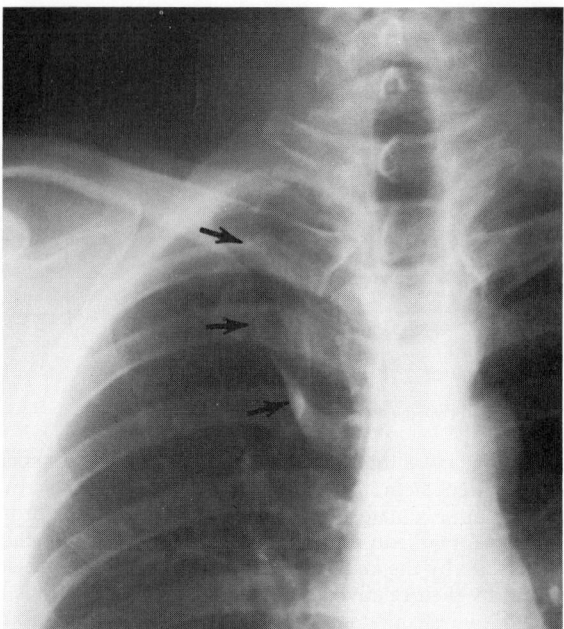

Figure 4. This is a posterior PA chest film that is normal except for the appearance of an azygos lobe, indicated by the arrow marking the course of the vein. The remaining lobar anatomy in this patient is normal. (From Weibel, E. R.: Is the lung built reasonably? Am. Rev. Respir. Dis., *128:*752, 1983.)

and fibrous tunica propria. Like that of the trachea, the bronchial epithelium consists of pseudostratified ciliated and nonciliated cells, including goblet cells.[13] Peribronchial tissue consists of connective tissue that extends from the pulmonary hilus to the primary bronchioles. The peribronchium is continuous with the connective tissue investment of the arterial partners of the bronchi and the connective tissue sheath of the large veins. These connections form the basis for understanding the location and spread of certain types of edema and inflammation and the paths followed by air in and about the lung in interstitial emphysema. Interestingly, the peribronchium occupies a space in which subatmospheric pressure prevails. Von Hayek[14] believes that this subatmospheric pressure has an important role in the flow of venous blood, lymph, and alveolar fluid as well as in migration of inhaled particulate matter.

Ciliated, Goblet, and Brush Cells

It has been demonstrated that each cilium-bearing cell has approximately 270 cilia. Each cilium originates in a basal corpuscle just beneath the cell surface and measures approximately $0.5\ \mu$ in length and $0.14\ \mu$ in diameter. The cilium is round on cross section and contains a pair of separate central filaments and a peripheral ring of nine paired, closely branched filaments.

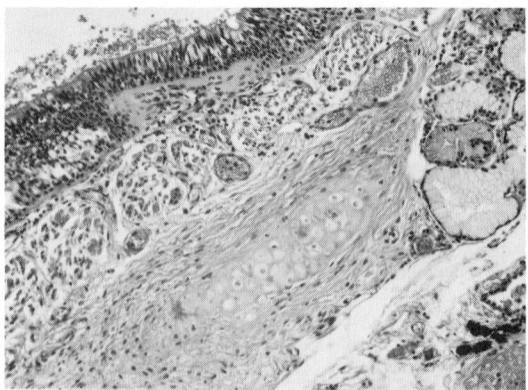

Figure 5. Section of a small bronchus. Note the prominence of the muscle layer, as compared with trachea and bronchi, and the rich vascular network between the muscular and cartilaginous fibrous layer. Magnification, ×100.

Cilia are phylogenetically ancient structures; and all cilia, whether in the plant or animal kingdom, have the same basic structure.[18,20,37]

Although the cilia are borne by separate cells, these many thousands of cilia beat in an organized, coordinated manner. Studies have shown that they beat in a whiplike manner, the cycle of activity being divided into a rapid forward propulsive stroke and a slower recovery stroke.[18,20,37] This propulsion is effective in moving a superimposed carpet of mucus along with a variable number of trapped particles and cells upward toward the larynx. The rate at which particulate matter is propelled by cilia varies according to species and that portion of the respiratory tree involved and has been recorded to be approximately 10 to 35 mm. per minute. The cilia do not beat within the viscous sheet of mucus but are bathed instead in fluid of considerably lower viscosity. The source of the fluid, factors controlling its viscosity, and rate of production are not known.[18,27,35] The ciliated cells disappear gradually as respiratory bronchioles are approached.

The nonciliated cells are the goblet and brush cells. Goblet cells occur singly and in groups between the ciliated epithelial cells. When filled with secretion, they are conspicuous by their bulging walls. In cases of chronic irritation of the tracheobronchial mucosa, there is marked increase in goblet cells at the expense of ciliated cells. It has been suggested that when mucus laden with particles of carcinogenic material has been carried to the branching point of an airway, there may be a temporary stasis at that site owing to the local paucity of cilia.[20]

The brush cells are tall, standing from the basement membrane of the lumen of the airway. Electron photomicrographs demonstrate dovetailed cytoplasmic processes rearing on their sides interlocking with neighboring goblet cells. This arrangement may serve to add mechanical stability to the epithelial sheet. Whether or not the brush cells are sustentacular in function or are the source of low-viscosity fluid that bathes the cilia is not known.[20,36]

Bronchioles

Bronchioles are said to have a diameter of 1 mm. or less and to be devoid of cartilage support. Of all the airways, bronchioles have the highest proportion of smooth muscle in their walls

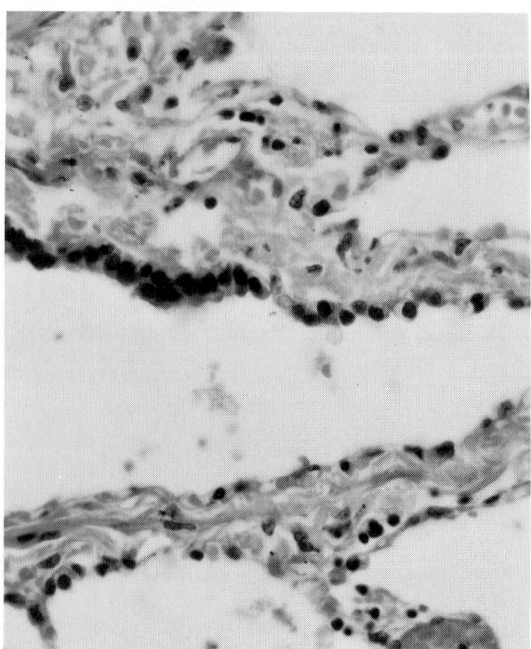

Figure 6. Section of a terminal bronchus, demonstrating the cuboidal epithelium, which grades off into a flat epithelium near the alveolar entrances. Also, a large amount of smooth muscle is evident. Magnification, ×400.

relative to the diameter of the lumen. Because small bronchi are also without connective tissue sheaths, the fibrous strands of the fibrocartilagines must extend peripherally into the mucous membrane of the bronchiole. The fibrous elements intermingle freely with the surrounding pulmonary parenchyma, exerting circumferential traction on the airway, maintaining its patency.

Bronchioles of the first order arise at the tip of the terminal bronchus and continue branching to produce three or four further divisions fully lined by cuboidal epithelium. The last to be lined is the terminal bronchiole. Estimates of the number of terminal bronchioles from a single bronchus vary between 10 and 20 (Fig. 6).

A terminal bronchiole usually divides at an angle of 60 to 90 degrees into respiratory bronchioles, which may give rise to further divisions. The branching of the terminal bronchiole is by no means uniform, because a single branch may be given laterally and two or more may follow (Fig. 7). Respiratory bronchioles vary also in size (in man ranging from 1 through 3.5 mm. in length and approximately 1.5 mm. in diameter). The cuboidal epithelium stops abruptly at the entrance of the alveoli, which are lined by extremely thin squamous epithelium not revealed by conventional light microscopes. The last in a series of respiratory bronchioles usually bifurcate to produce the first in a series of alveolar ducts (Fig. 8).

Alveoli

The alveolar ducts terminate in one of several rotunda-like enclosures termed alveolar sacs. The sacs bear a small and variable number of terminal alveoli. Like the alveolar ducts, the sacs lack proper walls and open on all sides into alveoli. Each alveolus shares an entrance frame and a wall with its neighbor similar to two rooms being separated by a single wall. Because the alveoli surrounding an alveolar duct are an integral part of the pulmonary parenchyma, they are subjected to all of the stages of the respiratory cycle and to tractional forces that hold them open.

Pulmonary alveoli vary considerably in shape and size with the various mammalian species, corresponding in general to body size. The determinants of the dimensions in specific species are not clearly understood but probably relate to a combination of factors, including the metabolic rate of the animal and the number and size of red blood cells. In man, the alveoli are approximately 160 μ in size (Fig. 9).[20]

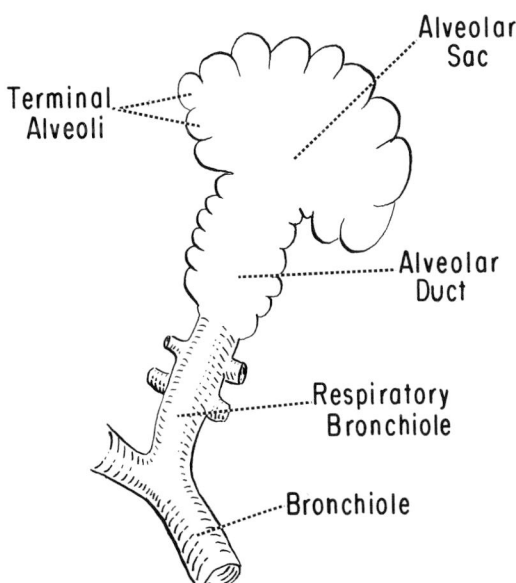

Figure 7. The relationship of the airway in the periphery of the respiratory tree. Bronchioles lead to the respiratory bronchioles, which then terminate in the alveolar duct and the alveolar sac.

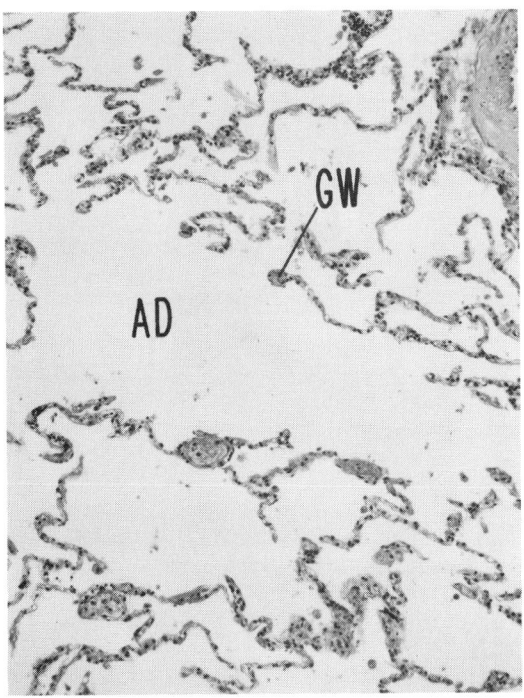

Figure 8. Section of lung demonstrating an alveolar duct (AD) with its contiguous alveoli. Note that the alveolar duct is not a structural entity in and of itself. Its walls are, in fact, alveolar septa. GW is a cross section of a collagen bundle. These bundles are important in maintaining patency of the alveolar ducts and the openings into the alveoli. They are analogous to guy wires.

Alveolar Epithelium

The alveolar epithelial sheet rests on a basement membrane that lies on or near the basement membrane of the adjacent capillary. The structural layers composing the air-blood barrier are the stratum of the alveolar epithelial cells, their basement

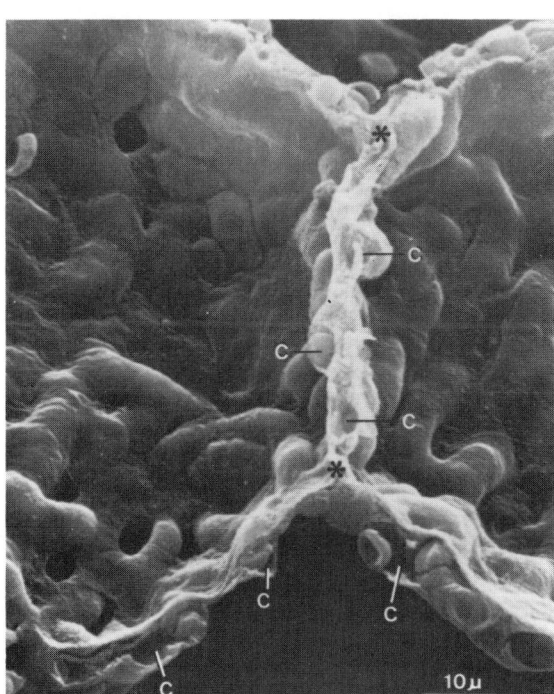

Figure 9. Scanning electron micrograph of *human lung* fixed near total lung capacity by instillation of fixative into the airways. Three alveolar septa and their triple junction line (*) are shown. Capillaries (C) alternate sides in the septal midplane marked by fibers. (From Weibel, E. R., and Bachoffen, H.: Structural design of the alveolar septum and fluid exchange. *In* Fishman, A. P., and Renkin, E. M. (Eds.). Pulmonary Edema. American Physiological Society Clinical Physiology Series, 1979, pp. 1–20.)

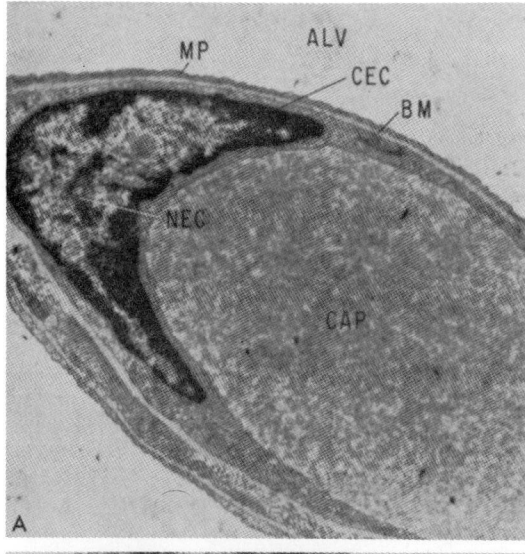

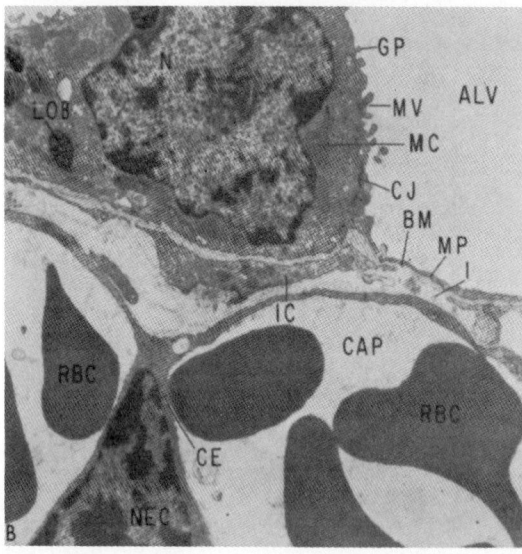

Figure 10. *A,* Electron photomicrograph of an alveolus. This demonstrates the structure of the thinnest part of the blood-air interface. Note that the blood is separated from the alveolar air only by the attenuated cytoplasm of an endothelial cell and a membranous pneumocyte joined by a basement membrane. Magnification, ×6700; print magnification, 13,725. *B,* Note the relationship of the granular pneumocyte to the alveolar wall. The granular pneumocyte is an integral part of the alveolar lining. This cell has been referred to as "Type II cell," "great alveolar cell," and "alveolar phagocyte." It is thought to produce surfactant: the laminated osmiophilic bodies illustrated here may be surfactant or surfactant precursors. Magnification, ×6700; print magnification, 13,725. N, Nucleus of granular pneumocyte; LO, laminated osmiophilic body (these cells thought to be the site of surfactant production); GP, granular pneumocyte (sometimes called the alveolar Type II or the great alveolar cell); MV, microvilli; ALV, alveolus; MC, mitochondria; CJ, cell junction; BM, basement membrane; MP, membranous pneumocyte; I, interstitium; IC, interstitial cell; CAP, capillary; RBC, red blood cell; CE, capillary endothelium; NEC, nucleus of the endothelial cell; CEC, cytoplasm of the endothelial cell.

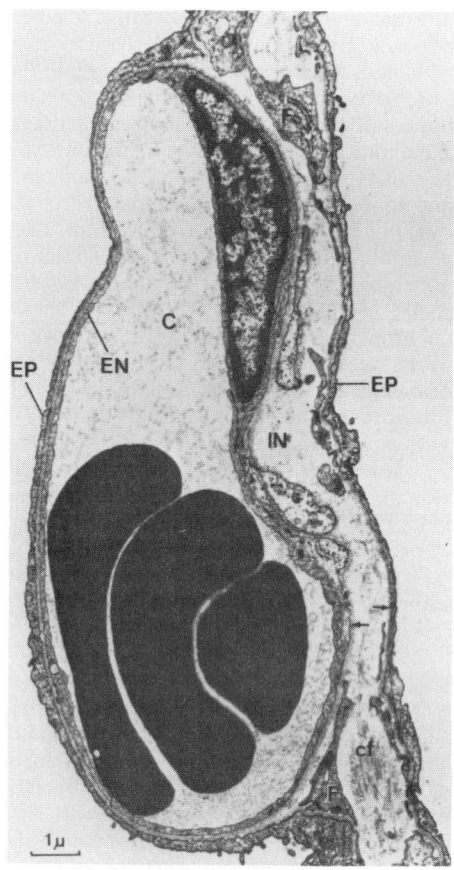

Figure 11. Transmission electron micrograph of the alveolar capillary (C) cross section from human lung. In the upper part of the air-blood barrier the basal laminae of epithelium (EP) and endothelium (EN) are fused, forming a restricted interstitial space; connective tissue fibers (cf) are found in the free interstitial space (IN) in the bottom part of the barrier, where the basal laminae (arrows) are separated. Note fibroblast processes (F) associated with fibers. (From Weibel, E. R., and Bachoffen, H.: Structural design of the alveolar septum and fluid exchange. *In* Fishman, A. P., and Renkin, E. M. (Eds.): Pulmonary Edema. American Physiological Society Clinical Physiology Series, 1979, pp. 1–20.)

membrane, the variable connective tissue layer, the basement membrane of the capillary, and the cells of the capillary endothelium (Figs. 10 and 11.).[2,19,25,26,33]

Knowledge of the structures separating the alveolar air and capillary blood is important. Alveolar epithelial cells are known to be sensitive to the noxious fumes and foreign particles that may be carried by the inspired air. Simple, rapid hypertrophy of the alveolar lining cell layer is possible, and the cells are able to undergo metamorphosis into at least one type of alveolar phagocyte.[3,14,20,29] The hypertrophy of the alveolar lining cells could provide the quantity of cells found in the pulmonary alveoli, in alveolar cell carcinoma, and in the lung disease of sheep jaagsiekte.

There is evidence that some of the alveolar lining cells elaborate secretion products, one of importance being the surface-active layer that lines pulmonary alveoli.[14,20,29]

Alveolar Capillary Network

Pulmonary capillary networks are the richest in the body, so dense that openings in them are frequently smaller than the diameter of the capillaries. Because the connective tissue fibers form the principal support of the capillary networks, any disease state, such as emphysema, in which there is destruction of the alveolar wall and supporting framework would permit stretching, attenuation, and destruction of the entire capillary bed (Figs. 12 to 14).[23]

Pulmonary and Bronchial Vessels

The surgical anatomy of pulmonary arteries and veins, particularly their relation to each other and to other structures of the pulmonary hilus, is of obvious importance in pulmonary surgery. Knowledge of the "anatomy" of the normal pulmonary angiogram is critical for recognition of pathologic conditions (Fig. 15).[6,12,38] Pulmonary arteries and their ramifications are invested in connective tissue sleeves, permitting continuous spatial adjustments to the changing position and volume of surrounding lung tissue. This permits marked dynamic changes in the arterial diameters while not imposing direct mechanical change on lung tissue.

Pulmonary veins do not travel the same course as their arte-

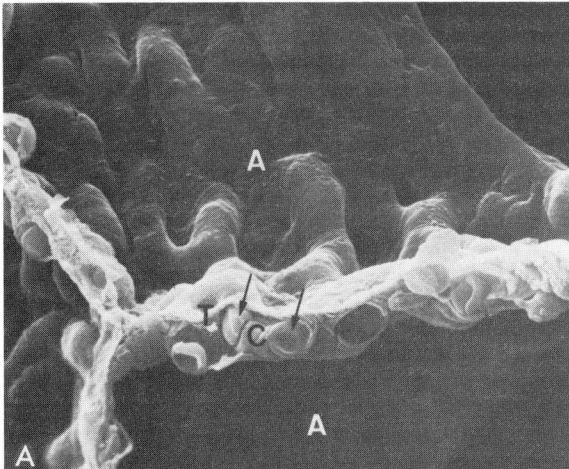

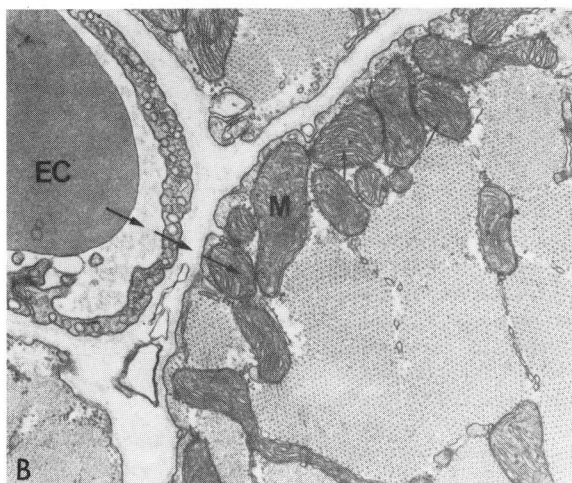

Figure 12. This figure demonstrates oxygen conductance in the lungs themselves. *A*, A scanning electron micrograph with gas exchanger of the human lungs consisting of capillary (C) between alveoli (A) with the blood separated from the air by a thin tissue barrier (T). *B*, The erythrocyte (EC) in the muscle capillary delivers oxygen to mitochondria (M) in the muscle cells. The oxygen transfer from the outside air is affected by convection in the pulmonary air spaces and in the bloodstream. Molecular diffusion is the process by which gas exchange occurs between air and blood and between blood and the cells. Finally, in the mitochondria, molecular oxygen disappears in water, the end product of oxidation.

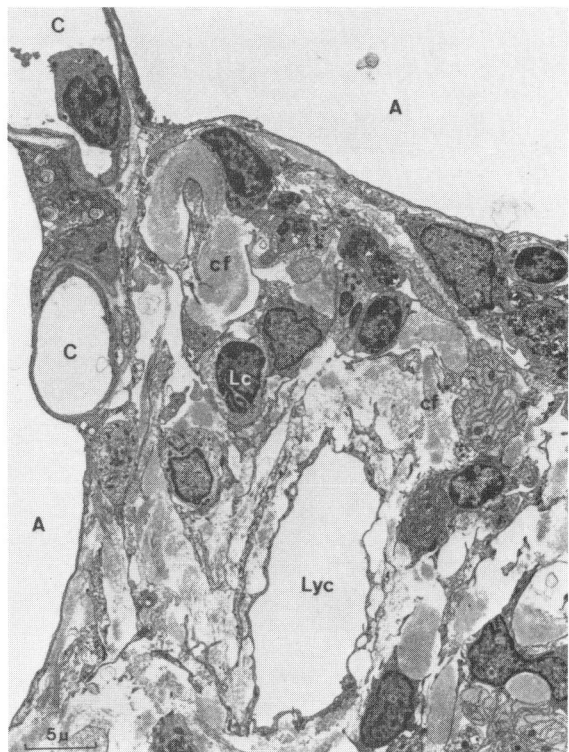

Figure 13. Juxta-alveolar fluid sump associated with connective tissue around small vessel from human lung. Note fluid-filled clefts among coarse fibers (cf) and free cells (Lc), as well as a lymphatic capillary (Lyc) with irregular scalloped endothelial lining. (From Weibel, E. R., and Bachoffen, H.: Structural design of the alveolar septum and fluid exchange. *In* Fishman, A. P., and Renkin, E. M. (Eds.): Pulmonary Edema. American Physiological Society Clinical Physiology Series, 1979, pp. 1–20.)

rial partners, as is the case in the systemic circulation. They course along interlobular connective tissue planes and adapt longitudinally to surrounding parenchyma but cannot withdraw from it. The direct connection of the vein to adjacent lung tissue by connective tissue fibers is the anatomic device that makes its diameter largely dependent on lung volume. This arrangement provides the mechanism for promoting venous return in the special situation of the low-pressure pulmonary circuit.

Although blood from the rich pulmonary capillaries undoubtedly supplies the metabolic needs of the pulmonary parenchyma, the many servant tissues (conducting airways, pulmonary vessels, lymphoid tissue, and so forth) require their own circulation supplied by vessels derived from the systemic circulation, the bronchial arteries.

Leonardo da Vinci was perhaps the first to dissect the bronchial vessels. Deffebach has recently reviewed the bronchial circulation, which has new importance with the resurgence of lung transplantation. The bronchials originate either directly from the aorta or indirectly via the intercostals. Bronchial arteries accompany the bronchial ramifications and eventually lose their identity along the respiratory bronchioles, where the capillaries that they supply drain into the alveolar capillary net-

work and into the pulmonary veins (Fig. 16). There is no bronchial vein corresponding to the bronchial artery; however, there is a rich peribronchial venous network. The bronchial veins that drain the first several orders of bronchi empty into the azygos and hemiazygos system via mediastinal tributaries. The bronchial microvascular plexus serves as a link between the systemic and pulmonary veins in the periphery of the lung. Under normal conditions most of the bronchial venous blood drains into the right side of the heart because of orientation of the valves and the higher pressure in the left atrium as compared with the right. The pressure differences are slight, however; and if the valves become incompetent, flow can reverse. Although the bronchial veins are described, their presence in normal individuals has been questioned. They may, however, appear as sizable vessels in those with diseases such as pulmonary emphysema and mitral stenosis.[11,23] In bronchiectasis, chronic pulmonary obstructive disease, or other conditions causing cor pulmonale, the bronchial venous plexus expands considerably, creating large shunts between systemic and pulmonary veins.[12]

Literature on pulmonary vascular anastomoses covers more than two centuries of anatomic studies. In Weibel's studies[42] it was concluded that pulmonary arteries and veins are end vessels and that there is no possibility for production of the collateral circulation. He found no precapillary arteriovenous pulmonary anastomosis that might permit blood to bypass the alveolar capillary net. Extensive studies of pulmonary vasculature and its anastomotic connection have been made by von Hayek.[14] He described arterioarterial communications between pulmonary arteries and bronchial arteries, which are distinguishable by their remarkable thickness and unusual corkscrew course in addition to the abundant longitudinal musculature. Nothing is known at present about their importance in the regulation of vascular perfusion in the lung.

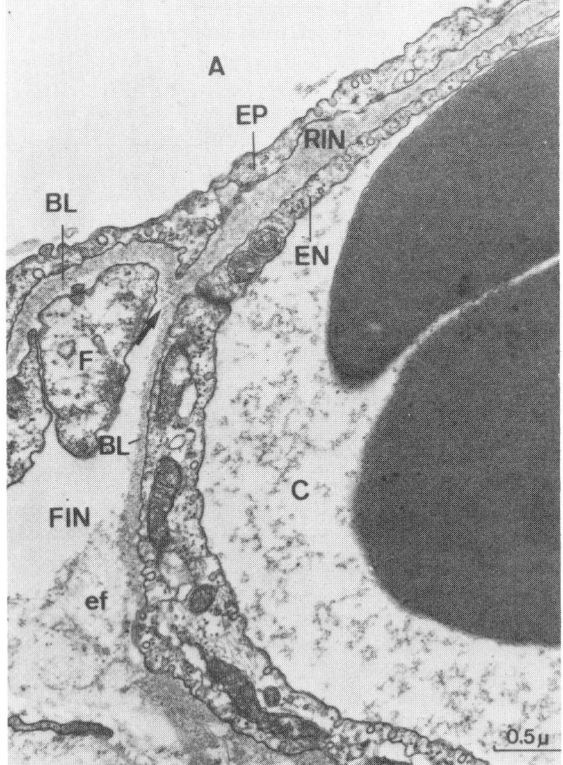

Figure 14. Higher-power view of air-blood barrier between an alveolus (A) and a capillary in human lung, showing transition (arrow) between free interstitial space (FIN) and restricted interstitium (RIN) due to fused basal laminae (BL) of epithelium (EP) and endothelium (EN). A small interstitial fluid pool is found between elastic fiber (ef) and fibroblast process (F). (From Weibel, E. R., and Bachoffen, H.: Structural design of the alveolar septum and fluid exchange. *In* Fishman, A. P., and Renkin, E. M. (Eds.): Pulmonary Edema. American Physiological Society Clinical Physiology Series, 1979, pp. 1–20.)

Pulmonary Lymphatics

Pulmonary lymphatic vessels enter the hilar region in the second month of fetal life and continue to ramify and produce plexiform channels along the bronchi and pulmonary arteries and veins and in the subpleural connective tissue.[14,20] According to Miller,[30] the lungs are more extensively supplied by lymphatics than the more metabolically active organs such as the liver and kidneys.

Studies of Tobin[39,40] have demonstrated that pulmonary lymphatics do extend as far as alveoli. In most instances, the distance between the alveolus and the nearest lymphatic is extremely small. At the pulmonary hilus, the lymphatics, having gained both connective tissue and smooth muscle fibers, are relatively thick-walled and bear a histologic resemblance to the thoracic duct.

Collectively, the lymph nodes found along the lobar branches are termed hilar nodes and are included in the great group of nodes along the root of the lung. The tracheobronchial nodes are usually larger on the right. On the left, one or more nodes are commonly related to the ligamentum arteriosum and thus to the recurrent laryngeal branch of vagus nerve and to the vagal contributions to the anterior pulmonary plexus. Tracheal nodes form chains and are intimately related to the recurrent nerves.

Nerve Supply

Histologic studies and physiologic experiments have shown both afferent and efferent fibers present in the nerves that follow the vessels and airways to the lung.[12,20] Right and left vagus nerves send one or more bronchial branches to the smaller anterior pulmonary plexus and many others to the rich posterior pulmonary plexus dorsal to the pulmonary hilus. A great many ganglion cells are found scattered along the cervical and thoracic portions of the vagus nerves. Those in the cervical vagus are thought to be sensory, whereas the thoracic vagus is considered to be motor in function. Ganglion cells often lie adjacent to bronchial mucous glands and send short fibers with nonterminal twigs to the cells of glandular epithelium.

Sympathetic nerves arise from the second to fourth thoracic sympathetic ganglia and join the vagi in formation of the pulmonary plexus. The clinical and experimental evidence points to the presence of sympathetic bronchodilator fibers having cells or origin in spinal cord levels T2 to T4.

The phrenic nerve, in addition to the usual fibers of origin in the third to fifth cervical nerves, has been found to receive various contributions from the cervical sympathetics. A number of afferent fibers from the diaphragm as well as the mediastinum also appear to ascend in the phrenic nerve (Fig. 17).

Collateral Ventilation

In airways less than 1 mm. in diameter (bronchioles), reduction of normal traction forces in the lungs by infection, inflam-

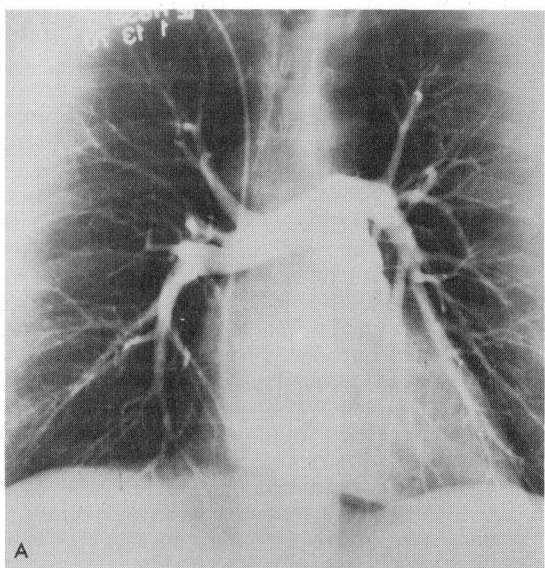

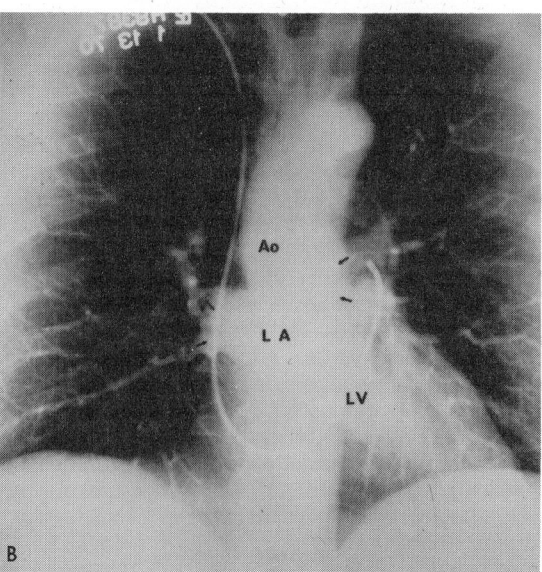

Figure 15. *A,* Normal pulmonary angiogram illustrating the branching of the pulmonary arteries in the right and left lungs to their respective lobes. *B,* Venous phase of the same arteriogram demonstrating the superior and inferior pulmonary veins entering the left atrium (arrows). Ao, Aorta; LA, left atrium; LV, left ventricle.

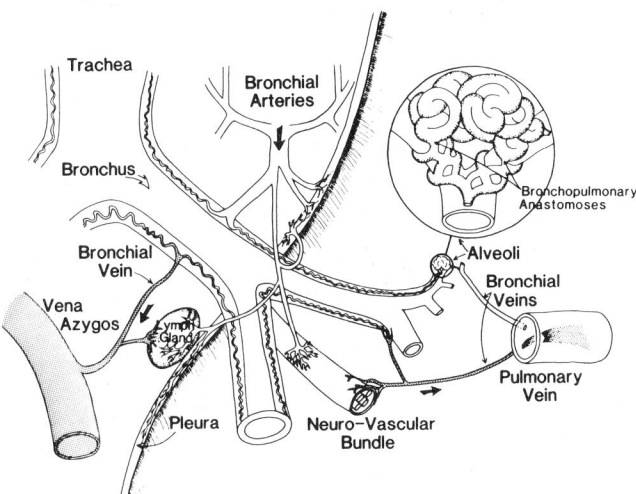

Figure 16. Schematic of the systemic blood supply to the lung. Note that the flow from the extrapulmonary airways and supporting structures returns to the right heart, whereas intrapulmonary flow becomes anastomotic with the pulmonary circulation and returns to the left heart. (From Deffebach, M. E., Charan, N. B., Lakshminarayan, S., and Butler, J.: The bronchial circulation: Small but vital attribute of the lung. Am. Rev. Respir. Dis., *135:*463, 1987.)

mation, fluid accumulation, or secretions singly or in combination may occlude the bronchial lumen. The consequences of such blockage may in some cases be offset by channels of collateral ventilation that form connections between well-aerated alveoli and those normally supplied by the occluded small airway. There are two principal mechanisms of collateral ventilation: interalveolar communications (pores of Kohn) and bronchial alveolar communications.

Alveolar pores are round to oval. Their shape and size are dictated by the delicate encirclements of elastic and other connective tissue fibers. As long as their fibrous framework is intact, the pores cannot enlarge beyond set limits. Alveolar pores may have the beneficial effect of preventing collapse of the lobules supplied by an occluded bronchiole. They may serve also as a temporary lodging place for alveolar phagocytes. Each communication may also provide pathways for the spread of fluid accumulations and for the transmission of bacteria between the communicating pulmonary lobules.[15,29,41]

In the past decade Lambert[22] described short, epithelium-like communications between distant bronchioles and neighboring alveoli. Such connections probably escaped discovery until recently because they are difficult or impossible to see in routine sections. They are approximately 30 μ in diameter, thus three or more times the diameter of most interalveolar pores. These communications are evidently able to remain open regardless of the degree of contraction of the bronchiolar smooth muscle. The benefit of pores may be shared only by the immediately adjacent alveoli, while the bronchiole-alveolar communications provide means of aerating hundreds of alveoli. Chen[9] has demonstrated the dynamic nature of the collateral ventilatory channels.

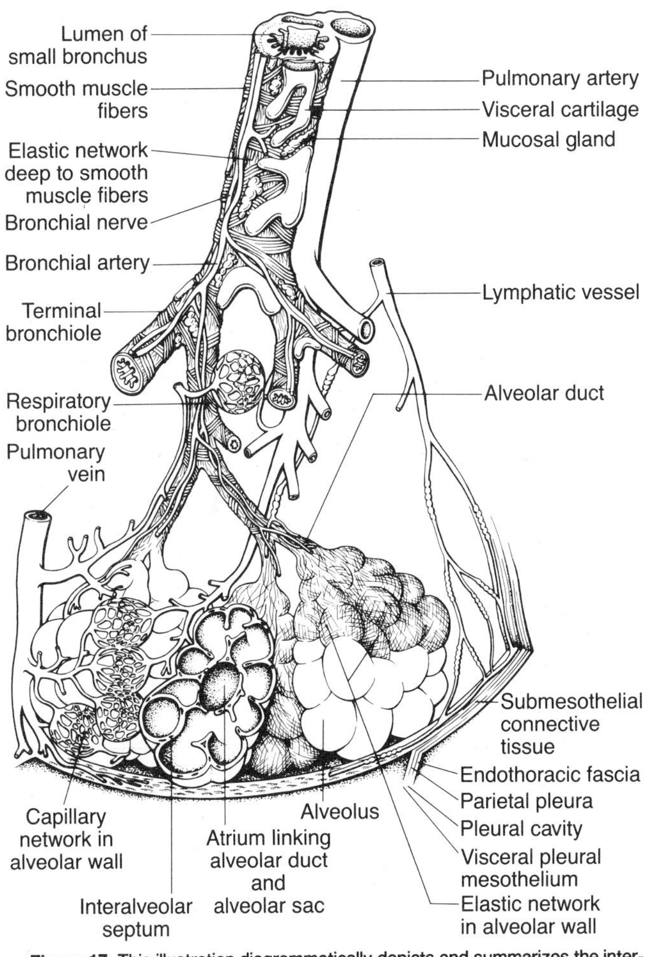

Figure 17. This illustration diagrammatically depicts and summarizes the interrelationships of all the anatomic structures involved in lung anatomy. (From Williams, P. L., Warwick, R., Dyson, M., and Bannister, L. H. (Eds.): Gray's Anatomy, 37th ed. Edinburgh, Churchill Livingstone, 1989, p. 1279.)

Labels for Figure 17:
Lumen of small bronchus
Smooth muscle fibers
Elastic network deep to smooth muscle fibers
Bronchial nerve
Bronchial artery
Terminal bronchiole
Respiratory bronchiole
Pulmonary vein
Capillary network in alveolar wall
Atrium linking alveolar duct and alveolar sac
Interalveolar septum
Pulmonary artery
Visceral cartilage
Mucosal gland
Lymphatic vessel
Alveolar duct
Alveolus
Submesothelial connective tissue
Endothoracic fascia
Parietal pleura
Pleural cavity
Visceral pleural mesothelium
Elastic network in alveolar wall

SELECTED REFERENCES

Boyden, E. A.: Segmental Anatomy of the Lungs, New York, McGraw-Hill Book Company, 1955.
This excellent monograph not only reviews the historical development of the segmental anatomy of the lungs, but provides the groundwork for basic concepts of functional anatomy as it can be applied surgically and to the physiology of respiration.

Deffebach, M. E., Charan, N. B., Lakshminarayan, S., and Butler, J.: The Bronchial Circulation: Small, but a Vital Attribute of the Lung. Am. Rev. Respir. Dis., 135:463, 1987.
This selected reference is clearly state-of-the-art, the most recent review of the structure and function of the bronchial circulation.

Hayek, H. von: The Human Lung. Translated by V. E. Krahl. New York, Hafner Publishing Company, 1960.
This monograph records the sophisticated anatomy of the respiratory system. It presents some of the newest concepts and findings in the functional anatomy of the lung and is one of the outstanding contributions to this field.

Krahl, V. E.: Anatomy of the mammalian lung. In American Physiological Society: Handbook of Physiology. Section 3, Respiration. Vol. I. Fenn, W. O., and Rahn, H. (Eds.). Baltimore, Williams & Wilkins, 1964, p. 213.
This chapter on the anatomy of the mammalian lung is one of the most complete treatises on the subject. It also contains more than 200 references, many of which are the original contributions that brought knowledge of the respiratory system to its present state.

Nagaishi, C.: Functional Anatomy and Histology of the Lung. Baltimore, University Park Press, 1972.
This magnificent volume combines studies of both the gross and the fine structures of the lung. The author is a thoracic surgeon who clearly recognizes the importance of basic knowledge in understanding and approaching the many difficult clinical problems involving the pulmonary system.

Supplement: Comparative Biology of the Lung. Am. Rev. Respir. Dis., 128, 1983.
This work reviews new and up-to-date techniques in the study of gross, histologic, electron microscopic, and biochemical anatomy of the lung.

Weibel, E. R.: Is the lung built reasonably? (The 1983 J. Burns Amberson Lecture). Am. Rev. Respir. Dis., 128:752, 1983.
This article by a leader in the field makes the continuing research in the anatomy and function of the lung exciting.

Williams, P. L., Warwick, R., Dyson, M., and Bannister, L. H. (Eds.): Gray's Anatomy, 37th ed. Edinburgh, Churchill Livingstone, 1989.
This is the classic of anatomy books.

REFERENCES

1. Arey, L. B.: Developmental Anatomy, Revised 7th ed. Philadelphia, W. B. Saunders Company, 1974.

2. Bertalanffy, F. D.: On the nomenclature of the cellular elements in respiratory tissue. Am. Rev. Respir. Dis., 91:605, 1965.
3. Bertalanffy, F. D., and Leblon, C. F.: The continuous renewal of the two types of alveolar cells in the lung of the rat. Anat. Rec., 115:515, 1953.
4. Blumenthal, B. J., and Boren, H. G.: Lung structure in three dimensions after inflation and fume fixation. Am. Rev. Tuberc., 79:764, 1959.
5. Boyden, E. A.: Segmental Anatomy of the Lungs. New York, McGraw-Hill Book Company, 1955.
6. Boyden, E. A.: The nomenclature of the bronchopulmonary segments and their blood supply. Dis. Chest. 39:1, 1961.
7. Brock, R. C.: The Anatomy of the Bronchial Tree with Special Reference to Surgery of Lung Abscess. 2nd ed. New York, Oxford University Press, 1954.
8. Brock, R. C.: The Anatomy of the Respiratory Tree. London, Oxford University Press, 1954.
9. Chen, C., Sealy, W. C., and Seaber, A. V.: The dynamic nature of collateral ventilation. J. Thorac. Cardiovasc. Surg., 59:518, 1970.
10. Churchill, E. D., and Belsey, R.: Segmental pneumonectomy in bronchiectasis. Ann. Surg., 109:481, 1939.
11. Ferguson, F. C., Kobilak, R. E., and Detrick, J. E.: Varices of bronchial veins as a source of hemoptysis in mitral stenosis. Am. Heart J., 28:445, 1944.
12. Goss, C. M. (Ed.): Gray's Anatomy of the Human Body. 28th ed. Philadelphia, Lea & Febiger, 1966.
13. Ham, A. W., and Wilson, T. S.: The Respiratory System in Histology, 4th ed. Philadelphia, J. B. Lippincott Company, 1961, p. 663.
14. Hayek, H. von: The Human Lung. Translated by V. E. Krahl. New York, Hafner Publishing Company, 1960.
15. Hesse, F. E., and Loosli, C. L.: The lining of the alveoli in mice, rats, dogs, and frogs following acute pulmonary edema produced by ANTU poisoning. Anat. Rec., 105:229, 1949.
16. Huber, J. F.: Practical correlative anatomy of the bronchial tree and lungs. J. Natl. Med. Assoc., 41:49, 1949.
17. Jackson, C. L., and Huber, J. F.: Correlated applied anatomy of the bronchial tree and lungs with a system of nomenclature. Dis. Chest, 9:319, 1943.
18. Kilburn, K. H.: A hypothesis for pulmonary clearance and its implications. Am. Rev. Respir. Dis., 98:449, 1968.
19. King, D. W. (Ed.): Ultrastructural Aspects of Disease. New York, Hoeber Medical Division, Harper & Row, 1966.
20. Krahl, V. E.: Anatomy of the mammalian lung. In American Physiological Society: Handbook of Physiology. Section 3. Respiration. Vol. I. Fenn, W. O., and Rahn, H. (Eds.). Baltimore, Williams & Wilkins, 1964, p. 213.
21. Kramer, R., and Glass, A.: Bronchoscopic localization of lung abscess. Ann. Otol., 41:1210, 1932.
22. Lambert, M. W.: Accessory bronchial alveolar channels. Anat. Rec., 127:472, 1957.
23. Liebow, A. A.: Pulmonary emphysema with special reference to vascular changes. Am. Rev. Respir. Dis., 80:67, 1959.

24. Loosli, C. G.: Intra-alveolar communications in normal and in pathologic mammalian lungs. Arch. Pathol., 24:743, 1937.
25. Low, F. N.: Electron microscopy of the rat lung. Anat. Rec., 113:437, 1952.
26. Low, F. N.: The pulmonary alveolar epithelium of laboratory mammals and man. Anat. Rec., 117:241, 1953.
27. Luchsinger, P. C., LaGarde, B., and Kilfeather, J. E.: Particle clearance from the human tracheobronchial tree. Am. Rev. Respir. Dis., 97:1046, 1968.
28. Macklin, C. C.: Alveolar pores and their significance in the human lung. Arch. Pathol., 21:202, 1936.
29. Macklin, C. C.: The alveoli of the mammalian lung. An anatomical study with clinical correlations. Proc. Inst. Med. Chicago, 18:78, 1950.
30. Miller, W. S.: The Lung, 2nd ed. Springfield, Ill., Charles C Thomas, Publisher, 1947.
31. Perkins, J. F.: Historical development of respiratory physiology. In American Physiological Society: Handbook of Physiology. Section 3, Respiration. Vol. I. Fenn, W. O. and Rahn, H. (Eds.). Baltimore, Williams & Wilkins, 1964, p. 62.
32. Pietra, G. G., Mango, M., Johns, L., and Fishman, P.: Bronchial veins and pulmonary edema. In Fishman, A. P., and Renkin, E. M. (Eds.). Pulmonary Edema. American Physiological Society Clinical Physiology Series. Baltimore, Williams & Wilkins, 1979, pp. 195–206.
33. Porter, K., and Bonneville, M. A.: Fine Structure of Cells and Tissues. Philadelphia, Lea & Febiger, 1968.
34. Pratt, P. C., and Klugh, G. A.: A technique for the study of ventilatory capacity, compliance, and residual volume of excised lungs and for fixation, drying, and serial sectioning in the inflated state. Am. Rev. Respir. Dis., 93:690, 1961.
35. Quinlan, M. F., Salman, S. D., Swift, D. L., Wagner, H. N., Jr., and Proctor, D. F.: Measurement of mucociliary function in man. Am. Rev. Respir. Dis., 99:13, 1969.
36. Rhodin, J. A. G.: An Atlas of Ultrastructure. Philadelphia, W. B. Saunders Company, 1963.
37. Spock, A., Heick, H. M. C., Cress, H., and Logan, W. S.: Abnormal serum factor in patients with cystic fibrosis of the pancreas. Pediatr. Res., 1:173, 1967.
38. Thorek, P.: Anatomy in Surgery. Philadelphia, J. B. Lippincott Company, 1962.
39. Tobin, C. E.: Lymphatics of the pulmonary alveoli. Anat. Rec., 120:625, 1954.
40. Tobin, C. E.: Pulmonary lymphatics with reference to emphysema. Am. Rev. Respir. Dis., 80:50, 1959.
41. Van Allen, C. M., and Lindskog, G. E.: Collateral respiration in the lung. Role in bronchial obstruction to prevent atelectasis and to restore patency. Surg. Gynecol. Obstet., 53:16, 1931.
42. Weibel, E. R., and Gomez, D. M.: Architecture of the human lung. Science. 137:577, 1962.
43. Weibel, E. R.: Is the lung built reasonably? (The 1983 J. Burns Amberson Lecture). Am. Rev. Respir. Dis., 128:752, 1983.

II

CLINICAL AND PHYSIOLOGIC EVALUATION OF PULMONARY FUNCTION

Richard A. Hopkins, M.D., and Walter G. Wolfe, M.D.

Evaluation and treatment of pulmonary dysfunction, whether related to chronic obstructive pulmonary disease (i.e., emphysema and bronchitis), pulmonary edema due to cardiac failure, or pulmonary insufficiency secondary to either a surgical procedure or traumatic injury, demands a careful history, a physical examination, and a complete physiologic evaluation. In an elective situation, these can be obtained prior to the operative procedure. However, when there is an acute emergency or traumatic injury, even during resuscitation of the patient, one should acquire the necessary pulmonary history from a family member. Environmental pollution, and a history of any exposure to asbestos or other toxic chemicals, and a pulmonary history with regard to allergies, emphysema, and bronchitis are extremely important, together with the patient's history of personal pollution, i.e., the number of cigarette pack years the patient has smoked.

MEASUREMENT OF PULMONARY FUNCTION

Air flows into the lungs because of differences in pressure.[61] Knowledge of these pressures is important in the management of respiratory insufficiency. One must consider oral, airway, alveolar, as well as pleural pressures. The act of breathing is complex, and disease affecting any part of the airway has an effect on ventilation and therefore the patient's physiologic performance after operation or injury.[60]

Understanding the factors that contribute to and alter pulmonary ventilation and gas exchange requires a detailed knowledge of lung function at the alveolar level.[50,54] Ventilation serves to replenish the gas in the lungs to maintain the high oxygen–low carbon dioxide pressure, producing maximal gradients. Distribution of gas is the delivery of air to the alveolar units by way of the bifurcating tracheobronchial tree. Diffusion is the

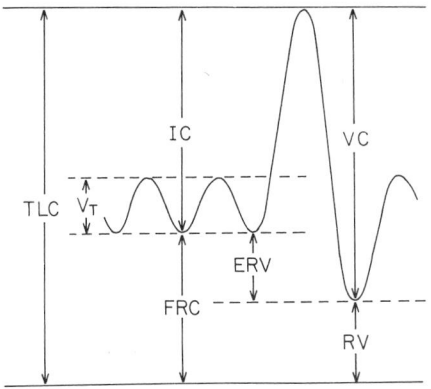

Figure 1. Spirometry. Subdivisions of lung volumes. TLC, total lung capacity; V$_T$, tidal volume; IC, inspiratory capacity; FRC, functional residual capacity, i.e., lung volume at end-expiration; ERV, expiratory reserve volume; RV, residual volume, i.e., lung volume after forced expiration from FRC; VC, vital capacity, i.e., the maximal volume of gas inspired from RV. For normal values in the adult, see Table 2.

transfer of gas molecules across the alveolar membranes in the region of high concentration. The blood-air surface of over 90 sq. m. in adults is condensed in a lung volume of only 5 liters. This is made possible by the small radius and the large number (300 million) of alveoli. Perfusion is the means by which desaturated blood is brought into intimate contact with the alveolar-capillary bed.

The necessity of measurement of lung function usually is obvious from the clinical evaluation. Initial tests are done for determining whether there is functional impairment. Later, the preoperative studies are used as a guide for determining whether the patient's condition has improved, is unchanged, or has deteriorated after illness or operation. When the history and physical examination do not suggest any evidence of lung disease, measurement of the vital capacity and forced expiratory volume in 1 second, combined with a normal chest film and normal blood gas determination, is sufficient to support the clinical impression that there is no underlying pulmonary disease. However, in patients with obvious or suspected lung disease, more detailed studies are necessary.[9,16,53]

PULMONARY FUNCTION TESTS. Pulmonary function tests are divided into the static volumes, flow rates, compliance, and resistance, and the measurement of arterial blood gases.[1,9,16,53] At times, diffusion capacity (D$_{LCO}$), right heart catheterization, and measurement of pulmonary diastolic pressure (PAD) are necessary as well as a ventilation-perfusion lung scan for evaluation of overall lung function.

The vital capacity (VC) permits detection of small changes in lung function (Fig. 1). However, variations between individuals are so great that vital capacity is not a very sensitive method for detection of disease with one measurement, although improvement or deterioration can be demonstrated in sequential measurements. Measurement of lung volumes allows the physician to determine physiologically an approximate index of the severity of some changes or dysfunction and to document the changes from time to time (Tables 1 and 2).

Respiratory excursion is the amount of air inspired and expired; this is termed tidal volume (V$_T$). The amount of gas contained in the lung at the end of quiet expiration is termed the functional residual capacity (FRC). When the patient makes a maximal inspiration and increases the lung volume, compared with that contained at the peak tidal volume, the inspiratory reserve capacity or volume (IRV) is reached. With forcible expiration, exhaling as much air as possible from the lung, the volume expired from maximal inspiration to maximal expiration is the vital capacity. The amount of air remaining in the lungs after maximal expiration is the residual volume (RV). All of these

lung volumes may be measured in the spirometer except the RV and the FRC. The FRC must be measured by other techniques. Three different methods may be used: inert gas dilution and washout, whole body plethysmography, and radioisotope techniques.

The RV is calculated by subtracting the expiratory reserve volume (ERV) from the FRC, since the respiratory midposition is believed to be more reproducible than the forced expiratory position. When FRC is measured by inert methods, helium or nitrogen is used. When helium is used, the patient rebreathes his own concentration of helium until it reaches a constant level (it equilibrates within the lung and spirometer). When nitrogen washout is performed to calculate FRC, the patient breathes 100 per cent oxygen. These two methods measure the residual volume of alveolar units in communication with an airway. The poorly ventilated units may be included in the overall calculation if helium equilibration and nitrogen washout are measured for sufficient periods of time. Although 7 minutes is considered the classic period used for nitrogen washout, a period in excess of 15 minutes may be necessary for patients with emphysema.

Body plethysmography measures all the gas in the lung and does not depend on communication with the airways. The volume is poorly termed thoracic gas volume (TGV), and the difference between thoracic gas volume and the FRC measured by dilution techniques is an index of maldistribution of ventilation. Discrepancy between thoracic gas volume and FRC is particularly striking in patients with bullous disease.

Boyle's law states that the product of the pressure and the volume of gas is constant for the same temperature. The patient is placed within a body plethysmograph, and the pressures within the plethysmograph and the mouth are measured. Any changes in the thoracic volume produce a reciprocal change in the plethysmograph volume that changes the plethysmograph pressure. Thus, an increase in the thoracic volume decreases plethysmograph volume and increases plethysmograph pressure. At the end of quiet expiration, the airway is occluded by an electrically operated shutter, and the patient is asked to continue panting against the obstructed airway. Because gas does not flow during the period of obstruction, the mouth pressure is assumed to be equal to alveolar pressure, and the increase is determined from the rise in the plethysmograph pressure.

MAXIMAL BREATHING CAPACITY. Maximal breathing capacity (MBC) is the largest volume of air that can be moved in and out of the chest per minute. The term *MBC* is reserved for the maximal breathing capacity of an individual, whereas the term *maximal voluntary ventilation (MVV)* indicates the maximal volume of gas breathed per minute under testing conditions. The analysis of vital capacity and of maximal breathing capacity permits differentiation of ventilatory abnormality as obstructive versus restrictive disease, since MBC is markedly decreased in obstructive disease.

SPECIFIC ABNORMALITIES OF LUNG VOLUME. In restrictive disease, the total lung capacity (TLC) and vital capacity are small; whereas in obstructive disease, uncomplicated by fibrosis, the residual volume is large. In emphysema, the FRC and TLC are increased, but the vital capacity may be equal to or less than normal. Certain restrictive diseases may have decreased FRC. These are muscular weaknesses, pulmonary granulomatosis, heart failure, and mixed restriction and obstruction. The patient with kyphoscoliosis typically has a small FRC. Obstructive diseases such as moderate asthma and acute bronchitis do not have marked increases in FRC.[8,49]

Patients with chronic emphysema and lung cysts have an increase in FRC. The ratio of residual volume to total lung capacity is also increased in emphysema but may also be increased in restrictive disease. Therefore, this ratio is of no value without simultaneous measurement of absolute figures for residual volume and total lung capacity.

TABLE 1. Predicted Values for Pulmonary Function Tests: Part A—Men

Height (cm.)	Age (yr.)	VC	FRC	RV	TLC	$FEV_{0.75} \times 40$ (L./min.)	$FEV_{1.0}$ (L)	MMFR (L./sec.)	$DLCOSS_2$	FICO − FEXCO FICO	DLCOSB	ME%
155	20	3.97	2.72	1.13	5.10	136	3.6	4.3	23.8	0.56	26.7	70
	30	3.65	2.72	1.30	4.95	121	3.3	3.9	21.0	0.52	23.7	65
	40	3.35	2.72	1.45	4.80	106	3.0	3.5	18.2	0.49	20.7	60
	50	3.04	2.72	1.61	4.65	91	2.7	3.1	15.4	0.45	17.7	55
	60	2.73	2.72	1.77	4.50	76	2.4	2.7	12.6	0.42	14.7	50
	70	2.42	2.72	1.91	4.35	61	2.1	2.3	9.8	0.39	11.7	45
160	20	4.30	2.98	1.27	5.57	141	3.8	4.4	24.1	0.55	29.0	70
	30	4.00	2.98	1.42	5.42	126	3.5	4.0	21.3	0.52	26.0	65
	40	3.70	2.98	1.57	5.27	111	3.2	3.6	18.6	0.48	23.0	60
	50	3.40	2.98	1.72	5.12	96	2.8	3.2	15.8	0.45	20.0	55
	60	3.10	2.98	1.87	4.97	81	2.5	2.8	13.0	0.41	17.0	50
	70	2.80	2.98	2.02	4.82	65	2.2	2.4	10.1	0.39	14.0	45
165	20	4.62	3.23	1.42	6.04	145	3.9	4.5	24.5	0.55	31.3	70
	30	4.32	3.23	1.57	5.89	130	3.7	4.1	21.7	0.52	28.3	65
	40	4.02	3.23	1.72	5.74	115	3.3	3.7	18.9	0.48	25.3	60
	50	3.72	3.23	1.87	5.59	100	3.0	3.3	16.1	0.44	22.3	55
	60	3.42	3.23	2.02	5.44	85	2.7	2.9	13.3	0.42	19.3	50
	70	3.12	3.23	2.17	5.29	70	2.4	2.5	10.6	0.38	16.3	45
170	20	4.94	3.48	1.57	6.51	150	4.1	4.6	24.9	0.54	33.6	70
	30	4.64	3.48	1.72	6.36	135	3.8	4.2	22.1	0.50	30.6	65
	40	4.35	3.48	1.86	6.21	120	3.5	3.8	19.3	0.47	27.6	60
	50	4.05	3.48	2.01	6.06	105	3.2	3.4	16.5	0.43	24.6	55
	60	3.74	3.48	2.17	5.91	90	2.9	3.0	13.7	0.40	21.6	50
	70	3.44	3.48	2.32	5.76	75	2.6	2.6	10.9	0.37	18.6	45
175	20	5.26	3.74	1.72	6.98	155	4.3	4.7	25.2	0.53	35.8	70
	30	4.96	3.74	1.87	6.83	140	4.0	4.3	22.4	0.50	32.8	65
	40	4.66	3.74	2.02	6.68	124	3.7	3.9	19.6	0.47	29.9	60
	50	4.36	3.74	2.17	6.53	110	3.4	3.5	16.9	0.43	26.9	55
	60	4.06	3.74	2.32	6.38	94	3.1	3.1	14.1	0.39	23.9	50
	70	3.76	3.74	2.47	6.23	79	2.8	2.7	11.3	0.36	20.9	45
180	20	5.58	3.99	1.87	7.45	159	4.5	4.8	25.6	0.52	38.1	70
	30	5.28	3.99	2.02	7.30	145	4.2	4.4	22.8	0.49	35.1	65
	40	4.98	3.99	2.17	7.15	129	3.9	4.0	20.0	0.46	32.1	60
	50	4.68	3.99	2.32	7.00	114	3.6	3.6	17.2	0.42	29.2	55
	60	4.38	3.99	2.47	6.85	99	3.3	3.2	14.2	0.39	26.2	50
	70	4.08	3.99	2.62	6.70	83	2.9	2.8	11.6	0.35	23.2	45
185	20	5.90	4.25	2.02	7.92	163	4.7	4.9	25.9	0.53	40.4	70
	30	5.60	4.25	2.17	7.77	148	4.3	4.5	23.2	0.48	37.4	65
	40	5.30	4.25	2.32	7.62	133	4.1	4.1	20.4	0.46	34.4	60
	50	5.00	4.25	2.47	7.47	118	3.7	3.7	17.6	0.42	31.4	55
	60	4.70	4.25	2.62	7.32	103	3.5	3.3	14.8	0.38	28.4	50
	70	4.40	4.25	2.77	7.17	88	3.1	2.9	12.0	0.35	25.5	45

Subdivisions of lung volume measured in seated subjects.
Ventilatory tests performed with subjects standing.
Diffusion capacity tests performed on seated subjects.

MMFR, maximal mid-expiratory flow rate; DLCOSS, diffusion capacity; steady-state carbon monoxide uptake with alveolar carbon monoxide measured from an end-tidal sample of gas; VC, vital capacity; FRC, functional residual capacity; RV, residual volume; TLC, total lung capacity; $FEV_{0.75}$, forced expiratory volume at 0.75 second (the $FEV_{0.75}$ multiplied by 40 gives an approximate indication of the maximal breathing capacity in liters per minute); $FEV_{1.0}$, forced expiratory volume at 1.0 second; FICO − FEXCO/FICO, fractional uptake of carbon monoxide where FICO equals the inspired and FEXCO equals the expired fraction of carbon monoxide; DLCOSB, diffusion capacity; single-breath method using helium and carbon monoxide, modified Krogh technique; ME%, closed circuit helium index; measure of FRC.

From Bates, D. V., Macklem, P. T., and Christie, R. V.: Respiratory Function in Disease, 2nd ed. Philadelphia, W. B. Saunders Company, 1971.

FLOW RATES. Measurements of dynamic properties of the lungs, i.e., flow rates, are extremely important. The patient inhales maximally and then exhales forcibly into a spirometer while the device records the volume versus the time. A common test of maximal expiratory airflow is the volume of air expired in 1 second (FEV_1). This number is decreased in the presence of bronchial obstruction, but the value may also be decreased in restrictive disease. For this reason, the FEV_1 is usually related to the total exhaled vital capacity. This ratio of FEV_1 to VC may be decreased in the presence of airway obstruction but normal in restrictive lung disease.

DIFFUSION OF GAS. A single-breath carbon monoxide (DLCO) diffusion capacity measurement should be considered a screening test. In this test, the patient is required to inhale low, nontoxic concentrations of carbon monoxide, hold the breath for 10 seconds, and then exhale. This test is rapid, simple, safe, and painless. DLCO is an estimate of the pulmonary capillary surface area.[19]

There are several factors that affect diffusion in a single alveolus. The thickness of the alveolar lining membrane is important, as is the thickness of the layer of plasma between the capillary wall and the red blood cell. In addition, the permeability of the erythrocyte to carbon monoxide or oxygen must be considered along with the reaction rate of hemoglobin with

TABLE 1. Predicted Values for Pulmonary Function Tests: Part A—Men

Height (cm.)	Age (yr.)	VC	FRC	RV	TLC	FEV$_{0.75}$ × 40 (L./min.)	FEV$_{1.0}$ (L)	MMFR (L./sec.)	DLCOSS$_2$	FICO − FEXCO FICO	DLCOSB	ME%
145	20	2.81	1.96	1.00	3.81	88	2.6	3.6	20.7	0.58	19.5	70
	30	2.63	1.96	1.08	3.71	80	2.4	3.3	18.2	0.55	16.9	65
	40	2.45	1.96	1.16	3.61	72	2.1	2.9	15.7	0.51	14.2	60
	50	2.27	1.96	1.24	3.51	64	1.9	2.5	13.2	0.48	11.7	55
	60	2.09	1.96	1.32	3.41	56	1.5	2.2	10.7	0.44	9.0	50
	70	1.91	1.96	1.40	3.31	48	1.4	1.8	8.2	0.41	6.4	45
150	20	3.08	2.20	1.05	4.13	92	2.7	3.7	21.1	0.57	21.7	70
	30	2.89	2.20	1.14	4.03	84	2.5	3.3	18.6	0.54	19.1	65
	40	2.71	2.20	1.22	3.93	76	2.2	3.0	16.0	0.51	16.4	60
	50	2.53	2.20	1.30	3.83	67	2.0	2.6	13.5	0.47	13.7	55
	60	2.35	2.20	1.38	3.73	60	1.6	2.3	11.0	0.43	11.1	50
	70	2.17	2.20	1.46	3.63	52	1.5	1.9	8.5	0.40	8.5	45
155	20	3.34	2.43	1.19	4.53	95	2.8	3.8	21.5	0.56	23.9	70
	30	3.15	2.43	1.28	4.43	88	2.6	3.4	18.9	0.52	21.2	65
	40	2.97	2.43	1.36	4.33	79	2.4	3.1	16.4	0.49	18.5	60
	50	2.79	2.43	1.44	4.23	71	2.1	2.7	13.9	0.45	15.8	55
	60	2.61	2.43	1.52	4.13	63	1.7	2.3	11.4	0.42	13.1	50
	70	2.43	2.43	1.60	4.03	55	1.6	2.0	8.9	0.39	10.5	45
160	20	3.60	2.67	1.32	4.92	99	2.9	3.9	21.9	0.55	26.0	70
	30	3.41	2.67	1.41	4.82	91	2.7	3.5	19.4	0.52	23.3	65
	40	3.22	2.67	1.50	4.72	83	2.5	3.2	16.8	0.48	20.6	60
	50	3.05	2.67	1.57	4.62	75	2.2	2.8	14.3	0.45	17.9	55
	60	2.87	2.67	1.65	4.52	67	1.8	2.4	11.8	0.41	15.2	50
	70	2.69	2.67	1.73	4.42	59	1.7	2.1	9.2	0.39	12.5	45
165	20	3.88	2.90	1.44	5.32	103	3.1	4.0	22.2	0.55	28.1	70
	30	3.68	2.90	1.54	5.22	95	2.8	3.6	19.7	0.52	25.4	65
	40	3.50	2.90	1.62	5.12	87	2.6	3.3	17.2	0.48	22.7	60
	50	3.32	2.90	1.70	5.02	79	2.3	2.9	14.6	0.44	20.0	55
	60	3.14	2.90	1.78	4.92	71	1.9	2.5	12.1	0.42	17.3	50
	70	2.96	2.90	1.86	4.82	63	1.8	2.2	9.6	0.38	14.6	45
170	20	4.13	3.14	1.58	5.71	107	3.2	4.1	22.6	0.54	30.3	70
	30	3.94	3.14	1.67	5.61	99	2.9	3.7	20.1	0.50	27.6	65
	40	3.76	3.14	1.75	5.51	90	2.7	3.3	17.5	0.47	24.9	60
	50	3.58	3.14	1.83	5.41	82	2.4	3.0	15.0	0.43	22.2	55
	60	3.40	3.14	1.91	5.31	74	2.0	2.6	12.5	0.40	19.5	50
	70	3.22	3.14	1.99	5.21	66	1.9	2.3	9.9	0.37	16.8	45
175	20	4.38	3.37	1.80	6.18	111	3.3	4.1	22.7	0.53	32.3	70
	30	4.20	3.37	1.90	6.10	102	3.0	3.8	20.0	0.50	29.6	65
	40	4.02	3.37	2.00	6.02	94	2.8	3.4	17.7	0.47	26.9	60
	50	3.84	3.37	2.10	5.94	86	2.5	3.1	15.2	0.43	24.2	55
	60	3.66	3.37	2.20	5.86	78	2.1	2.7	12.7	0.38	21.5	50
	70	3.38	3.37	2.40	5.78	70	2.0	2.3	10.2	0.36	18.8	45

Subdivisions of lung volume measured in seated subjects.
Ventilatory tests performed with subjects standing.
Diffusion capacity tests performed on seated subjects.
For abbreviations, see Table 1.
From Bates, D. V., Macklem, P. T., and Christie, R. V.: Respiratory Function in Disease, 2nd ed. Philadelphia, W. B. Saunders Company, 1971.

carbon monoxide or oxygen. In a single-breath diffusion capacity measurement using carbon monoxide, the presence of carbon monoxide hemoglobin in the pulmonary arterial blood diminishes the rate of carbon monoxide transfer.

A decrease in pulmonary diffusion capacity may be the earliest detectable abnormality in collagen disease such as sarcoidosis or in industrial diseases such as asbestosis. Also, a decreased DLCO is found in patients with pulmonary emboli, and a perfusion lung scan and/or arteriogram may be indicated for those patients in whom this diagnosis may be considered. Diffusion capacity is increased in mitral stenosis, left heart failure, and polycythemia.

AIRWAY RESISTANCE AND LUNG ELASTICITY. In emphysema, the lung compliance is high, and therefore the FRC is large. These lungs exhibit little elastic recoil at the measured FRC. As a result, the resting intrapleural pressure is not as negative as it would be normally. This absence of negative intrapleural pressure allows the bronchi to collapse at a volume of only slightly less than FRC because the bronchi do not have either a negative pleural pressure around them or the outwardly pulling force of the lung tissues surrounding them to keep them open. With collapsed bronchi, the emphysematous patient has difficulty emptying the air from the lungs to reach a volume much lower than the large FRC. Adequate measurement of the lung's elastic properties is done only by measurement of the static pressure-volume curve, in which absolute transpulmonary pressure is related to absolute lung volume over the whole vital capacity during both inflation and deflation. Airway resistance is increased in emphysema and may also be increased in patients with bronchitis. The degree of bronchitis is important because with appropriate therapy some of the increased resistance is reversible.

ARTERIAL BLOOD GASES. Not only is adequate pulmonary function necessary to maintain delivery of oxygen to the periph-

PREOPERATIVE PULMONARY PREPARATION

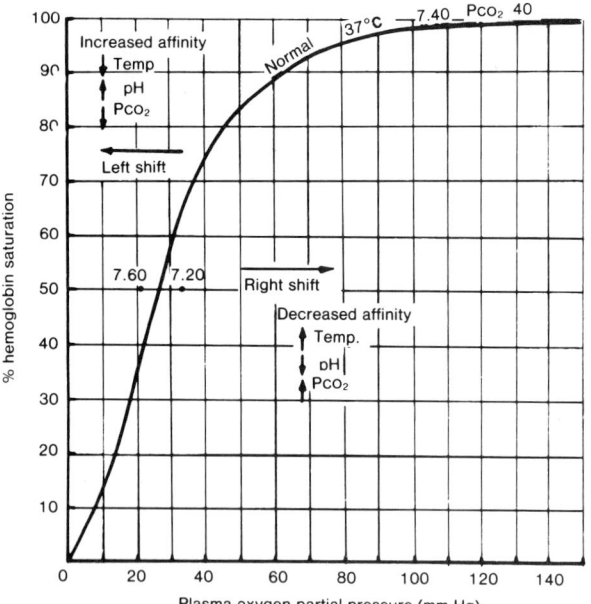

Figure 2. The oxygen-hemoglobin dissociation curve. This figure highlights the effects of temperature and acid-base as well as the effect of changes in the partial pressure of carbon dioxide on the curve. The points 7.6 and 7.2 represent the left and right shifts that occur secondary to pH. (From Margand, P. M. D., Brooks, C. G., Jr., and Hunter, J. W.: Preoperative Pulmonary Preparation: A Clinical Guide. Baltimore, Williams & Wilkins Company, 1981.)

ery as well as to remove carbon dioxide, but the hemoglobin must function to absorb and release oxygen (Fig. 2). It is important also that the hemoglobin be fully saturated and sufficiently available so that the cardiac output can deliver the quantity of oxygen necessary for aerobic metabolism. The hemoglobin should be maintained at normothermia and normal pH so that it can not only transport adequate oxygen but also unload it at the periphery.

The measurement of arterial blood gases is probably the most frequently used pulmonary function test. The interpretation of Pao_2 depends on the oxygen tension in the inspired air. One can then calculate first the alveolar oxygen tension and then the alveolar arterial oxygen tension gradient; if the Pao_2 and the $A-aDo_2$ are normal, there is no disturbance in oxygen transport.

ARTERIAL OXYGEN TENSION. The measurement of arterial Po_2 is very useful in evaluating pulmonary function. An alveolar-arterial Po_2 difference of about 10 torr is customarily found in young healthy adults, and a 20-torr difference is found in healthy older adults. Greater differences—that is, an arterial Po_2 of less than 80 torr in the absence of hypoventilation—require explanation. Possibilities include a right-to-left shunt, a diffusion barrier, or an uneven distribution of ventilation to blood flow. To test for right-to-left shunt, the patient is given 100 per cent oxygen, and the arterial Po_2 should increase to greater than 604. If the arterial Po_2 is less than predicted but greater than 150 torr, the percentage of right-to-left shunting can be calculated as follows:

$$\% \text{ shunt} = \frac{\dfrac{(673 - Pao_2)2.3}{760}}{\left(\dfrac{(673 - Pao_2)2.3}{760}\right) + 4.5} \times 100$$

This equation assumes 2.3 as the solubility of O_2 in plasma and 4.5 as the usual arteriovenous difference (see Table 10). The normal shunt is below 8 per cent; in obese patients this may approach 10 per cent; shunts greater than these are usually abnormal.

ARTERIAL CARBON DIOXIDE TENSION. The measurements of $Paco_2$ provide an immediate indication of the patient's alveolar ventilation (Fig. 3). A $Paco_2$ of less than 37 mm. Hg is hypocapnia, whereas hypercapnia is defined as greater than 43 mm. Hg (i.e., normal range, 38 to 42 mm. Hg). Any level of hypercapnia indicates severe disease, representing functional loss of perhaps more than 50 per cent of the lung. Acidosis is defined as a pH of less than 7.37, and alkalosis is a pH of greater than 7.43. Evaluation of acid base requires interpretation of both respiratory and metabolic determinants of pH. Potential aberrations include respiratory acidosis, respiratory alkalosis, metabolic acidosis, and metabolic alkalosis.

ACID BASE. The principal buffering systems in the body are bicarbonate, phosphates, and cells. During acute changes, the extracellular bicarbonate and the hemoglobin are the major buffers. In addition to chemical buffering, there are also physiologic responses to alteration in acid-base status that are very critical in minimizing changes in pH for each of the four types of acid-base disturbances. Wherever compensation occurs for primary respiratory acid-base disturbances, there must be a physiologically induced metabolic alteration, usually renal. Conversely, metabolic disturbances must be corrected by using the respiratory mechanism. Renal acid-base adjustments occur slowly because urinary secretion of acid, although beginning rapidly, may take 2 hours to days to complete.

RESPIRATORY ACIDOSIS. Respiratory acidosis is compensated by renal retention of bicarbonate and, thus, excretion of acid. Renal compensation begins immediately upon development of respiratory acidosis but takes days to weeks to become maximal. This mechanism can return blood pH completely to normal, given sufficient time, if the steady state of $Paco_2$ is 60 to 65 torr or less. Above this level of hypercapnia, the kidney cannot sufficiently increase its rate of reabsorption of bicarbonate. If the pH is low and the $Paco_2$ is below 60 torr, respiratory acidosis is likely to be acute or subacute.

The effect of respiratory acidosis on the sensorium is probably due to lowering of pH of the cerebrospinal fluid (CSF), with which blood CO_2 equilibrates rapidly. Since the CSF is corrected toward normal by accumulation of bicarbonate in CSF, within a

GAS EXCHANGE

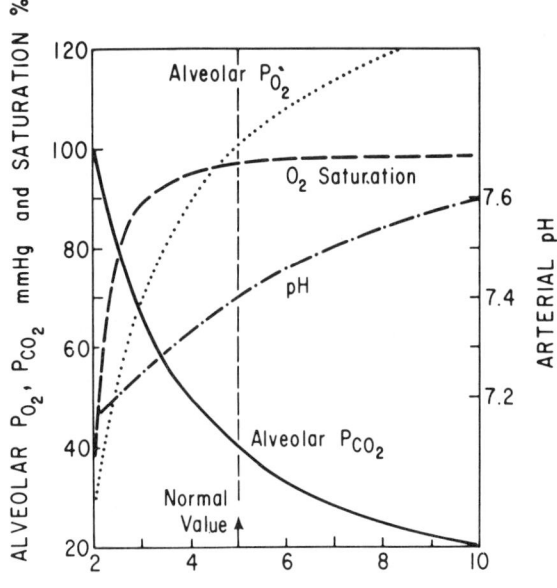

Figure 3. Changes in gas exchange during hypoventilation. Note the rapid rise in Pco_2 compared with the so-called slow fall in arterial oxygen saturation. (From West, J. B.: Pulmonary Pathophysiology: The Essentials. Baltimore, Williams & Wilkins, 1977.)

few days of the onset of hypercapnia, patients with chronic hypercapnia may have a clear sensorium at a level of $Paco_2$ that would cause coma if it should develop acutely. Thus, clinical observation of the patient with known hypercapnia often indicates whether hypercapnia is acute or chronic.

RESPIRATORY ALKALOSIS. Controversy remains as to whether or not the kidney compensates for chronic respiratory alkalosis by excretion of bicarbonate and retention of acid. There is suggestive evidence that such compensation occurs, at least in chronic situations, but it is probably incomplete.

METABOLIC ACIDOSIS. Metabolic acidosis is corrected by inducing respiratory alkalosis and stimulating chemoreceptors both in the aortic-carotid area and in the floor of the fourth ventricle, which represents at least half, and possibly much more, of the respiratory stimulation occurring during metabolic acidosis. The aortic-carotid chemoreceptors are affected rapidly by changes in the pH of the CSF. The maximal respiratory response to an acid load is delayed for a matter of hours or days. For any given blood pH during chronic metabolic acidosis, there is an appropriate lowering of $Paco_2$. A $Paco_2$ that is inappropriately above or below the response to uncomplicated metabolic acidosis suggests the presence of a superimposed primary respiratory acidosis or alkalosis.

METABOLIC ALKALOSIS. Metabolic alkalosis is compensated by the development of respiratory acidosis, but under ordinary circumstances $Paco_2$ does not increase above 50 torr no matter how severe the metabolic alkalosis, although exceptional cases in which severe hypercapnia occurred have been reported. The usual minimal effect on $Paco_2$ appears to follow the fact that ventilation is linked to the rate of oxygen consumption or CO_2 production in some unknown manner, and this link prevents development of more severe hypercapnia by taking precedence over the compensatory mechanism.

PREOPERATIVE EVALUATION

Pulmonary complications are not infrequent after major operative procedures.[3,4,12,13,24,53] Age, obesity, type of surgical procedure, cigarette smoking, and anesthesia impair pulmonary function and are preoperative risk factors.[32,36,37] With age, the lungs show gradual deterioration both in performance of the airways and in gas exchange (Fig. 4). Both flow-volume curves and position as well as blood gases change with age (Table 3).[55] Although a nonsmoker's pulmonary function deteriorates only slightly with time, age remains a relative factor.[26,27] The older patient with obstructive airway disease has a markedly increased risk. Obesity impairs lung and chest wall compliance. There may be a component of restrictive lung disease, and the work of breathing is increased. When abnormal closure of small airways occurs, this leads to significant ventilation-perfusion mismatches.[47] These changes become worse in the supine position, in which the weight of the abdomen and chest wall contributes to the impairment of pulmonary function (Fig. 5). These changes may be even more apparent if the patient is placed in a lateral position with one lung partially deflated. More effort is required for each breath, and the $Paco_2$ usually falls.

Smoking, even in the absence of detectable lung disease, is associated with increased postoperative atelectasis and infection.[14,15,23] The site of incision, whether abdominal or thoracic, also influences postoperative performance. With upper abdominal and thoracic incisions, the chest wall and diaphragmatic mechanics are altered. Incisional pain contributes to postoperative hypoventilation. These patients may cough ineffectively and experience difficulty in clearing secretions. With lower abdominal incisions, the changes in pulmonary function are less marked.[18]

Pulmonary function should be evaluated in relation to the operative procedure planned.[32–35,41,43] Patients can be divided into the following groups: (1) those undergoing thoracotomy for

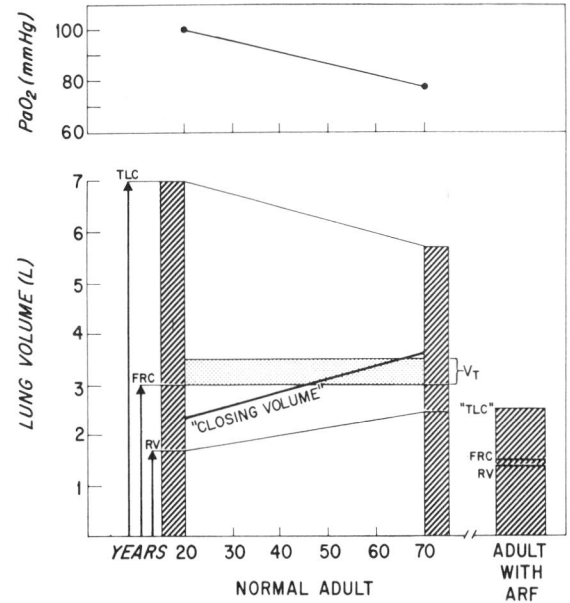

Figure 4. Demonstrates the changes in PaO_2 and lung volumes with age in normal adults in the supine position and the typical values for FRC and vital capacity in an adult patient with adult respiratory failure. RV, residual volume; FRC, functional residual capacity; TLC, total lung capacity. (From Pontoppidan, H., Geffin, G., and Lowenstein, E.: Acute Respiratory Failure in the Adult. Boston, Little, Brown and Company, 1973.)

removal of lung tissue, (2) those undergoing thoracotomy without excision of pulmonary tissue, (3) those undergoing abdominal surgery, and (4) those undergoing procedures on extremities or elsewhere.[17–20] It is apparent that each group responds differently to the effects of the operation, anesthesia, and pulmonary function (Table 4). Every effort should be made postoperatively to obtain maximal pulmonary function as soon as possible to ensure rapid return of the functional residual capacity to the preoperative level. Supplemental oxygen should be used as necessary to prevent hypoxemia. If the vital capacity and the FRC are returned to the preoperative level and hypoxemia is prevented, the ventilation-perfusion ratio is corrected. These are important guidelines, because all patients who are injured, undergo anesthesia, and have an operative procedure experience decreased lung volume with decreased ventilation, hypoxemia, and lowered FRC in the postoperative period. If these factors are not corrected and if hypoxemia progresses, respiratory insufficiency and failure may develop rapidly.[48,50,52]

RISK IN PATIENTS WITH PRE-EXISTING PULMONARY DISEASE. Obstructive pulmonary disease is the most important risk factor in the patient undergoing surgical therapy. The more severe the disease, the greater the risk of postoperative complications (Table 5). Restrictive lung disease is usually better tolerated; however, these patients cannot afford to lose much functioning lung. Because of better expiratory flow rates, cough is better preserved in these patients than in those with obstructive disease. In general, an FEV_1 of 1 to 2 liters is not associated with an increased operative risk; with an FEV_1 of less than 800 ml., there is clearly increased risk for severe pulmonary complications; those with less than 500 ml. have the greatest risk (Table 6). The presence of carbon dioxide retention is a marker for the patient at dramatically increased risk.[45,46,52,56]

Thoracotomy and pulmonary resection are not well tolerated in patients with obstructive airway disease. There is not only a loss of functional tissue in a patient with pulmonary disease, but the thoracotomy alters the mechanical and gas exchange properties of the lung. This may be accentuated if lung tissue is removed during operation. Thoracotomy produces pain in the

TABLE 3. The Effect of Age on Arterial P_{O_2} and P_{CO_2} While Breathing Ambient Air at Rest

Age Group (Years)	No. Observations	Mean PaO_2 (mm. Hg)	±SD	Mean $PaCO_2$ (mm. Hg)	±SD
<30 (median = 23)	38	94.2	3.31	39.0	1.8
31–40 (median = 36)	30	87.2	3.47	38.5	2.0
41–50 (median = 46)	30	83.9	4.07	39.6	2.4
51–60 (median = 55)	30	81.2	3.74	39.0	1.9
>60 (median = 71)	24	74.3	4.43	39.8	2.1

From Sorbini, C. A., et al.: Arterial oxygen tension in relation to age in healthy subjects. Respiration, 25:3, 1968.

postoperative period, which reduces the patient's ability to cough to clear secretions. If the airway disease is severe, the patient may not be able to tolerate the loss of even a single pulmonary segment. Thus, in these patients, preoperative evaluation is extremely important, and preparation of the patient by cessation of smoking and the use of a variety of drugs to improve airway function and ventilation is extremely helpful in decreasing operative risk.[14,15,26,43,52]

In patients with pulmonary hypertension and carbon dioxide retention, resective procedures may be contraindicated. For example, when the FEV_1 is less than 2 liters and the MVV or MBC less than 50 per cent, patients do not usually tolerate pneumonectomy.[29,37,41,45,50,56] Therefore, predicting postresection lung function can be helpful in preventing a surgically cured but pulmonary-crippled patient.

A reliable estimate of postoperative pulmonary function can be obtained by comparing the quantitative perfusion lung scan with the patient's preoperative FEV_1. As an example, if the preoperative FEV_1 is 2.2 liters and the quantitative perfusion scan indicates that 60 per cent of the total lung function is from the right lung, a left pneumonectomy may be associated with a postoperative FEV_1 of about 1.3 liters. In this situation, the patient could tolerate the operation. However, if the predicted postoperative FEV_1 is less than 800 ml., operation is not indicated. This method is less accurate when three or fewer segments of the lung are removed. In a marginal patient, another predictive test such as right heart catheterization and measurement of pulmonary artery pressures with balloon occlusion of one pulmonary artery can be accomplished for assessment of the patient for tolerance of a pneumonectomy.[45,53,54] Ferguson and colleagues have demonstrated that measurement of D_{LCO} is an important discriminator for postoperative morbidity and mortality following pulmonary resection; they reason that the D_{LCO} is a sensitive indicator of both structural and functional abnormalities because it is a measure of functional alveolar microarchitecture and can be an independent measure of physiologic capability apart from FEV_1 and FVC.[19]

PREOPERATIVE PREPARATION. When the risks have been defined, every effort should be made to eliminate or reduce postoperative complications. Patients should cease smoking; although the optimal time is unknown, there is a marked benefit from cessation of smoking even after only 5 to 7 days. Preoperative respiratory muscle conditioning is important, as is education of the patient about breathing patterns and effective coughing. Bronchial dilators should be used preoperatively and continued postoperatively in patients in whom their efficacy can be demonstrated (Table 7). Preoperative evaluation of the efficacy of or intolerance to medications is optimal. Many of these medications are associated with premature ventricular or atrial contractions; such arrhythmias may become a serious postoperative problem and may be accentuated when hypoxemia is present. Therefore, it may be important to administer intravenous antiarrhythmic agents in these patients. Every effort should be made to decrease the amount of secretions and assist the patient in coughing and deep breathing to clear secretions (e.g., postural drainage and chest percussion). In patients with asthma and severe chronic bronchitis, steroids may be used and can prevent accentuation of postoperative bronchospasm.

OPERATIVE AND POSTOPERATIVE CHANGES. The effects of anesthesia may increase venous admixture, increase ventilation and perfusion mismatching, change the cardiac output, and alter the mechanical properties of the chest wall or the lung itself, whether or not paralysis is used during anesthesia. Mucociliary transport may be decreased, and the hemoglobin concentration and function may change.[17,18,34,52,60] Diaphragmatic function may be impaired, and the position of the patient during operation may compound some of these difficulties. The dependent basilar segments, for example, are usually underventilated and therefore have a greater tendency to develop atelectasis. In general, the patient is ventilated with positive pressure, and the dependent areas of the lung, which have the smallest airway diameters and are the least compliant, are poorly ventilated. The more compliant and less perfused areas receive the greatest ventilation. This leads to ventilation-perfusion mismatching and to hypoxemia and atelectasis. Also, as discussed earlier, the FRC decreases in almost all anesthetized surgical patients as well as in injured patients regardless of whether the injury follows operation or trauma.[20] Therefore, the FEV_1 and VC are also reduced. These changes are maximal in the first and second postoperative days but remain abnormal for a week after operation. Decrease in the FRC leads to airway closure and ventilation-perfusion mismatching with resulting hypoxemia, which may be accentuated in the older patient.

To combat these changes, continuous airway pressure or positive end-expiratory pressure (PEEP) has been used.[17,20,43,57] PEEP acts to increase the FRC, but it may also reduce cardiac output by limiting preload to the left ventricle. Alveolar dead

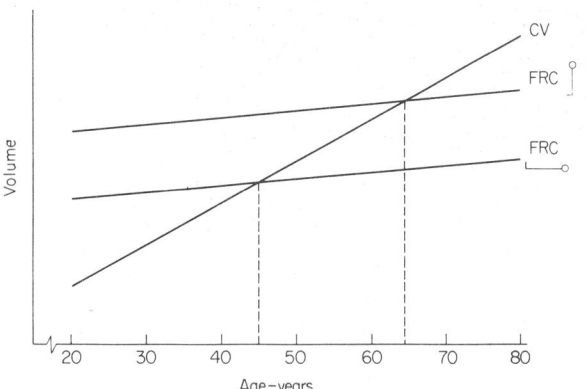

Figure 5. The effect of increasing age and closing volume in relation to FRC in both the erect and supine positions. (From Sykes, M. K., McNicol, M. W., and Campbell, E. J. M.: Respiratory Failure, 2nd ed. Oxford, Blackwell Scientific Publications, 1976.)

TABLE 4. Effect of Moderate and Heavy Exercise on the Oxygen Required for Breathing

Condition	External Work (kg.-m./min.)	Tidal Vol. (ml.)	Resp. Rate (breaths/min.)	Min. Vol. (L./min.)	O₂ Con-sumption (ml./min.)	Respiratory Work			
						kg.-m./min.	% Elastic	% Resistive	O₂ cost ml./min.
Quiet breathing	0	500	15	7.5	300	0.3	66	33	3
Moderate exercise	620	1600	23	37.0	1500	5.2	57	43	52
Heavy exercise	1600	2400	48	115.0	3500	35.2	39	61	352
Maximal voluntary ventilation	0	1500	120	180	—	65.0	20	80+	—

Heavy exercise is accompanied by a 10-fold increase in oxygen consumption. The distribution of work is reversed as compared with quiet breathing (elastic component falls from 66 to 39 per cent, and the resistive component rises from 33 to 61 per cent) and is associated with a fivefold rise in tidal volume but only a threefold increase in respiratory frequency. Maximal voluntary ventilation is achieved by a significantly greater increase in frequency than tidal volume. An increase in minute ventilation during the postoperative period represents an increase in work to overcome resistance to gas flow. Thus an increase in respiratory rate is indicative of inefficient respiration and incipient respiration failure.

TABLE 5. Evaluation of Risk of Pulmonary Resection in Patients with Pulmonary Disease

Function	Test	Patient at Risk — Needs Preoperative Optimization or Further Evaluation	Prohibitive Risk
Mechanical ventilatory	FEV₁ postoperative predicted	<1.01/sec.	<0.8 L./sec.
	FVC preoperative	<2.01	<1.5 L.
	MBC preoperative	<55%	<35%
Parenchymal pulmonary	Po₂ preoperative (rest)	50–60 mm. Hg	<50 mm. Hg
	Pco₂ preoperative (rest)	40–44 mm. Hg	>45 mm. Hg
	Qₛ/Qₜ preoperative	10%–20%	>20%
Cardiac	EKG at rest	Abnormal, especially ischemic changes	Acute MI, ventricular arrhythmias
	Exercise tolerance test (ETT)	Stage IV + (consider cardiac cath.)	Early + ETT
	Ventricular function (rest-exercise ejection fraction by radionuclide studies)	EF < 50% or deterioration with exercise	EF < 30%
Cardiopulmonary capacity	Chronic Hgb level	>17 gm./100 ml.	>20% gm./100 ml.
	Exercise tests: ETT	Unable to complete Stage IV secondary to dyspnea on exertion	Unable to complete Stage I (cardiac ischemia or arrhythmias)
	Stairwalking	Unable to complete three flights of stairs	Unable to walk one flight
	Postexercise arterial blood gases	Fall in Po₂	Fall in Po₂ to <49 mm. Hg or CO₂ retention

TABLE 6. Interpretation of Risk in Patients with Pulmonary Disease

Findings	Interpretation
Normal test	No increased risk demonstrated
Obstructive disorders	
FEV₁ >1.5 liters; MVV >50% Normal blood gases	Little increased risk if special precautions taken in patient management
FEV₁ = 1–1.5 liters; MVV = 35–50% Normal Paco₂; no more than slight hypoxemia; normal ECG	Definitely increased risk even with proper management; a relative contraindication to surgery
FEV₁ = 1–1.5 liters; MVV = 35–50% Normal Paco₂; slight hypoxemia; abnormal ECG	Greatly increased operative risk; a contraindication to major elective surgical procedures
FEV₁ <1 liter; MVV <35% Normal Paco₂; mild hypoxemia; normal ECG	Greatly increased operative risk; a contraindication to major elective surgical procedures; probably precludes extensive lung resection
FEV₁ <1 liter; MVV <35% Elevated Paco₂; severe hypoxemia or abnormal EKG	Extremely high operative risk; only mandatory surgery justifiable; probably precludes any pulmonary resection
Restrictive disorders	
VC > 50%; DL > 50% Normal blood gases	Little increased operative risk
VC = 35–50%; DL > 50% Slight hypoxemia on exertion	Some increase in operative risk but not a serious contraindication to surgery, except extensive lung resection
VC < 35%; DL < 50% or frank hypoxemia	Greatly increased operative risk, especially contraindicating extensive lung resection

MVV, maximum voluntary ventilation; VC, vital capacity; DL, diffusing capacity.

TABLE 7. Preoperative Pharmacologic Preparation

Category	Route	Typical Adult Dosage
Beta-agonist		
Isuprel	Nebulized	1/200 dilution 0.5 ml. in 4.5 ml. normal saline 2 to 4 times a day
Isoetharine	Nebulized	0.25% 0.5 ml. in 4.5 ml. normal saline 2 to 4 times a day
Ephedrine	PO	12–24 mg. every 6 hours
Racemic epinephrine	Nebulized	0.5 ml. in 4.5 ml. normal saline every 4 to 6 hours
Beta-selective		
Metaproterenol	Nebulized	5.0% 0.33 ml. in 4.5 ml. normal saline 2 to 4 times a day
Metaproterenol	PO	10–20 mg. 4 times a day
Albuterol	Nebulized	2 (90-μg.) inhalations 2 to 4 times a day
Albuterol	PO	12–24 mg. every 6 hours
Terbutaline	PO	2.5–5.0 mg. 3 times a day
Terbutaline	IM	0.25 mg. every 6 to 8 hours
Theophylline		
Aminophylline	PO	200 mg. 3 to 4 times a day
Aminophylline	IV	load 5.6 mg./kg., then 0.9 mg./kg/hr.
Theophylline	PO	200 mg. 3 to 4 times a day
Oxytriphylline	PO	100–200 mg. 3 to 4 times a day
Diphylline	PO	200 mg. 3 to 4 times a day
Mucolytics and expectorants		
Terpin hydrate elixir	PO	5–15 ml. every 4 to 8 hours
Robitussin	PO	5–15 ml. every 4 to 8 hours
SSKI	PO	10 drops in 50 ml. H_2O 2 times a day
Acetylcysteine	Nebulized	20% 1–3 ml. every 4 to 8 hours
Steroid		
Solu-Cortef	IM	100 mg. every 12 hours for 6 doses, begin night before surgery
Solu-Medrol	IV	25–40 mg. every 6 hours for 6 doses, begin with surgery
Prednisone	PO	40 mg. 4 times a day; begin 2–3 days prior to surgery
Beclomethasone	Inhalation	2 puffs (84 μg.) every 6 hours.

space generally increases with mechanical ventilation; therefore, there is a need for increased minute ventilation to maintain a normal $Paco_2$. All of these changes may lead to postoperative atelectasis, segmental lobar collapse, retained secretions, and pneumonia.

The patient should be encouraged to sit upright as soon as possible. Lung function is clearly improved with early ambulation. This is especially important in the obese and elderly. Early ambulation increases FRC and also reduces the risk of pulmonary embolism. Pulmonary embolism in the postoperative period is a dangerous postoperative complication in these higher risk patients with impaired pulmonary functions. Moreover, care must be taken to prevent aspiration. Careful attention to these preoperative and postoperative details significantly reduces the risks of pulmonary complications.[8,31,33]

RESPIRATORY FAILURE

The adult respiratory distress syndrome (ARDS) has many definitions. Essentially, there is impairment of effective gas ex-change, which is commonly defined in terms of findings on arterial blood gases. Usually there is arterial hypoxemia, a Pao_2 of less than 60, or hypercarbia (i.e., a $Paco_2$ of greater than 50 that is not associated with metabolic alkalosis). The usual presentation includes hypoxemia, a Pao_2 of less than 60, and respiratory alkalosis with a $Paco_2$ of less than 40. Other parameters associated with the respiratory distress syndrome include increased dead space, decreased vital capacity, decreased FRC, and a decrease in inspiratory force that is less than 30 cm. of water (Table 8).[2,21,44]

Respiratory failure has two components: (1) pulmonary parenchymal failure (failure of gas exchange, manifested by hypoxemia), and (2) pulmonary ventilatory failure, manifested by hypercapnia. Both components have a role in the pathogenesis of respiratory insufficiency: (1) difficulty in ventilating and getting air (air hunger), (2) hypoxemia, (3) stiff lungs requiring increasingly high ventilatory pressures, and (4) evidence of infiltration and consolidation by radiographic evaluation.

Normally, there is an approximately 8 per cent shunt within the lung. Factors that contribute to increased shunting are at-

TABLE 8. Indications for Respiratory Support

	Acceptable	PT/Monitor	Intubate
Mechanics			
Respiratory rate (breaths per minute)	12–25	25–35	>35
Vital capacity (ml./kg.)	70–30	30–15	<15
Inspiratory force (cm. H_2O)	100–50	50–25	<25
Parenchymal			
$AaDo_2$	50–200	200–350	>350
Vd/Vt	0.3–0.4	0.4–0.6	>0.6
$Paco_2$ torr	35–45	45–60	>60
Qs/Qt	8–12%	12–20%	>20%
Pao_2 torr	100–75 air		<65 on mask O_2

Adapted from Wilson, R. S., and Pontoppidan, H.: Acute respiratory failure: Diagnostic and therapeutic criteria. Crit. Care Med., 2:293, 1974. Reproduced with permission.

electasis, alveolar edema, abnormalities in hemoglobin, and the closing volumes of the airways.[5,10,40]

The FRC provides a mechanism for avoiding great fluctuations in arterial oxygen and carbon dioxide tensions. With a normal tidal volume, new air is added to the functional residual capacity, creating adequate alveolar ventilation. The normal lung has mismatched ventilation and perfusion. In the upright position, the upper segments are ventilated much better than they are perfused; the lower segments are ventilated less than the upper segments of the lung and have much greater perfusion. In the normal lung, although there are regional differences in ventilation and perfusion throughout, the net effect is a reasonable match of ventilation and perfusion. The pathologic changes of the respiratory distress syndrome include increased capillary permeability, interstitial edema, and congestive atelectasis.[2,16] With the development of interstitial edema, there is impaired gas flow to the fine terminal airways, and the FRC falls. With the reduction of the FRC, there is an increase in pulmonary shunting. As a result, when venous admixture increases, the arterial $Paco_2$ falls.

Awareness of the potential development of the respiratory distress syndrome is a prerequisite for reducing morbidity and mortality.[39,42] Often the chronic nature of pre-existing pulmonary disease is subtle. A history of increased sputum production, chronic cough, wheezing, orthopnea, multiple pulmonary infections, and the number and pack years of smoking is extremely important. Smoking associated with chronic bronchitis or chronic obstructive lung disease is a major factor in determining the risk of postoperative and posttraumatic pulmonary problems. Cessation of smoking for 1 or 2 weeks prior to elective operation is one of the most important factors in managing any patient.[14,15,23,24,32,48]

PATHOPHYSIOLOGY. Whatever the etiology for respiratory distress syndrome, whether it is postsurgical or posttraumatic or related to sepsis, hypovolemic shock, cardiogenic shock, or aspiration, the final common pathway is the same. Physiologically, there are two clinically significant components, that is, an abnormal pattern of gas distribution related to alveolar closure and interstitial edema caused by pulmonary vascular congestion or loss of endothelial integrity of the capillaries.[26,27] There are decreases in both FRC and compliance as well as ventilation-perfusion abnormalities.

Pulmonary dysfunction becomes critical when the arterial oxygen content falls so low that elevations in cardiac output can no longer compensate to deliver sufficient oxygen to maintain aerobic metabolism. Many precipitating causes have been associated with progressive pulmonary insufficiency: fluid overload, pneumonia, shock, thromboembolism, massive blood transfusions, sepsis, peritonitis, prolonged ventilatory therapy with high inspired oxygen concentrations, fat emboli, prolonged cardiopulmonary bypass. Regardless of the precipitating factors, there are four general categories of abnormalities in pulmonary function: (1) hypoventilation, (2) ventilation-perfusion, (3) diffusion defects, and (4) arteriovenous shunts.[1,39,40,42,44]

HYPOVENTILATION. The function of the pulmonary circulation is to expose the cardiac output to ventilation for the purpose of oxygenating hemoglobin and removing carbon dioxide. This gas exchange is less sensitive to variations in total pulmonary blood flow than to inequalities in the distribution of the blood flow as matched to regional alveolar ventilation. The relationship of the oxygen utilized by the body delivered to the periphery is known as the Fick principle:

$$O_2 \text{utilized} = \frac{\text{cardiac output}}{\text{a-}\bar{v}O_2 \text{ difference}}$$

This very simple but important relationship demonstrates the reciprocal behavior of the a-$\bar{v}O_2$ difference and the cardiac output. As cardiac output declines, the amount of oxygen extracted from the hemoglobin must increase if aerobic metabolism is to be maintained.

The total amount of oxygen delivered to the periphery depends on the cardiac output and the total oxygen content of arterial blood.

$$O_2 \text{ delivery periphery} = (O_2 \text{ content}) (\text{cardiac output})$$
$$O_2 \text{ content} = (\text{Hgb}) (O_2 \text{ sat}) (1.34) + (.0031) (Pao_2)$$

It can readily be seen that most of the oxygen is transported by the hemoglobin molecule.

Hypoventilation exists when the volume of alveolar ventilation is reduced to the point at which normal gas exchange cannot occur. It is simply defined as an inability to maintain a normal Pco_2, and this definition is related to the rapid carbon dioxide dissociation that makes it more sensitive to alveolar Pco_2. As alveolar ventilation falls, alveolar Pco_2 rises rapidly, which is reflected in the arterial partial pressure of CO_2 (see Fig. 3). In contrast, the oxygen saturation decreases only gradually with hypoventilation until hypoventilation is quite severe.

Simply enriching the oxygen concentration of the inspired gas limits the hypoxemia of hypoventilation. The converse of this is true as well, in that pure hypoventilation does not cause a dramatic fall in the arterial oxygen partial pressure. The effect of doubling the $Paco_2$ as a consequence of hypoventilation decreases the arterial Po_2 by only 40 mm. Hg. Although the patient is moderately hypoxemic, he is markedly acidotic, and the CO_2 relationship dominates the clinical situation.

Although hypoventilation is by definition alveolar hypoventilation, it can follow a number of factors. In patients who are spontaneously ventilating, depression of the respiratory center by narcotics can cause hypoventilation, neurologic damage to the neuromuscular respiratory axis can cause hypoventilation, and mechanical abnormalities of the chest (e.g., pneumothorax, flail chest, paralyzed diaphragm) can cause mechanical hypoventilation. Muscular fatigue due to chronic disease or malnutrition, myasthenia gravis, or exhaustion can lead to hypoventilation and eventually airway obstruction to airway gas flow that causes hypercarbia. Thus, the etiology of hypoventilation must be sought and corrected. Patients on ventilators can develop hypoventilation due to inappropriate adjustments or to mechanical problems with the gas exchange circuit such that the expected delivery of gases does not occur.

DIFFUSION IMPAIRMENT. Diffusion of oxygen between the alveolus and the pulmonary capillary blood is slower than that of CO_2. Even with increased cardiac output, sufficient transcapillary transit time exists for nearly total equilibration. However, if the blood gas barrier is increased and diffusion is impaired, oxygen equilibration is slowed and pulmonary venous hypoxemia can occur even at normal transit times. This usually occurs in chronic interstitial pulmonary diseases such as diffuse interstitial fibrosis, asbestosis, sarcoidosis, Goodpasture's syndrome, and collagen vascular diseases. Hypoxemia caused by diffusion impairment can be improved by administering higher Fio_2.

ARTERIOVENOUS SHUNTS. This category of causes for arterial oxygen desaturation includes congenital (anatomic) shunts that bypass the lungs, such as atrial or ventricular septal defects with right-to-left shunting or intrapulmonary shunts caused by arteriovenous fistulas. Perfusion of an unventilated portion of lung produces a physiologic shunt and is discussed in the next section on ventilation-perfusion abnormalities. With an anatomic shunt, no matter how high the Fio_2, the arterial Po_2 does not normalize. Physiologic shunting due to ventilation-perfusion abnormalities can be improved by altering the ventilation-perfusion ratio.

VENTILATION-PERFUSION ABNORMALITIES. The major cause of hypoxemia in postoperative patients is physiologic shunting due to ventilation-perfusion mismatching. All lungs have some ventilation-perfusion mismatching due to the regional variation in pulmonary blood flow. Mismatches of ventilation and perfusion occur in the lung as a consequence of atelectasis, alveolar edema, interstitial edema, bronchial obstruction, acidosis, and alveolar collapse.

Variations in regional matching of perfusion and ventilation can occur in three different situations. An area can experience overventilation in comparison with perfusion, a situation that does not necessarily cause any abnormalities if the amount of perfusion to the rest of the lung is normal. An area can be overperfused in relation to the amount of ventilation, which can lead to hypoxemia. When severe or total alveolar hypoventilation occurs, Pco_2 begins to rise. In addition, the ventilation-perfusion matching can be essentially one to one, which leads to normal blood gas values. The first situation causes wasted work of breathing but may not necessarily lead to a change in arterial blood gases. A mismatch of overperfusion to underventilation is the most common clinical problem. Thus, ventilation-perfusion abnormalities cause variable degrees of intrapulmonary physiologic shunting that can be accurately measured by means of the shunt equation (Table 9):

$$Qs/Q_T = \frac{Cc - Ca}{Cc - C\bar{v}} \times 100$$

This is an accurate measurement of the amount of blood traveling from the right heart to the left heart that does not equilibrate with the alveolar gases.

CLOSING VOLUMES. The closing volume is the remaining lung volume at the end of expiration below which alveolar collapse begins to cause "physiologic" shunting. In the normal young individual, this closing volume is well below the functional residual capacity (see Fig. 5). Age alone is associated with

TABLE 9. The Shunt Equation

A. Components of the shunt equation
 1. Constant anatomic shunts (normal 2%)
    Bronchial veins
    Pleural veins
    Thebesian veins
    Abnormal AV connections
 2. Variable intrapulmonary shunts (2 → 6%)
    $\dot{V}/\dot{Q}$ abnormalities (regional and changing)
    Alveolar wall interstitial edema
    RBC/capillary bed transit time
    Atelectasis
    Ventilation abnormalities
B. Shunt equation formula
 1. % intrapulmonary $\rightarrow$ $R \rightarrow L$ shunt $= Qs/Q_T = \dfrac{Cc - Ca}{Cc - C\bar{v}} \times 100$

    Where $Cc = O_2$ content leaving alveolar capillary bed
         $Ca = O_2$ content of arterial bed
         $C\bar{v} = O_2$ content of mixed venous blood

 2. Calculation of O_2 capacity
    $\dfrac{(Hgb) \, (1.34 \text{ cc. } O_2)(\% \text{ saturation}) + (Po_2)(.0031)}{gm. \, Hgb.}$

 3. e.g.,
    $Cc = \dfrac{(15 \text{ gm. Hgb.})(1.34 \text{ cc. } O_2)}{100 \text{ cc. blood gm. Hgb.}} \, (1.00) + (673)(.0031)$
      $= 21.99 \text{ vol.\%}$
    $Ca = (15)(1.34)(.985) + (200)(.0031) = 20.30 \text{ vol.\%}$
    $C\bar{v} = (15)(1.34)(.670) + (35)(.0031) = 13.51 \text{ vol.\%}$
    $\dfrac{Qs}{Q_T} = \dfrac{21.99 - 20.30}{21.99 - 13.50} \times 100 = 19.8\% \text{ shunt}$

C. Derivation of shunt equation
 1. Amount of O_2 in arterial blood = amount of O_2 in blood that has traversed the pulmonary capillaries + the amount of O_2 in shunted blood.
 2. Since the amount of $O_2 = Cc_2 \times \dot{Q}$, then
 3. $Ca \, Q_T = (Cco_2 \cdot Qc) + (C\bar{v} \cdot Qs)$
    Q_T = total blood flow
    Qc = blood flow through pulmonary capillaries
    Qs = blood flow (of mixed venous blood) through shunt
 4. Hence $Qc = Q_T - Qs$ or $Q_T = Qs + Qc$
 5. Therefore,
    $CaQ_T = Cc \, (Q_T - Qs) + C\bar{v} \cdot Qs$
 6. Clearing
    $Qs = \dfrac{Ca - Cc}{C\bar{v} - Cc} \times Q_T$

 If Q_T has been measured, then Qs can be calculated in absolute quantities.

If not, then
    Qs can be calculated as the fraction
    Q_T of the total cardiac output that flows through the shunt.
 7. As before
    a. $\dfrac{Qs}{Q_T} = \dfrac{Cao_2 - Cco_2}{C\bar{v}o_2 - Cco_2}$

    This is the value of the "physiologic shunt," which includes not only absolute anatomic shunts but also a quantity of blood coming from regions with low ventilation-perfusion ratios. The latter is included because the calculated "end-capillary" Po_2 is really a contrived end-capillary Pco_2
    b. When ventilated with 100% O_2
      $Pao_2 = P_B - Paco_2 - P_{H_2O}$ (e.g., 673
                    $= 760 - 40 - 47)$
    where $Paco_2 = (Hgb)(1.34)(1.00) + (.0031)(Pao_2)$

D. Variations on the shunt equation
 1. $\dfrac{Qs}{Q_T} = \dfrac{Cc - Ca}{Cc - C\bar{v}} = \dfrac{Ca - Cc}{C\bar{v}Cc}$

    if $Pao_2 > 150$, % Hgb. desaturation of Pao_2 may be disregarded and simplify the shunt equation to:

 2. $\dfrac{Qs}{Q_T} = \dfrac{(.0031)(Pao_2 - Pao_2)}{(Cao_2 - Cvo_2) + (.0031)(Pao_2 - Pao_2)}$

               or

 3. $\dfrac{Qs}{Q_T} = \dfrac{(.0031)(AaDo_2)}{(a-vo_2 \text{ diff}) + (.0031)(AaDo_2)}$

E. Alveolar-arterial O_2 gradient ($AaDo_2$)
 1. $AaDo_2 = (Pao_2 - Pao_2)$
 2. $Pao_2 = P_B - Paco_2 - P_{H_2O}$ as in equation C-7b
 3. Measure the gradient by ventilating the patient with $FIo_2 = 1.00 \times 20$ minutes and the above assumptions can be made
 4. $AaDo_2$ correlates with Qs/Q_T
 5. If the patient has a Swan-Ganz catheter in place and mixed venous samples are obtained simultaneously with Pao_2, and if the patient is preventilated with 100% O_2, then a specific $AaDo_2 : Qs/Q_T$ graphic relationship can be plotted and used after the Swan-Ganz catheter has been discontinued. This is better than making a-vo_2 diff assumptions unless cardiac outputs are obtained and an appropriate a-vo_2 diff is derived
 6. e.g.,
    $FIo_2 = 1.00$
    $Pao_2 = 200 \quad Pco_2 = 36$
    $AaDo_2 = 760 - 36 - 47 - 200 = 477$
 7. 40–50% shunt = 70% mortality
    >50 % shunt = 90% mortality

a decrease in the elastic properties of the lung, such that although functional residual capacity gradually increases with age, so does the effective closing volume. At some point these lines cross, and at end-expiration portions of alveoli are underventilated so that a physiologic right-to-left shunt occurs and the total oxygen saturation decreases. This is the reason the partial pressure of oxygen in the arterial blood gradually decreases with age. This process is accelerated by smoking and other causes of chronic pulmonary disease, leading to hypoxemia at a younger age. In addition, placing a patient supine, even at a young age, or other mechanical factors such as obesity may lead to an elevation in closing volume and relative hypoxemia.[47,55] Hypoxemia is common postoperatively because of this "closing volume effect."[34,42] The presence of interstitial pulmonary edema accentuates this effect. Applying end-expiratory pressure causes the return of FRC to normal and corrects the closing volume abnormality.[10]

MANAGEMENT OF RESPIRATORY DISTRESS SYNDROME

Awareness of the potential for development of the respiratory distress syndrome should lead to early aggressive treatment prior to the development of respiratory insufficiency. Excellent pulmonary care for postsurgical and injured patients is extremely important.

All postsurgical and traumatically injured patients have decreased vital capacity, decreased total lung capacity, decreased FRC, and a degree of hypoxemia. Therefore, it is important to return the lung volumes to normal as soon as possible and administer oxygen to correct the hypoxemia. These patients should be closely monitored with repeated clinical examinations and frequent blood gas determinations. If the patient has respiratory insufficiency and respiratory failure, a Swan-Ganz catheter should be inserted to monitor cardiac output and a-vO_2 difference.

Patients with respiratory insufficiency in whom sepsis develops present the greatest challenge. Careful sterile technique must be maintained in the management of an endotracheal tube; infiltrates on the chest film or change in the character of secretions dictates acquisition of multiple blood and sputum cultures so that specific organisms can be identified and treated. Narrowing of the a-vO_2 difference occurs early in sepsis at a time when there is normal or only slightly increased cardiac output. If this combination is present, sepsis should be strongly suspected.[2,7,10,28,42,57]

POSITIVE END-EXPIRATORY PRESSURE. Since the development of continuous positive airway pressure therapy for respiratory distress in the newborn, and later positive end-expiratory pressure (PEEP) by Ashbaugh and Petty,[6,7,10,49] this form of therapy has been used in all patients with respiratory insufficiency. It is apparent that the main positive effect of PEEP is an increase in FRC. As indicated earlier, all patients have loss of lung volume and decreased FRC. Therefore, return of FRC to near the pre-injury state is extremely helpful in improving oxygenation, stabilizing the airways, and correcting closing volume abnormalities. PEEP also decreases venous return and may decrease cardiac output.[21,51] Therefore, its use must be monitored by close observation of the patient's lung perfusion and cardiac output. In general, most patients are managed with variations in PEEP and manipulation of the inspired oxygen concentrations so that the PEEP can be kept below 20 cm. H_2O. Today there are few indications for "super" PEEP.[28,53]

COMPLICATIONS OF PEEP. The main complication of PEEP, other than its deleterious effects on cardiac function, is pneumothorax, which may subsequently develop into unrecognized tension pneumothorax. In any patient on PEEP with sudden circulatory collapse tension pneumothorax should be suspected. Although acute collapse is the usual presentation, absent breath sounds in one thorax may be another classic finding of tension pneumothorax. Frequently, there is no time for radiographic confirmation of this diagnosis; the insertion of a large-bore needle decompresses the tension pneumothorax while the surgeon is awaiting the opportunity to insert a chest tube. The presence of an intrathoracic tube does not preclude the possibility of tension pneumothorax, especially in newborns.

WEANING OF PATIENTS FROM PEEP. Patients with respiratory insufficiency are weaned first by a progressive decrease in the FIO_2 with rapidity determined by the PaO_2 to approximately 40 per cent. The mechanical ventilator rate is lowered and adjusted based on the PaCO_2. With intermittent mandatory ventilation, in combination with PEEP and airway pressure support, the ventilatory support rate may be lowered over a matter of hours or days. If the arterial pH remains normal and oxygenation is adequate at a rate below 8, most patients can be weaned from the respirator. Many patients who are being weaned have an increased PaCO_2 in excess of 40 to compensate for the metabolic alkalosis caused by the metabolism of lactic acid during times of decreased perfusion; a pH between 7.36 and 7.4 is within the acceptable range in these patients. During this time, the patient's respiratory mechanics should be measured, and if these fall within an acceptable range for the clinical status and pre-existing pulmonary disease, the patient then can be weaned from the ventilator and extubated (see Table 8).

OXYGEN THERAPY. Oxygen is a drug and therefore has benefits, indications, complications, and dosage schedules. The goal of oxygen therapy is to avoid tissue hypoxia. There are many methods of delivering oxygen, but most patients with acute respiratory insufficiency are intubated, and oxygen is provided through the ventilator and the endotracheal tube.

To avoid oxygen toxicity, the level of inspired oxygen concentration should be lowered to 0.4 or less as soon as possible.[38,54,59] There is high-dose oxygen toxicity as well as low-dose oxygen toxicity. It is clear that a high dosage level is required to produce toxicity when exposure is brief, but low dosage levels of oxygen when exposure is prolonged can also produce oxygen toxicity. At present it appears that the use of 100 per cent oxygen for less than 24 hours is not apt to produce oxygen toxicity. However, patients who receive 100 per cent oxygen for more than 60 hours will probably have a degree of oxygen toxicity, and concentrations of oxygen should be lowered to 40 per cent as soon as possible. This concentration of oxygen can be given for prolonged period without risk of physiologic and pathologic oxygen toxicity in man.

SELECTED REFERENCES

Bates, D. V., Macklem, P. T., and Christie, R. V.: Respiratory Function in Disease: An Introduction to the Integrated Study of the Lung, 2nd ed. Philadelphia, W. B. Saunders Company, 1971.
This is the second edition of an outstanding text that correlates respiratory physiology and pulmonary disease. Basic pulmonary function studies are reviewed, and individual disease processes that alter physiologic function presented. It also contains one of the most complete and updated bibliographies on this subject.

Comroe, J. H., Jr., Forster, R. E., II, Dubois, A. B., Broscoe, W. A., and Carlsen, E.: The Lung: Clinical Physiology and Pulmonary Function Tests, 2nd ed. Chicago, Year Book Medical Publishers, Inc., 1962.
This is a classic text written for medical students and physicians explaining with excellent diagrams and illustrations aspects of pulmonary physiology and presenting the rationale for treatment of acute and chronic disease.

Tisi, G. M.: Pulmonary Physiology in Clinical Medicine, 2nd ed. Baltimore, Williams & Wilkins Company, 1983.
This is the second edition of an outstanding monograph. It is well illustrated and provides an excellent clinical approach to the physiologic interpretation of pulmonary function in health and disease. This edition has been expanded and covers specific clinical situations commonly encountered in both medical and surgical patients.

REFERENCES

1. AHA Cardiopulmonary Council: Manual for Evaluation of Lung Function by Spirometry. Circulation, 65:644A, 1982.
2. Alexander, J. A., and Rodgers, B. M.: Diagnosis and management of pulmonary insufficiency: Symposium on Noncardiac Thoracic Surgery. Surg. Clin. North Am., 60:983, 1980.
3. Ali, M. K., Mountain, C. F., and Miller, J. M.: Regional pulmonary function before and after pneumonectomy using ^{133}xenon. Chest, 68:288, 1975.
4. Ali, M. K., Mountain, C. F., Ewer, M. S., et al: Predicting loss of pulmonary function after pulmonary resection for bronchogenic carcinoma. Chest, 77:337, 1980.
5. Ashbaugh, D. G., Bigelow, D. B., Petty, T. L., and Levine, B. E.: Acute respiratory distress in adults. Lancet, 2:319, 1969.
6. Ashbaugh, D. G., Petty, T. L., and Bigelow, D. B.: Continuous positive-pressure breathing (CPPB) in adult respiratory distress syndrome. J. Thorac. Cardiovasc. Surg., 57:31, 1969.
7. Ashbaugh, D. G., and Petty, T. C.: Positive end-expiratory pressure: Physiology, indications, and contraindications. J. Thorac. Cardiovasc. Surg., 65:165, 1973.
8. Barter, S. J., Cunningham, D. A., Lavender, J. P., Gibellino, F., Connellan, S. J., and Pride, N. B.: Abnormal ventilation scans in middle-aged smokers. Am. Rev. Respir. Dis., 132:148, 1985.
9. Bates, D. V., Macklem, P. T., and Christie, R. V.: Respiratory Function in Disease. An Introduction to the Integrated Study of the Lung, 2nd ed. Philadelphia, W. B. Saunders Company, 1971.
10. Bone, R. C.: Treatment of severe hypoxemia due to the adult respiratory distress syndrome. Arch. Intern. Med., 140:85, 1980.
11. Boushy, S. F., Billing, D. M., North, L. B., and Helgason, A. H.: Clinical course related to preoperative and postoperative pulmonary function in patients with bronchogenic carcinoma. Chest, 59:383, 1971.
12. Boysen, P. G., and Benfield, J. R.: Preoperative pulmonary evaluation and postoperative care. Clin. Challenge Cardiopul. Med., 3(1):1, 1980.
13. Bria, W. F., Kanarek, D. J., and Kazemi, H.: Prediction of postoperative pulmonary function following thoracic operations. J. Thorac. Cardiovasc. Surg., 86:186, 1983.
14. Buczko, G. B., Day, A., Vanderdoelen, J. L., Boucher, R., and Zamel, N.: Effects of cigarette smoking and short-term smoking cessation on airway responsiveness to inhaled methacholine. Am. Rev. Respir. Dis., 129:12, 1984.
15. Buist, A. S., Sexton, G. J., Nagy, J. M., and Ross, B. B.: The effect of smoking cessation and modification on lung function. Am. Rev. Respir. Dis., 114:115, 1976.
16. Comroe, J. H., Jr., Forster, R. E., II, Dubois, A. B., Biscoe, W. A., and Carlsen, E.: The Lung: Clinical Physiology and Pulmonary Function Tests, 2nd ed. Chicago, Year Book Medical Publishers, Inc., 1962.
17. Craig D. B.: Postoperative recovery of pulmonary function. Anesth. Analg., 60:46, 1981.
18. Fahey, P. J., and Hyde, R. W.: "Won't breathe" vs "can't breathe": Detection of depressed ventilatory drive in patients with obstructive pulmonary disease. Chest, 84:21, 1983.
19. Ferguson, M. K., Little, L., Rizzo, L., Popovich, K. J., Glonek, G. F., Leff, A., Manjoney, D., and Little, A. G.: Diffusing capacity predicts morbidity and mortality after pulmonary resection. J. Thorac. Cardiovasc. Surg., 96:894, 1988.
20. Fiser, W. B., Friday, C. D., and Read, R. C.: Changes in arterial oxygenation and pulmonary shunt during thoracotomy with endobronchial anesthesia. J. Thorac. Cardiovasc. Surg., 83:523, 1982.
21. Fulton, R. L., and Jones, C. E.: The cause of post-traumatic pulmonary insufficiency in man. Surg. Gynecol. Obstet., 140:179, 1975.
22. Hammon, J. W., Wolfe, W. G., Moran, J. F., Jones, R. H., and Sabiston, D. C., Jr.: The effect of positive end-expiratory pressure on regional ventilation and perfusion in the normal and injured primate lung. J. Thorac. Cardiovasc. Surg., 72:680, 1976.
23. Hammond, E. C., and Horn, D.: Smoking and death rates: Report on forty-four months of follow-up of 187,783 men. J.A.M.A., 251:2840, 1984.
24. Harman, E., and Lillington, G. A.: Pulmonary risk factors in surgery. Med. Clin. North Am., 63:1289, 1979.
25. Heinemann, H. O., and Goldring, R. M.: Bicarbonate and the regulation of ventilation. Am. J. Med., 57:361, 1974.
26. Hoeppner, V. H., Cooper, D. M., Zamel, N., Bryan, A. C., and Levinson, H.: Relationship between elastic recoil and closing volume in smokers and non-smokers. Am. Rev. Resp. Dis., 109:81, 1974.
27. Hyatt, R. E., and Rodarte, J. R.: Modern medical physiology: "Closing volume": one man's noise—other men's experiment. Mayo Clin. Proc., 50:17, 1975.
28. Kirby, R. R., Downs, J. B., Civetta, J. M., et al.: High level positive end-expiratory pressure (PEEP) in acute respiratory insufficiency. Chest, 67:156, 1975.

29. Lipscombe, D. J., and Pride, N. B.: Ventilation and perfusion scans in the preoperative assessment of bronchial carcinoma. Thorax, 32:720, 1977.
30. Lumb, P. D.: Perioperative Pulmonary Physiology. In Sabiston, D. C., Jr., and Spencer, F. C. (Eds.): Gibbon's Surgery of the Chest, 4th ed. Philadelphia, W. B. Saunders Company, 1983.
31. Matthay, M. A., and Wiener-Kronish, J. P.: Respiratory management after cardiac surgery. Chest, 95:427, 1989.
32. McCarthy, D. S., Craig, D. B., and Cherniack, R. M.: Effect on modifications of the smoking habit on lung function. Am. Rev. Respir. Dis., 114:103, 1976.
33. Menkes, H. A., Beaty, T. H., Cohen, B. H., and Weinmann, G.: Nitrogen washout and mortality. Am. Rev. Respir. Dis., 132:115, 1985.
34. Meyers, J. R., Lembeck, L., O'Kane, H., and Baue, A. E.: Changes in functional residual capacity of the lung after operation. Arch. Surg., 110:576, 1975.
35. Miller, J. I., Grossman, G. D., and Hatcher, C. R.: Pulmonary function criteria for operability and pulmonary resection. Surg. Gynecol. Obstet., 153:893, 1981.
36. Mittman, C.: Assessment of operative risk in thoracic surgery. Am. Rev. Respir. Dis., 84:197, 1961.
37. Mittman, C., and Bruderman, I.: State of the art: Lung cancer—to operate or not. Am. Rev. Respir. Dis., 116:477, 1977.
38. Moran, J. F., Robinson, L. A., Lowe, J. E., and Wolfe, W. G.: Effects of oxygen toxicity on regional ventilation and perfusion in the primate lung. Surgery, 89:575, 1981.
39. Murray, J. F.: The adult respiratory distress syndrome: "May it rest in peace." Am. Rev. Respir. Dis., 111:716, 1975.
40. Murray, J. F.: Mechanisms of acute respiratory failure. Am. Rev. Respir. Dis., 107:115, 1977.
41. Olsen, G. N., Block, A. J., Swenson, E. W., Castle, J. R., and Wyne, J. W.: Pulmonary function evaluation of the lung resection candidate: A prospective study. Am. Rev. Respir. Dis., 111:379, 1975.
42. Peters, R. M.: Lifesaving measures in acute respiratory distress syndrome. Am. J. Surg., 138:368, 1979.
43. Peters, R. M.: Management of surgically treated patients with limited pulmonary reserve. Am. J. Surg., 138:379, 1979.
44. Pontoppidan, H., Geffin, B., and Lowenstein, E.: Acute Respiratory Failure in the Adult. Boston, Little, Brown and Company, 1973.
45. Rams, J. J., Harrison, R. W., Fry, W. A., Moulder, P. V., and Adams, W. E.: Operative pulmonary artery pressure measurements as a guide to postoperative management and prognosis following pneumonectomy. Dis. Chest. 41:85, 1962.
46. Reichel, J.: Assessment of operative risk of pneumonectomy. Chest, 62:570, 1972.
47. Remolina, C., Khan, A. U., Santiago, T. V., and Edelman, N. H.: Positional hypoxemia in unilateral lung disease. N. Engl. J. Med., 304:523, 1981.
48. Shah, D. M., and Powers, S. R.: Prevention of pulmonary complications in high risk patients. Surg. Clin. North Am., 60:1359, 1980.
49. Shelhamer, J. H., Natanson, C., and Parrillo, J. D.: Positive end-expiratory pressure in adults. J.A.M.A., 251:2692, 1984.
50. Smith, P. K., Fuchs, J. C. A., and Sabiston, D. C., Jr.: Surgical management of aortic abdominal aneurysms in patients with severe pulmonary insufficiency. Surg. Gynecol. Obstet., 151:407, 1980.
51. Smith, P. K., Tyson, G. S., Jr., Hammon, J. W., Jr., Olsen, C. O., Hopkins, R. A., Maier, G. W., Sabiston, D. C., Jr., and Rankin, J. S.: Cardiovascular effects of ventilation with positive expiratory airway pressure. Ann. Surg., 195:121, 1982.
52. Smith, T. C., Cook, F. D., DeKornfeld, T. J., and Siebecker, K. L.: Pulmonary function in the immediate postoperative period. J. Thorac. Surg., 39:788, 1960.
53. Tisi, G. M.: Preoperative evaluation of pulmonary function. Am. Rev. Respir. Dis., 119:293, 1979.
54. Tisi, G. M.: Pulmonary Physiology in Clinical Medicine, 2nd ed. Baltimore, Williams & Wilkins, 1983.
55. Tucker, D. H., and Seiker, H. O.: The effects of change in body position on lung volumes and intrapulmonary gas mixing in patients with obesity, heart failure and emphysema. Am. Rev. Respir. Dis., 83:787, 1960.
56. Van Nostrand, D., Kjelsberg, M. O., and Humphrey, E. W.: Presectional evaluation of risk from pneumonectomy. Surg. Gynecol. Obstet., 127:306, 1968.
57. Waxman, K., and Shoemaker, W. C.: Management of postoperative and post-traumatic respiratory failure in the intensive care unit. Surg. Clin. North Am., 60:1413, 1980.
58. West, J. B.: Ventilation/Blood Flow and Gas Exchange, 3rd ed. Philadelphia, F. A. Davis Company, 1977.
59. Wolfe, W. G., Robinson, L. A., Moran, J. F., and Lowe, J. E.: Reversible pulmonary oxygen toxicity in the primate. Ann. Surg., 188:530, 1978.
60. Wolfe, W. G.: Preoperative assessment of pulmonary function: Quantitative evaluation of ventilation and blood-gas exchange. In Sabiston, D. C., Jr., and Spencer, F. C. (Eds.): Gibbon's Surgery of the Chest, 5th ed. Philadelphia, W. B. Saunders Company, 1990.

III _____

BRONCHOSCOPY

Ross M. Ungerleider, M.D.

In 1928, Chevalier Jackson described bronchoscopy as "looking into the living lungs."[11] Major advances in technology since that time have given the bronchoscopist of today not only the opportunity to view the fine details of the endobronchial anatomy but also the capability of diagnosing, understanding, and even treating diseases that were formerly "beyond the scope" of medical science. Bronchoscopy has become so intricately woven into the framework of treating diseases of the chest that it is now no longer possible for anyone to practice in this field of medicine or surgery without attaining some mastery of this procedure.

HISTORICAL ASPECTS

Sensing the obvious desirability of extending the usual limits of physical examination of the chest, Bozzini in 1806 created an endoscopic instrument utilizing a wax candle as a light source. Although he was able to examine the oropharynx, it is doubtful that he saw further than the cricopharyngeal sphincter. The development of Edison's miniature electric lamps lighted the pathway for modern bronchoscopy. In 1897, Gustav Killian (the "father of bronchoscopy") succeeded in removing an aspirated pork bone from the bronchus of a 63-year-old farmer under cocaine anesthesia. The worldwide sensation that this operation created was due not only to the feat itself but even more so to the demonstration that the trachea and bronchial tree could be safely intubated, because up to that time it was thought that these structures were rigid and stiff, precluding safe instrumentation. (It is somewhat ironic that Killian, in 1886, lost his bid to become head surgeon in Frankfurt to Ludwig Rehn, another pioneer who toppled an even more sacred surgical taboo by becoming the first to operate successfully on the heart!) Killian used an external light source and a head mirror for his bronchoscope. In 1898, Algernon Coolidge, Jr., became the first American to remove a foreign body from the endobronchial tree using an open urethroscope, a head mirror, and reflected sunlight.[11] In 1902, Einhorn produced an endoscope with tip illumination; and in 1904, Jackson incorporated suction into the end of a tip-illuminated bronchoscope.[10] The field of bronchoscopy rapidly developed into a science with the creation of better instruments and techniques. At the forefront remained Chevalier Jackson, who founded the Philadelphia School of Bronchoesophagology. This school attracted and trained students from all over the world in this new science and produced all of the leaders in the field. Jackson's monograph *Bronchoesophagology*, first published in 1950,[13] is a timely and experience-laden volume that is still fascinating and educational to read.

Recent developments with fiberoptics[8,10,20] and an interest in early diagnosis of lung cancer led Ikeda to develop a prototype for the flexible bronchofiberscope in 1964,[10] and after several improvements he introduced the first available flexible bronchoscope in 1967.[10] With the introduction of this instrument, bronchoscopy became a procedure that was easily mastered by all physicians, creating an explosion of trained bronchoscopists.

Finally, the development by the English physician, H. H. Hopkins, of the rod-lens optical telescopes, which could be used with rigid tube bronchoscopes, opened magnificent vistas through these instruments. Because many of the obstacles of early bronchoscopy are overcome by better instrumentation, one can only admire its pioneers, who, while literally groping in the dark, saw so much.

MODERN BRONCHOSCOPES

Bronchoscopes are either rigid or flexible. Each type has specific advantages and disadvantages, and the use of each requires specific training.

RIGID BRONCHOSCOPES. These hollow metal tubes are similar to the first bronchoscope developed. The standard Jackson-type adult instrument is 7 mm. in diameter and 40 cm long, but variable sizes are available down to a unit 3 mm. by 20 cm., designed for pediatric use.[4] These instruments usually have illumination at their tips as well as side holes near the tip to facilitate ventilation. They are always inserted transorally, and it obviously takes great skill and gentleness on the part of the surgeon to introduce these tubes safely into the airway. They can be inserted under topical anesthesia if the patient is cooperative, but general anesthesia is recommended for combative or pediatric patients.[20]

The view through these instruments is limited by the size of the lumen and dissipated by the length of the tube. The introduction of specially designed telescopes into the tube enhances the view without substantially reducing the airway. Moreover, these telescopes can be constructed in such a way that the endoscopist can view all major lobar orifices. A major improvement in these telescopes was the Hopkins rod-lens modification,[8] which reversed the air and lens interface in the standard telescope by providing highly polished glass rods in place of air spaces, leaving small "air lenses" in the position formerly occupied by glass. The results of these changes are greatly improved light transmission, a brighter image, and excellent resolution and depth of field.

The primary advantage of the rigid bronchoscope is that it provides a large, controlled airway that is of particular value in patients with excessive secretions or massive hemoptysis. This is the "battle-proven" instrument of choice for removal of foreign bodies.[1,6,13] Endobronchial surgery is also an indication for the rigid tube because it provides a large lumen for insertion of instruments or for control of significant bleeding. The usual indications for rigid, open-tube bronchoscopy are outlined in Table 1.

FLEXIBLE BRONCHOSCOPY. The flexible bronchofiberscope consists of a control section, a flexible insertion tube, and a bending tip[17] (Fig. 1). The control section contains the eyepiece, control lever, and a channel for aspiration or for introduction of solution and instruments. These bronchoscopes range in outside diameter from 1.8 mm. to 6 mm. with inner channels (on available models) ranging from 1.8 mm. to 2.6 mm. These instruments are highly maneuverable and, in conjunction with their smaller size, can reach areas in the endobronchial tree not accessible to their rigid predecessors.[10,22] These instruments are easy to use, are well tolerated by the awake patient, and can be inserted either transorally or transnasally.[1,20] Proponents of the transoral approach usually recommend placement of this bronchoscope through the temporary conduit of a rigid broncho-

TABLE 1. Bronchoscopic
Instruments of Choice

Rigid Tube

    Foreign bodies
    Massive hemoptysis
    Vascular tumors
    Use in small children
    Endobronchial resections

Flexible Instrument

    Mechanical problems of the neck
    Upper lobe and peripheral lesions
    Limited hemoptysis
    During mechanical ventilation
    Pneumonia, for selective cultures

Combination

    Positive cytology with negative
      chest x-ray

From Landa, J. F.: Indications for bronchoscopy. Chest, 73:686, 1978.

TABLE 2. Topical Anesthetics
for Bronchoscopy

Drug	Concentration (%)	Maximum Dose (mg.)
Cocaine	4–10	200
Tetracaine	1–2	80
Lidocaine	4	200

From Perry, L. B.: Topical anesthesia for bronchoscopy. Chest, 73:691, 1978.

scope or soft endotracheal tube.[1,22] This provides the additional safety of a large airway as well as a conduit for rapid removal and reinsertion of the flexible bronchoscope, which is of value in certain diagnostic procedures. This conduit, however, is not necessary and is thought to be undesirable by some practitioners. However, if no conduit is used, the patient should have some form of bite block to prevent damage to the instrument.

The major disadvantage of the flexible instrument is that, unlike the rigid open tube, it is a "closed" system that does not provide an airway, and the relatively small inner channel is considered by many to be incapable of allowing adequate suction when confronted with copious secretions or massive hemoptysis.[22] Some of the newer, extremely small flexible instruments (1.8, 2.3, and 2.7 mm.) do not even have a lumen for suctioning; this places special limitations on their usefulness.

TECHNIQUE AND ANATOMY

Regardless of the type of bronchoscope selected, the patient must be properly prepared for the examination. This usually entails at least 6 to 8 hours of NPO status to prevent aspiration.

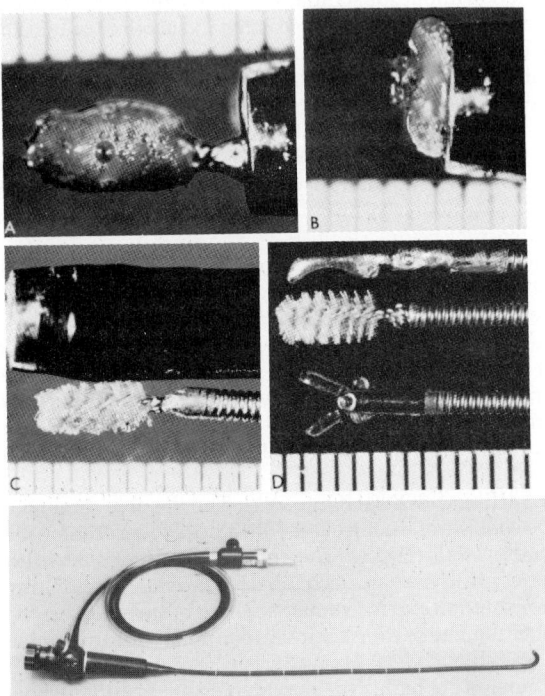

Figure 1. *A,* Brush with specimen. *B,* Brush being pulled into the bronchoscope. *C,* Brush nearly stripped of specimen after being pulled through the bronchoscope. *D,* Curet, brush, and biopsy forceps for use through the flexible bronchoscope. (From Marsh, B. M.: Advances in bronchoscopy. Otolaryngol. Clin. North Am., 2:371, 1978.) *E,* BF-B3 type fiberoptic bronchoscope (Olympus). (From Oho, K., and Ryuta, A.: Practical Fiberoptic Bronchoscopy. New York, Igaku-Shoin, 1980.)

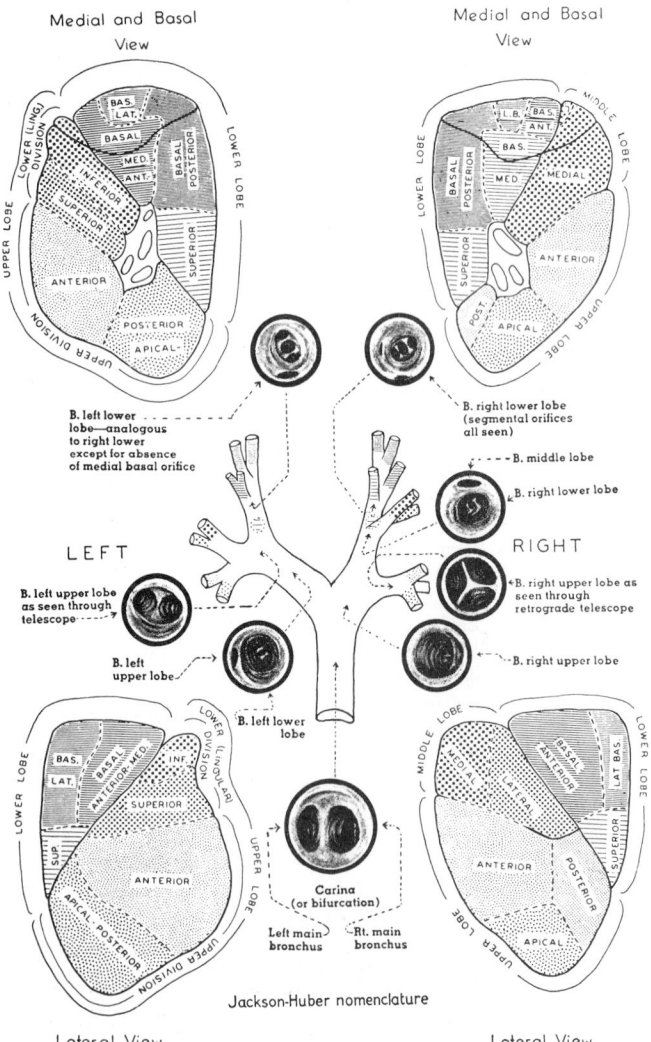

Figure 2. Drawings showing the pulmonary segments with lobar bronchi and segmental branches. The insets depict endoscopic landmarks at various points. The bronchial tree is "upside down" to show the structures in the same position as those observed by the bronchoscopist when the patient is examined in the usual position of dorsal recumbency. (From Jackson, C., and Jackson, C. L.: Bronchoesophagology. Philadelphia, W. B. Saunders Company, 1950.)

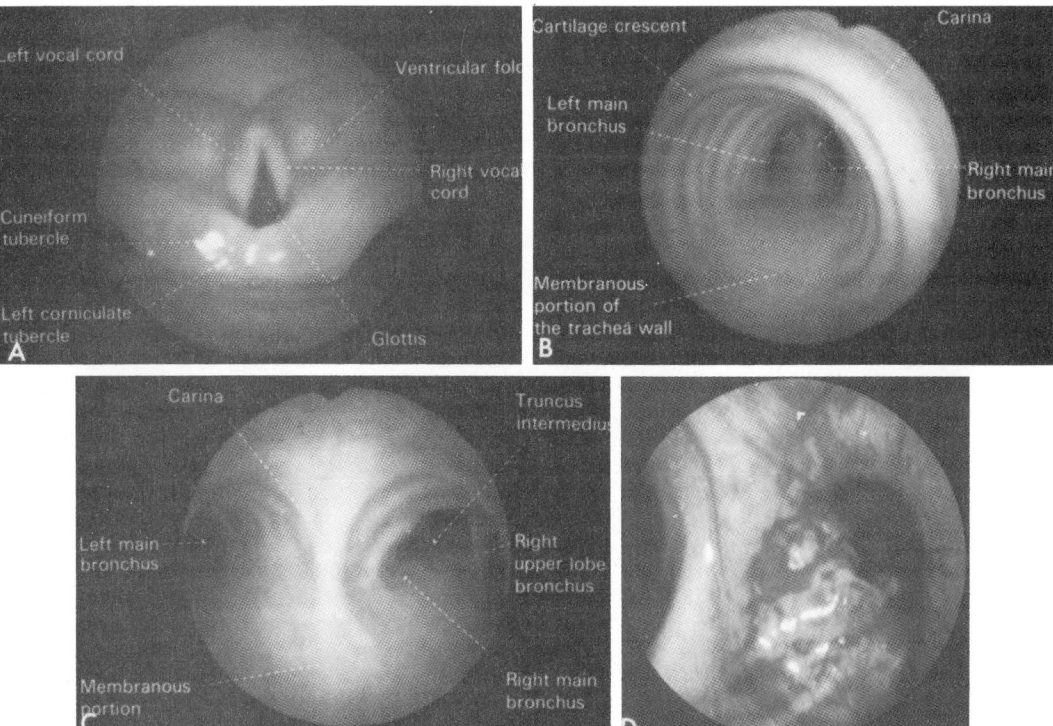

Figure 3. Photographs taken through the bronchoscope at certain important landmarks. *A,* The tip of the bronchoscope is poised above the vocal cords. This is the gateway to the tracheobronchial tree. The epiglottis, which is anterior (top), must be passed to obtain this view. *B,* Upon passing through the cords, the trachea is entered. The posterior membranous portion and the anterior cartilaginous rings are helpful for orientation. The carina can be seen in the distance. *C,* At the level of the carina, the endoscopist has the choice of pursuing the right or left main stem bronchus. The bronchus to the right upper lobe usually arises from the right main stem bronchus just below the carina. The left main stem bronchus is usually quite long and must be negotiated for visualizing its division into left upper and lower lobe branches. (From Oho, K., and Ryuta, A.: Practical Fiberoptic Bronchoscopy. New York, Igaku-Shoin, 1980.) *D,* A large tumor arising just below the carina in the right main stem bronchus. Although not visible on CXR, this lesion can be diagnosed easily by bronchoscopy. (From de Kock, M. A.: Dynamic Bronchoscopy. New York, Springer-Verlag, 1977.)

Adequate premedication is desirable to allay anxiety, dry secretions, and provide some mild analgesia. If the examination is to be performed under topical anesthesia, the choice of anesthetic becomes the primary responsibility of the endoscopist. The usual topical agents are cocaine, lidocaine, and tetracaine (Pontocaine). Tetracaine is also available in a convenient pressurized can as a 2 per cent solution (Cetacaine). Cocaine has the advantages of vasoconstriction (for nasal insertion) and a longer lasting effect. Lidocaine without epinephrine is shorter acting, and its lack of vasoconstriction allows more accurate assessment of mucosal color patterns. Whichever anesthetic is chosen, it is imperative that the bronchoscopist use only premeasured amounts and be acutely aware of each patient's toxic dose limit, because serious or even fatal reactions have occurred from the injudicious use of topical agents.[1] The usual maximal dose limits are listed in Table 2. The nasopharynx (for nasal insertion of the flexible instruments) and oropharynx should be anesthetized systemically. It is especially important to obtain adequate anesthesia of the vocal cords if intubation is to proceed without discomfort, and this is often done most easily through the bronchoscope under direct visualization prior to insertion.[20] The trachea and bronchial tree must also be anesthetized, by means of one of many available techniques. Transtracheal instillation of the anesthetic is effective but should probably be avoided in patients undergoing examination for location of the site of hemoptysis. During the procedure, additional amounts of the agent can be given through the bronchoscope, but care must always be taken not to exceed the safe dose for the agent used.

The technique of examination should follow a fairly routine system so that all parts of the endobronchial anatomy are consistently observed. It is wise to examine the area of disease first so that information will be obtained even if the procedure needs to be terminated before its completion. Excellent descriptions of a routine bronchoscopic examination can be found in the litera-

ture.[10,17,20] It should include evaluation of the vocal cords (for movement on phonation and for lesions), the trachea (mucosal pattern, masses, or evidence of compression), the carina (which should appear sharp and move freely with respiration), and both main stem bronchi and all of their lobar orifices (which should be free of masses, foreign bodies, compression, inflammation, bleeding, or excessive secretions).

An adequate examination mandates familiarity with endobronchial anatomy. The ability to translate bronchoscopic findings into reliable and understandable descriptions of the disease process requires a standard nomenclature. This was first provided by Jackson and Huber in 1943[12] and has been expanded in the era of flexible bronchofibroscopy.[10,17] It is important to understand the relationship and bronchoscopic appearance of the major lobar and segmental divisions (Fig. 2). Color photographs of exceptional quality abound in the literature[4,17] (Fig. 3). Despite the many atlases available, nothing can replace the experience of actually performing the procedure (or observing it through a teaching attachment), and the student is urged to view at least one examination from start to finish before embarking on a medical career.

INDICATIONS, USES, AND COMPLICATIONS

The indications for bronchoscopy are listed in Table 3. This list is by no means complete, because the value of bronchoscopy in diagnosing and treating pulmonary disease is growing rapidly. Still timely today is Jackson's 1915 statement: "In case of doubt as to whether bronchoscopy should be done or not, bronchoscopy should always be done."

Diagnostic Applications

NEOPLASMS. Perhaps the greatest contribution of bronchoscopy has been its utilization as a device in the early diag-

TABLE 3. Indications for Bronchoscopy

Diagnostic Indications

Cough
Hemoptysis
Wheeze
Atelectasis
Unresolved pneumonia
Positive cytology
Abnormal chest film findings
Diffuse lung disease
Recurrent nerve paralysis
Diaphragmatic paralysis
Selective bronchography
Acute inhalation injury
Immediately after intubation
During mechanical ventilation
Before extubation
After extubation
Assess local recurrence
Exclude foreign body
When in doubt

Therapeutic Indications

Foreign bodies
Accumulated secretions
Atelectasis
Aspiration
Lung abscess
Laser therapy
Facilitate intubation
Phototherapy

Preoperative Evaluation

Exclude multiple primary tumors
Metastases
Bronchiectasis (with bronchography)
Assess resectability

After Landa, J. F.: Indications for bronchoscopy. Chest, 73:690, 1978.

viewing range of the rigid bronchoscope that are easily uncovered in the extended reach of the bronchofiberscope. This experience has been shared by others.[6,22] Of equal importance are a number of devices developed for insertion through the flexible bronchoscope to obtain specimens from peripheral lesions (Fig. 1). It is critical that the bronchoscopist pay close attention to the details of handling the specimens obtained with these various devices,[14] because the procedure is futile if the skillfully obtained washing, brushing, or biopsy specimen is uninterpretable by the pathologist. Likewise, when brushing a lesion, it is important to remove the bronchoscope and brush as a unit, rather than withdrawing the brush through the channel in the bronchoscope. The latter practice may remove all diagnostic material from the brush (Fig. 1) and contaminate the channel for subsequent maneuvers.[16] If multiple brushings are to be performed, it is especially practical to insert the flexible scope through the conduit of an endotracheal tube as described earlier. If a radiologically demonstrable lesion is not visible through the bronchoscope, a brush (Fig. 5) or biopsy forceps can often be guided to the lesion under fluoroscopic control; yields as high as 97 per cent in the diagnosis of lung cancer with these techniques have been reported.[14] A good cytologist, working with a properly prepared specimen, can diagnose lung cancer from a single recovered cancer cell.[14] Transbronchial biopsy, a technique of pushing the forceps through the bronchial wall to obtain biopsy specimens of parenchymal lesions, is also quite useful if properly performed.[1] The examination of bronchial brush and washing cytology, combined with sputum cytology, transthoracic needle aspiration, and bronchoscopic forceps biopsy should allow preoperative diagnosis of 95 per cent of lung cancers.[15] In some patients, sputum cytology may provide the diagnosis of cancer when no lesion is evident on the chest radiograph. Bronchoscopy in these patients can often allow detection of very early cancers in the oropharynx or bronchial mucosa that might otherwise never be discovered until much later in their course.[1] Washings of selective bronchial segments can also be obtained to help isolate the origin of positive cytology.

Once the diagnosis of cancer is made, bronchoscopy is an essential procedure in the preoperative assessment of the resectability of the tumor, signs such as carinal or main stem bronchial involvement, vocal cord paralysis, bilateral lesions, and tumor location in relation to patient pulmonary function or tumor cell type (i.e., small cell) suggesting unresectable disease. More recently, several reports have appeared that document the value of transcarinal needle aspiration in the staging of bronchogenic carcinoma. These techniques entail aspiration of material from subcarinal lymph nodes by transbronchial insertion of an 18- or 21-gauge needle at the bifurcation of the main stem bronchi.

nosis of lung masses. Factors instrumental in this achievement include the advent of fiberoptic bronchoscopy and better technological procedures in acquiring and interpreting specimens. Ikeda found that the rigid bronchoscope was capable of detecting only 30 to 40 per cent of the tumors visible with his flexible instrument.[10] The reason for this is easily discerned in Figure 4, which demonstrates the large number of tumors outside the

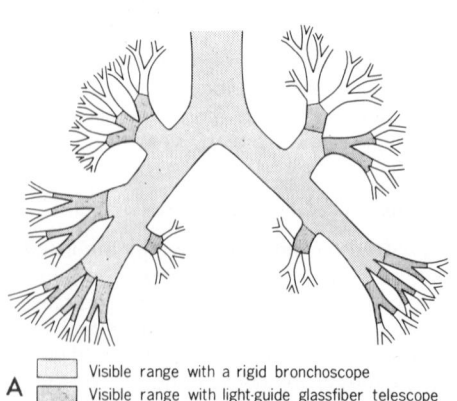
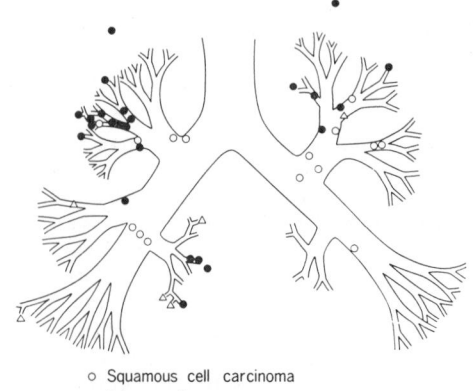

A — Visible range with a rigid bronchoscope
— Visible range with light-guide glassfiber telescope

B — ○ Squamous cell carcinoma
● Adenocarcinoma
△ Undifferentiated carcinoma

Figure 4. A, This illustration demonstrates the extended viewing range afforded by the flexible versus the rigid bronchoscope. B, The practical advantages of the flexible bronchoscope are easily appreciated when one is considering the location of 48 resected tumors less than 3 cm. in diameter. Many of these potentially curable lesions would not have been visualized with the rigid bronchoscope; thus their diagnosis is less likely. (From Ikeda, S.: Atlas of Flexible Bronchofiberoscopy. Baltimore, University Park Press, 1974.)

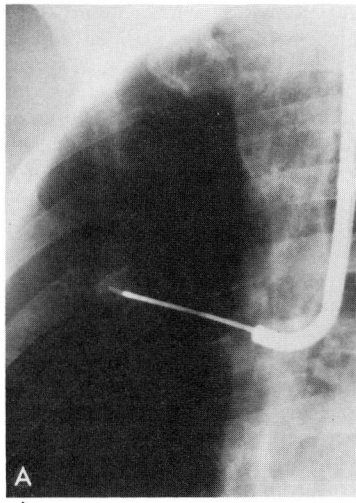
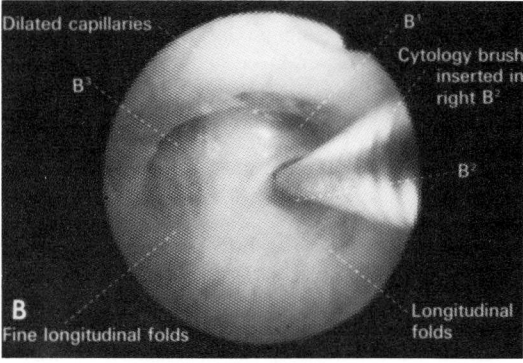
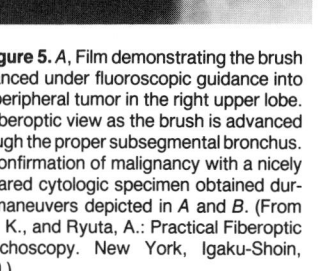
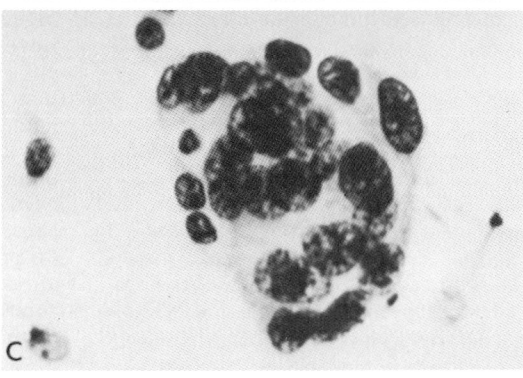

Figure 5. *A*, Film demonstrating the brush advanced under fluoroscopic guidance into the peripheral tumor in the right upper lobe. *B*, Fiberoptic view as the brush is advanced through the proper subsegmental bronchus. *C*, Confirmation of malignancy with a nicely prepared cytologic specimen obtained during maneuvers depicted in *A* and *B*. (From Oho, K., and Ryuta, A.: Practical Fiberoptic Bronchoscopy. New York, Igaku-Shoin, 1980.)

This can be safely performed through a flexible bronchoscope[24] and has been especially helpful in patients with subcarinal adenopathy (by CT scan), or in patients with confirmed endobronchial lesions or abnormal appearing carina at the time of bronchoscopy. Positive cytology from this maneuver contraindicates resection of a pulmonary tumor, and in as many as 69% of patients with documented cancer, it may provide the only indication of nonresectability.

HEMOPTYSIS. Bleeding from the endobronchial tree can be attributed to a number of causes, including tumors, chronic infection (e.g., tuberculosis), bronchiectasis, pulmonary infarction, mitral stenosis, pneumonia, and foreign body aspiration. If bleeding is mild or moderate (less than 600 ml. in 24 to 48 hours),[1] the flexible bronchoscope is valuable in identifying both the cause and the site of the bleeding. Most practitioners prefer the rigid endoscope for control of more massive hemoptysis because of its large airway and increased suctioning potential. However, proponents of the flexible scope in these patients claim better ability to diagnose more peripheral etiologic factors with no sacrifice in safety due to the ability to wedge the flexible bronchoscope in the diseased region, which thereby produces tamponade.[17]

OTHER DIAGNOSTIC USES. Bronchoscopy has proved a useful modality in the diagnosis of etiologic agents in pulmonary infections and diffuse interstitial pneumonitis. The ease and rapidity of flexible bronchoscopy have firmly established its use in emergency departments for the evaluation of smoke inhalation or acute airway obstruction, in outpatient clinics for the analysis of a variety of chronic pulmonary complaints, and in radiology departments for the performance of bronchography.

Therapeutic Applications

FOREIGN BODY REMOVAL. Since Killian's first successful application of bronchoscopy, the removal of foreign bodies by means of this translaryngeal approach has provided therapeutic benefit for literally thousands of patients.[1] The teachings of Jackson[13] elevated this technique to a delicate science, and his meticulous analysis of the mechanical problems related to foreign bodies and methodical approach to their extraction leave

little room for improvement. A large number of patients with aspirated foreign bodies cannot give a history (i.e., small children or comatose patients); and if the foreign body is not radiopaque, diagnosis may be made only with the bronchoscope. Presentation of coughing, wheezing, hemoptysis, or a chest film showing either atelectasis or hyperlucency of a portion of the lung may be reason enough to undertake bronchoscopy. Foreign body aspiration is usually not an emergency, and ample time can be allowed to prepare for extraction. Most practitioners prefer the rigid bronchoscope for this procedure and utilize a variety of specially designed forceps and grasping instruments.[1,13] Because it is easy to injure the bronchial anatomy during removal of a foreign body, a recommended practice is to obtain a duplicate of the aspirated object and become adept at grasping it in the safest manner (and selecting the most appropriate instrument) prior to attempting removal of the actual foreign body from the patient's airway. With skill and care, almost all foreign bodies can be removed in this manner. For foreign bodies out of range of the rigid bronchoscope, a number of instruments are available for use with the flexible scope, and foreign body removal can be accomplished with this instrument.[1,17]

ATELECTASIS. Whether atelectasis occurs as a postoperative complication or as part of the presentation of a pulmonary infection, it is critical to re-expand the atelectatic lung. Although this usually can be accomplished with good pulmonary toilet and endotracheal catheter suctioning, sometimes the lung is refractory to these conventional treatments. Many authorities report excellent success with bronchoscopically directed endotracheal suctioning in these patients. The advantages of this technique are its accuracy in effecting suction to specific regions of the lung under direct vision and its simplicity of performance at the bedside. The disadvantages are that the flexible bronchoscope may have inadequate suction capability for copious thick secretions, and the instrument's expense and relative fragility should prohibit its misuse as simply a "suction catheter." However, for properly selected patients, this can be a highly effective method of treating a difficult problem. A specially designed balloon-cuffed bronchoscope is also available to reinflate persistently collapsed segments.

OTHER THERAPEUTIC APPLICATIONS. The broncho-scope can provide a channel for endobronchial surgery. It is now recommended by most operators experienced in the use of endobronchial laser therapy that this technology be applied through rigid bronchoscopes to enhance efficiency and to improve safety. Proper application of these methods may provide a "cure" for "nonmalignant conditions" (i.e., fistulas or areas of stenosis) and significant palliation for patients with otherwise inoperable malignancies.[2]

Bronchoscopy is a valuable procedure in operating rooms and intensive care units for facilitating endotracheal intubation in difficult patients—here the bronchoscope is used as a visually guided stylet over which an endotracheal tube can be advanced into the proper position. In the same manner, the bronchoscope can be used to verify proper placement of an endotracheal tube above the carina.

Pediatric Bronchoscopy

The advanced technology of smaller flexible bronchoscopes and the Hopkins rod-lens telescopes for use with open-tube bronchoscopes have opened new vistas in the practice of pediatric endoscopy.[8] Because the tiny airway of small children and infants is susceptible to subglottic edema that could cause fatal obstruction to ventilation, selection of the proper-sized instrument and great gentleness and skill in performance of the procedure are imperative. In recent years, advances in the technology of flexible instruments have increased their popularity among specialists in pediatric endoscopy. Because they are easier to use than their rigid counterparts, flexible bronchoscopes may have a valuable role in screening patients with symptoms suggestive of foreign body aspiration to determine whether examination with a rigid instrument is warranted.[27,29] (These same authors agree that once its presence is confirmed, foreign body extraction in children should be attempted only through rigid endoscopes.) The major disadvantage of flexible instruments for the pediatric population is that they do not provide any form of airway; and despite their small size, they encroach upon a significant portion of the infant's own airway. Moreover, the view they afford is no better than that achieved with the rigid units that have Hopkins telescopes. Nevertheless, they can be quickly and safely inserted through small endotracheal tubes[26,28,30] and can be extremely useful in examining the airways of intubated patients within an intensive care unit without necessitating removal of the endotracheal tube or transfer of the critically ill young child to an operating room. When used in this manner, flexible instrumentation expands the potential application of bronchoscopy to the pediatric population.

Since the last issue of this textbook, several excellent articles have appeared outlining the indications for bronchoscopy in children.[26,30] With the advent of safer and smaller flexible instruments, indications parallel those outlined for adults, and bronchoscopy should be a frequently considered diagnostic and therapeutic modality. The majority of foreign bodies are extracted from the pediatric population.[1,8,13] Bronchoscopy has also been used in the diagnosis and preoperative respiratory stabilization of patients who have esophageal atresia with tracheoesophageal fistula[5] and in the localization of isolated tracheoesophageal fistulae to help in determining whether they can be better approached through a thoracic or a cervical incision. Most procedures should be performed in a controlled setting such as an operating room with the availability of general anesthesia.

Complications

When performed by properly trained individuals, bronchoscopy is an extraordinarily safe procedure. In 24,521 flexible bronchoscopic procedures,[3] the rate of minor and major complications was 0.2 per cent and 0.08 per cent, respectively. Mortality was 0.01 per cent. Experience with 1095 procedures in pediatric patients[26] provided equally excellent results with only four major complications (0.4 per cent) and no mortality. Most complications are related to premedication or to topical anesthesia and not to the procedure itself. However, a variety of other problems have been reported, including pneumothorax, bronchospasm, hemorrhage, bronchial perforation, subglottic edema, infections, arrhythmias, and, rarely, cardiopulmonary arrest. Because many of these are sequelae of biopsy procedures, prudence is advised during any bronchoscopic maneuver, and "exploratory thoracotomy" may be safer than "injudicious biopsy."[20] Meticulous cleaning of the bronchofiberscope between uses is mandatory because cases of endoscopy-related pneumonias have been suggested.[18] Even with adequate sterilization, bronchoscopy may impair mucociliary clearance, thus predisposing the patient to postprocedure infection.[18] It is controversial whether bronchoscopy causes arterial hypoxemia,[1] but supplemental oxygen for patients with a resting Pao_2 less than 70 torr is probably advisable. Some have advocated insufflating O_2 through the instrumentation channel during the procedure in these patients. There are few contraindications to bronchoscopy, and it is often more helpful than deleterious to even critically ill patients. Most agree, however, that rigid bronchoscopy is best avoided in the presence of cervical spine injury (to prevent hyperextension of the neck) and in patients with aneurysms of the thoracic aorta. Despite some reports to the contrary, flexible bronchoscopy is probably best avoided in patients with massive hemoptysis[22] or airway problems.

THE FUTURE

In 1928, Chevalier Jackson addressed the Boston Surgical Society on "Bronchoscopy: Past, Present and Future."[11] Now, 57 years later, the future continues to expand the uses of bronchoscopy. Students of multiple disciplines are acquiring competence with progressively newer instruments, and training in bronchoscopic techniques is required of those interested in treating diseases of the chest.[1,22] The bronchoscope is proving to be a valuable research instrument for the creation of animal models of lung cancer.[9,17] With this model (which employs endobronchial injections of the selected carcinogen through the bronchoscope), new ways of recognizing and treating lung cancer can be evaluated. Methods of achieving tumor fluorescence by either inhaled or injected[9] substances have been evaluated and show exciting promise as a way of easily recognizing early endobronchial lesions. In one study,[9] experimentally induced cancers were eradicated (using an argon laser) through the bronchoscope. More recent clinical experience with bronchoscopic phototherapy with hematoporphyrin derivative, though not yet approved by the Food and Drug Administration, shows exceptional promise for the local treatment of endobronchial lesions.[5]

As new methods of medical technology become available, the bronchoscope promises to become an instrument with applications limited only by the imagination.

SELECTED REFERENCES

Anderson, H. A., and Faber, L. P. (Eds.): Diagnostic and therapeutic applications of the bronchoscope. Chest, 73 (No. 5), May 1978.
This supplement to Chest is devoted entirely to bronchoscopy. It features several articles by well-known experts discussing a variety of topics. It provides an excellent overview of the various applications of bronchoscopy.

Ikeda, S.: Atlas of Flexible Bronchofiberscopy. Baltimore, University Park Press, 1974.
As the classic compilation of Ikeda's work that led to the development of the bronchofiberscope, this atlas is usually recommended by all experts in the field. This work not only contains a fine discussion of the principles of fiberoptics but also shows how these principles can enable visualization to fifth-order bronchi. An exceptional work both for its historic value and its value as a thorough atlas.

Jackson, C., and Jackson, C. L.: Bronchoesophagology. Philadelphia, W. B. Saunders Company, 1950.

Still a classic, this monograph by the "dean of American bronchoscopy" and his son is filled with wisdom regarding the presentation and treatment of foreign body aspiration. In addition, the work covers the experience of the Jackson Clinic with a variety of endoscopic procedures. Although it was written before the advent of fiberoptic technology, it remains an indispensable part of any education in the field of bronchoscopy.

Johnson, W. W., and Frable, W. J.: Diagnostic Respiratory Cytopathology. New York, Masson Publishing USA, Inc., 1979.

Although this superb monograph does not pertain to bronchoscopy per se, it describes the science that has enabled bronchoscopy to become such an effective diagnostic instrument — cytology. The authors, noted experts in this field, discuss the diagnosis of pulmonary disease from the material provided by the bronchoscopist. It is important for anyone who obtains bronchoscopic specimens to learn how to maximize the ability to prepare diagnostic material and how to recognize those diagnoses. This is probably the leading work toward accomplishing these goals.

Oho, K., and Ryuta, A.: Practical Fiberoptic Bronchoscopy. New York, Igaku-Shoin, 1980.

This magnificently photographed atlas covers the entire spectrum of bronchofibroscopy. Written by zealous proponents of the fiberoptic bronchoscope, it describes the use of this instrument for diagnosis and treatment of a broad range of problems and provides the reader with a true sense of the versatility of this instrument.

Sackner, M. A.: Bronchofiberoscopy. Am. Rev. Respir. Dis., 111:62, 1975.

This "state of the art" paper is a comprehensive review of the techniques of rigid and flexible bronchoscopy. The author provides a fair comparison of the two methods and discusses the various applications of each instrument.

Wood, R. E.: Medical progress. Endoscopy of the airway in infants and children. J. Pediatr., 112:1, 1988.

This article updates the current approach to bronchoscopy in infants and small children. Indications for use of the flexible and rigid instruments are provided as well as examples of the types of diagnostic and therapeutic uses for these instruments. The article summarizes the experience that this author has obtained in over 1000 bronchoscopic procedures in infants and children and provides the reader with a current understanding of the role that these procedures now have for this patient population.

REFERENCES

1. Anderson, H. A., and Faber, L. P. (Eds.): Diagnostic and therapeutic applications of the bronchoscope. Chest, 73, May 1978.
2. Cavaliere, S., Foccoli, P., and Farina, P. L.: Nd: YAG laser bronchoscopy. A five-year experience with 1,396 applications in 1,000 patients. Chest, 94:15, 1988.
3. Credle, W. F., Smiddy, J. F., and Elliott, R. C.: Complications of fiberoptic bronchoscopy. Am. Rev. Respir. Dis., 109:67, 1974.
4. de Kock, M. A.: Dynamic Bronchoscopy. New York, Springer-Verlag, 1977.
5. Edell, E. S.: Bronchoscopic phototherapy with hematoporphyrin derivative for treatment of localized bronchogenic carcinoma: A 5-year experience. Mayo Clin. Proc., 62:8, January 1987.
6. Faber, L. P., Monson, D. O., Amato, J. J., and Jensik, R. J.: Flexible fiberoptic bronchoscopy. Ann. Thorac. Surg., 16:163, 1973.
7. Filston, H. C., Rankin, J. S., and Grimm, J. K.: Esophageal atresia. Prognostic factors and contribution of preoperative telescopic endoscopy. Ann. Surg., 199:532, 1984.
8. Gans, S. L.: Pediatric Endoscopy. New York, Grune & Stratton, 1983.
9. Hayata Y., Kato, H., Konaka, C., Hayashi, N., Tahara, M., Saito, T., and Ono, J.: Fiberoptic bronchoscopic photoradiation in experimentally induced canine lung cancer. Cancer, 51:50, 1983.
10. Ikeda, S.: Atlas of Flexible Bronchoscopy. Baltimore, University Park Press, 1974.
11. Jackson, C.: Bronchoscopy: Past, present and future. N. Engl. J. Med., 199:759, 1928.
12. Jackson, C. L., and Huber, J. F.: Correlated applied anatomy of the bronchial tree and lungs with a system of nomenclature. Dis. Chest, 9:319, 1943.
13. Jackson, C., and Jackson, C. L.: Bronchoesophagology. Philadelphia, W. B. Saunders Company, 1950.
14. Johnston, W. W., and Frable, W. J.: The cytopathology of the respiratory tract. Am. J. Pathol., 84:372, 1976.
15. Landa, J. F.: Indications for bronchoscopy. Chest, 73:686, 1978.
16. Marsh, B. M.: Advances in bronchoscopy. Otolaryngol. Clin. North Am., 2:371, 1978.
17. Oho, K., and Ryuta, A.: Practical Fiberoptic Bronchoscopy. New York, Igaku-Shoin, 1980.
18. Pereira, W., Jr., Kovnat, D. M., and Snider, G. L.: A prospective cooperative study of complications following flexible fiberoptic bronchoscopy. Chest, 73:813, 1978.
19. Perry, L. B.: Topical anesthesia for bronchoscopy. Chest, 73:691, 1978.
20. Sackner, M. A.: Bronchofiberscopy. Am. Rev. Respir. Dis., 111:62, 1975.
21. Shure, D., and Fedullo, P. F.: The role of transcarinal needle aspiration in the staging of bronchogenic carcinoma. Chest, 86:693, 1984.
22. Taylor, F. H., Evangelist, F. A., and Barham, B. F.: The flexible fiberoptic bronchoscope: Diagnostic tool or medical toy? Ann. Thorac. Surg., 29:546, 1979.
23. Wang, K. P.: Flexible transbronchial needle aspiration biopsy for histologic specimens. Chest, 88:860, December 1985.
24. Wang, K. P., Brower, R., Haponik, E. F., and Siegelman, S.: Flexible transbronchial needle aspiration for staging of bronchogenic carcinoma. Chest, 84:571, 1983.
25. Wolfe, W. G., Cole, P. H., and Sabiston, D. C., Jr.: Experimental and clinical use of the YAG laser in the management of pulmonary neoplasms. Ann. Surg., 199:526, 1984.
26. Wood, R. E.: Splelunking in the pediatric airways: Explorations with the flexible fiberoptic bronchoscope. Pediatr. Clin. North Am., 31:785, 1984.
27. Wood, R. E., and Gauderer, M. W. L.: Flexible fiberoptic bronchoscopy in the management of tracheobronchial foreign bodies in children: The value of a combined approach with open tube bronchoscopy. J. Pediatr. Surg., 19:693, December 1984.
28. Wood, R. E.: Clinical application of ultrathin flexible bronchoscopes. Pediatr. Pulmonol., 1:244, 1985.
29. Wood, R. E.: The diagnostic effectiveness of the flexible bronchoscope in children. Pediatr. Pulmonol., 1:188, 1985.
30. Wood, R. E., and Postma, D.: Endoscopy of the airway in infants and children. J. Pediatr., 112:1, 1988.
31. Zollner, F.: Historical vignette. Gustave Killian: Father of bronchoscopy. Arch. Otolaryngol., 82:656, 1965.

IV

DIAGNOSTIC THORACOSCOPY

James W. Mackenzie, M.D.

Thoracoscopy is the examination of the pleural cavity with an endoscope. As a diagnostic procedure, its main use is in patients with pleural disease in whom simpler methods have not yielded a diagnosis. The safety of the procedure and the highly accurate results obtained suggest that one should consider thoracoscopy before resorting to diagnostic thoracotomy in all patients with pleural disease.

Historical Aspects

Hans Jacobaeus was the originator of thoracoscopy in about 1910.[12-14] He emphasized thoracoscopy as a therapeutic procedure to divide pleural adhesions during the era when induced pneumothorax was used for the control of tuberculosis. Diagnostic thoracoscopy continued to be largely ignored, even though there were reports in English that appeared to make a strong case for its selective use.[5,8,9] Delay in the acceptance of diagnostic thoracoscopy was caused by the mistaken impression that limited thoracotomy usually provided better evaluation of the pleural cavity and by fear of empyema. The reports of Sattler in 1961, Bergqvist and Nordenstam in 1966, DeCamp and associates in 1966 and 1973, and those of others stimulated interest in diagnostic thoracoscopy in the English-speaking world.[16,20] Although these investigators still favored the two-trocar system originated by Jacobaeus, their reports emphasized the safety and diagnostic accuracy of the technique. More recently, attention has focused on the use of a single instrument, such as a fiberoptic mediastinoscope, a rigid bronchoscope, a flexible bronchoscope, or specially designed thoracoscopes.[2,4,7,10,11,14,20] Miniaturized endoscopes have now been developed, as have specialized endoscopes particularly well-suited for children.[1,19]

Anatomic and Physiologic Considerations

The procedure may be performed under either general, regional, or local anesthesia.[6,14,18] If local or regional anesthesia is used, pre-existing pleural adhesions often prevent complete collapse of the lung and respiratory distress is not likely.[18] Careful closed techniques usually limit the size of the pneumothorax. Moreover, it is possible to re-expand the lungs at the completion of the procedure by asking the patient to perform the Valsalva maneuver or, preferably, by insertion of an intercostal tube. Nevertheless, general anesthesia is preferred, usually with endotracheal intubation, because it is at least as safe as local anesthesia and certainly is more acceptable to patients. Extensive inspection of the pleural cavity and the mediastinal surfaces may produce coughing with local anesthesia, limiting the effectiveness of the procedure. Ideal conditions for this study are provided by selective ventilation of the dependent lung. As with any anesthetic technique, care should be taken not to insufflate air into the pleural cavity, as gas emboli may result.

Surgeons accustomed to operating in the chest have little difficulty recognizing the normal structures. This procedure can be performed safely in almost all patients when the amount of pneumothorax is controlled by endotracheal intubation. If there is concern regarding the respiratory status of the patient, insertion of a cannula for sampling arterial blood gases is probably the best approach, although end-tidal carbon dioxide and transcutaneous oxygen measurements may suffice.

A hyperemic pleural reaction is highly suggestive of tuberculosis, as are the small tubercles that vary in size from 1 mm. to 4 or 5 mm. in diameter. Metastatic disease involving the pleura may be mistaken for miliary tuberculosis, but metastatic lesions are usually larger.

Indications and Contraindications

The clearest indication for diagnostic thoracoscopy is in the study of patients with pleural disease in whom simpler procedures have not provided a diagnosis. Such patients have usually undergone prior study of the pleural fluid, blind needle biopsy of the pleura, and bronchoscopy. Some of these patients have had mediastinoscopy as well.

There are other, less clear-cut indications for diagnostic thoracoscopy. It may be useful in the evaluation of patients with known bronchogenic carcinoma, if there is suspected chest wall involvement.[17] The many other uses of thoracoscopy include biopsy of discrete pulmonary lesions or infiltrates, evaluation of mediastinal masses, and as a method of obtaining tissue for estrogen-binding studies in carcinoma of the breast metastatic to the thoracic cavity.[3]

Absolute contraindications to thoracoscopy are rare. Lack of a free pleural space restricts use of thoracoscopy under local anesthesia, but with general anesthesia it is usually possible to divide the pleural adhesions and obtain adequate tissue in most patients. Most assuredly, thoracoscopy should not be employed in all patients with suspected or proved lung cancer.

Instrumentation and Technique

Many workers have recommended the use of a two-trocar technique for diagnostic thoracoscopy. In this method, the pleural cavity is inspected through one site, and manipulations

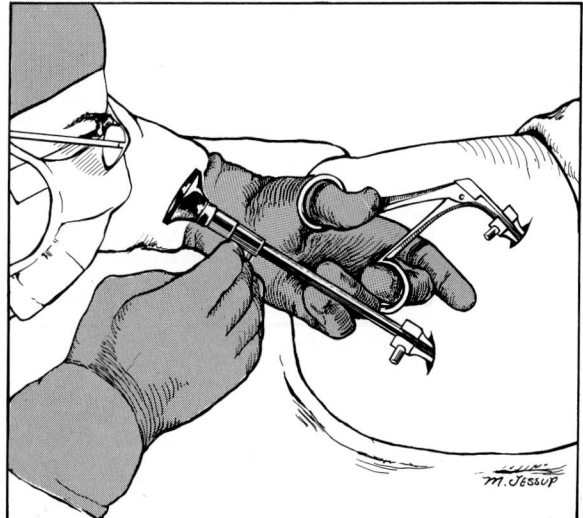

Figure 1. Two-trocar system of thoracoscopy.

are accomplished by insertion of forceps through another site (Fig. 1). Others advocate the use of the flexible fiberoptic bronchoscope as a thoracoscope.[6] The two-trocar system appears unduly complicated. The instruments are not readily available in most hospitals, nor is the technique familiar to most of the thoracic surgeons now practicing. The flexible bronchoscope, although more readily available, does not lend itself well to direction within the voluminous pleural cavity. For these reasons, the author prefers the technique illustrated in Figure 2.

The procedure often follows bronchoscopy and mediastinoscopy under the same anesthetic. In some patients, however, the surgeon may proceed directly to thoracoscopy. Although one may enter the pleural cavity at the time of mediastinoscopy and thereby perform thoracoscopy, access to the inferior portion of the pleural cavity is limited by this technique.[7] It is best to place the patient in the true lateral position; entry is then made into the pleural cavity at about the midaxillary line. Usually a 3- to 4-cm. incision is made at the fifth intercostal space, but adjustments are made depending upon the radiologic and clinical findings.

The extracostal muscles are separated in the direction of the fibers and, with use of an electrocautery, the intercostal muscles are incised. All the fluid within the pleural cavity is aspirated and aliquots sent for cytologic, bacteriologic, and biochemical studies. A finger is then inserted into the thoracic cavity to

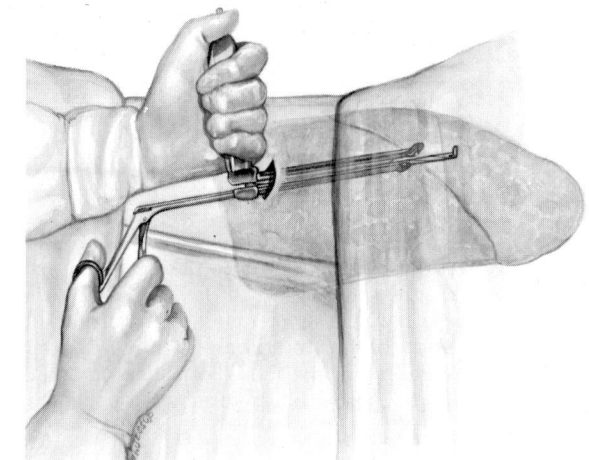

Figure 2. Use of fiberoptic mediastinoscope as thoracoscope. (From Lewis, R. J., Kunderman, P. J., Sisler, G. E., and Mackenzie, J. W.: Direct diagnostic thoracoscopy. Ann. Thorac. Surg., 21:536, 1976.)

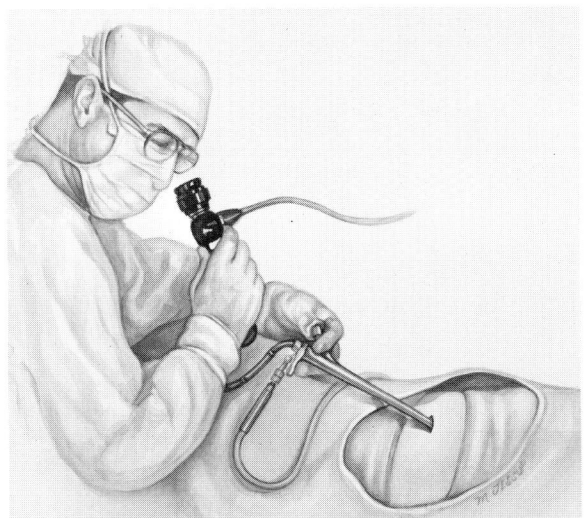

Figure 3. Insertion of flexible bronchoscope through rigid bronchoscope at thoracoscopy.

determine the extent of local adhesions; if any are present, they are carefully broken. The fiberoptic mediastinoscope or thoracoscope is then inserted into the pleural cavity and a careful sequential inspection is made of the surfaces of the pleural cavity. Large amounts of fibrin, if present, are sent for examination and any obvious nodules are sampled. In the region of the superior sulcus, insertion of a rigid bronchoscope may make the procedure easier and may be supplemented by a flexible bronchoscope inserted through the rigid bronchoscope (Fig. 3). Histologic specimens are sent for frozen section as well as for bacteriologic study. If gross inspection or frozen section suggests the possibility of active tuberculosis, antituberculosis drugs are started on the day of operation. No other antibiotics are used. The pleural cavity is drained to underwater seal drainage, and the chest tube is usually removed the next morning.

Although in this section emphasis has been placed on the use of thoracoscopy as a diagnostic procedure, it may also be helpful in treatment. Effusions or pneumothoraces may be treated by instillation of escharotics. Intrapleural foreign bodies, such as polyethylene catheters, may be removed, empyema spaces may be débrided, and blebs ablated by electrocautery.[15]

Thoracoscopy is a safe and diagnostically accurate procedure for many intrathoracic conditions. It is a worthwhile adjunct to thoracic surgery. Its greater use appears justified.

SELECTED REFERENCES

Bergqvist, S., and Nordenstam, H.: Thoracoscopy and pleural biopsy in the diagnosis of pleurisy. Scand. J. Respir. Dis., 47:64, 1966.
This report of 130 patients with pleurisy is carefully done and provides comparison with other techniques for diagnosis of pleural disease. There were no deaths or significant complications. The results were far more reliable than needle biopsy and "not inferior to open thoracotomy."

Bloomberg, A.: Thoracoscopy in perspective. Surg. Gynecol. Obstet., 147:433, 1978.
This recent excellent review article was written by an enthusiastic proponent of the technique. Accordingly, the author advocates thoracoscopy for a wide variety of conditions.

DeCamp, P., Moseley, P., Scott, M., and Hatch, B., Jr.: Diagnostic thoracoscopy. Ann. Thorac. Surg., 16:79, 1973.
This article reports a series of 126 patients who underwent thoracoscopy. The 95 per cent accuracy without any false-positive results was a strong stimulus for others to reconsider diagnostic thoracoscopy. Unfortunately, the two-trocar system used by the authors is not readily available nor, for that matter, is the expertise. Other techniques are easier and just as rewarding.

Jacobaeus, H. C.: The practical importance of thoracoscopy in surgery of the chest. Surg. Gynecol. Obstet., 34:289, 1922.
This article by the developer of thoracoscopy and laparoscopy is useful mainly for its historical aspects. It is primarily a discussion of the division of adhesions, in patients with pneumothorax induced for the treatment of pulmonary tuberculosis. However, diagnostic thoracoscopy is also discussed, including its use in 5 patients with intrathoracic tumor.

Lloyd, M.: Thoracoscopy and biopsy in the diagnosis of pleurisy with effusion. Q. Bull. Sea View Hosp., 14:128, 1953.
This is apparently the first report from the United States in which the combined procedure of thoracoscopy and biopsy is advocated for the diagnosis of pleural effusion of unknown etiology. It is remarkable that this report did not stimulate greater use of diagnostic thoracoscopy in this country.

Sattler, A.: Pleural biopsy: Results obtained and their practical significance. Ciba Symp., 9:109, 1961.
Although this report does not provide much statistical information, it is distilled from what is probably the largest personal experience with thoracoscopy. These observations were instrumental in establishing rupture of subpleural blebs as the usual cause of spontaneous pneumothorax. The style of the author and the excellent illustrations make the monograph a delight to read.

REFERENCES

1. Ash, A., and Manfredi, F.: Directed biopsy using a small endoscope. N. Engl. J. Med., 291:1398, 1974.
2. Ben-Isaac, F., and Simmons, D.: Fiberoptic pleuroscopy. Chest, 64:388, 1973.
3. Bonniot, J. P., Homasson, J. P., Roden, S. L., Angebault, M. L., and Renault, P. C.: Pleural and lung cryobiopsies during thoracoscopy. Chest, 95:492, 1989.
4. Boutin, C., Viallat, J. R., Cargnino, P., and Farisse, P.: Thoracoscopy in malignant pleural effusions. Am. Rev. Respir. Dis., 124:588, 1981.
5. Chandler, F. G., and Morlock, M. V.: Thoracoscopy in diagnosis. Br. Med. J., 2:982, 1938.
6. Davidson, A. C., George, R. J., Sheldon, C. D., Sinha, G., Corrin, B., and Geddes, D. M.: Thoracoscopy: Assessment of a physician service and comparison of a flexible bronchoscope used as a thoracoscope with a rigid thoracoscope. Thorax, 43:327, 1988.
7. Deslauriers, J., Beaulieu, M., Dufour, C., and Michaud, P.: Mediastinopleuroscopy: A new approach to diagnosis of intrathoracic diseases. Ann. Thorac. Surg., 22:265, 1976.
8. Fleishman, S., Lichter, A., Buchanan, G., and Sichel, R.: Investigation of idiopathic pleural effusions by thoracoscopy. Thorax, 11:324, 1956.
9. Geraci, C. L., and Brizzolara, L. G.: Use of the thoracoscope in the diagnosis of certain intrathoracic neoplasms. J. Thorac. Surg., 27:266, 1954.
10. Gwin, E., Pierce, G., Boggan, M., Kerby, G., and Ruth, W.: Pleuroscopy and pleural biopsy with the flexible fiberoptic bronchoscope. Chest, 67:5, 1975.
11. Gwin, E., Boggan, M., Pierce, G., Kerby, G., and Ruth, W.: Pleuroscopy and pleural biopsy with the bronchofiberscope. Am. Rev. Respir. Dis., 109:690, 1974.
12. Jacobaeus, H.: Ueber die Moglichkeit die Zystoscopie bei Untersuchung seroses Hohlungen anzuweden. Munch. Med. Wochenschr., 57:2090, 1910.
13. Jacobaeus, H.: Die Thorakoskopie und ihre praktische Bedeutung. Ergeb. Ges. Med. (Berlin), 8:112, 1925.
14. Lewis, R. J., Kunderman, P. J., Sisler, G. E., and Mackenzie, J. W.: Direct diagnostic thoracoscopy. Ann. Thorac. Surg., 21:536, 1976.
15. Oakes, D. D., Sherck, J. P., Brodsky, J. B., and Mark, J. B. D.: Therapeutic thoracoscopy. J. Thorac. Cardiovasc. Surg., 87:269, 1984.
16. Radigan, L. R., and Glover, J. L.: Thoracoscopy. Surgery, 82:425, 1977.
17. Rodgers, B. M., Ryckman, F. C., Moazam, F., and Talberg, J. L.: Thoracoscopy for intrathoracic tumors. Ann. Thorac. Surg., 31:414, 1981.
18. Rusch, V. W., and Mountain, C.: Thoracoscopy under regional anesthesia for the diagnosis and management of pleural disease. Am. J. Surg., 154:274, 1987.
19. Ryckman, F. C., and Rodgers, B. M.: Thoracoscopy for intrathoracic neoplasia in children. J. Pediatr. Surg., 17:521, 1982.
20. Senno, A., Moallem, S., Quijano, E., Adeyomo, A., and Clauss, R.: Thoracoscopy with the fiberoptic bronchoscope: A simple method in diagnosing pleuropulmonary diseases. J. Thorac. Cardiovasc. Surg., 67:606, 1974.

V

TRACHEOSTOMY AND ITS COMPLICATIONS

Hermes C. Grillo, M.D., and Douglas J. Mathisen, M.D.

Tracheostomy is one of the oldest operations and has long been used for the emergency management of upper airway obstruction. In the past two decades, tracheostomy has been increasingly employed to control secretions in severely ill patients. More recently, tracheostomy has provided a route for ventilatory support in respiratory insufficiency. This increased use of tracheostomy has reawakened recognition of the large number of serious complications that may follow the procedure. A spectrum of lesions, principally associated with its use for ventilatory support, has been identified.

INDICATIONS

The occurrence of serious complications has caused critical reappraisal of the three classic indications for tracheostomy: (1) relief of upper airway obstruction, (2) control of secretions, and (3) ventilatory support in respiratory failure. Tracheostomy often cannot be avoided in organic upper airway obstruction, although in some situations a tube may be inserted beyond an obstruction until definitive treatment can be provided. Emergency management of airway obstruction is best effected by skillful dilatation of inflammatory stenosis[12] or "coring-out" of tumor.[23] These techniques are preferable in safety, efficiency, and cost to use of the laser.[4,28]

The accumulation of secretions has increasingly been controlled by adequate humidification and by intensive pulmonary physiotherapy, consisting of expert instruction and assistance in cough, positional drainage, and thoracic percussion. Tracheal suctioning is used in conjunction with these measures, and, occasionally, transcricoid instillation of saline has been of assistance. Bronchoscopy, formerly used frequently, is rarely necessary. The flexible bronchoscope is employed at the bedside. "Minitracheostomy"—the insertion of a relatively small-bore catheter percutaneously through the cricothyroid membrane for repetitive suctioning over a prolonged period of time—has increasingly been recognized as a simple alternative to conventional tracheostomy for this purpose.[24] Unlike conventional cricothyroidostomy, it is effective and relatively free of complications,[29] because damage to the larynx is minimal.

Patients with respiratory insufficiency or impending failure are usually supported by a respirator with an endotracheal tube for varying lengths of time. If it appears that more than a day or so of support is required, a nasotracheal tube is generally preferred for the patient's comfort. Patients may thus be supported for a brief period of needed ventilatory support postoperatively without tracheostomy. There is no firm indication regarding the length of time an endotracheal tube may be employed. If it becomes clear that long-term support is needed, a tracheostomy is usually done as an elective procedure within 5 to 7 days. Such a transfer becomes necessary because of the dangers of tube obstruction, the discomfort to the patient of a nasal or oral tube, and the considerable damage to the larynx that may follow prolonged intubation. This injury occurs especially in the posterior commissure, with damage to the arytenoid and interarytenoid area. In a prospective study of the sequelae of endotracheal intubation, Whited[31] found three reversible laryngeal stenoses and one chronic posterior stenosis in 50 patients intubated for 2 to 5 days, five with chronic laryngotracheal stenosis in 100 patients intubated for 6 to 10 days, and six with complex laryngeal stenosis in 50 patients intubated for 11 to 24 days. Early conversion to tracheostomy prevented these injuries. The data support a policy of conversion from endotracheal tube to tracheostomy after 7 days.

TECHNIQUE

Tracheostomy is only rarely an emergency procedure. The safest method of establishing an emergency airway is insertion of an endotracheal tube or, if that fails, introduction of a ventilating bronchoscope. Even obstructing lesions can often be bypassed in this manner or sufficient ventilatory force applied beyond an obstruction through a tube so that a patient may be maintained until a more carefully considered procedure can be accomplished. For this reason, the simplest emergency surgical airway, an opening in the superficially located cricothyroid membrane, is rarely required.

Tracheostomy may be done under local anesthesia, with the patient supine and the neck hyperextended. An anesthetist should be in attendance to maintain a clear airway, to adjust the positioning of the endotracheal tube during the procedure, and to supply oxygen or other support as needed. The procedure should be performed in the operating room, so that the most sterile conditions are maintained and the operator is impressed with the need for meticulous technique. Blind tracheostomy procedures are unnecessary and are condemned because of the high incidence of associated complications. The rapidly made vertical cutaneous incision for emergency tracheostomy has been replaced by a carefully placed horizontal incision. This avoids the late tethering scars that may follow the vertical incision. Palpation of the extended neck always reveals the position of the cricothyroid membrane and the cricoid cartilage below. The incision is placed at the level of the second tracheal cartilage and extends through the platysma (Fig. 1). The strap muscles are separated vertically in the midline with minimal bleeding. The thyroid isthmus is usually divided between hemostats after careful dissection beneath it in the pretracheal plane. The thyroid tissue on either side is controlled with mattress sutures. Exact levels of the cartilaginous rings must be determined. The first cartilage must be left intact, and the opening in the trachea must be placed so that there is no tendency for the tube subsequently to erode the first ring or the adjacent cricoid cartilage by upward pressure. The second and third cartilages (and all or part of the fourth if necessary) are incised vertically in the midline so that the potential danger of upward pressure by the outside of the elbow of the tube is avoided. If there is any question, incision of a lower cartilage will avoid damage to a higher cartilage. Even after centuries of performance of tracheostomy, there is little controlled work to prove the superiority of the vertical incision over the cruciate or the horizontal incision, the excision of a disc or a segment of cartilage, or the

and supportive oxygenation given through a light-weight connector attached to the tube or to its inner cannula if it is a two-part tube. The skin is loosely closed with vertical mattress sutures on either side of the tracheostomy tube. Sutures on either side are passed through the flanges of the tracheostomy tube, securing it in place, in addition to the usual tracheostomy tapes. Such fixation is particularly important in the first few days, especially when a vertical incision in the trachea has been used, so that displacement of the tube does not occur at a time when replacement may be difficult. Too long a tube should be avoided to prevent placement in the right main bronchus. Cuffs must be firmly fixed or cemented, if they are not an integral part of the tube, to prevent dislodgement or prolapse over the end of the tube. Suctioning during tracheostomy and immediately after its completion helps to avoid postoperative atelectasis. Prolonged suctioning, which may cause hypoxia, is avoided.

COMPLICATIONS

Conversion of tracheostomy to a carefully performed elective procedure has largely eliminated the immediate and early complications of the procedure.[18,26] The longer-term complications of tracheostomy present mainly in three ways: (1) sepsis, (2) hemorrhage, and (3) obstruction of the airway. Additional complications are tracheoesophageal fistula and persistence of the stoma. In general, the longer a tracheostomy is in place (especially with an inflated cuff), the greater the chance that complications will occur.

SEPSIS. All tracheostomies are clinically contaminated, and *Staphylococcus aureus* (often a resistant strain), *Pseudomonas aeruginosa*, and a variety of other bacteria such as *Escherichia coli* and *Streptococcus* can be cultured. Despite this inevitability, sterile care and cleansing of the stoma and respiratory equipment must be maintained to minimize the possibility of invasive infection of the lower airway. Antibiotics are probably best reserved for use when there is evidence of tracheobronchitis, pneumonitis, or cellulitis, because premature use does not sterilize the stoma, but may merely permit other flora to be established.

HEMORRHAGE. The curve of the tube may erode the innominate artery and produce late hemorrhage, especially in children, in whom the trachea is small and the artery high. Massive hemorrhage also occurs from erosion by tracheostomy cuffs or even by the tip of a tube through the trachea into the innominate artery as it passes obliquely over the trachea. Bleeding from granulations or more superficial tracheal erosions is more common and usually less massive. Only immediate tamponade of a major arterial leak, digitally when due to erosion at the stoma, or with an inflated cuff when caused by cuff or tip injury lower in the trachea, and prompt surgical treatment lead to salvage. Resection of the injured artery with suture closure of both ends is one of the few possibilities in such a contaminated field. In the small number of cases in which this has been done successfully, there have been no neurologic problems. The trachea requires no treatment when arterial injury occurs at the stomal level. Injuries at the cuff level require resection and reconstruction.[9,27]

OBSTRUCTION. Airway obstruction may occur while the tube is in place. Cuff prolapse and avoidance have been discussed. If a tube with an inner cannula is used, crusts may be easily cleaned. With proper humidification, obstruction of single-lumen tubes is less commonly seen. Occasionally, a valve type of crust may form at the tip of a tube, so that a suction catheter may be easily passed without relieving the obstruction. If such a problem is suspected, the only course is to change the tube. If the change is necessary early after tracheostomy, it should be done over a guiding catheter with adequate instruments and personnel available to reinsert an endotracheal tube or a bronchoscope from above in the event that the tube is not

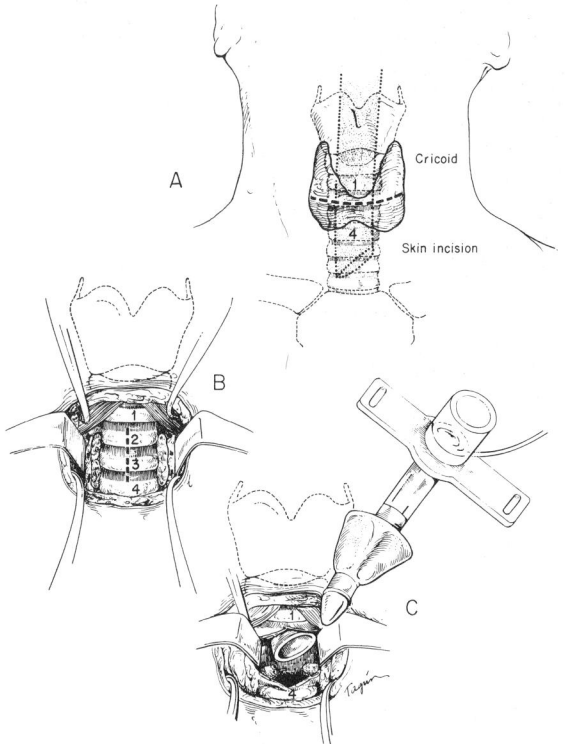

Figure 1. Technique of tracheostomy. *A,* An endotracheal airway is in place. With the patient's neck extended and centered in the midline, a short horizontal incision is made over the second or third tracheal ring after the level of the cricoid cartilage has been carefully palpated. The first and fourth tracheal cartilages are numbered. *B,* Following horizontal division of the platysma, the strap muscles are separated in the midline, the cricoid is identified, and the thyroid isthmus usually is divided and sutured to allow easy access to the second and third tracheal rings. The second and third rings are incised vertically. Occasionally an additional partial incision of the fourth ring is necessary. *C,* Smooth thyroid pole retractors are used to spread the opening in the trachea. The endotracheal tube is withdrawn to a point just above the incision. The tracheostomy tube is introduced with a small amount of water-soluble lubricant and with its large-volume cuff collapsed. The endotracheal airway is not removed until it is demonstrated that the tracheostomy tube is properly seated and permits suitable gas exchange. Closure is made with simple skin sutures. The flange of the tracheostomy tube is both sutured to the skin and tied with the usual tapes around the neck. On a rare occasion when an airway cannot be established from above, an emergency incision may be necessary over the cricothyroid membrane for rapid establishment of a temporary airway.

turning of a flap. The tracheal opening probably enlarges to the size of the tube in most cases after some days. It is important not to make too large an opening in the tracheal wall, whether with or without a flap, since the flap may well be destroyed or deformed. Any opening heals by cicatrization, and the larger the opening, the greater the likelihood of narrowing during stomal healing. If fine retractors are used in the open trachea, even a tube with a bulky low-pressure cuff may be inserted with ease with the assistance of water-soluble lubricant. Hemostasis should be precise throughout such an elective procedure.

Hypoxia and subsequent cardiac arrest, which formerly occurred during emergency tracheostomy, should not occur with this technique, because an airway has already been established. Formerly the site of tracheostomy was the suprasternal notch in the extended neck. In many, such an approach selects a midtracheal location and places the point of potential damage from cuff injury low in the trachea. The trachea is also farther away from the cervical skin surface at this level. In addition, it tends to further angulate the tube. In children and in some adults, a low incision also places the inner side of the elbow of the tube close to a high innominate artery, with greater potential for later erosive major hemorrhage.

Once the tube has been securely seated and any attached cuff is functioning satisfactorily, the endotracheal tube is withdrawn

easily replaced. Occasionally, obstructive granulations also form at the tip of a tube that is still in place.

A major syndrome of postintubation airway obstruction has been recognized (Fig. 2).[1,2,10,17,30] Improvements in cuffs and awareness of the problems have reduced its incidence. *Every patient with signs of upper airway obstruction—wheezing or stridor, dyspnea on effort, episodes of obstruction from secretions—who has been previously intubated with either an endotracheal tube or a tracheostomy tube must be considered to have organic obstruction until it is proved otherwise.* Unfortunately, many such patients who have been discharged from the hospital are still treated for asthma to the point of death or subtotal obstruction before the lesion is recognized.

Obstructive *laryngeal lesions* from prolonged endotracheal intubation may occur at the vocal cord level and consist of granulation tissue or cicatrix, particularly in the posterior commissure.[10,22,31] Large tubes relative to airway size especially may cause erosion at the subglottic and cricoid levels, with subsequent severe stenosis. Cricothyroidostomy, proposed to avoid the complications of tracheostomy,[3] fails to eliminate cuff lesions, of course, and transfers serious stomal lesions from the trachea to the subglottic larynx—where surgical treatment is more difficult, less satisfactory, and often impossible.[11]

At the stomal level, obstruction may be due to a polypoid granuloma that forms on the healing surface of the stomal site. Narrowing and indentation at the point of cicatrization of the stoma are often seen after tracheostomy. When the stoma is large—because of overgenerous initial surgical therapy or erosion by local infection or, most commonly, by the prying action of heavy-weight equipment that connects the tracheostomy to the ventilator—healing may produce clinically obvious obstruction. Such a stomal obstruction is usually three-sided, obstructing anteriorly and laterally, because the posterior wall is intact. Occasionally, some scarring occurs posteriorly as well. A combination of granuloma and stenosis may also produce obstruction. If the tracheostomy is placed too high, erosion of the cricoid cartilage may occur, with loss of substance and resultant subglottic stricture.

At the cuff site, pressure by the sealing cuff causes varying degrees of damage.[6] Prior to the introduction of true large-volume, low-pressure cuffs, damage of varying degrees occurred in all patients in whom a cuff was inflated for more than 48 hours.[7] In the days and weeks following, erosion frequently bared numerous cartilages, leading to their fragmentation and, eventually, total destruction (Fig. 3). Occasionally, the erosion pro-

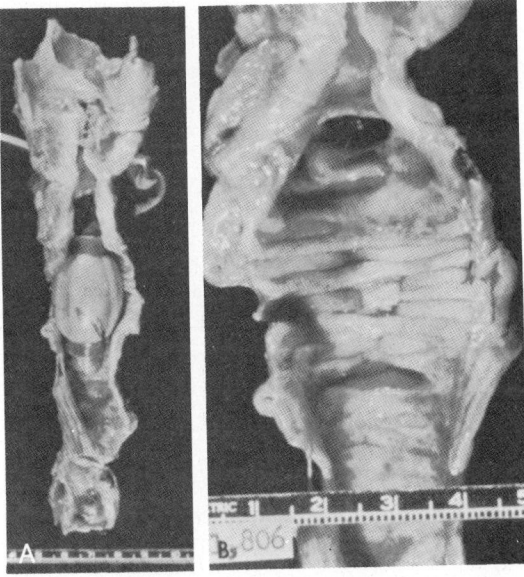

Figure 3. Tracheal injury due to a cuffed tracheostomy tube. Autopsy specimen of larynx and trachea. *A,* A metal tracheostomy tube with rubber cuff inflated had been in place for 16 days. *B,* Cartilaginous rings are exposed and fragmented at the cuff site. The tracheal wall is thinned and distended. Similar injuries occur with plastic tubes and cuffs. (From Cooper, J. D., and Grillo, H. C.: Ann. Surg., *169:*334, 1969.)

gresses anteriorly, through the wall of the innominate artery, or posteriorly, to produce a tracheoesophageal fistula. With lesser degrees of damage, healing occurs with variable deformity and narrowing. If the tracheal wall has been deeply eroded circumferentially, a circumferential stricture results during healing (Fig. 4). This may become arrested with partial closure and produce only dyspnea on effort, or it may go on to complete closure, with a fatal obstructive episode. The lengths of such strictures are extremely variable, extending from 0.5 to 4 cm. Such lesions may occur with either endotracheal tubes or tracheostomy tubes, because they are due to the cuff and not to the tube itself. A far greater number have followed cuffs on tracheostomy tubes, because there is greater long-term exposure to them. Other factors have been implicated in the etiology of cuff strictures, including periods of hypotension, which make it easier to compress the mucosal vascular supply; bacterial infection, which is always present; and toxic products from various materials and from ethylene oxide sterilization with inadequate aeration. However, clinical, pathologic, and experimental evidence clearly demonstrates that the common denominator is pressure.[1,7]

The tracheal cartilages *between the stoma and the cuff level* are often thinned, presumably by inflammatory changes, and this segment may become malacic. With respiratory effort, the malacic segment tends to collapse, contributing to the obstructive process. Granuloma may also form at the point of erosion by the *tip of the tracheostomy tube.* Children are more likely to show this lesion, because they are usually managed postoperatively without a cuff.

While most tracheostomies close spontaneously, a large and long *persistent stoma* fails to close occasionally and requires precise surgical repair.[21] This is apt to occur in aged or debilitated patients, in patients with metabolic disease, or in those who have been exposed to steroids. Once a clinical diagnosis of obstruction is made, confirmation is easily obtained by simple radiologic studies (Fig. 5).[25] Routine chest films most frequently show clear lung fields. The unwary physician may treat the patient for adult-onset asthma or other vague diagnoses. Lateral neck roentgenograms reveal tracheal deformities at the stomal level. Oblique views of the chest, which rotate the mediastinum to the side, reveal the entire trachea and demonstrate areas of

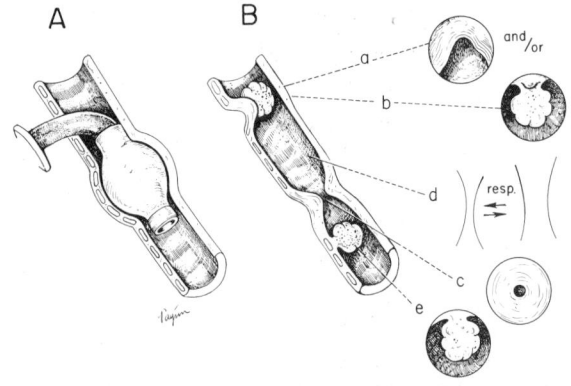

Figure 2. Obstructive lesions that may result from cuffed tracheostomy tubes. A conventional cuffed tube is in place at the left *(A).* Sagittal and cross-sectional (bronchoscopic) views of pathologic lesions are shown at the right *(B).* Anterolateral strictures are seen at the stoma (a), and granulomas also occur here (b). The lesions may occur concurrently. Circumferential stricture develops at the level of cuff injury (c). Between the stomal level and the cuff stricture, varying degrees of tracheal malacia may be seen; this leads to partial collapse during respiration (d). Granulomas may also occur at the level of the tip of the tube (e). (From Geffin, B., Grillo, H. C., Cooper, J. D., and Pontoppidan, H.: JAMA, *216:*1984, 1971.)

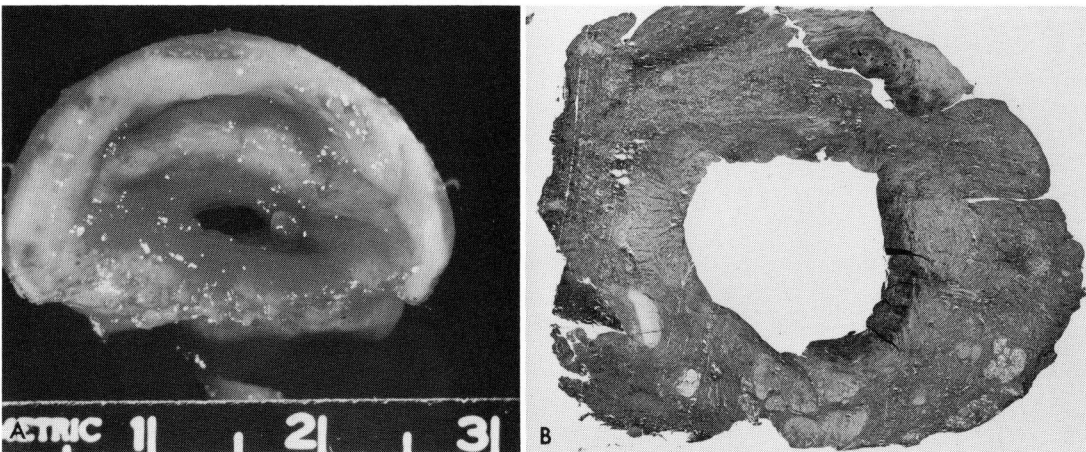

Figure 4. Tracheal stenosis from cuff damage. *A*, Gross specimen showing the typical circumferential fibrous and inflammatory lesion. *B*, Photomicrograph showing that the stricture in a severe case is composed almost entirely of scar tissue: little normal tracheal architecture is identifiable. Such strictures do not respond even to prolonged dilation or splinting. (From Grillo, H. C.: J. Thorac. Cardiovasc. Surg., *57:*52, 1969.)

narrowing at cuff level or elsewhere. A radiopaque marker taped to the skin at the site of an existing stoma or at the scar of such a stoma is helpful in pinpointing the level of a lesion. Fluoroscopy demonstrates the presence of malacia in the segment between the stoma and a cuff stricture. Tracheal laminagrams help to define the character, the level, and the extent of a lesion, facts that are necessary for planning correction. Contrast medium produces a crisper picture but is not necessary. Computed tomographic scans of the airway contribute little useful information about postintubation stenosis.

TREATMENT

With the development of techniques of tracheal surgery that permit safe end-to-end anastomosis after resection of lengthy segments, the majority of these patients may be returned to normal function by surgical excision of the obstructing lesion and anatomic reconstruction of the upper airway.[2,10,14]

If the patient is too ill for repair or has a disease that will soon require repeated tracheostomy, conservative management is recommended. This is possible in all but those cases in which the lesion is immediately above the carina, by reinstituting a tracheostomy, dilating the stricture, and passing a fenestrated tube or a Montgomery T-tube through it.[8,20] In an occasional patient in whom the original damage was small in amount, repeated dilations or prolonged splinting with an inlying tube may produce a satisfactory airway over a long period of time. In most, however, conservative treatment does not succeed despite prolonged attempts, and a permanent tracheostomy tube is required.

Two hundred seventy-nine patients with postintubation tracheal injuries were submitted to surgical reconstruction at the Massachusetts General Hospital from 1965 through 1982.[16] A small number were treated conservatively because their basic diseases did not suggest that reconstruction would be tolerated or, more often, because they were likely to require tracheostomy again in the near future for diseases such as severe myasthenia gravis. Of the 279 surgical cases, there were 98 postintubation lesions at the *stomal* level and 148 at the *cuff* level; 23 patients had stenoses at *both* levels, and in 10 the lesion was of uncertain origin. Six had malacia only, 11 had tracheoesophageal fistulas,[15] and 1 had an innominate artery fistula. Forty-four of the "cuff" stenoses were in patients who had had endotracheal intubation only, 1 for 18 hours. In 33 of the patients the strictures were incurred at the Massachusetts General Hospital.

The results of aggressive surgical treatment were good. Two hundred twenty-five patients had good to excellent results; in 25 the results were clinically satisfactory, although not ideal if the patients were to be put under physical stress. Twenty represented failures, but 9 attained good results with reoperation. There were five deaths. A number of deaths and failures were in patients with supracarinal stenoses impossible to manage conservatively and necessitating high risks. Four were lost to follow-up.

Postintubation stenosis involving the subglottic larynx is much more difficult to correct than are tracheal injuries, and a multitude of mainly multistaged procedures have been applied. However, one-stage laryngotracheoplastic procedures have been developed.[11] Acquired tracheoesophageal fistulas are successfully managed in a single operation also, after the patient is weaned from the respirator.[15]

Although the laser is widely used to treat post-intubation lesions, it rarely results in definitive correction except for granulomas or in the very rare and thin, web-like stenosis.[28] Scarring due to laser therapy, along with tracheal damage from a tracheostomy (often in conjunction with laser therapy), frequently complicates surgical repair.

PREVENTION

Prevention of tracheal stenosis is of key importance. Diminution in the incidence of stomal strictures was noted at the Toronto General Hospital when heavy connecting tubing was abandoned for light-weight swivel connectors.[1] A relatively low incidence of stomal strictures in a corresponding period at the Massachusetts General Hospital, where light-weight connectors were in use, confirms this observation. Obviously, the surgical stoma should not be excessively large.

Strictures have been associated with tubes of every material and with cuffs of varying types of materials. At cuff level, the principal preventive factor is elimination of pressure necrosis.[5,13,19] The large-volume, low-pressure cuffs, which occlude the irregularly shaped tracheal lumen by conforming to the shape of the trachea rather than by expanding to distend and so seal the airway, may accomplish this. Such a cuff was devised initially in animal experiments and then tested clinically in patients (Fig. 6).[13] The introduction of such cuffs has markedly reduced the occurrence of cuff injury. However, the inextensibility of plastic materials permits conversion of most "low-pressure" cuffs to high-pressure ones if a small excess of air is introduced beyond the maximal resting volume of the unstretched cuff. Additional safeguards are direct pressure monitoring and side balloons with pop-off valves to bleed excessive air. The lesions continue to occur despite these advances.

Substitution of cricothyroidotomy for tracheostomy[3] appears

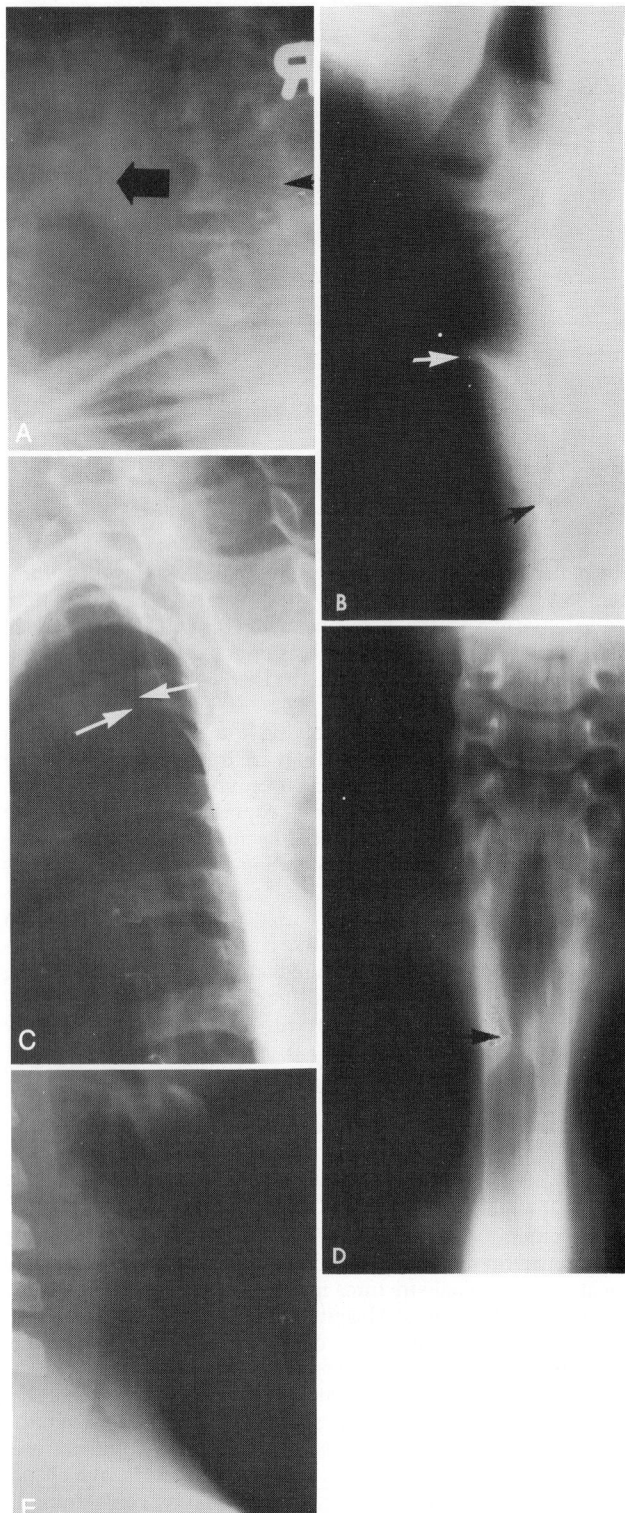

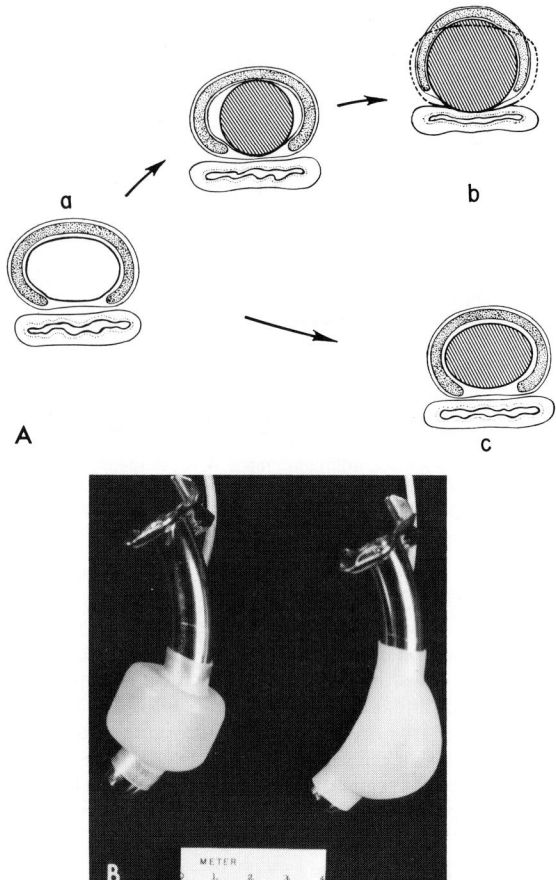

Figure 6. *A*, Diagram of the mechanism of cuff injury to the trachea and its avoidance. Above, a conventional cuff must be inflated under high pressure to effect a seal of the irregular tracheal airway. It distorts the trachea and exerts great pressure on the mucosa. Below, a cuff with large resting volume fills the irregular tracheal lumen by conforming to its shape at low intracuff pressures, below the point of elastic distention of the cuff. *B*, A low-pressure cuff and an old cuff mounted on standard Jackson tracheostomy tubes. The new cuff (left) is shown at its resting size. It must be collapsed with gentle syringe suction for insertion. The high-pressure cuff (right) has been inflated with 8 cc. of air. It has a high intracuff pressure, is asymmetrical, and is quite rigid. Unfortunately, overinflation of large volume cuffs converts them to high-pressure cuffs if they are made of relatively inextensible plastic. (From Grillo, H. C., Cooper, J. D., Geffin, B., and Pontoppidan, H.: J. Thorac. Cardiovasc. Surg., *62*:898, 1971.)

only to change the location of airway injury to a site more difficult to repair, despite the absence of complications in the experience of its original proponents.

SELECTED REFERENCES

Andrews, M. J., and Pearson, F. G.: The incidence and pathogenesis of tracheal injury following cuffed tube tracheostomy with assisted ventilation: An analysis of a two-year prospective study. Ann. Surg., *173*:249, 1971.
This excellent study correlates the factors attendant upon respiratory therapy, the gross pathologic observations at the time of extubation, and subsequent appearance of stenosis.

Cooper, J. D., and Grillo, H. C.: The evolution of tracheal injury due to ventilatory assistance through cuffed tubes: A pathologic study. Ann. Surg., *169*:334, 1969.
The pathogenesis of tracheal injuries is traced by means of study of autopsy specimens of tracheas from patients who died while in respiratory therapy and surgically resected specimens of fully developed strictures. Pressure necrosis is identified as the major etiologic factor.

Grillo, H. C.: Congenital lesions, neoplasms, and injuries of the trachea. *In* Sabiston, D. C., Jr., and Spencer, F. C. (Eds.): Gibbon's Surgery of the Chest, 5th ed. Philadelphia, W. B. Saunders Company, 1990.
The failure of conservative management is emphasized, and the successful application of new techniques of surgical reconstruction in the management of postintubation lesions is described in this current review of tracheal surgical problems.

Figure 5. Roentgenograms demonstrating tracheal lesions. *A*, Granuloma at stomal site. Circular radiopaque marker is on skin at site of prior stoma. Large arrow points to partially narrowed air column with large anterior granuloma visible. *B*, Stricture at tracheostomy site, shown in detail of lateral neck view. Larynx is clearly seen above. Arrows mark longitudinal limits of anterior stricture. The posterior wall of trachea is not involved. *C*, Cuff-level stenosis is demonstrated on oblique view of chest, which rotates mediastinal structures away from the trachea and shows its full length. Arrows indicate the narrowness of the airway. The lesion is circumferential. *D*, Cuff stricture shown on laminagram. The exact length of the stenosis, degree of airway narrowing, and level of stricture in relation to larynx and carina are detailed. *E*, Granuloma at level of anterior erosion by tip of tracheostomy tube, shown in lateral neck roentgenogram. In this child, a cuff had not been used.

Grillo, H. C.: Surgical treatment of post-intubation tracheal injuries. J. Thorac. Cardiovasc. Surg., 78:860, 1979.

A 14-year experience in management of 208 patients with postintubation injuries is described in detail, relating patient selection, diagnostic studies, categorization of lesions, treatment, and results.

Lindholm, C. E.: Prolonged endotracheal intubation. Acta Anesthesiol. Scand., Suppl. 33, 1969.

This exhaustive study of postintubation tracheal injury emphasizes the problems created by pressure of endotracheal tubes on the posterior commissural area of the larynx. It also describes posttracheostomy injury.

Whited, R. E.: A prospective study of laryngotracheal sequelae in long-term intubation. Laryngoscope, 94:367, 1984.

Replacing largely retrospective prior data, this careful study documents the frequency and severity of laryngeal and subglottic injuries due to endotracheal intubation. It demonstrates the validity of limiting endotracheal intubation to 7 to 10 days.

REFERENCES

1. Andrews, M. J., and Pearson, F. G.: The incidence and pathogenesis of tracheal injury following cuffed tube tracheostomy with assisted ventilation: An analysis of a two-year prospective study. Ann. Surg., 173:249, 1971.
2. Andrews, M. J., and Pearson, F. G.: An analysis of 59 cases of tracheal stenosis following tracheostomy with cuffed tube and assisted ventilation, with special reference to diagnosis and treatment. Br. J. Surg., 60:208, 1973.
3. Brantigan, C. O., and Grow, J. B., Sr.: Cricothyroidotomy. Elective use in respiratory problems requiring tracheostomy. J. Thorac. Cardiovasc. Surg., 71:72, 1976.
4. Brutinel, W. M., Cortese, D. A., McDougall, J. C., et al.: A two-year experience with the Neodymium-YAG laser in endobronchial obstruction. Chest, 91:159, 1987.
5. Carroll, R., Hedden, M., and Safar, P.: Intratracheal cuffs: Performance characteristics. Anesthesiology, 31:275, 1969.
6. Ching, N. P. H., Ayres, S. M., Spina, R. C., and Nealon, T. F., Jr.: Endotracheal damage during continuous ventilatory support. Ann. Surg., 179:123, 1974.
7. Cooper, J. D., and Grillo, H. C.: The evolution of tracheal injury due to ventilatory assistance through cuffed tubes: A pathologic study. Ann. Surg., 169:334, 1969.
8. Cooper, J. D., Pearson, W. G., and Todd, T. R., et al.: Use of silicone rubber stents in the management of airway problems. Ann. Thor. Surg., 47:371, 1989.
9. Grillo, H. C.: Complications of tracheal operations. In Cordell, A. R., and Ellison, R. G. (Eds.): Complications of Intrathoracic Surgery. Boston, Little, Brown and Company, 1979.
10. Grillo, H. C.: Surgical treatment of post-intubation tracheal injuries. J. Thorac. Cardiovasc. Surg., 78:860, 1979.
11. Grillo, H. C.: Primary reconstruction of airway after resection of subglottic laryngeal and upper tracheal stenosis. Ann. Thorac. Surg., 33:3, 1982.
12. Grillo, H. C.: The urgent management of tracheal obstruction. In Staudacher, V., and Bevilacqua, G. (Eds.): Eighth International Congress of Emergency Surgery, Milan, Monduzzi, 1987.
13. Grillo, H. C., Cooper, J. D., Geffin, B., and Pontoppidan, H.: A low pressure cuff for tracheostomy tubes to minimize tracheal injury: A comparative clinical trial. J. Thorac. Cardiovasc. Surg., 62:898, 1971.
14. Grillo, H. C., and Mathisen, D. J.: Surgical management of tracheal strictures. Surg. Clin. North Am., 68:511, 1988.
15. Grillo, H. C., Moncure, A. C., and McEnany, M. T.: Repair of inflammatory tracheoesophageal fistula. Ann. Thorac. Surg., 22:112, 1976.
16. Grillo, H. C., Zannini, P., Michelassi, F.: Complications of tracheal reconstruction: incidence, treatment and prevention. J. Thorac. Cardiovasc. Surg., 91:322, 1986.
17. Harley, H. R. S.: Laryngotracheal obstruction complicating tracheostomy or endotracheal intubation with assisted respiration. Thorax, 26:493, 1971.
18. Head, J. M.: Tracheostomy in the management of respiratory problems. N. Engl. J. Med., 264:587, 1961.
19. Knowlson, G. T. G., and Bassett, H. F. M.: The pressures exerted on the trachea by endotracheal cuffs. Br. J. Anaesth., 42:834, 1970.
20. Landa, L.: The tracheal T tube in tracheal surgery. In Grillo, H. C., and Eschapasse, H. (Eds.): International Trends in General Thoracic Surgery, Philadelphia, W. B. Saunders, 1987.
21. Lawson, D. W., and Grillo, H. C.: Closure of a persistent tracheal stoma. Surg. Gynecol. Obstet., 130:995, 1970.
22. Lindholm, C. E.: Prolonged endotracheal intubation. Acta Anaesthesiol. Scand., Suppl. 33, 1969.
23. Mathisen, D. J., and Grillo, H. C.: Endoscopic relief of malignant airway obstruction. Ann. Thorac. Surg., 48:469, 1989.
24. Matthews, H. R., and Hopkinson, R. B.: Treatment of sputum retention by minitracheostomy. Br. J. Surg., 71:147, 1984.
25. Momose, K. J., and MacMillan, A. S., Jr.: Roentgenologic investigations of the larynx and trachea. Radiol. Clin. North Am., 16:321, 1978.
26. Mulder, D. S., and Rubush, J. L.: Complications of tracheostomy: Relationship to long term ventilatory assistance. J. Trauma, 9:389, 1969.
27. Nelems, B.: Tracheoarterial fistula. In Grillo, H. C., and Eschapasse, H. (Eds.): International Trends in General Thoracic Surgery. Philadelphia, W. B. Saunders Company, 1987.
28. Toty, L., Personne, G., Colchen, A., et al.: Laser treatment of postintubation lesions. In Grillo, H. C., and Eschapasse, H. (Eds.): International Trends in General Thoracic Surgery. Philadelphia, W. B. Saunders Company, 1987.
29. Wain, J. C., Wilson, D. J., and Mathisen, D. J.: Clinical experience with minitracheostomy. Ann. Thorac. Surg., 49:881, 1990.
30. Weber, A. L., and Grillo, H. C.: Tracheal stenosis: An analysis of 151 cases. Radiol. Clin. North Am., 16:291, 1978.
31. Whited, R. E.: A prospective study of laryngotracheal sequelae in long-term intubation. Laryngoscope, 94:367, 1984.

VI ——————————————————

PULMONARY INFECTIONS

Stewart M. Scott, M.D.

LUNG ABSCESS

A lung abscess is a localized area of suppuration and cavitation in the lung. This definition includes such diverse etiologies as tuberculous, mycotic, or parasitic cavitation; bronchiectasis; infected cyst; and even pulmonary infarction with abscess formation. Cavitation of a tumor with an abscess may also occur. Most of these conditions are discussed in other chapters of the text. This section concerns primarily pyogenic lung abscesses secondary to aspiration pneumonitis. These have been termed "primary" or "simple" lung abscesses to distinguish them from those abscesses occurring in association with systemic diseases, malignant or nonmalignant, that follow the weakening of the natural defenses of the body to infection.[9] The former are declining in incidence, whereas the latter have achieved increasing prominence in recent years.

Pyogenic lung abscess has been recognized and even treated surgically for centuries. However, accurate diagnosis of lung abscess awaited approaches of modern medicine, such as the chest roentgenogram. In 1927, David Smith at Duke University observed that organisms seen in the walls of lung abscesses were also present in patients' mouths, especially patients with bad oral hygiene. He demonstrated in experimental animals that aspiration of these bacteria could cause lung abscess. At that time, the mortality from this disease was approximately 30 per cent and treatment often required surgical drainage or pulmonary resection. Once penicillin became available, however, the need for surgical therapy rapidly declined.[3]

Pathogenesis

Pyogenic lung abscesses usually occur as a result of aspiration of septic debris from the oropharynx into the lung in a patient with gingivodental disease or oral sepsis, during a period when the cough reflex is suppressed. Dental or tonsillar operations also commonly precede the development of lung abscesses.

Edentulous patients rarely have aspiration-type lung abscesses. Since episodes of aspiration occur during periods of unconsciousness from alcoholism or general anesthesia, epilepsy, cerebral vascular accident, or immersion, the victim is usually in a recumbent and often a supine position. The most direct route for the airway embolus to travel is into the right main bronchus, and the first dependent bronchus in a supine patient is that to the superior division of the right lower lobe. The posterior segment of the right upper lobe is also dependent and accessible. These two segments are therefore the most common sites of lodgment of septic emboli, and thus the usual sites of primary lung abscesses (Fig. 1). Esophageal disease that permits regurgitation and subsequent aspiration of esophageal contents into the lungs is another predisposing clinical setting. Rarely, septic pulmonary embolism causes infarction and lung abscess.

Following the development of severe pneumonitis in response to the embolus, liquefaction may occur. The microorganisms most commonly responsible are anaerobic bacteria, alpha- and beta-hemolytic streptococci, staphylococci, nonhemolytic streptococci, and *Escherichia coli*. Gram-negative rods and staphylococci are likely to occur in hospital-acquired lung abscess[31]; other organisms are isolated less often.[33] As the liquefied necrotic material empties through the bronchus, a necrotic cavity containing pus and air is formed. Clinically, lung abscesses present as indolent conditions in patients with a predilection for aspiration. Usually cough, foul-smelling sputum, fever, pleuritic chest pain, weight loss, and night sweats are noted.

In the suppurative pneumonias of infancy due to staphylococci, clinical symptoms and signs of abscess may be overshadowed by those of toxemia, dyspnea, cyanosis, and septic shock. These may appear suddenly, or they may be greatly intensified if pyopneumothorax due to rupture of a subpleural abscess ensues.

The chest film in lung abscess is not pathognomonic in the early stages. An area or areas of dense pneumonic consolidation precede the appearance of the characteristic cavitary lesion. Multiple abscesses may form multiple cavities. A distinguishing roentgenographic feature of lung abscess, the air-fluid level, is seen only on thoracic roentgenograms exposed in the upright position (or lateral decubitus, in a very sick patient). Accompanying pleural thickening, pneumothorax, or atelectasis may obscure or confuse this presentation. Computed tomography may be helpful in delineating the abscess (Fig. 2).[46] Staphylococcal pneumonia of infancy, which may lead to infected pneumo-

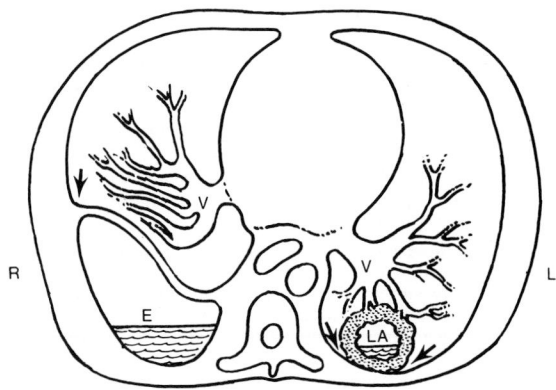

Figure 2. Diagram showing computed tomographic features of lung abscess and empyema. The lung abscess (LA) in the left lung is spherical, with thick, irregular walls and an irregular inner surface. The abscess forms acute angles with the chest wall (arrows). Pulmonary vessels (V) extend to the lung abscess. The empyema (E) in the right hemithorax is lenticular, with thin walls and smooth inner surfaces. It forms an obtuse angle with the chest wall (arrow). The pulmonary vessels (V) are compressed and distorted by the empyema. (From Williford, M. E., and Godwin, J. D.: Computed tomography of lung abscess and empyema. Radiol. Clin. North Am., 21:575, 1983.)

celes, differs in appearance from the classic lung abscess in that the lesions are characteristically thin-walled and cyst-like and are often accompanied by pleural effusion, empyema, or pyopneumothorax. Complete or partial opacification of the hemithorax may be the presenting roentgenographic presentation under these circumstances. With adequate therapy, even the most dramatic roentgenographic features may disappear completely.

Because of the availability of effective broad-spectrum antibiotics such as penicillin, lung abscesses can often be aborted in the stage of pneumonitis; therefore, the incidence of this type of abscess has declined in recent years.[9] However, much more difficult clinical problems are presented by patients, often at the extremes of age, who have serious associated diseases ranging from prematurity to malignant disease, in whom the normal defense mechanisms for successfully combating infections are lacking.[9] In such patients, lung abscess may occur as a complication of a systemic disease. Prematurity, bronchopneumonia, congenital defects requiring surgical treatment, the postoperative state itself, and the presence of other infections, blood dyscrasias, or systemic diseases are common predisposing conditions in early infancy. In addition to postoperative states, systemic diseases, malignant diseases (especially of the lung and oropharynx), and prolonged use of corticosteroid, immunosuppressive, or radiation therapy are the common conditions of the older age group associated with this type of lung abscess (Fig. 3). Such conditions often give rise to multiple abscesses, and the majority of these infections are acquired in the hospital. Bacteriologically, also, these abscesses differ somewhat from classic aspiration-type abscesses. *Staphylococcus aureus* is a common causative organism, but alpha-streptococci, *Neisseria catarrhalis*, pneumococci, *Pseudomonas*, *Proteus*, *E. coli*, and *Klebsiella* are all recognized, and, occasionally, after prolonged antibiotic treatment, rather unusual bacteria are all that remain to be cultured from the sputum.

Because of the unpredictability of these organisms, coupled with the urgent need to identify them in the very sick patient, invasive means for obtaining secretions for bacteriologic examination, including transtracheal and occasionally even percutaneous needle aspiration, may sometimes be justified.[11] Because these methods are not without hazard, alternative methods have recently been introduced, using specially designed protected brush catheters in association with fiberoptic bronchoscopy. There is no predilection for particular sites for these

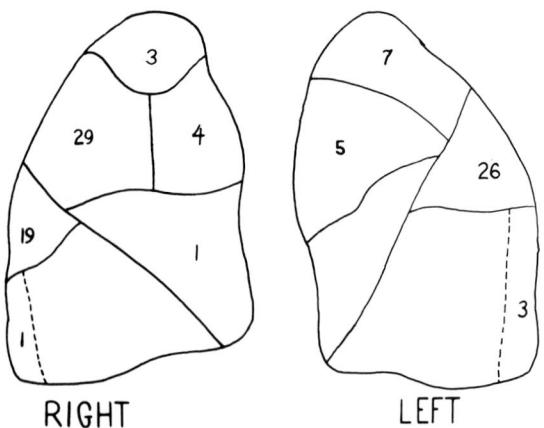

Figure 1. The segmental distribution in the two lungs of 98 lung abscesses caused by aspiration. Note the predilection for three principal sites: the superior segment of the right lower lobe, the posterior segment of the right upper lobe, and the superior segment of the left lower lobe. (From Bernhard, W. F., Malcolm, J. A., and Wylie, R. H.: Lung abscess: A study of 148 cases due to aspiration. Dis. Chest, 43:620, 1963.)

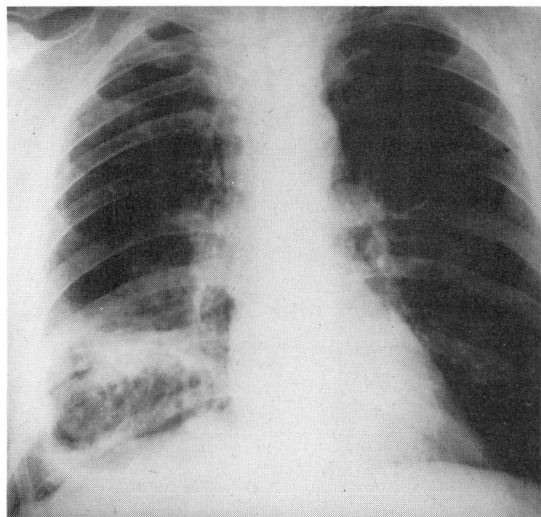

Figure 3. Thoracic roentgenogram of a patient with a huge lung abscess, right lower lobe, from which only the usually nonvirulent *Serratia marcescens* was cultured. This patient had had extensive corticosteroid therapy for severe asthma and multiple broad-spectrum antibiotics for superimposed infection, prior to operation. This type of abscess is currently being seen with greater frequency in similar clinical situations.

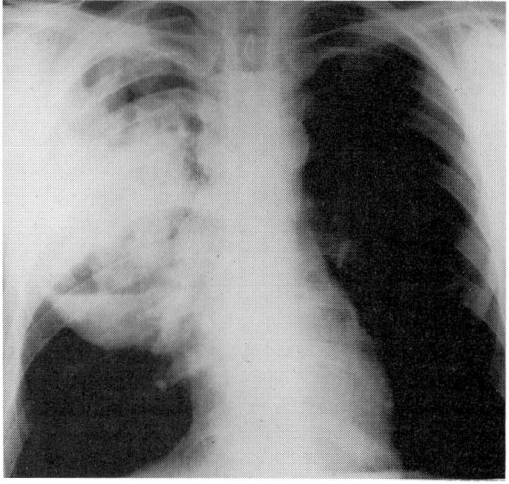

Figure 4. Posteroanterior thoracic roentgenogram of a patient with a pyogenic lung abscess, from which *Klebsiella pneumoniae* and alpha-streptococci were cultured. After a month of intensive antimicrobial therapy, a residual dense, thick-walled cavitary mass, 4 cm. in diameter, was resected by right upper lobectomy.

abscesses — they can occur almost anywhere, but the right lung is more commonly involved than the left.

Treatment

The treatment of classic primary aspiration lung abscess is prolonged antimicrobial therapy.[33] Penicillin G has traditionally been recommended as the antibiotic of choice and one that can be initiated even before the results of sputum cultures are known. However, in one randomized controlled trial, clindamycin was found to be more effective for community-acquired putrid lung abscess. Other antibiotics are used as indicated by subsequent bacteriologic studies. Bronchoscopy for diagnostic purposes, to remove a foreign body if one is present, and to provide drainage of the abscess by aspiration of the appropriate bronchus through the bronchoscope is also usually indicated. The refinement of transbronchial drainage by catheterization of the appropriate bronchus with or without fluoroscopic guidance has also been helpful.

Surgical treatment is reserved for the complicated problems of massive hemoptysis, lack of response to antibiotics, and presence of a cavity that is thick-walled or of large size (6 cm. or more).[9] (Fig. 4). When a malignant lesion is suspected or when empyema develops, surgical therapy may also be appropriate. In most instances, resective surgery is performed. Occasionally, percutaneous catheter drainage of a large abscess in a poor-risk patient may be justified. The need for surgical resection for primary lung abscess has declined markedly in recent years, because the effectiveness of antibiotics has increased.[9,31]

The complications of lung abscesses include empyema, septicemia, metastatic brain abscess, and bronchogenic spread. The most common complication is the development of chronicity. A residual cavity may be an indication for resection if symptomatic, or if infection recurs.

The mortality from aspiration-type lung abscess has declined appreciably in recent years and is currently reported at 5 to 6 per cent.[32] Surgical treatment, if required, carries an 11 per cent mortality.[9] In children, a zero per cent mortality is reported for lung abscesses treated medically. However, in patients whose abscesses complicate some other systemic disease, the mortality may be 35 to 90 per cent. Prompt recognition and urgently applied and appropriate antibiotic therapy may alter this dismal prognosis in the future.

FUNGAL INFECTIONS

Actinomycosis and nocardiosis have traditionally but mistakenly been classified as caused by fungal organisms. The etiologic agents are bacteria belonging to the Actinomycetaceae. The distinction is important, because the treatment of infections by these two organisms differs from the therapy for mycotic infections.

Actinomycosis

Actinomycosis in man is usually caused by *Actinomyces israelii*. Actinomycotic organisms were described by von Graefe in 1854. The disease, known as "lumpy jaw," was once more common in cattle (*Actinomyces bovis*) and in man before penicillin. It was associated with poor oral hygiene. The first description of thoracic actinomycosis was by Ponfic in 1882.[34]

The *Actinomyces* are anaerobic or microaerophilic organisms that require special techniques for culture and isolation. In pathologic material, organisms with branching filaments occur in clusters or microcolonies called granules. The much larger yellow-brown granules in draining material from abscesses or sinuses are called "sulfur granules" and are dense clusters of organisms.

Since *A. israelii* is a normal inhabitant of the oral cavity, it must be recovered from closed tissue spaces, draining sinuses, or abscesses or shown to be invasive in histopathologic sections.

Cervicofacial, thoracic, and abdominal forms of actinomycosis are recognized. Thoracic actinomycosis is most commonly due to bronchopulmonary invasion of infectious material from the oropharynx. The infection may be so indolent that symptoms may be few until pleural or chest wall involvement ensues.

Empyema and chronic draining chest wall sinuses, or roentgenographic evidence of involvement of the ribs or vertebrae, is characteristic. A nonspecific-appearing pulmonary infiltration, consolidation, or hilar mass strongly suggestive of bronchogenic carcinoma is also observed.[43] Primary actinomycetic empyema is rare.[23]

The drug of choice is penicillin. Because of the dense fibrous tissue surrounding the colonies of organisms and the concentration of organisms in clusters, high doses of pharmacologic agents must be used for long periods, and radical surgical excision should accompany antibiotic therapy if possible. The difficulties of establishing a diagnosis in this disease frequently result in surgical excision of the pulmonary lesions of

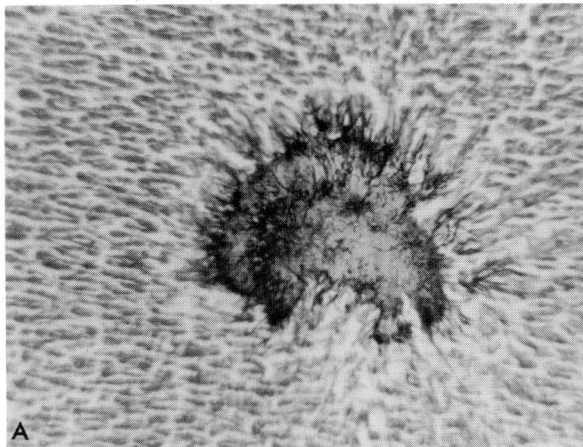

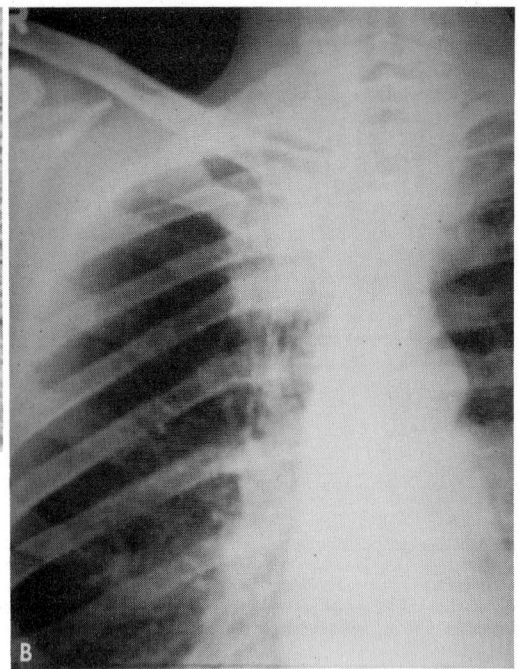

Figure 5. *A,* Actinomycotic granule showing branching filaments of a microscopic colony of *Actinomyces israelii.* Gomori stain. ×250. *B,* Thoracic roentgenogram of a patient who subsequently underwent right upper lobectomy for a suspected malignant lesion. Actinomycosis was found in the resected specimen.

actinomycosis or of chest wall abscesses (Fig. 5). Empyema may require decortication or pleural drainage.[23]

Nocardiosis

Like actinomycosis, nocardiosis was originally described in cattle (Nocar, 1888). Nocardiosis is usually caused by the aerobic actinomycete *Nocardia asteroides;* this organism has been isolated from the soil.[7] It occurs in pathologic material in clumps or granules, composed of short or long branching filaments that are gram-positive and acid-fast. This has led to confusion in the past with *Mycobacterium tuberculosis.*

Nocardiosis may mimic actinomycosis, tuberculosis, pneumonia, or lung abscess. In the last decade, most patients with nocardiosis have had some immunologic disorder associated with malignancy, organ transplantation, or immunosuppressive therapy. Thus, nocardiosis is often an opportunistic infection, with a grave prognosis. Nocardia occurs in patients with acquired immunodeficiency syndrome (AIDS), although the diagnosis may be concealed by the presence of *Pneumocystis carinii.*[36] The treatment is trimethoprim-sulfamethoxazole, continued on a long-term basis.[40] An alternative drug is minocycline. However, if the disease is resectable, a cure rate of 100 per cent is reported. In many instances, the diagnosis has been made for the first time from the resected specimen.

THORACIC MYCOTIC INFECTIONS

Formerly, blastomycosis, histoplasmosis, coccidioidomycosis, and cryptococcosis were considered to be rare, almost invariably fatal infections. Now it is recognized that benign, self-limited, and almost undetectable infections by all these organisms are much more common than had been previously thought. Millions of individuals exhibit evidence of subclinical histoplasmosis and coccidioidomycosis, with spontaneous healing.

The widespread use of antimetabolites, antibiotics, and steroids has given saprophytic fungi such as *Aspergillus, Candida,* and *Mucor* the opportunity to invade the host and cause disease. Thus, both true pathogens and saprophytes can cause opportunistic infection—that is, invasion of the host when body defenses have been weakened or altered by drugs or disease. The normally pathogenic fungi *Histoplasma, Blastomyces, Coccidioides, Paracoccidioides,* and *Sporothrix* are dimorphic. Because they exist in nature as molds that are not susceptible to

phagocytosis by leukocytes, they cause infection. In hosts, in response to the 37° C. temperature, they change into yeasts or spherules *(Coccidioides)* that are susceptible to phagocytosis, allowing the host to heal the infection they cause. Fungi, which exist only as opportunistic organisms, probably do not cause disease in normal hosts because they are susceptible to phagocytosis. They do cause disease in neutropenic patients. Both groups of fungi cause opportunistic infection in patients with suppressed cell-mediated immunity.[14]

The surgeon depends upon the pathologist for a definitive diagnosis, but the pathologist must rely upon the surgeon or physician to provide suspicion of fungal infection as well as appropriate samples of sputum or tissue to make positive identification possible. This is important because, for most of these diseases, serologic, immunologic, and skin tests cannot be relied upon for a definitive diagnosis, and specific but rather toxic antimycotic drugs are now available for treatment (Table 1).[20,42,44]

Epidemiology

Many of the fungi causing human infection are inhabitants of the soil. Most infections are believed to be caused by direct inhalation of the organisms in contaminated dust.

Three of these organisms are known to occur in the soil of specific geographic areas in North America (Fig. 6). These are *Histoplasma capsulatum* (histoplasmosis), *Coccidioides immitis* (coccidioidomycosis), and *Blastomyces dermatitidis* (North American blastomycosis). A soil reservoir is also accepted for *Cryptococcus, Aspergillus,* and *Mucor.* Candidiasis is considered an endogenous infection, since the yeast *Candida* is part of the normal flora of human beings and animals.

Histoplasmosis

Histoplasmosis, the most common of the pathogenic fungal infections, occurs in the valley of the Mississippi River and its tributaries. *Histoplasma capsulatum* is found in soil contaminated by pigeon, chicken, or bat droppings. It was first observed in Panama in 1905 by Darling, who mistakenly thought the organism was a plasmodium encapsulated in a histiocyte; hence its name. Some 30 million individuals have been infected, as judged from skin reactions to histoplasmin.[16]

The pathologic findings resemble those of pulmonary tuber-

TABLE 1. Antibiotic Therapy for Actinomycetes and Fungi

Disease	Antibiotic
Actinomycosis	Penicillin (may require 1 year or more). Erythromycin or tetracycline if patient is penicillin-sensitive
Nocardiosis	Trimethoprim - sulfamethoxazole or sulfadiazine for 3 to 6 months. Minocycline if patient is sulfa-sensitive
North American blastomycosis	Amphotericin B is effective (2 or more gm.); 2-hydroxystilbamidine, ketoconazole, and itraconazole are alternate drugs
Histoplasmosis	Amphotericin B is effective for most forms except endocarditis. Ketoconazole for CNS disease.
Coccidioidomycosis	Amphotericin B, 0.5 to 2.5 gm.; ketoconazole
Paracoccidioidomycosis	Amphotericin B; ketoconazole; itraconazole
Sporotrichosis	Potassium iodide is primary drug; amphotericin B, in combination with 5-fluorocytosine, and itraconazole are effective
Candidiasis	Amphotericin B alone or with 5-fluorocytosine
Zygomycosis	Amphotericin B
Pseudallescheriasis	Ketoconazole

See References 20, 38, 42, and 44.

culosis, except for the finding of the yeast cells of *H. capsulatum* in macrophages, or in the capsules of nonviable organisms of the necrotic center of granulomas. Most cases of infection are asymptomatic. Acute pulmonic infection may be accompanied by diffuse pulmonary infiltration or scattered nodular densities and may be characterized by an acute febrile course. Whereas this disease is mild in the normal host, in patients with AIDS it can be severe and even fatal unless aggressively treated.[22] By far the most common clinical presentation of histoplasmosis is an asymptomatic chronic granuloma, appearing on a thoracic roentgenogram as a solitary pulmonary nodule of undiagnosed etiology.

Chronic cavitary histoplasmosis resembles pulmonary tuberculosis both symptomatically and roentgenographically (Fig. 7). It appears to progress more slowly. In a considerable percentage of cases, pulmonary tuberculosis has been found to coexist in such patients. A wide variety of clinical manifestations of chronic histoplasmosis involving the mediastinal structures are also seen.[16]

The treatment of histoplasmosis depends upon the form of the disease that is encountered. For severe acute infections, therapy with amphotericin B, currently the only available effective drug, may be necessary. The solitary nodule may pose a problem in management. In a cooperative study of solitary pulmonary nodules resected in adult men, 53 per cent were found to be granulomas and 36 per cent malignant tumors. Fungi, either *H. capsulatum* or *C. immitis*, were isolated from the majority of these granulomas. Since malignancy was found in such a high percentage of cases, and since the presence of calcium in a nodule does not exclude carcinoma (unless calcification is concentric, dense, or unchanged for years), exploratory thoracotomy for the undiagnosed nodule is often indicated, especially in men over 40 years of age. If the diagnosis can be made by needle aspiration biopsy of the lesion, neither thoracotomy nor drug therapy may be necessary. Cavitary histoplasmosis, proved by culturing the organism in the sputum, should be treated primarily with either amphotericin B or ketoconazole.[42] Operative intervention is reserved for patients with large, thick-walled cavities who have not improved after one or two courses of amphotericin B of up to 2.0 gm. each. If resectional surgery is undertaken, amphotericin B should be used until a total dosage of at least 2 gm. is reached, over a period of a month before and a month after resection (if the diagnosis is established prior to operation). Surgical resection in Goodwin's series produced healed lesions in 95 to 100 per cent of patients.[16] The treatment of mediastinal forms of histoplasmosis is variable, complicated, and beyond the scope of this text.

For disseminated forms of histoplasmosis, amphotericin B is urgently needed to prevent death.

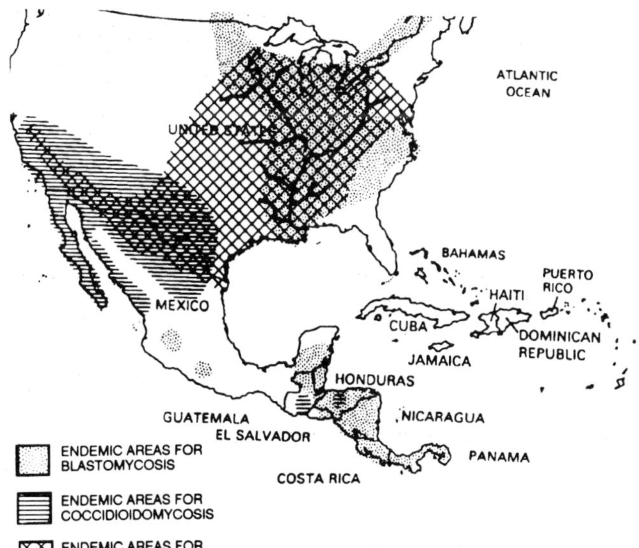

Figure 6. Areas of North America and Central America considered endemic for North American blastomycosis, histoplasmosis, and coccidioidomycosis.

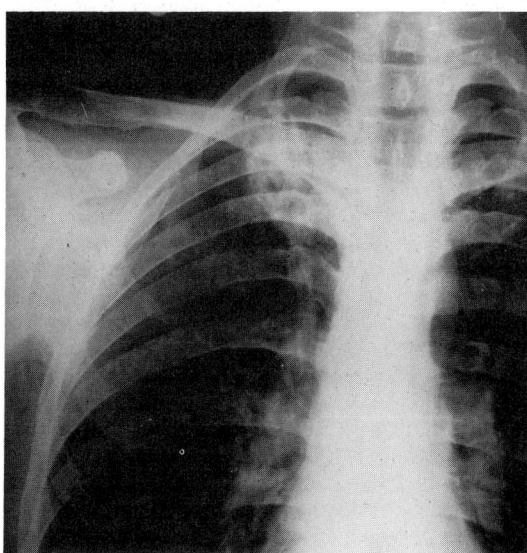

Figure 7. Thoracic roentgenogram of a patient with chronic cavitary histoplasmosis who underwent upper lobectomy prior to the availability of amphotericin B. (From Takaro, T.: Thoracic mycotic infections. *In* Lewis' Practice of Surgery. New York, Hoeber Medical Division, Harper & Row, 1968.)

Coccidioidomycosis

Coccidioidomycosis was first described by Posada in Buenos Aires in 1892, but Rixford and Gilchrist in San Francisco in 1896 incorrectly named the organism, believing it to be the protozoan *Coccidia*. Coccidioidomycosis is caused by the dimorphic fungus *Coccidioides immitis*, which may occur in tissues in the form of large spherules packed with endospores, but also as individual small endospores (following rupture of a spherule) or as mycelial elements or hyphae (in cavities) (Fig. 8).[12]

Coccidioidomycosis is an exogenous infection occurring in certain well-defined regions of California, Nevada, Arizona, New Mexico, Texas, and Mexico.[29] These regions are characterized by a dry, windy, dusty, hot climate. Irrigation has made these areas important both agriculturally and epidemiologically, since population growth has been rapid in the past several decades. Extensive travel through these areas has helped spread coccidioidomycosis to every part of the United States as well as to other countries. Some 10 million people in the United States are estimated to have been infected at some time in their lives with *C. immitis*.

The gross and microscopic lesions of coccidioidomycosis strongly resemble those of pulmonary tuberculosis, with two characteristic differences: the occurrence of thin-walled cavities and of suppuration. However, thick-walled cavities and chronic granulomas appearing as solitary nodules, as in histoplasmosis, are also common. Finally, apical or subapical infiltrates or cavities or both, indistinguishable roentgenographically from either chronic pulmonary tuberculosis or chronic pulmonary histoplasmosis, are also seen.

A history of "valley fever" during residence in an endemic area classically is obtainable, but often no clinical evidence is available as to the onset of the disease. With acute cavitation, hemoptysis is the most frequent symptom; with chronic infection, the presenting complaints are cough, weight loss, fever, and chest pain. Skin tests and complement fixation tests are almost always positive in active cases. The organisms can be recovered in the sputum and also by bronchial brushing.

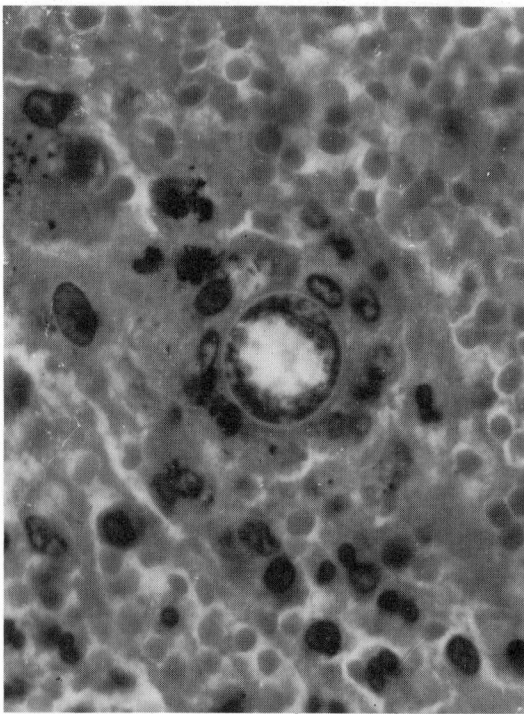

Figure 8. Spherules of *Coccidioides immitis*, packed with endospores, in a giant cell. Hematoxylin and eosin, × 500. (From Takaro, T.: Thoracic mycotic infections. *In* Lewis' Practice of Surgery. New York, Hoeber Medical Division, Harper & Row, 1968.)

The most effective specific therapy is amphotericin B, but many patients require no treatment at all. The drug should be reserved for acutely ill patients and those with cavitary disease and sputum cultures positive for *C. immitis*. Recently, ketoconazole has also proved to be effective for certain forms of chronic coccidioidomycosis.[17]

Although the majority of undiagnosed solitary pulmonary nodules occurring in patients in the endemic area prove to be coccidioidomas, 26 to 35 per cent are found to be malignant. Therefore, the indications for resection of solitary pulmonary nodules in this area may be difficult to define and must be individualized, as for histoplasmosis. For cavitary lesions, the indications are clearer. They include persisting cavities 2 cm. or greater in diameter; those that are enlarging, thick-walled, or ruptured; those associated with severe or recurrent hemoptysis; those occurring in diabetic[2] or pregnant patients; and those coexisting with pulmonary tuberculosis. Drug coverage with amphotericin B is recommended by some; but it is not clear that the use of amphotericin B has resulted in significantly fewer complications of bronchopleural fistula, empyema, and recurrent cavitation.

North American Blastomycosis

North American blastomycosis is endemic not only in the central United States and Canada but in parts of Central and South America, Africa, and Asia. It is caused by *Blastomyces dermatitidis*, a round, thick-walled, single-budding yeast first described by Gilchrist in 1894.[38] The disease often occurs in a cutaneous form, with chronic, indolent, usually enlarging papulopustules with thick adherent crusts and purple, raised edges. Biopsy in these areas may show microabscesses containing the organism. This form, with no evidence of systemic (including pulmonary) involvement, is the mildest. Pulmonary symptoms may be nonspecific. On the thoracic roentgenogram, cavitary, nodular, fibrotic, or disseminated lesions may be observed; the condition may mimic bronchogenic carcinoma. Occasionally, dissemination of blastomycosis may occur after operation on an undiagnosed blastomycotic lesion. Thus, a preoperative diagnosis is important to avoid an unnecessary operation. This may be aided by Papanicolaou smears of sputum and by serologic testing.[45] The standard therapy for blastomycosis is amphotericin B in a total dose of 1.5 to 2.0 gm. administered over 8 to 12 weeks.[42] Ketoconazole, however, has been found to be 79 per cent effective in curing patients with mild or moderately severe disease, and it is less toxic and can be taken orally.[25] Resectional surgery is rarely needed except for diagnosis, especially when cancer is suspected.

Cryptococcosis

Cryptococcosis was once considered a rare and fatal disease, often accompanied by meningitis. Benign and subclinical bronchopulmonary infections are now recognized with increasing frequency, and even the dreaded meningeal form is controllable by drug therapy.

Cryptococcus neoformans is found in nature in soil, dust, and pigeon dung. The organisms are round, budding yeast cells with thick gelatinous capsules, which until 1935 were confused with *Blastomyces*. Difficulty in classifying the organism has led to many confusing synonyms, e.g., *Torula histolytica*. Cryptococcosis is primarily an opportunistic infection. It is sometimes known as "malade signal" because it often signifies significant underlying disease, such as cancer.[34] It is the most common fungus infection seen in renal transplant patients.[47] Colonization of otherwise healthy individuals, without tissue invasion, can also occur. The roentgenographic features are nonspecific and may even include pleural effusion.

If cryptococci are cultured from sputum, with no demonstrable pulmonary lesion, or are isolated from lung tissue resected as an undiagnosed lesion, with no symptoms or signs of active disease (the most common way the diagnosis is made), opinions differ regarding the need for antifungal therapy.[18] Active treatment may not be necessary if there is no evidence of central nervous system involvement and no organisms are found in spinal fluid. However, now that two effective agents are available—the less toxic 5-fluorocytosine as well as amphotericin B—the proponents of treatment for proven disease have found additional support.[18]

There is little controversy regarding the need for definitive treatment if the presence of active cryptococcosis can be shown by evidence of progression of a pulmonary lesion and continued sputum positivity, or by evidence of meningeal involvement.

Aspergillosis

Aspergillosis has become the third most common systemic fungal infection (after histoplasmosis and coccidioidomycosis) and, in recent years, the one with the most rapidly rising incidence.[13] It is usually caused by *Aspergillus fumigatus,* a filamentous organism with coarse, septate, fragmented hyphae. Of interest is the tendency for this organism to invade pre-existing pulmonary cavities, there to form a rounded necrotic mass of matted hyphae, fibrin, and inflammatory cells, called an aspergilloma or fungus ball. This mass usually lies free in the cavity and can change its location as the patient moves from an upright to a recumbent position. On the chest film, a crescentic radiolucency adjacent to a rounded mass within a cavitary lesion is almost pathognomonic of an aspergilloma (Fig. 9). Chronic cystic lesions of the upper lobes that remain as residua of pulmonary tuberculosis, sarcoidosis, lung cyst, or bronchiectasis commonly harbor such fungus balls; hemoptysis, occasionally severe, is the usual presenting symptom.

The medical management of aspergillosis has been unsatisfactory. Iodides, nystatin, hydroxystilbamidine, and amphotericin B have all been used. Surgical excision of an aspergilloma is usually curative of symptoms of hemoptysis and should be undertaken if the patient's condition permits and pre-existing disease has not produced generalized lung damage.[1,4,8] However,

there is no unanimity about this view. If excisional surgery is contraindicated, as it often is because of pulmonary fibrosis and respiratory insufficiency, endocavitary or endobronchial treatment with sodium iodide or amphotericin B may be helpful. *Aspergillus* empyema is a serious complication requiring drainage and local instillations of amphotericin B or nystatin for effective management.[30] *Aspergillus* endocarditis occurs following cardiac surgery and on valves of immunocompromised patients. Treatment includes surgical therapy; no patient has survived without valve replacement.[27,48] *Aspergillus* pericarditis is a lethal infection.

Candidiasis and Fungal Endocarditis

The most common of fungal infections is candidiasis.[41] It is usually caused by *Candida albicans,* an opportunistic organism first identified as a fungus by Bergin in 1841. *Candida* species is a normal inhabitant of the gastrointestinal tract and the female genital tract, but overgrowth occurs with prolonged use of antibiotics. Candidemia and systemic infection occur in patients with suppressed immunity. Candidiasis is of interest to cardiac surgeons because of the occurrence of *Candida* endocarditis in association with cardiac (usually valvular) lesions, over 100 cases of which are already on record.[27] In a considerable number of patients, *Candida* endocarditis was diagnosed during or after prolonged and intensive antibiotic treatment for established subacute bacterial endocarditis. In another sizable group, fungal endocarditis (mainly due to *Candida,* but in some cases due to *Aspergillus*) has been reported following valve replacement. Heart operations offer a portal of entry through indwelling catheters, a damaged endocardial surface, and prolonged parenteral and antibiotic therapy, all of which favor the growth of this organism. The fungus is characterized by both budding yeast forms and mycelial elements (Fig. 10).

The clinical features of *Candida* endocarditis are almost indistinguishable from those of bacterial endocarditis, suspicion of and treatment for which may actually aggravate the fungal infection. The finding of sterile blood cultures when confronted

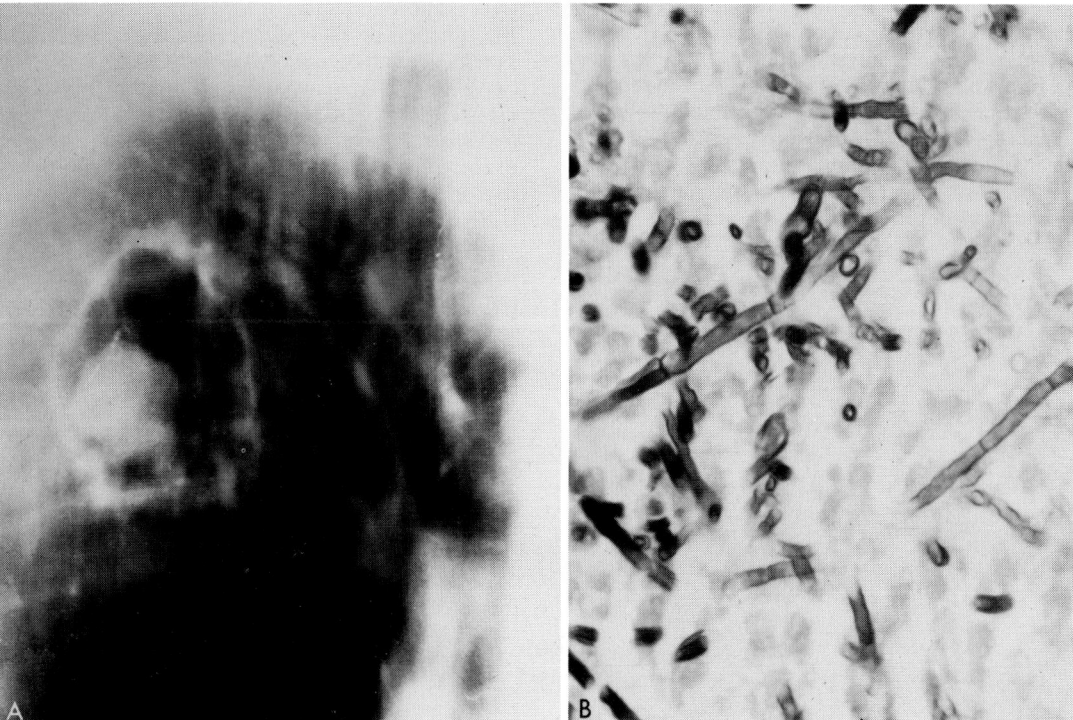

Figure 9. *A,* Laminagram showing typical aspergilloma ("fungus ball") lying free in a large cavitary lesion. This ball characteristically alters its location as the patient changes position. (From Aslam, P. A., Larkin, J., Eastridge, C. A., and Hughes, F. A., Jr.: Endocavitary infusion through percutaneous endobronchial catheter. Chest, 57:94, 1970.) *B,* Coarse, fragmented, septate mycelia of *Aspergillus fumigatus.* (From Takaro, T.: Thoracic mycotic infections. *In* Lewis' Practice of Surgery. New York, Hoeber Medical Division, Harper & Row, 1968.)

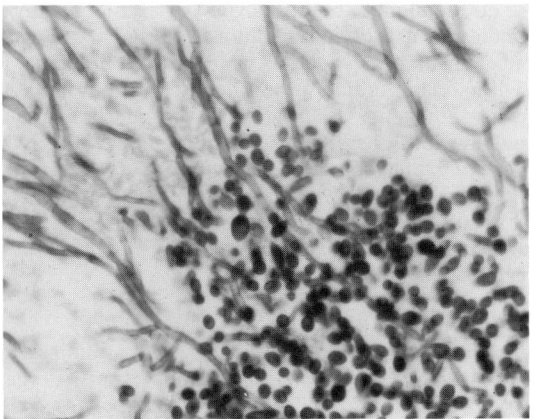

Figure 10. The organisms of *Candida albicans*, showing both mycelial and yeast forms. (From Takaro, T.: Thoracic mycotic infections. *In* Lewis' Practice of Surgery. New York, Hoeber Medical Division, Harper & Row, 1968.)

with a clinical presentation of bacterial endocarditis should dictate a search for *Candida; Candida* species found on blood culture must be interpreted as an indication of a potentially lethal infection. Distinguishing features of *Candida* endocarditis are embolic episodes to major vessels, due to the unusually large size of the mycotic valvular vegetations. Despite potentially beneficial treatment with the combination of 5-fluorocytosine and amphotericin B, the medical cure rate is still very low, and the mortality is between 80 and 90 per cent. Early surgical excision of vegetations or, when feasible, of an infected prosthetic valve, together with antifungal drug therapy, yields the best results (Fig. 11).[27] *Candida* lung abscess is uncommon and difficult to verify but has been diagnosed by needle aspiration biopsy and successfully treated with amphotericin B and flucytosine.[39]

Miscellaneous Fungal Infections

Sporotrichosis is caused by *Sporotrichum schenckii,* and pulmonary involvement is rare; the condition is usually encountered in its cutaneous or lymphatic manifestations. Agricultural workers and florists are especially susceptible. Localized cavities and other forms of pulmonary disease have been reported in over 150 cases thus far.[34] Iodides are sometimes effective in lymphocutaneous sporotrichosis, and amphotericin B is sometimes effective in the pulmonary forms. However, surgical excision of localized disease appears to be the most reliable method of treating pulmonary sporotrichosis.[32]

Zygomycosis (mucormycosis) is another rare and serious infection by any of the members of the phylum of fungi known as *Zygomycota.*[34] The organisms are characterized by broad, nonseptate hyphae; characteristically, blood vessel invasion, thrombosis, and infarction of organs are seen. Extensive necrosis of face, lungs, or brain may occur. Debilitated persons and uncontrolled diabetics appear to be especially prone to this infection. Control of the underlying disease, amphotericin B administration, and surgical excision of necrotic or infected tissue may prove helpful.[5]

Pulmonary pseudallescheriasis, also known as monosporosis, is a rare mycotic infection caused by *Pseudallescheriasis boydii.*[34] This inhabitant of soil appears to act as a secondary invader of previously damaged lung tissue, such as a cavity, cyst, or saccule. Sometimes a fungus ball is formed. The organism is resistant to amphotericin B and 5-flucytosine. Ketoconazole and miconazole have been effective in some instances, but pulmonary resection is indicated for cavitary lesions and sometimes to establish a diagnosis.

South American blastomycosis (paracoccidioidomycosis), a chronic granulomatous infection involving the skin, mucous membranes, lymph nodes, and visceral organs, is caused by *Paracoccidioides brasiliensis,* a soil saprophyte. Involvement of the lungs was once thought to be rare. It is now known that the infection occurs initially in the lungs and that, like histoplasmosis, subclinical and healed infections are common. It is endemic in South America and Central America, and it has been recognized in the United States as well. The organisms resemble *Blastomyces dermatitidis* in tissues. Cavitary lesions occur in about 15 per cent of patients with chronic pulmonary disease. Treatment with sulfonamides is suppressive but not curative. Amphotericin B, ketoconazole, and itraconazole are effective.[26] Surgical intervention usually is not required.

AIDS-Associated Pulmonary Infections

The acquired immune deficiency syndrome is a complex disease caused by one or possibly several retroviruses that are collectively known as the human immunodeficiency virus (HIV). The major effect of the HIV retrovirus is to interfere with the function of T4 lymphocytes. The opportunistic infections that most often occur in AIDS patients are those due to *Pneumocystis carinii,* cytomegalovirus, atypical mycobacteria, *Toxoplasma gondii, Candida,* herpes simplex virus, *Cryptococcus neoformans,* and *Cryptosporidium.* They involve the lung 80 per cent of the time. *Pneumocystis,* the most common opportunistic infection, occurs in 80 per cent of AIDS patients.[15]

PNEUMOCYSTIS CARINII *PNEUMONIA. Pneumocystis car-*

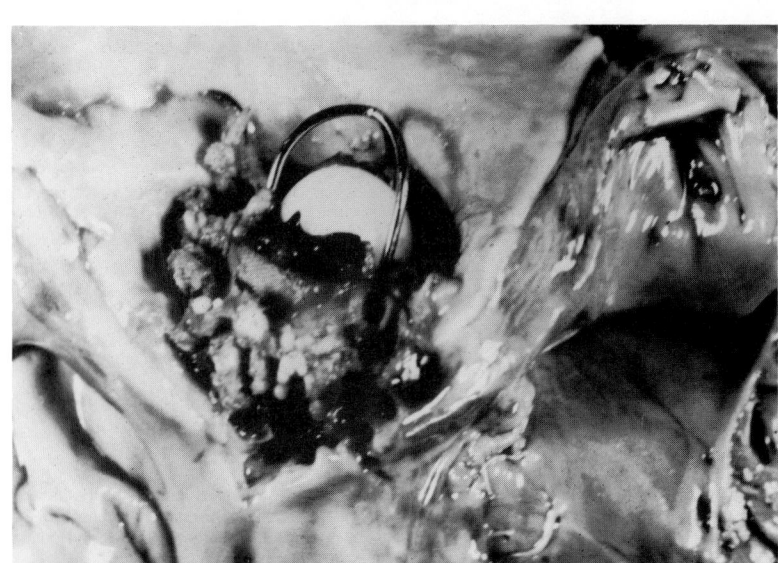

Figure 11. Fungal endocarditis caused by *Aspergillus* species, causing aortic prosthetic dehiscence due to perivalvular tissue necrosis. More commonly, *Candida albicans* has been the etiologic agent in opportunistic fungal infections following cardiac surgery. (From Ostermiller, W. E., Jr., Dye, W. S., and Weinberg, M.: Fungal endocarditis following cardiovascular surgery. J. Thorac. Cardiovasc. Surg., *61:*670, 1971.)

inii pneumonia is a diffuse interstitial pneumonitis that occurs as an opportunistic infection in marasmic or immunodeficient patients. It was first recognized in epidemic form in malnourished Central Europeans during World War II.

Until recently, most patients with *Pneumocystis* pneumonia were those who were immunosuppressed by chemotherapy for malignancies or were congenitally immunodeficient infants and children. A resurgence of interest in the disease occurred in the early 1980s when a new syndrome of *Pneumocystis* pneumonia in immunosuppressed homosexuals, bisexuals, and more recently the heterosexual population was recognized.[6,10,19,24,47]

The disease is caused by *P. carinii*, a protozoan named for its discoverer, Carini, who described it in 1910. This organism occurs in thick- or thin-walled cystic forms, 5 to 12 μ in diameter. It has a double-walled outer membrane, and within are three to eight intracystic bodies. The organism stains like a fungus with silver methenamine stains (Gomori stain) but responds to antiprotozoan drugs. The pneumonitis almost invariably occurs in patients with impaired cellular immunity caused by intensive drug therapy, usually for malignancies, or after organ transplantation. However, patients with primary immunodeficiency states are also susceptible, and, as noted, it occurs in patients with the acquired immunodeficiency syndrome (AIDS).[6,19,24]

In patients at risk, the combination of dyspnea, tachypnea, dry and nonproductive cough, fever, flaring of the nasal alae, intercostal retraction, and sometimes cyanosis, with minimal auscultatory signs, and the roentgenographic findings of unilateral or bilateral diffuse infiltrates radiating from the hilus or even localized areas of pneumonitis or consolidation should lead one to suspect *Pneumocystis* pneumonia.

Since the diagnosis depends on the demonstration of the organisms in lung tissue, either by transbronchoscopic lung or brush biopsy, by percutaneous needle biopsy, or by transthoracoscopic or open lung biopsy, the thoracic surgeon is often called upon. Neither needle biopsy nor open lung biopsy is entirely without risk in this disease. Therefore, bronchial brush biopsy, transbronchoscopic lung biopsy,[6] and bronchial lavage have been offered as less invasive and less risk-involved techniques. Transthoracoscopic lung biopsy has been advocated in children.[35]

However, open lung biopsy is still favored as the most certain method of making the diagnosis. It was successful in 32 of 33 patients in one series, 32 of 40 in another, and in 33 of 33 in a third. In another series comparing transbronchial with open lung biopsy in the same patients, 24 cases of a variety of pneumonias, including *Pneumocystis* pneumonia, were diagnosed by thoracotomy, compared with only 14 cases by transbronchoscopic lung biopsy. Moreover, bleeding, if it occurs, can be controlled under direct observation.

Clinical studies have shown that only two drug regimens have therapeutic value: trimethoprim/sulfamethoxazole and pentamidine isethionate.[19] Each is equally effective, but the former is preferred because of fewer side effects and less toxicity. Patients with AIDS and *Pneumocystis* pneumonia require longer treatment and have higher relapse rates than do other adults with known causes of immunosuppression, but the outcome should be similar.[19]

Other opportunistic infections may coexist with *P. carinii* pneumonia or may be important differential diagnostic possibilities. Some of these are cytomegalic inclusion virus infection, cryptococcosis, nocardiosis, and candidiasis. For some of these, specific treatment is also toxic. Therefore, it is important to make a definitive diagnosis so that appropriate drugs or combinations of drugs may be selected. However, one recommended strategy is to treat all immunocompromised pediatric patients who develop pneumonitis with trimethoprim/sulfamethoxazole while routine diagnostic tests are being obtained and to reserve open lung biopsy for diagnosis of those patients who do not respond

to these drugs.[21] Untreated, *P. carinii* pneumonia is often fatal. In patients treated early and adequately, approximately 65 to 75 per cent may survive.

Kaposi's Sarcoma of the Lung

Kaposi's sarcoma may be a viral-induced tumor. It occurs in 47 per cent of AIDS patients and when present is located in the lungs or airway in one third of afflicted patients. Kaposi's sarcoma appears as a painless purple or brown nodule.[37] Biopsy of these lesions should be done with caution because of the risk of hemorrhage.

SELECTED REFERENCES

Curry, W. A.: Human nocardiosis. A clinical review with selected case reports. Arch. Intern. Med., *140*:818, 1980.
This overview of nocardiosis emphasizes the microbiology, pathology, and epidemiology of the disease, with a description of the clinical manifestations and treatment.

DeVita, V. T., Jr., Hellman, S., and Rosenberg, S. A. (Eds.): AIDS Etiology, Diagnosis, Treatment, and Prevention, 2nd ed. Philadelphia, J. B. Lippincott Company, 1988.
The second edition of this monograph on the acquired immunodeficiency syndrome (AIDS) is thorough and up-to-date. The various chapters are written by authorities in the field. The text covers the basic virology, pathogenesis, epidemiology, clinical aspects, and prospects for future therapy.

Drutz, D. J., and Catanzaro, A.: Coccidioidomycosis. Parts I and II. Am. Rev. Respir. Dis., *117*:559, 727, 1988.
A complete presentation of the ecology, immunology, and epidemiology of coccidioidomycosis, with a fine section on clinical management and special emphasis on surgical aspects.

Goodwin, R. A., Loyd, J. E., and DesPrez, R. M.: Histoplasmosis in normal hosts. Medicine, *60*:231, 1981.
A comprehensive treatise on the epidemiology, pathology, clinical characteristics, and management of acute and chronic forms of pulmonary histoplasmosis.

Hammerman, K. J., Powell, K. E., Christianson, C. S., Huggin, P. M., Larsh, H. W., Vivas, J. R., and Tosh, F. E.: Pulmonary cryptococcosis. Am. Rev. Respir. Dis., *108*:1116, 1973.
This paper reviews the experience of the Centers for Disease Control Cooperative Mycoses Study (probably the largest series available for analysis), as well as experience reported in the literature.

Hermans, P. E., and Keys, T. F.: Antifungal agents used for deep-seated mycotic infections. Mayo Clin. Proc., *58*:223, 1983.
This is an up-to-date review of the principal antibiotics available, their pharmacologic properties, indications for use, and adverse effects.

Rippon, J. W.: Medical Mycology. Philadelphia, W. B. Saunders Company, 1988.
This is the third edition of this outstanding reference. It is current and provides in-depth descriptions of the pathogenic fungi and the actinomycetes.

Sarosi, G. A., and Davies, S. F. (Eds.): Fungal Diseases of the Lung. Orlando, Fla., Grune and Stratton, Inc., 1986.
This is a new volume devoted to the diagnosis and management of pulmonary infections caused by fungi and actinomycetes. It is current and provides a ready reference to the most recent experiences with medical and surgical treatment of these diseases.

REFERENCES

1. Allan, A., Sethia, B., and Turner, M. A.: Recent experience of the treatment of aspergilloma with a surgical stapling device. Thorax, *41*:483, 1986.
2. Baker, E. J., Hawkins, J. A., and Waskow, E. A.: Surgery for coccidioidomycosis in 52 diabetic patients, with special reference to related immunologic factors. J. Thorac. Cardiovasc. Surg., *75*:680, 1978.
3. Bartlett, J. G.: Anaerobic bacterial infections of the lung. Chest, *91*:901, 1987.
4. Battaglini, J. W., Murray, G. F., Keagy, B. A., Starek, P. J. K., and Wilcox, B. R.: Surgical management of symptomatic pulmonary aspergilloma. Ann. Thorac. Surg., *39*:512, 1985.
5. Bigby, T. D., Serota, M. L., Tierney, L. M., and Matthay, M. A.: Clinical spectrum of pulmonary mucormycosis. Chest, *89*:435, 1986.
6. Blumenfeld, W., Wagar, E., and Hadley, W. K.: Use of the transbronchial biopsy for diagnosis of opportunistic pulmonary infections in acquired immunodeficiency syndrome (AIDS). Am. J. Clin. Pathol., *81*:1, 1984.
7. Curry, W. A.: Human nocardiosis. A clinical review with selected case reports. Arch. Intern. Med., *140*:818, 1980.
8. Daly, R. C., Pairolero, P. C., Piehler, J. M., Trastek, V. F., Payne, W. S., and Bernatz, P. E.: Pulmonary aspergilloma. J. Thorac. Cardiovasc. Surg., *92*:981, 1986.
9. Delarue, N. C., Pearson, F. G., Nelems, J. M., and Cooper, J. D.: Lung abscess: Surgical implications. Can. J. Surg., *23*:297, 1980.

10. DeVita, V. T., Jr., Hellman, S., and Rosenberg, S. A. (Eds.): AIDS: Etiology, Diagnosis, Treatment, and Prevention, 2nd ed. Philadelphia, J. B. Lippincott Company, 1988.
11. Dobranowski, J., and Stringer, D. A.: Diagnosis of *Legionella* lung abscess by percutaneous needle aspiration. J. Can. Assoc. Radiol., 40:43, 1989.
12. Drutz, D. J., and Catanzaro, A.: Coccidioidomycosis. Parts I and II. Am. Rev. Respir. Dis., 117:559, 727, 1978.
13. Fraser, D. W., Ward, J. I., Ajello, L., et al.: Aspergillosis and other systemic mycoses: The growing problem. JAMA, 242:1631, 1979.
14. Fromtling, R. A., and Shadomy, H. J.: An overview of macrophage-fungal interactions. Mycopathologia, 93:77, 1986.
15. Gold, J. W. M.: Overview of infection with the human immunodeficiency virus: Infectious complications. Clin. Chest Med., 9:377, 1988.
16. Goodwin, R. A., Loyd, J. E., and DesPrez, R. M.: Histoplasmosis in normal hosts. Medicine, 60:231, 1981.
17. Graybill, J. R.: Treatment of coccidioidomycosis. Ann. N. Y. Acad. Sci., 544:481, 1988.
18. Hatcher, C. R., Jr., Sehdeva, J., Water, W. C., III, Schulze, V., Logan, W. D., Symbas, P., and Abbott, O. A.: Primary pulmonary cryptococcosis. J. Thorac. Cardiovasc. Surg., 61:39, 1971.
19. Haverkos, H. W.: Assessment of therapy for *Pneumocystis carinii* pneumonia. Am. J. Med., 76:501, 1984.
20. Herman, P. E., and Keys, T. F.: Antifungal agents used for deep-seated mycotic infections. Mayo Clin. Proc., 58:223, 1983.
21. Imoke, E., Dudgeon, D. L., Colombani, P., et al.: Open lung biopsy in the immunocompromised pediatric patient. J. Pediatr., 18:816, 1983.
22. Mandell, W., Goldberg, D. M., and Neu, H. C.: Histoplasmosis in patients with the acquired immune deficiency syndrome. Am. J. Med., 81:974, 1986.
23. Merdler, C., Greif, J., Burke, M., Sasson (Mizrachi), E., and Campus, A.: Primary actinomycotic empyema. South. Med. J., 76:411, 1983.
24. Murray, J. F., Felton, C. P., Garay, S. M., et al.: Pulmonary complications of the acquired immunodeficiency syndrome. (Report of a National Heart, Lung, and Blood Institute Workshop.) N. Engl. J. Med., 310:1682, 1984.
25. National Institute of Allergy and Infectious Disease Mycoses Study Group: Treatment of blastomycosis and histoplasmosis with ketoconazole. Ann. Intern. Med., 103:861, 1985.
26. Negroni, R.: Azole derivatives in the treatment of paracoccidioidomycosis. Ann. N.Y. Acad. Sci., 544:497, 1988.
27. Norenberg, R. D., Sethi, G. K., Scott, S. M., and Takaro, T.: Opportunistic endocarditis following open-heart surgery. Ann. Thorac. Surg., 19:592, 1975.
28. O'Driscoll, B. R. C., Cooke, R. D. P., Mamtora, H., Irving, M. H., and Bernstein, A.: *Candida* lung abscesses complicating parenteral nutrition. Thorax, 43:418, 1988.
29. Pappagianis, D.: Epidemiology of coccidioidomycosis. Curr. Topics Med. Mycol., 2:199, 1988.
30. Parry, M. F., Coughlin, F. R., and Zambetti, F. X.: *Aspergillus* empyema. Chest, 81:768, 1982.
31. Pennza, P. T.: Aspiration pneumonia, necrotizing pneumonia, and lung abscess. Emerg. Med. Clin. North Am., 7:279, 1989.
32. Pluss, J. L., and Opal, S. M.: Pulmonary sporotrichosis: Review of treatment and outcome. Medicine, 65:143, 1986.
33. Rienhoff, H. Y., Jr. (Ed.): Clinical Conferences, at The Johns Hopkins Hospital. Johns Hopkins Med. J., 150:141, 1988.
34. Rippon, J. W.: Medical Mycology. Philadelphia, W. B. Saunders Company, 1988.
35. Rodgers, B. M., Moazam, F., and Talbert, J. L.: Thoracoscopy. Early diagnosis of interstitial pneumonitis in the immunologically suppressed child. Chest, 75:126, 1979.
36. Rodriquez, J. L., Barrio, J. L., and Pitchenik, A. E.: Pulmonary nocardiosis in acquired immunodeficiency. Diagnosis with bronchoalveolar lavage and treatment with non-sulfa containing drugs. Chest, 90:912, 1986.
37. Safai, B., Johnson, K. G., Myskowski, P. L., Koziner, B., et al.: The natural history of Kaposi's sarcoma in the acquired immunodeficiency syndrome. Ann. Intern. Med., 104:744, 1988.
38. Sarosi, G. A., and Davies, S. F.: Blastomycosis. *In* Fungal Diseases of the Lung. Orlando, Grune & Stratton, Inc., 1986.
39. Schiffman, R. L., Johnson, T. S., Winberger, S. E., Weiss, S. T., and Schwartz, A.: *Candida* lung abscess: Successful treatment with amphotericin B and 5-flucytosine. Am. Rev. Respir. Dis., 125:766, 1982.
40. Smego, R. A., Jr., Moeller, M. B., and Gallis, H. A.: Trimethoprim-sulfamethoxazole therapy for *Nocardia* infections. Arch. Intern. Med., 143:711, 1983.
41. Sobel, J. D.: *Candida* infections in the intensive care unit. Crit. Care Clin. 4:325, 1988.
42. Stamm, A. M., and Dismukes, W. E.: Current therapy of pulmonary and disseminated fungal diseases. Chest, 83:911, 1983.
43. Stanley, S. L., Jr., and Lusk, R. H.: Thoracic actinomycosis presenting as a brachial plexus syndrome. Thorax, 40:74, 1985.
44. The Medical Letter: Drugs for treatment of systemic fungal infections. 28:41, 1986.
45. Turner, S., and Kaufman, L.: Immunodiagnosis of blastomycosis. Semin. Respir. Infect., 1:22, 1986.
46. Williford, M. E., and Godwin, J. D.: Computed tomography of lung abscess and empyema. Radiol. Clin. North Am., 21:575, 1983.
47. Wilson, W. R., Cockerill, F. R., III, and Rosenow, E. C., III.: Pulmonary disease in the immunocompromised host. Mayo Clin. Proc., 60:610, 1985.
48. Woods, G. L., Wood, R. P., and Shaw, B. W.: *Aspergillus* endocarditis in patients without prior cardiovascular surgery: Report of a case in a liver transplant recipient and review. Rev. Infect. Dis., 2:263, 1989.

VII

THE PLEURA AND EMPYEMA

Stewart M. Scott, M.D.

THE PLEURA

The pleura is the serous membrane lining of two complete and independent pleural sacs or potential cavities. Each extends into the neck, the retrosternal area, and the costophrenic sinuses, and also into the interlobar fissures. Familiarity with these ramifications of the pleural cavity can be extremely important, since unwitting violation of the pleural space, with its special anatomic and physiologic attributes, can be followed by serious consequences. Thus, the earliest surgical experiences with wounds penetrating into the pleural cavities, or with deliberate attempts to open into them, often resulted in disaster or near-disaster, from collapse of the lung, shift of the mediastinum, tension pneumothorax, and, later, infection.

A major surgical achievement occurred when the potential space between the two layers of the pleural cavity, measuring 10 to 27 μ, could at last be crossed safely. This was accomplished by Sauerbruch (1904), who placed his patient in a negative pressure chamber, leaving only the head and neck outside and exposed to atmospheric pressure, to achieve expansion of the lungs in the open chest. The entire surgical team had to

operate within this chamber. This cumbersome method became obsolete when Melzer and Auer introduced positive-pressure insufflation of the lungs. The Empyema Commission's findings during World War I marked another milestone, when it became understood that opening the pleural cavity to atmospheric pressure to drain an empyema could be catastrophic if adhesions had not formed that limited the extent of the infection. In the years that followed World War I, intrathoracic surgery gradually evolved. After World War II, this evolution progressed at a vastly accelerated pace. These surgical developments added greatly to the knowledge of pleuropulmonary physiology and pathology.[3]

ANATOMIC FEATURES. The pleural surface consists of a uniform layer of flattened mesothelial cells beneath which are layers of areolar connective tissue containing an abundance of blood vessels, nerves, and lymphatics. The visceral pleura is thinner, remarkably elastic, and intimately attached to the underlying lung by intrapulmonary fibrous prolongations of the deeper layer of connective tissue. The parietal pleura, however, is thicker and easily separable from the thoracic wall because of the loose layer of areolar tissue separating it from the endotho-

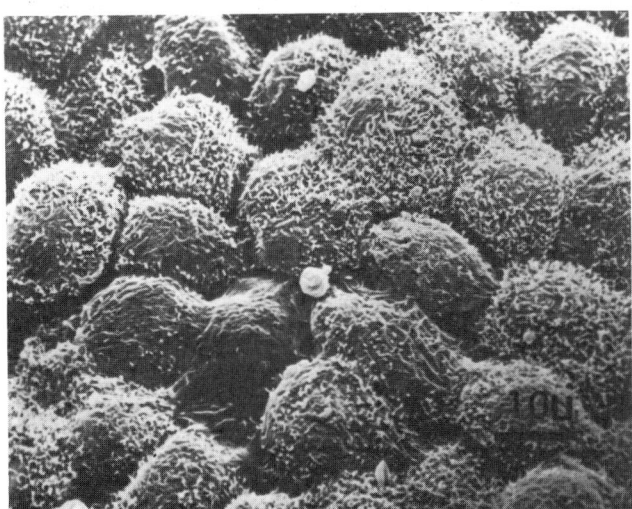

Figure 1. Many microvilli are present on the surface of cells forming the parietal pleura. Scanning electron microscopy. Original magnification × 1300. (From Wang, N.-S.: The regional difference of pleural mesothelial cells in rabbits. Am. Rev. Respir. Dis., *110*:623, 1974.)

racic fascia. It is supplied by the intercostal arteries. The visceral pleura is supplied largely by the bronchial arteries. Sensory nerve endings are present in the costal and diaphragmatic parietal pleura. Sensory fibers are absent in the visceral pleura.[25]

PHYSIOLOGIC CHARACTERISTICS. The two outstanding and interrelated features of the pleural cavities are (1) the subatmospheric pressures in the normally nonexistent pleural space, and (2) the serous secreting and absorbing surface of the pleural membranes. The elastic recoil of the lungs produces intrapleural negative pressures of −6 to −12 cm. H_2O during inspiration, and −4 to −8 cm. H_2O during expiration. Extremes of +40 cm. H_2O during the Valsalva maneuver, or −40 cm. H_2O during inspiratory effort against a closed glottis are also seen.

The secreting and absorbing properties of the pleura are substantial. Using special techniques, a rate of formation of 600 to 1000 ml. of fluid per day has been observed in patients, and an equal volume has been noted to be reabsorbed.[39] Increased capillary hydrostatic pressure, or a greater negative intrapleural pressure, tends to increase transudation into the pleural cavities. Loss of intrapleural negative pressure diminishes transudation, whereas increased diaphragmatic and intercostal activity increases its absorption. Resorption is made possible by numerous microvilli present on the mesothelial cells lining the pleura, particularly the visceral pleura. Scanning electron microscopy has demonstrated microvilli and pores in the parietal pleura that communicate with the lymphatics, through which proteins, cells, and particulate matter pass (Fig. 1).[44] Particulate matter, such as red blood cells, can be absorbed directly by the normal pleura. All these properties may be greatly altered by disease.

Pleural Effusions

Although pleural effusions are almost invariably secondary to some primary condition, they are often its first indication and therefore are always significant. Bloody effusions are ominous, for they may signify primary or secondary pleural tumor. Therefore, one should persist in attempts to make a precise diagnosis. The classic signs of fluid—flatness, absent tactile and vocal fremitus, diminished breath sounds, and mediastinal displacement—depend upon the size of the fluid collection and on the care with which the signs are sought.

A pleural effusion of up to 500 ml. may not be apparent clinically or roentgenographically in the adult in the upright position, since it ordinarily gravitates into the costophrenic sinuses and is obscured by the diaphragm. Thus, when a "small" effusion is noted on a thoracic roentgenogram, usually consid-

erable fluid is already present and can be obtained by a carefully performed thoracentesis (Fig. 2). Fluid may collect almost anywhere from the apex to the base of the pleural cavity in one or more loculated pockets, either in contact with the parietal pleura or in an interlobar fissure. Often bizarre roentgenographic features may result. Needle aspiration may be necessary to establish the presence of an effusion and to differentiate it from other thoracic conditions.

Major causes of effusions and their differentiation are outlined in Table 1. Infections, tumor, and congestive failure comprise 75 per cent of effusions in most patient populations. Less common causes such as pharmacologic agents should be borne in mind.[19,38] The differential diagnosis often depends upon obtaining samples of the fluid, the parietal pleura, or the lung and subjecting these to appropriate examinations. This does not always resolve the problem, however.

Sometimes a diagnosis can be made either from the pleural fluid alone or from cultures and smears for pathogenic organisms or cell blocks for tumor cells. If the pleural fluid is a transudate—that is, one low in protein and lactic acid dehydrogenase—the effusion is probably due to underlying systemic disease such as congestive heart failure, cirrhosis, or renal insufficiency. An exudative effusion is more likely to be associated with diseased pleura, which results in increased permeability of the pleura to proteins and decreased lymphatic clearance as seen in parapneumonic processes and malignancies. Pleural fluid analysis can be helpful even when not diagnostically specific. Normal pleural fluid pH in humans is 7.64; a low pH indicates significant inflammation. A pH of less than 7.20 is seen only in parapneumonic effusions, esophageal rupture, rheumatoid pleuritis, tuberculosis, malignancy, hemothorax, and systemic acidosis. A pH approaching 6.0 suggests esophageal rupture. A pleural fluid glucose of less than 60 mg. per 100 ml. is seen only in tuberculosis, malignancy, rheumatoid disease, or parapneumonic effusion. A pleural fluid amylase greater than that which is normal for serum is present only in pancreatitis, malignancy, and esophageal rupture. Cytologic examination of pleural fluid is positive in 50 per cent of patients with malignant disease. Chromosomal analysis of the malignant cells is particularly helpful in diagnosing pleural leukemia, lymphoma, and mesothelioma.[13,25]

Other studies of pleural fluid that may prove helpful include a white blood cell count and differential to help distinguish between a transudate and an exudate, and to identify the pres-

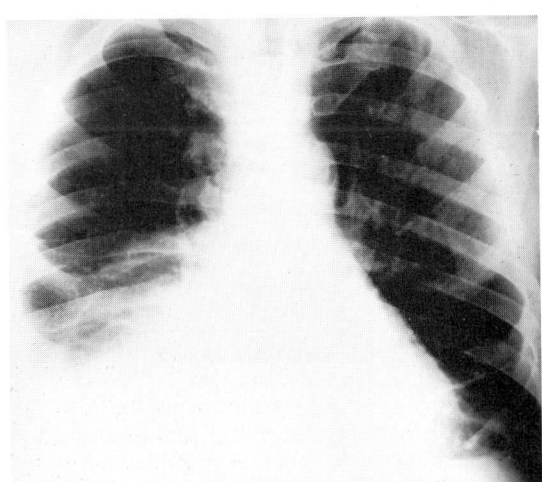

Figure 2. Pleural effusion, right base. After this thoracic roentgenogram was taken, 1300 ml. of straw-colored fluid was aspirated at thoracentesis. Surprisingly, large volumes of fluid may not be apparent clinically or roentgenographically when they gravitate into the costophrenic sinuses and are partially obscured by the diaphragm. A roentgenogram obtained in the lateral decubitus position may be more revealing.

TABLE 1. Etiologic Characteristics of Pleural Effusions

	Congestive Failure	Malignancy	Pneumonia and Other Nontuberculous Infections	Tuberculosis	Fungal Infection, Actinomycosis, Nocardiosis	Rheumatoid Arthritis and Collagen Disease	Pulmonary Embolism	Trauma	Chylothorax	Esophageal Rupture
Clinical	Signs and symptoms of congestive failure	Older patient, poor health prior to effusion	Signs and symptoms of respiratory tract infection	Younger patient, exposure to tuberculosis, good health prior	Exposure in endemic area	History of joint involvement may or may not be present, subcutaneous nodules	Postoperative patient, immobilized patient, venous disease	History of trauma	History of trauma, known malignancy	History of instrumentation or of vomiting
Gross appearance	Serous	Often sanguineous	Serous	Usually serous, may be sanguineous	Serous or purulent	Turbid or yellow-green	Often sanguineous	Sanguineous	Chylous or milky	Serous; may contain food particles
Microscopic examination	0	Cytology positive in 50 per cent	May or may not be positive for bacilli	Positive for acid-fast bacilli in 30 to 70 per cent of cases, cholesterol crystals	May or may not be positive for fungi	0	0	0	Fat droplets	Squamous epithelial cells
Cell count	10 per cent 10,000 erythrocytes; 10 percent over 1000 leukocytes	65 per cent bloody, over 40 per cent over 1000 leukocytes mainly leukolymphocytes	Polymorphonuclears predominate	Leukocytes, mainly lymphocytes; eosinophils more than 10 per cent excludes Tbc	Polymorphonuclear leukocytes or lymphocytes	Lymphocytes predominate	Erythrocytes predominate	Erythrocytes	0	Red blood cells and white blood cells
Culture	0	0	May or may not be positive	Less than 25 percent are positive	May or may not be positive	0	0	0	0	0
Specific gravity	90 per cent under 1.016 (unless pulmonary embolism)	75 per cent over 1.016	Over 1.016	75 percent over 1.016	Over 1.016	Over 1.016	Over 1.016	Over 1.016	Over 1.016	Over 1.016
Protein	75 per cent less than 3 gm.	90 per cent 3 gm. or more	3.0 gm or more	Usually 5.0 gm. per 100 ml. or more	3.0 gm. or more	3.0 gm. or more	3.0 gm. or more	3.0 gm. or more	Less than half plasma	3.0 gm. or more
Glucose	0	15 per cent have 60 mg. per 100 ml. or less	Occasionally less than 60 mg. per 100 ml.	Less than 50 per cent have 60 mg. per 100 ml. or less	0	78 per cent below 30 mg. per 100 ml. (rheumatoid)	0	0	0	0
pH	Greater than 7.20	May be 7.20 or less	May be 7.20 or less	May be less than 7.20	Greater than 7.20	May be 7.20 or less	Greater than 7.20	Greater than 7.20	Greater than 7.20	Usually less than 7.20; may be less than 6.00
Amylase	0	10 per cent are elevated	0	0	0	0	0	0	0	Elevated
Lactic acid dehydrogenase	Not elevated	May be elevated	May be elevated	May be elevated	May be elevated	May be elevated	May be elevated	0	0	0
Other	Right-sided in 55 to 70 per cent	If hemorrhagic fluid, 65 per cent will be due to tumor; tends to continue to form after removed	Associated with infiltrate on roentgenogram	Less than 5 per cent mesothelial cells; will be the cause in 75 per cent of men under 25 years; 50 per cent of men over 25 years; adenosine deaminase elevated	Skin and serologic tests may be helpful	Rapid clotting time; lupus erythematosus cell or rheumatoid factor may be present	Source of emboli may or may not be helpful	0	Fat content higher than plasma	0

Modified from Bessone, L. N., Ferguson, T. B., and Burford, T. H.: Chylothorax. Ann. Thorac. Surg., 12:527, 1971; and Light, R. W.: Pleural Diseases. Philadelphia, Lea & Febiger, 1983.

ence of empyema. IgE should be determined for suspected paragonimiasis; carcinoembryonic antigen for suspected adenocarcinoma; lactic acid dehydrogenase as an indicator of the severity of pleural inflammation; complement, rheumatoid factor, and LE cells for suspected systemic lupus erythematosus and rheumatoid arthritis; lipid analysis for a diagnosis of chylothorax; and countercurrent immunoelectrophoresis for a diagnosis of *Streptococcus pneumoniae, Staphylococcus aureus,* or *Haemophilus influenzae* in children.[25]

Often a specific diagnosis cannot be made from pleural fluid alone, despite cultures and smears for pathogenic organisms and cell blocks for tumor cells. Biopsy by needle or trephine may be expected to yield a specific diagnosis in fewer than half of the cases in which it is attempted (Fig. 3).[20] A small open thoracotomy may be necessary for a definitive diagnosis, to allow the surgeon to inspect both the visceral and the parietal pleura as well as the lung and to select the most promising areas for biopsy. Decortication of the lung, if indicated, may also be ac-

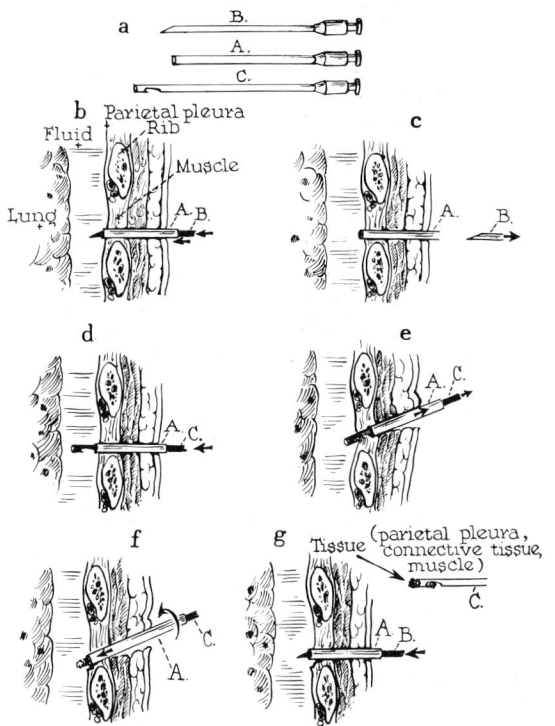

Figure 3. Diagrams illustrating methods of obtaining a pleural biopsy using the Cope needle. (From Levine, H., and Cugell, D. W.: Blunt-end needle biopsy of pleura and rib. Arch. Intern. Med., *109*:516, 1962.)

complished after enlargement of the incision. Thoracoscopy may still have a place in the definitive diagnosis of pleural effusions.[46]

Pleural effusions may occur from subdiaphragmatic or intra-abdominal processes, such as subphrenic or hepatic abscesses, cirrhosis of the liver, nephritis, pancreatitis, or ovarian fibroma. This last combination is called Meigs' syndrome.[30] Whether passage of fluid from the peritoneal into the pleural cavities occurs through the lymphatics or through recognized or unrecognized openings in the diaphragms is a matter of debate.

Thoracentesis is best done after careful localization of the effusion by roentgenograms in frontal, lateral, or oblique planes, or by the use of the fluoroscopic image intensifier. A syringe no larger than 20 ml., with a three-way stopcock interposed between needle and syringe, affords the most satisfactory control. After thorough infiltration of skin, intercostal muscle, and parietal pleura with a local anesthetic agent, the needle of appropriate caliber and length is directed just above the superior border of the lower rib of the appropriate interspace. It is allowed to penetrate the parietal pleura until fluid is reached, with constant moderate negative pressure applied to the syringe. During aspiration low in the costophrenic sinus, the needle tip should be directed cephalad to avoid puncture of the diaphragm. One may place a clamp on the needle at the level of the skin to prevent further penetration and thus avoid injuring the lung after the appropriate depth has been reached. The removal of all available fluid usually presents no difficulty unless a massive acute effusion is being completely evacuated. Under these circumstances, pain, discomfort, and severe coughing may be initiated in some instances. Rarely, transient unilateral pulmonary edema may occur. Thus, it may be wiser to evacuate no more than 1500 ml. of a massive effusion at the initial attempt.[42]

"Spontaneous" Pneumothorax

The accumulation of air in the pleural cavity without any apparent antecedent event, so-called *spontaneous pneumothorax*, is almost always due to rupture of a subpleural cyst, bleb,

or bulla, often in an otherwise apparently normal lung in a young adult (20 to 40 years of age), usually a male cigarette smoker (Fig. 4). The shape and dimensions of the chest cage may have a role in the occurrence of this condition.[34] However, it can also occur in the neonate, in whom vigorous resuscitative efforts may result in a pneumothorax, or in the elderly and emphysematous patient, in whom it may pose a very serious problem.[6] Occasionally, primary or metastatic tumor may be found in association with pneumothorax. Hemorrhage (hemopneumothorax) may accompany collapse of the lung due to a torn vascular adhesion and may be severe enough to warrant emergency thoracotomy for control.

Symptoms depend upon the degree of collapse of the lung and on its previous condition. There may be no symptoms whatsoever, or severe dyspnea, hypoxemia, and even shock may be observed. Chest pain may be prominent or absent. Hyperresonance and absent or diminished breath sounds are the characteristic physical findings.

The diagnosis is usually apparent from the roentgenogram of the chest. A film taken in expiration may help demonstrate a small pneumothorax more readily; appropriate laminagrams of the lung may aid in the differentiation of localized pneumothorax from a large, thin-walled pulmonary cyst or pneumatocele.

Treatment depends upon a variety of factors. An initial, small (5 to 20 per cent) asymptomatic pneumothorax may safely be kept under observation. Reabsorption of the pneumothorax is facilitated by the administration of supplemental oxygen, which, by lowering the pN_2 of capillary blood, increases the partial pressure difference between the pleural space and the pulmonary capillary. Intercostal tube thoracostomy with a closed drainage system is adequate for most patients with large pneumothoraces (Fig. 5).[45] Prevention of recurrences is said to be favored by keeping the tube in place for several days to foster a sterile pleuritis. Gentle suction on the catheter facilitates expansion of the lung. If air leakage persists or is larger than can be managed by a high-volume vacuum system, if the episode is a recurrent one, or if obvious bullae or cysts are seen in the collapsed lung, open thoracotomy is advocated, with suturing, ligation, or excision of the ruptured bleb or bulla and vigorous abrasion of especially the parietal, but also the visceral, pleura. This produces filmy adhesions and helps prevent recurrences. Excision of the parietal pleural is advocated by some, but the consensus is against its use as being unnecessary, more traumatic, and associated with a higher complication rate.[10] Subsequent thoracotomy, if it should become necessary, is rendered

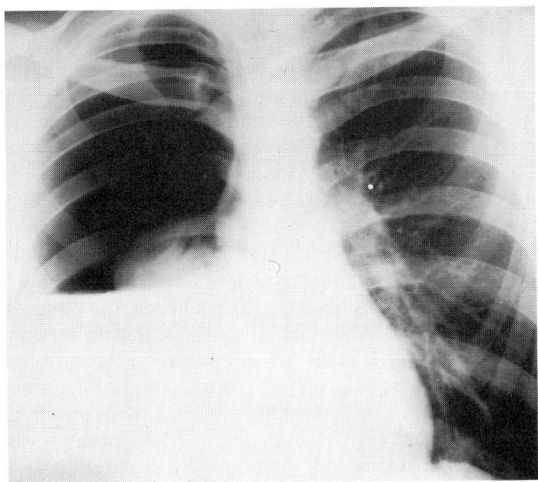

Figure 4. Thoracic roentgenogram illustrating spontaneous hemopneumothorax in a 22-year-old man. This was treated by closed-tube thoracostomy, and it responded with prompt and complete re-expansion of the lung. The etiology was undetermined.

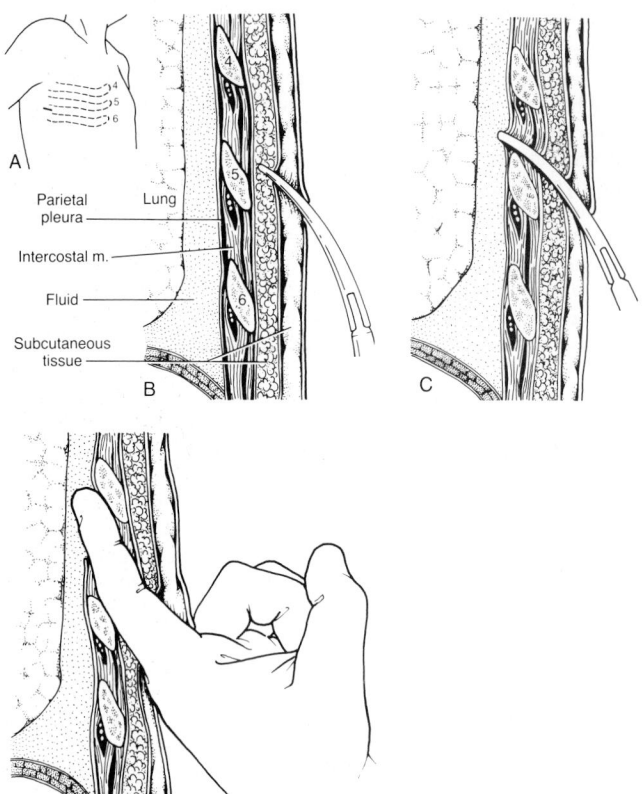

Parietal pleura
Lung
Intercostal m.
Fluid
Subcutaneous tissue

Figure 5. Insertion of a chest tube. *A*, Incision over intercostal space. *B*, Development of subcutaneous tract. *C*, Penetration of parietal pleura. *D*, Confirmation that lung is not adherent to the chest wall at the puncture site. (From Symbas, P. N.: Cardiothoracic Trauma. Philadelphia, W. B. Saunders Company, 1989.)

more difficult if an infectious process, such as tuberculosis, is present.

In tension pneumothorax, intrapleural pressures on one or both sides may rise precipitously. This is due to a valvelike mechanism that allows air to enter the pleural spaces from the lung parenchyma or airway during brief episodes of markedly elevated airway pressure, as occurs during cough. Because of collapse of the lung and shift of the mediastinum, severe respiratory distress may develop, requiring emergency needle aspiration followed by tube thoracostomy drainage. Physical findings of hyperresonance, absent breath sounds, and mediastinal shift away from the involved side are diagnostic.

Spontaneous pneumothorax, and especially tension pneumothorax, in the emphysematous patient with marginal respiratory function and cor pulmonale may present a grave problem in management. Monitoring of blood gases and the electrocardiogram, assisted ventilation, tracheostomy, appropriate cardiac drugs, multiple closed thoracotomies, and open thoracotomy may all be necessary. In one series from the Mayo Clinic, 10 of 57 such patients died, 5 before adequate therapy could be instituted.[6] Two of eleven succumbed following thoracotomy. The prognosis in the average patient with pneumothorax, however, is very good, with few recurrences if a sterile pleuritis has been successfully produced by closed-tube thoracostomy.[45]

Pneumothorax may occur in patients requiring mechanical ventilatory support (e.g., patients who have had cardiac surgery). This is more likely to occur in patients with emphysema, or cystic or cavitary disease of the lung. High airway pressures and positive end-expiratory pressure (PEEP) should be used with caution in these patients.[16]

Rarely, as with pleural effusions, rapid re-expansion of a complete pneumothorax using high negative pressure can be followed by ipsilateral pulmonary edema. A slower decompres-

sion, using lesser negative pressure, might obviate this complication.[17]

Closed pleural drainage systems should be simple but may be more complex, depending upon the particular clinical problem. Of primary importance is an understanding of the characteristics of the system used both by the responsible physician and by the attending nursing staff. When little or no continuing air escape is expected, and only fluid drainage is required, a simple underwater seal apparatus, or only a rubber flutter valve with a plastic bag arrangement, is adequate.[14] In the past, a "two-bottle" system, with the first bottle being a dry trap, provided a separate reservoir for collection of fluid in addition to the underwater seal, but this added to the volume of "dead space" between the pleural space and the water-seal surface. In small patients this may be of significance. When air leaks are expected, more complicated systems with active suction are recommended.[9] The large glass bottles with rubber stoppers and glass tubes have been replaced in most institutions with compact plastic drainage sets that require less space and are less likely to be damaged (Fig. 6). These sets may be used as simple underwater seals, or they can be attached to a vacuum source if needed. They are made with three plastic compartments that replace the three glass bottles. The first reservoir is a collecting chamber; the second, a water seal; and the third, a vacuum regulator with a long tube open to air and extending under water the specific distance that corresponds to the maximal negative suction in centimeters of water required (20 to 40 cm. H_2O).

Very strong suction has been advocated by some following pulmonary resections. Either a wall vacuum source or a high air-flow capacity, electrically driven turbine type of pump is effective.[9] Pumps with a low air-flow capacity should not be used when large air leaks, either continuous or intermittent (as

Underwater Seal Drainage System

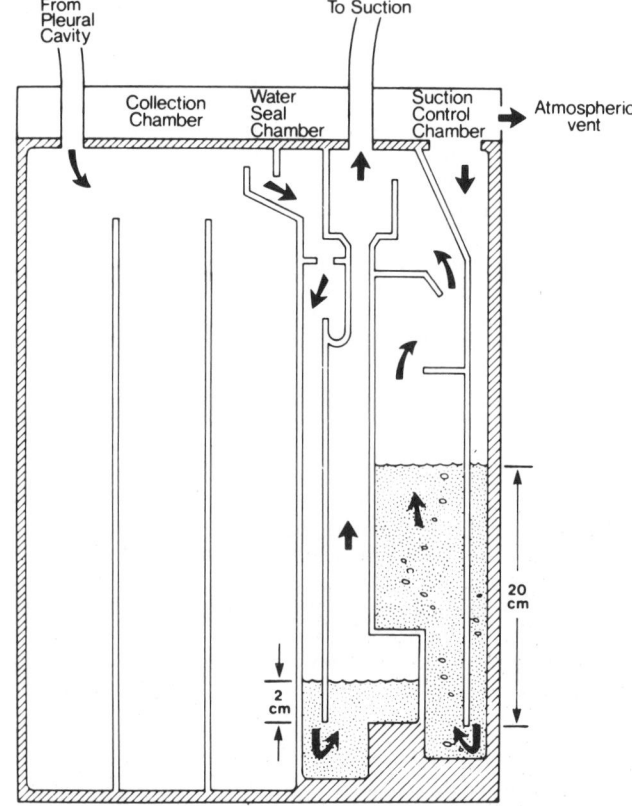

From Pleural Cavity
To Suction
Collection Chamber
Water Seal Chamber
Suction Control Chamber
Atmospheric vent
20 cm
2 cm

Figure 6. A commercial apparatus for chest drainage. (From Symbas, P. N.: Cardiothoracic Trauma. Philadelphia, W. B. Saunders Company, 1989.)

during coughing), may be expected. The drainage system should function to prevent ingress of air into the pleural cavity even when the vacuum source fails. It is equally important that the system allow egress of large volumes of air suddenly, whether the vacuum source is functioning or not. Time spent in understanding the physiologic and physical principles of pleural drainage systems and in communicating this understanding to attending nurses will be well spent.[9,41]

Hemothorax

An accumulation of blood in the pleural cavities (hemothorax) may result from trauma to the chest wall, the lung, the mediastinal structures, or the diaphragm. It may also be found with pulmonary infarction, pleural or pulmonary neoplasm, or following tearing of a pleural adhesion, as with spontaneous pneumothorax. It may occur as a complication of anticoagulant therapy. Hemothorax following thoracic surgery is also common. Partial defibrination of the blood may occur with deposition of fibrin on the pleural surface. A sterile hemothorax may be completely reabsorbed.[47] An infected hemothorax or hemothoracic empyema, however, can lead to the development of a fibrothorax, with serious compromise of pulmonary function. This is more likely after war wounds and gunshot wounds with underlying lung damage; it is less likely after a clean stab wound.[7] A hemopneumothorax is more likely to be followed by such a complication than is a hemothorax alone.

The management of hemothorax depends upon the rate of bleeding and the total volume bled as well as the underlying cause. If the hemothorax is small and bleeding has ceased, judged by clinical signs and serial roentgenograms, only observation is required. For moderate amounts of estimated blood accumulation (500 ml. or more), a closed thoracostomy with intercostal tube drainage for complete evacuation of blood allows observation of its reaccumulation plus re-expansion of the lung, and is preferable to needle aspiration. Continuing active bleeding (200 ml. per hour or more), as judged on serial thoracic roentgenograms, clinical signs, or output from chest tubes, demands open thoracotomy for control of hemorrhage. Massive bleeding such as from an intrathoracic vascular injury, may require rigorous blood volume replacement. Because blood in the pleural space tends to be defibrinated and slow to clot, it can be collected in a sterile drainage system and reinfused into the patient.[18] Postoperative bleeding may cease upon re-exploration and removal of blood clots, even if no active bleeding point is found.

To prevent the development of an imprisoning fibrothorax and to gain re-expansion of lung compressed by blood, some advocate early evacuation of clotted hemothorax or decortication, or both.[28] The fibrinous deposit peels off the visceral pleura readily (within 3 weeks of injury), and pulmonary expansibility can be restored. However, one should not resort to thoracotomy precipitously, since an uncomplicated hemothorax in most instances can be completely absorbed.[47]

Chylothorax

Chylothorax, or chyle in the pleural cavity, is most commonly due to trauma or tumor. The thin, fibromuscular thoracic duct, which transports chyle along the length of the mediastinum from the cysterna chyli to the left subclavian vein, may be ruptured anywhere along its course. Rupture above the fifth or sixth thoracic vertebra generally results in left-sided chylothorax; injury below that level often results in a right-sided collection. Because of excellent collateral pathways, the duct can be ligated with impunity.

Owing to the high fat and protein content of the milky white chyle (which are aids in diagnosis), loss of this material into the pleural cavity can be a serious matter from a nutritional standpoint. The large volume of the effusion may also cause severe respiratory embarrassment. The diagnosis may be confirmed by lymphangiography, and the location of the thoracic duct (although not the site of the rupture) may also thus be identified.

Chylothorax is readily distinguished from chyliform pleural effusion or pseudochylothorax by examining the milky pleural fluid for cholesterol crystals, which are absent in chylothorax. Pseudochylothorax occurs in long-standing pleural effusions and most often is due to rheumatoid pleuritis or tuberculosis.[25]

Of chylothorax due to traumatic causes, 80 per cent of cases are due to gunshot wounds, automobile accidents, stab wounds, and blunt trauma; 20 per cent are iatrogenic, mostly postsurgical and usually following operations for congenital cardiovascular abnormalities.[22] Conservative therapy includes decompression of the thoracic lymphatics (either by parenteral hyperalimentation or by oral medium-chain triglycerides),[21] as well as decompression of the pleural space (by thoracentesis and intercostal tube drainage).[1,22] If, after 3 to 4 weeks, chylothorax persists (most often as a result of malignancy), talc pleurodesis may be attempted.[1] Open thoracotomy is used if conservative treatment fails. Ligation of the thoracic duct at the site of leakage (if it can be identified with the aid of a fatty meal ingested just before surgical therapy) or low in the mediastinum, below the level of the eighth thoracic vertebra, should be effective when conservative treatment fails.[33] For adults with malignancies, surgical intervention may not be effective; in traumatic cases and in infants, operation will usually be unnecessary. When conservative management of chylothorax in infants fails, a pleuroperitoneal shunt can be attempted.[29]

EMPYEMA

Pleural empyema is a collection of purulent fluid in the pleural space (Fig. 7). It may be localized (encapsulated), or it may involve the entire pleural cavity. Empyemas are classified by some workers as "acute" or "chronic," depending upon duration and pathologic reaction, but there is no sharp division in either time or pathologic response between the two. A more informative but less popular differentiation among the stages of empyema may be that proposed by the American Thoracic Society. Exudative empyemas are characterized by thin fluid with low cellular content and an underlying lung that will re-expand readily. Fibrinopurulent empyemas are characterized by large numbers of polymorphonuclear leukocytes and by deposition of fibrin on both the visceral and the parietal surfaces of the involved pleura. In this transitional phase between "acute" and "chronic" empyema, there is a progressive tendency toward

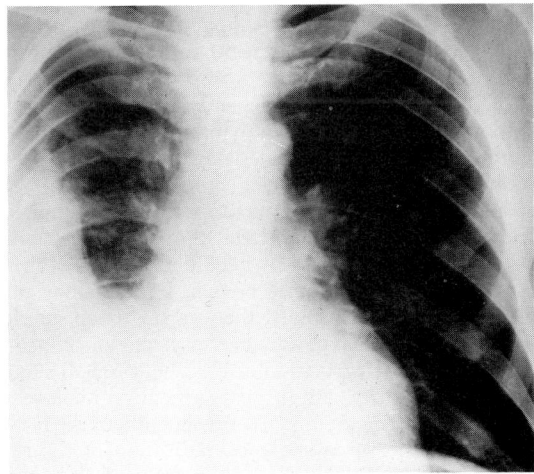

Figure 7. Roentgenogram of thoracic empyema of 2 months' duration, from which anaerobic streptococci and gram-negative *Bacteroides* bacilli were isolated. This patient was treated by open drainage following resection of a 2-inch segment of the seventh rib. The right lung re-expanded completely, and the empyema space was obliterated in approximately 2 weeks.

loculation and delimitation of the extent of the empyema space, accompanied by initial fixation of the lung. In organizing empyemas, fibroblasts appear in the now heavier fibrin coating of the pleural membranes, and the exudate is quite thick. Upon standing, over 75 to 80 per cent of the fluid consists of sediment. These distinctions are important because therapy differs with stage of the disease.

Despite antibiotics, there was an impressive increase in the incidence of both staphylococcal pneumonia and empyema in children in the late 1950s.[40] Such recrudescences of infections can be expected again.[42] Today, because of the increasing age and debility of patients with empyema who have underlying serious illness, this disease may still pose serious problems of diagnosis and management.[11] The incidence of hospital-acquired empyemas appears to be increasing.[11]

ETIOLOGY. Acute empyemas ordinarily result from primary disease elsewhere. Most commonly, the primary condition is a pneumonic process in the underlying lung, such as lobar pneumonia, pneumonitis, or lung abscess.[23] This may extend to the pleura directly, or by way of the lymphatics, or by hematogenous spread, or by rupture of necrotic pulmonary parenchyma. The pneumonic process may itself be secondary to other conditions, such as bronchial obstruction due to bronchogenic carcinoma or foreign body in an airway, or to bronchial infection, as seen in bronchiectasis. A ruptured emphysematous bleb with spontaneous pneumothorax may also occasionally result in an empyema. Less commonly, the source of infection may be a mediastinal structure, such as the trachea or bronchi (bronchopleural fistula); or the esophagus (perforation, leaking esophagogastric anastomosis); or an abscessed lymph node; or osteomyelitis of the dorsal spine. Subphrenic or intrahepatic abscesses may spread via the rich lymphatics of the diaphragm to cause empyema. Finally, infection may be introduced into the pleural spaces from without, for example, by trauma, needle aspiration, or operation. Chronic empyemas result from untreated or inadequately treated acute empyemas. This development should be prevented if possible. Empyema necessitatis, an encapsulated empyema discharging into the subcutaneous tissues of the chest wall, is now rarely reported but still occurs.

The most common bacteriologic agents formerly responsible for empyemas—the pneumococci and streptococci—have been displaced in importance and frequency in recent years by *Staphylococcus aureus*, *Streptococcus*, and a variety of gram-negative organisms: *Pseudomonas*, *Klebsiella pneumoniae*, *Escherichia coli*, *Aerobacter aerogenes*, *Proteus*, *Bacteroides*, and *Salmonella*. Anaerobic flora are common, *Bacteroides* especially, and usually occur in mixed flora. Special techniques are needed for identification.[16,23,43] Tuberculous empyema is now uncommon except in hospitals with large indigent populations or hospitals having a large number of immunocompromised patients.[16]

DIAGNOSIS. The diagnosis depends upon the detection of signs and symptoms of the underlying infectious process and the accumulation of purulent material in the pleural cavity. This is supported and localized by the clinical examination of the patient and the roentgenographic appearance of fluid, or of fluid and air, or of a pleural or interlobar opacification compatible with fluid. It is confirmed by needle aspiration of the empyema with the demonstration of pus. Bacteria may not be identified if intensive antibiotic therapy has been employed previously or if the etiologic agent is not bacterial.

TREATMENT. The objectives of treatment for all stages of empyema are (1) control of the primary infection and its secondary manifestation, the empyema; (2) evacuation of the purulent contents of the empyema sac and eradication of the sac, to prevent chronicity; and (3) re-expansion of the underlying lung in order to restore function. The methods used to achieve these objectives depend upon the stage of empyema being treated and the nature of the primary infection or source of contamination. These objectives are realized by the use of appropriate antibiotic therapy, based upon the bacteriologic diagnosis, and by prompt and adequate drainage.

Needle aspiration of an empyema at the time thoracentesis done for diagnosis may be all that is necessary if the pus is the very thin variety that is seen with streptococcal infections. Examination of the pus will reveal a pH above 7.20, a glucose above 40 mg. per 100 ml., and a lactate dehydrogenase (LDH) concentration below 1000 I.U. per liter.

An *intercostal tube* for closed drainage should be employed promptly if the purulent fluid is thick and therefore cannot be completely evacuated by thoracenteses, if the fluid reaccumulates, or if infection and toxicity are difficult to control. Thoracentesis or intercostal tube drainage is adequate for most children with empyema associated with staphylococcal pneumonia.[40] When intercostal tube drainage is elected, negative pressure may have to be applied to hasten pulmonary expansion, especially in the presence of bronchopleural fistula. The tube should be of a generous caliber commensurate with the material being evacuated and should not be permitted to become occluded. It should be placed in the most dependent part of the empyema pocket, with care to avoid perforation of the diaphragm. Accurate localization is greatly facilitated by the use of biplane roentgenograms of the chest or a fluoroscopic image intensifier. More than one tube may be necessary. Malecot or right-angle catheters, which can be inserted directly through a small incision and pulled flush with the parietal wall of the pleural cavity, are preferred by some surgeons.

Resection of a short segment of rib is necessary if the pus is thick and loculated or if the patient remains toxic after intercostal tube drainage. This technique provides adequate exposure, allowing one to evacuate the pus, break up loculations and adhesions, and assess the need for decortication. After washing the cavity, a tube may be placed in its most dependent portion and attached to underwater seal drainage. *Open drainage* may be necessary, in which case a wide-bore tube should be left in place, open to atmospheric pressure.[16,23,32] Another variation, the Eloesser skin flap, originally designed for tuberculous empyema, combines some of the virtues of open and closed drainage and eliminates the need for wide-bore tubes open to air.[8] With open drainage, the appropriate most dependent site must be carefully localized roentgenographically or fluoroscopically, and by repeated exploratory thoracenteses, before the rib is resected. The drainage tube is removed only when the empyema sac has been eliminated, as determined by measurement of its capacity, or radiographically, after introduction of contrast material.

In some instances, *decortication* will achieve the goals of therapy more efficiently than open drainage. This is more likely to be true in managing infected or noninfected hemothoraces, in which the lung has become imprisoned by its nonelastic fibrinopurulent coat but presumably remains expandable, and the patient is not toxic. Decortication may follow closed-tube drainage. Although advocated by some as primary treatment for empyema, it is used by others only under unusual circumstances, as in immunosuppressed patients.[12] Even here, closed drainage is usually used as a preliminary step. The exact place of decortication in the treatment of empyema has not been clearly defined. Infrequently, conventional thoracoplasty to obliterate the pleural space or Schede thoracoplasty to unroof an empyema pocket may be necessary. The use of skin flap open drainage or pedicled muscle flaps may be needed for complicated problems involving bronchopleural-cutaneous fistulas if simple open drainage fails to obliterate an empyema.

Approximately 25 per cent of all empyemas follow thoracic surgical procedures, most commonly pneumonectomy. An empyema may or may not be associated with a bronchopleural fistula. If a bronchopleural fistula occurs within the first week following operation, it is probably technical in origin, and an attempt should be made to close the fistula with a muscle flap.

The pleural space then should be irrigated with antibiotics. A bronchopleural fistula late in onset is most likely associated with residual tumor or some condition predisposing to poor healing, and open drainage likely will be necessary. Treatment of empyema following pneumonectomy has altered in recent years, with the observation that elimination of the empyema space is not necessary if it can be sterilized and if there is no underlying bronchopleural or esophagopleural fistula.[4] It can be accomplished in a variety of ways, involving instillation of a solution of antibiotics, with or without débridement of the lining of the empyema cavity.[35,36]

PLEURAL TUMORS

These are classified as primary and secondary. Primary pleural tumors are mostly mesotheliomas, of which localized benign and diffuse malignant types are recognized.[15] In both types, fibrous or fibrosarcomatous and epithelioid varieties are seen. Mixtures of the two histologic varieties also occur. Therefore, the pathologic classification of benign versus malignant as well as the differentiation from carcinoma is sometimes difficult.

Patients with localized fibrous mesotheliomas may be asymptomatic, or they may complain of symptoms of arthralgia, clubbing of the fingers, or fever.[31] Associated hypoglycemia also has been observed.[26] The solitary, often encapsulated, pedunculated, and usually easily removable tumor ordinarily arises from the visceral pleura. When it is excised, the symptoms and signs of arthralgia and pulmonary osteoarthropathy usually disappear, and longevity seems to be unaffected. These tumors may range in size from a few centimeters to 20 cm. or more in diameter.

Diffuse or malignant mesotheliomas, however, cause chest pain and bloody pleural effusion containing malignant mesothelial cells. These tumors are characterized by findings ranging from multiple papillary projections on both visceral and parietal pleurae to encasement of the entire lung in a thick rind of tumor, with similar findings on the parietal side. Part or all of the pleural space may be obliterated. Metastases are uncommon, except late in the disease, and are often limited to the regional lymph nodes. Extrathoracic metastases do occur, however. Death within 1 or 2 years generally occurs in most patients.

The evidence for a causal relationship between exposure to asbestos dust and the development of malignant mesothelioma is strong. It is based on occupational exposure, with a high incidence of both pleural mesothelioma and bronchogenic carcinoma in asbestos workers and those exposed to asbestos.[5]

Treatment of malignant mesothelioma has been unsatisfactory. There have been no cures. Palliation and a small number of long-term survivals have been achieved by "complete" pleurectomy or pleuropneumonectomy, but the great majority of patients have succumbed within 1 or 2 years of the diagnosis, regardless of the type of treatment used.[24] Radiation and chemotherapy, or combined treatment, is recommended if excisional surgery is impossible or incomplete. However, only a few of these treatment modalities have been studied in a systemic way.

Pleural involvement by metastatic disease is far more common than primary pleural tumor and is usually associated with implants involving the lung or with blockage of or interference with the lymphatic drainage of the visceral, parietal, diaphragmatic, or mediastinal pleura. The most common sites of primary tumor are the lung, breast, pancreas, and stomach. With direct involvement of the pleura by tumor implants, bloody fluid containing neoplastic cells can often be obtained. Various types of palliative treatment are advocated, depending upon the site of the primary tumor, the expansibility of the lung, the degree of disability from pleural effusion, and so forth.[37] Hormonal therapy, radiation or radioisotope therapy, multiple aspirations of the chest, closed-tube thoracostomy, and the insufflation of talc or the instillation of chemotherapeutic agents (especially quinacrine and tetracycline)[2] have all been reported, with varying degrees of palliation being achieved.[27] Pleurectomy is the most effective, but mortality (10 per cent) and morbidity (20 per cent) dictate careful patient selection.

SELECTED REFERENCES

Barrett, N. R.: The pleura — with special reference to fibrothorax. Thorax, 24:515, 1970.
The Tudor Edwards Memorial Lecture, 1970; Thoughts, observations, and interpretations that present a fresh insight into the structure and function of the pleura in health and disease.

Eloesser, L.: Milestones in chest surgery. J. Thorac. Cardiovasc. Surg., 60:157, 1970.
A brief but fascinating account of major landmarks in the development of thoracic and cardiovascular surgery, from Sauerbruch's chamber to Gibbon's pump-oxygenator.

Hillerdal, G.: Malignant mesothelioma 1982: Review of 4710 published cases. Br. J. Dis. Chest, 77:321, 1983.
A survey of the literature and an objective appraisal of current methods of management.

Hood, R. M., Antman, K., Boyd, A., Naidich, D., and Shemin, R.: Surgical Diseases of the Pleura and Chest Wall. Philadelphia, W. B. Saunders Company, 1986.
Recommended for a more detailed description of the surgical management of diseases of the pleura. Excellent illustrations of surgical techniques.

Light, R. W.: Pleural Diseases. Philadelphia, Lea & Febiger, 1983.
The most complete exposition to date on pleural diseases. An excellent reference for both the student and the experienced clinician.

REFERENCES

1. Adler, R. H., and Levinsky, L.: Persistent chylothorax: Treatment by talc pleurodesis. J. Thorac. Cardiovasc. Surg., 76:859, 1978.
2. Bayly, T. C., Kisner, D. L., Sybert, A., MacDonald, J. S., Tsou, E., and Schein, P. S.: Tetracycline and quinacrine in the control of malignant pleural effusions. Cancer, 41:1188, 1978.
3. Brock, L.: Evarts A. Graham: Recollections. Ann. Thorac. Surg., 9:272, 1970.
4. Clagett, O. T., and Geraci, J. E.: A procedure for the management of postpneumonectomy empyema. J. Thorac. Cardiovasc. Surg., 45:141, 1963.
5. Craighead, J. E., Abraham, J. L., Churg, A., Green, F. H. Y., Kleinerman, J., Pratt, P. C., Seemayer, T. A., Vallyathan, V., and Weill, H.: The pathology of asbestos-associated diseases of the lungs and pleural cavities: Diagnostic criteria and proposed grading schema. Arch. Pathol. Lab. Med., 106:544, 1982.
6. Dines, D. E., Clagett, O. T., and Payne, W. S.: Spontaneous pneumothorax in emphysema. Mayo Clin. Proc., 45:481, 1970.
7. Drummond, D. S., and Craig, R. H.: Traumatic hemothorax: Complications and management. Am. Surg., 33:403, 1967.
8. Eloesser, L.: Of an operation for tuberculous empyema. Ann. Thorac. Surg., 8:355, 1969.
9. Enerson, D. M., and McIntire, J.: A comparative study of the physiology and physics of pleural drainage systems. J. Thorac Cardiovasc. Surg., 52:40, 1966.
10. Ferguson, L. J., Imrie, C. W., and Hutchison, J.: Excision of bullae without pleurectomy in patients with spontaneous pneumothorax. Br. J. Surg., 68:214, 1981.
11. Finland, M., and Barnes, M. W.: Changing ecology of acute bacterial empyema: Occurrence and mortality at Boston City Hospital during 12 selected years from 1935–1972. J. Infect. Dis., 137:274, 1978.
12. Fishman, N. H., and Ellerston, D. G.: Early pleural decortication for thoracic empyema in immunosuppressed patients. J. Thorac. Cardiovasc. Surg., 74:537, 1977.
13. Good, J. T., Jr., Taryle, D. A., Maulitz, R. M., Kaplan, R. L., and Sahn, S. A.: The diagnostic value of pleural fluid pH. Chest, 78:55, 1980.
14. Heimlich, H. J.: Valve drainage of the pleural cavity. Dis. Chest, 53:282, 1968.
15. Hillerdal, G.: Malignant mesothelioma 1982: Review of 4710 published cases. Br. J. Dis. Chest, 77:321, 1983.
16. Hood, R. M., Antman, K., Boyd, A., Naidich, D., and Shemin, R.: Surgical Diseases of the Pleura and Chest Wall. Philadelphia, W. B. Saunders Company, 1986.
17. Humphreys, R. L., and Berne, A. S.: Rapid re-expansion of pneumothorax. Radiology, 96:509, 1970.
18. Jacobs, L. M., and Hsieh, J. W.: A clinical review of autotransfusion and its role in trauma. J.A.M.A., 251:3283, 1984.
19. Jurivich, D. A.: Iatrogenic pleural effusions. South. Med., J., 81:1417, 1988.
20. Kettel, L. J., and Cugell, D. W.: Pleural biopsy. J.A.M.A., 200:317, 1967.
21. Kosloske, A. M., Martin, L. W., and Schubert, W. K.: Management of chylothorax in children by thoracentesis and medium-chain triglyceride feedings. J. Pediatr. Surg., 9:365, 1974.
22. Kostiainen, S., Meurala, H., Mattila, S., and Appelqvist, P.: Chylothorax.

Clinical experience in nine cases. Scand. J. Thor. Cardiovasc. Surg., *17*:79, 1983.

23. Lemmer, J. H., Botham, M. J., and Orringer, M. B.: Modern management of adult thoracic empyema. J. Thorac. Cardiovasc. Surg., *90*:849, 1985.

24. Lewis, R. J., Sisler, G. E., and Mackenzie, J. W.: Diffuse, malignant pleural mesothelioma. Ann. Thorac. Surg., *31*:53, 1981.

25. Light, R. W.: Pleural Diseases. Philadelphia, Lea & Febiger, 1983.

26. Mandal, A. K., Rozer, M. A., Salem, F. A., and Oparah, S. S.: Localized benign mesothelioma of the pleura associated with a hypoglycemic episode. Arch. Intern. Med., *143*:1608, 1983.

27. Meyer, P. C.: Metastatic carcinoma of the pleura. Thorax, *21*:437, 1966.

28. Milfeld, D. J., Mattox, K. L., and Beall, A. C.: Early evacuation of clotted hemothorax. Am. J. Surg., *136*:686, 1978.

29. Murphy, M. C., Newman, B. M., and Rodgers, B. M.: Pleuroperitoneal shunts in the management of persistent chylothorax. Ann. Thorac. Surg., *48*:195, 1989.

30. Neustadt, J. E., and Levy, R. C.: Hemorrhagic pleural effusion in Meigs' syndrome. J.A.M.A., *204*:81, 1968.

31. Okike, N., Bernatz, P. E., and Woolner, L. B.: Localized mesothelioma of the pleura; Benign and malignant variants. J. Thorac. Cardiovasc. Surg., *75*:363, 1978.

32. Orringer, M. B.: Thoracic empyema—back to basics. Chest, *93*:901, 1988.

33. Patterson, G. A., Todd, T. R. J., Delarue, N. C., Ilves, R., Pearson, F. G., and Cooper, J. D.: Supradiaphragmatic ligation of the thoracic duct in intractable chylous fistula. Ann. Thorac. Surg., *32*:44, 1981.

34. Peters, R. M., Benirschke, B. A., and Friedman, P. J.: Chest dimensions in young adults with spontaneous pneumothorax. Ann. Thorac. Surg., *25*:193, 1978.

35. Provan, J. L.: Management of postpneumonectomy empyema. J. Thorac. Cardiovasc. Surg., *61*:107, 1971.

36. Rosenfeldt, F. L., McGibney, D., Braimbridge, M. V., and Watson, D. A.: Comparison between irrigation and conventional treatment for empyema and pneumonectomy space infection. Thorax, *36*:272, 1981.

37. Ruckdeschel, J. C.: Management of malignant pleural effusion: An overview. Semin. Oncol., *15*:24, 1988.

38. Sahn, S. A.: The pleura. Am. Rev. Respir. Dis., *138*:184, 1988.

39. Stewart, P. B.: The rate of formation and lymphatic removal of fluid in pleural effusion. J. Clin. Invest., *42*:258, 1963.

40. Stiles, Q. R., Lindesmith, G. G., Tucker, B. L., Meyer, B. W., and Jones, J. C.: Pleural empyema in children. Ann. Thorac. Surg. *10*:37, 1970.

41. Symbas, P. N.: Chest drainage tubes. Surg. Clin. North Am., *69*:41, 1989.

42. Trapnell, D. H., and Thurston, J. G. B.: Unilateral pulmonary edema after pleural aspiration. Lancet, *1*:1367, 1970.

43. Varkey, B., Rose, H. D., Kutty, C. P. K., and Politis, J.: Empyema thoracis during a ten-year period: Analysis of 72 cases and comparison to a previous study (1952–1967). Arch. Intern. Med., *141*:1771, 1981.

44. Wang, N. S.: The preformed stomas connecting the pleural cavity and the lymphatics in the parietal pleural. Am. Rev. Respir. Dis., *111*:12, 1975.

45. Watt, A. G.: Spontaneous pneumothorax: A review of 210 consecutive admissions to Royal Perth Hospital. Med. J. Aust., *1*:186, 1978.

46. Weissberg, D., and Kaufman, M.: Diagnostic and therapeutic pleuroscopy. Experience with 127 patients. Chest, *78*:732, 1980.

47. Wilson, J. M., Boren, C. H., Jr., Peterson, S. R., and Thomas, A. N.: Traumatic hemothorax: Is decortication necessary? J. Thorac. Cardiovasc. Surg., *77*:489, 1979.

VIII ———————————————————————————————

BRONCHIECTASIS

Donald D. Glower, M.D.

Although the incidence of bronchiectasis has decreased since the introduction of antibiotics, bronchiectasis continues to have importance for the surgeon. Laennec first described the pathologic findings of bronchiectasis in 1819,[13] and the term *bronchiectasis* was applied by Hasse in 1846.[18] The first successful operation for bronchiectasis was a partial lobe resection performed by Krause in 1898.[16] After Sicard and Forestier introduced bronchography for diagnosis of bronchiectasis in 1922,[22] bronchiectasis became one of the most common diseases treated operatively in the early days of pulmonary surgery. The first successful total pneumonectomy was performed by Nissen in 1931 for bronchiectasis in a child.[17] By 1937, Churchill reported a series of 38 lobectomies for bronchiectasis and cystic disease with a 2.6 per cent mortality.[5] Thereafter, mortality declined to under 1 per cent, and pulmonary resection for bronchiectasis remained a major portion of thoracic surgical practice in the 1950s. Although bronchiectasis has become relatively uncommon since the introduction of antibiotics, surgical therapy still has a role in the treatment of bronchiectasis today.

Etiology

Factors contributing to development of bronchiectasis may be grouped into two categories: congenital and acquired. At least 74 per cent of cases of bronchiectasis can be attributed to acquired causes, specifically airway infection, with impaired clearance of bronchial secretions causing bronchial injury and subsequent bronchiectasis.[10] The infections responsible may be bacterial or viral and include measles, whooping cough, pertussis, adenovirus, and tuberculosis. Bronchial obstruction from mucous obstruction, foreign body, neoplasm, or enlarged peribronchial lymph nodes may produce bronchiectasis of the distal airway. Bronchiectasis is present in up to 39 per cent of patients with chronic right middle lobe infection, or "middle lobe syn-drome," which may involve impaired clearance of secretions secondary to anatomic configuration of the right middle lobe airway, extrinsic airway compression by lymph nodes, or inadequate collateral ventilation.[4] Aspiration, heroin ingestion, and inhalational injury with noxious gases or chemicals may all injure the airway with resultant residual bronchiectasis.

Although congenital bronchiectasis is unusual, several congenital disorders may produce bronchiectasis. Congenital cystic bronchiectasis, with incomplete terminal airways, lack of alveolar tissue, and saccular bronchi, is now considered to be rare and the only truly congenital form of bronchiectasis.[1] In Williams-Campbell syndrome, annular bronchial cartilage is congenitally absent, causing bronchomalacia and bronchiectasis.[25] Genetic abnormalities in Ehlers-Danlos[20] and Mounier-Kuhn syndromes[9] may contribute to tracheobronchomegaly and tracheobronchiectasis. Kartagener's syndrome (bronchiectasis, situs inversus, and sinusitis) represents a genetic disorder with abnormal ciliary motility, impaired mucociliary transport, and resultant bronchiectasis.[6] In either partial or severe alpha$_1$-antitrypsin deficiency, enzyme deficiency may impair clearance of sputum elastase, producing airway damage and bronchiectasis in approximately 10 per cent of patients.[24] Patients with cystic fibrosis have abnormally viscid bronchial secretions and may be predisposed to bronchiectasis owing to impaired clearance of bronchial airways. Intralobar bronchopulmonary sequestration may occasionally be complicated by bronchiectasis.[3] Patients with panhypogammaglobulinemia have a clear predisposition to bronchiectasis, as may patients with other forms of immunodeficiency.[11]

Pathophysiology

Bronchiectasis is defined as persistent, abnormal dilation of the bronchi, generally beyond the subsegmental level (Fig. 1).

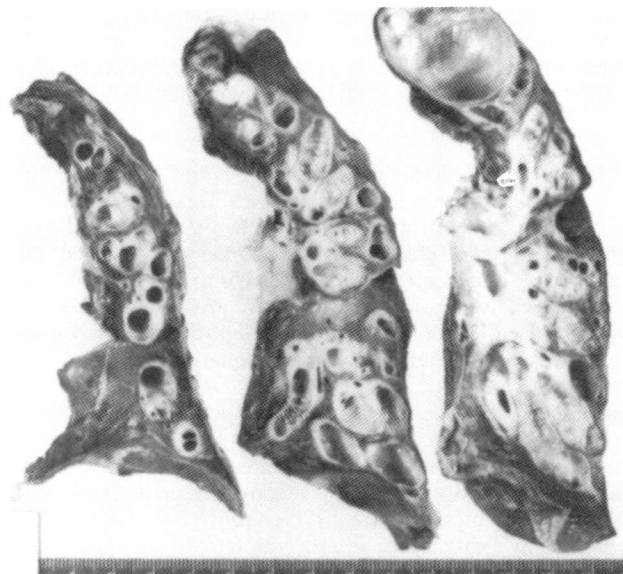

Figure 1. A lung specimen demonstrating grossly dilated subsegmental bronchi caused by bronchiectasis. (From Bolman, R. M., and Wolfe, W. G.: Bronchiectasis and bronchopulmonary sequestration. Surg. Clin. North Am. *60*:867, 1980.)

Reid classified the gross appearance of the bronchi into three types: cylindrical, varicose, and saccular, with the relative frequencies in surgically resected specimens of 27, 62, and 11 per cent, respectively.[19] Early mucosal changes may include thickening, followed later by ulceration, inflammation, and fibrosis. The ultimate result may be bronchiolitis obliterans, with little aeration of the distal alveoli and resultant atelectasis. Surrounding parenchyma is often involved with pneumonitis, and bronchial arteries may be enlarged, with increased collateral blood flow into the pulmonary arteries.

In a review of 3000 bronchograms demonstrating bronchiectasis, LeRoux and associates found the left lung to be involved more often than the right with a ratio of 9 to 7.[14] The left lower lobe was most frequently involved, followed by the right middle lobe, the lingula, the entire left lung, the right lower lobe, the entire right lung, the right upper lobe, and finally the left upper lobe.

Sealy and colleagues demonstrated that patients with bronchiectasis may be divided into two main groups: those with segmental disease and those with multisegmental disease.[21] Patients with bronchiectasis limited to a few isolated segments tended to have symptoms of shorter duration and more often related a clear inciting event, such as pneumonia or bronchial obstruction. Patients with multisegmental disease tended to have a more chronic presentation, often with over 10 years of symptoms. Multisegmental disease was associated with less symptomatic benefit from either medical or surgical therapy.

Clinical Manifestations

In most cases, the onset of bronchiectasis is in childhood, whereas symptoms generally appear in the second or third decades of life.[7,8] There is a female-to-male predominance of up to 2½ to 1.[7,21] Three quarters of the patients complain of a persistent cough productive of purulent sputum,[7,8] with fetor oris often being present and producing social disability in up to 46 per cent of patients.[7] As many as 50 per cent of patients have hemoptysis, which may at times be massive secondary to the intense neovascularity that can be present in the inflamed airways.[3,8,21] Repeated respiratory infection occurs in up to one third of the patients, with half of those relating episodes of pleurisy.[21]

The most common physical findings are audible rales over the involved lung fields, occurring in 55 to 91 per cent of patients.[15,21] Between 5 and 40 per cent of patients present with osteoarthropathy and some degree of clubbing, all of which may resolve entirely with adequate treatment.[14,15]

Diagnosis

A clinical history of chronic, productive cough and repeated respiratory infection should cause one to suspect the diagnosis of bronchiectasis, but distinction from other disorders, such as chronic bronchitis, may be difficult. The plain chest radiograph is abnormal but generally nondiagnostic in up to 90 per cent of patients having bronchiectasis, with common findings of increased lung markings, atelectasis, air fluid levels, or cystic spaces.[14]

The prime standard in diagnosing bronchiectasis is bronchography, which is most commonly performed today with the contrast agent Lipiodol (Fig. 2). Prior to bronchography, pulmonary toilet should be optimized with antibiotics and postural drainage, and any recent exacerbation should be allowed to clear for 4 to 6 weeks prior to bronchography. Reversible bronchodilation is known to occur after pulmonary infection and might otherwise be confused with bronchiectasis. Depending on institutional experience and preference, bronchography may be performed either with local anesthesia or under general anesthesia. Likewise, bronchography may be performed bilaterally or at two different times with each lung being studied individually.

In the initial experience, computed tomography of the chest lacked sensitivity in diagnosing bronchiectasis. However, recent application of high-resolution computed tomography with contiguous sections of 4 mm. or less has demonstrated a sensitivity and specificity of at least 95 per cent (Fig. 3).[12] Owing to its inherent noninvasiveness, computed tomography may assume some of the role of bronchography in screening for bronchiectasis. Bronchography will always be important in surgical candidates to define the bronchial anatomy for potential pulmonary resection.

Bronchoscopy should be performed in search of bronchial obstruction or endobronchial disease and to obtain sputum for culture. Depending upon institutional preference, bronchography may be done immediately after bronchoscopy or at a later date.[14] Bronchoscopy may also have some benefit in obtaining

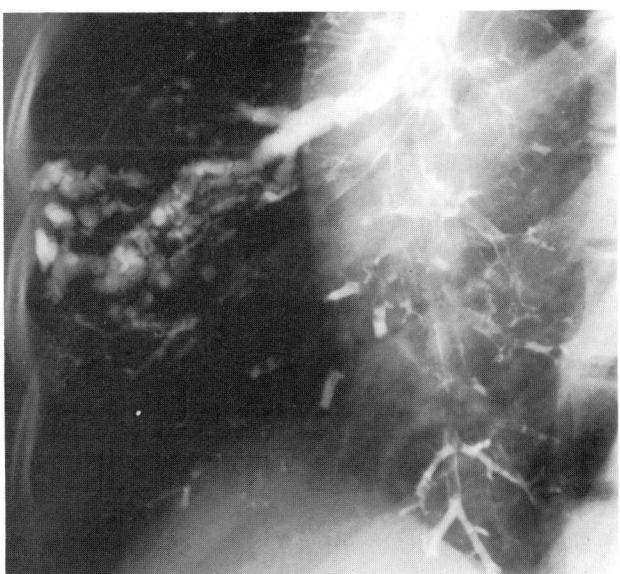

Figure 2. A bronchogram demonstrating saccular bronchiectasis of the right middle lobe in an 18-year-old woman.

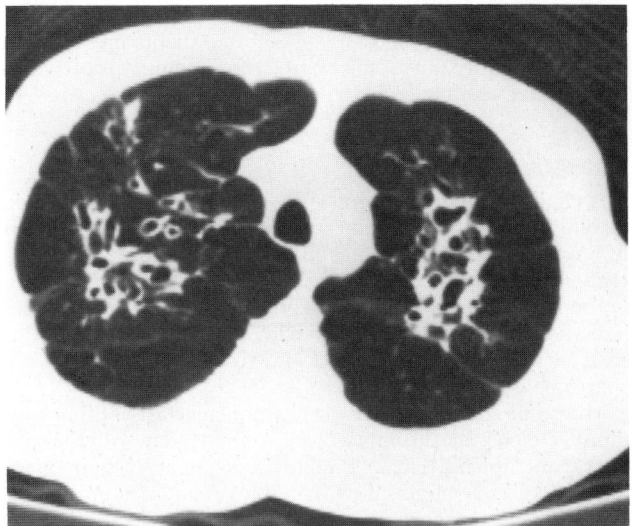

Figure 3. Computed tomogram of the chest in a 30-year-old man with multisegmental bronchiectasis involving both lungs. Note the abnormally dilated airways extending into the lung parenchyma bilaterally.

good tracheobronchial toilet. In general, however, bronchoscopic findings are not diagnostic of bronchiectasis.[14]

Additional diagnostic procedures of potential use in bronchiectasis include sinus radiographs seeking evidence of sinusitis that may require treatment. Although pulmonary function tests in bronchiectasis generally do not demonstrate more than mild airway obstruction,[7] spirometry should be performed in surgical candidates to evaluate tolerance for lung resection. Lung ventilation and perfusion scans often show areas of relatively normal perfusion but impaired ventilation and may be useful for screening, particularly in children.[15] Quantitative immunoglobulins or sweat chloride determination may be obtained if immunodeficiency or cystic fibrosis is suspected. Antibody titers for *Aspergillus* species may also be relevant to patients with an asthmatic component to their disease.[2]

Treatment

The mainstay of treatment for bronchiectasis is conservative medical therapy. A 2-week course of antibiotics such as amoxicillin is of proven benefit for acute exacerbations, shown by the decreasing organism count in the sputum and by decreasing sputum protein and elastase content. Long-term antibiotic therapy has been shown to decrease morbidity, but its use remains controversial and may follow the experience of cystic fibrosis, with chronic nebulized antibiotic therapy being of some benefit.[23]

Chest physiotherapy and postural drainage are generally beneficial in bronchiectasis, but long-term compliance may be difficult. Patients should avoid tobacco, and consideration should be given to pneumococcal and influenza vaccines. Several neutrophil elastase inhibitors, Egin C and alpha$_1$-antitrypsin, are now available from recombinant DNA technology, and these may ultimately have some role in long-term medical management.[23]

Operative procedures should be reserved for those patients who continue to have significant symptoms despite a prolonged medical trial. Operations are seldom performed on children under the age of 2 years because of the likelihood of improvement on medical therapy as the child grows. In those patients who can tolerate pulmonary resection, priority is given to preservation of lung parenchyma. Involved segments may be removed by segmentectomy, lobectomy, or pneumonectomy as indicated by anatomic involvement. For patients with bilateral disease, the side with greater involvement is resected first, with a common finding that symptoms are sufficiently improved to

preclude resection of the opposite side.[21] In those patients ultimately requiring bilateral resection, an interval between procedures of 6 to 12 months is generally recommended to allow adequate recovery and evaluation of symptoms.

Results

In studies prior to the use of antibiotics, life expectancy after the onset of bronchiectasis was 10 years. Death commonly ensued from septic complications such as meningitis and brain abscess.[18] After antibiotic therapy became prevalent, autopsy series reported a mean age of patients dying from bronchiectasis of greater than 50 years.[7] Those patients presenting with severe disease and debilitating symptoms often do progress despite therapy, with cor pulmonale or pulmonary infection as common causes of death.[7,8]

Although data are difficult to obtain, between 18 and 36 per cent of patients requiring hospitalization for bronchiectasis ultimately undergo operation, and the remaining majority are adequately managed with medical therapy. Of patients requiring operation for bronchiectasis, 95 per cent of the 140 patients reported by Sealy were either asymptomatic or improved at follow-up.[21] Progression of disease to other previously uninvolved lung segments occurs in fewer than 5 per cent of patients[7] after either surgical or medical therapy.[7,8] As demonstrated in the follow-up studies of Field, children tend to experience definite improvement in the second decade of life after medical therapy alone, with persistence of this improvement into at least the third and fourth decades. Patients with bronchiectasis secondary to tuberculosis may be less likely to progress to severe symptoms than patients with other etiologies. Up to a third of children followed by Field after either medical or surgical therapy ultimately became symptom-free.[8] Thus, selective application of modern surgical and medical therapy offers the patient with bronchiectasis opportunity for significant longevity and reduction in symptoms.[7]

SELECTED REFERENCES

Barker, A. F., and Bardana, E. J., Jr.: Bronchiectasis: Update of an orphan disease. Am. Rev. Respir. Dis., 137:969, 1988.
  This excellent review of the etiology and pathophysiology of bronchiectasis emphasizes a combination of host disorder and insult to the airways. A detailed protocol for diagnosis and evaluation of bronchiectasis is suggested.

Ellis, D. A., Thornley, P. E., Wightman, A. J., Walker, M., Chalmers, J., and Crofton, F. W.: Present outlook in bronchiectasis: Clinical and social study and review of factors influencing prognosis. Thorax, 36:659, 1981.
  One hundred and sixteen patients were followed for a mean of 14 years from the diagnosis of bronchiectasis. Outcomes are carefully analyzed in terms of symptoms, pulmonary function, disability, and survival.

LeRoux, B. T., Mohlala, M. L., Odell, J. A., and Whitton, I. D.: Suppurative diseases of the lung and pleural space. Part II: Bronchiectasis. Curr. Probl. Surg., 23:93, 1986.
  A thorough review of the history, anatomy, and surgical treatment for bronchiectasis. Supportive data come from a large South African experience of 2776 patients with bronchiectasis, of whom 1003 underwent pulmonary resection.

Stockley, R. A.: Bronchiectasis—New therapeutic approaches based on pathogenesis. Clin. Chest Med., 8,481, 1987.
  Recent developments are highlighted in understanding both the pathophysiology of bronchiectasis and newer therapeutic approaches, such as nebulized antibiotics, elastase inhibitors, anti-inflammatory drugs, inhibitors of chemotaxis, superoxide scavengers, and modifiers of the immune response.

REFERENCES

1. Aliabadi, P., and Shafiepoor, H.: Bronchography in the recognition of congenital cystic bronchiectasis. AJR, 131:255, 1978.
2. Barker, A. F., and Bardana, E. J., Jr.: Bronchiectasis: Update of an orphan disease. Am. Rev. Respir. Dis., 137:969, 1988.
3. Bolman, R. M., and Wolfe, W. G.: Bronchiectasis and bronchopulmonary sequestration. Surg. Clin. North Am., 60:(4):867, 1980.
4. Bradham, R. R., Sealy, W. C., and Young, W. G.: Chronic middle lobe infection. Factors responsible for its development. Ann. Thorac. Surg., 2:612, 1966.
5. Churchill, E. D.: Lobectomy and pneumonectomy in bronchiectasis and cystic disease. J. Thorac. Surg., 6:286, 1937.

6. Eliasson, R., Mossberg, B., Camner, P., and Afzelius, B. A.: The immotile-cilia syndrome. A congenital ciliary abnormality as an etiologic factor in chronic airway infections and male sterility. N. Engl. J. Med., 297:1, 1977.

7. Ellis, D. A., Thornley, P. E., Wightman, A. J., Walker, M., Chalmers, J., and Crofton, F. W.: Present outlook in bronchiectasis: Clinical and social study and review of factors influencing prognosis. Thorax, 36:659, 1981.

8. Field, C. E.: Bronchiectasis: Third report on a follow-up study of medical and surgical cases from childhood. Arch. Dis. Child., 44:551, 1969.

9. Gay, S., and Dee, P.: Tracheobronchomegaly—the Mounier-Kuhn syndrome. Br. J. Radiol., 57:640, 1984.

10. Glauser, E. M., Cook, D. C., and Hams, G. B. C.: Bronchiectasis—A review of 187 cases in children with followup pulmonary function studies in 58. Acta Pediatr. Scand., 165 (Suppl.):1, 1966.

11. Hilton, A. M., and Doyle, L.: Immunological abnormalities in bronchiectasis with chronic bronchial suppuration. Br. J. Dis. Chest, 72:207, 1978.

12. Joharjy, I. A., Bashi, S. A., and Abdullah, A. K.: Value of medium-thickness CT in the diagnosis of bronchiectasis. AJR, 149:1133, 1987.

13. Laennec, R. T. H.: De l'Auscultation Mediate ou Traite du Diagnostic des Maladies des Poumons et du Coeur. Paris, Brosson et Chaude, 1819.

14. LeRoux, B. T., Mohlala, M. L., Odell, J. A., and Whitton, I. D.: Suppurative diseases of the lung and pleural space. Part II: Bronchiectasis. Curr. Probl. Surg., 23:93, 1986.

15. Lewiston, N. J.: Bronchiectasis in childhood. Pediatr. Clin. North Am., 31(4):865, 1984.

16. Meade, R. H.: A History of Thoracic Surgery. Springfield, Ill., Charles C Thomas, 1961, p. 47.

17. Nissen, R.: Exstirpation eines ganzen Lungenflugels. Zentralbl. Chir., 58:3003, 1931.

18. Ochsner, A.: The development of pulmonary surgery, with special emphasis on carcinoma and bronchiectasis. Am. J. Surg., 135:732, 1978.

19. Reid, L. M.: Reduction in bronchial subdivision in bronchiectasis. Thorax, 5:233, 1950.

20. Robitaille, G.: Ehlers-Danlos syndrome and recurrent hemoptysis. Ann. Intern. Med., 61:716, 1964.

21. Sealy, W. C., Bradham, R. R., and Young, W. G., Jr.: The surgical treatment of multisegmental and localized bronchiectasis. Surg. Gynecol. Obstet., 123:80, 1966.

22. Sicard, J. A., and Forestier, J.: Methode generale d'explanation radiologique par l'huile iodee. Bull. Soc. Med. Hop. Paris, 46:463, 1922.

23. Stockley, R. A.: Bronchiectasis—New therapeutic approaches based on pathogenesis. Clin. Chest Med., 8:481, 1987.

24. Varpela, E., Koistinen, J., Korhola, O., and Keskinen, H.: Deficiency of alpha-1 antitrypsin and bronchiectasis. Ann. Clin. Res., 10:79, 1978.

25. Wayne, K. S., and Taussig, L.: Probable familial congenital bronchiectasis due to cartilage deficiency (Williams-Campbell syndrome). Am. Rev. Respir. Dis., 114:15, 1976.

IX

SURGICAL TREATMENT OF PULMONARY TUBERCULOSIS

Jon F. Moran, M.D.

The basic techniques of modern pulmonary surgery were developed during the first half of the twentieth century, primarily for the treatment of pulmonary tuberculosis. Surgical treatment of suppurative diseases of the lung, although required much less frequently today, has been largely unchanged since 1950.

It is estimated that 5 million new cases of active tuberculosis and 3.5 million deaths from tuberculosis occur worldwide each year. However, active tuberculosis has become an uncommon disease in North America and Europe. The incidence of mycobacterial infection in western Europe and the United States was declining prior to the discovery of effective chemotherapy (Fig. 1). The introduction of effective chemotherapy shortly after World War II dramatically decreased both the incidence of tuberculosis and the death rate. The total number of reported cases of tuberculosis in the United States in 1987 was 22,500.[23] Pulmonary tuberculosis represents 90 per cent of all cases of tuberculosis today. Despite modern antituberculous chemotherapy, approximately 2 per cent of all cases of pulmonary mycobacterial infection require surgical treatment.

HISTORICAL ASPECTS

Throughout history pulmonary tuberculosis has been recognized as a devastating disease. Hippocrates (470–376 B.C.) wrote extensively about clinical tuberculosis, or *phthisis*, as it was termed by the Greeks. *Phthisis* meant "a disease characterized by progressive weight loss and wasting." The Latin-based synonym was *consumption*. Tubercles (Fig. 2) were described within the lung by the Greeks, but it was not until 1839 that Schönlein used the term *tuberculosis* to describe the characteristic pathologic changes in the lungs.

Tuberculosis reached epidemic proportions in Europe and the United States during the eighteenth and nineteenth centuries. It has been estimated that tuberculosis caused approximately 20 per cent of all adult deaths in Europe during these two centuries.

In the United States in the 1920s tuberculosis was still the second leading cause of death, and most victims were young adults.

Understanding of the pathogenesis of pulmonary tuberculosis evolved during the latter half of the nineteenth century. Rokitansky (1804–1878) observed that over 90 per cent of individuals *not* dying of tuberculosis had evidence of prior tuberculous infection in their lungs. In 1865, Villeman, a French military surgeon, demonstrated that tuberculosis could be transmitted to guinea pigs or rabbits by injection of infected

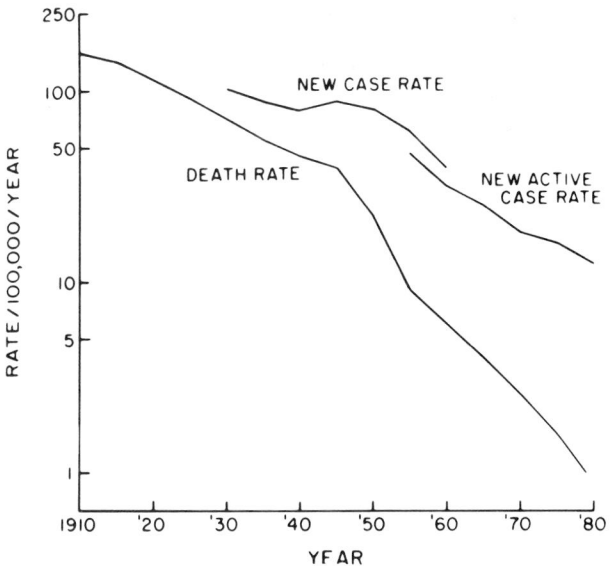

Figure 1. Tuberculosis death rates and new case rates in the United States, 1910 to 1980. (From Comstock, G. W.: Epidemiology of Tuberculosis. Am. Rev. Respir. Dis. 125 (Suppl):9, 1982.)

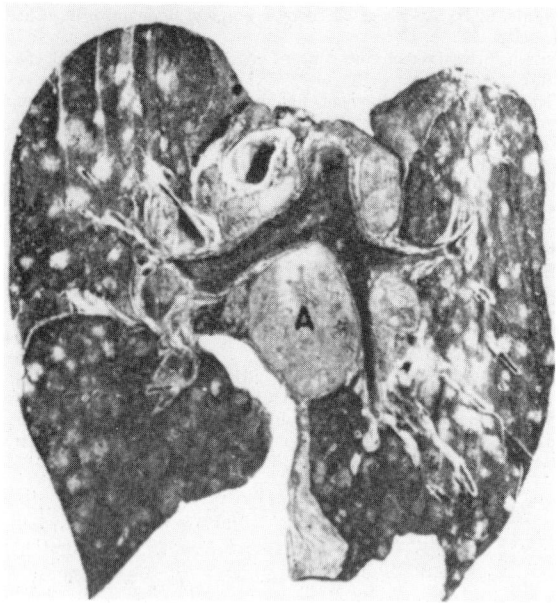

Figure 2. Large necrotic tubercles from generalized spread of tuberculosis with particular enlargement of the hilar lymph nodes (A). Tubercles or nodules such as these were the gross pathologic hallmark of phthisis or consumption. (From Auerbach, O.: The Natural History of the Tuberculous Pulmonary Lesion. Med. Clin. North Am. 43:239, 1959.)

material from either humans or cows. Robert Koch's announcement on March 24, 1882, of his isolation of the tubercle bacillus[16] was the key to understanding the etiology of tuberculosis and marked the beginning of a medical crusade against tuberculosis that led to its control in developed areas of the world within 100 years. Simultaneously, Koch enunciated his *postulates* for proving bacterial causation of disease: "to prove that tuberculosis . . . is caused by invasion of bacilli and . . . the growth and multiplication of the bacilli, it was necessary to isolate the bacteria from the body; to grow them in pure culture . . . ; and by administering the isolated bacilli to animals to reproduce the same morbid condition. . . ."

Tuberculin skin testing evolved from Koch's efforts to use "old tuberculin," a sterile filtrate of cultured tubercle bacilli, as therapy for tuberculosis. Tuberculin skin testing and the newly discovered chest roentgenogram together made mass screening for tuberculosis possible by 1940. By this time, it had been firmly established that transmission of disease was almost exclusively by airborne bacilli; and earlier case identification led to better case isolation, thereby reducing the spread of tuberculosis. The Nobel Prize–winning discovery of streptomycin in 1946 by Waksmann and the release of isoniazid (INH) in 1952 made pulmonary tuberculosis curable in most patients. During this same period (1875–1950), the clinical treatment of pulmonary tuberculosis had evolved rapidly. The first sanatorium specializing in the treatment of tuberculosis opened in 1854 in Görbersdorf, Germany. By 1952, there were over 100,000 sanatorium beds in the United States for the treatment of tuberculosis. The regimented routine of the sanatoria, stressing bed rest, diet, and fresh mountain air, was probably rarely effective in patients with advanced disease. Forms of collapse therapy such as therapeutic pneumothorax, phrenic nerve division, and pneumoperitoneum were widely employed during the early decades of the twentieth century. During this same period, Sauerbruch in Germany popularized thoracoplasty as treatment for pulmonary tuberculosis. John Alexander popularized thoracoplasty in the United States, and it soon was the standard treatment for cavitary pulmonary tuberculosis. Prior to effective chemotherapy, the yearly death rate from tuberculosis in the United States fell from 300 per 100,000 in 1880 to only 69 per

100,000 in 1935. This progress could be attributed to improved case screening, isolation, sanatorium care, and the introduction of various forms of collapse therapy.

Tuffier is credited with the first successful partial lung resection for tuberculosis. He resected the apex of the right lung in a 25-year-old man in 1891. Resectional pulmonary surgery for tuberculosis remained rare until the late 1930s. The first successful lobectomy for tuberculosis was performed in Cleveland by Freelander in 1934. Resectional surgery for tuberculosis carried a high mortality prior to the availability of effective chemotherapy. Effective chemotherapy made resectional surgery safer but simultaneously drastically reduced the need for surgical treatment of pulmonary tuberculosis.

BACTERIOLOGY

The name *Mycobacterium* was chosen for this genus by Lehmann and Neumann in 1896 because of the moldlike appearance of the bacteria when grown on nutrient broth. Mycobacteria are no more related to fungi than are other bacteria. Mycobacterial cell walls have a high lipid content that prevents permeation by aniline dyes; but once a dye binds, decolorization is difficult. Koch discovered this peculiar "acid-fast" staining property of mycobacteria. The modern staining technique that bears the names of Ziehl and Neelsen is essentially Ehrlich's original method. Acid-fast organisms stain red against a methylene blue counterstain.

Mycobacterium tuberculosis is responsible for most cases of clinically significant pulmonary mycobacterial disease and is an aerobic, nonmotile, slow-growing bacillus.[26] Many other species of mycobacteria were isolated during the first half of the twentieth century.[11] Several of these species can cause pulmonary infection, and they are referred to as "atypical mycobacteria."[5] Atypical mycobacteria (Table 1) are more frequently resistant to antituberculous drugs.[8,14] Because atypical mycobacteria are more resistant to chemotherapy, patients with atypical mycobacterial pulmonary infections represent nearly 50 per cent of all patients referred for surgical therapy of mycobacterial disease. The atypical mycobacteria were divided by Runyon, a botanist, into four separate groups according to growth rate and pigment production.[25]

Mycobacterium avium-intracellulare and *Mycobacterium kansasii* are the two atypical organisms that most frequently cause clinical pulmonary infection.[20] In the United States, clinical pulmonary infection with *M. avium-intracellulare* is most common in the Southeast. *M. avium-intracellulare* is usually resistant *in vitro* to most antituberculous drugs. *M. kansasii* has been found worldwide but in the United States occurs most frequently in the Midwest and Southwest. In contrast to *M. avium-intracellulare*, *M. kansasii* more often shows *in vitro* susceptibility to antituberculous drugs and less frequently requires surgical treatment.

Drug susceptibility testing is very important in the treatment of pulmonary mycobacterial infection.[7,14,24] Three to 4 weeks are necessary to isolate these slow-growing organisms and another 3 to 4 weeks to determine drug sensitivities. Because of the inevitable delay in precise speciation and susceptibility testing, therapy is often begun empirically as test results are awaited.

TABLE 1. Classification of Mycobacterial Species (Runyon)

Group I	Photochromogens	M. kansasii
Group II	Scotochromogens	M. scrofulaceum
Group III	Nonchromogens	M. tuberculosis
		M. avium-intracellulare
Group IV	Rapid growers	M. fortuitum
		M. chelonei

PATHOLOGY

The pathologic responses within the lung to the various common mycobacteria are identical.[2] *M. tuberculosis* is a virulent organism requiring a *very small* inoculum for infection to occur *even* in normal lung tissue, whereas the "less virulent" atypical mycobacteria more often invade abnormal lung tissue in compromised individuals. The tubercle bacillus generally gains entry to the body by inhalation of droplet nuclei less than 5 μ in diameter. A first infection in an unsensitized host causes a localized necrotizing pneumonia. Mycobacteria spread through the lymphatics to the hilar lymph nodes. The peripheral pneumonic process is characterized by "caseous necrosis" with formation of a granuloma containing mycobacteria with a rim of granulation tissue (Fig. 3). *Caseous* is descriptive of the gross appearance of the lesion with cheeselike material inside a thin capsule. The peripheral lung lesion accompanied by hilar nodal enlargement is termed the *primary Ghon complex*. Generally, the infection is contained at this stage by the body's immune responses. Any hematogenous spread that has occurred usually becomes inactive as the immune response mounts.

In children, primary tuberculosis occasionally progresses locally or by hematogenous dissemination. Childhood tuberculosis may present as a necrotizing pneumonia progressing to cavitation. When hematogenous spread is not halted by cell-mediated immunity, disease is found most commonly in the lung apices, the kidneys, the epiphyses of long bones, or the brain. These are locations favored by the strict aerobic growth requirement of mycobacteria. Hematogenous spread rarely leads to miliary tuberculosis. Miliary tuberculosis describes massive hematogenous spread, giving rise to thousands of 1- to 2-mm. (millet seed–sized) tubercles throughout the body. Most miliary tuberculosis seen today occurs in the elderly.

Adult pulmonary tuberculosis is the most common pattern of mycobacterial infection and is also called *reinfection,* or *postprimary,* tuberculosis. Adult tuberculosis begins as a segmental pneumonia in the apical or posterior segment of an upper lobe or the superior segment of a lower lobe. In adult pattern tuberculosis, it is relatively common for disease to be present bilaterally. The pneumonic infiltrate progresses to caseous necrosis, and cavity formation occurs when the area of liquefaction erodes into an adjacent bronchus. The cavities formed vary in

size from 2 to 20 cm., depending upon the amount of lung destruction prior to drainage. The cavity wall is composed of granulation tissue with organizing reaction in the rim of surrounding lung tissue. Erosion of a cavity into a bronchial vessel may cause severe hemoptysis. A Rasmussen aneurysm, a pulmonary artery aneurysm within or adjacent to a cavity, is found in about 4 per cent of advanced cavitary disease. There is usually intense inflammatory reaction in the rim of lung surrounding the tuberculous cavities. The overlying visceral pleura tends to contract, decreasing the volume of the involved segment of the lung. The visceral and parietal pleura are involved by this intense reaction; and as a result, the pleural space is completely obliterated and fused over these cavities. This intense pleural reaction makes operative separation of the two pleural surfaces overlying the diseased segments essentially impossible.

Cavity erosion into an airway permits infection of the proximal bronchial mucosa. Endobronchial tuberculosis may cause bronchostenosis with distal superimposed bacterial or fungal infection. Peripheral cavities can rupture into the pleural space, creating a tuberculous or mixed tuberculous and bacterial empyema. Tuberculous empyema can also occur secondary to hematogenous or lymphatic seeding of the pleural space. Pure tuberculous effusions are usually serofibrinous, whereas mixed effusions resemble a conventional bacterial empyema.

DIAGNOSIS

There is an important difference between mycobacterial infection and mycobacterial disease. Infection implies the entrance of a mycobacterial organism into the body without symptoms or overt clinical evidence of disease. The diagnosis of mycobacterial pulmonary disease depends upon the confirmation of active disease by appropriate radiographic and bacteriologic studies. Only 5 to 15 per cent of individuals infected with *M. tuberculosis* ever have clinically significant disease. The American Thoracic Society classification of tuberculosis infection recognizes four categories: 0, no tuberculosis exposure (no exposure history, negative skin test); I, tuberculosis exposure without infection (history of exposure, negative skin test); II, tuberculosis infection without disease (positive skin test without clinical disease); and III, tuberculosis disease proven by symptoms, roentgenographic studies, and bacteriologic studies.

The symptoms of pulmonary mycobacterial infection are frequently subtle. A chronic productive cough, a persistent "chest cold," easy fatigability, weight loss, chest pain, and fever all may be symptoms of tuberculosis. Hemoptysis and night sweats are more specific symptoms. A history of exposure or membership in a high-risk group should elevate the index of suspicion for mycobacterial disease. Pulmonary mycobacterial infection is more common in the immunosuppressed (secondary to corticosteroids, cancer chemotherapy, transplant immunosuppression, or acquired immunodeficiency syndrome [AIDS][12]); in diabetics; after gastrectomy; and in individuals with silicosis, pneumoconiosis, or reticuloendothelial malignancies.

Mycobacterial pulmonary disease causes a wide variety of roentgenographic abnormalities. The most frequent radiographic findings in pulmonary tuberculosis are apical upper or lower lobe infiltrates, often bilaterally, with frequent cavitation[9,31] (Fig. 4). The chest film findings in atypical mycobacterial disease are indistinguishable from those seen with tuberculosis.

SKIN TESTING. Skin testing was refined by Florence Siebert after she isolated the purified protein derivative (PPD) from *M. tuberculosis* organisms in 1939.[28] Skin testing was widely adopted as a screening test for mycobacterial infection. Most patients are sensitized to the protein fraction of the tubercle bacillus within several weeks after the onset of infection. Current standard tuberculosis skin testing involves the intracutaneous injection of five tuberculin units (TU) of PPD on the volar aspect of the forearm. This is termed an *intermediate PPD,* and

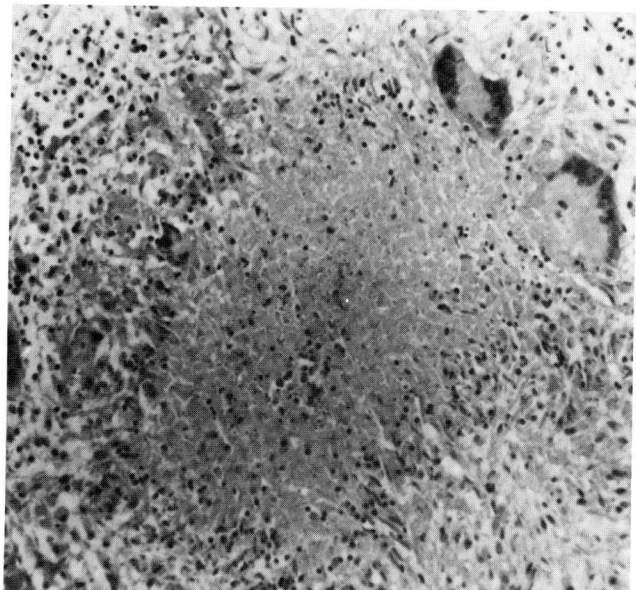

Figure 3. Typical tuberculous granuloma with central caseation and surrounding epithelioid and Langhans' giant cells. Hematoxylin and eosin, ×250. (From Dunnill, M.S.: Pulmonary Pathology, 2nd ed. Edinburgh, Churchill Livingstone, 1987, p. 447.)

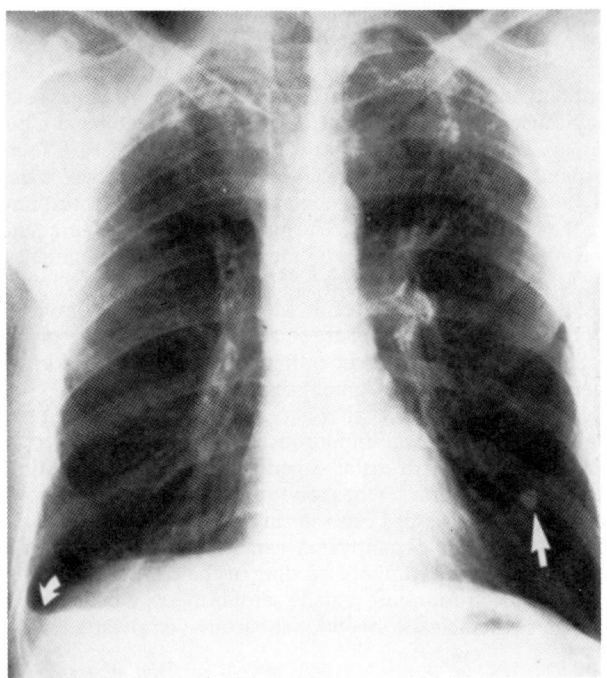

Figure 4. Bilateral apical and posterior segment upper lobe infiltrates typical of adult tuberculosis are seen in this 36-year-old man. Calcified Ghon focus in lingula (straight arrow) and blunting of right costophrenic angle (curved arrow) are the residua of earlier primary tuberculosis. (From Woodring, J. H., Vandiviere, H. M., Fried, A. M., and Dillon, M. L.: Update: The Radiographic Features of Pulmonary Tuberculosis. Am. J. Roentgenol. 146:502, 1986.)

the local reaction is evaluated after 48 to 72 hours. Greater than 10 mm. of induration defines a positive test. Tuberculin reactions may be blunted in the elderly or in seriously ill individuals, causing false-negative skin testing. A second intermediate PPD applied 1 week after the first is recommended to minimize false-negative tests. The intermediate PPD is positive in at least 90 per cent of cases of tuberculosis.

SMEAR AND CULTURE. The isolation of mycobacterial organisms from the sputum or lung tissue is required to confirm the diagnosis of pulmonary mycobacterial disease. Early morning sputum specimens or washings obtained by fiberoptic bronchoscopy are most helpful in establishing a diagnosis. The presence of acid-fast organisms on smear allows a rapid presumptive diagnosis. Subsequent cultures are necessary to document the specific type of mycobacterial disease. Approximately 10,000 organisms per milliliter of sputum are required for smear positivity. Mycobacterial cultures require 3 to 6 weeks to grow,

and it is often necessary to obtain multiple samples before a positive smear or culture is obtained. When the clinical pattern supports the diagnosis of pulmonary mycobacterial disease, antimycobacterial chemotherapy is often begun as a 1- to 2-month therapeutic trial during the wait for sputum cultures. Because patients referred for surgical treatment frequently are infected with organisms resistant to many antituberculous drugs, culture results with accurate sensitivity testing for most available antituberculous agents are particularly important in patients being considered for surgical intervention.

CHEMOTHERAPY

The vast majority of patients with pulmonary mycobacterial infection can be cured with appropriate chemotherapy. Many antimycobacterial drugs have been developed over the past 40 years.[21,30] Effective chemotherapy for tuberculosis has also improved the safety of surgical treatment.

Initial treatment of pulmonary mycobacterial disease is usually begun before precise identification of the causal organism. Treatment is generally initiated with two or three pharmacologic agents so as to avoid the emergence of drug-resistant organisms.[1,15] Mycobacterial organisms within the lung react differently to antimycobacterial drugs, depending upon whether the organisms are extracellular or intracellular. Extracellular organisms tend to multiply rapidly in the hyperoxic neutral pH environment of the pulmonary cavity. Organisms within activated macrophages grow slowly in their acidic environment. An effective treatment program halts mycobacterial growth, both intracellularly and extracellularly, promptly bringing about conversion of the patient to a sputum-negative status within 6 weeks. The five most commonly employed antimycobacterial agents are listed in Table 2. Atypical mycobacterial infections or drug-resistant M. tuberculosis infections may require the use of other antibiotics.[5,8,14]

Until recently the standard pharmacologic regimen for the treatment of pulmonary mycobacterial infection required 18 to 24 months of continuous therapy. Short course therapy (6 to 9 months) has now been shown to be equally effective. The two currently recommended regimens for treatment of pulmonary tuberculosis are (1) a 6-month course employing isoniazid, rifampin, and pyrazinamide for 2 months, followed by isoniazid and rifampin for 4 months; and (2) a 9-month course of isoniazid and rifampin.[1] With either regimen, ethambutol should be added initially if isoniazid resistance is suspected and continued until sensitivity testing has been completed. If either isoniazid or rifampin cannot be tolerated, streptomycin and pyrazinamide may be substituted. If resistance to isoniazid is documented, a 12-month course of rifampin and ethambutol is

TABLE 2. Commonly Used Antimycobacterial Drugs

Drug	Daily Dosage		Common Side Effects	Comments
	Children	*Adults*		
Isoniazid (INH)	10–20 mg./kg. PO or IM	5 mg./kg. PO or IM	Hepatitis; peripheral neuritis	Bactericidal to both intracellular and extracellular organisms; pyridoxine 10 mg./kg./day as prophylaxis for neuritis
Rifampin (RIF)	10–20 mg./kg. PO	10 mg./kg. PO	Hepatitis; febrile reaction	Bactericidal to both intracellular and extracellular organisms; colors urine orange; inhibits the effect of oral contraceptives, quinidine, digitalis, corticosteroids, and coumadin
Pyrazinamide (PZA)	15–20 mg./kg. PO	15–30 mg./kg. PO	Hepatotoxicity; hyperuricemia; arthralgia	Bactericidal to intracellular organisms; reduces total length of chemotherapy required
Streptomycin (SM)	20–40 mg./kg. IM	15 mg./kg. IM	8th cranial nerve damage; nephrotoxicity	Bactericidal to extracellular organisms within cavities; limit dose to 10 mg./kg. in elderly patients
Ethambutol (EMB)	15–25 mg./kg. PO	15–25 mg./kg. PO	Optic neuritis (reversible); skin rash	Bacteriostatic for both intracellular and extracellular organisms

PO, orally; IM, intramuscularly.

recommended, supplemented by pyrazinamide for the first 1 to 3 months.[7] Streptomycin is often included for the first 1 to 3 months of therapy as well.

The primary drug resistance rate for *M. tuberculosis* in the United States varies geographically and among ethnic groups, but is generally 7 to 10 per cent.[3] The increasing frequency of primary drug-resistant tuberculosis and of atypical mycobacterial pulmonary infection make accurate sensitivity testing to a wide spectrum of chemotherapeutic agents critical in order to optimize the chemotherapeutic regimen. Although atypical mycobacteria are frequently resistant *in vitro* to many or all of the usual drugs, four- and five-drug regimens may still be moderately effective.[8,14] Efficacy is increased by selection of drugs to which the particular atypical organism is susceptible.[14,29]

Coordination of chemotherapy and surgical intervention requires careful planning. Complications of resectional surgery are reduced in patients who have been converted to sputum-negative status.[18] Optimal pulmonary toilet, careful selection of appropriate chemotherapy, and the addition of one or two new drugs during the perioperative period are useful in reducing operative complications. In treating drug-resistant organisms (either *M. tuberculosis* or atypical mycobacteria), two or three chemotherapeutic agents to which the infecting organism is sensitive should be given perioperatively and for 6 to 9 months postoperatively. In the case of organisms that exhibit resistance to all chemotherapeutic agents, the administration of isoniazid and rifampin and an aminoglycoside perioperatively and isoni-

azid and rifampin for a period of 9 to 12 months postoperatively is still recommended.

COLLAPSE THERAPY

During the nineteenth century it was noted that when a pneumothorax occurred in a patient with pulmonary tuberculosis, an apparent remission of symptoms often followed. This led to the popular concept that collapsing the affected portion of lung would allow the infected area to rest and thereby recover. Artificially induced pneumothorax gained popularity at the beginning of the twentieth century, although it required repetitive instillations of gas in the pleural space at 2-week intervals. A wide variety of other techniques to encourage collapse of the infected portions of the lung were tried subsequently. Unilateral phrenic nerve division, pneumoperitoneum, thoracoplasty, and extraperiosteal thoracoplasty with plombage all were employed with varying degrees of success (Fig. 5). Surgical division of the phrenic nerve and pneumoperitoneum tended to preferentially collapse the lower lobes of the lung. Plombage thoracoplasty utilized filling materials such as paraffin or Lucite balls placed into the space between the apex of the rib cage and the parietal pleura, inducing selective collapse of the apex of the lung. Plombage thoracoplasty interfered relatively little with chest wall function or stability when compared with standard thoracoplasty. Plombage thoracoplasty was a nondeforming operation, because the shape of the overlying chest wall remained

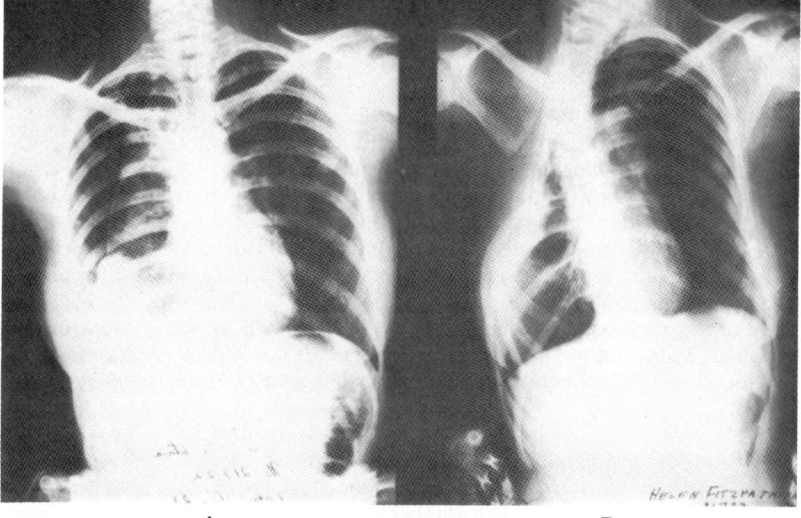

A   B

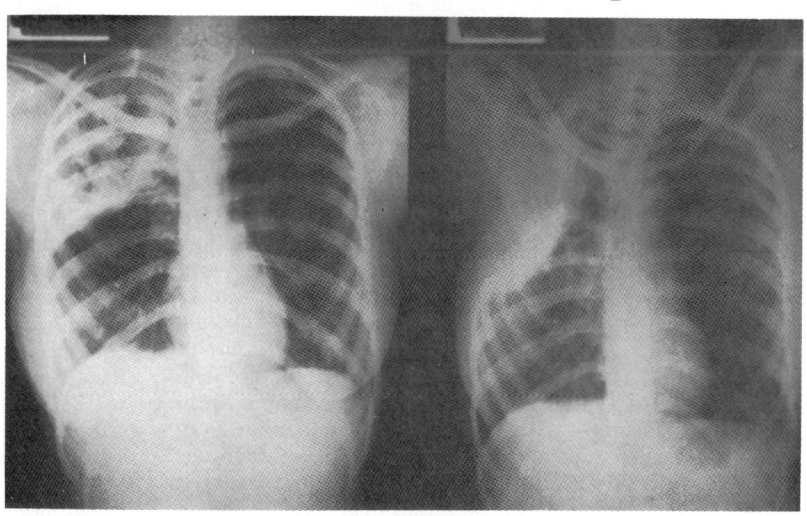

C   D

Figure 5. Examples of various types of collapse therapy for pulmonary tuberculosis. *A*, Chest film of a young woman with persistent cavitation after artificial pneumothorax therapy. *B*, The same patient after seven-rib thoracoplasty with excision of transverse processes and the entire first rib, causing scoliosis and severe chest wall deformity. *C*, Chest film of another young woman who underwent plombage thoracoplasty with Lucite spheres after artificial pneumothorax had failed to convert her sputum. *D*, Four months after sputum conversion by plombage for thoracoplasty, the patient underwent a modified thoracoplasty with preservation of the first rib and the transverse processes. This chest film shows the smaller degree of collapse with less chest wall deformity and scoliosis because of preservation of the first rib and the transverse processes. (From Gaensler, E. A.: The Surgery for Pulmonary Tuberculosis. Am. Rev. Respir. Dis. *125:*80, 1982.)

unchanged. Collapse of the apex of the lung was desirable in most patients, because this was the portion of the lung most frequently involved by tuberculosis. Sputum conversion was achieved in 30 to 60 per cent of patients. Unfortunately, later erosion of the plombage material into the lung proved to be relatively common. All forms of plombage thoracoplasty are now obsolete.

THORACOPLASTY

In the 50 years preceding the discovery of effective chemotherapy for tuberculosis in 1946, extrapleural paravertebral thoracoplasty was the most frequently employed surgical procedure for the treatment of pulmonary tuberculosis. Thoracoplasty achieved closure of tuberculous cavities in over 80 per cent of patients without chemotherapy with an operative mortality of approximately 10 per cent. Today thoracoplasty is rarely, if ever, indicated as primary treatment for pulmonary tuberculosis.[13] Paravertebral thoracoplasty remains an important operation for the treatment of tuberculous bronchopleural fistulas and empyemas and for bronchopulmonary fistulas complicating surgical resections in other settings. The resurgence of tuberculosis and atypical mycobacterial infections in immunocompromised patients, especially those with AIDS, has created a clinical setting similar to that in the era prior to effective chemotherapy. Many of these patients develop bronchopleural fistulas and empyemas despite chemotherapy. These patients are often debilitated and are not suitable candidates for aggressive resectional surgery. Thoracoplasty and other "outdated" surgical procedures from the pre-chemotherapy era will probably be employed with increasing frequency in this subgroup of patients.

Thoracoplasty should be considered when the virulence of the infecting organism or the poor overall condition of the patient makes resectional surgery hazardous. A modified or "tailoring" thoracoplasty, removing only four or five ribs, is indicated as a secondary procedure to obliterate an infected apical space and the accompanying bronchopleural fistula that may complicate a lung resection. The pleural reaction caused by tuberculosis inhibits shift of the mediastinum and upward movement of the diaphragm, predisposing to a postoperative "space problem" following pulmonary resections. Such a space problem increases the likelihood of a postresectional bronchopleural fistula.

In planning a thoracoplasty, it is important to remember that the operation causes an irreversible loss of ventilatory capacity on the operated side. Careful assessment of the patient's pulmonary function is mandatory. The number of ribs that need to be removed can be judged by carefully examining the patient's chest films. The thoracoplasty should remove a sufficient portion of the chest wall to allow complete collapse of the cavitated portion of the lung or obliteration of the entire residual pleural space (space problem). Originally it was recommended that no more than three to five ribs be removed at any stage to avoid excessive chest wall instability. With the availability of ventilators, more ribs can now be resected at one time without excessive postoperative complications. With the patient in a full lateral position, a high parascapular incision is made, extending from just below the upper edge of the trapezius along the posterior border of the scapula and turning anteriorly below the tip of the scapula. The trapezius and rhomboid muscles are divided, and the scapula is elevated off the chest wall. The insertion of the serratus onto the upper ribs is divided. The entire second rib and the posterior two thirds of the third rib are resected subperiosteally. One approaches the first rib subperiosteally from below, being careful to avoid damage to the subclavian vessels and the brachial plexus above the first rib. The entire first rib is removed in this manner. At the same time or at a second stage 2 weeks later, shorter segments of the fourth through sixth or seventh ribs are removed through the same incision. A five-rib

thoracoplasty reduces the size of the thoracic cavity by approximately 25 per cent. A seven-rib thoracoplasty is required to allow the scapula to collapse toward the mediastinum and achieve a severe degree of collapse of the underlying lung.

Intensive pulmonary toilet, nutritional support, and physiotherapy for generalized conditioning and for avoiding scoliosis are important in the postoperative care of these patients. Lying on the side of operation with a roll or sandbag positioned in the axilla improves posture and accentuates the collapsing effect.

PULMONARY RESECTION FOR MYCOBACTERIAL DISEASE

Operative treatment of pulmonary mycobacterial disease is rarely necessary. When an operation is required, resection of the diseased portion of the lung is the procedure of choice. Prior to the availability of effective chemotherapy, pulmonary resection for tuberculosis had an operative mortality of 20 to 40 per cent. Once effective chemotherapy for tuberculosis became available, pulmonary resection rapidly replaced thoracoplasty as the surgical treatment of choice. Compared with thoracoplasty, pulmonary resection had the advantage of achieving prompt conversion to sputum-negative status in a single stage without chest wall deformity or severe limitation of ventilatory capacity. By 1953, Chamberlain was able to report a series of 300 segmental resections for pulmonary tuberculosis with a 3 per cent mortality and a 93 per cent cure rate. Despite such excellent operative results, it was soon realized that pulmonary resection was not necessary in most cases of pulmonary mycobacterial infection.

The efficacy of modern antimycobacterial chemotherapy has reduced the indications for surgical intervention and pulmonary resection to the following:

1. *Persistently positive sputum cultures with cavitation* following 5 to 6 months of continuous chemotherapy with two or more drugs. The organism must be shown to be susceptible to the drugs used, or an alteration in the chemotherapy regimen is indicated.

2. *Localized pulmonary disease caused by M. avium-intracellulare* (or another mycobacterium with a similar broad resistance to chemotherapy). "Localized" disease is defined as any disease that can be encompassed by one or two pulmonary resections.

3. *A mass lesion* of the lung in an area of tuberclous involvement. This is an indication for resection for simultaneous diagnosis of the mass lesion and treatment of the mycobacterial disease.

4. *Massive life-threatening hemoptysis* or recurrent severe hemoptysis. This is an indication for resection of the portion of the lung that is the source of the hemorrhage. Pulmonary hemorrhage is a rare but frequently fatal complication of pulmonary mycobacterial disease. Massive hemoptysis is defined as greater than 600 ml. per 24 hours, whereas severe hemoptysis is defined as greater than 200 ml. per 24 hours. Asphyxiation, rather than hypovolemia, is the usual cause of death from hemoptysis. The site of bleeding is almost invariably a cavitary lesion. The bleeding arises from the abundant bronchial arterial circulation to the cavitated portion of the lung. Mild or moderate hemorrhage usually ceases with sedation, bed rest, and careful control of blood pressure. Bronchoscopy is performed for determination of the lobe from which the bleeding arises, because these patients frequently have bilateral cavitary changes on chest films. The source of bleeding should be resected on an urgent basis after an episode of massive or recurrent severe hemoptysis, because mortality when resection is not done is high.[4,6,10] Tuberculosis continues to be the most common cause of severe hemoptysis. Severe hemoptysis is unpredictable with frequent occurrence of sudden engulfing hemorrhage in previously stable patients awaiting endoscopy or operation.

5. *A bronchopleural fistula* secondary to mycobacterial infec-

tion that does not respond to tube thoracostomy. This requires surgical treatment and may require pulmonary resection. Pure tuberculous effusions normally resolve spontaneously or respond promptly to chemotherapy. Mixed tuberculous and pyogenic empyemas that occur when a bronchopleural fistula develops in a lung that is severely damaged by mycobacterial infection rarely respond to drug therapy alone. The efficacy of tube thoracostomy is limited by the dense pleural reaction that inhibits full re-expansion of the lung. Decortication may lead to full re-expansion with excellent recovery of pulmonary function, and localized areas of infection can be resected simultaneously. Often the pleural reaction is so intense and extends so far into the substance of the lung that decortication is impossible. Open drainage of the pleural space by creation of an Eloesser flap is a reasonable alternative procedure in such cases or when the patient's overall condition is marginal. When an entire lung is destroyed by infection and there is a surrounding empyema, pleuropneumonectomy as described below can be a dramatically effective treatment in carefully selected patients.

Several special situations may call for surgical treatment of pulmonary mycobacterial disease. Patients severely symptomatic because of a destroyed lobe or bronchiectatic area of the lung may benefit from resection. Unreliable patients or those with thick-walled cavities may require resection. A patient with a "trapped lung" after tuberculous empyema may benefit from decortication with or without resection in order to allow full expansion of the underlying lung and restoration of ventilatory capacity. Few specific contraindications to pulmonary resection for mycobacterial disease exist. Widespread pulmonary or endobronchial disease is generally a contraindication to resection. Children with mycobacterial disease rarely require resection.[17,19,27] Childhood primary disease often progresses to lobar tuberculous pneumonia with massive lymph node enlargement, but cavitation is rare. Even in advanced disease in children, chemotherapy is almost invariably curative, with complete resolution radiographically and excellent recovery of pulmonary function.

In planning an operation for mycobacterial infection, as in any other pulmonary surgery, it is important that the patient's cardiopulmonary reserve be adequate to sustain the patient through the contemplated procedure. Every effort should be made to convert the patient to sputum-negative status prior to operation, including the administration of additional antimycobacterial drugs perioperatively. Adequate nutritional support and physical therapy to encourage overall physical conditioning and optimal pulmonary toilet are beneficial preoperatively. Preoperative bronchoscopy should be done on all patients considered for pulmonary resection to exclude active proximal endobronchial disease. Active endobronchial disease interferes with healing of the bronchial stump following resection. Proximal endobronchial disease should be cleared by chemotherapy prior to pulmonary resection.

OPERATIVE MANAGEMENT

The use of a double-lumen endotracheal tube can make resection for tuberculosis technically easier and safer. The dependent lung can be protected from contamination by secretions from the infected upper lung while the patient is in the lateral position. In cases of severe hemoptysis, a double-lumen tube partially protects the dependent lung during the resection of portions of the upper lung.

The extent of pulmonary resection depends upon the extent of the mycobacterial disease and is guided by the principle that all gross evidence of disease should be resected. The extent of pulmonary involvement can be determined by careful examination of preoperative chest films or computed tomograms. Conservation of pulmonary tissue and pulmonary function is desirable; however, wedge resection and segmentectomy are not often applicable for the control of pulmonary mycobacterial disease. A generous wedge resection can be applied in the setting of a mass lesion that is being excised for excluding the presence of carcinoma or in the case of hemoptysis secondary to a localized peripheral cavity. The dense pleural reaction characteristic of mycobacterial disease makes separation of the segments within the lung difficult. For active mycobacterial disease, a lobectomy or pneumonectomy is usually required. It is occasionally necessary to combine upper lobectomy with wedge excision of the superior segment of the lower lobe to remove all gross disease.[18] Pneumonectomy is required only in the setting of a totally destroyed lung. It is possible for patients to tolerate bilateral staged upper lobectomies, even if the superior segment or right middle lobe has been resected in combination with the upper lobe on the same side.[18]

The operative techniques of lobectomy and pneumonectomy are covered elsewhere in this text and are not altered in the patient with tuberculosis. Because mycobacterial infection is a peripheral process with overlying dense pleural reaction, it is frequently necessary to mobilize portions of the lung in the extrapleural plane. Full re-expansion of the remaining lung tissue is important to avoid the complications of atelectasis, hemothorax, and apical space problems. Postoperative bronchoscopy may be required to clear infected secretions or blood from the proximal airway.

When extensive pulmonary parenchymal mycobacterial disease is complicated by a chronic empyema, an extrapleural pneumonectomy may be required. This is a difficult procedure and carries a significant morbidity and mortality. With the patient in a full lateral position, a standard posterolateral thoracotomy incision is made, resecting the fifth rib subperiosteally (Fig. 6). The goal is to resect the entire reactive pleura, underlying

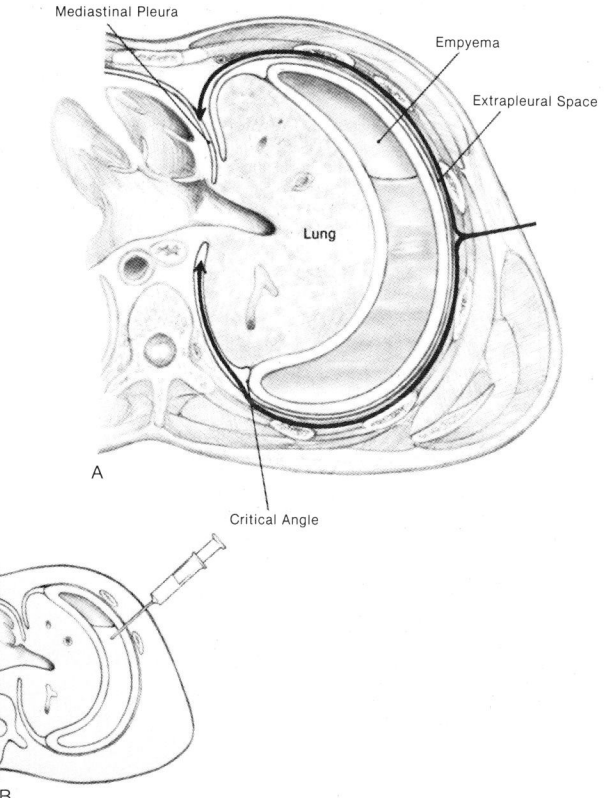

Figure 6. Technique of extrapleural pneumonectomy. *A*, Plane of dissection is developed in extrapleural space and carried beyond the empyema sac to the mediastinal surface of the lung. *B*, With a large empyema sac, aspiration is useful to allow more room within the chest for dissection. Aspiration also reduces the likelihood of endobronchial spillage during dissection and manipulation. (From Hood, R. M., Antman, K., Boyd, A., Naidich, D., and Shemin, R.: Surgical Diseases of the Pleura and Chest Wall. Philadelphia, W. B. Saunders Company, 1986, p. 126.)

empyema cavity, and lung without entering the empyema cavity itself. A dissection plane is developed along the extrapleural space, proceeding superiorly and inferiorly from the fifth rib incision. This plane is developed around the entire empyema cavity and the lung until the mediastinal surface of the lung is reached. The mediastinal surface of the lung tends to have less dense adhesions. The subclavian vessels and the brachial plexus must be carefully avoided near the apex of the lung. Care must be taken posteriorly to avoid damage to the esophagus. Once the entire lung has been mobilized to the hilum, the hilar structures are separated in the standard manner. The bronchus, pulmonary artery, and both pulmonary veins are divided and secured by means of standard techniques. Ligation of the hilar vessels often is required intrapericardially.

Administration of effective antimycobacterial drugs, judicious timing of operation, careful operative technique, and attentive postoperative care are the critically important factors in avoiding complications from pulmonary resection for mycobacterial disease.[18,22] Patients referred for operation generally have associated problems that predispose them to complications. Good pulmonary toilet and careful attention to the pleural drainage system are necessary to assure full re-expansion of the remaining lung in order to avoid apical space problems. Two specific complications of resection for mycobacterial disease are particularly worrisome: *empyema*, with or without bronchopleural fistula, and *bronchogenic spread* of the mycobacterial disease. Both of these complications occur more frequently in patients who are sputum-positive at the time of operation. The incidence of bronchopleural fistula after resection for mycobacterial disease is about 3 per cent, clearly higher than in pulmonary resections for other reasons. An apical space problem occurs after approximately 20 per cent of resections for mycobacterial disease, but only 10 to 15 per cent of these patients develop a bronchopleural fistula or empyema. Treatment of empyema in this setting is tube thoracostomy with later conversion to open drainage if a lung remnant remains. Subsequent thoracoplasty may be required. Bronchogenic spread of mycobacterial infection perioperatively is a rare complication. Appropriate chemotherapy and good pulmonary toilet perioperatively have essentially eliminated this complication.

Improved anesthetic techniques, better chemotherapy, careful patient selection, and the use of stapling devices have all contributed to the steadily decreasing morbidity and mortality of resectional surgery for pulmonary mycobacterial disease.[18,22] Resectional surgery is now employed in a selected group of patients who have failed chemotherapy or who have suffered complications such as massive hemoptysis or bronchopleural fistula. Mortality for pulmonary resection varies from 0 per cent with minimal morbidity when surgical intervention is elective[18,22] to 15 per cent[4,10] when resection is performed as an emergency procedure. The prognosis for long-term survival free of further mycobacterial disease is excellent in operative survivors, with 95 per cent of patients free of disease 5 to 8 years postoperatively.

SELECTED REFERENCES

Alexander, J.: The Collapse Therapy of Pulmonary Tuberculosis. Springfield, Ill., Charles C Thomas, 1937.
This text is a classic in the surgical treatment of pulmonary tuberculosis. The history of surgical treatment is covered extensively; and all forms of collapse therapy, including thoracoplasty, are presented in great detail.

Chapman, J. S.: The Atypical Mycobacteria and Human Mycobacteriosis. New York, Plenum Press, 1977.
This text is a thorough review of the development of knowledge of atypical mycobacteria. The relative responsiveness of each species to chemotherapy is presented, as well as an excellent review of surgical results in the treatment of atypical mycobacterial infection.

Des Prez, R. M., and Goodwin, R. A., Jr.: Mycobacterium Tuberculosis. *In* Mandell, G. L., Douglas, R. G., Jr., and Bennett, J. E. (Eds.): Principles and Practice of

Infectious Diseases, 2nd ed. New York, John Wiley & Sons, 1985, pp. 1383–1406.
This chapter provides an exhaustive current review of the bacteriology, pathophysiology, and chemotherapy of tuberculosis. It includes a particularly extensive bibliography.

Grange, J. M.: Mycobacteria and Human Disease. London, Edward Arnold, 1988.
This monograph provides a detailed review of the bacteriology of mycobacteria and the diseases caused by mycobacteria.

Green, G. M., Daniel, T. M., and Ball, W. C., Jr.: Koch Centennial Memorial. New York, American Lung Association, 1982.
This symposium contains both historical material and concise updates on all aspects of mycobacterial research and treatment.

Iseman, M. D., and Wallace, R. J.: Recent Advances in Mycobacterial Research and Management. Semin. Respir. Infect. 1(4), December 1986.
This volume contains excellent detailed reviews of the latest developments and research in the diagnosis and treatment of mycobacterial diseases.

Keers, R. Y.: Pulmonary Tuberculosis: A Journey Down the Centuries. London, A. Balliere Tindall, 1978.
An excellent up-to-date account of development of knowledge of tuberculosis from antiquity through the twentieth century. The impact of chemotherapy in the past 40 years throughout the world is detailed.

Snider, D. E., Jr.: Mycobacterial Diseases. Clin. Chest Med., 10(3), September 1989.
This volume presents recent reviews of the epidemiology of tuberculosis and atypical mycobacterial diseases. Recent advances in short course chemotherapy and the most current microbiologic diagnostic techniques are reviewed.

REFERENCES

1. American Thoracic Society/Centers for Disease Control: Treatment of tuberculosis and tuberculosis infection in adults and children. Am. Rev. Respir. Dis., 134:355, 1986.
2. Auerbach, O., and Dail, D. H.: Mycobacterial infections. *In* Dail, D. H., and Hammar, S. P. (Eds.): Pulmonary Pathology. New York, Springer-Verlag, 1988, pp. 173–188.
3. Bloch, A. B., Rieder, H. L., Kelly, G. D., Cauthen, G. M., et al.: The epidemiology of tuberculosis in the United States: Implications for diagnosis and treatment. Clin. Chest Med., 10:297, 1989.
4. Conlan, A. A., Hurwitz, S. S., Krige, L., Nicolaou, N., and Pool, R.: Massive hemoptysis: Review of 123 cases. J. Thorac. Cardiovasc. Surg., 85:120, 1983.
5. Contreras, M. A., Cheung, O. T., Sanders, D. E., and Goldstein, R. S.: Pulmonary infection with nontuberculous mycobacteria. Am. Rev. Respir. Dis., 137:149, 1988.
6. Corey, R., and Hla, K. M.: Major and massive hemoptysis: Reassessment of conservative management. Am. J. Med. Sci., 294:301, 1987.
7. Davidson, P. T.: Drug resistance and the selection of therapy for tuberculosis. Am. Rev. Respir. Dis., 136:255, 1987.
8. Etzkorn, E. T., Aldarondo, S., McAllister, C. K., Matthews, J., and Ognibene, A. J.: Medical therapy of *Mycobacterium avium-intracellulare* pulmonary disease. Am. Rev. Respir. Dis., 134:442, 1986.
9. Farman, D. P., and Speir, W. A., Jr.: Initial roentgenographic manifestations of bacteriologically proven mycobacterium tuberculosis: Typical or atypical? Chest, 89:75, 1986.
10. Garzon, A. A., Cerruti, M. M., and Golding, M. E.: Exsanguinating hemoptysis. J. Thorac. Cardiovasc. Surg., 84:829, 1982.
11. Grange, J. M.: Mycobacteria and Human Disease. London, Edward Arnold, 1988.
12. Hopewell, P. C.: Tuberculosis and human immunodeficiency virus infection. Semin. Respir. Infect., 4:111, 1989.
13. Hopkins, R. A., Ungerleider, R. M., Staub, E. W., and Young, W. G., Jr.: The modern use of thoracoplasty. Ann. Thorac. Surg., 40:181, 1985.
14. Horsburgh, C. R., Jr., Mason, U. G., III, Heifets, L. B., Southwick, K., LaBrecque, J., and Iseman, M. D.: Response to therapy of pulmonary *Mycobacterium avium-intracellulare* infection correlates with results of *in vitro* susceptibility testing. Am. Rev. Respir. Dis., 135:418, 1987.
15. Iseman, M. D., and Goble, M.: Treatment of tuberculosis. Adv. Intern. Med., 33:253, 1988.
16. Koch, R.: Die Aetiologie der Tuberculose. A translation by B. Pinner and M. Pinner. Am. Rev. Tuberc. 25:285, 1932.
17. Lowe, J. E., Daniel, T. M., Richer, C., and Wolfe, W. G.: Pulmonary tuberculosis in children. J. Thorac. Cardiovasc. Surg., 80:221, 1980.
18. Moran, J. F., Alexander, L. G., Staub, E. W., Young, W. G., Jr., and Sealy, W. C.: Long-term results of pulmonary resection for atypical mycobacterial disease. Ann. Thorac. Surg. 35:597, 1983.
19. Nemir, R. L., and Krasinski, K.: Tuberculosis in children and adolescents in the 1980's. Pediatr. Infect. Dis. J., 7:375, 1988.
20. O'Brien, R. J.: The epidemiology of nontuberculous mycobacterial disease. Clin. Chest Med., 10:407, 1989.
21. O'Brien, R. J., and Snider, D. E., Jr.: Tuberculosis drugs—old and new. Am. Rev. Respir. Dis., 131:309, 1985.
22. Reed, C. E., Parker, E. F., and Crawford, F. A., Jr.: Surgical resection for complications of pulmonary tuberculosis. Ann. Thorac. Surg., 48:165, 1989.

23. Rieder, H. L., Cauthen, G. M., Kelly, G. D., Bloch, A. B., and Snider, D. E. J., Jr.: Tuberculosis in the United States. J.A.M.A., 262:385, 1989.
24. Riley, L. W., Arathoon, E., and Loverde, V. D.: The epidemiologic patterns of drug-resistant Mycobacterium tuberculosis infections: A community-based study. Am. Rev. Respir. Dis., 139:1282, 1989.
25. Runyon, E. H.: Anonymous mycobacteria and pulmonary disease. Med. Clin. North. Am., 43:273, 1959.
26. Schlossberg, D.: Tuberculosis, 2nd ed. New York, Springer-Verlag, 1988.
27. Smith, M. H.: Tuberculosis in children and adolescents. Clin. Chest Med., 10:381, 1989.

28. Snider, D. E., Jr.: The tuberculin skin test. Am. Rev. Respir. Dis., 125(3)Pt. 2:108, 1982.
29. Tsukamura, M.: Evidence that antituberculosis drugs are really effective in the treatment of pulmonary infection caused by Mycobacterium avium complex. Am. Rev. Respir. Dis., 137:144, 1988.
30. Van Scoy, R. E., and Wilkowske, C. J.: Antituberculous agents. Mayo Clin. Proc., 62:1129, 1987.
31. Woodring, J. H., Vandiviere, H. M., Fried, A. M., and Dillon, M. L.: Update: The radiographic features of pulmonary tuberculosis. Am. J. Roentgenol., 146:497, 1986.

X

BENIGN TUMORS OF THE TRACHEA AND BRONCHI

James M. Douglas, Jr., M.D.

In 1767 Lieutaud first described at postmortem examination a tracheal fibroma.[28] Subsequently, in 1861, Türck identified a tracheal tumor within a living patient using indirect laryngoscopy.[44] Direct endoscopic visualization of a tracheal tumor was first documented by Killian in 1897[25]; and since that time, the incidence of benign tumors of the trachea and bronchi has remained exceedingly low. Caldarola and colleagues identified only 63 benign tumors and tumorlike conditions of the trachea and bronchi seen over a 30-year period from 1930 to 1960 at the Mayo Clinic.[5] In a study examining the Massachusetts General Hospital experience from 1969 to 1976, Weber and Grillo identified 84 tracheal tumors, only 8 of which were benign.[45] Despite their low incidence, these tumors represent potentially lethal phenomena that are eminently treatable when found prior to the occurrence of complications.

The majority of benign tumors of the trachea are also seen within the proximal bronchi. These tumors are three times more frequent in males than in females.[5] There is a peak incidence in the fifth and sixth decades. In children, 90 percent of upper airway tumors are benign, while in adults, malignant and benign tumors occur with equal frequency.[31] This chapter focuses on the truly benign tumors of the trachea and bronchi. The so-called bronchial adenomas, noted for their low-grade malignant potential, are reviewed in a subsequent chapter. Benign tumors of the trachea and bronchi are represented by a myriad of tumor types. Most of these tumors occur sporadically; and with the exception of squamous papillomas, which have been associated with viral infection, no consistent etiology for these tumors has been identified. Nonetheless, they do share similarities of clinical presentation and response to treatment. The usual features are explored, emphasizing differences as they occur, following which, a brief description of the various pathologic subtypes is presented.

CLINICOPATHOLOGIC FEATURES

Benign tumors of the trachea and bronchi are typically slow-growing, rounded masses under 2 cm. in length.[12] The surface of these tumors tends to be smooth, and ulceration is usually indicative of overlying inflammation. The presence or absence of calcium on radiographic examination does not reliably distinguish benign from malignant growth. Symptomatic presentation is a result of luminal obstruction or mucosal irritation, with or without bleeding. Greater than 75 per cent of the lumen may be obstructed before the development of symptoms.[45] The most common symptoms include dyspnea, cough, hemoptysis, and wheezing. More proximal tumors, particularly those in the subglottal area, may present with stridor. Symptoms may be positional. Pedunculated tumors can cause intermittent obstruction with varying degrees of respiratory symptoms. Persistent obstruction of the airway may result in distal atelectasis and/or pneumonia. The occurrence of any of the aforementioned symptoms should suggest the possibility of a tracheal or endobronchial tumor.

These tumors are identified by a variety of radiographic or endoscopic techniques. The presence of atelectasis or pneumonia may be indirect evidence of proximal airway obstruction. Occasionally, a large endotracheal tumor is visualized within the trachea on plain film (Fig. 1). More commonly, tomographic techniques, including linear tomography or computed tomography, are necessary for the actual radiographic visualization of these tumors[43] (Fig. 2). The detection of extrinsic compression or local invasion by potentially malignant lesions can be investigated noninvasively by means of barium swallow and computed tomography.[22] Newer techniques, including ultrafast computed tomography and nuclear magnetic resonance imaging, will become increasingly important as these techniques become more refined and generally available.[3] Clearly, the definitive diagnosis of these tumors is most easily made by endoscopic techniques, including laryngoscopy and bronchoscopy. However, in patients with severe airway compromise, endoscopy must be undertaken with caution for avoidance of further respiratory distress secondary to edema and bronchial constriction. It is prudent in extreme cases to have immediate access to tracheal intubation and surgical therapy. Cytologic evaluation is of little use in the diagnosis of benign tumors. Bronchoscopic biopsy may be definitive; however, in the presence of highly vascular tumors, e.g., hemangiomas, biopsy is contraindicated.

TREATMENT

The vast majority of benign tumors of the trachea or bronchi are best treated by segmental or sleeve resection. Pedunculated tumors may be excised with only partial removal of the tracheal or bronchial wall. Endoscopic removal is less reliable and requires follow-up evaluation for recurrence in most patients. Squamous papillomatosis is a particularly vexing problem because of the propensity for this tumor to recur after treatment. Laser ablation of these lesions has met with some success and is probably the current treatment of choice. Bronchoscopic fulguration has also been employed. Medical therapy has not generally been employed in the treatment of benign tumors of the

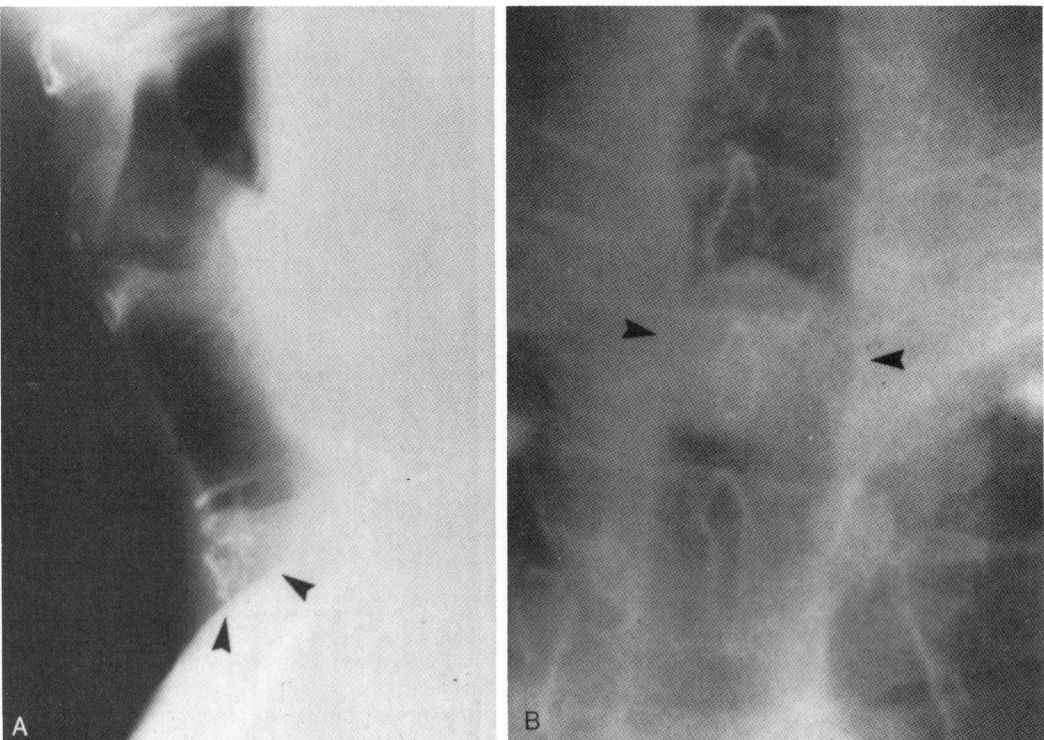

Figure 1. *A,* Lateral film of the neck demonstrating a chondroma of the middle third of the trachea with calcifications. *B,* Anteroposterior film of the trachea, revealing almost total occlusion of the tracheal lumen by the polypoid chondroma. (From Weber, A. L., and Grillo, H. C.: Tracheal tumors. Radiol. Clin. North Am. *16:*261, 1978.)

trachea and bronchi. Some authors have reported successful treatment of squamous papillomatosis with interferon.[20] However, steroid therapy was used at one time as adjunctive treatment of hemangiomas of the airways.[7] Presently, the majority

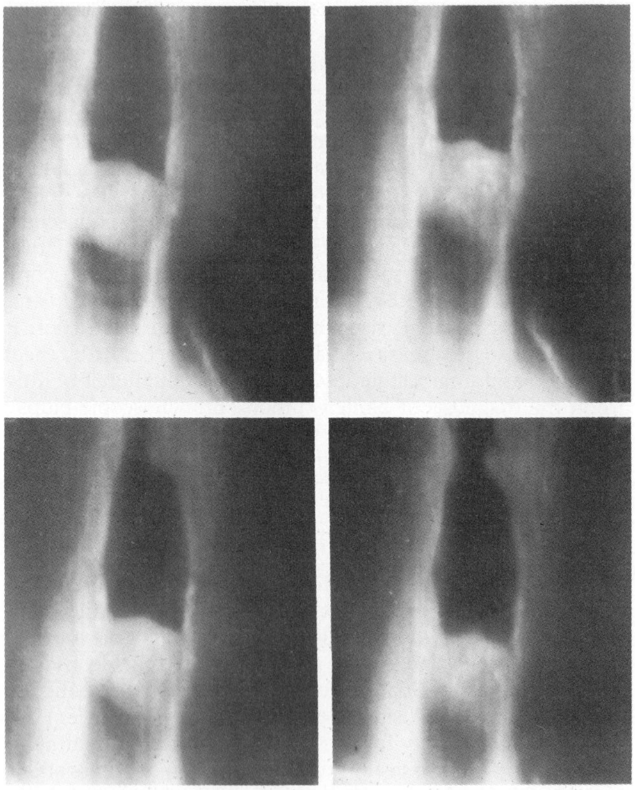

Figure 2. Tracheal tomograms of the chondroma from Figure 1, demonstrating increased resolution of this polypoid density occluding the trachea. (From Weber, A. L., and Grillo, H. C.: Tracheal tumors. Radiol. Clin. North Am. *16:*261, 1978.)

of endotracheal hemangiomas are treated by observation because of their propensity for spontaneous regression over time. Only resistant hemangiomas require surgical therapy. Radiation therapy is rarely indicated in the treatment of benign tumors. This mode of treatment is avoided because of the potential for inducing malignant degeneration and its lack of consistent efficacy.

The surgical treatment of proximal airway tumors presents some technical challenges specifically related to the maintenance of acceptable ventilation beyond the area of obstruction.[10,19] Techniques for distal intubation during the resection of proximal airway tumors are illustrated in Figures 3 and 4. The maintenance of a proper airway can also become problematic during the administration of endoscopic therapy. Percutaneous transtracheal ventilation has been used successfully for the laser endoscopic treatment of subglottic lesions.[32]

The surgical resection of tumors located in the distal portion of the main bronchi can be approached by standard posterolateral thoracotomies on the ipsilateral side. However, the management of tracheal tumors and tumors at the level of the carina require special considerations.[19] Tumors of the upper third of the trachea may be resected by a transcervical approach. This is typically accomplished by means of a standard collar incision. Occasionally, an incision parallel to the sternocleidomastoid is useful. Tumors of the middle third of the trachea may require a median sternotomy combined with a cervical extension. Tumors of the distal third of the trachea are typically approached through a right lateral thoracotomy for avoidance of the aortic arch. However, Perelman and Korolwa have described the resection of lower thoracic tracheal lesions via a left posterior thoracotomy through the bed of the resected fifth rib with the patient in the prone position.[35] In each approach, it is important that the tumor be accurately localized at the time of operation to ensure resection at the appropriate level. This becomes particularly important in the case of pedunculated tumors, in which the base may be located at a distance from the bulk of the tumor. Intraoperative bronchoscopy is useful for purposes of localization.

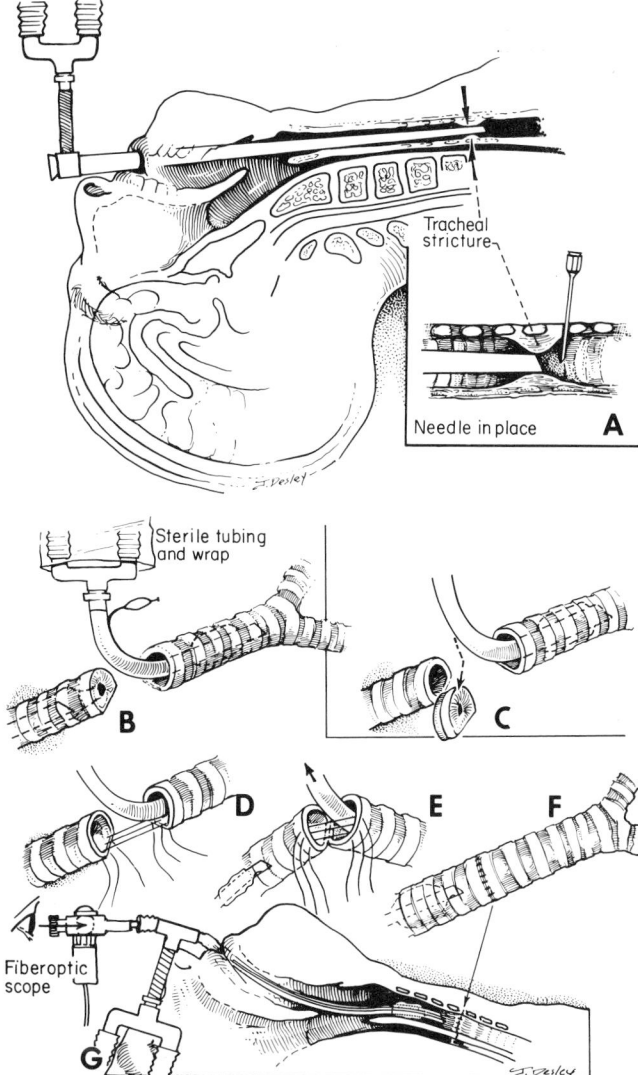

Figure 3. Technique for airway management and resection of occluding lesions of the middle trachea. *A*, Ventilating bronchoscope passed through the proximal trachea to the level of the obstructed mass. Needle localization of obstructing area may be useful. *B*, Sterile endotracheal tube passed into distal trachea after transection beyond the level of the obstruction. *C*, Excision of the obstructing lesion. *D* to *F*, Primary anastomosis of remaining trachea with removal of distal endotracheal tube. *G*, Ventilating bronchoscope passed for examination of result. (From Payne, W. S., Leonard, P. F., Miller, R. D., et al.: Physiologically based assessment and management of tracheal strictures. Surg. Clin. North Am., *53*:875, 1973.)

In the typical adult, primary anastomosis of the trachea can be safely accomplished after resection of 2 to 3 cm. of tracheal length without special efforts at mobilization.[18] However, primary anastomosis can be accomplished after resection of as much as 6 cm. of tracheal length if extensive mobilization techniques are employed. These techniques include division of the inferior pulmonary ligament, mobilization of the right mainstem bronchus from the pulmonary artery and vein and from the pericardium, and release of the larynx by separation of its thyrohyoid attachments.[18] After extensive tracheal resection, defects in the membranous portion may be closed with pericardium and reinforced with intrathoracic transposition of the serratus anterior muscle.[1] In all cases, Grillo has recommended that airway anastomoses be accomplished by means of absorbable 4–0 polyglactin (Vicryl) suture for minimizing granuloma formation.[19] In children, special techniques may be employed to avoid complete tracheal resection and subsequent stenosis.[33,37] This includes the use of rotational skin flaps as described by Daum and associates.[8]

SELECTED TRACHEAL AND BRONCHIAL TUMORS

Squamous Papillomatosis

Squamous papillomas are the most common benign tumors seen in the trachea. Most frequently they present as multiple lesions in children and are more commonly seen in the larynx in both children and adults. Only 2 to 3 per cent of papillomas occur in the lower respiratory tract. The typical appearance is that of multiple cauliflower-like lesions appearing on the larynx with associated lesions extending down the trachea and even mainstem bronchi. Pathologically, these tumors appear as irregular, papillary or villous processes comprised of branching stalks of loose fibrous tissue covered by thick squamous epithelium blending into the normal respiratory epithelium.[5] In adults, an isolated form that arises in the mucosa and is composed of squamous epithelium with a core of connective tissue is described.[12]

Squamous papillomatosis has been associated with human papilloma virus Types 6 and 11.[23] Approximately 2 per cent of patients with this entity develop malignant transformation.[11,30] The likelihood of malignant degeneration is increased in those patients with a history of previous radiation therapy. Isolated squamous papillomas in adults have been associated with a 50 per cent incidence of malignant degeneration.[42] Although papillomatosis is primarily associated with squamous cell carcinoma, a case of oat-cell carcinoma mimicking multiple papillomas was reported by Blackman and colleagues.[2]

Squamous papillomatosis occurs with equal frequency in both sexes. In its most frequent presentation in the larynx, voice change may be a presenting symptom. With more distal lesions, cough, recurrent infections, or upper airway obstruction can develop. In juvenile papillomatosis, there is a tendency toward regression with age, and by puberty the nodules usually subside. Occasionally, the onset of pregnancy has been accompanied by regression of lesions that later reappear following delivery. In some patients, the disease is relentless, and individuals are plagued with recurrent infections and upper airway symptoms.[26]

Squamous papillomas occurring in the bronchus frequently excavate. A pattern of multiple, large, smooth, thin-walled cavitary lesions in a young patient is essentially pathognomonic of papillomatosis.[12] These lesions may be differentiated from other cystic pulmonary diseases by their absence of fluid and their failure to fill on bronchography.[12]

The treatment of squamous papillomas is complicated by a recurrence rate as high as 90 per cent. Various methods have been used. Surgical resection may be indicated in localized lesions. Because of the frequently diffuse nature of the disease, bronchoscopic fulguration has been more often performed. Laser ablation is becoming the treatment of choice because it allows multiple treatments with a low incidence of complications.[47] Some experimental studies with medical therapy using interferon have been promising.[20] Because of the known association with malignant degeneration, the use of radiation therapy generally is not employed.

Angiomas

Hemangiomas are the most common tracheal neoplasms in children. They occur most often in the subglottic region and present with the early development of respiratory distress. Although the infants are asymptomatic at birth, 90 per cent become symptomatic prior to 3 months of age. These lesions vary in size depending upon engorgement. Symptoms of intermittent respiratory distress, often comparable to croup, may result in misdiagnosis. The tumors are sometimes associated with other vascular malformations, including hemangiomas of the skin, parotid gland, mediastinum, abdominal viscera, central nervous system, and retina. Tracheal hemangiomas are more

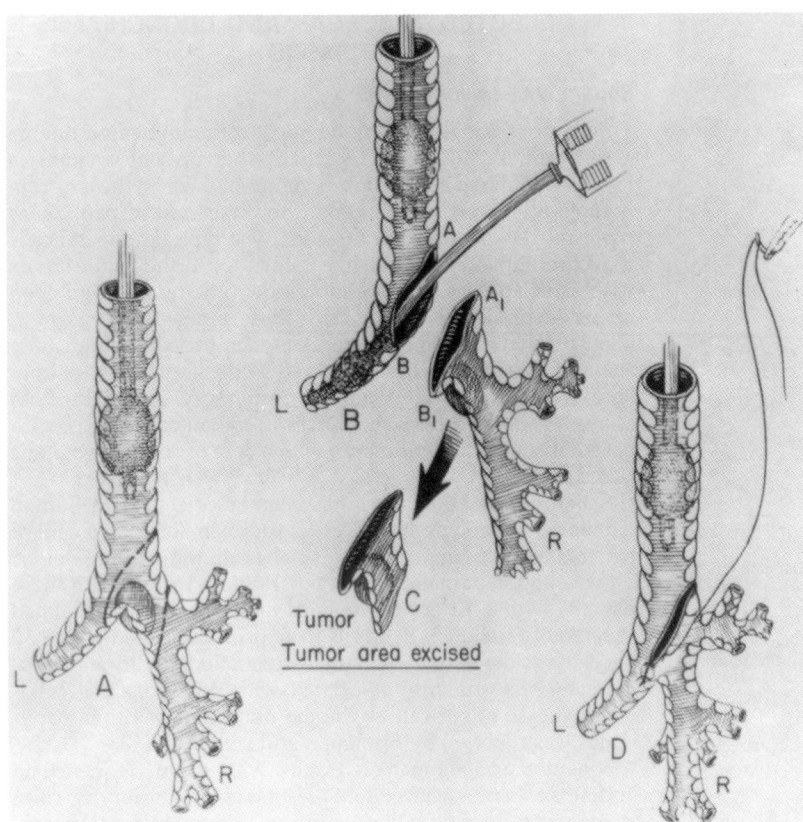

Figure 4. A technique for excision of a mass at the carina. *A,* Ventilation above the area of the tumor and the site of the proposed tumor excision. *B,* Division of the trachea and bronchus and insertion of the left-sided sterile endobronchial tube for ventilation. *C,* Removal of the tumor. *D,* Anastomosis of the remaining bronchus. (From Okike, N., Bernatz, P. E., Payne, W. S., et al.: Bronchoplastic procedures in the treatment of carcinoid tumors of the tracheobronchial tree. J. Thorac. Cardiovasc. Surg., 76:281, 1978.)

common in adults but when present occur most often in the supraglottal or laryngeal regions. Adults frequently present with the chief complaint of hoarseness. Tracheal hemangiomas are more common in females.[29] Pathologically, these hemangiomas are typically of the cavernous type. Nonetheless, the clinical course is characterized by spontaneous regression over time. Because of the frequency of regression, it is recommended that these tumors be treated conservatively with observation. Tracheostomy may be necessary when there is airway obstruction. Although steroids and radiation therapy have been used in the past, neither treatment is recommended.[4,7] Persistent, symptomatic hemangiomas require surgical excision.[29]

Hemangioendothelioma is an exceedingly rare vascular tumor of the trachea that appears grossly as a solid tumor and may be polypoid in appearance. It consists of a mass of endothelial cells with microscopic vascular channels. Local excision is adequate.[12,14]

Cartilaginous Tumors

Chondromas are slow-growing benign lesions of the trachea or bronchi arising from the cartilaginous plates. They appear grossly as gray to white firm masses with focal gritty areas secondary to calcification or ossification and are composed of both cartilage and bone cells with an intact overlying mucosa.[34] These tumors occur most commonly between the ages of 40 and 60 in both sexes, without any sexual predilection. There is a tendency toward malignant degeneration. Moreover, pathologic determination of malignancy is sometimes difficult.[46] Because of the tendency for local recurrence, treatment of these tumors should include complete segmental resection with end-to-end anastomosis.[27]

Hamartomas are usually seen in the bronchi but may occur in the trachea. These tumors typically contain cartilage along with fat, lymphoid tissue, or epithelial elements.[12] They characteristically present as asymptomatic solitary pulmonary nodules and comprise approximately 10 per cent of solitary pulmonary nodules described in large series. Approximately 20 per cent of hamartomas occur as endobronchial lesions and decrease in frequency with progression more proximally in the tracheobronchial tree. Peripheral hamartomas are frequently subpleural and may be evacuated from surrounding parenchyma with little loss of normal tissue. These tumors may also be treated by wedge excision; when more proximally located, sleeve resection is adequate.

Tracheobronchopathia osteoplastica is a pathologically distinctive lesion presenting as multiple submucosal tumors extending the entire length of the trachea. On endoscopic examination, it appears as multiple firm nodules. These tumors are composed of bone and cartilage. This process may extend into the bronchi, causing airway obstruction and distal infection. However, most commonly, it is asymptomatic or presents as mild dyspnea or cough. The peak incidence is at age 50 or greater. It is never found in children.[5] This process is most evident in the lower two thirds of the trachea.[5] Treatment is necessary only in the symptomatic patient and usually necessitates only bronchoscopic removal.[5]

Benign mixed tumor of the trachea is an extremely rare lesion. These tumors contain epithelial cells, mesenchymal cells, and cartilage. Histologically, they appear identical to the salivary gland tumors of the same name, and treatment is surgical excision.[24]

Fibroma

The first tracheal tumor described by Lieutaud in 1767 was probably a tracheal fibroma. These are unusual tumors typically found in the cervical trachea of children. They are solitary, well-defined masses composed of either pure acellular fibrous tissue or loose, cellular fibrous tissue.[12] Parenchymal fibromas may appear as coin lesions, and local surgical treatment is adequate.

Fibrous Histiocytoma

Fibrous histiocytoma is an unusual tumor that may have benign or malignant characteristics. Although this tumor is most commonly described in bone, it is occasionally seen within the tracheobronchial tree.[12]

Neurogenic Tumors

Neurogenic tumors of the lung were first described in the 1940s. These are rare tumors whose benign or malignant nature may be difficult to distinguish. Depending upon the predominant cell type, these tumors may be described as neurofibromas or neurilemomas. Intraluminal tracheal paragangliomas have been reported to secrete hormones.[12] Local excision of neurogenic tumors is the treatment of choice.

Leiomyoma

Leiomyoma of the trachea is a slow-growing, intramural tumor occurring most commonly in the lower third of the trachea. It may occur in the bronchus and usually appears as a smooth, broad-based sessile mass. Although this tumor must be distinguished from malignant leiomyosarcoma, local excision of the benign lesions is adequate.[12,38]

Granular Cell Myoblastoma

Granular cell myoblastoma was first described by Abrikossoff in 1926. Most commonly seen on the tongue,[45] it is a rare benign tumor of the larynx or major bronchi, less often found in the trachea. This tumor most frequently occurs in black women 30 to 50 years of age.[12] Histologically, it is characterized by large foamy cells in syncytial masses containing small hyperchromatic nuclei and numerous small eosinophilic granules.[6] They may be multiple or associated with subcutaneous lesions, and occasional malignant degeneration has been reported. Local removal is the treatment of choice.

Lipomas

Lipomas are rare tumors of the bronchus and trachea. They may present as pedunculated or sessile masses. They are typically soft but may be mucosal or mural, round or lobulated. Local removal is adequate.[40]

Ectopic Thyroid

Thyroid tissue occasionally occurs within the tracheal lumen and comprises approximately 7 per cent of all tracheal tumors.[17] These tumors occur three times more often in females, and two thirds are associated with goiter. They may connect with the trachea through the tracheal wall.[12] They most frequently occur in endemic areas of goiters, including Germany and Switzerland. Typically, the histologic features are normal; however, in approximately 10 per cent of these tumors, malignant degeneration develops.[36] Treatment is surgical therapy.

TUMORLIKE CONDITIONS

Numerous infectious, degenerative, and infiltrative diseases may present as tracheal or bronchial masses. Tuberculoma may simulate a neoplastic lesion. Other entities include scleroma, Wegener's granulomatosis, and xanthoma. Amyloid deposits in the tracheobronchial tree may present as irregular, nodular submucosal masses, which are stained with metachromatic dye and histologically contain eosinophilic, hyaline-like material. These deposits may be seen in the absence of systemic amyloidosis. Fungal diseases including histoplasmosis and coccidioidomycosis can also mimic airway tumors.[39]

SELECTED REFERENCES

Caldarola, V. T., Harrison, E. G., Clagett, O. T., and Schmidt, H. W.: Benign tumors and tumor-like conditions of the trachea and bronchi. Ann. Otol., 73:1042, 1964.
In this article, the authors provide a detailed description of one of the largest published compilations of benign tumors and tumorlike conditions of the trachea and bronchi. A report of 63 cases seen at the Mayo Clinic provides detailed descriptions of the clinical and pathologic findings in these patients.

Gilbert, J. J., Mazzarella, L. A., and Feit, L. J.: Primary tracheal tumors in the infant and adult. Arch. Otolaryngol., 58:1, 1953.
This is a classic study reviewing 546 cases of primary tracheal tumors in both infants and adults. It is well referenced and informative.

Grillo, H. C.: Tracheal surgery. Scand. J. Thorac. Cardiovasc. Surg., 17:67, 1983.
In this article, Grillo, a noted expert in the field of tracheal surgery, reports his 20-year experience with the treatment of disorders of the trachea. The article is filled with clinical and technical insights.

Grillo, H. C., Dignan, E. F., Miura, T., et al.: Extensive resection and reconstruction of the mediastinal trachea without prosthesis or graft: An anatomical study in man. J. Thorac. Cardiovasc. Surg., 48:741, 1964.
This anatomic study in cadavers provides important data demonstrating the allowable boundaries for tracheal resection and primary anastomosis. It is a carefully conducted study that provides useful data for all surgeons who operate on the trachea.

REFERENCES

1. Arnold, P. G., Pairolero, P. C., and Waldorf, J. C.: The serratus anterior muscle: Intrathoracic and extrathoracic utilization. Plast. Reconstr. Surg., 73(2):240, 1984.
2. Blackman, F., Chung, H. R., McDonald, R. J., et al.: Oat cell carcinoma with multiple tracheobronchial papillomatous tumors. Chest, 83:817, 1983.
3. Brasch, R. C., Gould, R. G., Goodling, C. A., et al.: Upper airway obstruction in infants and children: Evaluation with Ultrafast CT. Radiology, 165:459, 1987.
4. Calcaterra, T. C.: An evaluation of the treatment of subglottic hemangioma. Laryngoscope, 78:1956, 1968.
5. Caldarola, V. T., Harrison, E. G., Clagett, O. T., et al.: Benign tumors and tumor-like conditions of the trachea and bronchi. Ann. Otol., 73:1042, 1964.
6. Canalis, R. F., Dodson, T. A., Turkell, S. B., et al.: Granular cell myoblastoma of the cervical trachea. Arch. Otolaryngol., 102:176, 1976.
7. Cohen, S. R.: Unusual lesions of the larynx, trachea and bronchial tree. Ann. Otol. Rhinol. Laryngol., 78:476, 1969.
8. Daum, R., Denecke, H. J., and Roth, H.: Tumour-induced intraluminal stenoses of the cervical trachea: Tumour excision and tracheoplasty. Prog. Pediatr. Surg., 21:50, 1987.
9. Dedo, H. H., and Jackler, R. K.: Laryngeal papilloma: results of treatment with CO₂ laser and podophyllum. Ann. Otol. Rhinol. Laryngol., 91:425, 1982.
10. Ellis, D. J., Millar, W. L., and Karagianes, T. G.: Anesthesia for laser resection of a tracheal tumor in a woman pregnant with twins. Anesthesiology, 68:629, 1988.
11. Fechner, R. E., and Fitz-Hugh, G. S.: Invasive tracheal papillomatosis. Am. J. Surg. Pathol., 4:79, 1980.
12. Felson, B.: Neoplasms of trachea and mainstem bronchi. Semin. Roentgenol., 18:23, 1983.
13. Ferguson, C. F., and Flake, C. G.: Subglottic hemangioma as a cause of respiratory obstruction in infants. Ann. Otol. Rhinol. Laryngol., 70:1095, 1961.
14. Flege, J. B., Valencia, G., and Zimmerman, G.: Obstruction of a child's trachea by a polypoid hemangioendothelioma. J. Thorac. Cardiovasc. Surg., 56:144, 1968.
15. Frootko, N. J., and Rogers, J. H.: The treatment of juvenile multiple laryngeal papillomatosis by suction diathermy. J. Laryngol. Otol., 93:373, 1979.
16. George, P. J. M., Garrett, C. P. O., and Hetzel, M. R.: Role of the neodymium YAG laser in the management of tracheal tumours. Thorax, 42:440, 1987.
17. Gilbert, J. G., Mazzarella, L. A., and Feit, L. J.: Primary tracheal tumors in the infant and adult. A.M.A. Arch. Otolaryngol., 58:1, 1953.
18. Grillo, H. C., Dignan, E. F., Miura, T., et al.: Extensive resection and reconstruction of mediastinal trachea without prosthesis or graft: an anatomical study in man. J. Thorac. Cardiovasc. Surg., 48:741, 1964.
19. Grillo, H. C.: Tracheal Surgery. Scand. J. Thorac. Cardiovasc. Surg. 17:67, 1983.
20. Hendrickse, W. A., Irwin, B. C., Bailey, C. M., et al.: Regression of respiratory papillomatosis after treatment with interferon. Br. Med. J., 289:290, 1984.
21. Irwin, B. C., Hendrickse, W. A., Pincott, J. R., et al.: Juvenile laryngeal papillomatosis. J. Laryngol. Otol., 100:435, 1986.
22. Karlan, M. S., Livingston, P. A., and Baker, D. C.: Diagnosis of tracheal tumors. Ann. Otol. 82:790, 1973.
23. Kashima, H., Wu, T. C., Mounts, P., et al.: Carcinoma ex-papilloma: histologic and virologic studies in whole-organ sections of the larynx. Laryngoscope, 98:619, 1988.
24. Kay, S., and Brooks, J. W.: Benign mixed tumor of the trachea with seven-year follow-up. Cancer, 25:1178, 1970.
25. Killian: Quoted by Ellman, P., and Whittaker, H.: Primary carcinomas of the trachea. Thorax, 2:153, 1947.
26. LeRoux, B. T., Williams, M. A., and Kallichurum, S.: Squamous papillomatosis of the trachea and bronchi. Thorax, 24:673, 1969.
27. Le-Tian, X., Zhen-Fu, S., Ze-Jian, L., et al.: Tracheobronchial tumors: An eighteen-year series from Capitol Hospital, Peking, China. Ann. Thorac. Surg., 35:590, 1983.
28. Lieutaud, J.: Quoted by Ellman, P., and Whittaker, H.: Primary carcinomas of the trachea. Thorax, 2:153, 1947.
29. Maier, H. C.: Hemangiomas of the subglottic region, trachea, and mediastinum in infancy and childhood. Ann. Thorac. Surg., 3:514, 1967.
30. Matsuba, H. M., Thawley, S. E., Mauney, M., et al.: Laryngeal epidermoid carcinoma associated with juvenile laryngeal papillomatosis. Laryngoscope, 95:1264, 1985.
31. Miller, M. A. L., and Toma, G. A.: Fibroma of the trachea. Br. J. Dis. Chest, 53:177, 1959.
32. Monnier, P. H., Ravussin, P., Savary, M., et al.: Percutaneous transtracheal

ventilation for laser endoscopic treatment of laryngeal and subglottic lesions. Clin. Otolaryngol., 13:209, 1988.

33. Nakayama, D. K., Harrison, M. R., deLorimier, A. A., et al.: Reconstructive surgery for obstructing lesions of the intrathoracic trachea in infants and small children. J. Pediatr. Surg., 17:854, 1982.

34. Pairolero, P. C.: Benign and malignant neoplasms of the trachea. In Roth, J. A., Ruckdeschel, J. C., and Weisenburger, T. H. (Eds.): Thoracic Oncology. Philadelphia, W. B. Saunders Company, 1989.

35. Perelman, M. I., and Korolwa, N.: Surgery of the trachea. World J. Surg., 4:583, 1980.

36. Randolph, J., Grunt, J. A., and Vawter, G. F.: The medical and surgical aspects of intratracheal goiter. N. Engl. J. Med., 268:457, 1963.

37. Richardson, M. A., and Cotton, R. T.: Anatomic abnormalities of the pediatric airway. Pediatr. Clin. North Am., 31:821, 1984.

38. Sanders, J. S., and Carnes, V. M.: Leiomyoma of the trachea. N. Engl. J. Med., 264:277, 1961.

39. Scully, R. E., Mark, E. J., and McNeely, B. U.: Case records of the Massachusetts General Hospital, Case 43-1984. N. Engl. J. Med., 311:1105, 1984.

40. Scully, R. E., Mark, E. J., and McNeely, B. U.: Case records of the Massachusetts General Hospital, Case 45-1986. N. Engl. J. Med., 315:1277, 1986.

41. Shaha, A., DiMaio, T., Money, S., et al.: Prosthetic reconstruction of the trachea. Am. J. Surg., 156:306, 1988.

42. Spencer, H.: Rare pulmonary tumors. In Spencer, H. (Ed.): Pathology of the Lung, 3rd ed. New York, Pergamon Press, 1977.

43. Spizarny, D. L., Shepard, J. O., McLoud, T. C., et al.: CT of adenoid cystic carcinoma of the trachea. A.J.R. 146:1129, 1986.

44. Türck, L.: Quoted by Ellman, P., and Whittaker, H.: Primary carcinomas of the trachea. Thorax, 2:153, 1947.

45. Weber, A. L., and Grillo, H. C.: Tracheal tumors. Radiol. Clin. North Am., 16:227, 1978.

46. Weber, A. L., Shortsleeve, M., Goodman, M., et al.: Cartilaginous tumors of the larynx and trachea. Radiol. Clin. North Am., 16:261, 1978.

47. Wetmore, S. J., Key, J. M., and Suen, J. Y.: Complications of laser surgery for laryngeal papillomatosis. Laryngoscope, 95:798, 1985.

XI

BRONCHIAL ADENOMAS

James M. Douglas, Jr., M.D.

Bronchopulmonary carcinoids, mucoepidermoid tumors, and adenoid cystic carcinomas of the lung are all fundamentally different neoplasms that share certain clinical characteristics. Traditionally, these tumors have been grouped in the category of bronchial adenomas. However, each of these neoplasms has the potential for varying degrees of malignant behavior and, therefore, cannot be considered benign, as the term *adenoma* implies. The extremely rare true mucous gland adenoma has also been included, but it differs from the other three in that it *is benign.*

Bronchial carcinoids, adenoid cystic carcinomas of the bronchus, and mucoepidermoid tumors of the bronchus are typically slow-growing endobronchial neoplasms that collectively constitute approximately 5 per cent of all primary pulmonary neoplasms. Although they are much less aggressive than other carcinomas of the lung, they do retain the ability to invade locally and/or metastasize. In the majority of cases, surgical resection is the procedure of choice. There has been an increasing trend toward conservative resection whenever possible.

BRONCHOPULMONARY CARCINOIDS

Bronchial carcinoids were first described by Laennec in 1831.[16] The first clinical diagnosis was made by Kramer in 1930.[15] Carcinoids represent 0.6 to 2 per cent of all lung tumors and 83 per cent of bronchial adenomas.[6] They have been identified in a variety of patients with a wide age range and are seen in both children and the elderly. The median age was 55 years in a large study reported by McCaughan.[22] These tumors appear to have no sexual predilection.

Pathology

Bronchial carcinoids closely resemble the intestinal tumors of the same name (Fig. 1). They are composed of small, uniform cells with small nuclei and a reticular chromatin pattern. Characteristically, the cytoplasm contains neurosecretory granules, which may be identified by argyrophilic staining or electron microscopy.[17,19,29] In the bronchus, these tumors arise from the neuroendocrine argentaffin cells of the bronchial mucosa, called Kulchitsky's cells.[19] They are grouped among the APUD tumors (amine precursor uptake and decarboxylation). Immunohistochemical studies have demonstrated that these tumors

are capable of producing and storing a number of immunoreactive peptide hormones, including serotonin, kinin, histamine, bombesin, vasoactive intestinal peptide, gastrin, leu-enkephalin, growth hormone, corticotropin, glucagon, insulin, melanocyte-stimulating hormone, antidiuretic hormone, epinephrine, norepinephrine, somatostatin, substance P, calcitonin, and others.[4,29,33] Markers for two or more of these peptides can be demonstrated in most tumors. Immunoreactivity to neuron-specific enolase is seen in the vast majority of carcinoids.[19,33]

Most carcinoid tumors are slow-growing tumors with a favorable prognosis. Approximately 11 per cent of carcinoids behave aggressively and closely resemble the more common lung carcinomas.[2,34] The so-called atypical carcinoids were first suggested by Engelbreth-Holm in 1944 and more precisely defined by Vonalbertini in 1951.[2] Arrigoni in his 1972 report from the Mayo Clinic distinguished atypical carcinoids on the basis of features including increased mitotic activity, nuclear pleomorphism, nuclear hyperchromatism with prominent nucleoli, abnormal nuclear/cytoplasmic ratios, increased cellularity with disorganization of architecture, and tumor necrosis.[2] Ultrastructurally, these tumors generally have fewer neurosecretory granules and varying degrees of basal lamina deposition when compared with typical carcinoids.[34] Whereas the typical carcinoid tumors are most likely to be centrally located, the atypical carcinoids are frequently peripheral.[5,26] Detailed pathologic and

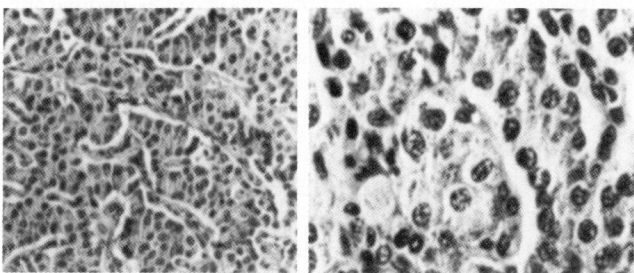

Figure 1. *A*, Photograph of a typical carcinoid tumor demonstrating islands of uniform, polyhedral cells with intervening fibrovascular stroma. Hematoxylin and eosin, ×80. *B*, High-power magnification of a typical carcinoid tumor demonstrating monotonous cells with uniform, round nuclei. Hematoxylin and eosin, ×500. (From Attar, S., Miller, J.E., Hankins, J., Thompson, B. W., Suter, C. M., Kleger, P. J., and McLaughlin, J. S.: Bronchial adenoma: A review of 51 patients. Ann. Thorac. Surg., 40:126, 1985.)

immunologic studies have recently suggested a close relationship among typical carcinoid tumors, atypical carcinoid tumors, and oat-cell carcinoma of the lung.[33,34] Each of these tumors is thought to originate from Kulchitsky cells. Varying degrees of differentiation are thought subsequently to result in a gradation of malignant behaviors, ranging from the more benign typical carcinoid to the extremely malignant oat-cell carcinoma. It has been recommended that typical carcinoids be categorized as Kulchitsky-cell Type I tumors, atypical carcinoids as Kulchitsky-cell Type II tumors, and small-cell carcinomas as Kulchitsky-cell Type III tumors.[25]

Clinical Presentation

Symptomatic bronchopulmonary carcinoid tumors typically present with cough, pneumonia, hemoptysis or dyspnea. Frequently, these signs and symptoms are present for months prior to definitive diagnosis. The more peripheral tumors are characteristically asymptomatic and are usually found on chest films. The carcinoid syndrome is rarely present and was seen in only 3 per cent of patients in a study from the Memorial Sloan-Kettering Cancer Center.[22] In addition to the episodes of flushing, diarrhea, and other systemic manifestations, the syndrome is characterized by lesions in the right side of the heart, including pulmonary stenosis and tricuspid insufficiency. Rarely, left valvular and endocardial lesions are seen. Although elevated levels of urinary 5-hydroxyindoleacetic acid (5-HIAA) may be diagnostic of the carcinoid syndrome, this metabolic end product of serotonin may be absent.[32] Bradykinin is a prime effector in the production of symptoms. Serotonin is inactivated by the liver but may be bound by platelets after its release and thereby inactivated throughout the circulation.[32]

Diagnosis

The chest radiograph is usually abnormal. The most common finding is some degree of distal atelectasis and/or pneumonia.[3,9] Occasionally, hyperinflated alveoli occur distal to an area of intermittent bronchial obstruction. Peripheral carcinoids present as isolated well-circumscribed, noncalcified parenchymal nodules. Large central masses may produce hilar enlargement; however, more often, these central tumors are discovered radiographically by means of tomography. Linear tomography can be particularly useful in defining such tumors. Computed tomography is useful not only for demonstrating intrabronchial tumors but also for evaluating nodal involvement, local invasion, and distal parenchymal changes.[23] Extension of the chest scan beneath the diaphragm is helpful in the evaluation of liver and adrenal metastases.

Bronchoscopy is extremely useful for biopsy of endobronchial lesions and the collection of washings for cytologic evaluation. Rarely, severe bleeding complications following broncho-

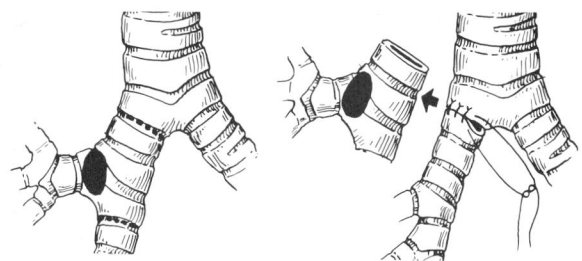

Figure 3. Technique for right upper sleeve lobectomy for a tumor at the right upper lobe orifice. (From Lowe, J. E., Bridgman, A. H., and Sabiston, D. C., Jr.: The role of bronchoplastic procedures in the surgical management of benign and malignant pulmonary lesions. J. Thorac. Cardiovasc. Surg., 83:227, 1982.)

scopic biopsy of carcinoid tumors have been reported.[31] However, flexible bronchoscopy with biopsy is thought by most to be a safe procedure that can be applied in most patients.

Therapy

Surgical resection of carcinoid tumors is the treatment of choice for all patients capable of tolerating surgical intervention.[3,18,22,26,27] The extent of resection is largely determined by the location of the tumor and the degree of distal parenchymal destruction. However, there has been an increasing trend toward conservative bronchoplastic procedures in those settings in which complete tumor removal can be assured while preserving pulmonary tissue[13] (Figs. 2 to 5). Because these tumors are malignant, lymph node sampling is still considered to be of prognostic value. Atypical carcinoids should be treated as other lung carcinomas are treated, because of their more malignant characteristics. Standard resection with inclusion of lymph node dissection is recommended.

Results

The overall prognosis for patients with carcinoid tumors is generally favorable. Because of the indolent growth characteristics of the typical carcinoid tumors, long-term survival has been demonstrated even in patients with malignant effusion who have undergone resection. Findings that indicate a poor prognosis include tumors greater than 3 cm. in diameter, lymph node metastases, and atypical histologic features. Patients with typical carcinoid tumors can expect a 95 per cent 5-year survival and a 90 per cent 10-year survival.[26] The prognosis is similar in children.[1,11] Atypical carcinoids carry a worse prognosis with a 66 per cent 5-year survival and a 60 per cent 10-year survival. A mean survival time of approximately 30 months was reported by both Arrigoni and Wilkins in separate studies.[2,35] Detailed studies of cytoarchitecture and chromosomal patterns have re-

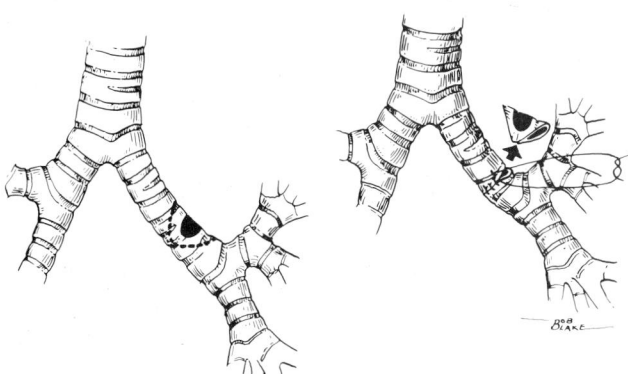

Figure 2. Technique for partial sleeve resection of a small tumor of the left main stem bronchus. (From Lowe, J. E., Bridgman, A. H., and Sabiston, D. C., Jr.: The role of bronchoplastic procedures in the surgical management of benign and malignant pulmonary lesions. J. Thorac. Cardiovasc. Surg., 83:227, 1982.)

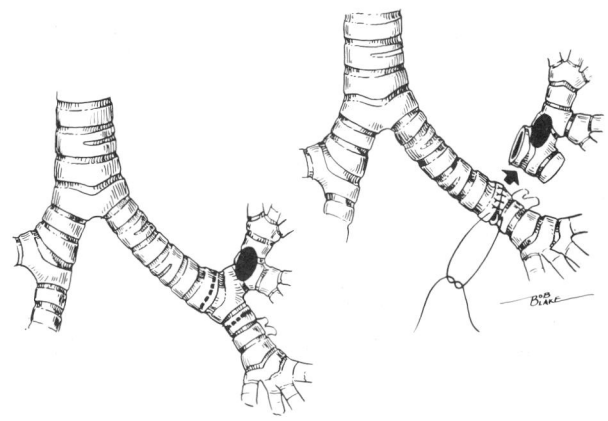

Figure 4. Left upper sleeve lobectomy for a tumor near the left upper lobe orifice. (From Lowe, J. E., Bridgman, A. H., and Sabiston, D. C., Jr.: The role of bronchoplastic procedures in the surgical management of benign and malignant pulmonary lesions. J. Thorac. Cardiovasc. Surg., 83:227, 1982.)

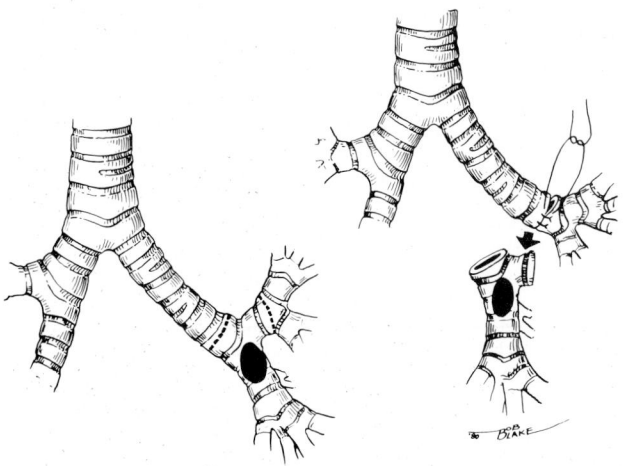

Figure 5. Left lower sleeve lobectomy for tumor arising near the left lower lobe orifice. (From Lowe, J. E., Bridgman, A. H., and Sabiston, D. C., Jr.: The role of bronchoplastic procedures in the surgical management of benign and malignant pulmonary lesions. J. Thorac. Cardiovasc. Surg., 83:227, 1982.)

vealed that DNA aneuploidy may be associated with increased malignant potential. However, this finding has not yet been shown to have clinical prognostic significance.[14]

ADENOID CYSTIC CARCINOMA

Adenoid cystic carcinomas of the bronchus, also known as cylindromas, are analogous to the tumors of the same name that arise from the salivary and lacrimal glands. In 1937, Hamperl categorized these tumors along with bronchopulmonary carcinoids as bronchial adenomas.[10] Although they are slow-growing tumors, they also share malignant characteristics and exhibit these tendencies more frequently than do carcinoid tumors. They represent approximately 12 per cent of all so-called bronchial adenomas. Adenoid cystic carcinomas are found throughout a broad range of ages and have been reported in children as young as 4 years of age and in the elderly.

Pathology

Adenoid cystic carcinomas are most often found in the distal trachea or proximal bronchi. Histologically, they may be divided into three distinguishable patterns. The tubular pattern is the most differentiated type and is characterized by single-lumen tubular units with small nests of cells (Fig. 6). The cribriform pattern consists of tumor cells arranged in nests or sheets fenestrated by round and oval spaces. The solid form consists of large cellular nests with no glandular spaces.[24] This is the most undifferentiated of the various histologic types. Similar patterns are also present in salivary gland and lacrimal gland tumors. The adenoid cystic carcinoma has a propensity for infiltration

within the submucosa or perineural lymphatic spaces along the tracheobronchial wall. This behavior is most characteristic of the tubular and cribriform subtypes. The solid subtype demonstrates more extensive extraluminal growth, and metastases are more common.[24]

Symptomatic presentations are directly related to the size and location of the adenoid cystic tumors. Within the trachea, these tumors may grow to near obstructive levels prior to being recognized symptomatically by the patient. Wheezing, cough, and dyspnea may occur. Hemoptysis may accompany superficial erosion of the tumor. Tumors located in the bronchus can become symptomatic earlier because of the relatively small diameter of the orifice. Recurrent pneumonia and a cough are common complaints.[24]

Diagnosis

Definitive diagnosis of adenoid cystic carcinoma of the bronchus may be made most expeditiously by bronchoscopic biopsy. Chest radiographs typically are nonspecific and most frequently show changes of parenchymal atelectasis, consolidation, or hyperinflation secondary to bronchial obstruction. Tomography may outline the tumor and indicate the degree of invasion.

Therapy

Surgical removal is the treatment of choice for all patients with resectable adenoid cystic carcinomas of the trachea and bronchi. Laser therapy has been used to open obstructed airways but is not considered curative.[20,30] Radiation therapy may be of some benefit in nonresectable tumors. Because of the rarity of these neoplasms, it is difficult to generate statistically significant numbers to attest to the relative value of adjunctive therapies.

Results

The prognosis in patients with adenoid cystic carcinoma of the trachea and bronchi is influenced by the tissue subtype and evidence for metastatic disease. Approximately 75 per cent of adenoid cystic carcinomas show evidence of lymph node involvement at the time of exploration. The most undifferentiated form of primary tumor is the solid subtype, and it is associated with a poor overall prognosis. Only 60 per cent of adenoid cystic carcinomas are totally resectable at the time of operation.[7] Even in the presence of local or distant spread, long-term survival can be predicted.

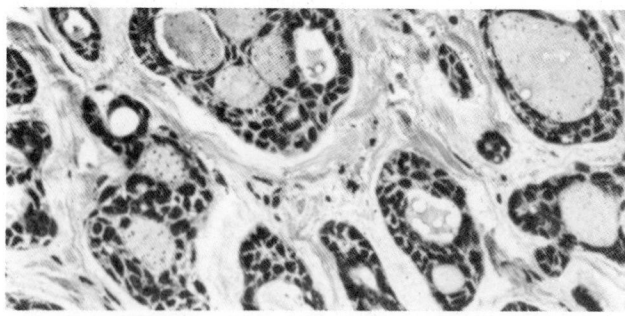

Figure 6. Cribriform subtype of adenoid cystic carcinoma. Hematoxylin and eosin, ×500. (From Nomori, H., Shizuka, K., Kobayashi, K., Ishihara, T., Yanai, N., and Torikata, C.: Adenoid cystic carcinoma of the trachea and main-stem bronchus. J. Thorac. Cardiovasc. Surg., 96:271, 1988.)

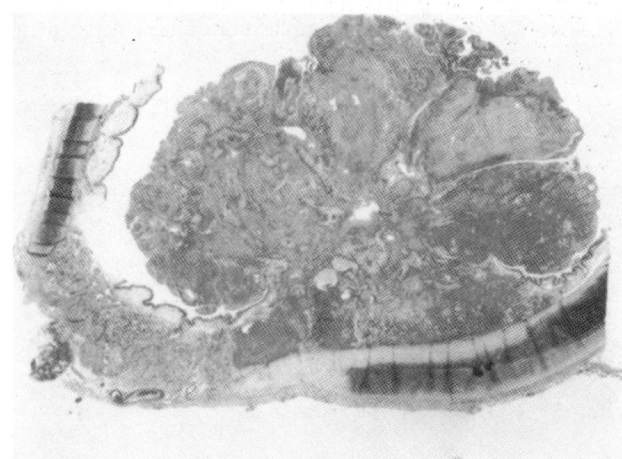

Figure 7. Mucoepidermoid tumor of the trachea. Hematoxylin and eosin, ×5. (From Heitmiller, R. F., Mathisen, D. J., Ferry, J. A., Mark, E. J., and Grillo, H. C.: Mucoepidermoid lung tumors. Ann. Thorac. Surg., 47:394, 1989.)

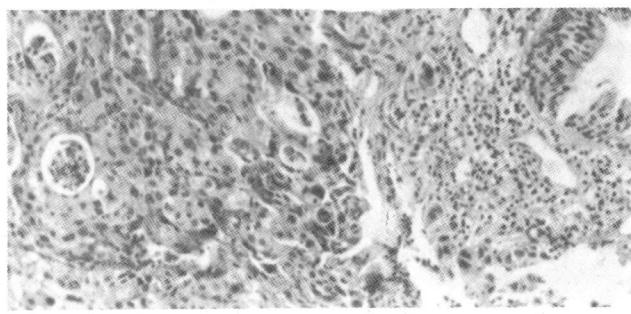

Figure 8. Photomicrograph of a low-grade mucoepidermoid tumor. Hematoxylin and eosin, ×125 before 3% reduction. (From Heitmiller, R. F., Mathisen, D. J., Ferry, J. A., Mark, E. J., and Grillo, H. C.: Mucoepidermoid lung tumors. Ann. Thorac. Surg., 47:394, 1989.)

MUCOEPIDERMOID CARCINOMA

Mucoepidermoid tumors of the lungs represent 0.2 per cent of all lung tumors. They constitute 1 to 5 per cent of all bronchial adenomas. Like other so-called bronchial adenomas, they are seen in a wide variety of patients and have no particular age, sex, or race predilection. These tumors were first described in autopsy cases by Smetana in 1952.[28]

Pathology

Mucoepidermoid lung tumors originate in the conducting airways (Fig. 7). Histologically, they are characterized by the presence of squamous or intermediate elements with intracellular bridges or cytoplasmic membranes. Glandular elements are present and are manifested by individual mucous cells, glandular cells, or ring cells. A mixture of cell types is seen, consisting of squamous, intermediate, and mucous cells. Broadly, the tumors may be divided into low-grade and high-grade tumors on the basis of mitotic activity, cellular necrosis, and nuclear pleomorphism[12] (Fig. 8). Most of the tumors are low-grade and slow-growing. The tumor grade does not appear to be directly related to the proportion of cell types present. Pathologically, it appears that mucoepidermoid and adenoid squamous carcinomas are the same entity. However, the latter tumors occur in the periphery of the lung and are usually of the high-grade type. These tumors are not related to bronchial carcinoids and histochemically may be differentiated by sparse monoamine oxidase activity.[8] No neurosecretory granules are seen on microscopic examination.

Diagnosis and Treatment

Patients with mucoepidermoid carcinoma present with signs of bronchial obstruction, bronchial irritation, constitutional symptoms, or no symptoms whatsoever. In a study by Heitmiller, 5 of 18 patients were asymptomatic upon presentation.[12]

These tumors may be visualized by chest films or computed tomographic scanning. However, definitive diagnosis is based upon biopsy specimens obtained at bronchoscopy or thoracotomy. Surgical extirpation is the treatment of choice. Radiation therapy has not been shown to be of value either as primary or adjuvant therapy, or as a treatment for metastatic disease. The overall prognosis for patients with mucoepidermoid lung tumors is generally favorable. However, survival is inversely related to tumor grade. Lymph node metastases are identified in 9 per cent of patients with these tumors.[21,22] Patients with low-grade tumors may experience 5-year survival approaching 100 per cent with therapy. However, high-grade tumors are associated with 66 per cent 4-year survival.[36]

SELECTED REFERENCES

Heitmiller, R. F., Mathisen, D. J., Ferry, J. A., et al.: Mucoepidermoid lung tumors. Ann. Thorac. Surg., 47:394, 1989.
This is an excellent reference on the clinical characteristics, pathologic findings, and surgical outcome of 18 patients with mucoepidermoid tumors of the lung. The authors provide clear separations between high-grade and low-grade tumor types and their associated prognoses.

Jensik, R. J., Faber, L. P., Brown, C. M., et al.: Bronchoplastic and conservative resectional procedures for bronchial adenoma. J. Thorac. Cardiovasc. Surg., 68:556, 1974.
This is a frequently quoted study of the surgical results for conservative resections of bronchial adenomas. The authors report an overall 5-year survival of 85 per cent and a 10-year survival of 78 per cent in 23 patients treated by bronchotomy and excision, segmental resection, or sleeve resection for bronchial adenomas. This was one of the major studies influencing the trend toward conservative resection for bronchial adenomas.

McCaughan, B. C., Martini, N., and Bains, M. S.: Bronchial carcinoids. J. Thorac. Cardiovasc. Surg., 89:8, 1985.
This is one of the largest series of bronchial carcinoid tumors reported in the literature and reviews the experience at the Memorial Sloan-Kettering Cancer Center over a 34-year period. It is a detailed study with significant survival data in patients with typical and atypical carcinoid tumors.

Nomori, H., Kaseda, S., Kobayashi, K., et al.: Adenoid cystic carcinoma of the trachea and main-stem bronchus. J. Thorac. Cardiovasc. Surg., 96:271, 1988.
Detailed clinical, histopathologic, and immunohistochemical data on 12 cases of adenoid cystic carcinoma of the trachea and main stem bronchus are presented.

Warren, W. H., Memoli, V. A., and Gould, V. E.: Immunohistochemical and ultrastructural analysis of bronchopulmonary neuroendocrine neoplasms. I. Carcinoids. Ultrastruct. Pathol. 6: 15, 1984.
The authors present an excellent discussion of the conventional staining, immunohistochemistry, and electron microscopic characteristics of 25 typical bronchopulmonary carcinoid tumors. The authors use this information to distinguish typical carcinoids from more aggressive, less differentiated neuroendocrine tumors.

Warren, W. H., Memoli, V. A., and Gould, V. E.: Immunohistochemical and ultrastructural analysis of bronchopulmonary neuroendocrine neoplasms. II. Well-differentiated neuroendocrine carcinomas. Ultrastruct. Pathol., 7:185, 1984.
This is the second part of the authors' extensive studies of neuroendocrine tumors. Excellent electron micrographs are presented along with standard hematoxylin and eosin photomicrographs. Extensive immunohistochemical studies were performed for characterization of the well-differentiated carcinomas.

REFERENCES

1. Archer, R. L., Grogg, S. E., and Sanders, S. P.: Mucoepidermoid bronchial adenoma in a 6-year old girl: A case report and review of the literature. Thorac. Cardiovasc. Surg., 94:453, 1987.
2. Arrigoni, M. G., Woolner, L. B., Bernatz, P. E.: Atypical carcinoid tumors of the lung. J. Thorac. Cardiovasc. Surg., 64:413, 1972.
3. Attar, S., Miller, J. E., Hankins, J., et al.: Bronchial adenoma: A review of 51 patients. Ann. Thorac. Surg., 42:126, 1985.
4. Blobel, G. A., Gould, V. E., Moll, R., et al.: Coexpression of neuroendocrine markers and epithelial cytoskeletal proteins in bronchopulmonary neuroendocrine neoplasms. Lab. Invest. 52:39, 1985.
5. Case Records of the Massachusetts General Hospital: Case 48-1987. N. Engl. J. Med., 317:1399, 1987.
6. Case Records of the Massachusetts General Hospital: Case 23-1989. N. Engl. J. Med., 320:1540, 1989.
7. Donahue, J. K., Weichert, R. F., and Ochsner, J. L.: Bronchial adenoma. Ann. Surg., 167:873, 1968.
8. Feldman, J. M., Benning, T. L., and Saltzman, H. S.: Biochemical and ultrastructural differences between muco-epidermoid and carcinoid tumors of the bronchus. J. Surg. Oncol., 37:227, 1988.
9. Halevy, A., Schachner, A., Nili, M., Moshe, N., et al.: Bronchial adenoma: Surgical experience with long-term follow-up (4–17 years). J. Surg. Oncol., 29:66, 1985.
10. Hamperl, H.: Über gutartige Bronchialtumoren (Cylindrome und Carcinoide). Virchows Arch. Pathol. Anat. 300:46, 1937.
11. Hartman, G. E., and Shochat, S. J.: Primary pulmonary neoplasms of childhood: A review. Ann. Thorac. Surg., 36:108, 1983.
12. Heitmiller, R. F., Mathisen, D. J., Ferry, J. A., et al.: Mucoepidermoid lung tumors. Ann. Thorac. Surg., 47:394, 1989.
13. Jensik, R. J., Faber, L. P., Brown, C. M., et al.: Bronchoplastic and conservative resectional procedures for bronchial adenoma. J. Thorac. Cardiovasc. Surg., 68:556, 1974.
14. Jones, D. J., Hasleton, P. S., and Moore, M.: DNA ploidy in bronchopulmonary carcinoid tumours. Thorax, 43:195, 1988.
15. Kramer, R.: Adenoma of bronchus. Ann. Otol. Rhinol. Laryngol., 39:689, 1930.
16. Laennec, R. T. H.: Traite de l'Auscultation mediate et des Maladres des Poumons et du Coeur, 3rd ed. Vol 1. Paris, Chard, 1831, p. 250.
17. Lehto, V.-P., Miettinen, M., Dahl, D., et al.: Bronchial carcinoid cells contain neural-type intermediate filaments. Cancer, 54:624, 1984.
18. Le-Tian, X., Zhen-Fu, S., and Ze-Jian, L.: Tracheobronchial tumors: An eighteen-year series from Capital Hospital, Peking, China. Ann. Thorac. Surg., 35:590, 1983.

19. Linnoila, R. I., Mulshine, J. L., Steinberg, S. M., et al.: Neuroendocrine differentiation in endocrine and nonendocrine lung carcinomas. Am. J. Clin. Pathol., 90:641, 1988.

20. Macha, H. N., Koch, K., Stadler, M., et al.: New technique for treating occlusive and stenosing tumours of the trachea and main bronchi: endobronchial irradiation by high dose iridium-192 combined with laser canalisation. Thorax, 42:511, 1987.

21. Markel, S. F., Abell, M. R., Haight, C., et al.: Neoplasms of bronchus commonly designated as adenomas. Cancer, 17:590, 1964.

22. McCaughan, B. C., Martini, N., and Bains, M. S.: Bronchial carcinoids. J. Thorac. Cardiovasc. Surg., 89:8, 1985.

23. Muller, N. L., and Webb, W. R.: Radiographic imaging of the pulmonary hila. Invest. Radiol., 20:661, 1985.

24. Nomori, H., Kaseda, S., Kobayashi, K., et al.: Adenoid cystic carcinoma of the trachea and main-stem bronchus. J. Thorac. Cardiovasc. Surg., 96:271, 1988.

25. Paladugu, R. R., Benfield, J. R., Pak, H. Y., et al.: Bronchopulmonary Kulchitzky cell carcinoma: A new classification scheme for typical and atypical carcinoids. Cancer, 55:1303, 1985.

26. Rea, F., Binda, R., Spreafico, G., et al.: Bronchial carcinoids: A review of 60 patients. Ann. Thorac. Surg., 47:412, 1989.

27. Rozenman, J., Pausner, R., Lieberman, Y., et al.: Bronchial adenoma. Chest, 92:145, 1987.

28. Smetana, H. F., Iverson, L., and Swan, L. L.: Bronchogenic carcinoma. Analysis of 100 autopsy cases. Milit. Surg., 3:335, 1952.

29. Stahlman, M. T., Kasselberg, A. G., and Orth, D. N.: Ontogeny of neuroendocrine cells in human fetal lung. II. An immunohistochemical study. Lab. Invest., 52:52, 1985.

30. Stanley, P. R. W., Anderson, T., and Pagliero, K. M.: Laser photoresection in the preoperative assessment of a bronchial adenoma. Thorax, 43:741, 1988.

31. Todd, T. R., Cooper, J. D., Weissberg, D., et al.: Bronchial carcinoid tumors. J. Thorac. Cardiovasc. Surg., 79:532, 1980.

32. Toole, A. L., and Stern, H.: Carcinoid and adenoid cystic carcinoma of the bronchus. Ann. Thorac. Surg., 13:63, 1972.

33. Warren, W. H., Memoli, V. A., and Gould, V. E.: Immunohistochemical and ultrastructural analysis of bronchopulmonary neuroendocrine neoplasms. I. Carcinoids. Ultrastruct. Pathol., 6:15, 1984.

34. Warren, W. H., Memoli, V. A., and Gould, V. E.: Immunohistochemical and ultrastructural analysis of bronchopulmonary neuroendocrine neoplasms. II. Well-differentiated neuroendocrine carcinomas. Ultrastruct. Pathol., 7:185, 1984.

35. Wilkins, E. W., Grillo, H. C., Moncure, A. C., et al.: Changing times in surgical management of bronchopulmonary carcinoid tumor. Ann. Thorac. Surg., 38:339, 1984.

36. Yousem, S. A., and Hochholzer, L.: Mucoepidermoid tumors of the lung. Cancer, 60:1346, 1987.

XII

CARCINOMA OF THE LUNG

David C. Sabiston, Jr., M.D.

The increasing incidence of primary carcinoma of the lung has been dramatic, especially because it was almost nonexistent until the twentieth century and now ranks first among malignant neoplasms in both men and women. Carcinoma of the breast was the most common malignant neoplasm in women until 1986, when it was surpassed by carcinoma of the lung. Cigarette smoking is regarded as the primary etiologic factor in the pathogenesis of carcinoma of the lung. Surgical extirpation remains the primary treatment except for small-cell ("oat cell") carcinoma, which is usually best managed by chemotherapy and radiation.

HISTORICAL ASPECTS

In 1895 Macewen did the first pneumonectomy, but it was performed in multiple stages by thermocoagulation.[28] The patient achieved a remarkable response and returned to the same hospital for a herniorrhaphy 45 years later. In 1933, Graham performed the first successful one-stage pneumonectomy.[12]

PATHOGENESIS

Cigarette smoke contains potent carcinogens, including polycyclic hydrocarbons (benzopyrenes) and N'-nitrosonornicotine is present in unburned tobacco and may also be significant. In a study of over 2000 patients with carcinoma of the lung, only 134 (5 per cent) were nonsmokers, which indicates again the highly significant relationship of cigarette smoking.[24] Further evidence of the link between cigarette smoking and carcinoma of the lung is found in a review of 6071 men 45 years of age or more, 805 of whom had bronchogenic carcinoma and were smokers. In another study, the *death rate* for lung cancer per 100,000 patients increased progressively in direct proportion to the amount of smoking. For example, in nonsmokers, the rate was 3.4 per 100,000, in those who smoked 10 to 20 cigarettes

daily it was 59 per 100,000, and in those smoking 40 cigarettes or more daily it was 217 per 100,000.

Auerbach described a landmark postmortem study involving 117 men, aged 22 to 88, two thirds being between 50 and 70.[1] The smoking history of each was documented, and studies were made of the entire tracheobronchial tree in each man at autopsy. Approximately 200 histologic sections were obtained, and microscopic evaluation was made by two or more pathologists. Of the 117 patients in the study, 34 died of bronchogenic carcinoma, and all were smokers. In the remaining 83 patients, death was due to a condition other than pulmonary carcinoma. In this group, 16 patients never smoked regularly or at all; 20 patients smoked a pack of cigarettes daily, and 47 patients smoked more than one pack daily. Four changes were evaluated in each histologic section, including (1) basal cell hyperplasia, (2) stratification, (3) squamous metaplasia, and (4) carcinoma *in situ*. This study showed that in those dying of conditions other than lung cancer, basal cell hyperplasia, stratification, and squamous cell carcinoma *in situ* were less frequent in the group who never smoked regularly and that there were progressive increases in the severity of the cytologic changes in those men who had been moderate to heavy smokers.

Additional evidence of cigarette smoking in the pathogenesis of lung cancer has been demonstrated in experimental studies that showed that in dogs that smoked cigarettes through tracheostomies for prolonged periods carcinoma of the lung developed, and in some, metastases to lymph nodes were present.[16] An example of such an invasive squamous carcinoma is shown in Figure 1.[16]

Combined cigarette smoking and exposure to asbestos is synergistic in carcinogenic effect. However, in nonsmokers exposed to asbestos, the incidence of pulmonary cancer was comparable to the incidence in the general population. Smoking and the use of tobacco are associated with other serious and often fatal diseases. In a study of 200,000 life-insurance holders who smoked

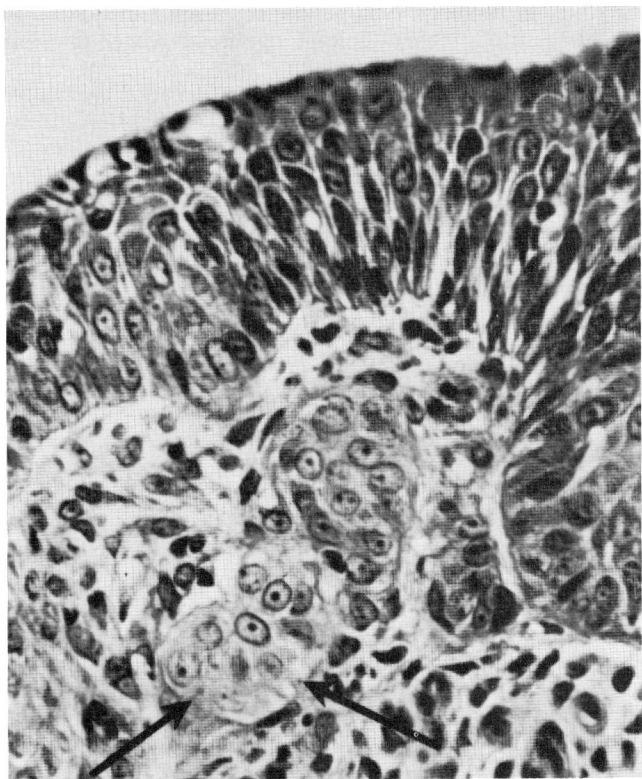

Figure 1. Invasive squamous cell carcinoma from the bronchus of a dog that had smoked 6210 cigarettes. The arrows indicate the area of invasion. Hematoxylin and eosin, ×560. (From Hammond, E. C., Auerbach, O., Kirman, D., and Garfinkel, L.: Effects of cigarette smoking on dogs. CA, 21:78, 1971. By permission of authors and the American Cancer Society, Inc.)

regularly, there was an increased incidence of death not only from lung cancer but also from cardiovascular disorders, respiratory diseases, and other ailments.[10]

PATHOLOGIC ASPECTS

A useful classification of carcinoma of the lung is as follows: (1) squamous cell carcinoma (epidermoid); (2) adenocarcinoma; (3) undifferentiated or anaplastic carcinoma (including small-cell, large-cell, and oat-cell carcinoma; and (4) bronchoalveolar carcinoma.

SQUAMOUS CELL CARCINOMA. The most common form is squamous cell carcinoma, and its incidence varies from 40 to 70 per cent of total lesions. It is usually associated with a history of prolonged smoking and is uncommonly seen in nonsmokers. With poorly differentiated forms of squamous cell carcinoma, the cytology merges into a pattern of anaplastic carcinoma. Most squamous cell carcinomas are located centrally in the large bronchi and frequently metastasize to the hilar, mediastinal, and (later) supraclavicular lymph nodes. Squamous cell carcinoma spreads to many distant organs but involves the brain and bone less frequently than adenocarcinoma. Squamous neoplasms are often large and discovered late.

ADENOCARCINOMA. In most series this type is present in 5 to 15 per cent of patients. The lesions are apt to be located in the periphery and occur more often in women. Adenocarcinoma tends to metastasize to the liver, brain, bone, and adrenals in addition to lymph nodes.

UNDIFFERENTIATED CARCINOMA. Undifferentiated cell types include small or round-cell, large-cell, and oat-cell lesions. In most series, this highly malignant type forms 20 to 30 per cent of the total. Such neoplasms must be diagnosed accurately because treatment is primarily by multiagent chemotherapy. In a group of patients considered to have bona fide small-cell carcinoma of the lung diagnosed by standard microscopy, those lesions with ultrastructural features of epithelial differentiation were defined by the presence of well-formed desmosomes that joined adjacent cells by additional features of squamous or glandular differentiation. By electron microscopy, 31 of 51 (60 per cent) cases were considered to be the typical oat-cell type, and 20 (40 per cent) showed features of epithelial differentiation.[22] Fifteen (75 per cent) tumors with epithelial features were considered to be operable, and 9 (45 per cent) were resected for cure. However, 26 (84 per cent) tumors regarded as typical oat-cell carcinomas by electron microscopy presented with extensive metastatic disease. The cancer-free 5-year survival rate of patients whose tumors showed features of epithelial differentiation was 25 per cent. The actual survival rate of nine patients with resected tumors with epithelial features was 38 per cent at 5 years, and only one patient whose tumor was considered typical of oat-cell carcinoma by electron microscopy survived for 5 years. Therefore, the significance of an examination by electron microscopy is apparent.

ALVEOLAR CELL CARCINOMA. Alveolar cell carcinoma is distinctive and has a more favorable prognosis than the other cell types. Evidence that it is increasing is drawn from a survey of the world literature. In a recent series of 205 patients at Duke University with alveolar cell carcinoma from 1970 to 1985, the presenting symptoms were most frequently productive cough and chest pain. Two radiologic types were identified; the first represented the "coin" lesion or nodule suspected of malignancy. These are usually located peripherally and may be involved in a previous scar. The second form is the "pneumonic" type and may be localized to a segment or generalized. Because this lesion may metastasize, computed tomograms of the chest with views of the adrenals and liver should be obtained. Among the 205 patients studied, 27 per cent underwent computed tomographic (CT) scanning, and evidence of metastatic disease was found in 32 per cent.[17]

The specific cytologic diagnosis of this type is very important. In the series of 205 patients, 29 had evidence of alveolar cell carcinoma by sputum analysis. Bronchial washings were positive in 26 per cent, and bronchial biopsy yielded positive results in 43 per cent of patients. Seventy-four per cent of transthoracic needle aspirations were positive. One quite promising test is immunohistochemical staining. With the use of specific antibodies to surfactant high-molecular-weight glycoprotein, alveolar cell carcinoma can be substantiated.

If metastases are not present, surgical excision of the primary lesion(s) is usually indicated. In the group of 205 patients, the resection varied from simple wedge excision in 22 per cent to pneumonectomy in 2 patients (1 per cent). Most often a lobectomy was done to provide cure (77 per cent). Radiation therapy is controversial, as is chemotherapy, in this group. A triple drug chemotherapy trial for advanced alveolar cell carcinoma using 5-fluorouracil (5-FU), vincristine, and mitomycin C showed a 33 per cent response rate and increased the rate of survival from 13 to 28 weeks, a rather impressive record. A 5-year survival of more than 50 per cent can be achieved when the disease is localized at the time of resection.

Giant-cell carcinoma can be considered separately since it has an unusually progressive clinical course.[34] A controversial subject is "scar carcinoma" of the lung, described as a secondary response to other primary disorders of the lung. Several authors have reported similar changes occurring in scars caused by tuberculosis, trauma, pulmonary infarction, pneumoconiosis, and other lesions. Various theories have been proposed to explain the development of malignancy in scars, including blockage of the lymphatics by scar tissue with concentrations of anthracotic pigments containing carcinogens. Among 32 patients with cancer in pulmonary scars, most were bronchoalveolar le-

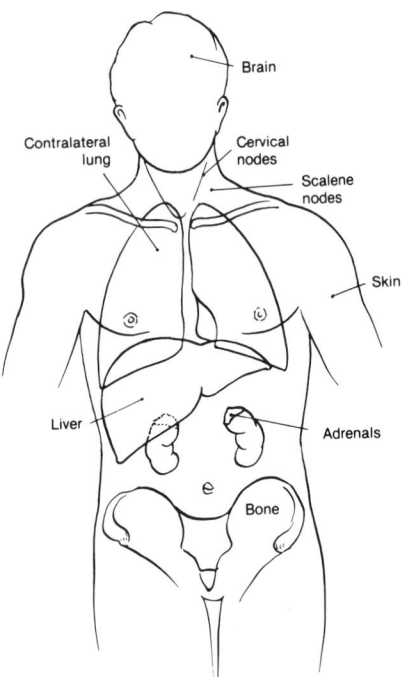

(1) different histologic type, (2) different lobe, (3) interval between the two tumors of at least 3 years. Moreover, the incidence of secondary primary tumors increases with survival and emphasizes the need for close follow-up for early detection.

METASTASES FROM CARCINOMA OF THE LUNG. Lymphatic spread to nodes in the hilum and the mediastinum is frequent. Other lymph nodes, including those in the paratracheal, paraesophageal, supraclavicular, and cervical regions, are well recognized. Metastases to other organs, in order of usual incidence, include the bones, adrenals, liver, kidneys, heart, and contralateral lung (Figs. 2 and 3; Table 1).

Solitary cerebral metastases from lung cancer were studied in 41 patients with resection of a primary pulmonary lesion and one or more metastases to the brain. In 19 patients, the cell type was adenocarcinoma; in 4, small-cell carcinoma; and in 2, large-cell carcinoma. Wedge resection was done in 4 patients; lobectomy, in 20; pneumonectomy, in 14; and bilobectomy, in 3. Cerebral radiation was used in 25 patients (61 per cent), with one survival 18.3 years after craniotomy. This 25-year experience with an aggressive approach to solitary cerebral metastases showed improved survival and justifies further use.[26]

CLINICAL MANIFESTATIONS

Patients may be asymptomatic or have severe disease with diffuse metastases. Symptoms are dependent upon the anatomic location of the lesions, extension to surrounding structures, metastases, and the systemic effects due to hormonal syndromes.[21] Lesions have been traced in previous chest films, and the neoplasm has been shown retrospectively from 5 years or more before the onset of clinical symptoms. A lesion was present in one series of operable patients an average of 3 years before surgical extirpation.[35,36] Cough, hemoptysis, anorexia, and weight loss are the most frequent clinical findings and are highly suggestive of primary bronchogenic carcinoma. If weight loss is considerable, there is a strong likelihood that metastases have occurred (Table 2). Although the disease is most frequent in the group 50 years of age and over, it may occur in young patients.

COUGH. The most common clinical symptom is cough, and it occurs in 75 per cent or more of patients. The lesions that produce cough are usually located in major bronchi and cause irritation by erosion. Sputum, often bloody, accompanies cough, and the amount depends on the degree of infection.

HEMOPTYSIS. One of the most alarming symptoms to the patient is hemoptysis, which frequently prompts consultation.

Figure 2. Common sites of metastases from carcinoma of the lung. (From Beahrs, O. H., and Myers, M. H. (Eds.): American Joint Committee on Cancer: Manual for Staging of Cancer, 2nd ed. Philadelphia, J. B. Lippincott Company, 1983.)

sions.[37] Although the use of the term scar carcinoma continues, there is no absolute proof that it exists, because the scarring may be caused by carcinoma.

Dual primary bronchogenic carcinoma has stimulated much interest and controversy. Among 2664 patients in a study of bronchogenic carcinoma, 34 were regarded as being dual primary lesions.[33] Five occurred simultaneously, and 20 had an interval between the appearance of the two lesions. Eight of the tumors were confined to the same side, and 26 were contralateral. It is interesting that bronchial mucus containing bronchogenic carcinoma has been shown to cause metastatic transfer of cells from a primary bronchogenic carcinoma to another portion of the lung.[4] In a recent study, in as many as 10 per cent of patients with primary carcinoma of the lung a second primary pulmonary cancer developed.[46] The criteria for diagnosing a second primary lung cancer were one or more of the following:

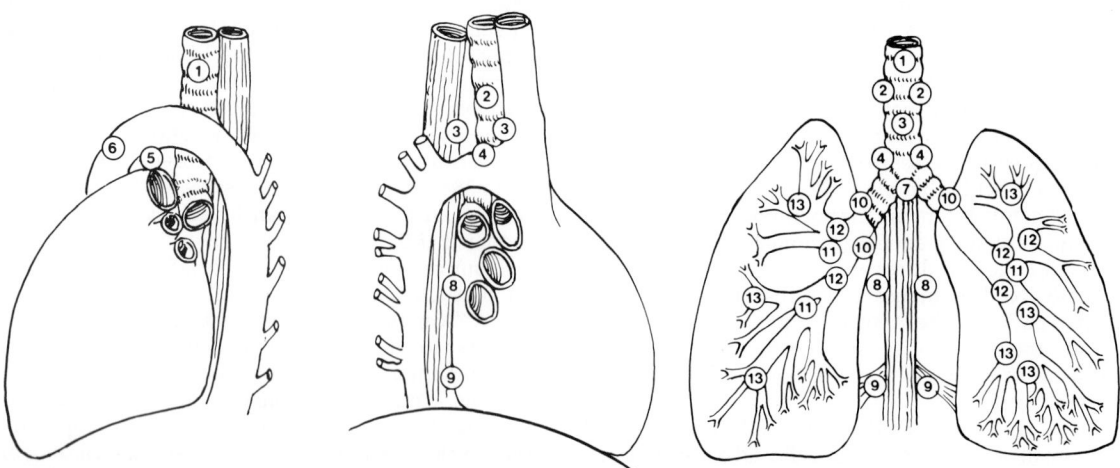

Figure 3. Sites of metastases in lymph nodes of mediastinum in carcinoma of the lung. N_2 *nodes. Superior mediastinal nodes:* 1, highest mediastinal; 2, upper paratracheal; 3, pre- and retrotracheal; 4, lower paratracheal (including azygos nodes). *Aortic nodes:* 5, subaortic (aortic window); 6, paraaortic (ascending aorta or phrenic). *Inferior mediastinal nodes:* 7, subcarinal; 8, paraesophageal (below carina); 9, pulmonary ligament. N_1 *nodes:* 10, hilar; 11, interlobar; 12, lobar; 13, segmental. (From Beahrs, O. H., and Myers, M. H. (Eds.): American Joint Committee on Cancer: Manual for Staging of Cancer, 2nd ed. Philadelphia, J. B. Lippincott Company, 1983.)

TABLE 1. Distribution of Metastases from Primary Carcinoma of the Lung

Organ	Per Cent
Lymph nodes	96
Bones	48
Adrenals	40
Liver	41
Kidneys	19
Heart	15
Contralateral lung	13

Adapted from Fried, B. M.: Tumors of the Lungs and Mediastinum. Philadelphia, Lea & Febiger, 1958.

This symptom varies from 6 to 52 per cent, although in most series it is present in approximately one third of patients. Rarely, hemoptysis may be massive and require emergent control.

CHEST PAIN. About half the patients with carcinoma of the lung have chest discomfort when first examined. It is often described as a "heaviness." Constant, severe pain is a poor prognostic sign, often signifying direct invasion of nerves and bone. Pain in the shoulder or arm may be associated with an apical (Pancoast's) pulmonary tumor.

DYSPNEA. Difficulty in breathing may occur in patients with carcinoma of the lung. Wheezing occurs in a few, usually caused by a lesion producing bronchial obstruction.

PLEURAL EFFUSION. Pleural effusion may be present and often suggests the presence of pleural metastases. Recurrence after aspiration is a poor prognostic sign. Blood-stained pleural fluid also strongly suggests direct involvement of the pleura with metastases. The superior vena cava syndrome occurs in approximately 5 per cent of patients and is generally indicative of extensive mediastinal spread. Radiation therapy produces a favorable response in approximately half of these patients.

CLUBBING. Clubbing of the fingers may be present and may disappear after resection of the tumor. Hypertrophic pulmonary osteoarthropathy occurs in 4 to 12 per cent of patients, produces symmetrical proliferative subperiosteal osteitis with new bone formation, and primarily affects the distal segments of the shafts of the long bones. Chronic synovitis may cause joint pain, with a diagnosis of rheumatoid arthritis. Prompt relief follows resection of the tumor.

HOARSENESS. Hoarseness is present in up to 8 per cent of patients and usually follows involvement of the recurrent laryngeal nerve by direct invasion of metastatic tumor. Cervical lymph node metastases occur in 15 to 20 per cent. Dysphagia occasionally occurs (1 to 5 per cent), indicating direct involve-

TABLE 2. Initial Symptoms of 2000 Patients with Bronchogenic Carcinoma

	VA Lung Cancer Group (1969–1972)
Cough	74%
Weight loss	68%
Dyspnea	58%
Chest pain	49%
Hemoptysis	29%
Lymphadenopathy	23%
Bone pain	25%
Hepatomegaly	21%
Clubbing	20%
Superior vena cava syndrome	4%

From Hyde, L., and Hyde, C. I.: Clinical manifestations of lung cancer. Chest, 65:299, 1974.

ment of the esophagus. Liver enlargement suggests metastatic spread.

Bronchogenic carcinoma is associated with some fascinating hormonal syndromes, including lesions producing clinical endocrinopathies such as adrenal hyperfunction, inappropriate diuresis, hypercalcemia, the carcinoid syndrome, and others. The most common of these is a type of Cushing's syndrome, usually with an oat-cell tumor. Antidiuretic hormone can be produced, especially from a poorly differentiated tumor or adenocarcinoma, with signs of mental confusion or coma and marked hyponatremia (100 to 120 mEq.). These patients can be managed by reduction of fluid intake to maintain appropriate levels of serum sodium. Parathormone secretion, usually from squamous cell lesions, occurs and may produce symptoms of

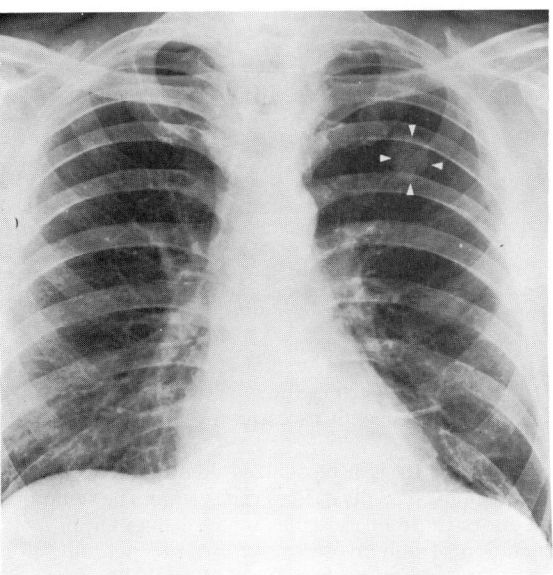

A

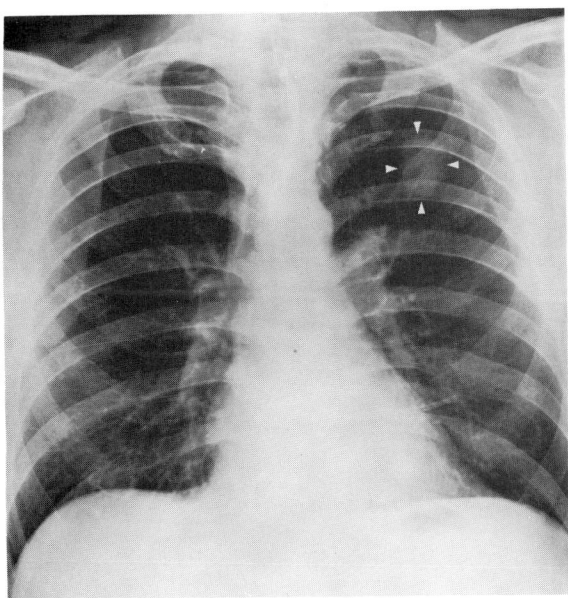

B

Figure 4. Growth of peripheral bronchogenic carcinoma: serial films. A, There is a poorly defined noncalcified nodule in the left upper lobe (arrowheads). B, Six months later there is a marked increase in the size of the nodule (arrowheads). The diameter of the nodule is 50 per cent greater, indicating tripling of the tumor volume. Doubling of tumor volume within 3 months to a year suggests a malignant lesion. (From Teplick, J. G., and Haskin, M. E.: Roentgenologic Diagnosis: A Complement in Radiology to the Beeson and McDermott Textbook of Medicine. Vol. 1. 3rd ed. Philadelphia, W. B. Saunders Company, 1976.)

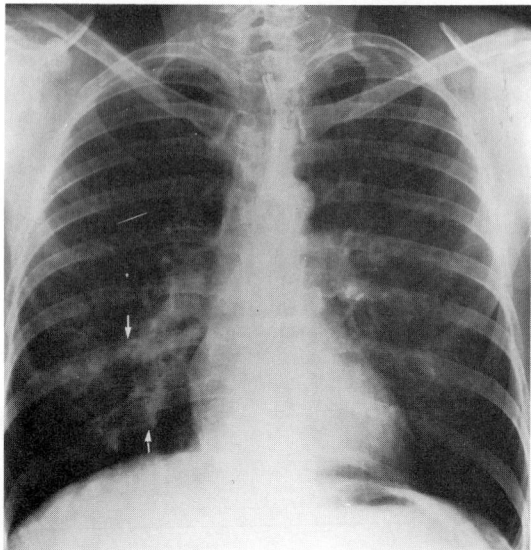

Figure 5. Bronchogenic carcinoma: pneumonic picture. Pneumonic consolidation (arrows) with irregular borders persisted with little change over 6 weeks. It was a small carcinoma in the segmental bronchus. Persisting, recurring, or unresolved pneumonia, especially in a patient over 40 years of age, should be investigated. (From Teplick, J. G., and Haskin, M. E.: Roentgenologic Diagnosis: A Complement in Radiology to the Beeson and McDermott Textbook of Medicine. Vol. 1. 3rd ed. Philadelphia, W. B. Saunders Company, 1976.)

hypercalcemia, including mental confusion. Additional features include hypoglycemia, the carcinoid syndrome, and gynecomastia associated with excessive production of gonadotropin.[30]

Neuromyopathy is a recognized complication of bronchogenic carcinoma (usually oat-cell carcinoma). The symptoms are divided into those of muscular origin, consisting of a clinical presentation of polymyositis, and those of neurologic origin, with sensory and motor loss. Cortical cerebellar degeneration with diffuse atrophy of the cerebellum and of the associated spinocerebellar tracts and systems can occur as a remote effect of carcinoma of the lung. Remissions may occur after the removal of the primary lesion.[31] Psychiatric problems may also be present.[29]

The superior sulcus tumor of Pancoast is an interesting lesion and consists of a neoplasm that infiltrates the upper mediastinum and involves the brachial plexus and cervical sympathetic nerves. Symptoms include pain in the shoulder and arm as well as the axilla, the inner aspect of the upper arm, and the scapular region. Horner's syndrome may be present on that side if the sympathetic nerves are involved.

DIAGNOSTIC TECHNIQUES

CHEST FILMS. The chest film is the primary tool in assessment of carcinoma of the lung. A mass is usually noted, and a pneumonic infiltrate may be present. Pleural effusion may be seen, as well as an elevated diaphragm, due to paralysis of the phrenic nerve. Osteolytic lesions may be seen in the ribs or other bones as metastases. Collapse of a lobe or segment may follow an obstructing bronchial lesion causing atelectasis. A common finding on the chest film is an isolated mass in the peripheral field of the lung and may be either a smooth-bordered coin-shaped lesion or an irregular defect varying in size. Frequently these lesions are asymptomatic and are first noted on a routine chest film. The radiographic features of several types of bronchogenic carcinoma are shown in Figures 4 to 11.[45]

Carcinoma of the lung can be roentgenographically occult. In a 10-year experience at the Mayo Clinic, 54 men were found to have carcinoma of the lung.[8] There were no initial changes seen on the chest films, but all patients had abnormal cytologic findings in the sputum. The lesion was localized in all patients by bronchoscopy, and pulmonary resection was performed. Among the 44 patients the 5-year survival with TIS N_0M_0 and $T_1N_0M_0$ neoplasms was 91 per cent. It is apparent that patients with occult lung cancer have a strong likelihood of long-term survival if the cancer is treated early. Careful follow-up is important because of the incidence of a second primary lung cancer, which was 22 per cent in this series.

COMPUTED TOMOGRAPHY. Scanning is useful in the detection of local spread of the primary lesion as well as in the demonstration of metastases.[5] CT scans of the thorax, including the adrenal glands, are important in establishing the appropriate staging of the lesion.

BIOPSY AND CYTOLOGIC STUDIES. A definite histologic diagnosis of carcinoma of the lung in 90 to 95 per cent of patients can be established by sputum cytology, bronchoscopy, bronchial biopsy, bronchial brushings, and/or bronchial washings.[6] Peripheral carcinomas of the lung may be diagnosed by bronchoscopic brushing techniques, and these lesions can be definitely diagnosed in 60 per cent of patients.[7]

PERCUTANEOUS TRANSTHORACIC ASPIRATION NEE-

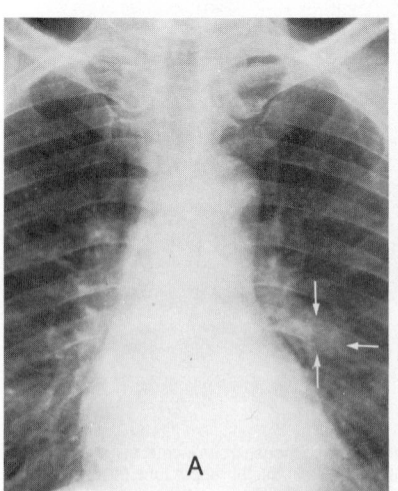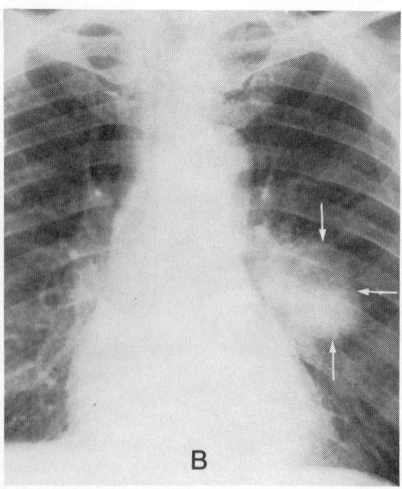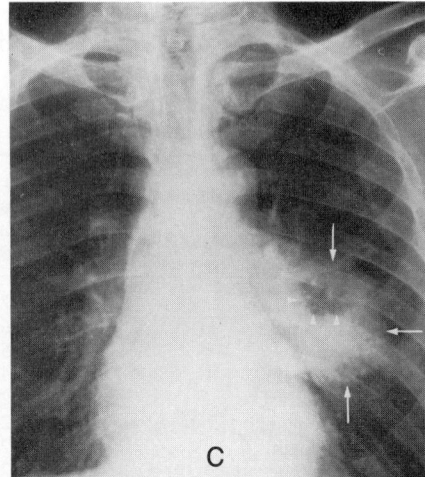

Figure 6. Bronchogenic carcinoma: progressive growth and cavitation. *A,* There is a small density in the lower left hilum (arrows). The patient was asymptomatic and refused surgery. *B,* Six months later there is a marked increase in the size of the mass (arrows). The mass was lobulated but still well demarcated. *C,* Two months later the mass is even larger (arrows) and has undergone central necrosis (arrowheads). Irregularity of the cavity, with protruding nodular densities, is characteristic of a cavitating bronchogenic carcinoma. (From Teplick, J. G., and Haskin, M. E.: Roentgenologic Diagnosis: A Complement in Radiology to the Beeson and McDermott Textbook of Medicine. Vol. 1. 3rd ed. Philadelphia, W. B. Saunders Company, 1976.)

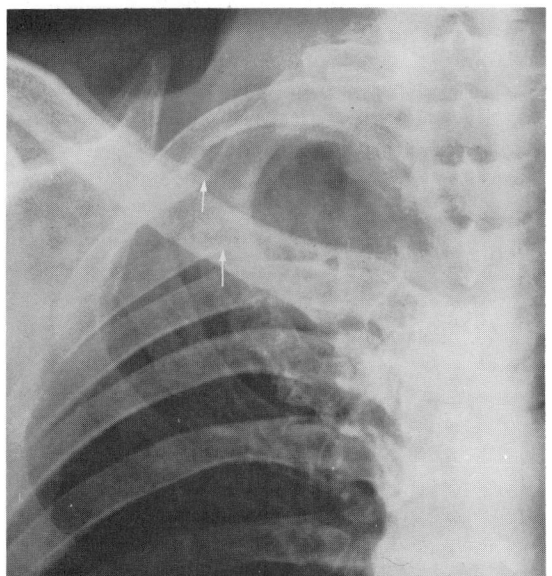

Figure 7. Superior sulcus tumor. The posterior portions of the third and fourth ribs (arrows) have been destroyed. The innocuous-appearing density in the right apex is due to an infiltrating anaplastic carcinoma that has destroyed the ribs. Tumors in the apical sulcus frequently simulate benign pleural thickenings, but rib erosion and the clinical symptoms of intractable shoulder pain and Horner's syndrome should aid in diagnosis. A superior sulcus lesion (Pancoast's tumor) may be either a squamous cell bronchogenic tumor or an anaplastic lesion. (From Teplick, J. G., and Haskin, M. E.: Roentgenologic Diagnosis: A Complement in Radiology to the Beeson and McDermott Textbook of Medicine. Vol. 1. 3rd ed. Philadelphia, W. B. Saunders Company, 1976.)

DLE BIOPSY. Aspiration needle biopsy is a useful approach for the diagnosis of bronchogenic carcinoma not visualized by bronchoscopy. Among 896 patients with malignant intrathoracic neoplasms, the needle aspirate showed malignant cells in 96 per cent.[40]

MEDIASTINOSCOPY. Direct observation of the mediastinum can be achieved by a small incision in the suprasternal fossa and passage of a mediastinoscope along the anterior course of the trachea. Lesions arising in the proximal bronchi are more likely to be associated with mediastinal metastases, whereas peripheral lesions do not usually metastasize to the mediastinum early in the clinical course.[20] An acceptable alternative to mediastinoscopy is a short anterior or lateral thoracotomy in preference to mediastinoscopy, since it is simple and also allows an assessment of operability for hilar lesions. The incision can be extended at the time, and pulmonary resection can be done if the lesion is operable. Occasionally, mediastinoscopy is associated with complications, including hemorrhage.

Bone marrow aspiration for detection of tumor cells in patients with bronchogenic carcinoma is helpful, particularly with oat-cell carcinoma. However, the overall incidence of identification of metastatic tumor by this technique is low.[14]

Differential Diagnosis

Other conditions that should be considered in the differential diagnosis of bronchogenic carcinoma include pneumonia, pulmonary abscess, tuberculosis, histoplasmosis, and other fungal infections. Metastatic lesions from a distant primary tumor can produce roentgenographic changes that suggest primary bronchogenic carcinoma. Lymphosarcoma of the lung may rarely simulate bronchogenic carcinoma, and a homogeneous mass is seen that may enlarge to fill almost the entire chest.

Signs of Inoperability

A bloody pleural effusion, Horner's syndrome, vocal cord paralysis, phrenic nerve paralysis, the superior vena cava syndrome, and distant metastases are usually considered contraindications to operation, and radiation or chemotherapy should be considered.

Operative Risk

Operative risk should be carefully assessed in all patients. Pulmonary function studies indicative of pulmonary insufficiency, cardiac disease, and age are known to be important factors. Combinations of these factors are associated with a high mortality. The mortality of pneumonectomy is generally less than 5 per cent, and most deaths after pulmonary resection are

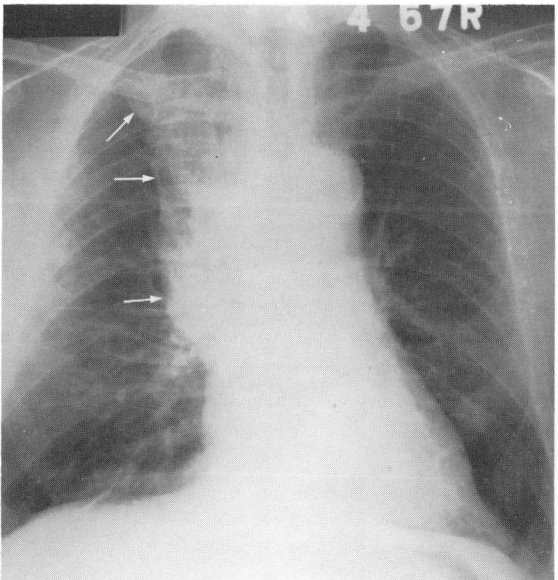 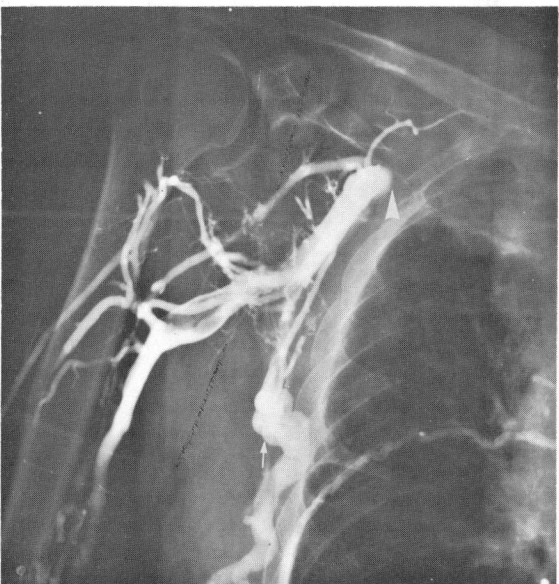

A **B**

Figure 8. Bronchogenic carcinoma: superior vena caval obstruction. A, There is enlargement of the right hilum and widening of the mediastinum on the right (arrows) due to mediastinal extension of a bronchogenic carcinoma. There was clinical evidence of superior vena caval obstruction. B, Venogram reveals complete blockage of the subclavian vein (arrowhead). There are large dilated and anastomotic channels (arrow) extending between the superior vena cava and subclavian vein. In the presence of such findings, the lesion is inoperable. (From Teplick, J. G., and Haskin, M. E.: Roentgenologic Diagnosis: A Complement in Radiology to the Beeson and McDermott Textbook of Medicine. Vol. 1. 3rd ed. Philadelphia, W. B. Saunders Company, 1976. By permission of Dr. Arlyne Shockman, Veterans Administration Hospital, Philadelphia.)

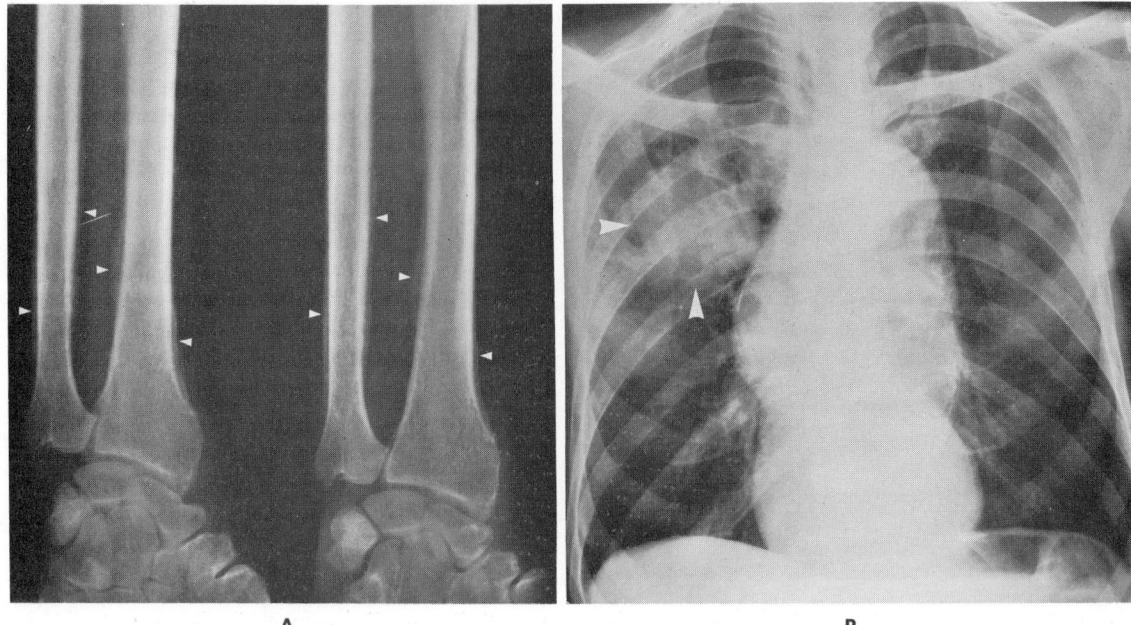

A   B

Figure 9. Bronchogenic carcinoma: pulmonary osteoarthropathy. *A,* There are linear irregular areas of subperiosteal new bone formation in the distal radius and ulna (arrowheads). *B,* A large bronchogenic carcinoma is apparent in the right upper lobe (arrowheads). Following resection, periosteal reaction cleared completely. Evidence of pulmonary osteoarthropathy may occasionally be the first clue to bronchogenic carcinoma. (From Teplick, J. G., and Haskin, M. E.: Roentgenologic Diagnosis: A Complement in Radiology to the Beeson and McDermott Textbook of Medicine. Vol. 1. 3rd ed. Philadelphia, W. B. Saunders Company, 1976.)

due to cardiac complications. The mortality for lobectomy is 2 per cent or less.

SURGICAL MANAGEMENT

Because about half of patients presenting with carcinoma of the lung have distant metastases, the remainder are candidates for surgical management. Of these, approximately half have disease in the chest at the time of operation beyond the limits of operability. In most patients, lobectomy is the treatment for bronchogenic carcinomas. Pneumonectomy is required for complete removal of the lesions that involve the left or right main bronchus or those with spread or fixation of the tumor to the hilum. For tumors in the periphery, especially in patients with reduced pulmonary reserve or those who are high risks for other reasons, local ("wedge") excision is an adequate procedure.[43] Most prefer a posterior thoracotomy (the standard thoracotomy) through the fifth or sixth intercostal space for pulmonary resection because it provides superior exposure.

In the technique of pulmonary resection, the automatic stapling device has become an important feature and provides a more secure bronchial closure. With its use, the postoperative

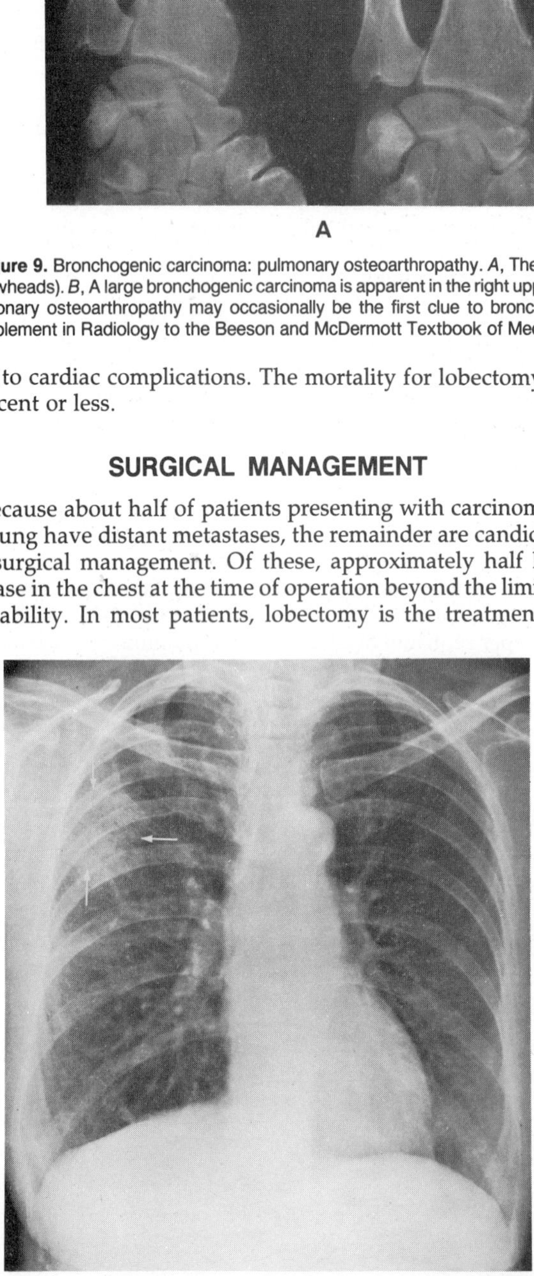

Figure 10. Alveolar cell carcinoma. Chest film in 55-year-old woman demonstrates an ill-defined density with an indistinct lower border (arrows) in the right upper lobe. The hilar nodes are not enlarged. This picture simulated pneumonitis but proved to be an alveolar cell carcinoma. (From Teplick, J. G., and Haskin, M. E.: Roentgenologic Diagnosis: A Complement in Radiology to the Beeson and McDermott Textbook of Medicine. Vol. 1. 3rd ed. Philadelphia, W. B. Saunders Company, 1976.)

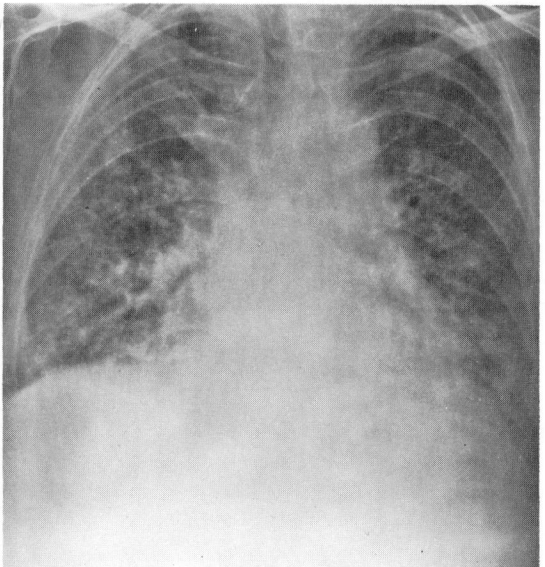

Figure 11. Diffuse alveolar cell carcinoma. There are diffuse irregular nodular infiltrates in both lung fields similar to the pattern of certain granulomatous diseases. These findings in an elderly female should suggest alveolar cell carcinoma as a possible diagnosis. (From Teplick, J. G., and Haskin, M. E.: Roentgenologic Diagnosis: A Complement in Radiology to the Beeson and McDermott Textbook of Medicine. Vol. 1. 3rd ed. Philadelphia, W. B. Saunders Company, 1976.)

TABLE 3. Stage Grouping in Carcinoma of the Lung

Occult Carcinoma

$T_xN_0M_0$ — An occult carcinoma with bronchopulmonary secretions containing malignant cells but without other evidence of the primary tumor or evidence of metastasis to the regional lymph nodes or distant metastasis.

Invasive Carcinoma

Stage I

$T_1N_0M_0$
$T_1N_1M_0$
$T_2N_0M_0$ — A tumor that can be classified T_1 without any metastasis or with metastasis to the lymph nodes in the ipsilateral hilar region only, or a tumor that can be classified T_2 without any metastasis to nodes or distant metastasis.

Stage II

$T_2N_1M_0$ — A tumor classified as T_2 with metastasis to the lymph nodes in the ipsilateral hilar region only.

Stage III

T_3 with any N or M
N_2 with any T or M
M_1 with any T or N — Any tumor more extensive than T_2, or any tumor with metastasis to the lymph nodes in the mediastinum or with distant metastasis.

From Beahrs, O. H., and Myers, M. H. (Eds.): American Joint Committee on Cancer: Manual for Staging of Cancer, 2nd ed. Philadelphia, J. B. Lippincott Company, 1983.

complication of bronchopleural fistula is uncommon, and experimental studies have shown that bronchial healing is better with metallic staples than with sutures. Following pulmonary resection, one or two catheters are left in the pleural cavity for drainage of blood, fluid, and air and are left in place until drainage ceases.

For patients requiring extensive pulmonary resection, a "sleeve" resection can be done, with removal of the lesion and anastomosis of the bronchus.

Inoperability at Surgical Exploration

At operation, the extent of spread of the primary neoplasm can be determined by examination of the parietal pleura, pericardium, heart, and mediastinal structure. If involvement of the chest wall is present, an *en bloc* resection of the chest wall can be done with fair survival in some patients.[11,13] Involvement of superior mediastinal nodes does not necessarily constitute a contraindication for pulmonary resection, because long-term survival has been accomplished in this group after resection.[32]

Metastases from bronchogenic carcinoma to the heart are seldom diagnosed before death, but an autopsy series confirms them to be frequent, and in one series 25 per cent had cardiac metastases.[44] Clinical signs of cardiac involvement include cardiomegaly, congestive heart failure, and electrocardiographic changes. Pericardial effusion also occurs and can be treated by pericardiocentesis.[3] If the fluid reaccumulates rapidly, pericardiectomy can be performed. The combined approach of systemic or local chemotherapy with precordial irradiation is also useful. The importance and usefulness of the American Joint Committee's System of Staging and End Results Reporting in long-term survival have been shown in several studies (Table 3).[2] Palliative resection may be done in certain cases, especially when the tumor has produced severe bronchial obstruction or a frank abscess distal to the lesion. In other cases, severe hemoptysis provides the basis for a palliative resection to remove the source of the hemorrhage.

RADIATION THERAPY

Surgical management remains the preferred treatment for carcinoma of the lung. Nevertheless, radiation has a useful role as an adjuvant and for those patients with primary lesions that are not resectable. Because many patients cannot be cured by resection, a number are candidates for radiation. Tremendous strides have been made in both the technique and the facilities available for radiation therapy with improved survival. Survival statistics in patients managed primarily by radiation therapy for carcinoma of the lung are shown in Table 4. Although

cure after radiotherapy alone is rare, some believe that it occurs in as many as 5 per cent or more of patients with non–small-cell carcinoma.

Patients selected for primary radiation treatment include (1) those with inoperable lesions, (2) those in whom operation is contraindicated for specific medical reasons or those who refuse operation, and (3) those in whom carcinoma recurs after previous surgical excision. Although several techniques for radiation therapy have been recommended, generally 5000 to 6000 rads are given five times a week for 5 to 6 weeks (180 to 200 rads per day). A split course, in preference to continuous daily fractions, has the advantage of accommodating the limited tolerance of the lungs for high doses of radiation. In this approach, 3000 rads are given over a 2-week period (300 rads per treatment), followed by a 2-week rest period; then an additional 2000 rads are given in a 1- to 2-week period.

Today radiation therapy is much improved, and complications primarily include radiation pneumonitis and esophagitis. Both are relatively mild and are frequently asymptomatic. Pneumonitis may be associated with a mild cough, fever, and occasionally minimal hemoptysis. Late pulmonary changes include interstitial fibrosis; damage to the spinal cord is prevented by reducing the amount of radiation over the spinal cord area to 4000 rads to avoid radiation myelitis. The exact role and indications for postoperative radiation remain controversial. It has had a limited trial in the past without significant evidence of benefit, but more recent reports suggest that in some patients, especially those in whom the risk of recurrence after surgical therapy is high, the addition of postoperative radiation therapy is beneficial. A dose of approximately 5000 rads is given over 5 weeks to the primary tumor and involved lymph nodes.

Radiation therapy for palliation can be useful for improving the quality of life of patients with hemoptysis, chest pain, and paroxysmal coughing. In addition, patients with the superior vena cava syndrome often respond dramatically to radiation therapy. This type of therapy can prolong survival. The re-

TABLE 4. Results of Radiation Therapy in the Primary Management of Carcinoma of the Lung

Number of Patients	Radiation Dose	Survival		
		1 yr.	3 yr.	5 yr.
93[18]	4000	22	5	
349[19]	5000	38	8	
150[15]	5000–6000	40		2.5
419[41]	5000–7000	62	14	6

sponse of bony metastases can be gratifying, and spinal cord compression can also be managed by radiation with decompression laminectomy if a neurologic deficit exists. Brain metastases can also be palliated by whole-brain radiation with doses of up to 4000 rads given during a 4-week period.

Studies of various chemotherapeutic agents have been evaluated in the treatment of patients with bronchogenic carcinoma. For extensive squamous cell carcinoma of the lung, several different combinations of drugs have been used. In a study in which bleomycin, doxorubicin (Adriamycin), vincristine, mechlorethamine, and nitrosourea (CCNU) were given, the response rate was 21 per cent. The median survival was 16 weeks for all patients who received the regimen. Toxicity caused a 4 per cent incidence of deaths related to treatment, and an additional 10 per cent of the patients were hospitalized because of life-threatening but reversible toxic effects. The results were not impressive.[25] For small-cell carcinoma of the lung (oat-cell), most agree that an aggressive combination of chemotherapy and radiation is preferred, because the brain, liver, lymph nodes, and bone marrow are common sites of initial metastatic spread. Because untreated patients with small-cell carcinoma die rapidly (with an average survival of only 1 to 3 months), combination chemotherapy is indicated to achieve remissions. Cyclophosphamide is probably the single most active agent, and vincristine and doxorubicin (Adriamycin) are potent additions. When these agents were administered in conjunction, a remission was achieved in 20 of 21 patients.[23]

To assess surgical management of small-cell carcinoma, the Veterans Administration Surgical Oncology group evaluated 132 patients with small-cell carcinoma who had potentially "curative" resections. The 5-year survival was 23 per cent. The effect of postoperative adjuvant chemotherapy was evaluated, but no beneficial effect could be determined. It was concluded that resection was definitely indicated in patients with $T_1N_0M_0$ lesions or $T_2N_0M_0$ lesions. However, with extension of the tumor, resection was not thought to be useful.[43]

In an evaluation of the role of resection in certain patients with small-cell differentiated carcinoma (oat-cell), 40 patients with limited-stage small-cell carcinoma of the lung underwent prospective evaluation for adjuvant surgical therapy after intensive chemotherapy for determination of resectability. The patients underwent postoperative evaluation after receiving two to four cycles of chemotherapy (cyclophosphamide, doxorubicin, and vincristine). Stage I tumors were present in 2 patients, Stage II in 12 patients, and Stage III in 25 patients. At the time of re-evaluation, 13 (33 per cent) were complete responders, 21 (54 per cent) were partial responders, and 5 (13 per cent) had stable disease. Eleven patients (28 per cent) of the 39 patients underwent thoracotomy with standard resection criteria for non–small-cell carcinoma. Eight of these 11 had resectable lesions. Twenty-eight were not candidates for operation for various reasons. The median survival for complete responders was 17 months. Therefore, a prospectively identifiable group of suitable candidates for adjuvant surgical therapy among the total group were identified.

IMMUNOLOGIC ASPECTS OF PATIENTS WITH BRONCHOGENIC CARCINOMA

A poor clinical prognosis is clearly associated with depressed cellular immunity in patients with all types of malignant tumors and has led to speculation that this unfavorable survival generally experienced with lung cancer may be related to defects in this mechanism. Immunoincompetence in patients with bronchogenic carcinoma has been clearly shown in both delayed cutaneous hypersensitivity skin testing and in vitro assays of lymphocyte function.

More encouraging has been the immunotherapeutic response in patients with advanced cancer and pulmonary metastases (Fig. 12), which shows complete regression of a hilar metastasis from a melanoma in a patient treated with LAK cells and interleukin-2.[39] In Figure 12, the illustrations are pretreatment chest films (7/21/1986) and posttreatment films (9/10/1986) that depict the disappearance of the hilar metastases. In this study,

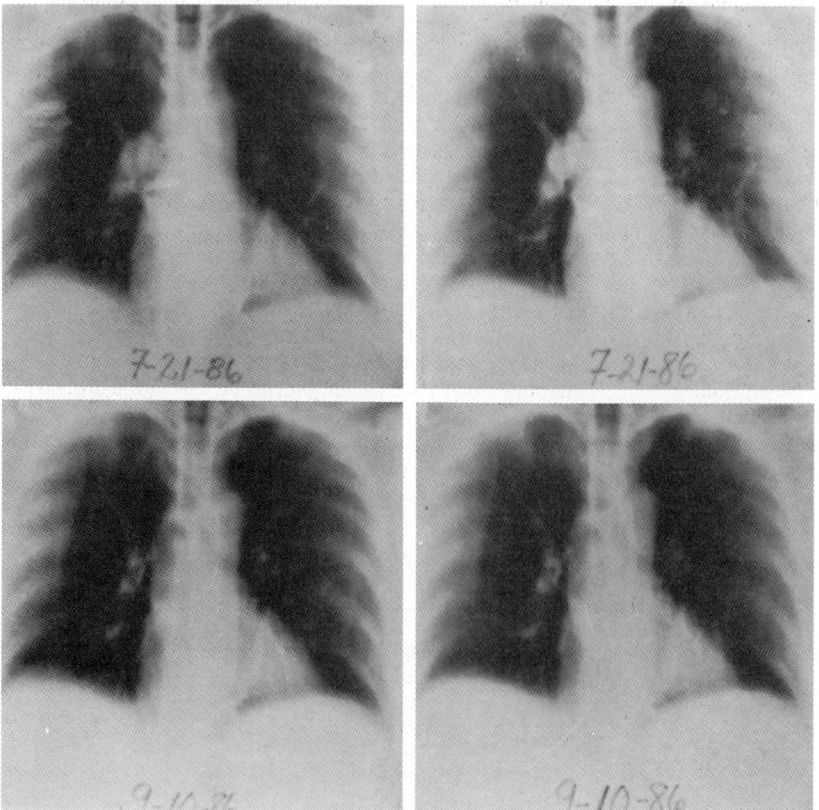

Figure 12. Complete regression of a hilar metastasis from melanoma in a patient treated with lymphokine-activated killer cells and interleukin-2. Pretreatment (top) and posttreatment (below). (From Rosenberg, S. A.: The development of new immunotherapies for the treatment of cancer using interleukin-2: A review. Ann. Surg., *208:*121, 1988.)

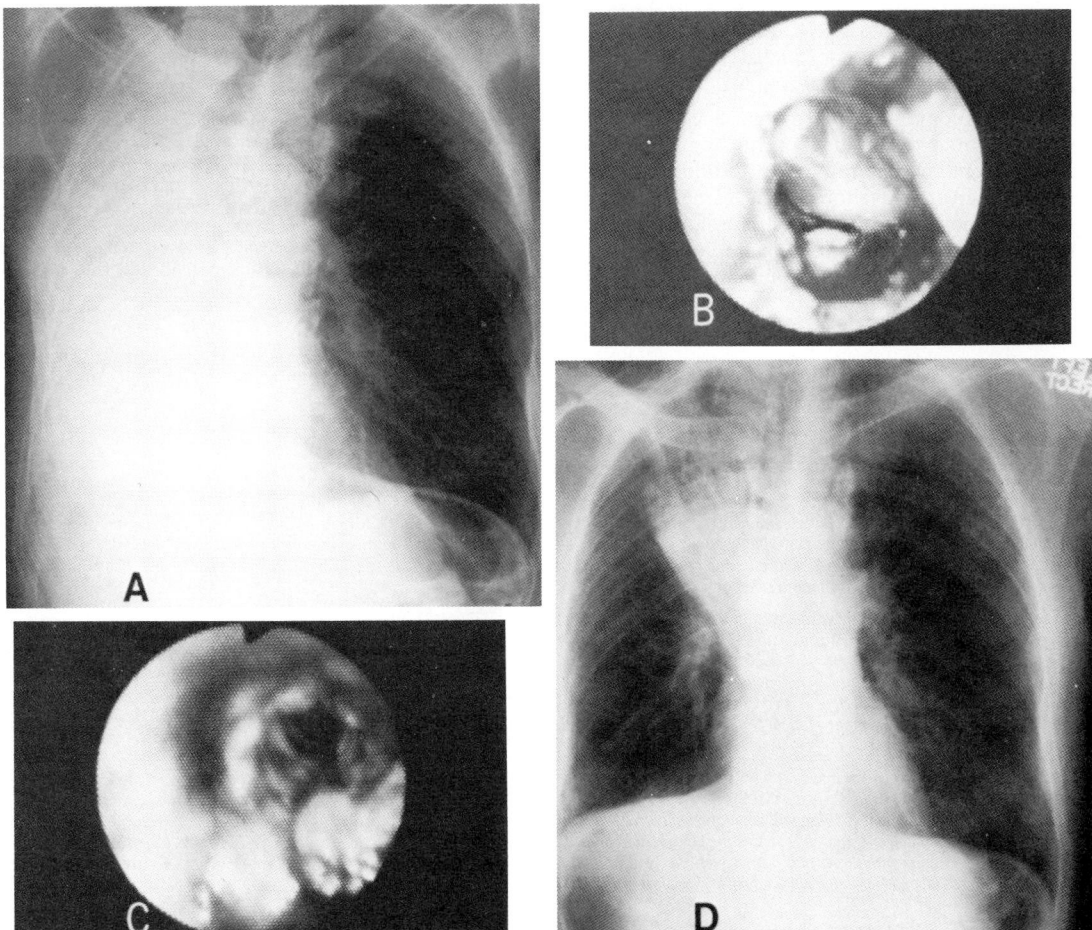

Figure 13. *A*, Chest film of 75-year-old man who presented with hemoptysis and fever secondary to obstructing carcinoma of the right main stem bronchus originating in the upper lobe. He was treated with antibiotics and radiation therapy was initiated. *B*, Endoscopic photograph of the obstructing tumor in the right main stem bronchus. The patient underwent two sessions of laser therapy. *C*, Endoscopic appearance at the completion of the first session of laser therapy. A second session produced complete resolution of the endobronchial tumor. *D*, Chest film at the time of discharge from the hospital demonstrates re-expansion of the lung. (From Wolfe, W. G., Cole, P. H., and Sabiston, D. C., Jr.: Experimental and clinical use of the YAG laser in the management of pulmonary neoplasms. Ann. Surg., *199*:526, 1984.)

34 patients with melanoma were described, 3 of whom had a complete response and 3 a partial response.[38]

LASER THERAPY. The yttrium-aluminum-garnet (YAG) laser and the carbon dioxide laser[27] have been used in the treatment of local malignant disease of the trachea and mainstem bronchi (Fig. 13).[47] Both short-term and long-term effects of the YAG laser have been evaluated. The laser is safe and produces effective results, especially in patients with inoperable lesions and those with primary symptoms of serious hemoptysis or even massive hemorrhage or for a lesion that obstructs the bronchus and causes infection distally. Airway patency can be reestablished and hemorrhage from the bronchus can be controlled by this technique.

RESULTS

The natural history of bronchogenic carcinoma is shown in a large study of more than 3800 patients in which those who were untreated had 95 per cent mortality within 1 year. It is usually stated that of each group of 100 patients with a diagnosis of carcinoma of the lung, half have inoperable lesions from the outset. Of the 50 per cent on whom exploratory thoracotomy is done, half (or 25 per cent of the original group) have such extensive disease that an operation for cure cannot be done. The remaining 25 per cent are candidates for a curative resection, and 25 to 35 per cent are alive at the end of 5 years. Therefore, for the series as a whole, survival is only 8 to 10 per cent at 5 years.

Survival in patients with carcinoma of the lung is primarily determined by the extent of the tumor at the time of operation and the degree of invasion of surrounding structures. Metastases to lymph nodes decrease survival significantly. The cell type bears less relation to survival except for the poor prognosis associated with small-cell (oat-cell) carcinoma and the improved results with alveolar cell carcinoma.[42]

The Solitary Pulmonary ("Coin") Lesions

A frequent problem is the evaluation of the patient with a solitary pulmonary nodule. Such "coin-shaped" lesions should be thoroughly investigated for establishment of the presence of malignancy. Large lesions with an irregular outline are apt to be carcinoma. Small lesions with smoothly circumscribed margins

TABLE 5. Incidence of Malignancy in Solitary Pulmonary Nodules Related to Age

Age (yr)	Malignant (%)
35–44	15
45–49	26
50–59	41
60–69	50
70–79	70
Over 80	Almost 100

From Sabiston, D. C., Jr., and Spencer, F. C. (Eds.): Surgery of the Chest, 5th ed. Philadelphia, W. B. Saunders Company, 1990.

with laminar or concentric calcifications are more likely to be benign. The younger the patient, the more apt the lesion is to be benign. If a lesion is followed and does not increase in size, it is also more likely to be benign. The differential diagnosis of these lesions includes tuberculoma, histoplasmoma, blastomycoma, coccidioidomycoma, primary carcinoma of the lung, metastatic carcinoma, and benign pulmonary tumors. In addition, vascular abnormalities, such as an arteriovenous fistula, can be causes of these radiographic abnormalities. Malignant lesions without metastases should be removed. The relationship of age to the incidence of malignancy in an isolated pulmonary nodule is shown in Table 5. If the diagnosis cannot be established, excision should be performed.

SELECTED REFERENCES

Katsuke, H., Shimada, K., Koyama, A., et al.: Long-term intermittent adjuvant chemotherapy for primary resected lung cancer. J. Thorac. Cardiovasc. Surg., 70:590, 1975.
Two chemotherapeutic agents were used to suppress local and distant recurrences following resection of carcinoma of the lung. Radiotherapy was given postoperatively to patients with known residual disease. Long-term, intermittent chemotherapy with mitomycin C and chromomycin A was administered. The results showed a difference between the treated and the untreated groups.

Kirsh, M. M., Dickerman, R., Fayos, J., et al.: The value of chest wall resection in the treatment of superior sulcus tumors of the lung. Ann. Thorac. Surg., 15:339, 1973.
The value of preoperative irradiation followed by extensive resection in the management of superior sulcus tumors was studied. The conclusions drawn from the data provide the reader with a different point of view from that of Paulson and Urschel.

Macumber, H. H., and Calvin, J. W.: Perfusion lung scan patterns in 100 patients with bronchogenic carcinoma. J. Thorac. Cardiovasc. Surg., 72:299, 1976.
The perfusion lung scans were classified into those with (1) perfusion defect larger than the mass lesion, (2) perfusion defect of the same size as the mass lesion, or (3) no focal defect seen. Among patients with larger perfusion defects 84 per cent had regional lymph node involvement, whereas among patients in whom a larger defect was not present only 23 per cent had this extension.

Paulson, D. L.: Superior sulcus carcinomas. In Sabiston, D. C., Jr., and Spencer, F. C. (Eds.): Gibbon's Surgery of the Chest, 4th ed. Philadelphia, W. B. Saunders Company, 1983.
Preoperative irradiation followed by radical excision is advocated in the treatment of superior sulcus tumors. Their results are excellent but differ from those reported by Kirsh and associates.

Rees, L. H.: The biosynthesis of hormones by non-endocrine tumours — A review. J. Endocrinol., 67:143, 1975.
A review of the hormonal syndromes associated with various primary neoplasms. In addition to detailed descriptions of various endocrine manifestations, there is an extensive and well-selected bibliography.

REFERENCES

1. Auerbach, O., Gere, J. B., Forman, J. B., et al.: Changes in the bronchial epithelium in relation to smoking and cancer of the lung. N. Engl. J. Med., 256:97, 1957.
2. Beahrs, O. H., and Myers, M. H. (Eds.): American Joint Committee on Cancer: Manual for Staging of Cancer, 2nd ed. Philadelphia, J. B. Lippincott Company, 1983.
3. Biran, S., Brufman, G., Klein, E., and Hochman, A.: The management of pericardial effusion in cancer patients. Chest, 71:182, 1977.
4. Cattaneo, S. M., Zipf, R. E., Johnson, O. E., and Everhart, L. S.: Transbronchial mucus transfer of bronchogenic carcinoma. J. Thorac. Cardiovasc. Surg., 75:585, 1978.
5. Chang, A. E., Schaner, E. G., Conkle, D. M., et al.: Evaluation of computed tomography in the detection of pulmonary metastases: A prospective study. Cancer, 43:913, 1979.
6. Chaudhary, B. A., Yoneda, K., and Burki, N. K.: Fiberoptic bronchoscopy: Comparison of procedures used in the diagnosis of lung cancer. J. Thorac. Cardiovasc. Surg., 76:33, 1978.
7. Cortese, D. A., and McDougall, J. C.: Biopsy and brushing of peripheral lung cancer with fluoroscopic guidance. Chest, 75:141, 1979.
8. Cortese, D. A., Pairolero, P. C., Bergstralh, E. J., et al.: Roentgenographically occult lung cancer: A ten-year experience. J. Thorac. Cardiovasc. Surg., 86:373, 1983.
9. Dorn, H. F.: Tobacco consumption and mortality from cancer and other diseases. Public Health Rep., 75:581, 1959.
10. Fried, B. M.: Tumors of the Lungs and Mediastinum. Philadelphia, Lea & Febiger, 1958.
11. Geha, A. S., Bernatz, P. E., and Woolner, L. B.: Bronchogenic carcinoma involving the thoracic wall: Surgical treatment and prognostic significance. J. Thorac. Cardiovasc. Surg., 54:394, 1967.
12. Graham, E. A., and Singer, J. J.: Successful removal of an entire lung for carcinoma of the bronchus. J.A.M.A., 101:1371, 1933.
13. Grillo, H. C., Greenberg, J. J., and Wilkins, E. W.: Resection of bronchogenic carcinoma involving the thoracic wall. J. Thorac. Cardiovasc. Surg., 51:417, 1966.
14. Gutierrez, A. C., Vincent, R. G., Sandberg, A. A., et al.: Evaluation of sternal bone marrow aspiration for detection of tumor cells in patients with bronchogenic carcinoma. J. Thorac. Cardiovasc. Surg., 77:392, 1979.
15. Guttmann, R.: Radical supervoltage therapy in inoperable carcinoma of the lung. In Deeley, T. J. (Ed.): Carcinoma of the Bronchus. New York, Appleton-Century-Crofts, 1971.
16. Hammond, E. C., Auerbach, O., Kirman, D., and Garfinkel, L.: Effects of cigarette smoking on dogs. CA, 21:78, 1971.
17. Harpole, D. H., Bigelow, C., Young, W. G., Jr., et al.: Alveolar cell carcinoma of the lung: A retrospective analysis of 205 patients. Ann. Thorac. Surg., 46:502, 1988.
18. Hocker, A. F., and Guttmann, R. J.: Three and one-half years' experience with the 1,000 kilovolt roentgen therapy unit at Memorial Hospital. A.J.R., 51:83, 1944.
19. Holsti, L. R.: Clinical experience with split-course radiotherapy: A randomized clinical trial. Radiology, 92:591, 1969.
20. Hutchinson, C. M., and Mills, N. L.: The selection of patients with bronchogenic carcinoma for mediastinoscopy. J. Thorac. Cardiovasc. Surg., 71:768, 1976.
21. Hyde, L., and Hyde, C. I.: Clinical manifestations of lung cancer. Chest, 65:299, 1974.
22. Iglehart, J. D., Wolfe, W. G., Vernon, W. B., et al.: Electron microscopy in selection of patients with small cell carcinoma of the lung for medical versus surgical therapy. J. Thorac. Cardiovasc. Surg., 90:351, 1985.
23. Johnson, R. E., Brereton, H. D., and Kent, C. H.: "Total" therapy for small cell carcinoma of the lung. Ann. Thorac. Surg., 25:510, 1978.
24. Kabat, G. C., and Wynder, E. L.: Lung cancer in nonsmokers. Cancer, 53:1214, 1984.
25. Livingston, R. B., Heilbrun, L., Lehane, D., et al.: Comparative trial of combination chemotherapy in extensive squamous carcinoma of the lung: A southwest oncology group study. Cancer Treat. Rep., 61:1623, 1977.
26. Magilligan, D. J., Jr., Duvernoy, C., Malik, G., et al.: Surgical approach to lung cancer with solitary cerebral metastasis: Twenty-five years' experience. Ann. Thorac. Surg., 42:360, 1986.
27. McElvein, R. B., and Zorn, G.: Treatment of malignant disease in trachea and mainstem bronchi by carbon dioxide laser. J. Thorac. Cardiovasc. Surg., 86:858, 1983.
28. Meade, R. H.: A History of Thoracic Surgery. Springfield, Ill., Charles C Thomas, 1961.
29. Morton, D. L., Itabashi, H. H., and Grimes, O. F.: Nonmetastatic neurological complications of bronchogenic carcinoma: The carcinomatous neuromyopathies. J. Thorac. Cardiovasc. Surg., 51:14, 1966.
30. Omenn, G. S., and Wilkins, E. W., Jr.: Hormone syndromes associated with bronchogenic carcinoma: Clues to histologic type. J. Thorac. Cardiovasc. Surg., 59:877, 1970.
31. Paone, J. F., and Jeyasingham, K.: Remission of cerebellar dysfunction after pneumonectomy for bronchogenic carcinoma. N. Engl. J. Med., 302:156, 1980.
32. Pearson, F. G., DeLarue, N. C., Ilves, R., et al.: Significance of positive superior mediastinal nodes identified at mediastinoscopy in patients with resectable cancer of the lung. J. Thorac. Cardiovasc. Surg., 83:1, 1982.
33. Razzuk, M. A., Pockey, M., Urschel, H. C., Jr., and Paulson, D. L.: Dual primary bronchogenic carcinoma. Ann. Thorac. Surg., 17:425, 1974.
34. Razzuk, M. A., Urschel, H. C., Jr., Albers, J. E., Martin, J. A., and Paulson, D. L.: Pulmonary giant cell carcinoma. Ann. Thorac. Surg., 21:540, 1976.
35. Rigler, L. G.: A roentgen study of the evolution of carcinoma of the lung. J. Thorac. Surg., 34:283, 1957.
36. Rigler, L. G., O'Loughlin, B. J., and Tucker, R. C.: The duration of carcinoma of the lung. Dis. Chest, 23:50, 1953.
37. Ripstein, C. B., Spain, D. M., and Bluth, I.: Scar cancer of the lung. J. Thorac. Cardiovasc. Surg., 56:362, 1968.
38. Rosenberg, S. A.: The development of new immunotherapies for the treatment of cancer using interleukin-2: A review. Ann. Surg., 208:121, 1988.
39. Rosenberg, S. A., Lotze, M. T., Muul, L. M., et al.: A progress report on the treatment of 157 patients with advanced cancer using lymphokine-activated killer cells and interleukin-2 or high-dose interleukin-2 alone. N. Engl. J. Med., 316:889, 1987.
40. Sagel, S. S., Ferguson, T. B., Forrest, J. V., et al.: Percutaneous transthoracic aspiration needle biopsy. Ann. Thorac. Surg., 26:399, 1978.
41. Schumacher, W.: The use of high-energy electrons in the treatment of inoperable lung and bronchogenic carcinoma. In Kramer, S., Suntharalingam, N., and Zinninger, G. F. (Eds.): High-Energy Photons and Electrons: Clinical Applications in Cancer Management. New York, John Wiley & Sons, 1978.
42. Shields, T. W., and Higgins, G. A.: Minimal pulmonary resection in treatment of carcinoma of the lung. Arch. Surg., 108:420, 1974.
43. Shields, T. W., Higgins, G. A., Jr., Matthews, M. J., and Keehn, R. J.: Surgical resection in the management of small cell carcinoma of the lung. J. Thorac. Cardiovasc. Surg., 84:481, 1982.

44. Strauss, B. L., Matthews, M. J., Cohen, M. H., et al.: Cardiac metastases in lung cancer. Chest, 71:607, 1977.
45. Teplick, J. G., and Haskin, M. E.: Roentgenologic Diagnosis: A Complement in Radiology to the Beeson and McDermott Textbook of Medicine. Vol. 1, 3rd ed. Philadelphia, W. B. Saunders Company, 1976.
46. van Bodegom, P. C., Wagenaar, S. S., Corrin, B., Baak, J. P., Berkel, J., and

Vanderschueren, R. G.: Second primary lung cancer: Importance of long term follow-up. Thorax, 44:788, 1989.
47. Wolfe, W. G., Cole, P. H., and Sabiston, D. C., Jr.: Experimental and clinical use of the YAG laser in the management of pulmonary neoplasms. Ann. Surg., 199:526, 1984.

XIII

THORACIC OUTLET SYNDROME

Alfred Harding, M.D., and Donald Silver, M.D.

Thoracic outlet syndrome is the preferred term for those syndromes—e.g., the cervical rib syndrome, scalenus anticus syndrome, hyperabduction syndrome, costoclavicular syndrome, pectoralis minor syndrome, and the first thoracic rib syndrome—that follow compression of the neurovascular structures to the upper extremities. The syndrome is caused by compression of the brachial plexus or subclavian-axillary artery and/or vein in the region between the thoracic outlet and the insertion of the pectoralis minor muscle onto the coracoid process. Symptoms may arise from neural, vascular, or combined neural and vascular compression, with neural compression representing approximately 90 to 95 per cent of the symptoms.

HISTORICAL ASPECTS

One of the earliest descriptions of the thoracic outlet syndrome appeared in 1860, when Willshire reported a pulsating subclavian artery (possibly an aneurysm) that crossed a presumed cervical rib.[34] In 1861, Coote excised a cervical rib to relieve pressure on the axillary vessels and nerves.[5] Murphy in 1905[15] and Keen in 1907[11] emphasized the role of cervical ribs in the compression of the neurovascular structures. In 1919, Stopford and Telford demonstrated that the brachial plexus and subclavian artery could be compressed by the first thoracic rib and indicated that resection of the rib would relieve symptoms.[26]

In 1927, Adson and Coffey emphasized the role of the scalene muscles in neurovascular compression and popularized scalenotomy as a method of therapy.[2] Various operative maneuvers were tried with varying degrees of success until 1962, when the role of the first rib, and the ligamentous and muscular attachments to it, in the pathogenesis of the thoracic outlet syndrome was re-emphasized.[4,9] Currently, scalenectomy and/or resection of the first rib is offered to the approximately 40 per cent of patients with the thoracic outlet syndrome who do not improve with a 4-month (or longer) trial of nonoperative management.

ANATOMY

An understanding of the sites of potential pressure in the thoracic outlet region is necessary for proper evaluation and management of this syndrome. The anterior rami of five spinal nerves, C5, C6, C7, C8, and T1 (C4 and T2 may also contribute to the brachial plexus), exit through the intervertebral foramina and form trunks that pass through the scalene triangle and then divide behind the clavicle. The divisions of the trunks reunite to form cords that surround the axillary artery as it passes behind the pectoralis minor tendon. The division of these cords into the major motor and sensory nerves of the upper extremity usually occurs distal to the pectoralis minor tendon.

Rami from C8 and T1 form the lowest trunk, which lies on the first rib behind the subclavian artery and is responsible for the groove in the rib (which is often attributed to the artery). The peripheral distribution of C8 and T1 fibers provides sensory perception from the fifth finger and medial half of the fourth finger and from the medial aspect of the forearm. The motor distribution of this trunk controls flexion of the wrist and fingers and innervates the intrinsic muscles of the hand.

Both subclavian arteries exit from the thorax behind the sternoclavicular joints and pass over the first ribs *between* the scalenus anticus and scalenus medius muscles. The arteries then course laterally behind the clavicles and become the axillary arteries. The axillary arteries pass posterior to the tendons of the pectoralis minor muscles and become the brachial arteries.

The axillary veins pass behind the costocoracoid ligaments and pectoralis minor tendons. At the edge of the first rib, each axillary vein becomes a subclavian vein that passes over the first rib *anterior* to the scalenus anticus muscle to join its respective jugular vein at the base of the neck.

The arteries, veins, and nerves that form the brachial plexus may be compressed in any of several areas as they pass from the neck or the thoracic outlet into the upper extremity. The anatomic sites of compression from medial to lateral include (1) the interscalene triangle (arteries and nerves); (2) the space between the scalenus anticus muscle and the clavicle (vein); (3) the first rib, or between the first rib and clavicle (nerves, arteries, and veins); (4) the costocoracoid fascia (nerves, arteries, and veins); and (5) the pectoralis minor tendon (nerves, arteries, and veins).

Other causes of compression of the neurovascular structures include the following:

1. Cervical ribs, which occur in approximately 1 per cent of the population and are bilateral in 80 per cent. Cervical ribs or fibrous bands associated with them may compress or irritate portions of the adjacent brachial plexus and compress or elevate the subclavian artery. However, fewer than 10 per cent of cervical ribs produce symptoms.

2. Long transverse processes of C7. These may function as cervical ribs.

3. Abnormal first thoracic ribs. These ribs frequently fail to reach the sternum, may be attached to the sternum or to the second rib by ligaments, and may cause distortion or compression of the lower components of the brachial plexus.

4. Variations of the scalene muscles. Roos has described at least 10 different fibromuscular anomalies in the thoracic outlet that may produce neurovascular compression.[21] He has suggested that these various congenital bands and muscular abnormalities are "almost invariably" present in patients who do not respond to conservative management. In addition, spasm, fibrosis, or inflammation of the scalene muscles may produce symptoms.

5. Postural changes during which there is downward dis-

placement of the upper extremity and shoulder girdle. Occupations that require hyperabduction, carrying heavy loads or working in narrow quarters so that the upper extremities are drawn forward and down, are frequently associated with thoracic outlet symptoms.

6. Acquired lesions such as fractures of the first rib or clavicle with deformity or callus formation.

7. Compression by tumor in the outlet spaces.[7]

8. Degenerative changes. Osteoarthritis of the spine[29] or cervicothoracic scoliosis[28] may cause nerve root compression and mimics the symptoms of the thoracic outlet syndrome.

SYMPTOMS

The symptoms of the thoracic outlet syndrome vary, depending on the vessels or nerves compressed, and may be neurologic or vascular or both. The syndrome occurs most often in the young to middle-aged female (70 to 75 per cent), although all age groups may be afflicted.[6] The clinical manifestations rarely indicate the site of compression.

Neurologic symptoms consist of pain, weakness, paresthesias, and numbness, usually in the fingers and hands in an ulnar distribution, but may occur anywhere in the upper extremity, neck, or shoulder girdle. Late neurologic sequelae include sensory loss, motor weakness, and atrophy.

Symptoms of arterial compression include ischemic pain, numbness, fatigue, paresthesias, coldness, and weakness in the arm or hand. These symptoms are accentuated by exercise and exposure to cold. Thromboses may occur in the compressed or poststenotic dilated areas of the subclavian or axillary arteries and, if occlusive, can produce distal ischemic changes. Recurrent, angina-like chest pain may occur in a few patients with the disorder. Distal embolization may be associated with vasomotor symptoms in the fingers, consisting of episodic pain with pallor and/or cyanosis. These symptoms are accentuated by cold exposure. If the embolization continues, advanced ischemia with ulceration or gangrene of the fingertips may occur.

Venous compression may produce upper extremity edema, pain, and cyanosis. The patients frequently complain of a sensation of heaviness and tightness in the arm.

DIAGNOSIS

A complete history and a thorough physical examination are essential in establishing the diagnosis of thoracic outlet syndrome. The symptom complexes plus a history of trauma with fracture(s) of the clavicle or ribs or both, a history of unusual exercise or occupation, poor posture, sagging bed, and so forth should suggest the thoracic outlet syndrome. A careful history also indicates whether or not the symptoms are part of a generalized process such as occurs with spinal cord tumors, peripheral embolizations, osteoarthritis, and connective tissue or metabolic disorders. Cervical intervertebral disc disease and the carpal tunnel syndrome may be confused with thoracic outlet syndrome.

The physical examination should be thorough, with special emphasis given to detecting the neural, arterial, and venous signs. Neural signs include sensory deficits, weakness, and atrophy. Most often the sensory and motor deficits occur in the distribution of the ulnar nerve. Occasionally, the symptoms may be reproduced by percussion of the supraclavicular fossa. Signs of arterial compression include weakened or absent brachial and radial pulses, a bruit in the supraclavicular or axillary space, delayed capillary blush, or occasional areas of distal gangrene. Signs of venous compression include distended superficial veins on the chest, arm, or hand, distal edema, and cyanosis.

The physical findings are not constant. Therefore, several examinations may be required before the thoracic outlet syndrome is suspected. The findings may vary according to the patient's position during the examination. Except when reproduced by hyperabduction of the arm, neural and/or vascular compression is rarely detected when patients are examined in the supine position, but is usually readily detected when the patient is sitting or standing. Diagnostic maneuvers for the thoracic outlet syndrome are listed below. The first three, which detect vascular compression *only*, may be abnormal in a large number (approximately 50 per cent) of patients who are asymptomatic.

1. Adson or scalene maneuver.[1,2] While the physician monitors the radial pulse, the patient takes a deep breath, extends the neck, and turns the chin toward the side being examined. Disappearance or reduction of the radial pulse constitutes a positive finding. During a positive test, a bruit frequently becomes audible in the supraclavicular fossa, and the hand may become cool and pale. The deep breath causes elevation of the first rib, and extending and turning the neck causes narrowing of the interscalene triangle. The symptoms are caused by compression of the subclavian artery and possibly the brachial plexus by the first rib and scalene muscles. If the pulse is altered before the head is turned, one should suspect the presence of a cervical rib.

2. Costoclavicular compressive maneuver.[8] While the radial pulse is monitored, the patient throws his shoulders back and downward into an exaggerated military position. Disappearance or reduction of the radial pulse or the appearance of a subclavian bruit constitutes a positive finding. The pulse changes are produced by compression of the subclavian artery between the clavicle and the first rib.

3. Hyperabduction maneuver.[33] The radial pulse is monitored while the arm is passively moved into a hyperabducted position. Reduction or cessation of the radial pulse and the appearance of an axillary bruit indicate arterial compression by the pectoralis minor tendon.

4. Three-minute elevated arm stress test.[21] The patient is asked to slowly open and close the hands while keeping both arms abducted, externally rotated, and flexed to 90 degrees at the elbow. Normal patients may experience fatigue but rarely have pain or paresthesias. In patients with a thoracic outlet syndrome, the test may reproduce their symptoms.

OBJECTIVE EXAMINATIONS. Roentgenograms of the neck and chest may demonstrate cervical ribs, anomalous first ribs, prominent transverse processes, bony exostoses, calluses, abnormalities of the clavicle, and so forth. The roentgenograms also yield information about narrowing of the intervertebral foramina and tumors. Myelograms may be necessary to demonstrate a cervical disc or other causes of cervical cord compression.

Arteriograms demonstrate sites of partial or complete arterial occlusion. Arteriography should be performed with the patient's arms by his side while he is performing the Adson, costoclavicular, and hyperabduction maneuvers. Occasionally, poststenotic dilatation or aneurysms of the subclavian artery distal to the site of compression are demonstrated. A normal arteriogram does not eliminate neural compression as a cause of the syndrome; neither does narrowing or obstruction of the subclavian-axillary arteries during the maneuvers confirm the diagnosis, because some obstruction of these arteries can be demonstrated in approximately half of the patients without symptoms of thoracic outlet syndrome. In general, arteriography is reserved for those few patients with suspected arterial aneurysms, obstruction, or distal embolization.

Phlebograms are useful to demonstrate sites of compression of the axillary or subclavian veins. If the veins become totally or partially occluded during the hyperabduction or costoclavicular

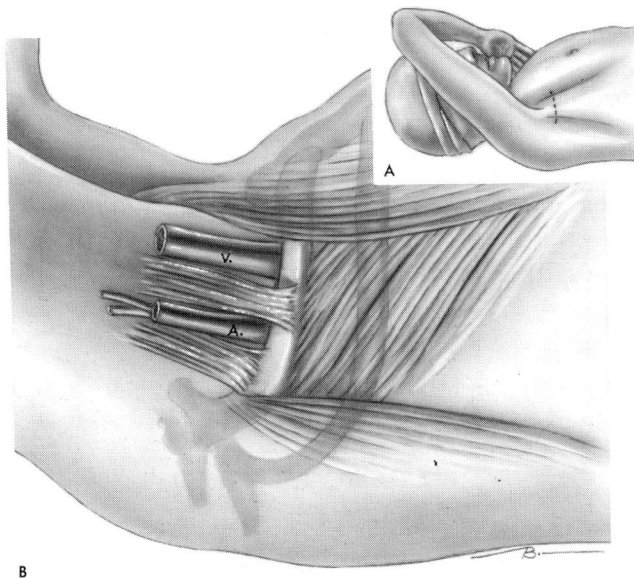

Figure 1. The transaxillary approach (*A*) to the first rib provides good exposure (*B*) of the first rib, scalene muscles, brachial plexus, and subclavian artery (A) and vein (V).

compression maneuvers, support is obtained for the diagnosis of thoracic outlet syndrome.

Plethysmography[24] has been used to document arterial compression. This technique records changes in digit volume that occur with each heartbeat and can demonstrate obstruction to arterial flow.[27] Electromyography is useful in detecting sites of compression of peripheral nerves by recording the altered response of the distal muscles to proximal electrical stimuli. Nerve conduction times across the thoracic outlet to the elbow and wrist may be prolonged; they have returned to the normal range after surgical relief of the compression.[30-31] However, the variability and unreliability of the nerve conduction studies have limited their usefulness in establishing the diagnosis of thoracic outlet syndrome.[12,21,23] Nerve conduction velocities are most important in determining whether a carpal tunnel syndrome is also present.

Recent evidence suggests that somatosensory evoked potentials (SEPs) may be useful in identifying those patients likely to respond to surgical therapy for thoracic outlet syndrome.[13] In addition to their diagnostic value, SEPs may provide objective evidence of persistent nerve dysfunction postoperatively. The technique consists of recording nerve action potentials at various sites along the central and peripheral nervous systems in response to electrical stimulation of the ulnar and median nerves at the wrist. By comparing the amplitudes of these various action potentials, the site of nerve dysfunction can be determined.

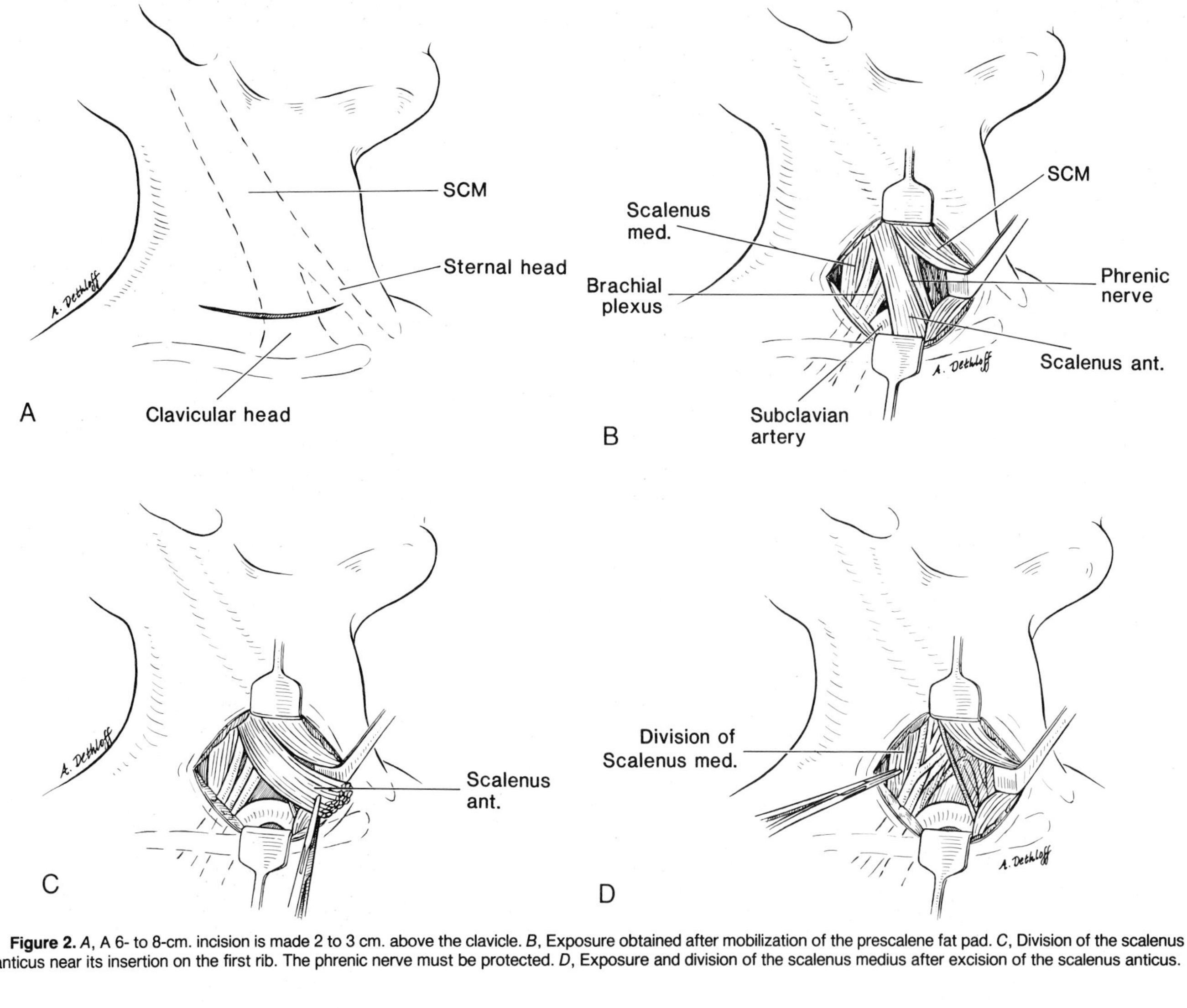

A

SCM

Sternal head

Clavicular head

B

Scalenus med.

Brachial plexus

SCM

Phrenic nerve

Scalenus ant.

Subclavian artery

C

Scalenus ant.

D

Division of Scalenus med.

Figure 2. *A*, A 6- to 8-cm. incision is made 2 to 3 cm. above the clavicle. *B*, Exposure obtained after mobilization of the prescalene fat pad. *C*, Division of the scalenus anticus near its insertion on the first rib. The phrenic nerve must be protected. *D*, Exposure and division of the scalenus medius after excision of the scalenus anticus.

MANAGEMENT

For all patients, except those with symptomatic complete vascular occlusion, distal embolization, or a poststenotic aneurysm, initial management should consist of a trial of weight reduction and an exercise program directed toward improving posture, strengthening the elevators of the shoulder girdle, and avoiding hyperabduction. These measures relieve symptoms in 50 to 70 per cent of patients.[10,16,28] Nonoperative management appears to be the most successful in the obese, young to middle-aged female with poor posture. When symptoms appear job-related, as in certain types of manual labor, a change in occupation may provide relief from the symptoms.

Patients with major neurologic or vascular complications and those who do not respond to a 4-month (or longer) trial of nonoperative management should be offered surgical intervention. Operative managment has included excision of a cervical rib, division of the scalenus anticus muscle, resection of the clavicle, and division of the pectoralis minor tendon.[17,25] Falconer and Li,[8] Clagett,[4] and Roos[21] emphasized that removal of the major portion of the first rib effectively decompresses the neurovascular structures. Subsequently, the removal of the first rib, and of a cervical rib if it is present, became the preferred surgical management for the thoracic outlet syndrome.

Clagett[4] suggested that the first rib be removed through a posterior incision along the medial border of the scapula. This approach provides good exposure for rib resection and for vascular reconstructive procedures. However, it produces a large scar and has increased morbidity. The posterior approach is uncommonly used today.

Nelson and Jenson[18] have employed an anterior extrapleural approach for excision of the first rib and have found this incision to be cosmetically acceptable with few complications. However, this approach is not suitable for removing cervical ribs or anomalous first ribs.

Roos[20] popularized the use of a transaxillary incision for removal of the first rib (Fig. 1). The vessels and nerves are lifted off the first rib when the arm is hyperabducted during operation. Of necessity, the scalene muscles are divided during removal of the rib. Although this procedure has proven effective for relieving neurovascular compression, it does not provide good exposure for vascular reconstructions. Brachial plexus injuries, pneumothorax, winged scapula, pleural effusion, and infection appear to be more common with the transaxillary approach than with supraclavicular decompression.[3] Up to 20 per cent of the operative injuries to the brachial plexus may be associated with significant residual disability.[5]

In recent years, increasing numbers of surgeons have chosen the supraclavicular approach for thoracic outlet decompression. This procedure consists of extensive anterior scalenectomy, middle scalenectomy, removal of the cervical rib if one is present, and, on occasion, first rib resection (Fig. 2).[24] Results of supraclavicular decompression are equivalent or superior to those achieved with transaxillary first rib resection. In a recent comparison of the two techniques by Cikrit and associates,[3] the supraclavicular procedure was accompanied by fewer complications, less blood loss, and shorter postoperative hospitalization. The average hospital stay is approximately 3 days with most patients returning to work in 7 to 10 days. Supraclavicular decompression is becoming accepted as the preferred operation for the surgical management of the thoracic outlet syndrome. Symptomatic improvement may be achieved in over 90 per cent of cases.[3,19,22]

Recurrent symptoms severe enough to require reoperation may occur in 1 per cent of patients after first rib resection.[30] Many of the patients with recurrent symptoms respond to physiotherapy and improvement in posture. A repeat supraclavicular decompression can be safely accomplished in the few patients who do not respond to physical therapy.[22]

Mild poststenotic dilatation of the subclavian artery usually does not progress once the compression is relieved and frequently remains of no clinical consequence. However, significant aneurysmal enlargement of the artery should be excised and replaced with a graft, preferably a vein graft. Thrombosis of the subclavian artery should be treated by thromboendarterectomy, by replacement, or by bypass grafting of the involved segment. Thrombosis of the subclavian-axillary vein requires elimination of the causative factors and treatment with a fibrinolytic agent and/or heparin, elevation, and an elastic sleeve until recanalization occurs. A thrombectomy, as suggested by Mahorner and associates,[14] may be useful in a few selected cases of acute total thrombotic obstruction of the upper extremity venous outflow. If chronic symptomatic thrombosis persists, a saphenous vein bypass from the axillary to the jugular vein provides symptomatic relief.

SELECTED REFERENCES

Clagett, O. T.: Research and prosearch. Presidential address. J. Thorac Cardiovasc. Surg., 44:153, 1962.
  In this paper, the author describes the classic features of the thoracic outlet syndrome. The posterior approach for removal of the first rib is carefully reviewed. It is a key reference source for this subject.

McGough, E. C., Pearce, M. B., and Byrne, J. P.: Management of thoracic outlet syndrome. J. Thorac. Cardiovasc. Surg., 77:169, 1979.
  The authors report 1200 patients with thoracic outlet syndrome managed between 1973 and 1978. Diagnosis was based on a careful history and detailed physical examination designed to establish the presence of brachial plexus irritation. The cervical spine was evaluated, and nerve conduction studies were obtained. All patients were initially treated with a comprehensive physical therapy program. One hundred thirteen patients had transaxillary first rib resections. Eighty per cent of surgical patients had complete relief of symptoms, and 13 per cent were improved. Seven per cent were unimproved, and none was made worse by the operation. There were no recurrences requiring operation.

Pang, D., Wessel, H. B.: Thoracic outlet syndrome. Neurosurgery, 22:105, 1988.
  This is an extensive review of the thoracic outlet syndrome.

Roos, D. B.: Transaxillary approach for the first rib resection to relieve thoracic outlet syndrome. Ann. Surg., 163:354, 1966.
  The author describes the transaxillary approach for first rib resection for relief of the thoracic outlet syndrome.

Sanders, R. J., Raymer, S.: The supraclavicular approach to scalenectomy and first rib resection: Description of technique. J. Vasc. Surg., 2:751, 1985.
  This paper includes a detailed description of supraclavicular thoracic outlet decompression. In addition, there is a brief discussion of the results of 145 cases.

REFERENCES

1. Adson, A. W.: Surgical treatment for symptoms produced by cervical ribs and the scalenus anticus muscle. Surg. Gynecol. Obstet., 85:687, 1947.
2. Adson, A. W., and Coffey, J. R.: Cervical rib. A method of anterior approach for relief of symptoms by division of scalenus anticus. Ann. Surg., 85:839, 1927.
3. Cikrit D. F., Haefner, R., Nichols, W. K., and Silver, D.: Transaxillary or supraclavicular decompression for the thoracic outlet syndrome: A comparison of the risks and benefit. Am. Surg., 55:347, 1989.
4. Clagett, O. T.: Research and prosearch. Presidential Address. J. Thorac. Cardiovasc. Surg., 44:153, 1962.
5. Coote, H.: Pressure on the axillary vessel and nerve by the exostosis from a cervical rib: Interference with the circulation of the arm: Removal of the rib and exostosis. Recovery Med. Tims Gaz., 2:108, 1861; cited in Clagett.
6. Dale, W. A.: Thoracic outlet compression syndrome, critique in 1982. Arch. Surg., 117:1437, 1982.
7. Van Echo, D. A., Sickles, E. A., and Wiernik, P. H.: Thoracic outlet syndrome, supraclavicular adenopathy, Hodgkin's disease (letter). Ann. Intern. Med., 78:608, 1973.
8. Falconer, M. A., and Li, F. W. P.: Resection of the first rib in costoclavicular compression of the brachial plexus. Lancet, 1:59, 1962.
9. Falconer, M. A., and Weddell, G.: Costoclavicular compression of the subclavian artery and vein: Relation to the scalenus anticus syndrome. Lancet, 2:539, 1943.
10. Haggart, G. E.: Value of conservative management in cervicobrachial pain. J.A.M.A., 137:508, 1948.
11. Keen, W.: The symptomatology, diagnosis and surgical treament of cervical ribs. Am. J. Med. Sci., 133:173, 1907.
12. Kremer, R. M., and Ahlquist, R. E., Jr.: Thoracic outlet compression syndrome. Am. J. Surg., 130:612, 1975.
13. Machleder, H. I., Moll, F., Nuwer, M., Jordan, S.: Somatosensory evoked

potentials in the assessment of thoracic outlet compression syndrome. J. Vasc. Surg., 6:177, 1987.

14. Mahorner, H., Castleberry, J. W., and Coleman, W. O.: Attempts to restore function in major veins which are the site of massive thrombosis. Ann. Surg., 146:510, 1957.

15. Murphy, J. B.: A case of cervical rib with symptoms resembling subclavian aneurism. Ann. Surg., 41:399, 1905.

16. Nelson, P. A.: Treatment of patients with cervicodorsal outlet syndrome. J.A.M.A. 163:1570, 1957.

17. Nelson, R. M., and Davis, R. W.: Thoracic outlet compression syndrome. Ann. Thorac. Surg., 8:437, 1969.

18. Nelson, R. M., Jensen, C. B.: Anterior approach for excision of the first rib. Ann. Thorac. Surg., 9:30, 1970.

19. Reilly, L. M., Stoney, R. J.: Supraclavicular approach of thoracic outlet decompression. J. Vasc. Surg., 8:329, 1988.

20. Roos, D. B.: Transaxillary approach for first rib resection to relieve thoracic outlet syndrome. Ann. Surg., 163:354, 1966.

21. Roos, D. B.: Congenital anomalies associated with thoracic outlet syndrome: Anatomy, symptoms, diagnosis, and treatment. Am. J. Surg., 132:771, 1976.

22. Roos, D. B.: The place for scalenectomy and first rib resection in thoracic outlet syndrome. Surgery, 92:1077, 1982.

23. Sadler, T. R., Jr., Rainer, W. G., and Twombley, G.: Thoracic outlet compression: Application of positional arteriographic and nerve conduction studies. Am. J. Surg., 130:704, 1975.

24. Sanders, R. J., Monsour, J. W., Gerber, W. F., Adams, W. R., and Thompson, N.: Scalenectomy versus first rib resection for treatment of the thoracic outlet syndrome. Surgery, 85:109, 1979.

25. Silver, D.: The thoracic outlet syndrome. In Goldsmith, H. S. (Ed.): Lewis' Practice of Surgery. New York, Harper & Row, 1975.

26. Stopford, J. S. B., and Telford, E. D.: Compression of the lower trunk of the brachial plexus by a first dorsal rib with a note on the surgical treatment. Br. J. Surg., 7:168, 1919.

27. Strandness, D. E., Jr., and Bell, J. W.: Peripheral vascular disease: Diagnosis and objective evaluation using a mercury strain gauge. Ann. Surg., 161(Suppl):3–34. 1965.

28. Tomsick, T. A., Ahlstrand, R. A., and Kiesel, T. M.: Thoracic outlet syndrome associated with rib fusion and cervicothoracic scoliosis. J. Can. Assoc. Radiol., 25:211, 1974.

29. Urschel, H. C., Jr., and Razzuk, M. A.: Management of the thoracic outlet syndrome. N. Engl. J. Med., 286:1140, 1972.

30. Urschel, H. C., Jr., Razzuk, M. A., Albers, J. E., Wood, R. E., and Paulson, D. L.: Reoperation for recurrent thoracic outlet syndrome. Ann. Thorac. Surg., 21:19, 1976.

31. Urschel, H. C., Jr., Razzuk, M. A., Wood, R. E., et al.: Objective diagnosis (ulnar nerve conduction velocity) and current therapy of the thoracic outlet syndrome. Ann. Thorac. Surg., 12:608, 1971.

32. Weinberg, H., Nathan H., Magora, F., Robin, G. C., and Aviad, L.: Arthritis of the first costovertebral joint as a cause of thoracic outlet syndrome. Clin. Orthop., 86:159, 1972.

33. Wright, I. S.: The neurovascular syndrome produced by hyperabduction of the arms: The immediate changes produced in 150 normal controls, and the effects on some persons of prolonged hyperabduction of the arms, as in sleeping, and in certain occupations. Am. Heart J. 29:1, 1945.

34. A mirror of the practice of medicine and surgery in the hospitals of London, clinical records, supernumerary first rib. Lancet, 2:633, 1860.

XIV

CONGENITAL DEFORMITIES OF THE CHEST WALL

David C. Sabiston, Jr., M.D.

The chest wall is the site of a number of congenital and acquired lesions that are associated with both physiologic and psychological abnormalities. For most of these, surgical management offers much to such patients, and the procedures can be performed with low risk and expectation of very favorable results.

PECTUS EXCAVATUM

The most common of the major congenital deformities of the sternum is pectus excavatum. This bony and cartilaginous malformation varies from a very mild and scarcely noticeable congenital deformity to those that are quite severe and symptomatic (Fig. 1). In the pectus excavatum defect, the primary problem is a deformity of the costal cartilages, which have developed in a concave position and thus depress the sternum toward the vertebral column. The most severe depression of the sternum is usually above the xiphoid process and usually extends to the sternomanubrial junction. Whereas this deformity varies widely in appearance, in the most extreme examples the sternum may be depressed close to the vertebral column. The heart is often displaced to the left. The extent of cardiac depression is clearly noted on the computed tomographic scan (Fig. 2). Most of these defects are apparent at birth but occasionally may not become noticeable until weeks or months later. In general, the defect increases with time. Although the defect may be familial and occur in siblings or in those with a familial history, most of those with this disorder do not provide such a history.

Clinical Manifestations

In most instances, patients with pectus excavatum have few, if any, symptoms. When questioned carefully, older children and teenagers are apt to recognize they do not have the same respiratory reserve, compared with peers of the same age and sex. This is especially found in those involved in competitive athletics, particularly when heavy and continuous exercise is necessary. After a corrective surgical procedure, it is common for such patients to become aware that they have gained a greater respiratory reserve although they were unaware preoperatively of limitation during exercise. In a few patients, serious cardiorespiratory problems have been described, which greatly improve after correction. A history may also be obtained of recurrent infections that are sometimes severe.[12]

Whereas respiratory and cardiac insufficiency was previously regarded as being uncommon in these defects, studies have

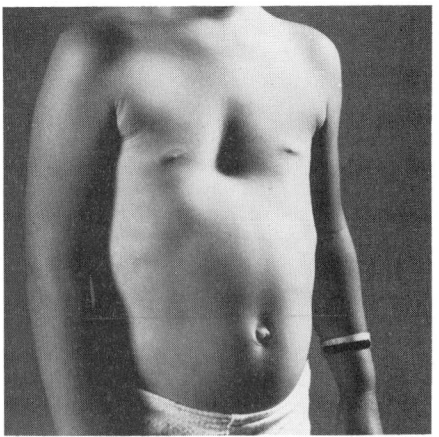

Figure 1. Pectus excavatum.

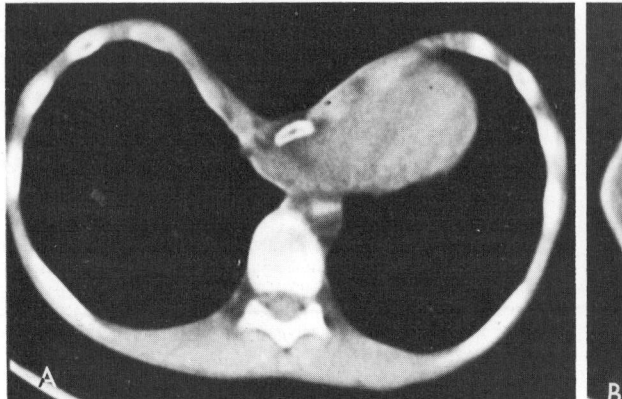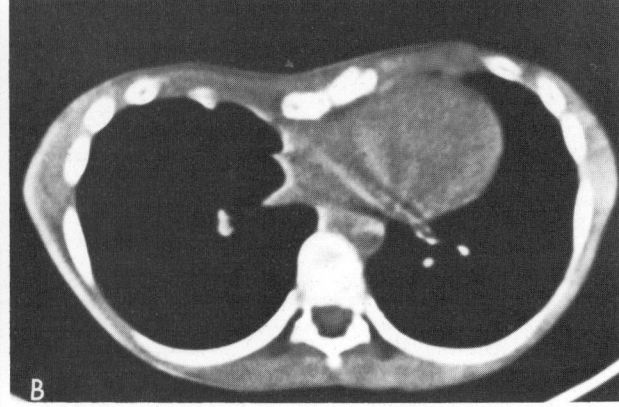

Figure 2. Pectus excavatum CT scan showing *(A)* the deformation and compression of the heart and *(B)* striking relief by operation.

provided evidence that both cardiac and respiratory function tend to be somewhat lower than normal. Among military trainees with pectus excavatum with exercise intolerance, significant decreases have been demonstrated in the force of expiratory flow and in maximal voluntary ventilation.[21] It has also been shown that the working capacity of patients with pectus excavatum is significantly lower in the sitting position, compared with the supine position, and the stroke volume did not increase as much as in normal subjects going from rest to exercise in the sitting position, a change thought to be due to impaired ventricular filling. A mild *restrictive* defect has also been observed. Cardiac catheterization at rest in the supine position showed normal atrial, right ventricular, pulmonary arterial, and pulmonary wedge pressures and a normal cardiac index. However, in some patients, the cardiac output during intense exercise when upright was below the normal range owing primarily to a subnormal increase in stroke volume. These studies were done at the National Heart, Lung, and Blood Institute and the following conclusion was drawn:

> Our results indicate that a mild to moderate pectus-excavatum deformity interferes importantly with cardiac function, primarily when exercise is performed in the upright position. These results appear to explain the disparity between operative reports describing marked clinical improvement of patients after correction of pectus-excavatum deformities and hemodynamic reports indicating little or no cardiac abnormality in such patients. Thus, if the supine catheterization data of the patients undergoing operation were analyzed, these patients would have been judged to have had normal hemodynamic function, which was unimproved by operation. However, in each the response of cardiac output during intense upright exercise was significantly enhanced after operation. It should be emphasized that the patients studied in this investigation did not have severe pectus-excavatum deformities.[2]

With use of the single-pass technique of radionuclide angiocardiography, changes in cardiac function were assessed during rest and exercise and following surgical correction of the deformity. Evaluations were made in the upright position with bicycle exercise for 6 months or more after correction of pectus excavatum and showed that the operation did not change the left ventricular ejection fraction or cardiac index at rest or exercise. However, the left ventricular end-diastolic volume index and stroke volume index increased at rest after surgical correction. The estimated right ventricular end-diastolic volume also increased greatly after operation and was associated with a reduction in ventricular ejection fraction. The increase in right and left ventricular volumes after operation suggests that cardiac compression improves following operation.[10]

Indications for Surgical Correction

For the majority of patients with pectus excavatum, the primary indication for operation is cosmetic. The poor self-image held by many patients with this disorder is especially notable when the child begins association with larger groups and play-

mates begin to be inquisitive or ridicule the defect. These patients rapidly recognize they are different because of their deformity. They usually cover the defect by wearing shirts at all times and are seldom comfortable when their chests are bare, even, for example, while swimming. Without surgical correction, many become withdrawn, are quite shy, and experience a significantly altered social life as contrasted with their peers. For these reasons, the presence of pectus excavatum is usually an indication for correction unless the defect is quite minimal. Patients with evidence of respiratory insufficiency, particularly during exercise, are also appropriate candidates for operation. The presence of Marfan's syndrome was formerly held by some to be a contraindication to operation, but those with this deformity respond well to a corrective procedure. The timing of the operation is important, and if a significant deformity is present at 1 or 2 years of age, operation can be done both safely and effectively. The best results are probably obtained at the age of 2 or 3 years. Whenever possible, correction should be done before the age of 5 years. Psychological complications may appear early in life. For these reasons, the earlier correction is performed, the less likely that such features will be as significant. The procedure is more easily performed in the young, since it can be done more effectively and with the best result.

Operative Technique

The general preference is for a technique now broadly used because the results are predictably excellent and there are few complications.[13] The incision is usually made in the midline in males as well as in older females.[12] However, if the patient prefers a more cosmetic type of incision, a transverse inframammary incision can be used but requires more dissection and may occasionally present difficulty with adequate exposure. Most of the dissection is preferably done with fine-needle electrocautery. With the midline approach, the incision is extended to the periosteum of the sternum, and the pectoral muscles are reflected laterally with exposure of the costal cartilages. The lower costal cartilages are often covered by the rectus muscles and should be dissected for adequate exposure. All involved cartilages are resected subperichondrially for the length of the deformed segments (Fig. 3A). The perichondrium is preserved to form new costal cartilages, and from this layer new cartilages regenerate within several months. A firm anterior wall is thereby developed and can be palpated adjacent to the sternum. After removal of the costal cartilages, the xiphoid joint is transected, and the finger can then be passed beneath the sternum to separate the parietal pleura bilaterally. The intercostal muscles are divided, and the sternum is entirely freed of all attachments except its junction with the manubrium (Fig. 3B). If it is not deformed, the second and at times the third costal cartilage may be divided obliquely, permitting the entire sternum to be lifted anteriorly. A transverse osteotomy is made through the sternomanubrial joint posteriorly. This permits a temporary

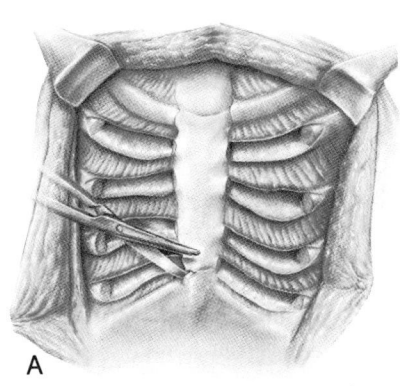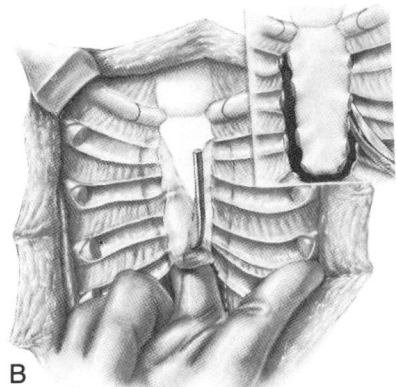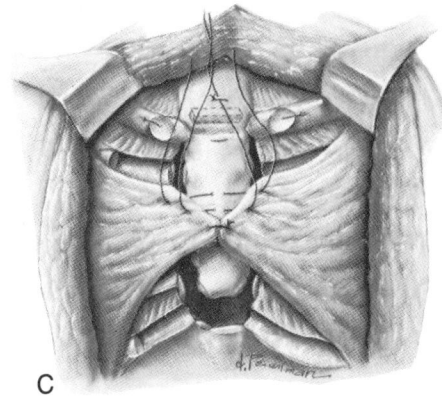

A   B   C

Figure 3. *A,* Division of the xiphoid. The deformed cartilages are removed subperichondrally for the full extent of their deformity, and the xiphoid is divided from the sternum. The sternum is elevated. The intercostal bundles are then completely divided from the sternum, and an attempt is made to incise medial to the internal mammary vessels. *C,* In older children and adults, a Steinmann pin may be placed such that the ends are in the subcutaneous tissue lateral to the nipples to prevent the sternum from becoming depressed. The pin is removed several months later under local anesthesia when the chest wall has healed and is firm. (From Ravitch, M. M.: Pectus excavatum. *In* Rob, C., and Smith, R. (Eds.): Operative Surgery: Cardiothoracic Surgery, 3rd ed. London, Butterworth & Co., (Publishers) Ltd., 1978. By permission.)

overcorrection of the sternum. For fixation of the sternum in correct position, a wedge of costal cartilage is placed in the osteotomy and secured with sutures. The pectoral fascia is then approximated with interrupted sutures, and the subcutaneous tissue is closed (Fig. 3C). In children over 12 years and adults, a Steinmann pin is placed such that the ends are in the subcutaneous tissue lateral to the nipples. The pin is removed several months later under local anesthesia when the chest wall has healed and is firm. A drain with multiple perforations is left in the mediastinum and is attached to sterile suction. Postoperatively, serous drainage may occur for several days. Blood transfusion is rarely necessary. Mild fever may be present postoperatively (38 or 39° C.), usually due to atelectasis. Wound infections are rare, and the patients are mobilized on the first day. At the time of discharge they are advised to avoid body-contact sports for several months or until after the Steinmann pin has been removed.

An alternative technique is the "sternal turnover" procedure, in which the entire deformed portion of the sternum with the associated costal cartilages is excised *en bloc* with the intercostal muscles. This free graft is then turned over and sutured in place.

STERNAL FISSURE

During embryologic development, the sternum originates in the lateral plate mesoderm that provides the pectoral muscles. At 6 weeks, the migrating cells form two bands and become fused by the tenth week. The manubrium is formed by primordia between the ventral ends of the developing clavicles, and rarely the sternal bars do not join or attach only in the lower portion, leaving a defect superiorly. There are three principal types of sternal fissure. In the *superior sternal cleft,*[15] the heart may appear to be in the cervical region, but it is primarily within the mediastinum. This defect is usually broad, has the appearance of a U or a V, and commonly extends to the fourth costal cartilages. In the surgical correction, the two sternal bands can usually be joined in the midline by encircling sutures after oblique chrondrotomies. In severe defects, oblique chrondrotomies may not be sufficient, and closure may cause excessive compression of the heart and produce hypotension and bradycardia. A prosthesis of Marlex or Gore-Tex is then required for correction.

Complete clefts of the sternum are more severe; an extensive procedure is necessary since there is usually no bone between the hyoid and the pubis. There is also a crescentic anterior defect in the diaphragm and a wide diastasis recti. This allows free communication between the pericardial and peritoneal cavities.

The third type of sternal deformity in this category is the *distal* *sternal cleft,* the most extensive of all.[4] This pentalogy is characterized by a cleft in the distal sternum, a ventral omphalocele, a crescentic deficiency of the anterior diaphragm, a deficiency of the diaphragmatic portion of the pericardium with free communication between the pericardial and peritoneal cavities, and the congenital heart defect that most often involves a ventricular septal defect, the tetralogy of Fallot, or a left ventricular diverticulum.

POLAND'S SYNDROME

Poland's syndrome is absence of the pectoralis major, absence or hypoplasia of the pectoralis minor, absence of costal cartilages, hypoplasia of breast and subcutaneous tissue, and brachysyndactyly. Poland said, "The whole of the sternal and costal portions of the pectoralis major muscle were deficient; . . . the pectoralis minor muscle was wholly absent; . . . the serratus-magnus muscle was also for the most part deficient . . . in the left hand the middle phalanges were absent in all the fingers . . . the web between the fingers extended to the third phalangeal articulation . . . the left hand was shorter than the right . . . no malformation was noticed in any other part." Various degrees of this malformation may be present from the simple absence of the costosternal portion of the pectoralis major to the fully developed syndrome. As children with this syndrome grow older, the defect usually becomes more severe. Several operative procedures have been described for its correction.[13,15,17,20]

PECTUS CARINATUM

Although less common than pectus excavatum, pectus carinatum ("pigeon breast") is not an infrequent malformation and should usually be corrected. It consists of protrusion of the sternum caused by an upward curve in the lower costal cartilages, generally the fourth to the eighth cartilages, pushing the sternum forward (Fig. 4). This defect is usually obvious. Symptoms occur in some patients and include exertional dyspnea and cardiac arrhythmias. It may be difficult for the chest to expand during inspiration.

Operative Technique

Correction is performed through a midline incision or a submammary transverse incision. The pectoral muscles are dissected laterally, and the rectus muscles are separated from the lower cartilages and the xiphoid. Each deformed cartilage is removed subperichondrially, and multiple reefing sutures are placed to remove the redundancy in the perichondrium. Protuberances are then excised, the muscles are approximated, and

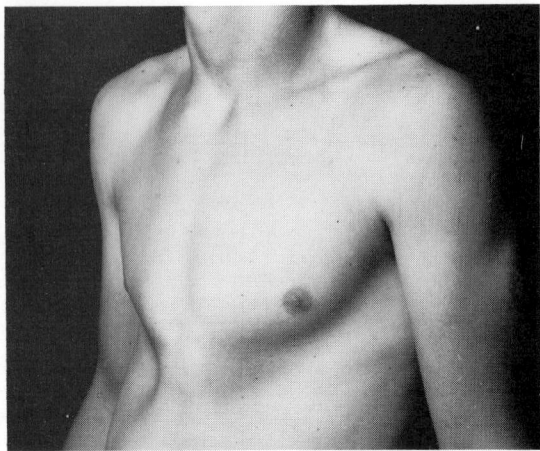

Figure 4. Pectus carinatum of the chicken breast type in a 16-year-old boy referred because of a prominent sternum. In fact, it is the depression of the rib on either side that causes the apparent prominence of the sternum. At operation, excision of four cartilages, subperichondrally, and reefing sutures in the now redundant perichondrium to provide a taut, straight course from the outer ends of the ribs to the sternum corrected the deformity very satisfactorily.

the incision is closed. The results are generally excellent with few if any complications, and very rare mortality. Few if any physiologic changes can be demonstrated postoperatively.[3]

NEOPLASMS OF THE CHEST WALL

The Sternum and Ribs

Benign and malignant neoplasms of the chest wall are not uncommon, and they may be in the sternum, ribs, and diaphragm. These lesions may be primary, metastatic, or the result of direct invasion of the chest wall from either a bronchogenic or breast neoplasm. Primary tumors arising in the chest represent approximately 8 per cent of all intrinsic bone tumors.[9,18]

Benign Neoplasms

Common benign neoplasms of the chest wall include chondromas, osteochondromas, bone cysts, fibrous dysplasia, and eosinophilic granuloma. Some lesions present with the appearance of a mass, at times tender, and show few clinical signs or symptoms to suggest the specific type of neoplasm. The chondroma is the most common benign tumor of the chest wall, with most appearing in the ribs and a minority in the sternum. Excision *en bloc* with a 4-cm. margin around the lesion is the appropriate operation. The same type of treatment applies to osteochondromas as well as bone cysts and eosinophilic granulomas. Among 53 primary chest wall tumors in one series, 26 were benign, with 49 occurring in the ribs and 4 in the sternum.[14] All patients with benign neoplasms were treated by excision with no recurrence or mortality. In general, it is not possible to distinguish benign neoplasms from malignant ones occurring in the chest wall unless *cortical* destruction and involvement of soft tissues are visualized. In management of benign as well as malignant lesions, these neoplasms should be considered malignant until proven otherwise, and wide excision with a 4- to 5-cm. margin is appropriate. With this approach, the largest number of patients will become long-term survivors as shown in Figure 5.[6]

Chondrosarcoma is generally the most common malignant lesion and appears as a lobulated, smooth, firm mass often showing destruction of cortex on radiographs. It should be removed by radical dissection *en bloc*. The survival of patients with chondrosarcoma of the chest wall managed by wide resection, local excision, and palliative excision is shown in Figure 6.[7]

Ewing's tumor is best evaluated by chest film and shows

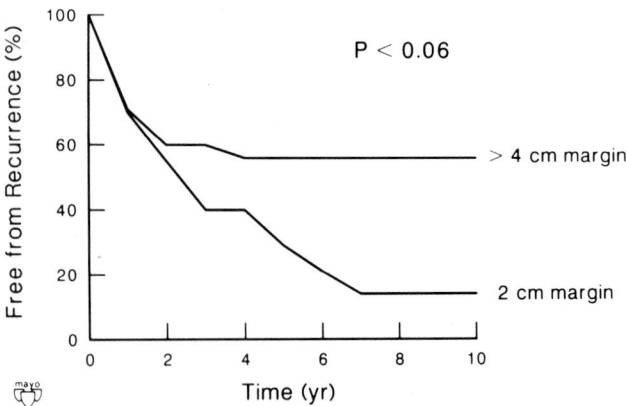

Figure 5. The percentage of patients with malignant chest wall tumors who are free from recurrent tumor is measured by the extent of the resection margin. Zero time on the abscissa represents the day of chest wall resection. (From King, R. M., Pairolero, P. C., Trastek, V. F., et al.: Primary chest wall tumors: Factors affecting survival. Ann. Thorac. Surg., *41*:597, 1986.)

evidence of destruction or lysis of bone with a diffuse, expanded bone lesion with little periosteal reaction in some of the patients. Surgical excision[14] and radiation and chemotherapy[8] are employed. Lymphomas are also managed primarily by chemotherapy and radiation.

Another primary malignant lesion is plasmacytoma, and radical excision, with or without radiation, is necessary. Clinical features suggesting that a neoplasm is malignant include recent and rapid increase in size, invasion of surrounding structures, and distant metastases. Whereas diagnostic biopsy has been described, most recommend wide excision of the neoplasm. In a series of 27 malignant primary chest wall tumors, the overall 5-year survival was 33 per cent and the 10-year survival 18 per cent.[14] Additional malignant neoplasms include osteogenic sarcoma, neurosarcoma, fibrosarcoma, liposarcoma, and angioplastic sarcoma.

Metastatic neoplasms may also involve the chest wall by extension or by metastases by blood-borne deposits. In general, surgical intervention in such lesions is palliative and should be done only to establish the diagnosis or in the management of otherwise uncontrollable discomfort. Although some neoplasms are amenable to radiotherapy, those that are radioresistant include chondrosarcoma, osteogenic sarcoma, neurosarcoma, fibrosarcoma, liposarcoma, angiosarcoma, and anaplastic neoplasms. Among the radiosensitive malignant tumors

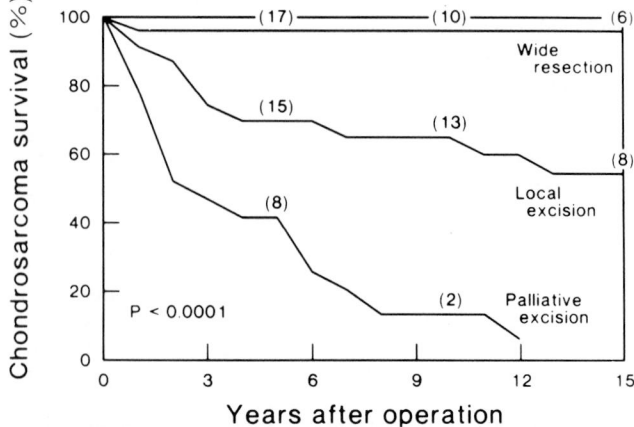

Figure 6. The survival of patients with chest wall chondrosarcoma is measured by the extent of operation. Zero time on the abscissa represents the day of chest wall resection. (From McAfee, M. K., Pairolero, P. C., Bergstralh, E. J., et al.: Chondrosarcoma of the chest wall: Factors affecting survival. Ann. Thorac. Surg., *40*:535, 1985.)

are Ewing's sarcoma, reticulum cell sarcoma, plasma cell myeloma, Hodgkin's disease, and lymphosarcoma.

Among 100 patients in one series with chest wall tumors, metastases were present in 32 instances, including 12 from sarcomas, 9 from the breast, 4 from the kidney, 3 from the lung, 3 from other genitourinary sources, and 1 from the thyroid gland.[8] The value of *en bloc* resection of the chest wall for patients with bronchogenic carcinoma has been demonstrated.[11] More controversial, however, is radical resection of breast cancer with metastases to the chest wall. Skin ulceration was present in 11 of 14 cases of breast cancer, and these were treated with excision and palliation.[8] Wide radical chest wall resection with immediate reconstruction, including the use of flaps and chest wall muscles as well as omentum and prosthetic materials (e.g., Prolene or polytetrafluoroethylene patch), is effective for many malignant lesions.

Neoplasms of the Diaphragm

Benign tumors of the diaphragm that have been reported include fibromas, lipomas, mesotheliomas, angiofibromas, and neurogenic tumors. In addition, congenital cysts of the diaphragm occur. Considerably more common have been malignant lesions, primarily metastatic, from neighboring structures such as the esophagus, lung, liver, and colon. Retroperitoneal malignant neoplasms may also extend to the diaphragm. Primary malignant lesions include fibrosarcomas and neurofibrosarcomas. Symptoms may be elusive, and the lesions are generally diagnosed by radiography. Computed tomography scans have also become quite useful in the diagnosis of these lesions.

The management of benign lesions is simple excision; for malignant primary lesions, wide removal with replacement by fascia lata or prosthetic material is required. Radiotherapy and chemotherapy are infrequently indicated.[5,16]

It has been reported that of the primary tumors of the diaphragm, the malignant lesions predominate in 60 per cent, whereas the remaining 40 per cent of neoplasms are benign.[1,19]

SELECTED REFERENCES

Groff, D. B., III, and Adkins, P. C.: Collective review: Chest wall tumors. Ann. Thorac. Surg., 4:260, 1967.
This is a collective review of a large number of cases of chest wall tumors with descriptions of the various types.

Morgan, R. F., Edgerton, M. T., Wanebo, H. J., Daniel, T. M., Spotnitz, W. D., and Kron, I. L.: Reconstruction of full thickness chest wall defects. Ann. Surg., 207:707, 1988.
A series of patients treated by wide en bloc resection of chest wall tumors with primary reconstruction is reviewed. All patients survived resection and reconstruction. Emphasis is placed on preservation of a portion of the innervated muscle

in situ or the transfer of the muscle with preservation of its resting length for maintenance of muscle function.

Pairolero, P. C., and Arnold, P. G.: Chest wall tumors: Experience with 100 consecutive patients. J. Thorac. Cardiovasc. Surg., 90:367, 1985.
A 10-year experience of 100 consecutive patients with neoplasms of the chest wall from the Mayo Clinic.

REFERENCES

1. Anderson, L. S., and Forrest, J. V.: Tumors of the diaphragm. Roentgenol. Radium Ther. Nucl. Med., 119:259, 1973.
2. Beiser, G. C., Epstein, S. E., Stampfer, M. D., et al.: Impairment of cardiac function with pectus excavatum with improvement after operative correction. N. Engl. J. Med., 287:267, 1972.
3. Cahill, J. L., Lees, G. M., and Robertson, H. T.: A summary of preoperative and postoperative cardiorespiratory performance in patients undergoing pectus excavatum and carinatum repair. J. Pediatr. Surg., 19:430, 1984.
4. Cantrell, J. R., Haller, J. A., Jr., and Ravitch, M. M.: A syndrome of congenital defects involving the abdominal wall, sternum, diaphragm, pericardium, and heart. Surg. Gynecol. Obstet., 107:602, 1958.
5. Claggett, O. T., and Johnson, M. A.: Tumors of the diaphragm. Am. J. Surg., 78:526, 1949.
6. King, R. M., Pairolero, P. C., Trastek, V. F., et al.: Primary chest wall tumors: Factors affecting survival. Ann. Thorac. Surg., 41:597, 1986.
7. McAfee, M. K., Pairolero, P. C., Bergstralh, E. J., et al.: Chondrosarcoma of the chest wall: Factors affecting survival. Ann. Thorac. Surg., 40:535, 1985.
8. Pairolero, P. C., and Arnold, P. G.: Chest wall tumors: Experience with 100 consecutive patients. J. Thorac. Cardiovasc. Surg., 90:367, 1985.
9. Pascuzzi, C. A., Dahlin, D. C., and Clagett, O. T.: Primary tumors of the ribs and sternum. Surg. Gynecol. Obstet., 104:390, 1957.
10. Peterson, R. J., Young, W. G., Jr., Godwin, J. D., et al.: Noninvasive assessment of exercise cardiac function before and after pectus excavatum repair. J. Thorac. Cardiovasc. Surg., 90:251, 1985.
11. Piehler, J. M., Pairolero, P. C., Weiland, L. H., Offord, K. P., Payne, W. S., and Bernatz, P. E.: Bronchogenic carcinoma with chest wall invasion: Factors affecting survival following en bloc resection. Ann. Thorac. Surg., 34:684, 1982.
12. Ravitch, M. M.: Pectus excavatum: Pectus carinatum. *In* Rob, C., and Smith, R. (Eds.): Operative Surgery, 3rd ed. London, Butterworth & Company, 1977.
13. Sabiston, D. C., Jr.: Disorders of the sternum and thoracic wall. *In* Sabiston, D. C., Jr., and Spencer, F. C. (Eds.): Surgery of the Chest, 5th ed. Philadelphia, W. B. Saunders Company, 1990.
14. Sabanathan, S., Salama, F. D., Morgan, W. E., and Harvey, J. A.: Primary chest wall tumors. Ann. Thorac. Surg., 39:4, 1985.
15. Salley, R. K., and Stewart, S.: Superior sternal cleft: Repair in the newborn. Ann. Thorac. Surg., 39:582, 1985.
16. Samson, P. C., and Childress, M. E.: Primary neurofibrosarcoma of the diaphragm. J. Thorac. Surg., 20:901, 1950.
17. Seyfer, A. E., Icochea, R., and Graeber, G. M.: Poland's anomaly: Natural history and long-term results of chest wall reconstruction in 33 patients. Ann. Surg., 208:776, 1988.
18. Teitelbaum, S. L.: Twenty years' experience with intrinsic tumors of the bony thorax at a large institution. J. Thorac. Cardiovasc. Surg., 63:776, 1972.
19. Trivedi, S. A.: Neurolemmoma of the diaphragm causing severe hypertrophic pulmonary osteoarthropathy. Br. J. Tuberculosis, 52:214, 1958.
20. Urschel, H. C., Jr., Byrd, S., Sethi, S. M., and Razzuk, M. A.: Poland's syndrome: Improved surgical management. Ann. Thorac. Surg., 37:204, 1984.
21. Weg, J. G., Krumholz, R. A., and Harkleroad, L. E.: Pulmonary dysfunction in pectus excavatum. Am. Rev. Respir. Dis., 96:936, 1967.

XV

EXTRACORPOREAL MEMBRANE OXYGENATION

Robert H. Bartlett, M. D.

The apparatus and techniques of extracorporeal circulation are routinely used for a few hours to permit surgical therapy on the heart. With modifications, extracorporeal circulation can be used for days or weeks to support the life of patients with severe cardiac or pulmonary failure. The procedure involves cannulation of major vessels without thoracotomy, carefully titrated partial anticoagulation with heparin, and continuous high-flow extacorporeal circulation through a membrane lung. Depending on the cannulation and application, this procedure has been called extracorporeal life support, extracorporeal CO_2 removal, extracorporeal heart assist, extracorporeal lung assist, and extracorporeal membrane oxygenation (ECMO). ECMO is not a therapy, but a mechanical support system that allows time for the damaged heart or lungs to heal in a milieu of normal perfusion and gas exchange while giving the damaged organs rest from the effects of mechanical ventilation and inotropic drugs. ECMO has been the most successful in neonatal respiratory failure and is considered standard therapy for that condition. It is the only method of mechanical cardiac support in children. It is a reasonable (albeit extraordinary) approach to the management of severe respiratory failure in children and adults.

HISTORICAL ASPECTS

Important steps in extending the use of extracorporeal circulation from hours to days were (1) the development of membrane artificial lungs[14]; (2) the titration of continuous low-dose heparin[5]; and (3) the elimination of gas interfaces, reservoirs, filters, and suction pumps from the extracorporeal circuit.[2] With these modifications in technique, prolonged extracorporeal circulation was developed and studied in animals by Kolobow,[15] Bartlett,[1] and others.[8] Hill reported the first successful use of ECMO in 1972.[12] The patient was a young man with the adult respiratory distress syndrome (ARDS) complicating multiple injuries from a motorcycle accident. Several other successful cases followed,[10] leading to an NIH-sponsored multicenter trial of ECMO for ARDS in 1975. Nine per cent of ECMO and control patients survived, and the study was terminated after 92 patients were entered with the conclusion that lung injury was usually irreversible, even if life was prolonged for a week or two with ECMO.[22] As a result of this study, clinical studies of ECMO for adult respiratory failure essentially ceased in 1978.

The first successful application of ECMO in neonatal respiratory failure was accomplished by Bartlett and colleagues in 1975.[3] By 1986 they had treated 100 patients, with 72 survivors.[4] Several centers corroborated these results and two prospective randomized studies proved that ECMO support improved survival results.[6,18] By 1986, 715 newborn patients had been treated in 18 centers, 82 per cent surviving.[20] Currently ECMO is used in more than 60 neonatal centers, the most experienced centers reporting 95 per cent survival.[17]

Not convinced by the results of the National Institutes of Health (NIH) ECMO adult trial, Gattinoni and Kolobow returned to the study of prolonged extracorporeal circulation in ARDS. In the NIH ECMO study, venoarterial bypass was used, bleeding was extensive (over 2 liters per day), and many patients were continued on high pressure and high oxygen during extracorporeal support. Gattinoni reasoned that ECMO should emphasize carbon dioxide removal, resting the lung from high-pressure ventilation, minimal heparin, and venovenous extracorporeal circulation to allow total pulmonary blood flow. With these modifications in the technique, they reported 50 per cent survival using the same patient selection criteria used for the NIH study.[9] These results have been corroborated in several other centers, primarily in Europe.[13]

In 1989, the centers using ECMO for respiratory failure formed a study group called the Extracorporeal Life Support Organization (ELSO). The purpose of this group is to design and perform multicenter clinical and laboratory studies, serve as a central source of information about extracorporeal life support for the medical public, and collect data on devices and treatment. ELSO maintains the ECMO Registry, a large data base that includes essentially all of the infants and children treated with ECMO since the procedure was devised.

ECMO PROCEDURE

Because most clinical applications of ECMO are currently in newborn infants, this description and discussion refers primarily to that group of patients. The basic principles of extracorporeal circulation, gas exchange, and systemic oxygen delivery

apply to patients of all sizes and ages. The pathophysiology of acute respiratory failure is quite different between newborn infants and older patients and is discussed later.

THE ECMO CIRCUIT AND MANAGEMENT. The circuit includes a servo-regulated roller pump, membrane lung, heat exchanger, tubing, and connectors (Fig. 1). Right atrial blood is drained via a right internal jugular vein cannula to a small distensible bladder. A microswitch on the bladder automatically regulates the roller pump, controlling blood flow based on venous drainage and preventing air embolism. Blood passes through the pump and is perfused through a membrane lung. The size of the artificial lung is selected to provide *total* cardiopulmonary support, even though partial support is adequate for most patients. Each artificial lung has a "rated flow" that specifies the blood flow rate at which 75 per cent saturated venous blood leaves the oxygenator 95 per cent saturated. The artificial lung chosen for a specific case must have a rated flow equivalent to or greater than the cardiac output of the patient. Routine blood flow rates are 70 to 90 ml. per kg. per minute in adults, 80 to 100 ml. per kg. per minute in children, and 120 to 170 mg. per kg. per minute in neonates. As the blood is oxygenated, CO_2 and water vapor are removed into the gas phase of the artificial lung. Blood then flows through a countercurrent heat exchanger and back into the patient. In *venoarterial* circulation, the blood is perfused through a carotid, femoral, or axillary artery cannula into the aortic arch. In *venovenous* circulation, blood is returned to the venous circulation. The circuit is primed sequentially with CO_2, electrolyte solution, albumin, and, finally, fresh blood. In neonates, the final prime is approximately 500 ml. in volume. This may be twice the newborn's blood volume and the prime must therefore be carefully adjusted for pH, temperature, and hematocrit.

Cannulation is performed at the bedside in the intensive care unit with an operating room team present. In neonates, the right common carotid artery and internal jugular vein are exposed via a right transverse cervical incision. Heparin (100 units per kg.) is administered intravenously after exposure of the vessels is com-

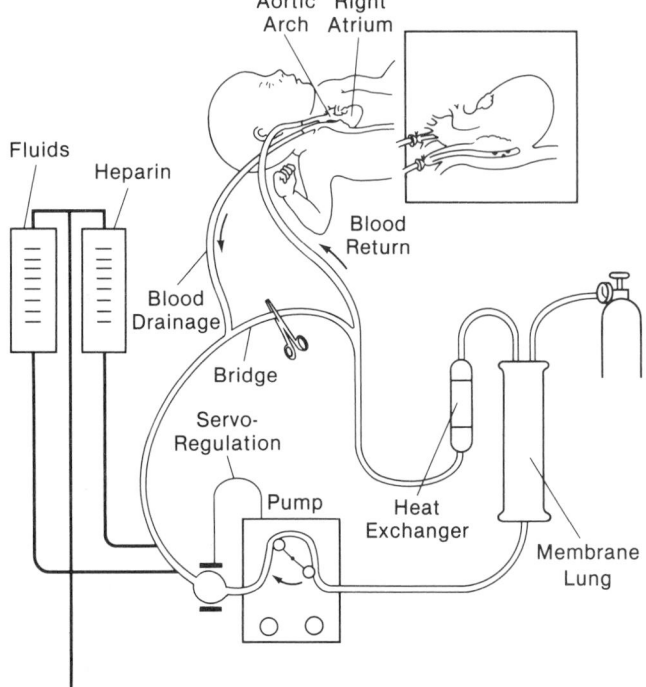

Figure 1. The typical ECMO circuit. This diagram illustrates venoarterial access in a newborn infant. The components of the circuit are the same for older children and adults. (Redrawn from Bartlett, R. H., Andrews, A. F., Toomasian, J. M., et al.: Extracorporeal membrane oxygenation for newborn respiratory failure: 45 cases. Surgery, 92:425, 1982.)

plete. The largest cannulas that may be easily advanced are placed with the tips in the aortic arch and the right atrium. The internal diameter of the venous catheter is the limiting factor that determines maximal flow. The venous catheter must be large enough to allow total cardiopulmonary bypass. Rarely, a second venous access site is necessary to achieve adequate flow. Cardiopulmonary bypass is initiated, and flow is gradually increased until levels of near total bypass are achieved.

Once the patient is on ECMO support, paralyzing agents, vasoactive drugs, and other infusions are generally discontinued. Ventilator settings are adjusted to minimal levels to allow "lung rest." Typical neonatal settings are as follows: pressure limit (PL), 20 cm. H_2O; positive end-expiratory pressure (PEEP), 4 cm. H_2O; rate, 10 per minute; and FIO_2, 30 per cent. The patient is usually awake and alert.

During venoarterial bypass, blood flow is maintained at a level sufficient to keep the venous saturation at approximately 75 per cent. Venous saturation is continuously monitored by a fiberoptic catheter in the venous line. A normal venous saturation ensures that the combined oxygen delivery from the patient's cardiopulmonary system and the circuit is adequate for oxygen consumption requirements. A continuous noninvasive arterial oxygen saturation monitor is placed on the patient in an area of postductal blood flow distribution. With this available monitoring, arterial blood gases need only be drawn occasionally once the patient is stable. The arterial saturation is maintained at 95 per cent and is manipulated by adjusting the extracorporeal blood flow rate. The PCO_2 is maintained between 35 and 50 and is inversely proportional to the flow rate of gas ventilating the membrane lung.

Heparin is infused continuously at 30 to 60 units per kg. per hour. The level of anticoagulation is monitored hourly by the whole blood activated clotting time (ACT). The heparin dose is adjusted to maintain the ACT between 200 and 240 seconds (normal is approximately 100 seconds). There is a fall in platelet count at onset of bypass, and platelet consumption continues during ECMO. In infants, platelet transfusions are required to maintain a level greater than 50,000 to 70,000. The hematocrit is maintained between 45 to 50 per cent, and occasional red blood cell transfusion is required. In general, hemolysis is minimal and free serum hemoglobin levels are usually less than 30 mg. per 100 ml. during an ECMO course (normal, less than 5 mg. per 100 ml.).

Patients are often edematous, and emphasis is placed on diuresis and return to approximate dry weight. If diuresis is not adequate after administration of furosemide and mannitol, a hemofilter is placed in the circuit to supplement urinary output. Crystalloid administration is minimized and given mainly in the form of parenteral nutrition. Red blood cells, 25 per cent albumin, or plasma is infused when an increase in intravascular volume is required. The patient is routinely placed on antibiotics.

The extracorporeal flow is gradually decreased as the native lung function increases. When the flow is approximately 20 ml. per kg. per minute, a trial off bypass at low ventilator settings is attempted. If tolerated for a 1- to 3-hour period, the cannulas are removed. Patients often are weaned from the ventilator and extubated over the subsequent 24 to 48 hours.

RESULTS

ECMO is used for patients with a very high mortality risk; so the results are measured as survival. The outcome for various age groups and diagnoses is shown in Table 1. Data on newborn infants and children are derived from the ECMO Registry maintained by the Extracorporeal Life Support Organization.[17] The best results are in neonates with respiratory failure. The most experienced centers routinely report survival of over 90 per cent in most diagnostic categories. The overall survival from congen-

TABLE 1. Survival Rates in Various Categories of Patients Supported with ECMO

	N	Survival (%)
Newborn infants	3094	83
Meconium aspiration syndrome	1215	92
Respiratory distress syndrome	474	82
Primary pulmonary hypertension	443	87
Congenital diaphragmatic hernia	493	63
Sepsis	351	76
Other causes	118	77
Children	73	38
Infection	26	38
Trauma, aspiration	8	50
Capillary leak syndrome	27	37
Other	12	33
Adults		
ARDS, all causes (1980–1989)	150	50

ECMO is used when the likelihood of survival is less than 10 per cent. Data from the Neonatal ECMO Registry[17] and Euroxy Congress on Respiratory Failure.[13]

ital diaphragmatic hernia has improved from 50 per cent in the pre-ECMO era to 76 per cent.[11] When death occurs during ECMO in newborn infants, it is caused by anoxic brain injury from the perinatal period or intracranial bleeding.[7]

Survival in children and adults is approximately 40 per cent in all categories of respiratory failure (infection, aspiration, trauma, or capillary leak syndromes). When death occurs in these patients, it is caused by diffuse pulmonary fibrosis with obliteration of alveoli and vasculature or by multiple organ failure and sepsis.

ECMO has been used for cardiac support in approximately 150 children, usually for cardiac failure following operation for congenital heart disease. Survival is approximately 40 per cent, and death is due to multiple organ failure from low cardiac output.

The reason that recovery occurs in 90 per cent of newborn infants but only 50 per cent of children and adults relates to the pathophysiology of pulmonary dysfunction. In the newborn infant, the problem is a functional problem related to pulmonary vasospasm and inadequate pulmonary blood flow. The lung is intrinsically normal, and there is no factor that predisposes to fibrosis except ventilator-induced lung injury. In children and adults, the primary disease usually affects the interstitium of the lung, leading to inflammation, fibrosis, and bacterial infection. All of these factors cause tissue destruction and scar formation, which obliterates lung parenchyma. The extent of fibrosis and necrosis determines the ability of the lung and the patient to recover.

COMPLICATIONS

The duration of the ECMO course is typically 4 days in neonates and 10 to 14 days in children and adults. Some patients have been supported by ECMO for more than 1 month with ultimate survival. The complication rate increases as the time on extracorporeal support increases.

Approximately two thirds of patients experience some type of physiologic complication (Table 2). Bleeding is the most common complication because of the systemic heparinization and thrombocytopenia. Data from the Neonatal ECMO Registry[20] show that 14 per cent experience intracranial bleeding (as detected by ultrasound examination), 14 per cent have bleeding from the surgical site, and 5 per cent have gastrointestinal bleeding. When bleeding occurs, it is managed by decreasing the systemic heparin dose to activated clotting times below 180 seconds, transfusing platelets until the platelet count is greater

TABLE 2. Physiologic and Mechanical Complications in the First 715 Newborn Infants Treated with ECMO

	Percentage of Series	Survival (%)
All patients (715 patients)	100	81
Physiologic complications	66	74
Intracranial bleed (ultrasound)	14	47
Surgical site bleed	14	69
Seizures	20	61
Renal failure	2	40
Hemolysis	7	79
Arrhythmia	4	74
Positive culture	6	73
Hypertension	7	87
Mechanical complications	23	80
Oxygenator change	7	72
Tubing rupture	3	87
Pump failure	2	87
Cannula problem	7	78

The overall survival rate in this series was 81 per cent. Physiologic complications are often associated with increased mortality, but mechanical complications are not.

than 150,000 per ml., and surgical control of bleeding if these measures are unsuccessful. In newborn infants, 20 per cent experience seizures, which are common in critically ill newborn infants and not necessarily associated with poor neurologic outcome. Two per cent of newborn infants experience renal failure, and 6 per cent have positive cultures. Organ failure (aside from respiratory failure) often occurs in children and adults and is generally due to the primary disease. In most adult and pediatric patients two or three organ systems fail before ECMO is instituted.

It is surprising that mechanical complications are unusual, considering the fact that all of the components of the ECMO circuit must work continuously for days or weeks (see Table 2). Twenty-three per cent of neonates had mechanical complications,[20] but none were associated with a decrease in survival. The most common mechanical complication is membrane lung failure requiring changing the device (7 per cent), or cannulation problems (7 per cent). The reason that mechanical complications do not increase mortality is that the system is continuously attended by an ECMO specialist who can recognize abnormalities and repair any circuit malfunction within minutes. The ECMO specialist is a unique medical professional who combines the role of nurse, respiratory therapist, perfusionist, bioengineer, and resident in managing the ECMO procedure.

FOLLOW-UP

Most of the ECMO survivors are normal.[21] Abnormalities in follow-up are related to the neurologic and pulmonary systems and are generally related to the primary disease, rather than the ECMO procedure. Twenty per cent of newborn infants have a detectable neurologic abnormality, such as hearing loss, weakness, spasticity or another motor-tone abnormality, or mental retardation. The incidence of neurologic handicaps is generally less than that found in follow-up studies of other critically ill newborns. Neurologic injury occurs primarily in those children who have prolonged ischemic or hypoxic episodes in the perinatal period, but some cases of right brain ischemic or hemorrhagic lesions have been identified that may be related to vascular ligation (either jugular vein or carotid artery). Pulmonary disability in the form of bronchopulmonary dysplasia, frequent pulmonary infection, or bronchospasm occurs in 10 per cent of infants treated with ECMO. Pulmonary symptoms usually subside by 1 year of age.

Follow-up examination in children and adults shows findings typical of recovery from severe pulmonary injury. Neurologic function is generally normal. Pulmonary function tests show a restrictive fibrotic pattern that may be associated with bronchospasm. This pulmonary abnormality usually subsides within 1 year from the time of discharge.

PATIENT SELECTION: MORTALITY CRITERIA, INDICATIONS, AND CONTRAINDICATIONS

ECMO is indicated when conventional management fails and mortality risk is high. In respiratory failure, the mortality risk is estimated by measuring the extent of pulmonary dysfunction and the level of ventilator support required to sustain gas exchange. In the neonate, the underlying pathophysiology is pulmonary arterial vasospasm, causing pulmonary hypertension and right-to-left shunting through the ductus arteriosus or foramen ovale (persistent fetal circulation syndrome, or PFC). This is true regardless of the primary diagnosis. Because of this pathophysiologic syndrome, the degree of vasospasm and right-to-left shunting is reflected in postductal hypoxia despite high Fio_2. In most neonatal centers, PFC is treated by hyperventilation to induce alkalosis and relax the vasospasm. Induced hyperventilation causes increased airway pressure so that Fio_2 and airway pressure are indirect measures of the degree of pulmonary dysfunction. These factors have been combined into measurements for estimating the severity of pulmonary dysfunction in the alveolar-arterial oxygen gradient ($AaDo_2$) or the oxygenation index (OI). The normal $AaDo_2$ is approximately 50 torr. When the $AaDo_2$ is consistently higher than 600 to 620, the mortality risk is 80 to 90 per cent. The OI is calculated as mean airway pressure $\times$ Fio_2 $\times$ 100/postductal Pao_2. An oxygenation index consistently greater than 40 is generally associated with 80 per cent or greater mortality risk. The usefulness of these measurements in any neonatal center is dependent upon the method and philosophy of ventilatory management, and each center must determine the mortality risk in that center, using $AaDO_2$, OI, or some other objective measurement.

Contraindications to ECMO in newborn infants are prematurity (less than 35 weeks' gestational age), pre-existing intracranial bleeding or other major neurologic injury, and mechanical ventilation longer than 10 days. Prematurity is associated with a high rate of intracranial bleeding.[7] Prior intracranial bleeding or neurologic injury may be made worse during ECMO. The incidence of severe bronchopulmonary dysplasia is high in children who have been ventilated with high pressures for a few days and is prohibitively high in infants who have been ventilated more than 10 days.

Failure of standard therapy and high mortality risk in adult patients with respiratory failure are identified by right-to-left shunting and poor compliance. The criteria for randomization in the NIH ECMO study identified a group of patients with 90 per cent mortality risk, and these physiologic milestones are used for selecting adult patients in most centers. These criteria are transpulmonary shunt consistently greater than 30 per cent despite optimal therapy, and static compliance consistently less than 30 ml. per cm. H_2O pressure. There are no epidemiologic studies to define high mortality risk criteria in children. Most centers that are employing ECMO for pediatric respiratory failure use the adult criteria defined previously.

Contraindications to ECMO in older children and adults include major brain injury, conditions incompatible with a favorable long-term prognosis, and active bleeding. Relative contraindications are systemic sepsis and failure of three or more organ systems (because of uniformly poor results), mechanical ventilation greater than 1 week (because of the high rate of irreversible pulmonary fibrosis), and immunosuppression (because of the high rate of bacterial infection).

THE PHYSIOLOGY OF EXTRACORPOREAL LIFE SUPPORT

ECMO is usually conducted as partial venoarterial bypass, taking 50 to 80 per cent of the venous return into the drainage catheter. The amount of venous drainage is determined by the amount of support required; the extracorporeal flow rate is regulated to the minimal level that supports gas exchange and perfusion. Extracorporeal flow is balanced against normal flow through the right ventricle and pulmonary artery. If the lung is not functioning at all, 80 per cent or more of the venous return must be diverted through the extracorporeal circuit. As lung function improves, the amount of extracorporeal flow can be decreased. The amount of oxygen that can be supplied through the extracorporeal circuit is a function of the flow, hemoglobin concentration, and saturation of the venous blood.

Obviously, the membrane lung can do no more than fully saturate the flowing blood; therefore the amount of oxygen that can be added per minute can be calculated as the difference in oxygen content from the inlet to the outlet of the membrane lung times the blood flow. For example, if the hemoglobin concentration is 15 gm. per 100 ml. and the venous blood is 75 per cent saturated with oxygen, the venous (oxygenator inlet) oxygen content is 15.5 ml. O_2 per 100 ml., and the arterial (oxygenator outlet) oxygen content is 21.5 ml. O_2 per 100 ml. The amount of oxygen that can be delivered to the patient is 6 ml. O_2 per 100 ml. of flow. The oxygen requirement for a 3-kg. newborn at rest is 15 ml. per minute, which would require 250 ml. per minute of blood flow. Oxygen delivery could be increased by increasing blood flow, or by increasing hemoglobin concentration, or by decreasing venous saturation. If, for example, oxygen consumption increased to 20 ml. per minute because of muscular activity or catecholamine effect, venous saturation would fall to approximately 50 per cent, and the arteriovenous oxygen content difference ($AVDo_2$) would increase to 11 ml. O_2 per 100 ml. Oxygen delivery could be increased by increasing blood flow or increasing hemoglobin. Oxygen consumption could be decreased by paralyzing or cooling the patient.

Although oxygen uptake is limited by the amount of unsaturated hemoglobin, CO_2 elimination is limited only by the gradient between the venous blood Pco_2 and the ventilating gas. CO_2 elimination is always more efficient than oxygenation during extracorporeal circulation. Because this gradient is relatively constant at about 45 torr, the amount of CO_2 elimination is essentially a function of the membrane lung surface area. Therefore, ECMO with the major intent of removing CO_2 can be conducted at relatively low blood flow with the use of a very large membrane lung surface area. This technique has been very successful in adult patients who retain most of their ability to oxygenate blood via the native lung.[9,13] However, in newborn infants the lung usually experiences a stage of no gas exchange; therefore, both CO_2 and oxygen requirements must be supplied.

With venoarterial bypass, systemic perfusion is controlled in addition to gas exchange. The arterial pulse contour and pulse pressure are minimal; but as long as the flow is adequate, this has no major physiologic side effect. When cardiac function is normal, it is possible to conduct ECMO in the venovenous mode. In this manner, the arterialized blood is returned to the venous circulation, rather than to the aorta, achieving prepulmonary gas exchange and leaving the patient totally dependent on his own cardiovascular system for systemic oxygen delivery. It is relatively simple to achieve total CO_2 elimination during venovenous bypass for the reasons discussed above. However, the ability to deliver oxygen is limited because the right atrial venous blood oxygen saturation is high, limiting the extracorporeal oxygen uptake capability. In venovenous ECMO, the native lung is relied upon to provide a significant portion of the systemic oxygen requirement. However, even if there is no oxygen uptake across the native lung, the total oxy-

gen requirement can be supplied during venovenous ECMO by using higher extracorporeal flow and accepting the fact that the patient's arterial saturation is between 80 and 90 per cent. For example, if the venous drainage saturation is 90 per cent and the hemoglobin is 15 gm. per 100 ml., the $AVDo_2$ is 3.3 ml. O_2 per 100 ml., and venovenous flow of 450 ml. per minute supplies 15 ml. O_2 per minute. Venovenous circulation can be achieved by continuous flow, through two separate catheters; continuous flow, through a single double-lumen catheter; or intermittent tidal flow, through a single catheter. The disadvantage of venovenous circulation is the requirement for higher extracorporeal blood flow rate, and the advantage is simplicity of vascular access.

THE FUTURE OF EXTRACORPOREAL LIFE SUPPORT

In 1990, ECMO is the treatment of choice for infants with severe respiratory failure who fail to respond to conventional management. It is a reasonable alternative when other therapy fails in children and adults. In the next decade, conventional management will undoubtedly improve, causing less lung injury and less mortality and decreasing the need for a radical approach such as extracorporeal life support. Simultaneously, however, ECMO will become safer and simpler, so that management of the critically ill newborn infant will probably include both mechanical ventilation and extracorporeal support. ECMO will be simplified by the use of single-catheter venovenous access and perhaps arteriovenous access via the umbilical vessels in some infants. A major complication of ECMO is bleeding, which is in part related to heparinization. The use of heparin-coated circuits has been demonstrated to be effective in the laboratory.[16,19] It is anticipated that neonatal ECMO with minimal systemic heparinization will decrease the risk of bleeding and expand the indications for use of ECMO.

Aside from these applications in respiratory failure, venoarterial ECMO will be commonly used to support systemic perfusion. As outlined in this discussion, this application is used primarily for children with postoperative cardiac failure but is also being used to support the circulation in patients with sudden left ventricular failure induced in the cardiac catheterization laboratory during attempted angioplasty or arteriography. In the next decade, this application will be extended to emergency room and intensive care unit resuscitation of patients in cardiac failure when the intra-aortic balloon pump is inadequate. In addition, the technique will be used for rewarming patients with systemic hypothermia and supporting patients with myocardial disease through difficult operations. The availability of ECMO without systemic heparinization will greatly expand the potential indications into areas such as trauma, intraoperative and postoperative support, and management of exsanguinating hemorrhage.

SUMMARY AND CONCLUSIONS

Extracorporeal life support has become standard treatment for term and near term newborn infants with severe respiratory failure that is unresponsive to conventional ventilator and pharmacologic management. Pulmonary hypertension with right-to-left shunting is the underlying pathophysiology in these infants, regardless of the primary diagnosis. With the lung rest provided by extracorporeal support, pulmonary hypertension resolves in 3 or 4 days and lung recovery occurs in almost all of these infants. The survival rate for 3094 cases in the Neonatal ECMO Registry was 82.6 per cent. The lesson learned from neonatal experience is that avoiding high-pressure, high-oxygen, mechanical ventilation by means of extracorporeal life support results in recovery of the lung and patient survival.

In severe respiratory failure in children and adults, the use of

ECMO enables survival in approximately 40 per cent. The pathophysiology of lung injury causes tissue necrosis and fibrosis leading to irreversible progressive pulmonary injury in many patients. The use of ECMO earlier in the course of disease decreases whatever component of progressive lung injury is related to high-pressure, high-oxygen mechanical ventilation. The use of heparin-coated circuits to eliminate systemic anticoagulation and simple access catheters will expand the applications of all types of extracorporeal life support during the next decade.

SELECTED REFERENCES

Gille, J. P. (Ed.): Neonatal and Adult Respiratory Failure. Paris, Elsevier, 1989.
This is the report of a symposium summarizing the activities of an extensive study of respiratory failure conducted in Europe and known as the Euroxy Program. It includes excellent contributions on adult and neonatal ECMO, other methods of respiratory support, and the pathophysiology and epidemiology of acute respiratory failure. Because it is the most recent and most inclusive publication, it is the best single source of information on extracorporeal support.

Reinhart, K., and Eyrich, K. (Eds.): Clinical Aspects of Oxygen Transport and Tissue Oxygenation. Berlin, Springer-Verlag, 1989.
This book includes the proceedings of a symposium on oxygen transport convened by the Steglitz University Clinic in 1989. It includes several excellent contributions summarizing the basic science background of extracorporeal support.

Bartlett, R. H., and Gazzaniga, A. B.: Extracorporeal circulation for cardiopulmonary failure. Curr. Probl. Surg., 15 (5), 1978.
This monograph is a good source of information on the bioengineering of extracorporeal circuits, the physiology and pathophysiology of extracorporeal circulation, and the development of prolonged extracorporeal support. An updated version will be published in 1991.

Toomasian, J. M., Snedecor, S. M., Cornell, R. G., et al.: National experience with extracorporeal membrane oxygenation (ECMO) for newborn respiratory failure: Data from 715 cases. Trans. ASAIO, 34:140, 1988.
This is the first formal report of the National ECMO Registry. It includes information on almost all the newborn patients treated with ECMO. The overall survival rate was 82 per cent. Results related to diagnoses, mechanical complications, physiologic complications, and the institutional learning curve are documented in this paper.

Bartlett, R. H., Roloff, D. W., Cornell, R. G., Andrews, A. F., Dillon, P. W., Zwischenberger, J. B.: Extracorporeal circulation in neonatal respiratory failure: A prospective randomized study. Pediatrics, 4:479, 1985.

O'Rourke, P. P., Krone, R., Vancanti, J., et al.: Extracorporeal membrane oxygenation and conventional medical therapy in neonates with persistent pulmonary hypertension of the newborn: A prospective randomized study. Pediatrics, 84:957, 1989.
Both of these papers report the results of prospective randomized controlled studies of ECMO in newborn respiratory failure. Both showed that the results with ECMO were much better than those with conventional treatment. Both studies used an adaptive design, and the statistical methodology is as interesting as the clinical studies.

Heiss, K., Manning, P. B., Oldham, K. T., Coran, A. G., Polley, T. Z., Wesley, J. R., Bartlett, R. H.: Reversal of mortality for congenital diaphragmatic hernia with ECMO. Ann. Surg, 209:225, 1989.
This study documents the full experience with newborn congenital diaphragmatic hernia at the University of Michigan and demonstrates that the use of ECMO in this condition has changed the natural history of the condition from 50 per cent to 76 per cent survival.

Taylor, G. A., Glass, P., Fitz, C. R., Miller, M. K.: Neurologic status of infants treated with extracorporeal membrane oxygenation: Correlation of imaging findings with developmental outcome. Radiology, 165;679, 1987.
This study from Children's Hospital National Medical Center in Washington, D. C. summarizes long-term follow-up studies for neonatal ECMO reported in the literature and reports results on 46 infants treated in that center. The correlation of neurologic imaging studies with neurologic outcome is a very important aspect of this paper. The incidence of abnormal neurologic function is approximately 20 per cent and is associated with brain injury from perinatal asphyxia and intracranial bleeding, often in unusual places.

REFERENCES

1. Bartlett, R. H., Fong, S. W., Burns, N. E., Gazzaniga, A. B.: Prolonged partial venoarterial bypass: Physiologic, biochemical and hematologic responses. Surg. Forum, 23:173, 1974.
2. Barlett, R. H., Gazzaniga, A. B., Huxtable, R. F., Schippers, H. C., O'Connor, M. J., Jefferies, M. R.: Extracorporeal circulation (ECMO) in neonatal respiratory failure. J. Thorac. Cardiovasc. Surg., 74:826, 1977.
3. Bartlett, R. H., Gazzaniga, A. B., Jefferies, M. R., et al.: Extracorporeal membrane oxygenation (ECMO) cardiopulmonary support in infancy. Trans. ASAIO, 22:80, 1976.
4. Bartlett, R. H., Gazzaniga, A. B., Toomasian, J. M., et al.: Extracorporeal membrane oxygenation (ECMO) in neonatal respiratory failure: 100 cases. Ann. Surg., 204:236, 1986.
5. Bartlett, R. H., Isherwood, J., Moss, R. A., Olszewski, W. L., Polet, H., Drinker, P. A.: A toroidal flow membrane oxygenator: Four day partial bypass in dogs. Surg. Forum, 20:152, 1969.
6. Bartlett, R. H., Roloff, D. W., Cornell, R. G., Andrews, A. F., Dillon, P. W., Zwischenberger, J. B.: Extracorporeal circulation in neonatal respiratory failure: A prospective randomized study. Pediatrics, 4:479, 1985.
7. Cilley, R. E., Zwischenberger, J. B., Andrews, A. F.: Intracranial hemorrhage during extracorporeal membrane oxygenation in neonates. Pediatrics, 78:699, 1986.
8. Dorson, W., Jr., Baker, E., Cohen, M. L., et al.: A perfusion system for infants. Trans. ASAIO, 15:155, 1969.
9. Gattinoni, L., Pesenti, A., Mascheroni, D., et al.: Low frequency positive pressure ventilation with extracorporeal CO_2 removal in severe acute respiratory failure. JAMA, 256:881, 1986.
10. Gille, J. P., Bagniewski, A. M.: Ten years of use of extracorporeal membrane oxygenation (ECMO) in treatment of acute respiratory insufficiency. Trans. ASAIO, 22:102, 1976.
11. Heiss, K., Manning, P. B., Oldham, K. T., Coran, A. G., Polley, T. Z., Wesley, J. R., Bartlett, R. H.: Reversal of mortality for congenital diaphragmatic hernia with ECMO. Ann. Surg., 209:225, 1989.
12. Hill, D., O'Brien, T. G., Murray, J. J., et al.: Extracorporeal oxygenation for acute post-traumatic respiratory failure (shock-lung syndrome): Use of the Bramson membrane lung. N. Engl. J. Med., 286:629, 1972.
13. Knoch, M.: Treatment of severe ARDS with extracorporeal CO_2 removal. In Gille, J. P. (Ed.): Neonatal and Adult Respiratory Failure. Paris, Elsevier, 1989, p. 123.
14. Kolobow, T., and Bowman, R. L.: Construction and evaluation of an alveolar membrane artificial heart-lung. Trans. ASAIO, 9:238, 1963.
15. Kolobow, T., Zapol, W., Sigman, R. L., et al.: Partial cardiopulmonary bypass lasting up to seven days in adult lambs with membrane lung blood oxygenation. J. Thorac. Cardiovasc. Surg., 60:781, 1970.
16. Mottaghy, K., Oedekoven, B., Schaich-Lester, D., and Poppel, K.: Non-heparin and heparin bonded systems for $ECCO_2R$: An experimental study. In Gille, J. P. (Ed.): Neonatal and adult respiratory failure. Paris, Elsevier, 1989, p. 209.
17. National Neonatal ECMO Registry, Ann Arbor, Michigan, October 1989.
18. O'Rourke, P. P., Krone, R., Vacanti, J., et al.: Extracorporeal membrane oxygenation and conventional medical therapy in neonates with persistent pulmonary hypertension of the newborn: A prospective randomized study. Pediatrics, 84:957, 1989.
19. Toomasian, J. M., Hsu, L. C., Hirschl, R. B., Heiss, K. F., Hultquist, K. A., Bartlett, R. H.: Evaluation of Duraflo II heparin coating in prolonged extracorporeal membrane oxygenation. Trans. ASAIO, 34:410, 1988.
20. Toomasian, J. M., Snedecor, S. M., Cornell, R. G., et al.: National experience with extracorporeal membrane oxygenation (ECMO) for newborn respiratory failure: Data from 715 cases. Trans. ASAIO, 34:140, 1988.
21. Towne, B. H., Lott, I. T., et al.: Long-term follow-up of infants and children treated with extracorporeal membrane oxygenation (ECMO): A preliminary report. J. Pediatr. Surg., 20:410, 1985.
22. Zapol, W. M., Snider, M. T., Hill, J. D., et al.: Extracorporeal membrane oxygenation in severe acute respiratory failure: A randomized prospective study. JAMA, 242:2193, 1979.

54

THE MEDIASTINUM

R. Duane Davis, Jr., M.D., and David C. Sabiston, Jr., M.D.

The mediastinum is an important and complex anatomic division of the thorax extending from the diaphragm to the thoracic inlet and is the site of many localized disorders as well as a number of systemic diseases. Localized disorders occurring in this region include infection, hemorrhage, emphysema, aneurysms, and many primary tumors and cysts. Systemic diseases include metastatic neoplasms, granulomas, and other general inflammatory disorders. Lesions that originate in the esophagus, great vessels, trachea, and heart may present as a mediastinal mass or may cause symptoms related to compression or invasion of adjacent mediastinal structures. Although these lesions are discussed in the sections covering the specific organ system of origin, they are relevant in the differential diagnosis of the various primary mediastinal disease processes. Mediastinal disorders present in a myriad of different clinical settings. Symptoms may be related to local involvement of adjacent structures, tumor secretory factors, or immunologic factors. In addition, many patients are asymptomatic and the disorder is identified on routine chest films. Technological advances in imaging including computed tomography (CT), magnetic resonance imaging (MRI), and various radioisotopic scans have enhanced the ability to assess the anatomic extent of disease. Combined with these imaging modalities, improvements in cytologic techniques, greater application of electron microscopy, and the monoclonal antibody revolution that has markedly improved immunohistochemical techniques and radioimmunoassays have made possible a more specific identification of the mediastinal disorder. Moreover, continued advances in anesthesia, surgical technique, perioperative patient management, chemotherapy, immunotherapy, and radiotherapy have reduced patient morbidity and increased survival and quality of life.

Historical Aspects

Prior to the introduction of endotracheal anesthesia and techniques for closed pleural drainage, few endeavors were made to intervene surgically in the mediastinum owing to the hazards inherent to entering the pleural cavity, particularly pneumothorax and subsequent respiratory insufficiency. The initial procedures involved processes in the anterior mediastinum that could be exposed through various sternal approaches. In 1893 Bastianelli excised a dermoid cyst from the anterior mediastinum after resecting the manubrium.[4] In 1897 Milton reported the removal of two caseous tuberculous lymph nodes from the anterior mediastinum.[37] He used a sternal splitting approach, which he developed after initially working on cadavers and subsequently goats, finding that it provided excellent exposure to the anterior mediastinum without entering the pleural cavities. Because of the involvement of the sternum by the disease process, Milton initially left the wound open, successfully utilizing a delayed primary closure on the second postoperative day.

With the introduction of endotracheal anesthesia, the safe performance of transpleural operations was possible. Harrington in 1929 and Heuer and Andrus in 1940 reported the first

series of patients documenting the safety and efficacy of the transpleural approach to a variety of mediastinal diseases.[23,24] In 1939, Blalock reported the excision of the thymus in a young woman with myasthenia gravis.[7] Subsequently, the patient had marked amelioration in symptoms. This success initiated the surgical treatment of myasthenia gravis. In the 1950s and 1960s, Kaplan and associates at Stanford introduced megavoltage radiation therapy and pioneered the treatment of Hodgkin's disease and a variety of other malignancies with this modality. Numerous groups have made significant contributions in the treatment of a large number of malignant diseases with chemotherapeutic agents with significant improvements in survival and cure, particularly in the treatment of the lymphomas and germ cell tumors.

Anatomy and Embryology

The mediastinum has the following anatomic borders: the thoracic inlet superiorly, the diaphragm inferiorly, the sternum anteriorly, the vertebral column posteriorly, and the parietal pleura laterally. Because many mediastinal tumors and cysts occur in characteristic locations, the mediastinum has been subdivided for the convenience of localizing specific types of lesions. The classic division of the mediastinum into four subdivisions, superior, anterior, middle, and posterior, utilizes a transverse plane from the sternal angle to the fourth intercostal space to divide the superior subdivision from the other inferior subdivisions. The inferior subdivisions are defined by their relationship to the pericardial sac. The anterior mediastinum is anterior to the pericardial sac; the middle mediastinum is contained within the pericardial sac; the posterior mediastinum is posterior to the pericardial sac.

However, many anterior mediastinal tumors also frequently occupy the anterior aspect of the superior mediastinum, and, similarly, many posterior mediastinal masses occupy the posterior aspect of the superior mediastinum. Therefore, a more frequently used and more helpful division of the mediastinum into three subdivisions, the anterosuperior, middle, and posterior, has been made (Fig. 1). The anterosuperior mediastinum is anterior to the pericardium and the pericardial reflection over the great vessels. The posterior mediastinum is posterior to the pericardium and the pericardial reflection. The middle mediastinum remains the same.

The contents of the anterosuperior mediastinum include the thymus gland, the aortic arch and its branches, the great veins, lymphatics, and fatty areolar tissue. The middle mediastinal contents include the heart, pericardium, phrenic nerves, tracheal bifurcation and main bronchi, the hila of each lung, and lymph nodes. The posterior mediastinum contains the esophagus, vagus nerves, sympathetic nervous chain, thoracic duct, descending aorta, azygous and hemiazygous systems, paravertebral lymphatics, and fatty areolar tissue (Fig. 2).

Development of mediastinal structures begins as early as the 5- to 6-mm. embryo stage. The pericardial cavity originates from the coalescence of mesenchymal spaces in the coelomic cavities on each side of the embryo. The pleural cavities develop

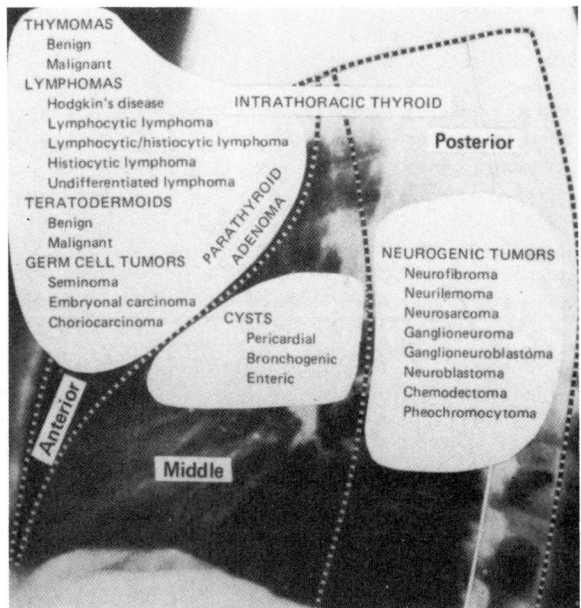

Figure 1. Lateral chest film divided into three anatomic subdivisions with the tumors and cysts that occur most frequently in each region. (From Davis, R. D., Jr., and Sabiston, D. C., Jr.: Primary mediastinal cysts and neoplasms. *In* Sabiston, D. C., Jr. (Ed.): Essentials of Surgery. Philadelphia, W. B. Saunders Company, 1987.)

into the epithelial lining of the esophagus. The cartilage, smooth muscle, and elastic tissue of the tracheobronchial tree and the fibromuscular tissue of the esophagus arise from mesenchymal tissue surrounding the foregut.

The thymus originates from the ventral aspect of the third branchial pouch; the dorsal aspect of the third branchial pouch gives rise to the inferior parathyroid glands. The thymus separates from the pharynx and migrates into the anterosuperior mediastinum; the inferior parathyroid glands usually remain attached to the thyroid gland. However, the common embryologic origin explains the frequent finding of the inferior parathyroid glands within the mediastinum closely associated with the thymus. Sympathetic ganglia, paraganglia, intercostal nerves, and the neurilemmal sheath cell have a neural crest origin.

MEDIASTINAL EMPHYSEMA

Air within the mediastinum produces mediastinal emphysema or pneumomediastinum. The source of the air may be from the esophagus, trachea, bronchi, neck, or abdomen. Common causes of pneumomediastinum include penetrating wounds and perforations of these structures, blunt trauma that causes fractured ribs or vertebrae, and barotrauma caused by either blunt trauma or positive-pressure ventilation. Blunt trauma due to compressive forces on the thorax, especially when the glottis is closed and ventilation occurs with high pressures, usually in the setting of decreased lung compliance, may cause sufficient pressures at the intra-alveolar region to rupture alveoli. Dissection through the visceral pleura causes a pneumothorax. However, dissection of the air along vascular structures into the hilum and mediastinum creates pneumomediastinum. Mediastinal emphysema may also be caused by intra-abdominal air dissecting through the diaphragmatic hiatus.

from the dorsal parietal recesses. Separation of the body cavity into the thorax and peritoneal cavities occurs with the development of the diaphragm from the septum transversum and the paired pleuroperitoneal membranes. During this period the primitive foregut differentiates into the respiratory and upper digestive tracts. The ventral foregut develops into the epithelial lining of the larynx and tracheobronchial tree as well as the alveolar respiratory epithelium. The dorsal foregut develops

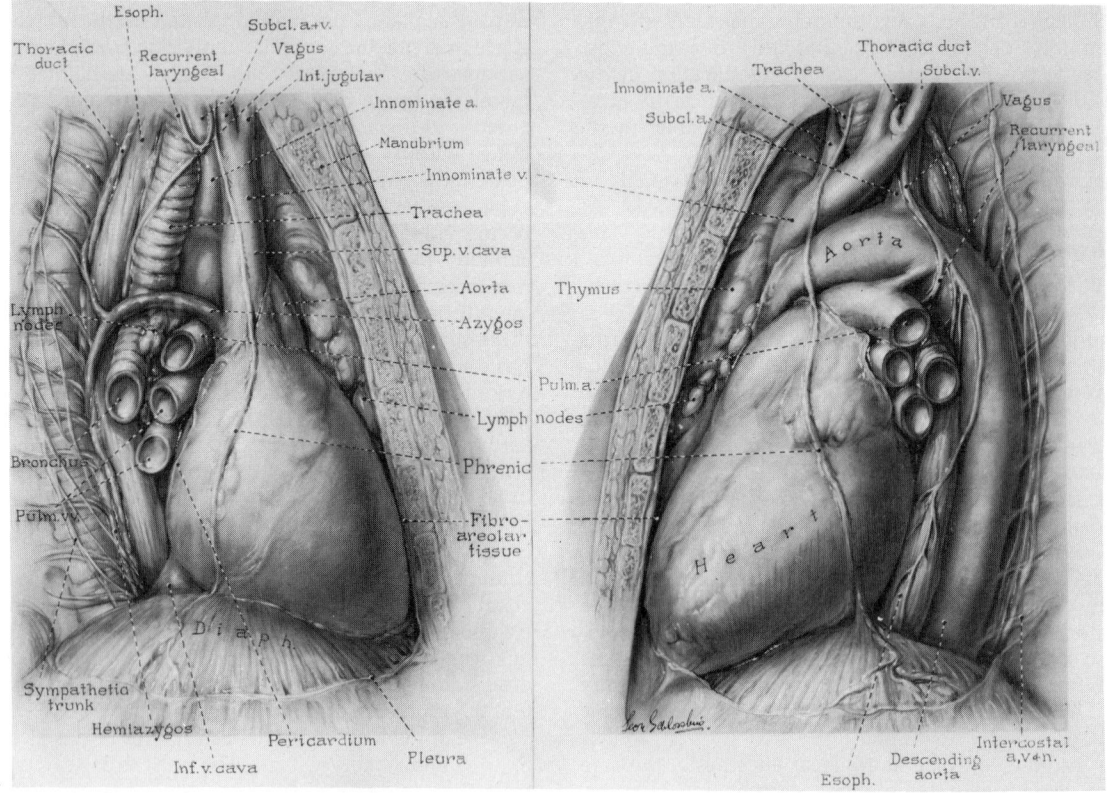

Figure 2. The anatomic structures of the mediastinum as seen from the right side *(A)* and from the left side *(B)*. (From Sabiston, D. C., Jr.: The esophagus and mediastinum. *In* Cooke, R. E., and Levin, S. (Eds.): The Biologic Basis of Pediatric Practice. New York, McGraw-Hill, 1968.)

Spontaneous pneumomediastinum is usually observed in patients with exacerbation of bronchospastic disease. In a similar manner to that caused by barotrauma, the pathophysiologic mechanism of spontaneous pneumomediastinum is thought to involve the rupture of a bleb within the pulmonary parenchyma creating interstitial emphysema. The air then dissects along vascular or bronchial planes into the mediastinum.

The clinical manifestations of this disorder were described initially by Hamman in 1939 and include substernal chest pain that may radiate into the back and crepitation in the region of the suprasternal notch, chest wall, and neck.[22] With increasing pressure, the air can dissect into the neck, face, chest, arms, abdomen, and retroperitoneum. Frequently, pneumomediastinum and pneumothorax occur simultaneously. The physical examination finding on auscultation of a characteristic crunching sound heard over the pericardium that is accentuated during systole is termed Hamman's sign. He stated that the crunching sound was similar to that made by walking on crusty snow. Only rarely does sufficient pressure develop to cause compression of venous structures so as to impair venous return. With impairment of venous return, clinical manifestations similar to the superior vena caval syndrome occur including cyanosis, prominence of neck and upper extremity veins, dyspnea, and, in severe cases, circulatory failure.

The diagnosis of pneumomediastinum is confirmed by the presence of air in the mediastinum. Air is usually also present in the pectoral muscles, neck, and upper extremities as visualized on the chest films. Treatment is directed toward correcting the cause when possible. In the majority, the spontaneous form resolves without sequelae. However, careful observation is required to recognize early the development of circulatory compromise. Supportive therapy with oxygen and analgesics is helpful. Surgical decompression is only rarely necessary. In patients with pneumomediastinum and pneumothorax, tube thoracostomy is indicated in the affected pleural space. Patients with pneumomediastinum secondary to barotrauma continuing to require high levels of pressure support may require bilateral tube thoracostomies as prophylaxis against development of tension pneumothorax.

MEDIASTINITIS

Infection of the mediastinal space is a serious and potentially fatal process. Etiologic factors responsible for the development of acute mediastinitis include perforation of the esophagus due to instrumentation, foreign bodies, penetrating or, more rarely, blunt trauma, spontaneous esophageal disruption (Boerhaave's syndrome), leakage from an esophageal anastomosis, tracheobronchial perforation, and mediastinal extension from an infectious process originating in the pulmonary parenchyma, pleura, chest wall, vertebrae, great vessels, or neck. The most frequent situation in which mediastinitis arises is following median sternotomy owing to the common use of this approach for cardiac operations as well as for exploration of the anterior mediastinum or thorax. Wound infections occur in approximately 2 per cent of patients following median sternotomy for cardiac operations; in half (1 per cent) of these patients the infection involves the mediastinum. Risk factors for the development of mediastinitis include prolonged operation, lengthy cardiopulmonary bypass, re-exploration for postoperative bleeding, dehiscence, external cardiac massage, postoperative cardiogenic shock, and the use of bilateral internal mammary arteries for coronary artery bypass grafting, especially in elderly patients or in patients with diabetes mellitus.

Mediastinitis is manifested clinically by fever, tachycardia, leukocytosis, and pain that may be localized to the chest, back, or neck, although in some patients the clinical course remains indolent for long periods. When mediastinitis is secondary to esophageal perforation following instrumentation, the pain is most frequently localized to the neck because the most common site of perforation is at the level of the cricopharyngeal muscle. In these cases, subcutaneous emphysema is almost invariably present.

Due to the added morbidity and mortality associated with delayed diagnosis, a high index of suspicion is paramount in establishing the diagnosis of mediastinitis. The lateral chest film is useful in evaluating air-fluid levels, abnormal soft tissue densities, and sternal dehiscence. In evaluating postoperative patients questionable for mediastinal infection, CT imaging can be useful. CT reliably distinguishes diffuse mediastinitis from a localized abscess. In addition, CT identifies an associated empyema or contiguous abscess (e.g., subphrenic abscess) and often reliably establishes whether continuity or communication exists between the mediastinal infection and the associated infection. CT, however, cannot differentiate mediastinitis from benign postoperative changes in the absence of mediastinal gas.[8] CT may also be useful in differentiating superficial soft tissue infections, which improve after wound opening and local wound care, from retrosternal infections that require aggressive intervention. Water-soluble contrast studies of the esophagus and esophagoscopy are important in evaluating a potential esophageal perforation or disruption. In patients with penetrating or blunt trauma, the use of both procedures has been necessary to minimize the number of overlooked esophageal injuries. Similarly, bronchoscopy is the optimal procedure to evaluate potential tracheobronchial disruption.

Treatment of mediastinitis requires correction of the inciting cause and aggressive supportive therapy. After obtaining cultures, appropriate antimicrobial coverage should be initiated with modification after culture reports and sensitivities are available. In patients with mediastinal infections in continuity or in communication with empyema, subphrenic abscess, or neck abscess, drainage of the empyema with tube thoracostomy or percutaneous drainage of the abscess in conjunction with appropriate antimicrobial therapy is frequently successful. Similarly, mediastinitis associated with catheter sepsis can often be treated with removal of the catheter and antimicrobial therapy. However, in patients with mediastinitis secondary to most other causes, thorough débridement of necrotic and infected tissue is necessary in conjunction with surgical drainage. When costal cartilage is infected, it is necessary to excise the cartilage until bleeding bone is present. Delay in making the diagnosis and subsequently initiating therapy, especially when the etiologic factor involves esophageal or tracheobronchial disruption, is associated with sharp increases in morbidity and mortality.

Postoperative mediastinitis following median sternotomy has been successfully treated with a number of different techniques. The simplest approach involves incision, débridement and drainage of the involved area in conjunction with local irrigation with antibiotics or antiseptic agents, and wound care using dressings soaked in dilute povidone-iodine, Dakin's solution, or acetic acid. Delayed closure is possible, however, although an unstable sternum is the usual result.

Improved results have been obtained after thoroughly débriding all affected tissue by using closed irrigation systems. Depending on the severity of the infection, the wound can be either closed or left open after the placement of large-bore drainage tubes through which continuous irrigation with antibiotic solution or diluted povidone-iodine is done (approximately 3 liters per day for 7 to 14 days). The tubes are removed gradually to minimize residual dead space.

The best results have been obtained using a variety of tissue flaps to obliterate dead space and to provide immediate coverage of the heart, bypass grafts, and great vessels following effective surgical control of the wound. This is generally the current preferred management, especially in cardiac cases. Débridement of infected and necrotic sternum, cartilage, and soft tissue in conjunction with wound care is often necessary to provide a clean wound to optimize results. This therapy has further reduced morbidity and mortality, usually produces a good long-term functional result, and has significantly reduced the duration of hospitalization. The pectoralis major and rectus abdominis muscles have been the most commonly used tissue flaps. Because the rectus abdominis flap is based on the superior epigastric artery, this flap is useful only when the internal mammary artery remains patent. In situations in which both internal mammary arteries have been used for bypass conduits or have been sacrificed during débridement, the omentum has been used successfully. Because the omentum is capable of enhancing neovascularization, relieving lymphedema, providing fibroblasts, and providing soft tissue coverage while allowing sternal closure, it is the tissue flap of choice in some centers.

Although chronic mediastinitis may be due to a chronic bacterial infection, more frequently chronic infections are granulomatous processes that follow tuberculosis or mycotic infections. Active infection requires treatment with antituberculosis or antifungal agents. With progressive cases of chronic infection, the granulomatous process within the mediastinal lymph nodes may compress adjacent structures, such as the venae cavae, trachea, bronchi, or esophagus. Of the mycotic infections, histoplasmosis has the greatest predilection for severe involvement of the mediastinal lymph nodes. Rarely, surgical decompression, excision, or bypass is necessary in addition to medical therapy to treat the resultant obstruction.

HEMORRHAGE

Mediastinal hemorrhage is most frequently caused by blunt or penetrating trauma, thoracic aortic dissection, rupture of aortic aneurysm, or surgical procedures within the thorax. Penetrating trauma to the thorax or cervical region may cause lacerations of major veins or arteries whereas blunt trauma may cause transection of the aorta or other great vessels. The usual site of aortic transection is immediately distal to the origin of the left subclavian artery, the second most common site occurring prior to the origin of the innominate artery, whereas the third most common site is distal to the aortic valve anulus. Most mediastinal hemorrhage associated with blunt trauma is due to rupture of small mediastinal veins; however, the possibility of aortic injury should be evaluated with arch aortography when mediastinal widening is present.

Significant hemorrhage may follow thoracic operations, particularly procedures involving the heart and great vessels that require cardiopulmonary bypass. Routine use of large-bore chest tubes for drainage usually prevents the development of mediastinal tamponade. Other iatrogenic causes of mediastinal hemorrhage include laceration of great vessels during angiography, placement of central venous or arterial catheters, erosion of indwelling vascular devices, and erosion of tracheostomy tubes into the great vessels.

Spontaneous mediastinal hemorrhage is a recognized entity with predisposing factors related to the following: (1) complication of a mediastinal mass of which thymoma, malignant germ cell tumor, parathyroid adenoma, retrosternal thyroid, and teratoma are the most common; (2) sudden sustained hypertension; (3) altered hemostasis due to anticoagulant therapy, thrombolytic therapy, uremia, hepatic insufficiency, or hemophilia; and (4) transient, sharp increases in intrathoracic pressure, which occur during coughing or vomiting, an entity initially described by Epstein in 1959.[17] The pathophysiologic mechanism of this disorder is thought to be associated with rupture of small mediastinal vessels. Usually, the clinical course is benign with resolution of symptoms without long-term sequelae.

The clinical presentation varies with the underlying etiologic factor. Retrosternal pain radiating to the back or neck is common. With increased accumulation of blood in the mediastinum, signs and symptoms related to compression of mediastinal structures, primarily the great veins, develop including dyspnea, venous distention, cyanosis, and cervical ecchymosis due to blood dissecting into soft tissue planes. Sufficient accumulation of blood causes mediastinal tamponade manifested by tachycardia, hypotension, reduced urinary output, equalization of right- and left-sided cardiac filling pressures, and diastolic collapse of the right ventricle. The development of mediastinal tamponade is more insidious than pericardial tamponade because of the larger volume of the mediastinum. However, because of the markedly poorer prognosis following the development of tamponade, the goal is diagnosis of mediastinal hemorrhage prior to the stage of circulatory compromise. Diagnostic measures include chest films that may indicate superior mediastinal widening, loss of the normal aortic contour, and soft tissue density in the anterosuperior mediastinum, echocardiography, and CT scanning, which may better characterize a mass as containing blood or clot and its relationship to vascular structures, particularly if a false lumen is present. Arteriography may be useful in localizing the site of bleeding or intimal disruption. Therapy is directed toward evacuation of existing clot and repairing the underlying process. In postoperative patients following cardiac operations, catheter drainage using CT guidance has been successful without significant morbidity.[47]

SUPERIOR VENA CAVA OBSTRUCTION

A number of benign and malignant processes may cause obstruction of the superior vena cava, and the superior vena caval syndrome may follow. The pathophysiologic process of the syndrome involves the increased pressure in the venous system draining into the superior vena cava producing the characteristic features of the syndrome, which include edema of the head, neck, and upper extremities; distended neck veins with dilated collateral veins over the upper extremities and torso; cyanosis; headache; and confusion. These findings are initially noted and remain more prominent when the patient is in a recumbent position. However, they are usually present to some extent in an upright position. With processes that slowly cause obstruction, these features develop insidiously. However, with rapid or sudden occlusion, the clinical presentation is often striking with rapid development of cerebral edema and intracranial thrombosis, which may cause coma and death.

The pathologic cause of the superior vena caval obstruction varies from compression to invasion as well as thrombosis. The cause may be the primary tumor or mass, or often it may be due to paratracheal lymph node metastases. Most frequently the etiologic factor is a malignant neoplasm. Bronchogenic carcinoma, most frequently of the right upper lobe, is the most common cause. Malignant germ cell tumors and thymomas, lymphomas, and primary mediastinal carcinomas as well as metastatic lesions are the common malignant etiologic processes. Less than 25 per cent of patients with superior vena caval obstruction have a benign cause. A large number of benign processes have been implicated including mediastinal granulomatous diseases, particularly histoplasmosis and tuberculosis, idiopathic mediastinal fibrosis, mediastinal goiter, bronchogenic cyst, teratoma, pleural calcification, and thoracic aortic aneurysm. Superior vena caval obstruction secondary to indwelling catheters or trauma to the vessel when placing the catheter has become more common. However, rarely does the superior vena caval syndrome result.

This syndrome is infrequently seen in children. The most frequent occurrence is following cardiac surgery (71 per cent), particularly after Mustard and, less frequently, Senning repairs for transposition of the great vessels.[25,26] Other significant causes of childhood superior vena caval syndrome include mediastinal neoplasm (16 per cent) (the majority are non-Hodgkin's lymphomas), ventriculoatrial shunts (5 per cent), and mediastinal fibrosis (3 per cent).

Contrast-enhanced CT scanning or MRI usually is adequate

to establish the diagnosis of superior vena caval obstruction and to assist in the differential diagnosis of probable etiology. Although venous angiography is rarely required to establish the diagnosis, it provides more accurate anatomic detail regarding the site of obstruction and collateral development, which is necessary if surgical bypass is required.

Because the malignant processes responsible for the superior vena caval syndrome are usually not surgically resectable, the initial attempt to establish a histologic diagnosis is usually a percutaneous needle biopsy technique. Histologic diagnosis is attempted prior to the initiation of empiric therapy because of the alteration of the morphologic appearance following therapy. In 42 per cent of patients receiving pre-biopsy radiation in one series, a histologic diagnosis could not be established.[35] Open biopsy in patients able to tolerate anesthesia may be necessary to establish a diagnosis. However, these patients are at an increased risk for cardiorespiratory compromise during general anesthesia. Preoperative screening and intraoperative management are discussed in a later section.

The most useful types of therapy include radiation, corticosteroids, and multiagent chemotherapy. The optimal therapeutic regimen is dependent on the histologic diagnosis. In patients in whom the syndrome develops rapidly or when neurologic symptoms are present, therapy may be necessary on an emergency basis. Improved success in the treatment of a number of the malignant causes of the superior vena caval syndrome has evolved, particularly with the lymphomas and germ cell tumors. When treating obstruction secondary to bronchogenic carcinoma, at least transient decompression can usually be obtained.

Historically, surgical bypass of obstructing lesions was associated with poor patency and high morbidity and mortality. However, improved patency using spiral vein grafts without tumor resection for palliation has been reported.[15] In addition, patency rates of 92 per cent at 1 year following resection of tumor and superior vena cava with interposition grafting using polytetrafluoroethylene grafts have been reported.[13] Of particular importance for success is the presence of adequate flow through either of the innominate veins, and this can be augmented by the creation of an arteriovenous fistula near the site. In conditions in which long-standing superior vena caval obstruction has been present with collateral development, the innominate veins are usually thrombosed, making them unsuitable for revascularization. Survival beyond 3 years is possible following resection with vascular reconstruction.[75] Superior vena caval syndromes caused by benign disease usually respond to medical therapy, which consists of diuretics, upright positioning, and fluid restriction until collateral channels develop that cause clinical regression.

PRIMARY NEOPLASMS AND CYSTS

A large number of different histologic neoplasms and cysts arise from multiple anatomic sites in the mediastinum and present a myriad of clinical signs and symptoms. The natural history varies from those that are asymptomatic, to those with benign slow growth that cause minimal symptoms, to aggressive, invasive neoplasms that are often widely metastatic, rapidly causing death. The increased use of chest films and the improved sensitivity of imaging techniques have enabled the diagnosis of a mediastinal mass at an earlier stage of disease, frequently in asymptomatic individuals. The number of patients with mediastinal masses has increased. The ability to cure many of these patients by surgical excision, chemotherapy, or radiation therapy underscores the importance of establishing a precise histologic diagnosis so that optimal therapy can be initiated. Observation of a mediastinal mass, except in rare circumstances, can rarely be justified when operative morbidity is less than 10 per cent and mortality is less than 1 per cent.[14]

A classification of primary mediastinal tumors and cysts is shown in Table 1. The relative incidence of occurrence in a series of 2431 patients is shown in Table 2. Although some differences in the relative incidence of neoplasms and cyst exist in some series, the most common mediastinal masses are neurogenic tumors (21 per cent), thymomas (19 per cent), primary cysts (18 per cent), lymphomas (13 per cent), and germ cell tumors (10 per cent).

Mediastinal masses are most frequently located in the anterosuperior mediastinum (54 per cent), with the posterior (26 per cent) and middle mediastinum (20 per cent) being less frequently involved. Many of the mediastinal lesions occur in characteristic sites within the mediastinum. The masses that occur most commonly in each of the three anatomic subdivisions and the relative incidence with which they occurred in a series of 441 patients from the Duke University Medical Center are shown in Table 3. In the anterosuperior mediastinum, the most frequent neoplasms are thymoma (31 per cent), lymphoma (23 per cent), and germ cell tumor (17 per cent). Posterior mediastinal lesions are usually neurogenic tumors (52 per cent), bronchogenic cysts (22 per cent), and enteric cysts (7 per cent). Middle mediastinal masses are usually pericardial cysts (35 per cent), lymphomas (20 per cent), and bronchogenic cysts (15 per cent). Because of the characteristic location of many mediastinal masses, the site of the mass establishes a useful differential diagnosis that aids in planning the diagnostic evaluation and possible operative procedure. In addition, the location of the mass explains some of the typical symptoms related to a mediastinal mass because of compression or invasion of adjacent mediastinal structures. Anterosuperior mediastinal masses are most likely to produce the superior vena caval syndrome; middle mediastinal masses are most likely to cause tamponade; posterior mediastinal masses are most likely to cause spinal cord compression syndromes. The common symptoms related to

TABLE 1. Classification of Primary Mediastinal Tumors and Cysts

Neurogenic tumors	Mesenchymal tumors
Neurofibroma	Fibroma/fibrosarcoma
Neurilemoma	Lipoma/liposarcoma
Neurosarcoma	Leiomyoma/leiomyosarcoma
Ganglioneuroma	Rhabdosarcoma
Neuroblastoma	Xanthogranuloma
Chemodectoma	Myxoma
Paraganglioma	Mesothelioma
	Hemangioma
Thymoma	Hemangioendothelioma
Benign	Hemangiopericytoma
Malignant	Lymphangioma
	Lymphangiomyoma
Lymphoma	Lymphangiopericytoma
Hodgkin's disease	
Lymphoblastic	
Large cell diffuse growth	Endocrine tumors
pattern	Intrathoracic thyroid
T immunoblastic sarcoma	Parathyroid adenoma/carcinoma
B immunoblastic sarcoma	Carcinoid
Sclerosing follicular cell	
	Cysts
	Bronchogenic
Germ cell tumors	Pericardial
Teratodermoid	Enteric
Benign	Thymic
Malignant	Thoracic duct
Seminoma	Nonspecific
Nonseminomas	
Embryonal	Giant lymph node hyperplasia
Choriocarcinoma	Castleman's disease
Endodermal	
	Chondroma
Primary carcinomas	
	Extramedullary hematopoiesis

TABLE 2. Primary Mediastinal Tumors and Cysts in 2431 Patients

Type of Tumor	Sabiston and Scott 1952	Heimburger et al. 1963	Burkell et al. 1969	Fontanelle et al. 1971	Benjamin et al. 1971	Conkle and Adkins 1972	Rubush et al. 1973
Neurogenic tumor	20	21	13	17	49	8	36
Thymoma	17	10	12	17	34	11	42
Lymphoma	11	9	12	16	32	10	14
Germ cell neoplasm	9	10	3	7	27	2	14
Primary carcinoma	10	11	0	2	0	10	3
Mesenchymal tumor	1	4	4	0	24	2	10
Endocrine tumor	2	8	4	0	24	0	13
Other	14	0	0	0	0	0	0
Cysts	17	24	13	23	19	0	21
Pericardial	2	4	4	2	3	0	10
Bronchogenic	5	12	9	13	11	0	6
Enteric	2	5	0	4	1	0	2
Other	8	3	0	4	4	0	3
Total	101	97	61	82	209	43	153

mechanical involvement with mediastinal structures are listed in Table 4.

Malignant neoplasms represent 25 to 42 per cent of mediastinal masses. Lymphomas, thymomas, germ cell tumors, primary carcinomas, and neurogenic tumors are the most common. The relative frequency of mediastinal mass malignancy varies with the anatomic site in the mediastinum. Anterosuperior masses are most likely malignant (59 per cent) relative to middle mediastinal masses (29 per cent) and posterior mediastinal masses (16 per cent). The relative percentage of lesions that are malignant also varies with age (Fig. 3). Patients in the second through fourth decades have a greater proportion of malignant mediastinal masses. This period corresponds with the peak incidence of lymphomas and germ cell tumors. In contrast, in the first decade of life, a mediastinal mass is most likely benign (73 per cent).

The incidence of various mediastinal masses varies in infants, children, and adults. In a series of 706 children with mediastinal masses (Table 5), neurogenic tumors (35 per cent), lymphomas (25 per cent), germ cell tumors (11 per cent), and primary cysts (16 per cent) were diagnosed most frequently. The neurogenic tumors in children most commonly originate from sympathetic ganglion cells, gangliomas, ganglioneuroblastomas, and neuroblastomas. In contrast, neurilemomas and neurofibromas are the most common neurogenic tumors in adults. The childhood lymphomas are usually of a non-Hodgkin's variety. The germ cell tumors are most frequently benign teratomas. Pericardial cysts and thymomas are uncommon in children.

Symptoms

The clinical presentation varies from those who are asymptomatic (the diagnosis is made by routine chest film), to those with symptoms related to mechanical effects of invasion or compression, to those who have systemic symptoms. These symptoms may be vague and nonspecific or they may be characteristic for a specific neoplasm, such as the relationship between myasthenia gravis and thymoma.

Of patients with a mediastinal mass, 56 to 65 per cent are symptomatic at presentation.[17] Patients with a benign lesion are more often asymptomatic (54 per cent) than are patients with a malignant neoplasm (15 per cent). The absence of symptoms is associated with a benign histologic diagnosis. In asymptomatic

TABLE 3. Anatomic Location of Primary Tumors and Cysts of the Mediastinum

Type of Tumor or Cyst	Percentage
Anterosuperior Mediastinum (n = 245)	
Thymic neoplasms	31%
Lymphomas	23%
Germ cell tumors	17%
Benign	9%
Malignant	8%
Carcinoma	13%
Cysts	6%
Mesenchymal	4%
Endocrine	5%
Other	1%
Middle Mediastinum (n = 83)	
Cysts	61%
Lymphomas	20%
Mesenchymal	8%
Carcinoma	6%
Other	5%
Posterior Mediastinum (n = 113)	
Neurogenic	52%
Benign	40%
Malignant	12%
Cysts	32%
Mesenchymal	10%
Endocrine	2%
Other	4%

TABLE 4. Clinical Manifestations of Anatomic Compression or Invasion by Neoplasms of the Mediastinum

Vena caval obstruction
Pericardial tamponade
Congestive heart failure
Dysrhythmias
Pulmonary stenosis
Tracheal compression
Esophageal compression
Vocal cord paralysis
Horner's syndrome
Phrenic nerve paralysis
Chylothorax
Chylopericardium
Spinal cord compressive syndrome
Pancoast's syndrome
Postobstructive pneumonitis

Vidne and Levy 1973	Ovrum and Birkeland 1979	Nandi et al. 1980	Adkins et al. 1984	Parish et al. 1984	Duke Medical Center 1988	Total	Incidence
9	19	27	8	212	61	500	21%
9	10	18	4	206	68	458	19%
6	11	4	7	107	75	314	13%
3	5	7	11	99	44	241	10%
2	9	0	5	25	37	114	5%
4	4	2	0	60	29	144	6%
2	21	6	2	56	13	151	6%
1	2	1	1	36	10	65	3%
8	10	9	0	196	104	444	18%
2	7	2	0	72	37	145	6%
2	0	0	0	54	39	151	6%
1	0	0	0	29	11	55	2%
3	3	7	0	41	17	93	4%
44	91	74	38	997	441	2431	

patients with a mediastinal mass at the Duke University Medical Center during the past 20 years, 76 per cent had a benign lesion. In contrast, 62 per cent of symptomatic patients had a malignant neoplasm during this period. The presenting symptoms in 441 patients are shown in Table 6. The most common symptoms were chest pain, cough, and fever. Although myasthenia gravis was present in only 7 per cent of patients from the overall series, in patients with thymoma 43 per cent had myasthenia gravis. Infants most likely present with symptoms or findings (78 per cent) because of the relatively small space within the mediastinum.[32] Paralleling the relative percentages of malignant neoplasms within the different anatomic regions, tumors of the anterosuperior mediastinum are most likely to cause symptoms (75 per cent) relative to the posterior mediastinum (50 per cent) and the middle mediastinum (45 per cent).

Symptoms related to compression or invasion of mediastinal structures, such as the superior vena caval syndrome, Horner's syndrome, hoarseness, and severe pain, are more indicative of a malignant histologic diagnosis, although patients with a benign lesion, on occasion, present in this manner.

A number of primary mediastinal lesions produce hormones or antibodies that cause systemic symptoms, which may characterize a specific syndrome (Table 7). Examples include Cushing's syndrome, which is caused by ectopic production of adre-

nocorticotropic hormone, most frequently by carcinoid tumors; thyrotoxicosis, which is caused by a mediastinal goiter; hypertension and a hyperdynamic state caused by pheochromocytoma; and hypercalcemia secondary to increased parathyroid hormone release from a mediastinal parathyroid adenoma.

In other syndromes, the pathophysiology is not as well understood (Table 8), such as the association of large mesenchymal tumors with episodic hypoglycemia, which is presumably related to production of circulating factors capable of insulin-like action (Doege-Potter syndrome). Autoimmune mechanisms have been implicated in the association of myasthenia gravis and red cell aplasia with thymoma. In other cases the pathophysiology is less defined: osteoarthropathy and neurogenic tumors; pain after ingestion of alcohol and the cyclic Pel-Ebstein fevers associated with Hodgkin's disease; the opsomyoclonus syndrome and neuroblastoma.

Diagnosis

The goal of the diagnostic evaluation is the precise histologic classification and staging of the lesion to determine optimal therapy. The initial diagnostic intervention should be a careful history and physical examination, especially when symptom complexes that are characteristic of a specific lesion or of involvement of an anatomic structure are present. Although a diagnosis is rarely possible after these examinations, important information regarding possible metastases or complications related to the mediastinal process may be obtained.

Advances in imaging, cytology, and immunobiology have altered the evaluation of patients with a mediastinal mass. A summary of the diagnostic procedures is shown in Table 9. Although many potentially useful diagnostic approaches are available, the evaluation should be determined by the location and nature of the mediastinal mass, the age and medical condition of the patient, and the results obtained from previous diagnostic procedures.

The initial diagnostic intervention should be posteroanterior and lateral chest films. These films can provide the following information: location within the mediastinum, size of the lesion, displacement and alteration of anatomic structures in the mediastinum and adjacent regions, relative density of the mass with regard to whether the lesion is cystic or solid, whether calcifications are present, and the pattern of the calcifications. Information regarding the anatomic location of the mediastinal mass narrows the differential diagnosis. Alterations in normal anatomy provide evidence of invasiveness and resectability of the mass. Additional information concerning the location, character, and anatomic structures involved can be obtained using

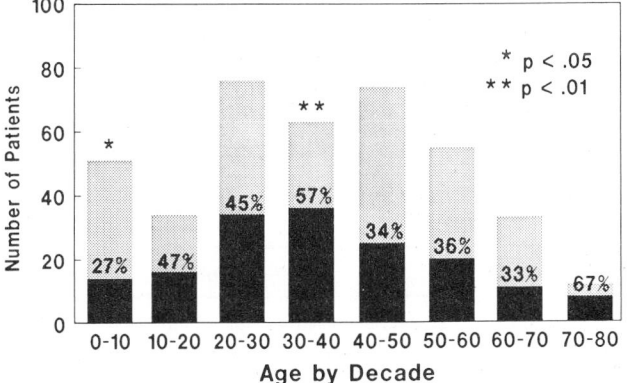

Figure 3. Age distribution and incidence of malignancy relative to age. The largest number of patients with a mediastinal mass were in the third through fifth decades. The fourth decade had a significantly greater proportion of malignant disease. The first decade had a significantly lower proportion of malignant disease. (From Davis, R. D., Jr., Oldham, H. N., Jr., and Sabiston, D. C., Jr.: Primary cysts and neoplasms of the mediastinum: Recent changes in clinical presentation, methods of diagnosis, management, and results. Ann. Thorac. Surg., 44:229, 1987.)

TABLE 5. Primary Mediastinal Tumors and Cysts in Children

Type of Tumor	Haller et al. 1969	Grosfeld et al. 1971	Whitaker and Lynn 1973	Pokorny and Sherman 1974	Heimburger and Battersby 1965	Bower and Kiesewetter 1977	King et al. 1982	Duke Medical Center 1988	Total	Incidence (%)
Neurogenic tumor	18	36	37	35	9	41	48	26	250	35
Lymphoma	9	20	9	27	3	12	87	13	180	25
Germ cell neoplasm	8	5	21	4	4	5	17	11	75	10
Primary carcinoma	10	0	0	6	0	0	0	1	17	2
Mesenchymal tumor	7	1	13	8	6	7	22	5	69	10
Other	0	0	0	0	0	6	4	6	16	2
Cysts	11	6	14	17	10	22	10	26	116	16
Pericardial	1	0	0	0	0	1	0	3	5	1
Bronchogenic	4	0	5	11	8	6	6	14	54	7
Enteric	6	6	7	3	2	11	2	5	42	6
Other	0	0	2	3	0	4	2	4	15	2
Total	63	68	94	97	32	93	188	88	723	100

fluoroscopy, barium swallow, and conventional tomography. The introduction of CT has decreased the use of these techniques; however, physiologic information obtained using these techniques, such as diaphragmatic movement and movement of the mass during swallowing, can be integral to the diagnostic evaluation.

CT scanning has altered the sensitivity and specificity of the diagnostic evaluation and has become the imaging modality of choice for further assessment of a mediastinal mass. CT imaging provides excellent spatial resolution and cross-sectional anatomy, which allows identification of small lesions that are often manifested as questionable abnormalities on chest films or the presence of which is suggested by local or systemic symptoms. More accurate anatomic information regarding the relationship of the mass to mediastinal structures is provided. Anatomic areas in the mediastinum not well seen on routine chest films are well visualized by CT imaging, such as the aortopulmonary window and the subcarinal region. CT imaging is useful when the chest film is not revealing: examining patients with myasthenia gravis for thymoma; evaluating children with recurrent respiratory tract infections for the presence of a subcarinal mass, caused most frequently by a bronchogenic cyst; staging patients with intrathoracic tumor for metastatic disease by more careful assessment of the aortopulmonary window and subcarinal region; and preoperatively evaluating patients with respiratory symptoms and an intrathoracic tumor to assess the risk of airway obstruction during anesthesia.[3,29,32] Contrast-enhanced CT accurately evaluates whether the mediastinal mass has a vascular origin, such as aortic, ventricular, and sinus of Valsalva aneurysms. This has greatly reduced the need for invasive angiographic techniques previously necessary to differentiate primary mediastinal masses from vascular lesions. Using CT, considerable information can be obtained regarding the relative invasiveness and malignant nature of the mediastinal mass. Tumor disruption of fat planes, irregularity of pleural, vascular, or pericardial margins by tumor, and infiltration into muscle or periosteum are useful in differentiating tumor compression from invasion. However, in a prospective series of 60 patients with anterosuperior mediastinal masses, the sensitivity, specificity, and accuracy by CT predicting resectability was 46 per cent, 85 per cent, and 64 per cent, respectively.[46] CT predicts resectability of a neoplasm more accurately than it does unresectability. Additional information obtained using CT not available from chest films includes the presence of chest wall invasion, differentiation of multiple masses from a single large mass (useful in differentiating lymphomas from other common solitary lesions), and possible extension from a posterior mediastinal mass into the spinal column. The CT images are also useful to determine radiation portals for the treatment of radiosensitive tumors such as Hodgkin's disease and seminoma, as well as evaluating response to therapy.

Several mediastinal masses can be diagnosed preoperatively because of their characteristic location, appearance, and attenuation values. For example, pericardial cysts usually occur at the cardiophrenic angle; they have smooth, circumscribed borders, and they have near-water attenuation values. Patients with pericardial cysts have been treated using needle aspiration and subsequent follow-up using serial CT scans and chest films to assess recurrence. Despite the accuracy of CT imaging, emphasis must remain on establishing the precise histologic diagnosis to avoid mistreating a potentially curable neoplasm. Using CT, the correct preoperative diagnosis is made in only approximately 68 per cent of patients.[46] Although CT scanning is sensitive in the evaluation of mediastinal masses and lymphadenopathy, it is not specific for tumor involvement. A histologic

TABLE 6. Presenting Symptoms in Patients with a Mediastinal Mass

Symptoms	Percentage of Patients (n = 441)
Chest pain	29%
Dyspnea	22%
Cough	18%
Fever	13%
Weight loss	9%
Superior vena caval syndrome	8%
Myasthenia gravis	7%
Fatigue	6%
Dysphagia	4%
Night sweats	3%

TABLE 7. Systemic Syndromes Caused by Mediastinal Neoplasm Hormone Production

Syndrome	Tumor
Hypertension	Pheochromocytoma, chemodectoma, ganglioneuroma, neuroblastoma
Hypoglycemia	Mesothelioma, teratoma, fibrosarcoma, neurosarcoma
Diarrhea	Ganglioneuroma, neuroblastoma, neurofibroma
Hypercalcemia	Parathyroid adenoma/carcinoma, Hodgkin's disease
Thyrotoxicosis	Thyroid adenoma/carcinoma
Gynecomastia	Nonseminomatous germ cell tumors

TABLE 8. Systemic Syndromes Associated with Mediastinal Neoplasms

Tumor	Syndrome
Thymoma	Myasthenia gravis
	Red blood cell aplasia
	White blood cell aplasia
	Aplastic anemia
	Hypogammaglobulinemia
	Progressive systemic sclerosis
	Hemolytic anemia
	Megaesophagus
	Dermatomyositis
	Systemic lupus erythematosus
	Myocarditis
	Collagen vascular disease
Lymphoma	Anemia, myasthenia gravis
Neurofibroma	von Recklinghausen's disease
Carcinoid	Cushing's syndrome
Carcinoid, thymoma	Multiple endocrine adenomatosis
Thymoma, neurofibroma, neurilemoma, mesothelioma	Osteoarthropathy
Enteric cysts	Vertebral anomalies
Hodgkin's disease	Alcohol-induced pain
	Pel-Ebstein fever
Neuroblastoma	Opsomyoclonus
	Erythrocyte abnormalities
Enteric cysts	Peptic ulcer

examination of abnormal mediastinal lymph nodes (greater than 1.5 cm.) determined by CT scanning in patients with known malignancies demonstrates that in more than one third of patients the lymph node was benign.[12]

Another useful imaging technique for evaluating mediastinal masses is MRI, which is noninvasive and provides excellent vascular delineation without the use of contrast agents. Because of poorer resolution than CT scanning, MRI is less sensitive in the evaluation of small lesions (less than 5 to 10 mm.), and small lymph nodes or separate masses appear as a single mass. Additionally, because MRI is not based on density, it does not determine tissue calcification. Although scanning times can be long, which may be a problem with infants and small children, and the current techniques are expensive, MRI offers more accurate information regarding vascular involvement, intracardiac pathology, and intraspinal extension from mediastinal tumor. Using cine-MRI, myocardial performance and valvular insufficiency can be assessed, which may be needed to determine operative risk in patients with concurrent intrathoracic and cardiac disease. Moreover, in patients with surgical clips, MRI provides better quality images than does CT. Although axial images provide the most information, coronal or sagittal images often provide additional anatomic information. Evaluation of airway compression appears to be equal to CT scanning. The initial hope of differentiating tumor histologic type based on charac-

TABLE 9. Diagnostic Evaluation of Mediastinal Masses

History	Ultrasonography
Physical examination	Radioisotope scanning
Radiology	Serology
Standard chest films	Endoscopy
Tomography	Bronchoscopy
Barium swallow	Needle aspiration and biopsy
Fluoroscopy	Operative procedures
Arteriography	Mediastinoscopy
Venography	Mediastinotomy
CT scanning	Thoracotomy
MRI	
Myelography	

teristic relaxation values has not been realized, although, in conjunction with clinical data, some specific lesions such as a parathyroid adenoma may be easily differentiated using MRI. Overall, CT and MRI are comparable in the evaluation and staging of mediastinal tumors. However, because CT currently is a less expensive modality, it is the imaging technique of choice except when a patient has an allergy to contrast dye or if possible myocardial involvement or intraspinal extension is present. Often when CT imaging is indeterminate, MRI is helpful in further delineating the process.

Echocardiography may be useful in the evaluation of mediastinal masses, especially tumors in the middle mediastinum, or in patients with tamponade or pulmonary stenosis. In patients with middle mediastinal masses, echocardiography is useful in differentiating primary masses from intracardiac or pericardial lesions. In patients with acquired pulmonary stenosis, the adjunctive use of color-flow Doppler helps to assess the physiologic significance of tumor encasement and compression. Echocardiography delineates the cystic nature of lesions, and it has been used to guide needle biopsy, especially with lesions adjacent to the chest wall. Compared with conventional chest films, echocardiography is more sensitive in evaluating the mediastinum for a mass, particularly in the presence of pericardial or pleural effusion. However, echocardiography is not as sensitive as MRI or CT.

A number of radioisotopic scans may be useful in evaluating a mediastinal mass. In patients with a superior mediastinal mass, radioisotopic iodine scans may identify a mediastinal goiter when functioning ectopic thyroid tissue is present. These scans can also determine if functioning cervical thyroid tissue is present. Examples of other useful nuclear scans include (1) ^{131}I-meta-iodobenzylguanidine (MIBG) for the identification of pheochromocytoma, which is particularly useful when the tumor is located in the middle mediastinum; (2) [99]technetium scans that show the presence of functioning gastric mucosa, which may be present in enteric cysts; and (3) technetium-thallium subtraction scan for the location of ectopic parathyroid adenomas.

Increased success has been reported in making a cytologic diagnosis preoperatively by using fine-needle biopsy techniques (22-gauge needle) with low morbidity and almost zero mortality. Fluoroscopic visualization is usually used to guide the biopsy. CT and echocardiography, because of better localization of the mass and improved placement of the needle, have increased the sensitivity of the technique. Although a precise histologic diagnosis is not always possible, a cytologic diagnosis of benign or malignant can be made in 80 to 90 per cent of patients. Complications related to the procedure include pneumothorax in 20 to 25 per cent of patients with approximately 5 per cent requiring tube thoracostomy; hemoptysis in 5 to 10 per cent, with rare occurrences of significant hemorrhagic complications; and tumor seeding along the needle track, which is a theoretic but extremely rare complication. An increased sensitivity in obtaining a precise histologic diagnosis has been reported using cutting-needle techniques (16-gauge needle) without an apparent increase in morbidity (23 per cent incidence of pneumothorax).[38] Needle biopsy techniques are particularly useful for evaluating patients with small cell carcinoma or metastatic carcinoma because of the possibility of obviating a thoracotomy or other invasive procedure to establish a histologic diagnosis. The use of electron microscopy to examine the cellular ultrastructure and immunohistochemical staining has increased the sensitivity of the various needle biopsy techniques.

Because of the marked associated desmoplastic changes, some tumors are rarely diagnosed by needle biopsy including nodular sclerosing Hodgkin's lymphoma. Additionally, needle biopsy rarely provides adequate tissue for precise immunotyping often necessary to determine optimal therapy, particularly with the non-Hodgkin's lymphomas. Poorly differentiated malignant tumors of the anterosuperior mediastinum, particularly thymomas, lymphomas, germ cell tumors, and primary carcinomas, can have remarkably similar cytologic and morphologic appearances. Diagnoses based on examination of frozen sections are therefore frequently incorrect, and, similarly, therapeutic decisions based on frozen section examination may be in error. In addition to light microscopy utilizing special staining techniques, immunostaining techniques and electron microscopy of multiple sections of the tumor may be necessary to establish an accurate diagnosis. The characteristic ultrastructural features as evaluated by electron microscopy are shown in Table 10. Monoclonal antibodies for surface antigens specific to a cell line of origin and for tumor secretory products can be useful in establishing a precise diagnosis. Immunotyping of non-Hodgkin's lymphomas has allowed accurate subtyping of these lesions, which has been important in predicting the natural history and optimal therapy.

Monoclonal antibodies have been used to develop radioimmunoassays to measure a number of tumor secretory products and antigens. Preoperative diagnosis is possible in some circumstances, such as malignant nonseminomal germ cell tumors in male patients with elevated alpha-fetoprotein and beta-human chorionic gonadotropin (β-HCG). These serologic measurements should be obtained in all male patients in the second through fifth decades of life with an anterosuperior mediastinal mass. However, serologic markers are most useful for monitoring the response to therapy and for diagnosing tumor relapse. Research continues in applying the monoclonal antibodies to imaging techniques as well as tumor-specific immunotherapy, chemotherapy, and radiotherapy.

Although surgical excision is not essential for the treatment of certain malignant neoplasms, the optimal therapeutic regimen often requires precise histologic subclassification. Because needle biopsy techniques do not usually produce sufficient tissue for this purpose, more invasive procedures are often required, such as mediastinoscopy, mediastinotomy, thoracotomy, and median sternotomy. Mediastinoscopy may be useful to evaluate and biopsy lesions of the anterosuperior mediastinum, particularly those located in the anterior aspect of the subcarinal space, around the proximal main stem bronchi, and around the lower trachea. Often it is used to evaluate associated lymphadenopathy in these regions. In centers commonly using mediastinoscopy (primarily to evaluate mediastinal lymph nodes in association with bronchogenic carcinoma), morbidity is usually minimal (2 per cent), with a 0.3 per cent incidence of significant hemorrhagic complications requiring emergency intervention, and only rare mortality.[19] In centers in which this procedure is done less routinely, a greater morbidity (16 per cent) and mortality (2 per cent) have been reported.[6]

Many use median sternotomy and anterolateral thoracotomy for anterosuperior mediastinal masses and posterolateral thoracotomy for middle and posterior masses as the initial surgical procedure for the following reasons: (1) these procedures can be done with morbidity and mortality similar to mediastinoscopy

or mediastinotomy; (2) these approaches provide adequate exposure to evaluate resectability and, when possible, to resect the mass; and (3) these approaches allow adequate exposure to safely biopsy the mass under optimal conditions. Although the choice of surgical procedure reflects individual preference, the incision should not be made in potential portals for radiotherapy.

Although most patients undergo surgical procedures safely, a subset of patients, particularly children with large anterosuperior or middle mediastinal masses, has an increased risk of developing severe cardiorespiratory complications during general anesthesia. Exacerbation of superior vena caval obstruction or extrinsic airway compression occurs during general anesthesia because of (1) the loss of negative intrathoracic pressure during respirations, (2) bronchial smooth muscle relaxation that increases the compressibility of the bronchi, and (3) reduced tidal volumes used for ventilation. Patients with posture-related dyspnea and superior vena caval syndrome are at increased risk. Useful techniques for identifying less symptomatic patients who have significant airway compromise include CT imaging, in which a reduction in tracheal cross-sectional area of more than 35 per cent is indicative of an increased risk with general anesthesia, and pulmonary flow mechanics, in which reductions in peak expiratory flow serve as a sensitive indicator of functional airway compression.[3,42] In patients with airway compression or superior vena caval obstruction, the risk of general anesthesia is prohibitive, and attempts to obtain a histologic diagnosis should be limited to needle biopsies or open procedures done under local anesthesia. If a histologic diagnosis cannot be obtained, treatment with radiation, corticosteroids, and, when appropriate, chemotherapy is based on a presumptive diagnosis to establish an adequate airway. When such treatment is necessary prior to biopsy, a histologic diagnosis may not be obtainable in as many as 40 per cent of patients. The majority of these lesions are malignant and unresectable, of which non-Hodgkin's lymphoma, Hodgkin's lymphoma, malignant germ cell tumors, neuroblastomas, and malignant mesenchymal tumors are the most frequent. Occasionally benign tumors, usually benign teratomas in young children and infants, may produce this clinical setting. In patients with large mediastinal masses who have an increased anesthetic risk but in whom a histologic diagnosis is needed before therapy, or for whom complete excision is the preferred treatment, recommendations for anesthetic management include (1) fiberoptic evaluation of the tracheobronchial system for evidence of severe extrinsic compression, (2) induction of anesthesia in Fowler's position with the ability to change to the lateral or prone position, (3) use of long endotracheal tubes to allow advancement of the tube beyond the site of obstruction, (4) standby rigid bronchoscopy to allow re-establishment of an adequate airway, (5) avoidance of muscle relaxants and use of spontaneous ventilation when possible, (6) lower extremity intravenous intubation to provide access to the systemic venous circulation if a sudden superior vena caval obstruction should occur, and (7) standby cardiopulmonary bypass with bilateral groin preparation.

Differential Diagnosis

A variety of intrathoracic and extrathoracic lesions have a similar roentgenographic appearance to a primary mediastinal mass. Several cardiovascular abnormalities, which include aneurysms, dilations, and abnormal locations of cardiac or vascular structures, may appear on chest films as a mediastinal mass (Table 11). CT and MRI usually differentiate a primary mediastinal mass from a cardiovascular lesion. However, angiography may be necessary for differentiation or, more typically, to better delineate the anatomy of the cardiovascular lesion and associated structures. Abnormalities of the spinal column, such as meningoceles, need to be differentiated from neurogenic tumors and other primary posterior mediastinal tumors. This

TABLE 10. Ultrastructural Characteristics of Mediastinal Tumors

Tumors	Ultrastructure
Carcinoid	Dense core granules, fewer tonofilaments and desmosomes
Lymphoma	Absence of junctional attachments and epithelial features
Thymoma	Well-formed desmosomes, bundles of tonofilaments
Germ cell	Prominent nucleoli, even chromatin, scant desmosomes, rare tonofilaments
Neuroblastoma	Neurosecretory granules, synaptic endings

TABLE 11. Mediastinal Masses Due to Cardiovascular Lesions

Mediastinal Location	Systemic Venous System	Pulmonary Arterial System	Pulmonary Venous System	Systemic Arterial System
Anterior				Aortic stenosis (poststenotic dilation) Ascending aortic aneurysm
Middle	Superior vena caval aneurysm Azygous vein enlargement	Pulmonary valve stenosis Idiopathic dilation of the pulmonary trunk Congenital absence of the pulmonary valve Pulmonary embolism Pulmonary arterial hypertension Anomalous left pulmonary artery	Pulmonary venous varix Pulmonary venous confluence Partial anomalous pulmonary venous return to the superior vena cava	Aortic stenosis Right aortic arch Transverse arch aortic aneurysm Aneurysm/fistula of the coronary artery
Posterior				Coarctation and pseudo-coarctation Descending aortic aneurysm Tortuous innominate artery
Superior	Aneurysms of the innominate veins Persistent left superior vena cava Hemiazygous vein enlargement	Aneurysm of the ductus	Partial anomalous pulmonary venous return to the innominate vein Total anomalous pulmonary venous return (supracardiac)	Cervical aortic arch Coarctation of the aorta Transverse arch aortic aneurysm

differentiation is particularly important in patients with neurofibromatosis who are at increased risk for the development of both meningoceles and neurofibromas. Other lesions that may resemble a mediastinal mass include esophageal lesions, such as esophageal diverticula, tumor, hiatal hernia, and achalasia, diaphragmatic herniations, pancreatic pseudocysts, herniations of peritoneal fat, mediastinitis, and a number of primary pulmonary parenchymal lesions and infections. The use of available diagnostic techniques should differentiate these lesions from primary mediastinal tumors or cysts prior to operative intervention.

Neurogenic Tumors

Neurogenic tumors are the most common neoplasm in the collected series of patients, comprising 21 per cent of all primary tumors and cysts. These tumors are usually located in the posterior mediastinum and originate from the sympathetic ganglia (ganglioma, ganglioneuroblastoma, and neuroblastoma), the intercostal nerves (neurofibroma, neurilemoma, and neurosarcoma), and the paraganglia cells (paraganglioma). Only rarely are these tumors located in the anterosuperior mediastinum. Although the peak incidence occurs in adults, neurogenic tumors comprise a proportionally greater percentage of mediastinal masses in children (35 per cent). Whereas the majority of neurogenic tumors in adults are benign, a greater percentage of neurogenic tumors are malignant in children.

Many of these tumors are discovered on routine chest films. When present, symptoms are usually caused by mechanical factors such as chest and back pain due to compression or invasion of intercostal nerve, bone, and chest wall; cough and dyspnea due to compression of the tracheobronchial tree; and Pancoast's syndrome and Horner's syndrome due to involvement of the brachial and the cervical sympathetic chain. Approximately 10 per cent of neurogenic tumors extend into the spinal column and are termed dumbbell tumors because of their characteristic shape due to the relatively large paraspinal and intraspinal portions connected by a narrow isthmus of tissue traversing the intervertebral foramen. Although 60 per cent of patients with such tumors have neurologic symptoms related to spinal

cord compression, the significant proportion of patients without symptoms underscores the importance of evaluating all patients with a posterior mediastinal mass for possible intraspinal extension. CT, MRI, and vertebral tomography are useful for indicating enlargement of the foramen, erosion of bone, and intervertebral widening. If these findings are present, CT with myelography or MRI is indicated to evaluate the presence and extent of the intraspinal component. The recommended surgical approach to dumbbell tumors is one-stage removal using a team of neurosurgeons and thoracic surgeons. Excision of the intraspinal component is performed prior to resection of the thoracic component to minimize any spinal column hematoma. Improved results with decreased morbidity have been reported using this approach.

Symptoms may be systemic and related to production of neurohormonal agents. Production of catecholamine by paragangliomas and neuroblastomas causes the constellation of symptoms that are characteristic of pheochromocytomas: hypertension, which is often severe and episodic, sweating, headaches, and palpitations. Production of vasoactive intestinal polypeptide by ganglioneuromas and neuroblastomas causes a syndrome of abdominal distention and profuse watery diarrhea. Secretion of an insulin-like factor or insulin-releasing factor by neurosarcomas causes the Doege-Potter syndrome characterized by episodic hypoglycemia.

The most common neurogenic tumor is the neurilemoma, which originates from the perineural Schwann cells. These tumors are well circumscribed and have a defined capsule. There are two morphologic patterns: Antoni Type A, which has organized architecture with a cellular pallisading pattern of growth, and Antoni Type B, which has a loose reticular growth pattern. The peak incidence of these tumors is in the third through fifth decades of life.

In contrast to neurilemomas, neurofibromas are poorly encapsulated and consist of randomly arranged spindle-shaped cells. These tumors originate as a proliferation of all the elements of the peripheral nerve. Although both neurilemomas and neurofibromas occur as a manifestation of neurofibromatosis (von Recklinghausen's disease), they must be differentiated from the two other common entities in the posterior mediastinum, meningioma and meningocele. With both neurilemoma and neurofibroma, surgical excision results in cure.

NEUROSARCOMA. Neurosarcomas originate by malignant degeneration of either neurilemomas or neurofibromas, in addition to developing *de novo*. These tumors usually occur in adults. However, patients with neurofibromatosis may develop neurosarcomas as children. These are rapidly growing tumors that frequently invade vital structures, preventing attempts at resection. On microscopic examination, neurosarcomas are extremely cellular tumors composed of spindle cells. Occasionally, these tumors have been associated with recurrent episodes of hypoglycemia that appears to be related to secretion of an insulin-like product. Control of the tumor has caused resolution of symptoms. Unless tumor excision is possible, the prognosis is extremely poor owing to the unresponsiveness to adjuvant therapies.

GANGLIONEUROMA. Ganglioneuromas are benign tumors originating from the sympathetic chain that are composed of ganglion cells and nerve fibers. These tumors typically present at an early age and are the most common neurogenic tumors occurring during childhood. The usual location is the paravertebral region. On the chest film, they have an elongated or triangular appearance with the broader base directed toward the mediastinum. Poorly defined on lateral projection, the inferior and superior margins are often indistinct. These tumors are well encapsulated, and when cross-sectioned, they frequently exhibit areas of cystic degeneration. Surgical excision provides cure.

GANGLIONEUROBLASTOMA. Ganglioneuroblastomas exhibit an intermediate degree of differentiation between ganglioneuromas and neuroblastomas (Fig. 4). They are composed of mature and immature ganglion cells. Stout defined two different histologic patterns that differed in their natural history: composite ganglioneuroblastoma, predominantly mature neuroblasts with focal areas containing primitive neuroblasts; and diffuse ganglioneuroblastoma, a diffuse mixture of well-differentiated and primitive neuroblasts. Composite ganglioneuroblastomas have a much greater incidence of metastasis with most series reporting an incidence between 65 and 75 per cent.[1] In contrast, less than 5 per cent of patients with the diffuse type develop metastases.

Ganglioneuroblastoma and neuroblastoma are staged as follows: Stage I, well-circumscribed, noninvasive tumor; Stage II, tumor invasion locally without extension across the midline; Stage III, tumor spread across the midline; Stage IV, tumor with metastasis. Younger patients who have a diffuse histologic appearance and a lower stage tumor have the best prognosis. Five-year survival of 88 per cent has been reported in patients with Stage I or Stage II disease treated solely by excision. Patients with Stage III or Stage IV disease, composite morphology, or age greater than 3 years are treated with multiagent chemotherapy.

NEUROBLASTOMA. Neuroblastomas originate from the sympathetic nervous system and therefore can occur wherever sympathetic nervous tissue is present. The most common location for a neuroblastoma is in the retroperitoneum; however, 10 to 20 per cent occur primarily in the mediastinum (Fig. 5). These are highly invasive neoplasms that have frequently metastasized prior to diagnosis. Common sites of metastases are the regional lymph nodes, bone, brain, liver, and lung. A majority of these tumors occur in children; 75 per cent occur in children under 4 years. The tumor is composed of small, round, immature cells organized in a rosette pattern. On ultrastructural examination, the presence of neurosecretory granules is characteristic. Patients are usually symptomatic, most commonly with cough, dyspnea, dysphagia, back or chest pain, and symptoms related to recurrent pulmonary infections. A number of paraneoplastic syndromes have been reported including "pheochromocytoma" syndrome due to catecholamine secretion, profuse watery diarrhea and abdominal pain related to vasoactive intestinal polypeptide production, and the opsoclonus-polymyoclonus syndrome—an unexplained symptom complex characterized by cerebellar and truncal ataxia with rapid, darting eye movements (dancing eyes) that is possibly related to an autoimmune mechanism. Successful treatment of the tumor or the use of corticosteroids relieves symptoms.

The immunobiology of neuroblastomas is unique. Well-documented cases of spontaneous regression or maturation of tumor have been reported. Lymphocytes collected from these patients have proved to be cytotoxic T cells capable of causing tumor lysis *in vitro*. Patients in whom tumor progression or relapse occurs appear to have suppressor T cells as well as circulating antigen-antibody complexes capable of inhibiting tumor regression.

Therapy is determined by the stage of the disease: Stage I, surgical excision; Stage II, excision and radiation therapy; Stage III and Stage IV, multimodality therapy using surgical debulking, radiation therapy, and multiagent chemotherapy as well as a second-look exploration to resect residual disease when necessary. Children less than 1 year have an excellent prognosis even when widespread disease is present. However, with increasing age and extent of involvement, the prognosis worsens. Interestingly, mediastinal neuroblastomas appear to have a better prognosis than does tumor occurring elsewhere. In patients with neuroblastomas resistant to therapy or in those who relapse, ablative chemotherapy with autologous bone marrow transplantation has been attempted with some success.

PARAGANGLIOMA (PHEOCHROMOCYTOMA). Mediastinal paragangliomas are rare tumors representing less than 1 per cent of all mediastinal tumors and less than 2 per cent of all pheochromocytomas. Although the majority are found in the paravertebral sulcus, an increasing number of middle mediastinal paragangliomas occur in the branchial arch structures, coronary and aortopulmonary paraganglia, atria, and islands of tissue in the pericardium. Because the clinical behavior of extra-adrenal paragangliomas is dependent on the site of origin, a division based on anatomic location, histochemical features, and innervation has been created:[20] (1) branchiomeric (chemodectoma) are associated with the arteries and cranial nerves derived from the branchial arches, including intercarotid (carotid body), jugulotympanic (glomus jugulare and glomus tympanic), orbital, laryngeal, subclavian, aortopulmonary, coronary, and pulmonary structures; (2) intravagal; (3) aortosympathetic, which are associated with the sympathetic chain and retroperitoneal ganglia; and (4) visceral autonomic, which include the atria, urinary bladder, liver hilum, and mesenteric vessels. The likelihood of functional activity of a paraganglioma is related to the site of origin: adrenal medulla, high likelihood; branchiomeric and intravagal, very low likelihood; aortosympathetic and visceral autonomic, intermediate likelihood. Catecholamine production causes the classic constellation of symptoms associated with pheochromocytomas including periodic or sustained hypertension, often accompanied by orthostatic hypotension, and hypermetabolism manifested by weight loss, hyperhidrosis, palpitations, and headaches. Measurement of elevated levels of urinary catecholamines or their metabolites, the metanephrines and vanillylmandelic acid, usually establishes the diagnosis. Although adrenal pheochromocytomas often produce both epinephrine and norepinephrine, extra-adrenal paragangliomas rarely secrete epinephrine.

Tumor localization has improved remarkably through the use of CT and [131]I-*meta*-iodobenzylguanidine (^{131}I-MIBG) scintigraphy, particularly when the tumors are hormonally active. Hormonally active tumors may be located with an 85 per cent sensitivity using the ^{131}I-MIBG scan. Owing to the high vascularity of these lesions, enhancement with contrast administration during CT imaging occurs, and in 30 per cent of cases, a tumor blush may be seen during thoracic arteriography. Selective venous

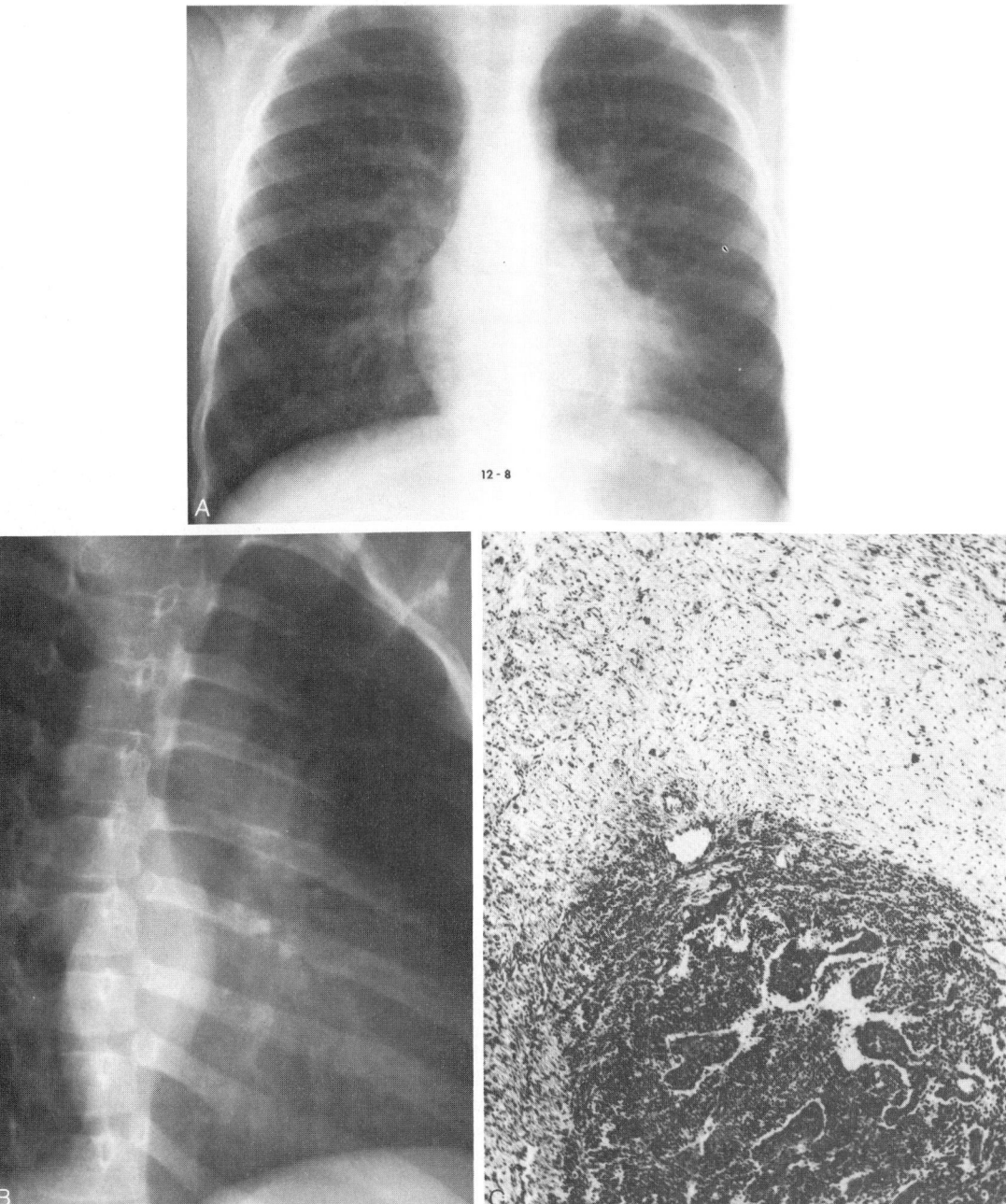

Figure 4. *A* and *B*, Chest films of a ganglioneuroblastoma. *C*, Example of a histologic specimen demonstrating the focal area of primitive neuroblasts (arrow) characteristic of the composite ganglioneuroblastoma. (From Adam, A., and Hochholzer, L.: Ganglioneuroblastoma of the posterior mediastinum: A clinicopathologic review of 80 cases. Cancer, *47*:373, 1981.)

angiography with serial sampling for catecholamine levels to observe a step-up is occasionally necessary for preoperative localization. Tumor localization using MRI has been reported.

When appropriate, surgical resection is the optimal therapy. In patients with tumors involving the middle mediastinum, cardiopulmonary bypass may be necessary to enable resection. Differentiation of benign from malignant tumors is determined by the patient's clinical course. Although 50 per cent of tumors appear malignant morphologically, metastatic disease develops in only 3 per cent of patients. In those with metastatic disease, alpha-methyltyramine, a tyrosine hydroxylase inhibitor that blocks the synthesis of catecholamines, is helpful in controlling symptoms.

Approximately 10 per cent of patients have multiple paragangliomas. They are more common in patients with the multiple endocrine neoplastic syndrome, a familial history of disease, and Carney's syndrome (pulmonary chondroma, gastric leiomyosarcoma, and extra-adrenal paraganglioma). In patients who have had excision of an adrenal pheochromocytoma and continue to have symptoms, a search for an extra-adrenal lesion should be undertaken with careful attention directed to the evaluation of the mediastinum.

Thymoma

Thymoma is the most common neoplasm of the anterosuperior mediastinum and the second most common of all mediastinal masses (20 per cent, Table 2). The peak incidence is in the third through fifth decades, but thymomas can occur throughout adulthood and are rare in the first two decades. Roentgenographically they may appear as a small, well-circumscribed mass or a bulky lobulated mass confluent with adjacent mediastinal structures (Fig. 6). Patients are usually symptomatic at

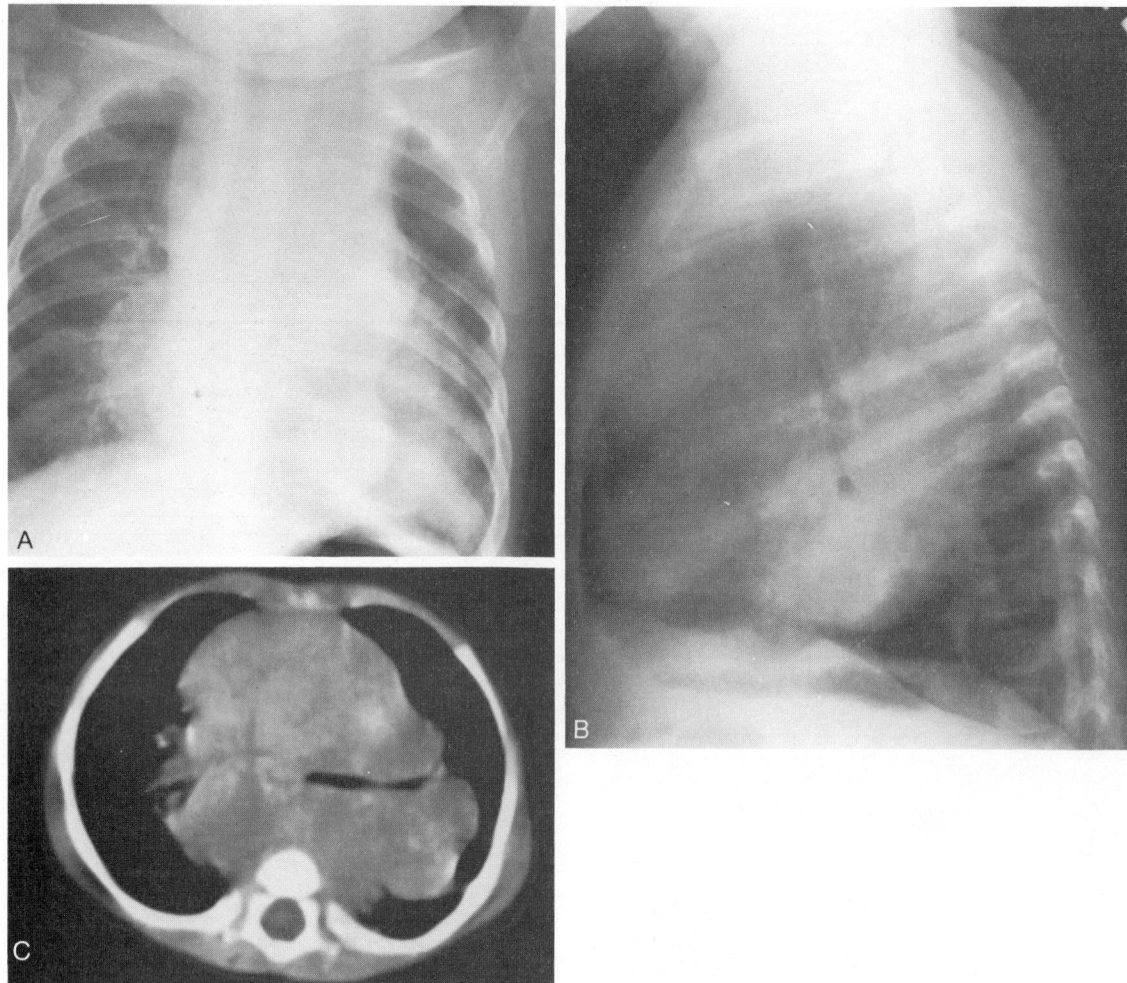

Figure 5. *A* and *B*, Chest films of a neuroblastoma in an 18-year-old female. *C*, CT image demonstrates the extensive nature of the tumor.

presentation and symptoms may be related to local mass effects causing chest pain, dyspnea, hemoptysis, cough, and the superior vena caval syndrome. However, thymomas frequently are associated with systemic syndromes presumably caused by an immunologic mechanism. The most common syndrome is myasthenia gravis. However, many other syndromes have been associated with thymomas including red cell aplasia, pure white cell aplasia, aplastic anemia, Cushing's syndrome, hypo- and hypergammaglobulinemia, dermatomyositis, systemic lupus erythematosus, progressive systemic sclerosis, hypercoagulopathy with thrombosis, rheumatoid arthritis, megaesophagus, and granulomatous myocarditis.

The etiologic factors involved in these syndromes have not been fully elucidated. Myasthenia gravis is characterized pathologically by destruction of postsynaptic nicotinic receptors. The mechanism is postulated to be an autoimmune process. In the majority of patients with myasthenia gravis, anti–acetylcholine receptor antibodies are present in high titers. Thymic lymphocytes isolated from these patients produce significant amounts of anti–acetylcholine receptor antibodies, and this production is enhanced by the addition of autologous or allogeneic thymic epithelial cells.[48] The thymic myoid cells bear complete acetylcholine receptors; the thymic epithelial cells and tumor epithelial cells contain acetylcholine receptor–related antigenic determinants, but not the complete acetylcholine receptor. These antigenic determinants are thought to be involved in the autosensitization; the varied antigenic determinants may be related to the heterogeneity of anti–acetylcholine receptor antibodies.

In patients with myasthenia gravis, there is an intimate relationship between the antigen-producing myoid cells and the interdigitating reticulum cells (potentially antigen-presenting) that are surrounded by T-helper (T3[+]) lymphocytes. In these patients, T lymphocytes reactive to acetylcholine receptors are present, and in the majority, acetylcholine receptor–specific T lymphocyte cell lines could be established that contain helper and inducer subsets.[36]

Similarly, the various hematologic abnormalities associated with thymomas appear to have an autoimmune basis. Serum from patients with red cell aplasia in the presence of complement, as well as T lymphocytes isolated from these patients, is able to suppress erythropoiesis colonies *in vitro*.[49] However, the mechanisms related to the development and maintenance of these syndromes have not been completely elucidated. The clinical phenomenon related to these syndromes is not well understood. The systemic syndromes often do not improve following successful control of the thymoma. Multiple associated syndromes may be present in a patient with a thymoma, suggesting a possible common etiologic factor. In regard to myasthenia gravis, the number of complete remissions achieved increases with increasing length of follow-up after thymectomy. In addition, the change in the acetylcholine receptor antibody titer following thymectomy does not correlate well with the patient's clinical response.

Myasthenia gravis occurs in 10 to 50 per cent of patients with thymoma and is characterized clinically by weakness and fatigue of the skeletal muscles, with sparing of cardiac or smooth

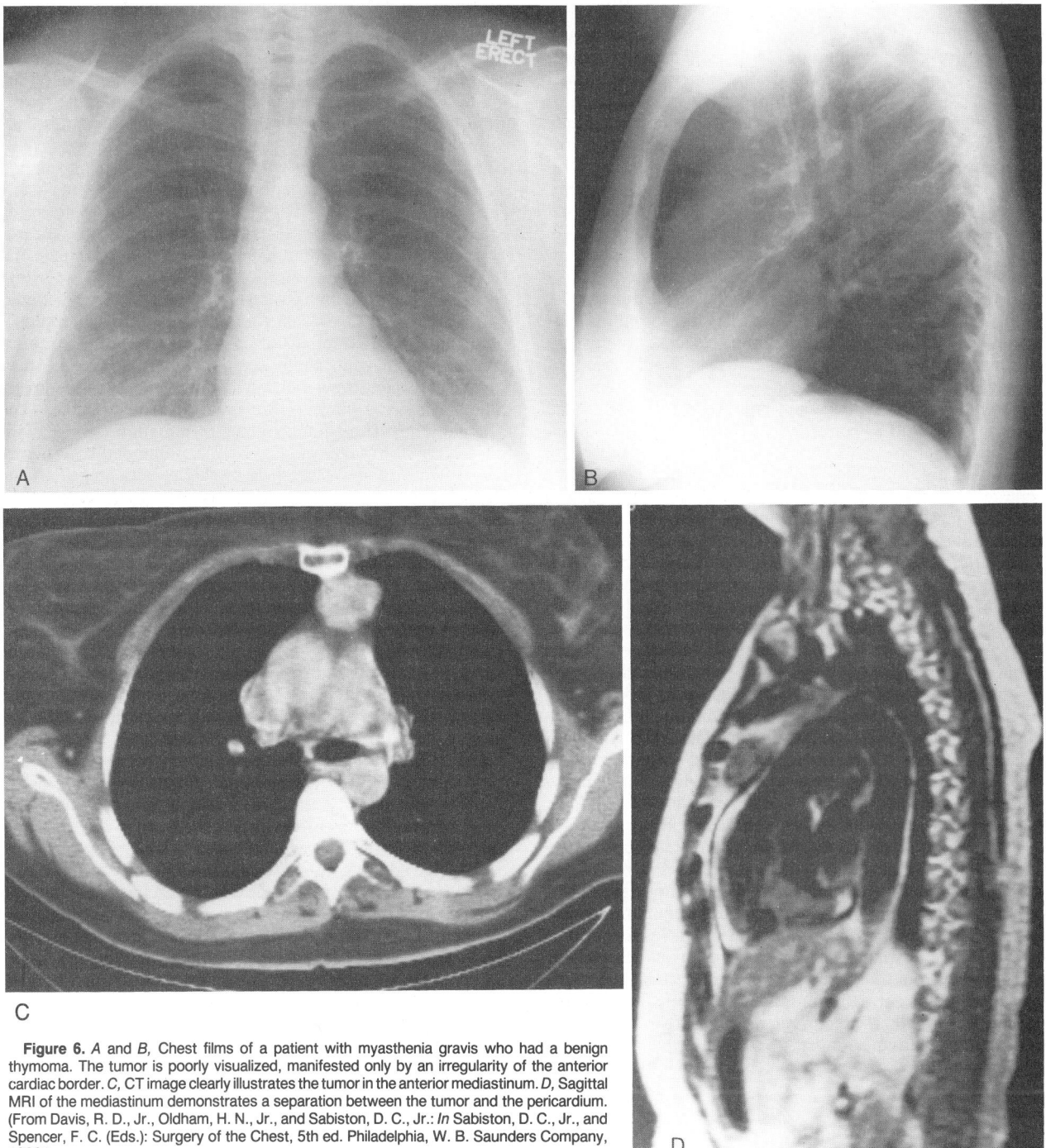

Figure 6. *A* and *B*, Chest films of a patient with myasthenia gravis who had a benign thymoma. The tumor is poorly visualized, manifested only by an irregularity of the anterior cardiac border. *C*, CT image clearly illustrates the tumor in the anterior mediastinum. *D*, Sagittal MRI of the mediastinum demonstrates a separation between the tumor and the pericardium. (From Davis, R. D., Jr., Oldham, H. N., Jr., and Sabiston, D. C., Jr.: *In* Sabiston, D. C., Jr., and Spencer, F. C. (Eds.): Surgery of the Chest, 5th ed. Philadelphia, W. B. Saunders Company, 1990.)

musculature. Muscles innervated by cranial nerves are the most frequently involved, particularly the extraocular muscles. However, generalized weakness occurs, and myasthenia crisis may cause respiratory failure. In only 14 per cent of patients does the disease remain localized to the extraocular muscles. In patients in whom the disease becomes generalized, it does so within the first year after onset of symptoms in 87 per cent. Peak severity is reached by 1 year in 55 per cent, by 3 years in 70 per cent, and in 85 per cent by 5 years. Male patients have more rapid progression of disease, fewer remissions, and less improvement with treatment than do females.[5]

The incidence with which myasthenia gravis occurs in patients with thymoma increases with the age of the patient. In males over 50 and females over 60 years of age, the incidence appears to be greater than 80 per cent. The majority of patients with myasthenia gravis do not have thymoma. The incidence is 10 to 42 per cent depending on the reporting medical center. Males with myasthenia gravis are 1.8 to 2 times more likely to have a thymoma than are females. Because of the significant association between thymoma and myasthenia gravis, an evaluation of the mediastinum with CT or MRI is recommended in all patients with myasthenia gravis.

The diagnosis of myasthenia gravis is usually confirmed by a transient increase in muscle strength following the administration of a short-acting anticholinesterase inhibitor such as edrophonium (Tensilon). Electromyographic testing is also used to make the diagnosis and to follow quantitatively the course of the disease. An abnormal loss of muscle contraction strength following multiple stimulations (usually 3 to 5 per second) of the appropriate motor nerve constitutes a positive test.

Since Blalock's pioneering work in 1939, thymectomy has been a significant part of the treatment of myasthenia gravis. The use of median sternotomy to perform extended thymectomy, which includes the removal of all anterior mediastinal fatty areolar tissue in addition to the thymus gland, has improved clinical benefit with fewer recurrences. This technique was developed to enable the extirpation of all ectopic foci of thymic tissue and to prevent recurrences that often followed transcervical thymectomy. In 85 to 96 per cent of patients, clinical improvement—defined as decreased symptoms, decreased use of medications, or remission—occurs following thymectomy.[18,27] Drug-free remission is achieved in 46 to 63 per cent. Remission rates increase with duration after thymectomy (up to 81 per cent at 89 months). Improved results and earlier remissions are associated with shorter duration of disease before thymectomy, decreased severity of disease, female sex (remission in 82 per cent of females, 46 per cent of males),[18] and absence of thymoma (remission rate 13 per cent, benefit rate 60 per cent).[27] Whereas red cell aplasia occurs in only 5 per cent of patients with thymoma, 33 to 50 per cent of adults with red cell aplasia have a thymoma.

Thymomas are histologically classified by the predominance of epithelial or lymphocytic cells (lymphocytic, epithelial, mixed, and spindle) or by the morphologic resemblance to cortical or medullary epithelium. Unfortunately, a wide variance in the cellular composition often is present within the tumor and a consistent relationship is not present between the microscopic appearance and biologic behavior, either with regard to tumor invasiveness or in association with systemic syndromes. However, in one series an improved 10-year survival was reported in patients with spindle cell or lymphocyte-rich thymomas (75 per cent) as compared with differentiated epithelial type (50 per cent) and undifferentiated (0 per cent).[50] Similarly, the differentiation into medullary and cortical types has been shown to offer no prognostic information in one series,[34] whereas in another series the presence of cortical morphologic appearance was associated with a malignant clinical course.[16]

The differentiation between benign and malignant disease is determined by the presence of gross invasion of adjacent structures, metastasis, or microscopic evidence of capsular invasion. However, using morphometric analysis of the nuclei of thymomas, invasive thymomas are histologically more malignant than are noninvasive thymomas. Of interest, nuclei in noninvasive thymomas from patients with associated myasthenia gravis are larger than from those patients without myasthenia gravis. Fifteen to 65 per cent of thymomas are benign. The relative percentage is partially related to early surgical treatment of myasthenia gravis; if thymectomy is performed early in the course of myasthenia gravis, a greater percentage of thymomas are benign.

Whenever possible, the therapy for thymoma is surgical excision without removing or injuring vital structures. Even with well-encapsulated thymomas, extended thymectomy with eradication of all accessible mediastinal fatty areolar tissue should be performed to ensure removal of all ectopic thymic tissue. This approach has been shown to lower the number of tumor recurrences. The best operative exposure is obtained using a median sternotomy. Because many thymomas are radiosensitive, the placement of surgical clips to outline the anatomic extent of disease aids in the determination of optimal radiation portals.

In patients with myasthenia gravis, perioperative patient management is extremely important to prevent complications. Discontinuation of anticholinesterase inhibitors decreases the amount of pulmonary secretions and prevents inadvertent cholinergic weakness. This is usually possible with the routine use of plasmapheresis within 72 hours of thymectomy. In the majority of patients, plasmapheresis is very effective in controlling generalized weakness. Also, careful attention to the mainte-

nance of pulmonary function with chest physiotherapy, endotracheal suctioning, and bronchodilators is the mainstay of postoperative management. Decision to extubate is based on evidence of adequate respiratory mechanics (e.g., vital capacity greater than 15 ml. per kg. and expiratory pressures greater than 40 cm. of water) rather than evidence of adequate ventilation as determined by analysis of arterial blood gases. Historically, myasthenic patients with thymoma had a poor prognosis. The introduction of plasmapheresis and improvements in anesthesia and medical therapy have eliminated the presence of myasthenia gravis as an adverse prognostic indicator. The prognosis in patients with thymoma is dependent on the stage of the disease.

Staging of thymoma is as follows: Stage I, tumor is well encapsulated without evidence of gross or microscopic capsular invasion; Stage II, tumor exhibits pericapsular growth into adjacent mediastinal fat, pleura, or pericardium; Stage III, tumor invades adjacent organs or intrathoracic metastasis is present; Stage IV, there is extrathoracic metastatic spread, which occurs uncommonly. The adjunctive use of radiation therapy with a dose of 3500 to 5000 rads is the recommended treatment for Stage II and Stage III disease. In one series with Stage II or Stage III disease following complete resection, the 5-year actuarial mediastinal relapse rate was 53 per cent in those patients not receiving radiation therapy, 0 per cent in those receiving radiation therapy, and 21 per cent in those with biopsy alone and radiation therapy.[11] In patients with resectable Stage III disease, excellent long-term results can be obtained with radiotherapy: 100 per cent 5-year survival and 95 per cent 10- and 15-year survival.[41] Preoperative radiation therapy is useful when superior vena caval obstruction is present or when extensive invasion is manifested by CT or MRI. Occasionally, tumors not resectable on initial exploration are resectable following therapy. In patients with Stage IV disease or recurrent disease that is unresponsive to prior therapy, multiagent chemotherapy (CHOP—cyclophosphamide, hydroxyl daunomycin, Oncovin, prednisone; CAP—doxorubicin, cyclophosphamide, and *cis*-platinum) has been used. Complete response rates of approximately 40 per cent with 3-year survival of 34 per cent have been achieved.[21] Aggressive multimodality therapy using radiation, chemotherapy, and surgical resection has been advocated by a number of groups for aggressive thymomas. The prognosis for patients with thymoma is dependent on clinical stage; 5-year survival is as follows: Stage I, 85 to 100 per cent; Stage II, 60 to 80 per cent; Stage III, 40 to 70 per cent; and Stage IV, 50 per cent.[40,50]

Germ Cell Tumors

Germ cell tumors are benign and malignant neoplasms thought to originate from primordial germ cells that fail to complete the migration from the urogenital ridge and come to rest in the mediastinum. These tumors are classified as teratomas and teratocarcinomas, seminomas, embryonal cell carcinomas, choriocarcinoma, and endodermal cell (yolk sac) tumors. Although these lesions are identical histologically to germ cell tumors originating in the gonads, they are not considered to be metastatic from primary gonadal tumors because mediastinal metastases from primary gonadal tumors are rare, and in over 95 per cent of patients with mediastinal germ cell tumors, no evidence of tumor was present in the testes in contrast to the high incidence of testicular involvement following therapy for apparently primary retroperitoneal tumor. Therapy restricted only to the mediastinum does not cause disease relapse in the testis. In patients with mediastinal germ cell tumors, the current recommendations for evaluating the testes are careful physical examination and ultrasonography. Biopsy is reserved for positive findings. Blind biopsy or orchiectomy is contraindicated.

Teratomas are neoplasms composed of multiple tissue elements derived from the three primitive embryonic layers foreign to the area in which they occur. The peak incidence is in the second and third decades of life. There is no sex predisposition. These tumors are located most commonly in the anterosuperior mediastinum, although 3 to 8 per cent occur in the posterior mediastinum. Symptoms when present are related to mechanical effects and include chest pain, cough, dyspnea, or symptoms related to recurrent pneumonitis. If a communication between the tumor and the tracheobronchial tree develops, the pathognomonic finding of a cough productive of hair or sebaceous material may result. Hematogenous infection of the cystic component of the tumor may cause symptoms of hemoptysis and recurrent infections due to contiguous spread. Unusual presentations include recurrent pericarditis or pericardial tamponade following invasion or rupture into the pericardium. Rupture into the pleural space may cause respiratory distress due to the markedly irritative nature of the cyst fluid. However, with the greater use of routine chest films, patients are diagnosed more frequently while asymptomatic and with much smaller tumors.

Although rare, the diagnosis of these tumors can be made on routine chest film by the identification of well-formed teeth. CT findings of a predominantly fatty mass with a denser dependent portion containing globular calcifications, bone, or teeth and a solid protuberance into a cystic cavity are considered specific. Despite occasional characteristic appearances using various imaging techniques, the diagnosis usually depends on microscopic examination.

The teratodermoid (dermoid) cyst is the simplest form. It is composed predominantly of derivatives of the epidermal layer including dermal and epidermal glands, hair, and sebaceous material. However, careful examination of the cyst wall usually reveals endodermal and mesodermal elements (Fig. 7). They are usually unilobular but occasionally are multilobular. Teratomas are histologically more complex. The solid component of the tumor contains well-differentiated elements of bone, cartilage, teeth, muscle, connective tissue, fibrous and lymphoid tissue, nerve, thymus, mucous and salivary glands, lung, liver, or pancreas. Pancreatic tissue appears to contain a greater volume of endocrine cells with a predominance of somatostatin-producing D cells. Malignant tumors are differentiated from benign by the presence of primitive or embryonic tissue. Therefore, diagnosis and therapy rely on surgical excision. For those benign tumors of such large size or involvement with adjacent mediastinal structures that complete resection is impossible, partial resection has relieved symptoms, frequently without relapse.

MALIGNANT GERM CELL TUMOR. Malignant germ cell tumors also occur predominantly in the anterosuperior mediastinum and represent approximately 4 per cent of the primary tumors and cysts in the collected series. Unlike the benign teratomas, there is a marked male predominance. The peak incidence is in the third and fourth decades of life. The majority of patients are symptomatic with chest pain, cough, dyspnea, and hemoptysis; the superior vena caval syndrome occurs commonly. The chest film usually demonstrates a large anterior mediastinal mass that is often multilobulated; frequently there is evidence of intrathoracic spread of disease. CT or MRI is most helpful in defining the extent of involvement for the purpose of providing a means of following response to therapy and diagnosing relapses. These imaging modalities are also useful in determining impingement on vital structures that may contraindicate general anesthesia. Serologic measurements of alpha-fetoprotein and β-HCG are useful for the following tasks: differentiating seminomas from nonseminomas, quantitatively assessing response to therapy in hormonally active tumors (plasma half-life of alpha-fetoprotein and β-HCG is 5 days and 12 to 24 hours, respectively), and diagnosing relapse or failure of therapy prior to changes that can be observed in gross disease. Seminomas rarely produce β-HCG (7 per cent) and never produce alpha-fetoprotein; in contrast, over 90 per cent of nonseminomas secrete one or both of these hormones. This differ-

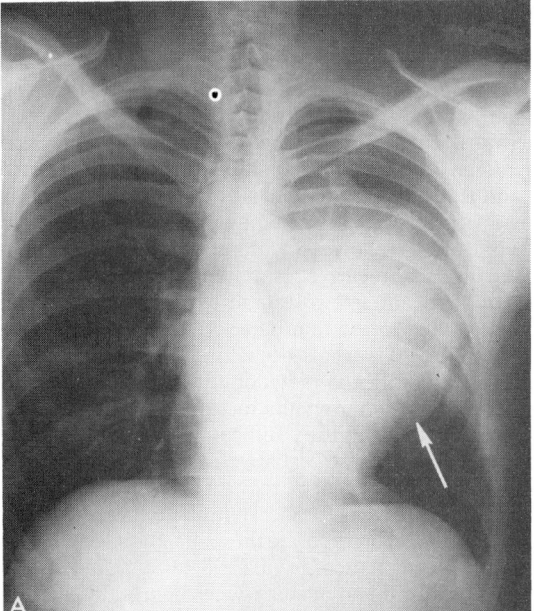
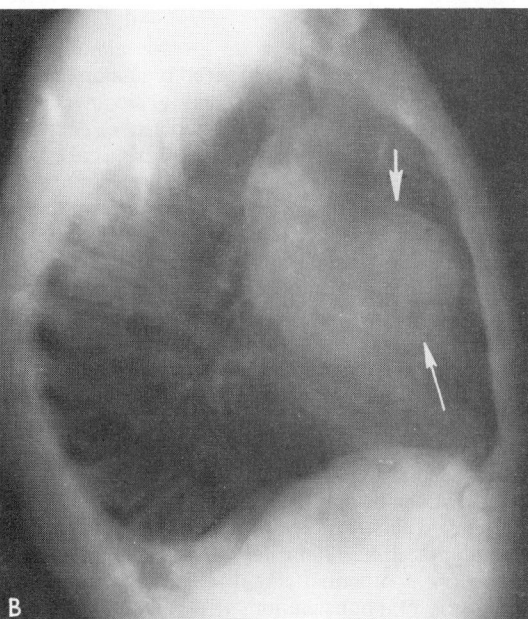

Figure 7. Chest films demonstrating teratoma of the anterior mediastinum.

entiation is important because of the marked radiosensitivity of seminomas and the relative radioinsensitivity of nonseminomas. In a multi-institutional study, 11 of 12 patients with mediastinal seminomas had local control with radiotherapy, whereas none of 13 patients with other germ cell histologic types had local control using radiotherapy.[31]

SEMINOMA. Seminomas comprise 50 per cent of malignant germ cell tumors and approximately 2 to 4 per cent of all mediastinal masses. These tumors predominantly occur in the anterosuperior mediastinum. Unlike other malignant germ cell tumors, seminomas usually remain intrathoracic with local extension to adjacent mediastinal and pulmonary structures. Although metastatic spread occurs first through lymphatics, hematogenous spread with extrathoracic involvement may develop late in the course of disease. Bone and lung are the most common sites of metastatic spread, although liver, brain, spleen, tonsil, and subcutaneous tissue also can be involved. Patients are usually symptomatic owing to the mechanical effects of the tumor on adjacent structures. The most common symptoms are chest pain, cough, lethargy, and weight loss. The superior vena caval syndrome occurs in 10 to 20 per cent of patients. The histologic appearance of this tumor is characterized by large cells with round nuclei, scant cytoplasm, and abundant glycogen.

Therapy is determined by the stage of the disease. Occasionally, excision is possible without injury to vital structures (22 per cent) and is recommended when possible. When complete resection is possible, the use of adjuvant therapy is unnecessary. However, careful follow-up with serial CT examinations is required to diagnose recurrences. When excision is not possible, a biopsy of sufficient size to establish the diagnosis should be obtained. Owing to the radiosensitivity of this tumor and the excellent control of local disease with radiation therapy, cytoreductive resection prior to radiation therapy is unnecessary and is contraindicated when vital structures are involved or when the procedure is technically difficult. The basis of therapy is megavoltage radiation to a shaped mediastinal field including the supraclavicular and neck regions (sites of initial lymphatic spread of disease). When cervical lymph nodes are involved, the field is expanded to incorporate the axilla, the site of subsequent lymphatic spread. A dosage of 4500 to 5000 rads (midplane dosage) is usually given over a 6-week course. In patients with extrathoracic disease, relapse following appropriate therapy, or sufficient intrathoracic disease to preclude the likelihood of a complete response using radiation therapy alone, multiagent chemotherapy has successfully induced remission in a majority of patients using either VBP (vinblastine, bleomycin, and *cis*-platinum, 59 per cent) or VAB-6 (vinblastine, dactinomycin, cyclophosphamide, and *cis*-platinum, 86 per cent). Etoposide and *cis*-platinum may be equally efficacious.

NONSEMINOMA. Malignant nonseminoma tumors include choriocarcinoma, embryonal cell carcinoma, malignant teratoma, and yolk sac (endodermal cell) tumors of which 40 per cent are a mixture of tissue types. The nonseminomas differ from seminomas in several aspects: (1) they are more aggressive tumors that are frequently disseminated at the time of diagnosis, (2) they are rarely radiosensitive, and (3) over 90 per cent produce either β-HCG or alpha-fetoprotein. All patients with choriocarcinoma and some patients with embryonal cell tumors have elevated levels of β-HCG, a hormone secreted by the syncytiotrophoblast. Alpha-fetoprotein is most commonly elevated in patients with embryonal cell carcinomas and yolk sac tumors. The presence of a significantly elevated titer of β-HCG or an elevated titer of alpha-fetoprotein is indicative of a nonseminoma germ cell component (Fig. 8). These tumors follow the natural history of a nonseminoma.

As with seminomas, the majority of patients with these neoplasms are symptomatic with chest pain, dyspnea, weight loss, cough, hemoptysis, fever and chills, and the superior vena caval syndrome (20 per cent). Patients are predominantly male and in the third or fourth decades. Chest films usually reveal a large anterior mediastinal mass with frequent extension into lung parenchyma and adjacent mediastinal structures. In addition to superior vena caval obstruction, they may cause pulmonary stenosis and coarctation of the aorta. Characteristically, these tumors have extensive intrathoracic involvement and frequently have metastasized outside of the thorax. Frequent sites of metastatic disease include brain, lung, liver, bones, and the lymphatic system, particularly the supraclavicular nodes. Chest wall involvement is common.

A number of chromosomal abnormalities are associated with an increased incidence of germ cell tumors, including Klinefelter's syndrome, trisomy 8, and 5q deletion. In one series of patients with germ cell tumors, the incidence of Klinefelter's syndrome was 22 per cent.[43] These patients were younger (median age of 15), and their tumors were nonseminomas. Additionally, mediastinal but not testicular germ cell tumors are associated with the development of rare hematologic malignan-

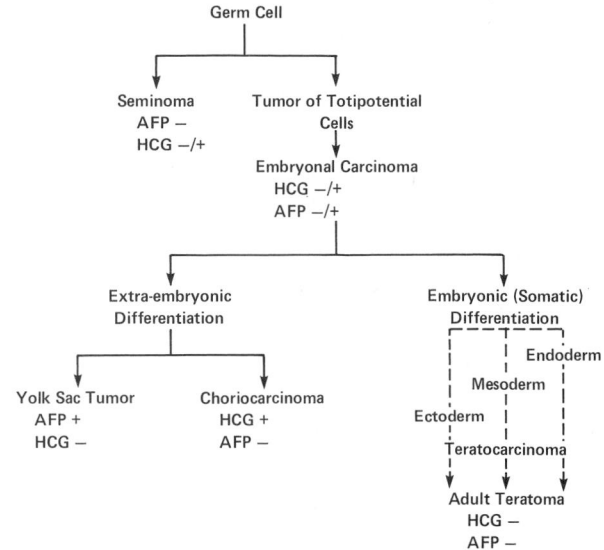

Figure 8. Interrelationships of germ cell tumors and tumor markers—alpha-fetoprotein (AFP) and beta-human chorionic gonadotropin (HCG). (Adapted from Sandhaus, I., Strom, R. L., and Mukai, K.: Primary embryonal choriocarcinoma of the mediastinum in a woman. Am. J. Clin. Pathol., 75:573, 1981.)

cies such as acute megakaryocytic leukemia and malignant histiocytosis as well as other hematologic abnormalities including the myelodysplastic syndrome and idiopathic thrombocytopenia refractory to treatment. One hypothesis for this association is the common derivation from a totipotent germ cell capable of hematopoietic differentiation that is dependent on the mediastinal environment for development.

The local invasiveness of these tumors and frequent metastases usually preclude surgical resection of all disease at the time of diagnosis. Initially, operative intervention is necessary only to establish the histologic diagnosis. Multiagent chemotherapy including *cis*-platinum is the basis of therapy. Other agents to which these tumors respond include vinblastine, bleomycin, methotrexate, etoposide, and doxorubicin. Following induction of therapy, operative exploration with removal of as much residual disease as possible without injuring vital structures is indicated. Patients with normalization of alpha-fetoprotein and β-HCG after induction chemotherapy (achievable in up to 60 per cent) have a good long-term prognosis.[30] The presence of residual disease following re-exploration portends an extremely poor prognosis. Using surgical resection as an adjuvant to multiagent chemotherapy, complete responses of 20 to 80 per cent have been reported.

A subset of these tumors also contains malignant tissue that is not germ cell in origin. The histology is adenocarcinoma or sarcoma. Malignant teratomas or other germ cell tumors with mature differentiated teratoma within the primary are most commonly involved. Non–germ cell malignant transformation occurred in 29 per cent of patients studied at autopsy.[2] Despite response of the germ cell component to chemotherapy, there is usually progression of the non–germ cell component. In these patients, the only effective treatment has been surgical resection, which is rarely possible. The overall prognosis is poor.

Lymphomas

Although the mediastinum is frequently involved in patients with lymphoma sometime during the course of the disease (40 to 70 per cent), it is infrequently the sole site of disease at the time of presentation. Only 5 to 10 per cent of patients with Hodgkin's and non-Hodgkin's lymphomas present solely with symptoms due to local mass effects, such as mediastinal involvement. Patients are usually symptomatic; chest pain, cough, dyspnea, hoarseness, and the superior vena caval syndrome are the most common clinical manifestations. Lymphomas also can cause a clinical pattern compatible with pulmonary stenosis and pulmonary embolism by encasement of the pulmonary artery. Nonspecific systemic symptoms of fever and chills, weight loss, and anorexia are frequently noted and are important in the staging of patients with Hodgkin's lymphoma. Symptoms characteristic of Hodgkin's lymphoma include chest pain after consumption of alcohol and the cyclic fevers that were first described by Pel and Ebstein.

Characteristically, these tumors occur in the anterosuperior mediastinum or in the hilar region of the middle mediastinum. CT and MRI are useful in delineating the extent of disease, determining invasiveness into contiguous structures, differentiating the lesions from cardiovascular abnormalities, aiding the selection of radiation portals, and following the response to therapy and diagnosing relapse. Also, differentiation from thymomas and germ cell tumors, which usually are solitary masses, is possible because lymphomas are usually composed of multiple involved nodes that appear as separate masses by CT.

HODGKIN'S LYMPHOMA. The Hodgkin's lymphomas are subdivided by histologic appearance into nodular sclerosing, lymphocyte predominant, mixed cellularity, and lymphocyte depleted. Mediastinal involvement is most common with nodu-

lar sclerosing (55 to 75 per cent) (Fig. 9) and lymphocyte predominant (40 per cent). Treatment of Hodgkin's lymphoma is determined by the stage of disease and is based on radiation therapy and chemotherapy (MOPP—nitrogen mustard, vincristine, procarbazine, prednisone; CHOP). Surgical excision of all disease is rarely possible, and the surgeon's primary role is to provide sufficient tissue for diagnosis and to assist in pathologic staging, a process frequently requiring staging exploratory laparotomy. Although extrathoracic lymph nodes are frequently involved and available for biopsy, when the sole site of involvement is the mediastinum, a needle biopsy is often unsuccessful because larger tissue samples are needed to make a histologic diagnosis particularly with nodular sclerosing lesions. Thoracotomy, mediastinoscopy, or mediastinotomy may be necessary to obtain sufficient tissue. Although surgical excision, when possible, provides adequate therapy, more often Stage IA and Stage IIA disease as defined by the Ann Arbor classification is treated with megavoltage external beam radiation with a total dose of 4500 rads. Ten-year survival greater than 90 per cent has been reported. Patients with Stage IIB, Stage III, and Stage IV disease are usually treated with chemotherapy. Patients with higher grade tumor, advanced stage of disease, persistence of an abnormal erythrocyte sedimentation rate, extensive mediastinal

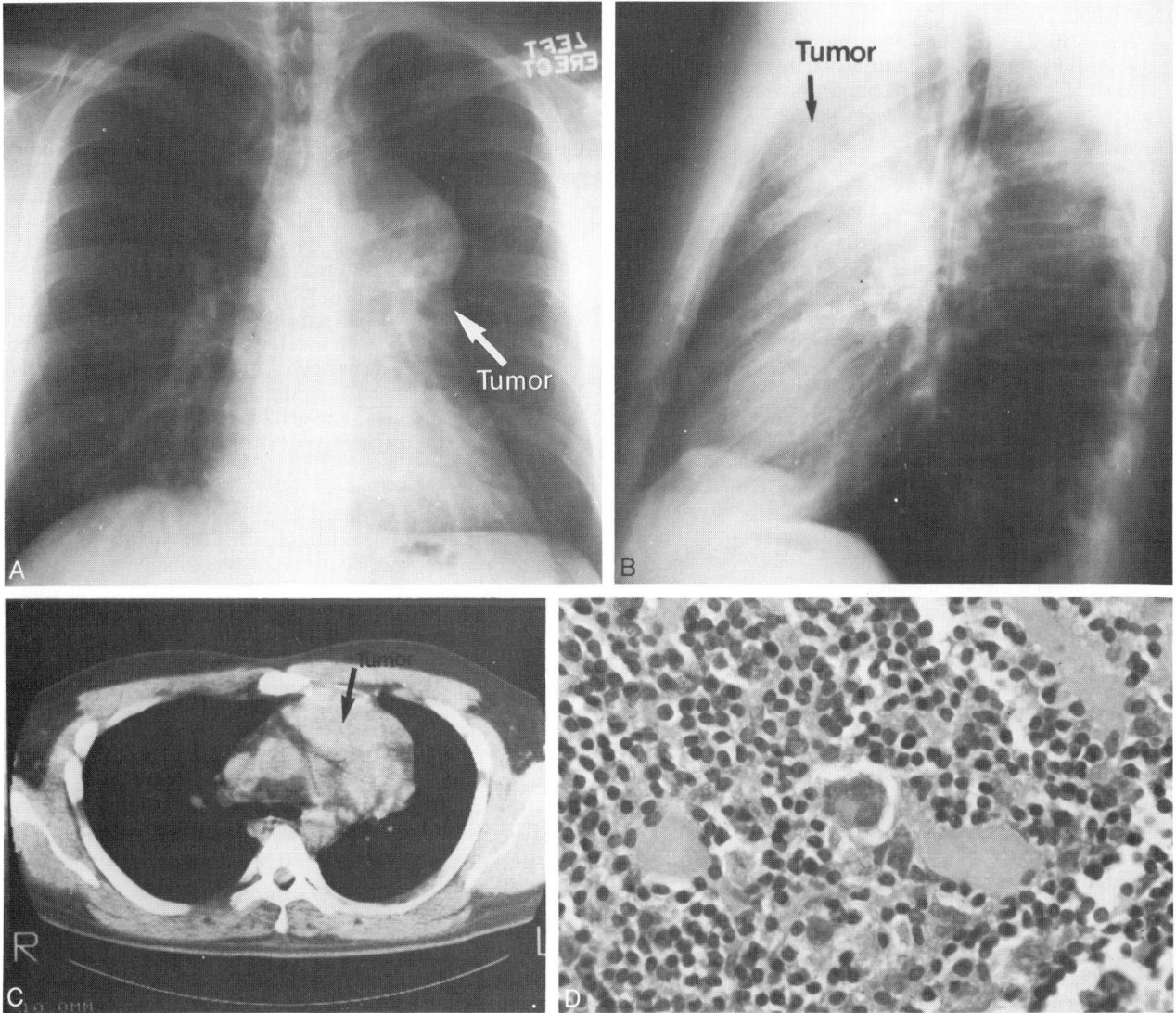

Figure 9. A and B, Chest films of an anterior mediastinal Hodgkin's tumor. C, CT image demonstrates the invasive nature of the tumor. D, The characteristic Reed-Sternberg cell is shown. (From Davis, R. D., Jr., Oldham, H. N., Jr., and Sabiston, D. C., Jr.: The mediastinum. In Sabiston, D. C., Jr., and Spencer, F. C. (Eds.): Surgery of the Chest, 5th ed. Philadelphia, W. B. Saunders Company, 1990.)

disease, and advanced age (greater than 50 years) are at an increased risk of disease relapse.

Controversy continues concerning the treatment of patients with extensive mediastinal disease as defined by tumor size greater than 35 per cent of the cardiothoracic diameter. These patients have a higher relapse rate when treated with radiation therapy alone. Although combining chemotherapy with radiation therapy reduces the relapse rate, prolongation of survival has not necessarily resulted because of the efficacy of salvage chemotherapy and the significant risk of secondary malignancies following the use of alkylating chemotherapeutic agents.

Residual abnormalities within the mediastinum are commonly noted radiographically following treatment of Hodgkin's disease (64 to 88 per cent).[28,45] These abnormalities include minimal mediastinal widening in 44 per cent of patients and widening greater than 6 cm. in 41 per cent. In 27 to 41 per cent of patients, radiographic abnormalities persist more than a year. Residual radiographic abnormality is more common in patients with initial bulky mediastinal disease. Residual mediastinal abnormalities were not significantly associated with eventual disease relapse except when treatment was with chemotherapy alone. In addition, benign thymic cysts appear to be more common following radiation therapy for anterior mediastinal neoplasms. Optimal therapy is surgical excision without additional chemotherapy or radiation therapy.

NON-HODGKIN'S LYMPHOMA. Non-Hodgkin's lymphomas are usually of lymphoblastic morphology (60 per cent) or large cell morphology with a diffuse pattern of growth (40 per cent). In 40 to 80 per cent of patients with lymphoblastic lymphoma, the mediastinum is involved. Although all ages may be afflicted, the peak incidence is in the second and third decades of life. Lymphoblastic lymphoma is characterized by (1) advanced stage of disease at presentation with 91 per cent of patients having Stage III or Stage IV disease, (2) early bone marrow involvement with frequent development of leukemia, (3) tumor cells that exhibit T lymphocyte antigens, (4) early metastatic spread to the leptomeninges, and (5) initial responsiveness to radiation therapy uniformly followed by relapse. Lymphoblastic lymphomas can be divided histologically into convoluted, nonconvoluted, and large cell, of which the convoluted and nonconvoluted preferentially involve the mediastinum. In the majority of lymphoblastic lymphomas, intermediate (CD1[+], CD4[+], or CD8[+]) or mature (CD3[+]) T-cell differentiation is present (62 per cent and 32 per cent, respectively). Those with an intermediate T cell differentiation are the subgroup most likely to have a mediastinal mass.[10] T cell acute lymphoid leukemia has morphologic and clinical similarities to lymphoblastic lymphoma, and approximately 70 per cent of patients manifest a mediastinal mass.

Operative intervention is limited to obtaining sufficient tissue to establish the diagnosis and, if necessary, to perform immunologic subtyping. The best results have been obtained using aggressive chemotherapy in conjunction with central nervous system prophylaxis of which the APO protocol (prednisone, vincristine, doxorubicin, 6-mercaptopurine, asparaginase, and methotrexate) has yielded the best results (nearly 100 per cent complete response following induction therapy with subsequent low rate of relapse). Patients with tumors exhibiting immature T cell differentiation (CD2[+] or CD7[+]) appear to have higher relapse rates.[53]

The large cell lymphomas of diffuse growth pattern (DHL) are a heterogeneous group differing in the cell type of origin, clinical presentation, natural history, and response to therapy. The DHL tumors can be subclassified into at least three diseases: T immunoblastic sarcoma, B immunoblastic sarcoma, and sclerosing variants of follicular cell lymphoma. The T immunoblastic sarcomas are characterized by morphologic appearance similar to peripheral T cell lymphomas, slight female predominance,

smaller, more confined masses that usually remain intrathoracic, and a higher incidence of causing the superior vena caval syndrome.

In comparison, the B immunoblastic and sclerosing follicular cell lymphomas are more aggressive tumors with more extensive intra- and extrathoracic involvement. The peak incidence is in the third and fourth decades with no clear gender predisposition. Operative intervention is useful in obtaining tissue for diagnosis, which often requires immunotyping, but is rarely important with regard to therapy. These tumors may be confused with thymomas, germ cell tumors, anaplastic carcinoid tumors, and Hodgkin's lymphoma if the light microscopic appearance alone is used. This is especially true if prior radiation therapy or chemotherapy has been administered. Although needle biopsy frequently does not provide sufficient tumor specimen to establish the diagnosis, extrathoracic tissue is often available for biopsy. Therapy is based on doxorubicin-containing chemotherapeutic protocols (CHOP ± bleomycin; ACOMLA—Adriamycin, cyclophosphamide, vincristine, methotrexate with leucovorin rescue, cytarabine; BACOP—bleomycin, Adriamycin, cyclophosphamide, vincristine, prednisone), which can induce complete responses in over 90 per cent of patients with relapse-free survival of 50 to 74 per cent after 2 years.

Primary Carcinoma

Primary carcinomas of the mediastinum comprise between 3 and 11 per cent of primary mediastinal masses in most series and represent 5 per cent of the mediastinal masses in the collected series. The origin of these tumors is unknown. However, it is important to differentiate them from malignant thymomas, germ cell tumors, carcinoid tumors, lymphomas, mediastinal extension of bronchogenic carcinomas, and metastatic tumors, which may have a similar light microscopic appearance. Metastatic disease in mediastinal lymph nodes is usually from bronchogenic or esophageal malignancies and rarely occurs with extrathoracic malignancies. Only 2.3 per cent of 1071 patients with extrathoracic neoplasms developed evidence of hilar or mediastinal lymph node involvement over a 2-year period as determined by serial chest films. The tumors most likely to metastasize to the mediastinum include those originating in the breast, head and neck, and genitourinary tract as well as melanomas. Primary carcinomas are usually of the large cell, undifferentiated morphologic type, although small cell and squamous cell have been described. Electron microscopic examination of the tumor ultrastructure and the increasing number of immunofluorescent stains for surface antigens and cellular proteins specific for a number of malignancies may define better the origin of some of these primary carcinomas.

These tumors occur with equal frequency in either sex. The majority of patients are symptomatic owing to the local mass effects of the tumor. These include chest pain, cough, dyspnea, hoarseness, dysphagia, and the superior vena caval syndrome. Extensive involvement within the thorax and often metastatic disease outside of the thorax characterize this disease. Surgical excision is rarely possible. Unfortunately, the routine use of radiation therapy and chemotherapy has been unsuccessful in prolonging survival. Only 2 of 32 patients treated at the Duke University Medical Center are alive at 6 and 11 years following surgical excision or biopsy and radiation therapy, respectively. Overall, the mean survival is less than 1 year.

Endocrine Tumors

THYROID TUMORS. Although substernal extension of a cervical goiter is common, totally intrathoracic thyroid tumors are rare and comprise only 1 per cent of all mediastinal masses in the collected series. In a series of 17,000 patients undergoing thyroidectomy, only 135 intrathoracic goiters were encountered. These tumors arise from heterotopic thyroid tissue that occurs most commonly in the anterosuperior mediastinum but may also occur in the middle mediastinum between the trachea and esophagus as well as in the posterior mediastinum. Although there may be a demonstrable connection with the cervical gland, usually a fibrous connective tissue band, a true intrathoracic thyroid gland derives its blood supply from thoracic vessels.

The peak incidence is in the sixth and seventh decades. Females are more commonly affected. When these lesions occur in the anterosuperior or middle mediastinum, symptoms related to tracheal compression often are present such as dyspnea, cough, wheezing, and stridor. When these tumors occur in the posterior mediastinum, esophageal compression manifested by dysphagia is common. Rarely, symptoms related to thyrotoxicosis may be the initiating factor for a patient to seek medical attention. On chest films, these lesions appear as sharply circumscribed, dense masses, occurring more frequently on the right. Intrathoracic goiters are contrast-enhancing lesions when visualized by CT. The administration of iodinated contrast material causes prolonged enhancement of thyroid tissue. When functioning thyroid tissue is present, the radioactive iodine (^{131}I) scan is usually diagnostic. However, some of these neoplasms are functionally inactive and are not identified by ^{131}I scanning. In asymptomatic patients with anterosuperior or posterosuperior masses, ^{131}I scanning should be performed to document the presence of functioning cervical thyroid tissue to prevent the removal of the sole functioning thyroid tissue.

The majority of these tumors are adenomas, but carcinomas have been reported. If the lesion is identified as the sole functioning thyroid tissue and the patient is asymptomatic, surgical exploration and excision is not indicated. In these patients, frequent follow-up radiographic examinations are indicated to evaluate changes in the size or nature of the lesion. Otherwise, these lesions should be resected because of the propensity to enlarge and compress adjacent structures. Because of thoracic derivation of the blood supply, intrathoracic thyroid tumors should be approached through the thorax, using either an anterolateral thoracotomy or median sternotomy for anterior lesions, or a posterolateral thoracotomy for posterior lesions. Substernal extensions of a cervical goiter can usually be excised using a cervical approach.

PARATHYROID TUMORS. Although parathyroid glands may occur in the mediastinum in 10 per cent of patients, they are usually accessible through the cervical incision. A sternotomy incision is necessary to excise a hyperfunctioning parathyroid gland in approximately 2.5 per cent of all patients and 15 per cent of those with a mediastinal gland.[9,51] Most often these adenomas are found in the anterosuperior mediastinum embedded in or near the superior pole of the thymus. This anatomic relationship is the result of the common embryogenesis of the inferior parathyroid glands from the third branchial cleft. The superior parathyroid glands and the lateral lobes of the thyroid gland are derived from the fourth branchial pouch. Because they migrate with the lateral lobes of the thyroid gland to a paraesophageal position, they are found in the posterior mediastinum when they migrate further caudad. Factors contributing to the caudal movement of parathyroid glands into the mediastinum include negative intrathoracic pressure, gravity, and the movement of the pharynx and larynx with deglutition.

The clinical manifestations of a mediastinal parathyroid tumor are similar to those that occur with tumors of the cervical region; symptoms are related to the excess secretion of parathyroid hormone causing the hyperparathyroid syndrome. Because of their small size, these neoplasms rarely cause symptoms related to mechanical effects and are not often visualized using conventional roentgenography. Using CT, MRI, thallium, and technetium scanning, venous angiography with selective sampling, and selective arteriography, preoperative localization of these tumors can be made in approximately 80 per cent of patients.

Most frequently, the mediastinal adenoma may be excised following a negative exploration of the cervical region through the existing cervical incision. Usually, the vascular supply to the adenoma extends from cervical blood vessels. Mediastinal exploration using a median sternotomy is indicated in those patients with persistent hyperparathyroidism producing severe biochemical or metabolic disease following an unsuccessful cervical exploration in which four normal glands have been identified.[51] Approximately 80 per cent of mediastinal parathyroids are located in the anterior mediastinum, with the majority of the remaining 20 per cent occurring in the posterior mediastinum.[9] Almost 75 per cent of the mediastinal parathyroids are found within or adjacent to the thymus. If an adenoma is not found following a systematic exploration of the mediastinum, which may require incision of the pleura and pericardium, removal of the thymus and the perithymic fatty areolar tissue is recommended.

Parathyroid carcinomas have been reported and are usually hormonally active. Patients differ in clinical presentation in that they often have higher serum calcium levels and manifest more severe symptoms of hyperparathyroidism. When possible, surgical resection is the optimal therapy.

Unlike parathyroid adenomas and carcinomas, parathyroid cysts are usually not hormonally active. These cysts are defined by the presence of parathyroid cells identifiable within the cyst wall. Because these lesions are frequently larger than adenomas, symptoms related to local mass effects are more common, as is visualization on chest films. Surgical excision yields a cure.

CARCINOID TUMORS. Mediastinal carcinoid tumors arise from cells of Kulchitsky located in the thymus. Occurring more often in male patients, these tumors usually are located in the anterosuperior mediastinum. Although these tumors originate from the thymus, they are not associated with myasthenia gravis or red cell aplasia, nor are they associated with the carcinoid syndrome. However, due to their origin from APUD cells, these tumors may be hormonally active, and they may occur as a variant of the multiple endocrine neoplastic syndromes. Mediastinal carcinoids have been most frequently associated with Cushing's syndrome due to production of adrenocorticotropic hormone. In a series of 15 patients with mediastinal carcinoid, 5 patients had clinical evidence of Cushing's syndrome, and a sixth had elevated adrenocorticotropic hormone levels without any clinical stigmata.[52] In addition, 1 of the 15 had Type I multiple endocrine neoplastic syndrome, whereas 3 others had variants of a multiple endocrine neoplastic syndrome.

In patients with hormonally inactive tumors, symptoms are related to local mass effects causing chest pain, dyspnea, cough, and the superior vena caval syndrome. Hormonally inactive carcinoids tend to be larger and frequently are invasive locally. In addition, metastatic spread to mediastinal and cervical lymph nodes, liver, bone, skin, and lungs occurs in the majority of patients. In the series of 15 patients, 73 per cent developed metastatic disease, with late development of metastases in 3 of the 15 patients (initial metastasis discovered at 5, 6, and 8 years, respectively).

Often, these tumors are difficult to differentiate from other common anterior mediastinal masses, particularly thymomas and germ cell tumors. However, carcinoids are characterized by the ultrastructural findings of dense core neurosecretory granules. Positive immunohistochemical staining for adrenocorticotropic hormone of these granules also is characteristic. Surgical removal when possible is the preferred treatment. When local invasiveness or metastasis precludes the successful use of operative therapy, radiation therapy and multiagent chemotherapy have been used, although no consistent benefit has been documented.

Mesenchymal Tumors

Mediastinal mesenchymal tumors originate from the connective tissue, striatal and smooth muscle, fat, lymphatic tissue, and blood vessels present within the mediastinum, producing a diverse group of neoplasms. Relative to other sites in the body, these tumors occur less commonly within the mediastinum. Mesenchymal tumors comprised 6 per cent of the primary masses in the collected series. There is no apparent difference in incidence between sexes. The soft tissue neoplasms include lipomas, liposarcomas, fibrosarcomas, fibromas, xanthogranulomas, leiomyomas, leiomyosarcomas, benign and malignant mesenchymomas, rhabdomyosarcomas, and mesotheliomas. These tumors have a similar histologic appearance and generally follow the same clinical course as the soft tissue tumors found elsewhere in the body. Fifty-five per cent of these tumors are malignant. Surgical resection remains the primary therapy, since poor results have been obtained using radiation and chemotherapy.

Similarly, the mesenchymal tumors derived from blood and lymph vessel are common elsewhere in the body, but rare in the mediastinum. Although these tumors occur anywhere in the mediastinum, the most frequent location is in the anterosuperior mediastinum. These tumors include the capillary, cavernous, and venous hemangiomas, hemangioendotheliomas, hemangiopericytomas, lymphangiomas, and derivatives of lymphangiomas. Symptoms are related to the size and invasiveness of the lesion. Occasionally, hemorrhage into the lesion may cause a rapid increase in the size. Significant compression and obstruction of mediastinal structures may result, causing a variety of clinical manifestations of which respiratory failure is the most dramatic. Rupture of hemangiomas into the pleural space may cause exsanguination; rupture into the mediastinum may cause tamponade.

Differentiation between the vascular tumors is based on the morphologic appearance: the size of the vascular space, the relative number and amount of pericytes, smooth muscle, and endothelial cells. Between 10 and 30 per cent of vascular tumors are malignant, although the differentiation may be difficult because the histologic appearance, the number of mitotic figures, and even the gross appearance are often similar. Vascular tumors are not well encapsulated, and even benign tumors may exhibit local invasion. However, the incidence of metastatic spread is low, approximately 3 per cent. Hemangiopericytomas have the highest incidence of malignancy, and these tumors usually occur in older patients. Vascular tumors have a variable roentgenographic appearance from a small discrete lesion to a large multilobulated lesion with ill-defined borders. Because these neoplasms are not supplied by large vessels, tumor opacification usually does not occur during angiographic studies. Excision remains the only effective means of therapy, although radiation therapy has been used with mixed results.

Tumors originating from lymphatic vessels are differentiated from tumors of blood vessel origin by using indirect evidence, such as the absence of red blood cells within the lumen of the tumor vasculature, the extrusion of chylous fluid from the cut edges, and the tumor's relationship to documented lymphatic tissue. Also, these tumors usually occur in the anterior mediastinum, appearing as round or lobulated cystic densities on chest films. The most common lymphatic tumor is the lymphangioma (also termed cystic hygroma, lymphatic cyst, and lymphatogenous cyst), which in the majority of patients occurs in the superior mediastinum as an extension of a cervical lesion. Only 17 per cent of mediastinal lymphangiomas are completely within the mediastinum, whereas 10 per cent of cervical lymphangiomas have a mediastinal extension. Lymphangiomas are usually diagnosed in children, and they frequently cause symptoms due to obstruction of the trachea, including stridor, dyspnea, recurrent pulmonary infection, and tachypnea. Growth of these tumors is by proliferation of endothelium-lined buds that spread along tissue planes. The local ingrowth of vessels and fibrous reaction to the endothelial buds prevent easy surgical removal owing to the lack of well-defined tissue planes. However, because radiation therapy and sclerotherapy have not been successful, resection is the optimal treatment.

Extramedullary Hematopoiesis

Extramedullary hematopoiesis occurs in all age groups usually following altered hematopoiesis. In the adult, this is typically due to massive hemolysis, myelofibrosis, spherocytic anemia, or thalassemia. These lesions appear as bilateral, asymmetric paravertebral masses. They are contrast-enhancing lesions as visualized by CT, a modality that is useful for determining the presence of intraspinal extension. Because these tumors are composed of hematopoietic tissue, they are readily visualized using either radioactive iron (^{59}Fe) or radioisotope-labeled gold scanning. These scanning modalities are useful in differentiating these tumors from other mediastinal lesions in patients with known hematologic abnormalities. Surgical resection is unnecessary unless there is invasion or compression of mediastinal structures. Radiation therapy can produce rapid shrinkage of these masses.

Giant Lymph Node Hyperplasia (Castleman's Disease)

Giant lymph node hyperplasia was initially described by Castleman in 1954. Although the mediastinum was the site of disease in the initial report and in the majority of patients, these tumors may develop wherever lymph nodes are present; the retroperitoneum and the cervical, axillary, and pelvic regions are the most frequent nonmediastinal sites. These lesions have been described using different terms including angiofollicular lymphoid hyperplasia, lymphoid hamartoma, follicular lymphoreticuloma, angiomatosis, and benign giant lymphomas. Although these tumors are usually located in the anterosuperior mediastinum, they also are found in the posterior mediastinum and at the pericardiophrenic angle where they may be confused with neurogenic tumors and pericardial cysts, respectively. Two distinct histologic entities exist: (1) hyaline vascular, characterized by small hyaline follicles and interfollicular capillary proliferation, and (2) plasma cell, characterized by large follicles with intervening sheets of plasma cells. The tumors most frequently appear as single, well-demarcated lesions. The hyaline vascular type represents 90 per cent of Castleman's tumors, and these are most often discovered in the asymptomatic patient on a routine chest film. Patients with the plasma cell type often exhibit systemic symptoms including fever, night sweats, anemia, and hypergammaglobulinemia. Surgical excision effects cure, although resection of the hyaline vascular type may be associated with significant hemorrhage due to extreme vascularity.

Multicentric Castleman's disease is characterized by generalized lymphadenopathy with morphologic features of giant lymph node hyperplasia. Patients are most often symptomatic with fever, chills, weight loss, and hepatosplenomegaly and exhibit disordered immunity and autoimmune phenomena. Unlike the benign clinical course of classic Castleman's disease, multicentric disease is a much more malignant disease with frequent deaths following infectious complications. It has also been reported in association with HIV infection.

Chondroma

Chondromas are rare tumors that occur in the posterior mediastinum originating from the primitive notochord. Males are affected twice as frequently as are females, with the peak age of incidence in the fifth through seventh decades. Chest pain, cough, and dyspnea are the most common symptoms. Spinal cord compression may follow extension into the spinal canal. Radical surgical excision is the only effective therapy; however, the majority of patients develop distant metastases. The mean survival is approximately 17.5 months.

Primary Cysts

Primary cysts of the mediastinum comprise 18 per cent of the mediastinal masses in the collected series. These cysts can be bronchogenic, pericardial, enteric, thymic, or of an unspecified nature. More than 75 per cent of patients are asymptomatic, and these tumors rarely cause morbidity. However, due to the proximity of vital structures within the mediastinum, with increasing size even benign cysts may cause significant morbidity. In addition, these masses need to be differentiated from malignant tumors.

BRONCHOGENIC CYSTS. Bronchogenic cysts are the most common primary cysts of the mediastinum, comprising 6.3 per cent of primary mediastinal masses and 34 per cent of cysts. They originate as sequestrations from the ventral foregut, the antecedent of the tracheobronchial tree. The bronchogenic cyst may lie within the lung parenchyma or the mediastinum. The cyst wall is composed of cartilage, mucous glands, smooth muscle, and fibrous tissue with a pathognomonic inner layer of ciliated respiratory epithelium. When bronchogenic cysts occur in the mediastinum, they are usually located proximal to the trachea or bronchi and may be just posterior to the carina. Rarely, a true communication between the cyst and the tracheobronchial tree exists, and an air-fluid level may be observed on the chest film.

Two thirds of patients with bronchogenic cysts are asymptomatic. In infants, these cysts may cause severe respiratory compromise by compressing the trachea or the bronchus; compression of the bronchus may cause bronchial stenosis and recurrent pneumonitis. Since tumors occurring below the carina are sometimes not well visualized using standard roentgenography, the routine use of CT has been recommended to evaluate children with recurrent pulmonary infections for possible bronchogenic cyst. More often, bronchogenic cysts occur in older children and adults, in whom these cysts may cause symptoms of chest pain, dyspnea, cough, and stridor. Bronchogenic cysts appear as a smooth density at the carina level that may compress the esophagus on barium swallow. Differentiation from hilar structures may be difficult.

Surgical excision is recommended in all patients to provide definitive histologic diagnosis, alleviate symptoms, and prevent the development of associated complications. Malignant degeneration has been reported, as well as the presence of a bronchial adenoma within the cyst wall.

PERICARDIAL CYSTS. Pericardial cysts are the second most frequently encountered cysts within the mediastinum and comprise 6 per cent of all lesions and 33 per cent of primary cysts (Table 2). These cysts classically occur in the pericardiophrenic angles (Fig. 10), with 70 per cent in the right pericardiophrenic angle, 22 per cent in the left, and the remainder in other sites in the pericardium. The embryogenesis of these cysts is thought to follow failure of fusion of one or more mesenchymal lacunae that coalesce to form the pericardium, or a persistent ventral parietal recess of the pericardial coelom. Pericardial cysts may or may not have a communication with the pericardium. Numerous reports have described the characteristic CT appearance of pericardial cysts: pericardiophrenic location, near-water attenuation value, and smooth borders. Patients with lesions and classic CT characteristics for pericardial cysts have been managed with needle aspiration and follow-up with serial CT rather than surgical excision. Surgical excision of pericardial cysts is indicated primarily for diagnosis and to differentiate these cysts from malignant lesions.

ENTERIC CYSTS. Enteric cysts (duplication cysts) arise from the posterior division of the primitive foregut, which develops into the upper division of the gastrointestinal tract. These cysts are found less frequently than bronchogenic or pericardial cysts and comprise 2 per cent of the mediastinal masses in the collected series. They are also known as inclusion cysts, gastric cysts, or enterogenous cysts and are most frequently located in the posterior mediastinum, usually adjacent to the esophagus (Fig. 11).

These lesions are composed of smooth muscle with an inner epithelial lining of esophageal, gastric, or intestinal mucosa. When gastric mucosa is present, peptic ulceration with perforation into the esophageal or bronchial lumen may occur producing hemoptysis or hematemesis. Erosion into the lung parenchyma may cause hemorrhage and cause lung abscess formation. Gastric mucosa within enteric cysts may be visualized using [99]technetium scanning. Usually, enteric cysts have an attachment to the esophagus and may be embedded within the muscularis layer. Symptoms are usually due to compression of the esophagus causing obstruction, commonly presenting as dysphagia. Compromise of the tracheobronchial tree with symptoms of cough, dyspnea, recurrent pulmonary infections, and chest pain may also result. The majority of enteric cysts are

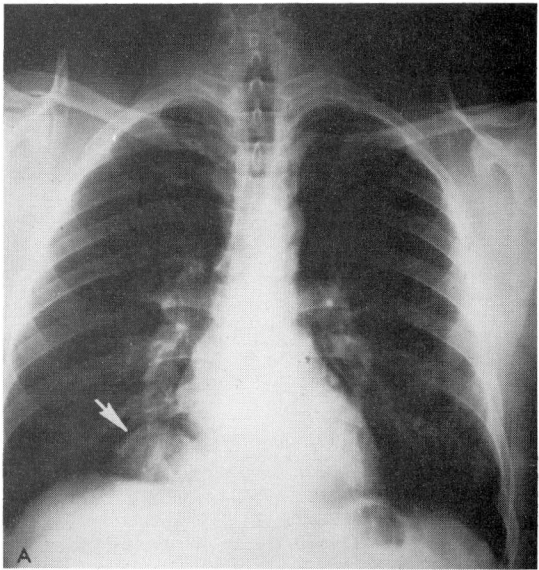

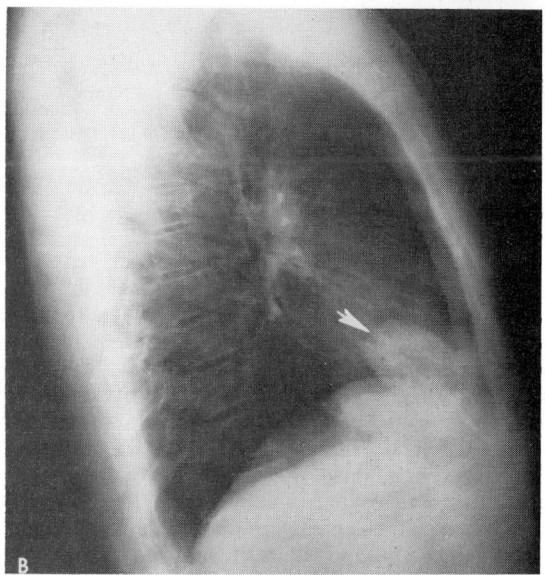

Figure 10. *A* and *B*, Chest films showing the typical location of a pericardial cyst in the right cardiophrenic angle. (From Sabiston, D. C., Jr., and Oldham, H. N., Jr.: The mediastinum. *In* Sabiston, D. C., Jr., and Spencer, F. C. (Eds.): Gibbon's Surgery of the Chest, 4th ed. Philadelphia, W. B. Saunders Company, 1983.)

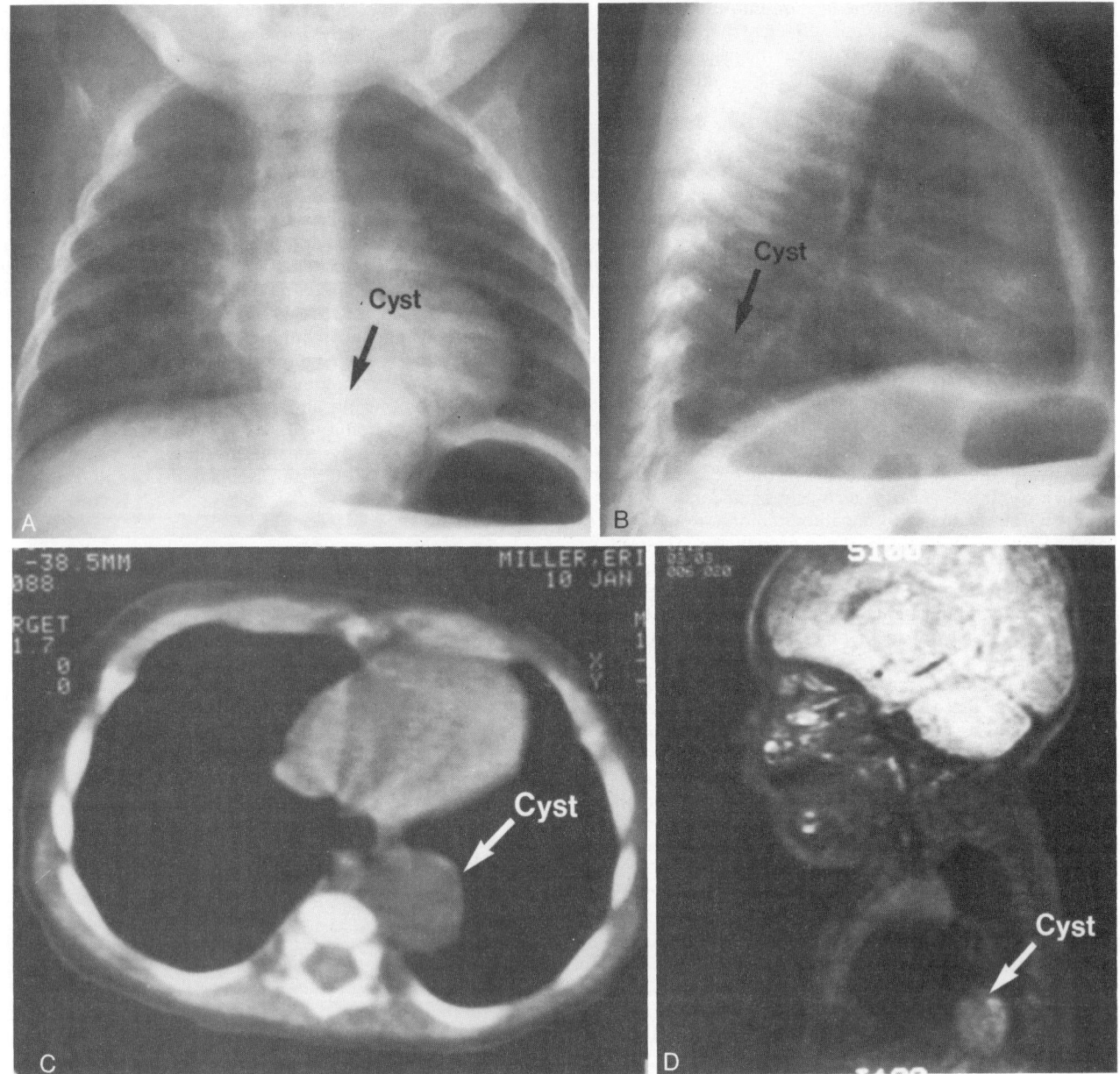

Figure 11. *A* and *B*, Chest films of a patient with an enteric cyst. *C*, CT delineates the anatomic location, but does not further differentiate the mass from a neurogenic tumor. *D*, MRI demonstrates the cystic nature of the mass and its relationship to the esophagus. (From Davis, R. D., Jr., and Sabiston, D. C., Jr.: Primary mediastinal cysts and neoplasms. *In* Sabiston, D. C., Jr.: Essentials of Surgery. Philadelphia, W. B. Saunders Company, 1987.)

diagnosed in children, who are also more likely to be symptomatic.

When enteric cysts are associated with anomalies of the vertebral column, they are referred to as neuroenteric cysts. Such cysts may be connected to the meninges, or, less frequently, a direct communication with the dural space may exist. In patients with neuroenteric cysts, preoperative evaluation for potential spinal cord involvement is mandatory. The vertebral anomalies associated with this syndrome include spina bifida, hemivertebrae, and widened neural canal. CT and myelography are useful in delineating the vertebral deformities, extension into the spinal column, and the possibility of a connection with the dural space. The embryogenesis of these tumors appears to be related to the failure of complete separation of the notochord from the primitive gut when these two structures are intimately juxtaposed during development. Rarely, multiple mediastinal enteric cysts may occur, or there may be an association with a duplication of the abdominal portion of the alimentary tract. In the latter, there may be a transdiaphragmatic connection between abdominal and mediastinal components. Treatment is surgical excision, providing a definite histologic diagnosis as well as alleviating symptoms and preventing potential complications.

THYMIC CYSTS. Thymic cysts may be inflammatory, neoplastic, or congenital lesions. Congenital cysts are thought to originate from the third branchial arch and are not usually related to thymomas. These cysts are defined by the presence of thymic tissue within the cyst wall. An apparent increase in the incidence of thymic cysts following treatment of malignant anterior mediastinal neoplasms has been reported.

NONSPECIFIC CYSTS. Nonspecific cysts include those lesions in which a specific epithelial or mesothelial lining cannot be identified. These lesions may originate in any of the aforementioned cysts by the destruction of the inner epithelial lining by an inflammatory or digestive process. Other causes include postinflammatory cysts and hemorrhagic cysts.

SELECTED REFERENCES

Azizkhan, R. G., Dudgeon, D. L., Buck, J. R., Colombani, P. M., Yaster, M., Nichols, D., Civin, C., Kramer, S. S., and Haller, J. A.: Life-threatening airway obstruction as a complication to the management of mediastinal masses in children. J. Pediatr. Surg., 20:816, 1985.
This article discusses the preoperative assessment of patients with a mediastinal mass to determine which patients are at an increased risk for cardiopulmonary complications during general anesthesia. Suggested perioperative management of those patients at an increased risk is also presented.

Blalock, A., Mason, M. F., Morgan, H. J., and Riven, S. S.: Myasthenia gravis and tumors of the thymic region: Report of a case in which tumor was removed. Ann. Surg., 110:544, 1939.
This classic paper presents the initial case report of an excision of a thymic tumor in a patient with myasthenia gravis producing symptomatic remission. In addition, the author presents 53 other cases from the literature with thymic abnormalities associated with myasthenia gravis. This established thymectomy as a treatment for myasthenia gravis in patients with associated thymic lesions.

Davis, R. D., Oldham, H. N., and Sabiston, D. C., Jr.: Primary cysts and neoplasms of the mediastinum: Recent changes in clinical presentation, methods of diagnosis, management, and results. Ann. Thorac. Surg., 44:229, 1987.
This paper reviews the changing pattern in clinical presentation, as well as the use of newer diagnostic techniques in the management of patients with a mediastinal mass. Changes in the results in treatment of patients with malignant mediastinal neoplasms are reported.

Ginsberg, R. J.: Evaluation of the mediastinum by invasive techniques. Surg. Clin. North Am., 67:1025, 1987.
Excellent review of the technical aspects, associated morbidity, and mortality of the various invasive techniques of evaluating mediastinal lesions.

Harrington, S. W.: Intrathoracic tumors. Arch. Surg., 19:1679, 1929.
This article presents the first large series of patients with mediastinal tumors and cysts. The success with resection demonstrated the feasibility of surgical therapy in patients with mediastinal masses.

Silverman, N. A., and Sabiston, D. C., Jr.: Primary tumors and cysts of the mediastinum. *In* Current Problems in Cancer. Chicago, Year Book Medical Publishers, 1977.
This monograph provides a concise, detailed description of the clinical presentation of patients with mediastinal tumors and cysts, in addition to recommended therapy.

Verley, J. M., and Hollmann, K. H.: Thymoma. A comparative study of clinical stages, histologic features, and survival in 200 cases. Cancer, 55:1074, 1986.
In this article, the clinical stage and histologic type of thymoma were evaluated for response to therapy and survival. With noninvasive tumors, 10-year survival was 80 per cent; whereas with invasive tumors, 10-year survival was 35 per cent. There was no significant difference in survival between moderately invasive and largely invasive tumors. Histologic typing correlated with survival.

Wychulis, A. R., Payne, W. S., Claggett, O. T., and Woolner, L. B.: Surgical treatment of mediastinal tumors. A 40-year experience. J. Thorac. Cardiovasc. Surg., 62:379, 1971.
This article presents the largest series of patients with primary mediastinal masses from a single institution. The experience with 1064 patients with mediastinal tumors and cysts treated at the Mayo Clinic over a 40-year period supports the treatment and provides information regarding prognosis for a large number of mediastinal lesions.

REFERENCES

1. Adam, A., and Hochholzer, L.: Ganglioneuroblastoma of the posterior mediastinum: A clinicopathologic review of 80 cases. Cancer, 47:373, 1981.
2. Aliotta, P. J., Castillo, J., Englander, L. S., Nseymo, U. O., and Huben, R. P.: Primary mediastinal germ cell tumors. Histologic patterns of treatment failures at autopsy. Cancer, 62:982, 1988.
3. Azizkhan, R. G., Dudgeon, D. L., Buck, J. R., et al.: Life-threatening airway obstruction as a complication to the management of mediastinal masses in children. J. Pediatr. Surg., 20:816, 1985.
4. Bastianelli, R., quoted by Meade, R. H.: A History of Thoracic Surgery. Springfield, Ill., Charles C Thomas, 1961.
5. Berrih-Aknin, S., Morel, E., Raimond, F., Safar, D., Gaud, C., Binet, J. P., Levasseur, P., and Bach, J. F.: The role of the thymus in myasthenia gravis: Immunohistologic and immunologic studies in 115 cases. Ann. N.Y. Acad. Sci., 505:50, 1841.
6. Best, L., Munichor, M., Ben-Shakkar, M., et al.: The contribution of anterior mediastinotomy in the diagnosis and evaluation of diseases of the mediastinum and lung. Ann. Thorac. Surg., 43:78, 1987.
7. Blalock, A., Mason, M. F., Morgon, H. J., and Riven, S. S.: Myasthenia gravis and tumors of the thymic region: Report of a case in which tumor was removed. Ann. Surg., 110:544, 1939.
8. Carrol, C. L., Jeffrey, R. B., Federle, M. P., and Vernacchia, F.: CT evaluation of mediastinal infections. J. Comput. Assist. Tomogr., 11:449, 1987.
9. Clark, O. H.: Mediastinal parathyroid tumors. Arch. Surg., 123:1096, 1988.
10. Crist, W. M., Shuster, J. J., Falletta, J., Pullen, D. J., Berard, C. W., Vietti, T. J.,

11. Alvarado, C. S., Roper, M. A., Prasthofer, E., and Grossi, C. E.: Clinical features and outcome in childhood T-cell leukemia-lymphoma according to stage of the thymocyte differentiation: A Pediatric Oncology Group Study. Blood, 72:1891, 1988.
11. Curran, W. J., Kornstein, M. J., Brooks, J. J., and Turrisi, A. T.: Invasive thymoma: The role of mediastinal irradiation following complete or incomplete surgical resection. J. Clin. Oncol., 6:1722, 1988.
12. Daly, B. D. T., Faling, J., Bite, G., et al.: Mediastinal lymph evaluation by computed tomography in lung cancer: An analysis of 345 patients grouped by TNM staging, tumor size, and tumor location. J. Thorac. Cardiovasc. Surg., 94:664, 1987.
13. Dartevelle, P., Chapelier, A., Navajas, M., Levasseur, P., Rojas, A., Khalife, J., Lafontaine, E., and Merlier, M.: Replacement of the superior vena cava with polytetrafluoroethylene grafts combined with resection of mediastinal-pulmonary malignant tumors. J. Thorac. Cardiovasc. Surg., 94:361, 1987.
14. Davis, R. D., Oldham, H. N., and Sabiston, D. C., Jr.: Primary cysts and neoplasms of the mediastinum: Recent changes in clinical presentation, methods of diagnosis, management, and results. Ann. Thorac. Surg., 44:229, 1987.
15. Doty, D. B.: Bypass of superior vena cava: Six years experience with spiral vein graft for obstruction of superior vena cava due to benign and malignant disease. J. Thorac. Cardiovasc. Surg., 83:326, 1982.
16. Elert, O., Buchwald, J., and Wolf, K.: Epithelial thymus tumors — therapy and prognosis. Thorac. Cardiovasc. Surg., 36:109, 1988.
17. Epstein, A. M., and Klassen, K. P.: Spontaneous superior mediastinal hemorrhage. J. Thorac. Cardiovasc. Surg., 39:740, 1960.
18. Fischer, D. E., Grinvalski, H. T., Nussbaum, M. S., Sayers, H. J., Cole, R. E., and Samaha, F. J.: Aggressive surgical approach for drug-free remission from myasthenia gravis. Ann. Surg., 205:496, 1987.
19. Ginsberg, R. J.: Evaluation of the mediastinum by invasive techniques. Surg. Clin. North Am., 67:1025, 1987.
20. Glenner, G. G., and Grimley, P. M.: Tumors of the extra-adrenal paraganglion system (including chemoreceptors). Atlas of Tumor Pathology, 2nd Series, Fascicle 9. Washington, D.C., Armed Forces Institute of Pathology, 1974.
21. Goldel, N., Boning, L. Fredrik, D., Holzel, D., Hartenstein, R., and Wilmanns, W.: Chemotherapy of invasive thymoma. A retrospective study of 22 cases. Cancer, 63:1493, 1989.
22. Hamman, L.: Spontaneous mediastinal emphysema. Bull. Johns Hopkins Hosp., 64:1, 1939.
23. Harrington, S. W.: Surgical treatment of intrathoracic tumors. Arch. Surg., 19:1679, 1929.
24. Heuer, G. J., and Andrus, W. D.: The surgery of mediastinal tumors. Am. J. Surg., 50:146, 1940.
25. Issa, P. Y., Brihi, E. R., Janin, Y., and Slim, M. S.: Superior vena cava syndrome in childhood: Report of ten cases and review of the literature. Pediatrics, 71:337, 1983.
26. Janin, Y., Becker, J., Wise, L., et al.: Superior vena cava syndrome in childhood and adolescence: A review of the literature and report of three cases. J. Pediatr. Surg., 17:290, 1982.
27. Jaretzki, A., Penn, A. S., Younger, D. S., Wolff, M., Olarte, M. R., Lovelace, R. E., and Rowland, L. P.: Maximal thymectomy for myasthenia gravis. J. Thorac. Cardiovasc. Surg., 95:747, 1988.
28. Jochelson, M., Mauch, P., Balikian, J., et al.: The significance of the residual mediastinal mass in treated Hodgkin's disease. J. Clin. Oncol., 3:637, 1985.
29. Jolles, P. R., Shin, M. S., and Jones, W. P.: Aortopulmonary window lesions: Detection with chest radiography. Radiology, 159:647, 1986.
30. Kay, P. H., Wells, F. C., and Goldstraw, P.: A multidisciplinary approach to primary nonseminomatous germ cell tumors of the mediastinum. Ann. Thorac. Surg., 44:578, 1987.
31. Kersh, C. R., Eisert, D. R., Constable, W. C., Hahn, S. S., Jenrette, J. M., Fitzgerald, R. H., and Grayson, J.: Primary malignant mediastinal germ-cell tumors and the contribution of radiotherapy: A southeastern multi-institutional study. Am. J. Clin. Oncol., 10:302, 1987.
32. King, R. M., Telander, R. L., Smithson, W. A., et al.: Primary mediastinal tumors in children. J. Pediatr. Surg., 17:512, 1982.
33. Kirks, D. R., Fram, E. K., Vock, P., and Effmann, E. L.: Tracheal compression by mediastinal masses in children: CT evaluation. Am. J. Radiol., 141:647, 1983.
34. Kornstein, M. J., Curran, W. J., Turrisi, A. T., and Brooks, J. J.: Cortical versus medullary thymomas: A useful morphologic distinction? Hum. Pathol., 19:1335, 1988.
35. Loeffler, J. S., Leopold, K. A., Recht, A., et al.: Emergency prebiopsy radiation for mediastinal masses: Impact on subsequent pathologic diagnosis and outcome. J. Clin. Oncol., 4:716, 1986.
36. Melms, A., Schalke, B. S., Kirchner, T., Muller-Hermelink, H. K., Albert, E., and Wekerle, H.: Thymus in myasthenia gravis. Isolation of T-lymphocyte lines specific for the nicotinic acetylcholine receptors from thymuses of myasthenic patients. J. Clin. Invest., 81:902, 1988.
37. Milton, H.: Mediastinal surgery. Lancet, 1:872, 1897.
38. Moinuddin, S. M., Lee, L. H., and Montgomery, J. H.: Mediastinal needle biopsy. Am. J. Radiol., 143:531, 1984.
39. Motzer, R. J., Bosl, G. J., Geller, N. L., Peneberg, D., Yagoda, A., Golbey, R., Whitmore, W. F., Fair, W. R., Sogani, P., Herr, H., Morse, M., Carey, R. W., and Vogelzang, N.: Advanced seminoma: The role of chemotherapy and adjunctive surgery. Ann. Intern. Med., 108:513, 1988.
40. Nakahara, K., Ohno, K., Hashimoto, J., Maeda, H., Miyoshi, S., Sakurai, M.,

Monden, Y., and Kawashima, Y.: Thymoma: Results with complete resection and adjuvant postoperative irradiation in 141 consecutive patients. J. Thorac. Cardiovasc. Surg., *95*:1041, 1988.

41. Nakahara, K., Ohno, K., Matsumura, A., Hirose, H., Mastuda, H., and Nakano, S.: Extended operation for lung cancer invading the aortic arch and superior vena cava. J. Thorac. Cardiovasc. Surg., *97*:428, 1989.

42. Neuman, G. G., Weingarten, A. E., Abramowitz, R. M., et al.: The anesthetic management of the patient with an anterior mediastinal mass. Anesthesiology, *60*:144, 1984.

43. Nichols, C. R., Heerema, N. A., Palmer, C., et al.: Klinefelter's syndrome associated with mediastinal germ cell neoplasms. J. Clin. Oncol., *5*:1290, 1987.

44. Normori, H., Horinouchi, H., Kaseda, S., Ishihara, T., and Torikata, C.: Evaluation of the malignant grade of thymoma by morphometric analysis. Cancer, *61*:982, 1988.

45. Radford, J. A., Cowan, R. A., Flanagan, M., Dunn, G., Crowther, D., and Eddleston, B.: The significance of residual mediastinal abnormality on the chest radiograph following treatment for Hodgkin's disease. J. Clin. Oncol., *6*:940, 1988.

46. Rendina, E. A., Venuta, F., Ceroni, L., Martelli, M., Gualdi, G., Caterino, M., and Ricci, C.: Computed tomographic staging of anterior mediastinal neoplasms. Thorax, *43*:441, 1988.

47. Rousou, J. A., Kirkwood, R., Engelman, R. M., and Breyer, R. H.: Catheter drainage of symptomatic postoperative mediastinal effusion guided by computed tomography. J. Thorac. Cardiovasc. Surg., *93*:715, 1987.

48. Safar, D., Berrih, A. S., and Morel, E.: In vitro anti–acetylcholine receptor antibody synthesis by myasthenia gravis patient lymphocytes: Correlations with thymic histology and thymic epithelial-cell interactions. J. Clin. Immunol., *7*:225, 1987.

49. Taniguchi, S., Shibuya, T., Morioka, E., Okamura, T., Okamura, S., Inaba, S., and Niho, Y.: Demonstration of three distinct immunological disorders on erythropoiesis in a patient with red cell aplasia and autoimmune haemolytic anaemia associated with thymoma. Br. J. Haematol., *68*:473, 1988.

50. Verley, J. M., and Hollman, K. H.: Thymoma: A comparative study of clinical stages, histologic features and survival in 200 cases. Cancer, *55*:1074, 1985.

51. Wang, C., Gaz, R. D., and Moncure, A. C.: Mediastinal parathyroid exploration: A clinical and pathologic study of 47 cases. World J. Surg., *10*:687, 1986.

52. Wick, M. R., Bernatz, P. E., Carney, J. A., and Brown, L. R.: Primary mediastinal carcinoid tumors. Am. J. Surg. Pathol., *6*:195, 1982.

53. Yumura, Y. K., Ishihara, S., Hara, J., Murata, M., Izumi, Y., Tawa, A., Sato, A., Matsumoto, Y., Kozaiwa, K., and Nishida, M.: Poor prognosis of mediastinal non-Hodgkin's lymphoma with an immature phenotype of CD2+, CD7+, CD3−, CD4−, and CD8−. Cancer, *63*:671, 1989.

I

SURGICAL MANAGEMENT OF SUPPURATIVE MEDIASTINITIS

Thomas J. Krizek, M.D., and John G. Lease, M.D.

The special construction of the chest wall serves a dual purpose: the rigid compartment *protects* the heart, lungs, and great vessels from injury and through *flexibility* allows expansion, which allows air to rush into the bronchi and alveoli with inspiration and to be forced out with expiration. Several anatomic features are reviewed. The upper sternum and clavicles are important structurally and physiologically for elevation of the upper rib cage and expansion of the chest volume. Removal of major portions of this part of the chest tends to promote collapse of the inferior ribs, with concomitant functional loss. Loss of the lower two thirds of the sternum tends to restrict the ability of the abdominal muscles to aid in expiration and coughing. Movement of the area is less paradoxical. Depending on the covering over the absent sternum, varying degrees of protection of the heart are lost.

Median Sternotomy

Although transecting the sternum provides unparalleled access with minimal interference with respiration, at the same time, it divides the superficially located sternum, a bone subject to the constant motion and stress of respiration. Techniques of closure have, in general, not involved rigid fixation as might be applied to other divided bones. The closed sternotomy wounds are large, often following long operations with considerable blood loss, often with hematoma, with bone that is difficult to immobilize even with large amounts of foreign body (wire); that some should become infected and that there should be dehiscence of bone is not surprising.

Scope of the Problem

Before open heart surgery and antibiotics, mediastinitis occurred occasionally in conjunction with tumors or granulomatous infections, usually tuberculosis. Resolution of the infection occasionally produced mediastinal fibrosis and possible constriction of vessels. Suppurative mediastinitis has been reported following closed chest cardiopulmonary resuscitation.[13] Sternal fracture from compression has been followed by hematogenous seeding, usually with *Staphylococcus aureus*, and has led to suppurative mediastinitis in the absence of any prior surgical therapy. Mediastinitis is currently almost always associated with surgical intervention.

Many series, some with large numbers of cases, indicate that the incidence is below 2 per cent and has remained approximately the same for more than 20 years (Table 1).

Patients who have undergone cardiac operative procedures are often quite ill and prone to a number of infection complications. The incidence of superficial wound infections is 4 to 6.3 per cent, but the incidence of deep, suppurative mediastinitis is less than 2 per cent.[15] In addition, patients experience infections in leg wounds (as high as 11.3 per cent), infections in the urinary tract (4.6 per cent), and pneumonia (2.5 per cent).[24] Although these are important, this section addresses the problem of deep sternal and mediastinal infections.

A slight difference in the incidence of deep infection has been noted in patients undergoing various cardiac surgical proce-

TABLE 1. Incidence of Mediastinitis

Series	Number of Patients	Mediastinitis (%)
Brown[3] (1969)	748	1.5
Engelman[8] (1973)	1042	1.6
Grmoljez[10] (1975)	1550	0.8
Culliford[7] (1976)	2594	1.5
Jurkiewicz[11] (1980)	3239	1.5
Sarr[19] (1984)	824	0.7
Rutledge[18] (1985)	2031	1.4
Verkkala[25] (1986)	1083	1.4
Ottino[16] (1987)	2579	1.86
Stiegel[22] (1988) (children)	2242	0.94

Review of major series of cardiac procedures and the incidence of suppurative mediastinitis over the last 2 decades. It is fairly constant at 1 to 2 per cent.

dures. The reported incidence in children with congenital defects is less than 1 per cent.[19] With a valve operation, the incidence of infection is about 1.8 per cent, slightly higher than that of coronary artery bypass procedures; but when the two are combined, the rate of mediastinitis is 2.5 to 3 per cent.[16] When the internal mammary artery is used, the incidence of infection increases; when both arteries are used, the infection rate is 8 per cent.[7]

PATHOGENESIS OF INFECTION

Many studies have demonstrated that surgical infections are not due to the mere presence of bacteria[17] but rather are the end result of a complex interplay between systemic and local host defense mechanisms and pathogenic microorganisms. Experience in burns and other contaminated wounds indicates that the presence of fewer than 10^5 microorganisms per gram of tissue is compatible with successful wound closure.[17] Levels greater than 10^5 microorganisms per gram cause wound breakdown, failure of graft take, and, as counts increase, invasive sepsis. Because 10^5 microorganisms per gram of tissue is the critical level, it is important to examine those factors in the patient and the operation that might allow levels to reach 10^5 microorganisms per gram.

Predisposing Patient Factors

Many studies, both of infection in general and of mediastinitis in particular, fail to identify age and sex as influencing the incidence of infection.[16] Obesity and diabetes increase infection rates in general. Those who are initially more ill, as manifested by poor nutrition and poor hemodynamics, and those who are undergoing reoperation have adverse factors related to infection.

Operating Factors

Patients with congenital heart defects have a lower incidence of infection (less than 1 per cent); those with coronary artery bypass have a higher infection rate, particularly when the internal mammary artery is used. A large series of operations on valves alone demonstrated an incidence of 1.4 per cent. There is a correlation between how the sternotomy is made and infection. Improvements from Gigli (hand-driven) saws to high-speed mechanical devices have reduced infection rates.[19] As with other operations and infections, there is a linear increase in infection with prolonged duration of the operation—a reflection of complexity and duration of potential lodgment of bacteria. In a series of 17 patients with mediastinitis, the length of operative procedures ranged from 6 to 17 hours and 9 patients were operated on for more than 10 hours.[8]

Most studies show increased sepsis with prolonged bypass (more than 3 hours). As mentioned, the presence of bacteria does not correlate with infection. There is evidence that cardiopulmonary bypass affects phagocytic capacity and there is decreased ability to clear bacteria, a problem that increases with prolonged bypass time.[19]

The technique of immobilizing the sternum postoperatively has improved from nylon or silk sutures to more rigid approximation with wire. The evolution of plating and other orthopedic techniques may be applicable, since each step toward more rigid immobilization has decreased complications.

PHYSIOLOGIC FACTORS

Low Flow. Low-flow states may cause decreased local host resistance to bacteria. Similarly, the use of both internal mammary arteries decreases the blood supply to the sternum and is accompanied by a four- to fivefold increase in mediastinitis.[2] As many as half of those with mediastinitis have had "low-flow" phenomena.

Hemorrhage. All studies of infection support the fact that bleeding and hematoma predispose to bacterial growth. Data confirm bleeding as a contributory factor; more than 53 per cent of patients with mediastinitis had postoperative blood loss of more than 1250 ml.[7] Those who require reoperation—either early or elective—are also predisposed, and 18 to 42 per cent of those with mediastinitis form this category.[7,18] Similarly, postoperative cardiopulmonary resuscitation, which clearly may disrupt the repair and cause bleeding, increases complication rates two to four times.

OTHER FACTORS

TECHNICAL ERRORS. Operating rooms rarely contain more than 60 to 70 microorganisms per cubic foot in the air, a level far below the critical 10^5 microorganisms that must lodge in the tissue for infection to occur.[17] Studies of the operative environment showed positive cultures from the heart-lung machine in an astounding 71 per cent of cases; 20 per cent of patients had multiple positive sites of culture. Cultures of prosthetic valves were positive in 50 per cent, and the cardiotomy site was positive in 64 per cent. However, in only 2 of the 66 patients did infection develop.[19] Other studies show Staphylococcus epidermidis in the nasal cultures of 80 per cent of operating room personnel, from 90 per cent of the inside of gloves, and from 80 per cent of wounds prior to closure. Diphtheroids also are found commonly.

DISTANT INFECTION. It is well known that individuals with infection elsewhere in the body are predisposed to mediastinal infection.[17] It is not surprising that those with tracheostomies or those on prolonged mechanical ventilation are susceptible to infection.[24] Intravenous catheters, urinary catheters, and other drainage tubes are sources for entry of microorganisms and hematogenous seeding of operative sites.

MICROBIOLOGY

The most common microorganisms causing infection are those most indigenous to patients and their environment: S. epidermidis and Pseudomonas aeruginosa.[19] Other gram-negative organisms are found, such as Escherichia coli, Klebsiella, Serratia, and Proteus species, and mixed infections represent approximately 40 per cent of cases.[7,8] Candida has also been identified, and several cases of pure anaerobic infection (Bacteroides fragilis) have been described.[19] The emergence of S. epidermidis rather than S. aureus, which was the most common organism a decade ago, can be attributed to the widespread use of the penicillinase-resistant antibacterials. Some 30 per cent of S. epidermidis is also resistant. The changing microbiologic environment is largely responsive to the changing pattern of antibacterial use.

ANTIBACTERIALS

Many studies have indicated that antibacterials, to be more effective, must be administered in adequate doses, in a timely manner, and by the proper route.[17] In surgical wounds, a timely manner means before, during, and within the first several hours of the wounding. Although the antibacterials reach therapeutic tissue levels at the margins in well-vascularized tissue and prevent invasive wound sepsis, it is believed most surgical wound infections and mediastinal infections are not preventable by antibacterial drugs administered after closure.

When infection has developed and when a wound is open, antibacterials are better delivered topically, since it is very difficult to achieve adequate tissue levels in the wound with systemic antibacterials. The opened sternotomy wound, the exposed mediastinum, and the granulating wound margins are biologically comparable to a burn wound, and lessons learned in burn therapy should be applied. Silver sulfadiazine and mafenide (Sulfamylon) are excellent antibacterials that penetrate well into granulating and infected tissue. Betadine-soaked materials deliver an agent that, albeit elegant for washing and skin decontamination, does not penetrate well into tissue. Many other agents can be delivered topically by constant or intermittent irrigation of the wound.

DIAGNOSIS

It is fitting to refer to redness and swelling with heat and pain since with these words Celsus introduced the cardinal signs of inflammation.[6] Bacteria lodged in the wound must reach 10^5 microorganisms per gram to survive and then must reach levels of 10^8 per gram before they are clinically manifest. In actuality, prophylactic antibacterials, as part of the postoperative management, may delay the clinical appearance for 2 to 3 months; most mediastinitis begins to be apparent between 4 days and 3 weeks.[19]

Although drainage of pus through the wound is a rather obvious sign, suspicions should be heightened with regard to patients whose pain increases rather than decreases toward the end of a week, and whose wounds become reddened and swollen. Warmth is usually present, but difficult to identify. A spiking fever suggests the presence of an abscess. Fever and leukocytosis are almost always present.

Those patients in whom fever and leukocytosis develop, in whom there is no other source of infection, must be suspected of harboring mediastinal sepsis, even if drainage has not appeared and the sternum is still stable. Aspiration of the mediastinitis is a simple diagnostic maneuver that is of value when it is positive. Any drainage must be immediately cultured anaerobically as well as aerobically and antibacterial sensitivity determined.[19] Routine chest films are difficult to interpret. Computed tomographic scans are valuable and are diagnostic when there is gas-forming infection or when distinct abscesses are present.

THERAPY

All surgical complications compromise the quality of the result or, in the case of suppurative mediastinitis, represent a proximate and real threat to life. Subsequent to valve procedures, mortality as high as 70 per cent has been reported.[8]

NONOPERATIVE THERAPY

Suppurative mediastinitis should be considered a surgical problem. Although nonsurgical supportive care to respiratory, vascular, and other systems is critical and systemic antibacterials are vital, they are strictly supportive, and do not constitute definitive therapy. The nonoperative decision in the algorithm (Fig. 1) is usually a preliminary step. Some patients may develop fever, leukocytosis, and other nonspecific signs, which resolve with nonoperative measures. Purulent drainage is an indication for surgical intervention.

OPERATIVE TECHNIQUE

The fundamental surgical approaches to infection include adequate débridement, proper irrigation, appropriate use of antibacterials by the proper route, and timely closure.

DÉBRIDEMENT. The wound should be opened; all foreign bodies in the form of suture material, wire, blood clots, and bits of bone must be removed. The costal cartilages are less vascular and may become devascularized as a consequence of infection, which demands their removal as well. The key to adequate débridement is usually the bone cartilage complex. The term *judgment* is appropriate here, emphasizing that damage is more often removal of too little than of too much.

IRRIGATION. The intraoperative irrigation should be performed under pressure. Large amounts of irrigation fluid are not nearly so important as is truly flushing out the microorganisms and debris from the interstices of the soft tissue where they are lodged. The pulsating jet lavage (70 pounds per square inch) is

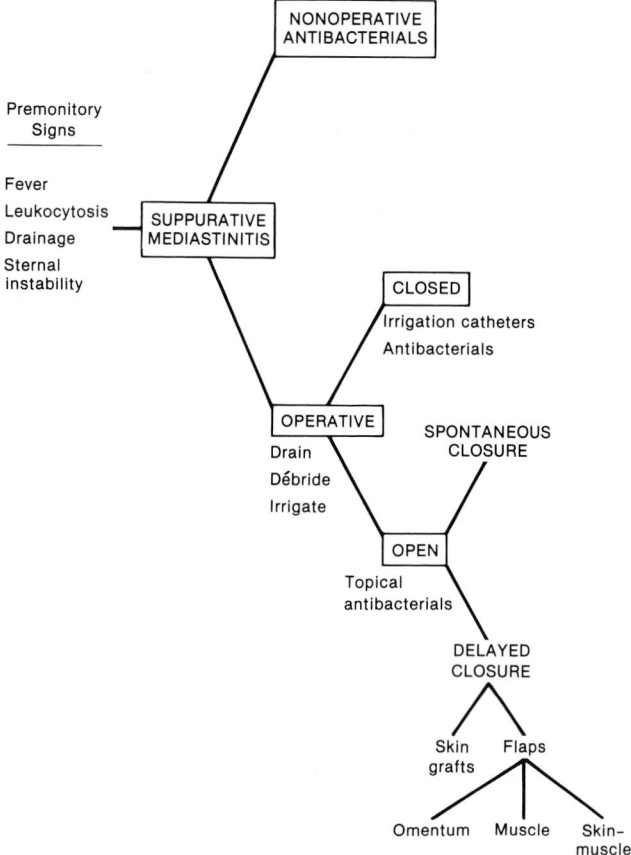

Figure 1. Algorithm of management of suppurative mediastinitis.

effective; a syringe with a fine needle directed to the wound is also. A bulb syringe is not adequate.

The term *irrigation* is also applied to a technique of postoperative management in which the contaminated but débrided wound is closed over irrigation catheters into which antibacterial or other irrigating solutions may be instilled. These or other catheters are used to collect the effluent with or without suction. This technique introduced by Shumaker in 1963 is of value in lesser infections, particularly where cavities ("dead space") are not a feature of the wound.[21]

ANTIBACTERIALS. Modern irrigation solutions include powerful antibiotics (polymyxin, bacitracin, and others) not readily available for systemic use.[4,20] The use of closed system drainage has been an effective management technique when performed early. The technique has been expanded during the last 2 decades.[1,4] Débridement and closed irrigation was used successfully in 16 patients. A more recent study comparing closed irrigation with open techniques found no difference in outcome.[20]

Open Technique

The alternative to débridement and closure with irrigation catheters is open treatment and is generally the preferred management. Wounds in which there is extensive necrosis or in which extensive bone or cartilage resection has been required may be better treated by leaving the wound open and employing topical antibacterials. The topical antibacterial is chosen, often packed in with gauze, which is then changed every 8 to 24 hours depending on the wound. The progress of the treatment can be monitored precisely by quantitative microbiologic techniques. Small amounts of tissue are biopsied to assess the number and variety of microorganisms within the wound. The rapid slide technique identifies whether the wound has more or fewer than 10^5 microorganisms per gram of tissue. This information can be available within 30 minutes and is of great value intraoperatively in determining the extent of débridement or deciding whether the wound can be closed. The traditional techniques provide the number and variety of organisms as well as antibacterial sensitivity in 18 to 24 hours. Experience gained from burn wounds suggests that topical sulfa agents (silver sulfadiazine, mafenide) would also be effective and have the advantage of thoroughly distributing in the wound, penetrating the tissue, and not requiring continuous application, since dressing changes every 8 to 24 hours may suffice.

The value of topical applications and dressing changes was confirmed in a study in which 19 patients were managed with topical application of granulated sugar, changed every 3 to 4 hours.[23] Long used in pressure sores and other contrary wounds, sugar destroys microorganisms and prevents their growth in a manner not well known, but much of sugar's value in preserving such foods as jam and jelly might be inferred. Its mechanical characteristics promote drainage and serve a débridement function.

CLOSURE

The most appropriate technique for wound closure is the use of local tissue when it is available. It has been reported that delayed closure done purposefully in the absence of infection is quite successful.[9] This is appropriate when possible after infection as well. The modern techniques of tissue transfer aided this very modern infection complication. Tissue may be transferred from nearby, maintaining vascularity, and serve to obliterate the cavity. In actuality, the availability of these techniques

should buoy the spirits of the surgeon responsible for the débridement. There is no need to be concerned about preserving marginally viable tissue because it can be replaced. It would be unwise to débride inadequately and waste valuable vascularized tissue in an inadequately prepared wound.

Omentum

The "policeman of the abdomen" can be rotated to an extraabdominal position. Many have demonstrated that the omentum could be freed from the colon and then rotated on either the left or the right gastroepiploic vessel (Fig. 2). The extent of the area of rotation is adjustable by subdividing the vascularity and thus lengthening it.

Muscle Flaps

The use of regional muscle to close the defect offers the exciting opportunity to fill the cavity with well-vascularized tissue and then closing over the skin margins or applying a graft. Each of these muscle flaps provides vascularity to territories of skin of varying size and configuration overlying the muscle, which may be transferred at the same time, thus serving a dual purpose.

PECTORALIS MAJOR MUSCLE. The pectoralis muscle is used in reconstructing the anterior mediastinum (Fig. 3).[2] It is easily mobilized medially and dressed into or turned over into cavitary defects and is particularly valuable for the upper three fourths of the anterior mediastinum; because its arc of rotation is away from the xiphoid, it is a little less effective in the most inferior defects. Closure may be completed either by applying skin grafts to the muscle or, when possible, by approximating the original skin margins.

RECTUS ABDOMINIS MUSCLE. Much experience with this flap has been gained from its use for breast reconstruction after mastectomy. Its unpredictability, particularly its skin territories, in patients who smoke or are obese is well known. Its use also

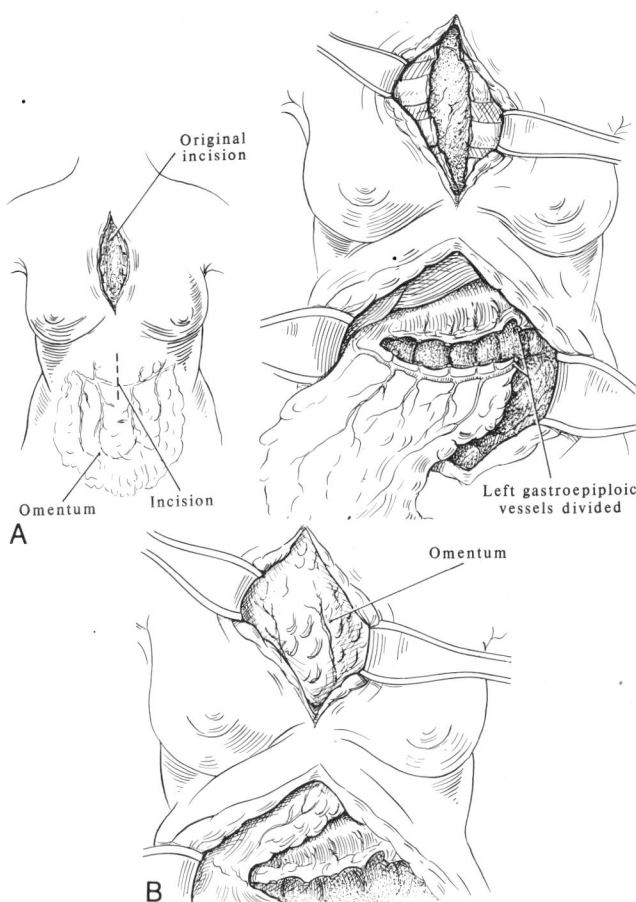

Figure 2. Omental flap technique. *A, left,* Relative position of omentum to defect; *right,* omentum may be transferred on either the right (illustrated) or left gastroepiploic vessel. *B,* Omentum in defect. The skin is then approximated, if possible, or a skin graft is applied.

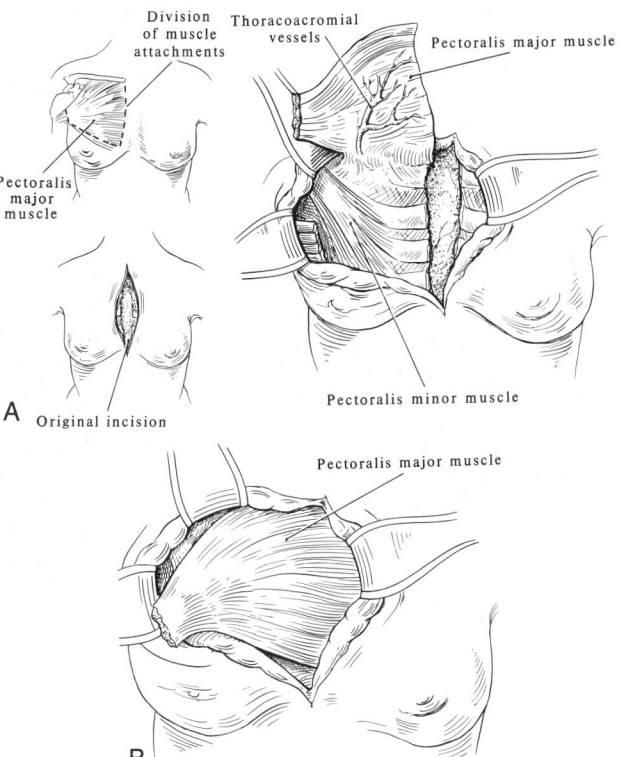

Figure 3. Pectoralis muscle transfer. *A, left,* Location of pectoralis sternal defect; *right,* pectoralis major muscle with both origin and insertion released, carried on dominant vasculature, thoracoacromial vessels. *B,* Transferred into defects. Both pectoralis major muscles may be used.

weakens the abdominal wall, and hernia is an unfortunate hazard. This flap has become the flap of choice for some. Majure has used the rectus flap on 14 patients and prefers this flap because of ease, dependability, and aesthetic considerations.[12] In Nahai's large series, the rectus was used on 145 occasions with only 3.3 per cent complications.[14]

RECONSTRUCTION

The goal of the wound closure is to obliterate the cavity, to eliminate residual infection, and to provide bulky, thick, durable tissue to cover the underlying vascular structures. Aesthetic appearances are important but not the critical issue. The concepts of omentum and muscle flap closures evolved when closed wounds over irrigation catheters failed. They have now been used as the primary treatment more often. In the large Emory series, there were 211 of 15,595 cases with deep infection which have been treated with flap closure. There was usually no interval between débridement and definitive closure, and wounds in all surviving patients healed (mortality was 5.3 per cent).

The choices in order are probably (1) single pectoralis major muscle, (2) single rectus abdominis muscle, (3) omentum, (4) bilateral pectoralis muscles, and (5) other.

Structural Support

The thorax is both semirigid and flexible; removal of large segments of the sternum, costochondral areas, and ribs may be accomplished without major functional loss. When instability causes paradoxic motion, the defect may be bridged with autologous material such as fascia or rib from elsewhere. Alloplastic material such as Marlex may also be used. In general, both the cardiac and the reconstructive surgeon wish to preserve the sternum and to reconstitute continuity when the edges move. When the bone is infected or marginally viable, it is far better to remove it. As final healing occurs, there is usually sufficient scarring to stabilize the chest functionally.

RESULTS

The mortality from untreated suppurative mediastinitis is staggering, and no series includes these untreated controls. In one study, before early open débridement, 73 per cent of the patients died. The accuracy of diagnosis and the precision with which superficial infections are differentiated from sternal dehiscence or true suppurative mediastinitis are often unclear. In one large series, 48 of 2579 cases were so diagnosed (1.86 per cent).[16] Of these, 19 died (40 per cent of infected cases, but only 0.7 per cent of all cases). Because of selection of cases, it is difficult to compare "open" with "closed" techniques; certainly, the worse the infection, the more likely it is that open treatment is used. In another large series of 2491 cases, 36 patients developed suppurative mediastinitis (1.4 per cent).[6] Twelve of these were considered to be high risk because of other problems not related to infection, of whom 10 (83.3 per cent) died. In the remaining 24, there were 8 who were managed before techniques of débridement, open management, and flap closure were readily available; 2 of these patients (25 per cent) died. The subsequent 16 patients were managed by débridement, topical therapy, and flap closure, and 3 underwent valve replacement; of these, only 1 (6 per cent) died.

SUMMARY

Suppurative mediastinitis is a modern problem, largely the consequence of extensive cardiac surgery. These patients are often ill before operation, the operative procedure is often prolonged, and cardiopulmonary bypass appears to dispose to infection. When infection results, it is difficult to manage; an incidence of 1 to 2 per cent has been constant for more than 20 years. Principles of management include early and aggressive débridement, followed by closed treatment with antibacterial irrigation or open treatment, topical antibacterials, and delayed closure. Muscle flaps are valuable in filling cavitary defects and obliterating dead space and can be used immediately after débridement or secondarily to close open wounds. These techniques have reduced mortality from 73 to 100 per cent with nonoperative management to less than 5 per cent at present.

REFERENCES

1. Acinapura, A. J., Godfrey, N., Romita, M., et al.: Surgical management of infected median sternotomy: Closed irrigation vs. muscle flaps. J. Cardiovasc. Surg., 26:443, 1985.
2. Arnold, P. G., and Pairolero, P. C.: Use of pectoralis major muscle flaps to repair defects of anterior chest wall. Plast. Reconstr. Surg., 52:205, 1979.
3. Brown, A. H., Braimbridge, M. V., Panagopoulos, P., et al.: The complications of median sternotomy. J. Thorac. Cardiovasc. Surg., 58:189, 1969.
4. Bryant, L. R., Spencer, F. C., and Trinkle, J. K.: Treatment of median sternotomy infection by mediastinal irrigation with an antibiotic solution. Surgery, 169:914, 1969.
5. Celsus, DeMedicina as described and amplified in Majno, G.: The Healing Hand. Cambridge, Harvard University Press, 1975; p. 370.
6. Cheung, E. H., Craver, J. M., Jones, E. L., et al.: Mediastinitis after cardiac valve operations. J. Thorac. Cardiovasc. Surg., 90:517, 1985.
7. Culliford, A. T., Cunningham, J. N., Zeff, R. H., et al.: Sternal and costochondral infections following open-heart surgery. J. Thorac. Cardiovasc. Surg., 72:714, 1976.
8. Engelman, R. M., Williams, C. D., Gouge, T. H., et al.: Mediastinitis following open-heart surgery. Arch. Surg., 107:772, 1973.
9. Fanning, W. J., Vasko, J. S., and Kilman, J. W.: Delayed sternal closure after cardiac surgery. Ann. Thorac. Surg., 44:169, 1987.
10. Grmoljez, P. F., Barner, H. H., Willman, V. L., et al.: Major complications of median sternotomy. Am. J. Surg., 130:679, 1975.
11. Jurkiewicz, M. J., Bostwick, J., III, Hester, T. R., et al.: Infected median sternotomy wound. Ann. Surg., 191:738, 1980.
12. Majure, J. A., Albin, R. E., O'Donnell, R. S., et al.: Reconstruction of the infected median sternotomy wound. Ann. Thorac. Surg., 42:9, 1986.
13. Mensah, G. A., Gold, J. P., Schreiber, T., et al.: Acute purulent mediastinitis and sternal osteomyelitis after closed chest cardiopulmonary resuscitation: A case report and review of the literature. Ann. Thorac. Surg., 46:353, 1988.
14. Nahai, F., Rand, R. P., Hester, T. R., et al.: Primary treatment of the infected sternotomy wound with muscle flaps: A review of 211 consecutive cases. Plast. Reconstr. Surg., 84:434, 1989.
15. Nelson, J. C., and Nelson, R. M.: The incidence of hospital wound infection in thoracotomies. J. Thorac. Cardiovasc. Surg., 54:586, 1969.
16. Ottino, G., DePaulis, R., Pansini, S., et al.: Major sternal wound infection after open-heart surgery: A multivariate analysis of risk factors in 2,579 consecutive operative procedures. Ann. Thorac. Surg., 44:173, 1987.
17. Robson, M. C., Krizek, T. J., and Heggers, J. P.: Biology of surgical infection. In Ravitch, M. M., Austen, W. G., Scott, H. W., Thal, A. P., Wangensteen, O. H., and Steichen, F. M. (Eds.): Current Problems in Surgery. Chicago, Year Book Medical Publishers, 1973; pp. 1–62.
18. Rutledge, R., Applebaum, R. E., and Kim, B. J.: Mediastinal infection after open heart surgery. Surgery, 97:88, 1985.
19. Sarr, M. G., Gott, V. L., and Townsend, T. R.: Mediastinal infection after cardiac surgery. Ann. Thorac. Surg., 38:415, 1984.
20. Scully, H. E., Leclerc, Y., Martin, R. D., et al.: Comparison between antibiotic irrigation and mobilization of pectoral muscle flaps in treatment of deep sternal infections. J. Thorac. Cardiovasc. Surg., 90:523, 1985.
21. Shumaker, H. B., Jr., and Mandelbaum, I.: Continuous antibiotic irrigation in the treatment of infection. Arch. Surg., 86:384, 1963.
22. Stiegel, R. M., Beasley, M. E., Sink, J. D., et al.: Management of postoperative mediastinitis in infants and children by muscle flap rotation. Ann. Thorac. Surg., 46:45, 1988.
23. Trouillet, J. L., Fagon, J. Y., Domart, Y., et al.: Use of granulated sugar in treatment of open mediastinitis after cardiac surgery. Lancet, 2:180, 1985.
24. Verkkala, K.: Occurrence of and microbiological findings in postoperative infections following open-heart surgery. Ann. Clin. Res., 19:170, 1987.
25. Verkkala, K., and Jarvinen, A.: Mediastinal infection following open-heart surgery. Scand. J. Thorac. Cardiovasc. Surg., 20:203, 1986.

II _____

SURGICAL MANAGEMENT OF MYASTHENIA GRAVIS

C. Warren Olanow, M.D., and Andrew S. Wechsler, M.D.

Myasthenia gravis is a disorder of neuromuscular transmission that is characterized by weakness and fatigue of voluntary muscles. It is now reasonably established to be due to an autoimmune attack directed against the postsynaptic nicotinic acetylcholine (ACh) receptors of voluntary muscles. Many detailed accounts of the clinical pattern have been recorded before this century. The similarity of the clinical features of myasthenia gravis to those following curare poisoning and the beneficial effect of prostigmine, shown by Mary Walker in 1934, focused attention on impaired neuromuscular·transmission as the basis of the disorder.

Interactions between quanta of ACh released from the presynaptic terminal at the neuromuscular junction and acetylcholine receptors (AChRs) on the postsynaptic membrane determine the likelihood of muscular contraction. The excessive number of potential interactions beyond that necessary to provide for maximal muscle contraction is referred to as the "safety factor" for neuromuscular transmission. Elmqvist and associates (in 1964) showed that patients with myasthenia gravis had reduced miniature endplate potential amplitudes, reflecting fewer interactions between ACh and AChR and thus a reduced safety factor.[11a] Initially, this was thought to be due to inadequate release of ACh. More recent studies using specific neurotoxins (prepared from snake venom) have shown a reduction in the number of AChR in patients with myasthenia gravis, which has been confirmed by histologic and electron microscopic studies. In 1960, Simpson proposed that myasthenia gravis was due to an autoimmune disorder. The identification by Patrick and Lindstrom in 1973 of an experimental allergic myasthenia gravis after immunization of rabbits with purified AChR and the detection of specific AChR antibodies in 90 per cent of patients with myasthenia gravis support this hypothesis.[30a]

A relationship between myasthenia gravis and the thymus gland has been appreciated since at least 1901. In 1912, Sauerbruch removed an enlarged thymus gland from a patient with myasthenia gravis who subsequently improved.[33a] In 1939, Blalock removed an enlarged thymus from a young woman with generalized myasthenia gravis. Encouraged by her response, in 1941, he made the important demonstration that removal of nontumorous thymus glands could provide clinical improvement in patients with myasthenia gravis.[4a] His success stimulated subsequent investigators to examine the role of thymectomy in the treatment of myasthenia gravis. Although the role of the thymus gland in myasthenia gravis is incompletely defined, numerous reports suggest that thymectomy is an effective therapy. Studies in the authors' clinic have shown that the use of thymectomy as the sole method of treatment provides dramatic clinical improvement in many patients and suggests that a specific thymic factor contributes to the development of clinical weakness in myasthenia gravis.

CLINICAL FEATURES

Myasthenia gravis has a prevalence in the population of 1:75,000. There is a biphasic mode of distribution, with a tendency for populations of young women and older men to be affected. Women are affected twice as often as men, and in

younger patients this ratio is increased to 4.5:1. The mean age of onset of symptoms is 26 years. Men tend to be affected at a later age and tend to have a higher incidence of thymoma. A genetic predisposition to develop myasthenia gravis is suggested by a high incidence of specific human leukocyte antigens (HLAs).

Weakness and fatigue with activity are the hallmarks of myasthenia gravis (Fig. 1). Almost any muscle group in the body may be involved, and fluctuation in strength from hour to hour is common. Individual muscle groups may be selectively involved. Weakness tends to be more pronounced as the day progresses and after exercise. It may develop gradually or rapidly, and recovery may be total or incomplete. The ocular muscles are the most frequently affected muscle group, and ocular disturbances are the presenting feature in 50 to 60 per cent of patients with myasthenia gravis, and they are ultimately involved in 90 per cent of patients. This is most often manifested by ptosis and diplopia and may be exaggerated by repetitive testing or sustained exercise. Ptosis may fluctuate during the course of the examination, and Cogan's sign (a downward fall of the levator palpebrae superioris after upward gaze) may be demonstrated. Weakness of the orbicularis oculi is a frequent accompanying feature of ocular muscle involvement. Other cranial nerves may also be affected, and cause potentially fatal complications due to dysphagia and respiratory distress. Impaired chewing, dysarthria, and nasal speech are particularly common in patients with late-onset myasthenia gravis. Facial weakness with a transverse smile and involuntary grimace may

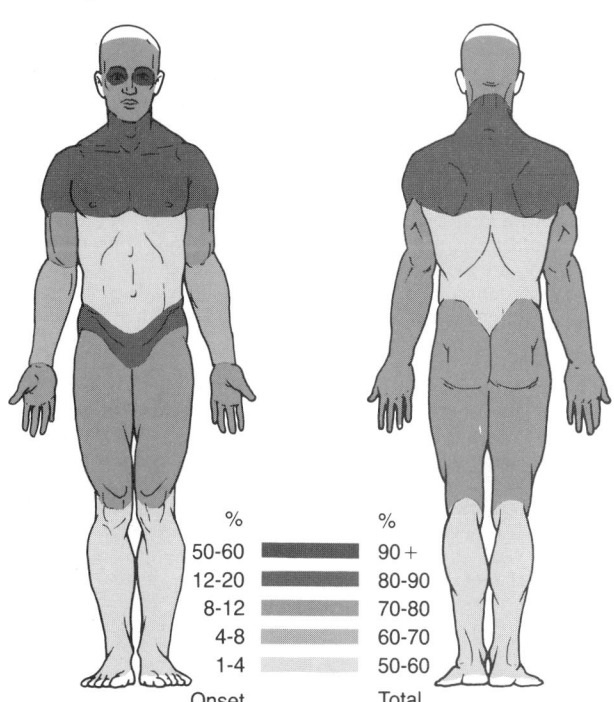

%		%	
50-60		90 +	
12-20		80-90	
8-12		70-80	
4-8		60-70	
1-4		50-60	
Onset		Total	

Figure 1. Involvement of muscle groups in patients with myasthenia gravis at time of onset *(left column)* and during course of illness *(right column)*.

develop. The tongue may become atrophic, with a characteristic triple furrow. Weakness of the flexor or extensor muscles of the neck may require that patients support their heads with their hands.

In the extremities, there is generally symmetrical weakness, involving proximal muscles more than distal groups and the arms more than the legs. This pattern varies considerably; and in a specific patient, there may be asymmetrical involvement, with any muscle group or even an isolated muscle being affected. The deep tendon reflexes tend to be preserved but may temporarily disappear with repetitive stimulation. The results of sensory examination are within normal limits, although patients may complain of nonspecific sensations. Autonomic nervous system involvement with pupillary changes, bladder disturbances, and increased sweating have all been described but are uncommon.

The onset of symptoms may be insidious or sudden, spontaneous or precipitated by emotional stress, exercise, allergies, vaccinations, or pregnancy. Myasthenia gravis may also become manifest as prolonged weakness after the use of relaxant drugs or anesthesia during surgical therapy. Symptoms may be confined to the ocular muscles, but more than 80 per cent of patients develop generalized weakness within 1 year of the onset of ocular disturbances. Grading systems to monitor clinical status are handicapped by difficulty in quantifying muscular strength and the variation that occurs in myasthenic patients, particularly after exposure to heat, exercise, stress, and drugs that interfere with neuromuscular transmission. The most widely used scale is the Osserman classification, which is given in Table 1. This is a clinical classification that is limited by its failure to consider dependency on medication or to reflect subtle clinical change, thus creating difficulty in monitoring response to treatment.

TABLE 1. Modified Clinical Classification of Patients with Myasthenia Gravis

Group I
  Ocular Myasthenia
    Ocular muscles are involved, with ptosis and diplopia.
    Its form is very mild; no mortality is present.
Group II
  A. Mild Generalized
      Onset is slow and frequently ocular, gradually spreading to skeletal and bulbar muscles.
      Respiratory system is not involved. Response to drug therapy is good. Mortality rate is low.
  B. Moderate Generalized
      Onset is gradual with frequent ocular presentations, progressing to more severe generalized involvement of the skeletal and bulbar muscles. Dysarthria, dysphagia, and difficult mastication are more prevalent than in mild generalized myasthenia gravis. Respiratory muscles are not involved. Response to drug therapy is less satisfactory; patients' activities are restricted, but mortality is low.
  C. Severe Generalized
      1. Acute fulminating. Onset of severe bulbar and skeletal muscle weakness is rapid with early involvement of respiratory muscles. Progress is normally complete within 6 months. Percentage of thymomas is highest in this group. Response to drug therapy is less satisfactory, and patients' activities are restricted, but mortality is low.
      2. Late severe. Severe myasthenia gravis develops at least 2 years after most of Group I or Group II symptoms. Progression of myasthenia gravis may be either gradual or sudden. The second highest percentage of thymomas occurs in this group. The response to drug therapy is poor, and the prognosis is poor.

From Olanow, C. W., and Wechsler, A. S.: Surgical management of myasthemia gravis. In Sabiston, D. C., Jr., and Spencer, F. C.: Surgery of the Chest, 5th ed. Philadelphia, W. B. Saunders Company, 1990.

The incidence of spontaneous remission without drug or other therapy is not known, but it is thought to be uncommon and short-lasting and to occur primarily in patients with ocular involvement. The ultimate course cannot be predicted with certainty; and many variations, including spontaneous remission in patients with long-standing disease or sudden deterioration in patients who have been asymptomatic for many years, have been recorded. Myasthenia gravis generally progresses in more than 80 per cent of patients within 3 years of onset. Before 1958 the mortality was in excess of 30 per cent, and only 39 per cent of patients improved with existing therapy. More modern management allows the majority of patients to remain functionally intact, and death as a consequence of myasthenia gravis is extremely rare. A fixed myopathy late in the course of the disorder with permanent muscle weakness has been described. The authors have been concerned that this may be due to chronic anticholinesterase administration, but it has also been recorded in patients who have not received such medication.

A transient neonatal myasthenia gravis has been reported in infants of mothers with myasthenia gravis. Symptoms usually include diffuse weakness, impaired crying and sucking, poor swallowing, and, occasionally, feeble respiration. Symptoms are self-limited and generally resolve within 6 weeks. There are no long-term consequences as long as the initial symptoms are recognized and managed appropriately. Passive transfer of immunoglobulin across the placenta (presumably anti-AChR antibodies) is thought to be responsible. Interestingly, there is little correlation between the clinical status of the infant and that of the mother, despite comparable AChR antibody titers, which supports the hypothesis that host factors contribute to the development of clinical weakness.

A congenital myasthenia gravis that is more common in males has been described; it is often familial, but the mother is usually unaffected. The clinical configuration is usually not severe, and improvement occurs after 6 to 10 years of symptoms. Drugs and thymectomy are generally not effective. It has been postulated that a delay in the maturation of the neuromuscular apparatus causes a prolonged reduction of the safety factor for neuromuscular transmission. Another congenital myasthenic syndrome, due to a reduction of acetylcholinesterase in the subneural apparatus of the end-plate, has also been described. These patients do not have AChR antibodies and do not respond to anticholinesterase medications.

The myasthenic, or Lambert-Eaton, syndrome (LES) is a disorder of peripheral cholinergic transmission characterized by weakness and fatigability of proximal muscles, particularly in the lower extremities. Ocular and bulbar involvement is mild or absent. Deep tendon reflexes tend to be depressed or absent. Characteristic electromyographic (EMG) abnormalities include small amplitude muscle evoked potentials and facilitation of the amplitude following repetitive stimulation. This can also be observed clinically where repetitive muscle contraction can cause some augmentation of muscle strength. LES is often seen in association with underlying carcinoma, predominantly oat-cell carcinoma of the lung. Symptoms of LES often antedate recognition of the tumor. LES may also occur in association with chronic disease states and occasionally even in combination with myasthenia gravis. The condition is due to a deficient release of quanta of ACh from nerve terminals. Recent evidence indicates that this condition is an autoimmune disorder, and auto-antibodies have been identified. In LES, unlike myasthenia gravis, anticholinesterase agents are generally not effective. Agents that facilitate the release of ACh from the presynaptic terminals, such as guanidine, calcium, or 4-aminopyridine, may be helpful. More recently, improvement has been reported following immunosuppression with prednisone or azathioprine coupled with plasma exchange.

In general, the diagnosis of myasthenia gravis is not difficult to make if it is considered. Hysteria, thyroid disease, neuromyopathies, and other myasthenic conditions are occasionally mistaken for myasthenia gravis; but a Tensilon test, single-fiber electromyography, and determination of AChR antibody levels allow a definitive diagnosis to be made in most patients.

Associated Conditions

A number of conditions have been associated with myasthenia gravis. Many of these, such as rheumatoid arthritis, systemic lupus erythematosus, polymyositis, Sjögren's syndrome, and ulcerative colitis, are thought to be autoimmune. An association with vitamin B_{12} deficiency, thyroid disorders, diabetes mellitus, parathyroid disease, adrenal disorders, and vitiligo has been described as part of a polyglandular failure syndrome. These may be predetermined genetically, based on their linkage with histocompatibility antigens, particularly HLA-A1, HLA-B8, and HLA-Dw3. These may constitute genetic risk factors for autoimmune diseases whereby a specific exposure activates an abnormal immune response in a patient with a particular haplotype. This theory is supported by studies of monozygotic twins in which only one of the twins has been affected.

Thyroid dysfunction has been reported in 5 per cent of patients with myasthenia gravis, and the overall incidence may be much higher. It may sometimes be difficult to distinguish features of thyroid disease from those of myasthenia gravis, because each can cause proximal muscle weakness and ocular disturbances. These conditions appear to be distinct, however, because it has been shown that increased quantities of thyroid hormone *per se* do not cause myasthenia gravis and that the relationship is more likely to be immunologic or genetic than hormonal. All forms of thyroid disease, including goiter, myxedema, Graves' disease, and Hashimoto's thyroiditis, have been associated with myasthenia gravis.

Thymic Abnormalities

Disorders of the thymus gland are found in 75 to 85 per cent of patients with myasthenia gravis, and new staining techniques suggest that this incidence may be even higher. Ten to 15 per cent of patients with myasthenia gravis have thymomas. In most cases, these are benign, well-defined, encapsulated lesions that may be cystic or calcified. They are generally composed of epithelial or lymphoid cells. However, two thirds of thymomas have no association with myasthenia gravis and contain mainly spindle cells. Malignancy is usually defined by tumor infiltration into surrounding tissue such as pleura and pericardium rather than by changes in the histologic pattern. As many as 43 per cent of thymomas were malignant in one series. However, in the authors' experience, malignancy is a rare occurrence, perhaps reflecting the tendency to perform thymectomy earlier in the course of myasthenia gravis. Thymomas have not been described in children and are generally not seen before the age of 30 years. They are more common in male patients. A high-quality computed tomographic (CT) scan of the mediastinum can detect almost all thymomas (Fig. 2). The authors have occasionally had a false-positive CT scan. In a study of patients with myasthemia gravis, all of whom underwent thymectomy, there were no false-negative CT scans.

Lymphoid hyperplasia of both the cortex and medulla is found in the thymus gland of most young patients with myasthenia gravis. The number of germinal centers may increase, but this is not unique to myasthenia gravis, and its significance is uncertain. Attempts to relate the numbers of germinal centers to the duration and severity of the disease and the response to treatment have been inconclusive. The T-cell composition of the thymus gland, in terms of both numbers and subsets, is generally normal. However, there is an increased number of B cells in the thymus glands of patients with myasthenia gravis.

Patients with late-onset myasthenia gravis (after the age of 55 years) most often have an atrophic involuted thymus gland.

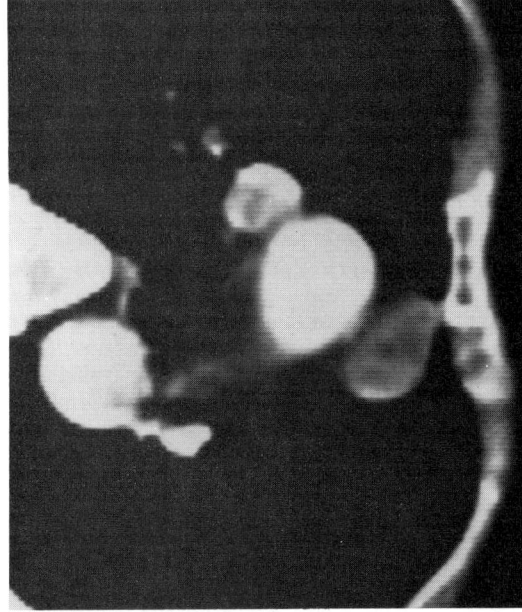

Figure 2. CT scan from a patient with a thymoma. The anterior mediastinal mass is easily visualized. With increasing experience, this test has become progressively more helpful in separating patients with thymomas from those with normal thymus glands and has even been able to identify islands of functioning thymus tissue within generally atrophic glands. (From Olanow, C. W., and Wechsler, A. S.: Surgical management of myasthenia gravis. *In* Sabiston, D. C., Jr., and Spencer, F. C.: Surgery of the Chest, 5th ed. Philadelphia, W. B. Saunders Company, 1990.)

Occasionally these can be recognized on CT scan by the presence of a low density throughout the anterior mediastinum (presumably fat) punctuated by dots of high density (presumably thymic tissue). There is evidence to suggest that an atrophic thymus gland may still be immunologically active, and thymic cells can be identified within the anterior mediastinal fat. This is important when one is considering the role of thymectomy in patients with late-onset myasthenia gravis. Older patients with myasthenia gravis have a relative lymphopenia in their peripheral blood consisting primarily of a reduction in T lymphocytes and 3A1[+] and OKT4 T-cell subsets. These changes are rapidly reversed after thymectomy and the removal of the "involuted" thymus gland.

DIAGNOSTIC STUDIES

Pharmacologic Agents

Anticholinesterase agents block the hydrolysis of ACh in the synaptic cleft, prolonging its action and increasing the likelihood of an interaction between ACh and the postsynaptic AChR. The result is an increase in the miniature end-plate potential and in the safety factor for neuromuscular transmission. These agents may temporarily reverse or improve the clinical and electrical abnormalities of myasthenia gravis. The most widely used anticholinesterase agent for diagnosis is edrophonium hydrochloride (Tensilon). This drug is short-acting and improves clinical and/or electrical abnormalities in 90 to 95 per cent of patients with myasthenia gravis. Its use is widespread, and before more sophisticated laboratory evaluations were available, a positive response was central to the definition of myasthenia gravis. The response in individual patients varies from dramatic improvement to little or no change. The ocular muscles are least sensitive to Tensilon, which occasionally makes it difficult to diagnose myasthenia gravis confined to the ocular muscles. Failure to respond to Tensilon does not exclude the diagnosis of myasthenia gravis. False-positive tests are uncommon, but have been reported in patients with brain stem gliomas, superior orbital fissure syndromes, myositis, and advanced amyotrophic lateral sclerosis (ALS). It is recommended that the Tensilon test be done at the end of the day or after exercise, when the patient's weakness is maximal.

The Tensilon test is performed by gradually injecting 2 to 10 mg. intravenously over approximately 2 minutes. It is recommended that 2 mg. be injected initially in order to minimize the possibility of inducing cholinergic weakness in patients already receiving anticholinergic medications. Additionally, some patients show a response to 2 mg. but not to 10 mg., because of cholinergic-induced weakness with the higher dose. Facilities to treat anaphylactic and respiratory complications should be available. A positive response to Tensilon generally develops within 30 to 60 seconds and lasts for approximately 1 to 5 minutes. It has been the authors' practice to do the Tensilon test in a triple-blind manner using saline and nicotinic acid as control agents. Tensilon generally causes a light-headed, hot sensation associated with lacrimation and flushing that patients or physicians may learn to recognize. Nicotinic acid reproduces some of these features without influencing neuromuscular transmission and thus serves as a suitable control substance.

Long-lasting anticholinesterase agents may be used when responses are too transient to record by standard bedside techniques. These agents have a longer latency and duration. Neostigmine may be used in a dosage of 1.5 mg. administered intramuscularly. Improvement is seen within 10 to 30 minutes and lasts up to 4 hours. When the response is still equivocal, a long-term trial of oral anticholinesterase agents over several weeks can be considered.

Patients with myasthenia gravis are highly sensitive to the neuromuscular blocking effect of curare and curare-like drugs. This heightened sensitivity has previously been used as a test to confirm the diagnosis. One-tenth of a curarizing dose may cause the patient to become significantly weak. An anesthetist must be present at this test because of the risk of respiratory decompensation. This test is now rarely used.

An abnormal "dual response" after administration of decamethonium has been described, consisting of brief depolarization after a longer period of curare-like competitive block. Although interesting pharmacologically, this test is no longer used in practice.

Electrophysiologic Studies

The hallmark of myasthenia gravis is failure of neuromuscular transmission, which is characterized electrically by a reduction in the amplitude of the miniature end-plate potential. In 1895, Jolly recognized that faradic stimulation of a peripheral nerve resulted in muscle fatigue. He reported that in patients with myasthenia gravis supramaximal repetitive stimulation of the nerve caused a gradual decrease in the amplitude of the evoked action potential without a change in antidromic conduction. The Jolly test consists of recording muscle action potentials induced by repetitive stimulation of the peripheral nerve. In normal patients, the safety margin is of such magnitude that repeated stimulations at rates of up to 40 to 50 per second can be tolerated without a change in amplitude. In patients with myasthenia gravis, abnormal decrementation of the amplitude of the evoked action potential (greater than 10 per cent) develops at stimulation rates of 2 to 3 per second, particularly when the test is performed after tetanic contraction of muscle or after the administration of regional curare. The Jolly test has the advantage of being simple and inexpensive; but unfortunately, it is not very sensitive. Changes are not detected in more than 50 per cent of patients with myasthenia gravis, particularly in the early stages, when diagnosis is most difficult.

The development of single-fiber electromyography has provided a more sensitive method of detecting impaired neuromuscular transmission. A single-fiber needle electrode is placed between two muscle fibers innervated by the same motor unit. The variation in the latency between the two action potentials is

referred to as jitter. The variation of neuromuscular transmission in myasthenia gravis causes increased jitter or blocking of one of the action potentials in severe cases. Jitter measurements are abnormal in 95 per cent of patients with myasthenia gravis if multiple muscle groups are studied. In patients with purely ocular symptoms, the frontalis or levator palpebrae superioris muscle should be examined. Jitter measurements must be analyzed in light of the clinical features, because abnormalities can be seen in disorders other than myasthenia gravis. Because jitter is a function of the amplitude of the miniature end-plate potential, this test can be used to monitor the clinical course of patients with myasthenia gravis. Although it has the advantage of being sensitive in the early detection of myasthenia gravis, it requires expensive complex machinery and neurophysiologic expertise.

Stapedial reflex decay has been used as a diagnostic study in myasthenia gravis. Preliminary results indicate a high sensitivity in patients with ocular dysfunction, but results are less encouraging in patients with generalized weakness.

Serum Antibodies

The isolation of specific neurotoxins from the venom of elapid snakes such as cobras and kraits allowed the identification of specific serum anti-AChR antibodies. Alpha-bungarotoxin, a specific neurotoxin from the banded krait, has been found to bind specifically and irreversibly to the active site of the AChR. This toxin can be used in measuring the number of receptors, purifying receptors, and assaying for serum anti-AChR antibody. The assay consists of a reaction between the test serum and AChR antigen derived from human muscle that has been incubated with ^{125}I-labeled α-bungarotoxin. If serum AChR antibodies are present, they bind to the AChR and form a complex with the ^{125}I-labeled α-bungarotoxin, which is bound to an adjacent site on the receptor. Anti-human globulin then precipitates this complex, and the radioactivity in the precipitant allows estimation of the quantitative AChR antibody level. Serum AChR antibodies are present in 85 to 90 per cent of patients with myasthenia gravis. These antibodies are highly specific for myasthenia gravis and have been reported otherwise only after the administration of penicillin or inoculation with snake venom but not in other disease states. AChR released from damaged muscle does not evoke the development of anti-AChR antibody. Anti-AChR antibody levels do not precisely correlate with the clinical status of patients with myasthenia gravis, but patients with purely ocular disease tend to have low or negative antibody titers. Antibodies that "block" α-bungarotoxin by binding to AChR have also been described. Blocking antibodies are most pronounced in patients with generalized myasthenia and particularly severe disease. By contrast, blocking antibodies are generally not detected in patients with ocular myasthenia gravis. There is little correlation between the blocking and binding antibodies. In general, it appears that patients with generalized myasthenia gravis are more likely to have blocking antibodies.

Antibodies directed against the AChR are thought to induce receptor damage by (1) accelerating degradation of the AChR by way of cross-linking of the antibody with the receptor; (2) blocking active sites on the receptor; and (3) inducing antigenic modulation and AChR degradation, possibly by inducing complement-mediated lysis.

PATHOGENESIS

Considerable evidence has accumulated since the original hypothesis by Simpson (1960) to support the concept that myasthenia gravis is an autoimmune disorder involving the postsynaptic nicotinic AChR.[33b] Histologically, the postsynaptic membrane is simplified and disorganized (Fig. 3). Alpha-bungarotoxin binding studies have shown quantitative reduction in the amount of AChR correlating with the reduction in the

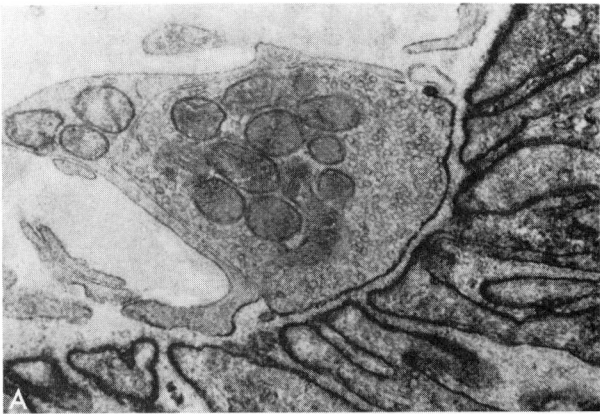
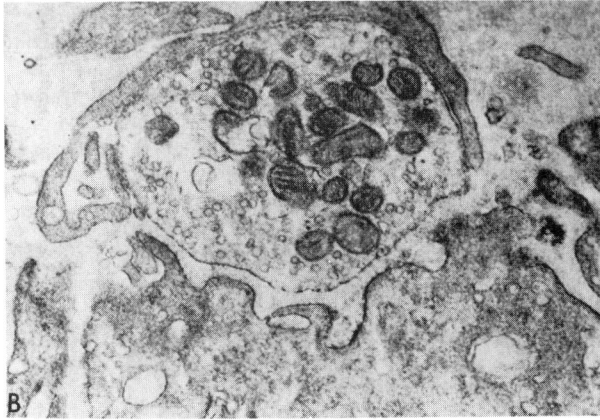

Figure 3. Neuromuscular junction with AChR stained by the peroxidase-labeled α-bungarotoxin technique. *A,* Normal neuromuscular junction with normal quantity of AChR. *B,* Neuromuscular junction in a patient with moderately severe myasthenia gravis. Note the disorganization and destruction of the postsynaptic membrane, with reduction in staining for AChR. (Courtesy of A. G. Engel.) (From Olanow, C. W., and Wechsler, A. S.: Surgical management of myasthenia gravis. *In* Sabiston, D. C., Jr., and Spencer, F. C.: Surgery of the Chest, 5th ed. Philadelphia, W. B. Saunders Company, 1990.)

amplitude of the miniature end-plate action potential and the clinical severity of the condition. The detection of specific anti-AChR antibodies in the serum of approximately 90 per cent of patients with myasthenia gravis has focused attention on this antibody in the pathogenesis of myasthenia gravis. It has been postulated that these antibodies induce clinical weakness by reducing the number of functioning AChRs, thus impairing neuromuscular transmission. Mechanisms proposed include (1) accelerated degradation of AChR in the postsynaptic membrane, (2) immunopharmacologic blockade in which the antibody hinders interactions between ACh and the AChR, (3) modulation or accelerated internalization with intracellular degradation of the AChR-AChR antibody complex, and (4) reduced synthesis of AChR.

Passive transfer of serum, more specifically immunoglobulin (Ig) G from patients with myasthenia gravis to experimental animals, can induce a myasthenic syndrome characterized by clinical, electrical, and pharmacologic features similar to those of human myasthenia gravis. This syndrome may also be caused by specific monoclonal AChR antibodies. Passive transfer among animal species has been shown. Moreover, IgG from patients with myasthenia gravis accelerates the degradation of AChR in myotubule tissue culture. In human myasthenia gravis, plasma exchange and steroids provide clinical benefit in association with a reduction in the serum anti-AChR antibody titer. The removal of thoracic duct lymph containing immunoglobulin also provides clinical improvement, and the readministration of this material causes rapid clinical deterioration. These observations support the hypothesis that AChR an-

tibodies contribute to and may be the major mechanism responsible for receptor damage in myasthenia gravis.

Nevertheless, it is by no means clear that the anti-AChR antibody is the sole factor responsible for clinical weakness. In studies at Duke University in which all patients were treated with thymectomy as the sole therapy and in which all drugs, including anticholinesterase agents, were avoided, dramatic clinical benefit was seen in most patients without a reduction in the anti-AChR antibody titer. There was no direct correlation between the serum anti-AChR antibody level and the clinical status of individual patients. The authors hypothesized that a thymic factor was essential to the development of clinical weakness in myasthenia gravis. This is supported by the development of transient neonatal myasthenia gravis in the infant of an asymptomatic thymectomized mother, with comparable levels and bioactivity of anti-AChR antibody in each. Although steroids and plasma exchange provide dramatic clinical improvement in many patients, the corresponding reduction in anti-AChR antibody titer may be an independent phenomenon. It is presumptive to assume that this reduction is essential for clinical improvement; and clearly, more than anti-AChR antibodies is removed by plasma exchange. Furthermore, the reduction in the anti-AChR antibody titer after plasma exchange is often short-lived, whereas clinical benefit may persist for weeks or months.

Different anti-AChR antibodies that react to different sites on the AChR have been identified, and it is possible that current techniques fail to identify the specific subset that would better correlate with the clinical status of patients with myasthenia gravis. Moreover, anti-AChR antibody titers may not accurately reflect antibody activity at the neuromuscular junction. In the Duke drug-free group, no patient converted to a negative antibody titer after thymectomy, despite clinical improvement, and when antibody titers did fall, they did so gradually over a period of years rather than in direct correlation with the clinical status.

In an elegant series of experiments, Engel and associates (1977) showed deposits of IgG and C3 on segments of the postsynaptic membrane in the distribution of the AChR and on fragments of degenerating junctional folds in the synaptic space.[12a] More severely affected myasthenic patients bind relatively smaller amounts of IgG and C3, presumably because there are fewer residual AChRs. The presence of C3 indicates activation of the complement reaction. Subsequent activation of the major or alternate pathway could then effect a complement-mediated lysis of the membrane.

Sahashi and associates (1980), by using an immunoperoxidase method, showed the presence of the C9 terminal and lytic complement component at the postsynaptic junctional folds and in debris within the synaptic clefts in the same basic distribution as C3. Once again, there was an inverse relationship between the structural integrity of the junctional folds and the abundance of C9. The areas of involvement were discrete and widely separated, supporting the concept of an autoimmune attack. C3 does not necessarily cause membrane damage and may be found over long portions of junctional membrane. Activation to C9, however, causes irreversible damage to the membrane. Demonstration of C9 over only short portions of junctional folds and in abundance in the degenerated material of the synaptic cleft supports the role of the complement-mediated lysis as the mechanism of membrane damage in myasthenia gravis. This differs from other conditions such as Duchenne's muscular dystrophy in which degeneration of junctional folds occurs in the absence of IgG or C9. It is possible that the anti-AChR antibody marks the receptor for complement-mediated lysis.

Although most attention has been focused on humoral immune mechanisms, cell-mediated immune mechanisms have not been excluded from having a role in the pathogenesis of myasthenia gravis. Studies in the authors' laboratories have shown a reduction in the number of peripheral blood T cells in patients with late-onset myasthenia gravis. This reduction consists primarily of T-cell subsets 3A1 and OKT4, and these changes normalize rapidly after thymectomy. Lymphocyte transformation has been described in several laboratories after exposure of peripheral blood and thymic lymphocytes to purified AChR antigen. This stimulation index has also been reported to be reduced after thymectomy. Alterations in mixed lymphocyte reactions and autologous lymphocyte reactions have also been observed in patients with myasthenia gravis. Although not a consistent finding, lymphorrhages, which are small groups of lymphocytes within muscle, are occasionally detected. All of these changes suggest that a cell-mediated mechanism has some role in the pathogenesis of myasthenia gravis, but its importance has not yet been defined. The possibility of multiple mechanisms and heterogeneous populations of patients must be considered.

Experimental Allergic Myasthenia Gravis

Using α-bungarotoxin derived from snake venom, Patrick and Lindstrom (in 1973) were able to isolate AChR from homogenized muscle. Purified receptor was then injected into rabbits in an effort to provoke specific anti-AChR antibodies.[30a] Several weeks after this immunization, the rabbits became weak and died. The weakness had clinical, electrical, and pharmacologic features resembling those seen in human myasthenia gravis, and this disorder is now known as experimental autoimmune myasthenia gravis. It is thought to be the result of AChR antibodies generated by immunization with AChR cross-reacting with the rabbits' own AChR, leading to impaired neuromuscular transmission. Histologic changes seen at the neuromuscular junction are similar to those seen in human patients, and passive transfer of serum or lymphocytes from these animals can induce the disease when injected into normal animals. An acute state occurs approximately 1 week after immunization and is characterized by severe muscle weakness and a cellular invasion of the neuromuscular junction with breakdown of the postsynaptic membrane and AChR. Approximately 3 weeks after immunization, a chronic stage develops in association with a rising anti-AChR antibody titer. The postsynaptic membrane becomes decreased in area and simplified, with a consequent reduction in the total number of AChRs. The chronic phase of experimental autoimmune myasthenia gravis is almost identical to that in the human disorder, but the experimental autoimmune condition differs from human myasthenia gravis in that the acute transient phase is not seen in human patients. This may reflect a differing nature of the immunizing event, with the human patient not being exposed to a massive bolus of antigen at one time, or differences in host response. It has also been suggested that the acute phase may be related to the adjuvant rather than the AChR.

Significantly, experimental autoimmune myasthenia gravis does not develop in animals that have been thymectomized before immunization. A thymic factor may be essential to the development of clinical weakness in this condition. Moreover, C3 deficiency also attenuates the clinical and electrical features of experimental autoimmune myasthenia gravis and supports the hypothesis that complement-mediated lysis may be the mechanism leading to membrane damage.

Role of the Thymus Gland

A relationship between the thymus gland and myasthenia gravis has been appreciated since the beginning of the twentieth century. Seventy-five to 85 per cent of patients with myasthenia gravis have pathologic changes in the thymus gland, and for 50 years thymectomy has been known to influence the clinical course of the disease. It is therefore not surprising that the thymus gland has been suggested to have a role in the pathogenesis of myasthenia gravis. The exact role of the thymus

gland, however, must still be defined. Within the thymus gland there are (myoid) cells that have a striking similarity to embryonic muscle cells. These cells express AChR epitopes on the surface and react with anti-AChR antibodies. Thymic cells in culture can produce anti-AChR antibody, and irradiated thymic cells that have been rendered functionally inactive can augment the production of anti-AChR antibody from peripheral lymphocytes. The thymus gland has a major role in lymphocyte maturation and is capable of influencing almost all humoral and cellular immune reactions. It has been proposed that an initiating event, possibly viral in origin, induces a "thymitis." Because of the proximity of myoid cells to maturing lymphocytes, it is possible that T cells, at a critical stage of maturation, could be activated to react against AChR epitopes. T cells could then be disseminated to the periphery and cross-react with peripheral AChR epitopes on postsynaptic membranes, causing interference with neuromuscular transmission. The altered thymus gland might also generate a population of T4 helper cells that could stimulate the production of anti-AChR antibodies by peripheral lymphocytes. In fact, the T4/T8 ratio is increased in patients with myasthenia gravis. This peripheral imbalance is not found in the thymus gland itself and persists even when patients improve. Increased B cells are observed in the thymus gland of patients with myasthenia gravis and could also produce anti-AChR antibodies. The thymus gland could generate killer T cells that damage the neuromuscular junction. Additionally, thymic hormones have been identified that bind to the AChR with a high affinity and may have a role in activating the complement pathway, ultimately causing AChR damage.

The mechanism by which thymectomy provides clinical benefit has not yet been elucidated. It has been shown that thymectomy influences cell-mediated immunity and peripheral T-cell counts in patients with late-onset myasthenia gravis. The clinical relevance of this finding is not established. Thymectomy may serve to remove a source of (1) AChR antigen, which is a source of autoactivation against AChR antigenic determinants; (2) anti-AChR antibody production; (3) sensitized helper T cells that facilitate the production of anti-AChR antibody by peripheral lymphocytes; (4) sensitized killer T cells directed against the neuromuscular junction; and (5) a putative thymic factor that may act directly at the acetylcholine receptor or may activate complement-mediated lysis at antibody-labeled receptor sites. It is also possible that thymectomy acts by multiple or unknown mechanisms and has different effects in individual patients.

Failure of thymectomy to induce clinical remission might be due to (1) incomplete thymectomy, (2) permanent irreparable damage to the neuromuscular junction, (3) immune complexes from damaged end-plates perpetuating the immune response in lymphocytes within the spleen and lymph nodes that are unaffected by thymectomy, and (4) the influence of long-lived peripheral T cells.

The association of myasthenia gravis with other autoimmune disorders, particularly the polyglandular failure syndrome, suggests that in some patients the immunologic attack may be more widely directed than at the AChR alone. The relationship with HLA antigens in some patients with myasthenia gravis also suggests that there is a genetically predisposed population of patients whose immunologic tolerance may be altered in such a manner that a specific exposure causes an altered immunologic response.

TREATMENT

Numerous methods of treatment have been used in the management of myasthenia gravis. Variations in the natural history and the lack of prospective controlled studies of the different treatment modalities prevent an absolute determination of the preferred form of treatment for a particular patient at the

TABLE 2. Drugs That Interfere with Neuromuscular Transmission Under Experimental Conditions

Antibiotics	Psychotropics
Amikacin	Amitriptyline
Paramycin	Amphetamines
Polymyxin A	Droperidol
Sisomicin	Haloperidol
Viomycin	Imipramine
	Paraldehyde
Antiarrhythmics	Trichloroethanol
Ajmaline	
	Others
Antirheumatics	Amantadine
Colchicine	Diphenhydramine
	Emetine
	Pindolol
Anticonvulsants	Sotalol
Ethosuximide	

From Olanow, C. W., and Wechsler, A. S.: Surgical management of myasthenia gravis. *In* Sabiston, D. C., Jr., and Spencer, F. C.: Surgery of the Chest, 5th ed. Philadelphia, W. B. Saunders Company, 1990.

present time. In addition, it has been suggested that the natural history of myasthenia gravis as it is seen today follows a more benign course than that seen in previous decades. Improvement in supportive measures and surgical technique may contribute to the improved statistics on patients, independent of the specific therapy chosen. The large number of variables to be controlled and physician bias favoring one form of therapy over another make it unlikely that an answer will be forthcoming, and at least for the present, judgment is required in instituting therapy.

The authors have favored thymectomy performed as early as possible after the development of generalized weakness as the preferred form of therapy, particularly for younger patients. Anticholinesterase medications have been avoided whenever possible and immunosuppressant therapy used only when necessary, rather than as a routine treatment. Patients were evaluated in a prospective, standardized treatment protocol to minimize variables and to avoid physician bias. After follow-up of approximately 5 years, more than 80 per cent of patients were free of generalized weakness, and more than 60 per cent were on no medication. This protocol did not compare thymectomy with other forms of treatment, but the excellent results obtained and the advantage of avoiding the side effects associated with medication prompt the authors to recommend this form of treatment, particularly in younger patients with generalized myasthenia gravis. Before a more detailed discussion of thymectomy is presented, the advantages and disadvantages of the major forms of treatment currently being used are considered. In all cases, drugs that interfere with neuromuscular transmission (Table 2) should be avoided or used cautiously because they might cause deterioration in myasthenic status.

Medical Treatment

ANTICHOLINESTERASE AGENTS. Anticholinesterase agents have been a standard form of medical treatment for myasthenia gravis since their introduction in the mid 1930s. They act by preventing the hydrolysis of ACh and increase the likelihood of interactions between ACh and the AChR. The safety margin for neuromuscular transmission is thus increased, providing temporary improvement in the clinical and electrical features of myasthenia gravis. These agents may provide considerable improvement with restoration of muscle strength. However, this response is only symptomatic and these drugs in and of themselves do not lead to remission. Side effects of anticholinesterase drugs include abdominal colic, diarrhea, nausea, salivation, and lacrimation as a result of smooth muscle and glandular stimulation. These symptoms may be controlled by atropine. This is not recommended, however, because the

symptoms may forewarn the patient and physician of developing "cholinergic crisis." Cholinergic crisis is the result of excessive stimulation of AChRs due to prolonged depolarization of receptors. Consequent muscle weakness is not directly related to myasthenia gravis. Cholinergic weakness can be differentiated from myasthenic weakness by administration of a test dose of Tensilon, because symptoms fail to respond or deteriorate after the administration of additional anticholinesterase medication. Treatment consists of discontinuation of anticholinesterase agents and appropriate supportive measures.

Neostigmine (Prostigmin) and pyridostigmine (Mestinon) are the most commonly used anticholinesterase agents. Neostigmine is available in 15-mg. tablets, which are usually administered every 4 hours or more frequently when required. There is usually a 30-minute delay before maximal efficacy, and the optimal dosage is determined by trial and error. Parenteral administration of 0.5 mg. is equivalent to 15 mg. orally. Pyridostigmine is the more popular medication because it is thought to have a smoother effect and to be longer-acting, with a less abrupt loss of efficacy. Sixty milligrams of pyridostigmine is approximately equivalent to 15 mg. of neostigmine. A 180-mg. timed-release capsule is available for more prolonged use, such as at night.

Despite the popularity of the anticholinesterase agents, the authors have preferred not to use them whenever possible. The symptomatic benefit they provide may delay the introduction of more definitive therapies, such as thymectomy or immunosuppression, that are believed to be more effective when initiated within the first few years of symptoms. Anticholinesterase agents increase bronchial and oropharyngeal secretions, which may cause respiratory complications, particularly in the perioperative period. After thymectomy, there appears to be an increased sensitivity to anticholinesterase medications, wherein the same dose that was used preoperatively may cause cholinergic weakness postoperatively. Cholinergic weakness may also be induced during the postoperative period by failure to appreciate that much smaller doses of anticholinesterase agent are required when administered parenterally. For these reasons, anticholinesterase agents have been avoided in patients undergoing thymectomy without an evident loss of clinical benefit and what appears to be a smoother operative and postoperative course.

Evidence in experimental animals indicates that chronic exposure to anticholinesterase agents independently causes AChR damage and electron microscopic alterations identical to those seen in myasthenia gravis. Although there is no proof that a similar phenomenon occurs in human patients, there has been the concern that long-term use of these agents may cause a fixed myopathic state unrelated to the myasthenia.

CORTICOSTEROIDS. There have been many studies demonstrating the beneficial effect of corticosteroids in patients with myasthenia gravis. Clinical response may be dramatic, and total remission may occur. However, it is important to appreciate that the introduction of steroids may be associated with a transient but profound clinical deterioration. This usually occurs between the fourth and eighth days after introduction; and for this reason, the authors generally initiate high doses of steroids in a hospital setting, where provisions for respiratory assistance are available. High-dose prednisone therapy is initiated at approximately 60 mg. per day and is generally reserved for patients with severe generalized weakness or bulbar dysfunctions. When an adequate response has been obtained, patients are switched to an alternate-day dosage schedule. The authors recommend that the alternate-day dosage be tapered by 10 mg. monthly as clinically appropriate. When the alternate-day dosage has been reduced to 60 mg., it is recommended that reductions in dosage not exceed 5 mg. every other day and that changes be made no more frequently than once every month to minimize the risk of inducing a myasthenic crisis. When patients have myasthenia gravis confined to the ocular muscles or only slight generalized weakness, some prefer to initiate prednisone at a dose of 5 mg. every other day and increase the alternate-day dosage by 5 mg. every 2 to 4 weeks as necessary. The advantage of this approach is that it may avoid higher doses and patients can be managed on an outpatient basis.

Although many authorities use steroids as a primary mode of therapy, the authors prefer to use them only in patients who cannot or will not undergo a thymectomy or in patients who have had a clinically unsatisfactory response to thymectomy. Corticosteroids have been used to prepare patients for thymectomy, but the same effect can now be accomplished with plasma exchange without the risk of clinical deterioration and the difficulty of withdrawing steroid medication.

The mechanism of action of corticosteroids is not understood. Most attention has focused on immunosuppression because steroids suppress all immunocompetent cells. Several groups have reported a reduction in the anti-AChR antibody titer that correlates with clinical improvement in patients with myasthenia gravis, raising the possibility that suppression of immunoglobulin is responsible for clinical benefit. However, studies of thymectomy as the sole treatment modality have failed to confirm a direct correlation between clinical status and the anti-AChR antibody titer. Although these studies suggest that an essential thymic component contributes to the development of clinical weakness, the possibility exists that steroids and thymectomy act by different mechanisms. Steroids may have a thymolytic effect, although it is noteworthy that they may be effective in patients who have already undergone thymectomy. A direct effect on neuromuscular transmission has also been suggested by the transient deterioration during the off day reported by patients on alternate-day steroid schedules.

When steroids have been initiated, they may be difficult to discontinue. Although the dosage may be substantially reduced, in many patients steroids have to be maintained indefinitely. Aside from the risk of clinical deterioration related to dosage change, there are many side effects associated with sustained administration of steroids. These side effects include cataracts, psychosis, gastrointestinal bleeding, carbohydrate intolerance, hypertension, obesity, osteoporosis, growth failure in the juvenile population, and decreased resistance to infection. In one large series, as many as 50 per cent of patients developed cushingoid features. Although the benefit of the steroids is not questioned, prospective control studies showing that they are superior to other forms of therapy such as thymectomy do not exist, and the authors have preferred to use these drugs only when necessary, rather than on a routine basis, in an effort to avoid these potential complications.

PLASMA EXCHANGE. Plasma exchange is a technique that permits the selective removal of plasma or plasma components by a centrifugal method. The remaining red blood cells are then suspended in a solution such as lactated Ringer's solution and reintroduced into the patient. The procedure, which is easy to accomplish, produces rapid transient clinical improvement in patients with myasthenia gravis. The authors have used plasma exchange primarily to optimize the medical status of patients before thymectomy. One to 3 liters of plasma is removed per run on an alternate-day basis until the maximal clinical benefit has been obtained (usually four to six runs). This clinical improvement facilitates perioperative management while avoiding the need for additional medications. Except for occasional hypotension during the first or second run, plasma exchange is generally well tolerated. Hypocalcemia and hypoalbuminemia may follow repeated runs and need to be identified and treated appropriately. Surgical intervention is not recommended within 24 hours of the last run of plasma exchange to minimize the risk of bleeding and infection due to removal of clotting factors or immunoglobulins.

Plasma exchange is an accepted treatment that provides temporary clinical benefits for patients with myasthenia gravis. The mechanism of action is related to the removal of specific plasma factors. The serum anti-AChR antibody has been implicated because levels are reduced by 50 to 60 per cent at the time of plasma exchange in conjunction with clinical improvement. Clinical benefit, however, may persist substantially longer than the anti-AChR antibody remains depressed, and some patients demonstrate response to plasma exchange who have no detectable serum anti-AChR antibodies. Current techniques are nonselective and involve the risk of transferring infectious agents such as hepatitis and the acquired immunodeficiency syndrome (AIDS) virus. Attempts have been made to define a more selective procedure in which there is specific immunoadsorption of the anti-AChR antibody. Protein A–Sepharose gels provide a high degree of selective IgG adsorption, causing reductions in anti-AChR antibodies comparable to those obtained with conventional plasma exchange techniques.

Plasma exchange induces rapid but temporary clinical benefit, and generally immunosuppressant drugs must be used in conjunction with it in order to obtain a stable clinical improvement. It has not been established that plasma exchange increases the likelihood of clinical remission, compared with the use of immunosuppressant drugs alone. The authors use plasma exchange primarily to prepare patients for operation, as discussed in the next section. In addition, plasma exchange can be used to provide temporary benefit for patients whose symptoms are refractory to thymectomy or who have had an acute deterioration after thymectomy. Plasma exchange can also be used in conjunction with the introduction of high-dose steroids to prevent the clinical deterioration associated with their introduction.

IMMUNOSUPPRESSANT AGENTS. The evidence supporting an immunologic basis for myasthenia gravis and the response to plasma exchange have fostered an interest in immunosuppressant drugs as a possible therapy for myasthenia gravis. Formerly, these drugs were primarily used in patients refractory to more conventional therapies such as thymectomy or steroids. Azathioprine has been widely used in a dose of 1.5 to 3 mg. per kg. There is a latent period of 6 to 12 weeks before the onset of benefit, and maximal effect may not be obtained for 1 year or longer. European physicians have extensive experience with this drug and report favorable responses in most patients, although serious complications such as marrow suppression, gastrointestinal bleeding, decreased resistance to infection, and death have been infrequently reported. The possibility of delayed side effects such as the development of a malignancy should also be considered. Occasionally patients experience nausea, vomiting, and diarrhea with the introduction of azathioprine, but otherwise the drug is generally well tolerated, and exacerbations of myasthenia with manipulation of dosage such as occurs with steroids are generally not observed.

There has been considerable interest recently in the possibility that cyclosporine, a potent immunosuppressant agent, may have a role in the treatment of myasthenia gravis. Cyclosporine has been widely used to achieve immunosuppression in patients undergoing renal, cardiac, and hepatic transplantation. Cyclosporine inhibits T-cell–dependent immune responses and reduces tolerance across major histocompatibility barriers through the expansion and functional activation of lymphocyte subsets. Although it appears to have its primary effect on cellular immunity, it is likely that it has an influence on humoral immunity as well. Cyclosporine induces a reduction in interleukin-1 and interleukin-2 as well as gamma interferon. Introduction before or during immunization provides a better response in laboratory animals, and it is thought to be more beneficial if introduced early in the course of myasthenia gravis.

Tindall performed a double-blind placebo-controlled study of cyclosporine in patients with early-onset myasthenia gravis. At both 6 and 12 months, patients randomized to cyclosporine demonstrated improved strength and a greater, although not statistically significant, decline in anti-AChR antibody titers than patients randomized to placebo. Clinical benefits evolved rapidly and were particularly noteworthy for patients with visual and bulbar dysfunction. Beneficial responses were observed in patients who were both anti-AChR antibody–negative and –positive, which suggests that cyclosporine may work in myasthenia gravis by influencing both cellular and humoral immunity. Studies are currently under way for assessing the role of cyclosporine in patients with more advanced myasthenia gravis as well as in those who are already receiving steroids. The authors have been particularly interested in the use of cyclosporine in patients with late-onset myasthenia gravis, where bulbar symptoms predominate and thymectomy provides less predictable benefit than in younger patients.

Nephrotoxicity is the major side effect of cyclosporine. Morphologic changes have been described in the proximal tubule, but it is not clear whether this is on the basis of toxic or hemodynamic effects. Generally, nephrotoxicity is nonprogressive with reduction in dosage and reversible if the drug is discontinued. Risks are greater in older patients and those with hypertension. It is generally recommended that the lowest clinically effective dose of cyclosporine be employed. Although the specific role of cyclosporine in the treatment of myasthenia gravis has not yet been established, it is an extremely promising drug.

The ideal immunotherapy for myasthenia gravis would selectively delete the autoimmune reaction directed at the AChR in a permanent manner without toxicity. Exciting new immunologic strategies designed to provide a treatment that might "cure" myasthenia gravis include (1) attempts to inhibit the accelerated degradation of the AChR using methylation inhibitors (designed to block the endocytosis of the AChR induced by anti-AChR antibodies that cross-link with the receptor); (2) elimination of specific B cells that produce anti-AChR antibodies by using toxins that bind to epitopes for AChRs that are present on AChR antibody–producing B cells; (3) total body lymphoid irradiation, designed to kill mature lymphocytes while protecting immunologic precursor cells, on the basis of evidence that immunologic tolerance may develop during and immediately after lymphoid irradiation (antigen-specific tolerance may be induced by presenting AChR antigens during or after lymphoid irradiation); (4) selective proliferation of anti-idiotype antibodies directed against the anti-AChR antibody, which may downregulate the immune response, and (5) generation of antigen-specific suppressor cells, which may have the capacity to suppress the immune response directed against a specific antigen.

Myasthenia gravis is one of the best studied and characterized of the immunologic disorders. Subunits of the AChR have been identified and have been cloned. Several "myasthenic" sites within the alpha subunit of the AChR have been defined that activate either T or B cells in patients with myasthenia gravis and initiate the specific stimulatory sequences critical to the development of myasthenia gravis in a specific patient. New immunologic strategies may soon permit immunologic therapy directed against a specific region within the AChR in individual patients with myasthenia gravis.

Surgical Treatment

THYMECTOMY. The central role of the thymus gland in myasthenia gravis, combined with current deficiencies in medical management, has caused increasing interest in the role of thymectomy in the management of myasthenia gravis. The authors employ thymectomy as a primary mode of treatment for myasthenia gravis. Patients with myasthenia are considered for thymectomy as soon as possible after the development of generalized weakness. Plasma exchange is used to optimize medical status prior to thymectomy if patients have significant weakness. Patients on anticholinesterase medications have these

agents slowly withdrawn during the time of plasma exchange. It is rare to encounter a patient who cannot be withdrawn from anticholinesterase agents during plasma exchange. As a result, patients are operated upon without these medications and consequently have a less complex perioperative course.

Patients receiving corticosteroids are maintained on them throughout the perioperative period for prevention of adrenal insufficiency; after this period attempts are made to gradually lower the dosage over the ensuing months as described above.

Thymectomy should be done in an institution with an experienced treatment team. There must be a close working relationship between the neurologist, the anesthesiologist, the surgeon, and the intensive care unit personnel. When thymectomy is done under these conditions, the operative mortality should be below 1 per cent and should occur only in high-risk patients with profound clinical weakness. Preoperative sedation may be given, but doses should be less than in patients without myasthenia gravis. Atropine is avoided. Most anesthesiologists use short-acting barbiturates for induction of anesthesia and maintain anesthesia with an inhalation agent. Succinyl chloride and curare are rarely necessary and are best avoided. Patients who have experienced significant respiratory difficulty or profound weakness before operation are generally managed with nasotracheal intubation, because it is more comfortable if ventilator support is required. When early extubation is anticipated, an orotracheal tube is used, which is easier to place and avoids trauma to the nasal mucosae.

SURGICAL ANATOMY OF THE THYMUS GLAND. Knowledge of the surgical anatomy of the thymus gland begins with an understanding of its embryonic differentiation. Human thymic primordium arises primarily from the third branchial pouch in close association with the inferior parathyroid gland, which affixes to the posterior side of the thyroid gland, whereas the thymus descends into the thorax. A portion of the thymic primordium may also develop from the fourth branchial pouch in association with the superior parathyroid gland. In the branchial complex stage, the pharyngobranchial duct closes and the communication between the pharynx and the thymus is loosened. Ultimately, the lobes of the thymus separate from the parathyroid glands and descend into the thorax. Controversy remains regarding ectopic portions of the thymus gland found in the neck, cephalad to the main body of the thymus gland. This thymic tissue may derive from the fourth branchial pouch along with parathyroid tissue. An alternative postulate suggests that this thymic tissue originates from the third branchial pouch but breaks off during its descent into the thorax. This complex migratory pattern of the thymus gland is thought to be responsible for the finding of ectopic thymic tissue in locations such as the left main bronchus, the parenchyma of the lung, the posterior mediastinum, and the hilum of the lung.

After the thymus gland has migrated into the anterior mediastinum, it relates to the major mediastinal structures. It overlies the pericardium and great vessels at the base of the heart and is in proximity to the left innominate vein. The thymus gland has an H-shaped configuration, with variable fusion of the right and left lobes at about the mid-portion of the gland. The superior poles of the gland are thinner than the inferior poles. The upper portion of the gland attenuates into the thyrothymic ligament, which connects the thymus gland to the thyroid gland. There are many variations in the regional anatomy of the thymus gland. It may lie posterior or anterior to the left innominate vein, and the superior pole of the gland may extend along the pretracheal fascia into the root of the neck. At the lateral extent of the gland, there is a fine capsule that separates it from the pleura and the parapleural mediastinal fat that lies proximal to the phrenic nerve. The arterial supply to the thymus gland is derived from the internal mammary arteries via their pericardiophrenic branches. Venous drainage is through one or two large veins that drain into the anterior aspect of the left innominate vein. When the thymus gland lies posterior to the left innominate vein, drainage may be into the posterior portion of that vein. The thymus gland is largest relative to body size within the first or second year of life, when it may attain as much as 50 per cent of its ultimate weight. The mass of the gland is usually greatest at the time of puberty, when it weighs 25 to 50 gm. After puberty, there is gradual replacement of the densely packed lymphocyte architecture of the gland by adipose tissue, and in late life, thymic remnants may be detected only microscopically. Normally, there is a distinct thymic capsule that allows its separation from surrounding mediastinal and cervical structures. The degree of fusion and the extent of upper pole development vary to a great extent.

SURGICAL TECHNIQUE. Various surgical techniques are available for the performance of thymectomy. The particular choice of technique varies as dictated by the personal preference of the surgeon and his beliefs concerning the pathogenesis of myasthenia and the role of thymectomy in the treatment of myasthenia gravis. Thymic tissue has been documented to be a normal component of perithymic fat; and if a diligent search for this tissue is made, it can be found approximately 75 per cent of the time. Thymic tissue is frequently located in multiple sites within the anterior mediastinum, and thus the median sternotomy approach for thymectomy is preferred because it allows the most complete approach for total removal of thymic tissue. Surgical approaches for thymectomy include the following:

1. Transcervical thymectomy
2. Median sternotomy
3. Partial median sternotomy
4. Median sternotomy plus cervical incision
5. Upper median sternotomy combined with transsternal sternotomy

The technique of cervical thymectomy was initially described by Crotti in 1938, was reintroduced by Crile, and was extended by Kark and Kirschner. The technique is preferred by some surgeons because of the cosmetic incision, low morbidity, and minimal stay in the hospital. It has been advocated as particularly useful in patients with significant respiratory distress and in whom no tracheostomy has been done. When cervical thymectomy is done, the patient is prepared and draped for a median sternotomy in the event of the occurrence of an intrathoracic complication requiring exploration or an unanticipated problem in removing the gland. The procedure is initiated by making a curvilinear incision approximately 2 cm. above the suprasternal notch and then extending this incision to the level of the strap muscles. After retraction of the strap muscles, the cervical fascia covering the thymus gland is entered, and the manubrium can be raised anteriorly. Special retractors have been devised that allow anterior traction to be placed on the sternum to facilitate the dissection. The thymus is mobilized from the innominate vein, and its venous attachment is divided between silver clips. By traction on the upper pole of the gland, it is possible to continue mobilization, and the arterial supply to the gland is then divided by using electrocautery. Resection is generally limited to that portion of the gland enclosed within the thymic capsule. If the wound is dry, drainage is generally not necessary. Inadvertent pleural entry can be treated by hyperinflation of the lungs as the deep tissue planes are closed. If the wound is not entirely free from bleeding at termination of the procedure, a small drainage catheter can be introduced into the superior mediastinum for several hours to a day for collection of any residual blood. Advocates of this procedure generally cite remission rates for their patients comparable to those using the transsternal approach, although patients are usually preselected and the studies are neither standardized nor controlled. Further residual mediastinal thymic tissue has been found in up to 60 per cent of patients after transcervical sternotomy. Recurrent myasthenia associated with significant

amounts of residual thymic tissue and even thymomas have been reported after transcervical thymectomy. Although it is an aesthetically pleasing and technically feasible procedure, transcervical thymectomy achieves a less complete thymectomy than transsternal thymectomy. The importance of total thymectomy is unknown, but there is concern that incomplete removal of the thymus may be associated with a higher recurrence of myasthenia gravis.

The initial concern with median sternotomy for thymectomy is related to impaired pulmonary mechanics after a major chest incision. Splinting of the chest, damage to the phrenic nerves, mediastinal infection, a higher pain medication requirement, a cosmetically less appealing incision, and postoperative pulmonary complications such as atelectasis and pneumonia have all been cited as disadvantages to the transsternal approach. Several factors have changed this situation. Patients are referred for thymectomy earlier in the course of their disease and tend to be less ill. Medical status can usually be improved by plasma exchange before thymectomy so that even patients having respiratory difficulty come to thymectomy with good ventilatory potential. The better clinical state of patients before thymectomy has allowed early mobilization and has reduced the incidence of pulmonary complications after the procedure. For patients requiring tracheostomy, an incision can be used that is anatomically separated from the tracheostomy stoma and that minimizes the risk of contamination and mediastinal sepsis.

A composite drawing constructed from the work of Jaretzki and associates (1977), who did a careful anatomic and histologic examination of the mediastinal and cervical regions at the time of thymectomy, is shown in Figure 4. The normal location of the thymus gland is shown along with the variety of other locations for thymic tissue that were noted. The wide range of locations of thymic tissue in the mediastinum emphasizes the need for good exposure of both the mediastinal contents and the cervical extent of the thymus gland if thymectomy is to be attempted. This exposure can be obtained with a median sternotomy. In men, a

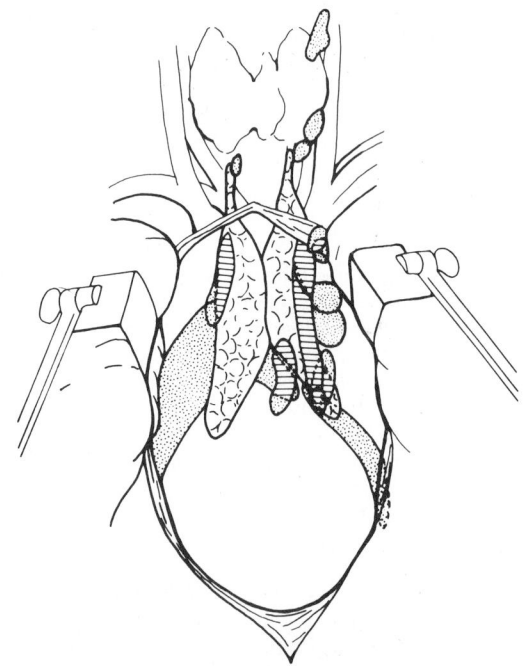

Figure 4. "Classic" location of the thymus gland. Based on the work of Jaretzki and associates (1977), the location of other thymic tissue is shown in the stippled or lined areas. Of particular importance is the location of thymic tissue deep in the lateral mediastinum and also superiorly in relation to the thyroid gland and frequently not in continuity with the remainder of the thymus gland. (From Olanow, C. W., and Wechsler, A. S.: Surgical management of myasthenia gravis. *In* Sabiston, D. C., Jr., and Spencer, F. C.: Surgery of the Chest, 5th ed. Philadelphia, W. B. Saunders Company, 1990.)

short vertical skin incision can be made and can be mobilized adequately cephalad and caudad to allow median sternotomy, sternal separation, and adequate cervical exposure by retraction of the skin. In women, a median sternotomy with excellent exposure of the superior extent of the thymus gland and the lower cervical region can be obtained by using supramammary or inframammary incisions that leave a cosmetically excellent scar. In these approaches, a curvilinear incision is made just over the breast and is extended inferiorly in the midline (supramammary incision) or beneath the breasts (inframammary incision).

By using skin hooks and electrocautery, it is possible to establish a bloodless plane of dissection that allows elevation of the anterior chest wall to well above the suprasternal notch superiorly and to the xiphoid inferiorly. The sternotomy is then done by using a saw and by taking care to remain in the midline of the sternum. This approach affords an excellent visualization of the thymus gland and its vascular attachments and is a cosmetically acceptable incision. It also allows extensive removal of perithymic tissue and mediastinal fat.

The pleural reflections onto the thymus gland are pushed gently to the sides by blunt dissection. A plane is then established between the inferior aspect of the thymus gland and the anterior aspect of the pericardium. Starting in the midline and working toward the pleural spaces, each lobe of the inferior thymus gland is freed from its superficial pericardial attachments. As the gland gradually assumes form, gentle traction separates it from the pleura. Efforts are made not to enter the pleural space, but if this occurs it is not a significant complication. As the dissection proceeds cephalad, the thymus gland is retracted superiorly to identify the thymic vein or veins on the posterior surface of the gland as they enter the left innominate vein. These veins are divided between silver clips, and the gland is separated from the innominate vein. Each of the superior poles of the thymus gland is then dissected from the surrounding fascial tissue until it is identified as an attenuated fibrous cord. Both fibrous cords are transected and the thymus is removed.

Placement of a warm cotton pad in the anterior mediastinum for a few moments generally provides excellent hemostasis, after which a No. 28 chest tube is positioned in the mediastinum and the sternum is reapproximated. If the pleural space has been entered, the tip of the chest tube may be advanced into the pleural space, but a separate pleural drainage catheter is rarely necessary. Postoperative bleeding is usually minimal, and the tube can be removed several hours after the operation. The sternotomy wound is closed in layers, with a subcuticular skin closure.

MODIFICATION OF THYMECTOMY FOR THYMOMA. When the thymus gland appears to be unusually firm or is adherent to any of the surrounding structures, the surgeon should be highly suspicious that a thymoma is present. This may not have been appreciated in the preoperative assessment, even if CT scanning of the mediastinum was done. If a thymoma is present, infiltration into surrounding structures must be searched for carefully, because this is the major criterion for malignancy. Because there may be recurrences even after removal of a benign thymoma, a complete and careful dissection of the tumor mass is required. Care should be taken to avoid injury to the phrenic nerve; however, if it is incorporated within the tumor mass and complete resection is otherwise impossible, it may be sacrificed. Extensive involvement of the left innominate vein or of the internal surface of the pericardium is an ominous prognostic sign, and complete resection may not be possible. If a malignancy is suspected, however, an aggressive attempt at removal of the tumor is warranted, and removal of a portion of the pericardium, the left innominate vein, one of the phrenic nerves, and the pleural reflections should be done. Total surgical extirpation offers the best likelihood for long-

term cure in cases of malignant thymoma. If removal of the tumor is impossible, radiation therapy is generally used, and the field can be better defined by marking the peripheral extent of tumor involvement with surgical clips. Frozen-tissue biopsies are of little help in diagnosing malignant thymomas because the determination of malignancy is primarily from the biologic behavior of the tumor. Biopsy may, however, disclose the presence of cell types other than those of thymoma.

POSTOPERATIVE CARE. After thymectomy, the patient is returned to the intensive care unit to be observed by the physician and nursing team. The effects of the anesthetic agents are allowed to dissipate while the patient is supported with a ventilator, usually using intermittent mandatory ventilation at low-rate settings. The decision of when to extubate the patient is based mainly on the preoperative condition. In patients with disease of relatively short duration and mild symptoms, extubation is considered several hours after operation. Patients with more severe myasthenia gravis may require intubation for longer periods. Extubation is done when the patient is alert and shows a satisfactory vital capacity. The patient should be able to generate inspiratory negative pressure greater than 20 cm. H_2O. After extubation, frequent measurements of vital capacity should be obtained by using a bedside digital spirometer. Patients must be watched carefully, because deterioration of ventilatory status may occur several days postoperatively. Preoperative preparation reduces the likelihood of prolonged intubation or subsequent ventilatory deterioration. The patient may be ambulated the morning after operation and, in most cases, is prepared for discharge within a few days.

RESULTS OF THYMECTOMY. Improvement after thymectomy has been reported in 57 to 86 per cent of patients and permanent remission in 20 to 36 per cent. This clinical improvement may be delayed 3 to 5 years from the time of operation. Analysis of these data is hampered by differences in patients selected for operation, timing of thymectomy, choice of route, underlying pathologic conditions, and perioperative care. Moreover, it is known that even without treatment, spontaneous remission may occasionally occur. There are no prospective controlled studies that allow comparison of the results of thymectomy versus medical therapy versus the natural history of myasthenia gravis in a particular population. Nonetheless, in reviewing most published articles, it has not been possible to find any reported series in which patients treated medically fared better than those treated surgically. A retrospective, controlled, matched, computerized study (Fig. 5) favored thymectomy over medical therapy with respect to remission and survival (Buckingham and associates, 1976).[4b] It is difficult to determine which patients with delayed improvement after thymectomy might have experienced spontaneous remission without therapy. Although the data are confusing, it is the impression of most groups that the greatest likelihood for permanent remission is seen after thymectomy. In general, patients with nonthymomatous myasthenia gravis have better remission rates and long-term survival than those with thymomatous myasthenia gravis.[29]

Only 10 per cent of patients with a noninvasive thymoma are reported to have remission. When the tumor is invasive, remission is less likely, and more than 50 per cent of patients die within 5 years. Most of these deaths occur in the first year after operation and are related to myasthenic complications. Because the primary feature of malignancy in thymoma is local invasion, the argument for early thymectomy has been advanced in an attempt to perform thymectomy before infiltration of surrounding tissues. This approach may result in a lesser percentage of malignant thymomas. The present ability to perform thymectomy safely and to potentially avoid long-term drug side effects causes many experts to consider thymectomy as the treatment of choice for myasthenia gravis.

The authors introduced a prospective management plan for

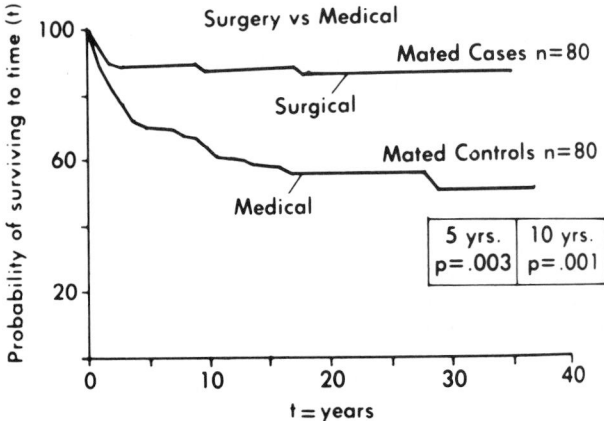

Figure 5. A matched, computerized, retrospective analysis of medical versus surgical management in myasthenia gravis. This work done at the Mayo Clinic provides the longest comparative follow-up for patients treated both medically and surgically in which the patients were matched for severity of disease as well as for their personal characteristics. The improved survival in the surgical group of patients was statistically significant at both 5 and 10 years, and this difference was maintained with additional passage of time. (From Buckingham, J. M., Howard, F. M., Bernatz, P. E., et al.: The value of thymectomy in myasthenia gravis: A computer-assisted matched study. Ann. Surg., *184:*453, 1976.)

patients with myasthenia gravis at Duke University Medical Center. All patients with evidence of generalized myasthenia gravis, regardless of severity, had thymectomy. Preoperative plasma exchange was used to optimize medical status if necessary. Efforts were made to use thymectomy as the sole treatment modality and to use medications only if necessary, rather than routinely. The results have been most gratifying and are indicated in Table 3. Thymectomy was not withheld because of age, and good results were obtained in all age groups with all types of thymic pathology. Residual myasthenic symptoms have been confined mainly to the ocular muscles. Forty-six of 47 patients were improved after thymectomy, compared with their prethymectomy, preplasmapheresis state (mean follow-up, 25.5 months). Thirty patients were functionally intact and free of generalized weakness at normal levels of activity. Nine patients had only residual ocular dysfunction. Thus 83 per cent of patients were free of significant generalized weakness. The majority of these patients require no medication. Before thymectomy, anti-AChR antibody titers generally correlated with the severity of the myasthenia. Postoperatively, there was no direct relationship between anti-AChR antibody titer and clinical status, because anti-AChR antibody levels did not change significantly, but there was dramatic clinical improvement in the patients.

Because the early results were encouraging, the series was continued and a second group of patients was analyzed in which 55 patients were treated for myasthenia gravis by using thymectomy as the primary therapy.[28] None of these 55 patients were receiving long-term medical management for myasthenia gravis at the time of entry into the study, and all patients were prepared for operation in an individualized manner by using plasma exchange as the interim treatment modality when indicated. None of the patients had isolated ocular myasthenia, and excluded from the study were patients with long-standing myasthenia thought to have a fixed neurologic deficit. Clinical status was assessed by using a modified Osserman grading system, and patients were followed for a mean of 39.3 months.

Sixty-four per cent of the patients (35 of 55) were asymptomatic and had no functional neurologic deficit. Sixteen per cent (9 patients) had residual ocular dysfunction, but no generalized weakness. Thus 80 per cent of the patients (44 of 55) were free of generalized weakness an average of 39.3 months after thymectomy. Ten patients continued to have mild generalized weakness, but none had residual bulbar dysfunction. Ninety-two per cent of the patients (50 of 55) were improved by at least one stage in comparison with their prethymectomy, pre-plasma exchange baseline status. Seventy-one per cent of patients (39 of 55) improved by two or more stages. Four patients did not improve; and there was one death related to management of an acute exacerbation with high-dose steroids, later development of a cushingoid state, and later pulmonary embolism. Thymic pathology included thymic hyperplasia, atrophic thymic involution, thymoma, and thymic cysts. Improvement in patients was the rule regardless of the underlying thymic pathology. After thymectomy, drug therapy was avoided whenever possible and fifty-five per cent of the patients (30 of 55) were not taking any medication at 39.3 months of follow-up.

By using thymectomy as primary treatment for generalized myasthenia gravis, 92 per cent of patients enrolled in the series were improved and 80 per cent were free of generalized weakness at the time of latest medical follow-up (mean, 39.3 months). Fifty-five per cent of patients were receiving no medical therapy, and 38 per cent never received medical therapy in the course of their treatment. Particularly important for surgeons is the awareness that early use of thymectomy with this approach avoided perioperative problems associated with the use of anticholinesterase and corticosteroid therapy. Specifically, slow wound healing, difficult postoperative management, and occasional postoperative deterioration were avoided.

Benefits were observed in patients of all age groups; but improvement was least likely in older patients, particularly if they had bulbar dysfunction. The authors have therefore preferred to initiate treatment with immunosuppressive agents such as azathioprine or cyclosporine in older patients with bulbar dysfunction and to reserve thymectomy for treatment failures.

There has not been a prospective randomized study that

TABLE 3. Clinical Status of Patients Who Underwent Thymectomy for Treatment of Myasthenia Gravis in the Duke Medical Center Series

| Clinical State | Before Thymectomy | | No. of Patients After Thymectomy | | | | | |
	No. of Patients	No. Receiving Medication	Normal	I	IIA	IIB	IIC	Died
IIA	28	21	24	4				
IIB	9	8	4	2	3			
IIC	10	10	2	3	3	1		1
Number of patients receiving antimyasthenia drugs after thymectomy according to post-thymectomy clinical state			1	1	3	1		

From Olanow, C. W., and Wechsler, A. S.: Surgical management of myasthenia gravis. *In* Sabiston, D. C., Jr., and Spencer, F. C.: Surgery of the Chest, 5th ed. Philadelphia, W. B. Saunders Company, 1990.

compares the effects of thymectomy with the effects of other forms of management for myasthenia gravis. The Duke Medical Center study is unique in its use of thymectomy as the primary mode of therapy for all patients when they enter the program. It is difficult to compare these results with those of other thymectomy series, because in some institutions thymectomy is used only when medical management for treatment of myasthenia gravis has failed or when a thymoma is suspected. Because of the strict treatment protocol in the Duke series, no physician bias with regard to which patient should have thymectomy entered into the treatment decision. Rather than pursuing medical management, every effort was made to avoid the use of antimyasthenic medications. Optimization of the clinical state was by plasma exchange without immunosuppression, rather than with drug therapy. All thymectomies were done in a standardized manner, were radical in nature, and were performed by the same surgeon. This approach showed that in most patients, thymectomy alone could provide dramatic and sustained clinical improvement without the need for additional medications. Moreover, reduction in the anti-AChR antibody titer was not essential for clinical improvement. These observations support the hypothesis that a factor elaborated by or in the thymus gland has a role in AChR destruction. Further studies to identify, isolate, and characterize a putative thymic factor are necessary, because the identification of such a "thymic factor" could allow the development of special techniques to provide for its removal or neutralization.

Because data continue to emerge relating the effects of thymectomy on the course of myasthenia gravis, it appears to be particularly important that a thymectomy that is as complete as possible be performed. Assessment of long-term data should not be confused by uncertainty regarding the presence of residual thymic tissue.

Algorithms for Management of Patients with Myasthenia Gravis

Because of success with the ongoing treatment plans discussed in this chapter, a summary for the diagnosis and management of patients with myasthenia gravis is provided here.

As outlined in Figure 6, when a patient presents with myasthenic symptoms a careful history is obtained and physical examination performed. One of the primary goals at this time is to determine whether the patient has myasthenia gravis or weakness associated with another clinical condition. The response to Tensilon, the Jolly and jitter tests, and determination of the level of the anti-AChR antibodies identify the disease correctly in more than 95 per cent of cases. The patient is then placed in a subgroup according to functional classification, and a distinction is made as to whether the patient has ocular or generalized myasthenia gravis. Many patients who seek the attention of a physician because of ocular symptoms have generalized myasthenia gravis but are unaware of it. Because the method of treatment for each type differs at this time, it is important to make this differentiation. Various laboratory tests are designed to determine whether there are associated conditions in addition to clinical myasthenia gravis; and when present, these conditions are specifically treated. Radiographic studies are used to detect the presence of a thymoma.

When the diagnosis of generalized myasthenia gravis has been made, a therapeutic decision must be made. If the patient has evidence of generalized weakness, the authors advocate thymectomy as the primary treatment. Plasma exchange is used to prepare the patient for thymectomy by minimizing weakness and permitting anticholinesterase agents to be withdrawn. If weakness is minimal, and the patient is not on anticholinesterase agents, thymectomy can be performed directly. Medical therapy is employed for patients who cannot or will not undergo thymectomy or for patients with late-onset myasthenia gravis (usually over the age of 60). If myasthenic symptoms are confined to the ocular muscles (ocular myasthenia gravis), a conservative treatment program is followed in which patients are carefully monitored for the development of features of generalized weakness. At that time, patients are managed in the same way as are those who present with features of generalized myasthenia gravis. If necessary, the ocular symptoms can be treated with low-dose prednisone employed on an alternate-day schedule.

It is the opinion of the authors that this approach provides the greatest likelihood of providing remission to patients with myasthenia gravis while minimizing the adverse effects of pharmacologic therapies.

By using this overall treatment plan, the systemic complications of pharmacologic management of myasthenia gravis can be avoided or minimized. Thymectomy as the primary therapy for myasthenia gravis yields remission in most patients and allows reduced pharmacologic requirements in patients with residual symptoms after thymectomy.

APPROACH TO MYASTHENIA PATIENT

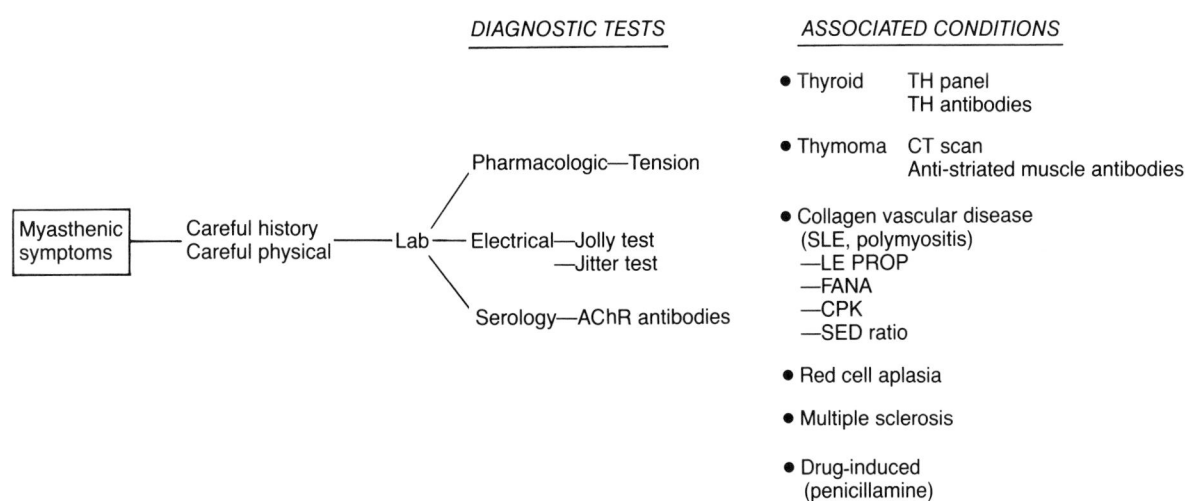

Figure 6. An algorithm for evaluating patients with myasthenia gravis. Identification of associated conditions is important for optimal management of patients with myasthenia gravis. (Redrawn from Olanow, C. W., and Wechsler, A. S.: Surgical management of myasthenia gravis. *In* Sabiston, D. C., Jr., and Spencer, F. C.: Surgery of the Chest, 5th ed. Philadelphia, W. B. Saunders Company, 1990.)

SELECTED REFERENCES

Blalock, A., Mason, M. F., Morgan, H. J., and Riven, S. S.: Myasthenia gravis and tumors of the thymic region. Ann. Surg., 110:544, 1939.
Blalock reported the first successful removal of a thymic tumor for the treatment of myasthenia gravis. He used this case as the impetus for reviewing the literature and provides an excellent summary of the rationale for surgical extirpation of the thymus gland in the treatment of myasthenia gravis. The comments from the audience at the end of the manuscript are well worth reading.

Drachman, D. B.: Myasthenia gravis. N. Engl. J. Med., 298:136, 186, 1978.
This is a broad review of myasthenia gravis in which the disease process is discussed from the basic concepts of neuromuscular transmission to specific therapy. It serves as a good source of reference for the reader interested in pursuing certain areas of the subject in greater depth. It differs slightly from the views presented in this chapter in that treatment depends more on medical therapy and indications for thymectomy are more conservative.

Jaretzki, A., Bethea, M., Wolff, M., et al.: A rational approach to total thymectomy in the treatment of myasthenia gravis. Ann. Thorac. Surg., 24:120, 1977.
This article is important for physicians interested in the surgical technique of thymectomy. The authors explore the completeness of thymectomy done by transcervical, median sternotomy, and combined transcervical and median sternotomy routes in a group of their own patients. There are extremely well done anatomic drawings that show some of the atypical thymus gland locations encountered in the course of their clinical experience. There is also an excellent discussion that includes comments by proponents of other techniques of thymectomy and the reasons behind their arguments.

Lindstrom, J. M., Lennon, V. A., Seybold, M. E., et al.: Experimental autoimmune myasthenia gravis and myasthenia gravis: Biochemical and immuno-chemical aspects. Ann. N.Y. Acad. Sci., 274:254, 1976.
This is a well-presented and comprehensive review of experimental work considering immune mechanisms in myasthenia gravis. It provides an excellent background for the understanding of current therapies designed to interfere with humoral and cell-mediated immunity.

Olanow, C. W., Wechsler, A. S., and Roses, A. D.: A prospective study of thymectomy and serum acetylcholine receptor antibodies in myasthenia gravis. Ann. Surg., 196:113, 1982.
This study, done at Duke University Medical Center, is unique in that every patient admitted with the diagnosis of myasthenia gravis was treated in accordance with a strict clinical protocol. For most patients, thymectomy was used as the primary and frequently the only method of therapy. High remission rates were reported with minimal reliance on drug therapy.

REFERENCES

1. Abdou, N. I., Lisak, R. P., Sweiman, B., et al.: The thymus in myasthenia gravis: Evidence for altered cell populations. N. Engl. J. Med., 291:1271, 1974.
2. Abramsky, O., Aharonov, A., Teitelbaum, D., et al.: Myasthenia gravis and acetylcholine receptor: Effect of steroids in clinical course and cellular immune response to acetylcholine receptor. Arch. Neurol., 32:684, 1975.
3. Appel, S. H., Almon, R. R., and Levy, N.: Acetylcholine receptor antibodies in myasthenia gravis. N. Engl. J. Med., 293:760, 1975.
4. Argov, Z., and Mastaglia, F. L.: Disorders of neuro-muscular transmission caused by drugs. N. Engl. J. Med., 301:409, 1979.
4a. Blalock, A., Harvey, A., Ford, F. R., and Lileuthal, J. L.: The treatment of myasthenia gravis by removal of the thymus gland. J.A.M.A., November 1941.
4b. Buckingham, J. M., Howard, F. M., Bernatz, P. E., et al.: The value of thymectomy in myasthenia gravis: A computer-assisted matched study. Ann. Surg., 184:453, 1976.
5. Castleman, B.: The pathology of the thymus gland in myasthenia gravis. Ann. N.Y. Acad. Sci., 135:496, 1966.
6. Chang, C. C., Chen, T. F., and Chuang, S. T.: Influence of chronic neostigmine treatment on the number of acetylcholine receptors and the release of acetylcholine from the rat diaphragm. J. Physiol., 230:613, 1973.
7. Dau, P. C., Lindstrom, J. M., Cassel, C. K., et al.: Plasmapheresis and immunosuppressive drug therapy in myasthenia gravis. N. Engl. J. Med., 297:1134, 1977.
8. Drachman, D. B.; Myasthenia gravis. N. Engl. J. Med., 298:136, 186, 1978.
9. Drachman, D. B., Kao, I., Pestronk, A., et al.: Myasthenia gravis as a receptor disorder. Ann. N.Y. Acad. Sci., 274:226, 1976.
10. Drachman, D. B., McIntosh, K. R., De Silva, S., et al.: Strategies for the treatment of myasthenia gravis. Ann. N.Y. Acad. Sci., 12:176, 1987.
11. Early thymectomy for myasthenia gravis (Editorial). Br. Med. J., 3:262, 1975.
11a. Elmqvist, D., Hoffman, W. W., Kugelberg, J., Quastel, D. M. J.: An electro-physiological investigation of neuromuscular transmission in myasthenia gravis. J. Physiol. (Lond..), 174:417, 1964.
12. Emeryk, B., and Strugalska, M. H.: Evaluation of results of thymectomy in myasthenia gravis. J. Neurol., 211:155, 1976.
12a. Engel, A. G., Lambert, E. H., and Howard, F. M., Jr.: Immune complexes (IgG and C3) at the motor end-plate in myasthenia gravis. Mayo Clin. Proc., 52:267, 1977.
13. Frambrough, D. M., Drachman, D. B., and Satyamurti, S.: Neuromuscular junction in myasthenia gravis: Decreased acetylcholine receptors. Science, 182:293, 1973.
14. Genkins, G., Papatestas, A. E., Horowitz, S. H., et al.: Studies in myasthenia gravis. Early thymectomy: Electrophysiologic and pathologic correlations. Am. J. Med., 58:517, 1975.
15. Goldman, A. J., Hermann, C., Jr., Keesey, J. C., et al.: Myasthenia gravis and invasive thymoma: A 20-year experience. Neurology, 25:1021, 1975.
16. Haynes, B. F., Harden, E. A., Olanow, C. W., et al.: Effective thymectomy on peripheral lymphocytes subsets in myasthenia gravis: Selective effect on T-cells in patients with thymic atrophy. J. Immunol., 131:773, 1983.
17. Jaretzki, A., Bethea, M., Wolff, M., et al.: A rational approach to total thymectomy in the treatment of myasthenia gravis. Ann. Thorac. Surg., 24:120, 1977.
18. Koelle, G. B.: Anticholinesterase agents. In Goodman, L. S., and Gilman, A., (Eds.): The Pharmacological Basis of Therapeutics, 5th ed. New York, Macmillan Company, 1975, p. 445.
19. Langman, J.: Medical Embryology. Baltimore, Williams & Wilkins Co., 1969.
20. Legg, M. A., and Brady, W. J.: Pathology and clinical behavior of thymomas: A survey of 51 cases. Cancer, 18:1131, 1965.
21. Lindstrom, J. M., Lennon, V. A., Seybold, M. E., et al.: Experimental autoimmune myasthenia gravis and myasthenia gravis: Biochemical and immunochemical aspects. Ann. N.Y. Acad. Sci., 274:254, 1976.
22. Matell, G., Bergstrom, K., Franksson, C., et al.: Effects of some immuno-suppressive procedures on myasthenia gravis. Ann. N.Y. Acad. Sci., 274:659, 1976.
23. Mittag, T., Kornfeld, P., Tormay, A., et al.: Detection of antiacetylcholine receptor factors in serum and thymus from patients with myasthenia gravis. N. Engl. J. Med., 294:691, 1976.
24. Mulder, D. G., Hermann, C., and Buckberg, G. D.: Effect of thymectomy in patients with myasthenia gravis: A sixteen year experience. Am. J. Surg., 128:202, 1974.
25. Namba, T., Brown, S. B., and Grob, D.: Neonatal myasthenia gravis: Report of two cases and review of the literature. Pediatrics, 45:488, 1970.
26. Noda, M., Furutani, Y., Takahashi, H., et al.: Cloning and sequence analysis of calf cDNA and human genomic DNA in coding alpha-subunit precursor of muscle acetylcholine receptor. Nature, 305:818, 1983.
27. Olanow, C. W., Wechsler, A. S., and Roses, A. D.: A prospective study of thymectomy and serum acetylcholine receptor antibodies in myasthenia gravis. Ann. Surg., 196:113, 1982.
28. Olanow, C. W., Wechsler, A. S., Sirotkin-Roses, M., et al.: Thymectomy as primary therapy in myasthenia gravis. Ann. N.Y. Acad. Sci., 505:595, 1987.
29. Papatestas, A. E., Alpert, L. I., Osserman, K. E., et al.: Studies in myasthenia gravis. Effects of thymectomy: Results on 185 patients with nonthymomatous and thymomatous myasthenia gravis, 1941–1969. Am. J. Med., 50:465, 1971.
30. Papatestas, A. E., Genkins, G., Horowitz, S. H., et al.: Thymectomy in myasthenia gravis: Pathologic, clinical, and electrophysiologic correlations. Ann. N.Y. Acad. Sci., 274:555, 1976.
30a. Patrick, J., Lindstrom, J., Culp, B., and McMillan, J.: Studies on purified eel acetylcholine receptor and anti-acetylcholine receptor antibody. Proc. Natl. Acad. Sci., 70:3334, 1973.
31. Pinching, A. J., Peters, D. K., and Newsom, D. J.: Remission of myasthenia gravis following plasma-exchange. Lancet, 2:1373, 1976.
32. Roses, A. D., Olanow, C. W., McAdams, M. W., and Lane, R. J. M.: There is no direct correlation between serum antiacetylcholine receptor and antibody levels and the clinical status of individual patients with myasthenia gravis. Neurology, 31:220, 1981.
33. Rowland, L. P.: Controversies about the treatment of myasthenia gravis. J. Neurol. Neurosurg. Psychiatry, 43:644, 1980.
33a. Schuhmacher and Roth: Thymektomie bei einem Fall van Morbus Basedowi mit myasthenia. Mitt. Grenzgeb. Med. Chir., 25:746, 1913.
33b. Simpson, J. A.: Myasthenia gravis: A new hypothesis. Scot. Med. J., 5:419–436, 1960.
34. Stalberg, E., Trontel, J. V., and Schwartz, M. S.: Single muscle fiber recording of jitter phenomenon in patients with myasthenia gravis and in members of their families. Ann. N.Y. Acad. Sci., 274:189, 1976.
35. Tindall, R. S. A., Rollins, J. A., Phillips, J. T., et al.: Preliminary results of a double-blind randomized placebo controlled trial of cyclosporin in myasthenia gravis. N. Engl. J. Med., 316:719, 1987.
36. van der Geld, H. W. R., and Strauss, A. J. L.: Myasthenia gravis: Immunological relationship between striated muscle and thymus. Lancet, 1:57, 1966.
37. Wechsler, A. S., and Olanow, C. W.: Myasthenia gravis. Surg. Clin North Am., 60:946, 1980.

55

SURGICAL DISORDERS OF THE PERICARDIUM

Thomas L. Spray, M.D.

Historical Aspects

Ancient people gained knowledge of the pericardium primarily by observations of corpses during war. Homer spoke of "hairy hearts" (presumably posttraumatic fibrinous pericarditis) in heroes who died on the battlefield.[10,77] Hippocrates (460 B.C.) described the pericardium as "a smooth mantle surrounding the heart and containing a small amount of fluid resembling urine." Galen (A.D. 131–201) named the pericardium and suggested its protective role.

In the seventeenth century, Richard Lower made accurate observations about the physiology of constrictive pericarditis and cardiac tamponade. In 1649, J. Riolan suggested pericardiotomy by trephination of the sternum for relief of effusion. William Harvey demonstrated to King Charles that a large part of the pericardium is insensitive to pain by palpating the heart of a nobleman who had sustained a large chest wound. Lancisi in 1728 described the clinical findings in constrictive pericarditis and correlated these with necropsy findings. Morgagni (1761) described seven cases of constrictive pericarditis and described the heart as "so constricted and confined that it could not receive a proper quantity of blood to pass on."[52] He also noted that these patients had relatively few symptoms prior to death. Romero (1819) reported the first successful pericardiotomy to relieve pericardial effusion through an approach in the fifth left intercostal space. Three patients were described, two of whom recovered.[65] Successful pericardiocenteses for massive pericardial effusions were described by Schuh and Karanaeff in 1840.[36]

The physiologic mechanism of constrictive pericarditis was accurately described by Norman Chevers of Guy's Hospital of London: "The principal cause of dangerous symptoms . . . appears to arise from the occurrence of gradual contraction in the layer of adhesive material which has been deposited around the heart, compressing its muscular tissue, and embarrassing its systolic movements, but more particularly the latter."[15] Kussmaul (1873) described the classic physical signs of pericardial tamponade: neck vein distention and pulsus paradoxus, which he defined as paradoxical because the palpated pulse disappeared during inspiration even though the heart continued to beat at the apex.[39] He also noted an inspiratory increase in central venous pressure in constrictive pericarditis (Kussmaul's sign). Rose (1884) described the effects of effusion or hemorrhage on the heart and coined the term "herz tamponade."[66]

Early surgical approaches to the pericardium were reported by Larrey, a surgeon in Napoleon's army, who performed the subxiphoid pericardiotomy.[44] Pericardial resection for constriction was introduced by Hallopeau and by Rehn and Sauerbruch early in the twentieth century.[62,69]

Significant advances have been made in the understanding of the physiologic mechanism of the normal and diseased pericardium by Isaacs and by Parsons and Holman.[33,57,58] Beck's experimental studies demonstrated that extensive fibrosis rather than obliteration of the pericardial space by adhesion was required to produce the syndrome of constriction, and that removal of the scarred pericardium would relieve the constrictive process.[3,5] Several authors have advocated extensive and radical pericardial excision for prevention of recurrence of constriction.[9,25,72]

Anatomy

The pericardium is a strong flask-shaped tissue sac that attaches and fuses to the great arteries, the proximal pulmonary veins, and the vena cava. Ligamentous attachments anchor the parietal pericardium anteriorly to the sternum and xiphoid process, posteriorly to the vertebral column, and inferiorly to the diaphragm. Arterial blood supply is from small branches of the aorta, internal mammary, and musculophrenic arteries. Innervation is via the vagus, left recurrent laryngeal, and esophageal plexus. Rich sympathetic innervation is derived from the stellate and first dorsal ganglia and the cardiac, aortic, and diaphragmatic plexuses. The phrenic nerves course along the pericardium laterally to the diaphragm and appear to carry afferent pain perception entering the spinal cord at C4 to C5.[31,76] The anterior portion of the parietal pericardium is sensitive to pain. The parietal pericardium consists of a layer of dense collagen and elastin fibers with an inner serous membrane composed of a single layer of mesothelial cells. The visceral pericardium is the surface of the heart itself and consists of a thin layer of loose fibrous tissue covered by mesothelial cells. The parietal and visceral pericardia are continuous at or near sites of attachment of the great vessels to the heart.

Electron microscopy reveals exuberant microvilli and long single cilia projecting from the serous mesothelium of the visceral and parietal pericardia (Fig. 1). The microvilli are believed to increase the surface area for fluid absorption, and the surface specializations of the mesothelial cells provide decreased friction during cardiac motion.[34]

The human pericardium normally contains up to 50 ml. of clear fluid, which is believed to be produced from the visceral pericardial surface.[64] The fluid appears to be an ultrafiltrate with protein concentration approximately one third that of plasma.[29] Lymphatic drainage of the pericardial space occurs by both the thoracic duct via the parietal pericardium and the right lymphatic duct in the right pleural space.

FUNCTIONS OF THE PERICARDIUM

The pericardium reduces friction between the heart and surrounding organs. In addition, it is a firm, fibrous sac with ligamentous attachments that fix the heart anatomically to prevent motion with change in body position. The fibrous tissue also provides a barrier against infection from contiguous structures. Hemodynamic functions of the pericardium are controversial, because congenital absence or surgical excision of the pericardium is not associated with clinical symptoms. Experimental observations suggest that the pericardium may have a role in (1) equalization of hydrostatic forces on the heart, (2) limitation of

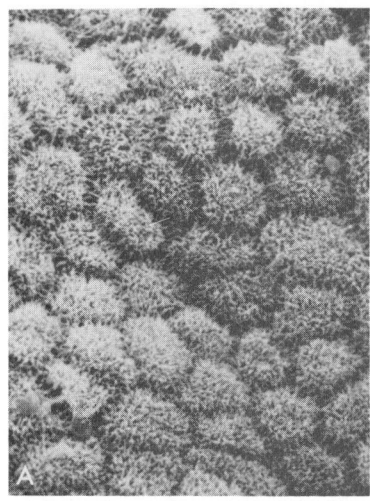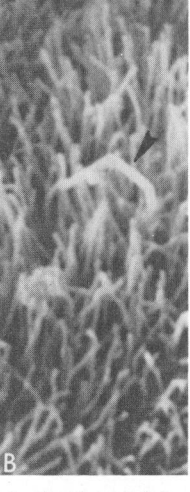

Figure 1. Scanning electron micrographs of parietal pericardium. *A*, Polygonal mesothelial cells are covered with surface microvilli (×2000). *B*, High magnification view of canine parietal pericardium (× 10,000). Single cilia (arrowhead) are present in addition to the surface microvilli. (From Ferrans, V. J., Ishihara, T., and Roberts, W. C.: Anatomy of the pericardium. *In* Reddy, P. S., Leon, D. F., and Shaver, J. A. (Eds.): Pericardial Disease. New York, Raven Press, 1982.)

cardiac distention, and (3) diastolic hemodynamic coupling of the two ventricles.[80]

Normal pericardial pressures equal intrapleural pressures and vary from −5 to +5 cm. H_2O. The pressure is transmitted uniformly throughout the intrapericardial space, minimizing gravitational and inertial forces on the circulation.[2] The normal parietal pericardium is noncompliant, and therefore, when the pericardium is filled, intrapericardial pressure rises sharply as volume of the pericardium increases (Fig. 2).[31] The transmural pressure (the difference between intracardiac and intrapericardial pressure), however, may fall, leading to decreased diastolic volume and preload. As pericardial fluid is removed, intrapericardial pressure is lower at any specific volume than during fluid addition (hysteresis).[53]

The noncompliant pericardium may also restrain ventricular dilation and, therefore, limit acute distention of the heart.[7,38] Hearts unsupported by the pericardia rupture at lower pressures than do hearts with intact pericardia.[8] The pericardium also contributes to diastolic coupling between the two ventricles. The distention of one ventricle alters the distensibility of the other, and this effect is markedly accentuated by the presence of an intact pericardium.[68] Elevation of right ventricle filling pressures causes shifting of the ventricular septum to the left and leads to a decrease in left ventricular volume and distensibility.[11,12]

ACUTE PERICARDITIS

Acute pericarditis due to inflammation of the pericardium is characterized by chest pain, pericardial friction rub, and electrocardiographic abnormalities. The most common causes of the syndrome of acute pericarditis include idiopathic or viral pericarditis, uremia, bacterial pericarditis, acute myocardial infarction, tuberculosis, trauma, or neoplastic infiltration of the pericardium.[73] Viral or idiopathic pericarditis is commonly seen in outpatients; however, patients admitted to hospitals more commonly have pericarditis due to trauma, neoplasm, uremia, or postpericardiotomy syndromes.[46] The pathologic changes in the pericardium consist of acute inflammation with polymorphonuclear leukocytes, increased pericardial vascularity, and fibrin deposition. Fibrinous adhesions between the pericardial parietes and exudation of fluid into the pericardial space are typical features. A wide range of etiologic factors produce the common pathologic features of pericarditis (Table 1).[63]

HISTORY. Chest pain is the most frequent complaint of patients with acute pericarditis, and it is variable in location. Often it is localized to the retrosternal or left precordial regions and radiates to the neck. The pain is often exacerbated by lying supine, coughing, deep inspiration, or swallowing and is eased by sitting up and leaning forward. Occasionally, pericardial pain may be induced by stretching of the pericardium from a contained effusion. Dyspnea occurs primarily because of the need to take shallow breaths to avoid the pleuropericardial pain.[19]

PHYSICAL EXAMINATION. The pathognomonic physical finding of acute pericarditis is a pericardial friction rub, which is classically of three components related to cardiac motion during atrial systole, ventricular systole, and rapid ventricular filling in diastole. The rub may be variable and evanescent.

ELECTROCARDIOGRAM. Four stages of electrocardiographic changes occur in acute pericarditis.[78,79] In Stage 1, ST segment elevation is present in all leads except aVR and V_1. T waves are usually upright. The Stage 1 changes accompany the onset of chest pain and are nearly diagnostic of pericarditis. In Stage 2 several days later, the ST segments return to the baseline accompanied by T wave flattening. In Stage 3, the T waves are inverted but are not associated with loss of R wave voltage or appearance of Q waves, differentiating this nonspecific T wave inversion from evolution of myocardial infarction. In Stage 4, the T waves revert to normal; this may occur weeks or months after the initial pericardial insult. All four stages of electrocardiographic changes can be observed in up to 50 per cent of patients with acute pericarditis. Intermittent atrial fibrillation, supraventricular tachycardia, or atrial flutter occurs in approximately 20 per cent of patients and is related to the proximity of the sinus node and perinodal tissue to the overlying inflamed pericardium.[35]

The chest film is of little diagnostic value unless it is accompanied by a large pericardial effusion, which may enlarge the cardiac silhouette. The most sensitive test for evaluation of pericardial effusion is the echocardiogram, which can localize and quantify the effusion in most patients. Additional information on the thickness of the pericardium may also be obtained. Nonspecific indicators of inflammation, including elevation of the sedimentation rate and leukocytosis, are often present.

NATURAL HISTORY. Most acute pericarditis is self-limited, with gradual improvement over 2 to 6 weeks. The most common causes are viral pericarditis due to coxsackieviruses A and B, idiopathic pericarditis, postmyocardial infarction pericarditis, or postpericardiotomy syndrome. The pericardial inflammation

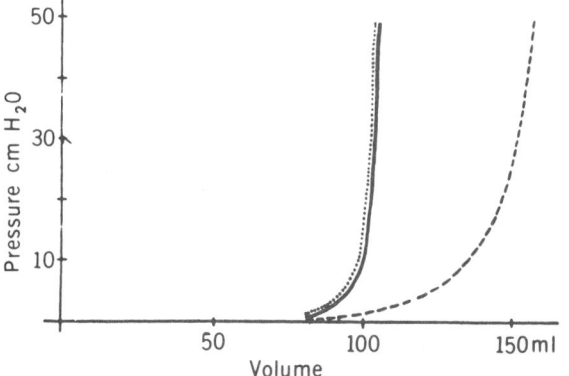

Figure 2. Pressure-volume curves before *(left)* and after *(right)* removal of the pericardium of a dog heart. On the left, the solid line is pericardial volume; the dotted line is heart volume within the pericardium. On the right, the dashed line is heart volume after the removal of the pericardium. Note the steep slope of the pressure-volume curve with the intact pericardium and the lesser rise in pericardial pressure with increasing volume in the absence of the pericardium. (From Hort, W.: Herzbentel und Herzgrosse. Arch. Kreislaufforsch., *44*:21, 1964.)

TABLE 1. Etiologic and Morphologic Classifications of Pericarditis

Etiologic	Morphologic							
	Fibrinous	Effusion	Infective	Fibrous	Neoplastic	Granulomatous	Calcific	Cholesterol
Idiopathic	++	+	0	++	0	0	++	++
Infective								
Pyogenic	+	+	++	+	0	0	0	0
Tuberculous	+	+	+	++	0	++	+	+
Viral or "acute benign nonspecific"	++	0	+	+	0	0	0	0
Parasitic	+	+	++	+	0	+	+	0
Fungal	+	+	++	+	0	+	+	0
Associated with systemic disease								
Collagen disease								
Rheumatic fever	++	0	0	0	0	0	0	0
Rheumatoid arthritis	+	0	0	++	0	+	0	+
Systemic lupus erythematosus	+	+	0	++	0	0	0	0
Scleroderma	+	0	0	++	0	0	0	0
Renal disease	++	+	0	+	0	0	0	0
Thyroid disease	0	+	0	0	0	+	+	++
Sarcoidosis	0	0	0	0	0	++	0	0
Associated with other disease of heart or aorta								
Acute myocardial infarction	++	0	0	+	0	0	0	0
Ascending aortic aneurysm	+	++	0	0	0	0	0	0
Trauma and iatrogenic								
Penetrating and nonpenetrating injury	+	++	0	++	0	0	0	+
Cardiac catheterization	++	+	0	0	0	0	0	0
Cardiac operation and postpericardiotomy syndrome	+	+	++	++	0	0	0	0
Resuscitation	+	+	++	++	0	0	0	0
Radiation	+	+	++	++	0	0	0	0
Drugs and hypersensitivity states	++	+	0	0	0	0	0	0
Talc	+	0	+	+	0	++	0	0
Neoplastic	+	+	0	0	++	0	0	0
Congenital								
True and false (diverticula) cysts	—	—	—	—	—	—	—	—
Complete and partial absence	—	—	—	—	—	—	—	—

From Roberts, W. C., and Ferrans, V. J.: A survey and the causes and consequences of pericardial heart disease. *In* Reddy, D. S., et al. (Eds.): Pericardial Disease. New York, Raven Press, 1982.

may recur weeks or months after the initial episode, with remissions and exacerbations lasting several months.

THERAPY. Treatment includes bed rest until the pain and fever subside, exclusion of an underlying etiologic factor that requires specific management, and control of the pain with nonsteroidal anti-inflammatory agents such as aspirin, ibuprofen, or indomethacin. However, when the pain does not respond within 48 hours, corticosteroids (60 to 80 mg. of prednisone daily) may be given. Gradual tapering of the anti-inflammatory agents to the smallest dose that controls symptoms is recommended. In patients with severe recurrent pain, left stellate ganglion block occasionally relieves symptoms. Development of life-threatening hemodynamic complications may occur as a result of cardiac compression, including (1) development of cardiac tamponade by pericardial effusion, (2) development of calcification or fibrosis leading to constriction, and (3) a combination of both effusive and constrictive disease.

PERICARDIAL EFFUSION

Pericardial effusion may develop in nearly all cases of acute pericarditis. Symptoms of cardiac tamponade develop if accumulation of the fluid causes a rise in intrapericardial pressure. The development of this complication depends on the volume of the effusion, the rate of accumulation of the fluid, and the relative thickness and elasticity of the pericardium itself. Often, development of a pericardial effusion may occur with no symptoms. Some patients complain of pressure in the chest related to

stretching of the pericardial sac. On physical examination, the heart sounds may be distant or muffled, and rales may be heard over the lung fields secondary to compression of the lung. Enlargement of the cardiac silhouette on chest roentgenogram does not occur until at least 250 ml. of fluid is present in the pericardial space, and therefore, moderate effusions may not be apparent. With a large effusion, the heart may assume a water bottle shape, with increased separation of the pericardial and epicardial fat layers.[14] The electrocardiogram may demonstrate nonspecific reduction in QRS voltage and flattening of the T waves.[85] The most accurate diagnostic test currently is echocardiography, which may be sufficiently sensitive to detect as little as 20 ml. of pericardial fluid.[32] Two-dimensional echocardiography may be necessary for locating loculated pericardial effusions. Pericardial effusions do not require treatment unless there is hemodynamic embarrassment from increased pericardial pressure or unless aspiration of the fluid is required for diagnosis of an underlying disease. Aspiration of acute pericardial effusions with symptoms may be curative; however, chronic pericardial effusion with significant or recurrent symptoms may require subxiphoid pericardiotomy or total pericardiectomy for control.

CARDIAC TAMPONADE

An increase in intrapericardial pressure secondary to accumulation of fluid or blood in the pericardial space due to trauma or progressive effusion may lead to cardiac tamponade. Tamponade is characterized by an elevation of the intrapericardial pressure, which may rise to the level of right atrial and right ventricular diastolic pressures. Intrapericardial pressures of this magnitude lead to decline in the transmural filling pressures and, therefore, decreased cardiac output (Fig. 3).[27] The initial reduction in stroke volume is compensated by an increase in adrenergic tone and heart rate; however, as these compensatory mechanisms fail, systemic arterial pressure drops and perfusion of the coronary circulation and vital organs becomes impaired.[71] The pathognomonic finding in cardiac tamponade is *pulsus paradoxus*, an inspiratory fall of aortic systolic pressure greater than 10 mm. Hg. Pulsus paradoxus appears to follow exacerbation of the normal inspiratory fall in intrapericardial and right atrial pressure, causing an increase in flow from the venae cavae to the right atrium and right ventricle and, therefore, increasing pulmonary blood flow.[26,67] The resulting increase in right ventricular dimensions causes flattening and displacement of the ventricular septum toward the left ventricle with decrease in the ventricular volume on the left side of the heart.[17] Left atrial and left ventricular diastolic pressures decrease, accompanied by a fall in systemic flow and aortic pressure. An additional factor may be an inspiratory increase in left ventricular afterload due to a rise in transmural aortic pressure during inspiration.[50] Cardiac tamponade may occur in almost any type of pericarditis and is commonly associated with chest trauma or penetrating injury of the myocardium. Jugular venous pressure is usually markedly elevated, precordial cardiac activity is often not palpable and heart sounds are distant or inaudible, and blood pressure is depressed. These signs are classically known as Beck's triad.[4] Tachypnea and tachycardia may be apparent clinically, and the electrocardiogram may demonstrate signs of electrical alternans, a phasic alteration of the amplitude of the R wave. The development of electrical alternans is highly suggestive of cardiac tamponade.[56] In acute cardiac tamponade, the patient is clinically in shock. The skin is moist and cool, and venous distention is striking at a time when other signs of circulatory failure are similar to those seen in hemorrhagic shock.

The *y* descent of the jugular venous pulse waves disappears in the presence of cardiac tamponade since almost all cardiac filling occurs during systole. The *x* descent is often exaggerated. Prompt treatment of acute tamponade is mandatory. Measurement of venous pressure should be obtained immediately, and elevation of venous filling pressure by infusion of blood or colloid often temporarily improves peripheral perfusion. Immediate pericardial aspiration may be lifesaving. In the presence of

significant chest trauma, immediate thoracotomy and direct repair of cardiac injury is often preferable to attempts to aspirate intrapericardial hemorrhage. Often the aspiration of only a small amount of pericardial fluid or blood may cause a striking reduction in intrapericardial pressure and improvement in cardiac output.

CONSTRICTIVE PERICARDITIS

Constrictive pericarditis occurs when fibrosis and adherent pericardium restrict diastolic filling of the cardiac chambers. The process is usually symmetric, producing uniform restriction of all cardiac chambers; however, localized constricting bands surrounding the atrioventricular groove or one or both ventricles have been reported.[49,64] Although tuberculosis was a leading cause of constrictive pericarditis in the past, today most cases of constrictive pericarditis are of unknown etiology and are infrequently preceded by a known episode of acute pericarditis.[59] Specific associated causes of pericarditis leading to constriction include idiopathic or viral pericarditis; chronic renal failure; connective tissue disorders, including rheumatoid arthritis and systemic lupus erythematosus; deposition of blood in the pericardial space due to trauma, cardiac surgery, or pacemaker implantation; purulent pericarditis; and drug- or radiation- induced pericardial inflammation. Previous cardiac operation is only rarely associated with constrictive pericarditis, but

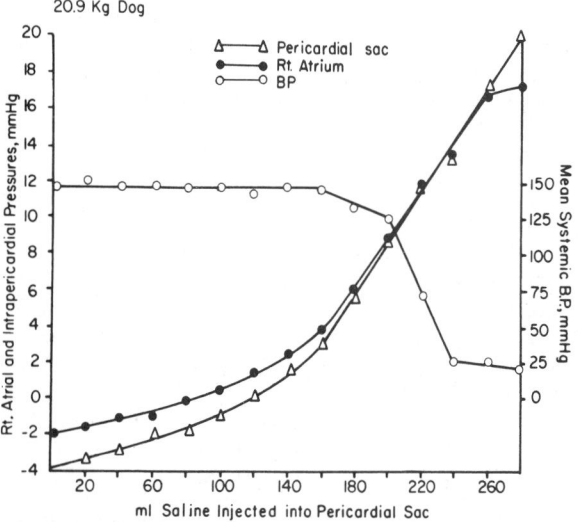

Figure 3. Production of experimental cardiac tamponade by injection of saline into the pericardium of an anesthetized dog. As the intrapericardial volume increases, right atrial and intrapericardial pressures rise and equilibrate, concomitant with an abrupt fall in blood pressure. (From Fowler, N. O.: Physiology of cardiac tamponade and pulsus paradoxus. Mod. Conc. Cardiovasc. Dis., 47:109, 1978.)

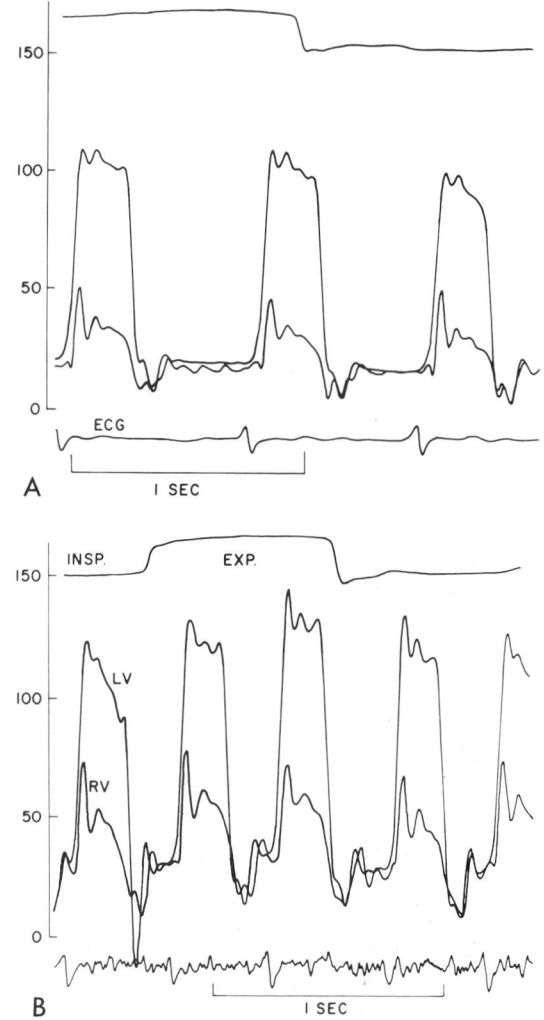

Figure 4. Hemodynamic tracings in constrictive pericarditis. *A*, Characteristic diastolic dip and early plateau contour of the diastolic waveforms of right ventricular and left ventricular pressure tracings. *B*, Tachycardia obscures the diastolic dip and plateau although diastolic pressures are equilibrated. (From Shabetai, R.: The Pericardium. New York, Grune & Stratton, 1981, p. 181.)

the interval from operation to the development of symptoms may be as rapid as 2 weeks to 6 months.[39]

PATHOPHYSIOLOGY. In classic constrictive pericarditis, the pericardial scarring restricts diastolic filling of the heart, causing elevation and equilibration of diastolic pressures in all four cardiac chambers. In early diastole, filling is unimpeded and occurs rapidly owing to elevation in venous pressures. When the intracardiac volume reaches the limits set by the non-compliant pericardium, diastolic filling rapidly ceases, creating the characteristic early diastolic dip and plateau waveforms in right and left ventricular pressure tracings (Fig. 4).[54] Because intrathoracic pressure changes during respiration cannot be transmitted to the obliterated pericardial space, systemic venous and right atrial pressures do not fall with inspiration, in contrast to the situation seen in cardiac tamponade. Occasionally, venous pressure may actually increase with inspiration. Usually systolic contraction of the ventricles is normal, although in severe cases myocardial systolic function can be depressed owing to myocardial atrophy, inflammation and fibrosis of underlying myocardial tissue, or interference with coronary artery blood flow.[18,45,86]

Symptoms include weakness, easy fatigability, and shortness of breath with exertion. Unlike in congestive heart failure, patients with constrictive pericarditis often develop significant ascites without evidence of peripheral edema. Syncope is occasionally seen as a result of low cardiac output. The primary physical finding is elevation of jugular venous pressure, occasionally with an increase on inspiration (Kussmaul's sign). The precordium is quiet with no right ventricular lift. Occasionally, a distinct diastolic precordial beat may be palpated during rapid filling in the presence of an elevated venous pressure. This has been correlated with a rapid diastolic heart sound (pericardial knock).[55] The liver may be enlarged and tender with a prominent hepatojugular reflex. Arterial blood pressure is often low, and pulse pressure is often narrow. Atrial fibrillation is present in approximately one third of patients. On the chest film, the heart is usually normal or mildly enlarged, and occasionally calcium deposits may be observed in the pericardium. The electrocardiogram often demonstrates low-voltage QRS complexes with flat or inverted T waves, and atrial arrhythmias are common.[48,82] Serum proteins may be low owing to a loss of protein throughout the gastrointestinal tract, with elevation of venous and portal pressures; congestion of the intestinal wall mucosa also diminishes absorption of ingested protein.[89]

Confirming the diagnosis of constrictive pericarditis may be difficult because of similar findings in familial or acquired cardiomyopathy. Cardiac catheterization offers the most reliable technique for differentiating myocardial and pericardial disease. In constrictive pericarditis, the diastolic pressure curve of the right ventricle shows an early diastolic dip and rapid plateau with a very small A wave. Right atrial pressure is elevated with a systolic pulmonary pressure rarely above 45 mm. Hg. Left ventricular end-diastolic pressure is usually normal, unlike the elevated end-diastolic pressure observed in most cardiomyopathies. Restrictive cardiomyopathy is most likely present when right ventricular systolic hypertension is present and left ventricular diastolic pressure exceeds right ventricular diastolic pressure at rest by more than 5 mm. Hg.[83] In contrast to patients with constrictive pericarditis, patients with cardiac tamponade often show marked pulsus paradoxus, a fall in right atrial pressure during inspiration, elevation of intrapericardial pressure, a right atrial pressure tracing with a predominant x descent and attenuated or absent y descent, and lack of a prominent dip and plateau pattern in the right and left ventricular pressure tracings. Computed tomographic scans may demonstrate pericardial thickening in up to 80 per cent of patients with constrictive pericarditis, although the presence of pericardial thickening is not diagnostic without other hemodynamic signs of constriction.[48]

Nuclear magnetic resonance imaging can be very useful,

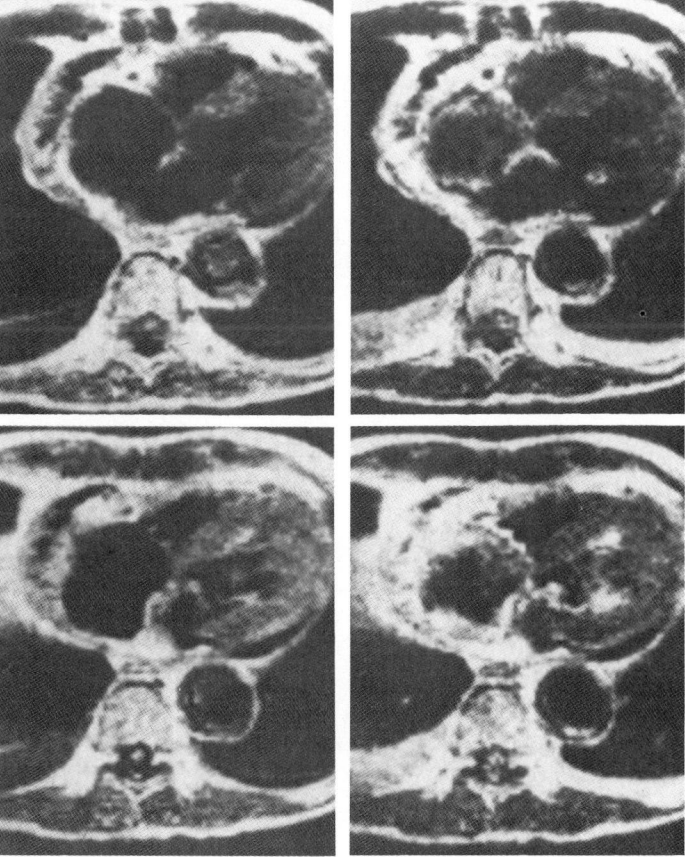

Figure 5. Constrictive uremic pericarditis. First *(left)* and second *(right)* spin echo images. Sequential axial images show irregularly thickened visceral and parietal pericardium of increased intensity, separated by low-intensity fluid, surrounding the enlarged right atrium. The second echo image shows a further increase in intensity, in keeping with a long T2. The right ventricle is normal in size, the left ventricle hypertrophied, the septum straight. Pericardial fluid is also seen behind the left ventricle where abnormalities of the pericardium itself are less marked. Bilateral pleural effusions are present. (From Soulen, R. L., Stark, D. D., and Higgins, C. B.: Magnetic resonance imaging of constrictive pericardial disease. Am. J. Cardiol., 55:480, 1985.)

since it permits evaluation of the thickening of the pericardium and demonstrates the dilation of the hepatic veins and right atrium and the small right ventricle characteristic of constriction[75] (Fig. 5).

Constrictive pericarditis is a progressive disease, although a minority of patients may survive for years with the use of diuretics or ganglionic blockade to decrease venous filling pressures. However, the majority of patients become progressively more disabled by weakness, ascites, and cardiac cachexia. Optimal treatment for constrictive pericarditis is complete resection of the pericardium.

SURGICAL TECHNIQUES

PERICARDIOCENTESIS. Aspiration of the pericardial sac can be lifesaving therapy in the case of cardiac tamponade or a diagnostic procedure for determining the etiologic basis of pericarditis or effusion. Pericardiocentesis is performed by the left parasternal approach in the fourth or fifth intercostal space or via the subxiphoid route under local anesthesia. The patient's thorax and head are tilted upward, enhancing the pooling of the effusion anteriorly and inferiorly. A long needle is attached to a stopcock and syringe and inserted just beneath and to the left of the xiphoid process. A precordial electrocardiogram lead is attached to the needle by a small clip, and the needle is inserted at a 30- to 45-degree angle posteriorly toward a point midway between the scapulae. The needle is then advanced slowly until fluid is encountered or the electrocardiogram demonstrates contact with the surface of the heart (Fig. 6). Use of a pacemaker connected to the exploring needle may provide a more accurate indication of contact with cardiac structures before injury occurs.[84] Echocardiography-guided aspiration of the pericardium is the preferred approach when the equipment is available (Fig. 7).[13] Aspirated fluid is reserved for bacteriologic and cytologic examination and protein determination. Blood aspirated from the pericardial sac does not clot because of rapid defibrination by cardiac motion. Aspiration of blood that subsequently clots suggests that it was obtained directly from a cardiac chamber. Introduction of a small amount of contrast material under fluoroscopic guidance may confirm intracardiac or intrapericardial location of the needle. If continued drainage of the pericardial space is required, a polyethylene catheter may be passed over a guidewire into the pericardial sac and left in place for several hours.[88]

Although the risk of developing a life-threatening complication from pericardiocentesis is approximately 5 per cent, the procedure is much safer than in the past.[37,90] Complications include lacerations of the heart or coronary arteries, internal mammary artery, or lung; aspiration of blood from cardiac chambers; and possible contamination of the pericardial or pleural cavities. Rarely, laceration of the liver or perforation of

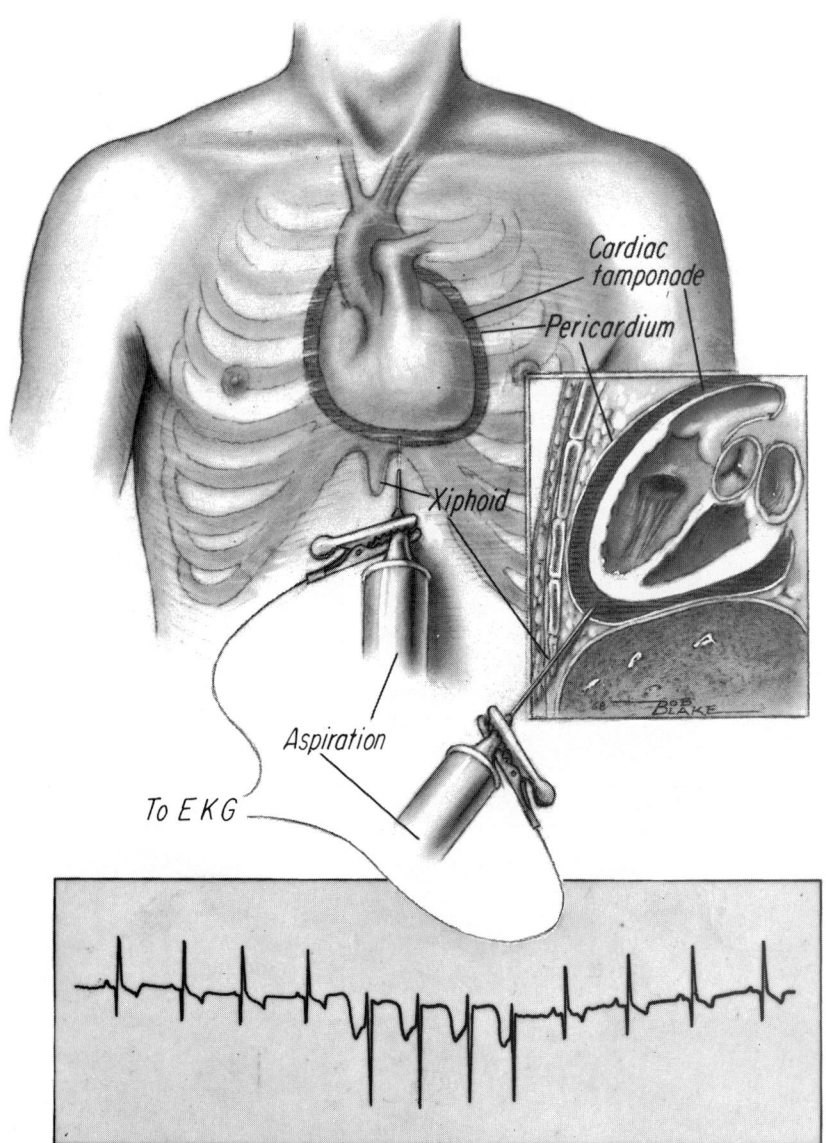

Figure 6. Technique of pericardiocentesis. Negative deflection of the QRS complex indicates contact with the epicardium. (From Ebert, P.: The pericardium. *In* Sabiston, D. C., and Spencer, F. C. (Eds.): Gibbon's Surgery of the Chest, 4th ed. Philadelphia, W. B. Saunders Company, 1983, p. 996.)

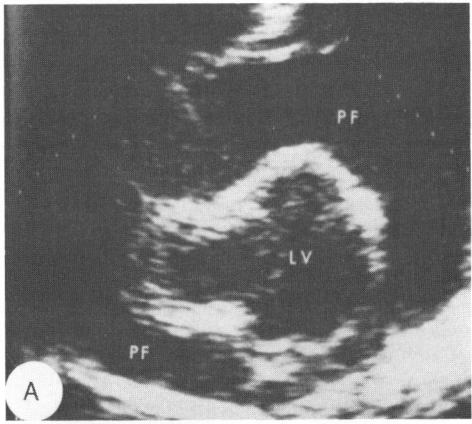

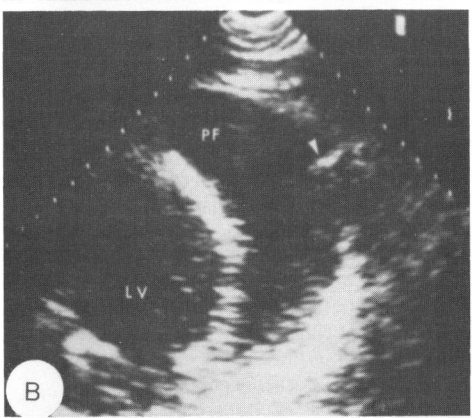

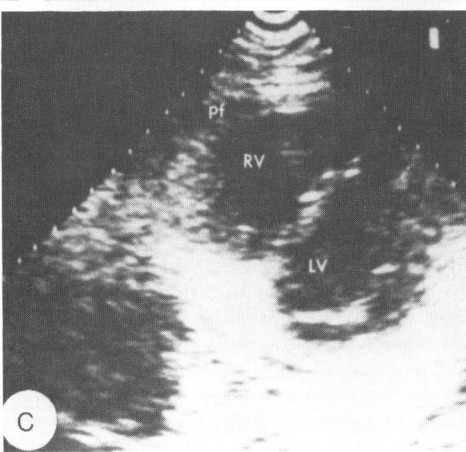

Figure 7. Two-dimensional echocardiograms. *A*, Still frame showing large pericardial effusion surrounding left ventricle. *B*, Still frame during pericardiocentesis. Note diminished volume of pericardial fluid and position of needle (arrowhead). *C*, Modified four-chamber view showing small amount of pericardial fluid remaining after pericardiocentesis. LV, left ventricle; PF, pericardial fluid; RV, right ventricle. (From Callahan, J. A., Seward, J. B., and Tajik, A. J.: Cardiac tamponade: Pericardiocentesis directed by two-dimensional echocardiography. Mayo Clin. Proc., *60*:344, 1985.)

abdominal organs may occur, and occasionally a shocklike state may follow penetration of the pericardium.

PERICARDIOTOMY AND PERICARDIAL BIOPSY. Open drainage of the pericardium is often required in the presence of chronic pericardial effusion or purulent pericarditis. Pericardiotomy with pericardial biopsy may be required for establishing the cause of pericardial disease.

The subxiphoid approach to the pericardium is by an incision just to the left of the xiphoid process extended through the rectus muscle to the transversus abdominis fibers (Fig. 8).[81] Dissection is then carried beneath the costal margin, exposing the inferior surface of the pericardial sac without encountering the peritoneum or diaphragm. The subxiphoid approach is com-

monly used for drainage of large effusions, especially in the presence of infection. Dependent drainage is effectively established, and drainage catheters can also be placed via this approach for irrigation and chronic drainage. In addition, small portions of pericardium for biopsy can be obtained. An alternative approach is through an anterior thoracotomy incision in the fourth intercostal space on the left (Fig. 9). The left pleura may be reflected laterally and entered, if desired, for drainage of chronic effusions into the left pleural space for absorption. This incision permits excision of an adequate piece of pericardium for bacteriologic and microscopic examination, and a more complete pericardiectomy to prevent the recurrence of effusion or the development of late constriction.[61] Alternative approaches include excision of the fifth or sixth costal cartilage for wide access to the pericardium. Complete excision of the costal cartilage should be performed in the presence of purulent pericarditis to prevent costochondritis.

The superior results of more extensive excision of the pericardium via the thoracotomy approach suggest that subxiphoid or subcostal drainage of large effusions should be limited to patients with malignant disease of limited survival and who are in poor condition.[61]

PERICARDIECTOMY. Pericardiectomy for constrictive pericarditis or effusive disease has an operative mortality of 4 to 15 per cent with long-term improvement in at least 75 per cent of the patients who survive the operation.[48,74,92] Preoperative preparation of the patient with efforts to correct ascites from cardiac failure and to optimize nutritional status is important, and antituberculous therapy should be initiated preoperatively in patients in whom a tuberculous etiology is suspected. Complete excision of the pericardium is required in most cases of constrictive pericarditis and can be performed via the left anterior thoracotomy, the greater exposure obtained with a median sternotomy, or bilateral thoracotomy. Attempts should be made

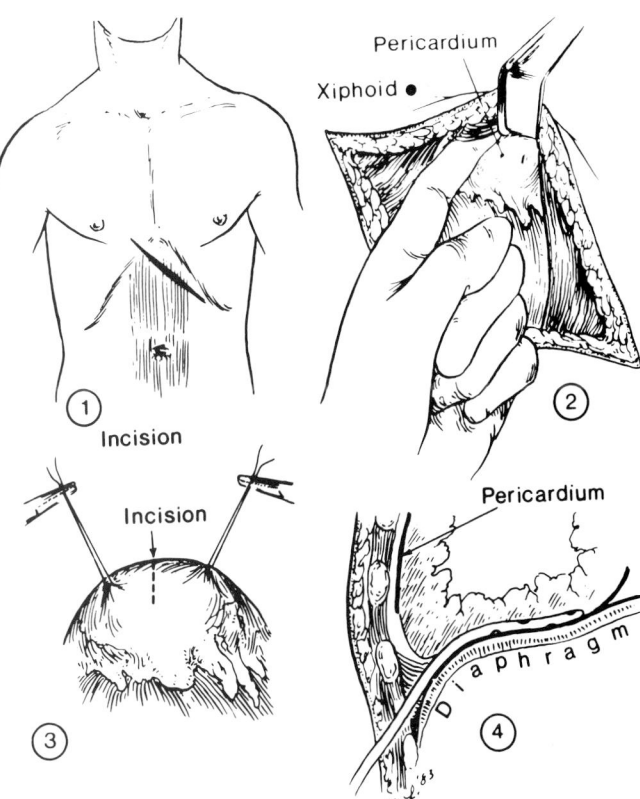

Figure 8. Subcostal approach to pericardium. *1*, Site of skin incision. *2*, Retractor elevating the xiphoid. The pericardium is dissected bluntly. *3*, Incision of pericardium between two silk sutures. *4*, Drain in the pericardial cavity. (From Steiger, Z., McAlpin, G., and Wilson, R. F.: Left subcostal approach to the pericardium. Surg. Gynecol. Obstet., *160*:414, 1985.)

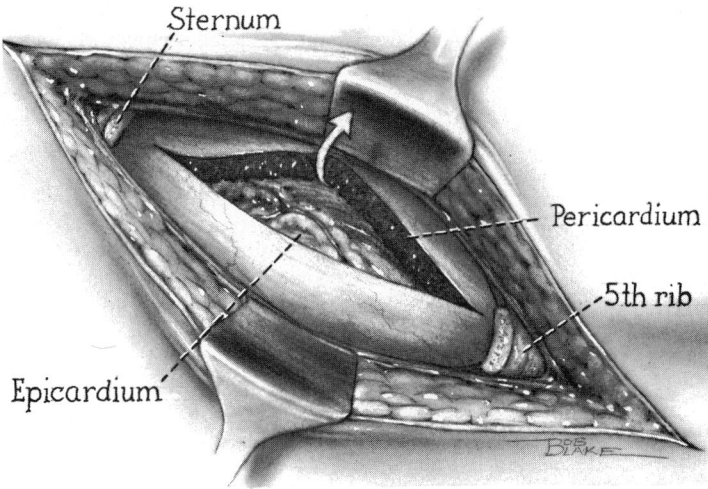

Figure 9. Left anterior thoracotomy for pericardial biopsy. Incision in the fourth or fifth intercostal space or excision of the fifth costal cartilage provides access to the thickened pericardium. The pleura on the left may be opened for drainage of effusion. (From Ebert, P., and Najafi, H.: The pericardium. *In* Sabiston, D. C., and Spencer, F. C. (Eds.): Surgery of the Chest, 5th ed. Philadelphia, W. B. Saunders Company, 1990, p. 1242.)

to locate the correct plane of dissection between the epicardial surface and the adherent organized exudate and pericardium. If this plane is identified, bleeding is surprisingly small. It may be important to first free the left ventricle in order to prevent pulmonary congestion from the increase in right-sided output,[20] findings that support use of the thoracotomy approach routinely. The phrenic nerves should be elevated from the pericardium and carefully protected, and care should be taken to free the ventricles completely. Occasionally, cardiopulmonary bypass may be used to control bleeding from friable areas of the heart, although this is rarely necessary. In most patients, prompt hemodynamic and symptomatic improvement is apparent after operation, but in some, resolution of the elevated jugular venous pressure may be delayed for weeks or months[16,48] (Fig. 10). The low cardiac output syndrome occurs in the immediate postoperative period in approximately 25 per cent of patients and may be related to underlying myocardial atrophy. Use of inotropic support or intra-aortic balloon counterpulsation in addition to intravenous fluid therapy may permit survival of many of these patients.

SPECIFIC PERICARDIAL DISEASES

TUBERCULOUS PERICARDITIS. Tuberculous pericarditis probably follows early dissemination from a primary infection and appears to reach the pericardium from the blood or by

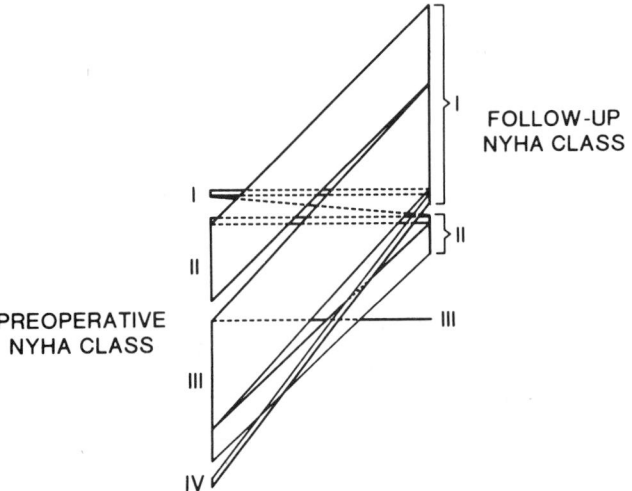

Figure 10. Long-term follow-up of 141 patients demonstrated marked symptomatic improvement after pericardiectomy for constrictive pericarditis. (From McCaughan, B. C., Schaff, H. V., Piehler, J. M., Danielson, G. K., Orszulak, T. A., Puga, F. J., Pluth, J. R., Connolly, D. C., and McGoon, D. C.: Early and late results of pericardiectomy for constrictive pericarditis. J. Thorac. Cardiovasc. Surg., 89:340, 1985.)

retrograde lymphatic spread from infected mediastinal glands.[6] Rarely, the infection may spread directly from infected lung or pleura. Symptoms are often nonspecific, with malaise, fever, sweats, and cough, and pericarditis may not be suspected in the absence of a friction rub. The early stage of fibrinous pericarditis gradually leads to the slow development of pericardial effusions, which may be massive. The fluid may be clear, straw-colored, or sanguineous. In the effusive stage, acid-fast bacilli may be found on pericardiocentesis.[60] Skin tests may be negative owing to the massive amounts of antigen present and are, therefore, unreliable.

It is important to treat tuberculous pericarditis early, because gradual fibrosis and scarring of the pericardium prevents effective delivery of antibiotics to the pericardial space. The healing of the pericardium may lead to fibrosis and calcification, with eventual constriction. Wood has emphasized that pericardial constriction is common if treatment is delayed for more than 4 months from the onset of the disease; therefore, early pericardiocentesis is often warranted to determine the specific cause of large pericardial effusion.[91] Combination chemotherapy with two and usually three agents should be initiated, and, in most patients, clinical improvement is seen in 2 to 3 weeks. Because as many as half of treated patients with tuberculous pericarditis eventually develop constriction, early operative resection of the pericardium is warranted and should be performed at a time when the patient is clinically well.[30] In its end stage, tuberculous pericarditis may cause calcified thickened pericardium, and occasionally the calcification may be localized and may burrow into the ventricular myocardium.

UREMIC PERICARDITIS. Uremic pericarditis is a frequent complication of chronic renal failure and may be detected in approximately 50 per cent of patients with untreated chronic renal disease.[87] Although uremic pericarditis often improves with initiation of dialysis, there is no clear correlation between the development of pericarditis and the levels of blood urea nitrogen. Pericarditis can develop in patients undergoing regular dialysis with normal creatinine and urea nitrogen levels.[70] The incidence appears to be decreased in patients who are on peritoneal dialysis, suggesting that repeated anticoagulation during hemodialysis may lead to hemorrhage into the pericardial space from pericardial granulation tissue, exacerbating the pericarditis. No treatment is required for small effusions; however, large effusions in symptomatic patients may resolve by increasing the frequency of dialysis. Only half of the patients recover with this therapy alone.[47] Management of symptoms of fever and chest pain may include use of a nonsteroidal anti-inflammatory agent and occasionally administration of steroids.[41] Pericardiectomy should be reserved for patients with pericardial constriction or recurrent cardiac tamponade that has not responded to conservative therapy.[21] Hemodynamically unstable patients may be initially treated by percutaneous pericardiocentesis with catheter drainage of the pericardium for 24 to 48 hours. Although some authors have advocated instillation of steroids into the pericardial space, this has been associated with an increased incidence of infection.[24,28]

PURULENT PERICARDITIS. Purulent pericarditis occurs as a result of direct contamination of the pericardium following penetrating injury or pneumonia. It may also occur from septicemia, from rupture of subphrenic or hepatic abscesses into the pericardial space, or as a complication of operations on the heart, lungs, or esophagus.

Severe chest pain and fever are common, and the rapid accumulation of fluid in the inflamed pericardial space may develop into cardiac tamponade. Currently, the most common infectious agents are *Staphylococcus* or gram-negative bacteria in adults and *Staphylococcus* or *Haemophilus influenzae* in children. Pericardial aspiration confirms the diagnosis, and treatment with antibiotics, repeated pericardiocentesis, and, on occasion, subxiphoid pericardial drainage with catheter irrigation of the pericardial space are indicated. Late development of constriction is not infrequent, and if loculated effusions or persistent sepsis occurs, pericardiectomy should be performed.

POSTPERICARDIOTOMY SYNDROME. Postpericardiotomy syndrome is suspected by the appearance of fever, pericarditis, and pleuritis 2 to 4 weeks after cardiac operation during which the pericardium has been opened. The incidence of this syndrome is 10 to 40 per cent. The sedimentation rate is elevated, and leukocytosis, often accompanied by an increase in lymphocytic cells, is usually present. The electrocardiogram may demonstrate the typical changes of acute pericarditis. The etiologic basis of postpericardiotomy syndrome is thought to be an autoimmune reaction directed against the epicardium at a time of active or recurrent viral infection. Studies by Engle and associates have demonstrated antiheart antibodies in the serum of patients undergoing pericardiotomy and noted a correlation between the level of the titers and the incidence of the syndrome.[22] Antiheart antibody titers are often associated with elevation of antiviral titers, suggesting that viral infection may be a triggering or permissive factor.[23]

There are no pathognomonic histopathologic features of postpericardiotomy syndrome; the pericardia are thickened from the presence of blood in the pericardial space, associated with serous or serosanguineous effusion (Fig. 11).

Symptoms of fever, malaise, and pleuritic chest pain may be self-limited, and salicylates, nonsteroidal anti-inflammatory drugs, and rest lead to improvement in most patients. Severe

cases may require the use of corticosteroids, which commonly produce improvement within 72 hours. Rebound of symptoms may occur with cessation of steroid treatment. A low serum albumin has been associated with the development of clinical symptoms, and administration of albumin intravenously and improvement in nutritional status have led to clinical improvement.[1] Recurrent effusions or cardiac compromise may require pericardiocentesis or pericardiectomy in rare patients.

NEOPLASTIC PERICARDITIS

The heart is involved in approximately 10 per cent of patients with malignant neoplasms, and of the patients with cardiac involvement, 85 per cent have tumor in the pericardium. The most common neoplasms in absolute numbers with cardiac metastases are lung (in males) and breast (in females), followed by leukemia and lymphoma. Almost any tumor, however, may metastasize to the heart. Among specific neoplasms, the highest percentage of metastases to the heart is seen in melanoma (70 per cent), leukemia (37 per cent), and lymphoma (24 per cent). Spread of these tumors appears to be by the hematogenous route. Signs and symptoms of pericarditis do not correlate well with the presence of tumor in the pericardium, and often the neoplastic pericarditis is found incidentally at necropsy examination.

Primary pericardial neoplasms are extremely rare and approximately half are benign. The most common is teratoma, and although this tumor is histologically benign, it may produce fatal compression of cardiac chambers. Hemangioma, leiomyofibroma, lipoma, and fibroma are other benign pericardial neoplasms. Mesothelioma is by far the most frequent primary malignant pericardial neoplasm. It may totally encase the heart and lead to fatal myocardial restriction.[64]

CONGENITAL PERICARDIAL DEFECTS

CONGENITAL ABSENCE OF THE PERICARDIUM. Partial or complete absence of the parietal pericardium may be classified into three major types: (1) heart and left lung in a common cavity (60 per cent); (2) defect or foramen in parietal pericardium providing communication between the pericardial sac and the pleural space (20 per cent); and (3) total absence or rudimentary parietal pericardium (20 per cent).[51] When small defects are present in the parietal pericardium or when there is partial absence of the pericardium, the left side is usually involved. It has been postulated that premature obliteration of the left duct of

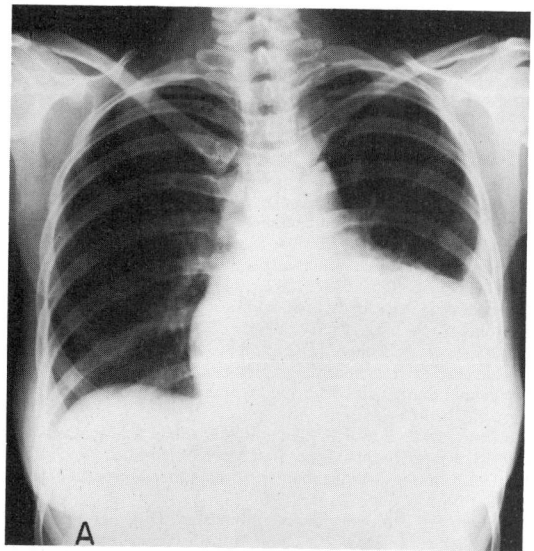
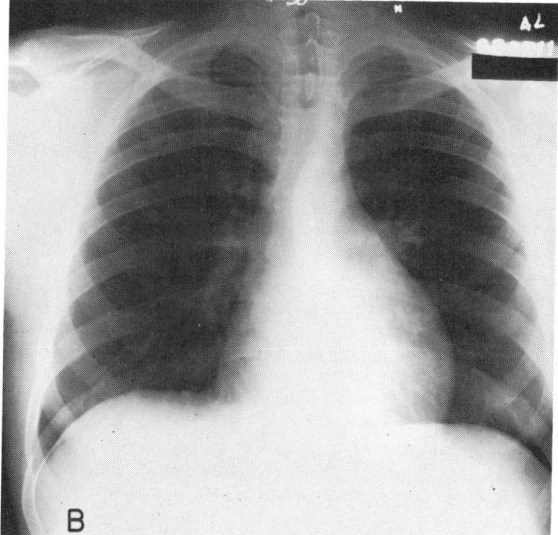

Figure 11. Postpericardiotomy syndrome. *A*, Ten days after open heart surgery, the patient developed fever, friction rub, and left pleural effusion. *B*, After treatment with steroids and salicylates, clearing of the effusion is present and symptoms have resolved. (From Ebert, P., and Najafi, H.: The pericardium. *In* Sabiston, D. C., and Spencer, F. C. (Eds.): Surgery of the Chest, 5th ed. Philadelphia, W. B. Saunders Company, 1990, p. 1246.)

Cuvier produces deficiency of the blood supply to the pleuro-pericardial membrane in the fifth week of gestation, causing failure of formation or incomplete formation of the parietal pericardium. These defects may be associated with anomalies of the heart in 30 per cent of patients or anomalies of the lungs, pleura, peritoneum, or kidney.[64] All of these congenital defects are more common in males than in females. Cardiac enlargement occurs in about half the patients, and commonly the heart is displaced to the left and is abnormally mobile. Total absence of the parietal pericardium has not been associated with any functional disturbances. Partial defects in the parietal pericardium, however, may lead to herniation of the entire heart or atrial appendage through the defect (which can occasionally be life-threatening) or may permit extension of pulmonary infection to the pericardial space.

PERICARDIAL CYSTS. The pericardium is postulated to develop from coalescence of lacunae that appear early in fetal life and fuse with the pericardial coelom.[43] Pericardial cysts are uncommon and are typically located at the right costophrenic angle. They are usually unilocular and filled with clear liquid. Occasionally the wall of the cysts can calcify. Pericardial cysts are usually asymptomatic and are found incidentally; however, chest pain may occur with torsion of the cyst pedicle. In rare instances, they may become life-threatening because of their space-occupying characteristics.[42] Partial fusion of developmental lacunae and communication with the pericardial space or protrusion of the pericardial sac at points of weakness are described as pericardial diverticula. They are usually more frequent on the right side and are rarely symptomatic.

SELECTED REFERENCES

Engle, M. A., Ehlers, K. H., O'Loughlin, J. E., Jr., Linday, L. A., and Fried, R.: The postpericardiotomy syndrome: Iatrogenic illness with immunologic and virologic components. *In* Engle, M. A. (Ed.): Pediatric Cardiovascular Disease. (Cardiovascular Clinics.) Philadelphia, F. A. Davis, 1981, pp. 381–391.
This report documents the appearance of antiheart antibodies in the serum of patients undergoing surgical therapy in which the pericardium has been opened and correlates the titers with clinical evidence of the syndrome. In addition, the association of a significant rise in viral titers in 70 per cent of patients with the syndrome is presented. The decreased incidence of postpericardiotomy syndrome in infants is compared with that seen in adults, and it is suggested that the short exposure period of children to viruses or viral illnesses may decrease the incidence of the clinical syndrome.

Isaacs, J. P., Carter, B. N., II, and Haller, J. A., Jr.: Experimental pericarditis: The pathologic physiology of constrictive pericarditis. Bull. Johns Hopkins Hosp., 90:259, 1952.
This experimental study of constrictive pericarditis emphasizes the effects of constriction of the atria on elevation of venous pressure. A review of the hemodynamic changes associated with constrictive pericarditis and the effects on the peripheral organs are presented in detail. Experimental production of localized pericardial constriction by placing plastic casts in the pericardium showed that pericardial constriction of one or both ventricles was associated with a reduction in cardiac output. Removal of scar over the right or left side of the heart individually led to a hemodynamic situation consistent with isolated constriction of the left or right ventricle, respectively. Only with removal of scar from both ventricles did hemodynamic values return to normal. Removal of scar over the right atrium alone did not lead to improvement in hemodynamics, confirming ventricular constriction as the clinically important feature. A well-detailed experimental study.

McCaughan, B. C., Schaff, H. V., Piehler, J. M., Danielson, G. K., Orszulak, T. A., Puga, F. J., Pluth, J. R., Connolly, D. C., and McGoon, D. C.: Early and late results of pericardiectomy for constrictive pericarditis. J. Thorac. Cardiovasc. Surg., 87:340, 1985.
In this extensive series of 231 patients who underwent pericardiectomy for constrictive pericarditis at the Mayo Clinic, 28 per cent of the patients experienced low cardiac output syndrome postoperatively, causing 70 per cent of all early deaths. Operative risk but not long-term survival was significantly influenced by preoperative disability classification. The authors recommend early pericardiectomy for constrictive pericarditis before significant disability occurs and preferably by the transthoracic approach.

Piehler, J. M., Pluth, J. R., Schaff, H. V., Danielson, G. K., Orszulak, T. A., and Puga, F. J.: Surgical management of effusive pericardial disease. Influence of extent of pericardial resection on clinical course. J. Thorac. Cardiovasc. Surg., 90:506, 1985.
This large series of 145 patients treated at the Mayo Clinic for effusive pericardial disease was divided into three groups according to the extent of pericardial resection: complete in 72 (49.7 per cent), partial in 36 (24.8 per cent), and window in 37

(25.5 per cent). Although survival was not influenced by the extent of pericardial resection, 15 patients (10 per cent) had recurrent effusion or developed constriction and 6 required reoperation. All reoperations were in patients who had window procedures. The authors conclude that complete transthoracic pericardiectomy is the preferred procedure for effusive pericardial disease.

Roberts, W. C., and Spray, T. L.: Pericardial heart disease: A study of its causes, consequences and morphologic features. *In* Spodick, D. H. (Ed.): Pericardial Diseases. Philadelphia, F. A. Davis, 1976, pp. 11–65.
This extensive pathologic study compares the etiologic classifications of pericardial disease with the morphologic changes observed during surgical procedures or necropsy examination. The authors emphasize the fact that pericarditis is relatively uncommon clinically when compared with its relatively frequent presence at necropsy. In most patients with chronic constrictive pericarditis, the etiology is not apparent even after histologic examination of the pericardia. Extensive illustrations of the morphologic aspects of the various pericardial diseases are presented.

Spodick, D. H.: Medical history of the pericardium. The hairy hearts of hoary heroes. Am. J. Cardiol., 26:477, 1970.
This article provides an excellent summary of the history of the knowledge of the pericardium, written by an authority in the field. Observations on the pericardium from antiquity through the Renaissance and eighteenth century, when accurate observations of the clinical signs of pericardial disease and the pathology of tamponade and constriction were made, are presented.

Spodick, D. H.: The normal and diseased pericardium: Current concepts of pericardial physiology, diagnosis, and treatment. J. Am. Coll. Cardiol., 1:240, 1983.
A concise summary of the relevant contributions of the past quarter century to knowledge and understanding of pericardial heart disease and a summary of the current state of the science. Excellent summaries of the physiology of normal pericardium, cardiac tamponade and its compensatory mechanisms, and pulsus paradoxus are presented in tabular form.

REFERENCES

1. Aronstam, E. M., and Cox, W. A.: A new concept of the pleuropericardial syndrome. Postpericardiotomy or postcardiotomy syndrome. J. Thorac. Cardiovasc. Surg., 51:341, 1966.
2. Avasthey, P., and Wood, E. H.: Intrathoracic and venous pressure relationships during responses to changes in body position. J. Appl. Physiol. 37:166, 1974.
3. Beck, C. S.: The surgical treatment of pericardial scar. J.A.M.A., 97:824, 1931.
4. Beck, C. S.: Two cardiac compressor triads. J.A.M.A., 104:714, 1935.
5. Beck, C. S., and Griswold, R. A.: Pericardiectomy in the treatment of the Pick syndrome: Experimental and clinical observations. Arch. Surg., 21:1064, 1930.
6. Bellett, S., McMillan, T. M., and Gouley, G. A.: Tuberculous pericarditis: Clinical and pathological study based upon a series of 17 cases. Med. Clin. North Am., 18:201, 1934.
7. Berglund, E., Sarnoff, S. J., and Isaacs, J. P.: Ventricular function: Role of the pericardium in regulation of cardiovascular hemodynamics. Circ. Res., 3:133, 1955.
8. Bernard, H. L.: The functions of the pericardium. J. Physiol., 22:43, 1898.
9. Bigelow, W. G., Dolan, F. G., Wilson, D. R., and Gunton, R. W.: The surgical treatment of chronic constrictive pericarditis. Can. Med. Assoc. J., 75:814, 1956.
10. Boyd, L. J., and Elias, H.: Contribution to diseases of the heart and pericardium. Historical introduction. Bull. N. Y. Med. Coll., 18:1, 1955.
11. Brenner, J. I., and Waugh, R. A.: Effect of phasic respiration on left ventricular dimension and performance in a normal population. Circulation, 57:122, 1978.
12. Brinker, J. A., Weiss, J. L., Lappe, D. L., Rabson, J. L., Summer, W. R., Permutt, S., and Weisfeldt, M. L.: Leftward septal displacement during right ventricular loading in man. Circulation, 61:626, 1980.
13. Callahan, J. A., Seward, J. B., and Tajik, A. J.: Cardiac tamponade: Pericardiocentesis directed by two-dimensional echocardiography. Mayo Clin. Proc., 60:344, 1985.
14. Carsky, E. W., Mauceri, R. A., and Azimi, F.: The epicardial fat pad sign: Analysis of frontal and lateral chest radiographs in patients with pericardial effusion. Radiology, 137:303, 1980.
15. Chevers, N.: Observations on the disease of the orifice and valves of the aorta. Guys Hosp. Rep., 7:387, 1842.
16. Collins, H. A., Woods, L. P., and Daniel, R. A., Jr.: Late results of pericardiectomy. Arch. Surg., 89:921, 1964.
17. D'Cruz, I. A., Cohen, H. C., Prabhu, R., and Glick, G.: Diagnosis of cardiac tamponade by echocardiography: Changes in mitral valve motion and ventricular dimensions, with special reference to paradoxical pulse. Circulation, 52:460, 1975.
18. Dines, D. E., Edwards, J. E., and Burchell, H. B.: Myocardial atrophy in constrictive pericarditis. Proc. Staff Meet. Mayo Clin., 33:93, 1958.
19. Dunn, M., and Rinkenberger, R. L.: Clinical aspects of acute pericarditis. Cardiovasc. Clin., 7:131, 1976.
20. Ebert, P.: The pericardium. *In* Sabiston, D. C., and Spencer, F. C. (Eds.): Gibbon's Surgery of the Chest, 4th ed. Philadelphia, W. B. Saunders Company, 1983, p. 1004.
21. Engelman, R. M., Levitsky, S., Konchigeri, H. N., Wyndham, C. R. C., Roper,

K., and Kurtzman, N. A.: Total pericardiectomy for uremic pericarditis. World J. Surg., 1:769, 1977.

22. Engle, M. A., Gay, W. A., Jr., Kaminsky, M. E., Zabriskie, J. B., and Senterfit, L. A.: Postpericardiotomy syndrome then and now. Curr. Probl. Cardiol. 3:1, 1978.

23. Engle, M. A., Ehlers, K. H., O'Loughlin, J. E., Jr., Linday, L. A., and Fried, R.: The postpericardiotomy syndrome: Iatrogenic illness with immunologic and virologic components. In Engle, M. A. (Ed.): Pediatric Cardiovascular Disease. (Cardiovascular Clinics.) Philadelphia, F. A. Davis, 1981, pp. 381–391.

24. Feinroth, M. V., Goldstein, E. J., Josephson, A., and Friedman, E. A.: Infection complicating intrapericardial steroid instillation in uremic pericarditis. Clin. Nephrol. 15:331, 1981.

25. Fitzpatrick, D. P., Wyso, E. M., Bosher, L. H., and Richardson, D. W.: Restoration of normal intracardiac pressures after extensive pericardiectomy for constrictive pericarditis. Circulation, 25:484, 1962.

26. Fowler, N. O.: Physiology of cardiac tamponade and pulsus paradoxus. I. Mechanisms of pulsus paradoxus in cardiac tamponade. Mod. Conc. Cardiovasc. Dis., 47:109, 1978.

27. Fowler, N. O.: Physiology of cardiac tamponade and pulsus paradoxus. Physiological, circulatory, and pharmacologic responses in cardiac tamponade. Mod. Conc. Cardiovasc. Dis., 47:115, 1978.

28. Fuller, T. J., Knochel, J. P., Brennan, J. P., Fetner, C. D., and White, M. G.: Reversal of intractable uremic pericarditis by triamcinolone hexacetonide. Arch. Intern. Med., 136:979, 1976.

29. Gibson, A. T., and Segal, M. B.: A study of the composition of pericardial fluid, with special reference to the probable mechanism of fluid formation. J. Physiol. (Lond.), 277:367, 1978.

30. Hageman, J. H., D'Esopo, N. D., and Glenn, W. W. L.: Tuberculosis of the pericardium: A long-term analysis of forty-four cases. N. Engl. J. Med., 270:327, 1964.

31. Holt, J. P.: The normal pericardium. Am. J. Cardiol., 26:455, 1970.

32. Horowitz, M. S., Schultz, C. S., and Stinson, E. B.: Sensitivity and specificity of echocardiographic diagnosis of pericardial effusion. Circulation, 50:239, 1974.

33. Isaacs, J. P., Carter B. N., II, and Haller, J. A., Jr.: Experimental pericarditis: The pathologic physiology of constrictive pericarditis. Bull. Johns Hopkins Hosp., 90:259, 1952.

34. Ishihara, T., Ferrans, V. J., Jones, M., Boyce, S. W., Kawanami, O., and Roberts, W. C.: Histologic and ultrastructural features of normal human parietal pericardium. Am. J. Cardiol., 46:744, 1980.

35. James, T. N.: Pericarditis and the sinus node. Arch. Intern. Med., 110:305, 1962.

36. Karanaeff: Paracentese des Brustkastens und des Pericardiums. Med. Ztg., 9:251, 1840.

37. Krikorian, J. G., and Hancock, E. W.: Pericardiocentesis. Am. J. Med., 65:808, 1978.

38. Kuno, Y.: The significance of the pericardium. J. Physiol., 50:1, 1915.

39. Kussmaul, A.: Über schwielige Mediastion-Perikarditis und den paradoxen Puls. Berl. Klin. Wochenschr., 10:433, 461, 1873.

40. Kutcher, M. A., King, S. B., III, Alimurung, B. N., Craver, J. M., and Logue, R. B.: Constrictive pericarditis as a complication of cardiac surgery: Recognition of an entity. Am J. Cardiol., 50:742, 1982.

41. Kwasnik, E. M., Koster, J. K., Lazarus, J. M., Sloss, L. J., Mee, R. B. B., Cohn, L. H., and Collins, J. J.: Conservative management of uremic pericardial effusions. J. Thorac. Cardiovasc. Surg. 76:629, 1978.

42. Lam, C. R.: Pericardial celomic cyst. Radiology, 48:239, 1947.

43. Lambert, A. V.: Etiology of thin-walled thoracic cysts. J. Thorac. Surg., 10:1, 1940.

44. Larrey, D. J.: New surgical procedure to open the pericardium and determine the cause of fluid in its cavity. Clin. Chirurg., 36:393, 1829.

45. Levine, H. D.: Myocardial fibrosis in constrictive pericarditis. Electrocardiographic and pathologic observations. Circulation, 48:1268, 1973.

46. Lorrell, B. H., and Braunwald, E.: Pericardial disease. In Braunwald, E. (Ed.): Heart Disease. A Textbook of Cardiovascular Medicine. Philadelphia, W. B. Saunders Company, 1984, p. 1474.

47. Masson, J. F., Maes, M. L., and Zilberman, C.: Pericarditis in chronic renal insufficiency treated by periodic hemodialysis. Rev. Med. Intern., 2:447, 1981.

48. McCaughan, B. C., Schaff, H. V., Piehler, J. M., Danielson, G. K., Orszulak, T. A., Puga, F. J., Pluth, J. R., Connolly, D. C., and McGoon, D. E.: Early and late results of pericardiectomy for constrictive pericarditis. J. Thorac. Cardiovasc. Surg., 89:340, 1985.

49. McGaff, F. J., Haller, J. A., Jr., Leight, L., and Towery, B. T.: Subvalvular pulmonic stenosis due to constriction of the right ventricular outflow tract by a pericardial band. Am. J. Cardiol., 34:142, 1963.

50. McGregor, M.: Current concepts: Pulsus paradoxus. N. Engl. J. Med., 301:480, 1979.

51. Moore, R. L.: Congenital deficiencies of the pericardium. Arch. Surg., 11:765, 1925.

52. Morgagni, G. B.: De Sedibus et Causis Morborum per Anatomen Indagatis, Venetiis, Typ. Remondiniana, 1761.

53. Morgan, B. C., Guntheroth, W. G., and Dillard, D. H.: Relationship of pericardial to pleural pressure during quiet respiration and cardiac tamponade. Circ. Res. 16:493, 1965.

54. Moscovitz, H. L.: Pericardial constriction versus cardiac tamponade. Am. J. Cardiol., 26:546, 1970.

55. Mounsey, P.: The early diastolic sound of constrictive pericarditis. Br. Heart J., 17:143, 1955.

56. Niarchos, A. P.: Electrical alternans in cardiac tamponade. Thorax, 30:228, 1975.

57. Parsons, H. G., and Holman, E.: Experimental Ascites. (Surgical Forum, 1950.) Philadelphia, W. B. Saunders Company, 1951, p. 251.

58. Parsons, H. G., and Holman, E.: Experimental segmental pericarditis. Arch. Surg., 70:479, 1955.

59. Paul, O., Castleman, B., and White, P. D.: Chronic constrictive pericarditis: A study of 53 cases. Am. J. Med. Sci., 216:361, 1948.

60. Peel, A. A. F.: Tuberculous pericarditis. Br. Heart J., 10:195, 1948.

61. Piehler, J. M., Pluth, J. R., Schaff, H. V., Danielson, G. K., Orszulak, T. A., and Puga, F. J.: Surgical management of effusive pericardial disease: Influence of extent of pericardial resection on clinical course. J. Thorac. Cardiovasc. Surg., 90:506, 1985.

62. Rehn, L.: Zur experimentellen Pathologie des Herzbeutels. Ver. Deutsch. Ges. Chir., 42:339, 1913.

63. Roberts, W. C., and Ferrans, V. J.: A survey of the causes and consequences of pericardial heart disease. In Reddy, D. S., et. al. (Eds.): Pericardial Disease. New York, Raven Press, 1982, p. 56.

64. Roberts, W. C., and Spray, T. L.: Pericardial heart disease: A study of its causes, consequences and morphologic features. In Spodick, D. H. (Ed.): Pericardial Diseases. Philadelphia, F. A. Davis, 1976, pp. 11–65.

65. Romero, cited by Baizeau: Memoire sur le fonction du pericarde au point de vue chirurgical. Gaz. Med. Chirc., 1868, p. 565.

66. Rose, E.: Herz Tamponade (Ein Beitrag zur Herzchirurgie). Dtsch. Z. Chir., 20:329, 1884.

67. Ruskin, J., Bache, R. J., Rembert J. C., and Greenfield, J. C., Jr.: Pressure-flow studies in man: Effect of respiration on left ventricular stroke volume. Circulation, 48:79, 1973.

68. Santamore, W. P., Lynch, P. R., Meier, G., Heckman, J., and Bove, A. A.: Myocardial interaction between the ventricles. J. Appl. Physiol., 41:362, 1976.

69. Sauerbruch, F.: Die Chirurgie der Brustorgane. Vol. II. Berlin, 1925.

70. Shabetai, R.: Uremia, dialysis, and metabolic causes of pericardial disease. In Shabetai, R. (Ed.): The Pericardium. New York, Grune & Stratton, 1981, pp. 385–389.

71. Shabetai, R., Fowler, N. O., and Guntheroth, W. G.: The hemodynamics of cardiac tamponade and constrictive pericarditis. Am. J. Cardiol., 26:480, 1970.

72. Shumacker, H. B., Jr., and Roshe, J.: Pericardiectomy. J. Cardiovasc. Surg., 1:65, 1960.

73. Sodeman, W. A., and Smith, R. H.: A re-evaluation of the diagnostic criteria for acute pericarditis. Am. J. Med. Sci., 235:672, 1958.

74. Somerville, W.: Constrictive pericarditis: With special reference to the change in natural history brought about by surgical intervention. Circulation, 38(Suppl. V):102, 1968.

75. Soulen, R. L., Stark, D. D., and Higgins, C. B.: Magnetic resonance imaging of constrictive pericardial disease. Am. J. Cardiol. 55:480, 1985.

76. Spodick, D. H.: Acute pericarditis. New York, Grune & Stratton, 1959.

77. Spodick, D. H.: Medical history of the pericardium. The hairy hearts of hoary heroes. Am. J. Cardiol., 26:447, 1970.

78. Spodick, D. H.: Pathogenesis and clinical correlations of the electrocardiographic abnormalities of pericardial disease. Cardiovasc. Clin. 8:201, 1977.

79. Spodick, D. H.: Acute pericarditis: ECG changes. Primary Cardiol., 8:78, 1982.

80. Spodick, D. H.: The normal and diseased pericardium: Current concepts of pericardial physiology, diagnosis and treatment. J. Am. Coll. Cardiol., 1:240, 1983.

81. Steiger, Z., McAlpin, G., and Wilson, R. F.: Left subcostal approach to the pericardium. Surg. Gynecol. Obstet., 160:414, 1985.

82. Surawicz, B., and Lasseter, K. C.: Electrocardiogram in pericarditis. Am. J. Cardiol., 26:471, 1970.

83. Swanton, R. H., Brooksby, I. A. B., Davies, M. J., Coltart, D. J., Jenkins, B. S., and Webb-Peploe, M. M.: Systolic and diastolic ventricular function in cardiac amyloidosis. Studies in six cases diagnosed with endomyocardial biopsy. Am. J. Cardiol., 39:658, 1977.

84. Tweddell, J. S., Zimmerman, A. N. E., Stone, C. M., Rokkas, C. K., Schuessler, R. B., Boineau, J. P., and Cox, J. L.: Pericardiocentesis guided by a pulse generator. J. Am. Coll. Cardiol., 14:1074, 1989.

85. Unverferth, D. V., Williams, T. E., and Fulkerson, P. K.: Electrocardiographic voltage in pericardial effusion. Chest, 75:157, 1979.

86. Vogel, J. H. K., Horgan, J. A., and Strahl, C. L.: Ventricular function in chronic constrictive pericarditis: Observations on fiber shortening rate. Cardiol. Digest, 6:21, 1971.

87. Wacker, W., and Merrill, J. P.: Uremic pericarditis in acute and chronic renal failure. J.A.M.A., 156:764, 1954.

88. Wei, J. Y., Taylor, G. J., and Aschuff, S. C.: Recurrent cardiac tamponade and large pericardial effusion: Management with an indwelling pericardial catheter. Am. J. Cardiol., 42:281, 1978.

89. Wilkinson, P., Pinto, B., and Senior, J. R.: Reversible protein-losing enteropathy with intestinal lymphangiectasia secondary to chronic constrictive pericarditis. N. Engl. J. Med., 273:1178, 1965.

90. Wong, B., Murphy, J., Chang, C. J., Hassenein, K., and Dunn, M.: The risk of pericardiocentesis. Am. J. Cardiol., 44:1110, 1979.

91. Wood, P.: Diseases of the Heart and Circulation, 2nd ed. Philadelphia, J. B. Lippincott Company, 1956.

92. Wychulis, A. R., Connolly, D. C., and McGoon, D. C.: Surgical treatment of pericarditis. J. Thorac. Cardiovasc. Surg., 62:608, 1971.

56

THE HEART

CARDIAC CATHETERIZATION AND PERCUTANEOUS CORONARY ANGIOPLASTY

Christopher Buller, M.D., Daniel Mark, M.D., M.P.H.,
Harry R. Phillips, M.D., and Richard S. Stack, M.D.

The utility of diagnostic cardiac catheterization lies in its capacity to combine high-resolution dynamic imaging of the cardiac chambers, great vessels, and coronary arteries with versatile quantitative hemodynamic measurements. The combination of structural, functional, and prognostic information that it can provide complements the clinical and modern noninvasive evaluation. In this context, findings at cardiac catheterization are often pivotal in patient management, guiding the selection of appropriate medical and surgical therapy in ischemic, valvular, myopathic, and congenital heart diseases.

Interventional cardiology has broadened the scope of cardiac catheterization. The safety and efficacy of percutaneous coronary angioplasty are widely recognized. Aortic and mitral valvuloplasty offer an alternative to surgical treatment in selected patients with valvular stenosis. Catheterization procedures have evolved as definitive treatment in some forms of congenital heart disease and are palliative in others. Until precise indications for interventional catheterization procedures are established, management of individual patients continues to require input from both cardiologists and cardiac surgeons.

HISTORICAL ASPECTS

Catheterization originated with the study of cardiovascular physiology in experimental animals. In 1726, Stephen Hales inserted a rigid tube into the femoral artery of a horse for measurement of its systemic blood pressure. In 1844, Claude Bernard was the first to perform retrograde catheterization of the right and left ventricles of a horse for comparison of the temperature of blood in the two chambers. He later repeated the procedure to measure pressure in the ventricles. Intracardiac pressures were studied in greater detail by Cheaveau and Marey, who, in 1863, published the first systematic description of the cardiac cycle. By the end of the nineteenth century, catheterization of the animal heart was performed routinely in many physiology laboratories.

Forssmann initiated human cardiac catheterization in 1929 by inserting a 4-French ureteral catheter into his own brachial vein and advancing it under fluoroscopic control to his right atrium.[80] He then walked to the radiology department to document the position of the catheter (Fig. 1). Forssmann perceived this technique as a method of introducing medication to the central circulation and was subsequently the first to inject contrast media into the heart.

Refinement of right heart catheterization for the study of pathophysiology was made by Cournand, Richards, Stead, and others. Forssmann, Cournand, and Richards shared the 1956 Nobel Prize in medicine for their work. Early clinical studies of congenital heart disease were performed during this period by Warren, Baldwin, and Dexter. The introduction of retrograde left heart catheterization by Zimmerman in 1950 and selective coronary arteriography by Sones in 1958 advanced cardiac catheterization from the role of an investigative technique to that of a clinical diagnostic method. Work by Dotter and Grüntzig culminated in the first percutaneous coronary angioplasty by 1977 and initiated the current era of interventional cardiac catheterization.

INDICATIONS

Cardiac catheterization is indicated when the information obtained by the study is likely to meaningfully influence patient management and is not otherwise reliably available by clinical and noninvasive evaluation. The inherent risks and discomfort of the procedure demand thoughtful consideration of the risk : benefit ratio for each patient.

Catheterization may be performed for *diagnosis* of symptoms. Patients with chest pain suggestive of angina but without conclusive evidence for myocardial ischemia on treadmill testing or thallium scintigraphy form the largest such group. The utility of demonstrating normal versus diseased coronary arteries in this circumstance is obvious. Similarly, symptoms following cardiac surgery are often problematic. Altered perception of symptoms, pre-existing abnormalities, surgical wounds, or prosthetic valves can make clinical and echocardiographic assessment unreliable. Common dilemmas include chest pain following coronary bypass surgery, dyspnea following mitral commissurotomy, and the infant with failure to thrive following a palliative shunt procedure.

When a diagnosis is previously established, catheterization may be indicated *for the determination of severity of disease and the selection of optimal therapy.* In particular, referral of patients to cardiac surgery is frequently based in part on the findings at cardiac catheterization. Patients with known coronary artery disease, few or absent symptoms, but severe ischemia are a common example. Coronary arteriography can identify subsets in whom coronary bypass surgery is indicated for prolonging life.[26,62,66] Cardiac catheterization remains the standard for

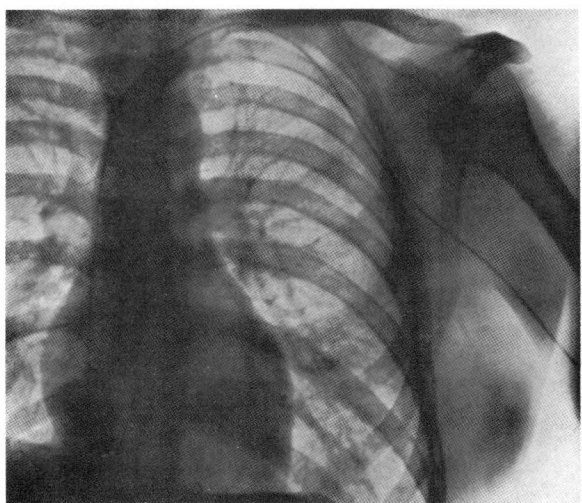

Figure 1. Photograph of the chest film of Forssmann documenting passage of a catheter from his left antecubital vein in his right atrium. (From Forssmann, W.: Klin. Wochenschr., 8:2085, 1929.)

quantitation of stenoses, regurgitant lesions, ventricular function, and shunts. Thus, the asymptomatic individual with aortic stenosis and borderline Doppler echocardiographic aortic valve gradients is likely to require invasive measurement of aortic valve area for determination of the need for surgical therapy.

Even when surgical therapy is indicated by clinical data, catheterization is usually required for *planning the operative approach and excluding coexistent disease.* For correction of complex congenital lesions, the surgeon must have the detailed anatomic information provided by angiocardiography. Adults over age 40 years (and those with multiple risk factors) undergoing noncoronary cardiac surgery require preoperative coronary angiography for the exclusion of unrecognized coronary disease. If significant disease is discovered, surgical therapy should include bypass grafting.

Invasive hemodynamic measurements may be required for the *evaluation of the efficacy of medical therapy.* This is the most common indication for pulmonary artery catheterization in the intensive care unit, where it allows rapid, objectively based titration of fluids and vasoactive medications. Similarly, evaluation of the response to vasodilators can guide chronic therapy for pulmonary hypertension.[70] Coronary arteriography following thrombolytic therapy for acute myocardial infarction can document reperfusion and aid selection of patients for salvage angioplasty when necessary.[79]

In addition, some catheterizations are performed primarily for *therapeutic intervention.* Percutaneous coronary angioplasty is discussed separately at the end of this section.

TECHNIQUES

Patient Preparation

Successful cardiac catheterization is aided by a cooperative and relaxed patient. The patient should appreciate why the procedure has been recommended. A thorough and understandable explanation of what occurs during and after the procedure must be provided. Instructional pamphlets and video presentations are helpful but should not replace direct interaction with the responsible physician. In addition, patients must be told of the risks of the procedure (see Complications of Cardiac Catheterization), and informed consent must be obtained.

Patients should avoid eating for at least 6 hours before an elective cardiac catheterization. Necessary medications should be continued as usual. Premedication routines vary between institutions, but the drugs and dosages chosen should have minimal hemodynamic and cardiodepressant effects. Particular

caution is needed for patients with cyanotic heart disease or poor left ventricular function. In most adults, a small dose of a benzodiazepine or meperidine is sufficient for light sedation. In children, deeper sedation is desirable, which necessitates the participation of an anesthesiologist. A combination of meperidine, chlorpromazine, and promethazine is often used. Prophylaxis for infective endocarditis is not required before cardiac catheterization.

Certain patients require special precatheterization preparation. The adult with renal insufficiency or diabetes should be well hydrated so that the risk of contrast-induced acute renal failure is reduced. The use of nonionic contrast agents does not, however, appear to reduce nephrotoxicity.[76] The child with cyanotic polycythemia requires hydration for the prevention of the consequences of hypovolemia. The patient with known or suspected allergy to radiocontrast media should receive corticosteroids and H_1- and H_2-blocking agents for a 24-hour period before the procedure.[37] Individuals on oral anticoagulants *in whom arterial cannulation is anticipated* should have their anticoagulants held for reduction of their prothrombin time below 1.5 times control. Those at high risk for thromboembolism during this period require hospitalization for administration of heparin.

Traditionally an inpatient procedure, diagnostic cardiac catheterization is increasingly performed on an outpatient basis. This approach may reduce cost, inconvenience to the patient, and delays in therapy, and it appears safe in selected patients.[9] Patients with unstable symptoms, congestive heart failure, a bleeding diathesis, significant renal dysfunction, a history of possible contrast allergy, or advanced age are unsuitable candidates for outpatient studies.

Planning the Procedure

Each cardiac catheterization must be planned to ensure that vital information is obtained with minimum catheter manipulation and radiation exposure. This requires the cardiologist performing the procedure to be familiar with the patient's clinical and noninvasive evaluation. Questions answered by the test can then be clearly articulated and prioritized. Thus, in an older patient with unequivocal clinical and Doppler echocardiographic evidence of critical aortic stenosis, *demonstration of coronary anatomy* is the principal indication for preoperative cardiac catheterization. In a child with a ventricular septal defect, it is insufficient merely to confirm its presence and quantify the shunt. Management requires precise demonstration of the location of the defect, the coexistence of associated lesions, and the condition of the pulmonary vasculature.

Inadequate planning leads to incomplete studies, possibly necessitating repeat catheterization with its attendant risks, discomfort, and cost. The review of complex cases with knowledgeable surgical colleagues can provide the cardiologist with important information and can therefore contribute to the quality of studies performed.

Vascular Access

Most diagnostic and interventional catheterizations are performed percutaneously via the right femoral artery and vein from a site 2 to 3 cm. below the inguinal ligament. In patients with advanced peripheral vascular disease or recent catheterization, the left side may be used. The femoral vessels offer ready access, are large enough to accept standard diagnostic and interventional catheters without threat to immediate or long-term vessel patency, and are easily compressed to attain hemostasis.

The femoral artery or vein, as required, is cannulated by use of the Seldinger technique. In a sterile field, the overlying skin and subcutaneous tissue are infiltrated with 1 to 2 per cent xylocaine, and a small skin puncture wound is made. A Seldinger or similar needle is then advanced at 45 degrees inclination until vessel cannulation is confirmed by the free return of blood (many operators prefer single-wall puncture needles to conventional Seldinger needles, particularly if thrombolytic therapy has been administered). A guidewire advanced through the needle secures access to the vessel lumen, and the needle is withdrawn. Catheterization may then proceed by direct exchange of catheters over the guidewire or through an indwelling sheath.

The brachial artery and vein provide alternative access for both diagnostic and interventional procedures. This approach (often termed Sones' technique) is most useful in patients with occlusive peripheral vascular disease involving the aorta, both iliac arteries, or both femoral arteries. It may also be used when morbid obesity or a bleeding tendency raises concerns about postprocedure hemostasis at a femoral artery puncture site. Although percutaneous puncture is possible, direct vessel exposure through a transverse antecubital incision permits the use of larger catheters. After withdrawal of the catheters, the arteriotomy is repaired and the vein repaired or ligated. With care, meticulous hemostasis can be obtained.

Access via the internal jugular or subclavian veins is reserved for bedside insertion of flow-directed pulmonary artery catheters. Their corresponding arteries cannot be safely cannulated.

Transseptal Left Heart Catheterization

Normally, left heart catheterization is performed retrogradely from the arterial access site, whereas right heart and pulmonary artery catheterization is performed antegradely from the venous access site. In some patients, however, retrograde left heart catheterization is undesirable. In 5 per cent of patients with aortic stenosis, difficulty crossing the aortic valve may prolong the procedure and expose the patient and operator to unnecessary radiation.[39] Tilting disc type aortic valve prostheses may be damaged if crossed by a catheter.[38] In such circumstances, the left side of the heart may be reached from a venous access site by advancing a catheter across the atrial septum from right to left.

This maneuver usually requires the use of a specialized Brockenbrough catheter. This device consists of a tapered end-hole catheter snugly fitted over a removable steel needle. The catheter tip is positioned in the right atrium against the fossa ovalis, and the needle is then abruptly advanced into the left atrium by puncturing the atrial septum. When correct positioning is confirmed, the catheter is advanced over the needle to the left atrium and the needle is removed. In 25 per cent of adults, the foramen ovale is potentially patent[43] and can sometimes be crossed by simply probing the area with a catheter and guidewire. Other applications of transseptal catheterization include measurement of mitral gradients (when the pulmonary wedge tracing is of poor quality) and mitral valvuloplasty procedures. The Brockenbrough technique is contraindicated if a patient has received anticoagulants, since inadvertent perforation of the atrium occasionally occurs. Suspicion of left atrial thrombus or tumor contraindicates left atrial catheterization because of the risk of systemic embolism.

HEMODYNAMICS

General Considerations

Cardiac catheterization allows several hemodynamic measurements to be recorded simultaneously or in close temporal proximity. The known relationships between these measurements may then be used to infer or calculate parameters of ventricular function, valvular stenosis or regurgitation, vascular resistance, shunts, and pericardial defects. Interpretation of hemodynamic data first requires familiarity with normal measurements. The range of normal measured and derived hemodynamic variables is given in Table 1.

Diagnostic catheterization provides a pattern of hemodynamics at a particular point in time. This "snapshot" must be viewed in light of the conditions present at the time of study. Routine cardiac medications, particularly diuretics, vasodilators, or inotropic drugs, may dramatically influence measurements. Other medications, pacemakers, and active pulmonary or metabolic disease may also introduce bias. In addition, it is important to recognize that hemodynamic measurements are subject to considerable physiologic variation. In patients, confounding factors beyond normal variability may also be present.

TABLE 1. Normal Hemodynamic Values (Recumbent Adults)

Pressure Site	Systolic (mm. Hg)	Diastolic (mm. Hg)	Mean (mm. Hg)
Right atrium	—	—	0–8
Right ventricle	5–30	0–8	—
Pulmonary artery	15–30	5–15	10–18
Pulmonary artery wedge	—	—	1–12
Left ventricle	90–140	2–12	—
Aorta	90–140	60–90	70–105

Fick Cardiac Output Parameter	Normal Range
AV O$_2$ difference	30–50 ml./L.
O$_2$ consumption	140–390 ml./min.
O$_2$ consumption index	110–150 ml./min./ sq. m.
Cardiac output	3.5–8.5 L./min.
Cardiac index	2.5–4.5 L./min./sq. m.

Vascular Resistances	
Systemic vascular resistance	8–15 units*
Pulmonary vascular resistance	≤2.0 units*

Value Gradients	
Aortic valve	<10 mm. Hg
Mitral valve	Negligible

Valve Areas	
Aortic valve	2.0–3.0 sq. cm.
Mitral valve	4.0–6.0 sq. cm.

AV, arteriovenous.
* To convert Wood units to dyne-sec.-cm.$^{-5}$, multiply by 80.

Abnormal circulatory reflexes, transient myocardial ischemia or rhythm disturbances, and the administration of fluids, oxygen, or vasoactive medications during the procedure may materially affect hemodynamics. These factors must be documented in order for surgeons and cardiologists *not present at the time of catheterization* to interpret hemodynamic data correctly.

Elevation of ventricular diastolic pressure is most commonly due to systolic ventricular dysfunction. Other causes include diastolic ventricular dysfunction (acute ischemia, ventricular hypertrophy), pericardial disease (constriction, tamponade), and regurgitant lesions (particularly acute aortic regurgitation). The conventional *direct* measurement of ventricular filling pressure is taken at the end of diastole after the *a* wave and is termed left or right ventricular end-diastolic pressure (LVEDP or RVEDP). Assessment of left ventricular filling pressures may also be made by measuring left atrial or pulmonary artery wedge pressure. Validity of these *indirect* measurements precludes abnormal gradients across the mitral valve or pulmonary venous bed present in mitral stenosis, cor triatriatum, and pulmonary veno-occlusive disease. Further substitution of pulmonary artery diastolic pressure for pulmonary wedge pressure is valid only if pulmonary vascular resistance is normal. In addition, it should be emphasized that normal end-diastolic pressure does not exclude ventricular dysfunction. This measurement is insensitive for mild impairment and may be normalized by diuretics or vasodilators despite severe impairment.

The *sine qua non* of significant stenosis is the presence of an abnormal pressure gradient. Although some gradient is necessary to produce forward flow within the cardiovascular system, such physiologic gradients are generally too small to detect. Mitral stenosis is characterized by a diastolic gradient from the left atrium (or pulmonary artery wedge position) to the left ventricle (Fig. 2). Conditions such as left atrial myxoma or cor

triatriatum, which also impede ventricular filling, may produce similar findings. Tricuspid stenosis causes analogous right heart pressure gradients.

Stenosis of the ventricular outflow tracts may occur at the valvular, subvalvular, or supravalvular level. Obstruction to outflow creates a systolic gradient between the involved ventricle and great vessel, which can be demonstrated upon catheter "pull-back" (Fig. 3). Since beat-to-beat variability is common, quantitation of gradients is best performed by simultaneous recording above and below the stenosis with two catheters and pressure transducers (Fig. 4). In some patients, uncertainty exists regarding the level of outflow obstruction. Slow withdrawal of a pressure-monitored end-hole catheter across the outflow tract can help localize the stenosis. Dynamic gradients, such as those observed in hypertrophic cardiomyopathy, may be labile.[33] Obstruction can be provoked in the catheterization laboratory by spontaneous or catheter-induced extrasystoles or administration of amyl nitrate (Fig. 5).

Several conventions for reporting valve gradients exist. This potential source of confusion is easily eliminated by familiarity with the various methods. Outflow tract gradients recorded in the catheterization laboratory are commonly expressed as the difference between peak ventricular and peak aortic or pulmonary artery pressures. This "peak-to-peak" value is artificial, since peak pressures in the ventricle and great vessel do not occur simultaneously when outflow tract obstruction is present (Fig. 4). The actual gradient across a stenosis at any point in time is referred to as the instantaneous gradient. The peak instantaneous gradient is the maximal instantaneous gradient within a cardiac cycle. Mean gradients may be obtained by manually or electronically planimetering the area between superimposed tracings and dividing by the interval during which the gradient exists. This method is preferred when calculating valve area (see Calculation of Stenotic Orifice Area). Electronically averaged instantaneous gradients from continuous wave Doppler echocardiography correlate well with mean gradients from catheterization.[20]

Valvular regurgitation may be reflected in pressure tracings. With mitral or tricuspid incompetence, normal atrial filling is augmented by the regurgitant volume. This partial ventricularization of atrial pressure manifests as a giant atrial V wave, or *CV wave* (Fig. 6). Since the magnitude of a CV wave is determined

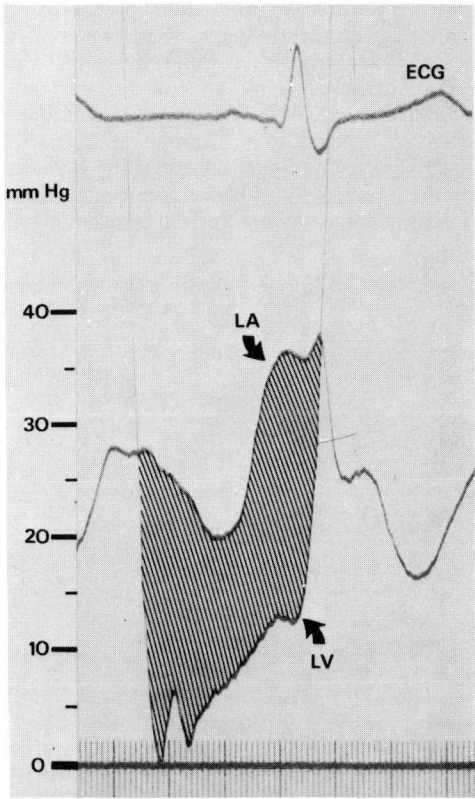

Figure 2. Simultaneous recordings of left atrial (LA) and left ventricular (LV) pressures in a patient with mitral stenosis. The hatched area represents the diastolic mitral valve gradient. (From Fowles, R. E.: Interpretation of cardiac catheterization. *In* Ream, A. K., and Fogdall, R. P. (Eds.): Acute Cardiovascular Management. Philadelphia, J. B. Lippincott Company, 1982.)

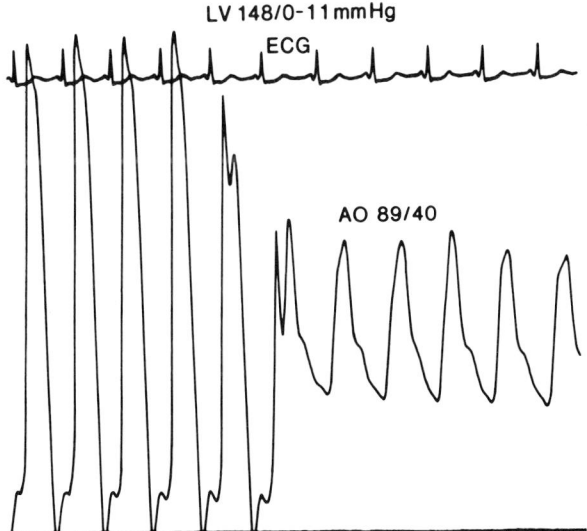

Figure 3. "Pull-back" recording of left ventricular (LV) and aortic (AO) pressures in a patient with aortic stenosis. There is a 59 mm. Hg difference between peak LV and peak AO tracings. (From Goolsby, J. P.: Cardiology. *In* Reller, L. B., et al. (Eds.): Clinical Internal Medicine. Boston, Little, Brown & Company, 1979. Copyright 1979.)

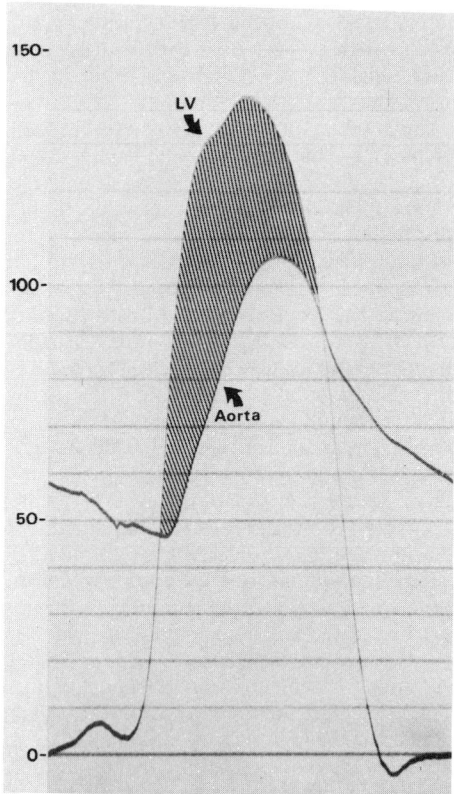

Figure 4. Simultaneous recordings of left ventricular (LV) and aortic pressures in a patient with aortic stenosis. The systolic aortic valve gradient is represented by the hatched area. Note that peak aortic pressure occurs measurably later than does peak LV pressure. The peak instantaneous gradient may be determined by finding the point in time at which the difference of LV and aortic pressure is maximal. The peak instantaneous gradient systematically exceeds the peak to peak gradient. (From Fowles, R. E.: Interpretation of cardiac catheterization. *In* Ream, A. K., and Fogdall, R. P. (Eds.): Acute Cardiovascular Management. Philadelphia, J. B. Lippincott Company, 1982.)

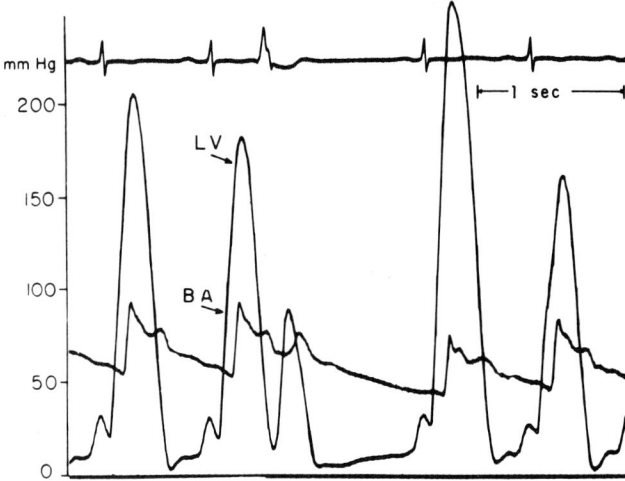

Figure 5. Simultaneous pressures recorded in the left ventricle (LV) and brachial artery (BA) in a patient with hypertrophic cardiomyopathy. During the post-extrasystole beat, a dynamic increase in obstruction causes a rise in LV peak pressure but a fall in BA pressure. (From Braunwald, E., et al.: Idiopathic hypertrophic subaortic stenosis. Circulation, *30*(Suppl. IV): 78, 1964, by permission of the American Heart Association, Inc.)

both by regurgitant volume and by compliance of the receiving atrium, AV regurgitation cannot be reliably quantified by pressure tracings alone. Mitral regurgitation also augments *diastolic* mitral flow and may increase the physiologic mitral gradient present in early diastole.[63] The delay inherent in pulmonary wedge tracings further exaggerates the apparent diastolic gradient when pulmonary wedge tracings are superimposed on left ventricular tracings. This phenomenon is distinguished from true mitral stenosis by the equilibration of pulmonary wedge and left ventricular pressures by mid-diastole. Abnormalities such as ventricular septal defects and left ventricular failure may elevate left atrial V waves and thereby masquerade as mitral regurgitation.

Chronic aortic and pulmonary incompetence increase diastolic filling of the respective ventricle. An adaptive change in ventricular compliance, however, minimizes elevation of end-diastolic pressure until ventricular dysfunction develops. When, however, aortic incompetence develops acutely (as in aortic dissection, infective endocarditis, or prosthetic dysfunction), the normal left ventricle cannot adapt, and elevation of LVEDP is recorded. In severe cases, LVEDP may approach aortic diastolic pressure.[69] Premature closure of the mitral valve may make indirect measurements of LVEDP inaccurate.[56]

In some circumstances, absence of an expected pressure difference is noteworthy. When an atrial septal defect is present, approximation of left and right mean atrial pressures to within 5 mm. Hg predicts a significant shunt. With a ventricular septal defect, equalization of ventricular systolic pressures implies unrestricted bidirectional shunting and, unless pulmonary steno-

sis coexists, progressive or established pulmonary vascular disease.

Pericardial disease can produce stereotypical pressure tracings. Constriction allows rapid early diastolic filling of the ventricles, which ends abruptly as the volume of pericardial constraint is reached with production of a characteristic dip-and-plateau waveform. End-diastolic pressures are elevated and equal in all chambers (Fig. 7) and increase further during inspiration. Constrictive physiology may be obscured by volume depletion. Rapid administration of intravenous saline during catheterization may expose such "occult" constriction.[17]

Tamponade is characterized by systemic hypotension and elevation of left and right heart filling pressures. Unlike constriction, the continuous compression of the heart produced by tamponade *slows* early diastolic filling and attenuates atrial y descents. Since transmission of negative intrathoracic pressure during inspiration enhances right heart filling at the expense of left heart filling, pulsus paradoxus is recorded. Conclusive evidence of tamponade is obtained when pericardiocentesis per-

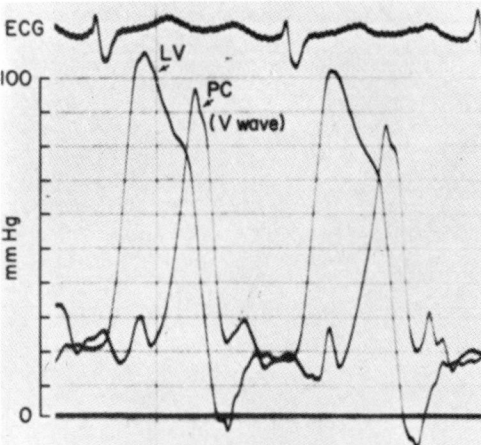

Figure 6. Left ventricular (LV) and pulmonary capillary wedge (PC) pressure tracings taken in a patient with ruptured chordae tendineae and acute mitral insufficiency. The giant V wave follows regurgitation of blood into a relatively small and noncompliant left atrium. The apparent diastolic gradient between PC and LV is due primarily to the inherent time delay present in PC tracings. (From Grossman, W.: Cardiac Catheterization and Angiography, 4th ed. Philadelphia, Lea & Febiger, 1991.)

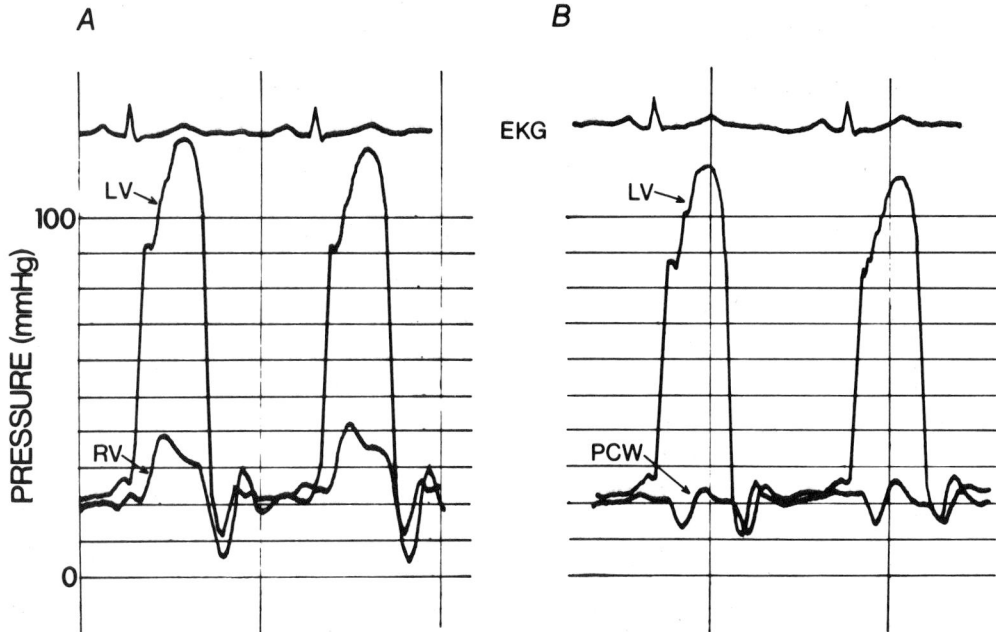

Figure 7. Pressure waveforms in a patient with constrictive pericarditis. *A,* Right (RV) and left (LV) ventricular diastolic pressures are elevated and equal with typical "dip-and-plateau" pattern. *B,* Pulmonary wedge (PCW) tracing shows same pattern with prominent y descent. (From Grossman, W.: Cardiac Catheterization and Angiography, 3rd ed. Philadelphia, Lea & Febiger, 1986.)

formed during right heart catheterization restores normal hemodynamics.

Measurement of Cardiac Output

There are three main methods for measurement of cardiac output during cardiac catheterization: the Fick method, indicator-dilution methods, and the angiographic method.

In 1870, Fick proposed the principle that subsequently became the basis for the Fick method of cardiac output measurement.[46] This principle states that the amount of oxygen extracted by the lungs from air is equal to the amount taken up by blood in its passage through the lungs. Therefore, by measuring the *rate* of lung oxygen extraction and the oxygen *content* of pulmonary arterial and pulmonary venous blood, the *rate* of pulmonary blood flow can be calculated. Unless a shunt is present, pulmonary blood flow equals cardiac output.

Traditionally, the rate of lung oxygen extraction (oxygen consumption) is measured by collecting *at steady state* a patient's expired gas over a known period of time in a Douglas bag. The concentration of oxygen in inspired and expired gas is measured, corrected to standard temperature and pressure, and expressed as oxygen content (milliliters O_2 per liter of gas). The total volume of expired gas is then measured with a spirometer, corrected for standard temperature and pressure, and divided by the duration of collection to obtain minute ventilation. The difference between inspired and expired oxygen content times the minute ventilation equals oxygen consumption in milliliters per minute. Recently, less cumbersome electronic methods of measuring oxygen consumption have become commercially available. These methods employ continuous sampling of exhaled gas diluted with a known quantity of ambient air for derivation of the lung oxygen extraction.[61] In addition, when oxygen consumption has not been measured, assumed oxygen consumptions calculated from body surface area are sometimes substituted. Assumed oxygen consumptions are prone to error introduced by age, sex, disease, and nonbasal conditions. In a study of 108 patients, "basal" oxygen consumption index varied widely between individuals (126 ± 26 ml. per minute per sq. m.).[21]

The oxygen content of pulmonary arterial (PA) and pulmonary venous (PV) blood is derived by measuring the fractional oxygen saturation of blood samples and applying the formula

O_2 content (ml. O_2/liter)
$$= (\text{saturation}) \times ([\text{hemoglobin, gm./liter}] \times K)$$

where K equals 1.36 ml. O_2 per gm. hemoglobin. Arteriovenous oxygen difference is then simply

AV O_2 diff. (ml. O_2/liter)
$$= (O_2 \text{ content PV}) - (O_2 \text{ content PA})$$

and cardiac output (CO) follows:

$$\text{CO (liter/min.)} = \frac{O_2 \text{ consumption (ml./min.)}}{\text{AV } O_2 \text{ diff. (ml./liter)}}$$

In practice, systemic arterial or left ventricular samples are substituted for pulmonary venous samples. This introduces a systematic but clinically insignificant overestimation of cardiac output owing to admixing of bronchial and thebesian venous blood in the left ventricle.

The indicator-dilution technique for measurement of cardiac output was first outlined in 1897 by Stewart.[81] It is based on the simple principle that *the dilution of an indicator is proportional to the volume of fluid to which it is added.* Thus, if the amount and concentration of indicator is known, the volume of fluid in which it is diluted can be calculated:

$$\text{Volume} = \frac{\text{Amount of indicator}}{\text{Concentration of indicator}}$$

This relationship is easily modified for circulating fluids. When a known bolus of indicator is added, the time-concentration curve generated at a point downstream is related to flow as follows:

$$\text{Flow} = \frac{\text{Amount of indicator}}{C \times T}$$

where C is the mean concentration of indicator and T is the time for first pass. (The reader may note that the Fick method is really a specific application of this principle in which the indicator [oxygen] is added continuously rather than as a bolus.) Whereas several specific indicator methods have been proposed, only two are used clinically—thermodilution and indocyanine green.

Thermodilution is now widely used in both the catheterization laboratory and intensive care unit. A known amount (usually 10 ml.) of iced 5 per cent dextrose (approximately 0° C.) is injected rapidly through the right atrial port of a thermistor-tipped pulmonary artery catheter. The temperature of blood passing the catheter tip is then used to generate a time-concentration curve from which cardiac output is calculated.[31] The popularity of this method can be attributed to its thermal indicator, which is nontoxic, has no significant recirculation, and does not accumulate. These properties permit frequent measurements to be performed.

Indocyanine green dye is usually reserved for the catheterization laboratory. With this method, 5 mg. of dye in 1 ml. diluent is injected into the main pulmonary artery, and the catheter is flushed with saline. Time-concentration curves are derived by sampling from a peripheral arterial site. Blood is withdrawn from this site at a constant rate (20 ml. per minute) through a densitometer cuvette, which records the concentration of indicator. Since indocyanine green is cleared slowly, recirculation occurs. This causes a discontinuity of concentration decay, which can lead to incorrect calculation of cardiac output. Extrapolation of the primary decay curve avoids this error.[51]

Comparisons of Fick, indocyanine green, and thermodilution methods have demonstrated good agreement.[88] The Fick method, however, is the most accurate method in patients with reduced cardiac output. For purposes of measuring cardiac output, the presence of a shunt or regurgitant lesion between the indicator injection site and the sampling site invalidates the time-concentration curve. Therefore, tricuspid or pulmonary regurgitation invalidates thermodilution measurements, and mitral or aortic regurgitation invalidates green dye measurements. The Fick method provides direct measurement of pulmonary (but not systemic) blood flow despite intracardiac shunts. Measurement of cardiac output by ventriculography is discussed later (see Quantitative Left Ventriculography).

Vascular Resistance

The opposition to blood flow created by frictional and other losses within a vascular bed is termed vascular resistance. It is defined by analogy to Ohm's law for electrical currents:

$$\text{Resistance} = \frac{\text{Driving pressure (volts)}}{\text{Flow (current)}}$$

Effects of viscosity, turbulent flow, pulsatile flow, and vessel elasticity introduce nonlinearity, which this equation ignores. Despite this, values for systemic and pulmonary vascular resistance derived by this relation remain clinically useful.

Systemic (peripheral) vascular resistance (SVR) is calculated as follows:

$$\text{SVR} = \frac{P_{Ao} - P_{Ra}}{Q_s}$$

where P_{Ao} is mean aortic pressure (mm. Hg), P_{Ra} is mean right atrial pressure, and Q_s is systemic blood flow (liters per minute). Measurement of systemic vascular resistance is most useful in the management of critically ill patients with shock. In this setting, the profile of SVR, cardiac output, and ventricular filling pressures obtained with a pulmonary artery catheter can help distinguish cardiogenic, hypovolemic, and vasodilatory causes. Sequential measurements allow objective assessment of specific therapeutic interventions.

Pulmonary vascular resistance (PVR) is calculated similarly:

$$\text{PVR} = \frac{P_{Pa} - P_{La}}{Q_p}$$

where P_{Pa} is mean pulmonary artery pressure (mm. Hg), P_{La} is mean left atrial or pulmonary artery wedge pressure, and Q_p is pulmonary blood flow (liters per minute). Measurement of pulmonary vascular resistance is most useful when pulmonary artery pressure is elevated. Pulmonary arterial hypertension may follow pulmonary venous hypertension (normal PVR), arteriolar vasoconstriction (elevated PVR that responds to administration of oxygen or vasodilators), or structural pulmonary vascular disease (fixed elevation of PVR). Correct medical and surgical management of mitral valve disease, shunt lesions, and cardiomyopathy (when transplantation is considered) often depend on the nature and potential reversibility of pulmonary hypertension as defined by pulmonary vascular resistance.

Calculation of Stenotic Orifice Area

Decisions regarding surgical intervention for aortic or mitral stenosis depend substantially on measurements of valve cross-sectional area.[12] The pressure gradient produced by a stenotic valve, although inversely proportional to valve area, is also proportional to the *square* of blood flow across the valve. Therefore, whereas abnormal pressure gradients may identify a stenosis, the magnitude of the gradient is at best a semiquantitative measure of valve area. Reliance on gradients alone can be frankly misleading in some circumstances. For example, poor left ventricular function with reduced cardiac output may cause an unimpressive aortic valve gradient despite critical stenosis. Conversely, augmentation of flow by shunts or nonbasal conditions may produce large gradients across only moderately stenotic pulmonary or aortic valves. (Fig. 8)

In 1950, Gorlin and co-workers proposed a method of calculating valve orifice cross-sectional areas on principles borrowed from fluid hydraulics. Gorlin's formula is based on the assumption that a stenosis can be modeled as a short rigid tube with a circular orifice through which fluid flows at a constant rate. The general form of this equation is

$$A = \frac{Q}{C(P^{1/2})}$$

where A is valve orifice area (square centimeters), Q is flow rate across valve (milliliters per minute), P is mean pressure gradient across valve (mm. Hg), and C is an empiric constant (C = 37.7 for mitral valve, C = 44.5 for aortic valve).

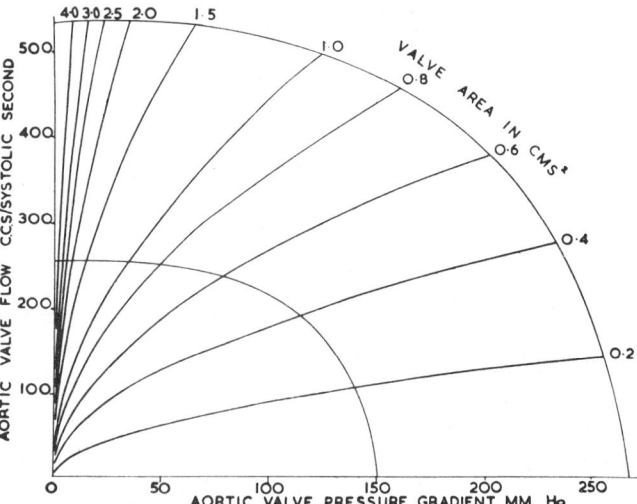

Figure 8. Schematic diagram of the relationship of valve orifice area, transvalvular pressure gradient, and blood flow across the aortic valve. Note that the aortic pressure gradient may be elevated by increases in blood flow despite a constant valve area. This is particularly true with moderate to severe stenosis (valve area less than 1.0 sq. cm.). (From Grossman, W.: Cardiac Catheterization and Angiography, 2nd ed. Philadelphia, Lea & Febiger, 1980.)

Cardiac valves open for only a portion of the cardiac cycle, yet the entire cardiac output must cross the valve during this abbreviated period. Valve flow rates (Q) are therefore calculated by dividing the cardiac output (milliliters per minute) by the fraction of time the valve is open (seconds per minute).

$$Q = \frac{CO}{DFP \text{ or } SEP}$$

where CO is cardiac output (milliliters per minute), DFP is diastolic filling period (seconds per minute), and SEP is systolic ejection period (seconds per minute). Diastolic filling periods (for atrioventricular valves) and systolic ejection periods (for semilunar valves) are derived by multiplying the appropriate systolic or diastolic interval measured from pressure tracings (seconds per beat) by the heart rate (HR, beats per minute). Thus, the final equations are as follows:

$$\text{Mitral valve} \quad A = \frac{\dfrac{CO[ml./min.]/(HR[beats/min.])}{(sec./beat)}}{37.7\,(P^{1/2})}$$

$$\text{Aortic valve} \quad A = \frac{\dfrac{CO[ml./min.]/(HR[beats/min.])}{(sec./beat)}}{45.5\,(P^{1/2})}$$

It is important to realize that cardiac output as used in the formula must represent the flow across the valve in question. In mixed stenotic and regurgitant mitral valve disease, for example, diastolic mitral flow is equal to the sum of forward cardiac output *plus* regurgitant output. Use of Fick or thermodilution outputs systematically underestimates diastolic mitral flow and therefore mitral valve area. Instead, cardiac output measured by left ventriculography should be used (see later). Similar considerations apply when a shunt is present.

Shunts

Evaluation of shunts requires their *detection, classification* (i.e., left-to-right, right-to-left, or bidirectional), *localization,* and *quantitation.* Both oxygen analysis (oximetry) and indocyanine green dilution techniques are used clinically for detecting and localizing shunts. Oximetry was first used systematically in 1947 by Dexter and colleagues in a series of classic studies on congenital heart disease and remains the most commonly employed method. With oximetry, orderly sampling of blood oxygen saturation is performed proximal and distal to a suspected shunt. An abnormal increase (step-up) or decrease (step-down) is detected immediately distal to the shunt, with the magnitude of the change being proportional to the size of the shunt. Indocyanine green dilution technique provides a more sensitive means of detecting shunts. This method is considerably more complex (see Measurement of Cardiac Output) and is therefore reserved for detection of shunts too small to be demonstrated by oximetry.

Left-to-right shunts are characterized by two basic abnormalities: mixing of saturated (systemic arterial or pulmonary venous) with desaturated (systemic venous or pulmonary arterial) blood on the right side of the circulation, producing an abnormal oxygen *step-up,* and an *increase* in pulmonary blood flow relative to systemic blood flow. Common causes are atrial septal defects, ventricular septal defects, and persistent ductus arteriosus. Other causes include anomalous pulmonary venous return, atrioventricular canal defects, aortopulmonary windows, coronary fistulas, and surgically constructed shunts (Blalock-Taussig, Potts, or Waterston types).

For detecting an oxygen step-up, saturation is measured sequentially in the pulmonary artery, right ventricle, right atrium, superior and inferior venae cavae, and aorta. The position of the catheter should be confirmed at each site by both fluoroscopy and the pressure waveform. The use of an end-hole catheter (Cournand or Swan-Ganz) ensures that samples are representative of conditions at the catheter tip. Before each sampling, several milliliters of blood are withdrawn and discarded for avoidance of contamination with blood from other sites. An additional 2 ml. is then aspirated and subjected to oximetry. Abnormalities should be assessed with multiple samples.

Some normal variability in right heart oxygen saturations occurs owing to incomplete mixing of venous blood from different locations and beat-to-beat changes. Step-ups of less than 5 to 7 per cent may reflect normal physiology and cannot be relied on as evidence for a shunt (Table 2). Streaming of venous and shunted blood may also interfere with shunt detection. Step-ups are often first detected in the chamber or vessel immediately distal to the shunt. When step-ups are detected, localization may be refined by comparing samples in various right ventricular and right atrial positions or in the proximal, right, and left pulmonary arteries.

The magnitude of a left-to-right shunt may be expressed as a ratio of pulmonary to systemic flow ($Q_p:Q_s$) or as an absolute shunt flow (Q_{shunt}) calculated as the difference between pulmonary and systemic blood flows derived by the Fick method (see Measurement of Cardiac Output):

$$Q_{shunt} = Q_p - Q_s$$

where

$$Q_p = \frac{O_2 \text{ consumption}}{(O_2 \text{ content Ao}) - (O_2 \text{ content PA})}$$

and

$$Q_s = \frac{O_2 \text{ consumption}}{(O_2 \text{ content Ao}) - (O_2 \text{ content MV})}$$

Mixed venous (MV) oxygen content is estimated from superior (SVC) and inferior vena caval (IVC) saturations as follows:

$$O_2 \text{ content MV} = \frac{1(O_2 \text{ content SVC}) + 2(O_2 \text{ content IVC})}{3}$$

Error introduced by this estimate of mixed venous oxygen content is seldom of clinical significance.

Small shunts ($Q_p:Q_s$ less than 1.3:1) may be missed by oximetry but are detectable by indocyanine green injection. Injection of the indicator into the pulmonary artery or right ventricle is followed by continuous sampling from a systemic artery. The shunt causes early recirculation, producing a characteristic de-

TABLE 2. Criteria for Oximetric Detection of Left-to-Right Shunts

Site of Step-up	Step-up in Oxygen Saturation (%)	Example
SVC to RA	≥7	ASD, anomalous pulmonary venous drainage
RA to RV	≥5	VSD, or ASD
RV to PA	≥5	PDA, or VSD

SVC, superior vena cava; RA, right atrium; PA, pulmonary artery; ASD, atrial septal defect; VSD, ventricular septal defect; PDA, patent ductus arteriosus.

formation in the downslope of the indicator-dilution curve. A left-to-right shunt may be localized by injection of dye sequentially into the left atrium, left ventricle, and aorta while sampling for premature appearance of the dye in the pulmonary artery. The first injection that is not followed by premature appearance of the dye identifies the chamber immediately distal to the shunt.

The two basic characteristics of right-to-left shunts are the mixing of desaturated (systemic venous or pulmonary arterial) with saturated (systemic arterial or pulmonary venous) blood on the left side of the circulation, creating an oxygen *step-down*, and a *decrease* in pulmonary blood flow relative to systemic blood flow. Common causes are tetralogy of Fallot, pulmonary atresia, and atrial or ventricular septal defects with severe pulmonary hypertension.

Right-to-left shunting is implied by the presence of systemic arterial desaturation (arterial oxygen saturation below 95 per cent) without significant pulmonary disease. Administration of supplemental oxygen fails to correct desaturation due to shunting. The absence of a coexistent oxygen step-up in the right heart indicates that shunting is unidirectional. The level at which shunting is occurring is often evident from clinical or echocardiographic findings, or may be suggested by inadvertent passing of a catheter across a septal defect. However, by adapting the technique described for left-to-right shunts, serial oximetric sampling of pulmonary venous, left atrial, left ventricular, aortic, and pulmonary arterial (or mixed venous) blood confirms the suspected site and allows quantitation of the shunt:

$$Q_{shunt} = Q_s - Q_p$$

where

$$Q_p = \frac{O_2 \text{ consumption}}{(O_2 \text{ content PV}) - (O_2 \text{ content PA})}$$

and

$$Q_s = \frac{O_2 \text{ consumption}}{(O_2 \text{ content Ao}) - (O_2 \text{ content PA})}$$

If pulmonary venous sampling is not practical, pulmonary venous oxygen content may be estimated by substituting pulmonary wedge oxygen saturation or using an assumed pulmonary venous oxygen saturation of 98 per cent.

Indocyanine green may also be employed to screen for right-to-left shunts. A bolus of dye is injected into the vena cava while sampling is done continuously from a systemic artery. Shunting causes early appearance of indicator in the arterial circulation. If necessary, localization of the shunt can be accomplished by performing serial injections in the inferior vena cava, right atrium, right ventricle, and pulmonary artery. The first injection site that does not produce early arterial circulation of indicator is the chamber immediately distal to the shunt.

Malformations such as single ventricle, double outlet right ventricle, tricuspid atresia, and hypoplastic left heart cause free mixing of systemic and pulmonary venous blood in a common chamber or vessel. The resulting bidirectional shunt is characterized by both an oxygen step-up between systemic venous and pulmonary arterial blood and a step-down between pulmonary venous and systemic arterial blood. Individuals with an atrial septal defect or ventricular septal defect complicated by moderately severe pulmonary hypertension also display bidirectional shunting. In such circumstances, the dominant direction of shunting may be labile and depend on dynamic changes in pulmonary and systemic vascular resistance. Quantification of shunt flow in each direction can be approximated with the following formulas:

$$\text{left to right } Q_{shunt} = \frac{Q_p (O_2 \text{ content PA} - O_2 \text{ content MV})}{(O_2 \text{ content PV} - O_2 \text{ content MV})}$$

$$\text{right to left } Q_{shunt} = \frac{\begin{array}{c} Q_p (O_2 \text{ content PV} - O_2 \text{ content Ao}) \cdot \\ (O_2 \text{ content PV} - O_2 \text{ content PA}) \end{array}}{\begin{array}{c} (O_2 \text{ content Ao} - O_2 \text{ content MV}) \cdot \\ (O_2 \text{ content PV} - O_2 \text{ content MV}) \end{array}}$$

CARDIAC ANGIOGRAPHY

Left Ventriculography

A contrast cineangiogram of the left ventricle is a routine part of most left heart catheterization studies. It permits evaluation of chamber dimensions, global and segmental systolic function, and the presence and severity of mitral regurgitation. Left ventriculography may also demonstrate congenital defects, aortic stenosis, mitral valve prolapse, and abnormal mitral valve motion in hypertrophic cardiomyopathy.[77]

Usually, the ventriculography catheter is advanced retrogradely across the aortic valve and positioned in the midportion of the ventricular cavity, free of the mitral apparatus. However, the catheter may also be advanced antegradely across the mitral valve by use of transseptal technique (see Techniques), or directly across a ventricular septal defect. In patients with severe aortic regurgitation, contrast aortography may permit adequate opacification of the left ventricle.

The volume of contrast required for ventriculography is determined by the patient's weight, hemodynamics, and the anticipated size of the ventricle; 0.6 to 0.8 ml. per kg. is appropriate for most images. Thus, approximately 50 ml. of contrast delivered by power injection over 4 seconds is nominal for most adults. Patients with elevated LVEDP are prone to pulmonary edema following the volume challenge induced by hyperosmolar contrast, and ventriculography should be performed cautiously with reduced volumes (0.4 to 0.5 ml. per kg.) of nonionic contrast. Patients with enlarged ventricles, regurgitant lesions, or shunts may require larger volumes for adequate images to be produced.

The standard camera angle for left ventriculography is 30 degrees right anterior oblique (RAO). This projects the ventricle close to its long axis with the beam passing at right angles to the trabeculated muscular interventricular septum (Fig. 9). The anterior, apical, and inferoposterior wall segments as well as the mitral anulus are therefore viewed tangentially. For assessment

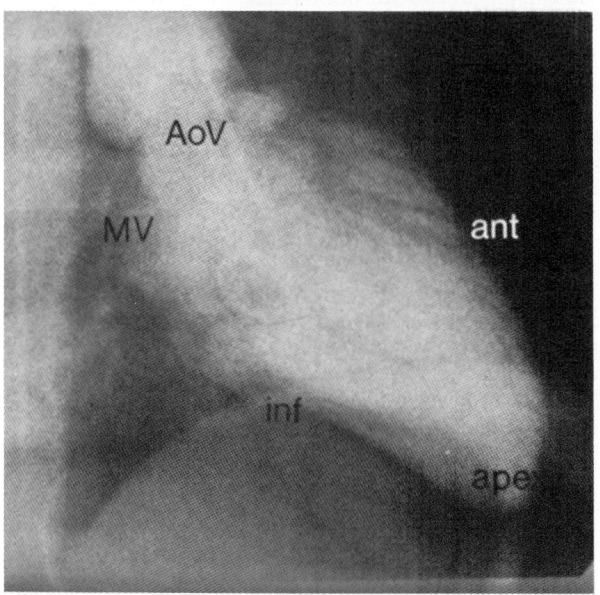

Figure 9. Right anterior oblique view of a left ventriculogram at end diastole demonstrating anterior (ant) wall, apex, and inferior (inf) wall, plus the location of the aortic (AoV) and mitral (MV) valves. (From Hillis, L. D., et al.: Cardiac Catheterization. *In* Kloner, R. A. (Ed.): The Guide to Cardiology. New York, Churchill Livingstone, 1984.)

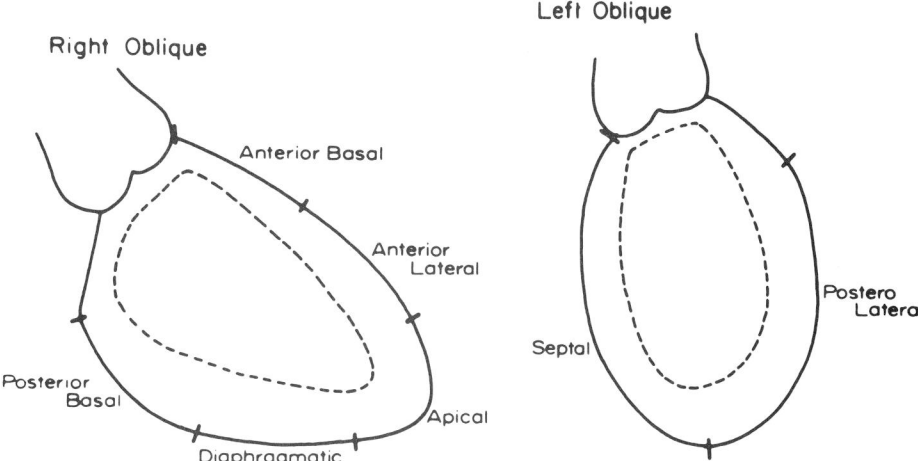

Figure 10. Left ventriculogram wall segments in right and left anterior oblique views. In the authors' laboratory, the anterior basal and anterior lateral segments are considered together as the anterior wall, and the posterior basal and diaphragmatic segments are considered together as the inferior wall. (From Franch, R. H., et al.: Techniques of cardiac catheterization including coronary arteriography. *In* Hurst, J. W. (Ed.): The Heart, 5th ed. New York, McGraw-Hill Book Company, 1982.)

of septal and posterolateral wall motion, however, a 60-degree left anterior oblique (LAO) view that projects the ventricle close to its short axis is required. Orthogonal RAO and LAO images may be obtained simultaneously if biplane equipment is employed. To define the anatomy of the ventricular septum and outflow tract fully, compound angulations are required[78] (see Congenital Heart Disease).

Global left ventricular function may be assessed semiquantitatively by examining the ventriculogram. A subjective impression of overall systolic function can be translated into an ordinal scale such as normal, mildly depressed, moderately depressed, or severely depressed. If an ejection fraction is not available, this summary impression of function can provide similar information.

Regional wall motion abnormalities are typical of coronary artery disease but may be observed in other disease processes that produce nonuniform damage to the myocardium. For the purpose of describing systolic regional wall motion, the left ventricle is divided into standard segments in both the RAO and LAO views (Fig. 10). Each segment is then described as normal, hypokinetic—reduced movement, akinetic—no movement, or dyskinetic—outward or paradoxic movement (Fig. 11). The term *aneurysm* is often misapplied to any wall segment exhibiting dyskinesia. This term is best reserved for dyskinetic segments that demonstrate persistent deformity in diastole. Asso-

ciated angiographic features include calcification within the wall of the aneurysm and intraventricular filling defects due to adjacent thrombus. *Pseudoaneurysms* (or false aneurysms), which occur when ventricular rupture is contained by adherent pericardium, are distinguished angiographically from true aneurysms by a narrow neck at the site of communication with the ventricle.

In ischemic heart disease, contrast left ventriculography can distinguish reversible from irreversible dysfunction. Wall motion abnormalities improved transiently by post-extrasystolic potentiation or nitroglycerin infusion may demonstrate sustained improvement following revascularization.[5]

Quantitative Left Ventriculography

Calculation of left ventricular volume is based on the modeling of left ventricular geometry as half a prolate ellipsoid (the shape produced by an ellipse rotated in space about its long axis). The area-length method described by Dodge and associates is commonly employed.[25] By planimetering the area (A, square centimeters) of left ventricular images in RAO and LAO projections, left ventricular volume (V, milliliters) can be calculated as follows;

$$V = \frac{8 \, A_{RAO} A_{LAO}}{3 \, \pi \, L}$$

where L is the long axis of the ventricle (centimeters). The derivation of this formula, single-plane formulas, and correction factors are discussed extensively elsewhere.[27]

By calculating left ventricular volume at end diastole (EDV) and end systole (ESV), the ejection fraction (EF) may be calculated as follows:

$$EF = \frac{EDV - ESV}{EDV}$$

Since its introduction in the early 1960s, the ejection fraction has become the most widely used measure of left ventricular systolic performance. Its limitations, however, should be recognized. The ejection fraction varies inversely with afterload and to some extent directly with preload. Thus, conditions that decrease afterload (e.g., mitral regurgitation, vasodilator therapy) or increase preload (e.g., aortic regurgitation, mitral regurgitation) may misleadingly normalize the ejection fraction despite important deterioration of ventricular function. A discussion of load-*independent* measures of ventricular function can be found elsewhere.[60] Irregular rhythms pose a problem because loading conditions, the interval-strength relation,[13] and ventricular activation may change from beat to beat. Extrasystolic and post-extrasystolic beats should therefore be ignored when evaluating basal ventricular function.

Angiographic measurements of ventricular volumes also per-

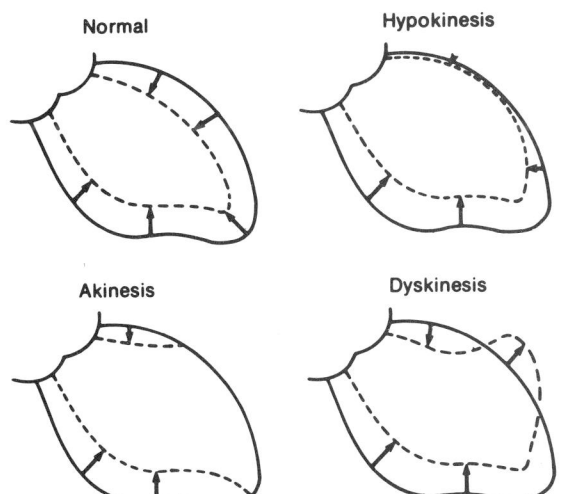

Figure 11. Left ventricular wall motion abnormalities. End diastole is demonstrated in solid lines. End systole is represented by dashed lines. The arrows show the direction of wall movement during systole. (From Ross, J., et al.: Cardiac Catheterization and angiography. *In* Petersdorf, R. G., et al. (Eds.): Harrison's Principles of Internal Medicine, 10th ed. New York, McGraw-Hill Book Company, 1983.)

mit calculation of cardiac output. Since cardiac output (CO) is the product of stroke volume (SV) and heart rate (HR), and SV is the difference of EDV and ESV:

$$CO(ml./min.) = HR(beats/min.) \times [EDV(ml.) - ESV(ml.)]$$

In selected patients with optimal biplane images, close agreement between angiographic and Fick measurements of cardiac output can be obtained.[73]

Right Ventriculography

Right ventricular function is less amenable to quantification because of the complex and irregular geometry of the chamber. Whereas quantitative methods using biplane angiography have been proposed,[32,35] subjective evaluation is sufficient for most clinical purposes.

Some forms of congenital heart disease cause ambiguous positioning of left and right ventricles. The anatomic right ventricle can be distinguished angiographically from the anatomic left ventricle by its trapezoidal shape, coarse trabeculation, and discontinuity between inlet and outlet valves created by the right ventricular muscular infundibulum. Isolated right ventricular wall motion abnormalities and aneurysms usually reflect congenital disorders (including arrhythmogenic right ventricular dysplasia), postoperative changes, or blunt trauma rather than myocardial infarction.

Valvular Disease

Normal semilunar valves are composed of three symmetrical and pliable leaflets occasionally visible during ventriculography as fine linear lucencies that open widely in systole. Dysplastic or degenerative valves are identified by thickening, irregular surfaces, and valvular calcification. "Doming" and reduced cusp mobility are characteristic of stenosis and may be recognized during ventriculography or aortography.[7] Mitral stenosis is most easily identified angiographically during RAO left ventriculography. In this view, an irregular scalloped lucency on the ventricular aspect of the mitral anulus is observed in diastole.[23] This represents the thickened leaflets surrounding nonopacified atrial blood. Reduced excursion of the anterior mitral leaflet may also be apparent.

Angiographic assessment of the severity of valvular regurgitation is an important factor in determining the need for surgical correction. Mitral regurgitation is assessed during left ventriculography. Care must be taken to ensure that the catheter is free of the mitral apparatus, and therefore not contributing to valvular incompetence. Extrasystoles may also cause factitious mitral regurgitation. Aortic regurgitation is assessed during aortography. Attention to correct catheter position (within 2 cm. of the aortic valve) prevents underestimation of severity, which occurs when contrast is flushed downstream. It follows that when reviewing films, surgeons should note the technical factors that may have influenced the apparent severity of regurgitant le-

sions. Subjective grading of both mitral regurgitation and aortic regurgitation is done on a 1 to 4+ scale (Table 3).

Quantification of valvular regurgitation is based on the comparison of angiographic and Fick (or thermal dilution) measurements of cardiac output. Angiographic measurements of cardiac output are based on stroke volume and are therefore the sum of forward ("effective") and regurgitant volumes. The Fick method, however, measures only effective cardiac output. The difference between the two measurements is the regurgitant output. The regurgitant output divided by heart rate is the regurgitant stroke volume. The *regurgitant fraction* is simply regurgitant stroke volume divided by angiographic stroke volume.

Congenital Heart Disease

The angiographic study of congenital heart disease is a particularly complex subject about which entire textbooks have been written.[29] The advent of two-dimensional and Doppler echocardiography has changed the primary role of angiography from diagnosis to the precise demonstration of surgical anatomy.

Suggested injection sites and projection angles for common lesions have been summarized by Criley and French.[19] The numerous permutations and combinations of lesions possible, however, require that studies be individualized based on clinical, echocardiographic, and hemodynamic data. Contrast injections should be made upstream of stenotic lesions for identification of the nature and level of obstruction. The dominant direction of shunting should be established hemodynamically so that the choice of injection site demonstrates septal defects in positive contrast. When Eisenmenger physiology has been identified, angiography should be avoided in order not to provoke peripheral vasodilation and hypercyanosis.

Compound projection angles (oblique with cranial or caudal angulation) are often employed. For example, cranial angulation reduces foreshortening of both left[48] and right[28] ventricular outflow tracts and the proximal pulmonary arteries. Left anterior oblique projection with cranial angulation minimizes overlap between the cardiac chambers and is useful in distinguishing ventricular from atrial septal defects when an endocardial cushion defect is present. Membranous and muscular ventricular septal defects are best demonstrated when viewed tangentially. Since the interventricular septum subtends a 100-degree arc from its posterior to anterior segments, the degree of obliquity must be adjusted to correspond to the position of the defect.

The extent of pulmonary vascular disease in children with lesions associated with increased pulmonary blood flow may also be assessed angiographically. Pulmonary wedge angiography, in which high-resolution images of a subsegmental pulmonary artery and its radicals are evaluated quantitatively, has been correlated with morphometric studies at lung biopsy.[68] This technique may identify children with left-to-right or bidirectional shunts who are poor surgical candidates.

TABLE 3. Subjective Grading of Valvular Regurgitation

Grade	Aortic Regurgitation*	Mitral Regurgitation†
1+	Small jet of contrast into LV that clears with each beat	Small jet of contrast into LA that clears with each beat
2+	Moderate opacification of LV but less than AO; incomplete clearing with each beat	Moderate opacification of LA but less than LV; incomplete clearing with each beat
3+	Persistent marked opacification of LV, equal to AO after three beats	Persistent marked opacification of LA, equal to LV after three beats
4+	Persistent marked opacification of LV, equal to AO with three beats	Persistent marked opacification of LA, equal to LV within three beats; systolic reflux into pulmonary veins may be observed

LV, left ventricle; LA, left atrium; AO, aorta.
* Assessed by aortography.
† Assessed by left ventriculography.

CORONARY ANGIOGRAPHY

In 1958, Sones and colleagues performed the first selective coronary angiograms. By use of an angled catheter inserted through an exposed brachial artery, they first injected contrast into the sinuses of Valsalva adjacent to the coronary ostia. As the technique evolved, it became apparent that direct cannulation of the coronary ostia was feasible and safe. A percutaneous femoral approach to selective coronary angiography was first performed by Ricketts and Abrams in 1962. The subsequent development of preformed left and right coronary catheters by Judkins, Amplatz, and others was followed by routine application of the technique.

Normal Coronary Anatomy

An appreciation of three-dimensional coronary anatomy is helpful when performing or interpreting coronary angiograms. The left and right coronary ostia are located approximately a centimeter above the aortic valve within the left and right sinuses of Valsalva. The proximal left coronary artery—or left main coronary artery—courses horizontally leftward between the pulmonary trunk anteriorly and the left atrial appendage posterosuperiorly. The length of the left main coronary varies from 1 mm. to almost 3 cm. before it bifurcates to form the left anterior descending and left circumflex arteries (Fig. 12). In one third of patients,[54] the left main artery trifurcates, producing an additional intermediate branch—the ramus intermedius.

The left anterior descending (LAD) artery turns gently anteriorly from the left main to lie in the anterior interventricular groove, parallel to the long axis of the left ventricle. From it arise two important types of branches. From one to three diagonal arteries branch leftward to traverse the epicardial surface of the anterolateral free wall of the left ventricle. A variable number of septal arteries branch inferoposteriorly and rightward from the LAD to enter the ventricular septum. The LAD usually wraps around the apex to end in the distal posterior interventricular groove, but in one quarter of cases it is smaller, ending at or just proximal to the apex.[67]

The left circumflex (LCX) artery turns sharply posterior from the left main to course in the left atrioventricular groove along the plane of the atrioventricular valves. From one to three obtuse marginal arteries arise from it and course apically to supply the lateral free wall. More distally, similar posterolateral branches supply the posterior wall.

The right coronary artery (RCA) points anteriorly and rightward in its proximal portion, then arcs 180 degrees as it follows the right atrioventricular groove diametrically opposite the LCX (Fig. 13). The sinoatrial node artery arises near the origin of the RCA in 60 per cent of patients. In the remaining 40 per cent, it is a branch of the LCX. Small right ventricular and acute marginal arteries supply the right ventricular free wall.

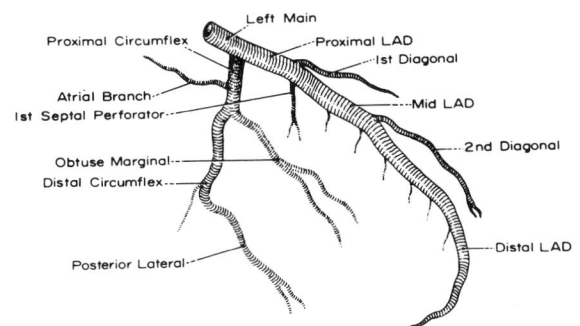

Figure 12. Normal left coronary artery anatomy observed from a right anterior oblique orientation. (From Franch, R. H., et al.: Techniques of cardiac catheterization including coronary arteriography. *In* Hurst, J. W. (Ed.): The Heart, 5th ed. New York, McGraw-Hill Book Company, 1982.)

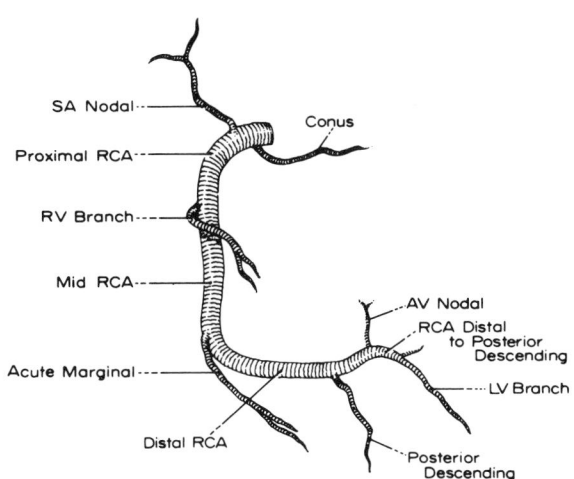

Figure 13. Normal right coronary artery anatomy observed from a left anterior oblique orientation. (From Franch, R. H., et al.: Techniques of cardiac catheterization including coronary arteriography. *In* Hurst, J. W. (Ed.): The Heart, 5th ed. New York, McGraw-Hill Book Company, 1982.)

In approximately 85 per cent of individuals, the RCA is *dominant*. Dominance is assigned to the vessel traversing the posterior crux of the heart, thus giving rise to the posterior descending and atrioventricular node arteries. In approximately 10 per cent of individuals, these branches arise from the distal LCX, and the left coronary is therefore dominant. In the remaining 5 per cent, a codominant pattern exists in which one or two posterior descending arteries are supplied by both the RCA and LCX. The posterior descending artery lies in the posterior interventricular groove opposite but parallel to the LAD and supplies *inferior* septal branches.

Technique of Coronary Angiography

In most laboratories, coronary arteries are opacified by hand injection of 4 to 8 ml. of contrast over several seconds through selective left and right coronary catheters. Between injections, pressure at the catheter tip is monitored to ensure that its tip is positioned safely and to document the effect of coronary injections on the patient's blood pressure. The coronary ostia are not infrequently involved with atherosclerosis. For this reason, manipulation of the catheter tip must always be delicate to prevent coronary dissection. Clues to the presence of ostial disease include difficulty seating the catheter, wedging of the catheter tip (with ventricularization of pressure tracings), and absence of "blow-back" of contrast proximal to the tip. Some operators prefer to identify ostial disease before engaging the coronary by first performing a flush injection within the sinus of Valsalva.

The purpose of coronary angiography is to demonstrate the severity and distribution of coronary stenoses. To accomplish this, each segment of the coronary tree should be demonstrated in at least two views in order to prevent overlooking important sites (Fig. 14). Left coronary angiograms are usually performed first. Initial views usually include a shallow RAO or LAO for assessment of the left main coronary, a 45- to 60-degree LAO, and a 30-degree RAO. On the basis of the preliminary findings, additional compound views are tailored for demonstration of particular regions of the left coronary tree. For example, the left main and its bifurcation are demonstrated by LAO/steep cranial angulation. Foreshortening of the proximal and mid LAD is reduced by RAO/cranial or left lateral/cranial projections. The proximal LCX can be isolated by steep LAO/caudal angles; the mid LCX and its obtuse marginal branches are displayed by RAO/steep caudal views. Initial RCA views also consist of 60-degree LAO and 30-degree RAO projections. The distal RCA and the origin of the posterior descending artery are demonstrated with cranial angulation.

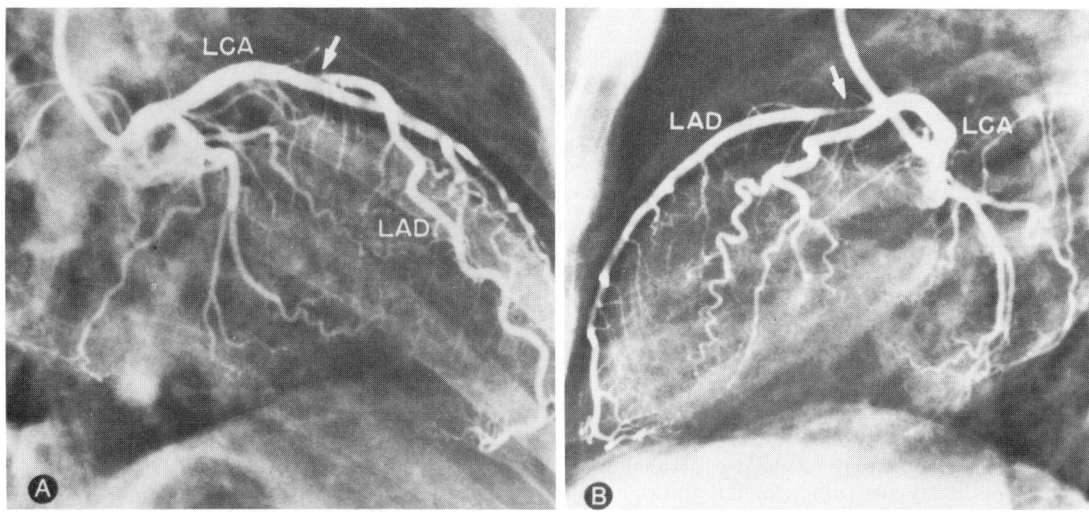

Figure 14. *A,* Right anterior oblique angiogram of the left coronary artery. A severe stenosis of the proximal left anterior descending artery (LAD, arrow) is almost completely obscured by overlapping branches. *B,* Left lateral view of the same artery demonstrates the stenosis (arrow) clearly. LCA, left circumflex artery. (From Mitchell, W.: Clinical angiographic description of the coronary artery anatomy. *In* Boucek, R. J., et al. (Eds.): Coronary Artery Disease. Baltimore, Williams & Wilkins, 1984.)

Interpretation of Coronary Angiograms

A simple and widely used convention for grading the severity of discrete coronary lesions compares the minimal luminal diameter of the lesion with that in adjacent normal vessels. The degree of stenosis is expressed as percentage reduction of luminal diameter or cross-sectional area. The accuracy with which these measurements can be made is influenced by several factors. Unrecognized narrowing within the adjacent "normal" vessel is common. This leads to systematic underestimation of lesion severity.[3,47] Eccentric coronary lesions that produce noncircular residual lumens are also common. The apparent diameter of such lesions varies with the angle of projection. In addition, visual quantification of stenoses is subject to considerable interobserver variability.[90] This may be due in part to imperfect resolution of vessel borders. Disagreement between observers is most likely to occur with lesions of intermediate severity.

Determining the functional significance of a coronary stenosis is even more problematic. Measurement of flow through arteries narrowed by extrinsic compression suggests that significant obstruction to maximal flow begins when luminal diameter is narrowed by 50 per cent. Greater narrowing produces a proportional decrement in flow as predicted by Poiseuille's law.[75] Unfortunately, extrapolation of these observations to atheromatous coronary lesions has proved to be an oversimplification.[86] Unlike experimental stenoses, atheromatous stenoses may be irregular, eccentric, of variable length, and situated in angulated or branching vessel segments. The increased obstruction to flow produced by this complex morphologic pattern cannot be predicted by measurements of minimal luminal diameter alone.[16] Computed methods that calculate the resistance and pressure-flow characteristics of coronary lesions from orthogonal coronary angiograms have been validated.[34]

Some morphologic features of the lesion on angiographic examination have been correlated with the clinical presentation. In particular, lesions characterized by multiple irregularities, overhanging edges, intraluminal filling defects, or persistent staining with contrast are much more likely to be observed in the setting of unstable angina[2,15] or following myocardial infarction.[1] These changes are thought to represent plaque rupture or ulceration and intraluminal thrombus.

Whereas computed interpretation is not yet in widespread clinical use, these observations underscore the need to consider both numeric and morphologic descriptors when interpreting angiograms visually. Attention should also be paid to sequential lesions that have additive obstructive effects. The presence of angiographically visible collateral supply to a distal vessel is sound evidence that a proximal stenosis is functionally significant. Common patterns of collateralization have been summarized by Levin.[53] Integration of angiographic findings with information from noninvasive testing may be necessary for the determination of the hemodynamic significance of questionable lesions.

Whereas left ventricular function is the most important predictor of outcome in patients with ischemic heart disease, the extent and distribution of angiographically apparent coronary disease have independent prognostic value. The most common convention for describing the extent of coronary disease is categorization of patients according to the *number* of major coronary vessels (LAD, LCX, RCA, or their large branches) containing a significant stenosis. In the Duke Cardiovascular Disease Databank (DCDD) registry, 5-year mortality of medically treated patients ranged nearly threefold depending on the presence of single-, double-, or triple-vessel disease at the time of index angiography (Fig. 15). Patients with left main coronary stenosis are at highest risk and are categorized separately regardless of the distribution of lesions in other vessels.[82]

Failure of this classification system to distinguish proximal from distal coronary lesions adequately, and therefore the amount of myocardium at risk, has prompted the development of angiographic coronary artery risk scoring systems. The "jeopardy score" proposed by Johnson and colleagues divides the coronary tree into six segments and assigns two points to each segment containing or distal to a 75 per cent diameter stenosis. Applied to patients without left main coronary artery stenosis, this score appears to improve prognostic accuracy.[18]

Categorizing the distribution of coronary disease is central to predicting whether bypass surgery will improve prognosis. Patients with left main coronary obstruction enjoy longer survival regardless of symptoms.[26,62] The benefit is greatest in those with severe left main coronary artery stenosis and those with coincident ventricular dysfunction. Patients with triple-vessel disease and moderate left ventricular dysfunction or severe ischemia also live longer after bypass surgery.[66] Finally, there is some evidence that bypass surgery improves prognosis in those with double-vessel disease involving the proximal LAD.[85]

When surgical revascularization is being considered, interpretation of the coronary angiogram must include an assessment of the distal coronary bed. Grafting to small (less than 1.5 mm.) or diseased distal vessels is less likely to produce long-

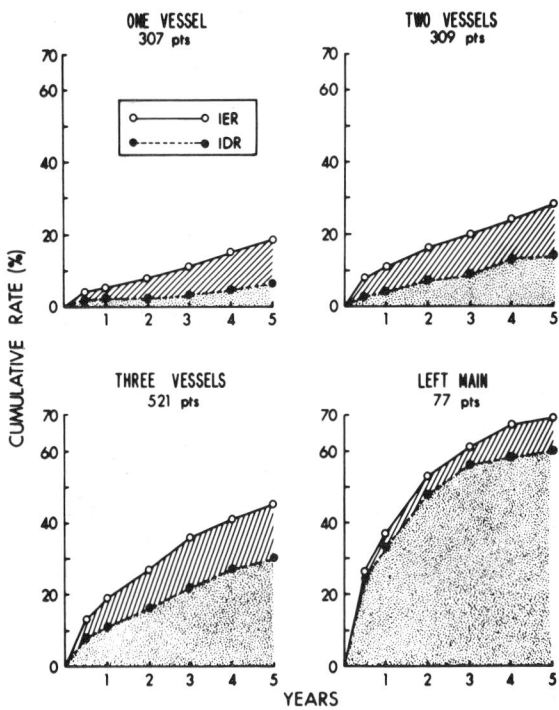

Figure 15. Cumulative ischemic event rates for medically treated patients with coronary artery disease stratified by the number of diseased vessels. IDR, ischemic death rate; IER, total ischemic event rate (death plus nonfatal myocardial infarction). As the number of involved vessels increases, both death (speckled area) and nonfatal myocardial infarction (hatched area) rates rise, and the proportion of events that are fatal increases. (Reprinted by permission of the American Heart Association from Harris, P. H., et al.: Circulation, 62:718, 1980.)

term graft patency.[52] Distal vessels may be sized by comparing them with the caliber of the diagnostic catheter.

COMPLICATIONS OF CARDIAC CATHETERIZATION

Cardiac catheterization can be performed with very low risk in the majority of patients. The experience of the angiographer, the volume of procedures performed in the laboratory, and the patient's underlying cardiac disease are the important determinants of the complication rate.

Right Heart Catheterization

The risk of death from right heart and pulmonary artery catheterization in patients who are not moribund at the time of the procedure is extremely low. Nonfatal complications are listed in Table 4. The principle risks during catheter insertion concern inadvertent puncture of a structure in the region of the vein (e.g., the carotid artery or lung with jugular insertions, and the subclavian artery or lung with subclavian insertions). In patients with pre-existing left bundle branch block, there is a small risk of inducing transient complete heart block by traumatizing the superficially located right bundle as the catheter passes through the right ventricle. Insertion of a prophylactic temporary pacemaker before catheterization is recommended in this situation.

Use of balloon-tipped pulmonary artery catheters for extended periods is associated with a small risk of infection and superior vena caval thrombosis. Correct positioning of the catheter tip just beyond the mediastinal shadow must be confirmed by chest films at the time of insertion and at least daily thereafter (or whenever the catheter is manipulated) for prevention of the more serious complications of pulmonary infarction and pulmonary artery rupture. Damped or spontaneously wedged

TABLE 4. Complications of Right Heart Catheterization

Insertion Complications
Local hematoma
Inadvertent arterial puncture
Pneumothorax
Hemothorax
Right bundle branch block
Dysrhythmias (atrial and ventricular)
Intracardiac catheter knotting*
Cardiac perforation*

Maintenance Complications
Dysrhythmias (especially ventricular)
Venous thrombosis
Pulmonary artery rupture*
Infection
Air embolism
Balloon rupture
Endocarditis*

* Rare.

pressure tracings often signal migration of the catheter tip to an undesirable distal position. The appearance of ventricular arrhythmias in patients with indwelling pulmonary artery catheters should always raise concern that the arrhythmia may be catheter-induced. This is particularly true if the arrhythmia fails to respond to usual measures.

Left Heart Catheterization

Reliable data regarding the nature and frequency of complications during left heart catheterization are available from the registry of the Society for Cardiac Angiography.[49] This report is based on nearly 54,000 procedures performed in 66 teaching, nonteaching, adult, and pediatric laboratories during 1979 and 1980. The major complications and their frequencies as established by the registry are listed in Table 5.

Death as a function of age demonstrates a bimodal distribution. Children less than 1 year are at highest risk (1.7 per cent), reflecting the severity of disease that leads to catheterization during the neonatal and infant period. The elderly, *particularly women*, are also at increased risk. Other characteristics associated with death include severe left ventricular dysfunction, left main coronary disease, valvular heart disease, and intercurrent noncardiac disease. Not uncommonly, the mechanism of death involves hypotension or intractable pulmonary edema associated with the combined negative inotropism and volume effect of hyperosmolar contrast. Careful patient preparation,

TABLE 5. Major Complications of Cardiac Catheterization

Complication	Percentage of Total Cases
Death	0.14
Nonfatal myocardial infarction	0.07
Stroke	0.07
Major arrhythmia	0.56
Vascular	0.57
Other	0.41
Total	1.82

Data from Kennedy,. J. W.: Complications associated with cardiac catheterization and angiography. From the Registry Committee of the Society for Cardiac Angiography. Cathet. Cardiovasc. Diagn., 8:5, 1982.

use of nonionic contrast,[74] avoidance of unnecessary contrast injections, and selective use of circulatory assist devices can prevent hemodynamic deterioration in those at highest risk. Left main coronary dissection or occlusion is another, often fatal complication. Avoidance of this hazard is discussed in Technique of Coronary Angiography.

Idiosyncratic immediate generalized contrast reactions may occur unpredictably, often without a history of previous contrast reaction. These reactions appear *not* to be mediated by IgE[36] and are therefore best categorized as anaphylactoid. Patients who must undergo angiography despite a history of suspected or documented previous contrast reaction should be pretreated for a full 24 hours with H_1- and H_2-blocking agents and corticosteroids.

Nonfatal myocardial infarction occurs in less than 0.1 per cent of cases involving coronary angiography.[10] Mechanisms include coronary dissection, embolism, and transient hypotension. The incidence and mechanisms of stroke during catheterization are similar to those of myocardial infarction. Careful manipulation and flushing of catheters, removal of blood from guidewires, and prompt treatment of hypotension during and after the procedure reduce the likelihood of these events.

The most common local vascular complication is the development of a hematoma at the site of arterial access. This can usually be managed with bed rest and local pressure. The advancing border of a hematoma should be outlined for monitoring of continued expansion. Vascular complications that require surgical intervention include uncontrolled hemorrhage, arterial thrombosis, and the formation of false aneurysms or arteriovenous fistulas.

PERCUTANEOUS CORONARY ANGIOPLASTY

Andreas Grüntzig first performed percutaneous angioplasty of human coronary arteries in 1977. His subsequent report of 50 consecutive cases in 1979 ignited widespread interest in the procedure.[40] Advances in technology have removed many of the early procedural barriers. By 1987, the use of the percutaneous transluminal coronary angioplasty (PTCA) in the United States had increased to nearly 175,000 cases per year.[11]

Indications

The clearest indication for angioplasty exists in patients with angina pectoris *resistant* to full medical therapy, who in addition have documented ischemia and single-vessel disease. However, whether PTCA should be offered to patients with angina pectoris as an alternative to *effective* medical therapy is controversial. This approach is most easily justified if medications produce side effects, or if residual ischemia precludes employment.

Patients with angina and *multivessel* disease who fail medical therapy comprise a heterogeneous group. PTCA has not yet been demonstrated to prolong survival in any patient subgroup with angina pectoris. For this reason, it is clearly contraindicated at the present time in those subsets who gain survival benefit from bypass surgery (see Interpretation of Coronary Angiograms). In others, bypass surgery is contraindicated by distal coronary disease or other medical illnesses. In the majority, however, the decision is not straightforward and must presently be individualized based on local expertise, details of coronary anatomy,[44] and the patient's expressed preference. For complex cases, a formal surgical consultation may be useful. This practice underscores the need for cardiovascular surgeons to be familiar with basic technical aspects of coronary angioplasty.

Case series suggest that multivessel PTCA can be performed successfully in over 85 per cent of patients[22,44] with an acceptable complication rate. Incomplete revascularization is common but is usually due to chronic occlusions subserving infarcted regions.[22] In addition, angioplasty avoids potential complica-

tions of anesthesia and cardiopulmonary bypass, can be repeated if necessary, and does not preclude subsequent bypass surgery if required. Several large randomized studies comparing PTCA with coronary artery bypass surgery in multivessel coronary artery disease are currently under way. One such study, the Bypass Angioplasty Revascularization Investigation (BARI) sponsored by the National Institutes of Health, is presently enrolling patients in 14 North American centers. Five-year end points will include mortality, myocardial infarction, residual ischemia, and quality of life.

In the setting of acute myocardial infarction, PTCA may be used *directly* as the primary reperfusion strategy, as an *adjunct* to successful thrombolytic therapy, or to *salvage* patency when thrombolytic therapy has failed. Direct angioplasty is at least as effective as thrombolysis in re-establishing vessel patency.[64,71] However, the resources required to treat myocardial infarction routinely using this approach are not widely available. In most centers, direct angioplasty is reserved for patients with acute myocardial infarction in whom a contraindication to thrombolysis exists, and for coronary thrombosis complicating cardiac catheterization. Anticipation that adjunctive angioplasty immediately following thrombolysis would improve outcome was not substantiated by randomized trials.[83,84] If thrombolytic therapy has successfully established reperfusion, a policy of deferred PTCA is currently favored. Since a reliable noninvasive marker of reperfusion is not presently available, routine identification of patients for salvage angioplasty requires 24-hour facilities for emergency coronary arteriography.

Mechanism of Angioplasty

Angioplasty reduces atherosclerotic stenosis by causing controlled injury of the plaque and adjacent arterial wall (Fig. 16). The hallmark of this injury is intimal plaque fracture and disruption (Fig. 17).[8] Stretching of elastic components in the media and adventitia also occurs and contributes to expansion of the artery. As the artery heals, a remodeling process involving dissolution of atheromatous material, retraction of the split plaque, and progressive dilation under physiologic pressure may further reduce the stenosis.[89]

Local endothelial denudation and exposure of plaque constituents create a powerful thrombogenic nidus. Despite antiplatelet and antithrombotic therapy, acute coronary thrombosis can occur. If gross disruption extends deeply into the media, coronary dissection may propagate, threatening patency of the true lumen.

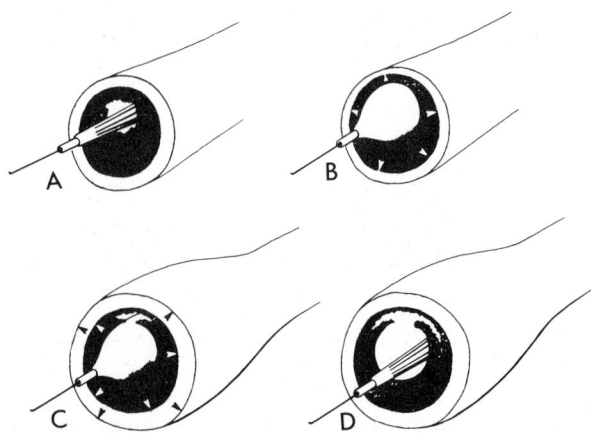

Figure 16. Changes in the arterial wall produced by a successful PTCA. The balloon catheter is positioned across the stenosis (A), and the balloon is inflated (B). The atherosclerotic plaque splits at its weakest point (C), and the media and adventitia of the artery are stretched to accommodate the expanded balloon. The balloon is then deflated and removed (D), leaving the plaque split and the media and adventitia expanded. The size of the arterial lumen is increased. (From Block, P. C.: Mechanism of transluminal angioplasty. Am. J. Cardiol., 53:69C, 1984.)

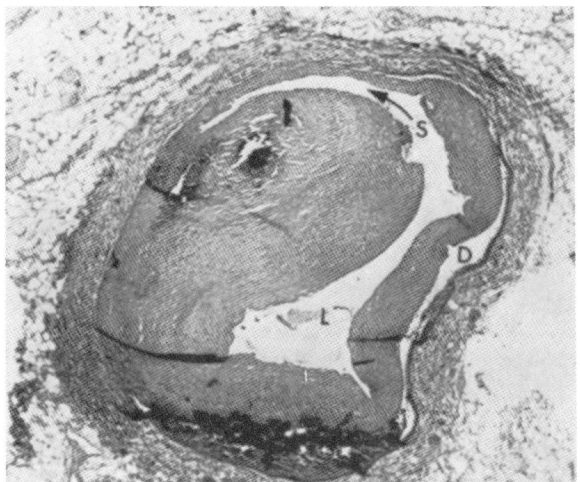

Figure 17. Section of left anterior descending artery at the site of angioplasty, revealing splitting (S, arrow), of the artherosclerotic plaque and a dissecting hematoma of the outer media (D). The split has enlarged the original lumen (L). (From Block, P. C., Myler, R. K., Stertzer, S., and Fallon, J. T.: Morphology after transluminal angioplasty in human beings. N. Engl. J. Med., *307*:382, 1981.)

Equipment

There are three major pieces of equipment that compose the angioplasty system; the balloon catheter itself, coronary guidewires, and guide catheters. Angioplasty catheters typically consist of a flexible double-lumen shaft fitted with an expandable balloon near its distal tip. Like other catheters, the central lumen allows insertion over a removable or integral guidewire. The second lumen permits inflation and deflation of the balloon by an external "indeflator." Angioplasty catheters are described by their *size* (nominal inflated balloon diameter), *profile* (deflated diameter), *pushability* (transmission of longitudinal force), and *trackability* (ability to advance freely around curves).

A major advance in guidewire design was the introduction of fine, 0.14 to 0.18 inch diameter steerable wires capable of transmitting rotation at their proximal end to their distal tip. When the tip is curved appropriately, the wire can be made to select specific branches as it is advanced through the coronary tree.

The other major component of angioplasty equipment is the guide catheter. These catheters are modified diagnostic coronary angiography catheters large enough to accommodate the angioplasty catheter and guidewire within their lumen. Their increased stiffness is used to support the angioplasty catheter as it is moved through tortuous vessels and across tight stenoses.

Procedure

Patient preparation is similar to that for diagnostic catheterization. Aspirin and a calcium entry blocker are administered before angioplasty for reduction of the risk of thrombosis, spasm, and acute closure at the site of dilation.[6] Because emergency operation may be required to manage complications of elective PTCA, consent for possible bypass surgery is often obtained, and patients receive nothing by mouth overnight. Guidelines for PTCA established by a joint task force of the American College of Cardiology and the American Heart Association state that "an experienced cardiovascular surgical team should be available within the institution for emergency surgery for all angioplasty procedures."[72] The former practice of maintaining a dedicated on-call surgical team and operating room, however, is neither practical nor necessary.

Femoral (or brachial) arterial access is secured with insertion of an 8-French or 9-French sheath. Insertion of a prophylactic temporary transvenous pacemaker is often recommended when right coronary or dominant left coronary dilation is planned. Intravenous heparin is administered to prevent the formation of thrombus at the site of dilation or on the guidewire

and catheters. Activated clotting time should be measured in the angioplasty laboratory to ensure adequate anticoagulation.

The guide catheter is positioned in the appropriate coronary ostium, and baseline coronary angiograms are obtained for balloon sizing and reference during the procedure. The prepared angioplasty catheter and guidewire are advanced via a Y coaxial connector to rest just proximal to the tip of the guide. The guidewire alone is then steered across the lesion and positioned with its tip in the distal coronary artery. The angioplasty catheter can then be advanced so that its balloon straddles the lesion.

Optimal durations and pressures of inflation are currently unknown, but dilations continuing 1 to 3 minutes at 6 to 10 atmospheres are typical. After several fully expanded inflations, the angioplasty catheter (but not the guidewire) is withdrawn. Repeat angiography is performed and compared with the baseline images. *Minimal* criteria for a satisfactory angiographic result are a 20 per cent change in luminal diameter narrowing such that the residual stenosis is less than 50 per cent.[72] When an acceptable result is obtained, the guidewire and guide catheter are removed. The arterial sheath is usually removed on the same day after normalization of the prothrombin time.

Results

Advances in technique and equipment have improved the procedural success of PTCA despite a concurrent increase in the difficulty of cases attempted. In a registry of cases performed during 1985 to 1986, 88 per cent of all lesions attempted were successfully dilated.[24] In-hospital mortality for this cohort was 1 per cent, and the nonfatal myocardial infarction rate was 4.3 per cent.

When PTCA is successful, a marked improvement in symptoms can be anticipated. Improvement in objective measures of myocardial ischemia,[57] systolic function,[50] and coronary reserve[65] usually accompanies symptomatic improvement. Long-term follow-up is now available for patients treated during the early days of the procedure. Of the 133 patients with initial procedural success, 67 per cent were asymptomatic 7 to 10 years later.[41]

Restenosis remains the primary limitation of PTCA, occurring in approximately one third of patients during the 6-month period after angioplasty.[42] Restenosis may be defined angiographically as loss of *half* the original improvement. The pathologic basis for this phenomenon is intimal proliferation of smooth muscle cells at the site of dilation.[4] Its exact pathogenesis, however, is uncertain.[55] Both mechanical and pharmacologic strategies for preventing restenosis have been proposed, but none are currently effective.[59] Repeat angioplasty appears to offer a safe and effective approach to management of recurrent angina due to restenosis.[87]

Spasm, thrombosis, and dissection lead to abrupt vessel closure in 4 per cent of patients undergoing PTCA.[14] This largely unpredictable event is the most common cause of death and myocardial infarction complicating the procedure. Failure of repeat dilations and intracoronary nitroglycerin to re-establish patency must prompt consideration of emergency bypass surgery. Factors favoring bypass surgery include proximal coronary occlusion, absence of collaterals, electrocardiographically extensive ischemia, and hemodynamic deterioration. Intracoronary reperfusion catheters have been demonstrated to reduce ischemia while the patient is being prepared for emergency bypass surgery.[45]

SELECTED REFERENCES

Freedom, R. M., Culham, J. A. G., and Moes, C. A. F.: Angiocardiography of Congenital Heart Disease. New York, Macmillan, 1984.
This extensively illustrated text covers angiographic diagnosis of congenital heart disease comprehensively on a lesion by lesion basis. An excellent discussion of radiologic, pathologic, and hemodynamic correlates is provided.

Grossman, W.: Cardiac Catheterization and Angiography, 3rd ed. Philadelphia, Lea & Febiger, 1986.
This standard reference text provides a thorough review of theoretic, technical, and clinical aspects of diagnostic cardiac catheterization. The third edition contains additional chapters concerning interventional catheter techniques.

Kutcher, M. A.: Evaluation of the coronary angiogram in the selection of patients for coronary angioplasty. *In* Hurst, J. W. (Ed.): Clinical Essays on the Heart. Vol. 3. New York, McGraw-Hill, 1985.
A clear discussion of the various views used for coronary arteriography is presented, with emphasis on axial compound views. The insights into interpretation of coronary angiography are equally valuable for cardiac surgeons.

Ryan, T. J., et al.: Guidelines for percutaneous transluminal coronary angioplasty. Circulation, 78:486, 1988.
This position paper provides a well-referenced overview of the results of coronary angioplasty. Morphologic features of coronary lesions that predict outcome with PTCA are reviewed.

Topol, E. J. (Ed.): Textbook of Interventional Cardiology. Philadelphia, W. B. Saunders Company, 1990.
A comprehensive textbook of modern adult interventional cardiology with contributions from many leaders in the field. Important specific issues such as multivessel PTCA, chronic total occlusions, PTCA of coronary grafts, supported angioplasty, and restenosis are assigned individual, well-referenced chapters. In addition, emerging technologies including atherectomy, stents, laser, and thermal angioplasty are covered in detail. Six chapters covering applications of balloon valvuloplasty are included.

REFERENCES

1. Ambrose, J. A., Winters, S. L., Arora, R. R., Haft, J. I., Goldstein, J., Rentrop, K. P., Gorlin, R., and Fuster, V.: Coronary angiographic morphology in myocardial infarction: A link between the pathogenesis of unstable angina and myocardial infarction. J. Am. Coll. Cardiol., 6:1233, 1985.
2. Ambrose, J. A., Winters, S. L., Stern, A., Eng, A., Teichholz, L. E., Gorlin, R., and Fuster, V.: Angiographic morphology and the pathogenesis of unstable angina. J. Am. Coll. Cardiol., 5:609, 1985.
3. Arnett, E. N., Isner, J. M., Redwood, D. R., Kent, K. M., Baker, W. P., Ackerstein, H., and Roberts, W. C.: Coronary artery narrowing in coronary heart disease. Comparison of cineangiographic and necropsy findings. Ann. Intern. Med., 91:350, 1979.
4. Austin, G. E., Ratliff, N. B., Hollman, J., Tabei, S., and Phillips, D. F.: Intimal proliferation of smooth muscle cells as an explanation for recurrent coronary artery stenosis after percutaneous transluminal coronary angioplasty. J. Am. Coll. Cardiol., 6:369, 1985.
5. Banka, V. S., Bodenheimer, M. M., Shah, R., and Helfant, R. H.: Intervention ventriculography: Comparative value of nitroglycerin, post-extrasystolic potentiation, and nitroglycerin plus post-extrasystolic potentiation. Circulation, 53:632, 1976.
6. Barnathan, E. S., Schwartz, J. S., Taylor, L., Laskey, W. K., Kleaveland, J. P., Kussmaul, W. G., and Hirshfeld, J. W.: Aspirin and dipyridamole in the prevention of acute coronary thrombosis complicating coronary angioplasty. Circulation, 76:125, 1987.
7. Baron, M. G.: The angiocardiographic diagnosis of valvular stenosis. Circulation, 44:143, 1971.
8. Block, P. C., Myler, R. K., Stertzer, S., and Fallon, J. T.: Morphology after transluminal angioplasty in human beings. N. Engl. J. Med., 305:382, 1981.
9. Block, P. C., Ockene, I., Goldberg, R. J., Butterly, J., Block, E. H., Degon, C., Beiser, A., and Colton, T.: A randomized trial of outpatient versus inpatient cardiac catheterization. N. Engl. J. Med., 319:1251, 1988.
10. Bourassa, M. G., and Noble, J.: Complication rate of coronary arteriography. Circulation, 53:106, 1976.
11. Bourassa, M. G., et al.: Report of the joint ISFC/WHO task force on Coronary Angioplasty. Circulation, 78:780, 1988.
12. Braunwald, E.: Valvular heart disease. *In* Braunwald, E. (Ed.): Heart Disease, A textbook of Cardiovascular Medicine, 3rd ed. Philadelphia, W. B. Saunders Company, 1988.
13. Braunwald, E., Sonnenblick, E. H., Frommer, P. L., and Ross, J., Jr.: Paired electric stimulation of the heart: Physiologic observations and clinical implications. Adv. Intern. Med., 13:61, 1967.
14. Bredlau, C. E., Roubin, G., Leimgruber, P., Douglas, J., King, S., and Grüntzig, A.: In-hospital morbidity and mortality in patients undergoing elective coronary angioplasty. Circulation, 72:1044, 1985.
15. Bresnahan, D. R., Davis, J. L., Holmes, D. R., and Smith, H. C.: Angiographic occurrence and clinical correlates of intraluminal coronary artery thrombus: Role of unstable angina. J. Am. Coll. Cardiol., 6:285, 1985.
16. Brown, B. G., Bolson, E. L., and Dodge, H. T.: Arteriographic assessment of coronary atherosclerosis. Review of current methods, their limitations, and clinical applications. Arteriosclerosis, 2:2, 1982.
17. Bush, C. A., Stang, J. M., Wooley, C. G., and Kilman, J.: Occult constrictive pericardial disease. Diagnosis by rapid volume expansion and correction by pericardiectomy. Circulation, 56:924, 1977.
18. Califf, R. M., Phillips, H. R., II, Hindman, M. C., Mark, D. B., Lee, K. L., Behar, V. S., Johnson, R. A., Pryor, D. B., Rosati, R. A., Wagner, G. S., and Harrell, F. E., Jr.: Prognostic value of a coronary artery jeopardy score. J. Am. Coll. Cardiol., 5:1055, 1985.
19. Criley, J. M., and French, W. J.: Cardiac catheterization in adults with congenital heart disease. Cardiovasc. Clin., 10:196, 1979.
20. Currie, P. J., Seward, J. B., Reeder, G. S., Vliestra, R. E., Bresnahan, D. R., Bresnahan, J. F., Smith, H. C., Hagler, D. J., and Tajik, A. J.: Continuous-wave Doppler echocardiographic assessment of severity of calcific aortic stenosis: A simultaneous Doppler-catheterization correlative study in 100 adult patients. Circulation, 71:1162, 1985.
21. Dehmer, G. J., Firht, B. G., and Hillis, L. D.: Oxygen consumption in adult patients during cardiac catheterization. Clin. Cardiol., 5:436, 1982.
22. Delignoal, U., Vandormael, M. G., Kern, M. J., Zelman, R., Galan, K., and Chaitman, B. R.: Coronary angioplasty: A therapeutic option for symptomatic patients with two and three vessel coronary disease. J. Am. Coll. Cardiol., 11:1173, 1988.
23. Demany, M. A., Kay, E. B., and Zimmerman, H. A.: An angiocardiographic sign for the evaluation of the stenotic mitral valve. Am. J. Cardiol., 18:843, 1966.
24. Detre, K., Holubkov, R., Kelsey, S., Cowley, M., Kent, K., Williams, D., Myler, R., Faxon, D., Holmes, D., Bourassa, R., Block, P., Gosselin, A., Bentivoglio, L., Leatherman, L., Dorros, G., King, S., Galichia, J., Al-Bassam, M., Leon, M., Robertson, T., and Passamani, E.: Percutaneous transluminal coronary angioplasty in 1985–1986 and 1977–1981. N. Engl. J. Med., 318:265, 1988.
25. Dodge, H. T., Sandler, H., Ballew, D. W., and Lord, J. D., Jr.: The use of biplane angiocardiography for the measurement of left ventricular volumes in man. Am. Heart J., 60:762, 1960.
26. European Coronary Surgery Study Group: Long-term results of a prospective randomized study of coronary artery bypass surgery in stable angina pectoris. Lancet, 2:1173, 1982.
27. Fifer, M. A., and Grossman, W.: Measurement of ventricular volumes, ejection fraction, mass, and wall stress. *In* Grossman, W. (Ed.): Cardiac Catheterization and Angiography, 3rd ed. Philadelphia, Lea & Febiger, 1986.
28. Freedom, R. M., and Olley, P. M.: Pulmonary arteriography in congenital heart disease. Cathet. Cardiovasc. Diagn., 2:309, 1976.
29. Freedom, R. M., Culham, J. A. G., and Moes, C. A. F.: Angiocardiography of congenital heart disease. New York, Macmillan, 1984.
30. Friesinger, G. C., Adams, D. F., Bourassa, M. G., Carlsson, E., Elliot, L. P., Gessner, I. H., Greenspan, R. H., Grossman, W., Judkins, M. P., Kennedy, J. W., and Sheldon, W. C.: Optimal resources for the evaluation of the heart and lungs: Cardiac catheterization and angiographic facilities. Circulation, 68:893A, 1983.
31. Ganz, W., Donoso, R., Marcus, H. S., Forrester, J. S., and Swan, H. J. C.: A new technique for measurements of cardiac output by thermodilution in man. Am. J. Cardiol., 27:392, 1971.
32. Gentzler, R. D., Briselli, M. F., and Gault, J. H.: Angiographic estimation of right ventricular volume in man. Circulation, 50:324, 1974.
33. Glancy, D. L., Shephard, R. L., Beiser, G. D., and Epstein, S. E.: The dynamic nature of left ventricular outflow obstruction in idiopathic hypertrophic subaortic stenosis. Ann. Intern. Med., 75:589, 1971.
34. Gould, K. L.: Identifying and measuring severity of coronary artery stenosis. Circulation, 78:237, 1988.
35. Graham, T. P., Jr., Jarmakani, J. M., Atwood, G. F., and Canent, R. V., Jr.: Right ventricular volume determination in children. Normal values and observations with pressure or volume overload. Circulation, 47:144, 1973.
36. Greenberger, P. A.: Contrast media reactions. J. Allergy Clin. Immunol., 74:600, 1984.
37. Greenberger, P. A., and Patterson, R.: Adverse reactions to contrast media. Prog. Cardiovasc. Dis., 31:239, 1988.
38. Grossman, W.: Catheter passage across prosthetic valves. *In* Grossman, W. (Ed.): Cardiac Catheterization and Angiography, 3rd ed. Philadelphia, Lea & Febiger, 1986.
39. Grossman, W., and Barry, W. H.: Cardiac catheterization. *In* Braunwald, E. (Ed.): Heart Disease, A Textbook of Cardiovascular Medicine, 3rd ed. Philadelphia, W. B. Saunders, 1988.
40. Grüntzig, A. R., Senning, A., and Siegenthaler, W. E.: Nonoperative dilatation of coronary artery stenosis. Percutaneous transluminal coronary angioplasty. N. Engl. J. Med., 301:61, 1979.
41. Grüntzig, A. R., King, S. B., Schlumpf, M., and Siegenthaler, W.: Long-term follow-up after percutaneous transluminal coronary angioplasty. The early Zurich experience. N. Engl. J. Med., 316:1127, 1987.
42. Guiteras, V. P., Bourassa, M. G., and David, P. R.: Restenosis after successful percutaneous transluminal coronary angioplasty: The Montreal Heart Institute experience. Am. J. Cardiol., 60(Suppl.):50B, 1987.
43. Hagen, P. T., Scholz, D. G., and Edwards, W. D.: Incidence and size of patent foramen ovale during the first ten decades of life: An autopsy study of 965 normal hearts. Mayo Clin. Proc., 59:17, 1984.
44. Hartzler, G. O.: Coronary angioplasty is the treatment of choice for multivessel coronary artery disease. Chest, 90:877, 1986.
45. Hinohara, T., Simpson, J. B., Phillips, H. R., and Stack, R. S.: Transluminal intracoronary reperfusion catheter: A device to maintain coronary perfusion between failed angioplasty and emergency coronary bypass surgery. J. Am. Coll. Cardiol., 11:977, 1988.
46. Hoff, H. E., and Scott, H. J.: Physiology (continued). N. Engl. J. Med., 239:120, 1948.
47. Isner, J. M., Kishel, J., Kent, K. M., Ronan, J. A., Ross, A. M., and Roberts, W. C.: Accuracy of angiographic determination of left main coronary artery narrowing. Circulation, 63:1056, 1981.

48. Kelley, M. J., Higgins, C. B., and Kirkpatrick, S. E.: Axial left ventriculography in discrete subaortic stenosis. Radiology, 135:77, 1980.

49. Kennedy, J. W.: Complications associated with cardiac catheterization and angiography. Cathet. Cardiovasc. Diagn., 8:5, 1982.

50. Kent, K. M., Bonow, R. O., Rosing, D. R., Ewels, C. J., Lipson, L. C., MacIntosh, C. L., and Bacharach, S. L.: Improved myocardial function during exercise in patients following percutaneous transluminal coronary angioplasty. N. Engl. J. Med., 306:441, 1982.

51. Kinsman, J. M., Moore, J. W., and Hamilton, W. F.: Studies on the circulation. I. Injection method. Physical and mathematical considerations. Am. J. Physiol., 89:322, 1929.

52. Lesperance, J., Bourassa, M. G., Biron, P., Campeau, L., and Saltiel, J.: Aorta to coronary artery saphenous vein grafts. Preoperative angiographic criteria for successful surgery. Am. J. Cardiol., 30:459, 1972.

53. Levin, D. C.: Pathways and functional significance of the coronary collateral circulation. Circulation, 50:831, 1974.

54. Levin, D. C., Harrington, D. P., Bettman, M. A., Garnic, J. D., Davidoff, A., and Lois, J.: Anatomic variations of the coronary arteries supplying the anterolateral aspect of the left ventricle. Possible explanation for the "unexplained" anterior aneurysm. Invest. Radiol., 17:458, 1982.

55. Liu, M. W., Roubin, G. S., and King, S. B.: Restenosis after coronary angioplasty. Potential biologic determinants and role of intimal hyperplasia. Circulation, 79:1374, 1989.

56. Mann, T., McLaurin, L., Grossman, W., and Craige, E.: Acute aortic regurgitation due to infective endocarditis. N. Engl. J. Med., 293:108, 1975.

57. Manyari, D. E., Knudston, M., Kloiber, R., and Roth, D.: Sequential thallium-201 perfusion studies after successful percutaneous transluminal coronary angioplasty: Delayed resolution of exercise induced scintigraphic abnormalities. Circulation, 77:86, 1988.

58. Marco, R., and Paulin, S.: Angiography; principles underlying proper utilization of radiologic and cineangiographic equipment. In Grossman, W. (Ed.): Cardiac Catheterization and Angiography, 3rd ed. Philadelphia, Lea & Febiger, 1986.

59. Mcbride, W., Lange, R. A., and Hillis, L. D.: Restenosis after successful coronary angioplasty. Pathophysiology and prevention. N. Engl. J. Med., 318:1734, 1988.

60. Mehmel, H. C., et al.: The linearity of the end-systolic pressure volume relationship in man and its sensitivity for assessment of left ventricular function. Circulation, 63:1216, 1981.

61. Metabolic Rate Meter, Waters Instruments, Rochester, Minnesota.

62. Murphy, M. L., Hultgren, H. N., Detre, K., Thompson, J., Takaro, T., and participants of the VA cooperative study: Treatment of chronic stable angina: A preliminary report of survival data of the Randomized Veterans Administration Cooperative Study. N. Engl. J. Med., 297:621, 1977.

63. Nixon, P. G. F., and Wooler, G. H.: Left ventricular filling pressure gradient in mitral incompetence. Br. Heart J., 25:382, 1963.

64. O'Neill, W., Timmis, G. C., Bourdillon, P. D., Lai, P., Ganghadarhan, V., Walton, J., Jr., Ramos, R., Laufer, N., Gordon, S., Schork, A., and Pitt, B.: A prospective randomized trial of intracoronary streptokinase versus coronary angioplasty for acute myocardial infarction. N. Engl. J. Med., 314:812, 1986.

65. O'Neill, W. W., Walton, J. A., Bates, E. R., Colfer, H. T., Aueron, F. M., LeFree, M. T., Pitt, B., and Vogel, R. A.: Criteria for successful coronary angioplasty as assessed by alterations in coronary vasodilatory reserve. J. Am. Coll. Cardiol., 3:1382, 1984.

66. Passamani, E., Davis, K. B., Gillespie, M. J., Killip, T., and the CASS principal investigators and their associates: A randomized trial of coronary artery bypass surgery: Survival of patients with a low ejection fraction. N. Engl. J. Med., 312:1665, 1985.

67. Perlmutt, L. M., Jay, M. E., and Levin, D. C.: Variations in the blood supply of the left ventricular apex. Invest. Radiol., 18:138, 1983.

68. Rabinovitch, M., Keane, J. F., Fellows, K. E., Castaneda, A. R., and Reid, L.: Quantitative analysis of the pulmonary wedge angiogram in congenital heart defects. Circulation, 63:152, 1981.

69. Rees, J. R., Epstein, E. J., Criley, J. M., and Ross, R. S.: Hemodynamic effects of severe aortic regurgitation. Br. Heart J., 26:412, 1964.

70. Rich, S., Martinez, J., Lam, W., Levy, P. S., and Rosen, K. M.: Reassessment of the effects of vasodilator drugs in primary pulmonary hypertension. Guidelines for determining a pulmonary vasodilator response. Am. Heart J., 105:119, 1983.

71. Rothbaum, D. A., Linnemeier, T. J., Landin, R. J., Steinmetz, E. F., Hillis, J. S., Hallam, C. C., Noble, R. J., and See, M. R.: Emergency percutaneous transluminal angioplasty in acute myocardial infarction: A 3 year experience. J. Am. Coll. Cardiol., 10:264, 1987.

72. Ryan, T. J., Faxon, D. P., Gunnar, R. M., Kennedy, J. W., King, S. B., Loop, F. D., Peterson, K. L., Reeves, T. J., Williams, D. O., and Williams, W. L.: Guidelines for percutaneous transluminal coronary angioplasty. Circulation, 78:486, 1988.

73. Saksena, F. B.: Hemodynamics in Cardiology: Calculations and Interpretations. New York, Praeger Publishers, 1983.

74. Salem, D. N., Konstam, M. A., Isner, J. M., and Bonia, J. D.: Comparison of the electrocardiographic and hemodynamic responses to ionic and non-ionic radiocontrast media during left ventriculography: A randomized double blind study. Am. Heart J., 111:533, 1986.

75. Shipley, R. E., and Gregg, D. E.: The effect of external constriction of a blood vessel on blood flow. Am. J. Physiol., 141:289, 1944.

76. Schwab, S. J., Hlatky, M. A., Pieper, K. S., et al.: Contrast nephrotoxicity: Non-ionic versus ionic agents. A randomized prospective trial. N. Engl. J. Med., 320:149, 1989.

77. Simon, A. L.: Angiographic diagnosis of idiopathic hypertrophic subaortic stenosis. Radiol. Clin. North Am., 6:423, 1968.

78. Soto, B., Coghlan, C. H., and Bargeron, L. M.: Present status of axially angled angiocardiography. Cardiovasc. Intervent. Radiol., 7:156, 1984.

79. Stack, R. S., Califf, R. M., Hinohara, T., Phillips, H. R., Pryor, D. B., Simonton, C. A., Carlson, E. B., Morris, K. G., Behar, V. S., Kong, Y., Peter, R. H., Hlatky, M. A., O'Connor, C. M., and Mark, D. B.: Survival and cardiac event rates in the first year after emergency coronary angioplasty for acute myocardial infarction. J. Am. Coll. Cardiol., 11:1141, 1988.

80. Steckelberg, J. M., Vleistra, R. E., Ludwig, J., and Mann, R. J.: Werner Forssmann (1904–1979) and his unusual success story. Mayo Clin. Proc., 54:746, 1979.

81. Stewart, G. N.: Researches on the circulation time and on the influences which affect it. IV. The output of the heart. J. Physiol., 22:159, 1987.

82. Takaro, T., Peduzzi, P., Detre, K. M., Hultgren, H. M., Murphy, M. L., Van der Belh-Khan, J., Thomsen, J., and Meadows, W. R.: Survival in subgroups of patients with left main coronary artery disease. Veterans Administration Cooperative Study for Coronary Arterial Occlusive Disease. Circulation, 66:14, 1982.

83. The TIMI Research Group: Immediate vs. delayed catheterization and angioplasty following thrombolytic therapy for acute myocardial infarction; TIMI IIA results. J.A.M.A., 260:2849, 1988.

84. Topol, E. J., Califf, R. M., George, B. S., Kereiakes, D. J., Abbottsmith, C. W., Candela, R. J., Lee, K. L., Pitt, B., Stack, R. S., and O'Neill, W. W.: A randomized trial of immediate versus delayed elective angioplasty after intravenous tissue plasminogen activator in acute myocardial infarction. N. Engl. J. Med., 317:581, 1987.

85. Varnauskas, E., and the European Coronary Surgery Study Group: Twelve year follow-up of survival in the randomized European Coronary Surgery Study. N. Engl. J. Med., 319:332, 1988.

86. White, C. W., Creighton, B. W., Doty, D. B., Hiratza, L. F., Eastman, C. L., Harrison, D. G., and Marcus, M. L.: Does visual interpretation of the coronary arteriogram predict the physiologic significance of a coronary stenosis? N. Engl. J. Med., 310:819, 1984.

87. Williams, D. O., Gruñtzig, A. R., Kent, K. M., Detre, K. M., Kelsey, S. F., and To, T.: Efficacy of repeat percutaneous transluminal coronary angioplasty for coronary restenosis. Am. J. Cardiol., 53:32C, 1984.

88. Yang, S. S., Bentivoglio, L. G., Maranhao, V., and Goldberg, H.: From Cardiac Catheterization to Hemodynamic Parameters, 2nd ed. Philadelphia, F. A. Davis Company, 1978.

89. Zarins, C. K., Lu, C. T., Gewertz, B. L., Lyon, R. T., Rush, D. S., and Glagov, S.: Arterial disruption and remodeling following balloon dilatation. Surgery, 92:1086, 1982.

90. Zir, L. M., Miller, S. W., Dinsmore, R. E., Gilbert, J. P., and Harthorne, J. W.: Interobserver variability in coronary angiography. Circulation, 53:627, 1976.

II

CARDIOPULMONARY RESUSCITATION

J. Scott Rankin, M.D.

Sudden cardiac death can be defined as an unexpected circulatory arrest from cardiac causes preceded by no apparent symptoms or with symptoms of less than 1 hour in duration.[19,29] In the United States alone, approximately 400,000 sudden deaths occur each year, and the absolute incidence has been rising. An estimated 80 per cent are due to atherosclerotic coronary artery disease, representing the majority of deaths in that disorder. It is interesting that sudden death occurs as the *initial* clinical presentation in 20 to 25 per cent of individuals with symptomatic coronary atherosclerosis. As with most other manifestations of coronary disease, males predominate, and the average age is in excess of 60 years. The majority of episodes occur outside of the hospital during normal daily activity and usually without acute antecedent symptoms. Given the aging of the population of the United States and the projected increase in absolute prevalence of coronary atherosclerosis, this conspicuous problem is likely to become even more important in future clinical practice. Based on experiences in coronary care units and supervised exercise programs, it is likely that a majority of sudden death victims could be salvaged by immediate cardiopulmonary resuscitation (CPR) and defibrillation at the scene of the arrest. Thus, it is essential that a large portion of the public be trained to initiate CPR immediately and that paramedical teams be organized to respond with a defibrillator within 3 minutes.[7,8] With this type of system, over 40 per cent of out-of-hospital arrest victims with documented ventricular fibrillation can be resuscitated, and it is estimated that 100,000 lives could be saved annually by providing effective on-site CPR.[10,15]

HISTORICAL DEVELOPMENT

Attempted resuscitation of the dead has been described in various forms since antiquity.[13] Biblical references to ancient Hebrew practices exist in the book of Kings,[36] and at the peak of the Roman Empire, Galen employed bellows to inflate the lungs of dead animals.[13] During the eighteenth century, methods for performing mouth-to-mouth ventilation were standardized, and in 1786, Sherwin suggested that "the surgeon should go on inflating the lungs and alternately compressing the sternum."[24] Koenig, professor of surgery at Göttingen, Germany, is credited as the father of external cardiac compression and reported in 1885 six successful resuscitations in man.[22] Further application of the closed-chest method was reported by Maas in 1892,[23] and Igelsrud successfully employed open-chest direct cardiac massage in 1901.[24] For the next 60 years, open-chest cardiac massage became standard practice. Crile[11] studied adrenaline injections in the treatment of cardiac arrest induced by chloroform anesthesia and later applied this method to the resuscitation of battle casualties in World War I.

Wiggers investigated the physiology of ventricular fibrillation in the 1930s and 1940s, developing experimental methods of electrical defibrillation in the dog.[39] In 1947, Claude Beck, a student of Wiggers and a pioneering thoracic surgeon at Case Western Reserve University, reported the first successful internal electrical defibrillation in man,[3] which was followed by the development of external cardioversion by Zoll in 1956.[42] While studying external electrical defibrillation of the heart in the surgical laboratories of Blalock in 1960, Kouwenhoven, Jude, and Knickerbocker rediscovered that an arterial pressure pulse could be generated by external chest compression.[22,23,28] These investigations soon combined external cardiac massage, mechanical ventilation, and electrical defibrillation to initiate the modern era of CPR. After positive experiences with early clinical trials, the American Heart Association in 1963 formed the Committee on Cardiopulmonary Resuscitation, which published guidelines for CPR in 1974, 1980, and 1986. These reports provided a standardized approach to CPR and stressed the importance of extensive training at the community level.[1,33]

ETIOLOGY

The most common cause of sudden cardiac arrest is ventricular fibrillation associated with ischemic heart disease.[8] Fibrillation may follow acute cardiac decompensation during myocardial infarction or may be a primary electrical event coincident with coronary thrombosis or transient coronary insufficiency. Asystole, profound bradycardia, and complete heart block are other dysrhythmias that can cause circulatory arrest and require specific therapy for the underlying disorder in addition to normal resuscitative measures. Recurrent ventricular tachycardia represents a very small proportion of the overall cardiac arrest population but necessitates referral to a tertiary care center that is equipped for electrophysiologic studies.

Another common etiologic factor of sudden cardiac arrest is inadequate ventilation or pulmonary gas exchange. The resultant hypoxia, hypercarbia, and systemic acidosis produce acute circulatory decompensation and ventricular fibrillation. Many such conditions are encountered in daily practice, such as suffocation, drowning, drug overdosage, foreign body aspiration, electrocution, or hypoventilation from primary pulmonary or neurologic disease. Early recognition of pulmonary insufficiency in hospitalized patients is essential so that ventilatory support can be provided before the development of cardiac arrest. With adequate intensive care monitoring of (1) ventilatory patterns, (2) work of breathing, (3) mental alertness, (4) arterial blood gases, and (5) capillary pulse oxymetry, respiratory support should be initiated before cardiac decompensation occurs. In the case of foreign body aspiration, a high index of suspicion and early diagnosis can effect dislodgment of the obstruction by one of several methods.[1]

The final general causes of cardiopulmonary arrest are metabolic disorders. Hyperkalemia causing ventricular fibrillation or asystole is associated with a very low rate of recovery and is best treated by prevention. Whenever the serum potassium approaches 6.0 mg. per 100 ml. or the rate of increase in serum potassium is rapid, aggressive therapy with intravenous glucose (25 gm.) and insulin (20 units) or sodium bicarbonate (44 mEq.) is indicated. At that point, the situation can be assessed further, the cause corrected, and ion exchange resin therapy (Kayexalate) or dialysis initiated. Other metabolic disturbances such as hypocalcemia or metabolic acidosis are more rarely associated

Supported by NIH Grants HL-09315, HL-29536, HL-17670.

with cardiac arrest but also should be treated at an early stage before circulatory standstill.

Independent of the causative factor, cardiopulmonary arrest is manifested by ineffective cardiac output and arterial blood pressure. Cessation of oxygenated blood flow to the body is associated with rapid progression of tissue hypoxia and acidosis. Because of high metabolic demands, the central nervous system is most vulnerable and can tolerate no more than 5 to 7 minutes of normothermic ischemia in adults before permanent neurologic injury ensues. After longer arrest periods, successful resuscitation may produce recovery of other organs, but return of central nervous system function is unlikely. Thus, one important goal of initial cardiopulmonary resuscitation is preservation of neurologic integrity until cardiac function can be restored.

DIAGNOSIS

The diagnosis of cardiac arrest should be considered whenever a previously alert individual collapses or appears to lose consciousness. The first step in approaching the patient is direct questioning and documentation of total loss of consciousness. Complete arrest also may be accompanied by initial tonic muscular movements and rolling back of the eyes. After transient agonal respiratory motion, spontaneous breathing ceases if the sequence progresses untreated. In a mechanically ventilated patient, thoracic motion and breath sounds obviously persist after cardiac arrest, and respiratory movements are of little value. If a question exists of ventilator malfunction, the patient should be removed from the ventilator and manually ventilated with 100 per cent oxygen.

The presumptive diagnosis of cardiac arrest is made whenever a previously palpable central arterial pulse is lost. Palpation of either the carotid or femoral artery is adequate for establishing the diagnosis, and in monitored patients, loss of the electrocardiogram or arterial pressure waveform is confirmatory. Occasionally, patients continue to have a normal-appearing electrocardiogram, even though the pulse is absent and systolic blood pressure diminished. In this event, resuscitation should be initiated because of ineffective circulatory performance. On more than one occasion, however, resuscitation has been instituted because electrocardiographic leads became disconnected or for other erroneous reasons. Inappropriate resuscitation should be avoided whenever possible by approaching each patient slowly and thoughtfully. A 15-second period of careful diagnostic attention is prudent, including the documentation of absent pulses. In emergency situations, the tendency often is to proceed with haste; however, a short evaluation does not delay therapy significantly, and the potentially harmful complications of an unnecessary resuscitation can be avoided. This concept is especially important in postoperative cardiac surgical patients in whom chest compression can produce sternal disruption, suture line hemorrhage, or perforation of the ventricles by artificial valves. Conversely, if a firm indication of arrested circulation exists, resuscitation should be initiated while further evaluation is pursued. Coincidentally, a call for help is issued, since effective CPR requires the coordinated efforts of multiple individuals.

RESUSCITATION METHODS

As defined by the subcommittee on Emergency Cardiac Care of the American Heart Association,[1,33] cardiopulmonary resuscitation can be divided into two phases: (1) Basic Life Support, and (2) Advanced Cardiac Life Support. During in-hospital resuscitation, basic and advanced techniques are not distinct but proceed simultaneously. For the sake of clarity, however, each is discussed individually as if utilized sequentially.

BASIC LIFE SUPPORT

Ventilation

After the diagnosis of cardiac arrest has been made, initial efforts are directed toward maintaining cardiopulmonary function and flow of oxygenated blood to the body. If evidence exists of isolated airway obstruction, such as produced by laryngeal meat impaction, a combination of back blows and abdominal thrusts frequently can dislodge the impaction. Otherwise, the patient is placed supine in a hospital bed or on the ground. With a complete cardiopulmonary arrest, the mouth is opened and inspected; foreign objects such as dentures or chewing gum are removed. An airway is established by extending the neck and tilting the victim's head backward. If difficulty is encountered in opening the airway, the jaw can be extended by applying forward pressure behind the mandibular angles. Ventilation is begun with a valved mask system, with care to maintain an airtight seal around the face. If a mask is unavailable, mouth-to-mouth breathing is employed while the patient's nostrils are occluded with one hand. With either technique, respirations should be delivered at 12 to 15 breaths per minute.

Ventilatory pressure should be sufficiently great to raise the chest and produce satisfactory breath sounds, but not forceful enough to distend the stomach. Gastric dilation can produce vomiting, aspiration, and long-term pulmonary complications. It should be emphasized that mask ventilation is *entirely satisfactory* in most cases, and intubation should not be attempted until satisfactory mask ventilation first has been established and until trained personnel are available. Unsuccessful attempts at endotracheal intubation can diminish the likelihood of resuscitation or directly injure the patient by lacerating the pharynx or vocal cords.

Endotracheal intubation in a semiconscious patient usually is performed nasally, and this method is preferred if ventilatory efforts are still present. In an arrest victim, intubation is accomplished orally with the aid of a laryngoscope.[9] The blade of the laryngoscope is inserted into the mouth and upper pharynx while the instrument is held delicately (Fig. 1A). By use of steady forward pressure, the blade is advanced in the midline until the epiglottis comes into view (Fig. 1B). At that point, the laryngoscope is passed further until the tip lies behind the epiglottis, and the entire tongue and mandible are elevated by a gentle upward and forward movement of the laryngoscope (Fig. 1C). Excessive force or a prying motion should never be necessary, and with proper technique, the glottis and vocal cords should

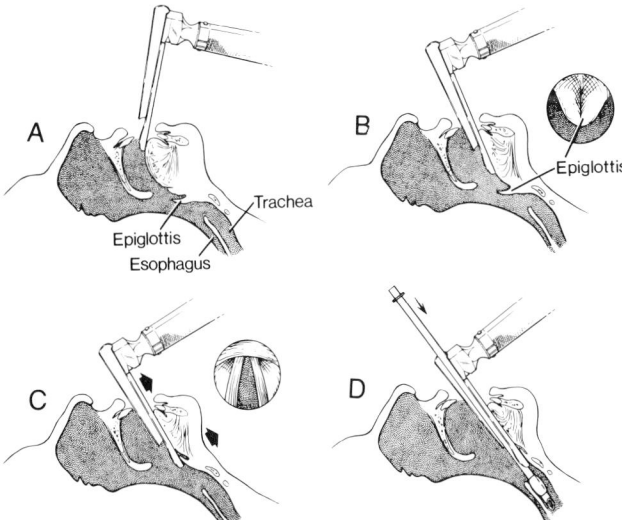

Figure 1. The standard technique of laryngoscopic endotracheal intubation. *A,* The laryngoscope is inserted into the mouth. *B* and *C,* The blade is advanced to expose the epiglottis and vocal cords. *D,* The trachea is intubated.

come clearly into view just beyond the tip of the blade. It is often helpful to have a suction catheter available for clearing secretions. With the balloon cuff deflated, the endotracheal tube is passed precisely through the vocal cords into the upper trachea (Fig. 1D). Care is taken to advance the tube only 5 to 6 cm. beyond the vocal cords so that the right main stem bronchus is not intubated. The cuffed endotracheal balloon is inflated until an airtight seal with the trachea is obtained, the chest is auscultated for the presence of bilateral breath sounds, and the patient is ventilated manually throughout the resuscitation with 100 per cent oxygen at 12 breaths per minute. Mechanical ventilatory support with a respirator is initiated only after restoration of stable cardiovascular performance.

Circulation

Before chest compression is begun in a patient with documented cardiac arrest, a precordial thump is delivered in an effort to restore cardiac rhythm. If the thump is unsuccessful, circulatory support is initiated with external cardiac massage. The patient is placed supine in the horizontal position, and a board or other rigid surface is interposed behind the back to provide support. The heel of one hand is placed over the other, and force is applied rhythmically over the lower half of the sternum (Fig. 2). The resuscitator's arms are locked to transmit the full momentum of the upper body to the patient's chest.

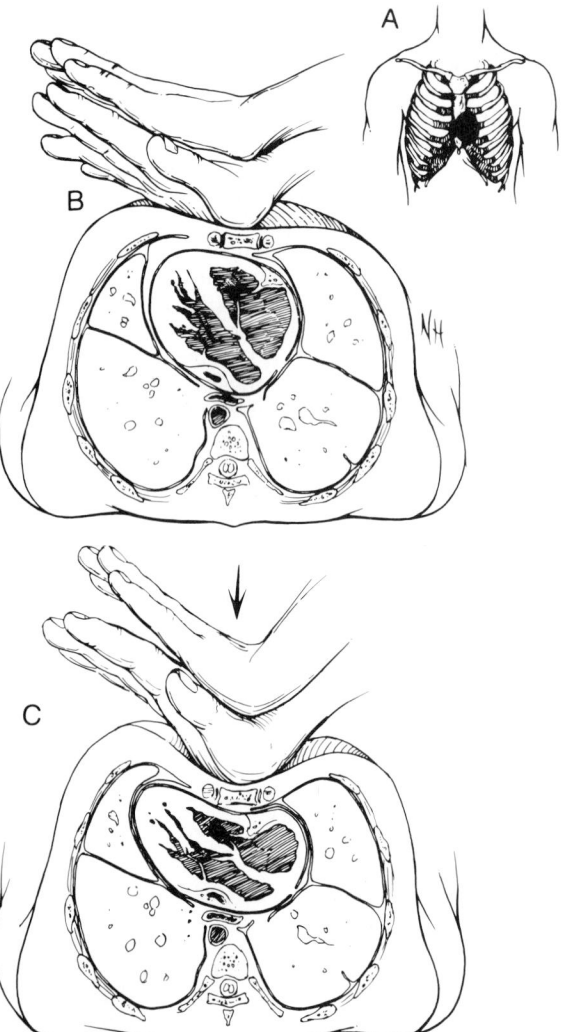

Figure 2. Manual compression is performed over the lower sternum (A). The position of the hands on the sternum is shown in B. External cardiac massage is performed with high-velocity compressions of moderate force and brief duration (C).

Several important studies over the past decade have clarified the physiology of circulatory support during CPR. It is now clear the *effective* external cardiac massage transmits pressure and flow energy to the cardiovascular system by a *direct cardiac compression* mechanism. The pressure-flow product (stroke work or circulatory energy) is generated through force and displacement of the chest wall, which then compresses the ventricular chambers, closes the mitral valve, opens the aortic valve, and produces unidirectional arterial pressure and flow. Thus, the heart acts as a valved pump that transmits the energy of chest wall compression to the cardiovascular system.

For illustration of the physiology of external chest compression, measurements of ventricular dimensions, aortic blood flow, and cardiac chamber pressures from an anesthetized dog are shown in Figure 3 in the control state (left panel) and during manual external chest compression with an arrested circulation (right panel). Several important observations can be made.[30,31] First, a flattening of ventricular shape is observed with external massage, consistent with direct ventricular chamber compression. Second, peak aortic flow velocity and stroke volume are reduced significantly during CPR, compared with control; however, a finite stroke volume occurs during compression similar to normal physiology and consistent with a cardiac pump mechanism. Third, peak ventricular and aortic pressures approach normal values with external compression, but diastolic and mean aortic perfusion pressures remain low because of reduced cardiac output. Intrathoracic pressure is less than 25 per cent of cavitary cardiac pressures. Thus, circulatory support provided by external cardiac massage is reduced, compared with normal physiology, but the mechanisms for maintaining the unidirectionality of blood flow appear similar to normal.

Cardiac stroke volume during external cardiac massage is optimized by compressions of *high velocity, moderate force,* and *brief duration* (high-impulse CPR). When compression rate is increased (Fig. 4), ventricular filling is not impaired, and, in fact, the heart remains distended because of ineffective chamber emptying. Significantly, compression stroke volume remains constant with *increasing manual compression rate* so that cardiac output and diastolic aortic pressure are significantly improved as compression rate increases.[30,31]

Coronary blood flow occurs primarily during noncompres-

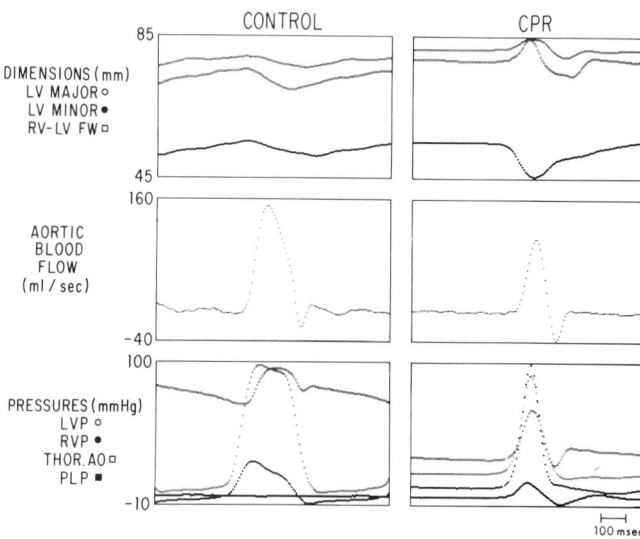

Figure 3. Digitized measurements of left ventricular dimensions, aortic blood flow, and cardiac chamber pressures during control (left panels) and during CPR in the arrested state (right panels) in a chronically instrumented dog. LV, left ventricular; Major, major axis diameter; Minor, minor axis diameter; RV-LV FW, right to left ventricular free wall diameter; PL, pleural; P, pressure. (From Maier, G. W., Tyson, G. S., Jr., Olsen, C. O., Kernstine, K. H., Davis, J. W., Conn, E. H., Sabiston, D. C., Jr., and Rankin, J. S.: The physiology of external cardiac massage: High impulse cardiopulmonary resuscitation. Circulation, 70:86, 1984.)

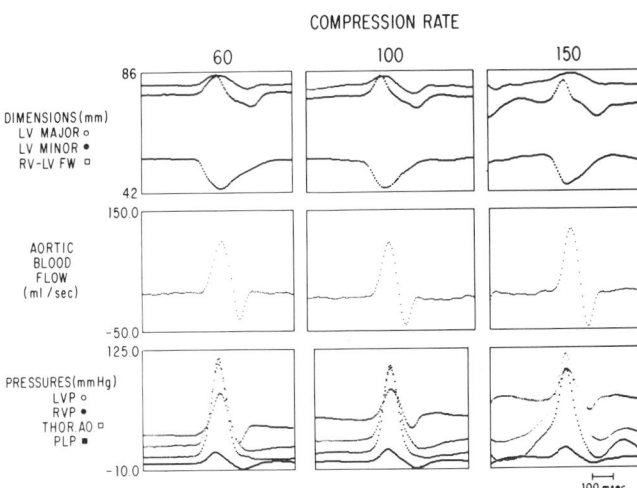

Figure 4. Representative digitized data from a compression rate study in an arrested chronically instrumented dog. Rate of manual compression was varied from 60 to 100 to 150 per minute while compression force was held constant at moderate levels. Abbreviations are the same as in Figure 3. See text for details. (From Maier, G. W., Tyson, G. S., Jr., Olsen, C. O., Kernstine, K. H., Davis, J. W., Conn, E. H., Sabiston, D. C., Jr., and Rankin, J. S.: The physiology of external cardiac massage: High impulse cardiopulmonary resuscitation. Circulation, 70:86, 1984.)

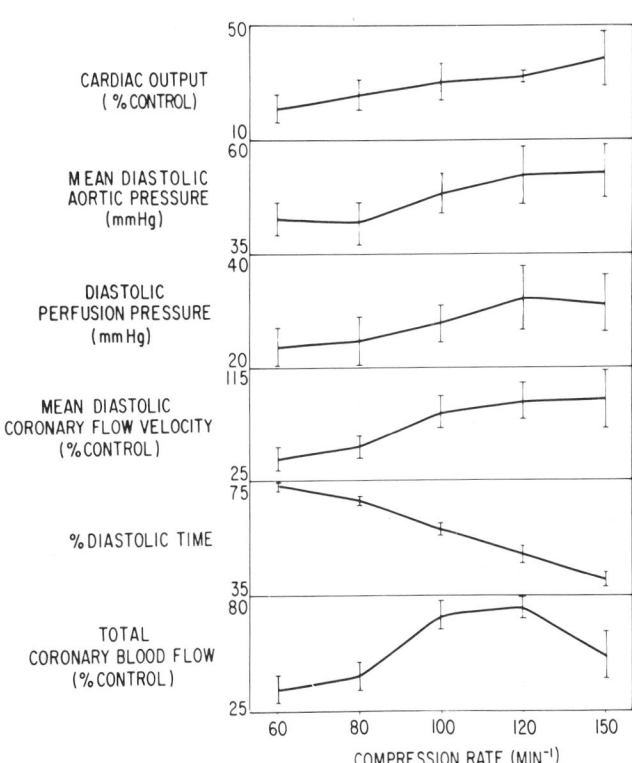

Figure 5. Cumulative hemodynamic data from compression rate study (mean ± standard error of the mean). Changes in cardiac output, percentage diastolic time, and total coronary blood flow with each increase in rate were significant by multivariate analysis (p < 0.05). Changes in other parameters were not significant. (From Wolfe, J. A., Maier, G. W., Newton, J. R., Glower, D. D., Tyson, G. S., Spratt, J. A., Rankin, J. S., and Olsen, C. O.: Physiologic determinants of coronary blood flow during external cardiac massage. J. Thorac. Cardiovasc. Surg., 95:523, 1988.)

sion or diastolic periods and falls to zero or even slightly negative values during compression.[41] This finding reflects a vascular waterfall phenomenon—pressure generated in the ventricular cavity acts as a resistance to coronary blood flow through the ventricular wall. Because of this finding, chest compression should not be prolonged but should be brief to provide sufficient diastolic time for coronary perfusion. Increasing the rate of manual chest compression improves overall cardiac output, aortic perfusion pressure, and coronary blood flow velocity. However, diastolic perfusion time declines linearly with increasing rate so that total coronary blood flow is optimized at a manual compression rate of 100 to 120 per minute (Fig. 5). The values for coronary blood flow observed with high-impulse CPR at 120 per minute are the best achievable with any closed resuscitation technique, and improved coronary perfusion may be especially important in providing the best possible conditions for successful early defibrillation.[41]

Mitral valve motion is a key factor in obtaining optimal hemodynamic support during external cardiac massage.[16,17] With the onset of sternal compression, left ventricular and left atrial pressures both rise as force is transmitted across the chest wall to the heart. Soon into the compression phase, a pressure gradient develops from the left ventricle to the left atrium. This gradient effects mitral valve closure, as observed with transesophageal echocardiography.[17] The aortic valve opens during compression to eject a "stroke volume" as illustrated in Figures 3 and 4. During the release phase, the aortic valve closes and maintains a coronary arterial perfusion gradient, whereas the mitral valve opens, allowing left ventricular filling. Thus, cardiac valve function during chest compression is essentially physiologic, again supporting the dominance of the direct cardiac compression mechanism during manual CPR. Significantly, it is mitral valve closure that directs the transthoracic energy of compression into forward perfusion pressure and blood flow, maintaining the efficient unidirectionality of the circulation.

When manual external chest compression with the high-impulse technique was compared with other types of CPR, the high-impulse method produced significantly better cardiac output, brachiocephalic blood flow, and coronary perfusion.[34] As a result, early and late survival in dogs arrested for 30 minutes was significantly improved with high-impulse CPR, compared with conventional methods at 60 compressions per minute.[18] Again, the primary factors associated with improved survival

appeared to be better cardiac output and mean coronary perfusion pressure. More recent animal studies have positively correlated mitral valve closure with success of resuscitation, again supporting a direct cardiac compression mechanism.[14] Although such a number of quantitative measurements are presently impossible in man, several papers have confirmed direct cardiac compression and mitral valve closure in patients undergoing therapeutic CPR.[6,21] In addition, hemodynamic measurements in man during high-impulse CPR confirm the efficacy of increasing compression rate in improving mean and diastolic arterial blood pressure.[30] These studies led the American Heart Association to increase the recommended rate of external chest compression from 60 per minute to approximately 100 per minute.[1]

In summary, available data suggest that sternal compression during manual CPR should be of *high velocity, moderate force,* and *brief duration.* A compression rate of *100 to 120 per minute* and a compression duration of 250 msec. (50 per cent duty cycle) have been shown to optimize cardiac output and coronary blood flow. High-impulse techniques introduce a fatigue factor for the resuscitator, and with in-hospital arrests, frequent changes of personnel are required. In current practice, ventilations are interspersed randomly at 12 to 15 breaths per minute.

In hospitalized arrest victims, successful resuscitation occasionally cannot be achieved with external chest compression. In this case, or if a question of pericardial tamponade exists, open-chest cardiac massage should be initiated. It has been clearly demonstrated that cardiac output and diastolic aortic perfusion pressure are better with open chest techniques,[2] and manual cardiac massage provides the ultimate direct cardiac compression. Open methods are used commonly when arrest occurs after cardiac surgery, where access to the heart is available

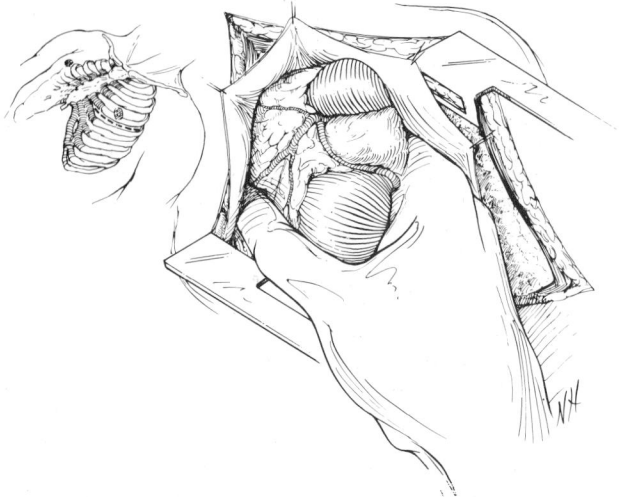

Figure 6. Open cardiac massage is performed through a short left anterior thoracotomy. The ventricles are compressed directly with the hands at 60 to 80 per minute.

through the sternotomy incision. In other situations, the left anterior chest is entered surgically after application of antiseptic solution, and a rib retractor is inserted (Fig. 6). The heart is compressed directly by squeezing the ventricles with the hands, and pericardiotomy is not always necessary. Ventricular emptying is more complete with open massage so that a compression rate of 60 to 80 per minute is utilized to allow adequate diastolic filling. Defibrillation is accomplished by direct application of cardioversion paddles to the heart, and if resuscitation is successful, the patient is taken to the operating room for chest closure. A surprisingly low incidence of thoracic infection exists with this technique, and little is lost by converting to the open-chest method. Recent data suggest that after 15 minutes of unsuccessful closed-chest CPR, one should convert to open-chest resuscitation, and resuscitation success can be improved by this policy.[26,27] A wider application of open-chest CPR as a backup to closed techniques probably is indicated.

When cardiac arrest occurs in the community with only one witness, single-rescuer CPR can be performed after a call for help has been made. With the single-rescuer method, it is more difficult to optimize resuscitation conditions, since the same individual performs mouth-to-mouth ventilation and external cardiac massage. Sternal compression proceeds at a rate of 80 to 100 per minute, and after each five compressions, two breaths are interposed by the rescuer during a brief pause in compressions. Obviously, this method is suboptimal and should be used only as a last resort. In addition, it should be emphasized that external cardiac massage, even under ideal conditions, is relatively ineffective, providing only 25 to 40 per cent of the normal cardiac output. Therefore, the goal of every resuscitation should be early defibrillation and restoration of a normal heart beat as soon as possible.

ADVANCED LIFE SUPPORT

In an organized in-hospital setting, the senior physician or most experienced individual coordinates the resuscitation. An electrocardiogram is obtained for documentation of the cardiac rhythm. In most cases, the paddles of the defibrillator also serve as electrocardiographic electrodes, and the rhythm can be assessed initially without other equipment. If ventricular tachycardia or fibrillation is present, an immediate attempt at cardioversion is made by using a maximal energy setting of 400 joules. Direct current countershock across the chest simultaneously depolarizes all myocardial cells and interrupts disorganized electrical activity. After repolarization, sinus node pacemaker activ-

ity resumes, and a coherent wavefront of depolarization spreads over the heart. Most defibrillators have two hand-held paddles that are positioned to the right of the upper sternum and to the left of the nipple in the anterior axillary line. For maximal current transmission to the heart, a low-impedance gel is applied to the paddle-skin interface. Occasionally, placing one defibrillator paddle behind the back improves the efficacy of cardioversion. Chest compression should be discontinued for no more than 5 to 10 seconds during diagnosis or defibrillation. So that the likelihood of inadvertent electrical shock is diminished, all personnel should stand well away from the patient during defibrillation. If initial cardioversion is unsuccessful, CPR is continued, and further interventions to increase the probability of cardioversion are initiated. During complex resuscitations or after defibrillation, a standard electrocardiogram monitor should be employed.

Venous access is obtained by inserting a large-bore plastic catheter into the subclavian or femoral vein; a large antecubital vein also can be used. If central or pulmonary artery lines are present, pharmacologic agents are administered directly into them to diminish the transit time to the coronary circulation. Because of the transit time, 30 seconds of CPR are provided after drug administration before further cardioversions are attempted. Periodically, CPR is discontinued briefly for assessment of changes in electrocardiographic rhythm and hemodynamics.

Restoration of coronary blood flow by CPR and correction of myocardial hypoxia and acidosis often improve the coarseness of fibrillation and make successful cardioversion more likely. As a routine, sodium bicarbonate is administered intravenously to correct metabolic acidosis. Arterial blood gases are drawn periodically for evaluation of the adequacy of bicarbonate therapy as well as arterial gas exchange. Intravenous or intracardiac cardiotonic drugs such as calcium chloride and epinephrine may improve the success of defibrillation. Both drugs produce arterial vasoconstriction, which increases arterial blood pressure at a given cardiac output and thereby improves coronary blood flow. If ventricular tachycardia or fibrillation persists, intravenous antiarrhythmic agents may be helpful. Intravenous lidocaine and/or procainamide are employed as first-line drugs; in especially refractory cases, bretylium may be required. Detailed dosages and protocols for drug therapy are provided elsewhere.[1,33,37]

If cardiac arrest occurs during induction of anesthesia for noncardiac operations, resuscitation is accomplished (by use of open-chest techniques if necessary), and the operation is terminated. The patient is transferred to an intensive care unit where hemodynamics are monitored with a thermodilution Swan-Ganz catheter for measurement of pulmonary capillary wedge pressure and cardiac output. When the patient is stabilized, cardiologic consultation is obtained, and coronary arteriography is considered when evidence of coronary artery disease exists. When cardiac arrest occurs during anesthetic induction for cardiac procedures, the operation is initiated immediately, and the patient is placed rapidly on cardiopulmonary bypass. Similarly, if arrest occurs after the conclusion of a cardiac operation, bypass is reinstituted as quickly as possible. When circulatory dynamics have been stabilized by the bypass circuit, the cause of the problem is investigated, and further therapy is initiated accordingly. In many ways, cardiopulmonary bypass is the ultimate resuscitation technique and should be used primarily whenever it is available.

MANAGEMENT AFTER RESUSCITATION

The goal of CPR is the early restoration of circulatory dynamics so that little permanent damage occurs to the patient. If this goal is attained, subsequent in-hospital care becomes important. In patients with acute coronary thrombosis who are

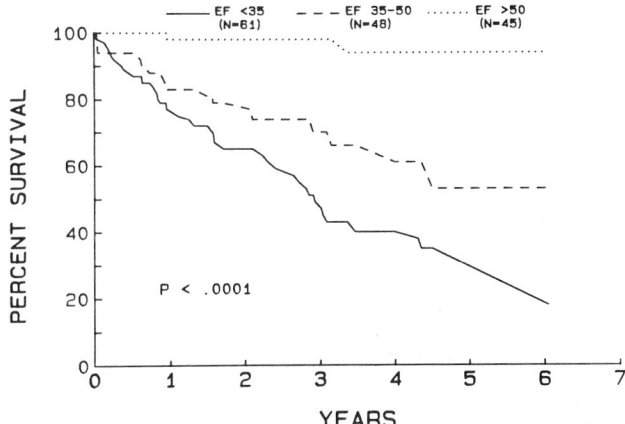

Figure 7. Survival of successfully resuscitated victims of sudden death as a function of resting left ventricular ejection fraction (EF). Survival decreased dramatically as ventricular function worsened. (From Ritchie, J. L., Hallstrom, A. P., Trobaugh, G. B., et al.: Out-of-hospital sudden coronary death: Rest and exercise radionuclide left ventricular function in survivors. Am. J. Cardiol., 55:645, 1985.)

appropriate candidates, thrombolytic therapy[4] can be used to re-establish coronary blood flow in the infarct-related artery. Successful reperfusion should be followed by interval cardiac catheterization and coronary revascularization if significant quantities of jeopardized myocardium remain. In survivors of cardiac arrest, the incidence of recurrent sudden death increases with the severity of coronary disease and ventricular dysfunction (Fig. 7).[35] Given the documented efficacy of coronary by-pass surgery in improving survival[5] and also in reducing the incidence of sudden death,[20,32,38] early therapeutic intervention with coronary revascularization should be strongly considered in appropriate arrest victims. Thus, the development of methods for treating acute ischemic heart disease have made successful resuscitation even more important than ever. Current efforts also should be directed toward identifying patients with ischemic heart disease who are at risk for sudden death and applying appropriate elective therapy at an earlier stage.

Primary cardiac dysrhythmic causes of sudden death, such as ventricular tachycardia or fibrillation associated with acute ischemia, left ventricular aneurysms, or Wolff-Parkinson-White syndrome, also should be managed aggressively after successful resuscitation. A recent study of 166 survivors of out-of-hospital arrest not associated with myocardial infarction revealed that 79 per cent had inducible ventricular dysrhythmias.[40] By use of multivariate analysis, successful suppression of inducibility significantly reduced long-term mortality ($p < 0.001$), as did appropriate cardiac surgery ($p = 0.05$). Patients with suppression of inducibility achieved survival characteristics comparable to those patients who were noninducible. Thus, aggressive diagnosis and management of possible primary rhythm disturbances is prognostically beneficial.

RESULTS

Two of the most important factors determining the success of resuscitation are (1) the severity and reversibility of the patient's underlying disease and (2) the time from arrest to defibrillation. With improved intensive care monitoring of high-risk patients with myocardial infarction, and with more rapid response times for defibrillation, the incidence of in-hospital sudden death from primary cardiac electrical events is now extremely low. In the overall hospital population, approximately half of the patients sustaining sudden cardiac arrest can be resuscitated, and half of these survive to discharge. Likewise, because of improved paramedical response times and better public education in providing immediate bystander CPR, resuscitation rates for outpatient arrests have been enhanced. With paramedical re-

sponse times averaging 2.9 minutes in the Seattle program, 60 per cent of out-of-hospital arrest victims could be resuscitated and transported to the hospital for further evaluation.[7] Half of this group survived to discharge. Hospital management after admission should be designed to diagnose and effectively treat the underlying cause of the cardiac arrest, as described before.

External cardiac massage is associated with a significant incidence of costochondral fractures, which increase with lengthening time of resuscitation. Occasionally, a flail sternal segment is produced and interferes with subsequent ventilatory function. Lacerations of the liver, spleen, lung, or other viscera also can occur. Vascular suture line disruption and perforation of the ventricular myocardium by prosthetic valves are important considerations during or soon after operation. These risks have to be incurred if the patient is to be saved after sudden cardiac arrest, and experienced personnel can minimize complications by exercising care with external chest massage. As shown experimentally,[30] additional stroke volume is not generated by using excessive force, so that compressions performed with brief, high-velocity, high-frequency strokes and only *moderate* compression force are effective and potentially less injurious. In addition, adequate training and proficiency with other techniques, such as central line placement and intubation, minimize the well-known complications of these procedures.

Because of ineffective circulatory maintenance with CPR, the likelihood of resuscitation diminishes directly with time after arrest. Therefore, as stated previously, the goal of every resuscitation should be restoration of the patient's cardiac function as quickly as possible. As the time of arrest increases, progressive and generalized ischemic injury occurs throughout the body, causing permanent organ dysfunction and worsening vasodilation. As systemic arterial resistance deteriorates, the aortic blood pressure attainable with CPR also diminishes, and, consequently, coronary and cerebral perfusion decline. In general, persistent cardiac arrest after 1 hour of full CPR (including open-chest techniques when feasible) is unlikely to be reversible, and resuscitation should be discontinued at that point. In summary, CPR has evolved into a highly technical and effective form of therapy for sudden cardiopulmonary arrest. With acquisition of additional knowledge in the future and with better physician and community training, the results should improve even further.

SELECTED REFERENCES

American Heart Association Committee on Emergency Cardiac Care: Standards and guidelines for cardiopulmonary resuscitation (CPR) and emergency cardiac care (ECC). J.A.M.A., 255:2905, 1986.
This publication is an important reference on current topics in CPR. Detailed information about CPR techniques is provided, as well as exact dosage schedules for pharmacologic therapy. Every physician should be familiar with this paper.

Cobb, L. A., Werner, J. A., and Trobaugh, G. B.: Sudden cardiac death. I. Experience with out-of-hospital resuscitation. II. Outcome of resuscitation, management, and future directions. Mod. Concepts Cardiovasc. Dis., 49:31, 1980.
This paper is a good review of an extensive clinical experience with CPR by leaders in the field. Detailed information about current results of CPR is provided along with recommendations for future development.

DeBard, M. L.: The history of cardiopulmonary resuscitation. Ann. Emerg. Med., 9:273, 1980.
This review describes the detailed history of CPR from antiquity to the present. Additional historical references are provided.

Kouwenhoven, W. B., Jude, J. R., and Knickerbocker, G. G.: Closed chest cardiac massage. J.A.M.A., 173:1064, 1960.
This paper initiated the modern era of cardiopulmonary resuscitation. The history of CPR to that date is provided, as well as the original experimental data on modern closed-chest cardiac massage. The methods of artificial ventilation, external chest compression, and external defibrillation were combined in five patients and reported for the first time. This is a landmark paper, which is highly recommended.

Maier, G. W., Tyson, G. S., Jr., Olsen, C. O., Kernstine, K. H., Davis, J. W., Conn, E. H., Sabiston, D. C., Jr., and Rankin, J. S.: The physiology of manual external cardiac massage: High impulse cardiopulmonary resuscitation. Circulation, 70:86, 1984.
This manuscript reviews the physiology of closed-chest cardiac massage. Instru-

mented dog models were utilized to investigate ventricular dynamics, cardiac output, and coronary blood flow during a number of different compression techniques. In this study, the method of high-impulse chest compression was developed.

REFERENCES

1. American Heart Association Committee on Emergency Cardiac Care: Standards and guidelines for cardiopulmonary resuscitation (CPR) and emergency cardiac care (ECC). J.A.M.A., 255:2905, 1986.
2. Badylak, S. F., Kern, K. B., Tacker, W. A., Ewy, G. A., Janas, W., and Carter, A.: The comparative pathology of open chest vs. mechanical closed chest cardiopulmonary resuscitation in dogs. Resuscitation, 13:249, 1986.
3. Beck, C. S., Pritchard, W. H., and Feil, H. S.: Ventricular fibrillation abolished by electric shock. J.A.M.A., 135:985, 1947.
4. Califf, R. M.: Fibrinolytic therapy in the management of acute myocardial infarction. In Sabiston, D. C., Jr., and Spencer, F. C. (Eds.): Surgery of the Chest, 5th ed. Philadelphia, W. B. Saunders Company, 1990.
5. Califf, R. M., Harrell, F. E., Lee, K. L., Rankin, J. S., Hlatky, M. A., Mark, D. B., Jones, R. H., Muhlbaier, L. H., Oldham, H. N., and Pryor, D. B.: The evolution of medical and surgical therapy for coronary artery disease: A 15-year perspective. J.A.M.A., 261:2077, 1989.
6. Clements, F. M., DeBruijn, N. P., and Kisslo, J. A.: Transesophageal echocardiographic observations in a patient undergoing closed-chest massage. Anesthesiology, 64:826, 1986.
7. Cobb, L. A., and Weaver, W. D.: Exercise: A risk for sudden death in patients with coronary heart disease. J. Am. Coll. Cardiol., 7:215, 1986.
8. Cobb, L. A., Werner, J. A., and Trobaugh, G. B.: Sudden cardiac death. I. Experience with out-of-hospital resuscitation. II. Outcome of resuscitation, management, and future directions. Mod. Concepts Cardiovasc. Dis., 49:31, 1980.
9. Collins, V. J.: Endotracheal anesthesia: II. Technical considerations. In Principles of Anesthesiology. Philadelphia, Lea & Febiger, 1976.
10. Copley, D. P., Mantle, J. A., Rogers, W. J., Russell, R. O., Jr., and Rackley, C. E.: Improved outcome for prehospital cardiopulmonary collapse with resuscitation by bystanders. Circulation, 56:901, 1977.
11. Crile, G.: Anemia and resuscitation; an experimental and clinical research. Daniel Appleton & Company, 1914.
12. Davies, M. J., and Thomas, A.: Thrombosis and acute coronary artery lesions in sudden cardiac ischemic death. N. Engl. J. Med., 310:1137, 1984.
13. DeBard, M. L.: The history of cardiopulmonary resuscitation. Ann. Emerg. Med., 9:273, 1980.
14. Deshmukh, H. G., Weil, M. H., and Gudipati, C. V.: Mechanism of blood flow generated by precordial compression during CPR: 1. Studies on closed chest precordial compression. Chest, 95:1092, 1989.
15. Eisenberg, M. S., Gergner, L., and Hallstrom, A.: Cardiac resuscitation in the community: Importance of rapid provision and implication for program planning. J.A.M.A., 241:1905, 1979.
16. Feneley, M. P., and Rankin, J. S.: Mechanisms of blood flow during cardiopulmonary resuscitation: Analysis of recent experimental observations concerning the importance of the chest compression technique. In Califf, R. M., and Wagner, G. S. (Eds.): Acute Coronary Care in the Thrombolytic Era. Boston, Martinus Nijhoff Publishers, 1988.
17. Feneley, M. P., Maier, G. W., Gaynor, J. W., Gall, S. A., Kisslo, J. A., Davis, J. W., and Rankin, J. S.: Sequence of mitral valve motion and transmitral blood flow during manual cardiopulmonary resuscitation in dogs. Circulation, 76:363, 1987.
18. Feneley, M. P., Maier, G. W., Kern, K. B., Gaynor, J. W., Gall, S. A., Sanders, A. B., Raessler, K., Muhlbaier, L. G., Rankin, J. S., and Ewy, G. A.: Influence of compression rate on initial success of resuscitation and 24 hour survival after prolonged manual cardiopulmonary resuscitation in dogs. Circulation, 77:240, 1988.
19. Goldstein, S.: Sudden Death Coronary Heart Disease. Mt. Kisco, New York, Futura Publishing Company, 1974.
20. Hammermeister, K. E., DeRouen, T. A., Murray, J. A., and Dodge, H. T.: Effect of aortocoronary saphenous vein bypass grafting on death and sudden death. Comparison of nonrandomized medically and surgically treated function. Am. J. Cardiol., 39:925, 1977.
21. Higano, S. T., and Jae, K. O.: The mechanism of forward blood flow during cardiopulmonary resuscitation: Transesophageal observations. Circulation, 82(Suppl. III): III-483, 1990.
22. Jude, J. R., Kouwenhoven, W. B., and Knickerbocker, G. S.: Cardiac arrest. J.A.M.A., 128:1063, 1961.
23. Jude, J. R., Kouwenhoven, W. B., and Knickerbocker, G. S.: External cardiac resuscitation. Monogr. Surg. Sci., 1:59, 1964.
24. Julian, D. G.: Cardiac resuscitation in the eighteenth century. Heart Lung, 4:46, 1975.
25. Keen, W. W.: Case of total laryngectomy (unsuccessful) and a case of abdominal hysterectomy (successful) in both of which massage of the heart for chloroform collapse was employed, with notes on 25 other cases of cardiac massage. Therap. Gaz., 28:217, 1904.
26. Kern, K. B., Sanders, A. B., and Ewy, G. A.: Open-chest cardiac massage after closed-chest compression in a canine model: When to intervene. Resuscitation, 15:51, 1987.
27. Kern, K. B., Sanders, A. B., Badylak, S. F., Janas, W., Carter, A. B., Tacker, W. A., and Ewy, G. A.: Long-term survival with open-chest cardiac massage after ineffective closed-chest compression in a canine preparation. Circulation, 75:498, 1987.
28. Kouwenhoven, W. B., Jude, J. R., and Knickerbocker, G. G.: Closed chest cardiac massage. J.A.M.A., 173:1064, 1960.
29. Kuller, L. H.: Sudden death—definition and epidemiologic considerations. Prog. Cardiovasc. Dis., 23:1, 1980.
30. Maier, G. W., Tyson, G. S., Jr., Olsen, C. O., Kernstine, K. H., Davis, J. W., Conn, E. H., Sabiston, D. C., Jr., and Rankin, J. S.: The physiology of external cardiac massage: High impulse cardiopulmonary resuscitation. Circulation, 70:86, 1984.
31. Maier, G. W., Newton, J. R., Wolfe, J. A., Tyson, G. S., Olsen, C. O., Glower, D. D., Spratt, J. A., Davis, J. W., Feneley, M. P., and Rankin, J. S.: The influence of manual chest compression rate on hemodynamic support during cardiac arrest: High impulse cardiopulmonary resuscitation. Circulation, 74(Suppl. IV):IV-51, 1986.
32. Mason, D. T., and Vismar, L. A.: Reduction of sudden death by aortocoronary bypass surgery. Am. J. Cardiol., 41:795, 1978.
33. McIntyre, K. M., and Parker, M. R.: Standards and guidelines for cardiopulmonary resuscitation (CPR) and emergency cardiac care (ECC). J.A.M.A., 244:453, 1980.
34. Newton, J. R., Glower, D. D., Wolfe, J. A., Tyson, G. S., Spratt, J. A., Feneley, M. P., Rankin, J. S., and Olsen, C. O.: A physiologic comparison of external cardiac massage techniques. J. Thorac. Cardiovasc. Surg., 95:892, 1988.
35. Ritchie, J. L., Hallstrom, A. P., Trobaugh, G. B., et al.: Out-of-hospital sudden coronary death: Rest and exercise radionuclide left ventricular function in survivors. Am. J. Cardiol., 55:645, 1985.
36. Rosen, Z., and Davidson, J. T.: Respiratory resuscitation in ancient Hebrew sources. Anesth. Analg., 51:502, 1972.
37. Safar, P.: Advances in Cardiopulmonary Resuscitation. New York, Springer-Verlag, 1977.
38. Vismara, L. A., Miller, R. R., Price, J. E., Karem, R., Demaria, A. N., and Mason, D. T.: Improved longevity due to reduction of sudden death by aortocoronary bypass in coronary atherosclerosis. Prospective evaluation of medical versus surgical therapy in matched patients with multivessel disease. Am. J. Cardiol., 39:919, 1977.
39. Wiggers, C. J.: The physiologic basis for cardiac resuscitation from ventricular fibrillation—method of serial defibrillation. Am. Heart J., 20:413, 1940.
40. Wilber, K. J., Garan, H., Finkelstein, D., et al.: Out-of-hospital cardiac arrest: Use of electrophysiologic testing in the prediction of long-term outcome. N. Engl. J. Med., 381:19, 1988.
41. Wolfe, J. A., Maier, G. W., Newton, J. R., Glower, D. D., Tyson, G. S., Spratt, J. A., Rankin, J. S., and Olsen, C. O.: Physiologic determinants of coronary blood flow during external cardiac massage. J. Thorac. Cardiovasc. Surg., 95:523, 1988.
42. Zoll, P. M., Paul, M. H., Linenthal, A. J., Norman, L. R., and Gibson, W.: The effects of external electric currents on the heart. Control of cardiac rhythm and induction and termination of cardiac arrhythmias. Circulation, 14:745, 1956.

III _____

PENETRATING CARDIAC INJURIES

Fred A. Crawford, Jr., M.D.

HISTORICAL ASPECTS

Penetrating chest injuries were described in the Smith papyrus in 3000 B.C.,[18] and Homer clearly described wounds of the heart in *The Iliad* in the ninth century B.C.[14] The subsequent history of cardiac injuries and their treatment were beautifully reviewed by Beck in 1926.[5] Both Hippocrates and Aristotle recognized the seriousness of cardiac wounds, and Galen noted that wounds of the heart in gladiators were often fatal. This concept persisted into the seventeenth century when Boerhraave said, "All wounds of the heart deep enough to penetrate into either of the ventricles are mortal."[5] In contrast, as early as the sixteenth century, Hollerius postulated that all cardiac wounds might not necessarily be fatal. Morgagni, in 1691, emphasized the consequences of pericardial tamponade, and Larrey in 1829 successfully treated a patient by drainage of pericardial tamponade.[5] By 1868, Fischer reported 452 patients with cardiac wounds, 10 per cent of whom recovered. Block in 1882 was the first to experimentally suture the heart in rabbits.[5] This concept was opposed by Billroth in 1883 with the famous statement that "the surgeon who should attempt to suture a wound of the heart would lose the respect of his colleagues".[5]

The first two attempts to suture a stab wound of the human heart by Cappalen in 1885 and Friria in 1896, were unsuccessful,[5] but these were followed by Rehn who in 1896 in Frankfurt successfully sutured a stab wound of the right ventricle with long-term survival.[26] Ten years later, he had compiled a series of 124 patients, 40 per cent of whom recovered. The first American to perform this feat was Lister Hill of Montgomery, Alabama, who repaired a stab wound in a 13-year-old boy by the light of a kerosene lamp on a kitchen table.[13] Over the next several decades, a number of series with an increasingly larger number of patients were reported in which survival rates of 30 to 50 per cent were obtained following thoracotomy and suture of a penetrating cardiac injury. In 1942, Blalock and Ravitch advocated the somewhat more conservative approach of pericardiocentesis and close observation of selected patients.[6] Several large series in the 1960s and early 1970s conclusively indicated that early thoracotomy and cardiorrhaphy are the most appropriate treatment in the management of patients with penetrating cardiac injury.[4,28,30,36]

INCIDENCE

The incidence of cardiovascular injuries has increased dramatically over the last several decades. In a series of 4459 patients with cardiovascular injuries treated over a 30-year period (1958–1987), the incidence increased from 27 patients per year in 1960 to 213 patients per year by the mid-1980s.[21] Paralleling this increase in numbers of injuries has been an increase in the relative frequency of injuries caused by gunshot wounds compared with stab wounds.[25,29] Previously, the overwhelming majority of penetrating cardiac injuries in reported series was due to stab wounds, but in more current series, gunshot wounds may equal or even outnumber stab wounds.[32,29] This is thought to be due to the ready availability of handguns and, in some

areas, to the increasing violence associated with illicit drug related activities. According to Naughton and colleagues, penetrating cardiac injuries occur most often in the home (70 per cent), by a known assailant (83 per cent), and are due to domestic or social disputes (73 per cent). The victims are predominantly male (83 per cent).[25]

In the past, most series of penetrating cardiac injuries originated from hospitals in large metropolitan areas. In the last decade, more series have been reported from smaller cities and war zones.[25,37] Trinkle emphasized the difficulties inherent in comparing different clinical series.[34] Significant differences in prehospital and inhospital mortality may exist because of (1) differing modes of injury (gunshot wound versus stab wound), (2) other associated injuries; and (3) availability or lack of availability of highly trained emergency medical personnel and well-organized rapid transport systems for trauma patients. For example, a series with a larger number of gunshot wounds compared with stab wounds usually has a higher mortality. Paradoxically, series from a city with an effective transport system may have a higher hospital or operative mortality because more seriously injured patients survived for admission to the hospital. Accordingly, Ivatury and associates have proposed an index for quantifying penetrating cardiac trauma (Penetrating Cardiac Trauma Index) and have shown that this index has a high correlation with survival.[15] Factors influencing mortality from penetrating cardiac injury, and which are incorporated into this index, include, in order of decreasing significance, (1) coronary artery injury; (2) multiple chamber injury or isolated left atrial or left ventricular injury; (3) comminuted tear of single chamber; (4) single right-sided chamber injury; and (5) tangential injuries that do not penetrate the endocardium. It follows that one must be cautious in comparing results from different series without carefully considering those factors that influence results. Most current series report survivals of 60 to 70 per cent for those patients who reach the hospital with vital signs present.[16,35,37]

ETIOLOGY

Penetrating injuries to the heart are most commonly associated with violence and are the result of stab wounds and gunshot wounds. However, such injuries have also been produced accidentally by nails, coat hangers, objects propelled by lawnmowers,[27] arrows,[9] and even iatrogenically by chest tubes and needles.[8] Despite the increasing sophistication of emergency medical services and rapid transportation to the hospital, some 60 to 80 per cent of those injuries cause death at the scene or prior to arrival at a trauma facility.[29,34]

DIAGNOSIS

Any patient with a penetrating injury to the chest, neck, upper abdomen, or back should be suspected of having a cardiac injury. The right ventricle occupies approximately 55 per cent of the anterior chest wall; the left ventricle, 20 per cent; the right atrium, 10 per cent; and the great vessels and venae cavae, 15 per cent.[29] One should therefore be especially suspicious of injuries to the anterior chest and of those adjacent to the sternum. The relative frequency of cardiac chamber injury corresponds somewhat to the aforementioned anatomy. Karrell and associates reviewed 20 series of penetrating cardiac injuries, consisting of a total of 1802 patients.[18] The right ventricle was injured in 42.4 per cent, the left ventricle in 32.9 per cent, the right atrium in 15.3 per cent, and the left atrium in 5.8 per cent. Great vessel injury occurred in 3.4 per cent.

Presenting signs and symptoms vary depending upon the mode of injury, the location of injury, and other associated injuries. In general, these patients present in two quite different states: cardiac tamponade or shock.[34,35] Patients with isolated stab wounds from smaller weapons (ice pick) to the left or right ventricle may present with normal hemodynamics and may have a relatively normal physical examination. Injuries to the ventricle may cause little or no bleeding or transient bleeding followed by sealing of the injury by the muscle fibers of the ventricle or by cardiac tamponade. Injuries to the atrium may cause bleeding followed by sealing of the injury by clot because of the lower pressure in the atrium. However, exsanguination may follow atrial injuries because of the inability of the thin-walled atrium to seal. Frequently in patients with stab wounds, the hole in the pericardium is small. If significant bleeding from the heart occurs, the blood is trapped in the pericardial cavity. These patients may present with classic cardiac tamponade, with the typical findings of hypotension, elevated venous pressure (distended neck veins), and decreased heart sounds (Beck's triad).[5] These typical physical findings may be hard to detect, however, in patients who are uncooperative, combative, or intoxicated. In addition, the loss of a significant amount of blood from the cardiac wound or other injuries may cause flat neck veins despite the presence of significant pericardial tamponade. In these patients, evidence of increased venous pressure may become obvious only after volume resuscitation. When hypotension and distended neck veins are present in a cooperative patient with a penetrating chest wound, one must assume some degree of cardiac injury and proceed accordingly. However, the absence of the classic findings of tamponade does *not* allow exclusion of a cardiac injury.

Chest films and fluoroscopy have been of little help in making the diagnosis and usually cause further delay of definitive diagnosis and treatment. The pericardium is relatively inelastic, and acute tamponade rarely causes significant cardiac enlargement on chest films. The electrocardiogram is rarely useful in making the diagnosis, but obvious ischemic changes might suggest a coronary artery injury. Echocardiography may occasionally be useful in patients in whom the diagnosis is in doubt. However, echocardiography requires a careful examination by a highly trained individual in a cooperative patient. Unfortunately, many patients present at a time when an echocardiogram is not rapidly available, and their condition may not permit a delay in treatment until it can be obtained.

The role of pericardiocentesis in the diagnosis and treatment of penetrating cardiac injuries has been widely debated. Pericardiocentesis is performed by inserting a large needle at the tip of the xyphoid and angling it posteriorly and superiorly toward the left shoulder. Some have advocated performing pericardiocentesis with the aid of electrocardiographic monitoring, but this is not necessary. Pericardiocentesis is a difficult technical procedure under optimal circumstances in a cooperative patient, and in the setting frequently associated with this type of injury (shock, intoxication, shivering, hypoxia, combativeness), it is nearly impossible. Blood in the pericardial cavity is frequently clotted and cannot be aspirated through the small needle, thus causing a false-negative diagnosis. Perhaps of equal frequency, the return of nonclotting blood may be due to needle penetration of a cardiac chamber or laceration of the heart or a coronary artery. In the acute setting, the pericardial cavity is nondistensible, and a relatively small amount of blood in this space can cause significant hemodynamic compromise. Accord-

ingly, removal of a small amount of blood from the pericardial space can produce rapid improvement in blood pressure. This improvement is most often transient but may be helpful in stabilizing the patient until transportation to the operating room.

Some investigators have advocated a subxiphoid pericardial window, created in the emergency room or the operating room under local or light general anesthesia.[7,23] If no blood is present in the pericardium, cardiac injury can almost certainly be excluded. However, if injury is present, opening the pericardium can result in release of tamponade and subsequent exsanguinating hemorrhage. Therefore, when this technique is employed, the surgeon should be ready to proceed immediately with a median sternotomy and/or thoracotomy for repair of the cardiac injury. It should be noted that a subxiphoid pericardial window is a particularly useful technique in patients undergoing laparotomy for penetrating injury when there is reason to believe that cardiac injury may have occurred in addition to the abdominal injuries.

Cardiac tamponade occurs in the majority (greater than 80 per cent) of stab wounds of the heart but in only 10 to 20 per cent of gunshot wounds. It is interesting that tamponade may have a protective effect and favorably influence survival. Moreno and co-workers found that survival occurred in 73 per cent of patients presenting with tamponade, compared to 11 per cent of those without tamponade.[24] This was true regardless of the mode of injury or the chambers involved. Although all the diagnostic techniques just discussed may be useful in selected patients who present in this manner, the emergency room physician and/or evaluating surgeon most often relies on clinical skills and a high degree of suspicion in making the diagnosis.

The second mode of presentation is that of *hemorrhagic shock* (hypotension, decreased venous pressure), which is secondary to exsanguination from the penetrating injury of the heart. This occurs most commonly following gunshot wounds but also may be seen in 20 per cent of patients with stab wounds. In these patients, the injury causes a large tear in the pericardium and in the underlying heart. Following the large defect in the pericardium, tamponade cannot occur. The more extensive injury to the heart is unable to seal spontaneously, and the patient may simply exsanguinate. Undoubtedly, such patients represent a large percentage of those who die before reaching medical care. Moreno and co-workers documented higher hospital mortality in this group.[24] The diagnosis of a significant injury is usually not difficult in patients who present with evidence of penetrating injury to the chest, hemorrhage, profound hypotension, and flat neck veins. These conditions usually demand immediate definitive treatment, and thus the diagnostic techniques mentioned earlier (chest films, echocardiography, and pericardiocentesis) are less useful.

TREATMENT

Patients with penetrating chest trauma and suspected cardiac injury should be supported with standard initial resuscitative measures upon arrival in the trauma facility. These include appropriate airway control, insertion of large central intravenous lines, and fluid replacement.[18] If the patient is stable and the diagnosis of cardiac injury is strongly suspected, prompt transportation to the operating room is mandatory for thoracotomy and prompt repair of the injury. Blalock and Ravitch advocated conservative management (pericardiocentesis and observation) in certain patients,[6] and this continues to be advocated by some.[22] However, Sugg and associates in 1968 reported in an analysis of 459 patients that in 23 per cent no blood was obtained by pericardiocentesis despite the fact that at operation 100 to 660 ml. of blood was noted in the pericardium.[28] In addition, 10 patients who had successful pericardiocentesis subsequently died of tamponade within 1 to 12 hours while being observed. All could have been saved by prompt thoracotomy.

They recommended immediate operation for all cardiac injuries and noted a decrease in overall mortality from 36 to 14 per cent after this policy was initiated.[28] In 1972, in a series of 269 patients with penetrating cardiac injury, Beall and colleagues also advised immediate operation with cardiorrhaphy for penetrating injuries.[4] As a result of these two papers, most institutions advocate early operation.[16,18,29,30,34,35] As previously noted, however, successful pericardiocentesis may stabilize the patient temporarily until definitive thoracotomy can be performed.

Among patients with suspected cardiac injuries, (1) some present initially in extremis with no blood pressure and agonal respirations, (2) some deteriorate rapidly immediately following arrival in the emergency room, and (3) some cannot be stabilized by the use of standard resuscitative measures. Emergency room thoracotomy has been advocated as providing the greatest likelihood of salvage in this last group. In a group of 37 patients, 67.5 per cent survived emergency room thoracotomy, resuscitation, and repair of the cardiac wound. Survival was 82 per cent with stab wounds and 68 per cent with gunshot wounds.[20] In another series of 37 consecutive emergency room thoracotomies, 57 per cent of patients survived.[28] Baker and colleagues noted a 50 per cent survival following emergency room thoracotomy in patients with cardiac injuries who had no signs of life on arrival.[3] They also noted a significant cost-benefit ratio in emergency room thoracotomy despite an extremely conservative method of calculating this benefit. Ivatury and associates documented survival in approximately one third of patients who arrived in extremis.[17] Survival in the entire series was related to the patients' status on arrival (73 per cent survival with stable vital signs; 29 per cent survival for those in extremis).

Most penetrating cardiac injuries occur in young, otherwise healthy individuals. It is clear that aggressive treatment, including emergency room thoracotomy is mandatory in the survival of a significant number of these patients whose conditions do not permit transportation to the operating room.[3,17,20,32] Complications (wound infection, neurologic injury) do occur with this approach, but they are relatively infrequent and must be accepted in view of the salvage of this population of patients.[17]

OPERATIVE TECHNIQUE

The patient with a documented or suspected penetrating cardiac injury who responds appropriately to resuscitation and is relatively stable may be transported to the operating room for thoracotomy under controlled conditions. Caution must be exercised during induction of anesthesia, since the initiation of positive-pressure ventilation in combination with an even moderate degree of tamponade may be sufficient to decrease venous return severely and cause rapid deterioration. Under such conditions, skin preparation and draping of the patient prior to induction may be useful. If not, one must be able to prepare and drape rapidly following induction. The operative approach may be through a left anterior thoracotomy in the fourth intercostal space or via a median sternotomy. The anterior thoracotomy can be performed rapidly and requires no special equipment. It provides perhaps better exposure to the posterior left ventricle as well as to the aorta and esophagus, but exposure of the right ventricle and right atrium is not as good. The thoracotomy incision may be extended across the sternum into the right chest, thus providing adequate exposure to all cardiac chambers. Most cardiac procedures today are performed through a median sternotomy, and this is the preferred incision of most for penetrating cardiac injuries. This approach requires division of the sternum and, although a sternal saw is preferred, the incision may also be made with a Lebsche knife. The cardiopulmonary perfusion team is routinely alerted as soon as the patient arrives so that cardiopulmonary bypass is available. However, it is rarely necessary for most simple injuries. Autotransfusion may be helpful, and this is facilitated by the pump team.

Once the pericardium is opened and blood is evacuated, control of the point of injury is usually possible with digital pressure. The laceration or hole may be closed with several interrupted sutures of silk or synthetic material (Fig. 1B). Teflon felt bolsters are preferred to prevent the sutures from tearing through the heart, but this is not always necessary. Injuries to the atrium or great vessels may be similarly repaired. Alternatively, for atrial or great vessel injury, a tangential side-biting clamp may be applied and the injury sutured (Fig. 1A). When the injury is adjacent to a major coronary artery, sutures should be placed beneath the coronary artery so that the injury is repaired without compromising blood flow in the coronary artery (Fig. 1C). More extensive or simple injuries that cannot be initially controlled by digital pressure may require prompt heparinization and institution of cardiopulmonary bypass and more definitive techniques of repair. When small coronary artery branches or distal coronary arteries are injured, they may be simply ligated, producing only a localized area of myocardial ischemia (Fig. 1D). More proximal coronary artery injuries require more definitive repair—either direct suture, which is rarely possible, or bypass utilizing a saphenous vein or internal mammary artery graft (Fig. 1E). Such proximal injuries to coronary arteries may be fatal if not repaired, or, if not fatal, may result in major myocardial infarction, subsequent loss of ventricular function, and/or development of a ventricular aneurysm.

In addition to simple injuries to cardiac chambers and to coronary arteries, penetrating cardiac wounds may cause injury to intracardiac valves and the development of intracardiac or extracardiac shunts.[2,19,33] It is estimated that arteriovenous fistulas or intracardiac shunts occur in up to 5 per cent of patients following penetrating cardiac injury.[2] Most commonly the shunt occurs between the left and right ventricles (ventricular septal defect) but it may also occur between the atria (atrial septal defect), the aorta and vena cava, aorta and pulmonary artery, or a coronary artery and a cardiac chamber.

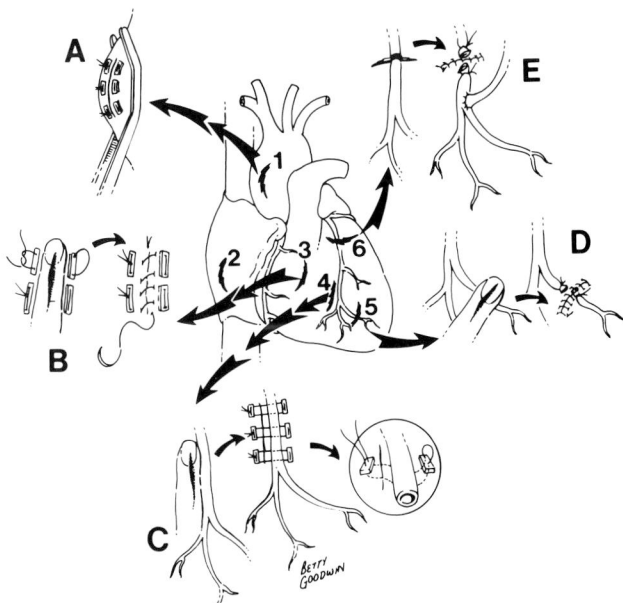

Figure 1. Penetrating injuries of the right atrium (2) or great vessels (1) may be initially controlled by digital pressure (B) and oversewn. An alternative way of managing this injury is to apply a tangential side-biting clamp and then to suture the laceration (A). Simple penetrating injuries to the left or right ventricle (3) may likewise be initially closed by digital pressure and oversewn (B). Injuries adjacent to a major coronary artery (4) may be closed with sutures placed in such a manner so as not to compromise coronary artery flow (C). Injuries to small coronary arteries (5) may be repaired in a similar manner and the small coronary artery ligated (D). Injuries that involve a proximal major coronary artery (6) require both repair of the injury and a bypass to the distal vessel (E).

Occasionally the fistula is sufficiently large to produce a murmur heard on initial examination in the emergency room. Most commonly, however, the fistula is initially small, and the associated murmur is not appreciated at the time the patient is first seen. When a murmur is identified on initial assessment, preoperative evaluation by two-dimensional echo/Doppler may be extremely valuable in assessing any intracardiac pathology.[10] If time and the patient's condition do not permit preoperative echocardiography, an intraoperative echo (either transesophageal or using a hand-held probe) may be useful in making the definitive diagnosis. Fortunately, most fistulas are initially small, and only rarely is it necessary to repair them definitively at the time of the initial operation. If the fistula is large or if a valve is severely damaged, the valve repair/replacement or closure of intracardiac defects should be performed using standard techniques.

Most intracardiac shunts first become obvious at some point following successful repair of the initial cardiac injury. Therefore, careful repeated physical examinations are required prior to discharge and subsequently in order to detect these defects. The physical examination should be supplemented by thorough two-dimensional echo/Doppler study prior to discharge and subsequently if an intracardiac defect or arteriovenous fistula is suspected. Small ventricular septal defects (less than 1.5 : 1 left-to-right shunt) may not require closure and may actually close spontaneously. Larger defects should be closed to prevent or to treat congestive heart failure. Again, standard techniques for the correlation of such defects are used at elective reoperation.

Gunshot wounds to the heart may result in whole or fragmented bullets in the pericardium, in the wall of the heart, or in a cardiac chamber. Such retained missiles may embolize, predispose to bacterial endocarditis, or erode into cardiac chambers or vessels. Harken described removal of retained foreign bodies in the heart in soldiers at the close of World War II and generally believed that such foreign bodies should be removed.[11] Symbas recently reviewed the world literature on this topic and, in addition, has reported with co-workers the series from Grady Hospital.[29,31] The fragment was removed in 7 patients, could not be found in 1 patient, and was not disturbed in another 12 patients. He indicated that small fragments in asymptomatic patients should not be disturbed. Generally, indications for operative removal include (1) large missiles; (2) symptomatic patients; and (3) an intracardiac location, especially on the left side. It is clear that not all retained missiles in or around the heart warrant removal and thus each patient must be evaluated individually. Echocardiography (by precise localization of the fragment) may be helpful in the decision regarding removal of the missile. When a decision is made to remove it, careful preoperative localization, including fluoroscopy and echocardiography, is necessary. Intraoperative echocardiography may also be useful in the localization of retained missiles at the time of operation.[12]

Finally, it has been shown that survivors of penetrating cardiac injuries may develop significant psychologic disturbances following recovery from the initial injury. In a study of 20 patients surviving penetrating cardiac injuries, Abbott and associates found that all had cardiac complaints.[1] Although stress testing showed work capacity to be normal in 90 per cent of these patients, only 40 per cent of them returned to work.

SELECTED REFERENCES

Antunes, M. J., Fernandes, L. E., and Oliveira, J. D.: Ventricular septal defects and arteriovenous fistulas, with and without valvular lesions, resulting from penetrating injury of the heart and aorta. J. Thorac. Cardiovasc. Surg., 95:902, 1988.
Intracardiac lesions that can occur at the time of a penetrating cardiac injury are described. Septal defects, arteriovenous fistula, and valve lesions, and the appropriate management, are described and discussed in detail.

Ivatury, R. R., Nallathame, M., Stahl, W., and Rohman, W.: Penetrating cardiac trauma. Ann. Surg. 205:61, 1987.
This is an analysis of 228 patients who sustained penetrating cardiac injury in a 20-year period extending from 1963 to 1983. All aspects of penetrating cardiac injury are reviewed in this very nice study.

Karrel, R., Shaffer, M. A., and Franaszek, J. B.: Emergency diagnosis, resuscitation, and treatment of acute penetrating cardiac trauma. Ann. Emerg. Med. 11:504, 1982.
This is an excellent review of all aspects of penetrating cardiac trauma. Included is a historical review, methods of diagnosis, techniques of treatment, and results that can be expected. Viewpoints of a variety of different authors are presented.

Naughton, M. J., Brissie, R. M., Bessey, P. Q., McEachern, M. M., Donald, J. M., Jr., and Laws, H. L.: Demography of penetrating cardiac trauma. Ann. Surg., 209:676, 1989.
This study covers a 2-year time span (1985–1986) in a medium-sized city. It includes all patients who sustained penetrating cardiac trauma, including those dying at the scene of injury as well as those treated in a hospital. It documents nicely the increasing frequency of gunshot wounds as well as the fact that rapid transport, aggressive resuscitation, and definitive repair remain the best treatment for cardiac injuries.

Symbas, P.N.: Cardiothoracic Trauma. Philadelphia, W. B. Saunders Company, 1989.
This relatively brief text reviews trauma to the contents of the thoracic cavity. It is current and complete. All aspects of penetrating cardiac injury, including diagnostic techniques, different modes of treatment, and associated injuries (septal defects, retained missiles) are discussed in detail.

Tavares, S., Hankins, J. R., Moulton, A. L., Attar, S., Ali, S., Lincoln, S., Green, D. C., Sequeira, A., and McLaughlin, J. S.: Management of penetrating cardiac injuries: The role of emergency room thoracotomy. Ann. Thorac. Surg., 38:183, 1984.
This article defines the role of emergency room thoracotomy in patients who have sustained cardiac injuries and shows that a significant number of individuals can be resuscitated by emergency room thoracotomy despite their presentation in extremis.

REFERENCES

1. Abbott, J. A., Cousineau, B. S., Cheitlin, J., Thomas, A. N., and Lim, R. C., Jr.: Late sequelae of penetrating cardiac wounds. J. Thorac. Cardiovasc. Surg., 75:510, 1978.
2. Antunes, M. J., Fernandes, L. E., and Oliveira, J. M.: Ventricular septal defects and arteriovenous fistulas, with and without valvular lesions, resulting from penetrating injury of the heart and aorta. J. Thorac. Cardiovasc. Surg., 95:902, 1988.
3. Baker, C. C., Thomas, A. N., and Trunkey, D. D.: The role of emergency room thoracotomy in trauma. J. Trauma, 20:848, 1980.
4. Beall, A. C., Jr., Patrick, T. A., Okies, J. E., Bricker, D. L., and DeBakey, M. E.: Penetrating wounds of the heart: Changing patterns of surgical management. J. Trauma, 12:468, 1972.
5. Beck, C. S.: Wounds of the heart: The technic of suture. Arch. Surg. 13:205, 1926.
6. Blalock, A., and Ravitch, M.: A consideration of the nonoperative treatment of cardiac tamponade resulting from wounds of the heart. Surgery, 14:157, 1943.
7. Brewster, S. C., Thirlby, R. C., and Snyder, W. H., III: Subxiphoid pericardial window and penetrating cardiac trauma. Arch. Surg., 123:937, 1988.
8. Casillas, J. A., de la Fuente, A.: Right atrium perforation by a pleural drain: Report of a case with survival. J. Thorac. Cardiovasc. Surg., 31:247, 1983.
9. Fingleton, L. J.: Arrow wounds to the heart and mediastinum. Br. J. Surg., 74:126, 1987.
10. Goldman, A., Kotler, M., Goldberg, S., Parameswaran, R., and Pairing, W.: The uses of two-dimensional Doppler echocardiographic techniques preoperatively and postoperatively in a ventricular septal defect caused by penetrating trauma. Ann. Thorac. Surg., 40:625, 1985.
11. Harken, D. E.: Foreign bodies in, and in relation to, the thoracic blood vessels and heart. I. Techniques for approaching and removing foreign bodies from the chambers of the heart. Surg. Gynecol. Obstet., 83:117, 1946.
12. Hassett, A., Moran, J., Sabiston, D. C., and Kisslo, J.: Diagnostic techniques: Utility of echocardiography in the management of patients with penetrating missile wounds of the heart. J. Am. Coll. Cardiol., 7:1151, 1986.
13. Hill, L. L.: Report of a case of successful suture of the heart. Med. Rec., Nov. 29, 1902, p. 846.
14. Homer: The Iliad, Book 16 (translated by Alexander Pope). New York, Heritage Press, 1934, p. 314.
15. Ivatury, R. R., Nallathame, M., Stahl, W., and Rohman, M.: Penetrating cardiac trauma. Ann. Surg., 205:61, 1987.
16. Ivatury, R. R., Rohman, M., Steichen, F. M., Gunduz, Y., Nallathambi, M., and Stahl, W. M.: Penetrating cardiac injuries: Twenty-year experience. Am. Surg., 53:310, 1987.
17. Ivatury, R. R., Shah, P. M., Ito, K., Ramirez-Shon, G., Suarez, F., and Rohman, M.: Emergency room thoracotomy for the resuscitation of patients with "fatal" penetrating injuries of the heart. Ann. Thorac. Surg., 32:377, 1981.
18. Karrel, R., Shaffer, M. A., and Franaszek, J. B.: Emergency diagnosis, resuscitation, and treatment of acute penetrating cardiac trauma. Ann. Emerg. Med., 11:504, 1982.
19. Lindenbaum, G., Larrieu, A. J., Goldberg, S. E., Wolk, L. A., Ghosh, S. C., Ablaza, S. G. G., and Fernandez, J.: Diagnosis and management of traumatic ventricular septal defect. J. Trauma, 27:1289, 1987.

20. Mattox, K. L., Beall, A. C., Jr., Jordan, G. L., Jr., and DeBakey, M. E.: Cardiorrhaphy in the emergency center. J. Thorac. Cardiovasc. Surg. 68:887, 1974.
21. Mattox, K. L., Feliciano, D. V., Burch, J., Beall, A. C., Jr., Jordan, G. L., Jr., and DeBakey, M. E.: Five thousand seven hundred sixty cardiovascular injuries in 4459 patients: Epidemiologic evolution, 1958 to 1987. Ann. Surg., 209:698, 1989.
22. Michelow, B. J., and Bremner, C. G.: Penetrating cardiac injuries: Selective conservatism—favorable or foolish? J. Trauma, 27(4):398, 1987.
23. Miller, F. B., Bond, S. J., Shumate, C. R., Polk, H. C., Jr., and Richardson, J. D.: Diagnostic pericardial window: A safe alternative to exploratory thoracotomy for suspected heart injuries. Arch. Surg., 122:605, 1987.
24. Moreno, C., Moore, E. E., Majure, J. A., and Hopeman, A. R.: Pericardial tamponade: A critical determinant for survival following penetrating cardiac wounds. J. Trauma, 26:821, 1986.
25. Naughton, M. J., Brissie, R. M., Bessey, P. Q., McEachern, M. M., Donald, J. M., Jr., and Laws, H. L.: Demography of penetrating cardiac trauma. Ann. Surg., 209:676, 1989.
26. Rehn, L.: Ueber penetrierende Herzwunden und Herznaht. Arch. f. klin. Chir. 55:315, 1897.
27. Rubio, P. A., and Reul, G. J.: Penetrating cardiac injury by wire thrown from a lawn mower. Int. Surg., 64:9, 1979.
28. Sugg, W. L., Rea, W. J., Ecker, R. R., Webb, W. R., Rose, E. F., and Shaw, R. R.: Penetrating wounds of the heart: An analysis of 459 cases. J. Thorac. Cardiovasc. Surg., 56:5312, 1968.
29. Symbas, P. N.: Cardiothoracic Trauma. Philadelphia, W. B. Saunders Company, 1989.
30. Symbas, P. N., Harlaftis, N., and Waldo, W. J.: Penetrating cardiac wounds: A comparison of different therapeutic methods. Ann. Surg., 183:377, 1976.
31. Symbas, P. N., Vlasis-Hale, S. E., Picone, A. L., and Hatcher, C. R., Jr.: Missiles in the heart. Ann. Thorac. Surg., 48:192, 1989.
32. Tavares, S., Hankins, J. R., Moulton, A. L., Attar, S., Ali, S., Lincoln, S., Green, D. C., Sequeira, A., and McLaughlin, J. S.: Management of penetrating cardiac injuries: The role of emergency room thoracotomy. Ann. Thorac. Surg., 38:183, 1984.
33. Thandroyen, F. T., and Matisonn, R. E.: Penetrating thoracic trauma producing cardiac shunts. J. Thorac. Cardiovasc. Surg., 81:569, 1981.
34. Trinkle, J. K.: Penetrating heart wounds: Difficulty in evaluating clinical series. Ann. Thorac. Surg., 38:181, 1984.
35. Trinkle, J. K., Toom, R., Franz, J., Jr., Arom, K., and Grover, F.: Affairs of the wounded heart: Penetrating cardiac wounds. J. Trauma, 19:467, 1979.
36. Wilson, R. F., and Bassett, J.: Penetrating wounds of the pericardium and its contents. J.A.M.A., 195:105, 1966.
37. Zakharia, A. T.: Analysis of 285 cardiac penetrating injuries in the Lebanon war. J. Cardiovasc. Surg., 28:380, 1987.

IV ──

PATENT DUCTUS ARTERIOSUS, COARCTATION OF THE AORTA, AORTOPULMONARY WINDOW, AND ANOMALIES OF THE AORTIC ARCH

J. William Gaynor, M.D., and David C. Sabiston, Jr., M.D.

PATENT DUCTUS ARTERIOSUS

Nature is neither lazy nor devoid of foresight. Having given the matter thought, she knew in advance that the lung of the fetus, a lung still contained in the uterus and in the process of formation and spared continual motion, does not require the same arrangements of a perfected lung endowed with motion. She has, therefore, anastomosed the pulmonary artery to the aorta.

Galen

Historical Aspects

Galen was the first to describe the ductus arteriosus. Harvey, in 1628, demonstrated the role of the ductus arteriosus in the fetal circulation. The eponym ductus Botalli is a misnomer following a mistranslation of Botallo's work. During the nineteenth century, the morbidity associated with patent ductus arteriosus (PDA) was recognized, and Gibson described the characteristic murmur in 1900. Munro, in 1907, first proposed surgical correction by ligating or crushing the ductus. In 1938 surgical intervention was attempted unsuccessfully in a patient with bacterial endocarditis by Graybiel and colleagues. Because of the friable tissues, the ductus was not able to be successfully ligated, and obliteration was attempted with plicating sutures. The patient survived the operation but with a persistent murmur and died 4 days postoperatively of gastric dilation and aspiration. In 1938, Gross successfully ligated a PDA in a 7-year-old girl, initiating the modern era. Touroff and Vesell in 1940 reported successful division of the ductus in a patient with bacterial endocarditis, curing the infection. An increased incidence of PDA in premature infants was reported by Burnard in 1959. Powell and DeCanq independently reported ligation of a PDA in premature infants in 1963. In 1966, Porstmann first described a nonoperative catheter technique for closure of a PDA using an Ivalon plug.[49] Successful closure of PDA in pre-mature infants by pharmacologic methods was reported independently in 1976 by Friedman and by Heymann.[29] Rashkind and Cuaso reported use of a transcatheter device to close a PDA in an infant. Wessel and co-workers recently reported the use of this device for closure of PDA as an outpatient procedure.

Embryology and Pathologic Anatomy

The ductus arteriosus is derived from the sixth aortic arch and normally extends from the main or left pulmonary artery to the descending aorta just distal to the origin of the left subclavian artery. The ductus is usually 5 to 10 mm. long but is variable, and the diameter varies from a few millimeters to 1 to 2 cm. The aortic orifice is usually larger than the pulmonary orifice. Rarely the ductus may be right-sided, bilateral, or completely absent. *In utero*, blood ejected by the right ventricle flows almost exclusively through the ductus to the lower extremities and placenta, bypassing the high-resistance pulmonary circulation. The relationship of the ductus and the ascending aorta is determined by the presence or absence of associated anomalies. In pulmonary atresia, the pulmonary circulation is ductus dependent; blood flows from the aorta to the pulmonary artery and the ductus may appear to be a downward-directed branch of the aorta. In isthmic hypoplasia or interruption of the aortic arch, the descending aorta may appear to be a continuation of the ductus.

Closure of the ductus occurs at birth during the transition from the fetal to the adult circulation. The lungs expand with the first breath, decreasing the pulmonary vascular resistance, causing increased pulmonary blood flow and arterial oxygen concentration. In normal full-term neonates, functional closure of the ductus occurs within the first 10 to 15 hours of life. Closure occurs after constriction of the smooth muscle layer, causing apposition of intimal cushions in the wall of the ductus, and is mediated by various substances that constrict or dilate ductal smooth muscle. There is proliferation of the intima and media causing mounds, mucoid-filled spaces, and disruption of the internal elastic membrane. Closure by Doppler echocardiography is complete in 96 per cent of full-term infants by 48 hours. In full-term infants, rising arterial oxygen tension causes constriction of the muscle fibers in the wall of the ductus. Prostaglandins of the E series dilate the ductus; therefore, the lower concentrations present after birth potentiate closure. Ductal smooth muscle in premature infants is less sensitive to oxygen-induced constriction and more sensitive to the vasodilatory effects of these prostaglandins. Various other substances may also be mediators of ductal closure. Anatomic closure by fibrosis produces the ligamentum arteriosum connecting the pulmonary artery to the aorta. Closure is complete in 88 per cent of newborns by the age of 8 weeks.

Delayed closure of the ductus is termed prolonged patency, and failure of closure causes persistent patency. Final closure may occur at any age but is uncommon after 6 months. Intermittent closure and reopening of the ductus may also occur. Persistent patency of the ductus may occur as an isolated lesion or may be associated with a variety of other congenital defects. Histologic examination of the wall of a persistently patent ductus reveals significant differences in the subendothelial elastic lamina when compared with a ductus that closes normally, suggesting that a primary defect in the composition of the ductal wall may be responsible for failure of closure. In infants with complex congenital heart disease, pulmonary or systemic blood flow may be dependent on the patency of the ductus, and these infants may suddenly decompensate as the ductus closes. Infusion of prostaglandins to dilate the ductus often produces dramatic improvement and allows stabilization prior to surgical intervention.

Prolonged or persistent patency of the ductus causes a left-to-right shunt of blood with pulmonary congestion and left ventricular volume overload. The magnitude of this shunt depends on the size of the ductus. With a large, nonrestrictive ductus, the level of pulmonary vascular resistance is important in determining the severity of shunting. Shunting occurs throughout systole and diastole and causes diastolic hypotension and possibly impaired perfusion of the brain, lower extremities, and abdominal organs. ST-T wave changes suggestive of subendocardial ischemia have been reported in infants with PDA. Myocardial dysfunction may result and lead to worsening left ventricular failure.

Incidence, Mortality, and Morbidity

Isolated PDA occurs approximately once in 2500 to 5000 live births. The incidence increases greatly with prematurity and with decreasing birth weight. The incidence may be more than 80 per cent in infants weighing less than 1000 gm. and is related to several factors including decreased smooth muscle in the ductal wall, diminished responsiveness of the ductal smooth muscle to oxygen, and possibly elevated circulating levels of vasodilatory prostaglandins. Persistent patency of the ductus occurs more commonly in females than in males, with a 2:1 ratio.

PDA is not a benign entity although prolonged survival has been reported. The mortality of infants with untreated PDA may be as high as 30 per cent. In her classic series, Abbott reported an average age at death of 24 years. In a study of the natural history of untreated PDA, Shapiro and Keys found that 80 per cent of patients with PDA would eventually die of their cardiac disease.[32] In their series, the life expectancy of patients alive at 17 years of age was a mean of 18 years. Forty per cent of patients with PDA died of bacterial endocarditis in the preantibiotic era, and most of the remainder died of congestive heart failure. Campbell calculated that 42 per cent of patients with untreated PDA are dead by 45 years of age. Patients surviving to adulthood may develop congestive heart failure or pulmonary hypertension, with reverse shunting through the ductus. Premature infants with PDA often have associated problems of

prematurity that are aggravated by the left-to-right shunting and abnormal hemodynamics. These problems include respiratory distress syndrome, necrotizing enterocolitis, and intraventricular hemorrhage. Congestive heart failure often results and may respond poorly to medical management. The incidence of long-term sequelae of prematurity such as bronchopulmonary dysplasia may be increased by the presence of a PDA. Young children with persistent patency of the ductus may demonstrate growth retardation. Infants with a large PDA may develop severe pulmonary hypertension at an early age. Calcification is often encountered in older patients and may complicate surgical repair.

Clinical Manifestations and Diagnosis

The signs and symptoms of PDA depend on the size of the ductus, the pulmonary vascular resistance, the age at presentation, and associated anomalies. Full-term infants usually do not become symptomatic until the pulmonary vascular resistance decreases at 6 to 8 weeks of life, allowing a significant left-to-right shunt. Because premature infants have less smooth muscle in the pulmonary arterioles, vascular resistance decreases earlier and symptoms may develop during the first week of life. In very-low-birth-weight infants (less than 1000 gm.), as many as 60 per cent may show ductal shunting echocardiographically at 2 and 3 days of life without the presence of a murmur or other clinical signs of a PDA. Approximately 40 per cent of these infants eventually develop a hemodynamically significant left-to-right shunt. Infants with a birth weight greater than 1000 gm. have a much lower risk of developing a clinically significant shunt even if a murmur is present.

A large, hemodynamically significant PDA usually presents in infancy with congestive heart failure. Afflicted infants are irritable, tachycardic, and tachypneic and take feedings poorly. Physical examination usually reveals evidence of a hyperdynamic circulation, with a hyperactive precordium and bounding peripheral pulses. The systolic blood pressure is usually normal, but diastolic hypotension may be present secondary to the large left-to-right shunt. Auscultation reveals a systolic or continuous murmur often termed a machinery murmur, which is heard best in the pulmonic area and radiates toward the middle third of the clavicle. The classic description of this murmur was provided by Gibson[23a]:

. . . a murmur which may be regarded as almost pathognomonic. Beginning distinctly after the first sound, it accompanies the latter part of that sound, occupies the short pause, accompanies the second sound, which may be accentuated in the pulmonary area, or may be, and often is, doubled, and finally dies away during the long pause.

Absence of the characteristic murmur does not, however, exclude the presence of a PDA, especially in premature infants. A mid-diastolic apical rumble may follow increased flow across the mitral valve. If cardiac failure is present, a gallop may also be heard. Hepatomegaly is frequently present. Cyanosis is not present in uncomplicated isolated PDA.

The diagnosis of PDA can often be made noninvasively, and the physical examination alone may be diagnostic. The chest film often shows cardiomegaly; and if cardiac failure is present, pulmonary congestion may be observed. In older infants, children, and adults, the electrocardiogram (ECG) may reveal left ventricular hypertrophy. Two-dimensional echocardiography may demonstrate the ductus and associated anomalies. The left atrial and aortic root diameters can be measured, and if their ratio is greater than 1.4 to 1.5, a left-to-right shunt is likely. However, this ratio may be normal in infants who have PDA and have been fluid restricted or treated with diuretics.[8] Continuous wave and pulsed Doppler echocardiography demonstrate abnormal aortic flow patterns and estimate the magnitude of ductal flow. Echocardiography may provide evidence of significant left-to-right shunting before it becomes clinically apparent.[26] Color-flow Doppler imaging also demonstrates flow in a

PDA and reveals the direction of shunting. Formal cardiac catheterization is not required in children and young adults with classic findings and should be reserved for older patients and those with atypical findings, suspicion of associated anomalies, or pulmonary hypertension. Echocardiography is especially useful to exclude associated anomalies.

Patients with a moderate-sized PDA may remain asymptomatic until the second or third decade of life when left ventricular failure occurs. The earliest symptom is usually dyspnea or exertion, followed by signs and symptoms of increasing congestive heart failure. Auscultation reveals the typical murmur. The ECG and chest film may show evidence of left ventricular enlargement and hypertrophy. A small PDA usually causes no symptoms or growth retardation. A systolic or continuous murmur is present and the ECG and chest film usually appear to be normal. Some patients with PDA present with bacterial endocarditis as the first clinical manifestation of their disorder. Bacterial endocarditis usually develops at the pulmonary orifice of the ductus.

Aneurysmal dilation and rupture of the ductus arteriosus, although rare, may occur in infants or adults. Ductal aneurysm was first described by Martin in 1827. Closure of the pulmonary orifice with delayed closure of the aortic orifice of the ductus, exposing the ductal tissue to systemic blood pressure, was proposed as the most likely etiologic factor by Taussig in 1947. Degenerative changes in the ductal wall may also be a factor. Ductus arteriosus aneurysm may present as a mediastinal mass and must be considered in the differential diagnosis.

The development of pulmonary hypertension in a patient with PDA is a serious prognostic sign. Pulmonary hypertension may be encountered in children who are under 2 years of age and have a nonrestrictive ductus with greatly increased pulmonary blood flow; however, significant pulmonary hypertension is usually noted only in older patients with PDA. The elevated pulmonary artery pressures may be secondary to the increased blood flow and may become normal after surgical closure of the PDA. In some patients, irreversible pulmonary vascular changes occur and pulmonary hypertension persists after closure of the PDA.

Management

The presence of a persistent PDA in a child or adult is sufficient indication for surgical closure because of the increased mortality and risk of endocarditis. In symptomatic patients, closure should be performed when the diagnosis is made. In asymptomatic children, intervention can be postponed, if desired, but should be done in the preschool years. Older patients should have the ductus closed when the diagnosis is made. However, if severe pulmonary hypertension has occurred with reversal of the ductal shunt, closure may not improve symptoms and is associated with a higher mortality. The management of PDA in premature infants remains controversial.

SURGICAL PROCEDURES. Gross initially used simple ligation to interrupt the PDA. Because of difficulties with recanalization, he attempted ligation and wrapping with cellophane to induce fibrosis; however, recanalization still occurred. Touroff and Vesell were the first to report division of a PDA. They were attempting to ligate a PDA in a patient with bacterial endocarditis and, when significant hemorrhage occurred, successfully divided the ductus to control the bleeding. Gross pioneered division of the PDA as a therapy of choice because of difficulties with recanalization. Blalock suggested ligation with multiple transfixion sutures as the preferred method because of concern about the safety of ductal division. In children, either division or multiple suture ligation of the ductus is appropriate. Ligation is usually done in neonates because of its simplicity and rare, if any, recurrences. In adults with a large ductus (10 mm. or more) or patients with pulmonary hypertension, division is indicated.

The operation may be done through either a left anterior or posterior thoracotomy. The lung is retracted, and an incision is

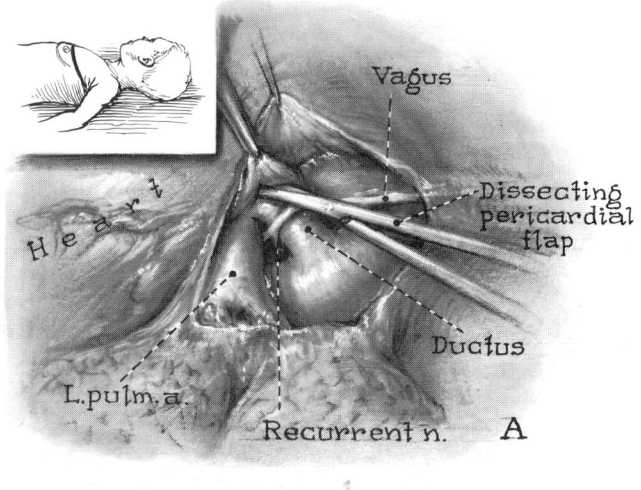

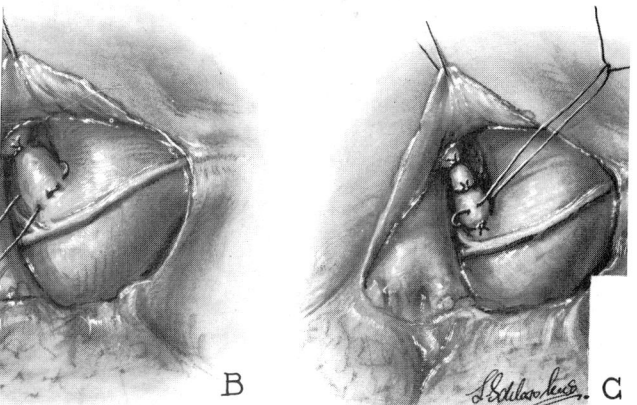

Figure 1. Operative treatment of PDA by ligation. Incision is anterolateral in the third interspace. In females, the incision circles beneath the breast. Elevation of pericardial lappet exposes the ductus. A pursestring suture, which does not enter the lumen, is placed at each end, and perforating mattress sutures are placed in between. The ductus should be obliterated over an 8- to 10-mm. distance.

made in the pleura overlying the pulmonary artery between the phrenic and vagus nerves. The ductus is exposed, taking care to avoid damage to the recurrent laryngeal nerve. After the ductus has been mobilized, it may be obliterated with multiple suture ligatures (Fig. 1) or divided (Fig. 2). If division is planned, vascular clamps are placed across the ductus, which is then divided. Closure of each end is accomplished with two rows of nonabsorbable suture. If the ductus is particularly short and wide, it may be necessary to cross-clamp the aorta above and below the ductus as in a coarctation repair. The pulmonary end of the ductus is clamped and the ductus is divided at the aorta, leaving a sufficient margin for closure. The opening in the aorta is closed and the cross-clamps are removed. The pulmonary end of the ductus is closed and the clamp is removed.

A calcified ductus in older patients presents a difficult surgical problem. Simple ligation or division may not be possible in patients with a PDA that has diffuse circumferential calcification. Several techniques using cardiopulmonary bypass and closure from within the aorta or pulmonary artery have been described.

In neonates, single or double ligation is usually the procedure of choice. Closure of the ductus in neonates by applying one or two surgical clips has also been described.[2] In recent years, several authors have advocated surgical closure of the ductus in the neonatal intensive care unit rather than transporting critically ill neonates to the operating room.

Closure of a PDA in patients with pulmonary hypertension presents special difficulties. In patients with pulmonary vascular changes, closure may cause further elevation of the pulmonary pressures, causing right ventricular failure. In 1956 Ellis

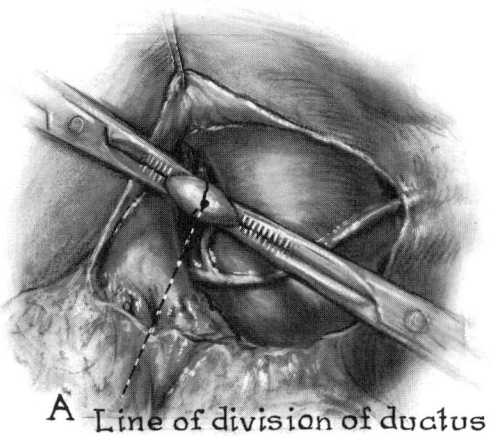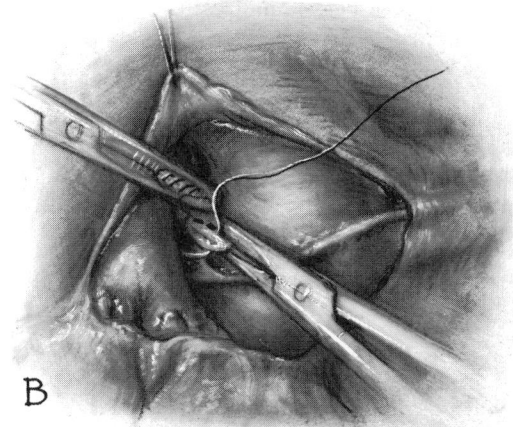

A Line of division of ductus   B

Figure 2. Treatment of PDA by division. Anterolateral third interspace incision is used for exposure, as for ligation. A thin occluding clamp is placed at each end, and the ductus is divided. Pressing the clamp against the pulmonary artery or aorta after division reduces the likelihood of slipping. Suture of the ductus is by a continuous mattress suture adjacent to the clamp, followed by whipstitch backup over the free edge. Suture of the pulmonary artery is easier when done from the patient's right side.

and associates reported closure of a PDA in 71 patients with pulmonary hypertension; overall mortality was 18 per cent and was 56 per cent in patients with a right-to-left shunt. John and co-workers in 1981 reported five deaths after PDA closure in 22 patients with pulmonary artery pressures greater than 70 mm. Hg.[31] Patients with marked pulmonary hypertension and right-to-left shunt who survive closure may not improve, and progressive cor pulmonale may develop.

Surgical closure of a PDA may be complicated by hemorrhage, pneumothorax, chylothorax, left recurrent nerve damage, and infection. Phrenic nerve paralysis has also been reported after closure of a PDA. Great care must be exercised in dissecting or placing clamps on the ductus, because the ductal tissue may be friable and a tear may cause hemorrhage that is difficult to control. Inadvertent ligation or division of the left pulmonary artery has been reported after attempted ductal ligation. In the early days of surgical closure of PDA, recanalization constituted a major problem; however, in the current era the incidence of recurrent ductal patency should approach zero after division or multiple suture ligation.

NONOPERATIVE THERAPY. In recent years there has been increasing interest in the nonoperative closure of PDA. Porstmann, in 1966, successfully used a transcatheter technique to block a PDA with an Ivalon plug.[49] Rashkind and Cuaso in 1979 used a double umbrella device inserted via a right-sided catheter to close the ductus.[39] In 1986 Porstmann reported long-term follow-up of 208 patients who had closure of a PDA with an Ivalon plug.[49] Ductal closure was successful in 94.7 per cent of the patients. There were no deaths, and no patient required thoracotomy for retrieval of a dislodged plug. Arterial complications occurred in 16 patients, 9 of whom required surgical intervention. In 1987 Rashkind and colleagues reported attempted ductal closure by using a double umbrella device in 146 patients.[39] Embolization occurred after release in 19 patients, 1 of whom required emergency operation. Wessel and co-workers reported transcatheter closure using Rashkind's device in 23 children, 19 of whom were discharged on the day of the procedure. Transcatheter techniques are potentially useful in patients who are poor candidates for surgical therapy. However, these techniques are still being investigated, and the exact role of transcatheter techniques in the management of PDA has not been determined.

MANAGEMENT OF PDA IN PREMATURE INFANTS. Premature infants face many problems, including immature lungs and hyaline membrane disease. These infants often require mechanical ventilation and oxygen therapy. An increased incidence of PDA is found with increasing prematurity and decreasing birth weight. The additional burden on the heart and lungs imposed by the left-to-right shunt may be poorly tolerated. The increased pulmonary blood flow causes increased pulmonary arterial pressures, decreased lung compliance, hypercarbia, and hypoxia often necessitating prolonged mechanical ventilation, which may cause an increased incidence of bronchopulmonary dysplasia and retrolental fibroplasia. The abnormal hemodynamics may potentiate other problems of prematurity such as necrotizing enterocolitis and intraventricular hemorrhage. It is sometimes difficult to differentiate the effects of a PDA from the underlying pulmonary disease. If the pulmonary disease is severe, ligation of the PDA may produce little or no improvement. A hemodynamically significant PDA is suggested by the presence of a hyperactive precordium, a continuous murmur, and bounding pulses. The chest film usually reveals cardiomegaly, pulmonary congestion, and the changes of hyaline membrane disease. Echocardiography is very useful in these patients in determining the presence of a significant left-to-right shunt.

Management of PDA in premature infants is controversial because the ductus may close as the child matures. There is an increased incidence of PDA in neonatal units in which fluids are not restricted. Some infants can be managed satisfactorily with fluid restriction and diuretics. Anemia worsens the heart failure, and transfusion of packed red blood cells may be necessary. Digitalis is rarely used in these infants because there is little evidence of therapeutic benefit and a high incidence of toxicity.

In some infants, conservative therapy fails. If a child with evidence of left-to-right shunting demonstrates persistent congestive heart failure, need for continuing mechanical ventilation, or inability to receive adequate nutrition secondary to fluid restriction, further intervention is indicated. Two therapeutic options are available. Pharmacologic closure can be attempted with prostaglandin inhibitors such as indomethacin.[29] Final closure may be achieved in more than 70 per cent of infants, although the ductus may reopen transiently in some children. Reopening occurs most frequently in the most premature infants and may be treated with a second course of indomethacin, but the success rate is lower. The success of therapy with indomethacin is related to the birth weight and postnatal age of the infant.[1] Side effects of indomethacin include renal dysfunction, hyponatremia, impaired platelet function, and gastrointestinal hemorrhage. Impaired left ventricular diastolic function has been reported following administration of indomethacin and may worsen pulmonary edema. No adverse long-term sequelae of successful indomethacin therapy have been identified. Surgical closure can be used if there is a contraindication to indomethacin or failure of the PDA to close. In some centers, surgical intervention is the primary therapy after conservative medical therapy fails. A national collaborative trial was done to compare methods of treatment.[23] Indomethacin as primary therapy was compared with indomethacin as reserve therapy for conventional medical treatment and with operation as primary therapy. The use of indomethacin significantly reduced the need for surgical closure of the PDA. There was an increased incidence of bleeding other than intraventricular hemorrhage in infants receiving indomethacin as primary therapy, but no other adverse results. The incidence of retinopathy of prematurity was higher in the group having primary surgical closure. There was no difference in outcome if the indomethacin was given as first-line therapy or after failure of conservative medical therapy.

Early closure of a PDA in premature infants has been shown to decrease the need for mechanical ventilation and to decrease complications such as bronchopulmonary dysplasia, necrotizing enterocolitis, and intolerance of enteral feeding. Closure with indomethacin is as effective as surgical ligation in preventing these complications. There has been a trend toward earlier intervention in premature infants, and the prophylactic use of indomethacin before the development of a hemodynamically significant shunt has been suggested.[14] Studies suggest that indomethacin is indicated in very-low-birth-weight infants (less than 1000 gm.) when clinical signs of a PDA first appear, because most of these infants develop significant shunting. In infants with a birth weight more than 1000 gm., there is no benefit to initiation of therapy before the development of significant shunting. If indomethacin fails to close the ductus or if the ductus closes and reopens, surgical ligation is indicated. A recent study has reported a 42 per cent failure rate with indomethacin in infants of very low birth weight and suggested that primary surgical closure is more predictable, with minimal morbidity.[38]

Results

Surgical closure of an isolated PDA has become a very safe procedure. Operative mortality approaches zero even in critically ill neonates. In premature infants, hospital mortality and long-term results depend primarily on associated pulmonary disease, coexistent anomalies, and the degree of prematurity. Mortality is increased and long-term results are poor in older patients with a calcified ductus and are poorest in those patients with severe pulmonary hypertension and reverse shunting. Most patients with PDA become functionally normal with a normal life expectancy after closure.

COARCTATION OF THE AORTA

Coarctation is derived from the Latin *coarctatio* (a drawing or pressing together) and is defined as a narrowing that diminishes the lumen and produces an obstruction to the flow of blood. The lesion may be a definite, localized obstruction or may be a diffusely narrowed segment, which is termed tubular hypoplasia. Localized coarctation and tubular hypoplasia may occur separately or may coexist. Isolated coarctation may occur at any site in the aorta, but the most common location is at the site of the insertion of the ductus (or ligamentum) arteriosus. Coarctation of the abdominal aorta is present in approximately 2 per cent of the patients. Externally the aorta appears to be sharply indented or constricted, and internally an obstructing diaphragm is present on the posterior wall (located preductally, postductally, or paraductally). The obstruction is usually more marked than is apparent by external appearance. The "shelf" consists of an infolding of the aortic media with a ridge of intimal hyperplasia. Tubular hypoplasia most often occurs in the aortic isthmus (the segment of aorta between the left subclavian artery and the insertion of the ductus arteriosus). Localized coarctation of the aorta and tubular hypoplasia are part of a spectrum of disorders ranging from pseudocoarctation (a kinking or buckling of the aorta without producing obstruction to flow) to complete interruption of the aorta.

Historical Aspects

Paris provided the first accurate description of coarctation of the aorta in 1791. Meckel, in 1750, and Morgagni, in 1760, had reported finding aortic narrowing at autopsy. Throughout the nineteenth century, coarctation of the aorta was considered a rare disorder. Legrand, in 1835, made the first premortem diagnosis of obstruction of the thoracic aorta. In 1903, Bonnet published an extensive review and distinguished between preductal coarctation (infantile) and postductal coarctation (adult). In 1928, Abbott documented 200 cases of coarctation in patients over 2 years of age. This historic report stimulated much interest in the disorder, and in 1944, Blalock and Park proposed anastomosis of the left subclavian artery to the descending aorta to bypass the obstruction.[10] In the same year, Crafoord and Nylin performed the first surgical correction with resection of the coarctation and end-to-end anastomosis. Gross and Hufnagel independently performed a similar procedure in 1945. Subsequently, Gross was the first to use aortic homografts to replace the narrowed segment of aorta. In 1951 Lynxwiler and colleagues reported the first successful repair of coarctation in an infant. The use of prosthetic onlay grafts was reported by Vossschulte in 1957, and in 1966 Waldhausen and Nahrwold described the subclavian flap aortoplasty. In recent years there has been increasing interest in the use of percutaneous transluminal angioplasty for native and recurrent coarctation.

Embryology and Pathologic Anatomy

The cause of coarctation of the aorta and tubular hypoplasia is still controversial. Two major theories have been proposed to explain the embryonic development of aortic narrowing. It has been proposed that in some patients, tissue from the ductus arteriosus extends circumferentially into the aortic wall; contraction and fibrosis of this tissue at the time of ductal closure could lead to a localized narrowing. A second hypothesis proposes that coarctation results from abnormal fetal blood flow patterns. In the normal fetus, blood flow across the aortic isthmus is much less than flow in either the ascending aorta or the descending aorta (which receives ductal blood flow), and thus the diameter of the isthmus is less than the diameter of either the ascending or descending aorta. An increased incidence of coarctation is found with certain ventricular septal defects (those producing left ventricular outflow tract obstruction), aortic stenosis, and mitral valve anomalies; all of these anomalies diminish ascending aortic flow and increase ductal flow. The resultant decrease in flow across the isthmus leads to abnormal narrowing of the isthmus.

Incidence and Associated Anomalies

Coarctation of the aorta represents 5 to 10 per cent of congenital heart disease, and the autopsy incidence is 1 per 3000 to 4000 autopsies. With isolated coarctation, males predominate; but there is no sex difference in patients with more complex lesions. Several anomalies occur commonly in patients with coarctation of the aorta: bicuspid aortic valve, ventricular septal defect, PDA, and various mitral valve disorders. Congenital aortic stenosis, aortic atresia, and the hypoplastic left heart syndrome may occur with coarctation, in addition to bicuspid aortic valves. A study by Moene and associates revealed that up to 70 per cent of ventricular septal defects occurring in association with coarctation are of types characterized by frequent spontaneous closure. Shone's syndrome is the complex of parachute mitral valve, cor triatriatum, subaortic stenosis, and coarctation. There are reports of familial occurrences of coarctation, and 15 to 36 per cent of patients with Turner's syndrome have a coarctation.[11] There is also an increased incidence of aortic arch anomalies, especially interrupted arch, in patients with Di-

George's syndrome. Patients with severe associated defects tend to have tubular hypoplasia, rather than isolated coarctation.

Clinical Manifestations

The age of presentation and the mode of presentation depend on the location of the coarctation and the associated anomalies. When the obstruction is preductal, there is an increased incidence of other cardiac defects and the patients usually present in infancy with congestive heart failure. Preductal coarctation usually consists of tubular hypoplasia terminating in an obstructing shelf. Paraductal and postductal coarctation are usually isolated obstructions and have a low incidence of associated defects. Preductal coarctation was considered by Bonnet to be the infantile form because of its usual presentation in infancy. However, the terms infantile and adult are inappropriate descriptions of preductal and postductal coarctation, because patients with the infantile form can survive to adulthood, and some patients with the adult type develop clinical manifestations in infancy.

Preductal coarctation and even interruption of the aortic arch may not seriously alter the normal fetal circulation and therefore do not provide a stimulus to the development of collateral circulation *in utero*. Infants with severe narrowing may appear normal at birth and have palpable femoral pulses because a PDA allows blood flow around the obstructing shelf. Symptoms usually develop as the PDA closes, resulting in significant aortic obstruction. The infant becomes irritable, tachypneic, and uninterested in feeding. A systolic murmur may be present over the left precordium and posteriorly between the scapulae. Although the blood pressure is difficult to record accurately in neonates, moderate upper extremity hypertension and an arm-leg systolic pressure gradient are usually present. These findings may be absent in critically ill infants with a low cardiac output. Hypotension, oliguria, and severe metabolic acidosis may be present in severely ill infants. In severe obstruction or complete aortic interruption, the pulmonary artery pulse may be palpated in the femoral arteries when the ductus is open, obscuring the diagnosis. Differential cyanosis may be present between the upper and lower extremities. In neonates, there are no signs of collateral circulation because collateral vessels become clinically apparent only with time.

Older children and adults often present with unexplained hypertension or complications of hypertension. Some may be entirely asymptomatic for many years and lead an active life. Presenting complaints include headache, epistaxis, visual disturbances, and exertional dyspnea. Some patients present with a cerebrovascular accident (secondary to an aneurysm of the circle of Willis), aortic rupture, dissecting aneurysm, or bacterial endocarditis. Many cases are discovered during evaluation of hypertension or of a murmur heard on routine examination.

Diagnosis

The diagnosis of coarctation can usually be made clinically and depends on evidence of obstruction to blood flow in the thoracic aorta. The findings include hypertension, a systolic pressure gradient between the arms and legs, a systolic murmur heard over the left precordium and posteriorly between the scapulae, and diminished or absent femoral pulses with a delayed upstroke. Presence of an anterior diastolic murmur may indicate aortic regurgitation secondary to a bicuspid aortic valve. Anomalous origin of the right subclavian artery can occur with the orifice distal to the coarctation. Blood pressure measurements must be obtained in both arms because the orifice of either subclavian artery may be involved in the coarctation. There may be evidence of collateral circulation in older children and adults. The collateral circulation involves branches of the subclavian arteries that are proximal to the obstruction, including the internal mammary, vertebral, thyrocervical, and costo-

cervical arteries. These vessels anastomose with intercostal vessels and other arteries distal to the obstruction. Enlarged collateral vessels may be observed or palpated in the infrascapular region; bruits may be audible as well. Aneurysmal dilation of the intercostal arteries can occur and may complicate surgical reconstruction. Poststenotic dilation of the descending aorta is common, and, rarely, an aneurysm of the ascending or descending aorta may occur.

The ECG in infancy may reveal right, left, or biventricular hypertrophy. In older children and adults, it may be normal or demonstrate evidence of left ventricular hypertrophy, often with a "strain" pattern. The chest film is usually helpful, demonstrating cardiomegaly with left ventricular hypertrophy. In infants with heart failure, extreme cardiomegaly and pulmonary congestion may be present. Rib notching secondary to the enlarged, tortuous intercostal vessels is almost pathognomonic (Fig. 3) and was first described by Meckel in 1827. Rosler, in 1928, and Railsback and Dock, in 1929, emphasized the presence of rib notching roentgenographically. These erosions occur on the underside of the rib and may be unilateral if the orifice of the left subclavian artery is narrowed by the coarctation or arises distal to the obstruction, or if there is anomalous origin of the right subclavian artery distal to the coarctation. Absence of rib notching in older patients may indicate a poor collateral circulation. The "3" sign may be present, consisting of proximal enlargement of the aorta, aortic constriction, and poststenotic dilation (Fig. 3).

Angiocardiography remains the most objective method of demonstrating the coarctation, providing evidence of the location and extent of narrowing, the involvement of the great vessels, and the extent of collateral circulation. The pressure gradient can be measured, and associated cardiac defects can be evaluated by cardiac catheterization. Newer methods of noninvasive imaging also provide valuable information. Two-dimensional echocardiography with spectral and color-flow Doppler echocardiography may demonstrate the site of obstruction, suggest or exclude associated anomalies, and provide an estimate of the arterial pressure gradient.[44] Computed tomography, digital subtraction angiography, and magnetic resonance imaging[45] are also helpful and can be used postoperatively to assess the result.

Natural History

The natural history of untreated coarctation of the aorta depends on the age at presentation and associated anomalies. Symptomatic infants have a high mortality, depending on the severity of the coarctation and the presence of associated defects. Patients surviving until adulthood have a greatly decreased life expectancy. In 1928, before the development of antibiotics and surgical correction of coarctation, Abbott reviewed 200 cases of coarctation confirmed at autopsy in patients older than 2 years of age. Death occurred in 74 per cent of the patients by 40 years of age, and the average age of death was 32 years. However, the lesion does not preclude prolonged survival, because one patient lived to the age of 92. The most common causes of death were spontaneous rupture of the aorta, bacterial endocarditis, and cerebral hemorrhage. Reifenstein and colleagues reported 104 cases of coarctation in 1947. The average age of death was 35 years; 23 per cent of the patients died of aortic rupture, 22 per cent of bacterial endocarditis or aortitis, 18 per cent of congestive heart failure, and 11 per cent of cerebrovascular accident. Rupture of the aorta or an intracranial aneurysm usually occurred in the second or third decade of life. Endocarditis was most commonly associated with a bicuspid aortic valve. Campbell in 1970 calculated that of patients with coarctation surviving the first 2 years of life, 25 per cent would die by 20 years of age, 50 per cent by 32 years of age, 75 per cent by 46 years of age, and 90 per cent by 58 years of age. The coronary arteries in patients with untreated coarctation show striking changes, with intimal degeneration, medial thick-

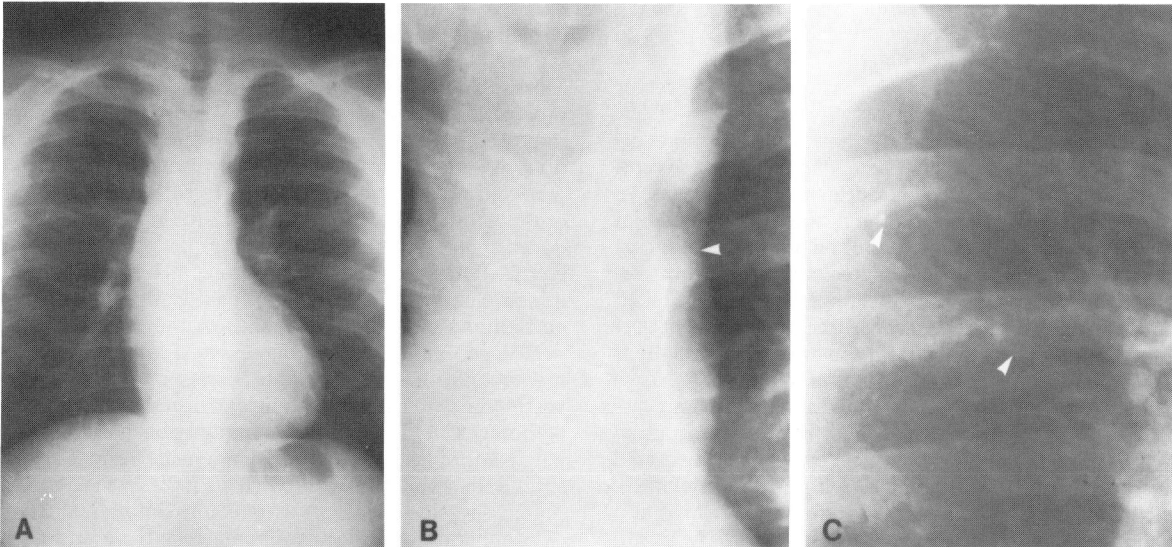

Figure 3. Patient with coarctation of the aorta. *A,* Chest roentgenogram. *B,* Detail demonstrating "3" sign formed by proximal dilated aorta, area of constriction (arrow), and distal dilated aorta. *C,* Detail demonstrating rib notching (arrows) secondary to dilated intercostal vessels. (Courtesy of Dr. James Chen.)

ening, and increased mineralization. These changes can be demonstrated even in young children and may predispose patients to early atherosclerosis. Hypertension secondary to the coarctation is thought to be the most important factor in the pathogenesis of these changes. The advent of surgical therapy has significantly increased the life expectancy of patients with coarctation, although they do not become fully normal.

Pseudocoarctation, first reported by Souders and associates in 1951, is a buckling or kinking of the aorta that does not produce an obstruction to flow. The chest film usually reveals an abnormal aortic contour mimicking a left superior mediastinal mass. There is no evidence of collateral circulation, and the diagnosis is confirmed by aortography demonstrating a tortuous, kinked aorta with no measurable pressure gradient.

Physiology of Hypertension

The pathogenesis of hypertension in coarctation is multifactorial, and the most prominent causes appear to be mechanical and renal factors. Abbott emphasized the importance of hypertension in coarctation of the aorta. Rytand and others noted an increase in vascular resistance proximal and distal to the narrowed segment causing diastolic hypertension and suggested that coarctation might be analogous to Goldblatt's model of hypertension. Gupta and Wiggers showed that it was necessary to diminish the aortic lumen by 45 to 55 per cent to cause an elevation in the blood pressure and suggested that mechanical factors alone were responsible for the hypertension. Scott and Bahnson in 1951 were the first to definitively demonstrate the role of the kidneys in the pathogenesis of the hypertension of coarctation. In experimental coarctation, they showed that hypertension could be eliminated by transplanting one kidney to the neck (proximal to the obstruction) with contralateral nephrectomy. Renal blood flow is usually normal in patients with coarctation, and studies of the renin-angiotensin system have yielded conflicting results. Renin and angiotensin levels have been reported to be normal in both experimental animals and patients with coarctation. However, Bagby and co-workers, using a canine model of coarctation, were able to show greater than expected elevation of plasma renin during sodium restriction.[5] During low, normal, and high sodium intake, plasma volume, extracellular volume, and plasma renin activity were higher in coarcted animals than in control animals. Alpert and colleagues showed significant increases in plasma renin activity during volume depletion in children with coarctation compared with normal individuals or patients with essential hyperten-

sion. Plasma renin activity is initially elevated and leads to an increase in plasma volume that restores renal perfusion to normal levels, normalizing plasma renin activity, and the hypertension is maintained by volume expansion. It is hypothesized that coarctation hypertension is a variant of the single-clip single-kidney Goldblatt model. Angiotensin blockade has not been consistently useful in treating the hypertension of coarctation. Ferguson and co-workers, by using a model of coarctation similar to that of Scott and Bahnson, showed that animals with coarctation developed generalized hypertension; but when a graft was used to re-establish renal blood flow, hypertension developed only proximal to the stenosis. Other investigators have shown abnormal rigidity of the prestenotic aortic wall and abnormal baroreceptor function.

Management

Nonsurgical therapy has only a small role in the management of patients with coarctation, and the presence of coarctation is generally sufficient indication for surgical correction. The major questions are the timing and method of repair. Symptomatic infants usually require intervention, although a few improve with conservative medical treatment of congestive heart failure and can then undergo elective surgical correction. A major advance in the treatment of critically ill neonates with coarctation and interrupted aortic arch has been the introduction of prostaglandin E_1 therapy.[28] Infusion of prostaglandin E_1 can reopen and maintain patency of the ductus arteriosus in many neonates and allow perfusion of the lower body with correction of the severe metabolic acidosis and oliguria that are often present. Stabilization of these severely ill patients allows surgical correction to be accomplished under more optimal conditions with decreased mortality.

The timing of elective repair of coarctation of the aorta is perhaps the most important determinant of surgical outcome. Repair in late childhood or adulthood, although providing relief of some symptoms, has an increased incidence of persistent hypertension with its associated morbidity. Repair in infancy using the classic method of resection and end-to-end anastomosis was reported to cause a high incidence (up to 60 per cent) of residual or recurrent stenosis, although recent series report a much lower incidence. Alternative techniques of repair were developed to allow repair at an earlier age with fewer recoarctations. The current trend is for elective repair at an early age, and some authors believe that repair should be undertaken at the time of diagnosis in symptomatic and asymptomatic infants to prevent development of complications.[13] Others prefer elective repair in asymptomatic children at the age of 1 to 6 years to decrease the recoarctation rate.

SURGICAL PROCEDURES. The classic method of repair used by Crafoord and by Gross is resection of the area of obstruction with primary end-to-end anastomosis. A left thoracotomy is performed, and an incision is made in the pleura overlying the coarctation. The proximal aorta, the left subclavian artery, the area of coarctation, and the ligamentum arteriosum are dissected first, with an effort to avoid damage to the recurrent laryngeal nerve (Fig. 4). The ductus or ligamentum is divided, greatly increasing the mobility of the aorta. Care is taken not to injure any enlarged intercostal arteries during the dissection. It may be necessary to divide these arteries, especially if aneurysmal dilation has occurred; but it is preferable to preserve all collaterals. The aorta is cross-clamped proximally and distally and the area of constriction is excised. To obtain an optimal result, it is absolutely necessary to resect the entire constricted segment and construct the anastomosis without tension (Fig. 5). Even in infants with tubular hypoplasia, the aorta is elastic and can usually be mobilized sufficiently to allow primary repair. The earliest repairs used a continuous silk suture. An unacceptable rate of restenosis resulted, probably secondary to failure of the anastomosis to grow. Most surgeons currently use interrupted sutures, fine nonabsorbable monofilament sutures (polypropylene), or fine absorbable monofilament sutures (polydioxane) to improve results. Several groups have recently reported excellent results with resection and primary anastomosis even in neonates.[15,34] Experimental work has shown that the use of the absorbable monofilament suture for end-to-end anastomosis permits significant growth of the suture line. Advantages of the classic repair include complete resection of abnormal tissue, preservation of normal vascular anatomy, and no requirement for prosthetic material.

In some patients with tubular hypoplasia and some older patients with inelastic aortas, it is not possible to resect the narrowed segment completely and restore aortic continuity by primary anastomosis. Gross pioneered the use of aortic homografts to bridge the gap in these patients. In 1962, he reported follow-up of 70 patients who had undergone homograft inser-tion. No complications other than calcification of the graft (which was present in less than 50 per cent of the patients) were reported, and there were no cases of aneurysmal formations. Morris, Cooley, DeBakey, and Crawford introduced the use of prosthetic interposition grafts in 1960. Tube grafts are rarely indicated but may be useful in patients with complex coarctation, recurrent coarctation, or aneurysmal formation.

Because of early unsatisfactory results, especially in infants, other techniques were developed. In 1957, Vossschulte introduced the prosthetic patch onlay graft technique. The area of constriction is incised, and a Dacron patch is used to enlarge the lumen. Yee and associates reported the use of Gore-Tex patches and emphasized the advantages of the technique, including decreased operative time, decreased dissection, maximal augmentation of the area of stenosis, preservation of the collateral vessels, and no need for sacrifice of normal vascular structures. A thoracotomy incision has commonly been used for synthetic patch aortoplasty. However, Ungerleider and Ebert demonstrated the applicability of patch aortoplasty via a median sternotomy in selected infants who require simultaneous correction of coarctation and intracardiac defects. Sade and co-workers have documented growth of the posterior wall of the aorta after patch aortoplasty. Patch aortoplasty is highly effective in relieving the aortic obstruction, with a low incidence of restenosis and persistent hypertension (at rest and following exercise). The use of prosthetic material may predispose to infection. Aneurysmal dilation of the posterior aortic wall opposite the prosthetic patch has been reported with increasing frequency (up to 38 per cent of patients followed long term), but the true incidence is unknown. Aneurysm formation may be related to weakening at the posterior wall following resection of the intimal shelf. Patch aortoplasty is very useful in surgical therapy of recurrent coarctation. All patients who have had patch aortoplasty must be followed closely for monitoring development of an aneurysm. A recent review of 29 children following patch aortoplasty reported a 29 per cent incidence of development of aneurysms. This study suggested that use of Gore-Tex, rather than Dacron, as the patch decreased the risk of development of aneurysm.[12] Children who underwent patch aortoplasty for recoarctation, rather than as a primary procedure, may have a diminished risk

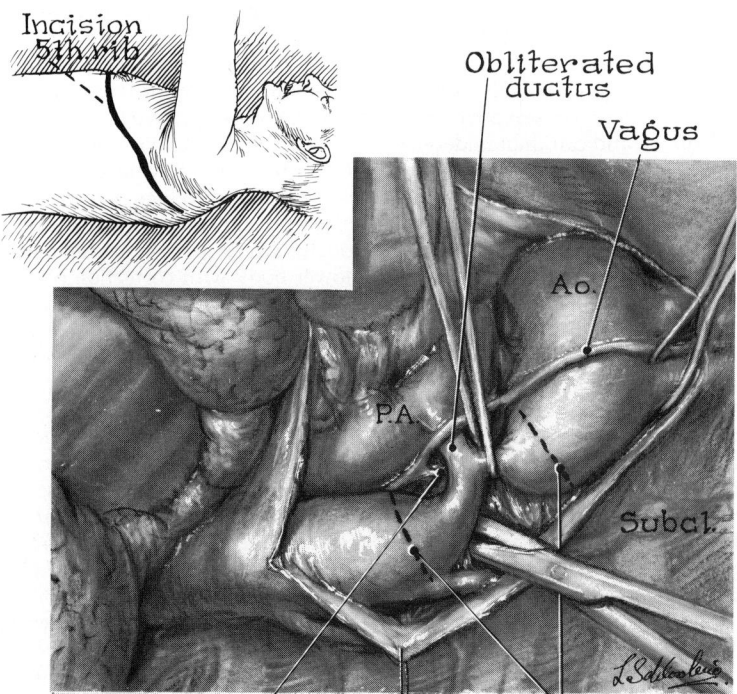

Figure 4. Operative exposure for resection of coarctation of the aorta is through the bed of the fifth rib. The entire rib is removed from neck to cartilage. The constricted segment is usually held medially by an obliterated ductus, division of which allows considerable mobility. The coarctation is held forward to facilitate dissection posteriorly. Large intercostal arteries must be carefully avoided. Division of the aorta should be through a point of normal diameter.

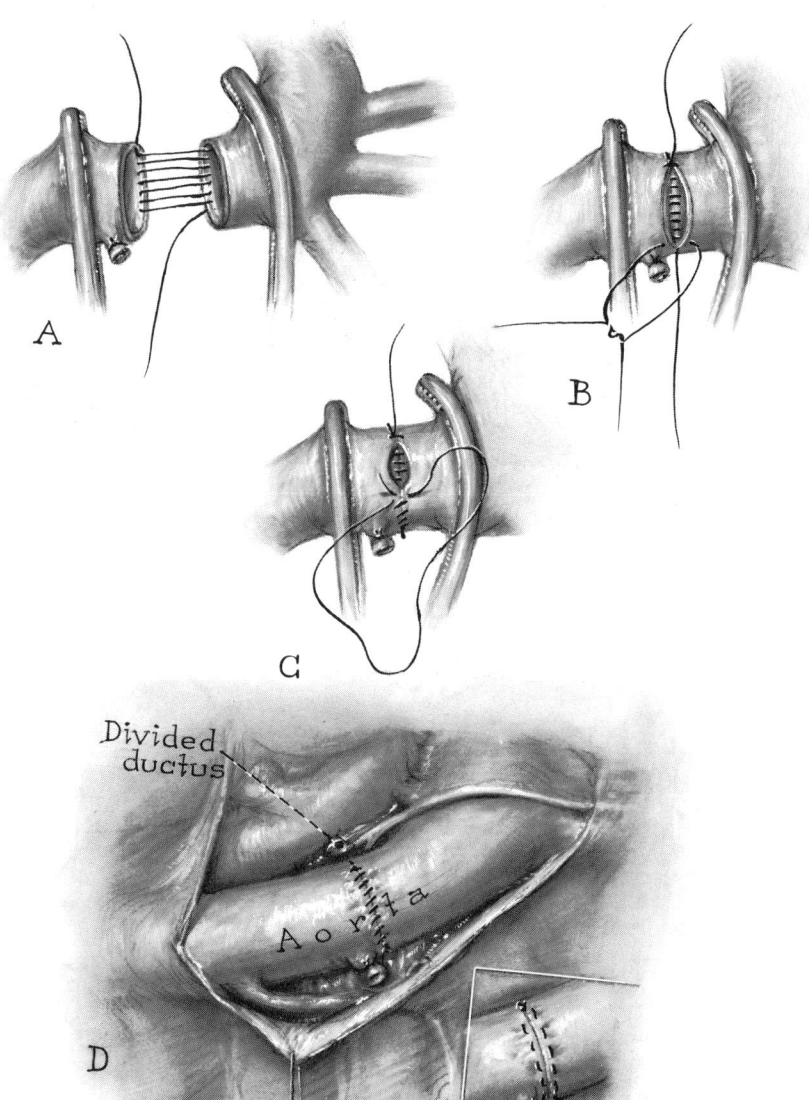

Figure 5. Anastomosis after excision of coarctation. *A*, An everting mattress suture is placed over about one third of the posterior row before the vessels are approximated and the suture is pulled up *(B)*. *C*, The anastomosis is completed with continuous over-and-over suture. Inset in *D* shows the everting mattress suture sometimes used. In children, interrupted mattress sutures are used for the entire anterior row.

of aneurysm formation. The chest film was found to be a very sensitive, although nonspecific, screening test for aneurysm formation.[12]

The subclavian flap aortoplasty was introduced by Waldhausen and Nahrwold in 1966 (Fig. 6). A left thoracotomy is performed, and the pleura overlying the aorta is incised. The left subclavian artery is dissected free and ligated at its first branch. The vertebral artery should be ligated to prevent a subclavian steal phenomenon. A longitudinal incision is made through the region of coarctation and continued onto the subclavian artery, which creates a flap. The posterior obstructing shelf is resected, and the flap of subclavian artery is turned down to enlarge the constriction. It is important that the flap be of sufficient length to bridge the obstruction completely. Advantages of this technique include avoidance of prosthetic material, decreased dissection, decreased aortic cross-clamp period, and increased anastomotic growth because there is no circumferential suture line. If the area of narrowing occurs proximal to the left subclavian artery, the flap may be directed proximally and a reversed subclavian flap aortoplasty done to enlarge the aortic arch. Campbell and associates reported the use of the subclavian flap repair in 53 patients under 1 year of age. Operative mortality was 4 per cent, and follow-up revealed no pressure gradient greater than 20 mm. Hg. Hamilton and co-workers reported 45 infants who underwent subclavian flap aortoplasty with an overall mortality of 24 per cent; all deaths occurred in children who had associated anomalies and who had repair before 2 months of age. There was no evidence of residual or recurrent coarctation in the survivors.

The subclavian flap aortoplasty has commonly been recommended for use in infants, although it is occasionally employed in older children as well. However, there has been concern that subclavian flap aortoplasty may not be the optimal method for coarctation repair in very young infants. Cobanoglu and co-workers in 1985 reported an increased incidence of early recoarctation in infants under 3 months of age after subclavian flap aortoplasty when compared with resection and primary anastomosis.[15] They proposed that the etiologic factor was inadequate resection of ductal tissue in the aortic wall, which continued to involute and fibrose. Sanchez and colleagues reported a 22 per cent incidence of early recoarctation secondary to a posterior shelf in infants less than 3 months old.[41] Restenosis was strongly correlated with younger age at the time of surgical correction and was thought to be secondary to the presence of ductal tissue in the aortic wall.

In addition to the possibility of early recoarctation in very young neonates, there is concern about sacrifice of the major vascular supply to the left upper extremity.[48] The subclavian

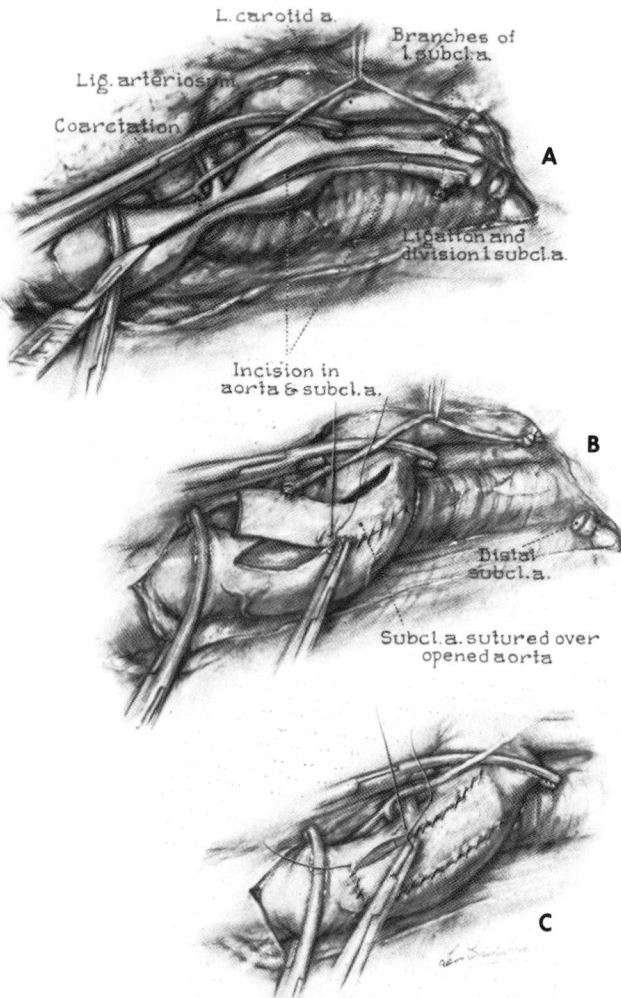

L. carotid a.

Branches of l.subcl.a.

Lig. arteriosum

Coarctation

A

Ligation and division l subcl.a.

Incision in aorta & subcl. a.

B

Distal subcl. a.

Subcl. a. sutured over opened aorta

C

Figure 6. *A,* Through a left posterolateral thoracotomy, the proximal and distal aorta are mobilized and the aorta is cross-clamped between the left subclavian and left carotid arteries. The aorta is also clamped distally. The subclavian artery is divided, and a longitudinal incision is made through the entire length of the subclavian artery and the coarctation segment. *B,* The subclavian artery is rolled down over the coarctation to enlarge the segment. *C,* The suture line is completed. Care must be taken to ensure that the length of the subclavian artery is adequate to cover the entire coarctation segment. (From Elbert, P. A.: Atlas of Congenital Cardiac Surgery. New York, Churchill Livingstone, 1989.)

artery is frequently divided for creation of systemic-to-pulmonary shunts, and adverse sequelae have been rare. There is some evidence of decreased growth of the extremity causing decreased length and mass, with rare reports of vascular insufficiency and gangrene of the arm, especially if branches of the subclavian artery distal to the vertebral artery are ligated.

In some infants with tubular hypoplasia, it is difficult to excise the narrowed segment completely and create a satisfactory anastomosis. In 1977, Amato and associates proposed anastomosis of the distal aorta to the inferior aspect of the arch with anastomosis of the contiguous walls of the left carotid and subclavian arteries if necessary to release the obstruction. Lansman and colleagues proposed an extended resection with primary anastomosis.[35] The coarcted segment is excised and the inferior aspect of the arch incised to provide a larger anastomosis. A more extensive procedure has been described by Elliott; the arch is completely dissected, the descending aorta is mobilized to the diaphragm, an incision is made on the inferior aspect of the arch as proximal as possible, and the anastomosis is completed. There have been no reports of neurologic complications. These techniques have not been widely applied, but the reported mortality is low.

Various other surgical reports have been proposed to correct coarctation. The Blalock-Park anastomosis involved division of the left subclavian artery with anastomosis to the descending aorta to bypass the obstruction.[10] Ascending aorta to descending aorta bypass grafts have been used and may be useful at the time of reoperation.

MANAGEMENT OF ASSOCIATED ANOMALIES. Outcome after surgical correction depends on the age at the time of operation, the method of repair chosen, and especially the presence of associated anomalies. The optimal management of infants with associated anomalies is still controversial. A PDA is frequently present and should be divided or ligated. A bicuspid aortic valve may be present but often requires no intervention at the time of correction of the coarctation. Appropriate management of an associated ventricular septal defect is less clear; several therapeutic options are available. Formerly, the pulmonary artery was often banded at the time of repair of the coarctation in infants with a nonrestrictive ventricular septal defect. However, ventricular septal defects associated with coarctation are often of a type with a high incidence of spontaneous closure. In infants with coarctation, a ventricular septal defect, and no other associated anomalies, some experts advocate repair of the coarctation alone. If congestive heart failure does not resolve, the septal defect is closed at a second operation. Hammon and associates reported improved survival with pulmonary artery banding at the time of coarctation repair and later closure of the ventricular septal defect.[27] Leanage and colleagues suggest that the banding should be done only in infants with an associated large ventricular septal defect. Goldman and co-workers found no survival benefit to pulmonary artery banding even in infants with a large ventricular septal defect.[25] They did, however, report decreased mortality with the use of pulmonary artery banding in patients with coarctation, ventricular septal defect, and associated intracardiac anomalies. Children with associated complex anomalies may improve sufficiently after coarctation repair to allow elective repair or palliation at a later date. Some authors advocate a one-stage repair of the coarctation and associated defects via a median sternotomy.

NONOPERATIVE THERAPY. In recent years, percutaneous transluminal balloon angioplasty has been introduced as an alternative therapy for coarctation. Initial results were encouraging; however, reports soon appeared of aneurysmal dilation of the aorta following balloon angioplasty. Balloon dilation of recurrent stenosis has been more successful, and there have been fewer reports of aneurysm formation, presumably secondary to surrounding scar tissue. Several centers have continued to use balloon angioplasty for native coarctation.[7,40] Morrow and co-workers in 1988 reported successful angioplasty in 31 of 33 patients with native coarctation. Follow-up angiography in 10 patients demonstrated no significant restenosis; however, aneurysmal dilation was present in 2 patients. Cystic medial necrosis has been described as a consistent histologic finding in patients with coarctation, suggesting that balloon-induced tears into an abnormal media may provide the substrate for aneurysm formation. The long-term results of balloon angioplasty for native coarctation in terms of recoarctation and especially aneurysm formation are unknown, and the technique must be considered investigational.[40] The results of angioplasty of postoperative recoarctation appear to be better, and angioplasty may be associated with less mortality and morbidity than reoperation; however, long-term follow-up is necessary.[17]

Complications

Correction of coarctation may be complicated by hemorrhage, chylothorax, recurrent nerve paralysis, infection, and suture line thrombosis. It has been suggested that patients with Turner's syndrome may be at increased risk for hemorrhage because of their friable tissues.[11] Postoperative paradoxical elevation of the blood pressure to greater than preoperative levels may occur. This is a two-phase phenomenon characterized by a rise in the systolic blood pressure during the first 24 to 36 hours after operation and a later increase in the diastolic pressure. The first phase is characterized by activation of the sympathetic nervous system with elevation of serum catecholamines. The late phase is characterized by elevation of plasma renin and angiotensin levels. Postoperative elevation of blood pressure has not been described in children undergoing thoracotomy for repair of other cardiac lesions. Paradoxical hypertension may be associated with the postcoarctectomy syndrome of abdominal pain and distention first reported by Sealy in 1953. Up to 20 per cent of patients having repair of coarctation experience abdominal pain and distention postoperatively. Laparotomy is occasionally indicated and may reveal evidence of mesenteric ischemia. On rare occasions, bowel resection may be necessary. Arteriography demonstrates changes in the mesenteric vessels, and pathologic examination reveals necrotizing mesenteric arteritis. The syndrome is possibly related to elevated renin levels. Aggressive therapy of hypertension appears to prevent full manifestation of the postcoarctectomy syndrome. Many drugs have been successfully used to control the postoperative hypertension, including sodium nitroprusside, propranolol, and reserpine.

A dreaded complication of coarctation repair is paraplegia, which occurs in 0.5 to 1 per cent of patients. Variations in the blood supply to the anterior spinal cord, poor collateral formation, anomalous origin of the right subclavian artery, distal hypotension during the period of aortic cross-clamping, and reoperation may predispose to paraplegia during the procedure. Brewer and colleagues reviewed 66 cases of paraplegia after 12,532 procedures for repair of coarctation, an incidence of 0.41 per cent. In this study, neither sacrifice of intercostals nor duration of aortic cross-clamping could be related to the occurrence of paraplegia. Brewer emphasized the marked variation in spinal cord blood supply and suggested that measurement of distal pressure after cross-clamping of the aorta be done to assess adequacy of the collateral circulation. A recent survey of surgeons in the United Kingdom and Ireland revealed that paraplegia occurred in 16 patients in 5492 operations or an incidence of 0.3 per cent. Hughes and Reemtsma, based on results in two patients, suggested monitoring distal perfusion pressure with use of bypass if the pressure fell below 50 mm. Hg. Others have recommended monitoring of cerebrospinal fluid pressure with the use of bypass and drainage of spinal fluid if necessary to maintain adequate perfusion pressure of the spinal cord. Spencer and associates have extensively investigated the use of somatosensory evoked potentials to assess adequacy of spinal cord perfusion, as have others.[18] Loss of somatosensory evoked potentials is a sensitive indicator of spinal cord ischemia. Maintenance of distal aortic pressure during aortic cross-clamping above 60 mm. Hg correlated with preservation of the somatosensory evoked potentials. Distal hypotension with loss of somatosensory evoked potentials for more than 30 minutes was associated with a greater than 70 per cent incidence of paraplegia. Except in small infants, distal aortic pressure should be measured during repair of coarctation and maintained above 60 mm. Hg with shunt or bypass techniques as necessary.

Results

The results of surgical correction depend on the age at repair, the type of repair used, and the associated anomalies. Operative mortality in neonates has decreased to 5 to 10 per cent and is lower in older children. Mortality is very low in patients with isolated coarctation. Classically, in patients who had resection and end-to-end anastomosis in infancy, the rate of recoarctation was as high as 60 per cent. There is a decreased incidence of recurrent coarctation with the subclavian patch aortoplasty and the prosthetic patch graft repair, compared with historical series. However, the most recent series using resection and end-

to-end anastomosis show, even in neonates, results that compare very favorably with other methods in terms of mortality and recoarctation. In 1986 Beekman and colleagues reported follow-up of 125 infants after repair of coarctation of the aorta by resection with end-to-end anastomosis or subclavian flap angioplasty.[16] The risk of reoperation at 5 and 10 years postoperatively was the same for both methods. Trinquet and associates in 1988 reported follow-up of 178 infants undergoing coarctation repair at less than 3 months of age.[47] Sixty-three infants had isolated coarctation, 47 had associated ventricular septal defects, and 68 had other associated anomalies. Actuarial survival at 5 years was 90 per cent for infants with isolated coarctation, 84 per cent for those with associated ventricular septal defects, and 40 per cent for those with complex anomalies. The rate of restenosis was the same for subclavian flap angioplasty, resection with primary anastomosis, and extended resection with anastomosis. Hopkins and co-workers in 1988 reported follow-up of 179 children under 1 year of age undergoing coarctation repair and found no difference between subclavian flap aortoplasty and resection with primary anastomosis with respect to mortality and recoarctation.[30] They recommended an individualized approach based on each patient's anatomy.

Any comparison of techniques for repair of coarctation must consider the historical time frame.[50] Advances in the care of critically ill infants such as the introduction of neonatal intensive care units and prostaglandin therapy have provided dramatic improvements in the preoperative condition of patients that may affect mortality as much as the choice of repair. Advances in suture materials and vascular surgical technique also make it difficult to compare results of different time periods. Circumferential arterial suture lines have been effectively used in the arterial switch operation for transposition of the great arteries and other congenital cardiac anomalies and, therefore, should be as successful in coarctation repair. Since a prospective, randomized trial of the various repair techniques has not been done, long-term results cannot be accurately compared. The optimal method for coarctation repair is unknown, and therapy should be individualized on the basis of each patient's anatomy, clinical condition, and associated anomalies and the experience of the surgeon.

Recoarctation usually manifests as persistent hypertension or arm-leg gradient. The arm-leg pressure gradient should be measured in the immediate postoperative period to differentiate residual stenosis secondary to an inadequate repair from true recoarctation. The causes of recoarctation include failure of growth of the anastomosis, inadequate resection of the narrowed segment, residual abnormal ductal tissue, and suture line thrombosis. Exercise testing with measurement of the arm-leg gradient should be obtained for serial evaluation of postoperative patients. Many patients who are normotensive at rest and who do not have a resting arm-leg gradient develop severe hypertension with a gradient following exercise.[36] These patients may have significant restenosis. The long-term consequences of exercise-induced hypertension after the correction of coarctation are unknown but may adversely affect the prognosis.

Reoperation is indicated if significant hypertension or other symptoms occur and a pressure gradient is demonstrated.[21] Reoperation is more difficult secondary to scarring and is associated with an increased morbidity and mortality. Lack of collaterals may cause an increased incidence of paraplegia. In patients who have had previous resection and end-to-end anastomosis, subclavian flap aortoplasty and prosthetic patch onlay grafting are appropriate methods for repair of the recoarctation. Balloon angioplasty may also be used for treatment of recoarctation.[17]

Some patients who have had a technically excellent repair may not have complete resolution of hypertension. The cause of this persistent hypertension is unclear but is related to the age at repair and the duration of preoperative hypertension. Follow-up of surgical patients indicates that they are not rendered entirely normal. Maron and associates, reporting in 1973 long-term follow-up of 248 patients who had correction of aortic coarctation, found an increased incidence of premature death usually secondary to cardiovascular disease and related this to the duration of preoperative hypertension. There is evidence of increased coronary atherosclerosis in patients with coarctation.[16] Koller and colleagues found that patients operated on between the ages of 2 and 4 years had the lowest risk for restenosis and persistent hypertension. There is evidence of abnormal left ventricular function despite relief of the obstruction. Kimball and associates found a persistent increase in ventricular contractility after successful coarctation repair, possibly secondary to cardiac ultrastructural changes following congenital pressure overload.[33] They have also documented abnormal thallium scans after successful coarctation repair, suggesting persistent changes in the coronary arteries. Aortic stenosis or regurgitation secondary to a bicuspid aortic valve may develop and necessitate valve replacement. As has been emphasized, the long-term prognosis of many patients is determined primarily by the associated anomalies.

INTERRUPTION OF THE AORTIC ARCH

Complete absence of a segment of the aortic arch without any anatomic connection between the proximal and distal segments is termed interruption of the aortic arch. If a fibrous strand connects the segments, the condition is termed aortic atresia. Interruption of the aortic arch at the aortic isthmus was first described by Steidele in 1778. Seidel, in 1818, reported absence of the segment between the left subclavian and left common carotid arteries. Interruption of the aortic arch between the left common carotid and the innominate arteries was reported by Weisman and Kesten in 1948. Samson and colleagues reported the first successful correction in 1955. Sirak and associates in 1968 were the first to successfully correct an interrupted aortic arch in a neonate. Barratt-Boyes and colleagues in 1972 reported the first simultaneous correction of interrupted aortic arch and all associated anomalies. In 1976, the introduction of prostaglandin therapy to maintain ductal patency allowed preoperative stabilization of infants with interrupted arch and greatly improved surgical results.

Incidence, Pathologic Anatomy, and Natural History

Interruption of the aortic arch is a rare anomaly constituting less than 1.5 per cent of congenital heart disease. Interrupted arch may be an isolated defect but is usually associated with other anomalies. Everts-Suarez and Carson noted the frequent association of interrupted arch, PDA, and ventricular septal defect. Interruption of the arch may be associated with a wide variety of cardiac anomalies including persistent truncus arteriosus and aortopulmonary window. Celoria and Patton classified interrupted aortic arch based on the absent segment. In Type A, the interruption occurs distal to the left subclavian artery; in Type B, the interruption occurs between the left subclavian and left common carotid arteries; and with Type C, the interruption occurs between the left common carotid and innominate arteries. In a review of 165 cases of interrupted aortic arch, Van Praagh and associates found that 43 per cent were Type A, 53 per cent were Type B, and 4 per cent were Type C.

The cause of interrupted arch is unclear. As with coarctation, there is an association with defects that decrease ascending aortic flow and increase ductal flow, implying that abnormal fetal blood flow patterns are an etiologic factor. Type B interrupted arch is frequently found in association with DiGeorge's syndrome (absence of the third and fourth pharyngeal pouches). In DiGeorge's syndrome the thymus and parathyroid glands are absent; thus, patients are hypocalcemic and suffer from defects in cellular immunity. Defects in the development of the neural crest may be responsible for DiGeorge's syndrome and Type B interrupted arch.

The prognosis of uncorrected interruption of the aortic arch is poor. The mean age at death has been reported to be 4 to 10 days. Ninety per cent of infants with interrupted arch die in the first year of life unless they undergo surgical intervention. Only in the rare case of interrupted arch with no associated anomalies is prolonged survival possible, presumably because of the development of a collateral circulation *in utero.*

Diagnosis and Management

Most infants with interrupted aortic arch present with congestive heart failure secondary to left-to-right shunting through a ventricular septal defect and increased left ventricular afterload. Lower body perfusion is maintained by right-to-left shunting through a PDA. When the ductus closes, perfusion of the lower body essentially ceases; the infants become anuric and severely acidotic, with nonpalpable femoral pulses. The congestive heart failure and acidosis are resistant to medical therapy, and death occurs within a few days. Since the advent of prostaglandin E_1 therapy, however, it is possible to maintain ductal patency, improve lower body perfusion, reverse the acidosis, and increase urinary output. The physical examination is not specific for interrupted arch, and there are no characteristic murmurs. The ECG is not useful, and the chest film reveals an enlarged heart with pulmonary congestion. Cardiac catheterization with angiography allows accurate diagnosis. Contrast injection must be done in both the proximal and distal segments to define the anatomy adequately. Echocardiography is also useful to clarify the anatomy and exclude associated anomalies. When the diagnosis has been made and the infant has been stabilized with prostaglandin therapy, surgical correction is undertaken. In infants with Type B interrupted arch, there is a high incidence of DiGeorge's syndrome, and great care must be taken to avoid hypocalcemia. Because of their immunologic defect, these patients should receive irradiated blood products to prevent the development of graft-versus-host disease.

Various procedures have been used to either palliate or correct interrupted arch. The ultimate goal is restoration of aortic continuity and correction of associated anomalies. Aortic continuity may be restored by direct anastomosis of the aortic segments, end-to-side anastomosis of an arch vessel to either the proximal or distal segment, or use of an interposition graft. If palliation is planned, a left thoracotomy may be utilized and aortic continuity restored by using one of the arch vessels as a conduit. In Type A interrupted arch, a Blalock-Park anastomosis is used; in Type B, the left common carotid artery is anastomosed to the distal segment, or a "reversed" Blalock-Park anastomosis may be created; and in Type C, the left common carotid artery may be anastomosed to the ascending aorta. The use of ductal tissue in the anastomosis should be avoided, because obstruction may occur if the tissue contracts and fibroses. Alternatively, interposition of a Dacron or Gore-Tex graft may be used to restore continuity. Simultaneous correction of intracardiac anomalies is not possible through a left thoracotomy; however, pulmonary artery banding may be performed if indicated. Repair of a ventricular septal defect and other anomalies may be undertaken at a later date through a median sternotomy.

Turley and colleagues in 1984 reported improved results with an anterior approach and total correction by primary anastomosis. Cardiopulmonary bypass with biaortic cannulation is used for cooling, with profound hypothermia and circulatory arrest during the arch repair. The ductus is divided, the aorta is mobilized to the diaphragm, and aortic continuity is restored by direct anastomosis of the proximal and distal aortic segments. The ventricular septal defect is repaired through a right ventriculotomy. Early mortality was 20 per cent, compared with 33 to 43 per cent mortality for staged procedures at the same institution. Development of subaortic stenosis has been reported after successful repair of interrupted aortic arch and may necessitate further surgical intervention.

Sell and associates reported 71 patients observed with interrupted aortic arch between 1974 and 1987.[43] In the early years of the series, tube graft repair was performed. More recently, direct anastomosis with repair of the ventricular septal defect was performed. Actuarial survival at 10 years was 47 per cent and mortality declined with increasing experience. Recurrent arch obstruction was managed with reoperation or balloon angioplasty. Left ventricular outflow tract obstruction occurred in approximately 50 per cent of patients undergoing repair. Improved results with direct anastomosis have also been reported by Scott and colleagues and by Munro and associates.[37,42]

Interrupted aortic arch remains a difficult surgical problem. Advances in surgical techniques and neonatal intensive care and the introduction of prostaglandin E$_1$ therapy have greatly increased survival. After stabilization of these critically ill infants, total correction of the interrupted arch and associated anomalies should be undertaken via a median sternotomy.

AORTOPULMONARY WINDOW

Aortopulmonary window is a rare congenital heart defect following abnormal septation of the truncus arteriosus into the aorta and pulmonary artery. Various other terms have been applied to this anomaly: *aortopulmonary fistula, aortic septal defect, aorticopulmonary septal defect,* and *aortopulmonary fenestration.* Elliotson first described aortopulmonary window in 1830. Abbott was able to include only 10 cases of aortopulmonary window in her classic review of 1000 cases of congenital heart disease. In 1948, Gross successfully ligated an aortopulmonary window but noted that this method would be dangerous in many patients because of the friability of the tissues. Scott and Sabiston described a closed method for division of an aortopulmonary window in 1953. Cooley and associates reported successful division of an aortopulmonary window by using cardiopulmonary bypass in 1957. In 1966, Putnam and Gross suggested a transpulmonary approach for closure of the defect. In 1968, Wright and associates reported direct suture closure of an aortopulmonary window via a transaortic approach. Deverall and colleagues subsequently described patch closure of the defect by using a transaortic approach.

Embryology, Pathologic Anatomy, and Natural History

In the truncus arteriosus, two conotruncal ridges form proximally and fuse to create the septum between the aorta and the pulmonary artery. More distally, the right and left sixth aortic arches fuse with the main pulmonary artery to form the right and left pulmonary arteries and complete formation of the aortopulmonary septum. Failure of fusion or malalignment of the conotruncal ridges may cause a defect in the aortopulmonary septum. Abnormal migration of the sixth aortic arches may cause aortic origin of a pulmonary artery. It is important to note that the aortic and pulmonic valves are normally formed, distinguishing these defects from persistent truncus arteriosus. Unlike persistent truncus arteriosus and Type B interrupted aortic arch, there is no association between aortopulmonary window and DiGeorge's syndrome. A closely related disorder is aortic origin of either the right or left pulmonary artery.

An aortopulmonary window is usually a single large defect beginning a few millimeters above the aortic valve on the left lateral wall of the aorta. Multiple defects have been rarely reported. The defect may occasionally be found more distally overlying the origin of the right pulmonary artery, and rarely absence of the entire aortopulmonary septum may be encountered. Origin of the right coronary artery and rarely the left from the pulmonary artery may occur and can complicate surgical correction. Associated anomalies include Type A interrupted aortic arch, ventricular septal defect, tetralogy of Fallot, and patent ductus arteriosus. An aortopulmonary window allows a large left-to-right shunt, causing pulmonary hypertension and congestive heart failure. As with a nonrestrictive ventricular septal defect, irreversible pulmonary vascular disease may occur at an early age.

Aortopulmonary window is a rare defect, and thus the natural history is not well defined. Patients with a large aortopulmonary window usually do not survive infancy. Children or young adults with an aortopulmonary window are encountered occasionally and usually have developed significant pulmonary vascular disease. The clinical course is thought to be similar to that of untreated patients with a large ventricular septal defect.

Diagnosis

Infants with aortopulmonary window usually present with congestive heart failure early in life. They often have growth retardation and recurrent pulmonary infections. Physical examination reveals a systolic murmur and occasionally a continuous murmur suggestive of PDA. The chest film reveals cardiomegaly, with pulmonary vascular engorgement or congestive heart failure. Aortopulmonary window must be differentiated from PDA, persistent truncus arteriosus, ventricular septal defect with aortic regurgitation, and ruptured aneurysm of the sinus of Valsalva.

Two-dimensional echocardiography can be used to visualize the defect. Cardiac catheterization reveals an oxygen saturation step-up at the level of the pulmonary artery, and the course of the catheter may suggest the diagnosis. Retrograde aortography provides accurate visualization of the defect. It is necessary to document the presence of normal aortic and pulmonic valves to confirm the diagnosis, and the location of coronary ostia must be carefully demonstrated before surgical intervention.

Surgical Correction

The presence of an aortopulmonary window is sufficient indication for repair unless severe pulmonary vascular disease has occurred. The preferred technique for repair is transaortic closure either by direct suture or patch closure. Simple ligation should not be done because of the risk of hemorrhage from the friable tissues. Division and primary closure may cause narrowing of the vessels. The transaortic approach is preferred to the transpulmonary method because it allows better visualization of the defect and the coronary ostia. The operation is undertaken via a median sternotomy, and either cardiopulmonary bypass or hypothermic circulatory arrest may be used. A transverse aortotomy at the level of the window is performed and the anatomy is carefully defined. Particular attention should be given to the location of the coronary ostia and the origin of the right pulmonary artery. Small defects may be closed by direct suture; larger defects should be closed with a Dacron patch. Care must be taken to place the patch so that the coronary ostia are on the aortic side. If the defect involves the origin of the right pulmonary artery, a teardrop-shaped patch extending along the right pulmonary artery may be used to repair the defect. Johansson and colleagues in 1978 described a method of repair by opening the anterior wall of the defect, suturing a patch to the posterior wall, and continuing this suture to close the incision, incorporating the patch with the suture line.

Operative mortality is low for repair of isolated aortopulmonary window or aortic origin of a pulmonary artery in infancy. Long-term results are good if there are no associated anomalies. In older infants and children, the results depend on the severity and reversibility of the pulmonary vascular disease.

ANOMALIES OF THE AORTIC ARCH

At length, by mere accident I discovered an extraordinary lusus naturae in the disposition of the right subclavian artery.[5a]

David Bayford

Vascular rings are developmental anomalies of the aorta and great vessels that encircle and may constrict the esophagus and trachea. In 1735, Hunauld reported the necropsy finding of anomalous origin of the right subclavian artery from the descending aorta. A persistent double aortic arch was described in 1737 by Hommel. In a case report read before the Medical Society of London in 1787 and published in 1794, Bayford presented the case history and autopsy findings of a 62-year-old woman who died of starvation secondary to severe dysphagia. An anomalous origin of the right subclavian artery from the descending aorta was present, and he attributed the woman's dysphagia to this anomaly, although the artery coursed between the trachea and esophagus rather than posterior to the esophagus. He termed the finding a lusus naturae, or "prank of nature," and coined the term dysphagia lusoria. Throughout the nineteenth century, aortic arch anomalies remained anatomic curiosities. Congdon greatly clarified the embryology of the aortic arches. The clinical syndrome of stridor and dysphagia in early infancy secondary to persistent double aortic arch was clearly delineated by Wolman. Surgical correction of constricting vascular rings was not reported until 1945, when Gross successfully divided a double aortic arch and an aberrant right subclavian artery. Neuhauser later pioneered the use of the barium esophagogram for diagnosis of vascular rings. Edwards in 1948 presented the concept of a hypothetical double arch, allowing classification of multiple possible arch anomalies (Figs. 7 and 8).

Embryology and Pathologic Anatomy

In the embryo, six pairs of aortic arches arise sequentially from the truncus arteriosus and join paired dorsal aortas. Persistence or regression of various segments of these arches results in the normal pattern of the aorta, pulmonary artery, and great vessels. In normal development, the third pair of arches form parts of the common carotid arteries. The left fourth arch forms the adult aortic arch, and the proximal portion of the right fourth arch persists as the innominate artery. The pulmonary arteries develop from the proximal right and left sixth aortic arches. The distal left sixth arch develops into the ductus arteriosus, whereas the distal right sixth arch normally regresses. Failure of a segment to regress normally may cause a vascular ring. Various anomalies occur and may be easily visualized by using the hypothetical scheme of Edwards, consisting of an ascending aorta, right and left aortic arches, a descending aorta on either the right or left, and bilateral ductus arteriosi. Associated cardiac defects may be encountered, especially in patients with a persistent right aortic arch, frequently tetralogy of Fallot.

Clinical Manifestations and Natural History

The natural history of vascular rings is obscured by the wide spectrum of anomalies and the range of symptoms. Vascular rings should be suspected in any infant with stridor, dysphagia, recurrent respiratory tract infections, difficult feeding, or failure to thrive. Vascular rings are not necessarily inconsistent with prolonged survival, and many patients are totally asymptomatic. Anomalies that become symptomatic usually present by 6 months of age, although some adults present when atherosclerosis causes dilation of the aorta and increasing constriction. Children with mild symptoms may show marked improvement as they grow. Afflicted infants most commonly present with respiratory difficulties; the breathing is stridorous and may be exacerbated by feeding. Hyperextension of the neck tends to

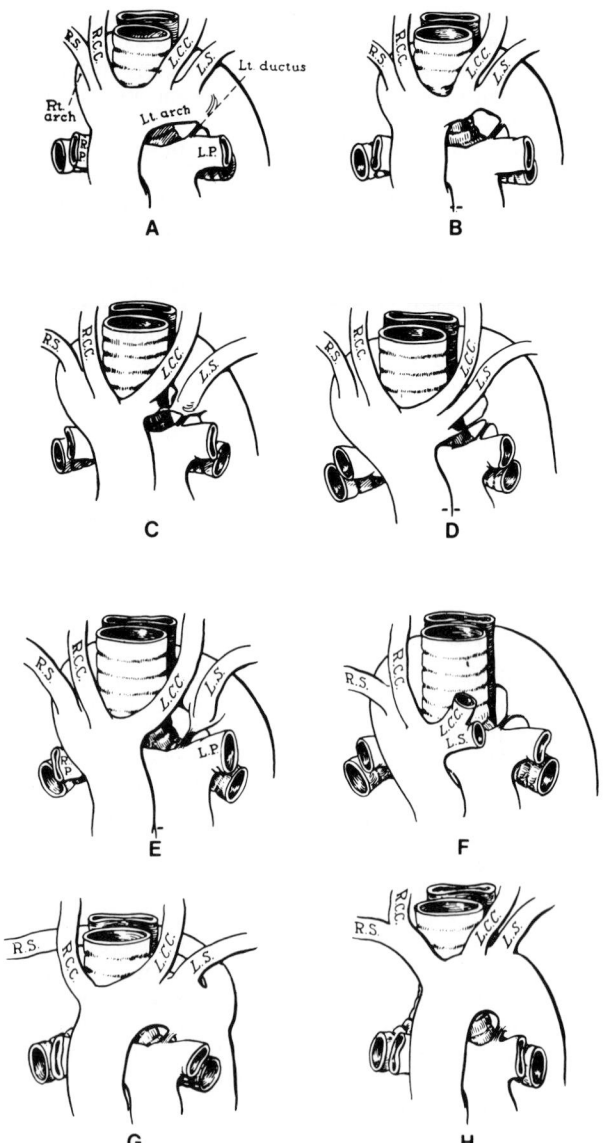

Figure 7. Aortic arch anomalies (left descending aorta and ligamentum arteriosum). *A*, Double aortic arch with equal anterior and posterior arches. *B*, Double aortic arch with smaller anterior (left) arch. *C*, Double aortic arch with atresia of anterior arch between the carotid and subclavian arteries. *D*, Double aortic arch with atresia of anterior arch distal to subclavian artery. *E*, Right aortic arch with retroesophageal segment and anomalous origin of the left subclavian artery from Kommerell's diverticulum. *F*, Right aortic arch with retroesophageal segment and mirror image branching. (Note the ligamentum arteriosum inserting onto the diverticulum of the descending aorta.) *G*, Left aortic arch with anomalous origin of the right subclavian artery. *H*, Normal pattern. (From Edwards, J. E.: Anomalies of the derivatives of the aortic arch system. Med. Clin. North Am., July:925, 1948.)

reduce the constriction, and marked respiratory difficulties may occur if the neck is flexed. The physical examination is usually nondiagnostic, although signs of associated cardiovascular defects may be found.

The plain chest film may be normal or may reveal pneumonia or occasionally compression of the air-filled trachea. A right aortic arch is observed in some anomalies. The barium esophagogram is a particularly valuable study. The combination of posterior compression of the esophagus on barium swallow and anterior tracheal compression is almost pathognomonic for a vascular ring. Angiocardiography accurately delineates the anatomy of vascular rings and allows evaluation of associated anomalies. Although most vascular rings can be divided without preoperative catheterization, many centers routinely perform catheterization because misdiagnosis can occur. Various

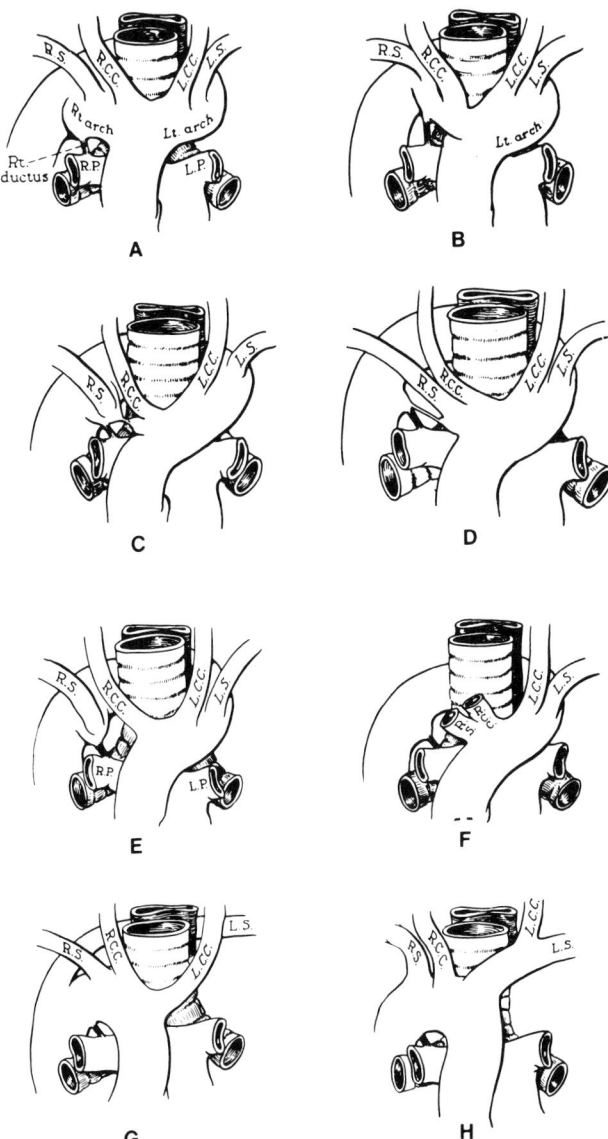

Figure 8. Aortic arch anomalies (right descending aorta and ligamentum arteriosum). *A,* Double aortic arch with equal anterior and posterior arches. *B,* Double aortic arch with smaller anterior (right) arch. *C,* Double aortic arch with atresia of anterior arch between carotid and subclavian arteries. *D,* Double aortic arch with atresia of anterior arch distal to subclavian artery. *E,* Left aortic arch with retroesophageal segment and anomalous origin of right subclavian artery from Kommerell's diverticulum. *F,* Left aortic arch with retroesophageal segment. (Note the insertion of the ligamentum arteriosum onto the diverticulum of the descending aorta.) *G,* Right aortic arch with a normal origin of the left subclavian artery. *H,* Right aortic arch with mirror image branching. (From Edwards, J. E.: Anomalies of the derivatives of the aortic arch system. Med. Clin. North Am., July:925, 1948.)

other diagnostic modalities may occasionally be useful, including echocardiography, magnetic resonance imaging, and digital subtraction angiography. Bronchoscopy is indicated in some patients, especially those with suspected anomalous origin of the innominate artery.

Management

Although a few patients with constricting vascular rings improve with growth, the long-term prognosis of medical therapy is poor in most symptomatic patients. Despite the wide spectrum of anomalies, the principles of surgical therapy are simple.[3,4,9] Surgical intervention should be undertaken at the time of diagnosis and is designed to divide the vascular ring, relieve the constriction, and preserve circulation to the aortic branches. Adequate exposure is an absolute necessity. Gross stated that all

vascular rings could be safely divided through a left thoracotomy; however, a few anomalies require approach via a right-sided thoracotomy.

The most common anomaly causing a true vascular ring is persistence of the right and left fourth aortic arches, forming a double aortic arch. In the usual situation, the right or posterior arch is larger, and there is a left descending aorta with a left ductus arteriosus (Fig. 7B). However, occasionally the arches are of equal size (Fig. 7A) or the anterior (left) arch is larger. Rarely, a right descending aorta is encountered, in which case the right arch is anterior (Fig. 7C and D). The right carotid and subclavian arteries arise from the right arch, whereas the left carotid and subclavian arteries arise from the left arch. Patients with double aortic arch usually present early in infancy and are severely symptomatic. The diagnosis of double aortic arch can be made easily from the barium esophagogram. In the most common situation, the anteroposterior projection shows right- and left-sided indentation of the barium-filled esophagus, the right indentation being higher and larger. The lateral projection shows posterior esophageal compression from the retroesophageal posterior arch. Arteriography may also be used to make the diagnosis, although atretic segments are not visualized. Surgical correction is indicated at the time of diagnosis. In the usual situation, a left-sided thoracotomy is done and the smaller anterior arch is divided and oversewn at its junction with the descending aorta so that the left carotid and subclavian arteries arise from the ascending aorta or may be divided at an atretic segment, if present. The ligamentum arteriosum is also divided, and the constricting vessels are dissected away from the trachea and esophagus. If necessary, the divided left arch may be suspended from the posterior surface of the sternum to further relieve the constriction. In patients with atresia of the posterior (right) arch, a right-sided thoracotomy provides optimal exposure.

Aberrant origin of the right subclavian artery is a very common anomaly but rarely causes symptoms (Fig. 7G). This defect follows regression of the right fourth aortic arch between the carotid and subclavian arteries, rather than distal to the subclavian. The artery may appear to arise from a diverticulum of the descending aorta (Kommerell's diverticulum), which is actually a remnant of the distal right aortic arch. The artery most often courses posterior to the esophagus but may pass between the trachea and esophagus or anterior to the trachea. An anomalous right subclavian artery does not constitute a true vascular ring. However, the aberrant artery or occasionally the diverticulum may compress the esophagus, causing dysphagia. The diagnosis of aberrant origin of the right subclavian artery can be made by a barium esophagogram. The lateral esophagogram shows an oblique posterior impression coursing upward from left to right, and arterial pulsations may be observed. This anomaly may be an incidental finding at the time of barium study for other indications. Gross pioneered surgical therapy for anomalous origin of the right subclavian artery. In children, the artery may be simply ligated and divided without sequelae. In adults, a subclavian steal syndrome may follow simple division, and anastomosis to the aorta is usually necessary.

Left aortic arch with a retroesophageal segment and a right descending aorta is a rare arch anomaly that was first reported by Paul in 1948 (see Fig. 8). The right subclavian artery arises from the descending aorta, and the ring is completed by a right ligamentum arteriosum. Most of the patients reported to have this anomaly have had minimal symptoms. However, a short ligamentum may cause a symptomatic constricting ring. The diagnosis may be suspected on the plain chest film and confirmed by barium swallow or arteriography. Surgical therapy consists of division of the ligamentum arteriosum through a right-sided thoracotomy.

Compression of the anterior trachea by an innominate artery originating farther to the left on the aortic arch than usual was first described by Gross and Neuhauser. Fearon and Shortreed in 1963 described 69 patients with compression of the airway by an anomalous innominate artery. They emphasized the importance of endoscopy as a diagnostic modality and described "reflex apnea" or respiratory arrest following stimulation of the compressed area of the trachea. Mustard and associates reported 285 cases of innominate artery compression in 1969. Less than 14 per cent of the patients required surgical intervention, and reflex apnea was the major indication for operation.

Children with anomalous origin of the innominate artery present with respiratory distress, stridor, and occasionally respiratory arrest. Dysphagia does not occur because the esophagus is not obstructed. Reflex apnea may follow irritation of the trachea by accumulated secretions or further compression of the trachea by a bolus of food in the esophagus. Recurrent pneumonia and atelectasis may also occur. The physical examination is not helpful in the diagnosis of anomalous origin of the innominate artery. The chest film may reveal only pneumonia or atelectasis, and the barium esophagogram is normal. Arteriography may demonstrate an abnormally leftward origin of the innominate artery, but this finding is not diagnostic of tracheal compression. Bronchoscopy is the optimal method for confirming tracheal compression and reveals buckling of the tracheal cartilages in affected patients.[20] Many infants with innominate artery compression have mild symptoms and improve as they grow. The primary indication for surgical intervention is reflex apnea. Aortopexy may be done via a median sternotomy or a right-sided anterior thoracotomy. By using multiple adventitial sutures, the aorta and innominate artery are suspended from the posterior aspect of the sternum. The innominate artery is not dissected free from the trachea, but suspended and allowed to exert traction on the buckled tracheal cartilages.

Fiorratti and Anglietta reported a right aortic arch in 1763, and Corvisart described a right aortic arch in a patient with tetralogy of Fallot in 1818. Persistence of the right aortic arch occurs commonly, but a vascular ring cannot result unless there is a retroesophageal segment or aberrant vessel. The right aortic arch with mirror image origin of the branches frequently accompanies tetralogy of Fallot (Fig. 8H). In some patients, the left subclavian artery arises aberrantly from the descending aorta and courses posterior to the esophagus (Fig. 8G). In either case, the presence of a left ligamentum arteriosum that attaches to the descending aorta constitutes a true vascular ring. In a symptomatic patient with a right aortic arch, retroesophageal segment, and left descending aorta or an aberrant left subclavian artery, a left ligamentum arteriosum usually must be present for significant tracheal and esophageal compression to occur. Surgical therapy requires division of the ligamentum arteriosum through a left-sided thoracotomy.

Cervical aortic arch is a rare anomaly in which the aortic arch rises to a point above the clavicle. Bevan and Fatti in 1947 reported the first case in a 9-year-old girl, who rapidly expired following ligation of a presumed carotid artery aneurysm. Cervical aortic arch is thought to represent persistence of the third rather than the fourth aortic arch. Cervical aortic arch may be an isolated finding or may occur in association with other arch anomalies. Presence of a cervical aortic arch can be confirmed if compression of a pulsatile neck mass causes loss of the femoral pulses. No intervention is indicated unless another symptomatic anomaly is present.

Results

Results in terms of both survival and relief of symptoms of surgical therapy are good in infants with isolated vascular rings. Operative mortality is low but not zero. Postoperative morbidity is often related to tracheomalacia secondary to the vascular compression. The infants may continue to have residual obstruction that causes recurrent respiratory distress and infection. These problems usually diminish as the child grows. In children with associated cardiac anomalies, the long-term outcome is related to the severity of the cardiac defect.

PULMONARY ARTERY SLING

Pulmonary artery sling is a rare cardiac anomaly occurring when the left pulmonary artery arises aberrantly from the right pulmonary artery and courses between the trachea and esophagus. A true vascular ring is not present; however, compression of the distal trachea and main stem bronchi usually occurs. Glaevecke and Doehle first described pulmonary artery sling in 1897. Scheid in 1938 reported a pulmonary artery sling with associated tracheal stenosis and complete cartilaginous rings. Welsh and Munro in 1954 reported a patient with aberrant left pulmonary artery and suggested that this anomaly would produce an anterior defect in the barium esophagogram, a finding later described by Wittenborg and colleagues. Potts and associates performed a thoracotomy in a child with a suspected vascular ring and discovered a pulmonary artery sling in 1954. They divided the anomalous left pulmonary artery and reanastomosed the artery to the proximal portion of the artery anterior to the trachea. A similar procedure was reported by Hiller and MacLean; however, they anastomosed the left pulmonary artery to the main pulmonary artery rather than to the proximal left pulmonary artery.

Pathologic Anatomy

The aberrant left pulmonary artery arises from the posterior aspect of the right pulmonary artery (Fig. 9). It then courses posteriorly over the right main stem bronchus and passes between the trachea and esophagus. The hilum of the left lung is lower than normal. Tracheal stenosis with complete cartilaginous rings and absence of the membranous portion of the trachea occurs frequently. Tracheal stenosis may extend proximally, may include the left main stem bronchus, and may be present in segments not actually compressed by the anomalous vessel. Tracheomalacia and origin of the right main stem bronchus from the trachea (bronchus suis) are also commonly associated with pulmonary artery sling.[24]

Clinical Findings and Diagnosis

Infants with pulmonary artery sling often present with respiratory symptoms at birth, and many are symptomatic by 1 month. It is impossible to estimate the number of asymptomatic patients with pulmonary artery sling. The most common findings are respiratory distress, wheezing, and expiratory stridor. Acute respiratory failure secondary to obstruction may occur, requiring intubation. Signs and symptoms of esophageal obstruction are rare. Repeated respiratory tract infections may occur.

The physical examination is not helpful in the diagnosis of pulmonary artery sling. The chest film may be normal or may show a number of findings suggestive of pulmonary artery sling, including hyperinflation of one lung (most commonly the right, but occasionally the left), anterior bowing of the tracheal air column, and a low hilum of the left lung (see Fig. 9). Infants may present at birth with opacification of one lung secondary to retention of fetal fluid. Pulmonary artery sling may present in adults as a mediastinal or paratracheal mass. The barium esophagogram is particularly useful and shows anterior pulsatile compression of the esophagus (see Fig. 9). This finding strongly suggests a pulmonary artery sling but can be observed if an anomalous subclavian artery courses between the trachea and esophagus. Mediastinal tumors, cysts, or lymph nodes may occasionally cause anterior esophageal compression, but these lesions are nonpulsatile. Angiocardiography is useful to demonstrate the aberrant vessel and evaluate associated anomalies (see Fig. 9). Newer techniques, including digital subtraction angiography, two-dimensional echocardiography, computed tomography, and magnetic resonance imaging, are proving useful

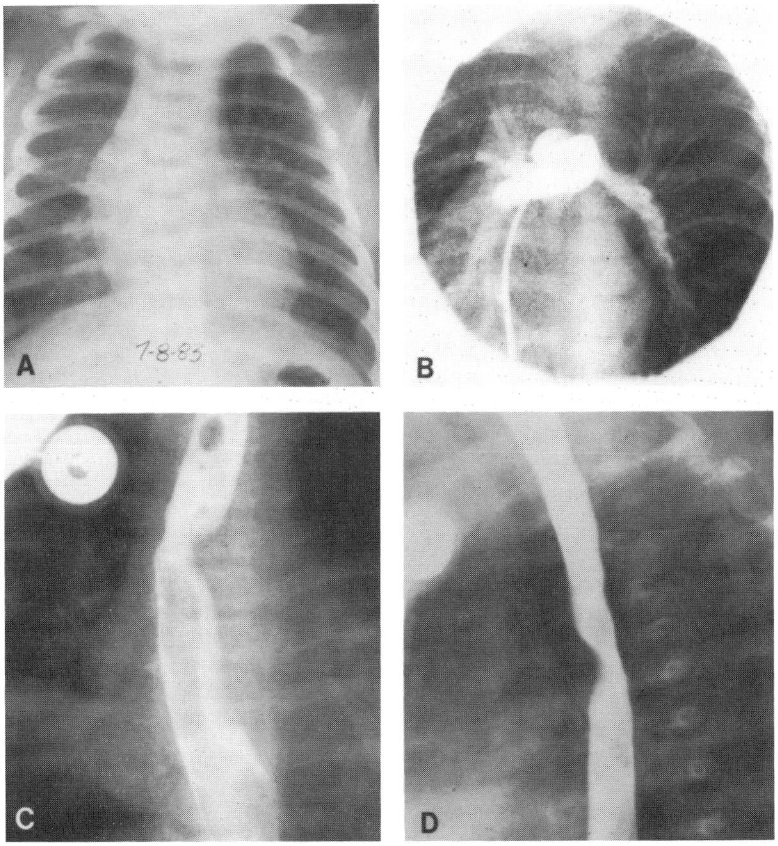

Figure 9. Infant with pulmonary artery sling. *A*, Plain chest film demonstrates hyperaeration of the left lung. *B*, Pulmonary arteriogram demonstrates anomalous origin of the left pulmonary artery from the right pulmonary artery. (Note the course of the left pulmonary artery around the tracheal air column.) *C*, Barium esophagogram (AP) showing compression of the esophagus. *D*, Barium esophagogram (lateral) showing characteristic anterior indentation of the esophagus behind the distal trachea. (Courtesy of Dr. Eric Effman and Dr. Bennett Pearce.)

in the diagnosis of pulmonary artery sling. Bronchoscopy is particularly useful in these patients for evaluation of associated tracheobronchial anomalies. Bronchography is now rarely indicated.

Natural History

The exact incidence of pulmonary artery sling is unknown. Patients may present with severe symptoms in infancy, but survival to an advanced age is also possible. The oldest reported patient was 78 years old, and he was asymptomatic until a few months before his death. There are increasing reports of children and adults who have pulmonary artery sling but minimal or no symptoms; the anomaly may be discovered during evaluation for unrelated complaints. The natural history of patients with pulmonary artery sling depends on the degree of respiratory obstruction and associated tracheobronchial and cardiac anomalies. Infants who present with respiratory obstruction may succumb to the acute event; if they survive, their prognosis is poor without surgical intervention. However, Phelan and Venables reported nonsurgical management in five patients (one patient had division of a ligamentum arteriosum), with resolution or marked diminution of symptoms in all of the patients. Three of these patients had associated tracheobronchial stenosis, which was thought to contribute to the residual symptoms.

Management and Results

Surgical intervention is indicated in any patient with a pulmonary artery sling and symptoms of significant respiratory obstruction. Nonsurgical management may be possible in patients with minor symptoms. The recommended procedure is division of the anomalous artery with anastomosis to the main pulmonary artery rather than to the proximal left pulmonary artery to avoid kinking. This may be done by using either a left thoracotomy or a median sternotomy with cardiopulmonary bypass. The management of associated tracheobronchial anomalies continues to be a difficult problem. If significant obstruc-

tion remains after correction of the pulmonary artery sling, resection of the stenotic segment of the trachea or tracheoplasty may be required.

Results of surgical therapy for pulmonary artery sling have been somewhat disappointing. Potts' first patient in 1953 fared very well and was discharged on the eleventh postoperative day. Follow-up 24 years later showed that the child had developed normally and had normal exercise tolerance. However, a ventilation-perfusion scan demonstrated minimal perfusion of the left lung. Sade and associates reviewed 40 cases of pulmonary artery sling that were treated surgically with a 50 per cent mortality. The survivors were generally asymptomatic; however, 9 of 10 patients studied had occluded left pulmonary arteries. Dunn and colleagues reported four patients who had repair of pulmonary artery sling.[19] Patency of the left pulmonary artery was documented in all patients. Mortality is usually related to the severity of the tracheobronchial stenosis and associated defects. Survivors generally have a benign course despite occlusion of the left pulmonary artery, and residual symptoms tend to decrease as the patients grow. Although there has been concern that patients with an occluded left pulmonary artery might develop pulmonary hypertension in the right lung or hemoptysis secondary to bronchial collaterals, neither has been encountered. Attempts to restore patency to occluded pulmonary arteries have not met with success and are not generally recommended.

SELECTED REFERENCES

Abbott, M. E.: Coarctation of the aorta of the adult type II: A statistical study and historical retrospect of 200 recorded cases, with autopsy, or stenosis or obliteration of the descending arch in subjects above the age of two years. Am. Heart J., 3:574, 1928.
 A classic series reporting the natural history, physical examination, and autopsy findings of 200 patients with coarctation of the aorta.
Brewer, L. A., III, Fosburg, R. G., Mulder, G. A., and Verska, J. J.: Spinal cord complications following surgery for coarctation of the aorta: A study of 66 cases. J. Thorac. Cardiovasc. Surg., 64:368, 1972.
 An extensive review encompassing 12,532 cases of repair of coarctation of the aorta

delineating the incidence of spinal cord complications and possible contributing factors.

Edwards, J. E.: Anomalies of the derivatives of the aortic arch system. Med. Clin. North Am., July:925, 1948.
First description of the hypothetical double aortic arch that forms the basis for classification of vascular rings.

Sade, R. M., Rosenthal, A., Fellows, K., and Castaneda, A. R.: Pulmonary artery sling. J. Thorac. Cardiovasc. Surg., 69:333, 1975.
Excellent review of embryology, natural history, and surgical correction of pulmonary artery sling.

Schuster, S. R., and Gross, R. E.: Surgery for coarctation of the aorta: A review of 500 cases. J. Thorac. Cardiovasc. Surg., 43:54, 1962.
A report by Gross, a pioneer in cardiac surgery, of his extensive experience with coarctation of the aorta.

Scott, H. W., Jr., and Bahnson, H. T.: Evidence for a renal factor in the hypertension of experimental coarctation of the aorta. Surgery, 30:206, 1951.
Classic experimental demonstration of the role of the kidney in the hypertension of coarctation.

Waldhausen, J. A., and Nahrwold, D. L.: Repair of coarctation of the aorta with a subclavian flap. J. Thorac. Cardiovasc. Surg., 51:532, 1966.
First report of the subclavian flap technique for repair of coarctation that is currently one of the most commonly used repairs.

Yee, E. S., Turley, K., Soifer, S., and Ebert, P. A.: Synthetic patch aortoplasty: A simplified approach for coarctation in repair during early infancy and thereafter. J. Surg., 148:240, 1984.
Review of the advantages of the prosthetic flap aortoplasty including decreased operative time, decreased need for dissection, and excellent hemodynamic result.

REFERENCES

1. Achanti, B., Yeh, T. F., and Pildes, R. S.: Indomethacin therapy in infants with advanced postnatal age and patent ductus arteriosus. Clin. Invest. Med., 9:250, 1986.
2. Adzick, W. S., Harrison, M. R., and Delorimier, A. A.: Surgical clip ligation of patent ductus arteriosus in premature infants. J. Pediatr. Surg., 21:158, 1986.
3. Arciniegas, E., Hakimi, M., Hertzler, J. H., et al.: Surgical management of congenital vascular rings. J. Thorac. Cardiovasc. Surg., 77:721, 1979.
4. Backer, C. I., Ilbawi, M. N., Idriss, P. S., and DeLeon, S. Y.: Vascular anomalies causing tracheoesophageal compression. J. Thorac. Cardiovasc. Surg., 97:725, 1989.
5. Bagby, S. P., and Mass, R. D.: Abnormality of the renin/body fluid–volume relationship in serially-studied inbred dogs with neonatally-induced coarctation hypertension. Hypertension, 2:631, 1980.
5a. Bayford, D.: An account of a singular case of obstructed deglutition. Memoirs of the Medical Society of London, 2:275, 1794.
6. Beekman, R. H., Rocchini, A. P., Behrendt, D. M., et al.: Long-term outcome after repair of coarctation in infancy: Subclavian angioplasty does not reduce the need for reoperation. J. Am. Coll. Cardiol., 8:1406, 1986.
7. Beekman, R. H., Rocchini, A. P., MacDonald, D., II, et al.: Percutaneous balloon angioplasty for native coarctation of the aorta. J. Am. Coll. Cardiol., 10:1078, 1987.
8. Bell, E. F., Warburton, D., Stonestreet, B. S., and Oh, W.: Effect of fluid administration on the development of symptomatic patent ductus arteriosus and congestive heart failure in premature infants. N. Engl. J. Med., 302:598, 1980.
9. Binet, J. P., and Langlois, J.: Aortic arch anomalies in children and infants. J. Thorac. Cardiovasc. Surg., 73:248, 1977.
10. Blalock, A., and Park, E. A.: The surgical treatment of experimental coarctation (atresia) of the aorta. Ann. Surg., 119:445, 1944.
11. Brandt, B., III, Heintz, S. E., Rose, E. F., et al.: Repair of coarctation of the aorta in children with Turner's syndrome. Pediatr. Cardiol., 5:175, 1984.
12. Bromberg, B. L., Beekman, R. H., Rocchini, A. P., et al.: Aortic aneurysm after patch aortoplasty repair of coarctation. A prospective analysis of prevalence. Screening tests and risks. J. Am. Coll. Cardiol., 14:734, 1989.
13. Campbell, D. B., Waldhausen, J. A., Pierce, W. S., et al.: Should elective repair of coarctation of the aorta be done in infancy? J. Thorac. Cardiovasc. Surg., 88:979, 1984.
14. Clyman, R. I., and Campbell, D.: Indomethacin therapy for patent ductus arteriosus: When is prophylaxis not prophylactic? J. Pediatr., 111:718, 1987.
15. Cobanoglu, A., Teply, J. F., Grunkemeier, G. L., et al.: Coarctation of the aorta in patients younger than three months. J. Thorac. Cardiovasc. Surg., 89:128, 1985.
16. Cokkinos, D. V., Leachman, R. D., and Cooley, D. A.: Increased mortality rate from coronary artery disease following operation for coarctation of the aorta at a late age. J. Thorac. Cardiovasc. Surg., 77:315, 1979.
17. Cooper, S. G., Sullivan, I. D., and Wren, C.: Treatment of recoarctation: Balloon dilation angioplasty. J. Am. Coll. Cardiol., 14:413, 1989.
18. Cunningham, H. N., Jr., Larchinger, J. C., and Spencer, F. C.: Monitoring of somatosensory evoked potentials during surgical procedures on the thoracoabdominal aorta. IV. Clinical observations and results. J. Thorac. Cardiovasc. Surg., 94:275, 1987.
19. Dunn, J. M., Gordon, I., Chrispin, A. R., et al.: Early and late results of surgical correction of pulmonary artery sling. Ann. Thorac. Surg., 28:230, 1979.
20. Filston, H. C., Ferguson, T. B., Jr., and Oldham, H. N.: Airway obstruction by vascular anomalies: Importance of telescopic bronchoscopy. Ann. Surg., 205:541, 1987.
21. Foster, E. D.: Reoperation for aortic coarctation. Ann. Thorac. Surg., 38:81, 1984.
21a. Gaynor, J. W., and Sabiston, D. C., Jr.: Patent ductus arteriosus, coarctation of the aorta, aortopulmonary window, and anomalies of the aortic arch. *In* Sabiston, D. C., Jr., and Spencer, F. C. (Eds.): Surgery of the chest, 5th ed. Philadelphia, W. B. Saunders Company, 1990.
22. Gersony, W. M.: Patent ductus arteriosus in the neonate. Pediatr. Clin. North Am., 33:54, 1986.
23. Gersony, W. M., Peckham, G. H., Ellison, R. C., et al.: Effects of indomethacin in premature infants with patent ductus arteriosus: Results of a national collaborative study. J. Pediatr., 102:895, 1983.
23a. Gibson, G. A.: Clinical lectures on circulating afflictions. Lecture I: Persistence of the arterial duct and its diagnosis. Edinb, Med. J., 8:1, 1900.
24. Gikonyo, B. M., Jue, K. L., and Edwards, J. E.: Pulmonary vascular sling: Report of seven cases and review of the literature. Pediatr. Cardiol., 10:81, 1989.
25. Goldman, S., Hernandez, J., and Pappas, G.: Results of surgical treatment of coarctation of the aorta in the critically ill neonate, including the influence of pulmonary artery banding. J. Thorac. Cardiovasc. Surg., 91:732, 1986.
26. Hammerman, C., Strates, E., and Valaitis, S.: The silent ductus: Its precursors and its aftermath. Pediatr. Cardiol., 7:121, 1986.
27. Hammon, J. W., Jr., Graham, T. P., Jr., Boucek, R. J., Jr., and Bender, H. W., Jr.: Operative repair of coarctation of the aorta in infancy: Results with and without ventricular septal defect. Am. J. Cardiol., 55:1555, 1985.
28. Heymann, M. A., Berman, W., Jr., Rudolph, A. M., and Whitman, V.: Dilation of the ductus arteriosus by prostaglandin E_1 in aortic arch abnormalities. Circulation, 59:169, 1979.
29. Heymann, M. A., Rudolph, A. M., and Silberman, N. H.: Closure of the ductus arteriosus in premature infants by inhibition of prostaglandin synthesis. N. Engl. J. Med., 295:530, 1976.
30. Hopkins, R. A., Kostic, I., Klages, U., et al.: Correction of coarctation of the aorta in neonates and young infants in an individualized surgical approach. Eur. J. Cardiothorac. Surg., 2:296, 1988.
31. John, S., Muralidharan, S., Jairaj, P. S., et al.: The adult ductus: Review of surgical experience with 131 patients. J. Thorac. Cardiovasc. Surg., 82:314, 1981.
32. Keys, A., and Shapiro, M. J.: Patency of the ductus arteriosus in adults. Am. Heart J., 25:158, 1943.
33. Kimball, B. P., Shurvell, B. L., Houle, S., et al.: Persistent ventricular adaptations in postoperative coarctation of the aorta. J. Am. Coll. Cardiol., 8:172, 1986.
34. Korfer, R., Meyer, H., Kleikamp, G., and Bircks, W.: Early and late results after resection and end to end anastomosis of coarctation of the thoracic aorta in early infancy. J. Thorac. Cardiovasc. Surg., 89:616, 1985.
35. Lansman, S., Shapiro, A. J., Schiller, M. S., et al.: Extended aortic arch anastomosis for repair of coarctation in infancy. Circulation, 74(Suppl. I):37, 1986.
36. Markel, H., Rocchini, A. P., Beekman, R. H., et al.: Exercise induced hypertension after repair of coarctation of the aorta: Arm versus leg exercise. J. Am. Coll. Cardiol., 8:165, 1986.
37. Munro, J. L., Brunton, R. W., Sutherland, G. R., and Keeton, B. R.: Correction of interrupted aortic arch. J. Thorac. Cardiovasc. Surg., 98:421, 1989.
38. Palder, S. B., Schwartz, M. Z., Tyson, K. R. T., and Marr, C. C.: Management of patent ductus arteriosus: A comparison of operative vs. pharmacologic treatment. J. Pediatr. Surg., 22:1171, 1987.
39. Rashkind, W. J., Mullins, C. E., Hellenbrand, W. E., and Tait, M. A.: Nonsurgical closure of patent ductus arteriosus: Clinical application of the Rashkind PDA occluder system. Circulation, 75:583, 1987.
40. Ritter, S. B.: Coarctation and balloons: Inflated or realistic? J. Am. Coll. Cardiol., 13:696, 1989.
41. Sanchez, G. R., Balsara, R. K., Dunn, J. M., et al.: Recurrent obstruction after subclavian flap repair of coarctation of the aorta in infants. J. Thorac. Cardiovasc. Surg., 91:738, 1986.
42. Scott, W. A., Rocchini, A. P., Bove, E. L., et al.: Repair of interrupted aortic arch in infancy. J. Thorac. Cardiovasc. Surg., 96:564, 1988.
43. Sell, J. E., Jonas, R. A., Mayer, J. E., et al.: The results of a surgical program for interrupted aortic arch. J. Thorac. Cardiovasc. Surg., 96:864, 1988.
44. Simpson, I. A., Sahn, D. J., Valdes-Cruz, C. M., et al.: Color Doppler flow mapping in patients with coarctation of the aorta: New observations and improved evaluation with color flow diameter and proximal acceleration as predictors of severity. Circulation, 77:736, 1988.
45. Simpson, I. A., Chung, K. J., Glass, R. E., et al.: Cine magnetic resonance imaging for evaluation of anatomy and flow relations in infants and children with coarctation of the aorta. Circulation, 78:142, 1988.
46. Tiraboschi, R., Salomone, G., Crupi, G., et al.: Aortopulmonary window in the first year of life: Report of 11 surgical cases. Ann. Thorac. Surg., 46:438, 1988.
47. Trinquet, F., Vouhe, P. O., Vernant, F., et al.: Coarctation of the aorta in infants: Which operation? Ann. Thorac. Surg., 45:186, 1988.
48. Van Son, J. A. M., Van Asten, W. N. J. C., Van Lier, H. J. J., et al.: Detrimental sequelae on the hemodynamics of the upper left limb after subclavian flap angioplasty in infancy. Circulation, 81:996, 1990.
49. Wierny, L., Plass, R., and Porstmann, W.: Transluminal closure of patent ductus arteriosus: Long-term results of 208 cases treated without thoracotomy. Cardiovasc. Intervent. Radiol., 9:279, 1986.
50. Ziemer, G., Jonas, R. A., Perry, S. B., et al.: Surgery for coarctation of the aorta in the neonate. Circulation, 74(Suppl. I):25, 1986.

V

ATRIAL SEPTAL DEFECTS, OSTIUM PRIMUM DEFECTS, AND ATRIOVENTRICULAR CANALS

Ross M. Ungerleider, M.D.

An atrial septal defect (ASD) is an opening in the atrial septum that enables mixing of blood from the systemic and pulmonary venous circulations. This opening may develop in a variety of locations because the embryologic causes of ASDs are numerous. Although functionally the same with respect to the physiology of shunting, these defects present the surgeon with several considerations that differ depending upon the precise nature and location of the defect.

Atrioventricular canal (AV canal) defects include defects in the atrial and ventricular septum immediately above and below the atrioventricular valves (tricuspid and mitral). These defects usually involve the valves, and the physiologic aspects depend upon the extent of shunting at both the atrial and ventricular levels, as well as regurgitation from the involved valves. Defects limited to the atrial septum are termed *ostium primum* atrial septal defects (or partial AV canal defects). Complete AV canal defects (also referred to as *complete atrioventricular septal defects* or *endocardial cushion defects*) combine deficiency of both the atrial and ventricular septum with severe abnormality of the mitral and tricuspid valves—creating what is in essence a common atrioventricular valve that serves both ventricles.

HISTORICAL ASPECTS

Because they are located in the relatively accessible upper chambers of the heart, ASDs were among the first intracardiac congenital heart defects to attract surgical correction. Surgeons were initally limited by their ability to open the heart, and several ingenious methods for external closure of ASDs by invagination and suturing of the wall of the right atrium into the defect were developed.[4,78,96] Because of the great variation in these defects as well as the inaccuracy of these methods, these techniques had limited usefulness and applicability. Certainly, a technique that would allow closure of these defects under more direct vision in the open atrium was more desirable. Gross[46,55] devised an ingenious funnel-type "well" that could be sewn to the atrium, allowing an atriotomy to be performed with the blood contained within the "well." The surgeon could then close the ASD through the "well" in the opened atrium by sewing to the rim of the palpated defect. The introduction of surface cooling with moderate induced hypothermia, coupled with short periods of inflow occlusion by vena caval occlusion to allow visualization of intracardiac anatomy, provided surgeons with a technique for safe direct vision intracardiac repair, and Lewis reported the first successful closure of an ASD using this system in 1953[64]; but the nature of this method limited its application to simple defects that could be quickly evaluated and repaired. With a daring characteristic of early attempts to correct congenital heart defects, Lillehei and colleagues[66,67] reported successful intracardiac surgery for a variety of defects, including ASDs and partial and complete AV canal defects, using a technique of "cross-circulation" in which the patient was connected to the circulation of another human being (often

a parent) who served as an oxygenator and blood reservoir to support the patient during intracardiac repair. Modern heart surgery began with the introduction by Gibbon[40] in 1953 of the mechanical pump-oxygenator. Using this device, which culminated a lifetime of dedicated research, Gibbon closed an atrial septal defect in a young woman. With rapid improvements in the techniques of extracorporeal circulation, open correction of ASDs (as well as most other forms of complex congenital heart disease) was routinely performed on cardiopulmonary bypass and this has supplanted all other methods.

ANATOMY

A variety of developmental factors influence normal development of the atrial septum and an understanding of the embryologic development of this portion of the heart facilitates appreciation for the nature of these various anomalies. Partitioning of the atrioventricular canal and the atrium begins about the middle of the fourth week and is essentially complete by the end of the fifth week.[77] The atrial septum is initially partitioned by a thin membrane (*septum primum*) which appears to extend toward the region of the atrioventricular valves from the superior aspect of the atrium. Simultaneously, endocardial cushion tissue extends upward to meet this septum and to close the intervening space (referred to as the *ostium primum*). Just prior to obliteration of the *ostium primum*, perforations appear near the middle of the *septum primum* to allow free flow of blood between the right and left sides of the atrium. These perforations coalasce to form the *ostium secundum*. A second ridge of tissue (*septum secundum*) begins to grow in a downward direction from the top of the atrium and to the right side of the *septum primum*. This *septum secundum* covers the *ostium secundum* in such a manner that the *septum primum* attaches to the left atrial side of the superior aspect of the *septum secundum* and completes the atrial partitioning. Because of the nature of this septation, the *septum primum* performs as a "flap valve" to allow flow of blood from the right to left direction across the septum through a small potential defect referred to as the *foramen ovale* (Fig. 1). The *septum primum*, as seen from the right atrial side, is termed the *fossa ovalis*.

All defects in the atrial septum in the region of the *fossa ovalis* are termed *secundum* atrial septal defects. Most of these are usually defects of the *septum primum* (Fig. 2*A, B,* and *D*) although they can also include deficient downward growth of the *septum secundum*, and in association with a normal *septum primum* can be termed a *foramen ovale* defect (Fig. 2*C*).

Concurrent with the septation of the atrium, thickenings of subendocardial tissue, i.e., *endocardial cushions*, develop in the dorsal and ventral walls of the heart in the region of the atrioventricular canal. During the fifth week, the atrioventricular endocardial cushions grow toward each other and fuse, dividing the atrioventricular canal into right and left sides.[77] These cushions provide a portion of the atrial septum (the part that

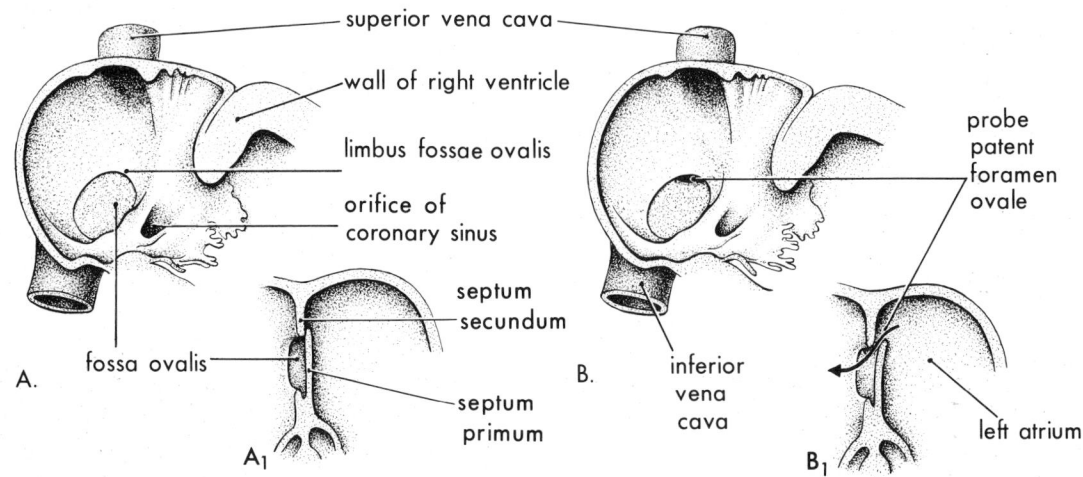

Figure 1. A, This depiction of the anatomy in the right atrium demonstrates that the fossa ovalis is closed by the septum primum, which attaches on the left atrial side of the septum secundum (A). The location of the fossa ovalis near the coronary sinus is a consistent anatomic feature. B, When the septum primum does not grow adequately to attach to the left atrial side of the septum secundum, a patent foramen ovale results, which permits intra-atrial shunting. The distinction between right and left atrium is easily made by observing the side to which the septum primum attaches, because that always identifies the left atrium. (From Moore, K. L.: The Developing Human: Clinically Oriented Embryology. Philadelphia, W. B. Saunders Company, 1977.)

grows upward to fuse with the septum primum), the ventricular septum (immediately below the tricuspid valve in the inlet to the right ventricle), and the septal leaflets of both the mitral and tricuspid valves. Therefore, abnormal growth in this region can produce a deficiency in the lowermost part of the atrial septum (often with associated abnormalities such as "clefts" of the mitral and tricuspid valves) (Fig. 2E). The most extensive form of this developmental anomaly produces a ventricular septal deficiency as well (Fig. 3) and what is essentially a hole in the middle of the heart (complete AV canal) with communication at this level between all four cardiac chambers.

Defects can also occur high in the superior aspect of the interatrial septum and are referred to as *sinus venosus* defects. Initially, the sinus venosus is a separate chamber of the heart and opens into the caudal wall of the right atrium. The left side of the *sinus venosus* becomes incorporated into the coronary sinus, and the right side merges with the upper portion of the right atrium. The *sinus venosus* represents the confluence of venous drainage to the heart, and a defect in this region can produce communication between the posterior aspect of the superior vena cava and the top of the left atrium (Fig. 2F). It is not uncommon for the right superior pulmonary veins to drain to the left atrium at the top of the *sinus venosus* and, if a *sinus venosus* defect is present, to appear to return anomalously to the right atrium at, or slightly above, its junction with the superior vena cava. Therefore, most *sinus venosus* atrial septal defects are associated with *partial* anomalous pulmonary venous return. Other rare types of defects in the atrial septum occur and are usually related to some definable abnormality during embryologic development. For example, a deficiency in the left horn of the sinus venosus, as it becomes incorporated into the coronary sinus, can cause an *unroofed coronary sinus* that drains into the left atrium or enables communication between the left atrium and the right atrium in the usual region of the coronary sinus — a *coronary sinus* type of ASD. It is also possible to observe a communication between the left and right atrium inferior to the substance of the septum primum located between the inferior vena cava and the coronary sinus. This rare type of defect is probably in the inferior aspect of the sinus venosus and can be considered a sinus venosus type defect. This region should be investigated in all cases of superior sinus venosus defects.

INCIDENCE AND ASSOCIATED DEFECTS

Atrial septal defects are among the most common congenital cardiac lesions and may be observed in association with almost any other type of cardiac anomaly. They are commonly present[11] in patients with ventricular septal defects; pulmonary stenosis; patent ductus arteriosus; coarctation of the aorta; mitral stenosis, which in association with an ASD is termed Lutembacher's syndrome,[98] and various anomalies of systemic venous return, such as a persistent left superior vena cava.[52] ASDs also appear to be more frequent with pericardial disease than would be expected.[39] Approximately 30 per cent of secundum ASDs occur with other cardiac defects.[111]

Physiologic flow communication at the level of the atrial septum is, in fact, essential for survival in some of the more complicated forms of congenital heart disease; and in this setting, the occurrence of an ASD is not always considered to be part of the pathologic entity. Examples of this include pulmonary atresia (or critical pulmonary stenosis) with intact ventricular septum, tricuspid atresia, mitral atresia, and total anomalous pulmonary venous return. In addition, creation of an atrial level shunt (by balloon catheter or catheter-guided blade septostomy in the cardiac catheterization laboratory or by surgical excision in the operating room) has an important role in the treatment of certain lesions such as transposition of the great vessels and palliation for hypoplastic left heart syndrome.

When ASDs occur as isolated congenital lesions, they still comprise a common entity and may be the fifth most common congenital cardiac lesion, occurring in as many as 13,500 children less than 14 years of age.[51] ASDs represent as many as 7 per cent of all cases of congenital heart disease.[37] Moreover, ASD is the most common heart defect detected in patients over 20 years of age[111]—in large part because of its benign and relatively obscure clinical course, which enables these patients to grow and develop normally with deceptively few clinical signs of heart disease.[35,38,47,48,80,89,97] It is of interest that secundum ASDs occur more frequently in females than in males, with a ratio of 3:1.[111]

Atrial septal defects may also be correlated to genetic factors and are clearly increased in incidence in syndromes such as Down's,[11] Turner's,[84] Ellis-van Creveld,[41] Marfan's,[39,111] and Ehler-Danlos.[111,113] It is not uncommon for the defects in these disorders to be extremely large, bordering on a common atrium. Familial inheritance on the basis of a dominant autosomal gene with incomplete penetrance has been reported[17] and may explain the appearance of ASDs in a family lineage. Varying degrees of AV block may be more common in the familial form of ASD and the risk to offspring of parents with ASDs is 21 times higher than to children of normal parents (although the overall risk is still less than 5 per cent).[17,111] Most ASDs are probably

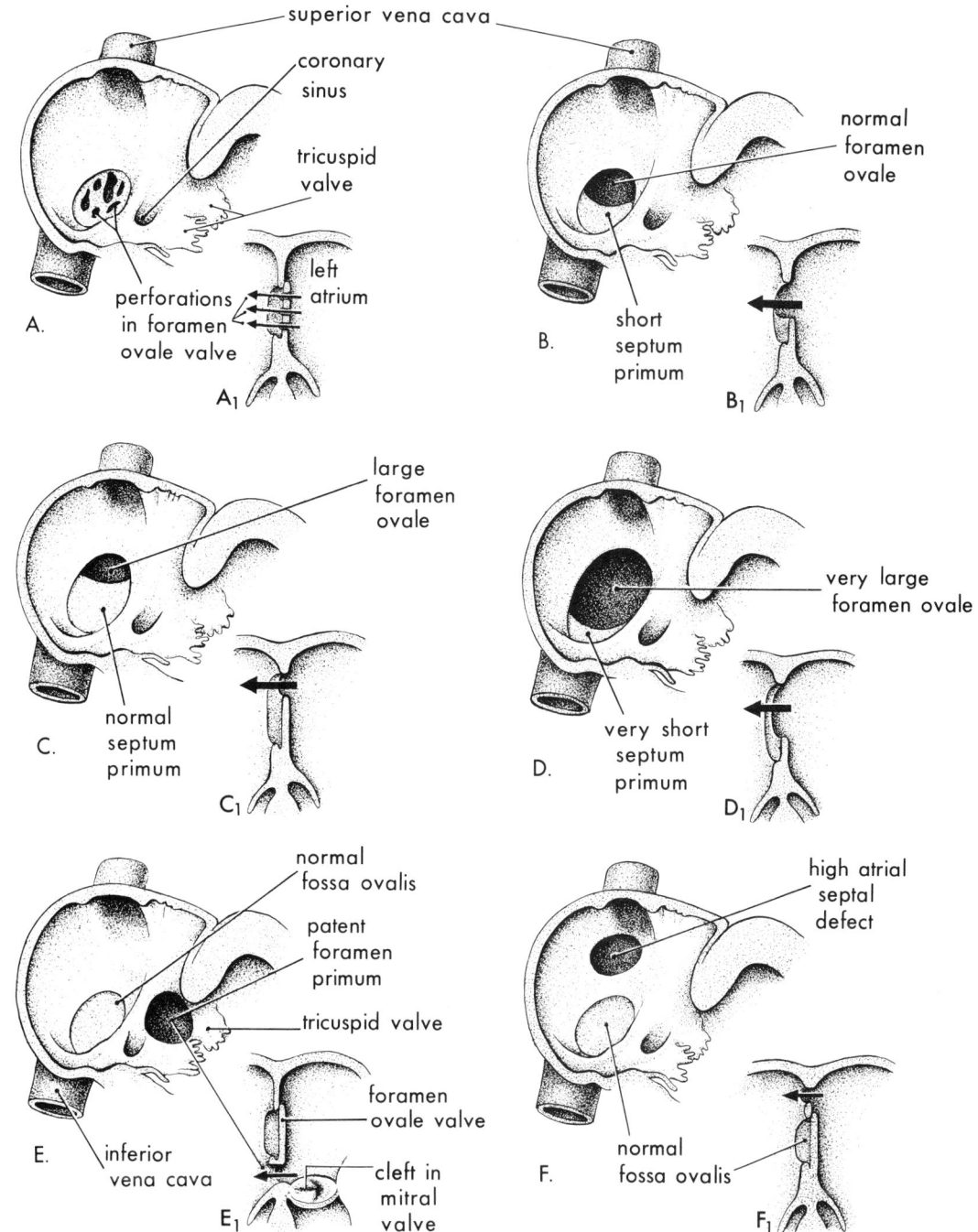

Figure 2. *A,* Perforations in the substance of the septum primum create a deficiency in the foramen ovale, which is commonly called a secundum type of ASD. *B,* A nonperforated but anatomically deficient septum primum allows communication between the atria below the limbus of the septum secundum, frequently referred to as foramen ovale type (secundum) ASD. *C,* A foramen ovale type of ASD can also occur when a normal-sized septum primum is unable to attach to the left atrial surface of the septum secundum. *D,* Likewise, a very short septum primum leaves a large opening through the foramen ovale, causing a large ASD. *E,* Deficiency of the atrioventricular (AV) septum (endocardial cushion tissue) near the coronary sinus and immediately adjacent to the anulus of the tricuspid and mitral valve produces a partial AV canal defect or ostium primum ASD. In this situation, the fossa ovalis is intact, and the atrial communication is just above the mitral and tricuspid valve orifices. These defects, as indicated, are often associated with a "cleft" in the mitral valve. *F,* A defect high in the limbus of the septum secundum can occur superior to the intact fossa ovalis and is referred to as a sinus venosus type ASD. This variety of ASD is commonly associated with partial anomalous pulmonary venous return of the right superior pulmonary veins. (From Moore, K. L.: The Developing Human: Clinically Oriented Embryology. Philadelphia, W. B. Saunders Company, 1977.)

caused by unknown and random disturbances in development. This impression is based on the lack of association of most ASDs with known hereditary abnormalities, the high incidence of associated nongenetic abnormalities of other structures, and the lack of concordance of cardiac defects in identical twins.[105,111] Exposure of the mother to rubella[96] or ingestion of thalidomide by the mother during the first few weeks of pregnancy appears to enhance the likelihood of the development of an ASD in the fetus.[111]

Sinus venosus defects are much less common than secundum ASDs and comprise about 10 per cent of ASDs. Unlike a secundum ASD, a sinus venosus ASD is not commonly associated with other forms of congenital heart disease, except for anomalies of pulmonary venous return, which really comprise part of the spectrum of this lesion. In some cases, the anomalies of pulmonary venous return constitute the most disturbing feature of the defect and may be associated with abnormalities of the ipsilateral lung.[52] Defects in the sinus venosus region are really a

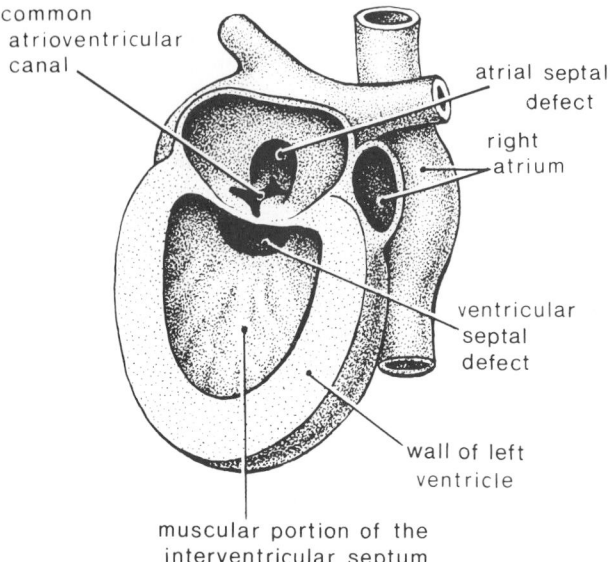

common
atrioventricular
canal

atrial septal
defect

right
atrium

ventricular
septal
defect

wall of left
ventricle

muscular portion of the
interventricular septum

Figure 3. When a defect of endocardial cushion tissue creates an atrial septal communication as well as a ventricular septal communication, the anomaly is referred to as a complete AV canal. This defect, depicted here as seen from the left side of the heart, creates communication between all four cardiac chambers at the level of a common AV valve orifice. (From Moore, K. L.: The Developing Human: Clinically Oriented Embryology. Philadelphia, W. B. Saunders Company, 1977.)

deficiency between the posterior portion of the superior vena cava and the anterior aspect of the left atrium, where these two structures share a "common wall" (Fig. 4).

Endocardial cushion defects that cause both partial and complete AV canal defects show no sex predilection, with an equal incidence in both males and females. As is true with secundum type ASDs, ostium primum ASDs (partial AV canal) and complete AV canals are frequently associated with other cardiac defects (ranging between 7 and 25 per cent).[99,111] AV canal defects (both partial and complete) are sometimes seen in association with more complex and severe forms of congenital heart disease, including the heterotaxy syndromes,[52] tetralogy of Fallot,[16,54] double outlet right ventricle,[16,52] total anomalous pulmonary venous return,[99] and transposition of the great arteries.[16] It is very common for patients with a complete AV canal also to have small secundum ASDs.[108] A patent ductus arteriosus is seen in as many as 10 per cent of these patients,[52,99,108] especially when the diagnosis is made in infancy. There is clearly an association between Down's syndrome and endocardial cushion defects, and some form of the defect may be present in as many as 30 per cent of children with this syndrome.[51]

NATURAL HISTORY

The natural history of untreated ASDs is related to the type of defect, the size of the shunt, and to associated anomalies.[3,22,26] Young patients usually do not have symptoms, although a tendency for increased pulmonary infections due to the increased pulmonary blood flow has been noted. As patients grow older, the impact of chronic intracardiac shunting can become apparent by development of congestive heart failure or atrial dysrhythmias. Pulmonary hypertension is a reported[26,52] but unusual long-term complication that can occur in up to 14 per cent of patients with ASDs. Because of the potential for bidirectional shunting at the atrial level, emboli from the systemic venous circulation (normally cleared by the lungs) can cross the atrial septum to the left-sided circulation and lead to systemic arterial embolization (paradoxical emboli)[103] and be the cause of a stroke, brain abscess, or renal failure. Long-term complications of an unrepaired ASD also include mitral and tricuspid valve incompetence,[52] pulmonary valve incompetence,[64] and systemic hypertension.[97] Of particular note is the well established fact that patients with ASDs have a shortened life expectancy. Although over 99.9 per cent of infants born with isolated ASDs reach the age of 1 year,[22,52] there is a substantial decrement in survival by the time these patients reach the third and fourth decade of life, due in large part to a combination of the various factors mentioned above (Fig. 5). Moreover, the functional status of patients with ASDs deteriorates with age, so that con-

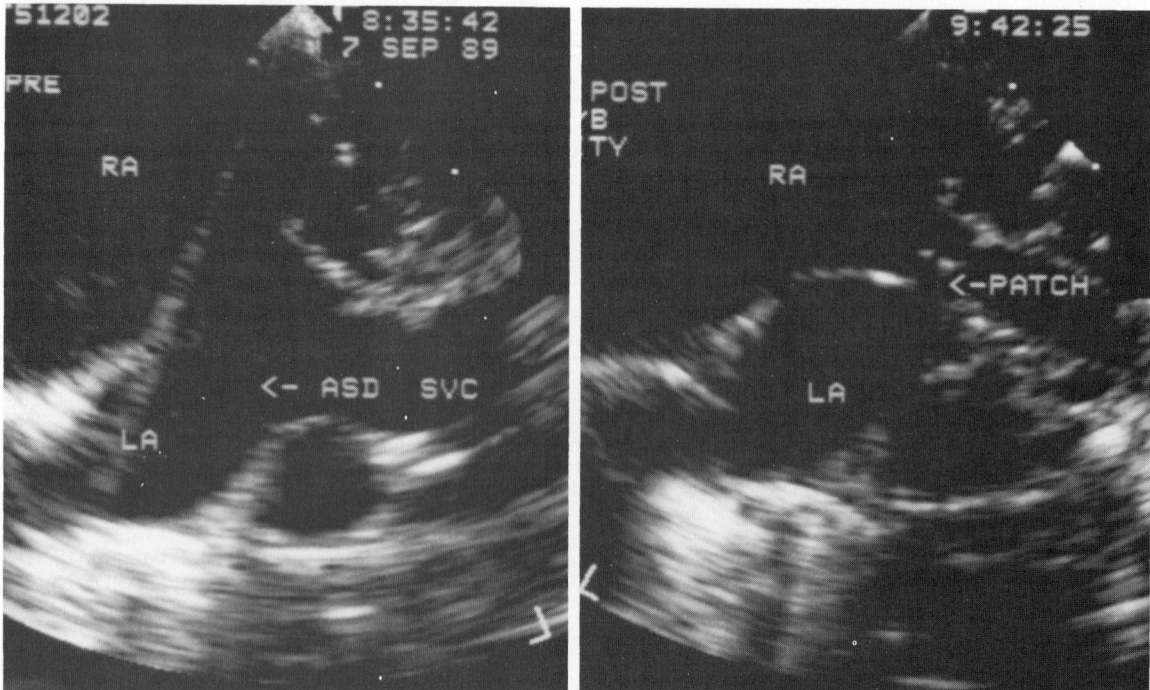

Figure 4. This two-dimensional echo obtained from the epicardial surface of the heart at the time of surgical therapy nicely demonstrates a sinus venosus ASD. It is easily appreciated that the superior vena cava (SVC) and left atrium (LA) share a common wall (arrow) and absence of this wall creates the sinus venosus defect. Panel 2 demonstrates reconstruction of this wall (patch) so that the left atrium is separated from the overlying SVC and right atrium (RA).

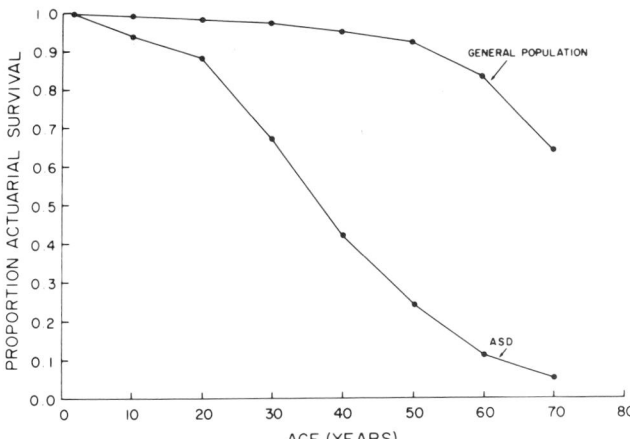

Figure 5. Actuarial survival for patients with unrepaired ASDs compared with an age-matched general population. These survival curves clearly demonstrate a marked increase in the mortality occuring beyond 20 years of age for these patients with unrepaired ASDs. (From Kirklin, J. W., and Barratt-Boyes, B. G.: Cardiac Surgery. New York, John Wiley & Sons, 1986.)

comitant with the decline in life expectancy, increasing symptoms of easy fatigability, exercise intolerance, and palpitations appear. Children with ASDs often have increased sweating with eating and the tendency to appear chronically tired. Slow growth rates are also attributed to ASDs, and it is not infrequent for a child to have a marked increase in growth after repair of the defect.

The natural history of patients with AV canal defects depends upon the extent of the lesion (partial versus complete), the degree of mitral insufficiency, and the nature of any associated lesions (both cardiac and noncardiac). Expectations for patients with partial AV canal defects (ostium primum ASD) and only mild mitral insufficiency parallel those for ASDs.[95] There is an accelerated tendency for these patients to develop atrial arrhythmias at the time of onset of symptoms. This may be due to

the location of this defect near (and displacing) the AV node as well as to the fact that most of these patients have large left-to-right shunts with distention of the right atrium and ventricle. When an ostium primum defect is associated with moderate to severe mitral insufficiency, the impact on natural history is more pronounced. As many as one fifth of these patients are symptomatic (congestive heart failure, dyspnea, arrhythmias) in infancy,[52] and several die during the first decade of life. This reflects the degree of intracardiac shunting as well as the diminished forward cardiac output secondary to mitral insufficiency.

The natural history for complete AV canal defects is not well understood, because it is unusual for these patients to be managed without surgical intervention. Nevertheless, the addition of an intracardiac shunt at the ventricular level, combined with the atrial level shunt and AV valve insufficiency, makes this a particularly morbid lesion with low expectation for acceptable untreated survival. A few small series have confirmed this suspicion[13,52,75] and suggest that 80 per cent of patients who do not undergo surgical intervention die by 2 years of age. Even infants who survive for 1 year have only a 15 per cent likelihood of living to the age of 5. These patients die of overwhelming congestive heart failure, with respiratory distress, arrhythmias, or pulmonary infections. Those who survive do so by elevation of pulmonary artery pressures for protection against the intracardiac shunt. Irreversible changes of pulmonary hypertension almost invariably develop at an early age,[79] and this can be expected in up to 90 per cent of patients who survive until their first birthday. Patients with Down's syndrome (a frequent association with complete AV canal defects) may demonstrate more rapid development of irreversible changes of pulmonary hypertension, and this has been described in these patients within the first 2 months of life.[2,117] Although patients in whom severe pulmonary hypertension develops have less intracardiac shunting and appear to be clinically improved, the outlook for the future is dismal, because corrective surgery becomes extremely hazardous, if not impossible. It is also of interest that 14 per cent of women with repaired AV canal defects who survive to have children risk a heritable congenital heart defect (usually tetral-

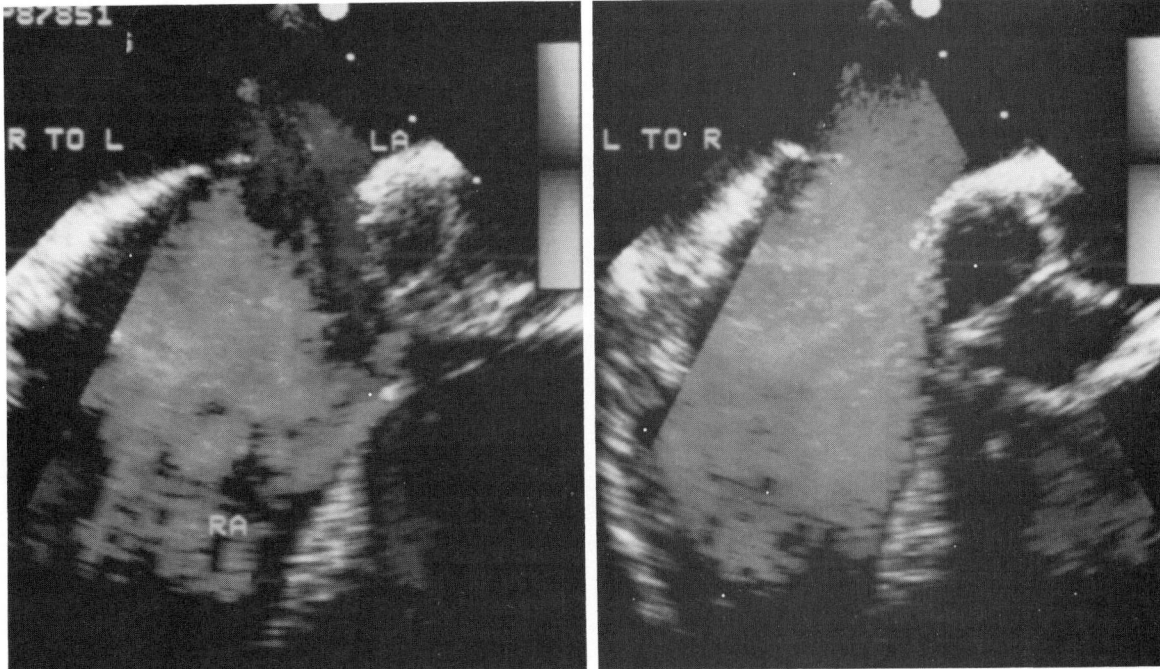

Figure 6. This transesophageal color flow Doppler image demonstrates the ability for ASDs to shunt right to left (*left panel*) as well as left to right (*right panel*) at various stages of the cardiac cycle. The phase of the cardiac cycle during which the image was obtained is demonstrated by placement of a bar over the ECG, which is reproduced at the lower portion of each image. In this case, flow toward the transducer (which is represented by the white dot at the top of each panel) appears to be red in color, whereas flow away from the transducer appears as blue. Therefore, right-to-left shunting appears as red flow (toward the transducer), and left-to-right shunting appears as blue flow (away from the transducer). RA, right atrium; LA, left atrium.

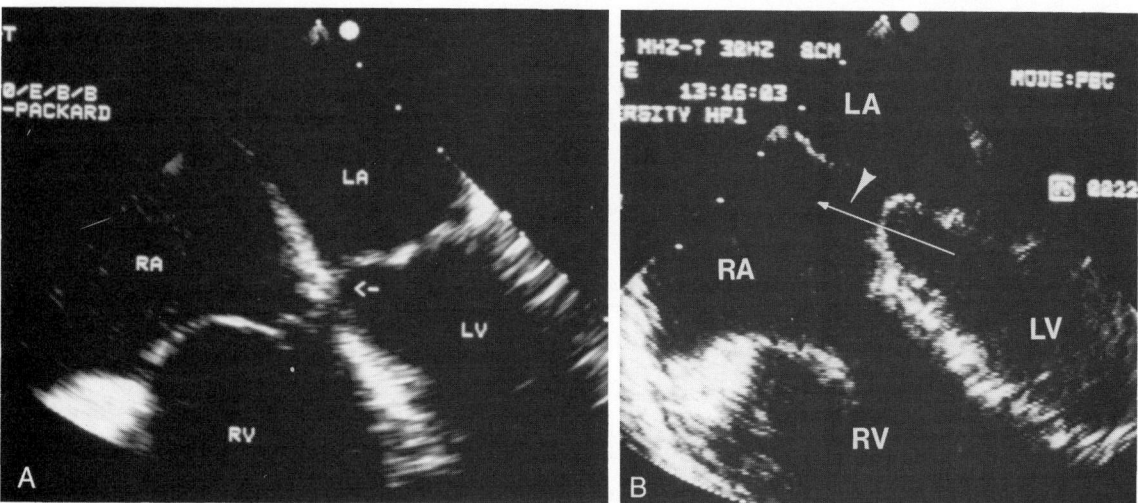

Figure 7. *A,* A four-chamber echo view of the heart obtained from a transesophageal probe demonstrates the left atrium (LA), the right atrium (RA), the right ventricle (RV), and the left ventricle (LV). It is clearly appreciated that the tricuspid valve attaches closer toward the apex of the heart than the mitral valve in this normal situation. This creates a septum between the left ventricle and right atrium (arrow), which is the normal atrioventricular (AV) *septum. B,* When the AV septum is absent, as in an ostium primum ASD, the mitral valve attaches further toward the apex at the crest of the ventricular septum. This displacement of the mitral valve is often associated with a cleft in the anterior leaflet, which enables direct regurgitant shunting between the left ventricle to the right atrium (thin arrow). In addition, the absence of the AV septum enables intra-atrial shunting to occur as well (thick arrow).

ogy of Fallot or an AV canal defect) in their offspring.[32] This is substantially higher than the 2 to 4 per cent risk that mothers with other types of congenital heart defects have of giving birth to a child with a heart lesion.[52]

PHYSIOLOGY

The natural history described above is created by abnormal blood flow patterns that cause excessive pulmonary blood flow, increased cardiac (especially right ventricular) work, and the potential risk of bidirectional intracardiac shunting with paradoxical emboli. The direction of an intracardiac shunt is predominantly determined by compliance of the downstream chamber. In the case of an ASD, the downstream chambers are the ventricles. Compliance is a reflection of distensibility, or the amount of pressure necessary to add volume to a chamber. In infants, the right and left ventricles are essentially equivalent in muscle mass and equally distensible. However, as pulmonary vascular resistance falls shortly after birth, the right ventricle

increases less than the left in hypertrophy of muscle mass and becomes a more compliant, or distensible, chamber. Flow through an ASD that occurs during diastole, with the AV valves open, moves toward the direction of "least resistance." The right ventricle offers less resistance to filling than does the left, and therefore most of the flow through an ASD moves from left to right across the atrial septum and causes volume loading of the right ventricle, which easily distends to accommodate this load.[20] Even during systole, with the AV valves closed, pressure differences between the left atrium and right atrium favor flow from left to right.[62] Despite this predominant left-to-right shunt, there are moments during the cardiac cycle when the instantaneous pressure gradient favors right to left flow across an ASD. In addition, the dynamics by which the inferior vena cava empties into the right atrium usually cause some "streaming" of inferior caval blood across the defect into the left atrium. This can be demonstrated easily with color flow Doppler mapping (Fig. 6) and is the reason that microcavitation studies are a sensitive indicator of atrial septal shunts.[1,7,36,62] The total shunt flow

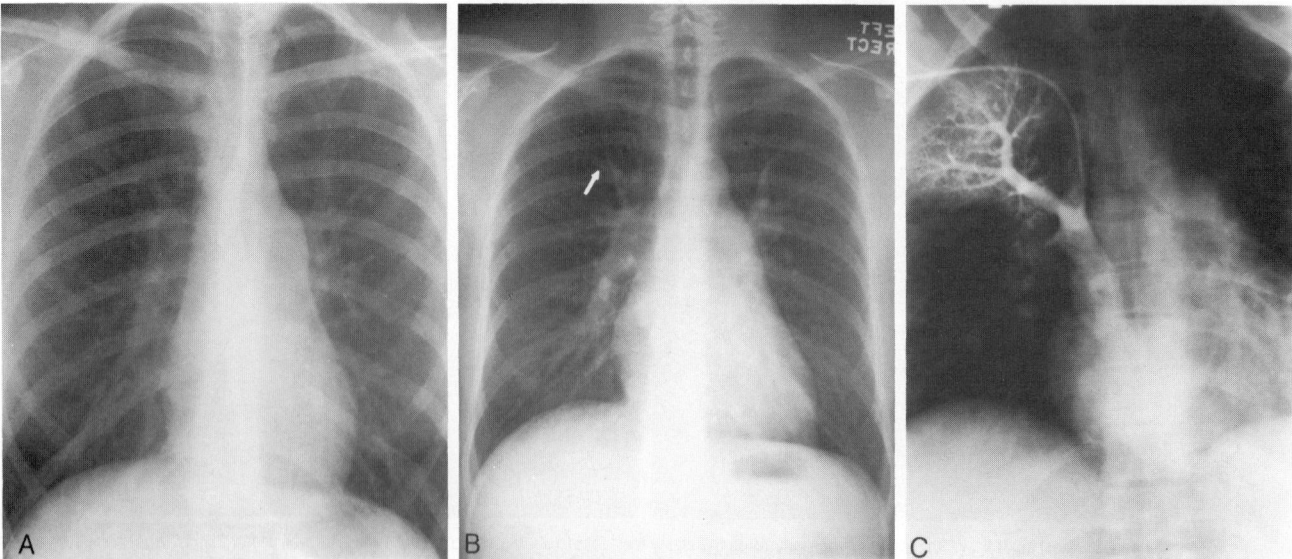

Figure 8. *A,* Posteroanterior chest film of a patient with a secundum atrial septal defect. Notice the prominence of the pulmonary artery shadow and the increased pulmonary blood flow. *B,* This film from a patient with a sinus venosus defect suggests anomalous drainage of the right superior pulmonary vein to the SVC (arrow). *C,* This latter suspicion is confirmed by direct injection of the anomalous right superior pulmonary vein.

across the defect is determined by the compliance of the ventricles[20] and not by the size of the defect (unless the defect is small and restrictive to free flow). Thus, quantitation of the shunt does not predict the size of the defect.[62] Pulmonary blood flow may be three to four times systemic flow (Q_p:Q_s = 3 or 4:1) in patients who are otherwise asymptomatic.

In patients with large shunts, the right ventricular volume is usually increased and the interventricular septum may be displaced into the left ventricle. Although this may appear to create some diminished left ventricular (LV) function, LV performance should be normal after closure of the defect,[19,112] unless it is abnormally small and "hypoplastic."[14] Right ventricular (RV) function, however, may be affected by the chronic volume loading and distention.[19,118]

The long-term ability of the right ventricle to recover normal function is probably related to the age of the patient at the time of repair, those undergoing ASD closure prior to 10 years of age having a better likelihood of achieving normal RV function.[65,81] In addition, the increase in RV stroke volume causes relative stenosis across the pulmonary valve,[111] which can produce gradients as high as 40 mm. Hg (although usually only as high as 15 to 20 mm. Hg), and this can cause some degree of RV hypertrophy. As the right ventricle hypertrophies, it becomes less compliant, and the size of the left-to-right intracardiac shunt decreases. Patients may then become less symptomatic, despite a heart that is more impaired.

In a small number of patients with ASDs, pulmonary hypertension may develop and lead to hypertrophy of the right ventricle and diminishment of the left-to-right shunt. Patients with ASDs living at lower altitudes can be expected to have comparatively lower pulmonary arterial pressures than those at higher altitudes. For example, the average mean pulmonary arterial pressure in a group of patients under 20 years old living below 2000 feet was 18.7 mm. Hg, whereas in a comparable group living at 4000 feet, the mean pressure was 30.4 mm. Hg.[28]

As the RV compliance begins to approach that of the LV, the intracardiac shunt may dissipate and the patient may have a Q_p:Q_s equal to 1:1. This shunt ratio actually reflects net pulmonary versus net systemic blood flow and does not mean that there is no shunting across the defect. In patients with pulmonary hypertension, which limits the left-to-right shunt flow,

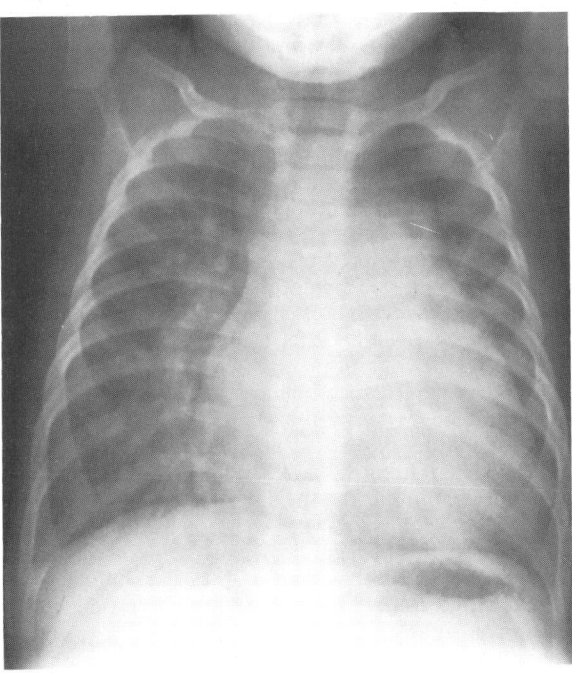

Figure 10. This infant with a complete AV canal defect has cardiomegaly, pulmonary overcirculation, and congestive heart failure. This pattern seen early in infancy is highly suggestive of a complete AV canal defect.

right-to-left shunting develops during some phases of the cardiac cycle that balances the left-to-right shunting, which continues during the remaining phases. Although they do not have a net increase in pulmonary flow versus systemic flow, they have bidirectional shunting of blood inside the heart, and the right-to-left component causes a significant quantity of desaturated (unoxygenated) blood to cross to the systemic circulation, producing mild cyanosis. This is often a sign that the defect is no longer correctable.

Without the development of significant RV hypertrophy from pulmonary stenosis or pulmonary hypertension, the intracardiac shunt continues to produce excessive pulmonary blood flow, with increased blood return to the left atrium. Most of this blood shunts across the ASD to produce volume loading of the right atrium and ventricle, with signs of congestive heart failure. Atrial arrhythmias occur and appear to be related to the right

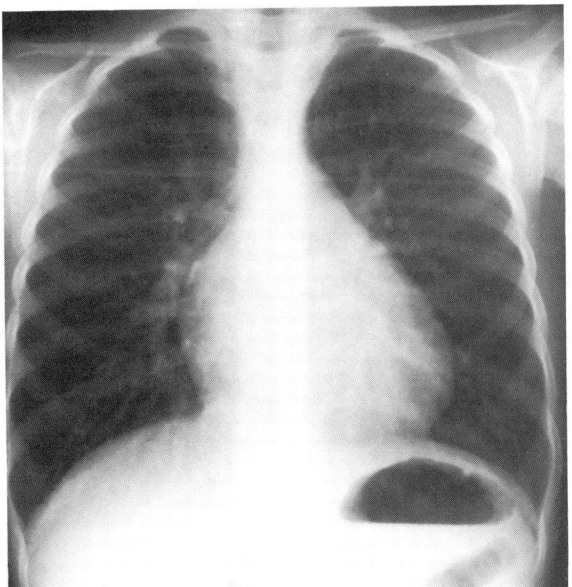

Figure 9. Posteroanterior chest film of a patient with an ostium primum atrial septal defect and moderate mitral regurgitation. Not only is the pulmonary artery shadow and pulmonary vascular pattern increased, but there is also left ventricular dilatation producing a pattern of biventricular hypertrophy and overall cardiomegaly.

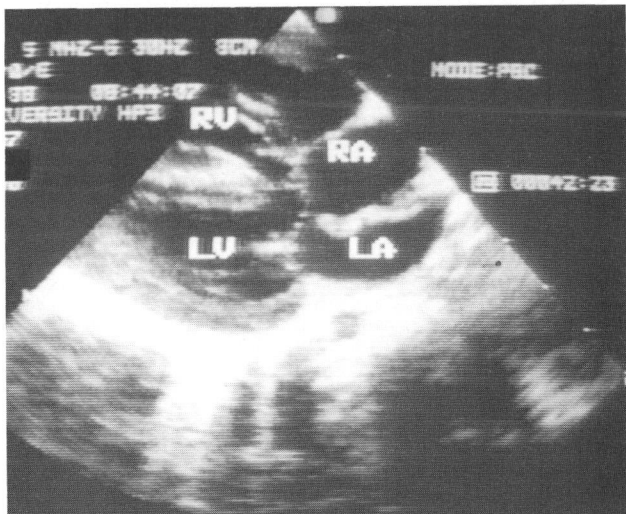

Figure 11. This four-chamber echocardiogram clearly reveals the distinguishing features of a complete AV canal defect with a large communication above the ventricular septum and below the atrial septum through which crosses the common AV valve.

atrial distention. Of interest is the fact that these arrhythmias do not appear to resolve after closure of the defect.[52,70,92,97] As patients with ASDs age, they may develop coronary artery disease, and the concomitant decrease of LV function and compliance may actually cause an increase in left-to-right shunting across a previously insignificant ASD.[52] The increase in RV work can exacerbate symptoms of coronary artery lesions, causing ischemia, infarction, or accelerated signs of congestive heart failure.[111]

The hemodynamics of sinus venosus ASDs are similar to those described for secundum ASDs. However, the fact that the pulmonary venous return is often directed into the right atrium contributes to the observation that sinus venosus ASDs are usually physiologically significant.

The hemodynamics of shunting in partial AV canal defects (ostium primum ASDs) are also similar to those of secundum ASDs, although the degree of mitral valve insufficiency has a large role in determining the severity of the lesion. The direction of the shunt is controlled by the differences between right and left ventricular compliance. However, when substantial mitral insufficiency occurs, the regurgitant jet is often directed into the right atrium across the absent atrioventricular septum (Fig. 7). This not only increases the shunt load to the right side but also requires an obligatory increase in LV stroke volume to maintain forward cardiac output. The resultant demands on left and right ventricular function can hasten the onset of biventricular heart failure, and patients with ostium primum defects and moderate to severe mitral insufficiency usually present with symptoms early in life.

Patients with a complete AV canal defect also have a large interventricular communication (ventricular septal defect [VSD]), which dramatically alters the hemodynamics of this lesion, compared with isolated atrial level defects. Atrial shunting occurs for all of the reasons cited above, and this shunt is increased in patients with severe AV valve incompetence. However, shunting at the ventricular level produces the more serious problems. This shunting occurs at systemic pressures and causes RV and pulmonary artery pressures that equal LV and systemic arterial pressures. To protect against massive pulmonary blood flow, pulmonary vascular resistance rapidly increases and may become fixed and permanent during the first months of life.[2,117] Although elevated pulmonary vascular resistance decreases the net left-to-right shunt at the ventricular level (by decreasing compliance of the pulmonary vascular bed), permanent histologic changes prevent the pulmonary arteries from resuming normal resistance when the shunt is surgically corrected and can impose an intolerable impedance to flow that prevents the right ventricle from performing acceptably as a pulmonary ventricle when the intracardiac defect is correctly partitioned. When the pulmonary vascular resistance is allowed to attain this level (greater than 12 units · m²),[52] the condition is usually considered to be inoperable, because the right ventricle is no longer capable of supporting pulmonary blood flow when the VSD is closed and the assistance of the left ventricle is blocked. Although the $Q_p:Q_s$ of a complete AV canal defect may not be higher than in a patient with a secundum ASD, the increase in pulmonary artery pressure (and resistance) makes the impact of the shunt far more deleterious over the short term.

PHYSICAL FINDINGS

Patients with secundum, sinus venosus, or ostium primum ASDs may have few physical findings. They may be smaller than normal, as seen on serial growth charts. The patient may otherwise appear healthy, without disturbing complaints. Pa-

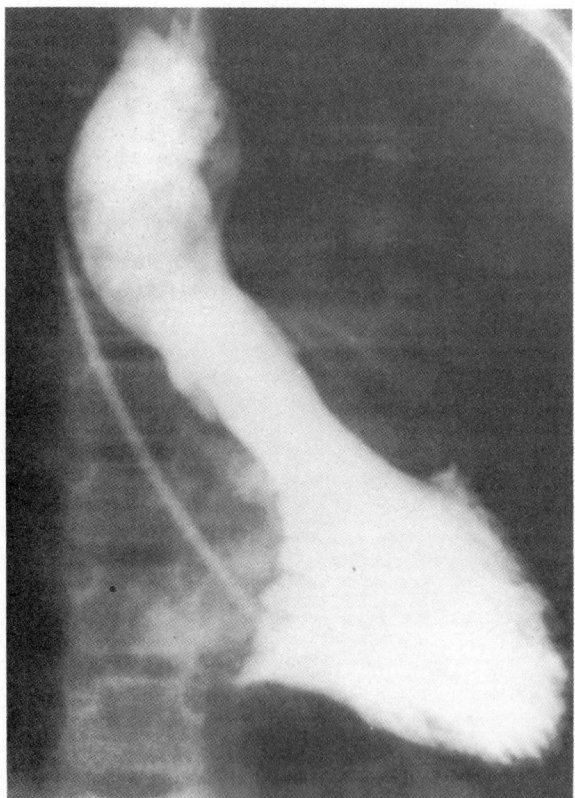

Figure 12. This cineangiogram of a patient with an AV canal defect shows scalloping of the AV valve and elongation of the left ventricular outflow tract ("gooseneck" deformity) which is characteristic of this lesion. (From Waldhausen, J. A., and Tyers, G. F. O.: Atrial septal defects, ostium primum defects, and atrioventricular canals. *In* Sabiston, D. C., Jr., (Ed.): Textbook of Surgery 13th ed. Philadelphia, W. B. Saunders Company, 1986.

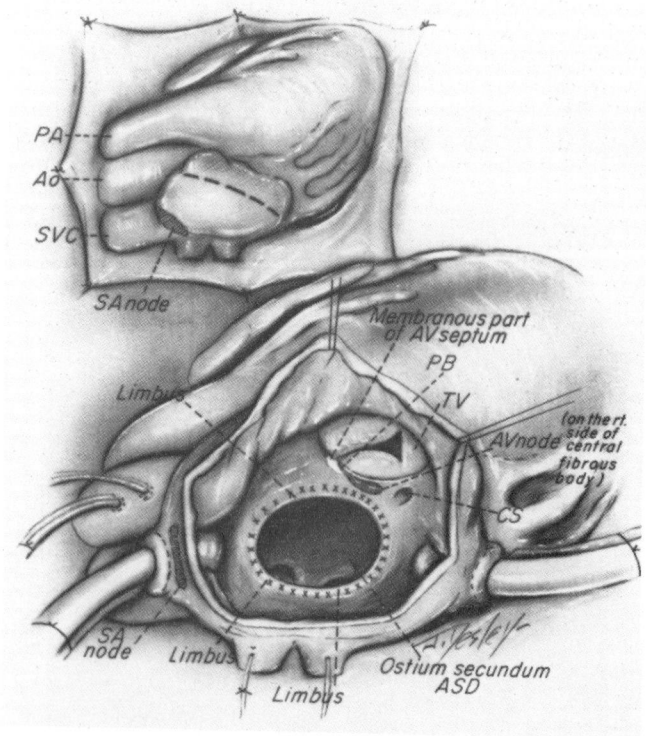

Figure 13. This diagram illustrates the location of the conduction tissue which must be appreciated by the surgeon during repair of an ASD. The sinoatrial node is located at the junction of the SVC and right atrium and should be avoided by atrial incisions. The AV node lies in the AV septum between the coronary sinus and the tricuspid anulus. This illustration demonstrates a large secundum ASD, and the Xs indicate the safe location for sutures placed to close this defect. (From Bharati, S., Lev, M., and Kirklin, J. W.: Cardiac Surgery and the Conduction System. New York, John Wiley & Sons, 1983.)

tients with sinus venosus defects may complain of palpitations, because it is not uncommon for this defect to be associated with supraventricular dysrythmias. If the intracardiac shunt is greater than 1.8:1, there may be a visible left parasternal heave with a palpable RV lift. In some patients, this can produce a localized chest wall deformity with protuberance of the costal cartilage in the left parasternal region. Auscultation reveals prominence of the first heart sound with fixed splitting of the second heart sound. (This fixed splitting of the second heart sound is not present in patients with partial anomalous pulmonary venous return if there is no associated ASD). A soft (Grade II or III) systolic ejection murmur is present in the second or third left intercostal space from the increased flow across the pulmonary valve. A middiastolic tricuspid flow rumble may also be audible in the fourth or fifth left intercostal space. If the patient is in congestive heart failure, there may be jugular venous distention, hepatomegaly, and cardiomegaly. Increased intensity of the RV lift with accentuation of the second heart sound suggests the presence of elevated pulmonary arterial pressures and alerts the clinician to the possibility of increased pulmonary vascular resistance. In patients with ostium primum defects and moderate to severe mitral insufficiency, there are usually more pronounced signs of heart failure, and pulmonary edema may be present and detected by the appearance of bibasilar rales. There is usually pronounced cardiomegaly; and auscultation discloses a distinct, apical pansystolic murmur of mitral regurgitation.

Patients with complete AV canal defects usually present with severe heart failure during the first year of life with tachypnea, poor feeding, failure to grow, and evidence of poor peripheral perfusion. This usually parallels a normal postnatal fall in pul-

monary vascular resistance. Occasionally, however, pulmonary vascular resistance does not fall to the point that the shunt becomes clinically apparent; and as changes of fixed pulmonary vascular disease dominate, the patient may appear clinically well. However, signs of RV overload (parasternal lift with signs of a hyperactive precordium), interventricular shunting (loud systolic murmur), and pulmonary hypertension (loud second heart sound) should be obvious and lead to correct diagnosis.

The risk of subacute bacterial endocarditis (SBE) from a simple secundum or sinus venosus ASD is slight; and when it occurs, it is usually on the pulmonary valve or RV outflow tract.[111] Patients with partial or complete AV canal defects present a greater risk for SBE because of the "jet" lesions created by the AV valve incompetence and the interventricular shunting. It is possible for these patients first to present with signs of intracardiac infection. Presentation with paradoxical emboli or cerebral infarction also occurs but is unusual.[52,83]

DIAGNOSIS

Patients in whom an ASD is suspected should have a chest film, which usually shows mild to moderate cardiomegaly, prominence of the pulmonary artery shadow, and increased pulmonary vascular markings (Fig. 8). The left ventricle and aorta should be normal or slightly smaller than normal. The roentgenographic appearance of a secundum ASD is indistinguishable from that of a sinus venosus ASD, unless the right superior pulmonary vein can be identified lying more superiorly than normal, in which case the diagnosis of sinus venosus ASD with partial anomalous pulmonary venous return can be considered (Fig. 8).[52] Patients with ostium primum ASDs have simi-

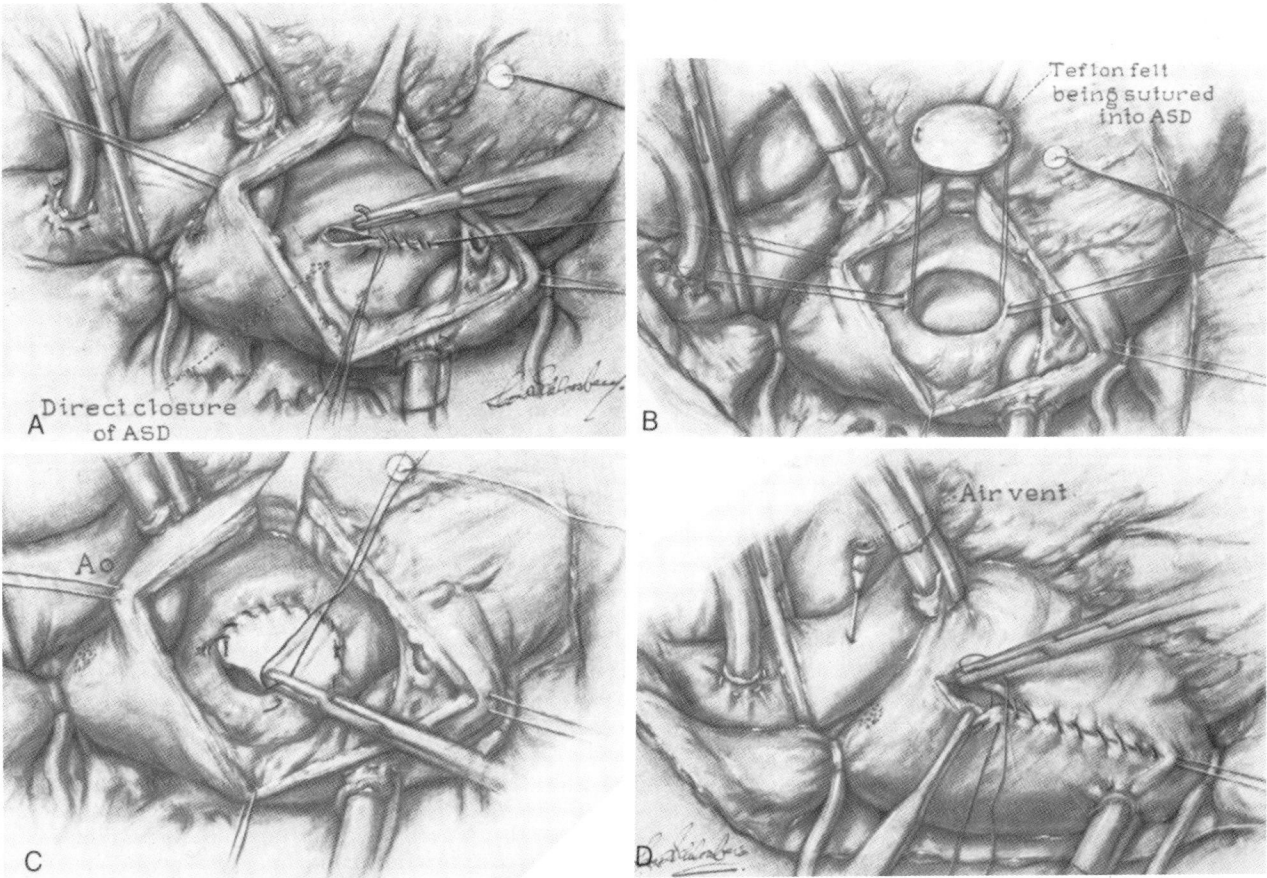

Figure 14. A secundum ASD (A) can be closed primarily with a running suture technique or (B) with a patch of prosthetic material or pericardium such that the sutures are placed around the entire rim of the defect (C). Before completing the ASD suture line, one evacuates air from the left atrium by filling it with saline. The atriotomy is then repaired (D). A needle vent to allow any air ejected by the left side of the circulation to escape from the aorta should be placed before one allows the heart to resume normal sinus rhythm (From Ebert, P. A.: Atlas of Congenital Cardiac Surgery. New York, Churchill Livingstone, 1989.)

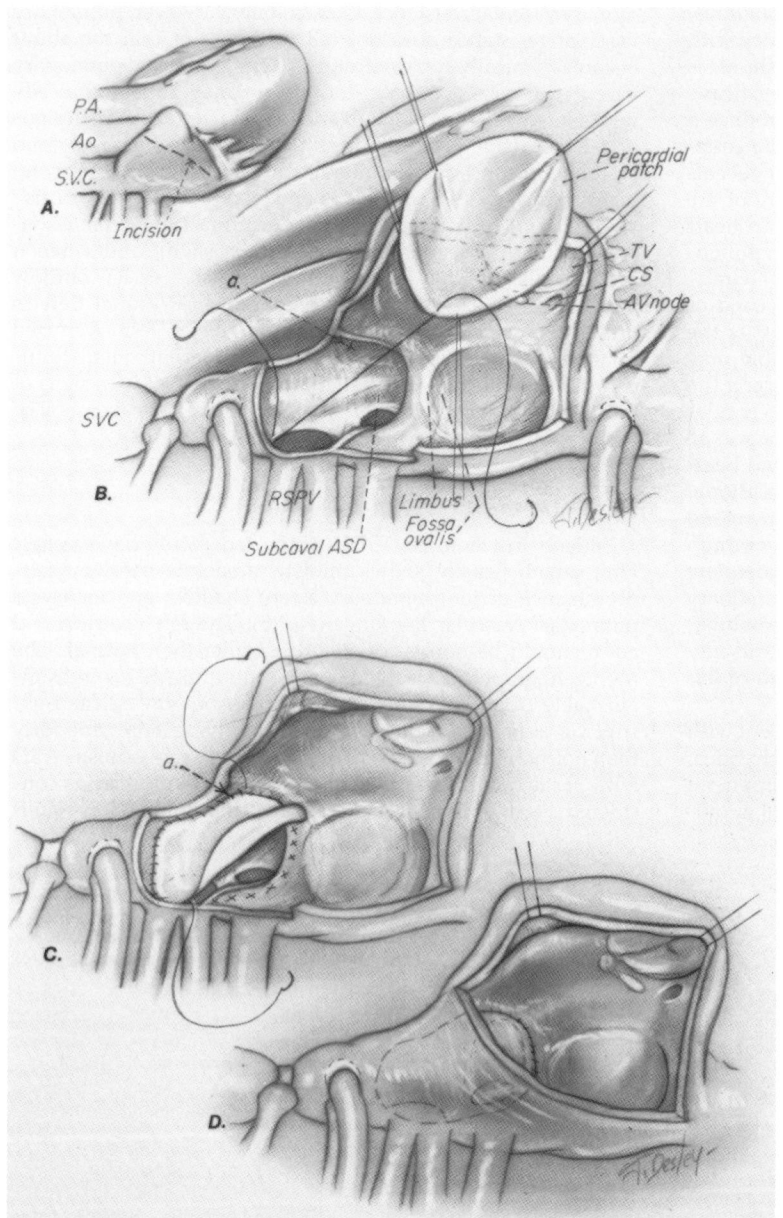

Figure 15. A sinus venosus ASD with anomalous return of the right superior pulmonary vein to the SVC (*A*) can be approached by an oblique atrial incision with direct caval cannulation. This defect is closed with a patch (usually of pericardium), which is placed in such a manner (*B* to *D*) to redirect the pulmonary veins below the patch into the left atrium and to partition the posterior aspect of the SVC so that there is no longer any atrial septal communication. (From Kirklin, J. W., and Barratt-Boyes, B. G., Cardiac Surgery. New York, John Wiley & Sons, 1986.)

lar appearing chest films although moderate or severe mitral insufficiency may produce prominence of the left ventricle with distinctive biventricular cardiomegaly and signs of pulmonary edema (Fig. 9). Patients with complete AV canal defects usually have a chest film consistent with severe heart failure during infancy with marked cardiomegaly and pulmonary overcirculation (Fig. 10). As pulmonary hypertension develops, the lung markings become clearer, and the central pulmonary arteries appear larger.

The electrocardiogram shows distinctive differences between these lesions. Patients with secundum ASDs almost invariably have some degree of incomplete right bundle branch block in lead V_1. Prominent P waves may suggest atrial enlargement. The vectorcardiogram reveals a clockwise loop directed inferiorly and to the right in the frontal projection.[34] Patients with AV canal defects (partial or complete) usually demonstrate marked RV hypertrophy with prolongation of the P-R interval. There may be LV hypertrophy as well. There is usually left axis deviation and the vector loop in the frontal plane is counterclockwise. Although left axis deviation and a counterclockwise loop strongly suggest an AV canal defect, this pattern can occur in about 10 per cent of patients with secundum ASDs.[52]

Diagnosis is clarified by two-dimensional echocardiography, and understanding of the physiologic alterations created by the defect is obtained with color flow mapping.[57] Secundum defects are easily distinguished from ostium primum defects, and it is possible to delineate both in the same patient. The direction of the intracardiac shunt can be visualized throughout the cardiac cycle (see Fig. 6). Although sinus venosus defects are difficult to visualize by transthoracic echo, the addition of microcavitation to the examination assists in detection of these defects. Echocardiography can be performed from the chest wall or with the use of specially created esophageal transducers which are inserted transorally into the esophagus and advanced until they lie directly posterior to the heart. Resolution from echo is so good with currently available instruments (especially with the transesophageal approach) that precise detail regarding the nature of the defect can be fully and uniquely appreciated. Echocardiography with color flow Doppler is now the diagnostic modality of choice to demonstrate secundum and ostium primum defects and usually obviates the necessity for cardiac catheterization prior to surgical intervention. In patients with ostium primum defects, the degree of mitral insufficiency is demonstrated, and the "cleft" in the mitral valve can usually be outlined.[10] Patients

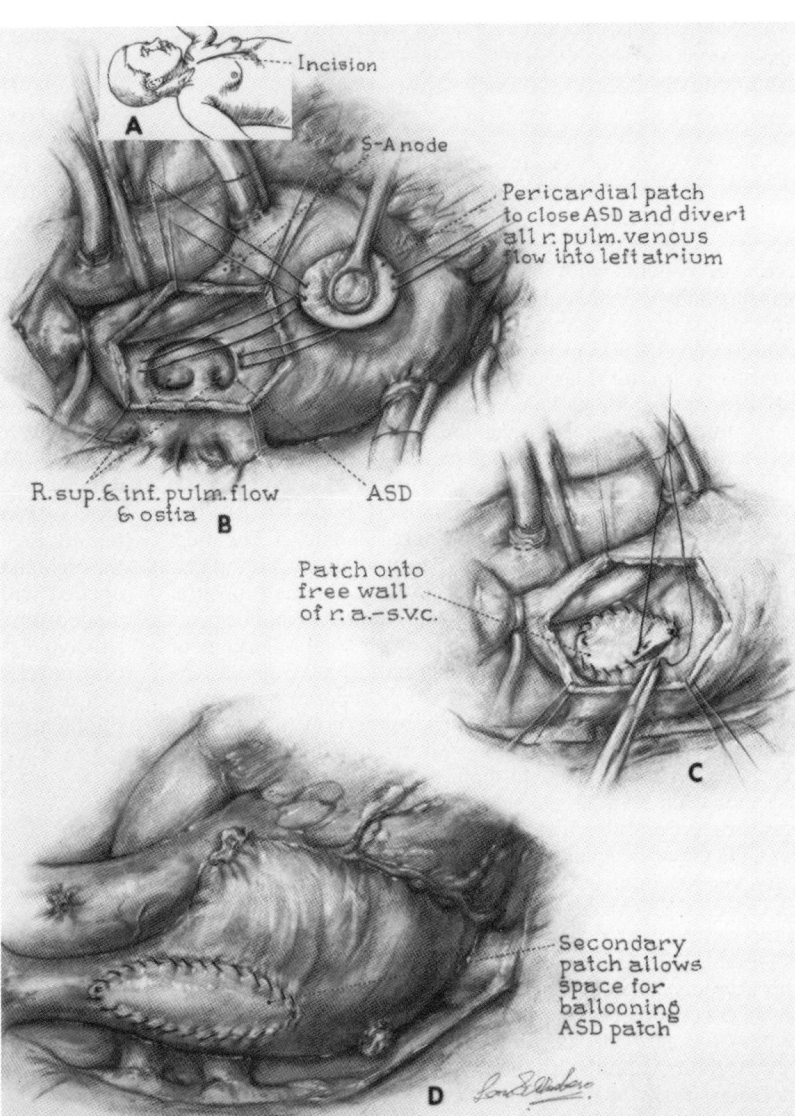

Figure 16. Another approach to a sinus venosus ASD is with a low, horizontally placed, atrial incision extending up onto the SVC (*A* and *B*). This enables easy visualization of the defect and placement of a patch (*C*) to redirect the anomalous pulmonary venous return as well as to close the ASD. This type of incision should often be repaired with a patch of pericardium (*D*) to prevent constriction of the SVC. (From Ebert, P. A.: Atlas of Congenital Cardiac Surgery. New York, Churchill Livingstone, 1989.)

with complete AV canal defects can also be evaluated with echocardiography alone. It is easy to disclose the presence of a ventricular level shunt, which distinguishes partial from complete forms of this lesion[108,114] (Fig. 11). Although Doppler techniques also predict gradients across areas of stenosis, patients in whom significant right or left ventricular outflow obstruction or aortic coarctation is suspected probably require cardiac catheterization. Infants with complete AV canal defects do not require cardiac catheterization prior to surgical therapy but patients older than 6 months (or older than 3 months in the presence of Down's syndrome) should probably undergo cardiac catheterization for measurement of pulmonary artery pressures and resistances.[2,117]

Cardiac catheterization with angiography is being performed less frequently in patients with ASDs because of the superior information provided by two-dimensional echocardiography. Patients with secundum and sinus venosus defects usually can proceed to operative therapy based on echo information alone. However, patients with ASDs who are older than 40, especially if chest pain is one of the presenting complaints, should be catheterized to exclude pulmonary hypertension (usually not present if the color flow Doppler shows predominantly left-to-right shunting) and undergo coronary angiography to evaluate the coronary arteries. Cardiac catheterization is also indicated for patients with secundum or primum defects who have a pronounced second heart sound. Catheterization provides data

that enables calculation of pulmonary and systemic blood flow so that the magnitude of the intracardiac shunt can be quantified. A $Q_p:Q_s$ of greater than 1.5:1 is usually considered an indication for surgical closure of an ASD.[42,52] Moreover, the degree of pulmonary hypertension, when present, can be measured, and an objective reflection of pulmonary vascular resistance can be calculated. Patients with pulmonary vascular resistance greater than 12 units $\cdot$ m^2 are considered inoperable. If the pulmonary vascular resistance is less than 6 units $\cdot$ m^2, the patient can usually be safely corrected, although long-term survival may be less in patients with elevated resistance, compared with those with normal values. Patients with pulmonary resistances between 6 and 12 units may benefit from measurement of pulmonary and systemic arterial pressure changes during exercise with simultaneous calculation of shunt fractions. The hearts of those patients whose systemic vascular resistance falls with an increase in right-to-left shunting during exercise may be best left uncorrected.[52] Finally, cardiac catheterization allows measurement of pressure gradients across the pulmonary and aortic outflow tracts so that in selected cases repair of clinically relevant valvular heart lesions can be accomplished during ASD closure.[30,59] In patients with AV canal defects, cineangiographic studies demonstrate the elongation of the left ventricular outflow tract in relationship to the inflow tract, which produces a characteristic "gooseneck" deformity (Fig. 12).[5,52] Although this finding is characteristic of AV canal defects, the anatomic detail provided by the less invasive echo technology has replaced the necessity of demonstrating this angiographic feature in establishing the diagnosis of AV canal defect.

TREATMENT

Spontaneous closure of ASDs may occur early in life[21,78] but is uncommon after the first year of life.[24,74,76] It is also unlikely to occur in patients with hemodynamically significant shunts which produce right ventricular enlargement and symptoms.[52] Specially designed umbrella-like devices can be placed in secundum level ASDs in the cardiac catheterization laboratory, but this procedure is largely experimental and is currently utilized for special indications in patients who cannot otherwise safely undergo surgical intervention. Surgical closure continues to be the method of choice for hemodynamically significant ASDs.[68]

The safety of modern cardiopulmonary bypass (CPB) has replaced previous approaches to atrial septal defects. The most common approach is through a median sternotomy, although a right anterolateral thoracotomy provides excellent exposure. Once the chest is opened, the exposed anatomy should be carefully inspected. Right atrial and right ventricular enlargement should be obvious, and the pulmonary artery may appear enlarged, compared with the aorta. The right superior pulmonary veins should be identified and their connection to the heart evaluated. If they appear to be more horizontal in position than normal, or if they appear to drain to the lateral aspect of the superior vena cava, it is likely that the patient has a sinus venosus defect and this information can help direct cannulation for CPB. Once the anatomy has been examined, and the pulmonary venous drainage evaluated, the patient is ready to be placed on CPB. Arterial perfusion is usually best obtained by direct cannulation of the aorta, although the femoral artery is an acceptable alternative, especially in older patients, if a right thoracotomy approach is being utilized. Usually both venae cavae are cannulated, so that the patient can be placed on total bypass for easy visualization of intracardiac anatomy. The venous return cannulas can be advanced into the cavae through insertion sites in the right atrium, or the cavae can be cannulated directly. Placement of the venous return cannulas depends, in part, upon the nature of the defect being repaired. Before CPB, it is helpful to perform epicardial echo with Doppler color flow imaging for clearly evaluating the nature of the defect and its precise location. This may be the best way to demonstrate a sinus venosus defect, and it also enables the surgeon to evaluate ventricular function, mitral and tricuspid valve competence and pulmonary outflow tract anatomy prior to operative repair.[106,107] It is not unusual for the pre-CPB echo to demonstrate previously unappreciated details of the patient's anatomy (including unsuspected associated defects such as a patent ductus arteriosus), and alter the operative procedure.[107] Once the patient has been stabilized on cardiopulmonary bypass, the surgeon can open the right atrium to expose the defect. For avoidance of the risk of the heart ejecting air into the systemic circulation, the heart should be electrically fibrillated before atriotomy. An alternative technique is to cross-clamp the aorta and infuse cold cardioplegia solution for electrically and mechanically arresting the heart.

Repair of secundum ASDs is best performed through an oblique atriotomy, to avoid injuring the sinoatrial node (Fig. 13). The intra-atrial anatomy is inspected for the presence of other defects. It is important that the surgeon understand the anatomy of the conduction system so that injury to the AV node is avoided (Fig. 13). Secundum ASDs can be closed primarily with running sutures (Fig. 14A) or with a patch of pericardium or prosthetic material (Fig. 14B and C). Large defects that require some tension for approximation of the borders are best closed

with patch material. Before completion of the suture line, the left atrium is filled with saline for help in reducing the risk of air embolus. The right atrium is then closed, a needle vent hole is made in the aorta (for venting any residual air that is ejected by the left ventricle), the aortic cross clamp is removed (if used), and the heart is defibrillated (Fig. 14D). The patient is then weaned from CPB, and the chest is closed in the usual manner over a chest tube. Because secundum defects are usually repaired with little difficulty, the CPB times are frequently short, and these patients can often have their endotracheal tubes removed before leaving the operating room.

Repair of sinus venosus ASDs is somewhat more complex. Because the defect is usually high in the atrium, over the top of the superior limbus of the septum secundum, it is sometimes helpful to cannulate the superior vena cava directly, so that this venous return cannula does not interfere with exposure of the defect. With this cannulation technique, most sinus venosus defects can be exposed by means of the same type of oblique atrial incision used in repairing secundum defects (Fig. 15). Alternatively, the superior vena cava cannula can be placed through the tip of the right atrial appendage and the atrium opened with a low-lying horizontal incision that can be extended superiorly onto the superior vena cava if necessary and still avoid the sinoatrial node (Fig. 16). It is essential to expose the orifices of the anomalous right superior pulmonary veins so that they can be redirected into the left atrium. These defects should always be closed with a patch (pericardium or prosthetic

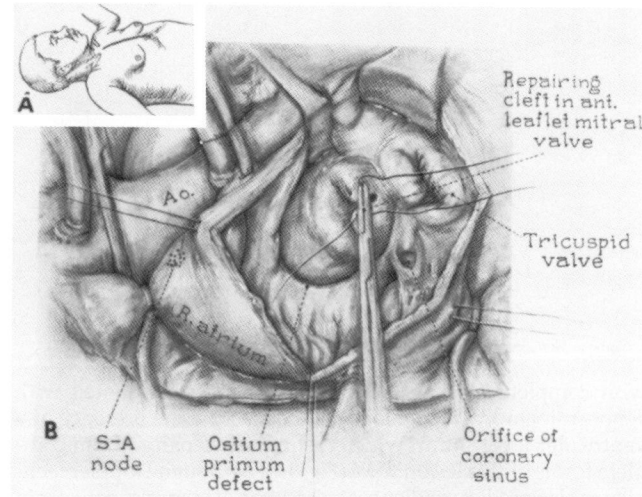

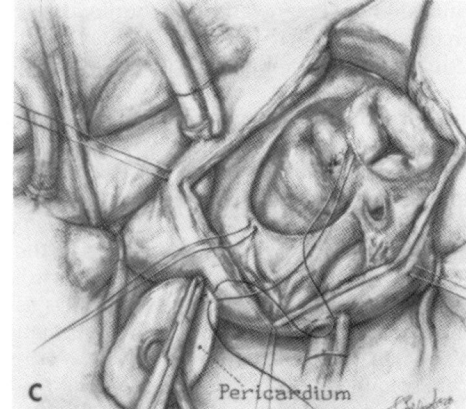

Figure 17. Exposure of an ostium primum ASD through an oblique atriotomy (A). The cleft in the anterior leaflet of the mitral valve is repaired with interrupted sutures (B). The defect is then closed with a patch of pericardium placed at the anulus between the mitral and tricuspid valves and sutured to the rim of the defect (C). [From Ebert, P. A.: Atlas of Congenital Cardiac Surgery. New York, Churchill Livingstone, 1989.]

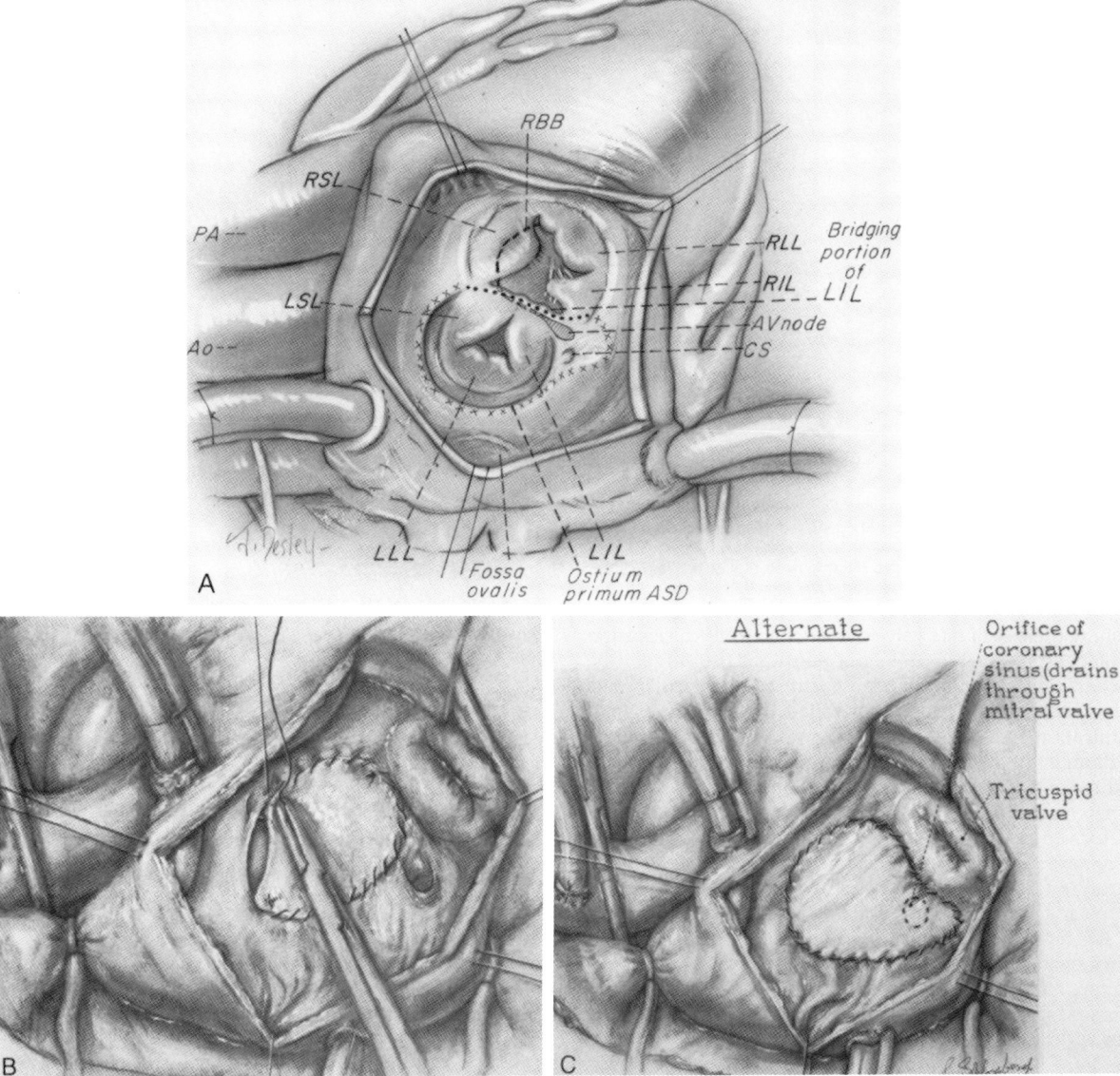

Figure 18. *A,* Location of the conduction system in an ostium primum ASD needs to be appreciated by the surgeon. The AV node is immediately adjacent to the coronary sinus and can be injured by sutures placed in this region. The Xs in this illustration demonstrate the location recommended by some for placement of sutures to secure the pericardial patch that closes the atrial level defect (see *C*). (From Bharati, S., Lev, M., and Kirklin, J. W.: Cardiac Surgery and the Conduction System. New York, John Wiley & Sons, 1983.) RBB, right bundle branch; RSL, right superior leaflet; LSL, left superior leaflet; LLL, left lateral leaflet; RIL, right inferior leaflet; RLL, right lateral leaflet (all of these pertain to the portions of the common atrioventricular valve); CS, coronary sinus. *B,* Placement of a pericardial patch to close an ostium primum ASD can be secured in such a manner as to keep the coronary sinus on the right atrial side. Sutures can be carefully placed for the purpose of avoiding injuring the AV node. *C,* Alternatively (and as demonstrated by the Xs in *A*), a pericardial patch can be placed for avoiding the AV node; utilizing this technique, the coronary sinus remains on the left atrial side of the circulation. The small right-to-left shunt created by this procedure is hemodynamically and clinically insignificant unless a left superior vena cava drains to the coronary sinus. (*B* and *C* from Ebert, P. A.: Atlas of Congenital Cardiac Surgery. New York, John Wiley & Sons, 1983.)

material) that is placed in such a manner that the superior pulmonary veins are kept below the patch and channeled through the venosus defect into the left atrium (see Figs. 15 and 16). If necessary, the superior vena cava is also patched so that unobstructed venous flow to the right atrium over this patch is possible.[31,52] It is also possible to augment the superior vena cava with a flap of right atrial tissue.[52] If an oblique atriotomy is utilized, augmentation of the vena cava is rarely necessary. The remaining steps are identical to those described above for secundum ASDs, although the potential for supraventricular arrhythmias makes it advisable to place temporary pacing wires on the heart before closing the chest. Because these procedures may take slightly longer than closure of an uncomplicated secundum defect, moderate hypothermia (28° C.) on CPB is usually recommended.

Repair of AV canal defects can be even more complicated,

depending on the extent of the defect. These defects are best approached through an oblique atriotomy (Fig. 17*B*). The intraatrial anatomy is then carefully inspected, because it is not unusual to have secundum level defects in association with defects of the atrioventricular septum. The mitral and tricuspid valves are inspected for "clefts." The inlet portion of the ventricular septum is also carefully examined. If a VSD is not present, the lesion is a partial AV canal (ostium primum ASD). The cleft in the mitral valve is repaired with interrupted sutures (Fig. 17*B* and *C*). Although some authorities believe that the "cleft" does not require repair[23,52] and that the mitral valve will function well as a "tri-leaflet" structure, the long-term failure rate of this approach is not trivial, especially if significant preoperative valvular regurgitation is present, and careful approximation of the cleft anterior leaflet provides excellent long-term results.[31,100] The "cleft" should be repaired with nonpledgeted sutures for

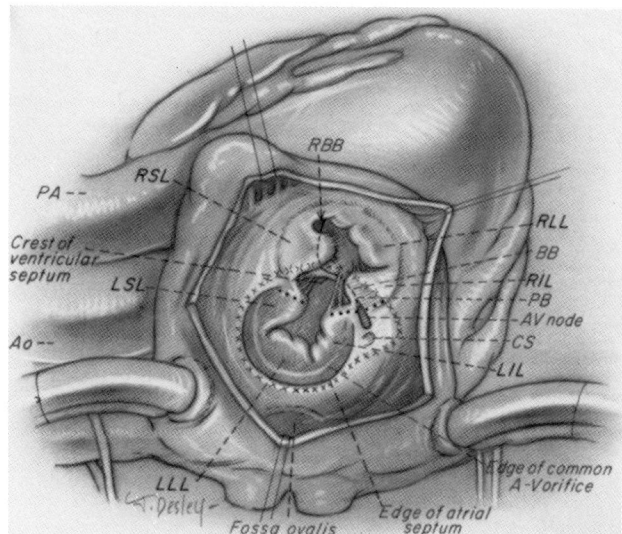

Figure 19. Location of the conduction system and anatomy of the AV valve in a patient with a complete AV canal defect. The legend is the same as for Figure 18A. The AV valve "bridges" the common atrial and ventricular chamber with free communication below and above the valve. (From Bharati, S., Lev, M., and Kirklin, J. W.: Cardiac Surgery and the Conduction System. John Wiley & Sons, 1983.)

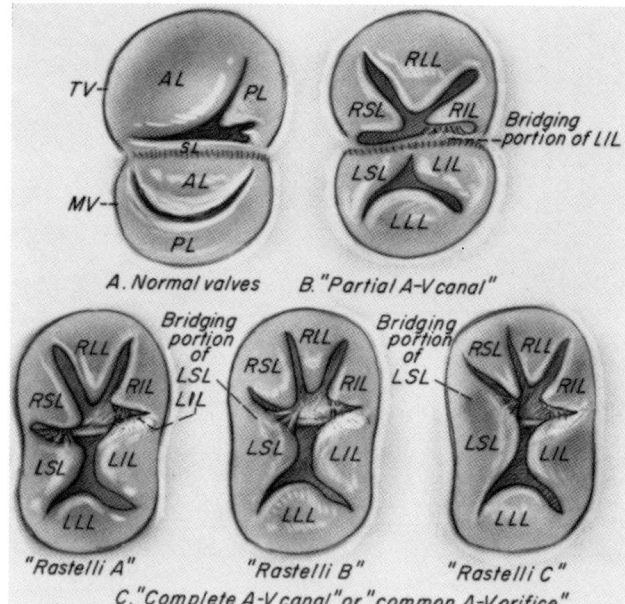

Figure 20. The anatomy of the AV valves as classified by Rastelli from the Mayo Clinic. A complete AV canal is classified as Rastelli Type A, B, or C, depending upon the attachment and nature of the superior bridging leaflet. Type A is distinguished by a superior bridging leaflet that is split in its middle and attached to the crest of the ventricular septum. A Rastelli Type B lesion has a superior bridging leaflet that is less evenly split but remains attached to the ventricular septal crest. A Rastelli Type C defect has an essentially unsplit superior bridging leaflet that is not attached to the crest of the ventricular septum. (From Kirklin, J. W., Pacifico, A. D., and Kirklin, J. K.: The surgical treatment of atrioventricular canal defects. In Arciniegas, E. (Ed.): Pediatric Cardiac Surgery. Chicago, Year Book Medical Publishers, 1985.)

diminishing the risk of late valve dysfunction from calcification of the pledget material.[100] It is important that the surgeon be aware that hemodynamically significant left ventricular outflow obstruction may follow after repair.[100] The atrial septal communication is carefully closed using a pericardial patch. Pericardium is the recommended material for closure, because residual mitral insufficiency directed against a patch of prosthetic material can cause significant hemolysis.[50,91,109] Location of the atrioventricular node must be appreciated (Fig. 18), and there are several techniques available to limit damage to this structure.[15,61] It is advisable to place temporary atrial and ventricular pacing wires for use, if necessary, in the postoperative period. It is rarely necessary to leave permanent pacing wires on the heart, even if the patient is in complete heart block at the completion of the procedure (from injury to the AV node), since this damage is rarely permanent and normal conduction usually resumes within a few days.[55]

If the defect is a complete AV canal, the anatomy can appear quite different from a partial AV canal. The single large AV valve bridges the canal defect and can be considered to have a superior and an inferior common leaflet (Fig. 19). Although the technique may vary, depending on the precise anatomy of the common AV valve (Rastelli classification)[56,85,87] (Fig. 20), the principles are essentially to close the VSD, to subdivide the common AV valves into a "tricuspid" and a "mitral" component, and to suspend these newly created valves from the top of the VSD patch. The atrial defect is then closed in the same manner as an ostium primum defect (Fig. 21). As with partial AV canal defects, placement of temporary pacing wires is advisable before closing the chest.

Regardless of the type of defect repaired, it is recommended that the adequacy of the surgical repair be evaluated before the patient leaves the operating room. This can be done by obtaining a right atrial and pulmonary artery oxygen saturation or by performing a dye-dilution curve. The introduction of intraoperative echo with Doppler color flow imaging for evaluating surgical results provides a more specific and sensitive method of

assessing the quality of the repair, for directing necessary revisions before allowing the patient to leave the operating room, and provides prognostic information regarding the likelihood of an optimal long-term outcome.[107,108] (Fig. 22).

Special Situations

AV canal defects are frequently repaired in infants and small children because of the severe and life-threatening symptoms that can exist in the first year of life. In these small patients, it is frequently helpful to use techniques of profound hypothermia (18° C.) with periods of total circulatory arrest (TCA). This enables the surgeon to operate in a bloodless field that is unencumbered by distortion produced from the cannula necessary to sustain cardiopulmonary bypass. Although the effects of these techniques on long-term neuropsychiatric development remain obscure, it appears that periods of TCA at 18° C. are well tolerated by infants for periods as long as 60 minutes,[52] and perhaps even longer. Recent clinical and experimental investigations continue to elucidate understanding of this fascinating alternative technique.[44,45]

Occasionally patients with ASDs have persistence of the left superior vena cava. This structure usually drains into the coronary sinus and can increase the intra-atrial venous return that confronts the surgeon once the right atrium is opened. Although this can usually be controlled with a cardiotomy sucker placed into the coronary sinus, another option is selective cannulation of the left superior vena cava—an alternative that might be considered if aortic cross-clamping is planned. With the patient on total CPB, the only blood entering the heart should be through the coronary sinus, and this can be elimi-

Figure 22. These intraoperative color flow Doppler examples illustrate the ability of this technology to provide anatomic detail of the defect before repair as well as to indicate the quality of the reconstruction prior to the patient's leaving the operating room. A, A large secundum level ASD with a substantial left-to-right shunt shown as red flowing toward the transducer. B, The same patient after placement of a patch to close the defect. There is no longer any residual shunting. C, This intraoperaive view nicely depicts a large aneurysm of the atrial septum that was also associated with an atrial level shunt. D, The same patient's heart before leaving the operating room. The aneurysm has been resected, and the ASD has been successfully closed with a patch.

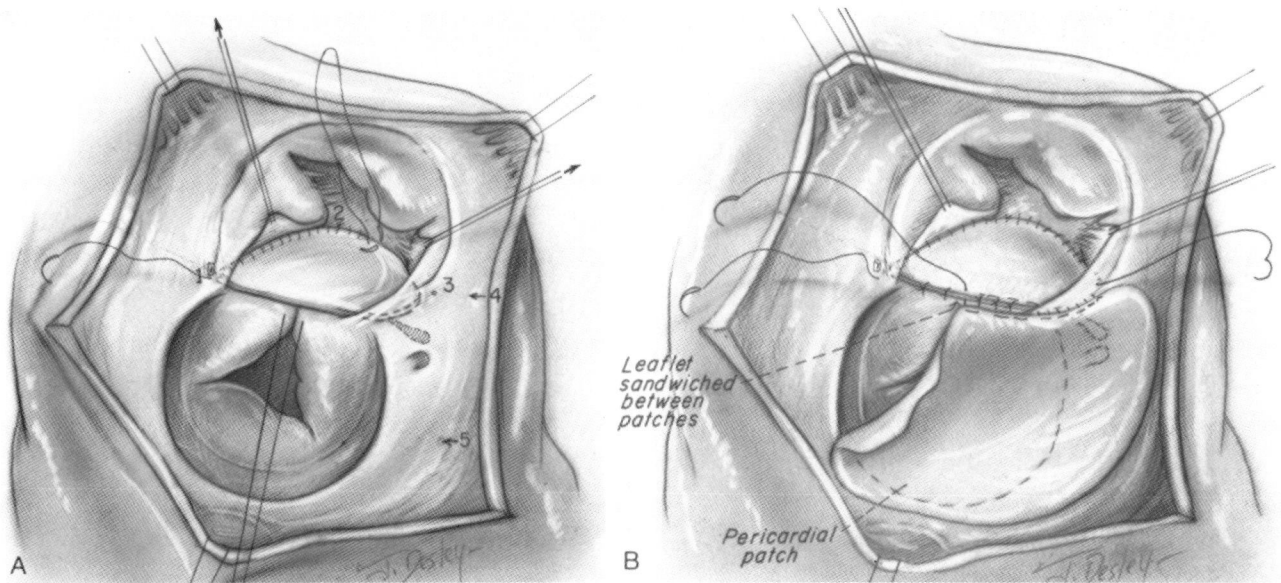

Figure 21. A complete AV canal can be closed by placing two separate patches to close the VSD (A) separately from the ASD (B). The valve leaflets are suspended from the point where these two patches are attached. (From Kirklin, J. W., and Barratt-Boyes, B. G.: Cardiac Surgery. New York, John Wiley & Sons, 1986.)

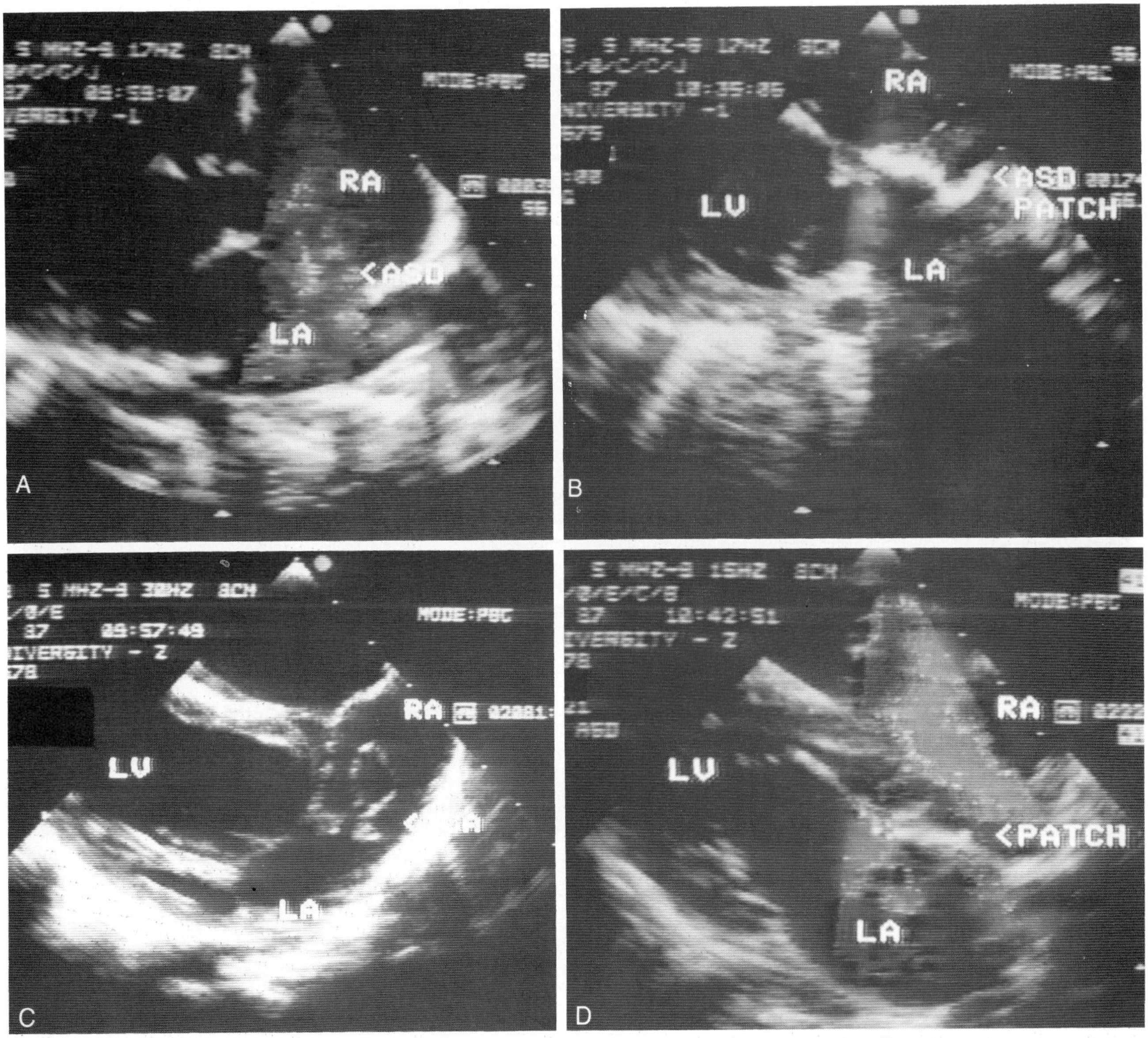

Figure 22. *See legend on opposite page*

Illustration continued on following page

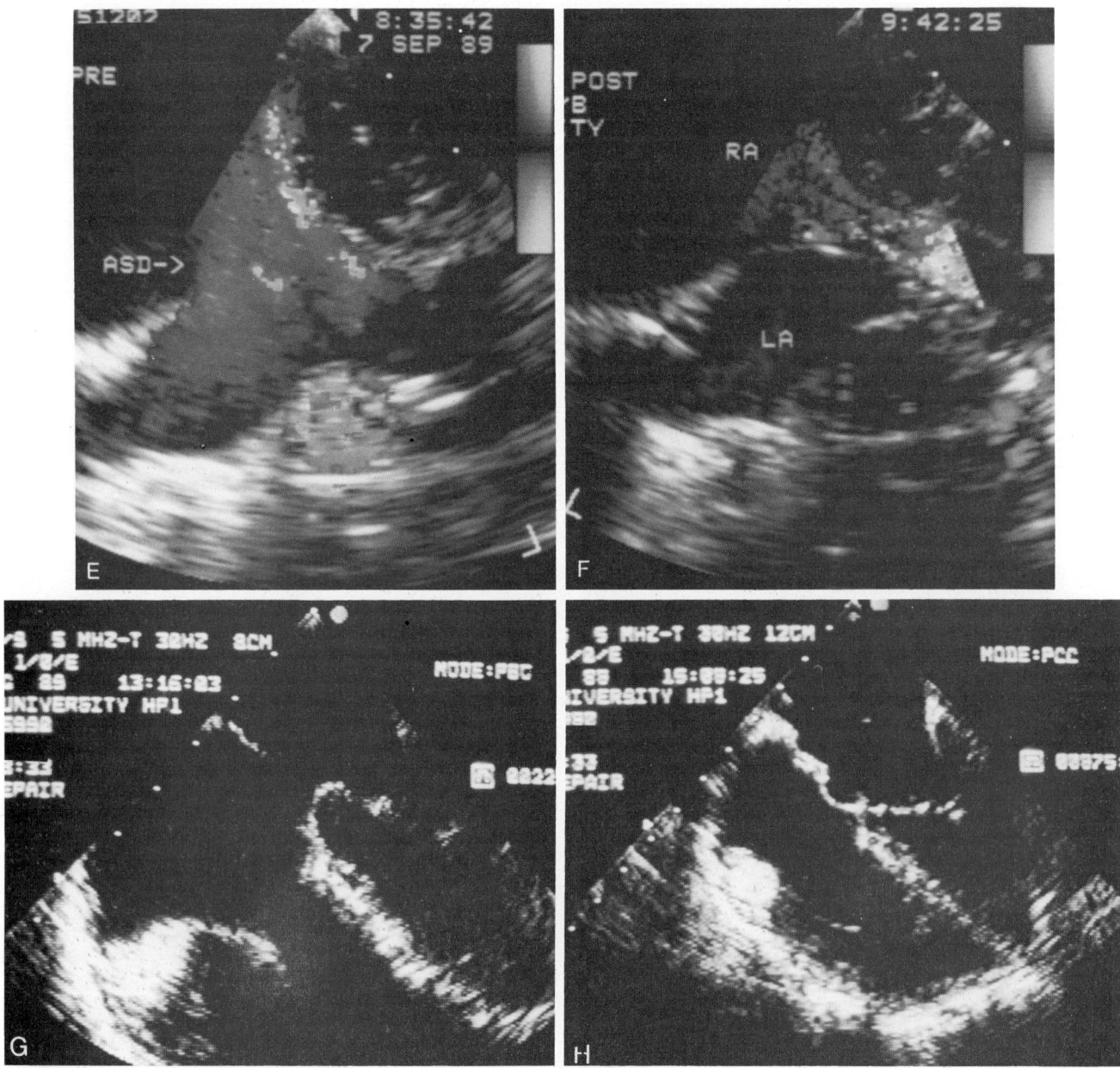

Figure 22 *Continued E*, This patient has a large sinus venosus ASD with a significant left-to-right shunt. *F*, The same patient is seen after completion of repair. A pericardial patch now separates the left atrium from the overlying SVC and right atrium. There is no residual shunting. *G*, A transesophageal image of an ostium primum ASD (see Figure 7B) shown prior to repair and, *H*, after repair. There is now a pericardial patch closing the atrial level communication, and the mitral valve has been reconstructed.

nated by aortic cross-clamping to abolish coronary flow. If the surgeon encounters an excessive amount of blood return to the heart with the patient on total CPB, and there is no persistent left SVC, it is important to seek a patent ductus arteriosus, a previously placed systemic-pulmonary shunt, bronchial collaterals, a pulmonary sequestration (intralobar), blood escaping around the snares on the caval cannulas, or (if the aorta is not clamped) a coronary fistula or aortic insufficiency.

Results

Operative mortality for closure of uncomplicated secundum and sinus venosus ASDs is extremely low, approaching 0 per cent, and should be no greater than 1 to 2 per cent, even in older patients.[6,25,32,52,58,93,110,111] Morbidity is also extremely low. In addition to the typical problems that can occur after open heart surgery, such as bleeding or infection, potential problems more specific to repair of these particular defects include thromboembolism (usually seen in older patients with chronic atrial arrhythmias),[46] mitral insufficiency,[8,60] neurologic deficits (most frequently from air embolism during CPB),[6,52] and arrhythmias[18,104] (especially in sinus venosus defects). The mortality risk is increased when the patient is older, with advanced congestive heart failure,[52] or when there is significant pulmonary hypertension with pulmonary vascular resistance approaching systemic resistance.[38,111] Moreover, patients with preoperative arrhythmias are likely to have persistence of this problem even after successful closure of the defect.[6,35,49,52] Long-term results are also very good, with survival statistics similar to those of a normal, age-matched population. This is especially true when repair if undertaken before the patient is 5 years of age[52] and less predictable if repair is delayed past the age of 60.[97,116] Symptoms, when present, almost invariably improve after repair; and even patients who had no symptomatic complaints recognize a substantial improvement in their health.[28,35,52,81,82,88,89,97] The likelihood of recurrence or the need for reoperation is less than 2 per cent.[52]

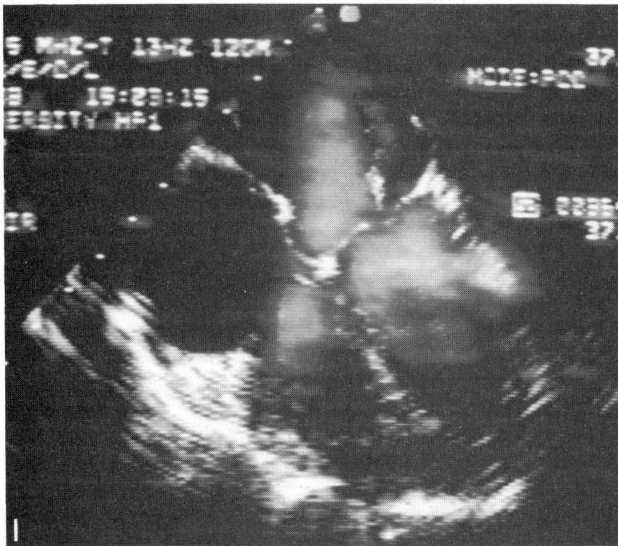

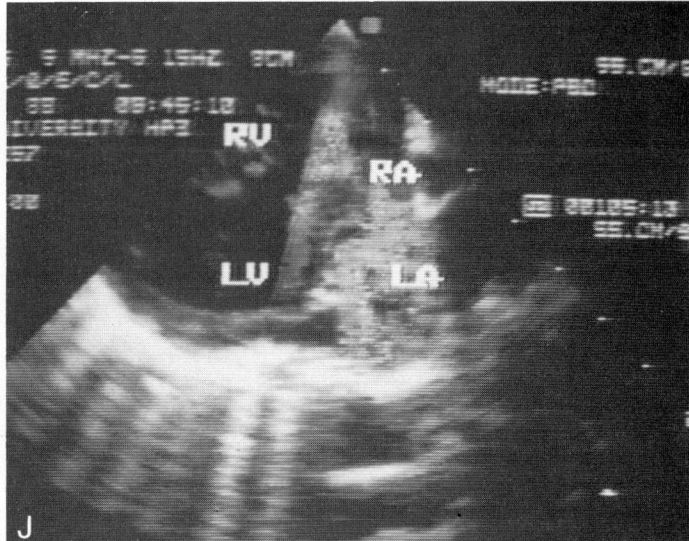

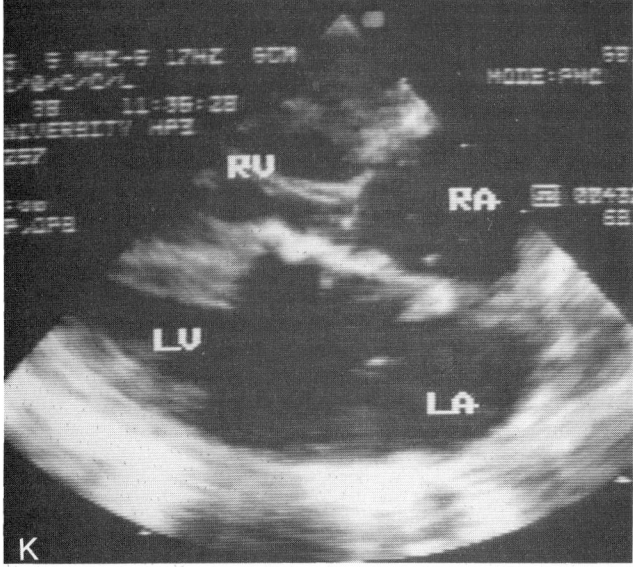

Figure 22 *Continued I,* This same patient shows no residual atrial level shunting and only mild residual mitral insufficiency (disclosed as the jet of red blood moving toward the transducer) after repair of the ostium primum defect. *J,* A color flow map of the large AV canal defect from the patient whose two-dimensional echocardiogram is shown in Figure 11. This image nicely demonstrates the free communication of blood between all chambers of the heart. *K,* The same patient after removal from cardiopulmonary bypass. This image shows that the patch now nicely divides the left and right sides of the heart, and the valve is resuspended from this patch. This patient had no significant residual shunting or valvular insufficiency at the completion of the repair (*J* and *K* from Ungerleider, R. M., et al: Intraoperative prebypass and postbypass epicardial color flow imaging in the repair of atrioventricular septal defects. J. Thorac. Cardiovasc. Surg. *98:*90, 1989.)

Repair of AV canal defects has a somewhat higher risk, depending on the nature and extent of the lesion, as well as the presence of any associated malformations. Uncomplicated partial AV canal defects, with minimal or no mitral incompetence, have a mortality risk that should approach 0 per cent and probably is no greater than 2 per cent.[52] The association of significant preoperative mitral insufficiency increases this risk to 4 per cent.[63,86] Long-term development of subaortic stenosis is reported and requires follow-up.[102] Overall long-term results are also affected by late mitral valve functional deterioration and arrhythmias.[43,69,73] The operative mortality for repair of complete AV canal defects is inconsistent because of the wide variation in the anatomic patterns of this anomaly. In addition, many of these patients are operated on as infants at a time when they are critically ill. Although operative mortality in some small series is reported as 0 per cent when current techniques are used to repair this defect in infants,[90,108] a more representative figure from larger series predicts the mortality risk to be between 5 and 13 per cent.[24,52] This risk is influenced by the nature of the common AV valve and the adequacy of the right and left ventricles.[52] Pulmonary hypertension with elevation of pulmonary vascular resistance can be an early occurrence in the natural history of complete AV canal defects[2,117] and influences operative mortality for patients coming to surgical correction beyond

6 months of age (or even earlier in patients with Down's syndrome).[37] Unless repair is undertaken by this age, it may be advisable to place a band around the pulmonary artery to limit pulmonary blood flow and protect the pulmonary vascular bed from progressing to irreversible damage. Although pulmonary artery banding is still applied with good success by some groups for small or seriously ill infants with complete AV canal defects (with repair then deferred for 1 to 2 years),[94,115] current techniques allow safe and effective complete repair of this defect in most small infants as a one-stage procedure.[9,12,24,52,53,71,72,108] Morbidity is similar to that cited for repair of ASDs, although there are more problems with mitral valve failure and arrhythmias (including complete heart block). AV valve failure occurs in as many as 10 per cent of these patients,[52] even when the preoperative valve function is good. This may be even more likely to occur in patients after repair of partial, as opposed to complete, AV canal defects.[52] With enhanced appreciation of the location of the conduction tissue, permanent complete heart block is becoming an unusual complication after repair of these defects,[52] but its likelihood is increased when AV valve failure causes the subsequent need for mitral valve replacement.[96] Long-term results are excellent, especially for patients with good mitral valve function, and survivors usually have excellent health with substantial improvement over their preoperative condition.

SELECTED REFERENCES

Arciniegas, E. (Ed.): Pediatric Cardiac Surgery. Chicago, Year Book Medical Publishers, 1985.
This excellent text of pediatric cardiac surgery has numerous authors who are experienced in the field. The chapters on ASDs and AV canal defects are superb overviews for the student attempting to gain a better understanding of these problems.

Bharati, S., Lev, M., and Kirklin, J. W.: Cardiac Surgery and the Conduction System. New York, John Wiley & Sons, 1983.
This carefully illustrated monograph depicts the location of important landmarks for conduction tissue in the normal heart as well as in a variety of common congenital heart defects. Careful review of these illustrations enables the surgeon to plan suture lines that will avoid damaging the important conduction tissue during intracardiac repair. This monograph is written by pioneers in the field.

Castaneda, A. R., Mayer, J. E., Jr., and Jonas, R. A.: Repair of complete atrioventricular canal in infancy. World J. Surg., 9:590, 1985.
The results of 48 patients undergoing repair for AV canal defects during infancy are reviewed. Operative mortality was 6 per cent, and late mortality was 4 per cent for an overall combined mortality of 10 per cent. Late functional results were excellent. The feasibility of performing total correction of AV canal defects in infancy is shown.

Ebert, P. A.: Atlas of Congenital Cardiac Surgery, New York, Churchill Livingstone, 1989.
This atlas contains exceptionally high quality illustrations from Leon Schlossberg and combines these artistic treasures with the text written by a truly exceptional contributor to the field of congenital heart surgery. These illustrations make it easier for the student to visualize surgical methods.

Kirklin, J. W., and Barratt-Boyes, B. G.: Cardiac Surgery. New York, John Wiley & Sons, 1986.
This thorough and exhaustively complete text should be read by students serious about the field of pediatric cardiac surgery. Kirklin and Barratt-Boyes present their extensive experience from several years of practicing surgical correction for these defects and provide important incremental risk tables describing the importance of various factors that might contribute to the overall outcome.

Lillehei, C. W., Varco, R. L., Cohen, M., Warden, H. E., Patton, C., and Moller, J. H.: The first open-heart repairs of ventricular septal defect, atrioventricular communis, and tetralogy of Fallot using extracorporeal circulation by cross-circulation: A 30-year follow-up. Ann. Thorac. Surg., 41:4, 1986.
This paper provides 30-year follow-up of some of the first patients undergoing repair of atrial septal defects and AV canal defects as well as other intracardiac lesions using Lillehei's dramatic technique of cross-circulation. Of particular interest in this article, is the discussion provided by many of Lillehei's students who established themselves as leaders in the field in congenital heart surgery. The poignancy of these remarks alone make this article well worth reading.

Rastelli, G. C.: Atrioventricular Canal Defects. Philadelphia, W. B. Saunders Company, 1976.
This monograph was written by Rastelli shortly before his death. The foreword by Dwight McGoon is a fitting memorial to this pioneer who contributed much to the field of congenital heart surgery prior to his death at 39. In this monograph, Rastelli clearly describes the anatomy of this defect and delineate many of the anatomic features that have enabled surgeons to develop successful surgical corrections.

Ungerleider, R. M., Kisslo, J. A., Greeley, W. J., Van Trigt, P., and Sabiston, D. C., Jr.: Intraoperative prebypass and postbypass epicardial color flow imaging in the repair of atrioventricular septal defects. J. Thorac. Cardiovasc. Surg., 98:90, 1989.
The utility of intraoperative epicardial Doppler color flow imaging for evaluating the repair of complete AV canal defects is described. The authors report on 18 patients undergoing such a repair (with a 0 per cent operative mortality) and demonstrate two examples of where the information generated by postrepair echo Doppler images enabled revision of residual ventricular septal defects, allowing the patient to leave the operating room with a better repair. The coupling of technology to surgical technique, leading to an era in which neonatal cardiac surgery can be performed with excellent results in the hope of yielding better long-term outcomes, is demonstrated.

REFERENCES

1. Alexander, J. A., Rembert, J. C., Sealy, W. C., and Greenfield, J. C.: Shunt dynamics in experimental atrial septal defects. J. Appl. Physiol., 39:28, 1975.
2. Alt, B., and Shikes, R. H.: Pulmonary hypertension in congenital heart disease: Irreversible vascular changes in young infants. Pediatr. Pathol., 1:423, 1983.
3. Andersen, M., Lyngborg, K., Moller, I., and Wennevold, A.: The natural history of small atrial septal defects: Long-term follow-up with serial heart catheterizations. Am. Heart J., 92:302, 1976.
4. Bailey, C. P., Nichols, H. T., Bolton, H. E., Jamison, W. L., and Gomez-Almedia, M.: Surgical treatment of forty-six interatrial septal defects by atrio-septo-pexy. Ann. Surg., 140:805, 1954.
5. Baron, M. G., Wolf, B. S., Steinfeld, L., and Van Mierop, L. H. S.: Endocardial cushion defects: Specific diagnosis by angiocardiography. Am. J. Cardiol., 13:162, 1964.

6. Behrendt, D. M.: Atrial septal defect. *In* Arciniegas, E. (Ed.): Pediatric Cardiac Surgery. Chicago, Year Book Medical Publishers, 1985.
7. Belkin, R. N., Waugh, R. A., Kisslo, J. A.: Interatrial shunting in atrial septal aneurysm. Am. J. Cardiol., 57:310, 1986.
8. Ben-Zvi, J., Hildner, F. J., and Samet, P.: Development of mitral insufficiency following closure of ostium secundum atrial septal defect. Am. Heart J., 91:83, 1976.
9. Bender, H. W., Jr., Hammon, J. W., Jr., Hubbard, S. G., Muirhead, J., and Graham, T. P.: Repair of atrioventricular canal malformation in the first year of life. J. Thorac. Cardiovasc. Surg., 84:515, 1982.
10. Beppu, S., Nimura, Y., Sakakibara, H., et al.: Mitral cleft in ostium primum atrial septal defect assessed by cross-sectional echocardiography. Circulation, 62:1099, 1980.
11. Berg, J. M., Crome, L., and France, N. E.: Congenital cardiac malformations in mongolism. Br. Heart J., 22:331, 1960.
12. Berger, T. J., Blackstone, E. H., Kirklin, J. W., et al.: Survival and probability of cure without and with surgery in complete atrioventricular canal. Ann. Thorac. Surg., 27:104, 1979.
13. Berger, T. J., Kirklin, J. W., Blackstone, E. H., Pacifico, A. D., and Kouchoukos, N. T.: Primary repair of complete atrioventricular canal in patients less than 2 years old. Am. J. Cardiol., 41:906, 1978.
14. Beyer, J.: Atrial septal defect: Acute left heart failure after surgical closure. Ann. Thorac. Surg., 25:36, 1978.
15. Bharati, S., Lev, M., and Kirklin, J. W.: Cardiac Surgery and the Conduction System. New York, John Wiley & Sons, 1983.
16. Bharati, S., Kirklin, J. W., McAllister, H. A., Jr., and Lev, M.: The surgical anatomy of common atrioventricular orifice associated with tetralogy of Fallot, double outlet right ventricle and complete regular transposition. Circulation, 61:1142, 1980.
17. Bizarro, R. O., Callahan, J. A., Feldt, R. H., et al.: Familial atrial septal defect with prolonged atrioventricular conduction: Syndrome showing autosomal dominant patterns of inheritance. Circulation, 41:677, 1970.
18. Bolens, M., and Friedli, B.: Sinus node function and conduction system before and after surgery for secundum atrial septal defect: An electrophysiologic study. Am. J. Cardiol., 53:1415, 1984.
19. Bonow, R. O., Borer, J. S., Rosing, D. R., et al.: Left ventricular functional reserve in adult patients with atrial septal defect: Pre- and postoperative studies. Circulation, 63:1315, 1981.
20. Brannon, E. S., Weens, H. A., and Warren, J. V.: Atrial septal defect: Study of hemodynamics by technique of right heart catheterization. Am. J. Med. Sci., 210:480, 1945.
21. Brody, H.: Drainage of the pulmonary veins into the right side of the heart. Arch. Pathol., 33:221, 1942.
22. Campbell, M.: Natural history of atrial septal defect. Br. Heart J., 32:820, 1970.
23. Carpentier, A: Surgical anatomy and management of the mitral component of atrioventricular canal defects. *In* Anderson, R. H., and Shinebourne, E. A. (Eds.): Pediatric Cardiology. London, Churchill Livingstone, 1978, p. 477.
24. Castaneda, A. R., Mayer, J. E., Jr., and Jonas, R. A.: Repair of complete atrioventricular canal in infancy. World J. Surg., 9:590, 1985.
25. Cayler, G. G.: Spontaneous functional closure of symptomatic atrial septal defects. N. Engl. J. Med., 276:65, 1967.
26. Cooley, D. A., Ellis, P. R., Jr., and Bellizzi, M. E.: Atrial septal defects of the sinus venosus type: Surgical considerations. Dis. Chest, 39:185, 1961.
27. Craig, R. J., Selzer, A.: Natural history and prognosis of atrial septal defect. Circulation, 37:805, 1968.
28. Dalen, J. E., Bruce, R. A., and Cobb, L. A.: Interaction of chronic hypoxia of moderate altitude on pulmonary hypertension complicating defect of the atrial septum. N. Engl. J. Med., 266:272, 1962.
29. Dave, K. S., Pakrashi, B. C., Wooler, G. H., and Ionescu, M. I.: Atrial septal defect in adults. Am. J. Cardiol., 31:7, 1973.
30. Ebels, T., Meijboom, E. J., Anderson, R. H., Schasfoort-van Leeuwen, M. J. M., Lenstra, D., Eijgelaar, A., Bossinia, K. K., and Homan vander Heide, J. N.: Anatomic and functional "obstruction" of the outflow tract in atrioventricular septal defects with separate valve orifices ("ostium primum atrial septal defect"): An echocardiographic study. Am. J. Cardiol., 54:843, 1984.
31. Ebert, P. A.: Atlas of Congenital Cardiac Surgery. New York, Churchill Livingstone, 1989.
32. Ellis, F. H., Jr., Brandenburg, R. O., and Swan, H. J. C.: Defect of the atrial septum in the elderly. Report of successful correction in five patients sixty years of age or older. N. Engl. J. Med., 262:219, 1960.
33. Emanuel, R., Somerville, J., Inns, A., and Withers, R.: Evidence of congenital heart disease in the offspring of parents with atrioventricular defects. Br. Heart J., 49:144, 1983.
34. Evans, J. R., Rowe, R. D., and Keith, J. D.: The clinical diagnosis of atrial septal defect in children. Am. J. Med., 30:345, 1961.
35. Forfang, K., Simonsen, S., Anderson, A., and Efskind, L.: Atrial septal defect of the secundum type in the middle-aged: Clinical results of surgery and correlations between symptoms and hemodynamics. Am. Heart J., 94:44, 1977.
36. Fraker, T. D., Jr., Harris, P. J., Behar, V. S., and Kisslo, J. A.: Detection and exclusion of interatrial shunts by two-dimensional echocardiography. Circulation, 54:379, 1979.
37. Frescura, C., Thiene, G., Franceschini, E., Talenti, E., and Mazzucco, A.: Pulmonary vascular disease in infants with complete atrioventricular septal defect. Int. J. Cardiol., 15:91, 1987.

38. Gault, J. H., Morrow, A. G., Gay, W. A., Jr., and Ross, J., Jr.: Atrial septal defect in patients over the age of forty years. Circulation, 37:261, 1968.
39. Gerbode, F., and Carr, I.: Surgery of congenital lesions of the heart and great vessels. In Gay, W. A., Jr., and Goldsmith, H. A. (Eds.): Cardiovascular Surgery. Philadelphia, Harper & Row, 1981.
40. Gibbon, J. H.: Application of a mechanical heart-lung apparatus to cardiac surgery. Minn. Med., 37:171, 1984.
41. Giknis, F. L.: Single atrium and the Ellis-van Creveld syndrome. J. Pediatr., 62:558, 1963.
42. Glenn, W. W. L., Stansel, H. C., Jr., Talner, N. S., Deren, M. M., and Van Heeckeren, D.: Surgical treatment of atrial septal defect: Analysis of 150 corrective operations. Am. J. Surg., 121:485, 1971.
43. Goldfaden, D. M., Jones, M., and Morrow, A. G.: Long-term results of repair of incomplete persistent atrioventricular canal. J. Thorac. Cardiovasc. Surg., 82:669, 1981.
44. Greeley, W. J., Ungerleider, R. M., Kern, F. H., Brusino, G. A., Smith, L. R., and Reves, J. G.: Effects of cardiopulmonary bypass on cerebral blood flow in neonates, infants and children. Circulation, 80(3):I-209, 1989.
45. Greeley, W. J., Ungerleider, R. M., Smith, L. R., and Reves, J. G.: The effects of deep hypothermic cardiopulmonary bypass and total circulatory arrest on cerebral blood flow in infants and children. J. Thorac. Cardiovasc. Surg., 97:737, 1989.
46. Gross, R. E., Pomeranz, A. A., Watkins, E., Jr., and Goldsmith, E. I.: Surgical closure of defects of the interauricular septum by use of an atrial well. N. Engl. J. Med., 247:455, 1952.
47. Hairston, P., Parker, E. F., Arrants, J. E., Bradham, R. R., and Lee, W. H., Jr.: The adult atrial septal defect: Results of surgical repair. Ann. Surg., 179:799, 1974.
48. Hanlon, C. R., Barner, H. B., Willman, V. L., Mudd, J. G., and Kaiser, G. C.: Atrial septal defect: Results of repair in adults. Arch. Surg., 99:275, 1969.
49. Hawe, A., Rastelli, G. C., Brandenburg, R. O., and McGoon, D. C.: Embolic complications following repair of atrial septal defects. Circulation, Suppl. 39:185, 1969.
50. Hines, G. L., Finnerty, T. T., Doyle, E., and Isom, O. W.: Near fatal hemolysis following repair of ostium primum atrial septal defect. J. Cardiovasc. Surg., 19:7, 1978.
51. Keith, J. D., Rowe, R. D., and Vlad, P.: Heart Disease in Infancy and Childhood. New York, Macmillan Company, 1978.
52. Kirklin, J. W, and Barratt-Boyes, B. G.: Cardiac Surgery. New York, John Wiley & Sons, 1986.
53. Kirklin, J. W., and Blackstone, E. H.: Management of the infant with complete atrioventricular canal. J. Thorac. Cardiovasc. Surg., 78:32, 1979.
54. Kirklin, J. W., Blackstone, E. H., Pacifico, A. D., Brown, R. N., and Bargeron, L. M., Jr.: Routine primary repair vs. two-stage repair of tetralogy of Fallot. Circulation, 60:373, 1979.
55. Kirklin, J. W., Ellis, F. H., Jr., and Barratt-Boyes, B. G.: Technique for repair of atrial septal defect using the atrial well. Surg. Gynecol. Obstet., 103:646, 1956.
56. Kirklin, J. W., Pacifico, A. D., and Kirklin, J. K.: The surgical treatment of atrioventricular canal defects. In Arciniegas, E. (Ed.): Pediatric Cardiac Surgery. Chicago, Year Book Medical Publishers, 1985.
57. Kisslo, J. A., Adams, D. B., and Belkin, R. N.: Doppler Color Flow Imaging. New York, Churchill Livingstone, 1988.
58. Kyger, E. R., Frazier, O. H., Cooley, D. A., Gillette, P. C., Reul, G. J., Jr., Sandiford, F. M., and Wukasch, D. C.: Sinus venosus atrial septal defect: Early and late results following closure in 109 patients. Ann. Thorac. Surg., 25:44, 1978.
59. Lappen, R. S., Muster, A. J., Idriss, F. S., Riggs, T. W., Ilbawi, M., Paul, M. H., Bharati, S., and Lev, M.: Masked subaortic stenosis in ostium primum atrial septal defect: Recognition and treatment. Am. J. Cardiol., 52:336, 1983.
60. Leachman, R. D., Cokkinos, D. V., and Cooley, D. A.: Association of ostium secundum atrial septal defects with mitral valve prolapse. Am. J. Cardiol., 38:167, 1976.
61. Lev, M.: The architecture of the conduction system in congenital heart disease. I. Common atrioventricular orifice. AMA Arch. Pathol., 65:174, 1958.
62. Levin, A. R., Spach, M. S, Boineau, J. P., Canent, R. V., Jr., Capp, M. P., and Jewett, P. H.: Atrial pressure-flow dynamics in atrial septal defects (secundum type). Circulation, 37:476, 1968.
63. Levy, S.: Long-term follow-up after surgical correction of the partial form of common atrioventricular canal (ostium primum). J. Thorac. Cardiovasc. Surg., 67:353, 1974.
64. Lewis, F. J., and Taufic, M.: Closure of atrial septal defects with the aid of hypothermia: Experimental accomplishments and the report of the one successful case. Surgery, 33:52, 1953.
65. Liberthson, R. R., Boucher, C. A., Strauss, H. W., Dinsmore, R. E., McKusick, K. A., and Pohost, G. M.: Right ventricular function in adult atrial septal defect. Am. J. Cardiol., 47:56, 1981.
66. Lillehei, C. W., Cohen, M., Warden, H. E., et al: Direct vision intracardiac surgery by means of controlled cross circulation or continuous arterial reservoir perfusion for correction of ventricular septal defects, atrioventricularis communis, isolated infundibular pulmonic stenosis, and tetralogy of Fallot. In Lam, C. R. (Ed.): Proceedings of Henry Ford Hospital Symposium. Philadelphia, W. B. Saunders Company, 1955, p. 371.
67. Lillehei, C. W., Varco, R. L., Cohen, M., Warden, H. E., Patton, C., and Moller, J. H.: The first open-heart repairs of ventricular septal defect, atrioventricular communis, and tetralogy of Fallot using extracorporeal circula-

tion by cross-circulation: A 30-year follow-up. Ann. Thorac. Surg., 41:4, 1986.
68. Lock, J. E., Rome, J. J., Davis, R., Van Praagh, S., Perry, S. B., Van Praagh, R., and Keane, J. F.: Transcatheter closure of atrial septal defects: Experimental studies. Circulation, 79:1091, 1989.
69. Losay, J., Rosenthal, A., Castaneda, A. R., Bernhard, W. H., and Nadas, A. S.: Repair of atrial septal defect primum: Results, course, and prognosis. J. Thorac. Cardiovasc. Surg., 75:248, 1978.
70. Magilligan, D. J., Jr., Lam, C. R., Lewis, J. W., Jr., and Davila, J. C.: Late results of atrial septal defect repair in adults. Arch. Surg., 113:1245, 1978.
71. Mavroudis, C., Weinstein, G., Turley, K., and Ebert, P. A.: Surgical management of complete atrioventricular canal. J. Thorac. Cardiovasc. Surg., 83:670, 1982.
72. McGrath, L. B., and Gonzalez-Lavin, L.: Actuarial survival, freedom from reoperation, and other events after repair of atrioventricular septal defects. J. Thorac. Cardiovasc. Surg., 94:582, 1987.
73. Meijboom, E. J., Ebels, T., Anderson, R. H., Schasfoort-van Leeuwen, M. J. M., Deanfield, J. E., Eijgelaar, A., and Homan vander Heide, J. N. H.: Left atrioventricular valve after surgical repair in atrioventricular septal defect with separate valve orifices ("ostium primum atrial septal defect"): An echo-Doppler study. Am. J. Cardiol., 57:433, 1986.
74. Menon, V. A., and Wagner, H. R.: Spontaneous closure of secundum atrial septal defect. NY State J. Med., 75:1068, 1975.
75. Mitchell, S. C., Korones, S. B., and Berendas, H. W.: Congenital heart disease in 56,109 births: Incidence and natural history. Circulation, 43:323, 1971.
76. Mody, M. R.: Serial hemodynamic observations in secundum atrial septal defect with special reference to spontaneous closure. Am. J. Cardiol., 32:978, 1973.
77. Moore, K. L.: The Developing Human: Clinically Oriented Embryology. Philadelphia, W. B. Saunders Company, 1977.
78. Murray G.: Closure of defects in cardiac septa. Ann. Surg., 128:843, 1948.
79. Newfeld, E. A., Sher, M., Paul, M. H., and Nikaidoh, H.: Pulmonary vascular disease in complete atrioventricular canal defect. Am. J. Cardiol., 39:721, 1977.
80. Pass, H. I., Crawford, F. A., Jr., Sade, R. M., Assey, M. E., and Usher, B. W.: Congenital heart disease in adults. Am. Surgeon, 50:36, 1984.
81. Pearlman, A. S., Borer, J. S., Clark, C. E., Henry, W. L., Redwood, D. R., Morrow, A. G., Epstein, S. E., Burn, C., Cohen, E., and McKay, F. J.: Abnormal right ventricular size and ventricular septal motion after atrial septal defect closure. Am. J. Cardiol., 41:295, 1978.
82. Phillips, S. J., Okies, J. E., Henken, D., Sunderland, C. O., and Starr, A.: Complex of secundum atrial septal defect and congestive heart failure in infants. J. Thorac. Cardiovasc. Surg., 70:696, 1975.
83. Rahimtoola, S. H., Kirklin, J. W., and Burchell, H. B.: Atrial septal defect. Circulation, 37, 38(Suppl. V):V-2, 1968.
84. Rainier-Pope, C. R., Cunningham, R. D., Nadas, A. S., and Crigler, J. F.: Cardiovascular malformation in Turner's syndrome. Pediatrics, 33:919, 1964.
85. Rastelli, G. C., Kirklin, J. W., and Titus, J. L.: Anatomic observations on complete form of persistent common atrioventricular canal with special reference to atrioventricular valves. Mayo Clin. Proc., 41:296, 1966.
86. Rastelli, G. C., Weidman, W. H., and Kirklin, J. W.: Surgical repair of the partial form of persistent common atrioventricular canal, with special reference to the problem of mitral valve incompetence. Circulation, 31, 32(Suppl. I):I-31, 1965.
87. Rastelli, G. C.: Atrioventricular Canal Defects. Philadelphia, W. B. Saunders Company, 1976.
88. Richmond, D. E., Lowe, J. B., and Barratt-Boyes, B. G.: Results of surgical repair of atrial septal defects in the middle-aged and elderly. Thorax, 24:536, 1969.
89. Saksena, F. B., and Aldridge, H. E.: Atrial septal defect in the older patient: A clinical and hemodynamic study in patients operated on after age 35. Circulation, 42:1009, 1970.
90. Santos, A., Boucek, M., Ruttenberg, H., Veasy, G., Orsmond, G., and McGough, E.: Repair of atrioventricular septal defects in infancy. J. Thorac. Cardiovasc. Surg., 91:505, 1986.
91. Sayd, H. M., Dacie, J. V., Handley, D. A, Lewis, S. M., and Cleland, W. P.: Hemolytic anemia of mechanical origin after open heart surgery. Thorax, 16:356, 1961.
92. Sealy, W. C., Farmer, J. C., Young, W. G., Jr., and Brown, I. W.: Atrial dysrhythmia and atrial secundum defects. J. Thorac. Cardiovasc. Surg., 57:245, 1969.
93. Sellers, R. D., Ferlic, R. M., Sterns, L. P., and Lillehei, C. W.: Secundum type atrial septal defects: Early and late results of surgical repair using extracorporeal circulation in 275 patients. Surgery, 59:155, 1966.
94. Silverman, N., Levitsky, S., Fisher, E., DuBrow, I., Hastreiter, A., and Scagliotti, D.: Efficacy of pulmonary artery banding in infants with complete atrioventricular canal. Circulation, 68(Suppl. II):II-148, 1983.
95. Somerville, J.: Ostium primum defects: Factors causing deterioration in the natural history. Br. Heart J., 27:413, 1965.
96. Sondergard, T.: Closure of atrial septal defects: Report of three cases. Acta Chir. Scand., 107:492, 1954.
97. St. John Sutton, M. G., Tajik, A. J., and McGoon, D. C.: Atrial septal defect in patients ages 60 years or older: Operative results and long-term postoperative follow-up. Circulation, 64:402, 1981.
98. Steinbrunn, W., Cohn, K. E., and Selzer, A.: Atrial septal defect associated

with mitral stenosis: The Lutembacher syndrome revisited. Am. J. Med., *48*:295, 1970.

99. Studer, M., Blackstone, E. H., Kirklin, J. W., Pacifico, A. D., Soto, B., Chung G. K. T., Kirklin, J. K., and Bargeron, L. M., Jr.: Determinants of early and late results of repair of atrioventricular septal (canal) defects. J. Thorac. Cardiovasc. Surg., *84*:523, 1982.

100. Sugimura, S., Okies, J. E., Litchford, B., and Starr, A.: Late results of mitral cleft closure for ostium primum atrial septal defect in adolescents and adults. Am. Surgeon, *45*:670, 1979.

101. Swan, C., Tostevin, A. L., Mayo, H., and Black, G. H. B.: Further observation on congenital defects in infants following infectious diseases during pregnancy with special reference to rubella. Med. J. Aust., *1*:409, 1944.

102. Taylor, N. C., and Somerville, J.: Fixed subaortic stenosis after repair of ostium primum defects. Br. Heart J., *45*:689, 1981.

103. Thompson, T., and Evans, W.: Paradoxical embolism. Q. J. Med., *23*:135, 1930.

104. Trusler, G. A., Kazenelson, G., Freedom, R. M., Williams, W. G., and Rowe, R. D.: Late results following repair of partial anomalous pulmonary venous connection with sinus venosus atrial septal defect. J. Thorac. Cardiovasc. Surg., *79*:776, 1980.

105. Uchida, I. A., and Rowe, R. D.: Discordant heart anomalies in twins. Am. J. Hum. Genet., *9*:133, 1957.

106. Ungerleider, R. M., Greeley, W. J., Sheikh, K. H., Kern, F. H., Kisslo, J. A., and Sabiston, D. C., Jr.: The use of intraoperative echo with Doppler color flow imaging to predict outcome after repair of congenital cardiac defects. Ann. Surg., *210*:526, 1989.

107. Ungerleider, R. M., Greeley, W. J., Sheikh, K. H., Philips, J., Pearce, F. B., Kern, F. H., and Kisslo, J. A.: Routine use of intraoperative, epicardial echo and Doppler color flow imaging to guide and evaluate repair of congenital heart lesions: A prospective study. J. Thorac. Cardiovasc. Surg., *100*:297, 1990.

108. Ungerleider, R. M., Kisslo, J. A, Greeley, W. J., Van Trigt, P., and Sabiston, D.

C., Jr.: Intraoperative prebypass and postbypass epicardial color flow imaging in the repair of atrioventricular septal defects. J. Thorac. Cardiovasc. Surg., *98*:90, 1989.

109. Verdon, T. A., Jr., Forrester, R. H., Crosby, W. H.: Hemolytic anemia after open heart repair of ostium primum defects. N. Engl. J. Med., *269*:643, 1963.

110. Verrier, E. D.: Secundum atrial septal defects. *In* Grillo, H. C., Austen, W. G., Wilkins, E. W., Jr., Mathisen, D. J., and Vlahakes, G. J.: Current Therapy in Cardiothoracic Surgery. Philadelphia, B. C. Decker, 1989.

111. Waldhausen, J. A., and Tyers, G. F. O.: Atrial septal defects, ostium primum defects, and atrioventricular canals. *In* Sabiston, D. C., Jr. (Ed.): Textbook of Surgery, 13th ed. Philadelphia, W. B. Saunders Company, 1986.

112. Wanderman, K. L., Orsysheher, I., and Gueron, M.: Left ventricular performance in patients with atrial septal defect: Evaluation with noninvasive methods. Am. J. Cardiol., *41*:487, 1978.

113. Wendet, V. E., Keech, M. K., Read, R. C., Bistue, A. R., and Bianchi, F. A.: Cardiovascular features of Marfan's syndrome: Family studies. Circulation, *32*(Suppl. 2):218, 1965.

114. Williams, R. G., and Rudd, M.: Echocardiographic features of endocardial cushion defects. Circulation, *49*:418, 1974.

115. Williams, W. H., Guyton, R. A., Michalik, R. E., Jones, E. L., Rhee, K. H., Plauth, W. H., Jr., and Hatcher, C. R., Jr.: Individualized surgical management of complete atrioventricular canal. J. Thorac. Cardiovasc. Surg., *86*:838, 1983.

116. Yalav, E., Brown, A. H., and Braimbridge, M. V.: Surgery for atrial septal defect in patients over 60 years of age. J. Thorac. Cardiovasc. Surg., *62*:788, 1971.

117. Yamaki, S., Horiuchi, T., and Sekino, Y.: Quantitative analysis of pulmonary vascular disease in simple cardiac anomalies with the Down syndrome. Am. J. Cardiol., *51*:1502, 1983.

118. Young, D.: Later results of closure of secundum atrial septal defect in children. Am. J. Cardiol., *31*:14, 1973.

VI ———————————————————————————————————————

DISORDERS OF PULMONARY VENOUS RETURN

Richard A. Jonas, M.D., and Aldo R. Castaneda, M.D.

Abnormalities of pulmonary venous return are most commonly due to anomalous connection of the pulmonary veins, which can involve all pulmonary veins, i.e., total anomalous pulmonary venous connection (TAPVC), or fewer than all pulmonary veins, so-called partial anomalous pulmonary venous connection (PAPVC). A critical determinant of the hemodynamic consequences of anomalous pulmonary venous connection is the presence of obstruction within the pulmonary venous pathway. Rarely, pulmonary venous obstruction can occur despite normal connection of the pulmonary veins to the left atrium in the form of individual pulmonary vein stenosis or an obstructive membrane within the left atrium, termed cor triatriatum (Fig. 1).

TOTAL ANOMALOUS PULMONARY VENOUS CONNECTION

Historical Aspects

TAPVC was first described by Wilson in 1798.[41] In 1951, Muller achieved surgical *palliation* by anastomosing the anomalous common pulmonary venous trunk to the left atrial appendage.[24] TAPVC was first *corrected* by Lewis and colleagues in 1956, using hypothermia and inflow occlusion.[22] Correction on cardiopulmonary bypass was described in the same year by Burroughs and Kirklin.[7] The application of deep hypothermic circulatory arrest, as popularized by Barratt-Boyes and coworkers,[1] has caused a progressive decrease in surgical mortality in infants, including neonates presenting *in extremis* because of obstructed TAPVC.

Embryology

The lungs develop as an outpouching from the foregut. They carry with them a plexus of veins derived from the splanchnic (systemic) venous plexus, which drains to the heart through the cardinal and umbilicovitelline veins. TAPVC occurs when the pulmonary vein evagination from the posterior surface of the left atrium fails to fuse with the pulmonary venous plexus surrounding the lung buds (Fig. 2). In this case, at least one connection of the pulmonary plexus to the splanchnic plexus persists and the pulmonary veins drain to the heart through a systemic vein.[27]

Pathologic Anatomy

TAPVC represents 2.5 per cent of all cases of congenital heart disease within the New England Regional Infant Cardiac Program.[11] Predictable from its embryologic origin, TAPVC consists of a wide spectrum of anatomic anomalies. Persistent

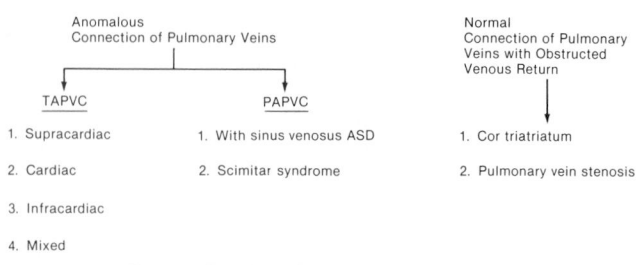

Figure 1. Disorders of pulmonary venous return.

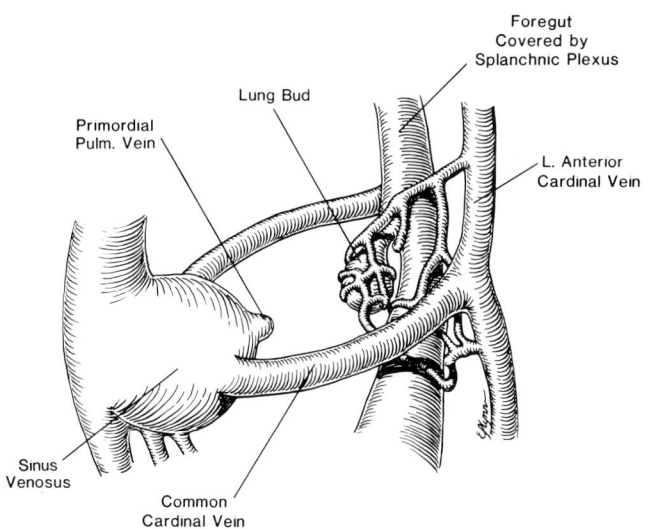

Figure 2. TAPVC results when the primordial pulmonary vein fails to unite with the plexus of veins that surrounds the lung buds and is derived from the splanchnic venous plexus, including the cardinal veins and umbilicovitelline veins.

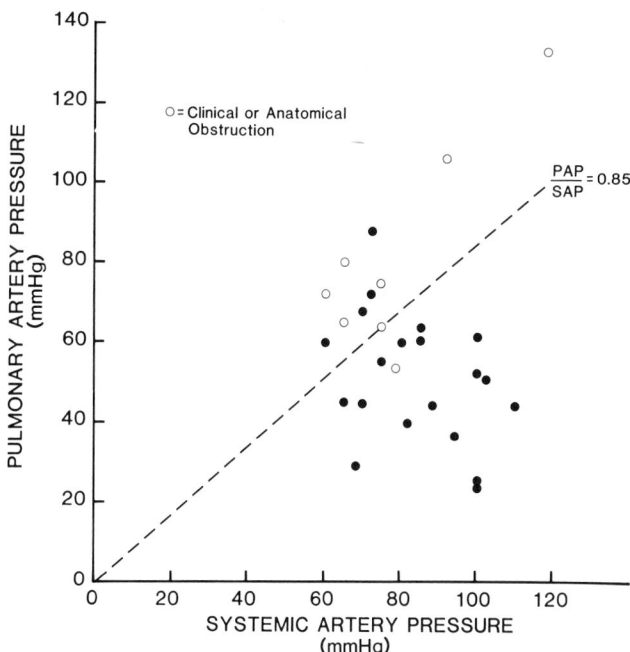

Figure 3. Pulmonary venous obstruction, demonstrated either at surgical correction or postmortem, is very likely in patients with TAPVC to the coronary sinus when right ventricular pressure is greater than 85 per cent of systemic pressure at cardiac catheterization.

splanchnic venous connections can occur to almost any point in the central cardinal or umbilicovitelline venous systems. In one classification described by Darling and associates,[9] TAPVC is described as *supracardiac* when the anomalous connection is to an ascending vertical vein, usually on the left connected to the left innominate vein; as *cardiac* when the pulmonary veins connect directly to the right atrium or to the coronary sinus; or as *infracardiac* when connection is to intra-abdominal veins. In a large autopsy series from Children's Hospital, Boston, approximately 45 per cent of cases of TAPVC were supracardiac, 25 per cent were cardiac, and 25 per cent were infracardiac.[10] In 5 per cent of patients, pulmonary venous connection was *mixed,* with at least one of the main lobar pulmonary veins connecting to a different systemic vein relative to the remaining veins (see Fig. 1).

Pulmonary venous obstruction can occur at any point in the anomalous pathway but is most commonly seen with infracardiac connection, where it is almost always present to some degree. When pulmonary venous obstruction is present, there are usually morphologic changes in pulmonary arterioles, with an increase in arterial muscularity and extension of muscle into smaller and more peripheral arteries.[14] Most patients with TAPVC have no associated major cardiac defects. However, many different associated anomalies have been reported, including tetralogy of Fallot and double outlet right ventricle.[10] Associated anomalies, particularly a single functional ventricle, are much more likely with heterotaxy syndrome.[3]

Left ventricular volume in patients with TAPVC is often at the lower limit of normal. This may be related to the leftward deviation of the ventricular septum, present with right ventricular hypertension.[13,40] Endocardial fibroelastosis of the left ventricle has also been reported.[21] The relative hypoplasia of the left ventricle is consistent with the low cardiac indices often seen in these patients postoperatively.[31]

Pathophysiology

Since both pulmonary venous blood and systemic venous blood return to the right atrium with all forms of TAPVC, survival of the child is dependent on the presence of a right-to-left intracardiac shunt. This almost always occurs through a patent foramen ovale that is rarely restrictive, i.e., there is no pressure gradient between the right and left atria.[12] Mixing of systemic and pulmonary venous return causes at least some degree of cyanosis in all patients. The degree of cyanosis is determined by the amount of pulmonary blood flow relative to systemic blood

flow, and this in turn is determined largely by the presence or absence of pulmonary venous obstruction. Pulmonary venous obstruction is amost always accompanied by pulmonary arterial and right ventricular hypertension. In fact, significant pulmonary venous obstruction is unlikely in the child with a right ventricular pressure of less than 85 per cent of systemic pressure[18] (Fig. 3). When no pulmonary venous obstruction is present, pulmonary blood flow is often increased, since pulmonary venous blood is returning to the compliant right heart. This increase in pulmonary blood flow may cause pulmonary hypertension to levels as high as systemic pressure. However, suprasystemic right ventricular pressure is unlikely in the absence of pulmonary venous obstruction. The observed muscularity of pulmonary arterioles is reflected in a tendency to have labile pulmonary vascular resistance postoperatively, resulting in so-called "pulmonary hypertensive crises."

The presence of pulmonary venous obstruction or of increased pulmonary blood flow is likely to cause an increase in extravascular lung water, which may be largely interstitial, although in severe cases of pulmonary venous obstruction this can progress to frank pulmonary edema with fluid extravasation into the alveoli.

An interesting feedback loop can occur in some cases of supracardiac TAPVC. The anomalous vertical vein carrying the entire pulmonary venous return may pass between the left main bronchus and left pulmonary artery. Some degree of pulmonary venous obstruction causes increased pressure within the left pulmonary artery, which further exacerbates the compression of venous return between the bronchus and left pulmonary artery. Ultimately, a severe degree of obstruction may ensue.[6]

Clinical Features

The presenting features of the child with TAPVC are determined by the degree of pulmonary venous obstruction. If obstruction is very severe, the child may be profoundly cyanosed and in respiratory distress within hours of birth. The child is tachycardic and hypotensive.

In children without serious pulmonary venous obstruction, the clinical status is determined by the level of pulmonary blood flow and degree of pulmonary hypertension. The child with significant pulmonary hypertension and greatly increased pulmonary blood flow fails to thrive and has tachypnea and diaphoresis, particularly when feeding. The degree of cyanosis is mild. If pulmonary artery pressure is only minimally elevated, the child may progress well for years with only a mild degree of cyanosis.

Diagnostic Studies

In the child with serious obstruction, arterial blood gas analysis reveals severe hypoxia, e.g., Po_2 less than 20 mm. Hg, often with an associated metabolic acidosis. Chest films show a normal heart size with generalized pulmonary edema. The electrocardiogram demonstrates right ventricular hypertrophy, but this is to be expected in the neonate. Two-dimensional echocardiography is very reliable in establishing the diagnosis of TAPVC. Ventricular septal position and Doppler assessment of any tricuspid regurgitant jet yield a useful estimate of right ventricular pressure. The avoidance of cardiac catheterization in the desperately ill neonate with obstructed TAPVC has been an important advance in the perioperative management of this condition.[34] The osmotic load induced by angiography in the past often exacerbated the degree of pulmonary edema.

In older children, cardiac catheterization may be indicated. The important hemodynamic data to be collected are the right ventricular pressure and pulmonary artery pressure, as well as a measure of the degree of pulmonary venous obstruction as determined by the pulmonary artery wedge pressure to right atrial gradient (there is generally minimal to no gradient across the foramen ovale). The point at which an increase in oxygen saturation is observed within the systemic venous system helps localize the point of connection of pulmonary venous return. Pulmonary arteriography demonstrates the anomalous pulmonary venous pathway during the levophase (which may be significantly delayed if obstruction is present).

Indications for and Timing of Surgical Therapy

OBSTRUCTED TAPVC. In the prostaglandin era, obstructed TAPVC remains perhaps the only true surgical emergency within the field of congenital heart disease. Other than intubation and positive-pressure ventilation with 100 per cent oxygen and correction of metabolic acidosis, no medical measures have been clearly demonstrated to adequately palliate this problem, although one recent report has suggested that maintenance of ductal patency with prostaglandin E_1 may be useful.[42] Surgical correction is indicated as soon as the diagnosis has been established.

NONOBSTRUCTED TAPVC. Since there is no possibility of spontaneous resolution of this entity, surgical correction should be undertaken during early infancy, before the secondary deleterious effects of an abnormal circulation have caused permanent damage to the lungs and brain, as well as to the heart itself.[5,28,32,38]

Management of TAPVC

THE NEONATE WITH OBSTRUCTED INFRACARDIAC TAPVC. The hypoxic, acidotic neonate with obstructed TAPVC requires meticulous perioperative management,[17] as well as an accurate and expeditious surgical procedure. Following endotracheal intubation, pulmonary resistance should be minimized by hyperventilation with 100 per cent oxygen. Anesthesia is induced with high-dose fentanyl (which decreases pulmonary vasoreactivity), as well as with a muscle relaxant. If an inotropic agent is required, isoproterenol is preferred because it decreases pulmonary vascular resistance. Metabolic acidosis is treated with bicarbonate or tromethamine (THAM). There may be a large calcium requirement, and blood glucose may be labile. Digoxin is probably not useful and lowers the threshold for ventricular fibrillation.

SURGICAL TECHNIQUE. The technique of deep hypothermic circulatory arrest is employed.[16] Adequate venous access and an arterial monitoring line, preferably in an umbilical artery, are essential. A pulse oximeter also provides extremely useful information. It is probably best to avoid surface cooling, because these desperately ill children may fibrillate at a relatively high core temperature. The chest is opened by a median sternotomy, and the thymus is partially excised. A pericardial patch is harvested that may be treated with glutaraldehyde. It is essential that there be minimal disturbance of the myocardium after the pericardium is opened. Even the slightest retraction of the ventricular myocardium can cause ventricular fibrillation.

After systemic heparinization, bypass is commenced with an arterial cannula in the ascending aorta and venous return via a single cannula inserted into the right atrial appendage. Immediately after bypass is begun, the ductus arteriosus is dissected free and ligated. During body cooling, the heart should be gently retracted out of the chest to allow dissection of the anomalous descending vertical vein. A heavy ligature is tied around the vertical vein at the point where it pierces the diaphragm. The vertical vein is divided and filleted proximally to the level of the superior pulmonary vein. The heart is now replaced in the pericardium. When the rectal temperature has fallen to 18° C., by which time the esophageal temperature is approximately 12° C. and tympanic membrane temperature is 15 to 16° C., the ascending aorta is cross-clamped. Cardioplegic solution is infused into the root of the aorta. Bypass is discontinued, and blood is drained from the child. The venous cannula is removed.

A transverse incision is made from the right atrial appendage and is carried posteriorly through the foramen ovale into the left atrium. Because the right pulmonary veins do not anchor the left atrium, excellent exposure of the previously dissected vertical vein is now obtained. The incision in the posterior wall of the left atrium is carried inferiorly parallel to the vertical vein (Fig. 4). It may also be extended superiorly into the base of the left atrial appendage. The common pulmonary vein–to–left atrium anastomosis is performed, using continuous 6-0 absorbable polydioxanone suture. Excellent exposure is obtained by the approach described, and there is no possibility of kinking or malalignment, as may be the case with the alternative technique of performing the anastomosis with the heart everted from the chest. The foramen ovale and the more posterior part of the right atriotomy can be closed with a pericardial patch. Direct suture closure of the foramen ovale has a tendency to narrow the anastomosis and should be avoided.

Before the atrial septal defect is closed, the left heart should be

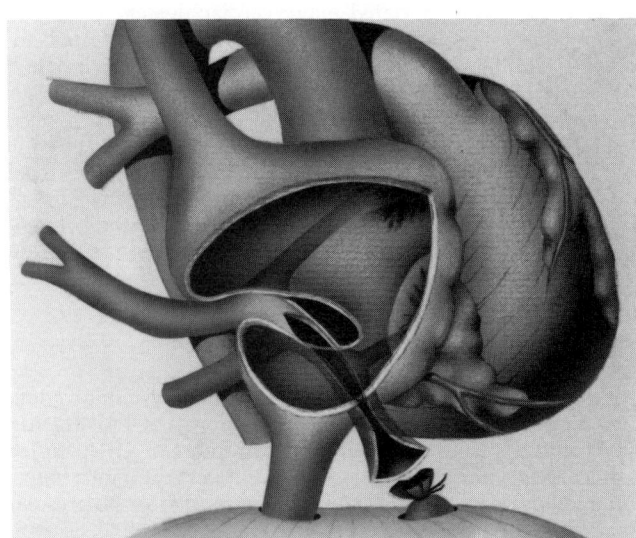

Figure 4. Surgical management of infracardiac TAPVC includes division of the anomalous vertical vein. The approach from the right allows a long anastomosis with the heart *in situ*.

filled with saline, and air can be vented through the cardioplegia site in the ascending aorta. After closure of the right atriotomy, the right heart is filled with saline, the venous cannula is reinserted, and bypass is recommenced. The aortic cross-clamp is released, with the cardioplegia site bleeding freely. During rewarming, a pulmonary artery monitoring line is inserted through a horizontal mattress suture in the infundibulum of the right ventricle. Insertion of a left atrial monitoring line through a pulmonary vein should be avoided, because of the small size of the pulmonary veins. However, it is possible to insert a left atrial line through the left atrial appendage.

Once rewarming to a rectal temperature of at least 35° C. is completed, the child can be weaned from cardiopulmonary bypass. Although this should be uneventful in any patient after elective surgical correction, it can be a critical phase in the management of one who is acutely ill and previously obstructed. Such patients tend to have markedly labile pulmonary vascular resistance. It is therefore useful to monitor pulmonary artery pressure at the time of weaning from bypass. It is not uncommon for pulmonary artery pressure to be close to systemic levels for the first 10 to 15 minutes after weaning from bypass. During this time, ventilatory management is critical. In the presence of a widely open anastomosis, pulmonary pressure should fall to less than two-thirds to one-half systemic pressure within 15 to 30 minutes of weaning from bypass. If pulmonary pressure remains elevated, a high suspicion of either an obstructed anastomosis or isolated pulmonary vein stenosis should be considered. Intraoperative two-dimensional echocardiography gives excellent visualization of this area.

ELECTIVE SURGICAL MANAGEMENT OF NONOBSTRUCTED SUPRACARDIAC TAPVC. The general operative approach to nonobstructed supracardiac TAPVC is similar to that for infracardiac TAPVC. Deep hypothermic circulatory arrest in the infant provides optimal exposure and therefore the most consistently wide open anastomosis. The horizontal pulmonary venous confluence is dissected free during the cooling period. In this case, after cessation of cardiopulmonary bypass and removal of the venous cannula, the right atrial transverse incision is carried across the atrial septum to the level of the foramen ovale into the left atrium. It is then continued transversely, extending into the base of the left atrial appendage. A longitudinal incision is made in the horizontal pulmonary venous confluence parallel to the incision in the posterior wall of the left atrium (Fig. 5A). A direct anastomosis is fashioned between the left atrium and pulmonary venous confluence, using continuous 6-0 polydioxanone suture. Once again, it is best to close the foramen ovale with a patch of autologous pericardium (Fig. 5B). Pulmonary hypertension is rare after such elective cases in which pulmonary artery pressure has usually been only mildly elevated before surgical correction.

ELECTIVE SURGICAL MANAGEMENT OF TAPVC TO THE CORONARY SINUS. It was previously thought that obstruction of TAPVC to the coronary sinus was extremely rare, but a recent review revealed a surprisingly high incidence of obstruction in 22 per cent of such cases.[18] Two-dimensional echocardiography, therefore, should carefully assess the point of junction between the pulmonary veins and the coronary sinus, which was the most common point of obstruction in the authors' series (Fig. 6A and B). If there is any doubt about this area, cardiac catheterization should be performed. In the absence of obstruction, a simple unroofing procedure of the coronary sinus suffices. The tissue between the foramen ovale and the coronary sinus is incised, and the incision in the coronary sinus is carried to the posterior wall of the heart. The resulting atrial septal defect is closed with an autologous pericardial patch (Fig. 7A and B). An alternative technique involves creation of a "fenestration" in the roof of the coronary sinus within the left atrium.[37] It was hoped that this method would decrease the incidence of arrhythmias, but this has not in fact been real-

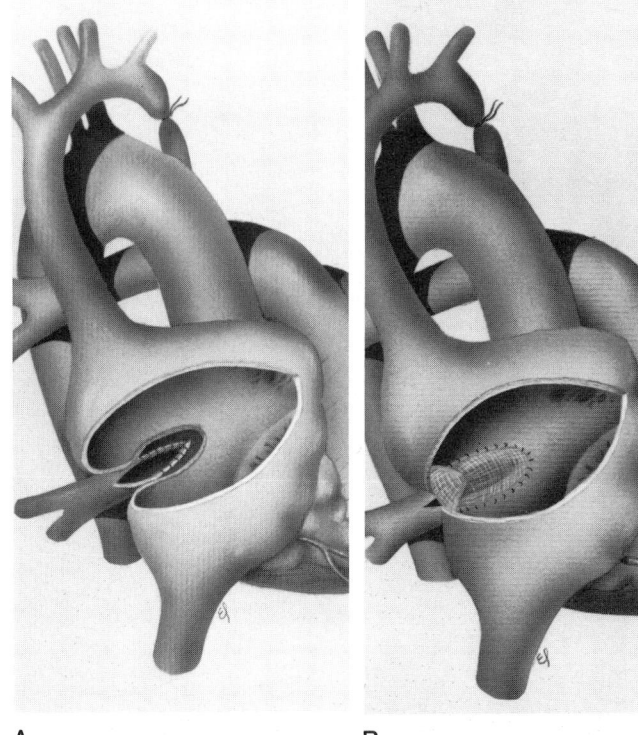

A   B

Figure 5. *A.* Excellent exposure of the horizontal pulmonary venous confluence is obtained by a single atrial incision through the foramen ovale into the left atrium for supracardiac TAPVC. *B,* Autologous pericardium is used to close the foramen ovale, supplement the anastomosis, and enlarge the left atrium in supracardiac TAPVC.

ized.[18] If two-dimensional echocardiography reveals a potential site of obstruction at the junction of the coronary sinus with the horizontal confluence, an operation similar to that for supracardiac TAPVC should be performed. The horizontal confluence should be filleted and a parallel incision made in the posterior wall of the left atrium, extending into the left atrial appendage. A direct anastomosis can be fashioned using continuous absorbable suture.[26]

Intensive Care Management

The heavily muscularized pulmonary arterioles of the child with obstructed TAPVC remain particularly labile for up to several days after corrective surgery. During this period, pulmonary resistance should be minimized by appropriate ventilatory management. The stress response of pulmonary vasoconstriction should be minimized by maintaining a constant state of anesthesia, using a fentanyl infusion supplemented with hourly boluses of pancuronium, 0.1 mg. per kg.[15] Arterial P_{CO_2} should be maintained at approximately 30 torr, and the inspired oxygen concentration should be titrated so as to achieve a pulmonary artery pressure of less than two-thirds systemic, as measured by the indwelling pulmonary artery line. A low-dose isoproterenol infusion of up to 0.1 μg. per kg. per minute may also be continued for 24 to 48 hours for its pulmonary vasodilatory effect. After 24 to 48 hours of hemodynamic stability, the level of anesthesia may be lightened, with careful observation for pulmonary hypertensive crises. These are particularly likely to occur in response to the stress of endotracheal tube suctioning, which should be performed carefully after hyperventilation. Assuming that the child remains hemodynamically stable, ventilatory weaning can be commenced. When an intermittent mandatory ventilation rate of 4 breaths per minute can be tolerated, the child usually withstands extubation. Throughout intensive care management it is essential that caloric intake be maintained at at least 125 per cent of basal requirements. Elec-

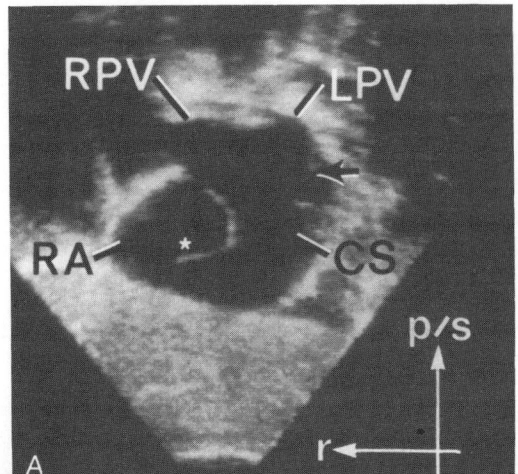

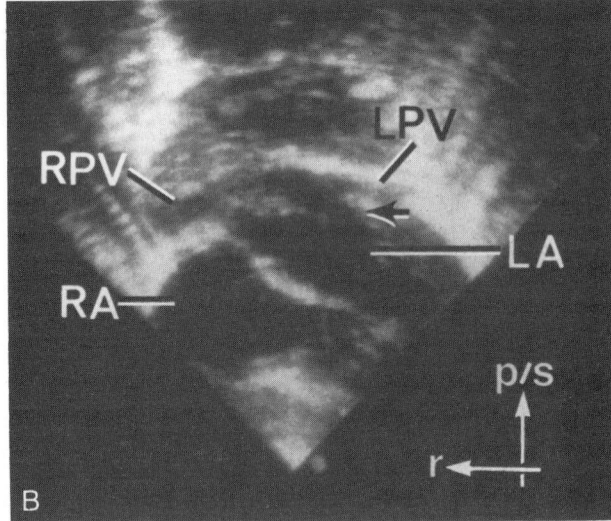

Figure 6. *A*, Two-dimensional echocardiography is now the diagnostic modality of choice for TAPVC. This subxiphoid long-axis cut shows the wide connection (arrow) between the pulmonary venous confluence and the dilated coronary sinus (CS). *B*, Preoperative two-dimensional echocardiogram of a patient with obstructed TAPVC to the coronary sinus. The subxiphoid long-axis cut shows a narrowed connection (arrow) between the pulmonary venous confluence and the mildly dilated coronary sinus. *, Eustachian valve; CS, coronary sinus; LA, left atrium; LPV, left pulmonary vein; p/s, posterior and superior; r, rightward; RA, right atrium; RPV, right pulmonary vein.

trolyte status, including ionized calcium levels, should be carefully monitored and proper levels maintained.

Long-Term Follow-up

Despite an initial satisfactory course, between 5 and 10 per cent of children develop pulmonary venous obstruction after surgical correction of TAPVC, often within 3 to 6 months.[20,34] Most commonly this takes the form of an obliterative intimal fibrous hyperplasia affecting the pulmonary veins close to their junction with the original common pulmonary vein and therefore somewhat remote from the actual line of anastomosis with the original true left atrium. This entity is particularly difficult to manage surgically and is also unresponsive to balloon dilation. Attempts at pericardial patch plasty have generally been unsuccessful. Patching techniques using flaps of atrial tissue may be more successful in relatively mild cases.[30]

Anastomotic obstruction caused by inadequate growth of suture lines can occur despite the use of absorbable sutures or interrupted suture techniques. This form of obstruction can usually be readily managed by repeat operation. Generally, there is dilatation of a secondary chamber behind the anastomosis. Simple incisions connecting the two chambers, followed by endo-

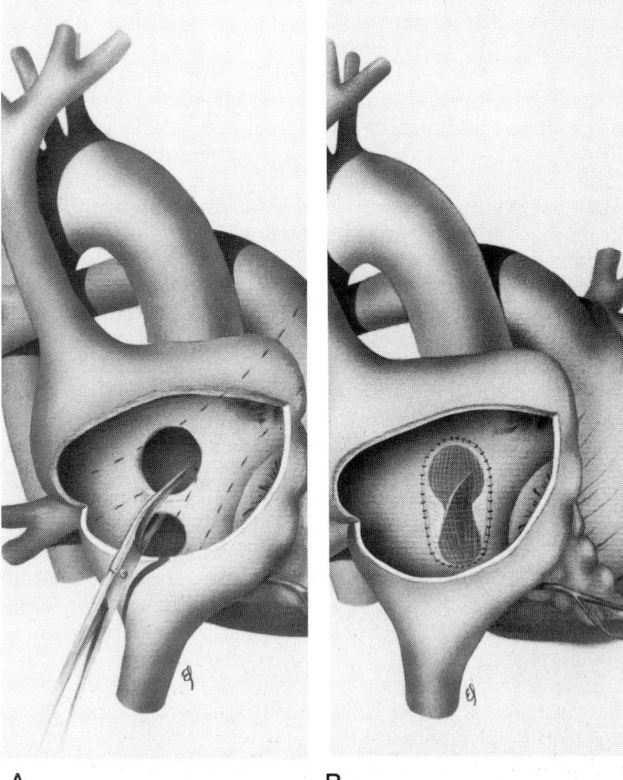

Figure 7. *A*, Unobstructed TAPVC to the coronary sinus is treated by incision of the tissue between the coronary sinus ostium and the foramen ovale, with complete unroofing of the coronary sinus. *B*, Autologous pericardium is used to close the resultant atrial septal defect in TAPVC to the coronary sinus.

cardial approximation, generally suffice to manage this problem.

Results of Surgical Management

Surgical results have improved dramatically over the last 3 decades. Before 1970, repair of TAPVC in infancy generally carried a mortality greater than 50 per cent.[2,25] Between 1970 and 1980, many centers reported mortality rates between 10 and 20 per cent.[29,40] Recent reports have described an early mortality of less than 10 per cent[18,23,34]

PARTIAL ANOMALOUS PULMONARY VENOUS CONNECTION

Pathologic Anatomy

WITH SINUS VENOSUS ATRIAL SEPTAL DEFECT (ASD). The pulmonary veins of the right upper and right middle lobes frequently connect to the superior vena cava in the presence of a sinus venosus ASD.[35] These veins also not uncommonly enter the superior vena cava as multiple small veins, some of which may enter relatively high in the superior vena cava above the level of the azygos vein.

SCIMITAR SYNDROME. The right pulmonary veins join to form a single vertical trunk, which descends in a curve (scimitar) to enter the inferior vena cava (IVC), generally close to the IVC/right atrial junction. Often a secundum ASD is present. The right lung may be hypoplastic, and the blood supply of the right lung (particularly the lower lobe) may be from aortopulmonary collaterals, rather than the true pulmonary artery.[19]

Pathophysiology

Obstruction of partially anomalous pulmonary veins is extremely rare. The hemodynamics, therefore, are similar to those of a left-to-right shunt at the atrial level.

Clinical Features

Like the child with an atrial septal defect, the child with PAPVC (usually in association with a sinus venosus ASD) is likely to be asymptomatic for many years. Diagnosis by two-dimensional echocardiography is generally possible, particularly since the advent of color Doppler.

Management

Surgical correction can be undertaken at any time convenient to the family in the preschool years. Careful consideration must be given to the placement of the venous cannulas to allow unimpeded access to the area of anomalous pulmonary venous connection. Where the anomalous veins enter close to the atriocaval junction, a pericardial baffle can be placed to direct pulmonary venous blood through the ASD to the left atrium. When the anomalous pulmonary veins enter high in the superior vena cava (SVC), the risk of creating SVC obstruction with this baffle technique is great. An alternative operation has been described that is technically straightforward and appears to have a low risk of pulmonary or systemic venous obstruction.[39]

Results

The risk of death or significant morbidity is less than 1 per cent. The incidence of caval obstruction should be very low with application of an appropriate operation, depending on the level of connection of the anomalous veins.

OBSTRUCTION OF PULMONARY VEINS DRAINING TO LEFT ATRIUM

Cor Triatriatum

This extremely rare anomaly is embryologically related to TAPVC. Although pulmonary venous blood drains appropriately to the left atrium, there is obstruction at the point of connection. This presumably represents a failure of completion of the normal process of communication between the pulmonary vein evagination from the posterior surface of the left atrium and the pulmonary venous plexus surrounding the lung buds. An upper common pulmonary vein chamber develops, which receives the pulmonary veins and a lower left atrium, including the left atrial appendage. The foramen ovale is generally present between the right atrium and common pulmonary vein chamber.[36] The diameter of the orifice in the fibrous membrane that separates the upper and lower chambers determines the degree of pulmonary venous obstruction. This also determines the age of presentation. The infant with severe obstruction presents with failure to thrive and respiratory distress. Chest films reveal pulmonary venous hypertension and the electrocardiogram demonstrates right ventricular hypertrophy from pulmonary arterial hypertension. Two-dimensional echocardiography, particularly with color Doppler, is usually diagnostic. It is useful for the small child with pulmonary congestion to avoid the osmotic load associated with pulmonary angiography, as required by cardiac catheterization diagnosis of cor triatriatum.

MANAGEMENT. Cor triatriatum is eminently suitable to surgical correction. This can be performed under deep hypothermic circulatory arrest in the small infant or on cardiopulmonary bypass in the larger child. The obstructive membrane is completely excised, working through the atrial septum.

RESULTS. Early mortality approaches zero.[8] There is probably a small risk that the pulmonary venous hypertension present before correction may lead to development of pulmonary vein stenosis, analogous to that seen after correction of TAPVC.

Pulmonary Vein Stenosis

This is also an extremely rare anomaly, which has a poor prognosis, either with or without surgical management. There is

generally fibrous intimal hyperplasia, which most commonly affects the point of junction between the pulmonary veins and left atrium but appears to be progressive in that with time the process extends upstream into the veins. The condition can progress to complete obliteration of the veins, which become fibrous cords.[4]

Diagnosis is generally made in infancy when the child presents with respiratory distress and failure to thrive. Chest films reveal pulmonary venous hypertension, and right ventricular hypertrophy is seen on electrocardiogram because of pulmonary hypertension. Two-dimensional echocardiography can usually provide excellent visualization of the stenotic veins, making cardiac catheterization unnecessary. Diagnosis with use of magnetic resonance imaging has also been reported.[33]

SURGICAL MANAGEMENT. Numerous surgical procedures have been attempted, but success has been rare. Although early survival can be achieved with satisfactory decompression of the veins at the point of obstruction, there is usually an inexorable progression of the disease process.[4] Probably the most promising procedure involves the use of a vascularized flap of atrial septum, which is rotated into the orifices of the pulmonary veins.[30]

SELECTED REFERENCES

Barratt-Boyes, B. G., Simpson, M., and Neutze, J. M.: Intracardiac surgery in neonates and infants using deep hypothermia with surface cooling and limited cardiopulmonary bypass. Circulation, 43 and 44 (Suppl. I):I25, 1971.
This landmark paper helped popularize the use of deep hypothermic circulatory arrest for complex neonatal repairs and described a quantum leap forward in results of neonatal repair of TAPVC.

Darling, R. C., Rothney, W. B., and Craig, J. M.: Total pulmonary venous drainage into the right side of the heart. Lab. Invest., 6:44, 1957.
The original description of the system of classification of TAPVC, which remains in general clinical use.

Gathman, G. E., and Nadas, A. S.: Total anomalous pulmonary venous connection: Clinical and physiologic observations of 75 pediatric patients. Circulation, 42:143, 1970.
An excellent analysis of the physiologic and clinical correlates of TAPVC and how they relate to survival.

Neill, C. A.: Development of the pulmonary veins: With reference to the embryology of anomalies of pulmonary venous return. Pediatrics, 18:880, 1956.
A lucid description of normal and pathologic development of the pulmonary veins, including the developmental anatomy of the various forms of TAPVC.

Sano, S., Brawn, W. J., and Mee, R. B. B.: Total anomalous pulmonary venous drainage. J. Thorac. Cardiovasc. Surg., 97:886, 1989.
A large recent series of surgical patients, demonstrating that a very low early mortality (2.3 per cent) can be achieved in the current era despite the desperately ill condition of many neonates at presentation.

REFERENCES

1. Barratt-Boyes, B. G., Simpson, M., and Neutze, J. M.: Intracardiac surgery in neonates and infants using deep hypothermia with surface cooling and limited cardiopulmonary bypass. Circulation, 43 and 44 (Suppl. I):I25, 1971.
2. Behrendt, D. M., Aberdeen, E., Waterson, D. J., and Bonham-Carter, R. E.: Total anomalous pulmonary venous drainage in infants. I. Clinical and hemodynamic findings, methods, and results of operation in 37 cases. Circulation, 46:347, 1972.
3. Bharati, S., and Lev, M.: Congenital anomalies of the pulmonary veins. Cardiovasc. Clin., 5:23, 1973.
4. Bini, R. M., Cleveland, D. C., Ceballos, R., Bargeron, L. M., Pacifico, A. D., and Kirklin, J. W.: Congenital pulmonary vein stenosis. Am. J. Cardiol., 54:369, 1984.
5. Borow, K. M., Green, L. H., Castaneda, A. R., and Keane, J. F.: Left ventricular function after repair of tetralogy of Fallot and its relationship to age at surgery. Circulation, 61:1150, 1980.
6. Burroughs, J. T., and Edwards, J. E.: Total anomalous pulmonary venous connection. Am. Heart J., 59:913, 1960.
7. Burroughs, J. T., and Kirklin, J. W.: Complete surgical correction of total anomalous pulmonary venous connection. Report of three cases. Proc. Staff Meet. Mayo Clin., 31:182, 1956.
8. Carpena, C., Colokathis, B., and Subramanian, S.: Cor triatriatum. Ann. Thorac. Surg., 17:325, 1974.
9. Darling, R. C., Rothney, W. B., and Craig, J. M.: Total pulmonary venous drainage into the right side of the heart. Lab. Invest., 6:44, 1957.
10. Delisle, G., Ando, M., Calder, A. L., Zuberbuhler, J. R., Rockenmacher, S., Alday, L. E., Mangini, O., Van Praagh, S., and Van Praagh, R.: Total anoma-

lous pulmonary venous connection: Report of 92 autopsied cases with emphasis on diagnostic and surgical considerations. Am. Heart J., *91*:99, 1976.

11. Fyler, D. C.: Personal communication, 1987.
12. Gathman, G. E., and Nadas, A. S.: Total anomalous pulmonary venous connection: Clinical and physiologic observations of 75 pediatric patients. Circulation, *42*:143, 1970.
13. Hammon, J. W., Jr., Bender, H. W., Jr., Graham, T. P., Jr., Boucek, R. J., Jr., Smith, C. W., and Erath, H. G., Jr.: Total anomalous pulmonary venous connection in infancy: Ten years' experience, including studies of postoperative ventricular function. J. Thorac. Cardiovasc. Surg., *80*:544, 1980.
14. Haworth, S. G., and Reid, L.: Structural study of pulmonary circulation and of heart in total anomalous pulmonary venous return in early infancy. Br. Heart J., *39*:80, 1977.
15. Hickey, P. R., Hansen, D. D., Wessel, D. L., Lang, P., Jonas, R. A., and Elixson, M. E.: Blunting of stress responses in the pulmonary circulation of infants by fentanyl. Anesth. Analg. *64*:1137, 1985.
16. Jonas, R. A., and Castaneda, A. R.: Total anomalous pulmonary venous connection. *In* Nelson, N. M. (Ed.): Current Therapy in Neonatal-Perinatal Medicine. Toronto, B. C. Decker, 1990, pp. 374–380.
17. Jonas, R. A., and Lang, P.: Open repair of cardiac defects in neonates and young infants. Clin. Perinatol., *15*:659, 1988.
18. Jonas, R. A., Smolinsky, A., Mayer, J. E., and Castaneda, A. R.: Obstructed pulmonary venous drainage with total anomalous pulmonary venous connection to the coronary sinus. Am. J. Cardiol., *59*:431, 1987.
19. Kiely, B., Filler, J., Stone, S., and Doyle, E. F.: Syndrome of anomalous venous drainage of the right lung to the inferior vena cava. Am. J. Cardiol., *20*:102, 1967.
20. Lamb, R. K., Qureshi, S. A., Wilkinson, J. L., Arnold, R., West, C. R., and Hamilton, D. I.: Total anomalous pulmonary venous drainage. J. Thorac. Cardiovasc. Surg., *96*:368, 1988.
21. Leblanc, J. G., Patterson, M. W., Taylor, G. P., and Ashmore, P. G.: Total anomalous pulmonary venous connection. J. Thorac. Cardiovasc. Surg., *95*:540, 1988.
22. Lewis, F. J., Varco, R. L., Taufic, M., and Nizai, S. A.: Direct vision repair of triatrial heart and total anomalous pulmonary venous drainage. Surg. Gynecol. Obstet., *102*:713, 1956.
23. Lincoln, C. R., Rigby, M. L., Mercanti, C., Al-Fagih, M., Joseph, M. C., Miller, G. A., and Shinebourne, E. A.: Surgical risk factors in total anomalous pulmonary venous connection. Am. J. Cardiol. *61*:608, 1988.
24. Muller, W. H.: The surgical treatment of transposition of the pulmonary veins. Ann. Surg., *134*:683, 1951.
25. Mustard, W. T., Keon, W. J., and Trusler, G. A.: Transposition of the lesser veins (total anomalous pulmonary venous drainage). Prog. Cardiovasc. Dis., *11*:145, 1968.
26. Myers, J. L., Campbell, D. B., and Waldhausen, J. A.: The use of absorbable monofilament polydioxanone suture in pediatric cardiovascular operations. J. Thorac. Cardiovasc. Surg., *92*:771, 1986.
27. Neill, C. A.: Development of the pulmonary veins: With reference to the embryology of anomalies of pulmonary venous return. Pediatrics, *18*:880, 1956.
28. Newberger, J. W., Silbert, A. R., Buckley, L. P., and Fyler, D. C.: Cognitive function and duration of hypoxemia in children with transposition of the great arteries. N. Engl. J. Med., *31*:1495, 1984.
29. Norwood, W. I., Hougen, T. J., and Castaneda, A. R.: Total anomalous pulmonary venous connection: Surgical considerations. Cardiovasc. Clin., *11*:353, 1981.
30. Pacifico, A. D., Mandke, N. V., McGrath, L. B., Colvin, E. V., Bini, R. M., and Bargeron, L. M.: Repair of congenital pulmonary venous stenosis with living autologous atrial tissue. J. Thorac. Cardiovasc. Surg., *89*:604, 1985.
31. Parr, G. V., Kirklin, J. W., Pacifico, A. D., Blackstone, E. H., and Lauridsen, P.: Cardiac performance in infants after repair of total anomalous pulmonary venous connection. Ann. Thorac. Surg., *17*:561, 1974.
32. Rabinovitch, M., Herrera-DeLeon, V., Castaneda, A. R., and Reid, L. M.: Growth and development of the pulmonary vascular bed in patients with tetralogy of Fallot with or without pulmonary atresia. Circulation, *64*:1234, 1981.
33. Ross, R. D., Bissett, G. S., Meyer, R. A., Hannon, D. W., and Bove, K. E.: Magnetic resonance imaging for diagnosis of pulmonary vein stenosis after "correction" of total anomalous pulmonary venous connection. Am. J. Cardiol., *60*:1199, 1987.
34. Sano, S., Brawn, W. J., and Mee, R. B. B.: Total anomalous pulmonary venous drainage. J. Thorac. Cardiovasc. Surg., *97*:886, 1989.
35. Swan, H. J. C., Kirklin, J. W., Becu, L. M., and Wood, E. H.: Anomalous connection of right pulmonary veins to superior vena cava with interatrial communications: Hemodynamic data in eight cases. Circulation, *16*:54, 1957.
36. Van Praagh, R., and Corsini, I.: Cor triatriatum: Pathologic anatomy and a consideration of morphogenesis based on 13 postmortem cases and a study of normal development of the pulmonary vein and atrial septum in 83 human embryos. Am. Heart J., *78*:379, 1969.
37. Van Praagh, R., Harken, A. H., Delisle, G., Ando, M., and Gross, R. E.: Total anomalous pulmonary venous drainage to the coronary sinus: A revised procedure for its correction. J. Thorac. Cardiovasc. Surg., *64*:132, 1972.
38. Walsh, E. P., Rochenmacher, S., Keane, J. F., Hougen, T. J., Lock, J. E., and Castaneda, A. R.: Late results in patients with tetralogy of Fallot repaired during infancy. Circulation, *5*:1062, 1988.
39. Warden, H. E., Gustafson, R. A., Tarnay, T. J., and Neal, W. A.: An alternative method for repair of partial anomalous pulmonary venous connection to the superior vena cava. Ann. Thorac. Surg., *38*:601, 1984.
40. Whight, C. M., Barratt-Boyes, B. G., Calder, A. L., Neutze, J. M., and Brandt, P. W.: Total anomalous pulmonary venous connection. Long-term results following repair in infancy. J. Thorac. Cardiovasc. Surg., *75*:52, 1978.
41. Wilson, J.: A description of a very unusual formation of the human heart. Philos. Trans. R. Soc. Lond., *88*:346, 1798.
42. Yee, E. S., Turley, K., Hsieh, W. R., and Ebert, P. A.: Infant total anomalous pulmonary venous connection: Factors influencing timing of presentation and operative outcome. Circulation, *76* (Suppl. III):III83, 1987.

VII

VENTRICULAR SEPTAL DEFECTS

Albert D. Pacifico, M.D., John W. Kirklin, M.D., and James K. Kirklin, M.D.

HISTORICAL ASPECTS

Ventricular septal defect (VSD), in its isolated form, is the most common congenital cardiac lesion and represents 30 to 40 per cent of all congenital heart malformations at birth.[18] In 1879, Roger described the clinical manifestations of ventricular septal defect and the underlying pathologic condition. The development of cardiac catheterization techniques by 1950 allowed precise delineation of the hemodynamic alterations produced by such defects. Muller and Dammann[35] first surgically managed VSD by banding the pulmonary artery to reduce the pressure and flow in the pulmonary vascular system and reduce the likelihood of development of irreversible pulmonary hypertension. Lillehei, Varco, and colleagues in 1954 first successfully repaired a ventricular septal defect using controlled cross circulation with an adult human being as the oxygenator.[31] Intracardiac repair using a pump oxygenator for cardiopulmonary support was first accomplished in 1955 by DuShane and colleagues.[11] Subsequent surgical refinements included the use of a transatrial approach to VSD closure in 1957 by Stirling and colleagues,[48] the use of the technique of profound hypothermia and total circulatory arrest, with rewarming by a pump oxygenator, by Okamoto in 1969,[37] the feasibility of primary repair of VSDs in infants by Kirklin in 1961[27] and Sigmann in 1967,[44] and the demonstration by Barratt-Boyes beginning in 1969 that routine primary repair of VSDs in symptomatic small infants was superior to pulmonary artery banding.[3]

ANATOMY

VSDs can be classified according to their location within the interventricular septum. The interventricular septum can be divided into a fibrous component, termed the membranous sep-

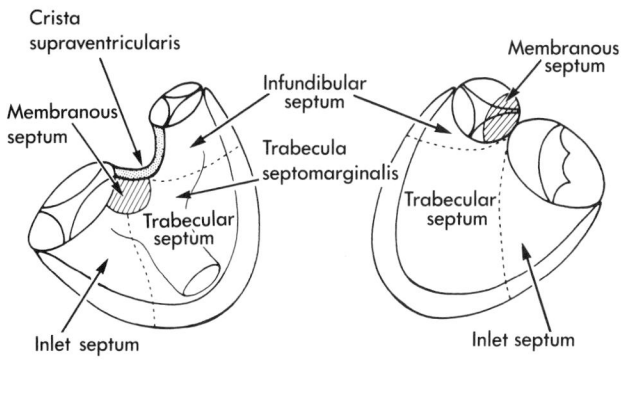

Crista supraventricularis
Membranous septum
Infundibular septum
Membranous septum
Trabecula septomarginalis
Trabecular septum
Trabecular septum
Inlet septum
Inlet septum

A Right Ventricle
B Left Ventricle

Figure 1. The components of the ventricular septum as observed from the right ventricle *(A)* and left ventricle *(B)*. (From Soto, B., Becker, A. E., Moulaert, A. J., et al.: Classification of ventricular septal defects. Br. Heart J., *43*:332, 1980.)

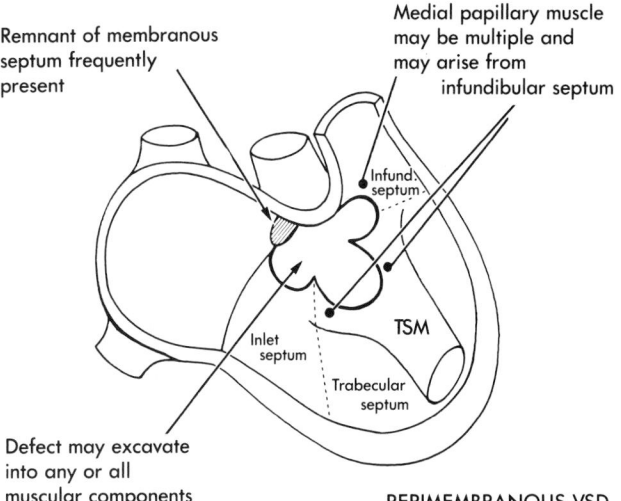

Remnant of membranous septum frequently present
Medial papillary muscle may be multiple and may arise from infundibular septum
Infund. septum
TSM
Inlet septum
Trabecular septum
Defect may excavate into any or all muscular components

PERIMEMBRANOUS VSD

Figure 3. The types of perimembranous ventricular septal defects are shown with excavation into the inlet, trabecular, and outlet septa. TSM, trabecula septomarginalis; Infund, infundibular. (From Soto, B., Becker, A. E., Moulaert, A. J., et al.: Classification of ventricular septal defects. Br. Heart J., *43*:332, 1980.)

tum, and three muscular components termed the inlet septum, the apical trabecular septum, and the outlet (or infundibular) septum (Fig. 1). The tricuspid and mitral valves in the normal heart are attached to the ventricular septum at different levels so that the tricuspid valve attachment is apically displaced, compared with that of the mitral valve. This portion of the ventricular septum separating the left ventricle from the right atrium is termed the atrioventricular septum. The atrioventricular septum has a fibrous component anteriorly and a muscular component posteriorly. The attachment of the tricuspid valve divides the area of the membranous septum into an interventricular component between the left and right ventricles and an atrioventricular component between the left ventricle and the right atrium.

A surgically useful classification of VSDs proposed by Soto and associates is depicted in Figure 2.[47] VSDs can have a partially fibrous rim or be completely surrounded by muscle. Defects with a partly fibrous rim are termed perimembranous when they are in the general area of the membranous septum or subarterial infundibular defects when either the aortic or pulmonary valve forms part of the rim of the defect within the infundibulum or outlet septum. Perimembranous defects can extend into the inlet, trabecular, or outlet septa and make them confluent with these areas (Fig. 3). The atrioventricular canal type of VSD is a perimembranous defect that extends into the inlet septum with the septal leaflet of the tricuspid valve forming its rightward border. Perimembranous defects are asso-

ciated with the anteroseptal commissure of the tricuspid valve and also with the aortic valve. The annulus of these valves often forms part of the rim of the defect, but in some patients it is separated from the VSD by a thin rim of muscular tissue.

Muscular defects are completely surrounded by muscular tissue and may be located in the infundibular, trabecular, or inlet portions of the ventricular septum. Most are located in the trabecular portion of the ventricular septum, where they may be single or multiple. Most commonly, multiple defects are located in the anterior portion of the trabecular septum. Approximately 10 per cent of VSDs are located in the infundibulum or outlet septum. When the aortic and pulmonary valve annuli form part of the rim of the defect, they are termed subarterial and form the majority of defects in this location. Less commonly, defects in the infundibular septum may be completely surrounded by muscle and are designated as infundibular muscular defects.

The size of VSDs can vary considerably, and their division into groups is arbitrary. A large VSD is approximately the size of the aortic orifice or larger and causes systemic right ventricular pressure. Small VSDs have insufficient size to raise right ventricular systolic pressure, and the pulmonary-systemic flow ratio ($Q_p:Q_s$) does not increase above 1.75. Moderate-sized VSDs are "restrictive" but have sufficient size to raise the right ventricular systolic pressure to approximately half of the left ventricular pressure and may cause a $Q_p:Q_s$ of 2 to 3.5. Several small defects may together appear as a large defect.

The location of the bundle of His must be known when surgical repair is undertaken to avoid production of heart block. With perimembranous defects, the bundle of His is located along the posterior and inferior margins of the defect (Fig. 4). A similar although displaced relation is present when the defect is of the atrioventricular canal type. The bundle of His is generally not in danger of being damaged when closure of defects in the trabecular septum or outlet infundibular septum is accomplished.

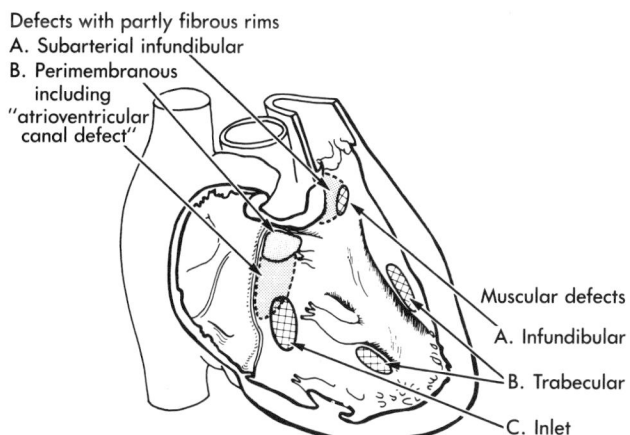

Defects with partly fibrous rims
A. Subarterial infundibular
B. Perimembranous including "atrioventricular canal defect"
Muscular defects
A. Infundibular
B. Trabecular
C. Inlet

Figure 2. Classification of ventricular septal defects according to their location within the septum. (From Soto, B., Becker, A. E., Moulaert, A. J., et al.: Classification of ventricular septal defects. Br. Heart J., *43*:332, 1980.)

ASSOCIATED LESIONS

In some patients with a subarterial VSD, aortic valve incompetence develops, presumably as a result of progressive prolapse of the right aortic cusp through the defect.[36,52] Abnormalities in the development of the aortic root may also contribute to the development of aortic incompetence. Systolic pressure gradients between the inlet portion of the right ventricle and the

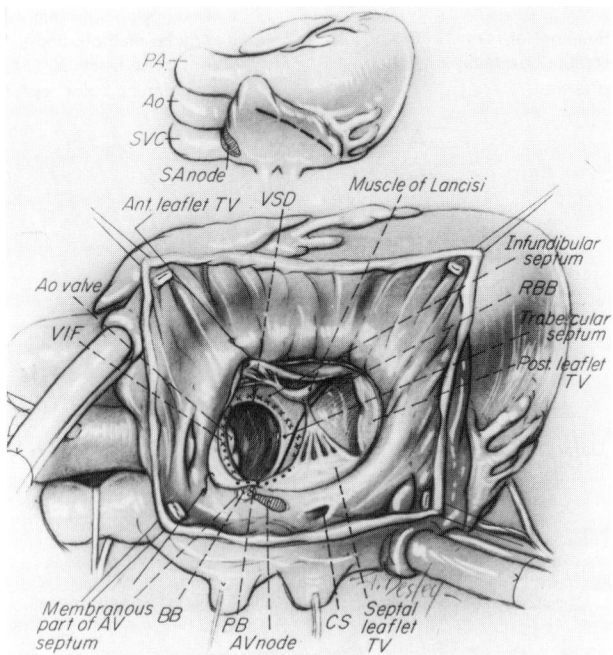

Figure 4. The sinus node and position of the right atriotomy are demonstrated above. Transatrial exposure of a perimembranous VSD is demonstrated below looking through the retracted tricuspid valve leaflets. The coronary sinus (CS) and the nearby atrioventricular (AV) node with the penetrating portion of the bundle of His (PB) and its branching portion (BB) as well as the right bundle branch (RBB) are demonstrated in relation to the VSD. The pathway of the suture line that secures the patch used to close the VSD is indicated by the xs along the muscular portion of the ventricular septum as well as the ventriculoinfundibular fold (VIF) and the dots shown in the base of the septal leaflet of the tricuspid valve (TV). The suture line remains well away from the inferior free edge of the VSD and on the tricuspid leaflet near its base to avoid the surgical creation of heart block. Ao, aorta; PA, pulmonary artery; SVC, superior vena cava; SA, sinoatrial. (From Bharati, S., Lev, M., and Kirklin, J. W.: Cardiac Surgery and the Conduction System. New York, John Wiley & Sons, 1983.)

pulmonary artery are present in approximately 50 per cent of patients with VSD and aortic valve incompetence. This follows associated displacement and hypertrophy of the infundibular portion of the septum and its parietal and septal insertions.[23] The prolapsed aortic leaflet may also contribute to the obstruction.[46]

Approximately 50 per cent of patients undergoing surgical treatment for primary VSD have an associated lesion.[3,4] A moderate- or large-sized patent ductus arteriosus is present in approximately 6 per cent of patients of all ages; but in infants with heart failure, it is present in approximately 25 per cent.[3] A VSD in combination with severe coarctation of the aorta occurs in approximately 12 per cent of patients. This combination is also more common among infants with large VSD undergoing operation under the age of 3 months.

Congenital valvular or subvalvular aortic stenosis occurs in approximately 4 per cent of patients undergoing operation for VSD. Subvalvular stenosis is more common and may be present when there is associated infundibular pulmonary stenosis.[28] In addition, it can develop from pulmonary artery banding[12] and may be a discrete fibromuscular bar on the inferior edge of the VSD within the left ventricular outflow tract. When leftward displacement of the infundibular septum occurs, the subaortic stenosis is superior to the location of the VSD. This type of subaortic stenosis is often associated with aortic arch anomalies.[9,34,51] Congenital mitral valve disease occurs in approximately 2 per cent of patients. Rarely, one pulmonary artery may be absent or severely stenotic, and severe peripheral pulmonary artery stenoses may be present.

Associated lesions of minor anatomic or functional significance were present in 47 per cent of patients undergoing closure

of a primary ventricular septal defect.[4] These included mild or moderate pulmonary stenosis in 20 per cent; atrial septal defect in 17 per cent; persistent left superior vena cava in 9 per cent; dextroposition of the aorta in 5 per cent; and aneurysm of the membranous septum, mild or moderate coarctation of the aorta, vascular ring, and tricuspid, mitral, or pulmonary valve incompetence in less than 1 per cent each.

PATHOPHYSIOLOGY

HEMODYNAMICS. The direction and size of the shunt in patients with VSD depend on the size of the defect and the differences in pressure between the ventricles during systole and diastole. When the VSD is small (restrictive), it offers considerable resistance to flow; and only a relatively large pressure difference between the two ventricles, such as occurs during mid and late systole, causes significant flow across the defect. In this circumstance, since pressure is higher in the left ventricle than in the right ventricle, the direction of the shunt is left to right. In contrast, when the defect is large (unrestrictive), it offers little resistance to flow and similar peak pressures are present in both the left and right ventricles. The direction and magnitude of flow through the defect is dependent on the small pressure differences that are present during systole between the left and right ventricles.[22,30] During mid and late systole, when most of the shunting occurs, the pressure differences between the two ventricles are primarily due to the relative resistance to ejection offered by the systemic and pulmonary vasculature. In diastole and early systole, a number of additional factors, including the relative compliance of each ventricle, their diastolic pressures, and the presence of asynchronous contraction, influence the magnitude and direction of the shunt.[30] The size of the VSD may vary during the various phases of the cardiac cycle, and this also may influence the degree of shunting.

When a left-to-right shunt is present at the ventricular level, pulmonary blood flow is increased above normal and above systemic blood flow. Thus, flow through the left atrium and mitral valve orifice is similarly increased, and greater work is done by both the left and the right ventricles. In the absence of a large atrial septal defect, the left atrium is enlarged to a degree corresponding to the magnitude of increase in pulmonary blood flow. A diastolic murmur may be heard over the apex of the heart, reflecting the increase in blood flow across the mitral valve. Left atrial pressure increases, and both the left and right ventricles are larger than normal.

EFFECTS ON THE PULMONARY VASCULATURE. Patients with a small (restrictive) VSD usually have normal right ventricular and pulmonary arterial pressures, slightly elevated pulmonary blood flow relative to systemic flow, and no pulmonary vascular disease as evidenced histologically or by the measurement of pulmonary vascular resistance. Alterations in these variables according to the size of the VSD are depicted in Table 1.

When the VSD is large, the hemodynamic state is determined by the pulmonary vascular resistance, which in these patients may be mildly, moderately, or severely elevated because of varying degrees of hypertensive pulmonary vascular disease. Pulmonary vascular resistance (R_p) is numerically expressed in resistance units, normalized to body surface area (BSA):

$$R_p \; (\text{units} \cdot \text{m}^2) = \frac{\text{Mean pulmonary artery pressure} - \text{Mean left arterial pressure}}{\text{Cardiac output/BSA}}$$

The absolute value for pulmonary vascular resistance may be a better predictor of operability than the ratio between the resistance in the pulmonary and systemic circuits, because of variations in the systemic vascular resistance. Some patients with large VSDs have a low pulmonary resistance and a large pulmo-

TABLE 1. Alterations in Pulmonary Arterial Pressure, Pulmonary Blood Flow, and Pulmonary Vascular Resistance

Size of Defect	Pulmonary Arterial Hypertension		Pulmonary Blood Flow		Pulmonary Vascular Disease		Resistance Units
	Degree	$P_p:P_s$*	Magnitude of Increase	$Q_p:Q_s$†	Severity	$R_p:R_s$‡	
Small	None	<0.25	Mild	<1.4	None	<0.25	<5
	None	<0.25	Moderate	1.4–1.8	None	<0.25	<5
Large	Mild	0.25–0.45	Large	>1.8	Mild	<0.25	5–7
	Moderate	0.45–0.75	Large	>1.8	Mild	<0.25	5–7
	Severe	>0.75	Large	>1.8	Mild	0.25–0.45	5–7
			Moderate	1.4–1.8	Moderate	0.45–0.75	8–10
			Small	<1.4	Severe	>0.75	>10

Modified from Pacifico, A.D., Kirklin, J.W., and Kirklin, J.K.: Surgical Treatment of Ventricular Septal Defect. *In* Sabiston, D. C., Jr., and Spencer, F. C. (Eds.): Gibbon's Surgery of the Chest, 3rd ed. Philadelphia, W. B. Saunders Company, 1976.

* $P_p:P_s$ refers to the ratio between peak pressure in the pulmonary artery and that in a systemic artery (ratio between mean pressures is more commonly used and is similar).

† $Q_p:Q_s$ refers to the ratio between pulmonary and systemic blood flow.

‡ $R_p:R_s$ refers to the ratio between pulmonary and systemic vascular resistance.

nary blood flow relative to systemic flow. In contrast, when the pulmonary resistance is between 8 and 10 units · m², indicating significant pulmonary vascular disease (see later discussion), pulmonary blood flow is only moderately elevated relative to systemic flow. When the resistance is greater than approximately 10 units · m², the flow across the defect is usually bidirectional or right-to-left and the pulmonary blood flow is similar to or less than systemic blood flow.

Intense exercise in a normal individual may cause a fourfold increase in pulmonary and systemic blood flow, without an increase in pulmonary artery pressure. In this circumstance, there is actually a decrease in pulmonary vascular resistance. In contrast, in patients with VSDs and moderate or severe pulmonary vascular disease, the pulmonary vasculature may lose the ability to accommodate to increases in pulmonary blood flow following physiologic stresses such as exercise by a decline in pulmonary vascular resistance. In this circumstance, the pulmonary resistance may become "fixed." When such a patient exercises, the increase in systemic blood flow is derived from a reduction in left-to-right shunting or an increase in right-to-left shunting. Closure of the VSD when the pulmonary vascular resistance is "fixed" is hazardous, since the fixed pulmonary vascular resistance prevents an increase in systemic blood flow during exercise postoperatively.

The elevations of pulmonary vascular resistance in patients with VSDs are associated with anatomic changes in the small arteries of the lungs.[16,17,53] The changes follow a decrease in the ratio between the diameter of the lumen and the total diameter of the small muscular pulmonary arteries and arterioles. In patients with moderately elevated pulmonary vascular resistance, the increase in vessel wall thickness is primarily due to increased thickness of the muscle of the media and to intimal fibrosis with actual occlusion of some of the vessels. In patients with severe elevation of pulmonary vascular resistance, the intimal proliferation is more pronounced, with widespread occlusion of the muscular pulmonary arteries and arterioles and plexiform dilation of many of the remaining vessels.[16]

NATURAL HISTORY

Many patients with VSDs have small defects and few or no symptoms, since the left-to-right shunt is small and pulmonary hypertension and vascular disease do not develop. It is estimated that only 10 to 20 per cent of patients have large defects and incur serious difficulties.[20]

Infants born with large VSDs have moderate elevation of pulmonary vascular resistance owing to persistence of the me-

dial thickening of the small pulmonary arteries present in the normal fetus. As the pulmonary vessels mature in the first few weeks of life, pulmonary resistance declines, the magnitude of the left-to-right shunt across the defect increases, and symptoms develop. Such infants may die of severe congestive heart failure during this period.[33] If they survive and the hemodynamic state stabilizes, the small systemic blood flow and breathlessness, which entails a large caloric expenditure and interferes with eating, can be the cause of growth failure. If operation is not performed, death may occur, usually from congestive failure or pneumonia and usually in the first year of life.[20]

In a small number of infants with large VSDs who survive the neonatal period, severe pulmonary vascular disease and a significant increase in pulmonary vascular resistance begin to develop by the age of 6 to 12 months. If operation is not performed and this condition progresses over the ensuing months or years until it becomes severe, these patients can no longer be considered candidates for operation because of the severity of the pulmonary vascular changes. When the shunting becomes dominantly right to left across the defect as a result of the hypertensive pulmonary vascular disease, the patients become cyanotic and can be considered to have Eisenmenger's complex. Operation is then contraindicated.

Another group of infants with large defects have only mild elevation in pulmonary vascular resistance in the first few years of life, although significant pulmonary hypertension and a large pulmonary blood flow are present. These children are usually of small stature and have significantly impaired exercise tolerance. If the defect is still open or unrepaired by the time the patient is approximately 10 years old, the pulmonary vascular disease usually begins to progress, and at the age of 15 to 20 years in these patients Eisenmenger's complex develops, with severe elevation of the pulmonary vascular resistance and predominant right-to-left shunting across the defect. Occasionally, severe pulmonary vascular disease does not develop, and the heart failure may occur in the second or third decade of life. Patients with Eisenmenger's complex become polycythemic and eventually succumb to the complications of hypoxia and polycythemia, usually by the age of 25 to 30 years.

In some infants, the VSD becomes smaller in size relative to the size of the heart as growth occurs. Pulmonary blood flow decreases because of the resistance to flow offered by the smaller defect, and pulmonary artery pressure also decreases. Although a left-to-right shunt is still present, severe pulmonary vascular disease does not develop. The growth and development of these children are quite normal. In a few of these patients bacterial endocarditis develops.[43]

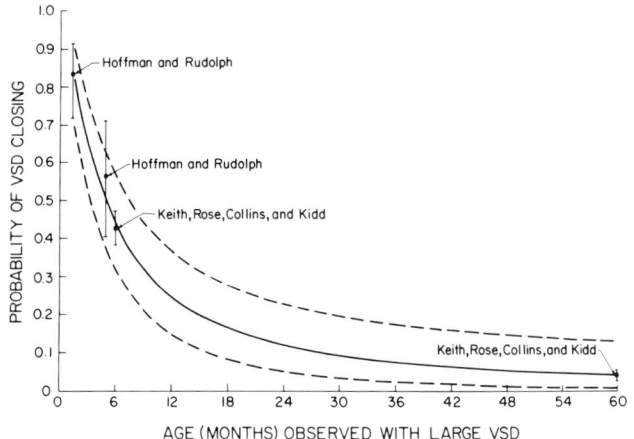

Figure 5. Probability of eventual spontaneous closure of a large VSD according to the age at which the patient is observed. The broken lines enclose the 70 per cent confidence limits around the solid probability line. The specific ratios, with the 70 per cent confidence limits reported by Hoffman and Rudolph[19] and Keith and associates[24] are demonstrated centered on the mean or assumed ages of patients in their reports (p < 0.0001). (From Blackstone, E. H., Kirklin, J. W., Bradley, E. L., et al.: Optimal age and results in repair of large ventricular defects. J. Thorac. Cardiovasc. Surg., 72:661, 1976.)

Spontaneous complete closure of VSDs, even large ones, has been estimated to occur in 25 to 50 per cent of patients during childhood.[20] The probability of eventual spontaneous closure is inversely related to the age at which the patient is observed (Fig. 5).[4] The mechanism of closure is usually related to ingrowth of fibrous tissue from the margins of the defect or adherence of the septal leaflet of the tricuspid valve to the margins of the defect.[20]

DIAGNOSIS

HISTORY. Infants with large VSDs do not usually have symptoms until they reach the age of 6 weeks to 3 months. At this time the pulmonary vascular resistance has decreased from the elevated levels present at birth, and maximal left-to-right shunting of blood across the defect and a marked increase in pulmonary blood flow occur. Tachypnea, poor feeding, growth failure, pneumonia, and severe cardiac failure may then develop.

Many patients with VSDs are asymptomatic. Generally these are patients whose defects are small. Children with moderate-sized or large septal defects may demonstrate growth failure and have limitations in exercise tolerance. The growth failure is related to the size of the defect and the magnitude of the left-to-right shunt.

Patients with markedly elevated pulmonary vascular resistance and predominant right-to-left shunting across the septal defect (Eisenmenger's complex) are cyanosed, polycythemic, and severely limited in their activities.

EXAMINATION. The infant with a large VSD and increased pulmonary blood flow characteristically presents with tachypnea and marked subcostal retraction. Severe growth failure and a lack of subcutaneous tissue are often evident. The jugular venous pulses are prominent even when the infant is held erect. On palpation, there is often a precordial bulge, and the heart is overactive with a rapid rate. A thrill is present in the third to fifth left intercostal space, and a loud systolic murmur is heard in this area. The second sound at the base is usually loud and may be split. The liver and spleen are usually enlarged, and the peripheral pulses are weak.

In older children with large ventricular septal defects, a protruding sternum or pigeon breast deformity is frequently present. Presumably this follows the enlarged right ventricle pushing the sternum anteriorly during the period of growth. The heart is hyperactive, there is a right ventricular lift, and the left ventricle is enlarged. A systolic thrill is often present over the left precordium. The characteristic murmur is harsh and pansystolic and is heard best in the left fourth interspace along the sternal border. If pulmonary blood flow is large, there may be a superimposed midsystolic ejection murmur in the area of the pulmonary valve.[29] A middiastolic murmur is present at the apex and indicates a large flow across the mitral valve. The first sound at the base is normal. The second sound is characterized by an abnormally wide split in expiration, and the splitting is accentuated in inspiration.[29]

Patients with small defects and small left-to-right shunts have only a systolic murmur. The heart is not hyperactive, and there is no enlargement of the left ventricle and no right ventricular lift. In patients with large defects and high pulmonary vascular resistance causing only small net left-to-right shunts or bidirectional shunts of equal magnitude, the systolic murmur is soft and short or may be absent. There is no apical diastolic rumble, and the second sound is markedly accentuated. There is no left ventricular enlargement, and a right ventricular lift is prominent.

CHEST ROENTGENOGRAMS. In patients with small VSDs and small left-to-right shunts, chest roentgenograms are usually normal. Patients with large VSDs, mild elevation of pulmonary vascular resistance, and large left-to-right shunts have large pulmonary arteries, both centrally and peripherally (Fig. 6). The right and left ventricles are enlarged, as is the left atrium. When marked enlargement of the left atrium is present in a patient suspected of having a VSD, the presence of coexisting mitral valvular regurgitation should be considered.

In patients with large VSDs and severe elevation of the pulmonary vascular resistance, the chest roentgenogram is quite different (Fig. 7). The central pulmonary arteries appear normal in size or are enlarged, but the peripheral pulmonary arteries appear normal. This suggests a normal or decreased pulmonary blood flow. The right ventricle appears somewhat enlarged, but there is no evidence of significant left atrial or left ventricular

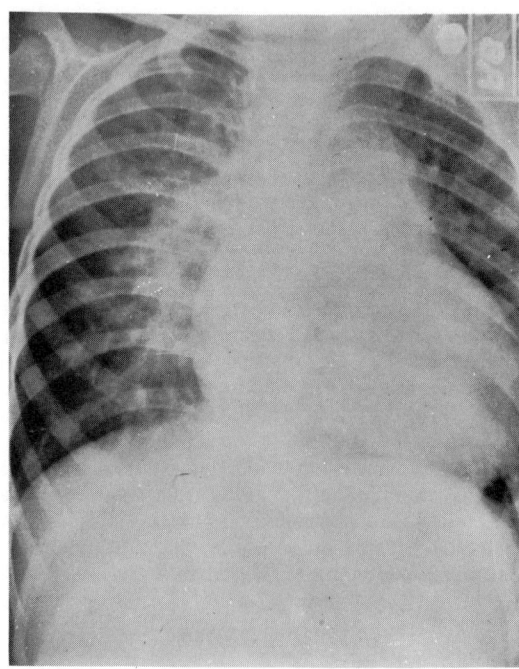

Figure 6. Chest roentgenogram of a child with a large ventricular septal defect, large pulmonary blood flow, and pulmonary hypertension, but only mild elevation of pulmonary vascular resistance. This is reflected in the evidence of left and right ventricular enlargement, enlargement of the main pulmonary artery, and marked increase in pulmonary blood flow. (From Pacifico, A.D., Kirklin, J.W., and Kirklin, J.K.: Surgical Treatment of Ventricular Septal Defect. In Sabiston, D. C., Jr., and Spencer, F. C. (Eds.): Surgery of the Chest, 5th ed. Philadelphia, W. B. Saunders Company, 1990.)

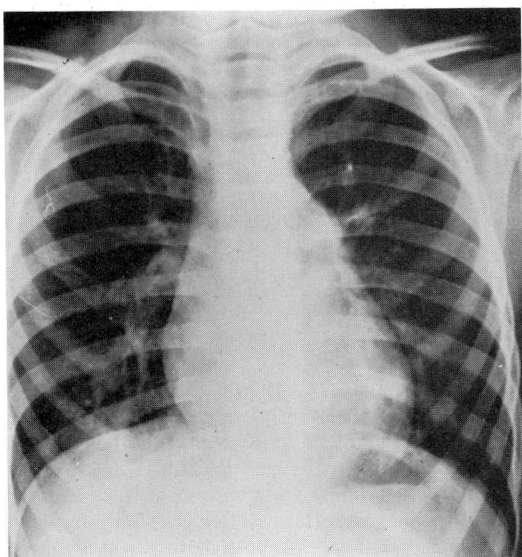

Figure 7. The chest roentgenogram is in contrast to that shown in Figure 6. The heart is not enlarged overall. The main pulmonary artery is enlarged; there is no evidence of increased pulmonary blood flow. This patient has a large ventricular septal defect, pulmonary hypertension, severe elevation of pulmonary vascular resistance, and pulmonary blood flow that is less than systemic blood flow. The condition is inoperable. (From DuShane, J. W., and Kirklin, J. W.: Selection for surgery of patients with ventricular septal defect and pulmonary hypertension. Circulation, 21:13, 1960. By permission of the American Heart Association.)

enlargement. Aside from the enlarged central pulmonary arteries, the cardiac silhouette may appear normal.

ELECTROCARDIOGRAM. In patients with small VSDs, the electrocardiogram may be normal. When the defect and shunt are slightly large ($Q_p:Q_s$ greater than approximately 1.8), the increase in left ventricular work from the large left ventricular stroke volume is evidenced by increased R wave voltage and tall peaked T waves from the left precordial leads. When the shunt is still larger, a pattern of mild right ventricular overload may be present as suggested by an RSR pattern in the V_1 lead.

If the VSD is large, and the left-to-right shunt is large ($Q_p:Q_s$ greater than 2), but the pulmonary vascular resistance is significantly less than the systemic vascular resistance ($R_p:R_s$ less than 0.75), there is evidence of increased work of both ventricles. The R wave from the right precordial leads is tall, and when the right ventricular peak pressure is similar to the left ventricular peak pressure, it is notched on the upstroke. The left precordial leads in this situation have the pattern of left ventricular overload previously described, although there may be a deeper S wave.

When the VSD is large and the pulmonary vascular resistance is equal to or greater than the systemic resistance, right axis deviation is usually present in the limb leads. The right precordial leads show the typical large, usually notched R waves of right ventricular hypertrophy, whereas the left precordial leads no longer show left ventricular overload.

The electrocardiogram supplements the physical findings and chest roentgenogram. Together they usually provide a useful categorization of patients as to the size of the VSD shunt and the magnitude of the pulmonary vascular resistance. Combined vectorgraphic and echocardiographic studies can provide additional noninvasive information and accurately identify infants with restrictive and nonrestrictive defects.[41]

DOPPLER ECHOCARDIOGRAPHY. Doppler echocardiography with color-flow mapping allows the noninvasive display of intracardiac anatomy cross-sectionally and the simultaneous display of real-time blood flow. This technique has become invaluable in the noninvasive diagnosis of VSDs as well as other forms of congenital cardiac malformations. Unidirectional as well as bidirectional shunting can be demonstrated. This method provides important information regarding the size and

location of a VSD. Often, an estimate of the pressure difference between the two ventricles can be made from knowledge of the velocity of flow through the defect. Although the general location of the defect can be defined by this technique, the presence of additional defects may not be ascertained. Therefore, some groups continue to advise cardiac catheterization studies and axial angiography to provide definitive information regarding the location and number of defects as well as information about the hemodynamic state.

CARDIAC CATHETERIZATION. Cardiac catheterization studies are useful to confirm the diagnosis and to detect secondary or multiple defects. In addition, the pulmonary and systemic arterial pressures and flows are measured and the pulmonary vascular resistance is calculated. These studies are also useful in excluding the presence of an associated cardiac defect.

ANGIOGRAPHY. Injection of radiopaque contrast media into the left ventricle at the time of cardiac catheterization is essential in any patient in whom operation is contemplated. This is particularly true for infants, in whom information regarding the location and number of defects is of value in planning the technical details of the operation. Axial angiography to provide a profile of the ventricular septum beautifully defines the number and location of the defect(s) (Fig. 8). These studies are also of value in defining associated defects such as aortic valve incompetence or pulmonary valvular or infundibular stenosis.

INDICATIONS FOR OPERATION. The decision to recommend operation for an individual patient is based on knowledge of the natural history of similar untreated patients and of the results of surgical correction. Important considerations in the natural history include the presence of congestive heart failure or growth failure, the likelihood of development of severe pulmonary vascular disease, and the possibility of spontaneous closure. The results of surgical therapy depend on the risk of operation, its effect on pulmonary vascular disease, and the incidence of complications such as heart block or incomplete repair.

At any age, the presence of pulmonary vascular disease so severe that the pulmonary vascular resistance is greater than 10 to 12 units $\cdot$ m^2 is considered a contraindication to operation. If the pulmonary vascular resistance is 8 to 10 units $\cdot$ m^2, operation is generally advised but with full knowledge of a possible unsatisfactory long-term result.[6] The presence of severe pulmonary hypertension is not a contraindication to operation if the resistance is less than 10 units $\cdot$ m^2.[2] Operation is usually not truly curative in older patients with established pulmonary vascular disease.

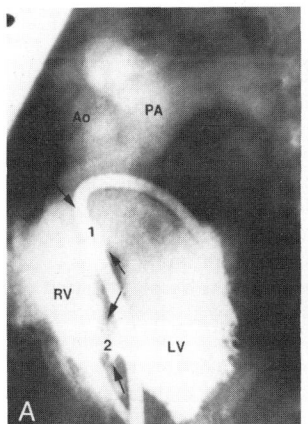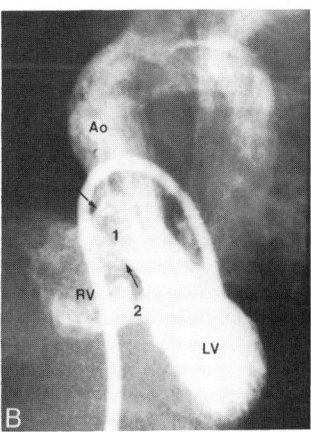

Figure 8. Axial angiography to profile the ventricular septum. *A*, Left ventriculogram in long axial view demonstrating a high perimembranous defect and a lower muscular defect in the trabecular septum. Ao, aorta; PA, pulmonary artery; RV, right ventricle; LV, left ventricle. *B*, Left ventriculogram in four-chamber view demonstrating a high perimembranous ventricular septal defect (VSD) and a lower muscular inlet VSD.

Prompt intracardiac repair is indicated in infants with large defects, large shunts, and pulmonary hypertension who present with left ventricular failure, recurrent pulmonary infections, severe growth failure, or evidence of increasing pulmonary vascular disease. The authors do not believe that pulmonary arterial banding has a place in the management of these patients unless a true "Swiss-cheese" septum is present.

VSDs have a tendency to close spontaneously, and this fact is relevant to decisions about operation.[4,7] Spontaneous closure can be complete by 1 year of age, or the defect may have only narrowed by then; complete closure takes considerably longer. The phenomenon of spontaneous closure or narrowing of VSDs explains the infrequency with which large VSDs are encountered in adults. An inverse relationship exists between the probability of eventual spontaneous closure and the age at which the patient is observed (Fig. 5).[4,19,24] This is highly relevant to clinical decisions concerning individual patients. According to these data, approximately 80 per cent of individuals observed at 1 month of age with large ventricular septal defects have eventual spontaneous closure, as do approximately 60 per cent of those observed at 3 months of age, approximately 50 per cent of those at 6 months of age, and 25 per cent of those at 12 months of age.

If the defect is small or moderate in size, the possibility of spontaneous closure and the general well-being of the patient support the decision to defer operation. If such defects remain patent in patients who reach the age of 10 to 12 years, the likelihood of spontaneous closure is small, and surgical repair is usually recommended when the $Q_p:Q_s$ is 1.5 or greater.

When aortic valvular incompetence develops in a child with a VSD, prompt closure of the defect should be undertaken to prevent further prolapse of the aortic cusps and progression of the aortic incompetence. When coexisting pulmonary infundibular or valvular stenosis is present, the VSD is generally large, and if the stenosis is severe, right-to-left shunting may be present. In these situations operation is also advisable. Mild or moderate mitral incompetence in association with VSD is not a contraindication to closure of the defect.

SURGICAL TREATMENT

Intracardiac Repair

A median sternotomy incision is employed. Careful exploration within the pericardial cavity is performed to determine the presence or absence of a patent ductus arteriosus, a left superior vena cava, and possible anomalies of pulmonary or systemic venous connection. The size of each cardiac chamber is noted from external examination. The presence of an enlarged left atrium and left ventricle is generally supportive of increased pulmonary blood flow. The right atrial approach is preferred for most perimembranous and midmuscular VSDs and for some apical and subarterial defects. The right ventricular approach provides good exposure through a transverse infundibular incision for subarterial and infundibular defects, through an apical ventriculotomy for apical muscular defects, and through a longitudinal anterior right ventriculotomy for some multiple muscular VSDs. Rarely, a left ventriculotomy is employed for multiple muscular defects in the trabecular septum.

Cardiopulmonary bypass is established by placing two appropriately sized thin-walled angled metal cannulas directly into each vena cava for venous return, and a cannula in the ascending aorta for arterial return from the pump oxygenator.[38] The perfusate temperature is adjusted to maintain moderate hypothermia at 24 to 28° C. The aorta is cross-clamped and cold potassium-containing cardioplegic solution is injected into the aortic root to protect the myocardium during the period of ischemia. Snares placed about the superior and inferior venae cavae are tightened around each respective venous cannula and the cardiotomy is performed. All VSDs are repaired with a patch. Although various methods of suturing are available, the authors prefer a continuous suturing technique with 4–0 polypropylene suture. The location of the specialized conduction tissue and its relation to the VSD must be clearly understood.

The right atriotomy used for transatrial repair and the view of a perimembranous VSD through the tricuspid valve are shown in Figure 4: the sinus node is shown in the intact heart above; the atrioventricular node and the penetrating portion of the bundle of His as well as its branching portion and right bundle in relation to the tricuspid valve and VSD are shown below. The continuous suturing technique used to close the VSD with a patch is shown in Figure 9.

In some cases, a perimembranous VSD is associated with an inlet muscular VSD, leaving an intact muscle bar between them (Fig. 10). Usually, they are exposed by tricuspid valve leaflet retraction; but where the chordal pattern is particularly complicated, exposure is facilitated by incising the anterior and septal leaflets near their base and retracting the leaflets anteriorly (Fig. 10). In this particular defect, the conduction tissue courses in the muscle bar and separates the two defects; its injury is avoided by using a single patch to cover both defects, leaving the muscle bar intact and placing the sutures in the path indicated.

The *atrioventricular canal type* of VSD and the course of the conduction tissue in relation to it are shown in Figure 11. No muscle tissue is present between the defect and the base of the septal tricuspid leaflet that is contiguous with the anterior mitral leaflet and usually with part of the aortic valve annulus superiorly. The conduction tissue is related to the inferior border of the defect, and the suture line used to attach the patch in this area is placed approximately 10 mm. inferior to the free edge of the VSD.

The specialized conduction tissue is not related directly to a muscular VSD in the trabecular septum (Fig. 12). In this case, the patch suture line is placed circumferentially on the free edge of the defect.

Subarterial and muscular defects in the infundibular septum can sometimes be approached through the right atrium. They are always exposed through a transverse incision in the right ventricular infundibulum and sometimes through a pulmonary arteriotomy operating through the retracted pulmonary valve and annulus.

Multiple anterior VSDs can be closed by mattress sutures placed over felt pledgets or strips operating transatrially through the tricuspid valve or through a vertical right ventriculotomy incision made near the septum.[5] A left ventriculotomy also provides excellent exposure,[1,45] but the authors prefer not to use it routinely in infants because it has been associated with left ventricular dysfunction early and late postoperatively in some of the small patients. In older patients, avoidance of a left ventriculotomy appears to be less important.

The rare Swiss-cheese septum usually requires a left ventricular approach. An associated perimembranous defect should be repaired through the right atrium, because its repair from the left ventricular side increases the risk of heart block.

When VSD closure is completed, rewarming is commenced, the vent is removed, and the atrial septal defect is closed after inflating the lungs to expel air from the left atrium. Air is aspirated from the ascending aorta, the aortic cross-clamp is released, and the right atriotomy is closed. De-airing is accomplished, and cardiopulmonary bypass is gradually discontinued. Decannulation is effected, and the incision is closed leaving temporary atrial and ventricular pacing electrodes.

When pulmonary infundibular or valvular stenosis coexists with a VSD, the authors prefer to perform the valvotomy operating through a pulmonary arteriotomy incision and begin the resection of the infundibular stenosis. The latter is completed through the right atrium and tricuspid valve, following which the VSD is closed with a patch.[39] When aortic valve incompe-

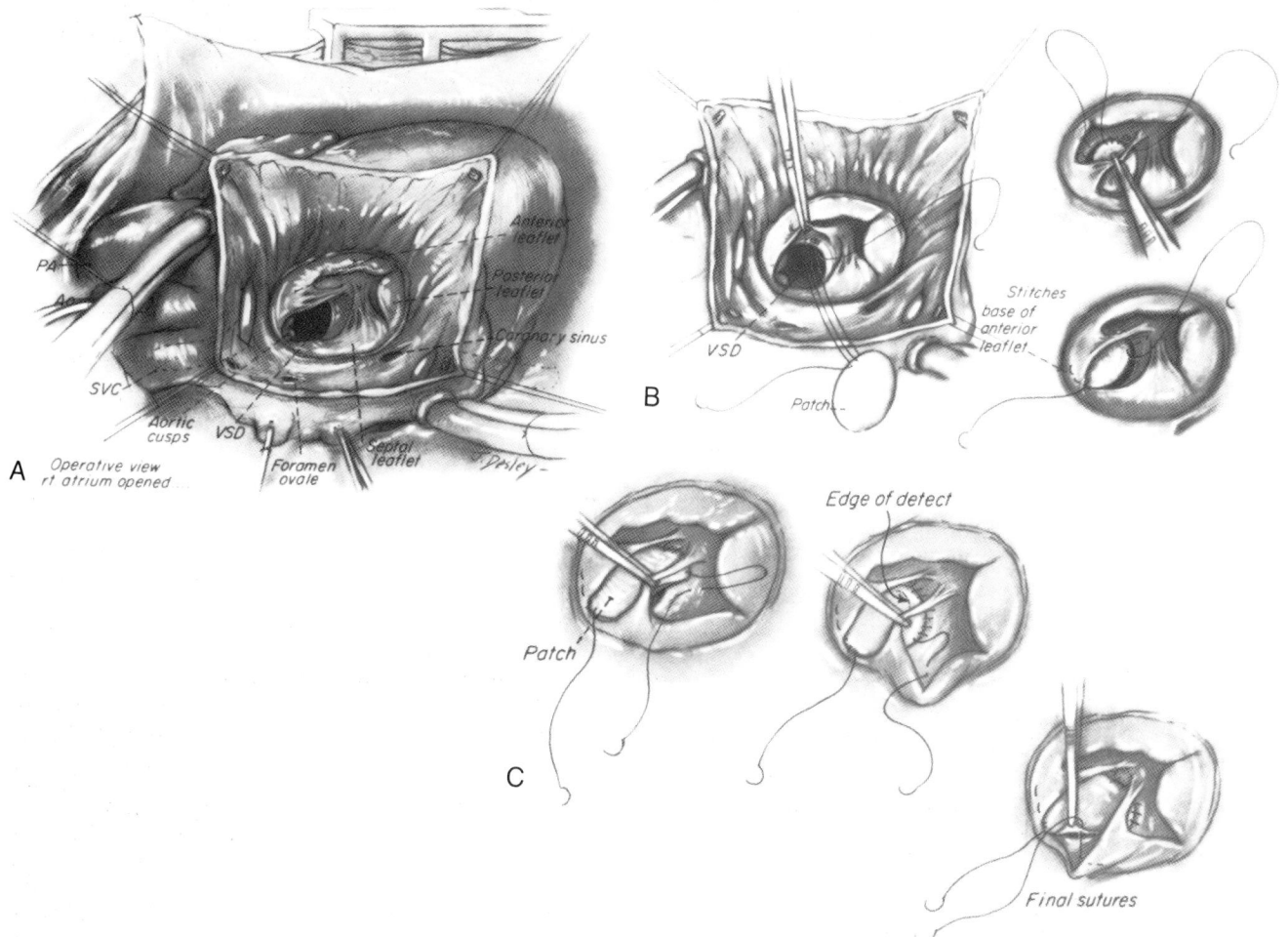

Figure 9. A, Right atrial incision and exposure of perimembranous VSD in the region of the tricuspid anteroseptal commissure. Stay sutures have been placed to slightly evert the atrial wall. Note that initially the superior edge of this typical perimembranous defect is not visible. The atrioventricular node is in the muscular portion of the atrioventricular septum, just on the atrial side of the commissure between the tricuspid septal and anterior leaflets. The bundle of His thus penetrates at the posterior angle of the VSD, where it is vulnerable to injury. B, The repair of the perimembranous VSD. This is initiated by placing a mattress suture of 4–0 Prolene with a small pledget at the 12 o'clock position in the defect as observed by the surgeon through the tricuspid valve. A piece of knitted Dacron velour is trimmed slightly larger than the approximate size of the defect, and one arm of the suture is passed through the Dacron patch, back through the septum, and again through the patch. Either now or after placing several more stitches, the sutures are snugged up as the patch is lowered into place. The suture line between the cephalad rim of the defect and the patch is continued. The traction on the suture exposes the next areas to be stitched and provides good visibility. When the junction of the superior muscular rim (ventriculoinfundibular fold) and tricuspid annulus has been reached, the suture is passed through the base of the contiguous portion of the tricuspid valve (usually the anterior leaflet) from the ventricular to the atrial side, then back from the atrial to the ventricular side of the valve and through the patch. After passing the stitch back through the leaflet, the suture is tagged. C, Operating now with the other limb of the suture, stitches are taken between the ventricular septum and the patch along the caudad side of the defect. These stitches are placed 3 to 5 mm. away from the edge of the defect to avoid the area most probably occupied by the bundle of His and more posteriorly 5 to 7 mm. back from the edge.

tence coexists with a VSD, the severity of the incompetence should be fully assessed preoperatively. If the incompetence is mild, only closure of the VSD is indicated. If the aortic incompetence is moderate or severe, plication of the aortic leaflets should be performed through an aortotomy before closure of the VSD.[49]

Although the authors continue to prefer standard perfusion techniques even in small infants, some surgeons prefer the use of a single venous cannula, deep hypothermia, and temporary total circulatory arrest during the repair.[3,38]

Pulmonary Artery Banding

The authors have not employed pulmonary arterial banding for uncomplicated VSDs for many years. It continues to have a place, however, in the management of some infants with multiple cardiac anomalies[20,50] and in some infants with severe heart failure from multiple (Swiss-cheese type) VSDs.

A left anterolateral thoracotomy incision in the third intercostal space is employed. The pericardium overlying the pulmonary artery is incised longitudinally and a plane developed between the pulmonary artery and the aorta. A Teflon-coated band 4 mm. wide is passed initially about the aorta. A right-angled clamp is then passed through the transverse sinus and the rightward limb of the band is grasped and delivered through the transverse sinus so that it is now around the pulmonary artery. This method ensures placement of the band on the main pulmonary artery and avoids the potential for exclusion of the right pulmonary artery. Although many methods are available to guide the degree of tightening of the band, the authors continue to employ the rule of Trusler and Mustard.[50] The circumference of the band in millimeters is determined from the weight of the infant in kilograms plus 20 mm. for an isolated ventricular septal defect or plus 24 mm. for more complex cardiac anomalies. The calculated length is initially marked on the band before it is placed around the pulmonary artery. The marked points are joined with a mattress suture of 4–0 Prolene. Tightening the band to this circumference usually causes a rise in systolic arterial pressure of 10 to 15 mm. Hg. Additional adjustment may be required in accordance with the change in systolic arterial pressure and alterations in the arterial oxygen saturation. The edges of the pericardial incision are then approximated and the thoracotomy incision is closed in the usual manner leaving a single chest tube for drainage.

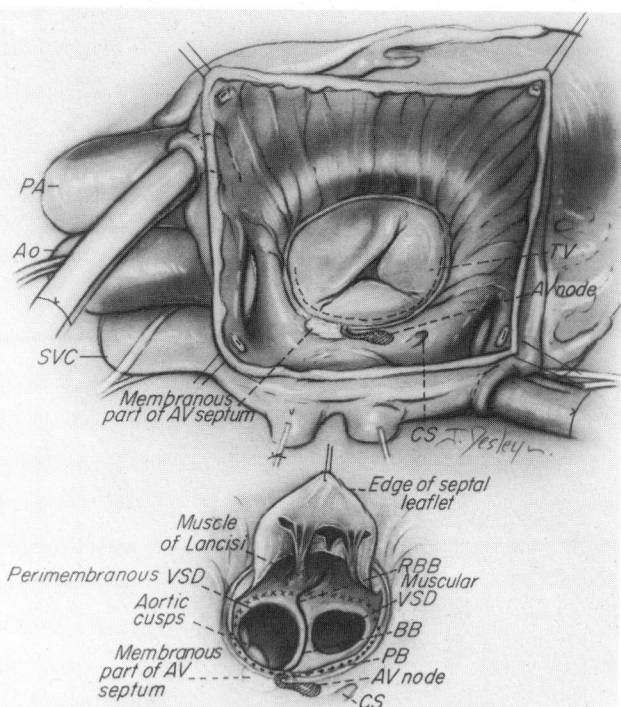

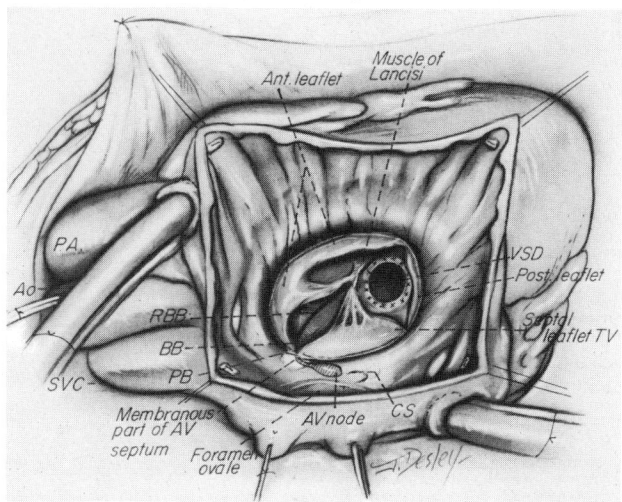

Figure 12. Transatrial exposure of a muscular defect in the trabecular portion of the septum is demonstrated. The pathway of the suture line used to attach the patch to close the defect is along its free edge and indicated by the *xs*. CS, coronary sinus; AV, atrioventricular; PB, penetrating portion of the bundle of His; BB, branching portion of the bundle of His; RBB, right bundle branch; Ao, aorta; SVC, superior vena cava; PA, pulmonary artery; TV, tricuspid valve. (From Bharati, S., Lev, M., and Kirklin, J. W.: Cardiac Surgery and the Conduction System. New York, John Wiley and Sons, 1983.)

Figure 10. Transatrial exposure for closure of a perimembranous VSD associated with an inlet muscular VSD. The coronary sinus (CS) and atrioventricular (AV) node as well as an incision in the base of the anterior and septal tricuspid valve (TV) leaflets is demonstrated above. The leaflets are retracted anteriorly in the lower part of the illustration to expose the two VSDs. The penetrating portion of the bundle of His (PB), its branching portion (BB), and the right bundle branch (RBB) are demonstrated in relation to the VSDs. The pathway of the suture line used to attach the Dacron patch along the muscular portion of the septum is indicated by *xs* and along the base of the tricuspid valve leaflet by dots. When repair is completed, the tricuspid leaflets are reattached to their basilar remnant by a continuous suture of fine polypropylene. PA, pulmonary artery; Ao, aorta; SVC, superior vena cava. (From Bharati, S., Lev, M., and Kirklin, J. W.: Cardiac Surgery and the Conduction System. New York, John Wiley & Sons, 1983.)

POSTOPERATIVE CARE

The majority of infants and small children convalesce normally after repair of VSD. Most are extubated within 24 hours of operation and do not require special supportive treatment. The outcome is primarily determined by events in the operating room and by proper preoperative selection of patients.

Sick small infants may be at risk for postoperative pulmonary

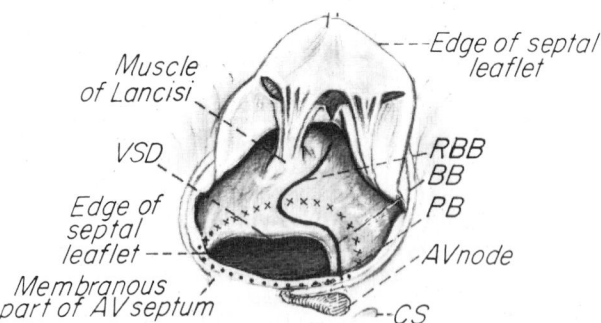

Figure 11. Transatrial exposure for repair of an atrioventricular canal type of VSD is demonstrated after incision of the base of the tricuspid valve and anterior traction as in Figure 10. The coronary sinus (CS), the atrioventricular (AV) node and its penetrating portion (PB) and branching portion (BB), and the right bundle branch (RBB) are shown in relation to the VSD. The *xs* indicate the path of the suture line used to attach the patch to the muscular portion of the septum and the dots along the base of the tricuspid leaflet. Most defects of this type can be closed without incision of the tricuspid leaflets; however, when the chordal pattern is complex, this maneuver aids in exposure. (From Bharati, S., Lev, M., and Kirklin, J. W.: Cardiac Surgery and the Conduction System. New York, John Wiley & Sons, 1983.)

hypertensive crises. These episodes are characterized by sudden marked increases in pulmonary vascular resistance and when severe may cause suprasystemic pulmonary artery pressure, which may cause severe acute cardiac failure. In these infants it is probably best to leave a monitoring catheter within the pulmonary artery for continuous measurement of postoperative pulmonary artery pressure. Management of pulmonary hypertensive crises can be difficult; but maintenance of alkalosis, hyperventilation, and the use of narcotic analgesia (fentanyl), prostaglandins, and tolazoline may be helpful.[21]

In the unusual case of low cardiac output after operation, in addition to the usual supportive treatment,[26] consideration should be given to the possibility of an overlooked or incompletely closed VSD. This possibility must especially be considered if the left atrial pressure is considerably higher than the right atrial pressure. A Doppler examination with color-flow mapping should be performed; and when secure information from this study is not obtained, urgent recatheterization is advisable. If complete atrioventricular dissociation was present for a time after cardiopulmonary bypass but sinus rhythm reappeared, a demand pacemaker attached to ventricular wires should be in place for 1 week postoperatively, because rarely the atrioventricular dissociation recurs temporarily in the early postoperative period.

RESULTS OF SURGICAL TREATMENT

HOSPITAL MORTALITY. Closure of VSDs can be safely accomplished in most centers properly prepared for this type of procedure, even in very small infants.[3,32,40,42] Hospital mortality and complications are directly related to the preoperative condition of the patient and to the conduct of the operative procedure. Hospital mortality now approaches zero. In earlier years, younger age was an incremental risk factor in the authors' experience, as it was in many centers, but this effect was neutralized by 1978[42] (Fig. 13). Multiple VSDs in earlier years were an important incremental risk factor for hospital mortality, but more recently the effect was only a minor one.[42] This improvement can be attributed primarily to better preoperative cineangiographic identification of the presence, size, and location of multiple VSDs that demand more complete surgical closure with little or no residual shunting. In earlier years, pulmonary artery pres-

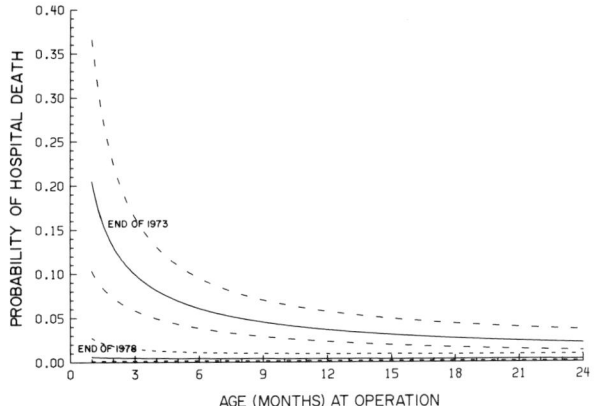

Figure 13. Probability of hospital death at the University of Alabama at Birmingham after repair of single large VSD in patients without major associated cardiac anomalies. Note that in 1971 and 1973 the risk was considerably increased in very young patients. By 1979, not only was the risk of hospital death less than 1 per cent, but an incremental risk in patients of young age was no longer apparent. (From Rizzoli, G., Blackstone, E. H., Kirklin, J. W., et al.: Incremental risk factors in hospital mortality after repair of ventricular septal defect. J. Thorac. Cardiovasc. Surg., *80:*494, 1980.)

sure and pulmonary vascular resistance were determinants of hospital mortality.[6] Currently this is no longer true probably because the upper limit of acceptable ("operable") pulmonary vascular resistance is better understood and management has improved.

Major associated lesions, particularly when present in symptomatic infants with large VSDs, do have an incremental risk effect on hospital mortality. At the University of Alabama at Birmingham, in 312 patients operated upon for VSD between 1967 and 1979, 16 (6.3 per cent) hospital deaths occurred among 254 patients with single or multiple VSDs but no major associated lesion, compared with 14 (24 per cent) among 58 patients with major associated lesions (p less than 0.0001).[42] Further scientific progress will probably reduce this incremental risk effect.

Although many VSDs can be closed through a right atrial approach, the precise route of surgical access, be it through the right atrium or right ventricle, has not been a determinant of hospital mortality after repair of a single VSD.[42] The same is true after repair of muscular or multiple VSDs through a left ventriculotomy, although the authors and others remain concerned regarding the long-term functional effects of a left ventriculotomy incision in infants.[25]

HEART BLOCK. Although permanent heart block occurred in a large percentage of patients in the very early years of cardiac surgery after repair of VSD, this complication is quite unusual at present. Its incidence in the current era continues to approach zero.[4]

INCOMPLETE REPAIR. High-quality left ventricular angiograms with angled views to profile the ventricular septum provide complete information regarding the size, location, and multiplicity of defects. Such studies minimize the chance of persistent (overlooked) defects after repair and have contributed significantly to the completeness of the surgical procedure.

Although small residual defects may sometimes be demonstrated by postoperative color Doppler studies, residual shunts of sufficient magnitude to indicate reoperation are uncommon. Only 1 (0.7 per cent) of 138 patients undergoing operation at the University of Alabama at Birmingham for repair of a large VSD has required reoperation, and this was for an overlooked second muscular VSD.[4] The technique used for reoperation for a residual or recurrent VSD has been nicely described.[8]

PULMONARY HYPERTENSION. Pulmonary artery pressure is more likely to be normal late postoperatively when operation is performed at a young age.[3,4,10] The relation is an inverse

one. Postoperative progression of pulmonary vascular disease is uncommon when the VSD is repaired before the age of 2 years. Closure of a VSD in small infants should be advised when there is evidence of increasing pulmonary vascular resistance even in the absence of symptoms.

Severe pulmonary hypertension postoperatively can increase with time[13] and cause premature late death, usually within 3 to 10 years of operation.[10,13,15] Some patients, however, with pulmonary hypertension and elevated pulmonary vascular resistance late postoperatively have neither progression nor regression of their disease for as long as 20 years, although there is some limitation in exercise tolerance.[10,14] It is presumed that life expectancy is reduced.

OVERALL RESULTS. Premature late death occurs rarely when pulmonary vascular resistance is low preoperatively. These deaths presumably follow arrhythmias, either ventricular fibrillation or the sudden late development of heart block. Patients with high pulmonary vascular resistance preoperatively have a tendency for this to progress and cause premature death. Approximately 25 per cent die within 5 years of operation when the preoperative pulmonary vascular resistance is more than 10 units · m².

Nearly all patients with large VSDs and mild elevation of pulmonary vascular resistance have an excellent prognosis. Improved physical development is a prominent feature of the late postoperative course after repair of large VSDs in infants.[40] There is an impressive increase in weight and usually complete relief of symptoms.[6] Cardiac function late postoperatively is essentially normal when repair is done in the first 2 years of life by modern techniques operating through the right atrium or right ventricle. Left ventricular end-diastolic volume, left ventricular systolic output, left ventricular mass, and left ventricular ejection fraction are normal approximately 1 year after operation in this subset. Persistent abnormalities of left ventricular size and function continue after repair of a large VSD at an older age, although patients remain asymptomatic. All of this information lends support to the advisability of surgical closure of a large VSD within the first 2 years of life.

SELECTED REFERENCES

Barratt-Boyes, B. G., Neutze, J. M., Clarkson, P. M., et al.: Repair of ventricular septal defect in the first two years of life using profound hypothermia–circulatory arrest techniques. Ann. Surg., 184:376, 1976.
This classic paper describes the results of primary repair of VSD in 57 patients less than 2 years of age, with many of the patients being less than 6 months old. Hospital mortality was 4 per cent in the patients without associated coarctation—a remarkable achievement. The late postoperative results are excellent. The method of profound hypothermia and total circulatory arrest and these superb results have had an important and worldwide impact on cardiac operations.

DuShane, J. W., and Kirklin, J. W.: Late results of the repair of ventricular septal defect on pulmonary vascular disease. In Kirklin, J. W. (Ed.): Advances in Cardiovascular Surgery. New York, Grune & Stratton, 1973, p. 9.
This paper analyzes the long-term course of 68 patients with large VSDs and severe pulmonary hypertension evaluated 5 or more years after operation with repeat cardiac catheterization, emphasizing the effects of operation on the pulmonary vasculature. Over 90 per cent of patients less than 2 years of age had normal or only mildly elevated pulmonary vascular resistance late postoperatively, even when pulmonary resistance was severely elevated preoperatively. Over 50 per cent of the older patients with moderate or severely elevated pulmonary resistance preoperatively had moderate or severely elevated resistance late postoperatively and potentially unsatisfactory long-term results. On the basis of these findings, the authors advise closure of large VSDs before the age of 2 years.

Hoffman, J. I. E., and Rudolph, A. M.: The natural history of isolated ventricular septal defect with special reference to selection of patients for surgery. Adv. Pediatr., 17:57, 1970.
This excellent article contains an enormous amount of information regarding the natural history of patients with isolated VSD. It extensively considers problems related to the severity of the disease, the frequency and the time course of spontaneous closure of VSDs, the incidence and importance of pulmonary vascular disease, and the changes in pulmonary vascular resistance that occur after surgical closure. In addition, a program is outlined for the management of patients with VSD, particularly infants, and the indications for operative intervention are given.

Rein, J. G., Freed, M. D., Norwood, W. I., and Castaneda, A. R.: Early and late results of closure of ventricular septal defect in infancy. Ann. Thorac. Surg., 24:19, 1977.

The superb results obtained by Castaneda and colleagues in the operation of primary repair of VSD in the first year of life in 50 infants are reported. The Kyoto–Barratt-Boyes technique of profound hypothermia and total circulatory arrest was used. Hospital mortality was 6 per cent, no late death occurred, and the late functional status was excellent. This paper provides strong supportive evidence for the excellence of the results that can be obtained from primary repair of VSD, even in very young infants.

Rizzoli, G., Blackstone, E. H., Kirklin, J. W., et al.: Incremental risk factors in hospital mortality after repair of ventricular septal defect. J. Thorac. Cardiovasc. Surg., 80:494, 1980.

This paper describes the incremental risk (degree of difficulty) of numerous factors in 312 patients having repair of VSD from 1967 to 1979. More important, it describes how these incremental risk factors have gradually been neutralized by scientific advances and minimization of human errors. Thus, in the era beginning in 1978, the hospital mortality of repair of single large VSDs is less than 1 per cent, no matter how young the patient (neutralization of the previous incremental risk of young age), and is approximately 5 per cent for multiple VSDs, again without an incremental risk of young age. Major associated cardiac anomalies or procedures (large patent ductus arteriosus, simultaneous repair of coarctation or interrupted arch, and important mitral valve abnormalities) still increase risk.

Soto, B., Becker, A. E., Moulaert, A. J., et al.: Classification of ventricular septal defects. Br. Heart J., 43:332, 1980.

Many anatomic studies of VSD have been reported through the years, but this study by Anderson and colleagues has been particularly helpful to surgeons. Their work, described in this paper, forms the basis for the description of morphology used in this chapter. The ventricular septum is divided into a membranous and muscular portion, and the latter is divided into an inlet, trabecular, and infundibular (outlet) portion. This paper introduces the advisable phrase "perimembranous VSD" for those in the region of the membranous septum, proximal to the tricuspid annulus. It also clarifies the fact that the atrioventricular canal type of VSD is really a perimembranous one and extends particularly beneath the septal tricuspid leaflet. Beautiful anatomic and cineangiographic plates clarify the description.

REFERENCES

1. Aaron, B. L., and Lower, R. R.: Muscular ventricular septal defect repair made easy. Ann. Thorac. Surg., 19:568, 1975.
2. Barratt-Boyes, B. G.: Complete correction of cardiovascular malformations in the first two years of life using profound hypothermia. *In* Barratt-Boyes, B. G., Neutze, J. M., and Harris, E. A. (Eds.): Heart Disease in Infancy: Diagnosis and Surgical Treatment. Proceedings of the Second International Symposium on Surgical Heart Disease. London, Churchill Livingstone, 1973, p. 25.
3. Barratt-Boyes, B. G., Neutze, J. M., Clarkson, P. M., et al.: Repair of ventricular septal defect in the first two years of life using profound hypothermia-circulatory arrest techniques. Ann. Surg., 184:376, 1976.
4. Blackstone, E. H., Kirklin, J. W., Bradley, E. L., et al.: Optimal age and results in repair of large ventricular septal defects. J. Thorac. Cardiovasc. Surg., 72:661, 1976.
5. Breckenridge, I. M., Stark, J., Waterston, D. J., and Bonham-Carter, R. E.: Multiple ventricular septal defects. Ann. Thorac. Surg., 13:128, 1972.
6. Cartmill, T. B., DuShane, J. W., McGoon, D. C., and Kirklin, J. W.: Results of repair of ventricular septal defect. J. Thorac. Cardiovasc. Surg., 52:486, 1966.
7. Collins, G., Calder, L., Rose, V., Kidd, L., and Keith, J.: Ventricular septal defect: Clinical and hemodynamic changes in the first five years of life. Am. Heart J., 84:695, 1972.
8. de Leval, M. R.: Reoperations after closure of ventricular septal defects. *In* Stark, J., and Pacifico, A. D. (Eds.): Reoperations in Cardiac Surgery. London, Springer-Verlag, 1989, p. 161.
9. Dirksen, T., Moulaert, A. J., Buis-Liem, T. N., and Brom, A. G.: Ventricular septal defect associated with left ventricular outflow tract obstruction below the defect. J. Thorac. Cardiovasc. Surg., 75:688, 1978.
10. DuShane, J. W., and Kirklin, J. W.: Late results of the repair of ventricular septal defect on pulmonary vascular disease. *In* Kirklin, J. W. (Ed.): Advances in Cardiovascular Surgery. New York, Grune & Stratton, 1973, p. 9.
11. DuShane, J. W., Kirklin, J. W., Patrick, R. T., et al.: Ventricular septal defects with pulmonary hypertension: Surgical treatment by means of a mechanical pump-oxygenator. J.A.M.A., 160:950, 1956.
12. Freed, M. D., Rosenthal, A., Plauth, W. H., Jr., and Nadas, A. S.: Development of subaortic stenosis after pulmonary artery banding. Circulation, 47, 48(Suppl. III):7, 1973.
13. Friedli, B., Kidd, B. S. L., Mustard, W. T., and Keith, J. D.: Ventricular septal defect with increased pulmonary vascular resistance. Late results of surgical closure. Am. J. Cardiol., 33:403, 1974.
14. Hallidie-Smith, K. A., Edwards, R. E., Wilson, R., and Zeidifard, E.: Long-term cardiorespiratory assessment after surgical closure of ventricular septal defect in childhood (abstract). Proc. Br. Cardiac Soc., 37:553, 1975.
15. Hallidie-Smith, K. A., Hollmann, A., Cleland, W. P., et al.: Effects of surgical closure of ventricular septal defects upon pulmonary vascular disease. Br. Heart J., 31:246, 1969.
16. Heath, D., and Edwards, J. E.: The pathology of hypertensive pulmonary vascular disease. A description of six grades of structural changes in the

17. Heath, D., Helmholz, H. F., Jr., Burchell, H. B., DuShane, J. W., and Edwards, J. E.: Graded pulmonary vascular changes and hemodynamic findings in cases of atrial and ventricular septal defect and patent ductus arteriosus. Circulation, 18:1155, 1958.
18. Hoffman, J. I. E.: Natural history of congenital heart disease: Problems in its assessment with special reference to ventricular septal defect. Circulation, 37:97, 1968.
19. Hoffman, J. I. E., and Rudolph, A. M.: The natural history of ventricular septal defects in infancy. Am. J. Cardiol., 16:634, 1965.
20. Hoffman, J. I. E., and Rudolph, A. M.: The natural history of isolated ventricular septal defect with special reference to selection of patients for surgery. Adv. Pediatr., 17:57, 1970.
21. Hopkins, R. A., Bull, C., Sumner, E., Haworth, S. G., de Leval, M. R., and Stark, J.: Pulmonary hypertensive crises following surgery for congenital heart defects in children. Circulation, 72:259, 1986.
22. Jarmakani, M. M., Edwards, S. B., Spach, M. S., Canent, R. V., Jr., Capp, M. P., Hagan, M. J., Barr, R. C., and Jain, V.: Left ventricular pressure-volume characteristics in congenital heart disease. Circulation, 37:879, 1968.
23. Keck, E. W. O., Ongley, P. A., Kincaid, O. W., and Swan, H. J. C.: Ventricular septal defect with aortic insufficiency. A clinical and hemodynamic study of 18 proved cases. Circulation, 27:203, 1963.
24. Keith, J. D., Rose, V., Collins, G., and Kidd, B. S. L.: Ventricular septal defect: Incidence, morbidity, and mortality in various age groups. Br. Heart J., 33(Suppl.):81, 1971.
25. Kirklin, J. K., and Kirklin, J. W.: Management of the cardiovascular subsystem after cardiac surgery. Ann. Thorac. Surg., 32:311, 1981.
26. Kirklin, J. K., Castaneda, A. R., Keane, J. F., et al.: Surgical management of multiple ventricular septal defects. J. Thorac. Cardiovasc. Surg., 80:485, 1980.
27. Kirklin, J. W., and DuShane, J. W.: Repair of ventricular septal defect in infancy. Pediatrics, 27:961, 1961.
28. Lauer, R. M., DuShane, J. W., and Edwards, J. E.: Obstruction of left ventricular outlet in association with ventricular septal defect. Circulation, 22:110, 1960.
29. Leatham, A., and Segal, B.: Auscultatory and phonocardiographic signs of ventricular septal defect with left to right shunt. Circulation, 25:318, 1962.
30. Levin, A. R., Spach, M. S., Canent, R. V., Jr., Boineau, J. P., Capp, M. P., Jain, V., and Barr, R. C.: Intracardiac pressure-flow dynamics in isolated ventricular septal defects. Circulation, 35:430, 1967.
31. Lillehei, C. W., Cohen, M., Warden, H. E., Ziegler, N., and Varco, R. L.: The results of direct vision closure of ventricular septal defects in eight patients by means of controlled cross circulation. Surg. Gynecol. Obstet., 101:446, 1955.
32. Lincoln, C., Jamieson, S., Joseph, M., et al.: Transatrial repair of ventricular septal defects with reference to their anatomic classification. J. Thorac. Cardiovasc. Surg., 74:183, 1977.
33. Morgan, B. C., Griffiths, S. P., and Blumenthal, S.: Ventricular septal defect. I. Congestive heart failure in infancy. Pediatrics, 25:54, 1960.
34. Moulaert, A. J., Bruins, C. G., and Oppenheimer-Dekker, A.: Anomalies of the aortic arch and ventricular septal defects. Circulation, 53:1011, 1976.
35. Muller, W. H., Jr., and Dammann, J. F., Jr.: Treatment of certain congenital malformations of the heart by the creation of pulmonic stenosis to reduce pulmonary hypertension and excessive pulmonary flow. A preliminary report. Surg. Gynecol. Obstet., 95:213, 1952.
36. Nadas, A. S., Thilenius, O. G., La Farge, C. G., and Hauck, A. J.: Ventricular septal defect with aortic regurgitation. Medical and pathological aspects. Circulation, 29:862, 1964.
37. Okamoto, Y.: Clinical studies for open heart surgery in infants with profound hypothermia. Arch. Jpn. Chir., 38:188, 1969.
38. Pacifico, A. D.: Cardiopulmonary bypass and hypothermic circulatory arrest in congenital heart surgery. *In* Grillo, H. C., et al. (Eds.): Current Therapy in Cardiothoracic Surgery. Toronto, B. C. Decker, 1988.
39. Pacifico, A. D., Sand, M. E., Bargeron, L. M., Jr., and Colvin, E. V.: Transatrial-transpulmonary repair of tetralogy of Fallot. J. Thorac. Cardiovasc. Surg., 93:919, 1987.
40. Rein, J. G., Freed, M. D., Norwood, W. I., and Castaneda, A. R.: Early and late results of closure of ventricular septal defect in infancy. Ann. Thorac. Surg., 24:19, 1977.
41. Riggs, T., Mehta, S., Hirschfield, S., Borkat, G., and Liebman, J.: Ventricular septal defect in infancy: A combined vectorgraphic and echocardiographic study. Circulation, 59:385, 1979.
42. Rizzoli, G., Blackstone, E. H., Kirklin, J. W., et al.: Incremental risk factors in hospital mortality after repair of ventricular septal defect. J. Thorac. Cardiovasc. Surg., 80:494, 1980.
43. Shah, P., Singh, W. S. A., Rose, V., and Keith, J.: Incidence of bacterial endocarditis in ventricular septal defects. Circulation, 34:127, 1966.
44. Sigmann, J. M., Stern, A. M., and Sloan, H. E.: Early surgical correction of large ventricular septal defects. Pediatrics, 39:4, 1967.
45. Singh, A. K., deLeval, M. R., and Stark, J.: Left ventriculotomy for closure of muscular ventricular septal defects. Ann. Surg., 186:577, 1977.
46. Somerville, J., Brandao, A., and Ross, D. N.: Aortic regurgitation with ventricular septal defect. Surgical management and clinical features. Circulation, 41:317, 1970.
47. Soto, B., Becker, A. E., Moulaert, A. J., et al.: Classification of ventricular septal defects. Br. Heart J., 43:332, 1980.
48. Stirling, G. R., Stanley, P. H., and Lillehei, C. W.: Effect of cardiac bypass and ventriculotomy upon right ventricular function. Surg. Forum, 8:433, 1957.

49. Trusler, G. A., Moes, C. A. F., and Kidd, B. S. L.: Repair of ventricular septal defect with aortic insufficiency. J. Thorac. Cardiovasc. Surg., 66:394, 1973.
50. Trusler, G. A., and Mustard, W. T.: A method of banding the pulmonary artery for large isolated ventricular septal defect with and without transposition of the great arteries. Ann. Thorac. Surg., 13:351, 1972.
51. Van Praagh, R., Bernhard, W. F., Rosenthal, A., et al.: Interrupted aortic arch: Surgical treatment. Am. J. Cardiol., 27:200, 1971.
52. Van Praagh, R., McNamara, J. J., and Gross, R. E.: Anatomic types of ventricular septal defect with aortic insufficiency. Circulation, 36(Suppl. 2):256, 1967.
53. Wagenvoort, C. A., Neufeld, H. N., DuShane, J. W., and Edwards, J. E.: The pulmonary arterial tree in ventricular septal defect. A quantitative study of anatomic features in fetuses, infants and children. Circulation, 23:740, 1961.

VIII ————————————————————————

THE TETRALOGY OF FALLOT

Ross M. Ungerleider, M.D., and David C. Sabiston, Jr., M.D.

The tetralogy of Fallot (TOF) is one of the most common congenital heart malformations. Depending on the criteria used to define this entity, it can be present in 3 to 6 infants for every 10,000 births.[98] It is probably proper to consider TOF within the spectrum of pulmonary stenosis (or atresia) with an accompanying ventricular septal defect (VSD). The condition usually has as its first symptom cyanosis shortly after birth, which attracts early medical attention. Diagnosis can be made with two-dimensional echocardiography or cardiac catheterization. Nearly all patients are candidates for surgical therapy, and several options exist that can provide excellent immediate and long-term outcomes for many of these children.

HISTORICAL ASPECTS

Although Stensen deserves credit for the first description (1672)[122] of what is now called tetralogy of Fallot, it is Etienne-Louis Arthur Fallot (1888)[39] of Marseille, France, whose name is characteristically attached to this congenital cardiac disorder. There were others prior to Fallot who described the malformation, including Sandifort (1777),[120] John Hunter (1784),[64] William Hunter (1784),[65] Farre (1814),[40] Gintrac (1824),[49] Hope (1839),[61] and Peacock (1866).[108] Most of these descriptions were case reports of comical curiosities. However, in his description of the disorder, Fallot was the first to describe accurately the clinical and complete pathologic manifestations of this deformity. He emphasized that with a knowledge of the clinical manifestations, one could diagnose the malformation accurately during life.

In the original description of this congenital anomaly, Fallot stated, "This malformation consists of a true anatomopathological type represented by the following tetralogy: (1) stenosis of the pulmonary artery; (2) interventricular communication; (3) deviation of the origin of the aorta to the right; (4) hypertrophy, almost always concentric, of the right ventricle. Failure of obliteration of the foramen ovale may occasionally be added in a wholly accessory manner." Fallot reported 55 patients with congenital heart disease of whom most had the tetralogy. In retrospect, it is remarkable that such a large number of patients could have been reported by a single author in that early day of the recognition of cardiac abnormalities.

Despite the fact that accurate clinical diagnosis could often be established after these contributions by Fallot, nevertheless, many years passed before definitive treatment of the condition became available. In 1944, Blalock operated on a severely ill infant with TOF who weighed only 4.5 kg. The child was severely cyanotic and had had multiple episodes of unconsciousness due to marked hypoxemia. A systemic-pulmonary anastomosis was achieved by joining the subclavian artery to the pulmonary artery, and the child was greatly benefited. Several months later, Blalock and Taussig[15] reported this patient together with two others, and a new era had been opened in the field of cardiac surgery. The first successful open repair was performed by Lillehei and Varco at the University of Minnesota in 1954 using "controlled cross circulation," with another patient serving as oxygenator and blood reservoir![87,89] The following year, Lillehei replaced this technique with the use of cardiopulmonary bypass and described repair of TOF using this technology.[88] Since that time, several advances in life-support technology as well as surgical methodology have evolved that have made surgical treatment of TOF one of the most interesting, and oftentimes most satisfying, procedures that surgeons perform.[126]

ANATOMY

There is wide morphologic variability in the spectrum of TOF. This can encompass the size of the right ventricle, the size and distribution of the pulmonary arteries, the location of the pulmonary stenosis (i.e., subvalvular, valvular, or peripheral) and additional sources of pulmonary blood flow (i.e., systemic-pulmonary collaterals) (Figs. 1 to 3).

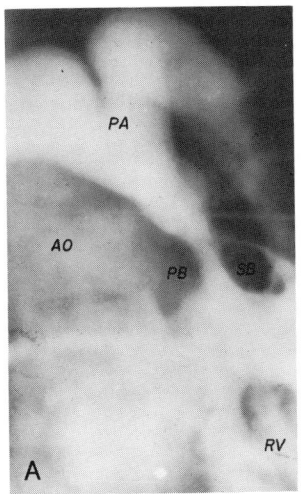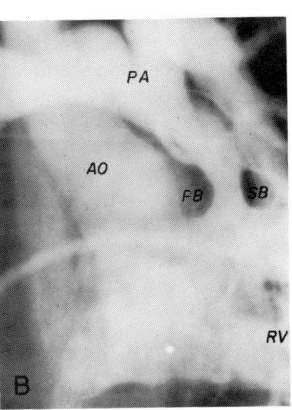

Figure 1. Obstruction in the region of the infundibulum. *A,* Frame made in systole. *B,* Frame made in diastole. The negative shadows of the hypertrophied parietal (PB) in septal (SB) bands are particularly well demonstrated. The pulmonary valve appears domed and at operation was bicuspid but not stenotic. The aorta (AO) is opacified by this right ventricular injection, and its diameter is three times that of the pulmonary artery. The underdevelopment of the infundibulum of the right ventricle, a basic characteristic of tetralogy of Fallot, is apparent in this angiocardiogram. This patient has anatomy suitable for total correction. RV, right ventricle; PA, pulmonary artery. (From Kirklin, J. W., and Karp, R. B.: The Tetralogy of Fallot from a Surgical Viewpoint. Philadelphia, W. B. Saunders Company, 1970.)

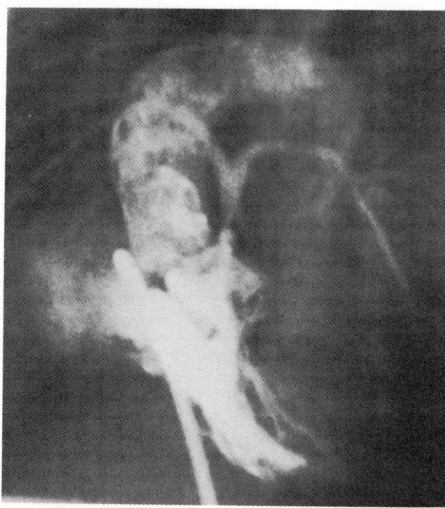

Figure 2. In this patient, the right ventricular outflow tract connects to a small main pulmonary artery with equally small branch pulmonary arteries. Because of the small size of these pulmonary arteries, total correction is not recommended, and palliative systemic-pulmonary artery shunting should be performed (From Kirklin, J. W., and Barratt-Boyes, B. G.: Ventricular septal defect and pulmonary stenosis or atresia. *In* Kirklin, J. W., and Brian, G. (Eds.): Cardiac Surgery. New York, Churchill Livingstone, 1986, p. 712.)

The lesion described by Fallot was believed to consist of four major defects: infundibular pulmonary stenosis, a ventricular septal defect, dextroposition of the aorta, and hypertrophy of the right ventricle. It is now recognized by most authorities that the two most important features of TOF are (1) the right ventricular (RV) outflow tract obstruction, which is nearly always infundibular and/or valvular in location,[3,5,77,85,142] and (2) the VSD, which is usually large, subaortic, adjacent to the membranous septum (perimembranous), and associated with misalignment of the conal septum.[77,85] A clinical definition of the tetralogy includes the basic principle that it is a congenital cardiac malformation with a VSD, the size of which approximates the aortic orifice, and with pulmonary stenosis of such a degree that approximately equal pressures occur in both ventricles.

From a physiologic point of view, most patients with TOF exhibit a high resistance to RV emptying owing to pulmonary outflow obstruction. The predominant shunt is from right to left with flow across the ventricular defect into the aorta, which produces cyanosis and an elevation of the hematocrit. When the pulmonary stenosis is less severe, bidirectional shunting may occur. In some patients, the infundibular stenosis is minimal and the predominant shunt is from left to right, producing what is called the pink tetralogy. Although such patients may not

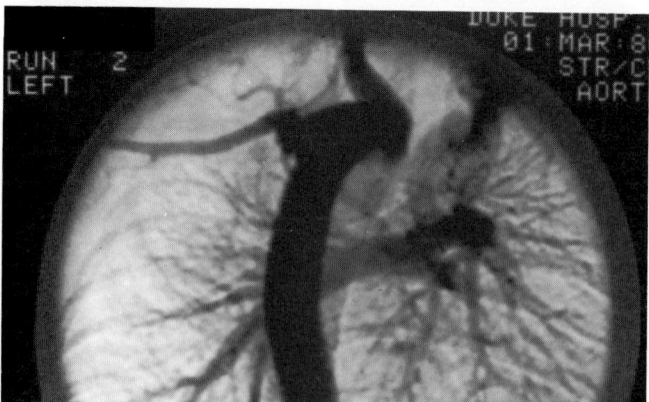

Figure 3. Digital subtraction angiography can demonstrate nicely the pulmonary artery anatomy as well as its source of flow in neonates. In this patient with pulmonary atresia, a ventricular septal defect and a right aortic arch, pulmonary flow is dependent on a large ductus arteriosus.

appear cyanotic, they often have oxygen desaturation in the systemic arterial blood.

The pulmonary arteries can also be variable in size and distribution. Occasionally, the left pulmonary artery may be absent (3 per cent), although this is rare for the right pulmonary artery. Many patients have some degree of stenosis of the peripheral pulmonary arteries, which further restricts pulmonary blood flow. There may be no communication between the right ventricle and main pulmonary artery (PA) (pulmonary atresia), and in this case pulmonary blood flow is maintained by a ductus arteriosus or some other form of bronchopulmonary collateral (Fig. 4). When both main pulmonary arteries are supplied by large bronchial collaterals, the condition is often classified as truncus arteriosus Type IV.

Aortic overriding is caused by true dextroposition and abnormal rotation of the aortic root, which causes an aorta that arises from the right ventricle to a varying degree. The aorta itself may have a right arch in as many as 25 to 30 per cent of patients with TOF; and in these situations, the branching pattern of the arch vessels may be abnormal. Occasionally, the ductus arteriosus persists on the side opposite the arch, or it may be completely absent. An aberrant subclavian artery coursing in a retroesophageal location may be present (5 to 10 per cent), although it is quite rare for the retroesophageal subclavian vessels to cause dysphagia. A persistent left superior vena cava occurs with about the same incidence.[101]

The coronary anatomy may have important variability. Most notable is the origin of the left anterior descending coronary artery from the proximal right coronary artery, which causes the RV outflow tract to be crossed by this important coronary at variable distances from the pulmonary valve anulus.[28,41,42] Occasionally, all coronaries arise from a single main coronary ostium (usually the left), or the left coronary arises from the pulmonary artery.[1]

Associated defects are not uncommon with TOF. The existence of an atrial septal defect is frequent enough to prompt its inclusion as "pentalogy" of Fallot. Other defects of importance include atrioventricular (AV) septal defects,[133,138] muscular VSDs,[42] anomalous pulmonary venous return,[77] and aortic incompetence.[94]

DIAGNOSIS

CLINICAL MANIFESTATIONS. The clinical presentation is dependent on the severity of the anatomic malformation. Infants with pulmonary atresia may become intensely cyanotic as the ductus arteriosus closes unless they have numerous bronchopulmonary collaterals. Heart failure is usually not a feature unless collaterals are extensive. Patients with RV-to-PA continuity are cyanotic in relation to their degree of stenosis and consequent pulmonary blood flow. This balance is also affected by flow through a ductus arteriosus, and symptoms usually increase when the ductus begins to close shortly after birth. Occasionally, children will have enough pulmonary blood flow that they do not appear cyanotic; and the lesion may go undetected until these children begin to outgrow their pulmonary blood flow.[16,51] A common way for these older children to augment pulmonary flow is to squat, increasing peripheral vascular resistance and thus decreasing the size of their right-to-left shunt across the VSD (Fig. 4). This position has diagnostic significance and is highly characteristic of TOF. There is usually increasing effort dyspnea with age.[74]

Not all children require early surgical therapy, although the natural history of the surgically untreated lesion is unfavorable. This natural history is heavily influenced by the severity of the anatomic defect.[95] Statistics demonstrate a 30 per cent mortality by age 6 months that increases to 50 per cent by 2 years. Only 20 per cent of patients can be expected to reach 10 years of age, and not more than 5 to 10 per cent live to reach 21.[10,47,79] Interest-

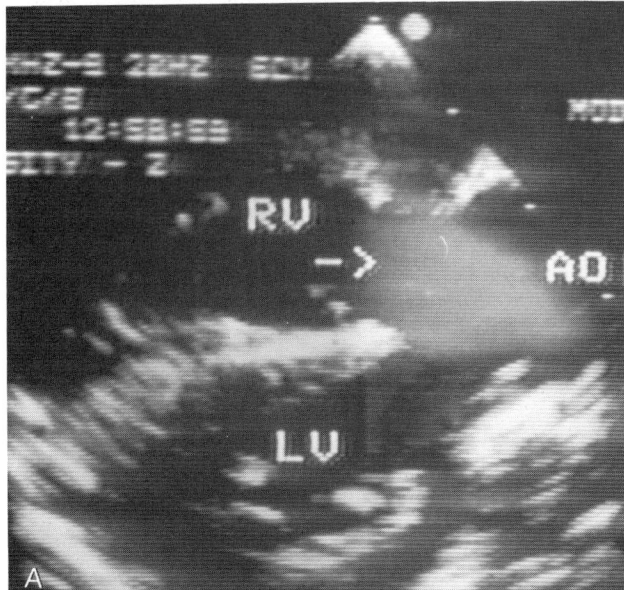

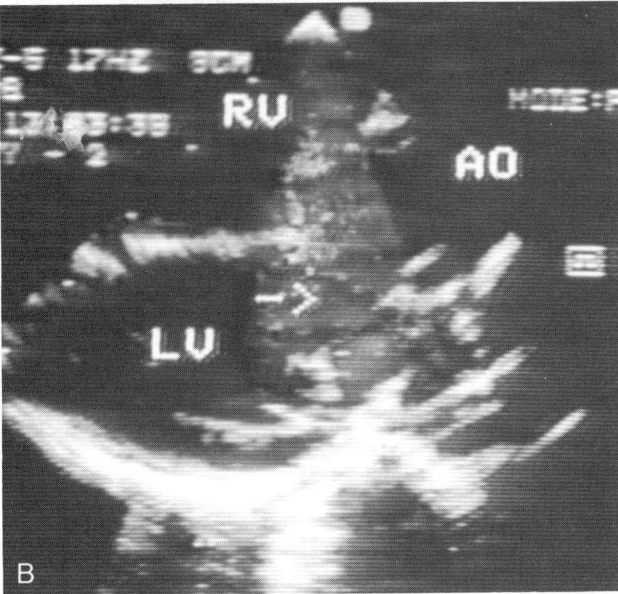

Figure 4. *A,* Intraoperative Doppler color flow image obtained during a tetralogy of Fallot symptomatic episode. There is increased right-to-left shunting across the ventricular septal defect as demonstrated (arrow) flowing from the right ventricle into the aorta. *B,* With increase of systemic vascular resistance, this right-to-left shunt is reversed thus improving systemic arterial oxygen saturation. (From Greeley, W. J., Stanley, T. E., Ungerleider, R. M., and Kisslo, J. A.: Intraoperative hypoxemic spells in tetralogy of Fallot: An echocardiographic analysis of diagnosis and treatment. Anesth. Analg., *68:*815, 1989.)

ingly, there are rare instances of patients whose shunts are so well balanced that they achieve a normal life span. One example of this is that of the American composer Gilbert, who lived to the age of 60 with TOF and led a relatively productive life without therapy.[139]

The greatest risks that these patients face are of paradoxical emboli (leading to stroke or end-organ failure), cerebral or pulmonary thrombosis (from increasing polycythemia), and subacute bacterial endocarditis.[8] Heart failure is uncommon in surgically untreated patients but does pose a greater risk after creation of a systemic-to-pulmonary artery shunt, especially if pre-existing collaterals are not considered.[47]

PHYSICAL EXAMINATION. The patient may appear to be smaller than expected for the age, and cyanosis of the lips and nail beds is usually apparent. The fingers and toes usually show clubbing (hypertrophic pulmonary osteoarthropathy). On pal-

pation of the chest, a thrill is usually present anteriorly. A harsh systolic murmur is audible over the pulmonary area and along the left sternal border. Absence of a murmur in a patient suspected of having the tetralogy is suggestive of pulmonary atresia. The second heart sound is usually single and rarely increased in intensity. During cyanotic episodes, murmurs may diminish, which is suggestive of less RV outflow to the pulmonary arteries. A continuous murmur suggests a collateral source of pulmonary blood flow (either a bronchopulmonary or a surgically created shunt).

LABORATORY STUDIES. The hemoglobin, hematocrit, and erythrocyte count are usually elevated. The magnitude of the increase is generally proportional to the cyanosis, with hematocrit values varying from normal to as high as 90 per cent, most being between 40 and 70 per cent. Similarly, the oxygen saturation in the systemic arterial blood is variable, usually between 65 and 70 per cent. However, in severe forms of the malformation, the arterial oxygen saturation during exercise may fall to as low as 25 per cent. A bleeding tendency is present in some patients with the TOF, especially those in whom cyanosis is marked. The usual finding is a diminution in a variety of the factors responsible for blood coagulation, but none of the factors are reduced to critical levels. The platelet count and total blood fibrinogen are frequently slightly diminished, and clot retraction is sometimes poor and associated with prolonged prothrombin and coagulation times. Despite the defects in the clotting mechanism in some patients, the changes are usually insufficient to explain the hemorrhagic tendency noted at the time of operation.[60,110] In infancy, the only significant alteration may be low arterial oxygen saturations.

ROENTGENOGRAMS. In the early stages, the chest film may be normal, but the chest film in the TOF usually shows diminished vascularity in the lungs and absence of prominence of the pulmonary artery. The shadow of the great vessels in the superior mediastinum is narrow, owing to the diminished caliber of the pulmonary artery. If cyanosis and dyspnea are quite prominent, the pulmonary vascular markings are usually markedly diminished. Later, the classic boot-shaped heart *(coeur en sabot)* may develop, and it is recognized as a hallmark of the TOF (Fig. 5*A*). Right ventricular enlargement is present and is best demonstrated in the left anterior oblique position. The barium swallow provides evidence of the side on which the aortic arch descends. This is of considerable importance, because approximately one fourth of the patients with TOF have a *right* aortic arch (Fig. 5*B*). In fact, the presence of a right aortic arch with cyanosis is strong evidence that the malformation is indeed TOF. Occasionally there is asymmetric pulmonary vasculature with unilateral oligemia in comparison with the opposite lung. This suggests absent pulmonary valve syndrome with unilateral pulmonary artery agenesis or anomalous origin of one pulmonary artery from the aorta.

ELECTROCARDIOGRAM. The electrocardiogram usually shows RV hypertrophy, usually apparent in the standard leads and most consistently found in the unipolar leads. The more commonly encountered findings include tall and peaked T waves, reversal of the RS ratio, and a normal PR interval and QRS duration. If right ventricular hypertrophy is absent, a diagnosis of TOF should be seriously questioned, and pulmonary atresia with hypoplastic right ventricle should be considered.

ECHOCARDIOGRAPHY. Recent advances in two-dimensional echocardiography and color flow Doppler have elevated the diagnostic capabilities of this technology. It is not uncommon for infants and children to be accurately diagnosed by echo prior to the performance of any laboratory tests, roentgenograms, electrocardiograms, or angiograms (Fig. 6). The addition of color flow mapping can sensitively detect the presence of a patent ductus arteriosus (PDA), additional muscular VSD, or small atrial septal defect (ASD). The physiology of a cyanotic episode with right-to-left shunting across a VSD that is reversed

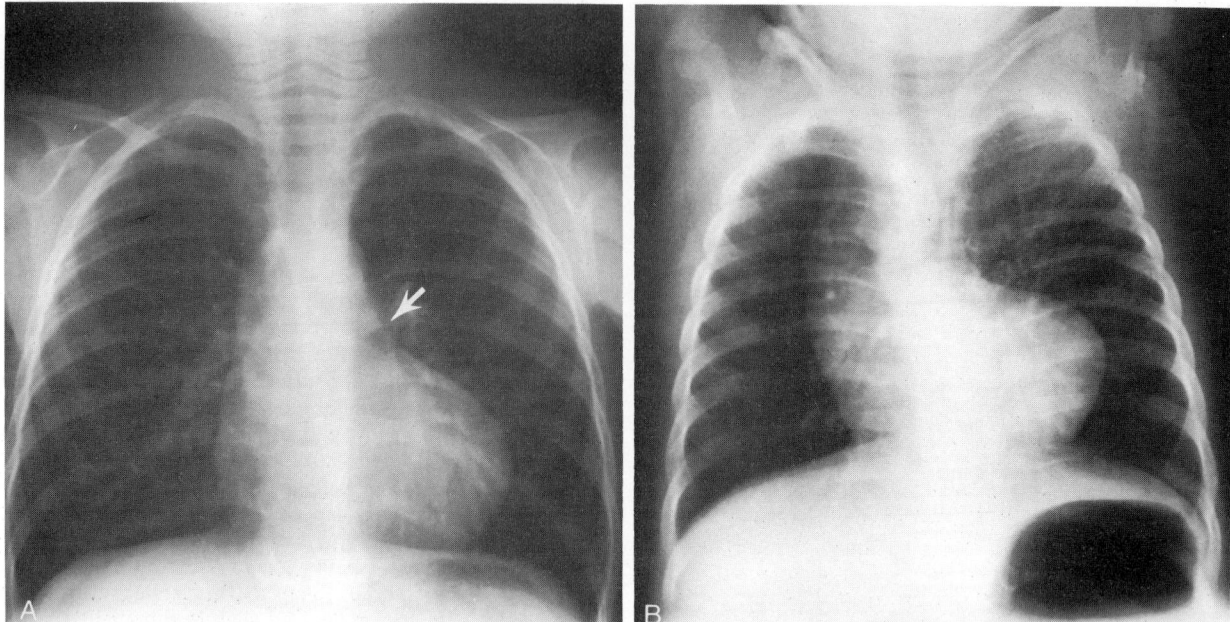

Figure 5. *A,* A chest film of a patient with a tetralogy of Fallot and a left aortic arch. The absence of the pulmonary artery shadow (arrow) gives the heart a characteristic "boot-shaped" appearance. *B,* In this patient, the "boot-shaped" appearance of the heart is made even more prominent because of the right aortic arch accentuating the absence of pulmonary arterial shadow.

by elevation of peripheral vascular resistance has been nicely demonstrated (see Fig. 4).[53] The coronary anatomy can be revealed with remarkable accuracy, and abnormalities of valvular apparatus (i.e., straddling chords) may be best delineated with this technology. It is not uncommon to take patients to the operating room for palliation or correction based on preoperative echo data alone.[79,93,131,132]

ANGIOCARDIOGRAM AND CARDIAC CATHETERIZATION. Cardiac catheterization provides angiographic demonstration of ventricular size, pulmonary artery size and, with aortic root injection, sources of pulmonary blood flow as well as anomalies of coronary artery anatomy. Some authors base prediction of the postrepair right-to-left ventricular pressure ratio

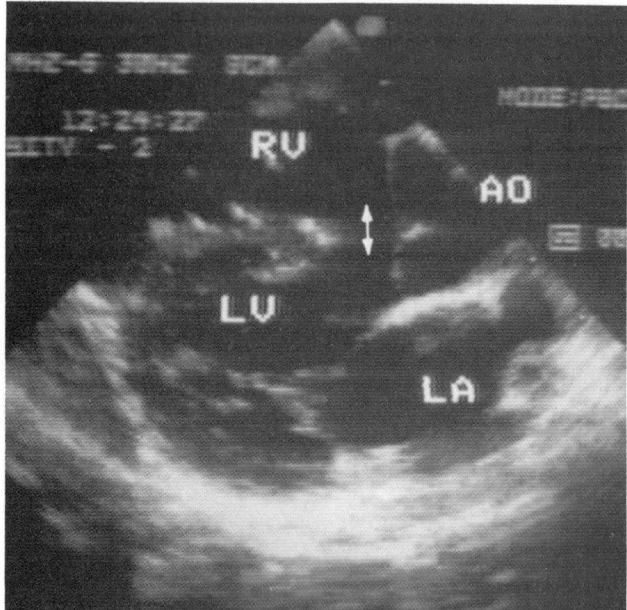

Figure 6. Long axis intraoperative echocardiogram demonstrating the typical features of tetralogy with a subaortic ventricular septal defect (VSD) and overriding of the aorta so that it appears to arise partially from the right ventricle. Arrow indicates VSD. (RV, right ventricle; LV, left ventricle; LA, left atrium; AO, aorta).

on data obtained from catheterization, thus assisting operative planning of the type of repair that should be performed.[12] Other pressure measurements should demonstrate equal pressures in both ventricles (distinguishing this condition from isolated pulmonary stenosis with an intact ventricular septum in which the right ventricular pressure may be considerably greater than that in the left ventricle). Angiograms are especially helpful after palliative shunt procedures prior to complete repair. These pictures define the anatomy of the pulmonary arteries as well as any iatrogenic distortion caused by the shunt that might need attention. If pressure data (i.e., cardiac catheterization) is not needed, digital subtraction techniques can supply excellent views (see Fig. 3) with minimal invasion—a worthwhile consideration, because it is not unusual for cyanotic episodes and seizures to occur in these children during intracardiac catheter manipulation.

INDICATIONS FOR OPERATION

As suggested by the natural history of this lesion, most patients require surgical intervention. Current trends are to provide surgical correction as soon as possible (often electively before the first year of life) and generally by the time the patient has reached the age of 2 years. The urgency with which surgery is performed is affected by numerous variables, including the symptoms at presentation, the age at presentation, and the associated lesions. The use of prostaglandins (PGE_1) to stabilize patients with diminished pulmonary blood flow has greatly influenced the emergent care of these patients.[31,45] Rather than performing systemic-to-pulmonary artery shunts on critically ill, hypoxemic, and acidotic neonates, surgeons have the luxury of more fully evaluating the patient's anatomy, while prostaglandins maintain ductal patency (and thus pulmonary blood flow), so that they can arrive at the most appropriate decision for each individual patient. Although controversy continues concerning the preferential operation during infancy, there has been a general trend toward open correction.[20,56,70,104,127,128,134] The groups who urge early total correction at any time emphasize that it avoids the necessity of a second operation and that the current results are sufficiently good to support this judgment. Some groups currently believe that corrective surgery should be performed in all patients with TOF irrespective of age or weight except for those with an anterior descending coronary artery arising from the right coronary artery or those who have associated pulmonary atresia.[21,23,56] Moreover, successful one-stage correction (using a valved homograft conduit) is feasible for patients with pulmonary atresia and VSD if pulmonary artery anatomy is favorable. Opposed to this approach are those who believe that palliation is preferable in infancy because the overall mortality is lower.[5,6,58,75,114] In addition, these observers are concerned about whether or not the small heart in infancy will remain corrected as growth continues, thinking perhaps that outflow tract obstruction of the right ventricle may recur.[78] Various factors that increase the risk for early repair have been described and include pulmonary artery problems, major associated anomalies, small size (early age), more than one previous operation, and absent pulmonary valve syndrome.[76] The type of palliation offered to infants, however, is variable and controversial. Although the Blalock-Taussig shunt has for years been the most popular palliative procedure, several groups now employ a modification of the Blalock-Taussig shunt using polytetrafluoroethylene (PTFE) interposition between the subclavian artery and pulmonary artery[29] or between the aorta and main pulmonary artery (central shunt).[2,33] In selected cases, RV outflow patching to promote RV-to-PA continuity, and symmetric PA growth has also been advocated.[34,127] Irrespective of the type of palliation chosen, the goal is simply to increase pulmonary blood flow, independent of ductal patency, to allow pulmonary artery growth and eventual total correction. Regardless of the philosophy chosen (one-stage versus two-stage), it does appear that the early use of prostaglandins has salvaged more infants with TOF and allowed them to be stabilized so that surgical decisions can be made.

SURGICAL TECHNIQUES

Palliative Procedures

The presence of pulmonary atresia or an anomalous left anterior descending coronary artery across the right ventricular outflow tract may preclude the possibility of establishing transanular RV-to-PA continuity if necessary, and require placement of a conduit. Although conduits can be used in infants,[32] patients with extremely small pulmonary arteries may not tolerate total correction in infancy. Likewise, patients with small left ventricular volumes (less than 60 per cent of normal) may do better with initial palliation.[103] Each patient must be individualized, but these considerations can provide adequate justification for performing a palliative rather than a corrective procedure when the diagnosis is first made.[117] Palliative procedures should be directed to increasing pulmonary blood flow without dependence on the ductus arteriosus. There are a number of systemic-to-pulmonary artery shunts being performed by various surgeons (Fig. 7), but the most common shunts are (1) the classic Blalock-Taussig shunt, (2) the modified Blalock-Taussig shunt,[29] and (3) a central aortopulmonary shunt using prosthetic graft material. The shunts popularized by Potts (1946),[111] Waterston (1962),[135] and Glenn (1954)[50] are no longer being widely used in this setting. This is because the Waterston anastomosis (ascending aorta to right pulmonary artery) can cause kinking and stenosis at the anastomotic site, and that may make subsequent open correction difficult[48,140]; and the Potts anastomosis (descending aorta to left pulmonary artery) can enlarge with time, producing an excessive shunt with pulmonary hypertension and often aneurysm formation at the site of anastomosis.[116,123] Moreover, a Potts anastomosis is more difficult to close at the time of subsequent correction. The Glenn anastomosis (which is between the superior vena cava and right pulmonary artery) can produce good results initially, with respect to symptoms in some patients, but more difficulty is experienced in the subsequent total correction. The majority of patients now receive one of the palliative shunts mentioned at the beginning of this section.

BLALOCK-TAUSSIG OPERATION. In performance of a subclavian-pulmonary anastomosis, the incision is generally made on the side opposite that on which the aorta descends[14] (Figs. 7C and 8). Ideally, the subclavian branch of the innominate artery is used for the anastomosis because the angle produced at its origin from its parent vessel is better than that formed when the subclavian artery is used.[118] The latter arises directly from the aorta and is apt to kink at its origin when

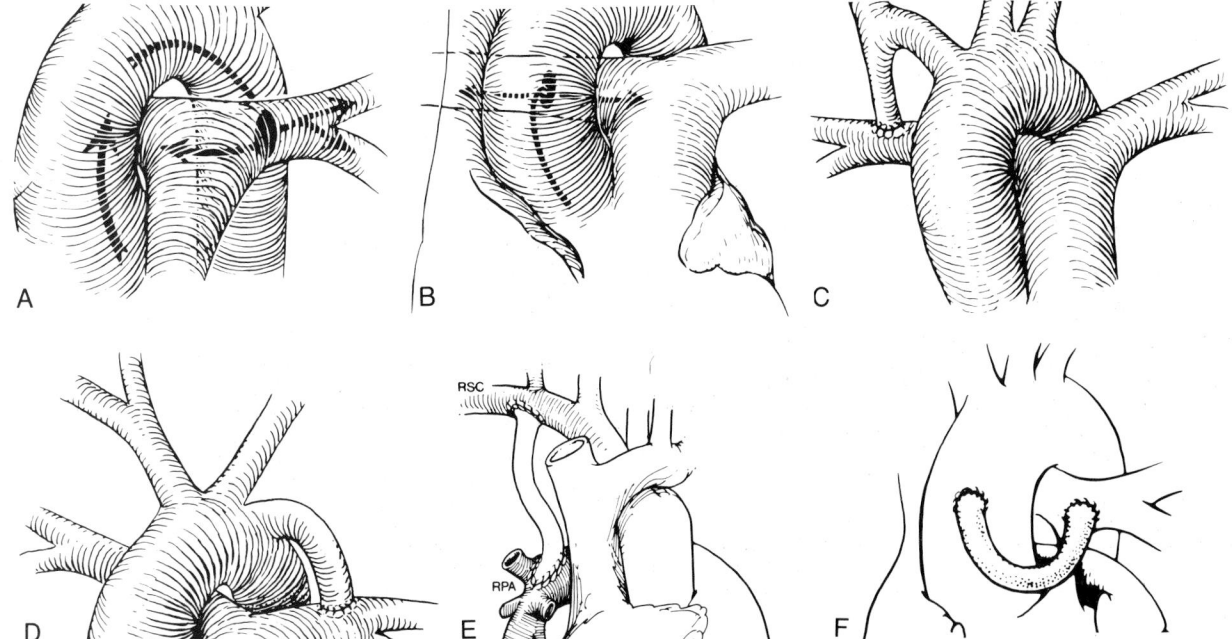

Figure 7. The most commonly encountered palliative shunts for increasing pulmonary blood flow in tetralogy of Fallot. *A*, A Potts' shunt. *B*, A Waterston shunt. *C*, A classic Blalock-Taussig shunt. *D*, A Blalock-Taussig shunt performed on the side of the aortic arch. *E*, A modified Blalock-Taussig shunt (After Cooley, D. A.: Techniques in Cardiac Surgery, 2nd ed. Philadelphia, W. B. Saunders Company, 1984). *F*, A central aortopulmonary shunt with prosthetic graft material. (From Turley, K., Tucker, W. Y., and Ebert, P. A.: The changing role of palliative procedures in the treatment of infants with congenital heart disease. J. Thorac. Cardiovasc. Surgery, 79:194, 1980.)

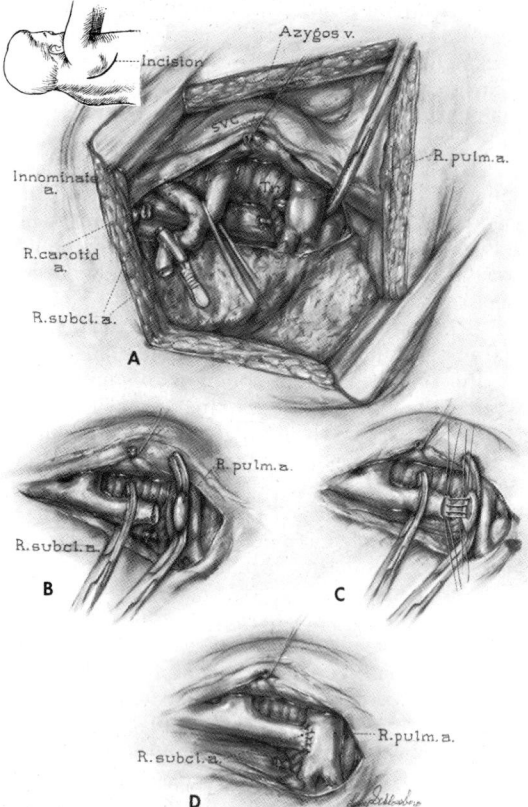

Figure 8. Performance of a classic Blalock-Taussig shunt. *A*, Initial dissection and exposure of the pulmonary artery for construction of a right subclavian-to-pulmonary artery anastomosis. The inset at the top shows the position of the patient on the operating table. The entry into the pleural cavity is through the second intercostal space. After the mediastinal pleura has been excised, the right pulmonary artery is easily identified and distinguished form the superior pulmonary vein. The vena cava is gently rolled anteriorly exposing the innominate artery with its termination in the subclavian and carotid arteries. The subclavian artery is dissected until its most prominent branch points are encountered; care is taken to protect the recurrent laryngeal nerve, which is located beneath the subclavian artery at this point. The subclavian artery is then divided, and the distal end is oversewn. The subclavian artery is removed from the sling made by the recurrent laryngeal nerve and lowered into position (*B*) toward the right pulmonary artery for subsequent anastomosis. *C*, The anastomosis is best completed with simple interrupted sutures so that the likelihood of scarring or stenosis is reduced. *D*, The completed anastomosis shows almost a straight-line configuration between the right subclavian artery and the right carotid artery. (From Ebert, P. A.: Atlas of Congenital Heart Surgery. New York, Churchill Livingstone, 1989.)

deflected inferiorly for an anastomosis to the pulmonary artery (Fig. 7*D*). If it is necessary to use the subclavian on the side of the arch, then the modification introduced by Laks and Castaneda[83] should be considered. Experimental studies have shown that approximately three fourths of the blood passing through a subclavian pulmonary shunt is directed to the lung on the side of the anastomosis.[44] There is evidence to suggest that growth of the pulmonary arteries after shunting is influenced by their structural composition and proportion of elastin as well as by differential blood flow.[115] Detailed attention must be given to performing the Blalock shunt, especially in construction of the anastomosis. Every effort must be made to prevent constriction of the anastomosis and meticulous technique is essential. In infants, it is preferable to use interrupted sutures to avoid a pursestring effect on the anastomosis. The advantages of the Blalock shunt are that it produces a reliable shunt with excellent flow characteristics and shunt flow that is ordinarily well matched to the size of the patient. Complications from transection of the subclavian artery are unusual.[4] The shunt employs no prosthetic material and is fairly easy to divide or ligate at the time of total correction. Disadvantages are that the shunt re-

quires meticulous and time-consuming dissection that may be difficult to justify in a severely ill infant. In addition, a Blalock shunt can cause distortion of the peripheral pulmonary artery, especially if technical difficulty is encountered during the procedure. As patients grow, one pulmonary artery may develop better than the others due to flow characteristics, especially if there is anastomotic distortion. This pulmonary artery distortion may make subsequent total correction more hazardous.[76] After creation of a Blalock-Taussig shunt, progression of the infundibular pulmonary stenosis has been encountered,[119] which also can influence the future operative approach (i.e., transatrial versus transventricular). Despite these features, the classic Blalock-Taussig shunt remains an excellent, time-proven option for increasing pulmonary blood flow in these patients.

MODIFIED BLALOCK-TAUSSIG SHUNT. With the advent of reliable prosthetic graft material, technically easier forms of systemic to pulmonary artery shunting as means of palliation have become popular. In addition, because most patients return within 2 years for total correction, the temporary nature of "palliation" justifies the use of an artificial conduit that may not have optimal longevity but does allow preservation of the subclavian arterial supply to the arm.[4,91,136] The "Great Ormond Street" shunt,[29] or "modified" Blalock-Taussig shunt, requires interposition of a segment of PTFE graft material (usually 4 or 5 mm. in diameter) between the subclavian artery and the pulmonary artery (Figs. 7*E* and 9). Each anastomosis can be performed with a partial occlusion clamp and continuous monofil-

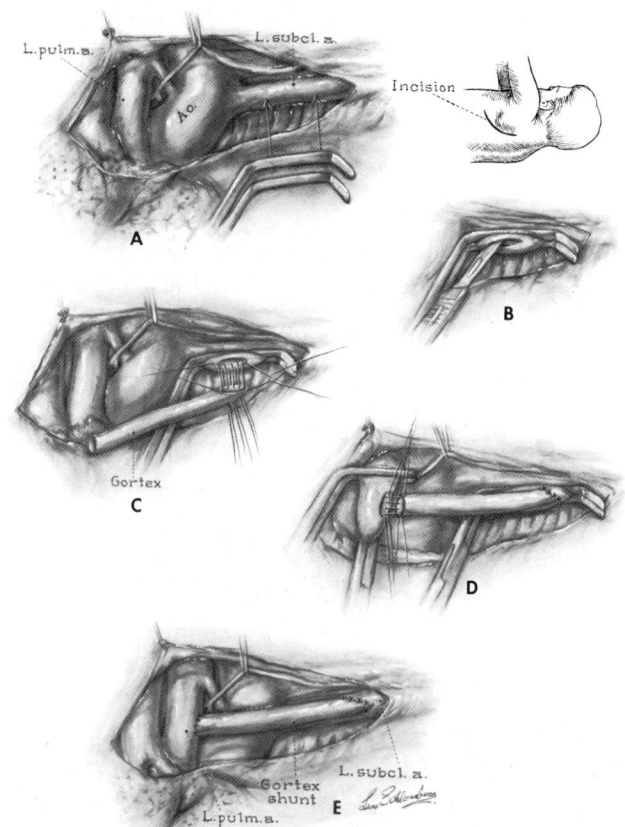

Figure 9. Performance of a modified Blalock-Taussig shunt. *A*, The left subclavian artery and left pulmonary artery are isolated through a left thoracotomy incision (inset). *B*, An occluding clamp is placed on the left subclavian artery, and a longitudinal incision is made. *C*, A beveled piece of 4- or 5-mm. Gore-Tex is sutured to the subclavian artery with fine, continuous sutures. With the Gore-Tex in place, occluding clamps are placed on the left pulmonary artery. *D*, A longitudinal incision is made in the left pulmonary artery, and the distal anastomosis is performed. *E*, The clamps are removed, and the graft lies in place without kinking either the graft or the left pulmonary artery. The left subclavian artery is preserved by this technique. (From Ebert, P.A.: Atlas of Congenital Heart Surgery. New York, Churchill Livingstone, 1989.)

ament suture. The shunts can be easily constructed on either side, because kinking of the subclavian artery is no longer a problem. Placement on the side of the aorta arch descent through a thoracotomy may be technically easier, although interposition of graft material between the innominate artery and ipsilateral pulmonary artery (usually right) through a median sternotomy is also technically feasible. Although flow through this shunt is still controlled by the size of the subclavian artery, a long segment of prosthetic graft nevertheless supplies its own unique amount of resistance, so that flow through these shunts can be more variable. Moreover, because the graft is fixed in size, distortion of the pulmonary artery by the shunt can be anticipated as the patient grows, although this has not been a universal experience.[84,129] These shunts can be slightly more difficult to take down than a classic Blalock-Taussig shunt and probably should be divided, rather than ligated, at the time of total correction. They have become the shunt of choice for some groups in infants less than 1 month of age.[68]

CENTRAL AORTOPULMONARY SHUNT. Several groups have been proponents of interposing a short segment of prosthetic graft material between the ascending aorta and main pulmonary artery.[9,33] This is an easy shunt to construct and can usually be performed without cardiopulmonary bypass (using partial occlusion clamps while pulmonary blood flow is maintained by the ductus arteriosus) (Figs. 7F and 10). Shunt flow is usually controlled by the size of prosthetic material used; and although there have been numerous suggestions as to how to construct the proper size graft, in most instances a 4-mm. graft is appropriate for small infants (less than 3 kg.) with a 5-mm. graft appropriate for larger neonates. These grafts have the advantage of creating symmetric pulmonary blood flow and growth without causing distortion of peripheral pulmonary arteries. Although subsequent total correction requires a repeat sternotomy, this is not usually a problem, and the shunts are easy to ligate or divide because of their anterior location. It is important when constructing these shunts to prevent kinking of the prosthetic graft material, because it does have a tendency to thrombose if flow through the graft is impeded.

The goal of all of these palliative procedures is to increase blood flow to the lungs. The decision as to which procedure to use can be based on many factors, including the experience and comfort that a particular surgeon has with each procedure. It must also be recognized today that these procedures in most cases are temporizing and that eventually total correction will be performed. Therefore, the shunt should be chosen that gives the best long-term preparation for repair. Individual problems with anatomy (such as proximal stenosis of the right or left pulmonary artery) should be considered, for in such an instance it may be more advantageous to perform a central aortopulmonary shunt (even if cardiopulmonary bypass is necessary) to enable concomitant enlargement of the area of pulmonary artery stenosis. A peripheral subclavian to pulmonary shunt in such a setting might otherwise limit flow to the contralateral pulmonary artery.

Total Correction

Total correction is the ideal operation for treatment of TOF and is accomplished with extracorporeal circulation. Prior to establishing cardiopulmonary bypass, previously placed systemic to pulmonary artery shunts should be identified so that they can be easily controlled. The patients are placed on cardiopulmonary bypass and usually cooled to 25° C. During this time, previously placed shunts are divided or ligated (Fig. 11A and B). The goal of operation once cardiopulmonary bypass has been established is to close the VSD, to resect the area of infundibular stenosis, and to relieve RV outflow obstruction (Fig. 12). The pulmonary valve should be sized; and if it is too small, the surgeon should not hesitate to perform transanular incision with enlargement of the right ventricular outflow tract out onto the pulmonary artery (Fig. 11D).[13,102,105] Although transanular patches have been considered to be an incremental risk factor for late surgical failure by leading to progressive RV dysfunction,[18,52,67] this association in the current era does not appear to be significant. Nevertheless, transanular patching should not be employed unless necessary to provide adequate RV outflow and, when performed, should be constructed in such a manner as to limit the degree of pulmonary insufficiency in order to preserve long-term RV dynamics.[55,69,80,97] The VSD can be approached transatrially[25,62,72,107] or transventricularly, although in patients with substantial infundibular stenosis, the transventricular approach is probably best, because a ventricular incision is usually necessary. The VSD should be closed with prosthetic patch material. Because these defects are large, it is unwise to attempt primary closure (see Fig. 12). Knowledge of the location of the conduction tissue is important, and sutures placed along the posteroinferior border of the defect should take this anatomy into consideration.[11,77,125] Several groups prefer to perform this part of the procedure under conditions of moderate hypothermia (25° C.) with cold potassium cardioplegic arrest, although the procedure can also be accomplished on the cold, non-cross-clamped, electrically fibrillating heart or during a period when the patient is in total circulatory arrest under profound hypothermic conditions (18° C.). The optimal method of myocardial protection remains controversial and probably depends on numerous factors related to the anatomy and physiology of each patient's lesion as well as to the patient's age at repair and the conduct of the operation itself.[30,77,141] After the

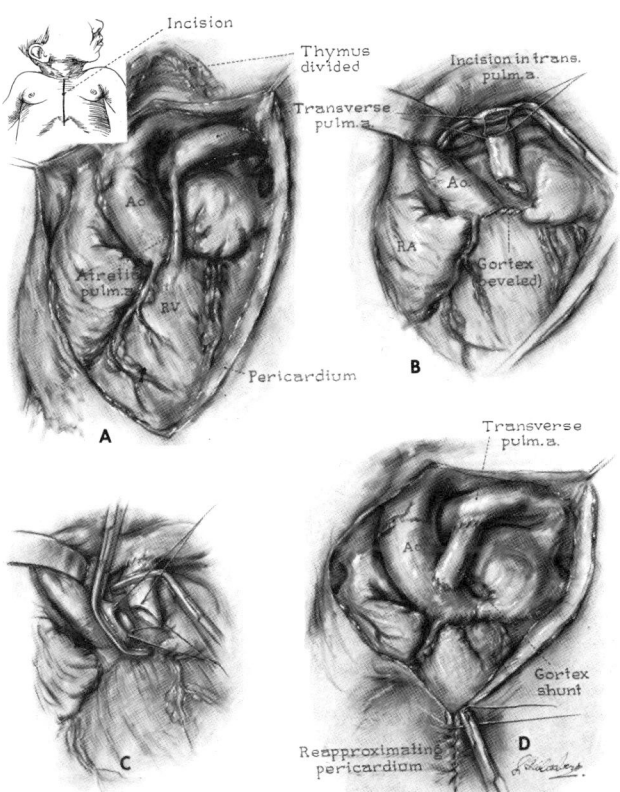

Figure 10. The aorta-pulmonary artery central shunt. *A,* Through a median sternotomy (inset), the anatomy is exposed. *B,* An occluding clamp is placed on the distal pulmonary artery at the location where a subsequent conduit repair is anticipated. The pulmonary artery flow is maintained through a ductus arteriosus, which is left unligated. A 4- or 5 mm. Gore-Tex graft is sutured to the pulmonary artery at this location. *C,* The clamp is released from the pulmonary artery and placed on the graft itself. A partially occluding clamp is placed on the ascending aorta, and a large entrance to the aorta is made. The graft is sutured to the ascending aorta with continuous fine suture material. *D,* The completed shunt is now opened, and the pericardium is reapproximated because future intracardiac repair is anticipated. (From Ebert, P. A.: Atlas of Congenital Heart Surgery. New York, Churchill Livingstone, 1989.)

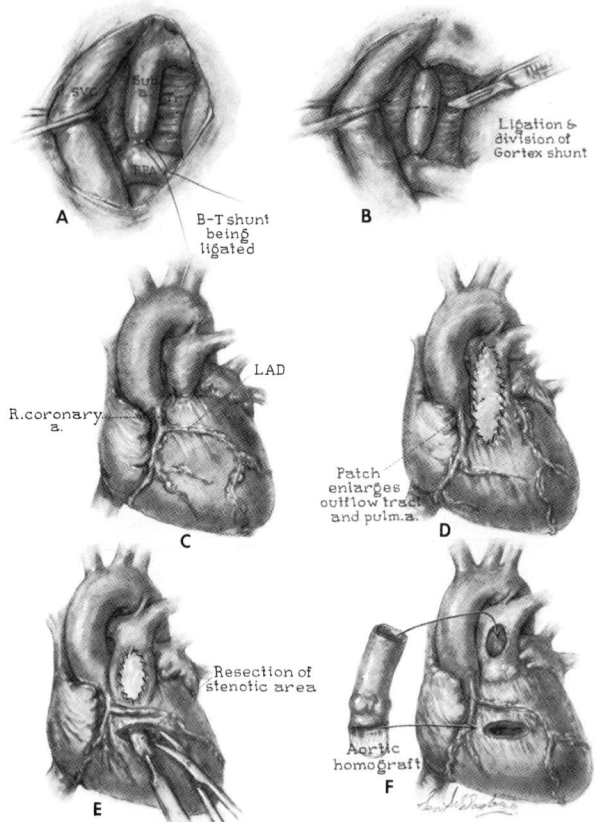

Figure 11. When performing total correction for tetralogy of Fallot previously performed, Blalock-Taussig shunts must be ligated *(A)* or divided if constructed of Gore-Tex *(B)*. The surface anatomy of the right ventricle should be inspected, and the presence of a left anterior descending coronary artery arising from the right coronary artery *(C)* should be noted if present. If there is no coronary anomaly crossing the right ventricular outflow tract, then transanular patching to enlarge the area of pulmonary stenosis can be safely performed *(D)*. The presence of an aberrant coronary artery across the right ventricular outflow tract necessitates an attempt to resect the pulmonary stenosis through two incisions, which can then be patched *(E)* or connected with an external conduit if there is concern that the underlying pulmonary stenosis remains significant *(F)*. (From Ebert, P. A.: Atlas of Congenital Heart Surgery. New York, Churchill Livingstone, 1989.)

defect has been adequately closed, attention must be given to relieving the RV outflow tract obstruction. Once all levels of obstruction have been relieved, the ventricular incision is patched (usually with pericardium although prosthetic material is acceptable). This patch may extend across the valve anulus out to the pulmonary artery bifurcation or may be more limited to a discrete area of infundibular obstruction (see Fig. 11). The patient is then rewarmed and removed from cardiopulmonary bypass. Even if conduction problems are not present, it is recommended that temporary atrial and ventricular pacing wires be left in place for the perioperative period. After the patient has been successfully weaned from cardiopulmonary bypass and the cannulas have been removed, several methods are available for testing for residual ventricular septal shunting. These include selective atrial, ventricular, and pulmonary artery oxygen saturations or pressure measurements. Green dye curves have also been used. Recent experience with intraoperative color flow Doppler, however, may provide a more sensitive and accurate way to assess the quality of the intracardiac repair.[57,130–132] When the surgeon is satisfied with the results of the repair, the chest is closed in the usual manner and the patient returned to an intensive care setting.

Special Situations

Because of the variability of anatomy in patients with TOF, numerous special situations deserve comment. When the left anterior descending coronary artery crosses the RV outflow

tract, a standard transanular enlargement is not feasible, because this would require transection of that coronary artery (see Fig. 11*C*, *E*, and *F*). In these instances (depending on the location of the stenosis), it may be possible to perform a transverse incision in the infundibulum below the coronary artery for closure of the VSD and resection of the infundibular stenosis. If the pulmonary valve requires commissurotomy or the pulmonary artery requires additional enlarging, this can be performed through a separate incision above the pulmonary anulus with patching of the pulmonary artery after valvotomy has been performed.[63,66] (see Fig. 11*E*). These two separate incisions may be preferable to dissection of the coronary artery from the outflow tract with placement of the patch beneath the coronary artery as described by Bonchek.[16] This is because RV distention, which is not uncommon in these patients, can cause coronary ischemia by stretching of the overlying coronary artery. Another alternative in patients with coronary anomalies that prohibit transanular patching is to place a systemic-to-pulmonary artery shunt and allow the patient to grow until such a time that the patient can accept a large enough conduit between the right ventricle and pulmonary artery that total correction by this method can be achieved (see Fig. 11*F*).

Patients with pulmonary atresia who may need a conduit to re-establish continuity between the right ventricle and pulmonary arteries can be palliated with shunts or RV-to-PA conduits until the pulmonary arteries are large enough to allow safe closure of the VSD. If pulmonary artery anatomy is acceptable, one-stage correction with VSD closure and placement of an RV-to-PA conduit can have excellent results. Although these conduits do not need to be valved, increasing experience with homografts has shown that they perform quite well in this situation because the material is easy to work with and more hemostatic than prosthetic conduits. Moreover, there is increasing recognition that pulmonary artery growth may be enhanced if pulmonary insufficiency is avoided.

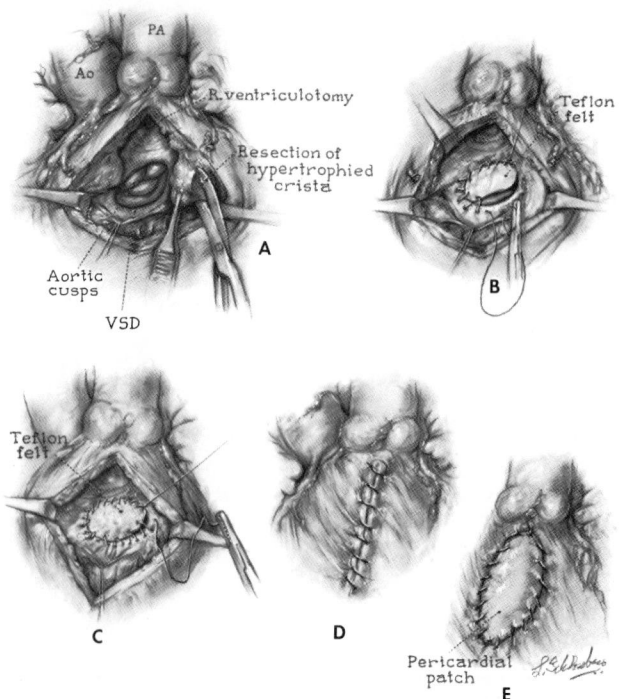

Figure 12. Correction of tetralogy requires adequate resection of infundibular muscle hypertrophy *(A)*, which can be performed through a ventriculotomy as shown as well as through the tricuspid orifice after a right atriotomy. *B* and *C*, The ventricular septal defect is closed with a prosthetic patch; care is taken to avoid the conduction tissue along the posterior-inferior border of the defect. The ventriculotomy is then oversewn *(D)* or more commonly repaired *(E)* with a patch of pericardium or prosthetic material. This patch can be carried across the pulmonary valve anulus if necessary to relieve the underlying outflow stenosis. (From Ebert, P. A.: Atlas of Congenital Heart Surgery. New York, Churchill Livingstone, 1989.)

POSTOPERATIVE MANAGEMENT

Many variables must be followed postoperatively. Pulmonary function is maintained by the use of an endotracheal tube and respirator until the patient's cardiac and respiratory status is stable, maintaining relatively normal values for the arterial Po_2, Pco_2, and pH. Maintenance of an adequate cardiac output is also of crucial importance. In small children, cardiac output may be difficult to measure, although techniques are evolving that will make such measurement easier.[73] It is essential that peripheral perfusion be followed as well as urinary output and acid-base status. It is not uncommon for these patients to have elevated RV pressures postoperatively, and some inotropic support may be necessary. Patients with this disease have small RV volumes and can increase their cardiac output more effectively by increasing heart rate, rather than stroke volume. Therefore, atrial pacing or isoproterenol to increase the heart rate may be useful. The patients should be maintained on a ventilator until they are hemodynamically stable and show good evidence of no longer requiring ventilatory support. Poor peripheral perfusion, indicative of low cardiac output, should be aggressively treated. Mechanical causes such as cardiac tamponade should be excluded and, if necessary, echocardiography performed in the intensive care unit can immediately assess ventricular function and/or the presence of pericardial fluid. Central venous pressure should be adequate, and in patients with poor right ventricular compliance, central venous pressure may be maintained at slightly higher than normal values. In infants and small children, palpation of the liver edge can be a useful indicator of volume status. If the patient has adequate volume status, there should be no hesitation in using an inotropic agent such as dobutamine or dopamine to improve cardiac function. It is not uncommon for these patients to increase their need for inotropic support throughout the course of their first postoperative night. The weight of the patient should be measured daily so that volume status can be followed. It is typical for these patients to show a tendency toward fluid retention, and diuretics can be useful. Because prosthetic materials are routinely used for palliation or correction of this lesion, perioperative broad-spectrum antibiotics should be commonplace. Arrhythmias, when they occur, can often be diagnosed by use of the temporary pacing wires so that treatment can be directed specifically to each individual arrhythmia. Patients with heart block should have AV sequential pacing until conduction returns to normal through the AV node.

If conduction has not returned in 5 to 6 days, it is likely that the patient requires placement of a permanent pacemaker. The hemodynamic results after intracardiac repair of the TOF have been assessed in several series. Surgical repair in infants under deep hypothermia has been compared hemodynamically with correction by conventional cardiopulmonary bypass with results equal to or better than those with deep hypothermia.[100] In a companion study, left ventricular dysfunction as determined after an afterload stress was found to be present postoperatively in those patients who had open correction at an older age but not in patients who underwent repair during infancy. This raises the possibility that early definitive repair may help to preserve postoperative left ventricular function.[17] In another study, the current status of a group of patients who had undergone surgical correction of tetralogy and had survived through adulthood was evaluated. For the 233 studied, it was concluded that clinical assessment alone is not predictive of the hemodynamic result and that for objective follow-up, cardiac catheterization should be performed in all patients. The combination of persistent elevation of right ventricular systolic pressure above 60 mm. Hg and ventricular premature depolarizations places the patient at risk of sudden death. However, 80 per cent of the patients lived a normal life without impairment of intellect, exercise tolerance, or fertility.[46]

With regard to the incidence of sudden death following correction of tetralogy, in a study of 243 patients evaluated with special emphasis on postoperative conduction disturbances, sudden death occurred in 7 patients, with an average follow-up of 12 years (range, 6.5 to 16.5 years). Among these patients, four deaths were in those with right bundle branch block, and 3 of these 4 patients had premature ventricular contractions for more than 1 month postoperatively. Premature ventricular contractions were documented in 10 of the 158 patients with right bundle branch block, and sudden death occurred in 3. Three of the 10 patients with the trifascicular block pattern died suddenly, but no deaths occurred in 24 patients with the bifascicular block pattern. The authors of this study concluded that the risk of sudden death in patients with right bundle branch block and premature ventricular contractions following tetralogy repair is high and warrants consideration of suppressive therapy.[113] With the advances in detection and surgical treatment of recurrent sustained ventricular tachycardia, a new approach to the therapy of these problems has arisen. Ventricular tachyarrhythmias are estimated to occur in from 0.3 to 3 per cent of patients following complete repair and have not appeared to be related to the hemodynamic success of the repair. A report in patients experiencing from 30 to 150 documented episodes of sustained ventricular tachycardia with failure of pharmacologic and pacing regimens indicated that the source of the arrhythmia was localized to the right ventriculotomy scar by electrophysiologic mapping.[59] The scar was surgically excised, and ventricular tachycardia was not inducible after operation and has not recurred following surgical excision of the scar in these patients. These data support the enthusiasm for transatrial repair of tetralogy when possible, although it remains to be proven that this will provide long-term protection from dysrhythmias. Contrary to these data are the findings of Garson and Cooley[47] that ventricular arrhythmias after repair of the TOF are primarily related to persistent RV outflow tract obstruction, suggesting that ventriculotomy with adequate patching to completely relieve the infundibular obstruction should provide (and has in their series) excellent long-term results with respect to freedom from ventricular ectopy. It appears that long-term success of repair is based on many factors that mandate continued investigation.[143]

Of increasing significance are those patients with TOF who also have major additional congenital cardiac anomalies. One of the more interesting associations is that with complete atrioventricular canal. Several studies have emphasized the fact that total correction of this combination consists of closure of the VSD as well as the ASD and reconstruction of the AV valve with relief of RV outflow tract obstruction.[7] A double-outlet right ventricle has also been reported with successful correction.[106] In addition, patients with TOF and associated aortic insufficiency[94] with aorticopulmonary window,[22] with anomalous origin of the left coronary artery from the pulmonary artery,[1] and with diverticulum of the right ventricle[92] have undergone successful repair.

It is possible to correct the tetralogy with extracorporeal circulation in patients with sickle cell anemia, including those with glucose-6-phosphate dehydrogenase deficiency. Intracardiac procedures can be performed safely on these patients if certain guidelines are observed, especially the avoidance of hypoxia, hypothermia, acidosis, and dehydration. The patient should be prepared for operation with transfusion of normal red cells.[124]

RESULTS

TOF is now being corrected with an ever diminishing mortality. The results with open correction during the recent past have been impressive. Nevertheless, it is important to realize that the spectrum of this disease with respect to the age at presentation as well as the severity of the anatomic derangements can greatly affect the outcome. Overall, the mortality in most series is between 1 and 5 per cent when the repair is done primarily or after

TABLE 1. Risks for Patients Undergoing Correction of Tetralogy of Fallot*

Category	n	Hospital Deaths		70% CL† (%)
		No. of Patients	Percentage of Patients	
Uncomplicated	89	2	2.2	0.7–5.3
Pulmonary arterial problems	22	3‡	14	6–26
Absent pulmonary valve	6	2§	33	12–62
Major associated cardiac anomalies	16	5‖	31	18–47
Multiple VSDs¶	4	2	50	18–82
Complete AV** canal defect	11	3	27	12–47
Others	1	0	0	0–85
More than one previous palliative operation	6	2††	33	12–62

*These risks increase with the problems listed. Patients with no risk factors have an overall operative mortality between 1 and 5 per cent in most centers.
†CL, confidence limit.
‡One patient was 10 months old; two patients were 30 months old.
§Ages were 7 and 15 days.
‖Ages were 8, 17, 17, 26, and 30 months.
¶VSD, ventricular septal defect.
**AV, atrioventricular.
††Ages were 17 and 69 months.
From Sabiston, D. C. Jr., and Spencer, F. C.: (Eds.) Surgery of the Chest. Philadelphia, W. B. Saunders Company, 1990, p. 1340.

a single systemic-to-pulmonary artery shunt. With improved techniques, excellent results with early one-stage repair in infants have been reported.[21,56] Likewise, the mortality for infants receiving palliative shunts is low and can be expected to be between 0.5 and 3 per cent, depending on the severity of the lesion and the type of shunt chosen.[77] Improved techniques of myocardial protection with hypothermia, cold cardioplegia, and even total circulatory arrest are enabling more precise anatomic repairs in younger infants with excellent results. Nevertheless, patients receiving total correction before 1 year of age have an increased risk, compared with patients over 1 year of age (Table 1).[6,8,76] This may be a reflection of the severity of their anatomy.

Early postoperative risks include the creation of heart block, which should occur in fewer than 1 per cent of patients of all ages, and residual ventricular septal defects, which should occur in fewer than 4 per cent of patients.[8,77]

PULMONARY STENOSIS WITH INTACT VENTRICULAR SEPTUM

Stenosis of the pulmonary valve with intact ventricular septum can be one of the most favorable congenital cardiac lesions from the point of view of treatment. It can also be a highly lethal lesion with dismal prognosis. Much of this depends on the size of the right ventricular chamber as well as the age of the patient at presentation.[36] For favorable cases, the symptoms are generally less pronounced than with TOF, although there are numerous examples of infants with extremely severe pulmonary stenosis producing congestive heart failure. Some infants require immediate valvotomy as an emergency procedure; but in the majority, the symptoms develop more slowly. In approximately three fourths of this group, the foramen ovale is patent. With development of increased pressure and decreased compliance in the right ventricle, blood is shunted to the left atrium, and cyanosis ensues. Clubbing of the fingers may appear later. The pulmonary valvar commissures are fused into a dome-shaped structure with a small central lumen. A jet of blood that is forced through the aperture under great pressure from the right ventricle into the pulmonary artery creates turbulence and a prominent thrill (Fig. 13). Poststenotic dilatation of the main pulmonary artery ensues. In many instances, infundibular stenosis may be associated with valvar stenosis and an intact ventricular septum.[109] Moreover, ASDs are also encountered, the latter

combination being called *the trilogy of Fallot*. The clinical findings are dependent on the severity of the valvar pulmonary stenosis and the patency of the foramen ovale.[37] In older children, exertional dyspnea is the most common complaint. Cyanosis is usually present in those patients with a patent foramen ovale or an ASD. A harsh systolic murmur and thrill are present over the pulmonary area; the thrill can be palpated in the suprasternal notch. The pulmonary second sound is characteristically weak or absent. The chest film is often typical, demonstrating prominence of the pulmonary artery due to poststenotic dilatation (Fig. 14). The angiocardiogram is also helpful in demonstrating the classic dome-shaped pulmonary valve with small aperture and poststenotic dilatation, or an ASD and infundibular stenosis combined with valvar stenosis. Cardiac catheterization demonstrates a gradient between the right ventricle and the pulmonary artery without evidence of a shunt at the ventricular level. In severe forms, the pressure gradient between the pulmonary artery and the right ventricle may exceed 200 mm. Hg.

Pulmonary atresia with an intact ventricular septum represents a very serious condition in infancy. Although this is not a common lesion, it usually demands urgent therapy quite early

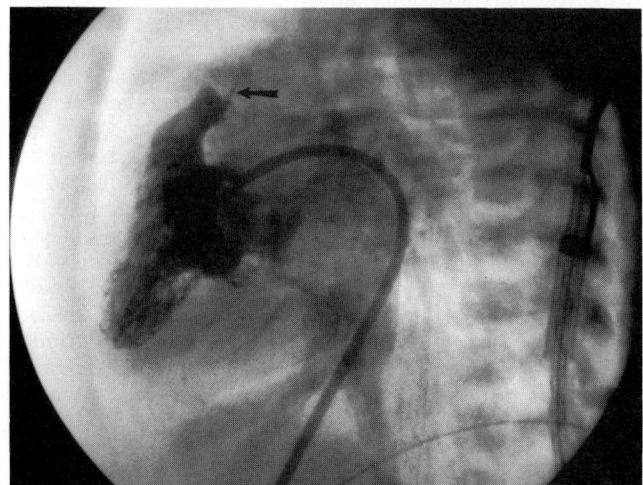

Figure 13. Angiocardiogram of a patient with critical pulmonary stenosis. Note the jet of blood (arrow) forced through the narrow pulmonary orifice. The main pulmonary artery demonstrates poststenotic dilatation.

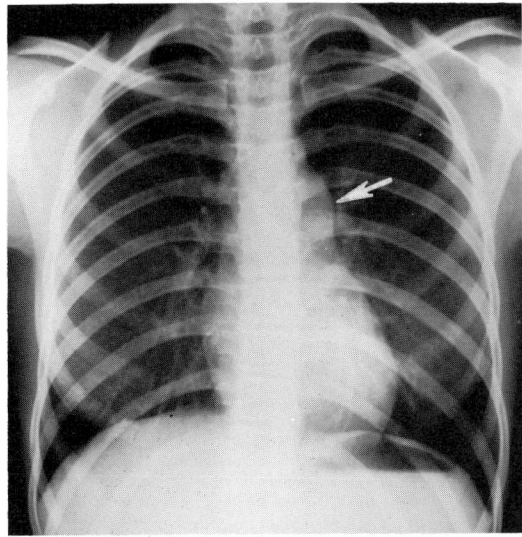

Figure 14. Chest film of a patient with isolated valvular pulmonary stenosis, demonstrating the typical appearance of poststenotic dilatation of the pulmonary artery (arrow).

in life. Infants with the combination of pulmonary atresia and an intact ventricular septum usually present within 24 to 48 hours of birth with dyspnea, tachypnea, and progressive cyanosis. A PDA is usually present, as well as a right ventricular heave and murmurs of tricuspid insufficiency. Ductal patency can be ensured by prostaglandin infusion while therapy is planned. Those in whom symptoms are not as prominent until several weeks or several months later usually have a widely patent ductus arteriosus. Arrhythmias, probably the result of right ventricular hypertension and right atrial dilatation, may be present. Cardiomegaly is demonstrated on the chest film together with diminished pulmonary vascular markings. The electrocardiogram usually shows a normal axis with left ventricular predominance in the precordial leads. The size of the right ventricular cavity can be assessed by echocardiography; the diagnosis together with details of anatomic and physiologic changes is best determined by cardiac catheterization and angiocardiography. Factors of considerable importance in planning therapy in these infants include the size of the main pulmonary artery and the right and left branches, the size and characteristics of the right ventricular cavity, the presence and relative size of a PDA.[71,99,137] Approximately 30 to 50 per cent of infants with pulmonary atresia and intact ventricular septum have fistulous connections between the right ventricle and the coronary arteries, and 30 per cent of these patients have significant coronary artery stenosis. Because these patients tend to

have small RV cavities with suprasystemic RV pressures, the coronary flow is often supplied from the right ventricle and decompression of the RV chamber can lead to coronary steal and myocardial ischemia. This subgroup of patients comprises a highly lethal spectrum of this disease for which cardiac transplantation may be warranted.

Treatment

Pulmonary valvotomy was introduced by Brock (1948)[19] and consisted of transventricular valvotomy. A valvulotome was passed through the wall of the right ventricle into the pulmonary artery to open the stenotic valve. Later, an improved valvulotome was designed for transventricular use.[112] Increasing success is now being reported by the use of percutaneous balloon valvuloplasty in the cardiac catheterization lab.[81,82,90] Nevertheless, open repair of valvular stenosis under direct vision produces excellent results when balloon valvotomy fails. Although some groups recommend valvotomy under inflow occlusion,[26] the use of extracorporeal circulation permits simultaneous correction of coexisting ASDs and of infundibular stenosis when indicated.[96,109] Moreover, the use of cardiopulmonary bypass allows stabilization of critically ill neonates and affords the time necessary for appropriate surgical treatment, since patients in whom balloon valvuloplasty fails often have more complex anatomy (Fig. 15).

Most infants with the combination of pulmonary atresia and intact ventricular septum become critically ill quite early in life and demand urgent therapy. In most, a patent ductus arteriosus is responsible for maintenance of life, and the infusion of PGE₁ can be helpful in preventing ductal closure and the associated severe hypoxemia and acidosis that would otherwise follow. Although closed valvotomy, systemic-pulmonary shunt, and combination procedures have been used, at present the preferred management appears to be combined open valvotomy and shunt.[71] Patients with normal size right ventricles may not need concomitant shunting,[24] but most groups have found that placement of a systemic-pulmonary shunt at the time of open valvotomy ensures adequate pulmonary blood flow after the ductus is allowed to close and until RV compliance improves to provide substantial antegrade flow.[99] If there is satisfaction over the degree of RV-to-PA continuity established, then temporary postoperative continuation of prostaglandins may ameliorate the necessity of placement of a shunt at the time of valvotomy.[43] Equal to the importance of ensuring pulmonary blood flow after valvotomy is the concept of establishing widely patent RV-to-PA continuity. Not only does this appear to prevent the development of sinusoids between the right ventricle and the coronary artery system, but it now appears fairly clear that it potentiates growth of the right ventricle to optimize its potential as a usable portion of the anatomy.[86,137] It also appears that with

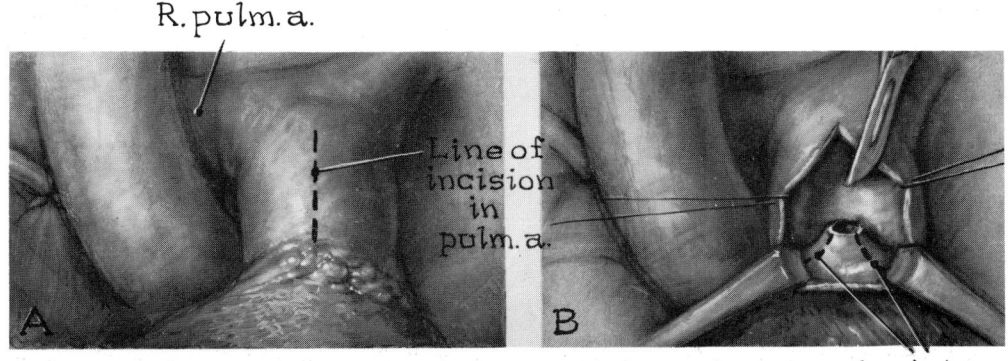

Figure 15. Pulmonary valvotomy can be performed during inflow occlusion or, preferably, on cardiopulmonary bypass. A, The pulmonary artery is opened above the valve anulus. B, The valve is inspected. It can then be incised along the areas of commissural fusion. In addition, the right ventricular chamber should be inspected and any areas of infundibular stenosis resected through the valvotomy. The pulmonary artery can be closed primarily or with a small patch of pericardium.

adequate relief of the RV outflow obstruction, infundibular hypertrophy resolves over time, producing a more normal right ventricle.[54] These considerations are important because failure to encourage growth of the right ventricle may result in its ultimate inability to provide normal function and require transformation of the circuit to a univentricular arrangement (Fontan's procedure).

Valvotomy by open correction of pulmonary valvar stenosis yields excellent results, and recurrence of the condition is rare. Moreover, the compensatory infundibular hypertrophy that frequently accompanies the valvar stenosis usually regresses with time. Although the gradient between the right ventricle and the pulmonary artery may not be totally abolished immediately after operation, regression of the secondary hypertrophy of the RV outflow tract occurs, and repeat catheterization later shows a marked reduction in the gradient.[38]

Isolated infundibular stenosis of the right ventricle may also occur as a congenital anomaly. The symptoms are quite similar to those of valvar stenosis, although the murmur may be located somewhat lower in the precordium. The angiocardiogram demonstrates the lesion with precision, and cardiac catheterization demonstrates two gradients: (1) between the pulmonary artery and (2) between the infundibulum and the right ventricle. Two-dimensional echocardiography can demonstrate this lesion beautifully and show why it is often referred to as "double-chamber right ventricle". Management of these cases is resection of the infundibular stenosis (which is often a hypertrophied moderator band) in the open heart employing extracorporeal circulation. The results are excellent.

SELECTED REFERENCES

Arciniegas, E., Farooki, Z. Q., Hakimi, J., and Green, E. W.: Results of a two-stage surgical treatment of tetralogy of Fallot. J. Thorac. Cardiovasc. Surg., 79:876, 1980.

This group reports 109 consecutive patients undergoing palliative shunt as the initial management for symptomatic tetralogy of Fallot. The total early shunt mortality, including the Blalock-Taussig as well as Waterston shunts, was 2.7 per cent. The mean patient age at the time of total repair was 4.8 years, and the second-stage corrective operation had a mortality of 1.6 per cent. They consider the Blalock-Taussig shunt to be the shunt of choice in all symptomatic infants and small children with tetralogy of Fallot and emphasize that the two-stage surgical approach compares favorably with primary total correction, particularly in infants under 1 year of age.

Bharati, S., Lev, M., and Kirklin, J. W.: Cardiac Surgery and the Conduction System. New York, John Wiley & Sons, 1983.

This beautifully illustrated monograph depicts the location of cardiac conduction tissue through a variety of standard surgical approaches. Increasing success with total repair of lesions such as tetralogy of Fallot is related to greater understanding of the location of specialized conduction tissue so that injury to this tissue can be routinely and reliably prevented during open cardiac procedures. The contribution toward that understanding by these authors is extensive.

Blalock, A., and Taussig, H. B.: The surgical treatment of malformations of the heart in which there is pulmonary stenosis or pulmonary atresia. J.A.M.A., 128:189, 1945.

In this paper, Blalock's first three operations for creation of a systemic-pulmonary anastomosis are reported. The first patient, a 15-month-old infant with severe cyanosis, had a history of multiple episodes of loss of consciousness. An anastomosis of the left subclavian artery to the left pulmonary artery was made, and the clinical improvement was striking. Two additional patients with successful results are also described. It is of interest that Blalock refers to earlier experimental work in which subclavian pulmonary anastomoses were performed in the dog in an effort to produce pulmonary hypertension. Although these experiments did not succeed in producing an elevated pulmonary arterial pressure, the operation was subsequently used for an entire different purpose. This procedure was the first of many additional cardiac surgical advances.

Castaneda, A. R., Freed, M. D., Williams, R. G., and Norwood, W. I.: Repair of tetralogy of Fallot in infancy: Early and late results. J. Thorac. Cardiovasc. Surg., 74:372, 1977.

These authors report a series of 41 consecutive infants operated on for primary correction of the tetralogy of Fallot with deep hypothermia and circulatory arrest. The infants ranged in age from 12 days to 1 year, with a mean age of 5 to 7 months. The authors conclude that the hospital mortality and early and late results justify continued evaluation of primary repair of tetralogy of Fallot in symptomatic infants, regardless of weight or age. The contraindications that they cite to reparative

operation in symptomatic infants with the tetralogy are an anterior descending coronary artery arising from the right coronary artery or associated congenital pulmonary atresia.

Foker, J. E., Braunlin, E. A., St. Cyr, J. A., Hunter, D., Molina, J. E., Moller, J. H., and Ring, W. S.: Management of pulmonary atresia with intact ventricular septum. J. Thorac. Cardiovasc. Surg., 92:706, 1986.

These authors report their clinical experience with 50 neonates with a diagnosis of pulmonary atresia with an intact ventricular septum. The goal of therapeutic intervention was to re-establish right ventricle-to-pulmonary artery continuity in order to encourage any potential right ventricular growth. In addition, placement of a systemic-to-pulmonary artery shunt was avoided in all patients by utilizing continued prostaglandin E_1 infusion in the postoperative period. This study suggests that patients with pulmonary atresia can be adequately managed by attempts at salvaging the right ventricle and that placement of an aortopulmonary shunt can often be avoided if one can patiently wait for the re-establishment of antegrade flow from the right heart. With successful application of this technique, management of pulmonary atresia with an intact ventricular septum can be accomplished as a one-stage procedure.

Gustafson, R. A., Murray, G. F., Warden, H. E., Hill, R. C., and Rozar, G. E.: Early primary repair of tetralogy of Fallot. Ann. Thorac. Surg., 45:235, 1988.

These authors report their experience with total correction of tetralogy of Fallot in 40 patients. Ten patients were less than 1 year of age, and the mean age of the other 30 patients was 24 months. Their operative mortality for this series was 0 per cent. The results of their study suggest that early primary repair of tetralogy of Fallot is justified in symptomatic children regardless of age or weight. In addition, they did not find any impact on operative mortality from the use of a transanular RVOT patch.

Kirklin, J. W., Blackstone, E. H., Kirklin, J. K., Pacifico, A. D., Aramendi, J., and Bargeron, L. M., Jr.: Surgical results and protocols in the spectrum of tetralogy of Fallot. Ann. Surg., 198:251, 1983.

This study reports the results that this outstanding group had with 1103 operations performed for tetralogy of Fallot of all types between 1967 and 1982. Analysis of this large number of patients allows description of incremental risk factors for operative mortality as well as recommendations for patients who should receive primary versus staged repair. Risks of correction ranged from 1.6 to 7.7 per cent, depending upon the age of the patient and the nature of the lesion.

Kirklin, J. W., and Barratt-Boyes, B. G.: Ventricular septal defect and pulmonary stenosis or atresia. In Cardiac Surgery. New York, John Wiley and Sons, 1986, p. 699.

This remarkable book catalogs the extraordinary experience of these two well known figures in the field of congenital heart surgery. The material included in this book is among the most comprehensive and well organized presentations available and should be read by anyone who desires in-depth reading in this field.

Lillehei, C. W., Varco, R. L., Cohen, M., Warden, H. E., Patton, C., and Moller, J. H.: The first open heart repairs of ventricular septal defect, atrioventricular communis and tetralogy of Fallot using extracorporeal circulation by cross-circulation: A thirty year follow-up. Ann. Thorac. Surg., 41:4, 1986.

More than just a 30-year follow-up of the first patients to successfully undergo open cardiac correction of complex cardiac lesions, this article provides a poignant recapitulation of the early days of open heart surgery. Dr. Lillehei's historical account of the frustrations and ingenious attempts by the intrepid individuals who began the era of open heart surgery that is now so commonplace should be read by anyone who has read this chapter. Of equal impact are the thoughts offered by the discussants, who include some of the more prominent figures in the field of cardiac surgery. Having read this paper, one will have a better understanding of the historical debt that is owed to those individuals with the insight and creativity to approach the problems of open cardiac surgery.

Moulton, A. L., Bowman, F. O., Jr., Edie, R. N., Hayes, C. J., Ellis, J., Gersony, W. M., and Malm, J. R.: Pulmonary atresia with intact ventricular septum. Sixteen-year experience. J. Thorac. Cardiovasc. Surg., 78:527, 1979.

This is a review of 30 patients with pulmonary atresia and intact ventricular septum treated by a variety of surgical approaches over a 16-year period. The authors conclude that in the majority of patients the preferred operation is combined pulmonary valvotomy (or outflow patch) together with a systemic-pulmonary shunt. This approach has yielded the best long-term results thus far.

Taussig, H. B.: Tetralogy of Fallot: Early history and late results. Neuhauser Lecture. Am. J. Roentgenol., 133:423, 1979.

This is a classic and updated reference written by a distinguished pediatric cardiologist. She summarizes the early and late results of the Blalock-Taussig operation in a large series of patients. In addition, an excellent historical review of the subject is included.

Turley, K., Tucker, W. Y., Ebert, P.A.: The changing role of palliative procedures in the treatment of infants with congenital heart disease. J. Thorac. Cardiovasc. Surg., 79:194, 1980.

These authors question the need for palliation in certain lesions, specifically transposition of the great arteries, tetralogy of Fallot, ventricular septal defect, and truncus arteriosus. Although previously palliated by many groups prior to the publication of this article, the feasibility of good results with early total correction is documented. In many ways, this landmark article encouraged numerous individuals to begin thinking about early total repair for complicated congenital heart defects.

REFERENCES

1. Akasaka, T., Itoh, K., Ohkawa, Y., Nakayama, S., Miyamoto, H., Nishi, T., Satoh, H., and Takarada, M.: Surgical treatment of anomalous origin of the left coronary artery from the pulmonary artery associated with tetralogy of Fallot. Ann. Thorac. Surg., 31:469, 1981.
2. Amato, J. J., Marbey, M. L., Bush, C., et al.: Systemic pulmonary polytetrafluoroethylene shunts in palliative operations for congenital heart disease: Revival of the central shunt. J. Thorac. Cardiovasc. Surg., 95:62, 1988.
3. Anderson, R. H., Path, M. R. C., Allwork, S. P., et al.: Surgical anatomy of tetralogy of Fallot. J. Thorac. Cardiovasc. Surg., 81:887, 1981.
4. Arciniegas, E., Blackstone, E. H., Pacifico, A. D., and Kirklin, J. W.: Classic shunting operations as part of two-stage repair for tetralogy of Fallot. Ann. Thorac. Surg., 27:514, 1978.
5. Arciniegas, E., Farooki, Z. Q., Hakimi, M., et al.: Results of two-stage surgical treatment of tetralogy of Fallot. J. Thorac. Cardiovasc. Surg., 79:876, 1980.
6. Arciniegas, E., Farooki, Z. Q., Hakimi, M., et al.: Early and late results of total correction of tetralogy of Fallot. J. Thorac. Cardiovasc. Surg., 80:770, 1980.
7. Arciniegas, E., Hakimi, M., Farooki, Z. Q., and Green, E. W.: Results of total correction of tetralogy of Fallot with complete atrioventricular canal. J. Thorac. Cardiovasc. Surg., 81:768, 1981.
8. Arciniegas, E.: Tetralogy of Fallot. In Pediatric Cardiac Surgery. Chicago, Year Book Medical Publishers, 1985.
9. Barragry, T. P., Ring, W. S., and Blatchford, J. W.: Central aortopulmonary artery shunts in neonates with complex cyanotic congenital heart disease. J. Thorac. Cardiovasc. Surg., 93:767, 1987.
10. Bertranou, E. G., Blackstone, E. H., Hazelrig, J. B., et al.: Life expectancy without surgery in tetralogy of Fallot. Am. J. Cardiol., 42:458, 1978.
11. Bharati, S., Lev, M., and Kirklin, J. W.: Cardiac Surgery and the Conduction System. New York, John Wiley & Sons, 1983.
12. Blackstone, E. H., Kirklin, J. W., Bertranou, E. G., et al.: Preoperative prediction from cineangiograms of postrepair right ventricular pressure in tetralogy of Fallot. J. Thorac. Cardiovasc. Surg., 78:542, 1979.
13. Blackstone, E. H., Kirklin, J. W., and Pacifico, A. D.: Decision-making in repair of tetralogy of Fallot based on intraoperative measurements of pulmonary arterial outflow tract. J. Thorac. Cardiovasc. Surg., 77:526, 1979.
14. Blalock, A.: Surgical procedures employed and anatomical variations encountered in the treatment of congenital pulmonic stenosis. Surg. Gynecol. Obstet., 87:385, 1948.
15. Blalock, A., and Taussig, H. B.: The surgical treatment of malformations of the heart in which there is pulmonary stenosis or pulmonary atresia. J.A.M.A., 128:189, 1945.
16. Bonchek, L. I., Starr, A., Sunderland, C. O., et al.: Natural history of tetralogy of Fallot. Circulation, 48:392, 1973.
17. Borow, K. M., Green, L. H., Castaneda, A. R., and Keane, J. F.: Left ventricular function after repair of tetralogy of Fallot and its relationship to age at surgery. Circulation, 61:1150, 1980.
18. Bove, E. L., Byrum, C. J., et al.: The influence of pulmonary insufficiency on ventricular function following repair of tetralogy of Fallot: Evaluation using radionuclide ventriculography. J. Thorac. Cardiovasc. Surg., 85:691, 1983.
19. Brock, R. C.: Pulmonary valvulotomy for the relief of congenital pulmonary stenosis: Report of 3 cases. Br. Med. J., 1:1121, 1948.
20. Calder, A. L., Barratt-Boyes, B. G., Brandt, P. W. T., and Neutze, J. M.: Postoperative evaluation of patients with tetralogy of Fallot repaired in infancy. J. Thorac. Cardiovasc. Surg., 77:704, 1979.
21. Castaneda, A. R., Freed, M. D., Williams, R. G., and Norwood, W. I.: Repair of tetralogy of Fallot in infancy: Early and late results. J. Thorac. Cardiovasc. Surg., 74:372, 1977.
22. Castaneda, A. R., and Kirklin, J. W.: Tetralogy of Fallot with aorticopulmonary window: Report of two surgical cases. J. Thorac. Cardiovasc. Surg., 74:467, 1977.
23. Castaneda, A. R., and Norwood, W. I.: Fallot's tetralogy. In Stark, J., and de Leval, M. (Eds.): Surgery for Congenital Heart Defects. New York, Grune & Stratton, 1983.
24. Cobanoglu, A., Metzdorff, M. T., Pinson, C. W., et al.: Valvotomy for pulmonary atresia with intact ventricular septum. J. Thorac. Cardiovasc. Surg., 89:482, 1985.
25. Coles, J. G., Kirklin, J. W., Pacifico, A. D., et al.: The relief of pulmonary stenosis by a transatrial versus a transventricular approach to the repair of tetralogy of Fallot. Ann. Thorac. Surg., 45:7, 1988.
26. Coles, J. G., Freedom, R. M., Olley, P. M., et al.: Surgical management of critical pulmonary stenosis. Ann. Thorac. Surg., 38:458, 1984.
27. Cooley, D. A.: Techniques in Cardiac Surgery, 2nd ed. W. B. Saunders Company, Philadelphia, 1984.
28. Dabizzi, R. P., Caprioli, G., and Alazzi, L: Distribution and anomalies of coronary arteries in tetralogy of Fallot. Circulation, 61:84, 1980.
29. de Leval, M. R., McKay, R., Jones, M., et al.: Modified Blalock-Taussig shunt: Use of subclavian artery orifice as flow regulator in prosthetic systemic-pulmonary artery shunts. J. Thorac. Cardiovasc. Surg., 81:112, 1981.
30. del Nido, P. J., Mickle, D. A., Wilson, G. J., et al.: Inadequate myocardial protection with cold cardioplegic arrest during repair of tetralogy of Fallot. J. Thorac. Cardiovasc. Surg., 95:223, 1988.
31. Donahoo, J. S., Roland, J. M., Kan, J., et al.: Prostaglandin E₁ as an adjunct to emergency cardiac operations in neonates. J. Thorac. Cardiovasc. Surg., 81:227, 1981.
32. Ebert, P. A., Robinson, S. J., Stanger, P., and Engle, M. A.: Pulmonary artery conduits in infants younger than six months of age. J. Thorac. Cardiovasc. Surg., 72:351, 1976.
33. Ebert, P.A.: Past, present, and future of palliative shunts. Adv. Cardiol., 26:127, 1979.
34. Ebert, P.A.: Discussion of Piehler, J. M., Danielson, G. K., McGoon, D. C., et al.: Management of pulmonary atresia with ventricular septal defect and hypoplastic pulmonary arteries by right ventricular outflow construction. J. Thorac. Cardiovasc. Surg., 80:552, 1980.
35. Ebert, P.A.: Atlas of Congenital Cardiac Surgery. New York, Churchill Livingstone, 1989.
36. Engle, M. A., Tomiko, I., and Goldberg, H. P.: The fate of a patient with pulmonic stenosis. Circulation, 30:554, 1964.
37. Engle, M. A., and Taussig, H. B.: Valvular pulmonic stenosis with intact ventricular septum and patent foramen ovale: Report of illustrative cases and analysis of clinical syndrome. Circulation, 2:481, 1950.
38. Engle, M. A., Holswade, G. R., Goldberg, H. P., et al.: Regression after open valvotomy of infundibular stenosis accompanying severe valvular pulmonic stenosis. Circulation, 17:862, 1958.
39. Fallot, E. L. A.: Contribution a fanatomic pathologique de la maladie bleue (cyanose cardiaque). Marseille Med., 25:77, 138, 207, 270, 341, 403, 1888.
40. Farre, J. R.: Pathological Researches. SA I. On malformations of the human heart: Illustrated by numerous cases, and preceded by some observations on the method of improving the diagnostic part of medicine. London, Longmans, Green & Co., 1814.
41. Fellows, K. E., Freed, M. K., Keane, J. R., et al.: Results of routine preoperative coronary angiography in tetralogy of Fallot. Circulation, 51:561, 1975.
42. Fellows, K. E., Smith, J., and King, J. F.: Preoperative angiocardiography in infants with tetrad of Fallot: Review of 36 cases. Am. J. Cardiol., 47:1279, 1981.
43. Foker, J. E., Braulin, E. A., St. Cyr, J. A., et al.: Management of pulmonary atresia with intact ventricular septum. J. Thorac. Cardiovasc. Surg., 92:706, 1986.
44. Fort, L., III, Morrow, A. G., Pierce, G. E., Saigusa, M., and McLaughlin, J. S.: The distribution of pulmonary blood flow after subclavian-pulmonary anastomosis: An experimental study. J. Thorac. Cardiovasc. Surg., 50:671, 1965.
45. Freed, M. D., Heymann, M. A., Lewis, A. B., et al: Prostaglandin E₁ in infants with ductus arteriosus–dependent congenital heart disease. Circulation, 64:899, 1981.
46. Garson, A., Nihill, M. R., McNamara, D. G., and Cooley, D. A.: Status of the adult and adolescent after repair of tetralogy of Fallot. Circulation, 59:1232, 1979.
47. Garson, A., Jr., McNamara, D. G., and Cooley, D. A.: Tetralogy of Fallot. In Roberts, W. C. (Ed.): Adult Congenital Heart Disease. Philadelphia, F. A. Davis Company, 1987.
48. Gay, W. A., Jr., and Ebert, P. A.: Aorta-to-right pulmonary anastomosis causing obstruction to the right pulmonary artery. Ann. Thorac. Surg., 16:402, 1973.
49. Gintrac, E.: Observations et Recherches sur la Cyanose, ou Maladie Bleue. Paris, J. Pinard, 1824.
50. Glenn, W. W. L., and Patino, J. F.: Circulatory bypass of the right heart. I. Preliminary observation on direct delivery of vena caval blood into pulmonary arterial circulation: Azygos vein–pulmonary artery shunt. Yale J. Biol. Med., 27:147, 1954.
51. Gotsman, M. S.: Increasing obstruction to the outflow tract in Fallot's tetralogy. Br. Heart J. 28:615, 1966.
52. Graham, T. P., Jr., Cordell, D., Atwood, G. F., et al.: Right ventricular volume characteristics before and after palliative and reparative operation in tetralogy of Fallot. Circulation, 54:417, 1976.
53. Greeley, W. J., Stanley, T. E., Ungerleider, R. M., and Kisslo, J. A.: Intraoperative hypoxemic spells in tetralogy of Fallot: An echocardiographic analysis of diagnosis and treatment. Anesth. Analg. 68:815, 1989.
54. Griffith, B. P., Hardesty, R. L., Siewers, R. D., et al.: Pulmonary valvulotomy alone for pulmonary stenosis: Results in children with and without muscular infundibular hypertrophy. J. Thorac. Cardiovasc. Surg., 83:577, 1982.
55. Guo-Wei, H., and Chia-Chiang, K.: Pulmonic regurgitation and reconstruction of right ventricular outflow tract with patch. J. Thorac. Cardiovasc. Surg., 92:128, 1986.
56. Gustafson, R. A., Murray, G. F., Warden, H. E., et al.: Early primary repair of tetralogy of Fallot. Ann. Thorac. Surg., 45:235, 1988.
57. Hagler, D. J., Tajik, A. J., Seward, J. B., et al.: Intraoperative two-dimensional Doppler echocardiography. J. Thorac. Cardiovasc. Surg., 95:516, 1988.
58. Hammon, J. W., Henry, C. L., Merrill, W. H., et al.: Tetralogy of Fallot: Selective surgical management can minimize operative mortality. Ann. Thorac. Surg., 40:280, 1985.
59. Harken, A. H., Horowitz, L. N., and Josephson, M. E.: Surgical correction of recurrent sustained ventricular tachycardia following complete repair of tetralogy of Fallot. J. Thorac. Cardiovasc. Surg., 80:779, 1980.
60. Hartmann, R. C.: Hemorrhagic disorder occurring in patients with cyanotic congenital heart disease. Bull. Johns Hopkins Hosp., 91:49, 1952.
61. Hope, J.: A treatise on the disease of the heart and great vessels, and on the affections which may be mistaken for them. London, J. Churchill & Sons, 1839.
62. Hudspeth, A. S., Cordell, A. R., and Johnston, F. R.: Transatrial approach to total correction of tetralogy of Fallot. Circulation, 27:796, 1963.

63. Humes, R. A., Driscoll, D. J., Danielson, G. K., et al.: Tetralogy of Fallot with anomalous origin or left anterior descending coronary artery: Surgical options. J. Thorac. Cardiovasc. Surg., 94:784, 1987.

64. Hunter, J.: Medical Observations and Inquiries by a Society of Physicians of London. London, 1757–1784.

65. Hunter, W.: Three cases of malformation of the heart. Case II. Medical Observations and Inquiries by a Society of Physicians in London, 6:291, 1784.

66. Hurwitz, R. A., Smith, W., King, H., et al.: Tetralogy of Fallot with abnormal coronary artery: 1967 to 1977. J. Thorac. Cardiovasc. Surg., 80:129, 1980.

67. Ilbawi, M. N., Idriss, F. S., Muster, A. J., et al.: Tetralogy of Fallot with absent pulmonary valve: Should valve insertion be part of the intracardiac repair? J. Thorac. Cardiovasc. Surg., 81:906, 1981.

68. Ilbawi, M. N., Grieco, J., DeLeon, S. Y., et al.: Modified Blalock-Taussig shunt in newborn infants. J. Thorac. Cardiovasc. Surg., 87:770, 1984.

69. Ilbawi, M. N., Idriss, F. S., DeLeon, S. Y., et al.: Factors that exaggerate the deleterious effects of pulmonary insufficiency on the right ventricle after tetralogy repair: Surgical implications. J. Thorac. Cardiovasc. Surg., 93:36, 1987.

70. Ilbawi, M. N.: Current status of surgery for congenital heart diseases. Clin. Perinatol. 16:157, 1989.

71. Joshi, S. V., Brawn, W. J., and Mee, R. B. B.: Pulmonary atresia with intact ventricular septum. J. Thorac. Cardiovasc. Surg., 91:192, 1986.

72. Kawashima, Y., Matsuda, H., Hirose, H., et al.: Ninety consecutive corrective operations for tetralogy of Fallot with or without minimal right ventriculotomy. J. Thorac. Cardiovasc. Surg., 90:856, 1985.

73. Keagy, B. A., Wilcox, B. R., Lucus, C. L., et al.: Constant postoperative monitoring of cardiac output after correction of congenital heart defects. J. Thorac. Cardiovasc. Surg., 93:658, 1987.

74. Kirklin, J. W., and Karp, R. B.: The Tetralogy of Fallot. Philadelphia: W. B. Saunders Company, 1970.

75. Kirklin, J. W., Blackstone, E. H., Pacifico, A. D., et al.: Routine primary repair vs two-stage repair of tetralogy of Fallot. Circulation, 60:373, 1979.

76. Kirklin, J. W., Blackstone, E. H., Kirklin, J. K., et al.: Surgical results and protocols in the spectrum of tetralogy of Fallot. Ann. Surg., 198:251, 1983.

77. Kirklin, J. W., and Barratt-Boyes, B. G.: Ventricular septal defect and pulmonary stenosis. In: Cardiac Surgery. New York, John Wiley & Sons, 1986, p. 699.

78. Kirklin, J. W., Blackstone, E. H., Colvin, E. V., and McConnell, M. E.: Early primary correction of tetralogy of Fallot. Ann. Thorac. Surg., 45:231, 1988.

79. Kisslo, J. A., Adams, D. V., and Belkin, R. N. (Eds.): Doppler Color Flow Imaging. New York, Churchill Livingstone, 1988.

80. Kurosawa, H., Imai, Y., Nakazawa, M., et al.: Standardized patch for infundibuloplasty for tetralogy of Fallot. J. Thorac. Cardiovasc. Surg., 92:396, 1986.

81. Kvelselis, D. A., Rocchini, A. P., Snider, A. R., Rosenthal, A., et al.: Results of balloon valvuloplasty in the treatment of congenital valvar pulmonary stenosis in children. Am. J. Cardiol. 56:527, 1985.

82. Lababidi, Z., and Wu, J. R.: Percutaneous balloon pulmonary valvuloplasty. Am. J. Cardiol., 52:560, 1983.

83. Laks, H., Castaneda, A. R.: Subclavian arterioplasty for the ipsilateral Blalock-Taussig shunt. Ann. Thorac. Surg., 19:319, 1975.

84. Lamberti, J. J., Carlisle, J., Waldman, J. D., et al.: Systemic-pulmonary shunts in infants and children. J. Thorac. Cardiovasc. Surg., 88:76, 1984.

85. Lev, M., and Eckner, F. A. Q: The pathologic anatomy of tetralogy of Fallot and its variations. Dis. Chest, 45:251, 1964.

86. Lewis, A. B., Wells, W., and Lindesmith, G. G.: Right ventricular growth potential in neonates with pulmonary atresia and intact ventricular septum. J. Thorac. Cardiovasc. Surg., 91:835, 1986.

87. Lillehei, C. W., Cohen, M., Warden, H. E., and Varco, R. L.: The direct-vision intracardiac correction of congenital anomalies by controlled cross circulation: Results in 32 patients with ventricular septal defects, tetralogy of Fallot, and atrioventricular communis defects. Surgery, 38:11, 1955.

88. Lillehei, C. W., Cohen, M., Warden, H. E., et al.: Direct vision intracardiac surgical correction of the tetralogy of Fallot, pentalogy of Fallot, and pulmonary atresia defects: Report of first ten cases. Ann. Surg., 142:418, 1955.

89. Lillehei, C. W., Varco, R. L., Cohen, M., et al.: The first open-heart repairs of ventricular septal defect, atrio-ventricular communis, and tetralogy of Fallot using extracorporeal circulation by cross-circulation: A thirty-year follow-up. Ann. Thorac. Surg., 41:4, 1986.

90. Lock, J. E., Keane, J. F., Fellows, K. E.: Diagnostic and interventional catheterization in congenital heart disease. Boston, Martinus Nijhoff Publishing, 1987.

91. Lodge, F. A., Lamberti, J. J., Goodman, A. H., et al.: Vascular consequences of subclavian artery transection for the treatment of congenital heart disease. J. Thorac. Cardiovasc. Surg., 86:18, 1983.

92. Magrassi, P., Chartrand, C., Guerin, R., et al.: True diverticulum of the right ventricle: Two cases associated with tetralogy of Fallot. Ann. Thorac. Surg., 29:357, 1980.

93. Marino, B., Corno, A., Pasquini, L., et al.: Indication for systemic-pulmonary artery shunts guided by two-dimensional and Doppler echocardiography: Criteria for patient selection. Ann. Thorac. Surg., 44:495, 1987.

94. Matsuda, H., Ihara, K., Mori, T., et al.: Tetralogy of Fallot associated with aortic insufficiency. Ann. Thorac. Surg., 29:529, 1980.

95. McCord, M. C., van Elk, J., Blount, G., Jr.: Tetralogy of Fallot clinical and hemodynamic spectrum of combined pulmonary stenosis and ventricular septal defects. Circulation, 16:736, 1957.

96. McGoon, D. C., and Kirklin, J. W.: Pulmonic stenosis with intact ventricular septum. Treatment utilizing extracorporeal circulation. Circulation, 17:180, 1958.

97. Misbach, G. A., Turley, K., and Ebert, P. A.: Pulmonary valve replacement for regurgitation after repair of tetralogy of Fallot. Ann. Thorac. Surg., 36:684, 1983.

98. Mitchell, S. C., Korones, S. B., and Berendes, H. W.: Congenital heart disease in 56,109 births. Incidence and natural history. Circulation, 63:323, 1971.

99. Moulton, A. L., Bowman, F. O., Jr., and Edie, R. N.: Pulmonary atresia with intact ventricular septum: Sixteen-year experience. J. Cardiovasc. Surg., 78:527, 1979.

100. Murphy, J. D., Freed, M. D., Keane, J. F., et al.: Hemodynamic results after intracardiac repair of tetralogy of Fallot by deep hypothermia and cardiopulmonary bypass. Circulation, 62(Suppl. I):168, 1980.

101. Nagao, G. I., Daoud, G. I., McAdams, A. J., et al.: Cardiovascular anomalies associated with tetralogy of Fallot. Am. J. Cardiol., 20:206, 1967.

102. Naito, Y., Fujita, T., Manabe, H., and Kawashima, Y.: The criteria for reconstruction of right ventricular outflow tract in total correction of tetralogy of Fallot. J. Thorac. Cardiovasc. Surg, 80:574, 1980.

103. Nomoto, S., Muraoka, R., Yokota, M., et al.: Left ventricular volume as a predictor of postoperative hemodynamics and a criterion for total correction of tetralogy of Fallot. J. Thorac. Cardiovasc. Surg., 88:389, 1984.

104. Norwood, W. I., and Pigott, J. D.: Recent advances in cardiac surgery. Pediatr. Clin. North Am., 32:1117, 1985.

105. Pacifico, A. D., Kirklin, J. W., and Blackstone, E. H.: Surgical management of pulmonary stenosis in tetralogy of Fallot. J. Thorac. Cardiovasc. Surg., 74:382, 1977.

106. Pacifico, A. D., Kirklin, J. W., and Bargeron, L. M., Jr.: Repair of complete atrioventricular canal associated with tetralogy of Fallot or double-outlet right ventricle: Report of ten patients. Ann. Thorac. Surg., 29:351, 1980.

107. Pacifico, A. D., Sand, M. E., Bargeron, L. M., Jr., and Colvin, E. C.: Transatrial-transpulmonary repair of tetralogy of Fallot. J. Thorac. Cardiovasc. Surg., 93:919, 1987.

108. Peacock, T. B.: On Malformations of the Human Heart, etc. with Original Cases and Illustrations, 2nd ed. London, J. Churchill and Sons, 1866.

109. Polansky, D. B., Clark, E. B., and Doty, D. B.: Pulmonary stenosis in infants and young children. Ann. Thorac. Surg., 39:159, 1985.

110. Porter, J. M., and Silver, D.: Alterations in fibrinolysis and coagulation associated with cardiopulmonary bypass. J. Thorac. Cardiovasc. Surg., 56:869, 1968.

111. Potts, W. J., Smith, S., and Gibson, S.: Anastomosis of the aorta to a pulmonary artery for certain types of congenital heart disease. J.A.M.A., 132:629, 1946.

112. Potts, W. J., Gibson, S., Riker, W. L., and Leninger, C. R.: Congenital pulmonary stenosis with intact ventricular septum. J.A.M.A., 144:8, 1950.

113. Quattlebaum, T. G., Varghese, P. J., Neill, C. A., et al.: Sudden death among postoperative patients with tetralogy of Fallot: A follow-up study of 243 patients for an average of twelve years. Circulation, 54:289, 1976.

114. Rittenhouse, E. A., Mansfield, P. B., Hall, D. G., et al.: Tetralogy of Fallot: Selective staged management. J. Thorac. Cardiovasc. Surg., 89:772, 1985.

115. Rosenberg, H. G., Williams, W. G., Trusler, G. A., et al.: Structural composition of central pulmonary arteries: Growth potential after surgical shunts. J. Thorac. Cardiovasc. Surg., 94:498, 1987.

116. Ross, R. S., Taussig, H. B., and Evans, M. H.: Late hemodynamic complications of anastomotic surgery for treatment of the tetralogy of Fallot. Circulation, 18:553, 1958.

117. Sabiston, D. C., Jr.: Role of the Blalock-Taussig operation in the hypoxic infant with tetralogy of Fallot. Ann. Thorac. Surg., 22:303, 1976.

118. Sabiston, D. C., Jr., and Blalock, A.: The tetralogy of Fallot, tricuspid atresia, transposition of the great vessels and associated disorders. In Derra, E. (Ed.): Encyclopedia of Thoracic Surgery, Vol. 2. Heidelberg, Springer-Verlag, 1959.

119. Sabiston, D. C., Jr., Cornell, W. P., Criley, J. M., et al.: The diagnosis and surgical correction of total obstruction of the right ventricle: An acquired condition developing after systemic-pulmonary artery anastomosis for tetralogy of Fallot. J. Thorac. Cardiovasc. Surg., 48:577, 1964.

120. Sandifort, E.: Observationes Anatomico-Pathologicae. Lugdunum Batavorum, P.v.d. Eyk et D. Vygh, 1777, Chapter 1, Figure 1.

121. Spencer, F.: Congenital heart disease. In Schwartz, S. I., Lillehei, R. C., Shires, G. T., Spencer, F. C., and Storer, E. H. (Eds.): Principles of Surgery, 2nd ed. New York, McGraw-Hill Book Company, 1974.

122. Stensen, H. (Nicholaus Steno). In Bartholin, T.: Acta Medica et Philosophica Hafnienca, 1671–72, Vol. 1, p. 302. Reprinted in Stenosis, N.: Opera Philosophica, Vol. 2. Copenhagen, Vilhelm Maar, 1910, pp. 49–53.

123. Stephens, H. B.: Aneurysm of the pulmonary artery following a Pott's shunt operation. J. Thorac. Cardiovasc. Surg., 53:642, 1967.

124. Szentpetery, S., Robertson, L., and Lower, R. R.: Complete repair of tetralogy associated with sickle cell anemia and G-6-PD deficiency. J. Thorac. Cardiovasc. Surg., 72:276, 1976.

125. Tamiya, T., Yamashiro, T., Matsumoto, T., et al.: A histological study of surgical landmarks for the specialized atrioventricular conduction system, with particular reference to the papillary muscle. Ann. Thorac. Surg., 40:599, 1985.

126. Taussig, H. B.: Tetralogy of Fallot: Early history and late results. Neuhauser Lecture. Am J. Roentgenol, *133*:423, 1979.
127. Tucker, W. Y., Turley, K., and Ullyot, D. J.: Management of symptomatic tetralogy of Fallot in the first year of life. J. Thorac. Cardiovasc. Surg., *78*:494, 1979.
128. Turley, K., Tucker, W. Y., and Ebert, P. A.: The changing role of palliative procedures in the treatment of infants with congenital heart disease. J. Thorac. Cardiovasc. Surg., *79*:194, 1980.
129. Ullom, R. L., Sade, R. M., and Crawford, F. A.:The Blalock-Taussig shunt in infants: Standard versus modified. Ann. Thorac. Surg., *44*:539, 1987.
130. Ungerleider, R. M., Kisslo, J. A., Greeley, W. J., Van Trigt, P., and Sabiston, D. C., Jr.: Intraoperative prebypass and postbypass epicardial color flow imaging in the repair of atrioventricular septal defects. J. Thorac. Cardiovasc. Surg., *98*:90, 1989.
131. Ungerleider, R. M., Greeley, W. J., Sheikh, K. H., Kern, F. H., Kisslo, J. A., and Sabiston, D. C., Jr.: The use of intraoperative echo with Doppler color flow imaging to predict outcome after repair of congenital cardiac defects. Ann. Surg., *210*:526, 1989.
132. Ungerleider, R. M., Greeley, W. J., Sheikh, K. H., Philips, J., Pearce, F. B., Kern, F. H., and Kisslo, J. A.: Routine use of intraoperative, epicardial echo and Doppler color flow imaging to guide and evaluate repair of congenital heart lesions: A prospective study. J. Thorac. Cardiovasc. Surg. *100*:297, 1990.
133. Vargas, F. J., Coto, E. O., Mayer, J. E., Jr., et al.: Complete atrioventricular canal and tetralogy of Fallot: Surgical considerations. Ann Thorac. Surg., *42*:258, 1986.
134. Walsh, E. P., Rockenmacher, S., Keane, J. F., Houghen, T. J., Lock, J. E., and Castaneda, A. R.: Late results in patients with tetralogy of Fallot repaired during infancy. Circulation, *77*:1062, 1988.
135. Waterston, D. J.: Treatment of Fallot's tetralogy in children under 1 year of age. Rozhl. Chir., *41*:181, 1962.
136. Webb, W. R., and Burford, T. H.: Gangrene of the arm following use of the subclavian artery in a pulmonosystemic (Blalock) anastomosis. J. Thorac. Surg., *23*:199, 1952.
137. Weldon, C. S., Hartmann, A. F., Jr., and McKnight, R. C.: Surgical management of hypoplastic right ventricle with pulmonary atresia or critical pulmonary stenosis and intact ventricular septum. Ann. Thorac. Surg., *37*:12, 1984.
138. Westerman, G. R., Norton, J. V., and Van Devanter, S. H.: A double-outlet right atrium associated with tetralogy of Fallot and common atrioventricular valve. J. Thorac. Cardiovasc. Surg., *91*:205, 1986.
139. White, P. D., and Sprague, H. B.: The tetralogy of Fallot: Report of a case in a noted musician who lived to his sixtieth year. J.A.M.A., *92*:787, 1929.
140. Wilson, J. M., Mack, J. W., Turley, K., and Ebert, P. A.: Persistence stenosis and deformity of the right pulmonary artery after correction of the Waterston anastomosis. J. Thorac. Cardiovasc. Surg., *82*:169, 1981.
141. Yamaguchi, M., Imai, M., Ohashi, H., et al.: Enhanced myocardial protection by systemic hypothermia in children undergoing total correction of tetralogy of Fallot. Ann. Thorac. Surg., *41*:639, 1986.
142. Zerbini, E. J., MacCruz, R., Bittencourt, D., et al.: Total correction of complex of Fallot under extracorporeal circulation: Immediate results in a group of 221 patients. J. Thorac. Cardiovasc. Surg., *49*:430, 1965.
143. Zhao, H., Miller, D. C., and Reitz, B. A., et al.: Surgical repair of tetralogy of Fallot. J. Thorac. Cardiovasc. Surg., *89*:204, 1985.

IX

DOUBLE OUTLET RIGHT VENTRICLE

Albert D. Pacifico, M.D., John W. Kirklin, M.D., and James K. Kirklin, M.D.

Double outlet right ventricle (DORV) is a congenital cardiac anomaly in which both great arteries arise wholly or in large part from the right ventricle. A ventricular septal defect (VSD) is the only outlet from the morphologic left ventricle. This malformation was first successfully corrected using the tunnel repair technique by Kirklin in 1956.[17] Considerable progress has since been made using a variety of surgical methods to repair more complex forms, including those coexisting with other major cardiac anomalies.

HEARTS WITH ATRIOVENTRICULAR CONCORDANCE

Definition and Morphology

DORV is present when more than 50 per cent of each great artery arises from the morphologic right ventricle.[23] There is considerable variability in the specific anatomy found within each heart. Often one (and rarely both) great arteries may overlie the ventricular septum, which may cause controversy in categorization. In general, when one great artery overlies the ventricular septum, it is assigned to the ventricle connected to its greater part. In hearts with tetralogy of Fallot, there is a variable degree of dextroposition of the aorta. Similarly, in the Taussig-Bing heart, there is often variability in the origin of the pulmonary trunk. At the University of Alabama at Birmingham (UAB), the authors have continued to categorize hearts as tetralogy of Fallot unless the aorta arises by more than 90 per cent from the right ventricle, in which case they are categorized as double outlet right ventricle with pulmonary stenosis. The authors categorize hearts within the Taussig-Bing category when the pulmonary trunk arises less than 90 per cent from the left ventricle; otherwise, they are classified as complete transposition with VSD. Others prefer to maintain the 50 per cent rule in each of these circumstances.

The definition of DORV is based solely on the origin of the great arteries and is exclusive of the presence or absence of continuity between the semilunar and atrioventricular (AV) valves. In some hearts there is a muscular conus beneath the aorta or the pulmonary artery, or both. Although some authors have used this anatomic variation in the basic definition of this malformation, the authors do not believe this consideration should be an essential part of the definition of DORV. A VSD is almost uniformly present but may vary in size and location.

Since the hemodynamics, clinical course, and specific type of operation employed depend on the relation of the VSD to either great artery, and the relation of the great vessels to each other, knowledge of the precise location of these structures is important. It is surgically useful to describe the commitment of the VSD to either or both great arteries as suggested by Lev and colleagues.[24] In hearts in which the aorta is to the right and either side-by-side or posterior to the pulmonary artery (i.e., great arteries more or less normally related), the VSD may be *subaortic, doubly committed, or noncommitted.* The location of the VSD within the ventricular septum does not uniformly predict its commitment to either great artery. Thus, in the authors' surgical series of 127 patients operated between 1967 and July 1984, a perimembranous VSD was present in 81 per cent of those with a subaortic defect, 30 per cent of those with a doubly committed defect, 35 per cent of those with a subpulmonary defect, and 58 per cent of those with a noncommitted defect.[20]

The *subaortic* VSD lies immediately beneath the aortic annulus or its subaortic muscular conus. It is usually perimembranous in location and extends to the commissure between the septal and anterior tricuspid valve leaflets. In some patients, it extends more inferiorly to include part of the septum at the base of the tricuspid valve septal leaflet. The *doubly committed* VSD lies immediately beneath both the aorta and the pulmonary artery, which in these hearts are often in a side-by-side and contiguous relationship. The *noncommitted* VSD does not occupy the perimembranous or outlet portion of the septum and is not immediately related to either great artery.[57] It may be located in the inlet portion of the ventricular septum beneath the septal leaflet of the tricuspid valve, or in the trabecular or apical portions of the muscular septum. The VSD may spontaneously undergo diminution in size and become restrictive to left ventricular outflow.[22,45] When DORV is associated with a complete AV canal defect, the VSD usually includes the perimembranous septum and is subaortic, although less commonly it is unrelated to either great artery and is noncommitted.[49]

DORV may exist with the aorta directly anterior to, or anterior and to the right or left of, the pulmonary artery. The VSD in these hearts is usually directly beneath the pulmonary valve annulus or its conus and is termed a subpulmonary defect. These hearts are generally categorized as the Taussig-Bing type of DORV, although Lev and colleagues have described additional morphologic characteristics peculiar to this entity.[25,53]

DORV can exist in hearts with the aorta to the left (l-malposition) and side-by-side with the pulmonary artery. In this rare malformation, the VSD is usually subaortic in location,[26,54] but this type of DORV with l-malposition of the aorta has also been described with a subpulmonary and with a noncommitted VSD.[2,46]

Although most hearts with atrioventricular concordance and DORV have two separate AV valves, the malformation also exists in the presence of a common AV valve.

The conduction tissue arises from a posterior AV node and courses along the inferior margin of the perimembranous VSD.[56] Defects in the outlet septum are separated from the major conducting pathways by a rim of septal musculature. Inlet muscular defects lie inferior to these pathways so that the His bundle is related to their anterosuperior margin. The AV canal type defects are superior to the conduction tissue, which is related to its inferior margin. This knowledge usually permits the placement of sutures away from the conduction tissue to avoid creation of surgical heart block.

DORV exists with or without valvular and/or subvalvular pulmonary stenosis (an important determinant of both clinical course and choice of operation) and is found in patients with levocardia, dextrocardia, and visceroatrial situs solitus, inversus, or ambiguus. Other important associated anomalies include mitral stenosis and atresia, coarctation and aortic arch interruption, and valvular and subvalvular aortic stenosis.[23] DORV has also been associated with straddling mitral or tricuspid valves.[30,35] Lev and associates, on morphologic grounds, have considered DORV within a spectrum of congenital cardiopathies beginning with isolated VSD and overriding aorta, proceeding through DORV with subaortic VSD, through the Taussig-Bing heart, and finally to complete transposition of the great arteries.[24]

Physiology, Clinical Course, and Diagnosis

The clinical course of patients with DORV depends primarily on the relation of the VSD to the great arteries and the presence and severity, or absence, of pulmonary stenosis. Those with a subaortic VSD without pulmonary stenosis remain acyanotic because of streaming of oxygenated left ventricular blood into the aorta. They are similar to patients with isolated large VSD.[7] In some, the large left-to-right shunt causes congestive heart failure early in life, whereas in others severe pulmonary vascular disease may develop within the first 2 years of life.[47]

In contrast, patients with a subpulmonary VSD and no pulmonary stenosis have a course more similar to that of patients with transposition of the great arteries with VSD. Cyanosis is present usually from birth, since streaming leads the desaturated systemic venous return toward the aorta and the oxygenated left ventricular blood into the pulmonary artery.[48] These patients tend to develop early congestive heart failure or severe

pulmonary vascular disease and usually have presenting symptoms in the first few months of life.[47] Pulmonary stenosis is usually present in those with subaortic VSDs and usually absent in those with subpulmonary defects.[24,28,47,52,57] Pulmonary stenosis protects the lungs from pulmonary vascular disease, effecting a more benign clinical course, which often resembles that of patients with the tetralogy of Fallot.

High-quality angiocardiograms, using axial projections after separate injection of contrast media into the left and right ventricles, offer the greatest diagnostic reliability.[3,6] These data coupled with hemodynamic information obtained during cardiac catheterization provide knowledge of the great artery relationship, size and location of the VSD, functional and anatomic status of each AV valve, and presence and severity, or absence, of pulmonary stenosis.[50] Two-dimensional ultrasonic imaging, particularly with color-flow mapping, is very useful in the noninvasive diagnosis of DORV and has eliminated much of the variable reliability previously found with M-mode echocardiography.[9–11,52]

Surgical Methods and Results

The goals of corrective surgery are to relieve pulmonary stenosis, to provide separate unobstructed outflow pathways from each ventricle to a great vessel, and to separate the pulmonary and systemic circulation. This is accomplished by appropriate use of intracardiac and extracardiac conduits and patches. The operation for DORV with subaortic or doubly committed VSD consists of an intraventricular tunnel repair designed to connect the VSD with the aorta.[11,12,17,18] When the VSD is restrictive, it must be enlarged anteriorly to avoid the conduction tissue. The intraventricular tunnel repair is shown in Figure 1. In some hearts, the tricuspid valve is so positioned that it interferes with construction of this tunnel, and alternative methods are required as described in the following.[32] When there is coexisting pulmonary stenosis, the same protocols are used as for the treatment of patients with tetralogy of Fallot.[34]

Although hospital mortality was formerly higher, there was 1 (4.4 per cent) hospital death among 23 patients with DORV and subaortic VSD operated at UAB between 1979 and 1984.[20] In earlier years, younger age was an incremental risk factor for hospital mortality, but this effect disappeared in 1978 and currently age at operation is unrelated to hospital mortality.[20] Late results were good in this subset. Thus, among 65 patients with subaortic or doubly committed defects who underwent repair by an intraventricular tunnel at UAB, late reoperation for tunnel dehiscence was required in 1, and no reoperations for tunnel stenosis were performed over a 16-year period of follow-up.[20] In addition, 13 patients underwent postoperative recatheterization and there were no gradients between the left ventricle and the aorta of greater than 10 mm. Hg. The actuarial freedom from reoperation for tunnel complications was 98 per cent at 14 years postoperatively for 56 patients who underwent tunnel repair for a subaortic VSD. In contrast, however, it was 40 per cent at 12 years for 34 patients with other variances of commitment of the ventricular septal defect.[20] Currently, tunnel repair of DORV with subaortic VSD is accomplished in most patients by a transatrial approach similar to that used for repair of most patients with classic tetralogy of Fallot.[37]

Repair of the Taussig-Bing type of DORV is more complex because the VSD is subpulmonary in location. The presence or absence of pulmonary stenosis as well as the relation of the great arteries to each other as well as to the interventricular septum affects the choice of operation. These relations should be assessed externally, and after establishing cardiopulmonary bypass, a right atriotomy is made and the position and interrelations of the VSD, the aortic and pulmonary valves, the tricuspid valve and its tensor apparatus, and the infundibular septum are carefully assessed. In the most common anatomic circumstance, the aorta is more or less anterior to the pulmonary artery and

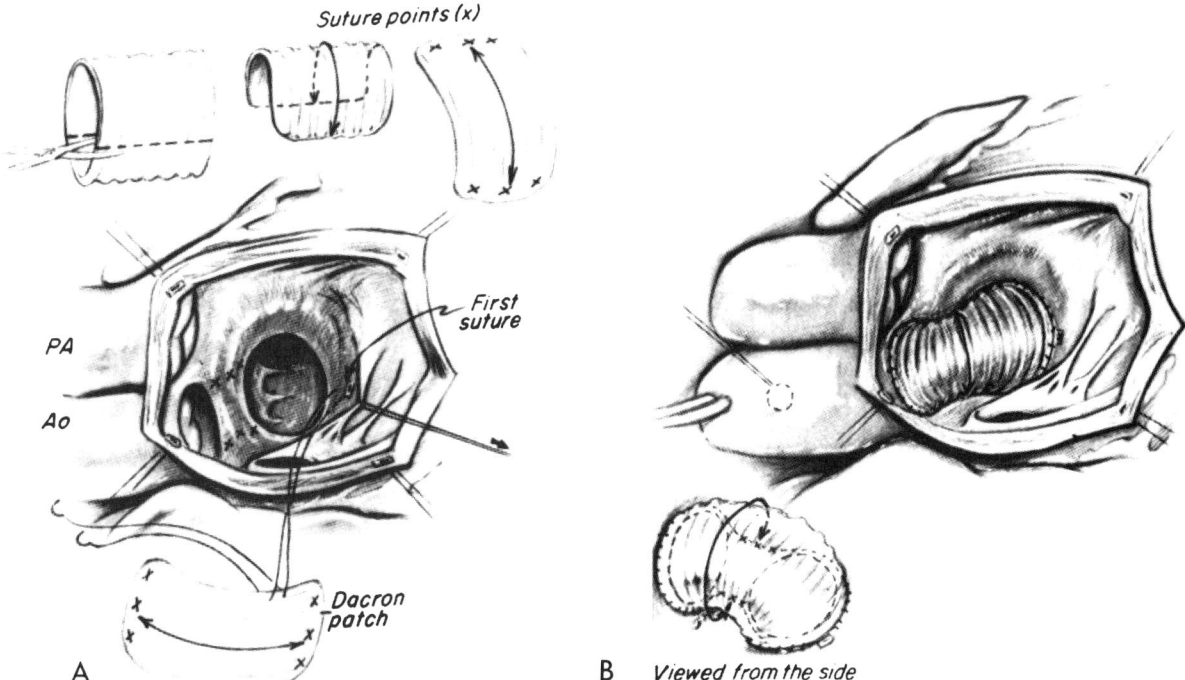

Figure 1. Construction of an intraventricular tunnel connecting VSD to aorta is depicted in a heart with DORV and subaortic VSD. *A*, The patch is tailored from a woven Dacron tube that forms the anterior two thirds of the tunnel. Its proper geometry and orientation during repair are essential to avoid subaortic stenosis. The first suture is placed well away from the edge of the VSD to avoid injury to conduction tissue. *B*, The completed repair is demonstrated leaving an unobstructed path through right ventricle to pulmonary artery. (From Stewart, R. W., Kirklin, J. W., Pacifico, A. D., et al.: Repair of double outlet right ventricle. An analysis of 62 cases. J. Thorac. Cardiovasc. Surg., 78:502, 1979.)

pulmonary stenosis is absent. In these hearts, the best definitive procedure consists of constructing an intraventricular tunnel connecting the subpulmonary VSD with the pulmonary artery (thus creating transposition of the great vessels), and restoring "veno-arterial concordance" with an arterial switch operation.[31,41,42] Although a venous switch operation at the atrial level can be accomplished by the technique described by Senning or Mustard,[14,29,30] early and late results are less favorable with atrial switching than with arterial switching in this entity.[20,42] When the great arteries are more or less side-by-side and chordae tendineae from the tricuspid valve do not insert upon the infundibular septum, resection of the infundibular septum and construction of a straight tunnel connecting the VSD with the aorta, leaving an unobstructed outlet from the right ventricle to the pulmonary artery (Kawashima's repair), is sometimes possible and remains an attractive surgical option for this specific subset.[16] These methods cannot be employed if severe pulmonary stenosis is present and cannot be surgically relieved.

When pulmonary stenosis is present, repair usually consists of constructing a tunnel that connects the VSD with the origin of the aorta (and includes the origin of the pulmonary artery since it is usually directly posterior to the aorta), closing the pulmonary artery, and using a valved extracardiac conduit to restore continuity between the right ventricle and the pulmonary artery. This is similar to the operation described by Rastelli and associates for repair of transposition, VSD, and pulmonary stenosis.[43,44]

A variety of other surgical methods have been employed in the past but have little place in current management. These include the Damus-Kaye-Stancil procedure (construction of an intraventricular tunnel connecting the VSD with the pulmonary artery, connection of the divided proximal main pulmonary artery with the aorta, and placement of an extracardiac conduit from the right ventricle to the distal pulmonary artery) and the spiral intraventricular tunnel arterial switch repair described by Patrick and McGoon.[36,39]

Hospital mortality for repair of this type of DORV is higher than when the VSD is in the subaortic location, but excellent

results when pulmonary stenosis is absent have been obtained using an intraventricular tunnel repair to the pulmonary trunk coupled with an arterial switch operation.[31,42]

Repair of hearts with DORV and noncommitted VSD can be accomplished by constructing an intraventricular tunnel (or Dacron patch partition) connecting the VSD (which usually must be enlarged anterosuperiorly) with the aorta, closing the pulmonary artery and placing a valved extracardiac conduit from the right ventricle to the pulmonary artery.[51] Alternative techniques consist of closing the VSD, closing the pulmonary artery, placing a valved extracardiac conduit from the left ventricle to the pulmonary artery, and constructing an interatrial transposition of venous return.[20] Additionally, repair including an arterial switch operation has been successfully accomplished.[42] In addition, when appropriate anatomic and hemodynamic criteria exist, repair can be accomplished by a modification of the operation described by Fontan.[13,27] Repair of this complex malformation generally has been associated with higher hospital mortality.[20,40,51]

DORV associated with complete atrioventricular canal has been repaired by constructing an intraventricular tunnel using a comma-shaped patch to connect the VSD with the aorta and concomitant repair of the common atrioventricular valve.[33] Although early results were associated with high hospital mortality, more recently encouraging success has been achieved.[38] Alternative methods of repair include mitral and tricuspid valve replacement, closure of the atrial and ventricular septal defect, and placement of a valved extracardiac conduit from the left ventricle to the aorta, or a modified Fontan procedure.[13,27]

Surgical Indications and Timing

The timing and type of operation for patients with DORV must balance their natural history with the early and late results of operation. The age and symptomatic state of the patient, the presence and degree of pulmonary vascular disease, the location of the VSD, the degree of pulmonary stenosis, and the type of operative repair are all important considerations. A plan of surgical management is summarized in Table 1.

TABLE 1. Surgical Management for Double Outlet Right Ventricle

Pulmonary Stenosis Absent

Subaortic VSD	Elective repair by 6 months of age
Subpulmonary VSD	Elective arterial switch repair by 3 months of age
Noncommitted VSD	Pulmonary artery banding by 6 months; repair at 2–5 years

Pulmonary Stenosis Present

Subaortic VSD	Manage as tetralogy of Fallot (see text)
Subpulmonary VSD or noncommitted VSD	Balloon atrial septostomy initially, systemic–pulmonary artery shunt if required; elective repair at 2–5 years

Patients with DORV and subaortic VSD without pulmonary stenosis have a natural history similar to those with isolated large VSD. Those who develop severe congestive heart failure early in life clearly require surgical therapy. As a group, they are prone to develop pulmonary vascular disease within the first few years of life, and if operation is further delayed, the risk of late death increases.[4,47] These considerations advise elective repair at approximately 6 months of age or sooner if poorly controlled heart failure is present.

Those with DORV and subaortic VSD with pulmonary stenosis clinically resemble patients with the tetralogy of Fallot. Elective repair is advised by the age of 2 years. If significant cyanosis or cyanotic episodes are present in infancy, definitive repair is usually advised although in some circumstances it is best to perform an initial systemic–pulmonary artery shunt, with later repair. This management policy is similar to that used for patients with classic tetralogy of Fallot.[19,37,40]

Patients with DORV and subpulmonary VSD have a natural history similar to those with transposition of the great arteries and large VSD. When pulmonary stenosis is absent, they tend to develop congestive heart failure or severe pulmonary vascular disease early in life. This poor natural history mandates elective operation within the first 3 months of life by methods that leave the left ventricle as the systemic ventricle. For the majority, this consists of constructing a tunnel connecting the VSD with the pulmonary artery and performing an arterial switch operation with translocation of the left and right coronary arteries.[31,42] Earlier experience with procedures leaving the right ventricle as the systemic ventricle have been poor.[14,20,40] When pulmonary stenosis is present, a balloon atrial septostomy is initially recommended within the first few weeks of life to improve mixing of systemic and pulmonary venous blood. Elective repair employing a cryopreserved homograft valve extracardiac conduit (Rastelli type procedure) is advised between ages 2 and 5 years. Some patients require a systemic–pulmonary artery shunt in the interim.

Patients with DORV, noncommitted VSD, and absent pulmonary stenosis should have pulmonary artery banding in the first 2 years of life to control heart failure and to prevent the development of advanced pulmonary vascular disease. In contrast to those with subpulmonary defects, severe cyanosis is usually absent and therefore does not require treatment. When pulmonary stenosis is present, an initial systemic–pulmonary artery shunt is performed to relieve cyanosis in patients less than approximately 2 years of age. Repair usually requires a valved extracardiac conduit or modifications of the Fontan operation and should be delayed until approximately 3 to 5 years of age.

Patients with DORV associated with complete atrioventricular canal defects can often be repaired with an intraventricular tunnel connecting the left ventricle with the aorta.[38] When this is possible and pulmonary stenosis is absent, repair should be accomplished by 6 months of age. When pulmonary stenosis is present, management is similar to that of patients with tetralogy of Fallot. When the interventricular communication is not related to the aorta, a valved extracardiac conduit is necessary as part of the repair. If pulmonary stenosis is absent, early pulmonary artery banding to control congestive heart failure and protect the pulmonary vasculature is advised. When pulmonary stenosis is present, an initial systemic–pulmonary artery shunt is constructed when needed and later repair at approximately 3 years employing an extracardiac conduit or by Fontan methods is accomplished.[38]

In a report of 62 consecutive patients from the Mayo Clinic undergoing operation for classic DORV (excluding those patients with subpulmonary VSDs, complete AV canals, AV discordance, and univentricular heart), 106 associated defects were present in 54 patients. Of these, 46 had pulmonary stenosis, and the age averaged 8 months to 37 years (median age 9 years). The early mortality was 11 per cent for those with pulmonary stenosis, 25 per cent for those without pulmonary stenosis, and 15 per cent for the entire series. The risk of mortality was related to the age of the patient. It was emphasized that there were 11 late deaths among the 53 operative survivors (21 per cent), and of these 10 were related to arrhythmia. Fortunately, all except one of the long-term survivors are now in functional Class I or Class II. These authors emphasize that whereas the mortality for repair of DORV continues to decrease, the late mortality is of concern, and the problem of late arrhythmia necessitates further study and analysis.[15]

HEARTS WITH ATRIOVENTRICULAR DISCORDANCE

DORV is less common in hearts with atrioventricular discordant connections. All of these patients have a VSD, the majority have associated pulmonary stenosis, and most have situs solitus of the atria and viscera with dextrocardia. In the typical heart, the right atrium lies to the right and connects to a morphologic left ventricle that is right-sided. The only outlet of this ventricle is a VSD that leads to the left-sided morphologic right ventricle, which also receives blood from the left atrium. Both great arteries arise from the morphologic right ventricle, and although relationship of each great artery is variable, the aorta is most commonly anterior and to the left (l-malposition) of the pulmonary artery. The VSD is usually in a subpulmonary position in those with l-malposition of the aorta and in a subaortic position when the aorta is to the right (d-malposition) or directly anterior to the pulmonary artery. The bundle of His and specialized conduction tissue are abnormally located, and in some, abnormalities of the left AV valve exist, similar to patients with corrected transposition of the great arteries.[1,55]

Kiser and associates first described the surgical repair of this entity in 1968 using a solely intraventricular repair connecting the VSD with the pulmonary artery in two patients and closing the VSD and pulmonary artery and placing a nonvalved extracardiac conduit from the left ventricle to the pulmonary artery in one.[21] The latter type of repair with the use of a valved extracardiac conduit from the left ventricle to the pulmonary artery is probably preferable, since it avoids an incision in the systemic (right) ventricle, can be used regardless of the location of the VSD, and avoids residual pulmonary stenosis.[5,8,52] The incidence of surgically induced complete heart block is high, approaching 30 per cent, and hospital mortality is approximately 15 per cent.[12,52]

SELECTED REFERENCES

Kirklin, J. W., Pacifico, A. D., Blackstone, E. H., Kirklin, J. K., and Bargeron, L. M., Jr.: Current risks and protocols for operations for double outlet right ventricle. J. Thorac. Cardiovasc. Surg., *92*:913, 1986.
This report of 127 patients who underwent repair of various types of DORV during an 18-year period thoroughly describes early and late results using various surgical methods. Results of tunnel repair of DORV with subaortic or doubly committed

VSD were excellent, and reoperation was required in only 1 of 56 patients. Predicted survival rates for intraventricular tunnel repair currently performed in a 6-month-old infant was 99 per cent at 2 weeks and 97 per cent at 10 years. Early and late results in patients with DORV and subpulmonary VSD were poor when an atrial switch operation was part of the repair. Results were least good in the subset of DORV with noncommitted VSD.

Lev, M., Bharati, S., Meng, C. C. L., Liberthson, R. R., Paul, M. H., and Idriss, F.: A concept of double-outlet right ventricle. J. Thorac. Cardiovasc. Surg., 64:271, 1972.

This classic article analyzes in detail the anatomic features of 91 hearts with DORV. The relation of each specific type of VSD to the great arteries is discussed, and the precise intracardiac anatomic details are presented. The differentiation of DORV with subaortic VSD and pulmonary stenosis from tetralogy of Fallot is considered, as are associated anomalies present in these specimens.

Musumeci, F., Shumway, S., Lincoln, C., and Anderson, R. H.: Surgical treatment for double-outlet right ventricle at the Brompton Hospital, 1973 to 1986. J. Thorac. Cardiovasc. Surg., 96:278, 1988.

Surgical results were thoroughly analyzed for 120 consecutive patients who underwent repair of various types of DORV. Best results were obtained when the VSD was subaortic or doubly committed, and the arterial switch operation was demonstrated to be the optimal approach when a subpulmonary VSD exists.

Sondheimer, H. M., Freedom, R. M., and Olley, P. M.: Double outlet right ventricle: Clinical spectrum and prognosis. Am. J. Cardiol., 39:709, 1977.

This paper reviews the natural history of 80 children with various types of DORV observed over a 19-year period at the Hospital for Sick Children in Toronto. Patients were grouped according to the location of the VSD and the presence or absence of pulmonary stenosis. Prognosis was significantly influenced by the associated presence of coarctation of the aorta or severe mitral valve abnormalities. The effect of palliative or corrective surgery on the prognosis of each group is presented.

Sridaromont, S., Ritter, D. G., Feldt, R. H., Davis, G. D., and Edwards, J. E.: Double-outlet right ventricle. Anatomic and angiocardiographic correlations. Mayo Clin. Proc., 53:555, 1978.

This article reports the angiocardiographic and anatomic features of various types of DORV in 72 patients. The paper contains excellent reproductions of angiocardiograms and anatomic specimens to illustrate the varying great artery relation and VSD location. The authors conclude that use of hemodynamic information regarding systemic and pulmonary arterial saturations, combined with right ventricular angiocardiograms, permits preoperative prediction of the location of the VSD in DORV.

Tabry, I. F., McGoon, D. C., Danielson, G. K., Wallace, R. B., Davis, Z., and Maloney, J. D.: Surgical management of double-outlet right ventricle associated with atrioventricular discordance. J. Thorac. Cardiovasc. Surg., 76:336, 1978.

A surgical series with 20 corrective operations performed for DORV with atrioventricular discordant connections is discussed. The various methods employed, the early and late results, and the abnormal location of the conduction system determined by electrophysiologic mapping are presented.

REFERENCES

1. Anderson, R. H., Becker, A. E., Arnold, R., and Wilkinson, J. L.: The conducting tissues in congenitally corrected transposition. Circulation, 50:911, 1974.
2. Anderson, R. H., Pickering, D., and Brown, R.: Double outlet right ventricle with l-malposition and uncommitted ventricular septal defect. Eur. J. Cardiol., 3:133, 1975.
3. Bargeron, L. M., Jr., Elliott, L. P., Soto, B., Bream, P. R., and Curry, G. C.: Axial cineangiography in congenital heart disease. I. Concept, technical and anatomic considerations. Circulation, 56:1075, 1977.
4. Blackstone, E. H., Kirklin, J. W., Bradley, E. L., DuShane, J. W., and Appelbaum, A.: Optimal age and results in repair of large ventricular septal defects. J. Thorac. Cardiovasc. Surg., 72:661, 1976.
5. DeLeval, M.: Surgery of double outlet right ventricle with atrioventricular discordance. *In* Anderson, R. H., and Shinebourne, E. A. (Eds.): Paediatric Cardiology. Edinburgh, Churchill Livingstone, 1977, p. 235.
6. Elliott, L. P., Bargeron, L. M., Jr., Bream, P. R., Soto, B., and Curry, G. C.: Axial cineangiography in congenital heart disease. II. Specific lesions. Circulation, 56:1084, 1977.
7. Engle, M. A., Steinberg, I., Lukas, D. S., and Goldberg, H. P.: Acyanotic ventricular septal defect with both great vessels from the right ventricle. Am. Heart J., 66:755, 1963.
8. Fox, L. S., Kirklin, J. W., Pacifico, A. D., Waldo, A. L., and Bargeron, L. M., Jr.: Intracardiac repair of cardiac malformations with atrioventricular discordance. Circulation, 54:123, 1976.
9. French, J. W., and Popp, R.: Variability of echocardiographic discontinuity in double outlet right ventricle and truncus arteriosus. Circulation, 51:848, 1975.
10. Goldberg, S. J., Allen, H. D., and Sahn, D. J.: Pediatric and Adolescent Echocardiography. Chicago, Year Book Medical Publishers, 1975, pp. 134–136.
11. Gomes, M. M. R., Weidman, W. H., McGoon, D. C., and Danielson, G. K.: Double-outlet right ventricle with pulmonic stenosis. Surgical considerations and results of operation. Circulation, 43:889, 1971.
12. Gomes, M. M. R., Weidman, W. H., McGoon, D. C., and Danielson, G. K.: Double-outlet right ventricle without pulmonic stenosis. Circulation, 43(Suppl. 1):31, 1971.
13. Gonzalez-Lavin, L., Blair, T. C., Chi, S., and Sparrow, A. W.: Orthoterminal correction of coexisting d-transposition of the great arteries, subpulmonary stenosis, and a complete form of atrioventricular canal. J. Thorac. Cardiovasc. Surg., 73:694, 1977.
14. Hightower, B. M., Barcia, A., Bargeron, L. M., Jr., and Kirklin, J. W.: Double-outlet right ventricle with transposed great arteries and subpulmonary ventricular septal defect. The Taussig-Bing malformation. Circulation, 39(Suppl. 1):207, 1969.
15. Judson, J. P., Danielson, G. K., Puga, F. J., Mair, D. D., and McGoon, D. C.: Double-outlet right ventricle. Surgical results, 1970–1980. J. Thorac. Cardiovasc. Surg., 85:32, 1983.
16. Kawashima, Y., Fugita, T., Miyamoto, T., and Manabe, H.: Intraventricular rerouting of blood for the correction of Taussig-Bing malformation. J. Thorac. Cardiovasc. Surg., 62:825, 1971.
17. Kirklin, J. W., cited by McGoon, D. C.: Origin of both great vessels from the right ventricle. Surg. Clin. North Am., 41:1113, 1961.
18. Kirklin, J. W., Karp, R. A., and McGoon, D. C.: Surgical treatment of origin of both vessels from right ventricle including cases of pulmonary stenosis. J. Thorac. Cardiovasc. Surg., 48:1026, 1964.
19. Kirklin, J. W., Blackstone, E. H., Kirklin, J. K., Pacifico, A. D., Aramendi, J., and Bargeron, L. M., Jr.: Surgical results and protocols in the spectrum of tetralogy of Fallot. Ann. Surg., 198:251, 1983.
20. Kirklin, J. W., Pacifico, A. D., Blackstone, E. H., Kirklin, J. K., and Bargeron, L. M., Jr.: Current risks and protocols for operations for double outlet right ventricle. J. Thorac. Cardiovasc. Surg., 92:913, 1986.
21. Kiser, J. C., Ongley, P. A., Kirklin, J. W., Clarkson, P. M., and McGoon, D. C.: Surgical treatment of dextrocardia with inversion of ventricles and double-outlet right ventricle. J. Thorac. Cardiovasc. Surg., 55:6, 1968.
22. Lavoie, R., Sestier, F., Gilbert, G., Chameides, L., Van Praagh, R., and Grondin, P.: Double outlet right ventricle with left ventricular outflow tract obstruction due to small ventricular septal defect. Am. Heart J., 82:290, 1971.
23. Lev, M., and Bharati, S.: Double outlet right ventricle, association with other cardiovascular anomalies. Arch. Pathol., 95:117, 1973.
24. Lev, M., Bharati, S., Meng, C. C. L., Liberthson, R. R., Paul, M. H., and Idriss, F.: A concept of double-outlet right ventricle. J. Thorac. Cardiovasc. Surg., 64:271, 1972.
25. Lev, M., Rimoldi, H. J. A., Eckner, F. A. O., Melhuish, B. P., Meng, C. C. L., and Paul, M. H.: The Taussig-Bing heart. Qualitative and quantitative anatomy. Arch. Pathol. Lab. Med., 81:24, 1966.
26. Lincoln, C., Anderson, R. H., Shinebourne, E. A., English, T. A. H., and Wilkinson, J. L.: Double outlet right ventricle with l-malposition of the aorta. Br. Heart J., 37:453, 1975.
27. McGoon, D. C.: Left ventricular and biventricular extracardiac conduits. J. Thorac. Cardiovasc. Surg., 72:7, 1976.
28. Mehrizi, A.: The origin of both great vessels from the right ventricle. I. With pulmonic stenosis. II. Without pulmonic stenosis. Johns Hopkins Hosp. Bull., 117:75, 1965.
29. Mustard, W. T., Keith, J. D., Trusler, G. A., Fowler, R., and Kidd, L.: The surgical management of transposition of the great vessels. J. Thorac. Cardiovasc. Surg., 48:953, 1964.
30. Muster, A. J., Bharati, S., Azia, K. U., Idriss, F. S., Paul, M. H., Lev, M., Carr, I., DeBoer, A., and Anagnostopoulos, C.: Taussig-Bing anomaly with straddling mitral valve. J. Thorac. Cardiovasc. Surg., 77:832, 1979.
31. Musumeci, F., Shumway, S., Lincoln, C., and Anderson, R. H.: Surgical treatment for double-outlet right ventricle at the Brompton Hospital, 1973 to 1986. J. Thorac. Cardiovasc. Surg., 96:278, 1988.
32. Pacifico, A. D., Kirklin, J. W., and Bargeron, L. M., Jr.: Complex congenital malformations. Surgical treatment of double-outlet right ventricle and double-outlet left ventricle. *In* Kirklin, J. W. (Ed.): Advances in Cardiovascular Surgery. New York, Grune & Stratton, 1973, p. 57.
33. Pacifico, A. D., Kirklin, J. W., and Bargeron, L. M., Jr.: Repair of complete atrioventricular canal associated with tetralogy of Fallot or double outlet right ventricle. Report of 10 cases. Ann. Thorac. Surg., 29:351, 1980.
34. Pacifico, A. D., Kirklin, J. W., and Blackstone, E. H.: Surgical management of the pulmonary stenosis in the tetralogy of Fallot. J. Thorac. Cardiovasc. Surg., 74:382, 1977.
35. Pacifico, A. D., Soto, B., and Bargeron, L. M., Jr.: Surgical treatment of straddling tricuspid valves. Circulation, 60:655, 1979.
36. Pacifico, A. D., Kirklin, J. K., Colvin, E. V., and Bargeron, L. M., Jr.: Intraventricular tunnel repair for Taussig-Bing heart and related cardiac anomalies. Circulation, 74(Suppl. I):I-53, 1986.
37. Pacifico, A. D., Sand, M. E., Bargeron, L. M., Jr., and Colvin, E. V.: Transatrial-transpulmonary repair of tetralogy of Fallot. J. Thorac. Cardiovasc. Surg., 93:919, 1987.
38. Pacifico, A. D., Ricchi, A., Bargeron, L. M., Jr., Colvin, E. V., Kirklin, J. W., and Kirklin, J. K.: Corrective repair of complete atrioventricular canal defects and major associated cardiac anomalies. Ann. Thorac. Surg., 46:645, 1988.
39. Patrick, D. L., and McGoon, D. C.: Operation for double-outlet right ventricle with transposition of the great arteries. J. Cardiovasc. Surg., 9:537, 1968.
40. Piccoli, G., Pacifico, A. D., Kirklin, J. W., Blackstone, E. H., Kirklin, J. K., and Bargeron, L. M., Jr.: Changing results and concepts in the surgical treatment of double outlet right ventricle. Am. J. Cardiol., 52:549, 1983.
41. Quaegebeur, J. M.: The optimal repair for the Taussig-Bing heart. J. Thorac. Cardiovasc. Surg., 85:276, 1983.

42. Quaegebeur, J. M., Rohmer, J., Ottenkamp, J., Buis, T., Kirklin, J. W., Blackstone, E. H., and Brom, A. G.: The arterial switch operation. An eight-year experience. J. Thorac. Cardiovasc. Surg., 92:365, 1986.
43. Rastelli, G. C., McGoon, D. C., and Wallace, R. B.: Anatomic correction of transposition of the great arteries with ventricular septal defect and subpulmonic stenosis. J. Thorac. Cardiovasc. Surg., 58:545, 1969.
44. Rastelli, G. C., Wallace, R. B., and Ongley, P. A.: Complete repair of transposition of the great arteries with pulmonary stenosis. A review and report of a case corrected by using a new surgical technique. Circulation, 39:83, 1969.
45. Serratto, M., Arevalo, F., Goldman, E. J., Hastreiter, A., and Miller, R. A.: Obstructive ventricular septal defect in double outlet right ventricle. Am. J. Cardiol., 19:457, 1967.
46. Shaffer, A. B., Lopez, J. F., Kline, I. K., and Lev, M.: Truncal inversion with biventricular pulmonary trunk and aorta from right ventricle (variant of Taussig-Bing complex). Circulation, 36:783, 1967.
47. Sondheimer, H. M., Freedom, R. M., and Olley, P. M.: Double outlet right ventricle. Clinical spectrum and prognosis. Am. J. Cardiol., 39:709, 1977.
48. Sridaromont, S., Feldt, R. H., Ritter, D. G., Davis, G. D., and Edwards, J. E.: Double outlet right ventricle: Hemodynamic and anatomic correlations. Am. J. Cardiol., 38:85, 1976.
49. Sridaromont, S., Feldt, R. H., Ritter, D. G., Davis, G. D., McGoon, D. C., and Edwards, J. E.: Double-outlet right ventricle associated with persistent common atrioventricular canal. Circulation, 52:933, 1975.
50. Sridaromont, S., Ritter, D. G., Feldt, R. H., Davis, G. D., and Edwards, J. E.: Double-outlet right ventricle. Anatomic and angiocardiographic correlations. Mayo Clin. Proc., 53:555, 1978.
51. Stewart, R. W., Kirklin, J. W., Pacifico, A. D., Blackstone, E. H., and Bargeron, L. M., Jr.: Repair of double outlet right ventricle. An analysis of 62 cases. J. Thorac. Cardiovasc. Surg., 78:502, 1979.
52. Tabry, I. F., McGoon, D. C., Danielson, G. K., Wallace, R. B., Davis, Z., and Maloney, J. D.: Surgical management of double-outlet right ventricle associated with atrioventricular discordance. J. Thorac. Cardiovasc. Surg., 76:336, 1978.
53. Taussig, H. B., and Bing, J. F.: Complete transposition of the aorta and a levoposition of the pulmonary artery. Clinical, physiological, and pathological findings. Am. Heart J., 37:551, 1949.
54. Van Praagh, R., Perez-Trevino, C., Reynolds, J. L., Moes, C. A. F., Keith, J. D., Roy, D. L., Belcourt, C., Weinberg, P. M., and Parisi, L. F.: Double outlet right ventricle (S, D, L) with subaortic ventricular septal defect and pulmonary stenosis. Report of six cases. Am. J. Cardiol., 35:42, 1975.
55. Waldo, A. L., Pacifico, A. D., Bargeron, L. M., Jr., James, T. N., and Kirklin, J. W.: Electrophysiological delineation of the specialized A-V conduction system in patients with corrected transposition of the great vessels and ventricular septal defect. Circulation, 52:435, 1975.
56. Wilkinson, J. L., Wilcox, B. R., and Anderson, R. H.: Anatomy of double outlet right ventricle. In Anderson, R. H., Macartney, F. J., Shinebourne, E. A., and Tynan, M. (Eds.): Paediatric Cardiology. Vol. 5. New York, Churchill Livingstone, 1983, pp. 397–407.
57. Zamora, R., Moller, J. H., and Edwards, J. E.: Double-outlet right ventricle. Anatomic types and associated anomalies. Chest, 68:672, 1975.

X

TRICUSPID ATRESIA

Harvey W. Bender, Jr., M.D.

The primary malformation in tricuspid atresia is the failure of development of the right atrioventricular valve. Associated with this are varying degrees of hypoplasia of the right ventricle and infundibulum and, in most patients, an atrial septal defect. This malformation may occur in patients with normally related great arteries or in patients with transposition of the great arteries. Ventricular septal defect can also occur with or without stenosis of the pulmonary outflow tract.

Tricuspid atresia represents 1 to 5 per cent of all congenital heart defects. The embryologic events that are altered to produce this complex are unknown. Two alternative explanations are offered.[9] The first is that differential growth occurs between the ventricle and bulbus cordis, with subsequent failure of adequate development of the right ventricle, with tricuspid atresia being a secondary event. The second possible etiologic mechanism is that the atrioventricular orifice fails to migrate from its initial position overlying the future left ventricle.

Various classifications for the spectrum of abnormalities found in tricuspid atresia are currently being used. An anatomic pathologic classification proposed by Tandon and Edwards[10] is based primarily on the relationships of the great arteries to the ventricles and secondarily on the presence or absence of obstruction to pulmonary blood flow. A clinical anatomic classification has been proposed by Rudolph.[9] Each of Rudolph's three classes has a characteristic clinical presentation. In Group I, tricuspid atresia with intact ventricular septum and hypoplastic right ventricle, infants present with hypoxemia and acidemia. Pulmonary blood flow is dependent on the presence of a patent ductus arteriosus. All systemic and pulmonary venous return mixes in the atria. The degree of cyanosis in these infants depends primarily on the size and patency of the ductus and the ratio of systemic to pulmonary vascular resistance. In Group II, tricuspid atresia with ventricular septal defect and normally related great arteries, cyanosis occurs during the first few days

of life and is then accompanied by left ventricular failure and pulmonary edema as pulmonary vascular resistance falls. Congestive heart failure develops in this group of infants within the first 2 to 3 weeks of life and increases as pulmonary vascular resistance decreases. In Group III, tricuspid atresia with ventricular septal defect and transposed great arteries, the infant may present with only mild cyanosis; however, the hypoplastic right (or systemic) ventricle is unable to sustain an adequate cardiac output in the absence of pulmonary stenosis and a ventricular septal defect.

All current treatment for infants with tricuspid atresia should be considered palliative. In the cyanotic infant, augmentation of pulmonary blood flow is required. This is accomplished by a shunt to increase pulmonary blood flow. This may be in the form of an aortopulmonary shunt, subclavian to pulmonary artery shunt, or superior vena cava to pulmonary artery shunt. Few infants in Rudolph's Group I survive the first 6 months without treatment. Operative mortality for shunts in these first few months of life has been high, and, as a result, there has been interest in performing more definitive surgical procedures in younger patients. However, after age 6 months palliative operations have a lower operative mortality and the long-term results have been good, with 50 per cent survival reported at 15 years of age.[11]

The various types of systemic pulmonary artery shunts are associated with their certain complications and results. With the improvement of operative techniques, particularly the use of magnification and fine monofilament suture, the subclavian to pulmonary artery anastomosis is now performed in newborns with increasing success. This appears to be the procedure of choice in patients who require a shunt in the first few weeks of life. In older children, the superior vena cava to right pulmonary artery shunt is quite satisfactory with good relief of symptoms for periods of several years.[8]

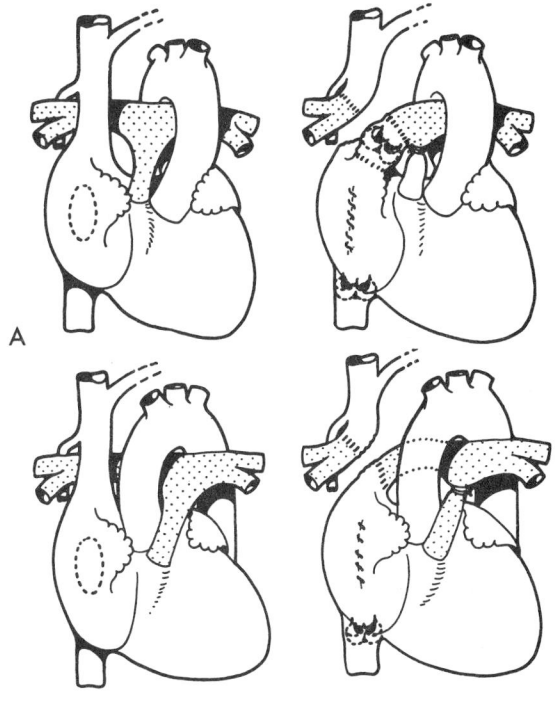

competence, and no obstruction in the pulmonary arterial tree. The essential feature of the procedure, however it is modified, is to provide a wide open, unimpeded connection between the right atrium or venae cavae and the pulmonary artery with subsequent closure of the atrial communication.

Although results of the intracardiac procedures for tricuspid atresia are encouraging, it must be recognized that they are a palliative procedure and that careful selection is essential to identify patients who might be candidates for intracardiac repair.[5] Whereas it has been shown that good results can be achieved outside Fontan's original criteria,[7] the criteria remain important in patient selection.[3]

SELECTED REFERENCES

Bowman, F., Malm, J., Hayes, C., and Gersony, W.: Physiological approach to surgery for tricuspid atresia. Cardiovasc. Surg., 58:83, 1977.
A modification of Fontan's procedure for the intracardiac repair for tricuspid atresia is reported. This technique takes advantage of right ventricular muscle by incorporating a valve-containing conduit as a roof to the right ventricle, so that right ventricular contraction aids in propelling blood through the pulmonary circulation.

Fontan, F., and Baudet, E.: Surgical repair of tricuspid atresia. Thorax, 26:240, 1971.
This is the first published report of attempts to correct tricuspid atresia; two of three patients survived. The details of the operation and indications for its applicability to older children who have received shunts are discussed.

Rudolph, A. M.: Congenital Diseases of the Heart. Chicago, Year Book Medical Publishers, 1974, pp. 424–461.
This monograph is a personal approach to understanding the physiology and clinical presentation of a variety of congenital cardiac defects. The natural history of tricuspid atresia, progressive changes in the hemodynamics of the circulatory system, and types of operative and nonoperative treatment are discussed clearly.

REFERENCES

1. Bjork, V. O., Olin, C. L., Bjarke, B. B., and Thoren, C. A.: Right atrial–right ventricular anastomosis for correction of tricuspid atresia. J. Thorac. Cardiovasc. Surg., 77:452, 1979.
2. Bowman, F., Malm, J., Hayes, C., and Gersony, W.: Physiological approach to surgery for tricuspid atresia. Cardiovasc. Surg., 58:83, 1977.
3. Choussat, A., Fontan, F., Besse, P., Vallot, F., Chauve, A., and Bricaud, H.: Selection criteria for Fontan's procedure. *In* Anderson, R. H., and Shinebourne, E. A. (Eds.): Pediatric Cardiology 1977. Edinburgh, Churchill Livingstone, 1978, p. 559.
4. de Leval, M. R., Kilner, P., Gewillig, M., and Bull, C.: Total cavopulmonary connection: A logical alternative to atriopulmonary connection for complex Fontan operations. Experimental studies and early clinical experience. J. Thorac. Cardiovasc. Surg., 96:682, 1988.
5. Fernandez, G., Costa, F., Fontan, F., Naftel, D. C., Blackstone, E. H., and Kirklin, J. W.: Prevalence of reoperation for pathway obstruction after Fontan operation. Ann. Thorac. Surg., 48:654, 1989.
6. Fontan, F., and Baudet, E.: Surgical repair of tricuspid atresia. Thorax, 26:240, 1971.
7. Gale, A. W., Danielson, G. K., McGoon, D. C., Wallace, R. B., and Mair, D. D.: Fontan procedure for tricuspid atresia. Circulation, 62:91, 1980.
8. Mathur, M., and Glenn, W. W. L.: Long-term evaluation of cava–pulmonary artery anastomosis. Surgery, 53:899, 1973.
9. Rudolph, A. M.: Congenital Disease of the Heart. Chicago, Year Book Medical Publishers, 1974, pp. 424–461.
10. Tandon, R., and Edwards, J. E.: Tricuspid atresia: A re-evaluation and classification. J. Thorac. Cardiovasc. Surg., 47:531, 1974.
11. Williams, W. G., Rubis, L., Trusler, G. A., and Mustard, W. T.: Palliation of tricuspid atresia. Arch. Surg., 110:1383, 1975.

Figure 1. *A,* Fontan's operation consists of the constriction of an end-to-side superior vena cava to right pulmonary artery anastomosis and an anastomosis between the right atrial appendage and the proximal stump of the right pulmonary artery, with interposition of a segment of aortic allograft with intact valve. The patient is then placed on cardiopulmonary bypass, the right atrium opened, the interatrial communication closed, and a pulmonary valve allograft inserted into the inferior vena cava. The main pulmonary artery is ligated, and bypass is discontinued. The last step of the procedure is division of the superior vena cava below the pulmonary anastomosis and suture closure of the two ends. *B,* In one patient, the same procedure was performed, but no allograft was used at the atrium to pulmonary artery anastomosis. (From Fontan, F., and Baudet, E.: Surgical repair of tricuspid atresia. Thorax, 26:240, 1971.)

In infants in Rudolph's Group II and Group III with increased pulmonary blood flow, medical management with digitalis and diuretics should be undertaken. If this treatment regimen fails, banding of the pulmonary artery may be necessary. In all groups, a satisfactory interatrial communication is necessary.

In 1971 Fontan and Baudet[6] reported an operative procedure to "correct" tricuspid atresia. This consisted of diverting all systemic venous return through a valve-containing conduit to the lungs with closure of the interatrial septal defect (Fig. 1). Originally they incorporated an aortic valve homograft into the inferior vena cava–right atrial junction to prevent reflux into the inferior vena cava. This is no longer employed, and the procedure has been modified in the last 2 decades with steadily improving results.[1,2,4] Predictable good results can be obtained with this procedure in patients with low pulmonary vascular resistance, good left ventricular function, no mitral valve in-

XI

HYPOPLASTIC LEFT HEART SYNDROME

William I. Norwood, M.D., Ph.D.

Hypoplastic left heart syndrome is the most common malformation in which there is only one ventricle and the fourth most common congenital cardiac anomaly presenting in the first year of life. Lev[46] first described the pathologic process of *hypoplasia of the aortic tract complexes* and included cases of (1) isolated hypoplasia of the aorta, (2) hypoplasia of the aorta with ventricular septal defect, and (3) hypoplasia of the aorta with aortic stenosis or atresia with or without mitral stenosis or atresia in this category. Noonan and Nadas[57] referred to these lesions as hypoplastic left heart syndrome. Whereas the anatomic associates involving the hypoplastic left heart syndrome are varied, the physiologic similarity of this collection of lesions made this term acceptable, but with the advent of surgical management for patients with hypoplastic left heart syndrome,* interest in a more precise anatomic definition has increased.

DEFINITION AND ANATOMY

Hypoplastic left heart syndrome is a collective term describing a group of cardiac malformations in which there is aortic valve hypoplasia, stenosis, or atresia with either hypoplasia or absence of the left ventricle and, as a consequence, hypoplasia of the ascending aorta. Most frequently, severe mitral hypoplasia or mitral atresia is also present. A less common variation includes malalignment of the common atrioventricular canal with the muscular ventricular septum over the right ventricle. Whereas 10 per cent of patients have double outlet right ventricle rather than the usual normally related great arteries, cases involving transposition of the great arteries with hypoplasia of the left ventricle and pulmonary artery, or hypoplasia of the right ventricle and aorta are not considered hypoplastic left heart syndrome.

The anatomy of patients with aortic stenosis/atresia has been thoroughly described.* The inferior vena cava and right superior vena cava enter the right atrium normally. In 2.5 to 4.3 per cent of patients, there is a persistent left superior vena cava.[13,64] The right atrium is dilated, and the tricuspid valve orifice is enlarged.[7,12,37,76] The right ventricle is enlarged[12,27,43,76,77] as well as the pulmonary orifice and main pulmonary artery. Bharati[12] reported 3 patients with aortic atresia with pulmonary valve abnormalities (thickened nodular leaflets). Two of 198 patients with hypoplastic left heart syndrome presenting to the Children's Hospital of Philadelphia since 1984 have had concurrent pulmonic stenosis. The left and right pulmonary arteries arise from the underside of the main pulmonary artery with the right branch orifice proximal to the left branch orifice. In patients dying before 2 weeks of age, there is no significant difference in the size and character of the small and medium-size pulmonary artery branches.[71] Pulmonary venous connection is usually normal, but occasionally there is anomalous or accessory pulmonary venous connection, usually through a persistent left vertical vein to the left innominate vein.[78] The left atrium is small and frequently hypertrophied.[12,27,43,64,76,78] An interatrial communication is usually present although there may be a congenitally small foramen ovale.[12,27,78,79] In an autopsy series, 65 per cent of patients had a posterior and leftward displacement of the superior attachment of the septum primum vis-à-vis septum secundum[79].

Mitral stenosis or hypoplasia is present in approximately 60 per cent of the patients, with the remaining 40 per cent having mitral atresia.[12,64] When there is mitral stenosis, the mitral valve leaflets are thickened with short, thick chordae attached to short papillary muscles.[12] In patients with mitral atresia, there may be a blind dimple on the floor of the left atrium at the usual site of the mitral valve with no grossly recognizable mitral valve tissue,[27,43] or there may be atretic mitral valve tissue.[80] The left ventricle does not form the apex of the heart. In patients with mitral hypoplasia or stenosis (patent left ventricular inflow), there is frequently prominent endocardial fibroelastosis[12,46,62,64,71] with myofiber disarray.[18]

In a study by Bharati,[12] 87 per cent of the patients had aortic atresia and 13 per cent aortic stenosis. The coronary arteries originate normally from the aortic root and have a normal distribution.[12] The ascending and transverse aorta are hypoplastic. With aortic atresia, the ascending aorta size is usually 1 to 3 mm. In rare cases with aortic stenosis, the mean size of the ascending aorta has been reported to be as large as 5 to 6 mm. True coarctation of the aorta is not a common finding. There is, however, a posterolateral intimal ridge at the junction of the aortic isthmus, ductus arteriosus, and thoracic aorta in the majority of patients.

EPIDEMIOLOGY

Hypoplastic left heart syndrome has been reported to occur in at least 0.016 per cent to 0.036 per cent of live births, making it the most common defect in which there is only one ventricle.[17,33] In pathologic series, it represents 1.4 to 3.8 per cent of congenital heart disease[1,25] and has been reported as causing 23 per cent of the deaths due to congenital heart disease in the newborn period.[78]

There is a slight male predominance in hypoplastic left heart syndrome. Currently, 57 per cent of the patients with hypoplastic left heart syndrome observed at the Children's Hospital of Philadelphia are male. The recurrence risk of siblings of patients with hypoplastic left heart syndrome has been reported as 0.5 per cent with a 2.2 per cent risk for other forms of congenital heart disease.[17,39,58]

ETIOLOGY

The abnormal development of the left-sided cardiac structures primarily follows atresia or marked hypoplasia of the aortic valve. When there is left ventricular outflow obstruction with an intact ventricular septum, the left ventricle is hypoplastic. In the rare case of left ventricular outflow obstruction with an unrestrictive ventricular septal defect, normal left ventricular development can occur. Thus, a primary myocardial abnormality is unlikely as the cause of hypoplastic left heart syndrome. The resultant elevation in left ventricular pressure that occurs with patent left ventricular inflow and obstructed left ventricu-

---

* See references 12, 16, 18, 27, 28, 37, 42, 43, 46, 54, 57, 62, 64, 71, and 76 to 80.

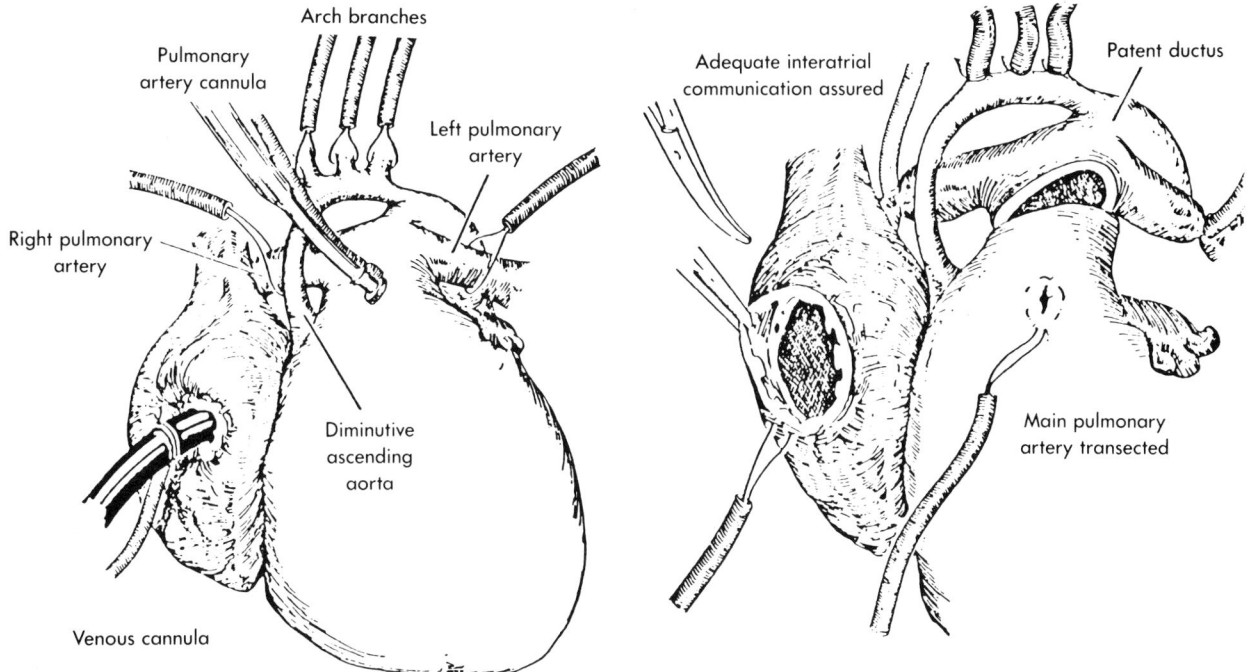

Figure 1. Cardiopulmonary bypass is established by arterial infusion in the proximal pulmonary artery. The branch pulmonary arteries are occluded with 2–0 Tevdek tourniquets. Through the atrial appendage the septum primum is excised. The main pulmonary artery is transected. (From Norwood, W. I., and Murphy, J. D.: Hypoplastic left heart syndrome. *In* Sabiston, D. C., Jr., and Spencer, F. C. (Eds.): Surgery of the Chest, 5th ed. Philadelphia, W. B. Saunders Company, 1989.)

lar outflow in the absence of a ventricular septal defect probably causes the endocardiofibroelastosis observed in some patients. Whereas a congenitally small or absent foramen ovale has been suggested as a possible cause of hypoplastic left heart syndrome,[10,12,47] this is more likely the result of increased left atrial pressure secondary to the left ventricular outflow obstruction.

PHYSIOLOGY

The left ventricle in hypoplastic left heart syndrome is a non-functional structure. Pulmonary venous return must therefore be to the right atrium. This occurs through an atrial septal defect, a stretched foramen ovale, or, rarely, an anomalous pulmonary venous connection. In the right atrium, systemic and pulmonary venous return mix. The right ventricle must maintain both the pulmonary and systemic output, and the ductus arteriosus must remain patent for systemic perfusion.

In utero, oxygenation occurs via the placenta. Because the right ventricle is able to maintain systemic output by the ductus arteriosus, the child develops normally *in utero.* After birth, systemic blood flow is maintained as long as the ductus arteriosus remains patent. Perfusion is retrograde through the transverse arch and ascending aorta to the carotid and coronary arteries. With the left and right pulmonary arteries connected parallel with the ductus arteriosus and descending aorta, the relative ratio of pulmonary to systemic blood flow depends on a delicate balance between pulmonary and systemic vascular resistances. In the majority of patients, balanced systemic and pulmonary perfusion can be maintained. In some, however, there is a low pulmonary to systemic resistance ratio causing excessive pulmonary blood flow. Although arterial oxygen saturation is elevated secondary to the high pulmonary blood flow, systemic perfusion is marginal in this circumstance and the child develops metabolic acidosis. In very rare cases, there is a high pulmonary to systemic resistance ratio secondary to a very restrictive interatrial communication. These patients appear markedly cyanotic because of inadequate pulmonary blood flow and can become acidotic because of hypoxemia with Pao_2 less than 20 mm. Hg.

CLINICAL FEATURES

When hypoplastic left heart syndrome presents within 24 hours of birth, it is usually secondary to severe obstruction to blood flow at the interatrial level (congenitally small or absent foramen ovale). More typically, however, Apgar scores are normal. Within 24 to 48 hours of birth, most patients with hypoplastic left heart syndrome develop a dusky cyanosis with evidence of tachypnea and respiratory distress.[27,57,64,71,78] When the ductus arteriosus begins to close, the patient develops metabolic acidosis. Prostaglandin must be administered at this stage to ensure patency of the ductus arteriosus and allow operative intervention. Both intravenous prostaglandin E_1 and oral prostaglandin E_2 have proved effective.[32,48,69,82]

Physical examination typically reveals a mildly cyanotic infant with tachypnea and tachycardia. Depending on the degree of ductal patency at the time of evaluation, peripheral pulses may be normal, diminished, or absent. Rales may be auscultated, although generally the lung fields are clear. Cardiac examination reveals a dominant right ventricular impulse on palpation[78] with a decreased left ventricular (apical) impulse. S_1 is normal and S_2 usually single and increased in intensity.[78]

The electrocardiogram frequently reflects the underlying pathologic process. Right atrial enlargement is observed in 30 to 41 per cent and right ventricular hypertrophy is found in 78 to 92 per cent of patients.[27,57,71] Approximately 56 per cent of patients have a QR pattern in lead V_1.[71,78] In patients with malaligned common atrioventricular canal, the QRS axis is leftward and superior.

The findings of the chest film in hypoplastic left heart syndrome are nonspecific. Cardiomegaly is reported in 75 to 85 per cent of the patients, and pulmonary vascular markings are increased in 68 to 82 per cent.[64,71]

Two-dimensional echocardiography is diagnostic in this lesion.[8,9,15,29,38,42,50,55,66,67,72,74] The intracardiac anatomy should be examined with subcostal frontal, sagittal, left oblique, and right oblique sweeps.[20,41,51]

With accurate diagnosis possible by two-dimensional and Doppler echocardiography, cardiac catheterization is no longer

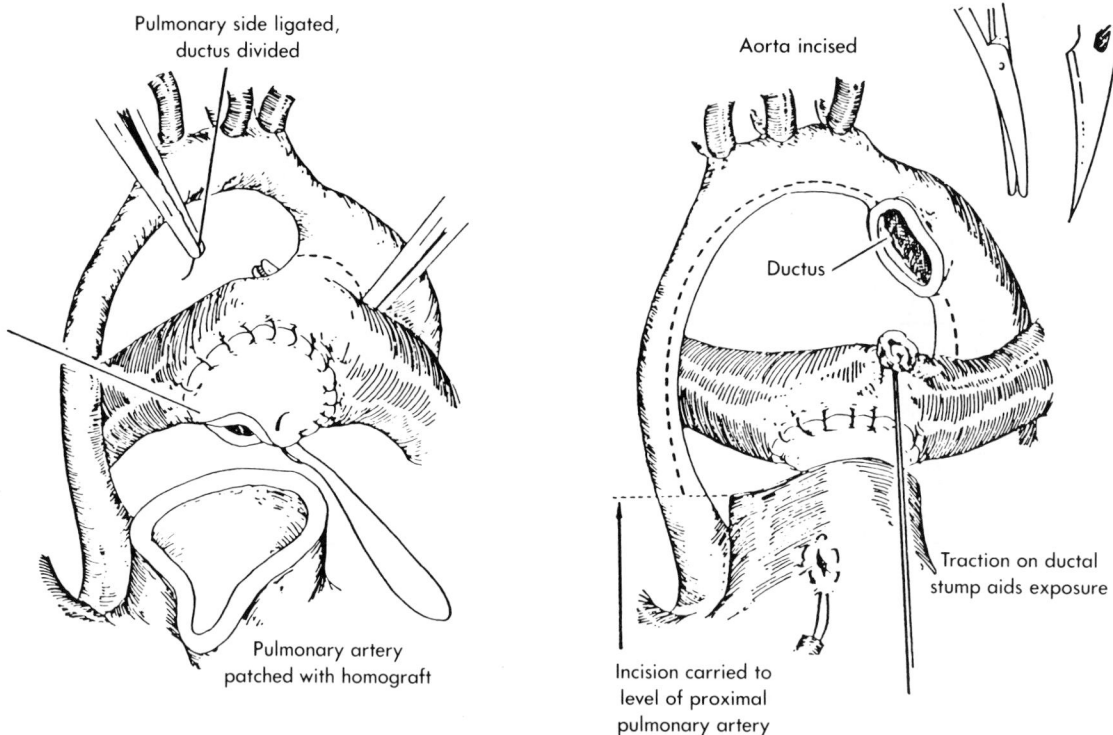

Pulmonary side ligated,
ductus divided

Aorta incised

Ductus

Pulmonary artery
patched with homograft

Traction on ductal
stump aids exposure

Incision carried to
level of proximal
pulmonary artery

Figure 2. The distal main pulmonary artery is closed with a patch. The ductus arteriosus is ligated and divided after patch closure of the distal main pulmonary artery. (From Norwood W. I., and Murphy, J. D.: Hypoplastic left heart syndrome. *In* Sabiston, D. C., Jr., and Spencer, F. C. (Eds.): Surgery of the Chest, 5th ed. Philadelphia, W. B. Saunders Company, 1989.)

routinely necessary in hypoplastic left heart syndrome. Moreover, because some obstruction to pulmonary venous return limits pulmonary overcirculation in patients with hypoplastic left heart syndrome, performance of a balloon atrial septotomy during cardiac catheterization may cause hemodynamic deterioration and should be avoided.

NATURAL HISTORY

Untreated, over 95 per cent of infants with hypoplastic left heart syndrome die within the first month of life.[34] Hypoplastic left heart syndrome represents approximately 25 per cent of cardiac deaths during the first week and 15 per cent of cardiac deaths during the first month of life.[57] Rarely, the ductus arteriosus remains patent. If pulmonary and systemic resistances are balanced, survival for 4 to 6 years has been reported sporadically.[26,53] These patients expire secondary to pulmonary vascular obstructive disease.

PREOPERATIVE CARE

The preoperative care of the child with hypoplastic left heart syndrome is the same regardless of the surgical approach chosen. When the diagnosis is made, a continuous infusion of prostaglandin E_1 intravenously at a dose of 0.05 to 0.10 μg. per kg. per minute should be administered. If available, orally administered prostaglandin E_2 may be used.[32,69] An arterial line should be inserted for monitoring of arterial oxygen saturation and acid-base status. If possible, the umbilical artery should be used to preserve the peripheral arteries for future use.

The major goal of the preoperative period is to ensure adequate systemic perfusion for the metabolic needs of the child. Systemic perfusion depends on a delicate balance between pulmonary and systemic vascular resistances. Usually the pulmonary resistance is less than systemic, and care must be taken not to further decrease pulmonary resistance. The primary metabolic factor that appears to influence pulmonary resistance in

this group of patients is PCO_2. For this reason, care must be taken not to hyperventilate these patients, and hyperoxic ventilation should be avoided. Patients with hypoplastic left heart syndrome often have no abnormality of oxygen transport across the alveolar membrane. The effect of supplemental oxygen is to decrease pulmonary resistance and increase systemic resistance causing increased pulmonary blood flow and decreased systemic perfusion. In this situation, the oxygen saturation of peripheral blood may be increased, but oxygen delivery decreases and metabolic acidosis can ensue. Similarly, inotropic agents often cause an unfavorable pulmonary to systemic resistance ratio. Whereas overall cardiac output may be increased, peripheral perfusion often decreases. Inotropic agents, although they may be necessary in cases of hypoplastic left heart syndrome with underlying abnormalities such as sepsis, are usually unnecessary and harmful in uncomplicated cases of hypoplastic left heart syndrome. When the pulmonary vascular resistance has decreased very low, it is often difficult to stabilize the systemic perfusion. One approach to increase pulmonary resistance, and thus systemic perfusion in these patients, is elective endotracheal intubation. The PCO_2 can then be adjusted to 45 to 50 mm. Hg. This elevates pulmonary resistance and increases peripheral perfusion. Some degree of pulmonary venous obstruction, usually at the level of a patent foramen ovale or atrial septal defect, is a frequent component of pulmonary resistance in this lesion. Mild to moderate interatrial obstruction is beneficial to preoperative hemodynamics. In the absence of PO_2 less than 25 mm. Hg, atrial septotomy should not be performed prior to surgical palliation.

Recently, two approaches to the surgical management of hypoplastic left heart syndrome have been advanced: reconstructive procedures and cardiac replacement. The rationale for reconstructive procedures is based on the fact that the lungs, coronary anatomy, and myocardial biochemistry are inherently normal in this condition. Thus, if one considers hypoplastic left heart syndrome as one of several cardiac malformations with only one effective ventricle, a surgical approach may be devised leading to a modification of Fontan's procedure. It has been demonstrated that a good functional result following Fontan's procedure can be expected when the pulmonary artery architecture is nearly normal, pulmonary vascular resistance is that of the normal mature lung, and ventricular function has been preserved (low end-diastolic pressure). However, since the systemic circulation in neonates with hypoplastic left heart syndrome is dependent on the patency of the ductus arteriosus that characteristically closes in the first days of life, an urgent operative procedure is necessary. The pulmonary vascular resistance of the newborn is prohibitively high for Fontan's procedure, and therefore surgical therapy is necessary. The general goals of the initial stage are to establish unobstructed systemic output from the right ventricle, to ensure normal maturation of the pulmonary vasculature by regulating pulmonary arterial blood flow and pressure, and to ensure a widely patent interatrial communication, thereby avoiding pulmonary venous hypertension. Although several approaches to these goals have been conceived, the surgical techniques outlined are designed to additionally incorporate as much as possible of the patient's own tissues and to avoid conduits or circumferential suture lines, thus minimizing the number of surgical interventions.

PALLIATION FOR HYPOPLASTIC LEFT HEART SYNDROME (STAGE I)

A conventional midline sternotomy incision is made and partial excision of the thymus undertaken to facilitate exposure of the diminutive aortic arch and its branch vessels. Cannulation for arterial infusion is most conveniently achieved in the proximal main pulmonary artery just above the sinuses of Valsalva by placing a single diamond-shaped pursestring suture through a small rubber tourniquet. Threading of the cannula through the ductus arteriosus is avoided because it is unnecessary and requires excessive manipulation of the cardiovascular structures. A 16-French venous cannula is placed through the right atrial appendage and cardiopulmonary bypass instituted. The right and left pulmonary artery branches are rapidly exposed and occluded with 2–0 Tevdek tourniquets to ensure systemic perfusion through the ductus arteriosus. The infant is cooled to 20° C. while esophageal, nasopharyngeal, and rectal temperatures are monitored. During this time, the branch vessels of the aortic arch are exposed and looped with 2–0 Tevdek tourniquets in preparation for circulatory arrest. Dissection is extended around the aortic arch onto the thoracic aorta in the posterior mediastinum. At this point, the branch vessels of the aortic arch are occluded, the circulation is discontinued, and the blood is drained into the venous reservoir. Through the right atrial cannulation site, the septum primum is identified and excised. Adjacent to the takeoff of the right pulmonary artery, the main pulmonary artery is transected and the distal stump of the main pulmonary artery is oversewn with a patch using a running monofilament suture technique (Fig. 1). Patch closure is recommended in order to better maintain continuity between the right and left pulmonary artery branches. The ductus arteriosus is then exposed, ligated, and transected at its entrance into the thoracic aorta. An incision in the aorta is extended distally 1 to 2 cm. into the thoracic aorta and also proximally into the aortic arch and ascending aorta to the level of the rim of the transected proximal main pulmonary artery (Fig. 2).

Because the isthmus of the aorta and the aortic arch actually function as a branch of the main pulmonary artery–ductus–thoracic aorta continuum, the junction of the isthmus and thoracic aorta should be gusseted with a patch and the intimal ridge excised in order to minimize the late development of distal aortic arch obstruction. Again, a monofilament running suture technique is used. At this point, the author favors the construction of a short central shunt of 4 mm. tube graft (polytetrafluoroethylene) between the inferior aspect of the augmented aortic

arch and the confluence of branch pulmonary arteries, although a right Blalock-Taussig shunt is also satisfactory. The rationale for a central shunt is to obtain more even distribution of flow and thus growth of the right and left pulmonary arteries. The remaining gusset is then extended to approximately 5 mm. above the end of the most proximal incision in the ascending aorta. The proximal anastomosis of the main pulmonary artery to the ascending aorta is initiated with multiple interrupted fine monofilament sutures to avoid pursestringing of the inlet into the diminutive aortic root. The reconstruction is completed by anastomosis of the ascending aorta, main pulmonary artery, and pulmonary homograft, thus creating outflow from the right ventricle to the augmented aorta through the pulmonary valve. Cardiopulmonary bypass is reinstituted and the patient is rewarmed to 37° C. Postoperatively, the ventilator may be used to adjust the pulmonary to systemic flow ratio by rapidly decreasing P_{CO_2} to decrease pulmonary resistance and increasing P_{CO_2} to increase pulmonary resistance.

FONTAN'S PROCEDURE (STAGE II)

Following the previously described palliative operation, the right ventricle is subjected to both a volume and pressure load. With a view to long-term preservation of ventricular function, assessment of suitability for Fontan's procedure is undertaken at 12 to 18 months of age. At this age, the pulmonary resistance is likely to be low (less than 2.5 Woods units) and ventricular end-diastolic pressure normal (less than 7 to 8 mm. Hg). The following surgical procedure may then be planned.

The systemic to pulmonary artery shunt is exposed and occluded as cardiopulmonary bypass is instituted and the patient's core temperature is reduced to 20° C. The aorta is then cross-clamped, and cardioplegia solution is infused as the circulation is arrested. The pulmonary arteries are opened by a single incision extending from behind the right superior vena cava across the midline to the left lower lobe branch. An incision is made in the dome of the right atrium adjacent to the right pulmonary artery, and this incision is extended into the posterior aspect of the right superior vena cava immediately adjacent to the most rightward aspect of the incision in the right pulmonary artery. A suture line is begun between the inferior lip of the incised right pulmonary artery and the posterior lip of the right superior vena caval–right atrial incision. This provides the floor for the anastomosis of the systemic venous return to the pulmonary arterial tree. An incision in the right atrium is made from the sulcus terminalis superiorly to the right lateral insertion of the eustachian valve inferiorly. A segment of polytetrafluoroethylene tubing 10 mm. in diameter of sufficient length to extend from the inferior vena caval–right atrial junction to the right superior vena caval–right atrial junction is cut in half lengthwise for use as a baffle to channel inferior vena caval flow along the right lateral aspect of the right atrium to the superior anastomosis between the right atrium and the pulmonary arterial tree. This particular baffling technique was introduced to minimize complications associated with tricuspid prolapse or regurgitation, or obstruction of pulmonary venous return to the right ventricle experienced early in this series with an alternative baffling technique. The construction of the systemic venous pulmonary arterial system is completed by gusseting the pulmonary arterial incision.

Results

In the 5 years 1984 to 1988, 198 newborns had palliative operative procedures similar to that described for hypoplastic left heart syndrome at the Children's Hospital of Philadelphia. The hospital mortality was 28 per cent, and the 18-month actuarial survival was 61 per cent. To date, 52 patients have undergone application of Fontan's procedure for the treatment of hypoplastic left heart syndrome. Among these, there were 16 early and 2 late deaths, with 2 deaths in the last 15 patients. The results continue to improve, both for initial palliation and for later reconstructive procedures as an ever-increasing knowledge of the anatomy and physiology of this complex group of patients is gained. Heart replacement is a modality considered in some centers as a primary treatment of this malformation. With an increasing understanding of all therapeutic procedures, an appropriate strategy for managing infants with this most complex and compelling malformation will be forthcoming.

SELECTED REFERENCES

Bailey, L., Concepcion, W., Shattuck, H., and Huang, L.: Method of heart transplantation for treatment of hypoplastic left heart syndrome. J. Thorac. Cardiovasc. Surg., 92:1, 1986.
  Technical details of the investigational orthotopic cardiac transplantation for management of hypoplastic left heart syndrome in the neonate are presented. A technique of extracorporeal perfusion and the need for extensive aortic arch reconstruction are emphasized. The source of donor graft in this case report was a subhuman primate but it is emphasized that the donor graft makes little difference with regard to the unique technical aspects of cardiac transplantation in a ductus dependent newborn infant with a diminutive aortic arch.

Bailey, L. L., et al.: Cardiac allotransplantation in newborns as therapy for hypoplastic left heart syndrome. N. Engl. J. Med., 315:949, 1986.
  These authors present the initial Loma Linda experience with heart replacement therapy for hypoplastic left heart syndrome. This report not only demonstrates the feasibility of heart replacement in patients with the aortic arch anatomy of hypoplastic left heart syndrome but also illustrates the complex circumstances surrounding heart procurement within a limited time frame of a heart sufficiently small to fit in the mediastinum of the newborn. Short-term results suggest that immunosuppressive management of the newborn and small infant is no more complicated than in the adult population.

Jonas, R. A., et al.: First-stage palliation of hypoplastic left heart syndrome: The importance of coarctation and shunt size. J. Thorac. Cardiovasc. Surg., 92:6, 1986.
  This report describes the experience with palliative surgery for 25 neonates between January 1984 and July 1985. During this time frame there were six deaths. The authors emphasize the importance of a posterior shelf at the junction of the isthmus of the aorta with the thoracic aorta, which can cause late coarctation of the aorta. Moreover, they emphasize the fact that careful ventilatory and pharmacologic management of the ratio of pulmonary to systemic vascular resistance is an essential part of the perioperative management of these neonates with two parallel competing circulations.

Norwood, W. I., Lang, P., and Hansen, D.: Physiologic repair of aortic atresia — hypoplastic left heart syndrome. N. Engl. J. Med., 308:23, 1983.
  This report outlines early experience with reconstructive surgical management of hypoplastic left heart syndrome beginning in 1979. This case report is of one patient in that series who underwent physiologic correction by modification of Fontan's operative procedure demonstrating the feasibility of reconstructive surgical management of hypoplastic left heart syndrome. The patient had physiologic correction at age 16 months, at which time the pulmonary vascular resistance was calculated to be 2 Woods units. The child was reported as clinically well during 6 months of follow-up after physiologically corrective surgery. In fact, the patient remains clinically well with a right atrial pressure of 11 mm. Hg determined by cardiac catheterization at age 7 years.

Noonan, J. A., and Nadas, A. S.: The hypoplastic left heart syndrome. Pediatr. Clin. North Am, 5:1029, 1958.
  This seminal paper coins the term hypoplastic left heart syndrome and outlines the anatomic-physiologic and natural historical features of this constellation of anatomic abnormalities in the development of the left heart structures. Although the modern concepts of hypoplastic left heart syndrome are somewhat more focused today, this report represents the initial specific categorization.

Pigott, J. D., Murphy, J. D., Barber, G., and Norwood, W. I.: Palliative reconstructive surgery for hypoplastic left heart syndrome. Ann. Thorac. Surg., 45:122, 1988.
  This report constitutes the experience from August 1985 through August 1987 with 104 consecutive nonselected neonates who underwent palliative surgery as newborns for hypoplastic left heart syndrome at the Children's Hospital of Philadelphia. It presents an evolution in technique to optimize pulmonary vascular development, minimize late aortic arch obstruction, and achieve a balanced pulmonary and systemic flow ratio. Such techniques were developed to achieve the best possible preparation for application of Fontan's procedure for the treatment of hypoplastic left heart syndrome.

REFERENCES

1. Abbott, M. E.: Atlas of Congenital Cardiac Diseases. New York, American Heart Association, 1936, pp. 48 and 61.
2. Anderson, R. H., Ho, S. Y., Zuberbuhler, J. R., et al.: Surgery for hypoplastic left heart syndrome: A fiction? Surgical anatomy and definition. In Marcelletti, C., Anderson, R. H., Becker, A. E., et al. (Eds.): Pediatric Cardiology. New York, Churchill Livingstone, 1986, pp. 111–121.
3. Bailey, L., Concepcion, W., Shattuck, H., and Huang, L: Method of heart transplantation for treatment of hypoplastic left heart syndrome. J. Thorac. Cardiovasc. Surg., 92:1, 1986.
4. Bailey, L. L., et al.: Cardiac allotransplantation in newborns as therapy for hypoplastic left heart syndrome. N. Engl. J. Med., 315:949, 1986.
5. Bailey, L. L., Nehlsen-Cannarella, S. L., Concepcion, W., and Jolley, W. B.: Baboon-to-human cardiac xenotransplantation in a neonate. J.A.M.A., 254:3321, 1985.
6. Barber, G., Helton, J. G., Aglira, B. A., et al.: The significance of tricuspid regurgitation in hypoplastic left heart syndrome. Am. Heart J., 116:1563, 1988.
7. Barber, G., Murphy, J. D., Pigott, J. D., and Norwood, W. I.: The evolving pattern of surgical following palliative surgery for hypoplastic left heart syndrome. J. Am. Coll. Cardiol., 2:139A, 1988.
8. Bash, S. E., Huhta, J. C., Vick, G. W., III, et al.: Hypoplastic left heart syndrome: Is echocardiography accurate enough to guide surgical palliation. J. Am. Coll. Cardiol., 7:610, 1986.
9. Bass, J. L., Ben-Shachar, G., and Edwards, J. E.: Comparison of M-mode echocardiography and pathologic findings in the hypoplastic left heart syndrome. Am. J. Cardiol., 45:79, 1980.
10. Benner, M. C.: Premature closure of the foramen ovale. Am. Heart J., 17:437, 1939.
11. Bharati, S., and Lev., M.: The spectrum of common atrioventricular orifice (canal). Am. Heart J., 86:553, 1973.
12. Bharati, S., and Lev., M.: The surgical anatomy of hypoplasia of aortic tract complex. J. Thorac. Cardiovasc. Surg., 88:97, 1984.
13. Bharati, S., Nordenberg, A., Brock, R. R., and Lev, M.: Hypoplastic left heart syndrome with dysplastic pulmonary valve with stenosis. Pediatr. Cardiol., 5:127, 1984.
14. Bidot-Lopez, P., Matisoff, D., Talner, N.S., et al.: Hypoplastic left heart in a patient with 45,X/46,XX/47,XXX mosaicism. Am. J. Med. Genet., 2:341, 1978.
15. Bierman, F. Z.: Two-dimensional echocardiography and its influence on cardiac catheterization. Cardiovasc. Intervent. Radiol., 7:140, 1984.
16. Bjerregaard, P., and Laursen, H. B.: Persistent left superior vena cava. Acta Paediatr. Scand., 69:105, 1980.
17. Brownell, L. G., and Shokeir, M. H.: Inheritance of hypoplastic left heart syndrome. Clin. Genet., 9:245, 1976.
18. Bulkley, B. H., D'Amico, B., and Taylor, A. L.: Extensive myocardial fiber disarray in aortic and pulmonary atresia. Circulation, 67:191, 1983.
19. Chin, A. J., Sanders, S. P., Sherman, F., et al.: Accuracy of subcostal two-dimensional echocardiography in prospective diagnosis of total anomalous pulmonary venous connection. Am. Heart J., 113:1153, 1987.
20. Chin, A. J., Yeager, S. B., Sanders, S. P., et al.: Accuracy of prospective two-dimensional echocardiographic evaluation of left ventricular outflow tract in complete transposition of the great arteries. Am. J. Cardiol., 55:759, 1985.
21. Cloez, J. L., Isaaz, K., and Pernot, C.: Pulsed Doppler flow characteristics of ductus arteriosus in infants with associated congenital anomalies of the heart or great arteries. Am. J. Cardiol., 57:845, 1986.
22. Cobanoglu, A., Metzdorff, M. T., Pinson, C. W., et al.: Valvotomy for pulmonary atresia with intact ventricular septum. J. Thorac. Cardiovasc. Surg., 89:482, 1985.
23. DiDonato, R. M., Fyfe, D. A., Puga, F. I., et al.: Fifteen-year experience with surgical repair of truncus arteriosus. J. Thorac. Cardiovasc. Surg., 89:414, 1985.
24. Doty, D. B., and Knott, H. W.: Hypoplastic left heart syndrome. Experience with an operation to establish functionally normal circulation. J. Thorac. Cardiovasc. Surg., 74:624, 1977.
25. Edwards, J. E.: Congenital malformation of the heart and great vessel. In Gould, S. E. (Ed.): Pathology of the Heart. Springfield, IL, Charles C Thomas, 1953, p. 407.
26. Ehrlich, M., Bierman, F. Z., Ellis, K., and Gersony, W. M.: Hypoplastic left heart syndrome: Report of a unique survivor. J. Am. Coll. Cardiol., 7:361, 1986.
27. Elliot, R. S., et al.: Mitral atresia. A study of 32 cases. Am. Heart J., 71:6, 1965.
28. Elzenga, N. J., and Gittenberger de Grott, A. C.: Coarctation and related aortic arch anomalies. Int. J. Cardiol., 8:379, 1985.
29. Farooki, Z. Q., Henry, J. G., and Green, E. W.: Echocardiographic spectrum of the hypoplastic left heart syndrome: A clinicopathologic correlation in 19 newborns. Am. J. Cardiol., 38:337, 1976.
30. Fontan, F., and Baudet, E.: Surgical repair of tricuspid atresia. Thorax, 26:240, 1971.
31. Friedman, S., Murphy, L., and Ash, R.: Congenital mitral atresia with hypoplastic nonfunctioning left heart. J. Dis. Child., 90:176, 1955.
32. Fujiseki, Y., Yamamoto, H., Hattori, M., et al.: Oral administration of prostaglandin E_2 in hypoplastic left heart syndrome. Jpn. Heart J., 24:481, 1983.
33. Fyler, D. C.: Report of the New England Regional Infant Cardiac Program. Pediatrics, 65(Suppl.):463, 1980.
34. Fyler, D. C., Rothman, K. J., Buckley, L. P., et al.: The determinants of five year survival of infants with critical congenital heart disease. In Engle, M. A. (Ed.): Pediatric Cardiovascular Disease. (Cardiovascular Clinics.) Philadelphia, F. A. Davis, 1981, pp. 393–405.
35. Harh, J. Y., Paul, M. H., Gallen, W. J., et al.: Experimental production of

hypoplastic left heart syndrome in the chick embryo. Am. J. Cardiol., 31:51, 1973.

36. Hastreiter, A. R., van der Horst, R. L., Dubrow, I. W., and Eckner, F. O.: Quantitative angiographic and morphologic aspects of aortic valve atresia. Am. J. Cardiol., 51:1705, 1983.

37. Hawkins, J. A., and Doty, D. B.: Aortic atresia: Morphologic characteristics affecting survival and operative palliation. J. Thorac. Cardiovasc. Surg., 88:620, 1984.

38. Helton, J. G., Aglira, B. A., Chin, A. J., et al.: Analysis of potential anatomic or physiologic determinants of outcome of palliative surgery for hypoplastic left heart syndrome. Circulation, 74(Suppl. I):I-70, 1986.

39. Holmes, L. B., Rose, V., and Child, A. H.: Comment on hypoplastic left heart syndrome. Birth Defects Original Article Series. In Bergsma, D. (Ed.): Clinical Delineation of Birth Defects. XVI: Urinary System and Others. Baltimore, Williams & Wilkins, 1974, pp. 228–30.

40. Hutchins, G. M.: Coarctation of the aorta explained as a branch point of the ductus arteriosus. Am. J. Pathol., 63:203, 1971.

41. Isaaz, K., Cloez, J. L., Danchin, N., et al.: Assessment of right ventricular outflow tract in children by two-dimensional echocardiography using a new subcostal view. Am. J. Cardiol., 56:539, 1985.

42. Jonas, R. A., et al.: First-stage palliation of hypoplastic left heart syndrome: The importance of coarctation and shunt size. J. Thorac. Cardiovasc. Surg., 92:6, 1986.

43. Kanjuh, V. I., Elliot, R. S., and Edwards, J. E.: Coexistent mitral and aortic valvular atresia. A pathologic study of 14 cases. Am. J. Cardiol., 15:611, 1965.

44. Kirklin, J. W., and Barratt-Boyes, B. G.: Cardiac Surgery, Morphology, Diagnostic Criteria, Natural History, Techniques, Results, and Indications. New York, John Wiley & Sons, 1986, pp. 843–856.

45. Lehman, E.: Congenital atresia of the foramen ovale. Am. J. Dis. Child., 33:585, 1927.

46. Lev, M.: Pathologic anatomy and interrelationship of hypoplasia of the aortic tract complexes. Lab. Invest., 1:61, 1952.

47. Lev, M., Arcilla, R., Remoldi, H. J. A., et al.: Premature narrowing or closure of the foramen ovale. Am. Heart J., 65:638, 1963.

48. Lewis, A. B., Freed, M., Heymann, M. A., et al.: Side effects of therapy with prostaglandin E₁ in infants with critical congenital heart disease. Circulation, 64:893, 1981.

49. Lumb, G., and Dawkins, W. A.: Congenital atresia of mitral and aortic valves with vestigial left ventricle (three cases). Am. Heart J., 60:378, 1960.

50. Mandorla, S., Narducci, P. L., Migliozzi, L., et al.: Fetal echocardiography. Prenatal diagnosis of hypoplastic left heart syndrome. G. Ital. Cardiol., 14:517, 1984.

51. Marino, B., Ballerini, L., Marcelletti, C., et al.: Complete transposition of the great arteries: Visualization of left and right outflow tract obstruction by oblique subcostal two-dimensional echocardiography. Am. J. Cardiol., 55:1140, 1985.

52. Milo, S., Ho, S. Y., and Anderson, R. H.: Hypoplastic left heart syndrome. Can this malformation be treated surgically? Thorax, 35:351, 1980.

53. Moodie, D. S., Gallen, W. J., and Friedberg, D. Z.: Congenital aortic atresia. Report of long survival and some speculation about surgical approaches. J. Thorac. Cardiovasc. Surg., 63:726, 1972.

54. Moodie, D. S., Gill, C. C., Sterba, R., et al.: The hypoplastic left heart syndrome: Evidence of preoperative myocardial and hepatic infarction in spite of prostaglandin therapy. Ann. Thorac. Surg., 42:307, 1986.

55. Mortera, C., and Leon, G.: Detection of persistent ductus in hypoplastic left heart syndrome by contrast echocardiography. Br. Heart J., 44:596, 1980.

56. Natowicz, M., and Kelley, R. I.: Association of Turner syndrome with hypoplastic left heart syndrome. Am. J. Dis. Child., 141:218, 1987.

57. Noonan, J. A., and Nadas, A. S.: The hypoplastic left heart syndrome. Pediatr. Clin. North Am., 5:1029, 1958.

58. Nora, J. J., and Nora, A. H.: Genetics and counseling in cardiovascular diseases. Springfield, IL, Charles C Thomas, 1978, p. 181.

59. Norwood, W. I., Kirklin, J. K., and Sanders, S. P.: Hypoplastic left heart syndrome. Experience with palliative surgery. Am. J. Cardiol., 45:87, 1980.

60. Norwood, W. I., Lang, P., Castaneda, A. R., and Campbell, D. N.: Experience with operations for hypoplastic left heart syndrome. J. Thorac. Cardiovasc. Surg., 82:511, 1981.

61. Norwood, W. I., Lang, P., and Hansen, D.: Physiologic repair of aortic atresia–hypoplastic left heart syndrome. N. Engl. J. Med., 308:23, 1983.

62. O'Connor, W. N., Cash, J. B. Cottrill, C. M., et al.: Ventriculocoronary connections in hypoplastic left hearts: An autopsy microscopic study. Circulation, 66:1078, 1982.

63. Oazi, Q. H., Kanchanapoomi, R., Cooper, R., et al.: Brief clinical report: Dup(12p) and hypoplastic left heart. Am. J. Med. Genet., 9:195, 1981.

64. Roberts, W. C., Perry, L. W., Chandra, R. S., et al.: Aortic valve atresia: A new classification based on necropsy study of 73 cases. Am. J. Cardiol., 37:753, 1976.

65. Sade, R. M., Fyfe, D., and Alpert, C. C.: Hypoplastic left heart syndrome: A simplified palliative operation. Ann. Thorac. Surg., 43:309, 1987.

66. Sahn, D. J., Allen, H. D., Goldberg, S. J., et al.: Pediatric echocardiography: A review of its clinical utility. J. Pediatr., 87:335, 1975.

67. Sahn, D. J., Shenker, L., Reed, K. L., et al.: Prenatal ultrasound diagnosis of hypoplastic left heart syndrome in utero associated with hydrops fetalis. Am. Heart J., 104:1368, 1982.

68. Schall, S. A., and Dalldorf, F. G.: Premature closure of the foramen ovale and hypoplasia of the left heart. Int. J. Cardiol., 5:103, 1984.

69. Schlemmer, M., Khoss, A., Salzer, H. R., and Wimmer, M.: Prostaglandin E₂ in newborns with congenital heart disease. Z. Kardiol., 71:452, 1982.

70. Silverberg, B.: Coexistent aortic and mitral atresia associated with persistent common atrioventricular canal. Am. J. Cardiol., 16:754, 1965.

71. Sinha, S. N., Rusnak, S. L., Sommers, H. M., et al.: Hypoplastic left ventricle syndrome. Analysis of thirty autopsy cases in infants with surgical consideration. Am. J. Cardiol., 21:166, 1968.

72. Skovranek, J., First, T., and Samanek, M.: Contribution of pulsed Doppler echocardiography to ultrasound diagnosis of congenital heart disease. Cor Vasa, 23:34, 1981.

73. Snider, A. R., and Silverman, N. H.: Suprasternal notch echocardiography: A two-dimensional technique for evaluating congenital heart disease. Circulation, 63:165, 1981.

74. Suzuki, K., Hitata, K., Eto, Y., et al.: Echocardiographic assessment of anatomical detail in patients with hypoplastic left heart syndrome. J. Cardiogr., 12:991, 1982.

75. Tuma, S., Samanek, M., Benesova, D., and Voriskova, M.: Premature closure of the foramen ovale with levoatriocardinal vein. Eur. J. Pediatr., 129:205, 1978.

76. van der Horst, R. L., Hastreiter, A. R., DuBrow, I. W., and Eckner, F. A. O.: Pathologic measurements in aortic atresia. Am. Heart J., 106:1411, 1983.

77. Von Reuden, T. J., Knight, L., Moller, J. H., and Edwards, J. E.: Coarctation of the aorta associated with aortic valve atresia. Circulation, 52:951, 1975.

78. Watson, D. G., and Rowe, R. D.: Aortic-valve atresia: Report of 43 cases. J.A.M.A., 179:14, 1962.

79. Weinberg, P. M., et al.: Postmortem echocardiography and tomographic anatomy of hypoplastic left heart syndrome after palliative surgery. Am. J. Cardiol., 58:1228, 1986.

80. Weinberg, P. M., Peyser, K., and Hackney, J. R.: Fetal hydrops in a newborn with hypoplastic left heart syndrome: Tricuspid valve stopper. J. Am. Coll. Cardiol., 6:1365, 1985.

81. Weldon, C. S., Hartman, A. F., and McKnight, R. C.: Surgical management of hypoplastic right ventricle with pulmonary atresia or critical pulmonic stenosis and intact ventricular septum. Ann. Thorac. Surg., 37:12, 1984.

82. Yabek, S. M., and Mann, J. S.: Prostaglandin E₁ infusion in the hypoplastic left heart syndrome. Chest, 76:330, 1979.

XII

TRUNCUS ARTERIOSUS

Robert B. Wallace, M.D., and Richard A. Hopkins, M.D.

HISTORICAL ASPECTS

Persistent truncus arteriosus is a rare congenital cardiac malformation constituting between 1 and 4 per cent of congenital cardiac defects in autopsy series. The condition is characterized by a single arterial vessel arising from the heart, receiving blood from both ventricles, and supplying blood to the aorta, lungs, and coronary arteries. The pathologic anatomy was first de-

scribed by Taruffi in 1875.[28] In 1949, Collett and Edwards classified the defect according to anatomic types, which is the basis for the surgical classification used today.[7] In 1965, Van Praagh and Van Praagh classified truncus arteriosus and termed it *common aorticopulmonary trunk*.[29] Although their classification more clearly defines the condition in relation to its embryology, it is not a practical surgical classification.

In 1968, McGoon and associates reported the first successful repair of truncus arteriosus.[18] They employed work of Rastelli and co-workers, in which a conduit consisting of a homograft of the ascending aorta and aortic valve was used to construct a pulmonary artery.[23] Subsequently, Bowman and co-workers suggested that a Dacron graft containing a porcine valve be used as the conduit.[4] Modifications of this technique represent the current definitive treatment for truncus arteriosus.

ANATOMY AND CLASSIFICATION

Truncus arteriosus is due to a lack of partitioning of the embryonic conus during the first few weeks of fetal development and is almost always associated with a ventricular septal defect. Collett and Edwards classified truncus arteriosus into four types, based on the origin of the pulmonary arteries (Fig. 1).[7] In Type I, a single arterial trunk gives rise to the aorta and main pulmonary artery. In Type II, the right and left pulmonary arteries arise immediately adjacent to one another from the dorsal wall of the truncus. In Type III, the right and left pulmonary arteries arise from either side of the truncus, and in Type IV, the proximal pulmonary arteries are absent and pulmonary blood flow is by way of bronchial arteries. Types I and II comprised 76 per cent of Collett and Edwards' series, and Type III, 13 per cent. Currently, Types II and III are grouped together. Type IV, in which there are no pulmonary artery trunks, more appropriately should be considered a severe form of tetralogy of Fallot with absence of the pulmonary trunks. Thus, for practical purposes, all cases of truncus arteriosus may be classified as either Type I or II of the Collet and Edwards' classification.

A ventricular septal defect immediately beneath the truncal valve has been present in all patients with truncus arteriosus except two reported by Van Praagh and Van Praagh.[29] The truncus most commonly overrides the ventricular septum or arises to the left of the plane of the septum. Collet and Edwards reported a 25 per cent incidence of common ventricle,[7] although this was not present in any of Van Praagh and Van Praagh's series and in only one of the 80 specimens studied by Bharati and associates.[1]

The truncal valve may have from two to six cusps, although most valves have three cusps. Four cusps have been noted in approximately 25 per cent of valves and two cusps in 5 per cent. Truncal valve incompetence was severe in 10 (6 per cent), moderate in 52 (31 per cent), and absent or minimal in 105 (63 per cent) of 167 patients operated on at the Mayo Clinic.[8] The aortic arch is to the right in approximately 20 per cent of patients with truncus arteriosus, and an interruption of the aortic arch occurs in 10 to 15 per cent.

The left or right pulmonary artery was absent in 2 per cent of

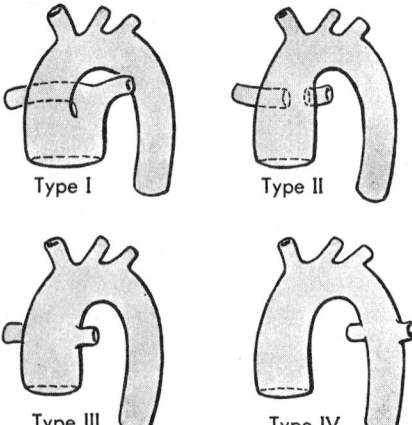

Figure 1. Anatomic types of truncus arteriosus. Collett and Edwards' classification. (From Keith, J. D., Rowe, R. D., and Vlad, P.: Heart Disease in Infancy and Childhood. New York, Macmillan Company, 1958, p. 521. By permission.)

Van Praagh and Van Praagh's series and in 4.5 per cent of Bharati and associates' series; however, DiDonato and associates reported a 9.6 per cent incidence of congenital unilateral absence of the pulmonary artery.[8] Other defects of surgical significance occurring with truncus arteriosus include patent ductus arteriosus in 15 to 30 per cent, persistent left superior vena cava in 10 to 15 per cent, and an atrial septal defect in 20 per cent.

The pathologic changes that may occur in the pulmonary vasculature are similar to those of other conditions in which a high-pressure, left-to-right shunt produces pulmonary vascular obstructive disease, as described by Heath and Edwards.[12]

HEMODYNAMICS

All the blood from both the left and the right ventricles is ejected into the truncus arteriosus. The systemic and pulmonary venous blood mixes, and the degree of arterial oxygen saturation depends on the amount of pulmonary blood flow. Pulmonary blood flow may be limited by stenosis of the pulmonary arteries, but this is uncommon. In most instances, pulmonary blood flow (and thus arterial oxygen saturation) is determined by the resistance to flow in the pulmonary vascular bed. As with isolated ventricular septal defect, the pulmonary vascular bed in truncus arteriosus is exposed to high flow at systemic pressure, a condition that may lead to progressive changes of pulmonary vascular obstructive disease. Mair and associates noted a high correlation between pulmonary vascular resistance and arterial oxygen saturation in truncus arteriosus.[16] In their series, patients with two pulmonary arteries and no pulmonary stenosis who had an arterial oxygen saturation of less than 85 per cent usually presented with a pronounced increase in pulmonary vascular resistance and advanced pulmonary vascular obstructive disease.

SYMPTOMS AND DIAGNOSIS

The symptoms associated with truncus arteriosus are related primarily to the amount of pulmonary blood flow. During the first few weeks of life, when pulmonary vascular resistance is normally increased, symptoms are usually absent unless there is associated significant truncal valve incompetence.[10] With maturation of the fetal pulmonary vascular bed, associated with a decrease in pulmonary vascular resistance and an increase in pulmonary blood flow, symptoms of congestive heart failure may develop. These include dyspnea, excessive perspiration, and failure to thrive. Cyanosis is not usually apparent, because the arterial oxygen saturation is generally greater than 85 per cent. With the progressive development of pulmonary vascular obstructive disease and the associated decrease in pulmonary blood flow, cyanosis becomes more evident. The condition then resembles tetralogy of Fallot or ventricular septal defect with severe pulmonary vascular obstructive disease.

Physical examination usually reveals a systolic thrill and murmur over the left third and fourth intercostal spaces parasternally. The apical impulse is prominent, and there are signs of cardiomegaly. The second heart sound is single and accentuated. When truncal valve incompetence is present, a diastolic murmur follows the second heart sound.

Chest roentgenography shows cardiomegaly with biventricular enlargement (Fig. 2). The aortic arch is to the right in 20 per cent of patients, and the left pulmonary artery may be elevated from the normal position. The peripheral pulmonary vasculature is increased, unless there is advanced pulmonary vascular obstructive disease. The electrocardiogram is nonspecific and usually indicates biventricular hypertrophy.

Right and left heart catheterization and angiocardiographic studies are indicated in all patients suspected of having truncus arteriosus in order to establish the diagnosis, define the anat-

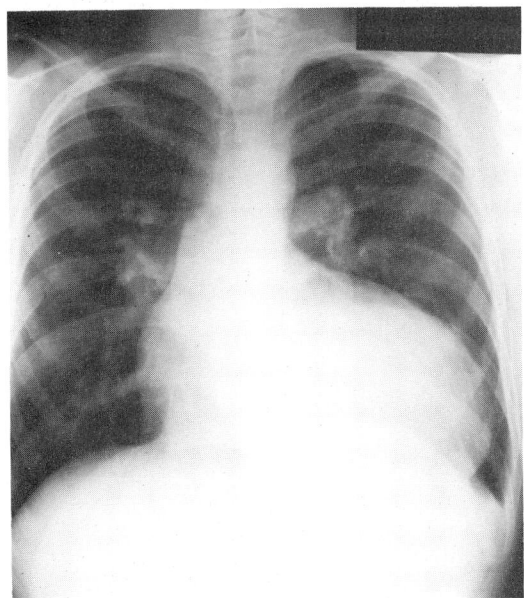

Figure 2. Chest roentgenogram of patient with truncus arteriosus showing cardiomegaly, increased pulmonary vasculature, and elevation of the left pulmonary artery relative to the right. (From Hallermann, F. J., Kincaid, O. W., Tsakiris, A. G., Ritter, D. G., and Titus, J. L.: Persistent truncus arteriosus: A radiographic and angiocardiographic study. Am. J. Roentgenol., *107*:827, 1969. By permission of Charles C Thomas, Publisher.)

omy, and determine the pulmonary vascular resistance. Ventricular pressures are equal, and in the absence of pulmonary artery stenosis there are equal pressures in the ventricles, truncus, and pulmonary arteries. Oxygen saturation studies indicate bidirectional shunting at the ventricular level, the predominant shunt being left-to-right. Pulmonary flow and resistance should be determined by measurement of pressures and oxygen saturations in both pulmonary arteries. In patients without left or right pulmonary artery, calculations of pulmonary blood flow are complicated by bronchial flow, and thus the amount of this flow must be considered in the calculations.

Angiocardiographic studies for defining the anatomy require the injection of large amounts of contrast medium.[11] Injection into the right ventricle shows the ventricle to be enlarged and hypertrophied (Fig. 3). The contrast medium outlines the ventricular septal defect beneath the truncal valve and traverses the defect, filling the left ventricle. Both ventricles eject into a single arterial trunk. Adequate visualization of the pulmonary arteries usually requires an injection into the truncus, which also allows assessment of the truncal valve.

PROGNOSIS

Most patients with persistent truncus arteriosus die from congestive heart failure in early infancy. Only 3 patients in Van Praagh and Van Praagh's autopsy series of 57 cases lived beyond 6 months of age. In Keith and associates' review of 89 patients, 22 per cent survived beyond 6 months of age, and 10 patients survived to the second or third decade.[14] The causes of death for those who survived the first 2 years of life were generally related to pulmonary vascular obstructive disease and decreased pulmonary blood flow.

TREATMENT AND RESULTS

Medical therapy is directed toward the treatment of congestive heart failure, the prevention of bacterial endocarditis, and, in older patients with pulmonary vascular obstructive disease, the complications of right-to-left shunts and the associated polycythemia. The high mortality in infants with unrepaired truncus arteriosus attests to the ineffectiveness of medical management in most patients.

Pulmonary Artery Banding

Banding of the pulmonary artery was proposed by Muller and Dammann to decrease pulmonary artery pressure and flow, in an attempt to control congestive heart failure, and to limit the progression of pulmonary vascular obstructive disease in patients with large left-to-right shunts.[19] This procedure has been used in truncus arteriosus, as reported by Smith and associates,[24] Oldham and co-workers,[20] and Stark and associates.[26] Although the mortality has been high in the reported series, a number of patients have been successfully palliated, and this has enabled them to undergo complete repair at a later age. It is currently reserved for patients with severe concomitant diseases (e.g., necrotizing enterocolitis) or with more complex forms of truncus arteriosus (e.g., multiple ventricular septal defects).

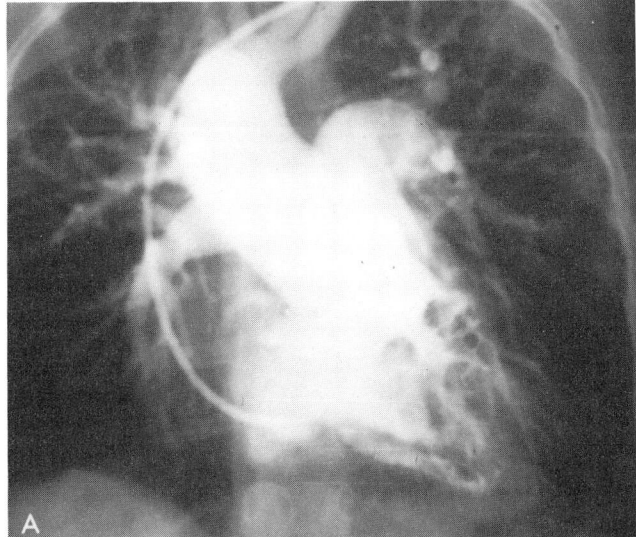
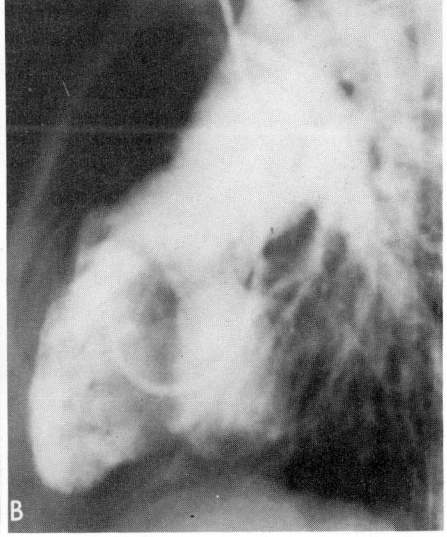

Figure 3. Angiocardiograms. Anteroposterior view *(A)* and left lateral view *(B)* after injection of contrast material into right ventricle. Both ventricles are enlarged; ventricular septal defect is present immediately beneath truncus. Right ventricular infundibulum is absent, and pulmonary arteries arise from truncus. (From Hallermann, F. J., Kincaid, O. W., Tsakiris, A. G., Ritter, D. G., and Titus, J. L.: Persistent truncus arteriosus: A radiographic and angiocardiographic study. Am. J. Roentgenol., *107*:827, 1969. By permission of Charles C Thomas, Publisher.)

Systemic-Pulmonary Shunts

Billig and associates have reported good palliation after a systemic-pulmonary shunting procedure.[2] The only indication for a shunt procedure is the presence of proximal pulmonary stenosis producing symptoms of inadequate pulmonary blood flow.

Complete Surgical Repair

TECHNIQUE. The operation is performed through a median sternotomy, using total cardiopulmonary bypass and deep hypothermia, either with total circulatory arrest or low flow. Myocardial protection is provided by cold cardioplegic arrest during aortic cross-clamping. Arterial cannulation is in the ascending aorta. The left ventricle is vented with a catheter introduced through the foramen ovale (Figs. 4 and 5).

In larger infants, the pulmonary arteries can be excised from the truncus as a single segment, even in Type II truncus. This occasionally can be facilitated by a short anterior aortotomy or division of the truncal root.[21] In smaller infants, the posterior defect is usually closed with a patch to avoid distortion of the semilunar valve pillars. The incision in the right ventricle is made high in the ventricle in the planned direction of the conduit. The aortic cross-clamp is temporarily released after air has been removed from the aortic root, and the competency of the valve is assessed. If incompetence is severe, valve replacement must be considered. A patch is used to close the ventricular septal defect. An appropriately sized valved Dacron or homograft conduit is cut to proper length and used to establish continuity between the right ventricle and the pulmonary arteries. The course of the conduit should be such that kinking is avoided and the closed sternum does not compress the conduit.

Although repairs have been performed successfully with valveless conduits for connection of the right ventricle to the pulmonary arteries,[25] most authorities recommend a valved conduit when there is high or reactive pulmonary vascular resistance, which also protects right ventricular function.[13] The 12-mm. porcine valved conduit has been used successfully for this reconstruction,[5] but the technical ease of insertion and perhaps greater durability of the homograft supports its use when available (Fig. 6).[3,6,13,15]

In patients in whom a previous pulmonary artery banding has been performed, the pulmonary arteries usually need to be incised to a point distal to the area of banding to relieve the stenosis produced by the band.[22] The distal end of the conduit is

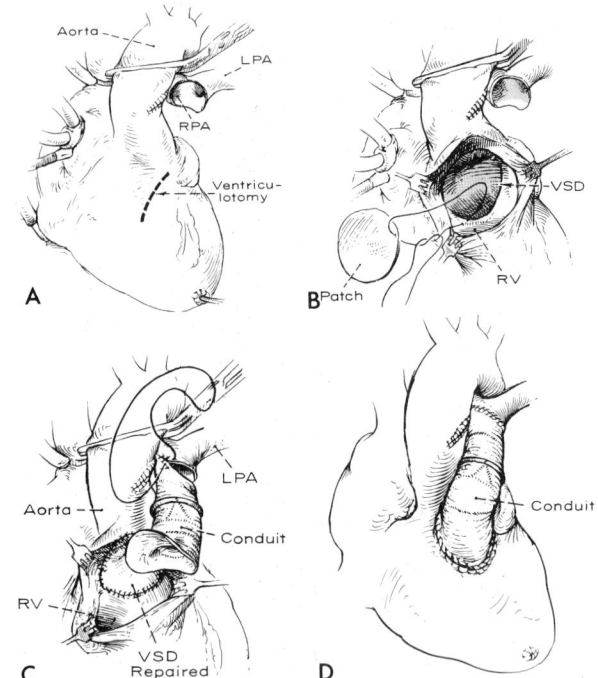

Figure 5. Surgical repair (continued). *A*, Incision made high in right ventricle. *B*, Ventricular septal defect closed with Teflon patch. *C*, Dacron graft with porcine valve sutured to pulmonary arteries. *D*, Proximal end of graft anastomosed to right ventricle. (LPA, left pulmonary artery; RPA, right pulmonary artery; VSD, ventricular septal defect; RV, right ventricle. (From Wallace, R. B.: Truncus arteriosus. *In* Sabiston, D. C., Jr., and Spencer, F. C. (Eds.): Gibbon's Surgery of the Chest, 3rd ed. Philadelphia. W. B. Saunders Company, 1976.)

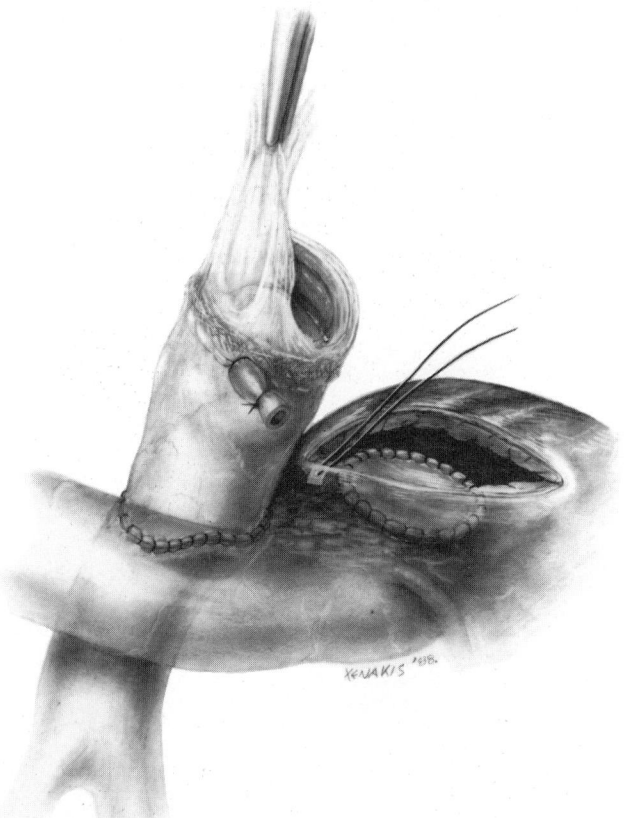

Figure 6. Homograft sutured to right ventriculotomy above VSD closure. Use a pledget at the start of the ventricular anastomosis when there is minimal muscular tissue remaining. Alternatively, the allograft can be sutured directly to the VSD patch at the midpoint. (From Hopkins, R. A.: Cardiac Reconstructions with Allograft Valves. New York, Springer-Verlag, 1989, p. 164. By permission.)

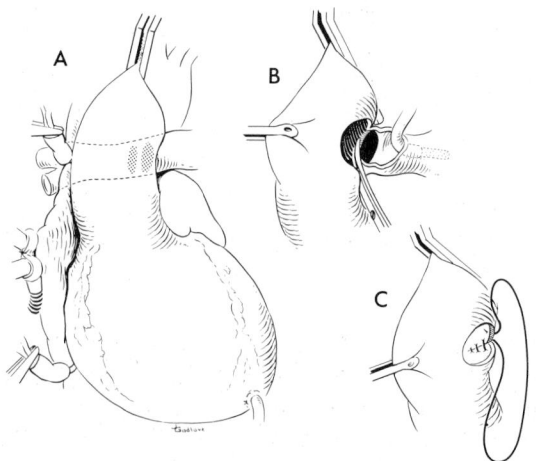

Figure 4. Surgical repair. *A*, Cardiopulmonary bypass, left ventricle vented at apex, aorta cross-clamped. *B*, Origin of pulmonary arteries excised from truncus. *C*, Closure of defect in truncus. (From Wallace, R. B., Rastelli, G. C., Ongley, P. A., Titus, J. L., and McGoon, D. C.: Complete repair of truncus arteriosus defects. J. Thorac. Cardiovasc. Surg., *57*:95, 1969. By permission of C. V. Mosby Company.)

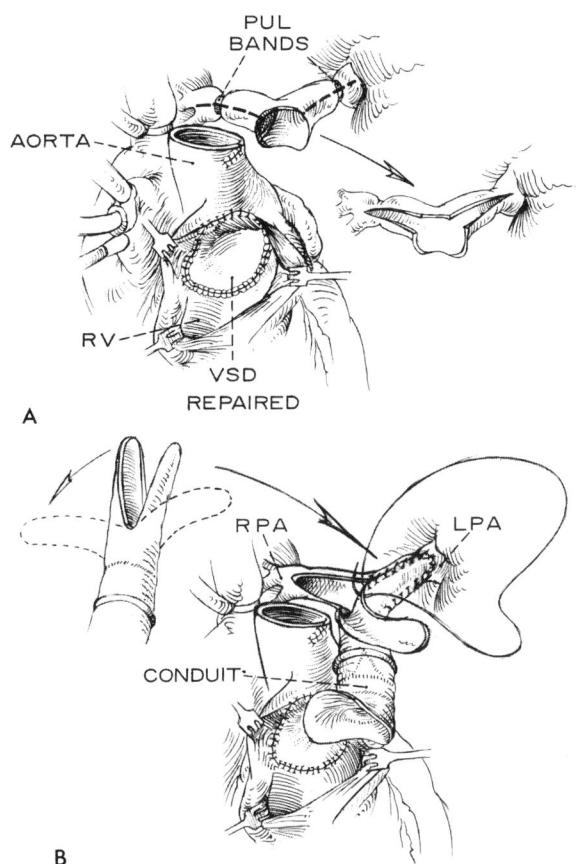

Figure 7. Complete repair with previous pulmonary artery banding. *A,* Pulmonary arteries are incised through areas of banding. *B,* Distal end of conduit tailored to enlarge the pulmonary arteries. (From Parker, R. K., McGoon, D. C., Danielson, G. K., and Wallace, R. B.: Repair of truncus arteriosus in patients with prior banding of the pulmonary artery. Surgery, *78:*761, 1975. By permission of C. V. Mosby Company.)

then tailored to produce an angioplastic enlargement of the pulmonary arteries (Fig. 7).

RESULTS. The Mayo Clinic experience with 167 patients with Type I and Type II truncus arteriosus who underwent surgical repair between 1965 and 1982 has been reported.[8] There were 48 hospital deaths (28.7 per cent). The most significant risk factors in this series were age less than 2 years at operation and a postrepair right ventricular/left ventriclar pressure ratio greater than 0.8. The operative mortality was 70 per cent for patients under 2 years, and 5 of 6 patients under 6 months of age died. During this period, children under 2 years were repaired only when medical management failed.

Late follow-up of the 119 hospital survivors ranged from 1.1 to 15.4 years, with a mean of 7 years, and revealed a 5-year survival of 84.4 per cent and a 10-year survival of 68.8 per cent. Thirty-six patients (30 per cent) required reoperation during the follow-up period, and in 32, an obstructive valve conduit was replaced. Nine of the patients required truncal valve replacement because of progressive valve incompetence. Of the 90 patients alive at the end of the follow-up period, 59 (66 per cent) were in functional NYHA Class I, 28 (31 per cent) in Class II, and 3 (3 per cent) in Class III.

Reported experiences from institutions in which elective repair in infancy has been performed indicate that this can be accomplished at an acceptable mortality.[6,27] Ebert reported an 11 per cent hospital mortality in 100 consecutive patients under 6 months of age who were operated on; 86 patients were alive at 16 months to 8 years postoperatively, and 55 of the survivors required conduit replacement (accomplished with no deaths).[9] At the time of follow-up, no survivors had evidence of pulmo-

nary vascular disease. Bove and colleagues have reported neonatal repairs in 11 patients, with a 9 per cent mortality.[3]

Indications for Operation

Definitive treatment for truncus arteriosus is complete repair. Ideally, operation should be performed in the first 3 to 6 months of life, during which time approximately 80 per cent of patients die without correction. Operation at this age also protects against the development of pulmonary vascular obstructive disease. Although conduit replacement will be required when operation is performed in infancy, it has been shown that this can be accomplished at a low risk.[9]

Although pulmonary artery banding can reduce pulmonary blood flow and protect against the development of pulmonary vascular obstructive disease without increasing operative mortality at the time of complete repair, the results achieved by performing complete repair in infancy clearly establish this as the practice of choice. There continues to be a need for a conduit that would not require replacement, and this suggests the use of tissue with the capacity to grow. It is possible that operation in infancy may prevent or reduce the rate of progression of truncal valve incompetence. Patients not operated upon in infancy who survive should probably undergo elective operation prior to 5 years of age. Operability at this stage is determined primarily by the severity of pulmonary vascular obstructive disease.

SELECTED REFERENCES

Collett, R. W., and Edwards, J. E.: Persistent truncus arteriosus: A classification according to anatomic types. Surg. Clin. North Am., Aug. 1949, p. 1245.
The anatomy, embryology, and criteria for diagnosis of truncus arteriosus based on 80 cases from the literature and the authors' material were reviewed. The embryologic discussion emphasized the development of the septal system that divides the ventricles, the conus arteriosus, and the truncus arteriosus to form two separate circulations. Two absolute criteria for the pathologic diagnosis of persistent truncus arteriosus were established: (1) that there be only one main arterial trunk leaving the base of the heart with no remnant of an atretic pulmonary trunk or aorta and (2) that this single arterial trunk supply branches to the coronary, pulmonary, and systemic circulations. An anatomic classification of truncus arteriosus was presented in which four types were identified, the classification being based on the embryologic development of the pulmonary arteries from the sixth aortic arch. In Type IV of this classification, the pulmonary blood flow is derived from bronchial arteries, and this type more appropriately should be classified as a severe form of tetralogy of Fallot with absence of the main pulmonary artery (pulmonary atresia).

DiDonato, R. M., Fyfe, D. A., Puga, F. J., Danielson, G. K., Ritter, D. G., Edwards, W. D., and McGoon, D. C.: Fifteen-year experience with surgical repair of truncus arteriosus. Annual Meeting of the Western Thoracic Surgical Association, Maui, Hawaii, June 20–23, 1984.
The authors review the experience at the Mayo Clinic of 167 patients operated on for correction of truncus arteriosus from 1965 to March 1982. The age at operation ranged from 18 days to 33 years (mean, 6 years). There were 48 hospital deaths (28.7 per cent). Age at operation of less than 2 years and a postrepair RV/LV pressure ratio of greater than 0.8 correlated with the possibility of operative mortality. There did not appear to be a significant correlation with pulmonary vascular resistance as shown in earlier publications.
One hundred and nineteen hospital survivors were followed for a mean of 7 years (range from 1.1 to 15.4 years). Survival at 5 years was 84.4 per cent and at 10 years, 68.8 per cent. Thirty-six patients required reoperation 0.8 to 13.7 years (mean, 6 years) following the initial operation, 32 of whom had replacement of an obstructed valve conduit and 9 had truncal valve replacement. There were no operative deaths in patients in whom conduit replacement was required. Fifty-nine of the 90 surviving patients (66 per cent) were in functional NYHA Class I, 28 (31 per cent) were in Class II, and 3 (3 per cent) were in Class III.

Ebert, P. A., Turley, K., Stanger, P., Hoffman, J. I. E., Heymann, M. A., and Rudolph, A. M.: Surgical treatment of truncus arteriosus in the first six months of life. Annual Meeting of the American Surgical Association, Toronto, Canada, April 25–27, 1984.
The results of a large series of infants with truncus arteriosus who underwent complete repair in the first 6 months of life are reviewed. The operative mortality was 11 per cent in 100 consecutive patients. Three late deaths occurred in the follow-up period of 16 months to 8 years. Fifty-five patients required reoperation for replacement of the conduit, and there was no associated mortality. No patient showed evidence of pulmonary vascular disease during the follow-up period. This report clearly documents the efficacy of repair of truncus arteriosus in infancy.

Mair, D. D., Ritter, D. G., Davis, G. D., Wallace, R. B., Danielson, G. K., and McGoon, D. C.: Selection of patients with truncus arteriosus for surgical correction: Anatomic and hemodynamic considerations. Circulation, *49*:144, 1974.

A series of 70 patients with Collett and Edwards' Types I and II truncus arteriosus underwent cardiac catheterization at the Mayo Clinic; 40 subsequently underwent surgical correction. Interruption of the aortic arch was present in 4 patients and 25 had some truncal valve incompetence; however, the incompetence was severe in only 4. In the series of 70 patients, 23 of 59 (39 per cent) with two pulmonary arteries were inoperable because of pulmonary vascular obstructive disease, and 8 of 11 (73 per cent) with a single pulmonary artery were inoperable for the same reason. Among the 40 patients who had surgical correction, a definite relationship was noted between operative mortality and the calculated pulmonary vascular resistance. For patients with calculated pulmonary resistances of less than 8.0 Wood units · m², the operative mortality was 18 per cent, whereas for those with resistances greater than 12 Wood units · m², the operative mortality was 100 per cent. There was good correlation between calculated pulmonary vascular resistance and degree of pulmonary vascular obstructive disease. There also was a relationship between aterial oxygen saturation and pulmonary stenosis; patients with arterial oxygen saturations greater than 85 per cent had pulmonary resistances greater than 12 Wood units · m². This review suggests that patients with two pulmonary arteries and a pulmonary resistance greater than 12 Wood units · m² are inoperable. A different criterion for operability must be used for patients with a single pulmonary artery.

REFERENCES

1. Bharati, S., McAllister, H. A., Jr., Rosenquist, G. C., Miller, R. A., Tatooles, C. J., and Lev, M.: The surgical anatomy of truncus arteriosus communis. J. Thorac. Cardiovasc. Surg., *67*:501, 1974.
2. Billig, D. M., Kreidberg, M. B., Chernoff, H. L., and Khan, M. A. A.: Systemic to pulmonary anastomosis in truncus arteriosus with reduced pulmonary blood flow. Am. J. Cardiol., *30*:228, 1972.
3. Bove, E. L., Beekman, R. H., Snider, A. R., Callow, L. B., Underhill, D. J., Rocchini, A. P., Dick, M., II., and Rosenthal, A.: Repair of truncus arteriosus in the neonate and young infant. Ann. Thorac. Surg., *47*:499, 1989.
4. Bowman, F. O., Jr., Hancock, W. D., and Malm, J. R.: A valve-containing Dacron prosthesis: Its use in restoring pulmonary artery–right ventricular continuity. Arch. Surg., *107*:724, 1973.
5. Boyce, S. W., Turley, K., Yee, E. S., Verrier, E. D., and Ebert, P. A.: The fate of the 12-mm. porcine valved conduit from the right ventricle to the pulmonary artery: A ten-year experience. J. Thorac. Cardiovasc. Surg., *95*:201, 1988.
6. Castaneda, A. R.: Truncus arteriosus. Ann. Thorac. Surg., *47*:491, 1989.
7. Collett, R. W., and Edwards, J. E.: Persistent truncus arteriosus: A classification according to anatomic types. Surg. Clin. North Am., Aug. 1949, p. 1245.
8. DiDonato, R. M., Fyfe, D. A., Puga, F. J., Danielson, G. K., Ritter, D. G., Edwards, W. D., and McGoon, D. C.: Fifteen-year experience with surgical repair of truncus arteriosus. Annual Meeting of the Western Thoracic Surgical Association, Maui, Hawaii, June 20–23, 1984.
9. Ebert, P. A., Turley, K., Stanger, P., Hoffman, J. I. E., Heymann, M. A., and Rudolph, A. M.: Surgical treatment of truncus arteriosus in the first six months of life. Annual Meeting of the American Surgical Association, Toronto, Canada, April 25–27, 1984.
10. Gelband, H., Van Meter, S., and Gersony, W. M.: Truncal valve abnormalities in infants with persistent truncus arteriosus: A clinicopathologic study. Circulation, *45*:397, 1972.
11. Hallerman, F. J., Kincaid, O. W., Tsakiris, A. G., Ritter, D. G., and Titus, J. L.: Persistent truncus arteriosus: A radiographic and angiocardiographic study. Am. J. Roentgenol., *107*:827, 1969.
12. Heath, D., and Edwards, J. E.: The pathology of hypertensive pulmonary vascular disease: A description of six grades of structural changes in the pulmonary arteries with special reference to congenital cardiac septal defects. Circulation, *18*:533, 1958.
13. Hopkins, R. A.: Right ventricular outflow tract reconstructions: The role of valves in the viable allograft era. Ann. Thorac. Surg., *45*:593, 1988.
14. Keith, J. D., Rowe, R. D., and Vlad, P.: Heart Disease in Infancy and Childhood. New York, Macmillan Company, 1958, p. 521.
15. Kirklin, J. W., Blackstone, E. H., Maehara, T., et al.: Intermediate-term fate of cryopreserved allograft and xenograft valved conduits. Ann. Thorac. Surg., *44*:598, 1989.
16. Mair, D. D., Ritter, D. G., Davis, G. D., Wallace, R. B., Danielson, G. K., and McGoon, D. C.: Selection of patients with truncus arteriosus for surgical correction: Anatomic and hemodynamic considerations. Circulation, *49*:144, 1974.
17. Marcelletti, C., McGoon, D. C., Danielson, G. K., Wallace, R. B., and Mair, D. D.: Early and late results of surgical repair of truncus arteriosus. Circulation, *55*:636, 1977.
18. McGoon, D. C., Rastelli, G. C., and Ongley, P. A.: An operation for the correction of truncus arteriosus. JAMA, *205*:69, 1968.
19. Muller, W. H., Jr., and Dammann, J. F.: The treatment of certain congenital malformations of the heart by the creation of pulmonic stenosis to reduce pulmonary hypertension and excessive pulmonary blood flow: A preliminary report. Surg. Gynecol. Obstet., *95*:213, 1952.
20. Oldham, N. H., Jr., Kakos, G. S., Jarmakani, M. M., and Sabiston, D. C., Jr.: Pulmonary artery banding in infants with complex congenital heart defects. Ann. Thorac. Surg., *13*:342, 1972.
21. Ott, D. A., Eren, E. E., Huhta, J. C., and Gutgesell, H. P.: Surgical treatment for the type II and III truncus: Complete division of the truncal root with primary repair using absorbable suture. Ann. Thorac. Surg., *40*:201, 1985.
22. Parker, R. K., McGoon, D. C., Danielson, G. K., Wallace, R. B., and Mair, D. D.: Repair of truncus arteriosus in patients with prior banding of the pulmonary artery. Surgery, *78*:761, 1975.
23. Rastelli, G. C., Titus, J. L., and McGoon, D. C.: Homograft of ascending aorta and aortic valve as a right ventricular outflow: An experimental approach to the repair of truncus arteriosus. Arch. Surg., *95*:698, 1967.
24. Smith, G. W., Thompson, W. M., Jr., Dammann, J. F., Jr., and Muller, W. H., Jr.: Use of the pulmonary artery banding procedure in treating type II truncus arteriosus. Circulation, *29* (Suppl. I):108, 1964.
25. Spicer, R. L., Behrendt, D., Crowley, D. C., Dick, M., Rocchini, A. P., Uzark, K., Rosenthal, A., and Sloan, H.: Repair of truncus arteriosus in neonates with the use of a valveless conduit. Circulation, *70* (Suppl. I):I-26, 1984.
26. Stark, J., Aberdeen, E., Waterston, D. J., Bonham-Carter, R. E., and Tynan, M.: Pulmonary artery constriction (banding): A report of 146 cases. Surgery, *65*:808, 1969.
27. Stark, J., Gandhi, D., de Leval, M., Macartney, F., and Taylor, J. F. N.: Surgical treatment of persistent truncus arteriosus in the first year of life. Br. Heart J., *40*:1280, 1978.
28. Taruffi, C.: Sulle malattie congenite e sulle anomalie del cuore. Mem. Soc. Med. Chir. Bologna, *8*:215, 1875.
29. Van Praagh, R., and Van Praagh, S.: The anatomy of common aorticopulmonary trunk (truncus arteriosus communis) and its embryologic implications: A study of 57 necropsy cases. Am. J. Cardiol., *16*:406, 1965.

XIII ————————————————————————

TRANSPOSITION OF THE GREAT ARTERIES

Gary K. Lofland, M.D.

Transposition of the great arteries, in the anatomically simplest form, is physiologically one of the most extreme of all congenital cardiac malformations. It is a lesion that is incompatible with life without intervention and an anomaly that over the past 3 decades has become completely correctable, both anatomically and physiologically, within the first few days to weeks of life. In many ways, the approach to the neonate with simple transposition is at the zenith of both technical expertise and an increasing understanding of the ever changing cardiopulmonary physiology of the neonate.

Whereas transposition of the great arteries may exist with nearly any cardiac lesion, this section is confined to complete transposition, complete transposition with ventricular septal defect (VSD), and complete transposition with left ventricular outflow tract obstruction. The Taussig-Bing anomaly is more appropriately considered with double outlet right ventricle.[52]

HISTORICAL ASPECTS

Although anatomic observation of transposition of the great arteries was made by Steno in 1672 and Morgagni in 1761, the first description of transposition of the great arteries is credited to Baillie in 1797.[4] The term *transposition of the aorta and pulmonary artery* was first used by Farre in 1814.[15] Rokitansky[55] reported analysis of the pathogenesis of transposition and attempted to classify the various types. The clinical recognition of transposition during life was emphasized by Fanconi[14] in 1932. In 1938, Taussig[46] described not only the clinical manifestations of the anomaly during life but also the pathologic anatomy and hemodynamic manifestations.

Surgical therapy for transposition began in 1950 when Blalock and Hanlon[8] reported a method of creating an atrial septal defect for the increase of mixing between systemic venous and pulmonary venous circulations. Although mortality for the operation was high, a method of palliation became feasible.

Mustard in 1952[31] attempted a reversal of the transposed great arteries, as did Bailey[3] in the same year, both without success. In 1952, Lillehei and Varco transferred the right pulmonary veins to the right atrium and the inferior vena cava to the left atrium in a partial correction. In 1954, Glenn and Patino[17] anastomosed the right pulmonary artery to the superior vena cava in patients with transposition and pulmonary stenosis. Baffes,[2] in 1956, successfully transferred the right pulmonary veins to the right atrium and grafted the right inferior vena cava to the left atrium. Kay and Cross[23] and Merendino[28] attempted interatrial diversionary procedures for redirection of the venous flow into respective ventricles. In 1959, Senning reported successfully transposing the atria by use of an ingenious procedure.[40] Barnard,[5] in 1961, excised the atrial septum and inserted a plastic prosthesis around the orifices of the pulmonary veins, connecting the other end of the orifice to the systemic or right ventricle. In 1964, Mustard[30] described excision of the entire atrial septum and placement of a pericardial baffle in the atrium for redirection of all the caval blood to the pulmonary ventricle, allowing the oxygenated blood returning by pulmonary veins to enter the systemic ventricle, which generated considerable enthusiasm. Indeed, the Mustard procedure remained the procedure of choice for transposition corrective surgery until the re-emergence of the Senning procedure in the 1970s. In 1975, Jatene reported switching of the great arteries in infants with reimplantation of the coronary arteries.[21] Enthusiasm for this technique was tempered by its high mortality in its initial applications. In recent years, the arterial switch procedure for transposition of the great arteries has become a mainstay of corrective surgery.

ANATOMIC ASPECTS

Data from the New England regional infant cardiac program indicate that complete transposition of the great arteries is the second most frequently encountered disorder in that registry. It was seen in 9.9 per cent of infants with congenital heart disease and occurred in a frequency of 0.206 per thousand live births. There is a distinct male preponderance. The lesion represents approximately 15 per cent of congenital cardiac anomalies seen at autopsy in infants less than 1 month of age.[13]

Complete transposition of the great arteries is characterized by the atria being connected to their appropriate ventricles but with inappropriate ventriculoarterial connections. Therefore, the aorta and pulmonary arteries are misplaced across the ventricular septum. The result is atrioventricular concordance and ventriculoarterial discordance (Fig. 1). This has been termed transposition, but there is controversy concerning this term.[49] This is in part because many use the term *transposition* to de-

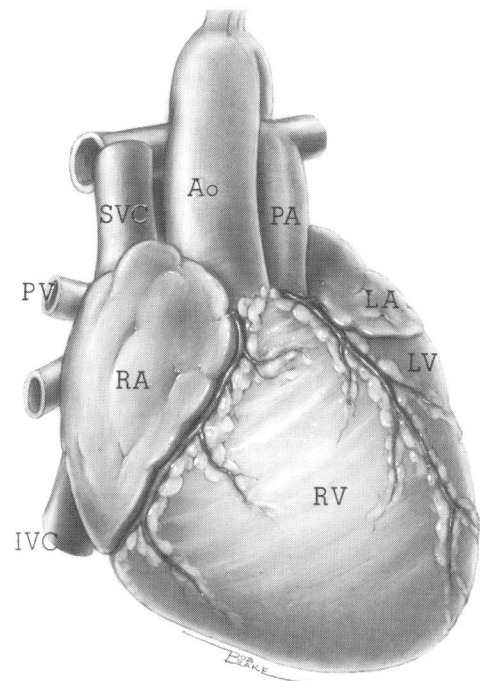

Figure 1. Frontal view of complete transposition. The aorta arises anteriorly from the right ventricle, the pulmonary artery arises posteriorly, and there is minimal if any rotation of the great vessels. The right and left ventricles have a nearly normal relationship. Although variations in this anatomic configuration may occur, this represents the most common form of complete transposition.

scribe a discordant ventriculoarterial connection,[54] whereas others use it to describe any heart with an anterior aorta.[51]

Those who use the term *transposition of the great arteries* to describe a discordant ventriculoarterial connection do not restrict it to the setting of atrioventricular concordance. When defined simply as a discordant ventriculoarterial connection, transposition can clearly coexist with double inlet ventricle or absent connection, and it is these last anomalies that then become the dominant features. Therefore, a term that describes only the chamber combinations of atrioventricular concordance and ventriculoarterial discordance is *complete transposition*.[56] There has been a vogue for using *d-transposition* to the same end, but this does not accurately describe those cases with the usual atrial arrangement, atrioventricular concordance, ventriculoarterial discordance, and left-sided aorta. Neither does d-transposition describe that majority of patients with these chamber combinations and mirror image atrial arrangement. It should also be noted that complete transposition as defined here refers only to patients with lateralized atria (usual and mirror image arrangements).[56] When ventriculoarterial discordance occurs in the setting of atrial isomerism, it is the venous and atrioventricular junctional anomalies that usually dominate the anatomic and clinical considerations, so these cases are also excluded from the author's category of complete transposition.[56]

Many theories of the morphogenesis of transposition have been proposed,[26] but the differential conal growth hypothesis has been favored.[20] It is postulated that in the normal heart, the subaortic segment of the conus does not grow, and that dominant growth of the left-sided pulmonary conus forces the pulmonary valve anteriorly and superiorly to the left; whereas in ordinary forms of transposition, growth of the subaortic part of the conus pushes the aorta anteriorly and disrupts the aortic valve continuity. Failure of the subpulmonary portion of the conus to develop maintains posterior location of the pulmonary artery and pulmonary-mitral valve continuity.[13]

Development of the conus determines truncal rotation, and the relationship of the great arteries proximally at the semilunar valves is similar to that at the arch. There is no twist in the great arteries simply because the aorta is anterior. In less common types of transposition, development of both right and left parts of the conus thrusts both the aortic and the pulmonary valves forward.[13]

PATHOPHYSIOLOGY

The physiologic abnormality in complete transposition is two separate circulations existing in parallel instead of in series, with nonoxygenated venous blood being pumped into the systemic circulation, and oxygenated blood being pumped into the pulmonary circulation. Without some means of systemic and pulmonary venous admixture, the most severe form of the lesion is completely incompatible with life. The intracirculatory shunts allowing admixture of oxygenated and nonoxygenated blood are illustrated in Figure 2. The greater the size or larger the number of shunts, the less the degree of cyanosis. Infants with smaller degrees of intracirculatory shunting are thus more cyanotic.

The degree of intracirculatory shunting that occurs is related to simple pressure gradients present at the sites of communication.[13] Both ventricles at this point are relatively noncompliant. Most infants with transposition have an increased pulmonary blood flow and pulmonary venous return. As the left atrium enlarges, the foramen ovale is stretched, and this causes greater admixture of oxygenated and nonoxygenated blood. Systemic-to-pulmonary shunts may also exist through the bronchial vessels and through a VSD or patent ductus arteriosus.

Neonatal pulmonary vascular resistance is normal in infants both with and without an associated VSD. Pulmonary vascular resistance falls progressively during the neonatal period with associated changes in ventricular compliance. With extreme pulmonary blood flows, pulmonary vascular resistance once again increases throughout infancy. Ferencz observed advanced histologic changes in the lungs of children over 2 years of age, and intimal fibrosis was noted as early as 1 month of age. These changes appear to be present in most children with transposition and suggest that this malformation may be associated with a more advanced and malignant form of pulmonary vascular disease than VSD with normal relationship of the great arteries. Severe pulmonary vascular disease is present in most older children with transposition of the great arteries with moderate to large VSDs. Although most VSDs are paramembranous in location, they may be muscular or subarterial. The location of various VSDs is illustrated in Figure 3.

Hemodynamic measurements may not completely support the histologic findings in children with an intact ventricular septum or small VSDs. It has been postulated that systemic hypoxemia stimulates sympathetic activity with a resultant increase in tone of pulmonary arterioles.[13]

The elevation of pulmonary vascular resistance that might be expected has been a problem in the postoperative management of patients undergoing an arterial switch procedure. However, a decrease in pulmonary vascular resistance following complete correction may be expected.

Left ventricular outflow tract obstruction may clearly exist in transposition of the great arteries and is an important consideration in the management of a neonate with complete transposition. Obstruction to the left ventricular tract may have multiple causes.[1,29,41,50] About 3 per cent of hearts with transposition of the great arteries have a bilateral infundibulum, with the subpulmonary infundibulum preventing pulmonary-mitral valve fibrous continuity.[53] Ventricular infundibular folds separate the semilunar valve from the atrioventricular valve; the infundibular septum separates the anterior outflow tracts. Subpulmonary obstruction potentially reflects a contribution from a malaligned infundibular septum; the narrowing may be fibromuscular or diffuse.

A fibrous membrane and abnormal anterior leaflet of the mitral valve can also, singularly or in combination, cause narrowing of the subpulmonary region. Posterior malalignment or displacement of the infundibular septum causes muscular subpulmonary stenosis and VSD and is probably the most common mechanism of subpulmonary obstruction in these patients. Isolated pulmonary valve stenosis can occur but is more commonly associated with abnormalities of the left ventricular outflow tract.[18] Aortic arch obstruction has also been observed in patients with transposition of the great arteries, left ventricular outflow tract obstruction, and VSD.[34] All of these are important considerations in determining whether a patient is suitable for anatomic correction.

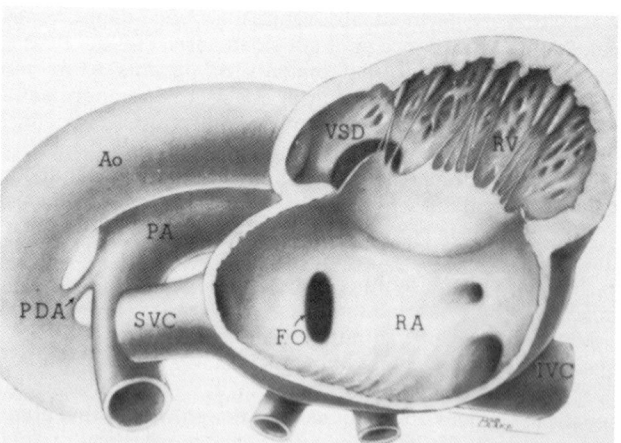

Figure 2. The more frequent anomalies associated with transposition of the great arteries are patent ductus arteriosus (PDA), ventricular septal defect (VSD), and patent foramen ovale (FO). These intra- and extracardiac communications facilitate mixing of arterial and venous blood between the parallel circulations. The size and number of these associated anomalies not only determine the degree of cyanosis but also contribute to the functional status of the morphologic left ventricle by allowing decompression of the left ventricle.

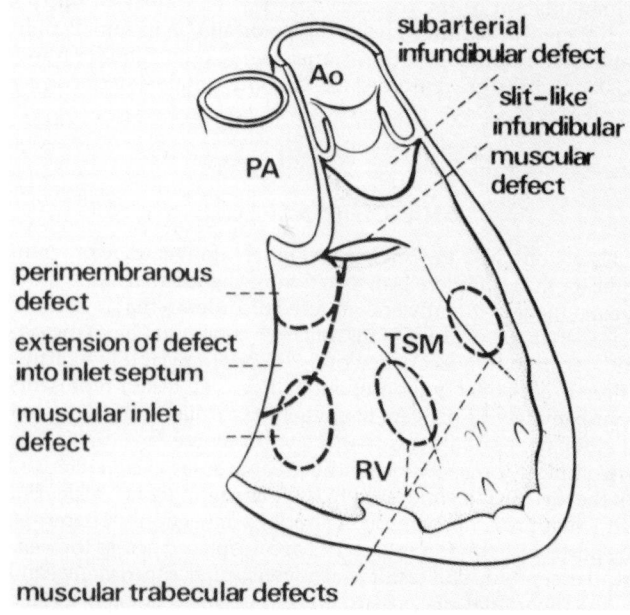

Figure 3. Although a paramembranous location is the most common, ventricular septal defects may occur anywhere in the ventricular septum.

CLINICAL FEATURES

The most common clinical findings in infants with complete transposition of the great arteries are cyanosis and congestive heart failure. The cyanosis is usually present at birth, is definitely observed by 1 week of age, and is more pronounced when the ventricular septum is intact. Late-appearing cyanosis is usually attributable to significant intracirculatory shunting through a large VSD or patent ductus arteriosus. Clubbing of the digits may appear, usually after the age of 6 months, but may be associated with rapid progression of pulmonary disease in the older infant.

Although birth weight may be normal or above normal, growth and subsequent physical development are usually retarded. Anoxic episodes are prominent and characterized by prolonged, labored breathing with increased cyanosis. Throughout these, the infant usually remains conscious and rarely has convulsions. These episodes are due to hypoxemia from inadequate intracirculatory shunting and metabolic acidosis. Symptoms of heart failure are present within the first week of life in about 10 per cent of patients but more commonly appear at about 1 month and are associated with the decline in pulmonary vascular resistance that would normally be expected. Seventy-five per cent of these infants have a systolic murmur even though the ventricular septum is intact. The second heart sound is single and loud because of the proximity of the aorta to the chest wall. End-diastolic gallops are commonly heard, and a mild diastolic atrial murmur may be noted in those with associated VSD. The second sound is usually loud and single, making assessment of pulmonary vascular obstructive disease impossible. The character of the murmur in children with pulmonary valvular or subvalvular stenosis is different and is associated with a long crescendo-decrescendo systolic murmur along the left sternal border transmitted to the right clavicular area.[13]

Common electrocardiographic findings are right atrial hypertrophy, right or combined ventricular hypertrophy, and right axis deviation. In early infancy, the electrocardiogram may appear normal for age because the newborn characteristically has right ventricular hypertrophy. These findings vary, depending on age, presence or absence of VSD, and presence or absence of pulmonary vascular resistance. Right axis deviation is usually associated with an intact ventricular septum, whereas in approximately 40 per cent of patients with a moderate size VSD the axis is normal.

The routine chest film is frequently diagnostic. The important features are progressive cardiomegaly in early infancy, an oval or egg-shaped cardiac configuration, a narrow superior mediastinum, and increased pulmonary markings. Characteristically, the heart is normal in size during the first 1 or 2 weeks of life, but then cardiac enlargement is observed in almost all infants with transposition of the great arteries and increased pulmonary blood flow. The pulmonary markings are prominent, and even pulmonary stenosis, unless unusually severe, does not significantly reduce the prominence of the pulmonary vasculature.

The advent of fetal echocardiography has enabled the diagnosis of transposition of the great arteries to be made *in utero*. Consequently, approximately 20 per cent of the patients in the author's series have been diagnosed antenatally. This has resulted in changes in the management of these patients as outlined subsequently.

MANAGEMENT

Most infants with transposition of the great arteries are cyanotic within the first week of life. Consequently, the majority are usually brought for treatment at a very early age. Indeed, the advent of fetal echocardiography has enabled antenatal establishment of diagnosis and institution of therapy before the infant's hemodynamic status is compromised. In the past, cardiac catheterization was undertaken for substantiation of the diagnosis and confirmation of the position of intracardiac chambers. Advances in echocardiography and echo Doppler have precluded this necessity in most patients with simple complete transposition. Cardiac catheterization need only be performed now in infants in whom there is inadequate intracirculatory shunting, or in infants who have other associated anomalies demanding clarification. Infants can now be diagnosed by echocardiography and managed without the necessity of cardiac catheterization if an early definitive anatomic and physiologic correction is undertaken with the arterial switch procedure. If inadequate intracirculatory shunting is present, cardiac catheterization is necessary to improve the degree of shunting by enlarging the interatrial septal communication.

Cardiac catheterization demonstrates left atrial pressure that is usually greater than the right atrial pressure. The pressure in the posterior or left ventricle depends on the presence or absence of a VSD, pulmonary valvular or subvalvular stenosis, and the state of the peripheral pulmonary vasculature. If catheterization is undertaken, it must be performed expediently, because any stress in these severely ill infants increases metabolic requirements, and a marked degree of cyanosis and subsequent metabolic acidosis may ensue. Likewise, maintenance of normothermia during cardiac catheterization is extremely important.

When the diagnosis is confirmed in the newborn period, decisions must be made concerning subsequent long-term management of the patient. It must be decided early whether the patient would best be served by an atrial diversion procedure or an arterial switch. If it is determined that the patient will ultimately have either a Senning or Mustard procedure, an atrial septostomy is usually necessary. In 1968, Rashkind and Miller[36] described a balloon septostomy that has since become the mainstay of management of patients with simple transposition. A balloon-tipped catheter is placed into a systemic vein and advanced into the right atrium and through the foramen ovale into the left atrium. This is usually an easy maneuver in the neonate with simple transposition. Should the atrial septum be somewhat thickened and the patent foramen ovale small because of concomitant congenital anomalies, a blade can be used for enlargement of the foramen ovale, allowing the subsequent passage of the balloon-tipped catheter. The balloon is then inflated with 1 to 3 ml. of contrast material so that it can be visualized on an image intensifier, and it is then pulled vigorously across the atrial septum to enlarge or tear the foramen ovale. This increases admixture of pulmonary and systemic venous blood at the atrial level. It has proved to be an excellent means of palliation in the very small infant. The septostomy can be repeated at subsequent intervals as cyanosis becomes unmanageable, but as the patient ages, thickening of the septum makes subsequent tearing of the septum much more difficult.

If it is determined that the patient is a good candidate anatomically for an arterial switch procedure, enlargement of the atrial septum has been found to be a disadvantage. If the atrial septal defect is sufficiently large to permit oxygen saturations that are acceptable, in the 80 to 90 per cent range, catheterization and balloon septostomy can be avoided. It has been found that the left ventricle is considerably decompressed by an atrial septostomy, with subsequent poor performance of the left ventricle following an arterial switch procedure. Consequently, if an arterial switch procedure is anticipated and will be performed within the first hours to days following life, catheterization and balloon septostomy can be eliminated.

Palliative Operations

Since the improvement of intracardiac repair in infants and the use of hypothermia, there is probably no role today for the performance of a palliative atrial septostomy as originally described by Blalock and Hanlon. There is an occasional patient, however, in whom this procedure is useful. With early recognition, prompt diagnosis, and early definitive correction, the Blalock-Hanlon atrial septostomy has been largely replaced by balloon septostomy or no septostomy.

Ventricular Septal Defect

Management of a patient with a small VSD and transposition of the great arteries is not different from management of a patient with a simple transposition. The presence of a small VSD and only moderate elevation of pressure in the left ventricle should not cause major concern, since irreversible pulmonary vascular disease is not likely to develop. Infants with large or significant VSDs present in the first few weeks of life with cyanosis and congestive heart failure. If congestive failure cannot be controlled adequately with medical therapy, repair is performed electively when the infant is 3 to 6 months of age, since after 6 months there is a high incidence of pulmonary vascular obstructive disease. When medical management is insufficient in an infant in the first few months of life, palliation can be accomplished by pulmonary artery banding. Banding of the pulmonary artery is a very delicate procedure in transposition of the great arteries. If the band is too tight, the pulmonary blood flow is reduced too much, and systemic hypoxia and metabolic acidosis ensue. However, if the band is too loose, it is physiologically inadequate and will not prevent the development of pulmonary vascular changes.

Since the advent of the arterial switch procedure and with improvement in clinical results, banding in many instances is not necessary because complete, definitive repair can occur early in infancy. In most instances, banding alone should not be considered.

Left Ventricular Outflow Obstruction

Left ventricular outflow tract obstruction was an important problem in transposition of the great arteries in a study of 210 postmortem cases of transposition reported by Van Praagh.[54] Eighty-four per cent of cases of transposition were found to have no stenosis, 14 per cent were found to have left ventricular outflow tract stenosis, and 1 per cent was found to have left ventricular outflow tract atresia. Of the 15 per cent of cases with left ventricular outflow tract obstruction, the anatomic types of obstruction were subpulmonary fibrous tissue in 45 per cent, malalignment of the conal septum in 42 per cent, both subpulmonary fibrous obstruction and conal malalignment in 9 per cent, and acquired myocardial hypertrophy in 3 per cent.

Left ventricular outflow tract obstruction remains a most perplexing problem with regard to subsequent total correction. Isolated left ventricular outflow tract obstruction can be approached through the pulmonary artery. However, if the extent of the obstruction is both valvular and fibrous, complete relief of obstruction can be difficult to obtain.[12,18,42] In patients undergoing an atrial switch procedure, the usual systemic or anatomic left ventricle is pumping blood beyond the stenosis to the lung, and the heart generally tolerates the obstruction or residual obstruction without difficulty. In the most severe forms of left ventricular outflow tract obstruction, if no direct approach or relief of stenosis can be accomplished in infancy, performance of a systemic–pulmonary artery shunt and enlargement of an inter-atrial communication is probably the best palliation. At a later time, the child will most probably require a conduit between the left ventricle and the pulmonary artery accompanied by an intra-atrial baffle correction.

If a VSD is present and pulmonary blood flow is severely restricted, a systemic-to-pulmonary shunt, preferably a Blalock-Taussig type, is indicated. The best subsequent procedure is most probably the Rastelli repair, in which blood is directed through the large VSD and out the aorta, and a valved conduit is placed between the right ventricle and a distal pulmonary artery. Other forms of shunts are generally not well tolerated, and a subsequent anatomic correction in an older child is usually very well tolerated.

Surgical Correction

Definitive surgical correction of transposition of the great arteries involves rerouting of systemic venous blood into the pulmonary circulation and pulmonary venous blood into the systemic circulation. This can be accomplished at either an atrial or a great arterial level. If it is accomplished at an atrial level, the systemic ventricle remains the morphologic right ventricle. If it is accomplished at an arterial level, the systemic ventricle becomes the morphologic left ventricle.

All definitive surgical corrections are accomplished through a median sternotomy incision and utilize cardiopulmonary bypass and hypothermia. Definitive correction in younger infants may also utilize profound hypothermia and circulatory arrest.

Diversion of venous inflow at the atrial level was first proposed by Senning in 1959.[40] In an ingenious operation utilizing autologous atrial tissue, he created two large channels crossing the systemic and pulmonary venous circulation. This was accomplished by incising, realigning, and suturing right atrial septal and free wall tissue for the creation of these channels.

Although conceptually elegant, the procedure proved to be difficult to perform and was largely abandoned in many institutions in favor of the Mustard procedure, which was conceptually and technically easier. With the recognition of the long-term complications following a Mustard type repair,[11,27,48] the Senning operation re-emerged as the procedure of choice in the late 1970s because of the lower incidence of atrial arrhythmias and caval obstruction.[6,10,38,39] Reasons for improved long-term success with the Senning operation were thought to be the use of autologous atrial tissue rather than a pericardial or a synthetic baffle for accomplishing the diversion of systemic venous drainage.

In 1964, Mustard described an operation for total correction based on principles proposed by Albert.[30] The Mustard operation utilizes an intra-atrial baffle for diversion of the systemic venous return to the posterior ventricle, allowing the pulmonary venous return to enter the more anteriorly located systemic ventricle (morphologic right ventricle).

The intra-atrial baffle is usually constructed from pericardium, but in the absence of pericardium, synthetic material may be used (Fig. 4). The entire atrial septum must be excised with special care taken to excise completely the interatrial groove in the cephalad area between the superior vena cava and the top of the ventricular septum. If the rim of the atrial septum is not completely excised, the residual ridge may be too close to the pericardial baffle and obstruct flow from the superior vena cava. Considerable care must also be taken in construction of the baffle so that a generous conduit is provided for unimpeded caval and systemic venous drainage.

Both procedures utilizing atrial diversion can be accomplished in the neonatal period, but there has proved to be little advantage for operations performed this early in a Mustard type repair. In general, successful palliation can be accomplished in early infancy by balloon septostomy; elective repair can be accomplished between the ages of 3 and 8 months. Early repair can be accomplished through the use of profound hypothermia and circulatory arrest, which is generally well tolerated by infants. Early repair decreases the incidence of cerebral thrombosis, hypoxic injury due to cyanotic episodes, peripheral emboli from right-to-left shunts, and other problems associated with severe, long-standing hypoxemia.

Success with the Mustard type operation has been as high as 95 per cent, with some series reporting a 1 to 2 per cent operative mortality. Because of excellent operative results accrued over a

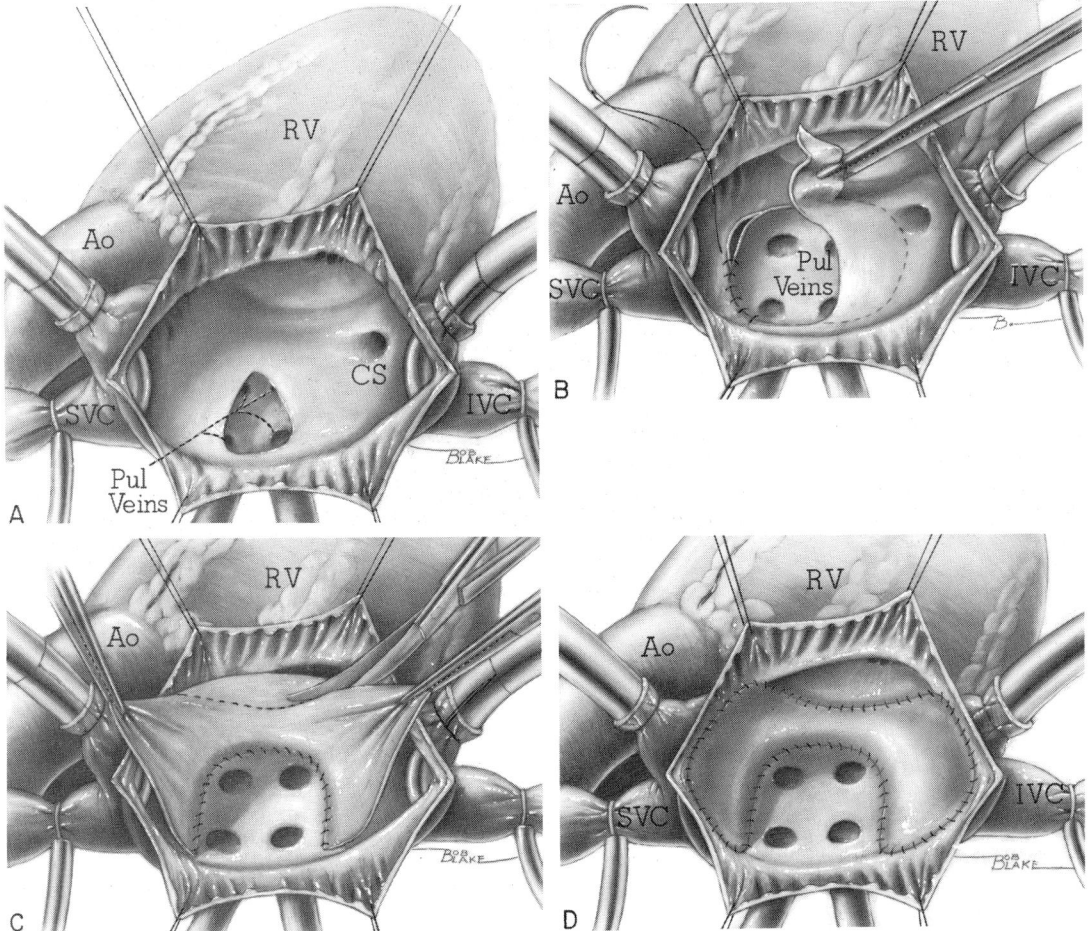

Figure 4. Total correction of transposition of the great arteries by intra-atrial diversion (Mustard's procedure). *A*, The right atrium is opened so that the atrial septum, coronary sinus, and atrial septal defect are exposed. *B*, The atrial septum is excised completely. If the excision of the atrial septum extends outside the heart in the interatrial groove, it may be repaired by direct suture. *C*, The pericardial or prosthetic patch is fashioned around the pulmonary veins and trimmed to fit the atrium. *D*, For completion of the repair, the baffle is sutured around the caval orifices into the remnant of tissue across the top of the ventricular septum. Caval blood is now diverted posteriorly into the left ventricle; pulmonary venous blood enters the right ventricle and then travels into the aorta.

period of years, some centers still perform a Mustard type repair, compared with a Senning or arterial switch.[44,47,48]

Both of the procedures discussed previously accomplish definitive correction at an atrial level, leaving residual ventriculoarterial discordance. Thus, the morphologic right ventricle remains the systemic ventricle. There has long been controversy and concern regarding the long-term fate of the right ventricle remaining as a systemic ventricle, and the belief that the right ventricle would eventually fail in this capacity. Morphologically, the right ventricle is thin-walled, heavily trabeculated, and of a geometric configuration different from the morphologic left ventricle. The morphologic right ventricle also has a tricuspid atrioventricular valve, which in its design and function is inherently less competent than is a mitral valve or a morphologic left ventricular atrioventricular valve.

These concerns have been realized in many institutions that have patients return years after a Mustard type repair, and now years after a Senning type repair, with intractable atrial arrhythmias and systemic ventricular (morphologic right ventricular) failure.[11] Because of these concerns, there has long been interest in achieving a definitive anatomic and physiologic correction of transposition of the great arteries. The realization of the concerns about the right ventricle have increased the enthusiasm in many institutions for achieving complete correction of transposition at an arterial level.

In 1975, Jatene[21] described anatomic correction of transposition of the great arteries in infants by dividing both the aorta and the pulmonary artery with removal of a "button" of aorta

around the origin of the coronary arteries for repositioning and anastomosis of the coronary arteries into the pulmonary artery. The neo-aorta was then anastomosed to the true aorta; the sinuses of Valsalva of the neo–pulmonary artery were reconstructed and anastomosed to the true pulmonary artery. Although of tremendous appeal, initial high mortality limited the application of this technique. In the past several years, reduced mortality in infancy has allowed more liberal application of the arterial switch procedure.

The initial application of the arterial switch procedure was in infants up to 6 months of age with VSD, which was closed at the time of switching of the great arteries.[7] In recent years, several institutions have applied the arterial switch technique to infants in the first month of life with an intact ventricular septum.[25,33,35,45] The rationale for this is the fact that all infants are born with an elevated pulmonary vascular resistance, and consequently the left ventricle at the time of birth is capable of supporting the systemic circulation. In 1986, Quaegebeur[35] published an 8-year experience in 66 patients, 23 of whom had intact ventricular septum. Eleven-month actuarial survival rate for the entire group of patients was 81 per cent, with no deaths occurring among 33 patients followed as long as 8 years. This publication and subsequent reports from other institutions[25,33,45] rekindled interest in the arterial switch procedure. The technique of the arterial switch operation, based on the methods described by Yacoub,[57] has evolved over the past decade and may vary from one institution to another. All techniques involve a median sternotomy, cardiopulmonary bypass,

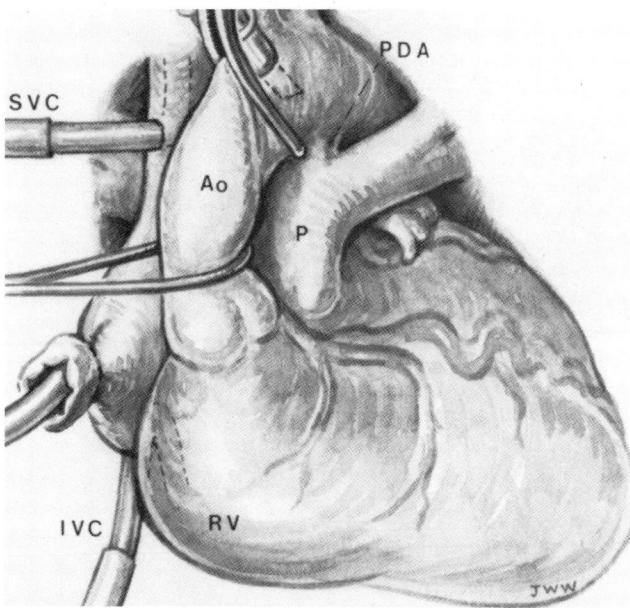

Figure 5. Considerable dissection has been accomplished, the aorta has been cannulated as close to the innominate as possible, and bicaval cannulation has also been utilized. Alternatively, the entire procedure can be performed by use of a single atrial cannula, profound hypothermia, and circulatory arrest.

and hypothermia. Some cardiothoracic surgeons prefer continuous cardiopulmonary bypass with variable flow, whereas others prefer to perform the entire procedure with use of circulatory arrest and profound hypothermia.

After the median sternotomy is made, the aorta and pulmonary artery are dissected apart as much as possible before the establishment of cardiopulmonary bypass (Fig. 5). The ligamentum or ductus arteriosus is dissected, and the branches of the right and left pulmonary arteries are mobilized into the hilum of the lung on each side. Adequate mobilization of the pulmonary arteries is essential for achieving no distortion of the pulmonary artery and aorta at the conclusion of the operation. If continuous cardiopulmonary bypass is employed, it is essential to cannulate the ascending aorta as far distal as possible to allow

appropriate transection of the aorta and subsequent manipulation. Following cannulation and establishment of bypass, the ductus arteriosus is divided between ligatures and the aortic end oversewn (Fig. 6). At the completion of cooling, the ascending aorta is clamped as far distally as possible and cold cardioplegic solution injected into the aortic root. Topical hypothermia may also be used at this point. The aorta is transected approximately 1.5 cm. above the sinuses of Valsalva, or a little more distally when the surgeon chooses not to perform the LeCompte maneuver. The aortic base is then retracted downward, and the anterior aspect of the proximal pulmonary artery is completely cleared up to its base (Fig. 7). The pulmonary artery is transected a few millimeters proximal to the bifurcation, with care taken not to deviate the incision into the origin of the left pulmonary artery. The bases of both great arteries may be stabilized with stay sutures. The most anterior coronary artery, which is usually the one on the patient's left side, is typically excised first (Fig. 8). The incision is begun at the aortic transection site and carried down toward the coronary ostium and then around the ostium for creation of as large a button of sinus wall tissue as is possible without damage to the valve leaflets. Alternatively, the entire sinus of Valsalva except for a rim of tissue above its base may be excised to provide a very large button. During excision of the coronary button, the anatomy is viewed primarily from within for good visualization of the ostium and the valve leaflets. The exact course of the coronary arteries originating from the button may be defined by gently probing from within, and only then is the very proximal portion of the artery mobilized, leaving the periarterial tissue around it. The dissection is done just enough to allow the coronary artery to fall upon a point on the extended proximal segment of the neo-aorta. At this point, a stab wound is made in the proximal neo-aorta; while the anatomy is viewed from within to protect the valve leaflets, a 4-mm. punch is used to create approximately a 5-mm. orifice. The coronary button is then anastomosed to this orifice with a continuous 7–0 polypropylene suture. The second coronary button is then mobilized and excised in a similar manner and reimplanted into the neo-aorta, with care being taken once again not to kink either of the

Figure 6. Control of the ductus arteriosus has been achieved, the pulmonary arteries have been dissected and mobilized into their hila, and considerable dissection has been accomplished between the aorta and the pulmonary artery in preparation for transection.

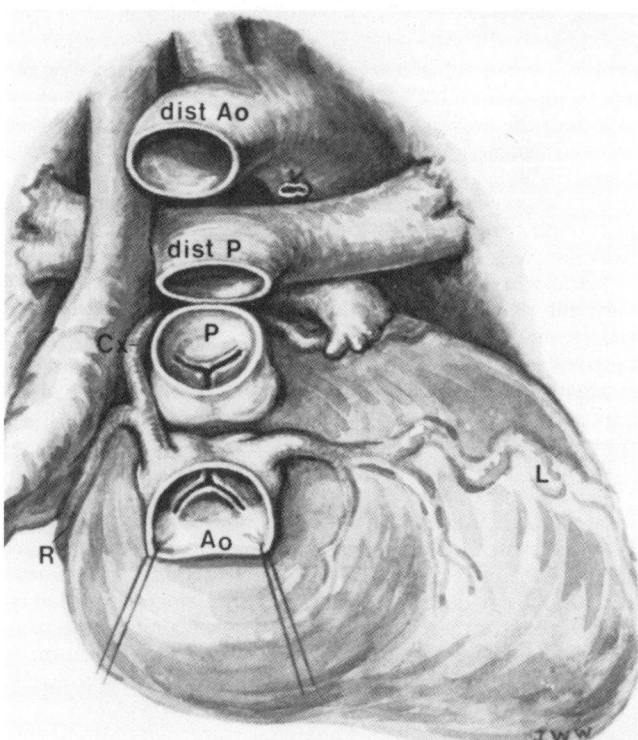

Figure 7. Both aorta and pulmonary artery have been transected. Stay sutures have been placed in the aorta to facilitate visualization.

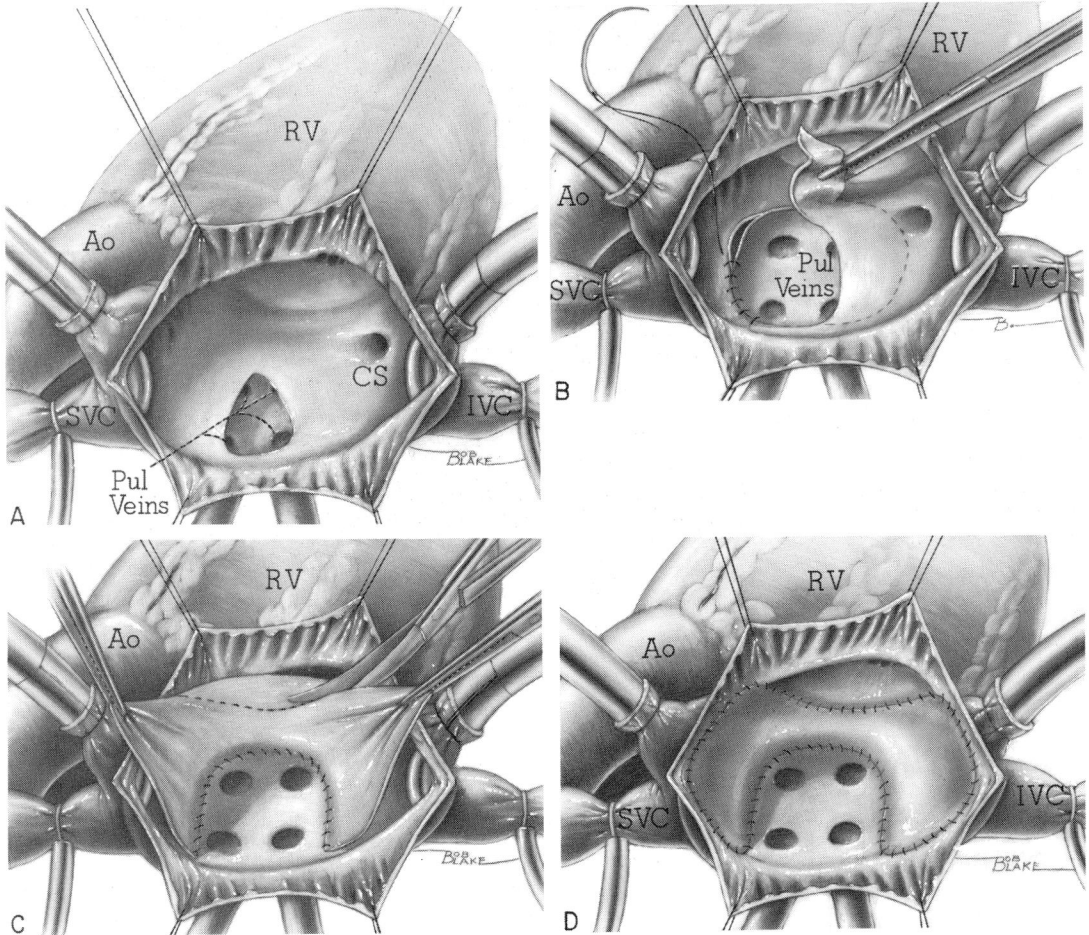

Figure 4. Total correction of transposition of the great arteries by intra-atrial diversion (Mustard's procedure). *A*, The right atrium is opened so that the atrial septum, coronary sinus, and atrial septal defect are exposed. *B*, The atrial septum is excised completely. If the excision of the atrial septum extends outside the heart in the interatrial groove, it may be repaired by direct suture. *C*, The pericardial or prosthetic patch is fashioned around the pulmonary veins and trimmed to fit the atrium. *D*, For completion of the repair, the baffle is sutured around the caval orifices into the remnant of tissue across the top of the ventricular septum. Caval blood is now diverted posteriorly into the left ventricle; pulmonary venous blood enters the right ventricle and then travels into the aorta.

period of years, some centers still perform a Mustard type repair, compared with a Senning or arterial switch.[44,47,48]

Both of the procedures discussed previously accomplish definitive correction at an atrial level, leaving residual ventriculoarterial discordance. Thus, the morphologic right ventricle remains the systemic ventricle. There has long been controversy and concern regarding the long-term fate of the right ventricle remaining as a systemic ventricle, and the belief that the right ventricle would eventually fail in this capacity. Morphologically, the right ventricle is thin-walled, heavily trabeculated, and of a geometric configuration different from the morphologic left ventricle. The morphologic right ventricle also has a tricuspid atrioventricular valve, which in its design and function is inherently less competent than is a mitral valve or a morphologic left ventricular atrioventricular valve.

These concerns have been realized in many institutions that have patients return years after a Mustard type repair, and now years after a Senning type repair, with intractable atrial arrhythmias and systemic ventricular (morphologic right ventricular) failure.[11] Because of these concerns, there has long been interest in achieving a definitive anatomic and physiologic correction of transposition of the great arteries. The realization of the concerns about the right ventricle have increased the enthusiasm in many institutions for achieving complete correction of transposition at an arterial level.

In 1975, Jatene[21] described anatomic correction of transposition of the great arteries in infants by dividing both the aorta and the pulmonary artery with removal of a "button" of aorta

around the origin of the coronary arteries for repositioning and anastomosis of the coronary arteries into the pulmonary artery. The neo-aorta was then anastomosed to the true aorta; the sinuses of Valsalva of the neo–pulmonary artery were reconstructed and anastomosed to the true pulmonary artery. Although of tremendous appeal, initial high mortality limited the application of this technique. In the past several years, reduced mortality in infancy has allowed more liberal application of the arterial switch procedure.

The initial application of the arterial switch procedure was in infants up to 6 months of age with VSD, which was closed at the time of switching of the great arteries.[7] In recent years, several institutions have applied the arterial switch technique to infants in the first month of life with an intact ventricular septum.[25,33,35,45] The rationale for this is the fact that all infants are born with an elevated pulmonary vascular resistance, and consequently the left ventricle at the time of birth is capable of supporting the systemic circulation. In 1986, Quaegebeur[35] published an 8-year experience in 66 patients, 23 of whom had intact ventricular septum. Eleven-month actuarial survival rate for the entire group of patients was 81 per cent, with no deaths occurring among 33 patients followed as long as 8 years. This publication and subsequent reports from other institutions[25,33,45] rekindled interest in the arterial switch procedure. The technique of the arterial switch operation, based on the methods described by Yacoub,[57] has evolved over the past decade and may vary from one institution to another. All techniques involve a median sternotomy, cardiopulmonary bypass,

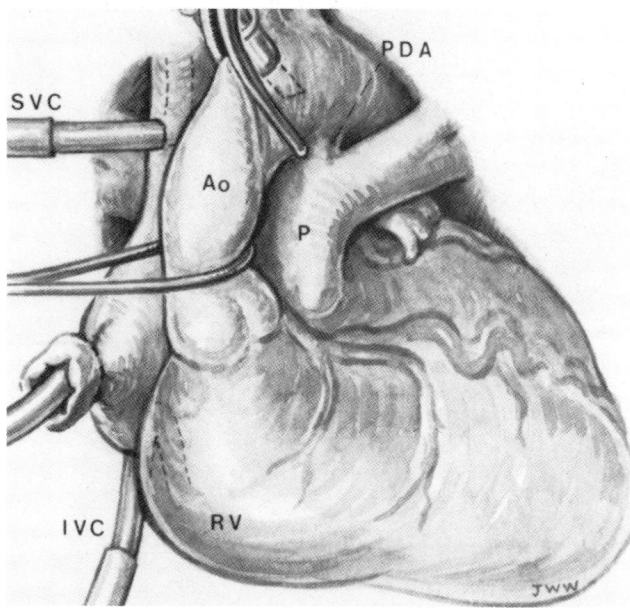

Figure 5. Considerable dissection has been accomplished, the aorta has been cannulated as close to the innominate as possible, and bicaval cannulation has also been utilized. Alternatively, the entire procedure can be performed by use of a single atrial cannula, profound hypothermia, and circulatory arrest.

and hypothermia. Some cardiothoracic surgeons prefer continuous cardiopulmonary bypass with variable flow, whereas others prefer to perform the entire procedure with use of circulatory arrest and profound hypothermia.

After the median sternotomy is made, the aorta and pulmonary artery are dissected apart as much as possible before the establishment of cardiopulmonary bypass (Fig. 5). The ligamentum or ductus arteriosus is dissected, and the branches of the right and left pulmonary arteries are mobilized into the hilum of the lung on each side. Adequate mobilization of the pulmonary arteries is essential for achieving no distortion of the pulmonary artery and aorta at the conclusion of the operation. If continuous cardiopulmonary bypass is employed, it is essential to cannulate the ascending aorta as far distal as possible to allow

appropriate transection of the aorta and subsequent manipulation. Following cannulation and establishment of bypass, the ductus arteriosus is divided between ligatures and the aortic end oversewn (Fig. 6). At the completion of cooling, the ascending aorta is clamped as far distally as possible and cold cardioplegic solution injected into the aortic root. Topical hypothermia may also be used at this point. The aorta is transected approximately 1.5 cm. above the sinuses of Valsalva, or a little more distally when the surgeon chooses not to perform the LeCompte maneuver. The aortic base is then retracted downward, and the anterior aspect of the proximal pulmonary artery is completely cleared up to its base (Fig. 7). The pulmonary artery is transected a few millimeters proximal to the bifurcation, with care taken not to deviate the incision into the origin of the left pulmonary artery. The bases of both great arteries may be stabilized with stay sutures. The most anterior coronary artery, which is usually the one on the patient's left side, is typically excised first (Fig. 8). The incision is begun at the aortic transection site and carried down toward the coronary ostium and then around the ostium for creation of as large a button of sinus wall tissue as is possible without damage to the valve leaflets. Alternatively, the entire sinus of Valsalva except for a rim of tissue above its base may be excised to provide a very large button. During excision of the coronary button, the anatomy is viewed primarily from within for good visualization of the ostium and the valve leaflets. The exact course of the coronary arteries originating from the button may be defined by gently probing from within, and only then is the very proximal portion of the artery mobilized, leaving the periarterial tissue around it. The dissection is done just enough to allow the coronary artery to fall upon a point on the extended proximal segment of the neo-aorta. At this point, a stab wound is made in the proximal neo-aorta; while the anatomy is viewed from within to protect the valve leaflets, a 4-mm. punch is used to create approximately a 5-mm. orifice. The coronary button is then anastomosed to this orifice with a continuous 7–0 polypropylene suture. The second coronary button is then mobilized and excised in a similar manner and reimplanted into the neo-aorta, with care being taken once again not to kink either of the

Figure 6. Control of the ductus arteriosus has been achieved, the pulmonary arteries have been dissected and mobilized into their hila, and considerable dissection has been accomplished between the aorta and the pulmonary artery in preparation for transection.

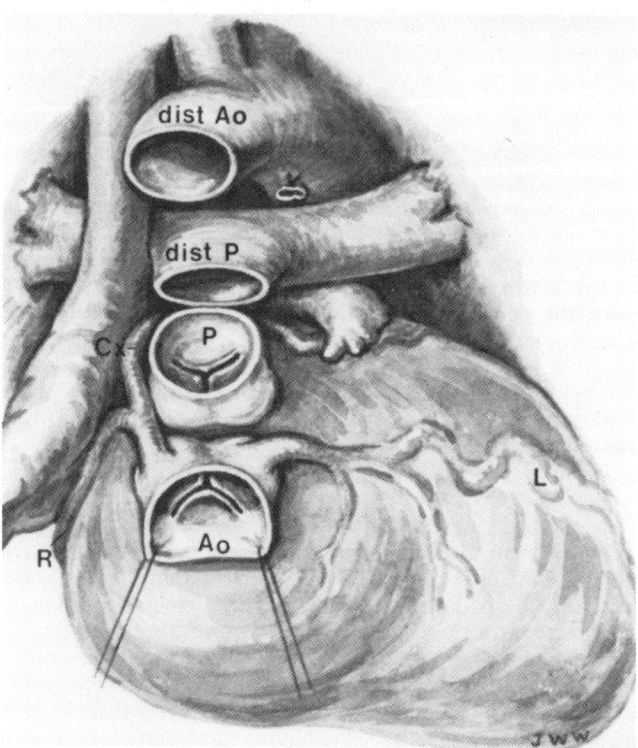

Figure 7. Both aorta and pulmonary artery have been transected. Stay sutures have been placed in the aorta to facilitate visualization.

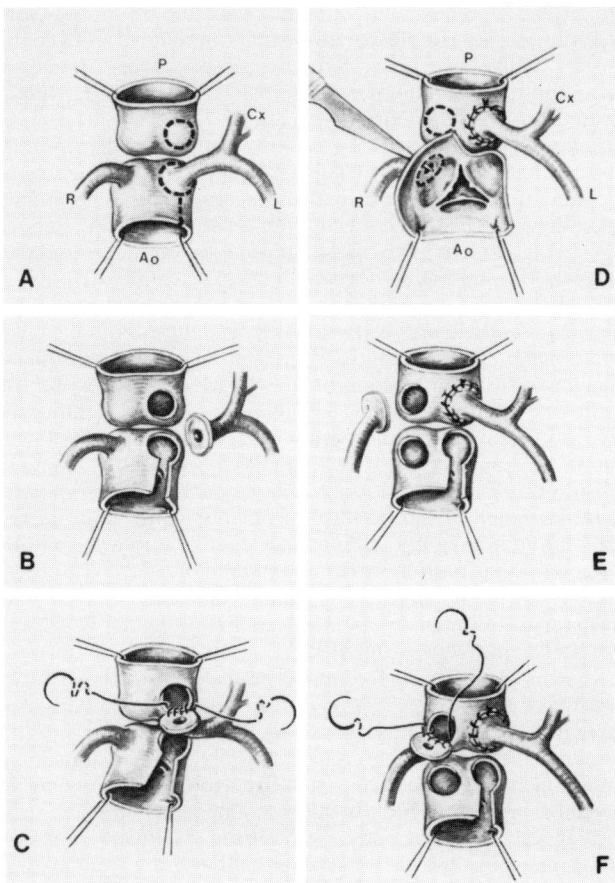

Figure 8. Steps involved in mobilization and excision of the coronary ostia as buttons of tissue from the sinus of Valsalva, with subsequent anastomosis to the neo-aorta. Care must be taken at each step to avoid kinking of the coronary arteries, damage to the valve leaflets, and narrowing of the coronary ostia.

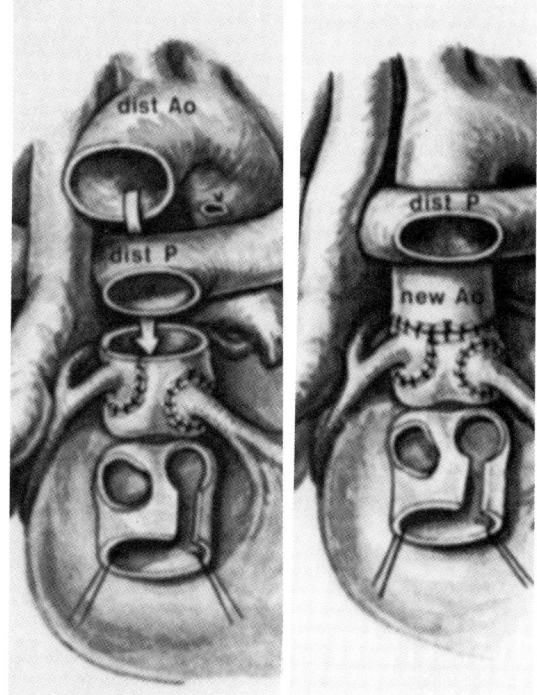

Figure 9. Following completion of the coronary anastomoses, the distal ascending aorta is passed posterior to the transected pulmonary artery and anastomosed to the neo-aorta. This is known as the LeCompte maneuver. (From Quaegebeur, J. M.: The arterial switch operation. Rationale, Results, Perspectives. Deerlijk, Belgium, Uitgeverij Rozengaard, 1986.)

coronary arteries. When two coronary ostia emerge from the same sinus, both ostia are included within the same button of sinus of Valsalva tissue that is removed.

The neo-aorta is then constructed. Unless the great arteries are side-by-side, the aorta is passed beneath the bifurcation of the pulmonary artery, the end of the aorta is grasped with a tissue forceps, and the aortic cross-clamp is released and subsequently replaced on the aorta inferior to the pulmonary artery bifurcation. This is known as the LeCompte maneuver (Fig. 9). Size mismatches between the neo-aorta and the native aorta may be corrected at this point.

In preparation for construction of the neo–pulmonary artery, the defects left by the button excision of the coronary ostia are filled by suturing into place pieces of autologous pericardium (Fig. 10). Some surgeons prefer to fix the autologous pericardium in glutaraldehyde to give the tissue more substance and make it easier to manipulate. Others prefer not to do this. An alternative to pericardium may be a bioprosthetic material such as porcine pericardium or a synthetic material. Autologous pericardium is far preferable to any other substitute, however. Size discrepancies between the neo–pulmonary artery and the native pulmonary arteries can once again be corrected at this point (Fig. 11).

When a VSD is present and in the perimembranous position, it is usually repaired by the transatrial approach before the actual arterial switch operation is commenced. Alternatively, very small VSDs may be repaired through the pulmonary artery (neo-aorta).

Atrial septal defects are usually repaired by direct suture, but a patch might be used if a previous Blalock-Hanlon operation

has been performed. Associated anomalies are managed in the manner most appropriate for them.

Following repair, all of these infants are prone to pulmonary hypertensive crises. Consequently, in the author's series, all infants were anesthetized, paralyzed, and mechanically ventilated for at least 24 hours after operation. If there is any degree of left ventricular dysfunction, left atrial pressures may be monitored. The cardiac subsystem was routinely supported in the early postoperative period with dopamine or dobutamine at approximately 5 μg. per kg. per minute, nitroprusside in low dosages (0.5 to 1 μg. per kg. per minute), and nitroglycerin at approximately 1 to 2 μg. per kg. per minute. Additionally, a continuous fentanyl or sufentanil infusion has proved most helpful in achieving appropriate sedation and analgesia for these patients. Duration of mechanical ventilation has ranged from 24 to 72 hours.

The management of pulmonary stenosis has been a most difficult problem in the child with transposition of the great

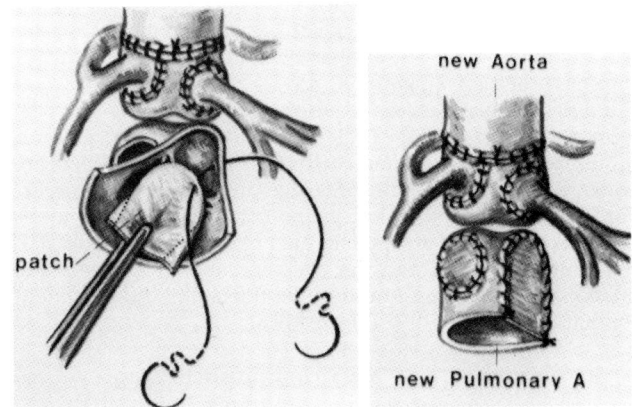

Figure 10. Defects in the sinus of Valsalva of the neo–pulmonary artery are repaired with utilization of autologous pericardium.

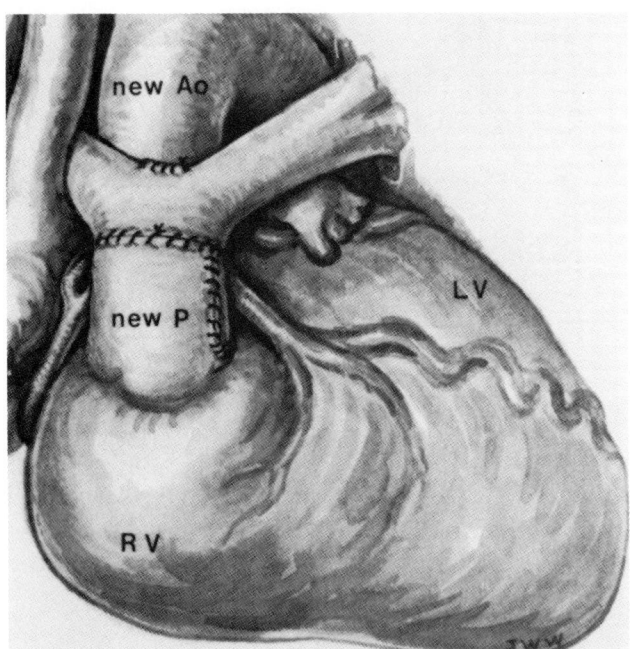

Figure 11. Completion of all anastomoses. The neo–pulmonary artery now lies directly anterior and emerges from the right ventricle, whereas the neo-aorta lies directly posterior and emerges from the left ventricle.

arteries.[13] In most cases, this is a subvalvular stenosis that incorporates a portion of the mitral valve into the stenotic fibrotic band. Because of the posterior location of the pulmonary outflow tract and the presence of a major coronary vessel overlying the tract, it is not impossible to patch the outflow tract, as is commonly done in repair of tetralogy of Fallot. Consequently, various attempts at resection have been undertaken, but complete relief of the stenosis may not be possible. Repeated operations for relief of pulmonary stenosis may be required as the child grows. Alternatively, the child may ultimately require a conduit from left ventricle to pulmonary arteries.

If a large VSD accompanies pulmonary stenosis, the technique described by Rastelli[37] can be utilized. The pulmonary artery is simply divided, and the end exiting from the heart is sutured closed. A ventriculotomy is then performed between the aortic outflow and the ventricular septum, and an intraventricular conduit patch is positioned for diversion of the posterior ventricle efflux through the VSD and out through the aorta. If the VSD proves small, it can be enlarged in its superior and cephalad area without risk of injury to the conduction system. A valved conduit is then placed over the ventriculotomy and connected to the pulmonary artery to carry the systemic venous blood into the lungs. Before the advent of aortic and pulmonary arterial allografts, conduits consisted of synthetic materials and porcine valves. Since the advent of aortic and pulmonary arterial allografts, either cryopreserved or fresh, the conduit of choice is a human allograft.

If a Rastelli procedure is required, the procedure is best performed at a later age if possible. The author prefers to perform this procedure at approximately the age of 4 years, but there are no large series to substantiate an age preference. If the procedure is performed in infancy, the conduit will need to be changed as the child grows. This has not proved to be a difficult procedure, however, and the operation should not be made unnecessarily simply because of the possibility of subsequent conduit changes.[13]

OPERATIVE AND POSTOPERATIVE COMPLICATIONS

As in any operative procedure when the systemic atrium and ventricles are open, air embolus must be prevented. Refilling of

the cardiac chambers with either blood or cold solutions before defibrillation is a simple maneuver that can remove air from the cardiovascular system. Careful hemostasis is also required, since children tolerate any degree of tamponade that might ensue from bleeding extremely poorly.

The mediastinum must be well drained; in smaller infants, this can be accomplished transthoracically, leaving the tips of the tubes in the superior mediastinum, and no tubes impinging upon the heart itself. These children, as are children with Fontan circulations, are extremely sensitive to any degree of mediastinal clot impinging upon the atria. The slightest compression of the right anterior atrial wall may impair filling of the systemic ventricle and cause low cardiac output and elevated pulmonary venous pressure. After an atrial correction of transposition, partial obstruction of the superior vena cava by the baffle may occur, but this is usually not of clinical significance because venous collaterals easily divert the return to the lower part of the body and into the inferior vena cava. One patient in the author's series has required enlargement of a superior vena caval cannulation site because of obvious constriction of the superior vena cava in the immediate postoperative period. Although this has been more common in the Mustard type procedure, it can be noticed in any patient undergoing one of the atrial repairs, or in any patient in whom the superior vena cava has been selectively cannulated.

Rhythm disturbances following complete correction of transposition of the great arteries have been quite common.[11] Most of these rhythm disturbances have been in patients undergoing an atrial type repair, although nodal rhythms and even junctional ectopic tachycardia have been noted in neonates undergoing an arterial switch procedure. In general, a nodal rhythm at a ventricular response rate of 80 to 90 has been well tolerated in any of the repairs. Complete heart block has been rare and has been more commonly found in children with associated VSD. Most of the atrial arrhythmias have proved relatively refractory to medical management. A notable exception that must be managed aggressively if discovered is junctional ectopic tachycardia. At the present time, digitalis is the drug of choice for this rhythm disturbance, and complete loading with digoxin must be accomplished very quickly. This rhythm has a tendency to continue to accelerate and causes significant hemodynamic deterioration unless controlled. A few patients prove refractory to pharmacologic intervention, and systemic cooling has proved most helpful in these patients. In Europe, amiodarone given intravenously has proved very effective in the management of junctional ectopic tachycardia.

Some degree of cardiac failure may be present in the immediate postoperative period and is usually manifested as mild pulmonary congestion and commonly as accumulation of fluid in the pleural cavity, usually the right pleural space. Close observation of body weight and judicious use of fluids are necessary for effective management of the cardiac failure. In general, fulminant cardiac failure has not been a major problem after correction of transposition of the great arteries, and whenever mild fluid accumulation occurs, it can usually be managed by diuretics. Although tracheostomy may have been utilized in the past, it is now extremely rare, although the majority of children require variable periods of endotrachial intubation.[13] Urinary output is generally a good index of cardiac output. The status of the fontanelle in a small infant, the amount of liver palpable below a costal margin, the warmth of the extremities, and the capillary filling time are all extremely useful indicators of cardiac output, thus proving that there is no substitute for hands-on care in the management of these infants and children.

RESULTS OF OPERATION

The results of operation utilizing either a Mustard or a Senning method have been most gratifying, with overall survival between 90 and 95 per cent for patients with an intact ventricular septum. One of the larger experiences with the Mustard operation in simple transposition of the great arteries is from the Hospital for Sick Children in Toronto.[47,48] Their experience in 329 infants and children demonstrated a 10.4 per cent operative mortality that had reduced to 0.9 per cent in the decade beginning in 1974. Likewise, 10-year actuarial survival was 73.4 per cent in their first 106 patients and 93.7 per cent in their second 223 patients. A majority of their patients, however, had sinus node dysfunction or other dysrhythmias. Similar results have been reported from other institutions. In addition, asymptomatic, dynamic left ventricular outflow tract obstruction has been reported despite what appears to be a good clinical result.[44] The long-term implications of this are not known. Bilateral phrenic nerve pulses have also been reported.[43] Excellent results of the Senning procedure have also been reported, with a much lower incidence of atrial arrhythmias and a much higher incidence of normal sinus rhythm.[6,10,11]

Age of operation does not appear to be a risk factor for operative success in either the Mustard or the Senning procedure. It appears that operations performed at an earlier age may have a better success rate than those performed between 1 and 2 years of age.[13] Clinical responses following operation have been excellent, with normal oxygen saturation and relatively unlimited activity.[47] The incidence of arrhythmias following the atrial correction remains of concern, however.

Pulmonary markings on chest films usually decrease over 6 to 12 months, and progressive pulmonary hypertension has been uncommon. Decreased contractility of the right ventricle has been found in a small number of children, and the question remains whether the right heart can maintain systemic pressure over a prolonged period.[27] The ultimate success of the intra-atrial baffle procedures depends greatly on the ability of the right heart to perform and the ability of the tricuspid valve to remain competent at systemic pressures.

Excellent results have also been obtained with the arterial switch procedure, although follow-up is obviously more limited. Late functional status has been excellent in several series,[9,25,35] with an incidence of rhythm disturbance that is less than 5 per cent. Neo-coarctation following a LeCompte maneuver has been reported but appears to be an infrequent complication.

Of primary concern is growth and development of the various anastomoses required for successful accomplishment of the arterial switch procedure. Laboratory experimentation examining growth and development of anastomoses accomplished with fine (7–0, 8–0) polypropylene sutures suggests that the suture material fragments and the anastomoses grow. This has been borne out by clinical experience.

In conclusion, the management of patients with transposition of the great arteries has undergone considerable evolution over the past 30 years. Satisfactory treatment options are available and can be tailored to the individual patient. A favorable outcome in patients presenting with this lesion can be expected.

SELECTED REFERENCES

Bender, H. W., Jr., Stewart, J. R., Merrill, W. H., Hammon, J. W., Jr., and Graham, T. P., Jr.: Ten years' experience with the Senning operation for transposition of the great arteries. Ann. Thorac. Surg., 47:218, 1989.
This article is a very concise and thoughtful analysis of a large, consecutive group of infants undergoing an atrial repair of simple transposition. Despite outstanding results achieved over a 10-year period, the authors abandoned the Senning procedure in favor of the more controversial arterial switch procedure. In this article, their rationale for doing so is explained.

Jatene, A., Fontes, V. F., Paulista, P. P., Souza, L. C. B., Neger, F., Galantier, M., and Sousa, J. E. M. R.: Anatomic correction of transposition of the great vessels. J. Thorac. Cardiovasc. Surg., 72:364, 1976.
This is a description of the concept of transposing the aorta and pulmonary artery in patients with transposition of the great vessels in order to achieve correction. The technique is very ingenious but requires reimplantation of the coronary arteries. Although ideal in concept, this procedure is associated with an operative mortality that has thus far prevented its widespread adoption.

Mustard, W. I., Keith, J. D., Trusler, G. A., Fowler, R., and Kidd, L.: The surgical management of transposition of the great vessels. J. Thorac. Cardiovasc. Surg., 48:953, 1964.
This excellent work describes the intra-atrial baffle procedure for total correction of transposition of the great vessels. The important details of the operation are well defined, and many subtle points are emphasized to allow a better understanding of its complexity. This paper was responsible for a complete change of thinking regarding the outlook for children with transposition of the great vessels.

Quaegebeur, J. M., Rohmer, J., Ottenkamp, J., Buis, T., Kirklin, J. W., Blackstone, E. H., and Brom, A. G.: The arterial switch operation. J. Thorac. Cardiovasc. Surg., 92:361, 1986.
This is a landmark article in which it was clearly shown that performance of the arterial switch operation in a very young, and sometimes anatomically very complex, group of patients was entirely feasible. The superb results achieved in this article with the complete anatomic and physiologic correction prompted re-emergence of the arterial switch procedure during a time when excellent short-term results with the Senning operation were being achieved.

Senning, A.: Surgical correction of transposition of the great vessels. Surgery, 45:966, 1959.
This original article describes the approach to the intra-atrial baffle (Senning) procedure. The technique is well described, and the illustrations are well developed. These procedures were performed on older children without the benefit of modern cannulation technique, thus making the accomplishment even more impressive.

Turley, K., and Ebert, P. A.: Total correction of transposition of the great arteries. J. Thorac. Cardiovasc. Surg., 76:312, 1978.
This article describes the low mortality possible in corrective procedures in early infancy. It is of interest that incidence of atrial arrhythmias with the Mustard operation was much lower in small infants than in older patients undergoing correction.

REFERENCES

1. Aziz, K. U., Paul, M. H., Idriss, F. S., et al.: Clinical manifestations of dynamic left ventricular outflow tract stenosis in infants with d-transposition of the great arteries with intact ventricular septum. Am. J. Cardiol., 44:290, 1979.
2. Baffes, T. G.: A new method for surgical correction of transposition of the aorta and pulmonary artery. Surg. Gynecol. Obstet., 102:227, 1956.
3. Bailey, C. P.: Surgery of the Heart. Philadelphia, Lea & Febiger, 1955.
4. Baillie, M.: The Morbid Anatomy of Some of the More Important Parts of the Human Body. London, Johnson & Nichol, 1797, p. 38.
5. Barnard, C. N., Schrire, V., and Beck, W.: Complete transposition of the great vessels: A successful complete correction. J. Thorac. Cardiovasc. Surg., 43:768, 1962.
6. Bender, H. W., Jr., Stewart, J. R., Merrill, W. H., Hammon, J. W., Jr., and Graham, T. P., Jr.: Ten years' experience with the Senning operation for transposition of the great arteries: Physiological results and late follow-up. Ann. Thorac. Surg., 47:218, 1989.
7. Bical, O., Hazan, E., LeCompte, Y., Fermont, L., Karam, J., Jarreau, M. M., Tran Viet, T., Sidi, D., Leca, F., and Neveux, J. Y.: Anatomic correction of transposition of the great arteries associated with ventricular septal defect: Midterm results in 50 patients. Circulation, 70:891, 1984.
8. Blalock, A., and Hanlon, C. R.: The surgical treatment of complete transposition of the aorta and pulmonary artery. Surg. Gynecol. Obstet., 90:1, 1950.
9. Colan, S. D., Trowitzsch, E., Wernovsky, G., Sholler, G. F., Sanders, S. P., and Castaneda, A. R.: Myocardial performance after arterial switch operation for transposition of the great arteries with intact ventricular septum. Circulation, 78:132, 1988.
10. Croto, E. O., Norwood, W. I., Lang, P., and Castaneda, A. R.: Modified Senning operation for treatment of transposition of the great arteries. J. Thorac. Cardiovasc. Surg., 78:721, 1979.
11. Deanfield, J., Camm, J., Macartney, F., Cartwright, T., Douglas, J., Drew, J., de Leval, M., and Stark, J.: Arrhythmia and late mortality after Mustard and Senning eight-year prospective study. J. Thorac. Cardiovasc. Surg., 96:569, 1988.
12. DeLeon, S. Y., Idriss, F. S., Ilbawi, M. N., Muster, A. J., Paul, M. H., Berry, T. E., Duffy, C. E., and Quinones, J.: The Damus-Stansel-Kaye procedure. J. Thorac. Cardiovasc. Surg., 91:747, 1986.
13. Ebert, P. A.: Transposition of the great arteries. In Sabiston, D. C. (Ed.): Textbook of Surgery, 14th ed. Philadelphia, W. B. Saunders Company, 1986, pp. 2249–2259.
14. Fanconi, G.: Die Transposition der grossen Gefuse (das Charakteristische Rontgenbild). Arch. Kinderheilk., 95:202, 1932.
15. Farre, J. R.: Pathological Researches. Essay 1: On malformations of the human heart. London, Longman, Hurst, Rees, Orme, Brown, 1814, p. 28.
16. Gittenberger-de Groot, A. C., Sauer, U., and Quaegebeur, J.: Aortic intramural coronary artery in three hearts with transposition of the great arteries. J. Thorac. Cardiovasc. Surg., 91:566, 1986.
17. Glenn, W. W. L., and Patino, J. F.: Circulatory bypass of the right heart. I. Preliminary observations on the direct delivery of vena caval blood into the pulmonary arterial circulation. Azygos vein–pulmonary artery shunt. Yale J. Biol. Med., 27:147, 1954.
18. Goor, D. A., and Ebert, P. A.: Left ventricular outflow obstruction in Taussig-Bing malformation. J. Thorac. Cardiovasc. Surg., 70:69, 1974.
19. Graham, T. P., Franklin, R. C. G., Wyse, R. K. H., Gooch, V., and Deanfield,

J. E.: Left ventricular wall stress and contractile function in transposition of the great arteries after the Rastelli operation. J. Thorac. Cardiovasc. Surg., 93:775, 1987.

20. Grant, R. P.: The morphogenesis of transposition of the great vessels. Circulation, 26:819, 1962.

21. Jatene, A., Fontes, V. F., Paulista, P. P., Souza, L. C. B., Neger, F., Galantier, M., and Sousa, J. E. M. R.: Anatomic correction of transposition of the great vessels. J. Thorac. Cardiovasc. Surg., 72:364, 1976.

22. Ilbawi, M. N., Idriss, F. S., DeLeon, S. Y., Muster, A. J., Gidding, S. S., Duffy, C. E., and Paul, M. H.: Preparation of the left ventricle for anatomical correction in patients with simple transposition of the great arteries. J. Thorac. Cardiovasc. Surg., 94:87, 1987.

23. Kay, E. B., and Cross, F. S.: Transposition of the great vessels corrected by means of atrial transposition. Surgery, 41:938, 1957.

24. Kurosawa, H., Imai, Y., Takanashi, Y., Hoshino, S., Sawatari, K., Kawada, M., and Takao, A.: Infundibular septum and coronary anatomy in Jatene operation. J. Thorac. Cardiovasc. Surg., 91:572, 1986.

25. Lange, P. E., Sievers, H. H., Onnasch, D. G. W., Yacoub, M. H., Bernhard, A., and Heintzen, P. H.: Up to 7 years of follow-up after two-stage anatomic correction of simple transposition of the great arteries. Circulation, 74:47, 1986.

26. Lev, M., and Saphir, O.: A theory of transposition of the arterial trunks based on the phylogenetic and ontogenetic development of the heart. Arch. Pathol., 39:172, 1945.

27. Mee, R. B. B.: Severe right ventricular failure after Mustard or Senning operation. J. Thorac. Cardiovasc. Surg., 92:385, 1986.

28. Merendino, K. A., Jesseph, J. E., and Herron, P. W.: Interatrial venous transposition, a one-stage intracardiac operation for the conversion of complete transposition of the aorta and pulmonary artery to corrected transposition: Theory and clinical experience. Surgery, 42:898, 1957.

29. Moene, R. J., and Oppenheimer-Dekker, A.: Congenital mitral valve anomalies in transposition of the great arteries. Am. J. Cardiol., 49:1972, 1982.

30. Mustard, W. T.: Successful two-stage correction of transposition of the great vessels. Surgery, 55:469, 1964.

31. Mustard, W. T., Chute, A. L., Keith, J. D., Sireck, A., Rowe, R. D., and Vlad, P.: A surgical approach to transposition of the great vessels with extracorporeal circuit. Surgery, 36:39, 1954.

32. Muster, A. J., Berry, T. E., Ilbawi, M. N., DeLeon, S. Y., and Idriss, F. S.: Development of neo-coarctation in patients with transposed great arteries and hypoplastic aortic arch after Lecompte modification of anatomical correction. J. Thorac. Cardiovasc. Surg., 93:276, 1987.

33. Nakazawa, M., Oyama, K., Imai, Y., Nojima, K., Aotsuka, H., Satomi, G., Kurosawa, H., and Takao, A.: Criteria for two-staged arterial switch operation for simple transposition of great arteries. Circulation, 78:124, 1988.

34. Pigott, J. D., Chin, A. J., Weinberg, P. M., Wagner, H. R., and Norwood, W. I.: Transposition of the great arteries with aortic arch obstruction. J. Thorac. Cardiovasc. Surg., 94:82, 1987.

35. Quaegebeur, J. M., Rohmer, J., Ottenkamp, J., Buis, T., Kirklin, J. W., Blackstone, E. H., and Brom, A. G.: The arterial switch operation. J. Thorac. Cardiovasc. Surg., 92:361, 1986.

36. Rashkind, W. J., and Miller, W. W.: Transposition of the great arteries: Results of palliation by balloon atrioseptostomy in 31 patients. Circulation, 38:453, 1968.

37. Rastelli, G. C., Wallace, R. B., and Ongley, P. A.: Complete repair of transposition of the great arteries with pulmonary stenosis. A review and report of a case corrected by using a new surgical technique. Circulation, 39:83, 1969.

38. Rubay, J. E., de Halleux, C., Jaumin, P., Moulin, D., Kestens-Servaye, Y., Lintermans, J., Stijns, J., Vliers, A., and Chalant, C.-H.: Long-term follow-up

of the Senning operation for transposition of the great arteries in children under 3 months of age. J. Thorac. Cardiovasc. Surg., 94:75, 1987.

39. Senning, A.: Correction of the transposition of the great arteries. Ann. Surg., 182:287, 1975.

40. Senning, A.: Surgical correction of transposition of the great vessels. Surgery, 45:966, 1959.

41. Shrivastava, S., Tadavarthy, S. M., Fukuda, T., et al.: Anatomic causes of pulmonary stenosis in complete transposition. Circulation, 54:154, 1976.

42. Snoddy, J. W., Parr, E. L., Robertson, L. W., Mauck, H. P., McCue, C. M., and Lower, R. R.: Successful intracardiac repair of the Taussig-Bing malformation in 2 children. Ann. Thorac. Surg., 25:158, 1978.

43. Stewart, S., Alexson, C., and Manning, J.: Bilateral phrenic nerve paralysis after the Mustard procedure. J. Thorac. Cardiovasc. Surg., 92:138, 1986.

44. Stewart, S., Harris, P. J., and Manning, J.: The midterm and long-term results of the Mustard operation in patients with transposition of the great vessels and dynamic left ventricular outflow tract obstruction. Ann. Thorac. Surg., 41:272, 1986.

45. Takahaski, M, and Van Praagh, R.: Anatomic varations in transposition of the great arteries. In Challenges in the treatment of congenital cardiac anomalies. Takahoshi, M., Wells, W. J., Lindesmith, G. G. (eds.) Mount Kisco, New York, Futura Publishing Company, 1986, p. 113

46. Taussig, H. B.: Complete transposition of the great vessels. Am. Heart J., 16:728, 1938.

47. Trusler, G. A., Williams, W. G., Duncan, K. F., Hesslein, P. S., Benson, L. N., Freedom, R. M., Izukawa, T., and Olley, P. M.: Results with the Mustard operation in simple transposition of the great arteries. Ann. Thorac., 206:251, 1987.

48. Trusler, G. A., Williams, W. G., Izukawa, T., and Olley, P. M.: Current results with the Mustard operation in isolated transposition of the great arteries. J. Thorac. Cardiovasc. Surg., 80:381, 1980.

49. Tynan, J. J., and Anderson, R. H.: Terminology of transposition of the great arteries. Paediatr. Cardiol., 2:341, 1979.

50. VanGils, F. A. W.: Left ventricular outflow tract obstruction in transposition with interventricular communication: Anatomical aspects. In Van Mierop, L. H. S., Oppenheimer-Dekker, A., and Bruins, C. L. D. (Eds.): Embryology and Teratology of the Heart and Great Arteries. The Hague, Leiden University Press, 1978, pp. 160–171.

51. Van Mierop, L. H. S.: Transposition of the great arteries. Am. J. Cardiol., 28:735, 1971.

52. Van Praagh, R.: What is the Taussig-Bing malformation? Circulation, 38:445, 1968.

53. Van Praagh, R., Layton, W. M., and Van Praagh, S.: The morphogenesis of normal and abnormal relationships between the great arteries and the ventricles: Pathologic and experimental data. In Van Praagh, R., and Takao, A. (Eds.): Etiology and Morphogenesis of Congenital Heart Disease. Mount Kisco, New York, Futura Publishing Company, 1980, pp. 271–316.

54. Van Praagh, R., Perez-Trevino, C., Lopez-Cuellar, M., et al.: Transposition of the great arteries with posterior aorta, anterior pulmonary artery, subpulmonary conus and fibrous continuity between aortic and atrioventricular valves. Am. J. Cardiol., 28:621, 1971.

55. Von Rokitansky, C.: Die Defekte der Scheidewande der Herzens. Vienna, Braumuller, 1875.

56. Wilcox, B. R., and Anderson, R. H.: Surgical Anatomy of the Heart. Lesions in Abnormally Connected Hearts. New York, Gower Medical Publishing Ltd., 1985, p. 7.7.

57. Yacoub, M. H., Radley-Smith, R., and Hilton, C. J.: Anatomical correction of complete transposition of the great arteries and ventricular septal defect in infancy. Br. Med. J., 1:1112, 1976.

XIV

CONGENITAL AORTIC STENOSIS

James D. Sink, M.D.

Anatomic malformations that cause obstruction of varying severity in the outflow of the left ventricle are not uncommon and occur in approximately 7 per cent of patients with congenital heart disease. Sites of obstruction, in decreasing order, are (1) valvular, (2) subvalvular, and (3) supravalvular. Although stenoses at various levels may coexist, they are considered separately.

No known genetic or etiologic factors are associated with valvular and discrete subvalvular aortic stenosis. Subaortic stenosis, however, has been associated with Turner's syndrome, Norman's syndrome, and congenital rubella.[20] Infantile hypercalcemia and derangements in vitamin D metabolism may occur with supravalvular aortic stenosis, whereas hypertrophic subaortic stenosis occurs in a familial form in approximately one third of patients.

HISTORICAL ASPECTS

Paget described congenitally obstructive bicuspid aortic valves in 1944. Carrel and Jeger, working independently, attempted to find a surgical solution to this malformation by experimentally attempting to place conduits between the left ventricular apex and the aorta. Marquis and co-workers reported the surgical treatment of congenital aortic stenosis by introducing dilators via the apex of the left ventricle in 1955. Downing reported a similar procedure in 1956. In 1955, Swan and Lewis, working independently, performed open valvotomy utilizing inflow occlusion and hypothermia. Spencer first reported aortic valvotomy for congenital aortic stenosis during cardiopulmonary bypass in 1958, although the procedure had been performed at the Mayo Clinic in 1956.

Discrete subvalvular aortic stenosis was first described by Chevers in 1842. Brock reported the results of treating subvalvular stenosis by transventricular dilation in 1956. Spencer reported the treatment of this condition using cardiopulmonary bypass in 1960. The tunnel type of subvalvular aortic stenosis was described by Spencer in 1960, and its effective treatment, aortoventriculoplasty, was introduced by Rastin and Konno[13] in 1975.

Mencarelli first described supravalvular aortic stenosis in 1930. The association of supravalvular aortic stenosis with unusual facies and mental retardation was reported by Williams in 1961. The association of supravalvular aortic stenosis and infantile hypercalcemia was noted in 1963. Successful surgical treatment for supravalvular stenosis using a patch to enlarge the noncoronary sinus of Valsalva was performed in 1956 and reported in 1961.

PATHOLOGY

In more than half of the patients with congenital aortic stenosis, the valve is bicuspid, with two commissures that are fused to various degrees with a slit-like orifice. The valve opening is usually eccentric. Stenosis can occur in bicuspid valves without fusion of the commissures if both leaflets are thickened and taut. Less frequently observed is a tricuspid valve with three recognizable commissures that are fused to varying degree.[18] Rarely, a unicuspid valve that is unicommissural or noncommissural is encountered.[18] The unicuspid type is more common in infants presenting with severe stenosis. Diffuse thickening of the leaflets, especially along the leaflet edge, is an important factor in causing stenosis of the orifice. This process can be particularly pronounced in neonates with cusps that are myxomatous and dysplastic, causing obstruction often in the absence of significant commissural fusion. The aortic valve anulus is usually normal, although it may be hypoplastic. Left ventricular hypertrophy is always associated with severe aortic stenosis. Particularly in infants, valvular aortic stenosis is often associated with coarctation of the aorta, patent ductus arteriosus, mitral valve abnormalities, endocardial fibroelastosis, and varying degrees of hypoplasia of the left ventricle and ascending aorta.

Discrete, localized subaortic stenosis is the second most common type of congenital obstruction of the left ventricular outflow tract. There are three types of subaortic stenosis. A localized fibrous shelf may be located at any level between the nadir of the aortic cusps to approximately 2 cm. beneath the aortic valve. The obstruction is usually more prominent anteriorly and laterally. The membrane may, however, be equally well developed across the anterior mitral valve leaflet, forming a complete ring with a central opening. The muscular ventricular septum beneath the right aortic cusp is variably prominent and may contribute to the obstruction. Fibromuscular type of subaortic obstruction is caused by a longer stenotic area with both a muscular and fibrous component. In its most severe form, the obstruction can extend for up to several centimeters and be associated with a small aortic anulus. There are gradations of obstruction between discrete subvalvular membrane obstruction and severe tunnel obstruction, and there is considerable evidence that progression from discrete to tunnel obstruction may occur. The aortic valve leaflets may become thickened as a

result of turbulence associated with subvalvular stenosis, causing aortic insufficiency.

Supravalvular aortic stenosis may be localized or diffuse. The localized form is most common, with narrowing usually at the level of the attachments of the aortic valve commissures to the aortic wall. The narrowing may, however, be diffuse, extending even beyond the ascending aorta. The outer diameter of the aorta may be normal or narrowed at the point of obstruction. The obstructing ridge is composed of fibrous tissue and may adhere to the valve cusps, producing valvular obstruction or insufficiency.[5] In addition to being associated with craniofacial abnormalities, supravalvular aortic stenosis is commonly observed with peripheral pulmonary stenosis and coronary artery abnormalities.

Asymmetric septal hypertrophy, although mainly described in adults, may also be seen in children and infants. First described by Brock in 1957, asymmetric septal hypertrophy is a genetically transmitted myocardial disease characterized by a disproportionate thickening of the ventricular septum as it relates to the left ventricular free wall. This type of obstruction is also referred to as hypertrophic obstructive cardiomyopathy and idiopathic hypertrophic subaortic stenosis and is discussed in another chapter.

PATHOPHYSIOLOGY

The primary hemodynamic alteration following left ventricular outflow tract obstruction is an increase in left ventricular pressure. This alteration is fairly well tolerated in utero, since most infants with this anomaly are well developed at birth. Obstruction of left ventricular outflow in utero causes an increase in right ventricular and ductus arteriosus blood flow. Following birth, an increase in pulmonary venous return causes the foramen ovale to close with a resultant increase in left atrial pressure. The increase in left atrial pressure increases left ventricular preload and stroke volume. As left ventricular compliance decreases, left atrial pressure increases and may cause pulmonary venous hypertension unless an intra-atrial communication remains.

When the ductus is closed, systemic blood flow depends entirely on left ventricular output. Severe obstruction to left ventricular output can cause impaired ventricular performance, decreased cardiac output, and decreased systemic blood pressure. The result is a decrease in peripheral perfusion causing metabolic acidosis and ultimately death.

In less severe cases of obstruction, the pressure overload is compensated by gradual concentric ventricular hypertrophy that preserves systolic myocardial performance. Hypertrophy, however, alters diastolic ventricular properties, causing reduced myocardial compliance. Myocardial oxygen consumption increases because there is an increase in systolic ventricular wall tension and prolonged duration of systole. Concomitantly, the decrease in diastolic time and the increase in diastolic intramural pressure decrease coronary perfusion. This combination of factors may ultimately cause left ventricular failure from myocardial ischemia.

VALVULAR AORTIC STENOSIS

Clinical Features

Congenital aortic stenosis is much more common in males than in females with a ratio of 4:1. Whereas approximately 7 per cent of infants and children born with congenital heart disease have left ventricular outflow tract obstruction, approximately 80 per cent of this group have valvular aortic stenosis. Severity of obstruction is judged by the peak systolic pressure gradient across the obstruction and the calculated aortic valve area. In valvular stenosis, if cardiac output is normal, a gradient greater than 75 mm. Hg or a calculated valve area of less than

0.5 sq. cm. per sq. m. is considered severe; a gradient between 50 and 75 mm. Hg or a valve area between 0.5 and 0.8 sq. cm. per sq. m. is considered moderate; and a gradient of less than 50 mm. Hg or a valve area greater than 0.8 sq. cm. per sq. m. is considered mild.

The clinical presentation is essentially identical in each type of outflow obstruction. Symptoms appear as the left ventricle is no longer able to compensate for its pressure overload at rest or at exercise. Children and young adults, even with severe aortic stenosis, may be essentially without symptoms at rest. As cardiac output decreases below demand, as may occur with exercise, patients develop symptoms of exertional syncope, angina pectoris, and congestive heart failure. Neonates with severe aortic stenosis may present at birth, or shortly thereafter, with pallor, perspiration, inability to feed, shortness of breath, and cyanosis. Infants presenting with congestive heart failure in the first 2 weeks of life are usually critically ill and represent true emergencies. Another small group of patients with less critical but severe stenosis develops symptoms within the first 6 months of life.

Most young patients, however, are asymptomatic, and the detection of a systolic murmur suggests the diagnosis of aortic stenosis. The murmur is harsh and most prominent at the second right intercostal space. A palpable thrill is often detectable along the left upper sternal border and radiates to the carotids. An early systolic ejection click at the apex is often present and helps distinguish valvular aortic stenosis from other forms of obstruction to left ventricular output. Although the peripheral pulses are usually normal in older infants, severe stenosis is characterized by a pulse with low volume and slow upstroke. Infants with critical aortic stenosis may have no palpable peripheral pulses.

The chest film usually shows overall heart size to be normal, but the left ventricle may be prominent. Cardiomegaly can be present, if congestive heart failure exists, and indicates severe disease. Post-stenotic dilation of the aorta is evident in approximately one half of the patients. Valvular calcification, evident on roentgenograms, is rare before the third decade of life.

In most patients, the electrocardiogram demonstrates left ventricular hypertrophy. Occasionally, however, the electrocardiogram is normal and therefore cannot be used to distinguish or determine appropriate patient management.

Characteristic M-mode and two-dimensional echocardiography patterns can distinguish valvular, subvalvular, supravalvular, and hypertrophic subaortic stenosis.[1,17] The addition of continuous wave Doppler echocardiography enables the velocity of flow across the aortic valve to be determined. From this information, the transvalvular gradient can be calculated.[7] For experienced surgeons, echocardiographic diagnosis is accurate enough that catheterization and angiography are unnecessary prior to surgical therapy.[9]

Definitive diagnosis is provided by demonstrating a systolic gradient across the aortic valve at cardiac catheterization. Cardiac output is also determined at catheterization so that the aortic valve area can be calculated. Increased left ventricular end-diastolic pressure is usually present and correlates with left ventricular failure. Angiography documents the site of obstruction. The aortic leaflets are typically thickened and domed with a central or eccentric jet of contrast during systole. Post-stenotic dilation of the aorta is usually seen. Catheterization and angiography are important to identify any accompanying cardiac defects.

Natural History and Operative Indications

Valvular aortic stenosis presenting in infancy is usually severe and may rapidly progress to congestive heart failure and death. Symptomatic infants require prompt surgical intervention. This fact, along with the frequent association of endocardial fibroelastosis and other intracardiac and extracardiac ab-

normalities, contributes to the significant mortality in this group of patients. Many survivors exhibit aortic regurgitation, and most eventually require further valve surgery.

In patients whose symptoms first appear after 1 year of age, a gradual progression in the severity of the pressure gradient can be documented in 30 to 40 per cent.[15] Noninvasive echo Doppler studies may now be employed in evaluating these patients. Associated lesions are less common in patients presenting beyond 1 year of age.

Sudden death has been reported in 1 to 19 per cent of children with aortic stenosis but has not been documented in patients without symptoms or abnormal physical findings. A careful recent study of the natural history of valvular aortic stenosis suggests that the risk of sudden death has been overemphasized and probably occurs in 1 per cent of the patients. Regular clinical assessment of patients is recommended as adequate protection from this catastrophic event. Spontaneous bacterial endocarditis, although serious, occurs in fewer than 1 per cent of patients with congenital valvular aortic stenosis.[8]

In newborns with severe valvular aortic stenosis, emergency surgical therapy is indicated as soon as the diagnosis is made. If the patient is moribund or has metabolic acidosis, administration of prostaglandin E_1 usually opens the ductus arteriosus, thereby improving systemic circulation and relieving the acidosis.[12]

In older infants or children, surgical therapy is indicated for a left ventricular to aortic systolic pressure gradient in excess of 75 mm. Hg and an abnormal pulse volume and contour, and for a calculated aortic valve index of less than 0.5 sq. cm. per sq. m. Angina and syncope are also indications for surgical intervention. Most would recommend surgical therapy for the patient with progressive symptoms, severe hypertrophy demonstrated on the electrocardiogram, or increasing cardiac enlargement even if the measured gradient is less than 50 mm. Hg.

Surgical Treatment

Valvular aortic stenosis is corrected by incising the fused commissures. In neonates and critically ill infants, several techniques have been suggested, including inflow occlusion, cardiopulmonary bypass, and closed transventricular dilation.[10] Profound hypothermic circulatory arrest may be employed, by which the temperature is lowered to 18° to 22° C. Cardiopulmonary bypass is used to lower the temperature after the heart is exposed through a median sternotomy. The circulation is then arrested, the aorta is cross-clamped, and the aortic valve is exposed through an incision in the aorta. Following completion of the commissurotomy, the aortotomy is closed, bypass is reinstituted, and the patient is rewarmed.

Others operate on this group of patients using cardiopulmonary bypass at normothermia with simple aortic cross-clamping. Excellent results have been reported from the Hospital for Sick Children in London with the use of inflow occlusion without cardiopulmonary bypass.[19] With this technique, the heart is exposed through a midline incision and tapes are passed around the superior and inferior venae cavae. The tapes are snugged down, and after the heart empties, the aorta is cross-clamped and opened. The commissures are then opened and the aortotomy is quickly closed as the cross-clamp is removed. The procedure is performed within 2 to 3 minutes, and the heart usually continues to beat throughout the procedure.

In older infants and children, the procedure is performed with the use of cardiopulmonary bypass, moderate hypothermia, and cold cardioplegic solution. A scalpel is used to divide fused commissures to within 1 mm. of the aortic wall (Fig. 1). Only true commissures with adequate leaflet attachment to the aortic wall are divided, since division of incomplete or false commissures can cause aortic insufficiency. The subvalvular area should be examined for associated pathologic conditions prior to closure of the aorta. Left ventricular and aortic pressures

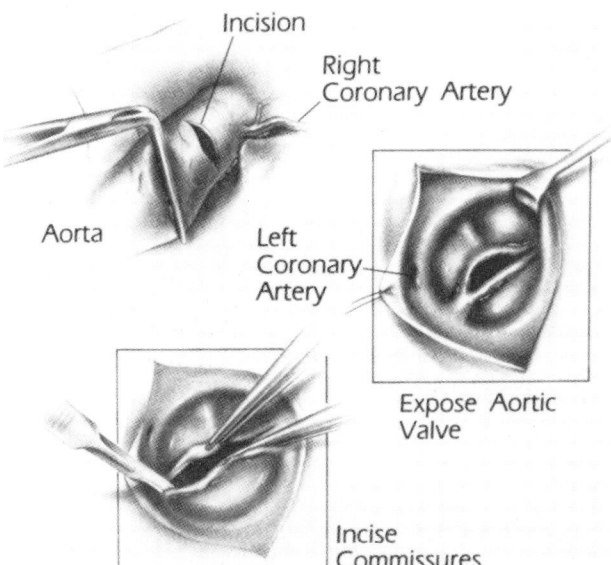

Figure 1. Valvular stenosis. After cardiopulmonary bypass has been established, the aorta is cross-clamped and cardioplegic solution is given. A transverse incision is then made in the ascending aorta above the sinuses of Valsalva. A retractor is placed into the right coronary sinus of Valsalva to expose the congenitally stenosed valve. The valve usually has a bicuspid configuration. Careful inspection of the valve will permit a decision as to which of the commissures to incise. The chosen commissures are then carefully incised to the wall of the aorta using a scalpel. This valvular area should also be examined for any associated pathologic conditions prior to closure of the aortotomy by continuous suture. (From Doty, D. B.: Cardiac Surgery. Chicago, Year Book Medical Publishers, 1985.)

are measured after cardiopulmonary bypass has been discontinued but before the chest is closed.

Repeat valvotomy may be attempted for recurrent or residual stenosis. It is rare that aortic valve replacement is necessary in primary operations in patients less than 10 years of age and is uncommon in patients less than 20 years old. Transluminal balloon dilation has been suggested as an alternative to valvotomy and can reduce the transvalvular gradient without causing severe aortic regurgitation in most patients.

Surgical Results

Operative mortality and morbidity following aortic valvotomy in the older infant or child are quite low, and the ventricular outflow tract obstruction is relieved.[2,11] Aortic valvotomy must be considered palliative, however, since recurrent aortic stenosis or progressive insufficiency is the usual late result. Reoperation is required in 25 to 35 per cent within 8 to 10 years of the original procedure. A satisfactory revalvotomy is possible in some patients, especially if the original procedure was performed during infancy. Calcification and restenosis eventually require aortic valve replacement in almost all patients who required valvotomy in infancy.

Unlike in older patients, the mortality following aortic valvotomy in critically ill infants remains high. Mortalities of 50 per cent to 100 per cent have been reported.[2,6] Subendocardial ischemia, endocardial fibroelastosis, small left ventricular volume, and small anular diameter are often present in this age group and probably influence mortality independently of age.[6]

SUBVALVULAR AORTIC STENOSIS

Clinical Features

Discrete subvalvular aortic stenosis is the second most common type of congenital left ventricular outflow tract obstruction, occurring in approximately 9 per cent of these patients. As in valvular obstruction, males are more frequently affected than are females with the ratio being 2.5 : 1. The symptoms of subvalvular stenosis are similar to those of valvular stenosis and

have the same implications. A systolic ejection murmur is heard similar to that of valvular stenosis but without the systolic ejection click. Also, an early diastolic murmur of aortic regurgitation is present in over 50 per cent of these patients. With severe stenosis, the peripheral pulse may be slow-rising.

The chest film is similar to that of valvular aortic stenosis except that post-stenotic dilation of the aorta is absent. The electrocardiogram usually shows left ventricular hypertrophy.

The obstructing membrane or fibromuscular ridge can be easily demonstrated with two-dimensional echocardiography. As in valvular stenosis, Doppler studies can estimate left ventricular to aortic pressure gradients.

Cardiac catheterization enables the severity of the gradient to be determined by a careful pull-back tracing. Angiography in axial as well in unconventional views visualizes the obstruction and its extent. Supravalvular aortography allows the determination of any aortic regurgitation. Since associated lesions are common, complete catheterization and angiography are recommended.

Natural History and Operative Indications

Discrete congenital subaortic stenosis, unlike valvular stenosis, is rarely a cause of symptomatic left ventricular outflow tract obstruction in infancy. A few patients become symptomatic by ages 3 to 5 years, but in most the obstruction becomes evident in early childhood or young adulthood. Obstruction is progressive and can be rapid. The associated aortic regurgitation is also progressive and may follow leaflet thickening associated with postobstructive turbulence.

Because subaortic stenosis can be rapidly progressive, operation is recommended when the left ventricular to aortic gradient is greater than 50 mm. Hg. By undertaking the operative procedure when moderate obstruction is present, it is hoped the risk of sudden death associated with severe obstruction is avoided.

Surgical Treatment

Membranous subvalvular aortic stenosis is exposed through the aortic root after cardiopulmonary bypass has been established and the heart has been arrested with cold cardioplegia following occlusion of the aorta. Care must be taken in operating through the aortic valve that the cusps are not injured. Small flat retractors are useful to protect the aortic leaflets. The fibromuscular ring between the commissure of the left and right coronary cusps of the aortic valve to the midportion of the right cusp should be safe for excision, with avoidance of the area of the His bundle. With a No. 11 scalpel, an incision is made into the fibromuscular ring below the center of the right coronary cusp, and a second incision is made beneath the commissure of the left and right coronary cusps. The depth of the incision is proportional to the estimated thickness of the septum. The tissue between these incisions may be removed as a wedge. If there is associated septal hypertrophy, the myotomy may be extended to the base of the anterior papillary muscle. The fibromuscular ridge is then resected with care. As the dissection is carried over the anterior mitral valve leaflet, only the fibrous ridge is removed so as not to damage the mitral leaflet. Also, care must be taken to excise only the fibrous ridge in the area to the right of the midportion of the right aortic cusp to prevent injury to the conduction tissue. Since the ventricular septum is always hypertrophied, it is important to excise a generous wedge of muscle to the left of the midpoint of the right coronary cusp (Fig. 2).

Local resection of tunnel subaortic obstruction has not been successful.[16] One of the most employed procedures for tunnel type subaortic obstruction is aortoventriculoplasty as first proposed by Konno and Rastan. Cardiopulmonary bypass is established with two caval cannulas. After the aorta is cross-clamped and cold cardioplegia is administered, a vertical incision is made in the aorta extending to the anulus in the right coronary sinus,

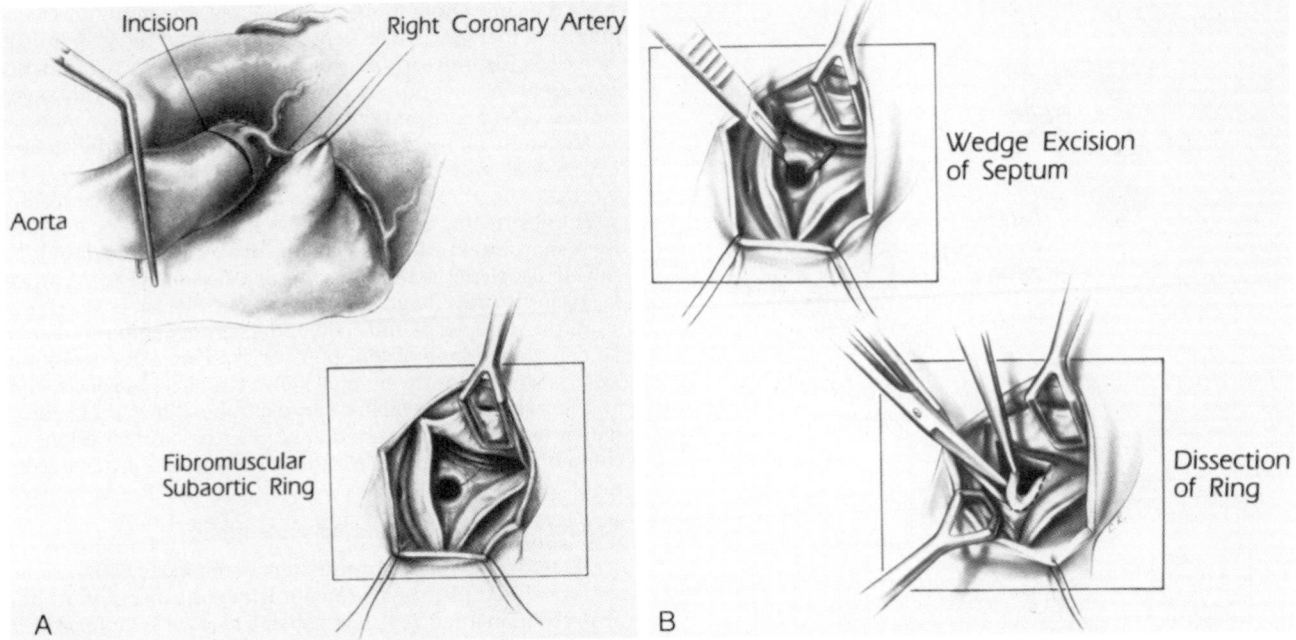

Figure 2. After cardiopulmonary bypass has been established, the aorta is cross-clamped and cold cardioplegic solution is given to protect the ischemic heart. *A,* A transverse incision is made in the ascending aorta, and the aortic valve is inspected for any associated abnormality. The right coronary cusp of the aortic valve is retracted anteriorly, exposing a subvalvular fibromuscular ring. Care must be taken in working through the aortic valve that the cusps of the valve are not injured. A retractor placed against the right coronary cusp provides exposure and protection of the right coronary cusp. The proposed area of septal excision should be placed anterior to the location of the membranous portion of the ventricular septum and away from the course of the His bundle. The portion of the fibromuscular ring from the commissure of the left and right coronary cusps of the aortic valve to the midportion of the right cusp should be safe for excision. *B,* Using a No. 11 scalpel, a wedge excision of the fibromuscular ring is performed anterior and to the left of the location of the conduction system. The center of the right coronary cusp is used as a reference point for the initial incision into the fibromuscular ring. The second point of penetration of the ring is below the commissure between the right and left coronary cusps. Deep incisions into the septum at these points provide a significant wedge of septum for excision. The scalpel is thrust into the fibromuscular obstruction and drawn posteriorly into the outflow tract to cut parallel grooves in the septum. The tissue between may be removed as a wedge. A septal myotomy may be continued to the base of the anterior papillary muscle of the mitral valve if there is associated septal hypertrophy. Débridement of the obstructing fibrous portion of the subvalvular ring must be performed with great care because the fibrous ring is attached to the anulus of the mitral valve. Deep excision of the fibrous ring may detach the anterior leaflet of the mitral valve, producing mitral valve insufficiency. Débridement of the subvalvular ring in the area of the anterior leaflet of the mitral valve must be superficial so as not to include full thickness of the mitral leaflet tissue or the anulus. (From Doty, D. B.: Cardiac Surgery. Chicago, Year Book Medical Publishers, 1985.)

just anterior to the commissure between the left and right coronary cusps. The aortotomy incision is extended into the right ventricle anteriorly. The ventricular septum is divided anterior and to the left of the conduction system. The outflow tract below the aorta is widened by these incisions, allowing the anulus to be separated widely. The aortic valve is then excised. The left ventricular outflow tract is reconstructed with a diamond-shaped Dacron patch. The diameter of the aortic anulus is measured and an appropriate-sized prosthetic valve is then used to replace the aortic valve. A second patch of Dacron or pericardium is then used to widen the right ventricular outflow tract (Fig. 3).

A modified Konno procedure can be used in patients with tunnel stenosis when the aortic anulus and valve are normal. The right ventricle is opened with a transverse incision. An incision is then made in the interventricular septum from the right ventricular side. The incision in the septum is extended across the stenotic area. A Dacron patch is then used to close the septum, enlarging the left ventricular outflow tract. The right ventriculotomy is closed with continuous sutures.

Other authors have suggested homograft replacement of the entire aortic root with reimplantation of the coronary arteries for diffuse subaortic obstruction,[14] whereas others report excellent results with apicoaortic conduits.[2] With this procedure, a valved conduit is placed through a left thoracotomy incision to the thoracic aorta or to the abdominal aorta through a midline laparotomy incision. Sutures are then placed into the left ventricular apex. A balloon-tipped catheter is introduced into the left ventricle through a stab wound and inflated with saline. An appropriate-sized cork-borer is placed over the catheter and a core of ventricle removed. The balloon-tipped catheter is used to occlude the resulting hole. A prosthetic graft is then anasto-

mosed to the apical opening with the previously placed sutures. The balloon is then removed and the graft is cross-clamped. The procedure is completed by anastomosing this graft to the previously placed graft on the aorta. This procedure can be performed with or without cardiopulmonary bypass.

Surgical Results

The surgical mortality for localized subvalvular aortic stenosis is between 2 and 4 per cent. Mortality for the more extensive Konno procedure has been reported as 6 to 12 per cent. Most patients have an excellent hemodynamic response to operative therapy with a dramatic decrease in the gradient and improvement persisting over a prolonged period. Several reports have suggested that patients with discrete subvalvular obstruction do not achieve long-term relief following surgical therapy. More recent series have not demonstrated a significant reoperative rate, which may be related to earlier operation or the resection of a generous amount of muscle from the septum.

Although it has been reported that valve-bearing conduits between the left ventricular apex and the thoracic or abdominal aorta frequently require replacement and may cause a number of late deaths,[3] others still prefer this technique for complex left ventricular outflow tract obstruction. Brown and co-workers cite this procedure because it is simple to perform, requires no cardiac ischemia for insertion, has no age or heart size restriction, contributes an additional outflow tract to the left ventricle, and does not require insertion of a large prosthetic valve into the aortic anulus. He also cites the advantage that the procedure does not violate the interventricular septum, which has been associated with coronary artery injury and conduction disturbances.[2]

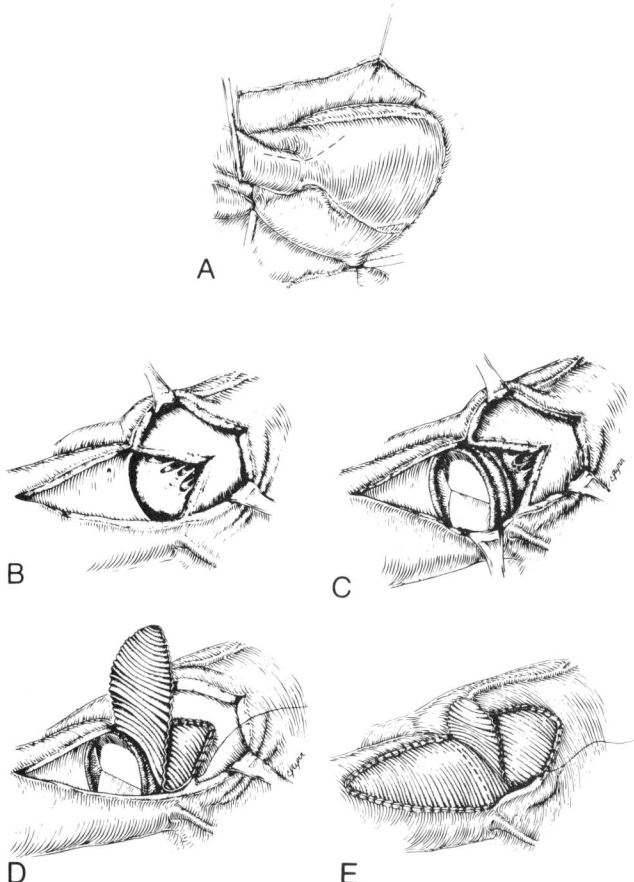

Figure 3. *A,* Augmentation of the aortic anulus. An aortotomy is made to the left of the right coronary artery and extended into the infundibulum of the right ventricle. *B,* After the aortic valve is excised, the aortotomy incision is extended into the ventricular septum. *C,* The aortic valve prosthesis is secured onto the widened aortic anulus. *D,* A tailored Dacron patch is placed in the ventricular septum at the level of the aortic anulus following insertion of the aortic prosthesis. The patch is secured to the sewing rim of the prosthetic valve and the remaining patch is used to close the aortotomy. *E,* A separate Dacron patch is used to close the right ventricular outflow tract. (From Castaneda, A., and Norwood, W.: Left ventricular outflow tract obstruction. *In* Arciniegas, E.: Pediatric Cardiac Surgery. Chicago, Year Book Medical Publishers, 1985.)

SUPRAVALVULAR AORTIC STENOSIS

Clinical Features

Supravalvular aortic stenosis rarely causes symptoms in infancy but frequently becomes evident in childhood. The symptoms are similar to those observed in other forms of congenital aortic stenosis. Angina pectoris may, however, be more common since stenosis of the coronary ostia is found not infrequently and there is an increased incidence of early atherosclerosis.

Supravalvular stenosis may be familial and associated with characteristic facies and mental retardation. Supravalvular stenosis may also be sporadic or follow congenital rubella. Mental retardation associated with supravalvular aortic stenosis is frequently referred to as Williams' syndrome. These cases, which are sporadic, are associated with depressed nasal bridge, anteverted nares, thick lips, mandibular recession, short palpebral fissures, and medial eyebrow flare. This syndrome has also been associated with idiopathic hypercalcemia of infancy. The most commonly associated anomaly is multiple stenoses of the peripheral pulmonary arteries, which may be extensive enough to cause pulmonary hypertension.

The systolic murmur of supravalvular aortic stenosis is similar to that of valvular aortic stenosis, but the ejection click is usually absent, and the murmur and thrill tend to be located somewhat

higher. A diastolic murmur is uncommon. A systolic blood pressure difference is occasionally noted in the upper extremities with the pressure being lower in the left arm. This may be due to stenosis at the origin of the left subclavian or to a jet effect.

The chest film demonstrates no dilation of the ascending aorta, and the electrocardiogram is similar to that in other forms of aortic stenosis. If pulmonary artery hypertension is present owing to pulmonary artery stenosis, right ventricular hypertrophy may be evident on the electrocardiogram.

Two-dimensional echocardiography can very clearly demonstrate this lesion and the extent of ascending aortic involvement. Cardiac catheterization can demonstrate the location of the stenosis by careful monitoring of the pull-back pressure. Angiography demonstrates the morphologic features of the lesion. Pulmonary artery pressures and pulmonary angiograms should be obtained for identifying associated pulmonary artery stenoses.

Natural History and Surgical Indications

Supravalvular aortic stenosis is the least common of the types of congenital aortic stenoses. Unlike the other forms, however, in this form there is no difference in the distribution between the sexes. In those patients with Williams' syndrome, sudden death early in life is common. The sequence of progressive stenosis with the appearance of symptoms and electrocardiographic changes has been demonstrated. Untreated patients probably die before reaching adulthood, because the lesion is rarely seen in adults. Operation is indicated at any age when the pressure gradient across the aorta is 50 mm. Hg or more. Coexisting pulmonary artery stenoses may be uncorrectable.

Surgical Treatment

In the localized type of supravalvular aortic stenosis, the lesion follows protrusion of an annular ridge into the lumen of the aorta just above the commissural attachment of the aortic valve cusps. Surgical relief of the localized type is performed on cardiopulmonary bypass by means of cold cardioplegia. An incision is made in the aortic root that crosses the stenotic region and extends well down into the noncoronary sinus of Valsalva.

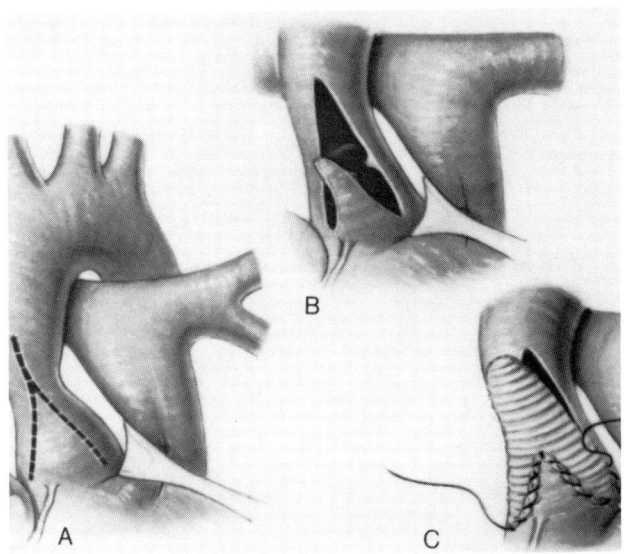

Figure 4. In the more extensive aortoplasty recommended by Doty, a Dacron prosthesis about the same diameter as the ascending aorta is divided longitudinally. *A,* The supravalvular ring is divided by extending the incision into the noncoronary and right coronary sinuses of Valsalva. *B,* The fibrous ring is excised posteriorly. The anterior flap contains the right coronary ostium. *C,* The prosthesis is then sutured into the aortotomy, the tips of the graft placed into the apex of each incision. This method of relieving supravalvular stenosis provides a symmetric reconstruction of the aorta with an expected improvement in aortic valve function. (From Stark, J., and deLeval, M.: Surgery for Congenital Heart Defects. London, Grune & Stratton, 1983.)

The stricture is excised, and a patch graft is used to close the aortotomy enlarging the stenotic area.

Doty has recommended a more extensive aortoplasty for this defect.[4] With this technique, the supravalvular ring is divided by extending the aortic incision into the noncoronary and right coronary sinuses of Valsalva. The fibrous ring is excised posteriorly, and the anterior flap contains the right coronary artery ostium. An inverted Y patch is then used to close the defect. This method of repair is designed to provide a more symmetrical reconstruction of the aorta (Fig. 4).

Diffuse supravalvular aortic stenosis requires a more complex repair. Cardiopulmonary bypass is established with arterial cannulation through the femoral artery. If the stenosis extends to the transverse arch, deep hypothermic circulatory arrest is employed after the body temperature has been lowered to 20° C. The aortotomy incision is extended from well down in the noncoronary sinus of Valsalva, up into the ascending aorta, and across the transverse aortic arch as far as the narrowing exists. Incisions are also made into the origin of the innominate and carotid arteries if stenoses are present. A patch of Dacron or pericardium is then used to close the defect, enlarging the area of stenosis. Cardiopulmonary bypass is then used to rewarm the patient, taking great care to avoid air emboli, especially to the cerebral circulation. A left ventricular apex to aorta conduit has also been suggested for patients with diffuse supravalvular stenosis.

Surgical Results

Surgical mortality in isolated supravalvular aortic stenosis is minimal.[2] Mortality is considerably greater, however, in patients with the diffuse form of stenosis. Late survival is improved, most patients being asymptomatic.

SELECTED REFERENCES

Brown, J. W., Stevens, L. S., Holly, B. S., Robison, R., et al.: Surgical spectrum of aortic stenosis in children: A thirty-year experience with 257 children. Ann. Thorac. Surg., 45:393, 1988.
This article is a retrospective review examining mortality and degree of gradient reduction following several surgical techniques used to treat all types of congenital aortic stenosis in children over a 30-year period. Two hundred and fifty-seven patients ranging in age from 1 day to 19 years were examined. Operative mortality for children older than 6 months of age was 4 per cent; neonates with critical aortic stenosis had a 60 per cent mortality. Eighty per cent of surviving patients have undergone cardiac catheterization following repair. There was an overall reduction of 57 mm. Hg in left ventricular to aorta gradient. Long-term results are documented. Interestingly, there was a nearly 5 per cent incidence of late bacterial endocarditis following repair with 6 of the 11 cases occurring in the group of patients who had discrete subvalvular aortic stenosis. Thirteen per cent of the 223 long-term survivors have had subsequent procedures for relief of residual or recurrent obstruction including 12 aortic valve replacements, 12 apicoaortic conduits, and 6 repeat valvotomies.

Ellis, F. H., Jr., and Kirklin, J. W.: Congenital valvular aortic stenosis: Anatomic findings and surgical technique. J. Thorac. Cardiovasc. Surg., 43:199, 1962.
This classic article describes 33 patients with valvular aortic stenosis, 3 with supravalvular stenosis, and 11 with subvalvular stenosis operated on from 1955 to 1960. Clinical results were good in 21 cases, fair in 7 cases, and unimproved in 1 case. There were two early deaths and two deaths following discharge. This article clearly outlines the technical aspects of aortic valvotomy, which remain sound and have withstood the test of time.

Messina, L. M., Turley, K., Stranger, P., Hoffman, J. I., and Ebert, P. A.: Successful aortic valvotomy for severe congenital valvular aortic stenosis in the newborn infant. J. Thorac. Cardiovasc. Surg., 88:92, 1984.
In this article the management of critical aortic stenosis in infants under 30 days of age is described. Eleven patients had emergency aortic valvotomy using hypothermic cardiopulmonary bypass with aortic cross-clamping. All but one of the patients presented with severe congestive heart failure, and five of the patients were in extremis at the time of operation. All patients had dramatic clinical improvement postoperatively, and only one patient died as a result of an acutely thrombosed ductus and a small left ventricular cavity. The 10 surviving patients were clinically free of heart failure at a mean follow-up of 2.2 years. One patient had residual valvular stenosis and underwent a successful repeat valvotomy. One patient also had evidence of aortic insufficiency at follow-up. The majority of patients in this series had a normal or enlarged left ventricular cavity, which favorably contributed to the excellent results achieved in this series. The authors agree that operative mortality for patients with small left ventricular cavity is usually considerably higher than that reported in this series.

Moses, R. D., Barnhart, G. R., and Jones, M.: The late prognosis after localized resection for fixed (discrete and tunnel) left ventricular outflow tract obstruction. J. Thorac. Cardiovasc. Surg., 87:410, 1984.
These authors reviewed the results of resection of fixed left ventricular outflow tract obstruction in 42 patients with discrete obstruction and in 14 patients with diffuse or tunnel left ventricular outflow tract obstruction. The details of the operative techniques for subaortic stenosis are clearly defined in this paper. The hospital mortality in cases of discrete subaortic obstruction was 2.4 per cent and there were three late deaths. Actuarial survival was 89 per cent at 10 years and 82 per cent at 20 years after operation. Hospital mortality was 14 per cent in the group with tunnel subaortic obstruction and there were two late deaths in this group. Actuarial survival in those patients with tunnel obstruction was 59 per cent at 10 years and 39.5 per cent at 20 years. The progressive nature of subaortic stenosis in less than ideal long-term results is clearly documented in this paper. The authors conclude that local resection of the fibrous membrane in discrete subvalvular stenosis should be considered a palliative procedure in many instances. Most patients operated on for discrete left ventricular outflow tract obstruction survive to the late postoperative period, but adverse effects are frequent. Less satisfactory results were found in the group with the tunnel form of left ventricular outflow tract obstruction, and more extensive procedures were recommended.

REFERENCES

1. Bolen, J. L., Popp, R. L., and French, J. W.: Echocardiographic features of supravalvular aortic stenosis. Circulation, 52:817, 1975.
2. Brown, J. W., Stevens, L. S., Holly, B. S., et al.: Surgical spectrum of aortic stenosis in children: A thirty-year experience with 257 children. Ann. Thorac. Surg., 45:393, 1988.
3. DiDonato, R. M., Danielson, G. K., McGoon, D. C., Driscoll, D. J., Julsrud, P. R., and Edwards, W. D.: Left ventricle-aortic conduits in pediatric patients. J. Thorac. Cardiovasc. Surg., 88:82, 1984.
4. Doty, D. B., Polansky, D. B., and Jenson, C. B.: Supravalvular aortic stenosis. J. Thorac. Cardiovasc. Surg., 74:362, 1977.
5. Flaker, G., Teske, D., Kilman, J., Hosier, D., and Wooley, C.: Supravalvular aortic stenosis. Am. J. Cardiol., 51:256, 1983.
6. Hammon, J. W., Parrish, M. D., Graham, T. P., Jr., Boucek, R. J., and Bender, H. W.: Risk factors for infants undergoing aortic valvotomy for critical aortic valvar stenosis. J. Am. Coll. Cardiol., 3:585, 1984.
7. Hatle, L., Angelsen, B. A., and Tromsdol, A.: Noninvasive assessment of aortic stenosis by Doppler ultrasound. Br. Heart J., 43:284, 1980.
8. Hossack, K. F., Neutze, J. M., Lowe, J. B., and Barratt-Boyes, B. G.: Congenital valvar aortic stenosis. Natural history and assessment for operation. Br. Heart J., 43:561, 1980.
9. Huhta, J. C., Glasow, P., Murphy, D. J., et al.: Surgery without catheterization for congenital heart defects: Management in 100 patients. J. Am. Coll. Cardiol., 9:823, 1987.
10. Huhta, J. C., Latson, L. A., Gutgesell, H. P., Cooley, D. A., and Kearney, D. L.: Echocardiography in the diagnosis and management of symptomatic aortic valve stenosis in infants. Circulation, 70:438, 1984.
11. Johnson, R. G., Williams, G. R., Razook, J. D., et al.: Reoperation in congenital aortic stenosis. Ann. Thorac. Surg., 40:156, 1985.
12. Jonas, R. A., Lang, P., Mayer, J. E., and Castaneda, A. R.: The importance of prostaglandin E in resuscitation of the neonate with critical aortic stenosis. J. Thorac. Cardiovasc. Surg., 89:314, 1985.
13. Konno, S., Imai, Y., Iida, Y., Nakajima, M., and Tatsuno, K.: A new method for prosthetic valve replacement in congenital aortic stenosis associated with hypoplasia of the aortic valve ring. J. Thorac. Cardiovasc. Surg., 70:909, 1975.
14. McKowen, R. L., Campbell, D. N., Woelfel, F., Wiggins, J. W., Jr., and Clarke, D. R.: Extended aortic root replacement with aortic allografts. J. Thorac. Cardiovasc. Surg., 93:366, 1987.
15. Mody, M. R., and Mody, G. T.: Serial hemodynamic observations in congenital valvular and subvalvular aortic stenosis. Am. Heart J., 89:137, 1975.
16. Moses, R. D., Barnhart, G. R., and Jones, M.: The late prognosis after localized resection for fixed (discrete and tunnel) left ventricular outflow tract obstruction. J. Thorac. Cardiovasc. Surg., 87:410, 1984.
17. Pelech, A. N., Dyck, J. D., Trusler, G. A., et al.: Critical aortic stenosis: Survival and management. J. Thorac. Cardiovasc. Surg., 94:510, 1987.
18. Roberts, W. C.: Valvular, subvalvular, and supravalvular aortic stenosis: Morphologic features. (Cardiovascular Clinics, series 5/1.) Philadelphia, F. A. Davis Company, 1973, p. 98.
19. Sink, J. D., Smallhorn, J. F., Macartney, F. J., Taylor, J. F. N., Stark, J., and de Leval, M. R.: Management of critical aortic stenosis in infancy. J. Thorac. Cardiovasc. Surg., 87:82, 1984.
20. Wright, G. B., Keane, J. F., Nadas, A. S., Bernhard, W. F., and Castaneda, A. R.: Fixed subaortic stenosis in the young: Medical and surgical course in 83 patients. Am. J. Cardiol., 52:830, 1983.

XV _____

THE CORONARY CIRCULATION

J. Scott Rankin, M.D., and David C. Sabiston, Jr., M.D.

> In certain cases of angina pectoris, when the mouth of the coronary arteries is calcified, it would be useful to establish a complementary circulation for the lower part of the arteries.
>
> *Alexis Carrel, 1910*

As the end of the twentieth century approaches, atherosclerotic coronary artery disease (CAD) continues to be the leading cause of death and lost life expectancy in the United States. It has been estimated that over one third of the population eventually will die from CAD, and 20 per cent will develop symptoms before the age of 60 years. Approximately 7 million Americans currently have symptomatic CAD, 1.5 million experience myocardial infarction annually, and over 500,000 die yearly from related complications. Estimates of the annual direct and indirect economic cost of CAD in the United States exceed 80 billion dollars, and similar data are available for most of the Western World.[28]

Whereas the age-adjusted mortality attributable to CAD per unit population of the United States has been falling since 1965, the absolute incidence continues to increase.[49] Assuming constant risk factors and therapeutic efficacies, epidemiologic models predict that aging of the population of the United States and especially maturation of the post–World War II baby-boom generation, will increase *absolute* CAD prevalence, annual incidence, total mortality, and economic cost by approximately 40 to 50 per cent by the year 2010 (Table 1). Thus, the medical significance of coronary atherosclerosis and the number of patients presenting for surgical intervention will, in all likelihood, continue to increase in coming decades. This section (1) reviews basic principles of coronary atherosclerosis and myocardial ischemia, (2) describes current techniques for surgical coronary revascularization, and (3) delineates, as precisely as possible, the prognostic efficacy of contemporary surgical therapy.

HISTORICAL ASPECTS

In the original description of angina pectoris, Heberden emphasized the chronic and progressive nature of ischemic chest pain and the propensity of affected patients for sudden death.

Heberden's remarkable clinical observations are as accurate today as they were 2 centuries ago:

> But there is a disorder of the breast marked with strong and peculiar symptoms, considerable for the kind of danger belonging to it, and not extremely rare, which deserves to be mentioned more at length. The seat of it, and sense of strangling, and anxiety with which it is attended, may make it not improperly be called angina pectoris.
>
> They who are afflicted with it, are seized while they are walking, (more especially if it be up a hill, and soon after eating) with a painful and most disagreeable sensation in the breast, which seems as if it would extinguish life, if it were to increase or to continue; but the moment they stand still, all this uneasiness vanishes.
>
> In all other respects, the patients are, at the beginning of this disorder, perfectly well, and in particular have no shortness of breath, from which it is totally different. The pain is sometimes situated in the upper part, sometimes in the middle, sometimes at the bottom of the os sterni, and often more inclined to the left than to the right side. It likewise very frequently extends from the breast to the middle of the left arm. The pulse is, at least sometimes, not disturbed by this pain, as I have had opportunities of observing by feeling the pulse during the paroxysm. Males are most liable to this disease, especially such as have passed their fiftieth year.
>
> After it has continued a year or more, it will not cease so instantaneously upon standing still; and it will come on not only when the persons are walking, but when they are lying down, especially if they lie on their left sides, and oblige them to rise up out of their beds. In some inveterate cases it has been brought on by the motion of a horse, or a carriage, and even by swallowing, coughing, going to stool, or speaking, or any disturbance of mind. . . .
>
> *The termination of the angina pectoris is remarkable. For if no accident intervene, but the disease go on to its height, the patients all suddenly fall down, and perish almost immediately. Of which indeed their frequent faintnesses, and sensations as if all the powers of life were failing, afford no obscure intimation.*[46]

The relationship between angina pectoris and atherosclerotic narrowing of the coronary arteries was established by Parry in 1799:

> The rigidity of the coronary arteries may act, proportionately to the extent of the ossification, as a mechanical impediment to the free motion of the heart; and though a quantity of blood may circulate through these arteries, sufficient to nourish the heart, yet there may probably be less than what is requisite for ready and vigorous action. Hence, though a

TABLE 1. Projections of Absolute Coronary Heart Disease Incidence, Prevalence, Mortality, and Cost

Year	Incidence	Prevalence	Mortality	Cost*
1980	692,117	5,977,405	432,613	$31.9
1985	729,235	6,700,639	486,428	35.3
1990	759,583	7,230,904	540,557	37.8
1995	792,006	7,625,001	567,798	39.9
2000	834,522	7,973,869	596,777	42.0
2005	888,438	8,385,046	608,434	44.4
2010	953,750	8,939,816	632,304	47.4

From Weinstein, M. C., et al.: Forecasting coronary heart disease incidence, mortality, and cost: The Coronary Heart Disease Policy Model. Am. J. Public Health, 77:1417, 1987.
* Billions of 1980 dollars, direct cost only.

heart so diseased may be fit for the purposes of common circulation, during a state of bodily and mental tranquility, and of health otherwise good, yet when an unusual exertion is required, its powers may fail, under the new and extraordinary demand.

Throughout the nineteenth century, the clinical manifestations of ischemic heart disease probably were rare. In 1910, Osler reviewed his personal experience and noted that angina pectoris frequently was compatible with long-term survival. The premortem clinical diagnosis of acute myocardial infarction was not made until 1912 by Herrick,[27] and in 1926, White described a 3.4-year average survival in 66 patients with angina while documenting several important risk factors. Thirty years later, White and associates reviewed the long-term follow-up on his original series of 601 patients with angina pectoris and reported an excess annual mortality of 7 per cent per year in males and 5.3 per cent per year in females (Fig. 1). The average duration of survival after onset of symptoms was 9.4 years, emphasizing the morbid nature of the disease.

Surgical therapy was first proposed by Francois-Franck, a professor of physiology in Paris, who theorized in 1899 that division of the cardiac sympathetic pain fibers would eliminate a patient's ability to perceive angina pectoris. Credit for performing the first sympathectomy for angina generally is given to Jonnesco. Thoracic sympathectomy proved to be effective in relieving angina in up to 75 per cent of patients but probably did little to modify the adverse prognosis.

In 1903, Thorel reported a postmortem case in which both coronary arteries were obliterated, the heart receiving its blood supply from vascular pericardial adhesions. Based on this observation, Beck devised several techniques for producing a new blood supply to the surface of the heart and, in 1935, successfully grafted a pedicle of pectoral muscle to the denuded epicardium of a patient with angina pectoris. Between 1936 and 1938, O'Shaughnessy and colleagues grafted omentum to the hearts of several patients and reported anginal improvement in all survivors. It was demonstrated subsequently, however, that myocardial blood flow was not significantly augmented, and these operations never achieved widespread acceptance. Further work by Beck in the 1940s attempted to increase intercoronary communications by obstructing coronary venous outflow. When this procedure proved ineffective, he grafted an artery from the descending thoracic aorta to the coronary sinus for the provision of a retrograde source of blood flow to the myocardium. Ultimately, this operation also failed and was abandoned.

Following several years of work in the experimental laboratory, Vineberg implanted the bleeding end of an internal mammary artery pedicle into the myocardium of a patient in 1948. During the next 15 years, this operation was performed extensively, and it was demonstrated that the implanted mammary artery developed anastomotic communications with the coronary vasculature. However, the functional adequacy of the communications was questionable, and with the advent of direct surgical approaches, mammary artery implantation was no longer performed. The first coronary endarterectomy was accomplished by Bailey in 1956, and Longmire subsequently modified the technique. The procedure was best used for localized proximal coronary lesions and was suitable for less than 10 per cent of patients. Long-term coronary patency after endarterectomy subsequently was shown to be suboptimal, and endarterectomy is rarely used today.

Vascular bypass of a coronary artery obstruction originally was proposed by Carrel, who performed several experimental procedures with limited success.[7] The first aortocoronary bypass graft in man utilizing a reversed segment of saphenous vein was performed in 1962 by Sabiston (Fig. 2), but the patient did not survive, because of a cerebrovascular accident.[45] Garrett and co-workers successfully constructed a vein bypass to the left anterior descending coronary artery in 1964.[18] Although the patient sustained a myocardial infarction postoperatively, he recovered and remained asymptomatic for many years; coronary arteriography in 1971 demonstrated prolonged graft patency in this patient. Favaloro and associates first applied bypass operations to a large series of patients, and the pioneering work of Johnson, Spencer, and their associates established firmly the role of coronary bypass in the treatment of ischemic heart disease.[30] Kolesoff, in 1967, reported six clinical cases of internal mammary artery (IMA) bypasses from the Soviet Union, and Green and associates initiated the first clinical series of IMA grafts in 1968 with documented excellent postoperative patency.[22] Since these first reports, coronary bypass procedures have gained general acceptance and have been utilized with ever-increasing frequency over the past 2 decades (Fig. 3).

ANATOMY OF THE CORONARY ARTERIES

The right and left coronary arteries are the first branches of the aorta and arise from the sinuses of Valsalva. The right coronary artery passes deep in the right atrioventricular groove and

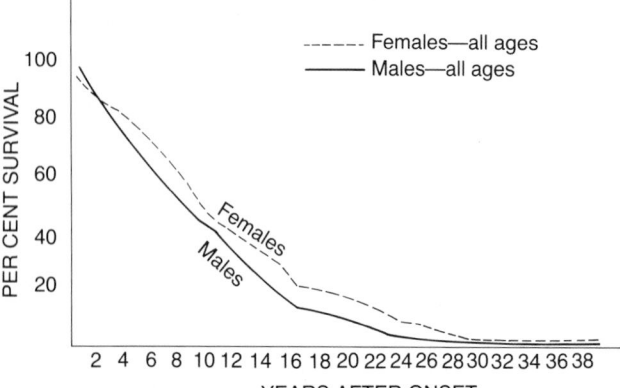

Figure 1. Survival after onset of angina pectoris in 456 patients. (From Richards, D. W., Bland, E. F., and White, P. D.: A completed 25-year follow-up study of 200 patients with myocardial infarction. J. Chronic Dis., *4:*423, 1950.)

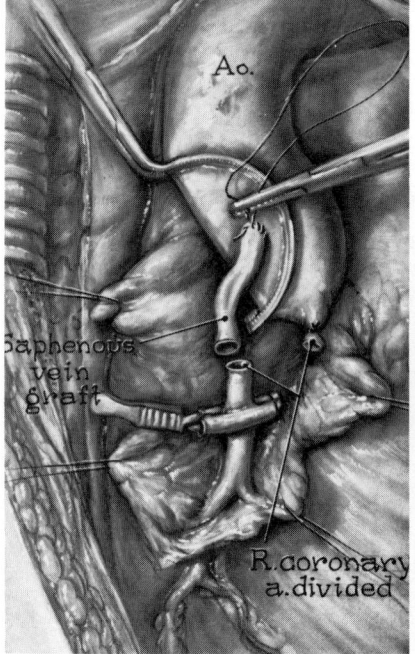
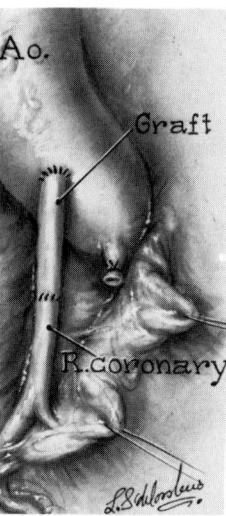

Figure 2. Illustration of use of the first saphenous vein autograft anastomosed from the ascending aorta to the right coronary artery for proximal coronary arterial occlusion in 1962 (see text). (From Sabiston, D. C., Jr.: The coronary circulation. The William F. Rienhoff, Jr. Lecture. Johns Hopkins Med. J., *134:*314, 1974.)

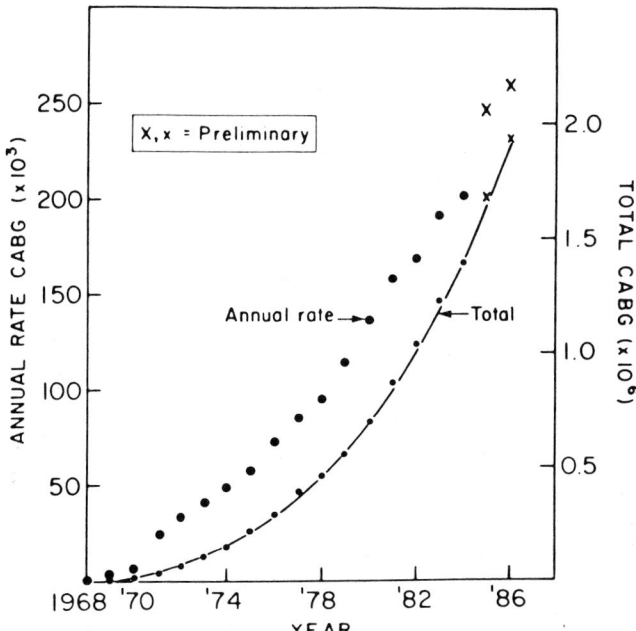

Figure 3. Numbers of annual coronary bypass procedures in the United States since 1968. (From Higgins, M. W., and Luepker, R. V. (Eds.): Trends in Coronary Heart Disease Mortality: The Influence of Medical Care. New York, Oxford University Press, 1988.)

proceeds over the anterior surface of the heart. At the superior end of the acute margin of the heart, the vessel turns posteriorly toward the crux and usually terminates as the posterior descending coronary artery in the posterior interventricular groove. The right coronary artery initially provides a number of small vessels, which anastomose on the anterior ventricle in the pulmonary conus region with corresponding branches from the left coronary artery (the arterial circle of Vieussens). It next supplies multiple right ventricular branches and the sinus node artery (the latter *may* arise from the left circumflex artery). Along the acute right border of the heart, the right marginal artery takes origin. In the 90 per cent of patients with *right coronary dominance*, the right coronary artery terminates in the posterior descending artery and, by an extension to the crux, branches into an atrioventricular nodal artery and several terminal posterolateral left ventricular branches.

The left main coronary artery is usually about 1 cm. in length and gives rise to the left anterior descending (LAD) and left circumflex coronary arteries. The LAD provides branches to the arterial circle of Vieussens and several diagonal branches to the anterior left ventricular wall. As it proceeds distally in the anterior interventricular groove, the LAD provides a number of anterior perforating branches to the interventricular septum and, in most patients, wraps the apex of the heart, anastomosing with the posterior descending artery. Thus, the LAD *usually* is the largest and most important of the coronary arteries, supplying the anterior wall of the left ventricle, the left margin of the right ventricle, the apex of the heart, and the majority of the interventricular septum.

The left circumflex artery lies in the left atrioventricular groove and proceeds laterally and posteriorly around the left lateral aspect of the left ventricle, usually terminating in several left marginal arteries. In the 10 per cent of patients with *left coronary dominance*, the circumflex system provides the posterior descending coronary artery. The first branch of the circumflex artery is usually the auricular anastomotic artery (Kugel's artery).

The venous drainage of the heart is via superficial and deep circuits. The superficial veins conduct most of the venous blood and accompany the respective coronary arteries. The surface coronary veins empty either into the coronary sinus (which drains into the right atrium) or into the anterior cardiac veins, the latter emptying individually into the right atrium. The deep veins communicate with both the atrial and ventricular cavities via thebesian and sinusoidal channels.

NORMAL PHYSIOLOGY

Coronary blood flow delivers oxygen and metabolic substrates to the myocardium and simultaneously removes carbon dioxide and metabolic by-products via transcapillary exchange. Normal coronary blood flow approximates 0.7 to 0.9 ml. per gm. myocardium per minute and delivers 0.1 ml. oxygen per gm. per minute to the heart; this is an extreme rate of energy utilization, compared with the rest of the body. The extraction of oxygen in the coronary bed is very high, averaging 75 per cent under normal conditions and increasing to nearly 100 per cent during stress. Coronary artery blood flow occurs primarily during diastole because systolic myocardial contraction increases intramyocardial vascular resistance.[45] Normally, mean coronary resistance is three to six times the totally vasodilated value, implying an extreme degree of vasodilatory reserve. During stress, increasing oxygen delivery is provided primarily by vasodilation because of the high baseline oxygen extraction. If adequate perfusion pressure is assumed, total and regional myocardial blood flow under normal conditions is determined by autoregulation of regional arteriolar resistance modulated by local metabolic demand.

The metabolic activity of heart muscle transfers the chemical energy provided by myocardial oxygen and substrate utilization into mechanical energy in the form of circulatory pressure and flow. With electrical depolarization of the myocardial cell membrane, ionized calcium fluxes into the cytoplasm, causing the myosin molecule to hydrolyze adenosine triphosphate (ATP) into adenosine diphosphate and inorganic phosphate. When ATP is split, a considerable amount of chemical energy is released from the ATP molecule and transferred into a conformational change in the myosin crossbridge. This chemomechanical alteration in the crossbridge produces sliding of myosin filaments relative to actin and shortening of the sarcomere.[48] Over the physiologic range of sarcomere lengths (1.6 to 2.0 μ), the surface area of available crossbridge interactions and, therefore, the metabolic energy transferred into mechanical work during sarcomere contraction are directly proportional to end-diastolic sarcomere length. This length-dependency of crossbridge interaction at the sarcomere level constitutes the fundamental basis for the Frank-Starling relationship. As a final step in the process, calcium is removed from the cell by active transport of the cytoplasmic reticulum, and ATP is regenerated at the mitochondrial level by aerobic metabolism of oxygen and substrates.

The intact cardiac ventricles appear to function as an integrated sum of their component sarcomeres. Mechanical energy production, in the form of external pressure and flow generation (stroke work), is a direct linear function of end-diastolic volume and is not influenced significantly by physiologic changes in afterload.[19] Therefore, short-term alterations in myocardial inotropism (defined as load-independent intrinsic myocardial performance) can be assessed by the slope of the stroke work/end-diastolic volume relationship. This fundamental Frank-Starling property of the heart is probably directly reflective of sarcomere and myosin crossbridge dynamics.

Energetically, cardiac metabolic activity over time can be assessed by myocardial oxygen consumption. Each milliliter of oxygen utilized by the heart provides 2.02 joules of energy to the contractile apparatus via aerobic metabolic pathways and ATP. Thus, oxygen consumption can be used for quantification of myocardial *energy utilization*. Myocardial *energy expenditure* has two components: (1) external energy, which is stroke work or the integral of the ventricular pressure (P)–volume (V) loop;

and (2) internal energy, which is the thermodynamic cost of maintaining systolic ventricular pressure at a given volume.[36] Internal energy expenditure can be estimated as the product of ventricular mean ejection pressure (P_{ME}) $\times$ end-diastolic volume (V_{ED}) and constitutes the sole mechanical energy production during isovolumic contraction. Total mechanical energy expenditure (TME) for each cardiac cycle can be calculated as

$$TME = \int PdV + (P_{ME} \cdot V_{ED})$$

Because 1 mm. Hg $\times$ ml. is equivalent to 1.333×10^{-4} joules, total mechanical energy expenditure can be compared with metabolic energy utilization for obtaining a measure of metabolic to mechanical energy transfer efficiency. Oxygen consumption is tightly coupled to mechanical energy expenditure, both on a steady-state and beat-to-beat basis.

PATHOLOGIC ANATOMY

Coronary atherosclerosis is a progressive disease, the earliest microscopic changes of which have been described in the newborn infant. The infantile lesions consist of rupture, degeneration, and regeneration of the internal elastic membrane together with deposition of mucopolysaccharide and proliferation of endothelial cells and fibroblasts. At this early stage, such lesions are quite minimal and solely microscopic. However, gross lesions subsequently appear within a few years in the form of small yellow deposits of lipoid material visible beneath the intima. These lesions are present in half the hearts examined at autopsy during the second decade of life. The presence of extensive coronary atherosclerosis in otherwise healthy young males was emphasized in routine autopsies on young military casualties in the Korean conflict, which demonstrated that 77 per cent had gross evidence of coronary atherosclerosis and 10 per cent showed advanced disease, with 70 per cent or greater occlusion of one or more major coronary arteries.[14] In a community study, coronary atherosclerosis (from 24 per cent to complete occlusion of one or more major arteries) was present in three fourths of the entire population. These figures indicate the extreme prevalence of the disorder, but unfortunately, its presence is usually not made manifest until serious symptoms appear. In the final stages of the disease, rupture of an intimal atherosclerotic plaque appears to be a dominant mechanism of worsening symptoms with deposition of platelets and thrombus progressing to thrombotic occlusion and acute myocardial infarction. Subtotal occlusions by "dynamic" thrombotic lesions appear to be of major importance in the pathogenesis of unstable angina.

Careful pathologic studies have been performed by a number of observers for assessing the incidence and degree of atherosclerosis in each of the major coronary arteries. Nearly all of the studies have shown that the anterior descending coronary artery is the most frequently involved, followed in incidence by the right coronary, the left circumflex, the left main, and, least

TABLE 2. Frequency of Obstructive Lesions in the Coronary Arteries Due to Atherosclerosis as Found in a Series of 300 Consecutive Patients with Coronary Atherosclerosis

Coronary Artery	Number of Cases	Percentage
Right	165	28.4
Left main	26	4.5
Left anterior descending	251	43.4
Left circumflex	134	23.7
Total	576	100.0

From Berger, R. L., and Stary, J. C.: Anatomic assessment of operability by the saphenous-vein bypass operation in coronary artery disease. N. Engl. J. Med. 285:248, 1971.

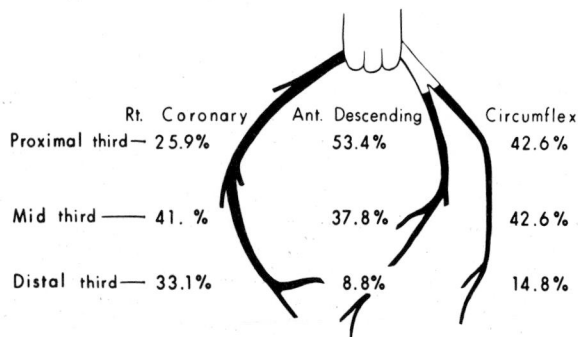

Figure 4. Localization of stenotic lesions in the three major coronary trunks. Each coronary artery is divided into three equal segments, and the percentage of the total number of lesions in each third is noted. In the anterior descending and circumflex arteries, the obstructions tend to be in the proximal two thirds, whereas the primary involvement is in the distal two thirds of the right coronary artery. (From Berger, R. L., and Stary, H. C.: Anatomic assessment of operability by the saphenous-vein bypass operation in coronary artery disease. N. Engl. J. Med., 285:248, 1971.)

frequently of all, the right posterior descending coronary artery (Table 2). It has also been noted that the more severe changes occur in the proximal third or half of the coronary arteries. In a thorough study of some 400 hearts, Schlesinger and Zoll concluded that most occlusions were less than 5 mm. in length and that the majority were in the proximal third of the vessel. In a review of atherosclerotic lesions in 300 hearts studied primarily for assessment of operability by direct bypass grafting, a definite anatomic pattern was identified. The usual pattern was one of multifocal lesions characteristically involving more than one major trunk in the same heart. The stenoses tended to be short but were contiguous with other areas of less severe coronary atherosclerosis. In general, lesions in the branches of the left coronary artery were usually proximal and originated at the bifurcation of the anterior descending and circumflex branches. However, appreciable numbers of distal lesions existed in most of the vessels. In the right coronary artery, the disease was more diffuse and involved primarily the proximal and middle portions of the artery. In this study, it was noted that 88 per cent of hearts with coronary atherosclerosis were anatomically suitable for grafts distal to the obstructing lesions. The most common sites of obstruction noted for each of the three major coronary vessels are shown in Figure 4.

ISCHEMIC PATHOPHYSIOLOGY

The pathophysiologic mechanisms of myocardial ischemia are complex. Reduction in myocardial oxygen supply during ischemia, or increasing oxygen demand during hemodynamic stress, produces regulatory coronary vasodilation. With decreasing arteriolar resistance, diastolic intramyocardial pressure becomes a more important determinant of mean myocardial perfusion. In the presence of adequate arterial pressure and low diastolic cavitary pressure, the modest transmural gradient of diastolic intramyocardial pressure has little effect on regional myocardial blood flow through the dilated vascular bed. However, transmural blood flow in this situation becomes pressure-dependent, and if aortic perfusion pressure decreases or diastolic intracavitary pressure increases, coronary perfusion may be redistributed away from the subendocardium where intramural compressive forces are the highest. This redistribution of flow can induce subendocardial ischemia, even in the presence of normal coronary arteries.

When an atherosclerotic plaque in a proximal coronary artery decreases the cross-sectional area by 75 per cent or more, the resistance to flow caused by the plaque becomes significant. The dominant point of coronary vascular resistance then becomes the critical stenosis that can limit myocardial perfusion to a fixed value. Whereas flow may be adequate at rest, exercise or other factors that increase myocardial oxygen demand can produce relative ischemia, a fall in the coronary pressure distal to the stenosis, and redistribution of blood flow away from the subendocardium. This appears to be the mechanism of exercise-induced angina pectoris and associated transient myocardial dysfunction. Superimposed on the phenomenon, coronary vasospasm and unstable thrombotic plaques can compound the obstructive physiologic process.

Because of high metabolic demand and tight coupling between energy utilization and expenditure, acute coronary occlusion produces an almost immediate decrement in myocardial segment shortening and work. Even when full reperfusion is accomplished after a 15-minute period of reversible ischemia, dysfunction can be prolonged, requiring up to 24 to 48 hours for complete recovery. Ischemic myocardial dysfunction in this setting is characterized by a diminished slope of the stroke work/end-diastolic segment length relationship together with a rightward shift of the x-intercept (l_0), termed *diastolic creep*.[20] With reperfusion, the slope recovers rapidly, but l_0 remains overstretched, diminishing the work capacity at any given preload. Subsequent recovery of systolic function occurs slowly and is associated with a reversal of creep. Catecholamine infusion,

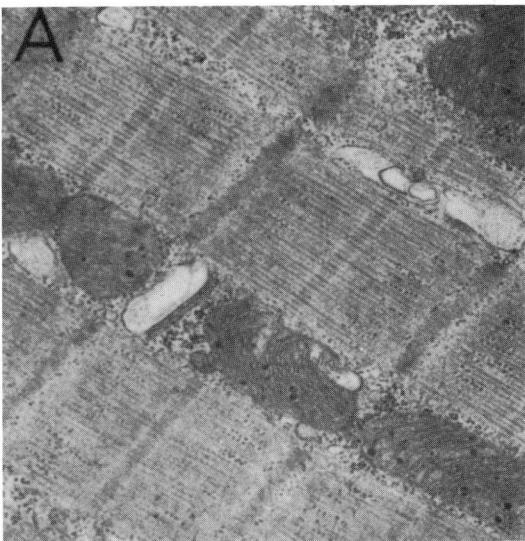

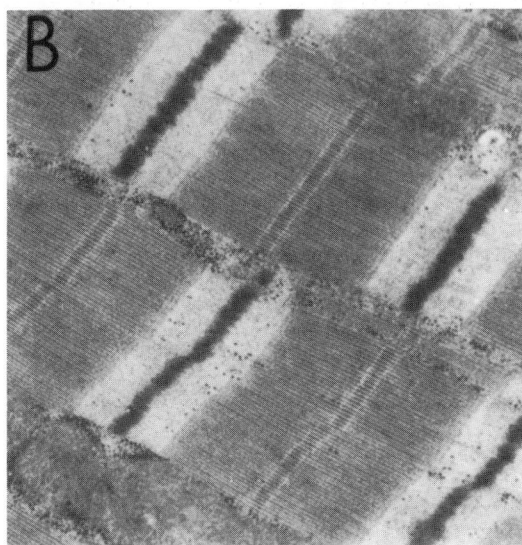

Figure 5. Typical electron micrographs of nonischemic *(A)* and ischemic *(B)* myocardium after 15 minutes of coronary occlusion. Ischemic tissue displays myofilament relaxation with increased Z-band separation and widening of bands. (From Glower, D. D., Schaper, J., Kabas, J. S., et al.: Relation between reversal of diastolic creep and recovery of systolic function after ischemic myocardial injury in conscious dogs. Circ. Res., *60:*850, 1987.)

increasing afterload, or a second ischemic event during early reperfusion can worsen dysfunction and prolong recovery.

Postischemic systolic dysfunction and diastolic creep can be correlated at an ultrastructural level with sarcomere overstretching, increased Z-band separation, and widening of the I-bands (Fig. 5). It appears that the sarcomeres become stretched beyond their normal working range, and disengagement of actin filaments from the M-band may reduce the number of possible crossbridge interactions and potentially be responsible for the mechanical findings. Moreover, diastolic properties during ischemia become insensitive to standard pharmacologic interventions, suggesting persistent crossbridge attachments during diastole or disarray of normal crossbridge cycling. This entire process undoubtedly will provide useful areas for investigation at the histochemical level in coming years and will yield further insights into ischemic pathophysiology.

CORONARY COLLATERAL CIRCULATION

The coronary collateral circulation has been studied extensively in both the experimental animal and man. The human heart has few natural collaterals of sufficient diameter for delivering a significant quantity of blood in the event of a major coronary occlusion. It is for this reason that sudden occlusion of an otherwise normal coronary artery is such a hazardous event. A number of collaterals the size of 200 μ or less are present in most hearts, but these channels require enlargement over a period of time, usually stimulated by the development of favorable pressure differentials in order to become functionally significant.

In the experimental animal, a slowly occluding obstructing device (ameroid constrictor) can be placed on a major coronary artery and used for total occlusion of the vessel over a period of weeks. Under these circumstances, the pressure and flow through the involved coronary artery are slowly reduced, during which time the natural collaterals concomitantly enlarge. As a result, the distal pressure following slow occlusion may progressively rise to essentially that of the preocclusion value. In the human, however, the coronary collateral circulation usually is less reliable and effective.

Stenotic lesions of 90 per cent or greater are required for production of significant collateral vessels in man. Under these circumstances, the mean back pressure at the time of operation for totally occluded arteries varies from 30 to 40 mm. Hg, and for those arteries with less than a 90 per cent stenosis, the average is only 18 to 20 mm. Hg. These findings indicate only marginal function, at best, of human collaterals. Angiographically defined coronary collaterals can appear and regress rapidly according to myocardial nutritional needs and pressure gradients, as may occur with the insertion of a bypass graft or its subsequent occlusion.

In addition, it should be remembered that some patients experience myocardial infarction with minimal or even absent coronary narrowing. Coronary arterial spasm may be responsible for this phenomenon (Prinzmetal's variant or atypical angina). Spasm can cause myocardial infarction in the absence of atherosclerotic lesions or can be superimposed on standard atherosclerotic stenoses, contributing to unstable pain patterns. Experience with the clinical spectrum of coronary spasm has indicated that patients with insignificant atherosclerosis are best managed by medical therapy (usually calcium channel–blocking agents) and those with coronary lesions by a surgical approach.

CLINICAL DIAGNOSIS

The most common symptom of myocardial ischemia is retrosternal chest pain, or angina pectoris, produced by a reduction in coronary blood flow. The discomfort generally is substernal in location and is often described by the patient as a pressure, choking sensation, or tightness. Early in the symptomatic course, a number of factors, such as exercise, cold exposure, eating, and emotional stress, can initiate the symptoms. The pain frequently radiates down the left arm and into the left neck, and occasionally to the right arm or mandible. The severity of chest pain can be graded by the New York Heart Association (NYHA) classification, with Class I indicating no symptoms; Class II, symptoms with severe exertion; Class III, chest pain with mild exertion; and Class IV, angina occurring at rest. Whereas minimal anginal symptoms often are easily tolerated and compatible with a fairly normal life-style (stable angina), the occurrence of an increasing NYHA class over a short period of time (progressive angina) worsens the clinical prognosis. In the late stages, ischemia occurs at rest and is refractory to medical therapy (unstable angina). Unstable pain patterns signify a particularly poor outlook, with an excessive early infarction and death rate. Significantly, a large proportion of patients do not follow the classic symptomatic progression and present initially with acute myocardial infarction or sudden death. Still others experience *no symptoms at all* during ischemia (silent myocardial ischemia), and coronary artery disease is discovered only in the late stage of congestive heart failure after severe ventricular damage has occurred.

The physical examination is frequently unremarkable, but a fourth heart sound can occasionally be heard on auscultation, reflecting an increase in the amplitude of the atrial systolic filling sound of the left ventricle. Although cardiac enlargement may be evident in patients with more advanced disease, the chest radiograph is normal in the majority. Left ventricular aneurysms can sometimes be detected radiographically as an isolated prominence of the left heart border. Although the electrocardiogram is within normal limits in at least half the patients, abnormal findings can be useful in establishing the diagnosis. Myocardial ischemia may be manifested by the presence of inverted T waves on the resting electrocardiogram or, alternatively, by transient ST segment and T wave changes during the course of an anginal episode. ST segment elevation or depression is an especially reliable sign and, if not present at rest, may be elicited by an exercise stress test. Exercise treadmill testing is most useful as a screening procedure for identifying the need for coronary angiography, although false-negative and false-positive responses can occur.

Cardiac catheterization and coronary arteriography are essential in defining the presence and extent of coronary atherosclerotic lesions. In recent years, a trend has favored early coronary arteriography in most patients with suspected coronary disease in order to define, as precisely as possible, individual prognostic characteristics. This approach has allowed a more objective application of medical therapy to low-risk subsets and selection of patients at high medical risk for elective surgical intervention. The general development of low-cost outpatient catheterization has facilitated this trend. At angiography, the major anatomic predictors of coronary death, such as the number of coronary vessels diseased and the resting left ventricular ejection fraction, are documented. Although the extent of disease can be underestimated in up to 10 per cent of patients, coronary arteriography has the highest sensitivity and specificity of any test available. Coronary angiography is clearly more precise, and even perhaps more cost-effective, than are other approaches. A comprehensive review of cardiac catheterization is provided in Part I. In patients with borderline anatomic indications for coronary bypass, physiologic assessment with radionuclide exercise ventriculography or stress thallium scanning can be useful in operative selection.

MEDICAL MANAGEMENT

If hypertension is present, it should be controlled, and smoking should be avoided, since the vasoconstrictive effects of nico-

tine and its influence on the coronary circulation are well established. It has also been demonstrated that cessation of smoking in patients with myocardial infarction tends to prevent reinfarction. Hyperlipidemias have a major role in the pathogenesis of coronary atherosclerosis, and clinical efforts should be directed toward aggressive management of lipid abnormalities by use of either dietary or pharmacologic means. After bypass grafting, risk factor modification and continued medical management are especially important, since atherosclerotic involvement of saphenous vein grafts is a major long-term risk.

When the choice is being made between medical and surgical therapy, the natural history of angina pectoris should be recalled. One study of the natural history of coronary atherosclerosis was obtained at a time when coronary arteriography was well established in the diagnosis of this disorder but when surgical therapy was rarely employed.[39] In a series of patients with proven coronary arterial lesions followed for 10 years, it was shown that the annual mortality was lowest in those with single-vessel disease, next lowest in those with double-vessel disease, and highest in patients with triple-vessel and left main coronary artery disease (Fig. 6). The degree of impairment in left ventricular function also was important (Fig. 7). In current practice, adverse prognostic characteristics that might suggest abandoning medical treatment and referral for coronary revascularization include severe or progressive angina on medical therapy, significant left main coronary disease, multivessel coronary obstruction (especially with proximal LAD involvement), ventricular impairment with a reduced ejection fraction, and evidence of exercise-induced ischemia. Although this topic is controversial and the decision in each patient has to be individualized, each of these factors, individually or in combination, significantly reduces survival with medical therapy and predicts improved longevity after coronary bypass grafting, as subsequently discussed. The recent addition of coronary balloon angioplasty as a therapeutic option has further complicated referral issues, and the evolving role of balloon angioplasty is discussed in Part I.

In patients with low-risk coronary anatomy, it is generally agreed that medical management is the treatment of choice, if anginal symptoms and exercise capacity can be maintained satisfactorily. Sublingual nitroglycerin remains a mainstay of ther-

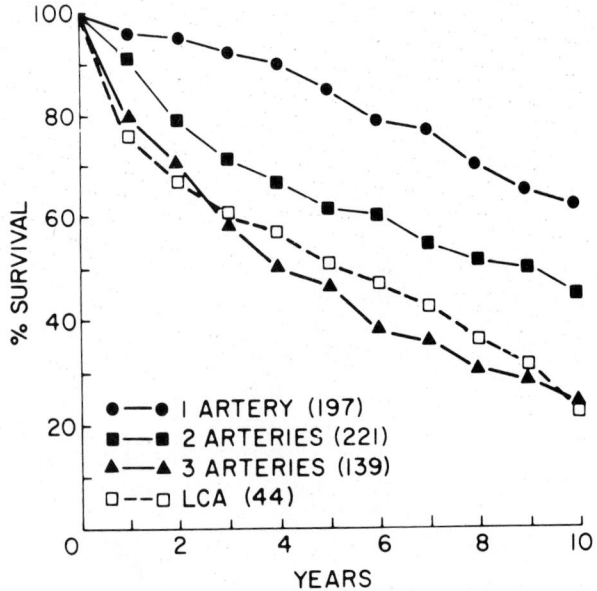

Figure 6. Survival in patients with significant lesions of one, two, and three coronary arteries and also the left main coronary artery (LCA). (From Bruschke, A. V. G.: Ten-year follow-up of 601 nonsurgical cases of angiographically documented coronary disease. Angiographic correlations. Cleve. Clin. Q., *45*:143, 1978.)

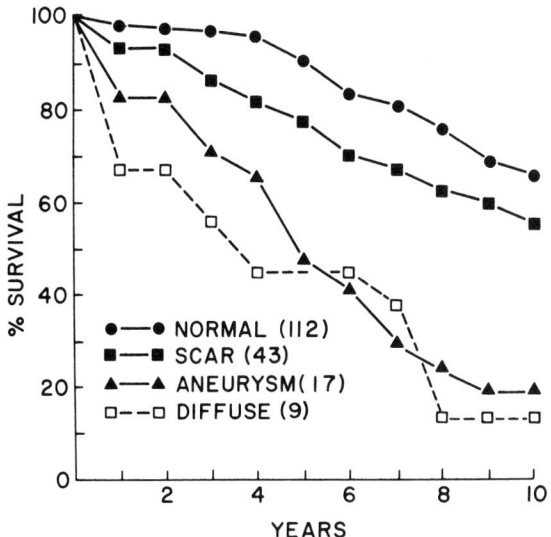

Figure 7. Survival according to ventriculographic estimates of resting left ventricular function in patients with ischemic heart disease. (From Proudfit, W. L., Bruschke, A. V. G., and Sones, F. M., Jr.: Natural history of obstructive coronary artery disease: Ten-year study of 601 non-surgical cases. Progr. Cardiovasc. Dis., 21:53, 1978.)

apy, and a response usually occurs within several minutes with one or two tablets. This drug also is useful in prophylaxis of stress known to produce angina. Long-acting nitrate preparations, such as isosorbide dinitrate, are available in different forms, and nitroglycerin ointment can be very useful.

Beta-adrenergic blocking agents, such as propranolol, atenolol, and timolol, are highly effective and safe in the chronic management of angina pectoris. These drugs act by lowering myocardial oxygen requirement through a reduction in heart rate with secondary effects on arterial blood pressure and myocardial contractility. Side effects include fatigue, gastrointestinal irritability, mental depression, and skin rash. If the patient has severe impairment of left ventricular function, beta-blocking agents can induce congestive heart failure and require cessation or the concomitant administration of digitalis. Calcium channel–blocking agents such as nifedipine, diltiazem, and verapamil are now well established in clinical practice and are quite effective in anginal management. There is evidence, however, that the symptomatic efficacy of these drugs may not be directly associated with an improvement in ultimate patient prognosis. Antiplatelet agents, such as aspirin, have a definite therapeutic role and have been shown to decrease coronary events significantly. Likewise, short-term heparinization has been effective in preventing coronary thrombosis and infarction in patients with unstable angina.

SURGICAL MANAGEMENT

Preoperative Preparation

It is essential that the goals and anticipated results of coronary bypass grafting are explained in detail to both the patient and family before the procedure. Potential risks and complications should be reviewed in a manner designed to be factual and yet to minimize fear and anxiety. All aspects of the physical examination, cardiac catheterization, and other special procedures should be reviewed, with emphasis on a full knowledge of cardiac anatomy and dynamics. Any neurologic deficits, including the presence of carotid bruits, should be fully evaluated, and respiratory status, renal function, and blood coagulation should be assessed. Aspirin should be discontinued, if possible, for 1 to 2 weeks prior to operation. In many patients, especially those with unstable angina, this may not be practical, and the increased risk of postoperative bleeding associated with aspirin

must be accepted.[16] Antianginal agents, including beta-blocking compounds, calcium channel–blocking drugs, isosorbide dinitrate, and nitroglycerin ointment, should be continued until the procedure. If further pharmacologic therapy is required for recurring angina, an intravenous nitroglycerin infusion can be employed. Intra-aortic balloon pumping can be particularly effective for preoperative stabilization of patients with unstable angina in the coronary care unit. Excellent cardiac anesthesia is essential for obtaining optimal results, and a complete review of contemporary anesthetic techniques is given in Chapter 9. Prophylactic broad-spectrum antibiotics are administered intravenously immediately before anesthetic induction and for 24 to 48 hours postoperatively.

Surgical Procedures

The majority of patients who are candidates for surgical management are treated with simple bypass of the obstructed coronary vessels by use of either the internal mammary artery or reversed segments of the saphenous vein. After a median sternotomy has been performed, the left internal mammary artery is dissected from the chest wall in the majority of patients. The procedure is conducted with extracorporeal circulation and cold potassium cardioplegia. Aortic arch cannulation is almost uniformly employed with the metal-tip Sarns cannula (Sarns, Inc., Ann Arbor, Michigan). For most coronary bypass procedures, single venous cannulation is utilized through the right atrial appendage, and direct cardiac venting is avoided. Cardiopulmonary bypass is initiated at 32° C., distal coronary grafting sites are visualized, and internal mammary artery flow is measured. As the cardioplegia cannula (DLP, Inc., Walker, Michigan) is inserted into the proximal ascending aorta, pump inflow temperature is reduced to 16° C. to "precool" the myocardium. Myocardial precooling with the bypass circuit allows better and more uniform myocardial hypothermia for a given volume of subsequent cardioplegia infusion. A silicone rubber catheter is placed in the posterior pericardium via the transverse sinus and connected to a cold saline lavage system. A metal coil submerged in an alcohol-ice mixture acts as a heat exchanger to cool the pericardial saline, and infusion is begun at 100 ml. per minute. A suction catheter at the inferior aspect of the incision collects the pericardial lavage and returns it to a cell-saver device to scavenge shed blood. A myocardial temperature needle is routinely positioned in the interventricular septum to ensure adequate myocardial hypothermia.

When myocardial temperature falls below 24° C., the aorta is occluded with a Fogarty clamp, and 1200 ml. of cold St. Thomas' Hospital cardioplegia solution (Table 3) is infused via the DLP cannula over 3 to 5 minutes.[25] A commercially prepared solution (Plegisol, Abbott Laboratories) is preferred so that the likelihood of bacterial contamination or human error during formulation is lessened. In addition, iced saline slush is applied topically; and a rapid reduction in myocardial temperature, well below 15° C., usually is achieved. If myocardial hypothermia is inadequate, additional volumes of cardioplegia solu-

TABLE 3. Composition of Modified St. Thomas' Hospital Cardioplegia Solution

Composition	Concentration
Sodium chloride	110.0 mmol./L.
Potassium chloride	16.0 mmol./L.
Magnesium chloride	16.0 mmol./L.
Calcium chloride	1.2 mmol./L.
Sodium bicarbonate	10.0 mmol./L.
Procaine	0.5 mmol./L.
Sodium heparin	1000 units/L.
Human serum albumin	12.5 gm./L.

324 mOsm./kg. of H_2O; pH 7.8.

tion are infused for attaining the desired temperature. Coincident with aortic clamping, systemic perfusate temperature is returned to 24° C., and flow is reduced to 1.0 to 1.5 liters per minute per sq. m. Systemic arterial pressure during the arrest period is maintained at approximately 40 mm. Hg so that cardiac rewarming due to noncoronary collateral blood flow is lessened. A side arm on the cardioplegia cannula is used for venting the aorta and left ventricle during aortic occlusion. The coronary bypass procedure then is performed, and additional 200- to 500-ml. volumes of cardioplegia solution are infused every 30 to 45 minutes for maintenance of myocardial temperature below 15° C. Five to 10 minutes before aortic unclamping, full rewarming is begun, and a 200-mg. dose of lidocaine is administered into the oxygenator for diminishing reperfusion arrhythmias. After aortic unclamping, additional procedures such as proximal aorta–vein graft anastomoses are completed, and cardiopulmonary bypass is discontinued after adequate rewarming.

All coronary arteries 1.5 mm. or greater in diameter with more than 50 per cent luminal narrowing are selected for bypass. In recent years, it has become possible to bypass all significant vessels in over 90 per cent of cases, and difficult grafts to septal perforating arteries, circumflex branches in the atrioventricular groove, and large right ventricular arteries have become routine when deemed clinically important. If a major vessel, such as the LAD, is completely occluded or diffusely diseased, an attempt at distal revascularization is still performed by utilization of single or sequential mammary artery grafting, intraoperative balloon dilation, or other techniques. In current practice, coronary endarterectomy is avoided whenever possible because of an appreciable incidence of distal intimal flaps and perioperative infarction. Approximately three to four grafts are inserted per patient, which reflects a philosophy of complete revascularization together with the tendency to reserve surgical therapy for symptomatic patients with multivessel disease. In general, the internal mammary artery is the graft of choice because of its superior long-term patency. At least one IMA graft is utilized in 95 per cent of coronary revascularization procedures, usually to the LAD coronary artery, and adjunctive saphenous vein grafts are used for additional vessels. In selected patients, multiple distal IMA anastomoses can be constructed by use of a combination of bilateral mammary artery dissection, sequential mammary anastomosis, and free mammary grafts.[43] Although the indications for multiple IMA procedures are not fully defined, conservative criteria include patients with limited or diseased saphenous veins, younger patients with extended life expectancy,[33] reoperative cases with previous early vein graft failure, and extensive atherosclerotic calcification of the ascending aorta precluding proximal vein graft anastomoses.

A standard method for distal saphenous vein–coronary artery anastomosis is illustrated in Figure 8. As a routine, the veins are dissected from the lower legs by use of gentle technique, and care is taken to prevent overdistention during preparation. A methylene blue stripe is placed along the vein for maintaining proper orientation and for avoidance of twisting. For distal anastomoses, a running 7–0 polypropylene suture and 8 to 12 stitches are employed, depending on the size of the vein graft and coronary artery. With the "toe" of the vein suspended by the first assistant, the anastomosis is begun on the side opposite the surgeon, and a continuous suture line is constructed around the "heel" of the vein. After the middle suture on the surgeon's side is placed, the suture line is tightened, pulling the vein onto the arteriotomy. With slight traction on the graft, the toe of the arteriotomy is exposed, which facilitates placement of the final sutures. Whereas deeper bites are performed on the sides for anchoring the vein, the toe and heel sutures are placed superficially so that no narrowing occurs. The polypropylene suture is sometimes tied with an appropriately sized probe lying within the vessel for elimination of the possibility of anastomotic nar-

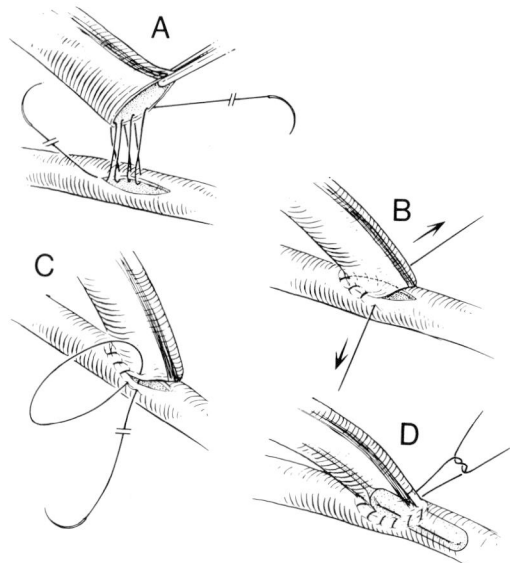

Figure 8. A standard method for distal vein graft anastomosis with use of a running suture technique. See text for details.

rowing. Because the surgeon never changes needles, temporal efficiency is maximized, and time also is saved by using smaller diameter lower leg veins, bevelling the vein grafts only slightly, and minimizing the length of the arteriotomy. Cardioplegia solution can be infused directly into the completed vein graft so that adequate myocardial hypothermia beyond severely obstructed coronary lesions is ensured.

A method for performing the aortic anastomosis is illustrated in Figure 9; a 6–0 polypropylene suture usually is employed. The beveled vein is sutured to a 4.5-mm. circular aortotomy by starting at the caudad aspect and progressing one half of the circumference around the heel with the vein suspended. After tightening of the suture line, the toe sutures are completed. Care is taken to obtain optimal graft lengths, where the graft is under no tension and makes a gentle curve to the coronary vessel without kinking.

Generally, circle grafts are avoided. Although overall early

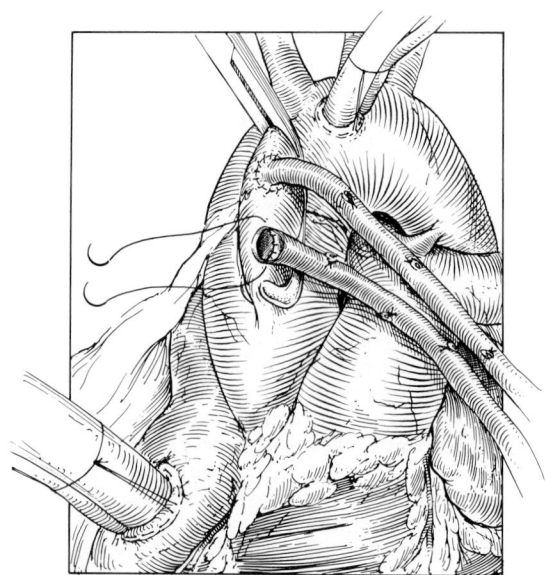

Figure 9. Method for performing proximal saphenous vein anastomoses to the aorta. A portion of the aorta is excluded by use of a partial occlusion clamp, and the vein grafts are anastomosed to circular aortotomies with running 6–0 polypropylene sutures. (Modified from Oschner, J. L., and Mills, N. L.: Coronary Artery Surgery. Philadelphia, Lea & Febiger, 1978.)

patency has been good with the circle graft, the occasional early or late graft thrombosis causes disastrous loss of the entire operation. When it is convenient, however, sequential saphenous vein graft anastomoses are performed to two distal coronary arteries, and a natural Y sequential method is preferred. This technique uses a short side branch of the vein for construction of the more proximal coronary anastomosis and has the advantages of minimizing distortion of the main vein while allowing more variation in interanastomotic distance without producing kinking. A large vessel with good run-off (not perfusing a previously infarcted segment) is used for the distal coronary anastomosis, and the vein side branch is usually sutured to a smaller, more proximal coronary artery. Although valves are rare in the proximal aspect of venous branches, the absence of valves should be documented by irrigating the vein before the anastomosis is undertaken.

As a first step, a standard running distal anastomosis is performed between the slightly beveled natural Y branch and the more proximal coronary arteriotomy. After completion of the middle anastomosis, cold cardioplegia solution is used for distending the vein to its ultimate size and length, and the distance to the distal coronary arteriotomy is determined, allowing a gentle curve between the two anastomoses. The distal vein graft is beveled to the appropriate length, and a standard anastomosis is performed to the distal coronary arteriotomy. The proximal aortic anastomosis usually is performed last, immediately after unclamping the aorta. In cases where adequate side branches are not available, a side-to-side "diamond" sequential method is utilized. Techniques are similar, except care is taken to perform a small (1.5 mm.) venotomy and arteriotomy for the middle anastomosis, which employs an eight-stitch technique. The vein usually is turned 90 degrees from parallel with the artery. With both methods, the methylene blue stripe on the vein is oriented to the opposite side of the distal anastomosis for prevention of interanastomotic kinking.

With increasing evidence of superior long-term mammary artery patency, at least one internal mammary graft is now em-ployed in most patients. In over 95 per cent of cases, mammary arteries are suitable, and in contrast to previous experiences, mammary grafts are used for emergency procedures, patients with poor ventricular function, and the elderly. Although arterial grafts may require slightly more operative time, current myocardial protection and cardiopulmonary bypass support are more than adequate so that mammary grafting has equivalently low mortality and morbidity, compared with other methods.

In all but the most hemodynamically unstable patients, the left internal mammary artery is gently dissected from the chest wall in a narrow pedicle by use of the low-current electrocautery. Arterial spasm is prevented by topical application of papaverine solution, and the distal coronary anastomosis is constructed with a technique similar to vein grafts (Fig. 10A). The pedicle is transected sharply at an appropriate length, and adequate flow capacity is documented on cardiopulmonary bypass before the heart is arrested. Usually, flow approaching 100 ml. per minute is required before the left IMA is accepted for grafting a large LAD. If the flow capacity is inadequate, the IMA is discarded, and a saphenous vein graft is utilized for avoidance of the disastrous consequences of a "bad" IMA graft. After turning the pedicle 180 degrees so that the pleura lies away from the heart, the graft is beveled on the undersurface for 2 to 3 mm. The pedicle rather than the graft is held with forceps by the first assistant, and the arterial wall is never grasped; a "no-touch" technique is utilized. After completion of the suture line with 7-0 or 8-0 polypropylene suture, the graft is opened, the suture is tied, and the pedicle is fixed to the epicardium for stabilization. If an important coronary artery beyond the reach of the in situ mammary artery needs to be grafted, extra length can be obtained by disconnecting the graft from its origin and suturing the proximal aspect to the aorta (free mammary grafting).

If necessary, more than one coronary artery can be bypassed with a given pedicle by use of sequential mammary techniques (Fig. 10B). After both coronary arteries have been opened and appropriate interanastomotic distances have been determined, the underside of the mammary vessel is freed of adventitial

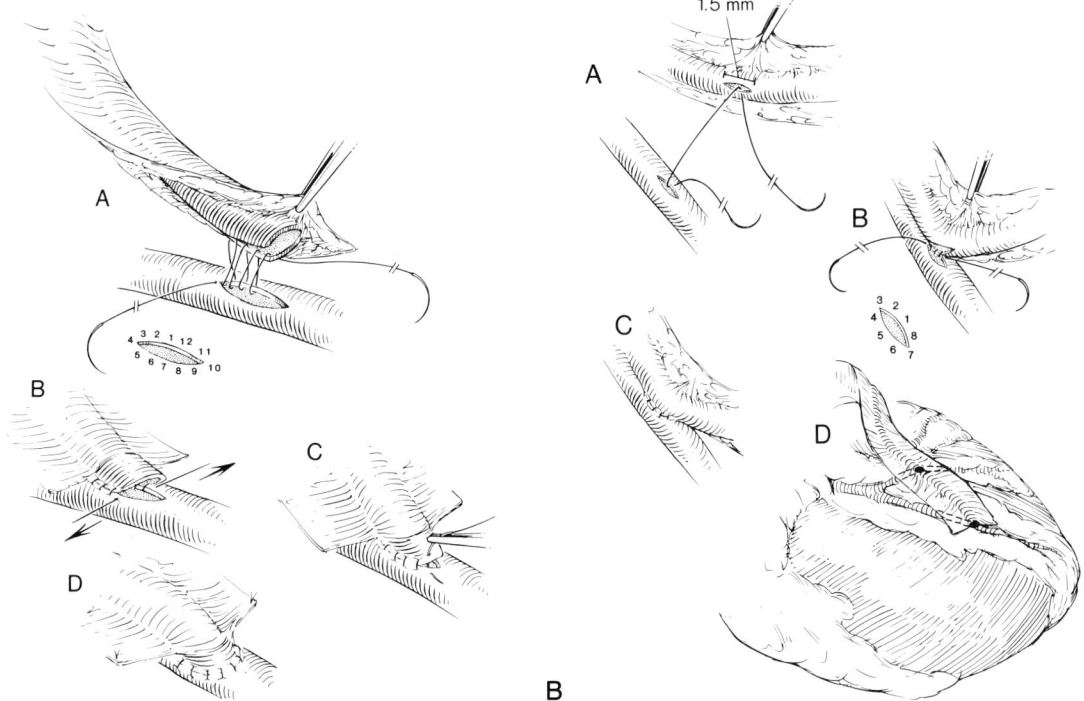

Figure 10. *A,* Technique of end-to-side IMA-coronary anastomosis. Stitches 1 to 6 are placed with the IMA elevated off the coronary (A). The assistant grasps the pedicle with a forceps in the right hand and controls the suture loops with a forceps in the left hand. After stitch 6, the suture line is tightened (B), and the remaining toe sutures are placed (C). The pedicle is sutured to the epicardium (D). For smaller coronary arteries, the IMA is beveled less, and (most commonly) 10 stitches (omitting 3 and 5) or 8 stitches (omitting 3, 5, 9, and 11) are used. *B,* Technique for sequential IMA-coronary grafting. See text for details.

tissue. A short 1.5-mm. arteriotomy is performed, and a running 8–0 polypropylene suture is employed with an eight-stitch technique. The anastomosis is begun on the side opposite the surgeon, and after the heel sutures are placed, the anastomosis is tightened. The toe sutures are completed, and the distal anastomosis is performed as described before. When the pedicle crosses the first artery at right angles, as in the circumflex system, the anastomosis is turned 90 degrees; otherwise, a parallel technique is used. The pedicle is carefully sutured to the epicardial surface at multiple points along its course for the prevention of torsion.

POSTOPERATIVE MANAGEMENT

Monitoring

The postoperative care of patients after coronary bypass procedures is of primary importance and is assuming a greater role as increasingly ill patients are selected for surgical therapy. Whereas most patients have a smooth and uncomplicated course, 5 to 10 per cent experience postoperative problems, and a number of parameters are monitored for warning of developing complications. Standard measurements include radial arterial blood pressure, central venous pressure, urinary output, a continuous electrocardiographic tracing, and periodic determinations of arterial blood gases (Po_2, Pco_2, and pH). In most patients, cardiac function is assessed with measurements of cardiac output and pulmonary capillary wedge pressure, as provided by a thermodilution Swan-Ganz catheter. Appropriate hematologic and blood chemistry studies, as well as chest radiographs, are obtained periodically. Body weight is recorded daily for monitoring potential fluid retention.

Postoperative Complications

With improving surgical techniques, and especially the introduction of cold potassium cardioplegia, postoperative *low cardiac output* is now uncommon in most centers. When it is encountered, however, all possible etiologic factors should be specifically considered, including hypovolemia, cardiac tamponade, concealed bleeding, dysrhythmias, myocardial insufficiency, and acidosis. If filling pressures are inadequate, appropriate volumes of crystalloid solutions, colloid-containing solution, or blood components are infused for raising pulmonary capillary wedge or left atrial pressure toward 15 mm. Hg. If low cardiac output persists despite adequate filling, optimization of afterload, or arterial blood pressure, should be considered by means of a continuous infusion of sodium nitroprusside. This agent acts directly on vascular smooth muscle for production of vasodilation independent of the autonomic nervous system. Infusion rates of up to 10 μg. per kg. per minute may be used transiently for treatment of hypertension, although potential complications such as methemoglobinemia should be borne in mind. Additionally, the mean arterial blood pressure should not be reduced below 65 to 75 mm. Hg for a prolonged period of time because of the possibility of multiorgan underperfusion.

If the cardiac index remains below 2.0 liters per minute per sq. m., pharmacologic support of the circulation usually is indicated. At this time, dopamine is the first-line catecholamine chosen in most units owing to its simultaneous enhancement of myocardial contractility and renal blood flow. Continuous central venous infusion rates of 5 to 20 μg. per kg. per minute are employed. Other catecholamines having beta-adrenergic activity increase heart rate, augment myocardial contractility, and produce arterial vasodilation. In contrast, pure alpha-adrenergic drugs do not influence heart rate or myocardial contractility but primarily produce peripheral vasoconstriction. Most clinically utilized adrenergic agents have varying degrees of mixed alpha and beta action, and drug selection should be based on

the desired physiologic effect. The relative merits to be considered in the selection of inotropic agents are discussed elsewhere. If circulatory insufficiency persists despite inotropic stimulation, placement of an intra-aortic balloon pump can be life-saving.

Cardiac tamponade can produce postoperative low cardiac output, and the characteristic hemodynamic finding is elevated and equalized central venous and pulmonary wedge pressures, usually in the setting of excessive mediastinal bleeding. The chest radiograph may demonstrate mediastinal widening or blood collection, but if a significant question of tamponade exists, reoperation should be considered. Excessive *mediastinal bleeding* in the setting of stable hemodynamics is managed by correction of clotting defects with blood component therapy and by autotransfusion of shed mediastinal blood.[10] Early reoperation is performed if bleeding remains excessive and is required in 2 to 3 per cent of patients after coronary bypass.

Atrial dysrhythmias are common following coronary revascularization. Premature atrial contractions, atrial fibrillation, or atrial flutter reflects postoperative atrial irritability and occurs in 10 to 30 per cent of patients. If atrial tachycardia occurs, control of ventricular response is achieved with intravenous digoxin, followed by attempts at pharmacologic cardioversion with atenolol, procainamide, or calcium channel–blocking agents. Rapid atrial pacing or direct current cardioversion can sometimes be effective in atrial flutter after initial drug therapy. Although transient atrial dysrhythmias are usually well tolerated, significant low cardiac output or systemic thromboembolism can occur rarely.

Ventricular irritability manifested by frequent or multifocal premature ventricular contractions, ventricular tachycardia, or ventricular fibrillation is managed by intravenous lidocaine and/or procainamide together with direct current cardioversion when necessary. Short periods of closed-chest cardiac massage may be necessary, but early cardioversion should be emphasized. Serious ventricular dysrhythmias are usually a manifestation of significant myocardial ischemia, and problems with the quality of revascularization should be considered. Beta-blocking agents and/or oral procainamide are used for long-term management of persistent ventricular ectopy.

After uncomplicated elective operations, most patients can be removed from ventilatory support and extubated within a few hours. After anesthetic recovery, criteria for early extubation include good pulmonary gas exchange, adequate ventilatory mechanics, a clear chest radiograph, absence of dysrhythmias and excess bleeding, and stable cardiac and neurologic function. Occasional patients exhibit prolonged *pulmonary dysfunction*, requiring controlled ventilation, positive end-expiratory pressure, diuresis, and transiently increased fractional inspired oxygen. If pulmonary infection is suggested by radiographic infiltrates, high white blood cell counts, or positive sputum cultures, appropriate antibiotic coverage is added. As the period of required ventilatory support via an endotracheal tube approaches 2 weeks, tracheostomy should be considered. Tracheostomy is especially useful for clearing pulmonary secretions and assisting ventilatory weaning.

Postoperative *renal dysfunction* can produce transient elevations in blood urea nitrogen and creatinine, with progression to oliguria or total renal shutdown. Ischemic renal injury can occur in the setting of low cardiac output or if excessively low perfusion pressures are encountered on cardiopulmonary bypass or perioperatively. Pre-existing renal artery stenosis or arteriolar nephrosclerosis predisposes certain patients to renal hypoperfusion. In the appropriate clinical setting, developing sepsis must also be considered as a cause of worsening renal performance. Therapy for renal dysfunction consists of maintaining higher arterial perfusion pressure (especially in patients with pre-existing hypertension), low-dose intravenous dopamine infusion, adequate free water hydration, and general support of cardiac output. Fluid balance and potassium intake are monitored carefully for the prevention of overhydration or hyperkalemia. If dialysis is required, peritoneal lavage is favored because patient survival associated with a policy of aggressive hemodialysis has been disappointing.

Sternal wound infection occurs in 1 to 2 per cent of patients after coronary bypass. Developing sternal instability, fever, leukocytosis, and wound drainage should suggest the diagnosis. Severity varies from a superficial subcutaneous infection with a stable sternum to an isolated sternal infection with no mediastinal involvement to fully developed septic mediastinitis. At the first suspicion of a major wound infection, broad-spectrum antibiotics should be instituted and cultures obtained. The combination of diabetes and bilateral IMA harvesting may predispose some patients to sternal infection. Infections producing sternal disruption are treated with a brief course of open wound care followed by wound closure with pectoral or omental pedicle flaps.[26] Mortality using this approach has been reduced to less than 10 per cent, although morbidity remains high.

With improvements in myocardial protection and coronary grafting techniques, *perioperative myocardial infarction* should occur in only 1 to 2 per cent of patients. The etiology varies from subclinical closure of an ungrafted small secondary coronary artery to failure of a major coronary bypass leading to cardiogenic shock. Therefore, the cause should be carefully evaluated, and most cases produce little clinical morbidity or deterioration of global ventricular function. Conversely, the development of serious problems might suggest early angiography or reintervention if it is deemed clinically feasible.

SURGICAL RESULTS

Analytic Methods

Clinical investigation of treatment efficacy is important in all areas of surgical therapy but is especially critical to the subject of coronary bypass. Survival analysis has been widely applied for this purpose and is a form of inductive reasoning with its origins in the philosophical discipline of logic. Prognostic analysis is useful in determining operative risk for each individual patient, as well as the appropriateness of surgical therapy in various patient subsets. Two methods generally have been employed: prospective randomized clinical trials[8,15,37] and retrospective observational analysis.[5] Both have advantages and limitations for a given question and require proper interpretation within the limits of clinical practice.

Risk Factors Influencing Surgical Results

Numerous risk factors are associated with increased early and late mortality after coronary revascularization. For illustration of this point, a multivariate observational analysis was performed for 1063 patients undergoing isolated coronary bypass in the most recent era for which long-term survival data are available (1984–1986). This series is representative of current surgical practice in which 93 per cent of patients received at least one IMA graft, and the data illustrated several important points. First, 90 per cent of patients referred for surgical therapy now have left main or multivessel disease (Table 4), half undergo operation under elective conditions, and half require emergency surgical therapy for refractory unstable angina or acute myocardial infarction. Approximately one third are older than 65 years, and over one fourth have severe left ventricular dysfunction.

Despite these adverse characteristics, the overall operative mortality averages 2 per cent, with a 92 per cent 4-year survival (Table 4). Better-risk patients with *either* elective operation, age less than 65 years, *or* ejection fraction greater than 0.40 experience an operative mortality of approximately 1 per cent with a 4-year survival exceeding 95 per cent. Only 0.9 per cent have required reoperation to an average of 4-years of follow-up. When the serious baseline illness profile displayed by these patients is considered, the long-term results are surprisingly good and represent the standard with which other emerging therapies must be compared.

By multivariate analysis, risk factors for long-term mortality include (in order of importance) severe left ventricular dysfunction, emergency operation for acute myocardial infarction, advanced age, and surgical indication of unstable angina (Table 4). In current series, the number of vessels diseased and female gender are only of marginal significance, whereas diabetes is a risk factor for late cardiac death possibly owing to accelerated vein graft atherosclerosis. Most analyses, including the authors', have suggested that performing one IMA graft independently reduces the probability of late cardiac death and reoperation.[6,32] However, consistent data demonstrating an additional survival advantage of multiple IMA grafting are not available at present.

Therapeutic Efficacy

The effects of bypass grafting on the clinical course of patients with coronary atherosclerosis can be assessed in several ways. Improvement in anginal *symptoms* is observed in the majority of patients in the first several postoperative years, and the rate of improvement is significantly better than that observed with medical therapy. In most series, long-term complete relief of angina is achieved in over two thirds of patients. In the Emory experience (Fig. 11), 92 per cent of patients had significant improvement in angina, and 62 per cent were completely pain-free at an average of 20 months postoperatively. In addition, the incidence of subsequent *myocardial infarction* is significantly reduced for many years in patients who undergo surgical therapy. Seven to 10 years postoperatively, however, the rate again increases, probably as a result of progression of the original disease or involvement of the vein grafts with atherosclerosis.

Whereas conflicting data have been reported in the past, consensus now exists that a primary physiologic effect of coronary

TABLE 4. Baseline and Survival Characteristics for 1063 Patients Undergoing Coronary Bypass, 1984–1986

Preoperative Data		Survival Data			Multivariate Analysis of Risk Factors for Survival		
			Survival				
Variable	Baseline Characteristics	Category	30-day	4-yr.	Variable	X^2	p
Left main, multivessel disease	90%	All patients	0.98	0.92	Ejection fraction	14.6	<0.001
Elective	53%	Elective	0.99	0.96	Acute myocardial infarction	7.1	0.008
Unstable angina	42%	Unstable	0.96	0.89			
Acute myocardial infarction	5%	Age ≥65 years	0.95	0.87	Age ≥65 years	6.7	0.009
Mean age (years)	60 ± 10	Age <65 years	0.99	0.95	Unstable angina	4.8	0.03
Age >65 years	34%	Ejection fraction ≥0.40	0.98	0.95			
Mean ejection fraction	50 ± 10	Ejection fraction <0.40	0.96	0.85			
Ejection fraction <0.40	26%	Nondiabetics	0.98	0.93			
		Diabetics	0.95	0.88			

DISEASED VESSELS

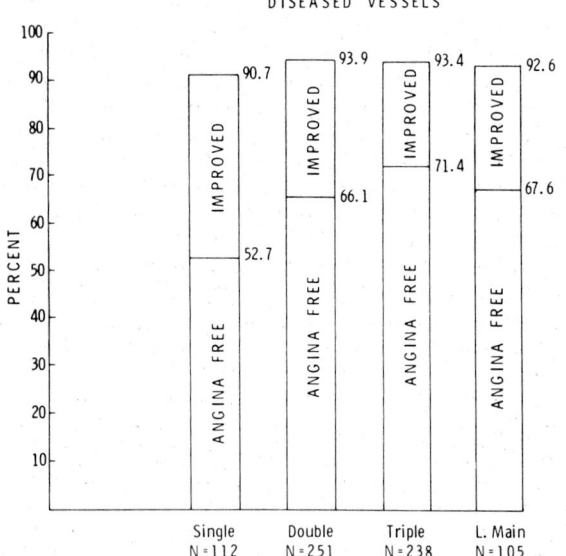

Figure 11. Percentage of patients free of angina and those who are improved in relationship to preoperative number of vessels diseased. (From King, S. B., III, and Hurst, J. W.: The relief of angina pectoris by coronary bypass surgery. *In* Hurst, J. W. (Ed.): Update II: The Heart. New York, McGraw-Hill, 1980.)

revascularization is maintenance or augmentation of *left ventricular function.*[13] Hemodynamic improvement can be demonstrated by comparison of preoperative and postoperative contrast ventriculograms or noninvasive radionuclide angiocardiograms obtained at rest, in which an increased ejection fraction, higher cardiac output, decreased diastolic volume, and improved left ventricular wall motion can be demonstrated in a significant proportion of patients (Fig. 12).[41] Moreover, im-

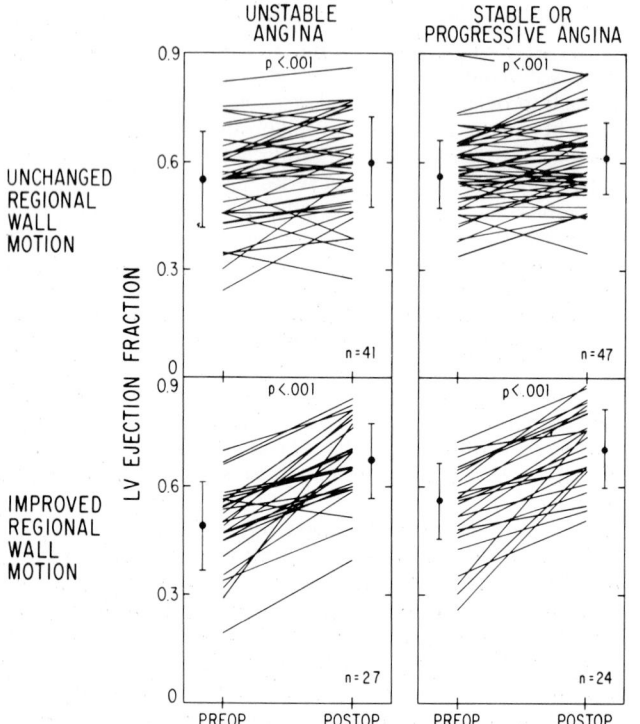

Figure 12. Perioperative ventriculographic ejection fraction data for 139 patients having coronary bypass with the technique described in this section. The categories are separated into unstable angina (left panels) and stable or progressive angina (right panels) and subdivided further according to the observed change in regional wall motion. Improvement in global ejection fraction was statistically significant in each category and in the entire group. (From Rankin, J. S., Newman, G. E., Muhlbaier, L. H., et al.: The effects of coronary revascularization on left ventricular function in ischemic heart disease. J. Thorac. Cardiovasc. Surg., 90:818, 1985.)

provement in exercise ventricular function has been demonstrated as early as 1 week postoperatively.[3] Clinical stabilization of exercise tolerance noted by the majority of patients following coronary bypass further supports the concept of improved ventricular function after revascularization.

Anatomic quality of revascularization can be assessed by angiographic studies of *graft patency.* With improvements in operative technique, saphenous vein graft patency in the first postoperative year should approximate 92 per cent, and 85 per cent of patients should have all grafts patent. A slow attrition rate then occurs over the next decade because of the development of graft atherosclerosis, so that 10-year vein graft patency averages approximately 50 per cent. Up to half of the patent vein grafts at 10 years are involved with the atherosclerotic process; thus, functional patency is somewhat less than 50 per cent. Persistent hyperlipidemias are a major risk factor for the development of vein graft atherosclerosis,[47] and aggressive lipid management is indicated postoperatively along with general risk factor modification. Evidence exists that pharmacologic therapy for hyperlipidemias can improve long-term graft patency and reduce the incidence of subsequent coronary events.[4] Aspirin also is administered indefinitely for its beneficial effects on graft patency.[21]

The long-term patency of IMA grafts is somewhat better.[23,34] In modern series, the early patency of IMA grafts, including the more complex sequential IMA grafts, approximates 95 to 99 per cent.[42] Because late atherosclerotic involvement of IMA grafts is rare, 10-year IMA patency averages 85 to 90 per cent, which translates into better survival, less anginal recurrence, and fewer reoperations.[6,11] It is for this reason that routine utilization of at least one IMA graft has been standard surgical policy in most medical centers since the early 1980s.

Whereas patient symptoms are important, perhaps the most objective measure of surgical outcome is *long-term survival.* As described in the preceding section, several methods exist for evaluating the survival benefits of coronary bypass procedures, from randomized prospective trials to retrospective observational statistical analysis. For the purposes of this discussion, observational information from the Duke Databank for cardiovascular disease is presented, although the results of this approach agree precisely with those of the randomized trials for similar patients treated over comparable time periods.

The most striking feature of the Duke Databank survival statistics over the past 2 decades is the improvement in absolute patient survival over time. The observed 2-year Kaplan-Meier survival rates for each year for all medical patients and for all surgical patients and their respective hazard scores as an estimate of baseline risk are shown in Figure 13. The smoothed curve superimposed on each panel represents the unadjusted Cox model survival estimate with date of entry as the independent variable. The data demonstrate that 2-year survival has improved progressively for both medically and surgically treated patients and that the magnitude of the trend was far greater with surgical therapy. Moreover, the improvement in late surgical survival was related not only to reduced operative mortality but also to a marked enhancement in long-term survival.

The results of the Cox model analysis are illustrated in Table 5. The magnitude of each survival trend is illustrated by the slope (the more negative, the greater the rate of improvement), and the significance of the trend is characterized by the chi-square statistic. The improvements in survival over time for both medically and surgically treated patients are summarized in the unadjusted Cox model results. The analyses adjusted for differences in baseline characteristics suggest different mechanisms were responsible for the improvements observed. The time trend in medical patients was greatly reduced after adjusting for baseline characteristics (Table 5). The slope markedly declined, and the trend was no longer significant. This finding

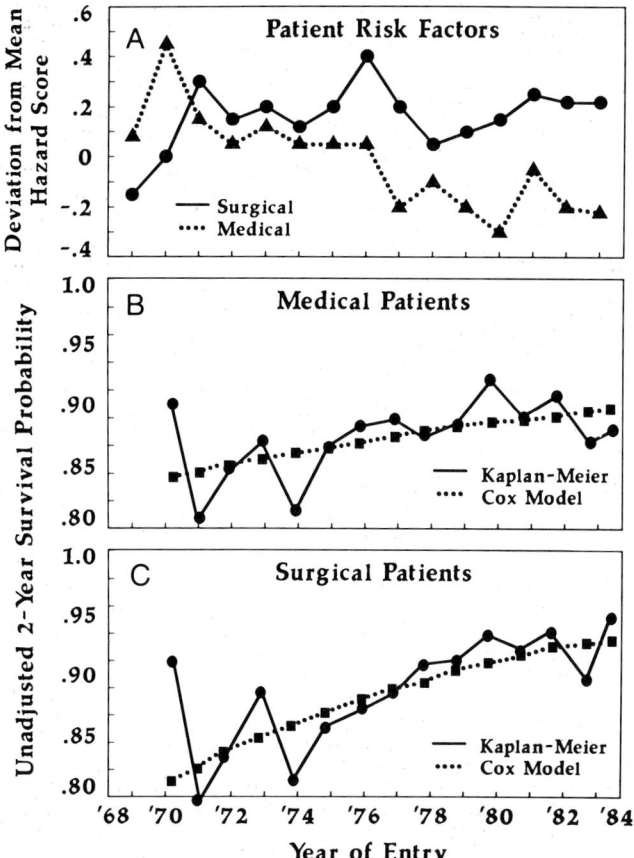

Figure 13. Kaplan-Meier observed 2-year survival (solid line) and estimated Cox model trends (dashed line) for each year of entry into the study for all medical patients and surgical patients and their relative hazard ratios as an index of baseline risk. (From Pryor, D. B., Harrell, F. E., Rankin, J. S., Lee, K. L., Muhlbaier, L. H., Oldham, H. N., Hlatky, M. A., Mark, D. B., Reves, J. G., and Califf, R. M.: The changing survival benefits of coronary revascularization over time. Circulation, 76(Suppl. V):V-13, 1987.)

methods of graft construction producing enhanced graft patency, and better intraoperative support. With more complete knowledge of pathophysiology, early anesthetic techniques designed only to maintain perfusion pressure and oxygenation yielded a more appropriate management that minimized myocardial oxygen consumption with depressant anesthetics and optimized oxygen delivery. Unacceptable anesthetic agents were replaced by high-dose opioid derivatives or inhalational compounds. The development of intravenous nitroglycerin and better methods of intraoperative cardiac monitoring are further examples of improved operative technology. Significant learning curves also exist after the introduction of new methods, and surgical experience is a major factor influencing operative results. It is likely that surgical survival has improved over time in most cardiac surgical centers.

For demonstration of the clinical implications of the selective improvement in surgical survival over time, estimated medical and surgical survival curves for 3 entry years (1970, 1977, and 1984) are illustrated in Figure 14 for patients with three-vessel disease. Although surgical therapy had a negative impact on survival in 1970 and equivocally positive effects in 1977, continued improvements in surgical results produced a clear survival benefit of surgical therapy by 1984. Similar findings were evident for all categories of multivessel and left main disease (Fig. 15). Thus, contemporary methods of coronary bypass grafting appear to significantly enhance overall patient survival as well as that of specific subsets across the spectrum of coronary disease severity.[5] Worsening left ventricular function appears to augment the survival benefit.

With the development of coronary balloon angioplasty and interventional cardiology, the focus of cardiologic practice appears to have shifted toward acute coronary care. However, it is important to bear in mind the excellent long-term results that are now possible with *elective* referral for coronary bypass grafting. Patients with high-risk coronary lesions should be considered for *early referral for elective coronary bypass* so that the best early and late therapeutic results can be achieved.

SPECIAL TOPICS

The Relative Roles of PTCA and Coronary Bypass

In 1977, Grüntzig introduced percutaneous transluminal coronary angioplasty (PTCA) as a means of dilating stenotic coronary arterial lesions in patients with angina pectoris.[24] This work demonstrated that atherosclerotic coronary stenoses could be dilated with relief of angina and improvement in myocardial perfusion. The topic of coronary angioplasty subsequently has expanded into a rapidly evolving discipline, which is reviewed in detail in Part I. After years of technological innovation, PTCA is now a mature, reproducible therapy. Early results have steadily improved, so that successful dilation rates per stenosis currently exceed 90 per cent. Major complication rates for elective angioplasty have fallen to about 4 per cent, and procedure-related myocardial infarction and death remain uncommon. Results of PTCA in patients with unstable angina or having incomplete revascularization have been somewhat less accept-

implies that most of the trend in medically treated patients was due to changes in the population mix, where less seriously ill patients were being selected for medical therapy. In contrast, the improvement in surgical survival was not markedly affected by adjustment for baseline characteristics. This observation suggests that the surgical survival trend represented refinements in the therapeutic efficacy of coronary revascularization and not changes in the patient mix. Thus, the survival benefit afforded by surgical therapy has increased dramatically, and the adjusted analysis for surgical survivors confirmed that the improvement was due not only to reduced operative mortality but also to an improved long-term survival.

The exact cause of the selective improvement in surgical survival cannot be precisely determined but may be due to a number of reasons. Refinements in surgical technique may be the most important factor, including improved myocardial preservation, more complete coronary revascularization, improved

TABLE 5. Cox Model Analyses

	Unadjusted		Adjusted	
	Slope	*Chi Square**	*Slope*	*Chi Square**
All medical patients	−0.0385	10.57	0.0014	0.01
All surgical patients	−0.0986	48.75	−0.1148	58.05
Surgical survivors	−0.1060	27.80	−0.1222	33.80
Operative mortality	−0.0941	20.74	−0.1244	24.72

* Chi square > 3.84; p < 0.05.

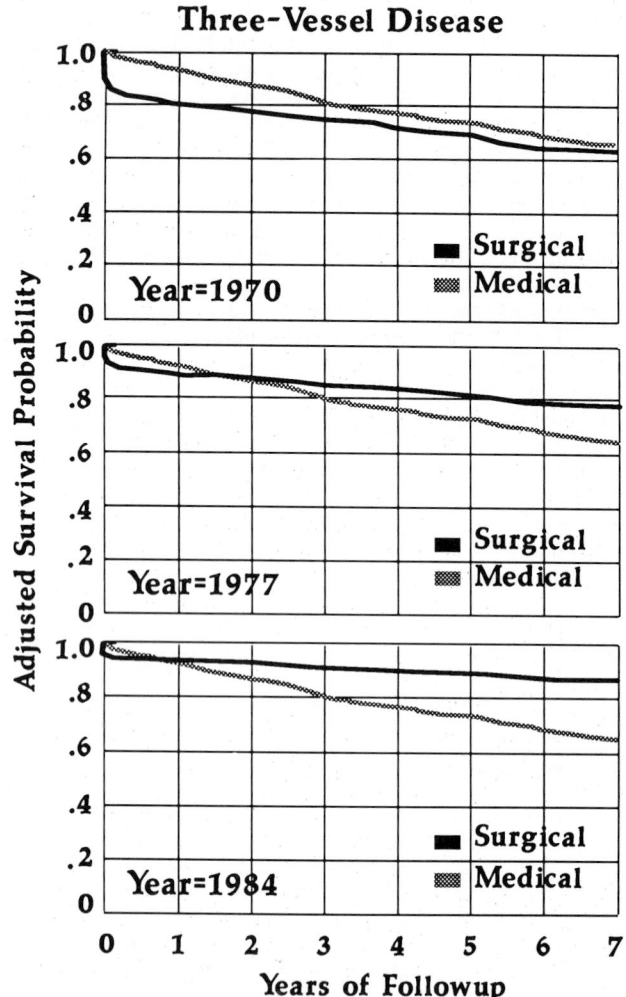

Three-Vessel Disease

Year=1970

■ Surgical
▦ Medical

Year=1977

■ Surgical
▦ Medical

Year=1984

■ Surgical
▦ Medical

Years of Followup

Figure 14. Estimated survival (adjusted Cox models) for medical and surgical patients with three-vessel disease treated in 1970, 1977, and 1984. (From Pryor, D. B., Harrell, F. E., Rankin, J. S., Lee, K. L., Muhlbaier, L. H., Oldham, H. N., Hlatky, M. A., Mark, D. B., Reves, J. G., and Califf, R. M.: The changing survival benefits of coronary revascularization over time. Circulation, 76(Suppl. V):V-13, 1987.)

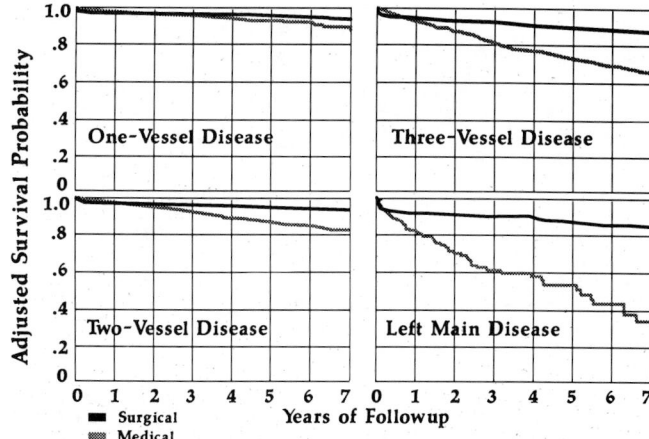

One-Vessel Disease

Three-Vessel Disease

Two-Vessel Disease

Left Main Disease

■ Surgical
▦ Medical

Years of Followup

Figure 15. Survival of patients treated medically or surgically in 1984 with one-vessel disease, two-vessel disease, three-vessel disease, and left main coronary artery disease. The survival curves are adjusted for all known important baseline characteristics. (From Califf, R. M., Harrell, F. E., Lee, K. L., Rankin, J. S., Hlatky, M. A., Mark, D. B., Jones, R. H., Muhlbaier, L. H., Oldham, H. N., and Pryor, D. B.: The evolution of medical and surgical therapy for coronary artery disease: A 15-year perspective. J.A.M.A., 261:2077, 1989.)

for patients having *either* elective CAB, ejection fraction greater than 0.40, *or* age less than 65 years, as described earlier, has been achieved. These current CAB results represent the standard with which PTCA must be compared.

Several retrospective analyses have examined the long-term results of PTCA versus CAB. Acinapura and associates in 1984 compared 198 single-vessel PTCA procedures with 143 patients undergoing single-vessel CAB.[1] Whereas long-term mortality in single-vessel disease was low in both groups (as expected), the incidence of acute myocardial infarction and symptomatic recurrence was significantly higher in PTCA patients. Similarly, an ingenious study design from the Mayo Clinic compared long-term results in 776 patients having successful PTCA with those observed in 146 patients requiring CAB for failed PTCA.[9] Anginal recurrence and event-free survival were significantly better in the CAB group despite similar entry criteria (Fig. 16). The more recent study from the Cleveland Clinic assessed long-term results in 781 patients with single-vessel disease having primary CAB or PTCA in the early 1980s.[31] Absolute survival (98 versus 95 per cent), event-free survival (93 versus 62 per cent), and the need for additional procedures was significantly better in the CAB group as compared with PTCA, consistent with other reports. At present, several randomized trials of PTCA versus CAB are under way but are likely to be fraught with the usual problems of unrepresentative patient selection and crossover. Nevertheless, future observational and randomized analyses should more clearly define the relative roles of PTCA versus CAB in the elective treatment of coronary disease. Both obviously will continue to have applications, and the goal should be conversion of currently competing therapies into complementary ones through scientific assessment.

In summary, a concept is emerging in the literature that the long-term results of primary PTCA will be significantly inferior to those achieved with contemporary CAB in stable and unstable forms of angina pectoris.[2,29] One might agree with Grüntzig[44] that until further long-term data are available, the currently accelerating enthusiasm for PTCA in complex forms of coronary disease should be assessed, and that the major application should be in patients at the prognostic ends of the spectrum. PTCA may be most useful in patients with severe symptoms from low-risk obstructions (such as single-vessel and mild double-vessel disease) that do not warrant CAB for prognostic reasons and in those at high risk for surgical intervention (patients with acute myocardial infarction, cardiogenic shock). It is hoped these issues will be clarified in coming years.

able. Recent enthusiasm for balloon dilation within the cardiology community has been accompanied by an increasing application to more complex forms of coronary artery disease and a dramatic increase in annual numbers of procedures. In many centers, PTCA now has become the most commonly applied invasive therapy for symptomatic coronary disease.[50] Whereas the initial results of PTCA have been considered acceptable by many, the major concern at present is long-term stability of revascularization. Significant restenosis occurs within the first year in up to 40 per cent of lesions, and both symptomatic recurrence and reintervention rates have been high during follow-up.

The impact of the PTCA trend on surgical practice has been significant, altering coronary artery bypass (CAB) patient profiles toward the higher-risk elderly population, and thus adversely influencing perioperative results to modest degrees.[12] Increasing numbers of patients requiring emergency CAB for failed PTCA have slightly increased overall surgical mortality and morbidity.[38] Simultaneously, the long-term results of CAB have become better defined. Because of steady improvements in surgical technique, a significant survival benefit now has been documented for patients undergoing CAB in the early 1980s, both in the overall coronary disease population and in all subgroups of multivessel/left main obstruction. With routine application of IMA grafting, results are continuing to improve for mid-1980s patients; a greater than 95 per cent 5-year survival

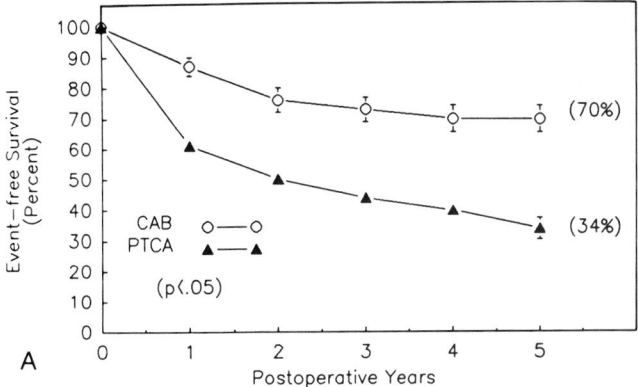

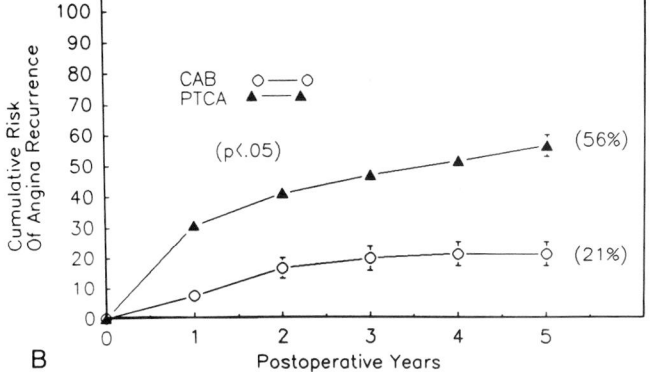

Figure 16. Event-free survival (A) and anginal recurrence (B) in patients having either PTCA or CABG for coronary disease. (From Connor, A. R., Vlietstra, R. E., Schaff, H. V., et al.: Early and late results of coronary artery bypass after failed angioplasty. J. Thorac. Cardiovasc. Surg., 96:191, 1988.)

Ventricular Septal Defect After Myocardial Infarction

Data obtained from postmortem studies indicate that 8 to 10 per cent of fatal cases of myocardial infarction are due to *rupture* of heart. In addition, infarction of the interventricular septum with subsequent formation of a ventricular septal defect causes death in 1 to 2 per cent of cases of acute myocardial infarction. The usual interval between the acute infarct and septal rupture is 4 to 12 days and correlates well with histologic findings of maximal cardiac muscle degeneration. When rupture has occurred, the prognosis is poor, as demonstrated in one series of 157 patients, of whom 24 per cent died on the first day after rupture, 65 per cent by the end of 2 weeks, and 81 per cent by 2 months. Only 7 per cent of these patients survived for a year.

This condition develops classically in a patient with myocardial infarction in whom shock or congestive heart failure suddenly occurs. A loud, holosystolic murmur is usually heard along the left sternal border, and two thirds of the patients demonstrate a palpable thrill. The differential diagnosis includes papillary muscle dysfunction, rupture of a papillary muscle with acute mitral insufficiency, and a pericardial friction rub secondary to myocardial infarction. Although clinical findings may be highly suggestive, the definitive diagnosis is made by cardiac catheterization and angiography. The oxygen saturation data classically demonstrate a left-to-right shunt at the ventricular level.

Since the natural history of the disease is dismal, surgical correction is indicated in nearly all cases with the possible exception of elderly patients with advanced multiorgan failure. In stable patients, it may be preferable to allow the infarct to heal, with operation deferred for 6 to 8 weeks. However, the condition of the patient usually does not permit delay, and early or even emergency operation should be the rule. An intra-aortic balloon pump is placed in most patients for stabilization while

an operating room is being prepared. Emergency coronary bypass and patch closure of the septal defect are then performed for preventing the consequences of intractable acute right ventricular overload and/or multiorgan failure.

The defects are often irregular, ragged tracts through the anterior apical septum with occlusion of the left anterior descending coronary artery or through the posterior septum in cases with right coronary occlusion. In the latter, right ventricular infarction may compound the problem. Multiple defects are present in approximately one third of patients. Cardiopulmonary bypass is instituted with bicaval cannulation, although a single right atrial cannula can be used for simple anterior defects. After cardioplegic arrest, an incision is made in the area of infarction, and good exposure of the interiors of both the left and right ventricles is obtained. A portion of the necrotic edge of the defect is resected, and a double patch technique is used for repair. For posterior defects, an identical procedure is performed with the apex elevated and the incision in the posterior interventricular groove. Coronary bypass grafts are constructed to all diseased vessels, including the right coronary artery in cases of right ventricular infarction. Fifty to 80 per cent of patients should survive the operative procedure, depending on the severity of preoperative shock and multiorgan failure.

REFERENCES

1. Acinapura, A. J., Cunningham, J. N., Jr., Jacobowitz, I. J., Rose, D. M., Kramer, M. D., Cappabianca, P., Elmquist, T. H., and Sanders, M.: Efficacy of percutaneous transluminal coronary angioplasty compared with single-vessel bypass. J. Thorac. Cardiovasc. Surg., 89:35, 1985.
2. Akins, C. W., Block, P. C., Palacious, I. F., Gold, H. K., Carroll, D. L., and Grunkemeier, G. L.: Comparison of coronary artery bypass grafting and percutaneous transluminal coronary angioplasty as initial treatment strategies. Ann. Thorac. Surg., 47:507, 1989.
3. Austin, E. H., Oldham, H. N., Jr., and Jones, R. H.: Early assessment of rest and exercise left ventricular function following coronary artery surgery. Ann. Thorac. Surg., 35:159, 1983.
4. Blankenhorn, D. H., Nessim, S. A., Johnson, R. L., Sanmarco, M. E., Azen, S. P., and Cashin-Hemphill, L.: Beneficial effects of combined colestipol-niacin therapy on coronary atherosclerosis and coronary venous bypass grafts. J.A.M.A., 257:3233, 1987.
5. Califf, R. M., Harrell, F. E., Lee, K. L., et al.: The evolution of medical and surgical therapy for coronary artery disease: A 15 year perspective. J.A.M.A., 261:2077, 1989.
6. Cameron, A., Davis, K. B., Green, G. E., et al.: Clinical implications of internal mammary artery bypass grafts: The Coronary Artery Surgery Study experience. Circulation, 77:815, 1988.
7. Carrel, A.: On the experimental surgery of the thoracic aorta and the heart. Ann. Surg., 52:83, 1910.
8. CASS Principal Investigators: Coronary artery bypass surgery: Survival data. Circulation, 68:939, 1983.
9. Connor, A., Vliestra, R. E., Schaff, H. V., et al.: Early and late results of coronary artery bypass after failed angioplasty. J. Thorac. Cardiovasc. Surg., 96:191, 1988.
10. Cosgrove, D. M., Amiot, D. M., and Meserko, J. J.: An improved technique for autotransfusion of shed mediastinal blood. Ann. Thorac. Surg., 40:519, 1985.
11. Cosgrove, D. M., Loop, F. D., Lytle, B. W., et al.: Predictors of reoperation after myocardial revascularization. J. Thorac. Cardiovasc. Surg., 92:811, 1986.
12. Davis, P. K., Parascandola, S. A., Miller, C. A., Campbell, D. B., Myers, J. L., Pae, W. E., Pierce, W. S., Wisman, C. B., and Waldhausen, J. A.: Mortality of coronary artery bypass grafting before and after the advent of angioplasty. Ann. Thorac. Surg., 47:493, 1989.
13. Dilsizian, V., Bonow, R. O., Cannon, R. O., Tracy, C. M., Vitale, D. F., McIntosh, C. L., Clark, R. E., Bacharach, S. L., and Green, M. V.: The effect of coronary artery bypass grafting on left ventricular systolic function at rest: Evidence for preoperative subclinical myocardial ischemia. Am. J. Cardiol., 61:1248, 1988.
14. Enos, W. F., Holmes, R. H., and Beyer, J.: Coronary disease among United States soldiers killed in action in Korea. Preliminary report. J.A.M.A., 152:1090, 1953.
15. European Coronary Surgery Study Group: Prospective randomized study of coronary artery bypass surgery in stable angina pectoris. Lancet, 2:491, 1980.
16. Ferraris, V. A., Ferraris, S. P., Lough, F. C., and Berry, W. R.: Preoperative aspirin ingestion increases operative blood loss after coronary artery bypass grafting. Ann. Thorac. Surg., 45:71, 1988.
17. Foster, E. D., Fisher, L. D., Kaiser, G. C., and Myers, W. O.: Comparison of operative mortality and morbidity for initial and repeat coronary artery bypass grafting: The Coronary Artery Surgery Study (CASS) registry experience. Ann. Thorac. Surg., 38:563, 1984.

18. Garrett, H. E., Dennis, E. W., and DeBakey, M. E.: Aortocoronary bypass with saphenous vein graft. J.A.M.A., 223:792, 1973.
19. Glower, D. D., Spratt, J. A., Snow, N. D., et al.: Linearity of the Frank-Starling relationship in the intact heart: The concept of preload recruitable stroke work. Circulation, 71:994, 1985.
20. Glower, D. D., Schaper, J., Kabas, J. S., et al.: Relation between reversal of diastolic creep and recovery of systolic function after ischemic myocardial injury in conscious dogs. Circ. Res., 60:859, 1987.
21. Goldman, S., Copeland, J., Moritz, T., Henderson, W., Zadina, K., Ovitt, T., Doherty, J., Reed, R., Chesler, E., Sako, Y., et al.: Saphenous vein graft patency 1 year after coronary artery bypass surgery and effects of antiplatelet therapy. Results of Veterans Administration Cooperative Study. Circulation, 80:1190, 1989.
22. Green, G. E., Stertzer, S. H., Gordon, R. B., and Tice, D. A.: Anastomosis of the internal mammary artery to the distal left anterior descending artery. Circulation, 41 and 42 (Suppl. II):I-79, 1970.
23. Grondon, C. M., Campeau, L., Lesperance, J., Enjalbert, M., and Bourassa, M. G.: Comparison of late changes in internal mammary artery and saphenous vein grafts in two consecutive series of patients 10 years after operation. Circulation, 70 (Suppl. I):I-208, 1984.
24. Grüntzig, A.: Transluminal dilatation of coronary-artery stenosis. Lancet, 1:263, 1978.
25. Hearse, D. J., Braimbridge, M. V., and Jynge, P.: Protection of the Ischemic Myocardium: Cardioplegia. New York, Raven Press, 1981.
26. Herrera, H. R., and Ginsberg, M. E.: The pectoralis major myocutaneous flap and omental transposition for closure of infected median sternotomy wounds. Plast. Reconstr. Surg., 70:465, 1982.
27. Herrick, J. B.: Clinical features of sudden obstruction of the coronary arteries. J.A.M.A., 59:2015, 1912.
28. Higgins, M. W., and Luepker, R. V. (Eds.): Trends in Coronary Heart Disease Mortality: The Influence of Medical Care. New York, Oxford University Press, 1988.
29. Hochberg, M. S., Gielchinsky, I., Parsonnet, V., Hussain, S. M., Mirsky, E., and Fisch, D.: Coronary angioplasty versus coronary bypass. Three-year follow-up of a matched series of 250 patients. J. Thorac. Cardiovasc. Surg., 97:496, 1989.
30. Johnson, W. D., Flemma, R. J., Lepley, D., Jr., and Ellison, E. H.: Extended treatment of severe coronary artery disease: A total surgical approach. Ann. Surg., 170:460, 1969.
31. Kramer, J. R., Proudfit, W. L., Loop, F. D., et al.: Late follow-up of 781 patients undergoing percutaneous transluminal coronary angioplasty or coronary artery bypass grafting for an isolated obstruction in the left anterior descending artery. Am. Heart J., 118:1144, 1989.
32. Loop, F. D., Lytle, B. W., Cosgrove, D. M., et al.: Influence of the internal mammary artery graft on 10-year survival and other cardiac events. N. Engl. J. Med., 314:1, 1986.
33. Lytle, B. W., Kramer, J. R., Golding, L. R., et al.: Young adults with coronary atherosclerosis: 10 year results of surgical myocardial revascularization. J. Am. Coll. Cardiol., 4:445, 1984.
34. Lytle, B. W., Loop, F. D., Cosgrove, D. M., Ratliff, N. B., Easley, K., and Taylor, P. C.: Long-term (5–12 years) serial studies of internal mammary artery and saphenous vein coronary bypass grafts. J. Thorac. Cardiovasc. Surg., 89:248, 1985.
35. Lytle, B. W., Loop, F. D., Cosgrove, D. M., et al.: Fifteen hundred coronary reoperations. J. Thorac. Cardiovasc. Surg., 93:847, 1987.
36. Maier, G. W., Owen, C. H., Feneley, M. P., et al.: The mechanical determinants of myocardial oxygen consumption in the conscious dog. Circulation, 73:II-67, 1988.
37. Murphy, M., Hultgren, H., Detre, K., et al.: Treatment of chronic stable angina. A preliminary report of survival data of the Randomized Veterans Administration Cooperative Study. N. Engl. J. Med., 297:621, 1977.
38. Parsonnet, V., Fisch, D., Gielchinsky, I., Kochberg, M., Hussain, S. M., Karanam, R., Rothfeld, L., and Klapp, L.: Emergency operation after failed angioplasty. J. Thorac. Cardiovasc. Surg., 96:198, 1988.
39. Proudfit, W. L., Bruschke, A. V. G., and Sones, F. M., Jr.: Natural history of obstructive coronary artery disease. Ten year study of obstructive coronary artery disease: Ten-year study of 601 non-surgical cases. Progr. Cardiovasc. Dis., 21:53, 1978.
40. Pryor, D. B., Harrell, F. E., Rankin, J. S., et al.: The changing survival benefits of coronary revascularization over time. Circulation, 76:V-13, 1987.
41. Rankin, J. S., Newman, G. E., Muhbaier, L. H., et al.: The effects of coronary revascularization on left ventricular function in ischemic heart disease. J. Thorac. Cardiovasc. Surg., 90:818, 1985.
42. Rankin, J. S., Newman, G. E., Bashore, T. M., et al.: Clinical and angiographic assessment of complex mammary artery bypass grafting. J. Thorac. Cardiovasc. Surg., 92:832, 1986.
43. Rankin, J. S., and Smith, L. R.: Utilization of the internal mammary arteries for coronary artery bypass. In Sabiston, D. C., Jr., and Spencer, F. C. (Eds.): Gibbon's Surgery of the Chest, 5th ed. Philadelphia, W. B. Saunders Company, 1989.
44. Roubin, G., and Grüntzig, A.: The coronary artery bypass surgery-angioplasty interface. Cardiology, 73:269, 1986.
45. Sabiston, D. C., Jr.: The coronary circulation. The William F. Reinhoff, Jr. Lecture. Johns Hopkins Med. J., 134:314, 1974.
46. Snellen, H. A.: A Disorder of the Breast. Rotterdam, Kooyker Scientific Publications, 1976.
47. Solymoss, B. C., Nadeau, P., Millette, D., and Campeau, L.: Late thrombosis of saphenous vein coronary bypass grafts related to risk factors. Circulation, 78:I140, 1988.
48. Squire, J.: The Structural Basis of Muscular Contraction. New York, Plenum Press, 1981.
49. Weinstein, M. C., Coxson, P. G., Williams, L. W., et al.: Forecasting coronary heart disease incidence, mortality, and cost: The coronary heart disease policy model. Am. J. Public Health, 77:1417, 1987.
50. Weintraub, W. S., Jones, E. L., King, S. B., et al.: Changing use of coronary angioplasty and coronary bypass surgery in the treatment of chronic coronary artery disease. Am. J. Cardiol., 65:183, 1990.

1. SURGICAL MANAGEMENT OF FAILED ANGIOPLASTY

Peter Van Trigt, M.D.

Percutaneous transluminal coronary angioplasty (PTCA) has gained increasing popularity as primary treatment for coronary atherosclerotic heart disease. Since 1977, when PTCA was an investigational technique in humans,[11] the number of procedures performed has dramatically increased. It is estimated that more than 400,000 PTCA procedures will be performed in 1990.[22]

The development of PTCA as a therapeutic modality has been associated with a concomitant rise in the need for emergency surgical myocardial revascularization for acute coronary angioplasty failure. Emergency coronary artery bypass grafting (CABG) in the setting of acute myocardial ischemia secondary to vessel dissection, thrombosis, or spasm causes significant morbidity and definite mortality. It is reasonable to assume that mortality and morbidity from failed angioplasty increase as the procedure is extended to patients with multivessel disease and more complex lesions. This progression appears inevitable, even though a decline in the need for emergency CABG has been documented as experience with angioplasty is acquired. The current incidence of failed PTCA requiring emergency CABG is reported at 4 to 5 per cent by most centers performing high-volume angioplasty.[5,6,18]

This discussion reviews the role of CABG following failed PTCA and examines determinants of risk in this patient population. Strategies to minimize ischemic injury to the myocardium after failed coronary angioplasty are also outlined.

Predictors of Acute Closure Following Coronary Angioplasty

Percutaneous transluminal coronary angioplasty utilizes intracoronary balloon inflation to approximately four atmospheres of pressure to produce localized trauma to the coronary artery wall; the intended result is atheroma fracture and arterial expansion that produce an increase in luminal area. Unfortunately, balloon inflation or guidewire and catheter manipulation can cause more extensive arterial wall damage with medial dissection and creation of an occlusive intimal flap. Thrombosis and spasm may also occur at the dilation site. In the absence of a well-developed collateral circulation, acute coronary occlusion causes severe myocardial ischemia and evolving myocardial infarction.

In a review of approximately 5000 PTCA procedures at Emory between 1982 and 1986,[7] a multivariate analysis found seven independent predictors of increased risk of vessel closure during PTCA: (1) stenosis length of two or more luminal diameters, (2) female gender, (3) stenosis at a bend point of the vessel, (4) stenosis at a branch point, (5) thrombus at the site of stenosis, (6) other stenoses in the same vessel, and (7) multivessel disease. The authors emphasize that although an estimation of risk for vessel closure can be made prior to PTCA, the most powerful

TABLE 1. Techniques to Minimize Ischemic Injury After Failed PTCA

Within Catheterization Laboratory

Coronary vasodilators
Intracoronary thrombolytic therapy
Repeat balloon inflations
Prolonged balloon inflation with perfusion balloon catheter
Reperfusion catheter placed across lesion
Insertion of intra-aortic balloon pump

Within Operating Room

Expeditious placement on cardiopulmonary bypass
Systemic hypothermia
Hyperkalemic hypothermic cardioplegic arrest
Internal mammary artery or saphenous vein bypass grafts
Rapid revascularization

predictors can be assessed only during the procedure (intimal tear following PTCA, persistent stenosis or gradient following PTCA, requirement for prolonged heparin infusion following angioplasty).

If coronary occlusion occurs, recrossing the occluded segment and repeating balloon inflation or using intracoronary thrombolytic or vasodilator agents can occasionally re-establish coronary artery patency and relieve ischemia (Table 1). However, prolonged maneuvers to this end are absolutely contraindicated since they inevitably delay emergency surgical revascularization. Rapid surgical revascularization after failed PTCA is the *only option* to reduce the associated mortality and morbidity.

Use of the Reperfusion Catheter and Intra-aortic Balloon Pump

The intracoronary reperfusion catheter has been introduced as a means of sustaining coronary flow past an occlusion following failed angioplasty.[8,12] The device is a 4.3-French catheter with 30 side holes over its distal 10 cm. and can maintain vessel flow in patients awaiting emergency coronary bypass surgery after failed coronary angioplasty. This causes reversal of active myocardial ischemia and can significantly contribute to clinical stabilization of the patient, allowing transport of the patient to the operating room under more controlled conditions. The utility of the reperfusion catheter to maintain coronary flow through a vessel closed during PTCA is illustrated in Figures 1 to 3. A pre-angioplasty arteriogram is shown in Figure 1 demonstrating a 95 per cent right ostial lesion. The angioplasty caused

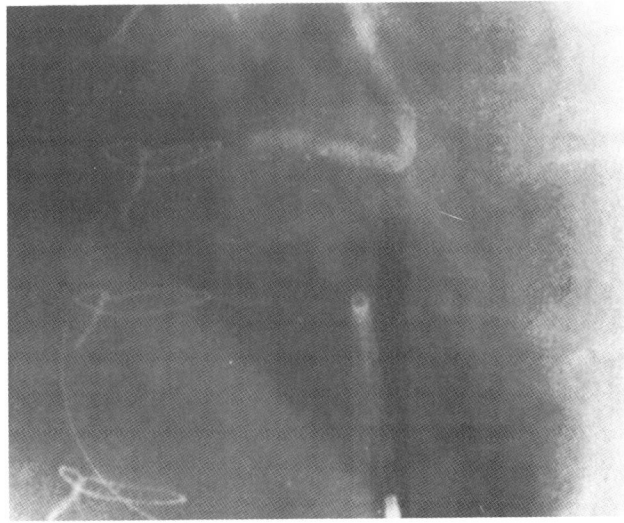

Figure 2. Angiogram made after angioplasty. The right coronary artery was dissected, which caused total distal occlusion.

dissection of the right coronary artery as shown in Figure 2. After placement of the reperfusion catheter across the lesion, blood flow is restored to the ischemic myocardium as demonstrated in Figure 3. Electrocardiographic changes after successful placement of a reperfusion catheter following PTCA and closure of a left anterior discending lesion are shown in Figure 4. Re-establishment of coronary flow through the reperfusion catheter and reduction of the duration of acute occlusion have a direct influence on reducing the extent of myocardial infarction that occurs in 30 to 40 per cent of angioplasty failures despite successful later surgical revascularization.[19,20] Reversal of acute ischemia also allows time to harvest the internal mammary artery for use in surgical revascularization.[8,9,14] An additional advantage of the reperfusion catheter is that cardioplegia can be delivered through the device after aortic cross-clamping directly to ischemic myocardium. The reperfusion catheter is then withdrawn through the aortic cross clamp, into the descending thoracic aorta, and then out the femoral artery sheath.

Routine use of the intra-aortic balloon pump following failed PTCA was advocated in two studies[2,17] published in 1984. The intra-aortic balloon pump was applied to patients with ST segment elevation following PTCA failure, and this intervention reduced the eventual development of Q wave infarction follow-

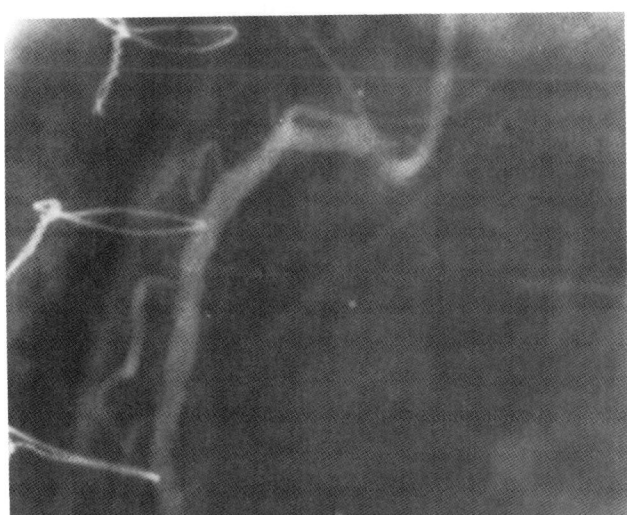

Figure 1. Angiogram made before angioplasty demonstrating 95 per cent ostial lesion of the right coronary artery.

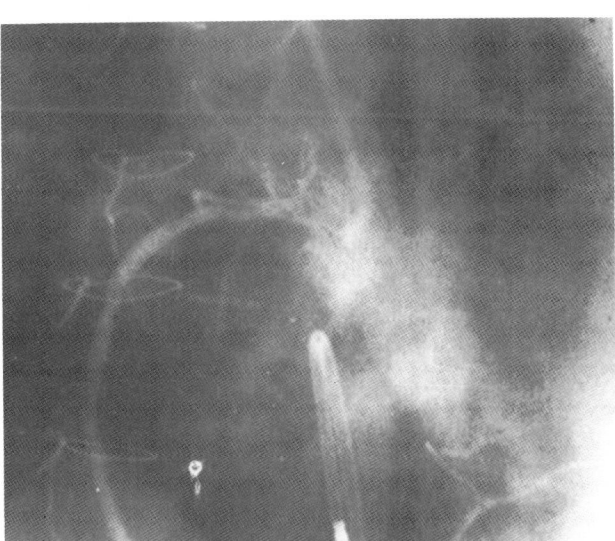

Figure 3. Angiogram performed after placement of the reperfusion catheter across the lesion. Blood flow was restored to the ischemic myocardium.

Pre PTCA

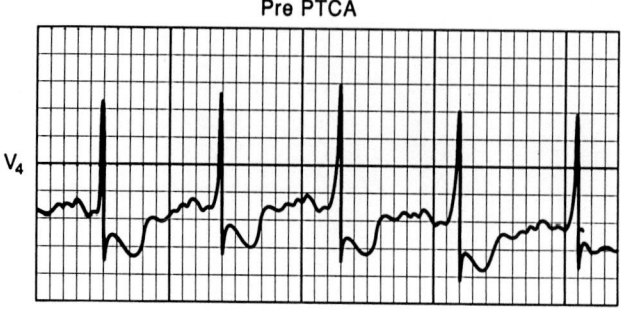

During Occlusion

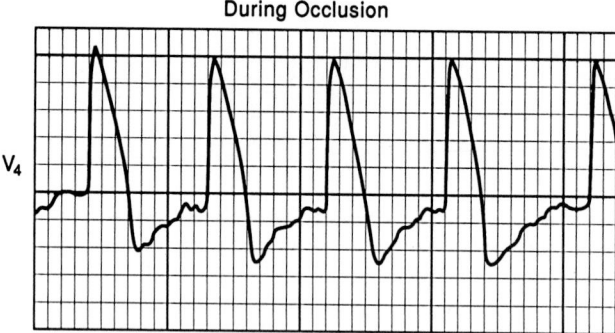

With RPC

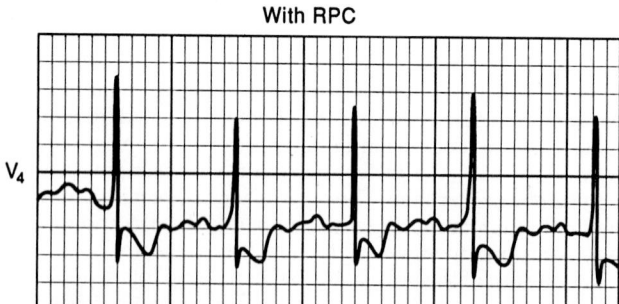

Figure 4. Total occlusion of the left anterior descending coronary artery following PTCA in lead V$_4$. Top, before PTCA; middle, during total occlusion; bottom, after placement of reperfusion catheter.

ing emergency CABG (however, not a statistically significant reduction). Despite these reports, intra-aortic balloon pumping has not been used routinely in subsequent reports of management of angioplasty failure, with its role limited to patients with hemodynamic instability. Balloon insertion does not greatly alter blood flow through diastolic augmentation to infarcting muscle, nor does afterload reduction reduce injury to ischemic, non-reperfused myocardium. If hemodynamic instability exists, then balloon insertion should be performed expeditiously with efforts directed toward the *main* priority of surgical revascularization.[4]

Surgical Considerations

When the patient leaves the catheterization laboratory, with or without a reperfusion catheter or intra-aortic balloon pump, expeditious placement on cardiopulmonary bypass with systemic cooling is the primary goal (Table 1). By converting the heart from a normothermic ejecting environment to a hypothermic empty beating state, oxygen demands are reduced significantly. The internal thoracic artery should be harvested if the patient has been stable and shows no evidence of ischemia by electrocardiographic or other clinical criteria. This can be readily

done after the patient is placed on cardiopulmonary bypass and the myocardial oxygen demands are minimized. In the Duke University Medical Center series of surgically treated angioplasty failures, the internal mammary artery was harvested and used as a graft conduit in 50 per cent of patients.[9]

Hypothermic hyperkalemic cardioplegia is then delivered into the aortic root through the reperfusion catheter if one has been placed in the catheterization laboratory. In the situation in which multiple grafts are required and no reperfusion catheter has been inserted preoperatively, the vessel occluded during PTCA should be the first vessel grafted, the cardioplegia delivered through the vein graft following distal coronary anastomosis.

In approximately 10 per cent of patients with angioplasty failure and acute coronary occlusion, the vessel has sustained a distal dissection, which requires special technical considerations. Extreme care is necessary in performing the arteriotomy, which when possible should be placed distal to the hematoma surrounding the vessel. If the arteriotomy must be placed through the dissection owing to a small distal vessel, delivery of cardioplegia as the opening is performed provides assistance in identifying the true lumen. Intracoronary probes should be avoided, and the vessel dissection is repaired in the course of performing the distal anastomosis by careful reapproximation of the intima to the media and adventitial layers of the coronary vessel.

In patients with multivessel coronary disease, other *major* vessels with greater than 50 per cent stenosis documented by preoperative catheterization should be grafted at the time of operation.

Mortality and Morbidity Associated with Emergency CABG After Failed Angioplasty

Most recent series of coronary angioplasty document an early failure rate of approximately 4 to 5 per cent. This contrasts remarkably to a 14 per cent incidence of emergency CABG required for PTCA failure in Grüntzig's first 50 patients.[11] Despite improved strategies that have been developed in managing patients with acute myocardial ischemia following PTCA failure (intracoronary thrombolysis, reperfusion catheter placement), the operative mortality, although less than 5 per cent, is still approximately three times the mortality for elective CABG at most centers.[1,10,15,27] Just as significant is a perioperative infarction incidence of over 30 per cent (Table 2). This infarction rate is consistent in nearly all series, despite successful surgical revascularization of the vessel occluded during PTCA.[24] This appears to be the result of the necessary time (approximately 120 minutes) required to transport the patient from the catheterization laboratory to the operating room, place the patient on cardiopulmonary bypass, and establish surgical revascularization. Golding[10] noted that if ischemia was present on the pre-surgical electrocardiogram following failed PTCA, the postoperative myocardial infarction rate was 57 per cent. In those patients without ischemia, the rate of perioperative infarction was reduced to 10 per cent. In 10 patients in whom cardiopulmonary bypass was established within 25 minutes of the onset of symptoms following PTCA failure, Reul and associates reported no perioperative deaths or infarctions.[21] The predictors of operative mortality in patients undergoing emergency CABG for failed PTCA include prior coronary bypass surgery, presence of multiple vessel disease, and cardiogenic shock.[15]

The effect of vessel closure requiring emergency CABG after elective coronary angioplasty versus emergent PTCA for acute myocardial infarction was reviewed at Duke University Medical Center.[9] Between 1984 and 1986, 1350 angioplasties were performed, 393 of these for acute myocardial infraction. Twenty-one patients (Group I) required emergency CABG following unsuccessful elective PTCA (failure rate 2.2 per cent), and 32 patients (Group II) underwent emergency CABG following un-

TABLE 2. Emergency Revascularization for Failed Angioplasty

Author	Years of Study	Year Reported	Number	Operative Mortality (%)	Perioperative Infarction
Talley	1980–1986	1989	202	5(2.5)	27.0%
Ferguson	1984–1986	1988	18	0(0.0)	23.8%
Barner	1986–1987	1989	31	1(3.2)	48.4%
Naunheim	1984–1987	1989	79	4(5.1)	35.9%
Golding	1981–1985	1986	79	0(0.0)	44.3%
Page	1981–1985	1985	26	2(7.7)	22.2%
Killen	1980–1984	1985	75	3(4.0)	43.5%
Pellitier	1980–1983	1985	30	0(0.0)	28.6%
Akins	1978–1983	1984	11	0(0.0)	9.1%
Cowley	1977–1982	1984	202	13(6.4)	41.0%
Murphy	1981–1983	1984	32	0(0.0)	53.0%
Reul	1979–1983	1984	63	1(1.4)	30.0%
Total			848	29(3.5%)	33.9%

successful emergent angioplasty (failure rate 8.1 per cent). All patients treated in Group II received thrombolytic therapy, and a reperfusion catheter was used in over half the patients in each group. There was no difference in mortality between the groups (4.7 per cent following elective PTCA failure versus 6.2 per cent following emergency PTCA failure, p = NS), and half of the patients in each group required postoperative inotropic support. The incidence of perioperative myocardial infarction was 24 per cent in Group I and 34 per cent in Group II. The internal mammary artery was used for grafting in 50 per cent of patients in each group, and both groups had similar bypass times and number of vessels bypassed. Hemorrhagic complications were significantly greater in the emergent PTCA failure group, in which 15.6 per cent of patients required re-exploration for bleeding versus none in Group I. The effects of thrombolytic therapy have been shown to affect operative morbidity up to 12 hours following administration.[16] This study concludes that emergency CABG can be performed when necessary in the setting of emergent failed PTCA with results comparable to CABG following failed elective angioplasty.

The in-hospital mortality and morbidity of patients who had failed elective PTCA and then underwent emergent or elective CABG was reviewed in a large series of 316 patients from Emory University between 1980 and 1986.[27] Emergency coronary bypass surgery was performed in 202 (64 per cent) of the patients with a 2.5 per cent operative mortality and a 27 per cent perioperative incidence of myocardial infarction. The internal mammary artery was used in only 20 per cent of the emergency CABG patients, and the intra-aortic balloon pump was used preoperatively in 24 per cent of the patients. These clinical parameters in the emergency CABG group were compared with 114 patients who underwent elective surgical revascularization following failed PTCA during the same hospitalization (Table 3). Although operative mortality in the elective CABG group was not statistically different from the elective CABG group, the perioperative myocardial infarction incidence was only 4 per cent in the patients requiring elective surgical revascularization.

The experience of the Cleveland Clinic in the surgical management of failed coronary angioplasty was reported in 1986.[10] Between 1981 and 1985, 81 patients required emergency surgi-

cal revascularization within 24 hours of failed PTCA (4.4 per cent of the total PTCA population). There were two early deaths in the series (2.5 per cent mortality) and a 43 per cent incidence of perioperative myocardial infarction. A significantly higher incidence of postoperative complications was encountered in this group of patients (Table 4) compared with a group of patients undergoing elective revascularization during the same time period.

A possible late complication of percutaneous coronary angioplasty not reported in other series was noted by Killen and associates in 1985.[15] In a group of 286 patients undergoing coronary bypass grafting for restenosis following PTCA, 7 patients had documented occurrence of severe left main stenosis during the interval between the initial PTCA and subsequent CABG. In 6 of the 7 patients, the interval was less than 1 year, and in 4 patients less than 6 months passed between the time of angioplasty and development of left main stenosis. The authors postulate that PTCA manipulations through the left main coronary artery cause arterial damage that leads to development of coronary stenosis. In each of the patients who developed left main stenosis, lesions in the left coronary arterial tree had been dilated but disease in the left main coronary artery at that time was only minimal. The mechanism may be similar to one that has been postulated in the evolution of left main coronary stenosis following cannulation and direct perfusion of the left coronary artery at the time of aortic valve replacement.

Newer percutaneous interventional techniques to treat coronary stenoses in an early stage of development include the coronary balloon laser[23] and the atherectomy catheter or transluminal extraction catheter, which mechanically removes plaque from the diseased coronary artery.[25,26] The use of laser devices in peripheral arteries has historically been associated with a relatively high rate of perforation and reocclusion, and these problems need to be resolved before application to the coronary circulation. Experience has been gained with the atherectomy catheter in a few centers, with early series reporting an 80 to 90 per cent early success rate in reduction of coronary stenosis.[13] These devices (Simpson atherectomy catheter, transluminal extraction catheter) can injure the coronary vessel wall with the cutting blade, causing the previously discussed complications

TABLE 3. Surgical Management of Failed PTCA (Emory)

Clinical Characteristics	Total Population (%)	Emergency CABG (%)	Elective CABG (%)	p
Patients	316	202	114	
Intra-aortic balloon pump	50(16)	48(24)	2(2)	<0.05
Internal mammary artery	75(24)	39(20)	36(32)	<0.05
Inotropic therapy	106(34)	84(42)	22(20)	<0.05

TABLE 4. Emergency CABG After Failed PTCA: Postoperative Morbidity (Cleveland Clinic)

	Emergency CABG (n = 81)	Elective CABG (n = 5000)
Myocardial infarction	43%	0.7%
Postoperative hemorrhage	11%	3.5%
Postoperative respiratory failure	9%	2.5%

associated with PTCA (dissection, thrombosis, and spasm) as well as distal embolization of atheromatous debris or actual perforation of the vessel wall. Emergency surgical revascularization in the setting of vessel perforation must consider the likelihood of cardiac tamponade. In order to allow safe transport to the operating room, a pericardial catheter may be required to decompress the pericardium, or, alternatively, the perforated vessel may require occlusion with a balloon catheter until surgical control of the site of bleeding. Still to be addressed is a high incidence of restenosis (greater than 30 per cent) in those patients undergoing percutaneous removal of atheroma.

Management of the patient who has sustained a failed coronary angioplasty and requires emergent CABG requires careful attention to strategies to minimize myocardial ischemia following vessel closure before surgical revascularization can be accomplished. Of paramount importance is rapid surgical revascularization, which requires well-coordinated cardiac anesthesia and surgical services working with the cardiac catheterization laboratory. Current experience has shown that operative mortality can be reduced to a low level (although not equivalent to elective surgical coronary mortality). However, the in-hospital morbidity remains quite high, specifically, a perioperative myocardial infarction rate of approximately 30 per cent. Further attempts to reduce this rate of perioperative infarction must involve intervention techniques to restore perfusion to the ischemic region preoperatively or to protect the myocardium from injuries associated with reperfusion.[3]

SELECTED REFERENCES

Barner, H. B., Lea, J. W., IV, Naunheim, K. S., and Stoney, W. S., Jr.: Emergency coronary bypass not associated with preoperative cardiogenic shock in failed angioplasty, after thrombolysis, and for acute myocardial infarction. Circulation, 79(Suppl. I):I-152, 1989.
The authors present an excellent literature review of emergent coronary bypass surgery for failed coronary angioplasty. A detailed review of the factors responsible for a high perioperative myocardial infarction rate is presented. Discussion is also directed to additional strategies that can be followed to reduce myocardial ischemia in these patients.

Ferguson, T. B., Muhlbaier, L. H., Salai, D. L., and Wechsler, A. S.: Coronary bypass grafting after failed elective and failed emergent percutaneous angioplasty—relative risks of emergent surgical intervention. J. Thorac. Cardiovasc. Surg., 95:761, 1988.
The authors compared clinical outcome of patients requiring emergency coronary artery bypass grafting (CABG) following failed angioplasty in the setting of elective PTCA (21 patients) versus PTCA for acute myocardial infarction (32 patients). All patients in the acute myocardial infarction group received thrombolytic therapy, and a reperfusion catheter was used in over half the patients in each group. The internal mammary artery was used as a conduit in 50 per cent of patients in each group. The operative mortality was no different in the two groups (5 per cent), and the perioperative myocardial infarction rates were also not significantly different. The authors conclude that emergency CABG can be performed in the setting of failed emergent PTCA with results comparable to coronary bypass after failed elective PTCA.

Talley, J. D., Jones, E. L., Weintraub, W. S., and King, S. B., III: Coronary artery bypass surgery after failed elective percutaneous transluminal coronary angioplasty. Circulation, 79(Suppl. I):I-126, 1989.
A large series of 316 patients from Emory University were reviewed who underwent emergent or elective CABG between 1980 and 1986. The majority (64 per cent) of the patients underwent emergency CABG with a perioperative mortality of 2.5 per cent and a perioperative infarction rate of 27 per cent. Although the operative mortality in the elective CABG group was not significantly different from the elective CABG group, the perioperative infarction rate was only 4 per cent in the patients having elective surgical revascularization. The authors emphasize

that rapid successful surgical revascularization after a failed PTCA is the main determinant in reducing in-hospital complications.

REFERENCES

1. Akins, C. W.: Early and late results following emergency myocardial revascularization during hypothermic fibrillatory arrest. Ann. Thorac. Surg., 43:131, 1987
2. Akins, C. W., and Block, P. C.: Surgical intervention for failed percutaneous transluminal coronary angioplasty. Am. J. Cardiol., 53:108C, 1984.
3. Allen, B. S., Okamoto, F., Buckberg, G. D., Bugyi, H., Young, H., Leaf, J., Beyersdorf, F., Sjostrand, F., and Maloney, J. V., Jr.: Immediate functional recovery after six hours of regional ischemia by careful control of conditions of reperfusion and composition of reperfusate. J. Thorac. Cardiovasc. Surg., 92:621, 1986.
4. Barner, H. B., Lea, J. W., IV, Naunheim, K. S., and Stoney, W. S., Jr.: Emergency coronary bypass not associated with preoperative cardiogenic shock in failed angioplasty, after thrombolysis, and for acute myocardial infarction. Circulation, 79(Suppl. I):I-152, 1989.
5. Cowley, M. J., Dorros, G., Kelsey, S. F., Raden, M. V., and Detre, K. M.: Emergency coronary bypass surgery after coronary angioplasty: The National Heart, Lung, and Blood Institute's percutaneous transluminal coronary angioplasty registry experience. Am. J. Cardiol., 53:22C, 1984.
6. Detre, K., Holubkov, R., Kelsey, S., et al.: Percutaneous transluminal coronary angioplasty in 1985–1986 and 1977–1981. The National Heart, Lung, and Blood Institute Registry. N. Engl. J. Med., 318:265, 1988.
7. Ellis, S. G., Roubin, G. S., King, S. B., III, Douglas, J. S., Jr., Weintraub, W. S., Thomas, R. G., and Cox, W. R.: Angiographic and clinical predictors of acute closure after native vessel coronary angioplasty. Circulation, 77:372, 1988.
8. Ferguson, T. B., Hinohara, T., Simpson, J., Stack, R. S., and Wechsler, A. S.: Catheter reperfusion to allow optimal coronary bypass grafting following failed coronary angioplasty. Ann. Thorac. Surg., 42:399, 1986.
9. Ferguson, T.B., Muhlbaier, L. H., Salai, D. L., and Wechsler, A. S.: Coronary bypass grafting after failed elective and failed emergent percutaneous angioplasty. J. Thorac. Cardiovasc. Surg., 95:761, 1988.
10. Golding, L. A. R., Loop, F. D., Hollman, J. L., Franco, I., Borsh, J., Stewart, R. W., and Lytle, B. W.: Early results of emergency surgery after coronary angioplasty. Circulation, 74(Suppl. III):III-26, 1986.
11. Grüntzig, A. R., Senning, A., and Siegenthaler, W. E.: Nonoperative dilatation of coronary-artery stenosis: Percutaneous transluminal coronary angioplasty. N. Engl. J. Med., 301:61, 1979.
12. Hinohara, T., Simpson, J. B., Phillips, H. R., and Stack, R. S.: Transluminal intracoronary reperfusion catheter: A device to maintain coronary perfusion between failed coronary angioplasty and emergency coronary bypass surgery. J. Am. Coll. Cardiol., 11:977, 1988.
13. Kaufmann, U. P., Garratt, K. N., Vlietstra, R. E., Menke, K. K., and Holmes, D. R., Jr.: Coronary atherectomy: First 50 patients at the Mayo Clinic. Mayo Clin. Proc., 64:747, 1989.
14. Kereiakas, J. R.: Emergent internal thoracic artery grafting following failed PTCA. Am. Heart J., 113:1018, 1987.
15. Killen, D. A., Hamaker, W. R., and Reed, W. A.: Coronary artery bypass following percutaneous transluminal coronary angioplasty. Ann. Thorac. Surg., 40:133, 1985.
16. Lee, K. F., Mandell, J., Rankin, J. S., Muhlbaier, L. H., and Wechsler, A. S.: Immediate versus delayed coronary grafting after streptokinase treatment. J. Thorac. Cardiovasc. Surg., 95:216, 1988.
17. Murphy, D. A., Craver, J. M., Jones, E. L., et al.: Surgical management of acute myocardial ischemia following percutaneous transluminal coronary angioplasty: Role of the intra-aortic balloon pump. J. Thorac. Cardiovasc. Surg., 87:332, 1984.
18. Naunheim, K. S. Fiore, A. C., Fagan, D. C., McBride, L. R., Barner, H. B., Pennington, D. G., Willman, V. L., Kern, M. J., Deligonul, U., Vandormael, M. C., and Kaiser, G. C.: Emergency coronary artery bypass grafting for failed angioplasty: Risk factors and outcome. Ann. Thorac. Surg., 47:816, 1989.
18a. Page, W. S., Okies J. E., Colburn, L. Q., et al.: Percutaneous transluminal angioplasty: A growing surgical problem. J. Thorac. Cardiovasc. Surg., 92:847, 1985.
19. Pellitier, L. C., Pardini, A., Renkin, J., David, P. R., Hebert, Y., and Bourassa, M. G.: Myocardial revascularization after failure of percutaneous transluminal coronary angioplasty. J. Thorac. Cardiovasc. Surg., 90:265, 1985.
20. Phillips, S. J., Kongtahworn, C., Zeff, R. H., Skinner, J. R., Toon, R. S., Grignon, A., Spector, M., and Iannone, L. A.: Disrupted coronary artery caused by

angioplasty: Supportive and surgical considerations. Ann. Thorac. Surg. 47:880, 1989.

21. Reul, G. J., Cooley, D. A., Hallman, G. L., Duncan, J. M., Livesay, J. J., Frazier, O. H., Ott, D. A., Angelini, P., Massumi, A., and Mathur, V. S.: Coronary artery bypass for unsuccessful percutaneous transluminal coronary angioplasty. J. Thorac. Cardiovasc. Surg., 88:685, 1984.

22. Ryan, T. J., et al.: Guidelines for percutaneous transluminal coronary angioplasty. J. Am. Coll. Cardiol., 12:529, 1988.

23. Spears, J. R., Reyes, V., Sinclair, I. N., Hopkins B., Schwartz, L., Aldridge, H., and Plokker, H. W. T.: Percutaneous coronary laser balloon angioplasty: Preliminary results of a multicenter trial. J. Am. Coll. Cardiol., 13(Suppl. A):61A, 1988.

24. Spencer, F. C.: A critique of emergency and urgent operations for complications of coronary artery disease. Circulation, 79(Suppl. 1):I-160, 1989.

25. Stack, R. S.: New interventional technologies in cardiology. Mayo Clin. Proc., 64:867, 1989.

26. Stack, R. S., Califf, R. M., Phillips, H. R., Pryor, D. B., Quigley, P. J., Bauman, R. P., Tcheng, J. E., and Greenfield, J. C., Jr.: Interventional cardiac catheterization at Duke Medical Center. Am. J. Cardiol., 62:3F, 1988.

27. Talley, J. D., Jones E. L., Weintraub, W. S., and King, S. B., III: Coronary artery bypass surgery after failed elective percutaneous transluminal coronary angioplasty. Circulation, 79(Suppl. I):I-126, 1989.

2. REOPERATION FOR CORONARY BYPASS

George S. Tyson, M.D.

The introduction of coronary bypass grafting into clinical practice over 2 decades ago provided direct revascularization of the coronary circulation. Based on the success in early series, widespread use of this procedure achieved symptomatic relief in large numbers of patients and increased longevity in certain subgroups.[3,17] Despite rapid improvements in the *operative* mortality, delayed failure of the operation was recognized early in the experience. Coronary angiography, performed after the recurrence of anginal symptoms, demonstrated the phenomenon of graft failure and the necessity for a second operation (Fig. 1). By 1972, repeat operation for coronary bypass grafting was a sufficiently common experience to allow series of patients to be reported.[1,18]

Since that time, both the patient population undergoing coronary artery bypass grafting and the procedure have been in a state of almost constant change. The effect of this evolution on the need for second and subsequent revascularization proce-

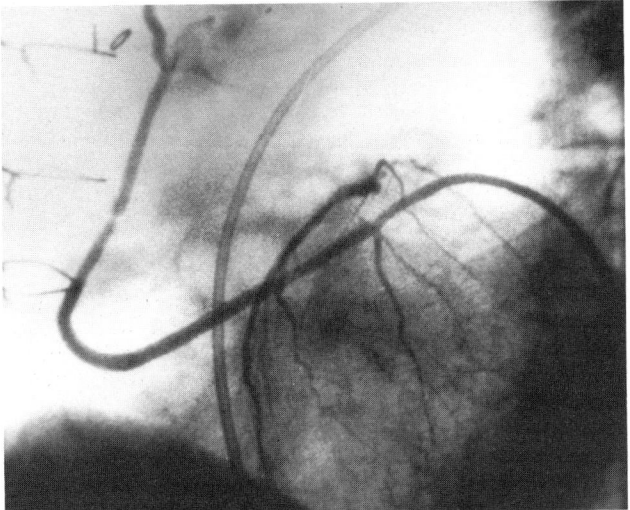

Figure 1. Coronary angiogram in a patient who developed recurrent angina accompanied by ischemic electrocardiographic changes across the precordium. His first operation 6 years previously had consisted of a single sequential saphenous vein graft. A tight stenosis can be seen in the body of the graft. He underwent successful reoperation using a left internal mammary graft to the anterior descending coronary in combination with multiple vein grafts.

TABLE 1. Incidence of Reoperation for Coronary Bypass

	Annual Incidence (%)	Cumulative Incidence (%)
5 yr.	1.1	2.7
10 yr.	3.2	11.4
12 yr.	3.9	17.3
15 yr.	—	38

Based on the Cleveland Clinic Experience.[9,24]

dures has been well documented in a series of reports from the Cleveland Clinic.[9,24,25,28] Whereas the interval between the first and second operation has continued to lengthen, the number of second operations has increased dramatically, both on an absolute basis and as a percentage of operations performed. Among patients at risk (Table 1), the annual incidence of reoperation increases from 1.1 per cent at 5 years after the first operation to 3.9 per cent at 12 years. As a consequence, the cumulative incidence reaches an astounding 38 per cent by the fifteenth postoperative year.[24] This inexorable increase in the incidence of second operations has occurred despite improved operative techniques, a clear trend toward complete revascularization at the initial procedure, and expanded use of the internal mammary graft.

The changing demographics of coronary artery disease as well as further advances in coronary surgery and invasive cardiology may alter this incidence. However, the number of primary operations performed over the past decade has produced an enormous number of patients at risk for coronary reoperation. Thus, the incidence of coronary reoperations will remain very high for the foreseeable future.

PATHOLOGY

Early graft closure generally has been attributed to thrombosis secondary to technical error, damage to the vein graft during preparation, or grafting a vessel with inadequate run-off. Late graft failure, particularly beyond 5 years, occurs most frequently as a result of atherosclerosis in the graft. Spray and Roberts[35] examined pathologic changes in vein grafts from patients autopsied up to 6 years after coronary artery bypass grafting. Most significantly, they noted atherosclerotic changes in various stages of development present in *all* grafts. The variability of this process within the same graft and among different grafts in the same patient was noted. Bulkley and Hutchins[2] observed similar changes in autopsy specimens. They confirmed that these were atherosclerotic changes rather than "arterialization" of the vein in response to chronic exposure to high pressure. In addition, they suggested that the process of atherogenesis may be accelerated in these vein grafts.

Campeau and colleagues[5] correlated the late recurrence of symptoms with atherosclerotic changes in a group of unselected patients undergoing serial coronary angiography. In patients surviving an initial coronary bypass procedure with improvement in symptoms 1 year postoperatively, over one third (36.1 per cent) deteriorated symptomatically by the sixth postoperative year. Of those with clinical deterioration, 27.3 per cent had stenosis or occlusion of a graft demonstrated by angiography, whereas 50 per cent had progression of atherosclerotic disease in the native coronary circulation. Subsequently, the same group demonstrated that atherosclerotic changes in vein grafts progressed to involve 36.4 per cent of grafts between the seventh and twelfth postoperative years.[4] In that study, the annual attrition rate for vein grafts reached 5.3 per cent per year between 7 and 12 years.

These data clearly indicate that the failure of existing vein

TABLE 2. Effect of Internal Mammary Artery (IMA) Graft on Actuarial Survival at 10 Years

Clinical Characteristic	IMA	No IMA
Single-vessel disease	93.4%	88.0%
Two-vessel disease	90.0%	79.5%
Three-vessel disease	82.6%	71.0%
Normal left ventricle; mild impairment	87.6%	78.5%
Moderate or severe impairment	76.5%	60.4%

Based on the Cleveland Clinic Experience reported by Loop[23] in which the left internal mammary artery was used to bypass the anterior descending coronary artery in combination with other grafts as necessary.

grafts due to atherosclerosis causes recurrent symptoms and ultimately necessitates a second operation. In view of these findings, the importance of the internal mammary artery as a conduit for bypass grafting cannot be overestimated. Atherosclerosis rarely occurs in this vessel, and many studies have demonstrated the superiority of this conduit, compared with the saphenous vein; both early and late patency rates are improved for both simple and complex grafts.[16,19,23,27,31,33] By the mid 1980s there was an emerging consensus that the mammary artery was the graft of choice and that, absent specific contraindications, every patient undergoing coronary bypass grafting should have at least one internal mammary utilized. Currently, the most commonly performed operation is the left mammary artery to the anterior descending coronary artery in combination with vein grafts as necessary. In a landmark paper, Loop[23] examined the effect of this particular graft configuration in a large group of patients in comparison with a similar group who received only vein grafts. In each subset of patients (Table 2), the 10-year actuarial survival was significantly increased for the internal mammary group, irrespective of the number of coronary arteries involved or the degree of impairment of left ventricular function. Moreover, the incidence of reoperation was increased in patients who received only vein grafts (Fig. 2).

NONSURGICAL MANAGEMENT

Medical management of the patient with recurrent symptoms after an initially successful coronary bypass procedure is similar to that used in patients prior to the first operation. Nitrates, beta blockade, calcium channel blockade, and antiplatelet therapy are utilized according to the same criteria as in patients prior to surgical therapy. Patients who develop *unstable* symptoms require admission to a coronary care unit. Invasive monitoring, intravenous nitroglycerin and heparin, and intra-aortic balloon counterpulsation may be indicated. This subset of patients presents particular problems, since emergency reoperation exacerbates the problems inherent with a previous sternotomy (see later). All possible measures must be undertaken to reverse the acute ischemia so that reoperation may be undertaken electively.

Percutaneous transluminal coronary angioplasty of patients who had undergone previous coronary artery bypass was performed early in the angioplasty experience.[12] Acceptable results have been obtained in selected patients with angioplasty both of the native coronary arteries and of saphenous vein grafts.[7,21] In a recent review, Kussmaul emphasized that percutaneous transluminal coronary angioplasty of vein grafts has been most successful when directed toward a lesion at or involving the distal anastomosis and somewhat less so when the lesion is in the body of the graft; the average restenosis rates at a mean follow-up of 10 months were 24 and 33 per cent, respectively. In contrast, an average restenosis rate of 50 per cent at the same

sis. The procedure is more likely successful when undertaken relatively early in the postoperative course, since the risk of distal embolization is greatly increased in older grafts. Other risks include bleeding and dissection or rupture of the graft. The possibility of converting an elective coronary reoperation to an emergency sternal re-entry must be considered. Nevertheless, percutaneous transluminal coronary angioplasty may represent an appropriate alternative to reoperation in highly selected patients.

INDICATIONS FOR REOPERATION

The indications for a second coronary bypass are similar to those for the initial coronary revascularization and are based on a correlation of the patient's symptoms with angiographic evidence of pathologic anatomy. Angina is the most common manifestation of coronary artery disease. In a patient previously asymptomatic or minimally symptomatic after coronary bypass surgery, recurrent angina or the progression of symptoms to Class III or Class IV frequently represents graft stenosis or occlusion. The angina may be unstable and debilitating; alternatively, the symptoms may be exertional and well controlled with medical therapy but cause an unacceptable decline in the satisfaction of the patient's life-style. In certain patients, the objective demonstration of myocardial ischemia by stress testing or radionuclide studies may be helpful in selecting patients for cardiac catheterization. Ultimately, because of recurrence or progression of symptoms, an assessment of the status of the bypass grafts is made by coronary angiography.

The angiographic indications for reoperation were described by Loop[25] and included, either singly or in combination, graft failure, progressive atherosclerosis in the native coronary circulation, and incomplete revascularization at the first operation. The early recognition that incomplete revascularization was a risk factor for recurrent symptoms and, thus, for the necessity of reoperation directed greater attention to the successful bypass of all vessels with significant stenoses. As a result, incomplete revascularization rarely occurs today in patients under consideration for reoperation, and primary graft failure due to atherosclerosis represents the overwhelming majority (85 per cent) of cases.[24,28]

Because of the recognition of increased risk with reoperation, the cardiovascular community as a whole appears to be somewhat more conservative in recommending surgical therapy.

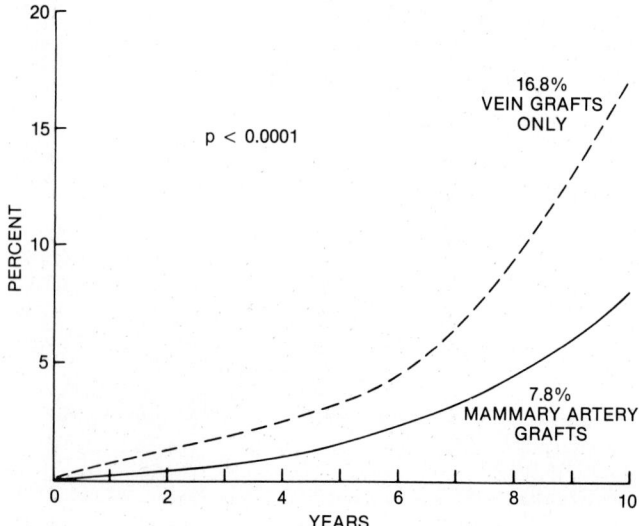

Figure 2. The cumulative incidence of reoperation demonstrates the significantly increased rate of reoperation in patients whose initial operation consisted of vein grafts only. Note that substantial divergence of the curves occurs after 5 years, coincident with the expected increased incidence of atherosclerotic graft failures. (From Cosgrove, D. M., Loop, F. D., Lytle, B. W., et al.: Predictors of reoperation after myocardial revascularization. J. Thorac. Cardiovasc. Surg., 92:811, 1986.)

Precisely analogous to patients presenting for initial coronary procedures in recent years, the patient population referred to cardiac surgeons for reoperation has changed substantially in recent years. In general, the patients are older with more diffuse coronary atherosclerosis, and there are more females in the group. There is a greater incidence of left main disease, a greater incidence of co-morbid conditions such as diabetes and peripheral vascular disease, and more severe impairment of left ventricular function.[24,28]

Based on logistic regression analysis of variables found to have a significant unvariate association with mortality, Lytle[28] found left main stenosis, Class III or Class IV symptoms, advanced age, and incomplete revascularization to be specific predictors of hospital mortality. From these and similar data, Parsonnet[32] calculated the additive risk for reoperation to be 5 per cent for each coronary surgical procedure beyond the initial operation. Quantification of risk in this manner defines subgroups of patients according to specific risk factors. The importance of such risk stratification in coronary surgery has become increasingly evident in recent years because of the need to enhance predictive ability and provide a rational basis for choosing among various therapies. Results may be assessed against the defined risk for a given subgroup.

OPERATIVE TECHNIQUES

Conceptually, the operation is identical to that for the initial procedure. The operation is technically more difficult and has higher risk for the patient. Specific challenges include gaining access to the heart in the presence of a previous sternotomy with the potential for fibrous adhesions between the heart and the sternum. Patent grafts traversing the anterior surface of the heart just below the site of the necessary sternotomy are of particular concern. The dissection necessary to sufficiently free the heart for cannulation and to perform the distal anastomoses can be time-consuming and hazardous. Diseased but patent grafts are at risk of embolizing atheromatous debris. Sufficient conduit may be difficult to obtain in patients who have undergone one or more previous coronary bypass procedures.

Anesthetic protocols are essentially the same as those for the primary operation. Intravenous access adequate for rapid transfusion is a necessity because of the potential for catastrophic hemorrhage upon sternal re-entry. Whereas flow-directed pulmonary artery catheters are not used uniformly for primary procedures, most cardiac surgeons and anesthesiologists advocate the use of invasive monitoring for reoperation. Even without catastrophic hemorrhage, the total blood loss may be expected to exceed that of the initial procedure. Therefore, all available means of blood conservation should be used in a combined, systematic approach.[8,10]

Given the increasing probability of reoperation for any specific patient, the possibility of sternal re-entry must be considered at the time of the primary operation. The use of plastic or bioprosthetic membranes to reduce adhesions has been advocated by some[11]; however, the safety and efficacy of these substances is not sufficiently well defined to advocate their routine use. Certainly, a vein graft to the right coronary system should be brought laterally over the right atrium and not anteriorly over the surface of the right ventricle.[22] Consideration should be given to the interposition of any available tissue over a right mammary graft traversing beneath the sternum to the anterior descending system. When reoperation requires only grafting of the circumflex and/or posterior descending branches, the heart may be approached through a left thoracotomy, obviating the need for sternotomy.[37] Cardiopulmonary bypass may be established with cannulation of the femoral artery and either the left atrium or the pulmonary artery.

The principles for sternal re-entry have been well defined[22] and, if followed, are likely to increase the safety of the procedure. These factors include (1) appreciation that a high-risk situation exists and assessment of the degree of risk for each particular patient; (2) cannulation of the femoral artery and vein before sternotomy in those cases estimated to be at highest risk for catastrophic bleeding; (3) use of the oscillating saw with division of each sternal table separately; (4) outward retraction of the sternum with deflation of the lungs during the sternotomy; (5) avoidance of blunt retrosternal dissection; (6) mobilization of each side of the sternum for several centimeters, by sharp dissection, before insertion of a sternal retractor; (7) mobilization of the innominate vein; and (8) gentle compression of any bleeding sites until adequate exposure is obtained. In general, examination of the lateral chest film provides the best assessment of the risk of sternal re-entry. The decision to expose or to cannulate the femoral artery and vein before sternotomy is attempted must be left to the surgeon.

After sternotomy, the aorta and right atrium should be exposed for cannulation, by use of sharp dissection only. The right atrium can nearly always be recannulated. Occasionally, because of aortic anatomy, severe aortic calcification, or number and placement of previous proximal anastomoses, sufficient room for aortic cannulation cannot be achieved. In those cases, the femoral artery is exposed and cannulated. Dissection of the remainder of the heart is accomplished with the heart decompressed after the institution of cardiopulmonary bypass. Some have advocated completion of the dissection during cardioplegic arrest after cross-clamping the aorta.

Generally, cardioplegia is administered in the usual manner, antegrade into the aortic root. However, diffuse multivessel disease in the native circulation and stenosis or occlusion of multiple vein grafts represents a situation in which retrograde delivery of cardioplegia may be superior. Before aortic cross-clamping and the administration of cardioplegia, a patent internal mammary graft must be identified and dissected free sufficiently to allow gentle occlusion by a bulldog clamp. Failure to occlude the mammary graft allows myocardial perfusion, generally of the anterior wall and septum, with relatively warm blood. Early restoration of electromechanical activity follows washout of cardioplegia in the perfused region. Maintenance of the desired degree of hypothermia in the entire heart is impaired. After the aorta is cross-clamped and cardioplegic arrest induced, the sites for anastomosis are identified and dissected free. Identification of the coronary arteries can be difficult in the presence of dense adhesions over the epicardial surface. Vessels previously grafted may be identified by following the vein graft to the coronary anastomosis.

For vessels previously grafted, the anastomosis is performed distal to the previous anastomosis. Some have advocated that proximal vein anastomoses be performed during cardioplegic arrest with the aorta cross-clamped. Irrespective of the timing of the proximal anastomoses, sufficient space on the ascending aorta may be difficult to achieve in a patient with multiple previous vein grafts. Sequential vein grafts reduce the number of proximal anastomoses necessary. The original proximal anastomoses may be taken down and those sites used again.

Many patients present for reoperation whose primary procedure consisted entirely of saphenous vein grafts. These patients should have at least one internal mammary artery graft. Lack of sufficient *standard* conduit (saphenous vein and internal mammary artery) is unfortunately observed with increasing frequency and may be a severe problem in a specific patient. Both mammary arteries may be used, and the lesser saphenous vein may be procured with results presumably similar to those obtained with the greater saphenous vein. Whereas the use of veins from the upper extremity should be avoided owing to a very high failure rate,[36] the right gastroepiploic artery has shown early promise as an *in situ* graft to the right coronary system and as a free graft.[26,30]

Patent vein grafts are a significant problem because of the possibility of embolization of atheromatous material from a diseased vein graft.[20] Marshall and colleagues[29] emphasized the discrepancy between the angiographic appearance of some vein grafts and the actual degree of intimal disease. Management of the patent graft has been controversial. However, there appears to be an emerging consensus that grafts implanted for 5 years or longer should be transected just proximal to the original coronary anastomosis and oversewn. Before transection, the patent grafts must not be disturbed during dissection. With use of this technique, postoperative survival and the perioperative infarction rate have been improved.[15]

POSTOPERATIVE CARE

Management of the patient in the intensive care unit after coronary reoperation does not differ from that of the patient undergoing a primary coronary procedure based on well-established principles discussed elsewhere in this text. Because of the potential for persistent oozing from raw epicardial and pericardial surfaces, the reinfusion of shed mediastinal blood postoperatively, which should be used in all cardiac surgical patients, is nearly mandatory after reoperation.[8]

Again, it must be emphasized that coronary artery bypass does not affect the underlying disease; the new grafts are as vulnerable to the development of atherosclerosis as were the previous grafts. Antiplatelet therapy should be undertaken.[6] Smoking cessation is a necessity. Diabetes and hyperlipidemic states should be controlled as with any patient with coronary artery disease.

RESULTS

Despite objective evidence that the patient population subjected to coronary reoperation has an increasingly severe risk profile, there have been continued decreases in the perioperative morbidity and mortality. The majority of perioperative deaths primarily are due to cardiac causes. These patients have limited functional reserve, and the effect of a perioperative myocardial infarction should not be underestimated. Myocardial protection reduced the incidence of perioperative infarction, as did the growing awareness of the special risks in managing patent but diseased vein grafts. Loop[24] documented a decrease in perioperative infarction to 4 per cent in patients undergoing reoperation in the period 1985 to 1987 in comparison with 7 to 8 per cent in previous years.

Other morbidity occurring perioperatively was reviewed by Lytle.[28] The incidence of neurologic complications ranged from 1.8 to 2.6 per cent and did not differ over time. This was also the case with wound complications, which ranged from 1.4 to 2.1 per cent. The incidence of re-exploration for bleeding differed significantly over time and was 11 per cent in patients undergoing reoperation from 1967 to 1978, 6.4 per cent from 1979 to 1981, and 4.2 per cent from 1982 to 1984.

In the initial experience with coronary reoperation, the operative mortality was approximately 10 per cent.[18] Improvements in operative technique and myocardial protection have reduced this to 3 to 5 per cent in current series. Thus, whereas most authors agree that reoperation independently increases the risk of operative mortality, the additive risk has been substantially reduced.[14,24,28,32,34]

Long-term results including survival and freedom from angina are directly related to graft patency. The few data available suggest that patency rates are comparable to those achieved after the initial operation, approximately 70 per cent for vein grafts and 90 per cent for mammary grafts at an average follow-up of 39 months.[28] The 5- and 10-year actuarial survival rates were 90 per cent and 75 per cent, respectively (Fig. 3). Emphasis has been directed to the importance of event-free survival, defined as freedom from reoperation, late myocardial infarction, and Class III or Class IV symptoms. In Lytle's series,[28] there was a reoperation rate of 2.6 per cent with the third operation occurring at a mean interval of 69 months after the initial reoperation. The incidence of late myocardial infarction was 5.8 per cent after a mean interval of 47 months. The postoperative functional class (New York Heart Association) of late survivors also was noted. Overall, 8 per cent of patients were Class III and 3 per cent were Class IV. Thus, event-free survival was 76 per cent at 5 years and 47.8 per cent at 10 years.

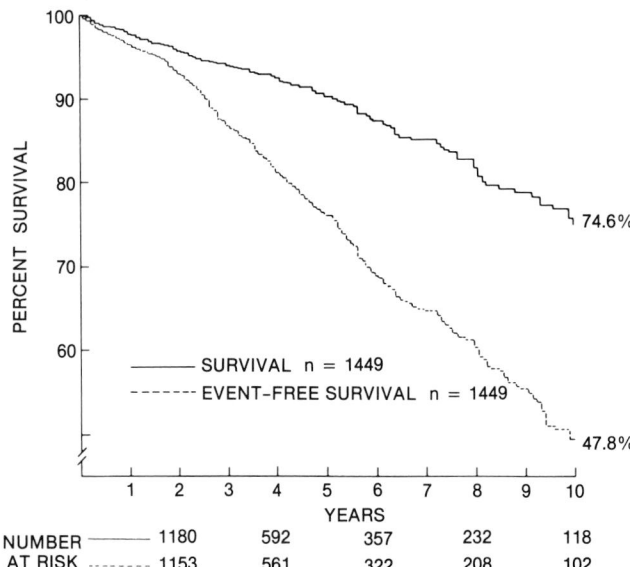

Figure 3. Late survival (Kaplan-Meier) and event-free survival are shown up to 10 years for patients surviving reoperation for coronary bypass. The survival and event-free survival rates at 5 years were 90 and 75 per cent respectively. (From Lytle, B. W., Loop, F. D., Cosgrove, D. M., et al.: Fifteen hundred coronary reoperations: Results and determinants of early and late survival. J. Thorac. Cardiovasc. Surg., 93:847, 1987.)

Thus, palliation of symptoms is adequate, and most patients are symptom-free or have only minimal symptoms. Survival does not match that obtained by primary coronary bypass; however, distinct improvements have been achieved since the earliest era of reoperative coronary surgery. Moreover, these results are impressive if survival after reoperation is considered to be a continuation of survival within the surgical group following initial coronary bypass.

REFERENCES

1. Adam, M. A., Geisler, G. F., Lambert, C. J., and Mitchell, B. F.: Reoperation following clinical failure of aorta-to-coronary bypass vein grafts. Ann. Thorac. Surg., 14:272, 1972.
2. Bulkley, B. H., and Hutchins, G. M.: Accelerated "atherosclerosis": A morphologic study of 97 saphenous vein coronary artery bypass grafts. Circulation, 55:163, 1977.
3. Califf, R. M., Harrell, F. E., Lee, K. L., Rankin, J. S., Hlatky, M. A., Mark, D. B., Jones, R. H., Muhlbaier, L. H., Oldham, H. N., and Pryor, D. B.: The evolution of medical and surgical therapy for coronary artery disease: A 15-year perspective. J.A.M.A., 261:2077, 1989.
4. Campeau, L., Enjalbert, M., Lesperance, J., Vaislic, C., Grondin, C. M., and Bourassa, M. G.: Atherosclerosis and late closure of aortocoronary saphenous vein grafts: Sequential angiographic studies at 2 weeks, 1 year, 5 to 7 years, and 10 to 12 years after surgery. Circulation, 68(Suppl. II):1, 1983.
5. Campeau, L., Lesperance, J., Hermann, J., Corbara, F., Grondin, C. M., and Bourassa, M. G.: Loss of the improvement of angina between 1 and 7 years after aortocoronary bypass surgery: Correlations with changes in vein grafts and in coronary arteries. Circulation, 60(Suppl. I):1, 1978.
6. Chesebro, J. H., Clements, I. P., Fuster, V., Elveback, L. R., Smith, H. L., Bardsley, W. T., Frye, R. L., Holmes, D. R., Vlietstra, R. E., Pluth, J. R., Wallace, R. B., Puga, F. S., Orszulak, T. A., Piehler, J. M., Schaff, H. V., and Danielson, G. K.: A platelet inhibitor drug trial in coronary artery bypass operations: Benefit of perioperative dipyridamole and aspirin therapy on early postoperative vein graft patency. N. Engl. J. Med., 307:73, 1982.
7. Cooper, I., Ineson, N., Demirtas, E., Cohart, J., Jenkins, S., and Webb-Peploe, M.: Role of angioplasty in patients with previous coronary artery bypass surgery. Cathet. Cardiovasc. Diagn., 16:81, 1989.
8. Cosgrove, D. M., Amiot, D. M., and Meserko, J. J.: An improved technique for autotransfusion of shed mediastinal blood. Ann. Thorac. Surg., 40:519, 1985.

9. Cosgrove, D. M., Loop, F. D., Lytle, B. W., Gill, C. C., Golding, L. A. R., Gibson, C., Stewart, R. W., Taylor, P. C., and Goormastic, M.: Predictors of reoperation after myocardial revascularization. J. Thorac. Cardiovasc. Surg., 92:811, 1986.

10. Cosgrove, D. M., Thurer, R. L., Lytle, B. W., Gill, C. C., Peter, M., and Loop, F. D.: Blood conservation during myocardial revascularization. Ann. Thorac. Surg., 28:184, 1978.

11. Dobell, A. R. C., and Jain, A. K.: Catastrophic hemorrhage during redo sternotomy. Ann. Thorac. Surg., 37:273, 1984.

12. Ford, W. B., Wholey, M. H., Zikria, E. A., Miller, W. H., Samadani, S. R., Koimattur, A. G., and Sullivan, M. E.: Percutaneous transluminal angioplasty in management of occlusive disease involving the coronary arteries and saphenous vein bypass grafts: Preliminary results. J. Thorac. Cardiovasc. Surg., 79:1, 1980.

13. Foster, E. D., and Kranc, M. A. T.: Alternative conduits for aortocoronary bypass grafting. Circulation, 79(Suppl. I):I34, 1989.

14. Foster, E. D., Fisher, L. D., Kaiser, G. C., Myers, W. O., and Cass investigators: Comparison of operative mortality and morbidity for initial and repeat coronary artery bypass grafting: The Coronary Artery Surgery Study (CASS) registry experience. Ann. Thorac. Surg., 38:563, 1984.

15. Grondin, C. M.: Reoperation in patients with coronary graft disease. Cardiovasc. Clin., 17:31, 1987.

16. Grondin, C. M., Campeau, L., Lesperance, J., Enjalbert, M., and Bourassa, M. G.: Comparison of late changes in internal mammary artery and saphenous vein grafts in two consecutive series of patients 10 years after operation. Circulation, 70(Suppl. I):208, 1984.

17. Isom, D. W., Spencer, F. C., Glassman, E., Cunninghan, J. N., Teiko, P., Reed, G. E., and Boyd, A. D.: Does coronary bypass increase longevity? J. Thorac. Cardiovasc. Surg., 75:28, 1978.

18. Johnson, W. D., Hoffman, J. F., Flemma, R. J., and Tector, A. J.: Secondary surgical procedure for myocardial revascularization. J. Thorac. Cardiovasc. Surg., 64:523, 1972.

19. Jones, J. W., Oschner, J. L., Mills, N. L., and Hughes, L.: Clinical comparison with saphenous vein and internal mammary artery as a coronary graft. J. Thorac. Cardiovasc. Surg., 80:334, 1980.

20. Keon, W. J., Heggtveit, H. A., and Leduc, J.: Perioperative myocardial infarction caused by atheroembolism. J. Thorac. Cardiovasc. Surg., 84:849, 1982.

21. Kussmaul, W. G.: Percutaneous angioplasty of coronary bypass grafts: An emerging consensus. Cathet. Cardiovasc. Diagn., 15:1, 1988.

22. Loop, F. D.: Catastrophic hemorrhage during sternal reentry. Ann. Thorac. Surg., 37:271, 1984.

23. Loop, F. D., Lytle, B. W., Cosgrove, D. M., Stewart, R. W., Goormastic, M., Williams, G. W., Golding, L. A. R., Gill, C. C., Taylor, P. C., Sheldon, W. C., and Proudfit, W. L.: Influence of the internal-mammary-artery graft on 10-year survival and other cardiac events. N. Engl. J. Med., 314:1, 1986.

24. Loop, F. D., Lytle, B. W., Cosgrove, D. M., Woods, E., Steward, R. W., Golding, L. A. R., and Taylor, P. C.: Reoperation for coronary atherosclerosis: Changing practice in 2,500 consecutive patients. Ann. Surg., 212:378, 1990.

25. Loop, F. D., Thurer, R. L., Lytle, B. W., and Cosgrove, D. M.: Reoperation for myocardial revascularization. World J. Surg., 2:719, 1978.

26. Lytle, B. W., Cosgrove, D. M., Ratliff, N. B., and Loop, F. D.: Coronary artery bypass grafting with the right gastroepiploic artery. J. Thorac. Cardiovasc. Surg., 97:826, 1989.

27. Lytle, B. W., Loop, F. D., Cosgrove, D. M., Ratliff, N. B., Easly, K., and Taylor, P. C.: Long-term (5 to 12 years) serial studies of internal mammary artery and saphenous vein coronary bypass grafts. J. Thorac. Cardiovasc. Surg., 89:248, 1985.

28. Lytle, B. W., Loop, F. D., Cosgrove, D. M., Taylor, P. C., Goormastic, M., Peper, W., Gill, C. C., Golding, L. A. R., and Stewart, R. W.: Fifteen hundred coronary reoperations: Results and determinants of early and late survival. J. Thorac. Cardiovasc. Surg., 93:847, 1987.

29. Marshall, W. G., Saffitz, J., and Kouchoukos, N. T.: Management during reoperation of aortocoronary saphenous vein grafts with minimal atherosclerosis by angiography. Ann. Thorac. Surg., 42:163, 1986.

30. Mills, N., and Everson, C. T.: Right gastroepiploic artery: A third arterial conduit for coronary artery bypass. Ann. Thorac. Surg., 47:706, 1989.

31. Okies, J. E., Page, U. S., Bigelow, J. C., et al.: The left internal mammary artery: The graft of choice. Circulation, 70(Suppl. I):213, 1984.

32. Parsonnet, V., Dean, D., and Bernstein, A. D.: A method of uniform stratification of risk for evaluating the results of surgery in acquired adult heart disease. Circulation, 79(6pt2):(Suppl. I):I3, 1989.

33. Rankin, J. S., Newman, G. E., Bashore, T. M., Muhlbaier, L. H., Tyson, G. S., Ferguson, T. B., Reves, J. G., and Sabiston, D. C.: Clinical and angiographic assessment of complex mammary artery bypass grafting. J. Thorac. Cardiovasc. Surg., 92:832, 1986.

34. Schaff, H. V., Orszulak, T. A., Gersh, B. J., Piehler, J. M., Puga, F. J., Danielson, G. K., and Pluth, J. R.: The morbidity and mortality of reoperation for coronary artery disease and analysis of late results with use of actuarial estimate of event-free interval. J. Thorac. Cardiovasc. Surg., 85:508, 1983.

35. Spray, T. L., and Roberts, W. C.: Changes in saphenous veins used as aortocoronary bypass grafts. Ann. Heart J., 94:500, 1977.

36. Stoney, W. S., Alford, W. C., Burrus, G. R., Glassford, D. M., Petracek, M. R., and Thomas, C. S.: The fate of arm veins used for aorta-coronary bypass grafts. J. Thorac. Cardiovasc. Surg., 88:522, 1984.

37. Ungerleider, R. M., Mills, N. L., and Wechsler, A. S.: Left thoracotomy for reoperative coronary bypass procedures. Ann. Thorac. Surg., 40:11, 1985.

38. Vouhe, P., and Grondin, C. M.: Reoperation for coronary graft failure: Clinical and angiographic results in 43 patients. Ann. Thorac. Surg., 27:328, 1979.

3. RADIONUCLIDE EVALUATION OF CORONARY ARTERY DISEASE

Robert H. Jones, M.D.

HISTORICAL ASPECTS

The first use of radioactive tracers to assess any biologic process in man was for evaluation of blood flow. More than 60 years ago, Blumgart and associates injected radon gas into veins of normal subjects and patients with a variety of cardiac disorders to measure transit times throughout the cardiovascular system.[3] The crude technology then available for detecting radiation and lack of an apparent clinical use for these measurements caused this early innovative work to lapse into obscurity. In 1948, Prinzmetal and colleagues used newly developed single-probe detectors to quantitate passage of a bolus of radioactive sodium through the heart and name this rediscovered procedure radiocardiography.[22] Continued improvement in technology renewed interest in use of radionuclide indicator-dilution curves for calculation of cardiac output and measurement of intracardiac shunts in patients.[21] Soon after development, gamma cameras were used to image individual cardiac chambers as tracer flowed through the heart.[2] The potential was soon recognized for these instruments to be interfaced with computers to obtain data with sufficient anatomic resolution to provide indicator-dilution curves from individual cardiac chambers.[14,18]

BASIC PRINCIPLES

Cardiac Function Measurements

Initial-transit radionuclide angiocardiography has evolved as a useful clinical modality applied primarily to measure left ventricular function.[15,27] This technique requires intravenous injection of a single bolus of radioactive tracer using a high-sensitivity gamma camera for precordial counting at brief intervals, usually 25 msec. Dynamic counting images blood flow through the right heart, lungs, and left heart (Fig. 1). To construct left ventriculograms, computer processing combines phasically related counts from within the left ventricle during several cardiac cycles into an averaged cardiac beat that has greater spatial and temporal resolution than the individual beats (Fig. 2). After subtraction of background counts arising outside the left ventricle, the remaining left ventricular count changes reflect relative left ventricular volume changes during the cardiac cycle (Fig. 3). Geometric assumptions commonly used to derive cardiac volumes from contrast ventriculograms can also be applied to radionuclide images to calculate absolute left ventricular volumes. Radionuclide measurements of ejection fraction and cardiac chamber volumes and volumetric cardiac output compare favorably with contrast ventriculogram measurements. Technology for performing initial-transit radionuclide angiocardiography has now been well standardized and is commercially available. Newer instrumentation, such as the Scinticor, is portable and can be taken into the operating room and intensive care units to measure cardiac function in surgical patients. Moreover, introduction of a high-fidelity micromanometer into the left ventricle to simultaneously record pressure during radionuclide volume measurement permits the construction of

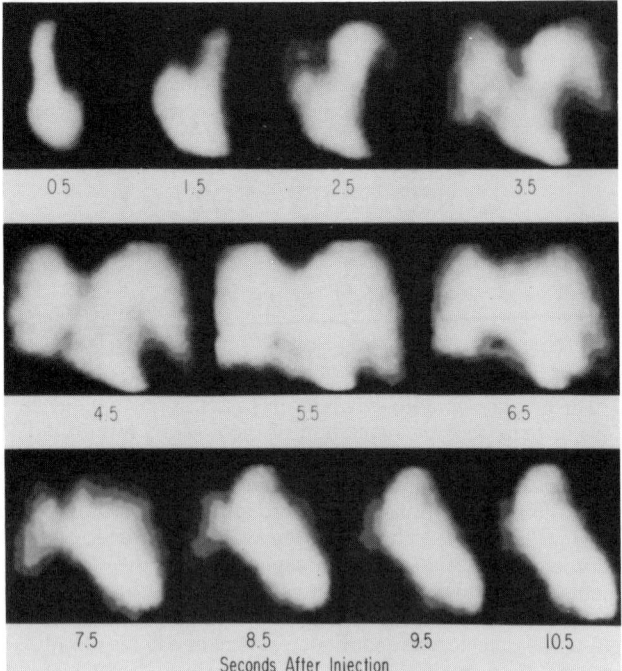

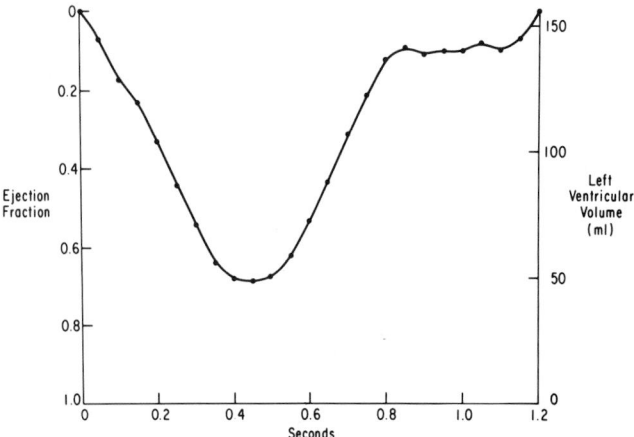

Figure 3. A representative cardiac cycle was constructed from radionuclide data obtained during several individual contractions during the initial passage of tracer through the left ventricle. The volume changes are expressed as fractional changes. In addition, planimetry of the end-diastolic image provides an end-diastolic volume in milliliters, so that the volume curve can also be calibrated as an absolute change in volume relative to time. The rapid increase in volume during end diastole reflects left atrial contraction.

Figure 1. Serial 1-second images each composed of 20 0.05-second data frames depict the progression of the tracer bolus through the central circulation in the anterior view. The rapid transit through the heart is apparent by the almost complete clearance of counts from the right ventricle during the time when count rates are maximal in the left ventricle.

pressure-volume loops that more completely characterize systolic and diastolic left ventricular function than use of either pressure or volume parameters alone (Fig. 4).[24]

Standard gamma cameras do not have sufficient counting sensitivity to image the heart from data recorded during the 5 to 10 cardiac beats when an injected tracer bolus first passes through the heart. An alternative approach of gated cardiac imaging acquires data after injected labeled red blood cells reach equilibrium within the blood pool. A simultaneous electrocardiogram synchronizes acquisition of radionuclide data with the appropriate phase of each of the 100 to 300 heartbeats as counts are added to form a single averaged cardiac beat, which is used to image cardiac motion and calculate ejection fraction. The advantage of gated equilibrium over initial-transit cardiac imaging is that it does not require specific instrumentation or a discrete bolus injection. However, the 2 to 3 minutes required to acquire the gated image made the approach less well suited than the initial-transit technique for measuring cardiac function during periods of rapid change in cardiac function, such as during exercise or pharmacologic intervention. Moreover, cardiac volume calculations are less accurate and reproducible using the gated technique because of higher back-

ground that results when tracer is at equilibrium in the blood pool. Measurement of cardiac volumes using the gated equilibrium technique also requires withdrawal of a blood sample at equilibrium to relate observed counts to absolute cardiac volumes, and this is not required using the initial-transit approach.

Myocardial Perfusion and Metabolism Measurements

Radionuclide methods for noninvasive regional myocardial blood flow measurement are based on the observation of Saperstein that tissue content of any tracer with a high extraction rate during initial capillary transit is primarily determined by blood flow.[25] This principle applies to potassium and the similar cationic tracers cesium, rubidium, and thallium, which accumulate in myocardium proportional to blood flow after intravenous injection. Love first reported use of rubidium 86 in dogs and humans for estimation of myocardial perfusion. Currently, the potassium analog thallium 201 with a half-life of 73 hours and photon energy of about 69 and 83 keV is the most widely used radionuclide for evaluation of regional myocardial perfusion. A large clinical experience with thallium 201 has documented the value and limitations of myocardial scintigraphy in patients with myocardial infarction and ischemia.[8] Other promising myocardial perfusion agents with superior physical characteristics for imaging may soon replace thallium 201 for measurements of the distribution of coronary blood flow.[5]

After intravenous injection, thallium 201 attains a high initial myocardial concentration as the initial bolus passes through the coronary circulation. The subsequent myocardial distribution changes continually as the intracellular tracer exchanges with that remaining in the blood pool. Therefore, the distribution of thallium 201 during the first few minutes after injection closely

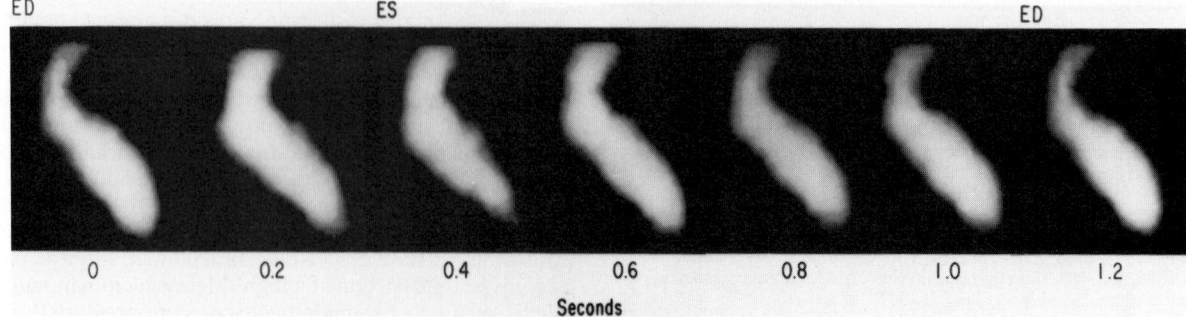

Figure 2. Serial images of the spatial distribution of counts taken from the representative cardiac cycle in Figure 3 depict normal left ventricular wall motion.

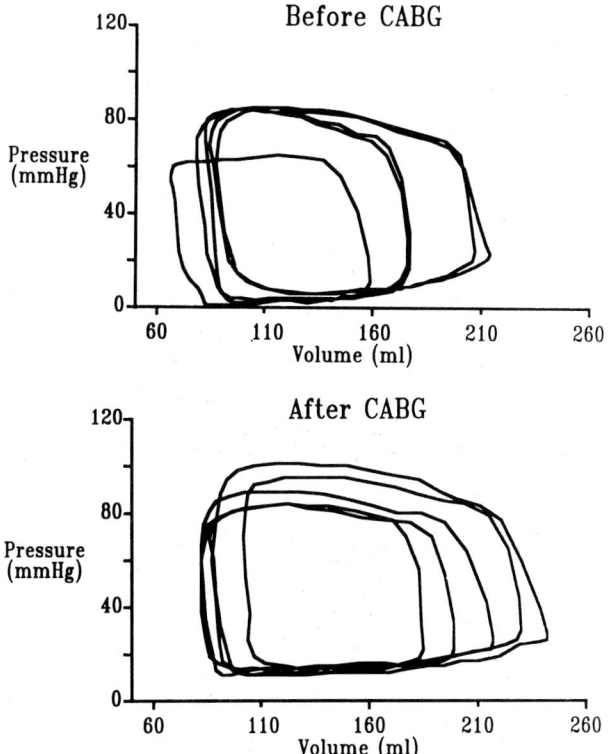

Figure 4. Pressure-volume loops obtained at different levels of filling before and immediately after coronary artery bypsss grafting (CABG) show minimal depression of left ventricular function immediately after myocardial revascularization.

reflects regional myocardial blood flow, but several hours after injection more closely resembles the potassium content of the heart. This characteristic of thallium 201 is used to obtain exercise and delayed redistribution images from a single tracer injection.

The interaction of specific radiopharmaceuticals with the heart may be used to study regional myocardial metabolism. During myocardial infarction, calcium ions accumulate within injured myocardial cells. The affinity of technetium-99m pyrophosphate for calcium causes a high accumulation of this tracer in infarcted myocardium.[4] More recently, labeled monoclonal antibodies that react with myosin and fibrin have been developed that show promise for detecting myocardial cell breakdown and intravascular thrombosis.[11] Cyclotron production of positron-emitting radiopharmaceuticals containing radioisotopes of carbon, oxygen, nitrogen, and fluorine now permit investigation of the full array of biochemical pathways in the myocardium.[26] In addition to measurement of blood flow, regional myocardial accumulation and utilization of glucose, fatty acids, and amino acids can be assessed. Future application of these techniques is certain to enhance understanding of abnormal cardiac metabolism in patients with cardiac disorders.

Images of the distribution of a radioactive tracer in the heart detected by a gamma camera represent two-dimensional projections of counts arising from three dimensions of the cardiac volume. Simultaneous interpretation of several images obtained from different projections offers reasonable approximation of the three-dimensional counts distribution in the heart. The most quantitative approach now available for imaging three-dimensional cardiac counts is single-photon emission computed tomography (SPECT). During SPECT imaging, the gamma camera detector encircles the patient, and data from these multiple projections is later reconstructed into a three-dimensional representation of counts. These counts matrices can be quantitated by comparison with normal standards or visually interpreted as a series of heart slice images. The accurate re-

gional quantitation of counts provided by SPECT imaging adds objectivity to radionuclide measurements of regional perfusion and metabolism.

Positron emission tomography is a technique that also uses a number of detectors encircling a patient to image positron-emitting tracers. Positron decay emits high-energy photons in opposite directions simultaneously, and this characteristic is used to accurately position the three-dimensional location of the original event. Positron emission tomography requires more expensive and complicated technology than does SPECT imaging, and present applications are primarily for cardiac metabolism research.

Applications of Radionuclide Techniques in Patients with Coronary Artery Disease

Proper selection of patients for interventional therapy for coronary artery disease requires accurate risk stratification. The large group of low-risk patients must be separated from the smaller subset of patients with a sufficiently high probability of a cardiac event in the near future to warrant evaluation for interventional therapy. Prior clinical studies of treatment of coronary artery disease have emphasized the anatomic severity and extensiveness of coronary atherosclerosis to be important predictors of natural history of the disease in an individual patient. Patients with severe proximal stenoses in coronary arteries have a greater amount of myocardium at jeopardy for ischemic events and a higher incidence of myocardial infarction and cardiac death than do other patients with less extensive disease. Patients with the most extensive forms of disease, such as left main coronary artery stenosis, derive the greatest benefit from revascularization procedures. Despite the prognostic importance of coronary angiographic definition of extensiveness of disease, this single parameter does not contain all information needed for risk stratification. For example, 70 per cent of patients with left main stenosis treated medically survive at least 5 years. Moreover, some patients with low risk suggested by single-vessel disease experience untoward events. Adding physiologic to anatomic information enhances risk stratification in patients with coronary artery disease.

Myocardial ischemia can be detected clinically by angina pectoris, electrocardiographically by ST segment depression, and functionally by regional perfusion abnormalities and segmental contraction abnormalities with associated hemodynamic alterations. Reversible left ventricular dysfunction as an indicator of ischemia was first demonstrated in man by Herman and associates,[12] who studied patients with unstable angina during and after periods of spontaneous pain. Sharma and associates in 1976 used contrast angiography to demonstrate reversible alterations of regional left ventricular function induced by exercise and cardiac pacing.[28] Exercise-induced left ventricular dysfunction is a very sensitive marker of ischemia that commonly occurs prior to electrocardiographic abnormality as ischemia progressively increases in an individual patient (Fig. 5).[30] Radionuclide techniques measuring ventricular function and myocardial perfusion reflect similar biologic processes because of the close link between myocardial integrity and blood flow. Therefore, perfusion defects on myocardial scintigraphy performed during exercise, which disappear after an interval adequate for thallium 201 redistribution, are also sensitive markers of ischemia. Myocardial infarction with subsequent fibrosis decreases resting regional and global ventricular function and also causes a resting perfusion defect due to loss of myocardial mass and the lower tissue blood flow rate of fibrotic myocardium.

Soon after introduction of radionuclide tests for detecting exercise-induced perfusion defects and functional abnormalities as indicators of myocardial ischemia, enthusiastic reports suggested these procedures were highly accurate for diagnosis of coronary artery disease. Further experience with broader populations of patients shows that rest/exercise perfusion and

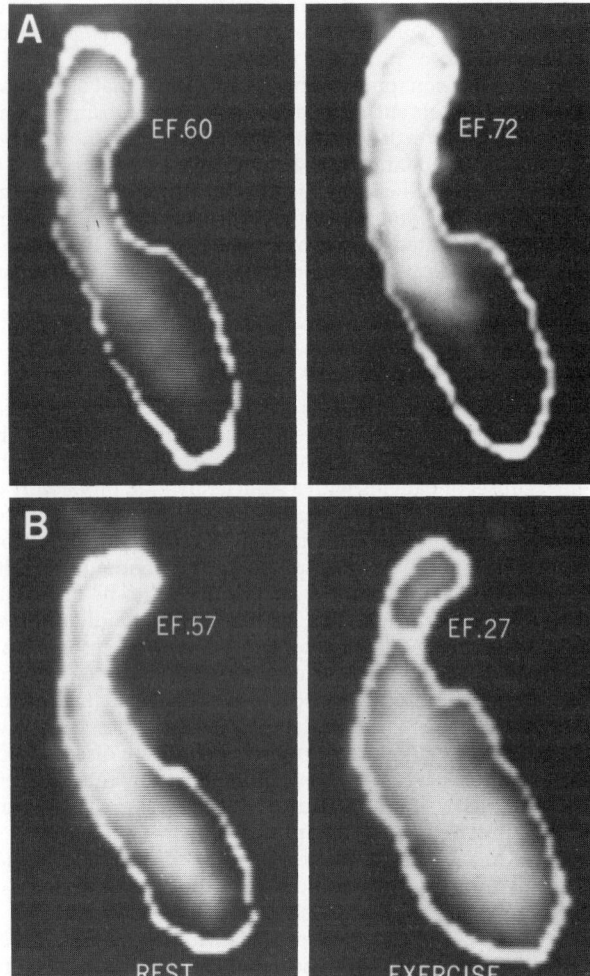

Figure 5. End-diastolic outlines and end-systolic images demonstrating wall motion at rest and at exercise in a normal subject (A) and a patient with coronary artery disease (B). Patients with myocardial ischemia show marked cardiac dilation and global hypokinesia with acute exercise.

function tests have an accuracy that ranges between 0.75 and 0.85 for the prediction of coronary disease.[17,29] Therefore, the severity of coronary artery disease reflected by the anatomic information from the coronary arteriogram correlates with that suggested by ischemia assessment of radionuclide stress tests in patient groups. However, consistent discrepancy occurs between the two approaches of assessment in 15 to 25 per cent of patients with coronary artery disease. The early disappointment in lack of complete agreement between radionuclide tests and coronary angiograms has more recently come to be interpreted as a benefit since the two forms of information appear to be complementary but independent.

Prognosis in Patients with Coronary Artery Disease

Radionuclide tests appear particularly well suited for screening large groups of patients, and individuals with the most severe abnormalities can be selected for cardiac catheterization and possible further intervention, whereas those defined to be very low risk would require catheterization in only special circumstances. Brown and colleagues[7] followed 100 medically treated patients without prior myocardial infarction for a mean of 3.7 years and documented a cardiac event rate of 3 per cent in patients with a normal thallium test and 33 per cent in patients with three or more defects. In 1689 consecutive patients with suspected coronary artery disease followed for 1 year, Ladenheim and associates[19] found three variables provided independent prognostic information: (1) the number of reversible thal-

lium defects, an extent variable; (2) the magnitude of initial reversible defect, a severity variable; and (3) the maximal heart rate achieved during exercise. Combining these variables into a prognostic model categorized risk of cardiac event from a low cardiac event rate of less than 1 per cent in patients with a normal exercise thallium study to a high event rate of 78 per cent in patients developing severe and extensive reversible defects at a low achieved heart rate.

Pryor and associates[23] used multivariate analysis of radionuclide variables to identify those which related to later myocardial infarction or cardiovascular death in 386 medically treated patients. The exercise ejection fraction was the most important radionuclide variable providing prognostic information in patients with coronary artery disease. These early observations have been extended by Lee and associates[20] in 571 medically treated patients followed for up to 10 years. This analysis documented the radionuclide angiocardiogram alone had as much prognostic information as the cardiac catheterization and added significant prognostic information even when all clinical and catheterization information was known. The exercise ejection fraction was the single most important radionuclide variable that contained 80 per cent of the prognostic information of the test. The amount of increase in heart rate and measurement of cardiac volume provided the remaining prognostic information. Analysis of the entire population of patients undergoing radionuclide angiocardiography for evaluation of coronary artery disease, including patients undergoing and not undergoing cardiac catheterization, demonstrated equivalent prognostic power in both patient populations.[16] Curves describing survival as a function of the exercise ejection fraction showed that patients with exercise ejection fractions greater than 0.50 have a low risk of cardiac death and that risk increases progressively as ejection fraction falls below 0.50 (Fig. 6).

Measurement of cardiac function during exercise, and especially documentation of the exercise ejection fraction, appears to provide a very sensitive index of the magnitude of myocardial ischemia. The amount of potential myocardial ischemia is the main determinant of survival in individual patients with coronary artery disease. Interventional therapy that is devised to reverse ischemia can be expected to benefit only patients with a significant amount of ischemic potential. Definition of the pathologic anatomy of the coronary arterial tree by angiography is indispensable for the planning of interventional procedures and provides some insight regarding the magnitude of myocardium at potential risk. However, radionuclide measurements of ventricular function during exercise provide important independent prognostic information useful in identifying patients likely to benefit from interventional therapy. Comparison of patient selection by different approaches used to assess individual patients for ischemic potential suggests radionuclide angiocardiography to be one of the most useful (Fig. 7).[13] The simplicity

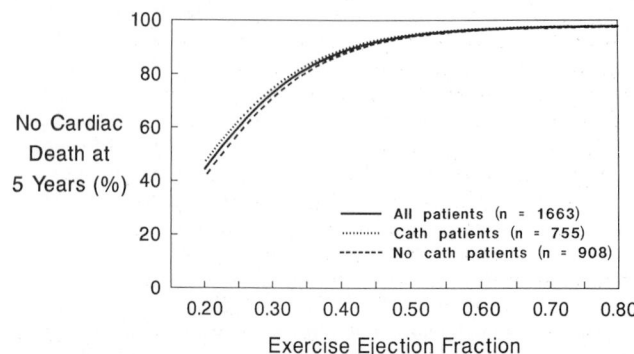

Figure 6. Comparison of probability of survival 5 years after radionuclide angiocardiogram as a function of exercise ejection fraction in 1663 patients evaluated for coronary artery disease including 908 patients without and 755 patients with cardiac catheterization.

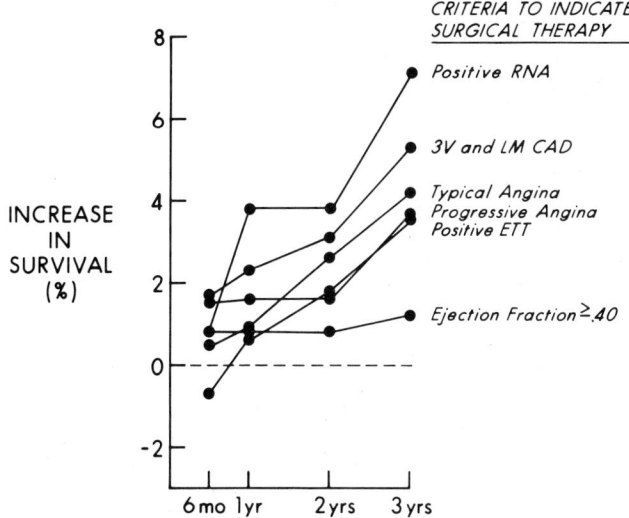

Figure 7. Data documenting the maximal percentage increase in survival of the total population that could be achieved at each time interval, using specific criteria to indicate surgical therapy and absence of those criteria to indicate medical therapy.

and low cost intrinsic to this radionuclide measurement also make it ideally suited as one of the first procedures to be performed in patients evaluated for stable chronic coronary artery disease.

Use of Radionuclide Angiocardiography to Document Outcome of Coronary Artery Bypass Grafting

Not every patient who survives coronary artery bypass grafting has an optimal functional result. Even the absence of angina after surgical therapy cannot be used as a valid end point since denervation of the heart or perioperative infarction of myocardium previously ischemic may decrease or obliterate anginal pain.

Patients with good anatomic results documented by angiography after coronary bypass grafting also improve exercise-induced myocardial dysfunction and perfusion deficits after successful bypass. However, coronary blood flow at rest and potential for flow augmentation during exercise cannot always be predicted from the coronary angiogram. Graft and vessel patency on arteriogram does not always correlate to improvements in regional function and perfusion. Therefore, as before operation, radionuclide tests provide important data that are complementary but do not always duplicate the information obtained from coronary angiography. Radionuclide procedures appear useful to objectively document improvement in myocardial perfusion and function to judge effectiveness of operative outcome and predict the future clinical course of individual patients.

Radionuclide measurements of resting left ventricular function before and after bypass operation show 10 to 20 per cent of patients to have a significant decrease in left ventricular function.[9] This documented loss in function is permanent and often occurs without clinical symptoms or changes suggestive of infarction on the electrocardiogram. A prospective study of 104 patients by Floyd and associates[10] showed a surprising lack of relationship between QRS change on the electrocardiogram and left ventricular function after coronary artery bypass grafting. Loss of left ventricular function did not relate to the duration of hypothermic cardioplegic arrest, and the etiology of this functional result probably relates to multiple causative factors that are now poorly understood. About 10 to 20 per cent of patients significantly improve resting function after myocardial revascularization, suggesting that reversible resting ischemic dysfunc-

tion was present before operation in the absence of resting pain. Although resting improvement in left ventricular function is modest in most patients, in some quite abnormal function observed before operation dramatically normalized after revascularization.

Physiologic improvement after myocardial revascularization is most consistently documented by radionuclide studies of myocardial function and perfusion during exercise. As early as 8 days after surgical therapy patients have been shown to greatly improve exercise left ventricular ejection fraction, and this improvement persists on later studies.[1] This early documentation of reversal of myocardial ischemia provides a useful baseline for patients who later become symptomatic. Subsequent radionuclide studies can quantify the amount of return of ischemia associated with disease progression or graft occlusion and provide a rational basis for selection of patients who might profit from repeat catheterization and consideration of another revascularization procedure.[6]

SELECTED REFERENCE

State-of-the-Art Symposium on Noninvasive Testing in the Diagnosis and Management of Patients with Suspect or Overt Cardiac Disease. Crawford, M. H. (Ed.). Press Circulation (Suppl.). In press.
This monograph includes papers presented at an American Heart Association State-of-the-Art Conference on Noninvasive Cardiac Imaging. Strengths and weaknesses of radionuclide and other noninvasive cardiac assessment techniques were compared, and their clinical applications were summarized.

REFERENCES

1. Austin, E. H., Oldham, H. N., Jr., Sabiston, D. C., Jr., and Jones, R. H.: Early assessment of rest and exercise left ventricular function following coronary artery surgery. Ann. Thorac. Surg., 35:159, 1983.
2. Bender, M. A., and Blau, M.: The autofluoroscope. Nucleonics, 21:52, 1963.
3. Blumgart, H. L., and Weiss, S.: Clinical studies on the velocity of blood flow. The pulmonary circulation time, the velocity of venous blood flow to the heart and related aspects of the circulation in patients with cardiovascular disease. J. Clin. Invest.,4:343, 1927.
4. Bonte, F. J., Parkey, R. W., Graham, K. D., Moore, J., and Stokely, E. M.: A new method for radionuclide imaging of myocardial infarcts. Radiology, 110:473, 1974.
5. Borges-Neto, S., Coleman, R. E., and Jones, R. H.: Perfusion and function at rest and treadmill exercise using Tc-99 sestamibi: Comparison of one- and two-day protocols in normal volunteers. J. Nucl. Med. 31:128, 1990.
6. Borges-Neto, S., Sell, T. L., Lee, K. L., and Jones, R. H.: Prediction of cardiac death after coronary artery bypass grafting. (abstract). Circulation, 80(Suppl.):II-49, 1989.
7. Brown, K. A., Boucher, C. A., Okada, R. D., Guiney, T. E., Newell, J. B., Strauss, H. W., and Pohost, G. M.: Prognostic value of exercise thallium-201 imaging in patients presenting for evaluation of chest pain. J. Am. Coll. Cardiol., 4:994, 1983.
8. Detrano, R., Janosi, A., Lyons, K. D., Marcondes, G., Abbassi, N., and Froelicher, V. F.: Factors affecting sensitivity and specificity of a diagnostic test: The exercise thallium scintigram. Am. J. Med., 84:699, 1988.
9. Floyd, R. D., Sabiston, D. C., Jr., Lee, K. L., and Jones, R. H.: The effect of duration of hypothermic cardioplegia on ventricular function. J. Thorac. Cardiovasc. Surg., 85:606, 1983.
10. Floyd, R. D., Wagner, G. S., Austin, E. H., Sabiston, D. C., Jr., and Jones, R. H.: Relation between QRS changes and left ventricular function after coronary artery bypass grafting. Am. J. Cardiol., 52:943, 1983.
11. Haber, E.: In vivo diagnostic and therapeutic uses of monoclonal antibodies in cardiology. Annu. Rev. Med., 37:249, 1986.
12. Herman, M. V., Heinle, R. A., Klein, M. D., and Gorlin, R.: Localized disorders in myocardial contraction. Asynergy and its role in congestive heart failure. N. Engl. J. Med., 277:222, 1967.
13. Jones, R. H., Floyd, R. D., Austin, E. H., and Sabiston, D. C., Jr.: The role of radionuclide angiocardiography in the preoperative prediction of pain relief and prolonged survival following coronary artery bypass grafting. Ann. Surg., 197:743, 1983.
14. Jones, R. H., Goodrich, J. K., and Sabiston, D. C., Jr.: Radioactive lung scanning in the diagnosis and management of pulmonary disorders. J. Thorac. Cardiovasc. Surg., 54:520, 1967.
15. Jones, R. H., Goodrich, J. K., and Sabiston, D. C., Jr.: Quantitative radionuclide angiocardiography in evaluation of cardiac function. Surg. Forum, 22:128, 1971.
16. Jones, R. H., Johnson, S. H., Bigelow, C., Pieper, K. S., Coleman, R. E., Cobb, F. R., Pryor, D. B., and Lee, K. L.: Exercise radionuclide angiocardiography predicts cardiac death in patients with coronary artery disease. (Submitted for publication.)

17. Jones, R. H., McEwan, P., Newman, G. E., Port, S., Rerych, S. K., Scholz, P. M., Upton, M. T., Peter, C. A., Austin, E. H., Leong, K., Gibbons, R. J., Cobb, F. R., Coleman, R. E., and Sabiston, D. C. Jr.: The accuracy of diagnosis of coronary artery disease by radionuclide measurement of left ventricular function during rest and exercise. Circulation, 64:586, 1981.
18. Jones, R. H., Sabiston, D. C., Jr., Bates, B. B., Morris, J. J., Anderson, P. A. W., and Goodrich, J. K.: Quantitative radionuclide angiocardiography for determination of chamber-to-chamber transit times. Am. J. Cardiol., 30:855, 1972.
19. Ladenheim, M. L., Pollock, B. H., Rozanski, A., Berman, D. S., Staniloff, H. M., Forrester, J. S., and Diamond, G. S.: Extent and severity of myocardial hypoperfusion as predictors of prognosis in patients with suspected coronary artery disease. J. Am. Coll. Cardiol., 7:464, 1986.
20. Lee, K. L., Pryor, D. B., Pieper, K. S., Harrell, F. E., Jr., Califf, R. M., Mark, D. B., Hlatky, M. A., Coleman, R. E., Cobb, F. R., and Jones, R. H.: The prognostic value of radionuclide angiography in medically treated patients with coronary artery disease: A comparison with clinical and catheterization variables. Circulation 82:1705, 1990.
21. MacIntyre, W. J., Pritchard, W. H., Eckstein, R. W., and Friedell, H. L.: The determination of cardiac output by a continuous recording system utilizing iodinated (I-131) human serum albumin. I. Animal studies. Circulation, 4:552, 1951.
22. Prinzmetal, M., Corday, E., Bergman, H. C., Schwartz, L., and Spritzler, R. J.: Radiocardiography: A new method for studying the blood flow through the chambers of the heart in human beings. Science, 108:340, 1948.
23. Pryor, D. B., Harrell, F. E., Jr., Lee, K. L., Califf, R. M., and Rosati, R. A.: An improving prognosis over time in medically treated patients with coronary artery disease. Am. J. Cardiol., 52:444, 1983.
24. Purut, C. M., Sell, T. L., and Jones, R. H.: A new method to determine left ventricular pressure-volume loops in the clinical setting. J. Nucl. Med., 29:1492, 1988.
25. Saperstein, L. A.: Regional blood flow by fractional distribution of indicators. Am. J. Physiol., 193:161, 1958.
26. Schelbert, H. R., and Buxton, D.: Insights into coronary artery disease gained from metabolic imaging. Circulation, 78:496, 1988.
27. Scholz, P. M., Rerych, S. K., Moran, J. F., Newman, G. E., Douglas, J. M., Jr., Sabiston, D. C., Jr., and Jones, R. H.: Quantitative radionuclide angiocardiography. Cathet. Cardiovasc. Diagn., 6:265, 1980.
28. Sharma, B., Goodwin, J. F., Raphael, M. J., Steiner, R. E., Rainbow, R. G., and Taylor, S. H.: Left ventricular angiography on exercise. A new method of assessing left ventricular function in ischaemic heart disease. Br. Heart J., 38:59, 1976.
29. Rozanski, A., and Berman, D. S.: The efficacy of cardiovascular nuclear medicine exercise studies. Semin. Nucl. Med., 17:104, 1987.
30. Upton, M. T., Rerych, S. K., Newman, G. E., Port, S., Cobb, F. R., and Jones, R. H.: Detecting abnormalities in left ventricular function during exercise before angina and ST-segment depression. Circulation, 62:341, 1980.

4. VENTRICULAR ANEURYSM

William A. Gay, Jr., M.D.

The majority of ventricular aneurysms are due to acute transmural myocardial infarction with its resultant muscle necrosis followed by scar formation. Rarely, however, aneurysms may follow trauma or congenital cardiac defects.[19,20,43] There are also false aneurysms, which may be due to previous surgical procedures,[36] trauma,[9] and bacterial endocarditis.[38] The typical ventricular aneurysm has been described as "a thinned-out transmural scar that has completely lost its trabecular pattern . . . always clearly delineated from the surrounding muscle."[25] Although this accurate description of ventricular aneurysms was given by John Hunter in the eighteenth century, it was more than 150 years later that the relationship of this entity with coronary occlusive disease was appreciated.[41] Moreover, it remained for Tennant and Wiggers to demonstrate the deleterious effects of acute coronary arterial occlusion on regional myocardial contractile function in 1935.[42]

In 1931, the famed German surgeon Sauerbruch accidentally entered an aneurysm of the right ventricle during the course of exploration of a patient believed to have a mediastinal tumor. He was able to resect the aneurysm sac and successfully suture its neck.[39] Beck, in 1944, used a fascia lata stent to reinforce the left ventricular wall of a patient with a ventricular aneurysm that was accurately diagnosed preoperatively.[5] In 1954, Bailey successfully resected a ventricular aneurysm by placing a large vascular clamp about its neck, excising the aneurysm, and oversewing the neck.[3] The use of cardiopulmonary bypass in operations for ventricular aneurysm was first described by Cooley in 1958.[12] The practice of simultaneous coronary revascularization became popular as direct coronary arterial operations became commonplace in the late 1960s and early 1970s.[19] Jatene, in 1985, described a technique for the geometric reconstruction of the left ventricle following aneurysmectomy with a significant reduction in operative mortality and improved postoperative ventricular performance.[27] Since that time others have been more attentive to reconstructive techniques with similar improvements in results.[11,17]

CLINICAL MANIFESTATIONS

The precise incidence of left ventricular aneurysm formation following acute myocardial infarction is not known. Retrospective clinical and autopsy analyses indicate an incidence of 10 to 15 per cent.[1,40] These figures were generated prior to the era of prompt interventional therapy for acute myocardial infarction such as thrombolysis and/or angioplasty or bypass surgery. It is hoped that the use of one or more of these therapeutic interventions combined with better hemodynamic and arrhythmia control has lowered the incidence of aneurysm formation.[24]

Although the relationship between coronary occlusion and aneurysm formation has been well established, until recently it was poorly understood why some infarctions caused aneurysms whereas others did not. A recent review of patients suffering their first myocardial infarction, all anterior, revealed that the absence of significant collateral circulation concomitant with total occlusion of the left anterior descending coronary artery was a significant determinant of aneurysm formation.[21] Another report evaluating the effectiveness of early reperfusion following myocardial infarction concluded that although collateral circulation to an area of anterior infarction did not improve global ventricular function in the absence of successful reperfusion, it did lower the incidence of left ventricular aneurysm.[24] Thus, it would seem that the presence of significant collateral circulation in the distribution of an acutely occluded coronary artery may lessen the likelihood of development of an aneurysm.

Prior to the establishment of special care units and use of sophisticated monitoring and aggressive therapy, many patients who developed left ventricular aneurysms succumbed in the early peri-infarction period. The typical patient who develops a left ventricular aneurysm has a turbulent postinfarction course, usually marked by overt or borderline congestive heart failure or recurring arrhythmias. In the absence of other hemodynamic lesions, such as mitral valve insufficiency or ventricular septal defect, the occurrence of congestive heart failure usually indicates that 20 per cent or more of the left ventricular mass is involved and that aneurysm formation is not unlikely.[28] Although some patients who have aneurysms of the left ventricle may not develop symptoms for several years after infarction,[15] this course of events represents the exception rather than the general course. The most common symptom in patients with ventricular aneurysm is dyspnea, with frequently associated palpitations and angina and manifestations of peripheral embolization occurring rarely (Table 1). Many patients have more than one symptom, for example, exertional dyspnea and angina or exertional angina and palpitations.

Although the presence of a ventricular aneurysm may be suspected from the above-described clinical course, substantiation of the diagnosis and therapeutic decision-making depend on further evaluation. An abnormal cardiac impulse is usually detectable at the apex and a ventricular gallop (S_3) is often audible. The aneurysm produces no cardiac murmurs, but coexisting

TABLE 1. Symptoms in 80
Patients with Ventricular
Aneurysm

Symptom	Number	Percentage
Dyspnea	61	75
Palpitations	36	45
Angina	32	40
Emboli	1	~1

valvular dysfunction (most commonly mitral regurgitation) produces characteristic findings.

The persistence of elevated ST segments following acute myocardial infarction is very suggestive of a developing left ventricular aneurysm, but this finding has not proved sufficiently reliable to be diagnostic.[10,22,23] Chest films most often reveal enlargement of the left ventricle and pulmonary congestion. Cardiac fluoroscopy may reveal systolic expansion (paradox) in the area of the aneurysm. The demonstration of abnormalities in segmental left ventricular wall motion using ultrasound and/or gated blood pool ventriculography is helpful in identifying patients for whom further study is indicated.[6,7,14,16,18,35] Whereas the diagnosis of left ventricular aneurysm may be confirmed by means of these minimally invasive techniques, left ventriculography and selective coronary arteriography most accurately outline the extent of the aneurysm, the presence of mural thrombus, the existence of valvular dysfunction, and the localization of coronary occlusive lesions.

TREATMENT

The treatment of left ventricular aneurysm is aneurysmectomy combined with correction of any significant valvular abnormalities and bypass of major coronary obstructive lesions. Operation is indicated in patients whose aneurysms cause symptoms. Additionally, those patients whose aneurysms were discovered during the course of coronary arteriography in anticipation of coronary bypass surgery should have aneurysmectomy at the time of bypass operation. Whereas the 3-year mortality following uncomplicated myocardial infarction is about 15 to 20 per cent, this figure rises to 70 to 75 per cent in patients with aneurysms and to nearly 90 per cent after 5 years.[33,40] In order to allow time for scar tissue to form in areas of necrotic myocardium, *elective* aneurysmectomy should not be undertaken earlier than 2 months from the time of infarction.

Operation for left ventricular aneurysm is best done through a midline sternotomy incision. An internal mammary artery and/or saphenous vein(s) should be prepared if coronary artery bypass grafting is planned as a part of the procedure. Cardiopulmonary bypass is begun and the core body temperature lowered to 26° to 28° C. Venting of the left ventricle is probably unnecessary but, if done, should be undertaken with extreme care so as not to dislodge any existing thrombotic material. Whereas most cardiac surgeons currently utilize aortic cross-clamping and myocardial protection with cold cardioplegia, Akins has had success in a large series of operations using hypothermia and induced ventricular fibrillation without aortic cross-clamping.[2,37]

The steps in excising the aneurysm and reconstructing the left ventricle are shown in Figure 1. The importance of geometric reconstruction of the left ventricle was emphasized by Hutching and Brawley[26] and made practical by Jatene.[27] The techniques have been modified by Dor and associates[17] and by Cooley[11] with steadily improving results. First, the aneurysm is opened and any mural thrombus is carefully and completely removed. The sac of the aneurysm is then inspected and followed back to its junction with healthy myocardium. This process allows identification of a circular or oval defect with a fibrous rim (Fig.

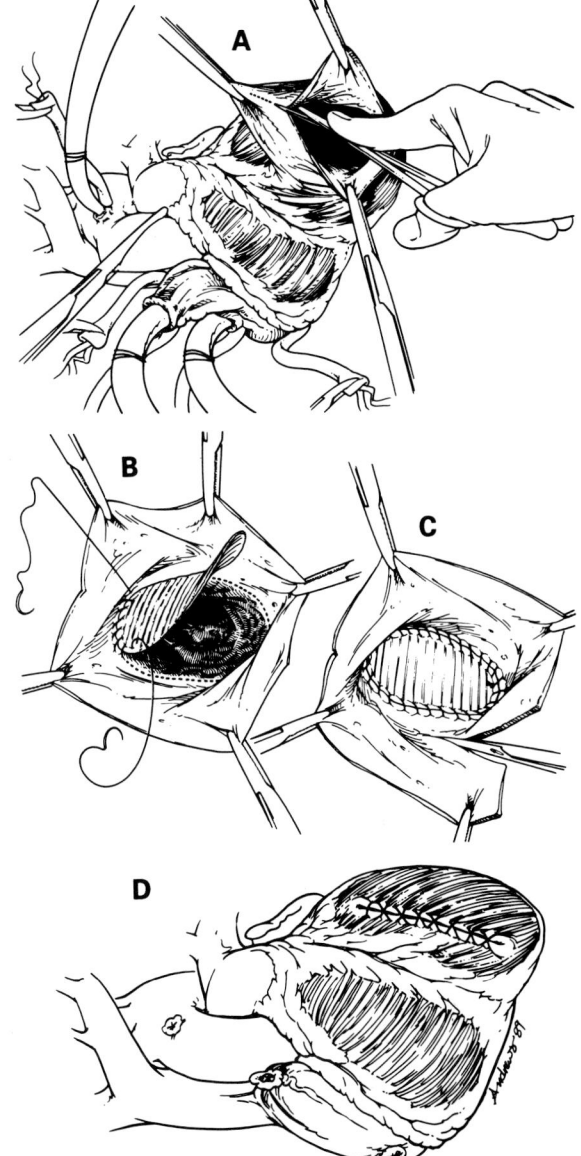

Figure 1. Steps for aneurysmectomy and reconstruction of the left ventricle. *A*, The aneurysm is opened and any mural thrombus carefully and completely removed. *B*, The fibrous rim of the aneurysm is identified from within the aneurysm and is closed using a patch fashioned to approximate the size of the defect. *C*, The remaining aneurysm sac is trimmed. *D*, The aneurysm sac is closed over the repair, usually without buttresses or pledgets. (From Cooley, D. A.: Ventricular endoaneurysmorrhaphy: Results of an improved method of repair. Tex. Heart Inst. J., *16*:72, 1989. Drawn by Bill Andrews.)

1*B*). A patch — the author prefers glutaraldehyde-prepared autologous pericardium (immersed in 0.5 per cent glutaraldehyde for 2 minutes, which makes the pericardium slightly stiff and easier to manage) — is then trimmed to approximate the size and shape of the defect and sewn into place with a continuous nonabsorbable suture (2-0 or 3-0 polypropylene). The aneurysm sac is then trimmed (Fig. 1*C*) and closed (Fig. 1*D*) over the repair. The use of buttressing strips or pledgets is usually not necessary. Although experience with this type of repair is not yet extensive, the improved functional results reported appear to justify its use whenever possible.[11,17]

The operative mortality for elective excision of left ventricular aneurysm is acceptable, even when combined with other procedures.[13] Most centers report operative mortalities in the 5 per cent range.[8,13,29,30] Moreover, it has been found that 80 per cent of the survivors are alive 4 years later. Factors influencing early mortality include advanced age (over 65 years), emergent operation, left main coronary disease, history of cardiogenic shock, renal failure, and NYHA Class IV status.[13,30] Factors that negatively affect long-term survival include the presence of extensive right coronary artery occlusive disease and evidence of posterobasal left ventricular dysfunction.[4]

Whereas there is little question that aneurysmectomy improves survival and causes subjective improvement, data documenting objective improvement are sparse. Nicolosi and Spotnitz used intraoperative echocardiography in 7 patients who had aneurysmectomy without geometric reconstruction and found no improvement in end-systolic function.[34] They concluded that elimination of paradoxically increased mechanical efficiency following aneurysmectomy may be responsible for the observed clinical improvement. A similar technique would be useful in the evaluation of geometric reconstruction as described earlier. Mangschau and associates, from Norway, recently studied 42 patients with radionuclide ventriculography prior to aneurysmectomy and again 10 months later, finding that global ejection fraction, both at rest and following exercise, had improved.[31] The resting cardiac index remained unchanged despite an NYHA functional Class I improvement along with an increased double product and workload.

Although aneurysms of the posterior and basilar aspects of the left ventricle are less common than those of the anterior and apical portions, they do occur. Resection and primary closure would cause significant distortion of ventricular geometry. This distortion in the posterobasal area, in addition to producing a disturbed and less effective contractile pattern, would probably lead to significant mitral valvular incompetence. Use of an adynamic patch, sometimes without closure of the aneurysm sac over it, is most often required to repair aneurysms in this area.[14]

COMPLEX VENTRICULAR ANEURYSMS

Some patients require consideration of operation soon after myocardial infarction because of hemodynamic deterioration producing refractory heart failure or, in some instances, cardiogenic shock. Whereas many of these critically ill patients die because the amount of residual functioning myocardium is inadequate to sustain circulation, in some operative intervention may prove lifesaving. In these patients, the plan of choice is temporary circulatory cardiac assistance with a device such as the intra-aortic balloon pump and evaluation of operability by ventriculography and coronary arteriography. If appropriate, operative repair of the existing hemodynamic lesion may be undertaken.[32] Acute, discrete left ventricular aneurysm, ruptured or dysfunctional papillary muscle causing acute mitral valve incompetence, and rupture of the interventricular septum represent lesions for which operative intervention is warranted. When there is no discrete area of ventricular dyskinesia, no ventricular septal defect, or no mitral incompetence or when the shock state has been prolonged so as to produce prolonged anuria or when the ventricle fails to respond even minimally to inotropic stimulation, operation is probably not indicated. For patients in this category, long-term ventricular support and/or cardiac transplantation probably represents the most favorable likelihood of survival.

Because of the severity of illness and the frequent presence of associated dysfunction of other organ systems, mortality is much higher in this group of patients than in those undergoing elective aneurysmectomy. If, however, hemodynamic improvement follows operation, many of these individuals who otherwise would not have survived may go on to a full recovery.

SELECTED REFERENCES

Cosgrove, D. M., Lytle, B. W., Taylor, P. C., Stewart, R. W., Golding, L. A. R., Mahfood, S., Goormastic, M., and Loop, F. D.: Ventricular aneurysm resection: Trends in surgical risk. Circulation, 79:I-97, 1989.

This is a retrospective analysis of 1183 patients operated upon at the Cleveland Clinic over a 15-year period. Significant risk factors included emergent procedures, advanced age (over 65 years), left main coronary disease, and congestive heart failure. Despite advancing patient age and the presence of more extensive coronary disease, operative mortality for ventricular aneurysm has remained in the 5 to 10 per cent range.

Forman, M. B., Collins, H. W., Kapelman, H. A., Vaughan, W. K., Parry, J. M., Virmani, R., and Friesinger, G. C.: Determinants of left ventricular aneurysm formation after anterior myocardial infarction: A clinical and angiographic study. J. Am. Coll. Cardiol., 8:1256, 1986.

This group studied 79 patients who experienced a transmural anterior infarction as their first myocardial infarction. Total occlusion of the left anterior descending coronary artery in the absence of collateral circulation was found to be a significant factor in the formation of a left ventricular aneurysm following anterior myocardial infarction.

Jatene, A. D.: Left ventricular aneurysmectomy: Resection or reconstruction. J. Thorac. Cardiovasc. Surg., 89:321, 1985.

Applying novel reconstructive techniques that cause less distortion of the normal ventricular geometry, this group of surgeons was able to reduce early operative mortality from 11.6 per cent to 4.3 per cent. More important, attention was called to the desirability of geometric reconstruction following aneurysmectomy.

REFERENCES

1. Abrams, D. L., Edelist, A., Luria, M. H., and Miller, A. S.: Ventricular aneurysm. A reappraisal based on a study of sixty-five consecutive autopsied cases. Circulation, 27:164, 1963.
2. Akins, C. W.: Resection of left ventricular aneurysm during hypothermic fibrillatory arrest without aortic occlusion. J. Thorac. Cardiovasc. Surg., 91:610, 1986.
3. Bailey, C. P., Holton, H. E., and Nichols, H.: Ventriculoplasty for cardiac aneurysm. J. Thorac. Cardiovasc. Surg., 35:37, 1958.
4. Barratt-Boyes, B. G., White, H. D., Agnew, T. M., and Wild, C. J.: The results of surgical treatment of left ventricular aneurysms. J. Thorac. Cardiovasc. Surg., 87:87, 1984.
5. Beck, C. S.: Operation for aneurysm of the heart. Ann. Surg., 120:34, 1944.
6. Borer, J. S., Bacharach, S. L., Green, M. V., Kent, K. M., Epstein, S. E., and Johnston, G. S.: Real-time radionuclide cineangiography in the noninvasive evaluation of global and regional left ventricular function at rest and during exercise in patients with coronary artery disease. N. Engl. J. Med., 296:839, 1977.
7. Borer, J. S., Jacobstein, J. G., Bacharach, S. L., and Green, M. V.: Detection of left ventricular aneurysm and evaluation of effects of surgical repair: The role of radionuclide cineangiography. Am. J. Cardiol., 45:1103, 1980.
8. Burton, N. A., Stinson, E. B., Oyer, P. E., and Shumway, N. E.: Left ventricular aneurysm: Preoperative risk factors and long-term postoperative results. J. Thorac. Cardiovasc. Surg., 77:65, 1979.
9. Candell, J., Valle, V., Paya, J., Cortadellas, J., Esplugas, E., and Rius, J.: Posttraumatic coronary occlusion and early left ventricular aneurysm. Am. Heart J., 97:509, 1979.
10. Cokkinos, D. V., Hallman, G. L., Cooley, D. A., Zamalloa, O., and Leachman, R. C.: Left ventricular aneurysm: Analysis of electrocardiographic features and postresection changes. Am. Heart J., 82:149, 1971.
11. Cooley, D. A.: Ventricular endoaneurysmorrhaphy: Results of an improved method of repair. Texas Heart Inst. J., 16:72, 1989.
12. Cooley, D. A., Colling, H. A., Morris, C. G., and Chapman, D. W.: Ventricular aneurysm after myocardial infarction: Surgical excision with use of temporary cardiopulmonary bypass. J.A.M.A., 167:557, 1958.
13. Cosgrove, D. M., Lytle, B. W., Taylor, P. C., Stewart, R. W., Golding, L. A. R., Mahfood, S., Goormastic, M., and Loop, F. D.: Ventricular aneurysm resection: Trends in surgical risk. Circulation, 79:I-97, 1989.
14. Daggett, W. M.: Surgical technique for early repair of posterior ventricular septal rupture. J. Thorac. Cardiovasc. Surg., 84:306, 1982.
15. Davis, R. W., and Ebert, P. A.: Ventricular aneurysm: A clinical-pathological correlation. Am. J. Cardiol., 29:1, 1972.
16. Dillon, J., Feigenbaum, H., Weyman, A., Peskoe, S., and Chang, S.: Echocardiography in the evaluation of patients for aneurysmectomy (abstract). Circulation, 52(Suppl. II):135, 1975.
17. Dor, V., Saab, M., Coste, P., Kornaszewska, M., and Montiglio, F.: Left ventricular aneurysm: A new surgical approach. Thorac. Cardiovasc. Surg., 37:11, 1989.
18. Dymond, D. S., Jarritt, P. H., Britton, K. E., and Spurrell, R. A. J.: Detection of postinfarction aneurysms by first-pass radionuclide ventriculography using a multicrystal gamma camera. Br. Heart J., 41:68, 1979.
19. Favaloro, R. G., Effler, D. B., Groves, L. K., Wescott, R. N., Saurez, E., and Lozada, J.: Ventricular aneurysm—clinical experience. Ann. Thorac. Surg., 6:227, 1968.
20. Flemma, R. J., Marx, L., Litwin, S. B., and Gallen, W. J.: Left ventricular aneurysmectomy in a child. Ann. Thorac. Surg., 19:457, 1975.
21. Forman, M. B., Collins, H. W., Kapelman, H. A., Vaughan, W. K., Parry, J. M., Virmani, R., and Friesinger, G. C.: Determinants of left ventricular aneurysm formation after anterior myocardial infarction: A clinical and angiographic study. J. Am. Coll. Cardiol., 8:1256, 1986.
22. Gorlin, R., Klein, M. D., and Sullivan, J. M.: Prospective correlative study of

ventricular aneurysm. Mechanistic concept and clinical recognition. Am. J. Med., 42:512, 1967.

23. Groden, B. M., and James, W. B.: Significance of persistent R-ST elevation after acute myocardial infarction. Br. Heart J., 31:34, 1969.

24. Hirai, T., Fujita, M., Nakajima, H., Asamoi, H., Yamanishi, K., Ohno, A., and Sasayama, S.: Clinical investigation: Importance of collateral circulation for prevention of left ventricular aneurysm formation in acute anterior myocardial infarction. Circulation, 79:791, 1989.

25. Hunter, J.: An account of the dissection of morbid bodys. London, Library of the Royal College of Surgeons, 32:30, 1757.

26. Hutching, G. M., and Brawley, R. K.: The influence of cardiac geometry on the result of ventricular aneurysm repair. Am. J. Pathol., 99:221, 1980.

27. Jatene, A.D.: Left ventricular aneurysmectomy: Resection or reconstruction. J. Thorac. Cardiovasc. Surg., 89:321, 1985.

28. Klein, M. D., Herman, M. V., and Gorlin, R.: A hemodynamic study of left ventricular aneurysm. Circulation, 35:614, 1967.

29. Loop, F. D., Effler, D. B., Navia, J. A., Sheldon, W. C., and Groves, L. K.: Aneurysms of the left ventricle: Survival and results of ten year experience. Ann. Surg., 178:399, 1973.

30. Magovern, G. J., Sakert, T., Simpson, K., Laug, G. W., Park, S. B., Liebler, G., Burkholder, J., Maher, T., Benkart, D., and Magovern, G. J., Jr.: Surgical therapy for left ventricular aneurysms—a ten year experience. Circulation, 79:I-102, 1989.

31. Mangschau, A., Forfang, K., Rootwelt, K., and Froysaker, T.: Improvement in cardiac performance and exercise tolerance after left ventricular aneurysm surgery—a prospective study. Thorac. Cardiovasc. Surg., 36:320, 1988.

32. Mundth, E. D., Buckley, M. J., Daggett, W. M., Sanders, C. A., and Austen, W. G.: Surgery for complications of acute myocardial infarction. Circulation, 45:1279, 1972.

33. Nagle, R. E., and Williams, D. O.: Natural history of ventricular aneurysm without surgical treatment. Br. Heart J., 36:1037, 1974.

34. Nicolosi, A. C., and Spotnitz, H. M.: Clinical investigation: Quantitative analysis of regional systolic function with left ventricular aneurysm. Circulation, 78:856, 1988.

35. Rakowski, R., Martin, R. P., Schapira, J. N., Wexler, L., Silverman, J. F., Cipriano, P. R., Guthaner, D. F., and Popp, R. L.: Left ventricular aneurysm: Detection and determination of resectability by two-dimensional ultrasound. Circulation, 55, 56(Suppl. III):153, 1977.

36. Rittenhouse, E. A., Sauvage, L. R., Mansfield, P. R., Smith J. C., Davis, C. C., and Hall, D. G.: False aneurysm of the left ventricle. Report of four cases and review of the surgical management. Ann. Surg., 189:409, 1979.

37. Rivera, R., and Dekan, J. L.: Factors influencing better results in operation for post infarction ventricular aneurysms. Ann. Thorac. Surg., 27:445, 1979.

38. Sapsford, R. N., Fitchett, D. H., Tarin, D., and Anderson, R. H.: Aneurysm of the left ventricle secondary to bacterial endocarditis. J. Thorac. Cardiovasc. Surg., 78:79, 1979.

39. Sauerbruch, F.: Erfolgreiche operative Beseitigung cines Aneurysm ab der rechten Herzkammer. Arch. Klin. Chir., 167:586, 1931.

40. Schlichter, J., Hellerstein, H. K., and Katz, L. N.: Aneurysm of the heart: A correlative study of one hundred and two proved cases. Medicine, 33:43, 1954.

41. Sternberg, M.: Das chronische partielle Herzaneurysma. Vienna and Leipsig, Franz Deutlicke, 1914.

42. Tennant, R., and Wiggers, C. J.: Effect of coronary occlusion on myocardial contraction. Am. J. Physiol., 112:351, 1935.

43. Turnia, M., Real, F., Meier, W., and Senning, Å.: Left ventricular aneurysmectomy in a four month old infant: Alternative method of treatment of anomalous left coronary artery. J. Thorac. Cardiovasc. Surg., 67:915, 1975.

5. KAWASAKI'S DISEASE

Thomas A. D'Amico, M. D.

Kawasaki's disease is a multisystemic disorder of undetermined etiology that is now the leading cause of acquired cardiac disease in children in both Japan and the United States.[81] Described in Japan by Kawasaki in 1967, the disorder was first presented in English in 1974.[41] This acute illness presents with fever, sterile conjunctivitis, cervical lymphadenopathy, mucocutaneous changes, and prominent vasculitic features.[29] Although usually indolent and self-limiting, in its advanced stage the syndrome is characterized by coronary and peripheral artery aneurysms, coronary stenoses, mitral valve insufficiency, and left ventricular dysfunction.[48] In Kawasaki's original description, the syndrome was thought to be limited to Japanese children. The syndrome was recognized in the United States in 1973[61]; and to date, more than 2200 cases have been reported nationally.[78] In addition, Kawasaki's disease has been described throughout North America,[77,81] Europe,[12,15,88,96] Australia,[9] and the Pacific, in addition to approximately 80,000 cases in Japan alone.[80]

Kawasaki's disease predominately affects infants and children, the highest incidence being at 12 to 16 months.[10] The overall incidence is 4.5 to 9.5 per 100,000 population; this contrasts with acute rheumatic fever, the incidence of which is 1 per 100,000. Kawasaki's disease has been found to be more common in males than in females (3:2), in Asians and blacks, and in siblings.[97] Various causative agents have been proposed, but the etiology of Kawasaki's syndrome is still unclear. The pathophysiology has been well described, but the infrequent progression to severe cardiovascular manifestation is not well understood. Increased awareness of the potential severity of Kawasaki's disease has contributed to more prompt diagnosis and earlier institution of therapy. Current management consists of antiplatelet agents and intravenous immunoglobulin, as well as surgical intervention in patients with advanced disease. An ideal treatment that ameliorates the early inflammatory symptoms, arrests the vasculitic progression, and prevents the formation of coronary aneurysms has not yet been found.

CLINICAL MANIFESTATIONS

Symptoms

Kawasaki's original description of the clinical features of the syndrome has been consistently supported by others. The diagnostic criteria, including the principal symptoms and associated findings, are shown in Table 1.[29,78,80] The diagnosis of Kawasaki's disease is secured by the presence of five of the six major criteria. The presentation of this syndrome is acute, and the symptoms evolve during a period of a few days, a stereotypical clinical pattern that usually leads to certain diagnosis. However, various reports of atypical presentations suggest that a high index of suspicion is required to prevent delayed diagnosis and late recognition of complications. Atypical patterns include presentation without rash,[6,87] with abdominal aortic aneurysm,[8] with otitis media,[18] and of Kawasaki's disease in an adult.[33]

The principal presenting symptom is fever, which usually has an abrupt onset, may be prolonged or intermittent, and does not respond to antibiotics.[24] The fever lasts from 7 to 14 days but may persist in more severe cases. The appearance of fever is

TABLE 1. Principal Symptoms and Associated Findings of Kawasaki's Disease

Principal Symptoms (5 of 6 needed for diagnosis)
1. Fever
2. Conjunctivitis
3. Changes in the mouth and oral cavity—at least one of the following:
   - dry, chapped, fissured, or reddened lips
   - prominent, reddened tongue
   - diffuse reddening of oral mucosa
4. Changes of the extremities—at least one of the following:
   - reddening of the palms and soles
   - indurative edema of the hands or feet
   - desquamation of fingertips or toes
5. Polymorphous truncal rash
6. Nonpurulent cervical adenopathy

Associated Findings
Arthralgia
Arthritis
Aseptic meningitis
Diarrhea
Hydrops of the gallbladder
Jaundice
Myocarditis
Pericarditis
Proteinuria
Urethritis

often accompanied by the presence of congested ocular conjunctivae, bilateral and sterile, a condition that does not respond to ocular preparations. After the appearance of conjunctivitis, several changes in the lips and oral cavity occur. Commonly, there is a reddening of the lips, which may then become dry and fissured. The tongue may appear prominently, with protuberant papillae ("strawberry tongue"), or there may be only diffuse reddening of the oropharyngeal mucosa.

By the third day of the illness, a polymorphous macular erythematous rash appears. The rash begins with reddening of the palms and soles; individual lesions may coalesce as the rash progresses proximally to spread over the trunk, usually over 48 hours. As the rash resolves, secondary changes in fingers and toes appear. A unique desquamation begins at the junction of the nails and the skin on the tips of the digits. In less than 50 per cent of patients, nonpurulent cervical lymphadenopathy develops.

Physical Examination

The principal physical findings are easily recognized. Elicitation of the more subtle physical findings early in the course of Kawasaki's disease may facilitate the prompt diagnosis of its numerous complications.

Examination of the heart may reveal tachycardia, distant heart sounds, or a gallop, suggestive of myocarditis or congestive failure. A holosystolic apical murmur signifies mitral valve insufficiency, which may be secondary to cardiomegaly, endocarditis, or papillary muscle dysfunction. The cardiac examination should be performed twice daily to ensure detection of cardiovascular abnormalities.[29] Palpation of the peripheral arteries, especially in the axillary and inguinal regions, may reveal an aneurysm (Fig. 1). Palpation of the abdomen may reveal hepatomegaly, secondary to congestive heart failure, or right upper quandrant tenderness, secondary to hydrops of the gallbladder.[70] Although infrequent, the presence of peritoneal signs suggests vascular compromise in the mesenteric arteries.[62] Auscultation of the abdomen may reveal the bruit of an aneurysm

of the renal, celiac, mesenteric, or iliac arteries. Neurologic examination may show meningeal signs, as well as emotional lability, irritability, stupor, or coma, secondary to aseptic meningitis. Examination of the neck in children often yields prominent cervical lymphadenopathy; however, this may be an early finding in patients, occurring prior to the other classic findings. It has been suggested that lymph node biopsy should be performed to ascertain the diagnosis of Kawasaki's disease and thereby institute therapy earlier.[27]

Laboratory Studies

Leukocytosis is invariably present and is often accompanied by a shift to the left. Anemia and thrombocytosis may be present.[4] Other findings include an increase in the red blood cell sedimentation rate, C-reactive protein, factor VII concentration, and fibrinogen level, as well as low antithrombin III concentration.[7] Hyperbilirubinemia, hyperamylasemia, and sterile pyuria are common but not invariably present.[58]

The electrocardiogram is abnormal in 70 per cent of patients.[75] The most common findings are sinus tachycardia, prolonged PQ and QR intervals, second-degree atrioventricular block, decreased voltage, ST segment changes, and T wave changes.[14]

Admission radiologic studies are often abnormal. Chest films may reveal cardiomegaly or pleural effusions. Echocardiograms are positive in 45 per cent of patients, providing early objective evidence of cardiovascular dysfunction.[11]

Natural History

There are three clinical stages of Kawasaki's disease.[29] The acute phase lasts approximately 10 days, during which fever and the development of the characteristic rash predominate. The subacute phase ensues, during which the cardiac complications commonly occur. The convalescent phase is defined as the period during which the red blood cell sedimentation rate remains elevated. Although the course of Kawasaki's disease is

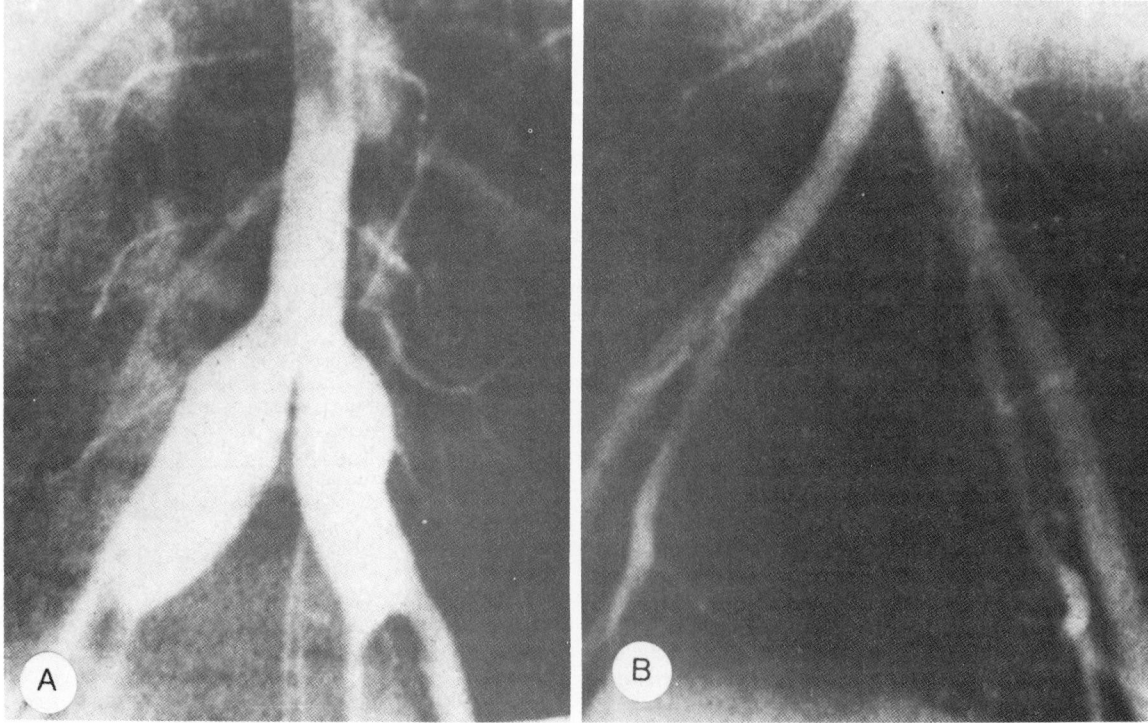

Figure 1. *A*, Aortogram in an infant with Kawasaki's disease demonstrates bilateral iliac artery aneurysms. *B*, After regression of the aneurysms 1 year later, the arteries appear radiographically normal. (From Chung, K. J., Fulton, D. R., Lapp, R., Spector, S., and Sahn, D. J.,: One-year follow-up of cardiac and coronary artery disease in infants and children with Kawasaki disease. Am. Heart J., *115:*1263, 1988.)

TABLE 2. Cardiac Manifestations of Kawasaki's Disease

Coronary aneurysms
Myocarditis
Mitral regurgitation
Aortic insufficiency
Valvulitis
Myocardial infarction
Sudden death

TABLE 3. Risk Factors for the Development of Coronary Aneurysms in Kawasaki's Disease

Male sex
Age under 1 year
Duration of fever greater than 16 days
WBC greater than 30
Erythrocyte sedimentation rate greater than 100
Elevated C-reactive protein
Thrombocytosis

typically acute, with resolution of symptoms and complications, it may recur with vasculitic symptoms[16] or with sudden death.[42]

A spectrum of cardiovascular manifestations may occur in Kawasaki's disease, although they are usually self-limited and benign (Table 2).[13,36] Myocarditis, diagnosed clinically and by electrocardiographic criteria, is present in as many as 50 per cent of patients.[92] One study, in which endomyocardial biopsies were taken during cardiac catheterization for coronary arteriography, showed inflammatory changes in each of 201 patients.[38] In the acute phase, myocarditis may cause exercise intolerance, congestive heart failure, or death, secondary to ischemia or diffuse hypokinesia.[48]

Mitral regurgitation occurs in only 5 per cent of patients with Kawasaki's disease;[24] however, in patients with coronary aneurysms, the incidence is 25 per cent.[49] Ischemia to the papillary muscles secondary to coronary artery involvement is responsible for most cases,[93] although diffuse myocardial inflammation and annular dilatation may also contribute.

Myocardial infarction, a rare complication of Kawasaki's disease, may occur after diffuse ischemia or a thromboembolic event.[98] Myocardial ischemia is due to profound fibrotic changes or is seconday to multiple stenotic lesions. The presence of collateral circulation usually preserves ventricular function, despite multiple stenotic lesions; however, left ventricular hypertrophy associated with diffuse hypokinesia sometimes develops.

The most serious complication of Kawasaki's disease is the formation of coronary artery aneurysms, which has an incidence of 20 to 40 per cent in the subacute phase.[39,42,74] Coronary aneurysms are responsible for at least 85 per cent of the mortality associated with Kawasaki's disease.[10] A spectrum of coronary artery involvement is associated with Kawasaki's disease.[59] Echocardiographic studies have demonstrated that coronary arterial wall changes occur in all patients, which progress to dilatation in half and true aneurysms in over one quarter of patients.[33] The aneurysms may be asymptomatic or may not become symptomatic until years later, whereas other aneurysms present initially with myocardial infarction, cardiogenic shock, or sudden death.[38]

Serial angiographic studies have shown "resolution" of aneurysms that are discovered as early as the second week; several studies have demonstrated resolution of 50 per cent of coronary aneurysms 1 year after initial presentation.[11,36,37] Pathologic analysis has shown that angiographic resolution may be caused by intimal proliferation rather than by healing, which leaves these arteries at further risk for stenosis and thromboembolism.[3,69] The risk of chronic coronary involvement and development of premature atherosclerosis is unknown.[34]

Coronary artery aneurysms follow inflammatory changes in the intima and adventitia, caused by perivasculitis of the major coronary arteries. As in atherosclerotic coronary artery disease, the most common locations for lesions are at the bifurcation of the left anterior descending (LAD) and circumflex vessels (found in 74 per cent of patients with coronary aneurysms) and at the origin of the right coronary artery (RCA) (48 per cent).[65,89] Most patients are found to have multiple aneurysms, but only aneurysms that reach 4 mm. in diameter are clinically significant.[22] Within the aneurysm, turbulence and stagnation pro-

duce platelet aggregation and thrombosis. Advanced thrombosis causes critical stenoses in the coronary arteries, the most common indication for surgical intervention. Thromboembolic phenomena are also common and sometimes produce acute myocardial infarction. Cardiac fatalities occur in less than 1 per cent of patients with Kawasaki's disease[60,90]; however, it is apparent that the heart may be extensively involved in those who survive.[17]

The diagnosis of Kawasaki's disease should be accompanied routinely by echocardiography, which has demonstrated a sensitivity of greater than 90 per cent in detecting coronary aneurysms.[14] However, echocardiography is not effective in detecting stenotic lesions.[37] To reduce the morbidity and mortality of Kawasaki's disease, early detection and treatment of coronary lesions are necessary.[67] In order to ensure prompt institution of therapy, evaluation of the severity of the disease in a particular patient is required at a stage before most aneurysms can be detected by echocardiography. Thus, many clinicians have developed a scoring system, using risk factors, to anticipate the major cardiac complications.[1,3,31,69] The accepted risk factors for the development of coronary aneurysms are listed (Table 3); however, some clinicians depend on only the duration of fever in determining the risk of coronary involvement.[53]

Selective coronary angiography is reserved for patients with complications of known coronary aneurysms (Fig. 2).[38] Analysis of these data has shown groups of patients who are most likely to develop aneurysms and who require serial echocardiograms, selective angiography, and possibly surgical intervention.[53,68] The indications for cardiac catheterization are shown in Table 4.[94]

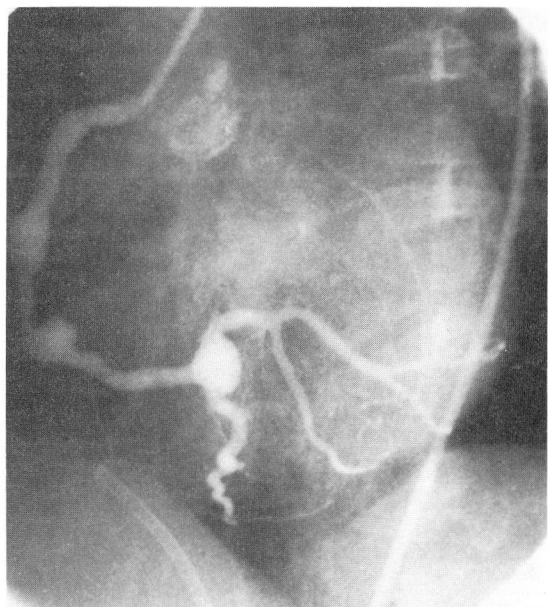

Figure 2. Coronary arteriogram demonstrating three aneurysms of the right coronary artery in a 10-year-old boy with Kawasaki's disease.

TABLE 4. Indications for Cardiac Catheterization in Kawasaki's Disease

Severe symptoms at onset
Symptoms of ischemic heart disease
Symptoms of congestive heart failure
Mitral regurgitation
Coronary calcifications evident on chest films
Persistent coronary aneurysms repeated on echocardiograms

PATHOLOGY

The pathologic basis of Kawasaki's disease is the progression of a nonspecific vasculitis that involves the microvasculature of the aorta and its major branches and is manifested by endarteritis of the vasa vasorum of the coronary, brachiocephalic, celiac, renal, and iliofemoral systems. As the inflammatory process of the intima and adventitia progresses, aneurysms form in these vessels and lead to stenosis, thromboembolism, ischemia, rupture, or asymptomatic healing. Pathologic analysis of hearts affected by Kawasaki's disease has helped elucidate the pathophysiology of the vasculitis.[23] Kawasaki's disease can be described in four stages: acute, subacute, convalescent, and chronic (Table 5).[20]

The acute phase, characterized by perivasculitis, corresponds to the febrile period and usually involves the first 10 days of the illness. During this period the oral changes, skin changes, and conjunctivitis also develop. On presentation, the patient may also have arthritis, myocarditis, pericarditis, mitral insufficiency, and meningitis. At this stage the perivasculitis affects the small vessels — arterioles, capillaries, and venules. There may be inflammation in the intima of medium and large arteries, as well as in the atrioventricular conduction system, but aneurysmal dilatation and stenosis are not observed. Death in the acute phase is usually secondary to advanced myocarditis but is rare.[22]

During the subacute phase, typically the second 10 days of the illness, most of the clinical findings may resolve, although fever and irritability often persist. Examination of arteries during this phase shows perivasculitis of the major coronary arteries, aneurysmal development, and early platelet thrombus formation (Fig. 3). Thrombotic occlusion may develop and cause myocardial ischemia, and thromboembolism may ensue with subsequent myocardial infarction. Myocarditis persists in the subacute stage, and coagulation necrosis may be found in the myocardium (especially in papillary muscles) and in the conduction system. Pericarditis may also persist, and endocar-

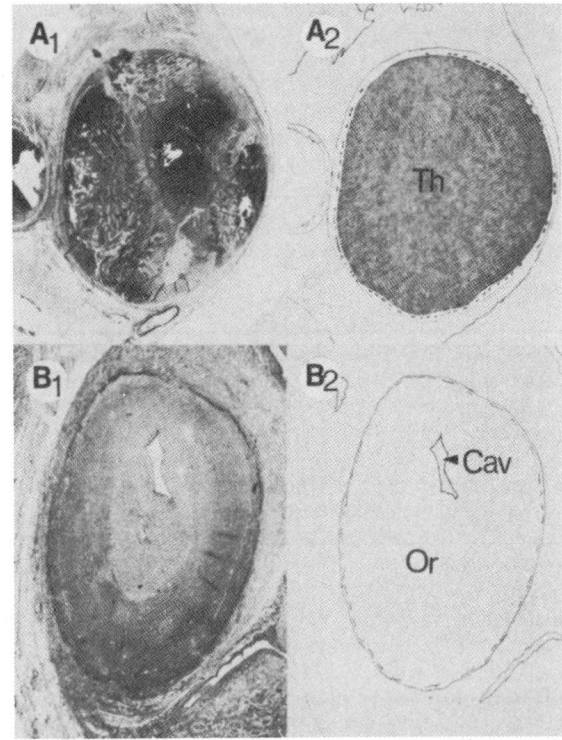

Figure 3. *A,* Coronary aneurysm with fresh occlusive thrombi, stained with elastic van Gieson's stain. A_1, original magnification $\times 6$; A_2, magnified 10 times by enlarger and sketched. *B,* Coronary aneurysms with organization or intimal thickening, stained with elastic van Gieson's stain. B_1, original magnification $\times 10$; B_2, magnified 10 times by enlarger and sketched. *Perforated line* indicates remnant elastic interna. Cav, cavity; Or, organization; Th, thrombi. (From Fujiwara, T., Fujiwara, H., and Hamashima, Y., Frequency and size of coronary arterial aneurysm at necropsy in Kawasaki disease. Am. J. Cardiol., *59:*808, 1987.)

ditis and valvulitis may develop. Death in the subacute stage is often caused by a ruptured coronary artery aneurysm.

The convalescent stage, which extends into the second month, is characterized by decreased arterial inflammation. Granulation changes are seen in this stage, as internal proliferation within the aneurysm may ameliorate luminal defects. Aneurysmal dilatation may persist and produce progressive stenosis and further risk of thromboembolism. Death in this stage is usually secondary to diffuse myocardial ischemia. The disease rarely enters a chronic phase, during which scarring continues, as does myocardial ischemia secondary to coronary stenoses. Resolution of the myocarditis may cause fibrous myocardial changes and endocardial fibroelastosis.

TABLE 5. The Four Stages of Kawasaki's Disease

Stage	Duration	Symptoms	Pathology
I	0–9 days	Fever Conjunctivitis Mucocutaneous changes	Myocarditis Perivasculitis of arterioles, capillaries, and venules Intimal inflammation of medium and large arterioles
II	10–20 days	Fever Palpable aneurysms	Panvasculitis Coronary and peripheral aneurysms, with early thrombosis
III	21–31 days	Arthritis (most symptoms resolved)	Coronary aneurysms Thrombosis and stenosis
IV	>40 days	Angina	Scarring Fibrosis Intimal thickening

From Fujiwara, H., and Hamashima, Y.: Pathology of the heart in Kawasaki disease. Pediatrics, *61:*100, 1978.

ETIOLOGY

Kawasaki's disease is the main cause of acquired heart disease in children in the United States and Japan.[81] Despite the prevalence of the disorder, investigations of the etiology have been unsuccessful; the pathogenesis of Kawasaki's syndrome has not yet been discovered. Many clinical aspects of the syndrome imply a communicable causative factor. The acute presentation of fever, rash, conjunctivitis, and lymphadenopathy in children suggests an infectious illness. That the disease exclusively affects children and spares adults suggests a mechanism of acquired immunity. Epidemiologic evidence supports the theory of an infectious etiology. In addition to geographic areas where it appears to be endemic, such as Japan, seasonal epidemic outbreaks are common.[2]

The search for a single causative agent has been unsuccessful. Possibilities include mite-associated antigens,[19] rickettsiae,[9,28] spirochetes,[57] *Propionibacterium*,[35] *Borrelia*,[56] *Pseudomonas*,[43] and Epstein-Barr virus,[76] all without confirmation. The lack of evidence for person-to-person transmissibility has made it difficult to isolate a single etiologic factor. Variable immunity or low communicability could explain this phenomenon.

Investigation of peripheral lymphocytes isolated from the blood during the acute stage of Kawasaki's disease showed increased helper T-lymphocyte activity and decreased suppressor T-lymphocyte activity, which suggests a retroviral component in the etiology of Kawasaki's disease.[86] In contrast to the human immunodeficiency virus (HIV), the helper-to-suppressor T-lymphocyte ratio is *increased*, which is compatible with a suppressor T-lymphotrophic virus.[78] That Kawasaki's disease is recurrent in 3 per cent of patients suggests a cell-associated agent, persistently infecting lymphocytes.[56] Reverse transcriptase, which synthesizes DNA from a template of RNA, is the hallmark of retroviral activity. Analysis of supernatants from cultures of lymphocytes from patients with Kawasaki's syndrome showed significantly increased reverse transcriptase activity compared with controls. Although this finding has been confirmed by multiple laboratories,[5,60,85] there has been no conclusive evidence of a specific viral agent, since cell lines and culture conditions have not been discovered, and there is no serologic evidence of a specific antiviral antibody.

TREATMENT

The mortality of Kawasaki's disease before 1976 was 1 to 2 per cent. Since 1976, the mortality has decreased to approximately 0.5 per cent,[90] because of earlier diagnosis and the evolution of effective treatment modalities, including surgical intervention. Optimal therapy depends ultimately on the discovery of the etiology of Kawasaki's disease. Early diagnosis and recognition of the appearance of the cardiovascular complications are critical in the successful management of patients with Kawasaki's disease, because death from congestive failure may occur in the first week. However, coronary inflammatory changes are not always evident.

Aspirin

When Kawasaki's disease is diagnosed, children are given a regimen of aspirin, 100 mg. per kg. per day, which is continued until defervescence. Thereafter, they are maintained on aspirin, 10 mg. per kg. per day, for 8 weeks or until the red blood cell sedimentation rate is normal. In children who develop aneurysms, low-dose aspirin therapy may be continued indefinitely; the risk of associated salicylate complications, including Reye's syndrome, is low. The goal of aspirin therapy is the amelioration of symptoms and the prevention of the thrombotic and embolic complications of Kawasaki's disease. Aspirin does *not* decrease the risk of the development of coronary aneurysms,[31,39] nor does it prevent obstruction in giant coronary aneurysms.

Gammaglobulin

Treatment with intravenous gammaglobulin has been shown to decrease the duration of fever,[25] to decrease the prevalence of coronary abnormalities,[64] and to prevent the progression to giant coronary aneurysms.[79] A cooperative study compared aspirin therapy alone for 14 days with the combination of intravenous gammaglobulin (400 mg. per kg. per day for 5 days) and aspirin for 14 days. A decreased incidence of cardiovascular complications at 14 days (8 versus 23.1 per cent) and at 49 days (3.8 versus 17.7 per cent) was reported in the group treated with both aspirin and gammaglobulin.[73] Further studies have demonstrated that 200 mg. per kg. per day is equally effective.[26] Moreover, gammaglobulin therapy improves cardiac function in patients with wall motion abnormalities secondary to diffuse myocarditis.[72] Proposed mechanisms to explain the efficacy of intravenous gammaglobulin therapy include competition for endothelial cell receptors, negative feedback on the B cell lymphocyte system, and the direct neutralization of a viral agent.[54] The side effects of this therapy are fever, chills, and urticaria,[82] and administration is usually well tolerated.

Surgical Management

Advanced cardiovascular complications require surgical intervention. Surgical treatment has included Vineberg's procedure,[45] coronary artery bypass grafting (CABG) with autologous saphenous vein grafts (SVG),[47,84] CABG with homologous SVG,[51] CABG with a right subclavian artery graft,[55] CABG with internal mammary artery grafts (IMAGs),[30,31,46] CABG with bilateral IMAG,[63] CABG with coronary artery aneurysmectomy,[44,90] mitral valve repair,[52] and mitral valve replacement.[49]

The first use of bypass grafting for obstructive coronary aneurysms in Kawasaki's disease was reported in 1976 by Kitamura and colleagues.[47] The procedure involved a 4-year-old boy with coronary aneurysms that obstructed the LAD and the RCA, which were diagnosed 10 months after presentation with Kawasaki's disease. Early follow-up showed the patient doing well. General problems with CABG became apparent with experience, however. Further use of homologous and autologous SVG showed frequent early occlusion of the grafts. In many patients, the distal coronary arteries appeared to be too small to accept vein grafts. In many children, autogenous SVG are not available. The potential for SVG to grow as the heart grows and the thoracic cavity expands is unknown.

Alternative graft choices were sought. Mains and associates reported the successful use of a right subclavian artery bypass to the LAD.[55] Kitamura and associates described the first successful use of IMAG to treat patients with coronary aneurysms in Kawasaki's disease.[46] Before the use of arterial bypass grafts, venous graft closure at 1 year was greater than 50 per cent. With the use of IMAG, patency is now 85 per cent at 1 year, and late patency is nearly 60 per cent. In a study by Hirose and associates of children over 4 years, the early patency rate with IMAG was 100 per cent and overall early patency with both IMAG and SVG was 83 per cent.[30] In that study, late patency of the IMAG was 50 per cent, compared with 38 per cent for the SVG. A more recent study by Kitamura (personal communication, 1988) showed 100 per cent early and late patency (more than 1 year) of the IMAG, compared with 90 per cent early patency and 50 per cent late patency of the SVG. In children younger than 8 years of age, patency of the SVG was 65 per cent, compared with 87 per cent in children older than 8 years of age.[50] The use of IMAG provides greater patency and the potential for growth, both elongation and dilatation. The operative indications are shown in Table 6.[91]

Mitral valve insufficiency in Kawasaki's disease is most often due to papillary muscle dysfunction, secondary to myocarditis and ischemia. Mitral regurgitation as a complication of this dis-

TABLE 6. Operative Criteria for Coronary Artery Bypass Grafting in Kawasaki's Disease

Progressively stenotic coronary lesions, demonstrated by selective coronary arteriography

No distal coronary aneurysms with stenosis

Localized aneurysm with significant stenosis in the left main coronary artery

Significant stenosis in two coronary arteries

The presence of collateral vessels arising from a coronary artery with a proximal aneurysm

Progressive stenosis in the left anterior descending coronary artery

Presence of left ventricular aneurysm

From Suzuki, A., Kamiya, T., Ono, Y., Takahashi, N., Naito, Y., and Kou, Y.: Indication of aortocoronary by-pass for coronary arterial obstruction due to Kawasaki disease. Heart Vessels, 1:94, 1985.

order is associated with high mortality when accompanied by poor left ventricular function. Survival is increased with the correction of valvular dysfunction, and both mitral valve repair and mitral valve replacement have been done. Surgical correction, in the presence of myocarditis and compromised left ventricular function, presents a more difficult problem than is usually encountered with valve replacement for rheumatic disease. Experience with ineffective valve repair has shown that mitral valve replacement is the most certain means of ensuring the management of severe mitral insufficiency, despite the absence of valvulitis.

SUMMARY

Kawasaki's disease is a fascinating disorder with many cardiovascular manifestations. Aspects of this disease yet to be explained include its etiology, selectivity for children, and ability to progress to severe stages in view of its usually benign and self-limited nature.

REFERENCES

1. Asai, T.: Evaluation method for the degree of seriousness in Kawasaki disease. Acta Paediatr. Jpn., 25:170, 1983.
2. Bell, D. M., Morens, D. M., Holman, R. C., Hurwitz, E. S., and Hunter, M. K.,: Kawasaki syndrome in the United States. Am. J. Dis. Child., 137:211, 1983.
3. Bierman, F. Z., and Gersony, W. M.: Kawasaki disease: Clinical perspective. J. Pediatr., 111:789, 1987.
4. Bligard, C. A.: Kawasaki disease and its diagnosis. Pediatr. Dermatol., 4:75, 1987.
5. Burns, J. C., Geha, R. S., Schneeberger, E. E., Newburger, J. W., Rosen, F. S., Glezen, L. S., Huang, A. S., Natale, J., and Leung, D. Y. M.: Polymerase activity in lymphocyte culture supernatants from patients with Kawasaki disease. Nature, 323:814, 1986.
6. Burns, J. C., Wiggins, J. W., Jr., Toews, W. H., Newburger, J. W., Leung, D. Y. M., Wilson, H., and Glode, M. P.: Clinical spectrum of Kawasaki disease in infants younger than 6 months of age. J. Pediatr., 5:759, 1986.
7. Burtt, D. M., Pollack, P., and Bianco, J. A.: Intravenous streptokinase in an infant with Kawasaki's disease complicated by acute myocardial infarction. Pediatr. Cardiol., 6:307, 1986.
8. Canter, C. E., Bower, R. J., and Strauss, A. W.: Atypical Kawasaki disease with aortic aneurysm. Pediatrics, 68:885, 1981.
9. Carter, R. F., Haynes, M. E., and Morton, J.: Rickettsia-like bodies and splenitis in Kawasaki disease (letter). Lancet, 2:1254, 1976.
10. Chabali, R., and Haynes, R. E.: Cardiovascular involvement in Kawasaki syndrome. South. Med. J., 76:359, 1983.
11. Chung, K. J., Fulton, D. R., Lapp, R., Spector, S., and Sahn, D. J.: One-year follow-up of cardiac and coronary artery disease in infants and children with Kawasaki disease. Am. Heart J., 6:1263, 1988.
12. Corbeel, L., Delmotte, B., Standaert, L., Casteels-Van Daele, M., and Eeckels, R.: Kawasaki disease in Europe (letter). Lancet, 1:797, 1977.
13. Crowley, D. C.: Cardiovascular complications of mucocutaneous lymph node syndrome. Pediatr. Clin. North Am., 31:1321, 1984.
14. Daniels, S. R., Specker, B., Capannari, T. E., Schwarts, D. C., Burke, M. J., and Kaplan, S.: Correlates of coronary artery aneurysm formation in patients with Kawasaki disease. Am. J. Dis. Child., 141:205, 1987.
15. Della Porta, G., and Alberti, A.: Kawasaki disease in Europe (letter). Lancet, 1:797, 1977.
16. Feild, C., Brady, S., and Lowe, B.: Relapsing Kawasaki's disease. Int. J. Cardiol., 15:241, 1987.
17. Fetterman, G. H., and Hashida, Y.: Mucocutaneous lymph node syndrome (MLNS): A disease widespread in Japan which demands our attention. Pediatrics, 54:268, 1974.
18. Friedman, A. D.: An atypical presentation of Kawasaki syndrome in an infant. Pediatr. Dermatol., 5:120, 1988.
19. Fujimoto, T., Kato, H., Ichiose, E., and Sasaguri, Y.: Immune complex and mite antigen in Kawasaki disease. Lancet, 2:980, 1982.
20. Fujiwara, H., and Hamashima, Y.: Pathology of the heart in Kawasaki disease. Pediatrics, 61:100, 1978.
21. Fujiwara, H., Kawai, C., and Hamashima, Y.: Clinicopathologic study of the conduction system in 10 patients with Kawasaki's disease (mucocutaneous lymph node syndrome). Am. Heart J., 96:744, 1978.
22. Fujiwara, T., Fujiwara, H., and Hamashima, Y.: Frequency and size of coronary arterial aneurysm at necropsy in Kawasaki disease. Am. J. Cardiol., 59:808, 1987.
23. Fujiwara, T., Fujiwara, H., and Nakano, H.: Pathological features of coronary arteries in children with Kawasaki disease in which coronary arterial aneurysm was absent at autopsy. Quantitative analysis. Circulation, 78:345, 1988.
24. Fukushige, J., Nihill, M. R., and McNamara, D. G.: Spectrum of cardiovascular lesions in mucocutaneous lymph node syndrome: Analysis of eight cases. Am. J. Cardiol., 45:98, 1980.
25. Furusho, K., Kamiya, T., Nakano, H., Kiyosawa, N., Shinomiya, K., Hayashidera, T., Tamura, T., Hirose, O., Manabe, Y., Yoloyama, T., Kawarano, M., Baba, K., Baba, K., and Mori, C.: High-dose intravenous gammaglobulin for Kawasaki disease. Lancet, 2:1055, 1984.
26. Furusho, K., Kamiya, T., Nakano, H., Kiyosawa, N., Shinomiya, K., Hayashidera, T., Tamura, T., Hirose, O., Manabe, Y., Yokoyama, T., Kawarano, M., Baba, K., Baba, K., Mori, C., Joho, K., and Seto, S.: Japanese gamma globulin trials for Kawasaki disease. Prog. Clin. Biol. Res., 250:425, 1987.
27. Giesker, D. W., Krause, P. J., Pastuszak, W. T., Hine, P., and Forouhar, F. A.: Lymph node biopsy for early diagnosis in Kawasaki disease. Am. J. Surg. Pathol., 6:493, 1982.
28. Hamashima, Y., Kishi, K., and Tasaka, K.: Rickettsia-like bodies in infantile acute febrile mucocutaneous lymph-node syndrome. Lancet, 2:42, 1973.
29. Hicks, R. V., and Melish, M. E.: Kawasaki syndrome. Pediatr. Rheumatol., 33:1151, 1986.
30. Hirose, H., Kawashima, Y., Nakano, S., Matsuda, H., Sakakibara, T., Hiranaka, T., Imagawa, H., Ogawa, M., and Harima, R.: Long-term results in surgical treatment of children 4 years old or younger with coronary involvement due to Kawasaki disease. Circulation, 74 (suppl. I):I-77, 1986.
31. Ichida, F., Fatica, N. S., Engle, M. A., O'Loughlin, J. E., Klein, A. A., Snyder, M. S., Ehlers, K. H., and Levin, A. R.: Coronary artery involvement in Kawasaki syndrome in Manhattan, New York: Risk factors and role of aspirin. Pediatrics, 80:828, 1987.
32. Ino, T., Iwahara, M., Boku, H., Akimoto, K., Shimura, N., Nishimoto, K., Yabuta, K., Yamamoto, K., Tanaka, A., and Hosoda, Y.: Aortocoronary bypass surgery for Kawasaki disease. Pediatr. Cardiol., 8:195, 1987.
33. Kamiya, T., and Suzuki, A.: Ischemic heart disease in Kawasaki disease. Prog. Clin. Biol. Res., 250:347, 1987.
34. Kato, H.: Cardiovascular involvement in Kawasaki disease: Evaluation and natural history. Prog. Clin. Biol. Res., 250:277, 1987.
35. Kato, H., Fujimoto, T., Inoue, O., Kondo, M., Koga, Y., Yamamoto, S., Shingu, M., Tominaga, K., Sasaguri, Y.: Variant strain of Propionibacterium acnes: A clue to the aetiology of Kawasaki disease. Lancet, 2:1383, 1983.
36. Kato, H., Ichinose, E., Inoue, O., and Akagi, T.: Intracoronary thrombolytic therapy in Kawasaki disease: Treatment and prevention of acute myocardial infarction. Prog. Clin. Biol. Res., 250:445, 1987.
37. Kato, H., Ichinose, E., Yoshioka, F., Takechi, T., Matsunaga, S., Suzuki, K., and Rikitake, N.: Fate of coronary aneurysms in Kawasaki disease: Serial coronary angiography and long-term follow-up study. Am. J. Cardiol., 49:1758, 1982.
38. Kato, H., Koike, S., Tanaka, C., Yokochi, K., Yoshioka, F., Takeuchi, S., Matsunaga, S., and Yokoyama, T.: Coronary heart disease in children with Kawasaki disease. Jpn. Circ. J., 43:469, 1979.
39. Kato, H., Koike, S., Yamamoto, M., Ito, Y., and Yano, E.: Coronary aneurysms in infants and young children with acute febrile mucocutaneous lymph node syndrome. J. Pediatr., 86:892, 1975.
40. Kawasaki, T.: Acute febrile mucocutaneous syndrome with lymphoid involvement with specific desquamation of the fingers and toes in children (Japanese). Jpn. J. Allergy., 16:178, 1967.
41. Kawasaki, T., Kosaki, F., Okawa, S., Shigematsu, I., and Yanagawa, H.: A new infantile acute febrile mucocutaneous lymph node syndrome (MLNS) prevailing in Japan. Pediatrics, 54:271, 1974.
42. Kegel, S. M., Dorsey, T. J., Rowen, M., and Taylor, W. F.: Cardiac death in mucocutaneous lymph node syndrome. Am. J. Cardiol., 40:282, 1977.
43. Keren, G., Barzilay, Z., Alpert, G., Spirer, Z., and Danon, Y. L.: Mucocutaneous lymph node syndrome (Kawasaki disease) in Israel. A review of 13 cases: Is pseudomonas infection responsible? Acta Paediatr. Scand., 72:455, 1983.
44. Kitamura, S.: Surgical treatment for coronary arterial lesions in Kawasaki disease. Prog. Clin. Biol. Res., 250:455, 1987.
45. Kitamura, S., Kawachi, K., Harima, R., Sakakibara, T., Hirose, H., and Kawashima, Y.: Surgery for coronary heart disease due to mucocutaneous lymph node syndrome (Kawasaki disease). Report of 6 patients. Am. J. Cardiol., 51:444, 1983.
46. Kitamura, S., Kawachi, K., Oyama, C., Miyagi, Y., Morita, R., Koh, Y., Kim, K.,

and Nishii, T.: Severe Kawasaki heart disease treated with an internal mammary artery graft in pediatric patients. A first successful report. J. Thorac. Cardiovasc. Surg., 89:860, 1985.

47. Kitamura, S., Kawashima, Y., Fujita, T., Mori, T., Oyama, C., Fujino, M., Kozuka, T., Nishzaki, K., and Manabe, H.: Aortocoronary bypass grafting in a child with coronary artery obstruction due to mucocutaneous lymph node syndrome. Report of a case. Circulation, 53:1035, 1976.

48. Kitamura, S., Kawashima, Y., Kawachi, K., Fujino, M., Kozuka, T., Fujita, T., and Manabe, H.: Left ventricular function in patients with coronary arteritis due to acute febrile mucocutaneous lymph node syndrome or related disease. Am. J. Cardiol., 40:156, 1977.

49. Kitamura, S., Kawashima, Y., Kawachi, K., Harima, R., Ihara, K., Nakano, S., Shimazaki, Y., and Mori, T.: Severe mitral regurgitation due to coronary arteritis of mucocutaneous lymph node syndrome. A new surgical entity. J. Thorac. Cardiovasc. Surg., 80:629, 1980.

50. Kitamura, S., Seki, T., Kawachi, K., Morita, R., Kawata, T., Mizuguchi, K., Kobayashi, S., Fukutomi, M., Nishii, T., Kobayashi, H., and Oyama, C.: Excellent patency and growth potential of internal mammary artery grafts in pediatric coronary artery bypass surgery. New evidence for a "live" conduit. Circulation, 78 (suppl. I):I-129, 1988.

51. Konishi, Y., Tatsuta, N., Miki, S., Matsuda, M., Ishihara, H., Taniguchi, T., Hikasa, Y., Hayashidera, T., Nishioka, K., and Ueda, T.: Simultaneous surgical treatment of tetralogy of Fallot and coronary artery aneurysm due to mucocutaneous lymph node syndrome in a 4-year-old child. Jpn. Circ. J., 43:749, 1979.

52. Konishi, Y., Tatsuta, N., Miki, S., Chiba, Y., Kao, C. T., Hikasa, Y., Yokota, M., Nishioka, K., Ueda, T., Kamiya, T., and Sugiyama, T.: Mitral insufficiency secondary to mucocutaneous lymph node syndrome: A case report of successful surgical treatment. Jpn. Circ. J., 42:901, 1978.

53. Koren, G., Lavi, S., Rose, V., and Rowe, R.: Kawasaki disease: Review of risk factors for coronary aneurysms. J. Pediatr., 108:388, 1986.

54. Leung, D. Y. M., Burns, J. C., Newburger, J. W., and Geha, R. S.: Reversal of lymphocyte activation in vivo in the Kawasaki syndrome by intravenous gammaglobulin. J. Clin. Invest., 79:468, 1987.

55. Mains, C., Wiggins, J., Groves, B., and Clarke, D.: Surgical therapy for a complication of Kawasaki disease. Ann. Thorac. Surg., 35:197, 1983.

56. Marchette, N. J., Ho, D., Kihara, S., Caplan, F., and Melish, M. E.: Search for the retroviral etiology of Kawasaki syndrome. Prog. Clin. Biol. Res., 250:131, 1987.

57. Marchette, N. J., Melish, J. F., James, J. F., Kihara, S., and Caplan, F.: Spirochetal studies in Kawasaki syndrome. Prog. Clin. Biol. Res.,250:87, 1987.

58. Meade, R. H. III, and Brandt, L.: Manifestations of Kawasaki disease in New England outbreak of 1980. J. Pediatr., 100:558, 1982.

59. Melish, M. E.: Kawasaki syndrome (the mucocutaneous lymph node syndrome). Annu. Rev. Med., 33:569, 1982.

60. Melish, M. E.: Kawasaki syndrome: A 1986 perspective. Rheum. Dis. Clin. North Am., 13:7, 1987.

61. Melish, M. E., Hicks, R. M., and Larson, E. J.: Mucocutaneous lymph node syndrome in the United States. Am. J. Dis. Child., 130:599, 1976.

62. Mercer, S., and Carpenter, B.: Surgical complications of Kawasaki disease. J. Pediatr. Surg., 16:444, 1981.

63. Myers, J. L., Gleason, M. M., Cyran, S. E., and Baylen, B. G.: Surgical management of coronary insufficiency in a child with Kawasaki's disease: Use of bilateral internal mammary arteries. Ann. Thorac. Surg., 46:459, 1988.

64. Nagashima, M., Matsushima, M., Matsuoka, H., Ogawa, A., and Okumura, N.: High dose gammaglobulin therapy for Kawasaki disease. J. Pediatr., 110:710, 1987.

65. Nakanishi, T., Takao, A., Nakazawa, M., Endo, M., Niwa, K., and Takahashi, Y.: Mucocutaneous lymph node syndrome: Clinical, hemodynamic and angiographic features of coronary obstructive disease. Am. J. Cardiol., 55:662, 1985.

66. Nakano, H.: Prediction of patients with a high risk of coronary artery aneurysm in Kawasaki disease: Indication for immunoglobulin therapy. Prog. Clin. Biol. Res., 250:287, 1987.

67. Nakano, H., Saito, A., Ueda, K., and Nojima, K.: Clinical characteristics of myocardial infarction following Kawasaki disease: Report of 11 cases. J. Pediatr., 108:198, 1986.

68. Nakano, H., Ueda, K., Saito, A., and Nojima, K.: Repeated quantitative angiograms in coronary arterial aneurysm in Kawasaki disease. Am. J. Cardiol., 56:846, 1985.

69. Nakano, H., Ueda, K., Saito, A., Tsuchitani, Y., Kawamori, J., Miyake, T., and Yoshida, T.: Scoring method for identifying patients with Kawasaki disease at high risk of coronary artery aneurysms. Am. J. Cardiol., 58:739, 1986.

70. Nehme, A. E., and Mikhail, R. A.: Kawasaki syndrome. An abdominal crisis. Am. Surg., 49:275, 1983.

71. Newburger, J. W.: U. S. gamma globulin trial. Prog. Clin. Biol. Res., 250:441, 1987.

72. Newburger, J. W., Sanders, S. P., Burns, J. C., Parness, I. A., Beiser, A. S., and Colan, S. D.: Left ventricular contractility and function in Kawasaki syndrome: Effect of intravenous gamma-globulin. Circulation, 79:1237, 1989.

73. Newburger, J. W., Takahashi, M., Burns, J. C., Beiser, A. S., Chung, K. J., Duffy, C. E., Glode, M. P., Mason, W. H., Reddy, V., Sanders, S. P., Shulman, S. T., Wiggins, J. W., Hicks, R. V., Fulton, D. R., Lewis, A. B., Leung, S. Y. M., Colton, T., Rosen, F. S., and Melish, M. E.: The treatment of Kawasaki syndrome with intravenous gamma globulin. N. Engl. J. Med., 315:342, 1986.

74. Novelli, V. M., Galbraith, A., Robinson, P. J., Smallhorn, J. F., and Marshall,

W. C.: Cardiovascular abnormalties in Kawasaki disease. Arch. Dis. Child., 59:405, 1984.

75. Onouchi, Z., Tomizawa, N., Goto, M., Nakata, K., Fukuda, M., and Goto, M.: Cardiac involvement and prognosis in acute mucocutaneous lymph node syndrome. Chest, 68:297, 1975.

76. Osato, T., Kikuta, H., Okano, M., Mizuno, F., Konno, M., Ishikawa, N., Hirai, K., and Matsumoto, S.: Kawasaki disease and Epstein-Barr virus infection. Prog. Clin. Biol. Res., 250:113, 1987.

77. Radford, D. J., Sondheimer, H. M., Williams, G. J., and Fowler, R. S.: Mucocutaneous lymph node syndrome with coronary artery aneurysm. Am. J. Dis. Child., 130:596, 1976.

78. Rauch, A. M.: Kawasaki syndrome: Review of new epidemiologic and laboratory developments. Pediatr. Infect. Dis. J., 6:1016, 1987.

79. Rowley, A. H., Duffy, E., and Shulman, S. T.: Prevention of giant coronary artery aneurysms in Kawasaki disease by intravenous gamma globulin therapy. J. Pediatr., 113:290, 1988.

80. Rowley, A. H., Gonzalez-Crussi, F., and Shulman, S. T.: Kawasaki syndrome. Rev. Infect. Dis., 10:1, 1988.

81. Rowley, A. H., and Shulman, S. T.: The search for the eitology of Kawasaki disease. Pediatr. Infect. Dis. J., 6:506, 1987.

82. Rowley, A. H., and Shulman, S. T.: What is the status of intravenous gamma-globulin for Kawasaki syndrome in the United States and Canada? Pediatr. Infect. Dis. J., 7:463, 1988.

83. Russell, A. S., Zaragoza, A. J., and Shea, R.: Mucocutaneous lymph node syndrome in Canada. Can. Med. Assoc. J., 112:1210, 1975.

84. Sandiford, F. M., Vargo, T. A. T., Shih, J. Y., Pelargonio, S., and McNamara, D. G.: Successful triple coronary artery bypass in a child with multiple coronary aneurysms due to Kawasaki's disease. J. Thorac. Cardiovasc. Surg., 79:283, 1980.

85. Schulman, S. T., Rowley, A. H., Fresco, R., and Morrison, D. C.: The etiology of Kawasaki disease: Retrovirus? Prog. Clin. Biol. Res., 250:117, 1987.

86. Shulman, S. T., and Rowley, A. H.: Does Kawasaki disease have a retroviral aetiology? Lancet, 2:545, 1986.

87. Sonobe, T., and Kawasaki, T.: Atypical Kawasaki disease. Prog. Clin. Biol. Res., 250:367, 1987.

88. Stephenson, S. R.: Kawasaki disease in Europe. Lancet., 1:373, 1977.

89. Suma, K., Takeuchi, Y., Shiroma, K., Tsuji, T., Inoue, K., Yoshikawa, T., Koyama, Y., Narumi, J., Asai, T., and Kusakawa, S.: Cardiac surgery of eight children with Kawasaki disease (mucocutaneous lymph node syndrome). Jpn. Heart J., 22:605, 1981.

90. Suma, K., Takeuchi, Y., Shiroma, K., Tsuji, T., Inoue, K., Yoshikawa, T., Koyama, Y., Narumi, J., Asai, T., and Kusakawa, S.: Early and late postoperative studies in coronary arterial lesions resulting from Kawasaki's disease in children. J. Thorac. Cardiovasc. Surg., 84:224, 1982.

91. Suzuki, A., Kamiya, T., Ono, Y., Takahashi, N., Naito, Y., and Kou, Y.: Indication of aortocoronary by-pass for coronary arterial obstruction due to Kawasaki disease. Heart Vessels, 1:94, 1985.

92. Takahashi, M.: Myocarditis in Kawasaki syndrome. A minor villain? Circulation, 79:1398, 1989.

93. Takao, A., Niwa, K., Kondo, C., Nakanishi, T., Satomi, G., Nakazawa, M., and Endo, M.: Mitral regurgitation in Kawasaki disease. Prog. Clin. Biol. Res., 250:311, 1987.

94. Takeuchi, Y., Suma, K., Shiroma, K., Asai, T., and Kusakawa, S.: Surgical experience with coronary arterial sequelae of Kawasaki disease in children. J. Cardiovasc. Surg., 22:231, 1981.

95. Tatara, K., and Kusakawa, S.: Long-term prognosis of giant coronary aneurysm in Kawasaki disease: An angiographic study. J. Pediatr., 111:705, 1987.

96. Valaes, T.: Mucocutaneous lymph node syndrome (MLNS) in Athens, Greece. Pediatrics, 55:295, 1975.

97. Yanagawa, H., Kawasaki, T., and Shigematsu, I.: Nationwide survey on Kawasaki disease in Japan. Pediatrics, 80:58, 1987.

98. Yanagisawa, M., Kobayashi, N., and Matsuya, S.: Myocardial infarction due to coronary thromboarteritis following acute febrile mucocutaneous lymph node syndrome (MLNS) in an infant. Pediatrics, 54:277, 1974.

6. CHANGES IN VENOUS AUTOGRAFTS USED AS AORTOCORONARY CONDUITS

William C. Roberts, M.D.

The most important contribution to therapy for patients with symptomatic myocardial ischemia has been the coronary bypass operation. Since its introduction over 2 decades ago, numerous patients have benefited from this procedure. Despite its benefits to most patients, coronary bypass is not free of complications. Stenosis or complete occlusion of venous grafts used as aortocoronary conduits still occurs too frequently. Whereas all venous grafts develop some morphologic changes, the degree and functional significance of the changes vary widely. The structural changes observed early and late in saphenous veins used as aortocoronary conduits are presented in this section.

Degrees of Narrowing of the Native Epicardial Coronary Arteries in Symptomatic Myocardial Ischemia

Before the changes in saphenous veins used as aortocoronary conduits are focused on, a brief discussion on the status of the native epicardial coronary arteries in patients likely to undergo aortocoronary bypass grafting appears appropriate. As summarized in Figure 1, examination at necropsy (or during life by intravascular ultrasonic imaging) of the four major (right, left main, left anterior descending, and left circumflex) epicardial coronary arteries in patients over 30 years of age with symptomatic myocardial ischemia and angiographic narrowing greater than 50 per cent in diameter of one or more major coronary arteries discloses that atherosclerotic plaques are present in nearly every 5-mm. segment of the entire length of the arteries.[17,18] In patients with angiographically "single-vessel dis-

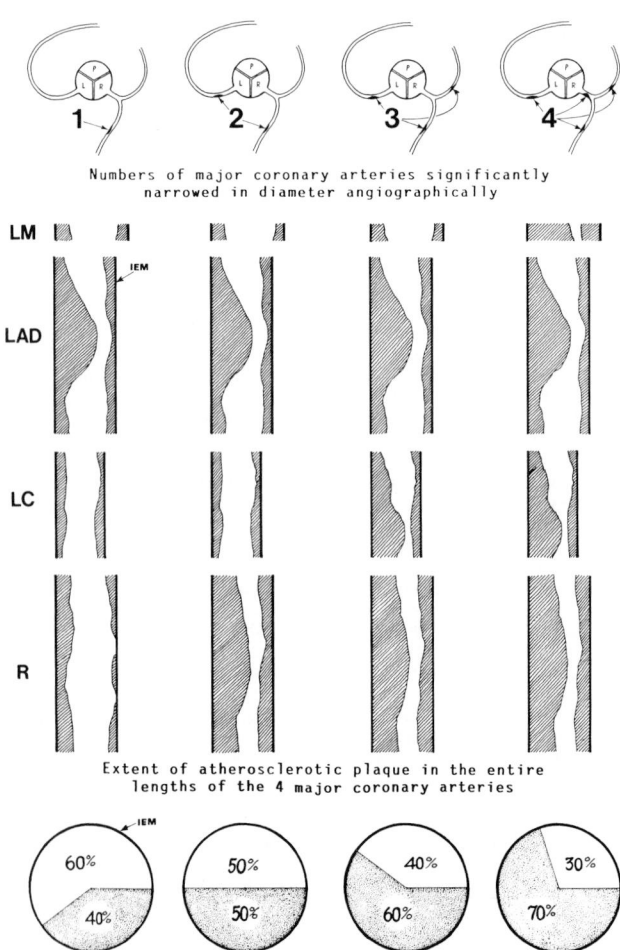

Figure 1. Diagram showing the number of major coronary arteries severely narrowed in diameter by angiogram *(upper)*; the average amount of atherosclerotic plaque in the left main (LM), left anterior descending (LAD), left circumflex (LC), and right (R) coronary arteries in full length according to the number of coronary arteries significantly narrowed by angiogram *(middle)*; and the average amount of cross-sectional area narrowing by atherosclerotic plaque in each 5-mm. segment of the four major epicardial coronary arteries *(lower)*. (From Roberts, W. C.: Coronary "lesion," coronary "disease," "single-vessel disease," "two-vessel disease": Word and phrase misnomers providing false impressions of the extent of coronary atherosclerosis in symptomatic myocardial ischemia. Am. J. Cardiol., 66:121, 1990.)

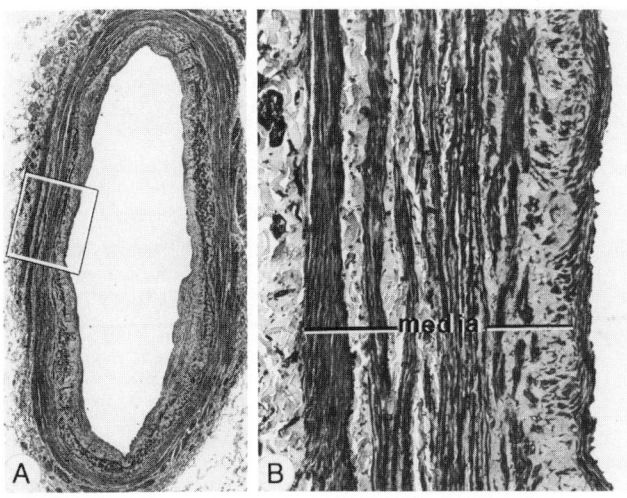

Figure 2. Normal saphenous vein. *A,* Low-power view showing medial circular and longitudinal smooth muscle layers (Movat stain, ×20). *B,* High-power view of area enclosed in box in *A* (Movat stain, ×130). Multiple layers of circular smooth muscle separated by layers of fibrous tissue form the media. Occasional longitudinal smooth muscle fascicles are present near the lumen. (From Spray, T. L., and Roberts, W. C.: Changes in saphenous veins used as aortocoronary bypass grafts. Am. Heart J., 94:500, 1977.)

ease," approximately 40 per cent of the lumen of each 5-mm. segment of the four major arteries (average of 54 segments per patient) is obliterated by plaque; in patients with angiographically "double-vessel disease," approximately 50 per cent of the total lumen is obliterated by plaque; in patients with "triple-vessel disease," approximately 60 per cent of the total lumen is filled with plaque; and in patients with "quadruple-vessel disease," approximately 70 per cent of the total lumen is filled with plaque. Thus, the greater the number of major coronary arteries significantly narrowed, the greater the total amount of atherosclerotic plaque in the major epicardial coronary arteries.

The Normal Saphenous Vein

The normal human saphenous vein contains a thin *intima* consisting of relatively acellular fibrous tissue covered by a single layer of endothelial cells and separated from the media by a rudimentary internal elastic membrane (Fig. 2). The *media* consists of multiple layers of smooth muscle cells, separated by bundles of collagen, ground substance, and occasional short elastic fibers. Most medial smooth muscle layers have a circular orientation; in areas near the venous valves, however, the middle circular layers have a more longitudinal arrangement. Frequently, longitudinally oriented smooth muscle fascicles form the innermost layers of the media. The *adventitia* is composed of bundles of collagen with scattered fascicles of longitudinally oriented smooth muscle cells. Broad loose bands of elastic fibers are present in abundance. Vasa vasorum are present and may extend into the outermost portion of the media.

Findings in Remnant Saphenous Veins Excised for Aortocoronary Conduits but Unused

Some degree of intimal fibrous thickening occurs commonly in saphenous veins excised but unused for aortocoronary bypass. Waller and Roberts[26] examined nearly 3500 cm. of unused but excised saphenous veins from 402 patients undergoing coronary bypass surgery. The length of the unused saphenous veins ranged from 0.5 to 52 cm. per patient (mean 8.5 cm.). A histologic section was examined from each of the 6788 5-mm. long segments: the lumen in 0.4 per cent of the sections was narrowed 76 to 100 per cent in cross-sectional areas by fibrous tissue; 0.6 per cent were narrowed 51 to 75 per cent in cross-sectional areas; 12 per cent were narrowed 26 to 50 per cent; and 87 per cent were narrowed 25 per cent or less in cross-sectional

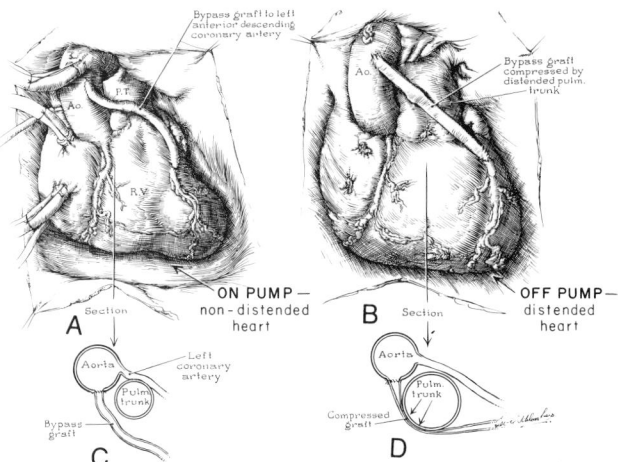

Figure 3. Schematic showing how a graft to the left anterior descending coronary artery can be placed under tension. (From Spray, T. L., and Roberts, W. C.: Tension on coronary bypass conduits. A neglected cause of real or potential obstruction of saphenous vein grafts. J. Thorac. Cardiovasc. Surg., 72:282, 1976.)

areas. The percentage of 5-mm. segments of unused vein narrowed more than 75 per cent in cross-sectional areas was similar in males and females, and it was similar in each of 5 decades (31 to 40, 41 to 50, 51 to 60, 61 to 70, and 71 to 80 years). Thus, approximately 1 per cent of saphenous veins excised for coronary bypass are narrowed more than 50 per cent in cross-sectional area by fibrous tissue before they are used as aortocoronary conduits.

Numbers of Aortic Anastomotic Sites, Conduits, and Coronary Anastomotic Sites

It is doubtful that any two surgeons perform the bypass operation in quite the same manner, and these individual variations may affect patient and graft outcome. The phrases "two bypasses" or "three bypasses" or "four bypasses" are commonly used, but their meaning is not always precise. It is suspected that most users of the phrase "three bypasses" are referring to the number of coronary anastomoses. A patient may have three coronary anastomotic sites and only one conduit ("round-the-world" bypass) or two or three conduits with similar numbers of aortic anastomotic sites. To prevent confusion, it might be best to always state the number of aortic anastomotic sites, the number of conduits, and the number of coronary anastomotic sites. To the author, it appears most reasonable for each of these three to be the same: if a patient is to have three coronary anastomotic sites, it might be ideal to have three conduits and three separate aortic anastomotic sites. If only one conduit is used with a single aortic anastomotic site and the single conduit is anastomosed to seven different coronary arteries, the outcome is not ideal if the single aortic anastomosis closes or the single conduit closes proximally. With similar numbers of aortic anastomotic sites, conduits, and coronary anastomotic sites, this circumstance is less likely to occur.

The location of the coronary anastomotic site appears to be relatively similar with most surgeons. The distal 1 cm. of the right coronary artery is probably ideal because the most severe narrowing of this artery tends to be its distal third rather than the proximal or middle third.[24] The most common anastomotic site of the left anterior descending is probably about two thirds down its length, and this location, of course, is logical because this artery tends to be more severely narrowed in its proximal third than in either its middle or distal thirds.[24] The same situation also appears reasonable for the first diagonal artery. Anastomoses in the obtuse marginal arteries are usually within 3 cm. of their origin from the left circumflex.

Of the various technical factors that can affect flow in aortocoronary conduits, *tension on the conduit* is one.[21] Abnormal

tension is indicated by grooving or indentation into the right atrial wall or right atrioventricular sulcus or by flattening of the graft passing anterior to the pulmonary trunk. Several explanations for the occurrence of this tension are probable and summarized in Figure 3. If the graft is under tension, leakage at the bypass anastomosis is probably more likely than it is without tension (Fig. 4). *Twisting of a conduit,* as illustrated in Figures 5 and 6, may prevent successful bypass grafting.[19]

Early Changes in Saphenous Veins Used as Aortocoronary Conduits

In 1906, Carrel and Guthrie[5] described intimal thickening of veins implanted into the arterial system in dogs and concluded that veins placed in the arterial circulation had a strong tendency to assume the character of an artery. In further vein transplantation experiments in 1908, Carrel[4] described four characteristic changes in veins used as arteries in the peripheral circulation: (1) intimal thickening, (2) adventitial thickening (from fibrosis), (3) loss of the inner third of the media, and (4) loss of elastic fibers producing a fibrous tube. In addition, medial hypertrophy was observed in some grafts. These changes have subsequently been confirmed in humans in saphenous veins used for femoropopliteal and aortocoronary bypass.

Spray and Roberts[22,23] studied a large number of saphenous vein grafts from patients dying within a year after aortocoronary bypass (Fig. 7). Vein grafts from patients dying intraoperatively showed minimal medial edema (clear spaces between layers of smooth muscle) and disrupted adventitia (occurring during excision of the vein before grafting). By 2 weeks, mural edema was more pronounced, some medial smooth muscle cells were necrotic, and inflammatory infiltrates were present. The endothelium often was disrupted, and the intimal surface usually was covered, either partially or completely, by fibrin. By 3 weeks, cells with characteristics of smooth muscle appeared in the subendothelial portion of the intima. The cells generally were oriented such that their longest diameter was parallel to the direction of blood flow. Thereafter, the subendothelial intimal lesions became more generalized and less cellular, ground substance appeared in abundance, and short elastic fibers and vascular channels occasionally were present. The smooth muscle fibers of the media gradually diminished in number and were replaced, in part or in whole, by fibrous tissue. Fibrous tissue also increased in the adventitia, and its elastic fibers became severely disrupted or disappeared completely. Organizing

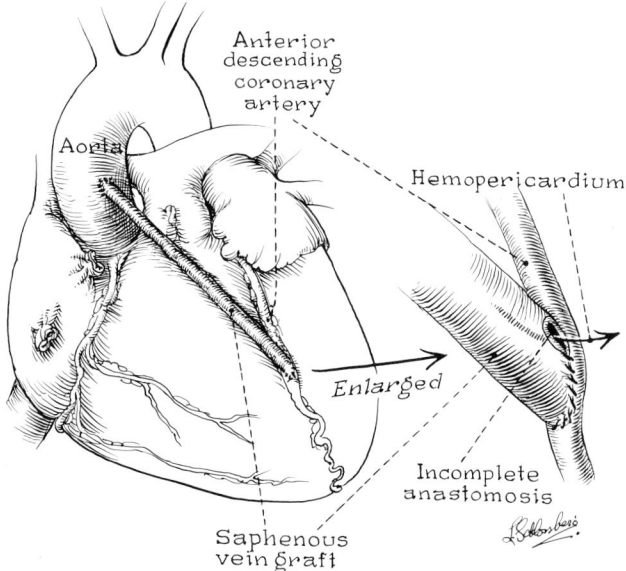

Figure 4. Schematic showing how tension on a graft might cause disruption of an anastomosis.

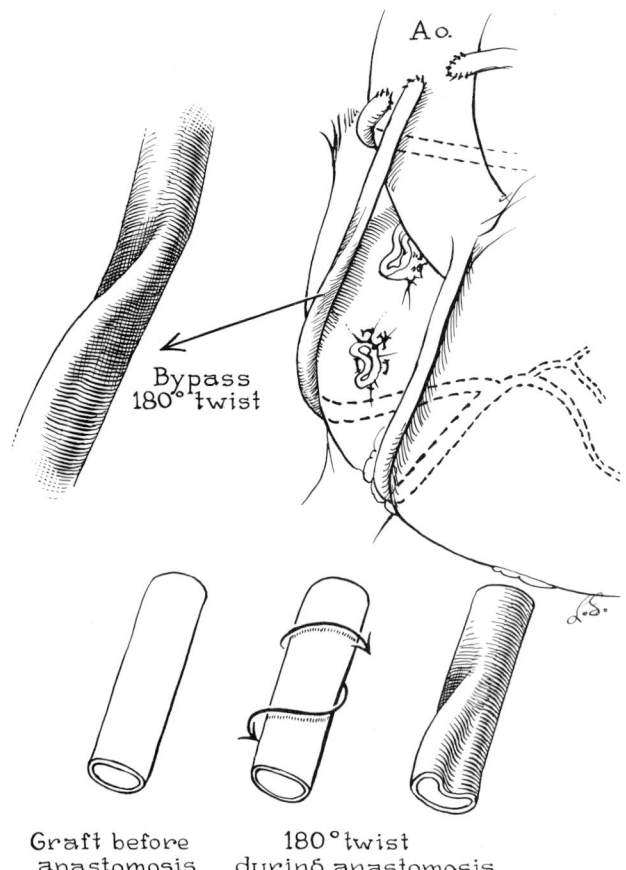

Figure 5. Schematic showing mild twisting of a graft to the right coronary artery. (From Roberts, W. C., Lachman A. S., and Virmani, R.: Twisting of an aorta-coronary bypass conduit. A complication of coronary surgery. J. Thorac. Cardiovasc. Surg., 75:772, 1978.)

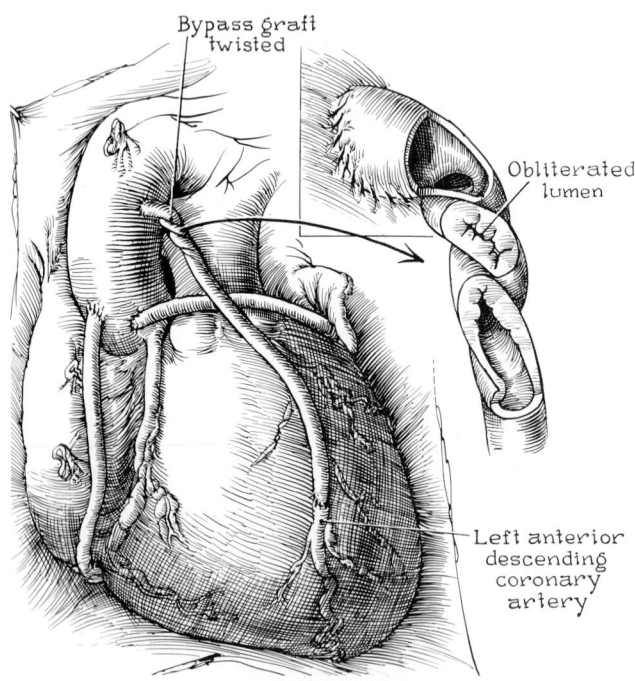

Figure 6. Schematic showing severe twisting of a graft to the left anterior descending coronary artery. (From Roberts, W. C., Lachman, A. S., and Virmani, R.: Twisting of an aorta-coronary bypass conduit. A complication of coronary surgery. J. Thorac. Cardiovasc. Surg., 75:772, 1978.)

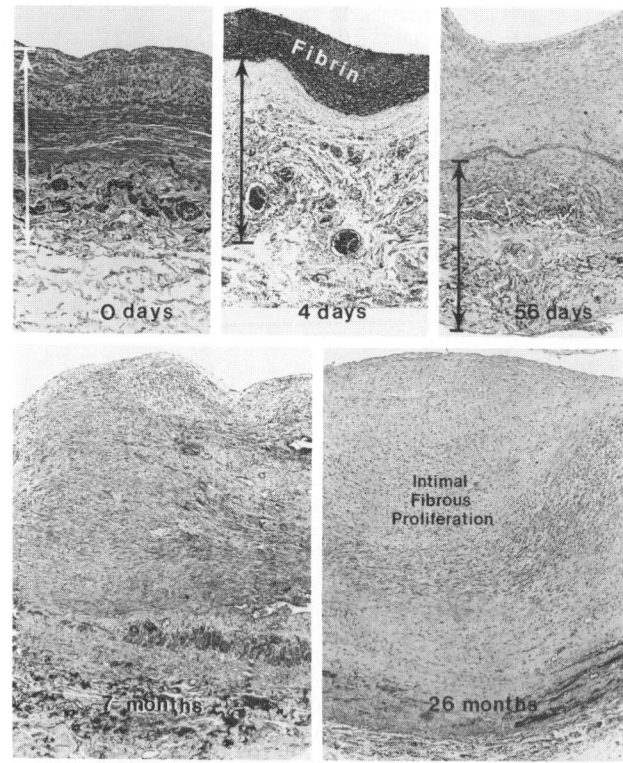

Figure 7. Composite of changes seen in saphenous vein aortocoronary grafts from 0 days (normal vein) to 26 months after implantation at the same magnification (×54). Arrows indicate normal wall thickness (media plus adventitia): 0 days, intima thin, marked medial smooth muscle layers in both circular and longitudinal directions, loose adventitial tissue; 4 days, large deposit of fibrin over slightly thickened intima, marked loss of medial smooth muscle with cellular infiltration; 56 days, thickened vein wall with marked intimal fibrous proliferation, medial smooth muscle cells depleted and replaced by fibrous tissue; 7 months, severe intimal fibrous proliferation is present containing some neovascular channels, and marked loss of medial smooth muscle and replacement fibrosis is present; 26 months, the vein wall has become almost completely replaced by fibrous tissue creating a fibrous tube, and only small areas of medial smooth muscle cells remain. (All Movat stains. From Spray, T. L., and Roberts, W. C.: Changes in saphenous veins used as aortocoronary bypass grafts. Am. Heart J., 94:500, 1977.)

fibrin on the external surface of the grafts probably contributed to the adventitial fibrosis. Capillaries were present in the adventitia, and they often extended into the fibrotic media. Thus, the saphenous vein used as an artery becomes a stiff, fibrous tissue conduit.

Late Changes in Saphenous Veins Used as Aortocoronary Conduits

Kalan and Roberts[9] described at necropsy findings in 123 saphenous vein grafts and in 1865 5-mm. segments of the grafts in 53 patients who had had a single aortocoronary bypass operation 13 to 185 months (mean 58 months) before death. Of the 53 patients, 32 (60 per cent) died from a cardiac cause, and of their 73 saphenous vein aortocoronary conduits, 36 (49 per cent) were narrowed at some point more than 75 per cent in cross-sectional area by atherosclerotic plaque; the remaining 21 patients (40 per cent) died of noncardiac causes, and of their 50 saphenous vein conduits, 10 (20 per cent) were narrowed at some point more than 75 per cent in cross-sectional area by plaque. Of the 53 patients, 31 (58 per cent) had at least one bypass graft maximally narrowed greater than 75 per cent in cross-sectional area at some point by fibromuscular tissue with or without lipid; 12 patients (23 per cent) had maximal graft narrowing of 51 to 75 per cent; 8 patients (15 per cent), 26 to 50 per cent; and 2 patients (4 per cent), 0 to 25 per cent. The percentage of patients with a graft narrowed over 75 per cent at necropsy did not increase as the interval from bypass surgery to death increased.

Of the 123 saphenous vein grafts, 47 (38 per cent) were maximally narrowed greater than 75 per cent in cross-sectional area; 44 (36 per cent), 51 to 75 per cent; 22 (18 per cent), 26 to 50 per cent; and 10 (8 per cent), 0 to 25 per cent. Of the 47 grafts narrowed over 75 per cent in cross-sectional area, 29 actually were narrowed greater than 95 per cent in cross-sectional area by fibrous tissue. The percentage of saphenous veins narrowed greater than 75 per cent at necropsy was not affected by sex (males 38 per cent, females 36 per cent), presence or absence of systemic hypertension (40 per cent versus 33 per cent), or presence or absence of diabetes mellitus (30 per cent versus 48 per cent). The percentage of grafts narrowed over 75 per cent in cross-sectional area did not correlate with the interval between bypass surgery and death or with the coronary artery to which the graft was connected.

The degree of narrowing of the saphenous vein graft was related to the degree of luminal narrowing of the native coronary artery at, or within 2 cm. distal to, the saphenous vein–coronary artery anastomosis. Of the 49 grafts attached to a coronary artery that was narrowed greater than 75 per cent at or distal to the anastomosis, 33 (67 per cent) were significantly narrowed. Of the 74 grafts attached to a coronary artery narrowed less than 75 per cent distal to the anastomotic site, 14 (19 per cent) were severely narrowed.

Analysis of the 1865 5-mm. long saphenous vein segments disclosed that 209 segments (11 per cent) were narrowed 96 to 100 per cent in cross-sectional area; 172 (9 per cent), 76 to 95 per cent; 407 (22 per cent), 51 to 75 per cent; 685 (37 per cent), 26 to 50 per cent; and 392 (21 per cent), 0 to 25 per cent. Similar percentages of segments were narrowed greater than 75 per cent in males and females (22 per cent versus 15 per cent); in diabetic and nondiabetic patients (18 per cent versus 26 per cent); and in hypertensive and nonhypertensive patients (21 per cent versus 20 per cent). Moreover, the interval from coronary bypass to death did not correlate with the percentage of segments severely narrowed.

Although the percentage of saphenous vein segments narrowed greater than 75 per cent in cross-sectional area at necropsy did not correlate with the interval from bypass grafting to death, it did relate to the mode of death. Of the 32 patients dying from a cardiac cause, 295 (27 per cent) of 1104 saphenous vein segments were narrowed greater than 75 per cent, whereas of the 21 patients dying from a noncardiac cause, 86 (11 per cent) of 761 saphenous vein segments were so narrowed. The percentage of segments of native coronary artery narrowed greater than 75 per cent was similar in patients with cardiac and noncardiac modes of death (673 of 1441 [47 per cent] versus 333 of 895 [37 per cent]).

Composition of Tissue Causing Luminal Narrowing Late in the Saphenous Veins Used as Aortocoronary Conduits

Lipid was present in the wall of a graft in 39 of the 53 patients (74 per cent). Fifteen had intracellular lipid alone (foam cells), and 24 had both foam cells and extracellular lipid. Extracellular lipid was not found in a saphenous vein graft until 26 months after bypass. Lipid was present in 69 (56 per cent) of the 123 saphenous vein grafts from the 39 patients. Intracellular lipid was present in all 69 grafts either alone (33 grafts) or along with extracellular lipid (36 grafts). The amount of lipid present appeared to increase as the interval from coronary bypass to death increased. Foam cells were located near the luminal surfaces of the intimal fibrous tissue, and they did not appreciably narrow the lumen. Extracellular lipid deposits were located deeper in the plaque separated from the lumen by a layer of fibrous tissue, and they often contributed significantly to luminal narrowing.

Hemorrhage into plaque (into the lipid portion only) was found in 26 (21 per cent) saphenous vein grafts from 17 (32 per cent) patients. It was observed as early as 24 months after bypass, and

it did not increase in frequency thereafter as the interval from bypass to death increased. Luminal narrowing greater than 75 per cent in cross-sectional area was significantly more common in grafts with than in those without plaque hemorrhage.

Luminal thrombus was present in 16 (13 per cent) saphenous vein grafts from 14 (26 per cent) patients. Thrombus was not seen until 32 months after bypass, and its frequency did not increase thereafter as the interval from bypass to death increased. Thrombus within the graft lumen was present in 16 of 69 grafts that had deposits of lipid in the walls and in none of 54 grafts devoid of lipid. In 14 of these 16 grafts, hemorrhage into plaque also was found.

Calcific deposits were present in 13 (11 per cent) of the 123 saphenous vein grafts from 11 patients, and they were first seen 34 months after coronary bypass. All the deposits were small. They were present in 18 (1 per cent) of the 1865 5-mm. saphenous vein segments.

The aforementioned data indicate that nearly all saphenous veins used as aortocoronary conduits for longer than a year develop atherosclerotic plaques in each 5-mm. segment of the entire length. Thus, the atherosclerotic plaquing late in saphenous veins used as aortocoronary conduits is diffuse, just as it is in native coronary arteries in patients with fatal myocardial ischemia.[17,18] The amount of luminal narrowing in the saphenous veins used as aortocoronary conduits was significantly greater in those patients who died from a cardiac cause, compared with those who died from a noncardiac cause. Surprisingly, the interval from coronary bypass to death did not correlate with either the percentage of vein conduits or the percentage of 5-mm. segments of vein conduit narrowed over 75 per cent in cross-sectional area by plaque. Moreover, the percentage of 5-mm. segments of saphenous vein conduit severely narrowed was similar in the 35 patients surviving up to 5 years, compared with the 18 patients surviving more than 5 years.

The composition of the plaques in the saphenous venous conduits is similar to that in the native coronary arteries. Fibrous tissue or fibromuscular tissue was the dominant component of the plaques in the saphenous vein conduits, just as it is the dominant component of plaques in the native coronary arteries in patients with fatal coronary artery disease without coronary bypass.[10,11]

The frequency of the various modes of death among the patients dying late after coronary bypass is different from that of patients with symptomatic myocardial ischemia without coronary bypass.[20] Of the 53 coronary bypass patients studied, only 32 (60 per cent) died from a cardiac cause, and 21 (40 per cent) died from a noncardiac cause. Among patients with symptomatic myocardial ischemia who do not have coronary bypass, approximately 95 per cent die from a cardiac cause. The fact that 40 per cent of the bypass patients studied died from a noncardiac cause supports the view that the bypass operation in many patients prolongs life, long enough in many to develop various fatal noncardiac conditions. Of the 53 bypass patients reported by Kalan and Roberts,[9] 10 (19 per cent) died from cancer, a percentage far higher than in patients with symptomatic myocardial ischemia not undergoing coronary surgery.

The study by Kalan and Roberts[9] re-emphasizes that coronary bypass is useful but that it does not deter progression of the underlying atherosclerotic process. In a minor way, the bypass operation might even cause acceleration of the atherosclerotic process because in about 25 per cent of individuals who undergo coronary bypass, the serum total cholesterol increases and the body weight increases substantially during the first year after operation. Because lowering of the serum (or plasma) total cholesterol level (and specifically the low-density lipoprotein cholesterol) decreases the likelihood of heart attack and may cause some portion of atherosclerotic plaques to regress and other portions to at least not progress, a strong case can be advanced for combined simultaneous initiation of both low-fat, low-cholesterol diet therapy and lipid-lowering drug therapy as soon as is reasonably feasible after a coronary bypass operation.[15]

Causes of Morphologic Changes in Saphenous Veins Used as Aortocoronary Conduits

Although the causes of the changes in saphenous vein grafts are in many ways similar to those of atherosclerotic plaques in native coronary arteries,[14,16] additional mechanisms almost surely have a role when a vein is switched to an arterial location. The changes in the saphenous veins are similar early to the phlebosclerotic lesions in venous varicosities, changes presumably caused by the response of the vein to increases in hydrostatic pressure. Arteriovenous shunts of any origin (congenital, traumatic, or iatrogenic) show intimal thickening, presumably the result of increased pressure and flow. Subendothelial proliferative lesions in the pulmonary arteries of patients with pulmonary hypertension and in the vena cava and portal veins in patients with chronic right-sided congestive cardiac failure or portal hypertension are also seen in the saphenous veins transferred to the aortocoronary position. Brody and colleagues[2,3] attempted to differentiate the effects of pressure and ischemia on femoral vein grafts in dogs. Vein segments were either left intact or dissected free from their adventitia, thereby severing the vasa vasorum and producing medial ischemia. The vein segments were then either left in the venous system or were arterialized by creation of an arteriovenous fistula. The presence of medial ischemia in the absence of elevated pressure and flow produced medial fibrosis in the vein without subendothelial intimal proliferative lesions. Elevated intravascular pressure alone, however, without alterations in blood supply to the media by the vasa vasorum, produced intimal lesions without evidence of medial fibrosis. The combination of both elevated intraluminal pressure and medial ischemia caused medial and intimal changes similar to the changes seen in human saphenous veins used as aortocoronary conduits (Table 1).

The intimal process in saphenous veins and specifically the degree of luminal narrowing in saphenous veins in the aortocoronary position is almost certainly accelerated when flow through the conduit is relatively poor. The major cause of poor flow is severe narrowing in the native coronary artery (to which the vein is attached) at or just distal to the site of anastomosis.[9,22,23,25] The smaller the native coronary arteries to which the graft is to be connected, the less the amount of atherosclerotic plaque necessary to cause significant luminal narrowing. Smaller sized hearts have smaller coronary arteries than do larger sized hearts.[13] Small patients tend to have smaller hearts than larger patients have. Thus, similar amounts of plaque cause more luminal narrowing in small patients than in large

patients. Females, on average, are smaller than males and, therefore, generally have smaller hearts and smaller coronary arteries. Coronary bypass might be expected therefore to have poorer results in females than in males because the smaller arteries might cause poorer flow through the conduits by plaque in the native coronary arteries. Kalan and Roberts[8] found this scenario to probably be the case. Their 121 necropsy patients dying within 60 days of a coronary bypass operation had significantly lower mean heart weights than did the 90 patients dying late, and this fact held true for both sexes. Most patients with normal sized hearts were in the early death group; conversely, most patients in the late death group had hearts of increased weight. Their findings suggest that patients with normal or near-normal sized hearts have a higher early mortality after coronary bypass than do those with hearts of increased weight. Moreover, more changes causing luminal narrowing of bypass conduits might be expected in individuals with small native coronary arteries (small hearts) because the run-off through the graft may not be as good as in patients with larger native coronary arteries (larger hearts).

Comparison of Morphologic Changes in Saphenous Veins to Those in Internal Mammary Arteries Used as Aortocoronary Conduits

For practical purposes, none of the aforedescribed changes in saphenous veins used as aortocoronary conduits are found in internal mammary arteries used in the coronary position. As emphasized by others, clinically[6,12] the patency rate both early and late is excellent with the mammary artery and much less with the saphenous vein. Although the internal mammary artery late after bypass remains much smaller than does the saphenous vein when each is utilized in the same patient, the internal mammary artery remains nearly devoid of intimal deposits, whereas the saphenous vein, although much larger, may develop severe atherosclerotic plaque in the lumen.[1,7]

TABLE 1. Effects of Pressure and Ischemia on Venous Conduits

Vasa Vasorum Intact

Low pressure (venous)	High pressure (arterial)
↓	↓
Normal histology	Intimal proliferation and fibrosis
Intact myocytes	Intact myocytes

Vasa Vasorum Interrupted

Low pressure (venous)	High pressure (arterial)
↓	↓
Medical fibrosis	Intimal Proliferation and fibrosis
Loss of myocytes	Medial fibrosis
	Loss of myocytes

After Brody, W. R., Kosek, J. C., and Angell, W. W.: Changes in vein grafts following aortocoronary bypass induced by pressure and ischemia. J. Thorac. Cardiovasc. Surg., 64:847, 1972.

REFERENCES

1. Barbour, D. J., and Roberts, W. C.: Additional evidence for relative resistance to atherosclerosis of the internal mammary artery compared to saphenous vein when used to increase myocardial blood flow. Am. J. Cardiol., 56:488, 1985.
2. Brody, W. R., Angell, W. W., and Kosek, J. C.: Histologic fate of the venous coronary artery bypass in dogs. Am. J. Pathol., 66:111, 1972.
3. Brody, W. R., Kosek, J. C., and Angell, W. W.: Changes in vein grafts following aortocoronary bypass induced by pressure and ischemia. J. Thorac. Cardiovasc. Surg., 64:847, 1972.
4. Carrel, A.: Results of transplantation of blood vessels, organs, and limbs. J.A.M.A., 51:1662, 1908.
5. Carrel, A., and Guthrie, C. C.: Results of biterminal transplantation of veins. Am. J. Med. Sci., 132:415, 1906.
6. Grondin, C. M., Campeau, L., Lesperance, J., Enjalbert, M., and Bourassa, M. G.: Comparison of late changes in internal mammary artery and saphenous vein grafts in two consecutive series of patients 10 years after operation. Circulation, 70(Suppl. I): I-208, 1984.
7. Kalan, J. M., and Roberts, W. C.: Comparison of morphologic changes and luminal sizes of saphenous vein and internal mammary artery after simultaneous implantation for coronary arterial bypass grafting. Am. J. Cardiol., 60:193, 1987.
8. Kalan, J. M., and Roberts, W. C.: Significance of cardiac weight in patients having coronary artery bypass grafting for angina pectoris. Am. J. Cardiol., 62:36, 1988.
9. Kalan, J. M., and Roberts, W. C.: Morphologic findings in saphenous veins used as coronary arterial bypass conduits for longer than 1 year: Necropsy analysis of 53 patients, 123 saphenous veins, and 1,865 five-millimeter segments of veins. Am. Heart J., 119:1164, 1990.
10. Kragel, A. H., Reddy, S. G., Wittes, J. T., and Roberts, W. C.: Morphometric analysis of the composition of atherosclerotic plaques in the four major epicardial coronary arteries in acute myocardial infarction and in sudden coronary death. Circulation, 80:1747, 1989.
11. Kragel, A. H., Reddy, S. G., Wittes, J. T., and Roberts, W. C.: Morphometric analysis of the composition of coronary arterial plaques in isolated unstable angina pectoris with pain at rest. Am. J. Cardiol., 66:562, 1990.
12. Loop, F. D., Lytle, B. W., Cosgrove, D. M., Stewart, R. W., Goormastic, M.,

Williams, G. W., Golding, L. A. R., Gill, C. C., Taylor, P. C., Sheldon, W. C., and Proudfit, W. L.: Influence of the internal-mammary-artery graft on 10-year survival and other cardiac events. N. Engl. J. Med., 314:1, 1986.

13. Roberts, C. S., and Roberts, W. C.: Cross-sectional area of the proximal portions of the three major epicardial coronary arteries in 98 necropsy patients with different coronary events. Relationship to heart weight, age, and sex. Circulation, 62:953, 1980.

14. Roberts, W. C.: Factors linking cholesterol to atherosclerotic plaques. Am. J. Cardiol., 62:495, 1988.

15. Roberts, W. C.: Lipid-lowering after an atherosclerotic event. Am. J. Cardiol., 64:693, 1989.

16. Roberts, W. C.: Atherosclerotic risk factors — are there ten or is there only one? Am. J. Cardiol., 64:552, 1989.

17. Roberts, W. C.: Qualitative and quantitative comparison of amounts of narrowing by atherosclerotic plaques in the major epicardial coronary arteries at necropsy in sudden coronary death, transmural acute myocardial infarction, transmural healed myocardial infarction and unstable angina pectoris. Am. J. Cardiol., 64:324, 1989.

18. Roberts, W. C.: Coronary "lesion," coronary "disease," "single-vessel disease," "two-vessel disease": Word and phrase misnomers providing false impressions of the extent of coronary atherosclerosis in symptomatic myocardial ischemia. Am. J. Cardiol., 66:121, 1990.

19. Roberts, W. C., Lachman, A. S., and Virmani, R.: Twisting of an aorta-coronary bypass conduit. A complication of coronary surgery. J. Thorac. Cardiovasc. Surg., 75:772, 1978.

20. Roberts, W. C., Potkin, B. N., Solus, D. E., and Reddy, S. G.: Mode of death, frequency of healed and acute myocardial infarction, number of major epicardial coronary arteries severely narrowed by atherosclerotic plaque, and heart weight in fatal atherosclerotic coronary artery disease: Analysis of 889 patients studied at necropsy. J. Am. Coll. Cardiol., 15:196, 1990.

21. Spray, T. L., and Roberts, W. C.: Tension on coronary bypass conduits. A neglected cause of real or potential obstruction of saphenous vein grafts. J. Thorac. Cardiovasc. Surg., 72:282, 1976.

22. Spray, T. L., and Roberts, W. C.: Status of the grafts and the native coronary arteries proximal and distal to coronary anastomotic sites of aortocoronary bypass grafts. Circulation, 55:741, 1977.

23. Spray, T. L., and Roberts, W. C.: Changes in saphenous veins used as aortocoronary bypass grafts. Am. Heart J., 94:500, 1977.

24. Vlodaver, Z., and Edwards, J. E.: Pathology of coronary atherosclerosis. Prog. Cardiovasc. Dis., 14:256, 1971.

25. Waller, B. F., and Roberts, W. C.: Amount of narrowing by atherosclerotic plaque in 44 nonbypassed and 52 bypassed major epicardial coronary arteries in 32 necropsy patients who died within 1 month of aortocoronary bypass grafting. Am. J. Cardiol., 46:956, 1980.

26. Waller, B. F., and Roberts, W. C.: Remnant saphenous veins after aortocoronary bypass grafting: Analysis of 3,394 centimeters of unused vein from 402 patients. Am. J. Cardiol., 55:65, 1985.

XVI

CONGENITAL LESIONS OF THE CORONARY CIRCULATION

James E. Lowe, M.D., and David C. Sabiston, Jr., M.D.

Congenital coronary arterial malformations have long been recognized, but the number of reported patients has increased markedly since the introduction of selective coronary arteriography by Sones in 1959.[79] In a review of 224 patients with coronary malformations, Ogden proposed three basic classifications: (1) major anomalies, in which there is an abnormal communication between an artery and a cardiac chamber or abnormal origin of a major coronary artery from the pulmonary artery; (2) minor anomalies, in which there is variation of the origin of the vessels from the aorta, but the distal circulation is normal; and (3) secondary anomalies, in which the coronary arterial variation probably represents a circulatory response to the primary intracardiac pathologic defect.[58]

Major anomalies that are amenable to surgical correction include congenital coronary fistulas, anomalous origin of either the left or right coronary artery from the pulmonary artery, congenital aneurysms of the coronary arteries, and congenital membranous obstruction of the ostium of the left main coronary artery. Minor anomalies, in which there is variation in the origin of the coronary arteries from the aorta with normal distal circulation, and secondary anomalies, associated with congenital heart defects, such as transposition of the great vessels, truncus arteriosus, and tetralogy of Fallot, seldom require surgical intervention.

Based on the authors' clinical experience and supported by that of others, it is recommended that most patients with major congenital coronary arterial malformations be considered candidates for surgical correction. In most cases, the natural history of these lesions is not associated with a normal life expectancy, with the possible exception of patients with congenital origin of the right coronary artery from the pulmonary artery. Because these malformations can now be safely corrected with excellent long-term results, surgical intervention should be recommended after a precise diagnosis has been established.

CORONARY ARTERY FISTULAS

Over 400 patients with coronary fistulas have been reported in the literature since Krause first described this malformation in 1865. Increasing numbers of patients with this anomaly are being recognized each year because of the widespread use of cardiac catheterization and selective coronary arteriography in the evaluation of cardiac disorders.

Congenital coronary artery fistulas are the most common of the congenital coronary malformations. They are characterized by normal origin of the involved coronary artery from the aorta with a fistulous communication with the atria or ventricles or with the pulmonary artery, coronary sinus, or superior vena cava without any interposed capillary bed. Coronary artery fistulas are found with no sex predilection in 1 of every 50,000 patients with congenital heart disease and in 1 of every 500 patients who have coronary arteriography.[89]

CLINICAL MANIFESTATIONS. In the past, it was commonly believed that most patients with coronary artery fistulas were asymptomatic. However, based on the authors' experience with 30 patients and supported by a review of 258 others reported in the literature, 55 per cent are symptomatic at the time of presentation.[48,49] Because the underlying pathophysiologic mechanism is essentially that of a left-to-right cardiac shunt, the most common manifestation is congestive heart failure[19] (Fig. 1). Other common symptoms are angina pectoris, secondary to a steal of coronary arterial flow through the fistulous communication, and subacute bacterial endocarditis. Bacterial endocarditis, anemia, and glomerulonephritis in the same patient have been reported.[73] Infants and children with this lesion may demonstrate a failure to thrive. Less commonly, patients present with acute myocardial infarction, aneurysm formation with subsequent rupture or embolization, or symptoms secondary to pulmonary hypertension.

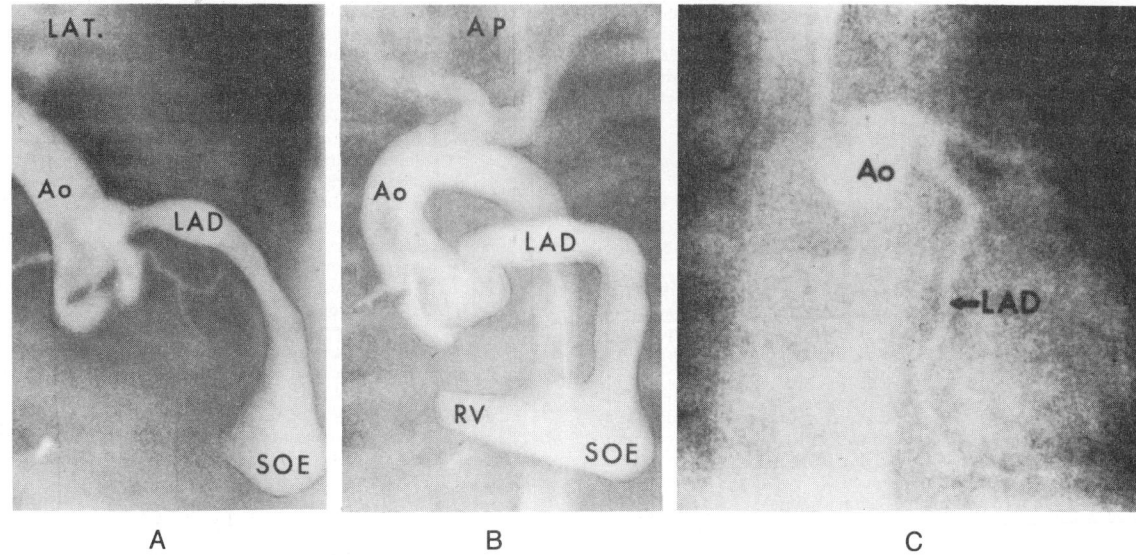

Figure 1. *A* and *B*, Ascending aortogram (lateral and anteroposterior views) in a 6-week-old infant who presented with severe congestive heart failure. The aortogram shows a left coronary artery–right ventricular fistula. Ao, aorta; LAD, left anterior descending coronary; SOE, site of entry of the fistula into the right ventricle; RV, incompletely opacified right ventricle. *C*, Repeat aortogram 1 year after successful surgical obliteration of the fistula. The left anterior descending coronary artery has returned to normal size. (From Daniel, T. M., Graham, T. P., and Sabiston, D. C., Jr.: Coronary artery–right ventricular fistula with congestive heart failure: Surgical correction in the neonatal period. Surgery, 67:985, 1970.)

In patients who are asymptomatic, the diagnosis is usually made after coronary angiography is performed for evaluation of asymptomatic murmurs, mild cardiomegaly discovered on a routine chest film, or electrocardiographic abnormalities.

The major clinical finding secondary to a coronary artery fistula is a continuous murmur over the site of the abnormal communication. This murmur may closely resemble that of a patent ductus arteriosus, and the first patient on whom closure was performed was operated on by Bjork and Crafoord in 1947 for a presumed patent ductus. Because a patent ductus was not found, the pericardium was opened, and a coronary artery fistula draining into the pulmonary artery was identified and obliterated.[8] The differential diagnosis of coronary artery fistulas, in addition to patent ductus arteriosus, includes congenital aortic-pulmonary fistulas, sinus of Valsalva fistulas, ventricular septal defect with aortic insufficiency, pulmonary arteriovenous malformations, and fistulas of systemic vessels, such as the subclavian and internal mammary arteries connecting to veins of the chest wall or to the lung.

The right coronary artery is most often involved in the development of congenital coronary artery fistula (56 per cent) and most commonly communicates with a chamber of the right side of the heart.[49] The fistula usually involves the right ventricle (39 per cent), followed closely in incidence by drainage into the right atrium (33 per cent), including the coronary sinus and superior vena cava, or the pulmonary artery (20 per cent). Left coronary artery fistulas are less common but usually drain into the right ventricle or right atrium. Rarely, coronary artery fistulas may drain into the left atrium or left ventricle.

EVALUATION. The successful surgical management of patients with congenital coronary artery fistulas depends on a thorough preoperative evaluation that precisely defines the anatomy and pathophysiology of the anomaly. Although echocardiography[7,60,65,75] and computed chest tomography[77] have been used to noninvasively identify coronary fistulas, the precise diagnosis requires arteriographic demonstration of the involved coronary artery, the recipient cardiac chamber, and the exact site of communication. In patients with a large fistula, injection of contrast medium into the aortic root may clearly delineate the lesion (see Fig. 1). In patients with a smaller fistula or fistulous communications from both coronary arteries, selective coronary arteriography is essential to establish the diagnosis.

Spontaneous closure of a coronary fistula is rare, and only 3 documented cases have been reported.[33,34,50] It should be emphasized that the ideal time for elective surgical closure is before the development of symptoms and major pathologic changes in the heart, the coronary arteries, and the pulmonary circulation. Liberthson and associates have shown that most patients with congenital coronary artery fistulas develop both symptoms and fistula-related complications with increased age and are subject to increased morbidity and mortality if surgical correction is done later in life.[46]

SURGICAL MANAGEMENT. Because patients with coronary artery fistulas have had a precise and detailed angiographic examination showing the involved coronary artery, the recipient cardiac chamber, and the exact site of communication, it can often be anticipated preoperatively whether cardiopulmonary bypass is required. Patients with a single communication that is easily dissected usually do not require bypass for suture obliteration. However, in patients with multiple communications or large, tortuous, draining channels, the fistula is best obliterated by opening the recipient cardiac chamber with the patient on bypass in order to completely close all fistulous tracts (Fig. 2).[47] Finally, if fistula obliteration in any way jeopardizes distal coronary arterial flow, a saphenous vein or internal mammary bypass graft should be placed under hypothermic potassium cardioplegic arrest. These procedures should be planned with pump standby, since the majority are now done using cardiopulmonary bypass.

RESULTS. Thirty patients with congenital coronary artery fistulas have been evaluated at the Duke University Medical Center. These patients were between 6 weeks and 76 years of age, with a mean age of 32 years and equal distribution between males and females. Half of the patients came to surgical attention because of symptoms such as congestive heart failure, angina, or failure to thrive. The remainder were asymptomatic and came to operation after evaluation of asymptomatic heart murmurs or cardiomegaly found on a routine chest film. Twenty-three of these patients have undergone surgical repair. All procedures were done through a median sternotomy, and 14 patients had suture obliteration of the fistula without bypass (61 per cent). Seven patients had cardiopulmonary bypass to open the recipient cardiac chamber and successfully occlude multiple draining fistulous tracts (30 per cent). Two patients had saphenous vein bypass grafting after fistula obliteration in order

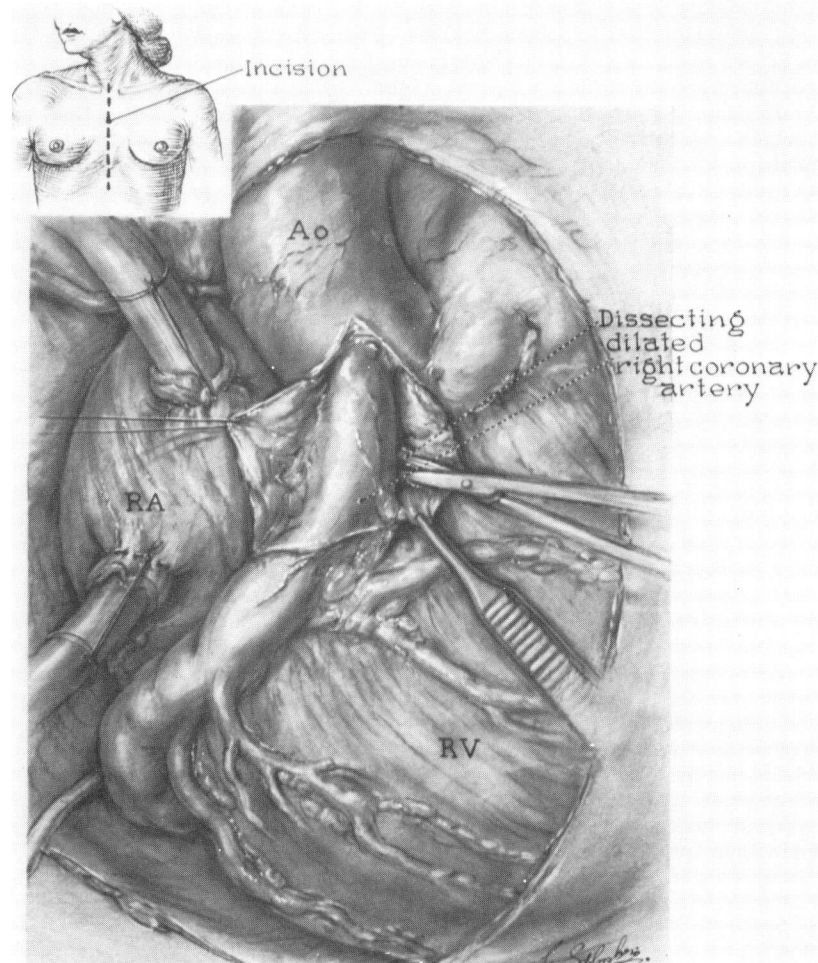

Figure 2. *A,* Right coronary–right atrial congenital coronary fistula as seen at operation in a 76-year-old woman who presented with severe congestive heart failure. Through a median sternotomy, the patient was placed on cardiopulmonary bypass with separate venous return cannulas placed in the superior and inferior venae cavae. (From Lowe, J. E., and Sabiston, D. C., Jr.: Congenital coronary malformations. *In* Cohn, L. H. (Ed.): Modern Technics in Surgery, Cardiac-Thoracic Surgery. Mt. Kisco, NY, Futura Publishing Company, 1981.)

Figure 2. *Continued. B,* Tapes are secured around the superior and inferior venae cavae to eliminate venous return to the right atrium. The heart is then made to fibrillate, and the right atrium is opened. A large fistulous opening is identified and closed with interrupted nonabsorbable pledged sutures (A). The site of entry into the right is shown in B. After closure of the site of entry into the right atrium, a second fistulous tract was found entering the aneurysm over the posterior surface of the heart (A and B). This fistulous tract was closed with multiple transfixion sutures. (From Lowe, J. E., and Sabiston, D. C., Jr.: Congenital coronary malformations. *In* Cohn, L. H. (Ed.): Modern Technics in Surgery, Cardiac-Thoracic Surgery, Mt. Kisco, NY, Futura Publishing Company, 1981.)

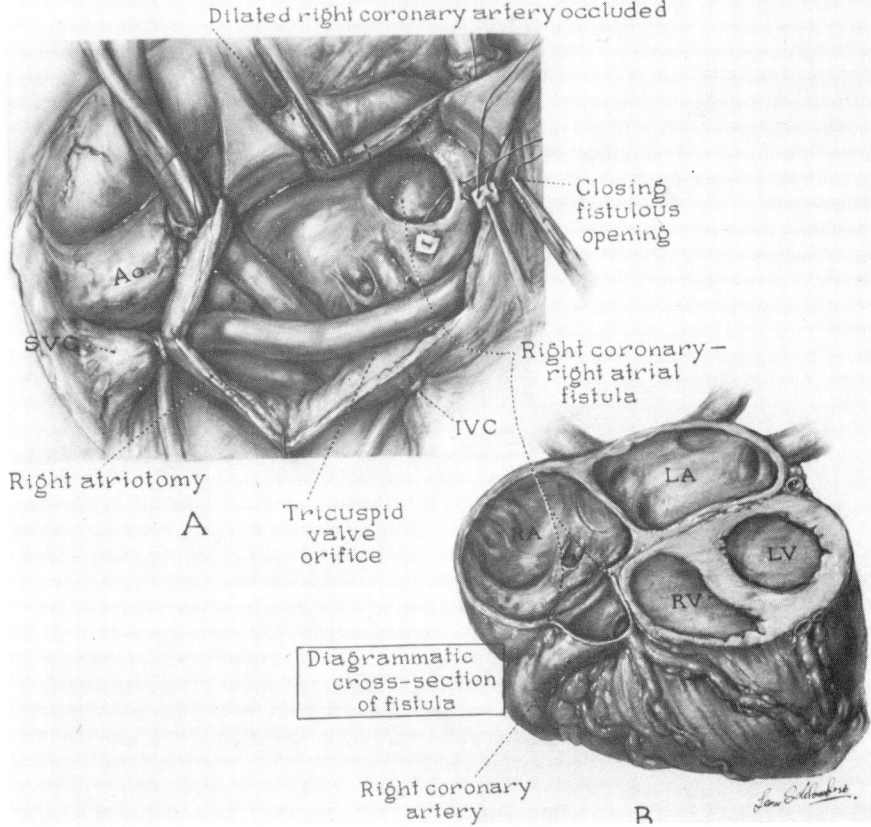

to reconstitute distal coronary flow (9 per cent). The mean time of follow-up for these 23 patients has been 10 years. There were no operative deaths, and all patients are well and do not have evidence of recurrent fistula formation, although one patient with a complex fistula of the circumflex coronary artery to the right ventricle has a small residual shunt.[48] Urrutia-S and associates reported similar surgical results in 56 patients with an overall survival of 98.3 per cent.[84]

ANOMALOUS ORIGIN OF THE LEFT CORONARY ARTERY FROM THE PULMONARY ARTERY

Ravi S. Chari, M.D., James E. Lowe, M.D., and David C. Sabiston, Jr., M.D.

Anomalous origin of the left coronary artery from the pulmonary artery is a rare but important cause of congestive heart failure, mitral insufficiency, and left ventricular infarction in infants and children. It has been reported to occur once in every 300,000 live births. Without surgical intervention, it has been estimated that 95 per cent of patients with the left coronary artery originating from the pulmonary artery die within the first years of life.[40] Thus, its early recognition and proper treatment are essential.

The first report of the left coronary artery originating from the pulmonary artery was made by Abbott in 1908.[1] In 1911, Abrikossoff described a 5-month-old infant who died of congestive heart failure and was found to have an aneurysm of the left ventricle at post mortem.[3] Photomicrographs of the ventricle revealed infarction, including areas of calcification. Bland and associates[9] in 1932 integrated clinical and pathologic data and recorded an electrocardiogram in a 3-year-old infant with this condition, showing that a diagnosis during life could be possible. Eidlow in 1948 reported the first patient in whom the condition was diagnosed ante mortem.[24]

The pathophysiologic mechanism of this condition was first suggested by Abbott[1] as a theory; she reasoned that the flow in the aberrant left coronary artery was toward the pulmonary artery, being derived via anastomotic vessels from the normally arising right coronary artery. However, these observations disappeared from view, and it was thought for many years that symptoms resulted from poorly oxygenated blood from the pulmonary artery flowing into the left coronary artery under low pressure. Edwards reviewed and re-established Abbott's original theory in 1958.[23] Numerous studies of postmortem specimens clearly reveal the presence of many collaterals originating from the right coronary and connecting to the left coronary artery. In fact, if the right coronary artery is injected in postmortem specimens, branches of the coronary rapidly fill in significant amounts.[15] At the time of operation, occlusion of the left coronary artery at its origin causes an increase in pressure within the coronary artery, suggesting that flow originates from the right coronary artery by collaterals.[71,72] Of additional significance is the fact that blood withdrawn from the coronary artery at the time of operation is fully saturated with oxygen. This is clear evidence that this blood originates from a systemic arterial source rather than the pulmonary artery, and that the direction of blood flow is from the right coronary artery by collaterals into the left coronary artery and then into the pulmonary artery. The resultant symptoms and clinical manifestations are secondary to left ventricular myocardial ischemia, which follows inadequate collateral flow from the right coronary artery to the left coronary artery or a steal of adequate collateral flow into the low-pressure pulmonary artery system.

CLINICAL MANIFESTATIONS. The vast majority of patients (90 per cent or more) with anomalous origin of the left coronary artery from the pulmonary artery develop symptoms during infancy. The infant usually appears normal at birth, since the pulmonary artery pressure at this age is elevated and allows perfusion of the left coronary from the pulmonary artery for a brief period of time. Symptoms may be present at birth, especially if there are associated cardiac defects. Symptoms are most likely to occur during the first several months of life as left ventricular ischemia becomes more pronounced. When symptoms appear, there is generally a course of progressive deterioration; progressive left ventricular dysfunction occurs, and unless operation is undertaken, death ensues. Nevertheless, some patients survive to adult life with few if any symptoms.[2,36,54,90] In a collected review, Harthorne and associates reported 28 adults with this condition,[36] and Moodie and associates studied 10 adult patients with this malformation and provided long-term follow-up after surgical correction.[54] Recently Purut and Sabiston described the oldest patient with this malformation, a 61-year-old female, who underwent surgical repair.[64] Of interest, only 7 patients over the age of 50 at the time of diagnosis have been reported.

SYMPTOMS. As described earlier, it has been shown that blood flow in the left coronary artery is retrograde from the right coronary artery via collaterals into the left coronary artery and subsequently into the pulmonary artery. Symptoms occur either from poor collateral flow from the pulmonary artery or secondary to a "steal" phenomenon of blood passing through well-developed collaterals into the left coronary arterial system with drainage into the pulmonary artery.[48] Because of the low pressures in the pulmonary artery, blood flow is selectively shunted into the pulmonary system instead of perfusing the left ventricular myocardium. The chief symptoms are intimately associated with the onset of heart failure and include dyspnea and tachycardia. Wheezing respirations, cough, and cyanosis usually follow. "Angina of feeding" is an interesting finding described as episodes of pain and distress during or immediately after feeding. Paroxysms of distress with pallor, sweating, and dyspnea have also been reported and are also thought to be anginal in origin. Often on presentation, the infant may have a respiratory infection that serves to precipitate the heart failure and often delays the proper diagnosis.

PHYSICAL EXAMINATION. The characteristic findings on physical examination include a rapid respiratory rate, tachycardia, and cardiac enlargement. A murmur is not usually present early in life, and congenital origin of the left coronary artery from the pulmonary artery is one of the few cardinal malformations that can cause congestive heart failure in infancy *without* a murmur. Evidence of a respiratory infection is commonly present with fever, cough, nasal discharge, or rales in the chest. In older infants and children, mitral regurgitation develops secondary to left ventricular dilation or chronic ischemia and/or infarction that causes papillary muscle dysfunction.[14] The liver is characteristically enlarged, and the spleen may be palpable in a small number of patients. Occasionally the presenting signs may be of collapse and shock, similar to those signs manifested by adults with sudden coronary artery occlusion.

EVALUATION. The chest film shows cardiomegaly predominantly involving the left ventricle. Aneurysmal dilation may be present as a result of marked thinning of the left ventricular wall, and in many instances, the left border of the heart extends to the lateral rib margin. As a result of left ventricular failure, the pulmonary vascular markings are usually exaggerated.

Considerable emphasis has been placed on the characteristic electrocardiographic changes that can establish the diagnosis. The first description of myocardial ischemia on the electrocardiogram of an infant with this condition was made in 1933 by Bland and associates.[9] Based on this work, congenital origin of the left coronary artery from the pulmonary artery has also been referred to as the Bland-White-Garland syndrome. Generally, it is possible to make a relatively firm diagnosis on the basis of electrocardiographic changes. Tachycardia is almost always present. The T waves are characteristically inverted in the standard limb leads and there may be slight ST segment elevation in lead I. The T waves in the precordial leads, especially V_5 and V_6 are usually inverted, and deep Q waves are frequently present. The body surface potential distribution has also been helpful in diagnosis and providing evidence of improved coronary blood flow following operation.[29]

Noninvasive tests to diagnose and evaluate anomalous origin of the left coronary artery from the pulmonary artery are receiving increasing attention and investigation. Two-dimensional echocardiography,[28] thallium scans,[27] pulsed-wave Doppler echocardiography,[42] and most recently magnetic resonance imaging[21] are diagnostic modalities that have been used to evaluate patients with anomalous left coronary artery. Experience with these techniques is limited, but preliminary reports suggest that although these serve as valuable adjuvants in the diagnosis of anomalous left coronary artery, they do not obviate the need for preoperative cardiac catheterization. Additionally, noninvasive studies can be used to assess the patient intraoperatively (Doppler)[81] and accurately assess and monitor postoperative patients.[30]

On angiography, the right heart is usually normal. The pulmonary vasculature may show subpectoral engorgement and enlargement. The most striking feature is enlargement of the left atrium and left ventricle. The wall of the left ventricle may be quite thin, especially on its anterolateral aspect near the apex. A true ventricular aneurysm with paradoxical pulsations may be present, and mitral insufficiency is quite common.

Injection of contrast medium into a catheter placed in the proximal aorta (or, when possible, directly into the right coronary ostium) demonstrates the classic findings (Fig. 3). Contrast enters the right coronary as it originates from the aorta and passes through dilated collaterals that communicate with the left coronary artery. The contrast can then be followed into the left anterior descending and circumflex coronary arteries where it converges to enter the left main coronary artery, with ultimate drainage into the pulmonary artery. Thus, retrograde flow of blood in the left coronary artery can be convincingly demonstrated in such a study, conclusively establishing the diagnosis.[70]

Cardiac catheterization is also helpful because the right ventricular and pulmonary artery pressures may be elevated. Moreover, it is usually possible to demonstrate left-to-right shunt at the pulmonary artery level by contrast. Although the oxygen saturation may at times show a significant increase from the right ventricle to the pulmonary artery, this is not always present, even when it can be demonstrated that the left coronary arises from the pulmonary artery. The ejection fraction in patients with anomalous origin of the left pulmonary artery was determined in 8 preoperative patients in whom it varied between 0.13 and 0.72. It is noteworthy that among those who died, the ejection fraction was less than 0.36, whereas in survivors, the ejection fraction was more than 0.55.[52]

PATHOLOGY. The major pathologic features of this condition are apparent at the time of operation. The left ventricle is characteristically greatly dilated, and the wall is thin. The left coronary artery is larger than normal, and numerous collateral vessels connect the right and left coronary arteries. These are usually tortuous and thin-walled. The right coronary artery arises in its normal position and is also enlarged. Its branches tend to be more tortuous than usual as they emit various collateral vessels. Over time, and especially in adults, the right coronary artery may become quite large and increasingly tortuous. Similarly, the left coronary artery may also enlarge, up to 10 mm. or more in diameter, at its origin. The left coronary artery arises from the left or posterior cusp of the pulmonary artery. The branches and course of the anterior descending and circumflex branches are usually otherwise normal. On section, the

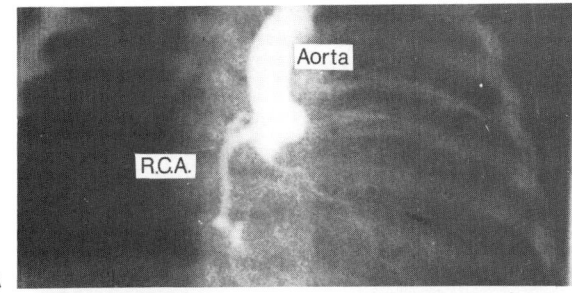

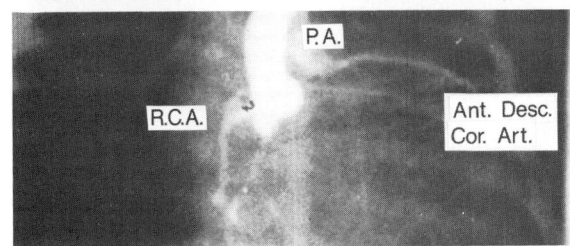

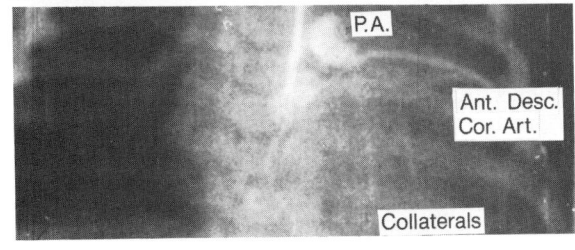

Figure 3. Several cine frames taken from a series illustrating coronary arterial filling during aortography. *A*, Filling of the right coronary artery as it arises normally from the aorta. Note that its size is slightly greater than normal. *B*, Filling of the branches of the left coronary artery through collaterals from the right coronary artery. *C*, Filling of the pulmonary artery by retrograde flow from the left coronary artery. (From Sabiston, D. C., Jr., and Orme, S. K.: Congenital origin of the left coronary artery from the pulmonary artery. J. Cardiovasc. Surg., 9:543, 1968.)

left ventricle may be very thin and in areas totally replaced by scar tissue. Various degrees of subendocardial fibroelastosis may also be present. Calcification is often present in the fibrotic portion of the left ventricle. Infarction of the ventricle may involve the papillary muscles, producing mitral insufficiency. If the left ventricle is dilated, the mitral ring may be sufficiently enlarged to prevent normal coaptation of the valve leaflets, also causing mitral insufficiency.

SURGICAL MANAGEMENT. The prime object of surgical correction in anomalous origin of the left coronary artery from the pulmonary artery is to establish adequate blood flow in the left coronary artery and its branches. Historically, several surgical procedures were advocated to accomplish this: Mustard's left common carotid artery anastomosis to the left coronary artery,[55] Potts' aortopulmonary anastomosis,[63] the pulmonary artery banding of Case,[15] and the technique of pericardial poudrage and de-epicardialization.[59] Disappointing results in these, however, led to their abandonment. In the modern era, two basic approaches are used in the surgical treatment of this malformation: simple ligation at the site of origin of the anomalous left coronary artery, and the establishment of a two-coronary artery system.

Simple ligation at the site of origin from the pulmonary artery is an effective treatment if enough collaterals from the right coronary exist to supply the left coronary system adequately.[38] Ligation prevents the "coronary steal" into the pulmonary artery, increases the coronary artery pressure, and improves myocardial blood flow.[70] Long-term follow-up of patients undergoing this procedure has demonstrated the beneficial effects of simple ligature with relief of symptoms and decrease in heart size.[76]

Simple ligature alone, however, has led to high mortality due to the variability in the number of intercoronary collaterals and to the inability of simple ligature to produce immediate and sufficient improvement in left ventricular myocardial perfusion in all patients.[91] Survivors of this procedure are left with a single–coronary artery system, which is theoretically less physiologic and at greater risk of atherosclerosis.[66] It has also been shown that the incidence of sudden death is higher in patients who have undergone simple ligation compared with those who have had a two–coronary artery system established.[91] Poorer performance on treadmill exercise testing[51] and higher late mortality[13] (not due to sudden death) have also been reported in patients with simple ligature or nonfunctioning grafts (ligature equivalent) compared with those with two–coronary artery systems. It is therefore recommended that simple ligature be reserved only for those critically ill patients in whom it may be lifesaving,[43,87] and creation of a two–coronary artery system can be accomplished later in life.[13]

Surgical re-establishment of a two–coronary artery system is the treatment of choice for anomalous left coronary artery arising from the pulmonary artery.[6,25,41,78] The surgical alternatives include left subclavian–left coronary artery anastomosis[41,53,61] or connection of the left coronary artery to the aorta. The latter can be performed by direct implantation,[32,56] autologous artery,[44,56] or venous[25,41] bypass grafting, or more recently by intrapulmonary tunneling. This transpulmonary aorta–left coronary artery continuity has been accomplished by using a flap of anterior pulmonary wall,[82] autogenous pericardium,[35] a free segment of left subclavian artery,[6] or polytetrafluoroethylene (PTFE, Gore-tex)[13] to connect a side-to-side aortopulmonary window to the left coronary ostium *within* the lumen of the pulmonary artery (Figs. 4 to 6).

In older children and adults, a two–coronary artery system can be reconstructed using saphenous vein graft[91] (Fig. 7) or internal mammary bypass grafting. These methods are technically difficult in infants and small children. Moreover, graft occlusion in infants is a problem.[6,51] Combined with its inability to grow with the child, bypass grafting with veins is considered

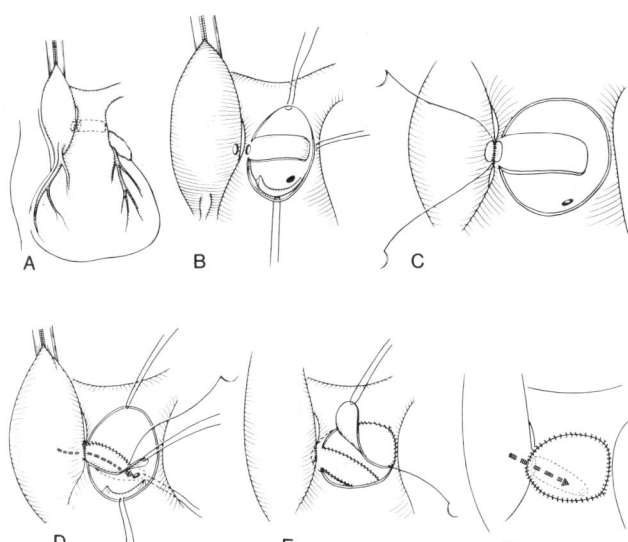

Figure 5. Following institution of hypothermic cardiopulmonary bypass, the aorta is cross-clamped and the heart is arrested by infusing cold potassium cardioplegia. An aortopulmonary window is created, and a flap of the anterior pulmonary wall is sutured to the aortopulmonary window (top). Using the pulmonary arterial flap, a tunnel is created inside the pulmonary artery between the aortopulmonary window and the anomalous left coronary ostium by suturing the pulmonary arterial flap to the posterior wall of the pulmonary trunk. The defect in the anterior wall of the pulmonary artery is then repaired using a pericardial patch (bottom). (From Takeuchi, S., Imamura, H., Katsumoto, K., et al.: New surgical method for repair of anomalous left coronary artery from pulmonary artery. J. Thorac. Cardiovasc. Surg., 78:7, 1979.)

an unsatisfactory method of reconstruction of a two–coronary vessel circulation in infants.[32]

Direct implantation of the anomalous left coronary artery into the root of the aorta is a method of establishing a two–coronary vessel circulation by recreating the normal anatomy. Excellent patency rates of 100 per cent have been reported in patients who survived direct aortic reimplantation,[44,87] but the operative mortality remains prohibitively high, especially in patients less than 1 year old. Technical difficulties with the inability to mobilize adequate length may also preclude the use of this technique. Moreover, reimplantation alters both the shape of the left coronary orifice and the angle it subtends with the aorta.[78] The clinical significance of these changes awaits further follow-up of survivors and detailed study of coronary blood flow and ventricular function in these infants.

The technique of subclavian–left coronary anastomosis was first described by Apley, Horton, and Wilson in 1951[4]; Meyer first performed this successfully in 1968[53] (Fig. 8). This procedure can be performed through a left posterolateral thoracotomy without cardiopulmonary bypass or with cardiopulmonary bypass through a median sternotomy or bilateral anterior thoracotomies with transverse sternotomy. Excellent results have been reported using this procedure in 6 patients between the ages of 2 and 76 months.[80] Technical advantages over other revascularizing techniques include the avoidance of aortic cross-clamping (which may increase the ischemic injury of the myocardium) and the avoidance of direct surgical procedures involving the pulmonary artery that may lead to late stenosis. In the infant group, however, the graft occlusion remains a problem, and occlusion rates as high as 50 per cent have been reported.[61] The tendency for the left subclavian artery to kink as it arises from the left aortic arch predisposes it to late graft occlusion. This technique may have a role in the establishment of a two–coronary artery system in critically ill infants, since it can be performed without cardiopulmonary bypass or aortic occlusion.[41]

In 1979, Takeuchi described a technique that involved the creation of a transpulmonary artery aortocoronary bypass in

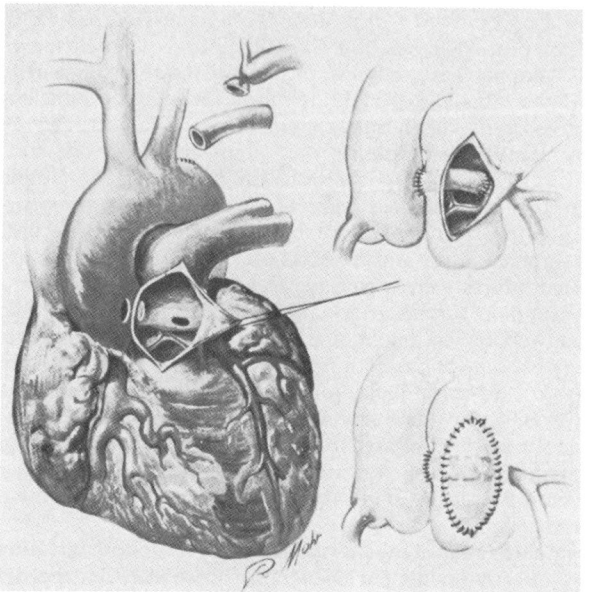

Figure 4. Transpulmonary arterial aortocoronary bypass grafting is performed with a free segment of the left subclavian artery (LSCA). A 4-mm. aortopulmonary window is constructed, and the LSCA segment is sutured within the pulmonary artery to the aortopulmonary anastomosis and around the ostium of the anomalous left coronary artery. A pericardial angioplasty prevents luminal compromise of the pulmonary artery containing the transpulmonary arterial bypass graft. (From Arciniegas, E. A., Farooki, Z. Q., Hakimi, M., and Green, E. W.: Management of anomalous left coronary artery from the pulmonary artery. Circulation, 62(Suppl. I):180, 1980.)

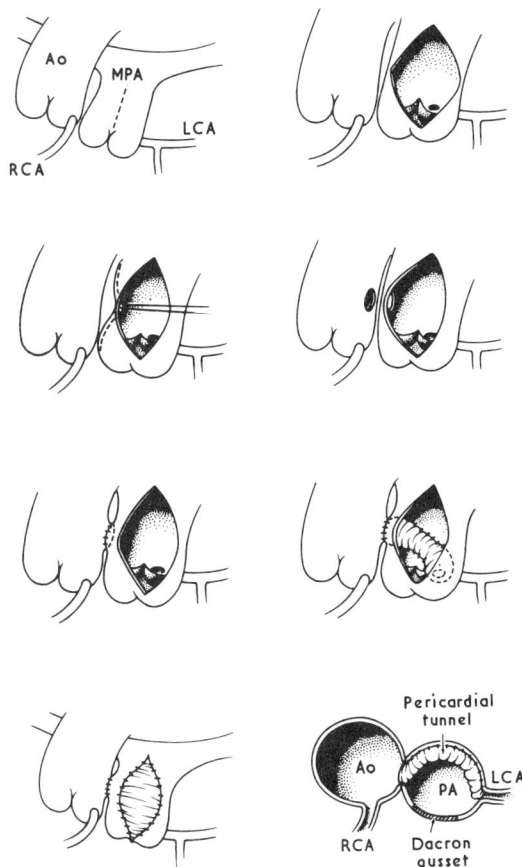

Figure 6. An opening is made in the pulmonary artery and an aortopulmonary window is created. A pericardial tunnel is then constructed and connects the aortopulmonary window within the pulmonary artery to the anomalous origin of the left main coronary artery from the pulmonary artery. The defect in the anterior pulmonary arterial wall is repaired using a Dacron patch. (From Hamilton, D. E., Ghosh, P. K., and Donnelly, R. J.: An operation for anomalous origin of left coronary artery. Br. Heart J., *41*:121, 1979.)

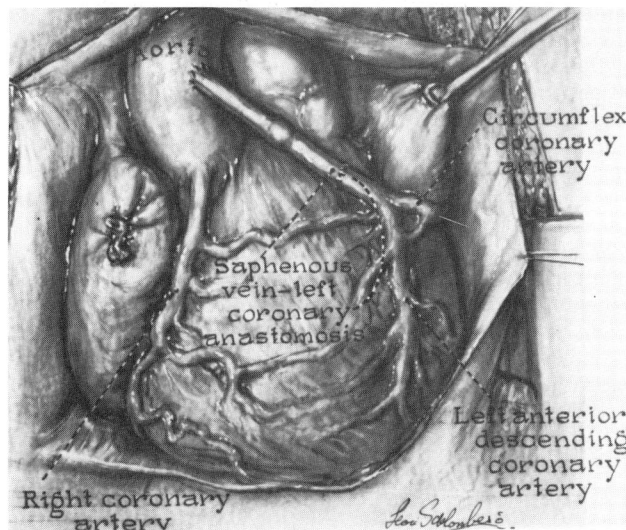

Figure 7. Congenital origin of the left coronary from the pulmonary artery can also be managed by division of the left coronary artery at its site of origin and reconstruction of a two-coronary system using a saphenous vein graft. Through median sternotomy, and with a patient on cardiopulmonary bypass, the saphenous vein graft is attached to the ascending aorta using a partial occluding clamp. The left coronary artery is then divided at its site of origin from the pulmonary artery. The saphenous vein graft is then anastomosed in end-to-end fashion to the left coronary artery using interrupted 7–0 nonabsorbable sutures. (From Lowe, J. E., and Sabiston, D. C., Jr.: Surgical correction of congenital malformations of the coronary circulation. South. Med. J., *75*:1508, 1982.)

which the anterior wall of the pulmonary artery was used as a tunnel flap to direct blood from a created aortopulmonary window into the anomalous left coronary artery ostium.[82] Modifications as noted previously have been made to this technique. Preliminary experience with this technique has shown it to be technically applicable to infants and small children (as well as adults) with favorable improvements in clinical status and left ventricular function.[13] Operative complications include aortic valve incompetence secondary to valve damage during creation of the aortopulmonary window and pulmonic stenosis as a result of pulmonary arteriotomy or the intrapulmonary conduit. Long-term patency and survival have shown this to be a simple and effective means of establishing a two–coronary artery system in this malformation. Transpulmonary arterial bypass is now considered by some to be the procedure of choice in infants since it is associated with low mortality and good patency rates.[6,13]

The best form of surgical treatment for this disorder is unknown. Clearly, the establishment of a two–coronary vessel circulation is superior to simple ligation. Simple ligation should be reserved for neonates whose critical illness precludes a lengthy cardiac bypass procedure. The Meyer operation serves as an alternative to this procedure because it can be performed without bypass. In older children and adults, a two–coronary artery system can be reconstructed by using saphenous vein or internal mammary artery by grafting. In young children, infants, and neonates, the surgical alternatives include direct implantation of the anomalous coronary artery into the aorta, intrapulmonary conduits, and left subclavian–left coronary

artery anastomosis. Bypass grafting with venous autograft or prosthetic graft is not a satisfactory option in this age group because of technical difficulty and poor graft patency. Intrapulmonary artery conduits are increasingly being used with good results and are rapidly becoming the procedure of choice in all age groups. Long-term results in significant numbers of patients, however, are still to be established.

RESULTS. The authors have evaluated 40 patients with anomalous origin of the left coronary artery from the pulmonary artery, and 30 have been surgically treated. Twenty-two had severe congestive heart failure. Five had angina, and 2 infants came to attention because of failure to thrive. The remaining 10 patients were evaluated for murmurs of uncertain

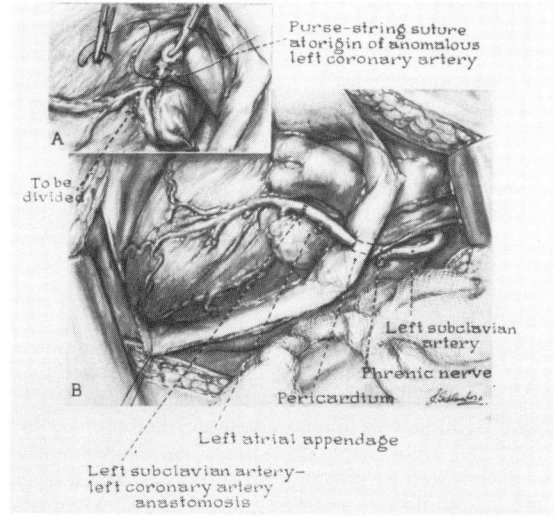

Figure 8. For congenital origin of the left coronary artery from the pulmonary artery, through a left anterior third interspace thoracotomy, the left coronary artery is occluded at its site of origin with suture ligatures and then is divided. The left subclavian artery is then anastomosed to the left coronary artery in end-to-end fashion with interrupted 7–0 nonabsorbable sutures. (From Lowe, J. E., and Sabiston, D. C., Jr.: Surgical correction of congenital malformations of the coronary circulation. South. Med. J., *75*:1508, 1982.)

cause, cardiomegaly on physical examination or chest films, or unexplained dyspnea. All 10 patients not operated on died within several hours to several months after diagnosis. Of the 30 patients undergoing repair, 17 had simple ligation at the origin of the left coronary artery from the pulmonary artery, with 6 operative deaths (35 per cent) and 1 additional death 4 months postoperatively. Seven patients had ligation of the left coronary artery followed by saphenous vein bypass grafting. There were no operative deaths and all 7 have been well 4 to 14 years after operation. Five of seven grafts were clotted on repeat angiography done 4 months to 2 years postoperatively. One patient treated with ligation of the left coronary artery from its origin had left subclavian–left coronary artery anastomosis at 14 months of age. This patient is a gymnast at age 13. One patient underwent a pulmonary artery tunnel procedure and died 1 hour postoperatively. Early in the authors' experience, 2 patients were treated with de-epicardialization and are long-term survivors. One early patient had pulmonary-aortic anastomosis and died shortly after operation, and 1 died during thoracotomy before a planned simple ligation. Among the 30 patients there were 9 operative deaths, with overall operative mortality of 30 per cent. Because of the 95 to 100 per cent mortality in those treated nonoperatively, surgical treatment is always recommended following diagnosis.

ORIGIN OF THE RIGHT CORONARY ARTERY FROM THE PULMONARY ARTERY

St. John Brooks in 1886 originally described this rare malformation in 2 cadavers studied in the anatomic dissection laboratory at the University of Dublin.[12] Both lesions occurred in adults, neither of whom had evidence of heart disease. Brooks noted dilated collaterals from the left coronary artery feeding the right coronary artery and correctly postulated, based on this observation, that flow in the right coronary artery might actually be retrograde into the pulmonary artery.[12]

CLINICAL MANIFESTATIONS. The clinical manifestations of this condition are usually minimal or absent. In the 17 cases collected from the literature (reviewed by Tingelstad and associates in 1972), the abnormal artery was discovered in individuals whose ages ranged from 17 to 90 years.[83] The malformation was thought to have been associated with death in only two cases. One of these was a 17-year-old female who died suddenly. Autopsy showed complete occlusion of the left coronary artery by thrombus with evidence of left ventricular infarction. The only other reported death occurred in a 55-year-old woman who presented with angina and congestive heart failure. In 3 additional patients, the anomaly was found in association with other congenital malformations.

Even though origin of the right coronary artery from the pulmonary artery is a rare anomaly with a benign natural history in most patients, it can lead to myocardial ischemia, infarction, congestive heart failure, and myocardial fibrosis.[16,67,74] Because it can be safely corrected when diagnosed, operative correction is indicated.

EVALUATION. In the rare patient with this condition who comes to medical attention, the diagnosis is established by aortography and selective coronary arteriography. The left coronary artery is found to be dilated, and large intercoronary collaterals feed the right coronary artery. As Brooks correctly suggested, flow in the right coronary artery is retrograde, emptying into the pulmonary artery. Contrasting with patients who have the more frequently occurring malformation of origin of the left coronary artery from the pulmonary artery, there are usually no electrocardiographic or radiographic abnormalities. The diagnosis is therefore established only in those who have selective coronary arteriography. Two-dimensional echocardi-

ography has been used to diagnose this malformation, which was confirmed later by coronary arteriography.[74,92]

SURGICAL MANAGEMENT AND RESULTS. A fascinating case was reported by Tingelstad of a 12-year-old boy who was asymptomatic but had a to-and-fro systolic and diastolic murmur along the left sternal border in the third intercostal space.[83] The chest film showed slight cardiac enlargement and normal pulmonary vasculature. Mild left ventricular hypertrophy was shown by a scalar electrocardiogram. An aortogram revealed a dilated left coronary artery arising normally from the left sinus of Valsalva of the aorta, and the right coronary artery was filled through tortuous intercoronary anastomoses from the left coronary artery and drained into the main pulmonary artery. At operation, a narrow rim of tissue from the pulmonary artery was removed with the origin of the right coronary artery, and this was successfully reimplanted into the ascending aorta.[83] This represents the ideal form of surgical management and has also been done successfully by others.[11,16,85] Other alternatives include simple ligation at the site of anomalous origin with or without saphenous vein bypass grafting.[68]

ORIGIN OF BOTH CORONARY ARTERIES FROM THE PULMONARY ARTERY

Twenty-five infants in whom both coronary arteries arose from the pulmonary artery have been reported. These patients have been reviewed in detail by Heifetz and colleagues.[37] The survival time ranged from 9 hours to 7 years. The patient who lived to the age of 7 years was able to do so because of severe pulmonary hypertension secondary to a ventricular septal defect and congenital mitral stenosis.[26] The pressure in the pulmonary artery was sufficient to force blood into the myocardial capillary bed, and the child lived for an amazingly long time. This malformation has been diagnosed by cardiac catheterization, and surgical repair has been attempted.[31,39,57]

ANEURYSMS OF THE CORONARY ARTERIES

In 1812, Bougon first reported an aneurysm of the coronary arteries.[10] These lesions have been reported from infancy to adult life.[18] Congenital aneurysms of the coronary arteries are rare and constituted only 15 per cent of coronary artery aneurysms reported by Daoud in 89 patients.[20] Other causes of aneurysms of the coronary arteries include atherosclerosis, mycotic aneurysms, syphilis, rheumatic heart disease, and mucocutaneous lymph node syndrome (Kawasaki's disease).

These lesions are most often asymptomatic until complications occur. Complications include thrombosis or embolization with subsequent myocardial ischemia or infarction or actual rupture of aneurysm. Wei and Wang reported a 26-year-old woman who presented with a 3-month history of cough, shortness of breath, and vomiting.[88] The patient was found to have a giant congenital right coronary aneurysm measuring 15 cm. in diameter. The aneurysm was excised, and symptoms resolved completely. An intramural coronary aneurysm has also been reported and produced reversed flow during systole owing to bulging of the thin-walled chamber into the left ventricular cavity. The narrow neck of the aneurysm was closed successfully at operation. An example of a congenital coronary artery aneurysm involving the left circumflex vessel is shown in Figure 9. In this patient, a mural thrombus occurred in the aneurysm; it embolized and produced acute myocardial infarction (Fig. 9B). The aneurysm was resected, and a saphenous vein autograft was inserted (Fig. 9C).[22] Surgical management of a coronary artery aneurysm is indicated if the aneurysm is symptomatic, especially if there is evidence of emboli arising from the aneurysm, producing myocardial ischemia in the distal coronary bed.

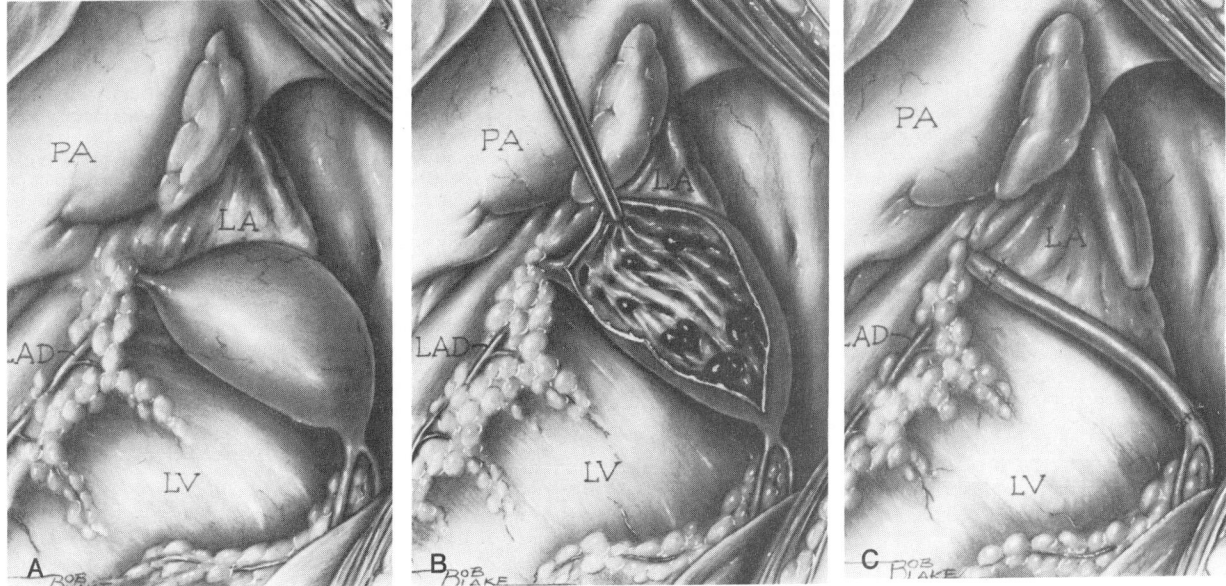

Figure 9. *A*, Congenital aneurysm of the left circumflex coronary artery as seen at operation on a 31-year-old female who presented with an acute myocardial infarction with subsequent disabling angina. PA, pulmonary artery; LAD, left anterior descending coronary artery; LV, left ventricle; LA, left atrium, *B*, Numerous small fresh thrombi are shown adherent to the rough, irregular surface of the aneurysm. The proximal opening into the aneurysm was a discrete, mildly dilated vessel of good quality and normal-appearing intima. The distal branches of the circumflex coronary artery were of normal size. *C*, The entire aneurysm was excised, and an interposition graft of saphenous vein was placed. There was only minimal discrepancy in the size of a saphenous vein graft and the ends of the circumflex coronary artery. A continuous 7–0 nonabsorbable suture was used at each anastomosis. (From Ebert, P. A., Peter, R. H., Gunnells, J. C., and Sabiston, D. C., Jr.: Resecting and grafting of coronary artery aneurysm. Circulation, *43*:593, 1971.)

MEMBRANOUS OBSTRUCTION OF THE OSTIUM OF THE LEFT MAIN CORONARY ARTERY

Hypoplasia, or atresia, of the coronary arteries in infancy and childhood has been reported and usually causes severe impairment of ventricular function and sudden death. Congenital atresia of the left main coronary artery has been reported in 9 patients, all of whom presented with signs and symptoms of myocardial ischemia, congestive heart failure, or both. Histopathologic studies in these patients showed that the left main coronary artery had been replaced by fibromuscular tissue and that the left coronary ostium was absent. These conditions are not surgically correctable. However, 3 patients have been reported with membranous obstruction at the ostium of the left main coronary artery, associated with a normal distal coronary artery. The first patient was a 6-month-old infant who died following myocardial infarction, and the diagnosis was established at the time of autopsy.[86] Josa and associates reported two cases diagnosed at the time of operation.[38] One patient, a 2-year-old child being operated on for congenital aortic stenosis, was found to have a membrane markedly obstructing the ostium of the left main coronary artery. The second patient was an 8-year-old boy with Type I truncus arteriosus who also had membranous obstruction of the ostium of the left main coronary artery at operation. Both of these patients showed evidence of myocardial ischemia preoperatively, and after excision of the membrane at operation, the symptoms were totally relieved. Grossly, the membranous structure appeared to be continuous with the aortic intima, and histologic studies revealed that its structure was similar to that of normal aortic root media. These two examples indicate the importance of careful evaluation of the origin and distribution of the coronary arteries in patients with congenital heart disease, especially when the signs and symptoms of ischemia and heart failure are disproportionate to the congenital lesion being evaluated.[38]

Lea and associates reported a patient with congenital ostial stenosis of the right coronary artery that was repaired successfully by vein patch angioplasty.[45]

SELECTED REFERENCES

Ebert, P. A., Peter, R. H., Gunnells, J. C., and Sabiston, D. C., Jr.: Resecting and grafting of coronary artery aneurysm. Circulation, *43*:593, 1971.
A congenital aneurysm of the circumflex coronary artery containing a thrombus that later embolized and produced myocardial infarction is reported. A review of the problem, the clinical manifestations, and management are discussed.

Heifetz, S. A., Robinowitz, M., Mueller, K. H., and Virmani, R.: Total anomalous origin of the coronary arteries from the pulmonary artery. Pediatr. Cardiol., *7*:11, 1986.
Four patients with total anomalous origin of the coronary arteries from the pulmonary artery are presented and compared with 21 previously reported patients. Of the 19 patients in whom a clinical history was available, 16 were symptomatic before 3 days of age. All patients died, 60 per cent before 2 weeks of age. Longer survival was associated with additional cardiovascular malformations that caused pulmonary hypertension, increased oxygen saturation, or both. Cardiomegaly was present in 56 per cent of patients, and most had myocardial fibrosis or infarction. Surgical correction has been attempted in 2 patients, but both attempts failed secondary to severe pre-existent myocardial injury.

Lowe, J. E., and Sabiston, D. C., Jr.: Congenital coronary malformations. *In* Cohn, L. (Ed.): Modern Technics in Surgery, Cardiac-Thoracic Surgery. Mt. Kisco, NY, Futura Publishing Company, 1981.
This review presents the surgical techniques used to correct congenital coronary artery fistulas, anomalous origin of the left or right coronary artery from the pulmonary artery, and congenital coronary artery aneurysms. The details of the preoperative evaluation, anesthetic management, and postoperative care are also reviewed.

Lowe, J. E., Oldham, N. H., Jr., and Sabiston, D. C., Jr.: Surgical management of congenital coronary artery fistulas. Ann. Surg., *194*:371, 1981.
This paper reports the clinical manifestations of 28 patients with congenital coronary artery fistulas seen at one institution and summarizes the results of surgical management in 22 patients. An additional 258 patients reported earlier are also reviewed. The natural history and pathophysiology of coronary fistulas are discussed, and the reason for early surgical intervention is presented.

Sabiston, D. C., Jr., and Orme, S. K.: Congenital origin of the left coronary artery from the pulmonary artery. J. Cardiovasc. Surg., *9*:543, 1968.
In this report, 23 patients with origin of the left coronary artery from the pulmonary artery are described. The youngest patient was 1 day of age and the oldest patient was 31 years of age. The natural history, clinical findings, laboratory data, and ultimate course are presented.

Stephenson, L. W., Edmunds, L. H., Jr., Friedman, S., et al.: Subclavian–left coronary artery anastomosis (Meyer operation) for anomalous origin of the left coronary artery from the pulmonary artery. Circulation, 64(Suppl. II):130, 1981.

Six patients, ages 2 to 76 months, had subclavian to coronary artery anastomosis for anomalous origin of the left coronary artery from the pulmonary artery. Five of the six patients had congestive heart failure and ongoing ischemia. All six had cardiomegaly, and preoperative left ventricular ejection fractions averaged 0.46 ± 0.171. Five patients survived operation and were alive at 8 to 92 months after operation, and four of the five anastomoses were patent at postoperative cardiac catheterization. None of the surviving patients have required cardiac medications, and all of them are symptom-free at follow-up. In addition to subclavian–left coronary anastomosis, multiple other surgical options including intrapulmonary shunts are discussed in detail.

Wei, J., and Wang, D.: A giant congenital aneurysm of the right coronary artery. Ann. Thorac. Surg., 41:322, 1986.

The authors report a 26-year-old patient who presented with shortness of breath and a chronic cough. A chest film showed a huge mass on the right ventricular border, and the patient was admitted with a tentative diagnosis of mediastinal tumor. Coronary arteriography showed a giant coronary aneurysm arising from the right coronary artery. At the time of operation, the aneurysm measured 15 cm. in diameter. The aneurysm was resected, and histologic examination of the aneurysmal wall showed no evidence of atheromatous change. The patient recovered, and symptoms resolved completely.

REFERENCES

1. Abbott, M. E.: Congenital cardiac disease. *In* Osler, W. (Ed.): Modern Medicine. Vol. 4. Philadelphia, Lea & Febiger, 1908.
2. Abbott, M. E.: Congenital cardiac disease. *In* Osler, W. (Ed.): Modern Medicine, 3rd ed. Philadelphia, Lea & Febiger, 1927.
3. Abrikossoff, A.: Aneurysma des linken Herzventrikels mit abnormer Abgangsstelle der linken Koronararterie von der Pulmonalis bei einem fünfmonatlichen Kinde. Virchows Arch. (Pathol. Anat.), 203:413, 1911.
4. Apley, J., Horton, R. E., and Wilson, M. G.: The possible role of surgery in the treatment of anomalous left coronary artery. Thorax, 12:28, 1951.
5. Anthony, C. L., Jr., McAllister, H. A., Jr., and Cheitlin, M. D.: Spontaneous graft closure in anomalous origin of the left coronary artery. Chest, 68:586, 1975.
6. Arciniegas, E., Farooki, Z. Q., Haimi, M., and Green, E. W.: Management of anomalous left coronary artery from the pulmonary artery. Circulation, 62(Suppl. I):168, 1980.
7. Barton, C. W., Snider, A. R., and Rosenthal, A: Two-dimensional and Doppler echocardiographic features of left circumflex coronary artery to right ventricle fistula: Case report and literature review. Pediatr. Cardiol., 7:167, 1986.
8. Bjork, G., and Craoford, C.: Arteriovenous aneurysm on the pulmonary artery simulating patent ductus arteriosus botalli. Thorax, 2:65, 1947.
9. Bland, E. F., White, P. D., and Garland, J.: Congenital anomalies of coronary arteries: Report of an unusual case associated with cardiac hypertrophy. Am. Heart J., 8:787, 1933.
10. Bougon: Bibl. Med., 37:183, 1812. Cited by Packard, M., and Wechsler, H. F.: Aneurysm of the coronary arteries. Arch. Intern. Med., 43:1, 1929.
11. Bregman, D., Brennan, J., Singer, A., et al.: Anomalous origin of the right coronary artery from the pulmonary artery. J. Thorac. Cardiovasc. Surg., 72:626, 1976.
12. Brooks, H. St. J.: Two cases of an abnormal coronary artery of the heart arising from the pulmonary artery. J. Anat. Physiol., 20:26, 1886.
13. Bunton, R., Jonas, R. A., Lang, P., et al.: Anomalous origin of the left coronary artery from pulmonary artery: Ligation versus establishment of a two coronary artery system. J. Thorac. Cardiovasc. Surg., 93:103, 1987.
14. Burchell, H. B., and Brown, A. L., Jr.: Anomalous origin of the coronary artery from the pulmonary artery masquerading as mitral insufficiency. Am. Heart J., 63:388, 1962.
15. Case, R. B., Morrow, A. G., Stainsby, W., and Nestor, J. O.: Anomalous origin of the left coronary artery: The physiologic defect and suggested surgical treatment. Circulation, 17:1062, 1958.
16. Coe, J. Y., Radley-Smith, R., and Yacoub, M: Clinical and hemodynamic significance of anomalous origin of the right coronary artery from the pulmonary artery. Thorac. Cardiovasc. Surg., 30:84, 1982.
17. Cooley, D. A., Hallman, G. L., and Bloodwell, R. D.: Definitive surgical treatment of anomalous origin of left coronary artery from pulmonary artery: Indications and results. J. Thorac. Cardiovasc. Surg., 52:798, 1966.
18. Crocker, D. W., Sobin, S., and Thomas, W. C.: Aneurysms of the coronary arteries. Report of three cases in infants and review of the literature. Am. J. Pathol., 33:819, 1957.
19. Daniel, T. M., Graham, T. P., and Sabiston, D. C., Jr.: Coronary artery–right ventricular fistula with congestive heart failure: Surgical correction in the neonatal period. Surgery, 67:985, 1970.
20. Daoud, A. S., Pankin, D., Tulgan, H., and Florentin, R. A.: Aneurysms of the coronary artery. Am. J. Cardiol., 11:228, 1963.
21. Duoard, H., Barat, J. L., Laurent, F., et al.: Magnetic resonance imaging of an anomalous origin of the left coronary artery from the pulmonary artery. Eur. Heart J., 9:1356, 1988.
22. Ebert, P. A., Peter, R. H., Gunnells, J. C., and Sabiston, D. C., Jr.: Resecting and grafting of coronary artery aneurysm. Circulation, 43:593, 1971.
23. Edwards, J. E.: Anomalous coronary arteries with special reference to arteriovenous-like communications. Circulation, 17:1001, 1958.
24. Eidlow, S., and MacKenzie, E. R.: Anomalous origin of the left coronary artery from the pulmonary artery: Report of a case diagnosed clinically and confirmed by necropsy. Am. Heart J., 32:243, 1948.
25. Elsaid, G. M., Ruzyllo, W., Williams, W. L., et al.: Early and late results of saphenous vein graft for anomalous origin of left coronary artery from pulmonary artery. Circulation, 48(Suppl.):382, 1973.
26. Feldt, R. H., Ongley, P. A., and Titus, J. L.: Total coronary arterial circulation from pulmonary artery with survival to age seven: Report of a case. Mayo Clin. Proc., 40:539, 1965.
27. Finley, J. P., Holman-Giles, R., Gilday, D. L., et al.: Thallium-201 myocardial imaging in anomalous left coronary artery arising from the pulmonary artery: Applications before and after medical and surgical treatment. Am. J. Cardiol., 42:675, 1978.
28. Fisher, E. A., Sepehri, B., Lendrum, B., et al.: Two-dimensional echocardiographic visualization of the left coronary artery in anomalous origin of the left coronary artery from the pulmonary artery. Circulation, 63:698, 1981.
29. Flaherty, J. T., Spach, M. S., Boineau, J. P., et al.: Cardiac potentials on body surface of infants with anomalous left coronary artery (myocardial infarction). Circulation, 36:345, 1967.
30. Fyfe, D. A., Sade, R. M., Gillette, P. C., and Kline, C. H.: Pre- and postoperative Doppler echocardiographic evaluation of anomalous left coronary artery arising from the pulmonary artery. J. Ultrasound Med., 6:101, 1987.
31. Goldblatt, E., Adams, A. P. S., Ross, I. K., et al.: Single-trunk anomalous origin of both coronary arteries from the pulmonary artery. J. Thorac. Cardiovasc. Surg., 87:59, 1984.
32. Grace, R. R., Angelini, P., and Cooley, D. A.: Aortic implantation of anomalous left coronary artery arising from pulmonary artery. J. Cardiol., 39:608, 1977.
33. Griffiths, S. P., Ellis, K., Hordof, A. J., et al: Spontaneous complete closure of a congenital coronary artery fistula. J. Am. Coll. Cardiol., 2:1169, 1983.
34. Hacket, D., and Hallidie-Smith, K. A.: Spontaneous closure of coronary artery fistula. Br. Heart J., 52:477, 1984.
35. Hamilton, D. E., Ghosh, P. K., and Donnelly, R. J.: An operation for anomalous origin of left coronary artery. Br. Heart J., 41:121, 1979.
36. Harthorne, J. W., Scannell, J. G., and Dinsmore, R. E.: Anomalous origin of the left coronary artery: Remediable cause of sudden death in adults. N. Engl. J. Med., 275:660, 1966.
37. Heifetz, S. A., Robinowitz, M., Mueller, K. H., and Virmani, R.: Total anomalous origin of the coronary arteries from the pulmonary artery. Pediatr. Cardiol., 7:11, 1986.
38. Josa, M., Danielson, G. K., Weidman, W. H., and Edwards, W. D.: Congenital ostial membrane of left main coronary artery. J. Thorac. Cardiovasc. Surg., 81:338, 1981.
39. Keeton, B. R., Keenan, D. J. M., and Monro, J. L.: Anomalous origin of both coronary arteries from the pulmonary trunk. Br. Heart J., 49:397, 1983.
40. Keith, J. D.: The anomalous origin of the left coronary artery from the pulmonary artery. Br. Heart J., 21:149, 1959.
41. Kessler, K. A., Pennington, G., Nouri, S., et al.: Left subclavian–left coronary artery anastomosis for anomalous origin of the left coronary artery: Long-term follow-up. J. Thorac. Cardiovasc. Surg., 98:25, 1989.
42. King, D. H., Danford, D. A., Huhta, J. C., and Gutgesell, H. P.: Noninvasive detection of anomalous origin of the left main coronary artery from the main pulmonary trunk by pulsed Doppler echocardiography. Am. J. Cardiol., 55:608, 1985.
43. Kirklin, J. W., and Barratt-Boyes, B. A.: Congenital anomalies of the coronary arteries. *In* Cardiac Surgery. New York, John Wiley & Sons, 1986, p. 945.
44. Laborde, F., Marchand, M., Leca, F., et al.: Surgical treatment of anomalous origin of the left coronary artery in infancy and childhood: Early and late results in 20 consecutive cases. J. Thorac. Cardiovasc. Surg., 82:423, 1981.
45. Lea, J. W., IV, Page, D. L., and Hammon, J. W., Jr.: Congenital ostial stenosis of the right coronary artery repaired by vein patch angioplasty. J. Thorac. Cardiovasc. Surg., 92:796, 1979.
46. Liberthson, R. R., Sagar, K., Behocoben, J. P., et al.: Congenital coronary arteriovenous fistula. Circulation, 59:849, 1979.
47. Lowe, J. E., and Sabiston, D. C., Jr.: Congenital coronary malformations. *In* Cohn, L. (Ed.): Modern Technics in Surgery, Cardiac-Thoracic Surgery. Mt. Kisco, NY, Futura Publishing Company, 1981.
48. Lowe, J. E., and Sabiston, D. C., Jr.: Surgical correction of congenital malformations of the coronary circulation. South. Med. J., 75:1508, 1982.
49. Lowe, J. E., Oldham, H. N., Jr., and Sabiston, D. C., Jr.: Surgical management of congenital coronary artery fistulas. Ann. Surg., 194:371, 1981.
50. Mahoney, L. T., Schieken, R. M., and Lauer, R. M.: Spontaneous closure of a coronary artery fistula in childhood. Pediatr. Cardiol., 2:311, 1982.
51. McNamara, D. G., and El Said, G.: Treatment of anomalous origin of the left coronary artery from the pulmonary artery. Eur. J. Cardiol., 1:497, 1973.
52. Menke, J. A., Shaher, R. M., and Wolff, G. S.: Ejection fraction in anomalous origin of the left coronary artery from the pulmonary artery. Am. Heart J., 84:325, 1972.
53. Meyer, W., Stefanik, G., Stiles, Q. R., et al.: A method of definitive surgical treatment of anomalous origin of left coronary artery. J. Thorac. Cardiovasc. Surg., 56:104, 1968.
54. Moodie, D. S., Fyfe, D., Gill, C. C., et al.: Anomalous origin of the left coronary

artery from the pulmonary artery (Bland-White-Garland syndrome) in adult patients: Long-term follow-up after surgery. Am. Heart J., 26:597, 1985.

55. Mustard, W. T.: Anomalies of the coronary artery. In Benson, C. D., Mustard, W. T., Ravitch, M. M., Synder, W. H., and Welch, K. J. (Eds.): Pediatric Surgery. Vol. 1. Chicago, Year Book Medical Publishers, 1962, p. 433.

56. Neches, W. H., Mathews, R. A., Park, S. C., et al.: Anomalous origin of the left coronary artery from the pulmonary artery. Circulation, 50:582, 1974.

57. Ogasawara, K., Aizawa, T., Fijii, J., et al.: A case with fistulas from both coronary arteries and the left bronchial artery to the pulmonary artery. Jpn. Heart J., 26:597, 1985.

58. Ogden, J. A.: Congenital anomalies of the coronary arteries. Am. J. Cardiol., 25:474, 1970.

59. Paul, R. M., and Robbins, S. G.: A surgical treatment proposed for either endocardial fibroelastosis or anomalous left coronary artery. Pediatrics, 16:147, 1955.

60. Pickoff, A. S., Wolff, G. S., Bennett, V. L., et al.: Pulsed Doppler echocardiographic detection of coronary artery to right ventricle fistula. Pediatr. Cardiol., 2:145, 1982.

61. Pinsky, W. W., Fagan, L. R., Kraeger, R. R., et al.: Anomalous left coronary artery. J. Thorac. Cardiovasc. Surg., 65:810, 1973.

62. Pinsky, W. W., Fagan, L. R., Mudd, J. F. G., and Willman, V. L.: Subclavian–coronary artery anastomosis in infancy for the Bland-White syndrome. J. Thorac. Cardiovasc. Surg., 72:15, 1976.

63. Potts, quoted by Kittle, C. F., Diehl, A. M., and Heilbrake, A.: Anomalous left coronary artery arising from the pulmonary artery. J. Pediatr., 47:198, 1955.

64. Purut, C. M., and Sabiston, D. C., Jr.: Anomalous origin of the left coronary artery from the pulmonary artery in the elderly. J. Thorac. Cardiovasc. Surg., 1991. In press.

65. Reeder, G. S., Tajik, A. J., and Smith, H. C.: Visualization of coronary artery fistula by two-dimensional echocardiography. Mayo Clin. Proc., 55:185, 1980.

66. Roberts, J. T., and Loube, S. D.: Congenital single coronary artery in man. Am. Heart J., 34:100, 1947.

67. Ross, T. C., Latham, R. D., and Craig, W. E.: Anomalous origin of the right coronary artery from the main pulmonary artery: Incidental finding in a case of dilated cardiomyopathy. South. Med. J., 80:783, 1987.

68. Rowe, G. G., and Young, W. P.: Anomalous origin of the coronary arteries with special reference to surgical treatment. J. Thorac. Cardiovasc. Surg., 39:777, 1960.

69. Sabiston, D. C., Jr., and Orme, S. K.: Congenital origin of the left coronary artery from the pulmonary artery. J. Cardiovasc. Surg., 9:543, 1968.

70. Sabiston, D. C., Jr., Floyd, W. L., and McIntosh, H. D.: Anomalous origin of the left coronary artery from the pulmonary artery in adults. Surgical management. Arch. Surg., 97:963, 1968.

71. Sabiston, D. C., Jr., Neill, C. A., and Taussig, H. B.: The direction of blood flow in anomalous left coronary artery arising from the pulmonary artery. Circulation, 22:591, 1960.

72. Sabiston, D. C., Jr., Pelargonio, S., and Taussig, H. B.: Myocardial infarction in infancy: The surgical management of a complication of congenital origin of the left coronary artery from the pulmonary artery. J. Thorac. Cardiovasc. Surg., 40:321, 1960.

73. Sabiston, D. C., Jr., Ross, R. S., Criley, J. M., et al.: Surgical management of congenital lesions of the coronary circulation. Ann. Surg., 157:908, 1963.

74. Saenz, C. B., Taylor, J. L., Soto, B., et al.: Acute myocardial infarction in a patient with anomalous right coronary artery. Am. Heart J., 112:1092, 1986.

75. Satomi, G., Endo, M., Takao, A., and Nakamura, K.: A case of right coronary artery to left ventricle fistula: Two-dimensional echocardiographic study. Pediatr. Cardiol., 4:229, 1983.

76. Shrivistava, S., Castaneda, A. R., and Moller, J. H.: Anomalous left coronary artery from pulmonary trunk. Long-term follow-up after ligation. J. Thorac. Cardiovasc. Surg., 76:130, 1978.

77. Slater, J., Lighty, G. W., Jr., Winer, H. E., et al.: Doppler echocardiography and computed tomography in diagnosis of left coronary arteriovenous fistula. J. Am. Coll. Cardiol., 4:1290, 1984.

78. Smith, A., Arnold, R., Anderson, R. H., et al.: Anomalous origin of the left coronary artery from the pulmonary trunk: Anatomic findings in relation to pathophysiology and surgical repair. J. Thorac. Cardiovasc. Surg., 98:16, 1989.

79. Sones, F. M., and Shirey, E. K.: Collateral arterial channels in living human with coronary artery disease. Circulation, 22:815, 1960.

80. Stephenson, L. W., Edmunds, L. H., Friedman, S., et al.: Subclavian–left coronary artery anastomosis (Meyer operation) for anomalous origin of the left coronary artery from the pulmonary artery. Circulation, 64(Suppl. II):130, 1981.

81. Swenson, R. E., Murillo-Olivas, A., Elias, W., et al.: Noninvasive Doppler color flow mapping for detection of anomalous origin of the left coronary artery from the pulmonary artery and for evaluation of surgical repair. J. Am. Coll. Cardiol., 11:659, 1988.

82. Takeuchi, S., Imamura, H., Katsumoto, K., et al.: New surgical method for repair of anomalous left coronary artery from pulmonary artery. J. Thorac. Cardiovasc. Surg., 78:7, 1979.

83. Tingelstad, J. B., Lower, R. R., and Eldredge, W. J.: Anomalous origin of the right coronary artery from the main pulmonary artery. Am. J. Cardiol., 30:670, 1972.

84. Urrutia-S, C. O., Falaschi, G., Ott, D. A., and Cooley, D. A.: Surgical management of 56 patients with congenital coronary artery fistulas. Ann. Thorac. Surg., 35:300, 1983.

85. van Meurs–van Woezik, H., Serruys, P. W., Reiber, J. H. C., et al.; Coronary artery changes 3 years after reimplantation of an anomalous right coronary artery. Eur. Heart J., 5:175, 1984.

86. Verney, R. N., Monnet, P., Arnaud, P., et al.: Infarctus du myocarde chez un nourrisson de cinq mois—ostium coronaire gauche punctiforme. Ann. Pediatr. (Paris), 16:260, 1969.

87. Voché, P. R., Baillot-Vernant, F., Trinquet, F., et al.: Anomalous left coronary artery from pulmonary artery in infants: Which operation? When? J. Thorac. Cardiovasc. Surg., 94:192, 1987.

88. Wei, J., and Wang, D: A giant congenital aneurysm of the right coronary artery. Ann. Thorac. Surg., 41:322, 1986.

89. Wenger, N. K.: Rare causes of coronary heart disease. In Hurst, J. W. (Ed.): The Heart. New York, McGraw-Hill, 1978.

90. Wesselhoeft, H., Fawcett, J. S., and Johnson, A. L.: Anomalous origin of the left coronary artery from the pulmonary trunk: Its clinical spectrum, pathology, and pathophysiology, based on a review of 140 cases with seven further cases. Circulation, 38:403, 1968.

91. Wilson, C. L., Dlabol, P. W., HoleyField, R. W., et al.: Anomalous origin of left coronary artery from pulmonary artery: Case report and review of literature concerning teen-agers and adults. J. Thorac. Cardiovasc. Surg., 73:887, 1977.

92. Worsham, C., Sanders, S. P., and Burger, B. M.: Origin of the right coronary artery from the pulmonary trunk: Diagnosis by two-dimensional echocardiography. Am. J. Cardiol., 55:232, 1985.

XVII

ACQUIRED DISORDERS OF THE AORTIC VALVE

Glenn J. R. Whitman, M.D., and Alden H. Harken, M.D.

AORTIC STENOSIS

Historical Aspects

In 1706, William Cowper wrote, "The dissections of morbid bodies not only instruct us in the seats and causes of diseases, but very often inform us in the true use of parts. . . ."[11] This enviably critical observer continued: "Anatomical inquiries in the true causes of diseases . . ." might lead us to an understanding of acute illnesses ". . . which have been ascribed to the want of spirits in some and radical moisture in aged people. . . ."[11] Cowper died at the age of 43, so his impression of "aged" may have been distorted, but his description of acute congestive failure as "radical moisture" is pathophysiologically eloquent. Cowper dissected several patients dying of congestive failure and found thickened nonpliable aortic valves harboring calcific vegetations (Fig. 1). This appears to be the first instance in which aortic valve disease was related to symptoms of heart failure.

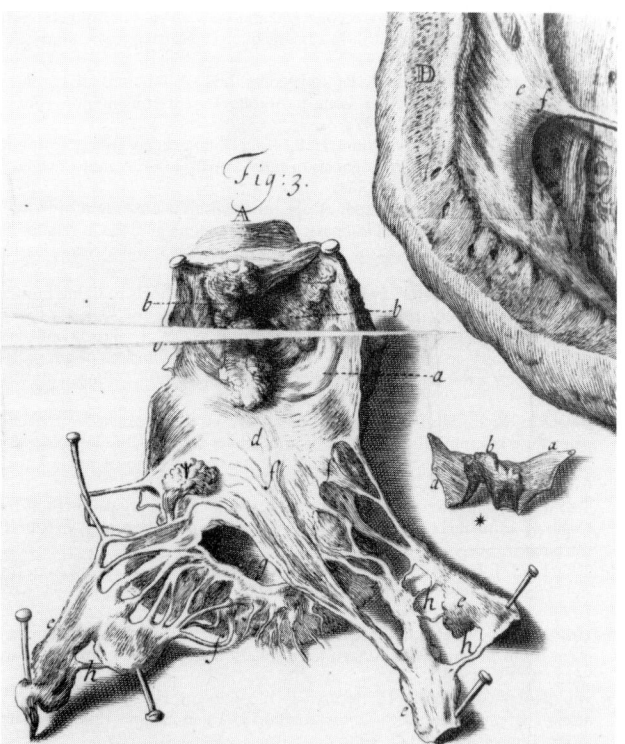

Figure 1. In 1706, William Cowper (1666–1709) published this drawing of "the three semilunar valves of the aorta which hinder the blood from returning to the heart . . . these valves in this case were somewhat thicker and not so pliable as naturally . . . but the stubbornness of these valves was owing to a bony or stony body, markt. b Fig:3." (From Cowper, W.: Of ossifications or petrifactions in the coats of arteries, particularly in the valves of the great artery. Philos. Trans. R. Soc. Lond., 24:1706. Photograph courtesy of the National Library of Medicine.)

Pathologic Anatomy

The normal aortic valve consists of three equal-sized leaflets attached to the aortic wall, forming the three aortic sinuses. Characteristically, the coronary arteries arise from the upper portion of two of these sinuses, thereby defining the left, right, and noncoronary cusps.

Obstruction to left ventricular outflow is most commonly caused by aortic valvular stenosis; supravalvular and subvalvular obstructions occur much less commonly. Aortic stenosis is the most common isolated valvular abnormality found in man and can be either congenital or acquired.[43] *Congenital valvular abnormalities* may cause stenosis immediately, as with unicuspid and dome-shaped valves.[14] However, *bicuspid* valves, usually asymptomatic at birth, generally lead to symptomatic stenosis in the sixth to eighth decades.[50] This occurs because of turbulent flow across the leaflets leading to fibrosis, calcification, and stiffening.[8] Acquired aortic stenosis is either rheumatic or degenerative in origin. In *rheumatic aortic stenosis,* inflammation leads to fusion of leaflet commissures and cusps with thickening and calcification. Retraction of the leaflet free borders often makes these valves both stenotic and regurgitant. Only rarely does the rheumatic process involve the aortic valve alone, usually being accompanied by mitral involvement. In *degenerative* or *senile aortic stenosis,* normal leaflet stress leads to calcification at the flexion points causing cusp immobility. This calcification can extend down onto the anterior mitral valve leaflet or upward along the aorta, occasionally causing coronary ostial stenosis (Fig. 2).

Pathophysiology

Diminution in left ventricular outflow diameter becomes important when it obstructs flow, generating a transvalvular pressure gradient. When this ventricular-aortic pressure gradient

reaches 60 mm. Hg in the presence of a normal cardiac output or causes a calculated valve area of less than 0.7 cm.[2], aortic stenosis is considered severe. In acquired aortic stenosis, obstruction to left ventricular outflow, which occurs over years, allows cardiac output to be maintained by left ventricular hypertrophy. This muscular hypertrophy may lead to diminished compliance and an elevation in left ventricular end-diastolic pressure. This rise in left ventricular end-diastolic pressure does not necessarily signify left ventricular failure but indicates a stiffer left ventricle. The decrease in left ventricular compliance may resolve after valve replacement.[34] With progressive hypertrophy and decrease in ventricular compliance, atrial contraction has an increasingly important role in diastolic loading. Loss of the normal sinus mechanism may cause acute decompensation in the patient with aortic stenosis.[49] Moreover, in severe aortic stenosis, oxygen delivery to hypertrophic, stiff muscle ceases to meet demand as the prolongation of ejection time and elevation in end-diastolic pressure conspire to limit diastolic coronary blood flow. The subendocardium becomes chronically ischemic, leading to cell death and fibrosis.[46] Heart failure follows owing to a decrease in stroke volume. The heart rate cannot increase sufficiently to maintain cardiac output. As cardiac output decreases, the transvalvular gradient also falls. As each cardiac catheterization is a stage in time, a low or decreasing aortic gradient must not be confused with resolving or stable aortic valvular disease.

The clinical course of aortic stenosis may therefore be divided into two stages. During the initial phase, the left ventricle can compensate for increasing afterload. Its hallmark is angina, which is the result of an imbalance in myocardial oxygen delivery and oxygen demand caused by increasing left ventricular

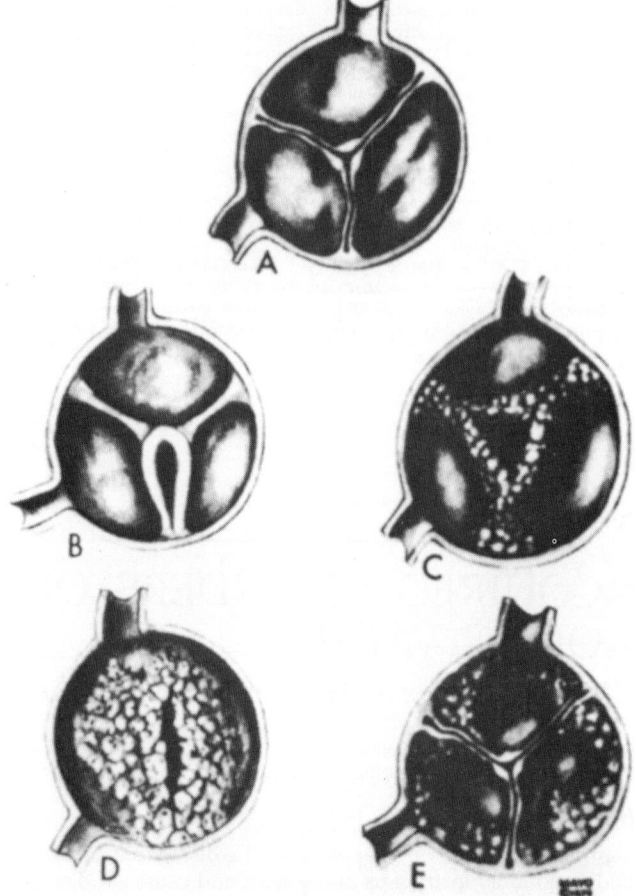

Figure 2. Types of aortic valve stenosis. *A,* Normal aortic valve. *B,* Congenital aortic stenosis. *C,* Rheumatic aortic stenosis. *D,* Calcific aortic stenosis. *E,* Calcific senile aortic stenosis. (From Brandenburg, R., et al.: Valvular heart disease—When should the patient be referred? Pract. Cardiol., 5:50, 1979.)

afterload with a concomitant decrease in coronary blood flow.[30] Along with angina, the patient may experience exercise-induced syncope, another and usually later symptom of aortic stenosis, probably the result of left ventricular baroreceptor dysfunction.[31,42] The second phase signals the onset of left ventricular dysfunction. The progressively stiff ventricle requires increasing preload for adequate filling; the resultant pulmonary hypertension translates into shortness of breath and dyspnea on exertion.

Diagnosis

Auscultation of the patient with aortic stenosis reveals a systolic murmur best heard at the base of the heart that radiates into the carotid arteries and to the cardiac apex. This murmur is associated with a slow, prolonged rise in the arterial pulse, "pulsus parvus et tardus." The severity of aortic obstruction may be estimated by echo Doppler, permitting calculation of the peak ventriculoaortic gradient by the following formula:[54]

$$\Delta = 4 V^2$$

where Δ is the peak ventriculoaortic gradient and V is the maximal measured blood velocity (meters per second) across the valve.

The most accurate measure of left ventricular outflow obstruction is determined invasively by cardiac catheterization. A careful catheter pullback from the left ventricle to the aorta yields pressure traces acceptable for determining the transvalvular pressure gradient. However, simultaneous aortic and ventricular pressure measurements (Fig. 3) are more precise and, in fact, are mandatory when the patient is in atrial fibrillation. These data may then be used to calculate the aortic valve area by the Gorlin formula:[17]

$$AVA = \frac{\text{aortic valve flow}}{C \times \sqrt{\text{aortic valve mean systolic gradient}}}$$

where aortic valve flow = cardiac output (ml./min.)/SEP (sec./min.); AVA is the aortic valve area in cm.²; and C is the empiric orifice constant (obtained by comparing calculated to measured aortic valve area at operation or postmortem) for the aortic valve. This constant is 1; 44.5 is the number derived from formulas that relate velocity of flow to the driving force; SEP is the systolic ejection period per minute expressed in seconds. For quick calculations, this simplifies to

$$AVA = \frac{C.O.}{\sqrt{\Delta}}$$

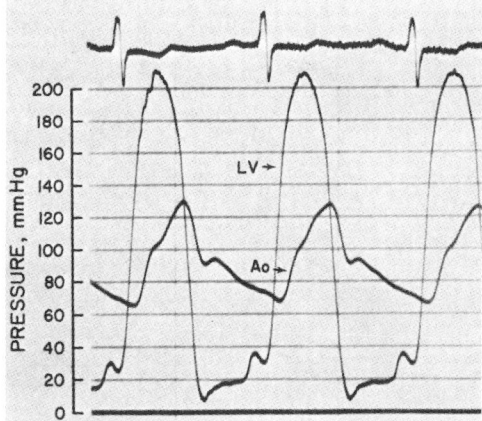

Figure 3. Pressure-time curve of simultaneous left ventricular (LV) and aortic pressure. Note that in this patient with severe aortic stenosis, a peak to peak gradient of 80 mm. Hg is present, suggesting a severely compromised aortic valve area. Also note the prolonged and delayed aortic upstroke ("parvus et tardus"). The A wave in the LV trace represents atrial contraction with filling of a noncompliant ventricle. (From Grossman, W.: Cardiac Catheterization, Angiography, and Intervention. 4th ed. Philadelphia, Lea & Febiger, 1991.)

where Δ is the measured aortic valve gradient. Patients are frequently symptomatic when the valve area is less than 1 cm². They are invariably symptomatic when the valve area is less than 0.7 cm².

Course and Prognosis

When the aortic valve area diminishes from the normal 3 to 4 cm.² to less than 1 cm.², patients are usually symptomatic.[26] Angina is usually the earliest symptom, and the mean survival of a patient with aortic stenosis and angina is 4.7 years. When a patient experiences syncope, survival is typically less than 3 years. Patients with dyspnea and congestive failure, in keeping with the associated left ventricular dysfunction, have a mean survival of 1 to 2 years[36] (Fig. 4). Failure may be the presenting symptom in nearly one third of patients.[25]

Treatment

Aortic stenosis is a mechanical condition obstructing outflow from the left ventricle. The only effective therapy is operative intervention. The existence of symptoms is an indication for valve replacement. Angina and syncope warrant elective surgical therapy, whereas dyspnea and failure mandate urgent intervention. The issue of aortic valve replacement in the asymptomatic patient with aortic stenosis is unanswered. The cardiologist/surgeon must balance the risk of surgical therapy against the risk of progressive irreversible myocardial fibrosis and dysfunction. Generally, in the patient with aortic stenosis, left ventricular hypertrophy resolves following surgical therapy, whereas left ventricular dilation does not. Asymptomatic patients are therefore considered candidates for aortic valve replacement when progressive cardiomegaly is documented. In this group, long-term survival with surgical therapy appears to be superior to medical therapy.[10] In patients with aortic stenosis, there is an inverse relationship between increasing wall stress (caused by afterload) and ejection fraction (Figs. 5 and 6). With end-stage aortic stenosis, contractility may decrease disproportionately to the increase in wall stress. This subset of patients with end-stage aortic stenosis appear to have irreversible left ventricular damage and derive little benefit from surgical therapy.[9,15]

In patients with good ventricular function, aortic valve replacement is associated with an operative mortality of 2 to 8 per cent.[10,25,47] Independent perioperative risk factors include age, left ventricular function, NYHA class, and pulmonary function. Following aortic valve replacement, the projected 5-year survival is 80 to 85 per cent. Symptoms are relieved in nearly all patients; however, improvement in ejection fraction and resolution of ventricular hypertrophy may require months to occur.[23,39] Surgical mortality increases exponentially with decreasing left ventricular contractility. Aortic valve replacement in patients with congestive heart failure has a mortality up to 24 per cent.[9,38] In patients with aortic stenosis and coronary artery disease, valve replacement and myocardial revascularization should be performed concurrently. Perioperative mortality is higher in those patients who do not undergo simultaneous coronary bypass grafting.[33]

Percutaneous aortic balloon valvuloplasty is an alternative in the treatment of aortic stenosis. In this procedure, either one or two balloon catheters are passed through the aortic orifice and then inflated in an effort to "crack" the calcium that is retarding leaflet motion. The patient population considered eligible for percutaneous aortic balloon valvuloplasty generally has been elderly, disabled, and not thought to be surgical candidates. The immediate results show an increase in the aortic valve area of only 50 per cent[45] with a 3 to 10 per cent[4,45] mortality. The long-term results are even more disappointing with an expected 1-year mortality of at least 25 per cent and a 30 to 35 per cent recurrence rate of symptoms.[4,45] Percutaneous aortic balloon valvuloplasty done in the operating room under direct vision[44]

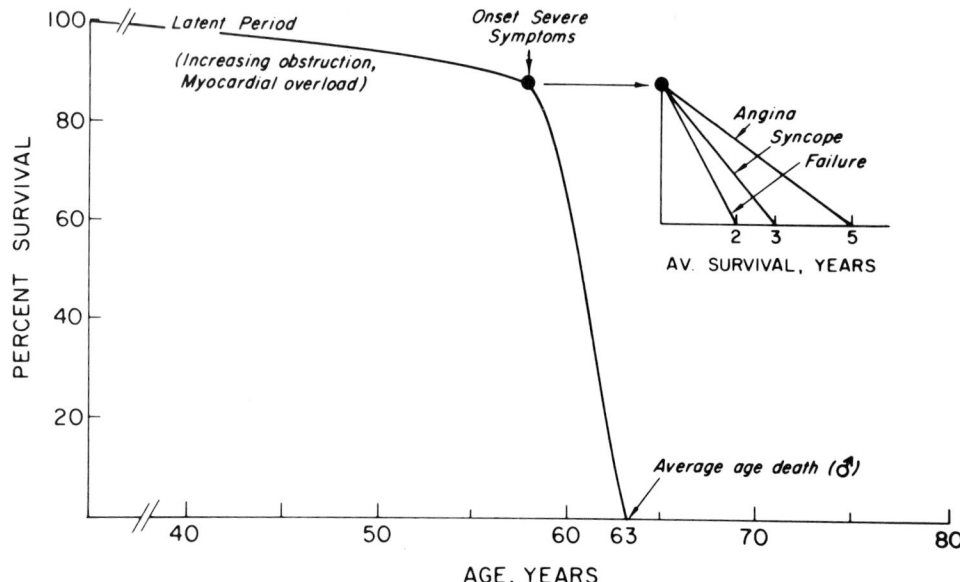

Figure 4. The natural history of medically treated aortic stenosis. One can understand the difficulty in deciding to operate on the asymptomatic patient (latent period). However, with the onset of symptoms, the issue becomes clear. (From Ross, R. S., and Braunwald, E.: Circulation, *37* (Suppl. V):61, 1968.)

has shown nearly no improvement in orifice size in two thirds of patients. With a recurrence of symptoms, death, hemodynamic evidence of restenosis, or a combination of these in over 50 per cent of patients at 6 months,[3] it appears clear that percutaneous aortic balloon valvuloplasty cannot compete with surgical valve replacement. If it has a role in the treatment of aortic stenosis, it may be limited to the aged, frail, and possibly senile patient whose long-term survival is abysmal.

AORTIC INSUFFICIENCY

Pathologic Anatomy

Incompetence of the aortic valve may be due to either primary valvular or aortic root disease.[37] As with aortic stenosis, *rheumatic fever* causes thickening of the valve leaflets, but in this situation, retraction of the cusps prevents adequate apposition causing a central leak. Commissural fusion, which so frequently accompanies this process, leads to physiologic stenosis. *Congenital bicuspid valves* generally lead to aortic stenosis. However, prolapse of a redundant leaflet may progress, leading to regurgitation. Similarly, *myxoid degeneration of the aortic valve* as seen

in Marfan's syndrome, Ehlers-Danlos syndrome, and cystic medial necrosis may lead to redundancy, progressive prolapse, and regurgitation. *Infective endocarditis* with bacterial destruction of the valve leaflets or scarring with leaflet retraction may cause valvular insufficiency. *Trauma* may cause an ascending aortic dissection, as can hypertensive atherosclerotic disease, leading to loss of commissural suspension and leaflet prolapse. In addition, *severe aortic dilation* such as seen in cystic medial necrosis, annuloaortic ectasia, syphilis, and ankylosing spondylitis may cause valvular insufficiency.

Pathophysiology

In aortic regurgitation, the increase in preload or end-diastolic volume is due to left ventricular filling both via the mitral valve and through the incompetent aortic valve. Ejection fraction remains normal as stroke volume and end-diastolic volume increase at the expense of a significant augmentation in left ventricular wall stress. This increased wall tension occurs following left ventricular dilation that produces a large increase in myocardial oxygen demand. Associated left ventricular wall thickening may maintain normal wall thickness to cavity radius

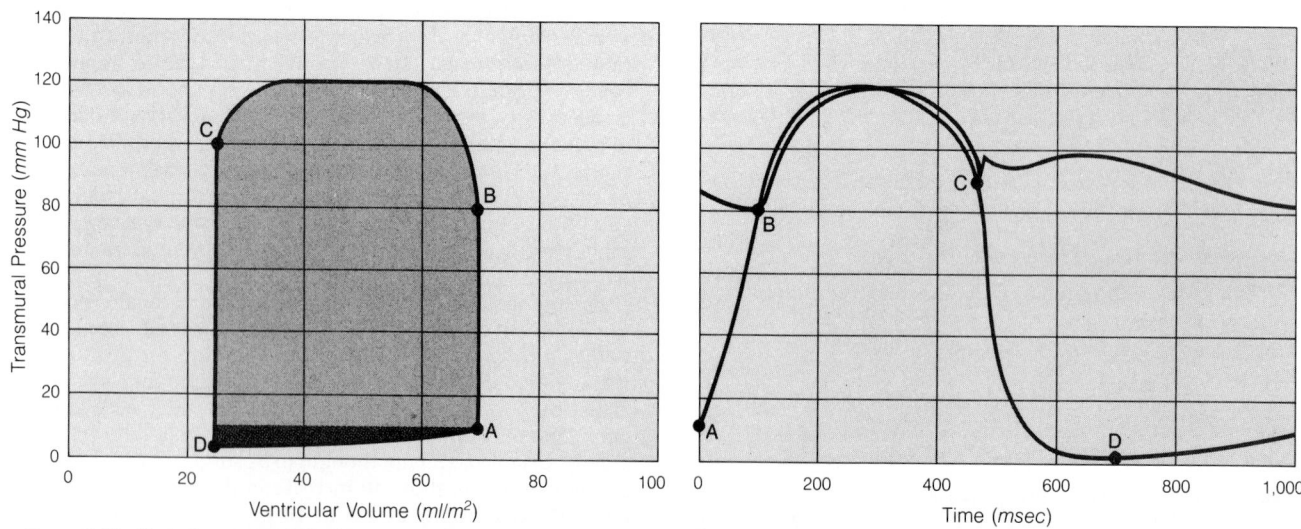

Figure 5. The illustration on the left is a pressure-volume loop. The illustration on the right represents a simultaneous left ventricular–aortic pressure time curve (the curved arrow marks aortic pressure, the straight arrow marks left ventricular pressure). In both curves, point A represents the commencement of isovolumetric contraction. At point B, the aortic valve opens and ejection begins. Despite the fact that contraction ceases in mid-systole, mass action continues to empty the ventricle until point C, which represents aortic valve closure and end-systole. Isovolumetric relaxation then occurs until ventricular pressure falls below left atrial pressure, at which time the mitral valve opens and ventricular filling begins. Thus, in the pressure-volume loop, B-C or A-D represents stroke volume. (From Wilmore, D., Brennan, M., Harken, A. H., Holcroft, J., and Meakins, J.: Care of the Surgical Patient. New York, Scientific American, 1989.)

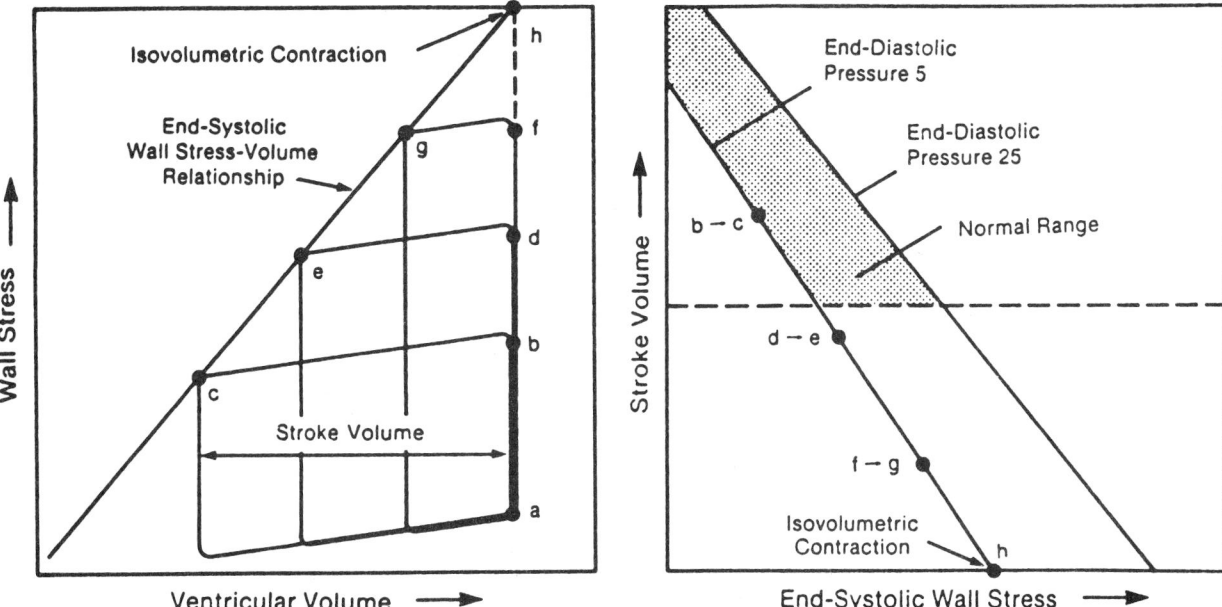

Figure 6. On the left a series of stress-volume loops is shown (as in Figure 5). As afterload is progressively increased, wall stress is increased such that ejection, which initially occurred at b, now occurs at d and then f. Stroke volume diminishes from b-c to d-e, and then f-g. At maximal wall stress h, there is no stroke volume but rather simply isovolumetric contraction.

On the right, the inverse relationship between stroke volume and end-systolic wall stress is portrayed. The two negative slopes represent families of stroke volumes generated with an LVEDP of 5 mm. Hg or an LVEDP of 25 mm. Hg. Note that a subnormal stroke volume of f-g at an LVEDP of 5 mm. Hg can be brought into the normal range by increasing preload to an LVEDP of 25 mm. Hg. Carabello[9] emphasizes that there is a group of patients who fall below and to the left of this curve whose stroke volume is diminished disproportionately to the increased wall stress. He suggests that it is this group who has the highest operative mortality and derives the least benefit from aortic valve replacement. (From Weber, K. T., et al.: The mechanics of ventricular function. Hosp. Pract., 18:113, 1983. Drawn by Alan Iselin.)

ratio.[20] As a result, aortic regurgitation may be associated with massive ventricular volumes, which interestingly does not initially cause a decrease in ventricular compliance. Consequently, end-diastolic volume may increase, whereas end-diastolic pressure remains normal. Exercise tolerance is maintained as peripheral vasodilation and a shorter diastolic time period combine to improve stroke volume with a decrease in the regurgitant fraction. However, as aortic incompetence progresses, wall thickness does not keep pace with diastolic volume, increased wall tension develops, and systolic dysfunction occurs.[18] At this point, left ventricular end-diastolic pressure may increase, and patients typically become symptomatic (Fig. 7). Significant cardiac dysfunction can occur, however, without symptoms.

In severe aortic regurgitation, an imbalance in myocardial oxygen supply and demand may cause ischemia despite normal coronary arteries. Increased left ventricular mass and wall tension occur with low diastolic pressures. Consequently, and particularly with exercise when the diastolic period shortens, coronary blood flow may not meet demand.[52]

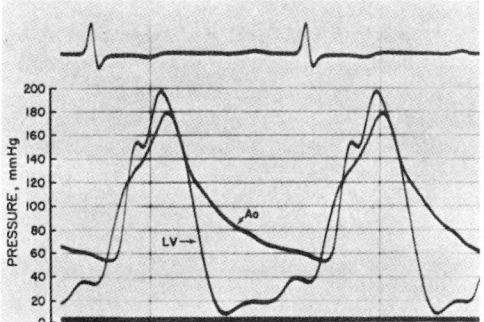

Figure 7. Simultaneous left ventricular and aortic pressure-time curves in a patient with severe aortic insufficiency. Note that in this trace the aortic and left ventricular end-diastolic pressures nearly equalize, suggesting the magnitude of this patient's regurgitant volume. (From Grossman, W.: Cardiac Catheterization, Angiography, and Intervention. Philadelphia, Lea & Febiger, 1991.)

Acute aortic regurgitation as occurs in a dissection or endocarditis leads to very high left ventricular end-diastolic pressures as the regurgitant volume exceeds the elastic limits of a small, unconditioned ventricle[40]; symptoms develop immediately.

Diagnosis

In patients with aortic insufficiency, the physical examination is very distinct owing to the wide pulse pressure. The peripheral pulses rise and fall abruptly (Corrigan's or water-hammer pulse), the head may bob with each systole (de Musset's sign), and the capillaries visibly pulsate (Quincke's sign). Auscultation reveals that aortic systolic closure is soft or absent. The high-frequency diastolic regurgitant murmur then commences and reaches an early peak, with an ensuing decrescendo. A mid to late diastolic rumble can be heard (Austin-Flint murmur) and represents rapid antegrade flow across the mitral valve that is closing because of rapid ventricular filling secondary to the aortic regurgitation. Echo Doppler is the most accurate noninvasive technique to determine aortic insufficiency.

Clinical Course

In chronic aortic regurgitation, left ventricular dilation and dysfunction can occur before the patient becomes symptomatic.[1] Symptoms, generally the result of an elevation in left atrial pressure, include dyspnea on exertion, orthopnea, and paroxysmal nocturnal dyspnea. Nocturnal angina occurs occasionally as a result of a slow heart rate and an exceedingly low diastolic pressure with resultant poor coronary flow. Acute aortic regurgitation, however, is poorly tolerated. These patients present with tachypnea, tachycardia, and peripheral vasoconstriction.

Management

Patients with symptomatic aortic insufficiency require surgical therapy since their prognosis treated medically is only a few years. The asymptomatic or mildly symptomatic patient with moderate or moderately severe aortic regurgitation may be managed with diuretics and afterload reduction for prolonged

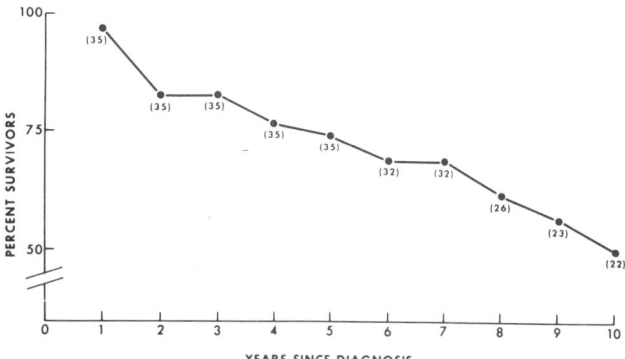

Figure 8. The natural history of medically treated aortic insufficiency. This curve is not too dissimilar from the results of surgically treated patients, although the two groups are not at all comparable. However, it supports the concept that the decision to operate on the asymptomatic patient with aortic insufficiency cannot be taken lightly. (From Rapaport, E.: Natural history of aortic and mitral valve disease. Am. J. Cardiol., *35*:221, 1975.)

periods of time (Fig. 8). Seventy-five per cent of patients survive 5 years and 50 per cent 10 years from the time of diagnosis.[41] Despite the lack of symptoms, irreversible myocardial dysfunction occurs. The end-systolic volume may help in determining management of these asymptomatic patients with aortic insufficiency.[7] When the end-systolic volume is less than 30 ml. per m.[2], prognosis after surgical therapy is excellent. Progressive systolic dysfunction with systolic volumes greater than 90 ml. per m.[2] is associated with poor operative results and frequent permanent postoperative disability. End-systolic volumes between 30 ml. per m.[2] and 90 ml. per m.[2] have intermediate short- and long-term results. The indications for surgical therapy in the asymptomatic patient with aortic insufficiency should be based on serial echography or radionuclide ventriculography to discern systolic dysfunction or a decreasing ejection fraction. When left ventricular dysfunction is noted in patients with diminished ejection fraction and good exercise tolerance, elective operation is recommended. Persistent medical management of these patients severely jeopardizes surgical outcome.[5]

The mortality associated with aortic valve replacement in aortic insufficiency is approximately 4 to 6 per cent.[5,19,27] Long-term survival is dependent on preoperative left ventricular function. Both early and late results are improved when surgical intervention precedes left ventricular decompensation.[5,16,51]

CHOICE OF VALVE PROSTHESES

The ideal heart valve clearly has yet to be designed. Currently surgeons have a choice of three broad categories of valves. The first are mechanical valves that include ball and cage prostheses or tilting disc prostheses. The second types are xenograft (porcine) prostheses (Carpentier-Edwards and Hancock). The third types are the free-sewn homografts, either antibiotic-sterilized or cryopreserved. At the University of Colorado Health Science Center, a tilting disc (St. Jude or the Medtronic-Hall) valve is the choice for a mechanical valve. These tilting disc prostheses function hemodynamically better in small sizes when compared with the high-profile Starr-Edwards ball and cage prosthesis. Consequently, they yield excellent results even in the patient with a small aortic root.

The Medtronic-Hall prosthesis was developed with changes directed specifically to increasing flow through the small orifice of the tilting disc by moving the pivot more centrally and allowing a disc excursion out of the housing during full opening. The valve housing was designed to rotate with the sewing ring so that after surgical implantation, valve orientation could be changed to avoid any supra- or subannular obstruction. The St. Jude valve has a lower profile than the Medtronic-Hall, and

rather than utilizing a single tilting disc, it has a bileaflet mechanism whereby each leaflet opens 85 degrees causing a very large effective orifice. Both of these valves have excellent hemodynamic profiles such that a prosthetic valve has an effective orifice area of approximately 1.5 cm[2]. Therefore, even at a very high cardiac output, transvalvular gradients of less than 15 to 20 mm. Hg can be expected.[12,48] The thromboembolic complication rate in these prostheses in the aortic position is 1 to 1.7 events per patient year, with freedom from emboli at 5 years being approximately 90 to 95 per cent. Anticoagulation is required in these patients, which has an associated complication rate of 5 per cent per year and an approximate 1 per cent yearly mortality.

The porcine bioprostheses (Hancock, Carpentier-Edwards valve) utilize the aortic valve of the pig, fixed with glutaraldehyde and mounted on a stent covered with Dacron or Teflon cloth. Xenograft prostheses do not require anticoagulation. This is their main appeal. In a prospective study, Hammermeister and associates[21] evaluated 575 patients randomized to either Bjork-Shiley (a mechanical tilting disc prosthesis) or Hancock (xenograft) valve replacement. In this Veterans Administration Cooperative Study in which the average follow-up was 5 years, the total number of embolic episodes was greater with tissue valves (20 of 196) than with mechanical valves (15 of 198). However, bleeding complications occurred in only 29 of 196 patients receiving tissue valves compared with 74 of 198 receiving the mechanical valve, a direct result of their need for anticoagulation. In this study, freedom from valve-related complications, fatal or nonfatal, was 63 per cent for the bioprosthetic versus 53 per cent for the mechanical valve in the aortic position. The advantage to the bioprosthetic group was due entirely to fewer bleeding complications.

The problem with the bioprosthetic valve, however, lies in its poor long-term durability. Borkon and associates[6] found that 99 per cent of over 500 patients with the Hancock valve were free of bioprosthetic failure at 5 years. However, at 9 years this had dropped to 70 per cent, and at 10 years to 61 per cent. Magilligan and associates[29] and Milano and colleagues[32] in similar studies showed that valve performance was excellent up to 60 months but then fell precipitously. Moreover, the bioprosthetic valve deteriorates even more rapidly in the younger age group.[53] About 40 per cent of patients less than 21 years old who have a porcine valve require replacement within 4 years,[39] and of patients less than 30 years old, 75 per cent require reoperation at 10 years[22] (Fig. 9). This increased risk of deterioration may

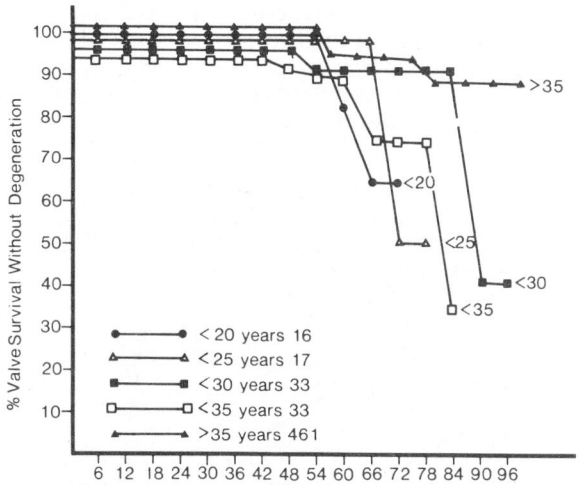

Figure 9. Porcine valve survival is excellent at 3 to 4 years. However, the age of the recipient has a major role thereafter, with valve degeneration most rapid in the youngest patients. (From Magilligan, D. J., Jr., et al.: Spontaneous degeneration of porcine bioprosthetic valves. Ann. Thorac. Surg., *30*:261, 1980.)

relate to the higher rate of calcification and stenosis in these valves in the younger population.

The hemodynamics of the Hancock and Carpentier-Edwards valves are not as good as in the mechanical valve prostheses. In small sizes the valves are intrinsically stenotic with an effective orifice area of less than 1 cm.[2] for 19-mm. valves. Although comparable *in vivo* data are not available for 19-mm. mechanical valves, the effective orifice area for a Medtronic-Hall or St. Jude 21-mm. valve is significantly larger than in a similarly sized bioprosthesis.[28] Consequently, in the authors' opinion, a bioprosthesis should be used with caution in sizes smaller than 23 mm.

The first free-sewn homograft valves were placed at Greenland Hospital, New Zealand, by Barratt-Boyes. Homograft valves are not stented but rather are sewn into the native annulus. This is a significantly more difficult and time-consuming operation than prosthetic aortic valve replacement with a mechanical or tissue bioprosthesis. The benefits of the homograft valve, however, may prove worth the added effort. In his series of over 250 antibiotic-sterilized valves, Barratt-Boyes[2] experienced a 77 per cent 5-year survival and a 57 per cent 10-year survival. Although only 15 patients received anticoagulation, there were no instances of valve-related thromboembolism. Moreover, the development of hemodynamically significant aortic stenosis was not noted. Long-term morbidity related nearly exclusively to valve degeneration leading to aortic regurgitation. Although freedom from significant incompetence was 95 per cent at 5 years, it was 78 per cent at 10 years, and only 42 per cent at 14 years. Analysis of donor and recipient factors affecting valve durability revealed that a donor age over 50 years, a recipient aortic root diameter greater than 30 mm., and a recipient age less than 15 years adversely affected valve survival. If grouped in this manner, those patients without any negative factors experienced a freedom from significant valve failure of 94 per cent at 9 years, although there was still a sharp decrease to 62 per cent at 13 years. Much more remarkable is O'Brien's report of a series of cryopreserved rather than fresh antibiotic-sterilized homografts[35] (Fig. 10). He reported a 92 per cent 10-year freedom from reoperation. Freedom from embolic events was 98 per cent at 10 years, again with no anticoagulation. Freedom from all valve-related complications at 10 years in his cryopreserved homograft group was 92 per cent. These tremendous results have generated enthusiasm for the cryopreserved valve. Until follow-up data significantly longer than 10 years are available, however, this may be premature. Regardless, viable homograft valves are very promising in view of freedom from anticoagulation and emboli and the predictably slow mode of failure.

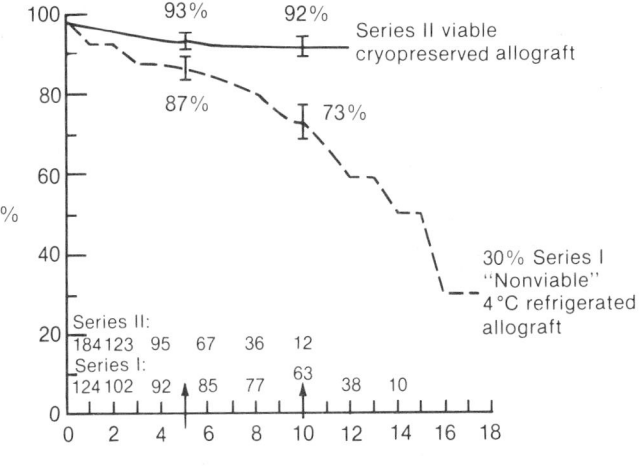

Figure 10. In a series of cryopreserved valves, O'Brien shows a freedom from complications at 10 years that is remarkable. However, only 12 patients are out 10 years. One must wait for longer follow-up to better evaluate this technique of homograft preservation. (From O'Brien, M. F., Stafford, G., Gardner, M., Pohlner, P., McGriffin, D., Johnston, N., Brosnan, A., and Duffy, P.: The viable cryopreserved allograft aortic valve. J. Cardiac Surg., 2(Suppl.):165, 1987.)

REFERENCES

1. Alpert, J. S.: Chronic aortic regurgitation. *In* Dalen, J. E., and Alpert, J. S. (Eds.): Valvular Heart Disease, 2nd ed. Boston, Little, Brown & Company, 1987, p. 283.
2. Barratt-Boyes, B. G., Roche, A. H. G., Subramanyan, R., Pemberton, J. R., and Whitlock, R. M. L.: Long-term follow-up of patients with the antibiotic-sterilized aortic homograft valve inserted free hand in the aortic position. Circulation, *75*:768, 1987.
3. Block, P. C.: Aortic valvuloplasty—a valid alternative? N. Engl. J. Med., *319*:169, 1988.
4. Block, P. C., and Palacios, I. F.: Clinical and hemodynamic follow-up after percutaneous aortic valvuloplasty in the elderly. Am. J. Cardiol., *62*:760, 1988.
5. Bonow, R. O., Picone, A. L., McIntosh, C. L., Jones, M., Rosing, D. R., Maron, B. J., Lakatos, E., Clark, R. E., and Epstein, S. E.: Survival and functional results after valve replacement for aortic regurgitation from 1976 to 1983: Impact of preoperative left ventricular function. Circulation, *72*:1244, 1985.
6. Borkon, M. A., McIntosh, C. L., Von Ruedon, T. J., and Morrow, A. G.: Mitral valve replacement with the Hancock bioprosthesis: Five to ten year follow-up. Ann. Thorac. Surg., *32*:127, 1981.
7. Borow, K., Green, L. H., Mann, T., Sloss, L. J., Braunwald, E., Collins, J. J., Cohn, L., and Grossman, W.: End-systolic volume overload from valvular regurgitation. Am. J. Med., *68*:655, 1980.
8. Braunwald, E., Goldblatt, A., Aygen, M. M., Rockoff, S. D., and Morrow, A. G.: Congenital aortic stenosis: Clinical and hemodynamic findings in 100 patients. Circulation, *27*:426, 1963.
9. Carabello, B. A., Green, L. H., Grossman, W., Cohn, L. H., Koster, J. K., and Collins, J. J., Jr.: Hemodynamic determinants of prognosis of aortic valve replacement in critical aortic stenosis and advanced congestive heart failure. Circulation, *62*:42, 1980.
10. Copeland, J. B., Griepp, R. B., Stinson, E. B., and Shumway, N. E.: Long-term follow-up after isolated aortic valve replacement. J. Thorac. Cardiovasc. Surg., *74*:875, 1977.
11. Cowper, W.: "Of ossifications or petrifications in the coats of arteries, particularly in the valves of the great artery." Philosophical Transactions of the Royal Society (London), Chapter 24, 1706.
12. Crawford, F. A.: The St. Jude valve. Cardiac Surgery: State of the Art Review, Vol. 1, No. 2, February 1987.
13. Kirklin, J. W., and Barratt-Boyes, B. G.: Aortic valve disease. *In* Cardiac Surgery, New York, John Wiley & Sons, 1986, p. 394.
14. Ellis, F. H., Jr., and Kirklin, J. W.: Congenital valvular aortic stenosis: Anatomic findings and surgical technique. J. Thorac. Cardiovasc. Surg., *43*:199, 1962.
15. Fifer, M. A., Gunther, S., Grossman, W., Mirsky, I., Carabello, B., and Barry, W. H.: Myocardial contractile function in the aortic stenosis as determined from the rate of stress development during isovolumic systole. Am. J. Cardiol., *44*:1318, 1979.
16. Fioretti, P., Roelandt, J., Bos, R. J., Meltzer, R. S., van Hoogenhuijze, D., Serruys, P. W., Nauta, J., and Hugenholtz, P. G.: Echocardiography in chronic aortic insufficiency: Is valve replacement too late when left ventricular end-systolic dimension reaches 55 mm? Circulation, *67*:216, 1983.
17. Gorlin, R., and Gorlin, S. G.: Hydraulic formula for calculation of area of stenotic mitral valve, other cardiac valves, and central circulatory shunts. Am. Heart J., *41*:1, 1951.
18. Greenberg, B., Massie, B., Thomas, D., Bristow, J. D., Cheitlin, M., Broudy, D., Szlachcic, J., and Krishnamurthy, G.: Association between exercise ejection fraction response and systolic wall stress in patients with chronic aortic insufficiency. Circulation, *71*:458, 1985.
19. Greves, J., Rahimtoola, S. H., McAnulty, J. H., DeMots, H., Clark, D. G., Greenberg, B., and Starr, A.: Preoperative criteria predictive of late survival following valve replacement for severe aortic regurgitation. Am. Heart J., *101*:300, 1981.
20. Grossman, W., Jones, D., and McLaurin, L. P.: Wall stress and patterns of hypertrophy in the human left ventricle. J. Clin. Invest., *56*:56, 1975.
21. Hammermeister, K. E., Henderson, W. G., Burchfiel, C. M., Sethi, G. K., Souchek, J., Opman, C., Cantor, A. B., Folland, E., Khuri, S., and Rahimtoula, S.: Comparison of outcome after valve replacement with bioprosthesis versus a mechanical prosthesis: Initial five year results of a randomized trial. J. Am. Coll. Cardiol., *10*:719, 1987.
22. Jamieson, W. R. E., Rosado, L. J., Munro, A. I., Gerein, A. N., Burr, L. H., Miyagishima, R. T., Janusz, M. T., and Tyers, G. F. O.: Carpentier-Edwards standard porcine bioprosthesis: Primary tissue failure (structural valve deterioration) by age groups. Ann. Thorac. Surg., *46*:155, 1988.
23. Kennedy, J. W., Doces, J., and Stewart, D. K.: Left ventricular function before and following aortic valve replacement. Circulation, *56*:944, 1977.
24. Kirklin, J. W., and Barratt-Boyes, B. G.: Mitral valve disease with or without tricuspid valve disease. *In* Cardiac Surgery. New York, John Wiley & Sons, 1986, p. 323.

25. Kirklin, J. W., and Barratt-Boyes, B. G.: Aortic valve disease. In Cardiac Surgery. New York, John Wiley & Sons, 1986, p. 373.
26. Lombard, J. T., and Selzer, A.: Valvular aortic stenosis: Clinical and hemodynamic profile of patients. Ann. Intern. Med., 106:292, 1987.
27. Lytle, B. W., Cosgrove, D. M., Loop, F. D., Taylor, P. C., Gill, C. C., Golding, L. A. R., Goormastic, M., and Groves, L. K.: Replacement of aortic valve combined with myocardial revascularization: Determinants of early and late risk for 500 patients, 1967–1981. Circulation, 68:1149, 1983.
28. Magilligan, D. J., Jr.: Porcine bioprosthesis. Cardiac Surgery: State of the Art Reviews, Vol. 1, No. 2, 1987.
29. Magilligan, D. J., Jr., Lewis, J. W., Jara, F. M., Lee, W. M., Alam, M., Riddle, J. M., and Stein, P. D.: Spontaneous degeneration of porcine bioprosthetic valves. Ann. Thorac. Surg., 30:259, 1980.
30. Marcus, M. L., Doty, D. B., Hiratzka, L. F., Wright, C. B., and Eastham, C. L.: Decreased coronary reserve: A mechanism for angina pectoris in patients with aortic stenosis and normal coronary arteries. N. Engl. J. Med., 307:1362, 1982.
31. Mark, A. L., Kioschos, J. M., Abboud, F. M., Heistad, D. D., and Schmid, P. G.: Abnormal vascular responses to exercise in patients with aortic stenosis. J. Clin. Invest., 52:1138, 1973.
32. Milano, A. D., Bortolotti, V., Mazzucco, A., Guerra, F., Stellin, G., Talenti, E., Thiene, G., and Gallucci, V.: Performance of the Hancock bioprosthesis following aortic valve replacement: Considerations based on a 15 year experience. Ann. Thorac. Surg., 46:216, 1988.
33. Miller, D. C., Sinson, E. B., Oyer, P. E., Rossiter, S. J., Reitz, B. A., and Shumway, N. E.: Surgical implications and results of combined aortic valve replacement and myocardial revascularization. Am. J. Cardiol., 43:494, 1979.
34. Murakami, T., Hess, O. M., Gage, J. E., Grimm, J., and Krayenbuehl, H. P.: Diastolic filling dynamics in patients with aortic stenosis. Circulation, 73:1162, 1986.
35. O'Brien, M. F., Stafford, G., Gardner, M., Pohlner, P., McGiffin, D., Johnston, N., Brosnan, A., and Duffy, P.: The viable cryopreserved allograft aortic valve. J. Cardiac Surg., 2(Suppl.):153, 1987.
36. Olesen, K. H., and Warburg, E.: Isolated aortic stenosis — the late prognosis. Acta Med. Scand., 160:437, 1957.
37. Olson, L. J., Subramanian, R., and Edwards, W. D.: Surgical pathology of pure aortic insufficiency: A study of 225 cases. Mayo Clin. Proc., 59:835, 1984.
38. O'Toole, J. D., Geiser, E. A., Reddy, P. S., Curtiss, E. I., and Landfair, R. M.: Effect of preoperative ejection fraction on survival and hemodynamic improvement following AVR. Circulation, 58:1175, 1978.
39. Pantely, G., Morton, M., and Rahimtoola, S. H.: Effects of successful, uncomplicated valve replacement on ventricular hypertrophy, volume and performance in aortic stenosis and in aortic incompetence. J. Thorac. Cardiovasc. Surg., 75:383, 1978.
40. Perloff, J. K.: Acute severe aortic regurgitation: Recognition and management. J. Cardiovasc. Med., 8:209, 1983.
41. Rapaport, E.: Natural history of aortic and mitral valve disease. Am. J. Cardiol., 35:221, 1975.
42. Richards, A. M., Nicholls, M. G., Ikram, H., Hamilton, E. J., and Richards, R. D.: Syncope in aortic valvular stenosis. Lancet, 2:1113, 1984.
43. Roberts, W. C.: Valvular, subvalvular and supravalvular aortic stenosis. Morphologic features. Cardiovasc. Clin., 5:97, 1973.
44. Robicsek, F., Harbold, N. B., Jr., Daugherty, H. K., Cook, J. W., Selle, J. G., Hess, P. J., and Gallagher, J. J.: Balloon valvuloplasty in calcified aortic stenosis: A cause for caution and alarm. Ann. Thorac. Surg., 45:515, 1988.
45. Safian, R. D., Berman, A. D., Diver, D. J., McKay, L. L., Come, P. C., Riley, M. F., Warren, S. E., Cunningham, M. J., Wyman, R. M., Weinstein, J. S., et al.: Balloon aortic valvuloplasty in 170 consecutive patients. N. Engl. J. Med., 319:169, 1988.
46. Schwarz, F., Flameng, W., Schaper, J., Langebartels, F., Sesto, M., Hehrlein, F., and Schlepper, M.: Myocardial structure and function in patients with aortic valve disease and their relation to postoperative results. Am. J. Cardiol., 41:661, 1978.
47. Sethig, K., Miller, D. C., Souchek, J., Oprian, C., Henderson, W. G., ul Hassan, Z., Folland, E., Khuri, S., Scotts, M., Burchfiel, C., and Hammermeister, K. D.: Clinical hemodynamic and angiographic predictors of operative mortality in patients undergoing single valve replacement. J. Thorac. Cardiovasc. Surg., 93:884, 1987.
48. Starek, P. J. K., Beaudet, R. L., and Hall, K. V.: The Medtronic-Hall valve: Development and clinical experience. Cardiac Surgery: State of the Art Reviews, Vol. 1, No. 2, February 1987, p. 233.
49. Tweedy, P. S.: The pathogenesis of valvular thickening in rheumatic heart disease. Br. Heart J., 18:173, 1956.
50. Tweedy, P. S.: Pathogenesis of aortic stenosis and its relation to age. Br. Heart J., 29:222, 1967.
51. Turina, J., Turina, M., Rothlin, M., and Krayenbuehl, H. P.: Improved late survival in patients with chronic aortic regurgitation by earlier operation. Circulation, 70(Suppl. I):147, 1984.
52. Uhl, G. S., Boucher, C. A., Oliveros, R. A., and Murgo, J. P.: Exercise-induced myocardial oxygen supply-demand imbalance in asymptomatic or mildly symptomatic aortic regurgitation. Chest, 80:686, 1981.
53. Williams, J. B., Karp, R. B., Kirklin, J. W., Kouchoucos, N. T., Pacifico, A. D., Zorn, G. L., Jr., Blackstone, E. H., Brown, R. N., Piantadosi, S., and Bradley, E. L.: Considerations in selection and management of patients undergoing valve replacement with glutaraldehyde-fixed porcine bioprosthesis. Ann. Thorac. Surg., 46:155, 1988.
54. Yeager, M., Yock, P. G., and Popp, R. L.: Companion of Doppler derived

pressure gradient to that determined at cardiac catheterization in adults with aortic valve stenosis: Implications for management. Am. J. Cardiol., 57:644, 1986.

1. SURGICAL TREATMENT OF HYPERTROPHIC CARDIOMYOPATHY

H. Newland Oldham, Jr., M.D.

Hypertrophic cardiomyopathy (HCM) has been recognized clinically since the late 1950s and has been extensively investigated by cardiac physiologists, cardiologists, electrophysiologists, and cardiovascular surgeons. The term *cardiomyopathy* describes a primary disorder of cardiac muscle that is divided by the World Health Organization classification into hypertrophic cardiomyopathy and dilated cardiomyopathy.[1] This terminology has replaced the earlier descriptive title of idiopathic hypertrophic subaortic stenosis that was popularized by reports from the National Institutes of Health (NIH).[5,52] Cardiomyopathy of all types represents less than 1 per cent of cardiac deaths in the United States, and less than 10 per cent of these are due to HCM.[1] The majority of patients with HCM have asymmetric hypertrophy with a marked increase in thickness of the upper ventricular septum.[67] Symptoms are related to dynamic systolic obstruction of left ventricular outflow, abnormalities of diastolic function, alterations in coronary blood flow, and cardiac arrhythmias. Most patients respond to medical therapy, and surgical therapy has been reserved for those with significant obstruction whose symptoms are unresponsive to medical treatment. Several centers have reported current results of surgical treatment of large numbers of patients with HCM.[29,30,43,44,49,50]

HISTORICAL ASPECTS

Brigden first used the term *cardiomyopathy* in 1956, and his recent editorial clearly describes the evolution of understanding of HCM.[6] Brock suggested that obstruction could be caused by the hypertrophied septum, and Teare described asymmetric septal hypertrophy in seven patients who died suddenly.[7,64] The early understanding of hemodynamic findings, clinical characteristics, and surgical treatment was based on reports from the NIH by Braunwald and Morrow and co-workers.[5,52] By 1964, there were 12 terms for this condition, and the concept of systolic obstruction was not accepted by all.[6] The evolution of surgical techniques for treatment of HCM is listed in Table 1. Morrow modified and refined the septal myotomy-myectomy (M-M) operation and accumulated a personal experience with this procedure in 350 patients.[42,51–53] This operation has remained a standard for comparison, although mitral valve replacement (MVR) is being recommended with increasing frequency.[30,42,44]

PATHOLOGIC ANATOMY

The two major pathologic features, which were initially described by Teare, are asymmetric septal hypertrophy and microscopic evidence of disorganized arrangement of muscle bundles.[64] Septal hypertrophy usually begins several centimeters below the aortic valve, and the maximal septal thickness is considerably greater than that of the left ventricular free wall (Fig. 1). Ninety-five per cent of patients have asymmetric septal hypertrophy, which involves the upper septum in 90 per cent, midventricular septum in 1 per cent, and apical septum in 3 per cent.[67] Atypical patterns of hypertrophy have been recognized

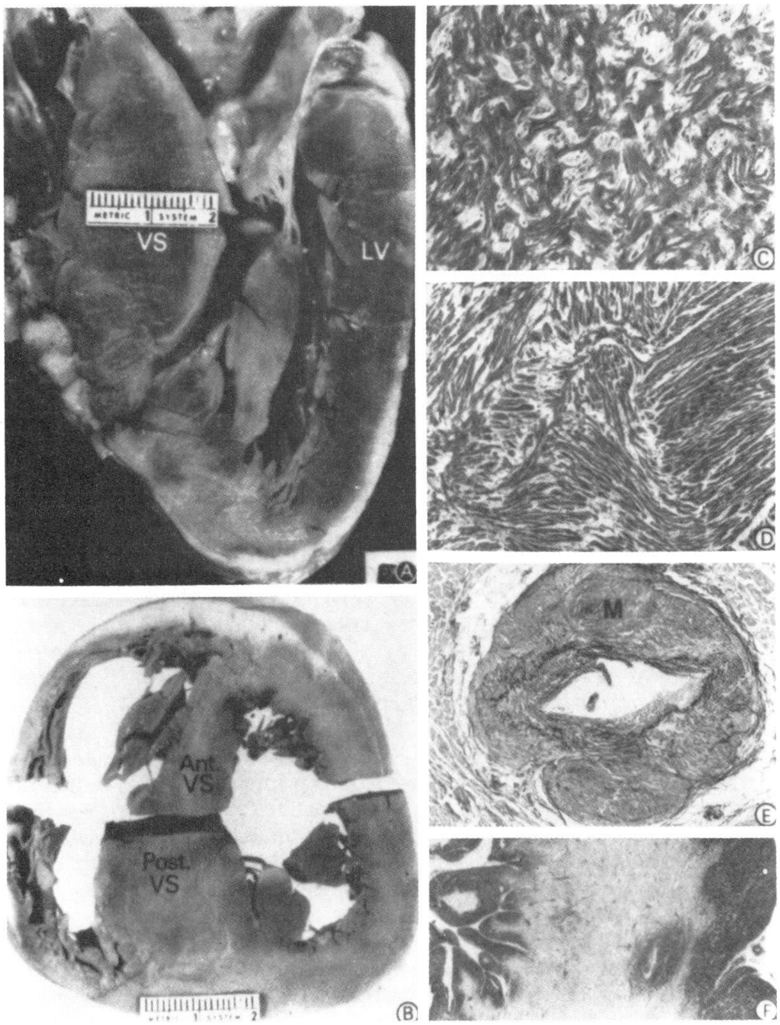

Figure 1. Pathologic features of hypertrophic cardiomyopathy. *A*, Heart specimen sectioned in a plane similar to the echocardiographic parasternal axis; the pattern of left ventricular hypertrophy is asymmetric, with wall thickening confined primarily to the anterior ventricular septum, which bulges into the left ventricular outflow tract. *B*, Left ventricular wall thickening is localized to the posterior portion of the ventricular septum, whereas the anterior is only minimally thickened. *C*, Disordered architecture with adjacent hypertrophied cardiac muscle cells arranged at perpendicular and oblique angles. *D*, Bundles of hypertrophied cells show a disorganized, interwoven arrangement. *E*, Intramural coronary artery with a narrowed lumen and thickened wall due to medial hypertrophy. *F*, Extensive transmural scarring of the septum. (From Maron, B. J., Bonow, R. O., Cannon, R. O., Leon, M. B., and Epstein, S. E.: Hypertrophic cardiomyopathy: Interrelations of clinical manifestations, pathophysiology, and therapy. Part I. N. Engl. J. Med., *316:*780, 1987.)

more frequently since the widespread use of echocardiography[43] (Figs. 1 and 4). Asymmetric septal hypertrophy is not unique to HCM as it occurs in 5 to 10 per cent of patients with other forms of congenital or acquired heart disease.[37] When the disease process occurs in infants, the right ventricle is commonly involved also.[2] Septal thickness is greatest at the level of the mitral valve, and the valve may be abnormally positioned in the left ventricular outflow tract. Recent reports of HCM have described uncommon variants ranging from localized apical hypertrophy found in Japan to hypertensive HCM in the elderly.[31,32,35] In elderly patients, calcification may displace the mitral valve anteriorly and contribute to obstruction. A change in cardiac shape is also usual in older patients, but the incidence of asymmetric septal hypertrophy and abnormal motion of the mitral valve are the same as in younger patients.[32]

Microscopically, the area of hypertrophy is composed of muscle fibers arranged in a disorganized pattern. Disagreement persists concerning the specificity of this disorganization, but it probably is not unique to HCM but only more extensive than in secondary types of hypertrophy.[1,20] Additional histologic features include myocardial scarring and abnormalities of the small intramural coronary arteries (Fig. 1.).

PHYSIOLOGY

Most investigators recognize the three basic pathophysiologic processes in HCM to be dynamic systolic subaortic obstruction, diastolic dysfunction, and myocardial ischemia. Only 25 per cent of patients with HCM have clinically significant obstruc-

tion, and diastolic dysfunction is, therefore, the most common and perhaps the most important mechanism. The relationships of these three processes to symptoms are quite variable, as described in detail in a recent review.[37,38] Initially there was considerable debate concerning the cause of obstruction and whether it was a real phenomenon or merely cavity obliteration produced by a hyperdynamic ventricle. Current evidence indicates that an outflow gradient is produced by obstruction caused by contact between the mitral valve and the ventricular septum.[37]

This dynamic subaortic obstruction may change spontaneously or by physiologic or pharmacologic provocation. A reduction in the gradient is caused by interventions that decrease myocardial contractility, increase ventricular volume, or increase arterial pressure. The gradient is increased by the opposite influences of increased contractility, decreased arterial pressure, or decreased ventricular volume.[37] Obstruction is caused by rapid ejection through a narrow outflow tract that is distorted by the asymmetric subaortic septal hypertrophy. This creates Venturi forces, which draw the anterior mitral leaflet toward the septum. This mechanism, first suggested in 1971, has now been extensively evaluated.[67] In addition to Venturi forces, abnormal papillary muscle support may contribute to systolic anterior motion of the mitral valve. Accumulated evidence including hemodynamic measurements, echocardiography, cineangiography, pulsed and continuous wave Doppler measurements, and color flow Doppler studies indicates that the systolic gradient is due to contact between the anterior leaflet of the mitral valve and the septum.[67]

Diastolic dysfunction of HCM is less well understood. Recent indices of myocardial relaxation have identified abnormalities in relaxation, compliance, and filling in the majority of these patients.[37,67] Improvement in diastolic function may be produced by calcium channel blockers.[14] Atrial fibrillation causes loss of atrial contribution to systolic filling and shortened diastole and may cause further clinical deterioration.

Myocardial ischemia is an important cause of chest pain and progression of the disease.[38,47] When obstruction is present, a high peak left ventricular pressure causes increased myocardial oxygen demand, producing ischemia. Ischemia may additionally be caused by alterations in capillary density, small vessel vasodilator reserve abnormalities, and abnormalities of the intramural myocardial arteries.[4,37] Exercise-induced ischemia has been documented by thallium scintigraphy in patients with angiographically normal coronary arteries.[9]

The pathophysiologic mechanisms are well recognized and described in recent reviews.[37,38] Interesting new experimental studies have demonstrated that mitral valve systolic anterior motion can cause a modest left ventricular outflow tract gradient, but that the additional creation of asymmetric septal hypertrophy produces a much greater obstruction.[55] Experimental models have also challenged the concept that the Venturi effect is the major cause of mitral valve systolic anterior motion. Alterations in the chordal support of the mitral valve and papillary muscle tension can displace the valve into the outflow tract.[33,34] Regional myocardial blood flow studies by positron emission tomography in 18 patients with HCM indicated an abnormal hyperemic response to dipyridamole. This was present in the hypertrophied septum and the free wall and was interpreted as a primary metabolic defect in HCM.[8] A contrasting study of 10 patients evaluated by positron emission tomographic scanning reported normal blood flow to the septum but found the metabolism of a glucose analog by the septum to differ from that of the remaining myocardium.[23,24] A recent study of 54 patients by echocardiography found a clear relationship between the severity of mitral regurgitation, the degree of outflow tract obstruction, and the incidence of systolic anterior motion.[56] A similar study of mitral regurgitation before and after surgical treatment reported that one half the total group had a reduction in mitral regurgitation, but all patients with severe mitral regurgitation demonstrated improvement.[19]

CLINICAL FEATURES

HCM may present at any time from infancy until old age. Clinical features at either end of the age spectrum are slightly atypical. Patients within the first year of life often have severe obstruction of the left and right sides of the heart.[2,39] When symptoms occur in the first year, death is common and usually from congestive heart failure rather than sudden death.[2] A form of obstructive HCM is more common in elderly patients than was previously recognized.[31,32,35] These patients are usually females and have severe distortion of left ventricular geometry and calcification of the mitral anulus. Symptoms do not respond well to medical therapy, and operative intervention has been required in many patients. The calcified mitral anulus contributes to the obstruction, and mitral valve replacement has been performed in a third of surgically treated patients.[32]

In more typical patients, the morphologic abnormalities are identified by 20 years of age, and symptoms are usually present by age 40. Patients frequently have a detectable cardiac murmur prior to the appearance of symptoms. The disease is more common in males and is familial in approximately 60 per cent of patients. It is not known whether the familial form is due to a single genetic defect or a combination of several separate defects.[1] The transmission of this pattern is consistent with an autosomal dominant trait.[37]

The classic symptoms of HCM are dyspnea, chest pain, and presyncope or syncope. In an extensive review of the NIH expe-

rience, Maron and colleagues described a poor relationship between symptoms and underlying pathophysiologic mechanisms. Symptoms may be caused by dynamic left ventricular outflow obstruction, alteration in diastolic myocardial function, myocardial ischemia, mitral regurgitation, or cardiac arrhythmias. An identical symptom complex may be caused by several mechanisms, and the severity of symptoms does not correlate with the magnitude of the pathophysiologic abnormality.[37,38] In the obstructive form of HCM, there is poor correlation between the magnitude of the outflow tract obstruction, the severity of symptoms, and improvement following pharmacologic treatment.[1,38] Dyspnea and exercise intolerance have been related to abnormalities of systolic function and to alterations in diastolic filling[13,14]

Sudden death is the most ominous clinical feature of HCM. There is no clear relationship between the incidence of sudden death and extent of hypertrophy, severity of symptoms, functional limitations, hemodynamic abnormalities, or degree of outflow tract obstruction.[1] The annual mortality for sudden death is 2 to 3 per cent with the incidence being slightly higher in younger patients.[38] Sudden death is thought to be due to an arrhythmia, and the most common type is probably ventricular tachycardia. The mechanism of this is unknown but may be related to disorganized myocardial cells, elevated left ventricular pressure, or areas of ischemia and fibrosis.[38] Hemodynamic measurements, clinical studies, and echocardiography have not been beneficial in identifying these patients. The most useful marker has been nonsustained ventricular tachycardia during 48-hour electrocardiographic monitoring.[45,54] Recent electrophysiologic studies have identified a wide variety of abnormalities that may be related to sudden death, but it is uncertain whether their detection will be beneficial in designing treatment that decreases the incidence of sudden death.[22,45]

DIAGNOSTIC EVALUATION

ECHOCARDIOGRAPHY. The development of echocardiography in the 1960s was of considerable benefit in understanding HCM. Myocardial thickness could be measured with echocardiography, and abnormalities of mitral valve motion could be identified. Thus, the characteristic findings of asymmetric septal hypertrophy and systolic anterior motion of the mitral valve could be recognized and followed serially.[6] With the introduction of two-dimensional echocardiography, the usual mechanism of obstruction was identified and unusual patterns of obstruction were localized. The presence of mitral valve systolic anterior motion has been identified in patients with other abnormalities of the left ventricular outflow tract, and asymmetric septal hypertrophy has been demonstrated occasionally in patients with valvular aortic stenosis.[12,26] The finding of asymmetric septal hypertrophy or systolic anterior motion in a patient with valvular or discrete subvalvular aortic stenosis should be a clear indication to inspect the outflow tract for a septal contribution to obstruction.

Two-dimensional echo has been helpful in identifying the mechanism by which mitral valve systolic anterior motion contributes to the subaortic gradient. The study by Maron and associates in 1985 demonstrated true obstruction of the left ventricular outflow tract and established septal M-M as a logical operation directed to normalization of left ventricular pressure.[40] A recent echo Doppler study demonstrated diastolic dysfunction in the majority of patients with HCM even in the absence of symptoms or subaortic gradients and indicated that impaired diastolic performance might be a common finding well before the occurrence of functional limitation.[41] Two-dimensional echocardiography has identified hypertrophy in regions other than the upper portion of the ventricular septum, and intraoperative echocardiography has been helpful in modifying the operation to match the specific type and location of obstruction[1,44] (Fig. 4).

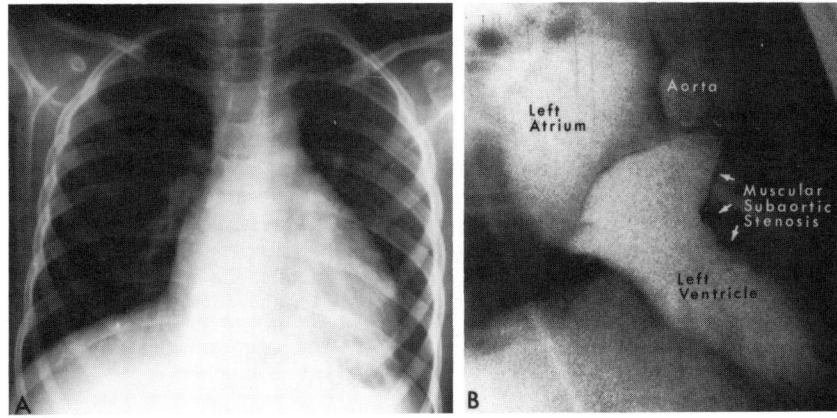

Figure 2. Hypertrophic cardiomyopathy. *A,* Chest film showing considerable enlargement of the left ventricle. *B,* Left ventricle cineangiogram illustrating a broad area of muscular obstruction. The left atrium is opacified as a result of associated mitral insufficiency. *C,* Pressure tracing showing an area of systemic pressure within the left ventricular outflow tract.

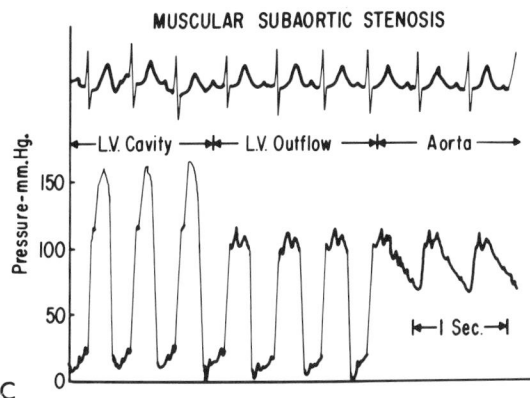

CARDIAC CATHETERIZATION. Complete cardiac catheterization was the original method of diagnostic evaluation of HCM, but since the development of echocardiography, catheterization has been employed less frequently (Fig. 2). Echo Doppler evaluation documents the location, mechanism, and magnitude of the obstruction as well as the presence of associated cardiac abnormalities. Coronary angiography is recommended to identify coronary artery obstruction, to aid in the medical management of patients, and to plan the proper combination of procedures for patients requiring operative intervention.

NATURAL HISTORY AND OPERATIVE INDICATIONS

The variable natural history of this disease makes the clinical course difficult to predict. Typical patients are symptom-free until midlife, although increasing numbers of elderly patients are now being recognized. Treatment is designed to alleviate symptoms and has not been documented to reverse the basic hypertrophic process or to reduce the incidence of sudden death.[6] The main medical treatment since the 1960s has been beta-blockers. Most patients respond to these drugs with improvement in angina, congestive failure, and presyncope. Beta-blockers are mainly helpful in patients with obstruction and cause a reduction in heart rate, contractility, systolic wall stress, and myocardial oxygen consumption.[38] Calcium channel blockers have been beneficial in patients with alterations in diastolic relaxation and filling. Recent information indicates that amiodarone improves the survival of patients with nonsustained ventricular tachycardia.[46] Amiodarone is, however, a very potent drug with serious side effects and is not of benefit to all patients.

Operative intervention is intended to relieve outflow tract obstruction and has been reserved for patients unresponsive to medical therapy. Thus, failure of pharmacologic agents to re-

TABLE 1. Evolution of Surgical Techniques for Hypertrophic Obstructive Cardiomyopathy

Reference	Year	Technique
Brock[7]	1957	Closed transventricular myotomy
Cleland[15]	1958	Transaortic myectomy
Kirklin and Ellis[27]	1961	Combined transaortic and transventricular myectomy
Morrow and Brockenbrough[52]	1961	Transaortic myectomy
Lillehei and Levy[36]	1963	Trans left atrial myectomy
Harken[25]	1964	Trans right ventricular myectomy
Binet et al.[3]	1968	Extended ventriculoaortic myotomy
Cooley et al.[18]	1971	Mitral valve replacement
Rastan and Koncz[57]	1976	Aortoventriculoplasty
Dembitsky and Weldon[21]	1976	Valved apicoaortic conduit

Modified from Walker, W. S., Reid, K. G., Cameron, E. W. J., Walbaum, P. R., and Kitchin, A. H.: Comparison of ventricular septal surgery and mitral valve replacement for hypertrophic obstructive cardiomyopathy. Ann. Thorac. Surg., *48*:528, 1989.

lieve symptoms of angina, cardiac failure, or syncope in the presence of a significant resting gradient usually indicates the advisability of surgical treatment. Treatment of asymptomatic patients with significant resting gradients and treatment of patients with gradients that can be demonstrated only by provocative measures remain more controversial. Proof that sudden death is reduced by surgical intervention in these patients is not currently available, but the recent assessment of surgical results in asymptomatic younger patients supports a more aggressive operative approach.[50] McIntosh reviewed 1700 operations performed in patients with obstructive HCM at 10 institutions. The indications for operation included severe symptoms unrelieved by adequate medical treatment with beta-blockers, calcium antagonists, or antiarrhythmics; obstruction to the left ventricular outflow tract of greater than 50 mm. Hg under basal conditions; and obstruction with provocative measures alone in a small number of patients. At the time of this review, surgical treatment of asymptomatic or mildly symptomatic patients with large gradients was considered investigational.[43]

SURGICAL TREATMENT

Two thirds of patients with HCM are managed adequately with calcium channel blockers, beta-blockers, and antiarrhythmic agents. Patients who remain symptomatic usually have dynamic outflow tract obstruction, diastolic dysfunction, or severe mitral regurgitation.[66] Surgical relief of obstruction is possible by eliminating abnormal mitral valve motion, reducing septal hypertrophy, or both. The two main treatments are septal myotomy-myectomy and mitral valve replacement, although numerous other approaches have been proposed (Table 1). The goals of surgical therapy are relief of symptoms and improvement in the quality of life, and these goals are attainable in 70 per cent of patients up to 25 years.[38]

The most commonly used procedure is septal M-M. This operation is described and illustrated in two excellent references by Morrow that should be read in original form[51,53] (Fig. 3). Septal M-M is performed using a transaortic approach and standard cardioplegic myocardial preservation. Two parallel incisions are made into the septal muscle and a strip of septum is excised, extending to below the site of mitral valve–septal contact. Muscle is removed from that area of the septum away from the conduction tissue. This classic operation has been slightly modified by McIntosh to begin the incision several millimeters below the aortic valve to maintain adequate support of the aortic anulus.[43] Removal of this rectangle of muscle enlarges the left ventricular outflow tract, which reduces the velocity of blood flow and decreases Venturi forces that cause apposition of the mitral valve to the septum. This, therefore, decreases the gradient and reduces left ventricular pressure and myocardial oxygen consumption.

Cooley and associates originally advocated MVR as another method to eliminate subaortic obstruction.[18] Because the gradient is due to systolic apposition of the mitral valve and the septum, removal of the anterior leaflet of the mitral valve relieves obstruction and MVR corrects any associated mitral insufficiency. Advantages of this operation include elimination of ventricular septal perforation and decreased injury to the conduction system. Technical considerations in MVR for HCM include the use of a smaller prosthesis because of the small size of the ventricular cavity and the need to excise both mitral leaflets.[42,66] This operation was not favored initially by many surgeons who preferred the classic Morrow procedure. Two recent reports, however, indicate that septal M-M is currently utilized in approximately two thirds of patients and MVR in approximately one third of patients.[30,43] Indications for MVR include severe mitral disease other than systolic anterior motion and reoperation following a previous septal M-M. Other relative

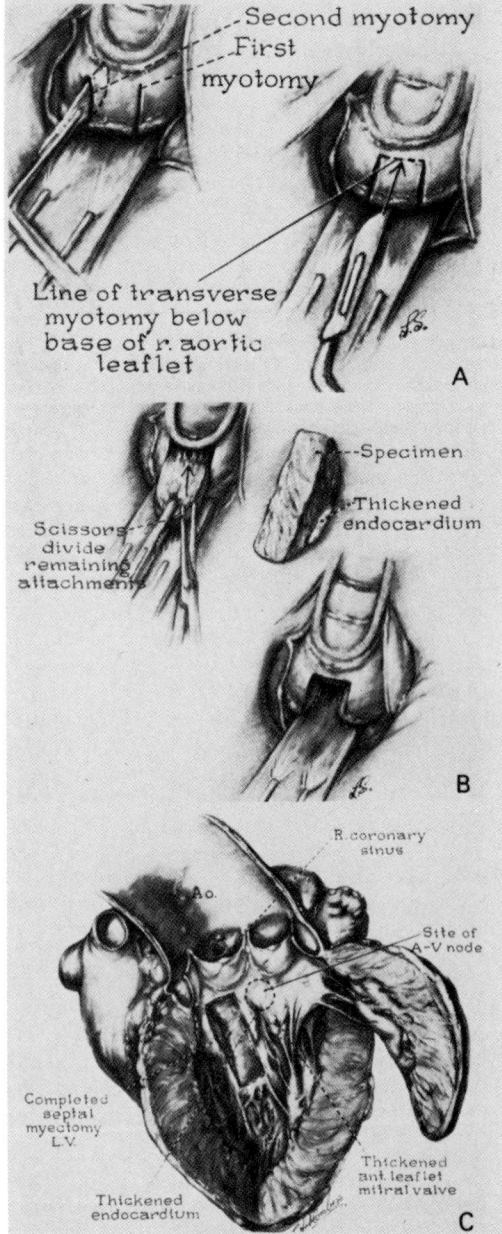

Figure 3. Septal myotomy-myectomy for hypertrophic cardiomyopathy. *A*, The aortic valve is retracted, and two parallel cuts are made in the ventricular septum. *B*, The portion of septum between the two incisions is excised, leaving a rectangular channel in the outflow tract. *C*, View of the open left ventricle and aorta demonstrating the relationships between the site of the myectomy, the aortic valve leaflets, and the conduction tissue. (From Morrow, A. G.: Operative methods utilized to relieve left ventricular outflow obstruction. J. Thorac. Cardiovasc. Surg., *76:*423, 1978.)

indications include older patients with severe mitral regurgitation or very large gradients.

The preferred method is currently not established. Most surgeons have based the decision on preoperative criteria, but the NIH group has emphasized the use of echocardiography. Preoperative evaluation with two-dimensional echocardiography has identified differing morphologic patterns of septal hypertrophy[43] (Fig. 4). The apparent increase in atypical patients may be related to the current trend of recommending surgical therapy only for the most severely involved patients.[65] The NIH experience with intraoperative echo mapping of septal morphology has provided criteria for choosing between septal M-M and MVR. The primary indications for MVR are inaccessible

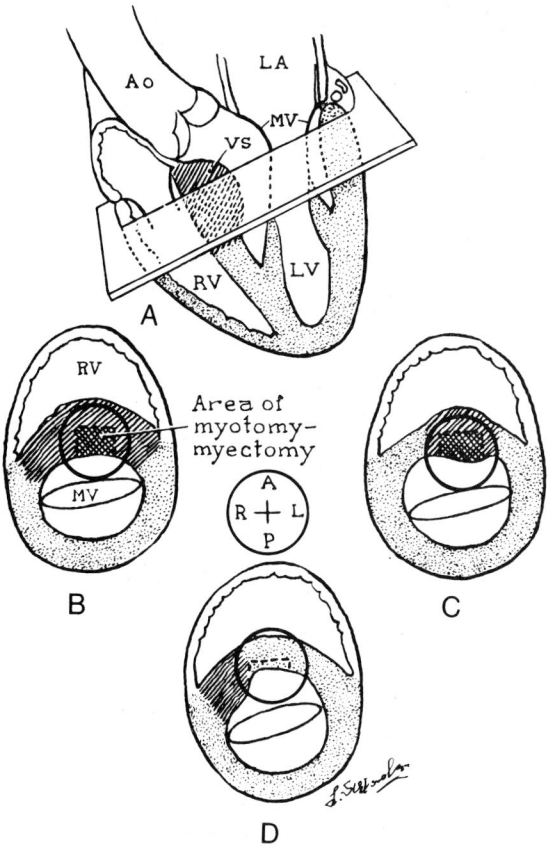

Figure 4. Morphologic spectrum of hypertrophic cardiomyopathy. *A*, Longitudinal cross-sectional plane through left ventricle showing hypertrophy of the ventricular septum. *B* to *D*, Short-axis views of left ventricle at mitral valve level shown in the echocardiographic orientation. *B*, Homogeneous thickening of anterior septum permits myectomy to be performed through conventional aortotomy (circle indicates superimposed aortic ring). *C*, Septal thickening is central. Myectomy can still be performed, but must be confined to the thickened segment. *D*, Thickening of anterior basal septum shows an inhomogeneous pattern. Myectomy cannot be performed in the conventional position because of the risk of septal perforation. Mitral valve replacement would be an alternative operation in such a patient. (From McIntosh, C. L., and Maron, B. J.: Current operative treatment of obstructive hypertrophic cardiomyopathy. Circulation, 78:487, 1988.)

septal hypertrophy and relative thinness of the basal septum of less than 18 mm. (Table 2).

Increasing numbers of patients require associated coronary artery bypass grafting.[49] A report of 28 patients undergoing coronary revascularization and septal M-M indicated a high incidence of ventricular septal defect due to septal ischemia or atypical septal morphology.[62] Other less well established or newer procedures should be mentioned. In children with bilat-

eral obstruction of the septum, thinning of the septum from the right ventricular side was reported in 1967.[17] Aortoventriculoplasty with opening of the aortic anulus through a commissure and without aortic valve replacement has been performed.[65] A recent report describes a patch septoplasty performed through the right ventricle without injuring the aortic valve.[16] Newer proposed procedures include transaortic plication of the mitral valve at the site of contact with the septum and transarterial laser myoplasty.[42,44,59] The effectiveness and safety of this latter procedure have not been established. The role of the automatic implantable cardiac defibrillator for HCM patients at increased risk of sudden death is currently being evaluated.[44]

RESULTS OF SURGICAL TREATMENT

Several large series report favorable initial and late results following surgical treatment of HCM.[30,42,44,49,50] The operative mortality is 5 to 8 per cent with no clear difference between septal M-M and MVR.[30,38,43,49] Operative mortality is increased in older patients and in those undergoing associated procedures such as coronary bypass grafting.[49] Complications of septal M-M include ventricular septal defect, complete heart block, and aortic or mitral valve damage. The incidence of these complications is usually less than 5 per cent.[43,49,66] Postoperative aortic insufficiency has been demonstrated in 54 per cent of patients by echo Doppler, although only 12 per cent were detected clinically. The degree of insufficiency was not progressive and was thought to be caused by leaflet trauma or loss of subvalvular support.[58] Aortic valve replacement has rarely been required.[49] These complications are not seen following MVR, but it is accompanied by the well-known sequelae of prosthetic valves, which include endocarditis, thromboembolism, anticoagulant-related bleeding, and deterioration of the prosthesis.[44]

Seventy per cent of 240 patients operated on by Morrow between 1960 and 1982 achieved long-lasting symptomatic relief; 123 of these were followed for up to 25 years, and two thirds maintained this improvement.[43] The mechanism of symptomatic improvement is relief of obstruction, and this has been documented in over 70 per cent of patients undergoing postoperative cardiac catheterization.[66] The resting gradient is effectively eliminated, but it is usually possible to provoke a postoperative gradient, which is of unknown significance.[43]

Mitral regurgitation is almost always improved by surgical therapy.[19] One third of patients in a recent series had significant mitral regurgitation preoperatively, and in 75 per cent it was greatly relieved or eliminated by septal M-M.[49] Postoperative echocardiographic studies demonstrate increased width of the outflow tract at the site of the septal M-M, decreased velocity of blood flow, decreased systolic anterior motion of the mitral valve, and reduced resting gradient[63] (Fig. 5). Measurements of myocardial oxygen consumption during exercise or atrial pacing

TABLE 2. Criteria for Mitral Valve Replacement in Patients with Obstructive Hypertrophic Cardiomyopathy

Criterion	Number of Patients
Interventricular septum < 18 mm. in usual region of resection	29
Atypical septal morphology	14
Previous left ventricular myomectomy with persistent obstruction and symptoms	15
Organic mitral valve disease and hypertrophic cardiomyopathy (excluded for this study)	(4)
Total	58

From McIntosh, C. L., Greenberg, G. J., Maron, B. J., Leon, M. B., Cannon, R. O., and Clark, R. E.: Clinical and hemodynamic results after mitral valve replacement in patients with obstructive hypertrophic cardiomyopathy. Ann. Thorac. Surg. 47:236, 1989.

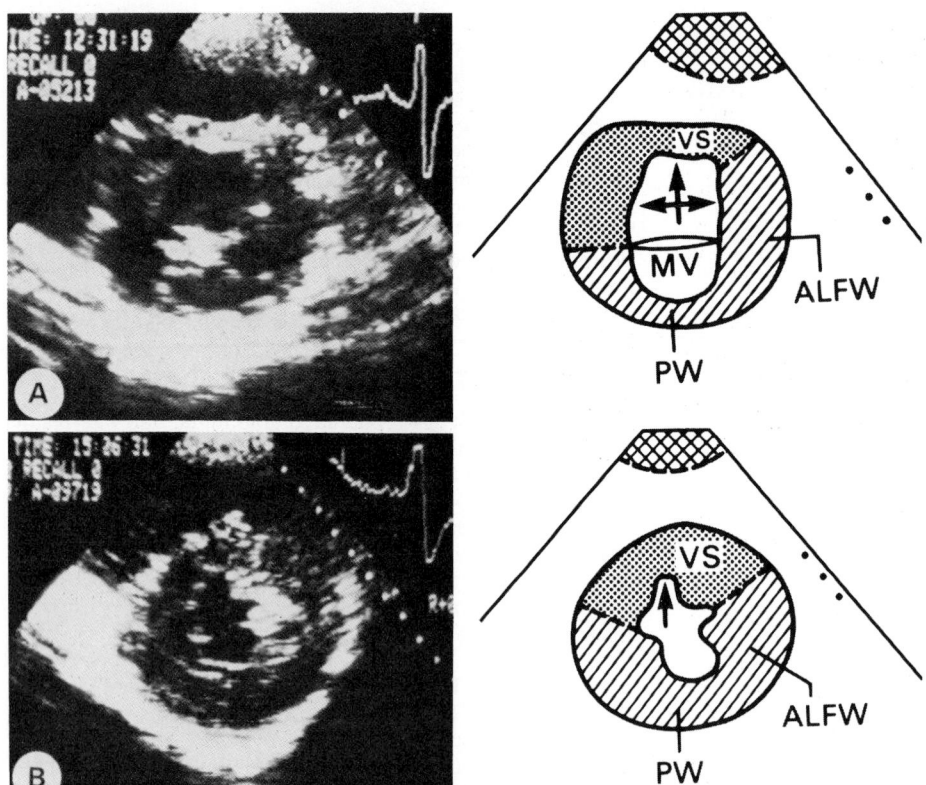

Figure 5. Two-dimensional echocardiograms illustrating the size and location of septal myotomy-myectomy. *A*, Echocardiogram from a patient with no postoperative basal or provocable gradient. An extensive myotomy-myectomy involving the central septum as well as adjacent segments has greatly increased the size of outflow tract. *B*, Echocardiogram from a patient with a postoperative basal gradient of 70 mm. Hg and a provocable gradient of 150 mm. Hg. The myotomy-myectomy (arrow) is limited to the medial portion of the ventricular septum. ALFW, anterolateral free wall; PW, posterior wall; VS, ventricular septum. (From Spirito, P., Maron, B. J., and Rosing, D. R.: Morphologic determinants of hemodynamic state after ventricular septal myotomy-myectomy in patients with obstructive hypertrophic cardiomyopathy: M mode and two-dimensional echocardiographic assessment. Circulation, 70:984, 1984.)

indicate that exercise capacity may be improved by reduction in the gradient and reduction in left ventricular end-diastolic pressure.[10] Coronary flow and myocardial oxygen consumption decrease after surgical relief of obstruction.[11]

There are no randomized comparisons of surgical and medical treatment, nor are there randomized studies comparing MVR with septal M-M. The earlier multicenter study by Shah and co-workers indicated a 3 to 4 per cent annual mortality following medical treatment although this was prior to currently available pharmacologic agents.[61] A subsequent study by McKenna and Camm reported the incidence of sudden death between 2 and 3 per cent annually.[45] The longest available surgical results are from Morrow's series with a 2.2 per cent annual mortality over an 11.5 year follow-up. These results are compared with recent findings of an annual mortality of 1 per cent in patients less than 65 years of age.[49,50] Based on these results, it has been recommended that symptomatic patients and asymptomatic patients with a resting or inducible gradient of greater than 80 mm. Hg be treated surgically.[50] Other authors have recently reported an improved late morality of 1.3 per cent per year following MVR and 0.7 per cent per year after septal M-M, and a sudden death rate of 0.3 per cent per year.[29] Additional studies indicate that amiodarone can reduce the incidence of sudden death.[47,48] A late survival study reports 56 per cent 10-year survival in control patients compared with 80 per cent in those treated with verapamil. The best results were in patients who were maintained on long-term verapamil after successful surgical therapy. These authors concluded that septal M-M improves systolic pressure overload, the addition of verapamil improves diastolic function, and the combination maximizes survival.[60]

The operation of choice continues to be septal M-M, based on recent excellent results.[49,50] Other groups, however, are currently treating between a quarter and a third of patients with MVR.[29,30,42,44] Based on these reports, there is no significant difference in operative mortality or 10-year survival, comparing the two operations. MVR is reserved for patients with severe hemodynamic obstruction, those with severe mitral regurgita-

tion, or those undergoing repeat operation.[30] Intraoperative echocardiographic findings of a thin basal ventricular septum or atypical obstruction also favors MVR.[44] MVR produces a more consistent decrease in diastolic pressure and may be the preferred operation for patients with alterations in diastolic function or ventricular compliance.[42,66] A more standardized approach for those centers encountering only an occasional patient with HCM may be MVR.[66] There are two acceptable operations for HCM that give comparable immediate and late results. The exact indications for each of these procedures await further studies including additional experience with intraoperative echocardiography.

SELECTED REFERENCES

Abelman, W. H., and Lorell, B. H.: The challenge of cardiomyopathy. J. Am. Coll. Cardiol., 13:1219, 1989.
"This article is part of a series of anniversary seminars of The American College of Cardiology attempting to set the stage for the future by describing current state-of-the-art management of selected major cardiovascular problems and the basic knowledge that will provide directions for advances in diagnosis and therapy." This purpose is admirably achieved by the authors in the review of the principal forms of cardiomyopathy. Over half of the article concerns hypertrophic cardiomyopathy and presents current concepts of pathogenesis and medical treatment, and emphasis is placed on recent developments and unresolved questions.

Krajcer, A., Leachman, R. D., Cooley, D. A., and Coronado, R.: Septal myotomy-myomectomy versus mitral valve replacement in hypertrophic cardiomyopathy. Circulation, 80:I-57, 1989.
The group of surgeons at the Texas Heart Institute initially recommended mitral valve replacement (MVR) as an alternative treatment for obstructive hypertrophic cardiomyopathy. This article summarizes their 22-year experience with 185 patients with about two thirds receiving septal myotomy-myectomy (M-M) and one third an MVR. No difference in mortality, symptomatic improvement, or hemodynamic benefit was found between the two methods of treatment. They recommend septal M-M as the procedure of choice and reserve MVR for severely symptomatic patients with a large outflow gradient, for those with severe mitral insufficiency, and for those who fail to improve after septal M-M.

Maron, B. J., Bonow, R. O., Cannon, R. O., Leon, M. B., and Epstein, S. E.: Hypertrophic cardiomyopathy: Interrelations of clinical manifestations, pathophysiology, and therapy. N. Engl. J. Med., 316:780(Part I); 844(Part II), 1987.
This two-part article is a portion of the Medical Progress Series and is an excellent review of the extensive experience from the National Institutes of Health. Empha-

sis is placed on the relationships between pathophysiologic mechanisms, the clinical manifestation, and the indications for and responses to therapy. The early and late surgical results in 240 patients treated by septal M-M are presented and support the recommendation that it is the preferred operation for most patients with obstructive hypertrophic cardiomyopathy.

McIntosh, C. L., and Maron, B. J.: Current operative treatment of obstructive hypertrophic cardiomyopathy.Circulation, 78:487, 1988.
This article from the Clinical Progress Series presents an excellent review of operative treatment of hypertrophic cardiomyopathy at the National Institutes of Health. The use of intraoperative echocardiography is described and the role of MVR is discussed. The results of Morrow's personal series of 240 patients operated on utilizing septal M-M are presented. These are contrasted to and compared with the experience with 156 patients treated after Morrow's death. One third of this recent group was treated by MVR, and the changing emphasis on this procedure is clearly summarized.

McIntosh, C. L., Greenberg, G. J., Maron, B. J., Leon, M. B., Cannon, R. O., and Clark, R. E.: Clinical and hemodynamic results after mitral valve replacement in patients with obstructive hypertrophic cardiomyopathy. Ann. Thorac. Surg., 47:236, 1989.
By 1989, the experience at the National Institutes of Health included 58 patients with hypertrophic cardiomyopathy treated by MVR. This is an interesting change over the short time span since the preceding two selected references. The criteria for MVR are clearly presented, and the use of intraoperative echocardiography is well described. Early results and complications are presented, but long-term results are not available. The discussion which followed the presentation of this material indicates that strong opinions exist concerning the role of MVR in treating this disease process.

Mohr, R., Schaff, H. V., Danielson, G. K., Puga, F. J., Pluth, J. R., and Tajik, A. J.: The outcome of surgical treatment of hypertrophic obstructive cardiomyopathy. J. Thorac. Cardiovasc. Surg., 97:666, 1989.
The 15-year experience at the Mayo Clinic with surgical treatment of 115 patients with hypertrophic cardiomyopathy is presented. In contrast to the preceding references, only six patients had MVR. Septal M-M is documented to be a low-risk procedure that effectively relieves symptoms in 90 per cent of patients. The late results in patients under 65 years of age indicate a linearized mortality of 1 per cent per year. This is one of the few reports suggesting that the late survival may actually be improved by surgical treatment in appropriately chosen patients.

Morrow, A. G.: Hypertrophic subaortic stenosis. J. Thorac. Cardiovasc. Surg., 76:423, 1978.
This article should be read in its entirety prior to performing any operation for hypertrophic cardiomyopathy. The report is a technical description of the operative methods developed by Morrow based on his large personal experience. Each step of the procedure is precisely described and clearly demonstrated by the lucid Schlossberg illustrations. The author's personal style is most apparent in the informative section entitled "Details considered to be of special importance." The article is a distillation of experience with 217 patients undergoing the operation by Morrow at the National Institutes of Health.

REFERENCES

1. Abelmann, W. H., and Lorell, B. H.: The challenge of cardiomyopathy. J. Am. Coll. Cardiol., 12:1219, 1989.
2. Barr, P. A., Celermajer, J. M., Bowdler, J. D., and Cartmill, T. B.: Idiopathic hypertrophic obstructive cardiomyopathy causing severe right ventricular outflow tract obstruction in infancy. Br. Heart J., 35:1109, 1973.
3. Binet, J. P., Langlois, J., Leiva-Semper, A., David, P., and Bigelow, W. G.: Ventriculomyotomy in hypertrophies of the left ventricle. J. Thorac. Cardiovasc. Surg., 56:469, 1968.
4. Bonow, R. O.: Left ventricular ejection dynamics and outflow obstruction in hypertrophic cardiomyopathy. J. Am. Coll. Cardiol., 13:1280, 1989.
5. Braunwald, E., Lambrew, C. T., Morrow, A. G., Pierce, G. E., Rockoff, S. D., and Ross, J., Jr.: Idiopathic hypertrophic subaortic stenosis. Circulation, 30:IV-1, 1964.
6. Brigden, W.: Hypertrophic cardiomyopathy. Br. Heart J., 58:299, 1987.
7. Brock, R. C.: Functional obstruction of the left ventricle. Acquired aortic subvalvar stenosis. Guy's Hosp. Rep., 106:221, 1957.
8. Camici, P., Chiriatti, G., Lorenzoni, R., Salvadori, P., Parodi, O., Guzzardi, R., Papi, L., and Bellina, C. R.: Regional myocardial blood flow in hypertrophic cardiomyopathy assessed by N23-ammonia and positron emission tomography. Circulation, 80:II-663, 1989.
9. Cannon, R. O., O'Gara, P., Udelson, J. M., and Bonow, R. O.: Significance of reversible thallium perfusion defects in hypertrophic cardiomyopathy. Circulation, 80:II-663, 1989.
10. Cannon, R. O., Schenke, W. H., and McIntosh, C. L.: Exercise capacity after surgery for obstructive hypertrophic cardiomyopathy. Circulation, 80:II-663, 1989.
11. Cannon, R. O., McIntosh, C. L., Schenke, W. H., Maron, B. J., Bonow, R. O., and Epstein, S. E.: Effect of surgical reduction of left ventricular outflow obstruction on hemodynamics, coronary flow, and myocardial metabolism in hypertrophic cardiomyopathy. Circulation, 79:766, 1989.
12. Charles, R., Makin, C., Coulshed, N., and Hamilton, D.: Echocardiography in combined discrete and hypertrophic subaortic stenosis. Thorax, 36:126, 1981.
13. Chikamori, T., Dickie, S., Poloniecki, J. D., Sugrue, D. D., Stewart, R., Myers,

M. J., Lavender, J. P., and McKenna, W. J.: Mechanism of exercise limitation in hypertrophic cardiomyopathy. Circulation, 80:II-664, 1989.
14. Choi, B. W., McCarthy, K. E., and Bacharach, S. L.: Left ventricular end diastolic volume response to exercise in hypertrophic cardiomyopathy. Circulation, 80:II-664, 1989.
15. Cleland, W. P.: The surgical management of obstructive cardiomyopathy. J. Cardiovasc. Surg., 4:489, 1963.
16. Cooley, D. A., and Garrett, J. R.: Septoplasty for left ventricular outflow obstruction without aortic valve replacement: A new technique. Ann. Thorac. Surg., 42:445, 1986.
17. Cooley, D. A., Bloodwell, R. D., Hallman, G. L., LaSorte, A. F., Leachman, R. D., and Chapman, D. W.: Surgical treatment of muscular subaortic stenosis. Circulation, 35-36:I-124, 1967.
18. Cooley, D. A., Leachman, R. D., Hallman, G. L., Gerami, S., and Hall, R. D.: Idiopathic hypertrophic subaortic stenosis: Surgical treatment including mitral valve replacement. Arch. Surg., 103:606, 1971.
19. Cooper, M. M., Tucker, E., McIntosh, C. L., Cannon, R. O., and Clark, R. E.: Effect of left ventricular septal myectomy on concurrent mitral regurgitation. Ann. Thorac. Surg., 48:251, 1989.
20. Davies, M. J.: The current status of myocardial disarray in hypertrophic cardiomyopathy. Br. Heart J., 51:361, 1984.
21. Dembitsky, W. P., and Weldon, C. S.: Clinical experience with the use of a valve-bearing conduit to construct a second left ventricular outflow tract in cases of unresectable intra-ventricular obstruction. Ann. Surg., 184:317, 1976.
22. Fananapazir, L., Tracy, C. M., Leon, M. B., Whinkler, J. B., Cannon, R. O., Bonow, R. O., Maron, B. J., and Epstein, S. E.: Electrophysiologic abnormalities in patients with hypertrophic cardiomyopathy. A consecutive analysis in 155 patients. Circulation, 80:1259, 1989.
23. Gould, K. L.: Myocardial metabolism by positron emission tomography in hypertrophic cardiomyopathy. J. Am. Coll. Cardiol., 13:325, 1989.
24. Grover-McKay, M., Schwaiger, M., Krivokapich, J., Perloff, J. K., Phelps, M. E., and Schelbert, H. R.: Regional myocardial blood flow and metabolism at rest in mildly symptomatic patients with hypertrophic cardiomyopathy. J. Am. Coll. Cardiol., 13:317, 1989.
25. Harken, D. E.: Discussion of Dobell, A. R. C., and Scott, H. J.: Hypertrophic subaortic stenosis: Evolution of a surgical technique. J. Thorac. Cardiovasc. Surg., 47:33, 1964.
26. Hess, O. M., Schneider, J., Turina, M., Carroll, J. D., Rothlin, M., and Krayenbuehl, H. P.: Asymmetric septal hypertrophy in patients with aortic stenosis: An adaptive mechanism or a coexistence of hypertrophic cardiomyopathy? J. Am. Coll. Cardiol., 1:783, 1983.
27. Kirklin, J. W., and Ellis, F. H.: Surgical relief of diffuse subvalvular aortic stenosis. Circulation, 24:739, 1961.
28. Koch, J-P., Maron, B. J., Epstein, S. E., and Morrow, A. G.: Results of operation for obstructive hypertrophic cardiomyopathy in the elderly. Septal myotomy and myectomy in 20 patients 65 years of age or older. Am. J. Cardiol., 46:963, 1980.
29. Krajcer, Z., Leachman, R. D., Cooley, D. A., Ostojic, M., and Coronado, R.: Mitral valve replacement and septal myomectomy in hypertrophic cardiomyopathy. Circulation, 78:I-35, 1988.
30. Krajcer, Z., Leachman, R. D., Cooley, D. A., and Coronado, R.: Septal myotomy-myectomy versus mitral valve replacement in hypertrophic cardiomyopathy. Circulation, 80:I-57, 1989.
31. Krasnow, N.: An acquired disease component in hypertrophic cardiomyopathy: New clinical clarifications. J. Am. Coll. Cardiol., 13:46, 1989.
32. Lever, H. M., Karam, R. F., Currie, P. J., and Healy, B. P.: Hypertrophic cardiomyopathy in the elderly. Distinctions from the young based on cardiac shape. Circulation, 79:580, 1989.
33. Levine, R. A., Gieseking, E., Lefebvre, X., Cape, E. G., Sung, H., and Yoganathan, A. P.: Increased outflow tract velocity fails to produce systolic anterior motion of a normally restrained mitral valve in vitro. Circulation, 80:II-662, 1989.
34. Levine, R. A., Viahakes, G. J., Gieseking, E., Cape, E. G., Guerrero, J. L., Yoganathan, A. P., and Weyman, A. E.: New insights into the mechanism of obstruction in hypertrophic cardiomyopathy: Experimental models. Circulation, 80:II-662, 1989.
35. Lewis, J. F., and Maron, B. J.: Elderly patients with hypertrophic cardiomyopathy: A subset with distinctive left ventricular morphology and progressive clinical course late in life. J. Am. Coll. Cardiol., 13:36, 1989.
36. Lillehei, C. W., and Levy, M. J.: Transatrial exposure for correction of subaortic stenosis. J.A.M.A., 186:8, 1963.
37. Maron, B. J., Bonow, R. O., Cannon, R. O., Leon, M. B., and Epstein, S. E.: Hypertrophic cardiomyopathy: Interrelations of clinical manifestations, pathophysiology, and therapy. Part I. N. Engl. J. Med., 316:780, 1987.
38. Maron, B. J., Bonow, R. O., Cannon, R. O., Leon, M. B., and Epstein, S. E.: Hypertrophic cardiomyopathy. Interrelations of clinical manifestations, pathophysiology, and therapy. Part II. N. Engl. J. Med., 316:844, 1987.
39. Maron, B. J., Tajik, A. J., Ruttenberg, H. D., Graham, T. P., Atwood, G. F., Victorica, B. E., Lie, J. T., and Roberts, W. C.: Hypertrophic cardiomyopathy in infants: Clinical features and natural history. Circulation, 65:7, 1982.
40. Maron, B. J., Gottdiener, J. S., Arce, J., Rosing, D. R., Wesley, Y. E., and Epstein, S. E.: Dynamic subaortic obstruction in hypertrophic cardiomyopathy: Analysis by pulsed Doppler echocardiography. J. Am. Coll. Cardiol., 6:1, 1985.
41. Maron, B. J., Spirito, P., Green, K. J., Wesley, Y. E., Bonow, R. O., and Arce, J.: Noninvasive assessment of left ventricular diastolic function by pulsed

Doppler echocardiography in patients with hypertrophic cardiomyopathy. J. Am. Coll. Cardiol., *10*:733, 1987.

42. McIntosh, C.: Commentary on comparison of ventricular septal surgery and mitral valve replacement for hypertrophic obstructive cardiomyopathy. Ann. Thorac. Surg., *48*:535, 1989.

43. McIntosh, C. L., and Maron, B. J.: Current operative treatment of obstructive hypertrophic cardiomyopathy. Circulation, *78*:487, 1988.

44. McIntosh, C. L., Greenberg, G. J., Maron, B. J., Leon, M. B., Cannon, R. O., and Clark, R. E.: Clinical and hemodynamic results after mitral valve replacement in patients with obstructive hypertrophic cardiomyopathy. Ann. Thorac. Surg., *47*:236, 1989.

45. McKenna, W. J., and Camm, A. J.: Sudden death in hypertrophic cardiomyopathy. Circulation, *80*:1489, 1989.

46. McKenna, W. J., Adams, K. M., Poloniecki, J. D., Dickie, S., Oakley, C. M., Kirkler, D. M., and Goodwin, J. F.: Long term survival with amiodarone in patients with hypertrophic cardiomyopathy and ventricular tachycardia. Circulation, *80*:II-7, 1989.

47. McKenna, W. J., Oakley, C. M., Kirkler, D. M., and Goodwin, J. F.: Improved survival with amiodarone in patients with hypertrophic cardiomyopathy and ventricular tachycardia. Br. Heart J., *53*:412, 1985.

48. McKenna, W. J., Harris, L., Towland, E., et al.: Amiodarone for long-term management of patients with hypertrophic cardiomyopathy. Am. J. Cardiol., *54*:802, 1984.

49. Mohr, R., Schaff, H. V., Danielson, G. K., Puga, F. J., Pluth, J. R., and Tajik, A. J.: The outcome of surgical treatment of hypertrophic obstructive cardiomyopathy. J. Thorac. Cardiovasc. Surg., *97*:666, 1989.

50. Mohr, R., Schaff, H. V., Puga, F. J., and Danielson, G. K.: Results of operation for hypertrophic obstructive cardiomyopathy in children and adults less than 40 years of age. Circulation, *80*:I-191, 1989.

51. Morrow, A. G.: Hypertrophic subaortic stenosis. Operative methods utilized to relieve left ventricular outflow obstruction. J. Thorac. Cardiovasc. Surg., *76*:423, 1978.

52. Morrow, A. G., and Brockenbrough, E. C.: Surgical treatment of idiopathic hypertrophic subaortic stenosis. Technic and hemodynamic results of subaortic ventriculotomy. Ann. Surg., *154*:181, 1961.

53. Morrow, A. G., Reitz, B. A., Epstein, S. E., Henry, W. L., Conkle, D. M., Itscoitz, S. B., and Redwood, D. R.: Operative treatment in hypertrophic subaortic stenosis. Techniques, and the results of pre and postoperative assessments in 83 patients. Circulation, *52*:88, 1975.

54. Nicod, P., Polikar, R., and Peterson, K. L.: Hypertrophic cardiomyopathy and sudden death. N. Engl. J. Med., *318*:1255, 1988.

55. O'Shea, J. P., Viahakes, G. J., Guerrero, J. L., Svizzero, T., Weyman, A. E., and

Levine, R. A.: Mechanism of obstruction of hypertrophic cardiomyopathy: Increasing septal thickness potentiates the effect of systolic anterior motion in an experimental echocardiographic model (Abstract). Circulation, *80*:II-269, 1989.

56. Pearce, B., Sheikh, K. H., and Kisslo, J.: Relationship of mitral regurgitation to left ventricular outflow obstruction in hypertrophic cardiomyopathy. Circulation, *80*:II-663, 1989.

57. Rastan, H., and Koncz, J.: Aortoventriculoplasty: A new technique for the treatment of left ventricular outflow tract obstruction. J. Thorac. Cardiovasc. Surg., *71*:920, 1976.

58. Sasson, A., Prieur, T., Skrobik, Y., Fulop, J. C., Williams, W. G., Henderson, M. A., Gresser, C., Wigle, E. D., and Rakowski, H.: Aortic regurgitation: A common complication after surgery for hypertrophic obstructive cardiomyopathy. J. Am. Coll. Cardiol., *13*:63, 1989.

59. Serruys, P. W., and den Boer, A.: What will be the requirement for acute interventional procedures in Europe? Eur. Heart J. (Suppl. F), *8*:55, 1987.

60. Seiler, C., Hess, O. M., Schoenbeck, M., Turina, J., Jenni, R., Turina, M., and Krayenbuehl, H. P.: Long-term follow-up in hypertrophic cardiomyopathy: Medical versus operative therapy. Circulation, *80*:II-6, 1989.

61. Shah, P. M., Adelman, A. G., Wigle, E. D., Gobel, F. L., Burchell, H. B., Hardarson, T., Curiel, R., de la Caizada, C., Oakley, C. M., and Goodwin, J. F.: The natural (and unnatural) history of hypertrophic obstructive cardiomyopathy: A multicenter study. Circ. Res., *35*:II-179, 1974.

62. Siegman, I. L., Maron, B. J., Permut, L. C., McIntosh, C. L., and Clark, R. E.: Results of operation for coexistent obstructive hypertrophic cardiomyopathy and coronary artery disease. J. Am. Coll. Cardiol., *13*:1527, 1989.

63. Spirito, P., Maron, B. J., and Rosing, D. R.: Morphologic determinants of hemodynamic state after ventricular septal myotomy-myectomy in patients with obstructive hypertrophic cardiomyopathy: M mode and two-dimensional echocardiographic assessment. Circulation, *70*:984, 1984.

64. Teare, D.: Asymmetrical hypertrophy of the heart in young adults. Br. Heart J., *20*:1, 1958.

65. Vouhe, P. R., Poulain, H., Bloch, G., Loisance, D. Y., Gamain, J., Lombaert, M., Quiret, J-C., Lesbre, J-P., Bernasconi, P., Pietri, J., and Cachera, J-P.: Aortoseptal approach for optimal resection of diffuse subvalvular aortic stenosis. J. Thorac. Cardiovasc. Surg., *87*:887, 1984.

66. Walker, W. S., Reid, K. G., Cameron, E. W. J., Walbaum, P. R., and Kitchin, A. H.: Comparison of ventricular septal surgery and mitral valve replacement for hypertrophic obstructive cardiomyopathy. Ann. Thorac. Surg., *48*:528, 1989.

67. Wigel, E. D.: Hypertrophic cardiomyopathy: A 1987 viewpoint. Circulation, *75*:311, 1987.

XVIII

MITRAL AND TRICUSPID VALVE DISEASE

J. Scott Rankin, M.D.

> There can be no more fascinating problem in surgery than the relief of pathological conditions of the valves of the heart.
>
> *Sir Henry Souttar, 1925*

Surgical therapy for acquired disorders of the atrioventricular valves has evolved rapidly since the first intracardiac operations were performed for mitral stenosis. Knowledge has progressed to allow prosthetic valve replacement or complex valve reconstructions to be performed on a routine basis. This chapter concerns the basic and clinical features of mitral and tricuspid valve disease with particular emphasis on surgical management.

HISTORICAL ASPECTS

Vesalius originally suggested the term *mitral* valve because of the resemblance to a bishop's miter, and Vieussens, in 1715, provided the earliest and most lucid description of the symptoms and pathologic process of calcific mitral stenosis. During the nineteenth and early twentieth centuries, most physicians believed that symptoms in mitral valve disease were caused by rheumatic myocarditis or myocardial failure, with valve lesions being of secondary importance. To quote Sir James Mackenzie,

"In chronic valvular affections, the subjective symptoms of heart failure only arise when exhaustion of the heart muscle sets in." Despite the prevailing attitude, Sir Lauder Brunton in 1902 suggested surgical enlargement of the stenotic mitral orifice and was immediately met with a barrage of controversy. In 1923, Elliot Cutler and associates performed the first successful intracardiac operation in man. Using a transventricular approach, they incised the anterior leaflet of a stenotic mitral valve with a tenotomy knife in a 15-year-old girl. The patient recovered, appeared to be improved symptomatically, but died 4 years later of progressive heart failure. The next six patients undergoing mitral valvotomy by Cutler expired, probably from acute mitral regurgitation, and the operation was thereafter abandoned.

Sir Henry Souttar of the London Hospital should be credited with suggesting the transatrial approach for valvotomy. Operating on a 19-year-old woman in 1925, and intending to incise the anterior leaflet, he encountered significant mitral regurgitation and only a "moderate degree" of stenosis after introducing his finger through the left atrial appendage. He instead performed "such dilatation as could be carried out by the finger," and the patient was said to be "greatly improved" postoperatively. There occurred, however, a reaction in the medical community against direct valve procedures (perhaps led by the physician-in-charge of the cardiac department of the London Hospital, Sir James Mackenzie), and Souttar received no more referrals of patients with mitral stenosis.

Although Murray, Smithy, and others attempted mitral procedures during the ensuing 20 years, the next breakthrough was attained by Bailey in 1948. After four fatal attempts, Bailey performed a successful transatrial mitral commissurotomy by use of a hooked knife blade attached to the index finger. Successful procedures by Harken and Brock followed shortly thereafter, and further refinements by Dubost, Edwards, and Logan established the use of mechanical dilators. With this work, and the subsequent introduction of cardiopulmonary bypass and open commissurotomy, the surgical treatment of mitral stenosis became firmly established.

Early attempts at correction of mitral incompetence involved the closed placement of intravalvular stents by Murray or external circumferential suture reduction of the mitral anulus by Glover and Davila. McGoon, Frater, Merendino, Gerbode, and others subsequently devised methods of repairing chordal or leaflet defects, and Wooler, Reed, Kay, and their associates developed lateral commissural suture techniques for mitral anuloplasty. Harken and Starr began the era of cardiac valvular replacement in 1960 by successfully replacing the aortic and mitral valves with totally mechanical prostheses.

NORMAL ANATOMY AND PHYSIOLOGY

The fibrous skeleton of the heart, to which the valves attach, is developmentally derived from the endocardial cushions. The fibrous anulus of the mitral valve is a thin, incomplete ring of fibrous tissue, which is most apparent at two points, the right and left fibrous trigones (Fig. 1). The left fibrous trigone is situated at the left anterior aspect of the mitral ring and consists of fibrous tissue joining the mitral ring to the base of the aorta. The right fibrous trigone, or central fibrous body, lies in the midline of the heart and represents confluence of fibrous tissue from the mitral valve, the tricuspid valve, the membranous septum, and the posterior aspect of the base of the aorta.

Although small portions of the anterior leaflets of the mitral and tricuspid valves are derived from the endocardial cushions, the majority of the valve tissue is elaborated from the internal layer of the muscular ventricular wall by the process of diverticularization and undermining. The valve tissue at first is a thick and muscular "skirt," originating from the atrioventricular junction and attaching lower to the ventricular walls. The mitral valve is initially quadricuspid, and as the cusps are transformed into thin fibrous leaflets, the accessory or commissural cusps become less prominent. In most adults, only two leaflets are

evident, the anterior leaflet and the posterior leaflet (Fig. 1). The commissures do not divide the leaflet tissue completely to the valve anulus, and the basal aspects at the commissures are composed of continuous valvular tissue. The anterior leaflet has a much longer base-to-margin length than does the posterior leaflet; however, the annular attachment of the posterior leaflet is twice as great, so that the surface areas of each leaflet are almost identical. Both leaflets are approximately the shape of a trapezoid, each attaching by thin fibrous chordae tendineae to *both* the anterior and posterior papillary muscles, that is, the chordae from each papillary muscle fan out and attach to nearly half of both cusp margins.

The papillary muscles arise from the ventricular walls, approximately two thirds of the distance toward the apex. The anterolateral papillary muscle is single in 75 per cent of patients, whereas its posteromedial counterpart commonly has multiple heads. Both papillary muscles have coronary arterial sources that are at some distance from the orifices of the coronary arteries. The anterolateral muscle is supplied by high lateral branches of the left anterior descending or circumflex system, and the posteromedial papillary muscle usually receives blood from posterolateral branches of the right coronary artery. In cases of left coronary dominance, posterolateral branches of the circumflex coronary artery supply the posterior papillary muscle. In 98 per cent of valves, the papillary muscle is an excellent guide to its corresponding commissure, and even in a severely fused valve, a single head generally points directly at the overlying commissure. With a bifid head, a groove is usually evident that is directly in line with the commissure. In most cases of double papillary muscles, the separation between the heads indicates the location of the corresponding commissure. In severely stenotic valves, a groove is often visible between the anterior and posterior sets of chordae arising from each papillary muscle. The groove is bordered by the chordae to each fan and has been termed the chordal gatepost because it forms a gateway to the overlying commissure. *First-order chordae* originate at or near the apices of the papillary muscles and insert into the free edges of the leaflets as fine strands. *Secondary chordae* also originate near the apices of the papillary muscles and insert into the ventricular surface of the leaflet 1 to 3 mm. from the free edge. Secondary chordae are usually thicker and less numerous than are the primary chordae. *Tertiary chordae* originate from the ventricular walls, insert along the basal aspects of the leaflets, and are more prominent in the posterior leaflet. The edges of the leaflets have a slightly serrated appearance owing to the insertion of chordae tendineae on the ventricular surface; these serrations mark the line of closure of the normal valve. Thus, the point of coaptation is not the free edge but is located a short distance proximally on the leaflet, and the leaflets coapt along a considerable area of their atrial surfaces.

The anatomy of the tricuspid valve apparatus is similar, except that three valve leaflets usually are evident: anterior, posterior, and septal (Fig. 1). The anterior leaflet commonly is the largest of the three, and the posterior the smallest, although multiple variations occur. The papillary muscles tend to be multiple but can be grouped into three components; anterior (arising from the right ventricular free wall), inferior (arising from the inferior septum), and septal (arising from the high septum in the area of the septal band). As in the mitral valve, papillary muscle groups tend to contribute chordae to multiple leaflets.

On histologic examination, the atrioventricular valve leaflets consist of a central fibrous layer that connects to the fibrous anulus. On each surface is an endocardial layer, composed of collagen, elastic tissue, and muscle cells, covered by a flat endothelial lining. Between the endocardial and fibrous layers is a matrix of loose connective tissue, the spongiosa. The central core of the chordae is collagen covered by endocardial cells contiguous with the lining of the ventricle. The layers of the chordae merge imperceptibly with those of the valve leaflets.

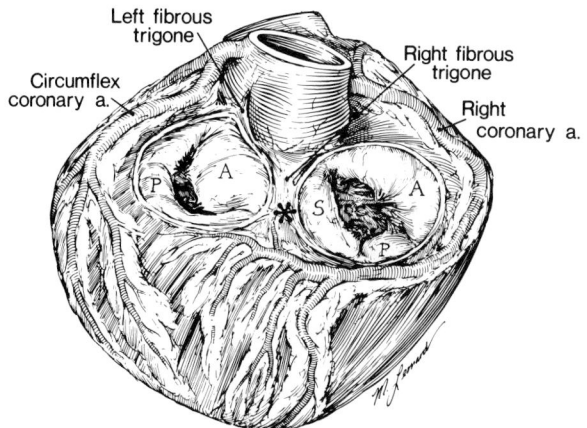

Figure 1. Anatomic interrelationships of the atrioventricular valves. A, anterior leaflet; P, posterior leaflet; S, septal leaflet; the asterisk represents the area of the bundle of His. (Redrawn from McAlpine, W. A.: Heart and Coronary Arteries. New York, Springer-Verlag, 1975.)

The function of the atrioventricular valves is to permit uninhibited flow of blood from the atria to the ventricles during ventricular diastole and to prevent reflux of blood into the atria during ventricular systole. The valves achieve this objective by a coordinated contraction of ventricular myocardium and the papillary muscles during the cardiac cycle. During systole, the valve is closed, and the left atrium serves as a reservoir for storing blood returning from the lungs. With isovolumic relaxation, left ventricular pressure falls, and when ventricular pressure becomes lower than that of the full atrium, the valve opens and initiates rapid filling of the ventricle. It is interesting to note that the highest filling velocities and the majority of diastolic ventricular filling occur during the rapid filling phase, before left ventricular pressure reaches its diastolic minimum. Early transmitral flow is produced not only by positive pressure gradients from the atrium to the ventricle, but also by active ventricular restorative forces related to myocardial relaxation.

Several factors contribute to mitral valve closure. First, deceleration of mitral flow during late rapid filling and after atrial systole is associated with partial closure of the valve leaflets. Flow deceleration produces positive pressure gradients from the ventricular to the atrial surfaces of the valve leaflets and initiates closure. Second, analyses of blood velocity patterns during filling demonstrate large asymmetric "ring vortices" produced by the incoming jet of blood striking the apex and spreading up the ventricular walls toward the base. These vortices then strike the ventricular surface of the leaflets and contribute to closure. There tends to be an asymmetry in the size of the vortices, with the larger being located behind the anterior leaflet. Flow deceleration and vortex strength have been shown to be of nearly equal importance to valve closure, achieving almost complete leaflet apposition by the onset of ventricular contraction. Finally, as ventricular systole begins, rising left ventricular pressure completely closes the valve with minimal retrograde flow. If it were not for flow deceleration and vortices, the magnitude of regurgitation during normal valve closure would be substantially greater.

The active motions of the mitral anulus and papillary muscles also contribute to valve competence. Anular area, determined by echocardiography, changes significantly during the cardiac cycle, decreasing by one third from end diastole to mid systole. The dynamic valve area curve appears similar to the ventricular volume curve, suggesting that active shortening of circumferential muscle bundles at the base reduces valve orifice area during systole and contributes to leaflet competence. Since the atrioventricular valves have no intrinsic structure, intact chordae and normal papillary muscle function are necessary for proper leaflet closure. During systole, contraction of each papillary muscle shortens the subvalvular apparatus and compensates for inward displacement of the ventricular walls. The systolic shortening characteristics of both papillary muscles are quite similar to segmental ventricular fiber shortening in the circumferential plane. With dilation of the mitral anulus, chordal rupture, or papillary muscle disruption, competence of the mitral valve is lost despite intact leaflets.

MITRAL STENOSIS

PATHOPHYSIOLOGY. A common etiologic factor of mitral stenosis remains rheumatic fever (RF). For nearly a century, the relationship between RF and an antecedent episode of Group A streptococcal pharyngitis has been documented, but the exact mechanism is still unclear. On serologic analysis, the magnitude of the immune response to the streptococcal infection, as assessed by antistreptolysin O testing, correlates with the clinical incidence of RF, which approaches 10 per cent in patients with strong antistreptolysin O responses. However, this remains only an association, and more investigation is necessary to verify autoimmune or other causal relationships.

There is often a disparity between the clinical severity of RF and the extent of pathologic changes. Clinically, RF is characterized by diffuse exudative and proliferative inflammatory reactions in the heart, joints, and skin. In the acute phase, myocarditis is associated with fibrinous degeneration and diffuse interstitial cellular infiltrates, predominantly lymphocytic. The exudative-degenerative phase continues for 2 to 3 weeks, followed by the development of the most characteristic histologic lesion of RF, the *Aschoff nodule*. The proliferative and healing phase then begins and may persist for many years. Gradual healing of Aschoff nodules leaves interstitial fibrous scars; however, the nodules may persist in surgical biopsies of the atrial appendage for many years after resolution of RF or streptococcal infections. Persistence of Aschoff bodies appears to correlate with progressive fibrosis and stenosis of the mitral valve.

The early valvular lesions of RF also are characterized by an acute inflammatory infiltrate that gradually heals by organization, producing fibrous tissue. Chronically, the leaflets become thickened by the fibrotic process, so that pliability and surface area are reduced. Fusion of the anterior and posterior leaflets may be severe, and in many cases, the commissures can no longer be identified. The scarring process may involve one or both commissures. Calcification may occur in the leaflets or in the fused commissures, being more common on the posteromedial aspect. The chordae are thickened, shortened, and fused by the same type of fibrosis, and occasionally the subvalvular apparatus may be calcified. The entire process transforms the mitral complex into a rigid funnel-shaped structure with a "fishmouth" opening. Occasionally, shortening, thickening, and fusion of the chordae predominate, even when valvular changes are minimal, producing primarily a subvalvular stenosis. Fibrosis may involve the fibrous anulus, which also may be calcified.

After an episode of RF, at least 2 years are required for severe mitral stenosis to develop, and most patients remain in an asymptomatic latent phase for 2 decades before the onset of symptoms. As obstruction to mitral flow develops, the left atrium becomes dilated and hypertrophied and frequently contains thrombi. The thrombi may be confined to the left atrial appendage or may laminate the entire atrial wall. Occasionally, thrombi are pedunculated or loosely attached to the valve apparatus. Any of the thrombotic material may embolize, and it appears to do so in a somewhat random manner, which is one treacherous feature of mitral stenosis. Embolization is most common soon after the development of atrial fibrillation.

As the incidence of RF diminishes in the United States because of early control of streptococcal infections with antibiotics, rheumatic valve disease is less frequent. Concurrently, the elderly population is increasing, and degenerative causes of mitral stenosis are now more common. Calcification of the mitral anulus occurs as a frequent autopsy finding in elderly patients. Narrowing of the mitral orifice may occur, and when accompanied by degenerative fibrosis or extension of calcific deposits onto the valve leaflets, the process may produce severe mitral stenosis. Congenital mitral stenosis occasionally persists into adulthood and may be mistaken for acquired disease. In the congenital "parachute" deformity, all chordae originate from a single papillary muscle (like the lines of a parachute), and obstruction to flow can occur. Congenital fibrous rings may exist just above the true mitral anulus and create a point of narrowing and obstruction. Rarer causes of mitral stenosis include malignant carcinoid, systemic lupus erythematosus, rheumatoid arthritis, and endomyocardial fibrosis.

The most significant pathophysiologic effects of mitral stenosis occur on the pulmonary vasculature and right ventricle. Congestion of the pulmonary vessels is characteristic with distention and thickening of pulmonary capillaries. Intimal fibrosis of the pulmonary veins and arterioles also is observed, and in advanced cases, medial thickening and fibrosis are common. Pulmonary hypertension progresses with time on the basis of two mechanisms: (1) retrograde transmission of left atrial hypertension to the pulmonary arteries and (2) reactive elevation of pulmonary vascular resistance. Pulmonary vascular resistance may increase to the point of producing systemic levels of systolic blood pressure in the right ventricle.

Pulmonary venous hypertension caused by valve obstruction produces the most prominent symptom in mitral stenosis, which is *dyspnea*. Initially, dyspnea is observed only with effort, but with time and progressive valve obstruction, dyspnea begins to occur at rest or at night, and is worsened by lying flat (orthopnea). Left atrial hypertension is related not only to valve area, but to the rate of blood flow across the valve. Thus, in many cases, symptoms can be improved by diuretic therapy and contraction of the blood volume only to be accompanied by reduced cardiac output, easy fatigability, and the characteristic *cardiac cachexia*. Atrial contraction augments transmitral flow significantly in mitral stenosis, so that development of atrial fibrillation increases mean left atrial pressure and reduces cardiac output by approximately 20 per cent. In addition, a more rapid ventricular rate decreases diastolic filling time, further exacerbating the problem. Therefore, it is common for the clinical status of a patient to deteriorate when atrial fibrillation develops. The exact cause of atrial fibrillation is unknown but probably relates to atrial dilation and alterations in normal atrial conduction patterns. In clinically progressive cases, patients usually experience worsening cardiac disability or hemoptysis and eventually die from acute pulmonary edema. It is important to note that the left ventricle has little role in the pathophysiologic mechanism of mitral stenosis, and left ventricular size is usually normal or slightly atrophic.

A variant clinical pattern is observed, however, where extreme elevations in pulmonary vascular resistance appear to "protect" the lungs and reduce the clinical signs of pulmonary congestion. In these cases, severe pulmonary hypertension progresses to right ventricular enlargement and failure, commonly associated with dilation of the tricuspid valve anulus and functional tricuspid incompetence. In the final stages of this syndrome, right ventricular failure is manifested by severe peripheral edema, pulsatile hepatic engorgement, cardiac cirrhosis, renal failure, and anasarca.

CLINICAL DIAGNOSIS. The clinical diagnosis of mitral stenosis, along with an assessment of physiologic severity, usually can be made without invasive procedures. A history of rheumatic fever is present in half of the cases. Progressive exertional dyspnea, orthopnea, and easy fatigability are common. Occasionally, hoarseness may develop from encroachment of a dilated left pulmonary artery on the left recurrent laryngeal nerve (Ortner's syndrome). Dysphagia may occur with esophageal obstruction by an enlarged left atrium. In some patients, symptoms may begin with pregnancy or with the onset of atrial fibrillation. Occasionally, patients are encountered who gradually adjust their life-styles to accommodate their cardiac condition and volunteer little disability. However, precise questioning about symptoms relative to activity often produces a history consistent with severe mitral stenosis.

On physical examination, the patient characteristically appears thin and cachectic with a washed-out and sallow "mitral facies." Ruddiness of the cheeks and peripheral cyanosis are often evident due to reduced cardiac output. Jugular venous pulsations may be prominent with fluid overload or with secondary tricuspid incompetence. If the cardiac rhythm is atrial fibrillation, irregularities in the jugular pulse and prominent V waves are observed. Peripheral edema and hepatic enlargement may be present, as well as the classic "hepatojugular reflux" or jugular venous distention observed with application of pressure over the right upper quadrant. In the presence of pulmonary edema, respirations are rapid and shallow, the work of breathing is increased, and rales are present to varying degrees from the lung bases up the chest. Palpation of the chest provides useful information. A sternal heave indicates right ventricular enlargement and suggests pulmonary hypertension. In severe cases of pulmonary hypertension, the pulmonary component of the second heart sound is often palpable in the second or third left intercostal space parasternally. The apical impulse usually is not displaced, indicating normal left ventricular size and insignificant mitral or aortic regurgitation. In the left lateral recumbent position, the diastolic murmur is palpable in some patients as a low-frequency thrill at the apex.

Auscultation of the heart reveals accentuation of the first heart sound, or mitral closure sound, in the early stages when the valve leaflets are pliable (Fig. 2). Calcification or severe thickening of the leaflets reduces the amplitude of the first heart sound. With development of pulmonary hypertension, the pulmonary component of the second heart sound becomes accentuated and widely transmitted, and the splitting of the second heart sound narrows. An opening snap of the mitral valve is common and appears to be due to sudden tensing of the valve leaflets by chordae after the valve cusps complete their opening excursion. The opening snap is best heard at the apex with the diaphragm of the stethoscope and is associated with reduced pliability of the valve leaflets. The mitral opening snap follows the second heart sound by 40 to 120 msec., with a shorter interval indicating severe left atrial hypertension. The diastolic murmur of mitral stenosis has a low-pitched rumbling quality best heard at the apex with the bell of the stethoscope. Because of its low frequency, the murmur can be difficult to detect, but in most cases, its amplitude can be accentuated by having the patient perform sit-ups in bed; the cardiac apex then is auscultated during expiration with the patient in the left lateral recumbent position. The murmur usually commences immediately after the opening snap, and its duration is directly related to the severity of valve obstruction. In sinus rhythm, a presystolic accentuation of the murmur is characteristic as blood is accelerated across the valve by atrial contraction (Fig. 2). Presystolic accentuation is lost with development of atrial fibrillation. It is important to remember that left atrial myxoma may produce auscultatory findings that are quite similar to rheumatic mitral valve stenosis. Pulmonary hypertension and extreme right ventricular enlargement can displace the left ventricular apex posteriorly and make the diastolic murmur extremely difficult to detect ("silent mitral stenosis").

Ninety per cent of patients in sinus rhythm with significant mitral stenosis exhibit a broad, notched P wave on the electrocardiogram in lead II, the "P mitrale." This finding correlates with left atrial enlargement and often regresses after successful commissurotomy. In later stages of the disease, atrial fibrillation and right ventricular hypertrophy are cardinal electrocardiographic signs. Rightward deviation of the QRS axis in the frontal plane beyond 60 degrees generally indicates significant right ventricular hypertrophy and a valve area of less than 1.3 sq. cm.

The radiographic findings in mitral stenosis are clinically useful and can be diagnostic. The overall cardiac silhouette may be normal, with the exception of left atrial enlargement (Fig. 3). The classic radiographic signs of left atrial enlargement include prominence of the left atrial appendage, elevation of the left main stem bronchus, a round or ovoid double density through the central heart shadow on the posteroanterior projection, and posterior displacement of the left atrium on the lateral projection. Pulmonary venous hypertension is accompanied by engorged, transversely oriented superior pulmonary veins, a finding that usually is termed *cephalization of pulmonary blood flow*. In the presence of pulmonary hypertension, the pulmonary arteries and right ventricle become enlarged with displacement of the right ventricle toward the sternum on the lateral projection. Severe valvular obstruction is manifested by Kerley B lines, short horizontal densities observed in the costophrenic angles of the lungs and corresponding to hypertrophied pulmonary lymphatics (Fig. 3).

At present, cardiac catheterization is performed in most patients with mitral stenosis who are being considered for surgical therapy. Coronary arteriography also is obtained in patients

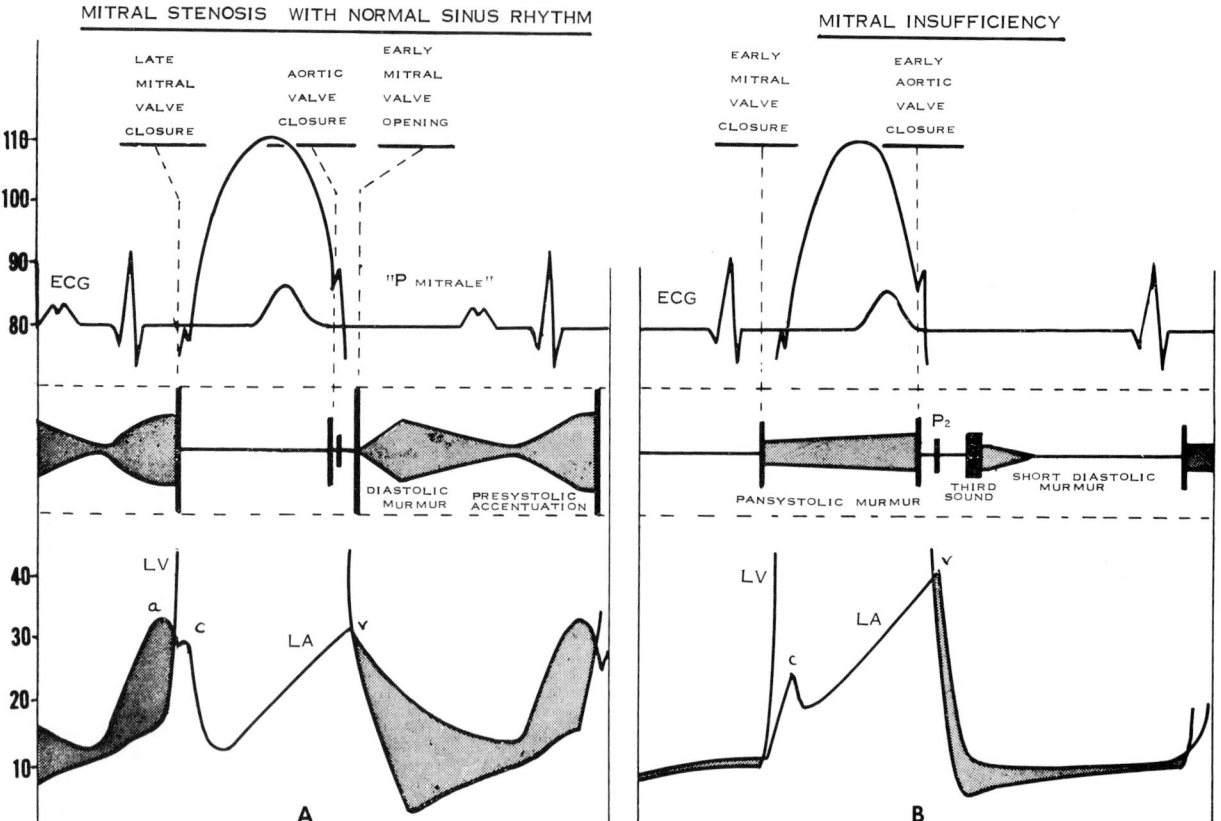

Figure 2. Classic illustration of clinical and hemodynamic features of mitral stenosis and regurgitation. *A*, Mitral stenosis in sinus rhythm. *B*, Mitral insufficiency in atrial fibrillation. (From Hamer, N. A. J.: *In* Glover, R. P., and Davilla, J. C.: The Surgery of Mitral Stenosis. New York, Grune & Stratton, 1961.)

over 35 years of age or in the presence of angina. Measuring the diastolic gradient across the mitral valve (Fig. 2) provides useful information about the physiologic severity of the stenosis. Usually, the left atrium is cannulated by means of transseptal methods, and the left ventricle is entered retrogradely across the aortic valve. In most laboratories, pulmonary artery pressures and cardiac output are measured with a thermodilution Swan-Ganz catheter. By use of the Gorlin formula, mitral valve orifice area can be derived from measurements of mean diastolic mitral gradient (ΔP) in mm. Hg and average diastolic mitral flow (F) in ml. per second:

$$\text{mitral valve area (sq. cm.)} = \frac{F}{38\sqrt{\Delta P}}$$

The normal mitral orifice area is 3 sq. cm. per square meter body surface area, and significant mitral stenosis is suggested when the calculated area approaches 1 sq. cm. per sq. M. Estimation of valve orifice area is subject to some error, however, particularly at low flow rates or in the presence of valvular regurgitation. Moreover, a well diuresed patient with a contracted blood volume occasionally exhibits a larger valve area and a lower left atrial pressure than is suggested by the clinical evaluation. Thus, it should be emphasized that catheterization findings are only supplemental, and the entire clinical status must be considered when therapeutic decisions are being made.

OPERATIVE INDICATIONS. The recommendation of surgical therapy in mitral stenosis is based on the natural history of medically treated patients as well as the observed benefits of the various operative procedures. After an episode of rheumatic fever in Wood's study, the latent period to the onset of symptoms in mitral stenosis averaged 19 years. Over the next 7 years, the clinical severity progressively worsened to the point of total incapacity. In half of the patients, clinical deterioration is gradual and is associated with progressive valvular obstruction. In

the remaining patients, symptomatic status degenerates rapidly after the onset of atrial fibrillation or systemic embolization. Long-term survival is depressed in mitral stenosis and is related to symptomatic status. In Olesen's analysis (Fig. 4), only patients with Class II symptoms and sinus rhythm (Group A) had a relatively good prognosis; worse symptoms or the presence of atrial fibrillation severely decreased longevity. The overall 10-year survival rate was 34 per cent, and after 20 years, only 14 per cent of patients were still alive. Sixty-two per cent died from congestive heart failure, 22 per cent from thromboembolic complications, and 8 per cent from infectious endocarditis. Ninety-two per cent of the total deaths were attributable to complications of mitral stenosis. Similar data were observed by Rowe and associates in a group of 250 patients with pure mitral stenosis followed for 20 years. Half of the patients were less than 30 years of age at the inception of the study, and 52 per cent of the patients were asymptomatic. After the first 10 years, 39 per cent of the patients had expired, primarily from cardiac causes. After 20 years, 80 per cent of the patients were dead, and only 13 per cent remained unchanged. Of patients with asymptomatic mitral stenosis in sinus rhythm, 59 per cent remained asymptomatic at 10 years, 25 per cent had worsened clinically, and 16 per cent had expired. In patients with mild symptoms or with atrial fibrillation, the mortality increased to 58 per cent at 10 years, and only 21 per cent remained stable. Moderate symptoms or congestive heart failure had an even worse prognosis.

A persistent and insidious risk in mitral stenosis is systemic embolization. In Bannister's series, 105 patients with clinically moderate stenosis and mild symptoms were followed with medical therapy over a 4.5-year period. Systemic embolization occurred in 22 of the patients, causing five deaths. Because half of the patients older than 40 years and in atrial fibrillation experienced emboli, the author concluded that it was safe to follow patients with mitral stenosis and mild symptoms only in the

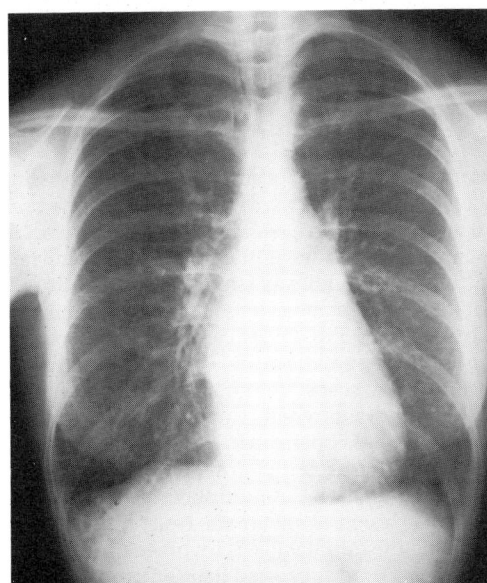

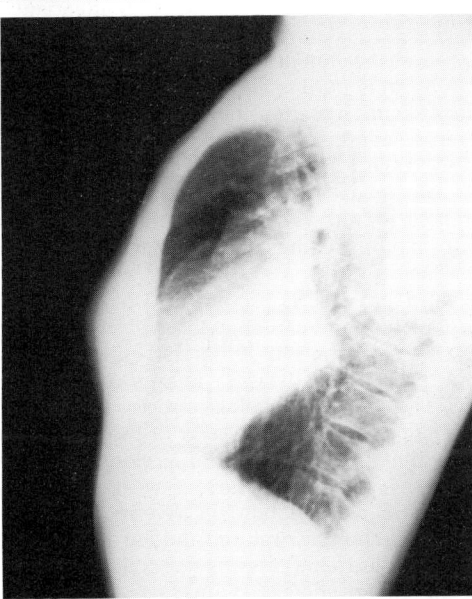

Figure 3. Posteroanterior and lateral chest radiographs of a patient with moderate mitral stenosis. Minimal overall cardiac enlargement is present, even though the left atrium is severely displaced toward the spine in the lateral view. A suggestion of a "double density" on the right heart border, right ventricular enlargement, and Kerley B lines in the right costophrenic angle are evident. (Courtesy of James T. T. Chen, M.D.)

younger age groups in sinus rhythm. Similar findings were published by Neilson and associates. In most studies, 50 to 75 per cent of emboli were cerebral, and the mortality after embolization approximated 50 per cent. Overall, systemic embolization occurred in 15 to 30 per cent of untreated patients with mitral stenosis but was rare in mitral regurgitation. Roberts concluded that the natural history of mitral stenosis is especially poor relative to other forms of acquired valvular disease, ranking second in terms of mortality only to aortic stenosis. Thus, as discussed by several authors, available data support the early application of surgical therapy in patients with mitral stenosis. To quote Wood's classic 1954 paper, "There can be little point in delaying mitral valvotomy long in anatomically suitable cases once unmistakable symptoms of stenosis have developed; to do so is to invite complications such as embolism and to deprive patients of good physical health at a time in life when they have the right to expect it." In the presence of clinically or hemodynamically significant valvular obstruction, firm indications for

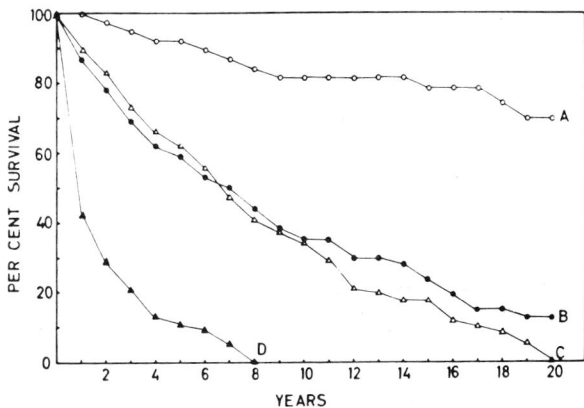

Figure 4. Survival in mitral stenosis after first observation in Olesen's study. Group A is patients with sinus rhythm and Class II symptoms. Group B represents sinus rhythm and Class III symptoms. Group C is atrial fibrillation with Class II or Class III symptoms. Group D is Class IV symptoms.

operation include NYHA Class III or Class IV symptoms, the onset of atrial fibrillation (independent of symptoms), worsening pulmonary hypertension, an episode of systemic embolization, and infective endocarditis. Class II patients who are over the age of 40 years, who have severe reduction in valve area at catheterization, or who experience undesired limitations in lifestyle also should be recommended surgical therapy. Most would agree that asymptomatic patients should be treated medically and carefully observed. Recently, percutaneous balloon mitral valvuloplasty has been introduced as an alternative approach to surgical therapy. At present, however, the exact role of balloon valvuloplasty remains to be defined.

SURGICAL RESULTS. Operations for mitral stenosis are designed to relieve the valvular obstruction and include closed commissurotomy, open commissurotomy, and mitral valve replacement. These procedures are discussed in a later section. Current operative mortality ranges from 1 to 5 per cent, depending on the severity of preoperative symptoms, the presence of severe pulmonary hypertension or right ventricular failure, and the need for mitral valve replacement.

Although scientific comparison of medical and surgical therapy is impossible, most would agree that contemporary operative procedures improve the natural history of mitral stenosis. The study of Rowe and associates was the first to address this question. Although differences in baseline variables may have existed between medical and surgical groups, a striking improvement in longevity was evident after commissurotomy (Fig. 5), with the surgically treated patients being twice as likely

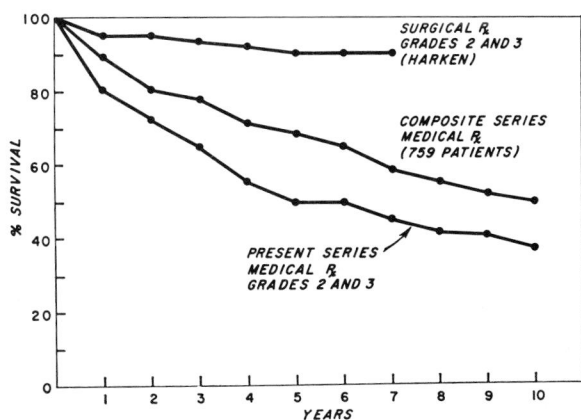

Figure 5. Medical versus surgical survival in comparable groups of patients with mitral stenosis. (From Rowe, J. C., Bland, E. F., Sprague, H. B., and White, P. D.: The course of mitral stenosis without surgery: Ten- and twenty-year perspectives. Ann. Intern. Med., 52:741, 1960.)

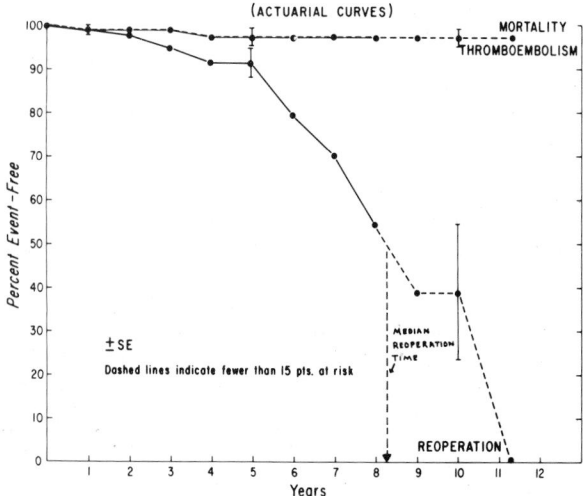

Figure 6. Analysis of late results after open commissurotomy in 100 patients. (From Housman, L. B., Bonchek, L., Lambert, L., et al.: Prognosis of patients after open mitral commissurotomy: Actuarial analysis of late results in 100 patients. J. Thorac. Cardiovasc. Surg., 73:742, 1977.)

to survive 5 years. Almost identical data were published by Munoz and co-workers. With more effective valve repairs, better patient follow-up, and aggressive reoperation when necessary, the long-term surgical survival may be even better at present.

Operations for mitral stenosis are not curative. Most patients experience significant improvement in symptoms after mitral commissurotomy but then develop progressive clinical deterioration with time, primarily due to recurrent valvular dysfunction (residual stenosis, restenosis, or induced regurgitation). Thus, in the series of Montoya and others, 67 per cent of patients were in NYHA Class III or Class IV preoperatively, whereas 95 per cent reverted to Class I or Class II after open commissurotomy. Similar excellent early results were reported by Housman and Gross and their associates with open commissurotomy, compared with earlier series of closed procedures; the difference may reflect, in part, selection of valves with less leaflet disease as well as more effective relief of obstruction with the open operation. At any rate, the probabilities of systemic embolization and infective endocarditis are lessened significantly after valvulotomy, and patients experiencing atrial fibrillation for less than 1 year have an excellent likelihood of reverting to sinus rhythm with quinidine therapy alone or in conjunction with cardioversion.

Elevated pulmonary vascular resistance usually diminishes after successful commissurotomy or valve replacement. Persistent pulmonary hypertension is observed, however, in patients with end-stage valvular disease, emphysema, or previous pulmonary emboli. Even with a competent tricuspid valve, continued pulmonary hypertension can impair complete resolution of symptoms and cause persistent mild right ventricular failure. Thus, the development of pulmonary hypertension is an important indication for surgical management in preventing these late sequelae. All surgical results tend to deteriorate with time, and the likelihood of a poor late postoperative result is predicted by the surgeon's operative assessment of leaflet condition. The median time to significant recurrent symptoms or reoperation in recent series is 8 to 10 years, whereas the 10-year survival exceeds 90 per cent (Fig. 6). In order to achieve optimal late survival rates, good medical follow-up is required, and when significant symptoms reappear, the patients should be evaluated for early reoperation. Mitral valve replacement generally is required as a second procedure, although good results can be obtained with a second commissurotomy if the valve leaflets remain pliable. In addition, it should be emphasized that a

"myocardial factor" related to rheumatic myocarditis and fibrosis exists and can limit the long-term prognosis in some patients.

MITRAL REGURGITATION

PATHOPHYSIOLOGY. As described in the preceding, competence of the mitral valve depends on an integrated section of the mitral anulus, the valve leaflets, the chordae tendineae, the papillary muscles, and the ventricular wall. Incompetence can be caused by abnormalities of any of these structures. Rheumatic heart disease remains a significant cause of mitral regurgitation, representing 35 to 45 per cent of cases. Involvement of the leaflets by the rheumatic process causes shortening, rigidity, and retraction of the cusps. The chordae tendineae also become fibrotic, fused, and shortened. Commissural fusion occurs so that the cusps are held open, and secondary calcification of the leaflets is common. Varying degrees of valvular stenosis may coexist with regurgitation. Interestingly, the most common significant valvular lesion of rheumatic heart disease is mitral regurgitation, and the mitral valve is involved in 85 per cent of all rheumatic cases. Wood suggested that the propensity for mitral involvement was due to the higher stresses attendant with mitral valve closure.

Idiopathic calcification of the mitral valve and anulus in the elderly can be an important cause of regurgitation and is associated with systemic hypertension, aortic stenosis, diabetes, and chronic renal failure. Calcification may involve the entire anulus and project into adjacent ventricular myocardium. Masses of calcium also may protrude into the subvalvular region, immobilizing the valve or preventing leaflet coaptation, and calcium can invade the conduction system or the adjacent coronary artery.

Mitral valve prolapse is present in 3 to 4 per cent of the general population and can be associated with a mid-systolic click and late systolic murmur. Progressive and clinically significant mitral regurgitation develops in approximately 5 per cent of patients. The primary pathologic process usually is *myxomatous degeneration* of the fibrous layer of the valve leaflets and chordae tendineae, producing thinning, elongation, and redundancy. In many patients, rupture of weakened chordae can cause acute mitral regurgitation, the severity of which depends on the size of the chordae ruptured and the degree of regurgitation produced. In extreme cases, severe congestive heart failure and acute pulmonary edema require emergency treatment. Less common causes of mitral valve prolapse include Marfan's syndrome, pseudoxanthoma elasticum, and Ehlers-Danlos syndrome.

Leaflet or chordal rupture also occurs as a consequence of chest trauma and infective endocarditis. The hemodynamic significance again is dependent on the degree of regurgitation, but symptoms can be especially severe in acute cases. Predominant regurgitation can occur with the congenital parachute mitral valve deformity or with cleft valves in atrioventricular canal defects. Mitral regurgitation also is observed in patients with hypertrophic obstructive cardiomyopathy. In this disorder, an enlarged and displaced anterior papillary muscle causes movement of the anterior mitral leaflet into the outflow tract during systole, rendering the valve incompetent.

The final category of mitral valve disease is ischemic mitral regurgitation, defined as moderate to severe valve incompetence precipitated by an acute myocardial infarction with no primary leaflet or chordal disease. This disorder is observed to a significant degree in 3 per cent of patients with coronary artery disease undergoing catheterization and is quite heterogeneous from both pathophysiologic and clinical viewpoints. Pathologically, the majority of patients exhibit posterior *papillary-annular dysfunction* in which regurgitation and congestive heart failure are coincident with the onset of a large posterior wall infarction. Combinations of posterior annular dilation, papillary muscle elongation, loss of papillary muscle shortening, and pre-existing congenital leaflet defects produce lateral valve incompetence at the posterior commissural region. Fluctuating mitral regurgitation in the setting of postinfarction unstable angina is a variant of this syndrome.

The least common type of ischemic incompetence is *papillary muscle rupture*, which occurs in only 0.1 per cent of patients with coronary disease undergoing catheterization. Congestive heart failure associated with a new murmur usually develops several days after infarction, and the majority have severe regurgitation requiring acute intervention. The infarction usually is posterior and often is small and localized; global ejection fraction is frequently maintained. The third type of ischemic mitral regurgitation occurs in patients with diffuse left ventricular infarctions or anterior aneurysms, and the regurgitation is secondary to *generalized annular dilation*. A history of multiple myocardial infarctions is common, and most present acutely with very low ejection fractions. Long-term prognosis in this group is poor, independent of therapy chosen.

Physiologic derangements caused by mitral regurgitation are similar to mitral stenosis. Left atrial hypertension is transmitted to the pulmonary vasculature, causing dyspnea and, in severe cases, pulmonary edema. Pulmonary arterial hypertension, right ventricular failure, and functional tricuspid regurgitation occur by similar mechanisms. However, unlike mitral stenosis, the left ventricle is subjected to a chronic volume overload, which ultimately causes myocardial failure.

The hemodynamic consequences of mitral regurgitation are interesting. Recent studies have focused on the reduced systolic ventricular afterload produced by the parallel low-resistance outflow circuit of the left atrium. Because of diminished afterload, left ventricular volume declines more rapidly as systole progresses, and total stroke volume and systolic emptying of the ventricle are augmented. The ratio of wall stress to cavitary pressure decreases as ejection proceeds because of smaller ventricular volumes. Velocity of shortening and ejection fraction increase and tend to maintain cardiac output and arterial blood pressure near normal. Because of reduced systolic wall tension, myocardial oxygen consumption increases minimally, and the enormous increment in total external work is accomplished with only minor energetic requirements.

However, chronic alterations in myocardial performance also occur that modify the physiologic process. With all volume overload lesions, a certain fraction of total work is wasted in regurgitation so that pump efficiency declines. End-diastolic ventricular pressure and volume increase because of augmented diastolic filling, and the magnitude of increase is proportional to the regurgitant volume. Chronically elevated diastolic filling pressure produces a time-dependent increase in unstressed ventricular volume, a process described as stress relaxation or creep. These alterations in diastolic properties and unstressed ventricular volume are the physiologic correlates of cardiac dilation. Associated with the creep process is an increasing radius of curvature and decreasing wall thickness as chamber dilation progresses. The radius : wall thickness ratio increases, and systolic wall stress is augmented for any systolic ventricular pressure. Thus, in chronic volume overload defects, systolic loading increases because of changes in diastolic properties and altered geometric determinants of wall stress. Increasing wall stress stimulates the hypertrophy process, wall thickness increases proportionately to the radius of curvature, and the radius : wall thickness ratio tends to normalize.

Simultaneously, inotropic reserves of the myocardium are depleted by undefined mechanisms, despite maximal activation of the sympathetic nervous system by baroreceptor reflexes. Further ventricular dilation, inadequate hypertrophy, or diminished inotropic state, along with possible myocardial fibrosis, then cause acute cardiac decompensation and irreversible myocardial damage. Without treatment, patients ultimately expire from biventricular cardiac failure, low cardiac output, and pulmonary edema.

CLINICAL DIAGNOSIS. Symptoms produced by mitral regurgitation are related to the level of pulmonary venous hypertension. Exertional dyspnea and orthopnea are common, and chronically reduced cardiac output produces easy fatigability and cardiac cachexia. Moderate to severe regurgitation can be tolerated for many years with relatively minor symptoms until irreversible left ventricular dysfunction develops. Therefore, the severity of symptoms cannot be used as the only criterion for intervention. Hemoptysis is rarely reported, and occasionally symptoms appear with the onset of atrial fibrillation, which complicates 75 per cent of severe cases. Systemic emboli can occur in patients with atrial fibrillation but are not as common as in mitral stenosis. Bacterial endocarditis should be suspected with symptoms of malaise, fever, chills, or a new or worsening murmur or when acute decompensation occurs in a previously stable patient. Angina secondary to mitral regurgitation is rare and should suggest coexisting coronary artery disease. Obviously, patients with ischemic mitral regurgitation usually manifest acute or chronic myocardial ischemic syndromes.

The physical signs of congestive heart failure are similar to those of mitral stenosis. Atrial fibrillation is observed in late cases, and the peripheral arterial pulse tends to have a rapid upstroke, reduced volume, and abbreviated ejection time. The apical impulse is displaced to the left in proportion to the degree of left ventricular enlargement, and an apical systolic thrill can be palpable. With significant right ventricular enlargement, a sternal heave is evident. On auscultation, the heart sounds usually are normal with the exception of a third heart sound with congestive heart failure or an increased second heart sound with pulmonary hypertension. The hallmark of mitral regurgitation is an apical, high-pitched, holosystolic murmur that radiates to the axilla and back (Fig. 2). On occasion, the murmur radiates to the base and has a musical quality. In mitral valve prolapse, the murmur usually occurs in late systole and is preceded by one or several mid-systolic clicks. The clicks are believed to be caused by abrupt systolic prolapse of the valve leaflets into the left atrium. In the presence of infectious endocarditis, peripheral signs such as splinter hemorrhages, Osler's nodes, clubbing, fever, and splenomegaly may be evident.

The electrocardiogram may show left ventricular hypertrophy from the chronic volume overload or biventricular hypertrophy with concomitant pulmonary arterial hypertension. In sinus rhythm, "P mitrale" may be present. The chest radiograph is extremely useful (Fig. 7). Left atrial enlargement is observed in chronic cases, but because of the volume overload, the left ventricle also is dilated. Right ventricular enlargement, pulmonary "cephalization," and Kerley B lines are common. Because of the biventricular and biatrial dilation, hearts with long-standing mitral regurgitation can exhibit the greatest cardiomegaly of any valvular disease.

Cardiac catheterization reveals prominent left atrial V waves due to retrograde ejection of blood across the valve (Fig. 2). With severe congestive heart failure, left ventricular end-diastolic pressure becomes elevated, and end-diastolic volume is increased. Pulmonary hypertension in mitral incompetence has the same prognostic implications as in mitral stenosis. A reduction in cardiac index below 2 liters per minute per square meter and a widened arteriovenous oxygen difference indicate severe hemodynamic impairment. Regurgitation can be graded on the basis of the left ventriculogram, with 1 + minor regurgitation, 2 + opacifying of the left atrial cavity with rapid clearing of dye, 3 + clear opacifying of the left atrial appendage with slow clearing of dye, and 4 + severe reflux of contrast into the pulmonary veins. Motion of the leaflets during the cardiac cycle and the presence of calcification are precisely documented. Most centers use the ventriculographic ejection fraction to assess left ven-

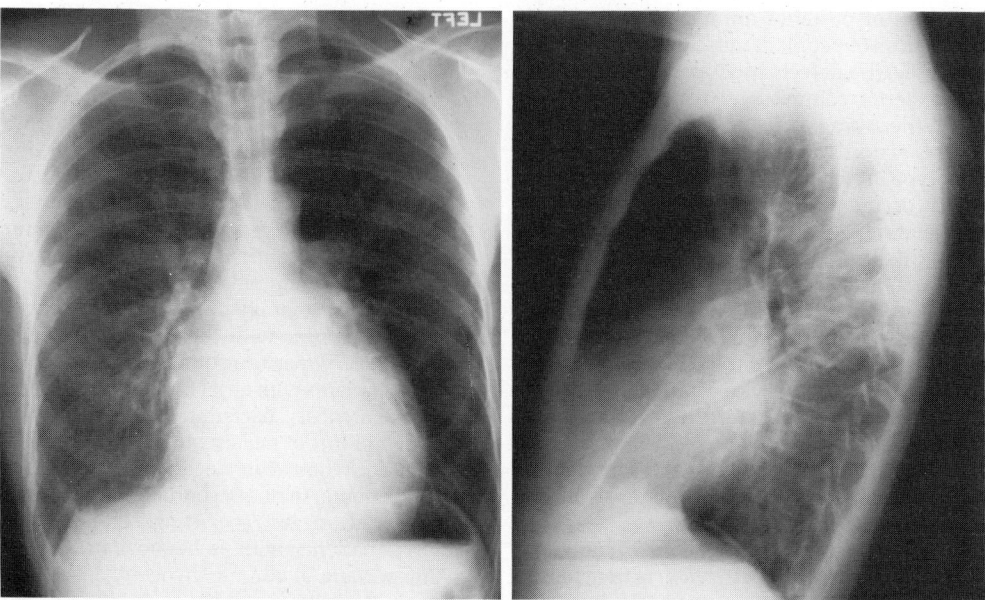

Figure 7. Posteroanterior and lateral chest radiographs in a patient with mitral regurgitation. Notice the generalized cardiomegaly, a double density on the right heart border, and posterior displacement of the left atrium. The left ventricle is enlarged on the lateral view, with the posterior left ventricular shadow crossing the inferior vena cava below the diaphragm. Pulmonary "cephalization" and mild pulmonary edema are evident. (Courtesy of James T. T. Chen, M.D.)

tricular function, although the ejection fraction usually is over-estimated owing to retrograde ejection into the low-resistance left atrium. Thus, an ejection fraction of less than 0.40 to 0.50 suggests severe myocardial impairment in mitral regurgitation.

OPERATIVE INDICATIONS. The natural history of mitral regurgitation is more variable than that of mitral stenosis because of the greater number of etiologic factors. The clinical course can range from asymptomatic patients with mild mitral regurgitation who remain stable for many years to patients experiencing a fulminant progression of overwhelming congestive heart failure. There are three main determinants of clinical severity: (1) the degree of regurgitation, (2) the status of left ventricular function, and (3) the cause of the valve disease.

Patients with mitral regurgitation due to rheumatic or myxomatous disease generally follow a slow and protracted course unless chordal rupture or infective endocarditis intervenes. In several series examining the natural history of pure mitral incompetence, significant symptoms were rare until the onset of heart failure, which usually appeared late in the overall course. After the appearance of heart failure, the clinical status generally deteriorated rapidly. Systemic embolization was rare, but the propensity for developing pulmonary hypertension was as high as in mitral stenosis. The excellent study of Hammermeister and associates assessed the problem of natural history with contemporary statistical methods in 72 medically treated patients. Interestingly, symptoms (NYHA functional class) and ejection fraction did not correlate with medical outcome when a multivariate Cox model was used. However, arteriovenous oxygen difference and left ventricular end-diastolic volume did predict medical survival (Fig. 8), with prognosis progressively deteriorating as end-diastolic volume increased. This finding suggests that symptoms alone are an unreliable guide to the timing of surgical intervention, and other factors, such as progressive cardiomegaly, need to be considered. This concept is further supported by the observation that operative mortality is higher and long-term survival is depressed in patients with severe cardiomegaly or Class IV symptoms. Thus, surgical intervention is recommended in chronic mitral regurgitation if symptoms significantly limit life-style or for NYHA Class III or Class IV congestive heart failure. In Class I or Class II patients, operation should be considered if pulmonary hypertension is

progressing, if atrial fibrillation occurs, or if the left ventricle is dilating. Similar criteria for surgical selection are used in patients with mixed stenosis and regurgitation, mitral valve calcification, or other forms of slowly progressive mitral incompetence.

Often a more acute clinical course is observed, particularly with infective endocarditis, trauma, or ruptured chordae tendineae. Emergency therapy commonly is required and can be lifesaving. In infective endocarditis, blood cultures and antibiotic therapy are indicated. If the patient's condition is stabilized by medical therapy and the infection is cleared with antibiotics, selection for operation can be made on an elective basis. Indications for emergency valve replacement in endocarditis include failure to respond to antibiotics, pulmonary or systemic emboli, evidence of an abscess involving the valvular ring, fungal endocarditis, and hemodynamic deterioration. In 90 per cent of patients, hemodynamic instability is the primary indication and is manifested by pulmonary edema, low cardiac output, hypoten-

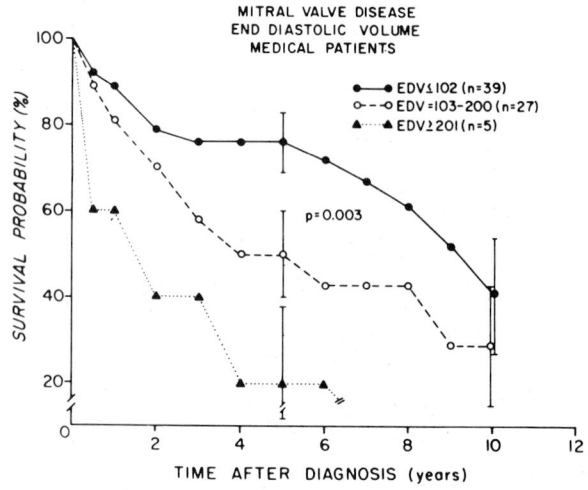

Figure 8. Survival curves of medically treated mitral valve disease according to left ventricular end-diastolic volume. (From Hammermeister, K. E., Fisher, L., Kennedy, J. W., et al.: Prediction of late survival in patients with mitral valve disease from clinical, hemodynamic, and quantitative angiographic variables. Circulation, 57:341, 1978.)

sion, and developing renal failure. Operation should not be delayed if the patient is unresponsive to medical therapy, since established pulmonary edema or renal failure significantly increases surgical risk. Similar selection criteria should be used for prosthetic endocarditis or other causes of acute mitral regurgitation. In patients with extreme hemodynamic compromise, insertion of an intra-aortic balloon pump can produce clinical stabilization as preparations are being made for a valve procedure. Obviously, operative and long-term survival are depressed in patients with impaired preoperative ventricular function, in those requiring operation under emergency conditions, or in elderly patients with pre-existing multiorgan failure.

Ischemic mitral regurgitation requires special consideration. In the 1970s, surgical treatment of this disorder was guided by two concepts. First, it was believed that a mitral valve procedure should be avoided whenever possible, with the anticipation that the regurgitation would subside with coronary revascularization alone. Second, when severe congestive heart failure mandated a valve procedure, prosthetic valve replacement usually was chosen to minimize the likelihood of residual regurgitation in these seriously ill patients. The postoperative results with these strategies were disappointing, however, with a hospital mortality of approximately 10 per cent for the coronary bypass *only* group, two thirds of which could be related to persistence of more significant valve dysfunction than anticipated preoperatively. Hospital mortality for patients requiring acute valve replacement approximated 50 per cent, with a correspondingly poor long-term survival (Fig. 9). Operative results at Duke University during this period were similar, with a 53 per cent operative mortality for acute mitral valve replacement at a time when the mortality was 8.6 per cent for nonischemic mitral valve procedures and 5.6 per cent for primary elective mitral valve replacement.

In the 1980s, surgical management changed significantly as intraoperative transesophageal Doppler echocardiography was introduced for prebypass valve assessment and assistance in the decision of whether to perform a valve procedure. Additionally, simplified methods of mitral valve repair became increasingly utilized when the valve was found to be severely incompetent. A better understanding of preoperative risk factors also allowed improvement in patient selection, with avoidance of operation

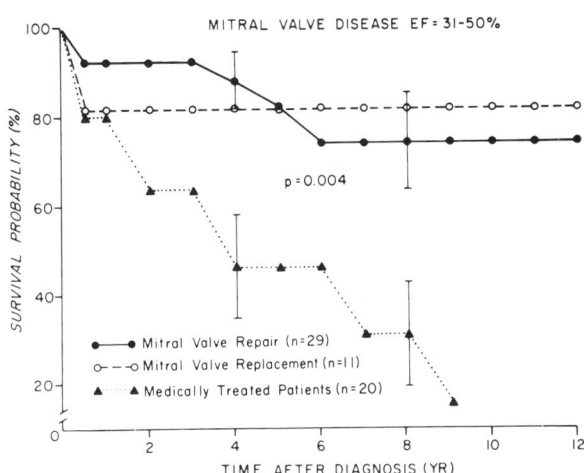

Figure 10. Survival curves for medical and surgical therapy of mitral valve disease with impaired ventricular function. (From Hammermeister, K. E., Fisher, L., Kennedy, J. W., et al.: Prediction of late survival in patients with mitral valve disease from clinical, hemodynamic, and quantitative angiographic variables. Circulation, 57:341, 1978.)

in subjects with diffusely infarcted left ventricles and in the extreme elderly group with multiple preoperative risk factors and multiorgan failure. All of these strategies combined to improve surgical results in ischemic mitral regurgitation, as discussed in the following section.

SURGICAL RESULTS. Surgical procedures used to correct mitral incompetence include mitral valve repair, usually consisting of anuloplasty, valvuloplasty, or chordal procedures, and prosthetic valve replacement with a bioprosthetic or mechanical valve. From available information, it is probable that patient longevity is improved after mitral valve procedures, although the variable of prosthesis-related complications is introduced. With use of a Cox multivariate regression model, Hammermeister and associates demonstrated a surgical survival benefit in all types of mitral valve disease, and the improved longevity was especially significant in patients with moderate ventricular dysfunction (Fig. 10). Hospital mortality and late survival after mitral valve procedures are related to preoperative symptomatic status (Fig. 11). In some reports, results were similar for stenotic and regurgitant lesions, whereas in most, mitral regurgitation had a worse postoperative prognosis. Ad-

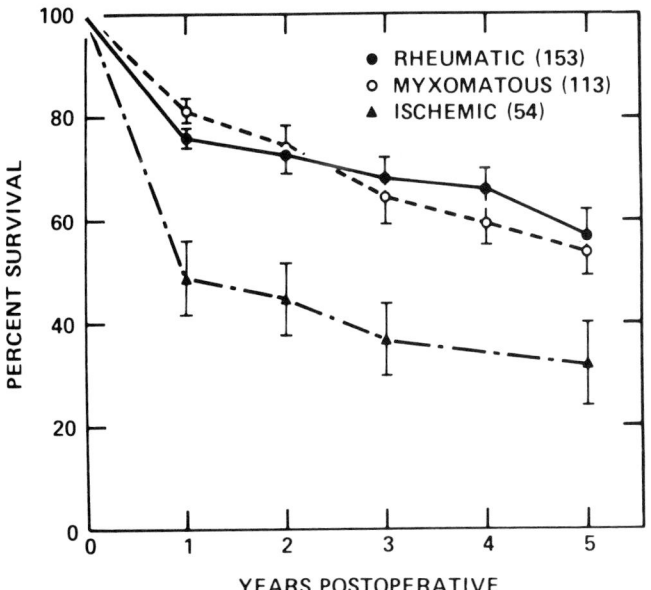

Figure 9. Influence of the primary cause of mitral valve disease on patient survival. (From Salomon, N. W., Stinson, E. B., Griepp, R. B., and Shumway, N. E.: Patient-related risk factors as predictors of results following isolated mitral valve replacement. Ann. Thorac. Surg., 24:519, 1977.)

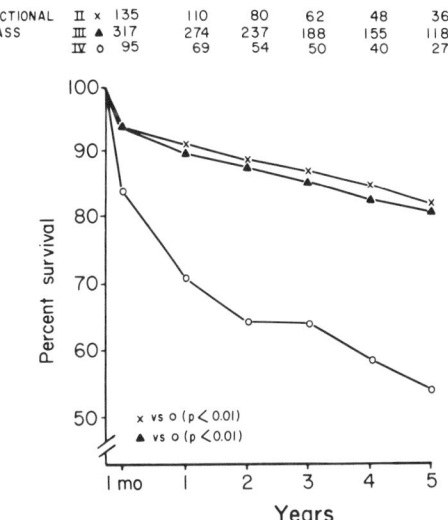

Figure 11. Overall survival after mitral valve replacement as a function of NYHA Class for congestive heart failure. (From Leply, D., Jr., Flemma, R. J., Mullen, D. C., et al.: Long-term follow-up of the Bjork-Shiley prosthetic valve used in the mitral position. Ann. Thorac. Surg., 30:164, 1980.)

vanced age is also an independent risk factor for mortality, being the primary influence on late survival in the Seattle experience. The overall operative mortality for elective isolated mitral valve procedures averages 3 to 10 per cent in most centers. However, in Class IV patients, the hospital mortality approaches 15 per cent, and emergency operations can have an even higher risk. As in mitral stenosis, pulmonary hypertension in mitral regurgitation usually resolves after a successful valve operation. Symptoms of congestive heart failure generally subside so that up to 95 per cent of survivors revert to NYHA Class I or Class II. Symptom-free survival is somewhat less uniform in patients with long-standing mitral regurgitation, Class IV symptoms, and cardiomegaly. Therefore, operation should be advised before this advanced stage of the disease.

In patients with ischemic mitral regurgitation, independent risk factors for hospital mortality include (1) the necessity for a valve procedure, (2) the year of therapy, with mortality decreasing significantly in recent years, (3) the sum of associated comorbid disorders, and (4) requirement of surgical intervention directly from the coronary care unit. During the 1980s, hospital mortality decreased significantly, so that in later years the mortality figures for each group were comparable to those observed for patients undergoing similar procedures without preoperative ischemic mitral regurgitation. Improved intraoperative selection of patients for coronary bypass *only* with transesophageal Doppler echocardiography was probably responsible for much of the mortality reduction in that group. The probable cause of the similarly decreasing mortality in the valve procedure group was the increasing use of simple and expeditious methods of mitral valve repair in the late 1980s, which reduced the risk of hospital mortality by approximately 50 per cent, compared with mitral valve replacement. Further evolution of therapeutic concepts should continue to improve results in the ischemic subgroup in coming years.

TRICUSPID VALVE DISEASE

PATHOPHYSIOLOGY. Pathologic disorders of the tricuspid valve can be either *functional* or *organic*. Tricuspid regurgitation usually is a functional derangement that is secondary to right ventricular dilation and enlargement of the free-wall tricuspid anulus (Fig. 1). The anulus in the area of the septal leaflet is spared, and the valve leaflets and chordae generally are normal. Causes of functional tricuspid regurgitation include mitral valve disease, cor pulmonale, primary pulmonary hypertension, right ventricular infarction, and congenital heart disease. In most cases, valve incompetence reflects the presence of, and further aggravates, severe right ventricular failure. Organic causes of tricuspid regurgitation affect the valve apparatus directly and include rheumatic fever, congenital malformations, papillary muscle rupture, trauma, Marfan's syndrome, infective endocarditis, carcinoid syndrome, and cardiac tumors.

Tricuspid stenosis is generally rheumatic in origin, usually accompanies mitral valve involvement, and is clinically significant in approximately 5 per cent of patients with rheumatic heart disease. Pathologic changes resemble those in the mitral valve, with thickening and fusion of the leaflets and chordae producing a stenotic, fixed tricuspid orifice. Other causes of tricuspid stenosis are rare and include carcinoid syndrome, congenital defects, and cardiac tumors. Carcinoid involvement of the tricuspid valve is characterized by deposition of fibrous carcinoid plaques on the leaflets and ventricular attachments. Both tricuspid stenosis and regurgitation produce right atrial hypertension, systemic venous engorgement, and hepatic congestion. Severe fluid retention, edema, and debility are characteristic. The process can progress to hepatic failure, cardiac cirrhosis, anasarca, and renal failure.

CLINICAL DIAGNOSIS. Symptoms in tricuspid stenosis or regurgitation are related to the degree of systemic venous hypertension. Fatigue and weakness are common, usually in the

absence of dyspnea or other signs of pulmonary congestion. Isolated tricuspid regurgitation is well tolerated in patients with normal pulmonary artery pressure, but when it is combined with mitral valve disease, pulmonary hypertension, and right ventricular failure, the clinical status deteriorates rapidly.

Tricuspid valve disease is easily overlooked, unless the observer has a high index of suspicion. In sinus rhythm, contraction of the right atrium against a stenotic valve produces a prominent A wave in the jugular venous pulse; with regurgitant lesions, the jugular V wave is accentuated. The liver is often enlarged and may be pulsatile, but in congestive cirrhosis, the liver may be firm and fibrotic. Whereas ascites and edema are common, the lung fields are clear despite engorged neck veins and other signs of congestive heart failure. A tricuspid opening snap may be present. Murmurs with tricuspid valve disease are similar to those observed in mitral disorders, and the two may be difficult to distinguish. Tricuspid murmurs usually are located more toward the left lower sternal border, and both the stenotic and regurgitant types are augmented by inspiration. Both murmurs may be difficult to hear, even when the physiologic defects are severe.

In sinus rhythm, tricuspid valve disease is suggested if the lead II P wave amplitude exceeds 0.25 mV. The key radiographic finding is marked cardiomegaly, with prominence of the right atrial shadow. At catheterization, *tricuspid stenosis* is confirmed by demonstrating a diastolic pressure gradient between the right atrium and right ventricle using simultaneous pressure measurements. The right atrial A wave is augmented, and the diastolic gradient increases during inspiration. A mean diastolic gradient of 5 mm. Hg is significant in tricuspid stenosis, and values as low as 3 mm. Hg may produce symptoms; the resting cardiac output is reduced. In *tricuspid regurgitation,* right atrial pressure is characterized by a prominent V wave, which in severe cases is described as "ventricularization" of atrial pressure. Occasionally, the atrial V wave may be normal despite severe regurgitation because of an enlarged, highly compliant systemic venous system. Pulmonary arterial hypertension favors a functional cause of tricuspid regurgitation, whereas normal pulmonary pressures suggest organic disease. Indicator-dilution curves or contrast ventriculography have been used to define the magnitude of the regurgitation. More recently, chest wall or transesophageal Doppler echocardiography has been employed and appears to be the most quantitative and reliable method of assessing tricuspid valve incompetence, both preoperatively and intraoperatively.

SURGICAL MANAGEMENT. Rheumatic tricuspid stenosis is treated by commissurotomy or valve replacement, depending on leaflet mobility, involvement of subvalvular structures, and the presence of regurgitation. Because residual gradients are tolerated poorly, valve replacement should be considered in significantly diseased valves. Most authors recommend that tissue valves be used exclusively for tricuspid valve replacement. Symptomatic cases of carcinoid valve disease require excision of the entire tricuspid apparatus and valve replacement.

Tricuspid endocarditis in drug addicts is a particularly difficult problem. For infections that cannot be eradicated with antibiotics, total excision of the valve has been recommended. Most patients tolerate loss of the tricuspid valve acutely, but valve replacement can be required at a later date. More recently, a number of reparative operations have been performed with good results.[50] If possible, prosthetic valve replacement should be avoided because of the risk of late prosthetic endocarditis. Functional tricuspid regurgitation secondary to mitral valve disease usually can be managed by tricuspid anuloplasty to obviate the early and late morbidity of residual tricuspid regurgitation.

OPERATIVE TECHNIQUE

Numerous methods exist for obtaining good results in mitral and tricuspid valve procedures, and only a few are covered in this section. Closed mitral commissurotomy is not discussed in detail. The more common procedures currently being performed on the mitral valve are presented, along with brief descriptions of their development, variations, and possible pitfalls. Mitral valve surgery requires great care, precision, and gentle operative technique.

Open Mitral Commissurotomy

The open approach to mitral commissurotomy originally was devised for less than optimal valves or for the complications of closed procedures. Nichols and associates first advocated open commissurotomy on a routine basis, and later reports from a number of centers firmly established the procedure. Most series suggest that operative mortality is equivalently low with the open approach and that the quality of the procedure is enhanced in terms of both hemodynamic improvement and operative complications. The likelihood of embolizing left atrial thrombus or creating serious regurgitation is lessened by direct visualization during commissurotomy. The hemodynamic results may be better for two reasons. First, the open operation probably is more effective in relieving obstruction, especially when mild calcification or subvalvular stenosis is present. Improved results also may reflect operative selection of valves with less leaflet disease for repair, and categories of valves previously shown to have poor long-term results (i.e., leaflet immobility or calcification) can be selected for valve replacement on the basis of the operative findings. This more precise intraoperative selection process is one important advantage of open procedures.

Open commissurotomy usually is performed for rheumatic mitral stenosis with good leaflet pliability, minimal or no leaflet calcification, and insignificant regurgitation. The operation is performed through a median sternotomy and with the support of cardiopulmonary bypass. After the aorta is cross-clamped, the heart is arrested by infusion of a cold potassium cardioplegia solution into the aortic root. The left atrium is opened to the left of the interatrial groove. Adequate exposure of the valve is extremely important and is facilitated by a generous atriotomy, by mobilizing the superior and inferior venae cavae, by direct caval cannulation, and by the Cosgrove retractor (Kapp Surgical, Cleveland, Ohio). The retractor blades apply traction to the atrial wall about 2 cm. superior to the mitral anulus; deeper insertion obscures exposure of the valve apparatus.

The left atrium is examined for thrombotic material, and some surgeons perform suture obliteration of the left atrial appendage to lessen the incidence of postoperative thromboembolism. If appendage closure is employed, care should be taken to avoid the circumflex coronary artery, which courses between the orifice of the atrial appendage and the valve ring. In severe mitral stenosis, the commissures can be fused to the point that leaflets cannot be delineated (Fig. 12). In addition, subvalvular chordal fusion and shortening can further obscure the anatomy. The heads of the papillary muscles usually "point" directly at the commissures, and traction on the adjacent chordae of the anterior leaflet creates a furrow at the commissure, allowing an incision to be performed in the endocardial layer. Occasionally, structures are sufficiently evident that the entire commissurotomy can be performed sharply, but, more often, a combination of sharp and blunt technique is required. After the endocardial incision has been made, the closed tips of DeBakey forceps can be used to develop the commissures, which usually split precisely along anatomic lines. Transatrial use of the Tubbs dilator is contraindicated because of the risk of perforating the ventricular wall as the tips are snapped open. It is often easier to begin the commissurotomy laterally, where less distortion is evident, and then to work medially toward the chordal insertions. Lateral commissural incisions are made to within 3 mm. of the anulus. Normal leaflet tissue is contiguous at the anulus, and the incision should not be extended all the way to the valve ring.

Minor amounts of calcium (especially when located in the

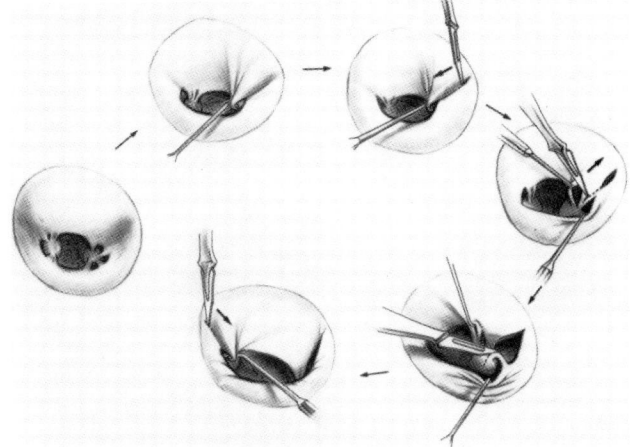

Figure 12. Operative techniques for open mitral commissurotomy. See text for details. (From Carpentier, A.: Cardiac valve surgery—the "French correction." J. Thorac. Cardiovasc. Surg., 86:323, 1983.)

fused commissures) can be débrided mechanically or with the aid of the CUSA device (Valley Labs CUSA, Boulder, Colorado). Significant leaflet calcification, however, is associated with a poor long-term result and should suggest valve replacement. If subvalvular fusion is evident, the chordae are separated carefully, again by combining sharp and blunt technique and being careful not to injure chordal attachments. If the chordae are severely shortened, the papillary muscle heads essentially insert into the leaflets, exacerbating the subvalvular obstruction. In this situation, the papillary muscle heads are incised to open the subvalvular apparatus further. Occasionally, secondary chordae are resected. Anular remodeling with a prosthetic ring may lessen the likelihood of early or late progressive regurgitation at the site of the commissurotomies. After completion of the procedure, valve competence is tested by injecting cold saline into the ventricle.

The atriotomy then is closed with a running polypropylene suture, the lungs are inflated, and residual intracardiac air is aspirated from the aortic root cardioplegia vent (DLP, Grand Rapids, Michigan) as the heart is filled by transiently occluding the venous return line. After aortic unclamping, the aortic cardioplegia cannula is placed to high cardiotomy suction throughout the reperfusion period for further assistance in removing air. Cardiac venting is no longer used for most valve procedures. The aortic vent is removed when ejection has been well established and the absence of significant intracardiac air documented by transesophageal echocardiographic monitoring. After cardiopulmonary bypass has been discontinued, it is helpful to monitor left atrial pressure with an indwelling fluid-filled catheter. Transesophageal Doppler echocardiography is employed routinely in the early post-bypass period.

Transatrial Carpentier Valve Repair

Methods for reconstructing incompetent mitral valves have existed for decades and yield good postoperative results. Valve repair most commonly is performed for the complications of myxomatous degeneration, such as annular dilation, leaflet prolapse, or chordal rupture. The most widely used method at present is that devised by Carpentier and associates. The valve is initially inspected during cold fibrillation, since some myocardial tone is helpful for proper assessment of pathologic valve geometry. Cold potassium cardioplegia is then instituted, and it should be remembered that flaccid arrest tends to make the degree of leaflet prolapse appear greater than in the normally functioning heart. In simple annular dilation, prosthetic ring anuloplasty is the only procedure required. A Carpentier obturator is chosen to match the length of the base of the anterior leaflet and the leaflet area. Mattress sutures of 2–0 Polydek (Deknatel, Queens Village, New York) are placed through the

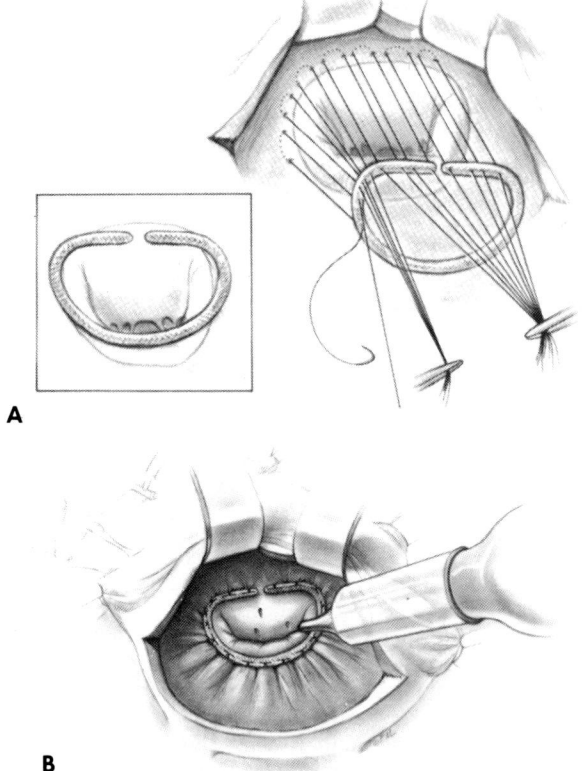

A

B

Figure 13. *A*, Placement of annuloplasty sutures. *B*, Testing competence of the reconstructed valve. See text for details. (From Carpentier, A.: Cardiac valve surgery—the "French correction." J. Thorac. Cardiovasc. Surg., 86:323, 1983.)

anulus of the anterior leaflet and then passed through the Carpentier ring, maintaining the same spacing for both (Fig. 13A). The posterior annular or free-wall sutures are then placed and passed through the ring with narrower spacing to selectively reduce the circumference of the posterior annulus. If asymmetric enlargement of one commissure is encountered, the ring spacing is specifically reduced in that area to compensate for the asymmetry. The ring is seated on the annulus, and the sutures are tied. In addition to reducing annular circumference, the shape of the orifice is restored, which assists in maintaining normal leaflet coaptation (Fig. 13A, inset). Insertion of too small a ring can cause buckling of the anterior leaflet and cause severe valve incompetence. Conversely, too large a ring can open the commissures and cause regurgitation; thus, proper ring sizing is

critical. Care is taken to place the sutures deeply into the valve anulus so that the likelihood of ring dehiscence is lessened, but the circumflex coronary artery, the aortic valve, or the conduction system is not injured (Fig. 1). After completion of the anuloplasty, competence of the valve is tested by injecting iced saline into the ventricle (Fig. 13B). Left atrial pressure and transesophageal Doppler echocardiographic monitoring are routinely utilized postoperatively. Minor left ventricular outflow tract gradients can be observed after mitral ring anuloplasty but are usually asymptomatic.

Frequently, mitral insufficiency is produced by a combination of dilation of the posterior annular circumference and elongation of chordae to both leaflets, which allows the valve to prolapse above the annular plane and into the left atrium (Figs. 14A and 15A). If extreme central redundancy of the posterior leaflet is encountered or if posterior chordae are ruptured, the central posterior leaflet between major chordal insertions is resected (Fig. 15B). This maneuver reduces the posterior anular circumference and moves the posterior anulus anteriorly. Elongated chordae are shortened into troughs in the papillary muscles to maintain both leaflets well below the annular plane (Fig. 14B). Occasionally, several sets of chordae require shortening. The Carpentier ring then is inserted and further moves the posterior anulus anteriorly, allowing coaptation of the leaflets over a substantial area of their atrial surface (Figs. 14C and 15C). Persistent fetal commissural clefts or other anatomic defects are common in this population and are closed with interrupted sutures when they appear to contribute to the incompetence. The long-term results of mitral valve repair have been good in most series. At present, mitral valve reconstruction probably should be performed in the majority of patients with myxomatous degeneration, rheumatic mitral regurgitation, and congenital valve incompetence.

Patients with papillary muscle rupture commonly present with florid congestive heart failure and require emergency intervention. Immediate operation should be performed in most cases. Since overall ventricular function is usually good in this disorder, the transatrial approach to valve repair should be employed most often, with transventricular repair reserved for patients with extensive posterior wall infarcts. The ruptured papillary head can be reimplanted into the ventricular wall or sutured to an adjacent papillary muscle. Whichever technique is utilized, the pledgeted horizontal mattress suture should be oriented in the long axis of the muscle and should incorporate the fibrous tip to obtain the best holding power. Remaining abnormalities in valve structure then are corrected as necessary by use of either the Carpentier or Kay technique. If reimplantation of

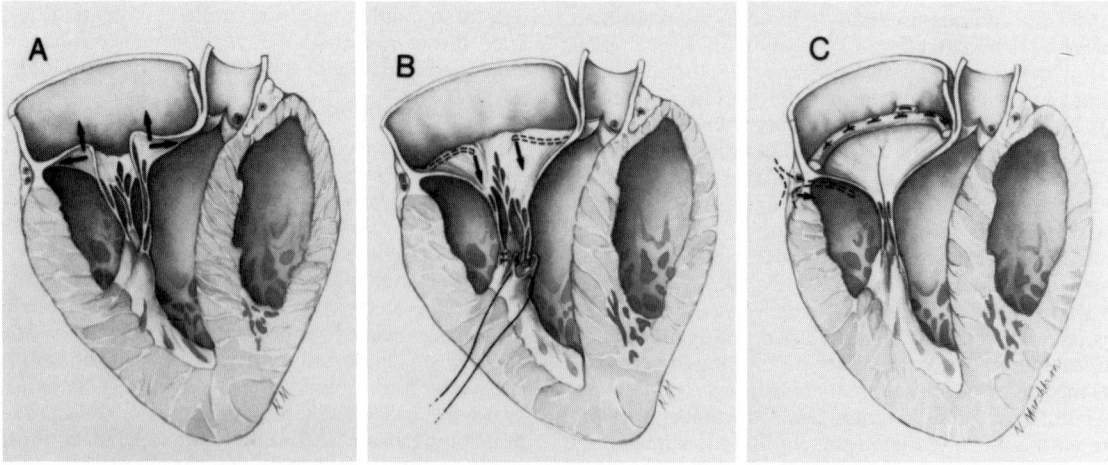

Figure 14. *A* to *C*, Sagittal views of sequential steps in a Carpentier mitral valve repair. See text for details.

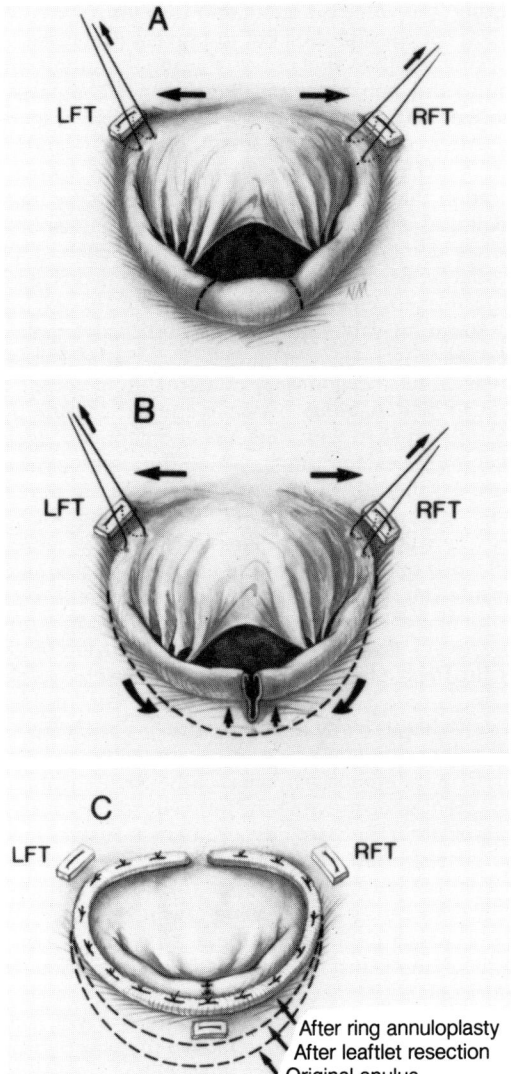

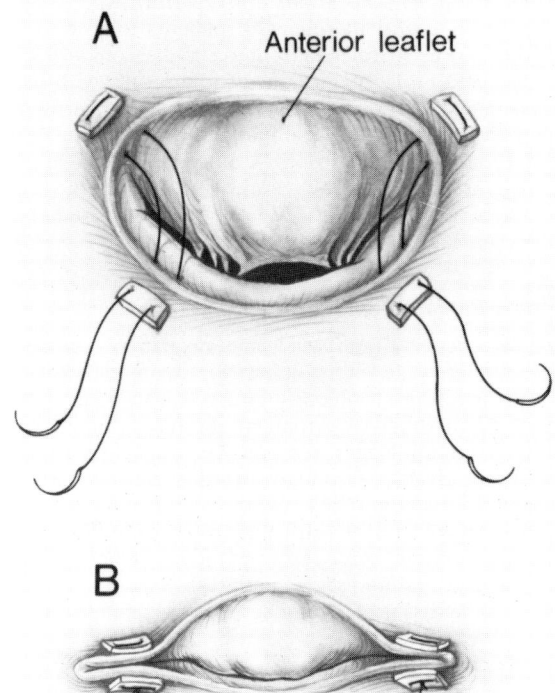

Figure 16. Atrial view of Kay annuloplasty. See text for details.

Figure 15. *A* to *C*, Atrial views of Carpentier mitral valve repair. See text for details.

the ruptured papillary muscle appears tenuous, prosthetic valve replacement is undertaken.

Transatrial Kay Annuloplasty

In patients with little leaflet prolapse or structural abnormality of valve tissue, such as those with posterior annular dilation after myocardial infarction, a transatrial lateral commissural annuloplasty is selected (Fig. 16). This procedure has been described by multiple authors but is now commonly termed the *Kay annuloplasty*. The operation is expeditious and effective when valves with appropriate anatomy are selected, and it is especially useful in patients with diminutive left atria in whom exposure for a standard valve replacement can be formidable. A valve with a dilated anulus but little prolapse is observed from the atrial surface in Figure 16*A*. Mattress sutures of 2–0 nonabsorbable material, supported with Teflon felt pledgets, are placed deeply into annular tissue at each commissure. The anterior bites of the annuloplasty sutures are placed into the right and left fibrous trigones, very close to the valve commissures. This maneuver leaves the anterior annulus intact as it attaches to the aortic root and fibrous skeleton of the heart. The posterior sutures are placed at some distance from the commissures so that the posterior anulus is selectively reduced in circumference. As with the Carpentier procedure, the posterior anulus then is

moved forward toward the anterior leaflet, which increases the surface area of leaflet coaptation (Fig. 16*B*).

Transventricular Mitral Valve Repair

In the presence of a thinned-out transmural infarct or aneurysm (again in the ischemic mitral regurgitation subgroup), a transventricular approach to the mitral valve is simple and provides excellent exposure. A longitudinal posterior ventriculotomy is performed to the left of the posterior descending coronary artery and toward the atrioventricular groove to avoid the bases of the papillary muscles. When the papillary muscles are identified, the incision is extended toward the apex, avoiding the papillary insertions. In most patients, a 5 cm. vertical incision, placed to within 1 cm. of the base, provides excellent visualization of the mitral valve and submitral apparatus. For isolated posterior papillary-annular dysfunction, a posterior commissural annuloplasty is performed. A pledgeted 2–0 horizontal mattress suture is placed deep to the valve anulus at the posterior commissure and tied firmly.

In most cases, the infarcted posterior papillary heads appear elongated, causing slack posterior chordae to both leaflets. For compensation of the elongation, the papillary muscles are sutured to the ventricular wall at a slightly more apical level by use of the fibrous tip of the muscle. The ventriculotomy then is closed with four to five large horizontal mattress sutures of No. 1 braided polyester suture buttressed with Teflon felt strips and oversewn with a running No. 1 polypropylene suture for hemostasis.

Long-term results after valve repair have been excellent; physiologic valve function is effectively restored, with minimal rates of thromboembolism or endocarditis. Residual minor regurgitation and apical systolic murmurs can occur and should not cause excessive concern. A low but definite incidence of progressive symptomatic mitral incompetence mandates reoperation in approximately 10 per cent of patients over the first several postoperative years. Occasionally, late valve failure is caused by interval chordal rupture or other events related to the myxomatous process and can be accompanied by severe hemolytic anemia. Doppler echocardiography, performed on a yearly basis, has been useful in following patients long-term. Although differences in selection criteria make comparison of valve repair and replacement difficult, the results with repair are at least as good and probably better. One can hardly disagree with the concept of using autologous tissue for any reconstruction, especially since the long-term complications of prosthetic valves are significant. Numerous variations on the theme of valve repair currently exist and have been described extensively.

Mitral Valve Replacement

Mitral valve repair is not feasible in many patients, even with current techniques. Severely deformed rheumatic valves or valves with significant leaflet or submitral calcification are best managed with prosthetic replacement. Ruptured primary chordae to the anterior leaflet occasionally can be repaired by transfer to an adjacent secondary chord or by transferring a posterior chord and adjoining leaflet tissue from the same papillary muscle. However, if the structural integrity of the anterior leaflet is questionable, valve replacement is prudent. Generalized bileaflet prolapse and segmentation associated with excessively thin leaflet tissue and chordae also can constitute indications for valve replacement.

In most centers, the mitral valve is replaced by means of a median sternotomy incision, although in reoperative circumstances, a right anterior thoracotomy is occasionally useful. The conduct of cardiopulmonary bypass and exposure through a left atriotomy are similar to those described earlier. With combined mitral and tricuspid disease, a right atrial/transseptal approach is advocated by some. Adequacy of myocardial protection is extremely important in mitral valve surgery, and a highly successful technique has combined (1) bicaval cannulation with occluding tapes, (2) myocardial precooling to 20 to 24° C. with the bypass circuit, (3) reduction in systemic flow during the arrest period to 1.0 to 1.5 liters per minute per square meter with systemic hypothermia of 24° C., (4) a 1200-ml. initial antegrade crystalloid cardioplegia infusion after aortic clamping, (5) combined topical pericardial and endocardial right atrial cold saline lavage, and (6) periodic antegrade reinfusion of 200 to 400 ml. of cardioplegia solution every 30 to 45 minutes to maintain myocardial temperature at approximately 10° C.

The valve is visualized, the pathologic anatomy assessed, and any thrombotic material removed. Usually, the anterior leaflet is grasped with a clamp, and the incision is initiated through the anterior leaflet, leaving a 2-mm. rim of cusp material attached to the anulus. Efficiency is enhanced by excising the valve at precisely this level over the entire circumference in one step. Care should be taken not to cut through the anulus, especially in the area of the posterior leaflet, since an atrioventricular rupture can be initiated. The chordae are cut at their origin, and it is important not to cut or otherwise damage the papillary muscles, since ventricular wall injury can cause myocardial rupture. To prevent prolapse of chordae through the prosthetic valve (which might interfere with valve function), tertiary chordae in the area of the posterior leaflet are carefully resected. Procedures designed to preserve mitral-papillary continuity have gained popularity recently but are avoided by the author because of potential problems with compromised prosthesis performance or ventricular outflow tract obstruction.

After adequate preparation of the annular circumference, the valve sutures are placed by use of a horizontal mattress technique and subannular pledgets. Usually, 2-0 Polydek sutures with small Teflon felt pledgets (¼ by ⅛ inch) are employed. The sutures are placed precisely into annular tissue and not beyond so as to avoid adjacent structures (Fig. 1). The suture line is begun at the superior commissure and continued in a clockwise manner, with spacing primarily within sutures rather than between them. The sutures then are passed through the valve sewing ring, the valve is seated, and the sutures are tied. The sutures are cut close to the knot to prevent prolapse of suture material through the valve orifice. Placing the sutures first into the annulus and then into the sewing ring in two steps requires a little more operative time but allows better matching of suture spacing. After completion, the annular tissue is "sandwiched" between the Teflon felt pledgets and the valve sewing ring, a configuration that has been shown experimentally to be very stable. Clinical experience with pledget techniques in several centers has demonstrated a negligible incidence of primary perivalvular dehiscence. If a concomitant aortic valve replacement is performed, the mitral valve is inserted after excision and sizing of the aortic valve, and then the aortic valve replacement is concluded.

If extensive calcification is encountered in the mitral anulus, removal can be dangerous. Minimal annular calcium deposits can be gently crushed with rongeurs and debrided, again with care taken not to extend the dissection through the heart wall. Severe bar calcification of the posterior anulus can pose serious problems for suture placement and valve seating. Rather than exposing the calcium, it is often easier to leave more leaflet tissue attached to the anulus in this area, and then to suture the valve to the imbricated leaflet. In the rare case in which an atrioventricular disruption occurs, it is important to recognize it intraoperatively and incorporate the ventricular and atrial borders into the pledgeted mattress sutures used for valve insertion.

Each valve has its own technical features. For example, Starr-Edwards valves should not be used in extremely small ventricles (as occur in mitral stenosis) because of the possibility of limiting ball movement or obstructing the left ventricular outflow tract. The struts of either the Starr-Edwards or tissue valves can perforate the posterior left ventricular wall as the sewing ring is seated. For this reason, it is important to move high-profile valves into the ventricle in a plane toward the apex, and not posteriorly, which might injure the heart wall. Excessive traction on the sutures during valve seating is avoided to prevent atrioventricular separation, and biologic valves should be irrigated with saline every few minutes to prevent drying. After the valve is inserted, the heart is not removed from the pericardium, again for the purpose of lessening the likelihood of atrioventricular dehiscence or ventricular perforation. With Medtronic Hall or St. Jude Medical valves, the major technical consideration is ensuring free mobility of the disc or leaflets. Leaving too much cusp tissue on the anulus or employing excessively large pledgets can cause the disc or leaflets to stick and should be avoided. Doppler echocardiography is useful intraoperatively and for long-term follow-up after prosthetic valve replacement.

Tricuspid Valve Annuloplasty or Replacement

Tricuspid valve annuloplasty should be performed during mitral valve procedures if Doppler evidence of significant functional tricuspid incompetence exists before or at the conclusion of cardiopulmonary bypass. Valve repair usually is performed during the reperfusion period of cardiopulmonary bypass as rewarming is accomplished after the mitral valve procedure. The right atrium is opened, and the valve apparatus is inspected. Functional incompetence is characterized by dilation of the right ventricular free-wall segment of the anulus, whereas the septal circumference usually is normal. After the area of the anterior leaflet and the base of the septal leaflet is sized with a Carpentier tricuspid obturator, the circumference is reduced with a Carpentier tricuspid ring,[11] bicuspidization annuloplasty, or a DeVega annuloplasty. Recent studies suggest that the Carpentier technique may be superior. Other authors prefer the DeVega method in terms of simplicity and clinical efficacy. Beginning at the superior commissure of the septal leaflet, deep bites are taken into the valve anulus using a pledgeted 2-0 polypropylene double-arm suture. Each suture enters the tissue very close to where it emerges from the previous bite, so that the suture is effectively buried within the anulus. The pursestring suture is continued to the posterior commissure of the septal leaflet, where it is tied over another pledget. The anulus is reduced exactly to the size of the obturator, restoring adequate competence without stenosis. Right atrial pressures are measured in the postoperative period.

If organic disease of the tricuspid valve is encountered, a tricuspid valve replacement is indicated. The procedure is performed with a technique similar to that of mitral valve replacement, with care being taken to avoid the right coronary artery and the bundle of His (Fig. 1). Because of thrombotic problems with mechanical valves in the tricuspid position, bioprostheses usually are employed. There is evidence that late bioprosthetic valve degeneration is uncommon in the tricuspid position because of the lower stresses associated with lower right ventricular pressures. The current status of multiple heart valve replacement has been reviewed by several authors.

Postoperative Care

The care of patients early after mitral valve replacement is similar to that in other types of cardiac surgery, except that specific factors related to the patient's valve disease and prosthetic valves require consideration. Whereas cardiac pump efficiency and forward stroke volume should improve after restoration of mitral competence, the ejection fraction usually decreases. Recent improvements in myocardial preservation, especially right ventricular protection, have reduced the incidence of low cardiac output significantly. If marginal cardiac output is encountered, familiarity with the management of postoperative cardiac dysfunction is required, including the use of inotropic agents and the intra-aortic balloon pump. Ventricular performance in patients with preoperative mitral regurgitation is particularly sensitive to arterial afterload, so that liberal administration of nitroprusside is indicated early postoperatively, and administration of hydralazine, prazosin, or captopril is useful later.

Temporary atrioventricular pacing wires and left atrial pressure lines are placed in most patients undergoing mitral valve surgery. Patients with tissue valves generally are anticoagulated with aspirin and dipyridamole, independent of cardiac rhythm. In all patients with mechanical valves in the mitral position, Coumadin anticoagulation is initiated on the fourth or fifth postoperative day and continued indefinitely. The prothrombin time ratio currently is maintained at approximately 1.5. Antibiotics are administered immediately before operation and then for 1 to 5 days postoperatively, depending on the clinical situation. Digoxin and diuretics are continued at preoperative doses for 4 to 6 weeks, since several weeks or months are required for resolution of the tendency toward fluid retention. If the patient has been in atrial fibrillation for less than 1 year, quinidine is begun postoperatively, and then cardioversion is attempted after 6 weeks if the rhythm does not revert spontaneously. Because of the high incidence of long-term valve-related complications, patients with prosthetic valves should be examined at least once yearly by a physician who is familiar with the associated problems.

VALVE SELECTION

The ideal prosthetic heart valve has not yet been developed, and the many valves currently available attest to that fact. Because each type of valve has advantages and disadvantages, selection should be individualized for each patient. As a group, bioprosthetic mitral valves (Fig. 17A and B) have low thromboembolic rates, do not require Coumadin anticoagulation, and have marginal flow characteristics in small sizes. The main concern with tissue valves is durability. Mechanical valves (Fig. 17C and D) for the most part are quite durable but have a higher incidence of thromboembolism, which requires Coumadin an-

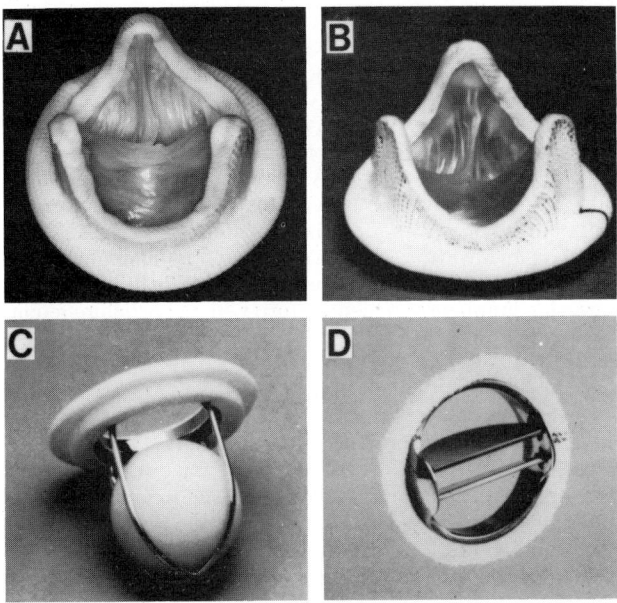

Figure 17. Commonly used prosthetic mitral valves. A, Hancock valve (Extracorporeal Medical Specialties, Inc., Anaheim, Ca.). B, Carpentier-Edwards valve (American Edwards Laboratories, Santa Ana, Ca.). C, Starr-Edwards 6120 valve (American Edwards Laboratories, Santa Ana, Ca.). D, St. Jude Medical valve (St. Jude Medical, St. Paul, Minn.).

ticoagulation and its associated independent risks. The advantages between valves must be considered individually, based on patient characteristics, intraoperative findings, and technical preferences of the surgeon.

Bioprosthetic Valves

The modern era of tissue valves began in the early 1970s when Hancock Laboratories and Edwards Laboratories introduced glutaraldehyde-fixed porcine heterografts for mitral valve replacement (Fig. 17A and B). This innovation was based on the work of Carpentier and co-workers, who demonstrated enhanced durability of biologic valves treated with glutaraldehyde. Subsequently, Ionescu introduced a valve consisting of bovine pericardium fixed with glutaraldehyde and mounted on a cloth-covered titanium frame. An excellent review of all aspects of bioprosthetic valves is edited by Cohn and Gallucci.

Bioprosthetic valves have certain common characteristics. They rarely induce hemolysis and are inaudible. The incidence of thromboembolism is low (0.1 to 2.0 per cent per patient year), so that Coumadin anticoagulation is not required. Earlier reports recommending Coumadin after mitral valve replacement in patients with atrial fibrillation have been superseded by the observation that aspirin and dipyridamole anticoagulation is equally effective. Valve thrombosis is rare, and all mitral bioprostheses have moderate diastolic pressure gradients in vivo. Thus, in sizes smaller than 27 to 29 mm. diameter, tissue valves may be distinctly stenotic, but the size of the patient and the need for physical exercise also should be considered. The incidence of postoperative prosthetic valve endocarditis is approximately the same as with mechanical valves (5 to 10 per cent over the valve lifetime), although evidence exists that tissue valve infections are more likely to be cured by antibiotic therapy alone. The diagnosis and management of prosthetic endocarditis have been reviewed by several authors.

The major concern with all tissue valves is durability.[8] Degeneration of leaflet tissue, calcification, and structural failure cause prosthetic valve dysfunction after an average of 7 to 10 years with porcine heterografts. The rate of valve failure is higher in the mitral than in the aortic position because of higher stresses associated with valve closure. The rate of valve failure is

2 to 5 per cent per patient year over the first 6 years and then accelerates, so that nearly every tissue valve requires replacement if the patient lives long enough. Frequently, biologic valves deteriorate slowly and can be replaced on a relatively elective basis. In other patients, valve failure is associated with a marked worsening of clinical status, which diminishes operative and long-term survival. A remarkably high incidence of sudden failure has been observed with the Ionescu-Shiley bovine pericardial valve, and this prosthesis has been removed from the American market. The problem of tissue valve durability is significant and becomes even more evident with time as increasing numbers of patients return with valve failure requiring reoperation.

Mechanical Valves

Current mechanical heart valves (Fig. 17C and D) offer better predictability of performance and durability than do tissue valves. However, all patients require Coumadin therapy, and valve thrombosis or thromboembolism can occur despite adequate anticoagulation. Although the quality of reporting has not been optimal, the thromboembolic rates for most mechanical valves (6120 Starr-Edwards and Medtronic Hall valves) with adequate anticoagulation approximate 2 to 5 per cent per patient year, although thromboembolism is less common with the St. Jude Medical (SJ) valve. Late valve thrombosis and strut fracture have been a problem with the Bjork-Shiley valve in the mitral position, and this valve has been removed from the American market. Recently, streptokinase thrombolysis has been employed successfully for thrombosed Bjork-Shiley mitral or aortic valves. With low-profile valves, late disc or leaflet obstruction also can occur from various causes. Anticoagulation complications are observed with all mechanical valves. The mortality attributable to Coumadin therapy approaches 1 per cent per year, being the major cause of late death after SJ valve replacement. Recent studies suggest that "modest" Coumadin anticoagulation of the SJ valve to a prothrombin time ratio of 1.3 to 1.5 is effective, but more follow-up of this regimen is necessary. The mitral SJ valve has the best flow characteristics, and the Starr-Edwards valve has the poorest. Severe hemolysis without perivalvular leak has been reported in three patients with the SJ mitral valve and has occurred once in the author's experience.

Specific Indications

In all tissue valves, the rate of leaflet calcification and degeneration is unacceptable in patients less than 20 to 30 years of age or in patients with chronic renal failure, which contraindicates bioprosthetic valve insertion. In children, the SJ valve is employed because of the necessity of good flow characteristics in small sizes. Coumadin anticoagulation is required in children, since recent trials of aspirin and dipyridamole anticoagulation with the SJ valve have reported an unacceptable thromboembolic rate. Young females desiring children may choose a tissue valve to reduce the complications of anticoagulation during pregnancy, with the understanding that the prosthesis eventually requires replacement. Patients with specific contraindications to anticoagulation also are candidates for tissue valves. Patients in the elderly age group generally are recommended mechanical valves by the author, since the return of an elderly patient 5 to 10 years later at an even older age with tissue valve failure is a difficult problem.

Patients undergoing complicated valve procedures such as aortic and mitral valve replacement or valve replacement–coronary bypass combinations should receive mechanical valves because of the higher mortality associated with reoperation in these groups. In difficult technical cases, such as small left atria or calcified anuli, a low-profile valve is implanted because of ease of insertion. Tricuspid valve replacement is performed exclusively with tissue valves. In most other patients, a mechanical valve is recommended, and presently the SJ valve is favored because of lower thromboembolic rates and better flow characteristics. It must be emphasized, however, that all prosthetic valves have significant long-term complications, which requires both the patient and referring physician to assume active roles in the decision-making process. In the final analysis, however, the thromboembolic and anticoagulation complications of mechanical valves are approximately equivalent to the durability problems of bioprostheses, so that late results after mitral valve replacement are similar with both types of valves. This realization has led to the increasing application of valve reconstruction to an expanding area of mitral valve disorders. However, more detailed analysis of long-term survival and complications is necessary to fully establish the relative indications and results of mitral valve repair, versus bioprosthetic valve replacement, versus mechanical valve utilization in the various subcategories of mitral valve disease.

REFERENCES

1. Abe, T., Tukamoto, M., Yanagiya, M., Morikawa, M., Watanabe, N., and Komatsu, S.: De Vega's annuloplasty for acquired tricuspid disease: Early and late results in 110 patients. Ann. Thorac. Surg., 48:670, 1989.
2. Angell, W. W., Oury, J. H., and Shah, P.: A comparison of replacement and reconstruction in patients with mitral regurgitation. J. Thorac. Cardiovasc. Surg., 98:665, 1987.
3. Antunes, M. J.: Valve replacement in the elderly. Is the mechanical valve a good alternative? J. Thorac. Cardiovasc. Surg., 89:485, 1989.
4. Armenti, F., Stephenson, L. W., and Edmunds, L. H., Jr.: Simultaneous implantation of St. Jude Medical aortic and mitral prostheses. J. Thorac. Cardiovasc. Surg., 94:733, 1987.
5. Arom, K. V., Nicoloff, D. M., Kersten, T. E., Lindsay, W. G., and Northrup, W. F., 3d: St. Jude Medical prosthesis: Valve-related deaths and complications. Ann. Thorac. Surg., 43:591, 1987.
6. Arom, K. V., Nicoloff, D. M., Kersten, T. E., Northrup, W. F., 3d, Lindsay, W. G., and Emery, R. W.: Ten years' experience with the St. Jude Medical valve prosthesis. Ann. Thorac. Surg., 47:831, 1989.
7. Bonchek, L. I.: Balloon valvuloplasty versus surgical commissurotomy (letter). Am. J. Cardiol., 62:1153, 1988.
8. Bortolotti, U., Milano, A., Thiene, G., Guerra, F., Mazzucco, A., Talenti, E., and Gallucci, V.: Long-term durability of the Hancock porcine bioprosthesis following combined mitral and aortic valve replacement: An 11-year experience. Ann. Thorac. Surg., 44:130, 1987.
9. Camara, M. L., Aris, A., Padro, J. M., and Caralps, J. M.: Long-term results of mitral valve surgery in patients with severe pulmonary hypertension. Ann. Thorac. Surg., 45:133, 1988.
10. Cammack, P. L., Edie, R. N., and Edmunds, L. H.: Bar calcification of the mitral anulus. J. Thorac. Cardiovasc. Surg., 94:399, 1987.
11. Carpentier, A.: Cardiac valve surgery—the "French correction." J. Thorac. Cardiovasc. Surg., 86:323, 1983.
12. Carpentier, A., Didier, L., Deloche, A., et al.: Surgical anatomy and management of ischemic mitral valve incompetence. Circulation, 76(Suppl.):1776, 1987.
13. Chavez, A. M., Cosgrove, D. M., 3d, Lytle, B. W., Gill, C. C., Loop, F. D., Stewart, R. W., Golding, L. R., and Taylor, P. C.: Applicability of mitral valvuloplasty techniques in a North American population. Am. J. Cardiol., 62:253, 1988.
14. Chidambaram, M., Abdulali, S. A., Baliga, B. G., and Ionescu, M. I.: Long-term results of DeVega tricuspid annuloplasty. Ann. Thorac. Surg., 43:185, 1987.
15. Cohn, L. H., Kowalker, W., Bhatia, S., DiSesa, V. J., St. John-Sutton, M., Shemin, R. J., and Collins, J. J., Jr.: Comparative morbidity of mitral valve repair versus replacement for mitral regurgitation with and without coronary artery disease. Ann. Thorac. Surg., 45:284, 1988.
16. Cohn, L. H., Peigh, P. S., Sell, J., and DiSesa, V. J.: Right thoracotomy, femorofemoral bypass, and deep hypothermia for re-replacement of the mitral valve. Ann. Thorac. Surg., 48:69, 1989.
17. Cortina, J. M., Martinel, J., Artiz, V. et al.: Surgical treatment of active prosthetic valve endocarditis. Results in 66 patients. Thorac. Cardiovasc. Surg., 35:209, 1987.
18. Cosgrove, D. M.: Valve reconstruction versus valve replacement. In Crawford, F. A., Jr. (Ed.): Cardiac Surgery: Current Heart Valve Prostheses. (Cardiac Surgery: State of the Art Reviews, Vol. 1, No. 2.) Philadelphia, Hanley & Belfus, 1987.
19. Cosgrove, D. M., and Stewart, W. J.: Mitral valvuloplasty. Curr. Probl. Cardiol., 14:353, 1989.
20. Czer, L. S., Matloff, J. M., Chaux, A., DeRobertis, M. A., and Gray, R. J.: Comparative clinical experience with porcine bioprosthetic and St. Jude valve replacement. Chest, 91:503, 1987.
21. DeBruijn, N. P., and Clements, F. M.: Transesophageal Echocardiography. Dordrecht, The Netherlands, Nijhoff, 1987.

22. DeBruijn, N. P., Clements, F. M., and Kisslo, J. A.: Applications of color flow imaging. Echocardiography, 4:557, 1987.

23. Duran, C. G., Revuelta, J. M., Gaite, L., Alonso, C., and Fleitas, M. G.: Stability of mitral reconstructive surgery at 10–12 years for predominantly rheumatic valvular disease. Circulation, 78:191, 1988.

24. Edmunds, L. H., Jr.: Thrombotic and bleeding complications of prosthetic heart valves. Ann. Thorac. Surg., 44:430, 1987.

25. Feld, H., and Roth, J.: Severe haemolytic anaemia after replacement of the mitral valve by a St. Jude medical prosthesis. Br. Heart J., 62:475, 1989.

26. Fiore, A. C., Naunheim, K. S., Barner, H. B., Pennington, D. G., McBride, L. R., Kaiser, G. C., and Willman, V. L.: Valve replacement in the octogenarian. Ann. Thorac. Surg., 48:104, 1989.

27. Galloway, A. C., Colvin, S. B., Baumann, F. G., Harty, S., and Spencer, F. C.: Current concepts of mitral valve reconstruction for mitral insufficiency. Circulation, 78:1087, 1988.

28. Galloway, A. C., Colvin, S. B., Baumann, F. G., Grossi, E. A., Ribakove, G. H., Harty, S., and Spencer, F. C.: A comparison of mitral valve reconstruction with mitral valve replacement: Intermediate-term results. Ann. Thorac. Surg., 47:655, 1989.

29. Goldman, M. E., Guarino, T., Fuster, V., and Mindich, B.: The necessity for tricuspid valve repair can be determined intraoperatively by two-dimensional echocardiography. J. Thorac. Cardiovasc. Surg., 94:542, 1987.

30. Harpole, D. H., Rankin, J. S., Wolfe, W. G., Smith, L. R., Young, W. G., Clements, F. G., and Jones, R. H.: Assessment of left ventricular functional preservation during isolated cardiac valvular operations. Circulation, 80(Suppl. III):III-1, 1989.

31. Herrmann, H. C., Wilkins, G. T., Bascal, V. M., Weyman, A. E., Block, P. C., and Palacios, I. F.: Percutaneous balloon mitral valvulotomy for patients with mitral stenosis. Analysis of factors influencing early results. J. Thorac. Cardiovasc. Surg., 96:33, 1988.

32. Kay, G. L., Kay, J. H., Mendez, M. A., Zubiate, P., and Yokoyama, T.: Long-term results of operations for mitral regurgitation secondary to coronary artery disease. Cardiovasc. Clin., 17:41, 1987.

33. Kay, G. L., Morita, S., Mendez, M., Zubiate, P., and Kay, J. H.: Tricuspid regurgitation associated with mitral valve disease: Repair and replacement. Ann. Thorac. Surg., 48:S93, 1989.

34. Kirklin, J. K., Naftel, D. C., Blackstone, E. H., Kirklin, J. W., and Brown, R. C.: Risk factors for mortality after primary combined valvular and coronary artery surgery. Circulation, 79:I185, 1989.

35. Kurzrok, S., Singh, A. K., Most, A. S., and Williams, D. O.: Thrombolytic therapy for prosthetic cardiac valve thrombosis. J. Am. Coll. Cardiol., 9:592, 1987.

36. McGrath, L. B., Gonzalez-Lavin, L., Eldredge, W. J., Colombi, M., and Restrepo, D.: Thromboembolic and other events following valve replacement in a pediatric population treated with antiplatelet agents. Ann. Thorac. Surg., 43:285, 1987.

37. Mok, P., Lieberman, E. H., Lilly, L. S., Schafer, A. I., DiSesa, V. J., and Rutherford, C. R.: Severe hemolytic anemia following mitral valve repair. Am. Heart J., 117:1171, 1989.

38. Myers, M. L., Lawrie, G. M., Crawford, E. S., Howell, J. F., Morris, G. C., Jr., Glaeser, D. H., and DeBakey, M. E.: The St. Jude valve prosthesis: Analysis of the clinical results in 815 implants and the need for systemic anticoagulation. J. Am. Coll. Cardiol., 13:57, 1989.

39. Okita, Y., Miki, S., Kusuhara, K., Ueda, Y., Tahata, T., Tsukamoto, Y., Komeda, M., Yamanaka, K., Shiraishi, S., Tamura, T., et al.: Early and late results of reconstructive operation for congenital mitral regurgitation in pediatric age group. J. Thorac. Cardiovasc. Surg., 96:294, 1988.

40. Rankin, J. S., and Sabiston, D. C., Jr.: Physiology of coronary blood flow, myocardial function, and intraoperative protection. In Sabiston, D. C., Jr., and Spencer, F. C. (Eds.): Gibbon's Surgery of the Chest, 5th ed. Philadelphia, W. B. Saunders Company, 1989.

41. Rankin, J. S., Hickey, M. St. J., Smith, L. R., et al.: A clinical comparison of mitral valve repair versus valve replacement in ischemic mitral regurgitation. J. Thorac. Cardiovasc. Surg., 95:165, 1988.

42. Rankin, J. S., Livesey, S. A., Smith, L. R., et al.: Trends in the surgical treatment of ischemic mitral regurgitation: Effects of mitral valve repair on hospital mortality. Semin. Thorac. Cardiovasc. Surg., 1:149, 1989.

43. Sand, M. E., Naftel, D. C., Blackstone, E. H., et al.: A comparison of repair and replacement for mitral valve incompetence. J. Thorac. Cardiovasc. Surg., 94:208, 1987.

44. Saour, J. N., Sieck, J. O., Mamo, L. A. R., et al.: Trial of different intensities of anticoagulation in patients with prosthetic heart valves. N. Engl. J. Med., 322:428, 1990.

45. Schoevaerdts, J. C., Buche, M., el-Gariani, A., et al.: Twenty years' experience with the model 6120 Starr-Edwards valve in the mitral position. J. Thorac. Cardiovasc. Surg., 94:375, 1987.

46. Scott, M. L., Stowe, C. L., Nunnally, L. C., Spector, S. D., Moseley, P. W., Schumacher, P. D., and Thompson, P. A.: Mitral valve reconstruction in the elderly population. Ann. Thorac. Surg., 48:213, 1989.

47. Sheikh, K. H., deBruijn, N. P., Rankin, J. S., et al.: The utility of transesophageal echocardiography and Doppler color flow imaging in patients undergoing cardiac valve operations. J. Am. Coll. Cardiol., 15:363, 1990.

48. Smith, R., Brender, D., and McCredie, M.: Percutaneous transluminal balloon dilatation of the mitral valve in pregnancy. Br. Heart J., 61:551, 1989.

49. Walley, V. M., and Keon, W. J.: Patterns of failure in Inescu-Shiley bovine pericardial bioprosthetic valves. J. Thorac. Cardiovasc. Surg., 93:925, 1987.

50. Yee, E. S., and Ullyot, D. J.: Reparative approach for right-sided endocarditis. Operative considerations and results of valvuloplasty. J. Thorac. Cardiovasc. Surg., 96:133, 1988.

XIX

EBSTEIN'S ANOMALY

James A. Alexander, M.D., and Daniel J. O'Brien, Ph.D.

Ebstein's anomaly is an extremely rare and variable defect of the tricuspid valve that represents less than 1 per cent of all congenital cardiac disorders. Two characteristic features of this anomaly are the redundancy of tricuspid valve tissue and adherence of a variable portion of the septal and posterior cusps to the right ventricular wall.

HISTORICAL ASPECTS

Ebstein's anomaly was first described by Wilhelm Ebstein in 1864 after the autopsy of a 19-year-old laborer.[27,39] At the time of hospital admission, 8 days before his death, the patient was noted to be emaciated with pronounced cyanosis of the face, hoarseness, and moderately edematous lower extremities. The pulse was 112 beats per minute, the respirations averaged 32 breaths per minute, and the jugular veins pulsed with each heart beat. Pulmonary edema was thought to be the cause of death. During the postmortem examination, Ebstein meticulously described the abnormality of the tricuspid valve. In-

cluded in this description was the pathologic downward displacement of the septal leaflet below the tricuspid annulus. Ebstein also established that the malformation had an embryologic origin and that the valve not only was insufficient but could also cause right-sided heart obstruction.

During Ebstein's lifetime, 8 similar cases of tricuspid malformation were reported. In 1900, MacCallum, of Johns Hopkins University, was the first to describe a similar tricuspid defect in the English literature. A case report by Arnstein was published in 1927. The case involved downward displacement of the tricuspid valve, and he suggested this type of congenital abnormality be designated *Ebstein's disease*. In 1937, Yata and Shapiro reported the first patient with Ebstein's anomaly to be examined with both radiographic and electrocardiographic techniques. Tourniaire, in 1949, used cardiac catheterization to make the diagnosis of Ebstein's malformation during life. The use of a prosthetic valve for total surgical correction of Ebstein's anomaly was first reported by Barnard and Schrire in 1963.[27]

EMBRYOLOGY

Ebstein's anomaly is better understood in the context of events that occur during the embryologic development of the tricuspid valve. Although it is somewhat controversial,[46,48] it is thought that the tricuspid valve is almost exclusively derived from the interior of the embryonic right ventricular myocardium and involves a process of undermining the right ventricular wall (Fig. 1). The inner layer of the ventricular myocardium is freed from the remainder of the right ventricular wall and forms a muscular skirt. The atrial side of this muscular skirt near the atrioventricular ostium is partially covered by endocardial cushion tissue. Openings form in the lower portion of the skirt, where papillary muscles and chordae tendineae remain. The chordae are initially muscular but later become fibrotic. The anterior cusp of the tricuspid valve is formed very early in embryonic development, and the posterior and septal cusps form much later, during the third month of gestation.

It is speculated that the characteristic sail leaflet of the tricuspid valve, which in some forms of Ebstein's anomaly is totally free, occurs because of much earlier embryologic development of that leaflet. In addition, given the lack of liberation of the posterior and septal leaflets, the corresponding right ventricular myocardium has no impetus to develop, causing a thinned atrialized portion of the right ventricle. During embryologic development, it is reasoned that the undermining process of the right ventricular wall did not reach the annulus of the tricuspid valve and the degree of undermining is responsible for the marked variations in appearance of the tricuspid valve seen in Ebstein's anomaly. These variations range from lack of undermining of all three valve cusps with only a small free valve edge at the apex of the right ventricle to an almost normal-appearing tricuspid valve with a small septal leaflet closely adherent to the ventricular septal surface[46] (Fig. 2).

ANATOMY AND PATHOPHYSIOLOGY

In Ebstein's malformation, the right atrium is dilated and, in advanced cases, may be enormous. Atrial septal defects are common and are usually of the patent foramen ovale type. The annulus of the tricuspid valve is generally quite dilated. The septal leaflet is small and firmly attached to the ventricular septum with cords that appear to enter the myocardium directly. The posterior leaflet may be firmly attached to the right

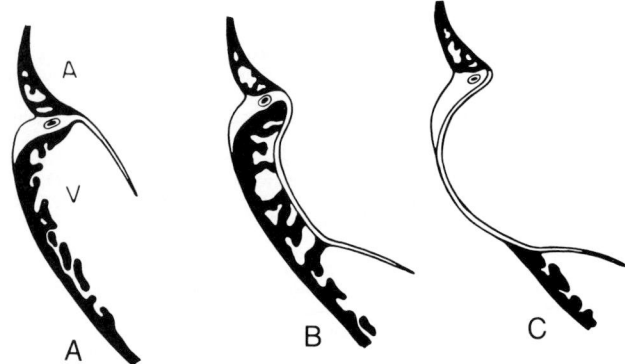

Figure 2. Section through the right atrioventricular junction. *A,* Normal heart. a, right atrium; V, right ventricle. *B,* Mild degree of Ebstein's anomaly. *C,* Severe Ebstein's anomaly. Note in *B* and *C* the apparent displacement of the tricuspid valve (From Ven Mierop, L. H. S., Kutsche, L. M., and Victorica, B. E.: Ebstein's anomaly. *In* Adams, F. H., Emmanouilides, G. C., and Riemenschneider, T. A. (Eds): Moss's Heart Disease in Infants, Children and Adolescents, 4th ed. Baltimore, Williams & Wilkins, 1987, p. 362.)

ventricular myocardium or, in some cases, may be absent. If undermining has occurred, the anterior leaflet of the tricuspid valve is generally redundant and has the appearance of a sail. The papillary muscles of the tricuspid valve are anomalous and may be malpositioned. The valve is generally incompetent. When the valve leaflets are displaced to the apex of the right ventricle, the atrialized portion of the right ventricle may be markedly thinned and dilated. In more severe cases, this atrialized portion has the appearance of a parchment right ventricle dissimilar to that seen in Uhl's anomaly. In other cases, the tricuspid valve leaflets may be attached at the apical portion of the right ventricle with only a perforation in the leaflet for an exit of blood flow to the infundibulum.[11,24,27,46,47]

A number of cardiac malformations may be associated with Ebstein's anomaly. In addition to a patent foramen ovale, other types of interatrial septal defects include ostium secundum, ostium primum, and sinus venosus defects.[47,48] Less frequently associated cardiac defects include patent ductus arteriosus, pulmonary valve stenosis or atresia, ventricular septal defects, tricuspid valve stenosis, transposition of the great vessels, and congenital mitral stenosis. Isolated cases of anomalous pulmonary venous connection to the coronary sinus, mitral valve prolapse, coarctation of the aorta, right aortic arch, and tetralogy of Fallot have also been reported.[34,36,46]

Ebstein's anomaly can occur in the tricuspid valve position of the left side of the heart. This is a relatively common feature in patients who have corrected transposition (atrioventricular discordance). Almost 30 per cent of left tricuspid valves are incompetent, but this is not necessarily due to an Ebstein's malformation.[24] Several reports have described Ebstein's anomaly of the mitral valve, that is, downward displacement of the mitral leaflets into the left ventricle. However, the authors do not consider this type of malformation to be part of the spectrum of Ebstein's anomaly.[7,15,26]

Pathophysiologic derangements associated with Ebstein's anomaly are generally dictated by the anatomic problems with the tricuspid valve in the presence of a patent foramen ovale or atrial septal defects. The combination of right ventricular dysfunction and coexistent tricuspid insufficiency and/or stenosis generally causes systemic venous hypertension with peripheral edema.

In the presence of an atrial septal defect, cyanosis develops as a result of increased right-to-left shunting of blood flow. In these patients, several mechanisms may contribute to the reappearance of cyanosis. These mechanisms include aneurysmal formation in the atrialized portion of the right ventricle that enhances tricuspid insufficiency,[24] increased pulmonary vascu-

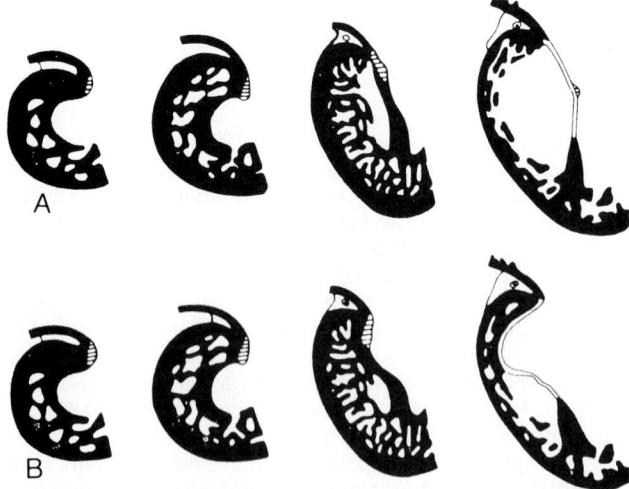

Figure 1. Concept of the pathogenesis of Ebstein's anomaly. *A,* Normal development of the atrioventricular valve cusp. *B,* Ebstein's anomaly. (From Van Mierop, L. H. S., Kutsche, L. M., and Victoria, B. E.: Ebstein's anomaly. *In* Adams, F. H., Emmanouilides, G. C., and Riemenschneider, T. A. (Eds): Moss's Heart Disease in Infants. Children and Adolescents, 4th ed. Baltimore, Williams & Wilkins, 1987, p. 362.)

lar resistance due to pulmonary embolism,[16] and atrial dysrhythmias.[38] Tachydysrhythmias such as atrial flutter and atrial fibrillation increase the degree of cyanosis and decrease cardiac output. With a stenotic tricuspid valve, right ventricular filling is decreased, and right-to-left shunting through the atrial septum is increased. With tricuspid valve insufficiency, an increase in heart rate increases mean right atrial pressure, which also causes an increase of right-to-left shunting. Obviously, higher heart rates reduce left ventricular filling, which causes lower systemic cardiac output. Aneurysmal dilation of the atrialized portion of the right ventricle may hamper loading of the trabecular and infundibular portions of the ventricle and contribute to increased right-to-left shunting and decreased pulmonary blood flow. Paradoxic emboli with cerebral embolization may also occur.[16,29]

CLINICAL MANIFESTATIONS

Patients who have Ebstein's anomaly are generally symptomatic during the newborn period and demonstrate signs of cyanosis, rapid respirations, cardiomegaly, and hepatomegaly. With the progressive reduction in pulmonary vascular resistance after birth, symptoms in patients with milder forms of Ebstein's disease may entirely disappear, only to return in childhood or early adult life. Depending on the extent of the tricuspid valve malformation, patients may die *in utero* or may not be diagnosed until adult life. The most common symptoms of Ebstein's anomaly are shortness of breath and fatigue. Palpitations are frequent, and cyanosis occurs in the majority of patients at some point during life. Dysrhythmias, especially atrial flutter, atrial fibrillation, and ventricular ectopy, occur in more than one half of patients with Ebstein's disease. Patients may also complain of dizziness and transient visual loss. In addition, patients may exhibit signs and symptoms of pulmonary or systemic embolization.[4,11,24,46]

On physical examination, signs may vary. Generally, patients who are not cyanotic have smaller hearts and a more localized cardiac impulse. Cyanotic patients with large hearts may have a diffuse point of maximal impulse and pulsations in the jugular veins. The liver is large, and there may be peripheral edema. On auscultation, the first and second heart sounds are generally normal. A systolic murmur is heard in a majority of patients and is attributable to either tricuspid insufficiency or right ventricular outflow tract obstruction. In patients with severe cyanosis and decreased pulmonary blood flow, the pulmonary component of the second heart sound may be diminished or absent. A diastolic murmur is occasionally heard, although its cause is unclear. In patients with long-standing cyanosis, clubbing is usually present.

The electrocardiogram is always abnormal. Usually present is a right ventricular bundle branch block with a characteristically prolonged PR interval. Generally, the P wave has an increased duration and increased amplitude owing to the generous size of the right atrium. Approximately 5 to 20 per cent of these patients have the Wolff-Parkinson-White syndrome, usually of the Type B pattern resembling left bundle branch block, and may experience increased frequency of supraventricular tachycardia.[11,24,38,46] Multiple accessory pathways may be present.[8,9,40]

Roentgenographic evaluation of the cardiac silhouette may vary from essentially normal to the classic globular heart. Cardiomegaly may be striking and extend from chest wall to chest wall. Even in patients with massive cardiomegaly, the pulmonary vasculature is either normal or decreased.[31]

For many years, cardiac catheterization has been the most effective method of diagnosing Ebstein's anomaly. The right atrium is usually massive, and there is a dominant V wave due to tricuspid insufficiency. A right ventriculogram demonstrates the abnormal attachment of the valve leaflets as well as insuffi-

ciency. The *sine qua non* of Ebstein's anomaly is a pull-back of an electrode catheter from the right ventricular outflow tract/apex with a ventricular complex associated with a ventricular pressure tracing.[46] Withdrawal of the catheter into the atrialized portion of the ventricle yields a ventricular complex with an atrial pressure tracing. However, when right ventricular and atrial pressures are similar in contour, interpretation of the electrical signals can be difficult. In patients with atrial septal defects, arterial desaturation may be present if there is a significant right-to-left shunt. Cardiac catheterization is helpful in identifying associated defects.

Two-dimensional echocardiography has greatly enhanced the ability to diagnose Ebstein's anomaly. Tricuspid valve mobility and valve attachments can be readily assessed. The degree of right ventricular wall thickness and paradoxic motion of the atrialized posterior right ventricular wall can also be visualized. Color-flow Doppler studies demonstrate stenosis of the displaced tricuspid valve as well as blood flow through the atrial septum.[28,33,42] During pregnancy, fetal echocardiography has been useful in diagnosing Ebstein's anomaly and accompanying cardiac defects.[37,41] Of note, females with exposure to lithium therapy in the first trimester have a 2 to 8 per cent risk of Ebstein's anomaly, compared with a risk of 1 in 20,000 for the general population.[2,18] These patients should undergo fetal echocardiography.

Currently, computed cine axial tomography does not provide sufficient anatomic detail.[17,25] Magnetic resonance imaging is useful in providing additional information about the relationship of the tricuspid valve to the right ventricular outflow tract.[21] Data from the cardiac catheterization and echocardiographic findings remain the most reliable information for surgical considerations.

In milder forms of Ebstein's anomaly, when the heart is of normal size, the differential diagnosis may include other forms of complex cyanotic heart disease such as tetralogy of Fallot, especially in association with an endocardial cushion defect. Other congenital malformations that may mimic Ebstein's anomaly include pulmonary atresia with intact septum and tricuspid insufficiency, right ventricular endomyocardial fibrosis without downward displacement of the tricuspid valve, and the rare Uhl's anomaly of the right ventricle.[3,46]

PATIENT MANAGEMENT

The anatomic variations of Ebstein's disease in addition to the presence of other cardiac defects require individualized therapeutic protocols. Irrespective of surgical therapy, children with Ebstein's anomaly should not be placed in competitive athletics, and these patients should receive antibiotics before dental or endoscopic procedures as prophylaxis against subacute bacterial endocarditis.

Patients with Ebstein's anomaly who are judged Class I or Class II according to the New York Heart Association (NYHA) Functional Classification System are generally followed and treated medically. Division of accessory pathways may be indicated if poor rate control is present despite reasonable dosages of antidysrhythmic medications. Other exceptions to following Class I and Class II patients include paradoxic emboli, right ventricular outflow tract obstruction, and moderate to severe cyanosis. Paroxysmal tachydysrhythmias such as atrial flutter, atrial fibrillation, or Wolff-Parkinson-White syndrome should be treated aggressively, including DC conversion, since pulmonary blood flow can be seriously compromised. In asymptomatic patients with the Wolff-Parkinson-White syndrome, surgical ablation of accessory tracts, with or without valve reconstruction or replacement, should be considered.[6,10-12]

Palliative surgical procedures for symptomatic patients with Ebstein's anomaly have generally produced poor results. Blalock-Taussig shunts should be avoided. Superior vena cava–

right pulmonary artery anastomosis (Glenn shunt) has been of some limited benefit to severely cyanotic patients. Isolated closure of atrial septal defects has been performed to reduce cyanosis and prevent paradoxic emboli.[11,46]

Patients with NYHA Class III or Class IV require surgical intervention for replacement or repair of the tricuspid valve and closure of the atrial septum. In 1963, Barnard and Schrire[5] first reported two patients treated surgically with prosthetic valve replacement and a valve ring sewn above the coronary sinus to prevent heart block. In 1964, Hardy and associates[19] reported the first successful valvuloplasty based on the approach of Hunter and Lillehei,[22] who suggested plication of the atrialized portion of the right ventricle to the true annulus of the tricuspid valve.

Despite less than ideal results, prosthetic valve replacement became the most frequently used method for surgical repair of Ebstein's anomaly. However, in the past decade, tricuspid valvuloplasty and reconstruction has become a significant part of the surgical armamentarium for Ebstein's anomaly.[1,13,20,30,32,35,43] Danielson[11] has employed plastic procedures in approximately 72 per cent of 134 consecutive patients undergoing surgical repair. In this series, the majority of patients had

tricuspid valve reconstruction by the creation of a monocusp tricuspid valve. This technique (Fig. 3) entails plication of the atrialized ventricular portion, reduction of the giant right atrium, closure of the atrial septal defect, and narrowing of the true tricuspid annulus.[12]

Recently, Carpentier and associates[6] introduced a slightly different approach to tricuspid valve reconstruction in which the atrialized ventricular portion is plicated on the long axis of the right ventricle in a vertical direction (Fig. 4). This procedure differs from the approach by Danielson in which the atrialized portion of the right ventricle is plicated in a horizontal or apex-to-base position, which shortens the long axis of the ventricle. Carpentier also recommends detaching the anterior leaflet and a portion of the posterior leaflet from the annulus as well as secondary cords. The leaflets are then resutured to the annulus after the appropriate vertical plication is performed. A tricuspid valvuloplasty ring is then inserted below the coronary sinus. Atrial plication is also performed.

Despite the trend toward repair rather than replacement of abnormal cardiac valves, some variations of Ebstein's anomaly require prosthetic valve replacement, which usually requires placement of the sewing ring above the coronary sinus. However, even in situations in which the atrialized ventricular portion is extremely thin, the efficacy of plication, as it relates to improvement of ventricular function, has been difficult to document. When valve replacement is necessary, the risk to benefit ratio of using bioprosthetic valves versus mechanical valves must be evaluated carefully, particularly in children. Although they are more durable, mechanical valves are subject to malfunction due to blood clotting, especially in patients with low-output states.[20] Additionally, there is an increased rate of morbidity and mortality from bleeding associated with

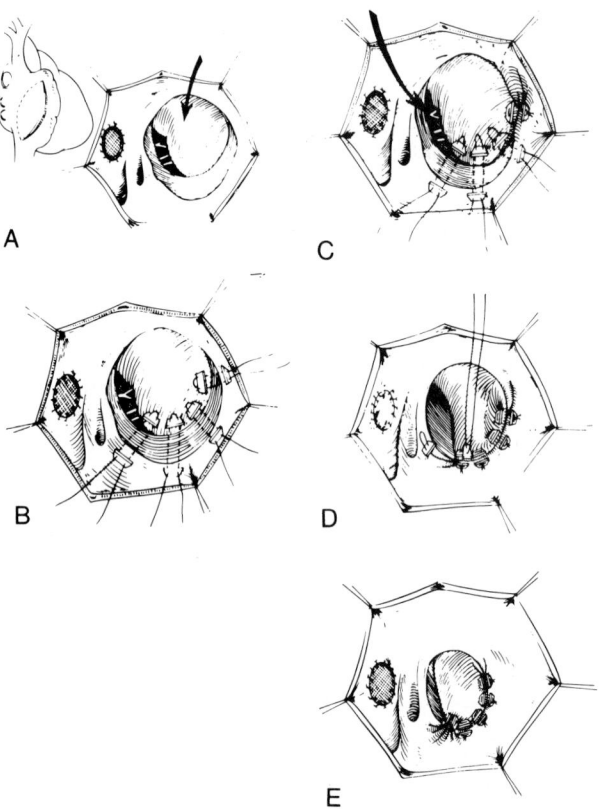

Figure 3. Diagram of repair. *A, left,* The right atrium is incised from atrial appendage to inferior vena cava. The redundant portion of the right atrium is excised (dotted line) so that the final size of the right atrium is normal. *Right,* The atrial septal defect is closed with a patch. Large anterior leaflet is indicated by arrow. The posterior leaflet is displaced down from annulus. The septal leaflet is hypoplastic and is not seen in this view. *B,* Mattress sutures passed through pledgets of Teflon felt are used for pulling the tricuspid annulus and tricuspid valve together. Sutures are placed in the atrialized portion of the right ventricle as shown so that when they are subsequently tied, the atrialized ventricle is plicated and the aneurysmal cavity is obliterated. *C,* Sutures are tied down sequentially. Hypoplastic, markedly displaced septal leaflets is now visible (arrow). *D,* A posterior anuloplasty is performed to narrow the diameter of the tricuspid annulus. Coronary sinus marks posteroleftward extent of the anuloplasty, which is terminated there so that injury to the conduction bundle is avoided. Occasionally, one or two additional mattress sutures are required to obliterate the posterior aspect of the anuloplasty repair in order to render the valve totally competent. The tricuspid annulus at this time will admit two or more fingers. *E,* Completed repair, which allows anterior leaflet to function as a monocusp valve. (From Danielson, G. K., and Fuster, V.: Surgical repair of Ebstein's anomaly. Ann. Surg., *196:*501, 1982.)

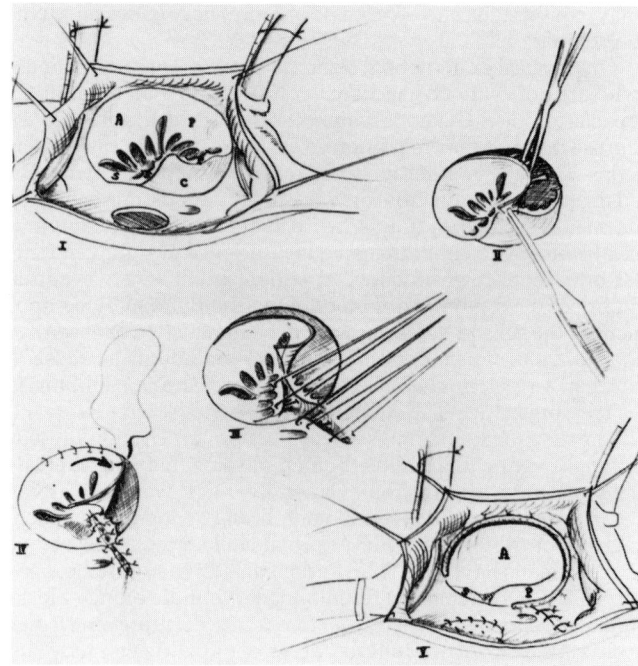

Figure 4. Surgical technique. *I,* Operative view. A, Anterior leaflet; P, posterior leaflet; S, Septal leaflet; C, atrialized chamber. *II,* Anterior leaflet and adjacent portion of posterior leaflet are detached from annulus. Leaflet time is mobilized by cutting fibrous bands attached to ventricular wall. Interchordal spaces are fenestrated if obliterated. *III,* Longitudinal plication of right ventricle by simple sutures passed through septal and posterior leaflet remnants. The tricuspid annulus and right atrium are plicated. *IV,* Anterior and posterior leaflets are sutured to the tricuspid annulus after clockwise rotation (arrow) to cover entire orifice area. *V,* A prosthetic ring is inserted for remodeling the orifice and reinforcing repair. The atrial septal defect is closed. (From Carpentier, A., Chauvaud, S., Macé, L., Relland, J., Milhaileanu, S., Marino, J. P., Abry, B., and Guibourt, P.: A new reconstructive operation for Ebstein's anomaly of the tricuspid valve. J. Thorac. Cardiovasc. Surg., *96:*95, 1988.)

anticoagulation in both children and adults.[44] Bioprosthetic valves are subject to more rapid deterioration, particularly in the younger age group. Whereas these valves fare better on the right side of the heart than on the left, they are associated with a significant likelihood of requiring replacement within the first decade of insertion.[14,23,35]

General postoperative concerns include maintaining adequate cardiac performance, reducing pulmonary vascular resistance, and optimizing the heart rate and rhythm. However, caution must be exercised. The need for catecholamine support must be carefully balanced against the dysrhythmogenic effects of inotropic agents. Conversely, the benefits of antidysrhythmic medications must be balanced against the myocardial depressant properties of these agents.

NATURAL HISTORY AND SURGICAL OUTCOME

Precise delineation of the natural history of Ebstein's anomaly is difficult given the extreme variability of the anatomy of the tricuspid valve. Approximately one third of the patients die before the age of 10 years, most in early infancy. The mean age of death is approximately the second decade of life, although a number of patients have survived into the sixth decade.[46,47] In a recent survey, patients with moderate Ebstein's anomaly were uninsurable by 93 per cent of the carriers who responded.[45] Patients who survive early infancy may do quite well and remain in NYHA Class I or Class II for many years. The presence of associated cardiac abnormalities significantly affects the prognosis, however. Sudden death from ventricular dysrhythmias can occur. Patients with paroxysmal tachydysrhythmias with or without the Wolff-Parkinson-White syndrome also experience more difficulties.

Mortality following surgical repair of Ebstein's disease has been reported to be as high as 50 per cent and, in one small series of nine patients, 0 per cent. Danielson[11] reported an overall operative mortality of 4.9 per cent for 134 patients undergoing either valve repair or replacement at the Mayo Clinic. In that series, the late mortality was an additional 3 per cent.

Pasque[35] reviewed 27 series of reported cases for tricuspid valve replacement in children. The total operative mortality was 24.4 per cent. The actuarial data demonstrated that late mortality, excluding operative risks, was 1.8 per cent per year for the first 10 years. The actuarial estimate of survival at 5 years, including operative deaths, was 68 per cent, and for 10 years, 59 per cent. In the series reviewed, 61 per cent of 129 children had tricuspid valves replaced for Ebstein's anomaly.

SELECTED REFERENCES

Carpentier, A., Chauvaud, S., Macé, L., Relland, J., Mihaileanu, S., Marino, J. P., Abry, B., and Guibourt, P.: A new reconstructive operation for Ebstein's anomaly of the tricuspid valve. J. Thorac. Cardiovasc. Surg., 96:92, 1988.
In this provocative paper, a new, innovative approach for surgical correction of Ebstein's anomaly is presented. With this procedure, the long axis of the right ventricular body is maintained and the anterior leaflet of the tricuspid valve is restructured. This technique may increase the number of patients for whom valvuloplasty may be applied. Also presented is a series of 14 cases with a mean follow-up of 37 months.

Danielson, G. K.: Ebstein's anomaly. In Sabiston, D. C., and Spencer, F. C. (Eds.): Gibbon's Surgery of the Chest, 5th ed. Philadelphia, W. B. Saunders Company, 1990, pp. 1485–1592.
This is an excellent chapter outlining the salient features of Ebstein's anomaly and, more significantly, presenting probably the largest single series of patients surgically treated for Ebstein's anomaly. One hundred thirty-four consecutive patients are presented; results and long-term follow-up are included. This chapter also outlines the basic surgical technique for tricuspid valve annuloplasty conceived by Lillehei and Hunter.

Van Mierop, L. H. S., Kutsche, L. M., and Victorica, B. E.: Ebstein's anomaly. In Adams, F. H., Emmanouilides, G. C., and Riemenschneider, T. A. (Eds.): Moss's Heart Disease in Infants, Children and Adolescents, 4th ed. Baltimore, Williams & Wilkins, 1987, pp. 361–371.
This chapter presents an outstanding discussion of the entire spectrum of Ebstein's anomaly. More important, the embryology, pathophysiology, and associated defects are clearly stated, which provides an understanding of this uncommon malformation of the tricuspid valve.

Watson, H.: Natural history of Ebstein's anomaly of tricuspid valve in childhood and adolescence: An international co-operative study of 505 cases. Br. Heart J., 36:417, 1974.
Watson has collected 505 cases of Ebstein's anomaly from 61 centers in 28 countries. It is an excellent review of the natural history of Ebstein's anomaly. With 505 cases, the spectrum of the disease can be appreciated. The author divides the entire group according to the severity of cardiac involvement and relates the severity to outcome in different age groups.

REFERENCES

1. Abe, T., and Komatsu, S.: Valve replacement for Ebstein's anomaly of the tricuspid valve: Early and long-term results of eight cases. Chest, 84:414, 1983.
2. Allan, L. D., Desai, G., and Tynan, M. J.: Prenatal echocardiographic screening for Ebstein's anomaly for mothers on lithium therapy. Lancet, 2:875, 1982.
3. Balakrishnan, K. G., Sapru, R. P., Sasidharan, K., and Venkitachalam, C. G.: A comparison of the clinical, haemodynamic and angiographic features in right ventricular endomyocardial fibrosis and Ebstein's anomaly of the tricuspid valve. Cardiology, 69:265, 1982.
4. Barber, G., Danielson, G. K., Heise, C. T., and Driscoll, D. J.: Cardiorespiratory response to exercise in Ebstein's anomaly. Am. J. Cardiol., 56:509, 1985.
5. Barnard, C. N., and Schrire, V.: Surgical correction of Ebstein's malformation with a prosthetic tricuspid valve. Surgery, 54:302, 1963.
6. Carpentier, A., Chauvaud, S., Macé, L., Relland, J., Mihaileanu, S., Marino, J. P., Abry, B., and Guibourt, P.: A new reconstructive operation for Ebstein's anomaly of the tricuspid valve. J. Thorac. Cardiovasc. Surg., 96:92, 1988.
7. Caruso, G., Cifarelli, A., Balducci, G., and Facilone, F.: Ebstein's malformation of the mitral valve in atrioventricular and ventriculoarterial concordance. Pediatr. Cardiol., 8:209, 1987.
8. Cox, J. L., Ferguson, B., Jr., Lindsay, B. D., and Cain, M. E.: Perinodal cryosurgery for atrioventricular node reentry tachycardia in 23 patients. J. Thorac. Cardiovasc. Surg., 99:440, 1990.
9. Crawford, F. A., Gilette, P. C., Zeigler, V., Case, C., and Stroud, M.: Surgical management of Wolff-Parkinson-White syndrome in infants and small children. J. Thorac. Cardiovasc. Surg., 99:234, 1990.
10. Danielson, G. K.: Ebstein's anomaly: Editorial comments and personal observations. Ann. Thorac. Surg., 34:396, 1982.
11. Danielson, G. K.: Ebstein's anomaly. In Sabiston, D. C., and Spencer, F. C. (Eds.): Gibbon's Surgery of the Chest, 5th ed. Philadelphia, W. B. Saunders Company, 1990, pp. 1485–1592.
12. Danielson, G. K., and Fuster, V.: Surgical repair of Ebstein's anomaly. Ann. Surg., 196:499, 1982.
13. Di Lello, F., Flemma, R. J., Mullen, D. C., Kleinman, L. H., and Werner, P. H.: Tricuspid valve replacement for Ebstein's anomaly in childhood with a Starr-Edwards caged-ball prosthesis. Chest, 94:1096, 1988.
14. Dunn, J.: Porcine valve replacement in children. Ann. Thorac. Surg., 32:357, 1981.
15. Dusmet, M., Oberhaensli, I., and Cox, J. N.: Ebstein's anomaly of the tricuspid and mitral valves in an otherwise normal heart. Br. Heart J., 58:400, 1987.
16. Fornace, J., Rozanski, L., and Berger, B.: Right heart thromboembolism and suspected paradoxical embolism in Ebstein's anomaly. Am. Heart J., 114:1520, 1987.
17. Garrett, J. S., Schiller, N. B., Botvinick, E. H., Higgins, C. B., and Lipton, M. J.: Cine-computed tomography of Ebstein anomaly. Case report. J. Comput. Assist. Tomogr., 10:664, 1986.
18. Gelenberg, A. J.: Lithium efficacy and adverse effects. J. Clin. Psychiatry, 49(Suppl. II):8, 1988.
19. Hardy, K., May, I., and Kimball, K.: Ebstein's anomaly: A functional concept and successful definitive repair. J. Thorac. Cardiovasc. Surg., 48:927, 1964.
20. Harjula, A., Kupari, M., Ventilä, M., and Mattila, S.: Failure of mechanical valves in Ebstein's malformation. Int. J. Cardiol., 11:265, 1986.
21. Herrera, M. A., D'Souza, V. J., and Formanek, A. G.: MR imaging of Ebstein anomaly: Results in four cases. Am. J. R., 159:363, 1988.
22. Hunter, S. W., and Lillehei, C. E.: Ebstein's malformation of the tricuspid valve: A case study, together with suggestions of a new form of surgical therapy. Dis. Chest, 33:297, 1958.
23. Ilbawi, M., Idriss, F., Deleon, S., Muster, A., Duffy, C., Gidding, S., and Paul, M.: Valve replacement for selection and timing of surgical intervention. Ann. Thorac. Surg., 44:398, 1987.
24. Kirklin, J., and Barratt-Boyes, B. G.: Ebstein's malformation. In Kirklin, J., and Barratt-Boyes, B. G.: Cardiac Surgery. New York, John Wiley & Sons, 1986, pp. 889–909.
25. Leung, M. P., Baker, E. J., Anderson, R. H., and Zuberbuhler, J. R.: Cineangiographic spectrum of Ebstein's malformation: Its relevance to clinical presentation and outcome. J. Am. Coll. Cardiol., 11:154, 1988.
26. Leung, M., Rigby, M. L., Anderson, R. H., Wyse, R. K. H., and Macartney, F. J.: Reversed offsetting of the septal attachments of the atrioventricular valves and Ebstein's malformation of the morphologically mitral valve. Br. Heart J., 57:184, 1987.
27. Mann, R. J., and Lie, J. T.: The life story of Wilhelm Ebstein (1836–1912) and his almost overlooked description of a congenital heart disease. Mayo Clin. Proc., 54:197, 1979.

28. Marino, J. P., Mihaileanu, S., Asmar, B. E., Chauvaud, S., Macé, L., Relland, J., and Carpentier, A.: Echocardiography and color-flow mapping evaluation of a new reconstructive surgical technique for Ebstein's anomaly. Circulation, 80(Suppl. I):I-107, 1989.

29. Matthews, J. L., Pennington, W. S., Isobe, J. H., Gaskin, T. A., Dumas, J. H., and Kahn, D. R.: Paradoxical embolization with Ebstein's anomaly. Arch. Surg., 118:1101, 1983.

30. McKay, R., Sono, J., and Arnold, R. M.: Tricuspid valve replacement using an unstented pulmonary homograft. Ann. Thorac. Surg., 46:58, 1988.

31. Mu-Sheng, T., Partridge, J., and Radford, D.: The plain chest radiograph in uncomplicated Ebstein's disease. Clin. Radiol., 37:551, 1986.

32. Nawa, S., Kioka, Y., Sano, K., Shirakawa, K., Ozaki, K., Beika, M., Nagase, H., Nakayama, Y., Mondori, E., Shigenobu, M., Murakami, T., Uchida, H., Senoo, Y., and Teramoto, S.: Surgical correction of Ebstein's anomaly by tricuspid valve replacement and its late problems. J. Cardiovasc. Surg., 25:142, 1984.

33. Nihoyannopoulos, P., McKenna, W. J., Smith, G., and Foale, R.: Echocardiographic assessment of the right ventricle in Ebstein's anomaly: Relation to clinical outcome. J. Am. Coll. Cardiol., 8:627, 1986.

34. Oh, J. K., Holmes, D. R., Jr., Hayes, D. L., Porter, C.-B. J., and Danielson, G. K.: Cardiac arrhythmias in patients with surgical repair of Ebstein's anomaly. J. Am. Coll. Cardiol., 6:1351, 1985.

35. Pasque, M., Williams, W. G., Coles, J. G., Trusler, G. A., and Freedom, R. M.: Tricuspid valve replacement in children. Ann. Thorac. Surg., 44:164, 1987.

36. Rebolledo, J. R.: Ebstein's anomaly with right aortic arch. J. Pediatr., 71:66, 1967.

37. Roberson, D. A., and Silverman, N. H.: Ebstein's anomaly: Echocardiographic and clinical features in the fetus and neonate. J. Am. Coll. Cardiol., 14:1300, 1989.

38. Rossi, L., and Thiene, G.: Mild Ebstein's anomaly associated with supraventricular tachycardia and sudden death: Clinicomorphologic features in 3 patients. Am. J. Cardiol., 53:332, 1984.

39. Schiebler, G. L., Gravenstein, J. S., and Van Mierop, L. H. S.: Ebstein's anomaly of the tricuspid valve. Am. J. Cardiol., 22:867, 1968.

40. Selle, J. G., Sealy, W. C., Gallagher, J. J., Fedor, J. M., Svenson, R. H., and Zimmern, S. H.: Technical considerations in the surgical approach to multiple accessory pathways in the Wolff-Parkinson-White syndrome. Ann. Thorac. Surg., 43:579, 1987.

41. Sharf, M., Abinader, E. G., Shapiro, S., Rosenfeld, T., and Eibschitz, I.: Prenatal echocardiographic diagnosis of Ebstein's anomaly with pulmonary atresia. Am. J. Obstet. Gynecol., 147:300, 1983.

42. Shiina, A., Seward, J. B., Edwards, W. D., Hagler, D. J., and Tajik, A. J.: Two-dimensional echocardiographic spectrum of Ebstein's anomaly: Detailed anatomic assessment. J. Am. Coll. Cardiol., 3:356, 1984.

43. Silver, M. A., Cohen, S. R., McIntosh, C. L., Cannon, R. O., III, and Roberts, W. C.: Late (5 to 132 months) clinical and hemodynamic results after either tricuspid valve replacement or annuloplasty for Ebstein's anomaly of the tricuspid valve. Am. J. Cardiol., 54:627, 1984.

44. Stewart, S., Cianciotta, D., Alexson, C., and Manning, J.: The long-term risk of warfarin sodium therapy and the incidence of thromboembolism in children after prosthetic cardiac valve replacement. J. Thorac. Cardiovasc. Surg., 93:551, 1987.

45. Truesdell, S. C., Skorton, D. J., and Lauer, R. M.: Life insurance for children with cardiovascular disease. Pediatrics, 77:687, 1986.

46. Van Mierop, L. H. S., Kutsche, L. M., and Victorica, B. E.: Ebstein's anomaly. In Adams, F. H., Emmanouilides, G. C., and Riemenschneider, T. A. (Eds.): Moss's Heart Disease in Infants, Children and Adolescents, 4th ed. Baltimore, Williams & Wilkins, 1987, pp. 361–371.

47. Watson, H.: Natural history of Ebstein's anomaly of tricuspid valve in childhood and adolescence: An international co-operative study of 505 cases. Br. Heart J., 36:417, 1974.

48. Zuberbuhler, J. R., Becker, A. E., Anderson, R. H., and Lenox, C. C.: Ebstein's malformation and the embryological development of the tricuspid valve. Case report. Pediatr. Cardiol., 5:289, 1984.

XX

SURGICAL TREATMENT OF CARDIAC ARRHYTHMIAS

James L. Cox, M.D.

Although the first definitive surgical treatment for a cardiac arrhythmia was accomplished over 20 years ago, cardiac arrhythmia surgery is still in its early stages of development and application. No other area of cardiac surgery requires more cooperation and teamwork than does the highly specialized field of cardiac arrhythmia surgery. It is essential for the arrhythmia surgeon to possess a basic understanding of cardiac electrophysiology, and it is just as mandatory for the clinical electrophysiologist to have a working knowledge of the surgical anatomy of the heart. During the past 2 decades, surgical intervention for the treatment of cardiac arrhythmias has evolved from an esoteric, experimental exercise to a well-established, and many times preferential, therapy for electrophysiologic abnormalities. This chapter is designed to acquaint the reader with the historical aspects, electrophysiologic basis, surgical indications and contraindications, preoperative electrophysiologic evaluation, intraoperative mapping procedures, surgical technique, and results of surgery for cardiac arrhythmias.

SURGICAL THERAPY FOR SUPRAVENTRICULAR TACHYARRHYTHMIAS

WOLFF-PARKINSON-WHITE SYNDROME

Historical Aspects

In 1893, Stanley Kent first demonstrated the presence of muscular connections between the atria and ventricles of mammals and erroneously concluded that those connections were multi-

ple, were always located on the right side of the heart, and represented the normal pathways of atrioventricular (AV) conduction.[95] In 1906, Tawara described, in clear and impeccable detail, the true anatomy and physiology of the specialized conduction system of the heart by identifying and characterizing the AV node, His bundle, bundle branches, and Purkinje system.[134] In the same year, Keith and Flack identified the sinoatrial (SA) node as the heart's normal pacemaker.[94]

The first description of what is now known as the Wolff-Parkinson-White (WPW) syndrome occurred in 1930,[144] when those three physicians identified a small group of young patients whose electrocardiogram (ECG) during normal sinus rhythm was characterized by a short P-R interval, a wide QRS complex, and an early deflection that preceded the QRS complex, which they called a "delta wave." Although the authors did not completely understand the anatomic basis of the abnormal ECG in these patients, they pointed out that such ECG abnormalities were frequently associated with sudden bouts of tachycardia. It remained for Wolferth and Wood to suggest first in 1933[143] and then to prove in 1943[145] that the ECG patterns in patients with the WPW syndrome were due to accessory anatomic connections between the atrium and ventricle similar to those previously described by Kent.

Despite the observations of Wolferth and Wood, the electrophysiologic basis for the WPW syndrome remained controversial for several decades, even though Durrer[46] was able to demonstrate eccentric electrical conduction across the AV groove by intraoperative mapping of a patient with the WPW syndrome in

1967. The final, unequivocal confirmation of the anatomic-electrophysiologic basis for the WPW syndrome occurred subsequently at Duke University and at the Mayo Clinic in the late 1960s. Boineau and colleagues at Duke performed epicardial mapping in animals with the WPW syndrome and documented the presence of an anatomic accessory AV connection located at the precise site of ventricular pre-excitation.[9] Subsequently, Burchell and colleagues temporarily ameliorated the WPW syndrome at the time of surgery by injecting procainamide into the AV groove at the site of ventricular pre-excitation in a patient undergoing surgery for an atrial septal defect.[13] Although conduction across the accessory AV connection resumed postoperatively, Burchell's experience confirmed that surgical intervention in these patients was feasible. Shortly thereafter, Sealy successfully divided an accessory pathway in a patient with the WPW syndrome and thereby initiated the new field of cardiac arrhythmia surgery.[17]

Since Sealy's original operative success, the surgical techniques employed for the treatment of the WPW syndrome have continued to evolve into the two primary surgical techniques that are employed today, the endocardial approach and the epicardial approach.

Anatomic-Electrophysiologic Basis

From the electrophysiologic standpoint, the WPW syndrome is the simplest of all arrhythmogenic abnormalities. Thus, it is no coincidence that the WPW syndrome was the first arrhythmogenic abnormality to be elucidated and reproducibly cured surgically.

Normally, the only connection between the atria and ventricles capable of conducting electrical activity is the AV node–His bundle complex. In patients with the WPW syndrome, the SA node and the AV node–His bundle complex are normal anatomically and functionally. In addition, however, these patients have an accessory connection between the atrium and ventricle that is capable of conducting electrical activity. On histologic examination, these accessory AV connections (accessory pathways) have the appearance of normal atrial muscle, and specifically they do not resemble either the specialized conduction system or nerve tissue. Accessory pathways may be located anywhere in the AV groove around the base of the heart except that region between the left fibrous trigone and the right fibrous trigone (Fig. 1). Since this region of the fibrous skeleton of the heart represents the site where the anterior leaflet of the mitral valve is contiguous with the aortic valve anulus, there is no ventricular myocardium immediately beneath the mitral anulus in this region. Thus, it is impossible for accessory AV connections to be located in that position.

Traditionally, the location of accessory pathways in the WPW syndrome has been based on the site of insertion of the ventricular end of the pathway. This arbitrary classification of accessory pathway locations into left free wall, posterior septal, right free wall, and anterior septal (in decreasing order of frequency) has proved to be advantageous, not only because of the dissimilarities of the electrophysiologic manifestations of pathways located in each of these four areas, but also because the surgical approach to each of these four spaces is unique. The four anatomic spaces in which a given accessory pathway may reside are identified by viewing the AV groove in the horizontal plane (see Fig. 1). Both the preoperative catheter electrophysiologic study and the intraoperative mapping procedure are directed toward localizing an accessory pathway to one of these four anatomic spaces. However, an appreciation of the potential for accessory pathways to be located at different *depths* in the vertical plane of the AV groove is necessary in order to understand many of the important principles that guide successful surgery for the WPW syndrome.[29] Because of the anatomic limitations imposed by the valve anulus and the epicardium overlying the AV groove externally (Fig. 2), all accessory pathways must connect to the

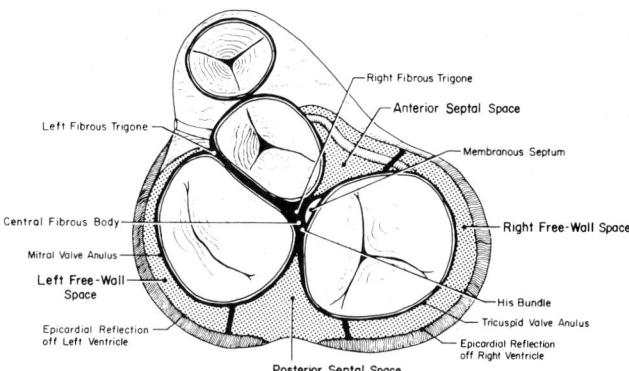

Figure 1. Diagram of the superior view of the heart with the atria cut away demonstrating the boundaries of each of the four anatomic areas where accessory pathways can occur in the Wolff-Parkinson-White syndrome. The boundaries of the *left free-wall* space are the mitral valve anulus and the ventricular epicardial reflection extending from the left fibrous trigone to the posterior septum. The boundaries of the *posterior septal* space are the tricuspid valve anulus, the mitral valve anulus, the posterior superior process of the left ventricle, and the ventricular epicardial reflection. The boundaries of the *right free-wall* space are the tricuspid valve anulus and the epicardial reflection extending from the posterior septum to the anterior septum. The boundaries of the *anterior septal* space are the tricuspid valve anulus, the membranous portion of the interatrial septum, and the ventricular epicardial reflection. All accessory atrioventricular connections must insert into the ventricle *somewhere* within these anatomic boundaries. (Modified from Cox, J. L., et al.: Experience with 118 consecutive patients undergoing surgery for Wolff-Parkinson-White syndrome. J. Thorac. Cardiovasc. Surg., 90:490, 1985.)

atrium somewhere between the valve anulus and the epicardial reflection off the atrium, and they must connect to the ventricle somewhere between the valve anulus and the epicardial reflection off the ventricle.[27] Thus, accessory pathways are confined (in the vertical plane) to locations (1) near the valve anulus, (2) within the fat pad of the AV groove, or (3) just beneath the epicardium overlying the AV groove.

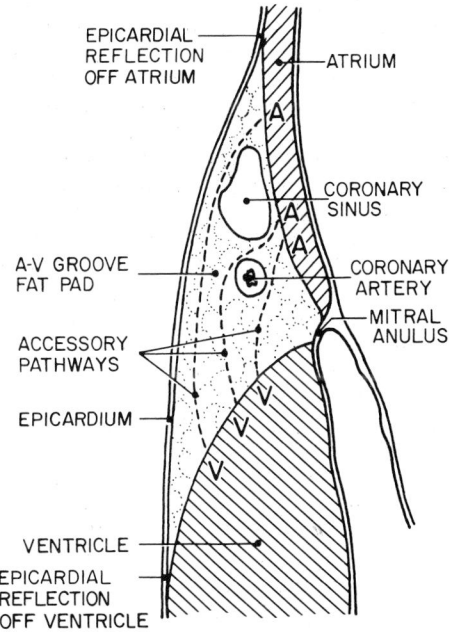

Figure 2. Diagrammatic representation of a cross section of the posterior left heart showing the different depths at which left free-wall pathways can be located in relation to the mitral anulus and the epicardium overlying the AV groove. Note that regardless of the depth of the accessory pathway in the vertical plane of the AV groove, the atrial end of the accessory pathway must attach to the atrium somewhere between the mitral valve anulus and the epicardial reflection off the atrium. Likewise, the ventricular end of the accessory pathway must connect to the ventricle somewhere between the mitral valve anulus and the epicardial reflection off the ventricle. (From Cox, J. L. and Ferguson, T. B., Jr.: Surgery for the Wolff-Parkinson-White syndrome: The endocardial approach. Semin. Thorac. Cardiovasc. Surg., 1:34, 1989.)

During sinus rhythm in a normal patient, AV conduction is delayed in the region of the AV node for approximately 100 msec. (Fig. 3A). During sinus rhythm in a patient with the WPW syndrome, AV conduction occurs through both the normal conduction system and the accessory pathway (Fig. 3B to D). Since accessory pathways do not usually exhibit the conduction delay characteristic of the AV node, the atrial impulse reaches the ventricle first across the accessory pathway. Thus, the earliest site of ventricular activation during normal sinus rhythm in patients with the WPW syndrome is at the site of insertion of the accessory pathway into the ventricular myocardium. This early activation of the ventricle prior to the time that it would normally have been activated by the impulse traveling antegrade through the AV node–His bundle complex is called *ventricular pre-excitation*. On the standard limb lead ECG, this pre-excitation of the ventricle causes an early deflection off the isoelectric line, the so-called delta wave. Thus, the rapid antegrade conduction across an accessory pathway with ventricular pre-excitation is responsible for the three ECG findings first described by Drs. Wolff, Parkinson, and White in 1930, namely, a short P-R interval, a wide QRS complex, and a delta wave.

Supraventricular tachycardia develops in patients with the Wolff-Parkinson-White syndrome when an antegrade conduction block occurs in the accessory pathway (Fig. 4A). Antegrade conduction still occurs normally through the AV node–His bundle complex, and the QRS complex on the standard ECG for that beat will be normal. As the electrical impulse then activates the ventricles from the apex to the base, it encounters the ventricular end of the accessory pathway that has not been activated. The electrical impulse thus continues to propagate in a retrograde (ventricular to atrial) direction across the accessory pathway to reactivate the atrium. This retrograde atrial activation then proceeds back into the AV node–His bundle complex in an antegrade fashion, and the re-entrant circuit is completed (Fig. 4B). Electrical activity usually travels around this re-entrant circuit between 3 and 4 times per second, or 180 to 240 times per minute. Thus, within the space of a single cardiac cycle, patients with the WPW syndrome may convert from a

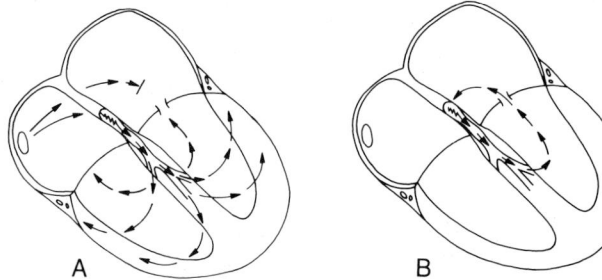

Figure 4. *A,* Antegrade conduction block across the accessory pathway in a patient with the WPW syndrome. *B,* Reciprocating tachycardia in a patient with the WPW syndrome. (From Cox, J. L.: The surgical management of cardiac arrhythmias. In Sabiston, D. C., Jr., and Spencer, F. C. (Eds.): Surgery of the Chest, 5th ed. Philadelphia, W. B. Saunders Company, 1990, pp. 1861–1900.)

normal heart rate of 80 beats per minute to a supraventricular tachycardia of 200 beats per minute.

Supraventricular tachycardias complicating the WPW syndrome are usually referred to as reciprocating tachycardias. The most common form of reciprocating tachycardia is that just described in which antegrade conduction occurs through the AV node–His bundle complex and retrograde conduction occurs across the accessory pathway (Fig. 4B). This type of reciprocating tachycardia is called orthodromic supraventricular tachycardia and accounts for over 90 per cent of the reciprocating tachycardias associated with the WPW syndrome. Infrequently, reciprocating tachycardia may occur in these patients in which antegrade conduction occurs across accessory pathways with retrograde conduction through the AV node–His bundle complex. This reciprocating tachycardia is referred to as antidromic supraventricular tachycardia and occurs in less than 10 per cent of patients with the WPW syndrome. As might be expected, the QRS complex is narrow during orthodromic reciprocating tachycardia (because the ventricles are activated via the AV node–His bundle complex), and the QRS complex is wide during antidromic reciprocating tachycardia (because the ventricles are activated via the accessory pathway).

Atrial flutter/fibrillation occurs in approximately 30 per cent of patients with the WPW syndrome. Depending on the conduction characteristics of the accessory pathway, the association of atrial fibrillation with the WPW syndrome may be a lethal combination. If the antegrade refractory period of accessory pathway is less than 220 msec., the accessory pathway is capable of conducting the chaotic atrial electrical impulses directly to the ventricles, resulting in ventricular fibrillation.[4,113] During this potentially lethal form of the WPW syndrome, the accessory pathway is activated passively and is not a direct component of the arrhythmia.

Finally, accessory pathways are classified as either "manifest" or "concealed." Manifest pathways, such as those described previously, are capable of conducting in both the antegrade and retrograde directions. Thus, during normal sinus rhythm, the ECG is abnormal because of antegrade conduction across the accessory pathway that pre-excites the ventricles, and during atrial fibrillation the ventricles may be vulnerable to fibrillation as well. Concealed accessory pathways conduct in only the retrograde (ventricular to atrial) direction. Therefore, the QRS morphologic pattern during sinus rhythm is normal, and during atrial fibrillation, AV conduction occurs exclusively through the AV node–His bundle complex. Thus, the ventricular rate response to atrial fibrillation in WPW patients with concealed accessory pathways is similar to that in patients without accessory pathways. Concealed accessory pathways compose the retrograde limb of the re-entrant circuit during orthodromic supraventricular tachycardia. In addition, on rare occasions, they may serve as the retrograde limb during antidromic tachycardia in patients with multiple accessory pathways.[14]

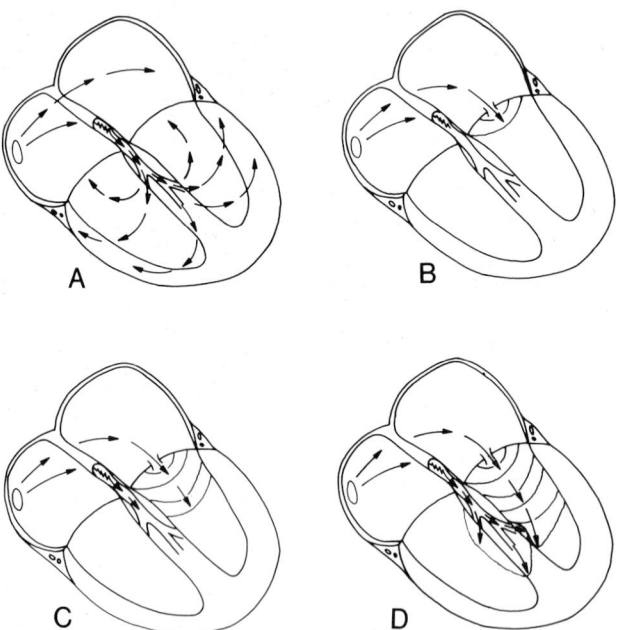

Figure 3. *A,* Normal spread of electrical activation in the heart during sinus rhythm. The electrical impulse is delayed approximately 100 msec. in the AV node. *B* to *D,* Spread of electrical activation during sinus rhythm in the WPW syndrome with an accessory pathway in the left free-wall position. (From Cox, J. L.: The surgical management of cardiac arrhythmias. In Sabiston, D. C., Jr., and Spencer, F. C. (Eds.): Surgery of the Chest, 5th ed. Philadelphia, W. B. Saunders Company, 1990, pp. 1861–1900.)

Surgical Indications and Contraindications

The major indication for surgical intervention in the WPW syndrome is medical refractoriness.[34,64,73,103,105] Other common surgical indications include patient intolerance to drug therapy, detrimental side effects of antiarrhythmic agents, and poor patient compliance. Major additions to these surgical indications in recent years have included (1) recurrent supraventricular tachycardia in young, otherwise healthy patients and (2) spontaneous atrial fibrillation that conducts rapidly enough antegrade across the accessory pathway to allow the induction of ventricular fibrillation from the atrium. The inclusion of young patients whose arrhythmias might be controllable with antiarrhythmic agents represents a liberalization of previous surgical indications.[22] However, surgery for the WPW syndrome is no longer an experimental procedure, and owing to its safety and curative nature, it should be considered as the conservative alternative to a lifetime of dependence on antiarrhythmic drugs.

Preoperative Electrophysiologic Evaluation

All patients who are to be subjected to surgery for the WPW syndrome must first undergo a preoperative catheter endocardial electrophysiologic study. Routinely, four multipolar catheters are inserted transvenously and positioned in the right atrium and right ventricle. A quadripolar or tripolar catheter is positioned at the AV junction to record the His bundle potential, and a decapolar catheter is positioned into the coronary sinus. The purposes of the preoperative electrophysiologic study are (1) to document that the arrhythmia is supraventricular in origin, (2) to evaluate the response of the supraventricular tachycardia to programmed electrical stimulation to determine if it is re-entrant or automatic in nature, (3) to establish the conduction properties of the normal specialized conduction system, (4) to document that the etiologic basis of the arrhythmia is the WPW syndrome rather than some other type of arrhythmia, and (5) to define the location of the accessory pathway responsible for the WPW syndrome. It is not within the scope of this chapter to describe the techniques for attaining all of these goals during a preoperative electrophysiologic study, but numerous excellent descriptions and reviews of this subject are available.[14]

Intraoperative Electrophysiologic Mapping

The availability of a computerized mapping system[97] in recent years has obviated the need to use cardiopulmonary bypass for the intraoperative mapping of patients with the WPW syndrome. Epicardial pacing and sensing electrodes are sutured onto the atrium and ventricle near the suspected site of the accessory pathway. The author employs an elastic band containing 16 bipolar electrodes for simultaneous multipoint mapping.[25,97] The band electrode is first placed around the ventricular side of the AV groove, and electrograms are recorded simultaneously from the 16 bipolar electrodes during normal sinus rhythm and during atrial pacing (Fig. 5). The digitized data are then displayed on a color graphics terminal in the operating theater. The electrogram recorded from the electrode located nearest the site of ventricular insertion of the accessory pathway shows the earliest activation (Fig. 6). This multipolar mapping system is particularly helpful in detecting the presence of multiple accessory pathways that are capable of conducting in the antegrade direction.

The band electrode is then moved to the atrial side of the AV groove, and reciprocating tachycardia (see Fig. 4B) is induced with programmed electrical stimulation. Only a few cycles of tachycardia are allowed to occur, since hemodynamic compromise is common and the patients are not on cardiopulmonary bypass. Atrial electrograms are recorded from the bipolar electrodes on the band, and again the digitized data are displayed on the graphics terminal, indicating the earliest site of *retrograde* atrial activity during the tachycardia. These retrograde atrial

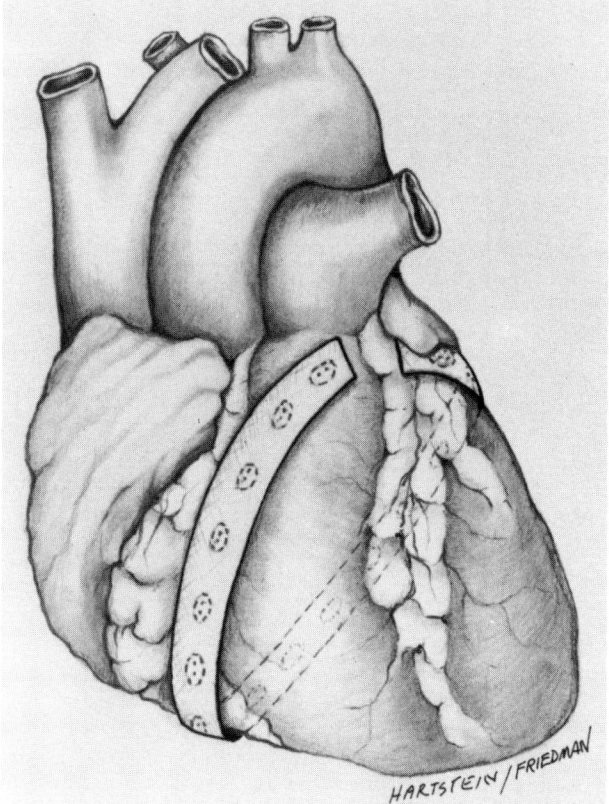

Figure 5. Diagrammatic sketch showing the placement of the band electrode around the ventricular side of the AV groove in a patient with the WPW syndrome during stable antegrade pre-excitation. (From Cox, J. L.: Intraoperative computerized mapping techniques. *In* Brugada, P., and Wellens, H. J. J.: Cardiac Arrhythmias: Where to Go From Here? Mount Kisco, NY, Futura Publishing Company, 1987.)

maps are especially important because they may demonstrate previously unsuspected concealed accessory pathways that would have gone undetected if only an antegrade map had been performed. If reciprocating tachycardia cannot be induced intraoperatively, the retrograde atrial map is performed during ventricular pacing. Since retrograde conduction is faster across the accessory pathway than through the AV node–His bundle complex, the atrium will still activate earliest at the site of atrial insertion of the accessory pathway.

These antegrade and retrograde epicardial mapping studies are capable of detecting not only free-wall pathways, but also anterior septal and posterior septal accessory pathways. However, if a septal pathway is detected during the epicardial mapping procedure, the patient is placed on cardiopulmonary bypass, a right atriotomy is performed, and endocardial mapping of the right atrium and atrial septum is completed using a hand-held, single-point mapping system prior to proceeding with surgical dissection. This endocardial procedure further localizes the septal pathways in preparation for surgical dissection of either the anterior or posterior septal space.

Surgical Technique

The objective of surgery for the WPW syndrome is to divide the accessory pathway(s) responsible for the syndrome. There are two surgical approaches that are commonly employed to divide these accessory pathways (Fig. 7). The endocardial technique[29,34,104] is designed to divide the ventricular end of the accessory pathway, and the epicardial technique[73,75,105] is directed toward division of the atrial end of the pathway. At the author's institution, the endocardial technique is preferred for all accessory pathways, regardless of location. Although some

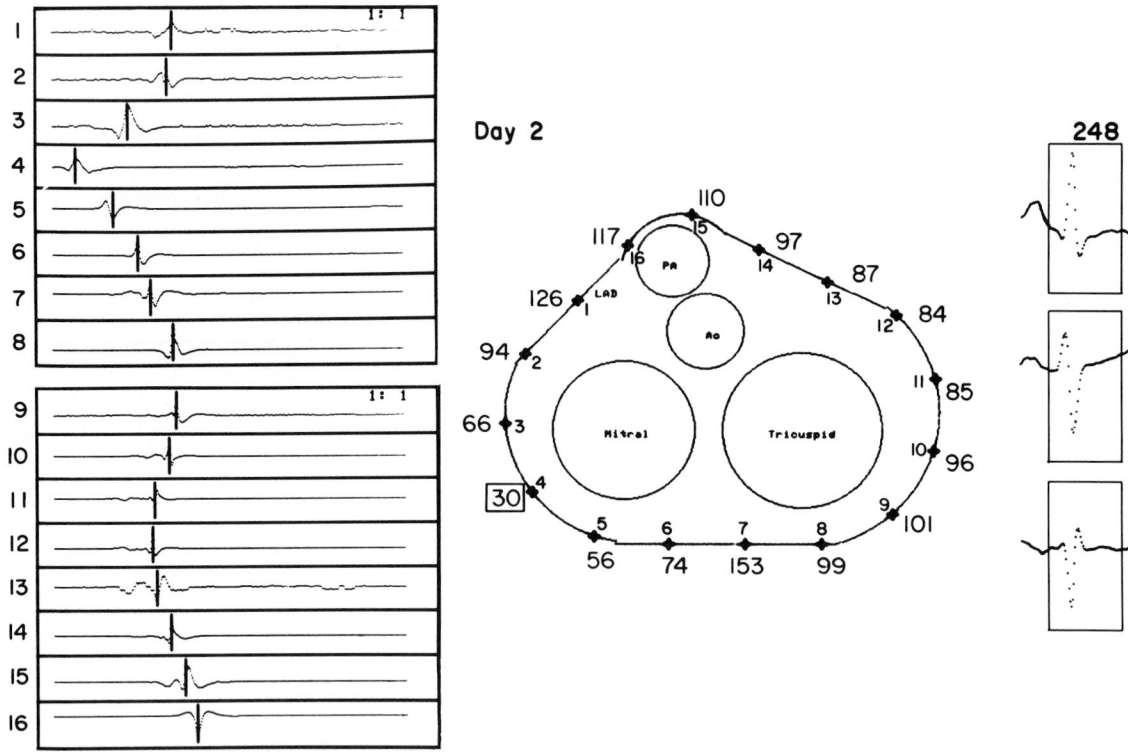

Figure 6. Left panel: Hard copy of the color graphics terminal display showing the activation sequence of the 16 electrodes contained in the band. Since this is an antegrade ventricular pre-excitation map and the band has been placed on the ventricular side of the AV groove, the electrode showing the earliest activation (electrode number 4) is located at the site of the ventricular insertion of the accessory pathway. Right panel: Hard copy of the color graphics terminal display showing the activation sequence of the base of the ventricles during antegrade pre-excitation. The designated window is displayed on the right side of the screen, and the activation sequence is related to a diagrammatic sketch of the base of the heart with the earliest site of ventricular activity during stable antegrade pre-excitation being enclosed in a box. (Modified from Cox, J. L.: Intraoperative computerized mapping techniques. *In* Brugada, P., and Wellens, H. J. J.: Cardiac Arrhythmias: Where to Go From Here? Mount Kisco, NY, Futura Publishing Company, 1987.)

controversy has arisen regarding which approach is preferable,[24] excellent results can be obtained with both techniques.

Left Free-Wall Accessory Pathways

If the endocardial technique is employed, accessory pathways on the left side of the heart are approached through a left atriotomy after the heart has been arrested with cold potassium cardioplegia. A supra-annular incision is placed 2 mm. above the mitral valve anulus, extending from the left fibrous trigone to the posterior septum. The entire space is dissected completely in every patient, regardless of the precise location of the accessory pathway within that space. After placing the supra-annular incision, a plane of dissection is established between the underlying AV groove fat pad and the top of the left ventricle throughout the length of the supra-annular incision. It is important to carry this plane of dissection all the way to the epicardial reflection off the posterior left ventricle in order to be certain to divide any accessory pathway that might be located in the subepicardial position in the AV groove. After this dissection, it is still theoretically possible for an accessory pathway located immediately adjacent to the valve anulus to remain intact unless the anulus has been cleaned meticulously with a sharp nerve hook or knife. In order to preclude this possibility, the two ends of the supra-annular incision are then "squared off" to the level of the mitral anulus so that even if such a juxta-annular pathway had survived the previous dissection, the small rim of atrial tissue to which it would be attached will be isolated from the remainder of the heart and, therefore, the potential conduction circuit would be interrupted.[34] This dissection exposes the entire left free-wall space and each of its boundaries, and therefore there is no other site in this space where an accessory pathway could insert into the ventricle.

The epicardial approach to left free-wall accessory pathways incorporates dissection from the atrial side of the AV groove.

The epicardial reflection off the atrium is opened, and a plane of dissection is established between the AV groove fat pad and the atrial wall. The plane of dissection is extended to the level of the posterior mitral valve anulus and carried slightly onto the top of the posterior left ventricle. This dissection divides the atrial end of all accessory pathways in this region except those that are located immediately adjacent to the mitral valve anulus. A cryosurgical lesion is placed at the level of the mitral anulus in order to interrupt such juxta-annular pathways that might have been missed during the prior surgical dissection. The atrial epicardial reflection is then reapproximated. In order to expose the atrial side of the AV groove on the left side of the heart for the epicardial approach, it is necessary to elevate the apex of the heart out of the pericardium (Fig. 8). This maneuver causes hypotension in the vast majority of patients to such an extent that cardiopulmonary bypass must be instituted in order to maintain stable hemodynamics.[73,105]

Posterior Septal Accessory Pathways

With the endocardial approach to posterior septal accessory pathways, normothermic cardiopulmonary bypass is instituted and a right atriotomy is performed. After completion of the endocardial mapping described before, a supra-annular incision is placed 2 mm. above the posterior medial tricuspid valve anulus, beginning at least 1 cm. posterior to the His bundle. The supra-annular incision is extended in a counterclockwise direction well onto the free wall of the posterior right atrium. This extension is important for two reasons: (1) it provides a larger incision for better exposure in the depths of the posterior septal space near the posterior superior process of the left ventricle, and (2) it simplifies identification of the epicardial reflection off the posterior right ventricle, a landmark that is to be followed across the crux of the heart to the posterior left ventricle during dissection of the posterior septal space. Once the fat pad occu-

ENDOCARDIAL TECHNIQUE

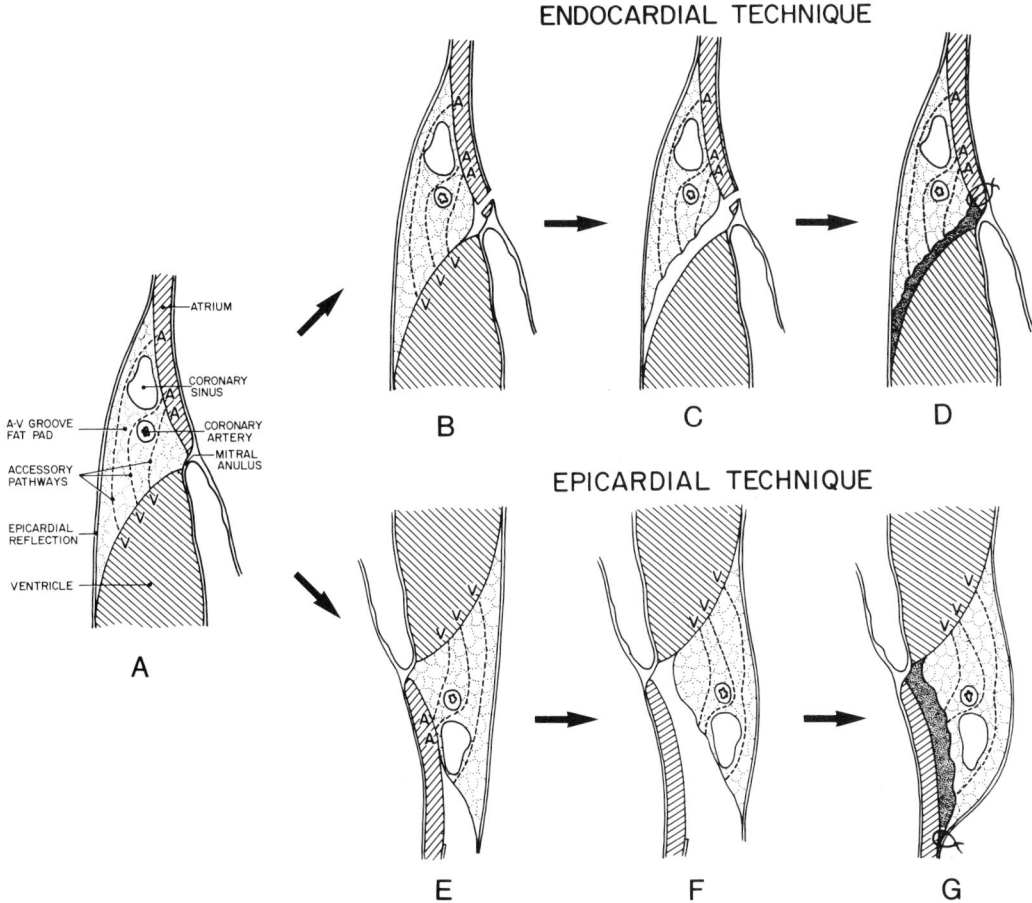

EPICARDIAL TECHNIQUE

Figure 7. Diagrammatic representation of a cross section of the posterior left heart showing the different depths at which left free-wall pathways can be located in relation to the mitral anulus and epicardial reflection (A). The endocardial surgical technique is depicted in B to D, and the epicardial technique in E to G. See text for further discussion. (From Cox, J. L.: The surgical management of cardiac arrhythmias. In Sabiston, D. C., Jr., and Spencer, F. C. (Eds.): Surgery of the Chest, 5th ed. Philadelphia, W. B. Saunders Company, 1990, pp. 1861–1900.)

pying the posterior septal space has been identified through the supra-annular incision, a plane of dissection is established between the fat pad and the top of the posterior ventricular septum. Prior to the institution of cardioplegic arrest, this plane is developed in the anterior portion of the posterior septal space closest to the His bundle, approaching the central fibrous body from the posterior aspect. The junction of the posteromedial mitral and tricuspid valve anuli forms an inverted V at the posterior edge of the central fibrous body, and the fat pad comes to a point at the apex of that V. The apex of the V is always posterior to the His bundle, although the distance between the apex of the V and the His bundle may vary. However, as long as the dissection in this region remains posterior to the central fibrous body, the His bundle will not be damaged. Once the anterior point of the fat pad is gently dissected away from the apex of the V (i.e., away from the posterior edge of the central fibrous body), the mitral valve anulus comes into view at the point where it joins the tricuspid valve to form the central fibrous body. The heart is usually arrested with cold potassium cardioplegia at this point, but it is not absolutely necessary to do so. If the plane of dissection is relatively bloodless and easily identified, the entire posterior septal space can be dissected with the heart beating.[103] On the other hand, if the plane is extremely vascular from the beginning, it is acceptable to perform the entire dissection under cardioplegic arrest.[29]

Since the epicardial reflection off the posterior right ventricle has already been identified, visualization of the mitral valve anulus in the anterior portion of the posterior septal space completes the identification of the boundaries of dissection of the space. The plane of dissection between the fat pad and the top

of the posterior ventricular septum is developed completely by following the mitral anulus over to the posterior superior process of the left ventricle and by following the epicardial reflection from the posterior right ventricle, across the posterior crux, onto the posterior left ventricle. It is absolutely essential to divide all structures penetrating the posterior ventricular septum and the posterior septal space, including, if necessary, the AV node artery. The author has found that the AV node artery does leave the posterior ventricular septum to enter the fat pad within the posterior septal space in approximately 50 per cent of patients with posterior septal accessory pathways.[34] In every case, it has been ligated, and no AV node dysfunction has been experienced as a result.

If the epicardial approach is used for posterior septal pathways, the posterior septal region, the adjacent inferior right ventricular region, and the left posterior paraseptal region are all dissected from the atrial epicardial aspect.[75] The AV groove fat pad is mobilized *en bloc*, and the inferior right ventricular wall–AV junction is exposed. The right coronary artery and its branches are identified. The midcardiac vein is ligated and divided. The right atrial–left ventricular fat pad is mobilized, and the posterosuperior process of the left ventricle is exposed. Complete exposure requires cauterization of small arteries and veins coursing over the ventricular process, including the AV node artery. The pericardium is incised anterior to the coronary sinus and the left AV junction, and the left posterior septal region is exposed. The right and the left AV junction are dissected, especially in the posterior septal region, to expose the whitish AV lamina. Ablation of epicardial pathways is secured by epicardial cryoblation of the exposed AV junction using

ADJUNCTIVE MEASURE WITH
ENDOCARDIAL TECHNIQUE

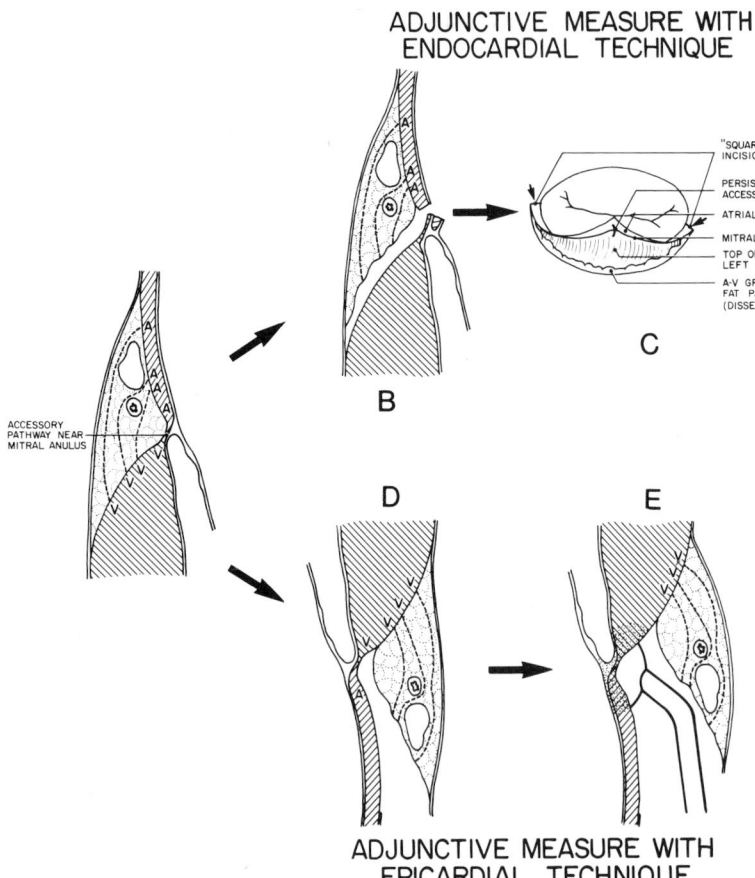

"SQUARING OFF"
INCISIONS

PERSISTENT
ACCESSORY PATHWAY

ATRIAL RIM

MITRAL ANULUS

TOP OF POSTERIOR
LEFT VENTRICLE

A-V GROOVE
FAT PAD
(DISSECTED)

Figure 8. Diagrammatic representation of the method for assuring that left free-wall accessory pathways located near the mitral anulus are inactivated using the endocardial technique (*B, C*) and the epicardial technique (*D, E*). (Modified from Cox, J. L.: The surgical management of cardiac arrhythmias. *In* Sabiston, D. C., Jr., and Spencer, F. C. (Eds.): Surgery of the Chest, 5th ed. Philadelphia, W. B. Saunders Company, 1990, pp. 1861–1900.)

ACCESSORY
PATHWAY NEAR
MITRAL ANULUS

B

C

D

E

ADJUNCTIVE MEASURE WITH
EPICARDIAL TECHNIQUE

overlapping applications of a cryoprobe while monitoring antegrade AV nodal conduction.

Right Free-Wall Accessory Pathways

This is the one condition, in the author's opinion, in which the epicardial technique without cardioplegic arrest is probably as easy to perform as the endocardial technique with cardioplegic arrest. In fact, the epicardial technique can usually be applied in these patients without cardiopulmonary bypass, making it a true closed-heart procedure in this case. However, we prefer to open the right atrium to perform endocardial mapping because there is frequently a large amount of fat in the AV groove on the right side, making the epicardial mapping less than optimal. After localizing the accessory pathway, the heart is cardioplegically arrested and a supra-annular incision is placed 2 mm. above the tricuspid valve anulus, extending around the entire right free wall. A plane of dissection is established between the underlying AV groove fat pad and the top of the right ventricle throughout the length of the supra-annular incision. This dissection plane is developed all the way to the epicardial reflection off the ventricle so that the entire right ventricular free wall that is in contact with the AV groove fat pad is free of any penetrating fibers from the fat pad.

When employing the epicardial approach for right free-wall pathways, an incision is made in the epicardium at the site of its reflection off the atrium to cover the AV groove fat pad of the right atrial free wall. A plane of dissection is established between the external right atrial wall and the AV groove fat pad down to the level of the tricuspid valve anulus. This plane of dissection is established throughout the entire length of the right atrial free wall. Numerous anterior cardiac veins frequently open into the right atrium over the anterior portion of the right free wall, making hemostasis difficult, which in turn makes precise anatomic dissection even more difficult. Never-

theless, the epicardial approach to right free-wall pathways can be safely and effectively accomplished in most patients.

There is an additional problem with right free-wall dissections, regardless of the surgical approach employed, that does not exist on the left side. The atrium and ventricle tend to "fold over" on one another at the tricuspid anulus much more than they do on the left side at the level of the mitral anulus[27] (Fig. 9). This condition results in right-sided pathways appearing to be located in a more "endocardial" position than those on the left side, but in fact they are not. Because of the "folding over" of the right atrial and ventricular walls at the annular level, the AV groove fat pad does not actually touch the true tricuspid valve anulus as it does the mitral anulus on the left. Therefore, when the fat pad is dissected away from the tricuspid anulus using the epicardial technique, the ventricular pre-excitation usually does not disappear. This observation has been reported on several occasions by the advocates of the epicardial technique who have erroneously attributed it to an "endocardial" accessory pathway.[73,74] Just as is the case on the left, right-sided accessory pathways must connect to the atrium somewhere between the valve anulus and the atrial epicardial reflection and to the ventricle somewhere between the valve anulus and the ventricular epicardial reflection. Unlike the left side, the "folded over" anatomy of the tricuspid anulus precludes the division of accessory pathways located adjacent to the anulus by the casual dissection of the fat pad away from the heart. In order to interrupt such right free-wall accessory pathways that reside too close to the valve anulus to be divided by routine dissection, one of three adjunctive measures must be added to the dissection: (1) mechanical "unfolding" of the atrium and ventricle so that the true valve anulus can be seen and freed of any adjacent fibers connecting the atrium and ventricle (applicable to both the epicardial and endocardial techniques); (2) application of a cryolesion to the tissues near the valve anulus to destroy the juxta-annular accessory pathway (applicable to both tech-

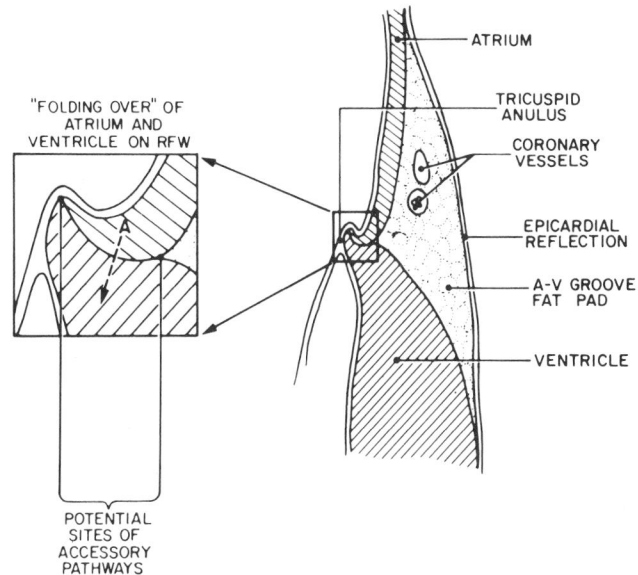

Figure 9. "Folding over" of the right atrium and right ventricle near the tricuspid anulus on the right free-wall. Note that simple dissection of the AV groove fat pad away from the ventricle (endocardial technique) or atrium (epicardial technique) will not divide accessory pathways connecting the atrium and ventricle if they are near the tricuspid anulus. This is a common location for right free-wall accessory pathways, accounting for the erroneous concept that they are "endocardial" pathways. (From Cox, J. L.: The surgical management of cardiac arrhythmias. *In* Sabiston, D. C., Jr., and Spencer, F. C. (Eds.): Surgery of the Chest, 5th ed. Philadelphia, W. B. Saunders Company, 1990, pp. 1861–1900.)

niques); or (3) "squaring off" of the supra-annular incision at both ends to isolate the atrial rim of tissue to which a juxta-anular accessory pathway would connect (applicable to the endocardial technique). This "folding over" of the atrium and ventricle at the level of the tricuspid anulus is much more pronounced in patients with Ebstein's anomaly, a condition present in 11 per cent of the patients in the author's surgical series. This is true whether the patient has the classic Ebstein's anomaly or only the forme fruste of the disease.

Anterior Septal Accessory Pathways

Epicardial mapping is excellent for documenting that an anterior septal pathway exists, but it does not localize these pathways very precisely because of the large fat pad covering both the atrium and ventricle and the anterior septal space. Therefore, endocardial mapping is especially important in these patients, particularly since these pathways are more frequently located adjacent to the His bundle (anteriorly) than are posterior septal pathways (posteriorly). After performing retrograde endocardial mapping, a supra-annular incision is placed just anterior to the His bundle, 2 mm. above the tricuspid anulus, and extended in a clockwise direction well onto the right anterior free wall. The initial endocardial incision frequently abolishes ventricular pre-excitation, but whether or not pre-excitation persists, the entire anterior septal space should be dissected. After the initial supra-annular incision is completed, a plane of dissection is established between the fat pad occupying the anterior septal space and the top of the right ventricle. This plane of dissection is developed completely to the aorta medially and to the epicardial reflection off the ventricle anteriorly. During this dissection, the fat pad must be retracted very gently to avoid injury to the proximal right coronary artery, which courses through the fat pad before entering the AV groove of the anterior right free wall (see Fig. 1). In addition, when the anterior medial portion of the anterior septal space is being dissected, extreme care should be taken to avoid injury to the aorta. This is actually the external surface of the right coronary sinus of Valsalva beneath the orifice of the right coronary artery and it is, therefore, quite thin.

Although the epicardial approach has been attempted for anterior septal pathways, poor surgical results have caused the advocates of the epicardial technique to switch to the endocardial approach for these pathways.[75]

Surgical Results

The incidence of successful surgical correction of the WPW syndrome now approaches 100 per cent, with an operative mortality that ranges from 0 to 0.5 per cent.[29,34,73,75,103,105] Both early and late recurrences following surgery, utilizing either the endocardial or epicardial technique, are extremely unusual. Previous problems, such as the inadvertent creation of heart block, are now of historical interest only. Whether one uses the endocardial or epicardial approach, these surgical results justify the liberalization of the previously mentioned indications for surgical intervention in this curable congenital cardiac abnormality.

AV NODE RE-ENTRY TACHYCARDIA

Historical Aspects

In 1926, Scherf and Shookhoff first observed reciprocating beats of AV nodal re-entry,[128] but it was not until 30 years later that Moe first characterized discontinuous AV node conduction over "fast" and "slow" pathways and associated this finding with reciprocating (echo) beats in response to premature stimulation.[109] In 1971, Goldreyer and Damato first inferred that AV node re-entry tachycardia was due to a re-entrant mechanism involving the AV node.[69] The role of AV node re-entry as a mechanism for paroxysmal supraventricular tachycardia in humans was subsequently confirmed by Bigger and Goldrey[5,68] and Denes.[43] Subsequent studies showed this to be the most common mechanism for paroxysmal supraventricular tachycardia in humans.[1,44,89,146]

During the 1970s, a few patients with medically refractory AV node re-entry tachycardia underwent surgical interruption of the His bundle, either by surgical dissection or by the application of cryolesions directly to the AV node–His bundle complex.[131] The objective of elective His bundle ablation was to protect the ventricles from the AV node re-entry. However, since the surgical block was created below the level of the AV node, AV node re-entry could persist at the atrial level. Thus, elective His bundle ablation represented perhaps the first surgical isolation procedure designed to control the detrimental effects of a medically refractory cardiac arrhythmia without actually ablating the arrhythmia. Since the procedure resulted in complete heart block, however, a permanent ventricular pacemaker was required postoperatively in all patients.

In 1982, Scheinman described a technique for ablating the His bundle by introducing an electrical shock through a catheter placed adjacent to the His bundle.[127] This closed-chest procedure immediately replaced the open-heart surgical method for interrupting the His bundle for obvious reasons. However, since the catheter fulguration technique of Scheinman also created complete heart block, all of these patients also required permanent pacemaker systems.

Although both the surgical technique and the catheter ablative technique for His bundle interruption ameliorated the unpleasant and detrimental effects of AV node re-entry tachycardia, both procedures replaced one type of arrhythmia (tachycardia) with another (heart block). No specific attempt at *curing* AV node re-entry tachycardia was made until a fortuitous occurrence in 1979.[122] During attempted surgical division of the His bundle in a patient with incessant AV node re-entry tachycardia, the tachycardia suddenly terminated but the patient maintained normal atrioventricular conduction. After observation of the patient for some time, the surgical procedure was terminated with the patient having normal atrioventricular conduction, and the patient subsequently remained tachycardia-free. This stimulated evaluation of the possibility of attaining this fortuitous result on a reproducible basis. Following several years of animal experimentation utilizing a discrete perinodal cryosurgical technique,[83-85] the first clinical cure of AV node re-entry tachycardia was attained utilizing this cryosurgical technique on August 13, 1982.[21] Ross, Johnson, and colleagues subsequently reported the cure of AV node re-entry tachycardia utilizing surgical dissection of the perinodal tissues.[124] Guiraudon and colleagues have reported success with a similar surgical dissection technique.[60] Thus, at the present time, there are two well-established techniques for curing patients with AV node re-entry tachycardia, perinodal cryosurgery[28,34] and perinodal surgical dissection.[60,88,124]

Anatomic-Electrophysiologic Basis

AV node re-entry tachycardia is caused by a re-entrant circuit that is confined to the AV node or to the perinodal tissues of the lower atrial septum. The anatomic-electrophysiologic basis for this re-entrant circuit is the presence of two functional conduction pathways, one slow and one fast, through the AV node, the so-called dual AV node conduction pathways (Fig. 10). The fast AV nodal pathway manifests rapid conduction but relatively long refractoriness. The slow AV nodal pathway manifests slow conduction but relatively short refractoriness. Although the complete dimensions of the re-entrant circuit have not been elucidated, the micro–re-entrant circuit is confined to the region of the AV node. During supraventricular tachycardia, antegrade conduction proceeds through the slow pathway and

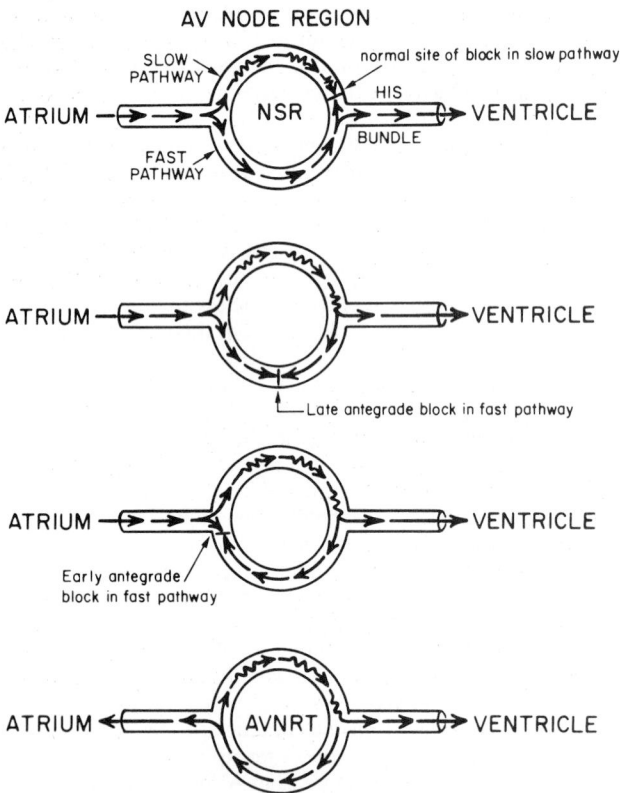

Figure 10. Schematic representation of dual AV node physiology and its relationship to AV node re-entry tachycardia. AV conduction during normal sinus rhythm (NSR) occurs preferentially through the fast pathway. However, because of longer refractoriness in the fast pathway, an atrial premature beat may block it (late antegrade block) and AV conduction occurs via the slow pathway, resulting in a prolonged P-R interval for that beat. If the antegrade block occurs more proximally (earlier) in the fast pathway, however, the retrograde impulse returning up the fast pathway may be able to reach the atrium causing a single atrial "echo" beat, or it may be able to continue antegrade down the slow pathway again, establishing the re-entrant circuit and tachycardia (AVNRT). (From Cox, J. L., et al.: Peri-nodal cryosurgery for AV node reentry tachycardia in 23 patients. J. Thorac. Cardiovasc. Surg., 99:440, 1990.)

retrograde conduction through the fast pathway, resulting in nearly simultaneous activation of the ventricles and atria. Whether these functionally distinct dual AV node conduction pathways have an anatomic correlate is a matter of some controversy. Perhaps even more controversial is whether the functionally distinct dual AV nodal pathways of conduction are confined to the anatomic AV node or also involve the perinodal tissues.[89] The fact that one of these dual AV nodal conduction pathways can be ablated by surgical dissection or cryosurgical techniques without altering the normal function of the AV node strongly suggests that the re-entrant circuit involves tissue lying outside the confines of the anatomic AV node. Moreover, detailed histologic studies in animals have documented preservation of the anatomic AV node following the perinodal cryosurgical procedure.[82]

Surgical Indications and Contraindications

Present indications for surgical intervention in patients with AV node re-entry tachycardia are similar to those applied to patients with the WPW syndrome. Medical refractoriness is certainly the most common indication, but as with the WPW syndrome, the successful surgical results in AV node re-entry tachycardia have justified a liberalization of the indications for surgery. Thus, the present surgical indications include medical refractoriness, drug intolerance, poor patient compliance, and patient preference for surgery as opposed to a lifetime of medical therapy.[28,88]

Another specific indication for surgical intervention either in patients with documented AV node re-entry tachycardia or in patients who simply exhibit the presence of dual AV node conduction physiology is the necessity for such patients to have surgery for the WPW syndrome.[36] A significant percentage of patients with the WPW syndrome also have either dual AV node physiology or documented AV node re-entry tachycardia in addition to the reciprocating tachycardia associated with the WPW syndrome. Obviously, patients who have experienced AV node re-entry tachycardia before surgical correction of their WPW syndrome can be expected to continue experiencing AV node re-entry tachycardia following WPW surgery if no concomitant attempt is made to cure the AV node re-entry tachycardia. Thus, we routinely perform perinodal cryosurgery for AV node re-entry tachycardia in such patients following completion of the WPW surgical procedure. Less obvious is the desirability of performing perinodal cryosurgery for ablation of dual AV node physiology in patients undergoing surgery for the WPW syndrome who have not previously experienced concomitant AV node re-entry tachycardia. Several patients in the author's WPW surgical series have been shown to have concomitant dual AV node conduction pathways in addition to the WPW syndrome, but they had never experienced AV node re-entry tachycardia clinically. Six of those patients did not undergo the perinodal cryosurgical procedure for the dual AV node pathways at the time of surgical correction of their WPW syndrome. Three of the six patients subsequently developed AV node re-entry tachycardia postoperatively even though they had never experienced it preoperatively. As a result, the author now routinely performs perinodal cryosurgery concomitantly with WPW surgery not only in patients who have had documented AV node re-entry tachycardia previously, but also in patients with dual AV node conduction pathways who have never experienced AV node re-entry tachycardia.

Preoperative Electrophysiologic Evaluation

Patients are instrumented with transvenous endocardial catheter electrodes in a manner identical to that used for the preoperative evaluation of the WPW syndrome. Programmed electrical stimulation of the atrium is performed, and standard criteria for the diagnosis of AV node re-entry tachycardia are employed.[90] The demonstration of disparate AV node conduction curves in response to programmed atrial extrastimuli documents the presence of dual AV node physiology. As the atria are paced faster (i.e., the pacing cycle length is decreased), the conduction time through the AV node (A-H interval) gradually prolongs. This normal characteristic of the AV node is termed decremental conduction. However, in patients with dual AV node conduction pathways, a sudden "jump" in the A-H interval occurs in response to a slight increase in the atrial pacing rate. This sudden, dramatic slowing of conduction through the AV node as the atria are paced faster is due to conduction block occurring in the fast pathway and continuing in the slow pathway.

Supraventricular tachycardia is then initiated with programmed atrial stimulation, and in order to establish the diagnosis of AV node re-entry tachycardia, the supraventricular tachycardia must be shown to be dependent on a critical A-H delay. AV node re-entry tachycardia can also be terminated by inducing AV nodal block. Finally, limited endocardial catheter mapping of the atrium during ventricular pacing and during induced AV node re-entry tachycardia shows concentric depolarization of the atrial septum, with the earliest atrial activation occurring in the region of the AV node–His bundle complex. The demonstration of dual AV node conduction curves and the initiation of supraventricular tachycardia with these characteristics will confirm that the patient has AV node re-entry tachycardia.

Intraoperative Electrophysiologic Mapping

It is not necessary to perform true isochronous electrophysiologic mapping intraoperatively in patients with AV node re-entry tachycardia in order to effect a surgical cure. However, the continuous monitoring of antegrade conduction through the AV node–His bundle complex is absolutely essential to avoid permanent conduction block.[36] Normal AV conduction is monitored by quadripolar epicardial plaque electrodes that are sutured to the right atrium and right ventricle for pacing and recording reference atrial and ventricular electrograms during the course of the operative procedure. A bipolar handheld electrode is used to identify the location of the His bundle. During the perinodal cryosurgical procedure, atrial pacing is instituted at a constant cycle length that results in stable AV conduction. The pacing spike is set to trigger the sweep of a standard storage oscilloscope. This timing dictates that the reference ventricular electrogram will be positioned at the same site on the oscilloscope screen during each cardiac cycle as long as the AV interval remains constant. After completion of cryothermia, but before disengagement from cardiopulmonary bypass, incremental atrial and ventricular pacing and programmed atrial stimulation are performed to assess AV conduction and ventricular-atrial conduction, to generate AV node refractory curves, and to attempt to initiate AV node re-entry tachycardia. Intraoperative mapping is not required to guide the cryosurgical procedure since it is performed in the same manner in all patients.

Surgical Technique

The objective of surgery for AV node re-entry tachycardia is to interrupt one of the two pathways of conduction through the AV node while leaving the other pathway of conduction intact. Experience has shown that the perinodal cryosurgical procedure as it is currently performed results in ablation of the slow conduction pathway and preservation of the fast conduction pathway through the AV node.[33,36] The heart is exposed through either a median sternotomy or a right anterior thoracotomy in the fourth intercostal space, the latter being preferred by some female patients for cosmetic reasons. The aorta and both venae cavae are cannulated for cardiopulmonary bypass, and epicardial plaque electrodes are sutured to the right atrium and right ventricle. Following incremental atrial pacing and induction and termination of AV node re-entry tachycardia as described previously, normothermic cardiopulmonary bypass is instituted, and a right atriotomy is performed (Fig. 11). After identification of the location of the His bundle, atrial pacing is

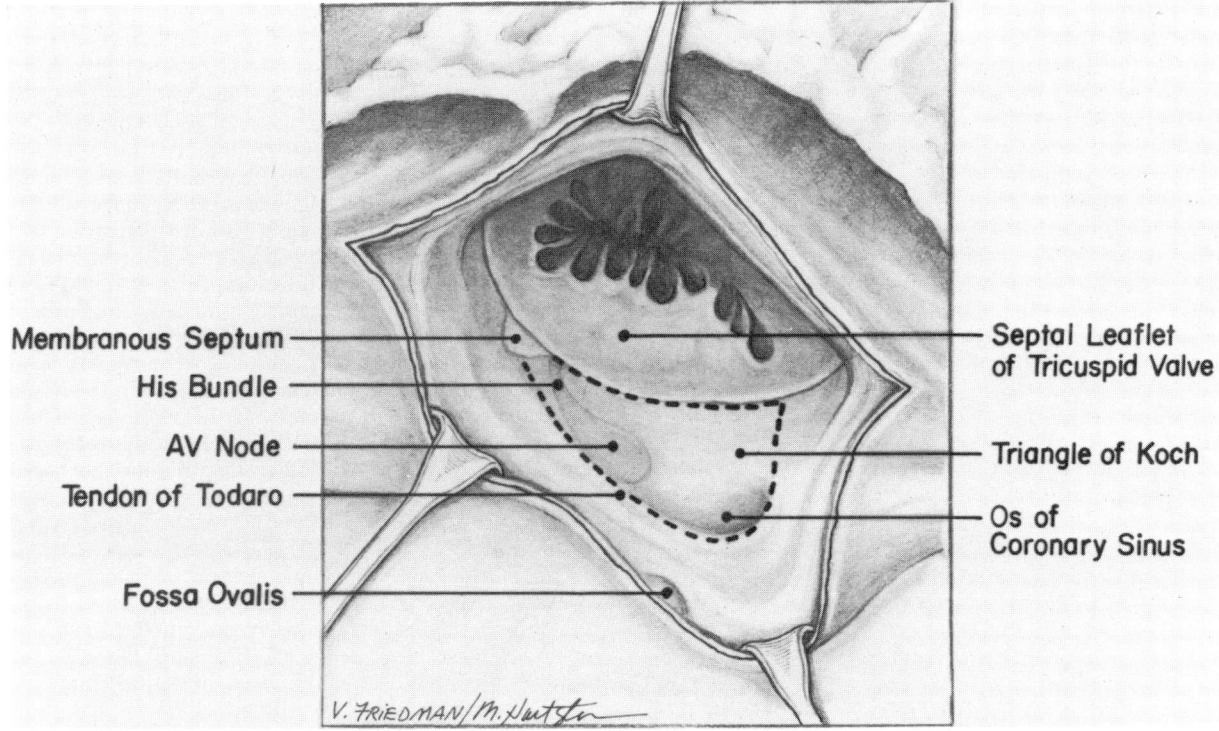

Figure 11. The right atrial septum viewed through a longitudinal right atriotomy. The patient's head is to the left and feet are to the right. The boundaries of the triangle of Koch are the tendon of Todaro, the tricuspid valve anulus, and a line connecting the two at the level of the os of the coronary sinus. Within the triangle of Koch reside the AV node and proximal portion of the His bundle, which enters the ventricular septum immediately posterior to the membranous portion of the interatrial septum. (From Cox, J. L., et al.: Cryosurgical treatment of atrioventricular node reentrant tachycardia. Circulation, 76:1329, 1987.)

instituted, and the AV interval is monitored on a beat-to-beat basis as described previously. A nitrous oxide cryoprobe with a 3-mm. diameter tip is then placed over the tendon of Todaro at the upper edge of the os of the coronary sinus. Cryothermia is applied at a temperature of −60° C. for 2 minutes. Three more cryolesions are placed along the tendon of Todaro, moving sequentially toward the apex of the triangle of Koch near the His bundle (sites 2, 3, and 4 in Fig. 12). Cryolesions are then placed along the anulus of the tricuspid valve, beginning just beneath the os of the coronary sinus (sites 5, 6, 7, and 8 in Fig. 12). Prolongation of the AV interval usually occurs during application of cryothermia at sites 7 or 8. The AV interval usually prolongs in a linear fashion during cryothermia application, allowing the electrophysiologist to notify the surgeon of the degree of AV interval prolongation with each succeeding beat. As the AV interval prolongs to approximately 200 to 300 msec., one can expect complete AV block to occur within the next few beats. Cryothermia is terminated instantly with the development of incomplete AV block, and the top of the cryoprobe is irrigated immediately with copious amounts of warm saline. AV conduction resumes invariably within 2 or 3 beats, and the AV interval returns to its control value during the ensuing 10 to 15 beats. The cryoprobe is then moved slightly more peripherally until cryothermia can be applied for the full 2 minutes to a given site without causing heart block. In this manner, cryolesions are placed at as many sites within the triangle of Koch as possible without creating permanent AV block, using the same end point of temporary block to terminate each cryolesion. In essence, the objective of this operation is to cryoablate as much of the perinodal tissue within the triangle of Koch as possible without causing permanent AV conduction block. This approach is feasible only because of the unique nature of cryosurgery, which allows a definitive end point (complete heart block) to be reached but only on a temporary, reversible basis.

In patients with AV node re-entry tachycardia and concomitant WPW syndrome, the WPW syndrome must be corrected

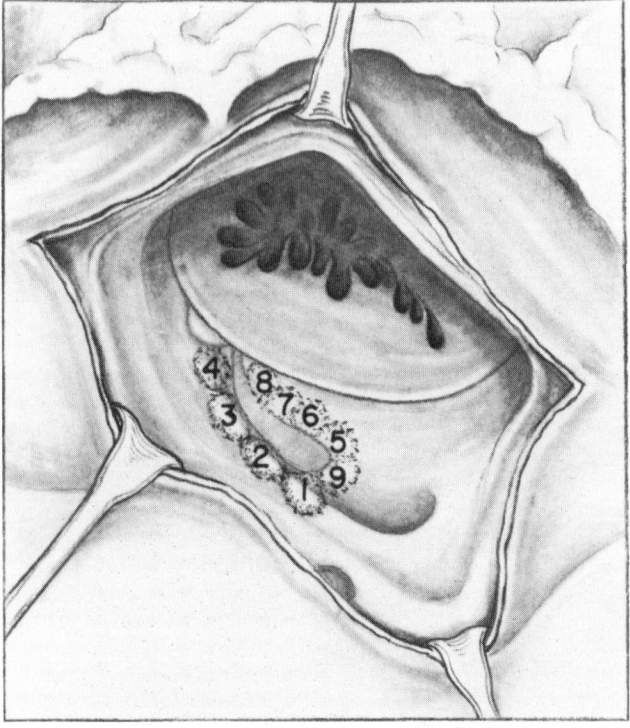

Figure 12. Cryolesions are placed in positions 1 to 4 as diagrammed, then in positions 5 to 8, and finally in position 9. During the application of cryothermia at positions 7 and 8, prolongation of the AV interval begins to occur. (From Cox, J. L., et al.: Cryosurgical treatment of atrioventricular node reentrant tachycardia. Circulation, 76:1329, 1987.)

first before any attempt is made to treat the AV node re-entry.[33,36] This sequence is essential because the discrete cryosurgical procedure for AV node re-entry depends on the ability to monitor exclusive conduction through the AV node–His bundle complex on a beat-to-beat basis. If the patient has a functioning accessory pathway that conducts in the antegrade direction, it is impossible to monitor the effects of cryosurgical modification of normal AV conduction during atrial pacing since the atrial impulse travels preferentially across the accessory pathway to the ventricles.

The surgical dissection technique for AV node re-entry tachycardia is also performed through a median sternotomy and on cardiopulmonary bypass.[88] Intraoperative mapping is usually performed prior to the surgical dissection technique with the aid of normothermic cardiopulmonary bypass. Using a hand-held bipolar electrode, earliest atrial activation during AV node re-entry tachycardia occurs just superior and medial to the AV node in those patients with Type A tachycardia and just superior and lateral to the AV node near the os of the coronary sinus in those patients with Type B tachycardia. Once the intraoperative mapping procedure has been completed, systemic temperature is decreased to 32° C. and the heart is arrested with cold potassium cardioplegia. Stay sutures are placed in the posterior tricuspid anulus to facilitate dissection and exposure. An incision is made through the right atrial wall immediately behind the tricuspid valve anulus, commencing just inferior and lateral to the os of the coronary sinus and extending superiorly and medially over the central fibrous body. The right atrial wall only is then reflected superiorly, using a knife to expose the posterior septal space. The AV node and central fibrous body are identified.

For Type A AV node re-entry tachycardia, the superolateral connections of the AV node to the atrium via the coronary sinus are left undisturbed. The tendon of Todaro is traced forward to the central fibrous body; then the tendon, along with all muscle over the central fibrous body and intra-atrial septum superior and medial to the AV node, down to the submucosa or fat, and the atrial septum is resected with a knife as far superiorly as the level of the coronary sinus. Inferior and lateral dissection stops before the AV node, but more posteriorly the dissection exposes the mitral anulus and the superior process of the left ventricle. Care is used not to dissect between the AV node and the central fibrous body, since this may divide the His bundle. The atrial incisions are then closed with a continuous suture.

In Type B AV node re-entry tachycardia, the superior and medial connections of the AV node to the atrium are left undisturbed. The free wall of the right ventricle is dissected with a knife from just inferior and lateral to the os of the coronary sinus to just lateral to the AV node and posterior to the AV nodal artery onto the interventricular septum, extending in depth to just beneath the epicardium. The inferior and posterior wall of the coronary sinus is then dissected to clean the epicardium from the os of the coronary sinus to the level of the left atrial wall, exposing the right coronary sinus. This dissection divides all connections between the AV node and the right atrium superior and lateral to the AV node. The atrial incisions are then closed.

Surgical Results

Although the surgical techniques designed to cure AV node re-entry tachycardia have been employed for only a short period of time, the results have been excellent.[28,88] The results of the three largest series reported are listed in Table 1. There have been no operative deaths in any of the series. Following the perinodal cryosurgical procedure, smooth AV node conduction curves through the remaining single conduction pathway have been demonstrated in all patients, and none of the patients have had inducible AV node re-entry tachycardia postoperatively. Moreover, all patients have maintained normal conduction

TABLE 1. Results of Surgery for AV Node Re-entry Tachycardia

Technique	Dates	Number of Patients	Operative Mortality	Early Failures	Heart Block	Late Failures	Patients Cured
Cryosurgery[33]	8/82–10/89	29	0	0%	0%	0%	100%
Dissection							
Johnson[88]	10/83–10/87	69	0	4%	3%	9%	84%
Guiraudon[76]	12/85–7/89	32	0	6%	6%	9%	79%

through the AV node–His bundle complex with no recurrent AV node re-entry tachycardia. The surgical dissection technique has been associated with a low incidence of permanent complete heart block and a low incidence of recurrent AV node re-entry tachycardia.

AUTOMATIC ATRIAL TACHYCARDIA

Historical Aspects

Automatic atrial tachycardias were first described by Sir Thomas Lewis in 1909.[101] The accumulation of scientific data on automatic atrial tachycardias since Lewis' time has been largely anecdotal. As a result of the paucity of information on these arrhythmias, the development of surgical procedures for their cure has been hampered. Moreover, since these arrhythmias cannot be initiated and terminated at will by pacing techniques, and because they are frequently suppressed by general anesthetic agents, automatic atrial tachycardias have been among the most difficult to treat surgically.

With the advent of intraoperative electrophysiologic mapping techniques during the late 1960s, it became feasible to attempt intraoperative localization of the automatic foci responsible for these arrhythmias. Thus, in 1973, Goldreyer and colleagues reported the first electrophysiologic demonstration of automatic atrial tachycardia in man.[70] Subsequently, attempts were made, sometimes successfully, to localize and ablate automatic atrial tachycardias intraoperatively.[61,66,119,147] However, because of the frequent suppression of the automatic atrial tachycardias by general anesthesia intraoperatively and the inability to induce the arrhythmias by pacing techniques, surgeons frequently had to resort to His bundle ablation and insertion of a permanent pacemaker system.[131] As mentioned in the previous section on AV node re-entry tachycardia, His bundle ablation in this setting represents a surgical isolation procedure designed to confine the automatic tachycardia to the atria. Since many of these tachycardias originate in the body of the left atrium, the concept of surgically isolating only the left atrium was introduced, leaving the remainder of the heart in normal sinus rhythm.[141] Since the sinus node, AV node, His bundle, and bundle branches are all located in the right atrium, atrial septum, or ventricular septum, surgical isolation of the left atrium does not interfere with the normal cardiac conduction system. Therefore, no pacemaker system is necessary postoperatively. The left atrial isolation procedure was first performed clinically for automatic left atrial tachycardia in 1982.[21] Currently, excision procedures, cryoablative procedure, and isolation procedures can be employed for automatic atrial tachycardias arising in the right or left atrium with excellent results.

Anatomic-Electrophysiologic Basis

Automatic atrial tachycardia is caused by an automatic focus of arrhythmogenic tissue lying outside the region of the normal anatomic SA node. Histologic examination of the atrial tissue excised at the site of origin of automatic atrial tachycardias has not revealed a specific finding common to all patients. In Lowe's excellent recent review of the world literature on this subject,[104] it was noted that a variety of pathologic findings have been

identified. Monocytic infiltrates,[121,147] focal myocyte hypertrophy,[67,98] islets of fatty tissue, fibrous tissue foci,[58] proliferation of abnormal cells,[92] and small atrial wall aneurysms[114] have been documented in the excised atrial myocardium responsible for the automatic atrial tachycardias.

Surgical Indications and Contraindications

Automatic atrial tachycardias frequently occur in pediatric patients in whom the tachycardia may be asymptomatic or may present with vomiting and epigastric pain. Adult patients more commonly present with palpitations, presyncope, syncope, or symptoms of congestive heart failure. One of the most common manifestations of automatic atrial tachycardia is cardiomegaly and congestive heart failure, with the overall incidence being 54 to 63 per cent.[11,65,67,120] Damiano demonstrated experimentally that chronic atrial tachycardia may lead to significant left ventricular enlargement and dysfunction and that restoration of normal rhythm following termination of the atrial tachycardia results in restoration of normal ventricular function.[41] Thus, the indications for surgical intervention in patients with automatic atrial tachycardias include medical refractoriness, intolerable side effects of antiarrhythmic drugs, poor patient compliance, patient preference to medical therapy, tachycardia-induced ventricular dysfunction, and congestive heart failure.

Preoperative Electrophysiologic Evaluation

In patients with automatic atrial tachycardia, the standard ECG demonstrates a P wave morphologic pattern that is different from that seen in sinus rhythm, suggesting the presence of an ectopic focus remote from the sinus node. Preoperative endocardial catheter electrophysiologic studies typically fail to initiate or terminate the tachycardia by programmed electrical stimulation techniques. However, either premature atrial extrastimuli or direct current countershock usually will reset, rather than terminate, the tachycardia.[14] Rapid atrial pacing may result in overdrive suppression of the underlying automatic atrial tachycardia, being manifest by a pause following termination of pacing or slowing of the automatic atrial tachycardia, which then accelerates to its previous rate.

Lowe reports that of the 125 patients with automatic atrial tachycardia reported to date, the location of the automatic focus was specified in 89 patients.[104] Sixty-one (68 per cent) were located in the right atrial free wall, 5 (6 per cent) within the atrial septum, and the remaining 23 (26 per cent) within the left atrium.

Intraoperative Mapping

If only a single-point, hand-held mapping system is available, it may be virtually impossible to identify the site of origin of an automatic atrial tachycardia intraoperatively because of the vulnerability of the tachycardia to suppression by general anesthesia.[62] The general anesthetic agents usually do not suppress the tachycardia completely, but they do frequently prevent the tachycardia from being sustained long enough intraoperatively to map and localize the site of origin with a single-point mapping system. However, the introduction of computerized multi-point mapping systems has alleviated this problem, since only one beat of an automatic tachycardia is necessary to localize its site of origin using such mapping systems.[16] The author currently employs three epicardial electrode templates containing a total of 156 bipolar electrode pairs. These templates, fashioned of silicone rubber, are designed to conform to the epicardial surfaces of the atria. The templates are attached to the epicardial surfaces of the atria by sutures placed at their periphery to avoid interference with data acquisition. As mentioned, once these electrode templates have been positioned on the atria, only a single beat of the automatic tachycardia is necessary to localize its site of origin.

Surgical Technique

If the site of origin of an automatic atrial tachycardia can be localized precisely by intraoperative mapping, the arrhythmogenic focus may be either excised or cryoblated. Automatic foci located in the free wall of the left atrium or in either of the atrial appendages are ideal for excision or cryoblation. Automatic atrial tachycardias arising near the orifices of the pulmonary veins are best treated either by pulmonary vein isolation or by left atrial isolation.

Theoretically, if intraoperative mapping properly localizes automatic foci in the free wall of the body of the right atrium, those foci can be either excised or cryoablated. However, automatic right atrial tachycardias are frequently multifocal in origin, and the ablation or excision of one automatic focus may be followed by the appearance of another at some later date. Thus, the recurrence rate following local excision or cryoablation of automatic right atrial tachycardias is unacceptably high, and as a result, the author prefers to perform a right atrial isolation procedure, even though the site of origin of the tachycardia may be well-defined by intraoperative computerized mapping.[78,79] The right atrial isolation procedure has now been performed in six patients, with uniform success and no recurrences during a 4-year follow-up period.

Surgical Results

Lowe reports that electrophysiologically guided operative procedures have been performed in 63 of the 125 patients available for review.[104] Fifty-six (89 per cent) have been completely cured without the need for permanent pacemaker implantation or postoperative antiarrhythmic therapy. One perioperative death occurred in a patient with severe congestive heart failure and dilated cardiomyopathy who arrested during the induction of anesthesia.

ATRIAL FLUTTER/FIBRILLATION

Historical Aspects

Elective His bundle ablation, either by open-heart surgical techniques[131] or by endocardial catheter fulguration,[127] has been the only effective means of treating atrial fibrillation nonpharmacologically. As mentioned in preceding sections, these two procedures do not actually ablate the supraventricular tachycardia (in this case atrial fibrillation), but rather they protect the ventricles from the adverse effects of the arrhythmias. Unfortunately, in the case of atrial fibrillation, His bundle ablation does not protect the patient from *all* of the detrimental effects of atrial fibrillation, as discussed later in this section. Nevertheless, a review of the international catheter ablation registry reveals that the most common indication for endocardial catheter ablation of the His bundle, since its introduction in 1982, is atrial fibrillation.[52]

The left atrial isolation procedure, first introduced experimentally in 1980[141] and clinically in 1982,[21] is capable of confining atrial fibrillation associated with mitral valve disease to the left atrium, but because the left atrium continues to fibrillate postoperatively, it has not been applied routinely to control the

detrimental effects of atrial fibrillation clinically. In 1985, Guiraudon introduced the "corridor procedure" in which a strip of atrial septum between the SA node and AV node was isolated from the remainder of the atrial myocardium in patients with atrial fibrillation.[71] Although this procedure has now been performed in several patients, it unfortunately alleviates only the rapid, irregular ventricular response to atrial fibrillation, but it does not restore AV synchrony, nor does it reduce the vulnerability of patients with atrial fibrillation to the development of thromboembolic problems.

The first surgical procedure designed specifically to cure atrial fibrillation, the so-called "maze procedure,"[38,40] is discussed later in this section.

Anatomic-Electrophysiologic Basis

Three theories have been proposed to explain the mechanism of atrial activation during atrial fibrillation: (1) a single automatic ectopic focus in the atrium, firing at an extremely rapid rate[125]; (2) multiple automatic foci in the atria, firing independently throughout the atria[51]; and (3) intra-atrial re-entry in which multiple re-entrant wavelets are present in the atria. This last multiple wavelet theory was originally proposed by Moe[108] and has subsequently been verified by the studies of Boineau[10] and Allessie.[2,3] These authors have demonstrated that atrial geometry, local refractory distribution, and the resultant local conduction velocity of the atrial tissues determine whether re-entry will occur, how many wavelets will form, and whether the process will be sustained. During the past four years, the author has employed epicardial template electrodes on the atria, both experimentally and clinically.[38,39] The results of these studies have documented complete re-entrant loops in some instances and partial loops in others, suggesting that the re-entrant wavefront moved through the septum around the pulmonary veins, inferior vena cava, or superior vena cava. The more complex patterns in which re-entrant loops were not documented were consistent with the multiple wavelet hypothesis of Moe[108] and the experimental data of Allessie.[2,3] Although anatomic obstacles, such as the pulmonary veins, inferior vena cava, and superior vena cava, were frequently involved in the apparent re-entrant loops, complete re-entrant circuits were frequently recorded in the absence of these anatomic obstacles. These re-entrant loops rotated around areas of functional conduction block, the most common site being along the sulcus terminalis. These studies confirmed that as atrial size increases, the number of wavefronts during atrial fibrillation and the duration of atrial fibrillation increase. As the cycle lengths decrease and become more variable, various regions of the atria are completely dissociated from one another. The importance of these experimental and clinical studies lies in the fact that they have documented unequivocally that atrial flutter/fibrillation is due to intra-atrial re-entry as first suggested by Moe and that the concept of multifocal automaticity is not operative in the genesis or perpetuation of atrial fibrillation in man.

Surgical Indications and Contraindications

The present indications for surgical intervention in patients with atrial fibrillation are extremely limited. However, the serious nature and life-threatening complications of atrial fibrillation would dictate that, should a safe and effective surgical technique be developed to cure atrial fibrillation,[53] the surgical indications would expand dramatically. Available statistics indicate that approximately 0.4 per cent of the United States population, 1 million people, suffer from atrial fibrillation.[15,45,80,115,126] There are three detrimental side effects when one converts from normal sinus rhythm to atrial fibrillation: (1) a rapid, irregular heartbeat, (2) impaired cardiac hemodynamics due to loss of AV synchrony, and (3) an increased vulnerability to thromboembolism. Thromboembolism occurs in approximately one third of patients with atrial fibrillation (330,000

United States citizens), approximately three fourths of all thromboembolic episodes associated with atrial fibrillation involve the brain (247,500 United States citizens), and approximately 60 per cent of those cerebroembolic events cause death or permanent severe neurologic deficit (148,200 United States citizens).[53] Thus, an effective surgical therapy for atrial fibrillation that restores normal AV synchrony would be indicated for medical refractoriness, intolerable drug side effects, poor patient compliance, preference to medical therapy, congestive heart failure due to atrial fibrillation, and thromboembolic episodes due to atrial fibrillation.

Preoperative Electrophysiologic Evaluation

Preoperative electrophysiologic studies are of limited value in patients with atrial fibrillation, since an accurate diagnosis can be made by standard ECG. Moreover, catheter mapping is not feasible in atrial fibrillation. Nevertheless, patients who are to be subjected to surgical intervention for atrial fibrillation should undergo a preoperative electrophysiologic study to rule out concomitant electrophysiologic abnormalities.

Intraoperative Electrophysiologic Mapping

Currently, the author employs the maze procedure for the surgical treatment of atrial fibrillation, which does not require intraoperative electrophysiologic mapping for its performance. Nevertheless, computerized atrial epicardial mapping is routinely performed in patients undergoing operation for atrial fibrillation because occasionally the atrial fibrillation may be dependent on a single macro–re-entrant circuit for its perpetuation. In such patients, a surgical procedure less complex in which the dominant re-entrant circuit is interrupted might be curative.

Surgical Technique

The left atrial isolation procedure is performed by placing a surgical incision just to the left of the atrial septum and extending it from the anterior mitral anulus to the posterior mitral anulus. This procedure causes electrical isolation of the left atrium from the rest of the heart, allowing the remainder of the heart to be in a normal sinus rhythm regardless of what is occurring in the left atrium. Loss of the left atrial kick has no effect on overall cardiac performance in the presence of a normal left ventricle, since the right atrial kick is preserved.[141] Preservation of the right atrial kick results in a normal right-sided cardiac output; therefore, the left ventricle simply adapts to the delivery of the same volume ouput, resulting in the left atrium becoming a passive conduit. Thus, two of the detrimental effects of atrial fibrillation, the irregular heartbeat and the impaired cardiac hemodynamics, are abolished by the left atrial isolation procedure. However, this procedure does not alleviate the risk of thromboembolism associated with chronic atrial fibrillation, since the left atrium may continue to fibrillate.

The corridor procedure[71] involves isolating a strip (or a corridor) or atrial septum from the SA node to the AV node so that the sinus impulse can travel down the corridor, through the AV node, to the ventricles. All atrial myocardium outside the SA node–AV node corridor is thus excluded from the ventricles. The corridor procedure abolishes only one of the three detrimental effects of atrial fibrillation, the irregular heartbeat. Since neither the left atrium nor the right atrium contracts in synchrony with its respective ventricle, the beneficial hemodynamic effect of the atrial kick is not restored. Moreover, since the atria remain free to fibrillate, the risk of thromboembolism is unaltered. Thus, the corridor procedure offers no advantage over catheter His bundle ablation and insertion of a physiologic ventricular pacemaker for the treatment of atrial fibrillation, a procedure that can be performed without opening the chest.

The maze procedure (Fig. 13) is performed on cardiopulmonary bypass after standard aortic and bicaval cannulation has been completed. The superior vena cava, inferior vena cava, and roof of the atrium between the aorta and superior vena cava are dissected free of all surrounding connective tissue and the interatrial groove is developed as completely as possible. Cardiopulmonary bypass is instituted and the right atrial incisions

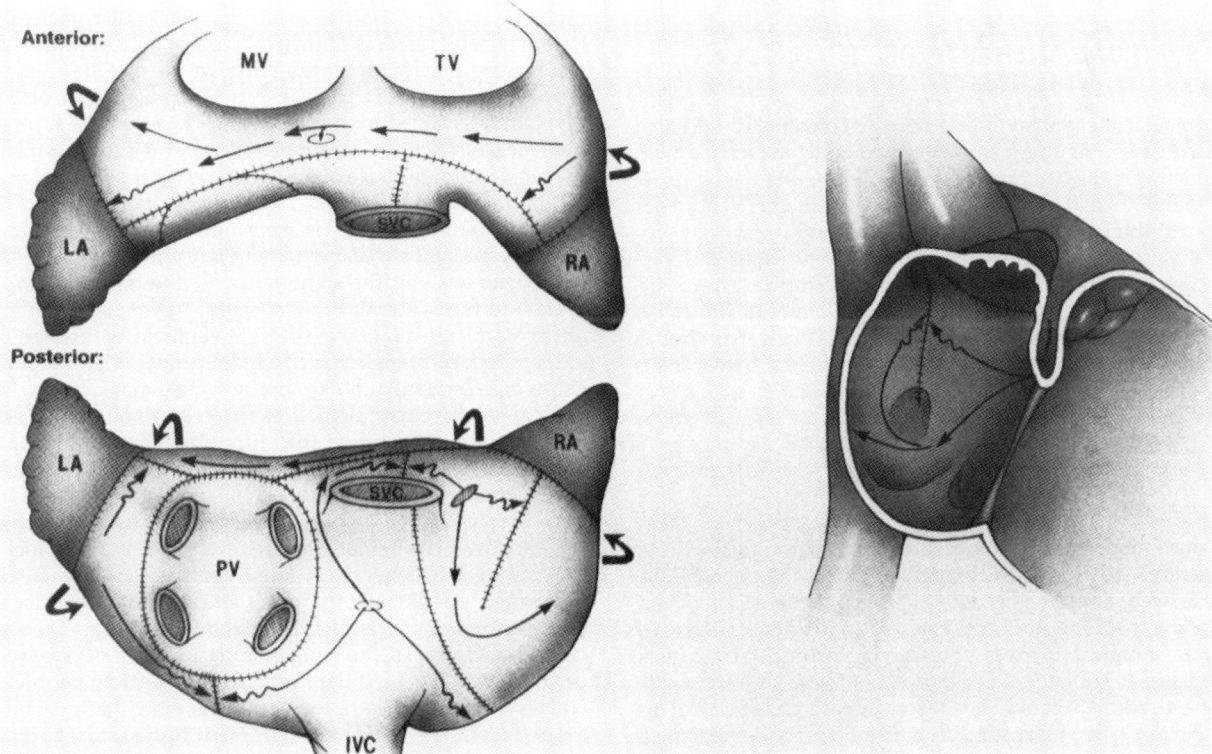

Figure 13. The maze procedure. See text for discussion. (Modified from Cox, J. L., et al.: The surgical treatment of atrial fibrillation: III. Development of a surgical cure. J. Thorac. Cardiovasc. Surg., *101*:402, 1991.)

are performed as diagrammed in Figure 13. The heart is then arrested with cold potassium cardioplegic solution and the left atrial incisions and cryosurgery are performed under cardioplegic arrest as described in Figure 13. After closure of the left atrial incisions and the atrial septal incision, the aortic cross-clamp is released and the left side of the heart is de-aired. The right atrial incisions are closed as the heart is being rewarmed. The effect of the maze procedure is to allow a normally generated impulse to propagate from the SA node and to activate the entire atrial myocardium except for the excised atrial appendages and the pulmonary veins. At the same time, it is impossible for a large macro–re-entrant circuit to exist, since the atrial impulses are precluded from turning back on themselves because of the refractory period of the tissue that has just been depolarized. Thus, regardless of the number of macro–re-entrant circuits responsible for the development and perpetuation of atrial fibrillation, they cannot occur following the maze procedure.

Surgical Results

As mentioned, although the left atrial isolation procedure has been applied clinically for the treatment of automatic left atrial tachycardias, it has not been applied routinely clinically for the treatment of atrial fibrillation. The corridor procedure has been employed in three patients with atrial fibrillation. The clinical results have confirmed the experimental findings, suggesting that the corridor procedure devascularizes the SA node and that a sick sinus syndrome is likely to ensue. Indeed, two of the three patients in whom the corridor procedure has been performed have required the insertion of permanent pacemakers.

The maze procedure has been performed in seven patients clinically, with no operative deaths. Complications have included drug-induced lupus erythematosus, left lower lobe pneumonia, and transient cholestasis. All patients have been cured of atrial fibrillation and none are on antiarrhythmic drugs postoperatively. Five of the seven patients are in continuous sinus rhythm and two of the patients who had sick sinus syndrome preoperatively have had DDD-R pacemakers implanted postoperatively. The longest follow-up is now $2\frac{1}{2}$ years.

SURGICAL THERAPY FOR VENTRICULAR TACHYARRHYTHMIAS

Ventricular tachyarrhythmias may be conveniently divided into two types, the more common type being associated with ischemic heart disease and the less common type being unrelated to myocardial ischemia. Virtually all ischemic ventricular tachyarrhythmias arise in the left ventricle and ventricular septum; the vast majority of nonischemic ventricular tachyarrhythmias arise in the free wall of the right ventricle. The difference in the clinical presentations and anatomic substrates responsible for these two types of ventricular tachyarrhythmias necessitates entirely different surgical approaches to their treatment.

NONISCHEMIC VENTRICULAR TACHYARRHYTHMIAS

Historical Aspects

Because nonischemic ventricular tachyarrhythmias occur only rarely, early scientific reports describing their clinical occurrence were entirely anecdotal. Perhaps the most important development leading to the eventual development of surgical therapies designed to treat nonischemic ventricular tachyarrhythmias was Fontaine's recognition that these seemingly disparate arrhythmias could be categorized and classified.[57] This provided the arrhythmia surgeon with a basis for developing a unified concept for treating all nonischemic right ventricular tachyarrhythmias, regardless of their etiology or associated pathologic anatomy.

The first attempts at surgical correction of nonischemic right ventricular tachyarrhythmias were performed by Fontaine's surgical colleague, Guiraudon, in the mid-1970s.[56] Surgical incisions and excisions were performed, on the basis of either electrophysiologic mapping or gross pathology, with an overall success rate of approximately 50 per cent. In 1979, the author began performing localized surgical isolation procedures for these arrhythmias arising in the right ventricular free wall and pulmonary outflow tract.[21] By combining the principles applied in these localized isolation procedures, a technique was eventually developed in which the entire free wall of the right ventricle could be isolated successfully.[30] Long-term follow-up of these patients has established the validity of the localized isolation procedures, but it is rarely, if ever, necessary presently to perform total isolation of the right ventricle. The availability of computerized intraoperative mapping systems has made it possible to localize the site of origin of right ventricular tachycardia in virtually all patients so that localized isolation or ablative procedures can be performed today with excellent expectation of a surgical cure.

Anatomic-Electrophysiologic Basis

Nonischemic ventricular tachyarrhythmias may be classified into five types based on their pathologic or clinical characteristics, or both.

Idiopathic ventricular tachycardia refers to patients in whom the only clinical manifestation of cardiac disease is the arrhythmia. Both the macroscopic appearance of the heart at operation and the pathologic data acquired at the time of autopsy in such patients failed to show any evidence of primary cardiac disease. The repetitive episodes of tachycardia produce functional heart failure and global dilation of the heart. A majority of these arrhythmias have been shown to arise in the septum, making surgical therapy difficult.

Patients with *diffuse cardiomyopathy* rarely present with sustained monomorphic ventricular tachycardia that is tolerated hemodynamically. These patients have angiographic and catheter data indicating some type of abnormal myocardial contractility associated with recurrent ventricular tachycardia. Pathologically, there is diffuse dilation of both ventricles, with widespread patchy myocardial fibrosis.

Fontaine described a previously unrecognized form of cardiomyopathy localized to the right ventricle, which he termed *arrhythmogenic right ventricular dysplasia*.[56] This abnormality is the most common cause of nonischemic ventricular tachycardia arising in the right ventricle. This congenital myopathy is remarkable pathologically for transmural infiltration of adipose tissue, resulting in weakness and aneurysmal bulging of three pathologic areas of the right ventricle, the infundibulum, the apex, and the posterior basilar region. Ventriculography demonstrates diffuse dilation of the right ventricle, with a significant reduction in contractility and marked delay in right ventricular emptying. Ventricular bulges or frank aneurysm are seen in one or all of the three pathologic areas noted previously, and hypertrophic muscular bands in the infundibulum and anterior right ventricular wall result in apparent pseudodiverticula, the so-called feathering appearance of the right ventricular outflow tract. Because the origin of the tachycardia is the right ventricle, the standard ECG demonstrates a left bundle branch block pattern during the tachycardia. Right ventriculography should be performed on all patients with ventricular tachycardia associated with an apparent left bundle branch block.

An adult form of the congenital lesion of *Uhl's syndrome*[135] occurs in which ventricular tachycardia is the dominant feature. Uhl's syndrome is a rare congenital anomaly that may be considered from the anatomic standpoint to be a more complete form of arrhythmogenic right ventricular dysplasia. There is complete absence of myocardium in the right ventricular free wall, resulting in the endocardial and epicardial layers being in direct contact without interposition of myocardial fibers. The right ventricle is dilated in this lesion, but the tricuspid valve remains in the normal position, differentiating it from Ebstein's anomaly.

Life-threatening ventricular tachyarrhythmias may occur as a result of familial or idiopathic *prolonged Q-T interval syndrome*.[87] This electrocardiographic abnormality has been associated with several congenital abnormalities[59,123,140] and it has also been detected as a sequela of acute myocardial infarction.[112,130] The ventricular tachycardia occurring in association with the long Q-T syndrome is frequently of a distinct type called torsade de pointes, which is characterized by inconsistent polarity of the tachycardia on standard ECG.[99] The arrhythmia is usually preceded by variations in the T wave during the last several beats before development of the tachycardia. One of the most frequent causes of torsade de pointes is the administration of medications that prolong ventricular repolarization, particularly quinidine.[112] These, and other data, suggest that torsade de pointes represents an abnormality of myocardial repolarization in contradistinction to other types of ventricular tachycardias that are thought to be abnormalities of myocardial depolarization.

Surgical Indications and Contraindications

Nonischemic ventricular tachyarrhythmias are notoriously resistant to medical therapy. Therefore, nearly all patients with nonischemic ventricular tachyarrhythmias who require surgical therapy do so because of medical refractoriness.

Preoperative Electrophysiologic Evaluation

Since the vast majority of nonischemic ventricular tachyarrhythmias arise in the right ventricle, the single distinguishing characteristic of these arrhythmias is the presence of a left bundle branch block pattern during the tachycardia. As mentioned, all patients with this morphologic type of tachycardia should undergo right ventriculography for suspected arrhythmogenic right ventricular dysplasia. If the patient is to be subjected to surgical intervention, a formal preoperative endocardial catheter electrophysiologic study should be performed. It is usually possible to localize the site of origin of the tachycardia by extensive catheter mapping during the preoperative electrophysiologic study. Generally, patients who are to undergo surgical intervention for the long Q-T syndrome do not require a formal preoperative electrophysiologic study.

Intraoperative Electrophysiologic Mapping

The materials and methods used for intraoperative mapping of nonischemic ventricular tachyarrhythmias are identical to those employed for ischemic ventricular tachyarrhythmias and are discussed in the section describing those arrhythmias. The objective of the intraoperative mapping procedure is to localize as precisely as possible the site of origin of the nonischemic ventricular tachycardia and to determine if more than one site of origin exists.

Surgical Technique and Results

LONG Q-T SYNDROME. Left cervical thoracic sympathectomy with removal of the left stellate ganglion and the first three to four left thoracic sympathetic ganglia has been advocated for patients requiring surgical intervention for the long Q-T syndrome.[130] Although some success has been reported with this surgical approach, others have found the results to be characterized by early success and late failure. Because of these equivocal surgical results, the author presently recommends implantation of an automatic internal cardioverter-defibrillator (AICD) as an adjunct to the sympathectomy to serve as a backup therapy for those patients with histories of life-threatening arrhythmias.

OTHER TYPES OF NONISCHEMIC VENTRICULAR TACHYCARDIA. If nonischemic ventricular tachycardia can be shown to originate from a single site in the right ventricular free wall, it may be treated by surgical excision, cryoablation, or surgical isolation. The author prefers to perform a localized surgical isolation procedure for these monomorphic tachycardias whether they are due to diffuse cardiomyopathy or to arrhythmogenic right ventricular dysplasia.[30] Unfortunately, ventricular tachycardia associated with arrhythmogenic right ventricular dysplasia frequently arises from multiple sites in the right ventricle free wall, and localized isolation or ablative procedures are inadequate for controlling the arrhythmia. In such patients, total isolation of the right ventricle may be necessary. The long-term follow-up on the few patients who have undergone total right ventricular isolation is both gratifying and disconcerting. Two 16-year old patients who underwent this procedure at the author's institution in 1982 have been free of subsequent ventricular tachycardia; they are now, interestingly enough, both well-trained weight lifters. However, both have experienced progressive and dramatic dilation of the right ventricular free wall. Thus, despite an 8-year follow-up, the longer term prognosis in these young patients remains unknown.

The only viable alternative at present for the treatment of these complex polymorphic ventricular tachycardias associated with arrhythmogenic right ventricular dysplasia is the implantation of an AICD or cardiac transplantation. The AICD would appear to be of limited value in such patients because of the frequency of occurrence of episodes of tachycardia in these patients and the limited battery power of the AICD units.

ISCHEMIC VENTRICULAR TACHYARRHYTHMIAS

Historical Aspects

Sir Thomas Lewis first noted the relationship between ventricular aneurysms and ventricular tachycardia in 1909 and he suggested the need for a controlled method of inducing tachycardia so that it could be studied in a systematic fashion.[102] Despite Lewis' foresight, no such technique existed even 50 years later, when Couch reported the performance of a simple aneurysmectomy for the treatment of intractable ventricular tachycardia.[18] However, Lewis' dream became a reality in 1967, when Durrer and associates[47] of Amsterdam and Coumel and colleagues[19] of Paris described programmed electrical stimulation, a technique that could induce and terminate tachycardia in a reproducible manner for the purposes of diagnosis and evaluation of interventional therapy.

Experimental studies in the mid- and late 1960s documented the heterogeneity of tissue injury in acute myocardial infarction,[37] and the re-entrant basis of ischemic ventricular tachyarrhythmias was subsequently confirmed.[7,31,48,50,77,129,139] Thus, with the advent of coronary artery bypass surgery in the late 1960s, it seemed apparent that ischemic ventricular tachycardia would be easily corrected by this new procedure, since the basis for the arrhythmia (myocardial ischemia) could be alleviated by myocardial revascularization. During the 1970s, however, it became apparent that neither revascularization nor resection of the injured myocardium resulted in acceptable cure rates, and in addition, the operative mortality reported when these procedures were performed primarily for ventricular tachycardia control was prohibitively high.[6]

Because of the lack of efficacy of myocardial revascularization and/or resection in controlling ischemic ventricular tachycardia, several groups began to approach the problem in a more direct surgical manner. In 1969, Daniel and associates[42] and Kaiser and colleagues[93] had independently reported intraoperative mapping in patients with ischemic heart disease to localize the area of ischemic injury. Fontaine and co-workers performed intraoperative mapping prior to performing a standard aneurysmectomy in 1974,[55] but Wittig and Boineau[142] and Gallagher and associates[63] first reported the use of intraoperative mapping specifically to guide the attempted surgical ablation of ischemic ventricular tachycardia. Subsequently, Guiraudon introduced the encircling endocardial ventriculotomy (EEV)[72] and Josephson and Harken[91] described the subendocardial resection procedure as specific surgical techniques for ablation of these malignant arrhythmias. Subsequent laboratory studies[136-138] and clinical experience[35] showed that the EEV was associated with a high incidence of postoperative left ventricular dysfunction, and it has now been essentially abandoned. However, subendocardial resection, with or without subsequent modifications, continues to be one of the most important procedures used for control of ischemic ventricular tachycardia. In 1982, Moran reported a modification of the original subendocardial resection procedure in which all of the endocardial fibrosis associated with aneurysm or infarct was resected, the so-called extended endocardial resection procedure.[110] Other modifications of the original direct surgical operations have included the addition of endocardial cryoablation as an adjunctive procedure[21,23,35] and the so-called partial EEV, which has been used by Ostermeyer with excellent results.[116,117] More recently, Selle and colleagues have reported promising results with the Nd-YAG laser in a small series of patients.[132,133]

Anatomic-Electrophysiologic Basis

Acute myocardial infarction results in juxtaposition of normal and injured myocardium, and ventricular irritability, tachycardia, and fibrillation frequently occur during the initial and early phases of the infarct.[8,20,31,37] These manifestations of acute ischemic injury are usually transient and tend to be responsive to medical management. On occasion, patients will develop life-threatening tachyarrhythmias during the setting of an acute myocardial infarction, during exercise-induced ischemia, or during episodes of angina pectoris. In this subset of patients, coronary revascularization as primary therapy has been quite successful.[12,148] In the majority of patients, however, there is subsequent progression of the acutely ischemic tissue to cell death, leaving a fibrous scar in place of the injured myocardium. The interlacing anisotropic pattern of the remaining scar and normal myocardium may harbor local areas of slow conduction, unidirectional block, uneven refractoriness, and nonuniform repolarization, the electrophysiologic substrates for the development of re-entrant circuits.[7,20]

Studies in animal models, and more recently in man,[86,142] suggest that most re-entrant ventricular tachycardias in ischemic heart disease are primarily myocardial and that they are more complex geometrically than previously thought. The arrhythmogenic regions are located primarily in the endocardium and subendocardium, especially at the periphery of myocardial infarcts or ventricular aneurysms. Re-entrant ischemic ventricular arrhythmias result from a complex interplay between (1) a nonuniform (heterogeneous) state of repolarization, (2) slow desynchronized conduction over abnormal myocardial pathways created by fibrotic or ischemic discontinuity, and (3) ventricular ectopy. Slow desynchronized conduction is a hallmark of myocardial injury or fibrosis.[8] Conduction velocity is dependent on the synchrony of the activation process. Since fibrosis is nonuniform at the borders of infarcts, it produces complex interdigitations between normal myocardium and scar.[6,8] A synchronous wavefront, upon approaching such an area, may become desynchronized, fragmenting into many individual wavelets. A slowing of conduction time accompanies the desynchronization.

Electrical activity is thought to be identifiable as part of the re-entrant tachycardia circuit if it precedes the onset of ventricular depolarization evident on the surface ECG and is required for the initiation and perpetuation of the tachycardia. The site of origin of the tachycardia is felt to be the area exhibiting the earliest presystolic electrical activity in the latter half of diastole and represents the region of myocardium that must be identified and removed at the time of surgery in order to prevent the arrhythmias.[106]

Surgical Indications and Contraindications

The decision regarding surgical therapy for ischemic ventricular tachycardia is based on a variety of preoperative clinical factors. The primary indication for surgery is refractoriness to medical therapy. Controversy exists, however, as to whether patients who have failed amiodarone therapy should be included in this group.[26] Amiodarone has been shown to depress left ventricular function, and this depressant effect is aggravated by ischemic cardioplegic arrest in the majority of patients on the drug.[96,100] Because therapy with amiodarone can complicate surgical intervention in patients requiring a procedure for ventricular tachycardia and coronary revascularization, and because it fails to control the arrhythmia in a significant number of patients,[81,96] it would appear logical to make the decision regarding surgical intervention before the institution of amiodarone therapy, after the patient has been proved to be refractory to all other medications.

The only absolute contraindication to surgery for ischemic ventricular tachycardia is left ventricular dysfunction so severe that the preoperative risk is judged to be prohibitive.[26] Because most patients with ischemic heart disease and ventricular tachycardia have a left ventricular aneurysm, accurate determination of the ejection fraction in these patients is often difficult, and the absolute number is not an accurate predictor of operative mortality. Poor systolic function in the nonaneurysmal portion of the ventricle increases the operative risk to the patient.

The availability of computerized mapping systems that permit localization of the majority of the areas of arrhythmogenic myocardium has made the presence of nonsustained polymorphic ventricular tachycardia no longer a contraindication to surgery.

Preoperative Electrophysiologic Evaluation

All patients who are to undergo surgical therapy for ventricular tachyarrhythmias should first undergo an endocardial catheter electrophysiologic study. The objectives of the preoperative study are: (1) confirmation that the arrhythmia is ventricular rather than supraventricular in origin, (2) demonstration that the ventricular arrhythmia can be induced and terminated by programmed electrical stimulation techniques (i.e., that it is a re-entrant arrhythmia), and (3) localization of the region of origin of the ventricular tachycardia by catheter mapping when possible. In addition to the preoperative electrophysiologic study, patients with ventricular tachyarrhythmias routinely undergo cardiac catheterization and coronary angiography prior to surgical intervention.

The preoperative electrophysiologic study may demonstrate the arrhythmia to be ventricular tachycardia of a single morphologic type, indicating that it is originating from a single region in the left or right ventricle. Following induction, these *monomorphic ventricular tachycardias* are usually sustained for a sufficient length of time to allow endocardial catheter mapping to determine their site of origin. However, monomorphic ventricular tachycardia may be nonsustained, thus precluding adequate mapping during the preoperative electrophysiologic study. The preoperative study may also document the arrhythmia to be *polymorphic ventricular tachycardia*. This term is applied not only to ventricular tachycardia that originates from several different regions of the left ventricle giving rise to different morphologic types of tachycardia, but also to tachycardia that originates from one general region of the left ventricle but is characterized electrophysiologically by excessive fragmentation such that individual depolarization complexes may be difficult to identify. Polymorphic ventricular tachycardia may also be either sustained or nonsustained , and it commonly deteriorates rather quickly into ventricular fibrillation. Electrophysiologic deterioration to ventricular fibrillation may be the result of primary electrical instability or it may occur because of hemodynamic compromise associated with the onset of polymorphic ventricular tachycardia. The third type of ventricular tachyarrhythmia that may be identified by the preoperative electrophysiologic study is *primary ventricular fibrillation*. This arrhythmia is characterized by the absence of any type of induced ventricular tachycardia prior to the onset of ventricular fibrillation following programmed electrical stimulation.

Intraoperative Electrophysiologic Mapping

All 160 channels of the computerized mapping system are used to map the heart in patients with ventricular tachycardia.[25,27] A sock electrode array is first used to determine the epicardial activation sequence in sinus rhythm and during induced ventricular tachycardia. The sock electrode used contains 96 electrodes. The earliest site of epicardial breakthrough is automatically cursored in red by the computer for rapid detection of the region of most interest. The epicardial map not only is helpful as an initial screening device that can be obtained in 2 to 3 minutes, but it is also useful in characterizing nonclinical arrhythmias that may be induced during programmed electrical stimulation.

Once the epicardial activation sequence during ventricular tachycardia has been established, multiple plunge needle electrodes containing four bipolar pairs of contacts along the needle shaft are inserted into the ventricle in the region of earliest epicardial activation. If the epicardial map has suggested that the tachycardia is arising from the ventricular septum, a right atriotomy is performed and up to 15 right-angle needle electrodes are inserted into the ventricular septum from the right side, access being gained across the tricuspid valve. This provides up to 60 transmural data points from the ventricular septum without the necessity for performing a ventriculotomy. As

many as 25 other needle electrodes can be placed in or near the arrhythmogenic region, yielding a total of 160 endocardial intramural and epicardial data points simultaneously from the septum and free wall without performing a ventriculotomy. The objective of the intraoperative mapping procedure in patients with ventricular tachycardia is to identify the site(s) of origin of the ventricular tachycardia(s).

Surgical Technique

The encircling endocardial ventriculotomy (EEV) was the first surgical procedure specifically designed to control ischemic ventricular tachycardia[72] (Fig. 14C). The objective of the encircling endocardial incision just outside the junction of endocardial fibrosis and normal myocardium was either to interrupt the re-entrant circuit or to encompass it entirely and isolate it from the remainder of the ventricle. Laboratory studies demonstrated, however, that the encompassed myocardium was made more ischemic, thus suppressing the re-entrant circuit responsible for the tachycardia.[136-138] This increased ischemia caused by the EEV resulted in depressed left ventricular function following the procedure in these studies, and clinically the EEV was associated with an unacceptable incidence of postoperative low-output syndrome and operative mortality.[35] As a result, the EEV has been largely abandoned.

The localized subendocardial resection introduced by Josephson and Harken has proved to be an effective means of controlling ischemic ventricular tachycardia (Fig. 14D).[91] The author's approach combines an extended endocardial resection (Fig. 15) with adjunctive cryosurgery.[26] A median sternotomy is performed, and the intraoperative mapping sequence described before is performed on cardiopulmonary bypass. Then, with the

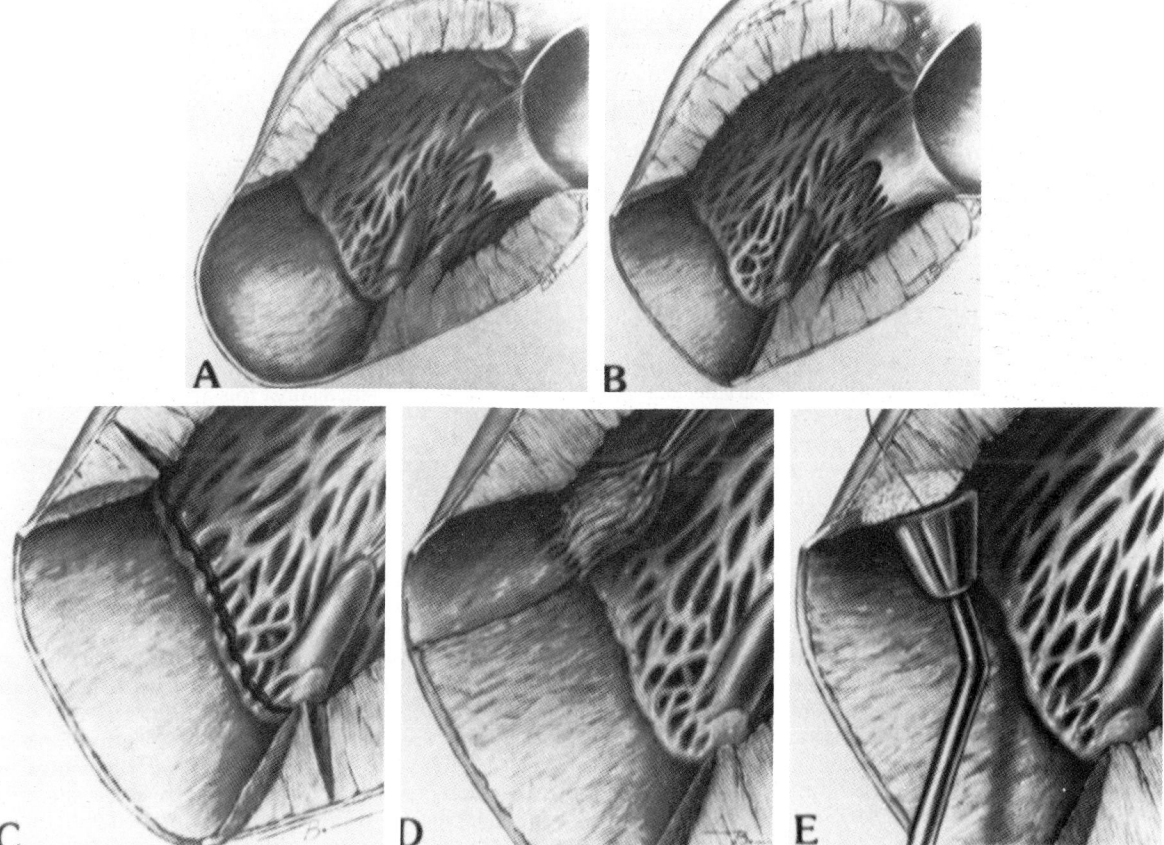

Figure 14. Diagrammatic cross section of an anterior left ventricular aneurysm showing more proximal extension of the associated fibrosis at the endocardial level than at the epicardial level (*A*). Since the re-entrant circuits responsible for ischemic ventricular tachycardia occur most commonly at the junction of this endocardial fibrosis and normal myocardium, a standard left ventricular aneurysm resection (*B*) does not ablate or remove them. The encircling endocardial ventriculotomy (*C*), localized endocardial (or "subendocardial") resection (*D*), and endocardial cryoablation (*E*) were all introduced specifically to ablate ventricular tachycardia associated with left ventricular aneurysms or infarcts. (Modified from Cox, J. L.: Anatomic-electrophysiologic basis for the surgical treatment of refractory ischemic ventricular tachycardia. Ann. Surg., *198*:119, 1983.)

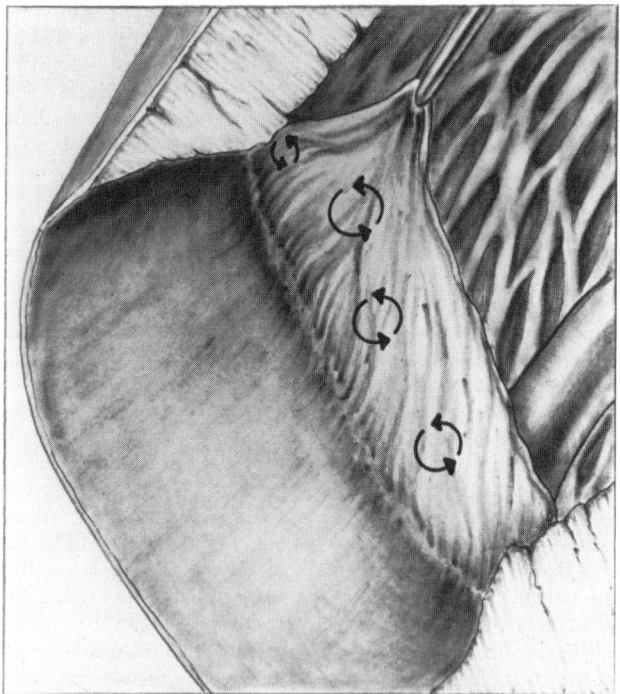

Figure 15. Diagrammatic sketch of an extended endocardial resection procedure in an anterior left ventricular aneurysm. The principle involved in this procedure is the same as that for a localized endocardial resection (Fig. 14D), but in this procedure *all* of the endocardial fibrosis associated with the aneurysm is resected except that involving the papillary muscles. (From Cox, J. L.: Surgical treatment of ischemic and non-ischemic ventricular tachyarrhythmias. *In* Cohn, L. H. (Ed.): Modern Technics in Surgery. Mount Kisco, NY, Futura Publishing Company, 1985.)

heart in the normothermic beating state and preferably in ventricular tachycardia, the ventricle is opened through the infarct or aneurysm and all of the associated endocardial fibrosis is resected, except that which extends onto the base of the papillary muscles. Approximately 10 per cent of patients will still have inducible tachycardia following resection of the fibrosis, indicating that the actual site of origin of the tachycardia in these patients is deeper in the myocardium than the visible border of the fibrosis. Endocardial cryolesions are applied to the site or sites of origin of the tachycardia as determined from the intraoperative mapping data, thus destroying the myocardium underneath the visible fibrosis responsible for the tachycardia. The endocardial fibrosis extending onto the base of the papillary muscles is not resected, but one or more cryolesions are placed directly on the base of the involved papillary muscle. Experience with this method of dealing with fibrosis extending onto the base of the papillary muscles argues strongly against the practice of resecting papillary muscles for ventricular tachycardia as has been reported in the past.[111]

Following completion of the extended endocardial resection and endocardial cryoablation, programmed electrical stimulation is applied in an attempt to induce the arrhythmia. If ventricular tachycardia is still inducible, mapping is again performed, and the remaining arrhythmogenic myocardium is cryoablated. If the arrhythmia is no longer inducible in this setting intraoperatively, there is a 98 per cent chance that it has been ablated.[26] If coronary bypass grafting or other procedures are to be performed, they are carried out after completion of the antiarrhythmic portion of the operation and confirmation of the result. The reason the use of cardioplegic solution is avoided in these patients is that the cardioplegia itself may temporarily alter the delicate re-entrant circuits causing the tachycardia. Therefore, if the antitachycardia procedure is performed under cardioplegic arrest, it is impossible to determine intraoperatively whether the surgical procedure has ablated the arrhythmia.

Ostermeyer has employed a variant of the original EEV in which an incision is placed at the base of the aneurysm or infarct in the region giving rise to the tachycardia.[116,117] Recently, promising results using endocardial mapping followed by ablation of the arrhythmogenic myocardium using the Nd-YAG laser have been reported.[132,133] This technique is easy and quick to perform and, as with the author's approach, can be applied in the normothermic beating heart, a major advantage in the ability to determine the efficacy of the procedure intraoperatively.

Surgical Results

A review of the cumulative experience with direct surgical procedures for the treatment of ventricular tachyarrhythmias during the past decade reveals that there are two problems that make ventricular tachycardia surgery less attractive as a therapeutic option than is surgery for supraventricular tachycardia.[26,118] The operative mortality has averaged 12.4 per cent (range, 0 to 21 per cent), and 23.8 per cent (range 0 to 38 per cent) of patients still have inducible ventricular tachycardia postoperatively. Although these figures are not comparable to those that can be attained for supraventricular tachycardia, the data must be weighed against the fact that during the decade that these procedures have been performed, the majority of patients coming to surgery for ventricular tachycardia have failed all forms of medical therapy and most have severely depressed left ventricular function. Despite the re-inducibility of ventricular tachycardia postoperatively in one of four survivors, the long-term follow-up reveals an extremely low incidence of sudden death in these patients. A review of the five series with over 50 patients and greater than a 5-year follow-up reported in the literature revealed that 96 per cent of the survivors were either cured by surgery alone or were able to have their arrhythmia controlled postoperatively by medical therapy,[26] a remarkable success rate in these patients with a life-threatening problem.

THE ROLE OF THE AUTOMATIC INTERNAL CARDIOVERTER-DEFIBRILLATOR (AICD) IN THE TREATMENT OF VENTRICULAR TACHYCARDIA

Because of the excessive operative mortality associated with application of the direct surgical procedures for the treatment of refractory ischemic ventricular tachycardia, some authors have advocated routine implantation of an AICD and performance of coronary artery bypass surgery as the primary therapy for essentially all patients with ventricular tachycardia.[54] Careful scrutiny of the operative and long-term follow-up results, however, argues strongly against this approach. The sudden death rate following AICD implantation is 1.5 to 2.0 per cent per year or 7.5 to 10.0 per cent over a 5-year period.[49,107] The sudden death rate in these survivors of ventricular tachycardia surgery is less than 1 per cent per year and less than 5 per cent for 5 years.[26] Thus, whereas the sudden death rate following AICD implantation is excellent, it remains approximately twice the sudden death rate following successful ventricular tachycardia surgery. Therefore, the argument for implanting the AICD routinely, rather than performing ventricular tachycardia surgery, should not be based on the contention that the AICD is more effective in preventing sudden death, since in fact it is less effective than ventricular tachycardia surgery.

The major reason for recommending routine implantation of the AICD for all patients with ventricular tachyarrhythmias rather than performing ventricular tachycardia surgery is based on the higher operative mortality associated with the ventricular tachycardia surgery. Although the operative mortality for implantation of an AICD is 2 to 3 per cent, as mentioned it is 12.3 per cent for the direct surgical procedures. However, the AICD was not routinely available to most surgeons performing ventricular tachycardia surgery during the first 5 to 8 years following the introduction of the direct surgical procedures. As a result, patients who were medically refractory had to be subjected to ventricular tachycardia surgery regardless of the degree of ventricular dysfunction present. Those essentially inoperable patients who had failed all forms of medical therapy and persisted in having intractable ventricular tachycardia accounted for the vast majority of operative deaths associated with the direct surgical procedures.[26] Paradoxically, the clinical availability of the AICD is perhaps the most important single development during the past decade that should decrease the operative mortality associated with ventricular tachycardia surgery during the next decade. The AICD represents the previously missing therapeutic option that can now be applied to patients with intractable, medically refractory ventricular tachycardia who are inoperable because of severe left ventricular dysfunction. By selecting such patients for AICD implantation, only those patients with acceptable levels of left ventricular dysfunction should now be subjected to the direct surgical procedures for the treatment of refractory ischemic ventricular tachycardia. Such a therapeutic approach should decrease the operative mortality for ventricular tachycardia during the next decade to less than 3 per cent, which is comparable to the operative mortality for AICD implantation. Since the long-term results of ventricular tachycardia surgery are superior to the long-term results of AICD implantation in terms of the prevention of sudden death, ventricular tachycardia surgery should be applied to any patient who is considered to be a candidate for operation. Thus, the two therapeutic modalities, ventricular tachycardia surgery and AICD implantation, should be viewed as complementary procedures for the treatment of medically refractory ischemic ventricular tachycardia.

REFERENCES

1. Akhtar, M.: Atrioventricular nodal reentry. Circulation, 75:26, 1987.
2. Allessie, M. A., Bonke, F. I. M., and Schopman, F. J. G.: Circus movement in rabbit atrial muscle as a mechanism of tachycardia. III. The "leading circle" concept. A new mode of circus movement in cardiac tissue without the involvement of an anatomical obstacle. Circ. Res., 41:9, 1977.
3. Allessie, M. A., Lammers, W. J. E. P., Bonke, F. I. M., et al.: Experimental evaluation of Moe's multiple wavelet hypothesis of atrial fibrillation. In Zipes, D. P., and Jalife, J. (Eds.): Cardiac Electrophysiology and Arrhythmias. Orlando, FL, Grune & Stratton, 1985, pp. 265–275.
4. Benditt, D. G., et al.: Characteristics of atrioventricular conduction and the spectrum of arrhythmias in the Lown-Ganong-Levine syndrome. Circulation, 57:454, 1978.
5. Bigger, J. T., and Goldreyer, B. N.: The mechanism of supraventricular tachycardia. Circulation, 42:673, 1970.
6. Boineau, J. P., and Cox, J. L.: Rationale for a direct surgical approach to control ventricular arrhythmias. Am. J. Cardiol., 49:381, 1982.
7. Boineau, J. P., and Cox, J. L.: Slow ventricular activation in acute myocardial infarction. A source of re-entrant premature ventricular contractions. Circulation, 48:702, 1973.
8. Boineau, J. P., and Cox, J. L.: Slow ventricular activation in acute myocardial infarction—a source of re-entrant premature ventricular contractions. Circulation, 48:702, 1973.
9. Boineau, J. P., and Moore, E. N.: Evidence for propagation of activation across an accessory atrio-ventricular connection in types A and B pre-excitation. Circulation, 41:375, 1970.
10. Boineau, J. P., Schuessler, R. B., Mooney, C. R., et al.: Natural and evoked atrial flutter due to circus movement in dogs: Role of abnormal atrial pathways, slow conduction, nonuniform refractory period distribution and premature beats. Am. J. Cardiol., 45:1167, 1980.
11. Borggrefe, M., and Breithardt, G.: Ectopic atrial tachycardia after transvenous catheter ablation of a posteroseptal accessory pathway. J. Am. Coll. Cardiol., 8:441, 1986.
12. Bryson, A. L., Parisi, A. F., Schechter, E., et al.: Life-threatening ventricular arrhythmias induced by exercise. Am. J. Cardiol., 32:995, 1973.
13. Burchell, H. B., Frye, R. L., Anderson, M. W., et al.: Atrial-ventricular and ventricular-atrial excitation in Wolff-Parkinson-White syndrome (type B): Temporary ablation at surgery. Circulation, 36:663, 1967.
14. Cain, M. E., and Lindsay, B. D.: The preoperative electrophysiologic study. In Cox, J. L. (Ed.): Cardiac Surgery: State of the Art Reviews. Philadelphia, Hanley & Belfus. In press.
15. Cameron, A., Schwartz, M. J., Kronmal, R. A., et al.: Prevalence and significance of atrial fibrillation in coronary artery disease (CASS Registry). Am. J. Cardiol., 61:714, 1988.
16. Canavan, T. E., Schuessler, R. B., Cain, M. E., Lindsay, B. D., Boineau, J. P., Corr, P. B., and Cox, J. L.: Computerized global electrophysiological mapping of the atrium in a patient with multiple supraventricular tachyarrhythmias. Ann. Thorac. Surg., 46:232, 1988.
17. Cobb, F. R., Blumenschein, S. D., Sealy, W. B., et al.: Successful surgical interruption of the bundle of Kent in a patient with Wolff-Parkinson-White syndrome. Circulation, 38:1018, 1968.
18. Couch, O. A., Jr.: Cardiac aneurysm with ventricular tachycardia and subsequent excision of aneurysm. Circulation, 20:251, 1959.
19. Coumel, P., Cabrol, C., Fabiato, A., et al.: Tachycardia permanente par rhythme réciproque. Arch. Mal Coeur, 60:1830, 1967.
20. Cox, J. L.: Anatomic-electrophysiologic basis for the surgical treatment of refractory ischemic ventricular tachycardia. Ann. Surg., 198:119, 1983.
21. Cox, J. L.: Surgery for cardiac arrhythmias. In Harvey, W. P. (Ed.): Current Problems in Cardiology. Chicago, Year Book Medical Publishers, 1983, p. 24.
22. Cox, J. L.: Editorial: Current status of cardiac arrhythmia surgery. Circulation, 71:413, 1985.
23. Cox, J. L.: Surgical treatment of ischemic and non-ischemic ventricular tachyarrhythmias. In Cohn, L. H. (Ed.): Modern Technics in Surgery. Mt. Kisco, NY, Futura, 1985.
24. Cox, J. L.: Manuscript reviewer's comment. J. Thorac. Cardiovasc. Surg., 92:411, 1986.
25. Cox, J. L.: Intraoperative computerized mapping techniques. In Brugada, P., and Wellens, H. J. J. (Eds.): Cardiac Arrhythmias: Where to Go From Here? Mt. Kisco, NY, Futura Publishing Company, 1987.
26. Cox, J. L.: Patient selection criteria and results of surgery for refractory ischemic ventricular tachycardia. Circulation, 79 (Suppl. I):I-163, 1989.
27. Cox, J. L.: The surgical management of cardiac arrhythmias. In Sabiston, D. C., Jr., and Spencer, F. C. (Eds.): Gibbon's Surgery of the Chest, 5th ed. Philadelphia, W. B. Saunders Company, 1989, pp. 1861–1900.
28. Cox, J. L., and Ferguson, T. B., Jr.: Surgery for atrioventricular node reentry tachycardia: The discrete cryosurgical technique. Semin. Thorac. Cardiovasc. Surg., 1:47, 1989.
29. Cox, J. L., and Ferguson, T. B., Jr.: Surgery for the Wolff-Parkinson-White syndrome: The endocardial approach. Semin. Thorac. Cardiovasc. Surg., 1:34, 1989.
30. Cox, J. L., Bardy, G. H., Damiano, R. J., et al.: Right ventricular isolation procedures for nonischemic ventricular tachycardia. J. Thorac. Cardiovasc. Surg., 90:212, 1985.
31. Cox, J. L., Daniel, T. M., Sabiston, D. C., Jr., and Boineau, J. P.: Desynchronized activation in myocardial infarction—a reentry basis for ventricular arrhythmias (Abstract). Circulation, 39 (Suppl. 3):63, 1969.
32. Cox, J. L., and Ferguson, T. B.: Cardiac arrhythmia surgery. Curr. Probl. Surg., 26(4):193, 1989.
33. Cox, J. L., Ferguson, T. B., Jr., Lindsay, B. D., and Cain, M. E.: Peri-nodal cryosurgery for AV node reentry tachycardia in 23 patients. J. Thorac. Cardiovasc. Surg. 99:440, 1990.
34. Cox, J. L., Gallagher, J. J., and Cain, M. E.: Experience with 118 consecutive patients undergoing surgery for the Wolff-Parkinson-White syndrome. J. Thorac. Cardiovasc. Surg., 90:490, 1985.
35. Cox, J. L., Gallagher, J. J., and Ungerleider, R. M.: Encircling endocardial ventriculotomy (EEV) for refractory ischemic ventricular tachycardia. IV. Clinical indications, surgical technique, mechanism of action, and results. J. Thorac. Cardiovasc. Surg., 83:865, 1982.
36. Cox, J. L., Holman, W. L., and Cain, M. E.: Cryosurgical treatment of atrioventricular node reentrant tachycardia. Circulation, 76:1329, 1987.
37. Cox, J. L., McLaughlin, V. W., Flowers, N. C., et al.: The ischemic zone surrounding acute myocardial infarction. Its morphology as detected by dehydrogenase staining. Am. Heart J., 76:650, 1968.
38. Cox, J. L., Schuessler, R. B., Cain, M. E., Corr, P. B., Stone, C. M., D'Agostino, H. J., Jr., Harada, A., Chang, B. C., Smith, P. K., and Boineau, J. P.: Surgery for atrial fibrillation. Semin. Thorac. Cardiovasc. Surg., 1:67, 1989.
39. Cox, J. L., Schuessler, R. B., D'Agostino, H. D., Jr., Harada, A., Eisenberg, S. B., Smith, P. K., and Boineau, J. P.: The surgical treatment of atrial fibrillation: II. Intraoperative electrophysiologic mapping. J. Thorac. Cardiovasc. Surg. (in press).
40. Cox, J. L., Schuessler, R. B., Stone, C. M., et al.: The surgical treatment of atrial fibrillation: III. Development of a surgical cure. J. Thorac. Cardiovasc. Surg. In press.
41. Damiano, R. J., Tripp, H. F., Asano, T., et al.: Left ventricular dysfunction and dilatation resulting from chronic supraventricular tachycardia. J. Thorac. Cardiovasc. Surg., 94:135, 1987.
42. Daniel, T. M., Cox, J. L., Sabiston, D. C., Jr., et al.: Epicardial and intramural mapping activation of the human heart. A technique for localizing infarction and ischemia of the myocardium (Abstract). Circulation, 40(Suppl. 3):III-66, 1969.
43. Denes, P., Delon, W., Dhingra, R. C., Chuquimia, R., and Rosen K. M.: Demonstration of dual AV nodal pathways in patients with paroxysmal supraventricular tachycardia. Circulation, 48:549, 1973.
44. Denes, P., Wu, D., Dhingra, R., Amat-y-Leon, F., and Wyndham, C.: Dual atrioventricular nodal pathways—a common electrophysiological response. Br. Heart J., 37:1069, 1975.
45. Diamantopoulos, E. J., Anthopoulos, L., Nanas, S., et al.: Detection of arrhythmias in a representative sample of the Athens population. Eur. Heart J., 8(Suppl. D):17, 1987.

46. Durrer, D., and Roos, J. P.: Epicardial excitation of the ventricles in a patient with Wolff-Parkinson-White syndrome (type B): Temporary ablation at surgery (Abstract). Circulation, 35:15, 1967.

47. Durrer, D., Schoo, L., Schuilenburg, R. M., et al.: The role of premature beats in the initiation and termination of supraventricular tachycardia in the Wolff-Parkinson-White syndrome. Circulation, 36:644, 1967.

48. Durrer, D., van Dam, R. T., Freud, G. E., et al.: Re-entry and ventricular arrhythmias in local ischemia and infarction of the intact dog heart. Proc. K. Ned. Akad. Wet. (Biol. Med.), 74:321, 1971.

49. Echt, D. S., Armstrong, K., Schmidt, P., Oyer, P. E., Stinson, E. B., and Winkel, R. A.: Clinical experience, complications, and survival in 70 patients with the automatic implantable cardioverter/defibrillator. Circulation, 71:289, 1985.

50. El-Sherif, N., Scherlag, B. J., Lazzara, R., and Hopen, R. R.: Reentrant ventricular arrhythmias in the late myocardial infarction period. I. Conduction characteristics of the infarction zone. Circulation, 55:686, 1977.

51. Engelmann, T. W.: Refractare Phase und compensatousche Ruhe in ihrer Bedeutung für den Herzrhythmus. Pflüger's Arch. Gesamte Physiol., 59:309, 1894–1895.

52. Evans, G. T., Jr., Scheinman, M. M., Scheinman, M. M., Zipes, D. P., Benditt, D., Breithardt, G., Camm, A. J., El-Sherif, N., Fisher, J., Fontaine, G., et al.: The Percutaneous Cardiac Mapping and Ablation Registry: Final summary of results. PACE, 11:1621, 1988.

53. Fisher, C. M.: Embolism in atrial fibrillation. In Kulbertus, H. E., Olsson, S. B., and Schlepper, M. (Eds.): Atrial Fibrillation. Molndal, Sweden, A B Hässle, 1982, pp. 192–210.

54. Fonger, J. D., Guarnieri, T., Griffith, L. S. C., Veltri, E., Levine, J. H., Mower, M., Mirowski, M., and Watkins, L., Jr.: Impending sudden cardiac death: Treatment with myocardial revascularization and automatic implantable cardioverter defibrillator. Ann. Thorac. Surg., 46:13, 1988.

55. Fontaine, G., Frank, R., and Guiraudon, G.: Surgical treatment of resistant re-entrant ventricular tachycardia by ventriculotomy: A new application of epicardial mapping. (Abstract). Circulation, 50(Suppl. 3):III-82, 1974.

56. Fontaine, G., Guiraudon, G., Frank, R., et al.: Epicardial mapping and surgical treatment in six cases of resistant ventricular tachycardia not related to coronary artery disease. In Wellens, H. J. J., Lie, K. I., and Janse, M. J. (Eds.): The Conduction System of the Heart. Philadelphia, Lea & Febiger, 1976, pp. 545–563.

57. Fontaine, G., Guiraudon, G., and Frank, R.: Stimulation studies and epicardial mapping in ventricular tachycardia: Study of mechanisms and selection for surgery. In Kulbertus, H. E. (Ed.): Reentrant Arrhythmias. Baltimore, University Park Press, 1977, pp. 334–350.

58. Frank, G., Baumgart, F., Klein, H., et al.: Successful surgical treatment of focal atrial tachycardia: A case report and review of the literature. Thorac. Cardiovasc. Surg. 34:398, 1986.

59. Fraser, G. R., and Froggatt, P.: Unexpected cot deaths. Lancet, 2:56, 1966.

60. Fujimura, O., Guiraudon, G. M., Yee, R., Sharma, A. D., and Klein, G. J.: Operative therapy of atrioventricular node reentry and results of an anatomically guided procedure. Am. J. Cardiol., 64:1327, 1989.

61. Gallagher, J. J., Cox, J. L., German, L. D., and Kasell, J. H.: Nonpharmacologic treatment of supraventricular tachycardia. In Josephson, M. E., and Wellens, H. J. J. (Eds.): Tachycardias: Mechanisms, Diagnosis, and Treatment. Philadelphia, Lea & Febiger, 1984, pp. 271–285.

62. Gallagher, J. J., Kasell, J. H., Cox, J. L., Smith, W. M., Ideker, R. E., and Smith, W. M.: The techniques of intraoperative electrophysiologic mapping. Am. J. Cardiol., 49:221, 1982.

63. Gallagher, J. J., Oldham, H. N., Jr., Wallace, A. G., et al.: Ventricular aneurysm with ventricular tachycardia. Report of a case with epicardial mapping and successful resection. Am. J. Cardiol., 35:696, 1975.

64. Gallagher, J. J., Sealy, W. C., Cox, J. L.: Results of surgery for pre-excitation caused by accessory atrioventricular pathways in 267 consecutive cases. In Josephson, M. E., and Wellens, H. J. J. (Eds.): Tachycardias: Mechanisms, Diagnosis, and Treatment. Philadelphia, Lea & Febiger, 1984, pp. 259–269.

65. Garson, G., and Gillette, P. C.: Electrophysiologic studies of supraventricular tachycardia in children. I. Clinical-electrophysiologic correlations. Am. Heart J., 102:223, 1981.

66. Gillette, P. C., Garson, A., Hesslein, P. S., et al.: Successful surgical treatment of atrial, junctional, and ventricular tachycardia unassociated with accessory connections in infants and children. Am. Heart J., 102:984, 1984.

67. Giorgi, L. V., Hartzler, G. O., and Hamaker, W. R.: Incessant focal atrial tachycardia: A surgically remediable cause of cardiomyopathy. J. Thorac. Cardiovasc. Surg., 87:466, 1984.

68. Goldreyer, B. N., and Bigger, J. T.: Site of reentry in paroxysmal supraventricular tachycardia in man. Circulation, 43:15, 1971.

69. Goldreyer, B. N., and Damato, A. N.: The essential role of atrioventricular conduction delay in the initiation of paroxysmal supraventricular tachycardia. Circulation, 43:679, 1971.

70. Goldreyer, B. N., Gallagher, J. J., and Damato, A. N.: The electrophysiologic demonstration of atrial ectopic tachycardia in man. Am. Heart J., 85:205, 1973.

71. Guiraudon, G. M., Campbell, C. S., Jones, D. L., et al.: Combined sino-atrial node atrio-ventricular node isolation: A surgical alternative to His bundle ablation in patients with atrial fibrillation. Circulation, 72:III-220, 1985.

72. Guiraudon, G., Fontaine, G., Frank, R., et al.: Encircling endocardial ventriculotomy: A new surgical treatment of life-threatening ventricular tachycar-

dias resistant to medical treatment following myocardial infarction. Ann. Thorac. Surg., 26:438, 1978.

73. Guiraudon, G. M., Klein, G. J., Sharma, A. D., et al.: Closed-heart technique for Wolff-Parkinson-White syndrome. Further experience and potential limitations. Ann. Thorac. Surg., 42:651, 1986.

74. Guiraudon, G. M., Klein, G. J., Sharma, A. D., et al.: Surgical ablation of posterior septal accessory pathways in the Wolff-Parkinson-White syndrome by a closed heart technique. J. Thorac. Cardiovasc. Surg., 92:406, 1986.

75. Guiraudon, G. M., Klein, G. J., Sharma, A. D., Yee, R., and McLellan, D. G.: Surgery for the Wolff-Parkinson-White syndrome: The epicardial approach. Semin. Thorac. Cardiovasc. Surg., 1:21, 1989.

76. Guiraudon, G. M., Klein, G. K., Sharma, A. D., Yee, R., Kaushik, R. R., and Fujimura, O.: Skeletonization of the atrioventricular node for AV node reentrant tachycardia: Experience with 32 patients. Ann. Thorac. Surg. 49:565, 1990.

77. Han, J., Gael, B. G., and Hansen, C. S.: Re-entrant beats induced in the ventricle during coronary occlusion. Am. Heart J., 80:778, 1970.

78. Harada, A., D'Agostino, H. J., Jr., Boineau, J. P., and Cox, J. L.: Right atrial isolation: A new surgical treatment for supraventricular tachycardia. I. Surgical technique and electrophysiologic effects. J. Thorac. Cardiovasc. Surg., 95:643, 1988.

79. Harada, A., D'Agostino, H. J., Jr., Boineau, J. P., and Cox, J. L.: Right atrial isolation: A new surgical treatment for supraventricular tachycardia. II. Hemodynamic effects. J. Thorac. Cardiovasc. Surg., 95:651, 1988.

80. Hirosawa, K., Sekiguchi, M., Kasanuki, H., et al.: Natural history of atrial fibrillation. Heart Vessels (Suppl.), 2:14, 1987.

81. Hockings, B. E., George, T., Mahrous, F., et al.: Effectiveness of amiodarone on ventricular arrhythmias during and after acute myocardial infarction. Am. J. Cardiol., 60:967, 1987.

82. Holman, W. L., Hackel, D. B., Lease, J. G., Ikeshita, M., and Cox, J. L.: Cryosurgical ablation of atrioventricular nodal reentry: Histologic localization of the proximal common pathway. Circulation, 77:1356, 1988.

83. Holman, W., Ikeshita, M., Lease, J., et al.: Elective prolongation of atrioventricular conduction by multiple discrete cryolesions: A new technique for the treatment of paroxysmal supraventricular tachycardia. J. Thorac. Cardiovasc. Surg., 84:554, 1982.

84. Holman, W. L., Ikeshita, M., Lease, J. G., et al.: Alteration of antegrade atrioventricular conduction by cryoablation of periatrioventricular nodal tissue. J. Thorac. Cardiovasc. Surg., 88:67, 1984.

85. Holman, W. L., Ikeshita, M., Lease, J. G., et al.: Cryosurgical modification of retrograde atrioventricular conduction: Implications for the surgical treatment of atrioventricular node reentry tachycardia. J. Thorac. Cardiovasc. Surg., 91:826, 1986.

86. Horowitz, L. N., Josephson, M. E., and Harken, A. H.: Epicardial and endocardial activation during sustained ventricular tachycardia in man. Circulation, 61:1227, 1980.

87. Jervell, A., and Lange-Nielsen, F.: Congenital deaf-mutism, functional heart disease with prolongation of the Q-T interval, and sudden death. Am. Heart J., 54:59, 1957.

88. Johnson, D. C., Nunn, G. R., and Meldrum-Hanna, W.: Surgery for atrioventricular node reentry tachycardia: The surgical dissection technique. Semin. Thorac. Cardiovasc. Surg., 1:53, 1989.

89. Josephson, M. E., and Kastor, J. A.: Paroxysmal supraventricular tachycardia — is the atrium a necessary link? Circulation, 54:430, 1976.

90. Josephson, M. E., and Seides, S. F.: Clinical cardiac electrophysiology: Techniques and interpretations. Philadelphia, Lea & Febiger, 1979, p. 163.

91. Josephson, M. E., Harken, A. H., and Horowitz, L. N.: Endocardial excision — a new surgical technique for the treatment of recurrent ventricular tachycardia. Circulation, 60:1430, 1979.

92. Josephson, M. E., Spear, J. F., Harken, A. H., et al.: Surgical excision of automatic atrial tachycardia: Anatomic and electrophysiologic correlates. Am. Heart J. 104:1076, 1982.

93. Kaiser, G. A., Waldo, A. L., Harris, P. D., et al.: New method to delineate myocardial damage at surgery. Circulation, 39(Suppl. 1):83, 1969.

94. Keith, A., and Flack, M.: The form and nature of the muscular connections between the primary divisions of the vertebrate heart. J. Anat. Physiol., 41:172, 1906–1907.

95. Kent, A. F. S.: Researches on structure and function of mammalian heart. J. Physiol., 14:233, 1893.

96. Klein, R. C., Machell, C., Rushforth, N., et al.: Efficacy of intravenous amiodarone as short-term treatment for refractory ventricular tachycardia. Am. Heart J., 115:96, 1988.

97. Kramer, J. B., Corr, P. B., Cox, J. L., et al.: Simultaneous computer mapping to facilitate intraoperative localization of accessory pathways in patients with Wolff-Parkinson-White syndrome. Am. J. Cardiol., 56:571, 1985.

98. Kuehl, K. S., Kapur, S., Toomey, K., et al.: Focal cardiomyopathy and ectopic atrial tachycardia in Beckwith syndrome. Am. J. Cardiol., 55:1234, 1985.

99. Kulbertus, H. E.: La torsades de pointes. Rev. Med. Liege, 33:63, 1978.

100. Landymore, R., Marble, A., MacKinnon, G., et al.: Effects of oral amiodarone on left ventricular function in dogs: Clinical implications for patients with life-threatening ventricular tachycardia. Ann. Thorac. Surg., 37:141, 1984.

101. Lewis, T.: Paroxysmal tachycardia, the result of ectopic impulse formation. Heart, 1:262, 1909–1910.

102. Lewis, T.: The experimental production of paroxysmal tachycardia and the effects of ligation of the coronary arteries. Heart, 1:98, 1909.

103. Lowe, J. E.: Surgical treatment of the Wolff-Parkinson-White syndrome and other supraventricular tachyarrhythmias. J. Cardiac Surg. 1:117, 1986.

104. Lowe, J. E., Hendry, P. J., Packer, D. L., and Tang, A. S.: Surgical management of chronic ectopic atrial tachycardia. Semin. Thorac. Cardiovasc. Surg., 1:58, 1989.

105. Mahomed, Y., King, R. D., Zipes, D. P., et al.: Surgical division of Wolff-Parkinson-White pathways utilizing the closed-heart technique: A 2-year experience in 47 patients. Ann. Thorac. Surg., 45:495, 1988.

106. Miller, J. E., and Josephson, M. E.: Intracardiac electrophysiologic studies in sustained ventricular tachycardia. In Iwa, T., and Fontaine, G. (Eds.): Cardiac Arrhythmias: Recent Progress in Investigation and Management. Amsterdam, Elsevier, 1988.

107. Mirowski, M.: The automatic implantable cardioverter-defibrillator: An overview. J. Am. Coll. Cardiol., 6:461, 1985.

108. Moe, G. K.: On the multiple wavelet hypothesis of atrial fibrillation. Arch. Int. Pharmacodyn., 140:183, 1962.

109. Moe, G. K., Preston, J. B., and Burlington, H.: Physiologic evidence for a dual A-V transmission system. Circ. Res., 4:357, 1956.

110. Moran, J. M., Kehoe, R. F., Loeb, J. M., et al.: Extended endocardial resection for the treatment of ventricular tachycardia and ventricular fibrillation. Ann. Thorac. Surg., 34:538, 1982.

111. Moran, J. M., Kehoe, R. F., Loeb, J. M., et al.: The role of papillary muscle resection and mitral valve replacement in the control of refractory ventricular arrhythmias. Circulation, 68(Suppl. II):154, 1983.

112. Moss, A. J., Schwartz, P. J., Crampton, R. S., et al.: The long QT syndrome: A prospective international study. Circulation, 71:17, 1985.

113. Myerburg, R. J., Sung, R. J., and Castellanos, A.: Ventricular tachycardia and ventricular fibrillation in patients with short PR intervals and narrow QRS complexes. PACE, 2:568, 1979.

114. Olsson, S. B., Blomstrom, P., Sabel, K., et al.: Incessant ectopic atrial tachycardia: Successful surgical treatment with regression of dilated cardiomyopathy picture. Am. J. Cardiol., 53:1465, 1984.

115. Onundarson, P. T., Thorgeirsson, G., Jonmundsson, E., et al.: Chronic atrial fibrillation—epidemiologic features and 14 year follow-up: A case control study. Eur. Heart J., 8:521, 1987.

116. Ostermeyer, J., Borggrefe, M., Breithardt, G., et al.: Direct operations for the management of life-threatening ischemic ventricular tachycardia. J. Thorac. Cardiovasc. Surg., 94:848, 1987.

117. Ostermeyer, J., Breithardt, G., Borggrefe, M., et al.: Surgical treatment of ventricular tachycardias. Complete versus partial encircling endocardial ventriculotomy. J. Thorac. Cardiovasc. Surg., 87:517, 1984.

118. Ostermeyer, J., Kirklin, J. K., Borggrefe, M., Cox, J. L., Breithardt, G., and Bircks, W.: Ten years electrophysiologically guided direct operations for malignant ischemic ventricular tachycardia—results. Thorac. Cardiovasc. Surg., 37:20, 1989.

119. Ott, D. A., Garson, A., Cooley, D. A., et al.: Definitive operation for refractory cardiac tachyarrhythmias in children. J. Thorac. Cardiovasc. Surg., 90:681, 1985.

120. Packer, D. L., Bardy, G. H., Worley, S. J., et al.: Tachycardia-induced cardiomyopathy: A reversible form of left ventricular dysfunction. Am. J. Cardiol., 57:563, 1986.

121. Perelman, M. S., and Krikler, D. M.: Termination of focal atrial tachycardia by adenosine triphosphate. Br. Heart J., 58:528, 1987.

122. Pritchett, E. L. C., Anderson, R. W., Benditt, D. G., Kasell, J., Harrison, L., Wallace, A. G., Sealy, W. C., and Gallagher, J. J.: Reentry within the atrioventricular node: Surgical cure with preservation of atrioventricular conduction. Circulation, 60:440, 1979.

123. Romano, C., Gemme, G., and Pongiglione, R.: Aritmie cardiache rare dell'eta pediatrica. Clin. Pediatr., 45:656, 1963.

124. Ross, D. L., Johnson, D. C., Denniss, A. R., et al.: Curative surgery for atrioventricular junctional ("A-V nodal") reentrant tachycardia. J. Am. Coll. Cardiol., 6:1383, 1985.

125. Rothberger, C. J., and Winterberg, H.: Über Vorhofflimmern und Vorhofflattern. Pflüger's Arch., 160:42, 1914.

126. Savage, D. D., Garrison, R. J., Castelli, W. P., et al.: Prevalence of submitral (anular) calcium and its correlates in a general population-based sample (the Framingham Study). Am. J. Cardiol., 51:1375, 1983.

127. Scheinman, M. M., Morady, F., Hess, D. S., and Gonzalez, R.: Catheter-induced ablation of the atrioventricular junction to control refractory supraventricular arrhythmias. J.A.M.A., 248:851, 1982.

128. Scherf, D., and Shookhoff, C.: Experimentelle Unterschungen über die Umkehrextrasystole. Wien. Arch. Inn. Med., 12:501, 1926.

129. Scherlag, B. J., El-Sherif, N., Hopen, R. R., et al.: Characterization and localization of ventricular arrhythmias resulting from myocardial ischemia and infarction. Circ. Res., 35:372, 1974.

130. Schwartz, P. J.: The idiopathic long QT syndrome. Ann. Intern. Med., 99:561, 1983.

131. Sealy, W. C., Gallagher, J. J., and Kasell, J. H.: His bundle interruption for control of inappropriate ventricular responses to atrial arrhythmias. Ann. Thorac. Surg., 32:429, 1981.

132. Selle, J. G., Svenson, R. H., Sealy, W. C., et al.: Successful clinical laser ablation of ventricular tachycardia: A promising new therapeutic method. Ann. Thorac. Surg., 42:380, 1986.

133. Svenson, R. H., Gallagher, J. J., Selle, J. G., et al.: Neodymium:YAG laser photocoagulation: A successful new map-guided technique for the intraoperative ablation of ventricular tachycardia. Circulation, 76:1319, 1987.

134. Tawara, S.: Das Reizleitungssystem des Säugetierherzens. Eine anatomisch-histologische Studie über das atrioventrikular-Bündel und die Purkinjeschen Fäden. Jena, Poland, Gustav Fisher, 1906.

135. Uhl, H. S.: A previously undescribed malformation of the heart: Almost total absence of the myocardium of the right ventricle. Bull. Johns Hopkins Hosp., 91:197, 1952.

136. Ungerleider, R. M., Holman, W. L., Calcagno, D., et al.: Encircling endocardial ventriculotomy (EEV) for refractory ischemic ventricular tachycardia. III. Effects on regional left ventricular function. J. Thorac. Cardiovasc. Surg., 83:857, 1982.

137. Ungerleider, R. M., Holman, W. L., Stanley, T. E., III, et al.: Encircling endocardial ventriculotomy (EEV) for refractory ischemic ventricular tachycardia. I. Electrophysiologic effects. J. Thorac. Cardiovasc. Surg., 83:840, 1982.

138. Ungerleider, R. M., Holman, W. L., Stanley, T. E., III, et al.: Encircling endocardial ventriculotomy (EEV) for refractory ischemic ventricular tachycardia. II. Effects on regional myocardial blood flow. J. Thorac. Cardiovasc. Surg., 83:850, 1982.

139. Waldo, A. L., and Kaiser, G. A.: A study of ventricular arrhythmias associated with acute myocardial infarction in the canine heart. Circulation, 47:1222, 1973.

140. Ward, O. C.: New familial cardiac syndrome in children. J. Ir. Med. Assoc., 54:103, 1964.

141. Williams, J. M., Ungerleider, R. M., Lofland, G. K., and Cox, J. L.: Left atrial isolation: New technique for the treatment of supraventricular arrhythmias. J. Thorac. Cardiovasc. Surg., 80:373, 1980.

142. Wittig, J. H., and Boineau, J. P.: Surgical treatment of ventricular arrhythmias using epicardial transmural and endocardial mapping. Ann. Thorac. Surg., 20:117, 1975.

143. Wolferth, C. C., and Wood, F. C.: The mechanism of production of short P-R intervals and prolonged QRS complexes in patients with presumably undamaged hearts: Hypothesis of an accessory pathway of auriculo-ventricular conduction (bundle of Kent). Am. Heart J., 8:297, 1933.

144. Wolff, L., Parkinson, J., and White, P. D.: Bundle branch block with short PR interval in healthy young people prone to paroxysmal tachycardia. Am. Heart J., 5:685, 1930.

145. Wood, F. C., Wolferth, C. C., and Geckler, G. D.: Histologic demonstration of accessory muscular connections between auricle and ventricle in a case of short P-R interval and prolonged QRS complex. Am. Heart J., 25:454, 1943.

146. Wu, D., Denes, P., Amat-y-Leon, F., Dhingra, R., Wyndham, C. R. C., Baurnfeind, R., Latif, P., and Rosen, K. M.: Clinical electrocardiographic and electrophysiologic observations in patients with paroxysmal supraventricular tachycardia. Am. J. Cardiol., 41:1045, 1978.

147. Wyndham, C. R. C., Arnsdorf, M. F., Levitsky, S., et al.: Successful surgical excision of focal paroxysmal atrial tachycardia. Circulation, 62:1365, 1980.

148. Zheutlin, T., Steinman, R., Summers, C., et al.: Long-term outcome in survivors of cardiac arrest with non-inducible ventricular tachycardia during programmed stimulation. Circulation, 70:1399, 1984.

XXI

CARDIAC NEOPLASMS

Norman A. Silverman, M.D., and David C. Sabiston, Jr., M.D.

Since Columbo's initial description in 1559, cardiac tumors have evolved from pathologic curiosities to, at present, a surgically curable form of heart disease. Significant early milestones in diagnosis and treatment include the first antemortem clinical recognition of a primary sarcoma of the heart by Barnes in 1934, successful surgical resection of a mural tumor by Maurer in 1951, and the first operative removal of an intracavitary tumor by Crafoord in 1954.[4] Although a left atrial myxoma was first demonstrated by angiography in 1951, the introduction of ultrasonic imaging modalities in 1968 has provided excellent detail of the origin and extent of intracavitary tumors.[2] Most recently, computed axial tomography, magnetic resonance imaging, and transesophageal echocardiography with color flow Doppler techniques have provided reliable and minimally invasive methods for diagnosing all primary and metastatic cardiac neoplasms. Whereas prior to 1960 over 60 per cent of these lesions were found at postmortem examinations, cardiac tumors are now recognized during life.[25]

INCIDENCE AND CLINICAL PRESENTATION

The rarity of primary cardiac tumors is evidenced by an autopsy incidence ranging between 0.002 and 0.33 per cent. With over 500 tumors, the Armed Forces Institute of Pathology has the largest series and reports approximately 80 per cent are benign, with myxoma being by far the most common.[17] Malignant tumors represent approximately 20 per cent of primary cardiac neoplasms and are predominantly various forms of sarcoma.[24] This incidence of malignancy varies with age, as malignant neoplasms are relatively more common in adults while comprising less than 10 per cent of primary cardiac tumors in children.[12,17] Metastatic neoplastic disease to the heart is 20 to 30 times more common than primary lesions, and when selecting patients having known cancers, nearly 10 per cent have secondary cardiac involvement at necropsy.[9,10]

The clinical manifestations of cardiac tumors are protean, producing symptoms by their mass effect, local invasion, embolization, or systemic constitutional signs.[12,23] Neoplastic pericarditis can cause effusion with tamponade or cardiac constriction. Cardiac performance is compromised when an intracavitary tumor obstructs blood flow through the cardiac chambers and prevents the normal function of the cardiac valves, or when an intramural tumor infiltrates and destroys ventricular myocardium. Systemic emboli from left heart lesions, especially left atrial myxoma, are common, but right heart tumors may embolize the pulmonary arteries. Certain patients with cardiac tumors, particularly in the pediatric age group, manifest only recurrent supraventricular or ventricular arrhythmias.[14] Less often, the conduction system is injured, resulting in heart block and Stokes-Adams attacks. Neural invasion by malignant tumors can cause pain, but rare instances of ischemic cardiac pain have been reported when the coronary circulation is compromised by tumor emboli or extrinsic compression.[4] Most intriguing are the systemic constitutional symptoms of fever, malaise, weight loss, polymyositis, hepatic dysfunction, Raynaud's phenomenon, hyperglobulinemia, and elevated erythrocyte sedimentation rate that have been noted in both benign and malignant lesions but in particular are associated with left atrial myxomas.[25] Such manifestations may reflect an autoimmune phenomenon or a systemic reaction to altered serum proteins and tumor breakdown products released into the circulation, since the symptoms and polyclonal hyperglobulinemia promptly abate with tumor extirpation. Finally, hemolytic anemia, polycythemia, and thrombocytopenia are recognized hematologic abnormalities associated with cardiac tumors.

DIAGNOSTIC MODALITIES

Echocardiography is the technique of choice in the initial evaluation of intracardiac tumors.[2,22] It is widely available at the bedside as well as in the laboratory, rapidly performed, noninvasive, and relatively inexpensive. The M-mode technique was introduced first and was most helpful for diagnosing mobile left atrial myxoma as a dense mass of reflected echoes moving during the cardiac cycle, behind but separate from the anterior mitral leaflet (Fig. 1). Additional findings are a decrease of the mitral E-F slope and delay between mitral valve opening and the appearance of the myxoma within the mitral orifice. Im-

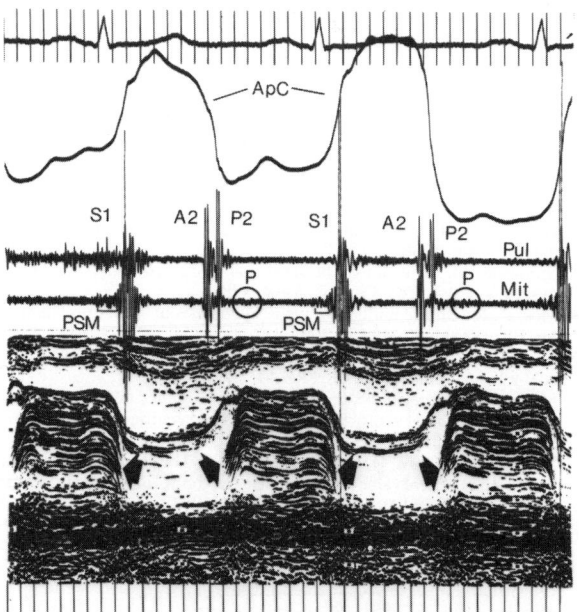

Figure 1. M-mode echocardiogram with simultaneous phonocardiogram demonstrating a mobile left atrial myxoma as dense echoes obstructing mitral valve orifice during ventricular diastole (large arrows). A delay between mitral valve leaflet opening and the appearance of the myxoma is seen during diastole. A classic "tumor plop" (P) follows an accentuated second heart sound (A2P2). A presystolic murmur (PSM) is noted. S1, first heart sound; Pul, pulmonary valve area; Mit, mitral valve area; ApC, apex cardiogram. (Courtesy of Ms. Carla Wolfe, Cardiac Graphics Laboratory, University of North Carolina Medical School. From Chitwood, W. R.: Cardiac neoplasms: Current diagnosis, pathology, and therapy. J. Cardiac Surg. 3:119, 1988.)

proved accuracy for real-time imaging of all cardiac chambers and more precise quantitation of tumor size, shape, location, consistency, and mobility are afforded by two-dimensional echocardiography (Fig. 2). A close correlation has been found between echo diameter and tumor specimens measured following surgical resection.[4] Moreover, concomitant Doppler color flow techniques can assess valvular dysfunction caused by tumor encroachment. Findings suggestive of myxoma occur in 95 per cent of patients examined by echocardiography and provide sufficient information to preempt the need, risk, and expense of further diagnostic studies prior to surgical intervention.

In selected patients, additional diagnostic studies are warranted. Bone and lung interference may limit ultrasonic imaging. Intramural tumors are nonechogenic, and extracavitary origin or extension may not be seen in its entirety by standard echocardiography. With the introduction of electrocardiographic gating and ultrafast scanners, computed tomography (CT) is a valuable alternative for imaging primary and metastatic cardiac tumors[8] (Figs. 3 and 4). Contrast enhancement allows cardiac and intracardiac structures to be differentiated from blood, and image reconstruction reveals cardiac anatomy in three dimensions. CT scanning is best utilized for showing the myocardial and intrapericardial extension of tumor. Magnetic resonance (MR) imaging is a newer technique that also enables high resolution tomography in three dimensions[7] (Fig. 5). Unlike CT scanning, MR is nonionizing and generates tissue contrast without the need for injecting contrast medium. Although an expensive and less widely available technology, histologic diagnosis by noninvasive tissue characterization is a potential future contribution of MR imaging.

Although obtained in all patients, the plain chest film and electrocardiogram show only indirect evidence of cardiac neoplasm by demonstrating chamber enlargement or rhythm disturbances.[3] On occasion, calcification will be noted by fluoroscopy in a right atrial myxoma. Historically, phonocardiography detected characteristic audible features of mobile left atrial myxomas but is seldom used today. Finally, cardiac cathe-

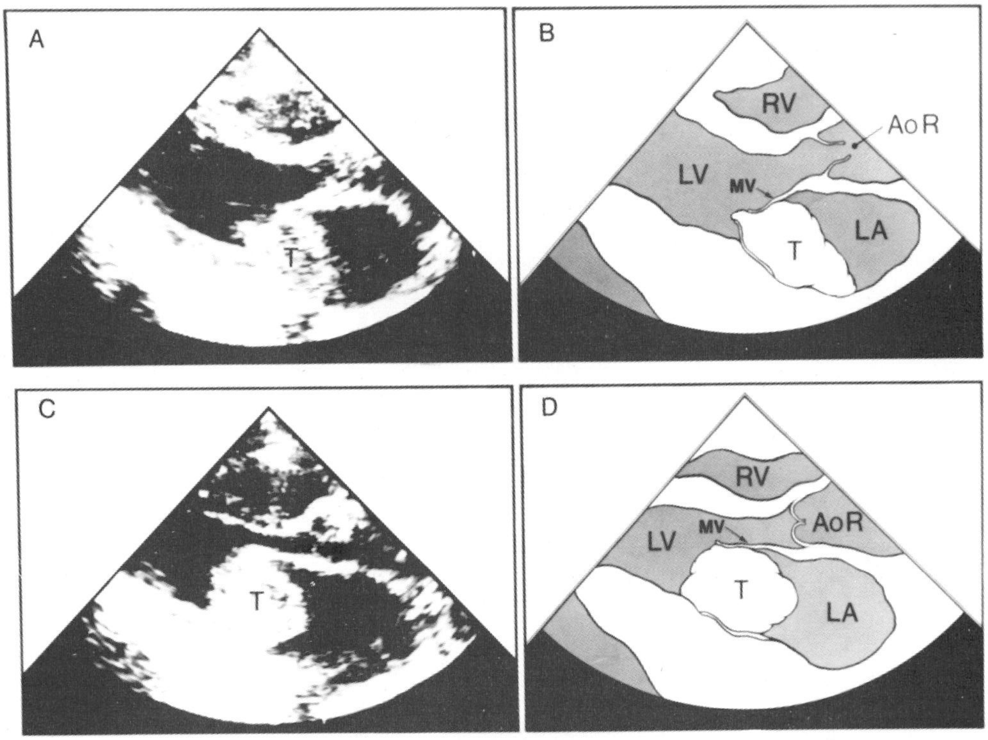

Figure 2. *A* and *B*, Parasternal two-dimensional echocardiogram of a large left atrial myxoma during ventricular systole. The left ventricle (LV), right ventricle (RV), aortic root (AoR), left atrium (LA), mitral valve (MV), and tumor (T) with attached stalk are shown. *C* and *D*, The same tumor is shown during ventricular diastole when the tumor (T) is prolapsing through the mitral valve (MV) orifice. (Courtesy of Dr. Wm. C. Reeves. From Chitwood, W. R.: Cardiac neoplasms: Current diagnosis, pathology, and therapy. J. Cardiac Surg., *3:*119, 1988.)

terization and angiography can provide helpful information by visualizing intracavitary defects and documenting the hemodynamic sequelae of valve dysfunction. However, echocardiography has supplanted this invasive procedure as the diagnostic modality of choice, and thus patients are no longer subjected to the inherent risk of tumor embolization associated with intracardiac manipulation.

BENIGN TUMORS

Myxomas constitute 50 per cent of benign primary cardiac tumors. Although reported to occur in neonates, they are most frequently found in adult females (70 per cent). Seventy-five per cent originate in the left atrium and 20 per cent occur in the right atrium. The majority of these lesions arise from the atrial septum in the region of the fossa ovalis. Ventricular myxomas are rare.[17] In the majority of patients, myxomas are solitary lesions recognized after 50 years of age. In a younger, predominantly male cohort of patients, associated skin myxomas, pigmented nevi, myxoid mammary fibroadenomas, Cushing's syndrome, pituitary adenoma, and/or Sertoli testicular tumors are found. Synchronous intracardiac myxomas are found in one half of these cases, and one third of these patients have a primary relative with an element of this complex. Familial and complex myxomas are more prone to recurrence (10 to 21 per cent).[15,18]

Grossly, most myxomas are friable, multilobulated, 5- to 8-cm. polypoid masses. Smaller tumors may have a smooth surface. Of surgical significance is the fact that myxomas rarely extend deeper than the endocardium, but grow as polypoid

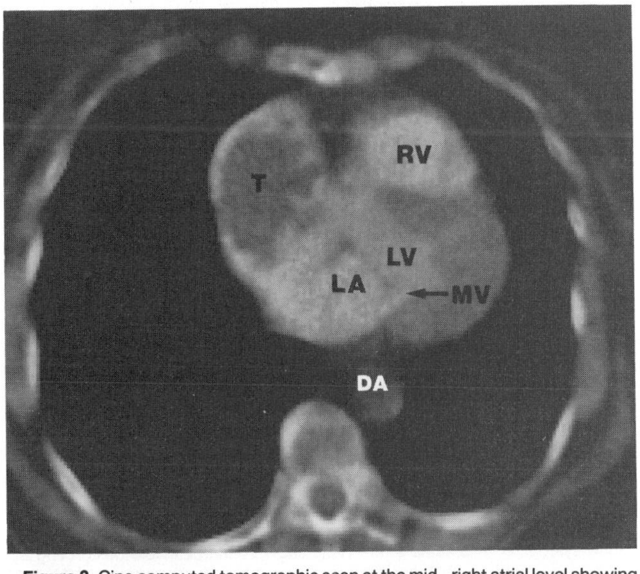

Figure 3. Cine computed tomographic scan at the mid–right atrial level showing a large tumor mass (T). This proved to be a myxoma. (LA, left atrium; RV, right ventricle; LV, left ventricle; MV, mitral valve; DA, descending aorta.) (From Seifert, P. S., et al.: Application of the cine computed tomographic scan for precise localization of the origin of an atrial myxoma. Ann. Thorac. Surg., *42:*469, 1986.)

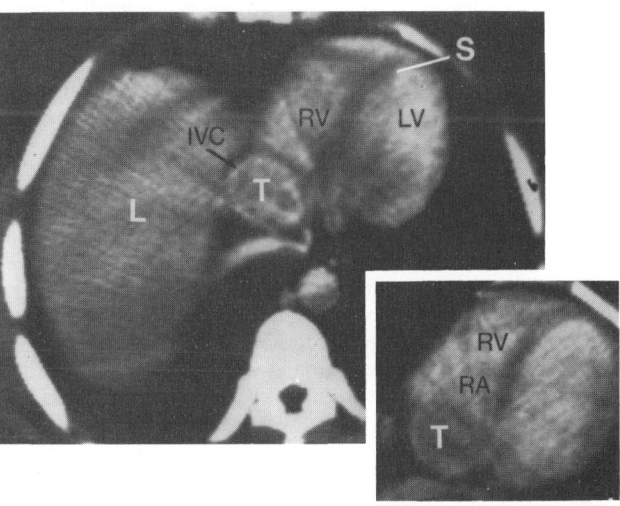

Figure 4. A computed tomographic scan shows extension of a renal cell tumor (T) into the inferior vena cava (IVC). The inset shows a more cephalad tomographic section with tumor obstruction of the right atrium (RA). RV, right ventricle; LV, left ventricle; S, septum; L, liver. (Courtesy of Dr. J. David Godwin. From Chitwood, W. R.: Cardiac neoplasms: Current diagnosis, pathology, and therapy. J. Cardiac Surg., *3:*119, 1988.)

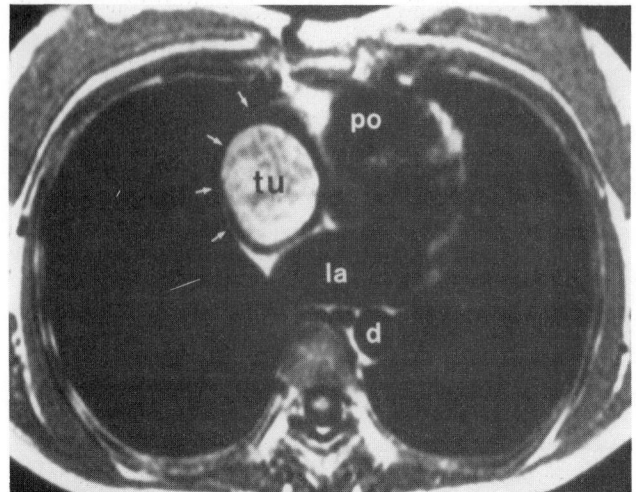

A

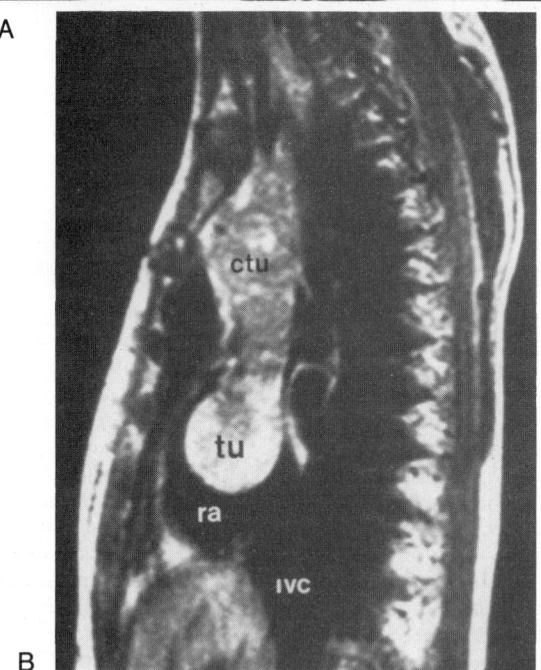

B

Figure 5. Magnetic resonance tomograms demonstrating extension of tumor (tu). *A*, Axial image through the atria showing a heterogeneous high signal tumor mass within the right atrium (arrows); d, descending aorta; la, left atrium; po, pulmonary outflow tract. *B*, Sagittal image showing the tumor mass within the right atrium (ra), with contiguous tumor (ctu) filling the superior vena cava. IVC, inferior vena cava. (From Freedberg, R. S., et al.: The contribution of magnetic resonance imaging to the evaluation of intracardiac tumors. Circulation, 77:96, 1988. Copyright 1988 by the American Heart Association.)

tumors to fill the cardiac chamber. All have a gelatinous consistency with frequent areas of hemorrhage and necrosis seen on cut section. Myxomas are usually pedunculated with attachment to the endocardial surface by a fibrovascular stalk that permits tumor mobility during the cardiac cycle. Microscopically, polyhedral cells with small, round nuclei are separated by an afibrillar, eosinophilic myxomatous stroma, which is predominantly an acid mucopolysaccharide. Although a "benign" tumor, myxomas can undergo malignant degeneration, and disseminated, systemic metastases have been documented, although this is an exceedingly rare occurrence.[4,17,25] Malignant change must be differentiated from local recurrence due to incomplete resection or multichamber involvement that is prevalent in the familial myxoma syndromes.

Because they often obstruct the mitral orifice and produce systemic emboli, left atrial myxomas frequently masquerade as rheumatic mitral stenosis. Although the physical findings of a "tumor plop" and positional alterations of the murmur are con-

sidered diagnostic, they are infrequently noted.[12,23] Up to one half of patients have some form of systemic emboli, most often to the brain. However, embolization to the kidneys, aortic bifurcation, lower extremities, and coronary arteries also occurs. Therefore, any specimen surgically removed from the arterial system should undergo pathologic examination, since this is often the presenting manifestation of a cardiac myxoma. In addition, any patient less than 40 years old who has evidence of arterial embolism and is in sinus rhythm should be screened for myxoma by echocardiography regardless of the presence or absence of precordial murmurs. When constitutional symptoms predominate, infective endocarditis, collagen vascular disease, and occult malignancy or infection enter the differential diagnosis.

Right atrial myxomas produce signs and symptoms of right heart failure by obstructing vena caval return or the tricuspid valve orifice (Fig. 6). Less often, tumor embolization to the pulmonary vasculature causes chest pain, cough, and dyspnea. Infrequently, systemic symptoms, as well as polycythemia and digital clubbing, predominate clinically. The differential diagnosis includes rheumatic tricuspid valve disease, constrictive pericarditis, myocardiopathy, Ebstein's anomaly, and carcinoid heart disease.

The rare ventricular myxomas arise from the outflow tract or interventricular septum and may induce syncope due to transient obstruction of ventricular ejection. Right ventricular lesions have a predilection for younger patients, whereas left ventricular myxomas have a high incidence of systemic emboli. Unlike atrial tumors, systemic constitutional symptoms rarely occur with ventricular lesions, which primarily must be differentiated from other causes of valvular or subvalvular stenosis.

Rhabdomyoma is a congenital, glycogen-rich hamartoma that

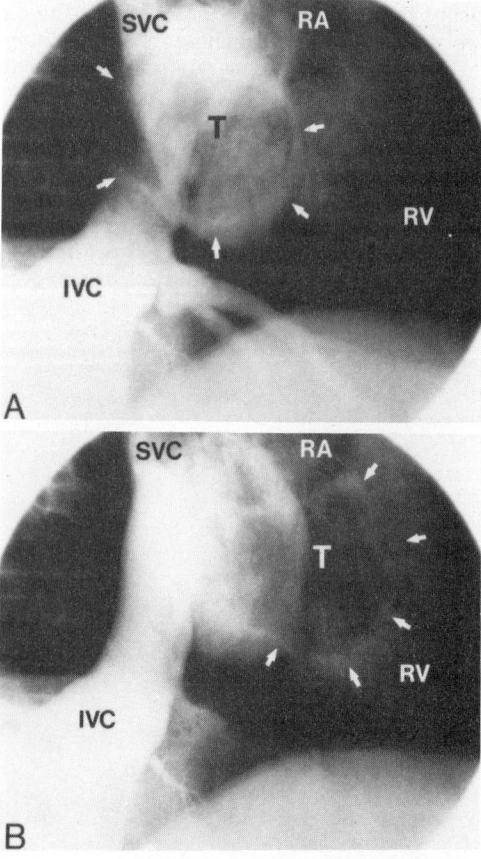

Figure 6. *A*, The large right atrial myxoma (arrows) is seen on cineangiography during systole. *B*, The same tumor (T) is shown during diastole obstructing the tricuspid valve orifice. SVC, superior vena cava; IVC, inferior vena cava; RA, right atrium; RV, right ventricle. (Courtesy of Dr. Tirone David, Toronto Western Infirmary. From Chitwood, W. R.: Cardiac neoplasms: Current diagnosis, pathological therapy. J Cardiac Surg., 3:119, 1988.)

is the most common cardiac tumor in children and represents 20 per cent of all benign primary cardiac tumors. Two thirds are diagnosed before 3 years of age, and one half of the patients have tuberous sclerosis. These tumors have a poor prognosis, with a majority of patients not surviving infancy. The lesions are most often multicentric, ventricular masses that cause recurrent tachyarrhythmias. On occasion, the tumor encroaches on the ventricular cavity to produce symptoms of outflow tract obstruction. These large, solitary lesions have been successfully removed.[6] Because of their usual multiplicity, poor encapsulation, and deep myocardial location, rhabdomyomas are most often unresectable by standard surgical techniques. However, electrophysiologic mapping has allowed local excision or cryoablation of arrhythmogenic foci in a small series of infants.[14] In contrast, the rare cardiac *fibromas* are well-circumscribed, solitary ventricular tumors in childhood that are more amenable to surgical cure.[20] *Mesothelioma* is a lethal congenital tumor that often is manifested in adult females and selectively destroys the atrioventricular node, producing sudden and complete heart block.[13] Lipoma, hemangioma, lymphangioma, teratoma, chemodectoma, neurilemoma, ganglioneuroma, and granular cell myoblastoma have also been reported to arise from the heart. Lambl's excrescences and simple cysts can arise from the cardiac valves but rarely are of physiologic consequence.[17]

MANAGEMENT

The diagnosis of primary cardiac tumor mandates prompt operative intervention. Minimal tumor manipulation during cannulation and prior to aortic cross-clamping and chemical cardioplegic arrest is mandatory to prevent perioperative tumor dislodgement and embolization. Right-sided myxomas are approached through the appropriate atriotomy or ventriculotomy. Left atrial myxoma can be approached through a left atriotomy posterior to the interatrial groove. However, small left atrial size and anterior positioning of the atrial septum may make operative exposure and/or closure of a septal defect difficult. Guided by intraoperative transesophageal echocardiography to determine the site of septal attachment, many surgeons prefer a right atriotomy with a transseptal approach.[4] Biatrial incisions have been utilized with the rationale of examining all cardiac chambers.[11] However, this exposure is also obtained by the transseptal technique. Adequate excision includes a margin of normal atrial septum around the tumor stalk. If a septal defect is created, it can be repaired primarily or with a patch. This margin of normal tissue is important to prevent local recurrence. An aortotomy with retraction of the aortic valve is the preferable access for removal of left ventricular lesions. However, an apical ventriculotomy may be needed for removing bulky or anteriorly situated tumors. All resections should be complete, but zealous removal of normal myocardium or trauma to intrinsically normal valvular apparatus should be avoided. On occasion, extensive reconstruction of the right atrial wall and prosthetic valve replacement are necessary for curative excision of large tumors. In addition, cardiac transplantation is a currently feasible alternative for otherwise unresectable tumors of the left ventricle.[5]

In recent studies comprising 226 patients, operative mortality was 2.2 per cent for excision of benign tumors.[5,11,15,18] The most common postoperative complication is supraventricular tachyarrhythmia; however, permanent rhythm disturbances are rare. After complete tumor resection, the prognosis is excellent with complete symptomatic relief and less than 1 per cent recurrence, except in patients with complex or familial myxoma.

MALIGNANT TUMORS

Malignant tumors are almost always some variant of a sarcoma.[1,21,24] Most often they originate from the right atrium, less frequently from the right ventricle, and rapidly grow to infiltrate all layers of the heart, invade adjacent mediastinal structures, and metastasize widely. Systemic metastases are present in 80 per cent of patients at the time of diagnosis. The characteristic clinical presentation is progressive, unrelenting congestive heart failure, cardiomegaly, chest pain, fever, hemopericardium, and arrhythmia. Sudden death or rapid vena caval obstruction is not uncommon. Angiosarcoma and rhabdomyosarcoma are the usual histologic types. Fibrosarcoma, liposarcoma, neurosarcoma, leiomyosarcoma, osteosarcoma, and chondrosarcoma have also been reported.[4,17] A precise histologic classification is not only difficult but also of little practical significance, because the clinical presentation and prognosis are comparable. The rare cases of lymphoma arising as a primary cardiac tumor, plasmacytoma, and malignant mesenchymoma have a similar clinical presentation.

Primary malignant cardiac tumors are less frequently diagnosed during life than are benign lesions. When the diagnosis is made at exploratory operation, the growth pattern of these lesions most often makes them unresectable. Two recent reviews comprising 39 patients treated by surgical resection yielded a median survival of approximately 9 months and no long-term survivors.[1,21] In general, mediastinal irradiation and systemic chemotherapy have been ineffective in controlling primary malignant tumors.

METASTATIC TUMORS

The heart and pericardium have been found to be involved by metastatic tumor in 0.1 to 6 per cent of consecutive unselected autopsies and in 2 to 21 per cent of patients dying of malignant disease.[26] Lately, an increase in cardiac metastases has occurred and probably relates to prolonged survival from prior surgical intervention and combined-modality therapy. Tumors that most frequently metastasize to the heart include lung and breast carcinoma as well as leukemia, lymphoma, and melanoma. Twenty-five to 50 per cent of these patients have cardiac involvement at necropsy. The myocardium and pericardium are involved with equal frequency by embolic hematogenous and retrograde lymphatic spread of tumor. The pericardium can also be invaded by direct extension of adjacent intrathoracic malignancies, in particular, bronchogenic carcinoma. Extension of tumor through the vena cava or the pulmonary veins can cause implantation of tumor on the endocardial surface. Metastases to the cardiac valves are extremely rare.[25]

Only 10 per cent of patients with cardiac metastases have cardiac symptoms. The clinical manifestations reflect the predominance of pericardial, myocardial, or endocardial involvement. Pericardial metastases produce inflammation, hemorrhagic effusion, tamponade, or cardiac constriction. The electrocardiographic findings include ST-T segment elevations and low voltage.[3] Myocardial metastases often cause rhythm disturbances or congestive heart failure if extensive infiltration of myocardial mass by tumor has occurred. Carcinomatous emboli or extrinsic compression of the coronary arteries can lead to myocardial ischemia and infarction. The rare endocardial lesions can obstruct ventricular filling or ejection in addition to causing valvular dysfunction. Noninvasive imaging by electrocardiography or, more recently, CT is helpful to delineate the feasibility of decompressing pericardial collections by the subxyphoid approach.

Treatment for cardiac metastases is almost always palliative. Limited benefit has accrued from systemic chemotherapy and radiation therapy. Surgical intervention is indicated to establish a tissue diagnosis, to effect electrical pacing, or to decompress symptomatic pericardial effusion. In carefully selected patients, surgical resection of solitary metastases to the right ventricular outflow tract has provided worthwhile survival.[4,16,25] However, operative intervention for tumors metastatic to the heart is best reserved for intra-atrial extensions of hypernephromas and Wilms' tumors.[19]

SELECTED REFERENCES

Chitwood, W. R.: Cardiac neoplasms. Current diagnosis, pathology and therapy. J. Cardiac Surg., 3:119, 1988.
This is a comprehensive review of all aspects of benign and malignant cardiac tumors. The illustrations are superb and the references are comprehensive and up-to-date. The newer imaging modalities are emphasized and operative techniques are detailed.

Dein, J. R., Frist, W. H., Stinson, E. B., Miller, D. C., Baldwin, J. C., Oyer, P. E., Jamieson, S., Mitchell, R. S., and Shumway, N. E.: Primary cardiac neoplasms. J. Thorac. Cardiovasc. Surg., 93:502, 1987.
This paper describes 42 patients who underwent surgical resection for benign and malignant cardiac neoplasms at Stanford University. Clinical and pathological features are detailed. Actuarial survival by histologic diagnosis is presented for a 5-year follow-up. One patient required cardiac transplantation for extirpation of a benign left ventricular tumor.

Freedberg, R. S., Kronzon, I., Rumancik, W. M., and Liebeskind, D.: The contribution of magnetic resonance imaging to the evaluation of intracardiac tumors diagnosed by echocardiography. Circulation, 77:96, 1988.
The role of MR imaging performed in 14 patients with intracavitary cardiac tumors is discussed. This paper is particularly important in outlining the relative roles of echocardiography, computerized axial tomography, and magnetic resonance imaging in the noninvasive diagnosis of cardiac neoplasms. MRI's potential for histologic diagnosis by tissue characterization is raised.

McAllister, A., and Fenoglio, J. J.: Tumors of the cardiovascular system. *In* Atlas of Tumor Pathology, Fasc. 15, 2nd series. Washington, D.C., Armed Forces Institute of Pathology, 1978.
This classic article remains the largest published modern series of benign and malignant primary neoplasms in adults and children. Data are derived from the collection of cardiac tumors at the Armed Forces Institute of Pathology. The authors are leading authorities on the subject, and this article is one of the definitive works on tumor pathology.

McCarthy, P. M., Piehler, J. M., Schaff, H. V., Pluth, J. R., Orszulak, T. A., Vidailler, H. J., and Carney, J. A.: The significance of multiple, recurrent and complex cardiac myxomas. J. Thorac. Cardiovasc. Surg., 91:389, 1986.
This article reviews the Mayo Clinic's experience with 56 patients who underwent operation for cardiac myxoma and 29 cases in which myxoma was found at autopsy. The synchronous nature and high recurrence rate of familial tumors and those tumors with associated syndromes are emphasized. The biologic behavior of "complex" myxoma is contrasted to "sporadic" myxoma.

REFERENCES

1. Bear, P. A., and Moodie, D. S.: Malignant primary cardiac tumors. Chest, 92:858, 1987.
2. Bogren, H. G., DeMaria, A. N., and Mason, D. T.: Imaging procedures in the detection of cardiac tumors with emphasis on echocardiography: A review. Cardiovasc. Intervent. Radiol., 3:107, 1980.
3. Cates, C. V., Virmani, R., Vaughn, W. K., and Robertson, R. M.: Electrocardiographic markers of cardiac metastasis. Am. Heart J., 112:1297, 1986.
4. Chitwood, W. R.: Cardiac neoplasms: Current diagnosis, pathology and therapy. J. Cardiac Surg., 3:119, 1988.
5. Dein, J. R., Frist, W. H., Stinson, E. B., Miller, D. C., Baldwin, J. C., Oyer, P. E., Jamieson, S., Mitchell, R. S., and Shumway, N. E.: Primary cardiac neoplasms. J. Thorac. Cardiovasc. Surg., 93:502, 1987.
6. Foster, E. D., Spooner, E. W., Farina, M. A., Shaher, R. M., and Alley, R. D.: Cardiac rhabdomyoma in the neonate: Surgical management. Ann. Thorac. Surg., 37:249, 1984.
7. Freedberg, R. S., Kronzon, I., Rumancik, W. M., and Liebeskind, D.: The contribution of magnetic resonance imaging to the evaluation of intracardiac tumors diagnosed by echocardiography. Circulation, 77:96, 1988.
8. Godwin, J. D., Axel, L., Adams, J. R., et al.: Computed tomography: A new method for diagnosing tumor of the heart. Circulation, 63:448, 1981.
9. Grenadier, E., Lima, C. O., Barron, J. V., et al.: Two-dimensional echocardiography for evaluation of metastatic cardiac tumors in pediatric patients. Am. Heart J., 107:122, 1984.
10. Hanfling, S. M.: Metastatic cancer to the heart: Review of the literature and report of 127 cases. Circulation, 22:474, 1960.
11. Hanson, E. C., Gill, C. C., Razavi, M., and Loop, F. D.: The surgical treatment of atrial myxomas. J. Thorac. Cardiovasc. Surg., 89:298, 1985.
12. Harvey, W. P.: Clinical aspects of cardiac tumors. Am. J. Cardiol., 21:328, 1968.
13. James, T. N., and Galakhov, I.: De Subitaneis Mortibus XXVI. Fatal electrical instability of the heart associated with benign congenital polycystic tumor of the atrioventricular node. Circulation, 56:667, 1977.
14. Kearney, D. L., Titus, J. L., Hawkins, E. P., Ott, D. A., and Garson, A.: Pathologic features of myocardial hamartomas causing childhood tachyarrhythmias. Circulation, 75:705, 1987.
15. Larsson, S., Lepore, V., and Kennergren, C.: Atrial myxomas: Results of 25 years' experience and review of the literature. Surgery, 105:695, 1989.
16. Leung, C. Y., Cummings, R. G., Reimer, K. A., and Lowe, J. E.: Chondrosarcoma metastatic to the heart. Ann. Thorac. Surg., 45:291, 1988.
17. McAllister, A., and Fenoglio, J. J.: Tumors of the cardiovascular system. *In* Atlas of Tumor Pathology, Fasc. 15, 2nd series. Washington, D. C., Armed Forces Institute of Pathology, 1978.
18. McCarthy, P. M., Piehler, J. M., Schaff, H. V., Pluth, J. R., Orszulak, T. A., Vidailler, H. J., and Carney, J. A.: The significance of multiple, recurrent and complex cardiac myxomas. J. Thorac. Cardiovasc. Surg., 91:389, 1986.
19. Nakayama, D. K., DeLorimier, A. A., O'Neill, J. A., Norkool, P., and D'Angio, G. J.: Intracardiac extension of Wilms' tumor. Ann. Surg., 204:693, 1986.
20. Parmley, L. F., Salley, R. K., Williams, J. P., and Head, G. B.: The clinical spectrum of cardiac fibroma with diagnostic and surgical considerations. Ann. Thorac. Surg., 45:455, 1988.
21. Poole, G. V., Jr., Meredith, J. W., Breyer, R. H., and Mills, S. A.: Surgical implications in malignant cardiac disease. Ann. Thorac. Surg., 36:484, 1983.
22. Salcedo, E. E., Adams, K. V., Lever, H. M., and Gill, C. C.: Echocardiographic findings in 25 patients with left atrial myxoma. J. Am. Coll. Cardiol., 1:1162, 1983.
23. Selzer, A., Sakai, F. J., and Popper, R. W.: Protean clinical manifestations of primary tumors of the heart. Am. J. Med., 52:9, 1972.
24. Shackell, M., Mitko, A., Williams, P. L., and Sutton, G. C.: Angiosarcoma of the heart. Br. Heart J., 41:498, 1979.
25. Silverman, N. A.: Primary cardiac tumors. Ann. Surg., 191:127, 1980.
26. Stark, R. M., Perloff, J. K., Glick, J. H., Hirshfield, J. W. Jr., and Devereux, R. B.: Clinical recognition and management of cardiac metastatic disease. Am. J. Med., 63:653, 1977.

XXII

CARDIAC PACEMAKERS

James E. Lowe, M.D.

Cardiac electrostimulation has a long and fascinating history beginning in the eighteenth century. However, the modern artificial cardiac pacemaker has followed technologic advances during the last 2 decades. The implantable pacemaker is one of modern medicine's greatest contributions to prolonging and improving human life. The exact number of individuals now living with an artificial pacemaker is unknown. However, estimates are that approximately 500,000 individuals now living in the United States have pacemakers, and each year 100,000 or more require permanent pacemaker implantation.[88] It is estimated that 1.5 to 2 million pacemakers have been implanted worldwide during the last 20 years.[23]

Advances in pacemaker design are now occurring so rapidly that refinements that previously required years of research and development are now achieved within months. Recent technologic improvements following the aerospace and computer industries are largely responsible for this progress.

HISTORICAL ASPECTS

Hyman developed a machine for controlled repetitive electrostimulation of the heart in 1932 and termed this device "the artificial cardiac pacemaker."[55] This device was used successfully in a number of animal experiments. By using a transthoracic needle electrode, the artificial cardiac pacemaker was subsequently used to resuscitate for brief intervals several patients with complete heart block and syncope. Unfortunately, these reports were never published because Hyman was subjected to abusive correspondence and even lawsuits from those who regarded his attempts to resuscitation by pacing as tampering with "Divine Providence."[101]

Zoll first described in 1952 successful pacing through external metal electrodes applied to the anterior chest wall in 2 patients.[126] The initial impulse generator was a Grass stimulator. This noninvasive technique was easy to apply and was much better accepted than the invasive techniques of Hyman or Bigelow and associates.[10,55] Zoll's continued work and many publications convinced the medical profession as well as the general public that cardiac pacing was both feasible and lifesaving.[127] Disadvantages of the external pacing technique included skin burns when inadequate electrode jelly was applied, painful chest wall muscle contractions in some patients, and inability to pace in thick-chested or emphysematous patients.

The new field of cardiac operations provided a major impetus in pacemaker development because complete heart block was sometimes created during operations such as pulmonic commissurotomy and closure of ventricular septal defect. Brockman and colleagues used a wire electrode in 1958 to successfully pace the heart of an infant who developed complete heart block after closure of a ventricular septal defect.[16] Although this patient died, pacing was effective and uninterrupted for 10 hours. Intramyocardial electrodes placed at the time of operation or introduced percutaneously through a needle were popularized in 1957 by investigators at the University of Minneapolis.[3,47,73,74,112,117–120] The electrodes were insulated silver-plated copper wires with exposed tips. These intramyocardial electrodes were connected to a self-contained external pacemaker containing transistors and a mercury battery. The disadvantages of this technique included lead dislodgment and steadily rising thresholds of the myocardial wire electrode.

In August of 1958, Furman and Schwedel used a right ventricular endocardial wire electrode connected to an external generator to successfully pace for 96 hours a 76-year-old patient with complete heart block.[37,38,41,103] This experience showed that prolonged cardiac pacing with low voltages could be accomplished with an endocardial right ventricular electrode connected to an external pacemaker. Other important and independent developments in the field of cardiac electrostimulation also occurred during this period. Elmquist and Senning in 1960 first implanted a rechargeable pacemaker in an epigastric pocket connected to electrodes that passed subcutaneously to the heart.[29] Glenn and associates developed a method of cardiac pacing in 1959 that used radiofrequency transmission.[44] This method required an external pulse generator but had the advantage of leaving the skin intact.

Chardack and colleagues in 1960 developed a transistorized, self-contained implantable pacemaker connected to modified Hunter-Roth epicardial electrodes.[21,54] This was the first implantable permanent pacemaker with the packing lead attached to the heart by thoracotomy. Other completely implantable units developed by Zoll and colleagues in 1961 and by Kantrowitz and associates in 1962 followed.[58,127] The technique for inserting a permanent transvenous bipolar pacemaker was developed in 1962 in the United States by Parsonnet and colleagues and in Sweden by Ekestrom and associates.[28,92] In the most common method of pacing, the permanent impulse generator is now implanted near the site where the lead enters the cephalic or subclavian vein.

These initial implantable permanent pacemakers were fixed-rate asynchronous devices that delivered the impulse independently of the underlying cardiac rate. Noncompetitive demand pacing of the ventricles was later introduced by Leatham and associates in 1956 and by Nicks and co-workers in 1962 using external pacemakers.[70,83] A brief period of asystole (1 to 2 seconds) triggered the onset of pacing, but deactivation of pacing required manual intervention. The use of implantable demand pacemakers that initiated pacing automatically in response to a single R-R interval prolongation with suppression on return of rhythm to a baseline R-R rate was first reported by Lemberg and associates in 1965.[71] Extensive clinical trials showing the efficacy of demand pacing were later reported in 1966 and 1967 by Goetz and associates, Parsonnet and colleagues, and Furman and co-workers.[39,45,93]

During the late 1960s, increased numbers of patients with sinus bradycardia and intact conduction were recognized. R wave–inhibited and synchronous pulse generators began to be applied to the atrium, and eventually bifocal pacemakers were designed to provide atrioventricular (AV) sequential pacing in patients with sinus bradycardia and heart block.[8,106] During the 1960s, new and improved pacemaker power sources were developed. Mercury-zinc batteries were used initially and usually lasted for less than 2 years. The mass of these cells represented two thirds to three quarters of the volume and even more of the weight of the pacemaker. Although various new power sources were tested, the lithium-iodine battery was soon recognized to be the best power source. In general, it is thought that the modern lithium-iodine battery may last for as long as 10 to 12 years. Nuclear-powered plutonium pacemakers are thought to last for a minimum of 10 to more than 20 years. However, cost and environmental restrictions have essentially eliminated their use in the United States.

NORMAL CARDIAC CONDUCTION SYSTEM

Impulse Formation

In the resting state, the myocardial cell maintains an electrical gradient or voltage potential across its cell membrane known as the resting membrane potential. The cell membrane is a semipermeable barrier through which ions can pass with various degrees of ease. In addition to the passive diffusion of ions along chemical or electrical gradients, active transport processes or "pumps" move ions against these gradients. The resting potential is the result of transmembrane differences in the concentrations of various ions, mainly sodium and potassium. The intracellular potassium concentration is much higher than that in the extracellular fluid. The opposite is true for sodium ions. The cell membrane is more permeable to potassium than to sodium, and potassium ions tend to pass outward through the cell membrane down the concentration gradient. This outward flow of positively charged ions causes a voltage gradient across the cell membrane. Because the flux of potassium ions is greater, potassium is the chief determinant of the voltage gradient at equilibrium. This equilibrium potential can be approximated by Nernst's equation, which relates the transmembrane potential to the ratio of extracellular and intracellular potassium concentrations:

$$V = \frac{RT}{F} \ln \frac{[K^+]_o}{[K^+]_i}$$

where R is the universal gas constant, T is the absolute temperature, and F is the Faraday constant. The cell membrane is a biologic system subject to variation, and the relationship between transmembrane potential and potassium levels becomes nonlinear at extremes of intra- or extracellular potassium concentrations. Changes in membrane permeability to other ions such as sodium at these extremes may also make their contribution to transmembrane potential more significant.

At equilibrium, when there is no net change in ion concentration across the cell membrane, the equilibrium or resting potential is constant. For myocardial cells, the equilibrium potential is approximately −90 mV. Depolarization refers to a change in membrane potential to a less negative value (toward zero). When cell membranes are depolarized to a particular critical value, the threshold potential, a chain reaction of events is triggered, causing complete, rapid depolarization followed by repolarization. When these events are recorded from a microelectrode placed inside the cell, an action potential is obtained (Fig. 1). The phases of action potential are the result of various transmembrane ionic currents, and rapid inward flux of sodium is mainly responsible for the rapid upstroke (phase 0) of the action potential recorded from myocardial cells and Purkinje fibers.

Certain cells, notably those in the sinoatrial (SA) node, display the property of automaticity. Automaticity refers to the spontaneous phase 4 depolarization noted in recordings from these cells. The resting membrane potential of these cells is considerably lower (less negative) than that in myocardial cells and Purkinje fibers, and phase 0 is slower. The depolarization of these cells depends on calcium as well as sodium ions. The transmembrane potential in cells displaying automaticity does not remain constant in phase 4, but undergoes spontaneous depolarization until the threshold potential is reached and an action potential is generated. A wave of depolarizing current then passes from one cell to another throughout the myocardium. Automaticity is normally a property of cells in the SA node and, to a lesser extent, cells of the AV node. Under abnormal conditions, Purkinje fibers and myocardial cells may also develop automaticity.

Myocardial cells can also be depolarized by means of artificially applied electrical stimuli. The stimulus must have sufficient strength to bring a critical number of cells up to the threshold potential, which causes a propagated impulse. When an activation wavefront is initiated by an artificial stimulus, it propagates throughout the myocardium. This unique property of myocardial cells forms the basis for artificial cardiac pacing.

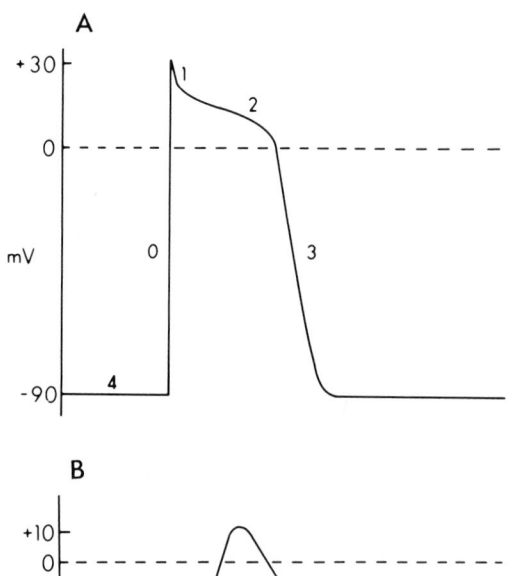

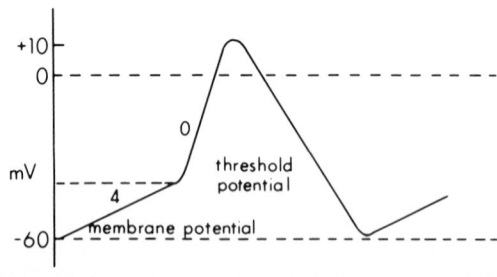

Figure 1. *A,* An action potential typical of a Purkinje fiber or ventricular myocardial cell. The resting membrane potential is −90 mV. and there is no spontaneous phase 4 depolarization. The upstroke (phase 0) is rapid. *B,* An action potential recorded from a cell displaying automaticity such as found in the SA and AV nodes. Spontaneous phase 4 depolarization is present. The resting membrane potential is lower (−60 mV.) and the upstroke is slower.

Functional Anatomy of the Conduction System

The SA node is a group of specialized cells located subepicardially at the lateral junction of the superior vena cava with the right atrium, although some anatomic variation may occur with extension of the node anteriorly across the caval-atrial junction. The SA node is especially vulnerable to surgical trauma because of its location. Three types of cells can be found in the human SA node, in addition to supporting elements of fibrocytes, nerves, and vessels.[75] Pacemaker or polygonal cells are polyhedral and contain prominent nuclei and sparse numbers of contractile elements. These cells are believed to be the site of impulse formation in the SA node, although electrophysiologic confirmation in humans is lacking. Transitional cells are found surrounding pacemaker cells and interposed between nodal cells and atrial myocardium. These cells have some features of both nodal cells and myocardial cells, with larger numbers of contractile elements. Atrial myocardial cells with prominent longitudinally oriented myofibrils may also be found in SA node tissue.[75]

The AV node is located subendocardially in the triangle of Koch, an anatomic region on the medial wall of the right atrium formed by the tendon of Todaro, the eustachian valve of the coronary sinus, and the tricuspid anulus. The AV node is composed of a transitional zone and compact zone. The cells of the compact zone are more distal and are arranged in fascicles that merge into the penetrating bundle of His.[5] The cells of the transitional zone are thought to provide distinct input pathways into the AV node from the atrium, and although the orientation of atrial muscle fibers appears to produce preferential pathways of conduction, evidence for functionally distinct conduction pathways across the atrium from the SA node (internodal tracts) is lacking.

Decremental conduction is a characteristic feature of conduction through the AV node. This refers to the normal slowing of conduction that occurs as impulses traverse the node from the atrium to the bundle of His. The AV node is the site of physiologic AV block (Wenckebach's or Mobitz Type I) that occurs when excessively rapid atrial rates (usually more than 150 to 160 beats per minute) are present. Conduction through the AV node depends heavily on autonomic tone. Withdrawal of vagal tone due to exercise or administration of atropine causes accelerated AV conduction, whereas increased vagal tone causes slower AV conduction or transient AV block.

The delay in conduction that occurs in the AV node is responsible for the majority of the P-R interval of the standard electrocardiogram as well as the A-H interval of the bundle of His recording. Normal conduction times across the AV node are between 60 and 120 msec., whereas conduction throughout the entire His-Purkinje system to the ventricles normally requires only 35 to 45 msec.

Conduction of impulses may proceed retrogradely from ventricle to atrium across the AV node. Retrograde conduction has become estimated to be intact in two thirds of normal humans.[2] Retrograde AV block often occurs in or below the bundle of His, compared with antegrade conduction block that normally occurs in the AV node.

When the cardiac impulse traverses the AV node, it rapidly courses down the bundle of His, which pierces the central fibrous body and divides into the left and right bundle branches. The bundle branches are composed of specialized cells oriented longitudinally with end-to-end connections. These conduction fibers traverse the subendocardium of the interventricular septum and carry the impulse to the distal ramifications of the Purkinje system where activation of ventricular myocardium occurs. The right bundle branch is a single distinct strand of fibers, whereas the fibers to the left ventricle divide into numerous ramifications with multiple interconnections.

INDICATIONS FOR PACEMAKER THERAPY

Artificial cardiac pacing has clearly led to the prolongation and improvement of the lives of thousands of patients with conduction system disorders. However, pacing is a costly type of therapy. In 1976, the average cost of pacing was estimated to be $102 per month per patient for the lifetime of the individual.[107] Inflation and rising hospital costs combined with the additional expense of improved pacing technology have further increased the overall cost of cardiac pacing. However, each advance in cardiac pacing has proved to be cost-effective.[46] Important advances containing the cost of permanent pacing have included improved electrodes and power sources, hermetic sealing of impulse generators, transtelephonic follow-up, and multiprogrammability of impulse generators. These advances have led to decreased rehospitalization and reoperation rates and lower follow-up costs. In fact, based on 1970 dollars, the current cost of pacing per patient year is approximately $40 per month.[46] A major challenge facing pacemaker manufacturers is the continued development of new products that provide improved clinical results with lower overall medical costs. Recent advances indicate that this goal is possible and should be a major consideration in the design of future pacing systems. Physicians, however, must be responsible for choosing the appropriate pacing system, either permanent or temporary, for the specific cardiac conduction disorder being treated. In the early 1960s, symptomatic complete AV block was almost the sole indication for permanent pacing. Although complete heart block is still a major indication, symptomatic patients with the sick sinus syndrome now represent the most common indication for permanent pacing.

Although there will always be controversy regarding indications for temporary and permanent cardiac pacing as well as the type of pacing system chosen, most would agree with the following guidelines.

Indications for Temporary Pacing

Three major factors that help to determine the indications for temporary pacing include (1) symptoms such as dizziness, near syncope, frank syncope, hypotension, and heart failure; (2) ventricular rate; and (3) clinical circumstances, which include the patient's underlying heart disease and the direct cause of the dysrhythmia being evaluated for temporary pacing. In general, ventricular rates less than 45 beats per minute produce symptoms and require temporary pacing. Acute dysrhythmias require temporary pacing more often than chronic arrhythmias. This appears to be particularly important in considering acute dysrhythmias associated with recent myocardial infarction. Indications for temporary pacing are shown in Table 1.

SYMPTOMATIC, SECOND-DEGREE, AND COMPLETE AV BLOCK. Wenckebach's (Mobitz Type I) AV block rarely requires temporary pacing unless the patient is symptomatic or

TABLE 1. Indications for Temporary Pacing

Symptomatic second-degree and complete AV block
Symptomatic bradyarrhythmias after acute myocardial infarction
New bifascicular or trifascicular block after acute myocardial infarction
Sick sinus syndrome (selected patients before permanent pacemaker insertion)
Symptomatic drug-induced bradyarrhythmias
Drug-resistant tachyarrhythmias (selected patients)
Carotid sinus syncope (selected patients)
Before permanent pacemaker implantation in selected patients
Therapeutic trial in patients with medically refractory low cardiac output
After cardiac surgery
Ventricular tachycardia (torsades de pointes) associated with long Q-T interval or bradycardia

the ventricular rate is slower than 45 beats per minute. Wenckebach's AV block is commonly due to enhanced vagal tone. In high-grade AV block, symptoms and the ventricular rate are the determining factors for insertion of a temporary pacemaker. Generally, temporary pacing is indicated in this group of patients who have symptoms that include dizziness, near syncope, frank syncope, hypotension, or congestive heart failure. Infranodal advanced or complete AV block frequently requires permanent pacing. Temporary pacing may be indicated before implantation of a permanent pacemaker, depending on the patient's ventricular rate and on the presence or absence of symptoms.

SYMPTOMATIC BRADYARRHYTHMIAS AFTER ACUTE MYOCARDIAL INFARCTION. Acute diaphragmatic myocardial infarction often leads to bradyarrhythmias that are usually transient and seldom require artificial pacing. However, when the ventricular rate is significantly slow (less than 45 beats per minute), or when the bradyarrhythmia becomes refractory to pharmacologic agents such as atropine and isoproterenol, or if symptoms develop, temporary pacing is indicated. Although less common, AV block due to anterior myocardial infarction usually represents infranodal block, which usually requires permanent cardiac pacing. However, a temporary pacemaker may be necessary before permanent pacing when the patient is symptomatic or the ventricular rate is inadequate.

NEW BIFASCICULAR OR TRIFASCICULAR BLOCK AFTER ACUTE MYOCARDIAL INFARCTION. In general, prophylactic temporary pacing should be considered in patients with acute bifascicular block or trifascicular block after acute infarction. Although some cardiologists have recommended prophylactic pacing for isolated acute left bundle branch block or for isolated left posterior hemiblock and right bundle branch block after infarction, the role of pacing in these disorders is still uncertain. Most physicians would agree that temporary pacing is not indicated in patients with myocardial infarction who display only acute left anterior hemiblock or in those with pre-existing bifascicular block.

SICK SINUS SYNDROME. Patients with advanced sick sinus syndrome often require permanent pacing. Many develop bradyarrhythmias as well as tachyarrhythmias and require a combination of pacemaker therapy and antiarrhythmic drug therapy. Temporary cardiac pacing is occasionally necessary before permanent pacemaker implantation in those patients who are symptomatic and have near syncope or syncope. In most of these patients, temporary pacing can be accomplished with conventional ventricular demand pacing. However, in those patients who require the atrial component to cardiac filling, temporary atrial pacing or dual-chamber pacing may be required.

SYMPTOMATIC DIGITALIS-INDUCED BRADYARRHYTHMIAS. Temporary cardiac pacing is indicated in symptomatic patients with marked bradyarrhythmia due to digitalis toxicity. Digitalis-induced bradyarrhythmias include sinus bradycardia, sinus arrest, second-degree AV block, and advanced or complete AV block.

DRUG-RESISTANT TACHYARRHYTHMIAS. When tachyarrhythmias, particularly ventricular tachycardia, become refractory to antiarrhythmic drug therapy, artificial overdrive pacing (80 to 120 beats per minute) is occasionally effective. Various modes of temporary pacing can be attempted, but atrial or coronary sinus pacing is usually ideal, particularly in patients in whom the atrial contribution to cardiac output is essential.

CAROTID SINUS SYNCOPE. Permanent pacemaker implantation is indicated in patients with cardiac sinus syncope or near syncope resulting from bradycardia. Syncope due to hypotension (vasodepressor syncope) does not respond to pacing. In some patients, hypersensitive carotid sinus reactions may be greatly exaggerated by drugs such as digitalis, methyldopa, guanethidine, and propranolol. Temporary pacing is occasionally indicated in this group while the offending drug is withdrawn.

BEFORE PERMANENT PACEMAKER IMPLANTATION. Most patients requiring permanent pacemaker implantation do not require a preoperative temporary pacemaker. However, temporary pacing is essential before permanent implantation in patients with acute arrhythmias, especially after acute myocardial infarction or in symptomatic patients with complete AV block.

THERAPEUTIC TRIAL FOR CONGESTIVE HEART FAILURE, CARDIOGENIC SHOCK, AND CEREBRAL OR RENAL INSUFFICIENCY. It is becoming increasingly apparent that some patients with intractable congestive heart failure, cardiogenic shock, and cerebral or renal hypoperfusion may be improved by an increased heart rate. Generally, atrial or coronary sinus pacing is chosen because the atrial contribution to cardiac output appears to be essential in patients with low perfusion states. Therefore, temporary pacing should be considered as a therapy in this difficult subgroup of patients. In patients who respond, permanent pacemaker implantation may be considered for long-term therapy.

AFTER CARDIAC SURGERY. Temporary atrial or AV sequential pacing through temporary epicardial electrodes may decrease the need for inotropic support in the perioperative period. Transient conduction disturbances are often encountered in the immediate perioperative period, and temporary epicardial pacing is essential. An additional advantage is that atrial dysrhythmias that occur perioperatively can be diagnosed more accurately through recording of electrograms from these temporary wires, and overdrive pacing can often be used to convert perioperative atrial flutter and occasionally atrial fibrillation.[116] Most cardiac surgeons routinely attach temporary atrial and ventricular pacing wires after major cardiac surgical procedures.

Indications for Permanent Pacing

Implantation of a permanent cardiac pacemaker commits the physician and patient to a lifetime of appropriate follow-up care and also exposes the patient to the possible complications of permanent pacing. In the early 1960s, after the introduction of the completely implantable pacing system, the major indication for permanent pacemaker therapy was complete AV block associated with presyncope or syncope. During the last several years, however, indications for implantation of permanent pacemakers have changed. Although complete AV block remains a definite indication for permanent pacing, most permanent pacemakers implanted are in patients with the sick sinus syndrome. Many patients with this syndrome have coexisting conduction disturbances, including AV block or fascicular block or both. When it has been decided that a patient is a candidate for a permanent pacemaker, the type and mode of the pacemaker most suitable for each patient must be determined. Factors involved in selecting an appropriate pacing system include the patient's age, general condition, underlying heart disease, and characteristics of the dysrhythmia being treated. When sinus rhythm predominates, a simple ventricular inhibited-demand pacemaker is often adequate. However, in patients in whom frequent or constant pacing is anticipated, a pacemaker that allows a changing heart rate according to physiologic demands with exercise should be used. Dual-chamber pacing is indicated in those who have shown that the atrial component of cardiac filling is essential for adequate cardiac output. The general trend now is toward the use of more dual-chamber or single-chamber rate-modulated pacemakers with multiprogrammable capability so that various pacing parameters can be adjusted noninvasively as the patient's need for pacing changes.

As with temporary pacing, opinions about the indications for permanent cardiac pacing differ. Indications for permanent pacing have been outlined in detail by a joint task force of the American College of Cardiology and the American Heart Association in 1984[48] and are shown in Table 2.

SICK SINUS SYNDROME AND BRADYCARDIA-TACHYCARDIA SYNDROME. Pharmacologic therapy alone is often ineffective in patients with the sick sinus syndrome, and permanent pacing is indicated in those who remain symptomatic because of bradycardia. The most common manifestation of the sick sinus syndrome is marked sinus bradycardia associated with intermittent sinus arrest or SA node block and episodes of AV junctional escape rhythm. In more advanced forms of the sick sinus syndrome, chronic atrial fibrillation may develop and may be associated with a slow ventricular rate secondary to advanced AV block. An additional group of patients develop various atrial tachyarrhythmias, which is a common result of advanced sick sinus syndrome.

In many patients, a ventricular inhibited-demand pacemaker is adequate therapy. However, in patients in whom the atrial contribution to cardiac output is essential, dual-chamber pacing should be used. Atrial arrhythmias can be suppressed occasionally by atrial pacing. In patients with the bradyarrhythmia-tachyarrhythmia syndrome, one or more antiarrhythmic agents are frequently required in addition to permanent pacemaker therapy.

MOBITZ TYPE II AV BLOCK. It is generally believed that permanent pacing is indicated for patients with Mobitz Type II AV block, associated with a wide QRS complex, regardless of whether the patient is symptomatic. It has been documented that Mobitz Type II AV block frequently leads to advanced AV block.[25]

COMPLETE AV BLOCK. Before pacemaker therapy became clinically available, 50 per cent of patients with complete heart block died within 1 year.[35,57] Complete heart block is frequently caused by sclerodegenerative disease of the cardiac skeleton or of the conduction system itself and is often preceded by the development of bifascicular blocks such as right bundle branch block with left- or right-axis deviation and left bundle branch block. Therefore, most surgeons would agree that complete AV block represents a definite indication for permanent cardiac pacing. In addition to sclerodegenerative diseases, other causes of acquired complete AV block include ischemic myocardial injury, infiltrative cardiomyopathies, Chagas' disease, traumatic injuries, and cardiac procedures. Permanent pacing is usually recommended for surgically induced complete heart block lasting more than 1 week after operation. Complete AV block associated with acute anterior wall myocardial infarction is often irreversible and requires permanent pacemaker implantation.[27,51] Conversely, complete AV block after a diaphragmatic myocardial infarction can usually be reversed and may require only temporary pacing. Permanent pacing is generally recommended in all patients with myocardial infarction when complete AV block continues for more than 10 to 14 days.

TABLE 2. Indications for Permanent Pacing

Complete AV block with:
  Syncope or presyncope
  Congestive heart failure
  Ventricular tachycardia
  Heart rate less than 40 or asystole greater than 3 seconds
  Cerebral hypoperfusion
Second-degree AV block with symptoms
Acute myocardial infarction with persistent second-degree AV block or complete AV block
Chronic bifascicular or trifascicular block with symptomatic intermittent complete or second-degree AV block
Sinus bradycardia or sinus pauses with symptoms
Hypersensitive carotid sinus syndrome with recurrent syncope
Atrial fibrillation with slow ventricular rate and symptoms

SYMPTOMATIC BIFASCICULAR AND TRIFASCICULAR BLOCK. Bifascicular or trifascicular block usually signifies extensive conduction system disease. Symptoms in patients with bundle branch block may be due to intermittent episodes of advanced or complete AV block or to ventricular tachycardia. Permanent pacing should be considered in symptomatic patients with bifascicular or trifascicular block and prolonged H-V intervals of 100 msec. or longer. In patients with documented episodes of complete AV block associated with bundle branch block, implantation of a permanent pacemaker should be an urgent consideration. Dual-chamber pacing is generally preferred in patients in whom progression to permanent complete AV block is likely.

BIFASCICULAR OR TRIFASCICULAR BLOCK WITH INTERMITTENT COMPLETE AV BLOCK AFTER ACUTE MYOCARDIAL INFARCTION. Clinical studies have shown that the potential risk of sudden death within 6 months after acute myocardial infarction increases in patients with bifascicular or incomplete trifascicular block associated with intermittent complete AV block during the peri-infarction period.[27,51] Therefore, it is now recommended that this group of patients be considered candidates for permanent pacemaker implantation before discharge from the hospital after their infarction.

CAROTID SINUS SYNCOPE. As mentioned earlier, a permanent pacemaker may be indicated in patients with carotid sinus syncope or near syncope when a significant cardioinhibitory component can be implicated.

RECURRENT DRUG-RESISTANT TACHYARRHYTHMIAS IMPROVED BY TEMPORARY PACING. Some patients with tachyarrhythmias, particularly paroxysmal ventricular tachycardia, can be managed successfully by temporary pacing. In patients who respond, permanent pacing techniques can be considered to be part of their therapy. Because of the excellent surgical results obtained in patients with the Wolff-Parkinson-White syndrome and ventricular tachycardia associated with left ventricular aneurysms and micro–re-entry, operation should be considered to be primary therapy. However, in patients who are not surgical candidates, various antitachycardia pacing techniques are useful. Torsades de pointes due to a long Q-T interval as encountered with drug toxicity or electrolyte imbalance can be managed successfully with temporary overdrive pacing.

INTRACTABLE CONGESTIVE HEART FAILURE AND CEREBRAL OR RENAL INSUFFICIENCY BENEFITED BY TEMPORARY PACING. As described earlier, patients with refractory congestive heart failure and decreased perfusion causing cerebral or renal insufficiency may be improved occasionally by increasing heart rate with temporary pacing. If temporary pacing has proved to be effective under these conditions and long-term therapy is indicated, permanent pacing should be considered. Most of these patients require atrial contraction to improve cardiac output. Therefore, dual-chamber atrial synchronous pacing is usually indicated in this subgroup. In patients with sinus bradycardia or atrial arrhythmias, single-chamber rate-modulated pacing should be considered. These examples show that choice of the exact mode of pacing depends on a thorough knowledge of the underlying conduction disturbance.

THE IMPULSE GENERATOR

An implantable cardiac pacemaker consists of an impulse generator, lead wire, and electrode (Fig. 2). The impulse generator contains a power source or battery, hybrid circuits, and a lead connector (Fig. 3). All of these components are kept in a hermetically sealed metal container. The size and weight of the impulse generator depend on the size of the battery and the number of electronic components. Impulse generators are usually placed in rectangular or oval packages with rounded edges and weigh between 32 and 135 gm.

Power Sources

The power source used in a totally implantable pacemaker may be biologic, rechargeable, nuclear, or chemical. Biologic

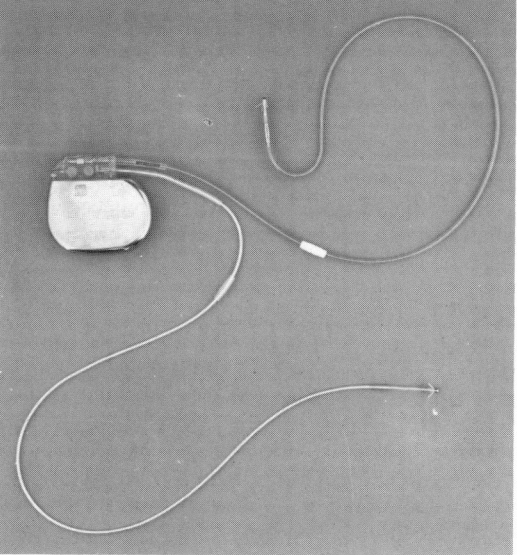

Figure 2. The modern implantable cardiac pacemaker consists of an impulse generator, lead wire, and electrode. A bipolar dual-chambered impulse generator is shown connected to an atrial J-tined lead and a ventricular-tined lead. Devices such as the system shown represent the current state of the art in pacemaker technology.

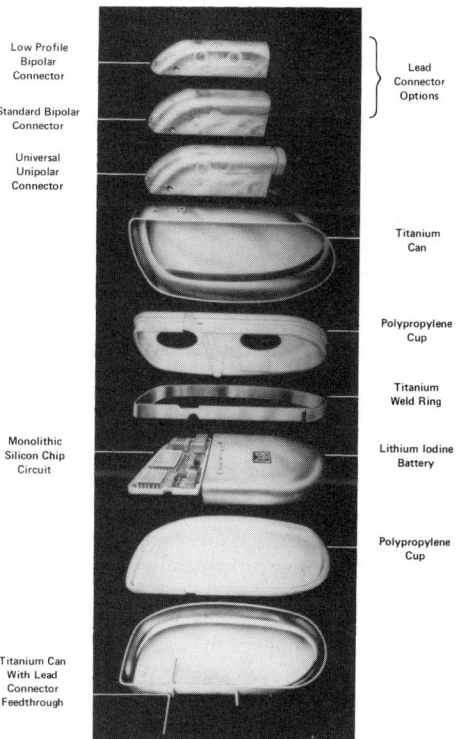

Figure 3. Exploded view of a modern multiprogrammable impulse generator. As shown, a variety of lead connectors are available to accept a variety of epicardial and transvenous leads. The battery and pacemaker electronics are enclosed in a titanium metal case. Hybrid circuit technology allows all components of the circuit including semiconductors, resistors, and capacitors to be diffused into a substrate to produce what is called a monolithic silicon chip. As shown, the major advantage of the silicon chip circuit is its extremely small size. This technology combined with the improved lithium power source has allowed modern multiprogrammable pacemakers to be much smaller, lighter, and more reliable than earlier pacemakers. (Courtesy of Paul Craven and Joe Hitselberger, Medtronic, Inc.)

power sources convert mechanical or chemical energy of the body into electrical energy using piezoelectric crystals, biogalvanic cells, or biofuel cells.[6,24,81] Theoretically, these power sources can be renewed potentially for the patient's lifetime, but they have not been developed to a point at which they are clinically practical. In 1973, a highly reliable, hermetically sealed, nickel-cadmium rechargeable pacemaker was developed at Johns Hopkins University and introduced commercially by Pacesetter, Inc.[32] The useful battery life of such a rechargeable pacemaker has been calculated to be 70 to 80 years. Rechargeable pacemakers, although reliable, are not widely used, primarily because of the necessity for weekly recharging. Nuclear-powered impulse generators have been implanted in more than 3000 patients worldwide. Their longevity is predicted to be longer than 20 years; however, nuclear generators are infrequently used because of cost, the improved longevity of newer chemical power sources, legislative restrictions, and concerns about the risk of chronic low-level radiation exposure. Chemical power sources continue to be the primary component of power cells in implantable pacemakers.

The modern power cell or battery is composed of an anode, a cathode, and an electrolyte. The power cell is generally named for the material used in the anode and cathode, for example, lithium-iodine. Current solid-state cells have a dry, crystalline electrolyte between the anode and cathode. Electric current is produced by ionization of the anode, causing migration of positively charged metallic ions through the electrolyte toward the cathode. Electrons are left behind on the anode, which becomes negatively charged relative to the cathode. When the anode and cathode are connected by a conductive pathway, a flow of electrons passes from the anode to the cathode. The higher the resistance in the conductor, the slower the flow of electrons and the longer the power cell will last. In the modern lithium-iodine power cell, the migrating or positively charged ions are lithium, which combines with iodine from the cathode to form a lithium-iodide electrolyte barrier.[113] Most currently available lithium-powered pacemakers contain a single power cell, unlike the original mercury-zinc generators, which were powered by multiple-cell batteries.

Lithium power cells are available in five chemical types: (1) lithium-iodine (polyvinyl pyridine), (2) lithium–lead sulfide, (3) lithium–silver chromate, (4) lithium–copper sulfide, and (5) lithium–thionyl chloride.[113] All of these lithium power sources have been extremely reliable and durable when compared with the earlier mercury-zinc systems. Most current pacemaker implants worldwide contain a solid-state lithium-iodine cell, which appears to be the power source of choice. Overall, pulse generator performance based on the type of power source is shown in Figure 4. The results with rechargeable impulse generators are essentially parallel to those of the nuclear power sources. The power source longevity of lithium pacemakers is estimated to be 10 to 12 years. However, because of wound, lead-electrode, and functional problems relating to pacing and sensing, it appears that approximately 20 per cent of patients have required reoperation 4 to 5 years after implantation of a lithium-powered pacemaker.[113] Therefore, it is unwise to suggest to a patient that the life of the pacemaker is governed only by the predicted life expectancy of the power cell. Even modern lithium-powered pacemakers have been associated with a small incidence of random failure.[121]

Pacemaker Electronics

The first implantable pacemakers contained individual or discrete components including resistors, capacitors, diodes, transistors, reed switches, and wire coils for induction. These individual components were mounted on or between printed circuit boards. A major advance in pacemaker electronics has been the development of "hybrid" circuits. Hybrid technology allows all components of the circuit including semiconductors,

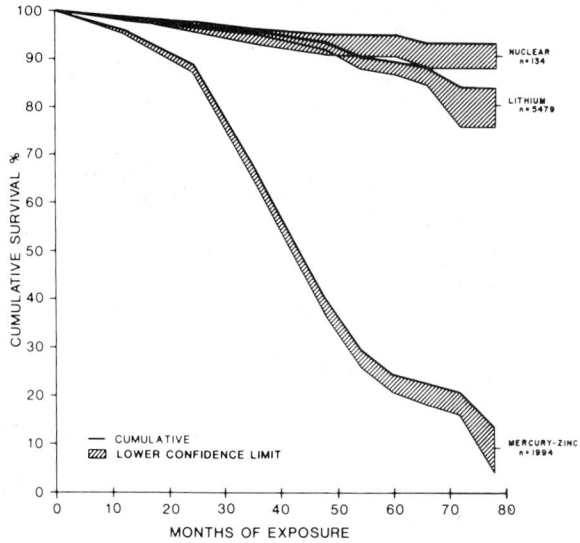

Figure 4. Impulse generator performance based on the type of power source. (From Bilitch, M., Hauser, R. G., Goldman, B. S., et al.: Performance of cardiac pacemaker pulse generators. PACE, 4:254, 1981.)

resistors, and capacitors to be diffused into a substrate to produce a monolithic silicon chip. The major advantage of the single-chip circuit is its small size. Customized digital, silicon, large-scale integrated circuits are used in almost all multiprogrammable pacemakers and may include as many as 40,000 transistors on a 4-sq. mm. wafer.[113] This technology combined with the improved lithium power source has allowed modern multiprogrammable pacemakers to be much smaller, lighter, and more reliable than earlier simpler pacemakers. The lithium-powered pacemaker containing a custom integrated circuit design is exceptionally reliable and capable of providing both multiprogrammable and physiologic pacing functions. However, its capacity for monitoring and data processing is limited.[113] Single-chip microcomputers are now available, although high-current drain and software limitations have prevented their widespread use in pacemakers. Future pacemakers will most likely use low-current drain, custom microcomputers consisting of a central processing unit, a memory unit, and an input-output circuit.[7] Pacemakers containing microcomputers are now capable of monitoring various physiologic changes to control pacemaker function in outline manner. Physiologic changes that can be monitored include cardiac output requirements as determined by online measurement of temperature, Q-T interval, oxygen saturation, body motion, and respiratory rate. Moreover, microcomputer-based pacemakers can automatically select an appropriate pacing technique for the control of various dysrhythmias. Future pacemakers will be able to automatically detect loss of capture due to threshold changes and adjust their output accordingly.

Hermetic Seal

The electronics and power source of the first totally implantable pacemakers were protected by epoxy resins and silicone rubber.[113] Gradually, however, moisture gained access to the interior of the pacemaker, causing short circuits, sudden cessation of pacing, battery explosion, pacemaker runaway, and occasionally even ventricular fibrillation. Fluid infiltration problems were responsible for the massive recalls that eventually terminated the use of mercury-zinc, epoxy-enclosed pacemakers. The modern pacemaker is hermetically enclosed, rendering it airtight and fluid-tight. Pacemaker manufacturers determine the quality of the hermetic seal in terms of a leak rate for an inert gas under standard conditions.[113] For example, an acceptable helium leak rate of 10^{-8} ml. per second at one atmosphere involves the passage of less than 0.01 ml. of helium per 24 hours. Permeability to fluid is many orders of magnitude lower. Hermetic seal is now achieved by encasing the power source and electronics in a sealed metal container, which usually requires laser welding. The materials chosen for enclosure have included stainless steel, Haynes' alloy, and titanium. Most modern pacemakers are enclosed in titanium.

Lead Connector

Impressive advances have been made in leads and electrodes and in pacemaker power sources and circuitry. As described by Tyers and Brownlee, the ideal pacemaker connector should be tangential to reduce electrode stress, universal to accept all available leads without adapters, simple, and short-circuit proof.[113] A standard coaxial bipolar connector that has been developed may represent an industry standard that eliminates incompatibilities between various leads and pacemakers. This universal lead connector is referred to as the VS-1 (voluntary standard) and is a 3.2-mm. diameter connector designed to fit potentially bipolar pacemakers[18] as well as to reduce the size of the connector itself (see Fig. 3).

LEAD-ELECTRODE

A pacemaker lead is an insulated wire used to connect the pacemaker impulse generator to the heart. The electrode is the uninsulated, electrically active metal tip that is in contact with the myocardium (see Fig. 2). The lead-electrode system in a demand pacemaker has two equally important functions: it conducts the electric stimulus from the impulse generator to the myocardium and transmits an endocardial electrogram from the heart to the pacemaker.[113] In unipolar systems, only the cathode is in the heart, and the indifferent electrode, or anode, which is a part of the metallic pacemaker case, is in soft tissue. In a bipolar system, a double wire runs from the pacemaker to the heart and the two electrodes are separated by approximately 1 cm. within the heart. The lead wire is most often a continuous helical coil or braided wire that is resistant to fracture caused by repeated flexion. Carbon leads as well as multistrand leads made of combinations of metals such as nickel alloy and silver are now under evaluation in Europe and in the United States. These new leads may offer improved flexibility and lower resistance, which will cause decreased energy consumption. In the past, the lead was most commonly insulated with silicone rubber. Polyurethane insulation has been introduced because of its greater elasticity and tensile strength, which allows lead diameter to be reduced with improved durability. In addition, polyurethane has a smoother surface, which improves handling characteristics during multilead placement and reduces the risk of venous thrombosis.[122]

The uninsulated electrically active metal tip of the lead in contact with the myocardium is the electrode. This exposed tip is usually made of platinum, iridium, nickel alloys, or activated carbon. Platinum-iridium electrodes are now the most common and may be either porous or solid.

Two general types of lead-electrode systems exist. The most common are the systems passed transvenously to embed within the subendocardium of the right atrium or right ventricle or both. The second group are those placed transthoracically; they are directly attached to the myocardium of any chamber. These leads have been referred to as epicardial leads, but this term is a misnomer because they are actually embedded within the myocardium and not just within the epicardium. Transthoracic leads are used primarily in small infants and children, after repeated failure of the transvenous approach, and sometimes when the chest is already open, such as after cardiac surgical procedures. Generally, transvenous lead-electrode systems are preferred because of their improved chronic thresholds and decreased incidence of lead failure.

Transvenous systems are referred to as active or passive. Passive leads have a small flanged expansion just proximal to the exposed distal electrode or have short, flexible tines. These tined leads are designed to catch beneath trabeculae and reduce the incidence of dislodgment, which should be less than 1 per cent.[38] Active fixation leads are designed for insertion into large, smooth-walled ventricular cavities as well as for lead placement in the atrial appendage. Currently used active fixation leads contain sharpened screws that may be remotely activated and retractable.[113] The author prefers polyurethane-coated tined leads for routine transvenous ventricular pacing and sharp corkscrew-type screw-in electrodes for placement in the right atrium or the right ventricle under adverse circumstances when the rate of dislodgment is increased. Leads designed primarily for placement in the atrial appendage by the transvenous route differ from ventricular leads in that when the stylet is withdrawn they assume a J shape, which allows them to be positioned well up into the atrial appendage (see Fig. 2).

As mentioned earlier, pacemaker lead-electrode systems are referred to as being either bipolar or unipolar. Possible advantages of a unipolar system include a more simple connection, slightly decreased energy requirements, lower risk of pacemaker-induced fibrillation, and decreased risk of anodal corrosion.[113] Advantages of bipolar pacing include reduced risk of skeletal muscle stimulation, lower susceptibility to electromagnetic interference, elimination of pacemaker suppression by skeletal myopotentials, decreased risk of "cross-talk" between atrial and ventricular stimuli, and increased sensing selectivity.[113] The advantages and disadvantages of unipolar and bipolar pacing should be considered when selecting the most appropriate pacemaker for a particular patient.

To a certain extent, decreasing electrode tip size causes lower thresholds, at the time of implant as well as chronically because of higher current density. However, better sensing function is directly related to electrode area and is adversely affected by small electrode size.[53] Therefore, a compromise between pacing and sensing efficiency is required. Typical electrode surface areas for pacing are between 8 and 10 sq. mm. The effective surface area for sensing is increased many times through the use of microporous electrodes. These porous-tip electrodes improve sensing for a specific electrode size because the interstices increase the sensing area without increasing overall electrode size and subsequent stimulation energy requirements.[68] Techniques such as platinization of the electrode or use of activated carbon cause lower stimulation thresholds by reducing polarizing currents at the electrode surface.

IMPLANTATION AND EVALUATION OF PACEMAKER FUNCTION

Operative Techniques

Implantation of a permanent impulse generator and lead-electrode system should be done in a fluoroscopic unit or a cardiac catheterization laboratory under sterile conditions. Various impulse generators and lead-electrodes as well as a pacing system analyzer should be readily available. Most commonly, the pacemaker lead-electrode is passed transvenously under local anesthesia to become embedded within the subendocardium of the right atrium or right ventricle. Transthoracic leads are used primarily in small infants and children, after repeated failure of the transvenous approach, and sometimes after cardiac procedures when a permanent pacemaker is indicated. In general, for elective permanent pacemakers, transvenous leads are preferred because of their improved chronic thresholds and decreased incidence of lead fracture.

Preoperatively, patients receive a therapeutic dose of an antistaphylococcal antibiotic based on the proven beneficial effects of prophylactic antibiotic administration in general and thoracic surgical procedures. Antibiotics are discontinued 24 hours postoperatively. Regardless of the planned approach for implantation, the entire anterior chest from the chin to the umbilicus should be prepared and draped as a sterile field. This wide field of preparation allows conversion from one transvenous approach to another and permits a limited anterior thoracotomy without interruption of the procedure.

Based on the work of Lagergren and Johansson (1963) in Sweden and by Furman and Schwedel (1959) and Chardack and colleagues (1965) in the United States, the transvenous approach under local anesthesia is now used in more than 90 per cent of patients requiring pacemakers.[20,38,68] The venous anatomy of the anterior chest wall is particularly well suited for implantation of pacing leads (Fig. 5). Generally, the pacemaker pocket is placed over the anterior side of the chest beneath the junction of the inner and middle thirds of the clavicle on the patient's nondominant side. The cephalic or subclavian veins are the preferred venous approaches for lead introduction. Implantation through the external or internal jugular veins requires a separate neck incision, and the lead must be tunneled over or under the clavicle to reach the pacemaker pocket and generator. Passing the lead over the clavicle predisposes to skin erosion and lead fracture; tunneling beneath the clavicle increases the risk of hemorrhage due to vascular injury.

An oblique incision on the anterior chest wall inferior to the deltopectoral groove provides excellent exposure to the cephalic vein and also allows introducer cannulation of the subclavian vein. The pacemaker pocket should be as far medial as is comfortable for the patient to minimize pectoral stimulation. It should be made only slightly larger than the impulse generator so that migration laterally, which tends to follow the curvature of the chest wall, is minimized. Small atrial and venous bleeders are ligated or electrocoagulated to avoid postoperative hematoma formation. The pacemaker generator pocket should be just superficial to the pectoralis major in thick-chested individuals or beneath the premuscular fascia or muscle itself in thin-chested patients.

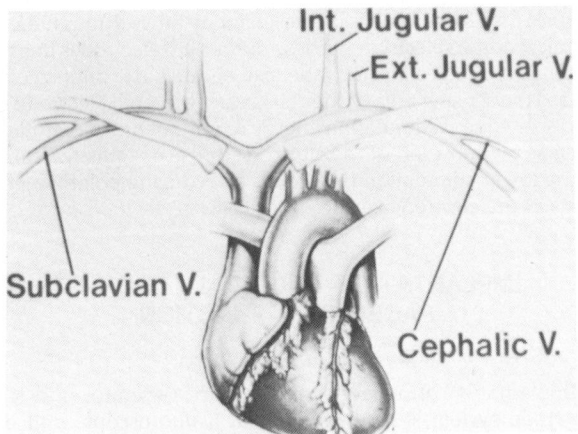

Figure 5. Anatomy for preferred venous approaches. Any vein in the neck, chest, or shoulder may be used for a permanent transvenous lead, but it is preferable to expose the vein through the same incision used for making the pocket. In order of preference, acceptable veins are as follows: (1) Cephalic vein, a tributary of the subclavian vein. It lies in the deltopectoral groove and is usually large enough to admit a lead up to No. 7 or 8 French. In 10 per cent of patients, it is quite delicate and may not be usable. It is occasionally absent. (2) Subclavian vein or tributary. If the cephalic vein cannot be used, it is always possible to expose another tributary of the subclavian or the subclavian vein itself through the same incision by freeing the pectoralis major from its lateral origin from the inferior surface of the clavicle. The subclavian vein is now commonly used as the primary choice for lead insertion with introducer techniques. (3) External jugular vein. This is usually the most prominent visible vein in the neck, although it may be absent in 10 per cent of patients. Because of the necessity of tunneling the electrode over or under the clavicle, with an increased incidence of fracture and erosion, this is a poor choice for permanent pacing. (4) Internal jugular vein. This is also a poor choice, except if there are purulent infections at every other potential site. (From Parsonnet, V.: Implantation of Transvenous Pacemakers. Tarpon Springs, FL, Tampa Tracings, 1972.)

A gentle, twisting motion is used to introduce the lead-electrode system into the right atrium. The guidewire is then exchanged for one with a J tip, which allows the lead to be passed across the tricuspid valve. The lead is then advanced across the pulmonary valve to confirm that the right ventricle has been cannulated and not the coronary sinus. The lead is then withdrawn into the cavity of the right ventricle, and the curved guidewire is replaced with a straight wire. The lead is then gradually withdrawn until the electrode falls and points toward the apex of the right ventricle. The guidewire is then withdrawn a few millimeters, and the lead is gently maneuvered to lodge the pacing and sensing electrode beneath right ventricular trabeculae. If a dual-chamber procedure is planned, ventricular lead placement is accomplished first, followed by placement of an atrial J lead, which is designed to lodge in the right atrial appendage. If stable positioning of an atrial J lead cannot be accomplished, an endocardial screw-in lead is placed into the wall of the right atrium. After transvenous positioning and testing of thresholds, the lead is anchored at the fascial or venous exit site to prevent dislodgment. After testing the impulse generator, the lead-electrode system is then connected to the impulse generator, which is then positioned in its pocket. Finally, the wound is irrigated with a dilute bacitracin-saline solution and closed in layers using absorbable suture.

Permanent transthoracic leads can be placed through either a small left anterior thoracotomy or a subxiphoid mediastinotomy. Generally, sutureless screw-in or hook leads are used and tunneled beneath the costal margin to the pacemaker pocket, which is created over the left upper quadrant of the abdomen well above the belt line or occasionally placed retroperitoneally in either lower quadrant in small infants. The electrode is placed by opening the pericardium and by identifying a fat-free area on the anterior or lateral aspect of the left ventricle. The electrode should not be placed too close to the apex of the heart because of its thinness and because increased motion in this area may cause electrode dislodgment or lead fracture. In addition, the electrode should not be placed in myocardium adjacent to the pericardial course of the phrenic nerve, which could cause diaphragmatic pacing.

Evaluation of Pacemaker Function

A thorough evaluation of pacing threshold energy requirements, atrial and ventricular endocardial electrograms, and impulse generator parameters should be done at the time of initial pacemaker implantation as well as at the time of replacement.[19,62,91,114] A pacing system analyzer stimulates the function of the pacemaker's output and sensing circuits and is also capable of evaluating the integrity of the impulse generator itself. The pacemaker's energy output and sensing circuits communicate with the myocardium through the implanted lead at the electrode-myocardial interface. The pacemaker impulse generator delivers an electrical discharge, which passes through its output circuit into the lead, to the electrode-myocardial interface, and back through body tissue to an indifferent electrode. This system is a simple series electrical circuit described by Ohm's law (resistance = voltage/current). The factors determining resistance are summarized.

The electrical pulse discharged by the impulse generator's output circuit is designed to initiate cardiac depolarization. The pacing threshold of the electrode-myocardial interface can be expressed in terms of energy, current, or voltage. The electrical energy discharged by the impulse generator is defined as follows: energy = voltage × current × time. This electrical energy has both an amplitude (voltage or current) and a time component (pulse width or duration). The lowest voltage or current that is delivered to the heart at a given pulse width and that causes cardiac depolarization is referred to as the stimulation threshold. A strength-duration curve (Fig. 6) is a graphic plot that shows the stimulation threshold for each pulse width. Any

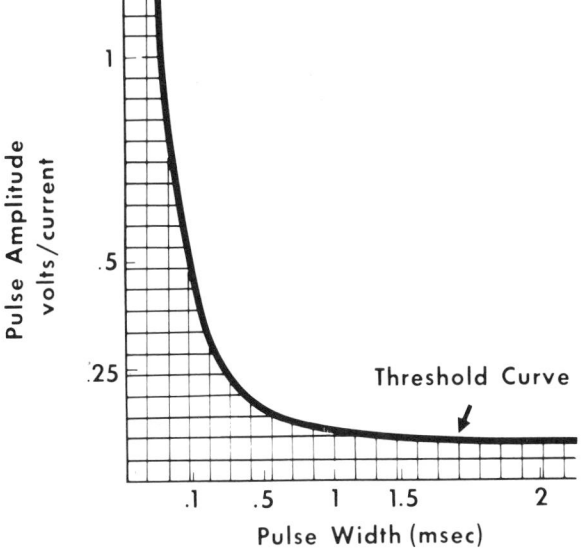

Figure 6. Strength-duration curve. A strength-duration curve demonstrates the relationship between the pulse amplitude (volts and current) and the pulse width. Each point on the curve is the stimulation threshold for that respective pulse amplitude and pulse width. The area above the strength-duration curve represents the pulse amplitude and pulse width combinations that stimulate an endocardial depolarization. The area below the curve represents the combinations of pulse amplitude and pulse width insufficient to stimulate a depolarization. (From Byrd, C.: Permanent pacemaker implantation techniques. *In* Samet, P., and El-Sherif, N. (Eds.): Cardiac Pacing, 2nd ed. New York, Grune & Stratton, 1980, p. 229.)

amplitude–pulse width combination on or above the strength-duration curve is sufficient to initiate cardiac depolarization. As shown in Figure 6, the amplitude component approaches an infinite value at very short pulse widths, such as less than 0.1 msec., and it approaches a minimal value at long pulse widths, such as greater than 1.5 msec. As can be seen from the strength-duration curve, at a short pulse width, the stimulation threshold may exceed the output of the pacemaker and cause loss of pacing. Conversely, excessively long pulse widths do not lower the pacing threshold and waste energy. In right ventricular implants using currently available transvenous electrodes, a pulse width of at least 0.5 msec. is usually used acutely to obtain a voltage threshold of less than or equal to 0.5 volt. Generally, an acute threshold greater than 1 volt is unsatisfactory. Atrial pacing thresholds are usually comparable with ventricular thresholds but may be slightly higher. Atrial thresholds greater than 2 volts are unsatisfactory. A low acute threshold provides a substantial safety margin because acute thresholds generally rise to higher values during the first several weeks and then decline slightly to their chronic levels secondary to maturation of the electrode-myocardial interface.

In addition to measuring pulse amplitude (voltage and current) and pulse width, resistance is also determined. As described by Ohm's law, resistance is calculated by dividing voltage by current. Resistance calculations are made at a voltage near that of the pacemaker's output. The calculated resistance at 5 volts should range from 300 to 800 ohms. Low resistances cause higher currents and are unsatisfactory for pacing. An unsatisfactorily low resistance can develop secondary to location of the electrode in the ventricular chamber or because of a separate competing electrical pathway (parallel circuit). If a competing pathway exists, current flows through a stimulating and nonstimulating pathway. The current flow through the non-stimulating pathway lowers the resistance and represents wasted energy. This phenomenon can be seen with poorly positioned endocardial electrodes as well as with epicardial electrodes. Very low acute resistance is unsatisfactory because current is wasted and battery life is shortened, which causes a potential for exit block or an increased incidence of muscle stimulation

due to increased current. Conversely, excessively high resistances (greater than 800 ohms) increase battery life but decrease the current delivered to the heart for both constant-voltage and constant-current pacemakers. For example, current flow from a 5-volt battery through a resistance greater than 1000 ohms is reduced below 5 mA., which is an inadequate safety margin to compensate for eventual chronic threshold elevation.

In addition to measuring stimulation thresholds and resistance, the sensing circuit of the pacemaker must be evaluated. The sensing circuit monitors spontaneous myocardial depolarizations. A cardiac depolarization waveform (P wave or R wave) passes from the myocardium into the electrode and is transmitted via the lead to the sensing circuit of the impulse generator. The sensing circuit is designed to detect electrical signals above a particular amplitude within the frequency range of endocardial electrograms. Measurements of amplitude and frequency are essential to ensure proper operation of the sensing circuit. As shown in Figure 7, an endocardial waveform has both an amplitude and a frequency component. The frequency component of the endocardial signal is approximated by the slew rate for the measured portion of the waveform. The slew rate is defined as

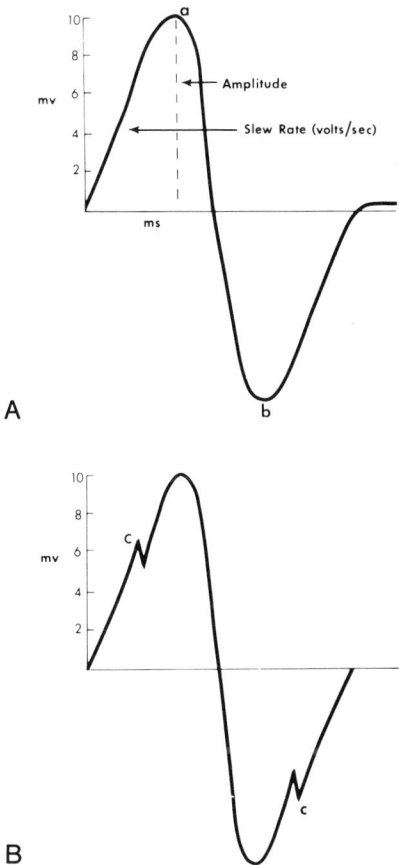

Figure 7. Endocardial waveform analysis. An endocardial waveform, as demonstrated on an electrogram, consists of deflections above and below the baseline. The pacemaker sensing circuit evaluates these deflections by rapidly determining the slew rate (rate of change of the amplitude with respect to time) and amplitude of that deflection. The amplitude is defined by a sensing circuit as the maximal uninterrupted excursion of the wave deflection at a constant slew rate (point a and point b). A change in the slew rate for a deflection such as a notch (point c) on the wave is interpreted as a point of maximal excursion (the amplitude or peak for that deflection). Modern sensing circuits can determine not only the peak deflections (points a, b, and c) from the baseline but also the peak-to-peak deflections across the baseline (point a to point b). The sensing circuit samples only a small portion of the waveform to determine the slew rate and amplitude. The slew rate obtained from a peak deflection above and below the baseline or a peak-to-peak analysis can be extrapolated into a frequency measurement assuming the entire waveform has that slew rate. (From Byrd, C.: Permanent pacemaker implantation techniques. *In* Samet, P., and El-Sherif, N. (Eds.): Cardiac Pacing, 2nd ed. New York, Grune & Stratton, 1980, p. 229.)

millivolts per millisecond (mV./msec.) and represents the rate of change of the amplitude with respect to time. The amplitude of the atrial or ventricular electrogram is measured in millivolts. As this waveform passes through the sensing circuit of the pacemaker, both the amplitude and the slew rate (rate of amplitude rise or frequency) must be acceptable for the signal to be detected. In general, ventricular endocardial electrograms greater than 4 mV. and atrial endocardial electrograms greater than 1.5 mV. in amplitude can be detected and provide a safety margin over time. A slew rate of 0.5 or greater is sufficient for detection of both types of signal.

A pacing system analyzer that is capable of simulating the function of a given pacemaker's output and sensing circuits is provided by each pacemaker manufacturer. In addition, the pacing system analyzer is used to evaluate the pacemaker's rate, interval, pulse width, voltage, current, sensitivity, refractory period, and A-V interval in dual-chamber devices. After complete testing of threshold energy requirements, atrial and ventricular endocardial signals, and pacemaker parameters, high-voltage settings are used to detect diaphragmatic or phrenic nerve stimulation, which requires lead repositioning. The patient is then asked to do deep-breathing and coughing exercises to attempt to produce electrode dislodgment before securing the pacemaker leads and implanting the generator.

PHYSIOLOGY OF PACING

Pacing Modes

Perhaps the most dramatic example of the advancement in pacemaker technology is the various ways in which the heart can be paced. The way in which an impulse generator functions is referred to as the pacing mode. An accurate description of the pacing mode must convey not only the chamber of the heart that is being paced, but also the chamber sensed by the pacemaker and the manner in which the pacemaker responds to sensed activity. Simple descriptive terms such as ventricular-demand pacemaker sufficed well for single-chamber devices but have become more awkward as the complexity of pacemakers increases. Devices that pace and sense both atrial and ventricular activity are now frequently implanted. To meet the need for a uniform method of describing pacemaker function, the Inter-Society Commission for Heart Disease Resources (ICHD) recommended a five-letter code that succinctly and accurately describes various pacing modes.[89] This code was updated in 1987 to accommodate newer pacemakers (Table 3).[9]

The ICHD code uses the letters A and V for atrium and ventricle. The letter D stands for "dual," indicating both chambers or, when indicating a mode of response, more than one mode. The two traditional response modes to sensed activity, either inhibition or triggering, are indicated by I and T. When no function or response is possible, the letter O is used. In the three-letter code system, the first letter designates the chamber(s) paced, the second letter the chamber(s) sensed, and the third letter the mode of response of the pacemaker to sensed activity. Thus, a pacemaker that paces only the ventricle, senses ventricular activity when intrinsic beats are present, and responds to the sensed activity by inhibiting its output (the well-known ventricular-demand pacemaker) is designated VVI in the ICHD code. An asynchronous ventricular pacemaker that does not sense but paces at a constant rate regardless of intrinsic cardiac rhythm would be designated VOO (the ventricle is paced, neither chamber is sensed, and there is therefore no response mode to sensed events). In the case of the standard AV sequential pacemaker in which both the atrium and ventricle are paced but only ventricular activity is sensed, the designation is DVI.

The five-letter code has a tremendous advantage in describing not only a certain pacemaker, but also various possible modes of function incorporated into a single programmable pacemaker. The magnet mode of a pacemaker may also be described. This is the test mode in which a pacemaker functions when the internal reed switch is closed by the external application of a strong magnet. Thus, a VVI pacemaker generally functions in the VOO (asynchronous) mode when an external magnet is applied. Likewise, a sophisticated DDD pacemaker, discussed later, may be programmed to function in one of many modes, including DVI, VVI, AAI, AOO, VDD, and many more.

Fourth and fifth letters are used to denote programmability and antitachycardia capabilities, respectively (Table 3). In this system, the letter P in the fourth position indicates the ability to program one or two parameters, and the letter M represents multiprogrammability. The letter R in the fourth position is used to designate a rate-modulated pacemaker (e.g., VVI-R); an O in the fourth position indicates a nonprogrammable pacemaker. In the fifth position, various antitachycardia functions may be indicated, including P for pacing, S for shock, and D (for both pacing and shock). These modes are discussed later in detail.

Multiple pacing modes are potentially feasible, although only seven modes have real significance in clinical practice. Of these, two (VVI and DVI) have comprised the majority of pacing applications until recently (Table 4).

VVI PACING. Single-chamber ventricular pacing has been the main type of cardiac pacing but is being replaced by more physiologic pacing modes. This mode, often referred to as ventricular-demand pacing, is the simplest of the pacing modes that are routinely used. As the ICHD code states, the pacemaker senses intrinsic ventricular activity and is inhibited when this activity exceeds the standby or escape rate of the pacemaker. When the intrinsic ventricular rate falls below the escape rate of the pulse generator, the pacemaker begins to function at its

TABLE 3. NBG (NASPE/BPEG) Generic Pacemaker Code

Position/ Category	I Chamber(s) Paced	II Chamber(s) Sensed	III Response to Sensing	IV Programmability, Rate Modulation	V Antitachyarrhythmia Function(s)
	O = None A = Atrium	O = None A = Atrium	O = None T = Triggers pacing	O = None P = Simple programmable	O = None P = Pacing (antitachyarrhythmia)
Letter Codes	V = Ventricle D = Dual (A + V)	V = Ventricle D = Dual (A + V)	I = Inhibits pacing D = Dual (T + I)	M = Multiprogrammable C = Communicating (telemetry) R = Rate modulation	S = Shock D = Dual (P + S)

Note: Positions I through III are used exclusively for antibradyarrhythmia pacing. Manufacturers may use "S" in positions I and II to indicate single chamber (A or V). A minimum of four positions is required to describe a pacemaker.

NASPE, North American Society of Pacing and Electrophysiology; BPEG, British Pacing and Electrophysiology Groups.

Adapted from Bernstein, A. D., Camm, A. J., Fletcher, R. D., et al.: The NASPE/BPEG Generic Pacemaker Code for antibradyarrhythmia and adaptive-rate pacing and antitachyarrhythmia devices. PACE, 10:794, 1987.

TABLE 4. Commonly Used Pacing Modes

ICHD Code	Description
VVI	Ventricular demand
VOO	Ventricular asynchronous
AAI	Atrial demand
AOO	Atrial asynchronous
DVI	AV sequential fixed rate
VDD	Atrial synchronous
DDD	AV "universal"
VVI-R	Ventricular rate-modulated

ICHD, Inter-Society Commission for Heart Disease.

programmed rate. The escape rate and the automatic rate (pacing rate) may be identical or may be different if hysteresis is programmed into the pacemaker.

Potential disadvantages of VVI pacing are the lack of AV synchrony and the inability to increase heart rate with physiologic stress. Loss of coordinated contraction of the atria and ventricles may cause unpleasant symptoms due to atrial contraction against a closed tricuspid valve and may produce symptoms of low cardiac output referred to as the pacemaker syndrome. The magnet code for VVI pacemakers (VOO) allows the function of the pacemaker to be observed even when an intrinsic rhythm is present that would otherwise inhibit pacemaker function.

Asynchronous ventricular pacing was used clinically before units capable of inhibition were available. Because of the potential dangers of asynchronous pacemaker function, with paced beats falling in the T wave of preceding spontaneous beats and inducing ventricular arrhythmias, VOO pacing is now relegated to the rare situation in which oversensing causes inappropriate inhibition that cannot be corrected by programming.

AAI PACING. Atrial pacing is potentially of great benefit in patients with intact AV conduction and sinus bradycardia, as in the sick sinus syndrome. Until recently, atrial pacing was not used extensively because of technical problems related to stability of endocardial atrial leads. In addition to achieving stable pacing, the atrial electrode must be able to sense an adequate atrial electrogram to avoid asynchronous atrial pacing, although this is not frought with the potential hazards of asynchronous ventricular pacing. Advances in electrode technology have led to preformed J-shaped atrial tined leads that may be placed in position in the atrial appendage and active fixation leads that can be screwed into the atrial endocardium in other locations. These leads are capable of providing reliable atrial pacing in most patients.

SINGLE-CHAMBER RATE-MODULATED PACING. Single-chamber rate-modulated pacing (VVI-R or AAI-R) has become an important and frequently used pacing mode with the commercial availability of pacemakers using various sensors to regulate the pacing rate. In rate-modulated pacing, the pacing rate is determined by a physiologic parameter, other than atrial rate, that is measured by a special sensor in the pacemaker or pacing lead. Examples of physiologic parameters that are currently used in rate-modulated pacing include body motion, venous blood temperature, the Q-T interval, and respiratory rate. Other parameters that are being developed include mixed venous oxygen saturation, contractility, and stroke volume. Although these pacing systems can theoretically respond to various physiologic stimuli with an increase in heart rate, their main use is to provide an increase in cardiac output with exercise.

Patients who have chronic or intermittent atrial fibrillation and in whom atrial synchronous pacing is impossible may be able to maintain normal heart rate responses to exercise through the use of ventricular rate-modulated pacing. In patients with normal AV conduction and sinus bradycardia that does not respond to exercise, rate-modulated atrial pacing may be indicated.

DVI PACING. Dual-chamber pacing has provided an important improvement over simple ventricular pacing in approximately 40 per cent of patients in whom optimal cardiac function depends on the atrial contribution to cardiac output. Before the development of atrial synchronous pacing, "bifocal" or AV sequential pacing was the only modality available.

In this mode, both the atrium and the ventricle are paced, with an artificial AV delay programmed between the atrial and ventricular impulses. In other respects, these devices function in a manner similar to VVI pacemakers. Only ventricular activity is sensed, thus atrial stimulation is asynchronous if the spontaneous atrial rate exceeds the paced rate. DVI pacemakers may be of two varieties: committed or noncommitted. Committed systems are those in which the ventricular output must be delivered when the atrial pulse has occurred. In these systems, a QRS appearing in the AV interval will not inhibit ventricular output, and the ventricular pulse falls in the QRS or ST segment (Fig. 8). The advantage of the committed system is that false inhibition of the ventricular output due to cross-talk from the atrial channel cannot cause inappropriate failure to pace. In noncommitted systems, ventricular activity occurring in the A-V interval causes inhibition of the ventricular output. Cross-talk from the atrial channel is prevented by means of a blanking period of approximately 20 to 30 msec. after atrial output during which the ventricular sensing circuits are closed. Some systems have used a compromise between these two modes in which sensed ventricular activity after the atrial output causes a paced beat with a shortened A-V interval, thus providing protection from failure to pace and diminishing the chance that the paced beat falls in the vulnerable period, causing an arrhythmia.

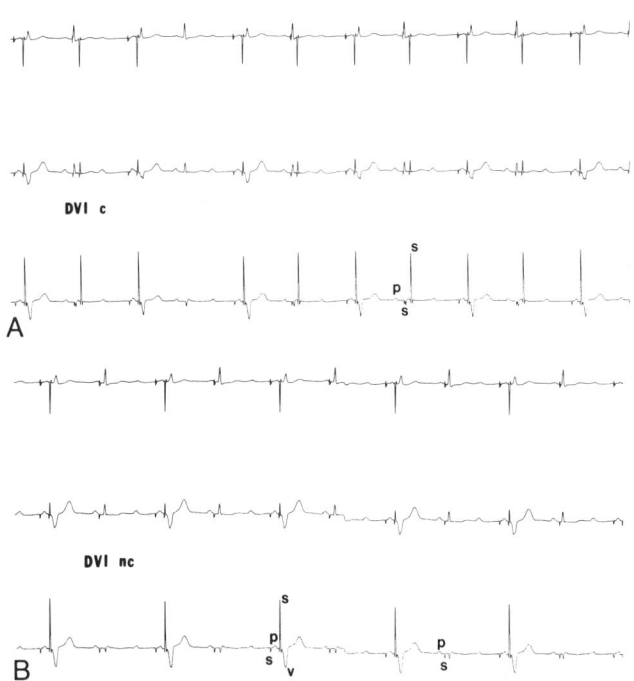

Figure 8. *A*, Simultaneous three-channel rhythm strip showing a normally functioning DVI pacemaker in the committed mode. Even though a normally conducted QRS occurs in the A-V interval (second, sixth, eighth, and tenth complexes), a ventricular pacing output occurs following the QRS. Note that there is no atrial sensing in the DVI mode. The pacemaker is completely inhibited only when a QRS occurs sufficiently early to inhibit both atrial and ventricular outputs (fourth complex). *B*, A normally functioning noncommitted DVI pacemaker. P waves are not sensed in the DVI mode (second, fourth, sixth, eighth, and tenth complexes), and atrial pacing artifacts occur in the P-R interval. Conducted QRS complexes that follow these P waves inhibit the ventricular output.

VDD PACING. One of the primary limitations of DVI pacing is its fixed rate and the need for pacing at a rate faster than the patient's intrinsic sinus rate if the benefits of AV synchrony are to be maintained. Atrial synchronous pacing allows the ventricle to be paced after sensed atrial activity. This method has the advantage of preserving AV synchrony and allowing the ventricular rate to vary as the sinus rate varies. VDD pacing is differentiated from an earlier form of atrial synchronous pacing (VAT) in which the ventricle was paced synchronously with atrial activity, but without sensing in the ventricle.

Advanced forms of dual-chamber pacing (VDD or DDD) have no fixed rate, but rather are programmed to lower and upper rate limits. The way in which the pacemaker functions when the atrial rate exceeds the upper rate limits is also an important feature of these devices.

The upper rate limit is the rate beyond which the pacemaker does not continue to track atrial activity. This is a programmable function that can be set according to the patient's needs. When the atrial rate reaches the upper rate limit, the pacemaker continues to pace at a constant rate (the upper rate), and an apparent Wenckebach's sequence appears.

When atrial activity decreases to the rate programmed as the lower rate limit of the pacemaker, the pacemaker responds in much the same manner as a VVI pacemaker at its escape interval. Because the VDD pacemaker cannot pace the atrium, VVI pacing occurs at the pacemaker's lower rate limit. Failure to sense in the atrium causes pacemaker function at lower rate limits despite the presence of faster atrial activity. A VDD pacemaker has no technologic advantage over present DDD units because both require atrial and ventricular leads, and devices capable only of VDD pacing are now obsolete.

DDD PACING. "Universal" or "automatic" pacing represents the height of pacing technology at the present time although, as discussed in the section on physiologic pacing, not necessarily the optimal form of pacing for every patient. The primary difference between early DDD pacemakers and VDD pacemakers was the ability to pace the atrium at the lower rate limit. Thus, instead of VVI pacing at the low rate, AV synchrony was maintained by DVI pacing. Newer and more sophisticated DDD pacemakers can now be programmed to almost every pacing mode conceivable in addition to DDD, including AAI, VVI, DVI, VVT, and VOO.

With atrial rates above the lower rate limit of the pacemaker, the atrial output is inhibited and the pacemaker tracks atrial activity and responds with ventricular pacing after the programmed AV delay. This method provides a range of rate variation between the lower and the upper rate limits. An upper rate limit is programmed to avoid excessive paced rates in the event of rapid atrial rhythms. When the patient's atrial rate exceeds the upper rate limit of the pacemaker, the pacemaker maintains a fixed ventricular rate, causing an apparent Wenckebach's sequence with gradually lengthening A-V intervals.

The fastest atrial rate the pacemaker can follow is also governed by the duration of total atrial refractoriness, composed of the A-V interval and the postventricular atrial refractory period. If the atrial rate becomes so rapid that alternating P waves fall during the pacemaker's period of atrial refractoriness, they will not be sensed at all and the pacemaker tracks only every other P wave. Injudicious programming of the atrial refractory period of the pacemaker may therefore cause abrupt reversion to 2:1 conduction by the pacemaker at or near the upper rate limit, and the patient has an abrupt decrease in heart rate.

UNIPOLAR VERSUS BIPOLAR PACING. The pacing configuration of any implanted system may be unipolar or bipolar. A unipolar system is one in which the cathode, or negative pole, of the pacemaker battery is connected to the stimulating electrode, and the anode, or positive pole, is connected to an indifferent electrode remote from the actual site being paced. In practice, this indifferent electrode is usually the exterior of the pulse generator. To prevent stimulation of the adjacent skeletal muscle, most of the surface of the pulse generator is insulated and only a small area is left bare.

A bipolar system is one in which two electrodes in proximity are connected to the anode and cathode of the pulse generator. Because cathodal stimulation requires lower energy than anodal stimulation, the electrode in best contact with myocardium is connected to the cathode in either unipolar or bipolar systems. In bipolar transvenous systems, the anode is usually the proximal electrode of the bipolar lead, and the cathode (negative pole) is connected to the distal or tip electrode.

In addition to pacing, sensing is also affected by the configuration of the pacing system. The bipolar system excludes remote electrical activity and is therefore less easily affected by extraneous electrical activity such as skeletal muscle potentials. When patients with unipolar systems are subjected to ambulatory monitoring, a significant incidence of sensing abnormalities is found, mainly related to oversensing of myopotentials with inappropriate inhibition of the pacemaker.[15,104]

Programmability

Programmability is defined as the ability to permanently and noninvasively change one or more of the operating characteristics of an implanted pacemaker. The advantages of modifying pacemaker function after implantation have been apparent for a long time. Early devices were made with the capability of changing rate by inserting a transcutaneous needle that turned a potentiometer in the pacemaker. Noninvasive programming was made possible originally through the use of an external magnet that activated a switch inside the pacemaker and changed its rate in incremental steps.

Almost all pacemakers implanted now have at least one programmable function. The use of programmability in terms of avoiding reoperation for pacing system malfunction and improving the patient's tolerance of the pacemaker has been documented, and essentially no indications exist for the implantation of nonprogrammable pacemakers.[12] Simple programmability usually includes the ability to change rate, pulse width, mode (usually from inhibited to asynchronous), and refractory period. The ability to change many parameters is called multiprogrammability (Table 5). The various programmable functions found in current devices are discussed in detail later in this section.

To effect programming of an implanted pacemaker, a signal must be sent from a programmer to the pacemaker. In practical terms, a programmer must be placed relatively close to the pacemaker to transmit coded information to the pacemaker that is specific for the change desired. The pacemaker must be able to reject inappropriate signals from the environment or from other programmers that could potentially cause unwanted changes in pacemaker functions. The pacemaker may respond by returning a signal to the programmer, indicating acceptance of the programming instructions.

Programming features that are desirable include the ability of the programmer to interrogate the pacemaker to retrieve two kinds of information: (1) the programmed settings of the pacemaker, that is, what the pacemaker is supposed to be doing; and (2) measured data from the pacemaker that indicate what the pacemaker is actually doing, what kind of sensed electrograms

TABLE 5. Commonly Programmable Functions of a Multiprogrammable Impulse Generator

Mode	Hysteresis
Rate	Polarity
Pulse width	A-H interval*
Output	Upper rate limit*
Sensitivity	Lower rate limit*
Refractory period	

* Dual-chamber devices only.

the pacemaker is receiving, and the state of the electrode and battery.

Most pacemakers now use radiofrequency signals to transmit coded information to and from the pacemaker. The functions that can be programmed in a given pacemaker vary considerably depending on the manufacturer and model. Obviously, the functions subject to programmability depend a great deal on the type of pacemaker (e.g., VVI, DVI, DDD). The most important functions for programmability are generally considered to be rate, pulse width, and sensitivity. Most of the potentially correctable problems encountered with implanted pacemakers can be managed by using these functions. Other functions that can be programmed in various models include refractory period, mode, and hysteresis. In dual-chamber pacemakers, the A-V interval, the upper and lower rate limits, and the mode of response to upper rate limit may be programmed. In sophisticated units, the pacemaker may actually be programmed off, blanking periods on atrial and ventricular channels can be changed, polarity can be programmed from bipolar to unipolar, and the pacemaker can even be programmed to respond or not respond to an external magnet.

RATE PROGRAMMABILITY. The ability to change the rate of an implanted pacemaker is the single most useful programmable function. In patients with chronic cardiac disease, cardiac output may be highly rate-dependent. The ability to increase rate allows the individual patient's heart rate to be changed to accommodate temporary changes in physical condition (e.g., cardiac procedures, heart failure, angina pectoris). Some patients develop an unpleasant sensation during pacemaker function or may actually have adverse hemodynamic effects from ventricular pacing. These situations may be remedied by lowering the pacing rate to allow more time in sinus rhythm. The ability to change rate also allows one pacemaker model to be used in all patient age groups, obviating the need for different models for use in pediatric patients who may require higher rates. In most pacemakers, rate can be programmed in steps from 40 to 130 pulses per minute.

OUTPUT PROGRAMMABILITY. The output of the pacemaker in terms of total pacing energy is a function of both voltage and pulse width. Standard lithium-iodine batteries have an output of approximately 2.5 volts. The nominal voltage output of most pacemakers is 5 volts, achieved by the use of a voltage multiplier circuit. The ability to program the voltage output down to the lower value may help greatly in prolonging the battery life when chronic lead thresholds permit a lower stimulation energy. In addition, some models have the capability of increasing voltage output to the 7- to 10-volt range, thus accommodating unusually high pacing thresholds.

Pulse width programmability also allows the output of the pacemaker to be lowered to prolong battery life. Lowering pulse width below 0.3 msec. is not generally recommended, because very high stimulation voltages may be required. Unfortunately, as evident from the strength-duration curve, increasing the pulse width beyond approximately 1 msec. does little to lower the stimulating threshold; thus, raising pulse width in situations of high threshold has little value (see Fig. 6).

SENSITIVITY PROGRAMMABILITY. The sensitivity setting of the pacemaker determines the amplitude of the patient's intrinsic cardiac activity required for proper sensing to occur. A balance must be reached between settings that are oversensitive, which may allow inhibition by extraneous signals such as myopotentials or T waves, and settings that are too insensitive and cause failure to sense intrinsic electrograms. Most pacemakers have a ventricular R wave sensitivity ranging from 1.25 to 5 mV. (the lower value representing the highest sensitivity). In the atrium, sensitivity values of 1.5 to 2.5 mV. are usual. Whether a given electrogram is sensed by a pacemaker depends not only on the actual amplitude of the electrogram, but also on the slew rate, or change in voltage over time (dv/dt). Thus, the programmed sensitivities do not necessarily guarantee adequate sensing of an electrogram based on its peak-to-peak amplitude. The ability to program sensitivity frequently corrects sensing problems that might otherwise require lead repositioning. Failure to sense premature ventricular contractions is a common example of a situation in which failure to sense may develop, despite proper sensing of sinus beats.

REFRACTORY PERIOD PROGRAMMABILITY. The refractory period of the pacemaker is the interval after a sensed or paced event during which the pacemaker is incapable of sensing any electrical activity. This feature prevents inappropriate inhibition of the pacemaker due to artifacts from the pacing stimulus and theoretically prevents sensing of other waveforms of the electrocardiogram such as the T wave. When electrodes are implanted in the atrium for AAI pacing, the refractory period should be extended to prevent sensing of far-field R waves. Occasionally, a pacemaker fails to sense closely coupled premature ventricular contractions that fall in the refractory period of the pacemaker. This problem can be managed by shortening the refractory period.

HYSTERESIS. Hysteresis is a feature that has more theoretic appeal than practical applicability. Hysteresis is usually expressed in terms of the number of pulses per minute below the programmed rate required to initiate pacing. Thus, the escape interval is longer than the automatic or pacing interval. A pacemaker programmed with 20 pulses per minute of hysteresis would remain inhibited until a sensed rate of 40 pulses per minute was present, at which time the pacemaker would begin to pace at a rate of 60 pulses per minute. The theoretic advantage of this function is that the patient is allowed to remain in sinus rhythm at intermediate rates between 40 and 60 beats per minute, but when pacing is required, the heart rate is maintained at the faster rate. A problem often encountered with hysteresis is that the patient's intrinsic rate must exceed the automatic rate to inhibit the pacemaker again. For patients who tend to maintain slow rates, hysteresis works well on the front end of the loop, but when pacing is initiated, patients may be unable to elevate their heart rate sufficiently to once again inhibit the pacemaker.

Physiologic Pacing

The term *physiologic pacing* is used to describe pacing modes that attempt to duplicate normally conducted sinus rhythm.[110,123] This concept assumes an understanding of the physiologic relationships between the conduction of the cardiac impulse and the hemodynamic events it initiates and implies that duplication of this physiology can be achieved with an artificial pacemaker. At best, current artificial pacemakers are only crude substitutes for normal sinus rhythm; therefore, the term physiologic pacing must be considered to be an oversimplification. Physiologic pacing has also been recognized as synonymous with dual-chamber pacing, although this is not necessarily true.

It has been well established that AV synchrony, that is, the contraction of the atria and the ventricles with normal sequence and timing, provides some margin of improved cardiac output when compared with ventricular pacing alone at comparable rates.[59,85,110,111,123] Appropriately timed atrial contraction has been shown to increase cardiac output by as much as 25 per cent.[59,96,100] This difference may be even greater during exercise or in certain pathologic states.[82,97,105] The deleterious effects of AV dissociation due to ventricular pacing vary greatly from one patient to another and depend on the heart's ability to compensate for a fixed rate, the presence of retrograde VA conduction, and the patient's overall level of activity.

The ability to increase heart rate to meet increased metabolic demand is also an important feature of normal cardiac conduction. Cardiac output is related directly to heart rate and stroke volume, and when cardiac disease impairs the ability to increase stroke volume, increased heart rate is the only mechanism remaining to increase cardiac output. Therefore, a physiologic pacing system has two aspects: the maintenance of AV synchrony and the preservation of rate variation. Obviously, these two features can be separated and may not be found in the same pacemaker. The familiar DVI pacemaker, for example, preserves AV synchrony without being able to vary rate in response to physiologic demands. Rate-modulated pacemakers can respond to physiologic stimuli including respiratory rate, Q-T interval, body motion during exercise, mixed venous oxygen saturation, and temperature.[97,123] These devices are particularly suited for patients with chronic atrial fibrillation. Thus, physiologic pacing should not be thought of as only dual-chamber pacing, but rather any pacing system that meets the physiologic needs of the patient.

The pacing modes that offer some preservation of normal physiologic relationships include AAI-R, DVI, VVI-R, and DDD. AAI-R pacing has the advantages of maintaining normal AV conduction, requiring only one electrode, and offering rate variation and is used in patients with chronic sinus bradycardia with intact AV conduction. DVI pacing obviates the concern for AV conduction but has the limitation of fixed rate. DDD pacing offers both rate variation and AV synchrony and is the optimal pacing mode when normal sinus mode function is present.

The acute benefits of AV sequential or atrial synchronous pacing compared with ventricular pacing have been well documented.[96] Numerous studies have also substantiated a sustained hemodynamic benefit of physiologic pacing modalities compared with fixed-rate ventricular pacing. Improvements in acute and chronic exercise capacity, symptoms (dyspnea and fatigue), and even survival have been attributed to rate-modulated and dual-chamber atrial synchronous pacing when compared with simple ventricular pacing.[4,31,59,64,66,67,72,95,97,111,115,123,124]

An often neglected aspect of dual-chamber pacing systems is the A-V interval. This function is programmable on most current models, but little is known regarding the effects of changes in programmed A-V interval. The optimal A-V interval must be defined in relationship to the pacing rate, because physiologically AV conduction shortens with increasing heart rate. A shorter A-V interval may be more appropriate for a patient with an atrial synchronous system in which optimal function during exercise is desired. The surgeon must also appreciate the differences in A-V interval with atrial synchronous pacing compared with DVI pacing. The latency from the atrial stimulus to the onset of atrial systole causes a longer A-V interval than occurs when ventricular pacing follows a sensed atrial event. The location of the atrial electrode also has an effect on the timing of ventricular systole in an atrial synchronous system.

It might be concluded that patients with normal cardiac function and potentially high levels of normal activity should benefit the most from physiologic pacing systems, whereas patients with limited exercise capacity should benefit the least. However, the former patients are probably best able to compensate for a fixed-rate ventricular pacing system through an increase in stroke volume, whereas patients with cardiac disease may depend completely on an increase in heart rate to increase their cardiac output.

An aspect of pacing that may also have significance in terms of physiologic pacing is the pacing site. Normal ventricular contraction is related to the sequence of myocardial depolarization. Ventricular dyssynergy is present during artificial ventricular pacing. This may cause an increase in myocardial oxygen consumption, inefficient ventricular emptying, and abnormal mitral valve function. The deleterious effects of artificial ventricular stimulation may depend on pacing site and are present even when AV synchrony is maintained with DVI pacing. Thus, in patients with intact AV conduction and sinus bradycardia, atrial pacing can be expected to be superior to both VVI and DVI pacing.

Indications for Pacing Modes

AAI PACING. Atrial fixed-rate pacing may be indicated in patients with resting sinus bradycardia and intact AV conduction. Patients with the sick sinus syndrome may be included in this category; however, the potential effects of antiarrhythmic drugs on AV conduction must be considered before an atrial pacing system is implanted. Likewise, the intermittent occurrence of atrial fibrillation would render this pacing mode ineffective. AAI-R (rate-modulated) pacing is indicated when a normal increase in sinus rate with exercise is absent.

Technical problems with atrial lead stability have been mainly overcome with the use of tined J leads, as well as the availability of endocardial screw-in leads. These active fixation leads make atrial pacing possible in patients who have had cardiac procedures with cannulation of the right atrial appendage. Screw-in leads may also be useful in other patients in whom a stable pacing site cannot be found in the atrial appendage. Atrial pacing from the coronary sinus has also been an effective method.[80]

VVI PACING. VVI pacing is indicated in patients who are receiving a pacemaker for the prevention of intermittent symptoms and who have normal sinus rhythm most of the time. VVI pacing systems should not be implanted in patients who would benefit from dual-chamber pacemakers because of unfamiliarity with these systems. The development and ready availability of more sophisticated pacing modalities compel the physician to implant a VVI unit in favor of a dual-chamber or rate-modulated system.

VVI-R pacing is indicated when dual-chamber pacing is not possible because of atrial arrhythmias and when a normal chronotropic response of heart rate to exercise is not present.

VVT PACING. Ventricular-triggered pacing is rarely indicated. Inappropriate inhibition causing failure to pace may be managed by using the VVT mode when reprogramming the sensing threshold is not successful. Another potential application of VVT pacing is in the treatment of re-entrant tachycardias. An external stimulator is used to trigger the pacemaker, causing interruption of the arrhythmia. To prevent sensing of T waves and pacing in the vulnerable period, the sensing refractory period should be extended in pacemakers programmed to the VVT mode.

DVI PACING. Fixed-rate AV sequential pacing devices are rapidly being replaced by pulse generators capable of atrial synchronous pacing. The indications for the use of these systems now are essentially limited to patients with chronic stable sinus bradycardia with unstable AV conduction. As a pacing mode within the capabilities of a DDD system, DVI may be useful when atrial sensing is unreliable or concomitant antiarrhythmic therapy causes sinus bradycardia.

DDD PACING. Atrial synchronous pacing systems are indicated in patients with chronic AV block (second-degree or third-degree) with stable sinus rhythm. Patients with exercise-induced second-degree AV block are also good candidates for a DDD pacemaker.

The pacemaker syndrome is an unusual problem associated with ventricular pacing, although, if carefully sought, symptoms that suggest suboptimal cardiac output may be found more frequently. It may be difficult to prove a causal relationship between nonspecific symptoms such as fatigue and ventricular pacing in patients who often have coexisting cardiopulmonary disease, and care should be taken before replacing a normally functioning VVI system with a dual-chamber system in an attempt to relieve these symptoms. Patients who clearly have hypotension or diminished exercise capacity with a fixed-rate VVI system or who are troubled by symptomatic jugular venous pulsations due to asynchronous atrial contractions may, however, benefit greatly from a dual-chamber pacing system.

Whenever an atrial synchronous system is contemplated, the

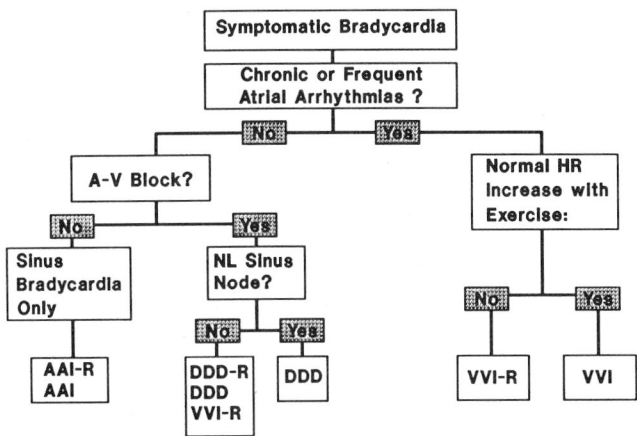

Figure 9. Algorithm for choosing a pacing mode. Patients with frequent atrial arrhythmias are generally not considered candidates for dual-chamber systems but may do well with a rate-modulated pacemaker if they do not increase their heart rate with exercise. Patients with an insufficient heart rate response to exercise and AV conduction abnormalities are candidates for the newer DDD-R pacemakers. Atrial pacing alone should be used only when AV conduction is known to be reliably intact.

presence of retrograde VA conduction must be considered. Retrograde conduction may be a particular problem in patients with the pacemaker syndrome. In these patients, retrograde conduction causing a reversed sequence of AV synchrony during ventricular pacing appears to exacerbate the hemodynamic abnormality. Most atrial synchronous devices have features designed to accommodate retrograde conduction and prevent the development of pacemaker-mediated tachycardia. Mechanisms built into atrial synchronous pacemakers to prevent sensing retrograde atrial activity and initiating pacemaker-mediated tachycardia include programmable atrial refractory period, automatic extension of the atrial refractory period after premature ventricular beats, and temporary reversion to the DVI mode after a premature ventricular beat. If the atrial sensing refractory period of the pacemaker exceeds the V-A interval of the retrograde P wave, the P wave is not sensed and pacemaker-mediated tachycardia cannot develop. Extending the atrial refractory period may be useful in this regard but necessarily limits the upper tracking rate of the pacemaker. Because retrograde VA conduction is likely after a premature ventricular beat, some devices attempt to prevent pacemaker-mediated tachycardia and at the same time preserve upper rate flexibility by keeping the atrial refractory period short normally, but automatically extending the atrial refractory period to a longer value when the pacemaker senses a ventricular event not preceded by an atrial event. Even extending the atrial refractory period cannot guarantee that the retrograde P wave always falls within that refractory period. A further extension of this principle is to totally disable the sensing function of the atrial circuit for one cycle after a premature ventricular beat. This causes the pacemaker to pace AV sequentially and, it is hoped, restores the normal atrial activation sequence.

The use of dual-chamber pacing systems in patients in whom pacemaker implantation is indicated for the prevention of syncope or presyncope due to carotid sinus hypersensitivity is controversial. In these patients, a VVI pacing system may not provide the required hemodynamic support during episodes of bradycardia and hypotension.[76,79,108]

An algorithm for choosing pacing modes based on the presence of atrial arrhythmias and AV conduction is shown (Fig. 9).

ANTITACHYCARDIA PACING

Mechanisms of Arrhythmias

Tachycardias are traditionally considered to follow one of three mechanisms: re-entry, triggered activity, or abnormal au-

tomaticity. Arrhythmias due to triggered activity are rarely documented clinically. Sinus rhythm is the prototype automatic rhythm, and although other arrhythmias due to abnormal automaticity are encountered occasionally, they are not generally amenable to termination by pacing. Arrhythmias due to re-entry are potentially amenable to termination by pacing.

Re-entry may occur around an anatomic circuit such as that created by the presence of an accessory AV pathway in Wolff-Parkinson-White syndrome, or may be created by functionally abnormal tissue such as in coronary artery disease with myocardial infarction or ischemia. The conditions that favor the development of re-entry are abnormally slow conduction in the re-entrant circuit and the presence of unidirectional block in one limb of the circuit. Re-entrant circuits that are large and anatomically defined are easily penetrated by pacing stimuli, whereas smaller re-entrant circuits that may exist within functionally abnormal regions of the heart may be relatively protected and difficult to interrupt.

Supraventricular re-entrant arrhythmias that may be terminated by pacing include reciprocating tachycardia due to the presence of an accessory AV pathway (Wolff-Parkinson-White syndrome), AV node re-entrant tachycardia, some cases of atrial flutter, and less commonly re-entrant tachycardias due to partial AV nodal bypass (Mahaim's) fibers. Ventricular tachycardia is also often amenable to termination by pacing, although the use of pacing techniques in treating ventricular tachycardia is limited by the frequent acceleration of the arrhythmia or the degeneration of the arrhythmia to ventricular fibrillation during attempts at termination.

Factors that determine the ease with which a re-entrant circuit is terminated by pacing include the size of the re-entrant circuit, the location of the pacing site relative to the re-entrant circuit, and the rate of the tachycardia. The functional properties of the myocardium between the site of stimulation and the site of the arrhythmia are also important. Termination of re-entrant tachycardia by pacing stimuli depends on the ability of the paced activation wavefront to penetrate the re-entrant circuit and create an area of refractoriness before the re-entrant wavefront. When the re-entrant wavefront collides with the area of refractoriness created by the paced impulse, the arrhythmia cannot propagate further and terminates. If the paced impulse fails to block the re-entrant circuit, it may instead penetrate the re-entrant circuit and advance or accelerate the tachycardia. Pacing during arrhythmia may also cause fibrillation. These complications are more serious when ventricular tachycardia is the arrhythmia being treated than in the case of supraventricular arrhythmias and may limit the use of pacing techniques in many patients. In addition, extensive electrophysiologic testing before implantation of the pacing device is mandatory to ensure safety and efficacy.

Some clinical considerations are important in the selection of an antitachycardia pacing device. The arrhythmia must be reliably terminated by the technique being considered. In addition, if the patient is to activate the device, the arrhythmia must be well tolerated hemodynamically, and the patient must be able to accurately sense the presence of the arrhythmia and distinguish between the arrhythmia and sinus tachycardia.

Modes of Antitachycardia Pacing

Several pacing techniques have been used successfully to terminate arrhythmias. These techniques include competitive or underdrive pacing, burst pacing, overdrive pacing, and critically timed premature stimuli.

Underdrive pacing was one of the first modalities to be applied and is easily accomplished by applying an external magnet to the implanted pulse generator, causing asynchronous pacing. Termination of the arrhythmia depends on the chance occurrence of an appropriately timed stimulus. Underdrive pacing can also be accomplished by extending the sensing refractory period of a VVI-AAI pacemaker to exceed the cycle length of the tachycardia. Thus, when the heart rate exceeds the refractory period of the pulse generator (spontaneous R-R interval is less than the pulse generator's refractory period), the pulse generator can no longer sense spontaneous activity and begins to function asynchronously. This "reverse" mode of pacing, response to a rapid heart rate as well as a slow one, is often called dual-demand pacing. To make this mode of tachycardia reversion feasible, a pulse generator with a refractory period programmable to greater than 400 msec. is necessary. Devices manufactured by Siemens-Elema and Telectronics have programmable refractory periods as long as 437 msec., causing dual-demand pacing when the heart rate exceeds 137 beats per minute.

Overdrive pacing (pacing at a rate less than 30 beats per minute faster than the tachycardia cycle length) is used frequently on a temporary basis to suppress both atrial and ventricular arrhythmias. Permanent overdrive pacing to suppress arrhythmias has been used most notably in patients with bradycardia-related ventricular tachycardia.

Burst pacing (defined as pacing at a rate greater than 30 beats per minute faster than the tachycardia) is often successful in terminating re-entrant tachycardias (Fig. 10).[33] Burst pacing may be activated by the patient or may be done automatically by an implanted device that senses the onset of tachycardia and responds with a preprogrammed pacing sequence. A device that has been available for routine use for a number of years is the Medtronic model 5998. This device consists of an implantable radiofrequency receiver that is connected to the pacing lead and an external transmitter that can easily be set to the desired pacing rate. The pacing burst is delivered as long as the external device is activated by the patient. This device has the advantages of not requiring an implantable battery (thus eliminating reoperation for battery changes), simplicity of operation, and ease of adjustment. The disadvantage of this system is the need for patients to be able to reliably sense their tachycardia and distinguish arrhythmia from sinus tachycardia. In addition, the tachycardia must be hemodynamically well tolerated to allow the patient time to use the transmitter. Pacing can be done at only one rate without readjustment of the transmitter, although the tachycardia rate may change under various conditions, rendering the device less effective at particular times.

A variation on patient-activated pacing is provided by pulse generators that can be programmed to the triggered mode. An external stimulator applied to the chest wall causes the pacemaker to respond to the transthoracic stimuli and pace the heart at whatever rate or stimulation sequence the external device is set to function. An advantage of this system is the ability of the external device to transmit not only pacing bursts but also timed extra stimuli.

The introduction of critically timed premature stimuli is also an effective method of terminating re-entrant tachycardias. Devices that function automatically to detect and terminate tachycardia are now commercially available. Stimuli may be delivered at present coupling intervals after recognition of tachycardia. In addition, the pacemaker automatically cycles through combinations of coupling intervals if the first sequence fails to terminate the tachycardia. The successful sequence is "remembered" by the device, which automatically begins with these coupling intervals with the next episode of tachycardia, causing prompt arrhythmia conversion. Newer devices also have backup pacing capability to manage the bradycardia that follows tachycardia termination in some patients.

The major limitation of the widespread use of antitachycardia pacemakers in the treatment of serious ventricular arrhythmias has been the potential for arrhythmia acceleration or fibrillation. With ventricular arrhythmias, these adverse effects can be fatal. Extensive preimplant testing has therefore been important to document the efficacy and safety of pacing techniques, because even the development of atrial fibrillation, although not often life-threatening, is usually undesirable.

COMPLICATIONS

As summarized in Table 6, pacemaker complications can be divided into four categories: immediate surgical complications, wound problems, delayed complications, and pacemaker malfunctions. Fortunately, all are relatively uncommon, making pacemaker insertion an exceptionally safe procedure when done by experienced surgeons.

Immediate Surgical Complications

As described earlier, perhaps the safest way of inserting a permanent transvenous lead-electrode system is via the cephalic vein. The risk of pneumothorax, vascular injury, air embolism, and air entrapment within the pacemaker pocket is increased when the subclavian vein access route is chosen. Air entrapment within the pacemaker pocket secondary to pneumothorax with subcutaneous emphysema or secondary to air entrapped during pacemaker pocket closure can cause pacemaker failure in unipolar systems secondary to insulation of the unipolar anodal plate (indifferent electrode) from the subcutaneous tissues.[50,63,69] Neural injury to both the phrenic and recurrent laryngeal nerves has been reported when the lead-electrode system is introduced through the internal jugular vein.[26]

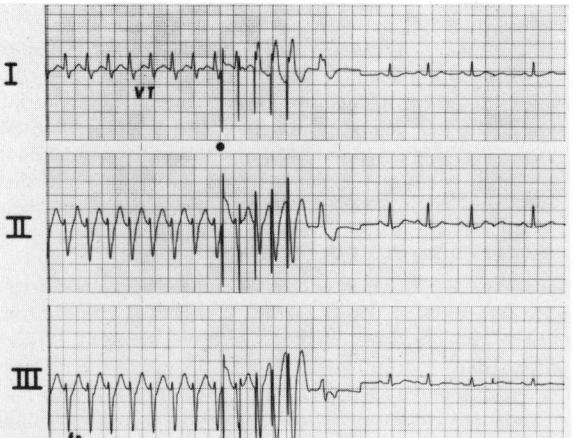

Figure 10. Termination of ventricular tachycardia (VT) with a manually activated radiofrequency pacemaker. A short burst of pacing stimuli causes interruption of the tachycardia. Extensive preimplantation testing was performed to demonstrate safety and efficacy.

TABLE 6. Pacemaker Complications

Immediate Surgical Complications	Delayed Complications
Pneumothorax	Venous thrombosis
Vascular injury	Pulmonary embolism
Air embolism	Twiddler's syndrome
Cardiac perforation	Constrictive pericarditis
Tamponade	Tricuspid insufficiency
Lead-electrode dislodgment	Pacemaker syndrome
Neural injury—phrenic, recurrent laryngeal	**Pacemaker Malfunctions**
Air entrapment in pocket	Radiation damage
	Runaway pacemaker
Wound Problems	Pacemaker-induced ventricular fibrillation
Hematoma	Irregular pacing
Infection	Failure of sensing
Skin erosion	Failure of capture
Migration of impulse generator	Electrode fracture
Skeletal muscle stimulation	Knotting of lead
	Inhibition of pacemaker by skeletal myopotentials
	Electromagnetic interference

Regardless of the venous access route chosen, cardiac perforation can occur but fortunately rarely leads to significant hemopericardium and tamponade.[56] A final complication is immediate electrode dislodgment. The risk of this complication can be reduced by doing provocative maneuvers such as coughing and deep breathing at the time of initial implantation. Transvenous electrode dislodgment problems have not been significantly increased in patients with congenitally corrected transposition of the great vessels, although this would have been expected because of the decreased trabeculation of the embryologic left ventricle, which is where the pacing lead lies.[30]

Wound Problems

Perhaps the most common wound problem associated with permanent pacemaker implantation is a hematoma. Obviously, this complication can be prevented by strict attention to hemostasis at the time of implantation. In patients who require impulse generator change, the pacemaker pocket should be débrided of excess pseudocapsule to prevent the formation of a sterile seroma. Fortunately, wound infection is a rare problem prevented by meticulous operative technique and the appropriate use of prophylactic antibiotics. In general, when infection occurs, the entire pacing system including the impulse generator and lead-electrode system should be removed, the patient should be treated with appropriate intravenous antibiotics, and a temporary pacemaker should be used for an interim period. When infection has completely cleared, a new pacemaker system is implanted through another access site. Skin erosion by either the impulse generator or lead can be prevented by proper positioning of pacemaker hardware deep within the subcutaneous tissues or beneath the fascia of the pectoralis major muscle. Unipolar impulse generators can cause muscle stimulation if placed immediately adjacent to skeletal muscle. However, bipolar impulse generators can be placed either in the subcutaneous tissue or beneath muscle. Migration of the impulse generator most commonly occurs in infraclavicular pacemaker pockets. Migration tends to follow the curvature of the chest wall, and the impulse generator tends to migrate laterally. This can be prevented by creating an anteromedial pocket sufficiently large to contain the impulse generator and lead. In susceptible individuals, the impulse generator can be further secured to the chest wall to prevent migration.

Delayed Complications

Unusual delayed complications associated with transvenous pacemakers include thrombosis of the superior vena cava with resultant superior vena caval syndrome, axillary vein thrombosis with upper extremity edema, cerebral venous sinus thrombosis, and right atrial and right ventricular thrombosis.[13,14,22,36,43,49,61,65,78,84,94,125] Pulmonary thromboembolism has also been recognized as a rare but lethal complication that occurs most often in patients with low cardiac output and underlying right atrial or right ventricular thrombi.[61] Constrictive pericarditis has been reported in patients who have received either transvenous or transthoracic electrodes.[34,102] Tricuspid insufficiency is rare, usually asymptomatic, and secondary to either lead placement or lead removal.[42,86] Electrode dislodgment and lead fracture can be caused by unconscious or habitual "twiddling" of the impulse generator. Twiddler's syndrome has been reported most commonly in patients with transvenous pacing systems but has also been reported in those with transmediastinal pacing systems.[98] Finally, several reports have suggested that permanent pacemaker implantation with the impulse generator lying over the infraclavicular area is associated with an increased risk of breast carcinoma in women. However, based on a careful review in 1980 by Magilligan and Isshak, the appearance of breast cancer in women with pacemakers is probably coincidental and is not related to materials, electrochemical stimulation, or chronic trauma.[77]

Pacemaker Malfunctions

Biomedical engineering improvements have led to exceptionally durable and reliable permanent pacemakers. However, random failures still occur and emphasize the need for appropriate long-term follow-up. Pacemaker malfunctions are secondary to alterations of the preset pacing rate (acceleration or slowing), irregular pacing, failure of sensing, failure of cardiac capture or depolarization, and various combinations of these events. Sudden acceleration of pacing rate, called "runaway pacemaker," causes pacemaker-induced ventricular tachycardia. This complication was most often a manifestation of malfunction of fixed-rate devices. Fortunately, the runaway pacemaker has been rarely encountered because demand ventricular pacemakers have gradually replaced fixed-rate models. In advanced runaway pacemaker syndrome, ventricular fibrillation may occur and lead to sudden death. The runaway pacemaker is a medical emergency and is treated immediately by placement of a new impulse generator.

Slowing of the pacing rate is a more common manifestation of pacemaker malfunction in modern demand impulse generators. Irregular pacing usually indicates an advanced form of malfunction and may be associated with acceleration or slowing of the pacing rate. Failure of sensing can occur as an isolated finding but is commonly associated with failure of cardiac capture. Failure of sensing leads to a demand unit that functions as a fixed-rate pacemaker when its sensing circuit does not work properly. Failure of cardiac capture may be complete but is usually intermittent. The most common cause of failure of capture is malposition of the pacemaker electrode or lead fracture. Electrode displacement may be observed at any time but most often occurs within the first few days after implantation. Late causes of failure of capture are fibrosis around the pacemaker electrode, advancement of underlying heart disease, severe hyperkalemia or hypokalemia, and drug toxicity, especially with quinidine and procainamide. If none of these factors is present, the pacemaker impulse generator itself is most likely malfunctioning.

Ventricular fibrillation can occur during insertion, especially when ventricular fibrillation thresholds are low, such as in patients with acute myocardial infarction. Ventricular fibrillation is uncommon because the R on T phenomenon should not occur in a properly functioning demand pacemaker.

Inhibition of demand pacemakers by myopotentials is always a possibility when unipolar pacing systems are used. Inhibition of bipolar demand pacemakers by noncardiac muscle potentials, however, is a relatively uncommon phenomenon. Transient pacemaker inhibition of unipolar pacemakers may also follow active contraction of the diaphragm, such as that created by deep inspiration, straining, and coughing.

It was previously thought that ionizing radiation did not have any adverse effect on the function of impulse generators. However, reports have suggested that ionizing radiation can cause malfunction of new-generation programmable pacemakers. No deleterious effects can be attributed to diagnostic x-ray exposure, but radiation for therapeutic purposes can cause permanent malfunction of susceptible programmable devices.[1,60] The mode of failure cannot be predicted.

The effect of magnetic resonance imaging (MRI) machines on pacemakers is unpredictable.[52] Pacemakers contain small amounts of ferrous metals and are therefore slightly attracted to magnetic fields. The presence of a strong magnetic field such as is present in MRI scanners causes closure of the reed switch, which would be expected. This leads to asynchronous operation of most pacemakers, except for those in which the magnetic mode of operation can be programmed "off." The radiofrequency pulses used during MRI may also affect pacemaker function, and some devices have for unknown reasons paced at the rapid rate of the radiofrequency pulse. However, permanent reprogramming or damage to pacemakers from MRI equipment has not been encountered. Patients with pacemakers who require MRI should be able to have this procedure done safely if they are monitored carefully for the possibility of rapid pacing during the procedure.

A syndrome that describes a complex of symptoms caused by pacemaker insertion has been recognized. This "pacemaker syndrome" is characterized by vertigo, lightheadedness, syncope, and hypotension occurring after implantation of a ventricular pacemaker. The cause has been attributed to a decrease in cardiac output during ventricular pacing secondary to loss of atrial contribution to ventricular end-diastolic volume. As discussed earlier, the pacemaker syndrome is most likely to occur in patients who require the atrial contribution to cardiac output. The symptoms can usually be relieved by placement of a dual-chamber pacing system that allows more physiologic pacing if lowering the demand pacing rate is ineffectual.

PACEMAKER FOLLOW-UP

An organized follow-up program for pacemaker patients should be provided by every clinic engaged in implanting permanent pacemakers. An adequate follow-up program must do more than merely document normal or abnormal function of a pacemaker, and the purpose of pacemaker follow-up is not just to detect pacemaker failure. Instead, a comprehensive program should provide preimplant and postimplant teaching, continued reassurance for the patient and family, transtelephonic monitoring of both the pacemaker and the patient's spontaneous rhythm, office or clinic visits when necessary, and assistance when admission to the hospital is required for complications, for routine battery changes, or for reasons not related to the pacemaker directly.

A properly designed follow-up program not only should provide support for the patient with a pacemaker but also should be capable of providing important information concerning the patient's pacemaker for the physicians who are involved in patient care. The functions of the pacemaker follow-up program may be summarized as involving the education of both the patient and the physician, documentation of normal and abnormal pacemaker function, detection of complications (surgical and related to pacemaker functions), facilitation of efficient medical care for the patient with the pacemaker, and storage of critical data regarding the pacemaker and electrodes for each patient in an organized system so that it is available to any physician who takes care of the patient. Commercial services can provide transtelephonic electrocardiographic tracings and monitor pacemaker function, but these services cannot substitute for a program that involves the medical personnel involved in pacemaker insertion and patient follow-up.

Although commonly thought to involve primarily transtelephonic electrocardiogram recording, pacemaker follow-up should be an integrated system of postimplant teaching, clinic visits, and telephone transmissions. The goals of teaching the patient when the pacemaker is implanted are to allay the patient's and family's concerns about the pacemaker, to inform the patient about the pacemaker, to inform the patient about the normal function of the pacemaker, and to teach the patient how to use the telephone transmission equipment. A schedule of call-in times should be arranged before discharge, and the use of the transmitter should be practiced with the personnel who will receive the calls. Baseline recordings should be made of the electrocardiogram with and without magnet and an overpenetrated chest film obtained to document lead position.

The patient should be examined as an outpatient at 6 weeks after implantation, at which time a noninvasive assessment of pacing thresholds should be made. This assessment is done in different ways, depending on the model and manufacturer of the pacemaker. Pulse generator output can be decreased in a stepwise manner by shortening pulse width in some generators and by lowering output voltage in others. By observing the point at which capture is lost, an estimation of the chronic pacing threshold can be obtained and the pacemaker's output programmed down to lower levels to prolong battery life. A margin of safety of at least 2:1 over the capture threshold should be maintained. Because pacing thresholds may rise during the first few weeks after implantation, decreasing pacing output, by reprogramming either pulse width or voltage, should not be done earlier than 4 to 6 weeks after implantation.

The return visit also provides an opportunity to carefully examine the surgical site for signs of excessive skin tension, inflammation, or improper wound healing.

Telephone transmissions should begin immediately after discharge and are done weekly for the first 4 weeks to document proper function. Subsequent telephone transmissions should be made regularly, but at longer intervals. In most patients, transmissions are probably not required more frequently than every 6 months in the absence of symptoms. At the time of the telephone transmission, recordings should be made of the spontaneous rhythm, and then with the application of the external magnet. Readings of pulse width and A-V interval (for dual-chamber devices) can also be obtained. These data are recorded in the follow-up files so that proper pacemaker function can be documented and any future malfunctions ascertained. Some pacemakers respond to magnet application with a change in rate and may also automatically begin a cycle of decreasing output to check pacing threshold. It should be borne in mind that the magnet response can be programmed off in some pacemakers.

As the pacemaker begins to approach its theoretic end of life, the frequency of telephone transmissions should be increased. In some models, the pulse width gradually extends before the pacemaker actually begins to change its rate. Thus, the approach of end of life can be monitored as pulse width extends, and the frequency of telephone transmissions can be increased when pulse width has doubled. When the pacemaker finally demonstrates its end of life indicator, usually a drop in rate, elective admission can be arranged and the generator can be replaced.

Finally, records of any reprogramming should be maintained in the follow-up files so that changes in pacemaker function that appear on routine tracings can be properly interpreted.

FUTURE TRENDS

Future trends in cardiac pacing will undoubtedly continue to follow the advances in technology that have characterized the field during the past decade. Improvements in lead-electrode technology can be expected in smaller leads and improved electrodes with lower chronic pacing thresholds causing lower energy requirements and longer battery life. The ability to pace with less energy output may permit the use of smaller batteries, and thus smaller pulse generators.

One of the predictable areas of continued progress is the field of antitachycardia pacing. Devices that can terminate supraventricular tachycardia are currently available and are being refined. Successful treatment of ventricular tachycardia requires the development of devices that incorporate both antitachycardia pacing and backup defibrillation.

The proliferation of programmable pacemakers has required pacemaker centers to stock an increasingly larger number of different manufacturers' programmers. At present, there is no compatibility between the various programmers. Unfortunately, it is unlikely that a device will be devised to program all existing pacemakers. In the future, it would appear to be in the best interests of efficiency and cost reduction to work toward a universal system for pacemaker programmability.

Finally, continued advances in physiologic pacing devices

can also be expected. Among these advances will be pacemakers that respond to various physiologic parameters and allow changes in heart rate that correspond with the patient's physiologic needs.[123]

With further technologic advances in the field of physiologic pacing, improved ways of determining which patients will benefit from these devices will be necessary. This analysis can be accomplished only through clinical databases located at centers that implant and closely monitor large numbers of patients with pacemakers.

SELECTED REFERENCES

Bernstein, A. D., Camm, A. J., Fletcher, R. D., et al.: The NASPE/BPEG generic pacemaker code for antibradyarrhythmia and adaptive-rate pacing and antitachyarrhythmia devices. PACE, 10:794, 1987.
Because of the variety of complex modes of operation available in pacemakers, letter codes were established in 1974 to indicate pacing modes in a condensed form. Recent technical advances in pacemakers have increased the need for an expanded code to reflect these developments. A new pacemaker code proposed by the North American Society of Pacing and Electrophysiology (NASPE) and the British Pacing and Electrophysiology Groups (BPEG) is called the NBG Generic Pacemaker Code. The NBG code expands on the previous Inter-Society Commission for Heart Disease (ICHD) code and was designed to meet two major needs previously not met by other codes. As described in detail in this report, the NBG pacemaker code shows the use of a rate-modulation mechanism to respond adaptively to changes in a physiologic variable, and it indicates the presence of one or more antitachyarrhythmia functions without identifying them specifically. The new five-digit NBG pacemaker code is an expansion of the three-digit ICHD code so that either code can be used with clarity.

Furman, S., Hayes, D. L., and Holmes, D. R.: A Practice of Cardiac Pacing. Mt. Kisco, NY, Futura Publishing Company, 1986.
This well-written, concise, and complete text presents all aspects of permanent and temporary cardiac pacing including electrophysiologic and hemodynamic concepts, indications, implantation techniques, and troubleshooting. Much practical information is provided and also answers to frequently posed questions with regard to pacemakers.

Mond, H. G.: The Cardiac Pacemaker: Function and Malfunction. New York, Grune & Stratton, 1983.
This comprehensive monograph discusses pacemaker function and malfunction in detail and also provides a great deal of historical and fundamental technical information on pacing leads, electrodes, batteries, and circuitry. This source is highly recommended for readers who desire more in-depth information regarding technical considerations in pacemaker design and function.

Morse, D., Steiner, R. M., and Parsonnet, V.: A Guide to Cardiac Pacemakers. Supplement, 1986–1987. Philadelphia, F. A. Davis, 1986.
Almost every modern pacemaker in current use is described in detail in this atlas. Radiographs of each pacemaker are included, and identification codes are thoroughly explained. Available pacemaker lead electrode systems and pacing system analyzers are also covered in detail.

Schechter, D. C.: Exploring the Origins of Electrical Cardiac Stimulation. Minneapolis, Medtronic, Inc., 1983.
This monograph contains selected works of Schechter on the history of electrotherapy. Areas covered in detail include the origins of electrotherapy, the background of clinical cardiac electrostimulation, and early observations on the pathophysiology of ventricular fibrillation. This special volume is exceptionally well illustrated and referenced and represents an outstanding source for those interested in the fascinating history of cardiac pacing.

REFERENCES

1. Adamec, R., Haefliger, J. M., Killisch, J. P., et al.: Damaging effect of therapeutic radiation on programmable pacemakers. PACE, 5:146, 1982.
2. Akhtar, M.: Retrograde conduction in man. PACE, 4:548, 1981.
3. Allen, P., and Lillehei, C. W.: Use of induced cardiac arrest in open heart surgery: Results in seventy patients. Minn. Med., 40:672, 1957.
4. Alpert, M. A., Curtis, J. J., San Felippo, J. F., et al.: Comparative survival after permanent ventricular and dual chamber pacing for patients with chronic high degree atrioventricular block with and without pre-existent congestive heart failure. J. Am. Coll. Cardiol., 7:925, 1986.
5. Anderson, R. H., Becker, A. E., Tranum-Jensen, J., and Janse, M. J.: Anatomico-electrophysiological correlations in the conduction system—a review. Br. Heart J., 45:67, 1981.
6. Armour, J. A., Roy, O. Z., Firor, W. B., et al.: A battery-less biological cardiovascular pacemaker. Surg. Forum, 17:164, 1966.
7. Barold, S. S., and Mugica, J.: Advances in technology and clinical applications. In Barold, S. S. (Ed.): The Third Decade of Cardiac Pacing. Mt. Kisco, NY, Futura Publishing Company, 1982.
8. Berkovits, B. V., Castellanos, A., Jr., and Lemberg, L.: Bifocal demand pacing. Circulation, 39:44, 1969.
9. Bernstein, A. D., Camm, A. J., Fletcher, R. D., et al.: The NASPE/BPEG generic pacemaker code for antibradyarrhythmia and adaptive-rate pacing and antitachyarrhythmia devices. PACE, 10:794, 1987.
10. Bigelow, W. G., Callaghan, J. C., and Hopps, J. A.: General hypothermia for experimental intracardiac surgery. The use of electrophrenic respirations, an artificial pacemaker for cardiac standstill, and radio-frequency rewarming in general hypothermia. Ann. Surg., 132:531, 1950.
11. Bilitch, M., Hauser, R. G., Goldman, B. S., et al.: Performance of cardiac pacemaker pulse generators. PACE, 4:254, 1981.
12. Billhardt, R. A., Rosenbush, S. W., and Hauser, R. G.: Successful management of pacing system malfunctions without surgery: The role of programmable pulse generators. PACE, 5:675, 1982.
13. Bradof, J., Sands, M. J., and Lakin, P. C.: Symptomatic venous thrombosis of the upper extremity complicating permanent transvenous pacing: Reversal with streptokinase infusion. Am. Heart J., 104:1112, 1982.
14. Branson, J. A.: Radiology of cardiac pacemakers and their complications with three cases of superior vena caval obstruction. Australas. Radiol., 22:125, 1978.
15. Breivik, K., and Ohm, O: Myopotential inhibition of unipolar QRS-inhibited (VVI) pacemakers, assessed by ambulatory Holter monitoring of the electrocardiogram. PACE, 3:470, 1980.
16. Brockman, S. K., Webb, R. C., Jr., and Bahnson, H. T.: Monopolar ventricular stimulation for the control of acute surgically produced heart block. Surgery, 44:910, 1958.
17. Byrd, C. C.: Permanent pacemaker implantation techniques. In Samet, P., and El-Sherif, N. (Eds.): Cardiac Pacing, 2nd ed. New York, Grune & Stratton, 1980, p. 229.
18. Calfee, R. V., and Saulson, S. H.: A voluntary standard for 3.2 mm unipolar and bipolar pacemaker leads and connectors. PACE, 9:1181, 1986.
19. Calvin, J. W.: Intraoperative pacemaker electrical testing. Ann. Thorac. Surg., 26:165, 1978.
20. Chardack, W. M., Gage, A. A., Federico, A. J., et al.: Five years clinical experience with an implantable pacemaker: An appraisal. Surgery, 58:815, 1965.
21. Chardack, W. M., Gage, A. A., and Greatbatch, W.: A transistorized self-contained, implantable pacemaker for the long-term correction of heart block. Surgery, 48:643, 1960.
22. Cholankeril, J. V., Joshi, R. R., and Ketyer, S.: Benign superior vena cava syndrome caused by transvenous cardiac pacemaker. Cardiovasc. Intervent. Radiol., 5:40, 1982.
23. Chung, E. K.: Artificial Cardiac Pacing: Practical Approach, 2nd ed. Baltimore, Williams & Wilkins, 1984.
24. Cywinski, J. K., Hahn, A. W., Nichols, M. F., et al.: Performance of implanted biogalvanic pacemakers. PACE, 1:117, 1978.
25. Dhingra, R. C., Denes, P., Wu, D., et al.: The significance of second degree atrioventricular block and bundle branch block: Observations regarding site and type of block. Circulation, 49:638, 1974.
26. Dieter, R. A., Jr., Asselmeier, G. H., Hamouda, F., et al.: Neural complications of transvenous pacemaker implantation: Hoarseness and diaphragmatic paralysis: Case reports. Milit. Med., 146:647, 1981.
27. Domenighetti, G., and Perret, C.: Intraventricular conduction disturbances in acute myocardial infarction: Short- and long-term prognosis. Eur. J. Cardiol., 11:51, 1980.
28. Ekestrom, S., Johansson, L., and Lagergren, H.: Behandling av Adams-Stokes syndrom med en intracardiell pacemaker elektrod. Opusc. Med., 7:1, 1962.
29. Elmquist, R., and Senning, A.: Implantable pacemaker for the heart. In Smyth, C. N. (Ed.): Medical Electronics. Proceedings on the Second International Conference on Medical Electronics, Paris, June 1959. London, Iliffe & Sons, Ltd., 1960.
30. Estes, N. A. M., III, Salem, D. N., Isner, J. M., and Gamble, W. J.: Permanent pacemaker therapy in corrected transposition of the great arteries: Analysis of site of lead placement in 40 patients. Am. J. Cardiol., 52:1091, 1983.
31. Faerestrand, S., and Ohm, O-J.: A time-related study of the hemodynamic benefit of atrioventricular synchronous pacing evaluated by Doppler echocardiography. PACE, 8:838, 1985.
32. Fischell, R. E., Lewis, K. B., Schulman, J. H., et al.: A long-lived, reliable, rechargeable cardiac pacemaker. In Schaldach, M. (Ed.): Advances in Pacemaker Technology. New York, Springer-Verlag, 1975, p. 357.
33. Fisher, J. D., Kim, S. G., Furman, S., and Matos, J. A.: Role of implantable pacemakers in control of recurrent ventricular tachycardia. Am. J. Cardiol., 49:194, 1982.
34. Foster, C. J.: Constrictive pericarditis complicating an endocardial pacemaker. Br. Heart J., 47:497, 1982.
35. Friedberg, C. K., Donoso, E., and Stein, W. G.: Nonsurgical acquired heart block. Ann. N.Y. Acad. Sci., 111:835, 1964.
36. Fritz, T., Richeson, J. F., Fitzpatrick, P., and Wilson, G.: Venous obstruction: A potential complication of transvenous pacemaker electrodes. Chest, 83:534, 1983.
37. Furman, S., and Robinson, G.: Stimulation of the ventricular endocardial surface in control of complete heart block. Ann. Surg., 150:841, 1959.
38. Furman, S., and Schwedel, J. B.: An intracardiac pacemaker for Stokes-Adams seizures. N. Engl. J. Med., 261:943, 1959.
39. Furman, S., Escher, D. J. W., Solomon, N., et al.: Electrocardiographic manifestation of standby pacing. J. Thorac. Cardiovasc. Surg., 54:723, 1967.

40. Furman, S., Pannizzo, F., and Campo, I.: Comparison of active and passive leads for endocardial pacing. II. PACE, 4:78, 1981.

41. Furman, S., Schwedel, J. B., Robinson, G., and Hurwitt, E. S.: Use of an intracardiac pacemaker in the control of heart block. Surgery, 49:98, 1961.

42. Gibson, T. C., Davidson, R. C., and DeSilvey, D. L.: Presumptive tricuspid valve malfunction induced by a pacemaker lead: A case report and review of the literature. PACE, 3:88, 1980.

43. Girard, D. E., Reuler, J. B., Mayer, B. S., et al.: Cerebral venous sinus thrombosis due to indwelling transvenous pacemaker catheter. Arch. Neurol., 37:113, 1980.

44. Glenn, W. W. L., Mauro, A., Longo, E., et al.: Remote stimulation of the heart by radiofrequency transmission: Clinical application to a patient with Stokes-Adams syndrome. N. Engl. J. Med., 261:948, 1959.

45. Goetz, R. H., Dormandy, J. A., and Berkovits, B.: Pacing on demand in the treatment of atrioventricular conduction disturbances of the heart. Lancet, 2:599, 1966.

46. Goldman, B. S., and Parsonnet, V.: Cardiac pacing, data collection, and world surveys. PACE, 2:115, 1979.

47. Gott, V. L., Sellers, R., and Lillehei, C. W.: The development of an epicardial-endocardial electrode for permanent placement in Stokes-Adams disease. Surg. Forum, 11:250, 1960.

48. Guidelines for Permanent Cardiac Pacemaker Implantation, May 1984. Subcommittee on Pacemaker Implantation–Joint AC/AHA Taskforce on Assessment of Cardiovascular Procedures. J. Am. Coll. Cardiol., 4:434, 1984.

49. Gundersen, T., Abrahamsen, A. M., and Jorgensen, I.: Thrombosis of superior vena cava as a complication of transvenous pacemaker treatment. Acta Med. Scand., 212:85, 1982.

50. Hearne, S. F., and Maloney, J. D.: Pacemaker system failure secondary to air entrapment within the pulse generator pocket: A complication of subclavian venipuncture for lead placement. Chest, 82:651, 1982.

51. Hindman, M. C., Wagner, G. S., Jo Ro, M., et al.: The clinical significance of bundle branch block complicating acute myocardial infarction. II: Indications for temporary and permanent pacemaker insertion. Circulation, 58:689, 1978.

52. Holmes, D. R., Jr., Hayes, D. L., Gray, J. E., and Merideth, J.: The effects of magnetic resonance imaging on implantable pulse generators. PACE, 9:360, 1986.

53. Hughes, J. C., Jr., Brownlee, R. R., and Tyers, G. F.: Failure of demand pacing with small surface area electrodes. Circulation, 54:128, 1976.

54. Hunter, S. W., Roth, N. A., Bernardez, D., et al.: A bipolar myocardial electrode for complete heart block. Lancet, 70: 506, 1959.

55. Hyman, A. S.: Resuscitation of the stopped heart by intracardial therapy. II: Experimental use of an artificial pacemaker. Arch. Intern. Med., 50:283, 1932.

56. Irwin, J. M., Greer, G. S., Lowe, J. E., et al.: Atrial lead perforation: A case report. PACE, 10:1378, 1987.

57. Johansson, B. W.: Longevity in complete heart block. Ann. N.Y. Acad. Sci., 167:1031, 1969.

58. Kantrowitz, A., Cohen, R., Raillard, H., et al.: The treatment of complete heart block with an implanted, controllable pacemaker. Surg. Gynecol. Obstet., 115:415, 1962.

59. Kappenberger, L., Gloor, H. O., Babotai, I., et al.: Hemodynamic effects of atrial synchronization in acute and long-term ventricular pacing. PACE, 5:639, 1982.

60. Katzenberg, C. A., Marcus, F. I., Heusinkveld, R. S., et al.: Pacemaker failure due to radiation therapy. PACE, 5:156, 1982.

61. Kinney, E. L., Allen, R. P., Weidner, W. A., et al.: Recurrent pulmonary emboli secondary to right atrial thrombus around a permanent pacing catheter: A case report and review of the literature. PACE, 2:196, 1979.

62. Kleinert, M., Elmqvist, H., and Strandberg, H.: Spectral properties of atrial and ventricular endocardial signals. PACE, 2:11, 1979.

63. Kreis, D. J., Jr., Licalzi, L., and Shaw, R. K.: Air entrapment as a cause of transient cardiac pacemaker malfunction. PACE, 2:641, 1979.

64. Kristensson, B. E., Arnmon, K., Smedgard, P., and Ryden, L.: Physiological versus single-rate ventricular pacing: A double-blind cross-over study. PACE, 8:73, 1985.

65. Krug, J., and Zerbe, F.: Major venous thrombosis: A complication of transvenous pacemaker electrodes. Br. Heart J., 44:158, 1980.

66. Kruse, I. B., and Ryder, L.: Comparison of physical work capacity and systolic time intervals with ventricular inhibited and atrial synchronous ventricular inhibited pacing. Br. Heart J., 46:129, 1981.

67. Kruse, I., Arnman, K., Conradson, T. B., and Ryden, L.: A comparison of the acute and long-term hemodynamic effects of ventricular inhibited and atrial synchronous ventricular inhibited pacing. Circulation, 65:846, 1982.

68. Lagergren, J., and Johansson, L.: Intracardiac stimulation for complete heart block. Acta Chir. Scand., 125:562, 1963.

69. Lasala, A. F., Fieldman, A., Diana, D. J., and Humphrey, C. B.: Gas pocket causing pacemaker malfunction. PACE, 2:183, 1979.

70. Leatham, A., Cook, P., and Davies, J. G.: External electric stimulator for treatment of ventricular standstill. Lancet, 2:1185, 1956.

71. Lemberg, L., Castellanos, A., Jr., and Berkovits, B.: Pacing on demand in AV block. J.A.M.A., 191:12, 1965.

72. Levy, S., Gerard, R., Jausseran, J. M., et al.: Long-term results of permanent atrioventricular sequential demand pacing. PACE, 2:175, 1979.

73. Lillehei, C. W., Gott, V. L., Hodges, P. C., Jr., et al.: Transistor pacemaker for

74. Lillehei, C. W., Levy, M. J., Bonnabeau, M. D., Jr., et al.: The use of a myocardial electrode and pacemaker in the management of acute postoperative and postinfarction complete heart block. Surgery, 56:463, 1964.

75. Lowe, J. E., Hartwich, T., Takla, M. W., and Schaper, J.: Ultrastructure of electrophysiologically identified human sinoatrial nodes. Basic Res. Cardiol. 83:401, 1988.

76. Madigan, N. P., Flaker, G. C., Curtis, J. J., et al.: Carotid sinus hypersensitivity: Beneficial effects of dual-chamber pacing. Am. J. Cardiol., 53:1034, 1984.

77. Magilligan, D. J., Jr., and Isshak, G.: Carcinoma of the breast in a pacemaker pocket. Simple recurrence of oncotaxis? PACE, 3:220, 1980.

78. Mitrovic, V., Thormann, J., Schlepper, M., and Neuss, J.: Thrombotic complications with pacemakers. Int. J. Cardiol., 2:363, 1983.

79. Morley, C. A., Perrins, E. J., Grant, P., et al.: Carotid sinus syncope treated by pacing: Analysis of persistent symptoms and role of atrioventricular sequential pacing. Br. Heart J., 47:411, 1982.

80. Moss, A. J., and Rivers, R. J., Jr.: Atrial pacing from the coronary vein: Ten-year experience in 50 patients with implanted pervenous pacemakers. Circulation, 57:103, 1978.

81. Myers, G. H., Parsonnet, V., Zucker, I. R., et al.: Biologically-energized cardiac pacemakers. Am. J. Med. Electron., 3:233, 1964.

82. Narahara, K. A., and Blettel, M. L.: Effects of rate on left ventricular volumes and ejection fraction during chronic ventricular pacing. Circulation, 67:323, 1983.

83. Nicks, R., Stening, G. F., and Hulme, E. C.: Some observations on the surgical treatment of heart block in degenerative heart disease. Med. J. Aust., 49:857, 1962.

84. Nicolosi, G. L., Charmet, P. A., and Zanuttini, D.: Large right atrial thrombosis: Rare complication during permanent transvenous endocardial pacing. Br. Heart J., 43:199, 1980.

85. Ogawa, S., Dreifus, L. S., Shenoy, P. N., et al.: Hemodynamic consequences of atrioventricular and ventriculoatrial pacing. PACE, 1:8, 1978.

86. Ong, L. S., Barold, S. S., Craver, W. L., et al.: Partial avulsion of the tricuspid valve by tined pacing electrode. Am. Heart J., 102:798, 1981.

87. Parsonnet, V.: Implantation of Transvenous Pacemakers. Tarpon Springs, FL, Tampa Tracings, 1972.

88. Parsonnet, V., Bernstein, A. D., and Norman, J. C.: Dual-chamber pacing for cardiac arrhythmias: Controversies in cloning the conduction system. Tex. Heart Inst. J., 11:208, 1984.

89. Parsonnet, V., Furman, S., and Smyth, N. P.: A revised code for pacemaker identification. PACE, 4:400, 1981.

90. Parsonnet, V., Myers, G. H., and Kresh, Y. M.: Characteristics of intracardiac electrograms. II: Atrial endocardial electrograms. PACE, 3:406, 1980.

91. Parsonnet, V., Werres, R., Atherley, T., et al.: Transvenous insertion of double set of permanent electrodes: Atraumatic technique for atrial synchronous and atrial ventricular sequential pacemakers. J.A.M.A., 243:62, 1980.

92. Parsonnet, V., Zucker, I. R., Gilbert, L., et al.: An intracardiac bipolar electrode for interim treatment of complete heart block. Am. J. Cardiol., 10:261, 1962.

93. Parsonnet, V., Zucker, I. R., Gilbert, L., et al.: Clinical use of an implantable standby pacemaker. J.A.M.A., 196:784, 1966.

94. Pauletti, M., Pingitore, R., and Contini, C.: Superior vena cava stenosis at site of intersection of two pacing electrodes. Br. Heart J., 42:487, 1979.

95. Perrins, E. J., Morley, C. A., Chen, S. L., and Sutton, R.: Randomized controlled trial of physiological and ventricular pacing. Br. Heart J., 50:112, 1983.

96. Reiter, M. J., and Hindman, M. C.: Hemodynamic effects of acute atrioventricular sequential pacing in patients with left ventricular dysfunction. Am. J. Cardiol., 49:687, 1982.

97. Rickards, A. F., and Donaldson, R. M.: Rate responsive pacing. Clin. Prog. Pacing Electrophysiol., 1:12, 1983.

98. Rodan, B. A., Lowe, J. E., and Chen, J. T. T.: Abdominal twiddler's syndrome. Am. J. Roentgenol., 131: 1084, 1978.

99. Samet, P., and El-Sherif, N.: Cardiac Pacing, 2nd ed. New York, Grune & Stratton, 1980, pp. 631–643.

100. Samet, P., Bernstein, W. H., Nathan, D. A., and Lopez, A: Atrial contribution to cardiac output in complete heart block. Am. J. Cardiol., 16:1, 1965.

101. Schechter, D. C.: Exploring the Origins of Electrical Cardiac Stimulation. Minneapolis, Medtronic, Inc., 1983, p. 91.

102. Schwartz, D. J., Thanavaro, S., Kleiger, R. E., et al.: Epicardial pacemaker complicated by cardiac tamponade and constrictive pericarditis. Chest, 76:226, 1979.

103. Schwedel, J. B., Furman, S., and Escher, D. J. W.: Use of an intracardiac pacemaker in the treatment of Stokes-Adams seizures. Prog. Cardiovasc. Dis., 3:170, 1960.

104. Secemsky, S. I., Hauser, R. G., Denes, P., and Edwards, L. M.: Unipolar sensing abnormalities: Incidence and clinical significance of skeletal muscle interferences and undersensing in 228 patients. PACE, 5:10, 1982.

105. Shapland, J. E., MacCarter, D., Tockman, B., and Knudson, M.: Physiologic benefits of rate responsiveness. PACE, 6:329, 1983.

106. Smyth, N. P. D., Basu, A. P., Bacos, J. M., et al.: Permanent transvenous synchronous cardiac pacing. Chest, 59:493, 1971.

107. Stoney, W. S., Alford, W. C., Jr., Burrus, G. R., et al.: Cost of cardiac pacing. Am. J. Cardiol., 37:23, 1976.

108. Stryjer, D., Friedensohn, A., and Schlesinger, Z.: Ventricular pacing as the

treatment of complete atrioventricular dissociation. J.A.M.A., 172:2007, 1960.

preferable mode for long-term pacing in patients with carotid sinus syncope of the cardioinhibitory type. PACE, 9:705, 1986.

109. Sutton, R., Morley, C., Chan, S. L., and Perrins, J.: Physiological benefits of atrial synchrony in paced patients. PACE, 6:327, 1983.

110. Sutton, R., Perrins, J., and Citron, P.: Physiological cardiac pacing. PACE, 3:207, 1980.

111. Sutton, R., Perrins, J., Morley, C., and Chen, S. L.: Sustained improvement in exercise tolerance following physiological cardiac pacing. Eur. Heart. J., 4:781, 1983.

112. Thevenet, A., Hodges, P. C., and Lillehei, C. W.: The use of a myocardial electrode inserted percutaneously for control of complete atrioventricular block by an artificial pacemaker. Dis. Chest, 34:621, 1958.

113. Tyers, G. F. O., and Brownlee, R. R.: Power pulse generators, electrodes and longevity. Prog. Cardiovasc. Dis., 23:421, 1981.

114. Venkataraman, K., and Bilitch, M.: Intracardiac electrocardiography during permanent pacemaker implantation: Predictors of cardiac perforation. Am. J. Cardiol., 44:225, 1979.

115. Videen, J. S., Huang, S. K., Bazga, I. D., et al.: Hemodynamic comparison of ventricular pacing, atrioventricular sequential pacing, and atrial synchronous ventricular pacing using radionuclide ventriculography. Am. J. Cardiol., 57:1305, 1986.

116. Waldo, A. L., and MacLean, W. A. H.: Diagnosis and treatment of cardiac arrhythmias following open heart surgery: Emphasis on the use of atrial and ventricular epicardial wire electrodes. Mt. Kisco, NY, Futura Publishing Company, 1980, p. 115.

117. Weirich, W. L., and Roe, B. B.: The role of pacemakers in the management of surgically induced complete heart block. Am. J. Surg., 102:293, 1961.

118. Weirich, W. L., Gott, V. L., and Lillehei, C. W.: The treatment of complete heart block by the combined use of myocardial electrode and an artificial pacemaker. Surg. Forum, 8:360, 1957.

119. Weirich, W. L., Paneth, M., Gott, V. L., and Lillehei, C. W.: Control of complete heart block by use of an artificial pacemaker and a myocardial electrode. Circ. Res., 6:410, 1958.

120. Weirich, W. L., Paneth, M., Gott, V. L., and Lillehei, C. W.: The treatment of complete heart block by the use of an artificial pacemaker and a myocardial electrode. Am. J. Cardiol., 2:250, 1958.

121. Welti, J. J.: Premature lithium batteries depletion. PACE, 4:349, 1981.

122. Williams, E. H., Tyers, G. F., and Shaffer, C. W.: Symptomatic deep venous thrombosis of the arm associated with permanent transvenous pacing electrodes. Chest, 73:613, 1978.

123. Wirtzfield, A., Schmidt, G., Himmler, F. C., and Stangl, K.: Physiologic pacing: Present status and future developments. PACE, 10:41, 1987.

124. Yee, R., Benditt, D. G., Kostuk, W. J., et al.: Comparative functional effects of chronic ventricular demand and atrial synchronous ventricular inhibited pacing. PACE, 7:23, 1984.

125. Youngson, G. G., McKenzie, F. N., and Nichol, P. M.: Superior vena cava syndrome: Case report. A complication of permanent transvenous endocardial cardiac pacing requiring surgical correction. Am. Heart J., 99:503, 1980.

126. Zoll, P. M.: Resuscitation of the heart in ventricular standstill by external electric stimulation. N. Engl. J. Med., 247:768, 1952.

127. Zoll, P. M., Frank, J. A., Zarsky, L. R. N., et al.: Long-term electric stimulation of the heart for Stokes-Adams disease. Ann. Surg., 154:330, 1961.

XXIII

THE USE OF CARDIOVASCULAR PHARMACOLOGIC AGENTS IN SURGICAL PATIENTS

Robert W. Anderson, M.D., and Kim M. Loria, M.D.

The changing population of patients who are older and have multiple associated diseases together with the rapid advances in biomedical technology requires that the surgeon be knowledgeable in a variety of basic and clinical sciences so that the best care for these patients can be provided. It is important to be familiar with the principles of clinical pharmacology. This chapter is limited to a consideration of the various drugs that are commonly employed in the management of cardiovascular problems that occur in patients requiring surgical therapy or may occur during the intraoperative or postoperative period. The preoperative patient who is hypertensive or has symptomatic coronary artery or valvular heart disease may take medication for modification of symptoms or prolongation of life. Some of these drugs have profound effects on the circulatory system and may significantly alter the safe conduct of an operation.

EVALUATION OF OPERATIVE RISK: CARDIOVASCULAR FACTORS

Operative risk is defined as the probability of morbidity or mortality from preoperative preparation, anesthesia, the surgical procedure, or postoperative convalescence. The decision as to whether to proceed with any therapeutic intervention, whether medical or surgical, must be determined by the potential risks and benefits of the intervention as contrasted with the natural history of the disorder. The cardiovascular system is particularly important in this evaluation, since myocardial infarction, stroke, and congestive heart failure are among the most common complications that occur in surgical patients.

In most cardiac patients undergoing noncardiac surgical procedures, the greatest potential risk arises from coronary artery disease. Data from three large series including 46,000 patients show the risk of perioperative myocardial infarction is 0.15 per cent in patients without prior clinical evidence of heart disease.[9,18,23] In those with a prior myocardial infarction, the incidence of reinfarction during a major noncardiac operation averages approximately 6 per cent.

It is important to emphasize that the risk of perioperative infarction is inversely related to the time between the preoperative myocardial infarction and the noncardiac surgical procedure, and that this risk follows a curvilinear, rather than a linear, relationship. A noncardiac surgical procedure performed within 3 months after an acute infarction has been associated with a reinfarction rate of approximately 30 per cent, whereas at 3 to 6 months after an infarction, the corresponding rate is approximately 14 per cent and falls to 4 per cent after 6 months.

Recently, Rao and colleagues[18] demonstrated a significant decrease in reinfarction rates with the implementation of aggressive and comprehensive perioperative management that was guided by noninvasive hemodynamic monitoring.

Despite multiple advances in intraoperative and postoperative care, the mortality from perioperative myocardial infarction remains high and averages approximately 50 per cent. The risk of cardiac death from reinfarction less than 6 months after a preoperative myocardial infarction is significantly greater than that observed after 6 months, at which time the risk of death is similar to that in patients with no history of cardiac disease who have a perioperative infarction. Factors that appear to be particularly important in evaluating the status of the patient with cardiac disease who is being considered for a major surgical procedure are outlined in Table 1.

TABLE 1. Cardiac Risk Factors in Noncardiac Surgical Patients

Historical Factors
Myocardial infarction (especially within the past 3 months)
Congestive heart failure (especially if refractory)
Angina pectoris
Poorly controlled hypertension
Symptomatic cardiac rhythm disturbance

Physical Examination Findings
Presence of third heart sound gallop or venous distention
Abnormal cardiac rhythm
Pulmonary rales
Significant valvular murmur
Hypertension

Laboratory Findings
Cardiomegaly on chest film
Ischemic changes on electrocardiogram (rest or stress)
Ventricular ectopy on electrocardiogram
Abnormal cardiac rhythm

Obtaining a thorough cardiovascular history is vital for noncardiac surgical procedures, and the findings must be correlated with the chest film and electrocardiogram. A history and the chronology of prior myocardial infarction should be elicited and evidence of left ventricular dysfunction carefully sought. Close attention should also be paid to the presence, severity, and pattern of angina pectoris and to the efficacy and appropriateness of the current medical program. Exercise stress testing may be useful in determining the functional limitation of a patient with suspected ischemic heart disease. Even if minimal symptoms of ischemic heart disease are present, stress testing should be undertaken before a major upper abdominal, intrathoracic, or peripheral vascular surgical procedure if the patient gives a prior history of myocardial infarction, demonstrates symptomatic left ventricular dysfunction, or has diabetes mellitus. Coronary arteriography should be performed if the patient is unable to exercise to an adequate workload because of ischemic symptoms or demonstrates other signs of an early positive high-risk stress test. In such a situation, coronary revascularization must be considered before the noncardiac surgical procedure.

Severe valvular heart disease should be evident on physical examination. The cause and severity of valvular heart disease can usually be clarified by echocardiography, but cardiac catheterization may be required in certain cases.

CARDIOVASCULAR DRUGS: MANAGEMENT IN THE PERIOPERATIVE PERIOD

During the past decade, there has been a substantial decrease noted in the mortality from cardiovascular diseases. Although there is a great deal of speculation as to the reasons for this decline, no definitive data are available for explaining this phenomenon. Modifications in dietary habits and an increasing awareness of physical fitness are most frequently cited as the reasons for the improvement in cardiovascular health. There is good evidence that the use of modern pharmacologic therapy for controlling hypertension, modifying the effects of ischemic heart disease, and altering the hemostatic mechanism on a chronic basis in order to prevent cerebrovascular events has had an important role in lowering cardiovascular disease mortality.[21] As a consequence, a larger number of patients are surviving the ravages of cardiovascular disease and are seen by surgeons for problems, both cardiovascular and noncardiovascular, requiring surgical treatment. Because of older age and associated illnesses, these patients present risks that must be carefully considered in the design of their overall surgical man-

agement plan. An important aspect of planning is the evaluation of how any essential preoperative pharmacologic agent may influence operative management.

There are many drugs that are employed in the management of cardiovascular diseases, but five general categories encompass the majority of commonly used agents: (1) antihypertensives and diuretics; (2) agents for the management of chronic congestive heart failure; (3) antianginal drugs; (4) inotropic drugs; and (5) antiarrhythmics. Overlap exists between these drugs, and the indications for their use may include several of the broader categories cited. Moreover, it is important to remember that both the drug and the disease for which it is prescribed influence the course of anesthetic and surgical management.

Antihypertensives and Diuretics

Hypertension is a common concern in patients seeking medical therapy, and the number of patients being treated for this disorder has increased substantially during the past 2 decades. In approximately 95 per cent of patients in whom hypertension is diagnosed, no single cause for the elevation in blood pressure can be identified. Although there are many popular theories for explaining the increased peripheral vascular resistance that appears to occur invariably in hypertension, the possibility that a single defect is responsible for all essential hypertension appears unlikely.

Despite an incomplete understanding of the pathophysiologic mechanism of essential hypertension, there has been very rapid growth in the use of pharmacologic agents for control of blood pressure, since it is well recognized from a number of therapeutic trials that many of the vascular complications that occur as a result of hypertension can be decreased by pharmacologic intervention. Five general classes of antihypertensive drugs are available for clinical use in the United States: (1) diuretics; (2) adrenergic inhibitors, including the beta-blockers; (3) vasodilators; (4) converting enzyme inhibitors; and (5) calcium antagonists.

A summary of these antihypertensive agents is presented in Table 2. In many instances, hypertension is most effectively controlled by a combination of two or more of these drugs, each of which may act by a different mechanism. Although the antihypertensive drugs are commonly used and have an important role in current medical therapy, they are all potentially toxic and

TABLE 2. Antihypertensive Agents

Diuretics
Thiazides and related drugs
Phthalimidines
Loop diuretics (furosemide and ethacrynic acid)
K+ sparing diuretics (spironolactone and triamterene)

Adrenergic Inhibitors
Peripheral (reserpine and guanethidine)
Central (methyldopa and clonidine)
Beta-receptor (propranolol, atenolol, metroprolol, nadolol, etc.)
Alpha-receptor (prazosin, phenoxybenzamine, phentolamine)

Vasodilators
Hydralazine
Minoxidil
Nitroprusside

Converting Enzyme Inhibitors
Captopril
Enalapril

Calcium Antagonists
Nifedipine
Verapamil
Diltiazem

work by inhibiting or modifying normal physiologic regulatory mechanisms. For this reason, they may be particularly troublesome and potentially dangerous in surgical patients in whom the stress of disease and the use of anesthetic agents may unmask potentially hazardous reactions and responses.

Although the list of drugs presented is incomplete and new antihypertensive agents are constantly being introduced into clinical practice, certain precautions related to each of the various classes of antihypertensive agents should be observed in surgical patients. The calcium antagonists are used in a variety of clinical situations, and their potential side effects in the surgical patient are discussed in a later section concerning their use in the management of angina pectoris.

DIURETICS. The thiazides and furosemide are usually the first agents employed for the treatment of mild or moderate hypertension. The thiazides act on the distal convoluted renal tubule for the inhibition of sodium transport, whereas furosemide acts on the ascending limb of Henle's loop for the inhibition of chloride transport. Since both of these drugs increase urinary excretion of salt and water, hypovolemia secondary to dehydration may be of particular concern in surgical patients. This causes tachycardia and also a predisposition to hypotension when anesthetics are administered that interfere with sympathetic function and therefore block the reflex increase in cardiac output or peripheral vascular resistance that are normal homeostatic responses to decreasing blood pressure. As a result, a minor blood loss during an operative procedure may cause profound hypotension and a severe decrease in cardiac output if pre-existing intravascular and extracellular deficits are present as a result of dehydration secondary to diuretic administration. By obtaining a careful history of diuretic use and observing clinical signs of volume depletion such as orthostatic hypotension or resting tachycardia, appropriate measures for restoration of volume before operation can be undertaken, and such problems can be avoided.

Since both furosemide and the thiazides increase delivery of sodium to the distal renal tubule where aldosterone-dependent sodium-potassium exchange occurs, potassium loss and hypokalemia may occur following administration of these agents.[22] In the presence of hypokalemia, the arrhythmogenic effects of digitalis or anesthetic agents that sensitize the myocardium may cause severe disturbances of cardiac rhythm and produce hemodynamic compromise or even fatal ventricular fibrillation. Such problems can be avoided or minimized by repleting diminished potassium before any extensive surgical procedure is undertaken. It is important to recognize that potassium depletion secondary to long-standing diuretic therapy may be quite severe in some patients. Although serum potassium levels generally indicate that hypokalemia exists, this value does not always reflect the severity of the intracellular deficit that is present. Repletion of diminished total body potassium stores before major surgical procedures, particularly cardiac operations, is essential in order to diminish cardiac rhythm disturbances, particularly if alkalosis or digitalis therapy coexists.

ADRENERGIC INHIBITORS. Antihypertensive drugs that act pharmacologically by inhibiting function of the sympathetic nervous system are classified according to the site at which they inhibit the sympathetic reflex arc. Each class of drug exhibits different forms of potential toxicity and may produce problems in surgical patients. The peripherally acting agents such as reserpine and guanethidine are capable of producing profound sympathoplegia by either blocking or inhibiting biogenic amine functions in both peripheral and central neurons. Although these actions are responsible for the success of the drugs in controlling hypertension, the problems of depressed cardiac output and hypotension due to mitigated sympathetic responses in the presence of volume depletion or exposure to anesthetic agents are often seen in surgical patients. Therefore, it is generally advisable to discontinue peripherally acting adrenergic blocking drugs for a period of time before an elective surgical procedure. Substitution of a more rapidly acting and easily managed agent may be required.

The centrally acting adrenergic inhibitors such as clonidine and methyldopa reduce sympathetic outflow from vasopressor centers in the brain stem. Since they allow these centers to retain their sensitivity to baroreceptor control, these drugs do not depress normal cardiovascular reflexes and do not depress cardiac output or produce the orthostatic hypotension observed with the peripherally acting agents. Abrupt withdrawal of clonidine may result in hypertensive crises or other evidence of profound sympathetic overactivity, and this drug should therefore be continued throughout the perioperative period or gradually withdrawn while other antihypertensive therapy is substituted.

Although beta-blocking agents were initially employed in the treatment of angina pectoris, it soon became apparent that they were extremely effective agents for the treatment of a variety of other disorders such as hypertension, thyrotoxicosis, migraines, arrhythmias, and glaucoma. Most treatment programs in patients with mild or moderately severe hypertension include one of the beta-blockers currently available in the United States. There was initial reluctance to administer a general anesthetic to a patient taking one of the beta-blocking drugs because of the rather frequent occurrence of bradycardia or hypotension secondary to a depression of cardiac output, but it is now considered safer to continue these agents throughout the surgical procedure and to utilize a specific beta-agonist or atropine if hypotension or bradycardia develops. The beta-blockers appear to be well tolerated in cardiac surgical patients and to offer a significant degree of protection from postoperative rhythm disturbance if continued without interruption throughout the perioperative period.[15] Although there has been much discussion about the "cardiac selectivity" of certain of the beta-blocking drugs, the clinical differences between the various beta-blockers are of minor importance from a surgical standpoint, and all are generally well tolerated. The most prudent policy may be to continue administration of these drugs during the perioperative period unless the dosage is very high, in which case they should be tapered to normal recommended dosages. Abrupt withdrawal of beta-blockers has been associated with acute myocardial infarction and should be avoided.

The alpha-receptor antagonists are rarely used for the management of uncomplicated hypertension. The most commonly employed agent is prazosin, which antagonizes alpha stimulation at the vascular alpha-receptors and appears to cause both arteriolar and venous vasodilation. Surgical patients who have been taking prazosin may develop a relative volume loss. A similar problem may be encountered with the other alpha-receptor antagonists, phenoxybenzamine and phentolamine. When possible, it is preferable to discontinue the alpha-receptor antagonists before any elective surgical procedure is performed unless specific indications exist for continuing use of these agents. An example would be in a patient with a pheochromocytoma in whom phenoxybenzamine or phentolamine may be important in the preoperative preparation. Careful management of the patient's volume status is mandatory when the alpha-receptor antagonists are used in surgical patients.

VASODILATORS. Peripheral vasodilators are usually employed in the management of hypertension only if a diuretic and adrenergic blocker do not control the blood pressure. Hydralazine is the only drug employed routinely as an oral agent. It is usually reserved for patients with severe hypertension and is often given in combination with a diuretic and beta-blocker. If given alone, hydralazine commonly elicits a number of reflex responses, such as tachycardia, that are troublesome and limit its usefulness. Other vasodilating agents used in the management of hypertension include minoxidil, which is usually reserved for the treatment of very severe hypertension in patients with renal insufficiency, and diazoxide and nitroprusside, two intravenous agents used in the management of malignant hypertension or in hypertensive emergencies. These agents act very rapidly and may need to be employed in patients with severe and refractory hypertension. They should be used only under carefully monitored circumstances because of their very rapid onset of action and propensity for inducing hypotension and tachycardia, which may aggravate pre-existing ischemic heart disease. Nitroprusside is presently the agent of choice for the control of acute hypertension in the operating room or during the postoperative period. It is rapid-acting and is easily titrated under conditions of proper monitoring, which allows the prompt detection and correction of fluid deficits.

CONVERTING ENZYME INHIBITORS. Captopril was the first orally effective inhibitor of angiotensin-converting enzyme, which is the enzyme responsible for conversion of inactive angiotensin I to the pressor peptide angiotensin II. Both captopril and the newer drug enalapril are potent and specific antihypertensive agents that lower total peripheral resistance and cause little change in cardiac output, heart rate, or pulmonary wedge pressure and are particularly effective in those hypertensive patients with elevated renin levels. They do not appear to interfere with normal cardiovascular homeostatic responses even when simultaneously administered with a diuretic. However, if significant volume depletion occurs as a result of a concomitantly administered diuretic, hypotension may develop. Abrupt withdrawal of angiotensin-converting enzyme inhibitors may cause severe hypertension that is difficult to manage, and these drugs should therefore be continued throughout the perioperative period.

Although certain antihypertensive agents may cause problems in surgical patients because of their particular mode of action, it is equally important to emphasize that uncontrolled hypertension in the surgical patient is a very serious problem. It is essential that a rational plan for the management and control of blood pressure in the operating room and postoperatively be formulated before any form of antihypertensive therapy is discontinued. After the period of hemodynamic instability surrounding the immediate operative period has ceased, the patient's normal antihypertensive regimen should be reinstituted in order to make the perioperative management less complex. Rapidly acting agents such as intravenous nitroprusside are the agents of choice for severe hypertension during the intraoperative or immediate postoperative period. It is mandatory that these agents be administered only under carefully monitored conditions because of their ability to produce profound hypotension.

Agents for the Management of Congestive Heart Failure

Traditional treatment for patients with evidence of cardiac failure has consisted of salt restriction, diuretics, and the administration of a digitalis preparation for cardiac rate control and an inotropic effect. It is now recognized that an increase in impedance to left ventricular ejection is an important factor in producing the left ventricular dysfunction that characterizes cardiac failure states. This increased impedance to ejection is the result of a complex series of peripheral vascular events produced by increased activity of the sympathetic system and the renin-angiotensin system.[3,6,24] The final result of this abnormal activity is narrowing of the arterioles, decreased arterial compliance, and a reduction in venous compliance that shifts blood into the central circulation and increases cardiac filling. The very logical concept has developed that instead of vigorously stimulating the failing heart with inotropic agents, one should attempt to reduce the cardiac load by means of vasodilators. The concept of afterload reduction by pharmacologic means is already well established for the treatment of hypertension and has now been extended to other disease states, including severe congestive

heart failure (particularly if due to hypertension), aortic or mitral valve incompetence, ischemic heart disease with accompanying congestive heart failure, and all of the cardiomyopathic states that produce cardiac failure.[3,4] It would appear illogical for the body to initiate responses in the presence of a failing myocardium that would increase the work of the ventricle, but this appears to be the situation. An increased level of peripheral vascular resistance and aortic impedance to ejection is characteristic of heart failure, and this reflex vasoconstriction, which probably was intended to manage intravascular volume depletion, becomes a deleterious feedback mechanism in the patient with cardiac failure due to impaired left ventricular function.[24] Although neuroendocrine responses are activated in congestive heart failure, as demonstrated by the striking variation in plasma norepinephrine and renin levels that are observed in patients with this disorder, the levels of these substances do not correlate well with the level of cardiac failure or the form of therapy employed.[3]

Drugs that produce vasodilation of vascular smooth muscle can favorably affect the performance of the heart in two ways.[2,19] First, by decreasing the peripheral vascular resistance through the mechanism of arteriolar relaxation, the ventricular ejection fraction improves, stroke volume improves, and end-systolic volume decreases. Second, the relaxation of venous smooth muscle shifts blood from the central circulation into the peripheral venous capacitance bed and thereby decreases the preload or end-diastolic volume, resulting in the following: (1) a reduction in myocardial wall stress and consequent lowering of myocardial oxygen requirements; (2) a shift to the more effective portion of the diastolic pressure-volume curve, where the flatness of the curve allows increasing amounts of volume with lesser increases in diastolic pressure; (3) a decrease in end-diastolic pressure in the left ventricle with a consequent decrease in pulmonary venous pressure and relief of pulmonary congestion; and (4) improved diastolic perfusion of the myocardium as a result of the lowered transmyocardial pressure gradient between epicardial and endocardial blood vessels. The facilitation of ventricular emptying leading to enhancement of stroke volume is the fundamental objective of any form of therapy for congestive heart failure secondary to cardiac dysfunction. The results of many trials of vasodilator therapy suggest that this approach to management is physiologically rational, although there are as yet no firm data in support of its clinical usefulness in long-term clinical efficacy or exercise capacity improvement.[4]

The surgical management of patients with evidence of congestive heart failure has been greatly improved with the addition of vasodilator drugs to the therapeutic armamentarium. This has been particularly evident in cardiac surgical patients, who can now be treated preoperatively and then brought to the operating room in a much more stable state than was previously possible. The deleterious effects of uncontrolled hypertension are well recognized, and drugs that are currently available allow precise regulation of cardiac function and blood pressure both preoperatively and during the intraoperative period. Although many agents are available that may act as vasodilators, only a few are currently commonly employed clinically (Table 3).

Any patient with cardiac disease sufficiently severe to produce symptoms or findings of congestive heart failure represents a substantial risk for any major surgical operation. A comprehensive evaluation of the patient's underlying cardiac disorder, the institution or continuation of appropriate therapy, and the judicious use of intraoperative monitoring of cardiac function are mandatory if surgical risk is to be reduced to an acceptable level. In almost all instances, pharmacologic agents that have successfully controlled symptoms of cardiac failure before surgical intervention should be continued or more appropriate agents utilized throughout the preoperative, operative, and postoperative periods. The vasodilator drugs discussed

TABLE 3. Vasodilator Drugs

Drug	Afterload Reduction	Preload Reduction	Indications
Nitroprusside (intravenous)	+++	++	Acute hypertension Cardiac failure Valvular insufficiency
Nitrates (intravenous, oral, patch)	+	+++	Ischemic failure
Hydralazine (oral or intravenous)	+++	0	Chronic cardiac failure
Prazosin (oral)	++	++	Hypertensive failure Pulmonary hypertension Chronic cardiac failure
Captopril (oral)	++	+	Chronic cardiac failure
Nifedipine (sublingual)	++	0	Acute left ventricular failure

+ present.

previously are generally short-acting and can usually be easily managed in the adequately monitored patient. However, abrupt termination of most of these drugs in the patient with severe cardiac compromise often produces significant hemodynamic instability and evidence of congestive heart failure.

Antianginal Drugs

It is generally appreciated that operative mortality and morbidity are significantly increased among patients with coronary artery disease. The optimal management of these patients is predicated on identifying those at significant risk, assessing their cardiac reserve and ability to withstand the stress of surgical therapy and anesthesia, and instituting suitable treatment before operation in an effort to minimize risk.

The most important cardiovascular risk factor in evaluating a patient for a major surgical procedure is the history of a recent myocardial infarction. Many institutions require a comprehensive cardiac evaluation, including stress testing and coronary angiography, if indicated, for patients with a history of recent infarction or severe angina pectoris. If necessary, myocardial revascularization should be performed before any major elective noncardiac surgical procedure. Although no definitive study has been reported that documents the ability of this plan to prevent myocardial infarction or cardiac death, there are isolated uncontrolled reports of the success of such an approach. In any event, patients undergoing major surgical procedures who have any history of ischemic cardiac disease must be optimally managed from a cardiac standpoint. Many take drugs for control of symptoms of angina pectoris, but others may have equally severe coronary disease despite minimal clinical symptoms. Patients undergoing surgical procedures for severe peripheral vascular disease have been found angiographically to have an incidence of coronary artery disease as high as 95 per cent, with many showing evidence of multivessel or inoperable disease. In nearly half of these patients, no clinical symptoms suggestive of coronary disease are present. A well-planned course of management may include either a surgical or a pharmacologic approach for the control of ischemic heart disease.

Three general classes of pharmacologic agents are specifically used for the treatment of angina pectoris: nitrates, beta-blockers, and calcium antagonists. A more complete list of the commonly used antianginal agents is presented in Table 4.

The short- and long-acting nitrates present no particular surgical problems and can be continued up to the time of operation. Either the paste or the intravenous form can be used at the time of operation if evidence of ischemic change is noted on the electrocardiogram or if signs of congestive heart failure develop. Patients who have been taking nitrates for a prolonged period of time, particularly the long-acting forms, may develop serious cardiac ischemia if the drugs are abruptly withdrawn, and suitable precautions must be taken to prevent this occurrence.

Unless patients show evidence of profound beta-blockade with a very low resting heart rate, have a history of or physical findings suggesting congestive heart failure, show evidence of a low cardiac output, or are having pulmonary symptoms such as wheezing, it is generally advisable to continue beta-blocking drugs up to the time of operation and then to reinstitute them immediately after the operation. Abrupt withdrawal of beta-blockers may cause ischemia during the stresses of anesthesia and operation that may cause serious arrhythmias or other ischemic complications.[15] If problems develop during the operative period that appear to be due to excessive beta-blockade, specific treatment should be instituted. Profound bradycardia can usually be managed with atropine, 1 to 2 mg. intravenously. Failure to increase the heart rate with atropine or evidence of a low cardiac output or hypotension secondary to these agents can be managed by the intravenous infusion of glucagon at a rate of 2.5 to 5 mg. per hour. This agent is the drug of choice because it stimulates formation of cyclic adenosine monophosphate by a route that bypasses the occupied beta-receptor.[13,15] The competitive beta-blockade may also be overcome by infusing dopamine or dobutamine. Isoproterenol would be a specific

TABLE 4. Antianginal Drugs

Agent	Route of Administration and Usual Dosage
Short-acting Nitrates	
Nitroglycerin	Sublingual, 0.3–0.6 mg. Intravenous, 0.6–12 mg./min.
Isosorbide dinitrate	Sublingual, 2.5–5 mg.
Long-acting Nitrates	
Isosorbide dinitrate	Oral, 10–40 mg., every 4–6 hr.
Nitroglycerin capsules	Oral, 2.5–9 mg., every 6–12 hr.
Nitroglycerin paste	Skin, ½–2 inches, every 6–12 hr.
Nitroglycerin patch	Transdermal, 5–10 mg., daily
Beta-blocking Agents	
Noncardioselective	
Propranolol	Oral, 20–80 mg., every 6–8 hr. Intravenous, 0.5–5 mg., slow infusion
Nadolol	Oral, 100 mg., daily
Timolol	Oral, 5–15 mg., 3 times/day
Pindolol	Oral, 2.5–7.5 mg., 3 times/day
Cardioselective	
Atenolol	Oral, 100 mg., daily
Metoprolol	Oral, 50–100 mg., 3 times/day
Calcium Antagonists	
Verapamil	Oral, 80–120 mg., every 8 hr.
Nifedipine	Oral, 10–20 mg., every 6–8 hr.
Diltiazem	Oral, 30–90 mg., every 6 hr.

agonist but is not a good choice in patients with ischemic heart disease because of its peripheral vasodilating effect, which may produce severe hypotension. Transvenous temporary pacing may be required in rare instances when pharmacologic therapy fails.

The calcium antagonists (calcium channel blockers) are an important group of agents utilized in the treatment of angina pectoris but also have antihypertensive and antiarrhythmic properties.[10,14] Whereas the beta-blockers tend to cause vasoconstriction of smooth muscle, the calcium antagonists cause vasodilation and therefore are not associated with such side effects as bronchospasm. They are thus very useful antianginal agents in patients with chronic obstructive pulmonary disease. The antianginal properties of the calcium channel blockers have been ascribed to three basic mechanisms: (1) an increase in coronary blood flow due to direct vasodilation of coronary arteries; (2) a decrease in myocardial oxygen demand as a result of a decrease in systolic ventricular wall stress or afterload and an improvement in diastolic relaxation; and (3) a cardioprotective effect during periods of transient ischemia. Some available evidence also suggests that the calcium channel antagonists inhibit platelet aggregation and help improve myocardial oxygen delivery by this mechanism in addition to the others mentioned.[14]

Although all of the calcium antagonists possess antianginal properties, their structural differences involve varying sites and modes of action. Verapamil has its most prominent effect on the atrioventricular (AV) node, slowing both antegrade and retrograde conduction through this node. As such, verapamil is also useful in the treatment of supraventricular tachycardias. Diltiazem also decreases AV nodal conduction and, like verapamil, may be used in the management of supraventricular tachycardia. Nifedipine has very little effect on the AV node. It is most noted for its potent peripheral vasodilating effect and thus may be used in patients with both ischemic heart disease and hypertension. Although all were initially thought to have profound negative inotropic effects, it has since become apparent that in the usual clinical dosages, their myocardial depressant properties are not great unless they are administered in combination with a beta-blocker or in the presence of pre-existing left ventricular dysfunction. The calcium antagonists act on vascular tissue in much lower concentrations than those required to produce myocardial depression.[16]

The calcium antagonists may, however, produce several problems in the surgical patient. Because of their peripheral vasodilating effects, these agents may unmask latent hypovolemia and cause profound hypotension after relatively minor amounts of volume loss. This is a particularly troublesome side effect with nifedipine, which has the strongest peripheral vascular vasodilating properties of the calcium channel blockers. As such, careful hemodynamic monitoring with attention to volume status must be undertaken in surgical patients who are maintained on these agents. Another problem that may be encountered is severe myocardial depression due to the combined use of a beta-blocker and a calcium antagonist, a combination often utilized in patients with angina pectoris. This depression follows blunting of normal reflex sympathetic responses to the depressant effects of the calcium antagonist and may be compounded by the use of inhalational anesthetic agents, which also have a negative inotropic effect on the myocardium. For these reasons, it is usually prudent to discontinue the calcium antagonist and continue the beta-blocker before major cardiac or general surgical procedures. The interaction between digitalis preparations and the calcium antagonists is safe in the absence of digitalis intoxication, but when toxic digoxin levels are present, lethal AV block may result.

At present, nitrates remain a first-line treatment for the relief or prevention of angina in patients with coronary artery disease. These agents present little problem for the surgical patient, since they have few serious limiting side effects and may be administered safely throughout the patient's operative course.

Inotropic Drugs

Inotropic drugs offer the most direct approach for improving cardiac performance. If a new pump (cardiac transplantation) is considered as a form of improving systolic or diastolic dysfunction, it is quite clear that the multiple abnormalities that develop as a result of heart failure (activation of the renin-angiotensin system, increased sympathetic nervous system activity, increased secretion of arginine, and so on) are reversible. The ideal myocardial-stimulating drug should improve myocardial contractile force without greatly increasing myocardial oxygen demand, without producing excessive afterload for the heart to work against by causing peripheral vasoconstriction, and without producing tachycardia or other cardiac arrhythmias. Unfortunately, none of the currently available inotropic agents fulfills these criteria.[5,13] Nonetheless, the inotropic drugs continue to have an important role in the management of heart failure patients and are particularly important in the management of surgical patients with cardiovascular instability on the basis of either primary cardiac dysfunction or peripheral vascular instability. The agents commonly employed for inotropic stimulation include the digitalis compounds, the sympathomimetic amines, and the phosphodiesterase inhibitors. The pharmacologic properties of these three classes of agents and potential problems that may cause the surgical patient following their administration are vastly different and are therefore discussed separately.

DIGITALIS COMPOUNDS. Digitalis has multiple direct and indirect cardiovascular effects that are both therapeutic and potentially toxic. At the molecular level, the digitalis compounds inhibit Na^+-K^+-ATPase, the membrane-bound enzyme associated with the sodium pump. This inhibition causes a loss of potassium from the myocardial cell and an increase in calcium released to the contractile proteins at the time of excitation-contraction coupling. The net result is an increase in myocardial contractility. The alterations in the mechanical and metabolic properties of the cardiac cell are accompanied by changes in the electrical properties that may cause rhythm disturbances as secondary toxic side effects. These same electrophysiologic properties of the digitalis compounds may also be employed therapeutically for the control of cardiac rhythm disturbances that are supraventricular in origin.

Because it has a moderately consistent inotropic effect and can be administered orally, digitalis is, in theory, a useful agent for the management of cardiac failure. Recently, there has been increasing controversy as to whether the proposed benefits of the drug outweigh its high toxic : therapeutic ratio.[13] The indications for digitalis are diminishing, particularly for the treatment of acute heart failure. Currently, the major indication for the administration of digitalis is the combination of congestive heart failure and atrial fibrillation.[17] Congestive heart failure in the presence of sinus rhythm may be more safely managed by diuretics or a combination of diuretics and a vasodilator, and acute left ventricular failure is generally treated by a combination of more potent inotropic drugs such as dopamine or dobutamine, a diuretic, and vasodilators before digitalis is considered. The issue of using digitalis for the treatment of chronic congestive heart failure remains questionable, but since it appears that some patients are substantially improved by this agent, the challenge is development of better methods of identifying patients who will have a good response and are at minimal risk for development of troublesome side effects.

Certain problems may arise in the course of an operation that predispose the surgical patient to toxic manifestations (usually arrhythmias) of the digitalis compounds. Both acute hypoxemia and hypokalemia increase susceptibility to digitalis-induced ventricular arrhythmias, and these disturbances require prompt and specific correction. Hypercalcemia, cardiac ischemia, certain anesthetic agents, and myocardial infarction are also responsible for a heightened sensitivity to the digitalis compounds. It is generally best to withhold digitalis compounds for a period of time before any surgical procedure and utilize safer pharmacologic agents throughout the operative and immediate postoperative period for the management of cardiac failure or rhythm disturbances.

SYMPATHOMIMETIC AMINES. The catecholamines increase contractility by stimulating beta-receptors located on the surface membrane, with subsequent augmentation of Ca^{++} availability to the contractile system and enhancement of myocardial contractility.[17] The beta$_1$-receptors normally respond to norepinephrine, which is released by cardiac sympathetic nerves. The norepinephrine stores in these nerves are depleted in chronic heart failure, and the sympathomimetic drugs that act by releasing norepinephrine stores may be ineffective. The receptors, however, are intact and respond to exogenously administered catecholamines.

The sympathomimetic drugs currently available in the United States as inotropic agents are delivered intravenously, and their overall effect on the circulatory system is influenced by their relative stimulatory effect on receptors other than those in the heart. The alpha-receptors in the peripheral circulation produce vasoconstriction, and the beta$_2$-receptors in the lungs and peripheral circulation produce bronchodilation and peripheral vasodilation.

Epinephrine and norepinephrine are prototypes of the class of sympathomimetic amines. Both drugs have potent beta$_1$-receptor stimulating properties and, thus, are powerful cardiac stimulants. As a result of beta$_1$-receptor stimulation, both drugs increase heart rate and myocardial oxygen consumption, which could prove to be detrimental to patients with coronary artery disease. In addition to the beta-receptor stimulation, both agents possess alpha-adrenergic effects and subsequently cause peripheral vasoconstriction at relatively low dosages. Renal blood flow is reduced because of the vasoconstrictive properties, and if these drugs are used for supporting the failing heart, an alpha-blocking drug should be administered simultaneously for minimizing the vasoconstriction. Because of these potential limitations, epinephrine and norepinephrine are usually employed in patients with refractory hypotension and low cardiac output as may be seen in various shock states.

Isoproterenol is a synthetic catecholamine with pure beta-adrenergic activity. Since its beta-receptor effects are unopposed by any alpha-receptor stimulation, isoproterenol produces significant peripheral vasodilation, which may be a very desirable feature in patients with severe vasoconstriction; but this same property could produce hypotension and limit its clinical usefulness. The most limiting feature of isoproterenol is that it increases myocardial oxygen demand, which may precipitate ischemia in patients with significant coronary artery disease. For this reason, isoproterenol should be used only in patients without evidence of ischemic disease.

Dopamine has become the drug of choice for patients with myocardial failure who require inotropic support for maintenance of hemodynamic stability. It is an intermediate compound in the synthesis of epinephrine and norepinephrine and also releases norepinephrine stores from nerve endings in the heart. It has both beta- and alpha-adrenergic effects; however, these effects are seen at different dosages. At the lower dosages of 2 to 10 μg. per kg. per minute, it increases cardiac contractility by beta-stimulation while causing widespread peripheral vasodilation and improving renal blood flow by selective stimulation of dopaminergic receptors.[13] It is less likely than other catecholamine drugs to produce ventricular irritability, tachycardia, or excessive increase in myocardial oxygen demands. In dosages

greater than 10 μg. per kg. per minute, the alpha-stimulating properties of dopamine become more prominent, and the resultant vasoconstriction may prove to be deleterious to the failing heart. Thus, vasodilators may be required for reversal of some of the vasoconstricting properties of the drug. The combination of dopamine and nitroprusside has proved to be particularly useful in the management of patients following cardiac surgery who demonstrate a persistent low cardiac output that is unresponsive to volume therapy alone.

Dobutamine is a synthetic analog of dopamine that acts directly on beta$_1$-adrenergic receptors, thus causing a stronger inotropic than chronotropic effect.[13] Although it has alpha$_1$-agonist effects, the beta$_2$-adrenergic effects tend to override these, producing a mild peripheral vasodilation. In contrast to dopamine, dobutamine does not release norepinephrine, nor does it stimulate the dopaminergic receptors in the kidneys. Since it does not rely on norepinephrine release for its inotropic action, dobutamine may be more effective than is dopamine in patients with long-standing myocardial failure in whom endogenous catecholamine levels are depressed. Dobutamine has been shown to decrease myocardial oxygen consumption by decreasing wall stress, and, thus, it is a useful inotropic agent in patients with coronary artery disease undergoing general or cardiac surgical procedures.

Attempts at developing and testing of oral sympathomimetic cardiac stimulants are being made because of the potential implications that such agents might have in the management of chronic congestive heart failure. Currently, however, all of these agents remain in clinical trial and are not widely available in the United States.[5]

PHOSPHODIESTERASE INHIBITORS. These are a relatively new class of agents, the beneficial hemodynamic effects of which are a result of the inhibition of phosphodiesterase Type III, which increases cyclic adenosine monophosphate levels. These drugs possess strong inotropic effects as well as direct arterial and venous vasodilatory properties.

The prototypical agent in this class of drugs is amrinone, which is available in intravenous form for the treatment of congestive heart failure. Amrinone produces an increase in cardiac output while reducing peripheral vascular resistance and left heart filling pressures. It has essentially no effect on heart rate or blood pressure. Because of its afterload-reducing properties, amrinone is useful in patients with low cardiac output and mitral or aortic insufficiency, since it tends to decrease the regurgitant volume during systole, thus increasing forward flow. It has also been used with success in patients with the low output syndrome following cardiac surgery. One important side effect with relatively long-term amrinone use is a nonimmunologic-mediated thrombocytopenia, which could prove to be deleterious in the preoperative or postoperative setting.

Milrinone is 20 times more potent than amrinone with a similar mechanism of action in addition to a prominent vasodilatory component. When milrinone is given acutely, its inotropic and vasodilatory effect is combined with an increase in heart rate. When it is given chronically, only some patients benefit, and there is risk of arrhythmias. Although amrinone in the oral form is no longer used, the intravenous preparation with its major inotropic and vasodilator effects should be especially useful in patients with beta-receptor downgrading, such as those in severe congestive heart failure or with prior prolonged therapy with dobutamine or other beta$_1$-stimulants. Milrinone is available in oral form, but its efficacy remains as yet undetermined.[5]

Antiarrhythmic Agents

The perioperative management of patients with cardiac arrhythmias and conduction disturbances is an important part of patient care. A knowledge of the preoperative drug ingestion history, electrocardiographic status, and cardiovascular history is mandatory and should be combined with an understanding of the intraoperative and postoperative factors that facilitate the occurrence of cardiac rhythm disturbances. A number of factors may be encountered perioperatively that predispose to the development of arrhythmias: (1) ventilatory problems that produce hypoxia or respiratory alkalosis; (2) hypokalemia and other electrolyte abnormalities; (3) toxic reaction to cardioactive anesthetics and other drugs; (4) hypotension; (5) hypertension; (6) reduced cardiac output; (7) anemia; (8) myocardial infarction; and (9) the cardiac trauma and pericarditis that invariably are associated with open cardiac surgical procedures. These factors must always be considered in the evaluation of a surgical patient with a cardiac rhythm disturbance, and initial treatment should always be directed toward correction of these abnormalities. Thus, the aim of modern antiarrhythmia therapy is reduction of ectopic pacemaker activity and modification of critically impaired conduction either by improving it in an area of depressed conduction or by suppressing it altogether.

As summarized by Harrison, investigators have categorized antiarrhythmic compounds by their effects on (1) the fast sodium current, (2) the sympathetic activity of the heart, (3) the repolarization current, and (4) the slow inward calcium current.[11] The sodium channel blockers are the most important group of agents and are similar to local anesthetics in that they exhibit membrane-stabilizing properties. This group is referred to as Class I agents and includes lidocaine, quinidine, procainamide, disopyramide, phenytoin, and the newer agents mexiletine, aprindine, tocainide, and encainide. These drugs are effective in the treatment of ventricular and supraventricular arrhythmias. All of these agents are capable of causing a variety of severe toxic side effects that either may directly affect the heart conduction system or may cause extracardiac manifestations.

Class II agents are the beta-antagonist drugs and include propranolol and similar drugs that have antiarrhythmic properties by virtue of their adrenergic receptor blocking action and direct membrane effects. The relative contributions of the beta-blocking and direct membrane effects are unknown, and these agents have also been shown in clinical trials to lower the incidence of recurrent infarction and sudden death in patients recovering from myocardial infarction. In addition, beta-adrenergic blocking drugs are particularly effective in suppressing ventricular premature beats and ventricular tachycardia that are increased by or occur from exercise or are associated with mitral valve prolapse syndrome.

The major effect of Class III drugs is widening of the action potential duration, and it appears that this group of drugs will emerge as the most significant for control of cardiac arrhythmias. The agents currently available in the United States classified as Class III agents are amiodarone and bretylium. Both are effective in the management of atrial flutter and fibrillation in association with the Wolff-Parkinson-White syndrome, and amiodarone has been used extensively in the treatment of sustained ventricular tachycardia that is refractory to other antiarrhythmic agents. There are reports of adverse effects of long-term amiodarone treatment. The most common side effects are corneal microdeposits, liver function abnormalities, and pulmonary fibrosis. Amiodarone noncompetitively blocks both alpha- and beta-adrenergic receptors *in vivo*. It increases coronary blood flow but reduces cardiac work and oxygen consumption as well as peripheral vascular resistance. Small intravenous doses in man do not affect cardiac contractility; however, at larger doses, contractility is depressed, and the left ventricular end-diastolic pressure is increased.

Class IV agents are the calcium channel blockers. The prototype Class IV drug is verapamil, which has become the agent of choice for the control of supraventricular arrhythmias because of its ability to slow conduction through the AV node with very few side effects and a low incidence of toxicity. Verapamil,

however, should not be used for treatment of atrial fibrillation in patients with the Wolff-Parkinson-White syndrome because conduction across the accessory pathway may increase as a result of inhibition of AV conduction, and this may cause hemodynamic collapse.

From a practical standpoint, the indications for the use of antiarrhythmic drugs in surgical patients must be based on a knowledge of the natural history of the rhythm disturbance and whether it is of physiologic significance in the overall management of the patient. Careful documentation and precise diagnosis of the type of rhythm disturbance are essential. There is a limited role for the prophylactic use of drug therapy in an attempt at preventing the development of arrhythmias, since all antiarrhythmic drugs have proarrhythmic effects and, therefore, may precipitate a rhythm disturbance.[11] In general, all cardiac rhythm disturbances that are potentially life-threatening, that can be shown to cause hemodynamic compromise, or that cause symptoms should be precisely diagnosed and specifically treated. Patients with no known structural heart disease usually do not require specific drug therapy for benign rhythm disturbances such as sinus tachycardia, premature atrial beats, or unifocal premature ventricular beats. The most prudent approach may be to define underlying etiologic factors such as fever, hypoxia, or anxiety and attempt to eliminate them. In some patients, the presence of heart disease may complicate the use of antiarrhythmic therapy. Heart failure and conduction problems are the most serious. Most of the antiarrhythmic drugs depress left ventricular function to a variable and dose-related degree, and patients with left ventricular dysfunction may tolerate these agents poorly. Drug therapy for patients with AV nodal disease or with conduction disease below the level of the AV node should be carefully monitored because of the potential for serious side effects and profound depression of cardiac conduction.

THE PHARMACOLOGIC MANAGEMENT OF SPECIFIC CARDIOVASCULAR PROBLEMS IN THE SURGICAL PATIENT

Arrhythmias and Conduction Disturbances

BRADYARRHYTHMIAS. Sinus bradycardia in the surgical patient is usually caused by increased vagal tone related to direct stimulation of the carotid sinus, stimulation of the vagus nerves, or pain. Myocardial ischemia should always be excluded as a cause for sudden cardiac slowing.

Bradycardia is best treated by administering atropine intravenously in 0.5 mg. boluses up to 2 mg. over a 30-minute period. If atropine therapy is unsuccessful, a continuous infusion of isoproterenol may be administered at a rate of 1 to 10 μg. per minute titrated to the heart rate responses. If pharmacologic therapy is unsuccessful, a temporary pacemaker should be placed.

VENTRICULAR ARRHYTHMIAS. This is a complex and changing area that cannot readily be simplified. The criteria for instituting therapy are not clear-cut, although patients with sustained ventricular tachycardia and those with symptomatic or hemodynamically compromising ventricular dysrhythmia require treatment.

Intraoperative or postoperative ventricular ectopy is often precipitated by hypoxia, hypercarbia, hypokalemia, anxiety, fever, or drug excess, and correction of these problems often resolves the ectopy without resorting to specific drug therapy. Ventricular ectopic activity that occurs in the absence of clinical heart disease or electrocardiographic abnormalities is generally benign and well tolerated.

In patients with a history of ischemic heart disease or with electrocardiographic or clinical evidence of perioperative ischemia or infarction in whom ventricular ectopic activity in the form of frequent multifocal ventricular beats or ventricular couplets develops, lidocaine therapy should be administered as a 100-mg. intravenous bolus followed by a continuous infusion at a rate 1 to 3 mg. per minute titrated for control of the ectopy. If lidocaine fails to control the rhythm, procainamide would be the second drug to administer, and bretylium may be required in cases that are particularly refractory to more conventional drugs.

SUPRAVENTRICULAR TACHYARRHYTHMIAS. The development of new supraventricular tachyarrhythmias in the surgical patient is usually associated with certain identifiable risk factors such as myocardial infarction or ischemia, congestive heart failure, electrolyte derangements, hypoxia, pulmonary embolism, the administration of arrhythmogenic drugs such as catecholamines, or fever associated with a major infection. Correction of these problems would obviate the need for specific drug therapy in about one third of the patients.

Atrial fibrillation is the most common supraventricular arrhythmia observed in surgical patients. The first goal of treatment is control of the rapid ventricular response rate, which is usually best done by administering digoxin. For patients who have not previously taken digoxin or any other digitalis agent, a total intravenous loading dose of 1 mg. should be administered over a 6- to 12-hour period, usually beginning with 0.5 mg. intravenously and then repeating 0.25-mg. doses at 2-hour intervals in order to lower the ventricular rate below 90 beats per minute. In patients with a rapid ventricular response to atrial fibrillation and no evidence of depressed ventricular function, verapamil can be administered in doses of 2.5 to 5 mg. intravenously every 15 minutes until a total dose of 10 mg. is given. For severe cardiac compromise due to tachycardia, synchronized cardioversion remains the treatment of choice.

Treatment of the underlying medical problems and control of the ventricular response to atrial fibrillation usually effect conversion to normal sinus rhythm. If the patient remains in atrial fibrillation for 48 hours despite adequate control of the ventricular response, a specific antiarrhythmic drug such as quinidine or procainamide should be administered in an attempt to achieve conversion into sinus rhythm.

Control of the ventricular rate in patients with atrial flutter is often more difficult than in those with atrial fibrillation. Although the treatment approach has traditionally been to digitalize the patient, there is good clinical evidence suggesting that the use of verapamil as the first drug may be more efficacious. Also, it is well known that atrial flutter is uniquely susceptible to cardioversion, and this form of treatment should be employed if there is any evidence of hemodynamic compromise.

Other forms of supraventricular tachyarrhythmia, including AV nodal re-entry tachycardia, sinus node re-entry tachycardia, intra-atrial tachycardia, automatic junctional tachycardia, or a re-entrant conduction pathway, may occur in surgical patients and may require pharmacologic treatment. In many instances, these arrhythmias may be terminated by vagotonic maneuvers, but if this is unsuccessful, intravenous verapamil in the same dosage recommended for atrial fibrillation is the agent of choice. Verapamil should be successful in about 80 per cent of cases, but in those patients in whom rate reduction is not achieved, the administration of propranolol is indicated.

Esmolol is an ultra short–acting cardioselective beta-blocker that has recently been introduced in the United States. Esmolol is rapidly converted to inactive metabolites by blood esterases, and full recovery from beta-blockade occurs within 30 minutes in patients with a normal cardiovascular system. The indications for esmolol are situations in which a rapid beta-blockade onset and termination are desired, such as in supraventricular tachycardia, perioperative tachycardia, or perioperative hypertension.[1] The dose range is 50 to 400 μg. per kg. per minute intravenously.

Low Cardiac Output Syndrome

The low cardiac output syndrome in surgical patients must be recognized and promptly treated before severe cellular and organ damage occurs. The syndrome represents a state of inadequate perfusion at the tissue level and may occur for a number of reasons. The clinical pattern is characterized by evidence of decreased organ perfusion with decreasing urinary output and an altered mental state in the awake patient. Acidosis is noted because of the decreased tissue perfusion.

A low cardiac output state in a surgical patient can best be managed by a methodic and physiologic approach. Careful clinical observation and serial monitoring of hemodynamic parameters such as heart rate, arterial blood pressure, cardiac filling pressures, and cardiac output are mandatory. The metabolic status of the patient should be followed by serial arterial blood gas measurements and mixed venous oxygen content analysis. Electrolyte abnormalities should be sought and corrected as required.

The most common cause of the low cardiac output state in surgical patients is hypovolemia, which follows unreplaced blood or extracellular fluid losses that occur as a result of both the underlying disease process and the losses incurred at the time of any surgical procedure. Typical features in these patients are low cardiac output and reduced filling pressures, particularly as noted from the measurement of pulmonary capillary wedge pressure, which reflects left-sided filling pressures. Because of sympathetic compensatory efforts, the peripheral circulation is profoundly vasoconstricted, and the peripheral vascular resistance is elevated.

The management of the low cardiac output state secondary to hypovolemia is straightforward and involves controlling blood and fluid loss while judiciously replacing deficits with appropriate solution or blood products. Therapy should be carefully guided by the measurements of left-sided filling pressures and repeated determinations of cardiac output.

Another cause of the low cardiac output syndrome is primary myocardial dysfunction, which is the result of the heart's failure to perform as a competent pump. The usual cause of primary myocardial dysfunction in noncardiac surgical patients is ischemic heart disease with regional dysfunction due to severe ischemia or infarction. The development of a dysfunctional state sufficiently severe to produce a low cardiac output syndrome suggests that at least 40 per cent of the ventricle is disabled. This type of injury may be related to pre-existing cardiac disease, recent myocardial infarction, or the residual effects of prolonged ischemia that may occur following cardiac surgical procedures in which preservation of the myocardium is unsuccessful in preventing injury to the myocardial muscle. Regardless of the etiologic factor, the principles of diagnosis and the approach to management are the same. The filling pressures of the ventricular chambers must be carefully optimized so as to take maximal advantage of the Frank-Starling mechanism without causing pulmonary edema. Cardiac rate and the normal synchrony between atrium and ventricle are important factors in the maintenance of cardiac pump function, and every attempt should be made to normalize them, including the use of pacing devices.

It is widely recognized that the impaired myocardium will function best if the afterload or systolic wall stress against which it must function is reduced. This afterload reduction is best achieved by the use of short-acting peripheral vasodilators such as nitroprusside or nitroglycerin. Both drugs are administered intravenously under carefully monitored conditions and are titrated for maintenance of a systemic vascular resistance in the low-normal range. Additional support for the poorly functioning myocardium can be achieved by the use of an inotropic agent that improves cardiac contractility without producing a pronounced increase in cardiac rate or significant increases in peripheral vascular resistance. The inotropic agents that appear to best achieve these goals are dopamine, dobutamine, and amrinone used either alone or in combination. In the patient with a chronically diseased and failing heart, epinephrine in small doses is occasionally beneficial. If pharmacologic and fluid therapy are unsuccessful in restoring myocardial function, mechanical support with a device such as the intra-aortic balloon pump must be considered.

An increasingly common cause of the low cardiac output syndrome in surgical patients is the presence of systemic sepsis. A wide range of microbial agents can cause profound cardiovascular alterations, leading to shock and death. The treatment of septic low-flow states is much more controversial than that of either hypovolemic or cardiogenic shock, and the mortality remains greater than 50 per cent in almost all reported series.

The most important factors in the management of the septic surgical patient are prompt recognition of the problem and careful monitoring of the hemodynamic status while a thorough search for the source of sepsis is commenced. Surgical drainage of sources of infection and the institution of antibiotics are crucial. In many instances, intravascular volume deficits are present and should be corrected. The hemodynamic interventions instituted in septic shock should augment cardiac output when demands for increased perfusion exist.

When perfusion cannot be improved further by expanding the intravascular volume and increasing the preload, afterload reduction and inotropic intervention with pharmacologic agents should be considered. In some forms of septic shock, the primary hemodynamic alteration appears to be intense peripheral vasoconstriction that eventually produces tissue and organ damage unless treated. In this setting, the use of a vasodilator such as nitroprusside or nitroglycerin is indicated under conditions of careful monitoring. A fall in blood pressure commonly occurs when these agents are used despite a rise in cardiac output. Some degree of hypotension is usually well tolerated by younger patients without pre-existing coronary artery or cerebrovascular disease, but the fixed and stenotic lesions often present in the coronary and cerebral circulation of older patients place them at substantial risk for myocardial infarction or stroke.

When afterload reduction fails to improve cardiac output, inotropic pharmacologic agents should be considered. The sympathomimetic agents dopamine, dobutamine, epinephrine, isoproterenol, and amrinone can provide inotropic support in association with the dose-related peripheral vascular effects previously discussed.

Patients with the hyperdynamic form of septic shock appear to have a unique problem and present a dilemma in management, since their cardiac output is usually more than sufficient to meet the peripheral metabolic demands of the body for the delivery of oxygen and substrate. Patients in this category are often refractory to pharmacologic interventions and by sustaining a very high cardiac output may eventually exhaust their cardiac reserves. The use of a vasoconstricting agent would appear to be physiologically appropriate, but this type of intervention usually severely depresses cardiac output and is not recommended. Treatment in this group of patients remains controversial, but the best available evidence suggests that it should be directed toward the metabolic abnormalities that appear to be the cause of this particular problem.

Acute Congestive Heart Failure and Pulmonary Edema

Current therapy for the management of congestive heart failure with associated pulmonary edema is a curious blend of the application of physiologic principles and the results of successful clinical trials. This situation reflects incomplete understanding of the pathophysiology of congestive heart failure and the mechanisms by which currently accepted therapeutic agents effect improvement.

In the case of cardiac arrest, standard recommendations for cardiopulmonary resuscitation must be instituted with recovery of reasonably stable cardiac rhythm and evidence of an adequate cardiac output.

Acid-base assessment, along with determination of blood gases, serum electrolytes, and calcium and glucose levels, must be rapidly performed when congestive heart failure becomes evident. Inotropic drug infusions may be started and titrated, and associated problems such as hypothermia and rhythm disturbances are aggressively corrected.

Acute pulmonary edema in the surgical setting is often the result of fluid overload in the presence of chronically compromised cardiac function or the occurrence of a recent myocardial infarction. Basic therapy involves the use of oxygen and an intravenous diuretic such as furosemide, which also acts as a vasodilator. Morphine, a narcotic possessing both venodilatory and vasodilatory properties, may be of benefit and may alleviate the anxiety often seen in awake patients. In some situations, it may be necessary to aid the failing ventricle by the use of intravenous vasodilators such as nitroprusside or nitroglycerin.

In the event that a rapid diuresis occurs, aggressive replacement of potassium is necessary for preventing hypokalemia. This is best accomplished by the intravenous route; however, care must be taken to avoid hyperkalemia, which may also cause life-threatening arrhythmias. For patients who develop pulmonary edema in association with marked renal insufficiency, the use of low-dose dopamine (2 to 3 μg. per kg. per minute) may improve renal blood flow and aid in diuresis. In those situations in which dopamine fails, aggressive therapy with ultrafiltration or dialysis may be required.

SELECTED REFERENCES

Freeman, W. K., Gibbons, R. J., and Shub, C.: Preoperative assessment of cardiac patients undergoing noncardiac surgical procedures. Mayo Clin. Proc., 64:1105, 1989.
An excellent review of the entire problem of assessing patients with all forms of cardiac disease and their management in the preoperative, operative, and postoperative period. Emphasis is placed on the physiologic assessment of such patients; an extensive bibliography covering all aspects of the problem is included.

Opie, L. H.: Drugs for the Heart. Philadelphia, W. B. Saunders Company, 1987.
A concise and up-to-date review of the major cardiovascular drugs employed in clinical practice. An extensive bibliography covers all areas of modern cardiovascular clinical pharmacology.

Waldhausen, J. A., and Biebuyck, J. F.: Surgery in the cardiac patient. Surg. Clin. North Am., 63:985, 1983.
A general discussion of the cardiovascular effects of surgical therapy and anesthesia on patients and particularly those with known cardiac risk factors. The discussion of the interacting of drugs and anesthesia on the patient with cardiac disease is particularly helpful.

REFERENCES

1. Byrd, R. C., Sung, R. J., Marks, J., and Parmley, W. W.: Safety and efficacy of esmolol (ASL-8052: an ultra short–acting beta-adrenergic blocking agent) for control of ventricular rate in supraventricular tachycardias. J. Coll. Cardiol., 3:394, 1984.
2. Chatterjee, K., and Parmley, W. W.: Vasodilator therapy for acute myocardial infarction and chronic congestive heart failure. J. Am. Coll. Cardiol., 1:133, 1983.
3. Cohn, J. N.: Physiologic basis of vasodilator therapy for heart failure. Am. J. Med., 71:135, 1982.
4. Cohn, J. N., Archibald, D. G., Phil, M., et al.: Effect of vasodilator therapy on mortality and chronic congestive heart failure. N. Engl. J. Med., 314:1547, 1986.
5. Colucci, W. S., Wright, R. F., and Brownwald, E.: New positive inotropic agents in the treatment of congestive heart failure. N. Engl. J. Med., 314:290, 349, 1986.
6. Curtiss, C., Cohn, J. N., Vrobel, T., and Franciosa, J. A.: Role of the renin angiotensin system in the vasoconstriction of congestive heart failure. Circulation, 58:763, 1978.
7. Edwards, C. R. W., and Padfield, P. L.: Angiotensin-converting enzyme inhibitors: Past, present and bright future. Lancet, 1:30, 1985.
8. Freeman, W. K., Gibbons, R. J., and Shub, C.: Preoperative assessment of cardiac patients undergoing noncardiac surgical procedures. Mayo Clin. Proc., 64:1105, 1989.

9. Goldman, L., Caldera, D., Nussbaum, S., et al.: Multifactorial index of cardiac risk in noncardiac surgical procedures. N. Engl. J. Med., 297:845, 1977.
10. Halperin, A. K., and Cubeddu, L. X.: The role of calcium channel–blockers in the treatment of hypertension. Am. Heart J., 111:363, 1986.
11. Harrison, D. C.: Antiarrhythmic drug classification: New science and practical applications. Am. J. Cardiol., 56:185, 1985.
12. Low, R. I., Takeda, P., Mason, D. T., and DeMaria, A. N.: The effects of calcium channel blocking agents on cardiovascular function. Am. J. Cardiol., 49:547, 1982.
13. Opie, L. H.: Drugs for the Heart. Philadelphia, W. B. Saunders Company, 1987.
14. Opie, L. H.: Calcium ions, drug action and the heart with special reference to calcium antagonist drugs. Pharmacol. Ther., 25:271, 1984.
15. Opie, L. H.: Drugs and the heart. I. Beta-blocking agents. Lancet, 1:693, 1980.
16. Opie, L. H.: Drugs and the heart. III. Calcium antagonists. Lancet, 1:806, 1980.
17. Opie, L. H.: Drugs and the heart. V. Digitalis and sympathomimetic stimulants. Lancet, 1:912, 1980.
18. Rao, T. L. K., Jacobs, K. H., and El-Etr, A. A.: Reinfarction following anesthesia in patients with myocardial infarction. Anesthesiology, 59:499, 1983.
19. Ribner, H. S., Bresnahan, D., and Hsieh, A. M.: Acute hemodynamics responses to vasodilator therapy in congestive heart failure. Prog. Cardiovasc. Dis., 25:1, 1982.
20. Richard, D., Ricome, J. L., Rimailho, A., et al.: Combined hemodynamic effects of dopamine and dobutamine in cardiogenic shock. Circulation, 67:620, 1983.
21. Stamler, J. L.: Lifestyles, major risk factors, proof and public policy. Circulation, 58:3, 1978.
22. Stewart, D. E., Ikram, H., Espiner, E. A., et al.: Arrhythmogenic potential of diuretic induced hypokalemia in patients with mild hypertension and ischemic heart disease. Br. Heart J., 54:290, 1985.
23. Tarhan, S., Moffitt, E. A., Taylor, W. F., et al.: Myocardial infarction after general anesthesia. J.A.M.A., 220:1451, 1972.
24. Zelis, R., Longhurst, J., Capone, R. J., and Lee, G.: Peripheral circulatory control mechanisms in congestive heart failure. Am. J. Cardiol., 32:481, 1973.

XXIV

CARDIOPULMONARY BYPASS FOR CARDIAC SURGERY

William L. Holman, M.D., and James K. Kirklin, M.D.

HISTORICAL ASPECTS

The concept of diverting the circulation to an extracorporeal oxygenator dates back to at least 1885 with the work of Frey and Gruber.[47] However, the development of devices for clinical use did not occur until the twentieth century when modern surgical and anesthetic techniques, new plastic materials, and the discovery of heparin made the development of these devices possible. As reviewed by Clowes,[27] the early methods for cardiopulmonary bypass included oxygenation using heterologous lung tissue, controlled cross-circulation, and artificial oxygenator devices.

Lillehei and colleagues at the University of Minnesota were the first to use "controlled cross-circulation" with another intact subject acting as the pump and oxygenator. In April of 1954, they began a spectacular series of cardiac operations using controlled cross-circulation.[80] Despite the eventual abandonment of this technique, their efforts initiated the era of modern open heart surgery.

Early work on the mechanical pump oxygenators was performed by many investigators including Gibbon,[52] Dennis,[34] Bjork,[10] and Senning.[108] Dennis and colleagues at the University of Minnesota were perhaps the first group to apply a pump oxygenator system to clinical cardiac surgery when they repaired what was thought to be an atrial septal defect in 1951. Unfortunately, the patient died, partly because of an imperfect repair of a partial atrioventricular canal defect.[34] In 1953, the pump oxygenator device developed by John Gibbon, who began initial experimental studies at the Massachusetts General Hospital in Boston and later at Jefferson Medical School in Philadelphia, was used by Gibbon to successfully repair an atrial septal defect.[51] Based on their experimental studies with cardiopulmonary bypass in the early 1950s,[36,64] Kirklin and colleagues at the Mayo Clinic began the world's first series of intracardiac operations using a pump oxygenator in March 1955, when they successfully repaired a ventricular septal defect.[72]

PUMP OXYGENATOR APPARATUS

The precise apparatus available for cardiopulmonary bypass (CPB) changes frequently, but the basic components remain

constant. A *venous reservoir* is usually present and is positioned to provide adequate siphonage of blood by gravity.[92] This provides storage of excess volume and allows escape of any air bubbles returning with venous blood.

The *oxygenator* provides oxygen to the blood and allows elimination of carbon dioxide. Currently bubble oxygenators, membrane oxygenators, and microporous hollow-fiber oxygenators are available for clinical use. In bubble oxygenators, gas is bubbled into the venous blood, and gas exchange occurs at the blood-gas interface. Antifoaming agents then cause the small bubbles to burst, and the gas escapes through exhaust portals. Membrane oxygenators utilize a semipermeable membrane between layers of blood and gas across which gas transfer occurs. The advantage of this type of oxygenator is the potential avoidance of the damaging effects of CPB related to the direct blood-gas interface of the bubble oxygenator. However, under most clinical conditions no clear-cut advantage of the membrane oxygenator has yet been demonstrated.[103] Microporous hollow-fiber oxygenators contain a mass of approximately 50,000 to 60,000 hollow fibers to provide a surface for gas exchange. The fibers have a diameter of 200 μ and are generally made of polypropylene or Teflon with an average pore size of 0.1 to 0.5 μ. The microporous hollow-fiber oxygenators share many of the theoretic advantages of the nonporous membrane oxygenating devices.

An efficient *heat exchanger* is necessary for control of the perfusate temperature in order to achieve systemic cooling and rewarming during CPB. Most heat exchanging devices are included as an integral part of the pump oxygenator.

The *arterial pump* is usually a roller pump,[32] which should be adjusted before each perfusion to be slightly nonocclusive. The pump tubing is either Silastic or latex, which, unlike the Tygon tubing, does not become stiff at low temperatures. The arterial pump should be calibrated at frequent intervals so that accurate perfusion rates can be established. Several nonocclusive vortex pumps are also available; however, their use is generally restricted to extracorporeal membrane oxygenator or ventricular assist device circuits.

The arterial line pressure in the pump oxygenator must be continuously monitored. When this pressure exceeds 300 mm. Hg, the risk of disruption of the arterial line or cavitation in the region of the arterial cannula increases. These risks are minimized by a properly positioned and adequately sized arterial cannula. An arterial bubble trap may be used as a safety device to remove air that enters the arterial line. A low-porosity arterial filter may be utilized, but a randomized study by Walker and colleagues at the University of Alabama in Birmingham failed to show any beneficial effects from such a filter.[131]

PHYSIOLOGIC RESPONSE TO CARDIOPULMONARY BYPASS

Many complex physiologic changes occur when a patient is temporarily supported by means of an oxygenator system. The term *total cardiopulmonary bypass* indicates that nearly all of the systemic venous blood is returned to the oxygenator. *Partial CPB* implies that some of the systemic venous blood returns to the heart and is ejected into the aorta. Two main types of physiologic variables exist during CPB, that is, *externally controlled variables*, which are controlled by the surgeon and perfusionist, and *patient variables*, which are less easily regulated.

Externally Controlled Variables

The *perfusion flow rate* is controlled by the perfusionist but should be actively established by the surgeon. Lactic acidosis occurs at flows of less than 1.6 liters per minute per sq. m. at normothermia.[28,35] Experimental and clinical data[79,86] indicate that normothermic perfusion flow rates of 1.7 liters per minute per sq. m. or greater are usually acceptable, but flow rates of 2.0 to 2.5 liters per minute per sq. m. provide a more secure margin of safety for organ perfusion. For large patients (body surface area 2.0 sq. m. or greater), the authors usually select a flow rate of 1.8 to 2.0 liters per minute per sq. m. to avoid the potential risks of exceeding the oxygenating capability of the pump oxygenator, exceeding the flow capacity of the venous cannulas, and increasing the damage to blood elements.

Because of the inherent individual variability of response to CPB, no absolute criteria exist for safe flow rates at a given temperature. Organ damage appears least likely to occur when the microcirculation is perfused at flows that maintain nearly normal tissue oxygen levels and maximal oxygen consumption. During hypothermic CPB, maximal perfusion of the microcirculation probably occurs near the asymptote of the temperature-specific curve relating flow to oxygen consumption ($\dot{V}o_2$) (Fig. 1).[68]

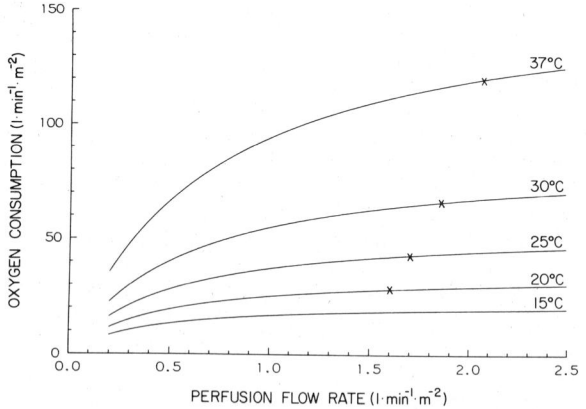

Figure 1. Nomogram of an equation expressing the relation of oxygen consumption ($\dot{V}o_2$) to perfusion flow rate ($\dot{Q}$) and temperature (T). The small x's represent the perfusion flow rates used by us at these temperatures. The equation is

$$1/(\dot{V}o_2) = 0.168 \ 10^{-387\,T} + 0.0378 \ \dot{Q}^{-1} \ 10^{-0.0253\,T}$$

(From Kirklin, J. W., et al.: Cardiopulmonary bypass for cardiac surgery. *In* Sabiston, D. C., Jr., and Spencer, F. C. (Eds.): Surgery of the Chest. 5th ed. Philadelphia, W. B. Saunders Company, 1990.)

The *temperature of the perfusate,* and secondarily of the patient, is controlled by the perfusionist via the heat exchanger.[16] This is one of the most important decisions made about each patient during CPB. Particularly in small infants, moderate and profound hypothermic perfusion allows the safe, temporary reduction in flow that is advantageous for the accurate intracardiac repair of many malformations (see Low-Flow Perfusion). The authors, and most other cardiac surgeons, utilize some degree of hypothermic perfusion for nearly all cardiac operations, since hypothermia provides an element of safety if a mechanical pump oxygenator failure requires a brief period of total circulatory arrest while the apparatus is being repaired. The commonly used roller pump provides nonpulsatile flow. Pulsatile flow during CPB can be achieved with pulsatile arterial pumps, the patient's own cardiac ejection, or the intra-aortic balloon pump.[94]

The systemic venous pressure is directly proportional to systemic blood flow and blood viscosity, and it is inversely proportional to venous cannula size, venous line diameter, and venous line suction. The systemic venous pressure should be maintained as close as possible to 0 during CPB and should certainly not exceed 10 mm. Hg because of the increased potential for cerebral edema and accumulation of extracellular fluid with high venous pressures. It is therefore advisable to use the largest venous cannulas consistent with satisfactory operative conditions. If a smaller than desired venous cannula must be used, the adverse effect on venous pressure can be overcome by reducing the perfusion flow rate.

Pulmonary venous pressure (left atrial pressure) should also be maintained near 0 during total CPB. High pulmonary venous pressure during bypass may result from excessive pulmonary collateral blood flow, an unrecognized extracardiac left-to-right shunt (e.g., patent ductus arteriosus), or incomplete venous drainage leading to increased pulmonary blood flow. Marked and prolonged elevation in pulmonary venous pressure during CPB promotes accumulation of extravascular lung water and probably contributes to postoperative pulmonary dysfunction.

The *hematocrit* of the patient-oxygenator system is determined by the body size and hematocrit of the patient, the composition and amount of the initial priming volume of the pump oxygenator, the amount of blood loss, and the composition and volume of solutions infused during CPB. The initial priming volume is determined by the volume required for the oxygenator and its reservoir, the pump lines, the bubble trap, and the cardioplegia apparatus.

At normothermia, a hematocrit of 40 to 50 per cent appears optimal for oxygen transport[24] and preserves the appropriate blood rheologic properties. Higher hematocrits cause increased oxygen content at the expense of increased viscosity and decreased blood flow.

During hypothermia, a lower hematocrit appears desirable because of the lower resultant viscosity and lower shear rates, theoretically providing improved perfusion of the microcirculation. Excessive hemodilution, however, is probably deleterious because of the greater extravascular extravasation of fluid secondary to the decreased intravascular osmotic pressure.[29] Since most pediatric and adult cardiac surgical patients are operated upon with hypothermic perfusion, it is probably advisable to maintain the "patient-machine" hematocrit between 25 and 30 per cent in order to take advantage of both of these effects.

Prior to operation a calculation is made of the mixed patient-machine hematocrit that would result if the pump oxygenator is primed with an asanguineous solution. The equation used is

$$\text{Hct}_{pm} = \frac{[\text{Body weight (kg.) f 1000}] [\text{Hct}_p]}{[\text{Body weight (kg.) f 1000}] + \text{machine BV}}$$

where Hct_{pm} is the hematocrit of combined patient-machine blood volume, Hct_p is the patient hematocrit, BV is blood volume, f equals 0.08 in infants and children (less than 12 years), and f equals 0.065 in older patients (more than 12 years).

If the hematocrit is in the desired range, an asanguineous prime is used with approximately 20 per cent of the prime as 5 per cent dextrose and 80 per cent as a balanced salt solution with sufficient human albumin added to make it colloidally isosmotic. If the calculated hematocrit is too low, an appropriate amount of blood or packed cells is added. In that instance, an additional equation is used:

$$\text{Hct} = \frac{\text{Patient red cell vol. (ml.)} + \text{machine red cell vol. (ml.)}}{\text{Patient BV} + \text{machine BV (ml.)}}$$

Packed red cells less than 5 days old are generally utilized. Because the blood is calcium-free and acidotic, heparin, calcium, and buffer are added (Table 1).

The *glucose concentration* is increased in the priming solution (about 350 mg. per 100 ml.) in order to provide an energy source as well as to promote an osmotic diuresis during and following cardiopulmonary bypass.

Arterial oxygen levels are usually maintained at a level of 100 to 250 mm. Hg with current bubble and membrane oxygenators. Shephard has shown that in dogs, arterial oxygen saturation levels less than 65 per cent at normothermia cause decreased $\dot{V}o_2$, indicating cellular hypoxia.[109] Hypothermic perfusion produces a decrease in $\dot{V}o_2$ and an increase in mixed venous oxygen pressure ($P\bar{v}o_2$), both of which cause increased Pao_2. During rewarming, the increasing $\dot{V}o_2$ causes relatively low $P\bar{v}o_2$ levels and a decreased Pao_2. This is the period of maximal demand on oxygenator reserves.[120,121]

The *arterial carbon dioxide pressure* ($Paco_2$) is determined by the ratio of gas flow to blood flow in the oxygenator, higher ratios causing a lower $Paco_2$. A $Paco_2$ of 30 to 40 mm. Hg (measured at 37° C.) is considered optimal during cardiopulmonary bypass. The optimal $Paco_2$ during profound hypothermia remains controversial. Reeves and Rahn[96,97] and Swan[116] have emphasized that at low temperatures ionic neutrality is associated with a higher pH than at normothermia because of the change in the dissociation constant of water. Thus, in a patient with a temperature of 20° C., the $Paco_2$ measured at 37° C. should be 30 to 40 mm. Hg, which is a $Paco_2$ of 14 to 20 mm. Hg at 20° C.[96,97] and a pH at 20° C. of nearly 7.6.[99] Rahn and Reeves reason that relative hyperventilation should be practiced during hypothermic cardiopulmonary bypass in order to maintain an alkalotic milieu.[96]

Patient Variables

The body's physiologic response to CPB is extremely complex and only partially understood. *Systemic vascular resistance* decreases abruptly with the onset of CPB. Thereafter it gradually increases throughout the period of bypass, although there is considerable variation among patients. The importance of maintaining a certain level of mean arterial perfusion pressure during bypass is controversial. Although some clinical[115,124] and experimental[61] studies suggest that decreased cerebral blood flow is associated with a mean perfusion pressure less than approximately 50 to 60 mm. Hg, studies by Ellis and associates[40]

TABLE 1. Additives to a Unit of CPD Blood for the Pump Oxygenator

CPD blood	500 ml.
Heparin	3 ml. (3000 units; mean 6 units/ml. of blood)
NaHCO₃	10 ml.
CaCl₂	5 ml. (added last)
	518 ml.

CPD, citrate-phosphate-dextrose.
From Kirklin, J. W., et al.: *In* Sabiston, D. C., Jr., and Spencer, F. C. (Eds.): Surgery of the Chest, 5th ed. Philadelphia, W. B. Saunders Company, 1990.

and Kolkka and associates[74] as well as the Alabama clinical experience indicate that pharmacologic manipulation of the resistance during hypothermic bypass is not necessary. During rewarming, however, it appears rational to increase arterial blood pressure pharmacologically if it persists at a level less than 50 or 55 mm. Hg, both to ensure adequate cerebral perfusion and to optimize coronary perfusion. Because of the theoretic potential for intracerebral bleeding with very high arterial perfusion pressures during bypass, it is probably desirable to reduce the mean arterial perfusion pressure pharmacologically if it exceeds 100 mm. Hg.

Total body $\dot{V}o_2$ and $P\bar{v}o_2$ levels are both partially controlled by the perfusion flow rate and the patient's temperature. Although individual variation occurs, it is generally assumed that the microcirculation is being effectively perfused if the mixed venous oxygen levels during bypass are 30 to 40 mm. Hg with a mixed venous O_2 saturation of 60 to 70 per cent.

Metabolic acidosis is almost always present during bypass, but lactate levels should not exceed 5 mEq. per liter if adequate perfusion flow rates are maintained.[59,81] Cardiopulmonary bypass is also associated with a massive release of epinephrine (primarily from the adrenal medulla). Plasma epinephrine levels rise in nearly all patients shortly after the onset of CPB and begin to fall after bypass.[132]

Changes in *body composition* also occur. During and after CPB, extracellular fluid is increased.[15,26] The major shift of fluid is from the intravascular space to the interstitial space, causing increased interstitial fluid pressure[26,98] and decreased plasma volume.[26] The magnitude of the increase in extravascular fluid volume is directly related to the duration of CPB, and it is further increased with hemodilution.[29] The amount of exchangeable potassium is decreased, whereas exchangeable sodium is increased.[91] Recent studies by Smith and associates[112] demonstrated that the increase in microvascular permeability during cardiopulmonary bypass probably is caused by an increase in the size of large pores in capillary walls. These large pores allow diffusion of macromolecules into the extravascular space, which reduces the colloid osmotic pressure gradient and promotes movement of fluid out of the microvasculature.

DAMAGING EFFECTS OF CARDIOPULMONARY BYPASS

"Safe" CPB is characterized by the absence of structural or functional damage after the perfusion. The vast majority of patients suffer no clinically apparent ill effects from CPB; however, an occasional patient develops severe multiorgan dysfunction despite an otherwise accurate and complete intracardiac repair.

In its most severe form, the "postperfusion syndrome" is characterized by a diffuse whole-body "inflammatory reaction," with elements of increased capillary permeability, extravascular extravasation of plasma, increased interstitial fluid, leukocytosis, fever, peripheral vasoconstriction, breakdown of red blood cells, and a diffuse bleeding diathesis. The fact that most patients convalesce normally after CPB attests not to the absence of these ill effects but rather to the ability of the organism to tolerate them. It is believed that much of the residual mortality and morbidity following CPB is related to these damaging effects.

Some incremental risk factors for an adverse clinical response to CPB have been identified, but the precise nature and magnitude of these effects have not been quantified. One is the *duration of bypass*.[70] In most adults, the probability of structural or functional damage appears to increase as the perfusion time extends beyond approximately 3 hours, and it probably sharply increases after 4 hours. Another incremental risk factor is *age*. The susceptibility to organ dysfunction after CPB appears to increase in neonates. The very elderly also appear less tolerant of the damaging effects of CPB, particularly in the presence of pre-existing renal dysfunction. These two risk factors undoubtedly interact, making the safe time constraints more rigid in the very young[70] and the elderly patient. *Increased levels of the anaphylatoxin C3a* also increase the probability of morbidity after CPB.[73]

Other factors undoubtedly interact, including the type of oxygenator, the composition of the perfusate, the perfusion flow rate, the presence or absence of pulsatile flow, and the patient's temperature. Certain cardiac malformations, particularly cyanotic congenital heart disease, may also be incremental risk factors. Although the importance of each of these factors has not yet been clarified, further research and development will likely lead to modifications of the bypass circuit that will improve its safety, particularly in high-risk situations.

The mechanisms for damage following CPB are most likely *altered arterial blood flow patterns and exposure of blood to abnormal events.* It is believed that the exposure of blood to abnormal events is the most powerful determinant of the two (Fig. 2).[69]

Altered Arterial Blood Flow Patterns

The standard roller pump for CPB produces nonpulsatile flow while the heart is empty on full bypass. This represents a marked deviation from the normal physiologic conditions in which the arterial pulse pressure is about one third the systolic pressure. *Pulsatile* perfusion during full bypass has been noted to provide lower vascular resistance, less red cell aggregation, improved renal function, and less cellular hypoxia than nonpulsatile flow during CPB.[50,53,84,134] However, clinical studies comparing pulsatile with nonpulsatile flow during CPB have been inconclusive. Some studies suggest a beneficial effect of pulsatile flow,[37,56,63,83,90,117-119,122,123,135] whereas other studies indicate no advantage over nonpulsatile perfusion.[92,110,111,133,136]

Exposure of Blood to Abnormal Events

During CPB, exposure of blood to abnormal events includes exposure to shear stresses, incorporation of abnormal substances, and, perhaps most important, exposure to unphysiologic (*nonendothelial*) surfaces.

Blood is a complex substance composed of both formed and unformed elements. The formed elements include red blood cells, white blood cells, and platelets. Among the unformed elements in blood, the plasma proteins appear particularly vulnerable during CPB. Plasma proteins include those proteins with primary osmotic effects (albumin), those acting as carrier vehicles for other blood-borne substances (albumin, lipoproteins, and immunoglobulin), and those constituting the humoral amplification system (coagulation, fibrinolytic, complement, and kallikrein cascades). *Shear stresses* are generated by blood pumps, by suction devices, and by cavitation around the end of the arterial cannula. Leukocytes appear to be particularly sensitive to shear stresses, which cause destruction of leukocytes or functional impairments such as decreased aggregation, decreased chemotactic migration, and impaired phagocytosis in surviving leukocytes.[85] During CPB, an initial leukopenia develops that returns to baseline values after approximately 2 hours of CPB.[75] This increase occurs in part secondary to active movement of leukocytes out of the vascular space.[76] Immediately following CPB, a leukocytosis is present and continues for several days.[101]

Lymphocytes, including both B cells and T cells, are decreased after CPB, and T cell function is depressed.[101] This depression of cellular immunity is specifically due to CPB and appears to resolve more rapidly in patients *not* exposed to blood transfusions.[60]

During CPB, red blood cells are damaged mainly by shear stresses. The result is either immediate hemolysis with release of free hemoglobin or a shortened red cell life span with delayed hemolysis. Hemolysis is less evident when an oxygenator is not in the system,[88] and bubble oxygenators generally produce more hemolysis than membrane oxygenators do.[5,25] The intracardiac suction lines are particularly damaging to erythrocytes. Levels of free hemoglobin have been noted to increase four-fold within 10 minutes after initiating CPB,[57] and the decreased erythrocyte survival time after bypass causes a progressive loss of red cell mass during the first 3 or 4 postoperative days.

The *incorporation of abnormal substances* during cardiopulmonary bypass includes air bubbles, fibrin, tissue debris, and platelet thrombi, as well as defoaming agents. Thromboplastinogen is activated when blood makes contact with injured tissues, and

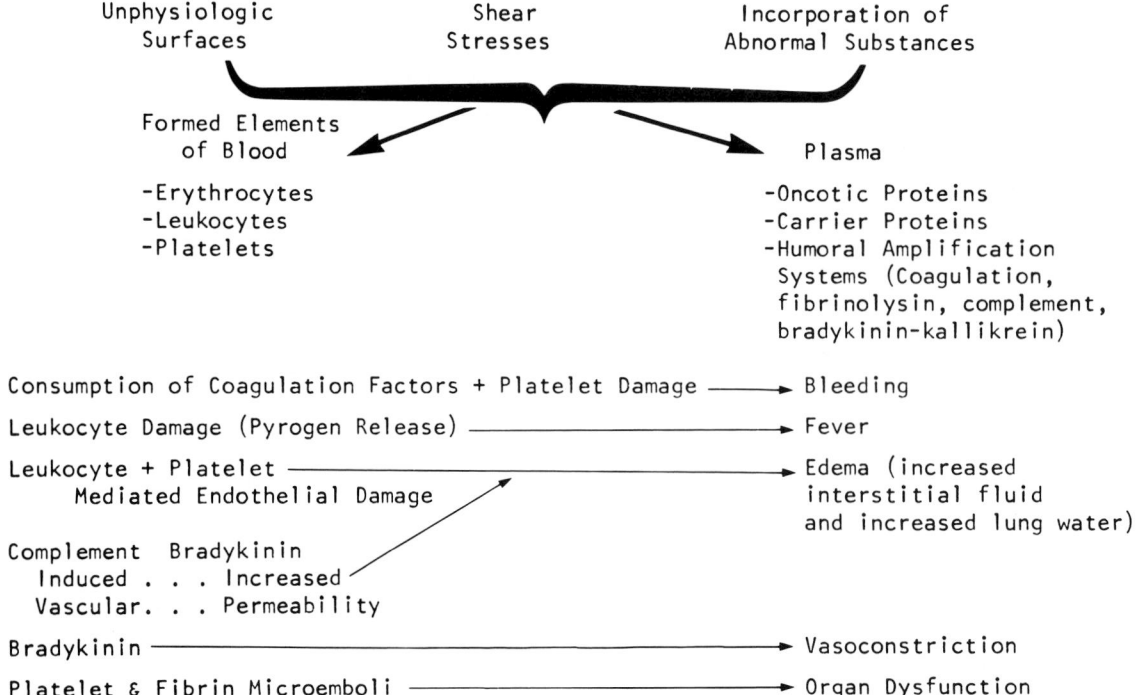

Figure 2. Schematic representation of a current concept of the damaging effects of cardiopulmonary bypass related to the exposure of blood to abnormal events. (From Kirklin, J. K., Kirklin, J. W., and Pacifico, A. D.: Cardiopulmonary bypass. *In* Arciniegas, E. (Ed.): Pediatric Cardiac Surgery. Chicago, Year Book Medical Publishers, 1985.)

this may contribute to intravascular coagulation and the formation of thrombin and platelet emboli. Recently, high circulating levels of plasticizing agents leached from polyvinyl chloride surfaces and have been documented in patients undergoing operations that include CPB,[7] and evidence for cerebral microembolization during CPB has been obtained from humans[12] and animals.[12,114]

It is the *exposure to unphysiologic surfaces* that produces the greatest damage during bypass. The most critical surfaces are probably those of the oxygenating device. The unphysiologic surface is gas in bubble, disc, and screen oxygenators and the membrane in a membrane oxygenator. The proportion of blood exposed to an unphysiologic surface is relatively small in the reservoirs, tubes, and cannulas. The effect on platelets is to promote platelet aggregation,[39,62] which causes platelet emboli as well as decreased platelet number[65] and function[8] after CPB. It is generally agreed that fibrinogen is rapidly adsorbed to the surfaces within the CPB circuit. Platelet surface glycoproteins (e.g., GPIIb-IIIa complex) then bind to these sites, producing platelet activation.[54] A portion of platelets exposed to the CPB circuit undergoes degranulation and is irreversibly damaged, whereas other platelets undergo partial degranulation and reversible aggregation. The precise sequence of events and proportions of impaired and destroyed platelets remain controversial.[33,38,49,54,87,137] Current investigations of this process are directed toward the development of methods to protect platelet function during bypass. Methods currently under investigation to attenuate platelet damage during CPB include protein "passivation" of oxygenator surfaces[3,54] and rendering platelets reversibly nonfunctional using prostanoids during CPB.[1-4,66] Recently, desmopressin acetate was shown to diminish bleeding after CPB[105]; however, this drug may be beneficial only in patients with a specific defect in platelet function related to low plasma levels of von Willebrand factor.[58] Aprotinin, a known inhibitor of plasmin and kallikrein, appears also to preserve platelets during CPB.[125] The effect of aprotinin on platelets has not yet been completely defined, but the results of several studies demonstrate markedly improved hemostasis with this drug.[9,125,126]

Denaturation of carrier proteins occurs during CPB, with breakdown of lipoproteins and generation of fat emboli.[77] Protein denaturation increases plasma viscosity and promotes clumping of erythrocytes; however, this effect can be attenuated by hemodilution.

The *humoral amplification system* is a complex system of plasma proteins that responds to a local stimulus with a self-perpetuating and expanding series of reactions. These normally involve an inflammatory reaction in a localized area of the body. The components of the humoral amplification system include the *coagulation cascade,* the *fibrinolytic cascade,* the *kallikrein system,* and the *complement system.* It is believed that the damaging effects of CPB are related in large degree to the humoral amplification system, which initiates a whole-body "inflammatory response" during CPB.

Hageman factor (factor XII) is activated almost immediately after the onset of CPB by the massive contact of blood with nonendothelial surfaces.[43,127] This activates the coagulation cascade and also other cascades. Even with appropriate heparinization during CPB, there is evidence of ongoing microcoagulation with consumption of clotting factors.[65]

The fibrinolytic cascade is also activated with the onset of CPB. Increased levels of serum plasmin (the active fibrinolytic agent) have been detected shortly after initiation of CPB.[6] Plasmin itself may serve as an activator of prekallikrein, the complement system, and possibly Hageman factor.

The kallikrein cascade may be activated by Hageman factor, which causes production of bradykinin. Bradykinin increases vascular permeability, dilates arterioles, initiates smooth muscle contraction, and elicits pain. Kallikrein can activate Hageman factor and activate plasminogen to form plasmin, again demon-

strating the complex interaction between these amplification systems. High levels of bradykinin are present during CPB.[41,93] Since bradykinin is metabolized mainly in the lungs, exclusion of the pulmonary circulation during CPB acts to sustain circulating bradykinin levels. In addition, very young infants appear to be less able to eliminate bradykinin.[48]

The complement system is composed of a group of circulating glycoproteins and forms a basic part of the body's response to immunologic, traumatic, or foreign body insult. Two pathways exist for activation of the complement sequence (Fig. 3).[55] The classic pathway is usually initiated via interaction with antigen-antibody complexes. The alternative or properdin pathway is activated by exposure of blood to foreign surfaces, and it is this pathway that is initially activated during CPB[23,67,129] with later activation of the classic pathway during protamine administration following CPB.[71]

In 1972, Parker and colleagues[95] noted that complement was consumed during CPB, and they hypothesized that the complement system may promote the increases in capillary permeability that are frequently seen following CPB. Chenoweth and colleagues[23] at the University of Alabama in Birmingham and Scripps Institute have demonstrated that the complement anaphylatoxin C3a is increased shortly after the onset of CPB, with continuing production throughout the duration of bypass (Fig. 4). In contrast, patients undergoing cardiac operations without CPB have normal levels of C3a at the end of the operation.[73] The anaphylatoxins C5a and C3a have physiologic effects similar to those observed in many patients after CPB, including vasoconstriction and increased capillary permeability.[11,89]

In addition to the direct microvascular effects of complement, neutrophil-mediated injury also occurs following complement activation (Fig. 5). Chenoweth and Hugli[22] in 1978 demon-

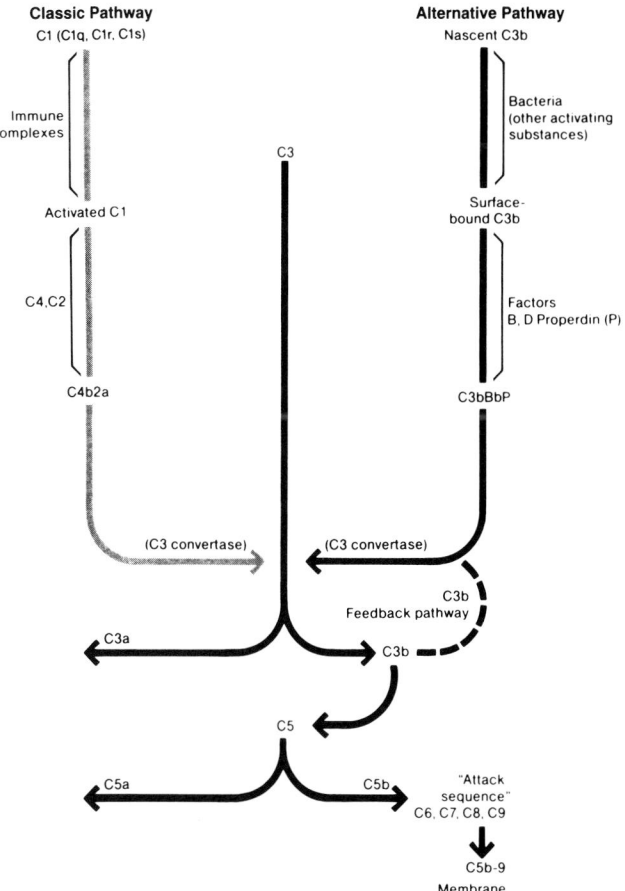

Figure 3. Pathways of complement activation (From Goldstein, I. M.: Complement in infectious diseases. Current Concepts, The Upjohn Company, 1980.)

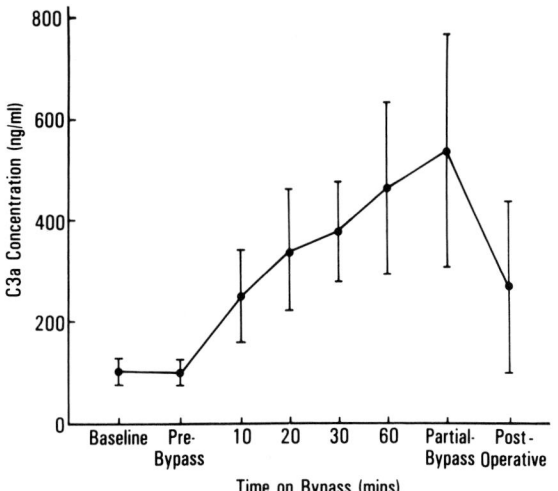

Figure 4. Plasma levels of C3a in patients undergoing cardiopulmonary bypass. (From Chenoweth, D. E., et al.: Complement activation during cardiopulmonary bypass: Evidence for generation of C3a and C5a anaphylatoxins. N. Engl. J. Med., *304*:497, 1981.)

strated specific C5a receptor sites on human neutrophils. Activation of the alternative pathway produces C5a that is rapidly bound to neutrophils, which are then deposited in the lungs as well as other organs. Neutrophil activation and degranulation during CPB has been demonstrated in humans[31,130] and may be responsible for some of the deleterious effects of CPB. Endothelial cell damage of oxygen radicals produced by complement-stimulated granulocytes has been demonstrated,[102] and Flick and colleagues[44] showed that leukocytes are required for the increased lung microvascular permeability seen after microembolization in sheep. Recently, several groups[14,42,100] have demonstrated associations during CPB between the generation of peroxidation products and pulmonary neutrophil sequestration, as well as between oxygen free radical generation and complement activation.[19] It is hypothesized that a portion of the pulmonary dysfunction after CPB is caused by complement activation with the elaboration of C3a and C5a. C5a then promotes pulmonary leukosequestration and release of superoxides and lysosomal enzymes, which in turn produce direct endothelial damage and alterations in permeability (Fig. 5).

Salama and colleagues have demonstrated deposition of the terminal C5b–9 complexes on erythrocytes (as well as neutrophils) during CPB. Intravascular hemolysis was noted in all patients, and C5b–9 was demonstrated on red cell ghosts but

not on intact erythrocytes, thus inferring a relationship between complement activation and hemolysis during CPB.[104]

Studies at the University of Alabama in Birmingham have correlated cardiac, pulmonary, renal, and hematologic dysfunction after CPB with higher levels of C3a after bypass, longer elapsed times of bypass, and younger age at operation.[73] An increased understanding of complement activation during CPB allows the development of methods to attenuate complement activation and diminish the deleterious effects of CPB. This may be achieved by designing oxygenator systems that produce less complement activation[20,128] or developing pharmacologic methods to inhibit complement activation during CPB.[129]

BLOOD CONSERVATION

During the past decade, efforts have been directed toward conservation of blood and avoidance of nonautologous transfusions in patients undergoing CPB. Autotransfusion of shed mediastinal blood after cardiac operations has been shown to be a safe and effective method for minimizing postoperative transfusion requirements.[30,106] Erythrocytes aspirated from the operative field can be separated by centrifugation and washing prior to reinfusion. Intraoperative ultrafiltration of blood using hollow-fiber hemofilters may also be used to conserve blood. Studies by Boldt and associates[13] and Solem and co-workers[113] have demonstrated that hemofiltration conserves the plasma fraction as well as erythrocytes. Hemofiltration or cell separation techniques can be used to conserve the blood that remains in the oxygenator after the termination of CPB.

Autologous blood donated prior to cardiac operations has been shown to reduce the need for homologous transfusion,[82] and the preoperative administration of human recombinant erythropoietin is currently under investigation as a means to diminish postoperative transfusion requirements. Ultimately, a much greater impact on postoperative hemostasis and transfusion requirements will result from the development of improved methods for platelet preservation during CPB.

LOW-FLOW PERFUSION

Particularly during infant intracardiac surgery, a nearly bloodless field can usually be achieved with hypothermic low-flow perfusion for a portion of the repair. At a nasopharyngeal temperature of 20° C., a flow rate of 1.2 to 1.6 liters per minute per m.² is well tolerated. A large clinical experience indicates that at 20° C. nasopharyngeal temperature, the perfusion flow rate can be safely reduced to 0.5 liter per minute per sq. m. for 30 to 45 minutes.

Oxygen consumption ($\dot{V}O_2$) is an important indication of the adequacy of perfusion to the microcirculation. The decrease in $\dot{V}O_2$ during low-flow perfusion probably results from closing down of portions of the microcirculation. The relationship between $\dot{V}O_2$ and the perfusion flow rate during hypothermic CPB (20° C.) is such that $\dot{V}O_2$ decreases rapidly only after flow is reduced below 1.0 liter per minute per sq. m. (Fig. 6).[45]

A series of hyperbolic curves can be generated from various experimental and clinical studies[21,45,77,86] that describe the relationship between $\dot{V}O_2$ and flow at various temperatures during CPB (see Fig. 1). Maximal perfusion of the microcirculation probably occurs near the asymptote of the curve, and from this a minimal safe flow rate at a given temperature can be selected during CPB.

The adequacy of cerebral perfusion during low-flow hypothermic perfusion has been examined in animal experiments.[46] Cerebral $\dot{V}O_2$ is well maintained as flow is reduced from 1.5 to 0.5 liter per minute per sq. m. on CPB at 20° C. (Table 2). In addition, calculated vascular resistance in the brain remains constant while overall systemic vascular resistance progressively increases as flow is reduced from 1.5 to 0.5 liter per min-

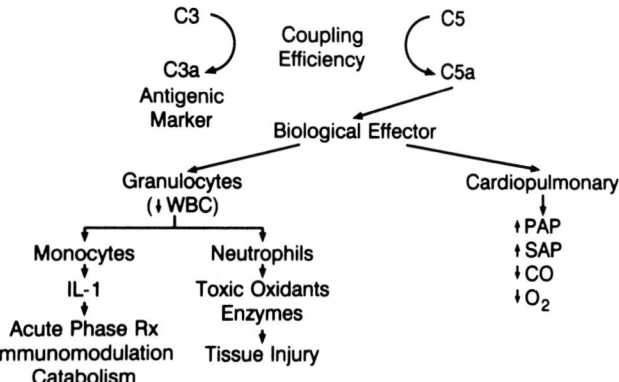

Figure 5. Diagram outlining the two modes of action for the human anaphylatoxins C3a and C5a produced during complement activation. The coupling efficiency refers to the relative quantity of C5a produced as compared with C3a. The coupling efficiency varies according to the activating or nonactivating character of the foreign surface in contact with blood. (From Chenoweth, D. E.: *In* Leonard, E. F., Turitto, V. T., and Vroman, L. (Eds.): Blood in Contact with Natural and Artificial Surfaces. New York, The New York Academy of Sciences, 1987.)

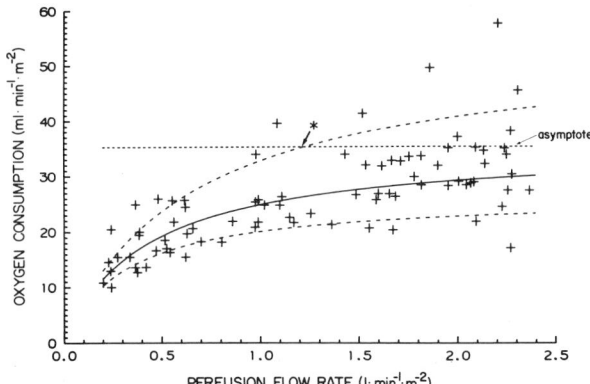

Figure 6. Relationship of oxygen consumption ($\dot{V}_{O_2}$) to perfusion flow rate ($\dot{Q}$) during nonpulsatile cardiopulmonary bypass at 20° C. Plus signs represent individual measurements. The solid line is the nomogram of the hyperbolic equation

$$\dot{V}_{O_2} = 35 \pm 2.03 \; (\dot{Q}/[\dot{Q} + 0.42 \pm 0.055])$$

The significance levels of coefficients are less than 0.0001. The dashed lines, also derived from the regression analysis, are the 70 per cent confidence limits for the observations (± 1 SD). The dotted line is the asymptote (35.3) representing the estimate of maximal $\dot{V}_{O_2}$. The asterisk indicates the flow rate (1.2 liters per minute per m.²) above which the upper 70 per cent confidence limit overlaps the asymptote. (From Fox, L. S., et al.: Relationship of whole body oxygen consumption to perfusion flow rate during hypothermic cardiopulmonary bypass. J. Thorac. Cardiovasc. Surg., 83:239, 1982.)

ute per sq. m. (Table 3). The contribution of autoregulation to the maintenance of cerebral perfusion during hypothermic low-flow perfusion has been confirmed in adult human studies.[17,45]

CLINICAL METHODOLOGY IN CARDIOPULMONARY BYPASS

Cardiopulmonary bypass should be used as a flexible clinical means, recognizing its physiologic limitations, risks, and damaging effects. Some degree of hypothermia is utilized for nearly all operations performed on CPB. Whenever possible, part of the repair is performed during the rewarming phase. An important advantage of hypothermia is that it allows a safe transient period of low-flow perfusion (0.5 to 1.0 liter per minute per sq. m.) if improved visibility is desired or a brief period of safe circulatory arrest if repair of an oxygenator malfunction is required.

The size of arterial (Table 4) and venous cannulas (Table 5) is determined primarily by the selected total perfusion flow rate. At any given patient size, there is an acceptable range of perfusion rates, which allows somewhat smaller cannulas to be utilized if the anatomic situation dictates. An arterial cannula is generally selected that provides a gradient across the cannula of

100 mm. Hg or less in order to minimize the risks of a high arterial line pressure (see Pump Oxygenator Apparatus). The constituents of the priming solution are reviewed with the perfusionist, and a decision is made regarding the addition of blood to the prime, depending on the desired "patient-machine" hematocrit (see Physiologic Response to CPB, Externally Controlled Variables).

After performing a median sternotomy and opening and tacking up the pericardium, the external cardiac anatomy is carefully assessed. Any dissection prior to CPB is usually accomplished before heparin is administered. Pursestring sutures are placed for arterial and venous cannulation and placement of the cardioplegic needle. The initial heparin dose is 3000 units per kg., and adequate anticoagulation is verified by an activated clotting time greater than 8 minutes.

Arterial Cannulation

The ascending aorta is generally utilized for arterial cannulation. The femoral artery is used under special circumstances, such as in patients undergoing resection of aneurysms or dissection of the ascending aorta and those undergoing closure of a previously constructed descending aorta–left pulmonary artery (Potts) anastomosis.

The hemodynamic advantages of entrance of the arterial inflow into the ascending aorta as opposed to the femoral artery have been debated. Most studies indicate that regional blood flow, including cerebral blood flow, is the same no matter which site is chosen.[18,78,107] The aortic cannula should be inserted proximal to the take-off of the innominate artery, and only a short length of cannula is introduced so that its tip cannot inadvertently enter a brachiocephalic vessel or lie near its orifice. The tapered plastic cannula is fitted for each patient with a small collar adjusted so that just the proper short length of cannula is beyond the collar. Care must be taken to ensure that enough cannula is beyond the collar to prevent inadvertent creation of an aortic dissection secondary to perfusion within the layers of the aortic wall rather than into its lumen. The cannula is inserted up to the collar. Alternatively, a long segment of the aortic cannula may be inserted into the aortic lumen, with the tip directed away from the orifice of the innominate artery.

The authors generally place two concentric pursestring sutures in the aortic adventitia and media at the proposed site of cannulation. The aorta is then incised with a stab wound within the pursestring suture, and the arterial cannula is directly inserted. The ends of the inner pursestring suture have previously been threaded through a long narrow rubber tube, and the tube is tucked down snugly and secured as a tourniquet and then tied to the cannula. After the cannula is connected to the arterial line in such a way as to exclude or remove any air bubbles, the line and cannula are secured so that the end of the cannula lies freely within the aortic lumen and the beveled end faces downstream,

TABLE 2. Oxygen Consumption During Profoundly Hypothermic, Nonpulsatile, Hemodiluted Cardiopulmonary Bypass in Monkeys

Organ	Oxygen Consumption (ml./min.⁻¹/100 gm.⁻¹)			p
	1.5*	1.0*	0.5*	
Whole body	0.119 ± 0.0077	0.086 ± 0.0045	0.056 ± 0.0029	<0.0001
	(17.3 ± 1.16)†	(12.5 ± 0.65)	(8.3 ± 0.44)	
Brain	0.51 ± 0.095	0.47 ± 0.076	0.45 ± 0.113	0.5
Whole body minus brain	0.114 ± 0.0074	0.081 ± 0.0085	0.0518 ± 0.00176	<0.0001

* Perfusion flow rate (L./min.⁻¹/m.⁻²).

† The numbers in parentheses are the whole-body oxygen consumption expressed as ml./min./m.².

From Fox, L. S., et al.: Relationship of brain blood flow and oxygen consumption to perfusion flow rate during profoundly hypothermic cardiopulmonary bypass: An experimental study. J. Thorac. Cardiovasc. Surg. 87:658, 1984.

TABLE 3. Resistance to Blood Flow in the Brain and Remainder of the Body at Various Perfusion Rates During Cardiopulmonary Bypass in Monkeys

Organ	Resistance (units/100 gm.)						p
	1.75*	1.5*	1.25*	1.0*	0.5*	0.25*	
Brain	1.2 ± 0.51	0.80 ± 0.080	0.8 ± 0.22	0.78 ± 0.126	0.80 ± 0.117	1.02 ± 0.173	0.4
Whole body minus brain	2.8 ± 0.157	3.3 ± 0.22	3.3 ± 1.21	3.9 ± 0.24	5.1 ± 0.49	9.5 ± 0.70	<0.0001

* Perfusion flow rate (L./min.$^{-1}$/m.$^{-2}$).
From Fox, L. S., et al.: Relationship of brain blood flow and oxygen consumption to perfusion flow rate during profoundly hypothermic cardiopulmonary bypass: An experimental study. J. Thorac. Cardiovasc. Surg., *87*:658, 1984.

the surgical field is uncluttered, and the line from the pump oxygenator is free from kinks.

As the cannula is removed after bypass, the assistant crosses the outer pursestring suture for hemostasis, and the surgeon ties the inner one. The outer pursestring suture is then tied. Rarely is anything further required to establish hemostasis.

Venous Cannulation

In infants and children, two angled, metal-tipped venous cannulas, which are inserted directly into each vena cava, are used for most operations, particularly if working through the right atrium or right ventricle. A single venous cannula is often used if working through the left atrium, left ventricle, or ascending aorta, and occasionally through the high right ventricle (e.g., changing a valved external conduit). A single venous cannula is also employed in those neonates in whom the entire repair is performed under total circulatory arrest.

In adults, a single large caval-atrial (two-stage) venous cannula with additional holes that come to lie in the right atrium while the tip is in the inferior vena cava may be used for coronary bypass grafting, aortic valve operations, mitral valve operations, and combinations of these. When operating in the right atrium, two venous cannulas are employed.

When a single venous cannula is used, a pursestring suture is placed around the right atrial appendage. When two venous cannulas are employed, tapes or large strings are placed around the superior or inferior vena cava. The superior vena caval pursestring suture is placed in an elliptical manner to avoid narrowing the superior vena cava when it is tied. The inferior vena caval pursestring suture is placed near the junction of the inferior vena cava with the diaphragm.

Conduct of Cardiopulmonary Bypass

After the patient is heparinized, cannulation is effected and CPB is established. The initial perfusate temperature is usually 30° C., which usually allows effective cardiac action if CPB needs to be discontinued abruptly because of an oxygenator system malfunction. The perfusion flow is gradually increased to approximately 2.2 liters per minute per sq. m., after which

perfusion cooling is initiated by decreasing the water temperature in the heat exchanger, either by decrements (to avoid ventricular fibrillation) or by direct reduction to 4° C. In operations performed through the right atrium or right ventricle in infants and small children, the left atrium is usually vented via the sump sucker placed across the atrial septum through the foramen ovale. In older children and adults undergoing aortic operations, a vent is generally placed directly into the left atrium through a pursestring suture positioned in the base of the right superior pulmonary vein.

The intracardiac portion of the operation is generally performed with the aorta cross-clamped and with cardioplegic-induced cardiac arrest. The precise perfusate temperature selected depends on the expected duration of the ischemic period as well as the anticipated needs for low perfusion flow rates or total circulatory arrest. In the absence of total circulatory arrest, perfusate temperature is generally maintained at 25° C. during the repair. When the nasopharyngeal temperature is reduced to 25 to 28° C., the perfusion flow rate can safely be reduced to 1.8 liters per minute per sq. m. When total circulatory arrest is planned, the nasopharyngeal temperature is reduced to 15° C.

Approximately 5 minutes before removing the aortic cross-clamp, rewarming is initiated by increasing the flow rate to 2.0 to 2.5 liters per minute per sq. m. and raising the temperature of the water in the heat exchanger to 42° C. The arterial line blood temperature should not exceed 39° C. to prevent heat damage to the blood elements. Air is evacuated from the cardiac chambers by needle aspiration or saline injection before the cross-clamp is removed. Suction is placed on the aortic needle vent as the cross-clamp is removed, and this is continued until cardiopulmonary bypass is discontinued. When the cardiac action is vigorous, the venous line is partially occluded for elevating the left atrial pressure to 10 to 14 mm. Hg to promote effective cardiac ejection for debubbling the heart. With strong suction on the aortic needle vent, the heart is gently massaged, and the left atrial appendage is gently inverted as the anesthesiologist inflates the lungs to force any residual air out of the pulmonary veins. Cardiopulmonary bypass is then gradually discontinued when the cardiac action is vigorous and the naso-

TABLE 4. Arterial Cannula Flow Chart: Pressure Gradient in Millimeters of Mercury (mm. Hg)

	Flow in Liters per Minute							
	0.5	1.0	1.5	2.0	2.5	3.0	3.5	4.0
10	60	175	350					
12	40	100	225	325				
14	25	60	140	240	350			
16		25	50	90	150	200	260	
18		20	40	60	80	120	150	200
20			25	40	60	80	100	120
22			25	40	50	60	75	90
24				40	50	60	70	80

TABLE 5. Venous Cannula Chart

Total Flow (L./min.)	Single Tygon	Single USCI*	Two Angled-Metal	
			SVC	IVC
<0.9	3/16 in.	20-Fr.	16-Fr.	20-Fr.
0.9–1.2	4/16 in.	24-Fr.	20-Fr.	20-Fr.
1.2–1.6			20-Fr.	24-Fr.
1.6–1.75			24-Fr.	24-Fr.
1.75–2.2		28-Fr.	24-Fr.	28-Fr.
2.2–3.2	5/16 in.		28-Fr.	28-Fr.
3.2–3.7	6/16 in.		28-Fr.	32-Fr.
>3.7	7/16 in.		32-Fr.	32-Fr.

* In adults, at the University of Alabama at Birmingham, USCI "two-stage" single cannula is used (46-French, tapering to 34-French).

pharyngeal temperature reaches 37° C. A polyvinyl catheter is usually placed in the left and right atria to facilitate postoperative hemodynamic management, and atrial and ventricular temporary pacing wires are usually placed for postoperative pacing and arrhythmia management.

SELECTED REFERENCES

Clowes, G. H. A.: Extracorporeal maintenance of circulation and respiration. Physiol. Rev., 40:826, 1960.
In this paper, the development of devices for cardiopulmonary bypass is reviewed; it was written shortly after completion of the basic research and development of extracorporeal pump oxygenators and their successful clinical application. In this review, Clowes notes that ". . . the single greatest factor in tissue damage during perfusion of the whole organism is no longer one of metabolic homeostasis, but rather, one of damage to blood elements which adversely affects the circulation and function of the various organs of the body."

Gibbon, J. H.: Application of a mechanical heart and lung apparatus to cardiac surgery. Minn. Med., 37:171, 1954.
This classic paper described the first successful use of a heart-lung machine in man to entirely support the circulation during open-heart surgery, with the closure of an atrial septal defect. The author discusses the physiologic response to cardiopulmonary bypass, including hemolysis, adequate tissue perfusion, and the problems of cardiac distention and air emboli. Gibbon concluded, "It seems to me that there will always be a place for an extracorporeal blood circuit because it permits a longer safe interval for opening the heart than can ever be obtained by any of the hypothermic methods."

Kirklin, J. K., Westaby, S., Blackstone, E. H., Kirklin J. W., Chenoweth, D. E., and Pacifico, A. D.: Complement and the damaging effects of cardiopulmonary bypass. J. Thorac. Cardiovasc. Surg., 86:845, 1983.
This prospective clinical study is one of the first rigorous attempts to identify those factors associated with cardiopulmonary bypass that contribute to organ system dysfunction after cardiac surgery. Complement levels remained normal in patients undergoing cardiac operations without cardiopulmonary bypass, in contrast to the marked complement activation that occurred during cardiopulmonary bypass. Cardiac, renal, pulmonary, and hemostatic dysfunction increased with higher levels of the complement anaphylatoxin C3a after bypass, younger age at operation, and longer time on bypass. The authors suggest that a more complete understanding of the biologic response to cardiopulmonary bypass may eventually lead to the neutralization of the damaging effects.

Kirklin, J. W., Dushane, J. W., Patrick, R. T., Donald, D. E., Hetzel, P. S., Harshbarger, H. S., and Wood E. H.: Intracardiac surgery with the aid of a mechanical pump-oxygenator (Gibbon type): Report of eight cases. Proc. Staff Meet. Mayo Clin., 30:201, 1955.
This is the first report of a series of patients successfully undergoing cardiac surgery with the use of a mechanical pump oxygenator. Four patients had ventricular septal defects, and two survived postoperatively. Two had atrioventricular canal defects, and one survived. One had tetralogy of Fallot and died. One patient had closure of an atrial septal defect and survived. At the time of this report, it was widely believed that a totally mechanical support system would not allow successful cardiac surgery.

Lillehei, C. W., Cohen, M., Warden, H. E., and Varco, R. L.: The direct vision intracardiac correction of congenital anomalies by controlled cross-circulation. Surgery, 38:11, 1955.
The authors report the first successful series of intracardiac operations using cardiopulmonary bypass. The experimental and physiologic basis for the use of another human being as the source of oxygenation and perfusion is discussed. Twenty-two patients had repair of a ventricular septal defect with 18 survivors, 6 had tetralogy of Fallot with 3 survivors, 2 had an atrioventricular canal defect with 1 survivor, and 2 had pulmonary stenosis with 1 survivor.

REFERENCES

1. Addonizio, V. P., Jr., Macarak, E. J., Niewiarowski, S., Colman, R. W., and Edmunds, L. H., Jr.: Preservation of human platelets with prostaglandin E_1 during in vitro simulation of cardiopulmonary bypass. Circ. Res. 44:350, 1979.
2. Addonizio, V. P., Jr., Strauss, J. F., III, Colman, R. W., and Edmunds, L. H., Jr.: Effects of prostaglandin E_1 on platelet loss during in vivo and in vitro extracorporeal circulation with a bubble oxygenator. J. Thorac. Cardiovasc. Surg., 77:119, 1979.
3. Addonizio, V. P., Jr., Macarak, E. J., Nicolaou, K. C., Edmunds, L. H., and Colman, R. W.: Effects of prostacyclin and albumin on platelet loss during in vitro simulation of extracorporeal circulation. J. Am. Soc. Hematol., 53:1033, 1979.
4. Addonizio, V. P., Jr., Strauss, J. F., III, Macarak, E. J., Colman, R. W., and Edmunds, L. H., Jr.: Preservation of platelet number and function with prostaglandin E_1 during total cardiopulmonary bypass in rhesus monkeys. Surgery, 83:619, 1978.
5. Alon, L., Turina, M., and Gattiker, R.: Membrane and bubble oxygenator: A

6. Backmann, F., McKenna, R., Cole, E. R., and Najafi, H.: The hemostatic mechanism after open-heart surgery. I. Studies on plasma coagulation factors and fibrinolysis in 512 patients after extracorporeal circulation. J. Thorac. Cardiovasc. Surg., 70:76, 1975.
7. Barry, Y. A., Labow, R. S., Keon, W. J., Tocchi, M., and Rock, G.: Perioperative exposure to plasticizers in patients undergoing cardiopulmonary bypass. J. Thorac. Cardiovasc. Surg., 97:900, 1989.
8. Bharadwaj, B. B., and Chong, G.: Effects of extracorporeal circulation on structure, function and population distribution of canine blood platelets. Presented at the Combined Meeting of the Royal Australasian College of Surgeons and Royal Australasian College of Physicians, Sydney, Australia, February 24–29, 1980.
9. Bidstrup, B. P., Royston, D., Sapsford, R. N., Taylor, K. M., and Cosgrove, D. M.: Reduction in blood loss and blood use after cardiopulmonary bypass with high dose aprotinin (Trasylol). J. Thorac. Cardiovasc. Surg., 97:364, 1989.
10. Bjork, V. O.: Brain perfusions in dogs with artificially oxygened blood. Acta Chir. Scand. (Suppl.), 137:1, 1948.
11. Bjork, J., Hugli, T. E., and Smedegard, G.: Microvasculature effects on anaphylatoxins C3a and C5a. J. Immunol. 134:1115, 1985.
12. Blauth, C. I., Arnold, J. V., Schulenberg, W. E., McCartney, A. C., and Taylor, K. M.: Cerebral microembolism during cardiopulmonary bypass. J. Thorac. Cardiovasc. Surg., 95:668, 1988.
13. Boldt, J., Kling, D., von Bormann, B., Zuge, M., Scheld, H., and Hempelmann, G.: Blood conservation in cardiac operations. J. Thorac. Cardiovasc. Surg., 97:832, 1989.
14. Braude, S., Nolop, K. B., Fleming, J. S., Krausz, T., Taylor, K. M., and Royston, D.: Increased pulmonary transvascular protein flux after canine cardiopulmonary bypass. Am. Rev. Respir. Dis., 134:867, 1986.
15. Breckenridge, I. M., Digerness, S. B., and Kirklin, J. W.: Validity of concept of increased extracellular fluid after open heart surgery. Surg. Forum, 20:169, 1969.
16. Brown, I. W., Smith, W. W., and Emmons, W. O.: An efficient blood heat exchanger for use with extracorporeal circulation. Surgery, 44:372, 1958.
17. Brusino, F. G., Reves, J. G., Smith, R., Prough, D. S., Stump, D. A., and McIntyre, R. W.: The effect of age on cerebral blood flow during hypothermic cardiopulmonary bypass. J. Thorac. Cardiovasc. Surg., 97:541, 1989.
18. Camishion, R. C., Scicchitano, C. P., Trotta, R., and Gibbon, J. H., Jr.: Blood flow through superior mesenteric artery during retrograde perfusion. Surgery, 54:651, 1963.
19. Cavarocchi, N. C., England, M. D., Schaff, H. V., Russo, P., Orszulak, T. A., Schnell, W. A., Jr., O'Brien, J. F., and Pluth, J. R.: Oxygen free radical generation during cardiopulmonary bypass: Correlation with complement activation. Circulation, 74:130, 1986.
20. Cavarocchi, N. C., Pluth, J. R., Schaff, H. V., Orszulak, T. A., Homburger, H. A., Solis, E., Kaye, M. P., Clancy, M. S., Kilff, J., and Deeb, G. M.: Complement activation during cardiopulmonary bypass. J. Thorac. Cardiovasc. Surg., 91:252, 1986.
21. Cheng, H. C., Kusunoki, T., Bosher, L. H., Jr., McElvein, R. B., and Blake, D. A.: A study of oxygen consumption during extracorporeal circulation. Trans. Am. Soc. Artif. Intern. Organs, 5:273, 1959.
22. Chenoweth, D. E., and Hugli, T. E.: Demonstration of specific C5a receptor on intact human polymorphonuclear leukocytes. Proc. Natl. Acad. Sci. U.S.A., 75:3943, 1978.
23. Chenoweth, D. E., Cooper, S. W., Hugli, T. E., Stewart, R. W., Blackstone, E. J., and Kirklin, J. W.: Complement activation during cardiopulmonary bypass: Evidence for generation of C3a and C5a anaphylatoxins. N. Engl. J. Med., 304:497, 1981.
24. Chien, S.: Present state of blood rheology. In Messemer, K., and Schmid-Schonbein, H. (Eds.): Hemodilution, Theoretical Basis and Clinical Application. New York, Karger, 1972, p. 145.
25. Clark, R. E., Beauchamp, R. A., Magrath, R. A., Brooks, J. D., Ferguson, T. B. and Weldon, C. S.: Comparison of bubble and membrane oxygenators in short and long perfusions. J. Thorac. Cardiovasc. Surg., 78:655, 1979.
26. Cleland, J., Pluth, J. R., Tauxe, W. N., and Kirklin, J. W.: Blood volume and body fluid compartment changes soon after closed and open intracardiac surgery. J. Thorac. Cardiovasc. Surg., 52:698, 1966.
27. Clowes, G. H. A., Jr.: Extracorporeal maintenance of circulation and respiration. Physiol. Rev. 40:826, 1960.
28. Clowes, G. H. A., Jr., Neville, W. E., Sabga, G. and Shibota, Y.: The relationship of oxygen consumption, perfusion rate, and temperature to the acidosis associated with cardiopulmonary circulatory bypass. Surgery, 44:220, 1958.
29. Cohn, L. H., Angell, W. W., and Shumway, N. E.: Body fluid shifts after cardiopulmonary bypass. I. Effects of congestive heart failure and hemodilution. J. Thorac. Cardiovasc. Surg., 62:423, 1971.
30. Cosgrove, D. M., Loop, F. D., Lytle, B. W., Gill, C. C., Golding, L. R., Taylor, P. C. and Forsythe, S. B.: Determinants of blood utilization during myocardial revascularization. Ann. Thorac. Surg., 40:380, 1985.
31. Craddock, P. R., Fehr, J., Brigham, K. L., Kronenberg, R. S., and Jacob, H. S.: Complement and leukocyte-mediated pulmonary dysfunction in hemodialysis. N. Engl. J. Med., 296:769, 1977.
32. Debakey, M. E.: Simple continuous flow blood transfusion instrument. New Orleans Med. Surg. J., 87:386, 1934.
33. Dechavanne, M., Ffrench, M., Pages, J., Ffrench, P., Boukerche, H., Bryon,

P. A., and McGregor, J. L.: Significant reduction in the binding of a monoclonal antibody (LYP 18) directed against the IIb/IIIa glycoprotein complex to platelets of patients having undergone extracorporeal circulation. Thrombosis Haemostasis, 57:106, 1987.

34. Dennis, C., Spreng, D. S., Jr., Nelson, G. E., Karlson, K. E., Nelson, R. M., Thomas, J. V., Eder, W. P., and Varco, R. L.: Development of a pump oxygenator to replace the heart and lungs; an apparatus applicable to human patients, and application to one case. Ann. Surg., 134:709, 1951.

35. Diesh, G., Flynn, P. J., Marable, S. A., Mulder, D. G., Schmutzer, K. J., Longmire, W. P., Jr., and Maloney, J. V., Jr.: Comparison of low (azygos) flow and high flow principles of extracorporeal circulation employing a bubble oxygenator. Surgery, 42:67, 1957.

36. Donald, D. E., Harshbarger, H. G., Hetzel, P. S., Patrick, R. T., Wood, E. H., and Kirklin, J. W.: Experiences with a heart-lung bypass (Gibbon type) in the experimental laboratory: Preliminary report. Proc. Staff Meet. Mayo Clin., 30:113, 1955.

37. Dunn, J., Kirsh, M. M., Harness, J., Carroll, H., Straker, J., and Sloan, H.: Hemodynamic, metabolic and hematologic effects of cardiopulmonary bypass. J. Thorac. Cardiovasc. Surg., 68:138, 1974.

38. Edmunds, L. H.: Invited letter concerning: Blood platelets and bypass. J. Thorac. Cardiovasc. Surg., 97:470, 1989.

39. Edmunds, L. H., Jr., Saxena, N. C., Hillyer, P., and Wilson, T. J.: Relationship between platelet count and cardiotomy suction return. Ann. Thorac. Surg., 25:306, 1978.

40. Ellis, R. J., Wisniewski, A., Potts, R., Calhoun, C., Loucks, P., and Wells, M. R.: Reduction of flow rate and arterial pressure at moderate hypothermia does not result in cerebral dysfunction. J. Thorac. Cardiovasc. Surg., 79:173, 1980.

41. Ellison, N., Behar, M., MacVaugh, H., III, and Marshall, B. E.: Bradykinin, plasma protein fraction and hypotension. Ann. Thorac. Surg., 29:15, 1980.

42. England, M. D., Cavarocchi, N. C., O'Brien, J. F., Solis, E., Pluth, J. R., Orszulak, T. A., Kaye, M. P., and Schaff, H. V.: Influence of antioxidants (mannitol and allopurinol) on oxygen free radical generation during and after cardiopulmonary bypass. Circulation, 74:134, 1986.

43. Feijen, J.: Thrombogenesis caused by blood foreign surface interaction. In Kenedi, R. M., Courtney, J. M., Gaylor, J. D. S., and Gilchrist, T. (Eds.): Artificial Organs. Baltimore, University Park Press, 1977, p. 235.

44. Flick, M. R., Perel, A., and Staub, N. C.: Leukocytes are required for increased lung microvasculature permeability after microembolization in sheep. Circ. Res., 48:344, 1981.

45. Fox, L. S., Blackstone, E. H., Kirklin, J. W., Steward, R. W., and Samuelson, P. N.: Relationship of whole body oxygen consumption to perfusion flow rate during hypothermic cardiopulmonary bypass. J. Thorac. Cardiovasc. Surg., 83:239, 1982.

46. Fox, L. S., Blackstone, E. H., Kirklin, J. W, Bishop, S. P., et al.: Relationship of brain blood flow and oxygen consumption to perfusion flow rate during profoundly hypothermic cardiopulmonary bypass: An experimental study. J. Thorac. Cardiovasc. Surg., 87:658, 1984.

47. Frey, M. V., and Gruber, M.: Untersuchungen über den Stoffwechsel isolierter Organe. Ein Respirations Apparat für isolierte Organs. Arch. Physiol., 9:519, 1885.

48. Friedli, B., Kent, G., and Olley, P. M.: Inactivation of bradykinin in the pulmonary vascular bed of newborn and fetal lambs. Circ. Res., 33:421, 1973.

49. George, J. N., Pickett, E. B., Sauceman, S., McEver, R. P., Kunicki, T. J., Keiffer, N., and Newman, P. J.: Platelet surface glycoproteins. J. Clin. Invest., 78:340, 1986.

50. German, J. C., Chalmers, G. S., Hirai, J., Mukherjee, N. D., Wakabayashi, A., and Connolly, J. E.: Comparison of nonpulsatile and pulsatile extracorporeal circulation on renal tissue perfusion. Chest, 61:65, 1972.

51. Gibbon, J. H., Jr.: The maintenance of life during experimental occlusion of the pulmonary artery followed by survival. Surg. Gynecol. Obstet., 69:602, 1939.

52. Gibbon, J. H., Jr.: Application of a mechanical heart and lung apparatus to cardiac surgery. Minn. Med., 37:171, 1954.

53. Giron, F., Birtwell, W. C., Soroff, H. S., and Deterling, R. A.: Hemodynamic effects of pulsatile and nonpulsatile flow. Arch. Surg., 93:802, 1966.

54. Gluszko, P., Rucinski, B., Musial, J., Wenger, R. K., Schmaier, A. H., Colman, R. W., Edmunds, L. H., Jr., and Niewiarowski, S.: Fibrinogen receptors in platelet adhesion to surfaces of extracorporeal circuit. Am. J. Physiol., 252:H615, 1987.

55. Goldstein, I. M.: Current Concepts: Complement in Infectious Diseases. Kalamazoo, The Upjohn Company, 1980, p. 7.

56. Habal, S. M., Weiss, M. B., Spotnitz, H. M., Parodi, E. N., Wolff, M., Cannon, P. J., Hoffman, B. F., and Malm, J. R.: Effects of pulsatile and nonpulsatile coronary perfusion on performance of the canine left ventricle. J. Thorac. Cardiovasc. Surg., 72:742, 1976.

57. Han, P., Turpie, A. G. G., Butt, R., LeBlanc, P., Genton, E., and Gunstensen, S.: The use of B-thromboglobulin release to assess platelet damage during cardiopulmonary bypass. Presented at the Combined Meeting of the Royal Australasian College of Surgeons and Royal Australasian College of Physicians, Sydney, Australia, February 24–29, 1980.

58. Harker, L. A.: Bleeding after cardiopulmonary bypass. N. Engl. J. Med., 314:1446, 1986.

59. Harris, E. A., Seelye, E. R., and Barratt-Boyes, B. G.: Respiratory and metabolic acid-base changes during cardiopulmonary bypass in man. Br. J. Anaesth., 42:912, 1970.

60. Hisatomi, K., Isomura, T., Kawara, T., Yamashita, M., Hirano, A., Yoshida, H., Eriguchi, N., Kosuga, K., and Ohishi, K.: Changes in lymphocyte subsets, mitogen responsiveness, and interleukin-2 production after cardiac operations. J. Thorac. Cardiovasc. Surg., 98:580, 1989.

61. Holly, M. M., Reemstma, K., and Creedi, O., Jr.: Cerebral blood flow metabolism and brain volume in extracorporeal circulation. J. Thorac. Surg., 36:506, 1958.

62. Hope, A. F., Adu, P., Lotter, M. G., van Reenan, O. R., de Kock, F., Badenhorst, P. N., Pieters, H., Kotze, H., Meyer, J. M., and Minnaar, P. C.: Kinetics and sites of sequestration of indium-111 labeled human platelets during cardiopulmonary bypass. J. Thorac. Cardiovasc. Surg., 81:880, 1981.

63. Jacobs, L. A., Klopp, E. H., Seamone, W., Topaz, S. R., and Gott, V. L.: Improved organ function during cardiac bypass with a roller pump modified to deliver pulsatile flow. J. Thorac. Cardiovasc. Surg., 58:703, 1969.

64. Jones, R. E., Donald, D. E., Swan, H. J. C., Harshbarger, H. G., Kirklin, J. W., and Wood, E. H.: Apparatus of the Gibbon type for mechanical bypass of the heart and lungs: Preliminary report. Proc. Staff Meet. Mayo Clin., 30:105, 1955.

65. Kalter, R. D., Saul, C. M., Wetstein, L., Soriano, C., and Reiss, R. F.: Cardiopulmonary bypass. Associated hemostatic abnormalities. J. Thorac. Cardiovasc. Surg., 77:428, 1979.

66. Kappa, J. R., Musial, J., Fisher, C. A., and Addonizio, V. P., Jr.: Quantitation of platelet preservation with prostanoids during simulated bypass. J. Surg. Res., 42:10, 1987.

67. Kirklin, J. K., Blackstone, E. H., and Kirklin, J. W.: Cardiopulmonary bypass: Studies on its damaging effects. Blood Purif., 5:168, 1987.

68. Kirklin, J. W., Kirklin, J. K., and Lell, W. A.: Cardiopulmonary bypass for cardiac surgery. In Sabiston, D. C., Jr., and Spencer, F. C. (Eds.): Gibbon's Surgery of the Chest, 4th ed. Philadelphia, W. B. Saunders Company, 1983, pp. 909–925.

69. Kirklin, J. K., Kirklin, J. W., and Pacifico, A. D.: Cardiopulmonary bypass. In Arciniegas, E. (Ed.): Pediatric Cardiac Surgery. Chicago, Year Book Publishers, 1985.

70. Kirklin, J. K., Blackstone, E. H., Kirklin, J. W., McKay, R., Pacifico, A. D., and Bargeron, L. M., Jr.: Intracardiac surgery in infants under 3 months: Incremental risk factors for hospital mortality. Am. J. Cardiol., 48:500, 1981.

71. Kirklin, J. K., Chenoweth, D. E., Naftel, D. C., Blackstone, E. H., Kirklin, J. W., Bitran, D. D., Curd, J. G., Reves, J. G., and Samuelson, P. N.: Effects of protamine administration after cardiopulmonary bypass on complement, blood elements, and the hemodynamic state. Ann. Thorac. Surg., 41:193, 1986.

72. Kirklin, J. W., DuShane, J. W., Patrick, R. T., Donald, D. E., Hetzel, P. S., Harshbarger, H. G., and Wood, E. H.: Intracardiac surgery with the aid of a mechanical pump-oxygenator system (Gibbon type): Report of eight cases. Proc. Staff Meet. Mayo Clin., 30:201, 1955.

73. Kirklin, J. K., Westaby, S., Blackstone, E. H., Kirklin, J. W., Chenoweth, D. E., and Pacifico, A. D.: Complement and the damaging effects of cardiopulmonary bypass. J. Thorac. Cardiovasc. Surg., 86:845, 1983.

74. Kolkka, R., and Hilberman, M.: Neurologic dysfunction following cardiac operation with low flow, low pressure cardiopulmonary bypass. J. Thorac. Cardiovasc. Surg., 79:432, 1980.

75. Kusserow, B. K., Larrow, R., and Nichols, J.: Perfusion and surface-induced injury in leukocytes. Fed. Proc., 30:1516, 1971.

76. Kusserow, B. K., Machanic, B., Collins, F. M., Jr., and Clapp, J. F., III: Changes observed in blood corpuscles after prolonged perfusions with two types of blood pumps. Trans. Am. Soc. Artif. Intern. Organs, 11:122, 1965.

77. Lee, W. H., Jr., Krumbhoar, D., Fonkalsrud, E. W., Schjeide, O. A., and Maloney, J. V., Jr.: Denaturation of plasma proteins as a cause of morbidity and death after intracardiac operations. Surgery, 50:29, 1961.

78. Lees, M. H., Herr, R. H., Hill, J. D., Morgan, C. L., Ochsner, A. J., III, Thomas, C., and Van Fleet, D. C.: Distribution of systemic blood flow of the rhesus monkey during cardiopulmonary bypass. J. Thorac. Cardiovasc. Surg., 61:570, 1971.

79. Levin, M. B., Theye, R. A., Fowler, W. S., and Kirklin, J. W.: Performance of the stationary vertical-screen oxygenator (Mayo-Gibbon). J. Thorac. Cardiovasc. Surg., 39:417, 1960.

80. Lillehei, C. W., Cohen, M., Warden, H. E., and Varco, R. L.: The direct-vision intracardiac correction of congenital anomalies by controlled cross-circulation. Surgery, 38:11, 1955.

81. Litwin, M. S., Panico, F. G., Rubivi, C., Harkin, D. E., and Moore, F. D.: Acidosis and lactic acidemia in extracorporeal circulation: The significance of perfusion respiratory alkalosis. Ann. Surg., 149:188, 1959.

82. Love, T. R., Hendren, W. G., O'Keefe, D. D., and Daggett, W. M.: Transfusion of predonated blood in elective cardiac surgery. Ann. Thorac. Surg., 43:508, 1987.

83. Maddoux, G., Pappas, G., Jenkins, M., Battock, D., Trow, R., Smith, S. C., Jr., and Steele, P.: Effect of pulsatile and nonpulsatile flow during cardiopulmonary bypass on left ventricular ejection fraction early after aortocoronary bypass surgery. Am. J. Cardiol., 37:1000, 1976.

84. Many, M., Soroff, H. S., Birtwell, W. C., Giron, F., Wise, H., and Deterling, R. A.: The physiologic role of pulsatile and nonpulsatile flow. II. Effects on renal function. Arch. Surg., 95:762, 1967.

85. Martin, R. R.: Alterations in leukocyte structure and function due to mechanical trauma. In Hwang, N. H. C., Gross, D. R., and Patel, D. J. (Eds.): Quantitative Cardiovascular Studies: Clinical and Research Applications of Engineering Principles. Baltimore, University Park Press, 1979, p. 419.

86. Moffitt, E. A., Kirklin, J. W., and Theye, R. A.: Physiologic studies during

whole-body perfusion in tetralogy of Fallot. J. Thorac. Cardiovasc. Surg., 44:180, 1962.

87. Mohr, R., Golan, M., Martinowitz, U., Rosner, E., Goor, D. A., and Ramot, B.: Effect of cardiac operation on platelets. J. Thorac. Cardiovasc. Surg., 92:434, 1986.

88. Mortenson, J. D.: Evaluation of ASAIO Blood Damage Test. Vol. I. Salt Lake City, Utah Biomedical Test Laboratory, University of Utah Research Institute, 1977.

89. Muller-Eberhard, H. J.: Complement. Am. Rev. Biochem., 44:697, 1975.

90. Nakayama, K., Tamiya, T., Yamamoto, K., Izumi, T., Akimoto, S., Hashizume, S., and Iimori, T.: High amplitude pulsatile pump in extracorporeal circulation with particular reference to hemodynamics. Surgery, 54:798, 1963.

91. Pacifico, A. D., Digerness, S., and Kirklin, J. W.: Acute alterations of body composition after open intracardiac operations. Circulation, 41:331, 1970.

92. Paneth, M., Sellers, R., Gott, V. L., Weirich, W. L., Allen, P., Read, R. C., and Lillehei, C. W.: Physiologic studies upon prolonged cardiopulmonary bypass with the pump oxygenator with particular references to (1) acid base balance, (2) siphon canal drainage. J. Thorac. Surg., 34:570, 1947.

93. Pang, L. M., Stalcup, S. A., Lipset, J. S., Hayes, C. J., Bowman, F. O., Jr., and Mellins, R. B.: Increased circulating bradykinin during hypothermia and cardiopulmonary bypass in children. Circulation, 60:1503, 1979.

94. Pappas, G., Winter, S. D., Kopriva, C. J., and Steele, P.: Improvement of myocardial and other vital organ function and metabolism using a simple method of pulsatile flow (IABP) during clinical CPB. Surgery, 77:34, 1975.

95. Parker, D. J., Cantrell, J. W., Karp, R. B., Stroud, R. M., and Digerness, S. B.: Changes in serum complement and immunoglobulins following cardiopulmonary bypass. Surgery, 71:824, 1972.

96. Rahn, H., Reeves, R. B., and Howell, B. J.: Hydrogen ion regulation temperature and evolution. Am. Rev. Respir. Dis., 112:165, 1975.

97. Reeves, R. B.: Temperature-induced changes in blood acid-base status: pH and PCO_2 in a binary buffer. J. Appl. Physiol., 40:752, 1976.

98. Rosenkranz, E. R., Utley, J. R., Menninger, F. J., III, Dembitsky, W. P., Hargens, A. R., and Peters, R. M.: Interstitial fluid pressure changes during cardiopulmonary bypass. Ann. Thorac. Surg., 30:536, 1980.

99. Rosenthal, T. B.: The effect of temperature on the pH of blood and plasma in vitro. J. Biol. Chem., 173:25, 1948.

100. Royston, D., Fleming, J. S., Desai, J. B., Westaby, S., and Taylor, K. M.: Increased production of peroxidation products associated with cardiac operations. J. Thorac. Cardiovasc. Surg., 91:759, 1986.

101. Ryhanen, P., Herva, E., Hollman, A., Nuutinen, L., Pihlajaniemi, R., and Saarela, E.: Changes in peripheral blood leukocyte counts, lymphocyte subpopulations, and in vitro transformation after heart valve replacement. J. Thorac. Cardiovasc. Surg., 77:259, 1979.

102. Sacks, T., Moldow, C. F., Craddock, P. R., Bowers, T. K., and Jacob, H. S.: Oxygen radicals mediate endothelial cell damage by complement stimulated granulocytes. Am. Soc. Clin. Invest., 21:1161, 1978.

103. Sade, R. H., Bartles, D. M., Dearling, J. P., Campbell, L. J., and Loadholt, C. B.: A prospective randomized study of membrane vs. bubble oxygenators in children. Ann. Thorac. Surg., 29:502, 1980.

104. Salama, A., Hugo, F., Heinrich, D., Hoge, R., Muller, R., Kiefel, V., Mueller-Eckhardt, C., and Bhakdi, S.: Deposition of terminal C5b-9 complement complexes on erythrocytes and leukocytes during cardiopulmonary bypass. N. Engl. J. Med., 318:408, 1988.

105. Salzman, E. W., Weinstein, M. J., Weintraub, R. M., Ware, J. A., Thurer, R. L., Robertson, L., Donovan, A., Gaffney, T., Bertele, V., Troll, J., Smith, M., and Chute, L. E.: Treatment with desmopressin acetate to reduce blood loss after cardiac surgery. N. Engl. J. Med., 314:1402, 1986.

106. Schaff, H. V., Hauer, J. M., Bell, W. R., Gardner, T. J., Donahoo, J. S., Gott, V. L., and Brawley, R. K.: Autotransfusion of shed mediastinal blood after cardiac surgery. J. Thorac. Cardiovasc. Surg., 75:632, 1978.

107. Schenk, W. G., Jr., Pollock, L. A., Kjarstansson, K. B., and Delin, N. A.: Influence of aortic perfusion on regional blood flow. Arch. Surg., 87:1059, 1963.

108. Senning, A.: Ventricular fibrillation during extracorporeal circulation: Used as a method to prevent air embolisms and to facilitate intracardiac operations. Acta Chir. Scand., 171:1, 1952.

109. Shephard, R. J.: Whole body oxygen consumption during hypoxemia and cardiopulmonary bypass circulation. Proceedings, Tenth International Symposium on Space Technology and Science, Tokyo, 1973, p. 1307.

110. Singh, R. K. K., Barratt-Boyes, B. G., and Harris, E. A.: Does pulsatile flow improve perfusion during hypothermic cardiopulmonary bypass? J. Thorac. Cardiovasc. Surg., 79:827, 1980.

111. Sink, J. D., Chitwood, R., Jr., Hill, R. C., and Wechsler, A. S.: Comparison of nonpulsatile and pulsatile extracorporeal circulation on renal cortical blood flow. Ann. Thorac. Surg., 29:57, 1980.

112. Smith, E. E. J., Naftel, D. C., Blackstone, E. H., and Kirklin, J. W.: Microvascular permeability after cardiopulmonary bypass. J. Thorac. Cardiovasc. Surg., 94:225, 1987.

113. Solem, J. O., Tengborn, L., Steen, S., and Luhrs, C.: Cell saver versus hemofilter for concentration of oxygenator blood after cardiopulmonary bypass. Thorac. Cardiovasc. Surg., 35:42, 1987.

114. Sorenson, H. R., Husum, B., Waaben, J., Andersen, K., Anderson, L. I., Gefke, K., Kaarsen, A. L., and Gjedde, A.: Brain microvascular function during cardiopulmonary bypass. J. Thorac. Cardiovasc. Surg., 94:727, 1987.

115. Stockard, J. J., Bickford, R. G., and Schauble, J. F.: Pressure dependent cerebral ischemia during cardiopulmonary bypass. Neurology, 23:521, 1973.

116. Swan, H.: Thermoregulation and Bioenergetics: Patterns for vertebrate survival. New York, American Elsevier Publishing Company, 1974, p. 183.

117. Taylor, K. M., Bain, W. H., Maxted, K. J., Hutton, M. M., McNab, W. Y., and Caves, P. K.: Comparative studies of pulsatile and nonpulsatile flow during cardiopulmonary bypass. I. Pulsatile system employed and its hematologic effects. J. Thorac. Cardiovasc. Surg., 75:569, 1978.

118. Taylor, K. M., Bain, W. H., Maxted, K. J., Hutton, M. M., McNab, W. Y., and Caves, P. K.: Comparative studies of pulsatile and nonpulsatile flow during cardiopulmonary bypass. II. The effects on adrenal secretion of cortisol. J. Thorac. Cardiovasc. Surg., 75:574, 1978.

119. Taylor, K. M., Wright, G. S., Bain, W. H., Caves, P. K., and Beastall, G. S.: Comparative studies of pulsatile and nonpulsatile flow during cardiopulmonary bypass. III. Response of anterior pituitary gland to thyrotropin releasing hormone. J. Thorac. Cardiovasc. Surg., 75:579, 1978.

120. Theye, R. A., Donald, D. E., and Jones, R. E.: The effect of geometry and filming surface on the priming volume of the vertical film oxygenator. J. Thorac. Cardiovasc. Surg., 43:473, 1962.

121. Theye, R. A., Kirklin, J. W., and Fowler, W. S.: Performance and volume of sheet and screen vertical film oxygenators. J. Thorac. Cardiovasc. Surg., 43:481, 1962.

122. Trinkle, J. K., Helton, N. E., Wood, R. E., and Bryant, L. R.: Metabolic comparison of a new pulsatile pump and a roller pump for cardiopulmonary bypass. J. Thorac. Cardiovasc. Surg., 58:562, 1969.

123. Trinkle, J. K., Helton, N. E., Bryant, L. R., and Griffen, W. O.: Pulsatile cardiopulmonary bypass. Clinical evaluation. Surgery, 68:1074, 1970.

124. Tufo, H. M., Ostfeld, A. M., and Shekelle, R.: Central nervous system dysfunction following open heart surgery. J.A.M.A., 212:1333, 1970.

125. van Oeveren, W., Janson, N. J. G., Bidstrup, B. P., Royston, D., Westaby, S., Neuhof, H., and Wildevuur, C. R. H.: Effects of aprotinin on hemostatic mechanisms during cardiopulmonary bypass. Ann. Thorac. Surg., 44:640, 1987.

126. van Oeveren, W., Eijsman, L., Roozendaal, K. J., and Wildevuur, C. R. H.: Platelet preservation by aprotinin during cardiopulmonary bypass. Lancet, 1:644, 1988.

127. Verska, J. J.: Control of heparinization by activated clotting time during bypass with improved postoperative hemostasis. Ann. Thorac. Surg., 24:170, 1977.

128. Vibeke, V., Fosse, E., Mollnes, T. E., Ellingsen, O., Pedersen, T., and Karlsen, H.: Different oxygenators for cardiopulmonary bypass lead to varying degrees of human complement activation in vitro. J. Thorac. Cardiovasc. Surg., 97:764, 1989.

129. Volanakis, J. E.: Invited letter concerning: Complement activation caused by different oxygenators. J. Thorac. Cardiovasc. Surg., 98:292, 1989.

130. Wachtfogel, Y. T., Kucich, U., Greenplate, J., Gluszko, P., Abrams, W., Weinbaum, G., Wenger, R. K., Rucinski, B., Niewiarowski, S., Edmunds, L. H., and Colman, R. W.: Human neutrophil degranulation during extracorporeal circulation. Blood, 69:324, 1987.

131. Walker, D. R., Blackstone, E. H., Kirklin, J. W., Karp, R. B., Kouchoukos, N. T., Pacifico, A. D., Shealy, A., Roe, C. R., and Bradley, E. L.: The effect of micropore filtration of the arterial return during cardiopulmonary bypass: A randomized clinical study (unpublished data).

132. Wallach, R., Karp, R. B., Reves, J. G., Paril, S., Smith, L. R., and James, T. N.: Pathogenesis of paroxysmal hypertension developing during and after coronary artery bypass surgery: A study of hemodynamic and humoral factors. Am. J. Cardiol., 46:559, 1980.

133. Wesolowski, S. A., Sauvage, L. R., and Pinc, R. D.: Extracorporeal circulation. The role of the pulse in maintenance of the systemic circulation during heart-lung bypass. Surgery, 37:663, 1955.

134. Wilkens, H., Regelson, W., and Hoffmeister, F. S.: The physiologic importance of pulsatile blood flow. N. Engl. J. Med., 267:443, 1962.

135. Williams, G. D., Seifen, A. B., Lawson, N. W., Norton, J. B., Readinger, R. I., Dungan, T. W., and Callaway, J. K.: Pulsatile perfusion versus conventional high-flow nonpulsatile perfusion for rapid core cooling and rewarming of infants for circulatory arrest in cardiac operation. J. Thorac. Cardiovasc. Surg., 78:667, 1979.

136. Wright, G., and Sanderson, J. M.: Brain damage and mortality in dogs following pulsatile and nonpulsatile blood flows in extracorporeal circulation. Thorax, 27:738, 1972.

137. Zilla, P., Fasol, R., Groscurth, P., Klepetko, W., Reichenspurner, H., and Wolner, E.: Blood platelets in cardiopulmonary bypass operations. J. Thorac. Cardiovasc. Surg., 97:379, 1989.

XXV

INTRA-AORTIC BALLOON COUNTERPULSATION: PHYSIOLOGY, INDICATIONS, AND TECHNIQUES

W. Randolph Chitwood, Jr., M.D.

HISTORICAL ASPECTS

The intra-aortic balloon pump (IABP) is the circulatory assist device used most frequently. In the last 10 years, major use of this device has transferred from the operating room to the catheterization suite and cardiac care unit. With the IABP, the salutary effects of diastolic coronary blood flow augmentation and systolic ventricular afterload reduction become additive with mild preload reduction. Together these features often enable jeopardized myocardium to function more efficiently.

In 1953 the brothers Kantrowitz found that coronary arterial blood flow could be increased by 20 to 40 per cent when perfused at a higher pressure during diastole.[26] Clauss and Birtwell first developed the concept of true counterpulsation in 1958 using an extracorporeal support device.[8] Blood was withdrawn during systole and reinfused during diastole employing a synchronized solenoid valve. This device had limited use; however, it was the progenitor of modern intra-aortic balloon pumping. In 1962 Moulopoulos, Topaz, and Kolff first developed a carbon dioxide–driven latex aortic balloon, obviating the need for extracorporeal exchange of blood.[42] Sones tested this technique first clinically during a futile resuscitation attempt.[55] Subsequently, Kantrowitz (1967) treated two patients and reported the first survival using his phase-shift IABP.[25] Later that year, he described seven long-term survivors pumped for cardiogenic shock.[27]

Other early studies suggested the IABP for treating patients with postinfarction cardiac failure.[7] Mundth (1970) popularized this technique for cardiogenic shock patients who were surgically revascularized.[43] During this era, pioneer studies by Powell and Buckley helped define the physiologic advantages of intra-aortic balloon pumping more clearly.[7,54] Therapy soon became expanded to patients with intractable failure following cardiopulmonary bypass procedures.[6,31] By 1978, the IABP was used for treating unstable angina (27 per cent) and postcardiotomy myocardial depression (52 per cent) primarily. Although the failing left heart has benefited most from this device, in 1980 Miller first used an IABP to support the right heart.[24,41]

More recently, the device has been used by almost all cardiac centers involved in percutaneous angioplasty and cardiac surgical procedures. These pumps have been used successfully for support of the patients up to 327 days following a cardiac operation.[2] Newer percutaneous techniques have expanded IABP use to clinical sites other than the operating room with relatively few complications.[17,45] Moreover, the IABP has made the failed angioplasty a much less formidable preoperative problem.[44] Some surgeons have advocated this method for myocardial protection even during noncardiac surgery.[20] Phillips has suggested alternative methods for aortic counterpulsation in patients in whom atherosclerosis prevents traditional passage of an IABP.[50]

PHYSIOLOGIC EFFECTS OF INTRA-AORTIC BALLOON PUMPING

Clinical use of the balloon pump has been based on several physiologic principles. Major determinants of myocardial oxy-

gen consumption in intact hearts include pulse rate, transmural wall stress, and intrinsic contractile properties. Systolic wall stress represents approximately 30 per cent of cardiac energy expenditure and is influenced by intraventricular pressure, afterload, end-diastolic volume, and wall thickness.[15] Moreover, myocardial oxygen consumption has been shown to relate linearly to peak systolic wall stress. Other factors contributing to cardiac energy expenditure include ventricular stroke work, the initiation of contraction, and basal cellular metabolism.[15] Sarnoff first fully appreciated the relationship between ventricular work and myocardial energetics.[59] His group determined that pressure work was more influential regarding myocardial oxygen demands than preload, heart rate, or left ventricular stroke work. The tension-time index emanated from his studies as a physiologic parameter reflecting systolic energy requirements.

Since intra-aortic balloon pumping modifies left ventricular ejection pressure significantly, and therefore afterload, determinants of transmural wall stress become altered effectively.[54] To compare these energy requirements with myocardial oxygen supply, the diastolic pressure-time index has been suggested as a hemodynamic correlate of coronary perfusion.[4] This parameter may be determined as the difference between the area under the diastolic aortic and left ventricular pressure curves. Thus, the tension-time and diastolic pressure-time indices serve to help illustrate supply and demand sides of myocardial metabolism utilization during balloon pumping. How intra-aortic balloon pumping can decrease tension-time index parameters and increase diastolic pressure-time index parameters in compromised hearts, causing improved cardiac function, is depicted in Figure 1.

The majority of ventricular oxygen requirements occur during isovolumic systole when wall stresses are maximal.[15] During periods of cardiac failure, ventricular dilation ensues and afterload enhancement causes augmented wall tension. Under these conditions, oxygen requirements have been shown to be at least 16 per cent higher than in normal hearts.[15,33] During counter-

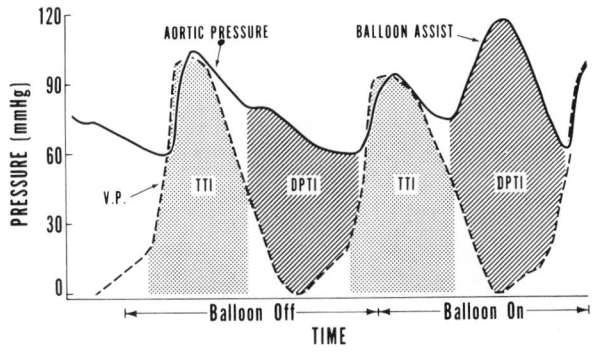

Figure 1. Effects of intra-aortic balloon pumping on myocardial oxygen supply and demand. DPTI, diastolic perfusion-time index. TTI, tension-time index. VP, ventricular pressure. During diastole, balloon assistance produced an elevated DPTI, suggesting an increase in myocardial oxygen supply. Simultaneously, ventricular work (TTI) decreased significantly. (From Bolooki, H.: Clinical Applications of the Intra-aortic Balloon Pump. Mount Kisco, NY, Futura Publishing Company, 1984.)

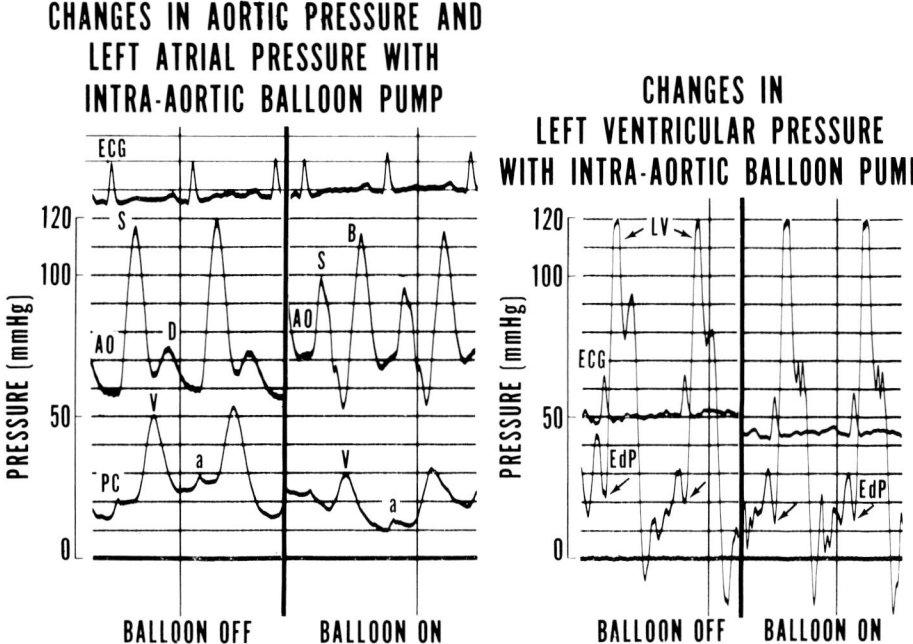

Figure 2. Left: With balloon augmentation, both aortic peak systolic and end-diastolic pressures decrease, suggesting a reduction in ventricular afterload. Simultaneously, the diastolic (D) aortic pressure is enhanced (B). AO, aortic pressure. PC, pulmonary capillary wedge. V, ventricular wave; a, atrial wave. Right: In a failing heart, the left ventricular end-diastolic pressure (EdP) markedly decreases with balloon pumping. LV, left ventricular pressure. (From Bolooki, H. K.: Clinical Applications of the Intra-aortic Balloon Pump. Mount Kisco, NY, Futura Publishing Company, 1984.)

pulsation, rapid collapse of the balloon reduces impedance to aortic flow in the proximal aorta. Thus, the aortic valve is allowed to open at a 10 to 15 per cent lower systolic pressure, reducing myocardial work and oxygen uptake (Fig. 2).[4] The additive effects often eventuate in decreased ischemia, decreased left ventricular end-diastolic pressure, elevated cardiac output by 20 to 50 per cent, and improved urinary output.[5] Secondary benefits include a decreased heart rate and diminished peripheral vascular tone. These and other physiologic benefits of intra-aortic balloon pumping in clinical situations have been detailed previously and are summarized in Table 1.[4,29,55,65]

Studies by Hill and co-workers, using regional ultrasonic crystals, compared pharmacologic afterload-reducing capabilities with those of the IABP (Fig. 3).[22] Data suggested that even though sodium nitroprusside may promote more significant ventricular unloading, segmental excursion was augmented more with counterpulsation.[22] With IABP implementation, segmental myocardial end-diastolic fiber lengths decreased, indicating a markedly reduced diastolic volume, and systolic excursion increased (Fig. 4). These data confirm earlier animal studies by Powell.[54]

In damaged hearts, many of the benefits of balloon pumping probably follow coronary flow augmentation. When adequate pharmacologic afterload reduction causes intolerable hypotension, IABP support must be instituted to provide effective myocardial perfusion along with the functional benefits similar to pharmacologic vasodilators. In most clinical situations, abnormal metabolic demands arise in hearts having severely impaired myocardial perfusion, and autoregulatory reserves become expended. Thus, transmural ventricular flow becomes almost entirely pressure-dependent. Simultaneously, the effective transmural coronary driving pressure continues to diminish during progressive ischemia as the influences of diastolic hypotension become compounded with a rising left ventricular end-diastolic pressure. The additive effects cause spiraling failure secondary to ventricular dilation, enhanced myocardial demands, and decreased cardiac output at a time when blood supply continues to diminish. Under these conditions, the IABP reduces left ventricular end-diastolic pressure, effectively augmenting the transmural coronary driving pressure (Fig. 2).[4] In a classic study, Powell showed that the balloon pump enhances coronary flow more in the presence of failure than in normal hearts.[54] Clinically, the diastolic pressure may increase to 90 per cent with the IABP. Despite this general concept, controversy exists suggesting that the major benefits of intra-aortic balloon pumping follow significant afterload reduction rather than diastolic pressure augmentation and coronary flow alterations.

INDICATIONS FOR INTRA-AORTIC BALLOON PUMPING

Current major indications (Table 2) for intra-aortic balloon pumping include (1) intractable cardiac failure following a cardiopulmonary bypass procedure (35 to 40 per cent); (2) refractory angina despite maximal medical management (15 to 25 per cent); (3) perioperative treatment of the complications of myocardial infarction (10 per cent) including acute ventricular septal defects, acute mitral regurgitation, arrhythmias, and ventricular aneurysms; (4) failed percutaneous coronary angioplasties; and (5) as a bridge to cardiac transplantation.[4,29,44] Compared with

TABLE 1. Physiologic Effects of Intra-aortic Balloon Pumping

Aortic systolic pressure	↓↓	Cardiac preload	↓
Aortic diastolic pressure	↑↑	Left ventricular wall tension	↓
Left ventricular systolic pressure	↓	Left ventricular volume	↓
Left ventricular end-diastolic pressure	↓	Left ventricular stroke work	↓
Cardiac output	↑	Coronary blood flow	↑
Cardiac afterload	↓↓	Renal blood flow	↑

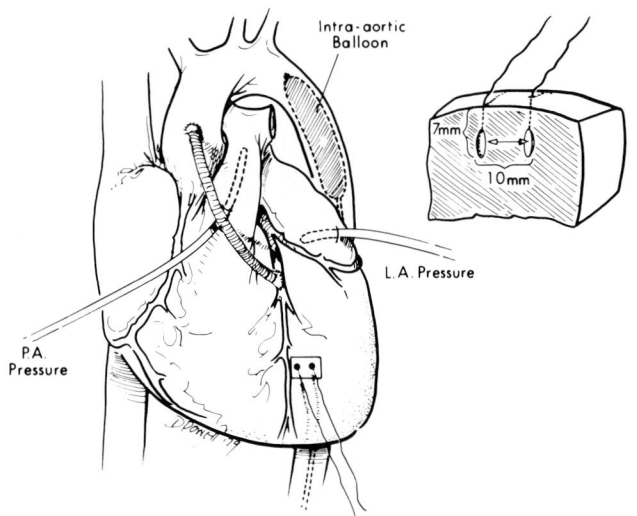

Figure 3. A clinical study comparing the afterload-reducing effects of intra-aortic balloon pumping versus sodium nitroprusside infusion. Mid-wall regional (2 mm.) ultrasonic crystals were placed in patients in postcardiotomy cardiac failure. In the postoperative intensive care unit, segmental diastolic and systolic function parameters were assessed and compared with pulmonary artery (P.A.) and left atrial (L.A.) mean pressures. (Courtesy of Dr. R. C. Hill.)

former years, the IABP is almost never used to treat postinfarction cardiogenic shock unless the potential of angioplasty or coronary surgery exists. With the evolution of newer monitoring, pharmacologic, and anesthetic techniques, prophylactic use in surgical patients with severe three-vessel and left main coronary disease has declined markedly. Conversely, counterpulsation has been expanded to use in children and occasionally in patients with isolated right ventricular failure.[41,52,64]

MYOCARDIAL INFARCTION AND CARDIOGENIC SHOCK. The major indication for use of the balloon pump in the early years of development was refractory cardiogenic shock following myocardial infarction.[4,6,7] Although some pa-

tients with profound ventricular failure improve transiently, only 15 to 20 per cent of patients who are not candidates for revascularization can be weaned from this device.[19,60] Moreover, the long-term survival for these few individuals ranges only between 10 and 30 per cent.[3,10] In a randomized group of patients having failure following transmural infarction, survival and infarct size reduction were not modified with IABP compared with pharmacologic support.[48] In comparison, patients who improve with IABP support so that they can undergo angiography and revascularization do markedly better.[10,51] Weiss has shown that global and segmental left ventricular function can be improved transiently using the IABP in cardiogenic shock patients with anterior infarctions.[67] Patients having postinfarction angina without shock also benefit significantly from intra-aortic balloon pumping.[32] The concept that intra-aortic balloon pumping can modify an infarct size remains controversial. Independent experimental studies by Maroko and Roberts suggest that areas of ischemic damage may be reduced using counterpulsation.[36,58] However, other investigators have shown no significant reduction in infarct area using this device. In stable anterior infarction, Flaherty and co-workers showed that the addition of IABP to nitroglycerin therapy did not reduce infarction size but may have prevented ventricular dilation.[13]

REFRACTORY ANGINA. The intra-aortic balloon pump is very effective for patients with pharmacologically refractory angina and has been extremely helpful in patients being readied for revascularization.[10,34,53,66] When persistent angina occurs in the presence of large doses of intravenous nitroglycerin, the IABP enables angiography and angioplasty to be done more safely. In this setting, balloon pumping has been shown objectively to decrease myocardial ischemia and improve left ventricular function significantly.[32,46,53] At least 80 per cent of patients obtain pain relief from balloon pumping. Survival in patients with medically refractory angina has been excellent using IABP support followed by surgical revascularization.[16,34,66]

FOLLOWING CARDIAC SURGERY. This technique remains extremely efficacious for weaning patients from cardiopulmonary bypass when cardiac failure follows a surgical pro-

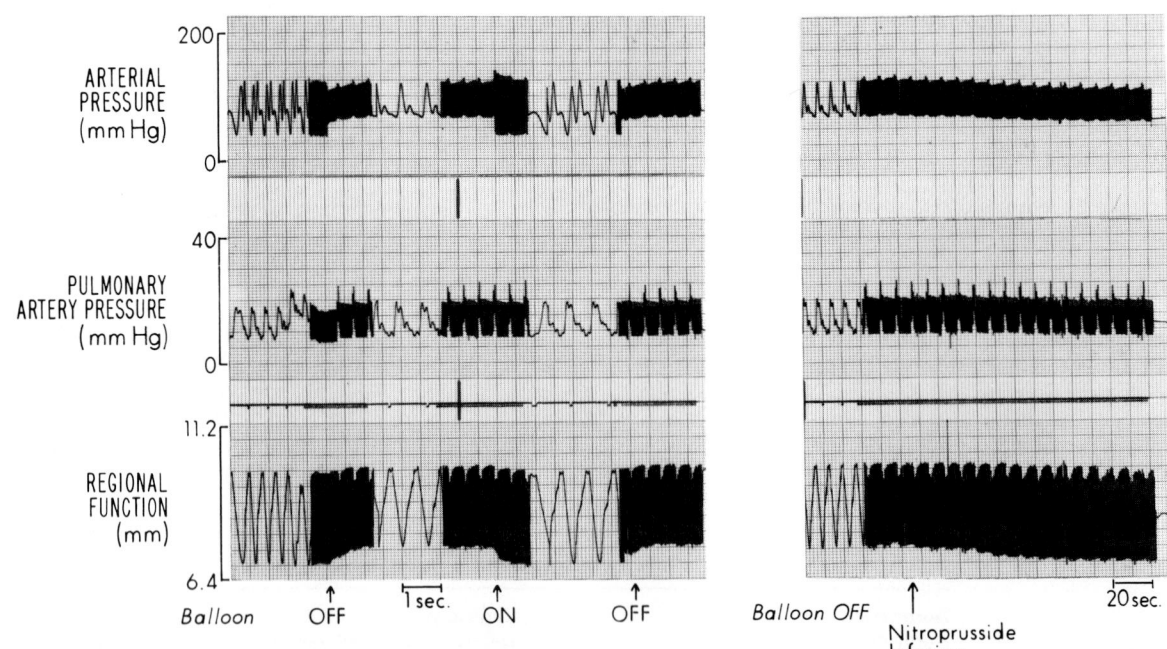

Figure 4. In a failing ventricle, ultrasonic crystals from the study shown in Figure 5 indicated an increase in segmental myocardial excursion with institution of balloon pumping (left). Simultaneously, the left ventricular end-diastolic length diminishes, suggesting a decrease in the overall end-diastolic volume. Balloon pumping effected as good a functional augmentation as nitroprusside (right) but without the associated hypotension. (Courtesy of Dr. R. C. Hill.)

TABLE 2. Indications for Intra-aortic Balloon Pump Support

Unstable angina: refractory pharmacologically
Intractable failure following cardiotomy
Cardiogenic shock prior to angioplasty or coronary bypass grafting
Balloon angioplasty failure: preoperative stabilization
Unstable patients with myocardial infarction undergoing thrombolysis
Complications of myocardial infarction including:
    Acute mitral insufficiency
    Acute ventricular septal defect
    Refractory arrhythmias
    Ventricular aneurysm
Postmyocardial infarction angina: coronary artery bypass candidate
Occasional prophylactic insertion:
    Poor ventricular function
    Tight left main coronary lesion
    Very severe three-vessel disease
    Combination of the preceding
Occasionally for high–cardiac risk noncardiac surgery

cedure.[38,49] Despite attention to intraoperative myocardial protection and maximal pharmacologic support after the period of required arrest, approximately 3 to 6 per cent of patients require an IABP for weaning from cardiopulmonary bypass.[38,49] In general, 75 to 85 per cent of patients who require IABP insertion during cardiopulmonary bypass can be weaned effectively.[5,47] Between 50 and 80 per cent of this group leave the hospital, and a majority of these have a significant long-term survival.[4,5,38,47]

Patients requiring IABP for weaning either have a severely damaged ventricle preoperatively and are exposed to transient but significant ischemia or have a relatively normal heart that experiences severe myocardial injury intraoperatively. The latter group do better, since cardiac function often improves in the early postoperative days if a large infarction has not occurred. Downing reported that individuals requiring balloon counterpulsation following valve operations may not benefit nearly as much as will coronary bypass patients.[11] Specific guidelines have been established to aid in instituting balloon pumping following operative procedures (Table 3).[5,29,47]

Balloon pumping should be compounded with optimal vasodilator and inotropic drug therapy to offer maximal reduction in peripheral vascular resistance, enhanced coronary perfusion, and augmentation of ventricular function. As the goal remains to provide adequate cardiac perfusion and minimize myocardial energy expenditures, many surgeons prefer to institute counterpulsation prior to infusing large doses of inotropic agents. With increased contractility and afterload associated with dopamine and epinephrine administration, ischemia may be aggravated, causing irreversible myocardial damage. Therefore, early IABP treatment may be a more reasonable alternative. Although left ventricular dysfunction occurs much more often, right ventricular or biventricular failure occasionally precludes removal from cardiopulmonary bypass. The IABP may improve right heart failure when inserted into the pulmonary artery. This method

TABLE 3. Indications for Beginning Intra-aortic Counterpulsation During Cardiopulmonary Bypass

Inability to discontinue bypass despite multiple interventions after 30 minutes
Inadequate hemodynamics in the presence of adequate inotropic support including:
    Persistent hypotension (systolic blood pressure <70 mm. Hg)
    Inadequate cardiac index (<2.0 L./min./m.²)
    Elevated left atrial pressure (>20 mm. Hg)
    High peripheral vascular resistance (>2500 dynes/sec./cm.⁻⁵)
Necessity of very large doses of cardiotonic drugs
Persistent malignant ventricular arrhythmias
Preoperative cardiogenic shock secondary to a myocardial infarction or complication of myocardial infarction and/or angioplasty failure

should be considered for patients being operated upon with intractable right ventricular infarctions.[24,41,62,63]

Previously, balloon counterpulsation of children and infants was considered impractical. Pollock has employed IABP to wean children between 1.5 and 18 years of age from bypass following congenital heart surgery.[52] Also, Veasy reported balloon use in infants as young as 6 weeks with significant functional improvement.[64] Dunn has treated 21 children following complex corrective procedures with success.[12] However, three children awaiting transplantation on an IABP have done poorly because of an inadequate organ supply. Single-lumen balloon catheters for infants and children are available in volumes from 2.5 to 20 ml. and are mounted on 4.5- to 7.0-French catheters. Extreme care must be used, especially in infants, to position these devices correctly because occlusion of intra-abdominal vessels may occur more easily. Moreover, in children and infants with heart failure, markedly elevated (190 to 200 beats per minute) heart rates may make timing and diastolic augmentation difficult. Dunn found that in children with heart rates above 160 beats per minute, augmentation of every other beat becomes more efficient.[12] Enhanced aortic elasticity has been implicated also in preventing optimal counterpulsation in children. However, satisfactory afterload reduction and diastolic augmentation have been effected even in very young children. This problem can be decreased slightly by selecting a slightly larger balloon size.

COMPLICATIONS OF MYOCARDIAL INFARCTION. Following myocardial infarction, circulatory deterioration may occur rapidly when either papillary muscle rupture or dysfunction produces severe mitral insufficiency. Moreover, the development of an acute ventricular septal defect following infarction may cause intractable failure. Patients with either of these conditions may require immediate surgical repair and benefit from early IABP support. Vasodilators usually reduce cardiac afterload significantly; however, they supplement the hypotension, aggravating already severe ischemia.

Acute mitral insufficiency following myocardial infarction often causes pulmonary edema, hypotension, and low cardiac output. Most commonly, papillary rupture follows an inferior myocardial infarction. Mitral regurgitation may cause cardiogenic shock in patients with *minimally* impaired left ventricular function. Patients having both severe left ventricular dysfunction and acute mitral insufficiency have a poor prognosis. In this clinical setting, accurate quantitation of preoperative cardiac function becomes impossible. Treatment with systemic vasopressors may augment afterload, causing even more shunting into the lower resistance left atrium. Institution of the IABP decreases cardiac afterload and usually augments forward left ventricular ejection, lessening the regurgitant fraction.[17,55] Under these conditions, balloon pumping effects a decrease in both pulmonary capillary wedge and left atrial pressures. Simultaneously, both the mean arterial pressure and cardiac output are increased (Fig. 5A).[17,56] Counterpulsation should be instituted relatively early in patients who are beginning to decompensate. In a recent review, long-term survival of patients undergoing mitral valve replacement was 78 per cent if the preoperative ejection fraction was greater than 35 per cent, and only 38 per cent if less.[56] Since the salutary effects of the IABP may be short-lived when treating both ischemic mitral regurgitation and ventricular septal rupture, catheterization and surgical therapy should proceed rapidly.[17,56]

Ventricular septal rupture occurs in 1 to 3 per cent of acute myocardial infarctions and is responsible for 5 per cent of preinfarction deaths in this group. Rapid hemodynamic deterioration occurs in approximately 60 per cent of patients. Without surgical therapy, nearly 80 per cent succumb within 2 months of infarction. Thus, nearly all patients should undergo immediate surgical repair.[57] Recent use of the IABP combined with early repair has eventuated in an operative mortality as low as 30 per

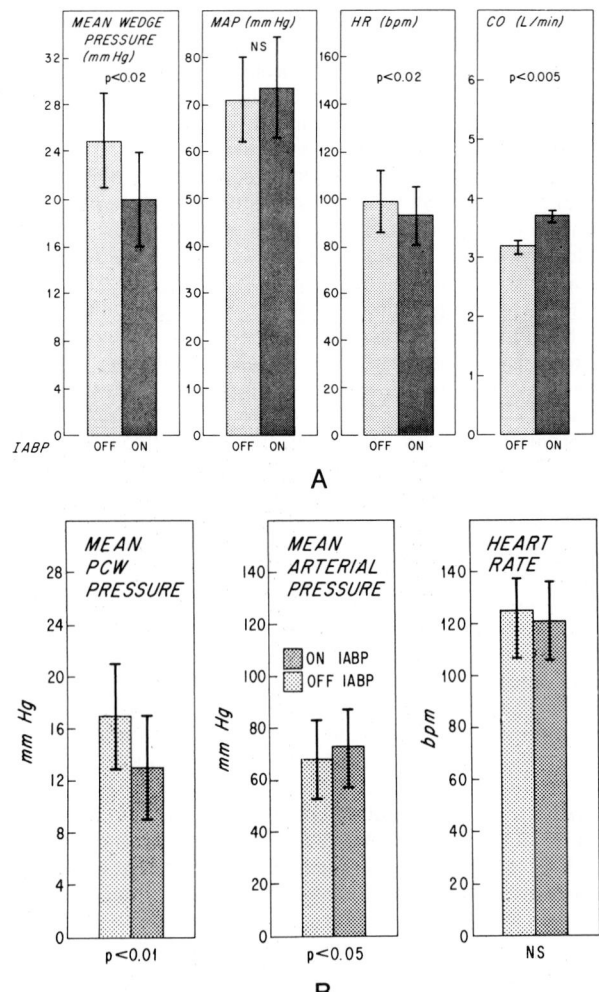

Figure 5. *A,* Patients with acute mitral insufficiency demonstrated a significant decrease in pulmonary capillary wedge pressure and an increase in cardiac output after introduction of balloon counterpulsation. *B,* In patients with an acute ventricular septal rupture, balloon pumping decreased the mean pulmonary capillary wedge pressure (PCW) while increasing mean arterial pressure. Simultaneously, abnormal shunting across the septal defect decreased significantly. (From Gold, H. K., Leinbach, R. C., Sanders, C. A., Buckley, M. J., Mundth, E. D., and Austen, W. G.: Intra-aortic balloon pumping for ventricular septal defect or mitral regurgitation complicating acute myocardial infarction. Circulation, *47:*1191, 1973.)

ever, individuals who sustain refractory ventricular irritability are at an extremely high risk with a very poor prognosis.[21] Both continuing ischemia and an altered myocardial substrate, such as an aneurysm, can initiate problematic arrhythmias. When ischemia persists as the major etiologic factor, institution of IABP effectively controls ventricular irritability in most patients. Hanson found an 86 per cent improvement in these ischemic patients and a 55 per cent total resolution of arrhythmias following institution of IABP.[21] In 90 per cent, anginal pain was completely resolved and in this group survival was markedly increased if IABP was followed by subsequent coronary artery bypass grafting. In contrast, when myocardial fibrosis is the inciting arrhythmogenic problem, IABP use appears less effective. Surgical alternatives such as endocardial resection, either alone or combined with coronary artery bypass grafting and the implantation of automatic internal defibrillators, have been helpful in these situations.

Ventricular aneurysms develop in as many as 20 per cent of patients following a myocardial infarction.[3] Acute ventricular aneurysms have been much more difficult to treat than chronic ventricular aneurysms. Ventricular irritability occurs in the former group in 7 to 41 per cent of cases; however, only 7 to 11 per cent require surgical intervention because of arrhythmias. In these surgical candidates, hemodynamic improvement usually results from IABP, since the salutary effects on heart failure and electrical irritability are usually additive.[3] Thus, when a chronic aneurysm causes severe failure, preoperative insertion of an IABP may be protective.

CORONARY ANGIOPLASTY FAILURES. For patients who require emergent revascularization because of a failed angioplasty, balloon counterpulsation has been demonstrated to provide optimal stabilization in the catheterization laboratory.[44] This is especially important with multivessel coronary disease or markedly impaired ventricular function. In most instances, the cardiologists can accomplish intra-aortic balloon insertion rapidly using guidewires placed during the diagnostic catheterization. The benefits of fluoroscopic control in the catheterization laboratory become obvious when considering severe coexisting aortofemoral arterial disease in many elderly patients. Modern reperfusion or "bail out" catheters may allow a counterpulsed IABP waveform to reach the distal segment of the jeopardized coronary artery. Small portable balloon consoles and dual-lumen balloon catheters with continuous central aortic pressure monitoring enable transport to the operating room with greater safety and speed. By minimizing ischemia following a failed angioplasty by use of a combination of these methods, most patients now can be revascularized emergently using the internal mammary artery instead of all vein grafts.

BRIDGE TO CARDIAC TRANSPLANTATION. For end-stage patients with cardiomyopathy awaiting transplantation, intra-aortic balloon counterpulsation has been helpful, especially for those refractory to inotropic drug therapy. The importance of IABP support has increased with the declining donor heart supply. The waiting period may be well over a month even for acutely deteriorating patients. A balloon pump may provide sufficient afterload reduction to obviate the need for a more invasive left ventricular assist device. At the University of Pittsburgh, 28 per cent of patients who required inotropic support prior to cardiac transplant also required an IABP as a bridge.[30] In these patients, there was no difference in survival at 3 years between those supported with the IABP and individuals transplanted electively.

OTHER INDICATIONS. Previously, prophylactic balloon pumping prior to cardiac surgery was popular in patients with left main artery disease, unstable angina, poor left ventricular function, and severe aortic stenosis. Presently, most cardiac surgeons and anesthesiologists believe that less than 1 per cent of patients require prophylactic IABP use.[29] Patients with either poor left ventricular function or severe left main coronary artery

cent.[9] In postoperative patients, long-term survival has been approximately 70 per cent when left ventricular function is good.

As with mitral regurgitation, an acute ventricular septal defect causing shock may occur with moderate to good left ventricular function. Many of the pathologic effects from an acute septal rupture may follow severe right ventricular failure induced by increased left-to-right shunting. Stabilization with the IABP markedly reduces both shunting and the pulmonary capillary wedge pressure with a concomitant increase in cardiac output and mean arterial pressure (Fig. 5*B*).[17,55] As with mitral regurgitation, these improvements follow afterload reduction, which provides less resistance to systemic ejection. Enhanced coronary perfusion may help reduce ischemic ventricular dysfunction simultaneously. In a recent study, 65 per cent of patients undergoing surgical repair of an acute septal defect required intra-aortic balloon pumping. Most clinicians institute balloon pumping prior to severe cardiac decompensation.

Ventricular arrhythmias that are significant occur in 10 to 50 per cent of patients following an acute myocardial infarction. The majority are well controlled with antiarrhythmic medications, cardioversion, and pacing alone or in combination. How-

disease who develop chest pain in the operating room prior to or during induction or who become hypotensive may require an IABP. However, nearly all of these patients can undergo induction of anesthesia safely using newer monitoring and pharmacologic techniques. Use of IABP for protection during noncardiac surgery is indicated rarely.[4,55] However, for patients with inoperable coronary artery disease who require urgent surgical therapy for other reasons, the IABP has been employed occasionally. Other infrequent indications include septic shock and massive pulmonary emboli.

CONTRAINDICATIONS FOR BALLOON PUMPING

With severe aortic insufficiency, balloon pumping enhances left ventricular regurgitation and cardiac failure. However, patients with minor degrees of insufficiency may be improved by IABP. Although the presence of a thoracic or abdominal aneurysm may be a relative contraindication to balloon insertion, intraoperative use may be feasible in specific situations. Most patients with coronary artery disease have some degree of diffuse atherosclerosis. Formerly, this precluded insertion via the femoral artery in approximately 10 to 25 per cent of patients. However, newer fluoroscopic percutaneous insertion techniques over a guidewire have aided in positioning IABP catheters even with diffuse atherosclerosis and tortuous vessels. The development of retrograde axillary artery and transthoracic introduction has rejuvenated the possibility of balloon pumping patients with totally occluded aortas. The previous administration of thrombolytic agents or anticoagulants has not posed any contraindication of IABP insertion.[14]

INSERTION TECHNIQUES

Percutaneous Insertion

In the majority of patients, intra-aortic balloon catheters can be inserted percutaneously via the femoral artery using a modified Seldinger technique.[49] This method precludes the necessity of a long arteriotomy, a patch closure, or a stump of graft material attached to the artery.

Percutaneous and surgical balloon catheters presently available from various manufacturers in this country are depicted in Tables 4 and 5. Currently, the smallest dual-lumen (inner guide-wire/arterial pressure channel) percutaneous catheter with a standard 40-ml. balloon has an outside diameter of 9.0-French. For single-lumen catheters, 8.5-French is the smallest

TABLE 4. Double-Lumen Percutaneous Intra-aortic Balloons

Volume (ml.)	Catheter Size (French)	Sheath Size Outside Diameter (French)	Manufacturer
50	11.0	13.0	A
50	10.5	12.5	D
50	10.0	S	K
50	11.5	13.0	M
40	11.0	S	A
40	10.0	12.5	D
40	9.0	S	K
40	9.5	11.5	D,M
34	9.5	11.5	D
30	11.0	13.0	A
30	9.0	S	K

A, Aires; D, Datascope; K, Kontron; M, Mansfield. S indicates that the introducer is withdrawn and the balloon catheter remains in the arterial lumen "sheathless" to provide less obstruction.

Size and technical information provided by manufacturers.

TABLE 5. Single-Lumen Percutaneous Intra-aortic Balloons

Volume (ml.)	Catheter Size (French)	Introducer Outside Diameter (French)	Manufacturer
40	9.0	11.0	A
40	8.5	11.5	D
30	9.0	11.0	A
20*	7.0	—	D
12*	7.0	—	D
7*	5.5	—	D
5*	5.5	—	D
2.5*	4.5	—	D

* Denotes that these balloons are for pediatric and infant patients and all require surgical introduction. The others are percutaneous single-lumen catheters.

with a 40-ml. balloon. For smaller patients, catheters for surgical insertion are available with balloon sizes ranging between 20 and 30 ml. Surgical balloons ranging between 2.5 and 20 ml. are manufactured for children and infants. Smaller catheters may help prevent untoward limb ischemia while still providing a balloon volume adequate for counterpulsation. In actuality the ratio between catheter size and balloon volume remains the limiting factor for helium exchange. Thus, even smaller catheters for the larger balloons may not be possible with the present technology. Overall, adult intra-aortic balloon catheters are approximately 70 cm. long with a 25 cm. long balloon at the tip. Many percutaneous balloons have an internal lumen that aids in passing the catheter over a guidewire during difficult insertion (Fig. 6). After balloon introduction, removal of this wire allows central aortic pressure measurement from the lumen.

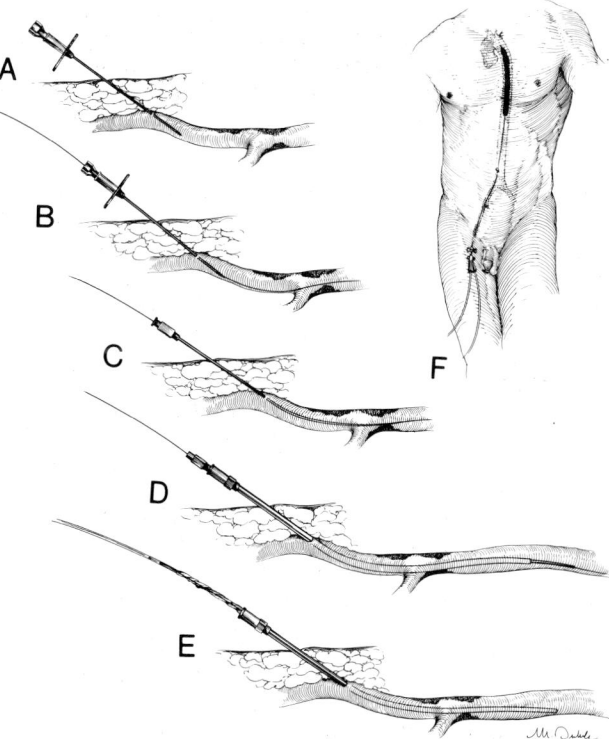

Figure 6. Percutaneous insertion technique. *A* and *B*, The Seldinger technique is used to insert the guidewire into the femoral artery. *C* and *D*, Subsequently, a dilator and introducing sheath are inserted over the guidewire and into the femoral artery. *E* and *F*, The guidewire and dilator are then removed, and the prewrapped catheter is inserted with a clockwise twisting motion until the balloon is passed to the premeasured length just distal to the subclavian artery.

For proper positioning of the catheter tip just distal to the subclavian artery origin, a prewrapped balloon should have vacuum applied to the catheter and be measured from the site of groin insertion to just below the sternal notch. A Cournard needle is used to puncture the common femoral artery just below the inguinal ligament. The needle should be inserted at a 45-degree angle to the skin. After pulsatile arterial flow returns, a guidewire should be passed above the iliac arterial bifurcation and the needle withdrawn. A vessel dilator then is positioned over the wire and passed into the arterial lumen (Fig. 6C). As shown in Figure 6D, the balloon introducer sheath then should be threaded over a larger dilator, and together the two are passed over the wire into the arterial lumen with a twisting motion. Long sheaths are available to make insertion with severely diseased or tortuous vessels easier. When the sheath is left at the iliac level and atherosclerotic narrowing exists, limb ischemia may cause occlusion.

Finally, as shown in Figure 6E, the dilator should be removed leaving the guidewire and sheath in the artery. When a dual-lumen balloon catheter is selected, it should be passed into the proximal aorta over the wire. Single-lumen catheters are smaller but require removal of the guidewire before introduction. Using a clockwise twisting motion, the prewrapped balloon should be placed in the sheath and advanced to the premeasured length (Fig. 6E and F). Care must be taken not to force the balloon against any obstruction, since iliac or aortic perforation may occur. Most balloons unwrap spontaneously in either the pulsatile aortic lumen or after the first inflation. After the balloon catheter is attached to the pump console, the gas exchange lumen should be purged. Balloon augmentation then can be timed appropriately from cutaneous electrocardiogram leads, a ventricular electrogram, or the arterial pressure tracing. Ventricular pacing wires provide an excellent source for electrocardiographic timing when all else fails.

Introducer sheaths should be withdrawn slightly to help prevent iliac obstruction; however, these should never slip beyond the arterial puncture site because hemorrhage occurs. Some catheters have a sterile positioning sleeve that becomes helpful after the surgical field removal. Extremity arterial pulses, temperature, and color should be assessed and documented frequently. In general, patients undergoing intra-aortic balloon pumping should be anticoagulated with heparin.[4]

Surgical Insertion: Femoral, Axillary, and Transthoracic

Formerly, balloon catheters were inserted through a 10-mm. Dacron/polytetrafluoroethylene graft sewn onto the femoral artery.[4] Although rarely required today, femoral surgical insertion techniques may become necessary. The lack of a palpable femoral pulse during nonpulsatile cardiopulmonary bypass may make percutaneous insertion difficult. Balloon catheters can be introduced surgically via a Dacron side graft sewn to a longitudinal iliac arteriotomy. At present, when an open technique is required, a pledgeted suture is placed around a small femoral arteriotomy with insertion of surgical balloons directly. This method is preferred for placement of catheters in children and very small adults.

The balloon catheters can be inserted into the axillary artery and passed toward the left subclavian artery. Surgeons at St. Louis University have used this method to enable ambulation of patients who require cardiac assist and are awaiting transplantation and are doing well. This method also provides access in the presence of an occluded aorta.

Occasionally, aortic occlusion or diffuse atherosclerosis may prevent retrograde femoral insertion of balloon catheters needed for weaning from cardiopulmonary bypass. In this situation, the transthoracic approach may be required.[4,39,49] As shown in Figure 7, balloons may be inserted into the ascending aortic arch via either a pursestring suture or attached 10-mm.

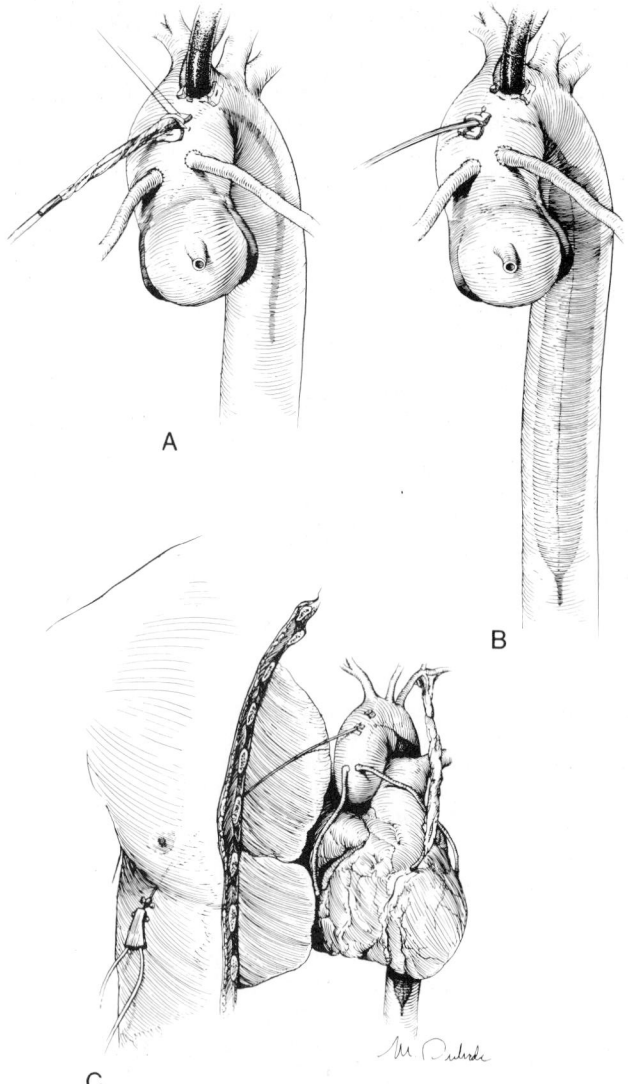

Figure 7. A to C, When an intra-aortic balloon catheter cannot be inserted by the femoral approach because of bilateral iliac obstruction, antegrade introduction via the thoracic aorta may be required. A pledgeted "pursestring" suture may be placed in the ascending aorta and the balloon introduced in an antegrade manner. The proximal catheter crosses the mediastinum and chest wall anterior to the right lung. With this particular method, removal requires return to the operating suite.

Dacron/polytetrafluoroethylene graft. Alternatively, an introducer sheath can be placed through the chest wall and the balloon passed into the aorta by the Seldinger method, described previously. Direct visualization of the insertion site remains paramount. The sheath should be withdrawn through the chest wall and a pursestring suture placed around the aortic entrance site to prevent leakage.

BALLOON CATHETER REMOVAL

Prior to balloon catheter removal, heparin should be discontinued 6 hours in advance. Both the platelet count and coagulation factors should be assessed and corrected if necessary. Surgical femoral balloons may be removed in the intensive care unit if appropriate sterile technique is available. Prior to removal, all balloons should be evacuated totally to reduce catheter size, minimizing trauma at the entrance site. During surgical removal, embolectomy catheters should be passed both proximally and distally to ensure arterial patency. Following withdrawal of percutaneous balloons, constant point-pressure should be applied to the groin for at least 30 minutes. Distal pulses should be palpated or examined by Doppler ultrasound to help prevent arterial thrombosis from occlusive pressure. Although methods have been reported that allow withdrawal of transthoracic balloon catheters through a long graft, the author's group has preferred to return to the operating room for removal.[39]

COMPLICATIONS

Major complications associated with insertion and use of intra-aortic balloon catheters include (1) limb ischemia from primary thrombosis, emboli, or vascular dissection; (2) intra-abdominal and intrathoracic hemorrhage from vascular perforation and/or dissection; (3) groin hematomas, lymph drainage, and femoral artery false aneurysms; (4) local wound infections and systemic sepsis; (5) renal failure and bowel infarction from balloon malposition; (6) device malfunction in IABP-dependent patients; and (7) neurologic complications including paraplegia. These complications may be enhanced by thrombolytic agents, including streptokinase, rTPA, and urokinase, as well as the relatively rare problem of heparin-induced thrombocytopenia. Kantrowitz has analyzed the complications in 733 IABP patients, and this review should be consulted.[28]

In up to 25 per cent of patients requiring an IABP, the balloon catheter cannot be advanced because of an atherosclerotic obstruction.[19,23,37,38] Complications of difficult insertions occur in 10 to 35 per cent of patients, and significant vascular problems occur in approximately 15 per cent.[1,37,61] Between 2 and 10 per cent of the latter group require vascular repair, which may include either patch angioplasty or femoral-femoral bypass grafting. The incidence of major IABP complications has been reported to be higher with percutaneous balloon catheters.[18,49] A balloon catheter may enter the aortic wall at an ulcerated

plaque, creating a dissection as depicted in Figure 8.[23] In most situations, ischemic complications can be obviated by early removal of the balloon catheter or partial withdrawal of the introducer sheath. The overall period of balloon counterpulsation and the sex of the patient appear to be the most significant determinants of complications.[61] Smaller balloon catheters (8.5- and 9.0-French) with 40 and 50 ml. volumes have been developed recently and help immensely in smaller female patients (Table 5). As noted previously, "sheathless" percutaneous balloons have recently been introduced and may have promise for these patients.

TIMING OF COUNTERPULSATION AND WEANING

After the intra-aortic balloon pump has been advanced to a satisfactory position, inflation and deflation must be timed carefully with either an electrocardiographic or arterial pressure tracing. The central aortic pressure channel in dual-lumen percutaneous balloon catheters enables optimal timing. Inflation delays of up to 50 and 120 msec. may occur with peripheral radial and femoral arterial monitoring catheters, respectively.[55] Moreover, radial arterial vasoconstriction accompanying low cardiac output and hypothermia may enhance timing problems. During periods of normal sinus rhythm, optimal counterpulsation is usually achieved without difficulty.

As shown in Figure 9, the balloon should inflate about 40 msec. before the arterial dicrotic notch (the ascending T wave) and deflate during early isovolumic contraction (after the P wave).[4] Total deflation must occur before ejection or the R wave. Usually, this provides excellent diastolic augmentation and optimal afterload reduction as reflected by a significant decrease in both the aortic systolic and end-diastolic pressures. Early inflation causes premature closure of the aortic valve with reduced stroke volume, and late inflation causes inadequate diastolic pressure augmentation. Early deflation effects poor afterload reduction; late deflation impedes systole, effecting increased cardiac work.

With either the initiation of electrical pacing or the development of atrial or ventricular arrhythmias, intra-aortic balloon timing may become difficult, causing inefficient augmentation. During pacing, a decrease in the pacer artifact amplitude may lessen the tendency for balloon pump dual sensing. However, most newer pump consoles have very good electrocautery suppression and pacemaker sensing capabilities. Older balloon pumps may be retrofitted to provide improved timing during pacing and extraneous electrical suppression. Timing from the

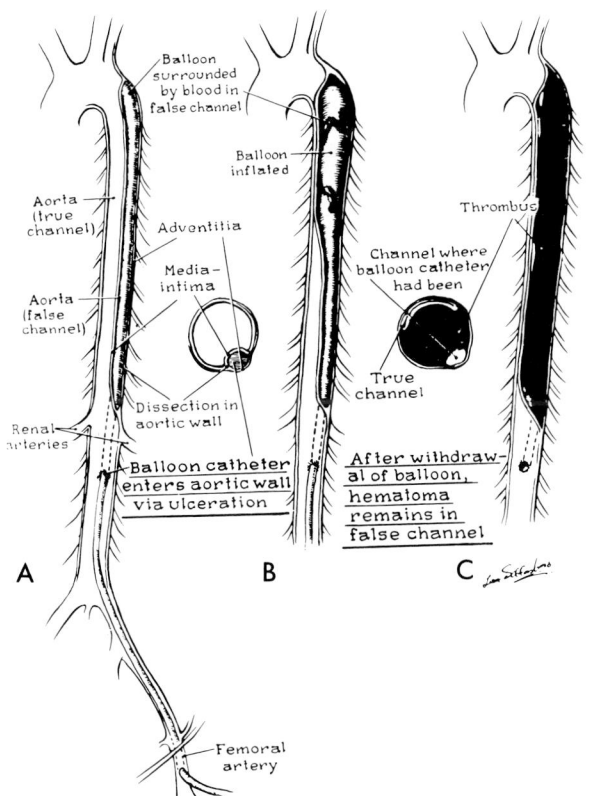

Figure 8. A balloon catheter may enter the aortic wall at an ulcerated plaque, creating a dissection and ultimate aortic occlusion. (From Isner, J. M., Cohen, S. R., Virmani, R., Lawrinson, W., and Roberts, W. C.: Complications of the intra-aortic balloon counterpulsation device: Clinical and morphologic observations in 45 necropsy patients. Am. J. Cardiol., 45:260, 1980.)

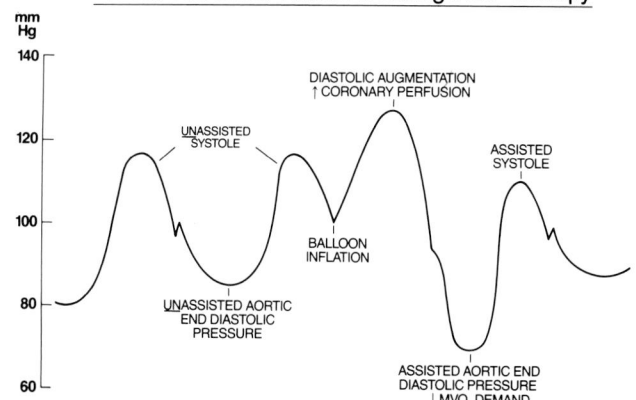

Figure 9. Correct timing of an intra-aortic balloon pressure tracing is shown. Diastolic augmentation should begin with closure of the aortic valve and proceed until isovolumic systole. (Courtesy of Datascope Corp., Paramus, NJ.)

ventricular pacing wires placed during operation may provide improved augmentation.

The author's group prefers to wean the majority of patients of inotropic medications before balloon catheter removal. This is predicated on the absence of peripheral vascular and groin problems. Usually, dopamine or dobutamine infusions have been decreased to below 5 μg. per kg. per minute, and no other vasopressors are present before establishing a 1:2 pumping ratio. Thereafter, the balloon pump inflation ratio and remaining inotropic support are weaned simultaneously. Counterpulsation also can be weaned by decreasing the balloon inflation volume gradually. However, the balloon must have some volume and motion while in the aorta to prevent thrombosis and emboli.

HELICOPTER AND AIR AMBULANCE IABP TRANSPORT

New smaller transport balloon consoles are optimal in the catheterization laboratory or operating room. The Datascope 90–T, Kontron KAAT, Aires 700, and Mansfield 3000 have all been tested for flight conditions but have different power requirements, purging characteristics, and Federal Aviation Administration requirements for motion security. These devices will fit in a variety of helicopters including the Aerospatiale Dauphin SA–365N, Bell 222 and 412, Messerschmitt-Bolkow-Blohm (MBB) BK117, Mitsubishi MU 2B–60, and Sikorsky S–76. Helicopters usually fly below 10,000 feet and do not require pressurization. However, during fixed-wing air transport, intra-aortic balloon characteristics are altered by aircraft pressurization. Because of constant balloon gas expansion and contraction (1.5 ml. per 1000 feet of altitude), it is recommended that the IABP operator be apprised constantly of changes in altitude to effect proper purging of the device. Mertlich and Quaal have outlined these changes as well as in-flight instructions for IABP users. Their work should be reviewed by individuals planning helicopter or fixed-wing air transport of IABP patients.[40] The group from Northwestern University of Evanston Hospital reported 50 IABP patients transported safely by helicopter.[35] At the University of Kentucky, a special team of cardiologists and nurses have inserted intra-aortic balloon catheters at regional emergency rooms in seven patients in cardiogenic shock. Subsequently, these patients were transported via helicopter to the university hospital without an in-flight or subsequent IABP complication. Although difficult to effect logistically, advanced outreach care and helicopter transport illustrate the wide application of balloon counterpulsation used presently for acute patient care.

SELECTED REFERENCES

Bolooki, H.: Clinical Application of Intra-aortic Balloon Pump. Mount Kisco, NY, Futura Publishing Company, 1984.
  This textbook provides a comprehensive overview of intra-aortic balloon counterpulsation. It details the technical aspects of surgical insertion as well as complications of this technique. This work represents a major reference illustrating the clinical indications and physiologic advantages of balloon pumping.

Clauss, R. H., Birtwell, W. C., Albertal, G., Lunzer, S., Taylor, W. J., Fosberg, A. M., and Harken, D. E.: Assisted circulation: The arterial counterpulsator. J. Thorac. Cardiovasc. Surg., 41:447, 1961.
  This is the first description of vascular counterpulsation, which was done by withdrawing blood from the aorta during systole with reinfusion during diastole via a solenoid-activated pump. The publication represents a milestone biomedical engineering collaborative effort.

Gold, H. K., Leinbach, R. C., Sanders, C. A., Buckley, M. J., Mundth, E. D., and Austen, W. G.: Intra-aortic balloon pumping for ventricular septal defect or mitral regurgitation complicating myocardial infarction. Circulation, 47:1191, 1973.
  This classic review describes the physiologic advantages of intra-aortic balloon pumping for either an acute ventricular septal defect or mitral regurgitation following myocardial infarction.

Kantrowitz, A., Wasfie, T., Freed, P. S., Rubenfire, M., Wajszuzuk, W., and Schork, M. A.: Intra-aortic balloon pumping 1967 through 1982: Analysis of complications in 733 patients. Am. J. Cardiol., 57:976, 1986.
  This modern paper analyzes complications relating to balloon counterpulsation in 733 patients over a 15-year period. The author is the progenitor of the technique as an assist device. This work should be consulted for a comprehensive understanding of problems associated with intra-aortic balloon pumping use.

Mertlich, G., and Quaal, S. J.: Air transport of the patient requiring intra-aortic balloon pumping. Crit. Care Nurs. Clin. North Am., 1:443, 1989.
  This paper is perhaps the definitive publication relating to balloon counterpulsation during air transport. Physiologic changes and physical properties of the balloon materials at higher altitudes are detailed. Specific patient transport and nursing issues are addressed very well.

Moulopoulos, S. D., Topaz, S., and Kolff, W. J.: Diastolic balloon pumping (with carbon dioxide) in the aorta: A mechanical assistance of the failing circulation. Am. Heart J., 63:669, 1962.
  This paper is the first description of diastolic augmentation using an inflatable intra-aortic balloon. This work emanated from the laboratory of Dr. Willem J. Kolff, the noted innovator in artificial organ support.

Pennington, D. G., Swartz, M., Codd, J. E., Merjavy, J. P., and Kaiser, G. C.: Intra-aortic balloon pumping in cardiac surgical patients: A nine year experience. Ann. Thorac. Surg., 36:125, 1983.
  This is a recent review of 378 patients requiring intra-aortic balloon pumping during cardiac surgery. Preoperative indications included unstable angina (5 per cent) and cardiogenic shock (9 per cent). In 252 patients (67 per cent), intra-aortic balloon pumping was required because of hemodynamic deterioration following surgical therapy. The overall survival in this group was 53 per cent, and the incidence of complications was 11.6 per cent. The article is an excellent overview of clinical indications, complications, and benefits of intra-aortic balloon pumping.

Powell, W. J., Daggett, W. M., Magro, A. E., Bianco, J. A., Buckley, M. J., Sanders, C. A., Kantrowitz, A. R., and Austen, W. G.: Effects of intra-aortic balloon counterpulsation on cardiac performance, oxygen consumption, and coronary blood flow in dogs. Circ. Res., 26:753, 1970.
  This article outlines classic experimental studies demonstrating the physiologic advantages of intra-aortic balloon pumping. The influences of balloon pumping on myocardial oxygen consumption, coronary blood flow, and left ventricular performance are detailed. These data documented that in the failing heart, afterload reduction effects a decrease in left ventricular end-diastolic pressure and peak systolic pressure while augmenting the aortic diastolic pressure and coronary blood flow simultaneously.

Radford, M. J., Johnson, R. A., Daggett, W. M., Fallon, J. T., Buckley, M. J., Gold, H. K., and Leinbach, R. C.: Ventricular septal rupture: A review of clinical and physiologic features and an analysis of survival. Circulation, 64:545, 1981.
  This paper is an excellent review of 41 patients who developed postinfarction ventricular septal rupture. Cardiac shock developed in 55 per cent of these patients, and intra-aortic balloon pumping was used prior to operative repair in 18 of the 22 patients in cardiogenic shock. This paper emphasizes the physiologic benefits of balloon pumping in preparing these patients for reparative cardiac surgery.

REFERENCES

1. Alderman, J. D., Gabliani, G. I., McCabe, C. H., Brewer, C. C., Lorell, B. H., Pasternak, R. C., Skillman, J. J., Steer, M. L., and Biam, D. S.: Incidence and management of limb ischemia with percutaneous wire-guided intraaortic balloon catheters. J. Am. Coll. Cardiol., 9:524, 1987.
2. Ashar, B., and Turcotte, L. R.: Analyses of longest IAB implant in a human patient (327 days). Trans. Am. Soc. Artif. Intern. Organs, 27:372, 1981.
3. Baudet, M., Rigaud, M., Rocha, P., Bardet, J., and Bourdarias, J. P.: Treatment of early postinfarction ventricular aneurysm by intra-aortic balloon pumping and surgery. J. Thorac. Cardiovasc. Surg., 78:445, 1979.
4. Bolooki, H.: Clinical Application of Intra-aortic Balloon Pump. Mt. Kisco, NY, Futura Publishing Company, 1984.
5. Bolooki, H., Williams, W., Thurer, R. J., Vargas, A., Kaiser, G. A., Mack, F., and Chahramani, A. R.: Clinical and hemodynamic criteria for use of the intra-aortic balloon pump in patients requiring cardiac surgery. J. Thorac. Cardiovasc. Surg., 72:456, 1976.
6. Buckley, M. J., Craver, J. M., Gold, H. K., Mundth, E. D., Daggett, W. M., and Austen, W. G.: Intra-aortic balloon assist for cardiogenic shock after cardiopulmonary bypass. Circulation, 48(Suppl. 3):III-90, 1973.
7. Buckley, M. J., Leinbach, R. C., Kastor, J. A., Laird, J. D., Kantrowitz, A. R., Madras, P. N., Sanders, C. A., and Austen, W. G.: Hemodynamic evaluation of intra-aortic balloon pumping in man. Circulation, 41–42(Suppl. 2):II-130, 1970.
8. Clauss, R. H., Birtwell, W. C., Albertal, G., Lunzer, S., Taylor, W. J., Fosberg, A. M., and Harken, D. E.: Assisted circulation: The arterial counterpulsator. J. Thorac. Cardiovasc. Surg., 41:447, 1961.
9. Daggett, W. M., Guyton, R. A., Mundth, E. D., Buckley, M. J., McEnany, M. T., Gold, H. K., Leinbach, R. C., and Austen, W. G.: Surgery for post-myocardial infarct ventricular septal defect. Ann. Surg., 186:260, 1977.
10. DeWood, A. M., Notske, R. N., Hensley, G. R., Shields, J. P., O'Grady, W. P., Spores, J., Goldman, M., and Ganji, J. H.: Intra-aortic balloon counterpulsation with or without reperfusion for myocardial infarction shock. Circulation, 61:1105, 1980.

11. Downing, T. P., Miller, D. C., Stofer, R., and Shumway, N. E.: Use of the intra-aortic balloon pump after valve replacement. J. Thorac. Cardiovasc. Surg., 92:210, 1986.

12. Dunn, J. M.: The use of intra-aortic balloon pumping in pediatrics patients. Cardiac Assists, 5:2, 1989.

13. Flaherty, J. T., Becker, L. C., Weiss, J. L., Brinker, J. A., Bulkley, B. H., Gerstenblith, G., Kallman, C. H., and Weisfeldt, M. L.: Results of a randomized prospective trial of intraaortic balloon counterpulsation and intravenous nitroglycerin in patients with acute myocardial infarction. J. Am. Coll. Cardiol., 6: 434, 1985.

14. George, B. S.: Thrombolysis and intra-aortic balloon pumping following acute myocardial infarction: Experience in four TAMI studies. Cardiac Assists, 4:1, 1988.

15. Gibbs, C. L., and Chapman, J. B.: Cardiac energetics. In Handbook of Physiology, Section 2, The Cardiovascular System. Vol. I, The Heart., Bethesda, MD, The American Physiological Society, 1979, pp. 775–804.

16. Gold, H. K., Leinbach, R. C., Buckley, M. J., Mundth, E. D., Daggett, W. M., and Austen, W. G.: Refractory angina pectoris: Follow-up after intra-aortic balloon pumping and surgery. Circulation, 54(Suppl. 3):41, 1976.

17. Gold, H. K., Leinbach, R. C., Sanders, C. A., Buckley, M. J., Mundth, E. D., and Austen, W. G.: Intra-aortic balloon pumping for ventricular septal defect or mitral regurgitation complicating acute myocardial infarction. Circulation, 47:1191, 1973.

18. Goldberg, M. J., Rubenfire, M., Kantrowitz, A., Goodman, G., Freed, P. S., Hallen, L., and Reimann, P.: Intraaortic balloon pump insertion: A randomized study comparing percutaneous and surgical techniques. J. Am. Coll. Cardiol., 9:515, 1987.

19. Goldberger, M., Tabak, S. W., and Shah, P. K.: Clinical experience with intra-aortic balloon counterpulsation in 112 consecutive patients. Am. Heart J., 111:497, 1986.

20. Grotz, R. L., and Yeston, N. S.: Intra-aortic balloon counterpulsation in high-risk cardiac patients undergoing noncardiac surgery. Surgery, 106:1, 1989.

21. Hanson, E. C., Levine, F. H., Kay, H. R., Leinbach, R. C., Gold, H. K., Daggett, W. M., Austen, W. G., and Buckley, M. J.: Control of postinfarction ventricular irritability with the intraaortic balloon pump. Circulation, 62(Suppl. 1):130, 1980.

22. Hill, R. C., Sink, J. D., Chitwood, W. R., Olsen, C. O., Jones, R. N., Cox, J. L., and Wechsler, A. S.: Effects of intra-aortic balloon diastolic augmentation and nitroprusside on postoperative regional left ventricular function. Am. J. Cardiol., 45:432, 1980.

23. Isner, J. M., Cohen, S. R., Virmani, R., Lawrinson, W., and Roberts, W. C.: Complications of the intraaortic balloon counterpulsation device: Clinical and morphologic observations in 45 necropsy patients. Am. J. Cardiol., 45:260, 1980.

24. Jett, G. K., Picone, A. L., and Clark, R. E.: Circulatory support for right ventricular dysfunction. J. Thorac. Cardiovasc. Surg., 94:95, 1987.

25. Kantrowitz, A.: Initial clinical experience with intra-aortic balloon pumping in cardiogenic shock. J.A.M.A., 203:113, 1968.

26. Kantrowitz, A., and Kantrowitz, A.: Experimental augmentation of coronary blood flow by retardation of arterial pressure pulse. Surgery, 34:678, 1953.

27. Kantrowitz, A., Tjonneland, S., Krakauer, J. S., Phillips, S. J., Freed, P. S., and Butner, A. N.: Mechanical intraaortic cardiac assistance in cardiogenic shock. Arch. Surg., 97:1000, 1968.

28. Kantrowitz, A., Wasfie, T., Freed, P. S., Rubenfire, M., Wajszuzuk, W., and Schork, M. A.: Intraaortic balloon pumping 1967 through 1982: Analysis of complications in 733 patients. Am. J. Cardiol., 57:976, 1986.

29. Kaplan, J. A., Craver, J. M., Jones, E. L., and Sumpter, R.: The role of the intra-aortic balloon in cardiac anesthesia and surgery. Am. Heart J., 98:580, 1979.

30. Kormos, R. L.: The role of the intra-aortic balloon as a bridge to cardiac transplantation. Cardiac Assists, 3:1, 1987.

31. Laird, J. D., Madras, P. N., Jones, R. T., Kantrowitz, A. R., Kothari, M. L., Buckley, M. J., and Austen, W. G.: Theoretical and experimental analysis of the intraaortic balloon pump. Trans. Am. Soc. Artif. Intern. Organs, 14:338, 1968.

32. Leinbach, R. C., Gold, H. K., Harper, R. W., Buckley, M. J., and Austen, W. G.: Early intraaortic balloon pumping for anterior myocardial infarction without shock. Circulation, 58:204, 1978.

33. Levine, H. J., and Wagman, R. J.: Energetics of the human heart. Am. J. Cardiol., 9:372, 1962.

34. Levine, F. H., Gold, H. K., Leinbach, R. C., Daggett, W. M., Austen, W. G., and Buckley, M. J.: Management of acute myocardial ischemia with intraaortic balloon pumping and coronary bypass surgery. Circulation, 58(Suppl. 1):69, 1978.

35. LoCicero, J., Hartz, R. S., Sanders, J. H., Hueter, D. C., McDonough, T. J., and Michaelis, L. L.: Interhospital transport of patients with ongoing intraaortic balloon pumping. Am. J. Cardiol., 56:59, 1985.

36. Maroko, P. R., Bernstein, E. F., Libby, P., DeLaria, G. A., Covell, J. W., Ross, J., and Braunwald, E.: Effects of intraaortic balloon counterpulsation on the severity of myocardial ischemic injury following acute coronary occlusion. Circulation, 45:1150, 1972.

37. Martin, R. S., Moncure, A. C., Buckley, M. J., Austen, W. G., Akins, C., and Leinbach, R. C.: Complications of percutaneous intraaortic balloon insertion. J. Thorac. Cardiovasc. Surg., 85:186, 1983.

38. McGee, M. G., Zillgitt, S. L., Trono, R., Turner, S. A., Davis, G. L., Fuqua, J. M., Edelman, S. K., and Norman, J. C.: Retrospective analyses of the need for mechanical circulatory support (intraaortic balloon pump/abdominal left ventricular assist device or partial artificial heart) after cardiopulmonary bypass. A 44 month study of 14,168 patients. Am. J. Cardiol., 46:135, 1980.

39. McGeehin, W., Sheikh, F., Donahoo, J. S., Lechman, M. J., and MacVaugh, H.: Transthoracic intraaortic balloon pump support: Experience in 39 patients. Ann. Thorac. Surg., 44:26, 1987.

40. Mertlich, G., and Quaal, S. J.: Air transport of the patient requiring intra-aortic balloon pumping. Crit. Care Nurs. Clin. North Am., 1:443, 1989.

41. Moran, J. M., Opravil, M., Gorman, A. J., Rastegar, H., Meyers, S. N., and Michaelis, L. L.: Pulmonary artery balloon counterpulsation for right ventricular failure: II. Clinical experience. Ann. Thorac. Surg., 38:254, 1984.

42. Moulopoulos, S. D., Topaz, S., and Kolff, W. J.: Diastolic balloon pumping (with carbon dioxide) in the aorta: A circulation. Am. Heart J., 63:669, 1962.

43. Mundth, E. D., Yurchak, P. M., Buckley, M. J., and Austen, W. G.: Circulatory assistance and emergency direct artery surgery for shock complicating myocardial infarction. N. Engl. J. Med., 283:1383, 1970.

44. Murphy, D. A., Craver, J. M., Jones, E. L., Curling, P. E., Guyton, R. A., King, S. B., Gruentzig, A. R., and Hatcher, C. R.: Surgical management of acute myocardial ischemia following percutaneous transluminal coronary angioplasty. J. Thorac. Cardiovasc. Surg., 87:332, 1984.

45. Naunheim, K. S., Kesler, K. A., Kanter, K. R., Fiore, A. C., McBride, L. R., Pennington, D. G., Barner, H. B., Kaiser, G. C., and Willman, V. L.: Coronary artery bypass for recent infarction: Predictors of mortality. Circulation, 78(Suppl. I):I-122, 1988.

46. Nichols, A. B., Pohost, G. M., Gold, H. K., Leinbach, R. C., Beller, G. A., McKusick, K. A., Strauss, H. W., and Buckley, M. J.: Left ventricular function during intra-aortic balloon pumping assessed by multigated cardiac blood pool imaging. Circulation, 58(Suppl. 1):1-176, 1978.

47. Norman, J. C., Cooley, D. A., Igo, S. R., Hibbs, C. W., Johnson, M. D., Bennett, J. G., Fuqua, J. M., Trono, R., and Edmonds, C. H.: Prognostic indices for survival during postcardiotomy intra-aortic balloon pumping: Methods of scoring and classification, with implications for left ventricular assist device utilization. J. Thorac. Cardiovasc. Surg., 74:709, 1977.

48. O'Rourke, M. F., Norris, R. M., Campbell, T. J., Chang, V. P., and Sammel, N. L.: Randomized controlled trial of intra-aortic balloon counterpulsation in early myocardial infarction with acute heart failure. Am. J. Cardiol., 47:815, 1981.

49. Pennington, D. G., Swartz, M., Codd, J. E., Merjavy, J. P., and Kaiser, G. C.: Intraaortic balloon pumping in cardiac surgical patients: A nine year experience. Ann. Thorac. Surg., 36:125, 1983.

50. Phillips, S. J.: Percutaneous cardiopulmonary bypass and innovations in clinical counterpulsation. Crit. Care Clin., 2:297, 1986.

51. Pierri, M. K., Zema, M., Kingfield, P., McCabe, J., Hoover, E., Gay, W., and Subramanian, V.: Exercise tolerance in late survivors of balloon pumping and surgery for cardiogenic shock. Circulation, 62(Suppl. 1):138, 1980.

52. Pollock, J. C., Charlton, M., Williams, W. G., Edmonds, J. F., and Trusler, G. A.: Intraaortic balloon pumping in children. Ann. Thorac. Surg., 29:522, 1980.

53. Port, S. C., Patel, S., and Schmidt, D. H.: Effects of intraaortic balloon counterpulsation on myocardial blood flow in patients with severe coronary artery disease. J. Am. Coll. Cardiol., 3:1367, 1984.

54. Powell, M. J., Daggett, W. M., Margo, A. E., Bianco, J. A., Buckley, M. J., Sanders, C. A., Kantrowitz, A. R., and Austen, W. G.: Effects of intra-aortic balloon counterpulsation on cardiac performance, oxygen consumption, and coronary blood flow in dogs. Circ. Res., 26:753, 1970.

55. Quaal, S. J.: Comprehensive Intra-aortic Balloon Pumping. St. Louis, C. V. Mosby, 1984.

56. Radford, M. J., Johnson, R. A., Buckley, M. J., Daggett, W. M., Leinbach, R. C., and Gold, H. K.: Survival following mitral valve replacement for mitral regurgitation due to coronary artery disease. Circulation, 60(Suppl. 1):39, 1979.

57. Radford, M. J., Johnson, R. A., Daggett, W. M., Fallon, J. T., Buckley, M. J., Gold, H. K., and Leinbach, R. C.: Ventricular septal rupture: A review of clinical and physiologic features and an analysis of survival. Circulation, 64:545, 1981.

58. Roberts, A. J., Alonso, D. R., Combes, J. R., Jacobstein, J. G., Post, M. R., Cahill, P. T., Ho, S. T., Abel, R. M., Subramanian, V. A., and Gay, W. A.: Role of delayed intra-aortic balloon pumping in treatment of experimental myocardial infarction. Am. J. Cardiol., 41:1202, 1978.

59. Sarnoff, S. J., Braunwald, E., Welch, G. H., Case, R. B., Stainsby, W. N., and Macruz, R.: Hemodynamic determinants of oxygen consumption of the heart with special reference to the tension-time index. Am. J. Physiol., 192:148, 1958.

60. Scheidt, S.: Preservation of ischemic myocardium with intraaortic balloon pumping: Modern therapeutic intervention or primum non nocere? Circulation, 58:211, 1978.

61. Shahian, D. M., Neptune, W. B., Ellis, F. H., and Maggs, P. R.: Intra-aortic balloon pump morbidity: A comparative analysis of risk factors between percutaneous and surgical techniques. Ann. Thorac. Surg., 36:644, 1983.

62. Spence, P. A., Peniston, C. M., Mihic, N., Jabr, A. K., and Salerno, T. A.: A rational approach to the selection of an assist device for the failing right ventricle. Ann. Thorac. Surg., 41:606, 1986.

63. Symbas, P. N., McKeown, P. P., Santora A. H., and Vlasis, S. E.: Pulmonary artery balloon counterpulsation for treatment of intraoperative right ventricular failure. Ann. Thorac. Surg., 39:437, 1985.

64. Veasy, L. G., Blalock, R. C., Orth, J. L., and Boucek, M. M.: Intra-aortic balloon pumping in infants and children. Circulation, 68:1095, 1983.

65. Weber, K. T., and Janicki, J. S.: Intraaortic balloon counterpulsation: A review of physiological principles, clinical results and device safety. Ann. Thorac. Surg., 17:602, 1974.
66. Weintraub, R. M., Aroesty, J. M., Paulin, S., Levine, F. H., Markis, J. E., LaRaia, P. J., Cohen, S. F., and Kurland, G. F.: Medically refractory unstable angina pectoris. Long term follow-up of patients undergoing intra-aortic balloon counterpulsation and operation. Am. J. Cardiol., 43:877, 1979.
67. Weiss, A. T., Engel, S., Gotsman, C. J., Shefer, A., Hasin, Y., Bitran, D., and

Gotsman, M. S.: Regional and global left ventricular function during intra-aortic balloon counterpulsation in patients with acute myocardial infarction shock. Am. Heart J., 108:249, 1984.
68. Williams, D. O., Korr, K. S., Gewirtz, H., and Most, A. S.: The effect of intraaortic balloon counterpulsation on regional myocardial blood flow and oxygen consumption in the presence of coronary artery stenosis in patients with unstable angina. Circulation, 66:593, 1982.

XXVI _____

THE ARTIFICIAL HEART

Wayne E. Richenbacher, M.D., Don B. Olsen, D.V.M., and William A. Gay, Jr., M.D.

HISTORY

Kolff and Akutsu were the first investigators to successfully implant a total artificial heart (TAH) in an experimental animal.[1] In 1957 they replaced a canine heart with a device made of polyvinyl chloride driven by an external air compressor and reported a survival time of 90 minutes. As work progressed during the 1960s, the calf became the standard experimental animal since it required comparable blood flows to man and was found to have relatively large intrathoracic dimensions that facilitated device implantation, good tolerance of cardiopulmonary bypass, and a docile nature that simplified postoperative care in chronic experiments.[32] By the mid 1960s, Kolff and Nose, using sac-type hearts, had extended calf survival to over 24 hours, and at the end of the decade survival times approaching 3 to 5 days were achieved.[25]

It became clear from these early experiments that the development of a nonthrombogenic blood-contacting surface and a control system that would balance the output of the two prosthetic ventricles and increase cardiac output with exercise were key to the future successful development of an implantable TAH. As blood flow dynamics and blood prosthesis interface interactions became better understood, blood sac construction and pump design underwent a number of modifications. Kwan-Gett, working with Kolff in 1967, designed a pneumatic TAH using two diaphragm pumps.[26] Use of the Kwan-Gett heart led to calf survival of 1 week in 1971 and 2 weeks in 1972. However, these blood sacs were originally constructed of smooth, low-tensile-strength, silica-filled silicone rubber, a surface that proved to be highly thrombogenic. Dacron-flocked blood-contacting surfaces were developed in an effort to promote and fix the deposition of a relatively nonthrombogenic fibrin layer.[29] Thick pseudoneointima, however, impaired sac flexibility, reduced cardiac output, and created substrata necrosis with dislodgment and embolization.

Nose introduced a TAH with blood-contacting surfaces constructed of glutaraldehyde-treated natural tissues such as pericardium.[24] These "biolized" hearts have functioned well in calves for periods of up to 145 days. Most contemporary blood pumps, however, contain blood-contacting surfaces of smooth segmented polyurethane. This high-strength, inert polyether polyurethane was introduced by Boretos and Pierce in 1967.[3] TAHs containing segmented polyurethane blood-contacting surfaces dramatically reduced thromboembolic complications in long-term implant experiments.

Currently, experimental animals with pneumatic TAHs routinely survive for up to 1 year.[2] Survival in growing calves is limited by inadequate cardiac output and elastomer blood sac calcification. Immature calves eat and gain weight normally when their natural hearts are replaced with a mechanical prosthesis. Weight gain can approach 0.5 to 1 kg. per day; 6 to 9 months following TAH implantation, the calves develop low-output cardiac cachexia manifested by exercise intolerance, fluid retention, and skeletal muscle wasting. Dystrophic blood sac calcification is attributed to the high calcium turnover observed in immature animals. Deposition of rough crystals limits diaphragm flexion and can lead to blood sac perforations. This problem is partially controlled by the administration of warfarin-sodium,[35] which blocks calcium-binding proteins, and etidronate disodium, which inhibits the formation and growth of hydroxyapatite crystals. Although neither problem has been encountered clinically, long-term animal studies can only continue following the development of an adult animal model.[16] Imachi and co-workers have successfully implanted pneumatic TAHs in goats,[20] and Olsen and colleagues have reported long-term survival in sheep.[36]

In 1969 Cooley and associates introduced the concept of staged cardiac replacement when they implanted a TAH in a 47-year-old man who was suffering from end-stage ischemic cardiomyopathy.[6,7] The device supported the patient's circulation for 64 hours until a donor heart was obtained and cardiac transplantation performed. The patient died of *Pseudomonas* pneumonia 32 hours after allografting.

In 1981, Cooley and associates bridged a second patient to cardiac transplantation using the Akutsu TAH.[5,14] In this case, a 36-year-old man received the TAH when he developed profound biventricular failure following unsuccessful coronary bypass surgery. Twenty-four hours following TAH implantation, the patient developed arterial desaturation secondary to a mechanical obstruction of the left pulmonary veins. Venovenous extracorporeal membrane oxygenation was instituted with a prompt increase in arterial hemoglobin saturations. Fifty-three hours following TAH insertion, the patient underwent cardiac transplantation.[4] He died 8 days later of multisystem failure secondary to gram-negative rod and *Candida* sepsis.

DeVries and co-workers at the University of Utah were the first to implant a pneumatic TAH as a permanent form of circulatory replacement.[22] In December 1982, the Jarvik–7 TAH was implanted in a 61-year-old man with end-stage idiopathic cardiomyopathy. The patient had been previously excluded from the cardiac transplant candidate pool secondary to advanced age, pulmonary hypertension, and chronic obstructive lung disease. Following TAH implantation, this patient was able to eat, exercise, and interact with his family, although he remained in the hospital bound to the external pneumatic drive unit. He died 112 days following TAH implantation of multisystem failure.

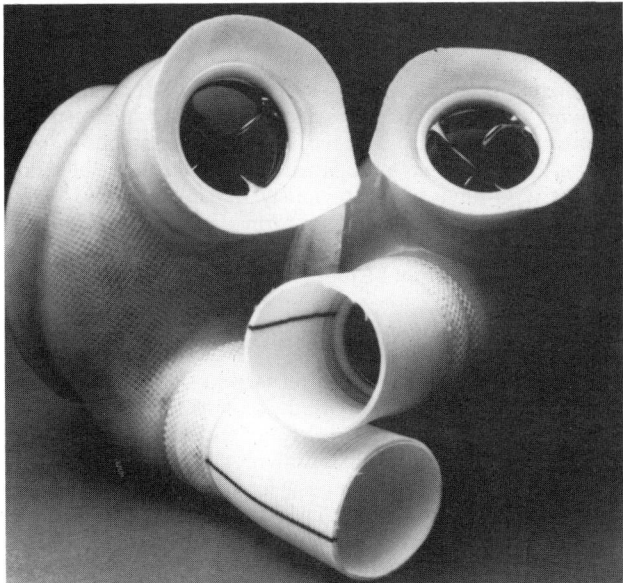

Figure 1. The Symbion–J–7 artificial heart. The wide skirts are trimmed and sutured to the patient's atrial remnants while the outflow grafts are anastomosed to the appropriate great vessel. Medtronic-Hall inflow and outflow valves are located in both the right and left prosthetic ventricles. (Courtesy of Symbion, Inc., Tempe, AZ.)

DEVICES AVAILABLE

Two pneumatic artificial hearts have been approved for clinical use in the United States by the Food and Drug Administration. The Symbion–J–7 TAH (Symbion Inc., Tempe, AZ) is commercially available with either a 70 ml. (J–7–70) or 100 ml. (J–7–100) ventricular stroke volume (Fig. 1).[17] The Penn State heart, which has been implanted only at the Pennsylvania State University, has a 70 ml. ventricular stroke volume (Fig. 2).[30] The Utah–100 TAH, which is being developed at the University of Utah, is currently under review by the Food and Drug Administration but has not as yet been approved for clinical use (Fig. 3).

All three pneumatic blood pumps share similar design ele-

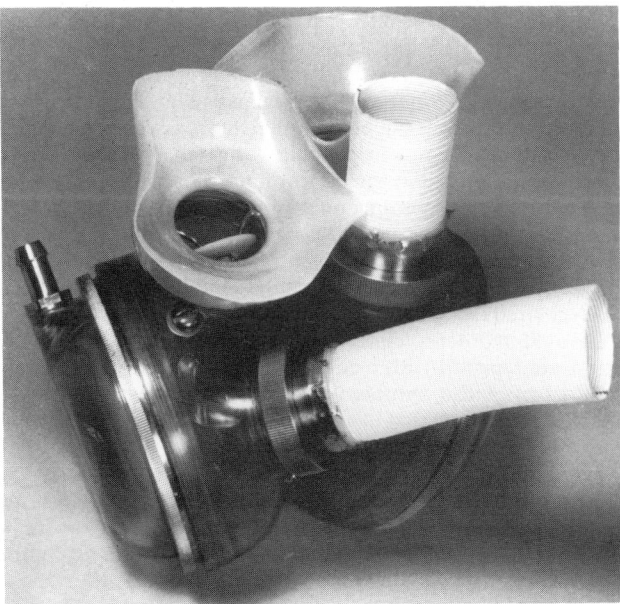

Figure 2. The pneumatic artificial heart developed at the Pennsylvania State University. This device employs coated Dacron outflow grafts that do not require preclotting. Bjork-Shiley inflow and outflow valves are located in both the right and left prosthetic ventricles. (Courtesy of William S. Pierce, M.D., Professor, the Pennsylvania State University, Hershey, PA.)

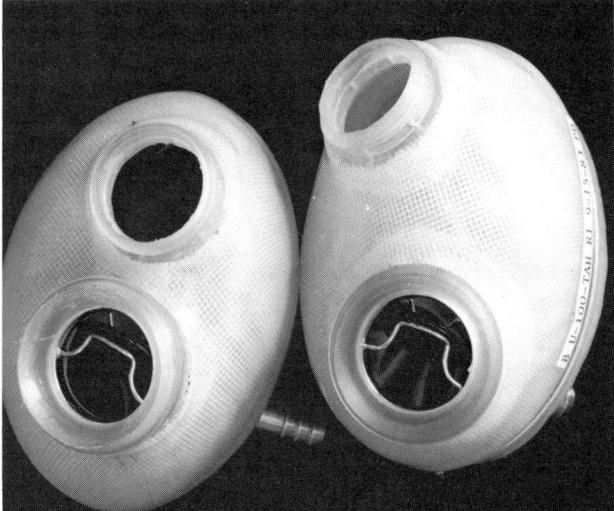

Figure 3. The Utah–100 is a diaphragm-type pneumatic artificial heart. The newest prototype employs threaded inlet and outlet connectors and a roll-sock flexing diaphragm-housing junction. The request for permission to use this device clinically is currently under consideration by the Food and Drug Administration.

ments. These artificial hearts are composed of independent right and left ventricles, each of which contains a mechanical inlet and outlet valve, smooth nonthrombogenic pumping chambers and detachable atrial cuffs, and arterial grafts (Fig. 4). The devices are tethered to external pneumatic drive units by percutaneous drive lines and are controlled in a manner that permits cardiac output to vary with physiologic need.

INDICATIONS FOR USE OF A TOTAL ARTIFICIAL HEART

The pneumatic TAH has been implanted in five patients as a permanent form of cardiac replacement.[10,37] These patients were categorized as New York Heart Association Class IV and failed to meet cardiac transplant selection criteria. Serious septic and thromboembolic complications were frequently observed and directly attributable to the presence of the chronic, indwelling cardiac prosthesis with its percutaneous drive lines. In addition, these patients were tethered to a relatively immobile drive unit, creating a life-style of questionable quality. Currently available pneumatic hearts are no longer considered to be a suitable form of long-term circulatory support.[34]

However, air-driven artificial hearts can provide temporary support of the circulation in patients with intractable heart fail-

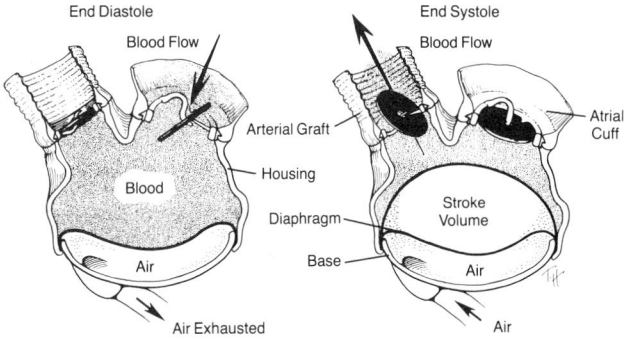

Figure 4. Cutaway view of the Symbion–J–7 diaphragm-type pneumatic artificial heart. Diastole, at left, occurs when air exits the prosthesis, permitting the inflow valve to open as blood fills the ventricle. During systole, at right, air enters the base plate, elevating the diaphragm. The inflow valve closes as the outflow valve opens, and blood is ejected into the outflow graft. (From Mays, J. B., Williams, M. A., Barker, L. E., et al.: Clinical management of total artificial heart drive systems. J.A.M.A., 259:881, 1988. Copyright 1988, American Medical Association. Reproduced with permission.)

TABLE 1. Cardiac Transplant Recipient Selection Criteria

End-stage heart disease unamenable to medical or surgical therapy
Prognosis for survival <12 months
Age <60–65 years
Normal renal function
Normal hepatic function
Absence of unresolved pulmonary infiltrate (other than pulmonary edema)
Absence of recent pulmonary infarction
Absence of infection
Absence of symptomatic peripheral or cerebrovascular disease
Pulmonary vascular resistance <5 Wood units
Stable psychological profile
Adequate support system and financial resources

ure who are awaiting a cardiac transplant but who decompensate hemodynamically prior to the availability of a donor allograft. In order to become a candidate for TAH implantation, the prospective recipient must meet two fairly rigid sets of criteria. First, the patient must be a suitable candidate for cardiac transplantation (Table 1). These patients must have advanced heart disease that is not amenable to current methods of medical or surgical therapy, associated with a prognosis for survival limited to less than 12 months. The patient must have normally functioning kidneys and liver; a history of malignancy, active infection, or pulmonary hypertension (more than 5 Wood units) excludes the individual from the transplant recipient pool. Age is a less rigid criterion, since clinical reports have now documented excellent results with cardiac transplantation in patients in their seventh decade.[15]

Patients who meet the selection criteria for cardiac transplantation but who deteriorate hemodynamically prior to the availability of a donor heart can be considered for an advanced form of mechanical circulatory assistance (Table 2). Patients who demonstrate a cardiac output index less than 2 liters per minute per m.[2] and left atrial pressure in excess of 25 mm. Hg despite cardiac pacing, maximal inotropic support, and intra-aortic balloon counterpulsation are ideal candidates for implantation of a ventricular assist device or artificial heart. Patients with single ventricle dysfunction are best managed with a ventricular assist pump. Patients with biventricular failure can be managed with two assist pumps or an artificial heart. In selecting the appropriate device, consideration should be given to the patient's cardiac rhythm, cardiac anatomy, and anteroposterior thoracic dimension. Patients with intractable arrhythmias or irreparable postinfarction ventricular septal defects or valvular dysfunction are best managed with a TAH. Absolute contraindications to the use of a TAH include patients with an anteroposterior thoracic dimension at the level of the tenth thoracic vertebra of less than 9 cm., as determined by computed tomography.[21] These patients are at risk for compression of the atrial connectors with resultant inflow obstruction and systemic and pulmonary venous hypertension. In addition, patients who develop end-stage congestive failure acutely (postpartum cardiomyopathy)

TABLE 2. Artificial Heart Recipient Selection Criteria

Fulfills cardiac transplant recipient selection criteria
Biventricular failure (cardiac index <2 L./min./m.[2]) despite:
    Adequate preload
    Corrected metabolism
    Maximal inotropic support
    Intra-aortic balloon pump
Absence of a coagulopathy or active gastrointestinal hemorrhage
Absence of coma or fluctuating neurologic examination
Adequate anteroposterior thoracic dimension
No previous sternotomy
? No previous cardiac transplant

have smaller intrapericardial dimensions and are at particular risk for great vessel compression and incomplete sternal approximation following TAH insertion.

Relative contraindications to insertion of a TAH include coma following cardiopulmonary resuscitation, due to concern over the potential for neurologic recovery, and a previous sternotomy, as the patient has a propensity for postoperative bleeding. Patients who have been previously transplanted and whose graft fails in the presence of preformed antibodies to human lymphocyte antigens may well be device-dependent when a second allograft cannot be identified.[18]

TECHNICAL CONSIDERATIONS

Informed consent is obtained; discussions involving the use of the TAH should involve both the patient and the immediate family. Baseline liver and renal function tests are performed, and a free serum hemoglobin is drawn. A brief, complete neurologic examination serves as a basis for comparison with subsequent examinations following TAH implantation. The patient is urgently transported to the operating room, and general anesthesia is induced routinely. If time permits, all previously indwelling catheters are removed and the tips sent for culture; otherwise all lines are replaced in the immediate postoperative period. The patient's anterior chest and abdomen are prepared and draped.

A standard median sternotomy is employed. The Dacron outflow grafts of the Symbion–J–7 TAH require preclotting. Baking the prostheses in the autoclave is avoided because the high temperatures can melt the snap-on connectors.[9] Heparin (3 mg. per kg.) is administered, and normothermic cardiopulmonary bypass is initiated using bicaval venous cannulas and an ascending aortic arterial cannula. The Swan-Ganz catheter, if present, should be withdrawn. Caval tapes are applied in order to eliminate blood flow into the right heart. The aortic cross-clamp is placed, and the cardiectomy is performed by transecting the atria along the atrioventricular groove and the great vessels just distal to the semilunar valves (Fig. 5). The ascending aorta is completely mobilized by developing the tissue plane between the aorta and main and right pulmonary arteries. The recipient cardiectomy mimics the technical approach to cardiac transplantation, since maximal preservation of both atrial and great vessel length facilitates both TAH insertion and subsequent donor heart implantation.

The atrial connectors are cut to an appropriate size and sutured in place. It is imperative that meticulous hemostasis be achieved throughout the procedure because anastomotic exposure is difficult, if not impossible, when the rigid prosthetic ventricles are placed in the pericardium. Double running rows of 3–0 or 4–0 polypropylene suture are employed, and each suture line should be leak tested. Atrial anastomoses in the Penn State heart are leak tested with an occlusive, threaded cap connected by a length of tubing to an intravenous bag of methylene blue–colored lactated Ringer's solution.[38] The intravenous bag is elevated in order to distend the atrium being tested, and leak points are repaired with pledgeted polypropylene sutures. The atrial cuffs of the Symbion–J–7 TAH are pressurized with blood-tinged saline that is administered through a snap-on injector.

The grafts to the great vessels are trimmed and sutured in place with running rows of 3–0 or 4–0 polypropylene suture. Aortic anastomotic leak testing is accomplished by cross-clamping the outflow graft while removing the cross-clamp from the native aorta. The patient should be in the Trendelenburg position during this maneuver, and care must be taken to avoid introducing air into the transverse arch. The pulmonary artery is usually accessible for inspection following TAH implantation. Levinson, however, recommends that the anastomosis be tested

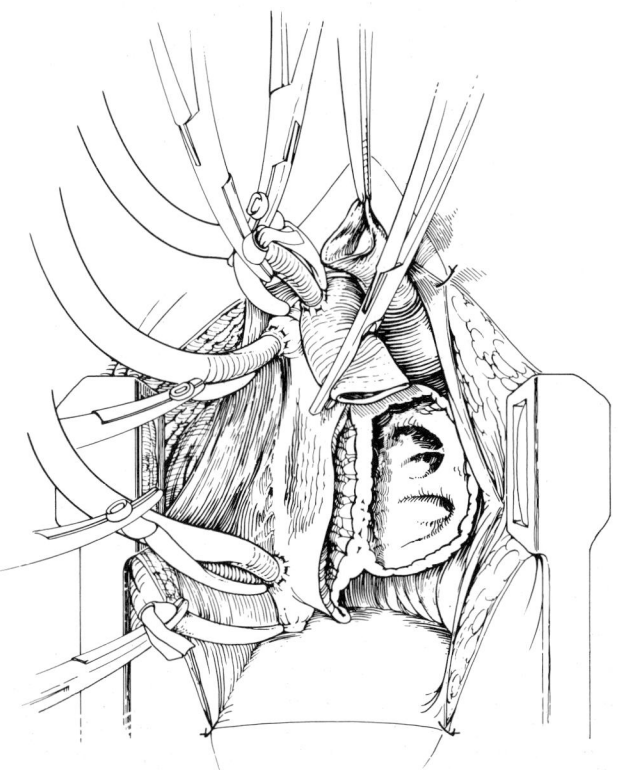

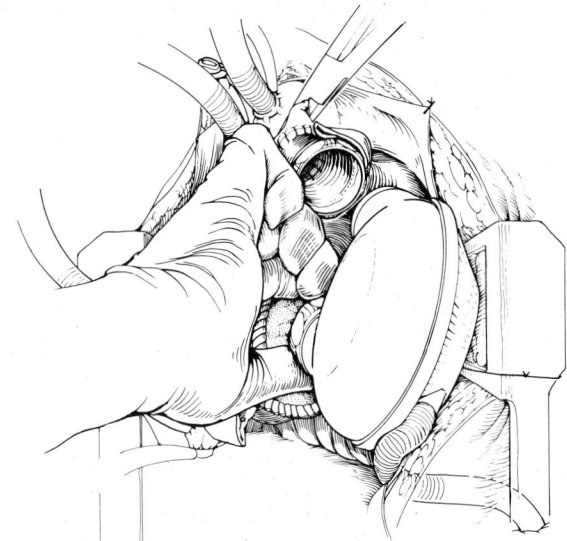

Figure 6. The left prosthetic ventricle is positioned toward the apex of the pericardium. The left atrial skirt is visible between the surgeon's thumb and index finger. The left ventricular outflow graft is anastomosed to the cross-clamped aorta. (From Richenbacher, W. E., Pennock, J. L., Pae, W. E., and Pierce, W. S.: Artificial heart implantation for end-stage cardiac disease. J. Cardiac Surg., 1:3, 1986. Reproduced with permission from Futura Publishing Company.)

Figure 5. Following recipient cardiectomy, the mediastinum appears exactly as at the time of de novo cardiac transplantation. Bicaval venous return cannulas and a single distal ascending aortic cannula are employed. By preserving maximal atrial and great vessel length, artificial heart implantation and subsequent cardiac transplantation are greatly simplified. (From Richenbacher, W. E., Pennock, J. L., Pae, W. E., and Pierce, W. S.: Artificial heart implantation for end-stage cardiac disease. J. Cardiac Surg., 1:3, 1986. Reproduced with permission from Futura Publishing Company.)

by cross-clamping the main pulmonary artery and injecting saline into the outflow graft through the specially designed snap-on injector, similar to that used in atrial anastomotic leak testing.[27]

Proper positioning of the prosthetic ventricles within the pericardium is key to the successful use of the TAH. Although the TAH is designed to fit within the pericardium, anteroposterior thoracic dimensions and the size of the pericardial space vary greatly from patient to patient. In trimming the atrial connectors and great vessel grafts, an effort should be made to orient the TAH toward the patient's left. By so doing, the anteroposterior blood pump dimension is reduced, minimizing the risk of vena caval and pulmonary vein compression at the time of sternal approximation. Orientation of the TAH toward the patient's left hemithorax is facilitated by mobilization of both cavae from their pericardial attachments, a left pleurotomy or pleurectomy, and placement of the drive lines toward the apex of the pericardium. Care should be taken to avoid compression of the left lower lobe of the lung.

The left blood pump is positioned first (Fig. 6). This ventricle can be inserted prior to performing the right atrial and pulmonary arterial anastomoses, a maneuver that simplifies right ventricular insertion. The drive line of the left ventricle is positioned at the apex of the pericardium; the right ventricular drive line exits the pericardium at a point midway between the left ventricular drive line exit site and the inferior vena cava. The Symbion–J–7 TAH was originally designed to have the drive lines exit the chest near the sixth intercostal space in the anterior axillary line.[27] Although extreme lateral placement of the drive lines further encourages the heart to lie toward the left chest,

transpleural percutaneous tubes were found to cause chest wall necrosis and increase the risk of pleural space infection and left lower lobe atelectasis. Ideally the pleura should remain intact and the drive lines brought through the skin in the left subcostal[38] or periumbilical region.[11]

When the left ventricle is connected to the atrial skirt and aortic graft, it must be de-aired. Air is withdrawn from the blood sac of the Penn State heart by passing a blunt catheter (modified Swan-Ganz catheter) through the atrial anastomosis, across the inflow valve into the most superior part of the blood sac. Air is removed as bronchial arterial return fills the sac. The aortic cross-clamp is removed and the left ventricle pulsed slowly, thereby avoiding pulmonary venous congestion.

The Symbion–J–7 TAH, with its diaphragm design, contains an integral aspiration port that facilitates ventricular de-airing.[27] When the atrial and aortic connectors are attached, air is aspirated from the blunt tip needle previously inserted by the manufacturer. When the needle is withdrawn, the de-airing port is secured with a no. 2 silk tie.

The right pump is inserted and de-aired in a manner identical to that used for the left ventricle (Fig. 7). Ventilation is resumed, biventricular pumping initiated, and cardiopulmonary bypass slowly discontinued. Initially passive diastolic filling usually suffices, and diastolic vacuum is reserved until sternal closure is complete in order to avoid air embolism. The patient is decannulated, the heparin reversed with protamine, and the sternum approximated. As the sternum is closed, blood pressure and ventricular filling curves should be monitored for evidence of inflow obstruction. A falling blood pressure, low cardiac output, and inadequate left pump filling in combination with complete right-sided filling and emptying suggest pulmonary venous compression. When a similar hemodynamic pattern occurs in the presence of reduced right pump filling, caval compression has occurred. Inferior vena caval compression can be correctly diagnosed by inserting a femoral venous line. Even though right pump filling may be adequate and the central venous pressure normal, as measured via a line in superior vena cava, a kink at the inferior cavoatrial junction can lead to a significant rise in inferior vena caval pressure with resultant renal failure, ascites, and hepatic congestion.

The implantation procedure is concluded by suturing the Da-

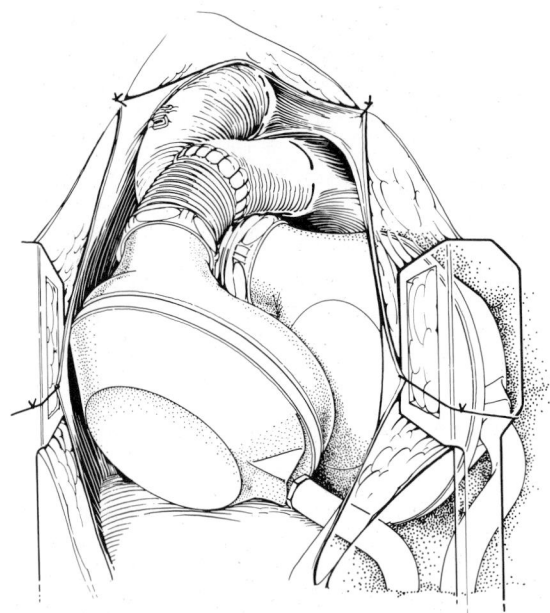

Figure 7. The appearance of the mediastinum following artificial heart insertion and the discontinuation of cardiopulmonary bypass. Orienting the prosthetic ventricles toward the patient's left avoids compression of the venae cavae and pulmonary veins at the time of sternal closure. (From Richenbacher, W. E., Pennock, J. L., Pae, W. E., and Pierce, W. S.: Artificial heart implantation for end-stage cardiac disease. J. Cardiac Surg., *1*:3, 1986. Reproduced with permission from Futura Publishing Company.)

cron cuffs around the drive lines to the skin. Motion of the drive lines with respect to the skin and soft tissues is reduced, thereby decreasing the risk of ascending drive line infections. The intraaortic balloon pump is removed, and the femoral arteriotomy is closed with polypropylene suture.

Postoperatively, the patient is maintained in reverse isolation in the intensive care unit. Prompt extubation and removal of all monitoring catheters reduce the incidence of iatrogenic catheter-related sepsis. Prophylactic antibiotics are continued 24 hours following mediastinal drain removal. The percutaneous drive lines are cleansed with hydrogen peroxide and covered with povidone-iodine ointment twice daily.

There is no consensus regarding the ideal postoperative anticoagulation regimen. It is agreed, however, that owing to the propensity for postoperative hemorrhage, anticoagulation be withheld for 12 to 24 hours following implantation. Most investigators believe that adequate protection from thromboembolic complications can be afforded by the continuous administration of heparin in order to maintain an activated clotting time at 200 seconds. Heparin is discontinued and its effect reversed within a few hours at the time of cardiac transplantation. Furthermore, the administration of blood products, with the alternative risk of transfusion-related infection and cytotoxic antibody production, is avoided. The use of antiplatelet agents in the postoperative period remains controversial.

Although it is clear that morbidity increases with the duration of TAH support,[13] most investigators agree that following TAH implantation, cardiac transplantation should be delayed until there is objective evidence of improvement in the patient's medical condition. With increased cardiac output and end-organ perfusion, most patients demonstrate rapid improvement in mild pre-implantation renal and hepatic dysfunction. This period of mechanical support can also allow time for diuresis and resolution of pulmonary congestion. Unfortunately, as time passes, the risk of sepsis and thromboembolic-related complications increases. The "window in time" when end-organ function has been optimized and cardiac transplantation can be most safely performed remains poorly defined.

When a donor heart is identified, anticoagulant therapy is discontinued and the patient returned to the operating room. As the sternum is reopened, random pericardial cultures are obtained. Hypothermic cardiopulmonary bypass is reinstituted using bicaval venous cannulation and aortic arterial return. The drive lines are transected at the pericardial exit points and all mediastinal instruments removed. The external drive lines are withdrawn from beneath the sterile drapes. Skin buttons are not exposed until sternal closure is complete. The pericardial drive line exit sites are oversewn, the arterial and great vessels are débrided, and the pericardium is irrigated with antibiotic solution. Donor heart insertion is accomplished in a manner identical to that for a *de novo* heart transplant.

Following sternal closure, the drive line skin sites are sharply débrided and the fascial layer is oversewn with absorbable suture. The skin and soft tissues are packed open and permitted to heal by second intention. Posttransplant patient care is the same as that for a transplant patient who did not require mechanical circulatory support.

CLINICAL RESULTS OF USE OF THE TOTAL ARTIFICIAL HEART

As of December 31, 1989, the combined registry for the clinical use of mechanical blood pumps included 92 patients who received a TAH as a bridge to cardiac transplantation (personal communication with Walter E. Pae, Jr., M.D., Associate Professor, the Pennsylvania State University, Hershey, PA). Seventy-two patients (78.3 per cent) had undergone transplantation; 36 patients (39.1 per cent) were discharged from the hospital (Table 3). Although the results of cardiac transplantation in this group do not compare favorably with the results of cardiac transplantation in patients who do not require mechanical blood pump support, it is clear that survival is increasing as additional clinical experience with the use of the TAH is gained. The third registry report notes that in 1988, 17 patients received a TAH as a bridge to transplantation.[33] Fourteen patients (82.4 per cent) underwent transplantation; 10 patients (58.8 per cent) were discharged from the hospital. The registry of the International Society for Heart Transplantation reports a 30-day mortality following cardiac transplantation alone of 8.9 per cent.[19]

Another large combined series reported in 1988 includes 116 TAHs implanted in 113 patients.[23] One hundred and eleven implants were performed as a bridge to cardiac transplantation. Eight different types of TAHs were included in this series. Seventy-two (66.7 per cent) of the 108 patients receiving the TAH for temporary circulatory support underwent transplantation; 34 (31.5 per cent) of the 108 patients were alive after transplantation.

Although 11 different pneumatically powered artificial hearts have been used in 14 countries, the most frequently employed blood pump is the Symbion–J–7 TAH (formerly the Jarvik–7 TAH). As of December 31, 1989, this device had been implanted in 157 patients as a bridge to cardiac transplantation (personal communication with Gary M. Cole, Vice President of Sales and Marketing, Symbion Inc., Tempe, AZ). While 5 pa-

TABLE 3. Clinical Results of Use of the Artificial Heart as a Bridge to Cardiac Transplantation

Reporting Group	Number Implanted	Transplanted	Survived
Registry of mechanical blood pumps	92	72(78.3%)	36(39.1%)
Registry of mechanical blood pumps (1988 alone)	17	14(82.4%)	10(58.8%)
Combined series[23]	108	72(66.7%)	34(31.5%)
Symbion, Inc.	152	111(73.0%)	80(52.6%)

tients still had a TAH in place at the time of the report, 111 patients (73 per cent) had undergone subsequent cardiac transplantation. Eighty (52.6 per cent) of the 152 patients survived for at least 30 days following cardiac transplantation. Eighty-five of these patients had received their Symbion–J–7 TAH at 17 centers in the United States. Seventy-two patients had their Symbion–J–7 TAH implanted at 11 centers abroad.

PERMANENT TOTAL ARTIFICIAL HEARTS

Patients with an irreversible end-stage cardiomyopathy who fail to meet cardiac transplantation selection criteria are ultimately candidates for insertion of a motor-driven TAH. These devices are more complex than their pneumatic counterparts in that they require an implantable motor and portable external battery pack. Because a single motor is responsible for driving both ventricles, a sophisticated control mechanism, which balances the output of the two blood pumps and varies output with physiologic need, is mandatory. Moreover, the potential for infection from chronic percutaneous pneumatic drive lines is obviated by the use of transcutaneous energy transmission techniques.[41] Portable battery packs eliminate the need for a bulky external drive unit, thereby increasing patient mobility and improving the quality of life.

Initial efforts to develop an implantable, motor-driven TAH occurred in the late 1960s under the auspices of the United States Atomic Energy Commission (now the Nuclear Regulatory Commission).[31] The nuclear-powered artificial heart program hoped to design an implantable TAH that employed a [238]plutonium heat source to operate a thermal engine. The engine would, in turn, drive the blood pumps. Radionuclide-powered artificial hearts proved to be quite costly and potentially unsafe, and long-term animal studies were never performed. Although an occasional report describing work with radioisotope-powered artificial hearts continues to appear in the literature,[40] most investigators have directed their efforts toward developing electrically driven implantable blood pumps.

In January 1988, the National Heart Lung and Blood Institute of the National Institutes of Health began funding four programs using contracts that extend through 1993. The four insti-

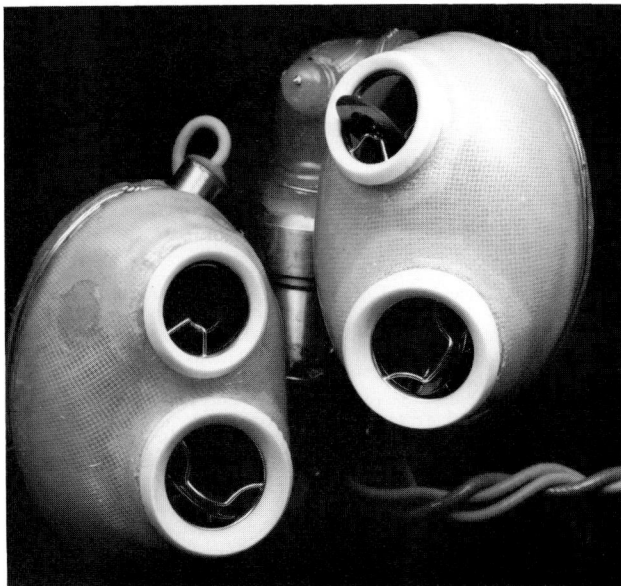

Figure 9. The single-energy convertor Utah–100 electrohydraulic artificial heart. The prosthetic ventricles are similar in design to those employed in the Utah–100 pneumatic artificial heart. The energy convertor is a high-speed reversing turbine that is located between the two ventricles.

tutions involved in this contract program (University of Utah, Pennsylvania State University, Abiomed, Inc., and Nimbus, Inc.) are developing devices driven by electric motors.[8] The Pennsylvania State University (Fig. 8)[39] and the University of Utah (Fig. 9)[28] have employed their devices *in vivo*.

Acknowledgment: The authors greatly appreciate the assistance of Martha L. Noll in the preparation of this manuscript.

SELECTED REFERENCES

Didisheim, P., Olsen, D. B., Farrar, D. J., et al.: Infections and thromboembolism with implantable cardiovascular devices. Trans. Am. Soc. Artif. Intern. Organs, 35:54, 1989.
Sepsis and thromboembolism are the two most serious complications that currently limit the long-term use of mechanical blood pumps. This workshop from the 34th annual meeting of the American Society for Artificial Internal Organs addresses the incidence of these problems at a number of leading centers and presents a detailed discussion of their etiology and potential interrelationship.

Joyce, L. D., Johnson, K. E., Cabrol, C., et al.: Nine year experience with the clinical use of total artificial hearts as cardiac support devices. Trans. Am. Soc. Artif. Intern. Organs, 34:703, 1988.
This manuscript summarizes the world experience with 116 total artificial heart implantations, the largest clinical series currently in the literature.

Levinson, M. M., and Copeland, J. G.: Technical aspects of total artificial heart implantation for temporary applications. J. Cardiac Surg., 2:3, 1987.
Patient selection and operative technique in large part determine the outcome of total artificial heart implantation. These authors present a very detailed discussion of the indications and contraindications to artificial heart implantation and the preoperative, intraoperative, and postoperative patient management.

Pierce, W. S.: The artificial heart—1986: Partial fulfillment of a promise. Trans. Am. Soc. Artif. Intern. Organs, 32:5, 1986.
The author provides an in-depth look at the development of both air-driven and electric artificial hearts. This article also describes all of the devices currently under evaluation in the United States and Europe.

REFERENCES

1. Akutsu, T., and Kolff, W. J.: Permanent substitutes for valves and hearts. Trans. Am. Soc. Artif. Intern. Organs, 4:230, 1958.
2. Aufiero, T. X., Magovern, J. A., Rosenberg, G., et al.: Long-term survival with a pneumatic artificial heart. Trans. Am. Soc. Artif. Intern. Organs, 33:157, 1987.
3. Boretos, J. W., and Pierce, W. S.: Segmented polyurethane: A new elastomer for biomedical applications. Science, 158:1481, 1967.
4. Cooley, D. A.: Staged cardiac transplantation: Report of three cases. Heart Transplant, 1:145, 1982.

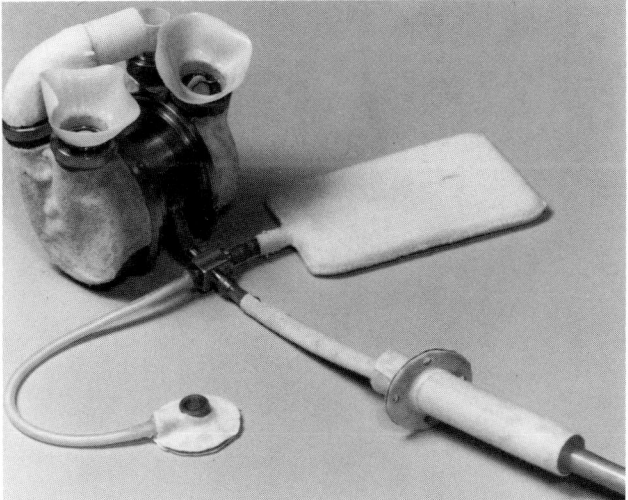

Figure 8. The Pennsylvania State University electric artificial heart as it appears prior to implantation in an experimental animal. Gases displaced from the motor housing are held in the intrathoracic compliance chamber, which can be accessed via the subcutaneous port. This prototype was powered by a percutaneous hard wire. Ultimate use of inductive coupling permits transcutaneous energy transmission, obviating the need for a break in the integument. (From Weiss, W. J., Rosenberg, G., Snyder, A. J., et al.: Permanent circulatory support systems at The Pennsylvania State University. IEEE Trans., to be published.)

5. Cooley, D. A., Akutsu, T., Norman, J. C., et al.: Total artificial heart in two-staged cardiac transplantation. Bull. Texas Heart Inst., 8:305, 1981.

6. Cooley, D. A., Liotta, D., Hallman, G. L., et al.: First human implantation of cardiac prosthesis for staged total replacement of the heart. Trans. Am. Soc. Artif. Intern. Organs, 15:252, 1969.

7. Cooley, D. A., Liotta, D., Hallman, G. L., et al.: Orthotopic cardiac prosthesis for two-staged cardiac replacement. Am. J. Cardiol., 24:723, 1969.

8. Davis, P. K., Rosenberg, G., Snyder, A. J., and Pierce, W. S.: Current status of permanent total artificial hearts. Ann. Thorac. Surg., 47:172, 1989.

9. DeVries, W. C.: Surgical technique for implantation of the Jarvik–7–100 total artificial heart. J.A.M.A., 259:875, 1988.

10. DeVries, W. C.: The permanent artificial heart. Four case reports. J.A.M.A., 259:849, 1988.

11. DeVries, W. C., and Joyce, L. D.: The artificial heart. CIBA Clin. Symp. 35:4, 1983.

12. Dew, P. A., Pantalos, G. M., Holfert, J. W., et al.: Mechanical failures of the pneumatic Utah–100 and Jarvik total artificial hearts. Trans. Am. Soc. Artif. Intern. Organs, 35:697, 1989.

13. Didisheim, P., Olsen, D. B., Farrar, D. J., et al.: Infections and thromboembolism with implantable cardiovascular devices. Trans. Am. Soc. Artif. Intern. Organs, 35:54, 1989.

14. Frazier, O. H., Akutsu, T., and Cooley, D. A.: Total artificial heart (TAH) utilization in man. Trans. Am. Soc. Artif. Intern. Organs, 28:534, 1982.

15. Frazier, O. H., Macris, M. P., Duncan, J. M., et al.: Cardiac transplantation in patients over 60 years of age. Ann. Thorac. Surg., 45:129, 1988.

16. Gaines, W. E., Pierce, W. S., Prophet, G. A., and Holtzman, K. L.: The goat: An animal model for implantable blood pumps. ASAIO J., 8:135, 1985.

17. Gaykowski, R., Taylor, K. D., and Yates, W. G.: Cumulative clinical experience with the Symbion J7 TAH. Trans. Am. Soc. Artif. Intern. Organs, 34:455, 1988.

18. Griffith, B. P.: Interim use of the Jarvik–7 artificial heart: Lessons learned at Presbyterian-University Hospital of Pittsburgh. Ann. Thorac. Surg., 47:158, 1989.

19. Heck, C. F., Shumway, S. J., and Kaye, M. P.: The registry of the International Society for Heart Transplantation: Sixth official report—1989. J. Heart Transplant, 8:271, 1989.

20. Imachi, K., Fujimasa, I., Miyake, H., et al.: Evaluation of polyurethane sac type blood pump after 232 and 288 days total artificial heart (TAH) pumping without anticoagulant. Trans. Am. Soc. Artif. Intern. Organs, 27:118, 1981.

21. Jarvik, R. K., DeVries, W. C., Semb, B. K. H., et al.: Surgical positioning of the Jarvik–7 artificial heart. J. Heart Transplant, 5:184, 1986.

22. Joyce, L. D., DeVries, W. C., Hastings, W. L., et al.: Response of the human body to the first permanent implant of the Jarvik–7 total artificial heart. Trans. Am. Soc. Artif. Intern. Organs, 29:81, 1983.

23. Joyce, L. D., Johnson, K. E., Cabrol, C., et al.: Nine year experience with the clinical use of total artificial hearts as cardiac support devices. Trans. Am. Soc. Artif. Intern. Organs, 34:703, 1988.

24. Kambic, H., Picha, G., Kiraly, R., et al.: Application of aldehyde treatments to cardiovascular devices. Trans. Am. Soc. Artif. Intern. Organs, 22:664, 1976.

25. Klain, M., Mrava, G. L., Tajima, K., et al.: Can we achieve over 100 hours' survival with a total mechanical heart? Trans. Am. Soc. Artif. Intern. Organs, 17:437, 1971.

26. Kwan-Gett, C., Zwart, H. H. J., Kralios, A. C., et al.: A prosthetic heart with hemispheric ventricles designed for low hemolytic action. Trans. Am. Soc. Artif. Intern. Organs, 16:409, 1970.

27. Levinson, M. M., and Copeland, J. G.: Technical aspects of total artificial heart implantation for temporary applications. J. Cardiac Surg., 2:3, 1987.

28. Lioi, A. P., Orth, J. L., Crump, K. R., et al.: In vitro development of automatic control for the actively filled electrohydraulic heart. Artif. Organs, 12:152, 1988.

29. Liotta, D., Hall, C. W., Akers, W. W., et al.: A pseudoendocardium for implantable blood pumps. Trans. Am. Soc. Artif. Intern. Organs, 12:129, 1966.

30. Magovern, J. A., Pennock, J. L., Campbell, D. B., et al.: Bridge to heart transplantation: The Penn State experience. J. Heart Transplant, 5:196, 1986.

31. Mott, W. E., and Cole, D. W.: Development of a nuclear-powered artificial heart. Trans. Am. Soc. Artif. Intern. Organs, 18:152, 1972.

32. Nose, Y., Topaz, S., SenGupta, A., et al.: Artificial hearts inside the pericardial sac in calves. Trans. Am. Soc. Artif. Intern. Organs, 11:255, 1965.

33. Pae, W. E., Miller, C. A., and Pierce, W. S.: Combined registry for the clinical use of mechanical ventricular assist pumps and the total artificial heart: Third official report—1988. J. Heart Transplant, 8:277, 1989.

34. Pierce, W. S.: Permanent heart substitution: Better solutions lie ahead. J.A.M.A., 259:891, 1988.

35. Pierce, W. S., Donachy, J. H., Rosenberg, G., and Baier, R. E.: Calcification inside artificial hearts: Inhibition by warfarin-sodium. Science, 208:601, 1980.

36. Razzeca, K., Olsen, D. B., Jarvik, R., et al.: Obstacles with sheep as the animal model in total artificial heart replacement. J. Artif. Organs 3(Suppl.):337, 1979.

37. Relman, A. S.: Artificial hearts—Permanent and temporary. N. Engl. J. Med., 314:644, 1986.

38. Richenbacher, W. E., Pennock, J. L., Pae, W. E., and Pierce, W. S.: Artificial heart implantation for end-stage cardiac disease. J. Cardiac Surg., 1:3, 1986.

39. Rosenberg, G., Snyder, A. J., Landis, D. L., et al.: An electric motor-driven total artificial heart: Seven months survival in the calf. Trans. Am. Soc. Artif. Intern. Organs, 30:69, 1984.

40. Shumakov, V. I., Griaznov, G. M., Zhemchuzhnikov, G. N., et al.: Implanted artificial heart with radioisotope power source. Artif. Organs, 7:101, 1983.

41. Weiss, W. J., Rosenberg, G., Snyder, A. J., et al.: In vivo performance of a transcutaneous energy transmission system with the Penn State motor driven ventricular assist device. Trans. Am. Soc. Artif. Intern. Organs, 35:284, 1989.

57

THE ROLE OF COMPUTERS IN SURGICAL PRACTICE

Peter K. Smith, M.D.

> Our present clinical clerk and house staff training takes a select group of people with the most expensive education in the world and wastes their time in the pursuit of more trivia, scheduling procedures and collecting results. . . . House officers must have strong legs, know whom to telephone, be expert sleuths, and be good at diplomatic negotiations. These data are then stored in a record devised a century ago. . . . The academic curse of wasting the talents of these skilled trainees with our obsolete systems leads to the present myth of deans and hospital administrators that house staff are an expensive luxury. Exploiting and wasting the time and talents of house staff is expensive because it fosters abysmally inefficient hospitals and clinics.[108]
>
> *R. M. Peters*

These statements apply equally well to all physicians and nurses as well as to deans and hospital administrators. In fact, all health care providers are in need of ready access to a wide variety of health care data, and they have turned to the computer to provide it.

The development of the electronic computer has been a complicated process in which the evolution of ideas (including logic and mathematics) has generally preceded the development of suitable technology. At the present time, however, it is apparent that *technology is advancing more rapidly than the application of ideas* and is thus no longer the limiting factor in the development of functional applications in health care.

This chapter reviews past accomplishments in computer applications and emphasizes ongoing developments that are essential for continued progress in the overall management of surgical patients.

ESTABLISHED COMPUTER APPLICATIONS

Most established computer applications can generally be defined as *databases*, wherein specific information is collected for refinement, organization, and reporting. Examples include the results of randomized clinical trials, private and federal insurance records, research registries, and quality assurance information. These databases are most often employed for studies of aggregate data, rather than for the care of individual patients. Two cases of databases that do serve the latter function are known broadly as Hospital Information Systems and Clinical Databases. In order to fully model disease states in terms of natural history, therapeutic needs, outcome, and cost, however, information may be needed from all database types.[103]

In this section, the advantages and disadvantages of application systems directly related to patient care are discussed. Emphasis is placed on databases with which surgeons interact on a daily basis and which can aid the surgeon to be more effective through such interaction.

HOSPITAL INFORMATION SYSTEMS

HISs have been successfully implemented in most large institutions. Their success has depended primarily on their ability to operate as accounting and inventory maintenance systems.[76] Successful installation has been widespread primarily because there has been a direct relationship between the funding of these computer applications and the limited uses for which they were intended.

The HIS operations generally utilize a mainframe computer with multiple "dumb" terminals. The data are entered predominantly by nonmedical personnel with secretarial or accounting backgrounds. Accordingly, they are very reliable in a highly structured environment. System architecture and software developments have been oriented toward maintaining the integrity of the database and the accuracy of the hospital balance sheet. Attempts to extend utility to the daily practice of medicine have yielded mixed results.

The Duke Hospital Information System (DHIS) was established in 1975 and is a prototype for over 60 HISs marketed by IBM as Patient Care System (PCS). It is currently based on an IBM 3090–200 mainframe computer and supports 550 terminals and 175 printers. It maintains information on approximately 1000 active inpatients daily and serves as the focal point for almost all patient service activities (Fig. 1).[71] The strengths of this HIS are (1) broad communication and convenient access (terminals and printers are installed in all patient care areas); (2) database of clinically relevant information generated as a by-product of accounting procedures (laboratory, pharmacy, and demographic data); and (3) large computing and storage capacity.

An institutional commitment to the HIS, however, is predicated on maintaining its business functions. The large capital investments necessary to ensure global communication are difficult to justify as technology advances rapidly. New application software is also costly, yet necessary to organize clinical data into usable formats. Unfortunately, the "system programming" skills necessary to accomplish these tasks are beyond the reach of the average clinician. An illustrative example of the underlying problems of a typical HIS can be found in detailing the processing of laboratory information.

In tracking a laboratory test from order entry to result reporting, the following individual data manipulation steps occur:

1. Handwritten entry of the order by the physician.
2. Transcription of this order by a data terminal operator.
3. Transmission of the order to the laboratory. Either a route sheet is printed locally for attachment to a physician-drawn sample, or the blood collection service is notified for phlebotomy and sample delivery. A standard multiple-chemistry test may be performed in any one of many different locations (sublaboratories), depending on the time of day and the urgency of the test.

DUKE HOSPITAL INFORMATION SYSTEM - Interactions

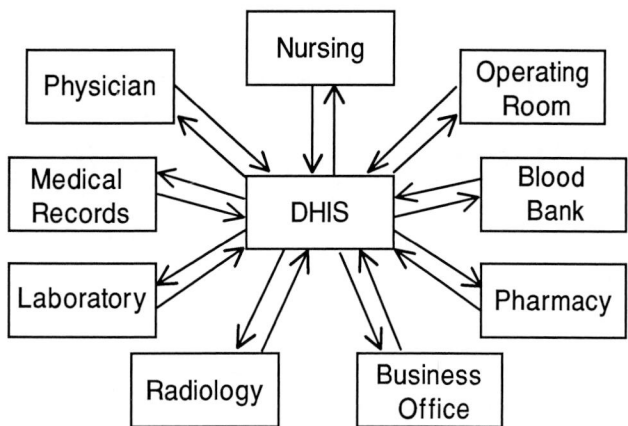

Figure 1. A diagrammatic representation of information flow in the Duke Hospital Information System (DHIS). Multiple interdepartmental two-way communication for data transfer and query is supported.

4. Performance of the test by an automated machine and verification of results against internal laboratory standards. The results are then entered into the HIS via a laboratory terminal along with the time, date, and initials of the laboratory technician.

5. Printing of the results at the terminal that originated the order and placement of the results in the patient chart or a local report bin.

From an administrative perspective, the transaction completely satisfies all needs. The system provides a clear record that the test was ordered and the blood was drawn. An audit trail is readily available should the result be erroneous or unavailable because of problems with the laboratory, the blood collection service, or the physician. Billing is assured, and differential billing for the same test is possible because the sub-laboratory site performing the test is known. For example, increased charges are possible for a test performed in the STAT laboratory as opposed to one performed in the routine chemistry laboratory. Moreover, printed paper reports delivered to the originating nursing station absolve the "system" of responsibility for notification. Internal surveys of particular machines for accuracy can be performed by batch jobs within the mainframe computer. Promptness of service can be assessed and rectified if necessary by comparison of the time of order entry, sample receipt in the laboratory, and result reporting.

From the physician's point of view, this system is adequate for the aggregate patient population but is less than adequate for optimal care of individual patients. Since there is no standard method of notification, the physician must periodically check the report bin or the HIS itself (through a terminal) to obtain results. Delays of variable length routinely accompany direct access to DHIS, and these delays are repeated for each different laboratory test ordered, regardless of whether the report contains normal or abnormal results. A common physician practice is to intentionally defer daily report gathering until such time as all test results are likely to be available.

The physician is then confronted with the problem of data analysis. The reports are not oriented toward efficient physician use and include extraneous details (such as which machine produced which set of results) of interest only to the accountant or the laboratory professional. This "electronic noise" and "transaction-oriented" format leaves to the physician the task of organizing the data logically in the diagnostic thought process and temporally for trend detection.

Physician-oriented organization and reporting are not performed by the HIS for two fundamental reasons. First, there is no obvious monetary gain. Second, these tasks are difficult to

implement because the architectural design of the database has been established to optimize the achievement of other goals. In general, one would not anticipate that a system designed for hospital billing (where time is measured in days to weeks) would respond in a timeframe appropriate for patient care (where time is measured in minutes). Because the original goals of the HIS are not usually directly related to patient care and do not take into consideration the need for such development, it is generally futile to expect improvement to occur at the mainframe level. It is probably also erroneous to expect the original funding agency (the hospital) to solely fund expansion of the clinical utility of the HIS, especially given the inevitable diminution in accounting or inventory power that would accompany such a shift in emphasis.

CLINICAL DATABASES

A clinical database can be described as a well-defined, discrete, and continuous series of data elements pertaining to patients.[111] These data elements are coupled with outcome descriptors. Those databases designed to aid in patient management have descriptors of the management process and have a primary emphasis placed on patient care assistance, data collection, report generation, and clinical research. Research databases contain additional descriptors that are useful for examining hypotheses, preferably defined in advance.

Information is collected, entered, and stored as data elements and subsequently recalled for either individuals or groups. The four processes common to all databases, data collection, entry, storage, and recall, have separate and conflicting attributes. In data collection, it must be decided which variables will be collected, how long they will be collected, and how they will be collected. Data entry should be efficient and utilize a *coding system* for efficiency and clarity. Some flexibility in data entry is desirable, but "free-text" data entry must be minimized. For maximal utility, data recall must be online, efficient, rapid, and addressable using common technology.

It is important that clinicians or end-users trained in the clinical arena be involved in clinical database design to ensure appropriate collection and relevance of data and to define long-term goals. Biostatisticians and computer scientists are necessary for the maintenance of data structure and quality, and the hardware and software. The *paucity of common ground between information scientists and clinicians* sometimes leads to insurmountable communication problems and serves as a major impediment to implementation.[111]

In general, clinical databases have been successfully implemented when the primary emphasis has been on a well-defined medical problem and when the impetus for establishing the database originates with the physician. When objectives are clearly defined, the database can be limited in size to contain only data of medical importance. Further simplification is possible by limiting the patient population involved.

The Medical Record

At Duke University Medical Center, The Medical Record (TMR) was developed in 1975 to support both inpatient and outpatient services and to act as a clinical database.[50,51,61,139] It operates on a VAX 6210 computer supporting 100 terminals. TMR provides the means by which the Cardiovascular Disease Databank is maintained at Duke University Medical Center and contains records on some 45,000 patients evaluated by the division of cardiology or the division of cardiothoracic surgery. Its operation, as opposed to that of an HIS, emphasizes the medical meaning of data rather than administrative functions.[137]

TMR is of modular design and contains demographic, financial, and appointment data as well as problem lists, procedures, subjective and physical findings, study results, and therapeutic interventions. Data can be retrieved in problem-oriented, time-oriented, or encounter-oriented formats. Six major groups use the patient record: (1) administration; (2) business office; (3) laboratory; (4) pharmacy; (5) nurses; and (6) physicians. The requirement that each group have access to all information despite their markedly different needs supports the concept that a consolidated system is mandatory to fully computerize the medical record.[137]

The system is designed upon interactive questionnaires and permits free-text data entry, exclusive response from a list, or multiple responses from a list. Data and application-independent programming are possible through the use of data definition tables or dictionaries. Over 90 per cent of the data are coded. Nonprogrammers may define the characteristics of a report using simple structured English.[52] The system is currently linked to the DHIS through IBM PCs using an IRMA connection.[53]

By developing a link to the DHIS, a TMR workstation can serve as the focal point in the development of a physician workstation.[71] Key aspects include time-oriented flow sheets, problem-oriented displays, and multiple formats for the same data elements.[140]

Other Clinical Databases

COSTAR (Computer-Stored Ambulatory Record)[11] was designed to replace the traditional medical chart and also to improve physician access to information in the medical record. This system includes both administrative and research functions. Alternative systems include the Regenstrief Medical Record System developed in 1973[94] and the HELP system[147] developed at Latter-Day Saints Hospital in conjunction with the faculty of the University of Utah. The latter is a comprehensive computer system designed to provide clinical information, medical decision-making, and administrative and research features.[25]

Microcomputer Clinical Databases

As microcomputer power has expanded and easy-to-use commercial software has become available, comprehensive medical databasing on local devices has become attractive.[8] A 250-element database for cardiac surgery that can be maintained on an IBM PC-AT has been developed,[100] with data entry performed by a medical secretary. Similar systems designed to monitor otolaryngology operative experience[40] and to maintain organ transplant results[28] have been described.

The operating room, as the central location for significant clinical interaction with surgical patients, has been the focus of much attention in computer application development. In the past, minicomputers or mainframe computers have been employed,[90] although the current generation of microcomputers have achieved sufficient power to be useful in this area.[9,21,56,93] Improved productivity has been one attractive aspect of these systems.[7]

Although several commercially available operating room scheduling programs exist,[113] the author has found it preferable to develop software specifically for personal use[135] based on Knowledgeman/2, a commercially available, general database program with a powerful programming language marketed by Micro Database Systems, Inc. All data commonly used to schedule surgical procedures (80 procedures per day, 30 operating rooms, 8 surgical divisions) are entered from a local area network of divisional workstations. Data elements are chosen from division-approved procedure libraries that are periodically updated by divisional quality assurance representatives. Thus, credentialing, monitoring of quality assurance through automatic linkage to pathology reports, infection control, clinical research, and administrative functions can all be derived from this one database. The most obvious advantages of this system are the reduction of errors and the ability to print a schedule in any desired format. Beyond this, are many potential and real-

ized features[57] such as uploading the schedule to the HIS for real-time distribution, instantaneous broad communication of schedule changes, and archiving.

THE NATIONAL LIBRARY OF MEDICINE

If practitioners attempted to keep up with the literature by reading two articles per day, by the end of one year, they would be 55 centuries behind.[12]

A large and expanding bibliographic database of medical literature exists and is a valuable resource in patient management. There are now more than 20,000 different biomedical journals published yearly[33] with an annual growth rate of 6 to 7 per cent.[110] Over 300,000 articles are indexed each year, with over 25,000 devoted primarily to surgical problems. The amount of diagnostic and procedural information gathered for an individual patient is similarly expanding and is now encoded using over 30,000 separate ICD and CPT codes. The correlation of this plethora of information involves the application of each individual physician's knowledge and thought processes, a task that simply cannot be accomplished without assistance.

Information gathering for individual patients often requires reference to published material. Ideally, the appropriate material itself would be incorporated in the medical record to document and justify diagnosis and therapy. That this is not a universal practice is reflective of the impracticality of locating appropriate information and the impossibility of placing it in the record.

Several methods exist to access the National Library of Medicine's (NLM) databases (MEDLARS and others) using a microcomputer, a telephone modem, and communication software. MEDLINE (MEDlars onLINE) can be accessed using NLM's GRATEFUL MED software package, which assists the user in formulating a search using the almost 16,000 MeSH terms (Medical Subject Headings). The query is submitted as a batch job directly to NLM's computers. Other searching aids have been developed,[1] including MicroMeSH, developed at the Massachusetts General Hospital Laboratory of Computer Science.[85] The information can be returned (title, author, abstract, and so on) for local viewing and disc storage. Other resources include Paperchase,[14,144] Dialogue, BRS/Information Technologies, and miniMEDLINE.[20]

In the department of surgery, BRS/Information Technologies has been used for the past 4 years. More than 100 individual accounts for the faculty and all levels of housestaff are supported. BRS leases NLM master data tapes for literature searches in addition to providing access to the full text of many prominent medical publications through contractual agreements. BRS provides front-end software (Colleague) to permit natural language queries as well as the use of standard MeSH terms. Interaction is online, as opposed to intermittent batch, and full data retrieval with local storage is supported. A local microcomputer is available 24 hours per day for housestaff use. Individuals, offices, or laboratories with individual passwords may access the system from any modem-equipped personal computer.

Commercially available software packages are available to organize citations and maintain practice- or disease-specific references. A relational database, such as DataEase, has been used to maintain over 3000 key references in vascular surgery.[68] A dedicated bibliographic data manager (Pro-Cite) has been used in a similar manner by combining citation material, abstract, and keywords downloaded from NLM with locally developed indexing terms to maintain the office filing system.

These microcomputer applications are well within the ability of the average surgeon with limited computer background. With modest effort, it is possible to create a large local reference library based on any area of interest. One can store search strat-

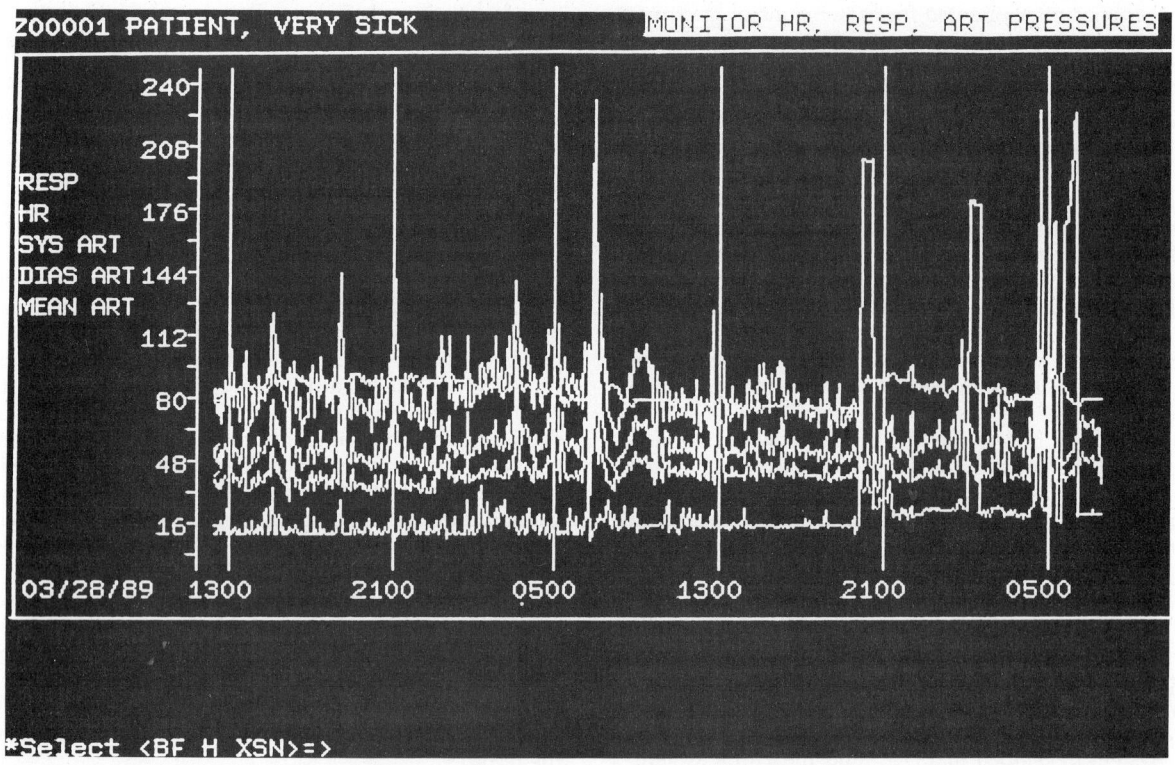

Figure 2. A monitor display of raw physiologic data acquired in the surgical intensive care unit over a 40-hour period. Heart rate, respiratory rate, systolic arterial pressure, diastolic arterial pressure, and mean arterial pressure are displayed as acquired from the monitor. Note that numerous artifacts (due to blood drawing, and so on) significantly detract from the information quality. (From Hammond, W. E., Grewal, R., Straube, M. J., and Stead, W. W.: Networking data sources for intensive care monitoring. Proceedings, American Association for Medical Systems and Informatics. Congress, 1989, pp. 277–281.)

egies, periodically query the NLM database, and add articles of interest from specialty journals as well.

INTENSIVE CARE UNIT COMPUTERIZATION

Intensive care unit (ICU) computer applications have been divided into five broad areas[91]: (1) monitoring of physiologic data; (2) controlling equipment; (3) interfacing with hospital laboratory computer system; (4) as terminals for commercially available databases; and (5) as stand-alone machines to maintain a multitude of individual programs for aid in drug interaction problems, blood gas interpretation, hemodynamic calculations, tutorials, and intravenous dosage calculations.

Historically, cardiac surgical ICUs implemented these functions as part of the earliest attempts to simplify patient care and reduce the intensity of specialized nursing support required. Sheppard and Kirklin, at the University of Alabama, are pioneers in this area, having developed a centralized minicomputer system that has enabled postoperative patient care to be highly streamlined and, to a large extent, data-driven. Their initial report outlined their experience with 124 patients from July 1, 1967, to March 15, 1968.[125] At their institution, one nurse is usually assigned to two postoperative cardiac surgical patients, in part because of the time savings engendered by an online computer system. Although a reduction in nurse staffing needs has not always followed successful installation of an ICU computer, an improvement in nursing efficiency is almost always noted.[29,81,98]

Although many other institutions and examples of all types of ICUs have followed this pathway with favorable results,[45,46,49,101,106,107,112,129,130,148] such applications have not yet been fully accepted.[38]

Acceptance and implementation will almost certainly be assured in the near future for a variety of reasons:

1. The growth in the number of all types of ICUs and other factors are creating a nationwide shortage of intensive care nurses. Moreover, legislative efforts are underway that will create a similar shortage of housestaff time-availability. Maintaining a high level of critical care will not be possible in the future without labor- and time-saving measures.

2. Such systems have been shown to improve the quality of intensive care and to diminish the average length of ICU stay.[127] Through prospective data collection, it has become possible to categorize patients to predict complications and outcome.[116,121,134,146,153] This information is useful in refining treatment strategies and containing costs.[59,97,114] The importance of computer monitoring in recognizing critical low-probability events was recognized early[87] and realized recently through demonstration of improved survival.[66]

3. The organization and storage of ICU information provides a superior environment for physician and nursing education[22] and can provide a better work environment.[64]

To facilitate computer interfacing, most manufacturers of monitoring systems have introduced microprocessor technology to provide digital output of monitor-derived information. A number of private companies have developed computer systems for direct connection to a number of monitors commonly used in the intensive care environment. These hardware and software packages are based on either a minicomputer with multiple terminals at the bedside or a distributed system with microcomputers at the bedside linked to a microcomputer server as a central databasing and data transmission point.[26,36,91,119,141]

The *networking* of various data sources, including clinical input from surgeons and nurses, is the major task accomplished by these systems. This is being accomplished in the Duke University Medical Center using TMR (described previously) in the surgical ICU.[55] Monitor-derived data are reformatted for easy

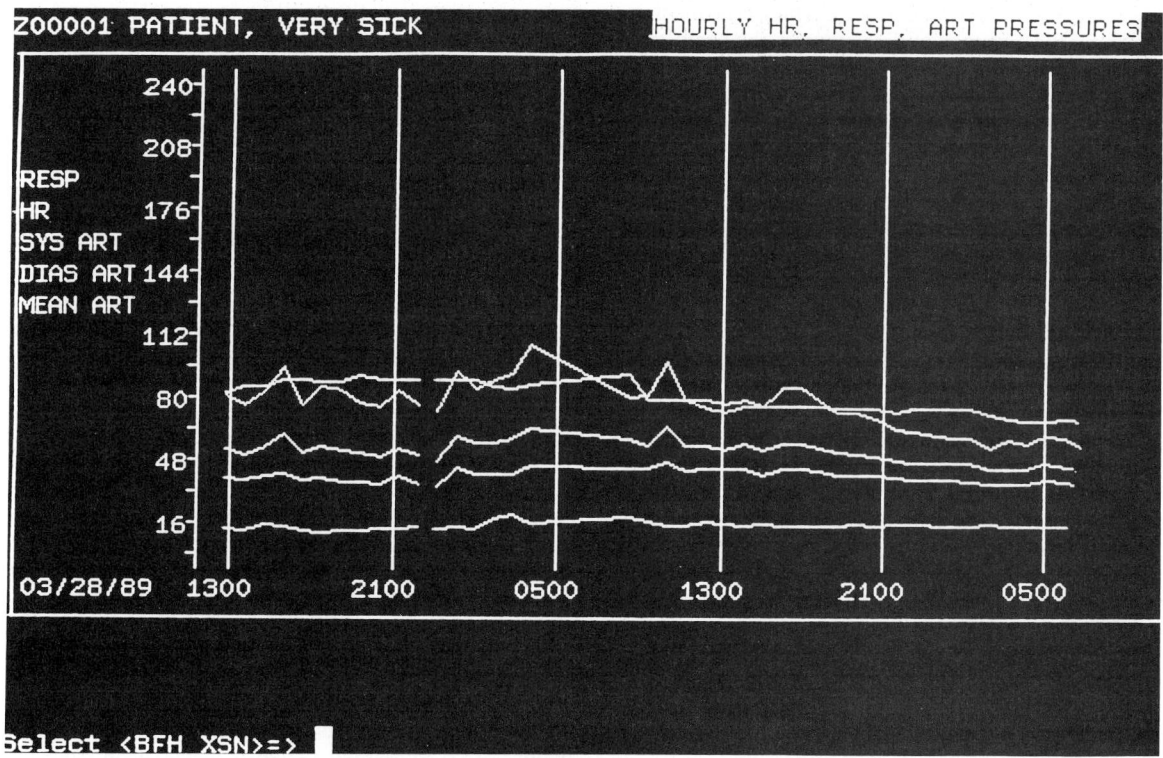

Figure 3. A similar display after "smoothing" of the data by algorithms designed to remove artifactual information. In practice, each parameter is color-coded for viewing, further enhancing the clarity of the data. (From Hammond, W. E., Grewal, R., Straube, M. J., and Stead, W. W.: Networking data sources for intensive care monitoring. Proceedings, American Association for Medical Systems and Informatics. Congress, 1989, pp. 277–281.)

viewing on bedside graphics workstations (Figs. 2 and 3). Each work station is linked to a central MicroVAX II (Digital Equipment Corporation), which is linked, in turn, to the HIS to collect demographic and laboratory data. Many specialty displays (Fig. 4) have been developed to enhance the medical meaning of the information acquired.

The computer provides the ability to perform multiple complex calculations for data reduction and simplification, and thus permits the recognition of adverse hemodynamic conditions that may not be apparent from raw physiologic data.[23,24,39,47,74,80,88,89,115,131,141] Monitor data coupled with laboratory information and automatically acquired intake and output values are used to generate the critical care flowsheet. These data can then be used to automate therapy with excellent results as has been accomplished for postoperative blood volume therapy,[75,127,128] the control of postoperative hypertension,[75,122,126,128] and the infusion of insulin for diabetic management.[150]

DEVELOPING COMPUTER APPLICATIONS

A variety of computer applications have been developed by highly motivated individuals for specialized (often entrepreneurial) purposes. These applications are often microcomputer-based and are currently approaching transition to broad application. Each application requires its own formal mechanism for information gathering and processing. Information processing by the computer compresses the massive amounts of data acquired, assesses accuracy, and sometimes highlights information that may be of critical importance. Physician interaction is required for implementation of changes in patient care based on these data.

In caring for the individual patient, a host of material is gathered that requires organization by the physician. These data include the results of the history and physical examination,

laboratory values, doctors' orders, and imaging results, all of which are quantifiable to some extent. In addition, variable amounts of basic physiologic data are recorded. The remainder consist of the impressions and thought processes of care providers as they evolve during the hospital admission.

These data are stored in a document (the medical record) that is now recognized as being poorly organized, incomplete, and "noisy" (that is, containing much material that is required for nonmedical, often legal, reasons).[4] The record does not include or make reference to other resource documents such as the medical literature, medical research databases, codification aids, pharmaceutical prescribing information, or drug interaction warnings. It does not provide a detailed enumeration of the

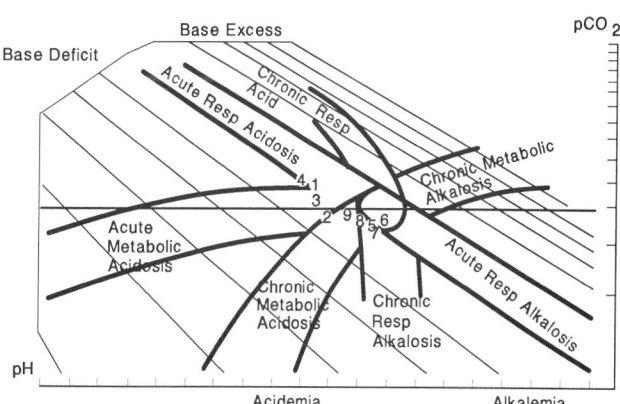

Figure 4. Bedside monitor display of a graphic acid-base nomogram to assist in the interpretation of arterial blood gas results. Data on individual determinations appear as sequential numbers displayed in this x-y coordinate system, assisting in the trend analysis and interpretation of individual results. (From Hammond, W. E., Grewal, R., Straube, M. J., and Stead, W. W.: Networking data sources for intensive care monitoring. Proceedings, American Association for Medical Systems and Informatics. Congress, 1989, pp. 277–281.)

thought processes guiding the patient's care. There is no mechanism for assessing the accuracy of data entered, the completeness of the document, or, finally, the appropriateness of any given entry.

Correction of these deficiencies is important and will be accomplished only with universal, general acceptance of computer assistance at all levels. Physician, nurse, and hospital action is necessary for the development of the required software (which is the present limiting factor) and for the purchase and installation of the hardware (which, it appears, will be accomplished last).

The Surgeon's Role

Several factors combine to make it likely that surgeons will be leaders in database development. The patient is highly defined in terms of pertinent anatomy and physiology. The number of potential principal diagnoses and outcomes is limited. The procedures performed are highly stylized, and thus relatively easy to encode. The complications of surgical therapy are limited in number and easily definable. All these features would tend to make the acquisition of a computerized patient database practical.

The practice of surgery is labor-intensive and information-intensive. An enormous amount of quantitative information is generated for each patient, and attention to each data item is critical for optimal results. The detection of low-probability events in such a setting is a job the computer performs well. Thus, computer assistance is likely to be well received and of practical value.

Finally and most importantly, surgeons have historically been leaders in the field of what can be termed "applied medical informatics." Regardless of the reasons, whether as outlined previously or because of an inherent attitude toward informa-

tion management, the surgical environment has tended to foster the development of computer applications.[149] It is this environment, more than any other factor, that is necessary for progress in this area.

In this section, evolving computer applications that concern the individual patient's management are reviewed. The methods used for information gathering, processing, and reporting are considered.

History and Physical Examination Databases

This fundamental evaluation of any patient must be codified (or encoded) in order to create a meaningful database. For the average patient, a myriad of signs and symptoms are possible. Those pertinent to surgical diseases are somewhat fewer and have been categorized for entry into databases. In cardiac surgery, this has been done using TMR as part of the ongoing effort of the Duke Cardiovascular Disease Databank.

The history and physical examination are performed by a Cardiology Fellow prior to cardiac catheterization. Forms are completed (Fig. 5), and data are entered and assessed by technicians. The catheterization results are entered similarly. The data are stored in a VAX computer in a framework established by TMR (previously described). The data can be reported in a variety of formats such as the history and physical examination (including demographic data), the full catheterization report, and a letter to the referring physician.

After the collection and coding of demographic patient information, physical findings, and historical information from the patient, each individual patient can be categorized based on these data. Patient outcome is tracked longitudinally during long-term follow-up. In the Cardiovascular Disease Databank, individual patients can be compared with cohorts of patients with similar clinical profiles based on demographic data and

---

DUKE MEDICAL CENTER
CORONARY ARTERY DISEASE (CAD) HISTORY AND PHYSICAL FORM

History

Reason(s) for Catheterization (indicate primary *one* by P):

1. ( ) chest pain
2. ( ) congestive heart failure
3. ( ) acute evolving myocardial infarction (MI)
4. ( ) old MI (>6 wk.), now asymptomatic
5. ( ) recent MI (≤6 wk.), now asymptomatic
6. ( ) post-MI angina (same admission)
7. ( ) arrhythmia
8. ( ) POS ETT
9. ( ) POS RNA
10. ( ) cardiac arrest
11. ( ) prior cardiac surgery
12. ( ) prior percutaneous transluminal coronary angioplasty
13. ( ) ICC 6-month Recath Protocol
14. ( ) ICC 7-day Protocol relook
15. ( ) ICC 24-hour Protocol relook
16. ( ) other_____

Cardiovascular Risk Factors: ( ) no change since last catheterization (this admission)

Hypertension   Y N
Type I diabetes (ketosis prone)   Y N
Type II diabetes (non-insulin-dependent)   Y N
Peripheral vascular disease   Y N
Hyperlipidemia   Y N
    If yes: ( ) cholesterol ( ) triglycerides
Cerebrovascular disease   Y N
Family history (first-degree relative, age <60) of CAD Y N
Smoking history   Y N
    If yes, average of _____ pk.(s)/day over _____
year(s)
    Quit _____ day(s)/wk.(s)/mo.(s)/
yr.(s) ago
    Date patient quit (if known): _____/_____/_____

Figure 5. Data entry form for the history and physical examination of a patient with coronary artery disease. The complete data form is several pages long but, as can be seen, requires primarily check-off data entry. Multiple entries are possible under many headings.

cardiac catheterization findings. In this manner, the anticipated results of either medical or surgical therapy are projected within certain confidence limits.

Procedural Databases

No patient encounter, except possibly the history and physical examination, more clearly defines a surgical patient's medical status than the nature and result of the procedures. This is particularly true in surgery, wherein the type of operation performed can forecast with reasonable accuracy the majority of potential outcomes, particularly with respect to complications.

The operative note for a cardiac operation generally consists of discrete factual data (the aortic cross-clamp time, cardiopulmonary bypass time, the vessels grafted, and the like), which are presented in a narrative format. To maintain consistency in reporting and to generate a database of the procedures performed, these data elements have been stored at Duke University Medical Center for the past 15 years. A form containing a series of questions is completed as the operation proceeds. The responsibility for data collection has been assumed by the perfusionists, who ascertain a limited amount of demographic and anesthetic information at the beginning of the procedure. They then record pertinent information regarding the conduct of extracorporeal circulation and query the operating surgeon at the termination of the procedure regarding the actual operative procedure itself. This information is incorporated into the Duke Cardiovascular Disease Databank, where it is matched with the patient's demographic information and cardiac catheterization results. A computerized operative note is generated at the termination of the procedure by the TMR system. A draft form of this note accompanies the patient to the ICU and is forwarded to the surgeon's office the next day. It is then reviewed, signed (or revised if necessary), and mailed to the referring physician.

Laboratory Databases

Laboratory reports include discrete data elements that can be of critical importance in patient management. Once acquired, categorized, and assessed for errors, these elements can be analyzed by relatively simple computer algorithms to identify values outside the physiologic range that would require medical

intervention. Either national or local laboratory standards may be applied before reporting of results.[82]

The results are usually stored in an HIS mainframe computer. In order to be incorporated into an electronic medium designed for patient evaluation and care, these data are reorganized to reflect physician analytic patterns. Report formats may be customized to suit various individuals. For example, the cardiac surgeon may wish to see the blood urea nitrogen, creatinine, potassium, hematocrit, and bilirubin levels at one time, even though these results are reported from three different locations. Time-oriented displays of serial results are essential (a fact that is usually considered only in accounting terms in most systems). Finally, the reported results should be presented to the physician in real time through computer-based surveillance of outstanding requests and receipt notification. This has been accomplished for the practice of outpatient nephrology (Fig. 6)[139] and is being implemented in ICUs using TMR.[54]

Image Databases

A wide variety of imaging methods, from the conventional radiograph to magnetic resonance imaging, are used in surgery. The electronic storage of the actual image can already be accomplished in echocardiography, computed tomography, magnetic resonance imaging, and many other modalities. Conventional radiographic studies can be digitally scanned and stored as well.[31,60]

The Department of Radiology at Duke University Medical Center in collaboration with AT&T and Philips has developed a radiographic image processing system that bypasses the production of a conventional film and electronically transmits images to the ICUs for local viewing (Figs. 7 and 8). This process utilizes special cassettes containing a reusable phosphor plate that is interrogated by laser in the radiology department. The information is digitally stored as a 1760 by 2140 pixel matrix and displayed locally at a graphics workstation (CommView). The images are maintained centrally in the radiology department and are electronically transmitted over an Ethernet network to critical care workstations in ICUs with 8 bits of information (256 levels of gray) per pixel, each distributed image requiring slightly less than 1 megabyte of memory for storage.

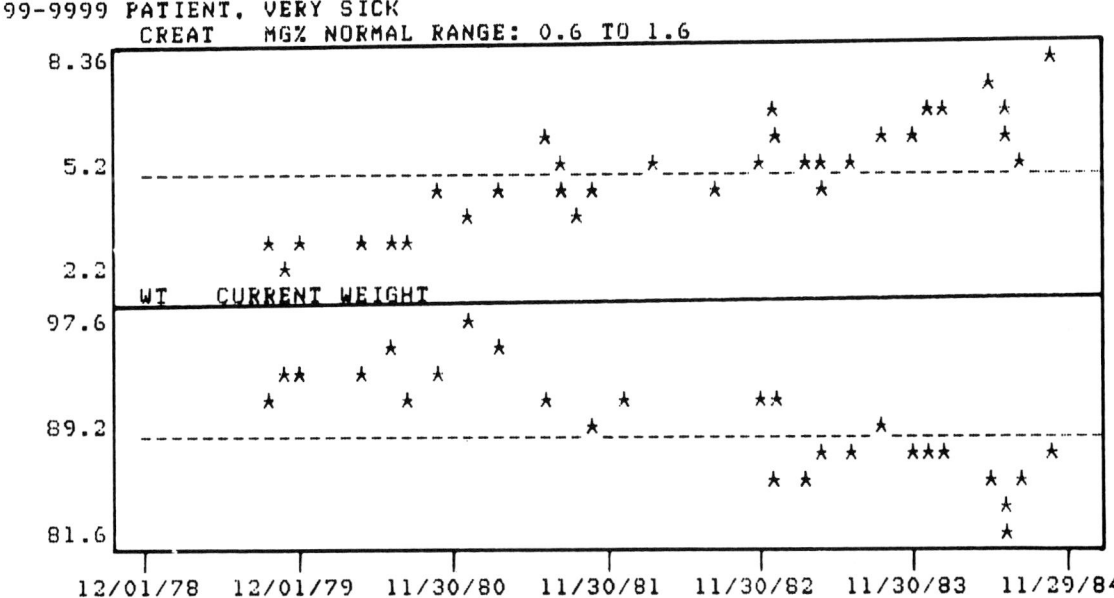

Figure 6. Graphic and time-oriented display of laboratory results (creatinine, upper panel) and objective physical examination data (patient weight, lower panel) that can be displayed as screen output using TMR. (From Jelovsek, F. R., and Stead, W. W.: Computerized medical records. *In* Javitt, J. (Ed.): Computers in Medicine: Applications and Possibilities. Philadelphia, W. B. Saunders Company, 1986, p. 234.)

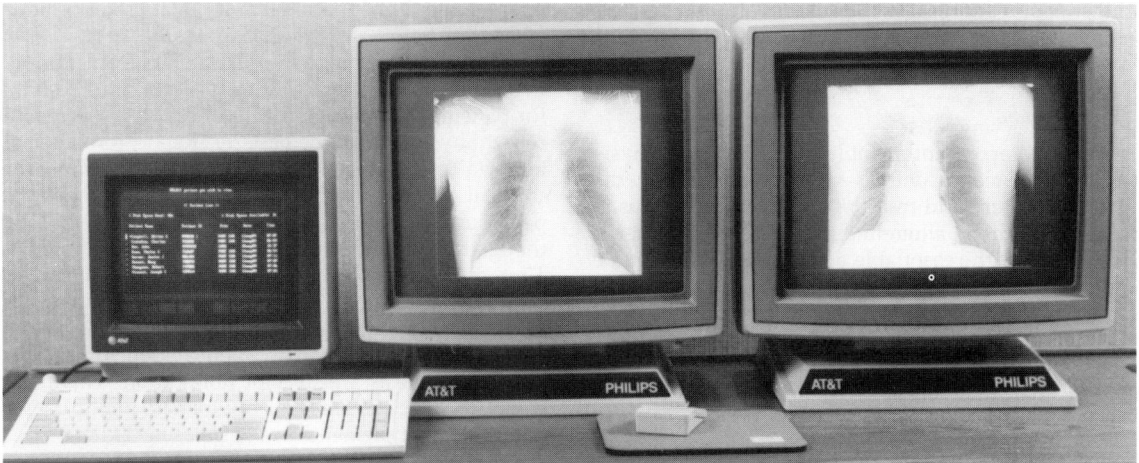

Figure 7. Components of the graphics workstation (CommView) that is physically located in an intensive care unit. The microcomputer is at the lower left. Note the ability to compare films side-by-side.

Approximately 8.5 seconds are required to fully display stored images.

Local imaging workstations allow physicians to view "x-rays" sequentially for all patients on an ICU and to compare recent films side-by-side. An interactive electronic mouse drives the system and enhances interpretation by allowing image brightness, contrast, and magnification to be varied at will. Since the data are digital, visual presentation of the information is possible in order to highlight specific information based on the clinician's reason for obtaining the study. For example, the chest film image can be enhanced to aid visualization of indwelling tubes or cannulas or to more clearly define a suspected pneumothorax.

An additional advantage of digital image storage is that it diminishes the time from the obtainment of a portable radiograph to viewing the radiograph at the patient's bedside. A fiberoptic network is in place between nodes in the radiology department and an Ethernet network is distributed to ICUs. As the image is processed centrally in the radiology department, the digital information is transmitted to the ICU monitoring station. Each image requires approximately 2 minutes to be reconstructed in the ICU setting. Thus, particularly critical films can be viewed simultaneously by clinicians at the bedside and by radiologists in the central imaging area.

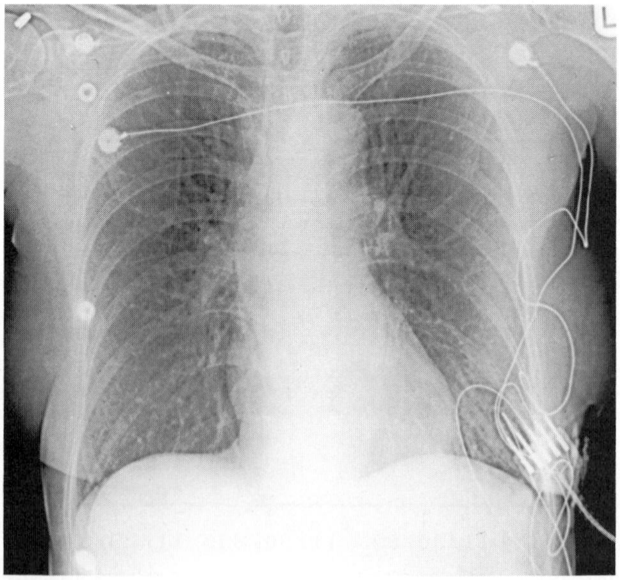

Although it is premature to believe that all imaging studies will soon be digitized and stored electronically,[65] advantages offered to surgical education may serve as an additional incentive in this area. Several applications have been described to link image data with text and to assist in planning operative procedures. The biomechanical effects of orthopedic procedures can be analyzed.[86] The reconstruction of craniofacial abnormalities can be planned and displayed three-dimensionally using digital computed tomographic data.[30] Residency training in the geometric relationships of organs and organ systems can be enhanced with pseudo–three-dimensional presentations, which can be developed for specific operative approaches (Fig. 9).[154]

Pharmaceutical Databases

Drug therapy information (drug type, dose, and dose interval) is maintained in the medical record in the form of drug

Figure 8. A digital chest radiograph, photographed as it is displayed on the graphics monitor.

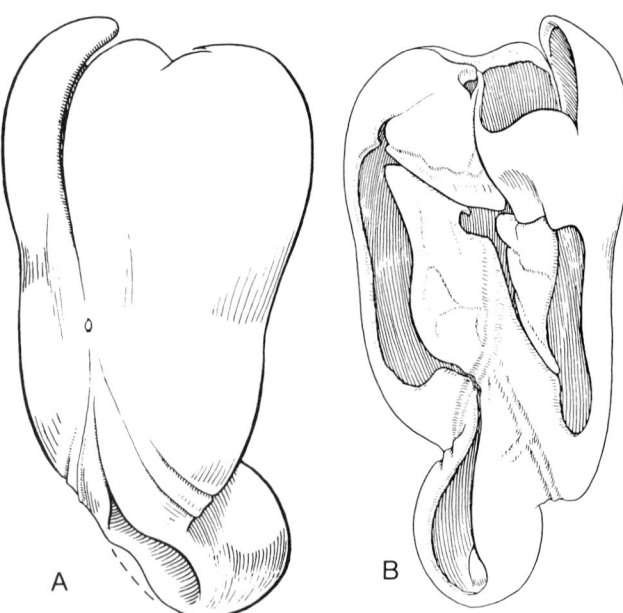

Figure 9. Anterior *(A)* and posterior *(B)* views of the parietal peritoneum drawn from computer graphic reconstructions. These displays reveal the complex infolding patterns of the parietal peritoneum and effectively demonstrate spatial relationships having surgical significance that are unattainable by conventional means. (From Wind, G., Dvorak, V. K., and Dvorak, J. A.: Computer graphic modeling in surgery. Orthop. Clin. North Am., *17:*657, 1986.)

orders and dispensation charting, as well as in the HIS for inventory, supply, and billing purposes. Pertinent results such as drug levels and values indicating adverse drug effects are located in the laboratory reports. Pharmaceutical information such as appropriate dosing schemes, pharmacokinetic information, and adverse reactions and incompatibilities can be found in manuals or through consultation with the pharmacy department. Currently, all of this information is encoded and could be incorporated in an individual database through the institution of direct physician order entry.[72]

Information is available on drug pharmacokinetics from a variety of studies of the volume of distribution of an individual drug and its clearance mechanism. Whereas these data can be accessed in relationship to any drug, a preferable method of information display would be a time-oriented projection of the effect of the drug on serum levels. The National Biomedical Simulation Resource has developed a program generator (SCoP) that can provide a general solution to this problem. For a variety of drugs, the dosage, dose frequency, volume of distribution, renal function, and function of other organs responsible for drug clearance can be defined. Utilizing published values of individual drug kinetics, the SCoP user interface is used to establish the appropriate pharmacokinetic formula and generate a graphic display of anticipated serum levels. This information assists the physician in initial dosing of a drug and allows anticipation of peak and trough levels. In addition, the proper timing of serum drug level measurements can be determined.[105,118]

Numerous microcomputer and calculator software packages are available for the evaluation of a variety of drugs and fluids as they relate to patient characteristics.[70,77] These can be obtained for Coumadin (private development), for theophylline (private development), or for any number of aminoglycosides (drug manufacturers). Private software developers have written software that evaluates several drugs commonly used in ICUs, thereby eliminating the need to repeatedly enter patient weight, height, creatinine, and other information for different drug regimens in the same patient. Unfortunately, a universal program that will assist in prescribing all common drugs is not available at this time, leaving the user in a position of maintaining a large library of disparate software to achieve this goal. Similar applications are available to write prescriptions automatically.[3]

Automated Discharge Summary

The provision of a timely, accurate automated discharge summary would benefit the care provider, both locally and in referral situations. In broad terms, the discharge summary is a simple list of patient problems expanded by subjective and objective information provided by the physician and the hospital. It chronicles the discovery of these problems and their resolution. As such, this instrument provides an important document to assess quality assurance. Moreover, the discharge summary is rapidly becoming the primary basis for both hospital and physician remuneration.

Several attempts have been made to automate the discharge summary. The Johns Hopkins Hospital has developed the AUTRES Report.[79] This pilot system produced discharge reports from database records created by user entries. Attempts were made to integrate work performed by ancillary services to automatically enter data into the system.

Lexical problems are one of the main impediments to the development of computerized report generators that will be necessary for the development of an automated discharge summary.[96] Various attempts have been made to overcome these problems, including natural language text processing. Gabrieli and Speth note that the inpatient chart is "an undisciplined diary without standards." They developed 362 formalized data fields and a word lexicon containing 126,000 different words.

They note that William Shakespeare used only 29,000 words in all his plays.[43]

It is probable that a system to generate an automated discharge summary would also generate progress notes and ensure daily input of information while at the same time providing work relief for physician users. This approach has been employed at the Ontario Cancer Treatment and Research Foundation.[92]

The benefits of computerized medical records are many, particularly if codification of diagnoses and treatments can be performed by the professional care provider, thus eliminating errors of translation now inherent when data are entered by coding clerks. When the interaction is made at the level of the care provider, all of the powerful features of computer memory and sorting ability are available to the individual most qualified to use them. Discrepancies between data entered and data previously acquired from patient cohorts can be made readily apparent. Completeness and accuracy of data should be enhanced. Less clerical work involving repetitive transcription and report collation, and more financial benefits due to fewer missing charges and improved cash flow, should result.[63] The major limiting factors appear to be the codification of diagnoses and physician acceptance and enthusiasm.

Decision-Making/Artificial Intelligence

> The underlying assumption that there is a well-defined, monolithic diagnostic process is almost certainly simplistic and fundamentally misleading.[10]

Decision-making regarding the care of an individual patient is the single area in which computer applications are most controversial. Diamond and colleagues[35] have noted the following relevant attributes of clinical decision-making: (1) lack of application of broader perspective to personal experience through ignorance of larger repositories of clinically relevant information; (2) hidden assumptions in decision-making that must be made explicit; (3) clinical decisions are made that do not appear consistent with reasonable or hidden assumptions.

When confronted with a patient who has a poorly characterized illness with a large differential diagnosis, the human mind is far superior to a computer in weighing the possibilities and eliminating the unlikely. Once the realm of clinical possibilities has been limited to a small subset, computerized decision-making supported by accurate data is far more efficient.[15,35] This is supported by the fact that 57 per cent of diagnostic errors are due to factors other than knowledge deficiencies.[17]

Computer-aided diagnosis of acute abdominal pain was successfully implemented in a multicenter trial. Initial diagnostic accuracy was raised from 45.6 per cent to 65.3 per cent, and the negative laparotomy rate was reduced by one half.[2] The overall accuracy of the diagnostic algorithm was 91.8 per cent.[32]

Cadenza, a microcomputer program based on Bayes' theorem, was developed to aid the physician in the interpretation of clinical data relative to the diagnosis and functional evaluation of coronary artery disease. Sensitivity and specificity estimates were derived from published medical experience encompassing over 60,000 patients.[34] Using this program, it was found that the higher the probability of disease, the greater the severity of angiographic disease. The program has been shown to be as effective as a cardiologist in the differential diagnosis of anginal pain.[58,156]

Numerous studies have shown that physicians are both intrigued and reluctant regarding computer assistance in decision-making.[35,78,84,132,133,151] In order to employ expert systems in diagnosis and management, it is imperative that the reasoning process used by the computer remain in full view of the physician at all times.[99] The method by which the computer makes the decision must be obvious and subject to "physician override."[48,102,152] Only in situations in which there is clear-cut and universal agreement (such as computation of a mean blood pressure from digital data describing an analog waveform) should the computer be allowed to manipulate data and present information without explanation or override capacity.

It has been found important that a computer application not attempt to alter the physician's thoughts about problems. The maintenance of the computer as "consultant" may enhance acceptance.[13] However, it is imperative that physicians using these aids be able to recognize that computers are not 100 per cent accurate.[69] The final requirement of a decision-making program is that it save the physician work.[151]

INHIBITORY FACTORS

Legal Considerations

A variety of medical-legal issues have arisen owing to the application of computers to patient care problems. Confidentiality is a broad issue that is not clearly defined for medical records even as they exist today.[18] Computer databases can be encrypted and protected by high levels of security. Such security can prevent access to the entire system or to selected subsets of the system according to privilege. Despite these capabilities, computer systems are generally regarded as being incapable of preventing determined access by unauthorized users. Progress in this area is required and can be anticipated.

Software designed to analyze patient data, to assist in medical diagnosis, and to advise in medical therapy can be expected to be less than 100 per cent accurate.[145] This leaves open the question of assignment of legal responsibility when an incorrect diagnosis or an unacceptable therapeutic result is attained.[109] The current tort system is likely to inhibit the growth of computer applications, particularly in the area of software design. Although numerous legal decisions have been rendered and, in general, software authors found to be strictly liable, this question has still not been answered completely.[1,19]

The Language of Medicine

The language of medicine must undergo several changes for the long-term success of computer implementation. An effort is under way at the National Library of Medicine (NLM) to create the Unified Medical Language System (UMLS) which incorporates features suitable for codification of the medical literature and reports of day-to-day care of patients.[104] Since the initial attempt to codify the medical literature in 1879 by John Shaw Billings, founder of the NLM, there have been two trends in this process.[83] The NLM, the American Society for Testing and Materials, and the American Association of Medical Systems and Informatics (AAMSI), in conjunction with practitioners of medical informatics, have attempted to structure the language of medicine to more easily translate medical terms into common denominators suitable for categorization.[41,42] The other trend, which has existed since the origin of medicine, has been driven by the perceived need of physicians and others to expand this vocabulary, thereby making it more descriptive, but at the same time more inaccessible. As a result of these two conflicting trends, an entire work force has been developed for the sole purpose of translating (codifying) medical information.

The problem is so large that many elements of the work force are involved in efforts that are highly redundant. For example, coding is performed in the NLM, in medical record departments for research purposes and for the assignment of diagnostic related groups (DRGs), in utilization review organizations, and in professional offices to assign fees for professional services. The overlap in effort is enormous, and the encoded information is not compatible.

The single largest difficulty in codification is the distance that separates the physician from the process. Codification procedures themselves are only recently becoming computerized and

then as an aid for trained encoders, not physicians. The protection of the physician from this effort is directly related to the lack of development of appropriate software to make physician encoding practical.[138] Direct physician encoding would greatly simplify the process and make it a self-correcting one. Physician encoding would ensure accuracy and timely availability of all medical information. This applies equally well at the level of individual patient care as to the indexing of the medical literature.

Academic Credit

Although the appropriate academic field has been defined as Medical Informatics since the early 1970s,[27] academic credit for software development is not yet a reality. This has tended to inhibit critically important physician participation in software development.

For over a decade, annual Symposia on Computer Applications in Medical Care (SCAMC) have been a major forum for this field. An analysis of the submissions in 1986 to this symposium[136] revealed a large degree of interest in artificial intelligence, systems and organizations, and database methods (Fig. 10). Clinical decision support and the development of computer-based medical records were predominant in the applications area (Fig. 11). Overall, 70 per cent of the submissions were in some way directed toward patient care or patient care facilities.[136]

Perceptions and Attitudes

Physician and nurse attitudes toward computer applications have served both as an impetus and as an inhibitor of their development. The situation can be expected to become more positive over time as health care professionals are exposed to computer applications through their training.[62] Whereas negative attitudes toward computer use in the past have been caused by premature implementations that caused more work without perceptible advantage, it is likely that current applications will have immediate and obvious advantages to users.

Numerous reviews of the subject of computer applications in patient care have demonstrated limited acceptance, particularly among practicing physicians.[142] When compared with residents, practicing physicians have evidenced concern about the potential effects of computers on their style of practice.[6] At the same time, physicians of a similar generation continue to complain of the mounting "data density" that is generated in current paper record processing.[4]

It has been shown that physicians who have intimate knowledge of computers are more likely to accept computer assistance in their practice.[5] It is clear that a physician entering practice

Medical Informatics Field

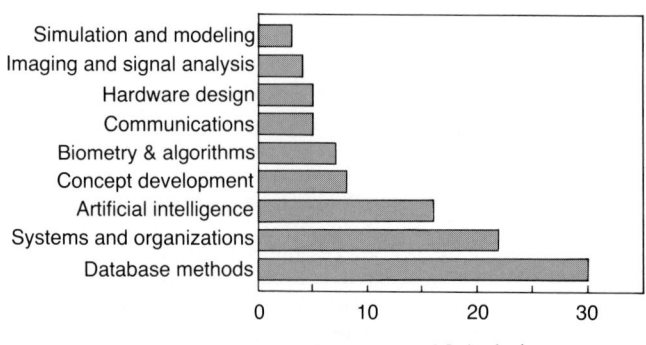

Figure 10. The number of separate submissions to the 11th SCAMC meeting, expressed as a percentage of total submissions and categorized according to major topics within the field of Medical Informatics. (From Stead, W. W.: A window on medical informatics. Proceedings, Symposium on Computer Applications in Medical Care, 1987, p. 3. © 1987 IEEE.

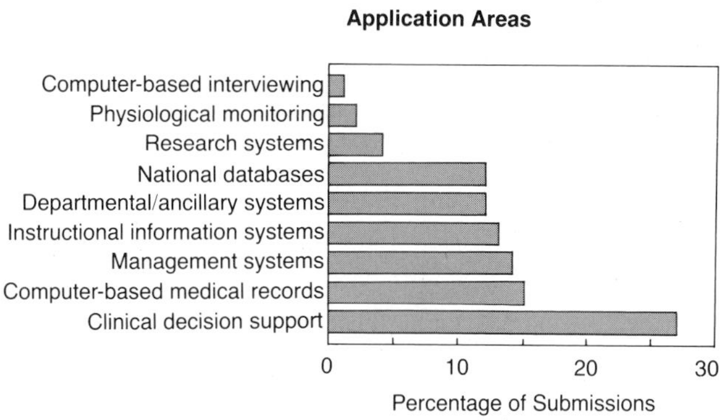

Application Areas

Computer-based interviewing
Physiological monitoring
Research systems
National databases
Departmental/ancillary systems
Instructional information systems
Management systems
Computer-based medical records
Clinical decision support

Percentage of Submissions

Figure 11. The number of articles submitted to the 11th SCAMC meeting, expressed as percentage of submissions, categorized according to the type of application area addressed by each article. (From Stead, W. W.: A window on medical informatics. Proceedings, Symposium on Computer Applications in Medical Care, 1987, p. 3. © IEEE.

today is more likely to have had formal education in computer programming and use, is more likely to own a personal computer, and is more likely to utilize a computer in practice. It is incumbent upon the profession to ensure that computer power at the bedside is available to this generation.

It is important that computer applications enhance rather than interfere with the physician's role as "chief architect" of patient management. The physician's judgment and autonomy should not be compromised, but augmented.[69,133] The issues of dehumanization, interference, and disruption of the doctor-patient relationship must be addressed.[67]

Funding Considerations

A final and extremely effective inhibitory factor is cost accountability. The financial benefits of "computerization" to the health care institution are distributed across traditional funding lines. Overall, the beneficiaries are not only the patients, but also physicians, nurses, other hospital employees, hospital administrators, insurance companies, granting agencies, and eventually the taxpayer. Each entity now tends to view computer applications with the narrow view of their area of interest, with a commensurate attitude toward partial funding. The development of an attitude of shared fiscal responsibility in advance of actual implementation is one that will be extremely difficult to cultivate. In the past, when computer costs were exorbitant and anticipated benefits subject to more rigid cost accounting procedures, this was an insurmountable problem. The current environment, with exponential increases of computer power accompanied by precipitous declines in hardware costs, should make shared fiscal responsibility a more realistic possibility. It is clear that the major costs of this development reside in the area of software development. Every effort should be made to foster such pursuits as both academic and proprietary achievements.

INTEGRATION OF DATA SOURCES

Potential Benefits of Computerization

The use of computers in hospital-wide applications can have a positive impact on the overall quality of care for all patients. At present, such applications are diverse and often use widely varying computer methods. They are not structured such that data flow and sharing are universal. Since a large proportion of hospital bed capacity and hospital income is related to surgical disease, the general management of these patients represents an attractive area in which to restructure these applications.

Utilization of Scarce Resources

The surgical patient utilizes a variety of scarce resources within the hospital. Not necessarily in the order of importance,

these include (1) physician time, (2) nursing time, (3) bed space, (4) investigational space, (5) operating room space, (6) laboratory resources, and (7) blood bank resources. In an era of cost-containment, efficiency of resource utilization is paramount. It is safe to say that in most hospitals the overall management of patients is dictated by a "check and balance" system, which essentially barters for resources on a first come–first served basis. Advance planning and scheduling are not the general situation, and communication between departments is inefficient and often obstructive.

The only attractive solution is to enroll individual patients in a centralized database from the time of first encounter to the time of discharge. Universal access to patient information at each step in the process by all individuals concerned would permit the development of scheduling algorithms that operate in near-real time and anticipate local needs. The central database would be periodically updated, thereby allowing all team members to adjust their schedules to fit changing needs. By permitting two-way communication with the database, physician requests, nursing requests, and patient needs can be globally communicated and addressed. By providing a time-oriented record of requests and response to services, overall resource utilization can be assessed in real time as well as in retrospect.

Communication

The presence and maintenance of the centralized database containing all relevant patient information are essential for efficient communication. For the most part, individuals need direct access to data. Communication with individuals is in reality a seeking of these data. By providing universal access to information electronically, interpersonal communication can be limited to that essential for decision-making. This process can be performed more efficiently if the individuals involved have equal and timely access to relevant information. Remote communication with the database would provide 24-hour access and would minimize interpersonal communication that crosses resource boundaries.

In no area is this more important than in the transition from hospitalization to home care. In surgical therapy, this eventually involves partial or complete transfer of the responsibility for patient care to another physician (the referring physician). As outlined previously, factual information transfer associated with discharge is currently in the form of the hospital discharge summary, a document with many serious limitations. An intermediate step in streamlining the process of communication is to generate the discharge summary from a computerized database. This would ensure quality and completeness of content and make the summary a timely one. The ultimate goal would be to supersede the printing of the discharge summary by providing direct access to the patient database for the referring physician and permitting query regarding all aspects of the patient's care.

Quality Assurance — Analyzed Results

It has been found that prospective assignment of risk is an effective method of quality assurance. SYN·OP·SYS is a computerized information system that is used for quality assurance and risk management and for meeting quality of care requirements for the Joint Commission Accreditation of Hospitals, PRO assessments, and liability concerns. It can also be used for institutional credentialing and cost-containment. This system was developed on a mainframe computer by the Medical Mutual Liability Insurance Society of Maryland. One important feature of this system is that it can organize occurrence data according to medical specialty.[143] There are many technical problems associated with the creation of large automated files of standards of compliance when such standards are treated as a hospital problem rather than as a specialty problem.[37]

Microcomputers have been used in infection control to provide surveillance of positive cultures. Because all data flow through a single point (the microbiology laboratory), accurate and complete case control is possible.[155] Moreover, statistical reports can be enumerated easily, and the hospital flora can be continually evaluated for the emergence of resistant strains or other unusual occurrences.

Quality control requires an extensive database to normalize morbidity and mortality and to enable identification of events outside of established norms.[120] In the surgical intensive care unit, an outcome score can be devised and converted to an outcome index to compare actual mortality with predicted mortality as a method of monitoring patient care.[44] It would appear that the fundamental problems in quality control issues relate to an inability to prospectively identify patient variables that can predict outcome and an incomplete ability to record these data in an ongoing manner to establish a normal-outcome database. It will be only through consistent, broad, and universal application of computer data collection that such norms will be established.

In the interim, reference to published statistics from large institutional studies remains the only standard available. In these situations, a relatively limited number of parameters have been recorded with which to define the control group. Comparisons are always subject to criticism regarding differences between the control patient population and that under study, and to differences in methods of patient enrollment and baseline characteristics.

In surgical patients, quality assurance is, in the main, an analysis of complications related to *patient selection* and *patient outcome*. In such a well-defined area, these complications can be defined prospectively. A centralized database containing salient features of a patient's diagnosis, evaluation, and treatment permits the analysis of individual outcome and comparison of this outcome to similar groups of patients. Potential outcomes are limited and can be predicted from preoperative diagnostic information and from operative procedural information. The prospective acquisition of a large demographic and medical database on each individual patient would allow the ability to clearly quantify the overall incidence and prevalence of any particular complication.

Administrative

The computerization of the operative schedule as well as operations performed provides many administrative functions inherent in the academic institution. It allows the divisional director to maintain an ongoing record of housestaff operative experience in order to ensure adequate training with minimal risk exposure. The categorization of departmental or divisional procedures provides important information regarding allocation of operating room facilities between various groups of operative surgeons.

The final administrative requirement is the development of cost-containment and marketing strategies related to preoperative diagnoses (leading to DRGs). When combined with outcome data and length of hospitalization, a positive feedback mechanism is provided to improve the overall financial status of the institution.[16]

INTEGRATION OF CURRENT TECHNOLOGY

The Local Workstation

The concept of distributed processing in local microcomputer workstations would provide immediate access to primary data regarding each patient at the bedside to the physician, nurse, or any health care provider.[117] The HIS could serve as the host computer. Distributed function of the Duke HIS is being implemented as MAPS (Micro-ADS Processing System).[71] Computer algorithms to address general problems would reside in the host computer, whereas algorithms related to specific groups of patients (i.e., general surgical patients only) would reside at the workstation level.

The patient database should reside in the host computer after data manipulation and entry at distributed stations. Therefore, the host computer would be responsible for maintaining the integrity of the overall database, considering such aspects as backup of information and disaster recovery. By structuring the system in this manner, data on individual patients can be preprocessed locally using specialized software to meet the specific needs of various users.

In the system envisioned, laboratory data would be entered into the hospital information system by the laboratory, downloaded to the workstation, and processed for display in a specially designed reporting format. The laboratory data could then be manipulated, reviewed, and compressed, and then returned to the individual patient's medical database on the HIS (separate from the patient's financial database). Another example of local entry would be the history and physical examination data, which would be entered at the bedside, processed, and uploaded to the HIS.

Through the use of such a system, any health care worker would have immediate access to all relevant information at the bedside. A reasonable goal for response time would be less than 1 second. Local data manipulations (for example, processing and display of physiologic waveforms) can be performed without burdening the HIS with excessive amounts of information.

The local workstation should be capable of display and manipulation of images. It should be incorporated in a local area network to allow the review of data on any patient from any workstation. The level of networking should be at the level of common care intensity and common service orientation. For instance, two local area networks would be necessary for surgery, one in the ICU and one at a ward having a lower level of care for either preoperative or predischarge patients. A number of shared peripheral devices would be supported by each network. These may include laser printers to generate hard copy information, modems to support remote communication (to physicians' offices or homes, or to national databases), and dedicated graphic monitors to display image results. Remote communication (from physicians' offices or homes) could be established through the local workstation network. The physician could access the patient database on the HIS to retrieve general information. More specific information could be gathered by a direct link to the bedside workstation, allowing access to more privileged information such as raw data or data manipulation results. Remote communication can logically be extended to include access for referring physicians to current inpatient data or to hospital-developed databases for informational purposes.

Microcomputers with faster response time, powerful local capabilities, superior "user-friendliness," and an increasing ability to be integrated into networks containing minicomputer and mainframe computers are likely to triumph as workstations in the fast-paced clinical environment.[95] The alternative solution of enlarging the HIS and adding terminals will likely fail because of poor response time for data retrieval and an inability to effectively develop software.

SELECTED REFERENCES

Angus, J. (Ed.): InfoWorld Consumer Product Guide. New York, Brady, 1989.
  This is a recent, comprehensive product guide that provides definitive ratings of personal computer hardware and software. It describes all the standard PCs and their clones and provides advice regarding speed, ease of use, and product support. Excellent sections on laser printers and video boards complement a comprehensive analysis of word processing and relational database software. This is an indispensable, up-to-date reference that can be used to guide decision-making at any level of sophistication.

Jelovsek, F. R., and Stead, W. W.: Computerized medical records. *In* Javitt, J. (Ed.): Computers in Medicine: Applications and Possibilities. Philadelphia, W. B. Saunders Company, 1986, p. 234.
  A recent review of progress toward computerizing the medical record. This article

summarizes the problems involved and offers many useful insights into the means by which they can be solved.

Maloney, J. V., Jr.: The trouble with patient monitoring. Ann. Surg., 168:605, 1968.
An early assessment of the impact of monitoring and computers on intensive care. Presented before the American Surgical Association in 1968, the discussion that follows this paper provides interesting insights into the thoughts of the time. The majority of comments have equal applicability to today's intensive care unit.

Pryor, D. B., Califf, R. M., Harrell, F. E., Jr., Hlatky, M. A., Lee, K. L., Mark, D. B., and Rosati, R. A.: Clinical data bases. Med. Care, 23:623, 1985.
An excellent review article describing clinical databases and their characteristics. This article contains a description of the Duke Data Bank for Cardiovascular Disease and comprehensive reviews of other available systems.

Sheppard, L. C., Kouchoukos, N. T., Kurtis, M. A., and Kirklin, J. W.: Automated treatment of critically ill patients following operation. Ann. Surg., 168:596, 1968.
The initial report of the continuous use of an automated intensive care unit monitoring system at the University of Alabama. In this report, the utility of this system in the management of 124 patients is described.

REFERENCES

1. Adams, E. S., and Gray, M. W.: Strict liability for the malfunction of a medical expert system. Proceedings, Symposium on Computer Applications in Medical Care, 1987, p. 93.
2. Adams, I. D., Chan, M., Clifford, P. C., Cooke, W. M., Dallos, V., de Dombal, F. T., et al.: Computer aided diagnosis of acute abdominal pain: A multicentre study. Br. Med. J., 293:800, 1986.
3. Allen, S. I., Johannes, R. S., Brown, C. S., Kafonek, D. R., and Plexico, P. S.: Prescription-writing with a PC. Proceedings IEEE, 1985, p. 54.
4. Anderson, B., Jr.: The "noisesome" hospital chart. N.C. Med. J., 49:105, 1988.
5. Anderson, J. G., Jay, S. J., Schweer, M. M., and Anderson, M. M.: Perceptions of the impact of computers on medical practice and physician use of a hospital information system. Proceedings IEEE, 1985, p. 565.
6. Anderson, J. G., Jay, S. J., Schweer, H. M., and Anderson, M. M.: Why doctors don't use computers: Some empirical findings. J. R. Soc. Med., 79:142, 1986.
7. Arnold, W. W., III, and King, S. S.: Recommendations for controlling costs in the university teaching hospital operating room. Perioper. Nurs. Q., 1:1, 1985.
8. Ball, M. J., Warnock-Matheron, A., and Hannah, K. J.: The case for using computers in the operating room. West. J. Med., 145:843, 1986.
9. Balzer, M. J.: Computerized systems for the OR. Management applications. AORN J., 43:187, 190, 193, 1986.
10. Barnett, G. O.: The computer and clinical judgment. N. Engl. J. Med., 307:493, 1982.
11. Barnett, G. O., Winickoff, R., Dorser, J. L., et al.: Communication: Quality assurance through automated monitoring and concurrent feedback using a computer-based medical information system. Med. Care. 16:962, 1978.
12. Bernier, C. L., and Yerkey, A. N. (Eds.): Cogent Communication: Overcoming Information Overload. Westport, Greenwood Press, 1979, p. 39.
13. Bleich, H. L.: The computer as a consultant. N. Engl. J. Med., 284:141, 1971.
14. Bleich, H. L., Jackson, J. D., and Rosenberg, H. A.: Paperchase: A program to search the medical literature. Proceedings IEEE, 1985, p. 595.
15. Blois, M. S.: Clinical judgment and computers. N. Engl. J. Med., 303:192, 1980.
16. Blum, B. I.: Clinical information systems—a review. West. J. Med., 145:791, 1986.
17. Bordage, G., and Allen, T.: The etiology of diagnostic errors: Process or content? An exploratory study. 21st Proceedings of Conference on Research in Medical Education, 1982.
18. Brannigan, V. M.: Patient privacy: A consumer protection approach. Proceedings IEEE, 1983, p. 648.
19. Brannigan, V.: The regulation of medical computer software as a "device" under the Food, Drug, and Cosmetic Act. Proceedings IEEE, 1986, p. 347.
20. Broering, N. C.: The miniMEDLINE System (TM) and the Library Information System. Proceedings IEEE, 1985, p. 601.
21. Brown, A. C.: Computer management of operating room time information with proposed standard definitions for the measurement of utilization. Symposium on Computer Applications in Medical Care (IEEE) 0195–4210, 1982, p. 246.
22. Burridge, P. W., and Skakun, E. N.: A computerized bedside clinical information system for an intensive care unit teaching service. Proceedings IEEE, 1983, p. 171.
23. Caceres, C. A., Steinberg, C. A., Abraham, S., Carbery, W. J., McBride, J. M., Tolles, W. E., and Rikli, A. E.: Computer extraction of electrocardiographic parameters. Circulation, 25:356, 1962.
24. Civetta, J. M.: Cardiopulmonary calculations: A rapid, simple and inexpensive technique. Intensive Care Med., 3:208, 1977.
25. Clayton, P. D., Delaplaine, K. H., Jensen, R. D., Bird, B., Evans, R. S., and Cannon, C. Y., III: Integration of surgery management and clinical information systems. Proceedings, Symposium on Computer Applications in Medical Care, 1987, p. 393.
26. Clochesy, J. M., and Henker, R. A.: Selecting computer software applications in critical care. Dimens. Crit. Care Nurs., 5:171, 1986.
27. Collen, M. F.: Origins of medical informatics. West. J. Med., 145:778, 1986.
28. Conser, C.: Transplant tracking. Data Based Advisor, September:114, 1989.
29. Crew, A. D., Stoodley, K. D. C., Old, S., Unsworth, W. N., and Kincaid, K.: A sampling study of bedside nursing activity in a cardiac surgical intensive care unit. Intensive Care Med., 13:119, 1987.
30. Cutting, C., Bookstein, F. L., Grayson, B., Fellingham, L., and McCarthy, J. G.: Three-dimensional computer-assisted design of craniofacial surgical procedures: Optimization and interaction with cephalometric and CT-based models. Plast. Reconstr. Surg., 77:877, 1986.
31. Dayhoff, R. E.: A medical image database system utilizing a write once optical disk. Proceedings, Symposium on Computer Applications in Medical Care, 1987, p. 549.
32. De Dombal, F. T., Leaper, D. J., Staniland, J. R., McCann, A. P., and Horrocks, J. C.: Computer-aided diagnosis of acute abdominal pain. Br. Med. J., 2:9, 1972.
33. Department of Clinical Epidemiology and Biostatistics, McMaster University Health Sciences Center: How to read clinical journals: I. Why to read them and how to start reading them critically. CMA J., 124:555, 1981.
34. Diamond, G. A., Staniloff, H. M., Forrester, J. S., Pollock, B. H., and Swan, H. J. C.: Computer assisted diagnosis in the noninvasive evaluation of patients with suspected coronary artery disease. J. Am. Coll. Cardiol. 1:444, 1983.
35. Diamond, G. A., Pollock, B. H., and Work, J. W.: Seminar on computer applications for the cardiologist. VI. Clinician decisions and computers. J. Am. Coll. Cardiol., 9:1385, 1987.
36. Diprose, G. K., Evans, D. H., and Levene, M. I.: A microcomputer monitoring and data-acquisition system for intensive care units. J. Med. Eng. Technol., 9:80, 1985.
37. Downey, J. E., Walczak, R. M., and Hohri, W. M.: Evaluating hospital compliance with the JCAH quality assurance standards. Proceedings IEEE, 1983, p. 94.
38. Edmunds, L. H., Jr., MacVaugh, H., III, Stevens, J., Wechsler, A. B., and Worthington, G. M.: Evaluation of computer-aided monitoring of patients after heart surgery. J. Thorac. Cardiovasc. Surg., 74:890, 1977.
39. Farrell, A. P., and Bruce, F.: Data acquisition and analysis of pulsatile signals using a personal computer: An application in cardiovascular physiology. Comput. Biol. Med., 17:151, 1987.
40. Feldman, M. D., Lowry, L. D., and Wisnicki, H. J.: Standardization of computer systems for logging operative cases. Arch. Otolaryngol. Head Neck Surg., 114:1178, 1988.
41. Gabrieli, E. R.: Standards for medical informatics. Proceedings, American Association for Medical Systems and Informatics Congress, 1989, p. 316.
42. Gabrieli, E. R.: A new biomedical nomenclature. Proceedings, American Association for Medical Systems and Informatics Congress, 1989, p. 336.
43. Gabrieli, E. R., and Speth, D. J.: Computer processing of discharge summaries. Proceedings, Symposium on Computer Applications in Medical Care, 1987, p. 137.
44. Gilbert, J., Schoolfield, J., and Gaydou, D.: Improved medical quality assurance in special care areas through computer management data collection. Proceedings, Symposium on Computer Applications in Medical Care, 1987, p. 662.
45. Glaeser, D. H., Trost, R. F., Brown, D. B., Kyle, A. C., Lenahan, M. S., Walker, C. K., Wilson, C. S., and DeBakey, M. E.: A hierarchical minicomputer system for continuous postsurgical monitoring. Comput. Biomed. Res., 8:336, 1975.
46. Goldwyn, R. M., Friedman, H. P., and Siegel, J. H.: Iteration and interaction in computer data bank analysis: A case study in the physiologic classification and assessment of the critically ill. Comput. Biomed. Res., 4:607, 1971.
47. Greenough, S. G.: Microcomputer program for the determination of haemodynamic indices using measurements obtained with a balloon-tipped pulmonary artery catheter. Eur. J. Anaesthesiol., 1:133, 1984.
48. Greenes, R. A., Pappalardo, A. N., Marble, C. W., et al.: Design and implementation of a clinical data management system. Comput. Biomed. Res., 2:469, 1969.
49. Halford, G., Pryor, T. A., and Burkes, M.: Measuring the impact of bedside terminals. Proceedings, Symposium on Computer Applications in Medical Care, 1987, p. 359.
50. Hammond, W. E., Stead, W. W., Straube, J. M., et al.: A clinical database management system. Policy Inform., 4:79, 1980.
51. Hammond, W. E., II, Stead, W. W., Straube, M. J., and Hammond, W. E., III: Adapting to the day to day growth of TMR. Proceedings, Seventh Annual Symposium on Computer Applications in Medical Care, 1983, p. 101.
52. Hammond, W. E., Stead, W. W., Straube, M. J., and Lutz, M.: TMR—Meeting the demand for the variety of report modalities. Proceedings, Symposium on Computer Applications in Medical Care, 1984, p. 421.
53. Hammond, W. E., and Stead, W. W.: The evolution of a computerized medical information system. Proceedings IEEE, 1986, p. 147.
54. Hammond, W. E., and Stead, W. W.: TLS—The Laboratory System: A networked patient care system and laboratory system. Proceedings, Symposium on Computer Applications in Medical Care, 1987, p. 778.
55. Hammond, W. E., Grewal, R., Straube, M. J., and Stead, W. W.: Networking data sources for intensive care monitoring. Proceedings, American Association for Medical Systems and Informatics Congress, 1989, p. 277.
56. Hanson, K. H.: Four years of computer assisted operating room scheduling.

Symposium on Computer Applications in Medical Care 0195–4210, 1982, p. 252.

57. Helsel, P., Smith, R. B., and Albin, M.: Computerized operating room information system. Proceedings, Seventh Annual Symposium on Computer Applications in Medical Care, 1983, p. 296.

58. Hlatky, M., Botvinick, E., and Brundage, B.: Diagnostic accuracy of cardiologists compared with probability calculations using Bayes' rule. Am. J. Cardiol., 49:1927, 1982.

59. Horn, S. D., and Sharkey, P. D.: Measuring severity of illness to predict patient resource use within DRGs. Inquiry, 20:314, 1983.

60. Huang, H. K.: Ten years progress in image processing technology related biomedical application. Proceedings IEEE, 1986, p. 203.

61. Jelovsek, F. R.: The Medical Record—session overview. Proceedings IEEE, 1983, p. 99.

62. Jelovsek, F. R.: Learning resources for medical computing. West. J. Med., 145:869, 1986.

63. Jelovsek, F. R., and Stead, W. W.: Computerized medical records. In Javitt, J. (Ed.): Computers in Medicine: Applications and Possibilities. Philadelphia, W. B. Saunders Company, 1986, p. 234.

64. Johnson, D. S., Burkes, J., Sittig, D., Hinson, D., and Pryor, T. A.: Evaluation of the effects of computerized nurse charting. Proceedings Symposium on Computer Applications in Medical Care, 1987, p. 363.

65. Jost, R. G., and Mankovich, N. J.: Digital archiving requirements and technology. Invest. Radiol., 23:808, 1988.

66. Jurado, R. A., Fitzkee, H. L., De Asla, R. A., Lukban, S. B., Litwak, R. S., and Osborn, J. J.: Reduction of unexpected, life-threatening events in postoperative cardiac surgical patients: The role of computerized surveillance. Circulation, 56(Suppl. 2):44, 1977.

67. Kaplan, B.: Barriers to medical computing: History, diagnosis, and therapy for the medical computing "lag." Proceedings IEEE, 1985, p. 400.

68. Kempczinski, R. F.: A microcomputer-based system for the management of vascular surgical references. J. Vasc. Surg., 6:542, 1987.

69. Kerr, C. P.: Computers in medicine. A Practitioner's comment. J.A.M.A., 249:2027, 1983.

70. Kievit, J.: Standardized diagnosis and treatment of fluid, acid-base and electrolyte disorders in the surgical patient with the aid of a programmable pocket calculator. Br. J. Surg., 70:282, 1983.

71. Kirby, J. D., Pickett, M. P., Boyarsky, M. W., and Stead, W. W.: Distributed processing with a mainframe-based hospital information system: A generalized solution. Proceedings, Symposium on Computer Applications in Medical Care, 1987, p. 764.

72. Klee, B. M., and Harris, R. B.: A microcomputer based pharmacy information system. Proceedings IEEE, 1985, p. 341.

73. Kootsey, J. M., Kohn, M. C., Feezar, M. D., Mitchell, G. R., and Fletcher, P. R.: SCoP: An interactive simulation control program for micro- and mini-computers. Bull. Math. Biol., 48:427, 1986.

74. Kouchoukos, N. T., Sheppard, L. C., McDonald, D. A., and Kirklin, J. W.: Estimation of stroke volume from the central arterial pressure contour in postoperative patients. Surg. Forum, 20:180, 1969.

75. Kouchoukos, N. T., Sheppard, L. C., and Kirklin, J. W.: Automated patient care following cardiac surgery. Cardiovasc. Clin., 3:109, 1971.

76. Kwon, I. W., Vogler, T. K., and Kim, J. H.: Computer utilization in health care. Proceedings, American Association for Medical Systems and Informatics Congress 83 (AAMSI: Bethesda, MD), 1983, p. 538.

77. Lamiell, J. M., and Wallis, J. G.: Computer-generated drug-dosing nomograms. Crit. Care Med., 16:1246, 1988.

78. Langlotz, C. P.: Advice generation in an axiomatically-based expert system. Proceedings, Symposium on Computer Applications in Medical Care, 1987, p. 49.

79. Lenhard, R., Jr., Patilla, J., Horbiak, P., Bergan, E., Tolchin, S., Volland, P., Weiner, M., Goldberg, H., and Achuff, S.: AUTRES: The Johns Hopkins Hospital automated clinical resume. Proceedings IEEE, 1985, p. 427.

80. Lewis, F. J., Shimizu, T., Scofield, A. L., and Rosi, P. S.: Analysis of respiration by an on-line digital computer system: Clinical data following thoracoabdominal surgery. Ann. Surg., 164:547, 1966.

81. Leyerle, B. J., Nolan-Avila, L. S., and Shabot, M. M.: Implementation of a comprehensive computerized ICU data management system. Proceedings IEEE, 1985, p. 386.

82. Lincoln, T. L., and Blume, P.: Laboratory medicine in the age of information. West. J. Med., 145:840, 1986.

83. Lindberg, D. A. B., and Schoolman, H. M.: The National Library of Medicine and Medical Informatics. West. J. Med., 145:786, 1986.

84. Long, W. J., Naimi, S., Criscitiello, M. G., and Jayes, R.: The development and use of a causal model for reasoning about heart failure. Proceedings Symposium on Computer Applications in Medical Care, 1987, p. 30.

85. Lowe, H. J., and Barnett, G. O.: MicroMeSH: A microcomputer system for searching and exploring the National Library of Medicine's medical subject headings (MeSH) vocabulary. Proceedings, Symposium on Computer Applications in Medical Care, 1987, p. 717.

86. MacModula-2: A Modula-2 development system for Apple Macintosh. Provo, Modula Corp., 1985.

87. Maloney, J. V., Jr.: The trouble with patient monitoring. Ann. Surg., 168:605, 1968.

88. Marino, P. L., and Krasner, J.: An interpretive computer program for analyzing hemodynamic problems in the ICU. Crit. Care Med., 12:601, 1984.

89. Martens, F., and Bertschat, F.: A BASIC program for calculation of often needed parameters in intensive care medicine. Comput. Biol. Med., 17:341, 1987.

90. Martin, J. B., Smith, R. F., Radoyevich, M., and Fichman, R. G.: Surgically-related applications of computerized operating room data. Surg. Gynecol. Obstet., 160:17, 1985.

91. Martin, L., and Jeffreys, B.: Microcomputers in intensive care. In Geisow, M. J., and Barrett, A. N. (Eds.): Microcomputers in Medicine. New York, Elsevier Science Publishers, 1987, p. 263.

92. Matte, W. B., and Murphy, B. A.: An automated progress note application. Proceedings IEEE, 1985, p. 431.

93. McColligan, E. E.: Operating room scheduling and utilization. Symposium on Computer Applications in Medical Care 0195–4210, 1982, p. 243.

94. McDonald, C. J.: Protocol-based computer reminders, the quality of care and the nonperfectability of man. N. Engl. J. Med., 295:1351, 1976.

95. McDonald, C. J., and Tierney, W. M.: The medical gopher—A microcomputer system to help find, organize and decide about patient data. West. J. Med., 145:823, 1986.

96. McGray, A. T., Sponsler, J. L., Brylawski, B., and Browne, A. C.: The role of lexical knowledge in biomedical text understanding. Proceedings, Symposium on Computer Applications in Medical Care, 1987, p. 103.

97. McMahon, L. F., Jr., and Newbold, R.: Variation in resource use within diagnosis-related groups. The effect of severity of illness and physician practice. Med. Care, 24:388, 1986.

98. Miller, J., Preston, T. D., Dann, P. E., Bailey, J. S., and Tobin, G.: Charting vs. computers in a postoperative cardiothoracic ITU. Nursing Times, August 24:1423, 1978.

99. Miller, R. A., Pople, H. E., Jr., and Meyers, J. D.: Internist-I, an experimental computer-based diagnostic consultant for general internal medicine. N. Engl. J. Med., 307:468, 1982.

100. Morin, J. E., Symes, J. F., Ralphs-Thibodeau, S., Tasse, S., Morin, A., Blanchard, G., and Lefebvre, C.: A microcomputer system for the practising cardiac surgeon. Can. J. Surg., 29:364, 1986.

101. Mortensen, J. D., and Anderson, L. H.: Clinical experiences with computerized monitoring of cardiovascular variables in the postoperative thoracic patient. J. Thorac. Cardiovasc. Surg., 56:510, 1968.

102. Moskowitz, A. J., and Pauker, S. G.: The decision to repair an abdominal aortic aneurysm in a patient with severe coronary artery disease. Proceedings IEEE, 1985, p. 212.

103. Muhlbaier, L. H., and Pryor, D. B.: Data for cardiovascular modeling. J. Am. Coll. Cardiol., 14:(3):60A, 1989.

104. National Library of Medicine Executive Summary, Long Range Plan, January 1987.

105. Nicholson, W. F., and Jelliffe, R. W.: "Smart" infusion apparatus for computation and automated delivery of loading, tapering, and maintenance infusion regimens of lidocaine, procainamide, and theophylline. Proceedings IEEE, 1983, p. 212.

106. Osborn, J. J., Beaumont, J. O., Raison, J. C. A., Russell, J., and Gerbode, F.: Measurement and monitoring of acutely ill patients by digital computer. Surgery, 64:1057, 1968.

107. Osborn, J. J., Beaumont, J. O., Raison, J. C. A., and Abbott, R. P.: Computation for quantitative on-line measurements in an intensive care ward. In Stacy, R. W., and Waxman, B. D. (Eds.): Computers in Biomedical Research. Vol. 3. New York, Academic Press, 1969, p. 207.

108. Peters, R. M.: Trivial pursuit or education? J. Thorac. Cardiovasc. Surg., 93:487, 1987.

109. Peterson, I.: A digital matter of life and death. Science News, 133:170, 1988.

110. Price, D. S.: The development and structure of the biomedical literature. Science News, 133:170, 1988.

111. Pryor, D. B., Califf, R. M., Harrell, F. E., Jr., Hlatky, M. A., Lee, K. L., Mark, D. B., and Rosati, R. A.: Clinical data bases. Med. Care, 23:623, 1985.

112. Robicsek, F., Masters, T. N., Reichertz, P. L., Daugherty, H. K., and Cook, J. W.: Three years experience with computer-based intensive care of patients following open heart and major vascular surgery. In Collected Works on Cardiopulmonary Disease. Vol. 21. Charlotte, N.C., The Heineman Medical Research Center, 1977, p. 48.

113. Robinson, L.: Computers to the OR . . . stat! Today's OR Nurse, 7:29, 32, 36, 1985.

114. Rypins, E. B., Khan, F., Collins-Irby, D., Sarfeh, I. J., Ashurst, J. T., and Stemmer, E. A.: Computer-derived equations for predicting survival postoperatively. Their usefulness and limitations. Arch. Surg., 123:354, 1988.

115. Schaber, D. C., and Carangio, F. C.: A simplified computer program for the performance of physiological calculations from cardiac catheterization data. Cleve. Clin. Q., 52:47, 1985.

116. Schneider, A. J.: Assessment of risk factors and surgical outcome. Surg. Clin. North Am., 63:1113, 1983.

117. Schneider, M., Tolchin, S. G., Kahane, S. N., Goldberg, H. S., and Barta, P.: A workstation-based inpatient clinical system in the Johns Hopkins Hospital. Proceedings IEEE, 1985, p. 388.

118. Seifert, S. A.: Computer-aided prescribing of aminoglycosides: Bedside determination of volume of distribution and elimination rate constant. Proceedings IEEE, 1985, p. 103.

119. Shabot, M. M., Carlton, P. D., Sadoff, S., and Nolan-Avila, L.: Graphical reports and displays for complex ICU data: A new, flexible and configurable method. Comput. Methods Programs Biomed., 22:111, 1986.

120. Shabot, M. M., LoBue, M., and Leyerle, B. J.: Use of automatic computerized intensity-intervention scores to measure the appropriateness of ICU utiliza-

tion. Proceedings, Symposium on Computer Applications in Medical Care, 1987, p. 671.

121. Shabot, M. M., Leyerle, B. J., and LoBue, M.: Automatic extraction of intensity-intervention scores from a computerized surgical intensive care unit flowsheet. Am. J. Surg., 154:72, 1987.

122. Sheppard, L. C.: Computer control of the infusion of vasoactive drugs. Ann. Biomed. Eng., 8:431, 1980.

123. Sheppard, L. C.: Computer control of blood and drug infusions in patients following cardiac surgery. J. Biomed. Eng., 2:83, 1980.

124. Sheppard, L. C.: Computer based clinical systems: Automation and integration. 39th Annual Conference in Engineering and Medicine in Biology, September 1986, p. 73.

125. Sheppard, L. C., Kouchoukos, N. T., Kurtis, M. A., and Kirklin, J. W.: Automated treatment of critically ill patients following operation. Ann. Surg., 168:596, 1968.

126. Sheppard, L. C., Kirklin, J. W., and Kouchoukos, N. T.: Computer-controlled interventions for the acutely ill patient. In Stacy, R. W., and Waxman, B. D. (Eds.): Computers in Biomedical Research. Vol. 4. New York, Academic Press, 1974, p. 135.

127. Sheppard, L. C., and Kouchoukos, N. T.: Automation of measurements and interventions in the systematic care of postoperative cardiac surgical patients. Med. Instrum., 11:296, 1977.

128. Sheppard, L. C., and Sayers, B. McA.: Dynamic analysis of the blood pressure response to hypotensive agents, studied in postoperative cardiac surgical patients. Comput. Biomed. Res., 10:237, 1977.

129. Shubin, H., and Weil, M. H.: Efficient monitoring with a digital computer of cardiovascular function in seriously ill patients. Ann. Intern. Med., 65:453, 1966.

130. Shubin, H., Weil, M. H., Palley, N., and Afifi, A. A.: Monitoring the critically ill patient with the aid of a digital computer. Comput. Biomed. Res., 4:460, 1971.

131. Siegel, J. H., Greenspan, M., Coh, J. D., and Del Guercio, L. R. M.: A bedside computer and physiologic nomograms. Arch. Surg., 97:480, 1968.

132. Siegel, J. H., and Strom, B. L.: An automated consultation system to aid the physician in the care of the desperately sick patient. In Stacy, R. W., and Waxman, B. D. (Eds.): Computers in Biomedical Research. Vol. 4. New York, Academic Press, 1974, p. 115.

133. Singer, J., Sacks, H. S., Lucente, F., and Chalmers, T. C.: Physician attitudes toward applications of computer data base systems. J.A.M.A., 249:1610, 1983.

134. Skaredoff, M. N.: Thorax—a program to assist in the preoperative risk assessment of patients undergoing thoracic surgery. Int. J. Clin. Monit. Comput. 3:245, 1986.

135. Smith, P. K., Dermer, M., Pickett, M., and Yaggy, D.: Implementation of a microcomputer operating room database. Proceedings, American Association for Medical Systems and Informatics, 1989, p. 204.

136. Stead, W. W.: A window on medical informatics. Proceedings, Symposium on Computer Applications in Medical Care, 1987, p. 3.

137. Stead, W. W., and Hammond, W. E.: Functions required to allow TMR to support the information requirements of a hospital. Proceedings, Seventh Annual Symposium on Computer Applications in Medical Care, 1983, p. 106.

138. Stead, W. W., Hammond, W. E., and Straube, M. J.: A chartless record—is it adequate? J. Med. Syst., 7:103, 1983.

139. Stead, W. W., Garrett, L. E., Jr., and Hammond, W. E.: Practicing nephrology with a computerized medical record. Kidney Int., 24:446, 1983.

140. Stead, W. W., and Hammond, W. E.: Demand-oriented medical records: Toward a physician work station. Proceedings, Symposium on Computer Applications in Medical Care, 1987, p. 275.

141. Stoodley, K. D., Crew, A. D., Lu, R., and Naghdy, F.: A microcomputer implementation of status and alarm algorithms in a cardiac surgical intensive care unit. Int. J. Clin. Monit. Comput., 4:115, 1987.

142. Teach, R. L., and Shortliffe, E. H.: An analysis of physician attitudes regarding computer-based clinical consultation systems. Comput. Biomed. Res., 14:542, 1981.

143. Thomas, D. J., Weiner, J., and Lippincott, R. C.: SYN·OP·SYS. A computerized management information system for quality assurance and risk management. Proceedings IEEE, 1985, p. 864.

144. Underhill, L. H., and Bleich, H. L.: Bringing the medical literature to physicians. West. J. Med., 145:853, 1986.

145. Victoroff, M. S.: Ethical report systems. Proceedings IEEE, 1985, p. 644.

146. Wagner, D. P., Knaus, W. A., and Draper, E. A.: Statistical validation of a severity of illness measure. Am. J. Public Health, 73:878, 1983.

147. Waki, R., Clayton, P. D., Jensen, R. L., et al.: HELP-based decision analysis applied to coronary artery disease. Comput. Biomed. Res., 15:188, 1982.

148. Warner, H. R., Gardner, R. M., and Toronto, A. F.: Computer-based monitoring of cardiovascular functions in postoperative patients. Circulation, 37(Suppl. 2):68, 1968.

149. Watson, R. J.: Medical staff response to a medical information system with direct physician-computer interface. In Anderson, J., and Forsythe, J. M. (Eds.): Medinfo 74. Oxford, North-Holland Publications. 1974, p. 299.

150. Watson, B. G., Elliott, M. J., Pay, D. A., and Williamson, M.: Diabetes mellitus and open heart surgery. Anaesthesia, 41:250, 1986.

151. Weaver, R. R.: Editorial Comments, 1974–1986: The case for and against the use of computer-assisted decision making. Proceedings, Symposium on Computer Applications in Medical Care, 1987, p. 143.

152. Weed, L. L., Hertzberg, R. Y., and Weed, C.: Construction and use of knowledge couplers and networks and a POMR on a personal computer. Proceedings IEEE, 1985, p. 600.

153. Weintraub, W. S., Jones, E. L., Craver, J., Guyton, R., and Cohen, C.: Determinants of prolonged length of hospital stay after coronary bypass surgery. Circulation, 80:276, 1989.

154. Wind, G., Dvorak, V. K., and Dvorak, J. A.: Computer graphic modeling in surgery. Orthop. Clin. North Am., 17:657, 1986.

155. Wise, W. S.: Microcomputers in infection control. In Geisow, M. J., and Barrett, A. N. (Eds.): Microcomputers in Medicine. New York, Elsevier Science Publishers, 1987, p. 115.

156. Wong, D. F., Tibbits, P., O'Donnell, J., et al.: Computer-assisted Bayesian analysis in the diagnosis of coronary artery disease (abstract). J. Nucl. Med., 23:P83, 1982.

Appendix

LABORATORY REFERENCE VALUES OF CLINICAL IMPORTANCE

Rex B. Conn, M.D.

REFERENCE VALUES IN HEMATOLOGY

	Percentage	Conventional Units	S.I. Units
Acid hemolysis test (Ham)		No hemolysis	No hemolysis
Alkaline phosphatase, leukocyte		Total score 14–100	Total score 14–100
Cell counts			
Erythrocytes			
Males		4.6–6.2 million/cu. mm.	$4.6–6.2 \times 10^{12}$/L.
Females		4.2–5.4 million/cu. mm.	$4.2–5.4 \times 10^{12}$/L.
Children (varies with age)		4.5–5.1 million/cu. mm.	$4.5–5.1 \times 10^{12}$/L.
Leukocytes, total		4500–11,000/cu. mm.	$4.5–11.0 \times 10^{9}$/L.
Leukocytes, differential	*Percentage*	*Absolute*	*Absolute*
Myelocytes	0	0/cu. mm.	0/L.
Band neutrophils	3–5	150–400/cu. mm.	$150–400 \times 10^{6}$/L.
Segmented neutrophils	54–62	3000–5800/cu. mm.	$3000–5800 \times 10^{6}$/L.
Lymphocytes	25–33	1500–3000/cu. mm.	$1500–3000 \times 10^{6}$/L.
Monocytes	3–7	300–500/cu. mm.	$300–500 \times 10^{6}$/L.
Eosinophils	1–3	50–250/cu. mm.	$50–250 \times 10^{6}$/L.
Basophils	0–0.75	15–50/cu. mm.	$15–50 \times 10^{6}$/L.
Platelets		150,000–350,000/cu. mm.	$150–350 \times 10^{9}$/L.
Reticulocytes		25,000–75,000/cu. mm.	$25–75 \times 10^{9}$/L.
		0.5–1.5% of erythrocytes	
Coagulation tests			
Bleeding time (template)		2.75–8.0 min.	2.75–8.0 min.
Coagulation time (glass tubes)		5–15 min.	5–15 min.
Factor VIII and other coagulation factors		50–150% of normal	0.5–1.5% of normal
Fibrin split products (Thrombo-Welco test)		<10 μg./ml.	<10 mg./L.
Fibrinogen		200–400 mg./dl.	2.0–4.0 gm./L.
Partial thromboplastin time (PTT)		20–35 sec.	20–35 sec.
Prothrombin time (PT)		12.0–14.0 sec.	12.0–14.0 sec.
Coombs' test			
Direct		Negative	Negative
Indirect		Negative	Negative
Corpuscular values of erythrocytes			
Mean corpuscular hemoglobin (MCH)		26–34 pg.	0.40–0.53 fmol.
Mean corpuscular volume (MCV)		80–96 cu. micra	80–96 fl.
Mean corpuscular hemoglobin concentration (MCHC)		32–36%	0.32–0.36
Haptoglobin		26–185 mg./dl.	260–1850 mg./L.
Hematocrit			
Males		40–54 ml./dl.	0.40–0.54
Females		37–47 ml./dl.	0.37–0.47
Newborn		49–54 ml./dl.	0.49–0.54
Children (varies with age)		35–49 ml./dl.	0.35–0.49
Hemoglobin			
Males		14.0–18.0 gm./dl.	2.17–2.79 mmol./L.
Females		12.0–16.0 gm./dl.	1.86–2.48 mmol./L.
Newborn		16.5–19.5 gm./dl.	2.56–3.02 mmol./L.
Children (varies with age)		11.2–16.5 gm./dl.	1.74–2.56 mmol./L.
Hemoglobin, fetal		<1.0% of total	<0.01 of total
Hemoglobin A_{1C}		3–5% of total	0.03–0.05 of total
Hemoglobin A_2		1.5–3.0% of total	0.015–0.03 of total
Hemoglobin, plasma		0–5.0 mg./dl.	0–0.8 μmol./L.
Methemoglobin		30–130 mg./dl.	4.7–20 μmol./L.

REFERENCE VALUES IN HEMATOLOGY *Continued*

	Conventional Units	S.I. Units
Sedimentation rate (ESR)		
Wintrobe, Males	0–5 mm./hr.	0–5 mm./h.
Females	0–15 mm./hr.	0–15 mm./h.
Westergren, Males	0–15 mm./hr.	0/15 mm./h.
Females	0–20 mm./hr.	0–20 mm./h.

REFERENCE VALUES FOR BLOOD, PLASMA, AND SERUM
(For some procedures, the reference values may vary depending on the method used.)

	Conventional Units	S.I. Units
Acetoacetate plus acetone		
Qualitative	Negative	Negative
Quantitative	0.3–2.0 mg./dl.	3–20 mg./L.
Acid phosphatase, serum	0.11–0.60 unit/L.	0.11–0.60 unit/L.
(Thymolphthalein monophosphate substrate)		
Adrenocorticotropin, plasma (ACTH)		
6:00 A.M.	10–80 pg./ml.	10–80 ng./L.
6:00 P.M.	<50 pg./ml.	<50 ng./L.
Alanine aminotransferase, serum (ALT, SGPT)	7–40 units/L.	7–40 units/L.
Albumin, serum	3.5–5.5 gm./dl.	35–55 gm./L.
Aldolase, serum	1.5–12.0 units/L.	1.5–12.0 units/L.
Aldosterone, plasma		
Supine	3–10 ng./dl.	0.08–0.30 nmol/L.
Standing		
Male	6–22 ng./dl.	0.17–0.61 nmol./L.
Female	5–30 ng./dl.	0.14–0.83 nmol./L.
Alkaline phosphatase, serum (ALP)	20–90 units/L. (30° C.)	20–90 units/L. (30° C.)
Ammonia nitrogen, plasma	15–49 μg./dl.	11–35 μmol./L.
Amylase, serum	25–125 units/L.	25–125 units/L.
Anion gap	8–16 mEq./L.	8–16 mmol./L.
Ascorbic acid, blood	0.4–1.5 mg./dl.	23–85 μmol./L.
Aspartate aminotransferase, serum (AST, SGOT)	7–40 units/L.	7–40 units/L.
Base excess, blood	0 ± 2 mEq./L.	0 ± 2 mmol./L.
Bicarbonate, venous plasma	23–29 mEq./L.	23–29 mmol./L.
arterial blood	18–23 mEq./L.	18–23 mmol./L.
Bile acids, serum	0.3–3.0 mg./dl.	3–30 mg./L.
Bilirubin, serum		
Conjugated	0.1–0.4 mg./dl.	1.7–6.8 μmol./L.
Unconjugated	0.2–0.7 mg./dl.	3.4–12 μmol./L.
Total	0.3–1.1 mg./dl.	5.1–19 μmol./L.
Calcium, serum	9.0–11.0 mg./dl.	2.25–2.75 mmol./L.
Calcium, ionized, serum	4.25–5.25 mg./dl.	1.05–1.30 mmol./L.
Carbon dioxide, total, serum or plasma	24–30 mEq./L.	24–30 mmol./L.
Carbon dioxide tension, blood, (P_{CO_2})	35–45 mm. Hg	35–45 mm. Hg
β-Carotene, serum	40–200 μg./dl.	0.74–3.72 μmol./L.
Ceruloplasmin, serum	23–44 mg./dl.	230–440 mg./L.
Chloride, serum or plasma	96–106 mEq./L.	96–106 mmol./L.
Cholesterol, serum or EDTA plasma		
Desirable range	<200 mg./dl.	<5.18 mmol./L.
LDL Cholesterol	60–180 mg./dl.	600–1800 mg./L.
HDL Cholesterol	30–80 mg./dl.	300–800 mg./L.
Copper		
Males	70–140 μg./dl.	11–22 μmol./L.
Females	85–155 μg./dl.	13–24 μmol./L.
Cortisol, plasma		
8:00 A.M.	6–23 μg./dl.	170–635 nmol./L.
4:00 P.M.	3–15 μg./dl.	82–413 nmol./L.
10:00 P.M.	<50% of 8 A.M. value	<0.5 of 8 A.M. value
Creatine, serum	0.2–0.8 mg./dl.	15–61 μmol./L.
Creatine kinase, serum (CK, CPK)		
Males	55–170 units/L.	55–170 units/L.
Females	30–135 units/L.	30–135 units/L.
Creatine kinase MB isoenzyme, serum	0.0–4.7 ng./ml.	0.0–4.7 μg./L.
Creatinine, serum	0.6–1.2 mg./dl.	53–106 μmol./L.

Table continued on following page

REFERENCE VALUES FOR BLOOD, PLASMA, AND SERUM *Continued*

	Conventional Units	S.I. Units
Ferritin, serum	20–200 ng./ml.	20–200 μg./L.
Fibrinogen, plasma	200–400 mg./dl.	2.0–4.0 gm./L.
Folate, serum	1.8–9.0 ng./ml.	4.1–20.4 nmol./L.
erythrocytes	150–450 ng./ml.	340–1020 nmol./L.
Follicle-stimulating hormone, plasma (FSH)		
Males	4–25 milliunits/ml.	4–25 units/L.
Females	4–30 milliunits/ml.	4–30 units/L.
Postmenopausal	40–250 milliunits/ml.	40–250 units/L.
γ-Glutamyltransferase, serum		
Male	5–38 units/L.	5–38 units/L.
Female	5–29 units/L	5–29 units/L.
Gastrin, serum	0–200 pg./ml.	0–200 ng./L.
Glucose (fasting), plasma or serum	70–115 mg./dl.	3.89–6.38 mmol./L.
Growth hormone, plasma (hGH)	0–10 ng./ml.	0–10 μg./L.
Haptoglobin, serum	26–185 mg./dl.	260–1850 mg./L.
Immunoglobulins, serum		
IgG	550–1900 mg./dl.	5.5–19.0 gm./L.
IgA	60–333 mg./dl.	0.60–3.3 gm./L.
IgM	45–145 mg./dl.	0.45–1.5 gm./L.
IgD	0.5–3.0 mg./dl.	5–30 mg./L.
IgE	<500 ng./ml.	<500 μg./L.
Insulin (fasting), plasma	5–25 microunits/ml.	36–179 pmol./L.
Iron, serum	75–175 μg./dl.	13–31 μmol./L.
Iron binding capacity, serum		
Total	250–410 μg./dl.	45–73 μmol./L.
Saturation	20–55%	0.20–0.55
Lactate, venous blood	4.5–19.8 mg./dl.	0.50–2.2 mmol./L.
arterial blood	4.5–14.4 mg./dl.	0.50–1.6 mmol./L.
Lactate dehydrogenase, serum (LD,LDH)	100–190 units/L.	100–190 units/L.
Lipase, serum	10–140 units/L.	10–140 units/L.
Lipids, total, serum	450–850 mg./dl.	4.5–8.5 gm./L.
Luteinizing hormone, serum (LH)		
Males	6–18 IU/L.	6–18 units/L.
Females, premenopausal	5–22 IU/L.	5–22 units/L.
midcycle	3 times baseline	3 times baseline
postmenopausal	>30 IU/L.	>30 units/L.
Magnesium, serum	1.8–3.0 mg./dl.	0.75–1.25 mmol./L.
Osmolality	286–295 mOsm./kg. water	285–295 mOsm./kg. water
Oxygen, blood		
Capacity (varies with hemoglobin)	16–24 vol. %	7.14–10.7 mmol./L.
Content, arterial	15–23 vol. %	6.69–10.3 mmol./L.
Saturation, arterial	94–100%	0.94–1.00
Tension, Po_2	75–100 mm. Hg	75–100 mm. Hg
P_{50}	26–27 mm. Hg	26–27 mm. Hg
pH, arterial blood	7.35–7.45	7.35–7.45
Phenylalanine, serum	<3 mg./dl.	<0.18 mmol./L.
Phosphate, inorganic, serum	3.0–4.5 mg./dl.	1.0–1.5 mmol./L.
Potassium, serum or plasma	3.5–5.0 mEq./L.	3.5–5.0 mmol./L.
Prolactin, serum		
Males	1–20 ng./ml.	1–20 μg./L.
Females	1–25 ng./ml.	1–25 μg./L.
Protein, serum		
Total	6.0–8.0 gm./dl.	60–80 gm./L.
Albumin	3.5–5.5 gm./dl.	35–55 gm./L.
Alpha$_1$-globulin	0.2–0.4 gm./dl.	2–4 gm./L.
Alpha$_2$-globulin	0.5–0.9 gm./dl.	5–9 gm./L.
Beta-globulin	0.6–1.1 gm./dl.	6–11 gm./L.
Gamma-globulin	0.7–1.7 gm./dl.	7–17 gm./L.
Pyruvate, blood	0.3–0.9 mg./dl.	0.03–0.10 mmol./L.
Sodium, serum or plasma	136–145 mEq./L.	136–145 mmol./L.
Testosterone, plasma		
Males	275–875 ng./dl.	9.5–30 nmol./L.
Females	23–75 ng./dl.	0.8–2.6 nmol./L.
Pregnant	38–190 ng./dl.	1.3–6.6 nmol./L.
Thyroid-stimulating hormone, serum (TSH)	0–7 microunits/ml.	0–7 milliunits/L.
Thyroxine, free, serum (FT$_4$)	1.0–2.1 ng./dl.	13–27 pmol./L.
Thyroxine, serum (T$_4$)	4.4–9.9 μg./dl.	57–128 nmol./L.
Triglycerides, serum	40–150 mg./dl.	0.4–1.5 gm./L.
Triiodothyronine, serum (T$_3$)	150–250 ng./dl.	2.3–3.9 nmol./L.
Triiodothyronine uptake, resin (T$_3$ RU)	25–38% uptake	0.25–0.38 uptake

REFERENCE VALUES FOR BLOOD, PLASMA, AND SERUM *Continued*

	Conventional Units	S.I. Units
Urate		
Males	2.5–8.0 mg./dl.	0.15–0.48 mmol./L.
Females	1.5–7.0 mg./dl.	0.09–0.42 mmol./L.
Urea, serum or plasma	24–49 mg./dl.	4.0–8.3 mmol./L.
Urea nitrogen, serum or plasma	11–23 mg./dl.	3.9–8.2 mmol./L.
Viscosity, serum	1.4–1.8 × water	1.4–1.8 × water
Vitamin A, serum	20–80 μg./dl.	0.70–2.80 μmol./L.
Vitamin B_{12}, serum	180–900 pg./ml.	133–664 pmol./L.

REFERENCE VALUES FOR URINE
(For some procedures, the reference values may vary depending on the method used.)

	Conventional Units	S.I. Units
Acetone and acetoacetate, qualitative	Negative	Negative
Albumin		
Qualitative	Negative	Negative
Quantitative	10–100 mg./24 hr.	0.15–1.5 μmol./24 h.
Aldosterone	3–20 μg./24 hr.	8.3–55 nmol./24 h.
δ-Aminolevulinic acid	1.3–7.0 mg./24 hr.	10–53 μmol./24 h.
Amylase	3–20 units/hr.	3–20 units/h.
Amylase : creatinine clearance ratio	1–4%	0.01–0.04
Bilirubin, qualitative	Negative	Negative
Calcium (usual diet)	<250 mg./24 hr.	<6.3 mmol./24 h.
Catecholamines		
Epinephrine	<10 μg./24 hr.	<55 nmol./24 h.
Norepinephrine	<100 μg./24 hr.	<590 nmol./24 h.
Total free catecholamines	4–126 μg./24 hr.	24–745 nmol./24 h.
Total metanephrines	0.1–1.6 mg./24 hr.	0.5–8.1 μmol./24 h.
Chloride (varies with intake)	110–250 mEq./24 hr.	110–250 mmol./24 h.
Copper	0–50 μg./24 hr.	0–0.80 μmol./24 h.
Cortisol, free	10–100 μg./24 hr.	27.6–276 nmol./24 h.
Creatinine	15–25 mg./kg. body weight/24 hr.	0.13–0.22 mmol./kg. body weight/24 h.
Creatinine clearance (corrected to 1.73 sq. m.² body surface area)		
Males	110–150 ml./min.	110–150 ml./min.
Females	105–132 ml./min.	105–150 ml./min.
Dehydroepiandrosterone		
Males	0.2–2.0 mg./24 hr.	0.7–6.9 μmol./24 h.
Females	0.2–1.8 mg./24 hr.	0.7–6.2 μmol./24 h.
Estrogens, total		
Males	4–25 μg./24 hr.	14–90 nmol./24 h.
Females	5–100 23 gm./24 hr.	18–360 nmol./24 h.
Glucose (as reducing substance)	<250 mg./24 hr.	<250 mg./24 h.
Hemoglobin and myoglobin, qualitative	Negative	Negative
17-Hydroxycorticosteroids		
Males	3–9 mg./24 hr.	8.3–25 μmol./24 h.
Females	2–8 mg./24 hr.	5.5–22 μmol./24 h.
5-Hydroxyindole acetic acid		
Qualitative	Negative	Negative
Quantitative	<9 mg./24 hr.	<47 μmol./24 h.
17-Ketosteroids		
Males	6–18 mg./24 hr.	21–62 μmol./24 h.
Females	4–13 mg./24 hr.	14–45 μmol./24 h.
Magnesium	6.0–8.5 mEq./24 hr.	3.0–4.2 mmol./24 h.
Metanephrines (see Catecholamines)		
Osmolality	38–1400 mOsm./kg. water	38–1400 mmol./kg. water
pH	4.6–8.0	4.6–8.0
Phenylpyruvic acid, qualitative	Negative	Negative
Phosphate	0.9–1.3 gm./24 hr.	29–42 mmol./24 h.
Porphobilinogen		
Qualitative	Negative	Negative
Quantitative	<2.0 mg./24 hr.	<9 μmol./24 h.

Table continued on following page

REFERENCE VALUES FOR URINE *Continued*

	Conventional Units	S.I. Units
Porphyrins		
Coproporphyrin	50–250 µg./24 hr.	77–380 nmol./24 h.
Uroporphyrin	10–30 µg./24 hr.	12–36 nmol./24 h.
Potassium	25–100 mEq./24 hr.	25–100 mmol./24 h.
Pregnanediol		
Males	0.4–1.4 mg./24 hr.	1.2–4.4 µmol./24 h.
Females, proliferative phase	0.5–1.5 mg./24 hr.	1.6–4.7 µmol./24 h.
luteal phase	2.0–7.0 mg./24 hr.	6.2–22 µmol./24 h.
postmenopausal	0.2–1.0 mg./24 hr.	0.6–3.1 µmol./24 h.
Pregnanetriol	<2.5 mg./24 hr.	<7.4 µmol./24 h.
Protein		
Qualitative	Negative	Negative
Quantitative	10–150 mg./24 hr.	10–150 mg./24 h.
Sodium	130–260 mEq./24 hr.	130–260 mmol./24 h.
Specific gravity	1.003–1.030	1.003–1.030
Urate	200–500 mg./24 hr.	1.2–3.0 mmol./24 h.
Urobilinogen	<4.0 mg./24 hr.	<6.8 µmol./24 h.
Vanillylmandelic acid (VMA)	1–8 mg./24 hr.	5–40 µmol./24 h.
(4-hydroxy-3-methoxymandelic acid)		

REFERENCE VALUES FOR THERAPEUTIC DRUG MONITORING

	Therapeutic Range	Toxic Levels	Proprietary Names
Antibiotics			
Amikacin, serum	25–30 µg./ml.	Peak >35 µg./ml.	Amikin
		Trough >5–7 µg./ml.	
Chloramphenicol, serum	10–20 µg./ml.	>25 µg./ml.	Chloromycetin
Gentamicin, serum	5–10 µg./ml.	Peak >12 µg./ml.	Garamycin
		Trough >2 µg./ml.	
Tobramycin, serum	5–10 µg./ml.	Peak >12 µg./ml.	Nebcin
		Trough >2 µg./ml.	
Anticonvulsants			
Carbamazepine, serum	5–12 µg./ml.	>12 µg./ml.	Tegretol
Ethosuximide, serum	40–100 µg./ml.	>100 µg./ml.	Zarontin
Phenobarbital, serum	10–30 µg./ml.	Vary widely because of developed tolerance	
Phenytoin, serum	10–20 µg./ml.	>20 µg./ml.	Dilantin
Primidone, serum	5–12 µg./ml.	>15 µg./ml.	Mysoline
Valproic acid, serum	50–100 µg./ml.	>100 µg./ml.	Depakene
Analgesics			
Acetaminophen, serum	10–20 µg./ml.	>250 µg./ml.	Tylenol
			Datril
Salicylate, serum	100–250 µg./ml.	>300 µg./ml.	
Bronchodilator			
Theophylline, serum	10–20 µg./ml.	>20 µg./ml.	
(aminophylline)			
Cardiovascular Drugs			
Digitoxin, serum	15–25 ng./ml.	>25 ng./ml.	Crystodigin
(specimen must be obtained 12–24 hours after last dose)			
Digoxin, serum	0.8–2.0 ng./ml.	>2.4 ng./ml.	Lanoxin
(specimen must be obtained 12–24 hours after last dose)			
Disopyramide, serum	2–5 µg./ml.	>5 µg./ml.	Norpace
Lidocaine, serum	1.5–5.0 µg./ml.	>6–8 µg./ml.	Xylocaine
Procainamide, serum	4–10 µg./ml.	>16 µg./ml.	Pronestyl
Measured as procainamide + *N*-acetyl procainamide	10–30 µg./ml.	>30 µg./ml.	
Propranolol, serum	50–100 ng./ml.	Variable	Inderal
Quinidine, serum	2–5 µg./ml.	>10 µg./ml.	Cardioquin
			Quinaglute
			Quinidex
			Quinora

REFERENCE VALUES FOR THERAPEUTIC DRUG MONITORING *Continued*

	Therapeutic Range	Toxic Levels	Proprietary Names
Psychopharmacologic Drugs			
Amitriptyline, serum (measured as amitriptyline + nortriptyline)	120–150 ng./ml.	>500 ng./ml.	Amitril Elavil Endep Entrafon Limbitrol Triavil
Desipramine, serum (measured as desipramine + imipramine)	150–300 ng./ml.	>500 ng./ml.	Norpramin Pertofrane
Imipramine, serum (measured as imipramine + desipramine)	150–300 ng./ml.	>500 ng./ml.	Antipress Imavate Janimine Presamine Tofranil
Lithium, serum (obtain specimen 12 hours after last dose)	0.8–1.2 mEq./L.	>2.0 mEq./L.	Lithobid
Nortriptyline, serum	50–150 ng./ml.	>500 ng./ml.	Aventyl Pamelor

REFERENCE VALUES IN TOXICOLOGY

	Conventional Units	S.I. Units
Arsenic, blood	3.5–7.2 µg./dl.	0.47–0.96 µmol./L.
Arsenic, urine	<100 µg./24 hr.	<1.3 µmol./24 h.
Bromides, serum	0	0
	Toxic above 17 mEq./L.	Toxic above 17 mmol./L.
Carboxyhemoglobin, blood	<5% saturation	<0.05 saturation
Symptoms occur	>20% saturation	>0.20 saturation
Ethanol, blood	<0.05 mg./dl.	<1.0 mmol./L.
	<0.005%	
Marked intoxication	300–400 mg./dl.	65–87 mmol./L.
	0.3–0.4%	
Alcoholic stupor	400–500 mg./dl.	87–109 mmol./L.
	0.4–0.5%	
Coma	>500 mg./dl.	>109 mmol./L.
	>0.5%	
Lead, blood	0–40 µg./dl.	0–2 µmol./L.
Lead, urine	<100 µg./24 hr.	<0.48 µmol./24 h.
Mercury, urine	<100 µg./24 hr.	<50 nmol./24 h.

REFERENCE VALUES FOR CEREBROSPINAL FLUID

	Conventional Units	S.I. Units
Cells	<5/cu. mm.	<5 × 10^6/L.
	All mononuclear	All mononuclear
Electrophoresis	Predominantly albumin	Predominantly albumin
Glucose	50–75 mg./dl.	2.8–4.2 mmol./L.
	(20 mg./dl. less than serum)	(1.1 mmol. less than serum)
IgG		
Children under 14	<8% of total protein	<0.08 of total protein
Adults	<14% of total protein	<0.14 of total protein
IgG index	0.3–0.6	0.3–0.6
CSF : serum IgG ratio		
CSF : serum albumin ratio		
Oligoclonal banding on electrophoresis	Absent	Absent
Pressure	70–180 mm. water	70–180 mm. water
Protein, total	15–45 mg./dl.	150–450 gm./L.

REFERENCE VALUES FOR SEMEN ANALYSIS

	Conventional Units	S.I. Units
Volume	2–5 ml.	2–5 ml.
Liquefaction	Complete in 15 min.	Complete in 15 min.
Leukocytes	Occasional or absent	Occasional or absent
Count	60–150 million/ml.	$60-150 \times 10^6$/ml.
Motility	>80% motile	>0.80 motile
Morphology	80–90% normal forms	0.80–0.90 normal forms
Fructose	>150 mg./dl.	>8.33 mmol./L.

REFERENCE VALUES FOR FECES

	Conventional Units	S.I. Units
Bulk	100–200 gm./24 hr.	100–200 gm./24 h.
Dry matter	23–32 gm./24 hr.	23–32 gm./24 h.
Fat, total	<6.0 gm./24 hr.	<6.0 gm./24 h.
Nitrogen, total	<2.0 gm./24 hr.	<2.0 gm./24 h.
Water	Approximately 65%	Approximately 0.65

REFERENCES

1. Brown, S. S., Mitchell, F. L., and Young, D. S. (Eds.): Chemical Diagnosis of Disease. Amsterdam, Elsevier/North-Holland Biomedical Press, 1979.
2. Conn, R. B. (Ed.): Current Diagnosis, 8th ed. Philadelphia, W. B. Saunders Company, 1991.
3. Goodman, A. G., Gilman, L. S., Rall, T. W., and Murad, F.: Goodman and Gilman's The Pharmacological Basis of Therapeutics, 7th ed. New York, Macmillan, 1985.
4. Henry, J. B. (Ed.): Todd-Sanford-Davidsohn Clinical Diagnosis and Management by Laboratory Methods, 18th ed. Philadelphia, W. B. Saunders Company, 1984.
5. Lundberg, G. D., Iverson, C., and Radulescu, G.: Now Read This: The SI Units Are Here. J.A.M.A., 255:2329, 1986.
6. Miale, J. B.: Laboratory Medicine-Hematology, 6th ed. St Louis, C. V. Mosby, 1982.
7. Tietz, N. W.: Clinical Guide to Laboratory Tests. 2nd ed. Philadelphia, W. B. Saunders Company, 1990.
8. Tietz, N. W.: Textbook of Clinical Chemistry. Philadelphia, W. B. Saunders Company, 1986.
9. Williams, W. J., Beutler, E., Erslev, A. J., and Lichtman, M. A.: Hematology, 3rd ed. New York, McGraw-Hill Book Company, 1983.

Some of these values have been established by the Clinical Laboratories at Thomas Jefferson University Hospital and have not been published elsewhere.

INDEX

Note: Page numbers in *italics* refer to illustrations; page numbers followed by t refer to tables.

Vertebral artery, traumatic injury of, 1613t
Vertigo, benign paroxysmal positional, 1194
in Meniere's disease, 1194
Vesalius, Andreas, 3–4
Vesicoenteric fistula, 1450
Vesicoumbilical fistula, 726, 728
Vesicovaginal fistula, 1450–1451
Vicary, Thomas, 3
Vicryl sutures, 216, 216
Villous adenoma, of small intestine, 802
VIPoma, 1102
Viral infection. See individual viral species.
Virchow, Rudolf, 10
Virchow's triad, 1502
Virilization, maternal, 1476
Virilizing tumors, adrenal, 638
Virus, oncogenic, 476
Viscera, sensory innervation of, 736, 737
Visceral ischemia, chronic, 1650–1651
Visceral pain, anatomy and physiology of,
736–737, 737
neurosurgical relief of, 1277–1281
Vision impairment, in diabetes mellitus,
142–143
Vital HN, 122t
Vitamin(s), in parenteral nutrition, 125, 125t
liver metabolism of, 988
Vitamin A deficiency, in wound healing, 171
Vitamin A excess, vitamin K effects of, 89
Vitamin B$_{12}$, malabsorption of, in Crohn's
disease, 850
Vitamin B$_{12}$-binding capacity, in hepatocellu-
lar carcinoma, 498t, 499
Vitamin C deficiency, in wound healing, 171
Vitamin D, in calcium metabolism, 600, 600t
photosynthesis of, in skin, 1385
Vitamin E excess, vitamin K effects of, 89
Vitamin K antagonists, hemostatic effects of, 89
Vitamin K deficiency, hemostatic effects of, 89
Vitaneed blenderized formula, 116t
Vivonex HN, 122t
Vivonex TEN, 123t
Vocal cords, anatomy of, 1202
nodules of, 1203
paralysis of, 1204
pathophysiology of, 1203
polyps of, 1203
speech mechanisms of, 1202–1203
true, structural changes in, 1203
Voit, Carl, 20
Volkmann's ischemic contracture, arterial
injury in, 1619–1620
Volume loss, due to blood loss, 23
due to salt loss, 23
due to water loss, 23
homeostasis in, 22–23
injury responses to, 28–29
isotonic, 23
Volume of distribution, of drug, 148
Volvulus, cecal, 835, 942–943, 942–943
midgut, 835
neonatal, 1161–1162
of colon, 835, 940–943
acute abdomen in, 751–752
splenic flexure, 943
transverse, 943
sigmoid, 835, 941, 941–942
Vomiting, bilious, 1152
metabolic alkalosis in, 65–66
von Haller, Albrecht, 8–9
von Langenbeck, Bernhard, 9, 10
von Recklinghausen's disease, gastrointestinal
tract in, 805, 925
pheochromocytoma in, 643
von Willebrand disease, 89
Vulva, 1413–1416

Vulva (Continued)
carcinoma in situ of, 1415
carcinoma of, 1415, 1415–1416
incidence of, 1415
metastasis of, 1415
subtypes of, 1415
treatment of, 1415–1416
condylomata acuminata of, 1414, 1414
degenerative disease of, 1414–1415
glandular lesions of, 1413–1414
physiology and endocrinology of, 1410
skin disorders of, 1413
varicose veins of, 1413
Vulvitis, 1414, 1414

Wangensteen, Owen, 12, 13
Warren, J. Mason, 5
Warts, perianal, 969
venereal, of penis, 1474
of vulva, 1414, 1414
perianal, 969
Wasp sting, 255
Water. See also Fluid entries.
average daily exchange of, 69, 69t
loss of, homeostatic response to, 23
insensible, in burns, 190
of solution, 69
total body, 57
WDHA syndrome, 1102
Weight, vs. height, standards for, 853–854,
854t
Weight loss, perioperative, parenteral
nutrition in, 127–128
surgical complications due to, 127–128
Wells, T. Spencer, 7
Whipple procedure (pancreaticoduodenectomy), 1095, 1095
Whipple's triad, 1099
White cells, in inflammatory reaction, 164–165
in surgical infection, 235
White phosphorus burns, 197
White shock, 42
Whole blood, storage of, 96, 96t
Whole blood clotting time, 91
Williams-Campbell syndrome, 1726
Wilms' tumor, 1179t, 1179–1180
diagnosis of, 1179
metastasis of, 1180
staging of, 1179t, 1179–1180
survival statistics in, 1180
treatment of, 1179
Wolff-Parkinson-White syndrome, 2048–
2055
accessory pathways in, anatomy of, 2049,
2049
manifest vs. concealed, 2050
anatomic-electrophysiologic basis of,
2049–2050, 2049–2059
antegrade conduction block in, 2050, 2050
atrial flutter/fibrillation in, 2050
AV conduction in, 2050, 2050
historical aspects of, 2048–2049
intraoperative electrophysiologic monitoring in, 2051, 2051–2052
preoperative electrophysiologic evaluation
in, 2051
supraventricular conduction block in, 2050,
2050
surgical indications and contraindications
in, 2051
surgical technique in, 2051–2052, 2053
for anterior septal accessory pathways,
2055

Wolff-Parkinson-White syndrome (Continued)
for left free-wall accessory pathways,
2052, 2054
for posterior septal accessory pathways,
2052–2054
for right free-wall accessory pathways,
2054–2055, 2055
results of, 2055
Wolffian duct persistence, 1413
Wounds, burn. See Burns.
care of, 172–174
contraction prevention in, 173–174
debridement and, 173, 212, 224
drains in, 218, 224
high pressure irrigation in, 211, 211
infection prevention in, 221–236. See
also Infection, surgical.
presurgical scrub and, 172–173, 211
secondary wound healing and, 174
sutures in, 173. See also Suture.
temporary skin grafting in, 213
tissue perfusion and, 172, 224
clean, definition of, 222t, 302
clean-contaminated, aseptic technique for,
223
definition of, 222t, 302
prophylactic antibiotics in, 225
closed, 164–168
burst strength of, 168, 168–169
chemical events in, 166–167
ground substance and, 167, 167t
inflammation as, 166–167
morphologic events in, 164–166
cellular phase in, 165, 166
epithelialization as, 165
fibroplasia as, 165–166, 166
inflammation as, 164–165
physical events in, 167–168, 168–169
tensile strength of, 168, 168–169
closure of, in decubitus ulcer, 1389
surgical techniques for, 1385–1386,
1386–1387
contaminated. See also Infection, surgical.
complication rate in, 301
dead space in, 224
debridement in, 173, 212, 224
definition of, 222t, 302
delayed closure of, 81, 168, 213, 224
drainage of, 224
prophylactic antibiotics in, 225
suction catheter antibiotic irrigation in,
224
sutures in, 224
dead space in, collapse of, 213, 224
failure of, 302–303
causes of, 303, 303t
dehiscence as, 302–303, 303t
incisional hernia as, 303
sutures in, 303–304
healing of, 164–175
anemia and, 172
anti-inflammatory agents and, 172
ascorbic acid deficiency and, 171
autogenous, 1385, 1386
biologic considerations in, 164–172
calcium levels and, 171
control of, 174–175
BAPN and, 175
cartilage powder for, 174
collagen cross-linking and, 174
ferrous iron chelation and, 174–175
fibrosis inhibition and, 174
penicillamine and, 175
proline analogues and, 175
scar tissue and, 175
tissue oxygen tension and, 174, 224